Sheryl G. A. Gabram-Mendola, MD, MBA, FACS
Surgeon-in-Chief
Grady Memorial Hospital
Emory University School of Medicine
Deputy Director
Georgia Cancer Center for Excellence
Director, AVON Comprehensive Breast Center at Grady
Director, High Risk Assessment Program
Winship Cancer Institute of Emory University
Georgia Cancer Coalition Distinguished Cancer Scholar
Atlanta, Georgia

Michele Gabree, MS
Certified Genetic Counselor
Center for Cancer Risk Assessment
Massachusetts General Hospital
Boston, Massachusetts

Patricia A. Ganz, MD
Distinguished University Professor
University of California, Los Angeles
Fielding School of Public Health
David Geffen School of Medicine at University of California, Los Angeles
Director, Cancer Prevention & Control Research
Jonsson Comprehensive Cancer Center
Los Angeles, California

Levi A. Garraway, MD, PhD
Associate Professor
Department of Medical Oncology
Dana-Farber Cancer Institute
Senior Associate Member
The Broad Institute of Massachusetts Institute of Technology and Harvard
Associate Physician
Brigham and Women's Hospital
Boston, Massachusetts

Jared J. Gartner, DO
Biologist, National Cancer Institute
Surgery Branch
National Institute of Health
Bethesda, Maryland

Juan C. Gea-Banacloche, MD
Head, Infectious Diseases Unit
Experimental Transplantation and Immunology Branch
National Cancer Institute
Chief, Infectious Diseases Consultation Service
National Institute of Allergy and Infectious Disease
Bethesda, Maryland

David M. Gershenson, MD
Professor and Chair
Department of Gynecologic Oncology
The University of Texas MD Anderson Cancer Center
Houston, Texas

Scott Nicholas Gettinger, MD
Associate Professor of Medicine
Thoracic Oncology Program
Developmental Therapeutics
Yale Cancer Center
New Haven, Connecticut

Alexander I. Geyer, MD
Assistant Clinical Member
Pulmonary Service
Department of Medicine
Memorial Sloan-Kettering Cancer Center
New York, New York

Juliet F. Gibson, BA
Research Fellow
Dermatology and Hematology
Yale University School of Medicine
New Haven, Connecticut

Hannah L. Gilmore, MD
Assistant Professor, Department of Pathology
Case Western Reserve University School of Medicine
Surgical Pathology Director
University Hospitals Case Medical Center
Cleveland, Ohio

Olivier Glehen, MD, PhD
Professor Lyon 1 University
Chief, Division of General Surgery
Hospices Civils de Lyon
Department of General and Oncologic Surgery
Centre Hospitalier Lyon Sud
Pierre-Bénite, France

Matthew P. Goetz, MD
Associate Professor of Pharmacology
Associate Professor of Oncology
Mayo Clinic
Rochester, Minnesota

Sarah B. Goldberg, MD, MPH
Assistant Professor of Internal Medicine
Medical Oncology
Yale Cancer Center
Yale University School of Medicine
New Haven, Connecticut

Donald P. Goldstein, MD
Professor of Obstetrics, Gynecology and Reproductive Biology
Harvard Medical School
Senior Obstetrician-Gynecologist
Brigham and Women's Hospital
Founder and Director Emeritus
New England Trophoblastic Disease Center
Dana-Farber and Brigham and Women's Cancer Center
Boston, Massachusetts

Leonard G. Gomella, MD, FACS
The Bernard W. Godwin Professor of Prostate Cancer
Chairman, Department of Urology
Associate Director
Jefferson Kimmel Cancer Center
Clinical Director, Jefferson Kimmel Cancer Center Network
Thomas Jefferson University
Philadelphia, Pennsylvania

Steven D. Gore, MD
Yale University School of Medicine
New Haven, Connecticut

Ramaswamy Govindan, MD
Professor of Medicine
Co-Director, Section of Medical Oncology
Division of Oncology
Washington University School of Medicine
St. Louis, Missouri

F. Anthony Greco, MD
Director, Sarah Cannon Cancer Center
Tennessee Oncology, PLLC and Sarah Cannon Research Institute
Nashville, Tennessee

Marcio L. Griebeler, MD
Fellow, Endocrinology, Metabolism and Nutrition
Mayo Clinic
Rochester, Minnesota

Ellen R. Gritz, PhD
Professor and Chair
Department of Behavioral Science
The University of Texas MD Anderson Cancer Center
Houston, Texas

Alessandro Gronchi, MD
Surgical Oncologist, Department of Surgery
Chief, Sarcoma Service
Fondazione IRCCS
Istituto Nazionale dei Tumori
Milan, Italy

Samuel D. Gross, MD
Professor and Chair, Department of Surgery
Jefferson Medical College of Thomas Jefferson University
Co-Director, Jefferson Pancreas, Biliary and Related Cancers Center
Philadelphia, Pennsylvania

José G. Guillem, MD, MPH
Department of Surgery
Memorial Sloan-Kettering Cancer Center
New York, New York

Caroline M. Gulati, MD
Fellow
Department of Medicine
Division of Pulmonary and Critical Care
New York Presbyterian Weill Cornell
    Medical Center
New York, New York

Jennifer Moliterno Günel, MD
Assistant Professor
Department of Neurosurgery
Yale University School of Medicine
New Haven, Connecticut

Murat Günel, MD
Nixdorff-German Professor
Chief, Yale Neurovascular Surgery
    Program
Co-Director, Yale Program on
    Neurogenetics
Director, Yale Program in Brain Tumor
    Research
Departments of Neurosurgery,
    Neurobiology and Genetics
Yale University School of Medicine
New Haven, Connecticut

Daphne A. Haas-Kogan, MD
Professor of Radiation Oncology and
    Neurological Surgery
Program Director and Vice Chair
Department of Radiation Oncology
Helen Diller Family Comprehensive
    Cancer Center
San Francisco, California

John D. Hainsworth, MD
Chief Scientific Officer
Sarah Cannon Research Institute
Nashville, Tennessee

Mehdi Hamadani, MD
Associate Professor of Medicine
Director-Myeloma & Lymphoma Service
Section of Hematology and Oncology
West Virginia University
Morgantown, West Virginia

Gary D. Hammer, MD, PhD
University of Michigan
Millie Schembechler Professor of Adrenal
    Cancer
Director Endocrine Oncology Program
Director, Center for Organogenesis
Ann Arbor, Michigan

Douglas Hanahan, PhD
Director
Swiss Institute for Experimental Cancer
    Research (ISREC)
Lausanne, Switzerland

Parameswaran N. Hari, MD
Professor Section Head, Hematological
    Malignancies and Transplantation
Division of Hematology Oncology
Department of Medicine
Medical College of Wisconsin
Milwaukee, Wisconsin

Jay R. Harris, MD
Professor and Chair
Department of Radiation Oncology
Dana-Farber Cancer Institute
Brigham and Women's Hospital
Harvard Medical School
Boston, Massachusetts

Lyndsay N. Harris, MD, FRCP(C)
Diana Hyland Chair in Breast Cancer
Director, Breast Cancer Program
Seidman Cancer Center
University Hospitals Case Medical Center
Professor of Medicine
Division of Hematology and Oncology
Case Western Reserve University
Cleveland, Ohio

Marc Haxer, MA, CCC-Sp
Departments of Speech Pathology and
    Otolaryngology/Head and Neck Surgery
University of Michigan Health System
Ann Arbor, Michigan

C. William Helm, MBBChir, FRCS
Northern Gynaecological Oncology Center
Queen Elizabeth Hospital, Gateshead
Tyne and Wear, United Kingdom

Lee J. Helman, MD
Scientific Director for Clinical Research
Center for Cancer Research National
    Cancer Institute
Bethesda, Maryland

James G. Herman, MD
Johns Hopkins University
Baltimore, Maryland

Paul J. Hesketh, MD
Professor, Department of Medicine
Tufts University School of Medicine
Boston, Massachusetts
Director Sophia Gordon Cancer Center
Lahey Hospital & Medical Center
Burlington, Massachusetts

Jay L. Hess, MD, PhD
Professor, Department of Pathology
Carl V. Weller Professor and Chair
Professor, Department of Internal
    Medicine
University of Michigan Health System
Ann Arbor, Michigan

Christopher J. Hoimes, DO
Assistant Professor
UH Case Medical Center
Department of Medicine-Hematology
    and Oncology
Cleveland, Ohio

Leora Horn, MD, MSc
Associate Professor, Department of
    Medicine
Vanderbilt University Medical Center
Nashville, Tennessee

Neil S. Horowitz, MD
Assistant Professor of Obstetrics,
    Gynecology, and Reproductive Medicine
Harvard Medical School
Director of Clinical Research
Division of Gynecologic Oncology
Brigham and Women's Hospital
Boston, Massachusetts

Ralph H. Hruban, MD
Professor, Department of Pathology
Director, The Sol Goldman Pancreatic
    Cancer Research Center
Johns Hopkins University School of
    Medicine
Baltimore, Maryland

Melissa M. Hudson, MD
Full Member
Director, Cancer Survivorship Division
Department of Oncology
St. Jude Children's Research Hospital
Memphis, Tennessee

Vanessa W. Hui, MD
Department of Surgery
Memorial Sloan-Kettering Cancer Center
New York, New York

Carolyn D. Hurst, BSc, MSc, PhD
Senior Postdoctoral Research Fellow
Section of Experimental Oncology
Leeds Institute of Cancer and Pathology
St. James's University Hospital
Leeds, United Kingdom

David H. Ilson, MD, PhD
Professor and Attending Physician
Department of Medicine
Memorial Sloan-Kettering Cancer Center
    and Weill Cornell Medical College
    Memorial Hospital
New York, New York

Caron A. Jacobson, MD, MSc
Instructor, Department of Medicine
Harvard Medical School
Brigham and Women's Hospital
Division of Medical Oncology
Hematologic Malignancies
Dana-Farber Cancer Institute
Boston, Massachusetts

Kory W. Jasperson, MS, CGC
Genetic Counselor
Department of Internal Medicine
Huntsman Cancer Institute
University of Utah
Salt Lake City, Utah

Peter Johnson, MD, FRCP
Professor of Medical Oncology
Cancer Research United Kingdom
    Centre
University of Southampton Faculty of
    Medicine
Southampton, United Kingdom

DeVita, Hellman, and Rosenberg's

Cancer

Principles & Practice of Oncology

10th Edition

Editors

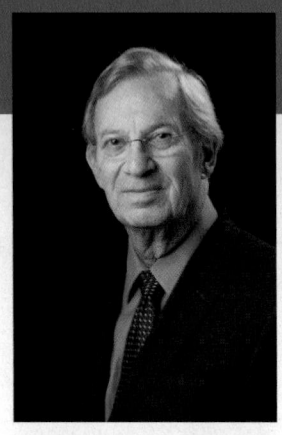

Vincent T. DeVita, Jr., MD

Amy & Joseph Perella Professor of Medicine
Yale Comprehensive Cancer Center and Smilow
    Cancer Hospital at Yale-New Haven
Professor of Epidemiology and Public Health
Yale University School of Public Health
New Haven, Connecticut

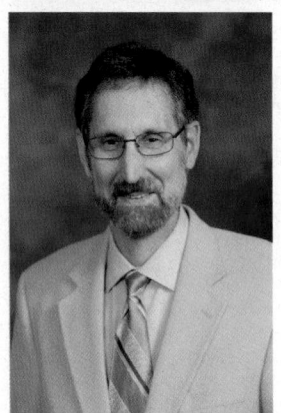

Theodore S. Lawrence, MD, PhD

Isadore Lampe Professor and Chair
Department of Radiation Oncology
University of Michigan
Ann Arbor, Michigan

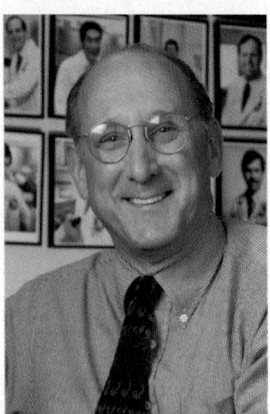

Steven A. Rosenberg, MD, PhD

Chief, Surgery Branch, National Cancer Institute, National Institutes of Health
Professor of Surgery, Uniformed Services University of the Health Sciences
School of Medicine
Bethesda, Maryland
Professor of Surgery
George Washington University School of Medicine
Washington, District of Columbia

With 403 Contributing Authors

DeVita, Hellman, and Rosenberg's

Cancer

Principles & Practice of Oncology

10th Edition

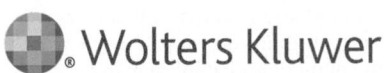 Wolters Kluwer

Philadelphia • Baltimore • New York • London
Buenos Aires • Hong Kong • Sydney • Tokyo

Acquisitions Editor: Julie Goolsby
Senior Product Development Editor: Emilie Moyer
Editorial Assistant: Brian Convery
Production Project Manager: David Orzechowski
Marketing Manager: Stephanie Kindlick
Senior Designer: Stephen Druding
Illustration Coordinator: Jennifer Clements
Illustrator: Jason M. Alexander, Electronic Publishing Services, Inc.
Manufacturing Coordinator: Beth Welsh
Prepress Vendor: Absolute Service, Inc.
Prepress Vendor Project Manager: Harold Medina

10th edition

9 8 7 6 5 4 3 2 1

Printed in the United States of America

Library of Congress Cataloging-in-Publication Data

Devita, Hellman, and Rosenberg's cancer : principles & practice of oncology / editors, Vincent T. DeVita, Jr., Theodore S. Lawrence, Steven A. Rosenberg ; with 404 contributing authors.—10th edition.
    p. ; cm.
    Cancer
    Includes bibliographical references and index.
    ISBN 978-1-4511-9294-0 (hardback)—ISBN 1-4511-9294-0 (hardback)
    I. DeVita, Vincent T., Jr., 1935- , editor. II. Lawrence, Theodore S., editor. III. Rosenberg, Steven A., editor. IV. Title: Cancer.
    [DNLM: 1. Neoplasms. QZ 200]
    RC261
    616.99'4—dc23

2014035783

LWW.com

In memoriam

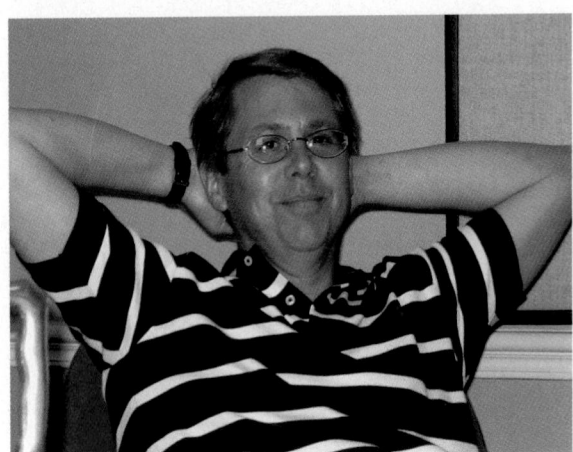

Jonathan W. Pine, Jr.
1957–2013

*We dedicate this edition to Jonathan Pine, our colleague and Senior
Executive Editor at Wolters Kluwer Health, whose relaxed style belied
his fierce dedication to turning out a quality book.*

Amy P. Abernethy, MD, PhD
Director, Center for Learning Health
   Care
Duke Clinical Research Institute
Director, Duke Cancer Care Research
   Program
Duke Cancer Institute
Associate Professor
Division of Medical Oncology
Department of Medicine
Duke University School of Medicine
Durham, North Carolina

Ghassan Abou-Alfa, MD
Associate Attending
Department of Medicine
Memorial Sloan-Kettering Cancer Center
Associate Professor
Department of Medicine
Weill Cornell Medical College
New York, New York

Ross A. Abrams, MD
Chairman and Hendrickson Professor of
   Radiation Oncology
Rush University Medical Center
Chicago, Illinois

Nadeem R. Abu-Rustum, MD
Professor
Weill Medical College of Cornell
   University
Chief, Gynecologic Oncology Service
Memorial Sloan-Kettering Cancer Center
New York, New York

Gregory P. Adams, PhD
Associate Professor Developmental
   Therapeutics Program
Director of Biological Research and
   Therapeutics
Fox Chase Cancer Center
Philadelphia, Pennsylvania

Anupriya Agarwal, PhD
Research Assistant Professor
The Knight Cancer Center
Oregon Health & Science University
Portland, Oregon

Bharat B. Aggarwal, PhD
Professor of Cancer Research
Professor of Cancer Medicine
   (Biochemistry)
Chief, Cytokine Research Laboratory
Department of Experimental
   Therapeutics
The University of Texas MD Anderson
   Cancer Center
Houston, Texas

Shahab Ahmed, MD
Data Analyst, Department of
   Gastrointestinal Medical Oncology
The University of Texas MD Anderson
   Cancer Center
Houston, Texas

Manmeet S. Ahluwalia, MD, FACP
Associate Professor, Department of
   Medicine
Cleveland Clinic Lerner College of
   Medicine of Case Western Reserve
   University
Associate Director, Clinical Trials,
   Operations
The Rose Ella Burkhardt Brain Tumor
   and Neuro-Oncology Center
Neurological Institute
Cleveland Clinic
Cleveland, Ohio

Kaled M. Alektiar, MD
Member Department of Radiation
   Oncology
Memorial Sloan-Kettering Cancer Center
New York, New York

James M. Allan, DPhil
Northern Institute for Cancer Research
Faculty of Medicine
Newcastle University
Newcastle-upon-Tyne, United Kingdom

**Matthew L. Anderson, MD, PhD,
   FACOG**
Assistant Professor
Division of Gynecology Oncology
Director of Clinical Research
   (Gynecology)
Department of Obstetrics & Gynecology
Research Member, Dan L. Duncan
   Cancer Center
Baylor College of Medicine
Houston, Texas

Kenneth C. Anderson, MD
Director, Jerome Lipper Multiple
   Myeloma Center and
Lebow Institute for Myeloma
   Therapeutics
American Cancer Society
Clinical Research Professor
Kraft Family Professor of Medicine
Dana-Farber Cancer Institute
Harvard Medical School
Boston, Massachusetts

Stephen Ansell, MD, PhD
Professor, Division of Hematology
Mayo Clinic
Rochester, Minnesota

Cristina R. Antonescu, MD
Attending Pathologist, Department of
   Pathology
Memorial Sloan-Kettering Cancer Center
Director, Bone and Soft Tissue Pathology
New York, New York

Shirin Arastu-Kapur, PhD
Associate Director
Biology at Onyx Pharmaceuticals
South San Francisco, California

**Luiz Henrique de Lima Araujo, MD,
   MSc**
Postdoctoral Researcher
James Cancer Center
The Ohio State University Medical
   Center
Columbus, Ohio

Alicia Y. Armstrong, MD, MHSCR
Chief, Gynecologic Services Program in
   Reproductive & Adult Endocrinology
Eunice Kennedy Shriver National
   Institute of Child Health and Human
   Development
Bethesda, Maryland

Alan Ashworth, FRS
Professor and Chief Executive
The Institute of Cancer Research
London, United Kingdom

Jon C. Aster, MD, PhD
Professor, Department of Pathology
Harvard Medical School
Head, Division of Hematopathology
Brigham and Women's Hospital
Boston, Massachusetts

David A. August, MD
Professor, Chief, Division of Surgical
    Oncology
Department of Surgery
Rutgers Robert Wood Johnson Medical
    School and the Rutgers Cancer
    Institute of New Jersey
New Brunswick, New Jersey

Itzhak Avital, MD, FACS
Professor of Surgery
Executive Medical Director
Bon Secours Cancer Institute
Richmond, Virginia

Jennifer E. Axilbund, MS, CGC
Cancer Risk Assessment Program
The Johns Hopkins Hospital
Baltimore, Maryland

Joachim M. Baehring, MD, DSc
Associate Professor
Departments of Neurology, Neurosurgery,
    and Medicine
Chief, Section of Neuro-Oncology
Yale Cancer Center
Yale University School of Medicine
New Haven, Connecticut

F. Amos Bailey, MD
Professor, Department of Medicine
Center for Palliative and Supportive Care
Division of Gerontology, Geriatrics, and
    Palliative Care
Department of Medicine
University of Alabama at Birmingham
Birmingham/Atlanta Geriatric, Research,
    Education, and Clinical Center
Birmingham Veterans Affairs Medical
    Center
Birmingham, Alabama

Sharyn D. Baker, PharmD, PhD
Associate Member
Pharmaceutical Sciences Department
St. Jude Children's Research Hospital
Memphis, Tennessee

Lodovico Balducci, MD
Program Leader, Senior Adult Oncology
    Program
Senior Member, H. Lee Moffitt Cancer
    Center & Research Institute
Professor of Oncologic Sciences &
    Medicine
University of South Florida College of
    Medicine
Tampa, Florida

Alberto Bardelli, MD
Laboratory of Molecular Genetics
Institute for Cancer Research and
    Treatment
University of Torino Medical School
Candiolo, Italy

Gene H. Barnett, MD, MBA
Professor and Director
Rose Ella Burkhardt Brain Tumor and
    Neuro-Oncology Center
Cleveland Clinic
Cleveland, Ohio

Tracy T. Batchelor, MD
Giovanni Armenise—Harvard Professor
    of Neurology
Harvard Medical School
Chief, Division of Neuro-Oncology
Massachusetts General Hospital Cancer
    Center
Co-Leader, Neuro-Oncology Program
Dana-Farber/Harvard Cancer Center
Boston, Massachusetts

Susan E. Bates, MD
Head, Molecular Therapeutics Section
Developmental Therapeutics Branch
Center for Cancer Research
National Cancer Institute
Bethesda, Maryland

Stephen B. Baylin, MD
Professor of Oncology
Professor of Medicine
Johns Hopkins University School of
    Medicine
Deputy Director of the Cancer Center
Baltimore, Maryland

Kevin P. Becker, MD, PhD
Assistant Professor
Department of Neurology
Section of Medical Neuro-Oncology
Yale Comprehensive Cancer
Yale University School of Medicine
New Haven, Connecticut

Andrew Berchuck, MD
Professor and Director
Gynecologic Oncology Program
Division of Gynecologic Oncology
Department of Obstetrics and
    Gynecology
Duke Cancer Institute
Duke University Medical Center
Durham, North Carolina

Jonathan S. Berek, MD, MMS
Laurie Kraus Lacob Professor
Director, Stanford Women's Cancer
    Center
Stanford Cancer Institute
Chair, Department of Obstetrics and
    Gynecology
Stanford University School of Medicine
Stanford, California

Ann M. Berger, MSN, MD
Pain and Palliative Care
Bethesda, Maryland

Ross S. Berkowitz, MD
William H. Baker Professor of
    Gynecology
Harvard Medical School
Director of Gynecology and Gynecologic
    Oncology
Brigham and Women's Hospital and
    Dana-Farber Cancer Institute
Co-Director of New England
    Trophoblastic Disease Center
Boston, Massachusetts

Leslie Bernstein, MS, PhD
Professor and Director
Division of Cancer Etiology
Department of Population Sciences
Beckman Research Institute
City of Hope Dean for Faculty Affairs
City of Hope National Medical Center
    and the Beckman Research Institute
Duarte, California

Bryan L. Betz, PhD
Assistant Professor
Department of Pathology
University of Michigan
Technical Director
Molecular Diagnostics Laboratory
University of Michigan Health System
Ann Arbor, Michigan

Smita Bhatia, MD, MPH
Professor and Chair
Department of Population Sciences
Associate Director, Population Research
City of Hope Comprehensive Cancer
    Center
Duarte, California

Ravi Bhatia, MD
Director, Division of Hematopoietic Stem
    Cell and Leukemia Research
Professor, Department of Hematology and
    Hematopoietic Cell Transplantation
City of Hope National Medical Center
Duarte, California

Michael J. Birrer, MD, PhD
Professor, Department of Medicine
Harvard Medical School
Director, Gynecologic Cancers Disease
    Center
Massachusetts General Hospital
Leader, Gynecologic Cancer Program
Dana-Farber Cancer Institute
Boston, Massachusetts

James S. Blachly, MD
Fellow, Division of Hematology
Department of Internal Medicine
The Ohio State University
Columbus, Ohio

Elizabeth M. Blanchard, MD
Director, Cancer Clinical Trials
Southcoast Centers for Cancer Care
Fairhaven, Massachusetts

Sharon L. Bober, PhD
Assistant Professor
Department of Psychiatry
Harvard Medical School Director
Sexual Health Program
Dana-Farber Cancer Institute
Boston, Massachusetts

Lawrence H. Boise, PhD
Professor
Winship Cancer Institute of Emory
    University
Departments of Hematology/Medical
    Oncology and Cell Biology
Emory School of Medicine
Atlanta, Georgia

Danielle C. Bonadies, MS, CGC
Director, Cancer Genetics Division
Gene Counsel, LLC
New Haven, Connecticut

Mitesh J. Borad, MD
Assistant Professor
Department of Medicine
Director, Phase I Drug Development
Mayo Clinic
Scottsdale, Arizona

Hossein Borghaei, MS, DO
Associate Professor
Chief, Thoracic Medical Oncology
Fox Chase Cancer Center
Philadelphia, Pennsylvania

Otis W. Brawley, MD, FACP
Chief Medical Officer
American Cancer Society, Inc.
Atlanta, Georgia

Rachel C. Brennan, MD
Assistant Member
Department of Oncology
Division of Solid Tumors
St. Jude's Children's Research Hospital
Memphis, Tennessee

Dean E. Brenner, MD
Kutsche Family Professor of Internal
    Medicine
Professor of Pharmacology
University of Michigan Comprehensive
    Cancer Center
Ann Arbor, Michigan

Jonathan R. Brody, PhD
Associate Professor
Director of Surgical Research
Department of Surgery
Jefferson Medical College of Thomas
    Jefferson University
Philadelphia, Pennsylvania

Paul D. Brown, MD
Professor
Co-Section Chief
Central Nervous System/Pediatrics
Director of Central Nervous System
Stereotactic Radiosurgery
Department of Radiation Oncology
The University of Texas MD Anderson
    Cancer Center
Houston, Texas

Christopher B. Buck, PhD
Investigator
Head, Tumor Virus Molecular Biology
    Section
Laboratory of Cellular Oncology
Center for Cancer Research
National Cancer Institute
Bethesda, Maryland

Harold J. Burstein, MD, PhD
Associate Professor of Medicine
Harvard Medical School
Susan F. Smith Center for Women's
    Cancers
Dana-Farber Cancer Institute
Boston, Massachusetts

Tim E. Byers, MD, MPH
Associate Dean for Public Health Practice
Colorado School of Public Health
Associate Director for Cancer Prevention
    and Control
University of Colorado Cancer Center
Aurora, Colorado

John C. Byrd, MD
D. Warren Brown Chair of Leukemia
    Research
Director, Division of Hematology
Department of Internal Medicine
The Ohio State Comprehensive Cancer
    Center
Columbus, Ohio

A. Hilary Calvert
Professor
Gynecologic Oncology
University College Hospitals (UCLH)
London, United Kingdom

Robert B. Cameron, MD
Professor, Cardiothoracic Surgery and
    Surgical Oncology
David Geffen School of Medicine
University of California, Los Angeles
Chief, Thoracic Surgery
West Los Angeles Virginia Medical
    Center
Los Angeles, California

Stephen A. Cannistra, MD
Professor of Medicine
Harvard Medical School
Program Director, Gynecologic Medical
    Oncology
Division of Hematology and Oncology
Beth Israel Deaconess Medical Center
Boston, Massachusetts

Daniel J. Canter, MD
Vice Chairman
Department of Urology
Urologic Institute of Southeastern
    Pennsylvania
Einstein Healthcare Network
Associate Professor, Urologic Oncology
Fox Chase Cancer Center
Philadelphia, Pennsylvania

Antonino Carbone, MD
Professor and Chairman of the
    Department of Pathology, Centro
    di Riferimento Oncologico Aviano
    (CRO)
Instituto Nazionale dei Tumori, IRCCS
Aviano, Italy

David P. Carbone, MD, PhD
Barbara J. Bonner Chair in Lung Cancer
    Research
Professor of Medicine
Director, James Thoracic Center
James Cancer Center
The Ohio State University Medical
    Center
Columbus, Ohio

Michele Carbone, MD, PhD
Director
University of Hawaii Cancer Center
Professor, Department of Pathology
John A. Burns School of Medicine
Honolulu, Hawaii

Thomas E. Carey, PhD
Professor of Otolaryngology and
    Pharmacology
Associate Chair for Research
Department of Otolaryngology-Head and
    Neck Surgery
Co-Director-Head and Neck Oncology
    Program
Comprehensive Cancer Center
The University of Michigan School of
    Medicine
Ann Arbor, Michigan

Paolo G. Casali, MD
Head
Adult Mesenchymal Tumor Medical
    Oncology Unit
Fondazione Instituto di Ricovero
    Carattere Scientifico
Instituto Nazionale dei Tumori
Milano, Italy

Eric J. Cassell, MD, MACP
Emeritus Professor
Department of Public Health
Weill Medical College of Cornell
    University
Attending Physician
New York Presbyterian Hospital
New York, New York
Adjunct Professor
Department of Medicine
McGill University Faculty of Medicien
Montreal, Quebec, Canada

Jan Cerny, MD, PhD
Assistant Professor of Medicine
Division of Hematology
Department of Medicine
Director, Leukemia Program
University of Massachusetts Medical
School
Associate Director, Cancer Research
Office
UMass Memorial Cancer Center
University of Massachusetts
Worcester, Massachusetts

Ronald S. Chamberlain, MD, MPA, FACS
Chairman and Surgeon-in-Chief
Department of Surgery
Saint Barnabas Medical Center
Livingston, New Jersey

Richard Champlin, MD
Professor of Medicine and Chairman
Department of Stem Cell Transplantation
and Cellular Therapy
The University of Texas MD Anderson
Cancer Center
Houston, Texas

Gayun Chan-Smutko, MS, CGC
Senior Genetic Counselor
Center for Cancer Risk Assessment
Massachusetts General Hospital
Boston, Massachusetts

Susan M. Chang, MD
Professor in Residence
Department of Neurological Surgery
Director, Division of Neuro-Oncology
Lai Wan Kan Endowed Chair
University of California, San Francisco
San Francisco, California

Samuel T. Chao, MD
Brain Tumor and Neuro-Oncology
Center
Radiation Oncology
Cleveland Clinic Main Campus
Cleveland, Ohio

Cindy H. Chau, PharmD, PhD
Scientist
Medical Oncology Branch
Center for Cancer Research
National Cancer Institute
National Institutes of Health
Bethesda, Maryland

Douglas B. Chepeha, MD, MSPH, FRCSC
Professor
Director of Microvascular Reconstructive
Surgery
Department of Otolaryngology-Head and
Neck Surgery
University of Michigan Health System
Ann Arbor, Michigan

Nathan I. Cherny, MBBS, FRACP, FRCP (Lon.)
Norman Levan Chair of Humanistic
Medicine
Associate Professor of Medicine (BGU)
Director, Cancer Pain and Palliative
Medicine Service
Department of Medical Oncology
Shaare Zedek Medical Center
Jerusalem, Israel

Arul M. Chinnaiyan, MD, PhD
Director, Michigan Center for
Translational Pathology
S.P. Hicks Endowed Professor of
Pathology
Investigator, Howard Hughes Medical
Institute
American Cancer Society Research
Professor
Professor of Urology
Ann Arbor, Michigan

Anu Chittenden, MS, CGC
Genetic Counselor
Center for Cancer Genetics & Prevention
Dana-Farber Cancer Institute
Boston, Massachusetts

Clifford S. Cho, MD
Associate Professor
Department of Surgery
University of Wisconsin School of
Medicine and Public Health
Madison, Wisconsin

Edward Chow, MBBS, MSc, PhD, FRCPC
Professor, Department of Radiation
Oncology
University of Toronto
Senior Scientist
Sunnybrook Research Institute
Chair, Rapid Response Radiotherapy
Program and Bone Metastases Site
Group
Sunnybrook Health Sciences Centre
Toronto, Ontario, Canada

Sean R. Christensen, MD, PhD
Assistant Professor Department of
Dermatology
Section of Dermatologic Surgery and
Cutaneous Oncology
Yale University School of Medicine
New Haven, Connecticut

Edward Chu, MD
Professor of Medicine and Pharmacology
& Chemical Biology
Chief, Division of Hematology-Oncology
Deputy Director, University of Pittsburgh
Cancer Institute
University of Pittsburgh School of
Medicine
Pittsburgh, Pennsylvania

Nicki Chun, MS, LCGC
Clinical Assistant Professor of Pediatrics/
Genetics
Stanford Cancer Genetics Clinic
Stanford, California

Jessica Clague, PhD, MPH
Assistant Research Professor
Division of Cancer Etiology
Department of Population Sciences
Beckman Research Institute
City of Hope National Medical Center
Duarte, California

Victoria Clark, MD
Departments of Neurosurgery and
Genetics
Yale Program in Brain Tumor Research
Yale School of Medicine
New Haven, Connecticut

Robert E. Coleman, MBBS, MD, FRCP
Professor of Medical Oncology
Academic Unit of Clinical Oncology
Weston Park Hospital Cancer Research
Yorkshire Cancer Research
Sheffield Cancer Research Centre
Sheffield, South Yorkshire, United
Kingdom

Louis S. Constine, MD, FASTRO
The Philip Rubin Professor of Radiation
Oncology and Pediatrics
Vice Chair, Department of Radiation
Oncology Director
Judy DiMarzo Cancer Survivorship
Program
James P. Wilmot Cancer Center
University of Rochester Medical Center
Rochester, New York

M. Sitki Copur, MD, FACP
Medical Director of Oncology
Saint Francis Cancer Treatment Center
Grand Island, Nebraska
Professor, Department of Medicine
Division of Hematology Oncology
Adjunct Faculty
University of Nebraska Medical Center
Omaha, Nebraska

Aimee M. Crago, MD, PhD, FACS
Assistant Attending Surgeon
Sarcoma Disease Management Team
Gastric and Mixed Tumor Service
Department of Surgery
Memorial Sloan-Kettering Cancer Center
New York, New York

Jennifer Cuellar-Rodriguez, MD
Staff Clinician
Laboratory of Clinical Infectious Diseases
National Institute of Allergy and
Infectious Diseases
National Institutes of Health
Bethesda, Maryland

Brian G. Czito, MD
Gary Hock and Lynn Proctor Associate
    Professor, Department of Radiation
    Oncology
Duke Cancer Institute
Duke University Medical Center
Durham, North Carolina

Bouthaina Dabaja, MD
Associate Professor and Section Chief,
    Hematology
Department of Radiation Oncology
The University of Texas MD Anderson
    Cancer Center
Houston, Texas

Douglas M. Dahl, MD, FACS
Associate Professor of Surgery
Harvard Medical School
Chief, Division of Urologic Oncology
Department of Urology
Massachusetts General Hospital
Boston, Massachusetts

Riccardo Dalla-Favera, MD
Professor of Pathology and Cell Biology
Director, Institute for Cancer Genetics
Columbia University
New York, New York

Molly S. Daniels, MS, CGC
Senior Genetic Counselor
Department of Clinical Cancer Genetics
The University of Texas MD Anderson
    Cancer Center
Houston, Texas

Caroline Davidge-Pitts, MB, BCh
Department of Endocrinology, Diabetes
    and Nutrition
Mayo Clinic
Rochester, Minnesota

Andrew M. Davidoff, MD
Professor Department of Surgery
University of Tennessee Health Science
    Center
Member and Chairman
Department of Surgery
St. Jude Children's Research Hospital
Memphis, Tennessee

Michael A. Davies, MD, PhD
Associate Professor
Department of Melanoma
Medical Oncology
Department of Systems Biology
The University of Texas MD Anderson
    Cancer Center
Houston, Texas

Marcos de Lima, MD
Professor of Medicine
University Hospitals
Case Medical Center
Case Western Reserve University
Cleveland, Ohio

Alan H. DeCherney, MD
Director, Program in Adult and
    Reproductive Endocrinology
National Institute of Child Health and
    Human Development
National Institutes of Health
Bethesda, Maryland

Roy H. Decker, MD, PhD
Associate Professor
Department of Therapeutic Radiology
Yale University School of Medicine
New Haven, Connecticut

Angelo Paolo Dei Tos, MD
Director, Department of Oncology
Director of Anatomic Pathology
Scientific Director
Veneto Region Cancer Registry
General Hospital of Treviso
Treviso, Italy

Marcello Deraco, MD
Peritoneal Surface Malignancies
Department of Surgery-Colorectal Unit
Fondazione IRCCS
Instituto Nazionale dei Tumori
Milano, Italy
Professor Postgraduation on Digestive
    Surgery
Tor Vergata University
Roma, Italy

Hari A. Deshpande, MD
Associate Professor of Medicine
Yale University School of Medicine
Section of Medical Oncology
Yale New Haven Hospital
New Haven, Connecticut

Frank C. Detterbeck, MD
Professor and Chief
Section of Thoracic Surgery
Yale University School of Medicine
New Haven, Connecticut

Khanh T. Do, MD
Senior Clinical Fellow
Division of Cancer Treatment and
    Diagnosis
National Cancer Institute
National Institutes of Health
Bethesda, Maryland

Jessica S. Donington, MD
Associate Professor
Department of Cardiothoracic Surgery
New York University School of Medicine
Director Thoracic Surgery
Bellevue Hospital
New York, New York

James H. Doroshow, MD
Director, Division of Cancer Treatment
    and Diagnosis
Deputy Director for Clinical and
    Translational Research
National Cancer Institute
National Institutes of Health
Bethesda, Maryland

Brian J. Druker, MD
Director, Oregon Health & Science
    University
Knight Cancer Institute
JELD-WEN Chair of Leukemia Research
Oregon Health & Science University
Investigator, Howard Hughes Medical
    Institute
Portland, Oregon

Steven G. DuBois, MD, MS
Associate Professor
Department of Pediatrics
University of California, San Francisco
    School of Medicine
University of California, San Francisco
Benioff Children's Hospital
San Francisco, California

Damian E. Dupuy, MD, FACR
Professor of Diagnostic Imaging
The Warren Alpert Medical School of
    Brown University
Director of Tumor Ablation
Rhode Island Hospital
Providence, Rhode Island

Craig C. Earle, MD, MSc, FRCP(C)
Director, Health Services Research
    Program
Cancer Care Ontario and the Ontario
    Institute for Cancer Research
Professor of Medicine
University of Toronto
Medical Oncologist
Sunnybrook Odette Cancer Centre
Toronto, Ontario, Canada

Richard L. Edelson, MD
Aaron B. & Marguerite Lerner Professor
    of Dermatology
Yale School of Medicine
New Haven, Connecticut

Jason A. Efstathiou, MD, DPhil
Assistant Professor
Department of Radiation Oncology
Massachusetts General Hospital
Harvard Medical School
Boston, Massachusetts

Christopher A. Eide, BA
Research Technician III
Howard Hughes Medical Institute
Division of Hematology and Medical
    Oncology
Oregon Health & Science University
Knight Cancer Institute
Portland, Oregon

Patricia J. Eifel, MD
Professor and Chief, Section of Gynecology
Department of Radiation Oncology
The University of Texas MD Anderson
 Cancer Center
Houston, Texas

Dominique M. Elias, MD, PhD
Professor, Department of Surgical
 Oncology
Villejuif, France

Tobias Else, MD
Assistant Professor
Department of Medicine
Division of Metabolism, Endocrinology &
 Diabetes
University of Michigan
Ann Arbor, Michigan

Cathy Eng, MD, FACP
Associate Professor
Associate Medical Director, Colorectal
 Center
Director, MD Anderson Cancer Center
 Clinical Trials Network
Gastrointestinal Medical Oncology
 Co-Chair
Southwest Oncology Group
Rectal Subcommittee
National Clinical Trials Network
 Institutional Grant
Lead Contact Principle Investigator
Department of Gastrointestinal Medical
 Oncology
The University of Texas MD Anderson
 Cancer Center
Houston, Texas

Charles Erlichman, MD
Professor, Department of Oncology
Deputy Director, Clinical Research
Peter and Frances Georgeson Professor of
 Gastroenterology Cancer Research
Mayo Clinic
Rochester, Minnesota

Elihu H. Estey, MD
Professor, Division of Hematology
University of Washington School of
 Medicine
Member and Director of Acute Myeloid
 Leukemia Clinical Research
 (Nontransplant)
Clinical Research Division
Fred Hutchinson Cancer Research
 Center
Seattle, Washington

Douglas B. Evans, MD
Professor and Chair
Department of Surgery
Medical College of Wisconsin
Milwaukee, Wisconsin

Jane M. Fall-Dickson, PhD, RN, AOCN
Associate Professor and Assistant Chair,
 Research
Department of Nursing
Georgetown University School of Nursing
 and Health Studies
Washington, District of Columbia

Adam S. Feldman, MD, MPH
Assistant Professor of Surgery
Harvard Medical School
Assistant in Urology, Department of
 Urology
Massachusetts General Hospital
Boston, Massachusetts

Steven A. Feldman, PhD
Staff Scientist
Director, Surgery Branch
Vector Production Facility
National Cancer Institute
Bethesda, Maryland

Mary Feng, MD
Associate Professor, Department of
 Radiation Oncology
University of Michigan Health System
Ann Arbor, Michigan

Felix Y. Feng, MD
Assistant Professor, Department of
 Radiation Oncology
Chief, Division of Translational
 Genomics
University of Michigan Health System
Ann Arbor, Michigan

William Douglas Figg, Sr., PharmD, MBA
Senior Investigator and Head of the
 Clinical Pharmacology Program
Clinical Director, Center for Cancer
 Research
Head of the Molecular Pharmacology
 Section
Medical Oncology Branch
Center for Cancer Research
National Cancer Institute
National Institutes of Health
Bethesda, Maryland

Paul T. Finger, MD
Clinical Professor of Ophthalmology
Director, Ocular Tumor Services
New York University School of Medicine
The New York Eye and Ear Infirmary
The New York Eye Cancer Center
New York, New York

Joel A. Finkelstein, MD, MSc, FRCS(C)
Division of Orthopaedic Surgery
Sunnybrook Health Sciences Centre
University of Toronto
Toronto, Ontario, Canada

Gini F. Fleming, MD
Professor, Department of Medicine
Director, Medical Gynecologic Oncology
Section of Hematology and Oncology
University of Chicago
Chicago, Illinois

Antonio Tito Fojo, MD, PhD
Medical Oncology Branch and Affiliates
Head, Experimental Therapeutics
 Section
Senior Investigator
Center for Cancer Research
National Cancer Institute
Bethesda, Maryland

Yuman Fong, MD
Chairman, Department of Surgery
Associate Director, International
 Relations
City of Hope Medical Center
Duarte, California

James M. Ford, MD
Associate Professor
Departments of Medicine, Pediatrics and
 Genetics
Divisions of Oncology and Medical
 Genetics
Director, Clinical Cancer Genomics
 Program
Stanford University School of Medicine
Stanford, California

Francine M. Foss, MD
Professor of Medicine, Hematology and
 Bone Marrow Transplantation
Yale University School of Medicine
New Haven, Connecticut

Arnold S. Freedman, MD
Associate Professor of Medicine
Harvard Medical School
Clinical Director, Lymphoma Program
Dana-Farber Cancer Institute
Associate Physician, Brigham and
 Women's Hospital
Boston, Massachusetts

Wayne L. Furman, MD
Member, Department of Oncology
St. Jude Children's Research Hospital
Professor, Department of Pediatrics
University of Tennessee Medical School
Memphis, Tennessee

Larissa V. Furtado, MD
Assistant Professor
Department of Pathology
Assistant Director
Division of Genomics and Molecular
 Pathology
University of Chicago
Chicago, Illinois

Matthew Kalady, MD
Associate Professor of Surgery
Krause-Lieberman Chair in Colorectal
    Surgery
Department of Colorectal Surgery
Digestive Disease Institute
Cleveland Clinic
Cleveland, Ohio

Kala Y. Kamdar, MD, MS
Assistant Professor
Department of Pediatrics
Hematology/Oncology Section
Baylor College of Medicine
Associate Clinical Director
Texas Children's Cancer and Hematology
    Center
Houston, Texas

Robert J. Kaner, MD
Associate Attending Physician
New York Presbyterian Weill Cornell
    Center
Associate Professor of Clinical Medicine
    and Genetic Medicine
Weill Cornell Medical College
New York, New York

Joyson J. Karakunnel, MD, FACP
Potomac, Maryland

Brian D. Kavanagh, MD, MPH
Professor, Department of Radiation
    Oncology
University of Colorado School of
    Medicine
Anschutz Medical Campus
Aurora, Colorado

Partow Kebriaei, MD
Associate Professor
Division of Cancer Medicine
Department of Stem Cell Transplant and
    Cellular Therapy
The University of Texas MD Anderson
    Cancer Center
Houston, Texas

David P. Kelsen, MD
Edward S Gordon Chair in Medical
    Oncology
Attending Physician, Department of
    Medicine
Memorial Sloan-Kettering Cancer Center
Professor of Medicine Weill Cornell
    Medical College
New York, New York

Scott E. Kern, MD
Everett and Marjorie Kovler Professor of
    Pancreas Cancer Research
Department of Oncology
Sidney Kimmel Comprehensive Cancer
    Center at Johns Hopkins
Baltimore, Maryland

Alok A. Khorana, MD, FACP
Professor of Medicine, Cleveland Clinic
    Lerner College of Medicine, Case
    Western Reserve University
Sondra and Stephen Hardis Chair in
    Oncology Research
Vice Chair for Clinical Services, Taussig
    Cancer Institute
Director, Gastrointestinal Malignancies
    Program
Cleveland Clinic
Cleveland, Ohio

Christopher J. Kirk, MD
Vice President of Research
Onyx Pharmaceuticals, Inc.
South San Francisco, California

Ann H. Klopp, MD, PhD
Assistant Professor
Section of Gynecology
Department of Radiation Oncology
The University of Texas MD Anderson
    Cancer Center
Houston, Texas

Margaret A. Knowles, PhD
Head, Section of Experimental Oncology
Leeds Institute of Cancer and Pathology
St. James's University Hospital
Leeds, United Kingdom

James N. Kochenderfer, MD
Investigator, Experimental
    Transplantation and Immunology
    Branch
National Cancer Institute
National Institutes of Health
Bethesda, Maryland

Manish Kohli, MD
Associate Professor of Oncology
Department of Oncology
College of Medicine
Mayo Clinic
Joint Appointment, Department of
    Urology
Mayo Clinic
Rochester, Minnesota

Rami S. Komrokji, MD
Clinical Director
Associate Member
Department of Malignant Hematology
H. Lee Moffitt Cancer Center &
    Research Institute
Tampa, Florida

**Panagiotis A. Konstantinopoulos, MD,
    PhD**
Assistant Professor of Medicine
Harvard Medical School
Gynecologic Medical Oncology Program
Dana-Farber Cancer Institute
Boston, Massachusetts

Vadim P. Koshenkov, MD
Assistant Professor of Surgery
Division of Surgical Oncology
Rutgers Cancer Institute of New Jersey
Robert Wood Johnson University Hospital
New Brunswick, New Jersey

Matthew J. Krasin, MD
Radiological Sciences
Radiation Oncology
St. Jude Children's Research Hospital
Memphis, Tennessee

Mark G. Kris, MD
Professor of Medicine
Weill Cornell Medical College
Attending Physician, Thoracic Oncology
    Service
Memorial Sloan-Kettering Cancer Center
New York, New York

Robert S. Krouse, MD, MS
Professor, Department of Surgery
University of Arizona College of
    Medicine
Staff General and Oncologic Surgeon
Surgical Care Line
Southern Arizona Veterans Affairs Health
    Care System
Tucson, Arizona

Lee M. Krug, MD
Associate Attending Physician
Department of Medicine
Memorial Sloan-Kettering Cancer Center
Associate Professor of Medicine
Weill Medical College of Cornell
    University
New York, New York

Shivaani Kummar, MD, FACP
Head, Early Clinical Trials Development
Office of the Director
Division of Cancer Treatment and
    Diagnosis
National Cancer Institute
Bethesda, Maryland

Pamela L. Kunz, MD
Assistant Professor of Medicine/Oncology
Stanford University School of Medicine
Division of Oncology
Stanford Cancer Institute
Stanford, California

John Kuruvilla, MD, FRCPC
Hematologist, Princess Margaret Cancer
    Centre
Assistant Professor Medicine
University of Toronto
Toronto, Ontario, Canada

Wendy Landier, PhD, RN, CPNP
Assistant Professor, Department of
    Population Sciences
Clinical Director, Center for Cancer
    Survivorship
City of Hope
Duarte, California

Brian R. Lane, MD, PhD
Associate Professor, Department of
    Surgery
Michigan State University College of
    Human Medicine
Betz Family Endowed Chair for Cancer
    Research
Spectrum Health Cancer Program
Grand Rapids, Michigan

Theodore S. Lawrence, MD, PhD
Isadore Lampe Professor and Chair
Department of Radiation Oncology
University of Michigan Health System
Ann Arbor, Michigan

Hillard M. Lazarus, MD, FACP
Professor of Medicine
Case Western Reserve University
Director, Novel Cell Therapy
The George & Edith Richman Professor
    and Distinguished Scientist in Cancer
    Research
University Hospitals
Case Medical Center
Cleveland, Ohio

Thomas W. LeBlanc, MD, MA
Assistant Professor, Division of
    Hematologic Malignancies and
    Cellular Therapy
Department of Medicine
Duke University School of Medicine
Durham, North Carolina

Richard J. Lee, MD, PhD
Assistant Professor, Department of
    Medicine
Harvard Medical School
Assistant Physician, Division of
    Hematology and Oncology
Massachusetts General Hospital
Boston, Massachusetts

Percy P. Lee, MD
Associate Professor of Radiation Oncology
Chief, Thoracic Radiation Oncology
Chief, Gastrointestinal Radiation Oncology
Director, Stereotactic Body Radiation
    Oncology Program
David Geffen School of Medicine at
    University of California, Los Angeles
University of California Los Angeles
    Jonsson Comprehensive Cancer Center
Los Angeles, California

Agnes Y. Y. Lee, MC, MSc, FRCPC
Associate Professor, Department of
    Medicine
Director, Thrombosis Program
University of British Columbia and
    British Columbia Cancer Agency
Vancouver, British Columbia, Canada

David J. Leffell, MD
David Paige Smith Professor of
    Dermatology & Surgery
Chief, Section of Dermatologic Surgery
    and Cutaneous Oncology
Department of Dermatology
Yale University School of Medicine
New Haven, Connecticut

Antonio M. Lerario, MD
Adrenal Disorders Unit
Department of Endocrinology and
    Metabolism
Hospital das Clinicas da Faculdade de
    Medicina da Universidade de Sao Paulo
Sao Paulo, Brazil

Rebecca A. Levine, MD
Assistant Professor, Department of
    Surgery
Montefiore Medical Center
Albert Einstein College of Medicine
Bronx, New York

Nancy L. Lewis, MD
Associate Professor
Department of Medical Oncology
Clinical Director
Experimental Therapeutics
Thomas Jefferson University
Kimmel Cancer Center
Philadelphia, Pennsylvania

Steven K. Libutti, MD, FACS
Director, Montefiore-Einstein Center for
    Cancer Care
Vice Chairman, Department of Surgery
Montefiore-Einstein Center for Cancer
    Care
Bronx, New York

Rogerio C. Lilenbaum, MD
Chief Medical Officer of Smilow Cancer
    Hospital
Thoracic Oncology Program
Yale University School of Medicine
New Haven, Connecticut

W. Marston Linehan, MD
Chief, Urologic Oncology Branch
Center for Cancer Research
National Cancer Institute
Bethesda, Maryland

Scott M. Lippman, MD
Director, Senior Associate Dean, &
    Associate Vice Chancellor
Cancer Research and Care
Chugai Pharmaceutical Chair
Professor of Medicine
University of California, San Diego
Moores Cancer Center
La Jolla, California

Roy Lirov, MD
Resident in General Surgery
Department of Surgery
University of Michigan Hospital and
    Health Systems
University of Michigan Health System
Ann Arbor, Michigan

Alan F. List, MD
President and CEO
Senior Member
H. Lee Moffitt Cancer Center
Tampa, Florida

Richard F. Little, MD, MPH
Senior Investigator
Head, Blood and AIDS Related Cancer
    Therapeutics
Clinical Investigations Branch
Cancer Therapy Evaluation Program
National Cancer Institute
Bethesda, Maryland

Mats Ljungman, PhD
Professor, Departments of Radiation
    Oncology and Environmental Health
    Sciences
Translational Oncology Program
University of Michigan Medical School
Ann Arbor, Michigan

Patrick J. Loehrer, Sr, MD
H. H. Gregg Professor of Oncology
Director, Indiana University Melvin and
    Bren Simon Cancer Center
Associate Dean for Cancer Research
Indiana University School of Medicine
Indianapolis, Indiana

Christopher J. Logothetis, MD
Principle Investigator
Genitourinary Medical Oncology
The University of Texas MD Anderson
    Cancer Center
Houston, Texas

Carlos López-Otin, PhD
Professor, Department of Biochemistry
    and Molecular Biology
Universidad de Oviedo
Principality of Asturias, Spain

Charles L. Loprinzi, MD
Regis Professor of Breast Cancer Research
Department of Oncology
Mayo Clinic
Rochester, Minnesota

Yani Lu, PhD
Assistant Research Professor
Division of Cancer Etiology
Department of Population Science
Beckman Research Institute of the City
    of Hope
Duarte, California

Samuel J. Lubner, MD
Assistant Professor
Department of Medicine
Hematology/Oncology Section
Associate Program Director
Hematology/Oncology Fellowship
University of Wisconsin
Madison, Wisconsin

Matthew A. Lunning, DO
Assistant Professor
Division of Hematology/Oncology
Department of Medicine
University of Nebraska Medical Center
Omaha, Nebraska

Teresa H. Lyden, MA, CCC-SLP
Speech Language Pathologist
Department of Otolaryngology-Head and
 Neck Surgery
University of Michigan Medical Center
Ann Arbor, Michigan

Xiaomei Ma, PhD
Associate Professor, Department of
 Chronic Disease Epidemiology
Yale University School of Public Health
New Haven, Connecticut

Krishnaraj Mahendraraj, MD
Resident, Department of Surgery
St. Barnabas Medical Center
Livingston, New Jersey

Ajay V. Maker, MD, FACS
Assistant Professor, Department of Surgery
Division of Surgical Oncology
Department of Microbiology and
 Immunology
University of Illinois at Chicago
Director of Surgical Oncology
Advocate Illinois Masonic Medical Center
Chicago, Illinois

David Malkin, MD
Staff Oncologist, Division of Hematology/
 Oncology
Senior Scientist, Genetics & Genome
 Biology Program
The Hospital for Sick Children
University of Toronto
Toronto, Ontario, Canada

Eddie W. Manning, III, MD
Senior Resident
Division of Cardiothoracic Surgery
The DeWitt Daughtry Family
 Department of Surgery
Miller School of Medicine
University of Miami
Miami, Florida

Judith F. Margolin, MD
Associate Professor
Department of Pediatrics
Baylor College of Medicine
Attending Oncologist
Texas Children's Cancer Center
Houston, Texas

David Marin, MD, DM, FRCP
Department of Stem Cell Transplantation
 and Cellular Therapy
The University of Texas MD Anderson
 Cancer Center
Houston, Texas

Jens U. Marquardt, MD
Resident Physician
Department of Medicine
University of Mainz
Mainz, Germany
Laboratory of Experimental
 Carcinogenesis
Center for Cancer Research
National Cancer Institute
National Institutes of Health
Bethesda, Maryland

Ellen T. Matloff, MS, CGC
President & CEO
Gene Counsel, LLC
New Haven, Connecticut

Peter Mauch, MD
Professor of Radiation Oncology
Department of Radiation Oncology
Harvard Medical School
Boston, Massachusetts

Susan T. Mayne, PhD
C.-E.A. Winslow Professor of Epidemiology
Chair, Department of Chronic Disease
 Epidemiology
Yale University School of Public Health
Associate Director for Population
 Sciences
Yale Cancer Center
New Haven, Connecticut

Howard L. McLeod, PharmD
Medical Director, DeBartolo Family
 Personalized Medicine Institute
Senior Member, Division of Population
 Sciences
H. Lee Moffitt Cancer Center
Tampa, Florida

Minesh P. Mehta, MBChB, FASTRO
Professor, Department of Radiation
 Oncology
Director, Maryland Proton Treatment
 Center
University of Maryland
Baltimore, Maryland

Laleh G. Melstrom, MD, MSCI
Assistant Professor, Department of Surgery
Rutgers Cancer Institute of New Jersey
Robert Wood Johnson School of
 Medicine
Robert Wood Johnson Hospital and the
 Rutgers Cancer Institute of New Jersey
New Brunswick, New Jersey

William M. Mendenhall, MD
Professor Department of Radiation
 Oncology
University of Florida
Shands Hospital at the University of
 Florida
Gainesville, Florida
University of Florida Proton Therapy
 Institute
Jacksonville, Florida

M. Dror Michaelson, MD, PhD
Associate Professor of Medicine
Harvard Medical School
Clinical Director, Urologic Oncology
Massachusetts General Hospital Cancer
 Center
Boston, Massachusetts

Karin B. Michels, ScD, PhD
Associate Professor
Obstetrician/Gynecologist
Epidemiology Center
Department of Obstetrics, Gynecology
 and Reproductive Biology
Brigham and Women's Hospital
Harvard Medical School
Boston, Massachusetts

Bruce D. Minsky, MD
Professor and Frank T. McGraw
 Memorial Chair
Deputy Head, Division of Radiation
 Oncology
The University of Texas MD Anderson
 Cancer Center
Houston, Texas

Sandra A. Mitchell, PhD, CRNP
Research Scientist and Program Director
Outcomes Research Branch
Applied Research Program
Division of Cancer Control and
 Population Sciences
National Cancer Institute
Rockville, Maryland

Jeffrey F. Moley, MD
Chief, Section of Endocrine and
 Oncologic Surgery
Professor of Surgery
Washington University School of
 Medicine
St. Louis, Missouri

Meredith A. Morgan, PhD
Research Assistant Professor
Department of Radiation Oncology
University of Michigan
Ann Arbor, Michigan

Daniel Morgensztern, MD
Associate Professor of Medicine
Director of Thoracic Oncology
Clinical Research Division of Oncology
Alvin J. Siteman Cancer Center
Washington University School of
 Medicine
St. Louis, Missouri

Monica Morrow, MD
Chief, Breast Service
Anne Burnett Windfohr Chair of Clinical
    Oncology
Department of Surgery
Memorial Sloan-Kettering Cancer Center
Professor of Surgery
Weill Cornell Medical College
New York, New York

Nikhil C. Munshi, MD
Associate Director, Jerome Lipper
    Multiple Myeloma Center
Department of Medical Oncology
Dana-Farber Cancer Institute
Associate Professor of Medicine
Harvard Medical School
Boston, Massachusetts

Rebecca Nagy, MS, LGC
Associate Professor
Clinical Internal Medicine
The Ohio State University
Department of Internal Medicine
Licensed Genetic Counselor
Division of Human Genetics
The Ohio State University Wexner
    Medical Center
Columbus, Ohio

Patrick Nana-Sinkam, MD
Associate Professor, Department of
    Internal Medicine
Division of Pulmonary, Allergy, Critical
    Care and Sleep Medicine
The Ohio State University
Columbus, Ohio

Fariba Navid, MD
Associate Member, Department of
    Oncology
Division of Solid Malignancies
St. Jude Children's Research Hospital
Memphis, Tennessee

Christian J. Nelson, PhD
Assistant Attending Psychologist
Department of Psychiatry and Behavioral
    Sciences
Memorial Sloan-Kettering Cancer Center
New York, New York

Anna C. Newlin, MS, CGC
Certified Genetic Counselor
Center for Medical Genetics
NorthShore University HealthSystem
Evanston, Illinois

Andrea Ng, MD, MPH
Associate Professor, Department of
    Radiation Oncology
Brigham and Women's Hospital
Dana-Farber Cancer Institute
Harvard Medical School
Boston, Massachusetts

**Dao M. Nguyen, MD, MSc, FRCSC,
    FACS**
The B. and Donald Carlin Endowed
    Chair of Thoracic Surgical Oncology
Professor and Chief
Section of Thoracic Surgery Section
Division of Cardiothoracic Surgery
The DeWitt Daughtry Family
    Department of Surgery
Miller School of Medicine
University of Miami
Miami, Florida

Torsten O. Nielsen, MD, PhD, FRCPC
Professor, Department of Pathology and
    Laboratory Medicine
University of British Columbia
Vancouver, British Colombia, Canada

Jeffrey A. Norton, MD
Professor, Department of Surgery
Chief, Section of Surgical Oncology and
    Division of General Surgery
Department of Surgery
Stanford University Hospital
Stanford, California

Susan M. O'Brien, MD
Professor, Department of Leukemia
The University of Texas MD Anderson
    Cancer Center
Houston, Texas

Richard J. O'Connor, PhD
Associate Member, Department of Health
    Behavior
Division of Cancer Prevention and
    Population Sciences
Roswell Park Cancer Institute
Buffalo, New York

Richard J. O'Donnell, MD
Professor of Clinical Orthopaedic Surgery
Chief, Orthopaedic Oncology Service
Director, Sarcoma Program
University of California, San Francisco
    Medical Center
University of California, San Francisco
Benioff Children's Hospitals
University of California, San Francisco
Bakar Cancer Hospital University of
    California, San Francisco
Helen Diller Family Comprehensive
    Cancer Center
San Francisco, California

Kunle Odunsi, MD, PhD
The M. Steven Piver Professor and Chair
Department of Gynecologic Oncology
    Director
Center for Immunotherapy
Professor of Obstetrics and Gynecology
Department of Gynecology-Obstetrics
School of Medicine and Biomedical
    Sciences
University at Buffalo-State University of
    New York
Buffalo, New York

Peter J. O'Dwyer, MD
Professor of Medicine
Abramson Cancer Center
University of Pennsylvania
Philadelphia, Pennsylvania

Kevin C. Oeffinger, MD
Director, Adult Long-Term Follow-Up
    Program
Co-Leader, Survivorship, Outcomes and
    Risk Program
Full Member, Departments of Medicine
    and Pediatrics
Memorial Sloan-Kettering Cancer Center
New York, New York

Brian O'Sullivan, MD, FRCPC
Bartley-Smith/Wharton Chair in
    Radiation Oncology
Professor, Department of Radiation
    Oncology
University of Toronto
Toronto, Ontario, Canada

Gregory A. Otterson, MD
Professor, Department of Internal
    Medicine
Division of Medical Oncology
Director, Hematology/Oncology
    Fellowship Program
The Ohio State University
    Comprehensive Cancer Center
Columbus, Ohio

Eric Padron, MD
Assistant Member
Malignant Hematology Section
Head, Genomics and Personalized
    Medicine
H. Lee Moffitt Cancer Center and
    Research Institute
Tampa, Florida

Lance C. Pagliaro, MD
Professor, Department of Genitourinary
    Medical Oncology
The University of Texas MD Anderson
    Cancer Center
Houston, Texas

Tara N. Palmore, MD
Hospital Epidemiologist
National Institutes of Health Clinical
    Center
Staff Clinician
National Institute of Allergy and
    Infectious Diseases
National Institutes of Health
Bethesda, Maryland

Alberto S. Pappo, MD
Member
Director, Solid Tumor Section
St. Jude Children's Research Hospital
Memphis, Tennessee

Howard L. Parnes, MD
Chief
Prostate and Urologic Cancer Research
    Group
Division of Cancer Prevention
National Cancer Institute
Rockville, Maryland

Mark Parta, MD
Clinical Research Directorate/Clinical
    Monitoring Research Program
Leodos Biomedical Research, Inc.
Frederick National Laboratory for Cancer
    Research
Frederick, Maryland

Laura Pasqualucci, MD
Associate Professor of Pathology and Cell
    Biology
Department of Pathology and Cell
    Biology
Institute for Cancer Genetics
Herbert Irving Comprehensive Cancer
    Center
Columbia University
New York, New York

Harvey I. Pass, MD
Stephen E. Banner Professor of Thoracic
    Oncology
Vice-Chairman, Research Department of
    Cardiothoracic Surgery
Director, General Thoracic Surgery
New York University Langone Medical
    Center
New York, New York

Tushar Patel, MBChB
Professor of Medicine
Mayo Clinic
Jacksonville, Florida

George Patounakis, MD, PhD
Clinical Fellow
Department of Reproductive
    Endocrinology and Infertility
National Institute of Child Health and
    Human Development
National Institutes of Health
Bethesda, Maryland

David M. Peereboom, MD, FACP
Professor of Medicine
Cleveland Clinic Lerner College of
    Medicine
Director, Clinical Research
The Rose Ella Burkhardt Brain Tumor &
    Neuro-Oncology Center
Solid Tumor Oncology
Cleveland Clinic
Cleveland, Ohio

Tanja Pejovic, MD, PhD
Associate Professor
Director, Gynecologic Cancer Research
Department of Obstetrics & Gynecology
Knight Cancer Institute
Oregon Health & Science University
Portland, Oregon

David G. Pfister, MD
Chief, Head and Neck Oncology Service
Memorial Sloan-Kettering Cancer Center
New York, New York

Giao Q. Phan, MD, FACS
Associate Professor
Division of Surgical Oncology
Massey Cancer Center
Virginia Commonwealth University
Richmond, Virginia

M. Catherine Pietanza, MD
Thoracic Oncology
Memorial Sloan-Kettering Cancer Center
New York, New York

Robert Pilarski, MS, LGC, MSW
Associate Professor
Clinical Internal Medicine
James Comprehensive Cancer Center
Department of Internal Medicine
The Ohio State University Wexner
    Medical Center
Columbus, Ohio

Peter W. T. Pisters, MD, FACS
Professor, Department of Surgical Oncology
Division of Surgery
The University of Texas MD Anderson
    Cancer Center
Houston, Texas

Mark N. Polizzotto, MB, BS, BMedSc
Assistant Clinical Investigator
HIV and AIDS Malignancy Branch
Center for Cancer Research National
    Cancer Institute
National Institutes of Health
Bethesda, Maryland

Yves Pommier, MD, PhD
Chief, Laboratory of Molecular
    Pharmacology
Head, DNA Topoisomerase/Integrase
    Group
Center for Cancer Research
National Cancer Institute
Bethesda, Maryland

David G. Poplack, MD
Elise C. Young Professor of Pediatric
    Oncology
Head, Hematology-Oncology Section
Department of Pediatrics
Baylor College of Medicine
Director, Texas Children's Cancer Center
Texas Children's Hospital
Houston, Texas

Edwin M. Posadas, MD, FACP, KM
Medical Director, Urologic Oncology
    Program
Assistant Professor, Department of
    Medicine
Samuel Ochsin Comprehensive Cancer
    Institute
Cedars-Sinai Medical Center
Los Angeles, California

Mitchell C. Posner, MD, FACS
Thomas D. Jones Professor of Surgery
    and Vice-Chairman
Chief, Section of General Surgery and
    Surgical Oncology
Professor, Radiation and Cellular Oncology
Medical Director, Clinical Cancer
    Programs
The University of Chicago Medicine
Chicago, Illinois

Sahdeo Prasad, PhD
Cytokine Research Laboratory
Department of Experimental
    Therapeutics
The University of Texas MD Anderson
    Cancer Center
Houston, Texas

Mark E. P. Prince, MD, FRCS(C)
Professor, Department of Otolaryngology-
    Head and Neck Surgery
Chief, Division of Head and Neck
    Surgery
University of Michigan Health System
Ann Arbor, Michigan

Ibrahim M. Qazi, PharmD
University of Maryland
Baltimore, Maryland

Karen R. Rabin, MD, PhD
Assistant Professor, Department of
    Pediatrics
Division of Pediatric Hematology and
    Oncology
Baylor College of Medicine
Houston, Texas

Glen D. Raffel, MD, PhD
Assistant Professor, Department of
    Medicine
Division of Hematology-Oncology
University of Massachusetts Medical
    School
Worcester, Massachusetts

Lee Ratner, MD, PhD
Professor Departments of Medicine and
    Molecular Microbiology
Co-Director, Medical & Molecular
    Oncology
Washington University School of
    Medicine
Barnes-Jewish Hospital
St. Louis, Missouri

Abram Recht, MD, FASTRO
Professor, Department of Radiation
    Oncology
Harvard Medical School
Deputy Chief, Department of Radiation
    Oncology
Beth Israel Deaconess Medical Center
Boston, Massachusetts

Michelle B. Riba, MD, MS
Professor and Associate Chair for
 Integrated Medical and Psychiatric
 Services
Department of Psychiatry
Director, PsychOncology Program
University of Michigan Comprehensive
 Cancer Center
Ann Arbor, Michigan

Antoni Ribas, MD, PhD
Professor of Medicine
Professor of Surgery
Professor of Molecular and Medical
 Pharmacology
Director, Tumor Immunology Program
Jonsson Comprehensive Cancer Center
David Geffen School of Medicine
University of California Los Angeles
Chair, Melanoma Committee
Southwest Oncology Group
Los Angeles, California

Stanley R. Riddell, MD
Member, Fred Hutchinson Cancer
 Research Center
Professor, Department of Medicine
University of Washington
Seattle, Washington

Andreas Rimner, MD
Assistant Professor, Department of
 Radiation Oncology
Assistant Attending, Department of
 Radiation Oncology
Memorial Sloan-Kettering Cancer Center
New York, New York

Brian I. Rini, MD, FACP
Professor of Medicine
Lerner College of Medicine
Department of Solid Tumor Oncology
Cleveland Clinic Taussig Cancer Institute
Glickman Urological Institute
Cleveland, Ohio

Paul F. Robbins, PhD
National Institutes of Health
Bethesda, Maryland

Matthew K. Robinson, PhD
Assistant Professor, Developmental
 Therapeutics Program
Fox Chase Cancer Center
Philadelphia, Pennsylvania

Steven A. Rosenberg, MD, PhD
Chief, Surgery Branch, National Cancer
 Institute, National Institutes of Health
Professor of Surgery, Uniformed Services
 University of the Health Sciences
School of Medicine
Bethesda, Maryland
Professor of Surgery
George Washington University School of
 Medicine
Washington, District of Columbia

Kenneth E. Rosenzweig, MD
Professor, Department of Radiation
 Oncology
Icahn School of Medicine at Mount Sinai
Chair, Department of Radiation
 Oncology
Mount Sinai Health System
New York, New York

Charles M. Rudin, MD, PhD
Chief, Thoracic Oncology Service
Memorial Sloan-Kettering Cancer Center
New York, New York

Anil K. Rustgi, MD
T. Grier Miller Professor of Medicine &
 Genetics
Chief of Gastroenterology
University of Pennsylvania Perelman
 School of Medicine
Philadelphia, Pennsylvania

Arjun Sahgal, MD
Associate Professor of Radiation Oncology
 and Surgery
Department of Radiation Oncology
Toronto, Ontario, Canada

M. Wasif Saif, MD, MBBS
Director, Gastrointestinal Oncology
 Program
Leader, Experimental Therapeutics
 Program
Tufts Medical Center
Tufts University School of Medicine
Boston, Massachusetts

Leonard B. Saltz, MD
Professor, Department of Medicine
Chief, Gastrointestinal Oncology Service
Memorial Sloan-Kettering Cancer Center
New York, New York

Yardena Samuels, PhD
Knell Family Professorial Chair
Department of Molecular Cell Biology
Weizmann Institute of Science
Rehovot, Israel

Charles L. Sawyers, MD
Investigator, Howard Hughes Medical
 Institute
Chair, Human Oncology and
 Pathogenesis Program
Memorial Sloan-Kettering Cancer Center
New York, New York

Peter T. Scardino, MD
Chairman, Department of Surgery
The David H. Koch Chair
Memorial Sloan-Kettering Cancer Center
New York, New York

Sanne B. Schagen, PhD
Division of Psychosocial Research and
 Epidemiology
The Netherlands Cancer Institute
Amsterdam, The Netherlands

Howard I. Scher, MD
Chief, Genitourinary Oncology Service
Member and Attending Physician
Department of Medicine
Memorial Sloan-Kettering Cancer Center
Professor of Medicine
Weill Cornell Medical College
New York, New York

Laura S. Schmidt, PhD
Principal Scientist
Leidos Biomedical Research, Inc.
Frederick National Laboratory for Cancer
 Research
Frederick, Maryland
Urologic Oncology Branch
National Cancer Institute
National Institutes of Health
Bethesda, Maryland

Meredith L. Seidel, MS, CGC
Genetic Counselor
Center for Cancer Risk Assessment
Massachusetts General Hospital
Boston, Massachusetts

Leigha Senter-Jamieson, MS, CGC
Director of Clinical Supervison
Associate Professor
Division of Human Genetics
Department of Internal Medicine
The Ohio State University
Columbuis, Ohio

Bijal Shah, MD
Associate Member
H. Lee Moffitt Cancer Center
Tampa, Florida

Syed Ammer Shah, MD
Postgraduate Year Four
Surgical Resident
Saint Barnabas Medical Center
Caldwell, New Jersey

Kristen M. Shannon, MS, CGC
Director, Cancer Center Genetics
 Program
Licensed Genetic Counselor
Massachusetts General Cancer Center
Massachusetts General Hospital
Boston, Massachusetts

Peter G. Shields, MD
Deputy Director, Comprehensive Cancer
 Center
Professor, College of Medicine
James Cancer Hospital
The Ohio State University
Columbus, Ohio

Ramesh A. Shivdasani, MD, PhD
Associate Professor, Department of
 Medical Oncology
Dana-Farber Cancer Institute
Department of Medicine
Harvard Medical School
Boston, Massachusetts

Richard M. Simon, DSc
Chief, Biometric Research Branch
National Cancer Institute
Rockville, Maryland

Samuel Singer, MD
Member, Department of Surgery
Chief, Gastric and Mixed Tumor Service
Vincent Astor Chair of Clinical Research
Memorial Sloan-Kettering Cancer Center
New York, New York

Craig L. Slingluff, Jr., MD
Joseph Helms Farrow Professor of Surgery
Division of Surgical Oncology
Vice-Chair for Research Director
Human Immune Therapy Center
University of Virginia
Charlottesville, Virginia

Eliezer Soto, MD, DABPM, FIPP
Anesthesia Pain Care Consultants
Tamarac, Florida

Alex Sparreboom, PhD
Associate Member, Department of
    Pharmaceutical Sciences
St. Jude Children's Research Hospital
Memphis, Tennessee

David Spiegel, MD
Willson Professor and Associate Chair
Department of Psychiatry & Behavioral
    Sciences
Director, Center on Stress and Health
Medical Director, Center for Integrative
    Medicine
Stanford University School of Medicine
Stanford, California

Thomas E. Stinchcombe, MD
Associate Professor, Division of
    Hematology/Oncology
University of North Carolina
Chapel Hill, North Carolina

Alexander Stojadinovic, MD
Bon Secours Cancer Institute
Richmond, Virginia

Diane E. Stover, MD
Professor of Clinical Medicine
Cornell University Medical College
Chief, Pulmonary Service
Department of Medicine
Memorial Sloan-Kettering Cancer Center
New York, New York

Michael D. Stubblefield, MD
Associate Attending Physiatrist
Rehabilitation Medicine Service
Department of Neurology
Memorial Sloan-Kettering Cancer Center
Associate Professor of Rehabilitation
    Medicine
Division of Rehabilitation Medicine
Weill Cornell Medical College
New York City, New York

Paul H. Sugarbaker, MD, FACS, FRCS
Medical Director, Center for
    Gastrointestinal Malignancies
Chief, Program in Peritoneal Surface
    Oncology
MedStar Washington Hospital Center
Washington, District of Columbia

John H. Suh, MD
Professor of Medicine
Chariman, Department of Radiation
    Oncology
Cleveland Clinic Taussig Cancer Institute
Burkhardt Brain Tumor and Neuro-
    ·Oncology Center
Cleveland Clinic
Cleveland, Ohio

Irene M. Tamí-Maury, DMD, DrPH, MSc
The University of Texas MD Anderson
    Cancer Center
Houston, Texas

Lynn Tanoue, MD
Professor of Internal Medicine
Medical Director
Yale Cancer Center
Thoracic Oncology Program
Yale University School of Medicine
New Haven, Connecticut

William D. Tap, MD
Associate Member, Department of
    Medicine
Section Chief, Sarcoma Oncology
    Melanoma and Sarcoma Service
Division of Solid Tumors
Memorial Sloan-Kettering Cancer Center
New York, New York

Michael D. Taylor, MD, PhD, FRCSC
Associate Professor
Departments of Surgery and of Laboratory
    Medicine and Pathobiology
University of Toronto
Hospital for Sick Children Research
    Institute
Toronto, Ontario, Canada

**Randall K. Ten Haken, PhD, FAAPM,
    FInstP, FASTRO, FACR**
Professor, Associate Chair, and Physics
    Division Director
Department of Radiation Oncology
University of Michigan Medical School
Ann Arbor, Michigan

Kenneth D. Tew, PhD, DSc
Chairman and John C. West Chair in
    Cancer Research
Cell and Molecular Pharmacology
Medical University of South Carolina
Charleston, South Carolina

**Geoffrey B. Thompson, MD, FACS,
    FACE**
Professor, Department of Surgery
Section Head, Endocrine Surgery
College of Medicine, Mayo Clinic
Consultant, Division of Gastroenterologic
    and General Surgery
Mayo Clinic
Rochester, Minnesota

Snorri S. Thorgeirsson, MD, PhD
Head, Center of Excellence in Integrative
    Cancer Biology and Genomics
Chief, Laboratory of Experimental
    Carcinogenesis Center for Cancer
    Research
National Cancer Institute
National Institutes of Health
Bethesda, Maryland

Benjamin A. Toll, PhD
Associate Professor of Psychiatry
Yale University School of Medicine
Yale Comprehensive Cancer Center
Program Director, Smoking Cessation
    Service
Smilow Cancer Hospital at Yale-New
    Haven
New Haven, Connecticut

Christopher W. Towe, MD
Chief Resident
Department of Cardiothoracic Surgery
New York University School of Medicine
New York, New York

Edouard J. Trabulsi, MD, FACS
Associate Professor, Department of
    Urology
Kimmel Cancer Center
Jefferson Medical College
Director, Division of Urologic Oncology
Thomas Jefferson University
Philadelphia, Pennsylvania

Lois B. Travis, MD, ScD
Director, Rubin Center for Cancer
    Survivorship
Professor and Chief, Division of Cancer
    Survivorship
Department of Radiation Oncology
University of Rochester Medical Center
Rochester, New York

William D. Travis, MD
Professor of Pathology
Weill Medical College of Cornell
    University
Memorial Sloan-Kettering Cancer Center
New York, New York

Brian B. Tuch, PhD
Associate Director, Translational
    Genomics
Onyx Pharmaceuticals
South San Francisco, California

Catherine E. Ulbricht, PharmD
Founder, Natural Standard
Vice President, Integrated Therapeutics
    & Clinical Solutions
Therapeutic Research Center
Senior Attending Pharmacist
Massachusetts General Hospital
Somerville, Massachusetts

Thomas S. Uldrick, MD, MS
Staff Clinician, HIV & AIDS Malignancy
    Branch
Center for Cancer Research
National Cancer Institute
Bethesda, Maryland

Robert G. Uzzo, MD
Professor and Chairman, Department of
    Surgery
Fox Chase Cancer Center
Temple University Health System
Philadelphia, Pennsylvania

Veronica Sanchez Varela, PhD
Assistant Professor
Department of Behavioral Sciences &
    Department of Internal Medicine
Section of Bone Marrow Transplant and
    Cell Therapy
Rush University Medical Center
Chicago, Illinois

Vic J. Verwaal, MD, PhD
The Netherlands Cancer Institute
Amsterdam, The Netherlands

Shaveta Vinayak, MD, MS
Instructor, Department of Medicine
Division of Oncology
Stanford University School of Medicine
Stanford, California

Michael A. Vogelbaum, MD, PhD,
    FAANS, FACS
The Robert W. and Kathryn B. Lamborn
    Chair for Neuro-Oncology
Professor of Surgery (Neurosurgery)
Cleveland Clinic
Lerner College of Medicine of Case
    Western Reserve University
Associate Director, Rose Ella Burkhardt
    Brain Tumor and Neuro-Oncology
    Center
Cleveland Clinic
Cleveland, Ohio

Christine M. Walko, PharmD, BCOP
Clinical Pharmacogenetic Scientist
DeBartolo Family Personalized Medicine
    Institute
Applied Clinical Scientist, Division of
    Population Science
H. Lee Moffitt Cancer Center and
    Research Institute
Tampa, Florida

Edus H. Warren, MD, PhD
Member, Clinical Research Division
Fred Hutchinson Cancer Research
    Center
Professor, Department of Medicine
University of Washington
Seattle, Washington

Graham W. Warren, MD, PhD
Associate Professor
Vice Chair for Research in Radiation
    Oncology
Department of Radiation Oncology
Department of Cell and Molecular
    Pharmacology
Hollings Cancer Center
Medical University of South Carolina
Charleston, South Carolina

Jeffrey S. Wefel, PhD, ABPP/CN
Associate Professor, Department of
    Neuro-Oncology
Chief, Section of Neuropsychology
The University of Texas MD Anderson
    Cancer Center
Houston, Texas

Robert A. Weinberg, PhD
Member, Whitehead Institute for
    Biomedical Research
Department of Biology
Massachusetts Institute of Technology
Director, Ludwig Center for Molecular
    Oncology
Whitehead Institute for Biomedical
    Research
Cambridge, Massachusetts

Louis M. Weiner, MD
Director, Lombardi Comprehensive
    Cancer Center
Professor and Chair, Department of
    Oncology
Francis L. and Charlotte G. Gragnani
    Chair
Georgetown University Medical Center
Washington, District of Columbia

Shelly M. Weiss, MS, CGC
Regional Medical Specialist
Myriad Genetics
Chicago, Illinois

Scott M. Weissman, MS, CGC
Certified Genetic Counselor
GeneDx
Gaithersburg, Maryland

Samuel A. Wells, Jr., MD
Adjunct Investigator, Medical Oncology
    Branch
Center for Cancer Research
National Cancer Institute
Bethesda, Maryland

Batsheva Werman, MD
Senior Physician
Oncology Department
Shaare Zedek Medical Center
Jerusalem, Israel

John W. Werning, MD, DMD
Associate Professor
Department of Otolaryngology
University of Florida, College of
    Medicine
Gainesville, Florida

William G. Wierda, MD, PhD
Professor, Department of Leukemia
The University of Texas MD Anderson
    Cancer Center
Houston, Texas

Elizabeth L. Wiley, MD
Professor and Director, Division of
    Surgical Pathology
Department of Pathology
University of Illinois Hospital and Health
    Sciences System
University of Illinois College of Medicine
Chicago, Illinois

Christopher G. Willett, MD
Professor and Chairman, Department of
    Radiation Oncology
Duke University
Durham, North Carolina

Walter C. Willett, MD, DrPH
Professor and Chair, Department of
    Nutrition
Harvard School of Public Health
Boston, Massachusetts

Terence M. Williams, MD, PhD
Assistant Professor, Department of
    Radiation Oncology
The Ohio State University
Arthur G. James and Richard Solove
    Research Institute
Columbus, Ohio

Lynn D. Wilson, MD, MPH
Professor, Vice Chairman, and Clinical
    Director
Department of Therapeutic Radiology
Yale University School of Medicine
New Haven, Connecticut

Jordan M. Winter, MD
Assistant Professor, Department of Surgery
Thomas Jefferson University
Philadelphia, Pennsylvania

Abraham J. Wu, MD
Assistant Attending Physician
Department of Radiation Oncology
Memorial Sloan-Kettering Cancer Center
New York, New York

Joachim Yahalom, MD
Vice Chairman for Academic Programs
Department of Radiation Oncology
Attending Physician and Member
Memorial Sloan-Kettering Cancer Center
Professor of Radiation Oncology
Weill Medical College of Cornell
    University
New York, New York

James C. Yao, MD
Professor Deputy Chairman, Department
    of Gastrointestinal Medical Oncology
The University of Texas MD Anderson
    Cancer Center
Houston, Texas

Robert Yarchoan, MD
Principal Investigator and Branch Chief
HIV and AIDS Malignancy Branch
Center for Cancer Research
National Cancer Institute
Bethesda, Maryland

Charles J. Yeo, MD
Samuel D. Gross Professor and Chair
Department of Surgery
Jefferson Medical College
Philadelphia, Pennsylvania

Anas Younes, MD
Professor, Department of Medicine
Chief, Lymphoma Service
Memorial Sloan-Kettering Cancer Center
New York, New York

Herbert Yu, MD, PhD
Professor and Director
Cancer Epidemiology Program
Associate Director for Population
    Sciences and Cancer Control
University of Hawaii Cancer Center
Adjunct Professor, Department of
    Chronic Disease Epidemiology
Yale School of Public Health
Honolulu, Hawaii

Stuart H. Yuspa, MD
Chief, Laboratory of Cancer Biology and
    Genetics
Center for Cancer Research
National Cancer Institute
Bethesda, Maryland

Michael J. Zelefsky, MD
Chief, Brachytherapy Service
Department of Radiation Oncology
Memorial Sloan-Kettering Cancer Center
New York, New York

Eric S. Zhou, PhD
Clinical Fellow, Dana-Farber Cancer
    Institute
Research Fellow, Harvard Medical School
Boston, Massachusetts

Anthony L. Zietman, MD
Jenot and William Shipley Professor of
    Radiation Oncology
Department of Radiation Oncology
Massachusetts General Hospital
Harvard Medical School
Boston, Massachusetts

Kenneth Zuckerman, MD
Senior Member
H. Lee Moffitt Cancer Center
Tampa, Florida

The first edition of *Cancer: Principles & Practice of Oncology* was published in 1982. Now, 32 years later, we present the 10th edition, a milestone of sorts. Our intention with the first edition was to publish a book that was comprehensive and balanced, covering not just one field, as had been the practice of cancer texts before 1982, but providing in-depth, expert coverage of all the specialties. In fact, a feature of the disease-oriented chapters then and now has been co-authorship by each of the major specialties.

Even in the early 1980s, it was apparent the field of cancer was changing rapidly and the regular production of new editions would be necessary to keep information fresh. Ten editions in 32 years has to be some kind of record for textbooks and accounts for the fact that *Cancer: Principles & Practice of Oncology* is the most popular cancer textbook in the world.

But times have changed. With the increase in the rate of new information and the digital information revolution, the text has changed too. Updates cannot wait for a new edition. Doctors need new information as it appears. For this reason, the 10th edition will be updated quarterly by a team of experts selected by the editors. The new information will be inserted and highlighted in the appropriate chapters, with references, and updates will be posted to the online version. This makes *Cancer: Principles & Practice of Oncology* the most up-to-date, easily searchable cancer text in the world, and the only comprehensive cancer text that is continuously updated. A perusal of how the contents have evolved from the first edition to the tenth shows the breathtaking pace of change in our understanding of the biology of cancer and the application of this information to the practice of medicine in the past 32 years. All these changes have been chronicled in the 10 editions of the book and the text has been a major vehicle for the translation of new information into practice. With the new flexible format of the 10th edition, we expect this will continue.

Vincent T. DeVita, Jr., MD
Theodore S. Lawrence, MD, PhD
Steven A. Rosenberg, MD, PhD

ACKNOWLEDGMENTS

To
Mary Kay,
Wendy, and
Alice

And to the invaluable Zia Raven

CONTENTS

PART III

Cancer Therapeutics

PART IV

Cancer Prevention and Screening

PART V

Practice of Oncology

SECTION 1. CANCER OF THE HEAD AND NECK

93. Molecular Biology of Cutaneous Melanoma 1337

Michael A. Davies and Levi A. Garraway

94. Cutaneous Melanoma 1346

Antoni Ribas, Craig L. Slingluff, Jr., and Steven A. Rosenberg

95. Genetic Testing in Skin Cancer 1395

Michele Gabree and Meredith L. Seidel

SECTION 10. NEOPLASMS OF THE CENTRAL NERVOUS SYSTEM

96. Molecular Biology of Central Nervous System Tumors 1403

Victoria Clark, and Jennifer Moliterno Günel, and Murat Günel

97. Neoplasms of the Central Nervous System . . . 1412

*Susan M. Chang, Minesh P. Mehta, Michael A. Vogelbaum,
Michael D. Taylor, and Manmeet S. Ahluwalia*

SECTION 11. CANCERS OF CHILDHOOD

98. Molecular Biology of Childhood Cancers . . . 1456

Lee J. Helman and David Malkin

PART VI

Palliative and Alternative Care

SECTION 1. SUPPORTIVE CARE AND QUALITY OF LIFE

PART I

Principles
of Oncology

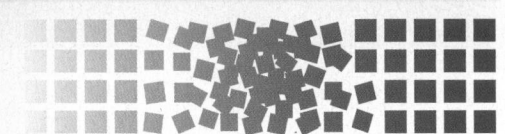

1 The Cancer Genome

Yardena Samuels, Alberto Bardelli, Jared J. Gartner, and Carlos López-Otin

INTRODUCTION

There is a broad consensus that cancer is, in essence, a genetic disease, and that accumulation of molecular alterations in the genome of somatic cells is the basis of cancer progression (Fig. 1.1).[1] In the past 10 years, the availability of the human genome sequence and progress in DNA sequencing technologies has dramatically improved knowledge of this disease. These new insights are transforming the field of oncology at multiple levels:

1. The genomic maps are redesigning the tumor taxonomy by moving it from a histologic- to a genetic-based level.
2. The success of cancer drugs designed to target the molecular alterations underlying tumorigenesis has proven that somatic genetic alterations are legitimate targets for therapy.
3. Tumor genotyping is helping clinicians individualize treatments by matching patients with the best treatment for their tumors.
4. Tumor-specific DNA alterations represent highly sensitive biomarkers for disease detection and monitoring.
5. Finally, the ongoing analyses of multiple cancer genomes will identify additional targets, whose pharmacologic exploitation will undoubtedly result in new therapeutic approaches.

This chapter will review the progress that has been made in understanding the genetic basis of sporadic cancers. An emphasis will be placed on an introduction to novel integrated genomic approaches that allow a comprehensive and systematic evaluation of genetic alterations that occur during the progression of cancer. Using these powerful tools, cancer research, diagnosis, and treatment are poised for a transformation in the next years.

CANCER GENES AND THEIR MUTATIONS

Cancer genes are broadly grouped into oncogenes and tumor suppressor genes. Using a classical analogy, oncogenes can be compared to a car accelerator, so that a mutation in an oncogene would be the equivalent of having the accelerator continuously pressed.[2] Tumor suppressor genes, in contrast, act as brakes,[2] so that when they are not mutated, they function to inhibit tumorigenesis. Oncogene and tumor suppressor genes may be classified by the nature of their somatic mutations in tumors. Mutations in oncogenes typically occur at specific hotspots, often affecting the same codon or clustered at neighboring codons in different tumors.[1] Furthermore, mutations in oncogenes are almost always missense, and the mutations usually affect only one allele, making them heterozygous. In contrast, tumor suppressor genes are usually mutated throughout the gene; a large number of the mutations may truncate the encoded protein and generally affect both alleles, causing loss of heterozygosity (LOH). Major types of somatic mutations present in malignant tumors include nucleotide substitutions, small insertions and deletions (*indels*), chromosomal rearrangements, and copy number alterations.

IDENTIFICATION OF CANCER GENES

The completion of the Human Genome Project marked a new era in biomedical sciences.[3] Knowledge of the sequence and organization of the human genome now allows for the systematic analysis of the genetic alterations underlying the origin and evolution of tumors. Before elucidation of the human genome, several cancer genes, such as *KRAS*, *TP53*, and *APC*, were successfully discovered using approaches based on an oncovirus analysis, linkage studies, LOH, and cytogenetics.[4,5] The first curated version of the Human Genome Project was released in 2004,[3] and provided a sequence-based map of the normal human genome. This information, together with the construction of the HapMap, which contains single nucleotide polymorphisms (SNP), and the underlying genomic structure of natural human genomic variation,[6,7] allowed an extraordinary throughput in cataloging somatic mutations in cancer. These projects now offer an unprecedented opportunity: the identification of all the genetic changes associated with a human cancer. For the first time, this ambitious goal is within reach of the scientific community. Already, a number of studies have demonstrated the usefulness of strategies aimed at the systematic identification of somatic mutations associated with cancer progression. Notably, the Human Genome Project, the HapMap project, as well as the candidate and family gene approaches (described in the following paragraphs), utilized capillary-based DNA sequencing (first-generation sequencing, also known as Sanger sequencing).[8] Figure 1.2 clearly illustrates the developments in the search of cancer genes, its increased pace, as well as the most relevant findings in this field.

Cancer Gene Discovery by Sequencing Candidate Gene Families

The availability of the human genome sequence provides new opportunities to comprehensively search for somatic mutations in cancer on a larger scale than previously possible. Progress in the field has been closely linked to improvements in the throughput of DNA analysis and in the continuous reduction in sequencing costs. What follows are some of the achievements in this research area, as well as how they affected knowledge of the cancer genome.

A seminal work in the field was the systematic mutational profiling of the genes involved in the RAS-RAF pathway in multiple tumors. This candidate gene approach led to the discovery that *BRAF* is frequently mutated in melanomas and is mutated at a lower frequency in other tumor types.[9] Follow-up studies quickly revealed that mutations in *BRAF* are mutually exclusive with alterations in *KRAS*,[9,10] genetically emphasizing that these genes function in the same pathway, a concept that had been previously demonstrated in lower organisms such as *Caenorhabditis elegans* and *Drosophila melanogaster*.[11,12]

In 2003, the identification of cancer genes shifted from a candidate gene approach to the mutational analyses of gene families. The first gene families to be completely sequenced were those that

A metastatic cancer genome requires decades to develop

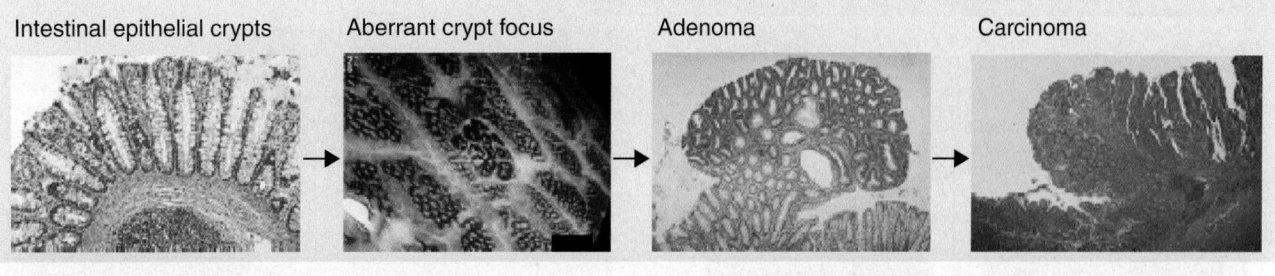

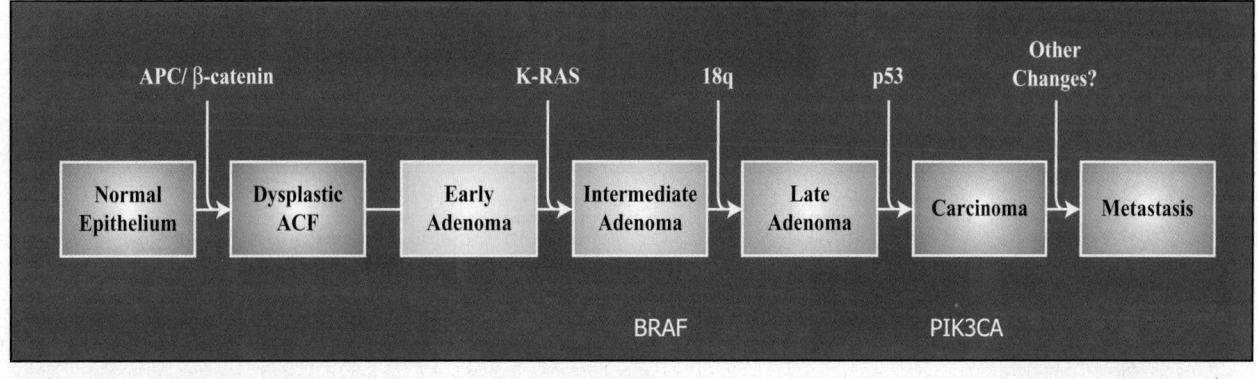

Figure 1.1 Schematic representation of the genomic and histopathologic steps associated with tumor progression: from the occurrence of the initiating mutation in the founder cell to metastasis formation. It has been convincingly shown that the genomic landscape of solid tumors such as that of pancreatic and colorectal tumors requires the accumulation of many genetic events, a process that requires decades to complete. This timeline offers an incredible window of opportunity for the early detection, which is often associated with an excellent prognosis, of this disease.

involved protein[13,14] and lipid phosphorylation.[15] The rationale for initially focusing on these gene families was threefold:

■ The corresponding proteins were already known at that time to play a pivotal role in the signaling and proliferation of normal and cancerous cells.
■ Multiple members of the protein kinases family had already been linked to tumorigenesis.
■ Kinases are clearly amenable to pharmacologic inhibition, making them attractive drug targets.

The mutational analysis of all the tyrosine-kinase domains in colorectal cancers revealed that 30% of cases had a mutation in at least one tyrosine-kinase gene, and overall mutations were identified in eight different kinases, most of which had not previously been linked to cancer.[13] An additional mutational analysis of the coding exons of 518 protein kinase genes in 210 diverse human cancers, including breast, lung, gastric, ovarian, renal, and acute lymphoblastic leukemia, identified approximately 120 mutated genes that probably contribute to oncogenesis.[14] Because kinase activity is attenuated by enzymes that remove phosphate groups called phosphatases, the rational next step in these studies was to perform a mutation analysis of the protein tyrosine phosphatases. A mutational investigation of this family in colorectal cancer identified that 25% of cases had mutations in six different phosphatase genes (*PTPRF*, *PTPRG*, *PTPRT*, *PTPN3*, *PTPN13*, or *PTPN14*).[16] A combined analysis of the protein tyrosine kinases and the protein tyrosine phosphatases showed that 50% of colorectal cancers had mutations in a tyrosine-kinase gene, a protein tyrosine phosphatase gene, or both, further emphasizing the pivotal role of protein phosphorylation in neoplastic progression. Many of the identified genes had previously been linked to human cancer, thus validating

the unbiased comprehensive mutation profiling. These landmark studies led to additional gene family surveys.

The phosphatidylinositol 3-kinase (*PI3K*) gene family, which also plays a role in proliferation, adhesion, survival, and motility, was also comprehensively investigated.[17] Sequencing of the exons encoding the kinase domain of all 16 members belonging to this family pinpointed *PIK3CA* as the only gene to harbor somatic mutations. When the entire coding region was analyzed, *PIK3CA* was found to be somatically mutated in 32% of colorectal cancers. At that time, the *PIK3CA* gene was certainly not a newcomer in the cancer arena, because it had previously been shown to be involved in cell transformation and metastasis.[17] Strikingly, its staggeringly high mutation frequency was discovered only through systematic sequencing of the corresponding gene family.[15] Subsequent analysis of *PIK3CA* in other tumor types identified somatic mutations in this gene in additional cancer types, including 36% of hepatocellular carcinomas, 36% of endometrial carcinomas, 25% of breast carcinomas, 15% of anaplastic oligodendrogliomas, 5% of medulloblastomas and anaplastic astrocytomas, and 27% of glioblastomas.[18–22] It is known that *PIK3CA* is one of the two (the other being *KRAS*) most commonly mutated oncogenes in human cancers. Further investigation of the *PI3K* pathway in colorectal cancer showed that 40% of tumors had genetic alterations in one of the *PI3K* pathway genes, emphasizing the central role of this pathway in colorectal cancer pathogenesis.[23]

Although most cancer genome studies of large gene families have focused on the kinome, recent analyses have revealed that members of other families highly represented in the human genome are also a target of mutational events in cancer. This is the case of proteases, a complex group of enzymes consisting of at least 569 components that constitute the so-called human degradome.[24] Proteases exhibit an elaborate interplay with kinases and

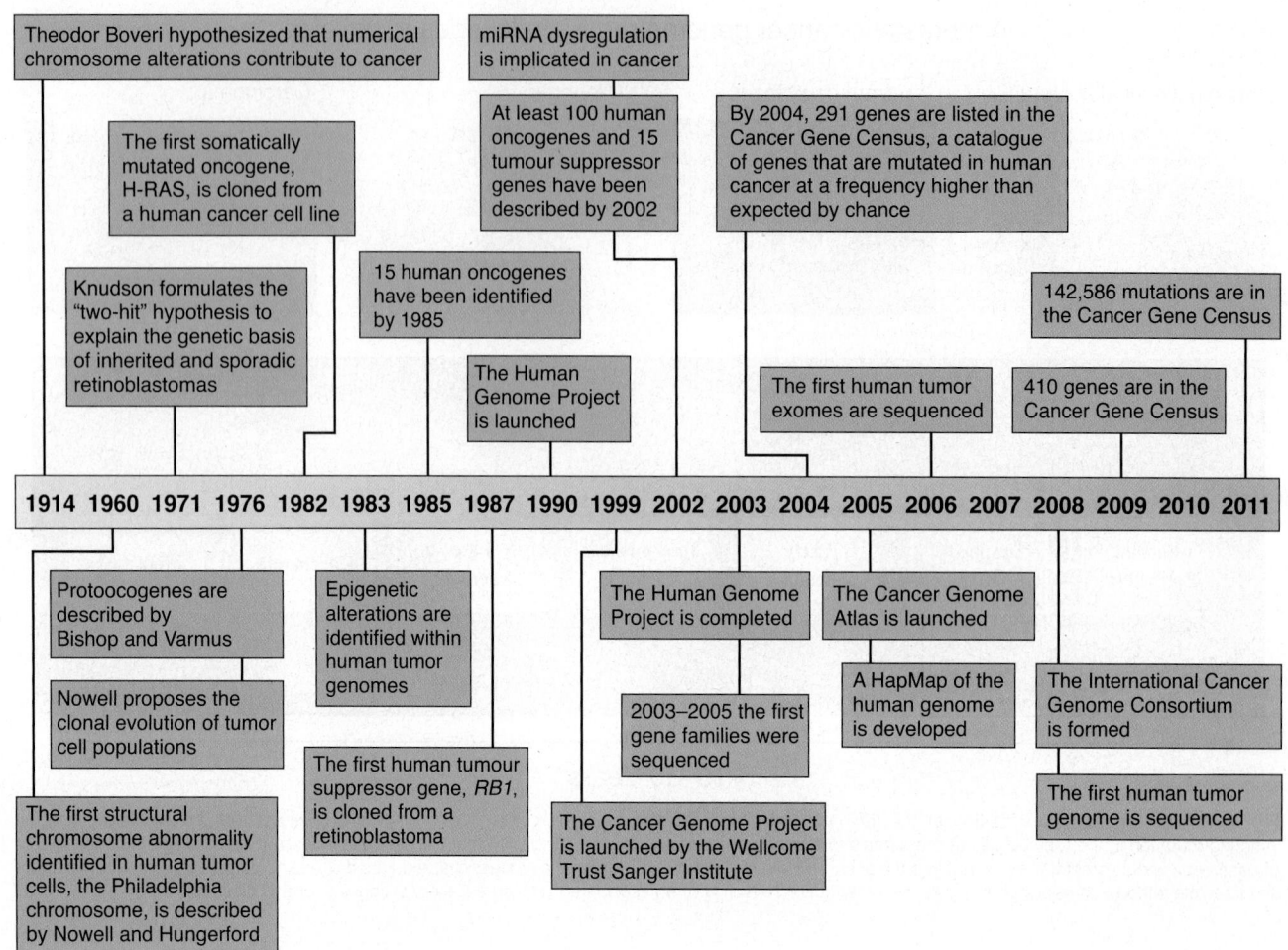

Figure 1.2 Timeline of seminal hypotheses, research discoveries, and research initiatives that have led to an improved understanding of the genetic etiology of human tumorigenesis within the past century. The consensus cancer gene data were obtained from the Wellcome Trust Sanger Institute Cancer Genome Project Web site (http://www.sanger.ac.uk/genetics/CGP). (Redrawn from Bell DW. Our changing view of the genomic landscape of cancer. *J Pathol* 2010;220:231–243.)

have traditionally been associated with cancer progression because of their ability to degrade extracellular matrices, thus facilitating tumor invasion and metastasis.[25,26] However, recent studies have shown that these enzymes hydrolyze a wide variety of substrates and influence many different steps of cancer, including early stages of tumor evolution.[27] These functional studies have also revealed that beyond their initial recognition as prometastatic enzymes, they play dual roles in cancer, as assessed by the identification of a growing number of tumor-suppressive proteases.[28]

These findings emphasized the possibility that mutational activation or inactivation of protease genes occurs in cancer. A systematic analysis of genetic alterations in breast and colorectal cancers revealed that proteases from different catalytic classes were somatically mutated in cancer.[29] These results prompted the mutational analysis of entire protease families such as matrix metalloproteinases (MMP), a disintegrin and metalloproteinase (ADAM), and ADAMs with thrombospondin domains (ADAMTS) in different tumors. These studies led to the identification of protease genes frequently mutated in cancer, such as *MMP8*, which is mutated and functionally inactivated in 6.3% of human melanomas.[30,31]

The mutational status of caspases has also been extensively analyzed in different tumors because these proteases play a fundamental role in the execution of apoptosis, one of the hallmarks of cancer.[32] These studies demonstrated that *CASP8* is deleted in neuroblastomas and inactivated by somatic mutations in a variety of human malignancies, including head and neck, colorectal, lung, and gastric carcinomas.[33-35] Other large protease families

whose components are often mutated in cancer are the deubiquitinating enzymes (DUB), which catalyze the removal of ubiquitin and ubiquitin-like modifiers of their target proteins.[36] Some DUBs were initially identified as oncogenic proteins, but further work has shown that other deubiquitinases, such as CYLD, A20, and BAP1, are tumor suppressors inactivated in cancer. *CYLD* is mutated in patients with familial cylindromatosis, a disease characterized by the formation of multiple tumors of skin appendages.[37] A20 is a DUB family member encoded by the *TNFAIP3* gene, which is mutated in a large number of Hodgkin lymphomas and primary mediastinal B-cell lymphomas.[38-41] Finally, the *BAP1* gene, encoding an ubiquitin C-terminal hydrolase, is frequently mutated in metastasizing uveal melanomas[42] and in other human malignancies, such as mesothelioma and renal cell carcinoma.[43]

Mutational Analysis of Exomes Using Sanger Sequencing

Although the gene family approach for the identification of cancer genes has proven extremely valuable, it still is a candidate approach and thus biased in its nature. The next step forward in the mutational profiling of cancer has been the sequencing of exomes, which is the entire coding portion of the human genome (18,000 protein-encoding genes). The exomes of many different tumors—including breast, colorectal, pancreatic, and ovarian clear cell carcinomas; glioblastoma multiforme; and medulloblastoma—have been analyzed using Sanger sequencing. For the first time, these large-scale analyses allowed researchers to describe and understand the genetic complexity of human cancers.[29,44–48] The declared goals of these exome studies were to provide methods for exomewide mutational analyses in human tumors, to characterize their spectrum and quantity of somatic mutations, and, finally, to discover new genes involved in tumorigenesis as well as novel pathways that have a role in these tumors. In these studies, sequencing data were complemented with gene expression and copy number analyses, thus providing a comprehensive view of the genetic complexity of human tumors.[45–48] A number of conclusions can be drawn from these analyses, including the following:

- Cancer genomes have an average of 30 to 100 somatic alterations per tumor in coding regions, which was a higher number than previously thought. Although the alterations included point mutations, small insertions, deletions, or amplifications, the great majority of the mutations observed were single-base substitutions.[45,46]
- Even within a single cancer type, there is a significant inter-tumor heterogeneity. This means that multiple mutational patterns (encompassing different mutant genes) are present in tumors that cannot be distinguished based on histologic analysis. The concept that individual tumors have a unique genetic milieu is highly relevant for personalized medicine, a concept that will be further discussed.
- The spectrum and nucleotide contexts of mutations differ between different tumor types. For example, over 50% of mutations in colorectal cancer were C:G to T:A transitions, and 10% were C:G to G:C transversions. In contrast, in breast cancers, only 35% of the mutations were C:G to T:A transitions, and 29% were C:G to G:C transversions. Knowledge of mutation spectra is vital because it allows insight into the mechanisms underlying mutagenesis and repair in the various cancers investigated.
- A considerably larger number of genes that had not been previously reported to be involved in cancer were found to play a role in the disease.
- Solid tumors arising in children, such as medulloblastomas, harbor on average 5 to 10 times less gene alterations compared to a typical adult solid tumor. These pediatric tumors also harbor fewer amplifications and homozygous deletions within coding genes compared to adult solid tumors.

Importantly, to deal with the large amount of data generated in these genomic projects, it was necessary to develop new statistical and bioinformatic tools. Furthermore, an examination of the overall distribution of the identified mutations allowed for the development of a novel view of cancer genome landscapes and a novel definition of cancer genes. These new concepts in the understanding of cancer genetics are further discussed in the following paragraphs. The compiled conclusions derived from these analyses have led to a paradigm shift in the understanding of cancer genetics.

A clear indication of the power of the unbiased nature of the whole exome surveys was revealed by the discovery of recurrent mutations in the active site of *IDH1*, a gene with no known link to gliomas, in 12% of tumors analyzed.[46] Because malignant gliomas are the most common and lethal tumors of the central nervous system, and because glioblastoma multiforme (GBM; World Health Organization grade IV astrocytoma) is the most biologically aggressive subtype, the unveiling of *IDH1* as a novel GBM gene is extremely significant. Importantly, mutations of *IDH1* predominantly occurred in younger patients and were associated with a better prognosis.[49] Follow-up studies showed that mutations of *IDH1* occur early in glioma progression; the R132 somatic mutation is harbored by the majority (greater than 70%) of grades II and III astrocytomas and oligodendrogliomas, as well as in secondary GBMs that develop from these lower grade lesions.[49–55] In contrast, less than 10% of primary GBMs harbor these alterations. Furthermore, analysis of the associated *IDH2* revealed recurrent somatic mutations in the R172 residue,

which is the exact analog of the frequently mutated R132 residue of *IDH1*. These mutations occur mostly in a mutually exclusive manner with *IDH1* mutations,[49,51] suggesting that they have equivalent phenotypic effects. Subsequently, *IDH1* mutations have been reported in additional cancer types, including hematologic neoplasias.[56–58]

Next-Generation Sequencing and Cancer Genome Analysis

In 1977, the introduction of the Sanger method for DNA sequencing with chain-terminating inhibitors transformed biomedical research.[8] Over the past 30 years, this first-generation technology has been universally used for elucidating the nucleotide sequence of DNA molecules. However, the launching of new large-scale projects, including those implicating whole-genome sequencing of cancer samples, has made necessary the development of new methods that are widely known as next-generation sequencing technologies.[59–61] These approaches have significantly lowered the cost and the time required to determine the sequence of the 3×10^9 nucleotides present in the human genome. Moreover, they have a series of advantages over Sanger sequencing, which are of special interest for the analysis of cancer genomes.[62] First, next-generation sequencing approaches are more sensitive than Sanger methods and can detect somatic mutations even when they are present in only a subset of tumor cells.[63] Moreover, these new sequencing strategies are quantitative and can be used to simultaneously determine both nucleotide sequence and copy number variations.[64] They can also be coupled to other procedures such as those involving paired-end reads, allowing for the identification of multiple structural alterations, such as insertions, deletions, and rearrangements, that commonly occur in cancer genomes.[63] Nonetheless, next-generation sequencing still presents some limitations that are mainly derived from the relatively high error rate in the short reads generated during the sequencing process. In addition, these short reads make the task of de novo assembly of the generated sequences and the mapping of the reads to a reference genome extremely complex. To overcome some of these current limitations, deep coverage of each analyzed genome is required and a careful validation of the identified variants must be performed, typically using Sanger sequencing. As a consequence, there is a substantial increase in both the cost of the process and in the time of analysis. Therefore, it can be concluded that whole-genome sequencing of cancer samples is already a feasible task, but not yet a routine process. Further technical improvements will be required before the task of decoding the entire genome of any malignant tumor of any cancer patient can be applied to clinical practice.

The number of next-generation sequencing platforms has substantially grown over the past few years and currently includes technologies from Roche/454, Illumina/Solexa, Life/APG's SOLiD3, Helicos BioSciences/HeliScope, and Pacific Biosciences/PacBio RS.[61] Noteworthy also are the recent introduction of the Polonator G.007 instrument, an open source platform with freely available software and protocols; the Ion Torrent's semiconductor sequencer; as well as those involving self-assembling DNA nanoballs or nanopore technologies.[65–67] These new machines are driving the field toward the era of third-generation sequencing, which brings enormous clinical interest because it can substantially increase the speed and accuracy of analyses at reduced costs and can facilitate the possibility of single-molecule sequencing of human genomes. A comparison of next-generation sequencing platforms is shown in Table 1.1. These various platforms differ in the method utilized for template preparation and in the nucleotide sequencing and imaging strategy, which finally result in their different performance. Ultimately, the most suitable approach depends on the specific genome sequencing projects.[61]

Current methods of template preparation first involve randomly shearing genomic DNA into smaller fragments, from which

TABLE 1.1

Comparative Analysis of Next-Generation Sequencing Platforms

Platform	Library/Template Preparation	Sequencing Method	Average Read-Length (Bases)	Run Time (Days)	Gb Per Run	Instrument Cost (U.S.$)	Comments
Roche 454 GS FLX	Fragment, mate-pair Emulsion PCR	Pyrosequencing	400	0.35	0.45	500,000	Fast run times High reagent cost
Illumina HiSeq 2000	Fragment, mate-pair Solid phase	Reversible terminator	100–125	8 (mate-pair run)	150–200	540,000	Most widely used platform Low multiplexing capability
Life/APG's SOLiD 5500xl	Fragment, mate-pair Emulsion PCR	Cleavable probe, sequencing by ligation	35–75	7 (mate-pair run)	180–300	595,000	Inherent error correction Long run times
Helicos BioSciences HeliScope	Fragment, mate-pair Single molecule	Reversible terminator	32	8 (fragment run)	37	999,000	Nonbias template representation Expensive, high error rates
Pacific Biosciences PacBio RS	Fragment Single molecule	Real-time sequencing	1,000	1	0.075	NA	Greatest potential for long reads Highest error rates
Polonator G.007	Mate pair Emulsion PCR	Noncleavable probe, sequencing by ligation	26	5 (mate-pair run)	12	170,000	Least expensive platform Shortest read lengths

NA, not available.
Data represent an update of information provided in Metzker ML. Sequencing technologies—the next generation. *Nat Rev Genet* 2010;11:31–46.

a library of either fragment templates or mate-pair templates are generated. Then, clonally amplified templates from single DNA molecules are prepared by either emulsion polymerase chain reaction (PCR) or solid-phase amplification.[68,69] Alternatively, it is possible to prepare single-molecule templates through methods that require less starting material and that do not involve PCR amplification reactions, which can be the source of artifactual mutations.[70] Once prepared, templates are attached to a solid surface in spatially separated sites, allowing thousands to billions of nucleotide sequencing reactions to be performed simultaneously.

The sequencing methods currently used by the different next-generation sequencing platforms are diverse and have been classified into four groups: cyclic reversible termination, single-nucleotide addition, real-time sequencing, and sequencing by ligation (Fig. 1.3).[61,71] These sequencing strategies are coupled with different imaging methods, including those based on measuring bioluminescent signals or involving four-color imaging of single molecular events. Finally, the extraordinary amount of data released from these nucleotide sequencing platforms is stored, assembled, and analyzed using powerful bioinformatic tools that have been developed in parallel with next-generation sequencing technologies.[72]

Next-generation sequencing approaches represent the newest entry into the cancer genome decoding arena and have already been applied to cancer analyses. The first research group to apply these methodologies to whole cancer genomes was that of Ley et al.,[73] who reported in 2008 the sequencing of the entire genome of a patient with acute myeloid leukemia (AML) and its comparison with the normal tissue from the same patient, using the Illumina/Solexa platform. As further described, this work allowed for the identification of point mutations and structural alterations of putative oncogenic relevance in AML and represented proof

of principle of the relevance of next-generation sequencing for cancer research.

Whole-Genome Analysis Utilizing Second-Generation Sequencing

The sequence of the first whole cancer genome was reported in 2008, where AML and normal skin from the same patient were described.[73] Numerous additional whole genomes, together with the corresponding normal genomes of patients with a variety of malignant tumors, have been reported since then.[56,63,74–86]

The first available whole genome of a cytogenetically normal AML subtype M1 (AML-M1) revealed eight genes with novel mutations along with another 500 to 1,000 additional mutations found in noncoding regions of the genome. Most of the identified genes had not been previously associated with cancer. However, validation of the detected mutations did not identify novel recurring mutations in AML.[73] Concomitantly, with the expansion in the use of next-generation sequencers, many other whole genomes from a number of cancer types started to be evaluated in a similar manner (Fig. 1.4).[87]

In contrast to the first AML whole genome, the second did observe a recurrent mutation in *IDH1*, encoding isocitrate dehydrogenase.[56] Follow-up studies extended this finding and reported that mutations in *IDH1* and the related gene *IDH2* occur at a 20% to 30% frequency in AML patients and are associated with a poor prognosis in some subgroups of patients.[79,80,88] A good example illustrating the high pace at which second-generation technologies and their accompanying analytical tools are found is demonstrated by the following finding derived from a reanalysis of the first AML whole genome. Thus, when improvements in sequencing

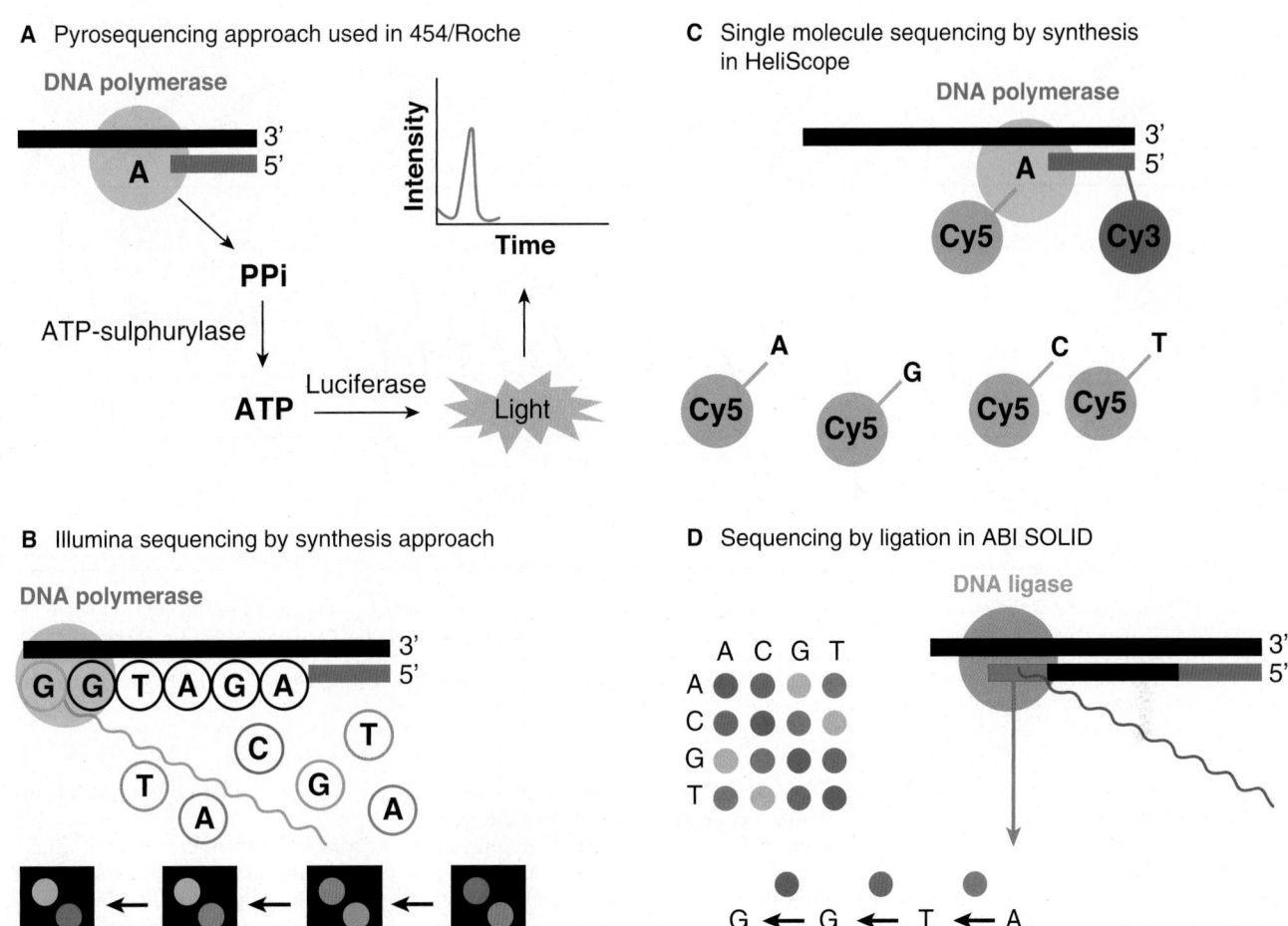

A Pyrosequencing approach used in 454/Roche

DNA polymerase

3'
5'

A

PPi

ATP-sulphurylase

ATP → Luciferase → Light

Intensity

Time

C Single molecule sequencing by synthesis in HeliScope

DNA polymerase

3'
5'

A

Cy5   Cy3

A   G   C   T

Cy5   Cy5   Cy5   Cy5

B Illumina sequencing by synthesis approach

DNA polymerase

3'
5'

G G T A G A

C   T

T   G   A

A   A

ATGG...

D Sequencing by ligation in ABI SOLID

DNA ligase

3'
5'

A C G T

A
C
G
T

G ← G ← T ← A

Figure 1.3 Advances in sequencing chemistry implemented in next-generation sequencers. **(A)** The pyrosequencing approach implemented in 454/Roche sequencing technology detects incorporated nucleotides by chemiluminescence resulting from PPi release. **(B)** The Illumina method utilizes sequencing by synthesis in the presence of fluorescently labeled nucleotide analogs that serve as reversible reaction terminators. **(C)** The single-molecule sequencing by synthesis approach detects template extension using Cy3 and Cy5 labels attached to the sequencing primer and the incoming nucleotides, respectively. **(D)** The SOLiD method sequences templates by sequential ligation of labeled degenerate probes. Two-base encoding implemented in the SOLiD instrument allows for probing each nucleotide position twice. (From Morozova O, Hirst M, Marra MA. Applications of new sequencing technologies for transcriptome analysis. *Annu Rev Genomics Hum Genet* 2009;10:135–151.)

PRINCIPLES OF ONCOLOGY

techniques were available, the first AML whole genome (described previously), which identified no recurring mutations and had a 91.2% diploid coverage, was reevaluated by deeper sequence coverage, yielding 99.6% diploid coverage of the genome. This improvement, together with more advanced mutation calling algorithms, allowed for the discovery of several nonsynonymous mutations that had not been identified in the initial sequencing. This included a frameshift mutation in the DNA methyltransferase gene *DNMT3A*. Validation of *DNMT3A* in 280 additional de novo AML patients to define recurring mutations led to the significant discovery that a total of 22.1% of AML cases had mutations in *DNMT3A* that were predicted to affect translation. The median overall survival among patients with *DNMT3A* mutations was significantly shorter than that among patients without such mutations (12.3 months versus 41.1 months; p <0.001).

Shortly after this study, complete sequences of a series of cancer genomes, together with matched normal genomes of the same patients, were reported.[56,78,83,84] These works opened the way to more ambitious initiatives, including those involving large international consortia, aimed at decoding the genome of malignant tumors from thousands of cancer patients. Thus, over the last 2 years, many whole genomes of different human malignancies have been made available.[74–76]

In addition to direct applications of next-generation sequencing technologies for the mutational analysis of cancer genomes, these methods have an additional range of applications in cancer research. Thus, genome sequencing efforts have begun to elucidate the genomic changes that accompany metastasis evolution through a comparative analysis of primary and metastatic lesions from breast and pancreatic cancer patients.[77,81,82,85] Likewise, massively parallel sequencing has been used to analyze the evolution of a tongue adenocarcinoma in response to selection by targeted kinase inhibitors.[89] Detailed information of several of these whole genome projects is found in the following paragraph.

The first solid cancer to undergo whole-genome sequencing was a malignant melanoma that was compared to a lymphoblastoid cell line from the same individual.[83] Impressively, a total of 33,345 somatic base substitutions were identified, with 187 nonsynonymous substitutions in protein-coding sequences, at least one order of magnitude higher than any other cancer type. Most somatic base substitutions were C:G > T:A transitions, and of the 510 dinucleotide substitutions, 360 were CC.TT/GG.AA changes, which is consistent with ultraviolet light exposure mutation signatures previously reported in melanoma.[14] Such results from the most comprehensive catalog of somatic mutations not only provide

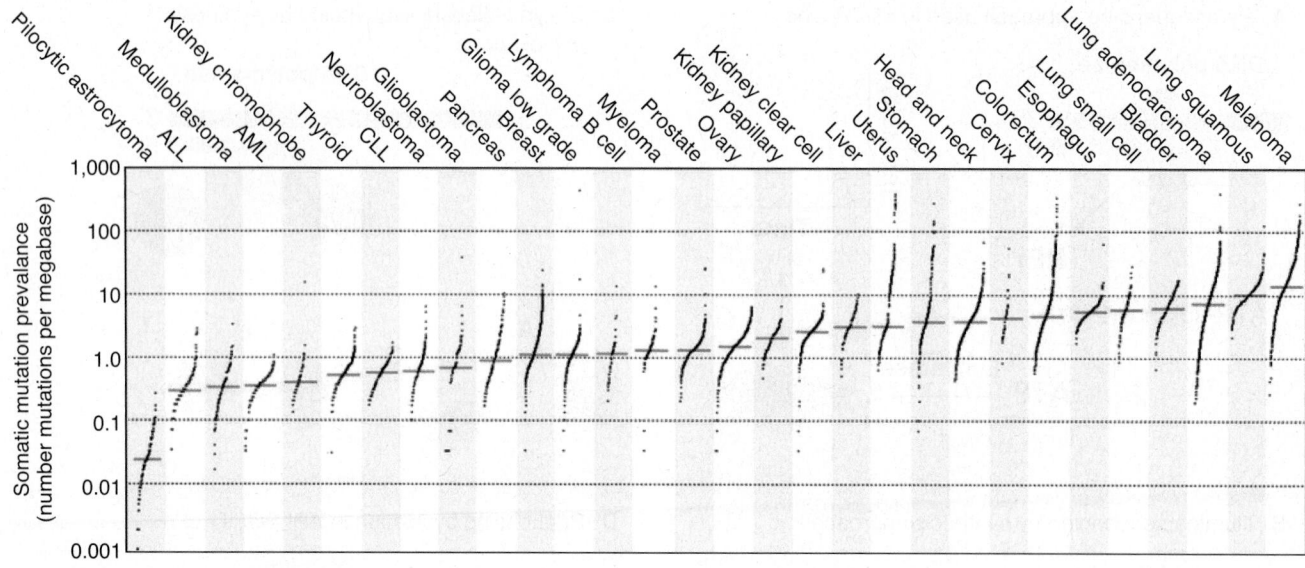

Figure 1.4 The prevalence of somatic mutations across human cancer types. Every *dot* represents a sample, whereas the *red horizontal lines* are the median numbers of mutations in the respective cancer types. The vertical axis (log scaled) shows the number of mutations per megabase, whereas the different cancer types are ordered on the horizontal axis based on their median numbers of somatic mutations. ALL, acute lymphoblastic leukemia; AML, acute myeloid leukemia; CLL, chronic lymphocytic leukemia. (Used with permission from Alexandrov LB, Nik-Zainal S, Wedge DC, et al. Signatures of mutational processes in human cancer. *Nature* 2013;500:415–421.)

insight into the DNA damage signature in this cancer type, but can also be useful in determining the relative order of some acquired mutations. Indeed, this study shows that a significant correlation exists between the presence of a higher proportion of C.A/G.T transitions in early (82%) compared to late mutations (53%). Another important aspect that the comprehensive nature of this melanoma study provided was that cancer mutations are spread out unevenly throughout the genome, with a lower prevalence in

regions of transcribed genes, suggesting that DNA repair occurs mainly in these areas.

An interesting and pioneering example of the power of whole-genome sequencing in deciphering the mutation evolution in carcinogenesis was seen in a study in which a basallike breast cancer tumor, a brain metastasis, a tumor xenograft derived from the primary tumor, and the peripheral blood from the same patient were compared (Fig. 1.5).[85] This analysis showed a wide range of

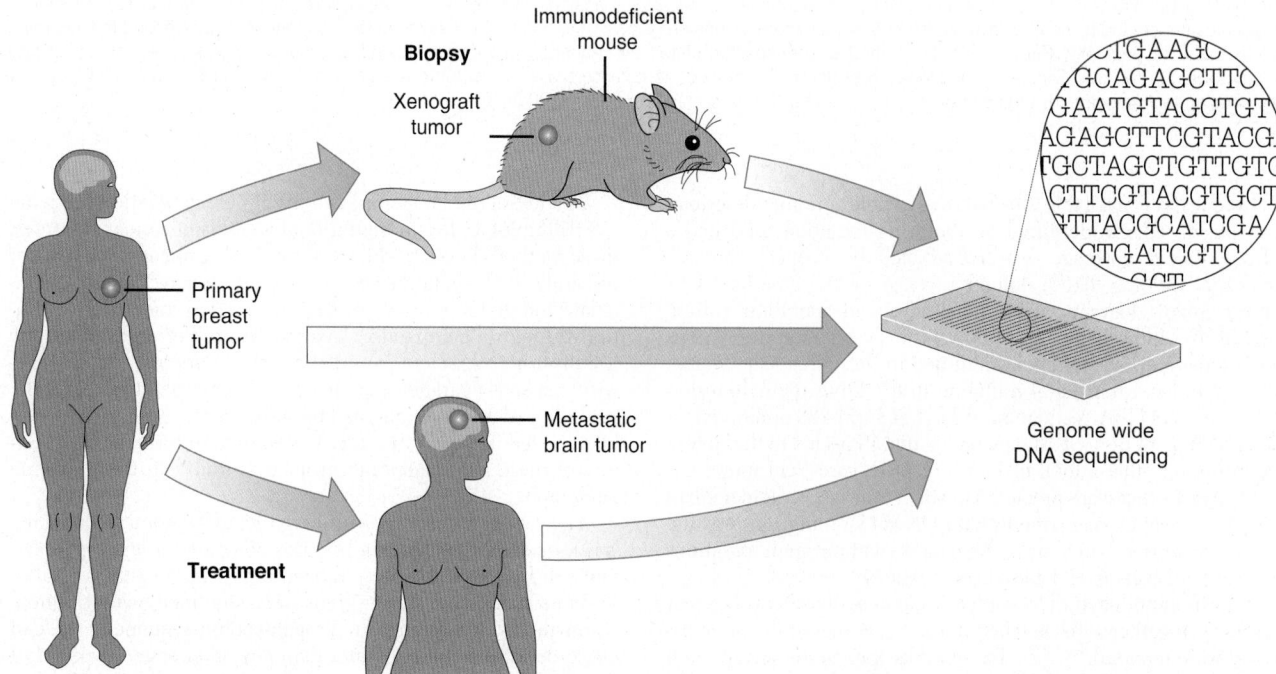

Figure 1.5 Covering all the bases in metastatic assessment. Ding et al.[85] performed a genomewide analysis on three tumor samples: a patient's primary breast tumor; her metastatic brain tumor, which formed despite therapy; and a xenograft tumor in a mouse, originating from the patient's breast tumor. They find that the primary tumor differs from the metastatic and xenograft tumors mainly in the prevalence of genomic mutations. (With permission from Gray J. Cancer: genomics of metastasis. *Nature* 2010;464:989–990.)

mutant allele frequencies in the primary tumor, which was narrowed in the metastasis and xenograft samples. This suggested that the primary tumor was significantly more heterogeneous in its cell populations compared to its matched metastasis and xenograft samples because these underwent selection processes whether during metastasis or transplantation. The clear overlap in mutation incidence between the metastatic and xenograft cases suggests that xenografts undergo similar selection as metastatic lesions and, therefore, are a reliable source for genomic analyses. The main conclusion of this whole-genome study was that, although metastatic tumors harbor an increased number of genetic alterations, the majority of the alterations found in the primary tumor are preserved. Interestingly, single-cell genome sequencing of a breast primary tumour and its liver metastasis indicated that a single clonal expansion formed the primary tumor and seeded the metastasis.[90] Further studies have confirmed and extended these findings to metastatic tumors from different types, including renal and pancreatic carcinomas.[91]

The importance of performing whole-genome sequencing has also been emphasized by the recent identification of somatic mutations in regulatory regions, which can also elicit tumorigenesis. In a study reviewing the noncoding mutations in 19 melanoma whole-genome samples, two recurrent mutations in 17 of the 19 cases studied within the *telomerase reverse transcriptase* (*TERT*) promoter region were revealed.[92] When these two mutations were investigated in an extension of 51 additional tumors and their matched normal tissues, it was observed that 33 tumors harbored one of the mutations and that the mutations occurred in a mutually exclusive manner. These two mutations generate an identical 11 bp nucleotide stretch that contains the consensus binding site for E-twenty-six (ETS) transcription factors. When cloned into a luciferase reporter assay system, it was shown that these mutations conferred a two- to fourfold increase in transcriptional activity of this promoter in five melanoma cell lines. Although this alteration is much more frequent in melanoma, it is also present in other cancer types because 16% of the cancers listed in the Cancer Cell Line Encyclopedia harbor one of the two *TERT* mutations. In combination, these *TERT* mutations are seen in a greater frequency than *BRAF*- and *NRAS*-activating mutations. They occur in a mutually exclusive manner and in regions that do not show a large background mutation rate, all suggesting that these mutations are important driver events contributing to oncogenesis. Further supporting this was another recent study that identified these same two mutations in the germ line of familial melanoma patients.[93]

As the *TERT* promoter mutation discovery shows, regions of the genome that do not code for proteins are just as vital in our understanding of the biology behind tumor development and progression. Another class of non–protein-coding regions in the genome are the noncoding RNAs. One class of noncoding RNAs are microRNAs (miRNA). Discovered 20 years ago, miRNAs are known to be expressed in a tissue or developmentally specific manner and their expression can influence cellular growth and differentiation along with cancer-related pathways such as apoptosis or stress response. miRNAs do this through either overexpression, leading to the targeting and downregulation of tumor suppressor genes, or inversely through their own downregulation, leading to increased expression of their target oncogene. miRNAs have been extensively studied in cancer and their functional effects have been noted in a wide variety of cancers like glioma[94] and breast cancer,[95] to name just a few.

Another class of noncoding RNAs (ncRNA) are the long noncoding RNAs (lncRNA). These RNAs are typically greater than 200 bp and can range up to 100 kb in size. They are transcribed by RNA polymerase II and can undergo splicing and polyadenylation. Although much less extensively studied when compared to miRNAs for their role in cancer, lncRNAs are beginning to come under much more scrutiny. A recent study of the steroid receptor RNA activator (SRA) revealed two transcripts, a lncRNA (SRA) and a translated transcript (steroid receptor RNA activator protein [SRAP]), that coexist within breast cancer cells. However, their expression varies within breast cancer cell lines with different phenotypes. It was shown that in a more invasive breast cancer line, higher relative levels of the noncoding transcript were seen.[96] Because this ncRNA acts as part of a ribonucleoprotein complex that is recruited to the promoter region of regulatory genes, it has been hypothesized that this shift in balance between both noncoding and coding transcripts may be associated with growth advantages. When this balance was shifted in vitro, it led to a large increase in transcripts associated with invasion and migration. The results of this study highlight the importance of the investigation into the roles of ncRNA in tumor development or progression and confirm again that the study of coding variants is not sufficient in determining the full genomic spectrum of cancer.

It must be also noted that the recent analysis of whole genomes of many different human tumors has provided additional insights into cancer evolution. Thus, it has been demonstrated that multiple mutational processes are operative during cancer development and progression, each of which has the capacity to leave its particular mutational signature on the genome. A remarkable and innovative study in this regard was aimed at the generation of the entire catalog of somatic mutations in 21 breast carcinomas and the identification of the mutational signatures of the underlying processes. This analysis revealed the occurrence of multiple, distinct single- and double-nucleotide substitution signatures. Moreover, it was reported that breast carcinomas harboring *BRCA1* or *BRCA2* mutations showed a characteristic combination of substitution mutation signatures and a particular profile of genomic deletions. An additional contribution of this analysis was the identification of a distinctive phenomenon of localized hypermutation, which has been termed *kataegis*, and which has also subsequently been observed in other malignancies distinct from breast carcinomas.[87]

Whole-genome sequencing of human carcinomas has also allowed for the ability to characterize other massive genomic alterations, termed *chromothripsis* and *chromoplexy*, occurring across different cancer subtypes.[97] Chromothripsis implies a massive genomic rearrangement acquired in a one-step catastrophic event during cancer development and has been detected in about 2% to 3% of all tumors, but is present at high frequency in some particular cases, such as bone cancers.[98] Chromoplexy has been originally described in prostate cancer and involves many DNA translocations and deletions that arise in a highly interdependent manner and result in the coordinate disruption of multiple cancer genes.[99] These newly described phenomena represent powerful strategies of rapid genome evolution, which may play essential roles during carcinogenesis.

Whole-Exome Analysis Utilizing Second-Generation Sequencing

Another application of second-generation sequencing involves utilizing nucleic acid "baits" to capture regions of interest in the total pool of nucleic acids. These could either be DNA, as described previously,[100,101] or RNA.[102] Indeed, most areas of interest in the genome can be targeted, including exons and ncRNAs. Despite inefficiencies in the exome-targeting process—including the uneven capture efficiency across exons, which results in not all exons being sequenced, and the occurrence of some off-target hybridization events—the higher coverage of the exome makes it highly suitable for mutation discovery in cancer samples.

Over the last few years, thousands of cancer samples have been subjected to whole-exome sequencing. These studies, combined with data from whole-genome sequencing, have provided an unprecedented level of information about the mutational landscape of the most frequent human malignancies.[74–76] In addition, whole-exome sequencing has been used to identify the somatic mutations characteristic of both rare tumors and those that are prevalent in certain geographical regions.[76]

Overall, these studies have provided very valuable information about mutation rates and spectra across cancer types and subtypes.[87,103,104] Remarkably, the variation in mutational frequency between different tumors is extraordinary, with hematologic and pediatric cancers showing the lowest mutation rates (0.001 per Mb of DNA), and melanoma and lung cancers presenting the highest mutational burden (more than 400 per Mb). Whole-exome sequencing has also contributed to the identification of novel cancer genes that had not been previously described to be causally implicated in the carcinogenesis process. These genes belong to different functional categories, including signal transduction, RNA maturation, metabolic regulation, epigenetics, chromatin remodeling, and protein homeostasis.[74] Finally, a combination of data from whole-exome and whole-genome sequencing has allowed for the identification of the signatures of mutational processes operating in different cancer types.[87] Thus, an analysis of a dataset of about 5 million mutations from over 7,000 cancers from 30 different types has allowed for the extraction of more than 20 distinct mutational signatures. Some of them, such as those derived from the activity of APOBEC cytidine deaminases, are present in most cancer types, whereas others are characteristic of specific tumors. Known signatures associated with age, smoking, ultraviolet (UV) light exposure, and DNA repair defects have been also identified in this work, but many of the detected mutational signatures are of cryptic origin. These findings demonstrate the impressive diversity of mutational processes underlying cancer development and may have enormous implications for the future understanding of cancer biology, prevention, and treatment.

SOMATIC ALTERATION CLASSES DETECTED BY CANCER GENOME ANALYSIS

Whole-genome sequencing of cancer genomes has an enormous potential to detect all major types of somatic mutations present in malignant tumors. This large repertoire of genomic abnormalities includes single nucleotide changes, small insertions and deletions, large chromosomal reorganizations, and copy number variations (Fig. 1.6).

Nucleotide substitutions are the most frequent somatic mutations detected in malignant tumors, although there is a substantial variability in the mutational frequency among different cancers.[60] On average, human malignancies have one nucleotide change per million bases, but melanomas reach mutational rates 10-fold higher, and tumors with mutator phenotype caused by DNA mismatch repair deficiencies may accumulate tens of mutations per million nucleotides. By contrast, tumors of hematopoietic origin have less than one base substitution per million. Several bioinformatic tools and pipelines have been developed to efficiently detect somatic nucleotide substitutions through comparison of the genomic information obtained from paired normal and tumor samples from the same patient. Likewise, there are a number of publicly available computational methods to predict the functional relevance of the identified mutations in cancer specimens.[60] Most of these bioinformatic tools exclusively deal with nucleotide changes in protein coding regions and evaluate the putative structural or functional effect of an amino acid substitution in a determined protein, thus obviating changes in other genomic regions, which can also be of crucial interest in cancer. In any case, current computational methods used in this regard are far from being optimal, and experimental validation is finally required to assess the functional relevance of nucleotide substitutions found in cancer genomes.

For years, the main focus of cancer genome analyses has been on identifying coding mutations that cause a change in the amino acid sequence of a gene. The rationale behind this is quite sound because any mutation that creates a novel protein or truncates an essential protein has the potential to drastically change the cellular environment. Examples of this have been shown earlier in the chapter with BRAF and KRAS along with many others. With the advancements in next-generation sequencing, larger studies are able to be conducted. These studies give the power to detect mutations occurring in the cancer genome at a lower frequency. Interesting to note is that these studies are leading to the discovery that recurrent synonymous mutations occur in cancer. Previously believed to be merely neutral mutations that maintain no functional role in tumorigenesis, these mutations were largely ignored, but a recent study shows[105] that simply dismissing these mutations as silent may be premature.

In a review of only 29 melanoma exomes and genomes, 16 recurring synonymous mutations were discovered. When these mutations were screened in additional samples, a synonymous mutation in the gene BCL2L12 was discovered in 12 out of 285 total samples. The observed frequency of this recurrent mutation is greater than expected by chance, suggesting that it has undergone some type of selective pressure during tumor development.[105] Noting that BCL2L12 had previously been linked to tumorigenesis, the mutation was further evaluated for its functional effect, with the finding that it led to an abrogation of the effect of a miRNA, leading to the deregulated expression of BCL2L12. BCL2L12 is a negative regulator of the gene p53, which functions by binding and inhibiting apoptosis in glioma.[106] Accordingly, the dysregulation observed in BCL2L12 led to a reduction in p53 target gene expression.

Small insertions and deletions (indels) represent a second category of somatic mutations that can be discovered by whole-genome sequencing of cancer specimens. These mutations are about 10-fold less frequent than nucleotide substitutions, but may also have an obvious impact in cancer progression. Accordingly, specific bioinformatic tools have been created to detect these indels in the context of the large amount of information generated by whole-genome sequencing projects.[107]

The systematic identification of large chromosomal rearrangements in cancer genomes represents one of the most successful applications of next-generation sequencing methodologies. Previous strategies in this regard had mainly been based on the utilization of cytogenetic methods for the identification of recurrent translocations in hematopoietic tumors. More recently, a combination of bioinformatics and functional methods has allowed for the finding of recurrent translocations in solid epithelial tumors such as TMPRSS2–ERG in prostate cancer and EML4–ALK in non–small-cell lung cancer.[108,109] Now, by using a next-generation sequencing analysis of genomes and transcriptomes, it is possible to systematically search for both intrachromosomal and interchromosomal rearrangements occurring in cancer specimens. These studies have already proven their usefulness for cancer research through the discovery of recurrent translocations involving genes of the RAF kinase pathway in prostate and gastric cancers and in melanomas.[110] Likewise, massively parallel paired-end genome and transcriptome sequencing has already been used to detect new gene fusions in cancer and to catalog all major structural rearrangements present in some tumors and cancer cell lines.[63,111–113] The ongoing cancer genome projects involving thousands of tumor samples will likely lead to the detection of many other chromosomal rearrangements of relevance in specific subsets of cancers. It is also remarkable that whole-genome sequencing may also facilitate the identification of other types of genomic alterations, including rearrangements of repetitive elements, such as active retrotransposons, or insertions of foreign gene sequences, such as viral genomes, which can contribute to cancer development. Indeed, a next-generation sequencing analysis of the transcriptome of Merkel cell carcinoma samples has revealed the clonal integration within the tumor genome of a previously unknown polyomavirus likely implicated in the pathogenesis of this rare but aggressive skin cancer.[114]

Finally, next-generation sequencing approaches have also demonstrated their feasibility to analyze the pattern of copy number

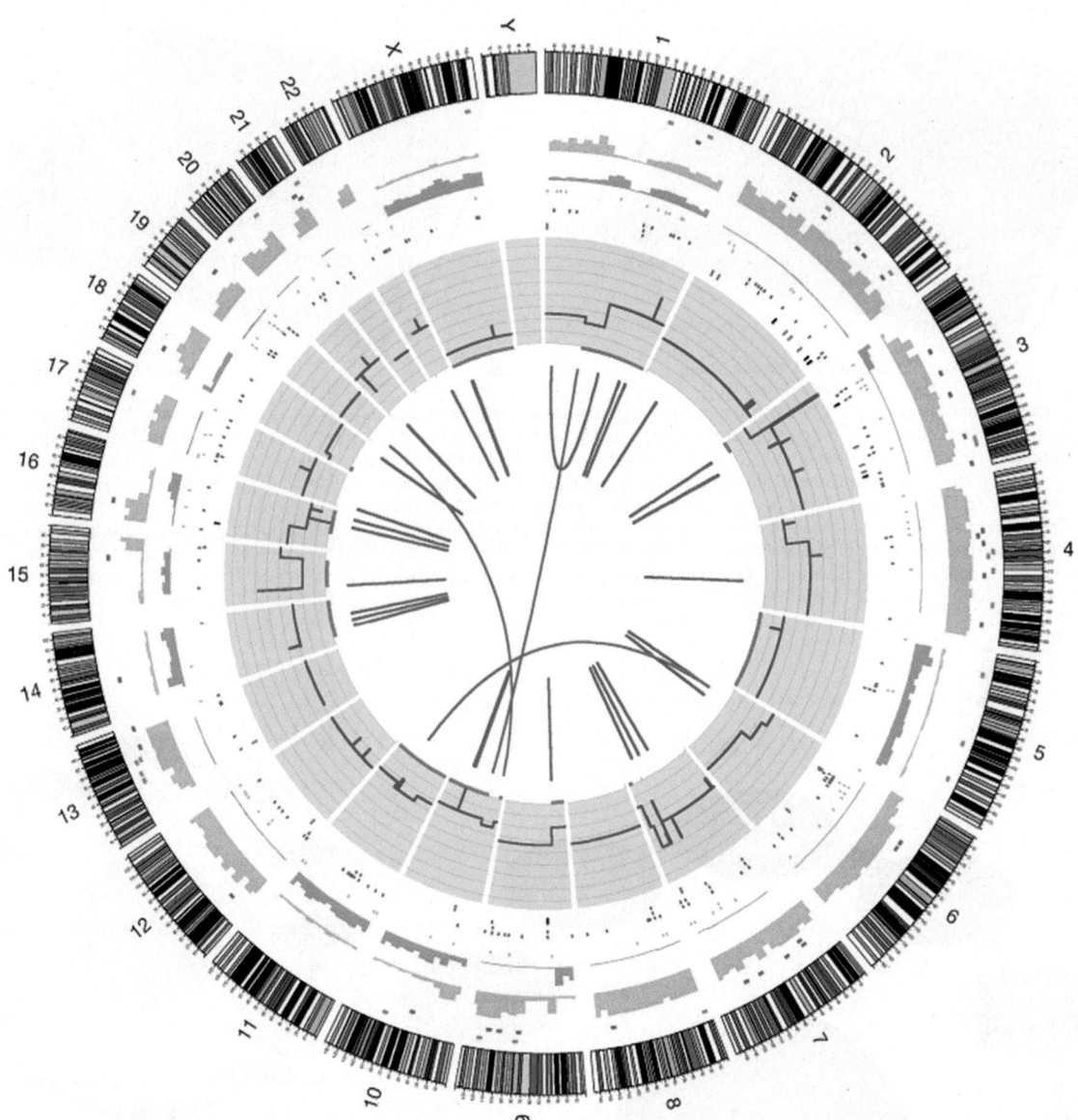

Figure 1.6 The catalog of somatic mutations in COLO-829. Chromosome ideograms are shown around the *outer ring* and are oriented pter–qter in a clockwise direction with centromeres indicated in *red*. Other tracks contain somatic alterations *(from outside to inside):* validated insertions *(light green rectangles);* validated deletions *(dark green rectangles);* heterozygous *(light orange bars),* and homozygous *(dark orange bars)* substitutions shown by density per 10 megabases; coding substitutions *(colored squares: silent in gray, missense in purple, nonsense in red, and splice site in black);* copy number *(blue lines);* regions of loss of heterozygosity (LOH) *(red lines);* validated intrachromosomal rearrangements *(green lines);* validated interchromosomal rearrangements *(purple lines).* (From Pleasance ED, Cheetham RK, Stephens PJ, et al. A comprehensive catalogue of somatic mutations from a human cancer genome. *Nature* 2010;463:191–196.)

alterations in cancer, because they allow researchers to count the number of reads in both tumor and normal samples at any given genomic region and then to evaluate the tumor-to-normal copy number ratio at this particular region. These new methods offer some advantages when compared with those based on microarrays, including much better resolution, precise definition of the involved breakpoints, and absence of saturation, which facilitates the accurate estimation of high copy number levels occurring in some genomic loci of malignant tumors.[60]

PATHWAY-ORIENTED MODELS OF CANCER GENOME ANALYSIS

Genomewide mutational analyses suggest that the mutational landscape of cancer is made up of a handful of genes that are mutated in a high fraction of tumors, otherwise known as *mountains*, and most mutated genes are altered at relatively low frequencies, otherwise known as *hills* (Fig. 1.7).[29] The mountains probably give a high selective advantage to the mutated cell, and the hills might provide a lower advantage, making it hard to distinguish them from passenger mutations. Because the hills differ between cancer types, it seems that the cancer genome is more complex and heterogeneous than anticipated. Although highly heterogeneous, bioinformatic studies suggest that the mountains and hills can be grouped into sets of pathways and biologic processes. Some of these pathways are affected by mutations in a few pathway members and others by numerous members. For example, pathway analyses have allowed for the stratification of mutated genes in pancreatic adenocarcinomas to 12 core pathways that have at least one member mutated in 67% to 100% of the tumors analyzed (Fig. 1.8).[45] These core pathways deviated to some that harbored one single highly mutated gene,

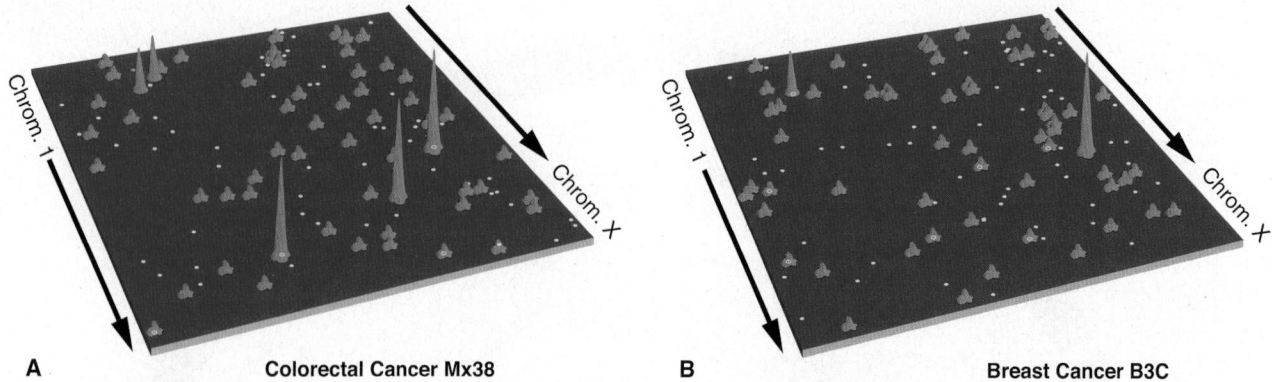

Figure 1.7 Cancer genome landscapes. Nonsilent somatic mutations are plotted in a two-dimensional space representing chromosomal positions of RefSeq genes. The telomere of the short arm of chromosome 1 is represented in the rear left corner of the *green plane* and ascending chromosomal positions continue in the direction of the arrow. Chromosomal positions that follow the front edge of the plane are continued at the back edge of the plane of the adjacent row, and chromosomes are appended end to end. Peaks indicate the 60 highest ranking CAN genes for each tumor type, with peak heights reflecting CaMP scores. The *dots* represent genes that were somatically mutated in the individual colorectal (Mx38) **(A)** or breast tumor (B3C) **(B)**. The *dots* corresponding to mutated genes that coincided with hills or mountains are black with white rims; the remaining *dots* are white with red rims. The mountain on the right of both landscapes represents *TP53* (chromosome 17), and the other mountain shared by both breast and colorectal cancers is *PIK3CA* (upper left, chromosome 3). (Redrawn from Wood LD, Parsons DW, Jones S, et al. The genomic landscapes of human breast and colorectal cancers. *Science* 2007;318:1108–1113. Reprinted with permission from the American Association for the Advancement of Science).

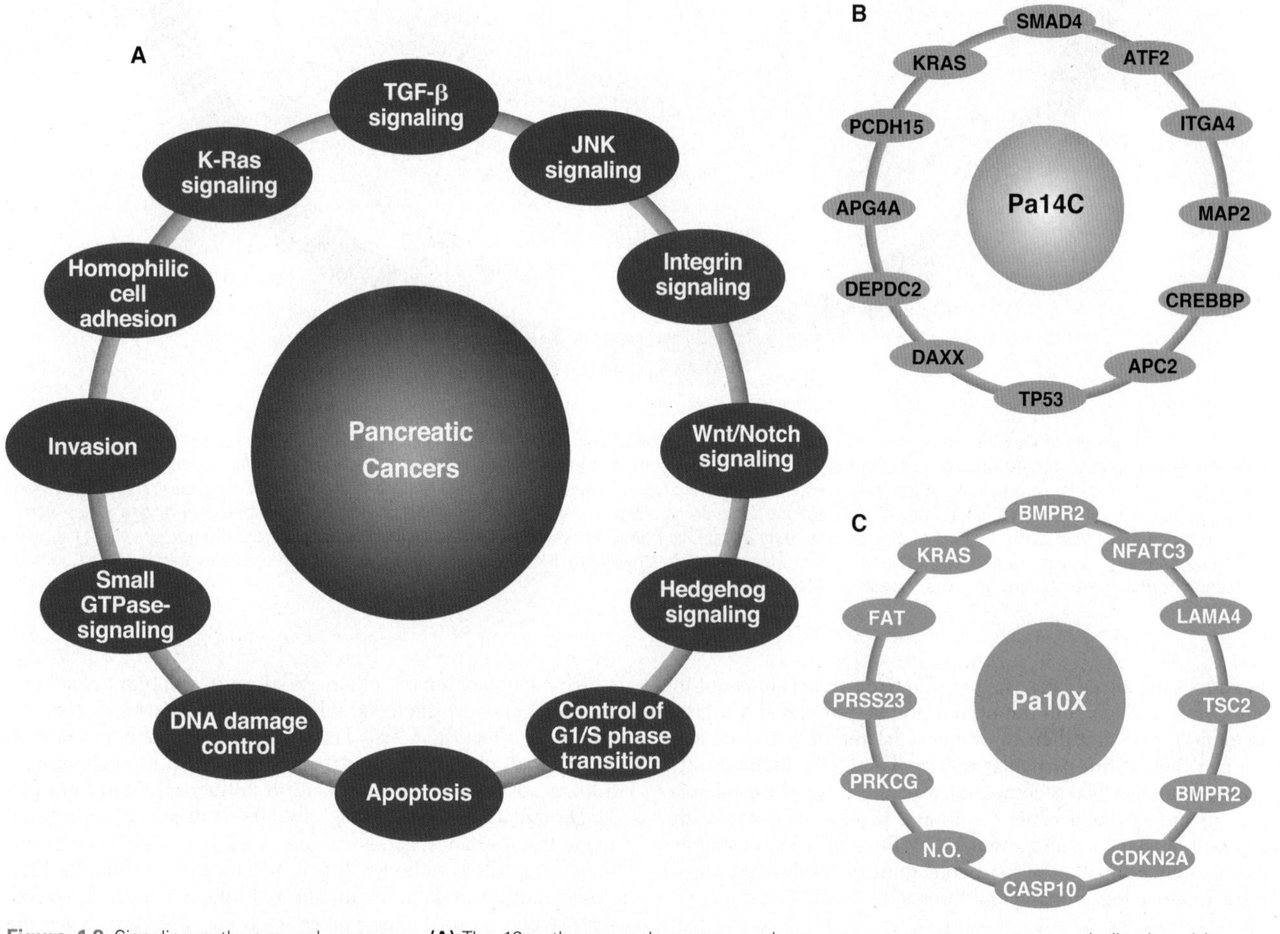

Figure 1.8 Signaling pathways and processes. **(A)** The 12 pathways and processes whose component genes were genetically altered in most pancreatic cancers. **(B,C)** Two pancreatic cancers (Pa14C and Pa10X) and the specific genes that are mutated in them. The positions around the circles in **(B)** and **(C)** correspond to the pathways and processes in **(A)**. Several pathway components overlapped, as illustrated by the BMPR2 mutation that presumably disrupted both the SMAD4 and Hedgehog signaling pathways in Pa10X. Additionally, not all 12 processes and pathways were altered in every pancreatic cancer, as exemplified by the fact that no mutations known to affect DNA damage control were observed in Pa10X. NO, not observed. (Redrawn from Jones S, Zhang X, Parsons DW, et al. Core signaling pathways in human pancreatic cancers revealed by global genomic analyses. *Science* 2008;321:1801–1806. Reprinted with permission from the American Association for the Advancement of Science).

such as in *KRAS* in the G1/S cell cycle transition pathway and pathways where a few mutated genes were found, such as the transforming growth factor (TGF-β) signaling pathway. Finally, there were pathways in which many different genes were mutated, such as invasion regulation molecules, cell adhesion molecules, and integrin signaling. Importantly, independent of how many genes in the same pathway are affected, if they are found to occur in a mutually exclusive fashion in a single tumor, they most likely give the same selective pressure for clonal expansion.

The idea of genetically analyzing pathways rather than individual genes has been applied previously, revealing the concept of mutual exclusivity. Mutual exclusivity has been shown elegantly in the case of *KRAS* and *BRAF*, where a *KRAS*-mutated cancer generally does not also harbor a *BRAF* mutation, because *KRAS* is upstream of *BRAF* in the same pathway.[9] A similar concept was applied for *PIK3CA* and *PTEN*, where both mutations do not usually occur in the same tumor.[23]

With the ever expanding amounts of genetic information being gathered, the ability to search for common pathways being affected in cancer is increasing. One new pathway that is beginning to emerge is the glutamate-signaling pathway. Glutamate dysregulation has been implicated in a number of cancers. In a study of pancreatic duct adenocarcinoma (PDAC), it was seen that glutamate levels were significantly higher in the tissue of individuals with chronic pancreatitis (CP) and PDAC when compared to normal pancreas tissue.[115] It was also observed that the increased glutamate levels led to proinvasion and antiapoptotic signaling through the activation of AMPA receptors.

Also in this regard, and through the use of whole-exome sequencing, it has been recently shown that the glutamate receptor gene *GRIN2A* is highly mutated in melanoma. The finding that many of these mutations are nonsense has suggested that *GRIN2A* is a novel tumor suppressor. Additional genes in the glutamate pathway have also found mutated in melanomas.[116] Pathway analyses and statistical testing on the whole-exome data have also revealed the glutamate signaling pathway to be dysregulated. These results have been further corroborated in another study reporting mutations in the metabotropic glutamate receptor *GRM3*[117,118] in melanoma. A functional analysis of mutations found in *GRM3* in melanoma tumor samples has shown an increased activation of MEK1/2 kinase, increased migration, and anchorage-independent growth.[117]

Passenger and Driver Mutations

By the time a cancer is diagnosed, it is comprised of billions of cells carrying DNA abnormalities, some of which have a functional role in malignant proliferation; however, many genetic lesions acquired along the way have no functional role in tumorigenesis.[14] The emerging landscapes of cancer genomes include thousands of genes that were not previously linked to tumorigenesis but are found to be somatically mutated. Many of these changes are likely to be *passengers*, or neutral, in that they have no functional effects on the growth of the tumor.[14] Only a small fraction of the genetic alterations are expected to drive cancer evolution by giving cells a selective advantage over their neighbors. Passenger mutations occur incidentally in a cell that later or in parallel develops a *driver* mutation, but are not ultimately pathogenic.[119] Although neutral, cataloging passengers mutations is important because they incorporate the signatures of the previous exposures the cancer cell underwent as well as DNA repair defects the cancer cell has. In many cases, the passenger and driver mutations occur at similar frequencies and the identification of drivers versus the passenger is of utmost relevance and remains a pressing challenge in cancer genetics.[120–122] This goal will eventually be achieved through a combination of genetic and functional approaches, some of which are listed as follows.

The most reliable indicator that a gene was selected for and therefore is highly likely to be pathogenic is the identification of recurrent mutations, whether at the same exact amino acid position or in neighboring amino acid positions in different patients. More than that, if somatic alterations in the same gene occur very frequently (mountains in the tumor genome landscape), these can be confidently classified as drivers. For example, cancer alleles that are identified in multiple patients and different tumors types, such as those found in *KRAS*, *TP53*, *PTEN*, and *PIK3CA*, are clearly selected for during tumorigenesis.

However, most genes discovered thus far are mutated in a relatively small fraction of tumors (hills), and it has been clearly shown that genes that are mutated in less than 1% of patients can still act as *drivers*.[123] The systematic sequencing of newly identified putative cancer genes in the vast number of specimens from cancer patients will help in this regard. However, even if examining large numbers of samples can provide helpful information to classify drivers versus passengers, this approach alone is limited by the marked variation in mutation frequency among individual tumors and individual genes. The statistical test utilized in this case calculates the probability that the number of mutations in a given gene reflects a mutation frequency that is greater than expected from the nonfunctional background mutation rate,[29,124] which is different between different cancer types. These analyses incorporate the number of somatic alterations observed, the number of tumors studied, and the number of nucleotides that were successfully sequenced and analyzed.

Another approach often used to distinguish driver from passenger mutations exploits the statistical analysis of synonymous versus nonsynonymous changes.[125] In contrast to nonsynonymous mutations, synonymous mutations do not alter the protein sequence. Therefore, they do not usually apply a growth advantage and would not be expected to be selected during tumorigenesis. This strategy works by comparing the observed-to-expected ratio of synonymous with that of nonsynonymous mutation. An increased proportion of nonsynonymous mutations from the expected 2:1 ratio implies selection pressure during tumorigenesis.

Other approaches are based on the concept that driver mutations may have characteristics similar to those causing Mendelian disease when inherited in the germ line and may be identifiable by constraints on tolerated amino acid residues at the mutated positions. In contrast, passenger mutations may have characteristics more similar to those of nonsynonymous SNPs with high minor allele frequencies. Based on these premises, supervised machine learning methods have been used to predict which missense mutations are drivers.[126] Additional approaches to decipher drivers from passengers include the identification of mutations that affect locations that have previously been shown to be cancer causing in protein members of the same gene family. Enrichment for mutations in evolutionarily conserved residues are analyzed by algorithms, such as SIFT (sorting intolerant from tolerant (SIFT),[127] which estimates the effects of the different mutations identified.

Probably the most conclusive methods to identify driver mutations will be rigorous functional studies using biochemical assays as well as model organisms or cultured cells, using knockout and knockin of individual cancer alleles.[128] Unfortunately, these methods are not well suited to the analysis of the hundreds of gene candidates that arise from every large-scale cancer genome project. In conclusion, it is fair to say that sequencing cancer genomes is only the beginning of a journey that will ultimately be completed when the thousands of the newly discovered alleles are annotated as being the drivers of this disease. A summary of the various next-generation applications and approaches for their analysis is summarized in Figure 1.9 and Table 1.2.

NETWORKS OF CANCER GENOME PROJECTS

The repertoire of oncogenic mutations is extremely heterogeneous, suggesting that it would be difficult for independent cancer genome initiatives to address the generation of comprehensive

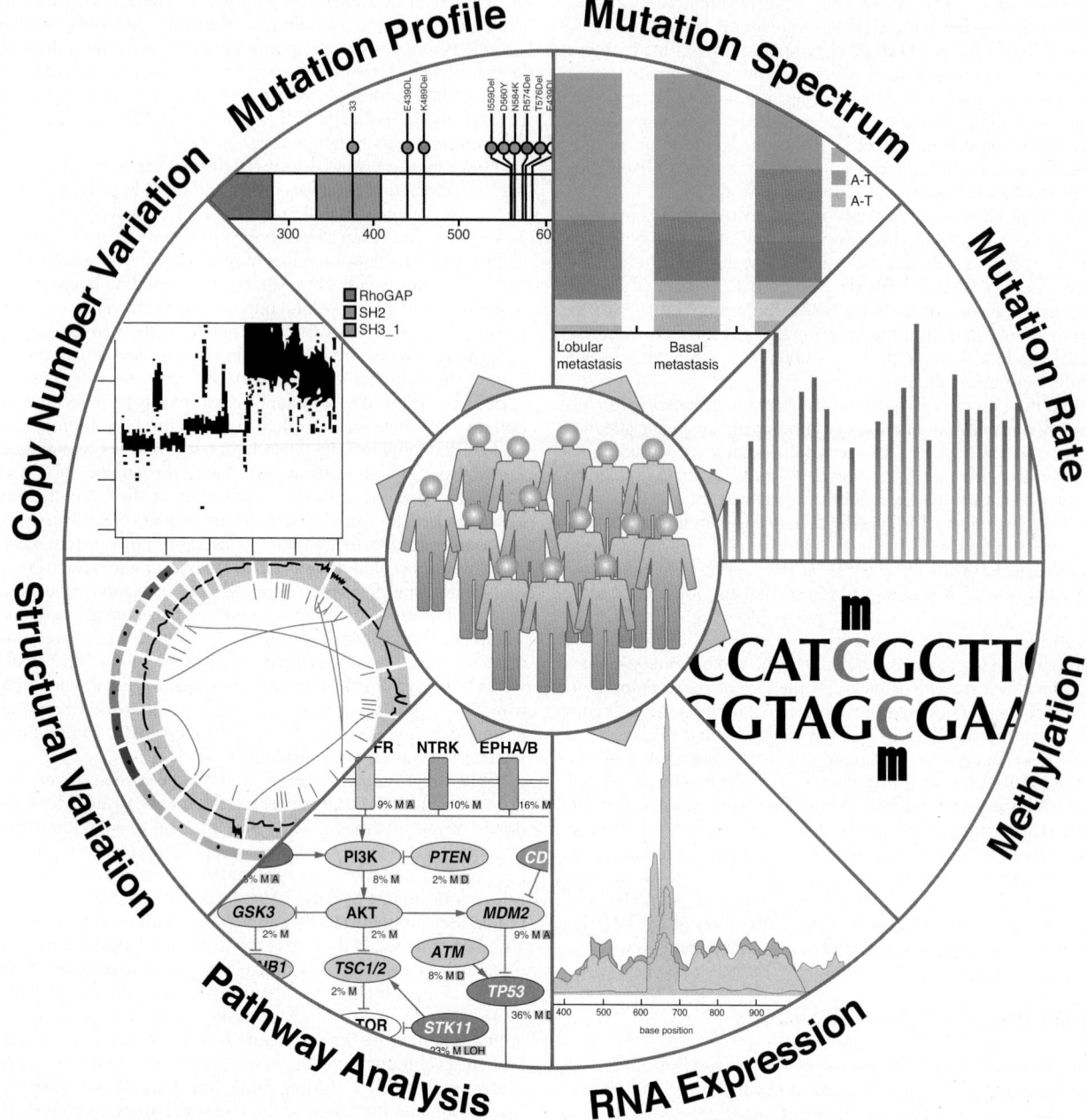

Figure 1.9 Landscape of cancer genomics analyses. NGS data will be generated for hundreds of tumors from all major cancer types in the near future. The integrated analysis of DNA, RNA, and methylation sequencing data will help elucidate all relevant genetic changes in cancers. (Used with permission from Ding L, Wendl MC, Koboldt DC, et al. Analysis of next-generation genomic data in cancer: accomplishments and challenges. *Hum Mol Genet* 2010;19:R188–R196.)

catalogs of mutations in the wide spectrum of human malignancies. Accordingly, there have been different efforts to coordinate the cancer genome sequencing projects being carried out around the world, including The Cancer Genome Atlas (TCGA) and the International Cancer Genome Consortium (ICGC). Moreover, there are other initiatives that are more focused on specific tumors, such as that led by scientists at St. Jude Children's Research Hospital in Memphis, and Washington University, which aims at sequencing multiple pediatric cancer genomes.[129]

TCGA began in 2006 in the United States as a comprehensive program in cancer genomics supported by the U.S. National Institutes of Health (NIH). The initial project focused on three tumors: GBM, serous cystadenocarcinoma of the ovary, and lung squamous carcinoma. These studies have already generated novel

and interesting information regarding genes mutated in these malignancies.[134] On the basis of these positive results, the NIH announced an expansion of the TCGA program with the aim to produce genomic data sets for at least 20 to 25 cancers during the next few years.

The ICGC was formed in 2008 to coordinate the generation of comprehensive catalogs of genomic abnormalities in tumors from 50 different cancer types or subtypes that are of clinical and societal importance across the world.[130] The project aims to perform systematic studies of over 25,000 cancer genomes at the genomic level and integrate this information with epigenomic and transcriptomic studies of the same cases as well as with clinical features of patients. At present, there are a total of 69 committed projects involving at least 16 different countries coordinated by

TABLE 1.2

Computational Tools and Databases Useful for Cancer Genome Analyses

Category	Tool/Database	URL
Alignment	Maq[a]	http://maq.sourceforge.net
	Burrows-Wheeler Aligner (BWA)[b]	http://bio-bwa.sourceforge.net
Mutation calling	SNVMix[c]	http://www.bcgsc.ca/platform/bioinfo/software/SNVMix
	SAMtools[d]	http://samtools.sourceforge.net
	VarScan[e]	http://varscan.sourceforge.net
	MuTect[f]	http://www.broadinstitute.org/cancer/cga/mutect
Indel calling	Pindel[g]	http://gmt.genome.wustl.edu/pindel/current/
Copy number analysis	CBS[h]	http://www.bioconductor.org
	SegSeq[i]	http://www.broadinstitute.org/cgi-bin/cancer/publications/pub_paper.cgi?mode=view&paper_id=182
Functional effect	SIFT[j]	http://sift.jcvi.org/
	PolyPhen-2[k]	http://genetics.bwh.harvard.edu/pph2
Visualization	CIRCOS[l]	http://mkweb.bcgsc.ca/circos
	Integrative Genomics Viewer (IGV)[m]	http://www.broadinstitute.org/igv
Repository	Catalogue of Somatic Mutations in Cancer (COSMIC)[n]	http://www.sanger.ac.uk/genetics/CGP/cosmic
	Cancer Genome Project (CGP)[o]	http://www.sanger.ac.uk/genetics/CGP
	dbSNP[p]	http://www.ncbi.nlm.nih.gov/SNP
	Gene Ranker[q]	http://cbio.mskcc.org/tcga-generanker/

[a] Li H, Durbin R. Fast and accurate short read alignment with Burrows–Wheeler transform. *Bioinformatics* 2009;25:1754–1760.
[b] Li H, Durbin R. Fast and accurate long-read alignment with Burrows–Wheeler transform. *Bioinformatics* 2010;26:589–595.
[c] Goya R, Sun MG, Morin RD, et al. SNVMix: predicting single nucleotide variants from next-generation sequencing of tumors. *Bioinformatics* 2010;26:730–736.
[d] Li H, Handsaker B, Wysoker A, et al. The Sequence Alignment/Map format and SAMtools. *Bioinformatics* 2009;25:2078–2079.
[e] Koboldt DC, Chen K, Wylie T, et al. VarScan: variant detection in massively parallel sequencing of individual and pooled samples. *Bioinformatics* 2009;25:2283–2285.
[f] Cibulski K, Lawrence MS, Carter SL, et al. Sensitive detection of somatic point mutations in impure and heterogeneous cancer samples. *Nat Biotechnol* 2013;31:213–219.
[g] Ye K, Schulz MH, Long Q, et al. Pindel: a pattern growth approach to detect break points of large deletions and medium sized insertions from paired-end short reads. *Bioinformatics* 2009;25:2865–2871.
[h] Venkatraman ES, Olshen AB. A faster circular binary segmentation algorithm for the analysis of array CGH data. *Bioinformatics* 2007;23:657–663.
[i] Chiang DY, Getz G, Jaffe DB, et al. High-resolution mapping of copy-number alterations with massively parallel sequencing. *Nature Methods* 2009;6:99–103.
[j] Ng PC, Henikoff S. Predicting deleterious amino acid substitutions. *Genome Res* 2001;11:863–874.
[k] Idzhubei IA, Schmidt S, Peshkin L, et al. A method and server for predicting damaging missense mutations. *Nature Methods* 2010;7:248–249.
[l] Krzywinski M, Schein J, Birol I, et al. Circos: an information aesthetic for comparative genomics. *Genome Res* 2009;19:1639–1645.
[m] Robinson JT, Thorvaldsdóttir H, Winckler W, et al. Integrative Genomics Viewer. *Nat Biotechnol* 2011;29:24–26.
[n] Forbes SA, Bhamra S, Dawson E, et al. The catalogue of somatic mutations in cancer (COSMIC). *Curr Protoc Hum Genet* 2008;Chapter 10:Unit 10.11.
[o] Futreal PA, Coin L, Marshall M, et al. A census of human cancer genes. *Nat Rev Cancer* 2004;4:177–183.
[p] Sherry ST, Ward MH, Kholodov M, et al. dbSNP: The NCBI Database of genetic variation. *Nucleic Acids Res* 2001;29:308–311.
[q] The Cancer Genome Atlas Research Network. Comprehensive genomic characterization defines human glioblastoma genes and core pathways. *Nature* 2008;455:1061–1068.
Based on Meyerson M, Stacey G, Getz G. Advances in understanding cancer genomes through second generation sequencing. *Nature Rev Genet* 2010;11:685–696, Table 2.

the ICGC. All of these projects deal with at least 500 samples per cancer type from cancers affecting a variety of human organs and tissues, including blood, the brain, the breast, the esophagus, the kidneys, the liver, the oral cavity, the ovaries, the pancreas, the prostate, the skin, and the stomach.[130]

All of these coordinated projects have already provided new insights into the catalog of genes mutated in cancer and have unveiled specific signatures of the mutagenic mechanisms, including carcinogen exposures or DNA-repair defects, implicated in the development of different malignant tumors.[83,84,87,131] Furthermore, these cancer genome studies have also contributed to define clinically relevant subtypes of tumors for prognosis and therapeutic management, and in some cases have identified new targets and strategies for cancer treatment.[74–76] The rapid technological advances in DNA sequencing will likely drop the costs of sequencing cancer genomes to a small fraction of

the current price and will allow researchers to overcome some of the current limitations of these global sequencing efforts. Hopefully, worldwide coordination of cancer genome projects, including Pan-Cancer initiative, with those involving large-scale, functional analyses of genes in both cellular and animal models will likely provide us with the most comprehensive collection of information generated to date about the causes and molecular mechanisms of cancer.

THE GENOMIC LANDSCAPE OF CANCERS

Examining the overall distribution of the identified mutations redefined the cancer genome landscapes whereby the *mountains* are the handful of commonly mutated genes and the *hills* represent the vast majority of genes that are infrequently mutated.

One of the most striking features of the tumor genomic landscape is that it involves different sets of cancer genes that are mutated in a tissue-specific fashion.[132,133] To continue with the analogy, the scenery is very different if we observe a colorectal, a lung, or a breast tumor. This indicates that mutations in specific genes cause tumors at specific sites, or are associated with specific stages of development, cell differentiation, or tumorigenesis, despite many of those genes being expressed in various fetal and adult tissues. Moreover, different types of tumors follow specific genetic pathways in terms of the combination of genetic alterations that it must acquire. For example, no cancer outside the bowel has been shown to follow the classic genetic pathway of colorectal tumorigenesis. Additionally, *KRAS* mutations are almost always present in pancreatic cancers but are very rare or absent in breast cancers. Similarly, *BRAF* mutations are present in 60% of melanomas, but are very infrequent in lung cancers.[1] Another intriguing feature is that alterations in ubiquitous housekeeping genes, such as those involved in DNA repair or energy production, occur only in particular types of tumors.

In addition to tissue specificity, the genomic landscape of tumors can also be associated with gender and hormonal status. For example, *HER2* amplification and *PIK3C2A* mutations, two genetic alterations associated with breast cancer development, are correlated with the estrogen-receptor hormonal status.[134] The molecular basis for the occurrence of cancer mutations in tissue- and gender-specific profiles is still largely unknown. Organ-specific expression profiles and cell-specific neoplastic transformation requirements are often mentioned as possible causes for this phenomenon. Identifying tissue and gender cancer mutations patterns is relevant because it may allow for the definition of individualized therapeutic avenues.

INTEGRATIVE ANALYSIS OF CANCER GENOMICS

The implementation of novel high-throughput technologies is generating an extraordinary amount of information on cancer samples in many different ways other than those derived from whole-exome or whole-genome sequencing. Accordingly, there is a growing need to integrate genomic, epigenomic, transcriptomic, and proteomic landscapes from tumor samples, and then linking this integrated information with clinical outcomes of cancer patients. There are some examples of human malignancies in which this integrative approach has been already performed, such as for AML, glioblastoma, medulloblastoma, and renal cell, colorectal, ovarian, endometrial, prostate, and breast carcinomas.[135–142] In these cases, the integration of whole-exome and whole-genome sequencing with studies involving genomic DNA copy number arrays, DNA methylation, transcriptomic arrays, miRNA sequencing, and proteomic profiling has contributed to improving the molecular classification of complex and heterogeneous tumors. These integrative molecular analyses have also provided new insights into the mechanisms disrupted in each particular cancer type or subtype and have facilitated the association of genomic information with distinct clinical parameters of cancer patients and the discovery of novel therapeutic targets.[143] Also in this regard, there has been significant progress in the definition of the mechanisms by which the cancer genome and epigenome influence each other and cooperate to facilitate malignant transformation.[144,145] Thus, many tumor-suppressor genes are inactivated by either mutation or epigenetic silencing, and in some cases such as colorectal carcinomas, both mechanisms work coordinately to create a permissive environment for oncogenic transformation.[146] Moreover, mutations in epigenetic regulators such as DNA methyl transferases, chromatin remodelers, histones, and histone modifiers, are very frequent events in many tumors,

including hepatocellular carcinomas, renal carcinomas leukemias, lymphomas, glioblastomas, and medulloblastomas. These genetic alterations of epigenetic modulators cause widespread transcriptomic changes, thereby amplifying the initial effect of the mutational event at the cancer genome level.[145]

The recent availability of different platforms for integrative cancer genome analyses will be very helpful in enabling the classification, biologic characterization, and personalized clinical management of human cancers (Table 1.3).[144,147]

THE CANCER GENOME AND THE NEW TAXONOMY OF TUMORS

Deciphering the cancer genome has already impacted clinical practice at multiple levels. On the one hand, it allowed for the identification of new cancer genes such as *IDH1*, a gene involved in glioma, which was discovered recently (see previous), and on the other hand, it is redesigning the taxonomy of tumors.

Until the genomic revolution, tumors had been classified based on two criteria: their localization (site of occurrence) and their appearance (histology). These criteria are also currently used as primary determinants of prognosis and to establish the best treatments. For many decades, it has been known that patients with histologically similar tumors have different clinical outcomes. Furthermore, tumors that cannot be distinguished based on an histologic analysis can respond very differently to identical therapies.[148]

It is becoming increasingly clear that the frequency and distribution of mutations affecting cancer genes can be used to redefine the histology-based taxonomy of a given tumor type. Lung and colorectal tumors represent paradigmatic examples. Genomic analyses led to the identification of activating mutations in the receptor tyrosine kinase *EGFR* in lung adenocarcinomas.[149] The occurrence of *EGFR* mutations molecularly defines a subtype of non–small-cell lung cancers (NSCLC) that occur mainly in non-smoking women, that tend to have a distinctly enhanced prognosis, and that typically respond to epidermal growth factor receptor (EGFR)-targeted therapies.[150–152] Similarly, the recent discovery of the *EML4-ALK* fusion identifies yet another subset of NSCLC that is clearly distinct from those that harbor *EGFR* mutations, that have distinct epidemiologic and biologic features, and that respond to ALK inhibitors.[109,153]

The second example is colorectal cancers (CRC), the tumor type for which the genomic landscape has been refined with the highest accuracy. CRCs can be clearly categorized according to the mutational profile of the genes involved in the *KRAS* pathway (Fig. 1.10). It is now known that *KRAS* mutations occur in approximately 40% of CRCs. Another subtype of CRC (approximately 10%) harbors mutations in *BRAF*, the immediate downstream effectors of *KRAS*.[10]

In CRCs and other tumor types, *KRAS* and *BRAF* mutations are known to be mutually exclusive. The mutual exclusivity pattern indicates that these genes operate in the same signaling pathway. Large epidemiologic studies have shown that the prognosis of tumors harboring wild-type *KRAS/BRAF* genes is distinct, and typically more favorable, than that of the mutated ones.[154,155] Of note, *KRAS* and *BRAF* mutations have been recently shown to impair responsiveness to the anti-EGFR monoclonal antibodies therapies in CRC patients.[156–158] Clearly distinct subgroups can be genetically identified in both NSCLCs and CRCs with respect to prognosis and response to therapy. It is likely that as soon as the genomic landscapes of other tumor types are defined, molecular subgroups like those described previously will also become defined.

Genotyping tumor tissue in search of somatic genetic alterations for *actionable* information has become routine practice in clinical oncology. The genetic profile of solid tumors is currently obtained from surgical or biopsy specimens. As the techniques

TABLE 1.3

Useful Information for the Description and Management of Cancer

Bioinformatic Tool or Webservices	Database Used	Webservice or Tool	Upload of Data Possible	Gene Search	Chromosomal Region Search	mRNA Expression	SNV	CNV	Methylation	miRNA Expression	Protein	Pathways
cBioPortal for Cancer Genomics	TCGA	Webservice	—	✓	—	✓	✓	✓	—	—	✓	✓
PARADIGM, Broad GDAC Firehose	TCGA	Webservice	✓	✓	—	✓	✓	✓	✓	—	—	✓
WashU Epigenome Browser	ENCODE	Webservice	✓	✓	✓	✓	✓	✓	✓	—	—	✓
UCSC Cancer Genomics Browser	UCSC	Webservice	✓	✓	✓	✓	✓	✓	✓	✓	—	—
The Cancer Genome Workbench	TCGA	Webservice	—	✓	✓	✓	✓	✓	✓	—	—	—
EpiExplorer	ENCODE and ROADMAP	Webservice	✓	✓	✓	—	—	—	✓	—	—	—
EpiGRAPH	ENCODE	Webservice	✓	✓	✓	✓	✓	✓	✓	—	—	—
Catalogue of Somatic Mutations in Cancer (COSMIC)	TCGA and ICGC	Webservice	—	✓	—	—	—	✓	—	—	—	—
PCmtl, MAGIA, miRvar, CoMeTa, etc.*	GEO and TCGA	Webservice	✓	✓	—	✓	—	—	✓	✓	—	✓
ICGC	ICGC	Webservice	—	✓	—	✓	✓	✓	—	—	—	—
Genomatix	User defined	Tool	—	✓	—	✓	✓	✓	✓	—	—	✓
Caleydo	TCGA	Tool	—	✓	✓	✓	✓	✓	✓	✓	—	✓
Integrative Genomics Viewer (IGV)	ENCODE	Tool	—	✓	✓	✓	✓	✓	✓	—	—	—
iCluster and iCluster Plus	User defined	Tool	—	✓	—	✓	—	✓	—	—	—	—

* Web Site with links for integrated analysis of microRNA and mRNA expression.
CNV, copy-number variation; ENCODE, Encyclopedia of DNA Elements; ICGC, the International Cancer Genome Consortium; GDAC, Genomic Data Analysis Center; GEO, Gene Expression Omnibus; miRNA, microRNA; SNV, single-nucleotide variation; TCGA, The Cancer Genome Atlas; USCS, University of California, Santa Cruz; Based on Plass C, Pfister SM, Lindroth AM, et al. Mutations in regulators of the epigenome and their connections to global chromatin patterns in cancer. *Nat Rev Genet* 2013;14:765–780, Table 1.

PRINCIPLES OF ONCOLOGY

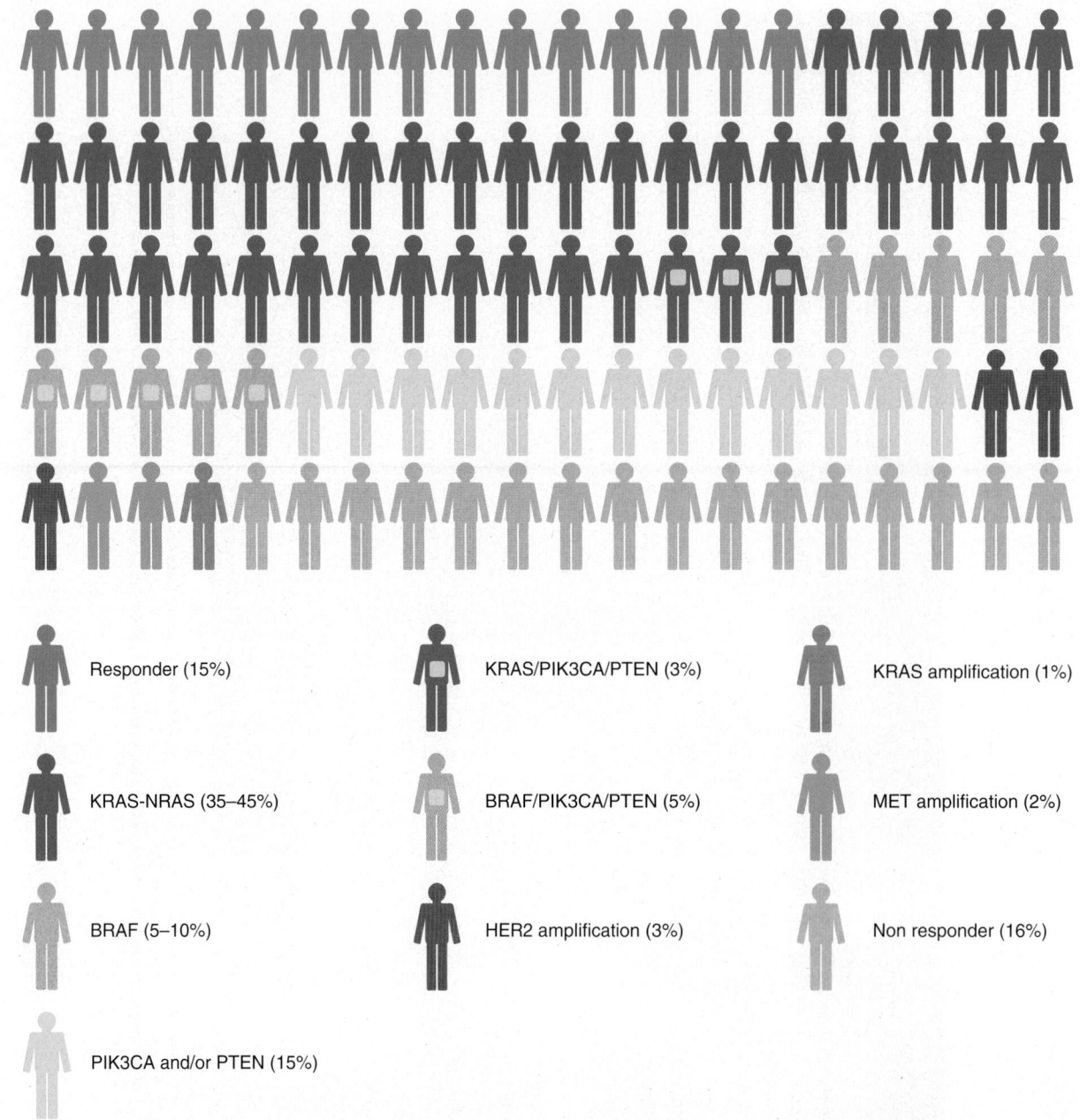

Figure 1.10 Graphic representation of a cohort of 100 patients with colorectal cancer treated with cetuximab or panitumumab. The genetic milieu of individual tumors and their impacts on the clinical response are listed. *KRAS, BRAF,* and *PIK3CA* somatic mutations as well as loss of PTEN protein expression are indicated according to different color codes. Molecular alterations mutually exclusive or coexisting in individual tumors are indicated using different color variants. The relative frequencies at which the molecular alterations occur in colorectal cancers are described. (Redrawn from Bardelli A, Siena S. Molecular mechanisms of resistance to cetuximab and panitumumab in colorectal cancer. *J Clin Oncol* 2010;28:1254–1261.)

that have enabled us to analyze tumor tissues become ever more sophisticated, we have realized the limitations of this approach. As previously discussed, cancers are heterogeneous, with different areas of the same tumor showing different genetic profiles (i.e., intratumoral heterogeneity); likewise, heterogeneity exists between metastases within the same patient (i.e., intermetastatic heterogeneity).[159] A tissue section (or a biopsy) from one part of a solitary tumor will miss the molecular intratumoral as well as intermetastatic heterogeneity. To capture tumor heterogeneity, techniques that are capable of interrogating the genetic landscapes of the overall disease in a single patient are needed.

In 1948, the publication of a manuscript describing the presence of cell-free circulating DNA (cfDNA) in the blood of humans offered—probably without realizing it—unprecedented opportunities in this area.[160] Only recently, the full potential of this seminal discovery has been appreciated. Several groups have reported that the analysis of circulating tumor DNA can, in principle, provide the same genetic information obtained from tumor tissue.[161] The levels of cfDNA are typically higher in cancer patients than healthy individuals, indicating that it is possible to screen for the presence of disease through a simple blood test. Furthermore, the specific detection of tumor-derived cfDNA has been shown to correlate with tumor burden, which changes in response to treatment or surgery.[162–164]

Although the detection of ctDNA has remarkable potential, it is also challenging for several reasons. The first is the need to discriminate DNA released from tumor cells (ctDNA) from circulating *normal* DNA. Discerning ctDNA from normal cfDNA is aided by the fact that tumor DNA is defined by the presence of mutations. These somatic mutations, commonly single base pair substitutions, are present only in the genomes of cancer cells or precancerous cells and are present in the DNA of normal cells of the same individual. Accordingly, ctDNA offers exquisite specificity as a biomarker. Unfortunately, cfDNA derived from tumor cells often represents a very small fraction (<1%) of the total cfDNA, thus limiting the applicability of the approach. The development and refinement of next-generation sequencing strategies as well as recently developed digital PCR techniques have made it possible to define rare mutant variants in complex mixtures of DNA. Using these approaches, it is possible to detect point mutations, rearrangements, and gene copy number changes in individual genes starting from a few milliliters of plasma.[165] Very recently, several groups have opened a new frontier by showing that exome analyses can also be performed from circulating DNA extracted from the blood of cancer patients.[166]

The detection of tumor-specific genetic alterations in patients' blood (often referred to as *liquid biopsies*) has several applications in the field of oncology, which are summarized as follows. Analyses of cfDNA can be used to genotype tumors when a tissue sample is not available or is difficult to obtain. Circulating tumor DNA fragments contain the identical genetic defects as the tumor themselves, thus the blood can reveal tumor point mutations (*EGFR*, *KRAS*, *BRAF*, *PIK3CA*), rearrangements (e.g., *EML4-ALK*), as well as tumor amplifications (*MET*).[167–169] *Liquid biopsies* may also be useful in monitoring tumor burden—a central aspect in the management of patients with cancer—that is typically assessed with imaging. In this regard, several investigational studies have shown that ctDNA can be a surrogate for tumor burden and that, much like viral load changes (e.g., HIV viral load), levels of ctDNA correspond with clinical course. Another application of ctDNA is the detection of minimal residual disease following surgery or therapy with curative intent.[163] Finally, *liquid biopsies* can be used to monitor the genomic drift (clonal evolution) of tumors upon treatment.[166] In this setting, the analysis of ctDNA in plasma samples obtained pretreatment, during, and posttreatment can lead to an understanding of the mechanisms of primary and, especially, acquired resistance to therapies.[170,171]

Importantly, the advances in sequencing technologies have made the idea of personalized treatment of cancer a reality, which is most evident in the field of adoptive cell therapy (ACT). Although already a treatment in use, the ability to use a patient's autologous tumor-infiltrating lymphocytes (TIL) is in position to benefit greatly from advances in sequencing technologies. A recent study demonstrated this when whole-exome data, along with a major histocompatibility complex (MHC)-binding algorithm, were utilized to identify candidate tumor epitopes that are recognized by the patients' TILs.[172] This study should allow for future work in which the information obtained from the direct sequencing of a patient's tumor can quickly be used to generate tumor-reactive T cells that can then be used for a personalized treatment.

In conclusion, the taxonomy of tumors is being rewritten using the presence of genetic lesions as major criteria. Genome-based information will improve the diagnosis and will be used to determine personalized therapeutic regimens based on the genetic landscape of individual tumors.

CANCER GENOMICS AND DRUG RESISTANCE

Cancer genomics has dramatically impacted disease management, because its application is helping researchers determine which patients are likely to benefit from which drug. As discussed in great detail in Chapter 22, good examples for such treatment include targeted therapy using imatinib for chronic myeloid leukemia (CML) patients and the use of gefitinib and erlotinib for NSCLC patients.

The key to the successful development and application of anticancer agents is a better understanding of the effect of the therapeutic regimens and of resistance mechanisms that may develop. In most tumor types, a fraction of patients' tumors are refractory to therapies (intrinsic resistance). Even if an initial response to therapies is obtained, the vast majority of tumors subsequently become refractory (i.e., acquired resistance), and patients eventually succumb to disease progression. Therefore, secondary resistance should be regarded as a key obstacle to treatment progress. The analysis of the cancer genome represents a powerful tool both for the identification of chemotherapeutic signatures as well as to understand resistance mechanisms to therapeutic agents. Examples for each of these are described as follows.

An important application of systematic sequencing experiments is the identification of the effects of chemotherapy on the cancer genome. For example, gliomas that recur after temozolomide treatment have been shown to harbor large numbers of mutations with a signature typical of a DNA alkylating agent.[173,174] Because these alterations were detected using Sanger sequencing, which as described previously has limited sensitivity, the data suggested that the detected alterations were clonal. The model that unfolds from this study indicates that although temozolomide has limited efficacy, almost all of the cells in a glioma respond to the drug. However, a single cell that was resistant to the chemotherapy proliferated and formed a cell clone. Later genomic analyses of the cell clone allowed for the identification of the underlying mutated resistance genes.[173,174]

Single-molecule–targeted therapy is almost always followed by acquired drug resistance.[175–177] Genomic analyses can be successfully exploited to decipher resistance mechanisms to such inhibitors. A few paradigmatic examples are presented as follows, which will be discussed extensively in other chapters. Despite the effectiveness of gefitinib and erlotinib in EGFR mutant cases of NSCLC,[178] drug resistance develops within 6 to 12 months after the initiation of therapy. The underlying reason for this resistance was identified as a secondary mutation in *EGFR* exon 20, T790M, which is detectable in 50% of patients who relapse.[179–181] Importantly, some studies have shown the mutation to be present before the patient was treated with the drug,[182,183] suggesting that exposure to the drug selected for these cells.[184] Because the drug-resistant *EGFR* mutation is structurally analogous to the mutated gatekeeper residue T315I in BCR-ABL, T670I in c-Kit, and L1196M in EML4-ALK, which have been shown previously to confer resistance to imatinib and other kinase inhibitors,[176,185,186] this mechanism of resistance represents a general problem that needs to be overcome.

A recent elegant study, which also represents the use of genomics in understanding drug-resistance mechanisms, focused on the inhibition of activating *BRAF* (V600E) mutations, which occur in 7% of human malignancies and in 60% of melanomas.[9] Clinical trials using PLX4032, a novel class I RAF-selective inhibitor, showed an 80% antitumor response rate in melanoma patients with *BRAF* (V600E) mutations; however, cases of drug resistance were observed.[187] The use of microarray and sequencing technologies showed that, in this case, the resistance was not due to secondary mutations in *BRAF*, but due rather to either upregulation of *PDGFRB* or *NRAS* mutations.[188]

It was, however, the introduction of two anti-EGFR monoclonal antibodies, cetuximab and panitumumab, for the treatment of metastatic colorectal cancer, that provided the largest body of knowledge on the relationship between tumors' genotypes and the response to targeted therapies. The initial clinical analysis pointed out that only a fraction of metastatic CRC patients benefited from this novel treatment. Different from the NSCLC paradigm, it was found that EGFR mutations do not play a major role in the response. On the contrary, from the initial retrospective analysis, it became clear that somatic *KRAS* mutations, thought to be present in 35% to 45% of metastatic colorectal cancers, are important negative predictors of efficacy in patients who are given panitumumab or cetuximab.[156–158] Among tumors carrying wild-type *KRAS*, mutations of *BRAF* or *PIK3CA*, or a loss of phosphatase and tensin homolog (PTEN) expression may also predict resistance to EGFR-targeted monoclonal antibodies, although the latter biomarkers require further validation before they can be incorporated into clinical practice. From these few examples, it is clear that a future, deeper genomic understanding of targeted drug resistance is crucial to the effective development of additional as well as alternative therapies to overcome this resistance.

PERSPECTIVES OF CANCER GENOME ANALYSIS

The completion of the human genome project has marked a new beginning in biomedical sciences. Because human cancer is a genetic disease, the field of oncology has been one of the first to be impacted by this historic revolution. Knowledge of the sequence and organization of the human genome allows for the systematic analysis of the genetic alterations underlying the origin and evolution of tumors. High-throughput mutational profiling of common tumors, including lung, skin, breast, and colorectal cancers, and the application of next-generation sequencing to whole genome, whole exome, and whole transcriptome of cancer samples has allowed substantial advances in the understanding of this disease by facilitating the detection of all main types of somatic cancer genome alterations. These have also led to historical results, such as the identification of genetic alterations that are likely to be the major drivers of these diseases.

However, the genetic landscape of cancers is by no means complete, and what has been learned so far has raised new and exciting questions that must be addressed. There are still important technical challenges for the detection of somatic mutations.[60] Clinical tumor samples often contain large amounts of nonmalignant cells, which makes the identification of mutations in cancer genomes more challenging when compared with similar analyses of peripheral blood samples for germ-line genome studies. Moreover, the genomic instability inherent to cancer development and progression largely increases the complexity and diversity of genomic alterations of malignant tumors, making it necessary to distinguish between driver and passenger mutations. Likewise, the fact that malignant tumors are genetically heterogeneous and contain several clones simultaneously growing within the same tumor mass raises additional questions regarding the quality of the information currently derived from cancer genomes. Hopefully, in the near future, advances in third-generation sequencing technologies will make it feasible to obtain high-quality sequence data of a genome isolated from a single cell, an aspect of crucial relevance for cancer research.

One of the next imperatives is the definition of the oncogenomic profile of all tumor types. In particular, the less common—although not less lethal—ones are still largely mysterious to scientists and untreatable to clinicians. For some of these diseases, few new therapeutically amenable molecular targets have been discovered in the past years. For example, the identification of drugable genetic lesions associated with pancreatic and ovarian cancers could help define new therapeutic strategies for these aggressive diseases. To achieve this, detailed oncogenomic maps of the corresponding tumors must be drafted. The latter will hopefully be completed in the coming years, thanks to the systematic cancer genome projects that are presently being performed.

Even in the case of common cancers, a lot of genomic profiling efforts still lay ahead. For example, in a significant fraction of breast and lung tumors, the mutations that are likely to be drivers have not yet been found. This is not surprising considering that even in these tumor types only a limited number of samples have been systematically analyzed so far. Therefore, low incidence mutations that could represent potentially key therapeutic targets in a subset of tumors might have escaped detection. Consequently, the scaling up of the mutational profiling to large numbers of specimens for each tumor type is warranted.

Finally, understanding the cellular properties imparted by the hundreds of recently discovered cancer alleles is another area that must be developed. As a matter of fact, compared to the genomic discovery stage, the functional validation of putative novel cancer alleles, despite their potential clinical relevance, is substantially lagging behind. To achieve this, high-throughput functional studies in model systems that accurately recapitulate the genetic alterations found in human cancer must be developed.

To conclude, the eventual goal of profiling the cancer genome is not only to further understand the molecular basis of the disease, but also to discover novel diagnostic and drug targets. One might anticipate that the most immediate application of these new technologies will be noninvasive strategies for early cancer detection. Considering that oncogenic mutations are present only in cancer cells, screening for tumor-derived mutant DNA in patients' blood holds great potential and will progressively substitute current biomarkers, which have poor sensitivity and lack specificity.[171] Further improvements in next-generation sequencing technologies are likely to reduce their cost as well as make these analyses more facile in the future. Once this happens, most cancer patients will undergo in-depth genomic analyses as part of their initial evaluation and throughout their treatment. This will offer more precise diagnostic and prognostic information, which will affect treatment decisions. Although many challenges remain, the information gained from next-generation sequencing platforms is laying a foundation for personalized medicine, in which patients are managed with therapies that are tailored to the specific gene mutations found in their tumors. Ultimately, these should lead to therapeutic successes similar to the ones attained for CML patients with imatinib,[189,190] melanoma patients with PLX4032,[187] and NSCLC patients with gefitinib and erlotinib.[178] Clearly, this is the absolute goal for all of this work.

ACKNOWLEDGMENTS

This work was supported by the Intramural Research Programs of the National Human Genome Research Institute, National Institutes of Health, USA, YS is supported by the Henry Chanoch Krenter Institute for Biomedical Imaging and Genomics, Louis and Fannie Tolz Collaborative Research Project, Dukler Fund for Cancer Research, De Benedetti Foundation-Cherasco 1547, Peter and Patricia Gruber Awards, Gideon Hamburger, Israel, Estate of Alice Schwarz-Gardos, Estate of John Hunter and the Knell Family. YS is supported by the Israel Science Foundation grant numbers 1604/13 and 877/13 and the ERC (StG-335377). A.B. is supported by the European Communityís Seventh Framework Programme under grant agreement no. 259015 COLTHERES, Associazione Italiana per la Ricerca sul Cancro (AIRC) IG grant no. 12812 and Fondazione Piemontese per la Ricerca sul Cancro–ONLUS. C.L-O. is an Investigator of the Botin Foundation supported by grants from Ministerio de Economía y Competitividad-Spain and Instituto de Salud Carlos III (RTICC), Spain.

1. Vogelstein B, Kinzler KW. Cancer genes and the pathways they control. *Nat Med* 2004;10:789–799.
2. Kinzler KW, Vogelstein B. Lessons from hereditary colon cancer. *Cell* 1996; 87:159–170.
3. International Human Genome Sequencing Consortium. Finishing the euchromatic sequence of the human genome. *Nature* 2004;431:931–945.
4. Stehelin D, Varmus HE, Bishop JM, et al. DNA related to the transforming gene(s) of avian sarcoma viruses is present in normal avian DNA. *Nature* 1976;260:170–173.
5. Rous P. Transmission of a malignant new growth by means of a cell-free filtrate. *J Am Med Assoc* 1911;56:198.
6. International HapMap Consortium. The International HapMap Project. *Nature* 2003;426:89–96.
7. International HapMap Consortium. A haplotype map of the human genome. *Nature* 2005;437:1299–1320.
8. Sanger F, Nicklen S, Coulson AR. DNA sequencing with chain-terminating inhibitors. *Proc Natl Acad Sci U S A* 1977;74:5463–5467.
9. Davies H, Bignell GR, Cox C, et al. Mutations of the BRAF gene in human cancer. *Nature* 2002;417:949–954.
10. Rajagopalan H, Bardelli A, Lengauer C, et al. Tumorigenesis: RAF/RAS oncogenes and mismatch-repair status. *Nature* 2002;418:934.
11. Moodie SA, Wolfman A. The 3Rs of life: Ras, Raf and growth regulation. *Trends Genet* 1994;10:44–48.
12. Hafen E, Dickson B, Brunner D, et al. Genetic dissection of signal transduction mediated by the sevenless receptor tyrosine kinase in Drosophila. *Prog Neurobiol* 1994;42:287–292.
13. Bardelli A, Parsons DW, Silliman N, et al. Mutational analysis of the tyrosine kinome in colorectal cancers. *Science* 2003;300:949.
14. Greenman C, Stephens P, Smith R, et al. Patterns of somatic mutation in human cancer genomes. *Nature* 2007;446:153–158.
15. Samuels Y, Wang Z, Bardelli A, et al. High frequency of mutations of the PIK3CA gene in human cancers. *Science* 2004;304:554.
16. Wang Z, Shen D, Parsons DW, et al. Mutational analysis of the tyrosine phosphatome in colorectal cancers. *Science* 2004;304:1164–1166.
17. Vivanco I, Sawyers CL. The phosphatidylinositol 3-Kinase AKT pathway in human cancer. *Nat Rev Cancer* 2002;2:489–501.
18. Broderick DK, Di C, Parrett TJ, et al. Mutations of PIK3CA in anaplastic oligodendrogliomas, high-grade astrocytomas, and medulloblastomas. *Cancer Res* 2004;64:5048–5050.
19. Lee JW, Soung YH, Kim SY, et al. PIK3CA gene is frequently mutated in breast carcinomas and hepatocellular carcinomas. *Oncogene* 2005;24:1477–1480.
20. Bachman KE, Argani P, Samuels Y, et al. The PIK3CA gene is mutated with high frequency in human breast cancers. *Cancer Biol Ther* 2004;3:772–775.
21. Oda K, Stokoe D, Taketani Y, et al. High frequency of coexistent mutations of PIK3CA and PTEN genes in endometrial carcinoma. *Cancer Res* 2005;65:10669–10673.
22. Samuels Y, Waldman T. Oncogenic mutations of PIK3CA in human cancers. *Curr Top Microbiol Immunol* 2010;2:21–42.
23. Parsons DW, Wang TL, Samuels Y, et al. Colorectal cancer: mutations in a signalling pathway. *Nature* 2005;436:792.
24. Lopez-Otin C, Overall CM. Protease degradomics: a new challenge for proteomics. *Nat Rev Mol Cell Biol* 2002;3:509–519.
25. Liotta LA, Tryggvason K, Garbisa S, et al. Metastatic potential correlates with enzymatic degradation of basement membrane collagen. *Nature* 1980;284:67–68.
26. Lopez-Otin C, Hunter T. The regulatory crosstalk between kinases and proteases in cancer. *Nat Rev Cancer* 2010;10:278–292.
27. Egeblad M, Werb Z. New functions for the matrix metalloproteinases in cancer progression. *Nat Rev Cancer* 2002;2:161–174.
28. Lopez-Otin C, Matrisian LM. Emerging roles of proteases in tumour suppression. *Nat Rev Cancer* 2007;7:800–808.
29. Wood LD, Parsons DW, Jones S, et al. The genomic landscapes of human breast and colorectal cancers. *Science* 2007;318:1108–1113.
30. Palavalli LH, Prickett TD, Wunderluch JR, et al. Analysis of the matrix metalloproteinase family reveals that MMP8 is often mutated in melanoma. *Nat Genet* 2009;41:518–520.
31. Lopez-Otin C, Palavalli LH, Samuels Y. Protective roles of matrix metalloproteinases: from mouse models to human cancer. *Cell Cycle* 2009;8:3657–3662.
32. Hanahan D, Weinberg RA. The hallmarks of cancer. *Cell* 2000;100:57–70.
33. Teitz T, Wei T, Valentine MB, et al. Caspase 8 is deleted or silenced preferentially in childhood neuroblastomas with amplification of MYCN. *Nat Med* 2000;6:529–535.
34. Mandruzzato S, Brasseur F, Andry G, et al. A CASP-8 mutation recognized by cytolytic T lymphocytes on a human head and neck carcinoma. *J Exp Med* 1997;186:785–793.
35. Soung YH, Lee JW, Kim SY, et al. CASPASE-8 gene is inactivated by somatic mutations in gastric carcinomas. *Cancer Res* 2005;65:815–821.
36. Fraile JM, Quesada V, Rodríguez D, et al. Deubiquitinases in cancer: new functions and therapeutic options. *Oncogene* 2012;31:2373–2388.
37. Bignell GR, Warren W, Seal S, et al. Identification of the familial cylindromatosis tumour-suppressor gene. *Nat Genet* 2000;25:160–165.
38. Schmitz R, Hansmann ML, Bohle V, et al. TNFAIP3 (A20) is a tumor suppressor gene in Hodgkin lymphoma and primary mediastinal B cell lymphoma. *J Exp Med* 2009;206:981–989.
39. Compagno M, Lim WK, Grunn A, et al. Mutations of multiple genes cause deregulation of NF-kappaB in diffuse large B-cell lymphoma. *Nature* 2009;459:717–721.
40. Kato M, Sanada M, Kato I, et al. Frequent inactivation of A20 in B-cell lymphomas. *Nature* 2009;459:712–716.
41. Novak U, Rinaldi A, Kwee I, et al. The NF-kappa B negative regulator TNFAIP3 (A20) is inactivated by somatic mutations and genomic deletions in marginal zone lymphomas. *Blood* 2009;113: 4918–4921.
42. Harbour JW, Onken MD, Roberson ED, et al. Frequent mutation of BAP1 in metastasizing uveal melanomas. *Science* 2010;330:1410–1413.
43. Carbone M, Yang H, Pass HI, et al. BAP1 and cancer. *Nat Rev Cancer* 2013; 13:153–159.
44. Sjöblom T, Jones S, Wood LD, et al. The consensus coding sequences of human breast and colorectal cancers. *Science* 2006;314:268–274.
45. Jones S, Zhang X, Parsons DW, et al. Core signaling pathways in human pancreatic cancers revealed by global genomic analyses. *Science* 2008;321:1801–1806.
46. Parsons DW, Jones S, Zhang X, et al. An integrated genomic analysis of human glioblastoma multiforme. *Science* 2008;321:1807–1812.
47. Jones S, Wang TL, Shih IeM, et al. Frequent mutations of chromatin remodeling gene ARID1A in ovarian clear cell carcinoma. *Science* 2010;330:228–231.
48. Parsons DW, Li M, Zhang X, et al. The genetic landscape of the childhood cancer medulloblastoma. *Science* 2011;331:435–439.
49. Yan H, Parsons DW, Jin G, et al. IDH1 and IDH2 mutations in gliomas. *N Engl J Med* 2009;360:765–773.
50. Bleeker FE, Lamba S, Leenstra S, et al. IDH1 mutations at residue p.R132 (IDH1(R132)) occur frequently in high-grade gliomas but not in other solid tumors. *Hum Mutat* 2009;30:7–11.
51. Hartmann C, Meyer J, Balss J, et al. Type and frequency of IDH1 and IDH2 mutations are related to astrocytic and oligodendroglial differentiation and age: a study of 1,010 diffuse gliomas. *Acta Neuropathol* 2009;118:469–474.
52. Hayden JT, Frühwald MC, Hasselblatt M, et al. Frequent IDH1 mutations in supratentorial primitive neuroectodermal tumors (sPNET) of adults but not children. *Cell Cycle* 2009;8:1806–1807.
53. Ichimura K, Pearson DM, Kocialkowski S, et al. IDH1 mutations are present in the majority of common adult gliomas but rare in primary glioblastomas. *Neuro Oncol* 2009;11:341–347.
54. Kang MR, Kim MS, Oh JE, et al. Mutational analysis of IDH1 codon 132 in glioblastomas and other common cancers. *Int J Cancer* 2009;125:353–355.
55. Watanabe T, Nobusawa S, Kleihues P, et al. IDH1 mutations are early events in the development of astrocytomas and oligodendrogliomas. *Am J Pathol* 2009;174:1149–1153.
56. Mardis ER, Ding L, Dooling DJ, et al. Recurring mutations found by sequencing an acute myeloid leukemia genome. *N Engl J Med* 2009;361:1058–1066.
57. Green A, Beer P. Somatic mutations of IDH1 and IDH2 in the leukemic transformation of myeloproliferative neoplasms. *N Engl J Med* 2010; 362:369–370.
58. Gross S, Cairns RA, Minden Md, et al. Cancer-associated metabolite 2-hydroxyglutarate accumulates in acute myelogenous leukemia with isocitrate dehydrogenase 1 and 2 mutations. *J Exp Med* 2010;207:339–344.
59. Mardis ER, Wilson RK. Cancer genome sequencing: a review. *Hum Mol Genet* 2009;18:R163–R168.
60. Meyerson M, Gabriel S, Getz G. Advances in understanding cancer genomes through second-generation sequencing. *Nat Rev Genet* 2010;11:685–696.
61. Metzker ML. Sequencing technologies - the next generation. *Nat Rev Genet* 2010;11:31–46.
62. Bell DW. Our changing view of the genomic landscape of cancer. *J Pathol* 2010;220:231–243.
63. Campbell PJ, Pleasance ED, Stephens PJ, et al. Subclonal phylogenetic structures in cancer revealed by ultra-deep sequencing. *Proc Natl Acad Sci U S A* 2008;105:13081–13086.
64. Kidd JM, Cooper GM, Donahue WF, et al. Mapping and sequencing of structural variation from eight human genomes. *Nature* 2008;453:56–64.
65. Drmanac R, Sparks AB, Callow MJ, et al. Human genome sequencing using unchained base reads on self-assembling DNA nanoarrays. *Science* 2010; 327:78–81.
66. Clarke J, Wu HC, Jayasinghe L, et al. Continuous base identification for single-molecule nanopore DNA sequencing. *Nat Nanotechnol* 2009;4: 265–270.
67. Schadt EE, Turner S, Kasarskis A. A window into third-generation sequencing. *Hum Mol Genet* 2010;19:R227–R240.
68. Dressman D, Yan H, Traverso G, et al. Transforming single DNA molecules into fluorescent magnetic particles for detection and enumeration of genetic variations. *Proc Natl Acad Sci U S A* 2003;100:8817–8822.
69. Fedurco M, Romieu A, Williams S, et al. BTA, a novel reagent for DNA attachment on glass and efficient generation of solid-phase amplified DNA colonies. *Nucleic Acids Res* 2006;34:e22.
70. Harris TD, Buzby PR, Babcock H, et al. Single-molecule DNA sequencing of a viral genome. *Science* 2008;320:106–109.

71. Morozova O, Hirst M, Marra MA. Applications of new sequencing technologies for transcriptome analysis. *Annu Rev Genomics Hum Genet* 2009;10: 135–151.

72. Pop M, Salzberg SL. Bioinformatics challenges of new sequencing technology. *Trends Genet* 2008;24:142–149.

73. Ley TJ, Mardis ER, Ding L, et al. DNA sequencing of a cytogenetically normal acute myeloid leukaemia genome. *Nature* 2008;456:66–72.

74. Garraway LA, Lander ES. Lessons from the cancer genome. *Cell* 2013;15: 17–37.

75. Vogelstein B, Papadopoulos N, Velculescu VE, et al. Cancer genome landscapes. *Science* 2013;339:1546–1558.

76. Watson IR, Takahashi K, Futreal PA, et al. Emerging patterns of somatic mutations in cancer. *Nat Rev Genet* 2013;14:703–718.

77. Campbell PJ, Yachida S, Mudie LJ, et al. The patterns and dynamics of genomic instability in metastatic pancreatic cancer. *Nature* 2010;467:1109–1113.

78. Lee W, Jiang Z, Liu J, et al. The mutation spectrum revealed by paired genome sequences from a lung cancer patient. *Nature* 2010;465:473–477.

79. Marcucci G, Maharry K, Wu YZ, et al. IDH1 and IDH2 gene mutations identify novel molecular subsets within de novo cytogenetically normal acute myeloid leukemia: a Cancer and Leukemia Group B study. *J Clin Oncol* 2010;28:2348–2355.

80. Paschka P, Schlenk RF, Gaidzik VI, et al. IDH1 and IDH2 mutations are frequent genetic alterations in acute myeloid leukemia and confer adverse prognosis in cytogenetically normal acute myeloid leukemia with NPM1 mutation without FLT3 internal tandem duplication. *J Clin Oncol* 2010;28: 3636–3643.

81. Shah SP, Morin Rd, Khattra J, et al. Mutational evolution in a lobular breast tumour profiled at single nucleotide resolution. *Nature* 2009;461:809–813.

82. Yachida S, Jones S, Bozic I, et al. Distant metastasis occurs late during the genetic evolution of pancreatic cancer. *Nature* 2010;467:1114–1117.

83. Pleasance ED, Cheetham RK, Stephens PJ, et al. A comprehensive catalogue of somatic mutations from a human cancer genome. *Nature* 2010;463:191–196.

84. Pleasance ED, Stephens PJ, O'Meara S, et al. A small-cell lung cancer genome with complex signatures of tobacco exposure. *Nature* 2010;463:184–190.

85. Ding L, Ellis MJ, Li S, et al. Genome remodelling in a basal-like breast cancer metastasis and xenograft. *Nature* 2010;464:999–1005.

86. Ley TJ, Ding L, Walter MJ, et al. DNMT3A mutations in acute myeloid leukemia. *N Engl J Med* 2010;363:2424–2433.

87. Alexandrov LB, Nik-Zainal S, Wedge DC, et al. Signatures of mutational processes in human cancer. *Nature* 2013;500:415–421.

88. Ward PS, Patel J, Wise DR, et al. The common feature of leukemia-associated IDH1 and IDH2 mutations is a neomorphic enzyme activity converting alpha-ketoglutarate to 2-hydroxyglutarate. *Cancer Cell* 2010;17:225–234.

89. Jones SJ, Laskin J, Lu YY, et al. Evolution of an adenocarcinoma in response to selection by targeted kinase inhibitors. *Genome Biol* 2010;11:R82.

90. Navin N, Kendall J, Troge J, et al. Tumour evolution inferred by single-cell sequencing. *Nature* 2011;472:90–94.

91. Vanharanta S, Massague J. Origins of metastatic traits. *Cancer Cell* 2013; 24:410–421.

92. Huang FW, Hodis E, Xu MJ, et al. Highly recurrent TERT promoter mutations in human melanoma. *Science* 2013;339:957–959.

93. Horn S, Figl A, Rachakonda PS, et al. TERT promoter mutations in familial and sporadic melanoma. *Science* 2013;339:959–961.

94. Ying Z, Li Y, Wu J, et al. Loss of miR-204 expression enhances glioma migration and stem cell-like phenotype. *Cancer Res* 2013;73:990–999.

95. Liang YJ, Wang QY, Zhou CX, et al. MiR-124 targets Slug to regulate epithelial-mesenchymal transition and metastasis of breast cancer. *Carcinogenesis* 2013;34:713–722.

96. Cooper C, Guo J, Yan Y, et al. Increasing the relative expression of endogenous non-coding Steroid Receptor RNA Activator (SRA) in human breast cancer cells using modified oligonucleotides. *Nucleic Acids Res* 2009;37:4518–4531.

97. Stephens PJ, Greenman CD, Fu B, et al. Massive genomic rearrangement acquired in a single catastrophic event during cancer development. *Cell* 2011;144:27–40.

98. Korbel JO, Campbell PJ. Criteria for inference of chromothripsis in cancer genomes. *Cell* 2013;152:1226–1236.

99. Baca SC, Prandi D, Lawrence MS, et al. Punctuated evolution of prostate cancer genomes. *Cell* 2013;153:666–677.

100. Turner EH, Lee C, Ng SB, et al. Massively parallel exon capture and library-free resequencing across 16 genomes. *Nat Methods* 2009;6:315–316.

101. Gnirke A, Melnikov A, Maguire J, et al. Solution hybrid selection with ultra-long oligonucleotides for massively parallel targeted sequencing. *Nat Biotechnol* 2009;27:182–189.

102. Levin JZ, Berger MF, Adiconis X, et al. Targeted next-generation sequencing of a cancer transcriptome enhances detection of sequence variants and novel fusion transcripts. *Genome Biol* 2009;10:R115.

103. Lawrence MS, Stojanov P, Polak P, et al. Mutational heterogeneity in cancer and the search for new cancer-associated genes. *Nature* 2013;499:214–218.

104. Kandoth C, McLellan MD, Vandin F, et al. Mutational landscape and significance across 12 major cancer types. *Nature* 2013;502:333–339.

105. Gartner JJ, Parker SC, Prickett TD, et al. Whole-genome sequencing identifies a recurrent functional synonymous mutation in melanoma. *Proc Natl Acad Sci U S A* 2013;110:13481–13486.

106. Stegh AH, Brennan C, Mahoney JA, et al. Glioma oncoprotein Bcl2L12 inhibits the p53 tumor suppressor. *Genes Dev* 2010;24:2194–2204.

107. Mullaney JM, Mills RE, Pittard WS, et al. Small insertions and deletions (INDELs) in human genomes. *Hum Mol Genet* 2010;19:R131–R136.

108. Tomlins SA, Rhodes DR, Perner S, et al. Recurrent fusion of TMPRSS2 and ETS transcription factor genes in prostate cancer. *Science* 2005;310:644–648.

109. Soda M, Choi YL, Enomoto M, et al. Identification of the transforming EML4-ALK fusion gene in non-small-cell lung cancer. *Nature* 2007; 448:561–566.

110. Palanisamy N, Ateeq B, Kalyana-Sundaram S, et al. Rearrangements of the RAF kinase pathway in prostate cancer, gastric cancer and melanoma. *Nat Med* 2010;16:793–798.

111. Leary RJ, Kinde I, Diehl F, et al. Development of personalized tumor biomarkers using massively parallel sequencing. *Sci Transl Med* 2010;2:20ra14.

112. Maher CA, Kumar-Sinha C, Cao X, et al. Transcriptome sequencing to detect gene fusions in cancer. *Nature* 2009;458:97–101.

113. Stephens PJ, McBride DJ, Lin ML, et al. Complex landscapes of somatic rearrangement in human breast cancer genomes. *Nature* 2009;462:1005–1010.

114. Feng H, Shuda M, Chang Y, et al. Clonal integration of a polyomavirus in human Merkel cell carcinoma. *Science* 2008;319:1096–1100.

115. Herner A, Sauliunaite D, Michalski CW, et al. Glutamate increases pancreatic cancer cell invasion and migration via AMPA receptor activation and Kras-MAPK signaling. *Int J Cancer* 2011;129:2349–2359.

116. Wei X, Walia V, Lin JC, et al. Exome sequencing identifies GRIN2A as frequently mutated in melanoma. *Nat Genet* 2011;43:442–446.

117. Prickett TD, Wei X, Cardenas-Navia I, et al. Exon capture analysis of G protein-coupled receptors identifies activating mutations in GRM3 in melanoma. *Nat Genet* 2011;43:1119–1126.

118. Krauthammer M, Kong Y, Ha BH, et al. Exome sequencing identifies recurrent somatic RAC1 mutations in melanoma. *Nat Genet* 2012;44:1006–1014.

119. Davies H, Hunter C, Smith R, et al. Somatic mutations of the protein kinase gene family in human lung cancer. *Cancer Res* 2005;65:7591–7595.

120. Bozic I, Antal T, Ohtsuki H, et al. Accumulation of driver and passenger mutations during tumor progression. *Proc Natl Acad Sci U S A* 2010;107:18545–18550.

121. Parmigiani G, Boca S, Lin J, et al. Design and analysis issues in genome-wide somatic mutation studies of cancer. *Genomics* 2009;93:17–21.

122. Kaminker JS, Zhang Y, Waugh A, et al. Distinguishing cancer-associated missense mutations from common polymorphisms. *Cancer Res* 2007;67:465–473.

123. Futreal PA. Backseat drivers take the wheel. *Cancer Cell* 2007;12:493–494.

124. Greenman C, Wooster R, Futreal PA, et al. Statistical analysis of pathogenicity of somatic mutations in cancer. *Genetics* 2006;173:2187–2198.

125. Baudot A, Real FX, Izarzugaza JM, et al. From cancer genomes to cancer models: bridging the gaps. *EMBO Rep* 2009;10:359–366.

126. Carter H, Chen S, Isik L, et al. Cancer-specific high-throughput annotation of somatic mutations: computational prediction of driver missense mutations. *Cancer Res* 2009;69:6660–6667.

127. Ng PC, Henikoff S. SIFT: Predicting amino acid changes that affect protein function. *Nucleic Acids Res* 2003;31:3812–3814.

128. Kohli M, Rago C, Lengauer C, et al. Facile methods for generating human somatic cell gene knockouts using recombinant adeno-associated viruses. *Nucleic Acids Res* 2004;32:e3.

129. Downing JR, Wilson RK, Zhang J, et al. The Pediatric Cancer Genome Project. *Nat Genet* 2012;44:619–622.

130. Hudson TJ, Anderson W, Artez A, et al. International network of cancer genome projects. *Nature* 2010;464:993–998.

131. Bignell GR, Greenman CD, Davies H, et al. Signatures of mutation and selection in the cancer genome. *Nature* 2010;463:893–898.

132. Sieber OM, Tomlinson SR, Tomlinson IP. Tissue, cell and stage specificity of (epi)mutations in cancers. *Nat Rev Cancer* 2005;5:649–655.

133. Benvenuti S, Frattini M, Arena S, et al. PIK3CA cancer mutations display gender and tissue specificity patterns. *Hum Mutat* 2008;29:284–288.

134. Karakas B, Bachman KE, Park BH. Mutation of the PIK3CA oncogene in human cancers. *Br J Cancer* 2006;94:455–459.

135. Brennan CW, Werhaak RG, McKenna A, et al. The somatic genomic landscape of glioblastoma. *Cell* 2013;155:462–477.

136. Cancer Genome Atlas Network. Comprehensive molecular characterization of human colon and rectal cancer. *Nature* 2012;487:330–337.

137. Cancer Genome Atlas Network. Comprehensive molecular portraits of human breast tumours. *Nature* 2012;490:61–70.

138. Cancer Genome Atlas Research Network. Integrated genomic analyses of ovarian carcinoma. *Nature* 2011;474:609–615.

139. Cancer Genome Atlas Research Network. Comprehensive molecular characterization of clear cell renal cell carcinoma. *Nature* 2013;499:43–49.

140. Cancer Genome Atlas Research Network. Integrated genomic characterization of endometrial carcinoma. *Nature* 2013;497:67–73.

141. Weischenfeldt J, Simon R, Feuerbach L, et al. Integrative genomic analyses reveal an androgen-driven somatic alteration landscape in early-onset prostate cancer. *Cancer Cell* 2013;23:159–170.

142. Cancer Genome Atlas Research Network. Genomic and epigenomic landscapes of adult de novo acute myeloid leukemia. *N Engl J Med* 2013; 368:2059–2074.

143. Dawson SJ, Rueda OM, Aparicio S, et al. A new genome-driven integrated classification of breast cancer and its implications. *EMBO J* 2013;32: 617–628.

144. Plass C, Pfister SM, Lindroth AM, et al. Mutations in regulators of the epigenome and their connections to global chromatin patterns in cancer. *Nat Rev Genet* 2013;14:765–780.

145. Shen H, Laird PW. Interplay between the cancer genome and epigenome. *Cell* 2013;153:38–55.

146. Yamamoto E, Suzuki H, Yamano HO, et al. Molecular dissection of premalignant colorectal lesions reveals early onset of the CpG island methylator phenotype. *Am J Pathol* 2012;181:1847–1861.

147. Gao J, Aksoy BA, Dogrusoz U, et al. Integrative analysis of complex cancer genomics and clinical profiles using the cBioPortal. *Sci Signal* 2013;6:pl1.

148. Bleeker FE, Bardelli A. Genomic landscapes of cancers: prospects for targeted therapies. *Pharmacogenomics* 2007;8:1629–1633.

149. Paez JG, Jänne PA, Lee JC, et al. EGFR mutations in lung cancer: correlation with clinical response to gefitinib therapy. *Science* 2004;304:1497–1500.

150. Ciardiello F, Tortora G. EGFR antagonists in cancer treatment. *N Engl J Med* 2008;358:1160–1174.

151. Janku F, Stewart DJ, Kurzrock R. Targeted therapy in non-small-cell lung cancer—is it becoming a reality? *Nat Rev Clin Oncol* 2010;7:401–414.

152. Pao W, Chmielecki J. Rational, biologically based treatment of EGFR-mutant non-small-cell lung cancer. *Nat Rev Cancer* 2010;10:760–774.

153. Gerber DE, Minna JD. ALK inhibition for non-small cell lung cancer: from discovery to therapy in record time. *Cancer Cell* 2010;18:548–551.

154. Andreyev HJ, Norman AR, Cunningham D, et al. Kirsten ras mutations in patients with colorectal cancer: the multicenter "RASCAL" study. *J Natl Cancer Inst* 1998;90:675–684.

155. Roth AD, Tejpar S, Delorenzi M, et al. Prognostic role of KRAS and BRAF in stage II and III resected colon cancer: results of the translational study on the PETACC-3, EORTC 40993, SAKK 60-00 trial. *J Clin Oncol* 2010;28:466–474.

156. Bardelli A, Siena S. Molecular mechanisms of resistance to cetuximab and panitumumab in colorectal cancer. *J Clin Oncol* 2010;28:1254–1261.

157. Siena S, Sartore-Bianchi A, Di Nicolantonio F, et al. Biomarkers predicting clinical outcome of epidermal growth factor receptor-targeted therapy in metastatic colorectal cancer. *J Natl Cancer Inst* 2009;101:1308–1324.

158. Tejpar S, Bertagnolli M, Bosman F, et al. Prognostic and predictive biomarkers in resected colon cancer: current status and future perspectives for integrating genomics into biomarker discovery. *Oncologist* 2010;15:390–404.

159. Gerlinger M, Rowan AJ, Horswell S, et al. Intratumor heterogeneity and branched evolution revealed by multiregion sequencing. *N Engl J Med* 2012;366:883–892.

160. Mandel P, Metais P. [Not Available]. *C R Seances Soc Biol Fil* 1948;142:241–243.

161. Crowley E, Di Nicolantonio F, Loupakis F, et al. Liquid biopsy: monitoring cancer-genetics in the blood. *Nat Rev Clin Oncol* 2013;10:472–484.

162. Diehl F, Li M, Dressman D, et al. Detection and quantification of mutations in the plasma of patients with colorectal tumors. *Proc Natl Acad Sci U S A* 2005;102:16368–16373.

163. Diehl F, Schmidt K, Choti MA, et al. Circulating mutant DNA to assess tumor dynamics. *Nat Med* 2008;14:985–990.

164. Frattini M, Gallino G, Signoroni S, et al. Quantitative and qualitative characterization of plasma DNA identifies primary and recurrent colorectal cancer. *Cancer Lett* 2008;263:170–181.

165. Chan KC, Jiang P, Zheng YW, et al. Cancer genome scanning in plasma: detection of tumor-associated copy number aberrations, single-nucleotide variants, and tumoral heterogeneity by massively parallel sequencing. *Clin Chem* 2013;59:211–224.

166. Murtaza M, Dawson SJ, Tsui DW, et al. Non-invasive analysis of acquired resistance to cancer therapy by sequencing of plasma DNA. *Nature* 2013;497:108–112.

167. Bardelli A, Corso S, Bertotti A, et al. Amplification of the MET receptor drives resistance to anti-EGFR therapies in colorectal cancer. *Cancer Discov* 2013;3:658–673.

168. Higgins MJ, Jelovac D, Barnathan E, et al. Detection of tumor PIK3CA status in metastatic breast cancer using peripheral blood. *Clin Cancer Res* 2012;18:3462–3469.

169. Leary RJ, Sausen M, Kinde I, et al. Detection of chromosomal alterations in the circulation of cancer patients with whole-genome sequencing. *Sci Transl Med* 2012;4:162ra154.

170. Misale S, Yaeger R, Hobor S, et al. Emergence of KRAS mutations and acquired resistance to anti-EGFR therapy in colorectal cancer. *Nature* 2012;486:532–536.

171. Diaz LA Jr, Williams RT, Wu J, et al. The molecular evolution of acquired resistance to targeted EGFR blockade in colorectal cancers. *Nature* 2012;486:537–540.

172. Robbins PF, Lu YC, El-Gamil M, et al. Mining exomic sequencing data to identify mutated antigens recognized by adoptively transferred tumor-reactive T cells. *Nat Med* 2013;19:747–752.

173. Hunter C, Smith R, Cahill DP, et al. A hypermutation phenotype and somatic MSH6 mutations in recurrent human malignant gliomas after alkylator chemotherapy. *Cancer Res* 2006;66:3987–3991.

174. Cahill DP, Levine KK, Betensky RA, et al. Loss of the mismatch repair protein MSH6 in human glioblastomas is associated with tumor progression during temozolomide treatment. *Clin Cancer Res* 2007;13:2038–2045.

175. Engelman JA, Zejnullahu K, Mitsudomi T, et al. MET amplification leads to gefitinib resistance in lung cancer by activating ERBB3 signaling. *Science* 2007;316:1039–1043.

176. Gorre ME, Mohmmed M, Ellwood K, et al. Clinical resistance to STI-571 cancer therapy caused by BCR-ABL gene mutation or amplification. *Science* 2001;293:876–880.

177. Heinrich MC, Corless CL, Blanke CD, et al. Molecular correlates of imatinib resistance in gastrointestinal stromal tumors. *J Clin Oncol* 2006;24:4764–4774.

178. Shepherd FA, Rodrigues Pereira J, Ciuleanu T, et al. Erlotinib in previously treated non-small-cell lung cancer. *N Engl J Med* 2005;353:123–132.

179. Kobayashi S, Boggon TJ, Dayaram T, et al. EGFR mutation and resistance of non-small-cell lung cancer to gefitinib. *N Engl J Med* 2005;352:786–792.

180. Kwak EL, Sordella R, Bell DW, et al. Irreversible inhibitors of the EGF receptor may circumvent acquired resistance to gefitinib. *Proc Natl Acad Sci U S A* 2005;102:7665–7670.

181. Pao W, Miller VA, Politi KA, et al. Acquired resistance of lung adenocarcinomas to gefitinib or erlotinib is associated with a second mutation in the EGFR kinase domain. *PLoS Med* 2005;2:e73.

182. Shih JY, Gow CH, Yang PC. EGFR mutation conferring primary resistance to gefitinib in non-small-cell lung cancer. *N Engl J Med* 2005;353:207–208.

183. Bell DW, Gore I, Okimoto Ra, et al. Inherited susceptibility to lung cancer may be associated with the T790M drug resistance mutation in EGFR. *Nat Genet* 2005;37:1315–1316.

184. Inukai M, Toyooka S, Ito S, et al. Presence of epidermal growth factor receptor gene T790M mutation as a minor clone in non-small cell lung cancer. *Cancer Res* 2006;66:7854–7858.

185. Daub H, Specht K, Ullrich A. Strategies to overcome resistance to targeted protein kinase inhibitors. *Nat Rev Drug Discov* 2004;3:1001–1010.

186. Choi YL, Soda M, Yamashita Y, et al. EML4-ALK mutations in lung cancer that confer resistance to ALK inhibitors. *N Engl J Med* 2010;363:1734–1739.

187. Flaherty KT, Puzanov I, Kim KB, et al. Inhibition of mutated, activated BRAF in metastatic melanoma. *N Engl J Med* 2010;363:809–819.

188. Nazarian R, Shi H, Wang Q, et al. Melanomas acquire resistance to B-RAF(V600E) inhibition by RTK or N-RAS upregulation. *Nature* 2010;468:973–977.

189. Pompetti F, Spadano A, Sau A, et al. Long-term remission in BCR/ABL-positive AML-M6 patient treated with Imatinib Mesylate. *Leuk Res* 2007;31:563–567.

190. Druker BJ, Builhot F, O'Brien SG, et al. Five-year follow-up of patients receiving imatinib for chronic myeloid leukemia. *N Engl J Med* 2006;355:2408–2417.

PRINCIPLES OF ONCOLOGY

2 Hallmarks of Cancer: An Organizing Principle for Cancer Medicine

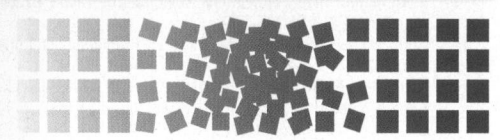

Douglas Hanahan and Robert A. Weinberg

INTRODUCTION

The hallmarks of cancer comprise eight biologic capabilities acquired by incipient cancer cells during the multistep development of human tumors. The hallmarks constitute an organizing principle for rationalizing the complexities of neoplastic disease. They include sustaining proliferative signaling, evading growth suppressors, resisting cell death, enabling replicative immortality, inducing angiogenesis, activating invasion and metastasis, reprogramming energy metabolism, and evading immune destruction. Facilitating the acquisition of these hallmark capabilities are genome instability, which enables mutational alteration of hallmark-enabling genes, and immune inflammation, which fosters the acquisition of multiple hallmark functions. In addition to cancer cells, tumors exhibit another dimension of complexity: They contain a repertoire of recruited, ostensibly normal cells that contribute to the acquisition of hallmark traits by creating the *tumor microenvironment*. Recognition of the widespread applicability of these concepts will increasingly influence the development of new means to treat human cancer.

At the beginning of the new millennium, we proposed that six *hallmarks of cancer* embody an organizing principle that provides a logical framework for understanding the remarkable diversity of neoplastic diseases.[1] Implicit in our discussion was the notion that, as normal cells evolve progressively to a neoplastic state, they acquire a succession of these hallmark capabilities, and that the multistep process of human tumor pathogenesis can be rationalized by the need of incipient cancer cells to acquire the diverse traits that in aggregate enable them to become tumorigenic and, ultimately, malignant.

We noted as an ancillary proposition that tumors are more than insular masses of proliferating cancer cells. Instead, they are complex tissues composed of multiple distinct types of neoplastic and normal cells that participate in heterotypic interactions with one another. We depicted the recruited normal cells, which form tumor-associated stroma, as active participants in tumorigenesis rather than passive bystanders; as such, these stromal cells contribute to the development and expression of certain hallmark capabilities. This notion has been solidified and extended during the intervening period, and it is now clear that the biology of tumors can no longer be understood simply by enumerating the traits of the cancer cells, but instead must encompass the contributions of the *tumor microenvironment* to tumorigenesis. In 2011, we revisited the original hallmarks, adding two new ones to the roster, and expanded on the functional roles and contributions made by recruited stromal cells to tumor biology.[2] Herein we reiterate and further refine the hallmarks-of-cancer perspectives we presented in 2000 and 2011, with the goal of informing students of cancer medicine about the concept and its potential utility for understanding the pathogenesis of human cancer, and the potential relevance of this concept to the development of more effective treatments for this disease.

HALLMARK CAPABILITIES, IN ESSENCE

The eight hallmarks of cancer—distinct and complementary capabilities that enable tumor growth and metastatic dissemination—continue to provide a solid foundation for understanding the biology of cancer (Fig. 2.1). The sections that follow summarize the essence of each hallmark, providing insights into their regulation and functional manifestations.

Sustaining Proliferative Signaling

Arguably, the most fundamental trait of cancer cells involves their ability to sustain chronic proliferation. Normal tissues carefully control the production and release of growth-promoting signals that instruct entry of cells into and progression through the growth-and-division cycle, thereby ensuring proper control of cell number and thus maintenance of normal tissue architecture and function. Cancer cells, by deregulating these signals, become masters of their own destinies. The enabling signals are conveyed in large part by growth factors that bind cell-surface receptors, typically containing intracellular tyrosine kinase domains. The latter proceed to emit signals via branched intracellular signaling pathways that regulate progression through the cell cycle as well as cell growth (that is, increase in cell size); often, these signals influence yet other cell-biologic properties, such as cell survival and energy metabolism.

Remarkably, the precise identities and sources of the proliferative signals operating within normal tissues remain poorly understood. Moreover, we still know relatively little about the mechanisms controlling the release of these mitogenic signals. In part, the study of these mechanisms is complicated by the fact that the growth factor signals controlling cell number and position within normal tissues are thought to be transmitted in a temporally and spatially regulated fashion from one cell to its neighbors; such paracrine signaling is difficult to access experimentally. In addition, the bioavailability of growth factors is regulated by their sequestration in the pericellular space and associated extracellular matrix. Moreover, the actions of these extracellular mitogenic proteins is further controlled by a complex network of proteases, sulfatases, and possibly other enzymes that liberate and activate these factors, apparently in a highly specific and localized fashion.

The mitogenic signaling operating in cancer cells is, in contrast, far better understood.[3–6] Cancer cells can acquire the capability to sustain proliferative signaling in a number of alternative ways: They may produce growth factor ligands themselves, to which they can then respond via the coexpression of cognate receptors, resulting in autocrine proliferative stimulation. Alternatively, cancer cells may send signals to stimulate normal cells within the supporting tumor-associated stroma; the stromal cells then reciprocate by supplying the cancer cells with various growth factors.[7,8] Mitogenic signaling can also be deregulated by elevating the levels of receptor proteins displayed at the cancer cell

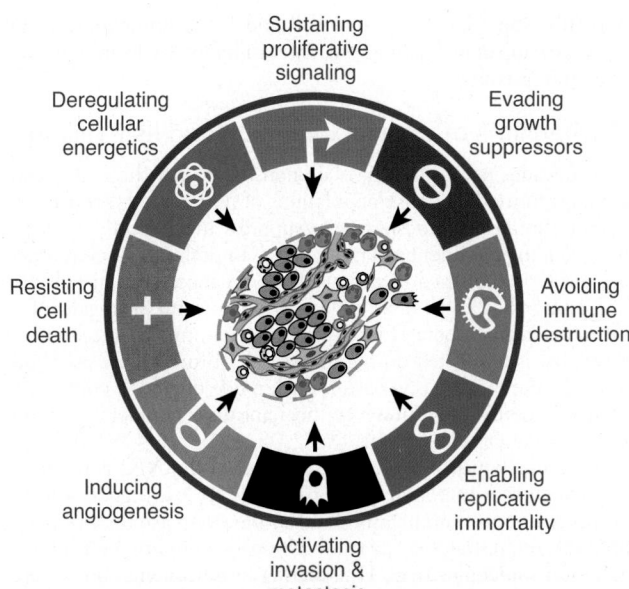

Figure 2.1 The hallmarks of cancer. Eight functional capabilities—the hallmarks of cancer—are thought to be acquired by developing cancers in the course of the multistep carcinogenesis that leads to most forms of human cancer. The order in which these hallmark capabilities are acquired and the relative balance and importance of their contributions to malignant disease appears to vary across the spectrum of human cancers. (Adapted from Hanahan D, Weinberg R. The hallmarks of cancer. *Cell* 2000;100:57–70; Hanahan D, Weinberg RA. Hallmarks of cancer: the next generation. *Cell* 2011;144:646–674.)

surface, rendering such cells hyperresponsive to otherwise limiting amounts of growth factor ligands; the same outcome can result from structural alterations in the receptor molecules that facilitate ligand-independent firing.

Independence from externally supplied growth factors may also derive from the constitutive activation of components of intracellular signaling cascades operating downstream of these receptors within cancer cells. These intracellular alterations obviate the need to stimulate cell proliferation pathways by ligand-mediated activation of cell-surface receptors. Of note, because a number of distinct downstream signaling pathways radiate from ligand-stimulated receptors, the activation of one or another of these downstream branches (e.g., the pathway responding to the Ras signal transducer) may only provide a subset of the regulatory instructions transmitted by a ligand-activated receptor.

Somatic Mutations Activate Additional Downstream Pathways

DNA sequencing analyses of cancer cell genomes have revealed somatic mutations in certain human tumors that predict constitutive activation of the signaling circuits, cited previously, that are normally triggered by activated growth factor receptors. The past 3 decades have witnessed the identification in tens of thousands of human tumors of mutant, oncogenic alleles of the *RAS* proto-oncogenes, most of which have sustained point mutations in the 12th codon, which results in RAS proteins that are constitutively active in downstream signaling. Thus, more than 90% of pancreatic adenocarcinomas carry mutant K-*RAS* alleles. More recently, the repertoire of frequently mutated genes has been expanded to include those encoding the downstream effectors of the RAS proteins. For example, we now know that ~40% of human melanomas contain activating mutations affecting the structure of the B-RAF protein, resulting in constitutive signaling through the RAF to the mitogen-activated protein (MAP)–kinase pathway.[9] Similarly, mutations in the catalytic subunit of phosphoinositide 3-kinase (PI3K)

isoforms are being detected in an array of tumor types; these mutations typically serve to hyperactivate the PI3K signaling pathway, causing in turn, excess signaling through the crucial Akt/PKB signal transducer.[10,11] The advantages to tumor cells of activating upstream (receptor) versus downstream (transducer) signaling remain obscure, as does the functional impact of cross-talk between the multiple branched pathways radiating from individual growth factor receptors.

Disruptions of Negative-Feedback Mechanisms that Attenuate Proliferative Signaling

Recent observations have also highlighted the importance of negative-feedback loops that normally operate to dampen various types of signaling and thereby ensure homeostatic regulation of the flux of signals coursing through the intracellular circuitry.[12–15] Defects in these negative-feedback mechanisms are capable of enhancing proliferative signaling. The prototype of this type of regulation involves the RAS oncoprotein. The oncogenic effects of mutant RAS proteins do not result from a hyperactivation of its downstream signaling powers; instead, the oncogenic mutations affecting *RAS* genes impair the intrinsic GTPase activity of RAS that normally serves to turn its activity off, ensuring that active signal transmission (e.g., from upstream growth factor receptors) is transient; as such, oncogenic RAS mutations disrupt an autoregulatory negative-feedback mechanism, without which RAS generates chronic proliferative signals.

Analogous negative-feedback mechanisms operate at multiple nodes within the proliferative signaling circuitry. A prominent example involves phosphatase and tensin homolog (PTEN), which counteracts PI3K by degrading its product, phosphatidylinositol 3,4,5-phosphate (PIP3). Loss-of-function mutations in PTEN amplify PI3K signaling and promote tumorigenesis in a variety of experimental models of cancer; in human tumors, PTEN expression is often lost by the methylation of DNA at specific sites associated with the promoter of the *PTEN* gene, resulting in the shutdown of its transcription.[10,11]

Yet another example involves the mammalian target of rapamycin (mTOR) kinase, a key coordinator of cell growth and metabolism that lies both upstream and downstream of the PI3K pathway. In the circuitry of some cancer cells, mTOR activation results, via negative feedback, in the inhibition of PI3K signaling. Accordingly, when mTOR is pharmacologically inhibited in such cancer cells (e.g., by the drug rapamycin), the associated loss of negative feedback results in increased activity of PI3K and its effector, the Akt/PKB kinase, thereby blunting the antiproliferative effects of mTOR inhibition.[16,17] It is likely that compromised negative feedback loops in this and other signaling pathways will prove to be widespread among human cancer cells, serving as important means by which cancer cells acquire the capability of signaling chronically through these pathways. Moreover, disruption of such normally self-attenuating signaling can contribute to the development of adaptive resistance toward therapeutic drugs targeting mitogenic signaling.

Excessive Proliferative Signaling Can Trigger Cell Senescence

Early studies of oncogene action encouraged the notion that ever-increasing expression of such genes and the signals released by their protein products would result in proportionately increased cancer cell proliferation and, thus, tumor growth. More recent research has undermined this notion, in that it is now apparent that excessively elevated signaling by oncoproteins, such as RAS, MYC, and RAF, can provoke counteracting (protective) responses from cells, such as induction of cell death; alternatively, cancer cells expressing high levels of these oncoproteins may be forced to enter into the nonproliferative but viable state called senescence. These responses contrast with those seen in cells expressing lower levels of these proteins, which permit cells to avoid senescence or cell death and, thus, proliferate.[18–21]

PRINCIPLES OF ONCOLOGY

Cells with morphologic features of senescence, including enlarged cytoplasm, the absence of proliferation markers, and the expression of the senescence-induced β-galactosidase enzyme, are abundant in the tissues of mice whose genomes have been reengineered to cause overexpression of certain oncogenes[19,20]; such senescent cells are also prevalent in some cases of human melanoma.[22]

These ostensibly paradoxical responses seem to reflect intrinsic cellular defense mechanisms designed to eliminate cells experiencing excessive levels of certain types of mitogenic signaling. Accordingly, the intensity of oncogenic signaling observed in naturally arising cancer cells may represent compromises between maximal mitogenic stimulation and avoidance of these anti-proliferative defenses. Alternatively, some cancer cells may adapt to high levels of oncogenic signaling by disabling their senescence- or apoptosis-inducing circuitry.

Evading Growth Suppressors

In addition to the hallmark capability of inducing and sustaining positively acting growth-stimulatory signals, cancer cells must also circumvent powerful programs that negatively regulate cell proliferation; many of these programs depend on the actions of tumor suppressor genes. Dozens of tumor suppressors that operate in various ways to limit cell proliferation or survival have been discovered through their inactivation in one or another form of animal or human cancer; many of these genes have been validated as bona fide tumor suppressors through gain- or loss-of-function experiments in mice. The two prototypical tumor suppressor genes encode the retinoblastoma (RB)-associated and TP53 proteins; they operate as central control nodes within two key, complementary cellular regulatory circuits that govern the decisions of cells to proliferate, or alternatively, to activate growth arrest, senescence, or the cell-suicide program known as apoptosis.

The RB protein integrates signals from diverse extracellular and intracellular sources and, in response, decides whether or not a cell should proceed through its growth-and-division cycle.[23–25] Cancer cells with defects in the RB pathway function are thus missing the services of a critical gatekeeper of cell-cycle progression whose absence permits persistent cell proliferation. Whereas RB transduces growth-inhibitory signals that largely originate outside of the cell, TP53 receives inputs from stress and abnormality sensors that function within the cell's intracellular operating systems. For example, if the degree of damage to a cell's genome is excessive, or if the levels of nucleotide pools, growth-promoting signals, glucose, or oxygenation are insufficient, TP53 can call a halt to further cell-cycle progression until these conditions have been normalized. Alternatively, in the face of alarm signals indicating overwhelming or irreparable damage to such cellular systems, TP53 can trigger apoptosis. Of note, the alternative effects of activated TP53 are complex and highly context dependent, varying by cell type as well as by the severity and persistence of conditions of cell-physiologic stress and genomic damage.

Although the two canonical suppressors of proliferation—TP53 and RB—have preeminent importance in regulating cell proliferation, various lines of evidence indicate that each operates as part of a larger network that is wired for functional redundancy. For example, chimeric mice populated throughout their bodies with individual cells lacking a functional *Rb* gene are surprisingly free of proliferative abnormalities, despite the expectation that a loss of RB function should result in unimpeded advance through the cell division cycle by these cells and their lineal descendants; some of the resulting clusters of *Rb*-null cells should, by all rights, progress to neoplasia. Instead, the *Rb*-null cells in such chimeric mice have been found to participate in relatively normal tissue morphogenesis throughout the body; the only neoplasia observed is of pituitary tumors developing late in life.[26] Similarly, *TP53*-null mice develop

normally, show largely normal cell and tissue homeostasis, and again develop abnormalities only later in life in the form of leukemias and sarcomas.[27]

Mechanisms of Contact Inhibition and Its Evasion

Four decades of research have demonstrated that the cell-to-cell contacts formed by dense populations of normal cells growing in 2-dimensional culture operate to suppress further cell proliferation, yielding confluent cell monolayers. Importantly, such *contact inhibition* is abolished in various types of cancer cells in culture, suggesting that contact inhibition is an in vitro surrogate of a mechanism that operates in vivo to ensure normal tissue homeostasis that is abrogated during the course of tumorigenesis. Until recently, the mechanistic basis for this mode of growth control remained obscure. Now, however, mechanisms of contact inhibition are beginning to emerge.[28]

One mechanism involves the product of the *NF2* gene, long implicated as a tumor suppressor because its loss triggers a form of human neurofibromatosis. Merlin, the cytoplasmic *NF2* gene product, orchestrates contact inhibition by coupling cell-surface adhesion molecules (e.g., E-cadherin) to transmembrane receptor tyrosine kinases (e.g., the EGF receptor). In so doing, Merlin strengthens the adhesiveness of cadherin-mediated cell-to-cell attachments. Additionally, by sequestering such growth factor receptors, Merlin limits their ability to efficiently emit mitogenic signals.[28–31]

Corruption of the TGF-β Pathway Promotes Malignancy

Transforming growth factor beta (TGF-β is best known for its anti-proliferative effects on epithelial cells. The responses of carcinoma cells to TGF-β's proliferation–suppressive effects is now appreciated to be far more elaborate than a simple shutdown of its signaling circuitry.[32–35] In normal cells, exposure to TGF-β blocks their progression through the G1 phase of the cell cycle. In many late-stage tumors, however, TGF-β signaling is redirected away from suppressing cell proliferation and is found instead to activate a cellular program, termed the epithelial-to-mesenchymal transition (EMT), which confers on cancer cells multiple traits associated with high-grade malignancy, as will be discussed in further detail.

Resisting Cell Death

The ability to activate the normally latent apoptotic cell-death program appears to be associated with most types of normal cells throughout the body. Its actions in many if not all multicellular organisms seems to reflect the need to eliminate aberrant cells whose continued presence would otherwise threaten organismic integrity. This rationale explains why cancer cells often, if not invariably, inactivate or attenuate this program during their development.[21,36–38]

Elucidation of the detailed design of the signaling circuitry governing the apoptotic program has revealed how apoptosis is triggered in response to various physiologic stresses that cancer cells experience either during the course of tumorigenesis or as a result of anticancer therapy. Notable among the apoptosis-inducing stresses are signaling imbalances resulting from elevated levels of oncogene signaling and from DNA damage. The regulators of the apoptotic response are divided into two major circuits, one receiving and processing extracellular death-inducing signals (the extrinsic apoptotic program, involving for example the Fas ligand/Fas receptor), and the other sensing and integrating a variety of signals of intracellular origin (the intrinsic program). Each of these circuits culminates in the activation of a normally latent protease (caspase 8 or 9, respectively), which proceeds to initiate a cascade of proteolysis involving effector caspases that are responsible for the execution phase of apoptosis. During this final phase, an apoptotic cell is progressively disassembled and then consumed, both by its neighbors and by professional phagocytic cells. Currently, the intrinsic apoptotic program is more widely implicated as a barrier to cancer pathogenesis.

The molecular machinery that conveys signals between the apoptotic regulators and effectors is controlled by counterbalancing pro- and antiapoptotic members of the Bcl-2 family of regulatory proteins.[36,37] The archetype, Bcl-2, along with its closest relatives (Bcl-XL, Bcl-W, Mcl-1, A1) are inhibitors of apoptosis, acting in large part by binding to and thereby suppressing two proapoptotic triggering proteins (Bax and Bak); the latter are embedded in the mitochondrial outer membrane. When relieved of inhibition by their antiapoptotic relatives, Bax and Bax disrupt the integrity of the outer mitochondrial membrane, causing the release into the cytosol of proapoptotic signaling proteins, the most important of which is cytochrome C. When the normally sequestered cytochrome C is released, it activates a cascade of cytosolic caspase proteases that proceed to fragment multiple cellular structures, thereby executing the apoptotic death program.[37,39]

Several abnormality sensors have been identified that play key roles in triggering apoptosis.[21,37] Most notable is a DNA damage sensor that acts through the TP53 tumor suppressor[40]; TP53 induces apoptosis by upregulating expression of the proapoptotic, Bcl-2-related Noxa and Puma proteins, doing so in response to substantial levels of DNA breaks and other chromosomal abnormalities. Alternatively, insufficient survival factor signaling (e.g., inadequate levels of interleukin (IL)-3 in lymphocytes or of insulinlike growth factors 1/2 [IGF1/2] in epithelial cells) can elicit apoptosis through another proapoptotic Bcl-2-related protein called Bim. Yet another condition triggering apoptosis involves hyperactive signaling by certain oncoproteins, such as Myc, which acts in part via Bim and other Bcl-2-related proteins.[18,21,40]

Tumor cells evolve a variety of strategies to limit or circumvent apoptosis. Most common is the loss of TP53 tumor suppressor function, which eliminates this critical damage sensor from the apoptosis-inducing circuitry. Alternatively, tumors may achieve similar ends by increasing the expression of antiapoptotic regulators (Bcl-2, Bcl-XL) or of survival signals (IGF1/2), by downregulating proapoptotic Bcl-2-related factors (Bax, Bim, Puma), or by short-circuiting the extrinsic ligand-induced death pathway. The multiplicity of apoptosis-avoiding mechanisms presumably reflects the diversity of apoptosis-inducing signals that cancer cell populations encounter during their evolution from the normal to the neoplastic state.

Autophagy Mediates Both Tumor Cell Survival and Death

Autophagy represents an important cell-physiologic response that, like apoptosis, normally operates at low, basal levels in cells but can be strongly induced in certain states of cellular stress, the most obvious of which is nutrient deficiency.[41–43] The autophagic program enables cells to break down cellular organelles, such as ribosomes and mitochondria, allowing the resulting catabolites to be recycled and thus used for biosynthesis and energy metabolism. As part of this program, intracellular vesicles (termed autophagosomes) envelope the cellular organelles destined for degradation; the resulting vesicles then fuse with lysosomes in which degradation occurs. In this fashion, low–molecular-weight metabolites are generated that support survival in the stressed, nutrient-limited environments experienced by many cancer cells. When acting in this fashion, autophagy favors cancer cell survival.

However, the autophagy program intersects in more complex ways with the life and death of cancer cells. Like apoptosis, the autophagy machinery has both regulatory and effector components.[41–43] Among the latter are proteins that mediate autophagosome formation and delivery to lysosomes. Of note, recent research has revealed intersections between the regulatory circuits governing autophagy, apoptosis, and cellular homeostasis. For example, the signaling pathway involving PI3K, AKT, and mTOR, which is stimulated by survival signals to block apoptosis, similarly inhibits autophagy; when survival signals are insufficient, the PI3K signaling pathway is downregulated, with the result that autophagy and/or apoptosis may be induced.[41,42,44,45]

Another interconnection between these two programs resides in the Beclin-1 protein, which has been shown by genetic studies to be necessary for the induction of autophagy.[41–44] Beclin-1 is a member of the Bcl-2 family of apoptotic regulatory proteins, and its BH3 domain allows it to bind the Bcl-2/Bcl-XL proteins. Stress sensor–coupled BH3-containing proteins (e.g. Bim, Noxa) can displace Beclin-1 from its association with Bcl-2/Bcl-XL, enabling the liberated Beclin-1 to trigger autophagy, much as they can release proapoptotic Bax and Bak to trigger apoptosis. Hence, stress-transducing Bcl-2–related proteins can induce apoptosis and/or autophagy depending on the physiologic state of the cell.

Genetically altered mice bearing inactivated alleles of the *Beclin-1* gene or of certain other components of the autophagy machinery exhibit increased susceptibility to cancer.[42,46] These results suggest that the induction of autophagy can serve as a barrier to tumorigenesis that may operate independently of or in concert with apoptosis. For example, excessive activation of the autophagy program may cause cells to devour too many of their own critical organelles, such that cell growth and division are crippled. Accordingly, autophagy may represent yet another barrier that needs to be circumvented by incipient cancer cells during multistep tumor development.[41,46]

Perhaps paradoxically, nutrient starvation, radiotherapy, and certain cytotoxic drugs can induce elevated levels of autophagy that apparently protect cancer cells.[45–48] Moreover, severely stressed cancer cells have been shown to shrink via autophagy to a state of reversible dormancy.[46,49] This particular survival response may enable the persistence and eventual regrowth of some late-stage tumors following treatment with potent anticancer agents. Together, observations like these indicate that autophagy can have dichotomous effects on tumor cells and, thus, tumor progression.[46,47] An important agenda for future research will involve clarifying the genetic and cell-physiologic conditions that determine when and how autophagy enables cancer cells to survive or, alternatively, causes them to die.

Necrosis Has Proinflammatory and Tumor-Promoting Potential

In contrast to apoptosis, in which a dying cell contracts into an almost invisible corpse that is soon consumed by its neighbors, necrotic cells become bloated and explode, releasing their contents into the local tissue microenvironment. A body of evidence has shown that cell death by necrosis, like apoptosis, is an organized process under genetic control, rather than being a random and undirected process.[50–52]

Importantly, necrotic cell death releases proinflammatory signals into the surrounding tissue microenvironment, in contrast to apoptosis, which does not. As a consequence, necrotic cells can recruit inflammatory cells of the immune system,[51,53,54] whose dedicated function is to survey the extent of tissue damage and remove associated necrotic debris. In the context of neoplasia, however, multiple lines of evidence indicate that immune inflammatory cells can be actively tumor-promoting by fostering angiogenesis, cancer cell proliferation, and invasiveness (discussed in subsequent sections). Additionally, necrotic cells can release bioactive regulatory factors, such as IL1α, which can directly stimulate neighboring viable cells to proliferate, with the potential, once again, to facilitate neoplastic progression.[53] Consequently, necrotic cell death, while seemingly beneficial in counterbalancing cancer-associated hyperproliferation, may ultimately do more damage to the patient than good.

Enabling Replicative Immortality

Cancer cells require unlimited replicative potential in order to generate macroscopic tumors. This capability stands in marked contrast to the behavior of the cells in most normal cell lineages in the body, which are only able to pass through a limited number of successive cell growth-and-division cycles. This limitation has been associated with two distinct barriers to proliferation: *replicative senescence*, a typically irreversible entrance into a nonproliferative but viable state, and *crisis*, which involves cell death. Accordingly, when cells are propagated in culture, repeated cycles of cell division lead first to induction of replicative senescence and then, for those cells that succeed in circumventing this barrier, to the crisis phase, in which the great majority of cells in the population die. On rare occasion, cells emerge from a population in crisis and exhibit unlimited replicative potential. This transition has been termed immortalization, a trait that most established cell lines possess by virtue of their ability to proliferate in culture without evidence of either senescence or crisis.

Multiple lines of evidence indicate that telomeres protecting the ends of chromosomes are centrally involved in the capability for unlimited proliferation.[55–58] The telomere-associated DNA, composed of multiple tandem hexanucleotide repeats, shortens progressively in the chromosomes of nonimmortalized cells propagated in culture, eventually losing the ability to protect the ends of chromosomal DNA from end-to-end fusions; such aberrant fusions generate unstable dicentric chromosomes, whose resolution during the anaphase of mitosis results in a scrambling of karyotype and entrance into crisis that threatens cell viability. Accordingly, the length of telomeric DNA in a cell dictates how many successive cell generations its progeny can pass through before telomeres are largely eroded and have consequently lost their protective functions.

Telomerase, the specialized DNA polymerase that adds telomere repeat segments to the ends of telomeric DNA, is almost absent in nonimmortalized cells but is expressed at functionally significant levels in the great majority (~90%) of spontaneously immortalized cells, including human cancer cells. By extending telomeric DNA, telomerase is able to counter the progressive telomere erosion that would otherwise occur in its absence. The presence of telomerase activity, either in spontaneously immortalized cells or in the context of cells engineered to express the enzyme, is correlated with a resistance to induction of both senescence and crisis/apoptosis; conversely, the suppression of telomerase activity leads to telomere shortening and to activation of one or the other of these proliferative barriers.

The two barriers to proliferation—replicative senescence and crisis/apoptosis—have been rationalized as crucial anticancer defenses that are hardwired into our cells and are deployed to impede the outgrowth of clones of preneoplastic and, frankly, neoplastic cells. According to this thinking, most incipient neoplasias exhaust their endowment of replicative doublings and are stopped in their tracks by either of these barriers. The eventual immortalization of rare variant cells that proceed to form tumors has been attributed to their ability to maintain telomeric DNA at lengths sufficient to avoid triggering either senescence or apoptosis, which is achieved most commonly by upregulating the expression of telomerase or, less frequently, via an alternative recombination-based (ALT) telomere maintenance mechanism.[59] Hence, telomere shortening has come to be viewed as a clocking device that determines the limited replicative potential of normal cells and, thus, one that must be overcome by cancer cells.

Reassessing Replicative Senescence

The senescent state induced by oncogenes, as described previously, is remarkably similar to that induced when cells are explanted from living tissue and introduced into culture, the latter being the replicative senescence just discussed. Importantly,

the concept of replication-induced senescence as a general barrier requires refinement and reformulation. Recent experiments have revealed that the induction of senescence in certain cultured cells can be delayed and possibly eliminated by the use of improved cell culture conditions, suggesting that recently explanted primary cells may be intrinsically able to proliferate unimpeded in culture up the point of crisis and the associated induction of apoptosis triggered by critically shortened telomeres.[60–63] This result indicates that telomere shortening does not necessarily induce senescence prior to crisis. Additional insight comes from experiments in mice engineered to lack telomerase; this work has revealed that shortening telomeres can shunt premalignant cells into a senescent state that contributes (along with apoptosis) to attenuated tumorigenesis in mice genetically destined to develop particular forms of cancer.[58] Such telomerase-null mice with highly eroded telomeres exhibit multiorgan dysfunction and abnormalities that provide evidence of both senescence and apoptosis, perhaps similar to the senescence and apoptosis observed in cell culture.[58,64] Thus, depending on the cellular context, the proliferative barrier of telomere shortening can be manifested by the induction of senescence and/or apoptosis.

Delayed Activation of Telomerase May Both Limit and Foster Neoplastic Progression

There is now evidence that clones of incipient cancer cells in spontaneously arising tumors experience telomere loss-induced crisis relatively early during the course of multistep tumor progression due to their inability to express significant levels of telomerase. Thus, extensively eroded telomeres have been documented in premalignant growths through the use of fluorescence in situ hybridization (FISH), which has also revealed the end-to-end chromosomal fusions that signal telomere failure and crisis.[65,66] These results suggest that such incipient cancer cells have passed through a substantial number of successive telomere-shortening cell divisions during their evolution from fully normal cells of origin. Accordingly, the development of some human neoplasias may be aborted by telomere-induced crisis long before they have progressed to become macroscopic, frankly neoplastic growths.

A quite different situation is observed in cells that have lost the TP53-mediated surveillance of genomic integrity and, thereafter, experience critically eroded telomeres. The loss of the TP53 DNA damage sensor can enable such cells to avoid apoptosis that would otherwise be triggered by the DNA damage resulting from dysfunctional telomeres. Instead, such cells lacking TP53 continue to divide, suffering repeated cycles of interchromosomal fusion and subsequent breakage at mitosis. Such breakage-fusion-bridge (BFB) cycles result in deletions and amplifications of chromosomal segments, evidently serving to mutagenize the genome, thereby facilitating the generation and subsequent clonal selection of cancer cells that have acquired mutant oncogenes and tumor suppressor genes.[58,67] One infers, however, that the clones of cancer cells that survive this telomere collapse must eventually acquire the ability to stabilize and thus protect their telomeres via the activation of telomerase or the ALT mechanism noted previously.

These considerations present an interesting dichotomy: Although dysfunctional telomeres are an evident barrier to chronic proliferation, they can also facilitate the genomic instability that generates hallmark-enabling mutations, as will be discussed further. Both mechanisms may be at play in certain forms of carcinogenesis in the form of transitory telomere deficiency prior to telomere stabilization. Circumstantial support for this concept of transient telomere deficiency in facilitating malignant progression has come from comparative analyses of premalignant and malignant lesions in the human breast.[68,69] The premalignant lesions did not express significant levels of telomerase and were marked by telomere shortening and chromosomal aberrations. In contrast, overt carcinomas exhibited telomerase expression concordantly with the reconstruction of longer telomeres and the fixation of the aberrant karyotypes that would seem to have been acquired after telomere failure but before the acquisition of telomerase activity. When portrayed in this way, the delayed acquisition of telomerase function serves to generate tumor-promoting mutations, whereas its subsequent expression stabilizes the mutant genome and confers the unlimited replicative capacity that cancer cells require in order to generate clinically apparent tumors.

Inducing Angiogenesis

Like normal tissues, tumors require sustenance in the form of nutrients and oxygen as well as an ability to evacuate metabolic wastes and carbon dioxide. The tumor-associated neovasculature, generated by the process of angiogenesis, addresses these needs. During embryogenesis, the development of the vasculature involves the birth of new endothelial cells and their assembly into tubes (vasculogenesis) in addition to the sprouting (angiogenesis) of new vessels from existing ones. Following this morphogenesis, the normal vasculature becomes largely quiescent. In the adult, as part of physiologic processes such as wound healing and female reproductive cycling, angiogenesis is turned on, but only transiently. In contrast, during tumor progression, an *angiogenic switch* is almost always activated and remains on, causing normally quiescent vasculature to continually sprout new vessels that help sustain expanding neoplastic growths.[70]

A compelling body of evidence indicates that the angiogenic switch is governed by countervailing factors that either induce or oppose angiogenesis.[71,72] Some of these angiogenic regulators are signaling proteins that bind to stimulatory or inhibitory cell-surface receptors displayed by vascular endothelial cells. The well-known prototypes of angiogenesis inducers and inhibitors are vascular endothelial growth factor-A (VEGF-A) and thrombospondin-1 (Tsp-1), respectively.

The VEGF-A gene encodes ligands that are involved in orchestrating new blood vessel growth during embryonic and postnatal development, in the survival of endothelial cells in already-formed vessels, and in certain physiologic and pathologic situations in the adult. VEGF signaling via three receptor tyrosine kinases (VEGFR1–3) is regulated at multiple levels, reflecting this complexity of purpose. VEGF gene expression can be upregulated both by hypoxia and by oncogene signaling.[73–75] Additionally, VEGF ligands can be sequestered in the extracellular matrix in latent forms that are subject to release and activation by extracellular matrix-degrading proteases (e.g., matrix metallopeptidase 9 [MMP-9]).[76] In addition, other proangiogenic proteins, such as members of the fibroblast growth factor (FGF) family, have been implicated in sustaining tumor angiogenesis.[71] TSP-1, a key counterbalance in the angiogenic switch, also binds transmembrane receptors displayed by endothelial cells and thereby triggers suppressive signals that can counteract proangiogenic stimuli.[77]

The blood vessels produced within tumors by an unbalanced mix of proangiogenic signals are typically aberrant: Tumor neovasculature is marked by precocious capillary sprouting, convoluted and excessive vessel branching, distorted and enlarged vessels, erratic blood flow, microhemorrhaging, leaking of plasma into the tissue parenchyma, and abnormal levels of endothelial cell proliferation and apoptosis.[78,79]

Angiogenesis is induced surprisingly early during the multistage development of invasive cancers both in animal models and in humans. Histologic analyses of premalignant, noninvasive lesions, including dysplasias and in situ carcinomas arising in a variety of organs, have revealed the early tripping of the angiogenic switch.[70,80] Historically, angiogenesis was envisioned to be important only when rapidly growing macroscopic tumors had formed, but more recent data indicate that angiogenesis also contributes to the microscopic premalignant phase of neoplastic progression, further cementing its status as an integral hallmark of cancer.

Gradations of the Angiogenic Switch

Once angiogenesis has been activated, tumors exhibit diverse patterns of neovascularization. Some tumors, including highly aggressive types such as pancreatic ductal adenocarcinomas, are hypovascularized and replete with stromal deserts that are largely avascular and indeed may even be actively antiangiogenic.[81] In contrast, many other tumors, including human renal and pancreatic neuroendocrine carcinomas, are highly angiogenic and, consequently, densely vascularized.[82,83]

Collectively, such observations suggest an initial tripping of the angiogenic switch during tumor development, which is followed by a variable intensity of ongoing neovascularization, the latter being controlled by a complex biologic rheostat that involves both the cancer cells and the associated stromal microenvironment.[71,72] Of note, the switching mechanisms can vary, even though the net result is a common inductive signal (e.g., VEGF). In some tumors, dominant oncogenes operating within tumor cells, such as *Ras* and *Myc*, can upregulate the expression of angiogenic factors, whereas in others, such inductive signals are produced indirectly by immune inflammatory cells, as will be discussed.

Endogenous Angiogenesis Inhibitors Present Natural Barriers to Tumor Angiogenesis

A variety of secreted proteins have been reported to have the capability to help shut off normally transitory angiogenesis, including thrombospondin-1 (TSP-1), fragments of plasmin (angiostatin) and type 18 collagen (endostatin), along with another dozen candidate antiangiogenic proteins.[77,84–88] Most are proteins, and many are derived by proteolytic cleavage of structural proteins that are not themselves angiogenic regulators.

A number of these endogenous inhibitors of angiogenesis can be detected in the circulation of normal mice and humans. Genes that encode several endogenous angiogenesis inhibitors have been deleted from the mouse germ line without untoward developmental or physiologic effects; however, the growth of autochthonous and implanted tumors is enhanced as a consequence.[84,85,88] By contrast, if the circulating levels of an endogenous inhibitor are genetically increased (e.g., via overexpression in transgenic mice or in xenotransplanted tumors), tumor growth is impaired.[85,88] Interestingly, wound healing and fat deposition are impaired or accelerated by elevated or ablated expression of such genes.[89,90] The data suggest that, under normal conditions, endogenous angiogenesis inhibitors serve as physiologic regulators modulating the transitory angiogenesis that occurs during tissue remodeling and wound healing; they may also act as intrinsic barriers to the induction and/or persistence of angiogenesis by incipient neoplasias.

Pericytes Are Important Components of the Tumor Neovasculature

Pericytes have long been known as supporting cells that are closely apposed to the outer surfaces of the endothelial tubes in normal tissue vasculature, where they provide important mechanical and physiologic support to the endothelial cells. Microscopic studies conducted in recent years have revealed that pericytes are associated, albeit loosely, with the neovasculature of most, if not all, tumors.[91–93] More importantly, mechanistic studies (discussed subsequently) have revealed that pericyte coverage is important for the maintenance of a functional tumor neovasculature.

A Variety of Bone Marrow-Derived Cells Contribute to Tumor Angiogenesis

It is now clear that a repertoire of cell types originating in the bone marrow play crucial roles in pathologic angiogenesis.[94–97] These include cells of the innate immune system—notably, macrophages, neutrophils, mast cells, and myeloid progenitors—that assemble at the margins of such lesions or infiltrate deeply within them; the tumor-associated inflammatory cells can help to trip the angiogenic switch in quiescent tissue and sustain ongoing angiogenesis associated with tumor growth. In addition, they can help protect the vasculature from the effects of drugs targeting endothelial cell signaling.[98] Moreover, several types of bone marrow–derived *vascular progenitor cells* have been observed to have migrated into neoplastic lesions and become intercalated into the existing neovasculature, where they assumed the roles of either pericytes or endothelial cells.[92,99,100]

Activating Invasion and Metastasis

The multistep process of invasion and metastasis has been schematized as a sequence of discrete steps, often termed the invasion–metastasis cascade.[101,102] This depiction portrays a succession of cell-biologic changes, beginning with local invasion, then intravasation by cancer cells into nearby blood and lymphatic vessels, transit of cancer cells through the lymphatic and hematogenous systems, followed by the escape of cancer cells from the lumina of such vessels into the parenchyma of distant tissues (extravasation), the formation of small nests of cancer cells (micrometastases), and finally, the growth of micrometastatic lesions into macroscopic tumors, this last step being termed *colonization*. These steps have largely been studied in the context of carcinoma pathogenesis. Indeed, when viewed through the prism of the invasion–metastasis cascade, the diverse tumors of this class appear to behave in similar ways.

During the malignant progression of carcinomas, the neoplastic cells typically develop alterations in their shape as well as their attachment to other cells and to the extracellular matrix (ECM). The best-characterized alteration involves the loss by carcinoma cells of E-cadherin, a key epithelial cell-to-cell adhesion molecule. By forming adherens junctions between adjacent epithelial cells, E-cadherin helps to assemble epithelial cell sheets and to maintain the quiescence of the cells within these sheets. Moreover, increased expression of E-cadherin has been well established as an antagonist of invasion and metastasis, whereas a reduction of its expression is known to potentiate these behaviors. The frequently observed downregulation and occasional mutational inactivation of the E-cadherin–encoding gene, *CDH1*, in human carcinomas provides strong support for its role as a key suppressor of the invasion–metastasis hallmark capability.[103,104]

Notably, the expression of genes encoding other cell-to-cell and cell-to-ECM adhesion molecules is also significantly altered in the cells of many highly aggressive carcinomas, with those favoring cytostasis typically being downregulated. Conversely, adhesion molecules normally associated with the cell migrations that occur during embryogenesis and inflammation are often upregulated. For example, N-cadherin, which is normally expressed in migrating neurons and mesenchymal cells during organogenesis, is upregulated in many invasive carcinoma cells, replacing the previously expressed E-cadherin.[104]

Research into the capability for invasion and metastasis has accelerated dramatically over the past decade as powerful new research tools, and refined experimental models have become available. Although still an emerging field replete with major unanswered questions, significant progress has been made in delineating important features of this complex hallmark capability. An admittedly incomplete representation of these advances is highlighted as follows.

The Epithelial-to-Mesenchymal Transition Program Broadly Regulates Invasion and Metastasis

A developmental regulatory program, termed the EMT, has become implicated as a prominent means by which neoplastic epithelial cells can acquire the abilities to invade, resist apoptosis, and disseminate.[105–110] By co-opting a process involved in various steps of embryonic morphogenesis and wound healing, carcinoma cells can concomitantly acquire multiple attributes that enable invasion and metastasis. This multifaceted EMT program can be activated transiently or stably, and to differing degrees, by carcinoma cells during the course of invasion and metastasis.

A set of pleiotropically acting transcriptional factors (TF), including Snail, Slug, Twist, and Zeb1/2, orchestrate the EMT and related migratory processes during embryogenesis; most were initially identified by developmental genetics. These transcriptional regulators are expressed in various combinations in a number of malignant tumor types. Some of these EMT-TFs have been shown in experimental models of carcinoma formation to be causally important for programming invasion; others have been found to elicit metastasis when experimentally expressed in primary tumor cells.[105,111–114] Included among the cell-biologic traits evoked by these EMT-TFs are loss of adherens junctions and associated conversion from a polygonal/epithelial to a spindly/fibroblastic morphology, concomitant with expression of secreted matrix-degrading enzymes, increased motility, and heightened resistance to apoptosis, which are implicated in the processes of invasion and metastasis. Several of these transcription factors can directly repress E-cadherin gene expression, thereby releasing neoplastic epithelial cells from this key suppressor of motility and invasiveness.[115]

The available data suggest that EMT-TFs regulate one another as well as overlapping sets of target genes. Results from developmental genetics indicate that contextual signals received from neighboring cells in the embryo are involved in triggering expression of these transcription factors in cells that are destined to pass through an EMT[111]; in an analogous fashion, heterotypic interactions of cancer cells with adjacent tumor-associated stromal cells have been shown to induce expression of the malignant cell phenotypes that are known to be choreographed by one or more of these EMT-TFs.[116,117] Moreover, cancer cells at the invasive margins of certain carcinomas can be seen to have undergone an EMT, suggesting that these cancer cells are subject to microenvironmental stimuli distinct from those received by cancer cells located in the cores of these lesions.[118] Although the evidence is still incomplete, it would appear that EMT-TFs are able to orchestrate most steps of the invasion–metastasis cascade, except perhaps the final step of colonization, which involves adaptation of cells originating in one tissue to the microenvironment of a foreign, potentially inhospitable tissue.

We still know rather little about the various manifestations and temporal stability of the mesenchymal state produced by an EMT. Indeed, it seems increasingly likely that many human carcinoma cells only experience a *partial EMT*, in which they acquire mesenchymal markers while retaining many preexisting epithelial ones. Although the expression of EMT-TFs has been observed in certain nonepithelial tumor types, such as sarcomas and neuroectodermal tumors, their roles in programming malignant traits in these tumors are presently poorly documented. Additionally, it remains to be determined whether aggressive carcinoma cells invariably acquire their malignant capabilities through activation of components of the EMT program, or whether alternative regulatory programs can also enable expression of these traits.

Heterotypic Contributions of Stromal Cells to Invasion and Metastasis

As mentioned previously, cross-talk between cancer cells and cell types of the neoplastic stroma is involved in the acquired capabilities of invasiveness and metastasis.[94,119–121] For example, mesenchymal stem cells (MSC) present in the tumor stroma have been found to secrete CCL5/RANTES in response to signals released by cancer cells; CCL5 then acts reciprocally on the cancer cells to stimulate invasive behavior.[122] In other work, carcinoma cells secreting IL-1 have been shown to induce MSCs to synthesize a spectrum of other cytokines that proceed thereafter to promote activation of the EMT program in the carcinoma cells; these effectors include IL-6, IL-8, growth-regulated oncogene alpha (GRO-α), and prostaglandin E2.[123]

Macrophages at the tumor periphery can foster local invasion by supplying matrix-degrading enzymes such as metalloproteinases and cysteine cathepsin proteases[76,120,124,125]; in one model system, the invasion-promoting macrophages are activated by IL-4 produced by the cancer cells.[126] And in an experimental model of metastatic breast cancer, tumor-associated macrophages (TAM) supply epidermal growth factor (EGF) to breast cancer cells, while the cancer cells reciprocally stimulate the macrophages with colony stimulating factor 1 (CSF-1). Their concerted interactions facilitate intravasation into the circulatory system and metastatic dissemination of the cancer cells.[94,127]

Observations like these indicate that the phenotypes of high-grade malignancy do not arise in a strictly cell-autonomous manner, and that their manifestation cannot be understood solely through analyses of signaling occurring within tumor cells. One important implication of the EMT model, still untested, is that the ability of carcinoma cells in primary tumors to negotiate most of the steps of the invasion–metastasis cascade may be acquired in certain tumors without the requirement that these cells undergo additional mutations beyond those that were needed for primary tumor formation.

Plasticity in the Invasive Growth Program

The role of contextual signals in inducing an invasive growth capability (often via an EMT) implies the possibility of reversibility, in that cancer cells that have disseminated from a primary tumor to more distant tissue sites may no longer benefit from the activated stroma and the EMT-inducing signals that they experienced while residing in the primary tumor. In the absence of ongoing exposure to these signals, carcinoma cells may revert in their new tissue environment to a noninvasive state. Thus, carcinoma cells that underwent an EMT during initial invasion and metastatic dissemination may reverse this metamorphosis, doing so via a mesenchymal-to-epithelial transition (MET). This plasticity may result in the formation of new tumor colonies of carcinoma cells exhibiting an organization and histopathology similar to those created by carcinoma cells in the primary tumor that never experienced an EMT.[128]

Distinct Forms of Invasion May Underlie Different Cancer Types

The EMT program regulates a particular type of invasiveness that has been termed *mesenchymal*. In addition, two other distinct modes of invasion have been identified and implicated in cancer cell invasion.[129,130] *Collective invasion* involves phalanxes of cancer cells advancing en masse into adjacent tissues and is characteristic of, for example, squamous cell carcinomas. Interestingly, such cancers are rarely metastatic, suggesting that this form of invasion lacks certain functional attributes that facilitate metastasis. Less clear is the prevalence of an *amoeboid* form of invasion,[131,132] in which individual cancer cells show morphologic plasticity, enabling them to slither through existing interstices in the ECM rather than clearing a path for themselves, as occurs in both the mesenchymal and collective forms of invasion. It is presently unresolved whether cancer cells participating in the collective and amoeboid forms of invasion employ components of the EMT program, or whether entirely different cell-biologic programs are responsible for choreographing these alternative invasion programs.

Another emerging concept, noted previously, involves the facilitation of cancer cell invasion by inflammatory cells that assemble at the boundaries of tumors, producing the ECM-degrading enzymes and other factors that enable invasive growth.[76,94,120,133] These functions may obviate the need of invading cancer cells to produce these proteins through activation of EMT programs. Thus, rather than synthesizing these proteases themselves, cancer cells may secrete chemoattractants that recruit proinvasive inflammatory cells; the latter then proceed to produce matrix-degrading enzymes that enable invasive growth.

The Daunting Complexity of Metastatic Colonization

Metastasis can be broken down into two major phases: the physical dissemination of cancer cells from the primary tumor to distant tissues, and the adaptation of these cells to foreign tissue microenvironments that results in successful colonization (i.e., the growth of micrometastases into macroscopic tumors). The multiple steps of dissemination would seem to lie within the purview of the EMT and similarly acting migratory programs. Colonization, however, is not strictly coupled with physical dissemination, as evidenced by the presence in many patients of myriad micrometastases that have disseminated but never progress to form macroscopic metastatic tumors.[101,102,134–136]

In some types of cancer, the primary tumor may release systemic suppressor factors that render such micrometastases dormant, as revealed clinically by explosive metastatic growth soon after resection of the primary growth.[87,137] In others, however, such as breast cancer and melanoma, macroscopic metastases may erupt decades after a primary tumor has been surgically removed or pharmacologically destroyed. These metastatic tumor growths evidently reflect dormant micrometastases that have solved, after much trial and error, the complex problem of adaptation to foreign tissue microenvironments, allowing subsequent tissue colonization.[135,136,138] Implicit here is the notion that most disseminated cancer cells are likely to be poorly adapted, at least initially, to the microenvironment of the tissue in which they have landed. Accordingly, each type of disseminated cancer cell may need to develop its own set of ad hoc solutions to the problem of thriving in the microenvironment of one or another foreign tissue.[139]

One can infer from such natural histories that micrometastases may lack certain hallmark capabilities necessary for vigorous growth, such as the ability to activate angiogenesis. Indeed, the inability of certain experimentally generated dormant micrometastases to form macroscopic tumors has been ascribed to their failure to activate tumor angiogenesis.[135,140] Additionally, recent experiments have shown that nutrient starvation can induce intense autophagy that causes cancer cells to shrink and adopt a state of reversible dormancy. Such cells may exit this state and resume active growth and proliferation when permitted by changes in tissue microenvironment, such as increased availability of nutrients, inflammation from causes such as infection or wound healing, or other local abnormalities.[49,141] Other mechanisms of micrometastatic dormancy may involve antigrowth signals embedded in normal tissue ECM[138] and tumor-suppressing actions of the immune system.[135,142]

Metastatic dissemination has long been depicted as the last step in multistep primary tumor progression; indeed, for many tumors, that is likely the case, as illustrated by recent genome sequencing studies that provide genetic evidence for clonal evolution of pancreatic ductal adenocarcinoma to a metastatic stage.[143–145] Importantly, however, recent results have revealed that some cancer cells can disseminate remarkably early, dispersing from apparently noninvasive premalignant lesions in both mice and humans.[146,147] Additionally, micrometastases can be spawned from primary tumors that are not obviously invasive but possess a neovasculature lacking in luminal integrity.[148] Although cancer cells can clearly disseminate from such preneoplastic lesions and seed the bone marrow and other tissues, their capability to colonize these sites and develop into pathologically significant macrometastases remains unproven. At present, we view this early metastatic dissemination as a demonstrable phenomenon in mice and humans, the clinical significance of which is yet to be established.

Having developed such a tissue-specific colonizing ability, the cells in metastatic colonies may proceed to disseminate further, not only to new sites in the body, but also back to the primary tumors in which their ancestors arose. Accordingly, tissue-specific colonization programs that are evident among certain cells within a primary tumor may originate not from classical tumor progression occurring entirely within the primary lesion, but instead from immigrants that have returned home.[149] Such reseeding is consistent with the aforementioned studies of human pancreatic cancer metastasis.[143–145] Stated differently, the phenotypes and underlying gene expression programs in focal subpopulations of cancer cells within primary tumors may reflect, in part, the reverse migration of their distant metastatic progeny.

Implicit in this *self-seeding* process is another notion: The supportive stroma that arises in a primary tumor and contributes to its acquisition of malignant traits provides a hospitable site for reseeding and colonization by circulating cancer cells released from metastatic lesions.

Clarifying the regulatory programs that enable metastatic colonization represents an important agenda for future research. Substantial progress is being made, for example, in defining sets of genes (*metastatic signatures*) that correlate with and appear to facilitate the establishment of macroscopic metastases in specific tissues.[139,146,150–152] Importantly, metastatic colonization almost certainly requires the establishment of a permissive tumor microenvironment composed of critical stromal support cells. For these reasons, the process of colonization is likely to encompass a large number of cell-biologic programs that are, in aggregate, considerably more complex and diverse than the preceding steps of metastatic dissemination that allow carcinoma cells to depart from primary tumors to sites of lodging and extravasation throughout the body.

Reprogramming Energy Metabolism

The chronic and often uncontrolled cell proliferation that represents the essence of neoplastic disease involves not only deregulated control of cell proliferation but also corresponding adjustments of energy metabolism in order to fuel cell growth and division. Under aerobic conditions, normal cells process glucose, first to pyruvate via glycolysis in the cytosol and thereafter via oxidative phosphorylation to carbon dioxide in the mitochondria. Under anaerobic conditions, glycolysis is favored and relatively little pyruvate is dispatched to the oxygen-consuming mitochondria. Otto Warburg first observed an anomalous characteristic of cancer cell energy metabolism[153–155]: Even in the presence of oxygen, cancer cells can reprogram their glucose metabolism, and thus their energy production, leading to a state that has been termed *aerobic glycolysis*.

The existence of this metabolic specialization operating in cancer cells has been substantiated in the ensuing decades. A key signature of aerobic glycolysis is upregulation of glucose transporters, notably GLUT1, which substantially increases glucose import into the cytoplasm.[156–158] Indeed, markedly increased uptake and utilization of glucose has been documented in many human tumor types, most readily by noninvasively visualizing glucose uptake using positron-emission tomography (PET) with a radiolabeled analog of glucose (^{18}F-fluorodeoxyglucose [FDG]) as a reporter.

Glycolytic fueling has been shown to be associated with activated oncogenes (e.g., RAS, MYC) and mutant tumor suppressors (e.g., TP53),[18,156,157,159] whose alterations in tumor cells have been selected primarily for their benefits in conferring the hallmark capabilities of cell proliferation, subversion of cytostatic controls, and attenuation of apoptosis. This reliance on glycolysis can be further accentuated under the hypoxic conditions that operate within many tumors: The hypoxia response system acts pleiotropically to upregulate glucose transporters and multiple enzymes of the glycolytic pathway.[156,157,160] Thus, both the Ras oncoprotein and hypoxia can independently increase the levels of the HIF1α and HIF2α hypoxia-response transcription factors, which in turn upregulate glycolysis.[160–162]

The reprogramming of energy metabolism is seemingly counterintuitive, in that cancer cells must compensate for the $\sim$18-fold lower efficiency of ATP production afforded by glycolysis relative to mitochondrial oxidative phosphorylation. According to one long-forgotten[163] and a recently revived and refined hypothesis,[164] increased glycolysis allows the diversion of glycolytic intermediates into various biosynthetic pathways, including those generating nucleosides and amino acids. In turn, this facilitates the biosynthesis of the macromolecules and organelles required for assembling new cells. Moreover, Warburg-like metabolism seems to be present in many rapidly dividing embryonic tissues, once again suggesting a role in supporting the large-scale biosynthetic programs that are required for active cell proliferation.

Interestingly, some tumors have been found to contain two subpopulations of cancer cells that differ in their energy-generating pathways. One subpopulation consists of glucose-dependent (Warburg-effect) cells that secrete lactate, whereas cells of the second subpopulation preferentially import and utilize the lactate produced by their neighbors as their main energy source, employing part of the citric acid cycle to do so.[165–168] These two populations evidently function symbiotically: The hypoxic cancer cells depend on glucose for fuel and secrete lactate as waste, which is imported and preferentially used as fuel by their better oxygenated brethren. Although this provocative mode of intratumoral symbiosis has yet to be generalized, the cooperation between lactate-secreting and lactate-utilizing cells to fuel tumor growth is in fact not an invention of tumors, but rather again reflects the co-opting of a normal physiologic mechanism, in this case one operative in muscle[165,167,168] and the brain.[169] Additionally, it is becoming apparent that oxygenation, ranging from normoxia to hypoxia, is not necessarily static in tumors, but instead fluctuates temporally and regionally,[170] likely as a result of the instability and chaotic organization of the tumor-associated neovasculature.

Finally, the notion of the Warburg effect needs to be refined for most if not all tumors exhibiting aerobic glycolysis. The effect does not involve a switching off oxidative phosphorylation concurrent with activation of glycolysis, the latter then serving as the sole source of energy. Rather, cancer cells become highly adaptive, utilizing both mitochondrial oxidative phosphorylation and glycolysis in varying proportions to generate fuel (ATP) and biosynthetic precursors needed for chronic cell proliferation. Finally, this capability for reprograming energy metabolism, dubbed to be an *emerging hallmark* in 2011,[2] is clearly intertwined with the hallmarks conveying deregulated proliferative signals and evasion of growth suppressors, as discussed earlier. As such, its status as a discrete, independently acquired hallmark remains unclear, despite growing appreciation of its importance as a crucial component of the neoplastic growth state.

Evading Immune Destruction

The eighth hallmark reflects the role played by the immune system in antagonizing the formation and progression of tumors. A long-standing theory of immune surveillance posited that cells and tissues are constantly monitored by an ever alert immune system, and that such immune surveillance is responsible for recognizing and eliminating the vast majority of incipient cancer cells and, thus, nascent tumors.[171,172] According to this logic, clinical detectable cancers have somehow managed to avoid detection by the various arms of the immune system, or have been able to limit the extent of immunologic killing, thereby evading eradication.

The role of defective immunologic monitoring of tumors would seem to be validated by the striking increases of certain cancers in immune-compromised individuals.[173] However, the great majority of these are virus-induced cancers, suggesting that much of the control of this class of cancers normally depends on reducing viral burden in infected individuals, in part through eliminating virus-infected cells. These observations, therefore, shed little light on the possible role of the immune system in limiting formation of the >80% of tumors of nonviral etiology. In recent years, however, an increasing body of evidence, both from genetically engineered mice and from clinical epidemiology, suggests that the immune system operates as a significant barrier to tumor formation and progression, at least in some forms of non–virus-induced cancer.[174–177]

When mice genetically engineered to be deficient for various components of the immune system were assessed for the development of carcinogen-induced tumors, it was observed that tumors arose more frequently and/or grew more rapidly in the immunodeficient mice relative to immune-competent controls. In particular, deficiencies in the development or function of either CD8+ cytotoxic T lymphocytes (CTL), CD4+ T_H1 helper T cells, or natural killer (NK) cells, each led to demonstrable increases in tumor incidence. Moreover, mice with combined immunodeficiencies in both T cells and NK cells were even more susceptible to cancer development. The results indicated that, at least in certain experimental models, both the innate and adaptive cellular arms of the immune system are able to contribute significantly to immune surveillance and, thus, tumor eradication.[142,178]

In addition, transplantation experiments have shown that cancer cells that originally arose in immunodeficient mice are often inefficient at initiating secondary tumors in syngeneic immunocompetent hosts, whereas cancer cells from tumors arising in immunocompetent mice are equally efficient at initiating transplanted tumors in both types of hosts.[142,178] Such behavior has been interpreted as follows: Highly immunogenic cancer cell clones are routinely eliminated in immunocompetent hosts—a process that has been referred to as *immunoediting*—leaving behind only weakly immunogenic variants to grow and generate solid tumors. Such weakly immunogenic cells can thereafter successfully colonize both immunodeficient and immunocompetent hosts. Conversely, when arising in immunodeficient hosts, the immunogenic cancer cells are not selectively depleted and can, instead, prosper along with their weakly immunogenic counterparts. When cells from such nonedited tumors are serially transplanted into syngeneic recipients, the immunogenic cancer cells are rejected when they confront, for the first time, the competent immune systems of their secondary hosts.[179] (Unanswered in these particular experiments is the question of whether the chemical carcinogens used to induce such tumors are prone to generate cancer cells that are especially immunogenic.)

Clinical epidemiology also increasingly supports the existence of antitumoral immune responses in some forms of human cancer.[180–182] For example, patients with colon and ovarian tumors that are heavily infiltrated with CTLs and NK cells have a better prognosis than those who lack such abundant killer lymphocytes.[176,177,182,183] The case for other cancers is suggestive but less compelling and is the subject of ongoing investigation. Additionally, some immunosuppressed organ transplant recipients have been observed to develop donor-derived cancers, suggesting that in ostensibly tumor-free organ donors, the cancer cells were held in check in a dormant state by a functional immune system,[184] only to launch into proliferative expansion once these *passenger cells* in the transplanted organ found themselves in immunocompromised patients who lack the physiologically important capabilities to mount immune responses that would otherwise hold latent cancer cells in check or eradicate them.

Still, the epidemiology of chronically immunosuppressed patients does not indicate significantly increased incidences of the major forms of nonviral human cancers, as noted previously. This might be taken as an argument against the importance of immune surveillance as an effective barrier to tumorigenesis and tumor progression. We note, however, that HIV and pharmacologically immunosuppressed patients are predominantly immunodeficient in the T- and B-cell compartments and thus do not present with the multicomponent immunologic deficiencies that have been produced in the genetically engineered mutant mice lacking both NK cells and CTLs. This leaves open the possibility that such

patients still have residual capability for mounting an anticancer immunologic defense that is mediated by NK and other innate immune cells.

In truth, the previous discussions of cancer immunology simplify tumor–host immunologic interactions, because highly immunogenic cancer cells may well succeed in evading immune destruction by disabling components of the immune system that have been dispatched to eliminate them. For example, cancer cells may paralyze infiltrating CTLs and NK cells by secreting TGF-β or other immunosuppressive factors.[32,185,186] Alternatively, cancer cells may express immunosuppressive cell-surface ligands, such as PD-L1, that prevent activation of the cytotoxic mechanisms of the CTLs. These PD-L1 molecules serve as ligands for the PD-1 receptors displayed by the CTLs, together exemplifying a system of *checkpoint* ligands and receptors that serve to constrain immune responses in order to avoid autoimmunity.[187–189] Yet other localized immunosuppressive mechanisms operate through the recruitment of inflammatory cells that can actively suppress CTL activity, including regulatory T cells (Tregs) and myeloid-derived suppressor cells (MDSC).[174,190–193]

In summary, these eight hallmarks each contribute qualitatively distinct capabilities that seem integral to most lethal forms of human cancer. Certainly, the balance and relative importance of their respective contributions to disease pathogenesis will vary among cancer types, and some hallmarks may be absent or of minor importance in some cases. Still, there is reason to postulate their generality and, thus, their applicability to understanding the biology of human cancer. Next, we turn to the question of how these capabilities are acquired during the multistep pathways through which cancers develop, focusing on two facilitators that are commonly involved.

TWO UBIQUITOUS CHARACTERISTICS FACILITATE THE ACQUISITION OF HALLMARK CAPABILITIES

We have defined the hallmarks of cancer as acquired functional capabilities that allow cancer cells to survive, proliferate, and disseminate. Their acquisition is made possible by two *enabling characteristics* (Fig. 2.2). Most prominent is the development of genomic instability in cancer cells, which generates random mutations, including chromosomal rearrangements, among which are rare genetic changes that can orchestrate individual hallmark capabilities. A second enabling characteristic involves the inflammatory state of premalignant and frankly malignant lesions. A variety of cells of the innate and adaptive immune system infiltrate neoplasias, some of which serve to promote tumor progression through various means.

An Enabling Characteristic: Genome Instability and Mutation

Acquisition of the multiple hallmarks enumerated previously depends in large part on a succession of alterations in the genomes of neoplastic cells. Basically, certain mutant genotypes can confer selective advantage to particular subclones among proliferating nests of incipient cancer cells, enabling their outgrowth and eventual dominance in a local tissue environment. Accordingly, multistep tumor progression can be portrayed as a succession of clonal expansions, most of which are triggered by the chance acquisition of an enabling mutation.

Indeed, it is apparent that virtually every human cancer cell genome carries mutant alleles of one or several growth-regulating genes, underscoring the central importance of these genetic alterations in driving malignant progression.[194] Still, we note that many heritable phenotypes—including, notably, inactivation of tumor suppressor genes—can be acquired through epigenetic

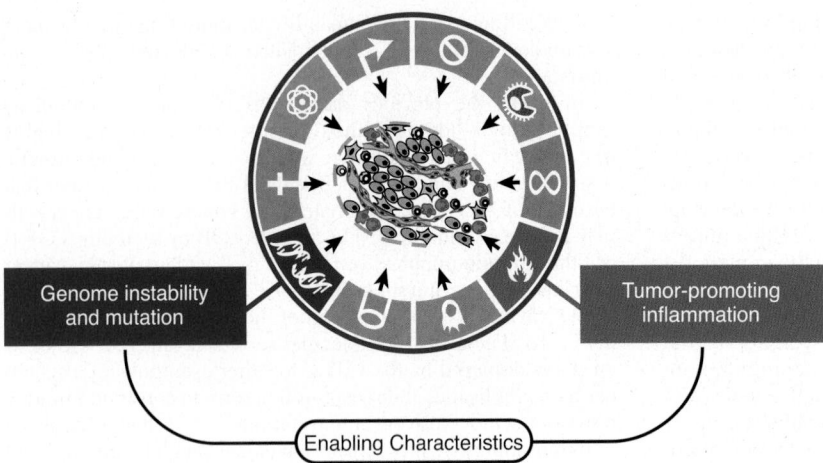

Figure 2.2 Enabling characteristics. Two ostensibly generic characteristics of cancer cells and the neoplasias they create are involved in the acquisition of the hallmark capabilities. First and foremost, the impairment of genome maintenance systems in aberrantly proliferating cancer cells enables the generation of mutations in genes that contribute to multiple hallmarks. Secondarily, neoplasias invariably attract cells of the innate immune system that are programmed to heal wounds and fight infections; these cells, including macrophages, neutrophils, and partially differentiated myeloid cells, can contribute functionally to acquisition of many of the hallmark capabilities. (Adapted from Hanahan D, Weinberg RA. Hallmarks of cancer: the next generation. *Cell* 2011;144:646–674.)

mechanisms, such as DNA methylation and histone modifications.[195–198] Thus, many clonal expansions may also be triggered by heritable nonmutational changes affecting the regulation of gene expression. At present, the relative importance of genetic versus heritable epigenetic alterations to the various clonal expansions remains unclear, and likely, varies broadly amongst the catalog of human cancer types.

The extraordinary ability of genome maintenance systems to detect and resolve defects in the DNA ensures that rates of spontaneous mutation in normal cells of the body are typically very low, both in quiescent cells and during cell division. The genomes of most cancer cells, by contrast, are replete with these alterations, reflecting loss of genomic integrity with concomitantly increased rates of mutation. This heightened mutability appears to accelerate the generation of variant cells, facilitating the selection of those cells whose advantageous phenotypes enable their clonal expansion.[199,200] This mutability is achieved through increased sensitivity to mutagenic agents, through a breakdown in one or several components of the genomic maintenance machinery, or both. In addition, the accumulation of mutations can be accelerated by aberrations that compromise the surveillance systems that normally monitor genomic integrity and force such genetically damaged cells into either quiescence, senescence, or apoptosis.[201–203] The role of TP53 is central here, leading to its being called the *guardian of the genome*.[204]

A diverse array of defects affecting various components of the DNA-maintenance machinery, referred to as the *caretakers* of the genome,[205] have been documented. The catalog of defects in these caretaker genes includes those whose products are involved in (1) detecting DNA damage and activating the repair machinery, (2) directly repairing damaged DNA, and (3) inactivating or intercepting mutagenic molecules before they have damaged the DNA.[199,201,202,206–208] From a genetic perspective, these caretaker genes behave much like tumor suppressor genes, in that their functions are often lost during the course of tumor progression, with such losses being achieved either through inactivating mutations or via epigenetic repression. Mutant copies of many of these caretaker genes have been introduced into the mouse germ line, resulting, not unexpectedly, in increased cancer incidence, thus supporting their involvement in human cancer development.[209]

In addition, research over the past decade has revealed another major source of tumor-associated genomic instability. As described earlier, the loss of telomeric DNA in many tumors generates karyotypic instability and associated amplification and deletion of chromosomal segments.[58] When viewed in this light, telomerase is more than an enabler of the hallmark capability for unlimited replicative potential. It must also be added to the list of critical caretakers responsible for maintaining genome integrity.

Advances in the molecular–genetic analysis of cancer cell genomes have provided the most compelling demonstrations of function-altering mutations and of ongoing genomic instability during tumor progression. One type of analysis—comparative genomic hybridization (CGH)—documents the gains and losses of gene copy number across the cell genome. In many tumors, the pervasive genomic aberrations revealed by CGH provide clear evidence for loss of control of genome integrity. Importantly, the recurrence of specific aberrations (both amplifications and deletions) at particular locations in the genome indicates that such sites are likely to harbor genes whose alteration favors neoplastic progression.[210]

More recently, with the advent of efficient and economical DNA sequencing technologies, higher resolution analyses of cancer cell genomes have become possible. Early studies are revealing distinctive patterns of DNA mutations in different tumor types (see: http://cancergenome.nih.gov/). In the not-too-distant future, the sequencing of entire cancer cell genomes promises to clarify the importance of ostensibly random mutations scattered across cancer cell genomes.[194] Thus, the use of whole genome resequencing offers the prospect of revealing recurrent genetic alterations (i.e., those found in multiple independently arising tumors) that in aggregate represent only minor proportions of the tumors of a given type. The recurrence of such mutations, despite their infrequency, may provide clues about the regulatory pathways playing causal roles in the pathogenesis of the tumors under study.

These surveys of cancer cell genomes have shown that the specifics of genome alteration vary dramatically between different tumor types. Nonetheless, the large number of already documented genome maintenance and repair defects, together with abundant evidence of widespread destabilization of gene copy number and nucleotide sequence, persuade us that instability of the genome is inherent to the cancer cells forming virtually all types of human tumors. This leads, in turn, to the conclusion that the defects in genome maintenance and repair are selectively advantageous and, therefore, instrumental for tumor progression, if only because they accelerate the rate at which evolving premalignant cells can accumulate favorable genotypes. As such, genome instability is clearly an *enabling characteristic* that is causally associated with the acquisition of hallmark capabilities.

An Enabling Characteristic: Tumor-Promoting Inflammation

Among the cells recruited to the stroma of carcinomas are a variety of cell types of the immune system that mediate various inflammatory functions. Pathologists have long recognized that some (but not all) tumors are densely infiltrated by cells of both the innate and adaptive arms of the immune system, thereby mirroring inflammatory conditions arising in nonneoplastic tissues.[211] With the advent of better markers for accurately identifying the distinct cell types of the immune system, it is now clear that virtually every neoplastic lesion contains immune cells present at densities ranging from subtle infiltrations detectable only with cell type–specific antibodies to gross inflammations that are apparent even by standard histochemical staining techniques.[185] Historically, such immune responses were largely thought to reflect an attempt by the immune system to eradicate tumors, and indeed, there is increasing evidence for antitumoral responses to many tumor types with an attendant pressure on the tumor to evade immune destruction,[174,176,177,183] as discussed earlier.

By 2000, however, there were also clues that tumor-associated inflammatory responses can have the unanticipated effect of facilitating multiple steps of tumor progression, thereby helping incipient neoplasias to acquire hallmark capabilities. In the ensuing years, research on the intersections between inflammation and cancer pathogenesis has blossomed, producing abundant and compelling demonstrations of the functionally important tumor-promoting effects that immune cells—largely of the innate immune system—have on neoplastic progression.[19,53,94,174,212,213] Inflammatory cells can contribute to multiple hallmark capabilities by supplying signaling molecules to the tumor microenvironment, including growth factors that sustain proliferative signaling; survival factors that limit cell death; proangiogenic factors; extracellular matrix-modifying enzymes that facilitate angiogenesis, invasion, and metastasis; and inductive signals that lead to activation of EMT and other hallmark-promoting programs.[53,94,116,212,213]

Importantly, localized inflammation is often apparent at the earliest stages of neoplastic progression and is demonstrably capable of fostering the development of incipient neoplasias into full-blown cancers.[94,214] Additionally, inflammatory cells can release chemicals—notably, reactive oxygen species—that are actively mutagenic for nearby cancer cells, thus accelerating their genetic evolution toward states of heightened malignancy.[53] As such, inflammation by selective cell types of the immune system is demonstrably an *enabling characteristic* for its contributions to the acquisition of hallmark capabilities. The cells responsible for this enabling characteristic are described in the following section.

THE CONSTITUENT CELL TYPES OF THE TUMOR MICROENVIRONMENT

Over the past 2 decades, tumors have increasingly been recognized as tissues whose complexity approaches and may even exceed that of normal healthy tissues. This realization contrasts starkly with the earlier, reductionist view of a tumor as nothing more than a collection of relatively homogeneous cancer cells, whose entire biology could be understood by elucidating the cell-autonomous properties of these cells (Fig. 2.3A). Rather, assemblages of diverse cell types associated with malignant lesions are increasingly documented to be functionally important for the manifestation of symptomatic disease (Fig. 2.3B). When viewed from this perspective, the biology of a tumor can only be fully understood by studying the individual specialized cell types within it. We enumerate as follows a set of accessory cell types recruited directly or indirectly by neoplastic cells into tumors, where they contribute in important ways to the biology of many tumors, and we discuss the regulatory mechanisms that control their individual and collective functions. Most of these observations stem from the study of carcinomas, in which the neoplastic epithelial cells constitute a compartment (the parenchyma) that is clearly distinct from the mesenchymal cells forming the tumor-associated stroma.

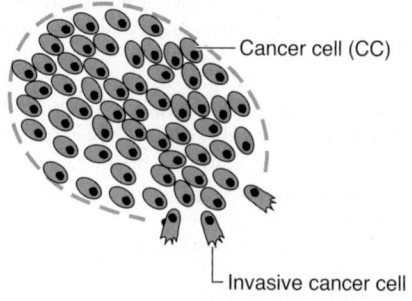

A simple view of cancer

Cancer cell (CC)

Invasive cancer cell

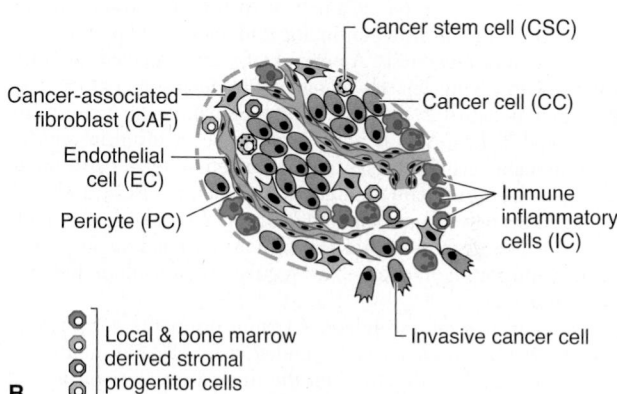

A more realistic view of cancer

Cancer stem cell (CSC)

Cancer-associated fibroblast (CAF)

Cancer cell (CC)

Endothelial cell (EC)

Pericyte (PC)

Immune inflammatory cells (IC)

Local & bone marrow derived stromal progenitor cells

Invasive cancer cell

Figure 2.3 Tumors as outlaw organs. Research aimed at understanding the biology of tumors has historically focused on the cancer cells, which constitute the drivers of neoplastic disease. This view of tumors as nothing more than masses of cancer cells **(A)** ignores an important reality, that cancer cells recruit and corrupt a variety of normal cell types that form the tumor-associated stroma. Once formed, the stroma acts reciprocally on the cancer cells, affecting almost all of the traits that define the neoplastic behavior of the tumor as a whole **(B)**. The assemblage of heterogeneous populations of cancer cells and stromal cells is often referred to as the tumor microenvironment (TME). (Adapted from Hanahan D, Weinberg R. The hallmarks of cancer. *Cell* 2000;100:57–70; Hanahan D, Weinberg RA. Hallmarks of cancer: the next generation. *Cell* 2011;144:646–674.)

Cancer-Associated Fibroblasts

Fibroblasts are found in various proportions across the spectrum of carcinomas, in many cases constituting the preponderant cell population of the tumor stroma. The term *cancer-associated fibroblasts* (CAFs) subsumes at least two distinct cell types: (1) cells with similarities to the fibroblasts that create the structural foundation supporting most normal epithelial tissues, and (2) myofibroblasts, whose biologic roles and properties differ markedly from those of the widely distributed tissue-derived fibroblasts. Myofibroblasts are identifiable by their expression of α-smooth muscle actin (αSMA). They are rare in most healthy epithelial tissues, although certain tissues, such as the liver and pancreas, contain appreciable numbers of αSMA-expressing cells. Myofibroblasts transiently increase in abundance in wounds and are also found in sites of chronic inflammation. Although beneficial to tissue repair, myofibroblasts are problematic in chronic inflammation, in that they contribute to the pathologic fibrosis observed in tissues such as the lung, kidney, and liver.

Recruited myofibroblasts and variants of normal tissue-derived fibroblastic cells have been demonstrated to enhance tumor phenotypes, notably cancer cell proliferation, angiogenesis, invasion, and metastasis. Their tumor-promoting activities have largely been defined by transplantation of cancer-associated fibroblasts admixed with cancer cells into mice, and more recently by genetic and pharmacologic perturbation of their functions in tumor-prone mice.[8,121,133,215–219] Because they secrete a variety of ECM components, cancer-associated fibroblasts are implicated in the formation of the desmoplastic stroma that characterizes many advanced carcinomas. The full spectrum of functions contributed by both subtypes of cancer-associated fibroblasts to tumor pathogenesis remains to be elucidated.

Endothelial Cells

Prominent among the stromal constituents of the TME are the endothelial cells forming the tumor-associated vasculature. Quiescent tissue capillary endothelial cells are activated by *angiogenic* regulatory factors to produce a neovasculature that sustains tumor growth concomitant with continuing endothelial cell proliferation and vessel morphogenesis. A network of interconnected signaling pathways involving ligands of signal-transducing receptors (e.g., the Angiopoeitin-1/2, Notch ligands, Semaphorin, Neuropilin, Robo, and Ephrin-A/B) is now known to be involved in regulating quiescent versus activated angiogenic endothelial cells, in addition to the aforementioned counterbalancing VEGF and TSP signals. This network of signaling pathways has been functionally implicated in developmental and tumor-associated angiogenesis, further illustrating the complex regulation of endothelial cell phenotypes.[220–224]

Other avenues of research are revealing distinctive gene expression profiles of tumor-associated endothelial cells and identifying cell-surface markers displayed on the luminal surfaces of normal versus tumor endothelial cells.[78,225,226] Differences in signaling, in transcriptome profiles, and in vascular *ZIP codes* will likely prove to be important for understanding the conversion of normal endothelial cells into tumor-associated endothelial cells. Such knowledge may lead, in turn, to opportunities to develop novel therapies that exploit these differences in order to selectively target tumor-associated endothelial cells. Additionally, the activated (*angiogenic*) tumor vasculature has been revealed as a barrier to efficient intravasation and a functional suppressor of cytotoxic T cells,[227] and thus, tumor endothelial cells can contribute to the hallmark capability for evading immune destruction. As such, another emerging concept is to normalize rather than ablate them, so as to improve immunotherapy[190] as well as delivery of chemotherapy.[228]

Closely related to the endothelial cells of the circulatory system are those forming lymphatic vessels.[229] Their role in the tumor-associated stroma, specifically in supporting tumor growth, is poorly understood. Indeed, because of high interstitial pressure within solid tumors, intratumoral lymphatic vessels are typically collapsed and nonfunctional; in contrast, however, there are often functional, actively growing (*lymphangiogenic*) lymphatic vessels at the periphery of tumors and in the adjacent normal tissues that cancer cells invade. These associated lymphatics likely serve as channels for the seeding of metastatic cells in the draining lymph nodes that are commonly observed in a number of cancer types. Recent results that are yet to be generalized suggest an alternative role for the activated (i.e., lymphangiogenic) lymphatic endothelial cells associated with tumors, not in supporting tumor growth like the blood vessels, but in inducing (via VEGF-C–mediated signaling) a lymphatic tissue microenvironment that suppresses immune responses ordinarily marshaled from the draining lymph nodes.[230] As such, the real value to a tumor from activating the signaling circuit involving the ligand VEGF-C and its receptor VEGFR3 may be to facilitate the evasion of antitumor immunity by abrogating the otherwise immunostimulatory functions of draining lymphatic vessels and lymph nodes, with the collateral effect of inducing lymphatic endothelial cells to form the new lymphatic vessels that are commonly detected in association with tumors.

Pericytes

Pericytes represent a specialized mesenchymal cell type that are closely related to smooth muscle cells, with fingerlike projections that wrap around the endothelial tubing of blood vessels. In normal tissues, pericytes are known to provide paracrine support signals to the quiescent endothelium. For example, Ang-1 secreted by pericytes conveys antiproliferative stabilizing signals that are received by the Tie2 receptors expressed on the surface of endothelial cells. Some pericytes also produce low levels of VEGF that serve a trophic function in endothelial homeostasis.[93,231] Pericytes also collaborate with the endothelial cells to synthesize the vascular basement membrane that anchors both pericytes and endothelial cells and helps vessel walls to withstand the hydrostatic pressure created by the blood.

Genetic and pharmacologic perturbation of the recruitment and association of pericytes has demonstrated the functional importance of these cells in supporting the tumor endothelium.[93,217,231] For example, the pharmacologic inhibition of signaling through the platelet-derived growth factor (PDGF) receptor expressed by tumor pericytes and bone marrow–derived pericyte progenitors results in reduced pericyte coverage of tumor vessels, which in turn destabilizes vascular integrity and function.[91,217,231] Interestingly, and in contrast, the pericytes of normal vessels are not prone to such pharmacologic disruption, providing another example of the differences in the regulation of normal quiescent and tumor vasculature. An intriguing hypothesis, still to be fully substantiated, is that tumors with poor pericyte coverage of their vasculature may be more prone to permit cancer cell intravasation into the circulatory system, thereby enabling subsequent hematogenous dissemination.[91,148]

Immune Inflammatory Cells

Infiltrating cells of the immune system are increasingly accepted to be generic constituents of tumors. These inflammatory cells operate in conflicting ways: Both tumor-antagonizing and tumor-promoting leukocytes can be found in various proportions in most, if not all, neoplastic lesions. Evidence began to accumulate in the late 1990s that the infiltration of neoplastic tissues by cells of the immune system serves, perhaps counterintuitively, to promote tumor progression. Such work traced its conceptual roots back to the observed association of tumor formation with sites of chronic inflammation. Indeed, this led some to liken tumors to "wounds that do not heal."[211,232] In the course of normal wound healing and the resolution of infections, immune inflammatory cells appear transiently and then disappear, in contrast to their persistence in sites of chronic inflammation, where their presence has been associated with a variety of tissue pathologies, including fibrosis, aberrant angiogenesis, and as mentioned, neoplasia.[53,233]

We now know that immune cells play diverse and critical roles in fostering tumorigenesis. The roster of tumor-promoting inflammatory cells includes macrophage subtypes, mast cells, and neutrophils, as well as T and B lymphocytes.[96,97,119,133,212,234,235] Studies of these cells are yielding a growing list of tumor-promoting signaling molecules that they release, which include the tumor growth factor EGF, the angiogenic growth factors VEGF-A/-C, other proangiogenic factors such as FGF2, plus chemokines and cytokines that amplify the inflammatory state. In addition, these cells may produce proangiogenic and/or proinvasive matrix-degrading enzymes, including MMP-9 and other MMPs, cysteine cathepsin proteases, and heparanase.[94,96] Consistent with the expression of these diverse signals, tumor-infiltrating inflammatory cells have been shown to induce and help sustain tumor angiogenesis, to stimulate cancer cell proliferation, to facilitate tissue invasion, and to support the metastatic dissemination and seeding of cancer cells.[94,96,97,119,120,234–237]

In addition to fully differentiated immune cells present in tumor stroma, a variety of partially differentiated myeloid progenitors have been identified in tumors.[96] Such cells represent intermediaries between circulating cells of bone marrow origin and the differentiated immune cells typically found in normal and inflamed tissues. Importantly, these progenitors, like their more differentiated derivatives, have demonstrable tumor-promoting activity. Of particular interest, a class of tumor-infiltrating myeloid cells has been shown to suppress CTL and NK cell activity, having been identified as MDSCs that function to block the attack on tumors by the adaptive (i.e., CTL) and innate (i.e., NK) arms of the immune system.[94,133,193] Hence, recruitment of certain myeloid cells may be doubly beneficial for the developing tumor, by directly promoting angiogenesis and tumor progression, while at the same time affording a means of evading immune destruction.

These conflicting roles of the immune system in confronting tumors would seem to reflect similar situations that arise routinely in normal tissues. Thus, the immune system detects and targets infectious agents through cells of the adaptive immune response. Cells of the innate immune system, in contrast, are involved in wound healing and in clearing dead cells and cellular debris. The balance between the conflicting immune responses within particular tumor types (and indeed in individual patients' tumors) is likely to prove critical in determining the characteristics of tumor growth and the stepwise progression to stages of heightened aggressiveness (i.e., invasion and metastasis). Moreover, there is increasing evidence supporting the proposition that this balance can be modulated for therapeutic purposes in order to redirect or reprogram the immune response to focus its functional capabilities on destroying tumors.[133,238,239]

Stem and Progenitor Cells of the Tumor Stroma

The various stromal cell types that constitute the tumor microenvironment may be recruited from adjacent normal tissue—the most obvious reservoir of such cell types. However, in recent years, bone marrow (BM) has increasingly been implicated as a key source of tumor-associated stromal cells.[99,100,240–243] Thus, mesenchymal stem and progenitor cells can be recruited into tumors from BM, where they may subsequently differentiate into the various well-characterized stromal cell types. Some of these recent arrivals may also persist in an undifferentiated or partially differentiated state, exhibiting functions that their more differentiated progeny lack.

The BM origins of stromal cell types have been demonstrated using tumor-bearing mice in which the BM cells (and thus their disseminated progeny) have been selectively labeled with reporters such as green fluorescent protein (GFP). Although immune inflammatory cells have been long known to derive from BM, more recently progenitors of endothelial cells, pericytes, and several subtypes of cancer-associated fibroblasts have also been shown to originate from BM in various mouse models of cancer.[100,240–243] The prevalence and functional importance of endothelial progenitors for tumor angiogenesis is, however, currently unresolved.[99,242] Taken together, these various lines of evidence indicate that tumor-associated stromal cells may be supplied to growing tumors by the proliferation of preexisting stromal cells or via recruitment of BM-derived stem/progenitor cells.

In summary, it is evident that virtually all cancers, including even the *liquid tumors* of hematopoietic malignancies, depend not only on neoplastic cells for their pathogenic effects, but also on diverse cell types recruited from local and distant tissue sources to assemble specialized, supporting tumor microenvironments. Importantly, the composition of stromal cell types supporting a particular cancer evidently varies considerably from one tumor type to another; even within a particular type, the patterns and abundance can be informative about malignant grade and prognosis. The inescapable conclusion is that cancer cells are not fully autonomous, and rather depend to various degrees on stromal cells of the tumor microenvironment, which can contribute functionally to seven of the eight hallmarks of cancer (Fig. 2.4).

Heterotypic Signaling Orchestrates the Cells of the Tumor Microenvironment

Every cell in our bodies is governed by an elaborate intracellular signaling circuit—in effect, its own microcomputer. In cancer cells, key subcircuits in this integrated circuit are reprogrammed so as to activate and sustain hallmark capabilities. These changes are induced by mutations in the cells' genomes, by epigenetic alterations affecting gene expression, and by the receipt of a diverse array of signals from the tumor microenvironment. Figure 2.5A illustrates some of the circuits that are reprogrammed to enable cancer cells to proliferate chronically, to avoid proliferative brakes and cell death, and to become invasive and metastatic. Similarly, the intracellular integrated circuits that regulate the actions of stromal cells are also evidently reprogrammed. Current evidence suggests that stromal cell reprogramming is primarily affected by extracellular cues and epigenetic alterations in gene expression, rather than gene mutation.

Given the alterations in the signaling within both neoplastic cells and their stromal neighbors, a tumor can be depicted as a network of interconnected (cellular) microcomputers. This dictates that a complete elucidation of a particular tumor's biology will require far more than an elucidation of the aberrantly functioning integrated circuits within its neoplastic cells. Accordingly, the rapidly growing catalog of the function-enabling genetic mutations within cancer cell genomes[194] provides only one dimension to this problem. A reasonably complete, graphical depiction of the network of microenvironmental signaling interactions remains far beyond our reach, because the great majority of signaling molecules and their circuitry are still to be identified. Instead, we provide a hint of such interactions in Figure 2.5B. These few well-established examples are intended to exemplify a signaling network of remarkable complexity that is of critical importance to tumor pathogenesis.

Coevolution of the Tumor Microenvironment During Carcinogenesis

The tumor microenvironment described previously is not static during multistage tumor development and progression, thus creating another dimension of complexity. Rather, the abundance and functional contributions of the stromal cells populating neoplastic lesions will likely vary during progression in two respects. First, as the neoplastic cells evolve, there will be a parallel coevolution occurring in the stroma, as indicated by the shifting composition of stroma-associated cell types. Second, as cancer cells enter into different locations, they encounter distinct stromal microenvironments. Thus, the microenvironment in the interior of a primary tumor will likely be distinct both from locally invasive breakout lesions and from the one encountered by disseminated cells in distant organs (Fig. 2.6A). This dictates that the observed histopathologic progression of a tumor reflects underlying changes in heterotypic signaling between tumor parenchyma and stroma.

We envision back-and-forth reciprocal interactions between the neoplastic cells and the supporting stromal cells that change during the course of multistep tumor development and progression, as depicted in Figure 2.6B. Thus, incipient neoplasias begin the interplay by recruiting and activating stromal cell types that assemble into an initial preneoplastic stroma, which in turn responds reciprocally by enhancing the neoplastic phenotypes of the nearby cancer cells. The cancer cells, in response, may then undergo further genetic evolution, causing them to feed signals back to the stroma. Ultimately, signals originating in the stroma of primary tumors enable cancer cells to invade normal adjacent tissues and disseminate, seeding distant tissues and, with low efficiency, metastatic colonies (see Fig. 2.6B).

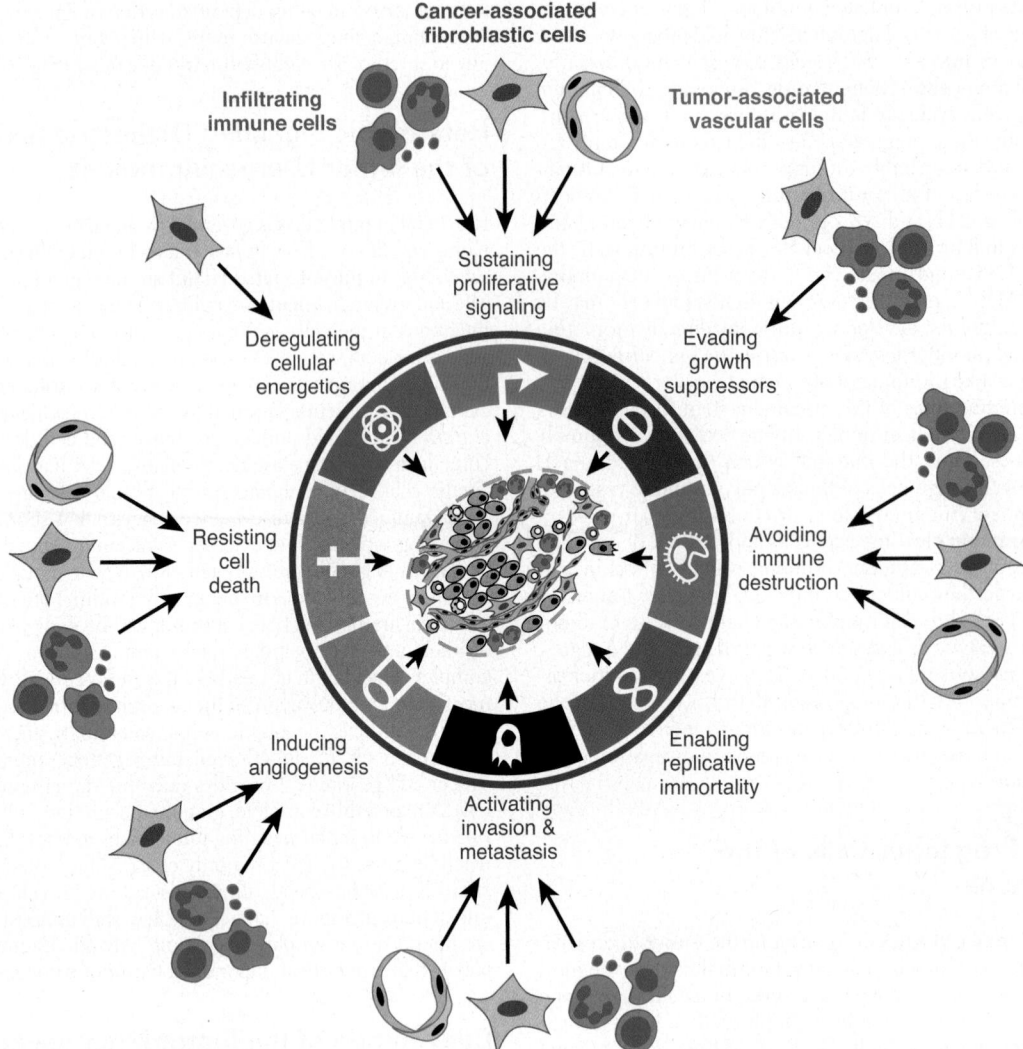

Figure 2.4 Diverse contributions of stromal cells to the hallmarks of cancer. Of the eight hallmark capabilities acquired by cancer cells, seven depend on contributions by stromal cells forming the tumor microenvironment.[2,213] The stromal cells can be divided into three general classes: infiltrating immune cells, cancer-associated fibroblastic cells, and tumor-associated vascular cells. The association of these corrupted cell types with the acquisition of individual hallmark capabilities has been documented through a variety of experimental approaches that are often supported by descriptive studies in human cancers. The relative importance of each of these stromal cell classes to a particular hallmark varies according to tumor type and stage of progression. (Adapted from Hanahan D, Coussens LM. Accessories to the crime: functions of cells recruited to the tumor microenvironment. *Cancer Cell* 2012;21:309–322.)

The circulating cancer cells that are released from primary tumors leave a microenvironment supported by this coevolved stroma. Upon landing in a distant organ, however, disseminated cancer cells must find a means to grow in a quite different tissue microenvironment. In some cases, newly seeded cancer cells must survive and expand in naïve, fully normal tissue microenvironments. In other cases, the newly encountered tissue microenvironments may already be supportive of such disseminated cancer cells, having been preconditioned prior to their arrival. Such permissive sites have been referred to as *premetastatic niches*.[146,244,245] These supportive niches may already preexist in distant tissues for various physiologic reasons,[101] including the actions of circulating factors dispatched systemically by primary tumors.[245]

The fact that signaling interactions between cancer cells and their supporting stroma are likely to evolve during the course of multistage primary tumor development and metastatic colonization clearly complicates the goal of fully elucidating the mechanisms of cancer pathogenesis. For example, this complexity poses challenges to systems biologists seeking to chart the crucial regulatory networks that orchestrate malignant progression, because much of the critical signaling is not intrinsic to cancer cells and instead operates through the interactions that these cells establish with their neighbors.

Cancer Cells, Cancer Stem Cells, and Intratumoral Heterogeneity

Cancer cells are the foundation of the disease. They initiate neoplastic development and drive tumor progression forward, having acquired the oncogenic and tumor suppressor mutations that define cancer as a genetic disease. Traditionally, the cancer cells within tumors have been portrayed as reasonably homogeneous cell populations until relatively late in the course of tumor progression, when hyperproliferation combined with increased genetic instability spawn genetically distinct clonal subpopulations. Reflecting such clonal heterogeneity, many human tumors are histopathologically diverse, containing regions demarcated by various

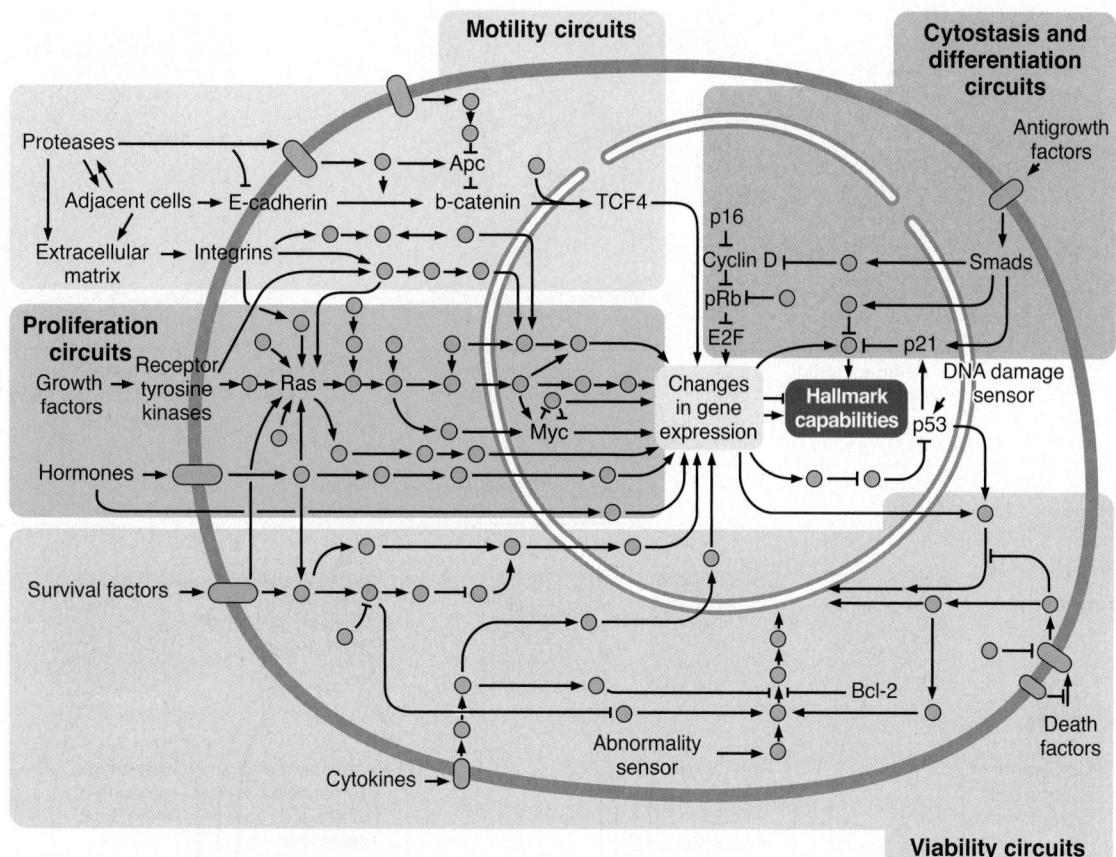

A

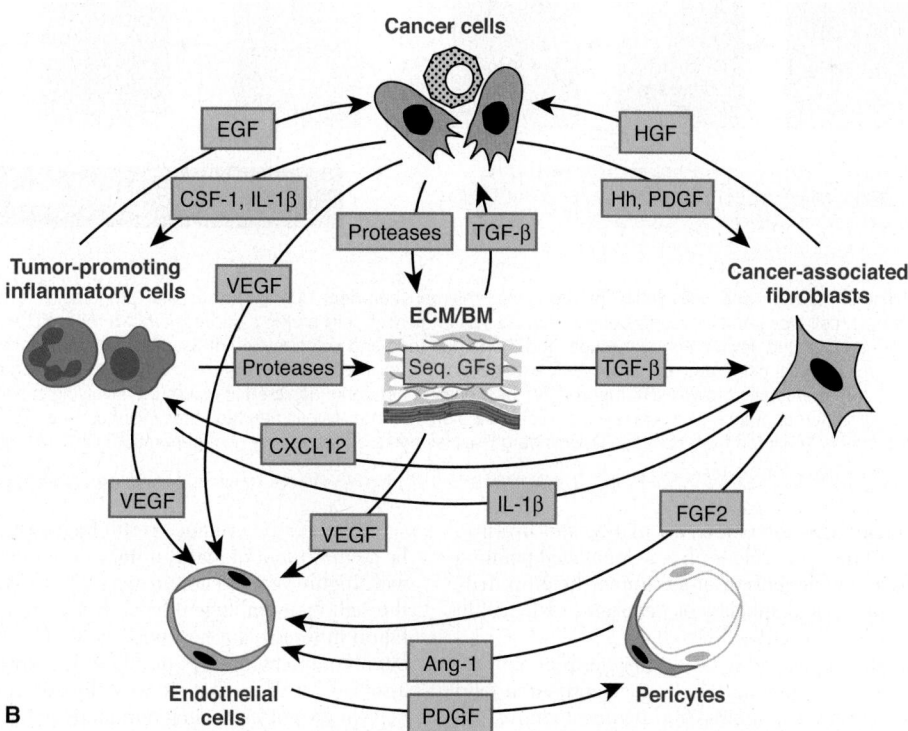

B

Figure 2.5 Reprogramming intracellular circuits and cell-to-cell signaling pathways dictates tumor inception and progression. An elaborate integrated circuit operating within normal cells is reprogrammed to regulate the hallmark capabilities acquired by cancer cells **(A)** and by associated stromal cells. Separate subcircuits, depicted here in differently colored fields, are specialized to orchestrate distinct capabilities. At one level, this depiction is simplistic, because there is considerable cross-talk between such subcircuits. More broadly, the integrated circuits operating inside cancer cells and stromal cells are interconnected via a complex network of signals transmitted by the various cells in the tumor microenvironment (in some cases via the extracellular matrix *[ECM]* and basement membranes *[BM]* they synthesize), of which a few signals are exemplified **(B).** HGF, hepatocyte growth factor for the cMet receptor; Hh, hedgehog ligand for the Patched (PTCH) receptor; Seq. GF, growth factors sequestered in the ECM/BM. (Adapted from Hanahan D, Weinberg RA. Hallmarks of cancer: the next generation. *Cell* 2011;144:646–674.)

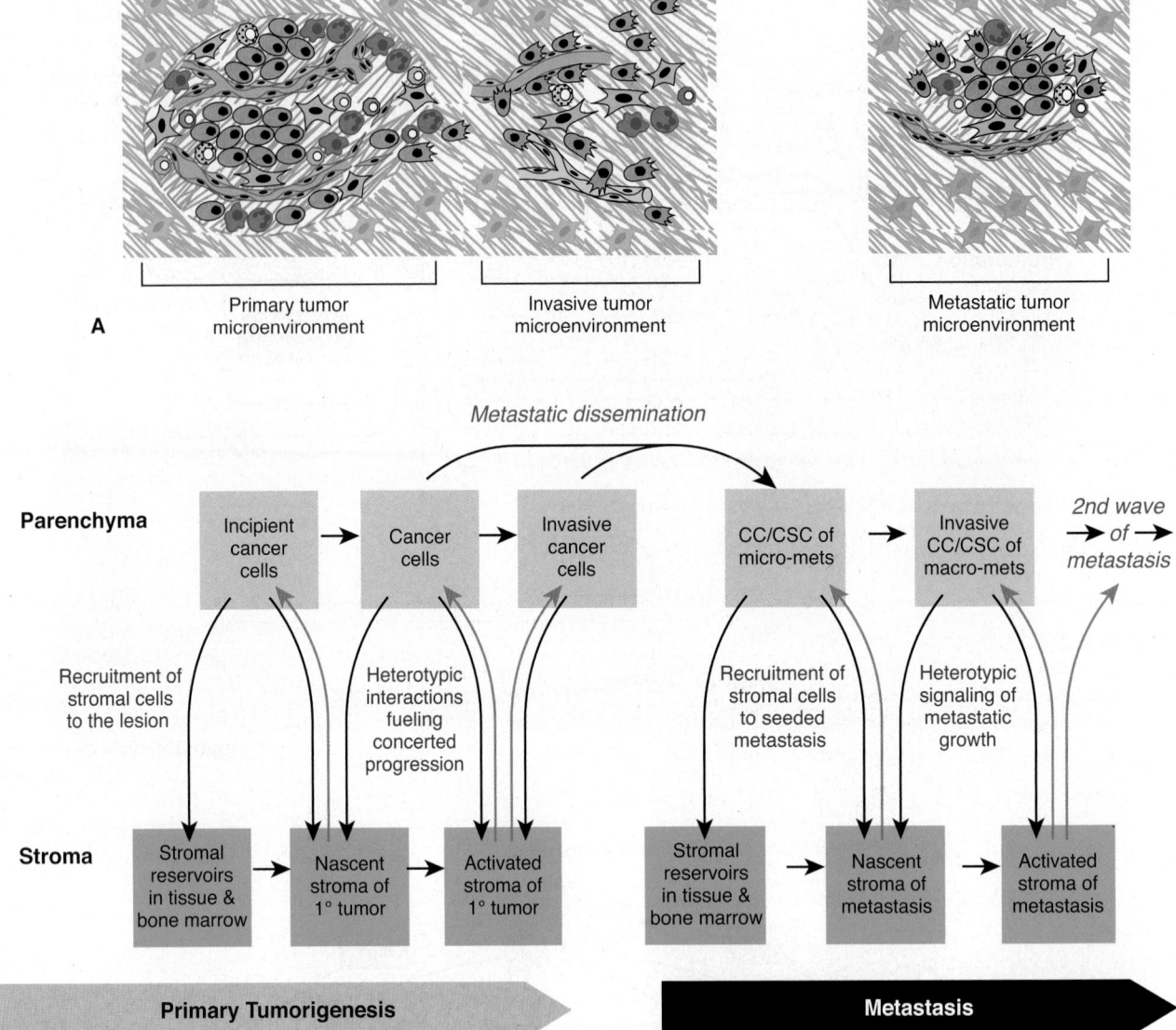

Figure 2.6 The dynamic variation and coevolution of the tumor microenvironment during the lesional progression of cancer. **(A)** Interactions between multiple stromal cell types and heterogeneously evolving mutant cancer cells create a succession of tumor microenvironments that change dynamically as tumors are initiated, invade normal tissues, and thereafter seed and colonize distant tissues. The abundance, histologic organization, and characteristics of the stromal cell types and associated extracellular matrix *(hatched background)* evolves during progression, thereby enabling primary, invasive, and then metastatic growth. **(B)** Importantly, the signaling networks depicted in Figure 2.5 involving cancer cells and their stromal collaborators change during tumor progression as a result of reciprocal signaling interactions between these various cells. CC, cancer cell; CSC, cancer stem cell; mets, metastases. (Adapted from Hanahan D, Weinberg RA. Hallmarks of cancer: the next generation. *Cell* 2011;144:646–674.)

degrees of differentiation, proliferation, vascularity, and invasiveness. In recent years, however, evidence has accumulated pointing to the existence of a new dimension of intratumor heterogeneity and a hitherto unappreciated subclass of neoplastic cells within tumors, termed cancer stem cells (CSC).

CSCs were initially implicated in the pathogenesis of hematopoietic malignancies,[246,247] and years later, were identified in solid tumors, in particular breast carcinomas and neuroectodermal tumors.[248,249] The fractionation of cancer cells on the basis of cell-surface markers has yielded subpopulations of neoplastic cells with a greatly enhanced ability, relative to the corresponding majority populations of non-CSCs, to seed new tumors upon implantation in immunodeficient mice. These, often rare, tumor-initiating cells have proven to share transcriptional profiles with certain normal tissue stem cells, thus justifying their designation as stemlike.

Although the evidence is still fragmentary, CSCs may prove to be a constituent of many, if not most tumors, albeit being present with highly variable abundance. CSCs are defined operationally through their ability to efficiently seed new tumors upon implantation into recipient host mice.[250–253] This functional definition is often complemented by profiling the expression of certain CSC-associated markers that are typically expressed by the normal stem cells in the corresponding normal tissues of origin.[249] Importantly, recent in vivo lineage-tracing experiments have provided an additional functional test of CSCs by demonstrating their ability to spawn large numbers of progeny, including non-CSCs within tumors.[250] At the same time, these experiments have provided the most compelling evidence to date that CSCs exist, and that they can be defined functionally through tests that do not depend on the implantation of tumor cells into appropriate mouse hosts.

The origins of CSCs within a solid tumor have not been clarified and, indeed, may well vary from one tumor type to another.[250,251,254] In some tumors, normal tissue stem cells may serve as the cells of origin that undergo oncogenic transformation to yield CSCs; in others, partially differentiated transit-amplifying cells, also termed progenitor cells, may suffer the initial oncogenic transformation, thereafter assuming more stemlike characters. Once primary tumors have formed, the CSCs, like their normal counterparts, may self-renew as well as spawn more differentiated derivatives. In the case of neoplastic CSCs, these descendant cells form the great bulk of many tumors and thus are responsible for creating many tumor-associated phenotypes. It remains to be established whether multiple distinct classes of increasingly neoplastic stem cells form during the inception and subsequent multistep progression of tumors, ultimately yielding the CSCs that have been described in fully developed cancers.

Recent research has interrelated the acquisition of CSC traits with the EMT transdifferentiation program discussed previously.[250,255] The induction of this program in certain model systems can induce many of the defining features of stem cells, including self-renewal ability and the antigenic phenotypes associated with both normal and cancer stem cells. This concordance suggests that the EMT program may not only enable cancer cells to physically disseminate from primary tumors, but can also confer on such cells the self-renewal capability that is crucial to their subsequent role as founders of new neoplastic colonies at sites of dissemination.[256] If generalized, this connection raises an important corollary hypothesis: The heterotypic signals that trigger an EMT, such as those released by an activated, inflammatory stroma, may also be important in creating and maintaining CSCs.

An increasing number of human tumors are reported to contain subpopulations with the properties of CSCs, as defined operationally through their efficient tumor-initiating capabilities upon xenotransplantation into mice. Nevertheless, the importance of CSCs as a distinct phenotypic subclass of neoplastic cells remains a matter of debate, as does their oft cited rarity within tumors.[254,257–259] Indeed, it is plausible that the phenotypic plasticity operating within tumors may produce bidirectional interconversion between CSCs and non-CSCs, resulting in dynamic variation in the relative abundance of CSCs.[250,260] Such plasticity could complicate a definitive measurement of their characteristic abundance. Analogous plasticity is already implicated in the EMT program, which can be engaged reversibly.[261]

These complexities notwithstanding, it is already evident that this new dimension of tumor heterogeneity holds important implications for successful cancer therapies. Increasing evidence in a variety of tumor types suggests that cells exhibiting the properties of CSCs are more resistant to various commonly used chemotherapeutic treatments.[255,262,263] Their persistence following initial treatment may help to explain the almost inevitable disease recurrence occurring after apparently successful debulking of human solid tumors by radiation and various forms of chemotherapy. Moreover, CSCs may well prove to underlie certain forms of tumor dormancy, whereby latent cancer cells persist for years or even decades after initial surgical resection or radio/chemotherapy, only to suddenly erupt and generate life-threatening disease. Hence, CSCs represent a double threat in that they are more resistant to therapeutic killing, and at the same time, are endowed with the ability to regenerate a tumor once therapy has been halted.

This phenotypic plasticity implicit in the CSC state may also enable the formation of functionally distinct subpopulations within a tumor that support overall tumor growth in various ways. Thus, an EMT can convert epithelial carcinoma cells into mesenchymal, fibroblast-like cancer cells that may well assume the duties of CAFs in some tumors (e.g., pancreatic ductal adenocarcinoma).[264] Intriguingly, several recent reports that have yet to be thoroughly validated in terms of generality, functional importance, or prevalence have documented the ability of glioblastoma cells (or possibly their associated CSC subpopulations) to transdifferentiate

into endothelial-like cells that can substitute for bona fide host-derived endothelial cells in forming a tumor-associated neovasculature.[265–267] These examples suggest that certain tumors may induce some of their own cancer cells to undergo various types of metamorphoses in order to generate stromal cell types needed to support tumor growth and progression, rather than relying on recruited host cells to provide the requisite hallmark-enabling functions.

Another form of phenotypic variability resides in the genetic heterogeneity of cancer cells within a tumor. Genomewide sequencing of cancer cells microdissected from different sectors of the same tumor[145] has revealed striking intratumoral genetic heterogeneity. Some of this genetic diversity may be reflected in the long recognized histologic heterogeneity within individual human tumors. Thus, genetic diversification may produce subpopulations of cancer cells that contribute distinct and complementary capabilities, which then accrue to the common benefit of overall tumor growth, progression, and resistance to therapy, as described earlier. Alternatively, such heterogeneity may simply reflect the genetic chaos that arises as tumor cell genomes become increasingly destabilized.

THERAPEUTIC TARGETING OF THE HALLMARKS OF CANCER

We do not attempt here to enumerate the myriad therapies that are currently under development or have been introduced of late into the clinic. Instead, we consider how the description of hallmark principles is likely to inform therapeutic development at present and may increasingly do so in the future. Thus, the rapidly growing armamentarium of therapeutics directed against specific molecular targets can be categorized according to their respective effects on one or more hallmark capabilities, as illustrated in the examples presented in Figure 2.7. Indeed, the observed efficacy of these drugs represents, in each case, a validation of a particular capability: If a capability is truly critical to the biology of tumors, then its inhibition should impair tumor growth and progression.

Unfortunately, however, the clinical responses elicited by these targeted therapies have generally been transitory, being followed all too often by relapse. One interpretation, which is supported by growing experimental evidence, is that each of the core hallmark capabilities is regulated by a set of partially redundant signaling pathways. Consequently, a targeted therapeutic agent inhibiting one key pathway in a tumor may not completely eliminate a hallmark capability, allowing some cancer cells to survive with residual function until they or their progeny eventually adapt to the selective pressure imposed by the initially applied therapy. Such adaptation can reestablish the expression of the functional capability, permitting renewed tumor growth and clinical relapse. Because the number of parallel signaling pathways supporting a given hallmark must be limited, it may become possible to therapeutically cotarget all of these supporting pathways, thereby preventing the development of adaptive resistance.

Another dimension of the plasticity of tumors under therapeutic attack is illustrated by the unanticipated responses to antiangiogenic therapy, in which cancer cells reduce their dependence on this hallmark capability by increasing their dependence on another. Thus, many observers anticipated that potent inhibition of angiogenesis would starve tumors of vital nutrients and oxygen, forcing them into dormancy and possibly leading to their dissolution.[86,87,268] Instead, the clinical responses to antiangiogenic therapies have been found to be transitory, followed by relapse, implicating adaptive or evasive resistance mechanisms.[220,269–271] One such mechanism of evasive resistance, observed in certain preclinical models of antiangiogenic therapy, involves reduced dependence on continuing angiogenesis by increasing the activity of two other capabilities: invasiveness and metastasis.[269–271] By invading nearby and distant tissues, initially hypoxic cancer cells gain access to normal,

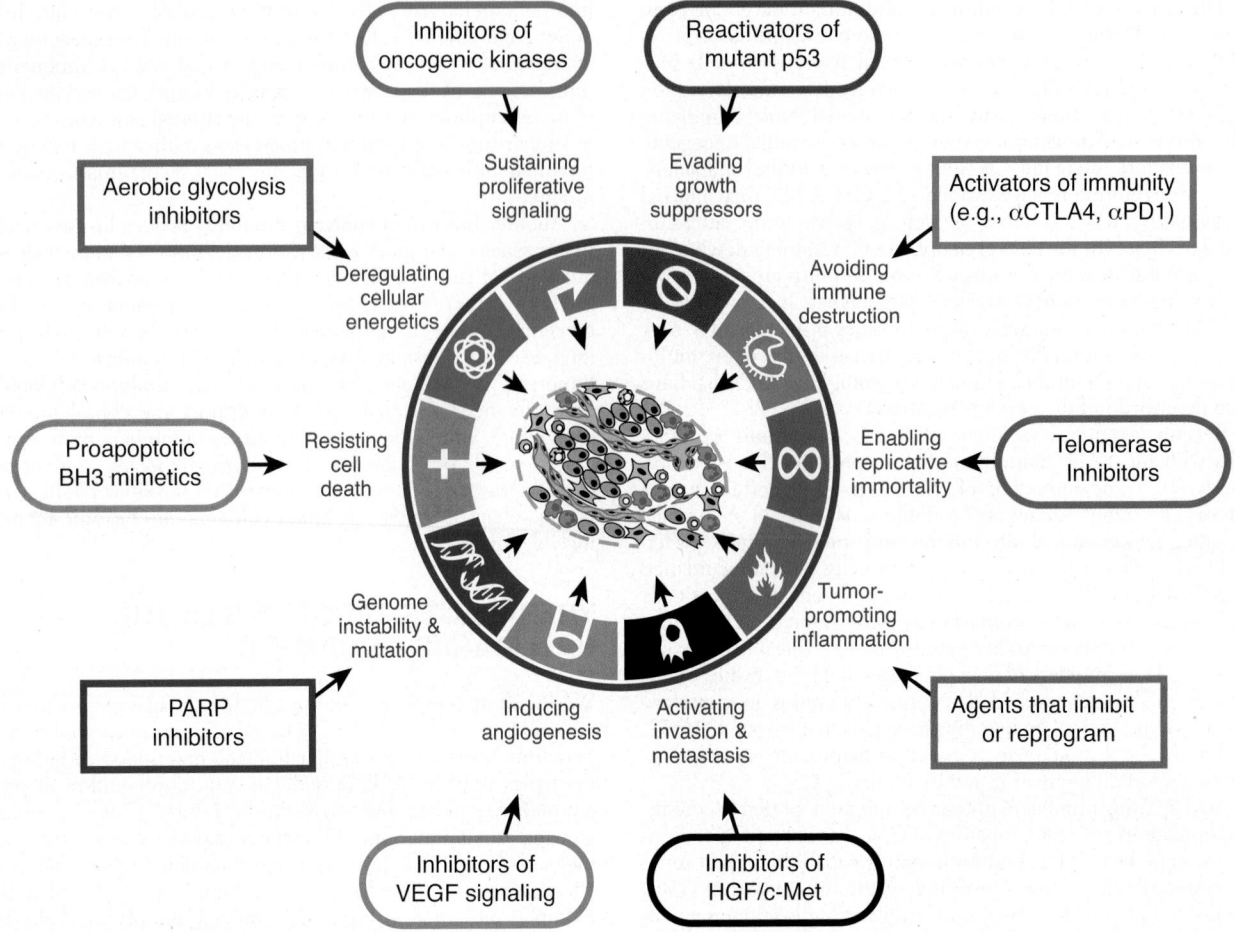

Figure 2.7 Therapeutic targeting of the hallmarks of cancer. Drugs that interfere with each of the hallmark capabilities and hallmark-enabling processes have been developed and are in preclinical and/or clinical testing, and in some cases, approved for use in treating certain forms of human cancer. A focus on antagonizing specific hallmark capabilities is likely to yield insights into developing novel, highly effective therapeutic strategies. PARP, poly ADP ribose polymerase. (Adapted from Hanahan D, Weinberg RA. Hallmarks of cancer: the next generation. *Cell* 2011;144:646–674.)

preexisting tissue vasculature. The initial clinical validation of this adaptive/evasive resistance is apparent in the increased invasion and local metastasis seen when human glioblastomas are treated with antiangiogenic therapies.[272–274] The applicability of this lesson to other human cancers has yet to be established.

Analogous adaptive shifts in dependence on other hallmark traits may also limit the efficacy of analogous hallmark-targeting therapies. For example, the deployment of apoptosis-inducing drugs may induce cancer cells to hyperactivate mitogenic signaling, enabling them to compensate for the initial attrition triggered by such treatments. Such considerations suggest that drug development and the design of treatment protocols will benefit from incorporating the concepts of functionally discrete hallmark capabilities and of the multiple biochemical pathways involved in supporting each of them. For these reasons, we envisage that attacking multiple hallmark capabilities with hallmark-targeting drugs (see Fig. 2.7), in carefully considered combinations, sequences, and temporal regimens,[275] will result in increasingly effective therapies that produce more durable clinical responses.

CONCLUSION AND A VISION FOR THE FUTURE

Looking ahead, we envision significant advances in our understanding of invasion and metastasis during the coming decade. Similarly, the role of altered energy metabolism in malignant growth will be

elucidated, including a resolution of whether this metabolic reprogramming is a discrete capability separable from the core hallmark of chronically sustained proliferation. We are excited about the new frontier of immunotherapy, which will be empowered to leverage detailed knowledge about the regulation of immune responses in order to develop pharmacologic tools that can modulate them therapeutically for the purpose of effectively and sustainably attacking tumors and, most importantly, their metastases.

Other areas are currently in rapid flux. In recent years, elaborate molecular mechanisms controlling transcription through chromatin modifications have been uncovered, and there are clues that specific shifts in chromatin configuration occur during the acquisition of certain hallmark capabilities.[195,196] Functionally significant epigenetic alterations seem likely to be factors not only in the cancer cells, but also in the altered cells of the tumor-associated stroma. At present, it is unclear whether an elucidation of these epigenetic mechanisms will materially change our overall understanding of the means by which hallmark capabilities are acquired, or simply add additional detail to the regulatory circuitry that is already known to govern them.

Similarly, the discovery of hundreds of distinct regulatory microRNAs has already led to profound changes in our understanding of the molecular control mechanisms that operate in health and disease. By now, dozens of microRNAs have been implicated in various tumor phenotypes.[276,277] Still, these only scratch the surface of the true complexity, because the functions of hundreds of microRNAs known to be present in our cells and to be altered in expression levels in different forms of cancer remain total mysteries. Here again, we are unclear whether future progress will cause fundamental shifts in our understanding of the pathogenic mechanisms of cancer, or only add detail to the elaborate regulatory circuits that have already been mapped out.

Finally, the existing diagrams of heterotypic interactions between the multiple distinct cell types that collaborate to produce malignant tumors are still rudimentary. We anticipate that, in another decade, the signaling pathways describing the intercommunication between these various cell types within tumors will be charted in far greater detail and clarity, eclipsing our current knowledge. And, as before,[1,2] we continue to foresee cancer research as an increasingly logical science, in which myriad phenotypic complexities are manifestations of an underlying organizing principle.

ACKNOWLEDGMENT

This chapter is modified from Hanahan D, Weinberg RA. Hallmarks of cancer: the next generation. *Cell* 2011;144(5):646–674.

SELECTED REFERENCES

The full reference list can be accessed at lwwhealthlibrary.com/oncology.

1. Hanahan D, Weinberg R. The hallmarks of cancer. *Cell* 2000;100:57–70.
2. Hanahan D, Weinberg RA. Hallmarks of cancer: the next generation. *Cell* 2011;144:646–674.
3. Lemmon MA, Schlessinger J. Cell signaling by receptor tyrosine kinases. *Cell* 2010;141:1117–1134.
7. Franco OE, Shaw AK, Strand DW, et al. Cancer associated fibroblasts in cancer pathogenesis. *Semin Cell Dev Biol* 2010;21:33–39.
9. Davies MA, Samuels Y. Analysis of the genome to personalize therapy for melanoma. *Oncogene* 2010;29:5545–5555.
11. Yuan TL, Cantley LC. PI3K pathway alterations in cancer: variations on a theme. *Oncogene* 2008;27:5497–5510.
12. Wertz IE, Dixit VM. Regulation of death receptor signaling by the ubiquitin system. *Cell Death Differ* 2010;17:14–24.
14. Amit I, Citri A, Shay T, et al. A module of negative feedback regulators defines growth factor signaling. *Nature Genet* 2007;39:503–512.
16. Sudarsanam S, Johnson DE. Functional consequences of mTOR inhibition. *Curr Opin Drug Discov Devel* 2010;13:31–40.
18. Dang CV. MYC on the path to cancer. *Cell* 2012;149:22–35.
20. Evan GI, d'Adda di Fagagna F. Cellular senescence: hot or what? *Curr Opin Genet Dev* 2009;19:25–31.
22. Mooi WJ, Peeper DS. Oncogene-induced cell senescence—halting on the road to cancer. *N Engl J Med* 2006;355:1037–1046.
23. Burkhart DL, Sage J. Cellular mechanisms of tumour suppression by the retinoblastoma gene. *Nat Rev Cancer* 2008;8:671–682.
28. McClatchey AI, Yap AS. Contact inhibition (of proliferation) redux. *Curr Opin Cell Biol.* 2012;24:685–694.
31. Stamenkovic I, Yu Q. Merlin, a "magic" linker between the extracellular cues and intracellular signaling pathways that regulate cell motility, proliferation, and survival. *Curr Protein Pept Sci* 2010;11:471–484.
32. Pickup M, Novitskiy S, Moses HL. The roles of TGFβ in the tumour microenvironment. *Nat Rev Cancer* 2013;13:788–799.
34. Massagué J. TGF-beta in cancer. *Cell* 2008;134:215–230.
36. Strasser A, Cory S, Adams JM. Deciphering the rules of programmed cell death to improve therapy of cancer and other diseases. *EMBO J* 2011;30:3667–3683.
40. Junttila MR, Evan GI. p53—a jack of all trades but master of none. *Nat Rev Cancer* 2009;9:821–829.
41. White E. Deconvoluting the context-dependent role for autophagy in cancer. *Nat Rev Cancer* 2012;12:401–410.
42. Levine B, Kroemer G. Autophagy in the pathogenesis of disease. *Cell* 2008;132:27–42.
48. Amaravadi RK, Thompson CB. The roles of therapy-induced autophagy and necrosis in cancer treatment. *Clin Cancer Res* 2007;13:7271–7279.
50. Vanden Berghe T, Linkermann A, Jouan-Lanhouet S, et al. Regulated necrosis: the expanding network of non-apoptotic cell death pathways. *Nat Rev Mol Cell Biol* 2014;15:135–147.
51. Galluzzi L, Kroemer G. Necroptosis: a specialized pathway of programmed necrosis. *Cell* 2008;135:1161–1163.
53. Grivennikov SI, Greten FR, Karin M. Immunity, inflammation, and cancer. *Cell* 2010;140:883–899.
57. Shay JW, Wright WE. Telomeres and telomerase in cancer. *Sem Cancer Biol* 2011;21:349–353.
58. Artandi SE, DePinho RA. Telomeres and telomerase in cancer. *Carcinogenesis* 2010;31:9–18.
59. Cesare AJ, Reddel RR. Alternative lengthening of telomeres: models, mechanisms and implications. *Nat Rev Genet* 2010;11:319–330.
63. Sherr CJ, DePinho RA. Cellular senescence: mitotic clock or culture shock? *Cell* 2000;102:407–410.
64. Feldser DM, Greider CW. Short telomeres limit tumor progression in vivo by inducing senescence. *Cancer Cell* 2007;11:461–469.
68. Raynaud CM, Hernandez J, Llorca FP, et al. DNA damage repair and telomere length in normal breast, preneoplastic lesions, and invasive cancer. *Am J Clin Oncol* 2010;33:341–345.
70. Hanahan D, Folkman J. Patterns and emerging mechanisms of the angiogenic switch during tumorigenesis. *Cell* 1996;86:353–364.
71. Baeriswyl V, Christofori G. The angiogenic switch in carcinogenesis. *Semin Cancer Biol* 2009;19:329–337.
75. Carmeliet P. VEGF as a key mediator of angiogenesis in cancer. *Oncology* 2005;69:4–10.
76. Kessenbrock K, Plaks V, Werb Z. Matrix metalloproteinases: regulators of the tumor microenvironment. *Cell* 2010;141:52–67.
78. Nagy JA, Chang SH, Shih SC, et al. Heterogeneity of the tumor vasculature. *Semin Thromb Hemost* 2010;36:321–331.
81. Olive KP, Jacobetz MA, Davidson CJ, et al. Inhibition of Hedgehog signaling enhances delivery of chemotherapy in a mouse model of pancreatic cancer. *Science* 2009;324:1457–1461.
84. Xie L, Duncan MB, Pahler J, et al. Counterbalancing angiogenic regulatory factors control the rate of cancer progression and survival in a stage-specific manner. *Proc Natl Acad Sci U S A* 2011;108:9939–9944.
91. Raza A, Franklin MJ, Dudek AZ. Pericytes and vessel maturation during tumor angiogenesis and metastasis. *Am J Hematol* 2010;85:593–598.
94. Qian BZ, Pollard JW. Macrophage diversity enhances tumor progression and metastasis. *Cell* 2010;141:39–51.
98. Ferrara N. Pathways mediating VEGF-independent tumor angiogenesis. *Cytokine Growth Factor Rev* 2010;21:21–26.
101. Talmadge JE, Fidler IJ. AACR centennial series: the biology of cancer metastasis: historical perspective. *Cancer Res* 2010;70:5649–5669.
103. Berx G, van Roy F. Involvement of members of the cadherin superfamily in cancer. *Cold Spring Harb Perspect Biol* 2009;1:a003129.
105. De Craene B, Berx G. Regulatory networks defining EMT during cancer initiation and progression. *Nat Rev Cancer* 2013;13:97–110.
107. Polyak K, Weinberg RA. Transitions between epithelial and mesenchymal states: acquisition of malignant and stem cell traits. *Nat Rev Cancer* 2009;9:265–273.
108. Thiery JP, Acloque H, Huang RY, et al. Epithelial-mesenchymal transitions in development and disease. *Cell* 2009;139:871–890.
113. Schmalhofer O, Brabletz S, Brabletz T. E-cadherin, beta-catenin, and ZEB1 in malignant progression of cancer. *Cancer Metastasis Rev* 2009;28:151–166.
114. Yang J, Weinberg RA. Epithelial-mesenchymal transition: at the crossroads of development and tumor metastasis. *Develop Cell* 2008;14:818–829.
116. Karnoub AE, Weinberg RA. Chemokine networks and breast cancer metastasis. *Breast Dis* 2006;26:75–85.
119. Egeblad M, Nakasone ES, Werb Z. Tumors as organs: complex tissues that interface with the entire organism. *Dev Cell* 2010;18:884–901.
120. Joyce JA, Pollard JW. Microenvironmental regulation of metastasis. *Nat Rev Cancer* 2009;9:239–252.
124. Palermo C, Joyce JA. Cysteine cathepsin proteases as pharmacological targets in cancer. *Trends Pharmacol Sci* 2008;29:22–28.
125. Mohamed MM, Sloane BF. Cysteine cathepsins: multifunctional enzymes in cancer. *Nat Rev Cancer* 2006;6:764–775.
128. Hugo H, Ackland ML, Blick T, et al. Epithelial-mesenchymal and mesenchymal-epithelial transitions in carcinoma progression. *J Cell Physiol* 2007;213:374–383.
129. Friedl P, Wolf K. Plasticity of cell migration: a multiscale tuning model. *J Cell Biol* 2009;188:11–19.
131. Madsen CD, Sahai E. Cancer dissemination—lessons from leukocytes. *Dev Cell* 2010;19:13–26.
133. Quail DF, Joyce JA. Microenvironmental regulation of tumor progression and metastasis. *Nat Med* 2013;19:1423–1437.
135. Aguirre-Ghiso JA. Models, mechanisms and clinical evidence for cancer dormancy. *Nat Rev Cancer* 2007;7:834–846.
137. Demicheli R, Retsky MW, Hrushesky WJ, et al. The effects of surgery on tumor growth: a century of investigations. *Ann Oncol* 2008;19:1821–1828.
141. Kenific CM, Thorburn A, Debnath J. Autophagy and metastasis: another double-edged sword. *Curr Opin Cell Biol* 2010;22:241–245.
142. Teng MW, Swann JB, Koebel CM, et al. Immune-mediated dormancy: an equilibrium with cancer. *J Leukoc Biol* 2008;84:988–993.
144. Luebeck EG. Cancer: genomic evolution of metastasis. *Nature* 2010;467:1053–1055.
147. Klein CA. Parallel progression of primary tumours and metastases. *Nat Rev Cancer* 2009;9:302–312.

148. Gerhardt H, Semb H. Pericytes: gatekeepers in tumour cell metastasis? *J Mol Med* 2008;86:135–144.

149. Kim MY, Oskarsson T, Acharyya S, et al. Tumor self-seeding by circulating cancer cells. *Cell* 2009;139:1315–1326.

152. Nguyen DX, Bos PD, Massagué J. Metastasis: from dissemination to organ-specific colonization. *Nat Rev Cancer* 2009;9:274–284.

158. Hsu PP, Sabatini DM. Cancer cell metabolism: Warburg and beyond. *Cell* 2008;134:703–707.

159. Ward PS, Thompson CB. Metabolic reprogramming: a cancer hallmark even warburg did not anticipate. *Cancer Cell* 2012;21:297–308.

160. Semenza GL. HIF-1: upstream and downstream of cancer metabolism. *Curr Opin Genet Dev* 2010;20:51–56.

162. Kroemer G, Pouyssegur J. Tumor cell metabolism: cancer's Achilles' heel. *Cancer Cell* 2008;13:472–482.

164. Vander Heiden MG, Cantley LC, Thompson CB. Understanding the Warburg effect: the metabolic requirements of cell proliferation. *Science* 2009;324:1029–1033.

165. Semenza GL. Tumor metabolism: cancer cells give and take lactate. *J Clin Invest* 2008;118:3835–3837.

166. Nakajima EC, Van Houten B. Metabolic symbiosis in cancer: refocusing the Warburg lens. *Mol Carcinog* 2013;52:329–337.

168. Feron O. Pyruvate into lactate and back: from the Warburg effect to symbiotic energy fuel exchange in cancer cells. *Radiother Oncol* 2009;92:329–333.

173. Vajdic CM, van Leeuwen MT. Cancer incidence and risk factors after solid organ transplantation. *Int J Cancer* 2009;125:1747–1754.

174. Elinav E, Nowarski R, Thaiss CA, et al. Inflammation-induced cancer: crosstalk between tumours, immune cells and microorganisms. *Nat Rev Cancer* 2013;13:759–771.

177. Galon J, Angell HK, Bedognetti D, et al. The continuum of cancer immunosurveillance: prognostic, predictive, and mechanistic signatures. *Immunity* 2013;39:11–26.

178. Kim R, Emi M, Tanabe K. Cancer immunoediting from immune surveillance to immune escape. *Immunology* 2007;121:1–14.

180. Bindea G, Mlecnik B, Fridman WH, et al. Natural immunity to cancer in humans. *Curr Opin Immunol* 2010;22:215–222.

183. Pagès F, Galon J, Dieu-Nosjean MC, et al. Immune infiltration in human tumors: a prognostic factor that should not be ignored. *Oncogene* 2010;29:1093–1102.

185. Yang L, Pang Y, Moses HL. TGF-beta and immune cells: an important regulatory axis in the tumor microenvironment and progression. *Trends Immunol* 2010;31:220–227.

186. Shields JD, Kourtis IC, Tomei AA, et al. Induction of lymphoidlike stroma and immune escape by tumors that express the chemokine CCL21. *Science* 2010;328:749–752.

189. Pardoll DM. The blockade of immune checkpoints in cancer immunotherapy. *Nat Rev Cancer* 2012;12:252–264.

190. Motz GT, Coukos G. Deciphering and reversing tumor immune suppression. *Immunity* 2013;39:61–73.

191. Gabrilovich DI, Nagaraj S. Myeloid-derived suppressor cells as regulators of the immune system. *Nat Rev Immunol* 2009;9:162–174.

192. Mougiakakos D, Choudhury A, Lladser A, et al. Regulatory T cells in cancer. *Adv Cancer Res* 2010;107:57–117.

195. You JS, Jones PA. Cancer genetics and epigenetics: two sides of the same coin? *Cancer Cell* 2012;22:9–20.

196. Berdasco M, Esteller M. Aberrant epigenetic landscape in cancer: how cellular identity goes awry. *Dev Cell* 2010;19:698–711.

199. Negrini S, Gorgoulis VG, Halazoneitis TD. Genomic instability—an evolving hallmark of cancer. *Nat Rev Mol Cell Bio* 2010;11:220–228.

201. Jackson SP, Bartek J. The DNA-damage response in human biology and disease. *Nature* 2009;461:1071–1078.

204. Lane DP. Cancer. p53, guardian of the genome. *Nature* 1992;358:15–16.

205. Kinzler KW, Vogelstein B. Cancer-susceptibility genes. Gatekeepers and caretakers. *Nature* 1997;386:761–763.

206. Ciccia A, Elledge SJ. The DNA damage response: making it safe to play with knives. *Mol Cell* 2010;40:179–204.

209. Barnes DE, Lindahl T. Repair and genetic consequences of endogenous DNA base damage in mammalian cells. *Annu Rev Genet* 2004;38:445–476.

210. Korkola J, Gray JW. Breast cancer genomes—form and function. *Curr Opin Genet Dev* 2010;20:4–14.

211. Dvorak HF. Tumors: wounds that do not heal. Similarities between tumor stroma generation and wound healing. *N Engl J Med* 1986;315:1650–1659.

213. Hanahan D, Coussens LM. Accessories to the crime: functions of cells recruited to the tumor microenvironment. *Cancer Cell* 2012;21:309–322.

214. de Visser KE, Eichten A, Coussens LM. Paradoxical roles of the immune system during cancer development. *Nat Rev Cancer* 2006;6:24–37.

215. Servais C, Erez N. From sentinel cells to inflammatory culprits: cancer-associated fibroblasts in tumour-related inflammation. *J Pathol* 2013;229:198–207.

217. Pietras K, Ostman A. Hallmarks of cancer: interactions with the tumor stroma. *Exp Cell Res* 2010;316:1324–1331.

220. Welti J, Loges S, Dimmeler S, et al. Recent molecular discoveries in angiogenesis and antiangiogenic therapies in cancer. *J Clin Invest* 2013;123:3190–3200.

221. Pasquale EB. Eph receptors and ephrins in cancer: bidirectional signalling and beyond. *Nat Rev Cancer* 2010;10:165–180.

224. Carmeliet P, Jain RK. Angiogenesis in cancer and other diseases. *Nature* 2000;407:249–257.

225. Ruoslahti E, Bhatia SN, Sailor MJ. Targeting of drugs and nanoparticles to tumors. *J Cell Biol* 2010;188:759–768.

227. Motz GT, Coukos G. The parallel lives of angiogenesis and immunosuppression: cancer and other tales. *Nat Rev Immunol* 2011;11:702–711.

228. Carmeliet P, Jain RK. Principles and mechanisms of vessel normalization for cancer and other angiogenic diseases. *Nat Rev Drug Discov* 2011;10:417–427.

229. Tammela T, Alitalo K. Lymphangiogenesis: Molecular mechanisms and future promise. *Cell* 2010;140:460–476.

230. Card CM, Yu SS, Swartz MA. Emerging roles of lymphatic endothelium in regulating adaptive immunity. *J Clin Invest* 2014;124:943–952.

231. Gaengel K, Genové G, Armulik A, et al. Endothelial-mural cell signaling in vascular development and angiogenesis. *Arterioscler Thromb Vasc Biol* 2009;29:630–638.

232. Schäfer M, Werner S. Cancer as an overhealing wound: an old hypothesis revisited. *Nat Rev Mol Cell Biol* 2008;9:628–638.

233. Karin M, Lawrence T, Nizet V. Innate immunity gone awry: linking microbial infections to chronic inflammation and cancer. *Cell* 2006;124:823–835.

234. Coffeldt SB, Lewis CE, Naldini L, et al. Elusive identities and overlapping phenotypes of proangiogenic myeloid cells in tumors. *Am J Pathol* 2010;176:1564–1576.

237. Mantovani A, Allavena P, Sica A, et al. Cancer-related inflammation. *Nature* 2008;454:436–444

238. DeNardo DG, Brennan DJ, Rexhepaj E, et al. Leukocyte complexity predicts breast cancer survival and functionally regulates response to chemotherapy. *Cancer Discov* 2011;1:54–67.

239. De Palma M, Coukos G, Hanahan D. A new twist on radiation oncology: low-dose irradiation elicits immunostimulatory macrophages that unlock barriers to tumor immunotherapy. *Cancer Cell* 2013;24:559–561.

240. Koh BI, Kang Y. The pro-metastatic role of bone marrow-derived cells: a focus on MSCs and regulatory T cells. *EMBO Rep* 2012;13:412–422.

243. Giaccia AJ, Schipani E. Role of carcinoma-associated fibroblasts and hypoxia in tumor progression. *Curr Top Microbiol Immunol* 2010;345:31–45.

244. Labelle M, Hynes RO. The initial hours of metastasis: the importance of cooperative host-tumor cell interactions during hematogenous dissemination. *Cancer Discov* 2012;2:1091–1099.

245. Peinado H, Lavothskin S, Lyden D. The secreted factors responsible for premetastatic niche formation: old sayings and new thoughts. *Semin Cancer Biol* 2011;21:139–146.

246. Reya T, Morrison SJ, Clarke MF, et al. Stem cells, cancer, and cancer stem cells. *Nature* 2001;414:105–111.

248. Gilbertson RJ, Rich JN. Making a tumour's bed: glioblastoma stem cells and the vascular niche. *Nat Rev Cancer* 2007;7:733–736.

250. Beck B, Blanpain C. Unravelling cancer stem cell potential. *Nat Rev Cancer* 2013;13:727–738.

251. Magee JA, Piskounova E, Morrison SJ. Cancer stem cells: impact, heterogeneity, and uncertainty. *Cancer Cell* 2012;21:283–296.

254. Meacham CE, Morrison SJ. Tumour heterogeneity and cancer cell plasticity. *Nature* 2013;501:328–337.

255. Singh A, Settleman J. EMT, cancer stem cells and drug resistance: an emerging axis of evil in the war on cancer. *Oncogene* 2010;29:4741–4751.

256. Brabletz T, Jung A, Spaderna S, et al. Opinion: migrating cancer stem cells—an integrated concept of malignant tumor progression. *Nat Rev Cancer* 2005;5:744–749.

258. Gupta P, Chaffer CL, Weinberg RA. Cancer stem cells: mirage or reality? *Nature Med* 2009;15:1010–1012.

260. Chaffer CL, Brueckmann I, Scheel C, et al. Normal and neoplastic nonstem cells can spontaneously convert to stem-like state. *Proc Natl Acad Sci U S A* 2011;108:7950–7955.

261. Thiery JP, Sleeman JR. Complex networks orchestrate epithelial-mesenchymal transitions. *Nat Rev Mol Cell Biol* 2006;7:131–142.

262. Creighton CJ, Li X, Landis M, et al. Residual breast cancers after conventional therapy display mesenchymal as well as tumor-initiating features. *Proc Natl Acad Sci U S A* 2009;106:13820–13825.

264. Rhim AD, Mirek ET, Aiello NM, et al. EMT and dissemination precede pancreatic tumor formation. *Cell* 2012;148:349–361.

265. Soda Y, Marumoto T, Friedmann-Morvinski D, et al. Transdifferentiation of glioblastoma cells into vascular endothelial cells. *Proc Natl Acad Sci U S A* 2011;108:4274–4280.

267. Wang R, Chadalavada K, Wilshire J, et al. Glioblastoma stem-like cells give rise to tumour endothelium. *Nature* 2010;468:829–833.

268. Folkman J, Kalluri R. Cancer without disease. *Nature* 2004;427:787.

270. Ebos JM, Lee CR, Kerbel RS. Tumor and host-mediated pathways of resistance and disease progression in response to antiangiogenic therapy. *Clin Cancer Res* 2009;15:5020–5025.

271. Bergers G, Hanahan D. Modes of resistance to anti-angiogenic therapy. *Nat Rev Cancer* 2008;8:592–603.

273. Norden AD, Drappatz J, Wen PY. Antiangiogenic therapies for high-grade glioma. *Nat Rev Neurol* 2009;5:610–620.

275. Hanahan D. Rethinking the war on cancer. *Lancet* 2014;383:558–563.

276. Pencheva N, Tavazoie SF. Control of metastatic progression by microRNA regulatory networks. *Nat Cell Biol* 2013;15:546–554.

277. Garzon R, Marcucci G, Croce CM. Targeting microRNAs in cancer: rationale, strategies and challenges. *Nat Rev Drug Discov* 2010;9:775–789.

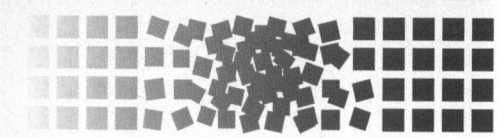

3 Molecular Methods in Cancer

Larissa V. Furtado, Jay L. Hess, and Bryan L. Betz

APPLICATIONS OF MOLECULAR DIAGNOSTICS IN ONCOLOGY

Molecular diagnostics is increasingly impacting a number of areas of cancer care delivery including diagnosis, prognosis, in predicting response to particular therapies, and in minimal residual disease monitoring. Each of these depends on detection or measurement of one or more disease-specific molecular biomarkers representing abnormalities in genetic or epigenetic pathways controlling cellular proliferation, differentiation, or cell death (Table 3.1). In addition, molecular diagnostics is beginning to play a role in predicting host metabolism of drugs—for example, in predicting fast versus slow thiopurine metabolizers using polymorphisms in the thiopurine methyltransferase (TPMT) allele and in use in dosing patients with thiopurine drugs.[1] Molecular diagnostics has also had a major impact on assessing an engraftment after bone marrow transplantation and in tissue typing for bone marrow and solid organ transplantation.

The ideal cancer biomarker is only associated with the disease and not the normal state. The utility of the biomarker largely depends on what the clinical effect the biomarker predicts for, how large the effect is, and how strong the evidence is for the effect. For clinical application, biomarkers need a high level of *analytic validity*, *clinical validity*, and *clinical utility*. Analytic validity refers to the ability of the overall testing process to accurately detect and, in many cases, measure the biomarker. Clinical validity is the ability of a biomarker to predict a particular disease behavior or response to therapy. Clinical utility, arguably the most difficult to assess, addresses whether the information available from the biomarker is actually beneficial for patient care.

Biomarkers can take many forms including *chromosomal translocations* and *other chromosomal rearrangements*, *gene amplification*, *copy number variation*, *point mutations*, *single nucleotide polymorphisms*, *changes in gene expression* (including micro RNAs), and *epigenetic alterations*. Most biomarkers in widespread use represent either gain of function or loss of function alterations in key signaling pathways. Those that occur early and at a high frequency in tumors tend to be *driver mutations*, whose function is important for the cancer cell's proliferation and/or survival. These are particularly useful as biomarkers because they often represent important therapeutic targets. However, cancer cells accumulate many genetic alterations, called *passenger mutations*, which tend to occur at a lower frequency overall and in a subset of a heterogeneous population of tumor cells that may contribute to the cancer phenotype but are not absolutely essential.[2] Distinguishing passenger from driver mutations using various functional assays has become a major focus of translational research in cancer. The same biomarker may have utility in a variety of settings. For example, the detection of the *BCR-ABL1* translocation, pathognomonic for chronic myelogenous leukemia (CML), is used for establishing the diagnosis, for the selection of therapy, and for monitoring for minimal residual disease during and after therapy.

Some of the most heavily used genetic biomarkers in cancer, particularly in hematologic malignancies, are *chromosomal translocations*. For certain diseases such as CML, detection of the *BCR-ABL1* translocation or in Burkitt lymphoma the immunoglobulin gene-*MYC* translocation is required, according to current World Health Organization (WHO) guidelines, to make the diagnosis. Identification of translocations is important in the diagnosis and subtyping of acute leukemias (e.g., detection of *PML-RARA* and variant translocations in acute promyelocytic leukemia) and is also extremely important for the diagnosis of sarcomas such as Ewing sarcoma. The discovery of chromosomal translocations, such as the *TMPRSS-ETS* in prostate cancer and *ALK* translocations in non–small-cell lung cancer, portends an importance of detecting translocations in solid tumors.[3] Chromosomal translocations, especially for hematologic malignancies, have been traditionally detected by classical karyotyping. This approach has limitations; in particular, it requires viable, dividing cells, which are often not readily available from solid tumor biopsies. In addition, a significant proportion of chromosomal translocations are not detectable by conventional karyotyping. For example, 5% to 10% of CML cases lack detectable t(9;22) by G banding. Such "cryptic" translocations require other approaches for detection, which are to be discussed, including *fluorescent in situ hybridization (FISH)*, *polymerase chain reaction (PCR)*, as well as *nucleic acid sequencing-based methods*.

In certain settings, it can be helpful to detect if a population of cells is clonal. For example, in some lymphoid infiltrates, the cells are well differentiated and it can be difficult to determine whether these represent a reactive or neoplastic infiltrate. If dispersed, cells are available and these could be analyzed by flow cytometer to detect whether a monotypic population expressing either immunoglobulin kappa or lambda light chains is present. In theory, immunohistochemical staining (IHC) for immunoglobulin light chains could be used to assess clonality; however, in practice this is done with more sensitivity using RNA in situ hybridization for immunoglobulin kappa and lambda light chain transcripts. The most sensitive way to detect clonality in a B-cell population is to analyze the size of the break point cluster region that arises as a result of VDJ recombination by *PCR*. Reactive B cells will show a distribution in the size of the VDJ recombination for the *IGH* or *IGK* or *IGL*, whereas clonal cells will show a predominant band that represents the size of the VDJ region of the dominant clone. Similarly, sometimes it can be difficult to distinguish neoplastic from reactive T-cell infiltrates. Given the large number of T-cell antigen receptors, it is not as simple to detect clonality by IHC or flow cytometry in T-cell proliferations. One approach is to use aberrant loss of T-cell antigen expression to aid in the diagnosis of T-cell neoplasms. Another is to detect clonal rearrangement of the VDJ region of the T-cell receptor gamma (*TCRγ*) gene, which can be done by PCR on both fresh and formalin-fixed paraffin-embedded (FFPE) tissue.

Gene amplification is another important mechanism in cancer that has been found to have high utility in a subset of cancers. *MYCN* amplification occurs in approximately 40% of undifferentiated or poorly differentiated neuroblastoma subtypes,[4,5] either appearing as double minute chromosomes or homogeneously

TABLE 3.1

Genomic Alterations as Putative Predictive Biomarkers for Cancer Therapy

Genes	Pathways	Aberration Type	Disease Examples	Putative or Proven Drugs
PIK3CA,[51,52] PIK3R1,[53] PIK3R2, AKT1, AKT2, and AKT3[54,55]	Phosphoinositide 3-kinase (PI3K)	Mutation or amplification	Breast, colorectal, and endometrial cancer	■ PI3K inhibitors ■ AKT inhibitors
PTEN[56]	PI3K	Deletion	Numerous cancers	■ PI3K inhibitors
MTOR,[57] TSC1,[58] and TSC2[59]	mTOR	Mutation	Tuberous sclerosis and bladder cancer	■ mTOR inhibitors
RAS family (HRAS, NRAS, KRAS), BRAF,[60] and MEK1	RAS–MEK	Mutation, rearrangement, or amplification	Numerous cancers, including melanoma and prostate cancers	■ RAF inhibitors ■ MEK inhibitors ■ PI3K inhibitors
Fibroblast growth factor receptor 1 (FGFR1), FGFR2, FGFR3, FGFR4[36]	FGFR	Mutation, amplification, or rearrangement	Myeloma, sarcoma, and bladder, breast, ovarian, lung, endometrial, and myeloid cancers	■ FGFR inhibitors ■ FGFR antibodies
Epidermal growth factor receptor (EGFR)	EGFR	Mutation, deletion, or amplification	Lung and gastrointestinal cancer	■ EGFR inhibitors ■ EGFR antibodies
ERBB2[61]	ERBB2	Amplification or mutation	Breast, bladder, gastric, and lung cancers	■ ERBB2 inhibitors ■ ERBB2 antibodies
SMO[62,63] and PTCH1[64]	Hedgehog	Mutation	Basal cell carcinoma	■ Hedgehog inhibitor
MET[65]	MET	Amplification or mutation	Bladder, gastric, and renal cancers	■ MET inhibitors ■ MET antibodies
JAK1, JAK2, JAK3,[66] STAT1, STAT3	JAK–STAT	Mutation or rearrangement	Leukemia and lymphoma	■ JAK–STAT inhibitors ■ STAT decoys
Discoidin domain-containing receptor 2 (DDR2)	RTK	Mutation	Lung cancer	■ Some tyrosine kinase inhibitors
Erythropoietin receptor (EPOR)	JAK–STAT	Rearrangement	Leukemia	■ JAK–STAT inhibitors
Interleukin-7 receptor (IL-7R)	JAK–STAT	Mutation	Leukemia	■ JAK–STAT inhibitors
Cyclin-dependent kinases (CDKs[67]; CDK4, CDK6, CDK8, CDKN2A, and cyclin D1 (CCND1)	CDK	Amplification, mutation, deletion, or rearrangement	Sarcoma, colorectal cancer, melanoma, and lymphoma	■ CDK inhibitors
ABL1	ABL	Rearrangement	Leukemia	■ ABL inhibitors
Retinoic acid receptor-α (RARA)	RARα	Rearrangement	Leukemia	■ All-trans retinoic acid
Aurora kinase A (AURKA)[68]	Aurora kinases	Amplification	Prostate and breast cancers	■ Aurora kinase inhibitors
Androgen receptor (AR)[69]	Androgen	Mutation, amplification, or splice variant	Prostate cancer	■ Androgen synthesis inhibitors ■ Androgen receptor inhibitors
FLT3[70]	FLT3	Mutation or deletion	Leukemia	■ FLT3 inhibitors
MET	MET–HGF	Mutation or amplification	Lung and gastric cancers	■ MET inhibitors
Myeloproliferative leukemia (MPL)	THPO, JAK–STAT	Mutation	Myeloproliferative neoplasms	■ JAK–STAT inhibitors
MDM2[71]	MDM2	Amplification	Sarcoma and adrenal carcinomas	■ MDM2 antagonist
KIT[72]	KIT	Mutation	GIST, mastocytosis, and leukemia	■ KIT inhibitors
PDGFRA and PDGFRB	PDGFR	Deletion, rearrangement, or amplification	Hematologic cancer, GIST, sarcoma, and brain cancer	■ PDGFR inhibitors
Anaplastic lymphoma kinase (ALK)[9,37,73,74]	ALK	Rearrangement or mutation	Lung cancer and neuroblastoma	■ ALK inhibitors

(continued)

TABLE 3.1

Genomic Alterations as Putative Predictive Biomarkers for Cancer Therapy *(continued)*

Genes	Pathways	Aberration Type	Disease Examples	Putative or Proven Drugs
RET	RET	Rearrangement or mutation	Lung and thyroid cancers	▪ RET inhibitors
ROS1[75]	ROS1	Rearrangement	Lung cancer and cholangiocarcinoma	▪ ROS1 inhibitors
NOTCH1 and *NOTCH2*	Notch	Rearrangement or mutation	Leukemia and breast cancer	▪ Notch signalling pathway inhibitors

PIK3CA, PI3K catalytic subunit-α; *PIK3R1*, PI3K regulatory subunit 1; *PI3K*, phosphoinositide 3-kinase; *AKT*, v-akt murine thymoma viral oncogene homolog; *PTEN*, phosphatase and tensin homolog; *mTOR*, mechanistic target of rapamycin; *TSC1*, tuberous sclerosis 1 protein; RAS–MEK, rat sarcoma; *MEK*, MAPK/ERK (mitogen-activated protein kinase/extracellular signal-regulated kinase) kinase; RAF, v-raf murine sarcoma viral oncogene homolog; *ERBB2*, also known as *HER2*; *SMO*, smoothened homolog; *PTCH1*, patched homolog; *MET*, hepatocyte growth factor receptor; *JAK*, Janus kinase; *THPO*, thrombopoietin; *STAT*, signal transducer and activator of transcription; RTK, receptor tyrosine kinase; *CDKN2A*, cyclin-dependent kinase inhibitor 2A; ABL, Abelson murine leukemia viral oncogene homolog 1; *FLT3*, FMS-like tyrosine kinase 3; *HGF*, hepatocyte growth factor; *MDM2*, mouse double minute 2; *KIT*, v-kit Hardy-Zuckerman 4 feline sarcoma viral oncogene homolog; GIST, gastrointestinal stromal tumor; PDGFR, platelet-derived growth factor receptor; *ROS1*, v-ros avian UR2 sarcoma virus oncogene homolog.
Reprinted by permission from Macmillan Publishers Limited: Nature Reviews Drug Discovery, Simon, R. and Rowchodhury, S. 12:358–369, 2013, ©2013.

staining regions. *MYCN* amplification is a very strong predictor of poor outcomes, particularly in patients with localized (stage 1 or stage 2) disease or in infants with stage 4S metastatic disease, where fewer than half of patients survive beyond 5 years.[6]

Use of *other chromosome abnormalities* has been largely limited to the diagnosis and prognostication of hematologic disorders. Roughly half of all myelodysplastic disorders show cytogenetically detectable chromosomal abnormalities, such as monosomy 5 or 7, partial chromosomal loss (5q-, 7q-), or complex chromosomal abnormalities. Certain abnormalities in isolation (e.g., 5q-) have a favorable prognosis, whereas many others (e.g., "complex" karyotypes with three or more abnormalities) carry a worse prognosis. Differences in ploidy have proven to be useful predictors in pediatric acute lymphocytic leukemia (ALL), with hyperdiploid cases (>50 chromosomes) showing a distinctly more favorable course compared with hypodiploid or near diploid cases.[7] Overall, DNA ploidy can be assessed by flow cytometry. Specific chromosomal copy number alterations can be detected by *conventional karyotyping, array hybridization methods*, or *FISH*.

Copy number variation (CNV) represents the most common type of structural chromosomal alteration. Regions affected by CNVs range from approximately 1 kilobase to several megabases that are either amplified or deleted. It is estimated that about 0.4% of the genomes of healthy individuals differ in copy number.[8] CNVs resulting in deletion of genes such as *BRCA1, BRCA2, APC*, mismatch repair genes, and *TP53* have been implicated in a wide range of highly penetrant cancers.[9,10] CNVs can be detected by a variety of means including *FISH, comparative or array genomic hybridization*, or *virtual karyotyping* using *single nucleotide polymorphism (SNP) arrays*. Increasingly, CNV is detected using *next-generation sequencing*.

Large-scale sequencing of tumors has identified many *mutations* that are of potential prognostic and therapeutic significance. As will be discussed further, a wide range of strategies is available for the detection of point mutations (Fig. 3.1). It is important to

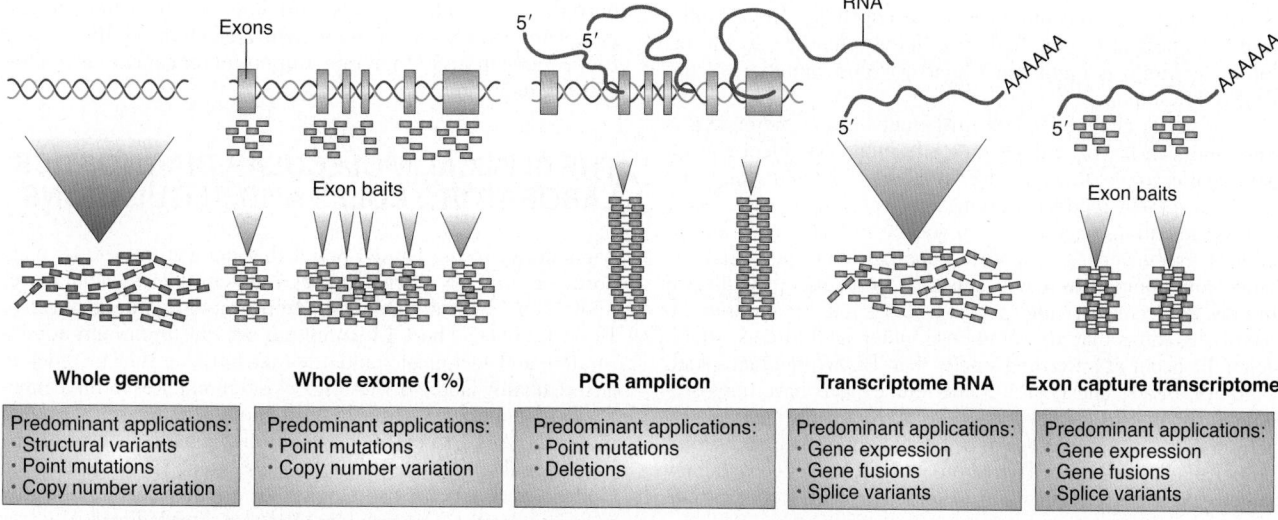

Whole genome	Whole exome (1%)	PCR amplicon	Transcriptome RNA	Exon capture transcriptome
Predominant applications: • Structural variants • Point mutations • Copy number variation	Predominant applications: • Point mutations • Copy number variation	Predominant applications: • Point mutations • Deletions	Predominant applications: • Gene expression • Gene fusions • Splice variants	Predominant applications: • Gene expression • Gene fusions • Splice variants

Figure 3.1 Strategies for the detection of mutations, translocations, and other structural genomic abnormalities in cancer. Whole genome sequencing, which involves determining the entire sequence of both introns and exons, is not only the most comprehensive, but also the most laborious and expensive approach. Exome sequencing uses *baits* to capture either the entire exome (roughly 20,000 genes [about 1% of the genome]) or else a subset of genes of interest. Amplicon-based sequencing uses PCR or other amplification techniques to amplify targets of interest for sequencing. Transcriptome sequencing, also known as RNAseq, is based on sequencing expressed RNA and can be used to detect not only mutations, but also translocations, other structural abnormalities, as well as differences in expression levels. This can be combined with exome capture techniques for a higher sensitivity analysis of genes of particular interest. (Reprinted by permission from Macmillan Publishers Limited: Nature Reviews Drug Discovery, Simon, R. and Rowchodhury, S. 12:358–369, 2013, ©2013.)

recognize that many nucleotide variations occur at any given allele in populations. Formally, the term *polymorphism* is used to describe genetic differences present in ≥1% of the human population, whereas *mutation* describes less frequent differences. However, in practice, *polymorphism* is often used to describe a nonpathogenic genetic change, and mutation a deleterious change, regardless of their frequencies.

Mutations can be classified according to their effect in the structure of a gene. The most common of these disease-associated alterations are single nucleotide substitutions (point mutations); however, many deletions, insertions, gene rearrangements, gene amplification, and copy number variations have been identified that have clinical significance. Point mutations may affect promoters, splicing sites, or coding regions. Coding region mutations can be classified into three kinds, depending on the impact on the codon: *missense mutation*, a nucleotide change leads to the substitution of an amino acid to another; *nonsense mutation*, a nucleotide substitution causes premature termination of codons with protein truncation; and *silent mutation*, a nucleotide change does not change the coded amino acid.

Loss of function mutations, either through point mutations or deletions in tumor suppressor genes such as *APC* and *TP53*, are the most common mutations in cancers. Tumor suppressor genes require two-hit (biallelic) mutations that inactivate both copies of the gene in order to allow tumorigenesis to occur. The first hit is usually an inherited or somatic point mutation, and the second hit is assumed to be an acquired deletion mutation that deletes the second copy of the tumor suppressor gene. Promoter methylation of tumor suppressor genes is an alternative route to tumorigenesis that, to date, has not been commonly employed for molecular diagnostics.

Oncogenes originate from the deregulation of genes that normally encode for proteins associated with cell growth, differentiation, apoptosis, and signal transduction (proto-oncogenes, [e.g., *BRAF* and *KRAS*]). Proto-oncogenes generally require only one gain of function or activating mutation to become oncogenic. Common mutation types that result in proto-oncogene activation include point mutations, gene amplifications, and chromosomal translocations. One example is mutations in the epidermal growth factor receptor (*EGFR*) that occur in lung cancer, which are almost exclusively seen in nonmucinous bronchoalveolar carcinomas. Somatic mutations of *EGFR* constitutively activate the receptor tyrosine kinase (TK). Importantly, responsiveness of tumors harboring these mutations to the inhibitor gefitinib is highly coordinated with a mutation of the EGFR TK domain.[11,12]

One of the challenges with using mutations as biomarkers is that there can be many nucleotide alterations that affect a given gene. For example, there are over 100 known different point mutations in *EGFR* reported in non–small-cell lung cancer. Many of these mutations occur at low frequency and have an unknown clinical significance.[13,14] Another important concept is that the same driver oncogene may be mutated in a variety of different tumors. For example, lung cancers harbor a number of other different alterations that are common in other solid tumors, which generally occur at lower frequencies than *EGFR* mutations such as *KRAS*, *BRAF*, and *HER2*. Some lung cancers have translocations involving the *ALK* kinase gene. *ALK*, interestingly, is also activated by point mutations in a neuroblastoma as by translocation in anaplastic large cell lymphoma (Fig. 3.2). Hence, a therapy targeted to a genetic alteration in one cancer may demonstrate efficacy in other cancers.

The detection of mutations is also important in the evaluation of chemotherapy resistance. Roughly a third of CML patients are resistant to the frontline ABL1 kinase inhibitor imatinib, either at the time of initial treatment or, more commonly, secondarily. In cases of primary failure or secondary failure, over 100 different *ABL1* mutations have been identified, including particularly common ones such as T315I and P loop mutations. While some

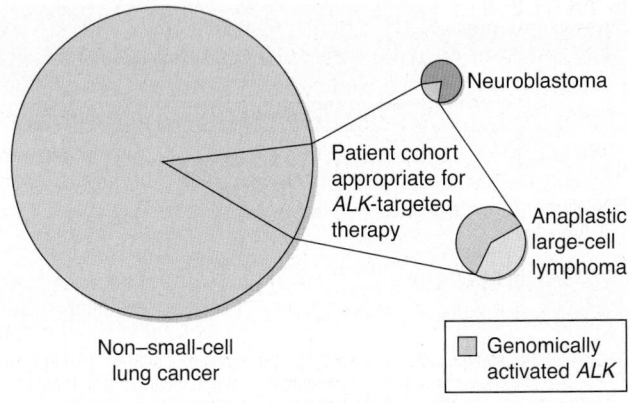

Figure 3.2 Activating genomic alterations occur in a variety of tumor types. *ALK* translocations, mutations, and amplifications occur in non–small-cell lung cancer, neuroblastomas, and in anaplastic large cell lymphomas. Such recurrent alterations in cancer, together with effective inhibitors of these pathways, are transforming oncologic therapies from organ-specific to pathway-specific interventions and are driving the use of molecular diagnostics in a wider range of tumor types (Reprinted with permission. © 2009 American Society of Clinical Oncology. All rights reserved. From McDermott, U. and Settleman, J. *J Clin Oncol* 2009;27:5650–5659.)

mutations, such as Y253H, respond to second generation TK inhibitors (TKI), others, such as the T315I mutation, are noteworthy because they confer resistance not only to imatinib, but also to nilotinib and dasatinib.

Mutations are also used as important predictive biomarkers (Table 3.1). Two of the most notable examples are the use of the *BRCA1* and *BRCA2* mutation analysis for women with a strong family history of breast cancer. Over 200 mutations (loss of function point mutations, small deletions, or insertions) occur in *BRCA* genes, which are distributed across the genes necessitating full sequencing for their detection. The overall prevalence of these occur in about 0.1% of the general population.[15,16] The lifetime risk of breast cancer for women carrying *BRCA1* mutations is in the range of 47% to 66%, whereas for *BRCA2* mutations, it is in the range of 40% to 57%.[17,18] In addition, the risk of other tumors including ovarian, fallopian, and pancreatic cancer is also increased. Detection of *BRCA1* and *BRCA2* mutations is, therefore, important for cancer prevention and risk reduction.

THE CLINICAL MOLECULAR DIAGNOSTICS LABORATORY: RULES AND REGULATIONS

Laboratories in the United States that perform molecular diagnostic testing are categorized as high-complexity laboratories under the Clinical Laboratory Improvement Amendments of 1988 (CLIA).[19] The CLIA program sets the minimum administrative and technical standards that must be met in order to ensure quality laboratory testing. Most laboratories in the United States that perform clinical testing in humans are regulated under CLIA. CLIA-certified laboratories must be accredited by professional organizations such as the Joint Commission, the College of American Pathologists, or another agency officially approved by the Centers for Medicare & Medicaid Services (CMS), and must comply with CLIA standards and guidelines for quality assurance. Although the regulation of laboratory services is in the U.S. Food and Drug Administration's (FDA) jurisdiction, the FDA has historically exercised enforcement discretion. Therefore, FDA approval is not currently required for clinical implementation of molecular tests as long as other regulations are met.[20,21]

SPECIMEN REQUIREMENTS FOR MOLECULAR DIAGNOSTICS

Samples typically received for molecular oncology testing include blood, bone marrow aspirates and biopsies, fluids, organ-specific fresh tissues in saline or tissue culture media such as Roswell Park Memorial Institute (RPMI), FFPE tissues, and cytology cell blocks. Molecular tests can be ordered electronically or through written requisition forms, but never through verbal requests only. All samples submitted for molecular testing need to be appropriately identified. Sample type, quantity, and specimen handling and transport requirements should conform to the laboratory's stated requirements in order to ensure valid test results.

Blood and bone marrow samples should be drawn into anticoagulated tubes. The preferred anticoagulant for most molecular assays is ethylenediaminetetraacetic acid (EDTA; lavender). Other acceptable collection tubes include ACD (yellow) solutions A and B. Heparinized tubes are not preferred for most molecular tests because heparin inhibits the polymerase enzyme utilized in PCR, which may lead to assay failure. Blood and bone marrow samples can be transported at ambient temperature. Blood samples should never be frozen prior to separation of cellular elements because this causes hemolysis, which interferes with DNA amplification. Fluids should be transported on ice. Tissues should be frozen (preferred method) as soon as possible and sent on dry ice to minimize degradation. Fresh tissues in RPMI should be sent on ice or cold packs. Cells should be kept frozen and sent on dry ice; DNA samples can be sent at ambient temperature or on ice.

For FFPE tissue blocks, typical collection and handling procedures include cutting 4 to 6 microtome sections of 10-micron thickness each on uncoated slides, air-drying unstained sections at room temperature, and staining one of the slides with hematoxylin and eosin (H&E). A board-certified pathologist reviews the H&E slides to ensure the tissue block contains a sufficient quantity of neoplastic tumor cells, and circles an area on the H&E slide that will be used as a template to guide macrodissection or microdissection of the adjacent, unstained slides. The pathologist also provides an estimate of the percentage of neoplastic cells in the area that will be tested, which should exceed the established limit of detection (LOD) of the assay.

MOLECULAR DIAGNOSTICS TESTING PROCESS

The workflow of a molecular test begins with receipt and accessioning of the specimen in the clinical molecular diagnostics laboratory followed by extraction of the nucleic acid (DNA or RNA), test setup, detection of analyte (e.g., PCR products), data analysis, and result reporting to the patient medical record (Fig. 3.3).

An extraction of intact, moderately high-quality DNA is essential for molecular assays. For DNA extraction, the preferred age for blood, bone marrow, and fluid samples is less than 5 days; for frozen or fixed tissue, it is indefinite; and for fresh tissue, it is overnight. Although there is no age limit for the use of a fixed and embedded tissue specimen for analysis, older specimens may yield a lower quantity and quality of DNA. Because RNA is significantly more labile than DNA, the preferred age for blood and bone marrow is less than 48 hours (from time of collection). Tissue samples intended for an RNA analysis should be promptly processed in fresh state, snap frozen, or preserved with RNA stabilizing agents for transport.

Dedicated areas, equipment, and materials are designated for various stages of DNA and RNA extraction procedures. DNA and RNA isolation can be done by manual or automated methods. Currently, most clinical laboratories employ commercial protocols based on liquid- or solid-phase extractions. Nucleated cells are isolated from biological samples prior to nucleic acid extraction.

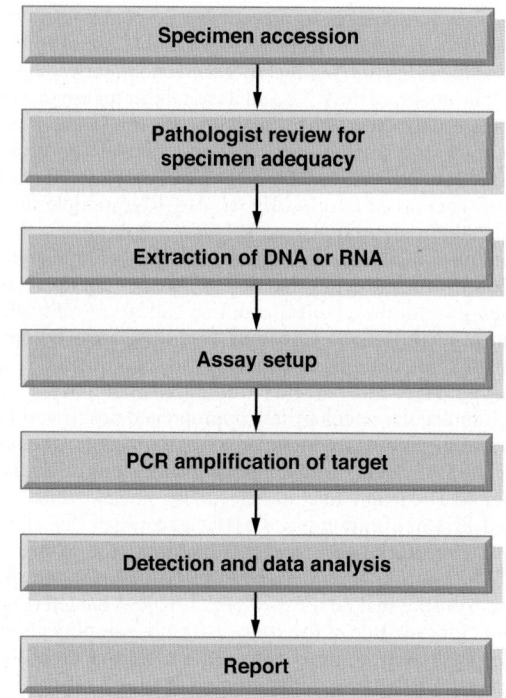

Figure 3.3 Simplified workflow of clinical molecular diagnostic testing.

White blood cells (WBC) can be isolated from blood and bone marrow samples by different methods. One method involves lysing the red blood cells with an ammonium chloride solution, which yields the total WBC population and other nucleated cells present. Another method involves a gradient preparation with a Ficoll solution, which yields the mononuclear cell population only. Sections of FFPE tissue blocks are prepared for DNA extraction by first removing the paraffin and disrupting the cell membranes with proteinase K digestion. Fresh and frozen tissues also undergo proteinase K digestion prior to nucleic acid extraction. DNA isolation protocols consist of several steps, including cell lysis, DNA purification by salting out the proteins and other debris (nonorganic method), or by solvent extractions of the proteins with phenol and chloroform solutions (organic method). The DNA is then precipitated out of the solution with isopropanol or ethanol. The pellet is washed with 70% to 80% ethanol and then solubilized in buffer, such as Tris-EDTA solution. Proteinase K can be added to assist in the disruption and to prevent nonspecific degradation of the DNA. RNase is sometimes added to eliminate contaminating RNA. The DNA yield is quantitated spectrophotometrically, and the DNA sample integrity is visually checked, if necessary, on an agarose gel followed by ethidium bromide staining. Intact DNA appears as a high–molecular-weight single band, whereas degraded DNA is identified as a smear of variably sized fragments. After extraction, the DNA is stored at 4°C prior to use in a PCR assay, and is then stored at −70°C after completion of the assay. Because the DNA extracted from formalin-fixed tissue is degraded to a variable extent, an analysis of the extraction product by gel electrophoresis is not informative. Yield and integrity of the extracted DNA is best assessed by an amplification control to ensure that the quality and quantity of input DNA is adequate to yield a valid result.

RNA isolation steps are similar to the ones described previously for DNA extraction. However, RNA is inherently less stable than DNA due to its single-strand conformation and susceptibility to degradation by RNase, which is ubiquitous in the environment. To ensure preservation of target RNA, special precautions are required, including the use of diethylpyrocarbonate (DEPC) water in all reagents used in RNA procedures, and special decontamination of work area and pipettes to prevent RNase contamination. The extracted RNA is usually degraded to a variable extent so that the analysis of the extraction product by gel electrophoresis is not informative. The quality of the RNA and its suitability for use in a reverse transcriptase polymerase chain reaction (RT-PCR)–based assay is assessed most appropriately by the demonstration of a positive result in an assay designed to detect the RNA transcripts for a "housekeeping gene," such as *ABL1* or *GAPDH*. Any RNA sample in which the 260/280-nm absorption ratio is below 1.9 or greater than 2.0 may contain contaminants and must be cleaned prior to analysis.

Following nucleic acid extraction, the assay is set up according to written procedures established during validation/verification of the assay by qualified laboratory staff. Dedicated areas, equipment, and materials are designated for various stages of the test (e.g., extraction, pre-PCR and post-PCR for amplification-based assays). For each molecular oncology test, appropriated positive and negative control specimens are included to each run as a matter of routine quality assessment. A no template (blank) control, containing the complete reaction mixture except for nucleic acids, is also included in amplification-based assays to evaluate for amplicon contamination in the assay reagents that may lead to inaccurate results. The controls are processed in the same manner as patient samples to ensure that established performance characteristics are being met for each step of the assay (extraction, amplification, and detection). All assay controls and overall performance of the run must be examined prior to interpretation of sample results. Following acceptance of the controls, results are electronically entered into reports. The final report is reviewed and signed by the laboratory director or a qualified designee who meets the same qualifications as the director, as defined by CLIA (see previous).

TECHNOLOGIES

Several traditional and emerging techniques are currently available for mutation detection in cancer (Table 3.2). In the era of personalized medicine, molecular oncology assays are rapidly moving from a mutational analysis of single genes toward a multigene panel analysis. As the number of "actionable" mutations such as *ALK*, *EGFR*, *BRAF*, and others increase, the use of next-generation sequencing platforms is expected to become much more widespread. Both traditional and emerging testing approaches have advantages and disadvantages that need to be balanced before a test platform is implemented into practice.

An important consideration when adding a new oncology test in the clinical laboratory menu is to define the intended use of the assay (e.g., diagnosis, prognosis, prediction of therapy response). The clinical utility of the assay, appropriate types of specimens, the spectrum of possible mutations that can be found in the genomic region of interest, and available methods for testing should also be determined. The laboratory director and ordering physicians should also discuss the estimated test volume, optimal reporting format, and required turnaround time for the proposed new test.[21–23]

Polymerase Chain Reaction

Polymerase chain reaction (PCR)[24,25] is widely used in all molecular diagnostics laboratories for the rapid amplification of targeted DNA sequences. The reaction includes the specimen template DNA, forward and reverse primers (18 to 24 oligonucleotides long), Taq DNA polymerase, and each of the four nucleotides bases (dATP, dTTP, dCTP, dGTP). During PCR, selected genomic sequences undergo repetitive temperature cycling (sequential heat and cooling) that allows for *denaturation* of double-stranded DNA template, *annealing* of the primers to the targeted complementary sequences on the template, and *extension* of new strands of DNA by Taq polymerase from nucleotides, using the primers as the starting point. Each cycle doubles the copy number of PCR

templates for the next round of polymerase activity, resulting in an exponential amplification of the selected target sequence. The PCR products (amplicons) are detected by electrophoresis or in real-time systems simultaneously to the amplification reaction (see real-time PCR, which follows).

PCR is specifically designed to work on DNA templates because the Taq polymerase does not recognize RNA as a starting material. Nonetheless, PCR can be adapted to RNA testing by including a reverse transcription step to convert a RNA sequence into its cognate cDNA sequence before the PCR reaction is performed (see reverse-transcription PCR, which follows). Multiplex PCR reactions can also be designed with multiple primers for simultaneous amplification of multiple genomic targets. PCR is a highly sensitive and specific technique that can be employed in different capacities for the detection of point mutations, small deletions, insertions and duplications, as well as gene rearrangements and clonality assessment. Limits of detection can reach 0.1% mutant allele or lower, which is important for the detection of somatic mutations in oncology because tumor specimens are usually composed of a mixture of tumor and normal cells. Reverse transcription PCR can also be used for the relative quantification of target RNA in minimal residual disease testing, such as *BCR-ABL1* transcripts in CML. Another advantage of PCR is its ability to amplify small amounts of low quality FFPE-derived DNA. However, applications of PCR can be limited because it cannot amplify across large or highly repetitive genomic regions. Also, the PCR reaction can be inhibited by heparin or melanin if present in the extracted DNA, which may lead to assay failure. Finally, the risk of false positives due to specimen or amplicon contamination is an important issue when using PCR-based techniques; therefore, stringent laboratory procedures, as described previously, are used to minimize contamination. With the exception of hybridization assays, such as fluorescence in situ hybridization and genomic microarrays, PCR is the necessary initial step in all current molecular oncology assays.

Targeted Mutation Analysis Methods

Real-Time PCR (q-PCR)

In real-time PCR (q-PCR), the polymerase chain reaction is performed with a PCR reporter that is usually a fluorescent double-stranded DNA binding dye or a fluorescent reporter probe. The intensity of the fluorescence produced at each amplification cycle is monitored in real time, and both quantification and detection of targeted sequences is accomplished in the reaction tube as the PCR amplification proceeds.

The intensity of the fluorescent signal for a given DNA fragment (wild type or mutant) is correlated with its quantity, based on the PCR cycle in which the fluorescence rises above the background (crossing threshold [Ct] or crossing point [Cp]).[26] The Ct value can be used for qualitative or quantitative analysis. Qualitative assays use the Ct as a cutoff for determining "presence" or "absence" of a given target in the reaction. A qualitative analysis by q-PCR is particularly useful for a targeted detection of point mutations that are located in mutational hotspots. Examples include the *JAK2* V617F mutation, which is located within exon 14, and is found in several myeloproliferative neoplasms (polycythemia vera, essential thrombocythemia, and primary myelofibrosis),[27] and the *BRAF* V600E,[28] which is located within exon 15, and is found in various cancer types including melanomas and thyroid and lung cancers.

For a quantitative analysis, the Ct of standards with known template concentration is used to generate a standard curve to which Ct values of unknown samples are compared. The concentration of the unknown samples is then extrapolated from values from the standard curve. The quantity of amplicons produced in a PCR reaction is proportional to the prevalence of the targeted sequence;

TABLE 3.2

Molecular Methods in Oncology

Method	Advantages	Disadvantages	Analytic Sensitivity	Examples of Applications in Oncology
Real-time PCR (q-PCR) Allele-specific PCR (AS-PCR) Reverse transcriptase PCR (RT-PCR)	Flexible platforms that permit detection of a variety of conserved hotspot mutations including nucleotide substitutions, small length mutations (deletions, insertions), and translocations High sensitivity is beneficial for residual disease testing and specimens with limited tumor content Adaptable to quantitative assays	Detects only specific targeted mutations/ chromosomal translocations Not suitable for variable mutations May not determine the exact change in nucleotide sequence	Very high	*KRAS, BRAF,* and *EGFR* mutations in solid tumors *JAK2* V617F and *MPL* mutations in myeloproliferative neoplasms *KIT* D816V mutation in systemic mastocytosis and AML Quantitation of *BCR-ABL1* and *PML-RARA* transcripts for residual disease monitoring in CML and APL, respectively
Fragment analysis	Detects small to medium insertions and deletions Detects variable insertions and deletions regardless of specific alteration Provides semiquantitative information regarding mutation level	Does not determine the exact change in nucleotide sequence Does not detect single nucleotide substitution mutations Limited multiplex capability	High	*NPM1* insertion mutations in AML *FLT3* internal tandem duplications in AML *JAK2* exon 12 insertions and deletions in PV *EGFR* exon 19 deletions in NSCLC
FISH	Detects chromosomal translocation, gene amplification, and deletion Morphology of tumor is preserved, allowing for a more accurate interpretation of heterogeneous samples	High cost Unable to detect small insertions and deletions Limited multiplex capability Does not determine the exact breakpoint and change in nucleotide sequence	High	*IGH/BCL2* translocation detection in follicular lymphoma and in a subset of diffuse large B-cell lymphoma *ALK* translocation in NSCLC *EWSR1* translocation in soft tissue tumors *HER2* amplification in breast cancer 1p/19q deletion in oligodendroglioma
High-resolution melting (HRM) curve analysis	Qualitative detection of variable single nucleotide substitutions and small insertions and deletions	Does not determine the exact mutation Result interpretation may require testing via an alternate technology Limited multiplex capability	Medium	*KRAS* and *BRAF* mutations in solid tumors *JAK2* exon 12 mutations in PV
Sanger sequencing	Detects variable single nucleotide substitutions and small insertions and deletions Provides semiquantitative information about mutation level Current gold standard for mutation detection	Low throughput Low analytic sensitivity limits application in specimens with low tumor burden Does not detect copy number changes or large (>500 bp) insertions and deletions	Low	*KIT* mutations in GIST and melanoma *CEBPA* mutations in AML *EGFR* mutations in NSCLC
Pyrosequencing	Higher analytical sensitivity than Sanger sequencing Detects variable single nucleotide substitutions and small insertions and deletions Provides quantitative information about mutation level	Short read lengths limit analysis to mutational hotspots Low throughput	Medium	*KRAS* and *BRAF* mutations in solid tumors
Single nucleotide extension assay (SNaPshot)	Simultaneous detection of targeted nucleotide substitution mutations Multiplex capability	Detects only targeted mutations	High	Small gene panels (3–10) for melanoma, NSCLC, breast cancer, and metastatic colorectal cancer

(continued)

Molecular Methods in Oncology *(continued)*

Method	Advantages	Disadvantages	Analytic Sensitivity	Examples of Applications in Oncology
Next-generation sequencing (NGS)	Quantitative detection of variable single nucleotide substitutions, small insertions and deletions, chromosomal translocations, and gene copy number variations Highly multiplexed High throughput	Requires costly investment in instrumentation and bioinformatics Technology is rapidly evolving Higher error rates for insertion and deletion mutations Limited ability to sequence GC-rich regions	High	Small to large gene panels (3–500) for solid tumor and hematologic malignancies
Genomic microarray	Simultaneous detection of copy number variation and LOH (SNP array)	Limited application to FFPE tissue Does not detect balanced translocations May not detect low-level mutant allele burden	Medium	Analysis of recurrent copy number variation and LOH in chronic lymphocytic leukemia and myeloproliferative neoplasms

AML, acute myelogenous leukemia; CML, chronic myelogenous leukemia; APL, acute promyelocytic leukemia; PV, polycythemia vera; NSCLC, non–small-cell lung carcinoma; GIST, gastrointestinal stromal tumor; GC, guanine-cytosine; LOH, loss of heterozygosity; FFPE, formalin-fixed paraffin-embedded.

therefore, samples with a higher template concentration reaches the Ct at earlier PCR cycles than one with a low concentration of the amplified target. Quantitative q-PCR has high analytical sensitivity for the detection of low mutant allele burden. For that reason, this method has been widely utilized for monitoring minimal residual disease.

Allele-Specific PCR

Allele-specific PCR (AS-PCR) is a variant of conventional PCR. The method is based on the principle that Taq polymerase is incapable of catalyzing chain elongation in the presence of a mismatch between the 3′ end of the primer and the template DNA. Selective amplification by AS-PCR is achieved by designing a forward primer that matches the mutant sequence at the 3′ end primer. A second mismatch within the primer can be introduced at the adjacent -1 or -2 position to decrease the efficiency of mismatched amplification products. This will minimize the chance of amplifying and, therefore, detecting the wild-type target. AS-PCR is usually performed as two PCR reactions: one employing a forward primer specific for the mutant sequence, the other using a forward primer specific for the correspondent wild-type sequence. In this case, a common reverse primer is used for both reactions. Following amplification, the PCR products are detected by electrophoresis (capillary or agarose gel) or in q-PCR systems. The detection of adequate PCR product in the wild-type amplification reaction is important to control for adequate specimen quality and quantity, particularly when the specimen is negative in the mutation-specific PCR reaction.

AS-PCR is particularly useful for the detection of targeted point mutations. Multiplex AS-PCR reactions can be designed for the simultaneous detection of multiple mutations by including several mutation-specific primers. The method has high analytical sensitivity and specificity and can be easily deployed in most clinical laboratories. However, an important limitation is that this approach will not detect mutations other than those for which specific primers are designed. Therefore, it is utilized for highly recurrent mutations that occur at specific locations within genes, rather than for the detection of variable mutations that may occur throughout a gene.

Examples of AS-PCR applications in oncology include the detection of *JAK2* V617F and *MPL* mutations in myeloprolifera-

tive neoplasms (primary myelofibrosis, essential thrombocythemia, and/or polycythemia vera),[29] the *BRAF* V600E mutation,[30] and *KIT* D816V mutations in cases of systemic mastocytosis and in acute myelogenous leukemia (AML).

Reverse Transcriptase PCR

RT-PCR is utilized for the detection and quantification of RNA transcripts. The first step for all amplification-based assays that use RNA as a starting material is reverse transcription of RNA into cDNA, because RNA is not a suitable substrate for Taq polymerase. In RT-PCR, RNA is isolated and reverse transcribed into cDNA by using a reverse transcriptase enzyme and one of the following: (1) random hexamer primers, which anneal randomly to RNA and reverse transcribe all RNA in the cell; (2) oligo dT primers, which anneal to the polyA tail of mRNA and reverse transcribe only mRNA; or (3) gene-specific primers that reverse transcribe only the target of interest. PCR is subsequently performed on the cDNA with forward and reverse primers specific to the gene(s) of interest. The RT-PCR products may then be analyzed by capillary electrophoresis or in real-time systems as in a standard PCR reaction.

RT-PCR is commonly used for detecting gene fusions during translocation analysis because breakpoints frequently occur within the intron of each partner gene and the precise intronic breakpoint locations may be variable. This variability complicates the design of primers used in DNA-based PCR assays. RT-PCR tests are advantageous because mature mRNA has intronic sequence spliced out, allowing for simplified primer design within the affected exon of each partner gene. In this setting, RT-PCR is useful in tests where both translocation partners are recurrent and only one or a few exons are involved in each partner gene. For instance, 95% of acute promyelocytic leukemia (APL) cases harbor the reciprocal t(15;17) chromosomal translocation and these breakpoints always occur within intron 2 of the *RARA* gene. By contrast, three distinct chromosome 15 breakpoints are involved, all occurring within the *PML* gene: intron 6, exon 6, and intron 3. Because the breakpoints in the two genes are recurrent, most of the reported *PML-RARA* fusions can be detected by targeting these three transcript isoforms.

RT-PCR is the method of choice when high sensitivity is required to detect gene translocations. For example, *PML-RARA*

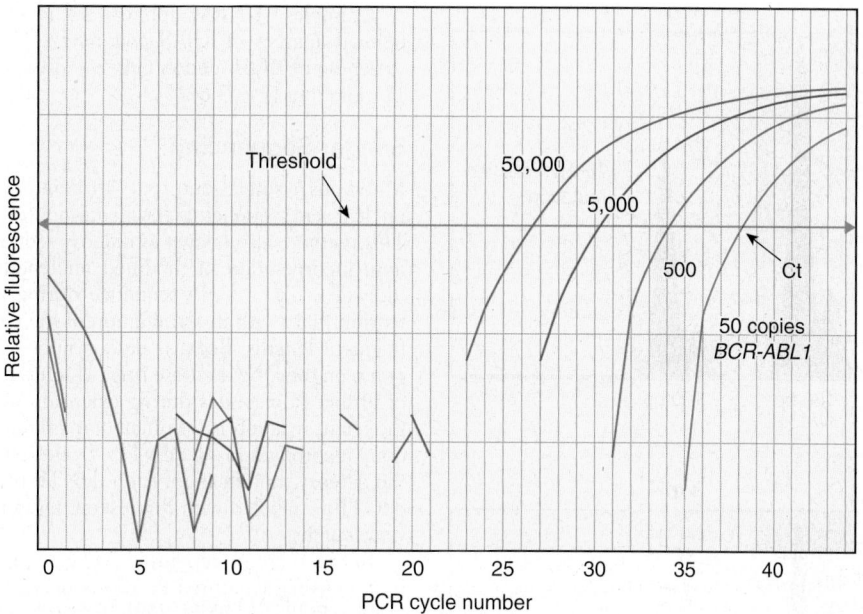

Figure 3.4 Reverse transcriptase PCR (RT-PCR) is a sensitive means to detect *BCR-ABL1* fusion transcripts in CML. RT-PCR can be combined with real-time PCR (q-PCR) to quantitate *BCR-ABL1* transcripts across four to six log range levels. Amplification products are detected during each PCR cycle using a fluorescent probe specific to the PCR product. The accumulated fluorescence in log(10) value is plotted against the number of PCR cycles. For a given specimen, the PCR cycle number is measured when the increase in fluorescence is exponential and exceeds a threshold. This point is called the Ct, which is inversely proportional to the amount of PCR target in the specimen (i.e., lower Ct values indicate a greater amount of target). Calibration standards of known quantity are used in standard curves to calculate the amount of target in a tested specimen. These are shown in the chart as different colored plots. Note that PCR increases the amount of amplification product by a factor of two with each PCR cycle. Therefore, specimens that produce a Ct value that is one cycle lower are expected to have a twofold higher concentration of target. Specimens that differ in target concentration by a factor of 10 (as shown) are expected to have a Ct value 3.3 cycles apart ($2^{3.3} = 10$).

transcript detection by RT-PCR can detect this fusion transcript down to 1 tumor cell in the background of 100,000 normal cells. Detecting low levels of fusion transcript can reveal relapse after consolidation and guide further treatment.[31] RT-PCR can also be used to quantitate the amount of expression of a gene. One major application of RT-PCR in this setting includes quantitative detection of *BCR-ABL1* fusion transcript for prognostication and minimal residual disease testing in CML (Fig. 3.4). In this setting, a three log decrease in *BCR-ABL1* levels is associated with an improved outcome.[32,33]

Fragment Analysis

A fragment analysis is a PCR amplicon-sizing technique that is relevant for the detection of small- to medium-length–affecting mutations (deletions, insertions, and duplications). This is typically performed by capillary electrophoresis, which is capable of resolving length mutations from approximately 1 to 500 base pairs in size.

Fragment analysis represents a practical strategy because it enables comprehensive detection of a wide variety of possible length mutations and has high analytic sensitivity. Further, it can provide semiquantitative information regarding the relative amount of mutated alleles. Limitations of this approach include the inability to objectively quantitate mutant allele burdens, the inability to determine the exact change in nucleotide sequence, and the inability to detect non–length-affecting mutations such as substitution mutations.

Examples of fragment analysis applications in oncology include the detection of *NPM1* insertion mutations (Fig. 3.5),[34] *EGFR* exon 19 deletions, *FLT3* internal tandem duplications, and *JAK2* exon 12 mutations.[35]

High-Resolution Melting Curve Analysis

A high-resolution melting (HRM) curve analysis is a mutation screening method that allows for the detection of DNA sequence variations based on specific sequence-related melting profiles of PCR products.[36] Because the melting property of DNA duplexes is dependent on the biophysical and chemical properties of the nucleotide sequences, mutant and wild-type DNA sequences can be differentiated from one another based on their melting characteristics.

An HRM analysis is preceded by a PCR. The reaction employs a pair of gene-specific forward and reverse primers, template DNA, and a reporter that can either be a double-stranded DNA binding dye or a fluorescent reporter probe. Following the last cycle of the PCR, the amplification products undergo a cooling step that generates homoduplexes (double-stranded molecules with perfect complementarity between alleles) and heteroduplexes (double-stranded molecules with sequence mismatch between alleles) followed by a heating step that denatures (i.e., melts) the double-stranded products. Heteroduplexes (mutant DNA) produce a melting profile different from that of wild-type samples (homoduplexes). In most cases, the reaction is performed in a q-PCR system that allows for an analysis of amplification and

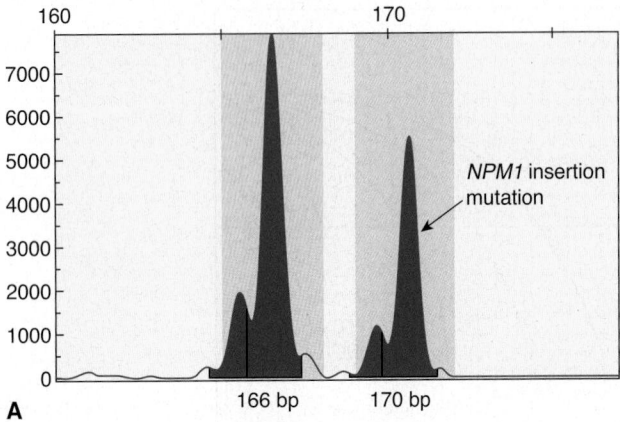

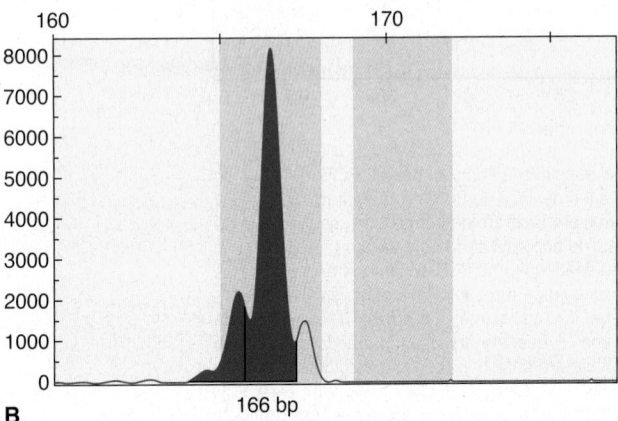

Figure 3.5 Fragment analysis. *NPM1* mutations are important prognostic markers in acute myeloid leukemia. Virtually all *NPM1* mutations result in a four nucleotide insertion within exon 12. Detection of these mutations can be accomplished by PCR utilizing primers that flank the mutation region. The amplification products are sized using capillary electrophoresis. A mutation is indicated by a PCR fragment that is 4 bp larger than the wild-type fragment. Mutation positive **(A)** and negative **(B)** cases are shown.

melting data in a close-tube format, thereby minimizing the risk of amplicon contamination.

An HRM analysis is useful for the qualitative detection of variable point mutations and small length-affecting mutations that occur within mutational hotspot regions. This method has high analytical sensitivity and can detect mutations even in a small fraction of alleles in a background of wild-type DNA. However, this assay does not characterize the specific sequence alteration in the mutant allele and may be challenging to interpret, especially for cases with mutation levels that approach the detection limit of the assay. Samples with a lower abundance of mutant alleles, and consequently a decreased fraction of heteroduplexes that produced fluorescence decay during the melting analysis, usually produce a melting curve that may not differ significantly from that of wild-type samples. Likewise, the detection of duplication mutations may be hampered by the similarity between the mutant and the duplicated wild-type genome sequences, which may produce only subtle differences in the melting behavior of the DNA duplexes, especially for samples with low mutant allele burden. Therefore, both the mutant sequence and the allelic burden play in the ability of an HRM analysis to detect mutations.[37] Poor quality and impurity of genomic DNA may also lower the sensitivity of an HRM analysis.[38] In instances of patients with a low mutant allelic burden, equivocal mutations identified by this approach may not be confirmable by an alternate method such as Sanger sequencing.

Examples of HRM applications in oncology include a mutational analysis of *KRAS* codons 12, 13, and 61[39]; a mutation screening of *BRAF* codon 600[39]; and the detection of *JAK2* exon 12 mutations (Fig. 3.6).[40]

Sanger Sequencing

Mutations in single gene assays are commonly analyzed by targeted nucleic acid sequencing, most commonly by Sanger sequencing.[41] This method, also known as dideoxy sequencing, is based on random incorporation of modified nucleotides (dideoxynucleotides [ddNTP]) into a DNA sequence during rounds of template extension that result in termination of the chain reaction at various fragment lengths. Because dideoxynucleotides lack a 3′ hydroxyl group on the DNA pentose ring, which is required for the addition of further nucleotides during extension of the new DNA strand, the chain reaction is terminated at different lengths with the random incorporation of ddNTPs to the sequence. In addition to the dideoxy modification, each ddNTP (ddATP, ddTTP, ddCTP, ddGTP) is labeled with fluorescent tags of different fluorescence wavelengths.

In this method, repetitive cycles of primer extension are performed using denatured PCR products (amplicons) as templates. Unlike PCR, in which both forward and reverse primers are added to the same reaction, in Sanger sequencing, the forward and reverse reactions are performed separately. Bidirectional sequencing is performed to ensure that the entire region of interest

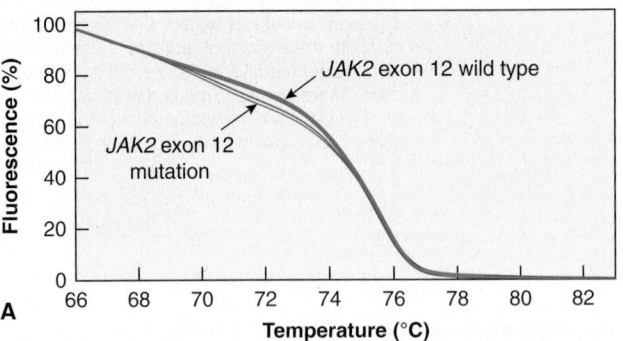

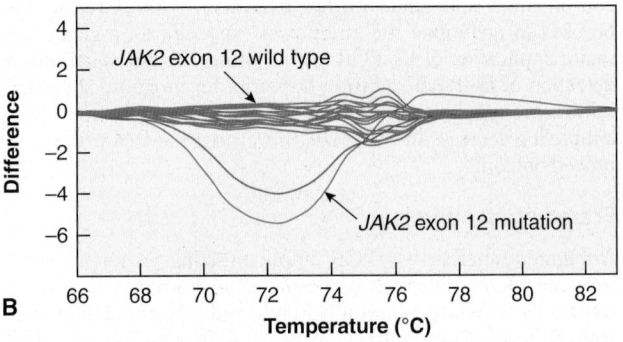

Figure 3.6 High resolution melting (HRM) curve analysis. An HRM analysis can be an efficient screening method for detecting a variety of mutations that may cluster in one or more hotspot regions, such as occurs with *JAK2* exon 12 mutations in polycythemia vera. PCR is utilized to amplify the target region in the presence of a fluorescent double-stranded DNA-binding dye. Following PCR, the product is gradually melted, and the emitted fluorescence is measured. **(A)** Plotting fluorescence versus temperature generates a melt curve characteristic of each amplicon. The presence of a mutation alters the melt profile due to mismatched double-stranded heteroduplexes of mutant and wild-type fragments. **(B)** A difference plot in which sample curves are subtracted from a wild-type control can accentuate the different melt profiles.

for each analysis is visualized adequately to produce unequivocal sequence readout. The sequencing products of increasing size are resolved by capillary electrophoresis, and the DNA sequence is determined by detection of the fluorescently labeled nucleotide sequences.

Sanger sequencing has the ability to detect a wide variety of nucleotide alterations in the DNA, including point mutations, deletions, insertions, and duplications. This technique is especially useful when mutations are scattered across the entire gene, when genes have not been sufficiently studied to determine mutational hot spots, or when it is relevant to determine the exact change in DNA sequence. Sanger sequencing can also provide semiquantitative information about mutation levels in a sample based on the evaluation of average peak drop values from forward and reverse mutant peaks on sequence chromatograms. Limitations of this approach include low throughput and limited diagnostic sensitivity. In general, heterozygous mutations at allelic levels lower than 20% may be difficult to detect by Sanger sequencing. This may be particularly problematic when testing for somatic mutations in oncogenes, such as *JAK2* exon 12 in polycythemia vera, which may occur at low levels.[35]

Examples of Sanger sequencing applications in oncology include the detection of *KIT* mutations for gastrointestinal stromal tumors (GIST) and melanomas that arise from mucosal membranes and acral skin, *EGFR* mutations for non–small-cell lung cancers, and *KRAS* mutations for colorectal and lung carcinomas (Fig. 3.7).

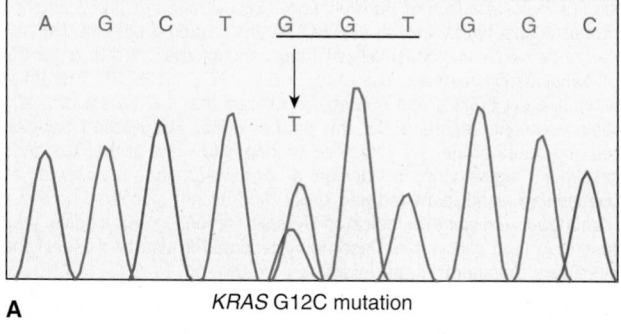

A   *KRAS* G12C mutation

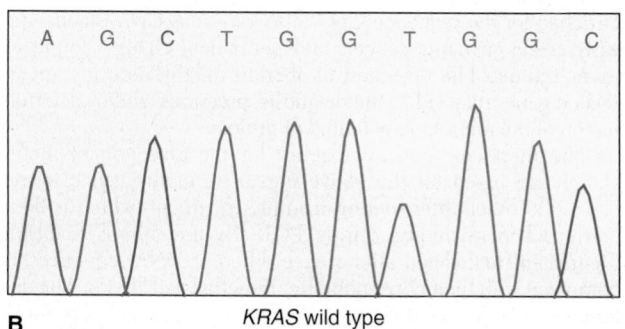

B   *KRAS* wild type

Figure 3.7 Sanger sequencing. *KRAS* mutation testing requires a technology like Sanger sequencing, which can detect the diverse variety of mutations that span multiple nucleotide sites. Overlapping peaks in the DNA sequence chromatogram indicate the presence of a mutation. The top panel **(A)** displays a G to T nucleotide substitution in codon 12. This results in a GGT to TGT codon change, leading to a glycine to cysteine (G12C) amino acid substitution. Activating mutations in *KRAS* such as G12C are associated with resistance to epidermal growth factor receptor (EGFR) targeted therapies in colon cancer. The bottom panel **(B)** displays a wild-type *KRAS* sequence.

Pyrosequencing

Pyrosequencing, also known as *sequencing by synthesis*, is based on the real-time detection of pyrophosphate release by nucleotide incorporation during DNA synthesis.[42] In the pyrosequencing reaction, as nucleotides are added to the nucleic acid chain by polymerase, pyrophosphate molecules are released and subsequently converted to ATP by ATP sulfurylase. Light is produced by an ATP-driven luciferase reaction via oxidation of a luciferin molecule. The amount of light produced is proportional to the number of incorporated nucleotides in the sequence. When a nucleotide is not incorporated into the reaction, no pyrophosphate is released and the unused nucleotide is degraded by apyrase. Light is converted into peaks in a charge-coupled device (CCD) camera. Individual dNTP nucleotides are sequentially added to the reaction, and the sequence of nucleotides that produce chemiluminescent signals allow the template sequence to be determined. Mutations appear as new peaks in the pyrogram sequence or variations of the expected peak heights.[43]

Pyrosequencing is particularly useful for the detection of point mutations and insertion/deletion mutations that occur at short stretches in mutational hotspots. This method has higher analytical sensitivity than Sanger sequencing and can provide quantitative information about mutation levels in a sample. Pyrosequencing can also be used for the detection and quantification of gene-specific DNA methylation and gene copy number assessments. A microfluidic pyrosequencing platform is available for massive parallel sequencing. However, this method is not well suited for detecting mutations that are scattered across the entire gene because pyrosequencing read lengths are limited to ~100 to 250 base pairs.[43]

Examples of pyrosequencing applications in oncology include the mutational analysis of *BRAF* (codon 600),[44,45] *KRAS* (codons 12, 13, 61),[45] *NRAS* (codon 61),[45] and the methylation analysis of *MGMT* in glioblastoma multiforme.[46,47]

Single Nucleotide Extension Assay (SNaPshot®)

The single nucleotide extension assay is a variant of dideoxy sequencing. This method consists of a single base extension of an unlabeled primer that anneals one base upstream to the relevant mutation with fluorophore-labeled dideoxynucleotides (ddNTP). Multiplexed reactions can be designed with multiple primers of differing lengths for simultaneous amplification of multiple genomic targets.[48] Mutations are identified based on amplicon size and fluorophore color via capillary electrophoresis. When a mutation is present, an alternative dideoxynucleotide triphosphate is incorporated, resulting in a different colored peak with a different amplicon length than the expected wild-type one.

The single nucleotide extension assay is particularly useful for the simultaneous detection of recurrent point mutations. Clinically, it has been employed for analyses of mutational hotspots in multiple genes involved in melanomas, non–small-cell lung cancers, breast cancers, and metastatic colorectal cancers.[49] The assay has higher analytical sensitivity than Sanger sequencing and can detect low-level mutations in FFPE-derived DNA, making it advantageous for biopsy specimens with limited tumor involvement. This assay, however, can only detect mutations that are immediately adjacent to the 3′ to the end of the primer.

Fluorescence In Situ Hybridization

FISH allows for the visualization of specific chromosome nucleic acid sequences within a cellular preparation. This method involves the annealing of a large single-stranded fluorophore-labeled oligonucleotide probe to complementary DNA target sequences within a tissue or cell preparation. The hybridization of the probe at the specific DNA region within a nucleus is visible by direct detection using fluorescence microscopy.

FISH can be used for the quantitative assessment of gene amplification or deletion and for the qualitative evaluation of gene rearrangements. Many oncologic FISH assays employ two probe types: *locus specific probes*, which are complementary to the gene of interest, and *centromeric probes*, which hybridize to the alpha-satellite regions near the centromere of a specific chromosome and help in the enumeration of the number of copies of that chromosome.

For the quantitative assessment of gene amplification, a locus-specific probe and a centromeric probe are labeled with two different fluorophores. The signals generated by each of these probes are counted and a ratio of the targeted gene to the chromosome copy number is calculated. The amount of signal produced by the locus-specific probe is proportional to the number of copies of the targeted gene in a cell. This type of gene amplification assay can be used for the detection of *HER2* gene amplification as an adjunct to existing clinical and pathologic information as an aid in the assessment of stage II, node-positive breast cancer patients for whom Herceptin treatment is being considered. It can also be used for an assessment of *MYCN* amplification in neuroblastoma.

For the detection of deletion mutations, dual-probe hybridization is usually performed using locus-specific probes. For instance, for the detection of 1p/19q codeletion in oligodendrogliomas, locus-specific probe sets for 1p36 and 19q13, and 1q25 and 19p13 (control) are used. The frequencies of signal patterns for each of these loci are evaluated. A signal pattern with 1p and 19q signals that are less than control signals is consistent with deletion of these loci.

Gene rearrangements/chromosomal translocations in hematologic or solid malignancies can be tested using locus-specific dual-fusion or break-apart probes. Dual-color, dual-fusion translocation assays employ two probes that are located in two separate genes involved in a specific rearrangement. Each gene probe is labeled in a different color. This design detects translocations by the juxtaposition of both probe signals. Dual-color, dual-fusion translocation assays are very specific for detecting a selected translocation. But, it can only be used for detecting translocations that involve consistent partners, where both partners are known. Alternate translocations with different fusion partners are not detected by this approach. Examples of application of dual-fusion probes in oncology include for the detection of the *IGH-BCL2* translocation that occurs in most follicular lymphomas and a subset of diffuse large B-cell lymphomas (Fig. 3.8) and for the detection of *IGH-CCND1* rearrangements in mantle cell lymphomas.

In break-apart FISH assays, both dual-colored probes flank the breakpoint region in a single gene that represents the constant partner in the translocation. By this approach, rearranged alleles show two split signals, whereas normal alleles show fusion signals. This design is particularly useful for genes that fuse with multiple translocation partners (e.g., *EWSR1* gene, which may undergo rearrangement with multiple partner genes, including *FLI1*, *ERG*, *ETV1*, *FEV*, and *E1AF* in Ewing sarcoma/primitive neuroectodermal tumor [PNET]; *WT1* in desmoplastic small round cell tumors; *CHN* in extraskeletal myxoid chondrosarcoma; and *ATF1* in clear cell sarcoma and angiomatoid fibrous histiocytoma).[50] The disadvantage of this approach is that break-apart FISH does not allow for the identification of the "unknown" partner in the translocation.

FISH has the advantage of being applicable to a variety of specimen types, including FFPE tissue. Because probes are hybridized to tissue in situ, the tumor morphology is preserved, which allows for an interpretation of the assay even in the context of heterogeneous samples. However, FISH is a targeted approach that will only detect specific alterations. Because most probes are large (e.g., >100 kb), small deletions or insertions will not be detected. In addition, poor tissue fixation, fixation artifacts, nuclear truncation on tissue slides, and nuclear overlaps are potential pitfalls of this technique that may hamper interpretation. Some intrachromosomal rearrangements (e.g., *RET-PTC* and *EML4-ALK*) may be challenging to interpret by FISH due to subtle rearrangements of the probe signals on the same chromosome arm.

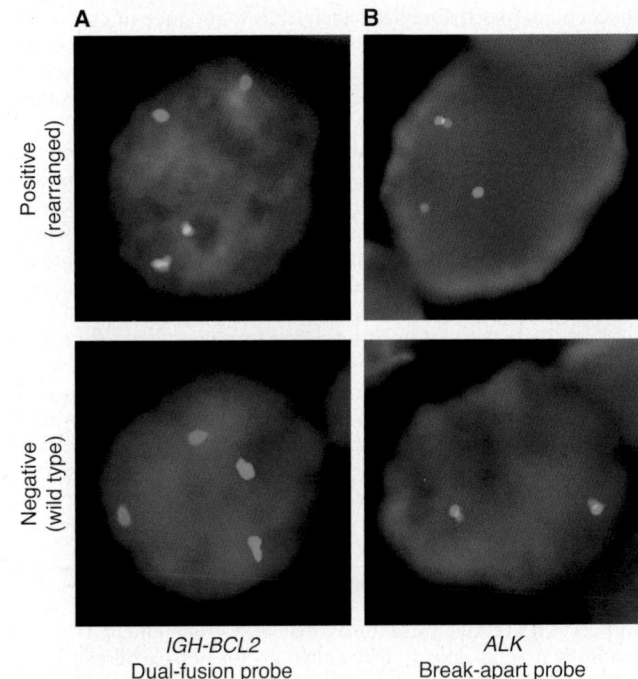

Figure 3.8 Fluorescence in situ hybridization (FISH). **(A)** Recurrent chromosomal translocations such as *IGH-BCL2* (occurring in B-cell lymphomas) can be effectively detected with a dual-fusion probe strategy. This design utilizes a green probe specific to the *IGH* locus and a red probe specific to the *BCL2* gene, with each probe spanning their respective breakpoint region. Individual green and red probe signals indicate a lack of translocation. Colocalization of green and red probes is observed when an *IGH-BCL2* translocation is present. **(B)** *ALK* rearrangements in non–small-cell lung cancers may involve a variety of translocation partners, including *EML4*, *TFG*, and *KIF5B*. Therefore, a break-apart FISH probe strategy is utilized that will detect any *ALK* rearrangement, regardless of the partner gene. Fluorescently labeled red and green probes are designed on opposite sides of the *ALK* gene breakpoint region. With this design, a normal *ALK* gene is observed as overlapping or adjacent red and green fluorescent signals, whereas a rearranged *ALK* gene is indicated by split red and green signals. *ALK* testing in lung cancer has become widespread in use because of the significant therapeutic implications.

Methylation Analysis

Changes in the methylation status of cytosine in DNA regions enriched for the sequence CpG (also known as CpG islands) are early events in many cancers and permanent changes found in many tumors. The detection of aberrant methylation of cancer-related genes may aid in the diagnosis, prognosis, and/or determination of the metastatic potential of tumors.

The most common approaches for the detection of methylation are based on the conversion of unmethylated cytosine bases into uracil after sodium bisulfite treatment, which is then converted to thymidine during PCR. By this approach, bisulfite-treated methylated alleles have different DNA sequences as compared with their corresponding unmethylated alleles. The differences between methylated and unmethylated DNA sequences can be evaluated by several methods, including methylation-sensitive restriction enzyme analysis, methylation-specific PCR, semiquantitative q-PCR, Sanger sequencing, pyrosequencing, and next-generation sequencing.

The methylation status of oncogenic genes can also be assessed by methylation-sensitive multiplex ligation-dependent probe amplification (MS-MLPA) assay.[51,52] MS-MLPA is a variant of multiplex PCR in which oligonucleotide probes hybridized to the targeted DNA samples are directly amplified using one pair of universal primers. This method is not based on bisulfite conversion of unmethylated cytosine bases into uracil. Instead, the target sequences detected by MS-MLPA probes contain a restriction site recognized by methylation-sensitive endonucleases. A probe amplification product will only be obtained if the CpG site is methylated because digested probes cannot be amplified during PCR. The level of methylation is determined by resolving PCR products by capillary electrophoresis and calculating the normalized ratio of each target probe peak area in both digested and undigested specimens. The ratio corresponds to the percentage of methylation present in the specimen.

Examples of applications of methylation analysis in oncology include an analysis of *MLH1* promoter hypermethylation in microsatellite unstable sporadic colorectal carcinomas, an analysis of *MGMT* promoter methylation status in glioblastoma multiforme patients treated with alkylating chemotherapy, and *SEPT9* promoter methylation in DNA derived from blood plasma in colorectal cancer patients.[53]

Microsatellite Instability Analysis

Microsatellites are short, tandem-repeated DNA sequences with repeating units of one to six base pairs in length. Microsatellites are distributed throughout the human genome, and individual repeat loci often vary in length from one individual to another. Microsatellite instability (MSI) is the change in length of a microsatellite allele due to either insertion or deletion of repeating units and a failure of the DNA mismatch repair (MMR) system to repair these replication errors. This genomic instability arises in a variety of human neoplasms where tumor cells have a decreased ability to faithfully replicate DNA. MSI is particularly associated with colorectal cancer, where 15% to 20% of sporadic tumors show MSI, in contrast to the more common chromosomal instability (CIN) phenotype, with MSI status being an independent prognostic indicator. MSI analysis is also clinically useful in identifying patients at increased risk of hereditary nonpolyposis colorectal cancer (HNPCC)/Lynch syndrome, where a germline mutation of an MMR gene causes a familial predisposition to colorectal cancer. MSI analysis alone is not sufficient to make a diagnosis of a germline MMR mutation given the high rate of sporadic MSI-positive colorectal tumors, but a positive result is an indication for follow-up genetic testing and counseling.

In an MSI analysis, DNA is extracted from tumor tissue and the corresponding adjacent normal mucosa. The DNA is subjected to multiplex PCR using fluorescent-labeled primers for coamplification of five mononucleotide repeat markers for MSI determination and two pentanucleotide markers for confirming tumor/normal sample identity. The resulting PCR fragments are separated and detected using capillary electrophoresis. Allelic profiles of normal versus tumor tissues are compared, and MSI is scored as the presence of novel microsatellite lengths in tumor DNA compared to normal DNA. Instability in two or more out of five mononucleotide microsatellite markers in tumor DNA compared to normal DNA is defined as MSI-H (high). MSI-L (low) is defined as instability in one out of five mononucleotide markers in tumor DNA compared to normal DNA. Tumors with no instability (zero out of five altered mononucleotide markers) are defined as microsatellite stable (MSS).[54,55]

Loss of Heterozygosity Analysis

Loss of heterozygosity (LOH) is a common event in cancer that usually occurs due to deletion of a chromosome segment and results in a loss of one copy of an allele. LOH is a common occurrence in tumor suppressor genes and may contribute to tumorigenesis when the second allele is subsequently inactivated by a second "hit" due to mutation or deletion.

LOH studies are used to identify genomic imbalance in tumors, indicating possible sites of tumor suppressor gene (TSG) deletion. LOH studies can be done by multiplex PCR analysis of microsatellites (short tandem repeats [STRs]), FISH, and genomic microarrays). By PCR, microsatellites located in the vicinity of a tumor suppressor gene are used as surrogate markers for the presence of the gene of interest. DNA is extracted from tumor tissue and corresponding adjacent normal mucosa. The DNA is subjected to multiplex PCR using fluorescent-labeled STR primers. Peak height ratio of informative (nonhomozygous) alleles at each locus is calculated from both normal and tumor tissues. LOH is defined as the decrease in peak height of one of the two alleles, relative to the allele peak heights of the normal sample.

An example of applications of LOH studies in oncology include an analysis of 1p/19q loss in oligodendrogliomas, and an analysis of 1p loss in parathyroid carcinomas.

Whole Genome Analysis Methods

Next-Generation Sequencing

Next-generation sequencing (NGS), also known as massive parallel sequencing or deep sequencing, is an emerging technology that has revolutionized the speed, throughput, and cost of sequencing and has facilitated the discovery of clinically relevant genetic biomarkers for diagnosis, prognosis, and personalized therapeutics. By way of this technology, multiple genes or the entire exome or genome can be interrogated simultaneously in multiple parallel reactions instead of a single-gene basis as in Sanger sequencing or pyrosequencing. Currently, the most common NGS approach for cancer testing in the clinical setting employs targeted sequencing of specific genes and mutation hotspot regions. This targeted approach increases sensitivity for the detection of low-level mutations by increasing the depth of sequence coverage.

Presently, there are numerous NGS platforms that employ different sequencing technologies. A comprehensive review and comparison of NGS platforms is beyond the scope of this chapter and has been reviewed elsewhere.[56,57] A generalized clinical workflow is shown (Fig. 3.9). Frequently, multiple DNA samples are individually barcoded and pooled together to leverage platform throughput. Pooled libraries are prepared and enriched, and single DNA molecules are arrayed in solid surfaces, glass slides, or beads and sequenced in situ using reversible DNA chain terminators or iterative cycles of oligonucleotide ligation. NGS signal outputs are based on luminescence, fluorescence, or changes in ion concentration. Robust bioinformatics pipelines are required for an alignment of reads to a reference genome sequence, variant calling, variant annotation, and to assist with result reporting.[58]

NGS can be used for the detection of single nucleotide variants, small insertions and deletions, translocations, inversions, alternative splicing, and copy number variations given sufficient depth of genomic DNA sequence (Fig. 3.10). Technical limitations of this technique include difficulty in sequencing guanine-cytosine (GC)–rich genomic regions, and erroneous sequencing of homologous DNA regions (e.g., pseudogenes) that may confound interpretation.

Examples of applications of NGS in oncology include small targeted panels (3 to 50 genes) for non–small-cell lung cancers, melanomas, colon cancers, and acute myeloid leukemias.[57,59–62] Larger panels (50 to 500 genes) are increasingly being utilized, particularly in both clinical trials and research.

Massively parallel sequencing of RNA (RNA-Seq) can be used for determining sequence variants, alternative splicing, gene rearrangements, and allelic expression of mutant transcripts. To date, this technique has been used primarily for discovery rather than clinical applications, but it is likely to play an increasing role in clinical diagnostics as the technology improves. For transcriptome sequencing, the RNA must first be converted to cDNA, which is then fragmented and entered into library construction. After sequencing, reads are aligned to a reference genome, compared with known transcript sequences, or assembled de novo

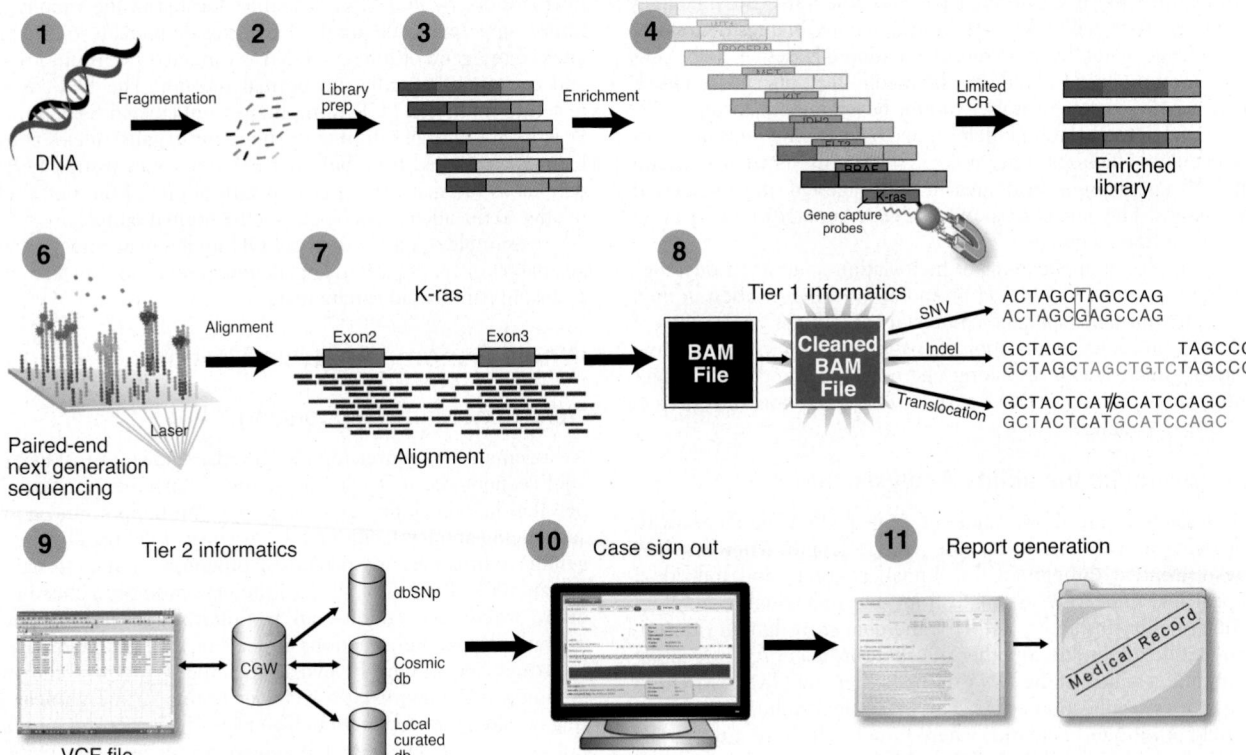

Figure 3.9 Next-generation sequencing (NGS) workflow in a clinical laboratory. Targeted-panel sequencing offers tremendous promise for cancer diagnostics due to the massive improvement in throughput, speed, and cost. NGS is a complex, multiday process that requires significant infrastructure and expertise to deploy in a clinical setting. The process begins with genomic DNA extraction, which is fragmented and to which linkers are ligated. In this targeted gene panel–based example, the sequencing libraries are enriched for the target genes, which are subjected to a limited PCR prior to sequencing. Sequence reads are mapped to a reference genome and subjected to several bioinformatics tools to provide variant calling results and variant annotation. Clinical interpretation and case sign out is performed by a physician with expertise in molecular pathology. BAM, Binary Sequence Alignment/Map; SNV, Single Nucleotide Variant; VCF, Variant Call Format; CGW, Clinical Genomicist Workstation; dbSNP, The Single Nucleotide Polymorphism Database. (Used with permission from Shashikant Kulkarni PhD and Eric Duncavage MD.)

to construct a genome-scale transcription map. Expression levels are determined from the total number of sequence reads that map to the exons of a particular gene, normalized by the length of exons that can be uniquely mapped.[56] Compared with genomic microarrays, RNA-Seq has a greater ability to distinguish RNA isoforms, determine allelic expression, and reveal sequence variants.

Chromatin immunoprecipitation with sequencing (ChIP-Seq) can be used to determine the genome-wide location of chromatin-binding transcription factors or specific epigenetic modifications of histones. This has proved to be a very powerful research tool, which to date has not been used for clinical diagnostics. Proteins in contact with genomic DNA are chemically cross-linked (usually with formaldehyde treatment) to their binding sites, the DNA is fragmented, and the proteins cross-linked with DNA are then immunoprecipitated with antibodies specific for the proteins (or specific epigenetic histone modification) of interest. The DNA harvested from the immunoprecipitate is converted into a library for NGS. The obtained reads are mapped to the reference genome of interest to generate a genome-wide protein binding map.[63,64] ChIP-Seq is rapidly replacing chromatin immunoprecipitation and microarray hybridization (ChIP-on-chip) technology[65] because of its higher sensitivity and resolution.[66]

Genomic Microarrays

High-density genomic microarrays are widely used for whole genome assessment of copy number changes, LOH, and geno-typing. In array comparative genomic hybridization (aCGH), cloned genomic probes are arrayed onto glass slides and serves as targets for the competitive hybridization of normal and tumor DNA. In the aCGH reaction, tumor DNA and DNA from a normal control sample are labeled with different fluorophores. These samples are denatured and hybridized together to the arrayed single-strand probes. Digital imaging systems are used to quantify the relative fluorescence intensities of the labeled DNA probes that have hybridized to each target probe. The fluorescence ratio of the tumor and control hybridization signals is determined at different positions along the genome, which provides information on the relative copy number of sequences in the tumor genome as compared to the normal genome.[67] This method is able to detect copy number variation, such as deletions, duplications, and gene amplification, but it cannot detect polymorphic allele changes.

An SNP array has the ability to detect LOH profiles in addition to high-resolution detection of copy number aberrations, such as amplifications and deletions. This method employs thousands of unique fluorescent-labeled nucleotide probe sequences arrayed on a chip to which a fragmented single-stranded specimen DNA binds to their complementary partners. Each SNP site is interrogated by complementary sets of probes containing perfect matches and mismatches to each SNP site. Each probe is associated with one of the two alleles of an SNP (also known as A and B). Relative fluorescence intensity depends on both the amount of target DNA in the sample, as well as the affinity between target and probe. An analysis of the raw fluorescence intensity is done by computational

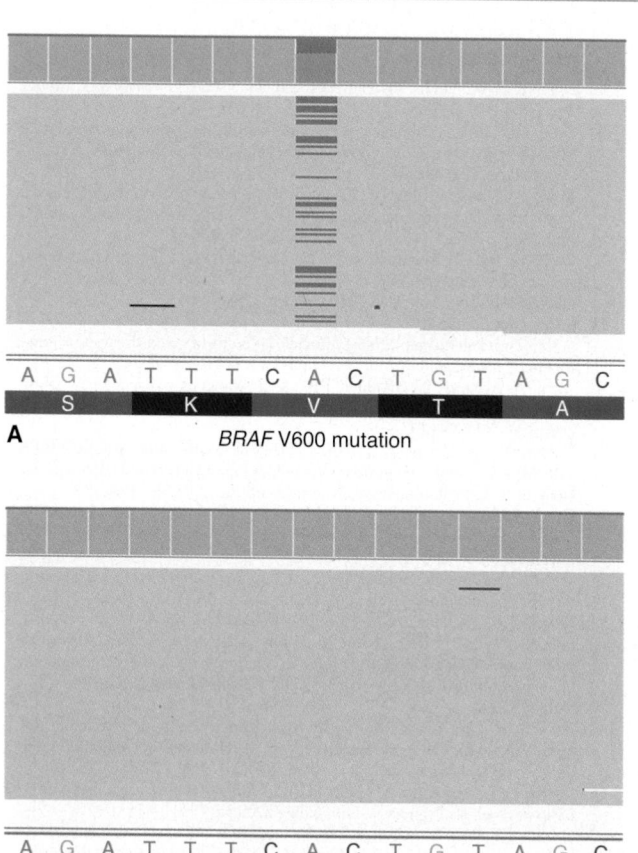

A   *BRAF* V600 mutation

A G A T T T C A C T G T A G C
S   K   V   T   A

B   *BRAF* wild type

A G A T T T C A C T G T A G C
S   K   V   T   A

Figure 3.10 Next-generation sequencing (NGS). Hundreds to thousands of sequence reads are mapped and horizontally aligned to specific targeted regions in the reference genome (sequence shown on *bottom* of each panel). A software-assisted analysis assists in the detection of mutations, displayed as colored bars in each read above the mutation site. A wild-type sequence within each read is displayed in *gray*. Mutation frequency correlates to the number of times the mutant sequence is detected compared to the total number of reads at that nucleotide position. Shown are sequencing results from *BRAF* V600E mutation positive **(A)** and negative **(B)** melanomas. The A to T base substitution that leads to the V600E mutation is displayed in red. Patients with metastatic melanoma that harbors the *BRAF* V600E mutation are candidates for targeted therapy.

algorithms that convert the set of probe intensities into genotypes. Deleted genomic regions are identified as having an LOH associated with copy number reduction. A copy-neutral LOH is detected when SNPs expected to be heterozygous in the normal sample are detected as homozygous in the tumor sample without copy number variation. A copy neutral LOH may arise from somatic homologous recombination of a mutated tumor suppressor allele and its surrounding DNA that replaces the other allele (uniparental disomy [UPD]). SNP microarrays are the only genomic microarrays that are able to identify UPD. Array technologies cannot detect true balanced chromosome abnormalities and low-level mosaicism.

Examples of genomic microarrays applications in oncology include the detection of copy number variations and LOH in chronic lymphocytic leukemia[68] and recurrent cytogenetic abnormalities in MDS (e.g., 5q-, -7 or 7q-, +8, 20q-).[69]

Expression Panels

Gene expression signatures of multiple cancer biomarkers are starting to be incorporated into clinical practice as an adjunct to clinical and pathologic information in diverse cancer management settings. An example of a multigene expression–based test in current use includes Oncotype DX, which is a quantitative RT-PCR–based assay that measures the expression of 21 genes in FFPE breast tumors. The test is designed to predict the potential benefit of chemotherapy and the likelihood of distant breast cancer recurrence in women with node negative or node positive, estrogen receptor (ER)-positive, and *HER2*-negative invasive breast cancer. This test has been in-corporated into current American Society of Clinical Oncology (ASCO) and National Comprehensive Cancer Network (NCCN) for breast cancer management.[70] Prospective trials are in progress to evaluate other multigene tests for early stage breast cancer.

With the rapid advances in molecular diagnostic technologies, it is likely that many mutation- and expression-based panels analyzing hundreds if not thousands of genes, or even the complete genome or transcriptome, will enter widespread use. Some of the many challenges to address will be to provide evidence-based, actionable reports that guide the oncologist to more effective therapies, to learn from the results of such testing to improve the algorithms guiding therapy, to handle the incidental findings in such testing in an ethically responsible way, and, ultimately, with the drugs available, to provide sufficient improvements in outcomes so that society will be willing to bear the costs.

PRINCIPLES OF ONCOLOGY

REFERENCES

1. Lennard L, Cartwright CS, Wade R, et al. Thiopurine methyltransferase genotype-phenotype discordance and thiopurine active metabolite formation in childhood acute lymphoblastic leukaemia. *Br J Clin Pharmacol* 2013;76(1):125–136.
2. Haber DA, Settleman J. Cancer: drivers and passengers. *Nature* 2007;446(7132):145–146.
3. Hayashi T, Sudo J. Relieving effect of saline on cephaloridine nephrotoxicity in rats. *Chem Pharm Bull (Tokyo)* 1989;37(3):785–790.
4. Brodeur GM, Seeger RC, Schwab M, et al. Amplification of N-myc in untreated human neuroblastomas correlates with advanced disease stage. *Science* 1984;224(4653):1121–1124.
5. Seeger RC, Brodeur GM, Sather H, et al. Association of multiple copies of the N-myc oncogene with rapid progression of neuroblastomas. *N Engl J Med* 1985;313(18):1111–1116.
6. Weinstein JL, Katzenstein HM, Cohn SL. Advances in the diagnosis and treatment of neuroblastoma. *Oncologist* 2003;8(3):278–292.
7. Pui CH, Crist WM, Look AT. Biology and clinical significance of cytogenetic abnormalities in childhood acute lymphoblastic leukemia. *Blood* 1990;76(8):1449–1463.
8. Lee JA, Lupski JR. Genomic rearrangements and gene copy-number alterations as a cause of nervous system disorders. *Neuron* 2006;52(1):103–121.
9. Kuiper RP, Ligtenberg MJ, Hoogerbrugge N, et al. Germline copy number variation and cancer risk. *Curr Opin Genet Dev* 2010;20(3):282–289.
10. Shlien A, Malkin D. Copy number variations and cancer. *Genome Med* 2009;1(6):62.
11. Lynch TJ, Bell DW, Sordella R, et al. Activating mutations in the epidermal growth factor receptor underlying responsiveness of non–small-cell lung cancer to gefitinib. *N Engl J Med* 2004;350(21):2129–2139.
12. Paez JG, Janne PA, Lee JC, et al. EGFR mutations in lung cancer: correlation with clinical response to gefitinib therapy. *Science* 2004;304(5676):1497–1500.
13. Forbes SA, Bindal N, Bamford S, et al. COSMIC: mining complete cancer genomes in the Catalogue of Somatic Mutations in Cancer. *Nucleic Acids Res* 2011;39(Database issue):D945–950.
14. Van Allen EM, Wagle N, Levy MA. Clinical analysis and interpretation of cancer genome data. *J Clin Oncol* 2013;31(15):1825–1833.
15. Newman B, Mu H, Butler LM, et al. Frequency of breast cancer attributable to BRCA1 in a population-based series of American women. *JAMA* 1998;279(12):915–921.
16. Ford D, Easton DF, Stratton M, et al. Genetic heterogeneity and penetrance analysis of the BRCA1 and BRCA2 genes in breast cancer families. The Breast Cancer Linkage Consortium. *Am J Hum Genet* 1998;62(3):676–689.
17. Antoniou A, Pharoah PD, Narod S, et al. Average risks of breast and ovarian cancer associated with BRCA1 or BRCA2 mutations detected in case series unselected for family history: a combined analysis of 22 studies. *Am J Hum Genet* 2003;72(5):1117–1130.

18. Chen S, Iversen ES, Friebel T, et al. Characterization of BRCA1 and BRCA2 mutations in a large United States sample. *J Clin Oncol* 2006;24(6):863–871.

19. Bachner P, Hamlin W. Federal regulation of clinical laboratories and the Clinical Laboratory Improvement Amendments of 1988—Part II. *Clin Lab Med* 1993;13(4):987–994.

20. Halling KC, Schrijver I, Persons DL. Test verification and validation for molecular diagnostic assays. *Arch Pathol Lab Med* 2012;136(1):11–13.

21. Jennings L, Van Deerlin VM, Gulley ML, College of American Pathologists Molecular Pathology Resource C. Recommended principles and practices for validating clinical molecular pathology tests. *Arch Pathol Lab Med* 2009;133(5):743–755.

22. Jennings LJ, Smith FA, Halling KC, et al. Design and analytic validation of BCR-ABL1 quantitative reverse transcription polymerase chain reaction assay for monitoring minimal residual disease. *Arch Pathol Lab Med* 2012;136(1):33–40.

23. Pont-Kingdon G, Gedge F, Wooderchak-Donahue W, et al. Design and analytical validation of clinical DNA sequencing assays. *Arch Pathol Lab Med* 2012;136(1):41–46.

24. Saiki RK, Gelfand DH, Stoffel S, et al. Primer-directed enzymatic amplification of DNA with a thermostable DNA polymerase. *Science* 1988;239(4839):487–491.

25. Mullis KB. The unusual origin of the polymerase chain reaction. *Sci Am* 1990;262(4):56–61, 64–65.

26. Bernard PS, Wittwer CT. Real-time PCR technology for cancer diagnostics. *Clin Chem* 2002;48(8):1178–1185.

27. Bench AJ, Baxter EJ, Green AR. Methods for detecting mutations in the human JAK2 gene. *Methods Mol Biol* 2013;967:115–131.

28. Halait H, Demartin K, Shah S, et al. Analytical performance of a real-time PCR-based assay for V600 mutations in the BRAF gene, used as the companion diagnostic test for the novel BRAF inhibitor vemurafenib in metastatic melanoma. *Diagn Mol Pathol* 2012;21(1):1–8.

29. Furtado LV, Weigelin HC, Elenitoba-Johnson KS, et al. Detection of MPL mutations by a novel allele-specific PCR-based strategy. *J Mol Diagn* 2013;15(6):810–818.

30. Lang AH, Drexel H, Geller-Rhomberg S, et al. Optimized allele-specific real-time PCR assays for the detection of common mutations in KRAS and BRAF. *J Mol Diagn* 2011;13(1):23–28.

31. Wang ZY, Chen Z. Acute promyelocytic leukemia: from highly fatal to highly curable. *Blood* 2008;111(5):2505–2515.

32. O'Brien SG, Guilhot F, Larson RA, et al. Imatinib compared with interferon and low-dose cytarabine for newly diagnosed chronic-phase chronic myeloid leukemia. *N Engl J Med* 2003;348(11):994–1004.

33. Hughes TP, Kaeda J, Branford S, et al. Frequency of major molecular responses to imatinib or interferon alfa plus cytarabine in newly diagnosed chronic myeloid leukemia. *N Engl J Med* 2003;349(15):1423–1432.

34. Szankasi P, Jama M, Bahler DW. A new DNA-based test for detection of nucleophosmin exon 12 mutations by capillary electrophoresis. *J Mol Diagn* 2008;10(3):236–241.

35. Furtado LV, Weigelin HC, Elenitoba-Johnson KS, et al. A multiplexed fragment analysis-based assay for detection of JAK2 exon 12 mutations. *J Mol Diagn* 2013;15(5):592–599.

36. Reed GH, Kent JO, Wittwer CT. High-resolution DNA melting analysis for simple and efficient molecular diagnostics. *Pharmacogenomics* 2007;8(6):597–608.

37. Palais RA, Liew MA, Wittwer CT. Quantitative heteroduplex analysis for single nucleotide polymorphism genotyping. *Anal Biochem* 2005;346(1):167–175.

38. Carillo S, Henry L, Lippert E, et al. Nested high-resolution melting curve analysis a highly sensitive, reliable, and simple method for detection of JAK2 exon 12 mutations—clinical relevance in the monitoring of polycythemia. *J Mol Diagn* 2011;13(3):263–270.

39. Ney JT, Froehner S, Roesler A, et al. High-resolution melting analysis as a sensitive prescreening diagnostic tool to detect KRAS, BRAF, PIK3CA, and AKT1 mutations in formalin-fixed, paraffin-embedded tissues. *Arch Pathol Lab Med* 2012;136(9):983–992.

40. Jones AV, Cross NC, White HE, et al. Rapid identification of JAK2 exon 12 mutations using high resolution melting analysis. *Haematologica* Oct 2008;93(10):1560–1564.

41. Sanger F, Nicklen S, Coulson AR. DNA sequencing with chain-terminating inhibitors. *Proc Natl Acad Sci U S A* 1977;74(12):5463–5467.

42. Ronaghi M, Uhlén M, Nyrén P. A sequencing method based on real-time pyrophosphate. *Science* 1998;281(5375):363, 365.

43. Ronaghi M, Shokralla S, Gharizadeh B. Pyrosequencing for discovery and analysis of DNA sequence variations. *Pharmacogenomics* 2007;8(10):1437–1441.

44. Shigaki H, Baba Y, Watanabe M, et al. KRAS and BRAF mutations in 203 esophageal squamous cell carcinomas: pyrosequencing technology and literature review. *Ann Surg Oncol* 2013;20:485–491.

45. Vaughn CP, Zobell SD, Furtado LV, et al. Frequency of KRAS, BRAF, and NRAS mutations in colorectal cancer. *Genes Chromosomes Cancer* 2011;50(5):307–312.

46. Everhard S, Tost J, El Abdalaoui H, et al. Identification of regions correlating MGMT promoter methylation and gene expression in glioblastomas. *Neuro Oncol* 2009;11(4):348–356.

47. Mikeska T, Bock C, El-Maarri O, et al. Optimization of quantitative MGMT promoter methylation analysis using pyrosequencing and combined bisulfite restriction analysis. *J Mol Diagn* 2007;9(3):368–381.

48. Dias-Santagata D, Akhavanfard S, David SS, et al. Rapid targeted mutational analysis of human tumours: a clinical platform to guide personalized cancer medicine. *EMBO Mol Med* 2010;2(5):146–158.

49. Su Z, Dias-Santagata D, Duke M, et al. A platform for rapid detection of multiple oncogenic mutations with relevance to targeted therapy in non–small-cell lung cancer. *J Mol Diagn* 2011;13(1):74–84.

50. Lazar A, Abruzzo LV, Pollock RE, et al. Molecular diagnosis of sarcomas: chromosomal translocations in sarcomas. *Arch Pathol Lab Med* 2006;130(8):1199–1207.

51. Nygren AO, Ameziane N, Duarte HM, et al. Methylation-specific MLPA (MS-MLPA): simultaneous detection of CpG methylation and copy number changes of up to 40 sequences. *Nucleic Acids Res* 2005;33(14):e128.

52. Hömig-Hölzel C, Savola S. Multiplex ligation-dependent probe amplification (MLPA) in tumor diagnostics and prognostics. *Diagn Mol Pathol* 2012;21(4):189–206.

53. Warren JD, Xiong W, Bunker AM, et al. Septin 9 methylated DNA is a sensitive and specific blood test for colorectal cancer. *BMC Med* 2011;9:133.

54. Boland CR, Thibodeau SN, Hamilton SR, et al. A National Cancer Institute Workshop on Microsatellite Instability for cancer detection and familial predisposition: development of international criteria for the determination of microsatellite instability in colorectal cancer. *Cancer Res* 1998;58(22):5248–5257.

55. Umar A, Boland CR, Terdiman JP, et al. Revised Bethesda Guidelines for hereditary nonpolyposis colorectal cancer (Lynch syndrome) and microsatellite instability. *J Natl Cancer Inst* 2004;96(4):261–268.

56. Voelkerding KV, Dames SA, Durtschi JD. Next-generation sequencing: from basic research to diagnostics. *Clin Chem* 2009;55(4):641–658.

57. Cronin M, Ross JS. Comprehensive next-generation cancer genome sequencing in the era of targeted therapy and personalized oncology. *Biomarker Med* 2011;5(3):293–305.

58. Coonrod EM, Durtschi JD, Margraf RL, et al. Developing genome and exome sequencing for candidate gene identification in inherited disorders: an integrated technical and bioinformatics approach. *Arch Pathol Lab Med* 2013;137(3):415–433.

59. Grossmann V, Kohlmann A, Klein HU, et al. Targeted next-generation sequencing detects point mutations, insertions, deletions and balanced chromosomal rearrangements as well as identifies novel leukemia-specific fusion genes in a single procedure. *Leukemia* 2011;25(4):671–680.

60. Marchetti A, Del Grammastro M, Filice G, et al. Complex mutations & subpopulations of deletions at exon 19 of EGFR in NSCLC revealed by next generation sequencing: potential clinical implications. *PloS One* 2012;7(7):e42164.

61. McCourt CM, McArt DG, Mills K, et al. Validation of next generation sequencing technologies in comparison to current diagnostic gold standards for BRAF, EGFR and KRAS mutational analysis. *PloS One* 2013;8(7):e69604.

62. Thol F, Kölking B, Damm F, et al. Next-generation sequencing for minimal residual disease monitoring in acute myeloid leukemia patients with FLT3-ITD or NPM1 mutations. *Genes Chromosomes Cancer* 2012;51(7):689–695.

63. Barski A, Cuddapah S, Cui K, et al. High-resolution profiling of histone methylations in the human genome. *Cell* 2007;129(4):823–837.

64. Schones DE, Zhao K. Genome-wide approaches to studying chromatin modifications. *Nat Rev Genet* 2008;9(3):179–191.

65. Ren B, Robert F, Wyrick JJ, et al. Genome-wide location and function of DNA binding proteins. *Science* 2000;290(5500):2306–2309.

66. Robertson G, Hirst M, Bainbridge M, et al. Genome-wide profiles of STAT1 DNA association using chromatin immunoprecipitation and massively parallel sequencing. *Nat Methods* 2007;4(8):651–657.

67. Shinawi M, Cheung SW. The array CGH and its clinical applications. *Drug Discov Today* 2008;13(17–18):760–770.

68. Iacobucci I, Lonetti A, Papayannidis C, Martinelli G. Use of single nucleotide polymorphism array technology to improve the identification of chromosomal lesions in leukemia. *Curr Cancer Drug Targets* 2013;13(7):791–810.

69. Ahmad A, Iqbal MA. Significance of genome-wide analysis of copy number alterations and UPD in myelodysplastic syndromes using combined CGH - SNP arrays. *Curr Med Chem* 2012;19(22):3739–3747.

70. Goncalves R, Bose R. Using multigene tests to select treatment for early-stage breast cancer. *J Natl Compr Canc Netw* 2013;11(2):174–182.

PART II

Etiology and Epidemiology of Cancer

4 Tobacco

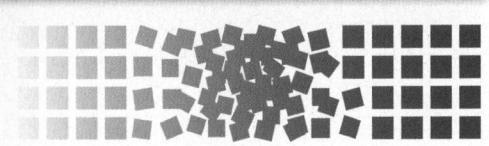

Richard J. O'Connor

INTRODUCTION

Regrettably, tobacco use remains one of the leading causes of death worldwide. It is projected to leave over 1 billion dead in the 21st century, after killing nearly 100 million during the course of the 20th century.[1] Data from the Global Adult Tobacco Survey (GATS), which conducted representative household surveys in 14 low- and middle-income countries (Bangladesh, Brazil, China, Egypt, India, Mexico, Philippines, Poland, Russia, Thailand, Turkey, Ukraine, Uruguay, and Vietnam), suggest 41% of men and 5% of women across these countries currently smoke.[2] Compare this to approximately 24% of men and 16% of women in the United States.[3] A preponderance of the death and disease associated with tobacco use is associated with its combusted forms, particularly the cigarette. However, all forms of tobacco use have negative health consequences, the severity of which can vary among products. From the introduction of the mass-manufactured, mass-marketed cigarette (e.g., Camel in 1913), smoking rates grew, first among men then among women, and peaked in Western countries in the 1960s to 1970s, before beginning a steady decline.[4] The smoking rate among US adults has dropped from its peak in 1965 of 42% to 19% in 2011.[3] Per capita consumption has been dropping almost continuously since the 1960s, although the rate of decline has slowed since the early 2000s.[5] Among youth, smoking rates have been in decline since the 1990s,[6,7] although there is some evidence of growth in use of other forms of tobacco (e.g., cigars, water pipes, electronic cigarettes) in 2011 to 2012 that may be displacing cigarette use.[8]

Tobacco control policy interventions can impact both smoking prevalence and lung cancer incidence.[9] For example, a recent analysis suggests that implementation of graphic health warnings in Canada in 1999 resulted in a significant reduction (up to 4.5 percentage points) in smoking prevalence over a decade.[10] Increases in tobacco taxes have long been shown to reduce youth smoking initiation and to prompt more attempts to quit smoking.[11] Evidence from state comparisons in the United States suggests that comprehensive tobacco control measures effectively implemented (such as in California and Massachusetts) can reduce lung cancer incidence.[12] Indeed, Holford and colleagues[13] have shown that since the seminal 1964 Report of the Surgeon General, an estimated 157 million years of life (approximately 20 years per person) have been saved by tobacco control activities in the United States over 50 years. That is, tobacco control activities are estimated to have averted 8 million premature deaths and extended mean life span by 19 to 20 years.[13] However, the marketing of cigarettes has since shifted focus to the developing world, where smoking rates are on the increase. In an attempt to head off an epidemic of smoking and associated diseases, the World Health Organization initiated a public health treaty, the Framework Convention on Tobacco Control (FCTC), to coordinate international efforts to reduce tobacco use.[14] The FCTC binds parties to enact measures to control the labeling and marketing of tobacco products, create a framework for testing and regulating product contents and emissions, combat smuggling and counterfeiting, and protect nonsmokers from secondhand smoke.[15] To date, the FCTC has been ratified by more than 150 countries. The FCTC provides governments the opportunity to regulate the marketing, labeling, and contents/emissions of tobacco products, as well as control the global trade in tobacco products. In the United States, which is currently not a party to FCTC, the U.S. Food and Drug Administration (FDA) has, since 2009, had authority to regulate tobacco products and their marketing along similar lines.[16]

EPIDEMIOLOGY OF TOBACCO AND CANCER

Linkages between tobacco use and cancers at various sites had been noted for several decades. In the late 1800s, it was believed that excessive cigar use created irritation that led to oral cancers.[17] In the 1930s, German scientists began to establish links between cigarette smoking and lung cancers.[18] However, it was not until the Doll and Hill[19] and Wynder and Graham[20] studies were published that the association was demonstrated in large samples and well-designed studies. Table 4.1 lists the cancers currently recognized by the U.S. Surgeon General as caused by smoking, along with their corresponding estimated mortality statistics.[21–23] Of these, the most well-publicized link is between smoking and lung cancer. In a recent examination of National Health and Nutrition Examination Survey (NHANES) data, Jha[24] showed a hazard ratio for lung cancer in smokers versus nonsmokers of 17.8 in women and 14.6 in men. However, smoking contributes substantially to overall cancer burden across multiple sites, including the oropharynx, cervix, and pancreas. Hazard ratios of 1.7 for women and 2.2 for men are seen for cancers other than in the lung in smokers versus nonsmokers.[24] Emerging evidence also links smoking with breast cancer, although the data are as yet insufficient to make causal conclusions.[23,25] Cancer risks associated with smoking, as well as outcomes and survival, depend on a number of factors. A common index of cancer risk is pack-years, or the number of packs of cigarettes smoked per day multiplied by the number of years smoked in the lifetime. In general, the higher the number of pack-years, the greater the cancer risk. Risks for lung cancer decline with smoking cessation, and the longer a former smoker remains off of cigarettes, the more the risk declines.[26] However, excepting those smokers who quit with relatively few pack years accumulated (typically before age 40), cancer risk rarely approaches that of a never smoker.[24,27]

A recent study using several large cohort studies examined death rates and the relative risks associated with smoking and smoking cessation for 3 epochs (1959 to 1965, 1982 to 1988, and 2000 to 2010).[27] Of most interest here is death from lung cancer. For men, the age-adjusted death rate from lung cancer increased from 1959 through 1965 to 1982 through1988, but then fell for 2000

TABLE 4.1

Level of Evidence for Smoking-Attributable Cancers According to the United States Office of the Surgeon General by Cancer Site and Yearly Smoking-Attributable Mortality at Sites with Available Estimates, United States, 2004

	Cancer Site	Yearly Smoking-Attributable Mortality
Evidence Sufficient to Infer Causal Relationship	Bladder	4,983
	Cervix	447
	Colon and rectum	N/A
	Esophagus	8,592
	Kidney	3,043
	Larynx	3,009
	Leukemia (AML)	1,192
	Liver	N/A
	Lung	125,522
	Oral cavity and pharynx	4,893
	Pancreas	6,683
	Stomach	2,484
Evidence Suggestive but Not Sufficient to Infer Causal Relationship	Breast	
Inadequate to Infer Presence or Absence of Causal Relationship	Ovary	
Evidence Sufficient to Infer No Causal Relationship	Prostate	

N/A, not available; AML, acute myeloid leukemia.

through 2010; for women, the age-adjusted death rate continued to rise over time, with the biggest increase between 1982 through 1988 to 2000 through 2010.[27] In relative risk terms, the likelihood of dying from lung cancer given current smoking has increased from 2.73 to 12.65 to 25.66 among women, and 12.22 to 23.81 to 24.97 for men. Equivalent risks for former smokers increased from 1.3 to 3.85 to 6.7 among women, versus 3.48 to 7.41 to 6.75 for men. These and other analyses suggest that the cancer risks from smoking may have increased with time.[27,28] The histologic subtypes of lung cancer seen in the US population have also shifted with time. Into the early 1980s, squamous cell carcinomas (SCC) were the most common manifestations of lung cancer. However, a rapid rise in adenocarcinomas has been noted, and by the 1990s, had overtaken SCC as the leading type of lung cancer.[23]

Tobacco Use Behaviors

The level of tobacco exposure is ultimately driven by use behaviors, including the number of cigarettes smoked, the patterns of smoking on individual cigarettes, and the number of years smoked. The primary driver of smoking behavior is nicotine—the major addictive substance and primary reinforcer of continued smoking.[29–31] Over time, smokers learn an *acceptable* level of nicotine intake that attains the beneficial effects they seek while avoiding negative withdrawal symptoms. Smokers can affect the amount of nicotine (and accompanying toxicants) they draw from a cigarette by altering the number of puffs taken, puff size,

frequency, duration, and velocity (collectively referred to as smoking topography).[32] Smokers tend to consume a relatively stable number of cigarettes per day and to smoke those cigarettes in a relatively consistent manner in order to maintain an acceptable level of nicotine in their system across the day.[33] The number of cigarettes smoked per day and the smoking pattern of an individual may be influenced by the rate of nicotine metabolism.[30] Nicotine is metabolized primarily to cotinine, which is further metabolized to trans-3'-hydroxycotinine (3HC), catalyzed by the liver cytochrome P450 2A6 enzyme.[34] Functional polymorphisms in the genes coding for these enzymes allow for the identification of *fast* metabolizers, who have more rapid nicotine clearance and show greater cigarette intake and more intensive smoking topography profiles relative to *normal* or *slow* metabolizers.[35–37] The ratio of 3HC to cotinine in plasma or saliva can be used as a reliable noninvasive phenotypic marker for CYP2A6 activity.[38,39] CYP2A6 activity is known to vary across racial/ethnic groups, with those of African or Asian descent showing slower metabolism than those of Caucasian descent.[40–42] Clinical trial data clearly show that the metabolite ratio can be used to predict success in quitting, and that the likelihood of quitting decreases as the ratio increases, such that slower metabolizers are more successful at achieving abstinence.[37,41,43] Despite their addiction to nicotine, most smokers in Western countries report that they regret ever starting to smoke and want to quit smoking, and there is evidence for similar regret in developing countries as well.[44–46] However, most smokers are unsuccessful in their attempts to quit smoking; the most effective evidence-based treatments increase the odds of quitting by 3 times, with 12-month cessation rates of approximately 40% relative to placebo.[47]

Evolution of Tobacco Products

Historically, tar was believed to be the main contributor to smoking-caused disease.[48] It is important to note that *tar* is not a specific substance, but simply the collected particulate matter from cigarette smoke, less water and nicotine (in technical reports, it is often referred to as nicotine-free dry particulate matter). Soon after the first studies were done showing that painting mice with cigarette tar caused cancerous tumors, it was theorized that reducing tar yields of cigarettes might also reduce the disease burden of smoking.[48] Concurrently, cigarette manufacturers were seeking to reassure their customers that their products were safe, that if hazardous compounds were identified they would be removed, and that product modifications could help to reduce risks.[4,49–51] Indeed, in the United States and United Kingdom, average tar levels of cigarettes dropped dramatically from the 1960s through the 1990s, and have since leveled off.[52,53] The European Union took the tar reduction mentality to heart in crafting maximum levels of tar in cigarettes that could be sold in member countries, beginning at 15 mg in 1992, then dropping to 12 mg in 1998, and 10 mg in 2005.[54] Unfortunately, these reductions in tar yields have not translated into changes in disease risks among smokers.[55] Despite initial optimism about these products, both laboratory-based and epidemiologic studies indicate neither an individual, nor a public health benefit from *low-tar* cigarettes as compared to *full-flavor* varieties.[56–58] The health consequences of mistakenly accepting the purported benefits of lower tar and nicotine products have been significant. The increases in adenocarcinoma of the lung observed in the United States over recent decades may reflect changes made to the cigarette, such as filters, filter ventilation, and tobacco-specific nitrosamines (TSNA) in smoke produced by the relatively high amount of burley tobacco used in the typical US cigarette blend.[23,59] Tobacco manufacturers engineered cigarettes be *elastic*; that is, cigarettes allow smokers to adjust their puffing patterns to regulate their intake of nicotine, regardless of how the cigarette might perform under the standard testing conditions that drove the labeling and advertising of the products.[55] Researchers have since come to determine that filter vents are the main design feature the industry relied on in creating elastic products.[54,55,60,61] Vents facilitate taking larger puffs and also contribute to sensory perceptions, because they dilute the smoke with air.[62] So, even with a larger puff, the same mass of toxins can seem less harsh and irritating because it is diluted by a proportionate amount of air, which may in turn underscore smokers' beliefs that they are smoking safer cigarettes.[62-64] Other smoke components (e.g., acetaldehyde, ammonia, minor tobacco alkaloids) and aspects of cigarette engineering (e.g., menthol, flavor additives) may further contribute to the addictiveness of cigarettes.[65]

Since the 1980s, manufacturers have introduced products that make more explicit claims about reduced health risks. Examples of modified cigarettelike products include Premier (RJ Reynolds), Eclipse (RJ Reynolds), Accord/Heatbar (Philip Morris), Omni (Vector Tobacco), and Advance (Brown and Williamson).[66] In the 2000s, as evidence of reduced lung cancer incidence and coincident increases in snus use in Sweden appeared,[67,68] manufacturers began to promote smokeless tobacco products as reduced harm alternatives. Most recently, electronic cigarettes, which vaporize a nicotine solution, have gained increasing popularity and generated concern among public health practitioners, particularly with regard to effects on youth.[8,69,70] In the United States, the FDA has authority to authorize marketing claims about reduced risk, which an Institute of Medicine panel concluded should be based on extensive testing of abuse liability, likely health effects, and effects on the whole population.[71]

CARCINOGENS IN TOBACCO PRODUCTS AND PROCESSES OF CANCER DEVELOPMENT

Cigarette smoke has been identified as carcinogenic since the 1950s, and efforts have continued to identify specific carcinogens in smoke and smokeless tobacco products. The International Agency for Research on Cancer (IARC) has classified both cigarette smoke and smokeless tobacco as Group 1 carcinogens.[72,73] IARC has also identified 72 measurable carcinogens in cigarette smoke where evidence is sufficient to classify them as Group 1 (carcinogenic to humans), 2A (probably carcinogenic to humans), or 2B (possibly carcinogenic to humans).[72] The IARC list, in addition to data from the U.S. Environmental Protection Agency (EPA), the National Toxicology Program, and the National Institute for Occupational Safety and Health (NIOSH), informed the FDA's development of a list of Harmful and Potentially Harmful Constituents (HPHC) in tobacco and tobacco smoke, which manufacturers will be required to report.[74] Table 4.2 illustrates the carcinogens listed as HPHC alongside their carcinogenicity classifications by IARC or the EPA.

Compounds of Particular Concern

Research groups have listed components of cigarette smoke theorized to impact health risk, often relying on carcinogenic potency indices and relative concentrations in smoke.[75,76] In these analyses, the N-nitrosamines, benzene, 1,3-butadiene, aromatic amines, and cadmium often rank highly. Polycyclic aromatic hydrocarbons (PAH), many of which are carcinogenic, consist of three or more fused aromatic rings resulting from incomplete combustion of organic (carbonaceous) materials, and are often found in coal tar, soot, broiled foods, and automobile engine exhaust.[77] A compound of particular concern in cigarette smoke historically has been benzo(a)pyrene (BaP), which has substantial carcinogenic activity and is considered carcinogenic to humans by the IARC.[77] In addition to PAH, other hydrocarbons found in significant quantities in cigarette smoke include benzene (a long-established cause

of leukemia), 1,3-butadiene (a potent multiorgan carcinogen), naphthalene, and styrene. Carbonyl compounds, such as formaldehyde and acetaldehyde, are found in copious amounts in cigarette smoke, primarily coming from the combustion of sugars and cellulose.[78] However, there are numerous other noncigarette exposures to these compounds, including endogenous formation during metabolism. Smoke contains a number of aromatic amines, such as known bladder carcinogens 2-aminonaphthalene and 4-aminobiphenyl, heterocyclic amines, and furans. Toxic metals, including beryllium, cadmium, lead, and polonium-210, are also present in cigarette smoke in measurable quantities,[79,80] levels of which may depend in part on the region of the world where the tobacco was grown.[81] Much attention has been focused on the N-nitrosamines, primarily because they are well-established carcinogens.[82-85] Nitrosamines form through reactions of nitrite with amino groups. In tobacco, two compounds of concern are 4-(methylnitrosamino)-1-(3-pyridyl)-1-butanone (NNK), which is derived from nitrosation of nicotine, and N'-nitrosonornicotine (NNN), which is derived from nitrosation of nornicotine. Both of these compounds are tobacco specific. NNN and NNK primarily form during the curing process for tobacco, where the leaves are dried through contact with combustion gases from heat (flue) curing or microbial activity in air curing.[78] NNK is known to be a potent lung carcinogen, but also shows tumor induction activity in the nasal cavity, the pancreas, and the liver, whereas NNN has been shown to induce tumors along the respiratory tract and esophagus in various animal models. Because they are produced in the curing process and transfer into smoke, rather than being formed by combustion, it is possible to reduce nitrosamines by changing curing and storage practices.[78,86,87]

Smokeless tobacco products, although they are not burned, nonetheless contain substantial levels of carcinogens, most prominently the N-nitrosamines.[73] Here, product type and composition has an enormous effect on nitrosamine levels. For example, US moist snuff has substantially higher levels than that sold in Sweden (snus), whereas smokeless products available in India are often far higher in nitrosamines.[88] US smokeless products also can contain PAH and carbonyl compounds, likely derived from fire curing the constituent tobacco.[89] Similar to cigarettes, smokeless products would also contain toxic metals.[79,80]

Although tobacco is an exceedingly complex mixture, it is possible to use animal model and epidemiologic evidence to postulate relationships between specific components and known tobacco-induced cancers.[90-92] There is strong evidence from multiple studies to suggest that PAH and N-nitrosamines are involved in lung carcinogenesis. For example, PAH–DNA adducts are observed in lung tissues, and p53 tumor suppressor mutations in lung tumors resemble the damage created by PAH diol epoxide metabolites in vitro.[93-96] NNK appears to preferentially induce lung tumors in the rat, regardless of the route of administration, and DNA–nitrosamine adducts are detectable in lung tissues.[97,98] Most importantly, nitrosamine metabolite levels measured in smokers were prospectively related to the risk of lung cancer in cohort studies, even adjusting for other indices of smoking exposure (e.g., cotinine, pack-years).[98-102] PAH and nitrosamines are also likely to be implicated in cancers along the respiratory tract and the cervix.[103,104] Considerable evidence exist that aromatic amines such as 4-aminobiphenyl and 2-naphthylamine are potent bladder carcinogens, and smokers are known to be at an elevated risk of bladder cancer, so these are presumed to be the primary causative agents.[105-107] Similarly, as benzene is a known cause of leukemia, it is presumed that this is the link to leukemia observed in smokers.

Important to examining the role of various smoke components in cancer is the ability to measure the exposure of smokers to these components. Biomarkers of exposure may also be crucial for examining products for their potential to reduce health risks associated with tobacco use.[71,108,109] Validation of tobacco exposure biomarkers is threefold: method validation, validation with respect to product use, and validation with respect to disease risk.[71]

TABLE 4.2

Carcinogens in Tobacco and Tobacco Smoke Identified as Harmful and Potentially Harmful by the U.S. Food and Drug Administration, with International Agency for Research on Cancer Carcinogenecity (IARC) Classifications as of 2013

Compound	CAS No.	IARC Group	IARC Volume	Year
1,3-Butadiene	106-99-0	1	100F	2012
2-Aminonaphthalene	91-59-8	1	100F	2012
4-(Methylnitrosamino)-1-(3-pyridyl)-1-butanone (NNK)	64091-91-4	1	100E	2012
4-Aminobiphenyl	92-67-1	1	100F	2012
Aflatoxin B1	1162-65-8	1	100F	2012
Arsenic	7440-38-2	1	100C	2012
Benzene	71-43-2	1	100F	2012
Benzo[a]pyrene	50-32-8	1	100F	2012
Beryllium	7440-41-7	1	100C	2012
Cadmium	7440-43-9	1	100C	2012
Chromium (Hexavalent compounds)	18540-29-9	1	100C	2012
Ethylene oxide	75-21-8	1	100F	2012
Formaldehyde	50-00-0	1	100F	2012
N-Nitrosonornicotine (NNN)	16543-55-8	1	100E	2012
Nickel (compounds)		1	100C	2012
o-Toluidine	95-53-4	1	100F	2012
Polonium-210	7440-08-6	1	100D	2012
Uranium (235, 238 Isotopes)	7440-61-1	1	100D	2012
Vinyl chloride	75-01-4	1	100F	2012
Acrylamide	79-06-1	2A	60	1994
Cyclopenta[c,d]pyrene	27208-37-3	2A	92	2010
Dibenz[a,h]anthracene	53-70-3	2A	92	2010
Dibenzo[a,l]pyrene	191-30-0	2A	92	2010
Ethyl carbamate (urethane)	51-79-6	2A	96	2010
IQ (2-Amino-3-methylimidazo[4,5-f]quinoline)	76180-96-6	2A	56	1993
N-Nitrosodiethylamine	55-18-5	2A	SUP 7	1987
N-Nitrosodimethylamine (NDMA)	62-75-9	2A	SUP 7	1987
2-Nitropropane	79-46-9	2B	71	1999
2,6-Dimethylaniline	87-62-7	2B	57	1993
5-Methylchrysene	3697-24-3	2B	92	2010
A-α-C (2-Amino-9H-pyrido[2,3-b]indole)	26148-68-5	2B	SUP 7	1987
Acetaldehyde	75-07-0	2B	71	1999
Acetamide	60-35-5	2B	71	1999
Acrylonitrile	107-13-1	2B	71	1999
Benz[a]anthracene	56-55-3	2B	92	2010
Benz[j]aceanthrylene	202-33-5	2B	92	2012
Benzo[b]fluoranthene	205-99-2	2B	92	2010
Benzo[b]furan	271-89-6	2B	63	1995
Benzo[c]phenanthrene	195-19-7	2B	92	2010
Benzo[k]fluoranthene	207-08-9	2B	92	2010
Caffeic acid	331-39-5	2B	56	1993
Catechol	120-80-9	2B	71	1999
Chrysene	218-01-9	2B	92	2010
Cobalt	7440-48-4	2B	52	1991

(continued)

ETIOLOGY AND EPIDEMIOLOGY OF CANCER

TABLE 4.2

Carcinogens in Tobacco and Tobacco Smoke Identified as Harmful and Potentially Harmful by the U.S. Food and Drug Administration, with International Agency for Research on Cancer Carcinogenecity (IARC) Classifications as of 2013 *(continued)*

Compound	CAS No.	IARC Group	IARC Volume	Year
Dibenzo[a,h]pyrene	189-64-0	2B	92	2010
Dibenzo[a,i]pyrene	189-55-9	2B	92	2010
Ethylbenzene	100-41-4	2B	77	2000
Furan	110-00-9	2B	63	1995
Glu-P-1 (2-Amino-6-methyldipyrido[1,2-a:3′,2′-d]imidazole)	67730-11-4	2B	SUP 7	1987
Glu-P-2 (2-Aminodipyrido[1,2-a:3′,2′-d]imidazole)	67730-10-3	2B	SUP 7	1987
Hydrazine	302-01-2	2B	71	1999
Indeno[1,2,3-cd]pyrene	193-39-5	2B	92	2010
Isoprene	78-79-5	2B	71	1999
Lead	7439-92-1	2B	SUP 7	1987
MeA-α-C (2-Amino-3-methyl)-9H-pyrido[2,3-b]indole)	68006-83-7	2B	SUP 7	1987
N-Nitrosodiethanolamine (NDELA)	1116-54-7	2B	77	2000
N-Nitrosomethylethylamine	10595-95-6	2B	SUP 7	1987
N-Nitrosomorpholine (NMOR)	59-89-2	2B	SUP 7	1987
N-Nitrosopiperidine (NPIP)	100-75-4	2B	SUP 7	1987
N-Nitrosopyrrolidine (NPYR)	930-55-2	2B	SUP 7	1987
N-Nitrososarcosine (NSAR)	13256-22-9	2B	SUP 7	1987
Naphthalene	91-20-3	2B	82	2002
Nickel	7440-02-0	2B	49	1990
Nitrobenzene	98-95-3	2B	65	1996
Nitromethane	75-52-5	2B	77	2000
o-Anisidine	90-04-0	2B	73	1999
PhIP (2-Amino-1-methyl-6-phenylimidazo[4,5-b]pyridine)	105650-23-5	2B	56	1993
Propylene oxide	75-56-9	2B	60	1994
Styrene	100-42-5	2B	82	2002
Trp-P-1 (3-Amino-1,4-dimethyl-5H-pyrido[4,3-b]indole)	62450-06-0	2B	SUP 7	1987
Trp-P-2 (3-Amino-1-Methyl-5H-pyrido[4,3-b]indole)	62450-07-1	2B	SUP 7	1987
Vinyl acetate	108-05-4	2B	63	1995
1-Aminonaphthalene	134-32-7	3	SUP 7	1987
Chromium	7440-47-3	3	49	1990
Crotonaldehyde	4170-30-3	3	63	1995
Dibenzo[a,e]pyrene	192-65-4	3	92	2010
Mercury	7439-97-6	3	58	1993
Quinoline	91-22-5	EPA Group B2		
Cresols (o-, m-, and p-cresol)	1319-77-3	EPA Group C		

Notes: Most recently published IARC monograph for each compound is listed.
Quinoline and cresols have not been evaluated by IARC, but have been evaluated by U.S. Environmental Protection Agency.
IARC Groups: 1, Carcinogenic to humans; 2A, Probably carcinogenic to humans; 2B, Possibly carcinogenic to humans; 3, Not classifiable as to its carcinogenicity to humans; http://monographs.iarc.fr/ENG/Classification/ClassificationsAlphaOrder.pdf
EPA Groups: B2, Likely to be carcinogenic in humans; C, Possible human carcinogen.
CAS No., Chemical Abstracts Service registry number. *CAS Registry Number is a Registered Trademark of the American Chemical Society.* EPA, Environmental Protection Agency.
Quinoline: http://www.epa.gov/iris/subst/1004.htm
Cresols: http://www.epa.gov/iris/subst/0300.htm; http://www.epa.gov/iris/subst/0301.htm; http://www.epa.gov/iris/subst/0302.htm

TABLE 4.3

Commonly Used Biomarkers of Exposure to Carcinogens in Tobacco Smoke

Biomarker	Tobacco Smoke Source	Matrices
Monohydroxy-30butenyl mercapturic acid (MHBMA)	1,3-butadiene	Urine
4-Aminobiphenyl-globin	4-aminobiphenyl	Blood
N-(2-hydroxypropyl)methacrylamide (HPMA)	Acrolein	Urine
Carbamoylethylvaline	Acrylamide	Blood
Cyanoethylvaline	Acrylonitrile	Blood
S-phenylmercapturic acid (SPMA)	Benzene	Urine
Cd	Cadmium	Urine
3-hydroxypropyl mercapturic acid (HBMA)	Crotonaldehyde	Urine
2-hydroxyethyl mercapturic acid (HEMA)	Ethylene oxide	Urine
Nicotine equivalents (nicotine, cotinine, trans-3'-hydroxycotinine, and their respective glucuronides)	Nicotine	Urine
Total 4-(methylnitrosamino)-1-(3-pyridyl)-1-butanol (NNAL) (NNAL + NNAL glucuronide)	NNK	Urine
Total NNN (NNN + NNN glucuronide)	NNN	Urine
1-Hydroxypyrene	Pyrene (representative of other PAH)	Urine

Adapted from Hecht SS, Yuan JM, Hatsukami D. Applying tobacco carcinogen and toxicant biomarkers in product regulation and cancer prevention. *Chem Res Toxicol* 2010;23:1001–1008.

Validation with respect to product use means that levels of a given biomarker differ substantially between users and nonusers, and that biomarker levels decrease substantially when product use is stopped. Validation with respect to disease risk implies that variation in biomarker levels in product users are predictive of variations in disease outcomes. Over the last decade, the development of modern high-throughput, high-resolution mass spectrometry has allowed for the measurement of multiple metabolites of tobacco carcinogens.[110–113] Commonly used biomarkers of tobacco exposure are listed in Table 4.3.

How Tobacco Use Leads to Cancer

A recent U.S. Surgeon General's report provides extensive detail on the current state of knowledge of how smoking causes cancer.[65] Therefore, only a brief overview is provided here. Hecht[101,113–116] has argued for a major pathway by which tobacco use leads to cancer: carcinogen exposure leads to the formation of carcinogen–DNA adducts, which then cause mutations that, if not repaired or removed by apoptosis, will eventually give rise to cancer. It is important to keep perspective that, whereas each cigarette may contain seemingly low levels of a given carcinogen, smoking is, for most people, a long-term addiction. Thus, a mixture of numerous carcinogens is administered multiple times per day over the course of decades. Further, compounds taken in during smokers can be metabolically activated, thus increasing their activity. Cigarette smoke compounds appear to induce the cytochrome P450 system, which facilitates the metabolic activation of carcinogens to electrophilic entities that are able to covalently bind DNA.[117,118] DNA adducts appear to be crucial to the cancer process, and numerous studies show that smoker tissues contain higher levels of DNA adducts than nonsmokers, and that DNA adduct levels are associated with cancer risk.[119,120] At the same time, other systems are involved in the detoxification and deactivation of smoke constituents, typically catalyzed by UDP-glucuronosyltransferases and glutathione-S-transferases, resulting in excretion of inactive compounds.[121,122] An individual's balance of activation and deactivation of toxicants

may be an important predictor of cancer risk, although evidence for this is mixed in the literature.[123,124] Similarly, DNA repair capacity is an important consideration, because, even if adducts are formed, processes exist to remove such perturbations to normalize DNA structure. Enzymatic processes of DNA repair include alkytransferases, nucleotide excision, and mismatch repair. Polymorphisms in genes coding for these enzymes may relate to individual cancer susceptibility. Table 4.4 outlines the metabolic activation/detoxification, DNA-adduct formation, and repair processes believed to be involved for four tobacco carcinogens (nitrosamines, PAH, benzene, 4-aminobiphenyl).[65,120]

Those DNA adducts that persist can cause miscoding during DNA replication. Smoke carcinogens are known to cause G:A and G:T mutations, and mutations in the *KRAS* oncogene and the *P53* tumor suppressor gene are strongly associated with tobacco-caused cancers.[95,114,125–127] Inactivation of *P53*, together with the activation of *KRAS*, appear to reduce survival in non–small-cell lung cancer.[65] Gene mutations that do not result in apoptosis may go on to influence a number of downstream processes, which may lead to genomic instability, proliferation, and eventually, malignancy.[128–130] Some smoke constituents may also act in ways that indirectly support the development of cancer. Nicotine, although not a carcinogen in itself, is known to reduce apoptosis and increase angiogenesis and transformation processes via nuclear factor kappa B (NF-κB).[65,131] Activation of nicotinic acetylcholine receptors (nAChR) in lung epithelium by nicotine or NNK is associated with survival and proliferation of malignant cells.[65] Nitrosamines also appear to have similar activities via the activation of protein kinases A and B.[132] NNK may bind β-adrenergic receptors to stimulate the release of arachidonic acid, which is converted to prostaglandin E2 by cyclooxygenase (COX)-2. Smoke compounds appear to activate epidermal growth factor receptor (EGFR) and COX-2, both of which are found to be elevated in many cancers.[133] Ciliatoxic, inflammatory, and oxidizing compounds, such as acrolein and ethylene oxide in smoke, may also impact the likelihood of cancer development. Epigenetic changes such as hypermethylation, particularly at P16, may also play a role in lung cancer development.[65]

TABLE 4.4

Key Pathways and Processes Where Selected Smoke Constituents Are Activated and Detoxified

	NNN, NNK	PAH	Benzene	4-ABP
Metabolic Activation	Alpha hydroxylation	Diol epoxide formation	Epoxide/oxepin formation	N-oxidation
Cytochrome P450 Enzymes Involved	2A6, 2A13, 2E1	1A1, 1B1	2E1	1A2
Enzymes Involved in Detoxification/ Activation	UGT	MEH, GST, UGT	MEH, GST	UGT, NAT
DNA Adduct Formation Sites				
Lung	*O6*-POB-deoxyguanosine	BPDE-N2-deoxyguanosine		
Bladder				C-8 deoxyguanosine
DNA Repair Pathways	AGT, BER	NER, MMR	BER, NER, NIR	NER

UGT, uridine-5′-diphosphate-glucuronosyltransferases; MEH, microsomal epoxide hydrolases; NAT, *N*-Acetyltransferases; GST, glutathione-S-transferases; AGT, *O6*-alkylguanine–DNA alkyltransferase; BER, base excision repair; NER, nucleotide excision repair; MMR, mismatch repair; NIR, nucleotide incision repair.

SELECTED REFERENCES

The full reference list can be accessed at lwwhealthlibrary.com/oncology.

1. World Health Organization, Research for International Tobacco Control. WHO Report on the Global Tobacco Epidemic, 2008: the MPOWER Package. Geneva: World Health Organization; 2008.
2. Giovino GA, Mirza SA, Samet JM, et al. Tobacco use in 3 billion individuals from 16 countries: an analysis of nationally representative cross-sectional household surveys. Lancet 2012;380:668–679.
9. Cummings KM, Fong GT, Borland R. Environmental influences on tobacco use: evidence from societal and community influences on tobacco use and dependence. Annu Rev Clin Psychol 2009;5:433–458.
10. Huang J, Chaloupka FJ, Fong GT. Cigarette graphic warning labels and smoking prevalence in Canada: a critical examination and reformulation of the FDA regulatory impact analysis. Tob Control 2014;1:i7–i12.
15. Liberman J. Four COPs and counting: achievements, underachievements and looming challenges in the early life of the WHO FCTC Conference of the Parties. Tob Control 2012;21:215–220.
21. US Department of Health and Human Services. The Health Consequences of Smoking: A Report of the Surgeon General. Atlanta: Department of Health and Human Services, Centers for Disease Control and Prevention, National Center for Chronic Disease Prevention and Health Promotion, Office on Smoking and Health; 2004.
23. US Department of Health and Human Services. The Health Consequences of Smoking—50 Years of Progress. A Report of the Surgeon General. Atlanta: U.S. Department of Health and Human Services, Centers for Disease Control and Prevention, National Center for Chronic Disease Prevention and Health Promotion, Office on Smoking and Health; 2014.
24. Jha P, Ramasundarahettige C, Landsman V, et al. 21st-century hazards of smoking and benefits of cessation in the United States. N Engl J Med 2013;368:341–350.
26. Peto R, Darby S, Deo H, et al. Smoking, smoking cessation, and lung cancer in the UK since 1950: combination of national statistics with two case-control studies. BMJ 2000;321:323–329.
27. Thun MJ, Carter BD, Feskanich D, et al. 50-year trends in smoking-related mortality in the United States. N Engl J Med 2013;368:351–364.
30. Benowitz NL. Pharmacology of nicotine: addiction, smoking-induced disease, and therapeutics. Annu Rev Pharmacol Toxicol 2009;49:57–71.
34. Benowitz NL, Hukkanen J, Jacob P. Nicotine chemistry, metabolism, kinetics and biomarkers. Handb Exp Pharmacol 2009;29–60.
40. Benowitz NL, Dains KM, Dempsey D, et al. Racial differences in the relationship between number of cigarettes smoked and nicotine and carcinogen exposure. Nicotine Tob Res 2011;13:772–783.
41. Dempsey DA, St Helen G, Jacob P, et al. Genetic and pharmacokinetic determinants of response to transdermal nicotine in white, black, and asian nonsmokers. Clin Pharmacol Ther 2013;94:687–694.
42. Zhu AZ, Renner CC, Hatsukami DK, et al. The ability of plasma cotinine to predict nicotine and carcinogen exposure is altered by differences in CYP2A6: the influence of genetics, race, and sex. Cancer Epidemiol Biomarkers Prev 2013;22:708–718.
44. Fong GT, Hammond D, Laux FL, et al. The near-universal experience of regret among smokers in four countries: findings from the International Tobacco Control Policy Evaluation Survey. Nicotine Tob Res 2004; 6:S341–S351.
47. Tobacco Use and Dependence Guideline Panel. Treating Tobacco Use and Dependence: 2008 Update. Rockville, MD: U.S. Department of Health and Human Services; 2008.
55. National Cancer Institute. Risks Associated with Smoking Cigarettes with Low Machine-Measured Yields of Tar and Nicotine. Bethesda, MD: The Institute; 2001.
56. Harris JE, Thun MJ, Mondul AM, et al. Cigarette tar yields in relation to mortality from lung cancer in the cancer prevention study II prospective cohort, 1982-8. BMJ 2004;328:72.
59. Burns DM, Anderson CM, Gray N. Do changes in cigarette design influence the rise in adenocarcinoma of the lung? Cancer Causes Control 2011;22:13–22.
62. Kozlowski LT, O'Connor RJ. Cigarette filter ventilation is a defective design because of misleading taste, bigger puffs, and blocked vents. Tob Control 2002;11:I40–I50.
65. Centers for Disease Control and Prevention, National Center for Chronic Disease Prevention and Health Promotion, Office on Smoking and Health. How Tobacco Smoke Causes Disease: The Biology and Behavioral Basis for Smoking-Attributable Disease: A Report of the Surgeon General. Rockville, MD: Centers for Disease Control and Prevetion; 2010.
66. Stratton KR. Clearing the Smoke: Assessing the Science Base for Tobacco Harm Reduction. Washington, DC: Institute of Medicine, National Academy Press; 2001.
70. Schaller K, Ruppert L, Kahnert S, et al. Electronic Cigarettes – An Overview. Heidelberg: German Cancer Research Center (DKFZ); 2013. http://www.dkfz.de/en/presse/download/RS-Vol19-E-Cigarettes-EN.pdf
71. Institute of Medicine. Scientific Standards for Studies on Modified Risk Tobacco Products. Washington, DC: National Academies Press; 2012.
72. International Agency for Research on Cancer. Tobacco Smoke and Involuntary Smoking. Vol 83. Lyon: International Agency for Research on Cancer, World Health Organization; 2004.
74. Center for Tobacco Products. Reporting Harmful and Potentially Harmful Constituents in Tobacco Products and Tobacco Smoke Under Section 904(a) (3) of the Federal Food, Drug, and Cosmetic Act. Rockville, MD: Department of Health and Human Services; 2012.
83. Hecht SS. Biochemistry, biology, and carcinogenicity of tobacco-specific N-nitrosamines. Chem Res Toxicol 1998;11:559–603.
84. Hoffmann D, Rivenson A, Hecht SS. The biological significance of tobacco-specific N-nitrosamines: smoking and adenocarcinoma of the lung. Crit Rev Toxicol 1996;26:199–211.
91. Hoffmann D, Stepanov I, Hecht SS, et al. Tobacco Carcinogenesis. New York: Academic Press; 1978.
93. Pfeiffer GP, Denissenko MF, Olivier M, et al. Tobacco smoke carcinogens, DNA damage and p53 mutations in smoking-associated cancers. Oncogene 2002;21:7435–7451.
113. Hecht SS, Yuan JM, Hatsukami D. Applying tobacco carcinogen and toxicant biomarkers in product regulation and cancer prevention. Chem Res Toxicol 2010;23:1001–1008.
116. Hecht SS. Lung carcinogenesis by tobacco smoke. Int J Cancer 2012;131:2724–2732.
120. Hang B. Formation and repair of tobacco carcinogen-derived bulky DNA adducts. J Nucleic Acids 2010;2010:709521.
125. Ahrendt SA, Decker PA, Alawi EA, et al. Cigarette smoking is strongly associated with mutation of the K-ras gene in patients with primary adenocarcinoma of the lung. Cancer 2001;92:1525–1530.

5 Oncogenic Viruses

Christopher B. Buck and Lee Ratner

ETIOLOGY AND EPIDEMIOLOGY OF CANCER

PRINCIPLES OF TUMOR VIROLOGY

Viral infections are estimated to play a causal role in at least 11% of all new cancer diagnoses worldwide.[1] A vast majority of cases (>85%) occur in developing countries, where poor sanitation, high rates of cocarcinogenic factors such as HIV/AIDS, and lack of access to vaccines and cancer screening all contribute to increased rates of virally induced cancers. Even in developed countries, where effective countermeasures are widely available, cancers attributable to viral infection account for at least 4% of new cases.[2,3]

Viruses thought to cause various forms of human cancer come from six distinct viral families with a range of physical characteristics (Table 5.1). All known human cancer viruses are capable of establishing durable, long-term infections and cause cancer only in a minority of persistently infected individuals. The low penetrance of cancer induction is consistent with the idea that a virus capable of establishing a durable productive infection would not benefit from inducing a disease that kills the host.[4] The slow course of cancer induction (typically over a course of many years after the initial infection) suggests that viral infection alone is rarely sufficient to cause human malignancy and that virally induced cancers arise only after additional oncogenic "hits" have had time to accumulate stochastically.

In broad terms, viruses can cause cancer through either (or both) of two broad mechanisms: direct or indirect. Direct mechanisms, in which the virus-infected cell ultimately becomes malignant, are typically driven by the effects of viral oncogene expression or through direct genotoxic effects of viral gene products. In most established examples of direct viral oncogenesis, the cancerous cell remains "addicted" to viral oncogene expression for ongoing growth and viability.

A common feature of DNA viruses that depend on host cell DNA polymerases for replication (e.g., papillomaviruses, herpesviruses, and polyomaviruses) is the expression of viral gene products that promote progression into the cell cycle. A typical mechanism of direct oncogenic effects is through the inactivation of tumor suppressor proteins, such as the guardian of the genome, p53, and retinoblastoma protein (pRB). This effectively primes the cell to express the host machinery necessary for replicating the viral DNA. The study of tumor viruses has been instrumental in uncovering the existence and function of key tumor suppressor proteins, as well as key cellular proto-oncogenes, such as Src and Myc.

In theory, viruses could cause cancer via direct hit-and-run effects. In this model, viral gene products may serve to preserve cellular viability and promote cell growth in the face of otherwise proapoptotic genetic damage during the early phases of tumor development. In principle, the precancerous cell might eventually accumulate enough additional genetic hits to allow for cell growth and survival independent of viral oncogene expression. This would allow for stochastic loss of viral nucleic acids from the nascent tumor, perhaps giving a growth advantage due to the loss of "foreign" viral antigens that might otherwise serve as targets for immune-mediated clearance of the nascent tumor. Although hit-and-run effects have been observed in animal models of virally induced cancer,[5] these effects are extremely difficult to address in humans. Currently, there are no clearly established examples of hit-and-run effects in human cancer.

In indirect oncogenic mechanisms, the cells that give rise to the malignant tumor have never been infected by the virus. Instead, the viral infection is thought to lead to cancer by attracting inflammatory immune responses that, in turn, lead to accelerated cycles of tissue damage and regeneration of noninfected cells. In some instances, virally infected cells may secrete paracrine signals that drive the proliferation of uninfected cells. At a theoretical level, it may be difficult to distinguish between indirect carcinogenesis and hit-and-run direct carcinogenesis, because, in both cases, the metastatic tumor may not contain any viral nucleic acids.

A variety of hunting approaches have been used to uncover etiologic roles for viruses in human cancer. The first clues that high-risk human papillomaviruses (HPVs), Epstein-Barr virus (EBV), Kaposi's sarcoma–associated herpesvirus (KSHV), and Merkel cell polyomavirus (MCPyV) might be carcinogenic were based on the detection of virions, viral DNA, or viral RNA in the tumors these viruses cause. A common feature of known virally induced cancers is that they are more prevalent in immunosuppressed individuals, such as individuals suffering from HIV/AIDS or patients on immunosuppressive therapy after organ transplantation. This is thought to reflect the lack of immunologic control over the cancer-causing virus. Studies focused on AIDS-associated cancers provided the first evidence for the carcinogenic potential of KSHV and MCPyV. A theoretical limitation of this approach is that some virally induced cancers may not occur at dramatically elevated rates in all types of immunosuppressed subjects, particularly if the virus causes only a fraction of cases (e.g., HPV-induced head and neck cancers). Fortunately, the unbiased analysis of nucleic acid sequences found in tumors has become substantially more tractable as deep-sequencing methods have continued to fall in price. In the coming years, it should be increasingly possible to search for viral sequences without making the starting assumption that all virally induced tumors are associated with immunosuppression.[6]

One limitation of tumor sequencing approaches is that they might miss undiscovered divergent viral species within viral families known to have extensive sequence diversity[7] and could miss viral families that have not yet been discovered.[8] Tumor-sequencing approaches might also miss viruses that cause cancer by hit-and-run or indirect mechanisms. It is conceivable that this caveat could be addressed by focusing on sequencing early precancerous lesions thought to ultimately give rise to metastatic cancer.

An additional successful approach to hunting cancer viruses involves showing that individuals who are infected with a particular virus have an increased long-term risk of developing particular forms of cancer. This approach was successful for identifying and validating the carcinogenic roles of high-risk HPV types, hepatitis B virus (HBV), hepatitis C virus (HCV), KSHV, and human T-lymphotropic virus 1 (HTLV-1). Although viruses that are extremely prevalent, such as EBV and MCPyV, are not amenable to this approach per se, it may still be possible to draw connections

TABLE 5.1

Oncogenic Viruses

Virus	Taxon	Viral Genome	Virion	Infection Rate	Site of Persistance	Diseases in Normal Hosts	Diseases in Immunocompromised Hosts	Associated Cancers
High-risk human papillomavirus types (e.g., HPV16)	*Alphapapillomavirus*	8 kb circular dsDNA	Nonenveloped	>70%	Anogential mucosa, oral mucosa	Carcinomas of the cervix, penis, anus, vagina, vulva, tonsils, base of tongue	Increased incidence of same diseases	610,000
Hepatitis B virus (HBV)	*Hepadnaviridae*	3 kb ss/dsDNA	Enveloped	2%–8%	Hepatocytes	Cirrhosis, hepatocellular carcinoma	Same diseases, increased incidence with AIDS	380,000
Hepatitis C virus (HCV)	*Flaviviridae*	10 kb +RNA	Enveloped	~3%	Hepatocytes	Cirrhosis, hepatocellular carcinoma, splenic marginal zone lymphoma	Same diseases, increased incidence with AIDS	220,000
Epstein-Barr virus (EBV, HHV-4)	*Gammaherpesvirinae*	170 kb linear DNA	Enveloped	90%	B cells, pharyngeal mucosa	Mononucleosis, Burkitt lymphoma, other non-Hodgkin lymphoma, nasopharyngeal carcinoma	Increased incidence of same diseases, lymphoproliferative disease, other lymphomas, oral hairy leukoplakia, leiomyosarcoma	110,000
Kaposi's sarcoma herpesvirus (KSHV, HHV-8)	*Gammaherpesvirinae*	170 kb linear DNA	Enveloped	2%–60%	Oral mucosa, endothelium, B cells	Kaposi's sarcoma (KS), multicentric Castleman disease (MCD)	Increased KS, MCD incidence, primary effusion lymphoma	43,000
Merkel cell polyomavirus (MCPyV, MCV)	*Orthopolyomavirus*	5 kb circular dsDNA	Nonenveloped	75%	Skin (lymphocytes?)	Merkel cell carcinoma (MCC)	Increased MCC incidence	1,500 (US)
Human T-cell leukemia virus (HTLV-1)	*Deltaretrovirus*	9 kb +RNA (RT)	Enveloped	0.01%–6%	T and B cells	Adult T-cell leukemia/lymphoma, tropical spastic paraparesis, myelopathy, uveitis, dermatitis	Unknown	2,100

Note: Ranges for infection rates imply major variations in prevalence among populations in different world regions. *Associated cancers* indicates the annual number of new cases clearly attributable to viral infection. An estimate for the worldwide incidence of Merkel cell carcinoma is not currently available and an estimate of the annual new cases in the United States alone is given instead.
ds, double-stranded; ss, single-stranded; HHV, human herpesvirus; RT, reverse transcriptase.

Adapted from de Martel C, Ferlay J, Franceschi S, et al. Global burden of cancers attributable to infections in 2008: a review and synthetic analysis. *Lancet Oncol* 2012;13(6):607–615; Schiller JT, Lowy DR. Virus infection and human cancer: an overview. *Recent Results Cancer Res* 2014;193:1–10; Chen CJ, Hsu WL, Yang HI, et al. Epidemiology of virus infection and human cancer. *Recent Results Cancer Res* 2014;193:11–32; and Virgin HW, Wherry EJ, Ahmed R. Redefining chronic viral infection. *Cell* 2009;138(1):30–50.

between cancer risk and either unusually high serum antibody titers against viral antigens or unusually high viral load. Relatively high serologic titers reflect either comparatively poor control of the viral infection in at-risk individuals or expression of viral antigens in tumors or tumor precursor cells.[9,10]

The finding that a virus causes cancer is good news, in the sense that it can suggest possible paths to clinical intervention. These can include the development of vaccines or antiviral agents that prevent, attenuate, or eradicate the viral infection and thereby prevent cancer; the development of methods for early detection or diagnosis of cancer based on assays for viral nucleic acids or gene products; or the development of drugs or immunotherapeutics that treat cancer by targeting viral gene products. Unfortunately, establishing the carcinogenicity of a given viral species is an arduous process that must inevitably integrate multiple lines of evidence.[11] The demonstration that the virus can transform cells in culture and/or cause cancer in animal models provides circumstantial evidence of the oncogenic potential of a virus. All known human cancer viruses meet this criterion. However, it is important to recognize that viruses can theoretically coevolve to be noncarcinogenic in their native host (e.g., humans) and cause cancer only in the dysregulated environment of a nonnative host animal. This caveat may apply to human adenoviruses.

Finding that viral DNA is clonally integrated in a primary tumor and its metastatic lesions helps address the caveat that the virus might merely be a hitchhiker that finds the tumor cell a conducive environment in which to replicate (as opposed to playing a causal carcinogenic role). This caveat is also addressed by the observation that, in most instances, viruses found in tumors have lost the ability to exit viral latency and are functionally unable to produce new progeny virions. An unfortunate consequence of this is that vaccines or antiviral agents that target virion proteins (e.g., vaccines against high-risk HPVs or HBV) or gene products expressed late in the viral life cycle (e.g., herpesvirus thymidine kinase, which is the target of drugs such as ganciclovir) are rarely effective for treating existing virally induced tumors.

Demonstrating that a vaccine or antiviral agent targeting the virus either prevents or treats human cancer is by far the strongest form of evidence that a given virus causes human cancer. This type of proof has fully validated the causal role of HBV in human liver cancer. Compelling clinical trial data also show that antiherpesvirus therapeutics can prevent KSHV- or EBV-associated lymphoproliferative disorders, and that vaccination against HPV can prevent the development of precancerous lesions on the uterine cervix.

PAPILLOMAVIRUSES

History

The idea that cancer of the uterine cervix might be linked to sexual behavior was first proposed in the mid 19th century by Dominico Rigoni-Stern, who observed that nuns rarely contracted cervical cancer, whereas prostitutes suffered from cervical cancer more often than the general populace.[12] Another major milestone in cervical cancer research was Georgios Papanikolaou's development of the so-called Pap smear for early cytologic diagnosis of precancerous cervical lesions.[13] This form of screening, which allows for surgical intervention to remove precancerous lesions, has saved many millions of lives in developed countries, where public health campaigns have made testing widely available.

Although observations in the early 1980s suggested the possibility of a hit-and-run carcinogenic role for herpes simplex viruses in cervical cancer,[14] this hypothesis was abandoned in light of studies led by Harald zur Hausen. Low-stringency hybridization approaches revealed the presence of two previously unknown papillomavirus types, HPV16 and HPV18, in various cervical cancer cell lines, including the famous HeLa cell line.[15,16] There is now

overwhelming evidence that a group of more than a dozen sexually transmitted HPV types, including HPV16 and HPV18, play a causal role in essentially all cases of cervical cancer. HPVs associated with a high risk of cancer also cause about half of all penile cancers, 88% of anal cancers, 43% of vulvar cancers, 70% of vaginal cancers,[2] and an increasing fraction of head and neck cancers (see the following). In 2008, zur Hausen was awarded the Nobel Prize for his groundbreaking work establishing the link between HPVs and human cancer.

The viral family *Papillomaviridae* is named for the benign skin warts (papillomas) that some members of the family cause. In the early 1930s, Richard Edwin Shope and colleagues demonstrated viral transmission of papillomas in a rabbit model system.[17] Using this system, Peyton Rous and others showed that cottontail rabbit papillomavirus-induced lesions can progress to malignant skin cancer.[18,19] This was the first demonstration of a cancer-causing virus in mammals, building on Rous' prior work demonstrating a virus capable of causing cancer in chickens (the Rous sarcoma retrovirus).

Tissue Tropism and Gene Functions

Although papillomaviruses can achieve infectious entry into a wide variety of cell types in vitro and in vivo, the late phase of the viral life cycle, during which the viral genome undergoes vegetative replication and the L1 and L2 capsid proteins are expressed, is strictly dependent on host cell factors found only in differentiating keratinocytes near the surface of the skin or mucosa. Interestingly, a majority of HPV-induced cancers appear to arise primarily at zones of transition between stratified squamous epithelia and the single-layer (columnar) epithelia of the endocervix, the inner surface of the anus, and tonsillar crypts. It is thought that the mixed phenotypic milieu in cells at squamocolumnar transition zones may cause dysregulation of the normal coupling of the HPV life cycle to keratinocyte differentiation.

There are nearly 200 known HPV types.[20] In general, each papillomavirus type is a functionally distinct serotype, meaning that serum antibodies that neutralize one HPV type do not robustly neutralize other HPV types. Various HPV types preferentially infect different skin or mucosal surfaces. Different types tend to establish either transient infections that may be cleared over the course of months, or stable infections where virions are chronically shed from the infected skin surface for the lifetime of the host. HPV infections may or may not be associated with the formation of visible warts or other lesions. High-risk HPV types, with clearly established causal links to human cancer, are preferentially tropic for the anogenital mucosa and the oral mucosa, are usually transmitted by sexual contact, rarely cause visible warts, and usually establish only transient infections in a great majority of exposed individuals. The lifetime risk of sexual exposure to a high-risk HPV type has been estimated to be >70%. Individuals who fail to clear their infection with a high-risk HPV type and remain persistently infected are at much greater risk of developing cancer. Polymerase chain reaction (PCR)-based screening for the presence of high-risk HPV types thus serves as a useful adjunct to, or even a replacement for, the traditional Pap test.[21]

A consequence of the strict tissue-differentiation specificity of the papillomavirus life cycle is that HPVs do not replicate in standard monolayer cell cultures. Papillomaviruses also seem to be highly species restricted, and there are no known examples of an HPV type capable of infecting animals.[22] Thus, the investigation of key details of papillomavirus biology has relied almost entirely on modern recombinant DNA and molecular biologic analyses.

Papillomavirus genomes are roughly 8 kb, double-stranded, closed-circular DNA molecules (essentially reminiscent of a plasmid). During the normal viral life cycle, the genome does not adopt a linear form, does not integrate into the host cell chromosome, and remains as an extrachromosomal episome or minichromosome.

All the viral protein-coding sequences are arranged on one strand of the genome. The expression of various proteins is regulated by differential transcription and polyadenylation, as well as effects at the level of RNA splicing, export from the nucleus, and translation. In addition to the late half of the viral genome, which encodes the L1 and L2 capsid proteins, all papillomaviruses encode six key early region genes: E1, E2, E4, E5, E6, and E7.

The master transcriptional regulator E2 serves as a transcriptional repressor, and loss of E2 expression (typically through integration of the viral episome into the host cell DNA) results in the upregulation of early gene expression. The most extensively studied early region proteins are the E6 and E7 oncogenes of HPV16 and HPV18. The E6 protein of high-risk HPV types triggers the destruction of p53 by recruiting a host cell ubiquitin–protein ligase, E6AP.[23–25] Another important oncogenic function of E6 is the activation of cellular telomerase.[26] A wide variety of additional high-risk E6 activities that do not involve p53 have been identified.[27]

Most E7 proteins, including those of many low-risk HPV types, contain a conserved LXCXE motif that mediates interaction with pRB and the related "pocket" proteins p107 and p130.[28] Interestingly, the LXCXE motif is present in a wide variety of other oncogenes, most notably the T antigens of polyomaviruses and the E1A oncogenes of adenoviruses. The interaction of E7 with pRB disrupts the formation of a complex between pRB and E2F transcription factors, thereby blocking the ability of pRB to trigger cell cycle arrest.[29] The E7 proteins of high-risk HPVs can also contribute to chromosomal mis-segregation and aneuploidy, which may in turn contribute to malignant progression.[30] Like E6, E7 interacts with a wide variety of additional cellular targets, the spectrum of which seems to vary with different HPV types.[27]

Some papillomavirus types express an E5 oncogene, which functions as an agonist for cell surface growth factor receptors such as platelet-derived growth factor beta (PDGF-β) and epidermal growth factor (EGF) receptor.[31] Because E5 expression is uncommon in cervical tumors, it is uncertain whether the protein plays a key role in human cancer.

Human Papilloma Virus Vaccines

Two preventive vaccines against cancer-causing HPVs, trade named Gardasil (Merck) and Cervarix (GSK), are currently marketed worldwide for the prevention of cervical cancer. Both vaccines contain recombinant L1 capsid proteins based on HPV16 and HPV18 that are assembled in vitro into virus-like particles (VLPs). Together, HPV16 and HPV18 cause about 70% of all cases of cervical cancer worldwide. Gardasil also includes VLPs based on HPV types 6 and 11, which rarely cause cervical cancer but together cause about 90% of all genital warts. The VLPs contained in the vaccines are highly immunogenic in humans, eliciting high-titer serum antibody responses against L1 that are capable of neutralizing the infectivity of the cognate HPV types represented in the vaccine. It appears that the current HPV vaccines may confer lifelong immunity against new infection with the HPV types represented in the vaccine.[32] The vaccines elicit lower titer cross-neutralizing responses against a subset of cancer-causing HPV types that are closely related to HPV16 and HPV18.[33] Although these cross-neutralizing responses can at least partially protect vaccinees against a new infection with additional high-risk types, such as HPV31 and HPV45, it remains unclear how durable the lower level cross-protection will be.[33]

Because L1 is not expressed in latently infected keratinocyte stem cells residing on the epithelial basement membrane, current HPV vaccines are very unlikely to eradicate existing infections.[34,35] Like keratinocyte stem cells, cervical cancers and precursor lesions rarely or never express L1. Thus, the existing L1-based vaccines seem unlikely to serve as therapeutic agents for treating cervical cancer.

Three types of next-generation HPV vaccines are currently in human clinical trials. Merck has recently announced that a newer version of Gardasil, which contains VLPs based on a total of nine different HPV types, remained highly effective against HPV16 and HPV18 and also prevented 97% of precancerous cervical lesions caused by a wider variety of high-risk HPV types.[36] Another class of second-generation vaccines targets the papillomavirus minor capsid protein L2. An N-terminal portion of L2 appears to represent a highly conserved "Achilles' heel", which contains conserved protein motifs required for key steps of the infectious entry process.[37] Anti-L2 antibodies can neutralize a broad range of different human and animal HPV types, and thus, L2 vaccines are hoped to offer protection against all HPVs that cause cervical cancer, all low-risk HPV types that cause abnormal Pap smear results, as well as the full range of HPV types that cause skin warts. Finally, a wide variety of vaccines that seek to elicit cell-mediated immune responses against the E6 and E7 oncoproteins are aimed at a therapeutic intervention for the treatment of cervical cancer.[38]

Oropharyngeal Cancer

It is well established that tobacco products and alcohol cause head and neck cancer. In the late 1990s, Maura Gillison and colleagues noted a surprising number of new cases of tonsillar cancer in nonsmokers.[39] Many of the tumors found in nonsmokers were found to have wild-type p53 genes, raising the possibility that the tumor might be dependent on a p53-suppressing viral oncogene (as seen in cervical cancer). Gillison and colleagues went on to show that nearly half of all tonsillar cancers contain HPV DNA, most commonly HPV16. Interestingly, HPV-positive oropharyngeal cancers tend to be less lethal than tobacco-associated HPV-negative tumors. This finding has important implications for treatment of HPV-positive head and neck cancers.[40]

Although the incidence of tobacco-associated head and neck cancer has been declining in recent decades due to decreased tobacco use, recent studies suggest an ongoing increase in the incidence of HPV-associated cancers of the tonsils and the base of the tongue. By 2025, the number of new HPV-induced head and neck cancer cases in the United States is expected to roughly equal the number of new cervical cancer cases.[39] Based in part on these observations, the U.S. Centers for Disease Control and Prevention recommends that boys, in addition to girls, should be vaccinated against high-risk HPVs.

Nonmelanoma Skin Cancer

Epidermodysplasia verruciformis (EV) is a rare immunodeficiency that is characterized by the appearance of numerous flat, wartlike lesions across wide areas of skin. The lesions typically contain genus betapapillomaviruses, such as HPV5 or HPV8. EV patients frequently develop squamous cell carcinomas (SCC) in sun-exposed skin areas (suggesting that ultraviolet [UV] light exposure is a cofactor). It is also well established that other immunosuppressed individuals, such as organ transplant recipients and HIV-infected individuals, are at increased risk of developing SCC.[41,42] Although the E6 and E7 proteins of betapapillomaviruses appear to exert a different spectrum of effects than the E6 and E7 proteins of HPV types associated with cervical cancer,[43–45] Betapapillomavirus oncogenes can transform cells in vitro.[46] Although these circumstantial lines of evidence suggest that infectious agents, such as Betapapillomaviruses, might play a causal role in SCC, recent deep sequencing studies have observed few or no viral sequences in SCC tumors.[47] Although the results argue against durable direct oncogenic effects of any known viral species in SCC, an animal model system using bovine papillomavirus type 4 strongly suggests that papillomaviruses can cause cancer by hit and run mechanisms.[5] Thus, the question of whether hit-and-run or indirect oncogenic effects of HPVs may be at play in human SCC remains open.

POLYOMAVIRUSES

History

In the early 1950s, Ludwik Gross showed that a filterable infectious agent could cause salivary gland cancer in laboratory mice.[48] Later work by Bernice Eddy and Sarah Stewart showed that the murine polyoma (Greek for "many tumors") virus caused many different types of cancer in experimentally infected mice.[49] The discovery that murine polyomavirus could be grown in cell culture helped rekindle research interest in tumor virology and interest in the question of whether viruses might cause human cancer.

Like papillomaviruses, polyomaviruses have a nonenveloped capsid assembled from 72 pentamers of a single major capsid protein (VP1). Both viral families also carry circular dsDNA genomes. These physical similarities initially led to the classification of both groups into a single family, *Papovaviridae*. When sequencing studies ultimately revealed that polyomaviruses have a unique genome organization (with early and late genes being arranged on opposing strands of the genome) and almost no sequence homology to papillomaviruses, the two groups of viruses were divided into separate families.

In the early 1960s, Bernice Eddy, Maurice Hilleman, and Benjamin Sweet reported the discovery of simian vacuolating virus 40 (SV40), a previously unknown polyomavirus that was found as a contaminant in vaccines against poliovirus.[50,51] SV40 was derived from the rhesus monkey kidney cells used to amplify poliovirus virions in culture.[52] SV40 rapidly became an important model polyomavirus, and studies of its major and minor tumor antigens (large T [LT]and small t [ST], respectively) have played an important role in understanding various aspects of carcinogenesis. Despite significant alarm about the possible risk SV40 might pose to exposed individuals, a comprehensive, decades long series of studies have failed to uncover compelling evidence that SV40 exposure is causally associated with human cancer.[53]

Two naturally human-tropic polyomaviruses, BK virus (BKV) and John Cunningham virus (JCV), were first reported in back-to-back publications in 1971.[54,55] BKV and JCV are known to cause kidney disease and a lethal brain disease called progressive multifocal leukoencephalopathy, respectively, in immunosuppressed individuals. Although both viruses can cause cancer in experimentally exposed animals, it remains unclear whether either virus plays a causal role in human cancer. Although BKV LT expression can frequently be observed in the inflammatory precursor lesions that are thought to give rise to prostate cancer,[56] there is no evidence for the persistence of BKV DNA in malignant prostate tumors.[57] There have been case studies finding BKV T-antigen expression in bladder cancer,[58] and some reports have indicated the presence of JCV DNA in colorectal tumors. The long history of conflicting evidence concerning possible roles for BKV or JCV in human cancer is reviewed elsewhere.[59,60]

Merkel Cell Polyomavirus

In 2008, Yuan Chang and Patrick Moore reported their lab's discovery of the fifth known human polyomavirus species, which they named Merkel cell polyomavirus (MCV or MCPyV) based on its presence in Merkel cell carcinoma (MCC).[61] The discovery used an RNA deep sequencing approach called digital transcriptome subtraction. Using classic Southern blotting, this report demonstrated the clonal integration of MCPyV in an MCC tumor and its distant metastases. Many other labs worldwide have independently confirmed the presence of MCPyV DNA in about 80% of MCC tumors.[11]

MCC is a rare but highly lethal form of cancer that typically presents as a fast-growing lesion on sun-exposed skin surfaces (Fig. 5.1).[62] The risk of MCC is dramatically higher in HIV/AIDS patients, offering an initial clue that MCC might be a virally induced cancer.[63] Although MCC tumors express neuroendocrine markers associated with sensory Merkel cells of the epidermis, one recent report has shown that some MCC tumors also express B-cell markers, including rearranged antibody loci.[64] Currently, there is no clear evidence for the involvement of MCPyV in other tumors with neuroendocrine features.

In 2012, the International Agency for Research on Cancer (IARC) concluded that MCPyV is a class 2A carcinogen (probably carcinogenic to humans).[10,53] It should be noted that IARC evaluations rely heavily on animal carcinogenicity studies, and the 2A designation was assigned prior to a recent report showing that MCV-positive MCC lines are tumorigenic in a mouse model system.[65]

A great majority of healthy adults have serum antibodies specific for the MCPyV major capsid protein VP1. A majority also shed MCPyV virions from apparently healthy skin surfaces, and there is a strong correlation between individual subjects' serologic titer against VP1 and the amount of MCPyV DNA they shed.[66-68] Interestingly, MCC patients tend to have exceptionally strong serologic titers against VP1.[69] MCC tumors do not express detectable amounts of VP1, so this is unlikely to reflect direct exposure to

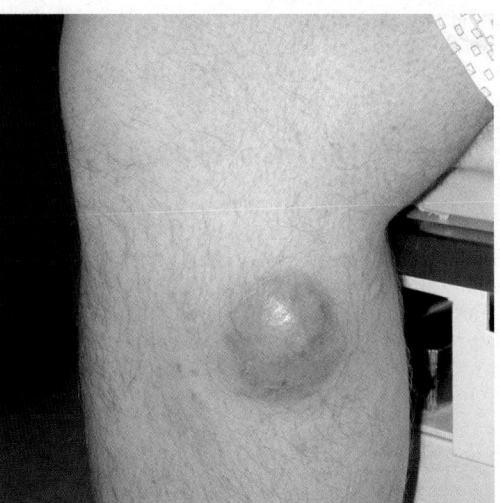
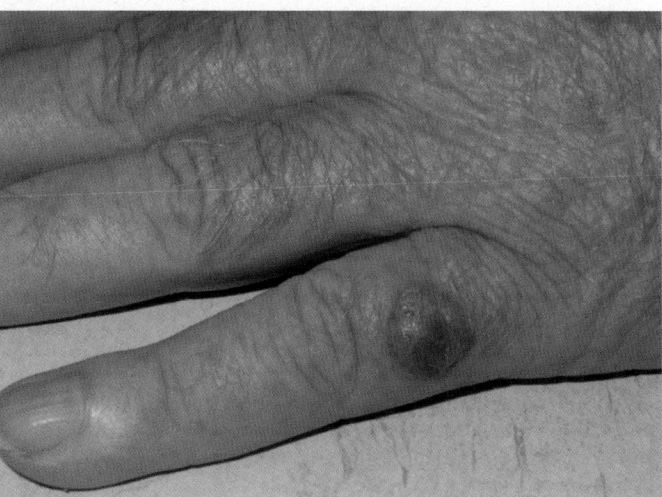

Figure 5.1 Merkel cell carcinoma (MCC). The *left panel* shows an MCC tumor on the calf. The *right panel* shows an MCC tumor on the finger. Photographs provided with permission by Dr. Paul Nghiem (University of Washington, www.merkelcell.org).

the tumor and instead likely represents a history of a high MCPyV load in MCC patients. A recent study of archived serum samples shows that unusually high serologic titers against MCPyV VP1 often precede the development of MCC by many years.[70]

Like the LT protein of SV40 (and the E7 proteins of high-risk HPVs), an N-terminal portion of the MCPyV LT protein contains an LXCXE motif that mediates inactivation of pRB function. In contrast to SV40 LT, which carries a p53-inactivation domain that overlaps the C-terminal helicase domain, MCPyV LT does not appear to inactivate p53 function.[71] Instead, the MCPyV LT helicase domain activates DNA damage responses and induces cell cycle arrest in cultured cell lines.[72] This may explain why the LT genes found in MCC tumors essentially always carry mutations that truncate LT upstream of the helicase domain. siRNA experiments indicate that most (although possibly not all) MCC tumors are "addicted" to the expression of MCPyV T antigens.[73–75] Interestingly, patients with higher levels of MCPyV DNA in their tumors, stronger T-antigen expression, and tumors that have been infiltrated by CD8+ T cells appear to have better prognoses.[76] This is consistent with the idea that cell-mediated immunity can help clear MCC tumors that express MCPyV antigens.

Recent work has shown that the pRB interacting domain of LT mediates increased expression of the cellular gene survivin. The knockdown of survivin using siRNAs results in MCC tumor cell death and YM155, a small molecule inhibitor of survivin expression, protects mice from MCC tumors in a xenograft challenge system.[77,78]

In contrast to SV40, where LT appears to be the dominant oncogene, the MCPyV ST protein appears to play a key role in cell transformation. In addition to modifying the signaling functions of the cellular proto-oncogene PP2A, ST triggers the phosphorylation of eukaryotic translation initiation factor 4E binding protein 1.[79] This results in dysregulation of cap-dependent translation and cellular transformation.

Although there is an intriguing epidemiologic correlation between MCC and chronic lymphocytic leukemia (CLL),[80] there are conflicting reports concerning the presence of MCPyV in CLL and other lymphocytic cancers.[81–83]

Other Human Polyomaviruses

In recent years, the number of known human polyomaviruses has expanded dramatically. Of the 12 currently known HPyV species, only MCPyV has been clearly linked to human cancer. One new HPyV, trichodysplasia spinulosa polyomavirus (TSV or TSPyV) has been found in association with abnormal spiny growths on the facial skin of a small number of immunocompromised individuals.

EPSTEIN-BARR VIRUS

History

In 1958, Denis Burkitt provided the first clear clinical description of an unusual B-cell–derived tumor that frequently affects the jawbones of children in equatorial Africa.[84] After hearing Burkitt give a 1961 lecture entitled "The Commonest Children's Cancer in Tropical Africa – A Hitherto Unrecognized Syndrome," Michael Epstein became interested in the idea that an insect vector-borne infection might account for the high incidence of Burkitt lymphoma in tropical Africa. Epstein, together with then PhD candidate Yvonne Barr, began examining tumor samples sent to them by Burkitt. Electron micrographs of lymphoid cells that grew out of the tumors in culture revealed viral particles with a morphology strikingly similar to herpes simplex viruses.[85] It was soon shown that Epstein-Barr herpesvirus (EBV, later designated human herpesvirus 4 [HHV-4]) can transform cultured B cells and is the agent responsible for infectious mononucleosis.[86–88]

Although the initial conjecture that tropically endemic Burkitt lymphoma depends on a geographically restricted infectious agent ultimately proved correct, it was quickly established that the EBV infection is not restricted to the tropics. It instead appears likely that the malaria parasite *Plasmodium falciparum* is a key geographically restricted cocarcinogen responsible for endemic Burkitt lymphoma.[53] In areas where children suffer repeated malaria infections, it appears that the parasite triggers abnormal B-cell responses, as well as weakened cell-mediated immune function, and these effects of recurring malaria infection in turn promote or allow the development of EBV-induced Burkitt tumors.[11]

Epstein-Barr Virus Life Cycle

EBV chronically infects nearly all humans. In a great majority of individuals, the infection is initially established in early childhood and is never associated with any noticeable symptoms. The infection is typically transmitted when virions, shed in the saliva of a chronically infected individual, come in contact with the oropharyngeal epithelium of a naïve individual. Although infected epithelial cells, such as keratinocytes, might serve to amplify the virus in some circumstances,[89] the establishment of chronic infection is ultimately dependent on mature B cells, as subjects with X-linked agammaglobulinemia (who lack mature B cells) appear to be immune to stable EBV infection.[90] Individuals who escape infection during childhood and instead first become infected during adolescence or adulthood often develop mononucleosis, which is associated with fevers and extreme fatigue lasting for weeks or sometimes months. Interestingly, late-infected individuals who experience mononucleosis and high EBV viral load are at increased risk of developing EBV-positive Hodgkin lymphoma.[91]

EBV-infected B cells can either go on to produce new virions, which are typically associated with cell lysis, or the virus can enter a nonproductive state known as latency. Viral latency is defined as a condition in which the virus expresses few (or possibly no) gene products but can, under some conditions, "reawaken" to express the full range of viral gene products and produce new progeny virions. Latently infected cells are highly resistant to immune clearance.

There are three recognized forms of EBV latency. In latency I, EBV nuclear antigen-1 (EBNA1), which is required for the stable maintenance of the circularized viral DNA minichromosome, is the only viral protein expressed. EBV-derived microRNAs (miRs) may also be expressed. At the other end of the spectrum, latency III is characterized by the expression of EBNA1–6, several latent membrane proteins (LMP1, 2A, and 2B), two noncoding RNAs (EBER1 and 2), the BCL-2 homolog BHRF1, BARF0, and multiple miRs. Although the initial discovery of EBV involved the visualization of virions, indicating that the virus had exited latency and entered the productive lytic phase of the life cycle, viral gene expression in EBV-induced cancers generally follows one of the three latent patterns. The oncogenic activities of various EBV gene products have recently been reviewed.[87,88]

In a great majority of healthy individuals, EBV exists almost exclusively in a latent state, with the occasional asymptomatic shedding of virions in the saliva. The infection is controlled, at least in part, by CD8+ T cells specific for various latency proteins. EBV, like other herpesviruses, expresses a variety of proteins that interfere with cell-mediated immune responses. Intriguingly, results from mouse model systems suggest that the chronic immunostimulatory effects of persistent gammaherpesvirus emergence (or abortive emergence) from latency in healthy hosts can nonspecifically boost immunity to other infections.[92]

Lymphomas

In addition to endemic Burkitt lymphoma, EBV is often present in sporadic cases of Burkitt lymphoma in individuals who have not been exposed to malaria. Although nearly all cases of endemic

Burkitt's lymphoma contain EBV DNA in the tumor (typically in a latency I–like state), only about 20% of sporadic cases arising in immunocompetent individuals contain EBV. Rates of Burkitt lymphoma are elevated in HIV-infected individuals, and HIV-associated Burkitt lymphomas contain EBV in about 30% of cases.

A common hallmark of all types of Burkitt's lymphomas is de-regulation of the cellular Myc proto-oncogene. A classic mutation involves chromosomal translocation of the Myc gene to the antibody heavy chain locus. Burkitt's lymphoma tumors that lack detectable EBV DNA tend to carry multiple additional mutations in host cell genes, raising the possibility that an originally EBV-positive precursor cell ultimately accumulated mutations that rendered it independent of viral genes.[88,93]

In addition to Burkitt lymphoma, EBV is associated, to varying extents, with a histologically diverse range of other lymphoid cancers, including Hodgkin lymphoma, natural killer (NK)/T-cell lymphoma, primary central nervous system (CNS) lymphoma, and diffuse large B-cell lymphoma. The incidence of these various forms of lymphoma is significantly increased both in AIDS patients as well as in iatrogenically and congenitally immunosuppressed individuals.[88] In particular, the essentially universal presence of EBV in CNS lymphomas in AIDS patients makes it possible to diagnose the disease with a PCR test for EBV that, together with radiologic findings, can obviate the need for a brain biopsy.

EBV is almost invariably associated with lymphoproliferative disorders, such as plasmacytic hyperplasia and polymorphic B cell hyperplasia, which are often observed in organ transplant recipients. These polyclonal lymphoproliferative responses can, in some instances, progress to oligoclonal or monoclonal lymphomas of various types. The occurrence of EBV-associated lymphoproliferative disease in immunosuppressed patients is generally heralded by the increased detection of EBV DNA in the peripheral blood and the oral cavity. This presumably reflects the failure of cellular immune responses to drive the virus into full latency and perhaps also a failure of cell-mediated immune responses targeting latency-associated EBV gene products present in the nascent tumor.

Carcinomas

In Southern China, NPC affects 25 out of 100,000 people, accounting for 18% of all cancers in China as a whole.[94] Most other world regions have a 25- to 100-fold lower rate of NPC. EBV is present in nearly all cases of NPC, both in endemic and nonendemic regions. Although there is support for the idea that dietary intake of salted fish and other preserved foods is a factor in endemic NPC, it remains possible that genetic traits or as yet unidentified environmental cocarcinogenic factors may play a role as well. Individuals with rising or relatively high IgA antibody responses to EBNA1, DNase, and/or EBV capsid antigens have a dramatically increased risk of developing NPC, offering an early detection method for at-risk individuals.[87]

EBV is also present in a small percentage (5% to 15%) of gastric adenocarcinomas and over 90% of gastric lymphoepithelioma-like carcinomas. In contrast to NPC, the prevalence of EBV-associated gastric cancer is similar in all world regions. As with NPC, elevated antibody responsiveness to EBV antigens may offer a method for identifying individuals at greater risk of gastric cancer.

Prevention and Treatment

The reduction of immunosuppression in response to increasing EBV loads is a standard approach to preventing EBV diseases in T-cell immunosuppressed individuals. Another approach to the prevention of EBV disease relies on ganciclovir (or related antiherpesvirus drugs), which can trigger the death of cells that express the EBV thymidine kinase gene. Pretreating at-risk individuals, such as organ transplant recipients, with ganciclovir has been shown to effectively prevent the development of EBV-induced

lymphoproliferative disorders.[95] However, it is important to note that thymidine kinase is only expressed in the lytic phase of the viral life cycle, and drugs of this class are not generally effective for treating existing tumors, presumably due to the fact that EBV gene expression in tumors is typically of a latent type.

Although a recently developed vaccine targeting the EBV gp350 virion surface antigen did not provide sterilizing immunity to EBV infection, vaccinees did experience lower peak EBV viral loads upon infection.[96] Given the strong correlation between high EBV loads and the development of EBV diseases, it is hoped that the vaccine's ability to merely blunt the acute infection may offer significant protection against disease.

Most forms of EBV-associated lymphoid cancers express the B-cell marker CD20, making rituximab (an anti-CD20 mAb) a potentially effective adjunct therapy.[97,98] An emerging treatment approach that has recently entered clinical trials involves stimulating T cells ex vivo against peptides based on EBV antigens or against autologous EBV-transformed B cells.

KAPOSI'S SARCOMA HERPESVIRUS

History and Epidemiology

In the late 19th century, Hungarian dermatologist Moritz Kaposi's described a relatively rare type of indolent pigmented skin sarcoma affecting older men.[99] Kaposi's sarcoma (KS) was later found to be more prevalent in the Mediterranean region and in eastern portions of sub-Saharan Africa.[100] An early clue to the emergence of the HIV/AIDS pandemic in the early 1980s was a dramatic increase in the incidence of highly aggressive forms of KS, particularly in gay men who were much younger than typical KS patients. After the discovery of HIV, it was briefly hypothesized that HIV might be a direct cause of KS. However, this hypothesis failed to explain the existence of KS long prior to the HIV pandemic and the low incidence of KS in individuals who became infected with HIV via blood products. This latter observation was more easily explained by the existence of a sexually transmitted cofactor other than HIV.[101]

Using a subtractive DNA hybridization approach known as representational difference analysis, Yuan Chang, Patrick Moore, and colleagues discovered the presence of a previously unknown herpesvirus in KS tumors.[102] The newly founded field of research rapidly established key lines of evidence supporting the conclusion that KSHV (later designated human herpesvirus-8 [HHV-8]) is a causal factor in KS.[11]

It is now clear that the rate of KSHV infection varies greatly in different world regions.[11,103] In North America and Western Europe, KSHV seroprevalence in the general population ranges from 1% to 7%. Seroprevalence among gay men in these regions is substantially higher (25% to 60%), suggesting a possible link to sexual transmission. KSHV infection is much more prevalent in the general population in central and eastern Africa, where seroprevalence ranges from 23% to 70%. In endemic areas, up to 15% of children are seropositive, suggesting either vertical transmission or transmission via nonsexual casual contact (presumably via saliva). In endemic regions, KS is estimated to be the third most common cancer among adults.[104]

Kaposi's Sarcoma-Associated Herpesvirus in Kaposi's Sarcoma

KS tumors are complex on a number of levels. In contrast to most other forms of cancer, where it is often clear that a single cell type has proliferated out of control, KS tumors are composed of cells from multiple lineages (Fig. 5.2). KSHV-infected cells in the tumor often have a spindle-shaped morphology. Interestingly,

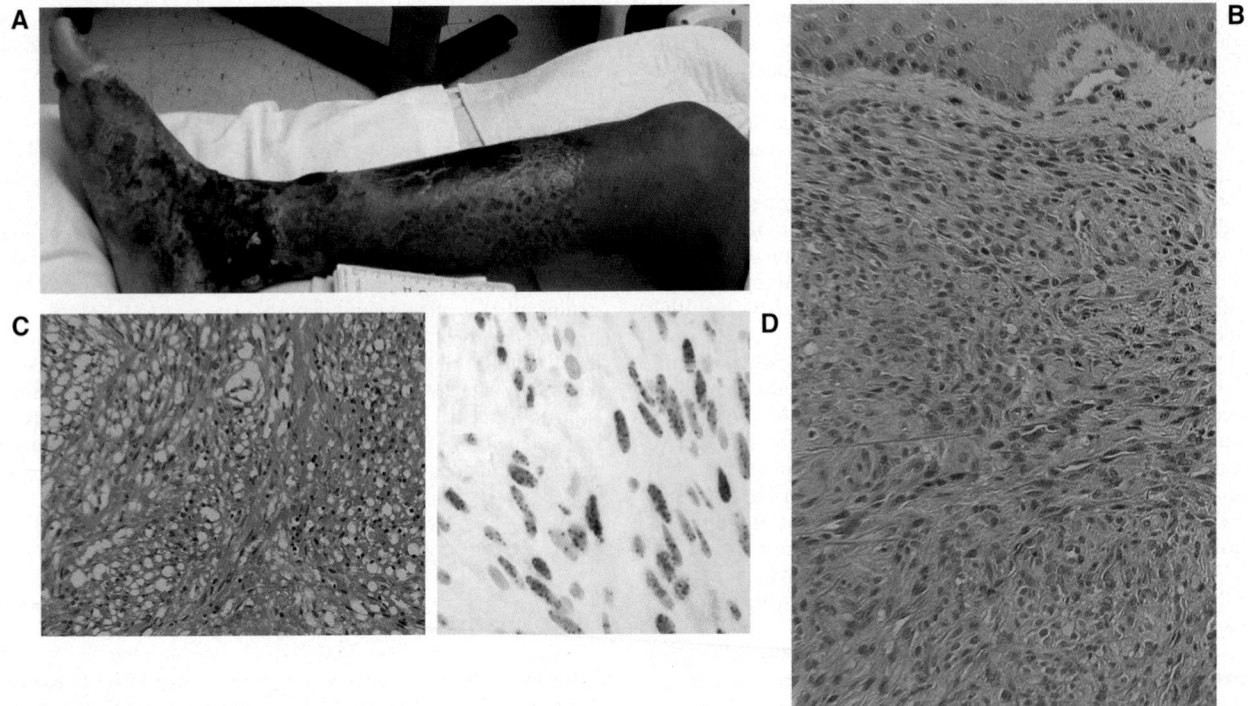

Figure 5.2 Kaposi's sarcoma (KS). **(A)** Photograph of the lower leg of an individual with severe, diffuse KS involving the lower leg. **(B)** Histology of the skin. **(C)** Lung shows a mixture of spindle to epithelioid cells, with slitlike vascular spaces intermixed with red blood cells and red blood cell fragments. **(D)** Immunohistochemical detection of KSHV LANA in the cutaneous tumor. Photographs provided with permission by Drs. Odey Ukpo and Ethel Cesarman.

spindle cells do not exhibit a highly transformed phenotype and tend to show relatively little chromosomal instability. In a culture, the cells are highly dependent on exogenous cytokines and other factors present in the tumor microenvironment in vivo. Although spindle cells express a number of markers of the endothelial lineage, it is uncertain whether they are derived from mature endothelial cells, the early precursor cells that give rise to smooth muscle and vascular endothelial cells, or cells of the lymphatic endothelial lineage. KS tumors also contain infiltrating lymphocytes and monocytes, as well as aberrant neovascular spaces lined with infected and uninfected endothelial cells. The aberrant blood vessels in KS lesion vessels rupture easily and leak red blood cells, giving KS tumors their classic dark red, brown, or purple color.

The latency status of KSHV in KS tumors is also complex, with the expression of gene products typical of latency (e.g., LANA) as well as lytic-phase genes (e.g., RTA/ORF50). Some of these gene products, such as the viral interleukin (IL)-6 homolog (vIL-6), trigger proliferation and secondary cytokine signaling in noninfected cells within the tumor. The tumorigenic effects of individual KSHV gene products have recently been reviewed.[88,103] In contrast to EBV, where tumorigenesis is driven by latency gene expression, it appears that KS pathogenesis is often dependent on lytic phase gene expression. This may explain why ganciclovir, which is not a particularly effective treatment for EBV tumors, was found to prevent the formation of new KS lesions in HIV-positive patients.[105] However, it should be noted that this outcome has more recently proven difficult to reproduce.[106] At present, there are no recommended preventive therapies for individuals at risk of KS, but this is an area of active investigation.

There are a variety of possible explanations for the need for lytic-phase KSHV gene expression during tumor development. For example, infected spindle cells may lose the viral DNA during cell division and require reinfection for ongoing tumorigenicity. Alternatively, factors secreted by a small fraction of tumor cells that enter the lytic phase may be required for tumorigenesis. An important area of current research focus is the role of KSHV gene products in the regulation of angiogenesis in KS lesions[107] and several current trials are investigating inhibitors of angiogenic pathways for the treatment of KS.

Lymphoproliferative Disorders

KSHV causes two forms of B-cell proliferative disorder: multicentric Castleman disease (MCD) and primary effusion lymphoma (PEL). Both diseases are most commonly found in association with HIV infection. In HIV-infected individuals, MCD tumors contain KSHV in nearly all cases, whereas in HIV-negative individuals, the tumor contains KSHV in only about 50% of cases.[108] KSHV in MCD tumors exhibits periodic activation of lytic replication and the expression of lytic phase genes.[109] The expression of vIL-6 during disease flare-ups appears to play a role in MCD pathogenesis, raising the possibility that tocilizumab (a mAb therapeutic that targets the IL-6 receptor) may be of therapeutic benefit.

PEL comprises about 4% of all HIV-associated non-Hodgkin lymphomas.[110] Typically, PEL tumors express markers of both plasma cells (akin to multiple myeloma tumors) and immunoblasts (similar to some EBV-induced tumors). In AIDS patients, essentially all PEL tumors are infected with KSHV and a great majority are also coinfected with EBV.[88] Although PEL is rare in HIV-negative individuals, PEL tumors in such individuals contain KSHV in about 50% of cases.

A common approach to the treatment of all KSHV-associated diseases is the restoration of immune function, either through antiretroviral therapy of HIV/AIDS or through a reduction of immunosuppressive therapy. The general success of immune reconstitution in many KSHV-associated diseases presumably involves an immune-mediated attack of cells expressing KSHV gene products, particularly the many lytic-phase gene products the virus can produce in various disease states.

ANIMAL AND HUMAN RETROVIRUSES

The first oncogenic retroviruses were discovered by Ellerman and Bang in 1908 and by Rous in 1911, but it was many years before the significance of these findings was appreciated.[111] One reason the field was stymied was the failure to identify RNA forms of the viral genome in infected cells. This led to the discovery of the reverse transcriptase independently by Baltimore and Temin in 1970. Another major development was the finding in 1976 of viral oncogenes derived from cellular genes, with the identification by Varmus and Bishop of the first dominant oncogene, *src*. With the discovery of IL-2 by Gallo in 1976, it became possible to culture the first human retrovirus, HTLV-1, from a form of adult T-cell leukemia/lymphoma (ATLL) that was first recognized by Takatsuki and coworkers.[112] These advances opened the door for Montagnier and colleagues' isolation of HIV-1 in 1983, a discovery confirmed independently by Gallo and Levy. This breakthrough led to the first licensed HIV test in 1985.

Retroviruses are positive single-strand RNA viruses that utilize transcription of their RNA genome into a DNA intermediate during virus replication.[111] This accounts for their name, retroviruses, because this is opposite to the normal flow of eukaryotic genetic information. They infect a wide range of vertebrate animal species and are distantly related to repetitive elements in the human genome, known as retrotransposons. Retroviruses are also related to hepadnaviruses, double-stranded DNA viruses, such as hepatitis B virus, which also undergo a reverse transcription step in their replication.

Retroviruses may be classified as *endogenous* or *exogenous* depending on whether they appear in the genome of the host species. There are approximately 100,000 endogenous retroviral elements in the human genome, making up nearly 8% of the genetic information, but their potential roles in disease are unclear.[113] Retroviruses may also be classified as *ecotropic*, *xenotropic*, or *polytropic* depending on whether they infect cells of the same animal species from which they are derived, infect cells of a different species, or both. *Amphotropic* retroviruses infect cells of the species of origin without producing disease, but infect cells of other species and may produce disease.

Retroviruses that produce disease after a long incubation period are termed *lentiviruses* and include human, simian, feline, ovine, caprine, and bovine immunodeficiency viruses. Another group of retroviruses that are not clearly associated with disease are known as *spumaviruses* and include human and simian foamy viruses. HTLV-1, which is classified in the genus Delta, is the only retrovirus known to be oncogenic in humans. A member of the retroviral genus Gamma identified in 2008, designated xenotropic murine leukemia virus-related virus (XMRV), was thought to be associated with human prostate cancer; however, more recent studies showed XMRV to be a lab-derived artifact.[114] A genus betaretrovirus related to the mouse mammary tumor virus has been suggested to be associated with biliary cirrhosis, but this finding requires independent validation.[115]

Retroviruses producing tumors in animals or birds are designated transforming viruses and may be classified as acute or chronic transforming retroviruses. Acute transforming retroviruses have acquired a mutated cellular gene, termed *oncogene*, and induce cancer in an animal within a few weeks. Many dominant acting proto-oncogenes in humans (e.g., *ras*, *myc*, and *erbB*), were first identified as retroviral oncogenes.

Chronic transforming retroviruses integrate almost randomly in the genome, but when integrated in the vicinity of specific genes disrupt their regulation and induce cell proliferation or resistance to apoptosis. Chronic transforming retroviruses induce malignancy only after many weeks to months of infection. The use of a murine leukemia virus vector for gene therapy in children with a form of severe combined immune deficiency syndrome characterized by defective expression of the common gamma chain of the IL-2 receptor resulted in T-cell acute lymphoblastic leukemia.

This was found to be the result of persistent expression of the LIM domain only 2 (LMO2) gene triggered by the nearby integration of the retroviral vector.[116]

In addition to acute or chronic transformation mechanisms, retroviruses can transform cells through direct effects on cell physiology mediated by structural or nonstructural viral proteins. Transforming genes of HTLV-1 are nonstructural viral proteins that activate host cell signaling pathways.[117] Because the oncogenic effects of HTLV-1 transforming genes generally take many years to cause cancer, the virus does not fit the precise definition of having either an acute or a chronic oncogenic mechanism.

HIV-1 infection is also associated with a variety of malignancies, but only by indirect effects of suppressing immunity to oncogenic virus infections, such as gammaherpesviruses, high-risk human papillomaviruses, and hepatitis viruses.

Human T-Cell Leukemia Virus Epidemiology

Four species of human T-cell leukemia virus have been identified. HTLV-1 was identified in 1980 as the first human retrovirus associated with cancer, and it is the focus of the remainder of this section.[118] HTLV-2 was discovered in 1982 and shares 70% genomic homology with HTLV-1.[119] HTLV-3 and -4 were sporadically isolated from individuals who had contact with monkeys.[120] HTLV-2, -3, and -4 do not appear to be associated with disease in humans.

HTLV-1 is present in 15 to 20 million individuals worldwide, most commonly in the Caribbean Islands, South America, southern Japan, and parts of Australia, Melanesia, Africa, and Iran.[121] In the United States, Canada, and Europe, 0.01% to 0.03% of blood donors are infected with HTLV-1. It is most commonly found in individuals who emigrated from endemic regions or among African Americans. HTLV-1 is transmitted sexually, by contaminated cell-associated blood products, or by breast-feeding.[122] Only 2% to 5% of HTLV-1–infected individuals develop disease, and ATLL only occurs in individuals who acquired HTLV-1 by breast-feeding.

Human T-Cell Leukemia Virus Molecular Biology

HTLV-1, like other retroviruses, encodes Gag, Protease, Pol, and Envelope proteins.[123] Gag proteins compose the inner nucleocapsid core of the virus. The Pol proteins include the reverse transcriptase and integrase. The reverse transcriptase copies the single-stranded viral RNA into double-stranded DNA, and it is inhibited by several nucleoside analogs, but not by the nonnucleoside reverse transcriptase inhibitors approved for HIV-1.[124] The integrase is responsible for inserting the linear double-stranded DNA product of reverse transcription into the host chromosomal DNA. At least one integrase inhibitor, raltegravir, now approved for HIV-1, is active against HTLV-1.[125] Integration occurs throughout the human genome, but there is preference for integration in transcriptionally active genomic regions.[126] The viral protease proteolytically processes Gag, Protease, and Pol precursor proteins to the mature individual proteins, but it is not affected by inhibitors of HIV-1 protease. The envelope proteins include the transmembrane protein, which anchors the surface envelope protein on the virion, which mediates binding to the viral receptor.[127]

The viral genome also encodes regulatory proteins, including Tax and HTLV-1 bZIP factor (HBZ).[117] Tax is a transcriptional transactivator protein that functions as a coactivator to induce members of the cAMP response element-binding protein/activating transcription factor (CREB/ATF) family, nuclear factor kappa B (NF-κB), and serum response factor (SRF) pathways. Tax activation of the CREB/ATF pathway is responsible for upregulation of the viral promoter. Tax induction of NF-κB promotes cell proliferation and resistance to apoptosis. Tax also binds and activates cyclin-dependent kinases and inhibits cell cycle checkpoint proteins. Tax is important for tumor initiation, whereas HBZ may be important in tumor maintenance.[128]

HTLV-1 preferentially immortalizes CD4+ T lymphocytes and induces tumors in mice.[129] Tax also promotes the leukemia-initiating activity of ATLL cells in mouse models.[130] In immunodeficient mice reconstituted with human hematopoietic cells, HTLV-1 causes CD4+ lymphomas.[131]

Clinical Characteristics and Treatment of HTLV-Associated Malignancies

The diagnosis of HTLV-1 is based on serologic assays.[132] HTLV-1 is associated with various inflammatory disorders, including uveitis, polymyositits, pneumonitis, Sjögren syndrome, and myelopathy. Infected patients are susceptible to certain infectious disorders (e.g. staphylococcal dermatitis) and opportunistic infections such as pneumocystis pneumonia, disseminated cryptococcosis, strongyloidiasis, or toxoplasmosis.[133] Vaccines have not been developed for HTLV infections.

T-lymphocyte proliferative disorders develop in 1% to 5% of infected individuals and are generally CD2+, CD3+, CD4+, CD5+, CD25+, CD29+, CD45RO+, CD52+, HLA-DR+, T-cell receptor αβ+, and variably CD30+, and lack CD7, CD8, and CD26 expression. The virus is clonally integrated in the malignant cells. Complex karyotypes are often found, and cytogenetic analysis is rarely useful. The histologic features of lymph nodes in ATLL may be indistinguishable from those of other peripheral T-cell lymphomas.[134] Circulating tumor "flower cells" are helpful in the diagnosis (Fig. 5.3).

ATLL is categorized in four subtypes.[135] (1) Smoldering ATLL is defined as 5% or more abnormal T lymphocytes and lactate dehydrogenase (LDH) levels up to 1.5× the upper limit of normal, with normal lymphocyte count, calcium, and no lymph node or visceral disease other than skin or pulmonary disease. (2) Chronic ATLL is characterized by lymphocytosis, LDH up to 2× the upper limit of normal, no hypercalcemia, and no CNS, bone, pleural, peritoneal, or gastrointestinal involvement, although the lymph nodes, liver, spleen, skin, or lungs may be involved. The mean survival of these forms of ATLL is 2 to 5 years.[136] No intervention in these subtypes of ATLL has been defined that prevents progression to the more aggressive forms of ATLL. Although chronic or smoldering ATLL may respond to zidovudine and interferon, randomized studies have not been conducted.[137] (3) Lymphoma-type ATLL is characterized by ≤1% abnormal T lymphocytes and features of non-Hodgkin lymphoma. (4) Acute-type ATLL includes the remaining patients. Even with optimal therapy, the median survival of lymphoma and acute-type ATLL is less than 1 year.[138] Lymphoma and acute types of ATLL are the most common presenting subtypes. Other major prognostic factors include performance status, age, the presence of more than three involved lesions, and hypercalcemia.[139]

Combination chemotherapy for lymphoma or acute-type ATLL with the infusional etoposide, prednisone, vincristine, and doxorubicin (EPOCH) regimen or the LSG-15 regimen results in complete remission rates of 15% to 40%.[140,141] However, responses are short lived, with <10% of patients free of disease at 4 years. The addition of anti-CCR4 antibody, mogamulizumab, may improve response rates, but studies are still underway.[142]

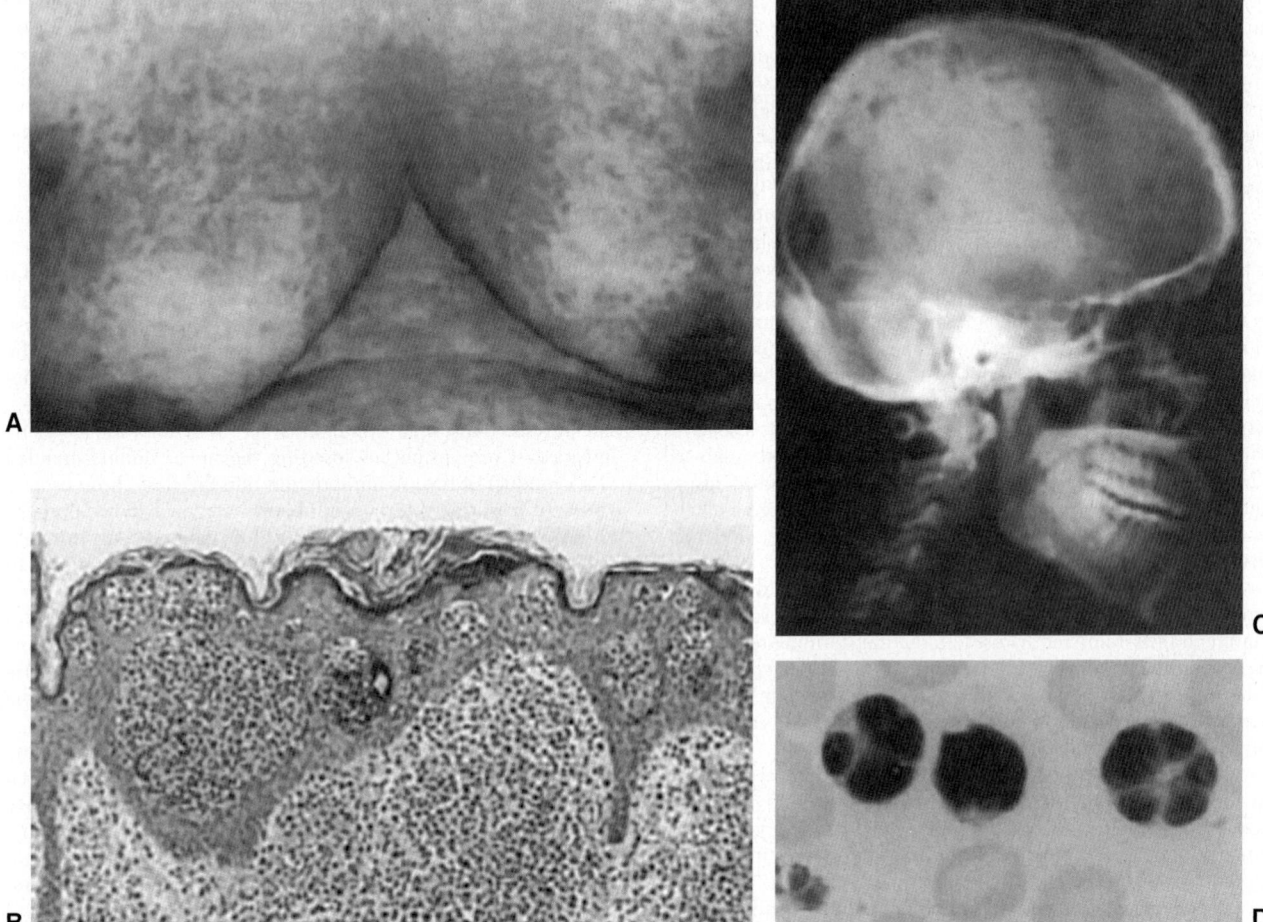

Figure 5.3 Clinical manifestation of adult T-cell leukemia/lymphoma. **(A–B)** Infiltration of malignant T lymphocytes into the skin. **(C)** Lytic bone lesions seen on lateral skull x-ray. **(D)** "Flower cells" in the blood.

The combination of interferon and zidovudine with or without arsenic may result in the remission of acute, but not lymphoma subtypes.[143] Allogenic transplantation may result in long-term, disease-free survival for patients with complete or near complete remission of disease, although infectious complications have been notable in these studies.[144]

HEPATITIS VIRUSES

The earliest record of an epidemic caused by a hepatitis virus was in 1885, occurring in individuals vaccinated for smallpox with lymph from other people.[145] The cause of the epidemic, HBV, was not identified until 1966, when Blumberg discovered the *Australian antigen* now known to be the hepatitis B surface antigen (HBsAg). This was followed by the discovery of the virus particle by Dane in 1970. In the early 1980s, the HBV genome was sequenced and the first vaccines were tested. In the mid 1970s, Alter described cases of hepatitis not due to hepatitis A or B viruses, and the suspected agent was designated non-A, non-B hepatitis virus, now known as HCV.[146] In 1987, Houghton used molecular cloning to identify the HCV genome and develop a diagnostic test, which was licensed in 1990.

Approximately 240 million people are chronically infected with HBV and 150 to 200 million people are infected with HCV worldwide, according to the World Health Organization (WHO). About 1 million deaths per year are attributed to the chronic diseases such as liver cirrhosis and hepatocellular carcinoma (HCC) that result from viral hepatitis infections. HBV and HCV are the leading cause of liver cancer in the world, accounting for almost 80% of the cases. In the United States, Europe, Egypt, and Japan, more than 60% of HCC cases are associated with HCV, and 20% are related to HBV and chronic alcoholism.[147] In Africa and Asia, 60% of HCC is associated with HBV, 20% related to HCV, and the remainder related to other risk factors, such as alcohol and aflatoxin. HCC is the sixth most common cancer worldwide and is the third most common cause of cancer death.[148]

In Asia and Africa, up to 70% of individuals have serologic evidence of current or prior HBV infection, and 8% to 15% of these subjects have a chronic active infection. Rates of HCV infection of >3.5% occur in Central and East Asia, North Africa, and the Middle East. In the United States, 0.8 to 1.4 million individuals are infected with HBV, and 3.2 million with HCV. The incidence of HCC in the United States tripled between 1975 and 2005, particularly in African American and Hispanic males.[149]

HBV is transmitted primarily through exposure to infected blood, semen, and other body fluids, whereas HCV is transmitted primarily by contact with contaminated blood. Acute HCV infection causes mild and vague symptoms in about 15% of individuals and resolves spontaneously in 10% to 50% of cases.[150] Liver enzymes are normal in 5% to 50% of individuals with chronic HCV infection.[151] After 20 years of an HCV infection, the likelihood of cirrhosis is 10% to 15% for men, and 1.5% for women.[152] Cofactors that increase the likelihood of cirrhosis is coinfection with both hepatitis viruses, persistently high levels of HBV or HCV viremia, HBeAg, certain viral genotypes, schistosoma, HIV, alcoholism, male gender, advanced age at the time of infection, diabetes, and obesity.[153,154]

Hepatitis B Virus

HBV is an enveloped DNA virus that is a member of the *Hepadnaviridae* family.[155] HBV has a strong preference for infecting hepatocytes, but small amounts of viral DNA can also be found in kidney, pancreas, and mononuclear cells, although it is not linked to extrahepatic disease. The viral genome is a relaxed circular, partially double-stranded (ds) DNA of 3.2 kb. The genome exists as an episomal covalently closed circular dsDNA (cccDNA)

molecule in the nucleus of infected cells, although chromosomal integration of viral genomic sequences can occur during cycles of hepatocyte regeneration and proliferation. In addition to 40 to 42 nm virions, HBV-infected cells also produce noninfectious 20-nm spherical and filamentous particles. The viral genome encodes four open reading frames. The presurface–surface (preS-S) region encodes three proteins from different translational initiation sites; these include the S (HBsAg), M (or pre-S2), and L (or pre-S1) proteins. The L protein is responsible for receptor binding and virion assembly. The precore–core (preC-C) region encodes the HBcAg and HBeAg. The P region encodes the viral polymerase, and the X (HBx) protein modulates host-signal transduction.

After infection, the viral genome is transcribed by host RNA polymerase II, and viral proteins are translated. Nucleocapsids assemble in the cytosol, incorporating a molecule of pregenomic RNA into the viral core, where reverse transcription occurs to produce the dsDNA viral genome. Viral cores are enveloped with intracellular membranes and viral L, M, and S surface antigens, which are exported from the cells.

HBV replication is not cytotoxic. Instead, liver injury is due to the host immune response, primarily T-cell and proinflammatory cytokine responses. Chronic HBV carriers exhibit an attenuated virus-specific T-cells response, although a vigorous humoral response is still evident. About 5% of infections in adults and up to 90% of infections in neonates result in a persistent infection, which may or may not be associated with symptoms and elevated serum aminotransferase levels. About 20% of such individuals develop cirrhosis. Immunosuppressed individuals also have a higher likelihood of a persistent infection.

With acute infection, viral titers of 10^9 to 10^{10} virions per mililiter are present, whereas levels of 10^7 to 10^9 virions per mililiter and HBsAg, and in some cases, HBeAg are present in the blood of individuals with a persistent infection. The resolution of infection, which is associated with declining viral DNA titers, is observed at a rate of 5% to 10% per year in persistently infected individuals. However, even subjects who have resolved the infection continue to have very low levels of viral DNA (10^3 to 10^5 copies per mililiter) for most of their lives.

HBV infection can be managed with alpha interferon or nucleos(t)ide analogs that inhibit the viral polymerase, such as lamivudine, telbivudine, entecavir, adefovir, and tenofovir.[156] Entecavir and tenofovir are both effective at inducing viral suppression, and may be used in combination in patients with high HBV DNA load or multidrug resistance. Because these agents are all associated with some toxicity, current guidelines recommend therapy only when liver disease is clinically apparent, with continued treatment for 6 to 12 months after clearance of HBeAg or HBsAg. Although these drugs effectively control HBV, they typically fail to cure the infection due to the long-term persistence of the cccDNA form of the viral genome. Other nucleos(t)ide analogs are currently in clinical trials, as well as a novel form of interferon (IFN-λ) and an inhibitor of virus release.[157]

Hepatitis D virus (HDV) occurs only in individuals coinfected with HBV. HDV is composed a single-stranded circular viral RNA genome of 1,679 nucleotides, a central core of HDAg, and an outer coat with all three HBV envelope proteins. HDV infection results in more severe complications than infection with HBV alone, with a higher likelihood and more rapid progression to cirrhosis and HCC.

Hepatits C Virus

HCV is an enveloped RNA virus associated with cancer, primarily HCC and, rarely, splenic marginal zone lymphoma.[158] HCV is a positive-sense, single-stranded RNA virus of the *Flaviviridae* family.[159] There are seven genotypes of HCV; in the United States, about 70% of infections are caused by genotype 1.[160] HCV replicates in the cytoplasm and does not integrate into the host cell genome. The viral RNA is 9.6 kb and encodes a single polyprotein of 3,010 amino acids that is proteolytically processed into structural and nonstructural proteins. In addition to the structural roles of the core (C) protein, it has also been reported to affect various host cell functions. The envelope glycoproteins E1 and E2 mediate infectious entry through tetraspanin CD81 and other receptors on hepatocytes and B lymphocytes.

HCV non structural proteins NS2, NS3, NS4A, NS4B, NS5A, NS5B, and p7 are required for virus replication and assembly. NS2 is a membrane-associated cysteine protease. NS3 is a helicase and NTPase that unwinds RNA and DNA substrates. The complex of NS3 with NS4A forms a serine protease. NS4B induces the formation of a membranous web associated with the viral RNA replicase. NS5A is an RNA-binding phosphoprotein, whereas NS5B is the RNA-dependent RNA polymerase. The p7 protein forms a cation channel in infected cells that has a role in particle maturation and release.

Treating an HCV infection typically utilizes 24 to 48 weeks of pegylated IFN-α and ribavirin.[161] Treatment with IFN and ribavirin alone produces sustained virologic responses in 70% to 80% of subjects with genotype 2 or 3 infections. Recently approved inhibitors of the NS3-4A protease (e.g., telaprevir, boceprevir, or simeprevir) may be included in IFN-based regimens, particularly if the patient has failed prior therapy. Protease inhibitors are currently approved for use in IFN/ribavirin combination therapy for HCV genotype 1 or 4 infection. Sofosbuvir, a nucleoside analog inhibitor of the viral NS5B polymerase, has recently been approved for use in combination with ribavirin alone for genotypes 2 or 3, or in triple therapy for genotypes 1 and 4. Recently, IFN-free regimens have also been approved. Additional protease and polymerase inhibitors are currently in development. A recent metaanalysis of eight randomized controlled trials comparing antiviral therapy with placebo suggested that antiviral therapy resulted in a 50% reduced risk of HCC.[162]

Hepatitis Virus Pathogenesis

HBV and HCV depress innate immune responses by inhibiting Toll-like receptor signaling through effects of HBx and NS3-4A.[147] In addition, HCV C inhibits the Janus kinase (JAK)-signal transducer and activator of transcription (STAT) signaling, and NS5A and E2 inhibit IFN signaling. Through an undefined mechanism, HBV can inhibit JAK-STAT signaling as well.

HBV and HCV induce HCC by direct and indirect mechanisms.[147] Both HBV and HCV encode proteins that have pro- and antiapoptotic properties. High levels of HBx block activation of the NF-κB pathway, whereas HCV C and NS5A block apoptosis by the activation of AKT and NF-κB, respectively. The C and NS5A proteins may also induce epithelial–mesenchymal transition (EMT), which is important for liver fibrosis, through effects on transforming growth factor β and Src signaling. Mice transgenic for NS5A develop steatosis and HCC.

HBx and HCV C are associated with mitochondria, where they trigger oxidative stress that induces apoptosis. In addition, HBs and HBx and NS3-4A alter calcium signaling and increase reactive oxygen species, which trigger endoplasmic reticulum (ER) stress, an unfolded protein response, and the production of proinflammatory cytokines that induce collagen synthesis, which drives the development of fibrosis. Autophagy is triggered by both viruses to restore ER integrity, which promotes cell survival and viral persistence.

HBV and HCV also disrupt tumor suppressor proteins. HCV NS5B recruits an ubiquitin ligase protein to modify pRB and induce its degradation, whereas HBx and HCV C proteins both inhibit p16INK4a and p21 cell cycle inhibitors, which leads to the inactivating phosphorylation of pRB. The HBx and HCV C, NS3, and NS5A proteins deregulate p53 tumor suppressor activity, by compromising p53-mediated DNA repair. HBV and HCV also induce alterations in micro-RNAs that are partially responsible for cell cycle effects.

Although not part of the normal virus replication cycle, the tendency of HBV genomic DNA sequences to integrate within the host cell chromosomes also contributes to the pathogenesis of HBV-associated HCC. In most hepatoma cells, HBV replication is extinguished, and integration at certain sites provides a growth or survival advantage, leading to tumors that are clonal with respect to viral integration. Whole-genome sequencing studies have identified a number of cellular loci, including *TERT* and *MLL*, where HBV integration is associated with HCC.[163,164]

Both HBV and HCV promote characteristics of cancer stem cells. HBx promotes the expression of Nanog, Kruppel-like factor 4, octamer-binding transcription factor 4, and Myc. These markers are also induced by HBV and HCV-induced hypoxia and hypoxia-induced factors.

Clinical Characteristics and Treatment of Hepatitis Virus-Associated Malignancies

HBV and HCV infections are diagnosed by serologic assays, and/or antigen assays in the case of HBV.[153] Quantitative HBV DNA and HCV RNA polymerase chain reactions are utilized to measure virus load. No vaccine has been identified that protects against HCV because infections consist of a genetically heterogenous "swarm" of virus particles, some of which escape neutralization. However, a vaccine, which now utilizes a recombinant HBsAg produced in yeast cells, has been available for HBV prevention for more than 30 years. The HBV vaccine reduces the risk of infection by more than 70%.[157] Factors associated with HBV vaccination failure in adults include increased age, obesity, smoking, diabetes, end-stage renal disease, HIV infection, alcoholism, or recipients of liver or kidney transplantation. There have been recent suggestions that emerging HBV strains may be evolving to escape neutralizing antibodies elicited by the current vaccine.[165] Novel vaccine adjuvants are currently in clinical trials, as well as studies of a therapeutic HBV vaccine.

Because an early diagnosis of HCC is key to a successful treatment, there has been extensive research on surveillance techniques in HBV- and HCV-infected individuals.[166] The U.S. Centers for Disease Control and Prevention has recently recommended that all individuals born between 1945 and 1965 be tested for HCV infection. The American Association for the Study of Liver Diseases, as well as the European and Asian Pacific Associations for the Study of the Liver, endorse surveillance in HCV-infected individuals with cirrhosis using ultrasound every 6 months. Viral eradication does not fully eliminate the risk of HCC, and thus, continued surveillance is still recommended in cirrhotic patients.

Therapeutic options for HCC are determined not only by the number and size of HCC nodules as well as the presence or absence of vascular invasion and metastases, but also by liver function and the presence or absence of portal hypertension.[167] HCC amenable to liver transplantation is usually defined as either one tumor measuring ≤50 mm in diameter or two to three tumors measuring ≤30 mm in diameter without vascular extension or metastasis (Milan criteria).[168] Up to 30% of all cases of HCC present with multiple nodules of HCC, suggesting a field carcinogenesis effect of HBV and HCV.[169] HBV- and HCV-infected patients may have a lower survival than noninfected patients after liver transplantation.[170] Hepatitis B immune globulin and nucleos(t)ide analogs are recommended for reinfection prophylaxis in the posttransplant period for HBV-infected individuals.[171] Studies are underway to examine the appropriate use of antiviral therapy for HCV-infected patients undergoing liver transplantation.

Reactivation of HCV can occur with chemotherapy or monoclonal antibody-based immunosuppressive therapies, but is less frequent as compared to HBV infection.[172] Individuals who appear to have cleared an HBV infection and who have an undetectable viral load can experience HBV reactivation on rituximab therapy. Monitoring hepatic function and virus load is indicated during chemoimmunotherapy of HBV- or HCV-positive patients.[173] Although there is controversy regarding the role of virus screening for patients undergoing chemotherapy, antiviral therapy is recommended for high-risk HBV-infected patients undergoing chemoimmunotherapy, such as rituximab-based chemotherapy regimens.[174]

An association between HCV and B-cell non-Hodgkin lymphoma (NHL) has also been demonstrated in highly endemic geographic areas.[175] Lymphoproliferation has been linked to type II mixed cryoglobulinemia in many of these individuals. In addition to diffuse large B-cell lymphoma, marginal zone lymphomas and lymphoplasmacytic lymphomas are the histologic subtypes most frequently associated with HCV infection. Antiviral treatment with IFNα with or without ribavirin has been effective in the treatment of HCV-infected patients with indolent lymphoma, but rarely in individuals with aggressive lymphomas.

CONCLUSION

Oncogenic viruses are important causes of cancer, especially in less industrialized countries and in immunosuppressed individuals. They are common causes of anogenital cancers, lymphomas, oral and hepatocellular carcinomas and are associated with a variety of other malignancies. Vaccines and antiviral agents play an important role in the prevention of virus-induced cancers. Studies of virus pathogenesis will continue to establish paradigms that are critical to our understanding of cancer etiology in general.

SELECTED REFERENCES

The full reference list can be accessed at lwwhealthlibrary.com/oncology.

1. de Martel C, Ferlay J, Franceschi S, et al. Global burden of cancers attributable to infections in 2008: a review and synthetic analysis. *Lancet Oncol* 2012;13(6):607–615.
2. Schiller JT, Lowy DR. Virus infection and human cancer: an overview. *Recent Results Cancer Res* 2014;193:1–10.
3. Chen CJ, Hsu WL, Yang HI, et al. Epidemiology of virus infection and human cancer. *Recent Results Cancer Res* 2014;193:11–32.
4. Virgin HW, Wherry EJ, Ahmed R. Redefining chronic viral infection. *Cell* 2009;138(1):30–50.
5. Campo MS, O'Neil BW, Barron RJ, et al. Experimental reproduction of the papilloma-carcinoma complex of the alimentary canal in cattle. *Carcinogenesis* 1994;15(8):1597–1601.
6. Khoury JD, Tannir NM, Williams MD, et al. Landscape of DNA virus associations across human malignant cancers: analysis of 3,775 cases using RNA-Seq. *J Virol* 2013;87(16):8916–8926.
8. Mizutani T, Sayama Y, Nakanishi A, et al. Novel DNA virus isolated from samples showing endothelial cell necrosis in the Japanese eel, Anguilla japonica. *Virology* 2011;412(1):179–187.
9. Paulson KG, Carter JJ, Johnson LG, et al. Antibodies to merkel cell polyomavirus T antigen oncoproteins reflect tumor burden in merkel cell carcinoma patients. *Cancer Res* 2010;70:8388–8397.
10. International Agency for Research on Cancer (IARC) Working Group. IARC Monographs on the Evalation of Carcinogenic Risks to Humans. Malaria and Some Polyomaviruses (SV40, BK, JC, and Merkel Cell Viruses), Vol. 104. Lyon, France: IARC; 2013.
11. Moore PS, Chang Y. The conundrum of causality in tumor virology: the cases of KSHV and MCV. *Semin Cancer Biol* 2013;26C:4–12.
21. Bosch FX, Broker TR, Forman D, et al. Comprehensive control of human papillomavirus infections and related diseases. *Vaccine* 2013;31 Suppl 8: I1–I31.
27. White EA, Howley PM. Proteomic approaches to the study of papillomavirus-host interactions. *Virology* 2013;435(1):57–69.
32. Schiller JT, Lowy DR. Understanding and learning from the success of prophylactic human papillomavirus vaccines. *Nat Rev Microbiol* 2012;10(10):681–692.
37. Wang JW, Roden RB. L2, the minor capsid protein of papillomavirus. *Virology* 2013;445(1–2):175–186.
38. Ma B, Maraj B, Tran NP, et al. Emerging human papillomavirus vaccines. *Expert Opin Emerg Drugs* 2012;17(4):469–492.
39. Scudellari M. HPV: sex, cancer and a virus. *Nature* 2013;503(7476):330–332.
40. Gillison ML, Alemany L, Snijders PJ, et al. Human papillomavirus and diseases of the upper airway: head and neck cancer and respiratory papillomatosis. *Vaccine* 2012;30 Suppl 5:F34–54.
44. White EA, Kramer RE, Tan MJ, et al. Comprehensive analysis of host cellular interactions with human papillomavirus E6 proteins identifies new E6 binding partners and reflects viral diversity. *J Virol* 2012;86(24): 13174–13186.
45. White EA, Sowa ME, Tan MJ, et al. Systematic identification of interactions between host cell proteins and E7 oncoproteins from diverse human papillomaviruses. *Proc Natl Acad Sci U S A* 2012;109(5):E260–267.
47. Arron ST, Ruby JG, Dybbro E, et al. Transcriptome sequencing demonstrates that human papillomavirus is not active in cutaneous squamous cell carcinoma. *J Invest Dermatol* 2011;131(8):1745–1753.
56. Das D, Wojno K, Imperiale MJ. BK virus as a cofactor in the etiology of prostate cancer in its early stages. *J Virol* 2008;82(6):2705–2714.
59. Abend JR, Jiang M, Imperiale MJ. BK virus and human cancer: innocent until proven guilty. *Semin Cancer Biol* 2009;19(4):252–260.
60. Maginnis MS, Atwood WJ. JC virus: an oncogenic virus in animals and humans? *Semin Cancer Biol* 2009;19(4):261–269.

61. Feng H, Shuda M, Chang Y, et al. Clonal integration of a polyomavirus in human Merkel cell carcinoma. *Science* 2008;319(5866):1096–1100.
66. Schowalter RM, Pastrana DV, Pumphrey KA, et al. Merkel cell polyomavirus and two previously unknown polyomaviruses are chronically shed from human skin. *Cell Host Microbe* 2010;7(6):509–515.
70. Faust H, Andersson K, Ekstrom J, et al. Prospective study of Merkel cell polyomavirus and risk of Merkel cell carcinoma. *Int J Cancer* 2014;134(4):844–848.
71. Cheng J, Rozenblatt-Rosen O, Paulson KG, et al. Merkel cell polyomavirus large T antigen has growth-promoting and inhibitory activities. *J Virol* 2013;87(11):6118–6126.
72. Li J, Wang X, Diaz J, et al. Merkel cell polyomavirus large T antigen disrupts host genomic integrity and inhibits cellular proliferation. *J Virol* 2013;87(16):9173–9188.
76. Paulson KG, Iyer JG, Tegeder AR, et al. Transcriptome-wide studies of merkel cell carcinoma and validation of intratumoral CD8+ lymphocyte invasion as an independent predictor of survival. *J Clin Oncol* 2011;29(12):1539–1546.
77. Arora R, Shuda M, Guastafierro A, et al. Survivin is a therapeutic target in Merkel cell carcinoma. *Sci Transl Med* 2012;4(133):133ra56.
79. Shuda M, Kwun HJ, Feng H, et al. Human Merkel cell polyomavirus small T antigen is an oncoprotein targeting the 4E-BP1 translation regulator. *J Clin Invest* 2011;121(9):3623–3634.
88. Cesarman E. Gammaherpesviruses and lymphoproliferative disorders. *Annu Rev Pathol* 2014;9:349–372.
89. Shannon-Lowe C, Rowe M. Epstein-Barr virus infection of polarized epithelial cells via the basolateral surface by memory B cell-mediated transfer infection. *PLoS Pathog* 2011;7(5):e1001338.
92. Barton ES, White DW, Cathelyn JS, et al. Herpesvirus latency confers symbiotic protection from bacterial infection. *Nature* 2007;447(7142):326–329.
93. Giulino-Roth L, Cesarman E. Molecular biology of Burkitt lymphoma. In: Robertson E, ed. *Burkitt's Lymphoma.* New York, NY: Springer; 2013: 211–226.
94. Chang ET, Adami HO. The enigmatic epidemiology of nasopharyngeal carcinoma. *Cancer Epidemiol Biomarkers Prev* 2006;15(10):1765–1777.
96. Cohen JI, Mocarski ES, Raab-Traub N, et al. The need and challenges for development of an Epstein-Barr virus vaccine. *Vaccine* 2013;31(Suppl 2):B194–196.
106. Krown SE, Dittmer DP, Cesarman E. Pilot study of oral valganciclovir therapy in patients with classic Kaposi's sarcoma. *J Infect Dis* 2011;203(8):1082–1086.
107. Sakakibara S, Tosato G. Regulation of angiogenesis in malignancies associated with Epstein-Barr virus and Kaposi's sarcoma-associated herpes virus. *Future Microbiol* 2009;4(7):903–917.
109. Polizzotto MN, Uldrick TS, Wang V, et al. Human and viral interleukin-6 and other cytokines in Kaposi's sarcoma herpesvirus-associated multicentric Castleman disease. *Blood* 2013;122(26):4189–4198.
111. Coffin JM, Hughes SH, Varmus HE, eds. The interactions of retroviruses and their hosts. *Retroviruses.* Cold Spring Harbor, NY: Cold Spring Harbor Laboratory Press; 1997.
112. Gallo RC. History of the discovery of the first human retroviruses: HTLV-1 and HTLV-2. *Oncogene* 2005;24:5926–5930.
116. Hacein-Bey-Abina S, VonKalle C, Schmidt M, et al. LMO2-associated clonal T cell proliferation in two patients after gene therapy for SCID-X1. *Science* 2003;302:415–419.
117. Matsuoka M, Jeang K-T. Human T-cell leukaemia virus type 1 (HTLV-1) infectivity and cellular transformation. *Nat Rev Cancer* 2007;7:270–280.
118. Poiesz BJ, Ruscetti FW, Mier JW, et al. T-cell lines established from human T-lymphocytic neoplasias by direct response to T-cell growth factor. *Proc Natl Acad Sci U S A* 1980;77:6815–6819.
120. Wolfe ND, Heneine W, Carr JK, et al. Emergence of unique primate T-lymphotropic viruses among central African bushmeat hunters. *Proc Natl Acad Sci U S A* 2005;102:7994–7999.
121. Goncalves DU, Prioietti FA, Ribas JGR, et al. Epidemiology, treatment, and prevention of human T-cell leukemia virus type 1-associated diseases. *Clin Microbiol Rev* 2010;23:577–589.

ETIOLOGY AND EPIDEMIOLOGY OF CANCER

122. Hino S, Sugiyama H, Doi H, et al. Breaking the cycle of HTLV-1 transmission via carrier mothers' milk. *Lancet Oncol* 1987;2:158–159.

123. Kannian P, Green PL. Human T lymphotropic virus type 1 (HTLV-1): molecular biology and oncogenesis. *Viruses* 2010;2:2037–2077.

124. Hill SA, Lloyd PA, McDonald S, et al. Susceptibility of human T cell leukemia virus type I to nucleoside reverse transcriptase inhibitors. *J Infec Dis* 2003;188:424–427.

125. Seegulam ME, Ratner L. Integrase inhibitors effective against human T-cell leukemia virus type 1. *Antimicrob Agents Chemother* 2011;55:2011–2017.

128. Matsuoka M, Green PL. The HBZ gene, a key player in HTLV-1 pathogenesis. *Retrovirology* 2009;6:71.

129. Grossman WJ, Kimata JT, Wong FH, et al. Development of leukemia in mice transgenic for the tax gene of human T-cell leukemia virus type I. *Proc Natl Acad Sci U S A* 1995;92:1057–1061.

135. Shimoyama M. Diagnostic criteria and classification of clinical subtypes of adult T-cell leukemia-lymphoma: a report from the Lymphoma Study Group. *Br J Hematol* 1991;79:426–437.

137. Bazarbachi A, Plumelle Y, Ramos JC, et al. Meta-analysis on the use of zidovudine and interferon-alfa in adult T-cell leukemia/lymphoma showing improved survival in the leukemic subtypes. *J Clin Oncol* 2010;28:4177–4183.

138. Katsuya H, Yamanka T, Ishitsuka K, et al. Prognostic index for acute- and lymphoma-type adult T-cell leukemia/lymphoma. *J Clin Oncol* 2012;30:1635–1640.

139. Tsukasaki K, Hermine O, Bazarbachi A, et al. Definition, prognostic factors, treatment, and reponse criteria of adult T-cell leukemia-lymphoma: a proposal from an international consensus meeting. *J Clin Oncol* 2009;27:453–459.

140. Yamada Y, Tomonaga M, Fukuda H, et al. A new G-CSF supported combination chemotherapy, LSG15, for adult T-cell leukaemia-lymphoma: Japan Clinical Oncology Group Study 9303. *Br J Hematol* 2001;113:375–382.

141. Ratner L, Harrington W, Feng X, et al. Human T cell leukemia virus reactivation with progression of adult T-cell leukemia-lymphoma. AIDS Malignancy Consortium. *PLoS One* 2009;4:e4420.

143. Bazarbachi A, Suarez F, Fields P, et al. How I treat adult T-cell leukemia/lymphoma. *Blood* 2011;118:1736–1745.

145. Blumberg BS. The discovery of the hepatitis B virus and the intervention of the vaccine: a scientific memoir. *J Gastroenterol Hepatol* 2002;17(Supplement s4):S502–S503.

146. Houghton M. Discovery of the hepatitis C virus. *Liver Int* 2009;29 (Supplement 1):82–88.

147. Arzumanyan A, Reis HM, Feitelson MA. Pathogenic mechanisms in HBV- and HCV-associated hepatocellular carcinoma. *Nat Rev Cancer* 2013;13:123–135.

148. Soerjomataram I, Lortet-Tieulent J, Parkin DM, et al. Global burden of cancer in 2008: a systematic analysis of disability-adjusted life-years in 12 world regions. *Lancet* 2012;380:1840–1850.

149. Altekruse SF, McGlynn KA, Reichman ME. Hepatocellular carcinoma incidence, mortality, and survival trends in the United States from 1975 to 2005. *J Clin Oncol* 2009;27:1485–1491.

158. Wang WK, Levy S. Hepatitis C virus (HCV) and lymphomagenesis. *Leuk Lymphoma* 2003;44:1113–1120.

159. Fernandez-Garcia MD, Mazzon M, Jacobs M, et al. Pathogenesis of flavivirus infections: using and abusing the host cell. *Cell Host Microbe* 2009;318:318–328.

160. Moradpour D, Penin F, Rice CM. Replication of hepatitis c virus. *Nat Rev Microbiol* 2007;5:453–463.

161. Liang TJ, Ghany MG. Current and future therapies for hepatitis C virus infection. *N Engl J Med* 2013;368:1907–1917.

162. Kimer N, Dahl EK, Gluud LL, et al. Antiviral therapy for prevention of hepatocellular carcinoma in chronic hepatitis C: systematic review and meta-analysis of randomised controlled trials. *BMJ Open* 2012;2:e001313.

165. Devi U, Locarnini S. Hepatitis B antivirals and resistance. *Curr Opin Virol* 2013;3:495–500.

167. Bruix J, Sherman M. Management of hepatocellular carcinoma: an update. *Hepatology* 2011;53:1020–1022.

171. Beckebaum S, Kabar I, Cicinnati VR. Hepatitis B and C in liver transplantation: new strategies to combat the enemies. *Rev Med Virol* 2012;23:172–193.

173. Huang Y-H, Hsaio L-T, Hong Y-C, et al. Randomized controlled trial of entecavir prophylaxis for rituximab-associated hepatitis B virus reactivation in patients with lymhoma and resolved hepatitis. *J Clin Oncol* 2013;31:2765–2772.

6 Inflammation

Sahdeo Prasad and Bharat B. Aggarwal

INTRODUCTION

Extensive research over the last half a century indicates that inflammation plays an important role in cancer. Although acute inflammation can play a therapeutic role, low-level chronic inflammation can promote cancer. Different inflammatory cells, the various cell signaling pathways that lead to inflammation, and biomarkers of inflammation have now been well defined. These inflammatory pathways, which are primarily mediated through the transcription factors nuclear factor kappa B (NF-κB) and signal transducer and activator of transcription 3 (STAT3), have been linked to cellular transformation, tumor survival, proliferation, invasion, angiogenesis, and metastasis of cancer. These pathways have also now been linked with chemoresistance and radioresistance. This chapter considers the role of inflammation in cancer and its potential for cancer prevention and treatment.

Inflammation is the complex biologic responses of the body to irritation, injury, or infection. The recognition of inflammation dates back to antiquity. As documented by Aulus Cornelius Celsus, a Roman of the 1st century AD, inflammation is characterized by the tissue response to injury that results in *rubor* (redness, due to hyperemia), *tumor* (swelling, caused by increased permeability of the microvasculature and leakage of protein into the interstitial space), *calor* (heat, associated with increased blood flow and the metabolic activity of the cellular mediators of inflammation), and *dolor* (pain, in part due to changes in the perivasculature and associated nerve endings). Rudolf Virchow subsequently added *functio laesa* (dysfunction of the organs involved) in the 1850s. The process includes increased blood flow with an influx of white blood cells and other chemical substances that facilitate healing. Inflammation is also considered the body's self-protective attempt to remove harmful stimuli, including damaged cells, irritants, or pathogens, and to begin the healing process.

The word inflammation is derived from the Latin *inflammo* (meaning "I set alight, I ignite"). Because inflammation is a stereotyped response, it is considered a mechanism of innate immunity, as compared with adaptive immunity. On the basis of longevity, inflammation is classified as acute or chronic. When inflammation is short term, usually appearing within a few minutes or hours and ceasing upon the removal of the injurious stimulus, it is called acute. However, if it persists longer, it is called chronic inflammation, which leads to simultaneous destruction from the inflammatory process. Inflammation is beneficial when it is acute; however, chronic inflammation leads to several diseases, including cancer. Cancer is primarily a disease of lifestyle, with 30% of all cancers having been linked to smoking, 35% to diet, 14% to 20% to obesity, 18% to infection, and 7% to environmental pollution and radiation (Fig. 6.1).[1] Smoking, obesity, infections, pollution, and radiation are all known to activate proinflammatory pathways.[2] Therefore, understanding how inflammation contributes to cancer etiology is important for both cancer prevention and treatment.[3]

MOLECULAR BASIS OF INFLAMMATION

Although it is clear that inflammation and cancer are closely related, the mechanisms underlying persistent and chronic inflammation in chronic diseases remain unclear. Numerous cytokines have been linked with inflammation, including tumor necrosis factor (TNF), interleukin (IL)-1, IL-6, IL-8, IL-17, and vascular endothelial growth factor (VEGF). Among various cytokines that have been linked with inflammation, TNF is a primary mediator of inflammation linked to cancer.[4] However, it has been shown that proinflammatory transcriptional factors (activator protein [AP]-1, STAT3, NF-κB, hypoxia-inducible factor [HIF]-1, and β-catenin/Wnt) are ubiquitously expressed and control numerous physiologic processes, including development, differentiation, immunity, and metabolism in chronic diseases. Although these transcription factors are regulated by completely different signaling mechanisms, they are activated in response to various stimuli, including stresses and cytokines, and are involved in inflammation-induced tumor development and its metastasis.[5] Interestingly, inflammation plays a role at all stages of tumor development: initiation, progression, and metastasis.[2] In initiation, inflammation induces the release of a variety of cytokines and chemokines that promote the release of inflammatory cells and associated factors. This further causes oxidative damage, DNA mutations, and other changes in the tissue microenvironment, making it more conducive to cell transformation, increased survival, and proliferation. Inflammation also contributes to tissue injury, remodeling of the extracellular matrix, angiogenesis, and fibrosis in diverse target tissues. Among all the inflammatory cell signaling pathways, NF-κB has been shown to play a major role in cancer,[6,7] and TNF is one of the most potent activators of NF-κB.[8,9]

ROLE OF INFLAMMATION IN TRANSFORMATION

Transformation is the process by which the cellular and molecular makeup of a cell is altered as it becomes malignant. Numerous factors are involved in the process of cell transformation, including inflammation. A clinical study has shown that chronic inflammation due to heavy metal deposition in lymph nodes leads to malignant transformation and, finally, to patient death.[10] More recently, chronic exposure to cigarette smoke extract[11] and arsenite[12] has been shown to induce inflammation followed by epithelial–mesenchymal transition and transformation of human bronchial epithelial (HBE) cells. Furthermore, activation of NF-κB and HIF-2α increased the levels of the proinflammatory IL-6, IL-8, and IL-1β, which are essential for the malignant progression of transformed HBE cells. Sox2, another important molecular factor, cooperates with inflammation-mediated STAT3 activation, which precedes the malignant transformation of foregut basal progenitor cells.[13] A clinical study reported that the p53 mutation is a critical event for the malignant transformation of sinonasal inverted papilloma. This p53 mutation resulted in cyclooxygenase (COX)-2–mediated inflammatory signals that contribute to the proliferation

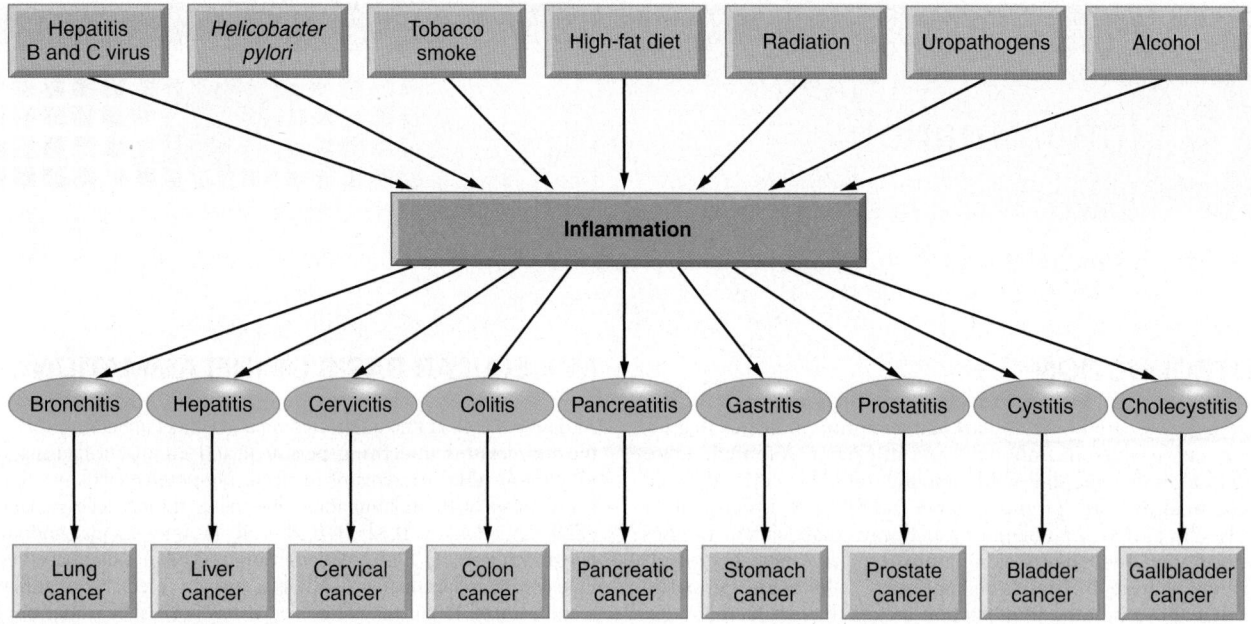

Figure 6.1 Origin of inflammation and its role in various cancers.

of advanced sinonasal inverted papilloma.[14] In another study in patients, the YKL-40 protein was found to be involved in chronic inflammation and oncogenic transformation of human breast tissues.[15] Inflammation-mediated transformation was also found to be regulated by MyD88 in a mouse model through Ras signaling.[16] In addition, inflammation contributed to the activation of the epidermal growth factor receptor (EGFR) and its subsequent interaction with PKCδ, which leads to the transformation of normal esophageal epithelia to squamous cell carcinoma.[17] Activation of Src oncoprotein triggers an inflammatory response mediated by NF-κB that directly activates Lin28 transcription and rapidly reduces let-7 microRNA levels. The inflammatory cytokine IL-6 mediates the activation of STAT3 transcription factor, which results in the transformation of cells.[18]

ROLE OF INFLAMMATION IN SURVIVAL

Numerous findings across different cancer populations have suggested that inflammation has an important role in carcinogenesis and disease progression.[19,20] The important markers of systemic inflammatory response in both in vitro findings and clinical outcomes include plasma C-reactive protein (CRP) concentration,[21,22] hypoalbuminemia,[23] and the Glasgow Prognostic Score (GPS), which combines CRP and albumin.[24,25] In addition to these, hematologic markers of systemic inflammatory response such as absolute white-cell count or its components (neutrophils, neutrophil-to-lymphocyte ratio [NLR]),[26–28] platelets, and a platelet-to-lymphocyte ratio[29,30] are also prognostic indicators for cancer clinical outcomes. Whether these inflammatory biomarkers influence the survival of cancer patients is discussed in this section.

In a study of 416 patients with renal cell carcinoma, with 362 patients included in the analysis, elevated neutrophil count, elevated platelet counts, and a high NLR were found. This inflammatory response was predictive for shorter overall patient survival.[31] Another study in unresectable malignant biliary obstruction (UMBO) found that patients with low GPS (0 and 1) had better postoperative survivals than did patients with a higher GPS. The 6-month and 1-year survival rates were 58.1% to 27.3%, respectively, for patients with low GPS and 25% to 6.2%, respectively, for patients with a higher GPS.[32] It has been also shown that prostate

cancer patients with aggressive, clinically significant disease and an elevated GPS[2] had a higher risk of death overall as well as high-grade disease.[33] Other than GPS, age and gastrectomy have also been shown to independently influence the disease-specific and progression-free survival of gastric cancer patients.[34] A biomarker of systemic inflammation, the blood NLR, predicted patient survival with hepatocellular carcinoma (HCC) after transarterial chemoembolization. Patients in whom the NLR remained stable or became normalized after transarterial chemoembolization showed improved overall survival compared with patients showing a persistently abnormal index of NLR.[35]

A further study found that inflammatory transcription factors and cytokines contribute to the overall survival of patients. One study found that 97% of patients with epithelial tumors of malignant pleural mesothelioma and 95% of patients with nonepithelial tumors expressed IL-4Rα protein, and this strong IL-4Rα expression was correlated with a worse survival. In response to IL-4, human malignant pleural mesothelioma cells showed increased STAT6 phosphorylation and increased production of IL-6, IL-8, and VEGF without any effect on proliferation or apoptosis. This finding indicates that high expression of STAT6 as well as STAT3 and cytokines is inversely correlated with survival in patients.[36,37] NF-κB, along with IL-6, contributes to the survival of mammospheres in culture, because NF-κB and IL-6 were hyperactive in breast cancer–derived mammospheres.[38] In addition, elevated CRP and serum amyloid A (SAA) were associated with reduced disease-free survival of breast cancer patients.[39] In gastroesophageal cancer, proinflammatory cytokines IL-1β, IL-6, IL-8, and TNF-α and acute phase protein concentrations (CRP) were found to be elevated, and these levels were associated with reduced survival of patients.[40] Additionally, the Bcl-2 family protein COX-2, which is regulated by inflammatory transcription factors, is also involved in the survival of cancer cells.[41,42] Thus, we conclude that inflammation in general contributes to poor survival of patients.

In contrast to these findings, an in vivo study of dogs with osteosarcoma showed that survival improvement was apparent with inflammation or lymphocyte-infiltration scores >1, as well as in dogs that had apoptosis scores in the top 50th percentile.[43] Also, in patients with epithelioid malignant pleural mesothelioma, a high degree of chronic inflammatory cell infiltration in the stromal component was associated with improved overall survival.[44]

ROLE OF INFLAMMATION IN PROLIFERATION

Several studies have shown that cell proliferation is affected by inflammation.[45] More significantly, proliferation in the setting of chronic inflammation predisposes humans to carcinoma in the esophagus, stomach, colon, liver, and urinary bladder.[46] In postgastrectomy patients, *Helicobacter pylori* induced inflammation and was associated with increased epithelial cell proliferation.[47] Even in the mouse model, chronic infection with *Helicobacter hepaticus* induced hepatic inflammation, which further led to hepatic cell proliferation.[48] Other reports found an increased expression of the cell proliferative markers PCNA and Ki-67 in the linings of inflamed odontogenic keratocysts compared with noninflamed lesions.[49,50] These findings suggest the existence of greater proliferative activity in the cells with inflammation. Wang et al.[51] showed an increased expression of cell proliferative markers PCNA and Ki-67 in a sample of 45 patients with benign prostatic hyperplasia.

The inflammatory biomarker COX-2 was also associated with the proliferation of cells. The highest proliferation index was found in COX-2–positive epithelium.[51] The association of COX-2 and proliferation was also reported in a rat model. The carcinogen dimethylhydrazine (DMH) induces an increase in epithelial cell proliferation and in the expression of COX-2 in the colon of rats.[52] Erbb2, a kinase, regulates inflammation through the induction of NF-κB, Comp1, IL-1β, COX-2, and multiple chemokines in the skin by ultraviolet (UV) exposure. This inflammation has been shown to increase the proliferation of skin tissue after UV irradiation.[53]

ROLE OF INFLAMMATION IN INVASION

A characteristic of invasive cancer cells is survival and growth under nonadhesive conditions. This invasion of cancer cells causes the disease to spread, which results in poor patient survival.[54] A strong relationship has been documented between inflammation and cancer cell invasion.[55,56] In a study of 150 patients with HCC, a high GPS score was associated with a high vascular invasion of cancer cells.[57] Another study of colorectal cancer also supports the links between inflammation and the invasion of cancer cells, with a finding that a high GPS increased the invasion of colorectal cancer cells.[58] In patients with esophageal squamous cell carcinoma, a high GPS score also showed a close relationship with lymphatic and venous invasion.[59]

At the molecular level, various proteins are known to be involved in tumor cell invasion. MMP-9, a gelatinase that degrades type IV collagen—the major structural protein component in the extracellular matrix and basement membrane—is thought to play an important role in facilitating tumor invasion, as it is highly expressed in various malignant tumors.[60,61] Additionally, the high expression of HIF-1α has been proposed as being associated with a greater incidence of vascular invasion of HCC. This expression of HIF-1α was further correlated with high expression of the inflammatory molecule COX-2.[62]

Breast cancer invasion has been linked to proteolytic activity at the tumor cell surface. In inflammatory breast cancer (IBC) cells, high expression of cathepsin B, a cell surface proteolytic enzyme, has been shown to be associated with invasiveness of IBC. In addition, a high coexpression of cathepsin B and caveolin-1 was found in IBC patient biopsies. Thus, proteolytic activity of cathepsin B and its coexpression with caveolin-1 contributes to the invasiveness of IBC.[63] In IBC, RhoC GTPase is also responsible for the invasive phenotype.[64] In addition, the PI3K/Akt signaling pathway is crucial in IBC invasion. The molecules involved in cell motility are specifically upregulated in IBC patients compared with stage-matched and cell-type-of-origin–matched non-IBCs patients. Distinctively, RhoC GTPase is a substrate for Akt1, and its phosphorylation is absolutely essential for IBC cell invasion.[65]

ROLE OF INFLAMMATION IN ANGIOGENESIS

Angiogenesis—the formation of new blood vessels from existing vessels—is tightly linked to chronic inflammation and cancer. Angiogenesis is one of the molecular events that bridges the gap between inflammation and cancer. Angiogenesis results from multiple signals acting on endothelial cells. Mature vessels control exchanges of hematopoietic cells and solutes between blood and surrounding tissues by responding to microenvironmental cues, including inflammation. Although inflammation is essential to defend the body against pathogens, it has adverse effects on the surrounding tissue, and some of these effects induce angiogenesis. Inflammation and angiogenesis are thereby linked processes, but exactly how they are related has not been well understood. Both inflammation and angiogenesis are exacerbated by an increased production of chemokines/cytokines, growth factors, proteolytic enzymes, proteoglycans, lipid mediators, and prostaglandins.

A close relationship has been reported between inflammation and angiogenesis in breast cancer. Tissue section staining showed increased vascularity with the intensity of diffuse inflammation.[66] Offersen et al.[67] found that inflammation was significantly correlated in bladder carcinoma with microvessel density, which is a marker of angiogenesis. Leukocytes have been described as mediators of inflammation-associated angiogenesis. In addition, the stable expression of TNF-α in endothelial cells increased angiogenic sprout formation independently of angiogenic growth factors. Furthermore, in work using the Matrigel plug assay in vivo, increased angiogenesis was observed in endothelial TNF-α–expressing mice. Thus, chronic inflammatory changes mediated by TNF-α can induce angiogenesis in vitro and in vivo, suggesting a direct link between inflammation and angiogenesis.[68] TNF-α–induced inhibitor of nuclear factor kappa kinase (IKK)-β activation also activates the angiogenic process. IKK-β activates the mammalian target of rapamycin (mTOR) pathway and enhances angiogenesis through VEGF production.[66] In addition to TNF-α, proinflammatory cytokines IL-1 (mainly IL-1β) and IL-8 were also found to be major proangiogenic stimuli of both physiologic and pathologic angiogenesis.[69,70] Recently, another cytokine macrophage migration inhibitory factor (MIF) was found to play a role in neoangiogenesis/vasculogenesis by endothelial cell activation along with inflammation.[71]

Benest et al.[72] found that a well-known regulator of angiogenesis, angiopoietin-2 (Ang-2), can upregulate inflammatory responses, indicating a common signaling pathway for inflammation and angiogenesis. TGF-β induction was also reported in head and neck epithelia and human head and neck squamous cell carcinomas (HNSCC), with severe inflammation that leads to angiogenesis.[73] The tumor-derived cytokine endothelial monocyte-activating polypeptide II (EMAP-II) has been shown to have profound effects on inflammation as well as on the processes involved in angiogenesis.[74] NF-κB plays an important role in inflammation as well as in angiogenesis, because the suppression of NF-κB and IkB-2A blocks basic fibroblast growth factor–induced angiogenesis in vivo. NF-κB regulates the angiogenic protein VEGF promoted by α5β1 integrin, which coordinately regulates angiogenesis and inflammation.[75] It has been also reported that a coculture of cancer cells with macrophages synergistically increased the production of various angiogenesis-related factors when stimulated by the inflammatory cytokine. This inflammatory angiogenesis was mediated by the activation of NF-κB and activator protein 1 (Jun/Fos), because the administration of either NF-κB–targeting drugs or COX-2 inhibitors or the depletion of macrophages blocked inflammatory angiogenesis.[76]

In a mouse model, cigarette smoke induced the inflammatory protein 5-lipoxygenase (5-LOX), and this induction activated matrix metalloproteinase 2 (MMP-2) and VEGF to induce the angiogenic process.[77] A cellular enzyme, Tank-binding kinase 1

(TBK-1), has been proposed as a putative mediator in tumor angiogenesis. TBK-1 mediates angiogenesis through the upregulation of VEGF and exerts proinflammatory effects via the induction of inflammatory cytokines. Thus, these pathways, including TBK-1, are an important cross-link between angiogenesis and inflammation.[78]

ROLE OF INFLAMMATION IN METASTASIS

Inflammation plays a regulatory role in cancer progression and metastasis. Chronic or tumor-derived inflammation and inflammation-related stimuli within the tumor microenvironment promote blood and lymphatic vessel formation and aid in invasion and metastasis.[79,80] The association of inflammation and metastasis has been observed in several cancer types. In an immunohistochemical analysis of lung cancer tissues, a remarkably high level of metastasis was observed with severe inflammation.[81] A mouse model of breast cancer found that mammary tumors increased the frequency of lung metastases, and this effect was associated with the recruitment of inflammatory cells to the lung as well as elevated levels of IL-6 in the lung airways.[82] In another murine model, implanting human ovarian tumor cells into the ovaries of severe combined immunodeficient mice resulted in peritoneal inflammation and tumor cell dissemination from the ovaries. In addition, enhancement of the inflammatory response with thioglycolate accelerated the development of ascites and metastases, and its suppression with acetylsalicylic acid delayed metastasis.[83] Thus, it can be concluded that inflammation facilitates ovarian tumor metastasis by a mechanism largely mediated by cytokines.

It has been shown that metastatic tumor cells entering a distant organ such as the liver trigger a proinflammatory response involving the Kupffer cell–mediated release of TNF-α and the upregulation of vascular endothelial cell adhesion receptors, such as E-selectin.[84] The physiologic expression of the selectins is tightly controlled to limit the inflammatory response, but dysregulated expression of selectins contributes to inflammatory and thrombotic disorders as well as tumor metastases.[85] Using P-selectin knockout mice, the importance of P-selectin–mediated cell adhesive interactions in the pathogenesis of inflammation and metastasis of cancers has been clearly demonstrated.[86]

Tumor-associated inflammatory monocytes and macrophages are essential promoters of tumor cell migration, invasion, and metastasis.[87] Macrophages and their mediators affect the multistep process of invasion and metastasis, from interaction with the extracellular matrix to the construction of a premetastatic niche. Monocytes are attracted by cytokines and chemokines (e.g., CSF-1, GM-CSF, and MCP-1), which are released by tumor cells or cells of the tumor microenvironment. These monocytes are then induced to express proangiogenic and metastatic factors, including VEGF, fibroblast growth factor (FGF)-2, platelet-derived growth factor (PDGF), intercellular adhesion molecule (ICAM)-1, vascular cell adhesion molecule (VCAM)-1, E-selectin, P- selectin, and MMP-9.[88] Versican, a large extracellular matrix proteoglycan, has been shown to activate tumor-infiltrating myeloid cells through Toll-like receptor (TLR) 2 and its coreceptors TLR6 and CD14 and to elicit the production of proinflammatory cytokines (including TNF-α), which enhance tumor metastasis. TLR2 increases the secretion of IL-8, which potentiates metastatic growth. Ligation of TLR2 by versican induces inflammatory cytokine secretion, providing a link between inflammation and cancer metastasis.[89]

IKK-α has been shown to be important in the inflammation-associated metastasis of cancer cells. Luo et al.[90] demonstrated that activation and nuclear localization of IKK-α by tumor-infiltrating immune cells in prostatic epithelial tumor cells leads to malignant prostatic epithelial cells with a metastatic fate. Src family kinases, when inappropriately activated, promote pathologic inflammatory processes and tumor metastasis, in part through their effects on the regulation of endothelial monolayer permeability.[91] Platelet-activating factor (PAF), an inflammatory biolipid, has also been

shown to increase metastasis. In particular, Melnikova et al.[92] demonstrated that PAF receptor antagonists can effectively inhibit the metastatic potential of human melanoma cells in nude mice. Mesenchymal stem cells promote HCC metastasis under the influence of inflammation through TGF-β.[93]

EPIGENETIC CHANGES AND INFLAMMATION

Epigenetics considers the heritable changes in the activity of gene expression without the alteration of DNA sequences, and such changes have been linked to many human diseases, including cancer.[94] DNA methylation and histone modification are well-known epigenetic changes that can lead to gene activation or inactivation.[94–96] DNA methylation occurs primarily at cytosine-phosphate-guanine (CpG) dinucleotides as well as at transcriptional regulatory sites on the gene promoter.[96–98] Epigenetic abnormalities result in dysregulated gene expression and function, which can further lead to cancer. Inflammation and epigenetic abnormalities in cancer are highly associated. Inflammation induces aberrant epigenetic alterations in a tissue early in the process of carcinogenesis, and accumulation of such alterations forms an epigenetic field for cancer. Yara et al.[99] have shown that increased inflammation, as evidenced by the activation of NF-κB, production of IL-6 and COX-2, as well as the decrease of IκB, leads to the promoter's methylation. However, preincubation of cells with a demethylating agent prevented inflammation.

Infectious agents also contribute to inflammation-induced epigenetic changes. Infectious agents such as *H. pylori* and hepatitis C virus as well as intrinsic mediators of inflammatory responses, including proinflammatory cytokines, induce genetic and epigenetic changes, including point mutations, deletions, duplications, recombinations, and methylation of various tumor-related genes. Interestingly, disturbances in cytokine and chemokine signals and the induction of cell proliferation are important ways that inflammation induces aberrant DNA methylation. A study has shown that infection of human gastric mucosae with *H. pylori* induces chronic inflammation and further gastric cancers.[100] This inflammation is associated with high methylation levels or high incidences of methylation.[101–103]

Furthermore, numerous reports have documented the fact that inflammation is linked with epigenetic changes in carcinogenesis. Recently, Achyut[104] reported that inflammation in stromal fibroblasts caused epigenetic silencing of p21 and further tumor progression. Chronic inflammation also led to epigenetic regulation of p16 and activation of DNA damage in a lung carcinogenesis model.[105]

A transient inflammatory signal has been shown to initiate an epigenetic switch from nontransformed cells to cancer cells via a positive feedback loop involving NF-κB, Lin28, let-7, and IL-6. This IL-6 induced STAT3, directly activated miR-21 and miR-181b-1, and further induced the epigenetic switch. Thus, STAT3 underlies the epigenetic switch of mir-21 and mir-181b-1 that links inflammation to cancer.[106] Another report also showed that transient activation of Src oncoprotein mediates an epigenetic switch from immortalized breast cells to a stably transformed line that contained cancer stem cells. Thus, inflammation activates a positive feedback loop that maintains the epigenetic transformed state for many generations in the absence of the inducing signal.[18]

DNA hypermethylation at promoter CpG islands is an important mechanism by which carcinogenesis occurs through the inactivation of tumor-suppressor genes. Aberrant CpG island hypermethylation is also frequently observed in chronic inflammation and precancerous lesions, which again suggests links between inflammation and epigenetic change.[107] In addition, inflammation induced the halogenation of cytosine nucleotide. Damage products of this inflammation-mediated halogenated cytosine interfere with normal epigenetic control by altering DNA-protein interactions that are critical for gene regulation and the heritable transmission of methylation patterns. These inflammation-mediated cytosine damage products also provide a mechanistic link between inflammation and cancer.[108]

ROLE OF INFLAMMATION IN CANCER DIAGNOSIS

Chronic inflammation plays an important role in the etiology and progression of chronic diseases, including cancer. Hence, chronic inflammation may have an important diagnostic role in cancer. Inflammation induced by inflammatory cells such as infiltrating cells and mesothelial cells is mediated via the release of various mediators and proteins, including PDGF, IL-8, monocyte chemotactic peptide (MCP-1), nitric oxide (NO), collagen, antioxidant enzymes, and the plasminogen activation inhibitor (PAI). Furthermore, several inflammatory mediators have been shown to be detected at increased concentrations, thereby aiding in the disease diagnosis.[109]

In one study, numerous inflammatory disorders were detected based on inflammation measured in gastric biopsies of patients by Fourier transform infrared spectroscopy (FT-IR). Using endoscopic samples, gastritis and gastric cancer were diagnosed.[110] Furthermore, the degree of prostate inflammation has been used to determine the level of incidental prostatitis.[111] An assessment of the expression of cytokines and other immune stimulatory molecules that drive B-cell activation provides insight into the etiology of cancers. It has been shown that the dysregulation of cytokine production precedes the diagnosis of non-Hodgkin lymphoma.[112]

Inflammation parameters have been used to diagnose cancer in patients. Inflammation parameters, including CRP, were found to differ in patients with cancer and in those without. In clinical practice, however, such parameters are considered to have modest diagnostic value for cancer.[113] In a study with 1,275 patients, granulomatous inflammation was identified in 154 patients (12.1%), of whom 12 out of 154 (7.8%) had a concurrent diagnosis of cancer.[114] In another study with 173 patients, 52% had lung adenocarcinoma. Patients with high systemic inflammation were more likely to have more than two sites of metastatic disease and to have poor performance status and less likely to receive any chemotherapy. Systemic inflammation at diagnosis is considered to be an independent marker of poor outcome in patients with advanced non-small cell lung cancer (NSCLC).[115]

INFLAMMATION AND GENOMICS

Recently, the genomic landscape of the most common forms of human cancer have been examined.[116] Almost 140 genes and 12 cell signaling pathways have been linked with most cancers. Several of these genes and pathways are directly or indirectly linked with inflammation. A cytokine pattern in patients with cancer has been identified.[117]

INFLAMMATION AND TARGETED THERAPIES

That inflammation can be used as a target for cancer prevention and treatment is indicated by the fact that several drugs approved by the U.S. Food and Drug Administration (FDA) actually modulate proinflammatory pathways. For instance, EGFR, HER2, VEGF, CXCR4, and proteasome have been shown to activate NF-κB–mediated proinflammatory pathways, and their inhibitors have been approved by the FDA for the treatment of various cancers. Similarly, steroids such as dexamethasone, nonsteroidal anti-inflammatory drugs (NSAIDs), and statins that are currently used for prevention or treatment have also been found to suppress the NF-κB pathway. Thus, these observations indicate that inflammatory pathways are excellent targets for cancer.

CONCLUSIONS

According to Colditz et al.,[118] almost 50% of all cancers can be prevented based on what we know today. All the studies summarized previously suggest that inflammation is closely linked to cancer, and the incidence of most cancers can be reduced by controlling inflammation. Proinflammatory conditions such as colitis, bronchitis, hepatitis, and gastritis can all eventually lead to cancer. Thus, one must find ways to treat these conditions before the appearance of cancer. All these studies indicate that an anti-inflammatory lifestyle could play an important role in both the prevention and treatment of cancer.

SELECTED REFERENCES

The full reference list can be accessed at lwwhealthlibrary.com/oncology.

52. Demarzo MM, Martins LV, Fernandes CR, et al. Exercise reduces inflammation and cell proliferation in rat colon carcinogenesis. *Med Sci Sports Exerc* 2008;40:618–621.
53. Madson JG, Lynch DT, Tinkum KL, et al. Erbb2 regulates inflammation and proliferation in the skin after ultraviolet irradiation. *Am J Pathol* 2006;169:1402–1414.
54. Bondong S, Kiefel H, Hielscher T, et al. Prognostic significance of L1CAM in ovarian cancer and its role in constitutive NF-kappaB activation. *Ann Oncol* 2012;23:1795–1802.
55. Wu Y, Zhou BP. Inflammation: a driving force speeds cancer metastasis. *Cell Cycle* 2009;8:3267–3273.
56. Aggarwal BB, Vijayalekshmi RV, Sung B. Targeting inflammatory pathways for prevention and therapy of cancer: short-term friend, long-term foe. *Clin Cancer Res* 2009;15:425–430.
57. Kinoshita A, Onoda H, Imai N, et al. The Glasgow Prognostic Score, an inflammation based prognostic score, predicts survival in patients with hepatocellular carcinoma. *BMC Cancer* 2013;13:52.
58. Toiyama Y, Miki C, Inoue Y, et al. Evaluation of an inflammation-based prognostic score for the identification of patients requiring postoperative adjuvant chemotherapy for stage II colorectal cancer. *Exp Ther Med* 2011;2:95–101.
59. Kobayashi T, Teruya M, Kishiki T, et al. Inflammation-based prognostic score, prior to neoadjuvant chemoradiotherapy, predicts postoperative outcome in patients with esophageal squamous cell carcinoma. *Surgery* 2008;144:729–735.
60. Nelson AR, Fingleton B, Rothenberg ML, et al. Matrix metalloproteinases: biologic activity and clinical implications. *J Clin Oncol* 2000;18:1135–1149.
61. Clark ES, Weaver AM. A new role for cortactin in invadopodia: regulation of protease secretion. *Eur J Cell Biol* 2008;87:581–590.
62. Dai CX, Gao Q, Qiu SJ, et al. Hypoxia-inducible factor-1 alpha, in association with inflammation, angiogenesis and MYC, is a critical prognostic factor in patients with HCC after surgery. *BMC Cancer* 2009;9:418.
63. Victor BC, Anbalagan A, Mohamed MM, et al. Inhibition of cathepsin B activity attenuates extracellular matrix degradation and inflammatory breast cancer invasion. *Breast Cancer Res* 2011;13:R115.
64. van Golen KL, Bao LW, Pan Q, et al. Mitogen activated protein kinase pathway is involved in RhoC GTPase induced motility, invasion and angiogenesis in inflammatory breast cancer. *Clin Exp Metastasis* 2002;19:301–311.
65. Lehman HL, Van Laere SJ, van Golen CM, et al. Regulation of inflammatory breast cancer cell invasion through Akt1/PKBalpha phosphorylation of RhoC GTPase. *Mol Cancer Res* 2012;10:1306–1318.
66. Lee DF, Kuo HP, Chen CT, et al. IKK beta suppression of TSC1 links inflammation and tumor angiogenesis via the mTOR pathway. *Cell* 2007;130:440–455.
67. Offersen BV, Knap MM, Marcussen N, et al. Intense inflammation in bladder carcinoma is associated with angiogenesis and indicates good prognosis. *Br J Cancer* 2002;87:1422–1430.
68. Rajashekhar G, Willuweit A, Patterson CE, et al. Continuous endothelial cell activation increases angiogenesis: evidence for the direct role of endothelium linking angiogenesis and inflammation. *J Vasc Res* 2006;43:193–204.

69. Voronov E, Carmi Y, Apte RN. Role of IL-1-mediated inflammation in tumor angiogenesis. *Adv Exp Med Biol* 2007;601:265–270.

70. Qazi BS, Tang K, Qazi A. Recent advances in underlying pathologies provide insight into interleukin-8 expression-mediated inflammation and angiogenesis. *Int J Inflam* 2011;2011:908468.

71. Asare Y, Schmitt M, Bernhagen J. The vascular biology of macrophage migration inhibitory factor (MIF). Expression and effects in inflammation, atherogenesis and angiogenesis. *Thromb Haemost* 2013;109:391–398.

72. Benest AV, Kruse K, Savant S, et al. Angiopoietin-2 is critical for cytokine-induced vascular leakage. *PLoS One* 2013;8: e70459.

73. Lu SL, Reh D, Li AG, et al. Overexpression of transforming growth factor beta1 in head and neck epithelia results in inflammation, angiogenesis, and epithelial hyperproliferation. *Cancer Res* 2004;64:4405–4410.

74. Berger AC, Tang G, Alexander HR, et al. Endothelial monocyte-activating polypeptide II, a tumor-derived cytokine that plays an important role in inflammation, apoptosis, and angiogenesis. *J Immunother* 2000;23:519–527.

75. Klein S, de Fougerolles AR, Blaikie P, et al. Alpha 5 beta 1 integrin activates an NF-kappa B-dependent program of gene expression important for angiogenesis and inflammation. *Mol Cell Biol* 2002;22:5912–5922.

76. Ono M. Molecular links between tumor angiogenesis and inflammation: inflammatory stimuli of hematopoiesis and cancer cells as targets for therapeutic strategy. *Cancer Sci* 2008;99:1501–1506.

77. Ye YN, Liu ES, Shin VY, et al. Contributory role of 5-lipoxygenase and its association with angiogenesis in the promotion of inflammation-associated colonic tumorigenesis by cigarette smoking. *Toxicology* 2004;203:179–188.

78. Czabanka M, Korherr C, Brinkmann U, et al. Influence of TBK-1 on tumor angiogenesis and microvascular inflammation. *Front Biosci* 2008;13:7243–7249.

79. Solinas G, Marchesi F, Garlanda C, et al. Inflammation-mediated promotion of invasion and metastasis. *Cancer Metastasis Rev* 2010;29:243–248.

80. Affara NI, Coussens LM. IKKalpha at the crossroads of inflammation and metastasis. *Cell* 2007;129:25–26.

82. Hobson J, Gummadidala P, Silverstrim B, et al. Acute inflammation induced by the biopsy of mouse mammary tumors promotes the development of metastasis. *Breast Cancer Res Treat* 2013;139:391–401.

83. Robinson-Smith TM, Isaacsohn I, Mercer CA, et al. Macrophages mediate inflammation-enhanced metastasis of ovarian tumors in mice. *Cancer Res* 2007;67:5708–5716.

84. Khatib AM, Auguste P, Fallavollita L, et al. Characterization of the host proinflammatory response to tumor cells during the initial stages of liver metastasis. *Am J Pathol* 2005;167:749–759.

85. McEver RP. Selectin-carbohydrate interactions during inflammation and metastasis. *Glycoconj J* 1997;14:585–591.

86. Geng JG, Chen M, Chou KC. P-selectin cell adhesion molecule in inflammation, thrombosis, cancer growth and metastasis. *Curr Med Chem* 2004;11:2153–2160.

87. Condeelis J, Pollard JW. Macrophages: obligate partners for tumor cell migration, invasion, and metastasis. *Cell* 2006;124:263–266.

88. Siegel G, Malmsten M. The role of the endothelium in inflammation and tumor metastasis. *Int J Microcirc Clin Exp* 1997;17:257–272.

89. Wang W, Xu GL, Jia WD, et al. Ligation of TLR2 by versican: a link between inflammation and metastasis. *Arch Med Res* 2009;40:321–323.

90. Luo JL, Tan W, Ricono JM, et al. Nuclear cytokine-activated IKKalpha controls prostate cancer metastasis by repressing Maspin. *Nature* 2007;446:690–694.

91. Kim MP, Park SI, Kopetz S, et al. Src family kinases as mediators of endothelial permeability: effects on inflammation and metastasis. *Cell Tissue Res* 2009;335:249–259.

92. Melnikova V, Bar-Eli M. Inflammation and melanoma growth and metastasis: the role of platelet-activating factor (PAF) and its receptor. *Cancer Metastasis Rev* 2007;26:359–371.

93. Jing Y, Han Z, Liu Y, et al. Mesenchymal stem cells in inflammation microenvironment accelerates hepatocellular carcinoma metastasis by inducing epithelial-mesenchymal transition. *PLoS One* 2012;7:e43272.

94. Jones PA, Baylin SB. The epigenomics of cancer. *Cell* 2007;128:683–692.

95. Esteller M. Aberrant DNA methylation as a cancer-inducing mechanism. *Annu Rev Pharmacol Toxicol* 2005;45:629–656.

96. Thiagalingam S, Cheng KH, Lee HJ, et al. Histone deacetylases: unique players in shaping the epigenetic histone code. *Ann N Y Acad Sci* 2003;983:84–100.

97. Li E, Beard C, Jaenisch R. Role for DNA methylation in genomic imprinting. *Nature* 1993;366:362–365.

98. Antequera F, Bird A. Number of CpG islands and genes in human and mouse. *Proc Natl Acad Sci U S A* 1993;90:11995–11999.

99. Yara S, Lavoie JC, Beaulieu JF, et al. Iron-ascorbate-mediated lipid peroxidation causes epigenetic changes in the antioxidant defense in intestinal epithelial cells: impact on inflammation. *PLoS One* 2013;8:e63456.

100. Uemura N, Okamoto S, Yamamoto S, et al. Helicobacter pylori infection and the development of gastric cancer. *N Engl J Med* 2001;345:784–789.

101. Maekita T, Nakazawa K, Mihara M, et al. High levels of aberrant DNA methylation in Helicobacter pylori-infected gastric mucosae and its possible association with gastric cancer risk. *Clin Cancer Res* 2006;12:989–995.

102. Nakajima T, Maekita T, Oda I, et al. Higher methylation levels in gastric mucosae significantly correlate with higher risk of gastric cancers. *Cancer Epidemiol Biomarkers Prev* 2006;15:2317–2321.

103. Perri F, Cotugno R, Piepoli A, et al. Aberrant DNA methylation in nonneoplastic gastric mucosa of H. Pylori infected patients and effect of eradication. *Am J Gastroenterol* 2007;102:1361–1371.

104. Achyut BR, Bader DA, Robles AI, et al. Inflammation-mediated genetic and epigenetic alterations drive cancer development in the neighboring epithelium upon stromal abrogation of TGF-beta signaling. *PLoS Genet* 2013;9:e1003251.

105. Blanco D, Vicent S, Fraga MF, et al. Molecular analysis of a multistep lung cancer model induced by chronic inflammation reveals epigenetic regulation of p16 and activation of the DNA damage response pathway. *Neoplasia* 2007;9:840–852.

106. Iliopoulos D, Jaeger SA, Hirsch HA, et al. STAT3 activation of miR-21 and miR-181b-1 via PTEN and CYLD are part of the epigenetic switch linking inflammation to cancer. *Mol Cell* 2010;39:493–506.

107. Suzuki H, Toyota M, Kondo Y, et al. Inflammation-related aberrant patterns of DNA methylation: detection and role in epigenetic deregulation of cancer cell transcriptome. *Methods Mol Biol* 2009;512:55–69.

108. Valinluck V, Sowers LC. Inflammation-mediated cytosine damage: a mechanistic link between inflammation and the epigenetic alterations in human cancers. *Cancer Res* 2007;67:5583–5586.

109. Kroegel C, Antony VB. Immunobiology of pleural inflammation: potential implications for pathogenesis, diagnosis and therapy. *Eur Respir J* 1997;10:2411–2418.

110. Li QB, Sun XJ, Xu YZ, et al. Use of Fourier-transform infrared spectroscopy to rapidly diagnose gastric endoscopic biopsies. *World J Gastroenterol* 2005;11:3842–3845.

111. Difuccia B, Keith I, Teunissen B, et al. Diagnosis of prostatic inflammation: efficacy of needle biopsies versus tissue blocks. *Urology* 2005;65:445–448.

112. Vendrame E, Martinez-Maza O. Assessment of pre-diagnosis biomarkers of immune activation and inflammation: insights on the etiology of lymphoma. *J Proteome Res* 2011;10:113–119.

113. Baicus C, Caraiola S, Rimbas M, et al. Utility of routine hematological and inflammation parameters for the diagnosis of cancer in involuntary weight loss. *J Investig Med* 2011;59:951–955.

114. DePew ZS, Gonsalves WI, Roden AC, et al. Granulomatous inflammation detected by endobronchial ultrasound-guided transbronchial needle aspiration in patients with a concurrent diagnosis of cancer: a clinical conundrum. *J Bronchology Interv Pulmonol* 2012;19:176–181.

115. Jafri SH, Shi R, Mills G. Advance lung cancer inflammation index (ALI) at diagnosis is a prognostic marker in patients with metastatic non-small cell lung cancer (NSCLC): a retrospective review. *BMC Cancer* 2013;13:158.

116. Vogelstein B, Papadopoulos N, Velculescu VE, et al. Cancer genome landscapes. *Science* 2013;339:1546–1558.

117. Lippitz BE. Cytokine patterns in patients with cancer: a systematic review. *Lancet Oncol* 2013;14:e218–228.

7 Chemical Factors

Stuart H. Yuspa and Peter G. Shields

INTRODUCTION

As early as the 1800s, initial observations of unusual cancer incidences in occupational groups provided the first indications that chemicals were a cause of human cancer, which was then confirmed in experimental animal studies during the early and mid 1900s. However, the extent to which chemical exposures contribute to cancer incidence was not fully appreciated until population-based studies documented differing organ-specific cancer rates in geographically distinct populations and in cohort studies such as those that linked smoking to lung cancer.[1] The most commonly occurring chemical exposures that increase cancer risk are tobacco, alcoholic beverages, diet, and reproductive factors (e.g., hormones). Today, it is recognized that cancer results not solely from chemical exposure (e.g., in the workplace or at home), but that a variety of biologic, social, and physical factors contribute to cancer pathogenesis.[2,3] For some common cancers, it also has been recognized that heritable factors also contribute to cancer risk from chemical exposure (e.g., genes involved in carcinogen metabolism, DNA repair, a variety of cancer pathways).[4] Twin studies show that for common cancers, nongenetic risk factors are dominant, and the best associations for genetic risks of sporadic cancers indicate that the risks for specific genetic traits are typically less than 1.5-fold.[5–7] The role of the tumor microenvironment, the cancer stem cells, and feedback signaling to and from the tumor also have been recently recognized as important contributors to carcinogenesis, although how chemicals affect these have yet been clearly demonstrated.[8–10]

The experimental induction of tumors in animals, the neoplastic transformation of cultured cells by chemicals, and the molecular analysis of human tumors have revealed important concepts regarding the pathogenesis of cancer and how laboratory studies can be used to better understand human cancer pathogenesis.[7,11,12] Chemical carcinogens usually affect specific organs, targeting the epithelial cells (or other susceptible cells within an organ) and causing genetic damage (genotoxic) or epigenetic effects regulating DNA transcription and translation. Chemically related DNA damage and consequent somatic mutations relevant to human cancer can occur either directly from exogenous exposures or indirectly by activation of endogenous mutagenic pathways (e.g., nitric oxide, oxyradicals).[13,14] The risk of developing a chemically induced tumor may be modified by nongenotoxic exogenous and endogenous exposures and factors (e.g., hormones, immunosuppression triggered by the tumor), and by accumulated exposure to the same or different genotoxic carcinogens.[7,15]

Analyses of how chemicals induce cancer in animal models and human populations has had a major impact on human health. Experimental studies have been instrumental in replicating hypotheses generated from human studies and identifying pathobiologic mechanisms. For example, animal experiments confirmed the carcinogenic and cocarcinogenic properties of cigarette smoke and identified bioactive chemical and gaseous components.[1] The transplacental carcinogenicity of diethylstilbestrol and the hazards of specific occupational carcinogens such as vinyl chloride,

benzene, aromatic amines, and bis(chloromethyl)ether led to a reduction in allowable exposures of suspected human carcinogens from the workplace and a reduction in cancer rates. Dietary factors that enhance or inhibit cancer development and the contribution of obesity to specific organ sites have been identified in models of chemical carcinogenesis, and alterations in diet and obesity are expected to result in reduced cancer risk. Experimental animal studies are the mainstay of risk assessment as a screening tool to identify potential carcinogens in the workplace and the environment, although these studies do not prove specific chemical etiologies as a cause of human cancer because of interspecies differences and the use of maximally tolerated doses that do not replicate human exposure.

THE NATURE OF CHEMICAL CARCINOGENS: CHEMISTRY AND METABOLISM

The National Toxicology Program, based mostly on experimental animal studies and supported by epidemiology studies when available, lists 45 chemical, physical, and infectious agents as known human carcinogens and about 175 that are reasonably anticipated to be human carcinogens (http://ntp.niehs.nih.gov/?objectid=035E57E7-BDD9-2D9B-AFB9D1CADC8 D09C1), whereas the International Agency for Research on Cancer (IARC) lists 113 agents as carcinogenic to humans and 66 that are probably carcinogenic to humans (http://monographs.iarc.fr/ENG/Classification/index.php). Table 7.1 provides a selected list of known human carcinogens, as indicated by the IARC, which are continuously updated.[16] Most chemical carcinogens first undergo metabolic activation by cytochrome P450s or other metabolic pathways so that they react with DNA and/or alter epigenetic mechanisms.[11,17] This process, evolutionarily presumed to have been developed to rid the body of foreign chemicals for excretion, inadvertently generates reactive carcinogenic intermediates that can bind cellular molecules, including DNA, and cause mutations or other alterations.[18] Recent data indicate that metabolizing enzymes also have the ability to cross-talk with transcription factors involved in the regulation of other metabolizing and antioxidant enzymes.[19] DNA is considered the ultimate target for most carcinogens to cause either mutations or gross chromosomal changes, but epigenetic effects, such as altered DNA methylation and gene transcription, also promote carcinogenesis.[20] The formation of DNA adducts, where chemicals bind directly to DNA to promote mutations, is likely necessary but not sufficient to cause cancer.

Genotoxic carcinogens may transfer simple alkyl or complexed (aryl) alkyl groups to specific sites on DNA bases.[18,21] These alkylating and aryl-alkylating agents include, but are not limited to, N-nitroso compounds, aliphatic epoxides, aflatoxins, mustards, polycyclic aromatic hydrocarbons, and other combustion products of fossil fuels and vegetable matter. Others transfer arylamine residues to DNA, as exemplified by aryl aromatic

89

TABLE 7.1

Known Chemical Carcinogens in Humans[a]

Target Organ	Agents	Industries	Tumor Type
Lung	Tobacco smoke, arsenic, asbestos, crystalline silica, benzo(a)pyrene, beryllium, bis(chloro)methyl ether, 1,3-butadiene, chromium VI compounds, coal tar and pitch, diesel exhaust, nickel compounds, soot, mustard gas, cobalt-tungsten carbide powders	Aluminum production, coal gasification, coke production, painting, hematite mining, painting, grinding in oil and gas	Squamous, large cell, and small cell cancer and adenocarcinoma
Pleura	Asbestos, erionite, painting	Insulation, mining	Mesothelioma
Oral cavity	Tobacco smoke, alcoholic beverages, nickel compounds, betel quid	–	Squamous cell cancer
Esophagus	Tobacco smoke, alcoholic beverages, betel quid	–	Squamous cell cancer
Gastric	Tobacco smoking	Rubber industry	Adenocarcinoma
Colon	Alcohol, tobacco smoking	–	Adenocarcinoma
Liver	Aflatoxin, vinyl chloride, tobacco smoke, alcoholic beverages	–	Hepatocellular carcinoma, hemangiosarcoma
Kidney	Tobacco smoke, trichloroethylene	–	Renal cell cancer
Bladder	Tobacco smoke, 4-aminobiphenyl, benzidine, 2-napthylamine, cyclophosphamide, phenacetin	Magenta manufacturing, auramine manufacturing, painting, rubber production	Transitional cell cancer
Prostate	Cadmium	–	Adenocarcinoma
Skin	Arsenic, benzo(a)pyrene, coal tar and pitch, mineral oils, soot, cyclosporin A, azathioprine, shale oils	–	Squamous cell cancer, basal cell cancer
Bone marrow	Benzene, tobacco smoke, ethylene oxide, antineoplastic agents, cyclosporin A, formaldehyde	Rubber workers	Leukemia, lymphoma

[a] The carcinogen designations are determined by the International Agency for Research on Cancer (http://monographs.iarc.fr/index.php). They do not imply proof of carcinogenicity in individuals. This table is not all inclusive. For additional information, the reader is referred to agency documents and publications.

amines, aminoazo dyes, and heterocyclic aromatic amines. For genotoxic carcinogens, the interaction with DNA is not random, and each class of agents reacts selectively with purine and pyrimidine targets.[7,18,21] Furthermore, targeting carcinogens to particular sites in DNA is determined by nucleotide sequence, by host cell, and by selective DNA repair processes (see later discussion), making some genetic material at risk over others. As expected from this chemistry, genotoxic carcinogens can be potent mutagens and particularly adept at causing nucleotide base mispairing or small deletions, leading to missense or nonsense mutations. Others may cause macrogenetic damage, such as chromosome breaks and large deletions. In some cases, such genotoxic damage may result in changes in transcription and translation that affect protein levels or function, which in turn alter the behavior of the specific host cell type. For example, there may be effects on cell proliferation, programmed cell death, or DNA repair. This is best typified by the signature mutations detected in the p53 gene caused by ingested aflatoxin in human liver cancer[22] and by polycyclic aromatic hydrocarbons human lung cancer caused by the inhalation of cigarette smoke.[15,23,24] Similarly, a distinct pattern of mutations is detected in pancreatic cancers from smokers when compared with pancreatic cancers from nonsmokers.[25]

Some chemicals that cause cancers in laboratory rodents are not demonstrably genotoxic. In general, these agents are carcinogenic in laboratory animals at high doses and require prolonged exposure. Synthetic pesticides and herbicides fall within this group, as do a number of natural products that are ingested. The mechanism of action by nongenotoxic carcinogens is not well understood, and may be related in some cases to toxic cell death and regenerative hyperplasia. They may also induce endogenous mutagenic mechanisms through the production of free radicals, increasing rates of depurination, and the deamination of 5-methylcytosine. In other cases, nongenotoxic carcinogens may have hormonal effects on hormone-dependent tissues. For example, some pesticides, herbicides, and fungicides have endocrine-disrupting properties in experimental models, although the relation to human cancer risk is unknown.

ANIMAL MODEL SYSTEMS AND CHEMICAL CARCINOGENESIS

Most human chemical carcinogens can induce tumors in experimental animals; however, the tumors may not be in the same organ, the exposure pathways may differ from human exposure, and the causative mechanisms may not exist in humans. In many cases, however, the cell of origin, morphogenesis, phenotypic markers, and genetic alterations are qualitatively identical to corresponding human cancers. Furthermore, animal models have revealed the constancy of carcinogen–host interaction among mammalian species by reproducing organ-specific cancers in animals with chemicals identified as human carcinogens, such as coal tar and squamous cell carcinomas, vinyl chloride and hepatic angiosarcomas, aflatoxin and hepatocellular carcinoma, and aromatic amines and bladder cancer. The introduction of genetically modified mice designed to reproduce specific human cancer syndromes and precancer models has accelerated both the understanding of the contributions of chemicals to cancer causation and the identification of potential exogenous carcinogens.[26,27] Furthermore, construction of mouse strains genetically altered to express human drug–metabolizing enzymes has added both to the relevance of mouse studies for understanding human carcinogen metabolism and the prediction of genotoxicity from suspected human carcinogens and other chemical exposures.[28] Together, these studies have indicated that carcinogenic agents can directly activate oncogenes, inactivate tumor suppressor genes, and cause the genomic changes that are associated with autonomous growth, enhanced survival, and modified gene expression profiles that are required for the malignant phenotype.[29]

Genetic Susceptibility to Chemical Carcinogenesis in Experimental Animal Models

The use of inbred strains of rodents and spontaneous or genetically modified mutant strains have led to the identification and characterization of genes that modify risks for cancer development.[30–32] For a variety of tissue sites, including the lungs, the liver, the breast, and the skin, pairs of inbred mice can differ by 100-fold in the risk for tumor development after carcinogen exposure. Genetically determined differences in the affinity for the aryl hydrocarbon hydroxylase (Ah) receptor or other differences in metabolic processing of carcinogens is one modifier that has a major impact on experimental and presumed human cancer risk.[33–35] The development of mice reconstituted with components of the human carcinogen–metabolizing genome should facilitate the extrapolation of metabolic activity by human enzymes and cancer risk.[27,28,36] Such mice also show that other loci regulate the growth of premalignant foci, the response to tumor promoters, the immune response to metastatic cells, and the basal proliferation rate of target cells.[30] In mice susceptible to colon cancer due to a carcinogen-induced constitutive mutation in the APC gene, a locus on mouse chromosome 4 confers resistance to colon cancer.[31] The identification of the phospholipase A2 gene at this locus and subsequent functional testing in transgenic mice revealed an interesting paracrine protective influence on tumor development.[31] This gene, and several other genes mapped for susceptibility to chemically induced mouse tumors (PTPRJ, a receptor type tyrosine phosphatase, and STK6/STK15, an aurora kinase), have now been shown to influence susceptibility to organ-specific cancer induction in humans.[30,31]

MOLECULAR EPIDEMIOLOGY, CHEMICAL CARCINOGENESIS, AND CANCER RISK IN HUMAN POPULATIONS

Molecular epidemiology is the application of biologically based hypotheses using molecular and epidemiologic methods and measures. New technologies continue to allow epidemiologic studies to improve the testing of biologically based hypotheses and to develop large datasets for hypothesis generation, most notably the application of various –omics technologies via next-generation sequencing (e.g., genomics, epigenomics, transcriptomics), proteomics, and metabolomics. The greatest challenge now is to develop methods that allow for analysis cutting across various technologies.[37–43] Recent advances now include the role of microRNA and long noncoding RNAs in tumor development and progression because of their impact on the regulation of gene expression.[44,45] Chemical effects on microRNAs and the resultant gene expression is currently being identified.[46] Using such technologies, emerging evidence is noting the importance of the microbiome and associated infections as a risk of human cancer.[47–50] The complexity of environmental exposure and how it interacts with humans to affect numerous biologic pathways has been characterized as the exposome, also expressed as a multidimensional complex dataset.[51] Therefore, the important goal remains: to characterize cancer risk based on gene–environment interactions. However, we remain challenged because cancer is a complex disease of diverse etiologies by multiple exposures causing damage in different genes; for example, $gene^n$–$environment^n$ interactions, for which the variable n is not known.

Two fundamental principles underlie current studies of molecular epidemiology. First, carcinogenesis is a multistage process, and behind each stage are numerous genetic events that occur either due to an exogenous insult such as a chemical exposure or an endogenous insult, such as from free radicals generated via cellular processes or errors in DNA replication. Therefore, identifying a cancer risk factor can be challenging because of the multifactorial nature of carcinogenesis, given that any one risk factor occurs within a background of many risk factors. Second, wide interindividual variation in response to carcinogen exposure and other carcinogenic processes indicate that the human response is not homogeneous, so that experimental models and epidemiology (e.g., the use of a single cell clone to study a gene's effect experimentally or the assumption that the population responds similarly to the mean in epidemiology studies), might not be representative of susceptible and resistant groups within a population.

Genetic Susceptibility

In humans, the determination of genetic susceptibility can be assessed by phenotyping or genotyping methods. Phenotypes generally represent complex genotypes. Examples of phenotypes include the assessment of DNA repair capacity in cultured blood cells, mammographic breast density, or the quantitation of carcinogen-DNA adducts in a target organ. Phenotypes now also include profiles of methylation that affect gene expression, a so-called epigenetic effect, for example, identified though next-generation sequencing or other methods.[52] The contribution of genetics to cancer risk from chemical carcinogens can range from small to large, depending on its penetrance.[4] Highly penetrant cancer-susceptibility genes cause familial cancers, but account for less than 5% of all cancers. Low-penetrant genes cause common sporadic cancers, which have large public health consequences.

A genetic polymorphism (e.g., single nucleotide polymorphisms) is defined as a genetic variant present in at least 1% of the population. Because of the advent of improved genotyping methods that have reduced cost and increased high throughput, haplotyping and whole genomewide association studies are ongoing. Although haplotyping studies, facilitated through the International HapMap Project (www.hapmap.org), have not proven useful for predicting human cancers; high-density, whole genomewide, single nucleotide polymorphism association studies have shown remarkable consistency for many gene loci, although the risk estimates are only 1.0 to 1.4, which are not useful in the clinic for individual risk assessment.[6] For example, the contribution of genetic polymorphisms to cancer risk, at least for breast cancer, appears to improve risk modeling by only a few percent; known breast cancer risk factors account for about 58% of risk, and adding 10 genetic variants increases the risk prediction only to 62%.[53] Genes under study are from pathways that affect behavior, activate and detoxify carcinogens, affect DNA repair, govern cell-cycle control, trigger apoptosis, effect cell signaling, and so forth.

Biomarkers of Cancer Risk

The evaluation of dose and risk estimates in epidemiologic studies can include four components: namely, external exposure measurements, internal exposure measurements, biomarkers estimating the biologically effective dose, and biomarkers of effect or harm. The latter three measurements are biomarkers that improve on the first by quantifying exposure inside the individual and at the cellular level to characterize low-dose exposures in low-risk populations, providing a relative contribution of individual chemical carcinogens from complex mixtures, and/or estimating total burden of a particular exposure where there are many sources.[54]

Chemicals cause genetic damage in different ways, namely in the formation of carcinogen-DNA adducts leading to base mutations or gross chromosomal changes. Adducts are formed when a mutagen, or part of it, irreversibly binds to DNA so that it can cause a base substitution, insertion, or deletion during DNA replication. Gross chromosomal mutations are chromosome breaks, gaps, or translocations. The level of DNA damage is the biologically effective dose in a target organ, and reflects the net result of carcinogen exposure, activation, lack of detoxification, lack of effective DNA repair, and lack of programmed cell death. A variety of assays have been used for determining carcinogen-macromolecular adducts in human tissues; for example, for assessing risk from tobacco smoking for lung cancer and aflatoxin and liver cancer.[55,56] Important considerations for the assessment of biomarkers include sensitivity, specificity, reproducibility, accessibility for human use, and whether it represents a risk measured in a target organ or surrogate tissue. No single biomarker has been considered to be sufficiently validated for use as a cancer risk marker in an individual as it relates to chemical carcinogenesis.[57] However, there is some evidence that DNA adducts are cancer risk factors in both cohort and case-control studies.[58]

People are commonly exposed to N-nitrosamine and other N-nitroso compounds from dietary and tobacco exposures, which are associated with DNA adduct formation and cancer. Exposure can occur through endogenous formation of N-nitrosamines from nitrates in food or directly from dietary sources, cosmetics, drugs, household commodities, and tobacco smoke. Endogenous formation occurs in the stomach from the reaction of nitrosatable amines and nitrate (used as a preservative), which is converted to nitrites by bacteria. The N-nitrosamines undergo metabolic activation by cytochrome P450s (CYP2E1, CYP2A6, and CYP2D6) and form DNA adducts. Biomarkers are available to assess N-nitrosamine exposure from tobacco smoke (e.g., urinary tobacco-specific nitrosamine levels) or DNA, including in target organs such as the lungs. Recent data indicate that increasing levels of tobacco-specific nitrosamine metabolites are associated with increased lung cancer risk.[55]

Heterocyclic amines are formed from the overheating of food with creatine, such as meat, chicken, and fish.[59] Heterocyclic amines, estimated based on consumption of well-done meat, have been associated with breast and colon cancer, presumably through metabolic activation mechanisms and DNA damage.[59] Aflatoxins, another food contaminant, are considered to be a major contributor to liver cancer in China and parts of Africa, especially interacting with hepatitis viruses, and urinary aflatoxin adduct levels are predictors of liver cancer risk.[56]

Aromatic amines are another class of human carcinogens. Aryl aromatic amines have been implicated in bladder carcinogenesis, especially in occupationally exposed cohorts (e.g., dye workers) and tobacco smokers.[60] These compounds are activated by cytochrome P4501A2 and excreted via the N-acetyltransferase 2 gene. They are genotoxic, and the quantitative assessment using biomarkers has been more difficult, but some persons have studied DNA adducts as well.[61]

Polycyclic aromatic hydrocarbons (PAH) are large, aromatic (three or more fused benzene rings) compounds that are a class of more than 200 chemicals. These compounds are ubiquitous in the environment and present in the ambient air. They are formed from overcooking foods, fireplaces, charcoal barbeques, burning of coal and crude oil, tobacco smoke, and can be found in various occupational settings. In order for PAHs to exert their toxic effect, they must undergo metabolic activation via cytochromes P4501A1 and P4503A4 to form DNA adducts, or are excreted via pathways involving the glutathione-S-transferase genes. PAHs are associated with an increased risk of lung and skin cancer in the occupational setting, although risk varies by type of industry and the individual being exposed.[62,63] Benzo(a)pyrene (BaP), the most frequently studied PAH, serves as a model for chemical carcinogens. The bay region diol epoxide binds to DNA, mostly as the N2-deoxyguanosine adduct. The evidence linking BaP-deoxyguanosine adducts with a carcinogenic effect in lung cancer is very strong, including site-specific hotspot mutations in the p53 tumor suppressor gene.[64-68] Various biomarkers of exposure have been developed for assessing PAH exposure. These include measuring DNA adducts, protein adducts, and urinary 1-hydroxypyrene; only the latter is a validated biomarker of exposure and no adducts have been validated as biomarkers of cancer risk. However, recent data indicate that PAH metabolites might be risk factors for lung cancer.[58]

Air pollution has been recently classified by the IARC as a known human lung carcinogen.[69] Studies that support the conclusion include cohort studies that use biomarkers of exposure.[70] Such markers include measurements of 1-hydroxypyrene, DNA adducts, chromosomal aberrations, micronuclei, oxidative damage to nucleobases, and methylation changes.[71]

Epidemiologic and experimental studies have linked benzene to hematologic toxicity, including aplastic anemia, myelodysplastic syndrome, and acute myeloid leukemia.[72-74] Benzene is metabolized by hepatic P4502E1 (CYP2E1), yielding benzene oxide and hydroquinone, among other reactive metabolites. Circulating hydroquinones may be further metabolized to reactive benzoquinones by myeloperoxidase in bone marrow white blood cell precursors and stroma. Benzene metabolites are reported to have a variety of biologic consequences on bone marrow cells, including covalent binding to DNA and protein, alterations in gene expression, cytokine and chemokine abnormalities, and chromosomal aberrations.[75] There are well-established biomarkers of exposure to benzene, but to date, biomarkers of toxicity have not been validated (except for high-level exposure workplaces and effects of peripheral blood counts).

ARISTOLOCHIC ACID AND UROTHELIAL CANCERS AS A MODEL FOR IDENTIFYING HUMAN CARCINOGENS

Aristolochic acids come from the Aristolochia genus of plants, which have been used for herbal remedies (e.g., birthwort, Dutchman's pipe). The case of the carcinogen aristolochic acid, which is identified as a Class 1 human carcinogen by the IARC (http://monographs.iarc.fr/ENG/Monographs/vol100A/mono100A-23.pdf), presents a powerful example of how the forces of epidemiology, classical chemical carcinogenesis, and genomics collaborate to unravel the pathogenesis and prevention of a specific human cancer.[76] In the 1990s, epidemiologists independently reported on three distinct unrelated population groups that developed nephrotoxicity (interstitial fibrosis) and an extraordinary high incidence of urothelial cancer of the upper urinary track after exposure for different reasons and in different parts of the world (Belgium, the Balkans, and China). In Belgian women ingesting an extract from plants of the Aristolochia species for weight reduction, which was provided to them in a weight loss clinic, nearly 50% developed this unusual syndrome. A similar clinical picture (so-called Balkan endemic nephropathy) was reported for residents farming around the Danube River and eating home-baked bread from wheat contaminated with seeds from Aristolochia weeds grown in the same fields. In China, the Aristolochia herbs have been used for centuries in Chinese medicine and are prominently prescribed in Taiwan, a nation with the highest incidence of urothelial cancer in the world, as remedies for ailments of the heart, liver, snake bites, arthritis, gout, childbirth, and others.

Common to all Aristolochia species are one of two major nitrophenanthrene carboxylic acid toxicants, namely, aristolochic acid I and II (http://monographs.iarc.fr/ENG/Monographs/vol100A/

mono100A-23.pdf).[77,78] The oral administration of aristolochic acid to rodents is highly carcinogenic, producing predominantly forestomach cancers and lymphomas, along with cancers of the lung, kidney, and urothelium (http://monographs.iarc.fr/ENG/Monographs/vol100A/mono100A-23.pdf). The major route of excretion of aristolochic acid is through the kidneys. These clinical and experimental observations inspired further analyses of the mechanism of action of these potent human carcinogens. Studies in intact mice and mice reconstituted with humanized P450 revealed that CYP1a and CYP2a were responsible for both the activation and the detoxification of aristolochic acid I and II, and that NAD(P)H:quinone oxidoreductase produced the ultimate reactive aristolactam I nitrenium species.[78] The molecular action of the ultimate carcinogen is remarkably specific, targeting purine nucleotides in DNA to form DNA adducts and binding at the exocyclic amino group of deoxyadenosine and deoxyguanosine with a far greater affinity for dA over dG (Fig. 7.1). DNA adducts from aristolochic acids have been found in both experimental animals and humans. Furthermore, unlike any other human carcinogen, the predominant mutagenic outcome is an A:T transversion with a marked preference for the nontranscribed strand of DNA, notably in the p53 gene.[77,79] The A:T to T:A transversions

are extremely uncommon among the mutation spectrum in all eukaryotes. These unique properties of aristolochic acid DNA adducts appear to elude DNA repair mechanisms that commonly focus on transcribing DNA, resulting in persistent carcinogen-DNA adducts in human tissues and surgical tumor specimens, thus confirming the association of exposure with a biologic effect.[80] In experimental models in mice where human p53 is substituted for the mouse gene, multiple sites on p53 are mutated, almost all of which are those unusual A:T transversions.[81] Modern genomic techniques have unraveled other selective properties of this unusual but potent human chemical carcinogen. Whole genome and exome sequencing of multiple aristolochic-associated kidney cancers from patients confirmed the high frequency of the unusual A:T to T:A transversion mutations. Furthermore, an unusual pattern emerges where there is selectivity for mutations at splice sites with a preferable consensus sequence of T/CAG. Among the many mutations detected, certain targets stand out, particularly in p53, MLL2, and other genes the products of which function in regulating gene expression through higher chromosome order.[82,83] This cancer story covers the gamut of all elements of chemical carcinogenesis, and its illumination has opened a door for cancer prevention.

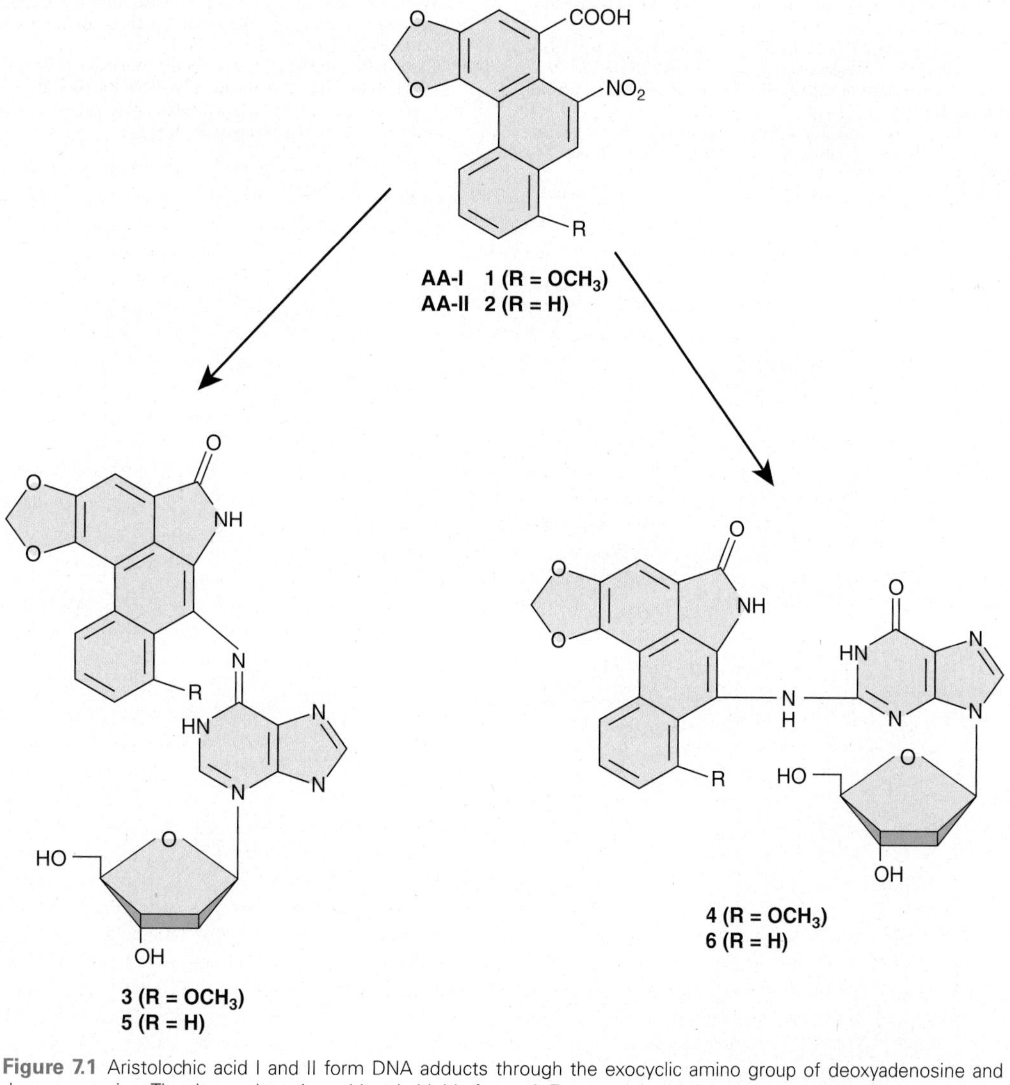

Figure 7.1 Aristolochic acid I and II form DNA adducts through the exocyclic amino group of deoxyadenosine and deoxyguanosine. The deoxyadenosine adduct is highly favored. For more detailed analysis of the complete metabolic profile, see Attaluri et al.[79]

SELECTED REFERENCES

The full reference list can be accessed at lwwhealthlibrary.com/oncology.

1. U.S. Department of Health and Human Services. *The Health Consequences of Smoking: 50 Years of Progress. A Report of the Surgeon General*. Atlanta: Author; 2014.
2. Colditz GA, Wei EK. Preventability of cancer: the relative contributions of biologic and social and physical environmental determinants of cancer mortality. *Annu Rev Public Health* 2012;33:137–156.
3. Lynch SM, Rebbeck TR. Bridging the gap between biologic, individual, and macroenvironmental factors in cancer: a multilevel approach. *Cancer Epidemiol Biomarkers Prev* 2013;22:485–495.
4. Rahman N. Realizing the promise of cancer predisposition genes. *Nature* 2014;505:302–308.
7. Luch A. Nature and nurture—lessons from chemical carcinogenesis. *Nat Rev Cancer* 2005;5:113–125.
8. Taddei ML, Giannoni E, Comito G, et al. Microenvironment and tumor cell plasticity: an easy way out. *Cancer Lett* 2013;341:80–96.
9. Fessler E, Dijkgraaf FE, De Sousa E Melo, et al. Cancer stem cell dynamics in tumor progression and metastasis: is the microenvironment to blame? *Cancer Lett* 2013;341:97–104.
10. Hanahan D, Coussens LM. Accessories to the crime: functions of cells recruited to the tumor microenvironment. *Cancer Cell* 2012;21:309–322.
11. Irigaray P, Belpomme D. Basic properties and molecular mechanisms of exogenous chemical carcinogens. *Carcinogenesis* 2010;31:135–148.
16. Baan R, Grosse Y, Straif K, et al. A review of human carcinogens—Part F: chemical agents and related occupations. *Lancet Oncol* 2009;10:1143–1144.
19. Anttila S, Raunio H, Hakkola J. Cytochrome P450-mediated pulmonary metabolism of carcinogens: regulation and cross-talk in lung carcinogenesis. *Am J Respir Cell Mol Biol* 2011;44:583–590.
20. Pogribny IP, Beland FA. DNA methylome alterations in chemical carcinogenesis. *Cancer Lett* 2012 [Epub ahead of print].
21. Shrivastav N, Li D, Essigmann JM. Chemical biology of mutagenesis and DNA repair: cellular responses to DNA alkylation. *Carcinogenesis* 2010;31:59–70.
22. Kew MC. Aflatoxins as a cause of hepatocellular carcinoma. *J Gastrointestin Liver Dis* 2013;22:305–310.
27. Boverhof DR, Chamberlain MP, Elcombe CR, et al. Transgenic animal models in toxicology: historical perspectives and future outlook. *Toxicol Sci* 2011;121:207–233.
29. Hanahan D, Weinberg RA. Hallmarks of cancer: the next generation. *Cell* 2011;144:646–674.
36. Jiang XL, Gonzalez FJ, Yu AM. Drug-metabolizing enzyme, transporter, and nuclear receptor genetically modified mouse models. *Drug Metab Rev* 2011;43:27–40.
37. Tuna M, Amos CI. Genomic sequencing in cancer. *Cancer Lett* 2013;340:161–170.
38. MacConaill LE. Existing and emerging technologies for tumor genomic profiling. *J Clin Oncol* 2013;31:1815–1824.
39. Watson IR, Takahashi K, Futreal PA, et al. Emerging patterns of somatic mutations in cancer. *Nat Rev Genet* 2013;14:703–718.
41. Adamski J, Suhre K. Metabolomics platforms for genome wide association studies—linking the genome to the metabolome. *Curr Opin Biotechnol* 2013;24:39–47.
42. Verma M, Khoury MJ, Ioannidis JP. Opportunities and challenges for selected emerging technologies in cancer epidemiology: mitochondrial, epigenomic, metabolomic, and telomerase profiling. *Cancer Epidemiol Biomarkers Prev* 2013;22:189–200.
43. Edwards SL, Beesley J, French JD, et al. Beyond GWASs: illuminating the dark road from association to function. *Am J Hum Genet* 2013;93:779–797.
44. Di LG, Garofalo M, Croce CM. MicroRNAs in cancer. *Annu Rev Pathol* 2014;9:287–314.
45. Cheetham SW, Gruhl F, Mattick JS, et al. Long noncoding RNAs and the genetics of cancer. *Br J Cancer* 2013;108:2419–2425.
46. Izzotti A, Pulliero A. The effects of environmental chemical carcinogens on the microRNA machinery. *Int J Hyg Environ Health* 2014 [Epub ahead of print].
50. Schwabe RF, Jobin C. The microbiome and cancer. *Nat Rev Cancer* 2013;13:800–812.
51. Wild CP, Scalbert A, Herceg Z. Measuring the exposome: a powerful basis for evaluating environmental exposures and cancer risk. *Environ Mol Mutagen* 2013;54:480–499.
52. Brennan K, Flanagan JM. Epigenetic epidemiology for cancer risk: harnessing germline epigenetic variation. *Methods Mol Biol* 2012;863:439–465.
76. Grollman AP. Aristolochic acid nephropathy: harbinger of a global iatrogenic disease. *Environ Mol Mutagen* 2013;54:1–7.

8 Physical Factors

Mats Ljungman

INTRODUCTION

Ionizing radiation (IR) and ultraviolet (UV) light have challenged the genetic integrity of all living organisms throughout time. By inducing DNA damage and subsequent mutations, these physical agents have promoted diversity through natural selection, and, as a result, organisms from all kingdoms of life carry genes that encode proteins that repair damaged DNA. In higher, multicellular organisms, many additional mechanisms of genome preservation have evolved, such as cell cycle checkpoints and apoptosis. Despite the many sophisticated mechanisms to safeguard the human genome from the mutagenic actions of DNA-damaging agents, not all exposed cells successfully restore the integrity of their DNA and some cells may subsequently progress into malignant cancer cells. Furthermore, through manmade activities, we are now exposed to many new physical agents, such as radiofrequency and microwave radiation, electromagnetic fields, asbestos, and nanoparticles, for which evolution has not yet had time to deliver genome-preserving response mechanisms. This chapter will highlight the molecular mechanisms by which these physical agents affect cells and how human exposure may lead to cancer.

IONIZING RADIATION

IR is defined as radiation that has sufficient energy to ionize molecules by displacing electrons from atoms. IR can be electromagnetic, such as x-rays and gamma rays, or can consist of particles, such as electrons, protons, neutrons, alpha particles, or carbon ions. Natural sources of IR make up about 80% of human exposure and medical sources make up about 20%.[1] The increased medical use of diagnostic x-rays and computed tomography (CT) scanning procedures likely translates into higher incidences of cancer. Of the natural sources, radon exposure is the most significant exposure risk to humans. Importantly, with better and more comprehensive screening techniques, the human exposure to radon could be dramatically lowered.

Mechanisms of Damage Induction

Linear Energy Transfer

The biologic effects of IR are unique in that the induced damage is clustered due to the local deposition of energy in radiation tracks. The distance between the depositions of energy is biologically very relevant and unique to the energy and the type of radiation. The term *linear energy transfer (LET)* denotes the energy transferred per unit length of a track of radiation. Electromagnetic radiation, such as x-rays or gamma rays, are sparsely ionizing and therefore classified as low LET radiation, whereas particulate radiation, such as neutrons, protons, and alpha particles, are examples of high LET radiation.[1]

Radiation Biochemistry

Radiation-induced damage to cellular target molecules, such as DNA, proteins, and lipids, can be either direct or indirect

(Fig. 8.1). The *direct action* of radiation, which is the dominant mode of action of high LET radiation, is due to the deposition of energy directly to the target molecule, resulting in one or more ionization events. The *indirect action* of radiation is due to the radiolysis of water molecules, which, after initial absorption of radiation energy, become excited and generate different types of radiolysis products where the reactive hydroxyl radical ($\bullet OH$), can damage both DNA and proteins. About two-thirds of the damage induced by low LET radiation is due to the indirect action of radiation. Since the hydroxyl radical is very reactive (half-life is 10^{-9} seconds), it does not diffuse more than a few nanometers after it is formed before it reacts with other molecules, and, thus, only radicals formed in close proximity to the target molecule will contribute to the damage of that target.[2] However, by chemical recombination of the primary radiolysis products, hydrogen peroxide (H_2O_2) is formed, which in turn can produce hydroxyl radicals at a later time through the Fenton reaction, involving free metals. Because H_2O_2 is not very reactive, it can diffuse long distances away from the initial site of energy deposition.

Radical scavengers normally present in cells, such as glutathione, can protect target molecules by reacting with the hydroxyl radical (see Fig. 8.1). Even after the target molecule has been hit and ionized, glutathione can contribute to cell protection by donating a hydrogen atom to the radical, allowing the unpaired electron present in the radical to pair up with the electron from the hydrogen atom. This is considered the simplest of all types of repair and is called *chemical repair.*[3] However, if oxygen molecules are present, they will compete with scavenger molecules for the ionized molecule, and if oxygen reacts with the ionized target molecule before the hydrogen donation occurs, the damage will be solidified as a peroxide, which is not amendable to chemical repair. Instead, this lesion will require enzymatic repair for the restoration of DNA. This augmenting biologic effect of oxygen is called the *oxygen effect* and is considered an important factor for the effectiveness of radiation therapy.[1]

Damage to DNA

The direct and indirect effects of radiation induce more or less identical types of lesions in DNA. However, the density of lesions induced in a stretch of DNA is higher for high LET radiation, and this increased complexity is thought to complicate the repair of these lesions. Radiation-induced lesions consist of more than 100 chemically distinct base lesions, such as the mutagenic lesions thymine glycol and 8-hydroxyguanine.[2,4,5] Furthermore, damage to the sugar moiety in the backbone of DNA and some types of base damage can result in single-strand breaks (SSB). Because the energy deposition of radiation is clustered even for low LET radiation, it is possible that two individual strand breaks are formed in close proximity on opposite strands, resulting in the formation of a double-strand break (DSB). It has been estimated that 1 Gy of ionizing radiation gives rise to about 40 DSBs, 1,000 SSBs, 1,000 base lesions, and 150 DNA-protein cross-links per cell.[2] For a similarly lethal dose of UV light, about 400,000 lesions are required, demonstrating that the lesions induced by IR are much more toxic

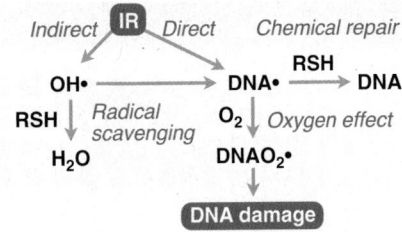

Figure 8.1 Factors affecting the induction of DNA damage by ionizing radiation (IR). Ionizing radiation can ionize DNA either by direct action or by indirect action, in which radiation energy is absorbed by neighboring molecules, such as water, leading to the generation of hydroxyl radicals that attack DNA. Sulfur-containing cellular molecules (RSH), such as glutathione, can scavenge hydroxyl radicals by hydrogen atom donations and thereby protect the DNA from the indirect action of radiation. Glutathione can also donate hydrogen atoms to ionized DNA, thereby restoring the integrity of DNA in a process termed *chemical repair*. Oxygen can compete with chemical repair in a process termed the *oxygen effect*, resulting in the enhancement of the biologic effect of ionizing radiation by the fixation of the initial DNA damage into DNA peroxides (DNAO$_2$•).

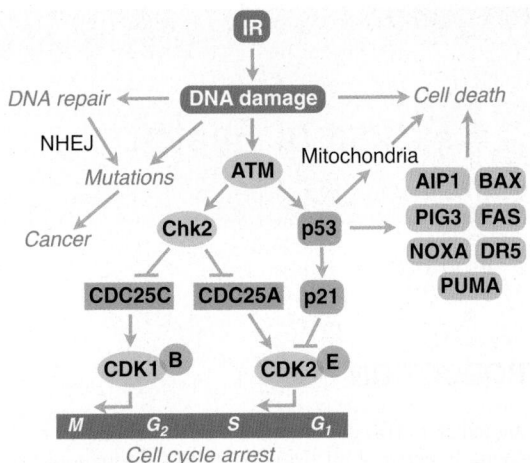

Figure 8.2 Cellular responses to ionizing radiation. Ionizing radiation induces predominantly base lesions and single- and double-strand breaks. Base lesions and single-strand breaks are repaired by base excision repair (BER), whereas double-strand breaks are repaired by nonhomologous end joining (NHEJ) and homologous recombination (HR). If DNA lesions are misrepaired by NHEJ or not repaired at all before cells enter S phase or mitosis, genomic instability is manifested as mutations or chromosome aberrations that promote carcinogenesis. In order for cells to assist DNA repair and safeguard against genetic instability and cancer, cells can induce cell cycle arrest or apoptosis. The ATM kinase is an early responder to DNA damage induced by ionizing radiation that activates the cell cycle checkpoint kinase Chk2 and the tumor suppressor p53. Chk2 inactivates the CDC25A and CDC25C phosphatases that are critical in promoting cell cycle progression by activating the cyclin-dependent kinases CDK2 or CDK1 and thereby arresting the cells at the G$_1$/S or G$_2$/M checkpoints. In addition, p53 can arrest cells at the G$_1$/S checkpoint by inducing the CDK inhibitor p21. p53 also plays a role in promoting apoptosis by inducing a number of proapoptotic proteins as well as translocating to mitochondria where it inhibits the actions of antiapoptotic factors. AIP1, actin interacting protein 1; BAX, bcl-2-like protein; PIG3, p53-inducible gene 3.

than lesions induced by UV light. It is believed that DSBs are the critical lesions that lead to cell lethality following exposure to ionizing radiation.[6]

Damage to Proteins

Although proteins and lipids are subject to damage following exposure to IR, the common belief is that DNA is the critical target for the biologic effects of radiation. Indeed, abrogation of DNA damage surveillance or repair processes in cells results in the enhanced induction of mutations and decreased cell survival following radiation.[5] However, studies of radiation-sensitive and radiation-resistant bacteria imply that mechanisms that suppress protein damage may also play important roles in radiation resistance.[7] *Deinococcus radiodurans* is a bacterium that can survive radiation exposures of up to 17,000 Gy, and its extreme radioresistance has been linked to high intracellular levels of manganese, which protect proteins from oxidation. The thought is that if a cell can limit protein oxidation, then its enzymes will remain active, and cellular functions such as DNA repair will be able to restore the integrity of DNA even after severe DNA damage.[8] It would be interesting to explore whether the concentration of manganese can be manipulated to sensitize tumor cells to radiation therapy. Furthermore, because protein damage due to reactive oxygen species (ROS) accumulate during the aging process, could supplements of manganese turn back the clock on aging?

Cellular Responses

DNA Repair

Ever since organisms started to utilize atmospheric oxygen for metabolic respiration many millions of years ago, they have been forced to deal with the cellular damage induced by ROS. Base excision repair (BER) evolved to remove many of the different types of oxidative base lesions and DNA SSBs induced by ROS. However, ROS seldom induce DSBs unless the generation of hydroxyl radicals is clustered near the DNA molecule. A more important source of intracellular generation of DSBs may instead be the process of DNA replication, and it is possible that homologous recombination (HR) repair primarily evolved to overcome DSBs sporadically induced during the replication process. The other major pathway of DSB repair is the nonhomologous end-joining (NHEJ) pathway, which is utilized by immune cells in the process of antibody generation. Although the HR pathway has high fidelity due to the utilization of homologous sister chromatids to ensure that correct DNA ends are joined, the NHEJ pathway lacks this

control mechanism and therefore occasionally rejoins ends incorrectly. Thus, the NHEJ pathway may contribute to the generation of mutations following radiation (Fig. 8.2). However, NHEJ is the only mechanism available for DSB repair in postmitotic cells and cells in the G$_1$ phase of the cell cycle because no sister chromatids are available in these cells to support HR repair.

Ataxia-Telangiectasia Mutated and Cell Cycle Checkpoints

Due to the enormous task of replicating the whole genome during the S phase and segregating the chromosomes during mitosis, proliferating cells are generally much more vulnerable to radiation than stationary cells. To prevent cells with damaged DNA from entering into these critical stages of the cell cycle, cells can activate cell cycle checkpoints (see Fig. 8.2). The major sensor of radiation-induced damage in cells is the ataxia-telangiectasia mutated (ATM) kinase, which, following activation, can phosphorylate more than 700 proteins in cells.[9] Two ATM substrates, p53 and Chk2, are critical for the activation of cell cycle arrests at multiple sites in the cell cycle.[10,11] The kinase p53 regulates the gene expression of specific genes such as *p21*, which inhibits cyclin-dependent kinase (CDK)2- and CDK4-mediated phosphorylation of the retinoblastoma protein, resulting in a block in the progression from the G$_1$ phase to the S phase of the cell cycle.[12,13] The Chk2 kinase promotes checkpoint activation in G$_1$ by targeting the cell division cycle 25 homolog A (CDC25A) phosphatase[14] and, in G$_2$/M, by targeting the CDC25C phosphatase.[15] The activation of a cell cycle arrest following DNA damage provides the cell with additional time to repair the DNA before entering critical cell cycle stages, which promotes genetic stability. Loss or defects in the *ATM* or *p53* genes result in abrogation of radiation-induced cell cycle checkpoints, which manifests itself as the highly cancer-prone human syndromes ataxia telangiectasia[16] or Li-Fraumeni,[17] respectively.

Radiation-Induced Cell Death

Terminally differentiated and stationary cells, such as kidney, lung, brain, muscle, and liver cells, are generally more resistant to radiation-induced killing than are cells with a high turnover rate, such as different epithelial cells, spermatogonia, and hair follicles. However, the spleen and thymus, which consist of mostly nondividing cells, are among the most radiosensitive tissues, implying that the rate of cell proliferation is not the sole determiner of the radiation sensitivity of a tissue. An important factor regulating the induction of programmed cell death (apoptosis) in tissues is the tumor suppressor p53.[18] The p53 protein is activated in cells following exposure to IR by the ATM kinase (see Fig. 8.2). When activated, it regulates the expression of multiple genes that have roles in DNA repair, cell cycle arrest, and apoptosis. p53 can also localize to mitochondria following irradiation, where it triggers apoptosis through the inactivation of antiapoptotic regulatory proteins.[19] Not all tissues induce the p53 response to the same degree after similar doses of IR, nor do they activate downstream pathways, such as DNA repair, cell cycle arrest, and apoptosis, in a similar way. For example, thymocytes have an intrinsic setting that favors apoptosis over cell cycle arrest following IR, whereas fibroblasts rarely induce apoptosis, but instead activate a strong and lasting cell cycle arrest.[18]

IR can induce cell death in tissues by many different mechanisms. Apoptosis can occur rapidly in a p53-dependent manner or later in a p53-independent manner. This later wave of radiation-induced apoptosis is often initiated by mitotic catastrophe, which occurs as a result of complications during chromosome segregation. Cell death induced by IR may in some cases be associated with autophagy, also called autophagocytosis, in which cells degrade cellular components via the lysosomal machinery. Whether autophagy is a programmed cell death or occurs in parallel with cell death is not clear. Interestingly, for some cell types, autophagy has been shown to actually protect the cells from radiation-induced death. Finally, tissue can undergo necrotic cell death following exposure to IR. Necrosis is a clinical problem following radiation therapy that can occur in normal tissues many months after treatment and can contribute to the inflammatory response.

Cancer Risks

It is clear from epidemiologic studies of radiation workers and atomic bomb and Chernobyl victims that IR can induce cancer.[20] Twenty years after the atomic bomb explosions in Japan during World War II, significant increases in the incidence of thyroid cancer and leukemia were observed. However, it took almost 50 years before solid tumors appeared in the population as a result of radiation exposure from the atomic bombs.[21] The incidences of solid tumors, such as breast, ovary, bladder, lung, and colon cancers, were estimated to have increased by a factor of 2 in the exposed group during this time period. The epidemiology studies following the nuclear power plant disaster in Chernobyl showed a clear increase in thyroid cancer as early as 4 years after the accident.[22] Young children were the most vulnerable to radiation exposure, with 1-year-old children being 237-fold more susceptible to thyroid cancer than the control group, while 10-year-old children were found to be sixfold more susceptible to thyroid cancer. Many of the thyroid cancers that developed following the Chernobyl disaster could have been prevented if the population had not consumed locally produced milk that was contaminated with radioactive iodine.

The molecular signatures of radiation-induced tumors are complex but involve point mutations that could lead to the activation of the *RAS* oncogene or inactivation of the tumor suppressor

gene *p53*. Furthermore, IR induces DNA DSBs that may be unfaithfully repaired by the NHEJ pathway, leading to chromosome rearrangements. One such rearrangement found in 50% to 90% of the thyroid cancers examined following the Chernobyl accident involved the receptor tyrosine kinase c-RET, which promotes cell growth when activated.[22] Furthermore, a great majority of the thyroid cancers found in the exposed children harbored kinase fusion oncogenes affecting the mitogen-activated protein kinase (MAPK) signaling pathway.[23]

The correlation between high exposure to IR and cancer following the atomic bomb explosions and the Chernobyl accident is clear. What about the cancer risk following lower radiation exposures occurring in daily life? There are four theoretical risk models of radiation-induced cancer to consider. First, the *linear, no threshold* (LNT) *model* suggests that the induction of cancer is directly proportional to the dose of radiation, even at low doses of exposure. Second, the *sublinear* or *threshold model* suggests that below a certain threshold dose the risk of radiation-induced cancers is negligible. At these lower doses of radiation exposure, the DNA damage surveillance and repair mechanisms are thought to be fully capable of safeguarding the DNA to avoid the induction of mutations and cancer. Third, the *supralinear* or *stealth model* suggests that doses below a certain threshold or radiation with sufficiently low dose rates may not trigger the activation of DNA damage surveillance and repair mechanisms, resulting in suboptimal activation of cell cycle checkpoints and repair. This would be expected to lead to a higher rate of mutations and cancers than predicted by the LNT model, but may be balanced by a higher incident of cell death. Fourth, the *linear-quadratic model* suggest that radiation effects at low doses are due to a single track of radiation hitting multiple targets, resulting in a linear induction rate, whereas at higher doses, multiple radiation tracks hit multiple cellular targets, resulting in a quadratic induction rate.

The Biological Effects of Ionizing Radiation (BEIR) VII report, released by the Committee on Biological Effects of Ionizing Radiation of the National Academy of Sciences and commissioned by the US Environmental Protection Agency (EPA), is a review of published data regarding human health and cancer risks from exposure to low levels of IR. Although this topic is controversial and not fully settled, the BIER VII report favored the LNT model.[24] Thus, the "official" view is that no level of radiation is safe; therefore, a careful consideration of risks versus benefits is necessary to ensure that the general population only receives radiation doses as low as reasonably achievable. Furthermore, the BIER VII committee concluded that the heritable effects of radiation were not evident in the published data, indicating that an individual is not likely to develop cancer due to radiation exposure of his or her parents.

The largest source of radiation exposure to the population is radon, which is a natural radioactive gas formed as a decay product of radium in the decay chain of uranium. Radon gas can accumulate to high levels in poorly ventilated basements in houses built on rock containing uranium. The major risk with radon is that some of its radioactive decay products can attach to dust particles that accumulate in the lungs, leading to a continuous exposure of the lung tissues to high LET alpha particles. Due to this radiation exposure, the EPA claims that radon is the second leading cause of lung cancer in the United States. Another important source of human exposure to IR is medical x-ray devices, and there is a growing concern about the dramatically increased use of whole body CT scans for diagnostic purposes. For a typical CT scan, a patient will receive about 100-fold more radiation than from a typical mammogram.[24] It is recommended that the use of whole body CT scans for children be very restricted due to the elevated risk of developing radiation-induced cancer for this age group.

Cancer patients who receive radiation therapy are at risk of developing secondary tumors induced by the radiation therapy treatment.[1] This is particularly a concern for young patients since (1) children are more prone to radiation-induced cancer,

(2) children have a relatively good chance of surviving the primary cancer and would have long life expectancies so a secondary tumor would have plenty of time to develop, and (3) many childhood cancers are promoted by genetic defects in DNA damage response pathways, making these patients highly prone to the genotoxic effects of radiation and subsequent secondary cancers. The most sensitive tissues for the development of secondary cancer have been found to be bone marrow (leukemia), the thyroid, breast, and lung.[1]

ULTRAVIOLET LIGHT

Depending on the wavelength, UV light is categorized into UVA (320 to 400 nm), UVB (290 to 320 nm), and UVC (240 to 290 nm) radiation. Most of the UVC light emitted from the sun is absorbed by the ozone layer in the atmosphere, and, thus, living organisms are mostly exposed to UVA and UVB irradiation.

Mechanisms of Damage Induction

UVC light is more damaging to DNA than UVA and UVB because the absorption maximum of DNA is around 260 nm. UVB and UVC induce predominantly pyrimidine dimers and 6-4 photoproducts, which consist of covalent ring structures that link two adjacent pyrimidines on the same DNA strand.[5] The formation of these lesions results in the bending of the DNA helix, resulting in the interference with both DNA and RNA synthesis. UVA light does not induce pyrimidine dimers or 6-4 photoproducts but can induce ROS, which in turn can form SSBs and base lesions in DNA of exposed cells.

Cellular Responses

DNA Repair

The nucleotide excision repair (NER) pathway removes pyrimidine dimers and 6-4 photoproducts from cellular DNA.[5] This pathway involves proteins that recognize the DNA lesions, nucleases that excise the DNA strand that contains the lesion, a DNA polymerase that synthesizes new DNA to fill the gap, and a DNA ligase that joins the backbone in the newly synthesized strand. Genetic defects in the NER pathway result in the human syndrome xeroderma pigmentosum, with individuals more than 1,000-fold more prone to sun-induced skin cancer than normal individuals. In addition, human polymorphisms in certain NER genes are thought to predispose individuals to cancers such as lung cancer, nonmelanoma skin cancer, head and neck cancer, and bladder cancer, indicating that NER is responsible for safeguarding the genome against many types of DNA adducts in addition to UV-induced lesions.[5]

UV-induced lesions formed in the transcribed strand of active genes block the elongation of RNA polymerase II, and if a cell does not restore transcription within a certain time frame, it may undergo apoptosis (Fig. 8.3).[25,26] To rapidly restore RNA synthesis and avoid cell death, NER enzymes are recruited to the sites of blocked RNA polymerase II and the lesions are removed in a process called transcription-coupled repair (TCR).[27] Individuals with Cockayne syndrome (CS), trichothiodystrophy, or the UV-sensitive syndrome, are unable to utilize the TCR pathway following UV irradiation.[5] Cells from these individuals do not recover RNA synthesis following UV irradiation and are therefore very prone to UV-induced apoptosis. Interestingly, despite a clear DNA repair defect, these individuals are not predisposed to UV-induced skin cancer. It is thought that the inability of CS cells to remove the toxic lesions that block transcription following UV irradiation results in the suppression of tumorigenesis by the elimination of damaged cells by apoptosis. However, while protecting against

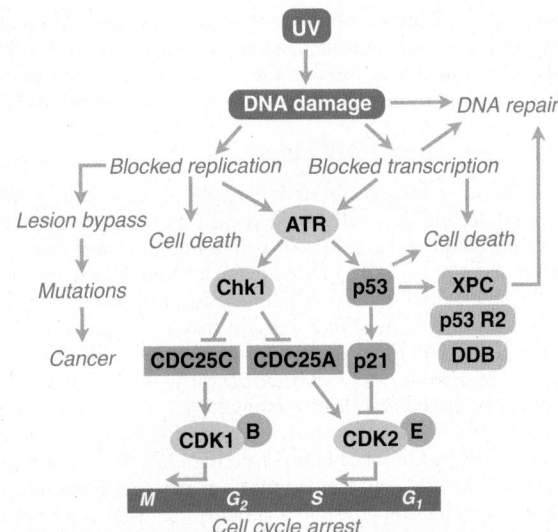

Figure 8.3 Cellular responses to ultraviolet (UV) light–induced DNA damage. UV light predominantly induces bulky DNA lesions that interfere with the processes of DNA replication and transcription. These lesions are removed from the global genome by global genomic nucleotide excision repair (GG-NER) and from transcribed DNA strands by transcription-coupled NER (TC-NER). Lesions blocking replication can be bypassed by exchanging processive DNA polymerases with less processive translesion DNA polymerases. While these polymerases allow cells to continue DNA synthesis and progress through the cell cycle, they have low fidelity, resulting in the potential induction of mutations promoting UV-induced carcinogenesis. To suppress mutations and support DNA repair efforts, the ataxia-telangiectasia and Rad3-related (ATR) kinase is activated in response to blocked replication or transcription. ATR activates the cell cycle checkpoint kinase Chk1, which, similar to Chk2, arrests cells in the G_1/S and G_2/M checkpoints by inhibiting CDC25A and CDC25C. ATR also activates p53, promoting G_1/S checkpoint activation via the induction of the Cdk-inhibitor p21. p53 also stimulates GG-NER by the transactivation of various NER genes and can promote apoptosis by the induction of proapoptotic factors and translocation to mitochondria. Finally, apoptosis is induced if cells do not recover transcription in a certain time frame, potentially due to the loss of survival factors or complications in the S phase when replication encounters stall the transcription complexes.

tumorigenesis, the elevated level of apoptosis in these cells leads to increased cell loss, which in turn may lead to neurologic degeneration.[25,28] Persistent transcription-blocking lesions in the genome have also been linked to aging.[29–31]

Translesion DNA Synthesis

Proliferating skin cells are very vulnerable to UV light because UV lesions block DNA replication (see Fig. 8.3). Cells that have entered the S phase and have initiated DNA synthesis have no choice but to finish replicating the whole genome or they will die. If DNA repair enzymes are not able to remove the blocking lesions from the template, the processive DNA polymerases may be exchanged for other, less processive DNA polymerases that can bypass the lesions. This is part of a "tolerance" mechanism, which allows cells to complete replication and eventually divide.[5] However, the translesion DNA polymerases do not have the same fidelity as the processive DNA polymerases; thus, mutations may occur. This is thought to be a major pathway by which UV light induces mutagenesis and, subsequently, cancer (see Fig. 8.3).

ATM and Rad3-Related Mediated Cell Cycle Checkpoints

In addition to utilizing the NER and BER pathways to repair UV-induced DNA damage, proliferating cells activate cell cycle checkpoints to allow more time for repair before entering critical parts of the cell cycle, such as the S phase and mitosis. The ATM and Rad3-related (ATR) kinase is activated following UV irradiation by blocked replication or transcription (see Fig. 8.3).[32] ATR phosphorylates a large number of proteins, many of which are the same as those phosphorylated by ATM after exposure to ionizing radiation.[9] Two important substrates of ATR are p53 and Chk1, which are critical in promoting cell cycle arrest. When induced by ATR, p53 transactivates the gene that encodes the cell cycle inhibitor p21, leading to the arrest of cells in the G_1 phase of the cell cycle, while Chk1 phosphorylates the CDK-activating phosphatases CDC25A and CDC25C, which targets them for degradation, resulting in an S-phase or G_2-phase arrest (see Fig. 8.3).[33]

Activation of Cell Membrane Receptors

In addition to triggering cellular stress responses by inducing DNA damage, UV light can directly induce membrane receptor signaling by receptor phosphorylation. This is thought to be due to the direct UV-mediated inhibition of protein-tyrosine phosphatases that regulate the phosphorylation levels of various membrane receptors.[34] In addition, membrane receptors may physically aggregate following UV irradiation, leading to the activation of signal transduction pathways that regulate cell growth[35] or apoptosis.[36]

Cell Death

UV light effectively induces apoptosis in skin cells. The mechanism by which UV light induces cell death is not fully understood, but failure to adequately resume RNA synthesis following UV light exposure is strongly linked to apoptosis (see Fig. 8.3).[25] Many potential mechanisms of how blocked transcription results in apoptosis have been suggested, such as a physical clash during the S phase between elongating replication machineries and transcription complexes stalled at UV lesions. Another possible mechanism involves the preferential loss of survival factors coded by highly unstable mRNAs.[37] The induction of p53 may also contribute to UV-induced apoptosis,[38] although p53 appears to protect human fibroblasts[39] and keratinocytes[40] from UV-induced apoptosis. Although complications induced by DNA damage may be the predominant mechanism by which cells die following UV irradiation, UV light may induce apoptosis in certain cell types by directly promoting the physical aggregation of the death receptor Fas/APO1.[36]

Cancer Risks

The incidence of sun-induced skin cancer, especially melanoma, is on the increase due to higher rates of sun exposure in the general population. The link between UV light exposure and skin cancer is very strong, but the role of UV light in the etiology of nonmelanoma and melanoma skin cancer differs. Although the risk of nonmelanoma cancer relates to the cumulative lifetime exposure to UV light, the risk of contracting melanoma appears to be linked to high sunlight exposure during childhood.[41] What makes UV light such a potent carcinogen is that it can initiate carcinogenesis by inducing DNA lesions as well as suppressing the immune system, resulting in a greater probability that initiated cells will survive and grow into tumors.[42,43]

Nonmelanoma Skin Cancer

Basal cell carcinoma (BCC) and squamous cell carcinoma (SCC) are the two most common skin cancer types. BCC and SCC occur predominantly in sun-exposed areas of the skin, but there are examples of these cancers forming in nonexposed areas as well (see Chapter 92). The tumor suppressor genes *p53* and *p16* are frequently inactivated in BCC and SCC, while the hedgehog-signaling pathway is activated primarily by mutations to the patched gene (percutaneous transhepatic cholangiography [*PTCH*]). This scenario promotes proliferation without the opposition of the cell cycle inhibitors p53 and p16.

Melanoma

Melanoma arises from mutations in epidermal melanocytes and is the most dangerous form of skin cancer because it has the highest propensity to metastasize (see Chapter 93). It is formed in both sun-exposed and shielded areas of the skin; therefore, the role of UV light as the major carcinogen in melanoma has been controversial.[41] Defects in the NER pathway do not seem to predispose the development of melanoma, suggesting that pyrimidine dimers or 6-4 photoproducts induced by UVB are not the initiators of melanoma carcinogenesis. Instead, ROS induced by UVA may be responsible for the development of melanoma.[41] However, a study using next-generation sequencing techniques to catalog all mutations in a melanoma cell line found a mutational spectrum of the over 33,000 mutations detected that strongly indicated that pyrimidine dimers and 6-4 photoproducts are the major mutagenic lesions in melanoma, whereas a subset of mutations may be induced by ROS.[44] The incidence of mutations in the *p16* and *ARF* genes is high, whereas *p53* and *RAS* mutations are fairly uncommon in melanoma (see Chapter 93).

Photoimmunosuppression

Studies of transplantation of mouse skin cancers into syngeneic mice revealed that prior UVB irradiation of recipient mice promoted tumor growth, whereas transplantation into naïve nonirradiated mice led to rejection.[43] These studies established that UV light has local immunosuppressing ability, and subsequent studies found that UV light preferentially depletes Langerhans cells from irradiated skin.[42] Langerhans cells play an important role in the immune response by presenting antigens to the immune cells, and, thus, depletion of these cells leads to local immunosuppression. In addition to local immunosuppression, UV light has been shown to promote systemic immunosuppression.[45] This response is complex, but it is known that UV-induced DNA lesions in skin cells contribute to the systemic immunosuppression response.[46] The secretion of the immunosuppressing cytokine interleukin (IL)-10 from irradiated keratinocytes as well as UV-induced structural alteration of the epidermal chromophore urocanic acid may mediate the long-range immunosuppressive effects of UV light.[42,45]

RADIOFREQUENCY AND MICROWAVE RADIATION

Radiofrequency radiation (RFR) is electromagnetic radiation in the frequency range 3 kHz to 300 MHz, whereas microwave radiation (MR) is in the frequency range between 300 MHz to 300 GHz. RFR and MR do not have sufficient energies to cause ionizations in target tissues. Rather, the radiation energy is converted into heat as the radiation energy is absorbed. Sources of radiofrequency and microwave radiation include mobile phones, radio transmitters of wireless communication, radars, medical devices, and kitchen appliances.

Mechanism of Damage Induction

Because human exposure to RFR has increased dramatically in recent years, it is important to know whether this type of radiation gives rise to genotoxic damage. Although there are many studies showing that RFR can induce ROS, leading to genetic damage in cell culture systems, other studies have generated conflicting results.[47] One confounding factor when assessing the genotoxic effect of RFR, and especially MR, is the heating effect that occurs in the tissue when the radiation energy is absorbed. A recent study controlling for the potential heating effect of exposure found that RFR induces ROS and DNA damage in human spermatozoa in vitro, which is an alarming finding considering the potential hereditary implications.[48] It has been suggested that MR may affect the folding of proteins in cells that promote new protein synthesis.[49] Furthermore, exposure of cells to MR has been shown to lead to the phosphorylation of numerous cellular proteins largely through the activation of the p38/MAPK stress response pathway.[50] However, the biologic consequences of these cellular changes are not clear. Epidemiology studies that monitored the genetic effects in individuals exposed to high levels of RF have revealed evidence of increased induction of chromosome aberrations in lymphocytes.[51] However, there is a level of uncertainty in these studies about exposure levels, making it difficult to come to meaningful conclusions.

Cancer Risks

Because the population's exposure to RFR and MR has dramatically increased in recent years, it is of great importance to assess the potential cancer risks of these types of radiation so that appropriate exposure limits can be implemented. A number of studies have focused on the potential cancer risks from mobile phone usage, and some of these studies indicate that long-term mobile phone usage may be associated with increased risks of developing brain tumors (see the following). Other epidemiologic studies of cancer incidences in populations living near radio towers or mobile phone base stations are inconclusive. Some studies have shown a connection between proximity to mobile phone base stations and increased cancer incidence,[52] whereas another study found no association between exposure to RFR from mobile phone base stations and early childhood cancers.[53]

ELECTROMAGNETIC FIELDS

An electromagnetic field (EMF) is a physical field produced by electrically charged objects that can affect other charged objects in the field. Typical sources of EMFs are electric power lines, electrical devices, and magnetic resonance imaging (MRI) machines.

Mechanisms of Damage Induction

A low frequency EMF does not transmit energy high enough to break chemical bonds; therefore, it is not thought to directly damage DNA or proteins in cells. The data obtained from studies to assess the potential genotoxic effects of EMF do not provide a clear conclusion. Some of the results obtained in cell culture studies suggest a harmful effect of EMFs, but the concerns are that these effects may be related to heat production induced by EMFs rather than from the magnetic field itself. A recent in vitro study detected DNA strand breaks in cells exposed to EMFs, but this induction was thought to not be the result of ROS production, but rather due to indirect effects through interference with DNA replication and induction of apoptosis in a subset of cells.[54] A study using an MRI found no evidence of an induced formation of DNA DSBs in cell cultures.[55] EMFs have been shown to induce nongenotoxic effects in cells, such as interference with cellular signaling pathways,[56] which could contribute to neurodegeneration.[57]

Cancer Risks

Studies with rodents have largely failed to detect an association between exposure to EMFs and cancer. This is also true for numerous epidemiology studies, with the only exception being the association between EMF exposure and childhood leukemia where

children exposed to doses of 0.4 mcT or above may have about a twofold increased risk of developing leukemia.[58,59] There is no strong link between EMF exposure and increased risks of contracting adult leukemia, brain tumors, or breast cancer.[60,61] Furthermore, a study investigating whether EMF exposure was associated with heritable effects found no correlation between parental exposure and childhood cancer.[62]

Potential Cancer Risks from Mobile Phone Usage

Mobile phones emit RFR and generate EMFs. The biggest health concern with mobile phone usage is its potential role in the development of brain tumors. During mobile phone use, the brain tissue is exposed to doses, giving peak specific absorption rates (SAR) of 4 to 8 W/kg. At these intensities, the induction of DNA damage has been detected in laboratory studies.[63] The current epidemiologic data are largely inconclusive on the association between mobile phone usage and brain tumor incidence. Meta-analysis studies of populations who had used mobile phones for more than 10 years concluded that mobile phone usage was associated with an elevated risk for brain tumors, such as acoustic neuroma and glioma cancer.[64–66] In contrast, other large prospective studies did not observe a correlation between mobile phone usage and incidences of glioma, meningioma, or non–central nervous system (CNS) cancers.[67,68] It is important to point out that, generally, it takes 30 to 40 years for brain tumors to develop, and because mobile phones have only been in general use for about 15 years, there has not been sufficient time to fully evaluate the brain cancer risks of mobile phone usage.

ASBESTOS

Asbestos is a class of naturally occurring silicate minerals that have been widely used in building materials for its heat, sound, and electrical insulating qualities. Asbestos becomes a serious health hazard if the fibers are inhaled over a long period of time, and these health effects are increased dramatically if the exposed individual is a smoker. It was first reported in 1935 that asbestos might be an occupational health hazard that could induce cancer.[69,70] However, it was not until 1986 that the International Labor Organization recommended banning asbestos.[71] The use of asbestos products peaked in the 1970s, yet remains a major health hazard in many places around the world today.

Mechanisms of Damage Induction

Asbestos fibers can enter cells and induce ROS, especially if they contain high levels of iron.[72] In addition, ROS can be generated by "frustrated" phagocytosis, and this in turn can lead to the release of proinflammatory cytokines with subsequent inflammation of the tissue. ROS have been implicated to originate from affected mitochondria leading to induction of SSBs and base damage, such as 8-hydroxyguanine in DNA.[73] Furthermore, if not successfully repaired, asbestos-induced DNA damage has been shown to result in chromosome aberrations, micronuclei formation, and increased rates of sister chromatid exchanges.[74]

Cellular and Tissue Responses

Asbestos-induced ROS cause base lesions and DNA strand breaks, which require base excision repair for the restoration of DNA and for minimizing mutagenesis. In addition to DNA repair, a number of cellular signaling pathways are activated by asbestos. These include the epidermal growth factor receptor (EGFR) and the MAPK pathway, leading to the activation of nuclear factor kappa B

(NF-κB) and transcription factor AP-1.[72,74] Activation of the NF-κB pathway leads to the induction of proinflammatory genes such as tumor necrosis factor (TNF), *IL-6, IL-8*, and proliferation-promoting genes such as *c-Myc*, leading to inflammation and increased cell proliferation. Asbestos exposure also stimulates the expression of the transforming growth factor beta (TGF-β), which, in turn, stimulates fibrogenesis in exposed tissues.[74]

Cancer Risks

Lung Cancer

Epidemiologic studies have found a strong link between asbestos exposure and lung cancer.[74] It has been estimated that about 5% to 7% of all lung cancers are attributable to asbestos exposure, and asbestos and tobacco smoking act in synergy to induce lung cancer. Mutational spectra due to 8-hydroxyguanine lesions formed by ROS can be linked to asbestos exposure, and point mutations in the tumor suppressor genes *p53* and *p16/INK4A* and in the *KRAS* oncogene have been found in tumors from asbestos-exposed individuals.

Mesothelioma

After being taken up by lung tissues, asbestos fibers can translocate into the pleura, the body cavity that surrounds the lungs. The pleura are covered with a protective lining, the mesothelium, which consists of squamouslike epithelial cells. Mesothelial cells can internalize asbestos fibers, resulting in the induction of ROS and inflammatory responses, subsequently leading to the initiation and progression of malignant mesothelioma.[75] Asbestos is considered one of the major causes of malignant mesothelioma, and frequent mutations are found in the *p16/INK4A* and *NF2* genes, whereas *p53* mutations are fairly rare.

NANOPARTICLES

Nanoparticles are defined as ultrafine particles of the size range 1 to 100 nm in diameter. Nanoparticle chemistry of a certain compound is different from bulk chemistry of that compound because of the high percentage of atoms at the surface of the particle. The production of nanoparticles has increased dramatically in recent years, and they are found in many industrial and consumer products such as paint, cosmetics, and sunscreens. They also have many potential medical applications, such as delivery vehicles for specific drugs to specific target tissues or tumors.

Mechanisms of DNA Damage Induction

Many of the cellular effects of nanoparticles are similar to the effects exerted by asbestos, such as the generation of ROS and inflammation.[72] Nanoparticles have been shown to induce oxidative DNA damage, such as DNA strand breaks and 8-hydroxyguanine lesions both in cell culture[76, 77] and in vivo.[78] Nanoparticle-induced DNA lesions are manifested as histone γ-H2AX nuclear foci, chromosome deletions, and micronuclei.

Cellular Responses

Nanoparticles induce ROS either directly or indirectly, resulting in DNA lesions, such as 8-hydroxyguanine–base damage and DNA strand breaks. These lesions are repaired by the base excision repair. The phosphorylation of histone H2AX has been shown to occur following exposure of cells to nanoparticles, suggesting that the DNA lesions trigger the activation of ATM or ATR stress kinases.[79] Nanoparticles have also been found to affect the immune system[80] and can induce the release of the proinflammatory cytokine TNF-α from cells.

Cancer Risks

Some nanoparticles, such as titanium dioxide, which is used as pigments in paint, have been classified by the International Agency for Research on Cancer (IARC) as a group 2B carcinogen, "possible carcinogenic to humans." However, rigorous epidemiologic data is lacking to fully evaluate the cancer-inducing potential of nanoparticles.[81]

SELECTED REFERENCES

The full reference list can be accessed at lwwhealthlibrary.com/oncology.

1. Hall E, Giaccia A. *Radiobiology for the Radiologist.* Philadelphia: Lippincott Williams & Wilkins; 2012.
2. Ward JF. DNA damage produced by ionizing radiation in mammalian cells: identities, mechanisms of formation, and repairability. *Prog Nucleic Acid Res Mol Biol* 1988;35:95–125.
4. Hutchinson F. Chemical changes induced in DNA by ionizing radiation. *Prog Nucleic Acid Res Mol Biol* 1985;32:115–154.
5. Friedberg E, Walker G, Siede W, et al. *DNA Repair and Mutagenesis.* 2nd ed. Washington, D.C.: ASM Press; 2006.
8. Krisko A, Radman M. Biology of extreme radiation resistance: the way of *Deinococcus radiodurans. Cold Spring Harb Perspect Biol* 2013;5.
9. Matsuoka S, Ballif BA, Smogorzewska A, et al. ATM and ATR substrate analysis reveals extensive protein networks responsive to DNA damage. *Science* 2007;316:1160–1166.
10. Kastan M, Onyekwere O, Sidransky D, et al. Participation of p53 protein in the cellular response to DNA damage. *Cancer Res* 1991;51:6304–6311.
13. El-Deiry W, Tokino T, Velculescu V, et al. WAF1, a potential mediater of p53 tumor suppression. *Cell* 1993;75:817–825.
16. Savitsky K, Bar-Shira A, Gilad S, et al. A single ataxia telangiectasia gene with a product similar to PI-3 kinase. *Science* 1995;268:1749–1753.
17. Srivastava S, Zou ZQ, Pirollo K, et al. Germ-line transmission of a mutated p53 gene in a cancer-prone family with Li-Fraumeni syndrome. *Nature.*1990;348:747–749.
18. Gudkov AV, Komarova EA. The role of p53 in determining sensitivity to radiotherapy. *Nat Rev Cancer* 2003;3:117–129.
21. Thompson DE, Mabuchi K, Ron E, et al. Cancer incidence in atomic bomb survivors. Part II: Solid tumors, 1958–1987. *Radiat Res* 1994;137:S17–67.
22. Williams D. Cancer after nuclear fallout: lessons from the Chernobyl accident. *Nat Rev Cancer* 2002;2:543–549.
23. Ricarte-Filho JC, Li S, Garcia-Rendueles ME, et al. Identification of kinase fusion oncogenes in post-Chernobyl radiation-induced thyroid cancers. *J Clin Invest* 2013;123:4935–4944.
24. National Research Council. *Health Risks from Exposure to Low Levels of Ionizing Radiation: BEIR VII Phase 2.* Washington, D.C.: National Academy Press; 2006.
25. Ljungman M, Zhang F. Blockage of RNA polymerase as a possible trigger for u.v. light-induced apoptosis. *Oncogene.*1996;13:823–831.
27. Hanawalt PC, Spivak G. Transcription-coupled DNA repair: two decades of progress and surprises. *Nat Rev Mol Cell Biol* 2008;9:958–970.
30. de Boer J, Andressoo JO, de Wit J, et al. Premature aging in mice deficient in DNA repair and transcription. *Science* 2002;296:1276–1279.
31. Garinis GA, Uittenboogaard LM, Stachelscheid H, et al. Persistent transcription-blocking DNA lesions trigger somatic growth attenuation associated with longevity. *Nat Cell Biol* 2009;11:604–615.
32. Derheimer FA, O'Hagan HM, Krueger HM, et al. RPA and ATR link transcriptional stress to p53. *Proc Natl Acad Sci U S A* 2007;104:12778–12783.
33. Kastan MB, Bartek J. Cell-cycle checkpoints and cancer. *Nature* 2004;432:316–323.
37. Ljungman M, Lane DP. Transcription - guarding the genome by sensing DNA damage. *Nat Rev Cancer* 2004;4:727–737.
42. Murphy GM. Ultraviolet radiation and immunosuppression. *Br J Dermatol* 2009;161(Suppl 3):90–95.
43. Fisher MS, Kripke ML. Systemic alteration induced in mice by ultraviolet light irradiation and its relationship to ultraviolet carcinogenesis. *Proc Natl Acad Sci U S A* 1977;74:1688–1692.

44. Pleasance ED, Cheetham RK, Stephens PJ, et al. A comprehensive catalogue of somatic mutations from a human cancer genome. *Nature* 2010;463:191–196.

46. Kripke ML, Cox PA, Alas LG, et al. Pyrimidine dimers in DNA initiate systemic immunosuppression in UV-irradiated mice. *Proc Natl Acad Sci U S A* 1992;89:7516–7520.

47. Vijayalaxmi, Prihoda TJ. Genetic damage in mammalian somatic cells exposed to radiofrequency radiation: a meta-analysis of data from 63 publications (1990–2005). *Radiat Res* 2008;169:561–574.

57. Consales C, Merla C, Marino C, et al. Electromagnetic fields, oxidative stress, and neurodegeneration. *Int J Cell Biol* 2012;2012:683897.

58. Ahlbom A, Day N, Feychting M, et al. A pooled analysis of magnetic fields and childhood leukaemia. *Br J Cancer* 2000;83:692–698.

60. Kheifets L, Monroe J, Vergara X, et al. Occupational electromagnetic fields and leukemia and brain cancer: an update to two meta-analyses. *J Occup Environ Med* 2008;50:677–688.

61. Chen C, Ma X, Zhong M, et al. Extremely low-frequency electromagnetic fields exposure and female breast cancer risk: a meta-analysis based on 24,338 cases and 60,628 controls. *Breast Cancer Res Treat* 2010;123:569–576.

64. Hardell L, Carlberg M, Hansson Mild K. Mobile phone use and the risk for malignant brain tumors: a case-control study on deceased cases and controls. *Neuroepidemiology* 2010;35:109–114.

66. Myung SK, Ju W, McDonnell DD, et al. Mobile phone use and risk of tumors: a meta-analysis. *J Clin Oncol* 2009;27:5565–5572.

67. Benson VS, Pirie K, Schuz J, et al. Mobile phone use and risk of brain neoplasms and other cancers: prospective study. *Int J Epidemiol* 2013;42:792–802.

68. Poulsen AH, Friis S, Johansen C, et al. Mobile phone use and the risk of skin cancer: a nationwide cohort study in Denmark. *Am J Epidemiol* 2013;178:190–197.

73. Liu G, Cheresh P, Kamp DW. Molecular basis of asbestos-induced lung disease. *Annu Rev Pathol* 2013;8:161–187.

76. Shukla RK, Kumar A, Gurbani D, et al. TiO(2) nanoparticles induce oxidative DNA damage and apoptosis in human liver cells. *Nanotoxicology* 2013;7:48–60.

77. Horie M, Nishio K, Endoh S, et al. Chromium(III) oxide nanoparticles induced remarkable oxidative stress and apoptosis on culture cells. *Environ Toxicol* 2013;28:61–75.

79. Prasad RY, Chastain PD, Nikolaishvili-Feinberg N, et al. Titanium dioxide nanoparticles activate the ATM-Chk2 DNA damage response in human dermal fibroblasts. *Nanotoxicology* 2013;7:1111–1119.

81. Shi H, Magaye R, Castranova V, et al. Titanium dioxide nanoparticles: a review of current toxicological data. *Part Fibre Toxicol* 2013;10:15.

9 Dietary Factors

Karin B. Michels and Walter C. Willett

INTRODUCTION

Over two decades ago, Doll and Peto[1] speculated that 35% (range: 10% to 70%) of all cancer deaths in the United States may be preventable by alterations in diet. The magnitude of the estimate for dietary factors exceeded that for tobacco (30%) and infections (10%).

Studies of cancer incidence among populations migrating to countries with different lifestyle factors have indicated that most cancers have a large environmental etiology. Although the contribution of environmental influences differs by cancer type, the incidence of many cancers changes by as much as five- to tenfold among migrants over time, approaching that of the host country. The age at migration affects the degree of adaptation among first-generation migrants for some cancers, suggesting that the susceptibility to environmental carcinogenic influences varies with age by cancer type. Identifying the specific environmental and lifestyle factors most important to cancer etiology, however, has proven difficult.

Environmental factors such as diet may influence the incidence of cancer through many different mechanisms and at different stages in the cancer process. Simple mutagens in foods, such as those produced by the heating of proteins, can cause damage to DNA, but dietary factors can also influence this process by inducing enzymes that activate or inactivate these mutagens, or by blocking the action of the mutagen. Dietary factors can also affect every pathway hypothesized to mediate cancer risk–for example, the rate of cell cycling through hormonal or antihormonal effects, aiding or inhibiting DNA repair, promoting or inhibiting apoptosis, and DNA methylation. Because of the complexity of these mechanisms, knowledge of dietary influences on risk of cancer will require an empirical basis with human cancer as the outcome.

METHODOLOGIC CHALLENGES

Study Types and Biases

The association between diet and the risk of cancer has been the subject of a number of epidemiologic studies. The most prevalent designs are the case-control study, the cohort study, and the randomized clinical trial. When the results from epidemiologic studies are interpreted, the potential for confounding must be considered. Individuals who maintain a healthy diet are likely to exhibit other indicators of a healthy lifestyle, including regular physical activity, lower body weight, use of multivitamin supplements, lower smoking rates, and lower alcohol consumption. Even if the influence of these confounding variables is analytically controlled, residual confounding remains possible.

Ecologic Studies

In ecologic studies or international correlation studies, variation in food disappearance data and the prevalence of a certain disease are correlated, generally across different countries. A linear association

may provide preliminary data to inform future research but, due to the high probability of confounding, cannot provide strong evidence for a causal link. Food disappearance data also may not provide a good estimate for human consumption. The gross national product is correlated with many dietary factors such as fat intake.[2] Many other differences besides dietary fat exist between the countries with low fat consumption (less affluent) and high fat consumption (more affluent); reproductive behaviors, physical activity level, and body fatness are particularly notable and are strongly associated with specific cancers.

Migrant Studies

Studies of populations migrating from areas with low incidence of disease to areas with high incidence of disease (or vice versa) can help sort out the role of environmental factors versus genetics in the etiology of a cancer, depending on whether the migrating group adopts the cancer rates of the new environment. Specific dietary components linked to disease are difficult to identify in a migrant study.

Case-Control Studies

Case-control studies of diet may be affected by recall bias, control selection bias, and confounding. In a case-control study, participants affected by the disease under study (cases) and healthy controls are asked to recall their past dietary habits. Cases may overestimate their consumption of foods that are commonly considered "unhealthy" and underestimate their consumption of foods considered "healthy." Giovannucci et al.[3] have documented differential reporting of fat intake before and after disease occurrence. Thus, the possibility of recall bias in a case-control study poses a real threat to the validity of the observed associations. Even more importantly, in contemporary case-control studies using a population sample of controls, the participation rate of controls is usually far from complete, often 50% to 70%. Unfortunately, health-conscious individuals may be more likely to participate as controls and will thus be less overweight, will consume fruits and vegetables more frequently, and will consume less fat and red meat, which can substantially distort associations observed.

Cohort Studies

Prospective cohort studies of the effects of diet are likely to have a much higher validity than retrospective case-control studies because diet is recorded by participants before disease occurrence. Cohort studies are still affected by measurement error because diet consists of a large number of foods eaten in complex combinations. Confounding by other unmeasured or imperfectly measured lifestyle factors can remain a problem in cohort studies.

Now that the results of a substantial number of cohort studies have become available, their findings can be compared with those of case-control studies that have examined the same relations. In many cases, the findings of the case-control studies have not been confirmed; for example, the consistent finding of lower risk of many cancers with higher intake of fruits and vegetables in case-control studies has generally not been seen in cohort studies.[4] These findings suggest that the concerns about biases in case-control studies of diet, and probably many other lifestyle factors, are justified, and findings from such studies must be interpreted cautiously.

Randomized Clinical Trials

The gold standard in medical research is the randomized clinical trial (RCT). In an RCT on nutrition, participants are randomly assigned to one of two or more diets; hence, the association between diet and the cancer of interest should not be confounded by other factors. The problem with RCTs of diet is that maintaining the assigned diet strictly over many years, as would be necessary for diet to have an impact on cancer incidence, is difficult. For example, in the dietary fat reduction trial of the Women's Health Initiative (WHI), participants randomized to the intervention arm reduced their fat intake much less than planned.[5] The remaining limited contrast between the two groups left the lack of difference in disease outcomes difficult to interpret. Furthermore, the relevant time window for intervention and the necessary duration of intervention are unclear, especially with cancer outcomes. Hence, randomized trials are rarely used to examine the effect of diet on cancer but have better promise for the study of diet and outcomes that require a considerably shorter follow-up time (e.g., adenoma recurrence). Also, the randomized design may lend itself better to the study of the effects of dietary supplements such as multivitamin or fiber supplements, although the control group may adopt the intervention behavior because nutritional supplements are widely available. For example, in the WHI trial of calcium and vitamin D supplementation, two-thirds of the study population used vitamin D or calcium supplements that they obtained outside of the trial, again rendering the lack of effect in the trial uninterpretable.

Diet Assessment Instruments

Observational studies depend on a reasonably valid assessment of dietary intake. Although, for some nutrients, biochemical measurements can be used to assess intake, for most dietary constituents, a useful biochemical indicator does not exist. In population-based studies, diet is generally assessed with a self-administered instrument. Since 1980, considerable effort has been directed at the development of standardized questionnaires for measuring diet, and numerous studies have been conducted to assess the validity of these methods. The most widely used diet assessment instruments are the food frequency questionnaire, the 7-day diet record, and the 24-hour recall. Although the 7-day diet record may provide the most accurate documentation of intake during the week the participant keeps a diet diary, the burden of computerizing the information and extracting foods and nutrients has prohibited the use of the 7-day diet record in most large-scale studies. The 24-hour recall provides only a snapshot of diet on one day, which may or may not be representative of the participant's usual diet and is thus affected by both personal variation and seasonal variation. The food frequency questionnaire, the most widely used instrument in large population-based studies, asks participants to report their average intake of a large number of foods during the previous year. Participants tend to substantially overreport their fruit and vegetable consumption on the food frequency questionnaire.[6] This tendency may reflect social desirability bias, which leads to overreporting healthy foods and underreporting less healthy foods. Studies of validity using biomarkers or detailed measurements of diet as comparisons have suggested that carefully designed questionnaires can have sufficient validity to detect moderate to strong associations. Validity can be enhanced by using the average of repeated assessments over time.[7]

THE ROLE OF INDIVIDUAL FOOD AND NUTRIENTS IN CANCER ETIOLOGY

Energy

The most important impact of diet on the risk of cancer is mediated through body weight. Overweight, obesity, and inactivity are major contributors to cancer risk. (A more detailed discussion is provided in Chapter 10.) In the large American Cancer Society Cohort, obese individuals had substantially higher mortality from all cancers and, in particular, from colorectal cancer, postmenopausal breast cancer, uterine cancer, cervical cancer, pancreatic cancer, and gallbladder cancer than their normal-weight counterparts.[8] Adiposity and, in particular, waist circumference are predictors of colon cancer incidence among women and men.[9,10] A weight gain of 10 kg or more is associated with a significant increase in postmenopausal breast cancer incidence among women who never used hormone replacement therapy, whereas a weight loss of comparable magnitude after menopause substantially decreases breast cancer risk.[11] Regular physical activity contributes to a lower prevalence of being overweight and obesity and consequently reduces the burden of cancer through this pathway.

The mechanisms whereby adiposity increases the risk of various cancers are probably multiple. Being overweight is strongly associated with endogenous estrogen levels, which likely contribute to the excess risks of endometrial and postmenopausal breast cancers. The reasons for the association with other cancers are less clear, but excess body fat is also related to higher circulating levels of insulin, insulin-like growth factor (IGF)-1, and C-peptide (a marker of insulin secretion), lower levels of binding proteins for sex hormones and IGF-1, and higher levels of various inflammatory factors, all of which have been hypothesized to be related to risks of various cancers.

Energy restriction is one of the most effective measures to prevent cancer in the animal model. While energy restriction is more difficult to study in humans, voluntary starvation among anorectics and situations of food rationing during famines provide related models. Breast cancer rates were substantially reduced among women with a history of severe anorexia.[12] Although breast cancer incidence was higher among women exposed to the Dutch famine during childhood or adolescence, such short-term involuntary food rationing for 9 months or less was often followed by overnutrition.[13] A more prolonged deficit in food availability during World War II in Norway was associated with a reduction in adult risk of breast cancer if it occurred during early adolescence.[14]

Alcohol

Aside from body weight, alcohol consumption is the best established dietary risk factor for cancer. Alcohol is classified as a carcinogen by the International Agency for Research on Cancer. The consumption of alcohol increases the risk of numerous cancers, including those of the liver, esophagus, pharynx, oral cavity, larynx, breast, and colorectum in a dose-dependent fashion.[15] Evidence is convincing that excessive alcohol consumption increases the risk of primary liver cancer, probably through cirrhosis and alcoholic hepatitis. At least in the developed world, about 75% of cancers of the esophagus, pharynx, oral cavity, and larynx are attributable to alcohol and tobacco, with a marked increase in risk among drinkers who also smoke, suggesting a multiplicative effect. Mechanisms may include direct damage to the cells in the upper gastrointestinal tract; modulation of DNA methylation, which affects susceptibility to DNA mutations; and an increase in acetaldehyde, the main metabolite of alcohol, which enhances the proliferation of epithelial cells, forms DNA adducts, and is a recognized carcinogen. The association between alcohol consumption and breast cancer is notable because a small but significant risk has been found even with one drink per day. Mechanisms may include an interaction with folate, an increase in endogenous estrogen levels, and an elevation of acetaldehyde. Some evidence suggests that the excess risk is mitigated by adequate folate intake possibly through an effect on DNA methylation.[16] Notably, for most cancer sites, no important difference in associations was found with the type of alcoholic beverage, suggesting a critical role of ethanol in carcinogenesis.

Dietary Fat

In recent years, reducing dietary fat has been at the center of cancer prevention efforts. In the landmark 1982 National Academy of Sciences review of diet, nutrition, and cancer, a reduction in fat intake to 30% of calories was the primary recommendation.

Interest in dietary fat as a cause of cancer began in the first half of the 20th century, when studies by Tannenbaum[17] indicated that diets high in fat could promote tumor growth in animal models. Dietary fat has a clear effect on tumor incidence in many models, although not in all; however, a central issue has been whether this is independent of the effect of energy intake. In the 1970s, the possible relation of dietary fat intake to cancer incidence gained greater attention as the large international differences in rates of many cancers were noted to be strongly correlated with apparent per capita fat consumption in ecologic studies.[2] Particularly strong associations were seen with cancers of the breast, colon, prostate, and endometrium, which include the most important cancers not due to smoking in affluent countries. These correlations were observed to be limited to animal, not vegetable, fat.

Dietary Fat and Breast Cancer

Breast cancer is the most common malignancy among women, and incidence has been increasing for decades, although a decline has been noted starting with the new millennium. Rates in most parts of Asia, South America, and Africa have been only approximately one-fifth that of the United States, but in almost all these areas rates of breast cancer are also increasing. Populations that migrate from low- to high-incidence countries develop breast cancer rates that approximate those of the new host country. However, rates do not approach those of the general US population until the second or third generation.[18] This slower rate of change for immigrants may indicate delayed acculturation; although because a similar delay in rate increase is not observed for colon cancer, it may suggest an origin of breast cancer earlier in the life course.

The results from 12 smaller case-control studies that included 4,312 cases and 5,978 controls have been summarized in a meta-analysis.[19] The pooled relative risk (RR) was 1.35 (P <.0001) for a 100-g increase in daily total fat intake, although the risk was somewhat stronger for postmenopausal women (RR, 1.48; P <.001). This magnitude of association, however, could be compatible with biases due to recall of diet or the selection of controls.

Because of the prospective design of cohort studies, most of the methodologic biases of case-control studies are avoided. In an analysis of the Nurses' Health Study that included 121,700 US female registered nurses, no association with total fat intake was observed, and there was no suggestion of any reduction in risk at intakes below 25% of energy.[20] Because repeated assessments of diet were obtained at 2- to 4-year intervals, this analysis provided a particularly detailed evaluation of fat intake over an extended period in relation to breast cancer risk. Similar observations were made in the National Institutes of Health (NIH)–American Association of Retired Persons (AARP) Diet and Health Study including 188,736 postmenopausal women[21] and in the European Prospective Investigation into Cancer and Nutrition (EPIC), which included 7,119 incident cases.[22] In a pooled analysis of seven prospective studies, which included 337,000 women who developed 4,980 incident cases of breast cancer, no overall association was seen for fat intake over the range of less than 20% to more than 45% energy (reflecting the current range observed

internationally).[23] A similar lack of association was seen for specific types of fat. This lack of association with total fat intake was confirmed in a subsequent analysis of the pooled prospective studies of diet and breast cancer, which included over 7,000 cases.[24] Therefore, these cohort findings do not support the hypothesis that dietary fat is an important contributor to breast cancer incidence.

Endogenous estrogen levels have now been established as a risk factor for breast cancer. Thus, the effects of fat and other dietary factors on estrogen levels are of potential interest. Vegetarian women, who consume higher amounts of fiber and lower amounts of fat, have lower blood levels and reduced urinary excretion of estrogens, apparently due to increased fecal excretion. A meta-analysis has suggested that a reduction in dietary fat reduces plasma estrogen levels,[25] but the studies included were plagued by the lack of concurrent controls, the short duration, and the negative energy balance. In a large, randomized trial among postmenopausal women with a previous diagnosis of breast cancer, a reduction in dietary fat did not affect estradiol levels when the data were appropriately analyzed.[26]

The WHI Randomized Controlled Dietary Modification Trial similarly suggested no association between fat intake and breast cancer incidence,[5] but these results are difficult to interpret.[27] The data on biomarkers that reflect fat intake suggest little if any difference in fat intake between the intervention and control groups.[28] Even if dietary fat does truly have an effect on cancer incidence and other outcomes, this lack of adherence to the dietary intervention could explain the absence of an observed effect on total cancer incidence and total mortality. In another randomized trial in Canada that tested an intervention target of 15% of calories from fat, a small but significant difference in high-density lipoprotein (HDL) levels was observed after 8 to 9 years of follow-up suggesting a difference in fat intake in the two groups.[29] The incidence of breast cancer in the intervention and the control group did not differ significantly.

Some prospective cohort studies suggest an inverse association between monounsaturated fat and breast cancer. This is an intriguing observation because of the relatively low rates of breast cancer in southern European countries with high intakes of monounsaturated fats due to the use of olive oil as the primary fat. In case-control studies in Spain, Greece, and Italy, women who used more olive oil had reduced risks of breast cancer.

In a report of findings from the Nurses' Health Study II cohort of premenopausal women, a higher intake of animal fat was associated with an approximately 50% greater risk of breast cancer, but no association was seen with intake of vegetable fat.[30] This suggests that factors in foods containing animal fats, rather than fat per se, may account for the findings. In the same cohort, an intake of red meat and total fat during adolescence was also associated with the risk of premenopausal breast cancer.[31,32]

Dietary Fat and Colon Cancer

In comparisons among countries, rates of colon cancer are strongly correlated with a national per capita disappearance of animal fat and meat, with correlation coefficients ranging between 0.8 and 0.9.[2] Rates of colon cancer rose sharply in Japan after World War II, paralleling a 2.5-fold increase in fat intake. Based on these epidemiologic investigations and on animal studies, a hypothesis has developed that higher dietary fat increases the excretion of bile acids, which can be converted to carcinogens or act as promoters. However, evidence from many studies on obesity and low levels of physical activity increasing the risk of colon cancer suggests that at least part of the high rates in affluent countries previously attributed to fat intake is probably due to a sedentary lifestyle.

The Nurses' Health Study suggested an approximately twofold higher risk of colon cancer among women in the highest quintile of animal fat intake than in those in the lowest quintile.[33] In a multivariate analysis of these data, which included red meat intake and animal fat intake in the same model, red meat intake remained significantly predictive of colon cancer risk, whereas the association with animal fat was eliminated. Other cohort studies have supported associations of colon cancer and the consumption of red meat and processed meats but not other sources of fat or total fat.[34-36] Similar associations were also observed for colorectal adenomas. In a meta-analysis of prospective studies, red meat consumption was associated with a risk of colon cancer (RR = 1.24; 95% confidence interval [CI], 1.09 to 1.41 for an increment of 120 g per day).[37] The association with the consumption of processed meats was particularly strong (RR = 1.36; 95% CI, 1.15 to 1.61 for an increment of 30 g per day).

The apparently stronger association with red meat consumption than with fat intake in most large cohort studies needs further confirmation, but such an association could result if the fatty acids or non-fat components of meat (e.g., the heme iron or carcinogens created by cooking) were the primary etiologic factors. This issue has major practical implications because current dietary recommendations support the daily consumption of red meat as long as it is lean.[38]

Dietary Fat and Prostate Cancer

Although further data are desirable, the evidence from international correlations, case-control[39] and cohort studies[40-44] provides some support for an association between the consumption of fat-containing animal products and prostate cancer incidence. This evidence does not generally support a relation with intake of vegetable fat, which suggests that either the type of fat or other components of animal products are responsible. Some evidence also indicates that animal fat consumption may be most strongly associated with the incidence of aggressive prostate cancer, which suggests an influence on the transition from the widespread indolent form to the more lethal form of this malignancy. Data are limited on the relation of fat intake to the probability of survival after the diagnosis of prostate cancer.

Dietary Fat and Other Cancers

Rates of other cancers that are common in affluent countries, including those of the endometrium and ovary, are also correlated with fat intake internationally. In prospective studies between Iowa and Canadian women, no evidence of a relation between fat intake and risk of endometrial cancer was found. Positive associations between dietary fat and lung cancer have been observed in many case-control studies. However, in a pooled analysis of large prospective studies that included over 3,000 incident cases, no association was observed.[45] These findings provide further evidence that the results of case-control studies of diet and cancer are likely to be misleading.

Summary

Largely on the basis of the results of animal studies, international correlations, and a few case-control studies, great enthusiasm developed in the 1980s that modest reductions in total fat intake would have a major impact on breast cancer incidence. As the findings from large prospective studies have become available, however, support for this relation has greatly weakened. Although evidence suggests that a high intake of animal fat early in adult life may increase the risk of premenopausal breast cancer, this is not likely to be due to fat per se because vegetable fat intake was not related to risk. For colon cancer, the associations seen with animal fat intake internationally have been supported in numerous case-control and cohort studies, but this also appears to be explained by factors in red meat other than simply its fat content. Further, the importance of physical activity and leanness as protective factors against colon cancer indicates that international correlations probably overstate the contribution of diet to differences in colon cancer incidence. At present, the available evidence most strongly suggests an association between animal fat consumption and risk of prostate cancer, particularly the aggressive form of this disease.

As with colon cancer, the possibility remains that other factors in animal products contribute to risk.

Despite the large body of data on dietary fat and cancer that has accumulated since 1985, any conclusions should be regarded as tentative, because these are disease processes that are poorly understood and are likely to take many decades to develop. Because most of the reported literature from prospective studies is based on fewer than 20 years' follow-up, further evaluations of the effects of diet earlier in life and at longer intervals of observation are needed to fully understand these complex relations. Nevertheless, persons interested in reducing their risk of cancer could be advised, as a prudent measure, to minimize their intake of foods high in animal fat, particularly red meat. Such a dietary pattern is also likely to be beneficial for the risk of cardiovascular disease. On the other hand, unsaturated fats (with the exception of *transfatty* acids) reduce blood low-density lipoprotein cholesterol levels and the risk of cardiovascular disease, and little evidence suggests that they adversely affect cancer risk. Thus, efforts to reduce unsaturated fat intake are not warranted at this time and are likely to have adverse effects on cardiovascular disease risk. Because excess adiposity increases the risk of several cancers and cardiovascular disease, balancing calories from any source with adequate physical activity is extremely important.

Fruits and Vegetables

General Properties

Fruits and vegetables have been hypothesized to be major dietary contributors to cancer prevention because they are rich in potential anticarcinogenic substances. Fruits and vegetables contain antioxidants and minerals and are good sources of fiber, potassium, carotenoids, vitamin C, folate, and other vitamins. Although fruits and vegetables supply less than 5% of total energy intake in most countries worldwide on a population basis, the concentration of micronutrients in these foods is greater than in most others.

The comprehensive report of the World Cancer Research Fund and the American Institute for Cancer Research, published in 2007 and titled *Food, Nutrition, Physical Activity, and the Prevention of Cancer: A Global Perspective*, reached the consensus based on the available evidence: "findings from cohort studies conducted since the mid-1990s have made the overall evidence, that vegetables or fruits protect against cancers, somewhat less impressive. In no case now is the evidence of protection judged to be convincing."[15]

Fruit and Vegetable Consumption and Colorectal Cancer

The association between fruit and vegetable consumption and the incidence of colon or rectal cancer has been examined prospectively in at least six studies. In some of these prospective cohorts, inverse associations were observed for individual foods or particular subgroups of fruits or vegetables, but no consistent pattern emerged and many comparisons revealed no such links. The results from the largest studies, the Nurses' Health Study and the Health Professionals' Follow-Up Study, suggested no important association between the consumption of fruits and vegetables and the incidence of cancers of the colon or rectum during 1,743,645 person-years of follow-up.[46] In these two large cohorts, diet was assessed repeatedly during follow-up with a detailed food frequency questionnaire. Similarly, in the Pooling Project of Prospective Studies of Diet and Cancer, including 14 studies, 756,217 participants, and 5,838 cases of colon cancer, no association with overall colon cancer risk was found.[47]

Fruit and Vegetable Consumption and Stomach Cancer

At least 12 prospective cohort studies have examined the consumption of some fruits and vegetables and the incidence of stomach cancer.[15] Seven of these studies considered total vegetable intake. Three found significant protection from stomach cancer, whereas three did not. All other comparisons were made for subgroups of vegetables and produced inconsistent results. Nine prospective cohort studies investigated the association between fruit consumption and stomach cancer risk. Four studies found an inverse association of borderline statistical significance.

Fruit and Vegetable Consumption and Breast Cancer

The most comprehensive evaluation of fruit and vegetable consumption and the incidence of breast cancer was provided by a pooled analysis of all cohort studies.[48] Data were pooled from eight prospective studies that included 351,825 women, 7,377 of whom developed incident invasive breast cancer during follow-up. The pooled relative risk adjusted for potential confounding variables was 0.93 (95% CI, 0.86 to 1.0; P for trend, .08) for the highest versus the lowest quartile of fruit consumption, 0.96 (95% CI, 0.89 to 1.04; P for trend, .54) for vegetable intake, and 0.93 (95% CI, 0.86 to 1.0; P for trend, .12) for total consumption of fruits and vegetables combined. The EPIC study confirmed this lack of association.[49] In a recent analysis within the Nurses' Health Study, an inverse association was seen between vegetable intake and the risk of estrogen receptor–negative breast cancer.[50] This observation was confirmed in the pooling project of prospective studies: The pooled relative risk for the highest vs. the lowest quintile of total vegetable consumption was 0.82 (95% CI 0.74 to 0.90) for estrogen-receptor negative breast cancer.[51]

Fruit and Vegetable Consumption and Lung Cancer

The relation between fruit and vegetable consumption and the incidence of lung cancer was examined in the pooled analysis of cohort studies.[52] Overall, no association was observed, although a modest increase in lung cancer incidence was evident among participants with the lowest fruit and vegetable consumption.

Fruit and Vegetable Consumption and Total Cancer

An analysis of the Nurses' Health Study and the Health Professionals' Follow-Up Study, including over 9,000 incident cases of cancer, did not reveal a benefit of fruit and vegetable consumption for total cancer incidence.[53] Observations from the EPIC cohort were essentially consistent with these findings.[54] Although there may be no or only a very weak protection conferred for cancer from consuming an abundance of fruits and vegetables, there is a substantial benefit for protection from cardiovascular disease.

Summary

The consumption of fruits and vegetables and some of their main micronutrients appear to be less important in cancer prevention than previously assumed. With an accumulation of data from prospective cohort studies and randomized trials, a lack of association of these foods and nutrients with cancer outcomes has become apparent. A modest association cannot be excluded because of an imperfect measurement of diet, and it remains possible that a high consumption of fruits and vegetables during childhood and adolescence is more effective at reducing cancer risk than consumption in adult life due to the long latency of cancer manifestation.

Conversely, it is possible that, with the fortification of breakfast cereal, flour, and other staple foods, the frequent consumption of fruits and vegetables has become less essential for cancer prevention. Nevertheless, an abundance of fruits and vegetables as part of a healthy diet is recommended, because evidence consistently suggests that it lowers the incidence of hypertension, heart disease, and stroke.

Fiber

General Properties

Dietary fiber was defined in 1976 as "all plant polysaccharides and lignin which are resistant to hydrolysis by the digestive enzymes of men."[55] Fiber, both soluble and insoluble, is fermented by the luminal bacteria of the colon. Among the properties of fiber that make it a candidate for cancer prevention are its "bulking" effect, which reduces colonic transit time, and the binding of potentially carcinogenic luminal chemicals. Fiber may also aid in producing short-chain fatty acids that may be directly anticarcinogenic. Fiber may also induce apoptosis.

Dietary Fiber and Colorectal Cancer

In 1969, Dennis Burkitt hypothesized that dietary fiber is involved in colon carcinogenesis.[56] While working as a physician in Africa, Burkitt noticed the low incidence of colon cancer among African populations whose diets were high in fiber. Burkitt concluded that a link might exist between the fiber-rich diet and the low incidence of colon cancer. Burkitt's observations were followed by numerous case-control studies that seemed to confirm his theories. A combined analysis of 13 case-control studies[57] as well as a meta-analysis of 16 case-control studies[58] suggested an inverse association between fiber intake and the risk of colorectal cancer. The inclusion of studies was selective, however, and effect estimates unadjusted for potential confounders were used for most studies. Moreover, recall bias is a severe threat to the validity of retrospective case-control studies of fiber intake and any disease outcome.

Data from prospective cohort studies have largely failed to support an inverse association between dietary fiber and colorectal cancer incidence. Initial analyses from the Nurses' Health Study and the Health Professionals' Follow-Up Study[36] found no important association between dietary fiber and colorectal cancer. A significant inverse association between fiber intake and incidence of colorectal cancer was reported from the EPIC study. The analysis presented on dietary fiber and colorectal cancer encompassed 434,209 women and men from eight European countries.[59] The analytic model used by the EPIC investigators included adjustments for age, height, weight, total caloric intake, sex, and center assessed at baseline and identified[60] a significant inverse association between fiber intake and colorectal cancer. Applying the same analytic model used in EPIC to data from the Nurses' Health Study and the Health Professionals' Follow-Up Study encompassing 1.8 million person-years of follow-up and 1,572 cases of colorectal cancer revealed associations similar to those found in the EPIC study.[61] After a more complete adjustment for confounding variables, however, the association vanished.[61] Results from the pooled analysis of 13 prospective cohort studies, including 8,081 colorectal cancer cases diagnosed during over 7 million person-years of follow-up, suggested an inverse relation between dietary fiber and colorectal cancer incidence in age-adjusted analyses, but this association disappeared after appropriate adjustment for confounding variables, particularly other dietary factors.[62] The NIH–AARP study, which included 2,974 cases of colorectal cancer, confirmed the lack of association between total dietary fiber and colorectal cancer risk.[63]

The association between dietary fiber and colorectal cancer appears to be confounded by a number of other dietary and nondietary factors. These methodologic considerations must be taken into account when interpreting the evidence. It is possible that other dietary factors such as folate intake are more important for colorectal cancer pathogenesis than dietary fiber.

Dietary Fiber and Colorectal Adenomas

In a few prospective cohort studies, the primary occurrence of colorectal polyps was investigated, but no consistent relation was found.

The study of fiber intake and colorectal adenoma recurrence lends itself to a randomized clinical trial design because of the relatively short follow-up necessary and because fiber can be provided as a supplement. A number of RCTs have explored the effect of fiber supplementation on colorectal adenoma recurrence. Evidence has fairly consistently indicated no effect of fiber intake.[64–68] In one RCT, an increase in adenoma recurrence was observed among participants randomly assigned to use a fiber supplement, which was stronger among those with high dietary calcium.[69]

Dietary Fiber and Breast Cancer

Investigators have speculated that dietary fiber may reduce the risk of breast cancer through a reduction in intestinal absorption of estrogens excreted via the biliary system.

Relatively few epidemiologic studies have examined the association between fiber intake and breast cancer. In a meta-analysis of 10 case-control studies, a significant inverse association was observed. However, these retrospective studies were likely affected by the aforementioned biases—selection and recall bias, in particular. Results from at least six prospective cohort studies consistently suggested no association between fiber intake and breast cancer incidence.[70–75]

Dietary Fiber and Stomach Cancer

The results from retrospective case-control studies of fiber intake and gastric cancer risk are inconsistent. In the Netherlands Cohort Study, dietary fiber was not associated with an incidence of gastric carcinoma.[76] Further investigations through prospective cohort studies must be completed before conclusions about the relation between fiber intake and stomach cancer incidence can be drawn.

Summary

The observational data presently available do not indicate an important role for dietary fiber in the prevention of cancer, although small effects cannot be excluded. The long-held perception that a high intake of fiber conveys protection originated largely from retrospectively conducted studies, which are affected by a number of biases, in particular, the potential for differential recall of diet, and from studies that were not well controlled for potential confounding variables.

OTHER FOODS AND NUTRIENTS

Red Meat

The regular consumption of red meat has been associated with an increased risk of colorectal cancer. In a recent meta-analysis, the increase in risk associated with an increase in intake of 120 g per day was 24% (95% CI, 9% to 41%).[37] The association was strongest for processed meat; the relative risk of colorectal cancer was 1.36 (95% CI, 1.15 to 1.61) for a consumption of 30 g per day.[37] No overall association has been observed between red meat consumption and breast cancer in a pooled analysis of prospective cohorts.[77] However, among premenopausal women in the Nurses' Health Study II, the risk for estrogen-receptor–positive and progesterone-receptor–positive breast cancer doubled with 1.5 servings of red meat per day compared to three or fewer servings per week.[78] No associations have been found in studies on poultry or fish.[15] Mechanisms through which red meat may increase cancer risk include anabolic hormones routinely used in meat production in the United States, heterocyclic amines, and polycyclic aromatic hydrocarbons formed during cooking at high temperatures, the high amounts of heme iron, and nitrates and related compounds in smoked, salted, and some processed meats that can convert to carcinogenic nitrosamines in the colon.

Milk, Dairy Products, and Calcium

Regular milk consumption has been associated with a modest reduction in colorectal cancer in both a pooling project[79] and a meta-analysis of cohort studies,[80] possibly due to its calcium content. In the pooling project of prospective studies of diet and cancer, a modest inverse association was also seen for calcium intake.[79] This finding is consistent with the results of a randomized trial in which calcium supplements reduced the risk of colorectal adenomas.[81] Associations with cheese and other dairy products have been less consistent.[79,80]

Conversely, in multiple studies, a high intake of calcium or dairy products has been associated with an increased risk of prostate cancer,[80,82–86] specifically fatal prostate cancer.[87,88] Similar observations were made in the NIH–AARP study, although the increase in risk there did not reach statistical significance.[89] While the Multiethnic Cohort[90] and the Prostate, Lung, Colorectal, and Ovarian Cancer Screening Trial[91] did not find an important association between dairy consumption and prostate cancer, these cohort studies did not specifically include fatal prostate cancer cases. A meta-analysis of prospective studies generated an overall relative risk of advanced prostate cancer of 1.33 (95% CI, 1.00 to 1.78) for the highest versus the lowest intake categories of dairy products.[92] In another meta-analysis, no significant association was found for cohort studies on dairy or milk consumption, but relative risk estimates suggested a positive association.[93] Thus, although the findings are not entirely consistent and are complicated by the widespread use of prostate-specific antigen (PSA) screening in the United States, the global evidence suggests a positive association between the regular consumption of dairy products and the risk of fatal prostate cancer. Consuming three or more servings of dairy products per day has been associated with endometrial cancer among postmenopausal women not using hormonal therapy.[94] A high intake of lactose from dairy products has also been associated with a modestly higher risk of ovarian cancer.[95]

These observations are particularly important in the context of national dietary recommendations to drink three glasses of milk per day.[38] Possible mechanisms include an increase in endogenous IGF-1 levels[96] and steroid hormones contained in cows' milk.[97]

Vitamin D

In 1980, Garland and Garland[98] hypothesized that sunlight and vitamin D may reduce the risk of colon cancer. Since then, substantial research has been conducted in this area supporting an inverse association between circulating 25-hydroxyvitamin D (25[OH]D) levels and colorectal cancer risk.[99–103] A meta-analysis, including five nested case-control studies with prediagnostic serum, suggested a reduction of colorectal cancer risk by about half among individuals with serum 25(OH)D levels of more than 82 nmol/L compared to individuals with less than 30 nmol/L.[104] A subsequent meta-analysis including eight studies confirmed these associations.[105] These observations are supported by similar findings for colorectal adenomas.[106] Vitamin D levels may particularly affect colorectal cancer prognosis; colorectal cancer mortality was 72% lower among individuals with 25(OH)D concentrations of 80 nmol/L or higher.[107]

The evidence for other cancers has been less consistent. High plasma levels of vitamin D have been associated with a decreased risk of several other cancers, including cancer of the breast[108–111]; prostate, especially fatal prostate cancer[112]; and ovary.[113,114] Whether vitamin D plays a role in pancreatic cancerogenesis remains to be determined with one pooling project, suggesting a positive association,[115] whereas other prospective studies[116] and a pooling project of cohort studies found inverse associations.[117]

The activation of vitamin D receptors by 1,25(OH)$_2$D induces cell differentiation and inhibits proliferation and angiogenesis.[118] Solar ultraviolet B radiation is the major source of plasma vitamin D, and dietary vitamin D without supplementation has a minor effect on plasma vitamin D. To achieve sufficient plasma levels through sun exposure, at least 15 minutes of full-body exposure to bright sunlight is necessary. Physical activity has to be considered as possible confounder of studies on plasma levels of vitamin D and cancer. Sunscreen effectively blocks vitamin D production. Populations who live in geographic areas with limited or seasonal sun exposure may benefit from a vitamin D supplementation of 1,000 IU per day.

Folate

Folate is a micronutrient commonly found in fruits and vegetables, particularly oranges, orange juice, asparagus, beets, and peas. Folate may affect carcinogenesis through various mechanisms: DNA methylation, DNA synthesis, and DNA repair. In the animal model, folate deficiency enhances intestinal carcinogenesis.[119] Folate deficiency is related to the incorporation of uracil into human DNA and to an increased frequency of chromosomal breaks. A number of epidemiologic studies suggest that a diet rich in folate lowers the risk of colorectal adenomas and colorectal cancer.[15] Because the folate content in foods is generally relatively low, is susceptible to oxidative destruction by cooking and food processing, and is not well absorbed, folic acid from supplements and fortification plays an important role. Pooled results from 13 prospective studies suggests that intake of 400 to 500 μg per day is required to minimize risk.[120]

Potential interactions among alcohol consumption, folic acid intake, and methionine intake have been described. Although alcohol consumption has been fairly consistently related to an increase in breast cancer incidence, the potential detrimental effect of alcohol seems to be eliminated in women with high folic acid intake.[16] A similar folic acid or methionine–alcohol interaction has been observed for colorectal cancer risk.[119]

Genetic susceptibility may also modify the relation between folate intake and cancer risk. A polymorphism of the *methylenetetrahydrofolate reductase (MTHFR)* gene (cytosine to thymine transition at position 677) may result in a relative deficiency of methionine. Individuals with the common C677T mutation appear to experience the greatest protection from high folic acid or methionine intake and low alcohol consumption.[121] Although the interaction between this polymorphism and dietary factors needs to be investigated further, the consistently observed association between this polymorphism and the risk of colorectal cancer supports a role of folate in the etiology of colorectal cancer.

Folate levels also affect the availability of methyl groups via S-adenosylmethionine in the one-carbon metabolism.[122] Low red blood cell folate levels are associated with low DNA methylation status among homozygous *MTHFR* 677T/T mutation carriers, whereas at high red blood cell folate levels, the amount of methylated cytosine in DNA is similar to that of the heterozygote *MTHFR* C677T genotype.[123]

Conversely, evidence from animal and human studies suggests that a high folate status may promote the progression of existing neoplasias.[122,124,125] The randomization of folic acid supplements among individuals with a history of colorectal adenoma resulted in either no effect on recurrent adenoma recurrence[126] or an increase in recurrence with over 6 to 8 years of follow-up.[127] The high proliferation rate of neoplastic cells requiring increased DNA synthesis is likely supported by folate, which is necessary for thymidine synthesis.[122,125] The effects of folate on de novo methylation and subsequent gene silencing have been insufficiently studied. An increase in colorectal cancer rates has been observed in the United States and Canada concurrent with the introduction of the folic acid fortification program, but this could be an artifact due to increased use of colonoscopies.[128] The lack of increase in mortality, but an acceleration in a long-term downward trend suggests the latter explanation (http://progressreport.cancer.gov/).

Carotenoids

Carotenoids, antioxidants prevalent in fruits and vegetables, enhance cell-to-cell communication, promote cell differentiation, and modulate immune response. In 1981, Doll and Peto[1] speculated that beta-carotene may be a major player in cancer prevention and encouraged testing its anticarcinogenic properties. Indeed, subsequent observational studies, mostly case-control investigations, suggested a reduced cancer risk—especially of lung cancer—with a high intake of carotenoids. In contrast, clinical trials randomizing the intake of beta-carotene supplements have not revealed the evidence of a protective effect of beta-carotene. In fact, beta-carotene was found to increase the risk of lung cancer and total mortality among smokers in the Finnish Alpha-Tocopherol, Beta-Carotene Cancer Prevention Study.[129] However, these adverse affects disappeared during longer periods of follow-up.[130] In a detailed analysis of prospective studies, no association was seen between the intake of beta-carotene and the risk of lung cancer.[131]

The pooled analysis of 18 cohort studies including more than 33,000 breast cancer cases suggested inverse associations between the intake of several carotenoids (beta-carotene, alpha-carotene, luteine/zeaxanthin) and estrogen-receptor–negative breast cancer incidence, whereas no association was found for estrogen-receptor–positive tumors.[132] Similarly, in a pooled analysis of data from eight prospective studies including about 3,055 breast cancer cases, blood levels of carotenoids were inversely related to estrogen-receptor–negative mammary tumor incidence.[133] Women in the highest quintile of beta-carotene levels had about half the risk of developing estrogen-receptor–negative breast cancer than women in the lowest quintile (hazard ratio [HR] = 0.52; 95% CI, 0.36 to 0.77).

The particularly pronounced antioxidant properties of lycopene, a carotenoid mainly found in tomatoes, may explain the inverse associations with some cancers. The frequent consumption of tomato-based products has been associated with a decreased risk of prostate, lung, and stomach cancers.[134] The bioavailability of lycopene from cooked tomatoes is higher than from fresh tomatoes, making tomato soup and sauce excellent sources of the carotenoid.

Selenium

Selenium has long been of interest in cancer prevention due to its antioxidative properties. Its intake is difficult to estimate because food content depends on the selenium content of the soil it is grown in. Selenium enriches in toenails, which provide an integrative measure of intake during the previous year and therefore are popular biomarkers in epidemiologic studies. Inverse associations with toenail selenium levels have been found in several prospective studies, especially for fatal prostate cancer.[135–137] In a recent meta-analysis, plasma/serum selenium was also inversely correlated with prostate cancer.[138] In the Selenium and Vitamin E Cancer Prevention Trial (SELECT), no protective effect of selenium was found for prostate cancer. However, the trial was terminated prematurely after 4 years, which is a short period in which to expect a reduction in cancer.[139]

Soy Products

The role of soy products has been considered for breast carcinogenesis. In Asian countries, which traditionally have a high consumption of soy foods, breast cancer rates have been low until recently. In Western countries, soy consumption is generally low, and between-person variation may be insufficient to allow meaningful comparisons. Soybeans contain isoflavones, which are phytoestrogens that compete with estrogen for the estrogen receptor. Hence, soy consumption may affect estrogen concentrations differently depending on the endogenous baseline level. This mechanism may also contribute to the equivocal results of studies on soy foods and breast cancer risk. In a recent meta-analysis of 18 epidemiologic studies, including over 9,000 breast cancer cases, frequent soy intake was associated with a modest decrease in risk (odds ratio = 0.86; 95% CI, 0.75 to 0.99).[140] Wu et al.[141] observed that childhood intake of soy was more relevant to breast cancer prevention than adult consumption.

Carbohydrates

The Warburg hypothesis postulated in 1924 that tumor cells mainly generate energy by the nonoxidative breakdown of glucose (glucolysis) instead of pyrovate.[142] Carbohydrates with a high glycemic load increase blood glucose levels after consumption, which results in insulin spikes increasing the risk for type 2 diabetes. Several cancers, including colorectal cancer[143] and breast cancer,[144] have been associated with type 2 diabetes. The evidence on the consumption of sucrose and refined, processed flour and cancer incidence is heterogeneous.[145] Whereas in some prospective cohort studies an increase in colon cancer incidence was observed,[146] this was not found in other studies.[147] In large cohort studies, associations have been observed for pancreatic[148] and endometrial[145] cancer risk, but not for postmenopausal breast cancer.[149] Especially in obese, sedentary individuals, abnormal glucose and insulin metabolism may contribute to tumorigenesis.

DIETARY PATTERNS

Foods and nutrients are not consumed in isolation, and, when evaluating the role of diet in disease prevention and causation, it is sensible to consider the entire dietary pattern of individuals. Public health messages may be better framed in the context of a global diet than individual constituents.

The role of vegetarian diets for cancer incidence has been examined in a few studies. In the Adventist Health Study-2, vegetarians had an 8% lower incidence of cancer than nonvegetarians (95% CI, 1 to 15%).[150] The protective association was strongest for cancers of the gastrointestinal tract with 24% (95% CI, 10 to 37%). Vegans had a 16% (95%, 1 to 28%) lower incidence of cancer, with a particular protection conferred to female cancers of 34% (95% CI, 8 to 53%). A combined analysis of data from the Oxford Vegetarian Study and EPIC similarly suggest a 12% (95% CI, 4 to 19%) reduction in cancer incidence among vegetarians compared to meat eaters.[151]

During the past decade, dietary pattern analyses have gained popularity in observational studies. The most commonly employed methods are factor analyses and cluster analyses, which are largely data-driven methods, and investigator-determined methods such as dietary indices and scores. The search for associations between distinct patterns such as the "Western pattern," which is characterized by a high consumption of red and processed meats; high fat dairy products, including butter and eggs; and refined carbohydrates, such as sweets, desserts, and refined grains, and the "prudent pattern," which is defined by the frequent consumption of a variety of fruits and vegetables, whole grains, legumes, fish, and poultry, and the risk of cancer has been largely disappointing. Notable exceptions were the link between a Western dietary pattern and colon cancer incidence and an inverse relation between a prudent diet[152] and estrogen-receptor–negative breast cancer.[153] These findings were subsequently in the California Teachers Study.[154] The general lack of association between global dietary patterns and cancer supports a more modest role of nutrition during adult life in carcinogenesis than previously assumed.

DIET DURING THE EARLY PHASES OF LIFE

Some cancers may originate early in the course of life. A high birth weight is associated with an increase in the risk of childhood leukemia,[155] premenopausal breast cancer,[156] and testicular cancer.[157] Tall height is an indicator of the risk of many cancers and is in part determined by nutrition during childhood.[15] Until recently, most studies focused on the role of diet during adult life. However, the critical exposure period for nutrition to affect cancer risk may be earlier, and because the latent period for cancer may span several decades, diet during childhood and adolescence may be important. However, relating dietary information during early life and cancer outcomes prospectively is difficult because nutrition records from the remote past are not available. Studies in which recalled diet during youth is used have to be interpreted cautiously due to misclassification, although recall has been found reasonably reproducible and consistent with recalls provided by participants' mothers.[158,159] The role of early life diet has been explored in only a few studies in relation to breast cancer risk. In a study nested in the Nurses' Health Study cohorts that used data recalled by mothers, frequent consumption of french fries was associated with an increased risk of breast cancer, whereas whole milk consumption was inversely related to risk.[160] Similarly, an inverse association with milk consumption during childhood was found among younger women (30 to 39 years), but not among older premenopausal women (40 to 49 years) in a Norwegian cohort.[161] Dietary habits during high school recalled by adult participants of the Nurses' Health Study II (but before the diagnosis of breast cancer) suggested a positive association of total fat and red meat consumption.[31,32] More data are needed in this promising area of research.[162]

DIET AFTER A DIAGNOSIS OF CANCER

The role of diet in the secondary prevention of cancer recurrence and survival is generally of great interest to cancer patients because they are highly motivated to make lifestyle changes to optimize their prognosis. The compliance of cancer patients makes the RCTs a more feasible design to evaluate the role of diet than among healthy individuals. However, concurrent cancer treatments may make any effect of diet more difficult to isolate.

Most evidence is available for breast cancer, colorectal, and prostate cancer. Observational data suggest a limited role of diet in the prevention of breast cancer recurrence and survival. The Life After Cancer Epidemiology (LACE) Cohort supported a beneficial role for vitamin C and E supplement use but the effect of other health-seeking behaviors is difficult to exclude.[163] In a pooled analysis, alcohol consumption after a diagnosis did not affect survival.[164] Several randomized trials have addressed the role of diet in breast cancer prognosis. In the Women's Intervention Nutrition Study (WINS), 2,437 women with early stage breast cancer were randomized to a dietary goal of 15% of calories from fat or maintenance of their usual dietary habits.[165] The intervention group received dietary counseling by registered dieticians and, according to self-reports, a difference of 19 g in daily fat intake was maintained between the intervention and the control group after 60 months of follow-up. However, at that time, women in the intervention group were also 6 pounds lighter, making it difficult to separate an effect of dietary fat from a nonspecific effect of intensive dietary intervention, which quite consistently produces weight loss. Breast cancer recurrence was 29% lower in the intervention group (95% CI, 6% to 47%), whereas overall survival was not affected. In the Women's Healthy Eating and Living (WHEL) RCT, 3,088 early stage breast cancer patients were randomly assigned to a target of five vegetable servings, three fruit servings, 30 g fiber per day, and 15% to 20% of calories from fat.[166] After 72 months, the intervention versus control group reports were 5.8 versus 3.6 servings of vegetables, 3.4 versus 2.6 servings of fruit, 24.2 versus 18.9 g fiber per day, and 28.9% versus 32.4% of calories from fat. The total plasma carotenoid concentration, a biomarker of vegetable and fruit intake, was 43% higher in the intervention group than the comparison group after 4 years (p<0.001). Neither recurrence rates nor mortality were affected by the intervention after the 7.3-year follow-up. Overall, diet is unlikely a major factor influencing breast cancer prognosis. However, because the prognosis for breast cancer is relatively good, women diagnosed with breast cancer remain at risk for cardiovascular disease and other causes of death that affect those without breast cancer. Thus, among women in the Nurses' Health Study diagnosed with breast cancer, a higher diet quality, which was assessed by the Alternative Healthy Eating Index, was not associated with mortality due to breast cancer but was associated with substantially lower mortality due to other causes.[167] Similarly, among over 4,000 women with breast cancer, intakes of saturated and trans fat, but not of total fat, were associated with significantly greater total mortality but not specifically breast cancer mortality. Thus, there is good reason for women with breast cancer to adopt a healthy diet even if it does not affect the prognosis of breast cancer.

In a systematic review, no consistent association between individual dietary components and colorectal cancer prognosis outcome was found.[168] However, in an observational study including 1,009 patients with stage III colon cancer, a Western dietary pattern was associated with lower rates of disease-free survival, recurrence-free survival, and overall survivals.[169] In the same patient population, higher dietary glycemic load and total carbohydrate intake were significantly associated with an increased risk of recurrence and mortality.[170] These findings support a possible role of glycemic load in colon cancer progression.

In the Physician's Health Study, whole milk consumption among men with incident prostate cancer was associated with double the risk of progression to fatal disease.[171] Among men with nonmetastatic prostate cancer in the Health Professionals' Follow-up Study, replacing 10% of energy intake from carbohydrates with vegetable fat was associated with a lower risk of lethal prostate cancer.[172] A marginally increased risk of progression of localized to lethal prostate cancer among these men was also associated with postdiagnostic poultry and processed red meat consumption,[173] whereas postdiagnostic consumption of fish and tomato sauce were inversely related with a risk of progression.[174] In an intervention study, 93 patients with early stage prostate cancer (PSA = 4 to 10 ng per mililiter and Gleason score <7) were randomized to comprehensive lifestyle changes, including a vegan diet based on 10% of calories from fat and consisting predominantly of vegetables, fruit, whole grains, legumes, and soy protein.[175] Other interventions included moderate exercise, stress management, and relaxation. After 1 year, PSA values decreased 4% in the intervention group, but increased 6% in the control group. Six patients in the control group, but none in the experimental group, underwent conventional prostate cancer treatment. Although the impact of the different intervention components are difficult to separate in this study, further data on diet and the prognosis for patients with localized prostate cancer are needed.

SUMMARY

A considerable proportion of cancers are potentially preventable through lifestyle changes. Besides a curtailment of smoking, the most important strategies are maintaining a healthy body weight and regular physical activity, which contribute to a lower prevalence of being overweight and obesity. The avoidance of a positive energy balance and becoming overweight are the most important nutritional factors in cancer prevention.

Although dietary patterns, including frequent fruit and vegetable consumption, appear to play a modest role in cancer prevention, knowledge gained about some specific foods and nutrients might inform a targeted approach. Vitamin D is a strong candidate to counter carcinogenesis, thus supplementation could be a feasible and safe route to avoid several types of cancer. Although the data on vitamin D and cancer incidence are not conclusive, the prevention of bone fractures is a sufficient reason to maintain good vitamin D status.

Limiting or avoiding red meat, processed meat, and alcohol reduces the risk of breast, colorectal, stomach, esophageal, and other cancers. Although the role of dairy products and milk remains to be more fully elucidated, current evidence suggests a probable increase in the risk of prostate cancer with frequent milk consumption, and possibly endometrial cancer, which raises concern regarding current dietary recommendations of three glasses of milk per day. The relation of calcium and dairy intake to cancer is complex, as the evidence for a reduction in the risk of colorectal cancer is strong, but high intakes appear likely to increase the risk of fatal prostate cancer. The consumption of tomato-based products may contribute to the prevention of prostate cancer. Finally, diet may influence the prognosis of colorectal and prostate cancer, but more data are needed in this area. Because most people with cancer remain at risk of cardiovascular disease and other common conditions related to unhealthy diets, an overall healthy diet can be recommended while further research on diet and cancer survival is ongoing.

LIMITATIONS

Studying the role of diet in health and disease requires overcoming a number of hurdles. Because biomarkers reflecting nutrient intake with sufficient accuracy are largely lacking, assessing nutrition in a population-based study has to rely on self-reports by individuals, which inevitably leads to imprecision or error in the diet assessment. Such misclassification may produce spurious associations in case-control studies or may lead to an underestimation of true associations in prospective cohort studies. Ideally, hypotheses relating dietary factors to cancer risks would be tested in large randomized trials. Besides being extremely expensive, maintaining adherence to assigned diets has been challenging; for example, in the WHI trial that focused on dietary fat reduction, there were no differences between intervention and control groups in blood lipid fractions that are known to change with a reduction in fat intake, indicating a failure to test the hypothesis.[28]

Most observational studies are conducted within populations or countries. Although reasonable variations in nutritional habits exist within populations, allowing for the detection of substantial dietary risk factors for cardiovascular disease and diabetes, these contrasts may be too limited to detect small relative risks as they may exist for cancer. The pooled analysis of large prospective cohort studies across countries and continents attempts to overcome this limitation. Studies taking advantage of the large between-population variation in diets across developed and developing countries would appear to be advantageous, but would be plagued by confounding by other differences in lifestyle factors that might be difficult to assess and control adequately.

Few epidemiologic studies repeatedly capture dietary habits over time and thus account for potential changes in diet over time. Furthermore, the length of follow-up in prospective studies may not be sufficient to capture the impact of diets assessed at baseline. In case-control studies, a recall of dietary habits prior to the disease onset may be influenced by current disease status; moreover, the relevant time for nutrition to act may be decades earlier, which is more difficult to remember.

Most epidemiologic studies of diet and cancer have assessed intake among adults. Due to greater susceptibility to genotoxic influences earlier in life, it is possible that data on diet during childhood or early adolescence are more relevant for carcinogenesis and cancer prevention. Studies that have collected dietary data during childhood and followed the subjects for cancer incidence would be most informative but are virtually nonexistent and will be challenging to conduct.

Finally, data on special diets including organic foods, whole foods, raw foods, and a vegan diet are limited.

FUTURE DIRECTIONS

Some of the most promising research at present is in the areas of vitamin D, milk consumption, and the effect of diet early in life on cancer incidence. Recent nutrition changes in countries previously maintaining a more traditional diet such as Japan and some developing countries have already been followed by increased rates of some cancers (but declines in stomach cancer), providing a setting to study the effect of change over time. Additional insight may come from studies on gene–nutrient interaction and epigenetic changes induced by the diet. To improve observational research methods, refined dietary assessment methods, including the identification of new biomarkers, will be advantageous.

RECOMMENDATIONS

A wealth of data are available from observational studies on diet and cancer, and the current evidence supports suggestions made by Doll and Peto[1] that approximately 30% to 40% of cancers may be avoidable with changes in nutrition; however, much of this risk of cancer is related to being overweight and to inactivity. Excessive energy intake and lack of physical activity, marked by rapid growth in childhood and being overweight, have become growing threats to population health and are important contributors to risks of many cancers. Nevertheless, the cumulative incidence for many cancers has decreased over the past decade, in part due to the decreasing prevalence of smoking and use of hormone therapy.

Dietary recommendations must integrate the goal of overall avoidance of disease and maintenance of health and, thus, should not focus singularly on cancer prevention. The strength of the evidence and magnitude of the expected benefit should also be considered in recommendations. With these considerations in mind, the following recommendations are outlined, which are largely in agreement with the guidelines put forth by the American Cancer Society in 2012:[176]

1. *Engage in regular physical activity.* Physical activity is a primary method of weight control and it also reduces risk of several cancers, especially colon cancer, through independent mechanisms. Moderate to vigorous exercise for at least 30 minutes on most days is a minimum and more will provide additional benefits.

2. *Avoid being overweight and weight gain in adulthood.* A positive energy balance that results in excess body fat is one of the most important contributors to cancer risk. Staying within 10 pounds of body weight at age 20 may be a simple guide, assuming no adolescent obesity.

3. *Limit alcohol consumption.* Alcohol consumption contributes to the risk of many cancers and increases the risk of accidents and addiction, but low to moderate consumption has benefits for coronary heart disease risk. The individual family history of disease as well as personal preferences should be considered.

4. *Consume lots of fruits and vegetables.* Frequent consumption of fruits and vegetables during adult life is not likely to have a major effect on cancer incidence, but will reduce the risk of cardiovascular disease.

5. *Consume whole grains and avoid refined carbohydrates and sugars.* A regular consumption of whole grain products instead of refined flour and a low consumption of refined sugars lower the risk of cardiovascular disease and diabetes. The effect on cancer risk is less clear.

6. *Replace red meat and dairy products with fish, nuts, and legumes.* Red meat consumption increases the risk of colorectal cancer, diabetes, and coronary heart disease and should be largely avoided. Frequent dairy consumption may increase the risk of prostate cancer. Fish, nuts, and legumes are excellent sources of valuable mono- and polyunsaturated fats and vegetable proteins and may contribute to lower rates of cardiovascular disease and diabetes.

7. *Consider taking a vitamin D supplement.* A substantial proportion of the population, especially those living at higher latitudes, are vitamin D deficient. Most adults may benefit from taking 1,000 IU of vitamin D_3 per day during months of low sunlight intensity. Vitamin D supplementation will, at a minimum, reduce bone fracture rates, probably colorectal cancer incidence, and possibly other cancers.

SELECTED REFERENCES

The full reference list can be accessed at lwwhealthlibrary.com/oncology.

1. Doll R, Peto R. The causes of cancer: quantitative estimates of avoidable risks of cancer in the United States today. *J Natl Cancer Inst* 1981;66:1191–1308.
2. Armstrong B, Doll R. Environmental factors and cancer incidence and mortality in different countries, with special reference to dietary practices. *Int J Cancer* 1975;15:617–631.
3. Giovannucci E, Stampfer MJ, Colditz GA, et al. A comparison of prospective and retrospective assessments of diet in the study of breast cancer. *Am J Epidemiol* 1993;137:502–511.
5. Prentice RL, Caan B, Chlebowski RT, et al. Low-fat dietary pattern and risk of invasive breast cancer: the Women's Health Initiative Randomized Controlled Dietary Modification Trial. *JAMA* 2006;295:629–642.
6. Michels KB, Bingham SA, Luben R, et al. The effect of correlated measurement error in multivariate models of diet. *Am J Epidemiol* 2004;160:59–67.
7. Willett W. *Nutritional Epidemiology.* 3rd ed. New York: Oxford University Press; 2013.
11. Eliassen AH, Colditz GA, Rosner B, et al. Adult weight change and risk of postmenopausal breast cancer. *JAMA* 2006;296:193–201.
12. Michels KB, Ekbom A. Caloric restriction and incidence of breast cancer. *JAMA* 2004;291:1226–1230.
13. Elias SG, Peeters PH, Grobbee DE, et al. Breast cancer risk after caloric restriction during the 1944–1945 Dutch famine. *J Natl Cancer Inst* 2004;96:539–546.
15. World Cancer Research Fund/American Institute for Cancer Research. *Food, Nutrition, Physical Activity, and the Prevention of Cancer: A Global Perspective.* Washington, D.C.: AICR; 2007.
16. Zhang S, Hunter DJ, Hankinson SE, et al. A prospective study of folate intake and the risk of breast cancer. *JAMA* 1999;281:1632–1637.
18. Kolonel L, Hinds M, Hankin J. *Cancer Patterns Among Migrant and Native-Born Japanese in Hawaii in Relation to Smoking, Drinking, and Dietary Habits.* Tokyo: Japan Scientific Societies Press; 1980.
23. Hunter DJ, Spiegelman D, Adami HO, et al. Cohort studies of fat intake and the risk of breast cancer—a pooled analysis. *N Engl J Med* 1996;334:356–361.
27. Michels KB. The women's health initiative—curse or blessing? *Int J Epidemiol* 2006;35:814–816.
28. Michels KB, Willett WC. The Women's Health Initiative Randomized Controlled Dietary Modification Trial: a post-mortem. *Breast Cancer Res Treat* 2009;114:1–6.
38. Dietary Guidelines for Americans. DietaryGuidelines.gov Web site. http://www.health.gov/dietaryguidelines/.
46. Michels KB, Edward G, Joshipura KJ, et al. Prospective study of fruit and vegetable consumption and incidence of colon and rectal cancers. *J Natl Cancer Inst* 2000;92:1740–1752.
61. Michels KB, Fuchs CS, Giovannucci E, et al. Fiber intake and incidence of colorectal cancer among 76,947 women and 47,279 men. *Cancer Epidemiol Biomarkers Prev* 2005;14:842–849.
62. Park Y, Hunter DJ, Spiegelman D, et al. Dietary fiber intake and risk of colorectal cancer: a pooled analysis of prospective cohort studies. *JAMA* 2005;294:2849–2857.
81. Baron JA, Beach M, Mandel JS, et al. Calcium supplements for the prevention of colorectal adenomas. Calcium Polyp Prevention Study Group. *N Engl J Med* 1999;340:101–107.
92. Gao X, LaValley MP, Tucker KL. Prospective studies of dairy product and calcium intakes and prostate cancer risk: a meta-analysis. *J Natl Cancer Inst* 2005;97:1768–1777.
98. Garland CF, Garland FC. Do sunlight and vitamin D reduce the likelihood of colon cancer? *Int J Epidemiol* 1980;9:227–231.

104. Gorham ED, Garland CF, Garland FC, et al. Optimal vitamin D status for colorectal cancer prevention: a quantitative meta analysis. *Am J Prev Med* 2007;32:210–216.

120. Kim D, Smith-Warner S, Spiegelman D, et al. Pooled analysis of 13 prospective cohort studies on folate and colon cancer. *Cancer Causes Control* 2010;21:1919–1930.

122. Osterhues A, Holzgreve W, Michels KB. Shall we put the world on folate? *Lancet* 2009;374:959–961.

123. Friso S, Choi SW, Girelli D, et al. A common mutation in the 5,10-methylenetetrahydrofolate reductase gene affects genomic DNA methylation through an interaction with folate status. *Proc Natl Acad Sci U S A* 2002;99:5606–5611.

124. Kim YI. Folate: a magic bullet or a double edged sword for colorectal cancer prevention? *Gut* 2006;55:1387–1389.

125. Mason JB. Folate, cancer risk, and the Greek god, Proteus: a tale of two chameleons. *Nutr Rev* 2009;67:206–212.

126. Wu K, Platz EA, Willett W, et al. A randomized trial on folic acid supplementation and risk of recurrent colorectal adenoma. *Am J Clin Nutr* 2009;90:1623–1631.

127. Cole BF, Baron JA, Sandler RS, et al. Folic acid for the prevention of colorectal adenomas: a randomized clinical trial. *JAMA* 2007;297:2351–2359.

128. Mason JB, Dickstein A, Jacques PF, et al. A temporal association between folic acid fortification and an increase in colorectal cancer rates may be illuminating important biological principles: a hypothesis. *Cancer Epidemiol Biomarkers Prev* 2007;16:1325–1329.

129. The effect of vitamin E and beta carotene on the incidence of lung cancer and other cancers in male smokers. The Alpha-Tocopherol, Beta Carotene Cancer Prevention Study Group. *N Engl J Med* 1994;330:1029–1035.

130. Virtamo J, Pietinen P, Huttunen JK, et al. Incidence of cancer and mortality following alpha-tocopherol and beta-carotene supplementation: a postintervention follow-up. *JAMA* 2003;290:476–485.

131. Mannisto S, Smith-Warner SA, Spiegelman D, et al. Dietary carotenoids and risk of lung cancer in a pooled analysis of seven cohort studies. *Cancer Epidemiol Biomarkers Prev* 2004;13:40–48.

134. Giovannucci E. Tomatoes, tomato-based products, lycopene, and cancer: review of the epidemiologic literature. *J Natl Cancer Inst* 1999;91:317–331.

138. Hurst R, Hooper L, Norat T, et al. Selenium and prostate cancer: systematic review and meta-analysis. *Am J Clinical Nutr* 2012;96:111–122.

155. Caughey RW, Michels KB. Birth weight and childhood leukemia: a meta-analysis and review of the current evidence. *Int J Cancer* 2009;124:2658–2670.

156. Michels KB, Xue F. Role of birthweight in the etiology of breast cancer. *Int J Cancer* 2006;119:2007–2025.

157. Michos A, Xue F, Michels KB. Birth weight and the risk of testicular cancer: a meta-analysis. *Int J Cancer* 2007;121:1123–1131.

158. Chavarro JE, Rosner BA, Sampson L, et al. Validity of adolescent diet recall 48 years later. *Am J Epidemiol* 2009;170:1563–1570.

160. Michels KB, Rosner BA, Chumlea WC, et al. Preschool diet and adult risk of breast cancer. *Int J Cancer* 2006;118:749–754.

162. Michels KB, Mohllajee AP, Roset-Bahmanyar E, et al. Diet and breast cancer: a review of the prospective observational studies. *Cancer* 2007;109:2712–2749.

165. Chlebowski RT, Blackburn GL, Thomson CA, et al. Dietary fat reduction and breast cancer outcome: interim efficacy results from the Women's Intervention Nutrition Study. *J Natl Cancer Inst* 2006;98:1767–1776.

166. Pierce JP, Natarajan L, Caan BJ, et al. Influence of a diet very high in vegetables, fruit, and fiber and low in fat on prognosis following treatment for breast cancer: the Women's Healthy Eating and Living (WHEL) randomized trial. *JAMA* 2007;298:289–298.

168. van Meer S, Leufkens AM, Bueno-de-Mesquita HB, et al. Role of dietary factors in survival and mortality in colorectal cancer: a systematic review. *Nutrition Rev* 2013;71:631–641.

169. Meyerhardt JA, Niedzwiecki D, Hollis D, et al. Association of dietary patterns with cancer recurrence and survival in patients with stage III colon cancer. *JAMA* 2007;298:754–764.

170. Meyerhardt JA, Sato K, Niedzwiecki D, et al. Dietary glycemic load and cancer recurrence and survival in patients with stage III colon cancer: findings from CALGB 89803. *J Natl Cancer Inst* 2012;104:1702–1711.

172. Richman EL, Kenfield SA, Chavarro JE, et al. Fat intake after diagnosis and risk of lethal prostate cancer and all-cause mortality. *JAMA Intern Med* 2013;173:1318–1326.

175. Ornish D, Weidner G, Fair WR, et al. Intensive lifestyle changes may affect the progression of prostate cancer. *J Urol* 2005;174:1065–1070.

176. Kushi LH, Doyle C, McCullough M, et al. American Cancer Society Guidelines on nutrition and physical activity for cancer prevention: reducing the risk of cancer with healthy food choices and physical activity. *CA Cancer J Clin* 2012;62:30–67.

ETIOLOGY AND EPIDEMIOLOGY OF CANCER

10 Obesity and Physical Activity

Yani Lu, Jessica Clague, and Leslie Bernstein

INTRODUCTION

Evidence showing that physical activity is associated with decreased cancer risk and that obesity is associated with increased cancer risk at certain sites is rapidly accumulating. It is not yet known whether these two factors are interrelated or independent. Physical activity may act to decrease cancer risk primarily by preventing weight gain and obesity. However, physical activity may also have independent effects on cancer risk. In this chapter, we present a summary of the current epidemiologic literature on the possible associations between physical activity and obesity and risk of cancer at several organ sites.

Physical activity is defined as any movement of the body that results in energy expenditure. In this chapter, we focus on recreational physical activity, also called leisure-time physical activity or exercise, and occupational physical activity, including household activity.[1] Occupational physical activity typically occurs over a longer period of time and generally requires less energy expenditure per hour than bouts of strenuous or moderate recreational physical activity. The distinction between recreational and occupational activity is important because increasing mechanization and technologic advances have led to decreased occupational physical activity in developed areas of the world, perhaps contributing to a decrease in overall physical activity.

Obesity is defined as the condition of being extremely overweight. In epidemiologic studies, the usual, but not necessarily the best, measure of body mass in adults is Quetelet's Index, or body mass index (BMI), which is measured as weight in kilograms (kg) divided by the square of height in meters (m^2). In the year spanning 2009 to 2010, the prevalence of obesity, defined by having a BMI of 30 kg/m^2 or greater, in the US population was 35.5% for adult men and 35.8% for adult women.[2] Physical inactivity has likely contributed to the high prevalence of obesity in the United States; data from the 2003 to 2004 National Health and Nutritional Examination Survey, a cross-sectional study of a sample of the civilian, noninstitutionalized population of the United States, has indicated that less than 5% of US adults achieve 30 minutes per day of physical activity, and that men are more physically active than women.[3]

Epidemiologic evidence on the associations of physical activity and obesity with cancer come from observational studies, including cohort studies, which follow populations forward in time after collecting exposure information, and case-control studies, which optimally identify a population-based series of newly diagnosed cases and healthy control subjects, collecting information retrospectively on exposures. In both study designs, physical activity information is usually self-reported and measures vary substantially with respect to timing and level of detail. Studies have measured lifetime or long-term physical activity, activity at defined ages or time points in life, and/or current or recent activity. Ideally, a study would capture activity by type (recreational, occupational, or other, such as an activity related to transportation), duration (minutes per session), frequency (sessions per day), and intensity (low, moderate, or strenuous as defined by examples of activity types) across the lifetime. These studies have often measured height and weight by self-report at one time point, such as at the time of study entry. Some studies have collected other or more detailed anthropometric information, such as waist circumference, hip circumference, or weight at an additional time point like age 18. Anthropometrics are directly measured by trained study personnel in only a few studies.

Epidemiologic evidence for a role of physical activity or obesity in relation to cancer risk exists for cancers of the breast, colon, endometrium, esophagus, kidney, and pancreatic cancer. Evidence is accumulating to link at least one of these "exposures" to the incidence of gallbladder cancer, non-Hodgkin lymphoma (NHL), and advanced prostate cancer. The evidence for an association between either physical activity or obesity and lung and ovarian cancer is inconclusive.

In addition to specific biologic mechanisms pertinent to physical activity or to obesity at each specific organ site, several global mechanisms have been implicated in both relationships across a number of these organ sites. The steroid hormone and insulin/insulinlike growth factor (IGF) pathways are two such global mechanisms hypothesized to be involved in the links between physical activity or obesity and cancer.[4] The role of steroid hormones as a mediator in these relationships is perhaps best understood in the context of breast cancer and endometrial cancer, and will be discussed in those sections. The roles of the insulin and IGF pathways have been discussed in depth with respect to colon cancer and, thus, will be presented in that context. Other global mechanisms have been proposed that have more generalized anticancer impacts and may explain associations between physical activity and several cancer sites; these include heightening immune surveillance, reducing inflammation, increasing insulin sensitivity, controlling growth factor production and activation, decreasing obesity and central adiposity, optimizing DNA repair capacity, and reducing oxidative stress.[5,6] Further, obesity has been shown to produce a proinflammatory state and, thus, inflammation may mediate the relationship between obesity and cancer risk.[7] It is highly plausible that several of these mechanisms act simultaneously and that they interact synergistically to mediate the associations between physical activity, obesity, and cancer.

BREAST CANCER

Low level of physical activity is an established breast cancer risk factor among postmenopausal women and, to a lesser extent, premenopausal women.[4,8,9] The evidence for an association between physical activity and breast cancer has been classified as convincing, with a 20% to 40% reduced risk among physically active women.[10] Obesity appears to have a paradoxical relationship with breast cancer risk in that it is an established breast cancer risk factor among postmenopausal women, but may offer some protection for breast cancer among premenopausal women.[4]

The epidemiologic literature has shown with relative consistency that breast cancer risk is reduced by increasing one's amount of physical activity.[4,8,9,11–13] One of the earliest studies, a case-control study of women age 40 years or younger, showed a dramatic reduction in risk of approximately 50% among women who averaged about 4 hours of activity per week during their reproductive years.[14] Similarly, among postmenopausal women, those with higher levels of recreational physical activity during their lifetimes have been shown to have lower breast cancer risk.[15] A meta-analysis of 29 case-control studies and 19 cohort studies published between 1994 and 2006 provided strong evidence for an inverse association between physical activity and risk of breast cancer, citing that the evidence for an association between physical activity and premenopausal breast cancer was not as strong as that for postmenopausal breast cancer.[8] The conclusion of the meta-analysis was that each additional hour of physical activity per week decreases breast cancer by approximately 6%.

Epidemiologists require that a risk factor demonstrate consistency across populations before considering it as accepted. Recently, studies have been published on the association between physical activity and breast cancer risk among Japanese,[16] Chinese,[17] Mexican,[18] Tunisian,[19] and African American women.[20] All studies showed a decreased risk of breast cancer with increasing physical activity. Interestingly, both Suzuki et al.[17] and Pronk et al.[21] observed the strongest associations among "heavier" women (BMI ≥ 25 kg/m^2 and 23.73 kg/m^2, respectively). In the California Teachers Study (CTS), a prospective cohort study of over 133,000 female public school professionals, a variable combining strenuous and moderate long-term recreational physical activity was associated with a reduced risk of estrogen receptor (ER)-negative but not ER-positive invasive breast cancer.[11] On the contrary, the Women's Health Initiative (WHI) observed decreases in breast cancer risk associated with recreational physical activity among postmenopausal women with ER-positive breast cancer and triple negative breast cancer, with only results for ER-positive breast cancer demonstrating a 15% statistically significant reduced risk (when comparing the highest versus lowest tertile of moderate-intensity physical activity).[22] Similar but not statistically significant results were observed for strenuous recreational physical activity.[22] A major limitation to this and previous studies stratifying by hormone receptor status is the inability to comprehensively classify triple negative breast cancer due to missing HER2 status (unknown in 40% of cases in the WHI study). The use of hormone therapy did not alter the inverse association between recreational physical activity and invasive breast cancer in the Women's Contraceptive and Reproductive Experiences (CARE) Study.[23] Most recently, in the American Cancer Society Cancer Prevention Study II Nutrition Cohort, it was observed that postmenopausal women who engage in at least 7 hours of walking over the course of a week had a modest decreased risk of breast cancer, even in the absence of more vigorous exercise.[24] Further, this association did not differ by ER status, BMI, adult weight gain, postmenopausal hormone therapy use, or time spent sitting.[24]

Lastly, whether physical activity reduces breast cancer risk by impacting preinvasive disease has been studied by assessing the associations with in situ breast cancer and benign breast disease. In the CTS cohort, increasing levels of long-term strenuous recreational physical activity were associated with a decreasing risk of in situ breast cancer.[11] Furthermore, a report from the Nurses' Health Study II cohort showed that lifetime recreational physical activity was associated with a decreased risk of benign breast disease and columnar cell lesions, which may be precursors to breast cancer.[25]

In summary, epidemiologic studies investigating the association between physical activity and breast cancer risk have produced relatively consistent results showing a reduction in breast cancer risk with increasing level of physical activity. Results to date suggest that moderate-to-strenuous activity may be required for the effect between physical activity and breast cancer risk to be clear; however, clarification of other key details, such as the importance of timing and intensity of activity or variation in effects by tumor characteristics, is pending.

Adult obesity and adult weight gain have both been associated with increased breast cancer risk among postmenopausal women, especially among women who were not current users of menopausal hormone therapy.[4,26,27] Most studies among postmenopausal women show a 1.5- to 2-fold increase in risk of invasive breast cancer when comparing the most obese women or those with the largest weight gain to normal-weight women (BMI: 18.5 to 24.9 kg/m^2) or those with the least weight gain.[4] Paradoxically, overweight or obese premenopausal women have a slightly decreased risk of breast cancer compared with normal-weight or thinner women. Whether larger waist circumference is more important than BMI has been studied in order to separate overall weight gain from abdominal obesity (i.e., visceral fat, which is one element of metabolic syndrome); however, most studies have reported a null association between waist circumference, used as a surrogate for visceral fat, and risk of postmenopausal breast cancer after adjustment for BMI.[26] In contrast to the results for postmenopausal women, waist circumference and a positive association with premenopausal breast cancer was found after adjustment for BMI.[26] A recent analysis of the Nurses' Health Study suggests that self-rated body fatness during youth and BMI at age 18 years are both inversely associated with breast cancer risk, with similar results for premenopausal and postmenopausal breast cancer.[28]

Hormones are central to the discussion of biologic mechanisms linking both physical activity and obesity with breast cancer risk. Physical activity can alter menstrual cycle patterns in premenopausal women, and hormone profiles in both premenopausal and postmenopausal women. Physical activity may lower body fat among children,[29] which in turn may delay age at menarche.[30] Later age at menarche has been associated with reduced breast cancer risk.[31] Physical activity may reduce the frequency of ovulatory cycles.[32] Having less frequent and therefore fewer cumulative ovulatory cycles is likely to reduce the lifetime exposure of the breast to endogenous ovarian hormones,[31] which are proven proliferative agents.[33] Physical activity also can have a direct impact on circulating estrogen levels among postmenopausal women.[34]

In the postmenopausal period, adipose tissue is the primary source of endogenous hormones via aromatization of androstenedione to estrone.[35] Thus, heavier postmenopausal women have higher levels of circulating estrogen than women with less adipose tissue. The involvement of estrogen in the relationship between obesity and breast cancer risk is supported by the observation that obesity does not independently increase breast cancer risk among menopausal hormone therapy users[27]; the obesity-related increase in estrogen over that provided by exogenous estrogens is negligible. The breast tissue of overweight or obese perimenopausal and postmenopausal women with relatively high risk of breast cancer has been shown to have cytologic abnormalities and higher epithelial cell counts than that of normal-weight women.[36] In contrast, obese premenopausal women experience menstrual cycle disturbances, including anovulatory cycles and secondary amenorrhea, thereby lowering their cumulative exposure to estradiol and progesterone.[31] A possible explanation for the inverse association between youth body fatness and breast cancer risk is that youth body size is inversely associated with adult IGF-1 levels.[28]

Other likely mechanisms that may link physical activity[37,38] and obesity[39,40] with breast cancer risk include aspects of immune function, inflammatory mechanisms, oxidative stress and DNA repair capability, metabolic hormones, and growth factors.

COLON AND RECTAL CANCER

An inverse association between physical activity and colon cancer risk has been consistently observed among epidemiologic studies; however, the evidence for rectal cancer remains inconclusive. Historically, comprehensive reviews have estimated that physical activity may reduce colon cancer risk by 20% to 25% when comparing individuals with the highest levels to those with the lowest levels of activity.[41] Risk reductions are greater for case-control studies (24%) than for cohort studies (17%), and risk reductions for occupational activity (22%) and recreational activity (23%) are similar.[41] In cohort studies, colon cancer risk reduction associated with physical activity is greater for men than for women, which may be due to the influence of hormone therapy on colon cancer risk,[42] although case-control studies suggest similar benefits for men and women.[43]

Whether physical activity preferentially protects against proximal or distal colon cancer is of interest. A meta-analysis including 21 cohort and case-control studies that examined associations between physical activity and the risks of proximal colon and distal colon cancers produced results suggesting that physical activity is associated with a reduced risk of both proximal colon and distal colon cancers, and that the magnitude of the association does not differ by subsite.[44]

Although the majority of previous studies have not found an association between physical activity and rectal cancer,[41] the National Institutes of Health (NIH)–AARP Diet and Health Study observed a modest reduction in rectal cancer risk for men but not for women after 6.9 years of follow-up.[45] Further, in a case-control study conducted in Australia, rectal cancer risk was reduced among men but not among women who participated in vigorous recreational physical activity averaging at least 6 metabolic equivalent task (MET)-hours per week during their adult years.[46]

An emphasis has been made on trying to identify risk factors for colon adenomas, which are considered precursor lesions for colon cancer; these are detected and removed during colonoscopy or sigmoidoscopy. Wolin et al. conducted a meta-analysis of 20 studies published through April 2010 that investigated the association between recreational physical activity and colon adenomas.[47] Adenoma risk was reduced by 19% among men and by 13% among women and, when combining men and women, the inverse association with physical activity was strongest for large/advanced polyps.

Obesity is an established risk factor for colon cancer in both men and women, although the relative risks for men have been higher than those for women.[4,26] The adverse impact of being overweight or obese on colon cancer risk is stronger for distal than for proximal colon cancers. In addition, visceral adiposity appears to confer greater risk than general adiposity.[26] In the European Prospective Investigation into Cancer and Nutrition (EPIC) study, abdominal obesity as well as adult weight gain were strongly associated with colon cancer risk in both men and women.[48,49] No association between these adiposity measures and colon cancer risk was evident among postmenopausal women who had used menopausal hormone therapy, and no association was observed between any measure of adiposity and rectal cancer risk.[48] The positive association between obesity and risk of colon cancer was further supported by the findings that both general obesity and abdominal obesity increase the risk of colon adenomas[47] with one study of women indicating that the distal colon is the main target site.[50]

Given that a higher BMI and lack of physical activity are both risk factors for colon cancer, several statistical approaches have been employed to tease apart their joint and independent effects on colon cancer risk. In the Netherlands Cohort Study,[51] colorectal cancer risk was increased at each subsite among larger women in the lowest recreational activity category (<30 minutes per day) than in smaller women in the highest recreational activity category (>90 minutes per day); however, the interaction between physical activity and body size was statistically significant only for proximal tumors. Using different fatness measures for men, the only similar finding was that men with low levels of physical activity whose trouser size was below the median of that for the cohort had an increased risk of distal colon cancer; no differences in risk were noted for other subsites or for men with larger trouser sizes.[51]

The mechanisms explaining the relationship between physical activity and colon cancer are not clearly established, but include the impact on insulin sensitivity and IGF profiles, and inflammation, as well as some colon-specific mechanisms. Physical activity may stimulate stool transit in the colon, thereby decreasing the exposure of colonic mucosa to carcinogens in the stool.[6] Alternatively, physical activity–induced decreases in prostaglandin E_2 may decrease colonic cell proliferation rates and increase colonic motility.[6] In addition to steroid hormones, which have been clearly implicated as biologic modifiers of the effect of physical activity and obesity on colon cancer risk, the insulin and IGF pathways may mediate the associations between these exposures and colon cancer risk. For obesity in particular, the link can be inferred because obesity can lead to insulin resistance,[52] a syndrome characterized by high circulating insulin levels. High insulin levels appear to promote cell proliferation and tumor growth in the colon[7] and may also suppress the expression of IGF-binding proteins 1 and 2, leading to increased bioavailable IGF-1 levels.[53] Another possible mechanism is obesity-enhanced inflammation in which increases in adipose tissue macrophages lead to the secretion of inflammatory cytokines associated with colon cancer risk (e.g., tumor necrosis factor [TNF]-α, monocyte chemoattractant protein [MCP]-1, and interleukin [IL]-6).

ENDOMETRIAL CANCER

The evidence for an association between physical activity and endometrial cancer risk is accumulating[4,54–58] but is not definitive. A meta-analysis of prospective cohort studies results published through 2009 indicates that recreational physical activity lowers endometrial cancer risk by 27%, and occupational activity lowers risk by 21%.[59] Adjustments for BMI minimally change relative risk estimates, suggesting that physical activity is independently associated with endometrial cancer. Although physical activity is associated with a decreased risk of endometrial cancer in both normal-weight and obese women, two recent studies have suggested that this association is more pronounced for obese women.[54,58]

Two meta-analyses of the association between physical activity and endometrial cancer have identified some inconsistencies in dose-response relationships, indicating the importance of differences in activity type and intensity.[55,56] Little evidence exists on how long-term or lifetime physical activity and activity patterns during different life periods might influence endometrial cancer risk; it has been suggested that recent or long-term activity might be more important than activity at early ages.[56] In the CTS, higher levels of recent (at cohort formation) strenuous recreational physical activity was associated with lower levels of endometrial cancer risk; among women exercising >3 hours per week per year, risk was approximately 25% lower than that of women exercising <0.5 hour per week per year.[60] This inverse association was limited to overweight and obese women (BMI ≥25 kg/m^2). Finally, sitting time has been independently associated with increased endometrial cancer risk.[59]

Epidemiologic studies have established a strong association between obesity and endometrial cancer risk.[26] Recent studies have suggested a linear trend between increasing body weight or BMI and increasing endometrial cancer risk among postmenopausal women, whereas among premenopausal women, no trend is observed, but rather, only obese women have an increased risk.[26] Furthermore, the strong association among postmenopausal women is only observed among those who are not using hormone therapy.[26] Finally, BMI appears to exert an effect on the risk of endometrial cancer that is independent of physical activity.[55]

Physical activity and obesity are likely to influence endometrial cancer risk by altering endogenous hormone profiles.[31,53] Heavier postmenopausal women have higher circulating levels of estrogen than do lighter postmenopausal women because of the aromatization of androstenedione to estrone in adipose tissue. This is pertinent to endometrial cancer risk because this aromatization occurs in the absence of progesterone, which opposes the proliferative effects of estrogen on endometrial tissue. Physical activity may counter the proliferative effects of estrogen either directly or by restricting weight gain. Some evidence also links elevated insulin levels and diabetes to endometrial cancer risk.[61] Physical inactivity and obesity play a role in the development of insulin insensitivity and diabetes, providing another mechanism by which they may influence endometrial cancer risk.

ADENOCARCINOMA OF THE ESOPHAGUS

Several case-control studies[62–64] and one cohort study[65] have examined the association between physical activity and risk of adenocarcinoma of the esophagus. Zhang et al.[62] reported a modest association between participation in recreational physical activity more than once per week and a decreased risk of all esophageal cancer (adenocarcinomas and squamous cell tumors), although the result was not statistically significant. Lagergren et al.[63] reported no association between total, usual recreational and occupational physical activity and esophageal adenocarcinoma. Vigen et al.[64] showed that lifetime occupational physical activity was modestly associated with a lower risk of adenocarcinoma of the esophagus: the average annual level of occupational physical activity before age 65 years was associated with an approximately 40% reduction in risk of esophageal adenocarcinoma when the highest was compared with the lowest occupational physical activity category. Results from the NIH–AARP Diet and Health Study also support the hypothesis that physical activity lowers the risk of esophageal adenocarcinoma, but no association between physical activity and the risk of squamous cell esophageal cancer was found.[65]

Obesity is strongly associated with an increased risk of esophageal adenocarcinoma.[66,67] A pooled analysis of existing data showed that individuals with severe obesity (BMI $\geq$40 kg/m^2) had a 4.8-fold greater risk than individuals who were not overweight (BMI <25 kg/m^2), with similar risk estimates for men and women.[68] Several studies have examined the effect of abdominal adiposity, which have suggested that the risk associated with obesity is driven primarily by abdominal fatness.[26]

It is likely that obesity impacts esophageal adenocarcinoma risk because it is associated with the risk of gastroesophageal reflux disease (GERD). GERD may cause changes in the esophageal epithelium, leading to Barrett esophagus, a well-established precancerous condition for esophageal adenocarcinoma. On the other hand, obesity is associated with a systemic inflammatory state, which includes the exposure to adipocytokines and procoagulant factors released by adipocytes in central fat, which may also contribute to the development of esophageal adenocarcinoma.[67] Physical activity may influence the risk of esophageal adenocarcinoma by increasing digestive track transit time, thus reducing exposure of the esophagus to putative cancer-causing agents.

KIDNEY/RENAL CELL CANCER

Physical activity has been studied in relation to renal cell carcinoma in part because of the known deleterious effects of high BMI and hypertension on the risk of renal cell cancer; however, no association has been firmly established. A review of physical activity and risk of genitourinary cancers noted significant protective effects in 8 of 15 studies of physical activity in relation to renal cell carcinoma, with an average 8% reduction in risk when comparing individuals with the highest level of physical activity to those with the lowest level of activity.[69] Reductions in risk were greater for recreational than for other forms of activity and for activity performed later in life.

Obesity, in addition to high blood pressure and diabetes, is an established risk factor for kidney cancer.[26] It is still uncertain whether a gender difference exists, however. A meta-analysis has suggested a similar impact of BMI on kidney cancer risk among women and men, with an approximate 7% increase in risk per unit increase in BMI.[26] The effect of obesity may differ by histology; a recent study reported an increased risk observed for clear cell and chromophobe cancers, but not papillary renal cell cancer.[70]

PANCREATIC CANCER

Pancreatic cancer is generally diagnosed at an advanced stage and is associated with high mortality rates. A meta-analysis of 28 stud-

ies of pancreatic cancer showed that higher total lifetime physical activity and occupational activity were associated with a lower risk.[71] Nonsignificant reductions in risk were observed for recreational physical activity and transportation (walking and cycling as a form of commuting). Significant heterogeneity was present across the studies, making it difficult to find a definitive answer.

Evidence indicating that obesity is a risk factor for pancreatic cancer is convincing. Three large pooled analyses and three of four meta-analyses that encompass a range of well-designed, independent observational epidemiologic studies have demonstrated a positive association between obesity and pancreatic cancer risk.[72,73] Effects were relatively consistent across studies, with an approximate 10% or greater increase in risk for every 5 kg/m^2 increase in BMI. Two of the pooled analyses and one of the meta-analyses assessed measures of adiposity such as waist circumference or waist-to-hip ratio (WHR); each of the results suggested positive associations with pancreatic cancer risk.[72,74,75] The pooled analyses reported at least a 35% greater risk when the fourth quartile of WHR was compared to the first quartile. The meta-analysis study reported an 11% increase in risk associated with each 10-cm increase in waist circumference and a 19% increase in risk for each 0.1-unit increment in WHR.

GALLBLADDER CANCER

Gallbladder cancer occurs more frequently in women than in men, and the major risk factor is a history of gallstones,[10] which has been associated with the use of exogenous estrogens.[76] To date, we have found no epidemiologic literature investigating the possible association of physical activity and gallbladder cancer, although several studies have suggested a positive association between obesity and gallbladder cancer. In a meta-analysis comprised of 3,288 cases derived from eight cohort studies and three case-control studies, obesity was associated with a 66% increased risk of gallbladder cancer, and the increase in risk was larger for women than for men.[77] Further, two studies found that WHR was positively associated with gallbladder cancer risk among men and women with and without a history of gallstones, suggesting that abdominal obesity may be important in the etiology of this disease.[78,79]

NON-HODGKIN LYMPHOMA

Studies addressing physical inactivity and obesity as potential risk factors for NHL have been mixed, in part because they have not had a sufficient number of cases to assess risk by NHL subtype. Generally, studies have shown no overall association between physical activity and NHL risk.[4] The results of four cohort studies, the CTS,[80] WHI,[81] EPIC,[82] and the American Cancer Society Prevention Study-II[83] have been unconvincing, with WHI showing a nonstatistically significant positive association, whereas the other studies showed no association.

In 2008, the International Lymphoma Epidemiology Consortium (InterLymph) published a pooled analysis of 18 case-control studies with more than 10,000 cases reporting no association between BMI around the time of diagnosis and NHL risk overall, but an increased risk of diffuse NHL for severe obesity (BMI $\geq$40 kg/m^2).[84] The results from meta-analyses of cohort studies suggested a weak positive association overall and for diffuse NHL.[85,86] An analysis of two cohort studies has suggested that body size in early adulthood may be more predictive of NHL risk than that later in life for all NHL and for the diffuse and follicular subtypes.[87]

PROSTATE CANCER

More than 20 studies have assessed the potential association between physical activity and prostate cancer.[4,88,89] Regardless of the different approaches used, the populations studied, or the sample sizes of the studies, the majority of studies have suggested a modest reduction in risk with an increased level of physical activity.[4] In a review of the literature, Friedenreich and Orenstein[88] concluded that prostate cancer risk is reduced 10% to 30% when comparing the most active with the least active men and suggested that it may be high levels of physical activity earlier in life that are most relevant to this disease. An update to this review, based on 22 additional studies, indicates that the majority of recent research studies observed protective effects.[90] Leitzmann and Rohrmann[91] added that the associations with reduced risk may be most apparent for fatal prostate cancer. A current systematic review and meta-analysis, including 19 cohort and 24 case-control studies, agrees.[92] A pooled 19% reduction in risk was observed for occupational physical activity, and a 5% reduction was observed for recreational physical activity comparing the most physically active men to the least active.[92] An issue that somewhat reduces our confidence in these estimates is that considerable heterogeneity between studies was observed. Further, it is not yet clear whether these results reflect a true causal association or whether they are due to confounding by prostate-specific antigen testing, which may be more common among physically active men.

The early epidemiologic literature on the potential association between obesity and prostate cancer provided no consistent evidence of any relationship.[4] Recent studies have suggested that obesity may have a dual effect on prostate cancer risk. One meta-analysis reported that the risk of early-stage prostate cancer decreased by 6%, whereas the risk of advanced prostate cancer increased 9% per 5-kg/m^2 increase in BMI.[93] Another possibility is that obesity may decrease the likelihood of diagnosis of less aggressive prostate cancer. Proposed mechanisms include the paradoxical effects of testosterone on low-grade versus more advanced prostate cancer and alterations in insulin and circulating IGF-1.[94]

LUNG CANCER

Physical activity may reduce lung cancer risk by 30% to 40%,[88] but no definitive conclusion can be drawn because one cannot ignore potential residual confounding or effect modification due to smoking as an explanation for any observed association. Recent studies have attempted to address this issue by estimating risk within subgroups defined by smoking status. A recent review suggests an inverse relationship between heavy lifetime physical activity and lung cancer in former and current smokers that is consistent across all histologies, but is not observed among never smokers.[5] A small case-control study of current and former smokers enrolled in the Cologne Smoking Study came to a similar conclusion, observing a lower risk of lung cancer among participants who were physically active compared to those who were not.[95] In the large NIH–AARP Diet and Health Study, no associations were observed between occupational or recreation physical activity and lung cancer risk among those who never smoked.[96]

Due to sex differences in lung cancer pathology, risk factors, and prognosis, current research has also begun to investigate the association for men and women separately.[97] The recent literature consists of small case-control studies,[98] which lack statistical power to examine risks in subgroups defined by histology, smoking status, or sex, and which may be affected by survival bias in that rapidly fatal cases or those who are too ill to be interviewed are excluded from the study population.

Several studies have suggested the existence of an inverse association between increasing BMI and lung cancer risk.[99–102] Nevertheless, this inverse effect may have been due to residual confounding by smoking because the inverse association was restricted to ever smokers. One meta-analysis showed an inverse association between BMI and lung cancer in nonsmokers[103]; however, caution should be exercised when interpreting the results due to concerns about heterogeneity of risk estimates across studies, the quality of the original studies, and confounding by smoking.[104]

OVARIAN CANCER

The literature on ovarian cancer risk in relation to physical activity and obesity has been inconclusive. More than 18 studies have assessed the impact of physical activity on ovarian cancer risk. A meta-analysis of 12 studies found an approximate 20% decrease in ovarian cancer risk associated with physical activity when the highest category of exercise was compared to the lowest.[105] Four[106–109] of five[110] additional studies found no association; the fifth study found a nonsignificant 10% to 20% reduction in ovarian cancer risk for women who participated in at least 1 hour per week of recreational aerobic activity.

The evidence for an association between obesity and increased ovarian cancer risk is weak, with few studies showing a statistically significant result.[4,111] A meta-analysis of 16 studies indicated that adult obesity increases the risk for ovarian cancer; the overall pooled effect estimate was a 30% increase in ovarian cancer risk associated with adult obesity with a possible dose-response effect, but no variation in risk estimates across histologic subtypes.[111] In contrast, the results from the Ovarian Cancer Association Consortium, based on original data from 15 case-control studies, suggest that obesity only increases the risk of the less common histologic subtypes of ovarian cancer; obesity does not increase risk of high-grade invasive serous cancers, the most common subtype.[112] A pooled analysis of 12 cohort studies reported that BMI was not associated with ovarian cancer risk in postmenopausal women, but was positively associated with risk in premenopausal women.[113] Another meta-analysis, using 47 studies, showed that the positive association between BMI and ovarian cancer was restricted to women who had never used hormone therapy; among these women, risk increased by 10% with every 5 kg/m^2 increase in BMI.[114]

CONCLUSIONS

Table 10.1 illustrates the strength of evidence regarding increased physical activity as a protective factor and obesity as a risk factor

---

TABLE 10.1

Summary of the Strength of the Observational Epidemiologic Evidence for Physical Activity as a Protective Factor and Obesity as a Risk Factor for Cancer, By Type of Cancer

	Physical Activity	Overweight/ Obesity
Breast, postmenopausal	+++	+++
Breast, premenopausal	++	++ (protection)
Colon	+++	+++
Endometrium	+	+++
Esophagus, adenocarcinoma	?	+++
Kidney/renal cell	?	+++
Gallbladder	?	++
Pancreas	?	+++
Non-Hodgkin lymphoma	?	+
Prostate, aggressive	+	+
Lung	+	?
Ovary	?	?

+++, evidence is convincing; ++, evidence is probable; +, evidence is possible; ?, evidence remains insufficient/inconclusive.

for cancer. The strength of evidence for each exposure is classified as convincing (+++), probable (++), possible (+), or insufficient and inconclusive (?). Overall, for physical activity, convincing evidence exists for an association with postmenopausal breast cancer and colon cancer; for obesity, the evidence is convincing for breast, colon, endometrial, esophageal, and kidney/renal cell cancer. Evidence for associations between these exposures and several other cancer sites is accumulating. Despite some convincing evidence of the effects of physical activity and obesity on the risk of certain cancers, it is difficult to make recommendations as to appropriate changes in lifestyle that will reduce a person's chances of developing cancer. We have no physical activity prescriptions to give at this time. Many questions remain to be answered: What are

the ages at which physical activity will provide the most benefit? What types of activity should one do and at what intensity, frequency (times per week), and duration (hours per week)? Similarly, for BMI, is there some threshold below which the individual will not have excess cancer risk? Does purposeful weight loss during the adult years lower the risk associated with being overweight or obese? Finally, necessary research is ongoing to identify the biologic mechanisms that account for these effects and to determine whether all persons are affected equally. For instance, it is possible that genetically defined subgroups of the population respond to physical activity or obesity differently. Understanding mechanisms and population variation in these effects will illuminate appropriate prescriptions for lifestyle change.

SELECTED REFERENCES

The full reference list can be accessed at lwwhealthlibrary.com/oncology.

4. Vainio H, Bianchini F, eds. *IARC Handbooks of Cancer Prevention Volume 6: Weight Control and Physical Activity.* Lyon, France: IARC Press; 2000.
7. Gunter MJ, Leitzmann MF. Obesity and colorectal cancer: epidemiology, mechanisms and candidate genes. *J Nutr Biochem* 2006;17(3):145–156.
8. Monninkhof EM, Elias SG, Vlems FA, et al. Physical activity and breast cancer: a systematic review. *Epidemiol* 2007;18(1):137–157.
9. World Cancer Research Fund/American Institute for Cancer Research. *Food, Nutrition, Physical Activity, and the Prevention of Cancer: A Global Perspective.* Washington, D.C.: World Cancer Research Fund/American Institute for Cancer Research; 2007.
26. Boeing H. Obesity and cancer—the update 2013. *Best Pract Res Clin Endocrinol Metab* 2013;27(2):219–227.
31. Bernstein L. Epidemiology of endocrine-related risk factors for breast cancer. *J Mammary Gland Biol Neoplasia* 2002;7(1):3–15.
40. Brown KA, Simpson ER. Obesity and breast cancer: progress to understanding the relationship. *Cancer Res* 2010;70(1):4–7.
41. Friedenreich CM, Neilson HK, Lynch BM. State of the epidemiological evidence on physical activity and cancer prevention. *Eur J Cancer* 2010; 46(14):2593–2604.
43. Wolin KY, Yan Y, Colditz GA, et al. Physical activity and colon cancer prevention: a meta-analysis. *Br J Cancer* 2009;100(4):611–616.
44. Boyle T, Keegel T, Bull F, et al. Physical activity and risks of proximal and distal colon cancers: a systematic review and meta-analysis. *J Natl Cancer Inst* 2012;104(20):1548–1561.
53. Calle EE, Kaaks R. Overweight, obesity and cancer: epidemiological evidence and proposed mechanisms. *Nat Rev Cancer* 2004;4(8):579–591.
55. Voskuil DW, Monninkhof EM, Elias SG, et al. Physical activity and endometrial cancer risk, a systematic review of current evidence. *Cancer Epidemiol Biomarkers Prev* 2007;16(4):639–648.
56. Cust AE, Armstrong BK, Friedenreich CM, et al. Physical activity and endometrial cancer risk: a review of the current evidence, biologic mechanisms and the quality of physical activity assessment methods. *Cancer Causes Control* 2007;18(3):243–258.
61. Kaaks R, Lukanova A, Kurzer MS. Obesity, endogenous hormones, and endometrial cancer risk: a synthetic review. *Cancer Epidemiol Biomarkers Prev* 2002;11(12):1531–1543.
66. Lepage C, Drouillard A, Jouve JL, et al. Epidemiology and risk factors for oesophageal adenocarcinoma. *Dig Liver Dis* 2013;45(8):625–629.

68. Hoyo C, Cook MB, Kamangar F, et al. Body mass index in relation to oesophageal and oesophagogastric junction adenocarcinomas: a pooled analysis from the International BEACON Consortium. *Int J Epidemiol* 2012;41(6):1706–1718.
69. Leitzmann MF. Physical activity and genitourinary cancer prevention. *Recent Results Cancer Res* 2011;186:43–71.
71. O'Rorke MA, Cantwell MM, Cardwell CR, et al. Can physical activity modulate pancreatic cancer risk? A systematic review and meta-analysis. *Int J Cancer* 2010;126(12):2957–2968.
72. Aune D, Greenwood DC, Chan DS, et al. Body mass index, abdominal fatness and pancreatic cancer risk: a systematic review and non-linear dose-response meta-analysis of prospective studies. *Ann Oncol* 2012;23(4): 843–852.
77. Larsson SC, Wolk A. Obesity and the risk of gallbladder cancer: a meta-analysis. *Br J Cancer* 2007;96(9):1457–1461.
84. Willett EV, Morton LM, Hartge P, et al. Non-Hodgkin lymphoma and obesity: a pooled analysis from the InterLymph Consortium. *Int J Cancer* 2008;122(9):2062–2070.
85. Larsson SC, Wolk A. Body mass index and risk of non-Hodgkin's and Hodgkin's lymphoma: a meta-analysis of prospective studies. *Eur J Cancer* 2011;47(16):2422–2430.
90. Young-McCaughan S. Potential for prostate cancer prevention through physical activity. *World J Urol* 2012;30(2):167–179.
92. Liu Y, Hu F, Li D, et al. Does physical activity reduce the risk of prostate cancer? A systematic review and meta-analysis. *Eur Urol* 2011;60(5):1029–1044.
93. Discacciati A, Orsini N, Wolk A. Body mass index and incidence of localized and advanced prostate cancer—a dose-response meta-analysis of prospective studies. *Ann Oncol* 2012;23(7):1665–1671.
97. Tardon A, Lee WJ, Delgado-Rodriguez M, et al. Leisure-time physical activity and lung cancer: a meta-analysis. *Cancer Causes Control* 2005;16(4): 389–397.
103. Yang Y, Dong J, Sun K, et al. Obesity and incidence of lung cancer: a meta-analysis. *Int J Cancer* 2013;132(5):1162–1169.
112. Olsen CM, Nagle CM, Whiteman DC, et al. Obesity and risk of ovarian cancer subtypes: evidence from the Ovarian Cancer Association Consortium. *Endocr Relat Cancer* 2013;20(2):251–262.
114. Collaborative Group on Epidemiological Studies of Ovarian Cancer. Ovarian cancer and body size: individual participant meta-analysis including 25,157 women with ovarian cancer from 47 epidemiological studies. *PLoS Med* 2012;9(4):e1001200.

11 Epidemiologic Methods

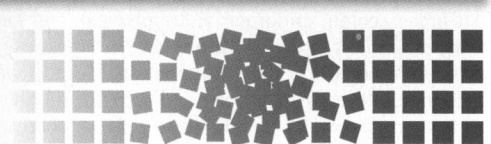

Xiaomei Ma and Herbert Yu

INTRODUCTION

Epidemiology is the study of the distribution and determinants of health-related states or events in specified populations and the application of this study to control health problems.[1] Epidemiologic principles and methods have long been applied to cancer research, with the assumptions that cancer does not occur at random and the nonrandomness of carcinogenesis can be elucidated through systematic research. An example of such applications is the lung cancer study conducted by Doll and Hill in the early 1950s, which linked tobacco smoking to an increased mortality of lung cancer in over 40,000 medical professionals in the United Kingdom.[2] The observation from this study and many other studies, in conjunction with laboratory findings regarding the underlying biologic mechanisms for the effect of tobacco smoking, helped establish the role of tobacco smoking in the etiology of lung cancer. Epidemiologic methods are also used in clinical settings, where trials are conducted to evaluate the efficacy of new treatment protocols or preventive measures and where observational studies of prognostic factors are done.

Epidemiologic studies can take different forms, but generally they can be classified into two broad categories, observational studies and experimental studies (Fig. 11.1). In experimental studies, an investigator allocates different study regimens to the subjects, usually with randomization (experimental studies without randomization are sometimes referred to as "quasi-experiments").[3] Experimental studies can be individual based or community based. An experimental study most closely resembles laboratory experiments in that the investigator has control over the study condition. Experimental studies can be used to evaluate the efficacy of a treatment protocol (e.g., low-dose compared with standard-dose chemotherapy for non-Hodgkin's lymphoma)[4] or preventive measures (e.g., tamoxifen for women at an increased risk of breast cancer).[5] Although experimental studies are often considered the "gold standard" because of well-controlled study situations, they are only suitable for the evaluation of effects that are beneficial or at least not harmful due to ethical concerns. Experimental studies are discussed in detail in other chapters of this book. This section will focus on observational studies.

Observational studies do not involve the artificial manipulation of study regimens. In an observational study, an investigator stands by to observe what happens or happened to the subjects, in terms of exposure and outcome. Observational studies can be further divided into descriptive and analytical studies (see Fig. 11.1). Descriptive studies focus on the *distribution* of diseases with respect to person, place, and time (i.e., who, where, and when), whereas analytical studies focus on the *determinants* of diseases. Descriptive studies are often used to *generate* hypotheses, whereas analytical studies are often used to *test* hypotheses. However, the two types of studies should not be considered mutually exclusive entities; rather, they are the opposite ends of a continuum. Descriptive studies are discussed in detail in other chapters of this book.

ANALYTICAL STUDIES

Ecologic Studies

As in experimental studies, the unit of analysis can be individuals or groups of people in observational studies. Studies that use groups of people as the unit of analysis are called ecologic studies, which are relatively easy to carry out when group level measures are available. However, a relationship observed between variables on a group level does not necessarily reflect the relationship that exists at an individual level. For example, the fraction of energy supply from animal products was found to be positively correlated with breast cancer mortality in a recent ecologic study, which used preexisting data on both dietary supply and breast cancer mortality rates from 35 countries.[6] Because the data were country based, no reliable inference can be made at an individual level. Within each country, it could be that the people who had a low fraction of energy supply from animal products were actually dying from breast cancer. Results from ecologic studies are useful for inference at an individual level only when the within-group variability of the exposure is low so that a group-level measure can reasonably reflect exposure at an individual level. Alternatively, if the implications for prevention or intervention are at a group level (e.g., taxation of cigarettes to reduce smoking), results from ecologic studies are very useful.

Cross-Sectional Studies

There are three main types of analytical studies in which the unit of analysis is individuals: cross-sectional, cohort, and case-control studies. In a cross-sectional study, the information on various factors is collected from the study population at a given point in time. From a public health perspective, data collected in cross-sectional studies can be of great value in assessing the general health status of a population and allocating resources. For example, the National Health and Nutrition Examination Survey has provided valuable national estimates of health and nutritional status of the US civilian, noninstitutionalized population.[7] Findings from cross-sectional studies can also help generate hypotheses that may be tested later in other types of studies. However, it should be noted that cross-sectional studies have serious methodologic limitations if the research purpose is etiologic inference. Because exposures and disease status are evaluated simultaneously, it is usually not possible to know the temporality of events unless the exposure cannot change over time (e.g., blood type, skin color, race, country of birth). If one observes that more brain cancer patients are depressed than people without brain cancer in a cross-sectional study, the correlation does not necessarily mean that depression causes brain cancer. Depression may simply have resulted from the pathogenesis and diagnosis of brain cancer, or depression may

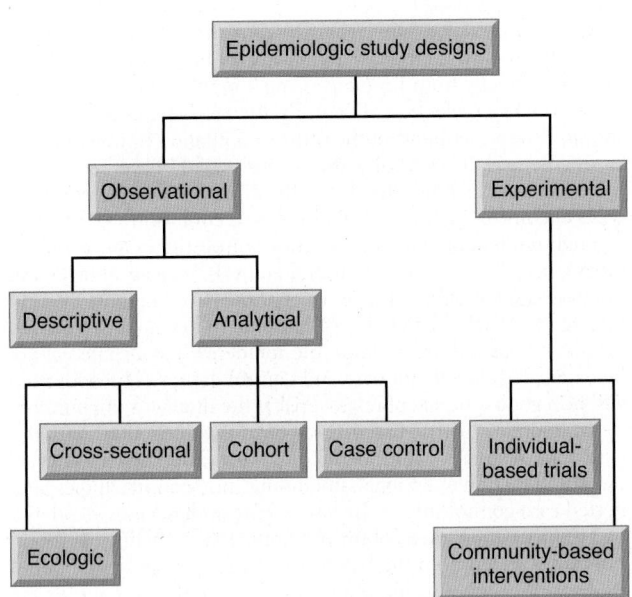

Figure 11.1 Classification of epidemiologic study designs.

have caused brain cancer in some patients and resulted from brain cancer in other patients. Without additional information on the timing of events, no conclusions can be made. Another concern in cross-sectional studies is the enrollment of prevalent cases, who survived different lengths of time after the incidence of disease. Factors that affect survival may also influence incidence. Prevalent cases may not be representative of incident cases, which makes etiologic inferences based on cross-sectional studies suspect at best.

Cohort Studies

In a cohort study, a study population free of a specific disease (or any other health-related condition) is grouped based on their exposure status and followed up for a certain period of time. Then the exposed and unexposed subjects are compared with respect to disease status at the end of the follow-up. The objective of a cohort study is usually to evaluate whether the incidence of a disease is associated with an exposure. The cohort design is fundamental in observational epidemiology and is considered "ideal" in that, if unbiased, cohort data reflect the real-life cause/effect sequence of disease.[8] Subjects in cohort studies may be a sample of the general population in a geographic area, a group of workers who are exposed to certain occupational hazards in a specific industry, or people who are considered at a high risk for a specific disease. A cohort study is considered prospective or concurrent if the investigator starts following up the cohort from the present time into the future, and retrospective or historical if the cohort is established in the past based on existing records (e.g., an occupational cohort based on employment records) and the follow-up ends before or at the time of the study. Alternatively, a cohort study can be ambidirectional in that data collection goes both directions.[9] Whether a cohort study is prospective, retrospective, or ambidirectional, the key feature is that all the subjects were free of the disease at the beginning of the follow-up and the study tracks the subjects from exposure to disease. Follow-up time, ranging from days to decades, is an essential element in cohort studies.

In a cohort study, the incidence of disease in the exposed group and the unexposed group is compared. The incidence measure can be cumulative incidence or incidence density, depending on the availability of data. When comparing the incidence in the two groups, both relative differences and absolute differences can be assessed. In cohort studies, the relative risk of developing the disease is expressed as the ratio of the cumulative incidence in the exposed group to that in the unexposed group, which is also called cumulative incidence ratio or risk ratio. If we have data on the exact person-time of follow-up for every subject, we can also calculate an incidence density ratio (also called rate ratio) in a similar way. The numeric value of the risk or rate ratio reflects the magnitude of the association between an exposure and a disease. For example, a risk ratio of 2 would be interpreted as exposed individuals have a doubled risk of developing a disease than unexposed individuals, whereas a risk ratio of 5 indicates that exposed individuals have 5 times the risk of developing a disease compared with unexposed individuals. To put in another way, a factor with a risk ratio of 5 has a stronger effect than another factor with a risk ratio of 2. In addition to risk ratio and rate ratio, another relative measure called probability odds ratio can be calculated in cohort studies. The probability odds of disease is the number of subjects who developed a disease divided by the number of subjects who did not develop the disease, and the probability odds ratio is the probability odds in the exposed group divided by the probability odds in the unexposed group. Many investigators prefer risk ratio or rate ratio to probability odds ratio in cohort studies, because the ability to directly measure the risk of developing a disease is one of the most significant advantages in cohort studies. In practice, however, a probability odds ratio is often used as an approximation for risk or rate ratio, especially when multivariate logistic regression models are employed to adjust for the effect of other factors that may influence the relationship between an exposure and a disease.

As for absolute differences, a commonly used measure is called attributable risk in the exposed, which is the incidence in the exposed group minus the incidence in the unexposed group. Attributable risk reflects the disease incidence that could be attributed to the exposure in exposed individuals and the reduction in incidence that we would expect if the exposure can be removed from the exposed individuals, provided that there is a causal relationship between the exposure and the disease. Another absolute measure called population attributable risk extends this concept to the general population; it estimates the disease incidence that could be attributed to an exposure in the general population. Because both relative and absolute differences can be assessed in cohort studies, a natural question to ask is what measures to choose. In general, the relative differences are used more often if the main research objective is etiologic inference, and they can be used for the judgment of causality. Once causality is established, or at least assumed, measures of absolute differences are more important from a public health perspective. This point can be illustrated using the following hypothetical example. Assume the following: toxin X in the environment triples the risk of bladder cancer and toxin Y doubles the risk of bladder cancer, the effects of X and Y are entirely independent of each other, the prevalence of exposure to toxin Y in the general population is 20 times higher than the prevalence of exposure to toxin X, and there are only resources available to reduce the exposure to one toxin. It would be more effective to use the resources to reduce the exposure to toxin Y instead of toxin X. This is because the population attributable risk due to Y is higher than that due to X, although the risk ratio associated with toxin Y is smaller than that associated with toxin X.

Cohort studies have many advantages. A cohort design is the best way to study the natural history of a disease.[9] There is usually a clear temporal relationship between an exposure and a disease because all the subjects are free of the disease at the beginning of the follow-up (it can be a problem if a subject has a subclinical disease such as undetected prostate cancer). Furthermore, multiple diseases can be studied with respect to the same exposure. On the other hand, cohort studies, especially prospective cohort studies, are costly in terms of both time and money. A cohort design requires the follow-up of a large number of study participants over a sometimes extremely lengthy period of time and usually extensive data collection through questionnaires, physical measurements, and/or biologic specimens at regular intervals. Participants may be

ETIOLOGY AND EPIDEMIOLOGY OF CANCER

"lost" during the follow-up because they became tired of the study, moved away from the study area, or died from some causes other than the disease under study. If the subjects who were lost during the follow-up are different from those who remained under observation with respect to exposure, disease, or other factors that may influence the relationship between the exposure and the disease, results from the study may be biased. To date, cohort studies have been used to study the etiology of a wide spectrum of diseases, including different types of cancer. If a cohort study is conducted to evaluate the etiology of cancer, usually the study sample size would need to be very large (such as the National Institutes of Health-AARP Diet and Health Study, which included more than half million subjects[10]) and the follow-up time would need to be long, unless the cohort selected is a high-risk population.

For simplicity, we have discussed cohort studies in which the outcome of interest is the incidence of a specific disease and there are only two exposure groups. In practice, any health-related event can be the outcome of interest, and multiple exposure groups can be compared.

Case-Control Studies

Case-control design is an alternative to cohort design for the evaluation of the relationship between an exposure and a disease (or any other health condition). A case-control approach compares the odds of past exposure between cases and noncases (controls) and uses the exposure odds ratio as an estimate for relative risk. A primary goal in a case-control study is to reach the same conclusions as what would have been obtained from a cohort study, if one had been done.[11] If appropriately designed and conducted, a case-control study can optimize speed and efficiency as the need for follow-up is avoided.[8] The starting point of a case-control study is a source population from which the cases arise. Instead of obtaining the denominators for the calculation of risks or rates in a cohort study, a control group is sampled from the entire source population. After selecting control subjects, who ideally would have become cases had they developed the disease, an investigator collects data on past exposures from both the cases and the controls and then calculates an odds ratio, which is the odds of exposure in the cases divided by the odds of exposure in the controls.

There are two main types of case-control studies: case-based case-control studies and case-control studies within defined cohorts.[8] Some variations of the case-control design also exist. For instance, if the effect of an exposure is transient, sometimes a case can be used as his/her own control (case cross-over design). In case-based case-control studies, cases and controls are selected at a given point in time from a hypothetical cohort (e.g., at the end of follow-up). A cross-sectional ascertainment of cases will result in a case group that mostly contains prevalent cases who may have survived for different lengths of time after disease incidence. Cases who died before an investigator began subject ascertainment would not be eligible to be included in the study. As a result, the cases finally included in the study may not be representative of all the cases from the entire hypothetical cohort. Another disadvantage of enrolling prevalent cases is that cases that were diagnosed a long time ago will likely have difficulties recalling exposures that occurred before the disease incidence. In case-control studies, it is preferable to ascertain incident cases as soon as they are diagnosed and to select controls as soon as cases are identified. Case-control studies that enroll only incident cases are sometimes called *prospective* case-control studies because the investigators need to wait for the incident cases to develop and get diagnosed. For cancer studies, the cases can be ascertained from population-based cancer registries or hospitals. A major advantage of using a cancer registry is the completeness of case ascertainment; however, the reporting of cancer cases to registries is usually not instantaneous. There could be a lag time of several months or even over a year, and some cases could have died during the lag time. If the cancer

under study has a poor survival rate and/or clinical specimens need to be obtained in a timely manner, it may be preferable to identify cases directly from hospitals using a rapid ascertainment protocol. As for the selection of controls, the key issue is that controls should be representative of the source population from which the cases arise and, theoretically, the controls would have been ascertained as cases had they developed the disease. The most common types of controls include population-based controls (often selected through random digit dialing in case-control studies of cancer etiology), hospital controls, and friend controls. The advantages and disadvantages of different types of controls have been nicely summarized by Wacholder et al.[12] Because no follow-up is involved in case-based case-control studies, the incidence risk or rate cannot be calculated directly for case and control groups. The odds ratio will be a good estimate of relative risk if the disease is uncommon.

In addition to case-based case-control studies, there are also case-control studies within defined cohorts (also known as hybrid or ambidirectional designs), including case-cohort studies and nested case-control studies. In case-cohort studies, cases are identified from a well-defined cohort after some follow-up time, and controls are selected from the baseline cohort. In nested case-control studies, cases are also identified from a cohort, but controls are selected from the individuals at risk at the time each case occurs (i.e., incidence density sampling).[8] In these types of designs, controls are a sample of the cohort and the controls selected can theoretically become cases at some point. The possibility of selection bias in case-control studies within defined cohorts is lower than that in case-based case-control studies because the cases and the controls are selected from the same source population. Because of an increased awareness of the methodological issues inherent in the design of case-based case-control studies and the availability of a growing number of large cohorts, case-control studies within defined cohorts have become more common in recent years. The advantage of case-control studies within cohorts over traditional cohort studies is mainly the efficiency in additional data collection. For instance, a recent nested case-control study evaluated the relationship between endogenous sex hormones and prostate cancer risk.[13] Instead of measuring the serum hormones levels of the entire cohort (over 12,000 subjects), investigators chose to measure 300 cases and 300 controls selected from the cohort. Doing so not only significantly reduced the cost of measurements and the time it took to address the research question, but also helped preserve valuable serum samples for possible analyses in the future. In a case-cohort design, an odds ratio estimates risk ratio; in a nested case-control design, an odds ratio estimates rate ratio. In both designs, the disease under study does not have to be rare for the odds ratio to be a good estimate of the risk ratio or rate ratio.[8,14]

The biggest advantage of a case-control design is the speed and efficiency of obtaining data. It is claimed that investigators implement case-control studies more frequently than any other analytical epidemiologic study.[15] Because most types of cancer are uncommon and take a long time to develop, to date, most epidemiologic studies of cancer have been case-control instead of cohort in design. A case-control study can be conducted to evaluate the relationship between many different exposures and a specific disease, but the study will have limited statistical power if the exposure is rare. In general, a case-control design tends to be more susceptible to biases than a cohort design. Such biases include, but are not limited to, selection bias when choosing and enrolling subjects (especially controls) and recall bias when obtaining data from the subjects. The status of the subjects—that is, case or control—may affect how they recall and report previous exposures, some of which occurred years or even decades ago. It is important for investigators to explicitly define the diagnostic and eligibility criteria for cases, to select controls from the same population as the cases independent of the exposures of interest, to blind data collection staff to the case or control status of subjects and/or the main hypotheses of the study, to ascertain exposure in a similar manner from cases and controls, and to take into account other factors that may influence the relationship between an exposure and a disease.[15]

INTERPRETATION OF EPIDEMIOLOGIC FINDINGS

We have discussed measures of effects in various study designs. However, a risk ratio of 3 from a cohort study or an odds ratio of 2.5 from a case-control study does not necessarily mean that there is an association between an exposure and a disease. Several alternative explanations need to be assessed, including chance (random error), bias (systematic error), and confounding. Potential interaction also needs be evaluated.

Statistical methods are required to evaluate the role of chance. A usual way is to calculate the upper and lower limits of a 95% confidence interval around a point estimate for relative risk (risk ratio, rate ratio, or odds ratio). If the confidence interval does not include one, one would say that the observed association is statistically significant; if the confidence interval includes one, one would say that the observed relationship is not statistically significant. The width of a confidence interval is directly related to the number of participants in a study, which is called sample size. A larger sample size leads to less variability in the data, a tighter confidence interval, and a higher possibility in finding a statistically significant association if one truly exists. A 95% confidence interval means that if the data collection and analysis could be replicated many times, the confidence interval should include the correct value of the measure 95% of the time.[16] It is better to consider a confidence interval to be a general guide to the amount of random error in the data but not necessarily a literal measure of statistical variability.[16]

Bias can be defined as any systematic error in an epidemiologic study that results in an incorrect estimate of the association between exposure and disease, and it can occur in every type of epidemiologic study design. There are two main types of bias: selection bias and information bias. Selection bias is present when individuals included in a study are systematically different from the target population. For example, a selection bias would occur if a study aimed to generate a sample representing all women in the United States, but of the women contacted, more with a family history of breast cancer agreed to participate. This sample would be at a higher risk for breast cancer than the target population. Refusal to participate poses a constant challenge in epidemiologic studies. As individuals have become more concerned about privacy issues and as studies have become more demanding of time, biologic specimens, and other impositions, participation rates have dropped substantially in recent years. If nonparticipants are different from the participants with respect to study-related characteristics, the validity of the study is threatened. Information bias occurs when the data collected from the study subjects are erroneous. Information bias is also known as misclassification if the variable is measured on a categorical scale and the error causes a subject to be placed in a wrong category. Misclassification can happen to both exposure and disease. For example, in a case-control study of previous reproductive history and ovarian cancer, a woman who had an extremely early pregnancy loss might not even realize that she was ever pregnant and would mistakenly report no pregnancy, and another woman who has only subclinical presentations of ovarian cancer might be mistakenly selected as a control. Misclassification can be differential or nondifferential. An exposure misclassification is considered differential if it is related to disease status and nondifferential if not related to disease status. Similarly, a disease misclassification is considered differential if it is related to exposure status and nondifferential if not related to exposure status. If a binary exposure variable and a binary disease variable are analyzed, a nondifferential misclassification will result in an underestimate of the true association. Differential misclassification can either exaggerate or underestimate a true effect. Usually not much can be done to control or correct bias at the data analysis stage; therefore,

it is important to establish research protocols that are not prone to bias. The evaluation of potential bias is critical to the interpretation of study results. An invalid estimate is worse than no estimate.

Confounding refers to a situation in which the association between an exposure and a disease (or any health-related condition) is influenced by a third variable. This third variable is considered a confounding variable or confounder. A confounder must fulfill three criteria: (1) be associated with the exposure, (2) be associated with the disease independent of the exposure, and (3) not be an intermediate step between the exposure and the disease (i.e., not on the causal pathway). Unlike bias, which is primarily introduced by the investigator or study participants, confounding is a function of the complex interrelationship between various exposures and disease.[17] In a hypothetical case-control study of the effect of alcohol drinking on lung cancer, we may observe an odds ratio of 2.5 (usually called a "crude" odds ratio in the sense that no other variables were taken into account), which indicates that alcohol drinking increases the risk of lung cancer by 1.5-fold. However, if we classify all study subjects into two strata based on a history of cigarette smoking and then calculate the odds ratio in the two strata (smokers and nonsmokers) separately, we may have two stratum-specific odds ratios both equal to one, indicating that alcohol drinking is not associated with lung cancer risk. In this example, the crude odds ratio calculated to estimate the association between alcohol drinking and lung cancer without considering smoking is simply misleading. Being associated with both the exposure (i.e., alcohol drinking) and the disease (i.e., lung cancer), smoking acted as a confounder in this example. A stratified analysis is needed to evaluate the potential confounding effect of a third variable, whether it is done with pencil and paper or statistical modeling. Usually data are stratified based on the level of a third variable. If the stratum-specific effect measures are similar to each other but different from the crude effect measure, confounding is said to be present. In this section, we have illustrated basic epidemiologic principles using an overly simplified scenario and only considered a single exposure. In practice, most if not all diseases, cancer included, have a multifactorial etiology. Consequently, it is usually necessary to assess the potential confounding effect of a group of variables simultaneously using multivariate statistical models. The effect measure derived from a multivariate model will then be called an "adjusted" one in the sense that the effect of other factors was also adjusted for. Without controlling for the potential effect of other variables, an investigator cannot really judge whether an observed association between a given exposure and a specific disease is spurious.

If the effect of an exposure on the risk of a disease is not homogeneous in strata formed by a third variable, the third variable is considered an effect modifier, and the situation is called interaction or effect modification. Put in other words, interaction exists when the stratum-specific effect measures are different from each other. In the lung cancer example given previously, if the odds ratio for alcohol drinking is 1 in smokers but 3 in nonsmokers, then there is interaction and smoking is an effect modifier. The evaluation of interaction is essentially a stratified analysis, which is similar to the evaluation of confounding. Confounding and interaction can be both present in a given study. However, when interaction occurs, the stratum-specific effect measures should be reported. It is no longer appropriate to report a summary measure in the presence of interaction. Unlike confounding, which is a nuisance that an investigator hopes to remove, interaction is a more detailed description of the true relationship between an exposure and a disease.

CANCER OUTCOMES RESEARCH

The discussion of epidemiologic methods in this section focuses primarily on etiological research, which aims at identifying the risk factors of cancer. However, similar principles and methods are applicable to cancer outcomes research, which aims at studying a variety of factors related to the early identification, treatment, prognosis, health related quality of life, and cost of care. Cancer outcomes research can be experimental or observational in nature. For example, randomized clinical trials have been conducted to assess the impact of screening on prostate cancer mortality[18] and to compare the effect of radical prostatectomy versus observation in patients with localized prostate cancer.[19] Observational studies of cancer outcomes, especially those that build upon preexisting resources,[20,21] can be carried out in a large group of patients with relatively little cost to capture the patterns and cost of care and to address many other research questions that have important clinical implications. Although the findings of such observation studies are subject to bias and confounding inherent in an observational design, these studies are complementary to experimental studies and have their unique value. Given an increasing interest in improving the effectiveness and value of cancer care, more cancer outcomes research is to be expected in the future.

MOLECULAR EPIDEMIOLOGY

Molecular epidemiology involves multidisciplinary and transdisciplinary research that entails not only traditional epidemiology and biostatistics, but also genetics, molecular biology, biochemistry, cellular biology, analytical chemistry, toxicology, pharmacology, and laboratory medicine. Unlike traditional epidemiology research of cancer, which focuses on exposures or risk factors ascertained through questionnaire-based interviews or surveys, molecular epidemiology studies expand the assessment of exposure to a much broader scope that includes an analysis of biomarkers underlying internal exposure of exogenous and endogenous carcinogenic agents or risk factors, molecular alterations in response to exposure, and genetic susceptibility to cancer. The biomarkers often measured in molecular epidemiology research include DNA, RNA, proteins, chromosomes, compound molecules (e.g., DNA and protein adducts), and various metabolites as well as other endogenous and exogenous substances (e.g., steroids, nutrients, chemical or biologic toxins, and phytochemicals). Molecular markers can reflect different aspects of the tumorigenic process, which include biomarkers of internal exposure, biomarkers of molecular or cellular changes in response to exposure, and biomarkers of precursor lesions or early diseases.[22,23] Depending on the source of molecules and location of diseases, surrogates are often used in epidemiologic studies. When using a surrogate marker or tissue, the relevance of a proxy to its underlying target needs to be established or justified.[23] This justification is especially important when conducting population-based epidemiologic studies that focus on organ-specific cancers, because assessing biomarkers in target tissue is difficult for controls; molecular markers from blood samples are often used as substitutes. If a biomarker in the blood does not travel to or act on the tissue or organ of interest, an association between the circulating marker and the cancer may not be relevant. Thus, establishing a close link between a surrogate and its target is crucial in molecular epidemiology research.

Gene-environment interaction plays an essential role in cancer development.[24] Common genetic variations are considered an important determinant of host susceptibility and are a major focus of molecular epidemiology research. Depending on the biologic mechanism involved, genetic variations can influence every aspect of the carcinogenic process, ranging from external and internal exposure to carcinogens or risk factors to molecular and cellular damage, alteration, and response.[22,23] Currently, single nucleotide polymorphisms (SNPs) are the most studied genetic variations. It is believed that even if SNPs confer a small risk, they may still be important at the population level because these variations are common in the general population. It is also important that the impacts of SNPs on cancer are considered under the context of gene–gene and gene–environment interactions. As genotyping technology has advanced substantially with respect to its analytic

quality, capacity, and cost, research of genetic polymorphisms has evolved rapidly from investigations of a single SNP to studies of haplotypes and tag SNPs, and from a pathway-based candidate gene approach to genome-wide association studies (GWAS).[25] A GWAS analyzes hundreds of thousands of SNPs simultaneously for hundreds or even thousands of study subjects. When these data are further combined with questionnaire information such as environmental exposures, lifestyle factors, dietary habits, and medical history, enormous information is generated, which requires a huge sample size to allow for a reliable and complete assessment of these variables individually and jointly. A single epidemiologic study can no longer provide sufficient power for this type of investigation. Multicenter investigations or study consortia that pool study information and specimens together are developed to address the sample size issue.[26] False-positive findings resulting from multiple comparisons constitute a major challenge in epidemiologic studies of genetic associations with cancer.[27] A meta-analysis or pooled analysis can be used to address this problem if sufficient studies are already published and available for evaluation. To address this issue at the time of study design, one may adopt a two- or multiphase study design in which study subjects are divided into two or multiple groups for genotyping and data analysis. Selected or genomewide SNPs are first screened in one group of the study subjects (discovery phase), and then the significant findings determined by stringent statistical criteria (usually p values less than 1×10^{-5} or 1×10^{-7}) are reanalyzed in one or several other groups of subjects for verification (validation phase). This study design also lowers the cost of genotyping. False-positive findings can also be addressed with various statistical methods, such as bootstrap, permutation test, estimate of false positive report probability, prediction of false discovery rate, and the use of a much more stringent p value to accommodate multiple comparisons. For epidemiologic studies that are not population based or not conducted strictly following epidemiology principles, population stratification is a potential source of bias that may distort genetic associations.[28]

A large number of GWAS have been completed in search for SNPs that influence host susceptibility to cancer. Considering that more than 5 million SNPs are present in the human genome, the numbers of SNPs that are found to be associated with cancer risk after rigorous validation are much fewer than what one would have anticipated. In addition, the risk associations detected are quite weak, with most of the odds ratios ranging from 1.1 to 1.5, and the functional relevance or biologic implications are unclear for most of the SNPs. Furthermore, not many SNPs associated with cancer risk are located in protein-coding regions, and even fewer are in the loci of candidate genes suspected to be involved in tumorigenesis, such as oncogenes, tumor suppressor genes, DNA repair genes, and xenobiotic metabolizing or detoxification genes. Genes where SNPs are found to be linked to cancer by GWAS include *FGFR2, MAP3K1, MRPS30, LSP1, TNRC9, TOX3, STXBP1,* and *RAD51L1* for breast cancer[29–31]; *JAZF1, HNF1B, MSMB, CTBP2,* and *KLK2/KLK3* for prostate cancer[29,32]; *SMAD7, CRAC1, EIF3H, BMP4, CDH1,* and *RHPN2* for colorectal cancer[29,33]; *CHRNA3* and *CHRNA5* for lung cancer[34,35]; *ABO* for pancreatic cancer[36]; *TACC3* and *PSCA* for bladder cancer[37,38]; and *KRT5* for basal cell carcinoma.[39] Among these genes identified by GWAS, two findings are considered especially interesting. One is the association of lung cancer with *CHRNA3* and *CHRNA5*, which encode neuronal nicotinic acetylcholine receptor subunits. Different genotypes of these receptor subunits appear to influence individual's addiction to tobacco, which further leads to different smoking exposure and lung cancer risk.[40,41] Another is the link of the *ABO* gene to pancreatic cancer. The association between pancreatic cancer risk and ABO blood type was observed 50 years ago. The GWAS finding not only confirms the relationship, but also provides new clues for understanding the underlying biologic mechanism.

Besides intragenic SNPs, GWAS also found many intergenic SNPs in association to cancer risk, which include those in the regions of 8q24, 5p15, 1p11, 1p36, 1q42, 2p15, 2q35, 3p12, 3p24,

3q28, 6p21, 6q25, 7q21, 7q32, 9p21, 9p22, 9p24, 9q22, 10p14, 11q13, 11q23, 14q13, 18q23, and 20p12.[29–31,33,39,42–48] Of these loci, SNPs in 8q24 are associated with several cancer sites, including prostate, breast, colon, and bladder.[29,31–33,47–49] Further analysis of 8q24 indicates that there are nine SNPs in five regions and each region is independently related to different types of cancer, with SNPs in regions 1, 4, and 5 associated exclusively with prostate cancer, a SNP in region 2 related to breast cancer, and SNPs in region 3 linked to prostate, colon, and ovarian cancers.[50] No known genes are located within the region of 8q24, but an oncogene *c-MYC* resides about 330 kb downstream of the region.[51] An initial investigation found no evidence of the SNPs' influence on *c-MYC* expression,[47] but a later study suggests that the SNPs in 8q24 may be distal enhancers of *c-MYC*, interacting with its promoter through a chromatin loop.[52] Another genomic region that is associated with the risk of multiple cancer sites is 5p15, a region involving telomerase reverse transcriptase (TERT) cleft lip and palate transmembrane protein 1–like protein (CLPTM1L). Five types of cancer are found to be linked to this region, including basal cell carcinoma, lung, bladder, prostate, and cervical cancers.[53] TERT extends the length of telomere and is associated with cell proliferation and abnormal telomere maintenance.[54] The risk alleles of TERT are associated with shorter telomere length among the elderly and with higher DNA adduct in the lungs.[53,55]

GWAS has demonstrated its value in identifying disease-related SNPs in unknown regions of the genome, which provides new clues for investigators to interrogate and understand different regions of the human genome, especially in the gene-desert areas. Despite the strength, the low yield of significant findings from the GWAS has raised concerns in several areas, including the SNP coverage in the genome (rare SNPs and SNP representativeness in unknown regions), associations with low statistical significance (p value between 0.01 and 1×10^{-5}, the GWAS cutoff), other forms of genetic variations (copy number variation and other structural variations), cancer subtypes, and genetic interplay with environmental factors (gene–environment interaction).[56,57] To address these issues, investigators propose to perform fine-mapping and re-sequencing to examine genetic regions more specifically and meticulously. Epidemiologists suggest that detailed environmental exposure and lifestyle factors should be included in the next wave of GWAS. Furthermore, to make the study more reliable and compelling, DNA specimens, instead of convenient samples, should come from well-designed and well-executed epidemiologic studies that pay close attention to the selection of study subjects and the measurement of environmental and lifestyle factors to eliminate or minimize selection bias and measurement errors.

As described earlier, analytical epidemiology has two major study designs: the case-control study and the cohort study. It is important that investigators choose an appropriate study design to investigate molecular markers in epidemiologic studies. Two types of molecular markers, genotypic and phenotypic markers, can be considered. Genotypic markers refer to nucleotide sequences of genomic DNA, and all other molecules are considered phenotypic markers, including most of the chemical modifications on DNA, such as cytosine methylation. The distinction between the two is a marker's status in relation to an outcome variable, usually a disease. Genotypic markers generally do not change over time and are not affected by the development of a disease, whereas phenotypic markers are likely to change over time or be influenced by the presence of a disease, either itself or the treatment associated with it. If measurements of a phenotypic marker are made from the specimens that are collected after or at the time of cancer diagnosis, investigators will have difficulties determining the status of the phenotypic marker before the cancer was diagnosed. A disease condition, however, does not affect genotypic markers such as SNPs; therefore, a temporal relationship can be easily established even if the samples are collected after the disease is diagnosed. Based on this distinction, one can evaluate genotypic markers either in case-control or cohort studies, but a case-control study would be

the design of choice because of efficiency and cost-effectiveness. A prospective cohort study design is ideal for phenotypic markers. Investigators, however, may use other study designs if they can demonstrate that the disease status does not influence the phenotypic markers of interest. To reduce study cost, investigators usually use nested case-control or case-cohort designs to avoid analyzing specimens from the entire cohort. The main purpose in choosing a cohort study design for a molecular epidemiology investigation is to ensure that biospecimens are collected before the development of a disease so that a temporal relationship between a marker and disease development can be established.

The differences between molecular epidemiology and genetic epidemiology are the scope of the molecular analysis and the emphasis on heredity. Sometimes molecular and genetic epidemiology both investigate genetic factors in association with cancer risk, but each has its own emphasis. The former assesses genetic involvement, but not necessarily inheritance, whereas the latter focuses mainly on heredity. Because of the difference in focus, study populations are different between the two types of investigation. Molecular epidemiology studies unrelated individuals, whereas genetic epidemiology investigates family members in the format of pedigrees, parent–child trios, or sibling pairs. Given the different research focus between genetic and molecular epidemiology, these investigations evaluate different genetic markers. Genetic epidemiology research is designed to identify genetic markers with high penetrance (strong association with an underlying disease) but low prevalence in the general populations, whereas a molecular epidemiology investigation targets low penetrance markers that are commonly present in the general population. Given the difference in study design, the analysis of genetic marker's link to cancer is also different between the studies. Relative risks or odds ratios are calculated in molecular epidemiology studies because study participants are unrelated individuals, whereas linkage analysis is used in genetic epidemiology because individuals in the study are genetically related family members. Recently, both genetic and molecular epidemiology study designs have been considered in GWAS to improve study validity and to minimize false positive findings. Another difference between genetic and molecular epidemiology research is that molecular epidemiology also studies nongenetic molecules. Thus, the scope of molecular analysis is much broader in molecular epidemiology research than in genetic epidemiology studies.

A laboratory analysis of molecular markers is another integral part of molecular epidemiology research, which has unique features that are different from basic science research. Collecting biologic specimens is difficult and expensive in population-based epidemiologic studies. It not only increases the study cost, but also imposes constraints to multiple areas of epidemiology research. Specimen collection may adversely influence the response rate of study participants, potentially compromising study validity. For organ-specific cancer research, investigating molecular markers in target tissue is difficult. Blood is the most common and versatile specimen used in molecular epidemiology research; other specimens used include urine, stool, nail, hair, sputum, buccal cells, and saliva. Tissue samples, either fresh frozen or chemically fixed, are also used, but the availability of these samples is highly limited to patients or selected subgroups of a general study population. Comparability and generalizability are always problems in epidemiologic studies involving tissue specimens, except for those investigations that focus on cancer prognosis or treatment in which only cancer patients are involved. Attempts have been made to use special body fluids for epidemiologic research, such as nipple aspirate and breast or pulmonary lavage, but the difficulty in specimen collection and preparation makes these samples impractical in large population-based studies.

Given the research value of biologic specimens and the difficulty in collecting them for population-based studies, technical issues related to specimen collection, processing, and storage become especially important in molecular epidemiology research.

These include time and conditions for specimen transportation and processing, a sample aliquot and labeling system, a sample special treatment for storage and analysis, a sample storage and tracking system, as well as backup plans and equipment for unexpected adverse events during long-term storage (e.g., power failure, earthquake, flooding). Laboratory methods used to analyze biomarkers are also important in molecular epidemiology. Because large numbers of specimens are involved, laboratory methods are required to be robust, reproducible, high throughput, low cost, and easy to use. These requirements are often met in the analysis of nucleotide sequences that serve as genotypic markers. However, for phenotypic markers, many methods do not readily meet these requirements. Moreover, many phenotypic markers, such as proteins, require both qualitative and quantitative assessments. An ideal laboratory method should be quantitative (able to measure a wide range of values), sensitive (able to detect a small amount of analyte), specific (able to detect only the molecule of interest, no other molecules), reproducible (high precision and low variation), and versatile (easy to use). In addition, investigators need to implement appropriate quality assurance procedures during sample processing and testing as well as include appropriate quality control samples in specimen analysis.

Host–environment interaction is believed to play a key role in the etiology of most types of cancer. Genetic factors, including mutations and polymorphisms, are initially considered important host factors, but recent developments in cancer research has indicated that epigenetic factors may also play a critical role in cancer as a host factor involved in host–environment interaction. Epigenetic factors, which regulate the function of human genome without altering the physical sequences of nucleotides, include pretranscription regulation through nucleotide modification (e.g., cytosine methylation at CpG sites), chromosome modification (e.g., histone acetylation), and posttranscription regulation by noncoding small RNA (e.g., microRNAs). These epigenetic factors have two unique features that have captured the attention of cancer researchers, especially cancer epidemiologists who are interested in the gene–environment interaction. It is known that epigenetic factors are heritable, but these inherited features are readily modifiable by environmental and lifestyle factors. Monozygotic twins have an identical genome as well as epigenome at birth, but the latter undergoes substantial changes over time, resulting in distinct epigenetic profiles that depend heavily on their environmental exposures.[58] Animal studies also indicated that the maternal intake of dietary nutrients involving one-carbon metabolism could influence offsprings' growth phenotypes, which are regulated by DNA methylation.[59] As evidence mounts on epigenetic involvement in cancer, molecular epidemiologists will start to look for clues in human populations that can link epigenetic factors to both lifestyle factors and cancer risk. Given that epigenetic regulation is tissue specific and time dependent, investigators face challenges in accurately assessing these phenotypic markers in etiologic studies. However, progress in the analysis of circulating methylation markers and microRNAs may provide an alternative to study epigenetic regulation in human cancer. Furthermore, methods for a genome-wide analysis of DNA methylation have been developed and applied in epidemiologic studies, which can substantially accelerate the search for cancer-related DNA methylation. Together with the high-throughput, high-dimensional analysis of DNA methylation, two other evolving fields that will have significant impacts on molecular epidemiology of cancer research are metagenomics and metabolomics. The former focuses on environmental genomics of the microbiome that resides in our body and influences one's biologic functions and health status. The latter refers to the analysis of hundreds or thousands of metabolites in a biologic specimen, including tissue, blood, urine, body fluids, and fecal samples. These new analyses will add tremendous value to epidemiologic studies.

SELECTED REFERENCES

The full reference list can be accessed at lwwhealthlibrary.com/oncology.

1. Last J. *A Dictionary of Epidemiology.* 3rd ed. New York: Oxford University Press; 1995.
2. Doll R, Hill AB. Lung cancer and other causes of death in relation to smoking: a second report on the mortality of British doctors. *Br Med J* 1956;12:1071–1081.
3. Kleinbaum D, Kupper L, Morgenstern H. *Epidemiologic Research.* New York: Van Nostrand Reinhold; 1982.
4. Kaplan LD, Straus DJ, Testa MA, et al. Low-dose compared with standard-dose m-BACOD chemotherapy for non-Hodgkin's lymphoma associated with human immunodeficiency virus infection. National Institute of Allergy and Infectious Diseases AIDS Clinical Trials Group. *N Engl J Med* 1997;336:1641–1648.
5. Dunn BK, Kramer BS, Ford LG. Phase III, large-scale chemoprevention trials. Approach to chemoprevention clinical trials and phase III clinical trial of tamoxifen as a chemopreventive for breast cancer—the US National Cancer Institute experience. *Hematol Oncol Clin North Am* 1998;12:1019–1036, vii.
6. Grant WB. An ecologic study of dietary and solar ultraviolet-B links to breast carcinoma mortality rates. *Cancer* 2002;94:272–281.
7. National Center for Health Statistics. Third National Health and Nutrition Examination Survey, 1988-1994, Plan and Operations Procedures Manuals (CD-ROM). Hyattsville, MD: U.S. Department of Health and Human Services (DHHS), Centers for Disease Control and Prevention; 1996.
8. Szklo M, Nieto F. *Epidemiology: Beyond the Basics.* Gaithersburg, MD: Aspen Publishers; 2000.
9. Grimes DA, Schulz KF. Cohort studies: marching towards outcomes. *Lancet* 2002;359:341–345.
10. Schatzkin A, Subar AF, Thompson FE, et al. Design and serendipity in establishing a large cohort with wide dietary intake distributions: the National Institutes of Health-American Association of Retired Persons Diet and Health Study. *Am J Epidemiol* 2001;154:1119–1125.
11. Mantel N, Haenszel W. Statistical aspects of the analysis of data from retrospective studies of disease. *J Natl Cancer Inst* 1959;22:719–748.
12. Wacholder S, Silverman DT, McLaughlin JK, et al. Selection of controls in case-control studies. II. Types of controls. *Am J Epidemiol* 1992;135:1029–1041.
13. Chen C, Weiss NS, Stanczyk FZ, et al. Endogenous sex hormones and prostate cancer risk: a case-control study nested within the Carotene and Retinol Efficacy Trial. *Cancer Epidemiol Biomarkers Prev* 2003;12:1410–1416.
14. Pearce N. What does the odds ratio estimate in a case-control study? *Int J Epidemiol* 1993;22:1189–1192.
15. Schulz KF, Grimes DA. Case-control studies: research in reverse. *Lancet* 2002;359:431–434.
16. Rothman K. *Epidemiology: An Introduction.* New York: Oxford University Press; 2002.
17. Hennekens C, Buring J. *Epidemiology in Medicine.* Boston: Little, Brown and Company; 1987.
18. Andriole GL, Crawford ED, Grubb RL 3rd, et al. Mortality results from a randomized prostate-cancer screening trial. *N Engl J Med* 2009;360:1310–1319.
19. Wilt TJ, Brawer MK, Jones KM, et al. Radical prostatectomy versus observation for localized prostate cancer. *N Engl J Med* 2012;367:203–213.
20. Yu JB, Soulos PR, Herrin J, et al. Proton versus intensity-modulated radiotherapy for prostate cancer: patterns of care and early toxicity. *J Natl Cancer Inst* 2013;105:25–32.
21. Ma X, Wang R, Long JB, et al. The cost implications of prostate cancer screening in the Medicare population. *Cancer* 2014;120(1):96–102.
22. Rundle A, Schwartz S. Issues in the epidemiological analysis and interpretation of intermediate biomarkers. *Cancer Epidemiol Biomarkers Prev* 2003;12:491–496.
23. Shields PG. Tobacco smoking, harm reduction, and biomarkers. *J Natl Cancer Inst* 2002;94:1435–1444.
24. Hunter DJ. Gene-environment interactions in human diseases. *Nat Rev Genet* 2005;6:287–298.
25. Hirschhorn JN, Daly MJ. Genome-wide association studies for common diseases and complex traits. *Nat Rev Genet* 2005;6:95–108.
26. Breast Cancer Association Consortium. Commonly studied single-nucleotide polymorphisms and breast cancer: results from the Breast Cancer Association Consortium. *J Natl Cancer Inst* 2006;98:1382–1396.
27. Wacholder S, Chanock S, Garcia-Closas M, et al. Assessing the probability that a positive report is false: an approach for molecular epidemiology studies. *J Natl Cancer Inst* 2004;96:434–442.

28. Clayton DG, Walker NM, Smyth DJ, et al. Population structure, differential bias and genomic control in a large-scale, case-control association study. *Nat Genet* 2005;37:1243–1246.

29. Easton DF, Eeles RA. Genome-wide association studies in cancer. *Hum Mol Genet* 2008;17:R109–115.

30. Ahmed S, Thomas G, Ghoussaini M, et al. Newly discovered breast cancer susceptibility loci on 3p24 and 17q23.2. *Nat Genet* 2009;41:585–590.

31. Thomas G, Jacobs KB, Kraft P, et al. A multistage genome-wide association study in breast cancer identifies two new risk alleles at 1p11.2 and 14q24.1 (RAD51L1). *Nat Genet* 2009;41:579–584.

32. Thomas G, Jacobs KB, Yeager M, et al. Multiple loci identified in a genome-wide association study of prostate cancer. *Nat Genet* 2008;40:310–315.

33. Le Marchand L. Genome-wide association studies and colorectal cancer. *Surg Oncol Clin N Am* 2009;18:663–668.

34. Hung RJ, McKay JD, Gaborieau V, et al. A susceptibility locus for lung cancer maps to nicotinic acetylcholine receptor subunit genes on 15q25. *Nature* 2008;452:633–637.

35. Amos CI, Wu X, Broderick P, et al. Genome-wide association scan of tag SNPs identifies a susceptibility locus for lung cancer at 15q25.1. *Nat Genet* 2008;40:616–622.

36. Amundadottir L, Kraft P, Stolzenberg-Solomon RZ, et al. Genome-wide association study identifies variants in the ABO locus associated with susceptibility to pancreatic cancer. *Nat Genet* 2009;41:986–990.

37. Kiemeney LA, Sulem P, Besenbacher S, et al. A sequence variant at 4p16.3 confers susceptibility to urinary bladder cancer. *Nat Genet* 2010;42(5):415–419.

38. Wu X, Ye Y, Kiemeney LA, et al. Genetic variation in the prostate stem cell antigen gene PSCA confers susceptibility to urinary bladder cancer. *Nat Genet* 2009;41:991–995.

39. Stacey SN, Sulem P, Masson G, et al. New common variants affecting susceptibility to basal cell carcinoma. *Nat Genet* 2009;41:909–914.

40. Thorgeirsson TE, Geller F, Sulem P, et al. A variant associated with nicotine dependence, lung cancer and peripheral arterial disease. *Nature* 2008;452:638–642.

ETIOLOGY AND EPIDEMIOLOGY OF CANCER

Trends in United States Cancer Mortality

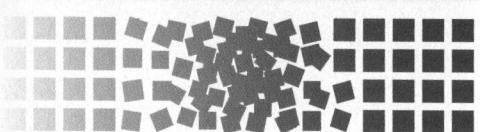

Tim E. Byers

INTRODUCTION

Cancer incidence registries now cover nearly all of the US population. State-based vital records systems and aggregate national systems regularly report trends in both cancer incidence and mortality, and national surveys routinely monitor cancer-related risk factors in the population. These surveillance systems have documented substantial changes in both risk factors for cancer and in cancer incidence and mortality rates in the United States over the past 3 decades. In 1996, the American Cancer Society (ACS) set an ambitious challenge for the United States: to reduce cancer mortality rates from their apparent peak in 1990 by 50% in the 25-year period ending in 2015.[1] In 1998, the ACS then challenged the United States to also reduce cancer incidence rates from their peak in 1992 by 25% by the year 2015.[2] In this chapter, we will examine trends in cancer risk factors as well as trends in cancer incidence and mortality rates in the United States over the 25-year period between 1990 and 2015.

CANCER SURVEILLANCE SYSTEMS

Collecting cancer incidence rates is largely a state-based activity in the United States, because cancer is a reportable disease in all states. The Centers for Disease Control and Prevention (CDC) organizes all state-based cancer registries within the National Program of Cancer Registries, which now reports collective data on cancer incidence from over 40 different state-based registries, providing data that meets strict quality standards.[3] The National Cancer Institute has supported high-quality cancer incidence and outcomes registration in selected states and cities since 1973 within the Surveillance, Epidemiology, and End Results (SEER) Program.[4] The most precise measures of long-term trends in cancer incidence come from SEER-9, a set of nine SEER registries that together include about 10% of the US population. The populations included in the SEER-9 registries document the most detailed history of cancer trends beginning in the 1970s based on highly standardized cancer case ascertainment, staging, treatment, and outcomes. Deaths from cancer are well ascertained in all states via state-based vital records, which are aggregated into annual national mortality reports by the CDC's National Center for Health Statistics.[5] Each year, the ACS, the National Cancer Institute, and the CDC publish a *Report to the Nation* on trends in cancer incidence and mortality in the United States.[6] Trends in the prevalence of behavioral factors that affect cancer risk are tracked by the Health Interview Survey, an ongoing, in-person interview of a nationally representative sample of adults, and in annual reports by the Behavioral Risk Factor Surveillance System, a continuously operating telephone-based survey operated by state departments of health and organized by the CDC.[7]

MAKING SENSE OF CANCER TRENDS

Understanding the reasons for cancer trends requires understanding trends in cancer-related risk factors. For factors like tobacco,

relating trends in exposure to trends in rates is easy, because those effects are large and single. However, for many other cancer risk factors, because effects are much smaller and multifactorial, simple correlations over time are less apparent. In most situations, all that maybe possible are crude qualitative relationships between temporal trends in cancer risk factors and subsequent trends in cancer rates. Statistical methods such as linear regression joinpoint analysis can tell us when inflections in cancer trends occur, but accounting for the precise reasons for changing rates is often impaired by our incomplete knowledge about the interacting impacts of variations in cancer screening, diagnosis, and treatment, and by uncertainties about latencies between interventions and outcomes.[8]

TRENDS IN CANCER RISK FACTORS AND SCREENING

Trends in major cancer risk factors have been mixed (Table 12.1). Although the downward trends in tobacco smoking among adults that began in the 1960s slowed after 1990, there has been a continuing downward trend in the number of cigarettes smoked per day by continuing smokers.[9] Obesity trends have been adverse among both men and women since the 1970s, with more than a doubling of the prevalence of obesity between 1990 and 2010. Long-term trends in the use of hormone replacement therapy (HRT) are not routinely monitored in the Behavioral Risk Factor Surveillance System (BRFSS), but HRT use increased substantially in the last 2 decades of the 20th century. Then, following the 2002 publication of the Women's Health Initiative trial, which showed clear adverse effects of HRT, there was a rapid and substantial drop in HRT use.[10,11] The use of endoscopic screening for colorectal cancer (sigmoidoscopy or colonoscopy) has increased substantially in recent years, approximately doubling since the mid 1990s, so that, as of 2010, about two-thirds of Americans age 50 and older reported ever having had an endoscopic examination. Mammography use increased progressively through the 1990s, but mammogram rates then leveled off after 2000.[12] Widespread prostate-specific antigen (PSA) testing began in the mid to late 1980s, then increased substantially during the 1990s. By 2002, a majority of US men age 50 and older reported having been tested.

CANCER INCIDENCE AND MORTALITY

In this chapter, we describe and discuss cancer trends for the time period 1990 through 2010 using cancer incidence data from the SEER-9 registry (Table 12.2 and Fig. 12.1) and US cancer mortality data from the National Center for Health Statistics (Table 12.3).[4,5] All rates were age-adjusted to the US 2000 standard population by the direct method, using 10-year age intervals.

Lung Cancer

The lung is the second leading site for cancer incidence and the leading site for cancer death among both men and women in the

TABLE 12.1

Trends in Risk Factors and Cancer Screening Practices in the United States, 1990–2010[a]

	Men		Women		Both Genders	
	Smoking	PSA Screening	Smoking	Mammography	Obesity	CRC Screening
1990	24.9	—	21.3	58.3	11.6	—
1991	25.1	—	21.3	62.2	12.6	—
1992	24.2	—	21.0	63.1	12.6	—
1993	24.0	—	21.1	66.5	13.7	—
1994	23.9	—	21.6	66.6	14.4	—
1995	24.8	—	20.9	68.6	15.8	29.4
1996	25.5	—	21.9	69.2	16.8	—
1997	25.4	—	21.1	70.3	16.6	32.4
1998	25.3	—	20.9	72.3	18.3	—
1999	24.2	—	20.8	72.8	19.7	43.7
2000	24.4	—	21.2	76.1	20.1	—
2001	25.4	—	21.2	—	21.0	—
2002	25.7	53.9	20.8	75.9	22.1	48.1
2003	24.8	—	20.2	—	—	—
2004	23.0	52.1	19.0	74.7	23.2	53.0
2005	22.1	—	19.2	—	24.4	—
2006	22.2	53.8	18.4	76.5	25.1	57.1
2007	21.2	—	18.4	—	26.3	—
2008	20.3	54.8	16.7	76.0	26.6	61.8
2009	19.5	—	16.7	—	27.1	—
2010	18.5	53.2	15.8	75.2	27.5	65.2

CRC, colorectal cancer; PSA, prostate-specific antigen.
[a] Median percent of the population across all states in the Behavioral Risk Factor Surveillance System. The survey covered such areas as body mass index and was based on self-reported height and weight. Questions included: Are you a regular cigarette smoker? Have you ever had a sigmoidoscopy or proctoscopic examination? For women age 40 and older, the following question was included: Have you had a mammogram in the past 2 years? For men aged 50 and older, the following question was included: Have you had a PSA test in the last 2 years? (From Centers for Disease Control and Prevention. Behavioral Risk Factor Surveillance System Web site. http://cdc.gov/brfss.)

ETIOLOGY AND EPIDEMIOLOGY OF CANCER

United States.[6] There are now more deaths from lung cancer in the United States than from the sum of colorectal, breast, and prostate cancers. Trends in lung cancer incidence and mortality have been nearly identical because there are few effective treatments for lung cancer, and survival time remains short. Lung cancer trends follow historic declines in tobacco use, lagged by about 20 years.[13] Between 1965 and 1985, tobacco use among US adults dropped substantially, and more in men than in women. Lung cancer mortality rates began to decline among men in 1990, but rates increased among women throughout the 1990s. The stabilization of lung cancer incidence trends among women from 2000 to 2005 and the beginning of a decline in the period 2005 to 2010 foretells a coming persistent decline in lung cancer mortality among women in the United States.

The effectiveness of annual examinations by use of chest radiographs in reducing lung cancer mortality was studied as part of the Prostate, Lung, Colorectal, Ovary (PLCO) trial, and the effectiveness of annual screening by low-dose computed tomography (LDCT) of the lung fields was studied in the National Lung Screening Trial (NLST).[14,15] In brief, screening with standard chest radiography finds more cancers earlier but does not affect mortality, whereas screening with LDCT reduces the risk of death from lung cancer by at least 20%.[14,15] Therefore, both the ACS and the US Preventive Services Task Force have issued recommendations that favor informed decision making for lung cancer screening using LDCT.[16,17]

The major factor that will determine lung cancer incidence in the coming decade is the past history of tobacco use, but future screening will also reduce future mortality rates. Considering all factors, it is likely that over the coming decade the downward trends in mortality from lung cancer will continue at about the same rate among men, and soon will become more apparent among women.

Colorectal Cancer

The colorectum is the third leading site for cancer incidence and the second leading site for cancer death in the United States.[6] Colorectal cancer incidence rates increased until 1985, when they began to decline. The reasons for this decline are not clear, but could be related to downward trends in cigarette smoking and the increasing use of both nonsteroidal anti-inflammatory drugs (NSAIDs) and HRT.[18] The rapid decline in HRT use following the publication of the Women's Health Initiative trial results in 2002 may adversely affect colorectal trends among women in the coming years, because HRT reduces the risk for colorectal cancer among women.[11] Recent trials have demonstrated the potential for NSAIDs to reduce colorectal neoplasia, but adverse effects from these agents will limit their widespread use for that explicit purpose. Nonetheless, even the common sporadic use of NSAIDs for other indications will contribute to continuing declines in colorectal cancer incidence in the coming years.

Screening with either sigmoidoscopy or colonoscopy leads to the identification and removal of adenomas, thus preventing the development of colorectal cancer.[19,20] Medicare included

TABLE 12.2

Trends in Age-Adjusted Cancer Incidence Rates in the United States by Cancer Site, 1990–2010[a]

	Men		Women		Both Genders	
	Lung	**Prostate**	**Lung**	**Breast**	**Colorectal**	**All Sites**
1990	96.9	171.0	47.8	131.8	60.7	482.0
1991	97.2	214.8	49.6	133.9	59.5	503.0
1992	97.2	237.4	49.9	132.1	58.0	510.6
1993	94.0	209.5	49.2	129.2	56.8	493.4
1994	90.9	180.3	50.5	131.0	55.6	483.5
1995	89.8	169.3	50.4	132.6	54.0	476.9
1996	88.0	169.5	50.2	133.7	54.8	479.1
1997	86.3	173.5	52.6	138.0	56.4	486.4
1998	88.0	171.0	53.0	141.4	56.8	488.2
1999	84.6	183.4	52.4	141.5	55.5	490.4
2000	82.1	183.0	51.2	136.4	54.1	486.0
2001	81.4	184.8	51.7	138.7	53.6	489.7
2002	80.4	182.2	52.5	135.6	53.1	487.5
2003	81.0	169.6	53.0	126.8	50.8	475.2
2004	76.2	165.7	52.0	128.0	50.0	476.1
2005	75.8	156.5	53.7	126.4	47.8	471.9
2006	74.2	171.5	53.4	126.0	46.8	475.0
2007	73.5	174.3	53.4	127.9	46.3	480.5
2008	72.0	157.0	51.6	128.0	45.2	473.4
2009	70.2	153.7	51.8	130.3	43.0	470.5
2010	66.8	145.1	49.2	126.0	40.6	457.5
Average annual % change 1990–2010	−1.8	−0.5	+0.2	−0.2	−2.0	−0.2

[a] Data source is the Surveillance, Epidemiology, and End Results-9 populations for cancer incidence. Rates are age-adjusted to the year 2000 population standard. The annual percent change is the mean percent change per year across the 20-year period, 1990 to 2010. (From National Cancer Institute. Surveillance, Epidemiology, and End Results Program Web site. http://seer.cancer.gov.)

coverage for all recommended colorectal screening methods in 2001, and national publicity has substantially increased public interest in screening.[21] Colorectal screening rates have increased over time, now with about two-thirds of adults over age 50 reporting having ever been screened by lower gastrointestinal endoscopy (see Table 12.1).

Decreasing rates of colorectal cancer incidence are occurring in spite of the obesity epidemic, which is an adverse force on colorectal cancer risk, because obesity may account for as much as 20% of colorectal cancer in the United States.[22] Recently, however, obesity trends have stabilized in the United States. [23] As a result of the increased use of lower gastrointestinal endoscopy for colorectal screening and this stabilization of obesity trends, the incidence of colorectal cancer may exceed the ACS goal for 2015 of a 25% reduction, and there is a high likelihood that the rate of decline in deaths from colorectal cancer will be steep enough to reach the 2015 ACS mortality reduction goal of 50%.

Breast Cancer

The breast is the leading site of cancer incidence and the second leading site for cancer death among women in the United States.[6] Over the period 1990 to 2001, no substantial changes in incidence rates were observed, but after 2000, breast cancer incidence began to decline. The decline in breast cancer incidence observed after 2002 seems to have been the result of the sudden decline in the use of HRT following the 2002 publication of the Women's Health Initiative results.[10,11] It is likely that persisting lower rates of HRT use will cause a continued decline in breast cancer incidence in the coming years. Countering this favorable trend, however, are the adverse effects of the obesity epidemic. Obesity, a major risk factor for postmenopausal breast cancer, increased substantially between 1990 and 2005, now with over 25% of US women being obese. However, the slowing of the obesity epidemic since 2005 may have substantial beneficial effects on the future trends in breast cancer incidence.

After persistent increases in the use of mammography over a 20-year period, mammography rates declined modestly between 2000 and 2004, and then leveled off. The downgrading of the evidence recommendations by the US Preventive Services Task Force for mammography for women age 40 to 49 and recommendations for every other year mammographies for women age 50 and older have resulted in lower mammogram utilization, which is likely to continue into the coming decade.[17] This trend will have an adverse effect on breast cancer mortality, but will tend to reduce breast cancer incidence somewhat because of a lack of detection of very early stage cancers.

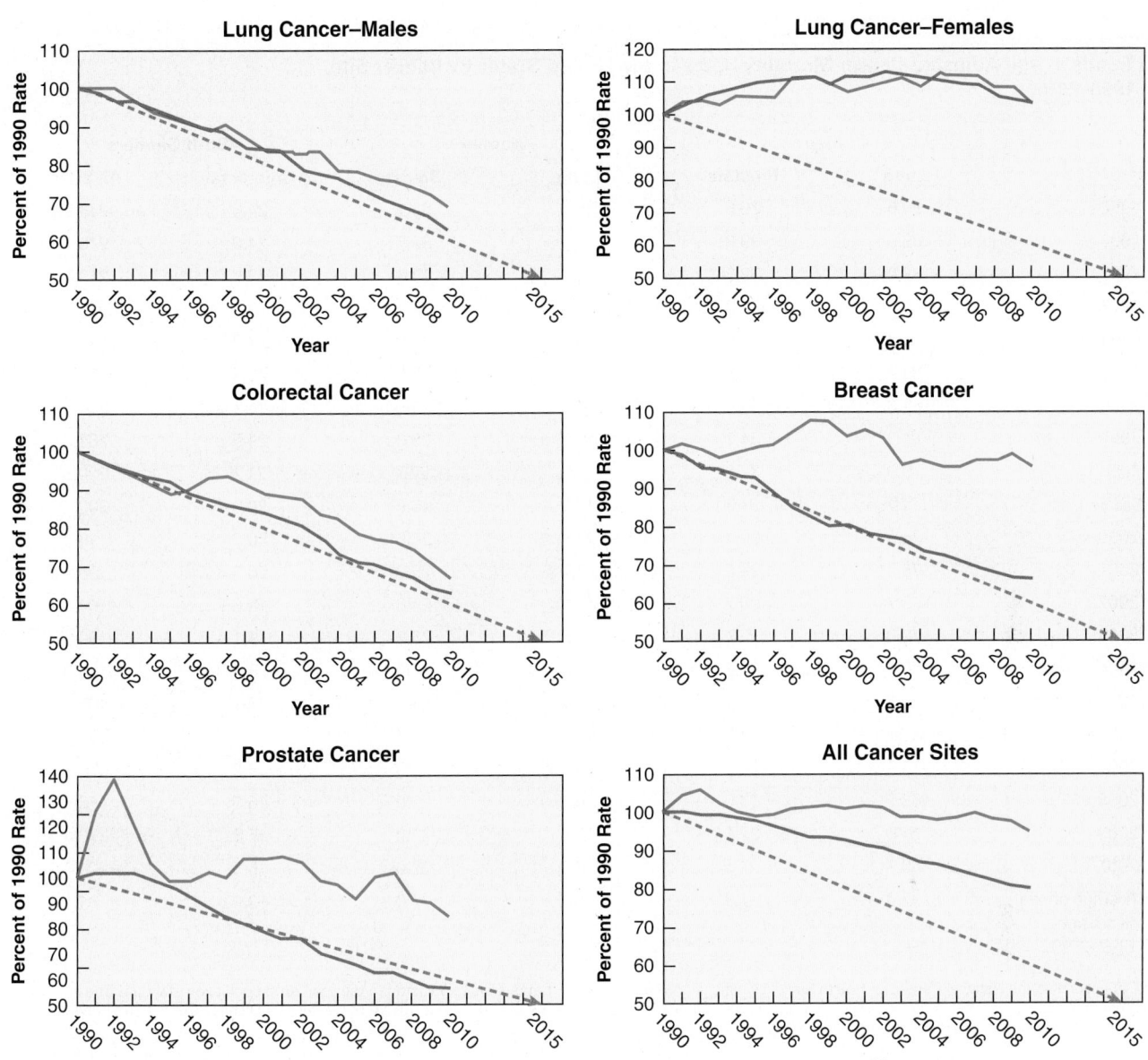

Figure 12.1 (A–F) Trends in cancer incidence and mortality between 1990 and 2010. Incidence rates are for the populations in the Surveillance, Epidemiology, and End Results Program; registries and mortality rates are for the entire United States. Rates are age-adjusted to the year 2000 standard. The y-axis rates are expressed as a percentage of the 1990 incidence and mortality rates. The *red lines* represent incidence rates, and the *blue lines* represent mortality rates. The *straight dotted green lines* represent the linear trend that would need to be followed to achieve a 50% mortality reduction between 1990 and 2015. (Data from National Cancer Institute. Surveillance, Epidemiology, and End Results Program Web site. http://seer .cancer.gov, and Centers for Disease Control and Prevention. U.S. mortality data. http://wonder.cdc.gov/ucd-icd10.html)

The antiestrogens tamoxifen and raloxifene have both been shown to reduce the risk of incident breast cancer.[24] The safety profile for tamoxifen discourages its widespread use, but there is a more favorable risk/benefit balance of raloxifene. Nonetheless, neither of these drugs is commonly used for breast cancer prevention among postmenopausal women in the United States.

The average decline in breast cancer death rates of 2% per year since 1990 is the combined result of earlier diagnosis and better treatment.[25] Progress in breast cancer treatment is continuing, especially in the development and application of hormone-targeted therapies. Aromatase inhibitors have largely replaced tamoxifen therapy for breast cancer treatment for postmenopausal women. Because all antiestrogens substantially reduce the incidence of second primary cancers in the contralateral breast, they impact both therapy and prevention. In the coming decade, the longer term effects of decreased HRT use, increased antiestrogen use, reversal

of the obesity trends, and continued improvements in therapies will likely lead to continued decreases in both the incidence and mortality rates from breast cancer.

Prostate Cancer

The prostate is the leading site for cancer incidence and the second leading site for cancer death among men in the United States.[6] The incidence of prostate cancer has been extremely variable over the period 1990 to 2010. The incidence spike observed in the early 1990s actually began in the late 1980s, coincident with the advent of PSA testing. The reasons for the 2.8% annual downward trend in prostate cancer mortality since 1990 are uncertain, however, because the ongoing PSA screening trials have not yet demonstrated a mortality benefit from screening anywhere as large as the downward mortality

TABLE 12.3

Trends in Age-Adjusted Cancer Mortality Rates in the United States by Cancer Site, 1990–2010[a]

	Men		Women		Both Genders	
	Lung	**Prostate**	**Lung**	**Breast**	**Colorectal**	**All Sites**
1990	90.6	38.6	36.8	33.1	24.6	214.9
1991	89.9	39.3	37.6	32.7	24.0	215.1
1992	88.0	39.2	38.7	31.6	23.6	213.5
1993	87.6	39.3	39.3	31.4	23.3	213.4
1994	85.7	38.5	39.6	30.9	22.9	211.7
1995	84.4	37.3	40.3	30.6	22.6	210.0
1996	82.8	36.0	40.4	29.5	21.9	207.0
1997	81.3	34.2	40.8	28.2	21.5	203.6
1998	79.9	32.6	41.0	27.5	21.2	200.8
1999	77.0	31.6	40.2	26.6	20.9	200.7
2000	76.5	30.4	41.1	26.6	20.7	198.8
2001	75.3	29.5	41.0	26.0	20.2	196.3
2002	73.7	28.7	41.6	25.6	19.8	194.4
2003	72.0	27.2	41.3	25.3	19.1	190.9
2004	70.4	26.2	41.0	24.5	18.1	186.8
2005	69.5	25.4	40.7	24.1	17.6	185.2
2006	67.4	24.2	40.3	23.6	17.3	182.0
2007	65.2	24.2	40.1	23.0	16.9	179.3
2008	63.7	23.0	39.1	22.6	16.5	176.3
2009	61.5	22.1	38.6	22.2	15.8	173.4
2010	60.1	21.8	38.0	22.0	15.5	171.8
Average annual % change 1990–2010	−2.0	−2.8	+0.2	−2.0	−2.3	−1.1

[a] Data source is the National Center for Health Statistics national mortality data set. Rates are age-adjusted to the year 2000 population standard. The average percentage change per year is the mean percent change per year across the 20-year period, 1990 to 2010. (From Centers for Disease Control and Prevention. U.S. mortality data. http://wonder.cdc.gov/ucd-icd10.html)

decline observed since 1990.[26,27] In fact, the US trial findings suggest that there was virtually no mortality benefit within the first decade following the initiation of screening.[28] Therefore, it is not possible to know how much of this favorable trend was related to early diagnosis, how much was related to improvements in treatment, or how much might have been related to other factors, such as changes in the way cause of death has been listed on death certificates.

The Prostate Cancer Prevention Trial provided an important proof of principle that antiandrogen therapies can reduce prostate cancer risk.[29] Although the net benefits of finasteride for prevention are not clearly demonstrated from this trial, other agents that interfere with androgen effects on prostate cancer growth could prove to be useful for prostate cancer chemoprevention in the future. Prostate cancer incidence trends will likely continue to be largely driven by rates of PSA screening in the coming decade. Longer term results of a clearer benefit to mortality from either the PLCO trial in the United States or the European PSA trial would help to better specify screening recommendations.

Other Cancers

Even though mortality rates have been declining by about 2% per year from the four most common causes of cancer death (lung,

colorectal, breast, and prostate), very little progress has been made in reducing death rates from the other half of all adult cancers in the United States. Continuing progress in tobacco control will have beneficial effects on many other types of cancer linked to tobacco, and stopping the obesity epidemic will have favorable effects on many obesity-related cancers that have been increasing in recent years, such as adenocarcinoma of the esophagus and renal cancer.[30] Melanoma incidence rates have been increasing substantially in recent years, likely the result of the combined effects of previous sun exposure and increased awareness and surveillance for pigmented skin lesions, but recent advances in therapy for metastatic melanoma may foretell future declines in melanoma morality. Declining rates of stomach cancer incidence and mortality over several decades may be related to the combined effects of historic improvements in nutrition and the declining prevalence of chronic infection with *Helicobacter pylori*. Liver cancer incidence has been substantially increasing in recent years, likely resulting from historic trends in chronic infection with hepatitis B and C viruses. As a result, liver cancer will likely continue to rise in the United States over the coming decade.

The incidence of thyroid cancer has been increasing in the United States for the past several decades, but thyroid cancer mortality rates have been stable, a pattern most likely due to increased detection from improved diagnostic techniques. Invasive cervical cancer is uncommon in the United States because of widespread screening using Pap smears. Although the vaccination for human papillomavirus (HPV) has been shown to be highly effective in protecting against the serotypes that together account for 70% of cervical cancer cases, so far, HPV vaccine coverage has been low among young women in the United States.[6] For many of the other cancers, such as cancers of the pancreas, brain, ovary, and the hematopoietic malignancies, risk factors are poorly understood, and there are no effective early detection methods. For these cancers, the current hope for improvement resides in the development of better methods for early cancer detection and treatment.

PREDICTING FUTURE CANCER TRENDS

In the United States, cancer is now the leading cause of death under age 85 years. Over the first half of the ACS 25-year challenge period, overall cancer incidence rates have declined by about 0.2% per year, and mortality rates have declined by about 1% per year. The trends in both incidence and mortality from the four leading cancer sites are summarized in Figure 12.1. Using simple linear extrapolation, it therefore seems that the ACS challenge goals of reducing cancer incidence by 25% and mortality by 50% over 25 years may be only half achieved.[31,32] Clearly, though, estimating future trends only by linear extrapolation is a crude way to foretell future events. Projecting cancer trends into the more distant future using complex modeling is possible, however, as knowledge about changes in major cancer risk factors can lead to reasonable predictions about the direction and approximate slope of future trends. One method to incorporate knowledge about trends in risk factors into estimates of future cancer trends is to estimate the impact of changes in the attributable risk (also called the *preventable fraction*) in the population for each risk factor. By making assumptions about latency period, then tying changes in factors to changes in cancer incidence and mortality, cancer trends resulting from risk factor changes can be predicted. For example, if there were a factor that explained 30% of a particular cancer, then cutting that exposure in half would eventually lead to a projected 15% reduction in rates (50% of 30%). This method was used to project cancer mortality trends to 2015 and seems to have projected trends that are quite similar to those observed in recent years.[33]

Progress in cancer prevention, early detection, and treatment since 1990 has been persistent, and there are many reasons to be optimistic about the future. Just how much steeper the future downward slope in cancer death rates can be driven will depend on the extent to which we can discover new factors causing cancer, and effectively deploy ways to better act on our current knowledge about how to prevent and control cancer. Especially important will be progress in reversing the epidemics of tobacco use and obesity, and ensuring that the coming improvements to health care access will lead to access to state-of-the-art cancer screening and therapy for all.

REFERENCES

1. American Cancer Society Board of Directors. ACS Challenge goals for U.S. Cancer Mortality for the Year 2015. *Proceedings of the Board of Directors.* Atlanta, GA: American Cancer Society, 1996.
2. American Cancer Society Board of Directors. ACS Challenge goals for U.S. Cancer Incidence for the Year 2015. *Proceedings of the Board of Directors.* Atlanta, GA: American Cancer Society, 1998.
3. Centers for Disease Control and Prevention. National Program of Cancer Registries (NPCR) Web site. http://cdc.gov/cancer/npcr.
4. National Cancer Institute. Surveillance, Epidemiology, and End Results Program Web site. http://seer.cancer.gov.
5. Centers for Disease Control and Prevention. U.S. mortality data. http://wonder.cdc.gov/ucd-icd10.html
6. Jemal A, Simard E, Dorell C, et al. Annual report to the nation on the status of cancer, 1975–2009, featuring the burden and trends in human papillomavirus (HPV)–associated cancers and HPV vaccination coverage levels. *J Natl Cancer Inst* 2013;105:175–201.
7. Centers for Disease Control and Prevention. Behavioral Risk Factor Surveillance System Web site. http://cdc.gov/brfss.
8. Ward E, Thun M, Hannan L, et al. Interpreting cancer trends. *Ann N Y Acad Sci* 2006;1076:29–53.
9. Centers for Disease Control and Prevention. Smoking & Tobacco Use Web site. http://cdc.gov/tobacco.
10. Rossouw JE, Anderson GL, Prentice RL, et al. Risks and benefits of estrogen plus progestin in healthy postmenopausal women: principal results from the Women's Health Initiative randomized controlled trial. *JAMA* 2002; 288:321–333.
11. Hersh A, Stefanick M, Stafford R. National use of postmenopausal hormone therapy: annual trends and response to recent evidence. *JAMA* 2004;291:47–53.
12. Ryerson AB, Miller J, Eheman CR, et al. Use of mammograms among women aged ≥40 years—United States, 2000–2005. *MMWR* 2007;56:49–51.
13. Giovino GA. Epidemiology of tobacco use in the United States. *Oncogene* 2002;21:7326–7340.
14. Oken M, Hocking W, Kvale P, et al. Screening by chest radiograph and lung cancer mortality. *JAMA* 2011;306:1865–1873.
15. The National Lung Screening Trial Research Team. Reduced lung-cancer mortality with low-dose computed tomographic screening. *N Engl J Med* 2011; 365:395–409.
16. Smith R, Brooks D, Cokkinides V, et al. Cancer screening in the United States, 2013: a review of current American Cancer Society guidelines, current issues in cancer screening, and new guidance on cervical cancer screening and lung cancer screening. *CA Cancer J Clin* 2013;63:88–105.
17. U.S. Preventive Services Task Force. U.S. Preventive Services Task Force Web site. http://uspreventiveservicestaskforce.org.
18. Martinez ME. Primary prevention of colorectal cancer: lifestyle, nutrition, exercise. *Recent Results Cancer Res* 2005;166:177–211.
19. Atkin W, Edwards R, Kralj-Hans I, et al. Once-only flexible sigmoidoscopy screening in prevention of colorectal cancer: a multicentre randomized controlled trial. *Lancet* 2010;375:1624–1633.
20. Schoen RE, Pinsky PF, Weissfeld JL, et al. Colorectal-cancer incidence and mortality with screening flexible sigmoidoscopy. *N Engl J Med* 2012; 366:2345–2357.
21. Cram P, Fendrick A, Inadomi J, et al. The impact of celebrity promotional campaign on the use of colon cancer screening: the Katie Couric effect. *Arch Intern Med* 2003;163(13):1601–1605.
22. World Cancer Research Fund/American Institute for Cancer Prevention. *Policy and Action for Cancer Prevention. Food, Nutrition, and Physical Activity: A Global Perspective.* Washington, DC: AICR; 2009.
23. Ogden CL, Carroll MD, Curtin LR, et al. Prevalence of overweight and obesity in the United States, 1999–2004. *JAMA* 2006;295:1549–1555.
24. Vogel V, Constantino J, Wickerham D, et al. Effects of tamoxifen vs raloxifene on the risks of developing invasive breast cancer and other disease outcomes: the NSABP Study of Tamoxifen and Raloxifene (STAR) P-2 trial. *JAMA* 2006;295:2727–2741.
25. Berry D, Cronin K, Plevritis S, et al. Effect of screening and adjuvant therapy on mortality from breast cancer. *N Engl J Med* 2005;353:1784–1792.
26. Andriole GL, Crawford ED, Grubb RL 3rd, et al. Mortality results from a randomized prostate-cancer screening trial. *N Engl J Med* 2009;360(13):1310–1319.
27. Schröder FH, Hugosson J, Roobol MJ, et al. Screening and prostate-cancer mortality in a randomized European study. *N Engl J Med* 2009;360(13):1320–1328.
28. Andriole G, Crawford D, Grubb R, et al. Prostate cancer screening in the randomized Prostate, Lung, Colorectal, and Ovarian Cancer Screening Trial: mortality results after 13 years of follow-up. *J Natl Cancer Inst* 2012;104:125–132.
29. Thompson I, Goodman P, Tangen C, et al. Long-term survival of participants in the prostate cancer prevention trial. *N Engl J Med* 2013;369:603–610.
30. International Agency for Cancer Research. *Weight Control and Physical Activity. Handbook 6.* Lyon, France: IARC Press; 2002.
31. Sedjo R, Byers T, Barrera E, et al. A midpoint assessment of the American Cancer Society challenge goal to decrease cancer incidence by 25% between 1992 and 2015. *CA Cancer J Clin* 2007;57:326–340.
32. Byers T, Barrera E, Fontham E, et al. A midpoint assessment of the American Cancer Society challenge goal to halve the U.S. cancer mortality rates between the years 1990 and 2015. *Cancer* 2006;107:396–405.
33. Byers T, Mouchawar J, Marks J, et al. The American Cancer Society challenge goals. How far can cancer rates decline in the U.S. by the year 2015? *Cancer* 1999;86:715–727.

ETIOLOGY AND EPIDEMIOLOGY OF CANCER

PART III

Cancer Therapeutics

13 Essentials of Radiation Therapy

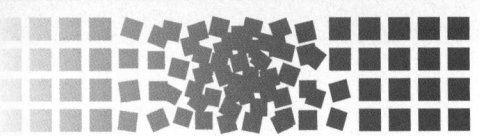

Meredith A. Morgan, Randall K. Ten Haken, and Theodore S. Lawrence

INTRODUCTION

The beneficial use of radiation was launched by the experiments of Wilhelm Roentgen, who, in 1895, found that x-rays could pass through materials that were impenetrable to light. Emil Grubbe provided one of the early examples of the therapeutic use of radiation by treating an advanced ulcerated breast cancer with x-rays in January 1896. We have made great progress since these early days, which has been strongly influenced by research in radiation chemistry, biology, and physics.

BIOLOGIC ASPECTS OF RADIATION ONCOLOGY

Radiation-Induced DNA Damage

Radiation is administered to cells either in the form of photons (x-rays and gamma rays) or particles (protons, neutrons, and electrons). When photons or particles interact with biologic material, they cause ionizations that can either directly interact with subcellular structures or they can interact with water, the major constituent of cells, and generate free radicals that can then interact with subcellular structures (Fig. 13.1).

The direct effects of radiation are the consequence of the DNA in chromosomes absorbing energy that leads to ionizations. This is the major mechanism of DNA damage induced by charged nuclei (such as a carbon nucleus) and neutrons and is termed *high linear energy transfer* (Fig. 13.2). In contrast, the interaction of photons with other molecules, such as water, results in the production of free radicals, some of which possess a lifetime long enough to be able to diffuse to the nucleus and interact with DNA in the chromosomes. This is the major mechanism of DNA damage induced by x-rays and has been termed *low linear energy transfer*.[1]

A free radical generated through the interaction of photons with other molecules that possess an unpaired electron in their outermost shell (e.g., hydroxyl radicals) can abstract a hydrogen molecule from a macromolecule such as DNA to generate damage. Cells that have increased levels of free radical scavengers, such as glutathione, would have less DNA damage induced by x-rays, but would have similar levels of DNA damage induced by a carbon nucleus that is directly absorbed by chromosomal DNA. Furthermore, a low oxygen environment would also protect cells from x-ray–induced damage because there would be fewer radicals available to induce DNA damage in the absence of oxygen, but this environment would have little impact on DNA damage induced by carbon nuclei.[2]

Cellular Responses to Radiation-Induced DNA Damage

Checkpoint Pathways

The cell cycle must progress in a specific order; checkpoint genes ensure that the initiation of late events is delayed until earlier events are complete. There are three principal places in the cell cycle at which checkpoints induced by DNA damage function: the border between G1 phase and S phase, intra-S phase, and the border between G2 phase and mitosis (Fig. 13.3). Cells with an intact checkpoint function that have sustained DNA damage stop progressing through the cycle and become arrested at the next checkpoint in the cell cycle. For example, cells with damaged DNA in G1 phase avoid replicating that damage by arresting at the G1/S interface. If irradiated cells have already passed the restriction point, a position in G1 phase that is regulated by the phosphorylation of the retinoblastoma tumor suppressor gene (*Rb*) and its dissociation from the E2F family of transcription factors, they will transiently arrest in S phase. The G1/S and intra-S phase checkpoints inhibit the replication of damaged DNA and work in a coordinated manner with the DNA repair machinery to permit the restitution of DNA integrity, thereby increasing cell survival.

The earliest response to radiation is the activation of ataxia-telangiectasia mutated (ATM), which involves a conformational change that results in the activation of its kinase domain and phosphorylation of serine 1981 (see Fig. 13.3).[3] This phosphorylation causes the ATM homodimer to dissociate into active monomers that phosphorylate a wide range of proteins such as 53BP1, the histone variant H2AX, Nbs1 (Nijmegen breakage syndrome; a member of the *MRN complex*, composed of Mre11, Rad50, and Nbs1), BRCA1, and SMC1 (structural maintenance of chromosomes), and these proteins coordinate repair with the cell cycle.[4] In response to DNA damage, H2AX is rapidly phosphorylated by ATM and localizes to sites of DNA double-strand breaks in multiprotein complexes described as foci (Fig. 13.4). Phosphorylation of H2AX by ATM results in the direct recruitment of Mdc1 and forms a complex with H2AX to recruit additional ATM molecules, forming a positive feedback loop.

The G1/S phase checkpoint is the best understood. In response to DNA damage, activated ATM can directly phosphorylate p53 and mdm2, the ubiquitin ligase that targets p53 for degradation. These phosphorylations are important for increasing the stability of the p53 protein. In addition to ATM, checkpoint kinase 2 (Chk2) also phosphorylates p53 and can enhance p53 stability. Activated p53 transcriptionally increases the expression of the *p21*^{WAF1/CIP1} gene, which results in a sustained inhibition of G1 cyclin/Cdk, and prevents phosphorylation of pRb and progression from G1 into S.[5] Mutations in p53 that are commonly found in solid tumors result in loss of transcriptional activity and compromised checkpoint function.

Control of the S-phase checkpoint is mediated in part by the Cdc25A phosphatase inhibiting Cdk2 activity and the loading of Cdc45 onto chromatin. If Cdc45 fails to bind to chromatin, DNA polymerase α is not recruited to replication origins and replicon initiation fails to occur.[6] A more prominent mechanism for S-phase arrest is signaled through the MRN complex and the cohesin protein SMC1 by ATM.[7] Loss of ATM, MRN components, or SMC1 leads to the loss of the intra-S phase checkpoint function and increased radiosensitivity. Both the CDC45 and ATM pathways represent parallel, but seemingly independent, pathways to protect replication forks from trying to replicate through DNA strand

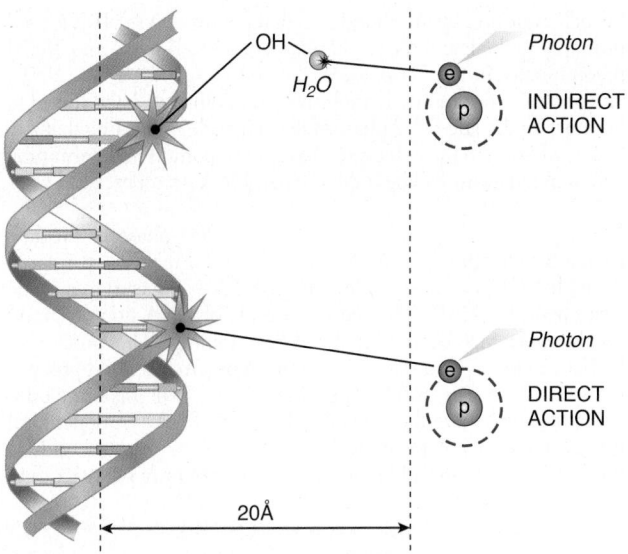

Figure 13.1 The direct and indirect effects of ionizing radiation on DNA. Incident photons transfer part of their energy to free electrons (Compton scattering). These electrons can directly interact with DNA to induce DNA damage, or they can first interact with water to produce hydroxyl radicals that can then induce damage.

breaks. Although ATM has received the lion's share of attention in signaling checkpoint activation in response to ionizing radiation, its family member ATR (ataxia telangiectasia and rad3-related) also plays a role in S-phase checkpoint responses.[8] ATM kinase activity is inducible by radiation, whereas ATR kinase activity is constitutive and does not significantly change with irradiation. (ATR is described in more detail in Chapter 19.) In contrast to Cdc45 and ATM, ATR is probably more important in monitoring

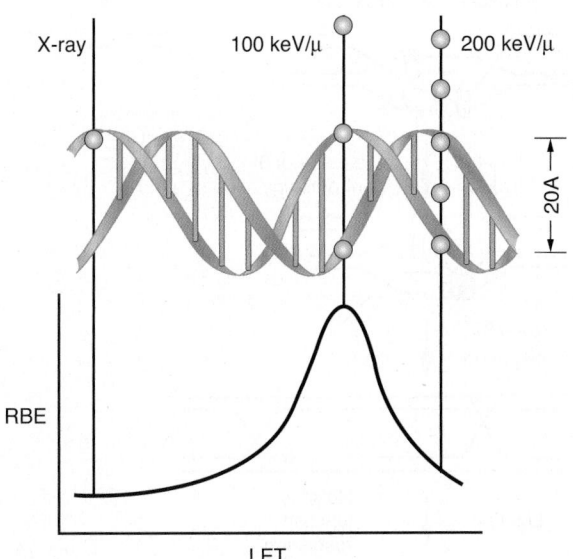

Figure 13.2 Linear energy transfer and DNA damage. Ionizing radiation deposits energy along the track (linear energy transfer [LET]), which causes DNA damage and cell killing. The most biologically potent (highest relative biologic effectiveness [RBE]) LET is 100 keV per μm because the separation between ionizing events is the same as the diameter of the DNA double helix (2 nm). (From Hall EJ, Giaccia AJ. *Radiobiology for the Radiologist*. Philadelphia: Lippincott Williams & Williams; 2012, with permission.)

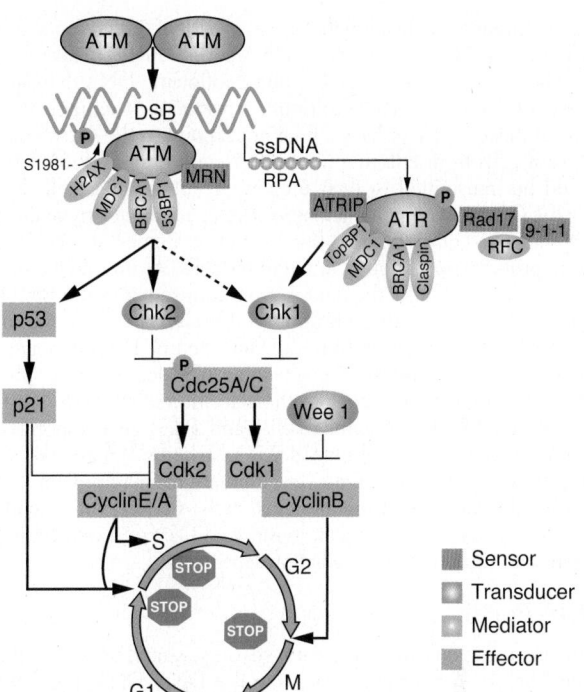

Figure 13.3 In response to DNA damage, the MRN complex—composed of MRE11, Rad50, and NBS1—together with ataxia-telangiectasia mutation (ATM) and H2AX are the earliest proteins recruited to the site of the break. ATM is released from its homodimer complex, activated by transautophosphorylation and, in turn, phosphorylates H2AX. Other members are recruited to the complex such as BRCA1 and 53BP1. As the DNA at the double-strand break (DSB) is resected, single-stranded DNA is formed and bound by replication protein A (RPA), resulting in the activation of the ataxia-telangiectasia and Rad3-related (ATR) pathway. The net result of ATM/ATR activation is the downstream activation of p53, leading to the transcription of the Cdk inhibitor, p21, and the activation of Chk1/Chk2, resulting in the degradation of Cdc25 phosphatases, Cdk-cyclin complex inactivation, and cell cycle arrest at phase G1, intra S, or G2. Note that ATM is also partially activated by changes in chromatin structure induced by DNA double-strand breaks.

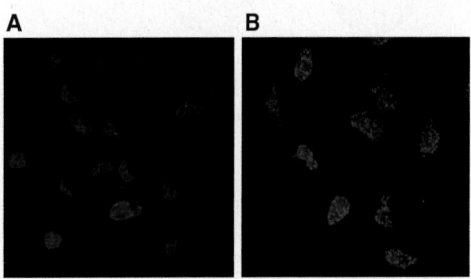

Figure 13.4 Phosphorylated histone variant H2AX as a marker of DNA damage. Phosphorylated histone variant H2AX (also called gamma H2AX) localizes to sites of DNA double-strand breaks, so that its appearance and disappearance correspond with induction and repair of breaks. The cells in panels **A** and **B** have been stained with DAPI (4′,6-diamidino-2-phenylindole) (*blue*) in order to visualize cell nuclei and stained with an antibody, which recognizes *gamma* H2AX (*red*). The cells in **A** are untreated and exhibit little to no gamma H2AX staining, whereas the cells in **B** are treated with 7.5 Gy radiation and exhibit strong gamma H2AX staining at punctate foci in the nuclei, which are thought to correlate with sites of DNA double-strand breaks. (Image provided by Dr. Leslie Parsels, University of Michigan.)

perturbations in replication that are the result of stalled replication forks to prevent the formation of DNA double-strand breaks.

The arrest of cells in the G2 phase following DNA damage is one of the most conserved evolutionary responses to ionizing radiation. It makes sense to have a final checkpoint in the G2 phase to prevent cells from entering into mitosis with damaged DNA that could be transmitted to their progeny. It follows that cells lacking the G2 checkpoint are radiosensitive because they try to divide with damaged chromosomes that cannot be aligned at metaphase to be properly apportioned to daughter cells. At the biochemical level, the regulation of the mitosis-promoting factor cyclin B/Cdk1 is the critical step in the activation of this checkpoint. At the molecular level, ATM and Chk1/2 are activated by DNA damage in the G2 phase and inhibit the activation of Cdc25A and C phosphatases, which are essential for the activation of cyclin B/Cdk1.[9,10] The pololike kinase family (Plk1 and Plk3) also responds to DNA damage and can inhibit Cdc25C activation.[11] A great deal of effort has been focused on the development of small molecules to inhibit checkpoint response proteins, such as Chk1, with the idea that they would inhibit radiation-induced G2 arrest and perhaps repair and thus be used as radiation sensitizers.[12]

DNA Repair

Ionizing radiation causes base damage, single-strand breaks, double-strand breaks, and sugar damage, as well as DNA–DNA, and DNA–protein cross-links. The critical target for ionizing radiation-induced cell inactivation and cell killing is the DNA double-strand break.[13,14] In eukaryotic cells, DNA double-strand breaks can be repaired by two processes: homologous recombination repair (HRR), which requires an undamaged DNA strand as a participant in the repair, and nonhomologous end joining (NHEJ), which mediates end-to-end joining.[15] In lower eukaryotes, such as yeast, HRR is the predominant pathway used for repairing DNA double-strand breaks, whereas mammalian cells use both HHR and non-HHR to repair their DNA. In mammalian cells, the choice of repair is biased by the phase of

the cell cycle and by the abundance of repetitive DNA. HRR is used primarily in the late S phase/G2 phases of the cell-cycle, and NHEJ predominates in the G1-phase of the cell cycle (Fig. 13.5). NHEJ and HRR are not mutually exclusive, and both have been found to be active in the late S/G2 phase of the cell cycle, indicating that factors in addition to the cell-cycle phase are important in determining which mechanism will be used to repair DNA strand breaks.

Nonhomologous End Joining. In the G1-phase of the cell cycle, the ligation of DNA double-strand breaks is primarily through NHEJ because a sister chromatid does not exist to provide a template for HRR. The damaged ends of DNA double-strand breaks must first be modified before rejoining. The process of NHEJ can be divided into at least four steps: synapsis, end processing, fill-in synthesis, and ligation (Fig. 13.6).[16] Synapsis is the critical initial step where the Ku heterodimer and the DNA-dependent protein kinase catalytic subunit (DNA-PKcs) bind to the ends of the DNA double-strand break. Ku recruits not only DNA-PKcs to

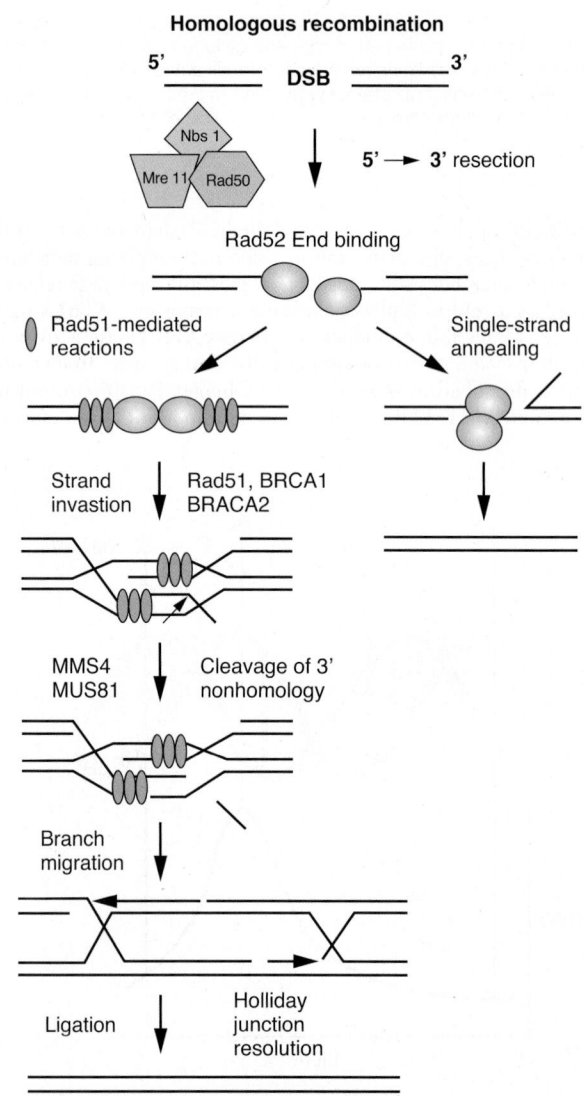

Figure 13.6 Schematic of the critical steps and proteins involved in homologous recombination repair (HRR). The process of HRR can be divided into the following steps: double-strand break (DSB) targeting by H2AX and the MRN complex, recruitment of the ataxia-telangiectasia mutation (ATM) kinase, end processing and protection, strand exchange, single-strand gap filling, and resolution into unique double-stranded molecules.

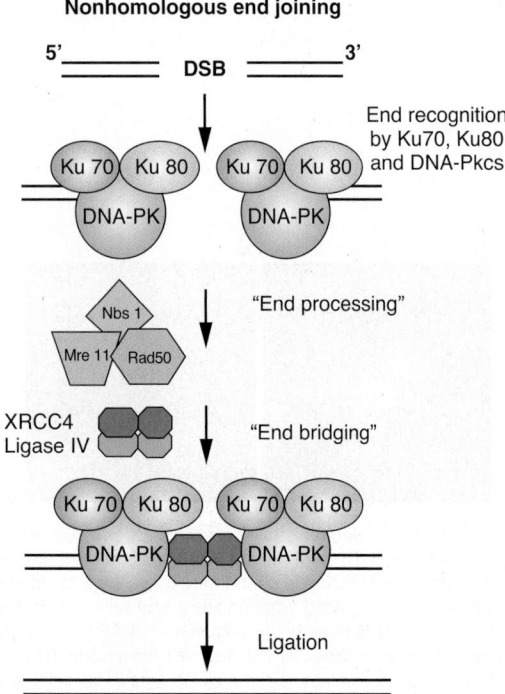

Figure 13.5 Schematic of the critical steps and proteins involved in nonhomologous end joining (NHEJ). The process of NHEJ can be divided into at least four steps: synapsis, end processing, fill-in synthesis, and ligation. DSB, double-strand break.

the DNA ends, but also artemis, a protein that possesses endonuclease activity for 5′ and 3′ overhangs as well as hairpins.[17] DNA-PKcs that is bound to the broken DNA ends phosphorylates artemis and activates its endonuclease activity for end processing. This role of artemis' endonuclease activity in NHEJ may not necessarily be required for the ligation of blunt ends or ends with compatible termini. DNA polymerase μ is associated with the Ku/DNA/XRCC4/DNA ligase IV complex, and is probably the polymerase that is used in the fill-in reaction. The actual rejoining of DNA ends is mediated by a XRCC4/DNA ligase IV complex, which is also probably recruited by the Ku heterodimer.[18,19] Although NHEJ is effective at rejoining DNA double-strand breaks, it is highly error prone. In fact, the main physiologic role of NHEJ is to generate antibodies through V(D)J rejoining, and the error-prone nature of NHEJ is essential for generating antibody diversity.

Homologous Recombination. HRR provides the mammalian genome a high-fidelity pathway of repairing DNA double-strand breaks. In contrast to NHEJ, HRR requires physical contact with an undamaged DNA template, such as a sister chromatid, for repair to occur. In response to a double-strand break, ATM as well as the complex of Mre11, Rad50, and Nbs1 proteins (MRN complex), are recruited to sites of DNA double-strand breaks (Fig. 13.6).[20] The MRN complex is also involved in the recruitment of the breast cancer tumor suppressor gene, BRCA1, to the site of the break.[21] In addition to recruiting BRCA1 to the site of the DNA strand break, Mre11 and as yet unidentified endonucleases resect the DNA, resulting in a 3′ single-strand DNA that serves as a binding site for Rad51. BRCA2, which is recruited to the double-strand break by BRCA1, facilitates the loading of the Rad51 protein onto replication protein A (RPA)-coated single-strand overhangs that are produced by endonuclease resection.[22] The Rad51 protein is a homolog of the *Escherichia coli* recombinase RecA, and possesses the ability to form nucleofilaments and catalyze strand exchange with the complementary strand of the undamaged chromatid, an essential step in HRR. Five additional paralogs of Rad51 also bind to the RPA-coated single-stranded region and recruit Rad52, which binds DNA and protects against exonucleolytic degradation.[23] To facilitate repair, the Rad54 protein uses its ATPase activity to unwind the double-stranded molecule. The two invading ends serve as primers for DNA synthesis, resulting in structures known as Holliday junctions. These Holliday junctions are resolved either by noncrossing over, in which case the Holliday junctions disengage and the DNA strands align followed by gap filling, or by crossing over of the Holliday junctions and gap filling. Because inactivation of most of the HRR genes discussed previously results in radiosensitivity and genomic instability, these genes provide a critical link between HRR and chromosome stability.

Chromosome Aberrations Result from Faulty DNA Double-Strand Break Repair

Unfaithful restitution of DNA strand breaks can lead to chromosome aberrations such as acentric fragments (no centromeres) or terminal deletions (uncapped chromosome ends). Radiation-induced DNA double-strand breaks also induce exchange-type aberrations that are the consequence of symmetric translocations between two DNA double-strand breaks in two different chromosomes (Fig. 13.7). Symmetrical chromosome translocations often do not lead to lethality, because genetic information is not lost in subsequent cell divisions. In contrast, when two DNA double-strand breaks in two different chromosomes recombine to form one chromosome with two centromeres and two fragments of chromosomes without centromeres or telomeres, cell death is inevitable. These types of chromosome aberrations are the consequence of asymmetrical chromosome translocations where the genetic material is recombined in what has been termed an *illegitimate* manner (e.g., a chromosome containing an extra centromere).

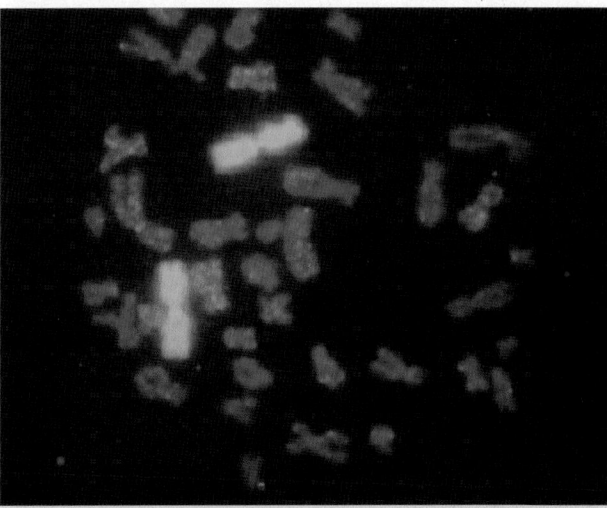
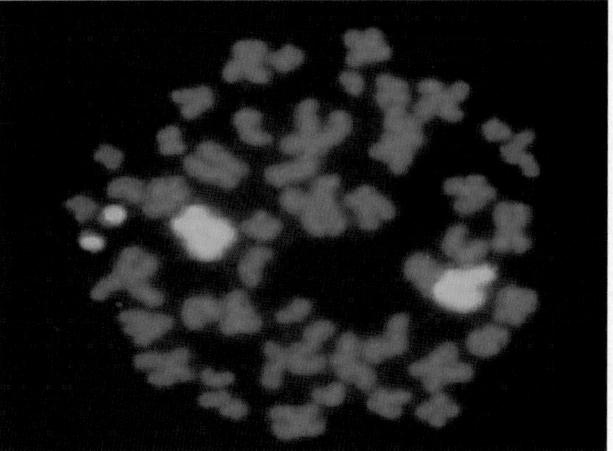

Figure 13.7 Fluorescent in situ hybridization of DNA probes that specifically recognize chromosome 4. In unirradiated cells **(top)**, two chromosome 4s are visualized. In irradiated cells **(bottom)**, one chromosome 4 illegitimately recombined with another chromosome to produce an asymmetrical chromosome aberration, with resulting acentric fragments that will be lost in subsequent cell divisions.

During mitosis, when a cell divides, aberrant chromosomes that have two centromeres, lack a centromere, or are in the shape of a ring have difficulty in separating, resulting in daughter cells with unequal or asymmetric distribution of the parental genetic material. The quantification of asymmetric chromosome aberrations induced by radiation is difficult and has to be performed by the first cell division because these aberrations will be lost during subsequent cell divisions. For this reason, symmetrical chromosome aberrations have been used to assess radiation-induced damage many generations after exposure because they are not lost from the population of exposed cells. In fact, symmetrical chromosome aberrations can be detected in the descendants of survivors of Hiroshima and Nagasaki, indicating that they are stable biomarkers of radiation exposure.[24]

Membrane Signaling

Apart from the direct of effects on DNA, radiation also affects cellular membranes. As part of the cellular stress response, radiation activates membrane receptor signaling pathways such as those initiated via epidermal growth factor receptor (EGFR) and transforming growth factor β (TGF-β).[25,26] Activation of these pathways promotes overall survival in response to radiation by promoting DNA damage repair and/or cellular proliferation. In addition,

Cellular Response to Genotoxic Stress

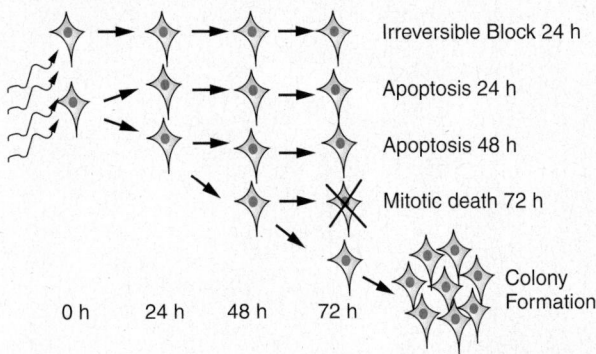

Irreversible Block 24 h

Apoptosis 24 h

Apoptosis 48 h

Mitotic death 72 h

Colony Formation

0 h   24 h   48 h   72 h

Figure 13.8 Consequences of exposure to ionizing radiation at the cellular level. Cells exposed to ionizing radiation can enter a state of senescence where they are unable to divide, but are still able to secrete growth factors. Alternatively, cells can die through apoptosis, mitotic linked cell death, or they can repair their DNA damage and produce viable progeny.

radiation also induces ceramide production at the membrane via activation of sphingomyelinases, which hydrolyze sphingomyelin to form ceramide. Ceramide production is linked to radiation-induced apoptosis.[27]

The Effect of Radiation on Cell Survival

The major potential consequences of cells exposed to ionizing radiation are normal cell division, DNA damage–induced senescence (reproductively inactive but metabolically active), apoptosis, or mitotic-linked cell death (Fig. 13.8). These manifestations of DNA damage can occur within one or two cell divisions or can manifest at later times after many cell divisions.[28] Effects that occur

at later times have been termed *delayed reproductive cell death* and may also be influenced by secreted factors that are induced in response to radiation.[29]

The ability to culture cells derived from both normal and tumor tissues has allowed us to gain insight into how radiosensitivity varies between tissues by analyzing the shape of survival curves. Survival curves of tumor cells often possess a shouldered region at low doses that becomes shallower as the dose increases and eventually becomes exponential. A shoulder on a survival means that these low doses of radiation are less efficient in cell killing, presumably because cells are efficient at repairing DNA strand breaks.[13,14] Killing at low doses of radiation can be described in the form of a linear quadratic equation: $S = e^{-\alpha D - \beta D2}$ (Fig. 13.9).[30] In this equation, S is the fraction of cells that survive a dose (D) of radiation, whereas α and β are constants. Cell killing by the linear and quadratic components are equal when $\alpha D = \beta D^2$ or $D = \alpha/\beta$. Over a larger dose range, the relationship between cell killing and dose is more complex and is described by three different components: an initial slope (D_1), a final slope (D_o), and the width of the shoulder (n, the extrapolation number) or Dq, the quasi-threshold dose (Fig. 13.10). The extrapolation number, n, defines the place where the shoulder intersects the ordinate when the dose is extrapolated to zero, and the quasithreshold dose, Dq, defines the width of the shoulder by cutting the dose axis when there is a survival fraction of unity. In contrast to photons, the shoulder on the survival curve disappears when cells are exposed to densely ionizing radiation from particles, indicating that this form of radiation is highly effective at killing cells at both low and high doses.

In Vivo Survival Determination of Normal Tissue Response to Radiation

Although much of our knowledge on the effects of radiation on cell survival has come from cell culture studies, investigators have also devised experimental approaches to assess the clonogenic survival of normal tissues. The earliest example came from McCulloch and Till,[31] who developed an assay to measure the

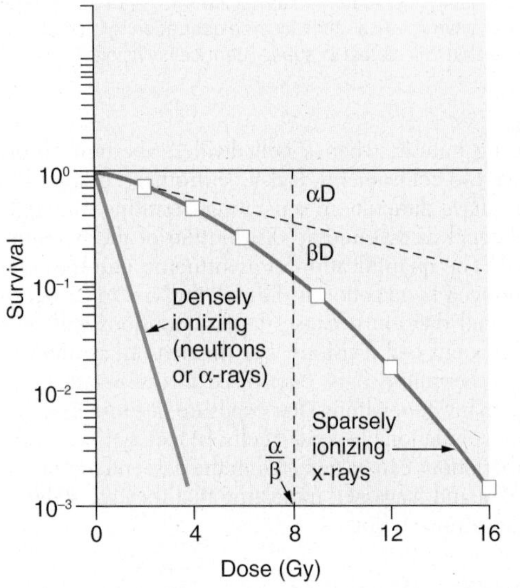

Figure 13.9 An analysis of survival curves for mammalian cells exposed to radiation by the linear quadratic model. The probability of hitting a critical target is proportional to dose (aD): the alpha component. The probability of hitting two critical targets will be the product of those probabilities; therefore, it will be proportional to dose[2] (βD^2): the beta component. The dose at which killing by both the alpha and beta components is equal is defined as $D = \alpha/\beta$. (From Hall EJ, Giaccia AJ. *Radiobiology for the Radiologist*. Philadelphia: Lippincott Williams & Williams; 2012, with permission.)

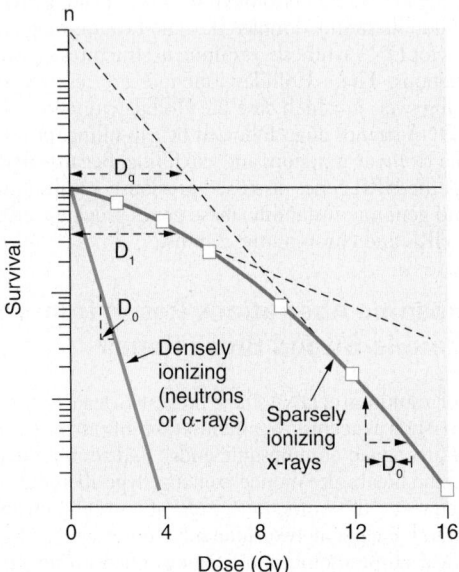

Figure 13.10 An analysis of survival curves for mammalian cells exposed to radiation by the multitarget model. This survival is described by an initial slope (D_1; dose to decreased survival to 37% on initial portion of the curve), a final slope (D_0; dose to decrease survival from starting point to 37% of that point on straight line portion of the curve), an extrapolation number (n; an estimate of the width of the shoulder), and a quasithreshold (D_q; a type of threshold dose below which radiation has no effect). (From Hall EJ, Giaccia AJ. *Radiobiology for the Radiologist*. Philadelphia: Lippincott Williams & Williams; 2012, with permission.)

clonogenic survival of bone marrow–derived cells in response to radiation by injecting them into a recipient mouse and quantifying the number of colonies that developed in the spleen. An analysis of these in vivo spleen assays indicated that bone marrow cells are highly radiosensitive (perhaps the most radiosensitive of all mammalian cells) in that their cell survival curve lacked a shoulder. These experiments represent two important firsts in the radiation sciences: They described the first development of an in vivo assay to assess normal tissue survival to radiation, and they demonstrated the first existence of normal tissue stem cells. Soon after, Withers and colleagues[32] developed an assay to assess the survival of skin stem cells, and Withers and Elkind[33] developed an assay to quantify the viability of small intestinal clonogens.

Because these ingenious approaches cannot be applied to all normal tissues, loss of tissue function instead of clonogenic survival has been used as an end point to assess radiation effects. Effects on tissue function can be grouped into the acute or late variety. Desquamation of skin by radiation is an example of an acute loss of function, whereas loss of spinal cord function is an example of a late functional effect. Acutely sensitive tissues such as skin, bone marrow, and intestinal mucosa possess a significant component of tissue cell division, whereas delayed sensitive tissues, such as spinal cord, breast, and bone, do not possess a significant amount of cell division or turnover and manifest radiation effects at later times.

In Vivo Determination of Tumor Response to Radiation

Assays have also been developed to assess the clonogenic survival of tumor cells in animals. Perhaps the most relevant of these assays is the tumor control dose 50% (TCD_{50}) assay,[34] in which the dose of radiation needed to control the growth of 50% of the tumors is determined in large cohorts of tumor-bearing animals. The TCD_{50} assay in animals most closely approximates the clinical situation because tumors are irradiated in animals and the ability to kill all viable tumor cells is assessed. Unlike assays in which tumor cells are irradiated ex vivo, the TCD_{50} assay takes into account the effects of the tumor microenvironment on tumor response. In contrast to the TCD_{50} assay, the tumor growth delay assay reflects the time after irradiation that a transplanted tumor reaches a fixed multiple of the pretreatment volume compared to an unirradiated control. This end point can be achieved by measuring tumor volume through the use of calipers or by a noninvasive measurement of tumor volume using bioluminescent molecules such as luciferase or fluorescent proteins. In the latter approach, all the tumor cells are stably transfected with a bioluminescent marker before implantation, and tumor growth is measured by bioluminescent activity.[35] The advantage of this approach is that tumor cells can be assessed even if they are orthotopically transplanted into their tissue of origin. In another approach, tumors or cells are first irradiated in vivo, the tumor is excised and made into a single-cell suspension, and these cells are then injected into a non–tumor-bearing animal. If the cells are injected subcutaneously under the skin, the end point is tumor formation.[36] If the tumor cells are injected in the tail vein of the mouse, the end point is colony formation in the lungs.[37] The major advantage of these assays is that the actual number of viable cells can be determined.

FACTORS THAT AFFECT RADIATION RESPONSE

The Fundamental Principles of Radiobiology

Studies on split-dose repair (SDR) by Elkind et al.[38] uncovered three of what we now recognize as the most fundamental principles of fractionated radiotherapy: repair, reassortment, and repopulation (Fig. 13.11). (Reoxygenation, described in the following paragraphs, is the fourth). SDR describes the increased survival

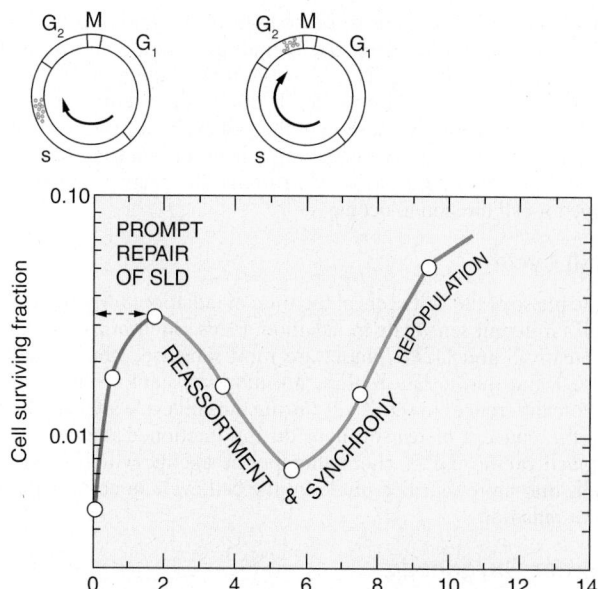

Figure 13.11 Idealized survival curve of rodent cells exposed to two fractions of x-rays. This figure illustrates how the time interval between doses alters the sensitivity of cells when exposed to multiple fractions. In this case, cells move from a resistant phase of the cell cycle (late S phase) to a sensitive phase of the cell cycle (G2 phase). This is known as *reassortment*. If longer periods of time occur between fractions of radiation, cells will undergo division. This latter process is called *repopulation*. SLD, sublethal damage. (From Hall EJ, Giaccia AJ. *Radiobiology for the Radiologist*. Philadelphia: Lippincott Williams & Williams; 2012, with permission.)

or tumor growth delay found if a dose of radiation is split into two fractions compared to the same dose administered in one fraction. This repair is likely due to DNA double-strand break rejoining. Elkind et al. found that the survival of cells increased with an increase in time between doses for up to a maximum of about 6 hours. This finding is consistent with the clinical observation that a separation of radiation treatments by 6 hours produces similar normal tissue injury as a 24-hour separation. The shoulder of a survival curve is strongly influenced by SDR: The broader the shoulder, the more SDR and the smaller α/β ratio.

Similar to repair, reassortment and repopulation are also dependent on the interval of time between radiation fractions. If cells are given short time intervals between doses, they can progress from a resistant portion of the cell cycle (e.g., S phase) to a sensitive portion of the cell cycle (e.g., G2 phase). This transit between resistant and sensitive phases of the cell cycle is termed *reassortment*. If irradiated cells are provided even longer intervals of time between doses, the survival of the population of irradiated cells will increase. This increase in split-dose survival after longer periods of time is the result of cell division and has been termed *repopulation*. Reassortment and repopulation appear to have more protracted kinetics in normal tissues than rapidly proliferating tumor cells, and thereby enhance the tumor response to fractionated radiotherapy compared to normal tissues.

Dose-Rate Effects

For sparsely ionizing radiation, dose rate plays a critical factor in cell killing. Lowering the dose rate, and thereby increasing exposure time, reduces the effectiveness of killing by x-rays because of increased SDR. A further reduction in dose rate results in more SDR and reduces the shoulder of the survival curve. Thus, if one plots the survival for individual doses in a multifraction experiment so that there is sufficient time for SDR to occur, the resulting survival curve would have little shoulder and appear almost linear.[39]

In some cell types, there is a threshold to the lowering of dose rate, and in fact, one paradoxically finds an increase, instead of a decrease, in cell killing. This increase in cell killing under these conditions of protracted dose rate is due to the accumulation of cells in a radiosensitive portion of the cell cycle. In summary, the magnitude of the dose rate effect varies between cell types because of SDR, the redistribution of cells through the cell cycle, and the time for cell division to occur.

Cell Cycle

The phase of the cell cycle at the time of radiation influences the cell's inherent sensitivity to radiation. Cells synchronized in late G1/early S and G2/M phases are most sensitive, whereas cells in G1 and mid to late S phase are more resistant to radiation.[1] These differences in sensitivity during the cell cycle are exploited by the concept of reassortment during fractioned radiotherapy as well by the use of chemotherapeutic agents, which reassort cells into more sensitive phases of the cell cycle in combination with radiation.

Tumor Oxygenation

The major microenvironmental influence on tumor response to radiation is molecular oxygen.[40] Decreased levels of oxygen (hypoxia) in tissue culture result in decreased killing after radiation, which can be expressed as an *oxygen enhancement ratio* (OER). Operationally, OER is defined as the ratio of doses to give the same killing under hypoxic and normoxic conditions. At high doses of radiation, the OER is approximately 3, whereas at low doses, it is closer to 2.[41] Oxygen must be present within 10 μs of irradiation to achieve its radiosensitizing effect. Under hypoxic conditions, damage to DNA can be repaired more readily than under oxic conditions, where damage to DNA is "fixed" because of the interaction of oxygen with free radicals generated by radiation. These changes in radiation sensitivity are detectable at oxygen ranges below 30 mm Hg. Most tumor cells exhibit a survival difference halfway between fully aerobic and fully anoxic cells when exposed to a partial pressure of oxygen between 3 and 10 mm Hg.[1] The presence of hypoxia has greater significance for single-dose fractions used in the treatment of certain primary tumors and metastases and is less important for fractionated radiotherapy, where reoxygenation occurs between fractions. Furthermore, most hypoxic cells are not actively undergoing cell division, thus impeding the efficacy of conventional chemotherapeutic agents that are targeted to actively dividing cells.

Although normal tissue and tumors vary in their oxygen concentrations, only tumors possess levels of oxygen low enough to influence the effectiveness of radiation killing. Although the variations in normal tissue oxygenation are in large part due to physiology governing acute changes in oxygen consumption, the variations in tumor oxygen can be directly attributed to abnormal vasculature that results in a more chronic condition. Thomlinson and Gray[42] observed that variations in tumor oxygen occur because there is insufficient vasculature to provide oxygen to all tumor cells. They hypothesized that oxygen is unable to reach tumor cells beyond 10 to 12 cell diameters from the lumen of a tumor blood vessel because of metabolic consumption by respiring tumor cells. This form of hypoxia caused by metabolic consumption of oxygen has been termed *chronic* or *diffusion-mediated hypoxia*. In contrast, changes in blood flow due either to interstitial pressure changes in tumor blood vessels that lack a smooth muscle component or red blood cell fluxes can cause transient occlusion of blood vessels resulting in *acute* or *transient hypoxia*. Chronically, hypoxic cells will only become reoxygenated when their distance from the lumen of a blood vessel decreases, such as during fractionated radiotherapy when tumor cords shrink. In contrast, tumor cells that are acutely hypoxic because of changes in blood flow or interstitial pressure often cycle in an unpredictable manner between oxic and hypoxic states as blood flow changes.

Based on studies demonstrating that hypoxia can alter radiation sensitivity and decrease tumor control by radiotherapy, strategies have been developed to increase tumor oxygenation. Most importantly, it appears that tumor oxygen levels increase during a course of fractionated radiation. This may be one of the most important benefits of fractionated radiation and is termed *reoxygenation* (the fourth of the four Rs of radiobiology). Tumor reoxygenation during a course of fractionated radiation may also offer an explanation for the general lack of clinical efficacy of hypoxic cell sensitizers despite the clear evidence that hypoxia causes radioresistance.

Aside from using fractionated radiation, the most direct approach to increasing tumor oxygenation is to expose patients receiving radiotherapy to hyperbaric oxygen therapy. The underlying concept is that increasing the amount of oxygen in the bloodstream should result in more oxygen being available for diffusion to the hypoxic regions of tumors. Experimentally, hyperbaric oxygen therapy increases the sensitivity of transplanted tumors to radiation. The results of clinical studies with hyperbaric oxygen therapy, when combined with radiotherapy, showed improvement for two sites—head and neck cancers, and cervix cancers—but failed to show an improvement with other sites, thus calling into question its general usefulness in radiotherapy.[43] In a related approach, erythropoietin (EPO), a hormone released by the kidney that increases red blood cell production, should also increase tumor oxygenation by increasing the delivery of hemoglobin-bound oxygen molecules. EPO has been effective at correcting anemia, but has not been successful in combination with radiation to control head and neck cancer and may, in fact, stimulate tumor growth.[44, 45]

Another strategy to increase tumor oxygenation has been the combined use of nicotinamide, which increases tissue perfusion and carbogen (95% O_2 and 5% CO_2) breathing (accelerated radiotherapy with carbogen and nicotinamide [ARCON] therapy). Recently, a randomized phase III clinical trial demonstrated improved regional but not local tumor control in larynx cancer patients treated with nicotinamide, carbogen, and radiation versus radiation alone.[46] Biologics such as antivascular endothelial growth factor (anti-VEGF) therapy have also been demonstrated to increase tumor oxygenation.[47] Anti-VEGF therapy may increase tumor oxygenation by eliminating abnormal vessels that are inadequate in perfusing tumor cells—the so-called *vascular normalization hypothesis*. Although there is solid experimental evidence to support this hypothesis, there appears to be only a short window of time in which it could be effectively combined with radiotherapy.

Because the presence of hypoxia has both prognostic and potential therapeutic implications, a substantial effort has been invested in trying to image hypoxia.[48] The goal of using imaging to "paint" radiation doses to different regions of tumors, although technically possible (as described in the next section, Radiation Physics), faces the problem that changes in oxygenation are dynamic.[49] In the future, hypoxia-directed treatment may evolve from the use of hypoxic cell cytotoxins to targeted drugs that exploit cellular signaling changes induced by hypoxia such as hypoxia-inducible factor 1α (HIF-1α). However, despite the strong rationale supporting their use, at this time, there are no agents used in the clinic that target hypoxia.

Immune Response

The abscopal effects of radiation (i.e., tumor cell killing outside of the radiation field) have been attributed to the activation of antigen and cytokine release by radiation, which subsequently activates a systemic immune response against tumor cells.[50,51] This response begins with the transfer of tumor cell antigens to dendritic cells and, subsequently, the activation of tumor-specific T cells and *immunogenic tumor cell death*. It is likely that radiation dose and fractionation influence the optimal immune response with higher doses and fewer fractions of radiation than those used in conventional fractionation schemes appearing superior in experimental models. Unfortunately, abscopal effects are uncommon because immune system evasion is an inherent characteristic of cancer cells that often dominates, even in the presence of a radiation-induced immune response. Strategies to amplify radiation-induced immune responses, and thus to overcome tumor cell evasion of the immune system, are under investigation. The combination of radiation with immune *checkpoint* modulators such as ipilimumab, an antibody against cytotoxic T-lymphocyte antigen 4 (CTLA-4), have shown promising, albeit anecdotal, clinical effects.

DRUGS THAT AFFECT RADIATION SENSITIVITY

For over 30 years now, chemotherapy and radiotherapy have been administered concurrently. In order to maximize the efficacy of radiochemotherapy, it is necessary to understand the biologic mechanisms underlying radiosensitization by chemotherapeutic agents. The several classes of standard chemotherapeutic agents as well as novel molecularly targeted agents that possess radiosensitizing properties will be discussed in this section.

Antimetabolites

5-fluorouracil is among the most commonly used chemotherapeutic radiation sensitizers. Given in combination with radiation, it has led to clinical improvements in a variety of cancers, including those of the head and neck, the esophagus, the stomach, the pancreas, the rectum, the anus, and the cervix. The combination of 5-fluorouracil with radiation is now a standard therapy for cancers of the stomach (adjuvant), the pancreas (unresectable), and the rectum. For other cancers such as head and neck, esophagus, or anal, 5-fluorouracil and radiation are combined with cisplatin or mitomycin C, respectively. Being an analog of uracil, 5-flourouracil is misincorporated into RNA and DNA. However, the ability of 5-fluorouracil to radiosensitize is related to its ability to inhibit thymidylate synthase, which leads to the depletion of thymidine triphosphate (dTTP) and the inhibition of DNA synthesis. This slowed, inappropriate progression through S phase in response to 5-fluorouracil is thought to be the mechanism underlying radiosensitization.[52] Similar to 5-fluorouracil, the oral thymidylate synthase inhibitor, capecitabine, is also being increasingly used in combination with radiation.

Gemcitabine (2′, 2′-deoxyfluorocytidine [dFdCyd]) is another potent antimetabolite radiosensitizer. Preclinical studies have demonstrated that radiosensitization by gemcitabine involves the depletion of deoxyadenosine triphosphate (dATP) (related to the ability of gemcitabine diphosphate (dFdCDP) to inhibit ribonucleotide reductase) as well as the redistribution of cells into the early S phase of the cell cycle.[53] The combination of gemcitabine with radiation in clinical trials has suggested improved clinical outcomes for patients with cancers of the lung, pancreas, and bladder. Gemcitabine-based chemoradiation has developed into a standard therapy for locally advanced pancreatic cancer. However, in some clinical trials, such as those in lung and head and neck cancers, the combination of gemcitabine with radiation has led to increased mucositis and esophagitis.[54] Thus, it should be emphasized that in the presence of gemcitabine, radiation fields must be defined with great caution. Such is the case with pancreatic cancer, where the combination of full-dose gemcitabine with radiation to the gross tumor can be safely administered if clinically uninvolved lymph nodes are excluded.[55] Conversely, the inclusion of the regional lymphatics in the treatment field in combination with full-dose gemcitabine produces unacceptable toxicities.[56]

Platinums and Temozolomide

Cisplatin is likely the most commonly used chemotherapeutic agent in combination with radiation. Although cisplatin was the prototype for several other platinum analogs, carboplatin is also frequently used in combination with radiation. Cisplatin, in combination with radiation, and sometimes in conjunction with a second chemotherapeutic agent, is indicated for cancers of the head and neck, esophagus (with 5-fluorouracil), the lung, the cervix, and the anus. Radiosensitization by cisplatin is related to its ability to cause inter- and intra-strand DNA cross-links. Removal of these cross-links during the repair process results in DNA strand breaks. Although there are multiple theories to explain the mechanism(s) of radiosensitization by cisplatin, two plausible explanations are that cisplatin inhibits the repair (both homologous and nonhomologous) of radiation-induced DNA double-strand breaks and/or increases the number of lethal radiation-induced double-strand breaks.[57]

Temozolomide in combination with radiation is standard therapy for glioblastoma. Temozolomide is an alkylating agent, which forms methyl adducts at the O^6 position of guanine (as well as at N^7 and N^3-guanine) that are subsequently improperly repaired by the mismatch repair pathway. Radiosensitization by temozolomide involves the inhibition of DNA repair and/or an increase in radiation-induced DNA double-strand breaks due to radiation-induced single-strand breaks in proximity to O^6 methyl adducts. Like cisplatin, temozolomide-mediated radiosensitization does not seem to require cell cycle redistribution.

Taxanes

The taxanes, paclitaxel and docetaxel, act to stabilize microtubules resulting in the accumulation of cells in G2/M, the most radiation-sensitive phase of the cell cycle. The radiosensitizing properties of the taxanes are thought to be attributable to the redistribution of cells into G2/M. Paclitaxel, in combination with radiation (and carboplatin), has demonstrated a clinical benefit in the treatment of resectable lung carcinoma.[58]

Molecularly Targeted Agents

Molecularly targeted agents are especially appealing in the context of radiosensitization because they are generally less toxic than standard chemotherapeutic agents and need to be given in multimodality regimens (given their often inadequate efficacy as single agents). The EGFR has been intensely pursued as a target; both antibody and small molecule EGFR inhibitors, such as cetuximab and erlotinib, respectively, have been developed. The head and neck seem to be the most promising tumor sites for the combination of EGFR inhibitors with radiation therapy. Preclinical data have demonstrated that the schedule of administration of EGFR inhibitors with radiation is important; EGFR inhibition before chemoradiation may produce antagonism.[59] In a randomized phase III trial, cetuximab plus radiation produced a significant survival advantage over radiation alone in patients with locally advanced head and neck cancer.[60] In a subsequent trial, however, cetuximab in combination with concurrent, cisplatin-based chemoradiation failed to produce a survival benefit in head and neck cancer patients.[61] The combination of EGFR inhibitor with cisplatin-radiation requires further preclinical investigation.

Although EGFR inhibition, concurrent with radiation, is by far the best established combination of a molecularly targeted agent with radiation, other exciting molecularly targeted agents are being developed as radiation sensitizers. Targeting DNA damage response pathways is one approach to radiosensitization. Recently, agents that abrogate radiation-induced cell cycle checkpoints, such as Wee1 and Chk1 inhibitors, have been shown to radiosensitize

CANCER THERAPEUTICS

tumor cells and are currently in clinical development in combination with chemotherapy, with clinical trials planned in combination with radiation.[62,63] In addition, poly(ADP-ribose) polymerase (PARP) inhibitors have been demonstrated to preclinically induce radiosensitization, and several clinical trials combining PARP inhibitors with radiation therapy are underway.[64]

Other Agents

Although the most common clinically used agents in combination with radiation have been shown to produce significant clinical benefit, as described previously, other agents with different mechanisms of action have been used as radiation sensitizers as well as radiation protectors. The vinca alkaloids, such as vincristine, possess radiosensitizing properties due to their ability to block mitotic spindle assembly and, thus, arrest cells in M phase. Although vincristine is used in combination with radiation to treat medulloblastoma, rhabdomyosarcoma, and brain stem glioma, its use is principally based on its lack of myelosuppressive side effects, which are dose limiting for radiation in these types of tumors, rather than its potential radiosensitizing properties.

Also worth mention in a discussion of modulators of radiation sensitivity are agents designed to radioprotect normal tissues. One such type of drug, amifostine, is a free radical scavenger with some selectivity toward normal tissues that express more alkaline phosphatase than tumor cells, the enzyme of which converts amifostine to a free thiol metabolite. Clinical trials in head and neck as well as lung cancers have shown a reduction in radiation-related toxicities such as xerostomia, mucositis, esophagitis, and pneumonitis, respectively.[65,66] However, further clinical investigations are necessary to conclusively demonstrate a lack of tumor protection and safety in combination with chemoradiotherapy regimens.

RADIATION PHYSICS

Physics of Photon Interactions

Tumors requiring radiation can be found at depths ranging from zero to 10s of centimeters below the skin. The goal of treatment is to deliver sufficient ionizing radiation to the tumor site, which can result in an absorbed dose. This involves both the availability of treatment beams and delivery techniques, and the methods to plan the treatments and ensure their safe delivery. This section will establish the general physical basis for the use of ionizing radiation in the treatment of tumors, briefly describe some of the treatment equipment, indicate physical qualities of the treatment beams themselves, and summarize the treatment planning process. Those who desire more in-depth details are referred to textbooks and other resources dedicated to medical physics and the technologic aspects of radiation oncology.[67] Most patients who are treated with radiation receive high-energy, external-beam photon therapy. Here, *external* indicates that the treatment beam is generated and delivered from outside of the body. High-energy (6 to 20 MV) photon beams (electromagnetic radiation) penetrate tissue, enabling the treatment of deep-seated tumors. Modern equipment generates these beams with sufficient fluence to ensure delivery of therapeutic fractions of dose in short treatment sessions. Other types of particles and beams also exist for use in treating tumors both externally and internally. They are mentioned briefly later. However, as external photon beams dominate the practice (and as common basic physics principles related to delivered dose exist among the modalities), the focus here will be on photon beam generation and interactions in tissue.

As mentioned earlier, ionizing radiation kills cells via both direct and indirect mechanisms. Radiation therapy aims to instigate those ionizations and events in the tumor cells. Photons are massless, uncharged packets of energy that primarily interact with matter via electromagnetic processes. As a consequence of those interactions, an incident photon can become either entirely absorbed (giving up its energy to the ejection of an atomic electron [photoelectric effect]), or create an energetic electron-positron pair (pair production), or scatter off an electron with a reduction in energy and a change in direction and subsequent transfer of parts of its energy to the free electron (Compton scattering). The secondary electrons generated as a consequence of these interactions have residual energy, mass, and, most importantly, electric charge. They slow down in matter through multiple interactions with (primarily) the electrons of atoms, leading to excitation and ionization of those atoms. These ionizations (hence the term *ionizing radiation*) lead to a local absorption of energy (i.e., dose = energy absorbed per unit mass) and the direct and indirect cell killing effects necessary to treat tumors.

Thus, the use of external photon beams for cancer therapy involves a two-step process: interaction (scattering) of the photons, with subsequent dose deposition via the secondary electrons. The probability of photon interactions is energy dependent. Photoelectric interactions dominate at lower photon energies. Whereas these beams are ideal for diagnostic procedures (for their preferential absorption by tissues of differing atomic number, leading to good subject contrast), they are attenuated too quickly in tissues to supply enough interactions to be useful for therapy for any but the most superficial tumors. Pair production interactions dominate at higher photon energies; however, the probability of interacting in tissues for those high-energy photons is so low as to preclude them from general use as well. In the 10s to 100s of kiloelectron volt (keV) to the few megaelectron volt (MeV) photon energy range, Compton scattering dominates. As will be shown, these beams have sufficient penetration and can be generated with sufficient intensity to be useful for tumor treatments, especially when combined in treatment plans that comprise multiple beams entering the patient from different directions but overlapping at the tumor.

It is useful to point out physical scales of reference for external photon beam therapy. A typical megavoltage photon beam may have an average photon energy near 2 MeV. Those photons primarily undergo Compton scattering with a mean free path in tissue of approximately 20 cm. An average Compton interaction results in a secondary electron with a mean energy near 0.5 MeV (and a Compton scattered photon near 1.5 MeV, which likely escapes or scatters elsewhere in the patient). A typical secondary electron of approximately 0.5 MeV will cause excitations and ionizations of atoms as it dissipates its energy over a path length of approximately 2 mm. This could be expected to lead to approximately 10,000 ionizations, or about 5 ionizations per micron of tissue. As can be seen, therapeutic damage to the DNA of cancer cells (2 nm; see Fig. 13.2) will require very many Compton scatterings with statistical interaction among the ionizations resulting from the slowing down of the secondary electrons.

Photon Beam Generation and Treatment Delivery

As previously mentioned, effective external-beam photon treatments require higher energy beams capable of reaching deep-seated tumors with sufficient fluence to make it likely that the dose deposition will kill the tumor cells. To spare normal tissues and maximize targeting, beams are arranged to enter the patient from several directions and to intersect at the center of the tumor (treatment isocenter). Although machines containing collimated beams from high-intensity radioactive sources (primarily cobalt 60 [^{60}Co]) are still in use, today's modern treatment machine accelerates electrons to high (MeV) energy and impinges them onto an x-ray production target, leading to the generation of intense beams of Bremsstrahlung x-rays. A typical photon beam treatment machine[68,69] (Fig. 13.12) consists of a high-energy (6 to 20 MeV) linear electron accelerator, electromagnetic beam steering and

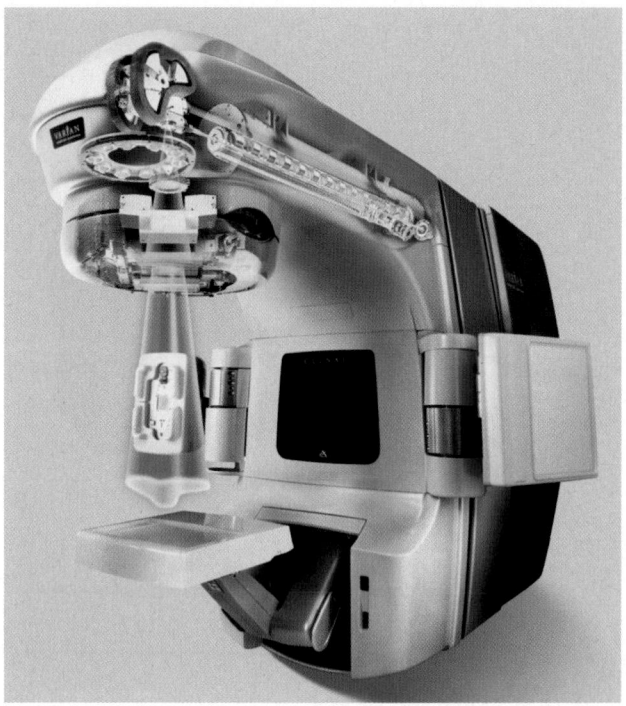

Figure 13.12 A shadow view of a C-arm linear accelerator. The electron beam (originating at upper right) is accelerated through a linear accelerator wave guide, selected for correct energy in a bending magnet, and then impinges on an x-ray production target. The x-ray beam (originating at target upper left) is flattened and collimated before leaving the treatment head. Also illustrated (downstream from the beam) is an electric portal imager that is used to measure (image) the beam exiting a patient. (From Varian Medical Systems, Palo Alto, CA, with permission.)

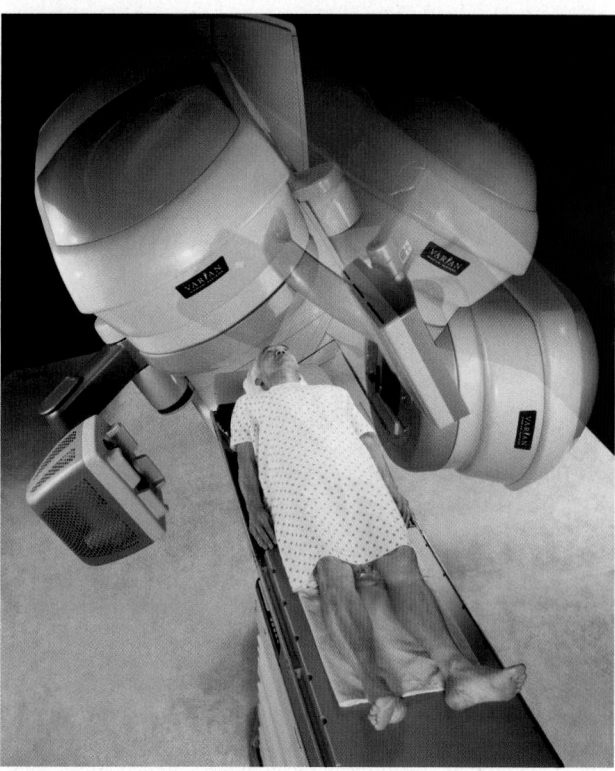

Figure 13.13 Model in treatment position on the patient support table. The treatment delivery head on the gantry's C-arm rotates about the patient, enabling the delivery of beams throughout 360 degrees of rotation. (From Varian Medical Systems, Palo Alto, CA, with permission.)

monitoring systems, x-ray generation targets, high-density treatment field-shaping devices (collimators), and up to a ton of radiation shielding on a mechanical C-arm gantry that can rotate precisely around a treatment couch (Fig. 13.13). These treatment-delivery machines routinely maintain mechanical isocenters for patient treatments to within a sphere of 1 mm radius. The development of *stereotactic radiotherapy*, which will be described in the section titled Clinical Application of Types of Radiation, depends on this level of machine precision.

X-ray production by monoenergetic high-energy electrons results in an x-ray (photon) beam that contains a continuous spectrum of energies with maximum photon energy near that of the incident electron beam. Lower energy photons appear with a much greater probability than do the highest energy ones, but they also become preferentially filtered out of the beam through the absorption in the target and the attenuation in the flattening filter. This generally results in a treatment beam energy spectrum with a mean photon energy of approximately one-third of the initial electron beam energy. In this energy range, the resulting photon beam exits the production target with a narrow angular spread focused primarily in the forward direction. These forward-peaked intensity distributions generally need to be modulated (flattened) to produce a large (up to 40 cm diameter at the patient) photon beam with uniform intensity across the beam. All modern treatment units take advantage of extensive computer control, monitoring, and feedback to produce highly stable and reproducible treatment beams.

The resulting photon beam requires beam shaping for conformal dose delivery. Some combination of primary, high-density field blocks (collimators) together with additional edge blocks generally provide the required shaping and shielding. Modern machines use computer-controlled multileaf collimators (Fig. 13.14)

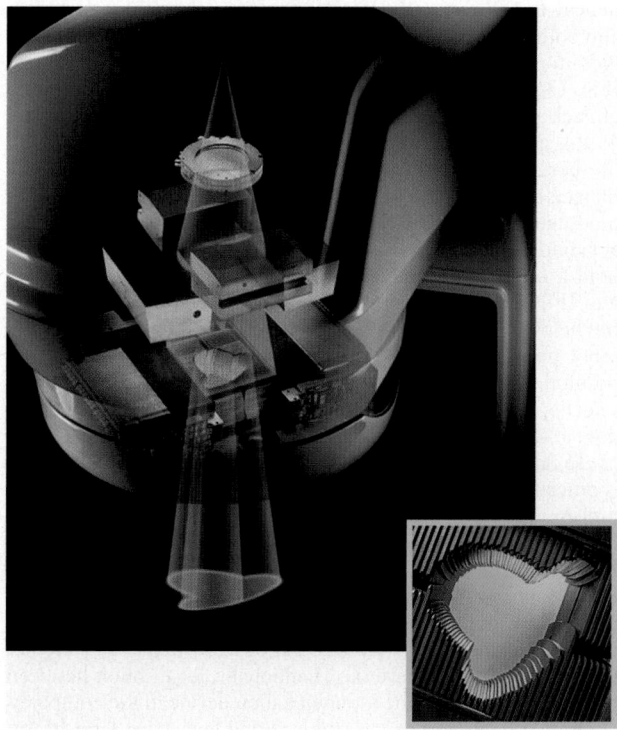

Figure 13.14 Multileaf collimator shaping of an x-ray treatment beam from a linear accelerator. *Inset* shows a view of the multileaf collimator. (From Varian Medical Systems, Palo Alto, CA, with permission.)

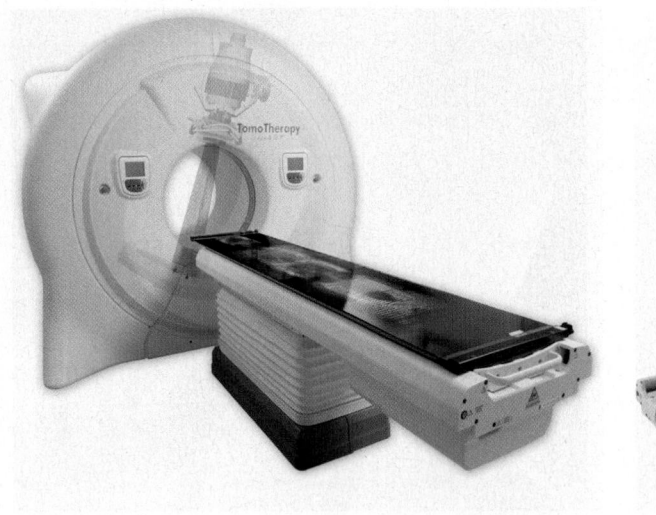
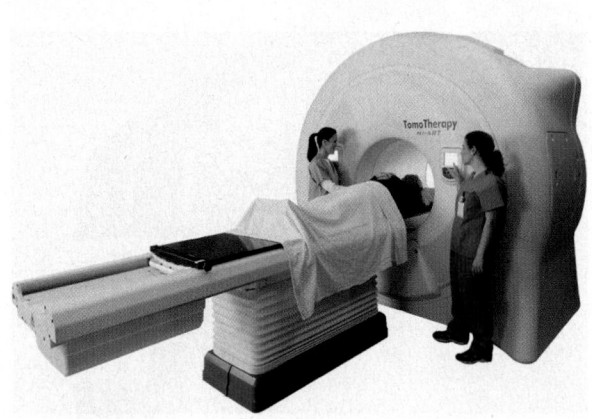

A   **B**

Figure 13.15 (A) A shadow view of linear accelerator, x-ray beam production system, and x-ray fan beam for helical tomotherapy treatment delivery. The beam production system rotates within its enclosed gantry. **(B)** The model patient on treatment table slides into the treatment unit. During treatment, the table moves as the collimated fan beam rotates about the patient, creating a modulated helical dose delivery pattern. (From TomoTherapy, Inc., Madison, WI, with permission.)

for the edge sculpting subsequent to setting the primary collimators for maximal shielding. This computer control provides high precision and reproducibility in the definition of field edges. Additionally, automation allows for a precise reshaping of the treatment beam for each angle of incidence, allowing not only conformation of irradiation to target volumes, but also modulation of the beam intensity patterns across the field (intensity-modulated radiation therapy [IMRT]).

Variations on the standard linear accelerator (linac) plus C-arm scenario that are being used for external-beam radiation treatments throughout the body include helical tomotherapy and nonisocentric miniature linac robotic delivery systems.[70] In helical tomotherapy, the accelerator, photon-production target, and collimation system are mounted on a ring gantry (similar to those found on diagnostic computed tomography [CT] scanners) (Fig. 13.15). It produces a fan beam of photons, and the intensity of each part of the fan being modulated by a binary collimator. As the gantry rotates, the patient simultaneously slides through the bore of the machine (again analogous to modern x-ray/CT imagers), which allows for the continuous delivery of intensity-modulated radiation in a helical pattern from all angles around a patient. Another delivery system uses an industrial robot to hold a miniature accelerator plus photon beam-production system (Fig. 13.16). The bulk of the system is reduced by keeping the field sizes small (spotlike). However, computer control of the robot provides flexibility in irradiating tumors from nearly any position external to the patient. The same control allows for the selection and use of many differing beam angles to build up the dose at the tumor location.

To take advantage of the precision of modern beam delivery, it is crucial to localize the patient's tumor and normal tissue.[71] This process can be divided into patient immobilization (i.e., limiting the motion of the patient) and localization (i.e., knowing the tumor and normal tissue location precisely in space). Although these concepts of immobilization and localization are related, they are not identical. Patients can be held reasonably comfortable in their treatment pose with the aid of foam molds and meshes (i.e., immobilization devices). Traditionally, localization has been achieved by indexing the immobilization device to the computer-controlled treatment couch and by using low-power laser beams aligned to skin marks. These techniques make it possible to reproducibly couple the surface of each patient with the treatment machine isocenter.

However, what is truly needed is to localize the tumor and normal tissues. The development of in-room, online x-ray, ultrasound, and infrared imaging equipment can now be used to ensure that the intended portions of each patient's internal anatomy are correctly positioned at the time of treatment. In particular, the development of rugged, low-profile, active matrix, flat-panel imaging devices, either attached to the treatment gantry or placed in the vicinity of the treatment couch, together with diagnostic x-ray generators or the patient treatment beam (see Fig. 13.13), allows the digital capture of projection x-ray images of patient anatomy with respect to the isocenter and treatment field borders. These digitized electronic images are immediately available for analysis. Software tools allow for a comparison to reference images and the generation of correction coordinates, which are in turn available for downloading to the treatment couch for automated fine adjustment of the patient's treatment position. Other precise localization systems rely on the identification of the positions of small, implanted radiopaque markers or other types of *smart* position-reporting devices. Careful use of these image-guided radiation

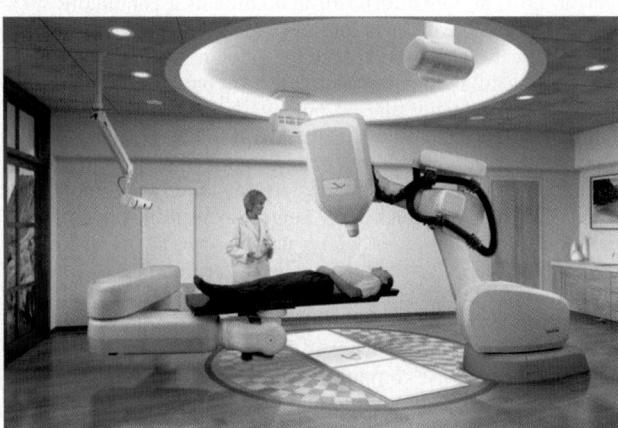

Figure 13.16 A miniature accelerator plus x-ray production system on a robotic delivery arm. Both the treatment table and the treatment head is set by a computer for multiple arbitrary angles of incidence. (From Accuray, Sunnyvale, CA, with permission.)

therapy (IGRT) systems[71, 72] can result in the repeated reducibility of patient position to within a few millimeters over a 5- to 8-week course of treatment.

The final part of external-beam patient treatment is dose delivery. All modern treatment units have computer monitoring (and often control) of all mechanical and dose-delivery components. Treatment-planning information (treatment machine parameters, treatment field configurations, dose per treatment field segment) is downloaded to a work station at the treatment unit that first assists with and then records treatment. This information, together with the readbacks from the treatment machine, are used to reproducibly set up and then verify each patient's treatment parameters, which prevents many of the variations that used to occur when all treatment was performed simply by following instructions written in a treatment chart.

Treatment Beam Characteristics and Dose-Calculation Algorithms

Beyond a basic understanding of the interactions of ionizing radiation with matter lies the requirement of being able to characterize the treatment beams for purposes of planning and verifying treatments. By virtue of a few underlying principles, this generally can be accomplished via a two-step process of absolute calibration of the dose at some reference point in a phantom (i.e., measurement media representative of a patient's tissues), with relative scaling of dose values in other parts of the beam or phantom with respect to that point.

As mentioned earlier, the predominant mode of interaction for therapeutic energy photon beams in tissuelike materials is through Compton scattering. The probability of Compton scattering events is primarily proportional to the relative electron density of the media with which they interact. Because many body tissues are waterlike in composition, it has been possible to make photon beam dosimetric measurements in phantoms consisting mostly of water (water tanks) or tissue-equivalent plastic and to then scale the interactions via relative electron density values (for example, as can be derived from computed x-ray/CT) to other waterlike materials. Thus, the relative fluence of photons in a therapeutic treatment beam is attenuated as it passes through a phantom, primarily via Compton scattering.

It was stated earlier that the photon beam is generated at a small region in the head of the machine. That fluence of photons spreads out through the collimating system before reaching the patient. Thus, without any interactions (e.g., if the beam were in a vacuum), the number of photons crossing any plane perpendicular to the beam direction would remain constant. However, the cross-sectional area of the plane gets larger the farther it is located from the source point. In fact, both the width and length of the cross-sectional area increase in proportion to the distance from the source, and thus the area increases in proportion to the square of the distance. This means that the primary photon fluence per unit area in a plane perpendicular to the beam direction of a pointlike source also decreases as one over the square of the distance, the so-called $1/r^2$ reduction in fluence as a function of distance, r, from the source.

Thus, we have two processes, attenuation and $1/r^2$ reduction, which reduce the photon fluence from an external therapeutic beam as a function of depth in a patient. There is also a process that can increase the photon fluence at a point downstream. Recall that Compton scattering interactions lead not only to secondary electrons (which are responsible for deposition of dose), but also to Compton scattered photons. These photons are scattered from the interaction sites in multiple, predominantly forward-looking directions. Thus, Compton-scattered photons originating from many other places can add to the photon fluence at another point. As the irradiated area (field size) increases, the amount of scattered radiation also increases.

As mentioned earlier, dose *deposition* is a two-step process of photon interaction (proportional to the local fluence of photons) and energy transfer to the medium via the slowing down of secondary electrons. Thus, the point where a photon interacts is not the place where the dose is actually deposited, which happens over the track of the secondary electron. Dose has a very strict definition of energy *absorbed* per unit mass (i.e., due to the slowing down charged particles) and should be distinguished from the energy released at a point, defined as kerma (e.g., energy transfer from the scattering incident photon). Thus, although the photon beam fluence will always be greatest at the entrance to a patient or phantom, the actual *absorbed dose* for a megavoltage photon beam builds up over the first couple of centimeters, reaching a maximum (d-max) at a depth corresponding to the range of the higher energy Compton electrons set in motion. This turns out to be a second desirable characteristic of these beams (beyond their ability to treat deep-seated lesions), because the dose to the skin (a primary dose-limiting structure in earlier times) is greatly reduced.

The relative distributions of dose, normalized to an absolute dose measurement (using a small thimblelike air ionization chamber at a standard depth and for a standard field size according to nationally and internationally accepted protocols), are the major inputs into treatment-planning systems. The major features of these distributions are (1) the initial dose buildup up to a depth of d-max, with a more gradual drop off in dose as a function of depth into the phantom due to the attenuation and $1/r^2$ factors at deeper depths (relative depth dose), and (2) the shape of the dose in the plane perpendicular to the direction of the beams; both as a function of field size. Central axis depth dose curves for typical external photon beams are shown in Figure 13.17 for two beam energies and for both a large and smaller field size. Notice both the expected increase in penetration with increasing beam energy and the increase in dose at a particular depth with increasing field size; the latter effect due to increased numbers of secondary Compton-scattered photons for larger irradiated areas. The change in dose perpendicular to the central axis is less remarkable, because the beams are designed to be uniform across a field as a function of depth.

It is useful to also point out the depth dose characteristics of clinical external treatment beams produced using ionizing

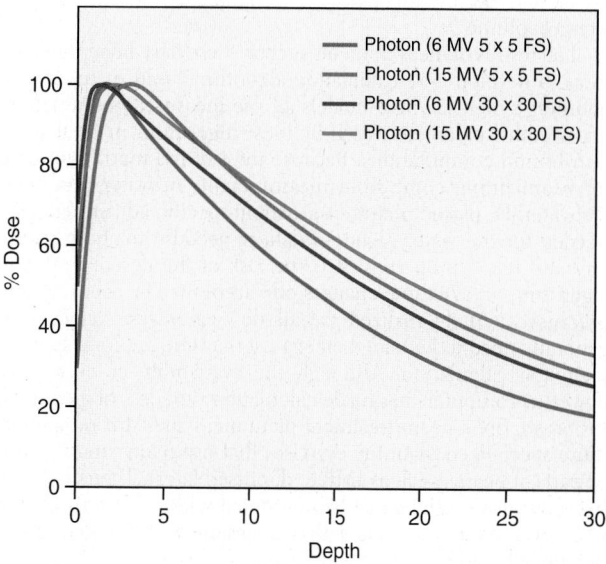

Figure 13.17 Sample depth-dose curves (change in delivered dose as a function of depth) along the central axis of some typical photon treatment beams for low (6 MV) and intermediate (15 MV) energy beams, and large (30×30 cm^2) and smaller (5×5 cm^2) field sizes (FS).

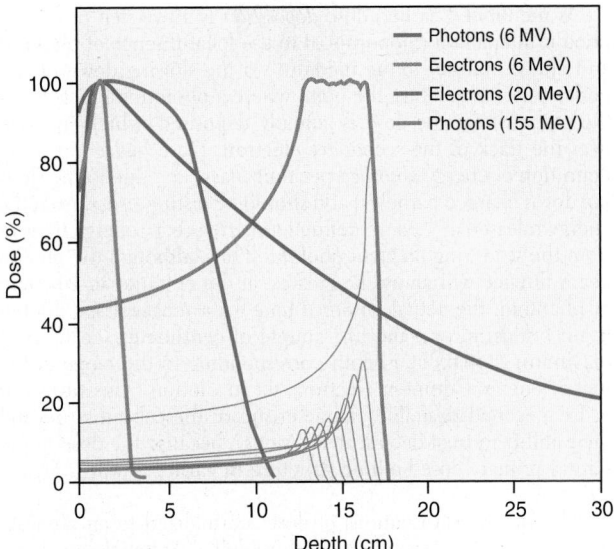

Figure 13.18 Sample depth-dose curves along the central axis of some typical charged particle treatment beams compared with that of a 6-MV proton beam. The spread out Bragg peak at the end of the 155-MeV proton beam (*thick pink curve*) is a composite dose deposition pattern from the addition of the multiple range-shifted proton curves (*thinner pink curves*).

radiations other than photons, primarily through the direct use of charged particles. Those beams (Fig. 13.18) illustrate interesting characteristics, which, when added to the options available for treatment planning (or used by themselves), can produce advantageous results. Relative to the photon beam, the direct use of electron beams leads to deposition of dose over a more localized range, but at the expense of a relative lack of penetration. Thus, electron beams are most widely used for treating, or boosting the treatment of, more superficial tumors and regions (see the section titled Clinical Application of Types of Radiation). The heavier charged particle beams (protons and carbon ions) appear to exhibit even more interesting *depth-dose* characteristics, with the advantage of both (when necessary) being highly penetrating and also lacking a significant dose beyond a certain depth (a depth that can be controlled and purposefully placed, for example, at the distal edge of a target volume).

The results of measurements such as these have been modeled so as to develop dose-calculation algorithms used in treatment-planning systems. These models all use measured beam data to set or adjust parameters used by those algorithms in their dose-distribution computations. Because most of the input data used for beam fitting come from measurements in water phantoms (or waterlike plastic phantoms), patient-specific adjustments are needed for the water phantom data to account for both geometry and tissue properties. It is the task of the dose-calculation algorithms to take those changes into account. The accuracy and precision actually realized for all dose-calculation algorithms generally need to be traded off against the time required to complete the calculation. Although the availability of ever more powerful computers has made calculation time less of a concern for broad, open-beam treatment planning, issues still remain for more specialized planning exercises that use many small beams or parts of beams such as IMRT (discussed later). Typically, relative dose distributions can be computed within patients on the scale of a few millimeters with a precision of better than a few percentage points.

An important area of research is the development of treatment-planning systems that calculate dose based on the principles of how radiation interacts with tissues, rather than simply by fitting data. These approaches use Monte Carlo techniques,[71,73] which

build a dose distribution by summing the calculated paths of thousands of photons and scattered electrons. This approach is more accurate than beam-fitting algorithms in regions of differing tissue densities, such as the lung, and therefore, will ultimately replace the current generation of treatment-planning systems, particularly for complex conditions. However, the time to perform these calculations is still prohibitive for a clinic, and it is anticipated that Monte Carlo calculations will be introduced over a period of years by balancing the need for accuracy in a particular clinical situation with the need to initiate patient treatment.

TREATMENT PLANNING

As discussed in the previous section, single-treatment beams usually deposit more of the dose closer to where they enter the patient than they do at depths corresponding to where a deep-seated tumor might be located. The use of multiple beams entering the patient from different directions that overlap at the target produces more dose per unit volume throughout the tumor volume than is received by normal tissues. In fact, as noted earlier, the treatment-delivery machines are designed to make this easy to accomplish. Planning patient treatments under these circumstances should be a somewhat trivial matter of first selecting a sufficient number of beam angles to realize the desired buildup of the dose in the overlap region relative to the doses in the upstream parts of each beam, and then second, designing beam apertures that shape the edges of the beams to match the target. However, dose-limiting normal tissues often also lie in the paths of one or more of the beams. These normal tissues are often more sensitive to radiation damage than the tumor, and regardless, it is best practice to minimize the dose in any case as a general principle. Computerized treatment-planning systems function to develop patient-specific anatomic or geometric models and then use these models together with the beam-specific dose deposition properties (derived from phantom measurements, as previously described) to select beam angles, shapes, and intensities that meet an overall prescribed objective. That is, modern radiation oncology dose prescriptions contain both tumor and normal tissue objectives, and the modern computerized treatment-planning systems make it possible to design treatments that meet these objectives.

The development and use of three-dimensional (3D) models of each patient's anatomy, treatment geometry, and dose distribution led to a paradigm shift in radiation therapy treatment planning. Computerized radiation treatment planning began in the 1980s as a mainly x-ray/CT–based reconstruction of 3D geometries from information manually contoured on multiple two-dimensional (2D) transverse CT images. Today, these models often incorporate imaging data from multiple sources. Geometrically accurate anatomic information from an x-ray/CT scan still anchors these studies (as well as provides tissue density information necessary for dose calculations). However, it is now quite common to also register the CT data set with other studies such as magnetic resonance imaging (MRI), which may add anatomic detail for soft tissues, or functional MRI or positron emission tomography (PET) studies,[74,75] which provide physiologic or molecular information about tumors and normal tissues. Once registered with each other, the unique or complementary information from each data set can be fused for inspection and incorporated into the design of each patient's target and normal tissue volumes (Fig. 13.19). Beyond the ability to more fully define the extent of the primary target volume (for instance, as the encompassing envelope of disease appreciated on all the imaging studies) lies the ability to define subvolumes of the tumor volume that might be appropriate for simultaneous treatment to higher dose. For example, it should soon become possible to define different biologic components of the tumor that could potentially be targeted and then monitored for response using these same imaging techniques.[76]

Current treatment planning makes the tacit assumption that the planning image yields "the truth" about the location and condition

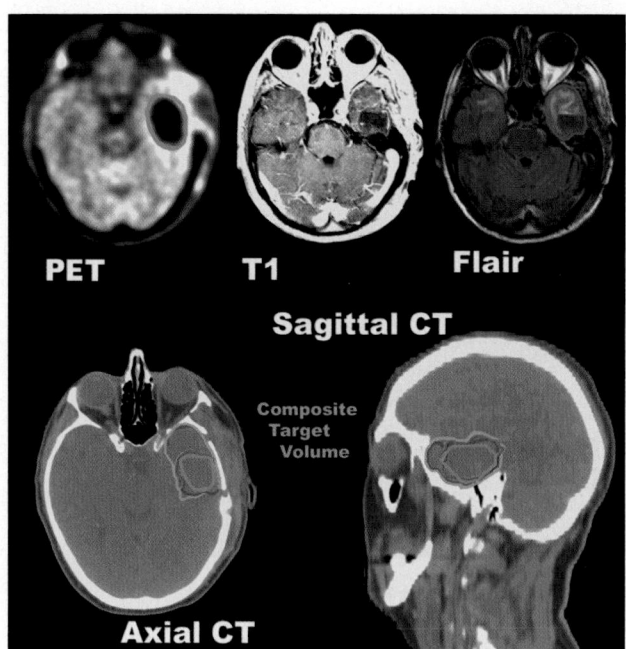

Figure 13.19 An illustration of the brain tumor target volume delineated on coregistered nuclear medicine and magnetic resonance imaging studies fused with computed tomography (CT) data for treatment planning. PET, positron emission tomography.

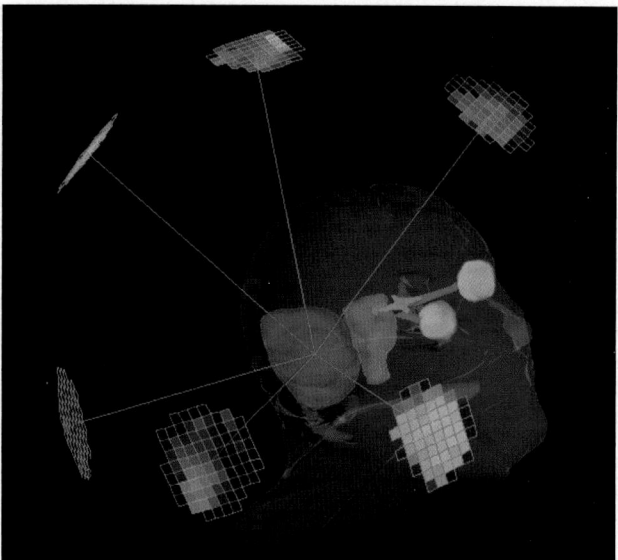

Figure 13.20 Six intensity-modulated treatment ports planned for treatment of a brain tumor (*large object in red*). Differing intensities of the 5 × 5 mm *beamlets* in each port illustrated by gray scale (brighter beamlet = higher intensity). The computer optimization of the beamlet intensities is designed to generate a delivered dose distribution that will conform to the tumor region, yet avoid critical normal tissues such as the brain stem (*dark pink*), optic chiasm (*green*), and optic nerves (*red tubular structures*).

of tumors and normal tissues throughout the course of treatment. However, this ignores the complexity inherent in attempting to build accurate 3D models from multimodality imaging for purposes of planning patient treatments. First, patients breathe and undergo other physiologic processes during a single treatment, changes that require dynamic modeling or other methods of accounting for the changes. Furthermore, the patient's condition may change over time (and hence their model). Thus, a complete design and assessment of a patient undergoing high-precision treatment requires the construction of four-dimensional (4D) patient models. Indeed, the recent ready availability of multidetector CT scanners with subsecond gantry rotations, and even more recently, the availability of cone-beam CT capabilities on the radiation therapy treatment simulators and treatment machines themselves, now makes it possible to construct 4D patient models. A very active area of physics research[72,75] deals with IGRT, including the formation of 4D patient models (including distortions and changes in anatomy) of the motion over time and the determination of the accumulated dose received by a moving tumor as well as the surrounding normal tissues such as uninvolved lung.

Complementary to the availability of these patient and dose models has come a much better understanding of the doses safely tolerated by normal tissues adjacent to a tumor volume (e.g., spinal cord) or surrounding it (e.g., brain, lung, liver).[77] Indeed, not only has knowledge of whole organ tolerances to irradiation been obtained, but it has also become possible to characterize in some detail the complex dependence of the probability of incurring a complication with respect to the highly (intentionally) inhomogeneous dose distributions these normal tissues receive as part of the planning process designed to avoid treating them. Modeling partial organ tolerances to irradiation is of great use in planning patient treatments because it enables[78] integration and manipulation of variable dose and volume distributions with respect to possible clinical outcomes.

Making the vast amount of tumor and normal tissue information useful for planning treatments requires equally sophisticated new ways of planning and delivering dose, potentially preferentially targeting subvolumes of the tumor regions or specifically

avoiding selected portions of adjacent organs at risk. As mentioned earlier, modern treatment machines are capable of either varying the intensity of the radiation across each treatment port or projecting many small beams at a targeted region. This modulation of beam intensities (IMRT) from a given beam direction, together with the use of multiple beams (or parts of beams) from different directions, gives many degrees of freedom to create highly sculpted dose distributions, given that a system for designing the intensity modulation is available. Much computer programming and computational analysis has gone into the design of treatment-planning optimization systems to perform these functions.[79,80]

In IMRT, as most often applied, each treatment beam portal is broken down into simple basic components called beamlets, typically 0.5 to 1 cm × 1 cm in size, evenly distributed on a grid over the cross-section of each beam. Optimization begins with precomputation of the relative dose contribution that each of these beamlets gives to every subportion of tumor and normal tissue that the beamlet traverses as it goes through the patient model. Sophisticated optimization engines and search routines then iteratively alter the relative intensities of each beamlet in all the beams to minimize a cost function associated with target and normal tissue treatment goals. These, often hundreds of beamlets (each with its own intensity) (Fig. 13.20), provide the necessary flexibility and degrees of freedom to create dose distributions that can preferentially irradiate subportions of targets and also produce sharp dose gradients to avoid nearby organs at risk (Fig. 13.21). The cost-function approach also facilitates the ability to include factors such as the normal tissue and tumor-response models, mentioned previously in the optimization process, thus integrating the overall effects of the complex dose distributions across whole organ systems or target volumes within the planning process.

OTHER TREATMENT MODALITIES

Other types of external-beam radiation treatments use atomic or nuclear particles rather than photons. Beams of fast neutrons have been used for some cancers,[81] primarily because of the

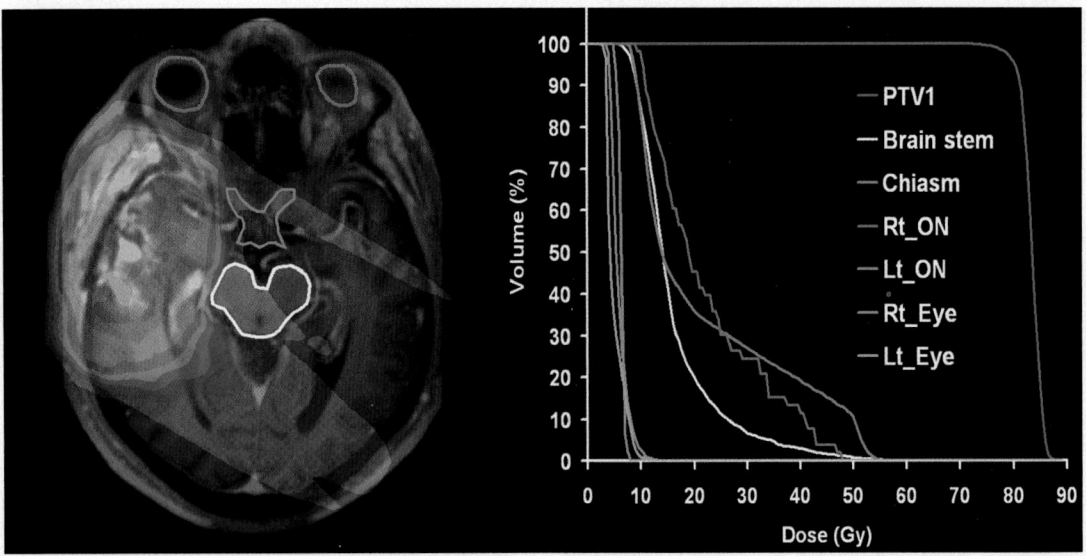

Figure 13.21 Resulting isodose distribution for an optimized intensity-modulated brain treatment. Dose-intensity pattern in the *left panel* is overlaid on the patient's magnetic resonance images used in planning. Also contoured are the optic chiasm (*green*), the brain stem (*white*), and the eyes (*orange*). In the *right panel,* the dose distribution throughout all slices of the patient's anatomy is summarized via cumulative dose-volume histograms for the various tissues and volumes that have been previously segmented. Each location on each curve represents the fraction of the volume of that tissue (%) that receives greater than or the same as the corresponding dose level.

dense ionization patterns they produce as they slow down in tissue (making cell killing less dependent on the indirect effect previously discussed). Being uncharged particles, neutron beams of therapeutic energy penetrate in tissue (have depth-dose characteristics) similar to photon beams, but with denser dose deposition in the cellular scale. Most other external-beam treatments use charged particles, primarily either electrons[82] (produced on the same machines used for photon beam treatments) or protons or heavier particles such as carbon ions.[83,84] The latter beams have desirable dose-deposition properties (see Fig. 13.18), because they can spare tissues downstream from the target volume and generally give less overall dose to normal tissue. There can also be some radiobiologic advantage to the heavier charged particle beams, similar to neutrons. The generation and delivery of proton beams and heavier charged particle beams generally requires an accelerator (in its own vault) plus a beam transport system and some sort of treatment nozzle, often located on an isocentric gantry. The cost of the accelerator is generally leveraged by having it supply beams to multiple treatment rooms, but these units still cost many times that of a standard linear accelerator.

Brachytherapy[85] is a form of treatment that uses direct placement of radioactive sources or materials within tumors (interstitial brachytherapy) or within body or surgical cavities (intracavitary brachytherapy), either permanently (allowing for full decay of short-lived radioactive materials) or temporarily (either in one extended application or over several shorter term applications). The ability to irradiate tumors from close range (even from the inside out) can lead to conformal treatments with low normal tissue doses. The radioactive isotopes most generally used for these treatments are contained within small tubelike or seedlike sealed source enclosures (which prevents direct contamination). They emit photons (gamma and x-rays) during their decay, which penetrate the source cover and interact with tissue via the same physical processes as described for external-beam treatments. The treatments have the advantage of providing a high fluence (and dose) very near each source that drops in intensity as 1 over the square of the distance from the source (1/r²). Radioactive sources decay in an exponential fashion characterized by their individual half-lives. After each half-life ($T_{1/2}$) the strength of each source decreases by half. Brachytherapy treatments are further generally classified into the two broad categories of low–dose-rate and

high–dose-rate treatments. Low–dose-rate treatments attempt to deliver tumoricidal doses via continuous irradiation from implanted sources over a period of several days. High–dose-rate treatments use one or more higher activity sources (stored external to the patient) together with a remote applicator or source transfer system to give one or more higher dose treatments on time scales and schedules more like external-beam treatments.

Isotopes for brachytherapy treatments are selected on the basis of a combination of specific activity (i.e., how much activity can be achieved per unit mass [i.e., to keep the source sizes small]), the penetrating ability of the decay photons (together with the 1/r² fall off determines how many sources or source location will be required for treatment), and the half-life of the radioactive material (which must be accounted for in computation of dose, but also determines how often reusable sources will need to be replaced). Table 13.1 lists those isotopes most commonly used, along with some of their primary applications.

The dose-deposition patterns surrounding each type of source can be measured or computed. These data (or the parameterization

TABLE 13.1

Common Isotopes for Brachytherapy Treatment

Isotope	Form	Primary Applications
[125]I	Implantable sealed seed	LDR: Permanent prostate implants, brain implants, tumor bed implants, eye plaques
[192]Ir	Implantable sealed seed	LDR: Interstitial solid tumor treatments
[192]Ir	High activity sealed source on a remote transfer wire	HDR: Intracavitary GYN treatments, intraluminal irradiations
[137]Cs	Sealed source tubes	LDR: Intracavitary GYN treatments

LDR, low-dose rate; HDR, high-dose rate; GYN, gynecologic; ^{137}Cs, caesium-137.

of same) can be stored within a computerized treatment-planning system. Planning a brachytherapy treatment-delivery scheme (desirable source strengths and arrangements) proceeds within the planning system by distributing the sources throughout the treatment area and having the computer add up the contributions of each source to designated tumor and normal tissue locations (e.g., obtained from a CT scan). Source strengths or spacing can be adjusted until an acceptable result is obtained. Indeed, optimization systems are now routinely used to fine tune this process.

Other types of therapeutic treatments with internal sources of ionizing radiation, generally classified as systemic targeted radionuclide therapy (STaRT), use antibodies or other conjugates or carriers such as microspheres to selectively deliver radionuclides to cancer cells.[86] Computing the effective dose to tumors and normal tissues via these techniques requires information on how much of the injected activity reaches the targets (biodistribution) as well as the energy and decay properties of the radionuclide being delivered. Imaging techniques and computer models are aiding in these computations.

CLINICAL APPLICATIONS OF RADIATION THERAPY

In contrast to surgical oncology and medical oncology, which focus on early- or late-stage disease, respectively, the field of radiation oncology encompasses the1p8.49 entire spectrum of oncology. Board certification requires 5 years of postdoctoral training, typically beginning with an internship in internal medicine or surgery, followed by 4 years of radiation oncology residency. Education, as defined by leaders in the field,[87] begins with a thorough knowledge of the biology, physics, and clinical applications of radiation. It also includes training in the theoretical and practical aspects of the administration of radiation protectors and anticancer agents used as radiation sensitizers and the management of toxicities resulting from those treatments. In addition, residents receive education in palliative care, supportive care, and symptom and pain management. This training is in preparation for a practice that, in a given week, might include patients with a 2-mm vocal cord lesion or a 20-cm soft tissue sarcoma, both of whom can be treated with curative intent, as well as a patient with widely metastatic disease who needs palliative radiation, medical care for pain and depression, and discussion of end-of-life issues. More than 50% of (nonskin) cancer patients receive radiation therapy during the course of their illness.[88]

Clinical Application of Types of Radiation

Electrons are now the most widely used form of radiation for superficial treatments. Because the depth of penetration can be well controlled by the energy of the beam, it is possible to treat, for instance, skin cancer, a small part of the breast while sparing the underlying lung, or the cervical lymph nodes but not the spinal cord, which lies several centimeters more deeply. Superficial tumors, such as of skin cancers, can also be treated very effectively with low-energy (kilovoltage) photons, but their use has decreased because a separate machine is required for their production.

The main form of treatment for deep tumors is photons. As described in the Radiation Physics section, photons spare the skin and deposit dose along their entire path until the beam leaves the body. The use of multiple beams that intersect on the tumor permit high doses to be delivered to the tumor with a relative sparing of normal tissue. The pinnacle of this concept is IMRT, which uses hundreds of beams and can treat concave shapes with relative sparing of the central region (see Figs. 13.20 and 13.21). However, as each beam continues on its path beyond the tumor, this use of multiple beams means that a significant volume of normal tissue receives a low dose. There has been considerable debate concerning the magnitude of the risk of second cancers produced

by radiating large volumes with low doses of radiation.[89] Charged particle beams (proton and carbon, in this discussion) differ from photons in that they interact only modestly with tissue until they reach the end of their path, where they then deposit the majority of their energy and stop (the Bragg peak; see Fig. 13.18). This ability to stop at a chosen depth decreases the region of low dose. The chief form of charged particle used today is the proton. In the decade from 1980 to 1990, proton therapy could deliver higher doses of radiation to the target than photon therapy because protons could produce a more rapid fall off of dose between the target and the critical normal tissue (e.g., tumor and brain stem). Therefore, initially, their main application was in the treatment uveal melanomas, base-of-skull chondrosarcomas, and chordomas. In contrast, today's IMRT photons are more conformal in the high-dose region than protons due to the range uncertainty of the latter.[90] Thus, it seems unlikely that protons will permit a higher target dose to be delivered than photons. In contrast, protons have the potential to decrease regions of low dose. This would be of particular advantage in the treatment of pediatric malignancies, where low doses of radiation would tend to increase the chance of second cancers and could affect neurocognitive function in the treatment of brain tumors.

A carbon ion beam has an additional potential biologic advantage over protons. As discussed in the section Biologic Aspects of Radiation Oncology, hypoxic cells, which are found in many tumors, are up to 3 times more resistant to photon or proton radiation than well-oxygenated cells. In contrast, hypoxia does not cause resistance to a carbon beam. Whether hypoxia is a cause of clinical resistance to fractionated radiation is still debated.[91] A carbon beam is available at a few sites in Europe and Japan.

Two major issues have affected the widespread acceptance of protons. The most widely recognized is cost. Proton (approximately $120 million) and carbon beam facilities (in excess of $200 million) are substantially more expensive than a similar-sized photon facility (approximately $25 million). The operating costs appear to be significantly higher as well. Although the majority of patients who have received proton therapy have prostate cancer, there is no evidence that protons produce superior results to those obtained with IMRT planned photons.[92,93] The lack of solid evidence that protons are superior to photons for any disease site and the magnitude of these costs are of societal importance.[94] Although less expensive single gantry proton units are under construction, there are no functioning units at the time of this writing. A second, less well-appreciated issue concerns the need to develop full integration of charged particle beams with IGRT, as has already been accomplished with photons, although this feature is being incorporated into second-generation proton units.

Neutron therapy attracted significant interest in the 1980s, based on the principle that it would be more effective than photons against hypoxic cells that some have thought are responsible for radiation resistance of tumors. The effectiveness of neutron therapy has been limited by initial difficulties with collimation and targeting, although there is evidence that they have a role in the treatment of refractory parotid gland tumors.[95]

Brachytherapy refers to the placement of radioactive sources next to or inside the tumor. The chief sites where brachytherapy plays a role are in prostate and cervical cancer, although it has applications in head and neck cancers, soft tissue sarcomas, and other sites. In the case of prostate cancer, most experience is with low–dose-rate permanent implants using iodine-125 (^{125}I) or, more recently, palladium-103 (^{103}Pd). Over the last 5 years, there has been an increasing emphasis on improving the accuracy of seed placement, guided by ultrasound and confirmed by CT or MRI, and in skilled hands, outstanding results can be achieved.[96] In the case of cervical cancer, high–dose-rate treatment, which can be performed in an outpatient setting, has essentially replaced low–dose-rate treatment, which typically requires general anesthesia and a 2-day hospital stay. The results from both techniques appear to be approximately equivalent.

Yttrium microspheres represent a distinct form of brachytherapy. These spheres carry yttrium-90 (^{90}Y), a pure beta emitter with a range of about 1 cm. These have been used to treat both primary hepatocellular cancer and colorectal cancer metastatic to the liver (hepatic arterial or systemic chemotherapy) by administration through the hepatic artery.

TREATMENT INTENT

Radiation doses are chosen so as to maximize the chance of tumor control without producing unacceptable toxicity. The dose of radiation required depends on the tumor type, the volume of disease (number of tumor cells), and the use of radiation-modifying agents (such as chemotherapeutic drugs used as radiation sensitizers). Except for a subset of tumors that are exquisitely sensitive to radiation (e.g., seminoma, lymphoma), doses that are required are often close to the tolerance of the normal tissue. A key fact driving the choice of dose is that a 1-cm^3 tumor contains approximately 1 billion cells. It follows that the reduction of a tumor that is 3 cm in diameter to 3 mm, which would be called a complete response by CT scan, would still leave 1 million tumor cells. Because each radiation fraction appears to kill a fixed fraction of the tumor, the dose to cure occult disease needs to be more similar to the dose for gross disease than one might otherwise expect. Thus, radiation doses (using the standard fractionation) of 45 to 54 Gy are typically used in the adjuvant setting when there is moderate suspicion for occult disease, 60 to 65 Gy for positive margins or when there is a high suspicion for occult disease, and 70 Gy or more for gross disease.

It is common during the course of radiation to give higher doses of radiation to regions that have a higher tumor burden. For example, regions that are suspected of harboring occult disease may be targeted to receive (in once daily 2-Gy fractions) 54 Gy, whereas, to control the gross tumor, the goal may be to administer a total dose of 70 Gy. Because the gross tumor will invariably reside within the region at risk for occult disease, it has become standard practice to deliver 50 Gy to the entire region, and then an additional *boost* dose of 20 Gy to the tumor. This sequence is called the *shrinking field technique*. With the development of IMRT, it has become possible to treat both regions with a different dose each day and achieve both goals simultaneously. For example, on each of the 35 days of treatment, the gross tumor might receive 2 Gy, and the region of occult disease 1.7 Gy, for a total dose of 59.5 Gy, which is of approximately equal biologic effectiveness to 54 Gy in 1.8-Gy fractions because of the lower dose per fraction (see the section Biologic Aspects of Radiation Oncology).

Radiation therapy alone is often used with curative intent for localized tumors. The decision to use surgery or radiation therapy involves factors determined by the tumor (e.g., is it resectable without a serious compromise in function?) and the patient (e.g., is the patient a good operative candidate?). The most common tumor in this group is prostate cancer, but patients with early-stage larynx cancer often receive radiation for voice preservation, and there are many patients with early-stage lung cancer who are not operative candidates. Control rates for these early-stage lesions are in excess of 70% (and as high as 90% for early-stage larynx cancer) and are usually a function of tumor size.

Stereotactic body radiation therapy (SBRT; sometimes called *stereotactic ablative radiation*) uses many (typically more than eight) cross-firing beams and provides an improved method of curing early-stage lung cancer[97] and liver metastases.[98] This approach uses precise localization and image guidance to deliver a small number (less than five) of high doses of radiation, with the concept of ablating the tumor, rather than using fractionation to achieve a therapeutic index (see the section title Fractionation). SBRT can provide long-term, local control rates of >90% for tumors less than 4 to 5 cm with minimal side effects.

Locally advanced or aggressive cancers can be cured with radiation alone or with a combination of radiation and chemotherapy

or a molecularly targeted therapy. The most common examples here are locally advanced lung cancer, head and neck, esophageal, and cervix cancers, with cure rates in the 15% to 40% range, and are discussed in detail in their own chapters. A general principle that has emerged during the last decade is that combination chemoradiation has increased the cure rates of locally advanced cancers by 5% to 10% at the cost of increased toxicity.

An important consideration in the use of radiation (with or without chemotherapy) with curative intent is the concept of organ preservation. Perhaps the best example of achieving organ preservation in the face of gross disease involves the use of chemotherapy and radiation to replace laryngectomy in the treatment of advanced larynx cancer. Combined radiation and chemotherapy does not improve overall survival compared with radical surgery; however, the organ-conservation approach permits voice preservation in approximately two-thirds of patients with advanced larynx cancer.[99] The treatment of anal cancer with chemoradiation can also be viewed in this light, with chemoradiotherapy producing organ conservation and cure rates superior to radical surgery used decades ago.[100] Multiple randomized trials have demonstrated that lumpectomy plus radiation for breast cancer produces survival rates equal to that of modified radical mastectomy, while allowing for the preservation of the breast.

In the last decade, it has become clear that some patients with metastatic disease can be cured with radiation (with or without chemotherapy). The concept underlying this approach was established by the surgical practice of resecting a limited number of liver or lung metastases. A significant fraction of patients have a limited number of liver metastases that cannot be resected because of location, but are able to undergo high-dose radiation (often combined with chemotherapy). This radical approach to *oligometastases*[101] can produce 5-year survivals in the range of 20% in selected patients.[102] Patients with a limited number of lung metastases from colorectal cancer or soft tissue sarcomas are now being approached with stereotactic body radiation with a similar concept as has been used to justify surgical resection.[102] In addition to the direct effect of radiation on metastatic tumor, there is now anecdotal but provocative evidence that radiation can stimulate the immune system so that tumors distant from the irradiated tumor can respond. Distant (abscopal) responses have been reported in patients who receive immune checkpoint inhibitors such as ipilimumab.[103]

Radiation therapy can also contribute to the cure of patients when used in an adjuvant setting. If the risk of recurrence after surgery is low or if a recurrence could be easily addressed by a second resection, adjuvant radiation therapy is not usually given. However, when a gross total resection of the tumor is still associated with a high risk of residual occult disease or if local recurrence is morbid, adjuvant treatment is often recommended. A general finding across many disease sites is that adjuvant radiation can reduce local failure rates to below 10%, even in high-risk patients, if a gross total resection is achieved. If gross disease or positive margins remain, higher doses and/or larger volumes may be required, which may be less well tolerated and are less successful in achieving tumor control.

Adjuvant therapy can be delivered before or after definitive surgery. There are some advantages to giving radiation therapy after surgery. The details of the tumor location are known and, with the surgeon's cooperation, clips can be placed in the tumor bed, permitting increased treatment accuracy. In addition, compared with preoperative therapy, postoperative therapy is associated with fewer wound complications. However, in some cases, it is preferable to deliver preoperative radiation. Radiation can shrink the tumor, diminishing the extent of the resection, or making an unresectable tumor resectable. In the case of rectal cancer, the response to treatment may carry more prognostic information than the initial TNM staging.[104] In patients who will undergo significant surgeries (particularly a Whipple procedure or an esophageal resection), preoperative (sometimes called neoadjuvant) therapy can be more reliably administered than postoperative therapy. Most importantly, after resection of abdominal or pelvic tumors (such as rectal cancers or retroperitoneal sarcomas), the small bowel may become fixed by adhesions in the region requiring treatment, thus increasing the morbidity of postoperative treatment. A randomized trial has shown that preoperative therapy produces fewer gastrointestinal side effects and has at least as good efficacy as postoperative adjuvant therapy for locally advanced rectal cancer.[105] Taken together, there appears to be a trend toward preoperative or neoadjuvant therapy in cancers of the gastrointestinal track (esophagus, stomach, pancreas, rectum), postoperative radiation seems to be favored in head and neck, lung, and breast cancer, and soft tissue sarcoma seems equally split.

The effectiveness of adjuvant therapy in decreasing local recurrence has been demonstrated in randomized trials in lung, rectal, and breast cancers. More recently, randomized trials have shown that postmastectomy radiation improved the survival for women with breast cancer and four or more positive lymph nodes, all of whom also received adjuvant chemotherapy. A fascinating analysis has revealed that, across many treatment conditions, each 4% increase in 5-year local control is associated with a 1% increase in 5-year survival.[106] It has been proposed that the long-term survival benefit of radiation in these more recent studies was revealed by the introduction of effective chemotherapy, which prevented such a high fraction of women from dying early with metastatic disease.[107] This concept has been developed into a hypothesis that the effect of adjuvant radiation on survival will depend on the effectiveness of adjuvant chemotherapy. If chemotherapy is either ineffective or very effective, adjuvant radiation may have little influence on the survival in a disease in which systemic relapse dominates survival. Radiation will have its greatest impact on survival when chemotherapy is moderately effective.[108]

In addition to these curative roles, radiation plays an important part in palliative treatment. Perhaps most importantly, emergency irradiation can begin to reverse the devastating effects of spinal cord compression and of superior vena cava syndrome. A single 8-Gy fraction is highly effective for many patients with bone pain from a metastatic lesion. There is increasing evidence of the effectiveness of body stereotactic radiation to treat vertebral body metastases in patients who have a long projected survival or who need retreatment after previous radiation.[109] Stereotactic treatment can relieve symptoms from a small number of brain metastasis, and fractionated whole-brain radiation can mitigate the effects of multiple metastases. Bronchial obstruction can often be relieved by a brief course of treatment as can duodenal obstruction from pancreatic cancer. Palliative treatment is usually delivered in a smaller number of larger radiation fractions (see the section titled Fractionation) because the desire to simplify the treatment for a patient with limited life expectancy outweighs the somewhat increased potential for late side effects.

FRACTIONATION

Two crucial features that influence the effectiveness of a physical dose of radiation are the dose given in each radiation treatment (i.e., the fraction) and the total amount of time required to complete the course of radiation. Standard fractionation for radiation therapy is defined as the delivery of one treatment of 1.8 to 2.25 Gy per day. This approach produces a fairly well-understood chance of tumor control and risk of normal tissue damage (as a function of volume). By altering the fractionation schemes, one may be able to improve the outcome for patients undergoing curative treatment or to simplify the treatment for patients receiving palliative therapy.

Two forms of altered fractionation have been tested for patients undergoing curative treatment: accelerated fractionation and hyperfractionation. Accelerated fractionation emerged from analyses of the control of head and neck cancer as a function of dose administered and total treatment time. It was found that with an increasing dose there was increasing local control, but that protraction of treatment was associated with a loss of local control that

was equivalent to about 0.75 Gy per day.[110] The data were best modeled by assuming that, approximately 2 weeks into treatment, tumor cells began to proliferate more rapidly than they were proliferating early in treatment (called *accelerated repopulation*).[111] In accelerated fractionation, the goal is to complete radiation before the accelerated tumor cell proliferation occurs. The most common method of achieving accelerated fractionation is to give a standard fraction to the entire field in the morning and to give a second treatment to the boost field in the afternoon (called *concomitant boost*). As in standard radiation, the boost would be given by extending the length of the treatment course; this concomitant boost approach can shorten treatment from 7 weeks to 5 weeks in head and neck cancer.

The second approach to altering fractionation is called *hyperfractionation*. Hyperfractionation is defined as the use of more than one fraction per day separated by more than 6 hours (see the section titled Biologic Aspects of Radiation Oncology), with a dose per fraction that is less than standard. Hyperfractionation is expected to produce fewer late complications for the same acute effects against both rapidly dividing normal tissues and tumors. Pure hyperfractionation might give 1 Gy twice a day, so that the total dose per day would be 2 Gy, and thus be equal to standard fractionation. In practice, hyperfractionated treatments are usually in the range of 1.2 Gy, which means that, compared with a standard fractionation, a somewhat higher dose is administered during the same period of time (so that most hyperfractionation also includes modest acceleration). The overall effect is to increase the acute toxicity (which resolves) and tumor response, while not increasing the (dose-limiting) late toxicity, which can improve cure rate. Both accelerated fractionation and hyperfractionation have been demonstrated in a meta-analysis to be superior to standard fractionation in the treatment of head and neck cancer with radiation alone.[112] However, a recent randomized trial has shown that there is no increase in control or survival, but there is an increase toxicity using chemotherapy with hyperfractionation compared to standard chemoradiation; therefore, the use of altered fractionation schemes has decreased dramatically during the last few years.[113]

Hypofractionation refers to the administration of a smaller number of larger fractions than is standard. Hypofractionation might be expected to cause more late toxicity for the same antitumor effect than standard or hyperfractionation. In the past, this approach was reserved for palliative cases, with the sense that a modest potential for increased late toxicity was not a major concern in patients with limited life expectancy. However, more recently, it has been proposed that the ability to better exclude normal tissue by using IGRT may permit hypofractionation to be used safely and that, in the specific case of prostate cancer, hypofractionation may have beneficial effects.[114]

ADVERSE EFFECTS

Radiation produces adverse effects in normal tissues. Although these are discussed in detail in later chapters as part of comprehensive discussions of organ toxicity, it is worth making some general comments here from the perspective of how radiation biology relates to the clinical toxicities. The term *radiation toxicity* is used to describe the adverse effects caused by radiation alone and radiation plus chemotherapy. Although this latter toxicity would be better labeled as *combined modality toxicity*, the pattern typically resembles a more severe form of the toxicity produced by radiation alone. Adverse effects from radiation can be divided into acute, subacute, and chronic (or late) effects. Acute effects are common, rarely serious, and usually self-limiting. Acute effects tend to occur in organs that depend on rapid self-renewal, most commonly the skin or mucosal surfaces (oropharynx, esophagus, small intestine, rectum, and bladder). This is due to radiation-induced cell death that occurs during mitosis, so that cells that divide rapidly show the most rapid cell loss. In the treatment of head and neck cancer,

CANCER THERAPEUTICS

mucositis becomes worse during the first 3 to 4 weeks of therapy, but then will often stabilize as the normal mucosa cell proliferation increases in response to mucosal cell loss. It seems likely that normal tissue stem cells are relatively resistant to radiation compared with the more differentiated cells, because these stem cells survive to permit the normal mucosa to reepithelialize. Acute side effects typically resolve within 1 to 2 weeks of treatment completion, although occasionally these effects are so severe that they lead to consequential late effects, as described later.

Because lymphocytes are exquisitely sensitive to radiation, there has been considerable investigation into the effects of radiation on immune function. In contrast to mucosal cell killing, which requires mitosis, radiation kills lymphocytes in all phases of the cell cycle by apoptosis, so that lymphocyte counts decrease within days of initiating treatment. These effects do not tend to put patients at risk for infection, because granulocytes, which are chiefly responsible for combating infections, are relatively unaffected.

Two acute side effects of radiation do not fit neatly into these models relating to cell kill: nausea[115,116] and fatigue.[117,118] The origin of radiation-induced nausea is not related to acute cell loss, because it can occur within hours of the first treatment. Nausea is usually associated with radiation of the stomach, but it can sometimes occur during brain irradiation or from large-volume irradiation that involves neither the brain nor the stomach. Irradiation typically produces fatigue, even if relatively small volumes are irradiated. It seems likely that the origins of both of these *abscopal* effects of radiation (i.e., effects that occur systemically or at a distance for the site of irradiation) are related to the release of cytokines, but little is known.

Radiation can also produce subacute toxicities in the form of radiation pneumonitis and radiation-induced liver disease. These typically occur 2 weeks to 3 months after radiation is completed. The risk of radiation pneumonitis and radiation-induced liver disease is proportional to the mean dose delivered.[119,120] Thus, the 3D tools that permit the calculation of dose-volume histograms (described in the physics section) are currently used to determine the maximum safe treatment that can be delivered in terms of dose and volume. These toxicities appear to be initiated subclinically during the course of radiation as a cascade of cytokines in which TGF-β, tumor necrosis factor α, interleukin 6, and other cytokines play a role.[121] High TGF-β plasma levels during a course of treatment have been found to be associated with a greater risk of radiation pneumonitis.[122] Thus, in the future, we might look toward a combination of physical dose delivery, measured by the dose-volume histogram, the functional imaging of normal tissue damage, and the detection of biomarkers of toxicity, such as TGF-β, to improve the ability to individualize therapy. Attempts to determine the genomic basis of radiation sensitivity, beyond the known rare genetic defects such as ataxia telangiectasia, have not yet been successful.[123]

Late effects, which are typically seen 6 or more months after a course of radiation, include fibrosis, fistula formation, or long-term organ damage. Two theories for the origin of late effects have been put forth: late damage to the microvasculature and direct damage to the parenchyma. Although the vascular damage theory is attractive, it does not account for the differing sensitivities of organs to radiation. Perhaps the microvasculature is unique in each organ.[124] Regardless of the mechanism of toxicity, the tolerance of whole-organ radiation is now fairly well established (Table 13.2). Late complications can also be divided into two categories: consequential and true late effects. The best example of a consequential late effect is fibrosis and dysphagia after high-dose chemoradiation for head and neck cancer. Here, late fibrosis or ulceration appears to be the result of the mucosa becoming denuded for a prolonged time period. Late consequential effects are distinct from true late effects, which can follow a normal treatment course of self-limited toxicity and a 6-month or more symptom-free period. Examples of true late effects are radiation myelitis, radiation brain necrosis, and radiation-induced bowel obstruction. In the past, radiation fibrosis was thought to be an irreversible condition. Therefore, an exciting recent development is that severe radiation-induced breast fibrosis is an active process that can be reversed by drug therapy (pentoxifylline and vitamin E).[125] Radiation therapy also causes second cancers, which is addressed in detail in Chapter 143.

TABLE 13.2

Radiation Tolerance Doses for Normal Tissues

Site	TD 5/5 (Gy)[a] Portion of Organ Irradiated			TD 50/5 (Gy)[b] Portion of Organ Irradiated			Complication End Point(s)
	$^1/_3$	$^2/_3$	$^3/_3$	$^1/_3$	$^2/_3$	$^3/_3$	
Kidney	50	30	23	—	40	28	Nephritis
Rain	60	50	45	75	65	60	Necrosis, infarct
Brain stem	60	53	50	—	—	65	Necrosis, infarct
Spinal cord	50 (5–10 cm)	—	47 (20 cm)	70 (5–10 cm)	—	—	Myelitis, necrosis
Lung	45	30	17.5	65	40	24.5	Radiation pneumonitis
Heart	60	45	40	70	55	50	Pericarditis
Esophagus	60	58	55	72	70	68	Stricture, perforation
Stomach	60	55	50	70	67	65	Ulceration, perforation
Small intestine	50	—	40	60	—	55	Obstruction, perforation, fistula
Colon	55	—	45	65	—	55	Obstruction, perforation, fistula, ulceration
Rectum	(100 cm³ volume)		60	(100 cm³ volume)		80	Severe proctitis, necrosis, fistula
Liver	50	35	30	55	45	40	Liver failure

[a]TD 5/5, the average dose that results in a 5% complication risk within 5 years.
[b]TD 50/5, the average dose that results in a 50% complication risk within 5 years.
Adapted from Emami B, Lyman J, Brown A, et al. Tolerance of normal tissue to therapeutic irradiation. *Int J Radiat Oncol Biol Phys* 1991;21:109–122.

PRINCIPLES OF COMBINING ANTICANCER AGENTS WITH RADIATION THERAPY

Combining chemotherapy with radiation therapy has produced important improvements in treatment outcome. Randomized clinical trials show improved local control and survival through the use of concurrent chemotherapy and radiation therapy for patients with high-grade gliomas and locally advanced cancers of the head and neck, lung, esophagus, stomach, rectum, prostate, and anus. There are least two proposed reasons why chemoradiotherapy might be successful. The first is radiosensitization. In the laboratory, radiosensitization is defined as a synergistic relationship, using mathematical approaches such as isobologram or median effect analysis.[126,127] The underlying concept is that the observed effect of using chemotherapy and radiation concurrently is greater than simply adding the two together. A second proposed reason to combine radiation and chemotherapy is to realize the benefit of improved local control radiation along with the systemic effect of chemotherapy, a concept called *spatial additivity*.[128]

Clinical results show that both radiosensitization and spatial additivity contribute to varying extents in different clinical settings. In the case of head and neck cancer, radiosensitization predominates. This conclusion is supported by the meta-analysis of head and neck cancer: sequential chemotherapy and radiotherapy produces little if any improvement in survival, whereas concurrent chemoradiation produces a significant increase in survival.[129] Furthermore, in the early positive studies using concurrent chemoradiation, systemic metastases were unaffected even though survival was improved. Radiosensitization may also predominate in the success of chemoradiotherapy for locally advanced lung cancer. For instance, although initial studies indicated that sequential chemotherapy and radiation had some benefit for lung cancer,[130] more recent work indicates that concurrent therapy is superior, and it is now the standard treatment.[131] However, there are also examples of spatial additivity. For example, both radiosensitization and spatial additivity is provided by the use of chemoradiation for locally advanced cervical cancer in that both local and systemic relapses are decreased by combined therapy.[132]

By targeting the aberrant growth factor or proangiogenic pathways that are specific to cancer cells rather than all rapidly proliferating cells, molecularly targeted therapies offer the potential to improve outcome without increasing toxicity. Even a selective cytostatic effect against the tumor would be predicted to act synergistically with radiation (Fig. 13.22). Although preclinical studies (summarized in the previous biology section) have highlighted the potential therapeutic gains that could be achieved by adding EGFR inhibitors to radiation, the best validation of this combination has been from the results of clinical trials in head and neck cancer. A phase III clinical trial demonstrated that, in a cohort of 424 patients with local–regionally advanced squamous cell carcinoma of the head and neck, the addition of cetuximab nearly doubled the median survival of patients (compared to radiotherapy alone), from 28 to 54 months. This study represents the first major success

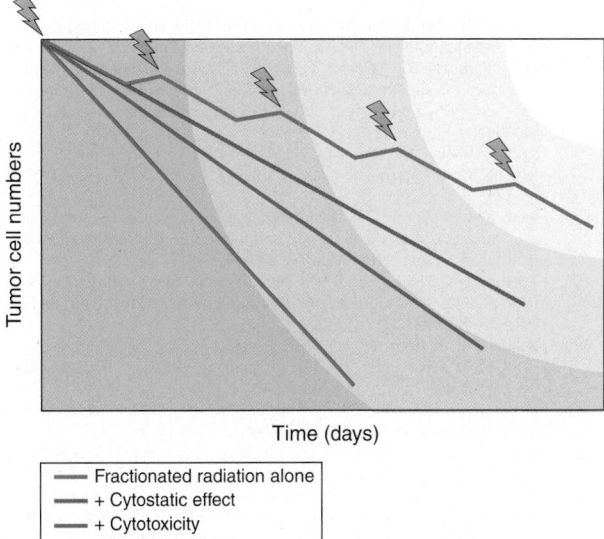

Figure 13.22 Potential mechanisms of synergy between epidermal growth factor receptor (EGFR) inhibitors and radiation. Although each daily radiation treatment kills a fraction of the cells, some cells grow back by the next day, which attenuates the effectiveness of radiation. If an EGFR inhibitor has only a selective cytostatic effect and blocks regrowth between fractions, the result would be a dramatic increase in radiation efficacy. The benefit of the inhibitor would be even greater if it caused tumor cell cytotoxicity or radiosensitization.

Legend for figure:
- Fractionated radiation alone
- + Cytostatic effect
- + Cytotoxicity
- + Radiosensitization

Axis labels: Tumor cell numbers (y-axis); Time (days) (x-axis)

achieved by the addition of an EGFR antagonist to radiotherapy. This improvement was achieved without enhanced toxicity. Notably, the rates of pharyngitis and weight loss were identical in the two arms.[60] Local control was improved rather than the development of metastases, suggesting synergy rather than spatial additivity. Thus, the principle that can be derived from this study is that in tumors expressing high EGFR levels and that are likely to depend on aberrant EGF signaling, combining a true cytotoxic agent such as radiation with a cytostatic agent such as cetuximab has considerable promise.

Because of the success of chemoradiotherapy, the natural tendency has not been to substitute molecularly targeted agents such as cetuximab for chemotherapy, but to add cetuximab to chemoradiotherapy. Thus, the combination of cisplatin, cetuximab, and radiation was recently found to have the same control rate as cisplatin and radiation for patients with locally advanced head and neck cancer, but the cetuximab arm had greater toxicity. Unfortunately, the triple therapy was never evaluated preclinically, and it has been shown preclinically that when EGFR inhibitors are given prior to chemotherapy, they can produce antagonism.[133] The principles of adding molecularly targeted therapy to chemoradiation are still evolving.[63]

SELECTED REFERENCES

The full reference list can be accessed at lwwhealthlibrary.com/oncology.

1. Hall EJ, Giaccia AJ. *Radiobiology for the Radiologist.* Philadelphia: Lippincott Williams & Williams; 2012.
2. Fowler JF. Developing aspects of radiation oncology. *Med Phys* 1981;8:427–434.
3. Lavin MF. Ataxia-telangiectasia: from a rare disorder to a paradigm for cell signalling and cancer. *Nat Rev Mol Cell Biol* 2008;9:759–769.
4. Thompson LH. Recognition, signaling, and repair of DNA double-strand breaks produced by ionizing radiation in mammalian cells: the molecular choreography. *Mutat Res* 2012;751:158–246.

5. Sherr CJ, McCormick F. The RB and p53 pathways in cancer. *Cancer Cell* 2002;2:103–112.
6. Bartek J, Lukas J. Chk1 and Chk2 kinases in checkpoint control and cancer. *Cancer Cell* 2003;3:421–429.
8. Abraham RT. Cell cycle checkpoint signaling through the ATM and ATR kinases. *Genes Dev* 2001;15:2177–2196.
12. Dai Y, Grant S. New insights into checkpoint kinase 1 in the DNA damage response signaling network. *Clin Cancer Res* 2010;16:376–383.
15. Helleday T, Lo J, van Gent DC, et al. DNA double-strand break repair: from mechanistic understanding to cancer treatment. *DNA Repair (Amst)* 2007;6:923–935.

16. Hefferin ML, Tomkinson AE. Mechanism of DNA double-strand break repair by non-homologous end joining. *DNA Repair (Amst)* 2005;4:639–648.

17. Ma Y, Pannicke U, Schwarz K, et al. Hairpin opening and overhang processing by an Artemis/DNA-dependent protein kinase complex in nonhomologous end joining and V(D)J recombination. *Cell* 2002;108:781–794.

22. Esashi F, Galkin VE, Yu X, et al. Stabilization of RAD51 nucleoprotein filaments by the C-terminal region of BRCA2. *Nat Struct Mol Biol* 2007;14:468–474.

23. Sleeth KM, Sorensen CS, Issaeva N, et al. RPA mediates recombination repair during replication stress and is displaced from DNA by checkpoint signalling in human cells. *J Mol Biol* 2007;373:38–47.

24. Littlefield LG, Kleinerman RA, Sayer AM, et al. Chromosome aberrations in lymphocytes—biomonitors of radiation exposure. *Prog Clin Biol Res* 1991;372:387–397.

25. Toulany M, Rodemann HP. Membrane receptor signaling and control of DNA repair after exposure to ionizing radiation. *Nuklearmedizin* 2010;49:S26–S30.

26. Barcellos-Hoff MH, Akhurst RJ. Transforming growth factor-beta in breast cancer: too much, too late. *Breast Cancer Res* 2009;11:202.

27. Deng X, Yin X, Allan R, et al. Ceramide biogenesis is required for radiation-induced apoptosis in the germ line of C. elegans. *Science* 2008;322:110–115.

28. Thompson LH, Suit HD. Proliferation kinetics of x-irradiated mouse L cells studied WITH TIME-lapse photography. II. *Int J Radiat Biol Relat Stud Phys Chem Med* 1969;15:347–362.

29. Sowa Resat MB, Morgan WF. Radiation-induced genomic instability: a role for secreted soluble factors in communicating the radiation response to non-irradiated cells. *J Cell Biochem* 2004;92:1013–1019.

30. Elkind MM. The initial part of the survival curve: does it predict the outcome of fractionated radiotherapy? *Radiat Res* 1988;114:425–436.

31. McCulloch EA, Till JE. The sensitivity of cells from normal mouse bone marrow to gamma radiation in vitro and in vivo. *Radiat Res* 1962;16:822–832.

32. Withers HR. Recovery and repopulation in vivo by mouse skin epithelial cells during fractionated irradiation. *Radiat Res* 1967;32:227–239.

33. Withers HR, Elkind MM. Microcolony survival assay for cells of mouse intestinal mucosa exposed to radiation. *Int J Radiat Biol Relat Stud Phys Chem Med* 1970;17:261–267.

34. Suit H, Wette R. Radiation dose fractionation and tumor control probability. *Radiat Res* 1966;29:267–281.

35. O'Neill K, Lyons SK, Gallagher WM, et al. Bioluminescent imaging: a critical tool in pre-clinical oncology research. *J Pathol* 2010;220:317–327.

36. Hewitt HB, Wilson CW. Survival curves for tumor cells irradiated in vivo. *Ann N Y Acad Sci* 1961;95:818–827.

39. Elkind MM, Whitmore GF. *Radiobiology of Cultured Mammalian Cells.* New York: Gordon and Breach; 1967.

40. Mottram JC. Factors of importance in radiosensitivity of tumors. *Br J Radiol* 1936;9:606.

43. Overgaard J, Horsman MR. Modification of hypoxia-induced radioresistance in tumors by the use of oxygen and sensitizers. *Semin Radiat Oncol* 1996;6:10–21.

44. Machtay M, Pajak TF, Suntharalingam M, et al. Radiotherapy with or without erythropoietin for anemic patients with head and neck cancer: a randomized trial of the Radiation Therapy Oncology Group (RTOG 99-03). *Int J Radiat Oncol Biol Phys* 2007;69:1008–1017.

45. Henke M, Laszig R, Rube C, et al. Erythropoietin to treat head and neck cancer patients with anaemia undergoing radiotherapy: randomised, double-blind, placebo-controlled trial. *Lancet* 2003;362:1255–1260.

46. Janssens GO, Rademakers SE, Terhaard CH, et al. Accelerated radiotherapy with carbogen and nicotinamide for laryngeal cancer: results of a phase III randomized trial. *J Clin Oncol* 2012;30:1777–1783.

47. Willett CG, Boucher Y, di Tomaso E, et al. Direct evidence that the VEGF-specific antibody bevacizumab has antivascular effects in human rectal cancer. *Nat Med* 2004;10:145–147.

48. Lapi SE, Voller TF, Welch MJ. Positron emission tomography imaging of hypoxia. *PET Clin* 2009;4:39–47.

49. Lee NY, Mechalakos JG, Nehmeh S, et al. Fluorine-18-labeled fluoromisonidazole positron emission and computed tomography-guided intensity-modulated radiotherapy for head and neck cancer: a feasibility study. *Int J Radiat Oncol Biol Phys* 2008;70:2–13.

50. Schaue D, Xie MW, Ratikan JA, et al. Regulatory T cells in radiotherapeutic responses. *Front Oncol* 2012;2:90.

51. Formenti SC, Demaria S. Combining radiotherapy and cancer immunotherapy: a paradigm shift. *J Natl Cancer Inst* 2013;105:256–265.

52. Lawrence TS, Davis MA, Tang HY, et al. Fluorodeoxyuridine-mediated cytotoxicity and radiosensitization require S phase progression. *Int J Radiat Biol* 1996;70:273–280.

53. Lawrence TS, Chang EY, Hahn TM, et al. Radiosensitization of pancreatic cancer cells by 2',2'-difluoro-2'-deoxycytidine. *Int J Radiat Oncol Biol Phys* 1996;34:867–872.

54. Eisbruch A, Shewach DS, Bradford CR, et al. Radiation concurrent with gemcitabine for locally advanced head and neck cancer: a phase I trial and intracellular drug incorporation study. *J Clin Oncol* 2001;19:792–799.

55. Ben-Josef E, Schipper M, Francis IR, et al. A phase I/II trial of intensity modulated radiation (IMRT) dose escalation with concurrent fixed-dose rate gemcitabine (FDR-G) in patients with unresectable pancreatic cancer. *Int J Radiat Oncol Biol Phys* 2012;84:1166–1171.

56. Wolff RA, Evans DB, Gravel DM, et al. Phase I trial of gemcitabine combined with radiation for the treatment of locally advanced pancreatic adenocarcinoma. *Clin Cancer Res* 2001;7:2246–2253.

57. Wilson GD, Bentzen SM, Harari PM. Biologic basis for combining drugs with radiation. *Semin Radiat Oncol* 2006;16:2–9.

58. Bradley JD, Paulus R, Graham MV, et al. Phase II trial of postoperative adjuvant paclitaxel/carboplatin and thoracic radiotherapy in resected stage II and IIIA non-small-cell lung cancer: promising long-term results of the Radiation Therapy Oncology Group—RTOG 9705. *J Clin Oncol* 2005;23:3480–3487.

59. Nyati MK, Morgan MA, Feng FY, et al. Integration of EGFR inhibitors with radiochemotherapy. *Nat Rev Cancer* 2006;6:876–885.

60. Bonner JA, Harari PM, Giralt J, et al. Radiotherapy plus cetuximab for locoregionally advanced head and neck cancer: 5-year survival data from a phase 3 randomised trial, and relation between cetuximab-induced rash and survival. *Lancet Oncol* 2010;11:21–28.

61. Ang KK, Zhang QE, Rosenthal DI, et al. A randomized phase III trial (RTOG 0522) of concurrent accelerated radiation plus cisplatin with or without cetuximab for stage III-IV head and neck squamous cell carcinomas (HNC). *J Clin Oncol* 2011;29.

62. Engelke CG, Parsels LA, Qian Y, et al. Sensitization of pancreatic cancer to chemoradiation by the Chk1 inhibitor MK8776. *Clin Cancer Res* 2013;19:4412–4421.

63. Morgan MA, Parsels LA, Maybaum J, et al. Improving the efficacy of chemoradiation with targeted agents. *Cancer Discov* 2014;4:280–291.

64. Chalmers AJ, Lakshman M, Chan N, et al. Poly(ADP-ribose) polymerase inhibition as a model for synthetic lethality in developing radiation oncology targets. *Semin Radiat Oncol* 2010;20:274–281.

66. Winczura P, Jassem J. Combined treatment with cytoprotective agents and radiotherapy. *Cancer Treat Rev* 2010;36:268–275.

67. Van Dyk J, ed. Radiation oncology medical physics resources for working, teaching, and learning. In: *The Modern Technology of Radiation Oncology.* Volume 3. Medical Physics Publishing Web site. http://www.medicalphysics.org/vandykch16.pdf. Madison, WI: Medical Physics Publishing; 2013.

68. Karzmark C, Nunan C, Tanabe E. *Medical Electron Accelerators.* New York: McGraw-Hill Ryerson; 1993.

69. Greene D, Williams P. *Linear Accelerators for Radiation Therapy.* 2nd ed. New York: Taylor and Francis Group; 1997.

70. Fenwick JD, Tome WA, Soisson ET, et al. Tomotherapy and other innovative IMRT delivery systems. *Semin Radiat Oncol* 2006;16:199–208.

71. Curran B, Balter J, Chetty I, eds. *Integrating New Technologies into the Clinic: Monte Carlo and Image-Guided Radiation Therapy.* Madison, WI: Medical Physics Publishing; 2006.

72. Bourland J, ed. *Image-Guided Radiation Therapy.* Boca Raton, FL: Taylor & Francis; 2012.

73. Seco J, Verhaegen F, eds. *Monte Carlo Techniques in Radiation Therapy.* Boca Raton, FL: Taylor & Francis; 2013.

74. Kessler ML. Image registration and data fusion in radiation therapy. *Br J Radiol* 2006;79:S99–S108.

75. Brock K, ed. *Image Processing in Radiation Therapy.* Boca Raton, FL: Taylor & Francis Group; 2014.

76. Sovik A, Malinen E, Olsen DR. Strategies for biologic image-guided dose escalation: a review. *Int J Radiat Oncol Biol Phys* 2009;73:650–658.

77. Marks LB, Ten Haken RK, Martel MK. Guest editor's introduction to QUANTEC: a users guide. *Int J Radiat Oncol Biol Phys* 2010;76:S1–S2.

78. Li A, Alber M, Deasy JO, et al. The use and QA of biologically related models for treatment planning: short report of the TG-166 of the therapy physics committee of the AAPM. *Med Phys* 2012;39:1386–1409.

79. Bortfeld T. IMRT: a review and preview. *Phys Med Biol* 2006;51:R363–R379.

80. Webb S. *Contemporary IMRT Developing Physics and Clinical Implementation.* London: IOP Publishing; 2005.

81. Maughan R, Yudelev M. Neutron therapy. In: Van Dyk J, ed. *The Modern Technology of Radiation Oncology.* Madison, WI: Medical Physics Publishing; 1999.

82. Hogstrom KR, Almond PR. Review of electron beam therapy physics. *Phys Med Biol* 2006;51:R455–R489.

83. Schlegel W, Bortfeld T, Grosu A, eds. *New Technologies in Radiation Oncology.* Heidelberg: Springer-Verlag; 2006.

84. Ma C-MC, Lomax T, eds. *Proton and Carbon Ion Therapy.* Boca Raton, FL: Taylor & Francis Group; 2012.

85. Venselaar J, Meigooni A, Baltas D, et al., eds. *Comprehensive Brachytherapy: Physical and Clinical Aspects.* Boca Raton, FL: Taylor & Francis Group; 2012.

86. Meredith RF. Systemic targeted radionuclide therapy symposium introduction. *Int J Radiat Oncol Biol Phys* 2006;66:S7.

87. Tripuraneni P, Watson RL, Ang KK, et al. Intersociety Radiation Oncology Summit-SCOPE II. *Int J Radiat Oncol Biol Phys* 2008;72:323–326.

88. Delaney G, Jacob S, Featherstone C, et al. The role of radiotherapy in cancer treatment: estimating optimal utilization from a review of evidence-based clinical guidelines. *Cancer* 2005;104:1129–1137.

89. Zelefsky MJ, Housman DM, Pei X, et al. Incidence of secondary cancer development after high-dose intensity-modulated radiotherapy and image-guided brachytherapy for the treatment of localized prostate cancer. *Int J Radiat Oncol Biol Phys* 2012;83:953–959.

90. Combs SE, Laperriere N, Brada M. Clinical controversies: proton radiation therapy for brain and skull base tumors. *Semin Radiat Oncol* 2013;23:120–126.

91. Overgaard J. Hypoxic radiosensitization: adored and ignored. *J Clin Oncol* 2007;25:4066–4074.

92. Mouw KW, Trofimov A, Zietman AL, et al. Clinical controversies: proton therapy for prostate cancer. *Semin Radiat Oncol* 2013;23:109–114.

93. Yu JB, Soulos PR, Herrin J, et al. Proton versus intensity-modulated radiotherapy for prostate cancer: patterns of care and early toxicity. *J Natl Cancer Inst* 2013;105:25–32.

94. Brada M, Pijls-Johannesma M, De Ruysscher D. Proton therapy in clinical practice: current clinical evidence. *J Clin Oncol* 2007;25:965–970.

96. Shilkrut M, Merrick GS, McLaughlin PW, et al. The addition of low-dose-rate brachytherapy and androgen-deprivation therapy decreases biochemical failure and prostate cancer death compared with dose-escalated external-beam radiation therapy for high-risk prostate cancer. *Cancer* 2013;119:681–690.

97. Iyengar P, Timmerman R. Stereotactic ablative radiotherapy for non-small cell lung cancer: rationale and outcomes. *J Natl Compr Canc Netw* 2012;10:1514–1520.

98. Lo SS, Moffatt-Bruce SD, Dawson LA, et al. The role of local therapy in the management of lung and liver oligometastases. *Nat Rev Clin Oncol* 2011;8:405–416.

99. Forastiere AA, Zhang Q, Weber RS, et al. Long-term results of RTOG 91-11: a comparison of three nonsurgical treatment strategies to preserve the larynx in patients with locally advanced larynx cancer. *J Clin Oncol* 2013;31:845–852.

100. Gunderson LL, Winter KA, Ajani JA, et al. Long-term update of US GI inter-group RTOG 98-11 phase III trial for anal carcinoma: survival, relapse, and colostomy failure with concurrent chemoradiation involving fluorouracil/mitomycin versus fluorouracil/cisplatin. *J Clin Oncol* 2012;30:4344–4351.

101. Hellman S, Weichselbaum RR. Oligometastases. *J Clin Oncol* 1995;13:8–10.

103. Stamell EF, Wolchok JD, Gnjatic S, et al. The abscopal effect associated with a systemic anti-melanoma immune response. *Int J Radiat Oncol Biol Phys* 2013;85:293–295.

104. Nagtegaal ID, Gosens MJ, Marijnen CA, et al. Combinations of tumor and treatment parameters are more discriminative for prognosis than the present TNM system in rectal cancer. *J Clin Oncol* 2007;25:1647–1650.

105. Sauer R, Becker H, Hohenberger W, et al. Preoperative versus postoperative chemoradiotherapy for rectal cancer. *N Engl J Med* 2004;351:1731–1740.

106. Clarke M, Collins R, Darby S, et al. Effects of radiotherapy and of differences in the extent of surgery for early breast cancer on local recurrence and 15-year survival: an overview of the randomised trials. *Lancet* 2005;366:2087–2106.

109. Wang XS, Rhines LD, Shiu AS, et al. Stereotactic body radiation therapy for management of spinal metastases in patients without spinal cord compression: a phase 1-2 trial. *Lancet Oncol* 2012;13:395–402.

112. Bourhis J, Overgaard J, Audry H, et al. Hyperfractionated or accelerated radiotherapy in head and neck cancer: a meta-analysis. *Lancet* 2006;368:843–854.

113. Bourhis J, Sire C, Graff P, et al. Concomitant chemoradiotherapy versus acceleration of radiotherapy with or without concomitant chemotherapy in locally advanced head and neck carcinoma (GORTEC 99-02): an open-label phase 3 randomised trial. *Lancet Oncol* 2012;13:145–153.

114. Adkison JB, McHaffie DR, Bentzen SM, et al. Phase I trial of pelvic nodal dose escalation with hypofractionated IMRT for high-risk prostate cancer. *Int J Radiat Oncol Biol Phys* 2012;82:184–190.

119. Dawson LA, Ten Haken RK. Partial volume tolerance of the liver to radiation. *Semin Radiat Oncol* 2005;15:279–283.

120. Kong FM, Hayman JA, Griffith KA, et al. Final toxicity results of a radiation-dose escalation study in patients with non-small-cell lung cancer (NSCLC): predictors for radiation pneumonitis and fibrosis. *Int J Radiat Oncol Biol Phys* 2006;65:1075–1086.

122. Hart JP, Broadwater G, Rabbani Z, et al. Cytokine profiling for prediction of symptomatic radiation-induced lung injury. *Int J Radiat Oncol Biol Phys* 2005;63:1448–1454.

123. Barnett GC, Coles CE, Elliott RM, et al. Independent validation of genes and polymorphisms reported to be associated with radiation toxicity: a prospective analysis study. *Lancet Oncol* 2012;13:65–77.

129. Blanchard P, Baujat B, Holostenco V, et al. Meta-analysis of chemotherapy in head and neck cancer (MACH-NC): a comprehensive analysis by tumour site. *Radiother Oncol* 2011;100:33–40.

131. De Ruysscher D, Belderbos J, Reymen B, et al. State of the art radiation therapy for lung cancer 2012: a glimpse of the future. *Clin Lung Cancer* 2013;14:89–95.

132. Klopp AH, Eifel PJ. Chemoradiotherapy for cervical cancer in 2010. *Curr Oncol Rep* 2011;13:77–85.

133. Chun PY, Feng FY, Scheurer AM, et al. Synergistic effects of gemcitabine and gefitinib in the treatment of head and neck carcinoma. *Cancer Res* 2006;66:981–988.

CANCER THERAPEUTICS

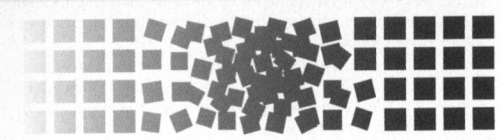

14 Cancer Immunotherapy

Steven A. Rosenberg, Paul F. Robbins, Giao Q. Phan,
Steven A. Feldman, and James N. Kochenderfer

INTRODUCTION

Progress in understanding basic aspects of cellular immunology and tumor–host immune interactions have led to the development of immune-based therapies capable of mediating the rejection of metastatic cancer in humans. Early studies of allografts and transplanted syngeneic tumors in mice demonstrated that it was the cellular arm of the immune response rather than the action of antibodies (humoral immunity) that was responsible for tissue rejection. Thus, studies of immunotherapy have focused on enhancing antitumor immune responses of T cells that recognize cancer antigens. Antibodies that recognize growth factors on the surface of tumors can contribute to tumor regression, primarily by interfering with growth signals rather than by the direct destruction of tumor cells. The use of monoclonal antibodies in cancer treatment will be considered in Chapter 29.

Evidence for specific tumor recognition by cells of the immune system was obtained in experiments first conducted in the 1940s using murine tumors generated or induced by the mutagen methylcholanthrene (MCA). Mice that received a surgical resection of previously inoculated tumors could be protected against a subsequent tumor challenge with the immunizing tumor but not generally protected against challenge with additional MCA tumors. The observation that CD8+ cytotoxic T cells were primarily responsible for mediating the rejection of MCA-induced tumors in mice led to the identification of genes that encoded tumor rejection antigens expressed on murine tumors as well as the subsequent identification of antigens recognized by human tumor-reactive T cells. The identification of widely shared nonmutated tumor antigens led to the expectation that effective vaccine therapies could be developed for the treatment of cancer patients; however, the response rates in clinical cancer vaccine trials targeting these antigens have, to this point, been disappointingly low. Vaccination with viruslike particles expressing human papilloma virus (HPV) proteins are successful in preventing the establishment of cervical cancer and immunization with peptides derived from the oncogenic HPV E6 and E7 proteins can mediate tumor regression in woman with high vulvar neoplasia.[1] Immune-based therapies have, however, been identified that mediate the regression of large, established tumor metastases. Nonspecific immune stimulation with interleukin-2 (IL-2) administration can lead to objective clinical responses in patients with melanoma and renal cancer,[2] and inhibition of regulatory pathways mediated by CTLA-4[3] or PD-1[4] can lead to tumor regression in patients with metastatic melanoma and lung cancer. The adoptive transfer of melanoma reactive T cells can mediate objective clinical responses in 50% to 70% of patients with melanoma,[5] and the ability to genetically modify antitumor lymphocytes is expanding this cell transfer therapy approach to the treatment of patients with other cancer histologies.[6] Studies aimed at identifying potent tumor rejection antigens, as well as mechanisms that regulate immune responses to cancer, are being actively pursued.

HUMAN TUMOR ANTIGENS

To be recognized by immune lymphocytes, intracellular proteins must be digested and the resulting peptides transported to the cell surface and bound to Class I or II main histocompatibility molecules (Fig. 14.1). A variety of approaches have been used to identify the antigens that are naturally processed and presented on tumor cells. These include evaluating the ability of cells transfected with tumor cDNA library pools along with genes encoding autologous major histocompatibility complex (MHC) molecules, as well as the ability of target cells pulsed with peptides eluted from tumor cell surface MHC molecules for their ability to stimulate tumor reactive T cells. Reverse immunology approaches that involve either repeated in vitro T cell sensitization or in vivo immunization with candidate peptides or proteins have also lead to the identification of tumor antigens. Candidate epitopes identified on the basis of their ability to bind to a particular MHC molecule, however, may not necessarily be naturally processed and presented on the tumor cell surface, and there are conflicting reports on the ability of T cells generated using some candidate epitopes to recognize unmanipulated tumor targets, as discussed further.

Additional tumor antigens have been identified using antisera from cancer patients to screen tumor cell cDNA libraries, a method that has been termed serological analysis of recombinant cDNA expression (SEREX).[7] Although some of the proteins identified using this technique are expressed in a tumor-specific manner, many of these antigens are simply expressed at higher levels in tumor cells than in normal cells. This may occur due to the release of normal self-proteins from necrotic and apoptotic tumor cells leading to the generation of antibodies against intracellular proteins that are normally sequestered from the immune system.

Finally, the use of recently described approaches involving whole exomic sequencing of tumor cells has led to the identification of mutated tumor antigens. These studies will be discussed further in the section devoted to mutated tumor antigens

Cancer/Germ-Line Antigens

The first antigen identified as a target of human tumor reactive T cells was isolated by screening a melanoma genomic DNA library with an autologous cytotoxic T lymphocyte (CTL) clone.[8] The gene that was isolated, termed *MAGE-1*, was found to be a nonmutated gene that was a member of a large, previously unidentified gene family, many of whose members encode antigens recognized by tumor reactive T cells.[9] Members of this family of antigens are expressed in the testes and placenta, both of which lack an expression of MHC molecules, but often not in other normal tissues, which has led to their designation as cancer germ-line (CG) antigens. Members of the MAGE gene family are expressed in a variety of tumor types, including melanoma, breast, prostate, and esophageal cancers. The expression patterns of three

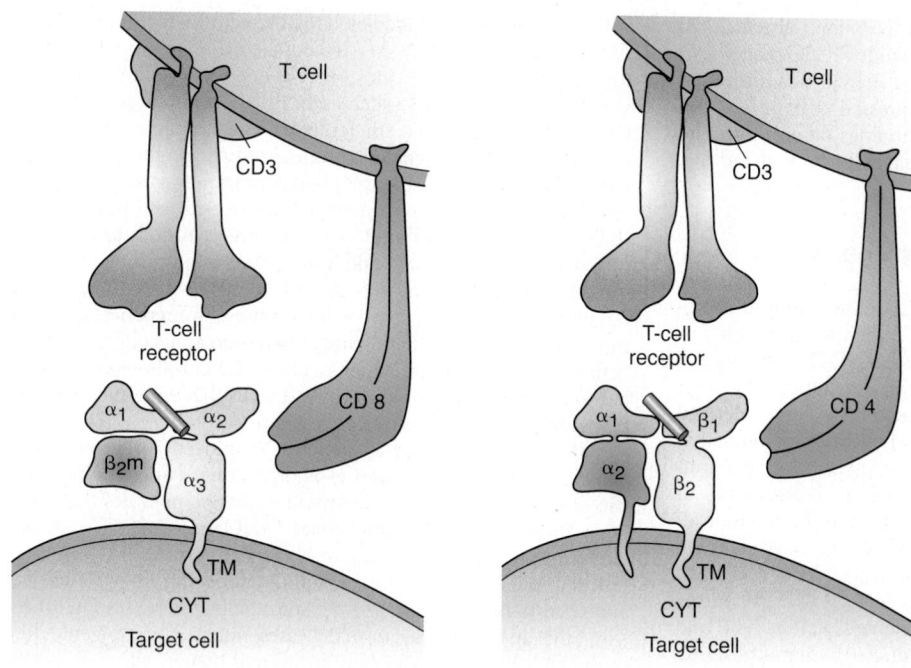

Figure 14.1 CD8 and CD4 cells use different molecules that interact with major histocompatibility complex (MHC) class I and II molecules respectively on the cell surface and serve to potentiate immune reactions.

different cancer/testes antigens in multiple tumor types is shown in Figure 14.2. The NY-ESO-1 antigen—a CG antigen that is unrelated to the MAGE family of genes—is expressed in approximately 30% of breast, prostate, and melanoma tumors, as well as between 70% and 80% of synovial cell sarcomas.[10]

Clinical adoptive immunotherapy trials targeting CG antigens have now been conducted in patients with melanoma as well as other tumor types. In a recent trial, objective clinical responses were seen in approximately 50% of patients with melanoma and 80% of patients with synovial cell sarcoma receiving autologous peripheral blood mononuclear cell (PBMC) transduced with a T-cell receptor directed against an HLA-A*02:01 restricted NY-ESO-1 epitope.[6] A trial targeting a MAGEA3

epitopes was recently carried out using a T-cell receptor (TCR) isolated from an HLA-A*02:01+ transgenic mouse immunized with the MAGEA3:112–120 peptide.[11] Objective clinical responses were observed in five of nine melanoma patients receiving the adoptively transferred PBMC that were transduced with the MAGEA3-reactive TCR.[12] Unexpectedly, neural toxicity was observed in three of the patients treated in this trial, two of whom lapsed into a coma and subsequently died. Autopsy samples of patients' brains revealed that *MAGEA12*, which encodes a cross-reactive epitope recognized by the MAGEA3 TCR, was expressed at low levels in patients' brains, which may have been responsible for the observed neurologic toxicities. In a recent trial carried out using an affinity-enhanced human TCR directed against the

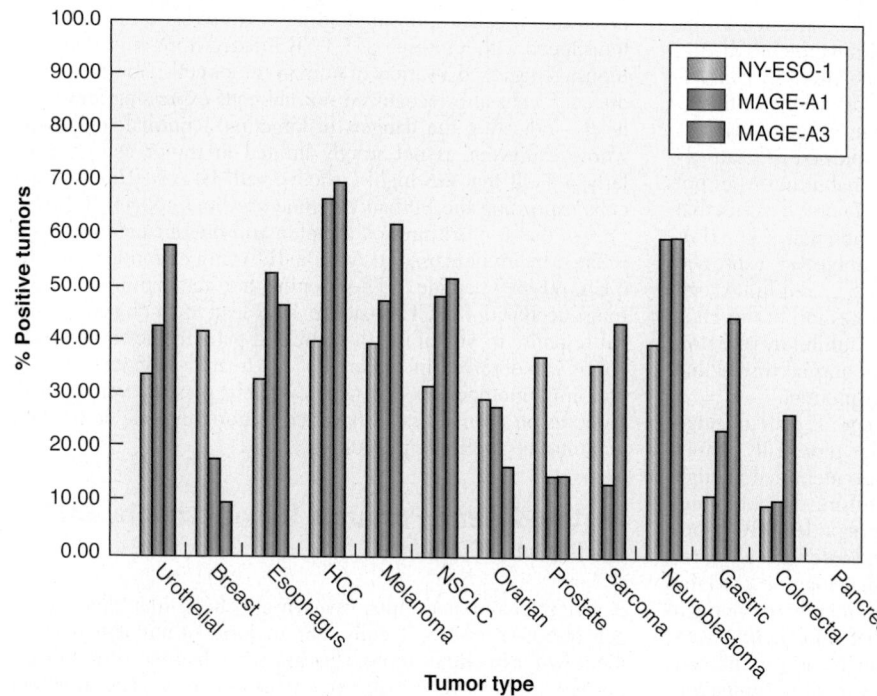

Figure 14.2 Expression of three different cancer/testes antigens in many different tumor types is shown. These data reflect reverse transcription–polymerase chain reaction measurements and is more sensitive than results obtained by immunohistochemistry. NSCLC, non–small-cell lung cancer. (Data compiled by Dr. J. Wargo. Massachusetts General Hospital.)

HLA-A*01:01-restricted, MAGEA3:168-176 epitope, the first two patients receiving TCR-transduced autologous PBMC died of cardiac arrest 4 to 5 days following infusion, which was attributed to cross-reactivity with titin, a protein expressed at high levels in cardimyocytes.[13] Taken together, these findings demonstrate the need for caution in evaluating cross-reactivity of high affinity TCRs recognizing tumor antigens.

Melanocyte Differentiation Antigens

Melanoma-reactive T cells have been frequently found to recognize gene products, termed melanocyte differentiation antigens (MDA), that are expressed in melanomas as well as in normal melanocytes present in the skin, eye, and ear but not in other normal tissues or tumor types. These include epitopes derived from gp100,[14,15] tyrosinase,[16] TRP-1,[17] and TRP-2,[18] proteins that had previously been found to play important roles in melanin synthesis. The screening of melanoma cDNA libraries with an HLA-A2–restricted tumor reactive T cells lead to the isolation of a previously unidentified gene, termed MART-1[19] or Melan-A.[20] The MART-1 antigen, which is expressed in 80% to 90% of fresh melanomas and cultured melanoma cell lines as well as normal melanocytes, represents an MDA of unknown function. The majority of melanoma reactive, HLA-A2–restricted tumor-infiltrating lymphocytes (TIL) recognize a single MART-1 epitope.[21] Studies carried out using a variety of approaches have also resulted in the identification of human leukocyte antigen (HLA) class II restricted epitopes of tyrosinase, TRP-1, TRP-2, and gp100.[9]

Overexpressed Gene Products

Gene products that are expressed at low levels in a variety of normal tissues but are overexpressed in a variety of tumor types have also been shown to be recognized by T cells. Screening of an autologous renal carcinoma cDNA library with a tumor reactive, HLA-A3–restricted T-cell clone resulted in the isolation of FGF5,[22] a protein that was expressed only at low levels in normal tissues but upregulated in multiple renal carcinomas as well as prostate and breast carcinomas. The peptide epitope recognized by FGF5-reactive T cells was generated by protein splicing, a process in which distant protein regions are joined together in the proteasome that had previously only been described in plants[23] and unicellular organisms.[24] Subsequent studies have led to the identification of multiple epitopes that result from protein splicing, suggesting that this represents a general mechanism for generating T-cell epitopes.[25-28] Screening of an autologous cDNA library led to the identification of a previously unknown gene that was termed PRAME.[29] This gene product was expressed in relatively high levels in melanomas as well as in additional tumor types but was also expressed at lower levels in a variety of normal tissues that included the testis, endometrium, ovary, and adrenals. The HLA-A24–restricted PRAME reactive T-cell clone, however, expressed the natural killer (NK) inhibitory receptor p58.2, and tumor cell recognition was dependent on the loss of expression of the HLA C*07 allele that represented the ligand for the inhibitory receptor, which may explain the lack of recognition of normal tissues that express relatively high levels of this HLA gene product.

Attempts have also been made to generate T cells directed against overexpressed candidate antigens by repeatedly stimulating PBMC in vitro with peptides that were identified as high binders for particular MHC molecules either using direct binding assays or in silico analysis carried out using peptide/MHC binding algorithms.[30,31] Using this approach, candidate epitopes have been identified from a variety of proteins that include prostate-specific antigen (PSA)[32] and prostate-specific membrane antigen (PSMA),[33] as well as Her-2/neu, a protein that is frequently overexpressed in a variety of tumor types, including breast carcinomas. Initial studies indicated that T cells derived by in vitro stimulation

with a peptide that was predicted to bind with high affinity to HLA-A*02:01, Her-2/neu:369–377, recognized the appropriate natural tumor targets.[34] In one study, T cells generated following two in vitro stimulations of postvaccination PBMC from three of the four patients who were tested efficiently recognized peptide-pulsed targets but failed to recognize appropriate tumor targets.[35] Similarly, although stimulation with a peptide corresponding to amino acids 540 through 548 of the human telomerase reverse transcriptase (hTERT) catalytic subunit was initially reported to generate tumor-reactive T cells,[36] additional observations indicated that T cells generated using this peptide failed to recognize tumor targets.[37] These factors responsible for these discrepancies remain unresolved, although the in vitro stimulation of T cells with target cells pulsed with relatively high peptide concentrations could have led to the generation of low-avidity T cells that were incapable of recognizing naturally processed antigens.

Alternative screening approaches employed for tumor antigen discovery that may help to address these issues include the use of tandem mass spectrometry to sequence peptides that have been eluted from tumor cell surface MHC molecules. Use of this technique, coupled with microarray gene expression profiling, resulted in the identification of peptides derived from proteins that appeared to be overexpressed in tumor cells.[38] Peptides identified using this approach may, in many cases, not be immunogenic due to the fact that their expression in normal tissues, although lower than in tumor cells, may be high enough to lead to central or peripheral tolerance. Nevertheless, one of the peptides that were identified in this study also appeared to be recognized by human tumor reactive T cells. Recently, a similar approach was used to identify candidate peptides presented on cell surface MHC molecules that appeared to be derived from proteins that were overexpressed on glioblastomas.[39] In a clinical trial involving vaccination of patients with pools of the identified peptides, overall survival was associated with the number of peptides in the vaccine pool that elicited immune response[40]; however, this may simply reflect the fact that T cells from healthier patients can more readily generate peptide-specific responses.

Transgenic mice that express human HLA molecules have also been immunized with candidate antigens in an attempt to identify high avidity tumor-reactive T cells. Immunization of transgenic mice expressing HLA-A*0201 with the native human p53:264–272 peptide that differed from the corresponding murine p53 sequence at a single position lead to the generation of T cells that recognized tumor cells expressing high levels of p53.[41] Human T cells transduced with a murine p53 TCR isolated from an immunized mouse recognized a variety of human tumor cells; however, transduced T cells also recognized normal cells expressing lower p53 levels, indicating the dangers of targeting a normal self-protein whose expression is not strictly limited to tumor cells.[42] Similarly, a TCR that was highly reactive with HLA-A*02:01+ tumor cells expressing the human carcinoembryonic antigen (CEA), a protein that is overexpressed in colon and breast carcinomas, was isolated by immunizing HLA-A*02:01+ transgenic mice with the CEA:691–699 peptide.[43] The adoptive transfer of human PBMC transduced with the CEA-reactive TCR lead to an objective clinical response in one of the three treated patients; however, severe colitis was observed in all three of the treated patients.[44] In general, immunotherapies that target antigens present even in small amounts on normal tissues have led to normal tissue destruction and must be applied with caution.

Mutated Gene Products Recognized by CD8+ and CD4+ T Cells

A variety of mutated antigens have also been identified as targets of tumor reactive T cells. The majority of mutated antigens identified using these approaches appear to be unique or only expressed in a relatively small percentage of cancers, and so do not represent targets that are broadly applicable to the treatment of multiple patients. Nevertheless, these studies have in some cases provided insights into mechanisms involved with tumor development, as the mutations may represent drivers of the transformed phenotype. The CDK4 gene product that was cloned using a CTL clone contained a point mutation that enhanced the binding to the HLA-A2 restriction element.[45] This mutation, which was identified in 1 of an additional 28 melanomas that were analyzed, led to the inhibition of binding to the cell cycle inhibitory protein p16^{INK4a} and may have played a role in the loss of growth control in this tumor cell. A point-mutated product of the β-catenin gene, containing a substitution of phenylalanine for serine at position 37, was isolated by screening a cDNA library with an HLA-24–restricted, melanoma reactive TIL.[46] This mutation was found to stabilize the β-catenin gene product by altering a critical serine phosphorylation site, and 2 of 24 additional melanoma cell lines were found to express transcripts with identical mutations.[47]

The observation that immunization against individual murine tumors did not generally cross-protect against challenge with additional syngeneic murine tumors has provided support for the hypothesis that mutant T-cell epitopes represent the predominant antigens responsible for tumor rejection.[48] Mutated epitopes also represent a foreign antigen, which may render them more immunogenic than the majority of normal self-antigens. Although many of the mutations are specific for individual tumors, T cells have been generated by carrying out in vitro sensitization with peptides encoded at mutational hot spots present in *driver* genes.[49]

Recently, novel approaches have been developed that involve the sequencing of tumor cell DNA to identify potential mutated epitopes. In one study, whole exome sequencing of the murine B16 melanoma led to the identification of mutated epitopes that elicited a T cell that appeared to specifically recognize the mutated but not the corresponding wild-type peptides.[50] In a second study, a mutated antigen was identified by screening candidate epitopes that were expressed by tumors derived from immunodeficient mice that regressed in immune-competent mice.[51] More recently, melanomas from three patients who responded to adoptive immunotherapy were subjected to whole exome sequencing, followed by in silico analysis using peptide/MHC binding algorithms to identify candidate epitopes that were predicted to bind to the patients' MHC molecules.[52] Using this approach, a total of seven peptides were identified as targets of the TIL that were administered to these patients. Two mutated epitopes were recently identified by whole exome sequencing of a melanoma from a patient who demonstrated a partial response to treatment with the anti–CTLA-4 antibody ipilimumab, followed by a screening of a panel of mutated candidate peptide/MHC tetramers that were predicted to bind to the patient's HLA-A and B alleles.[53] In addition, a mutated epitope expressed by a bile duct cancer was identified by screening tandem minigenes encoding all mutated epitopes that were identified by whole exome sequencing.[54] The adoptive transfer of T cells directed against this mutation-mediated regression of the patient's cancer. Mutations unique to each cancer represent ideal targets for immunotherapy and can potentially lead to the development of personalized therapies directed against these unique targets.

Antigens Identified in Viral-Associated Cancers

Viruses do not appear to play a role in the development of the majority of human cancers; however, an infection with HPV, a group of double-stranded DNA viruses that infect squamous epithelium, is highly associated with the development of a variety of genital lesions that range from warts to carcinomas, as well as the majority of oropharyngeal carcinomas. Recombinant vaccines have been produced by the generation of viruslike particles (VLP),

self-assembling particles that form following the expression of the HPV L1 protein in recombinant viral and yeast systems that were initially found to be protective in animal models. The results of a phase II trial in which 2,392 women between 16 and 23 years of age were immunized with HPV-16 VLPs indicated that 100% of those who were vaccinated were protected against infection with HPV-16.[55,56] Although vaccination with VLP does not lead to the regression of established disease, some success has been seen in therapeutic vaccination trials that target the oncogenic viral proteins E6 and E7. In a trial involving the vaccination of women with HPV-16–positive high-grade vulvar intraepithelial neoplasia with synthetic long peptides that encompass both HLA class I and class II restricted epitopes from the oncogenic HPV proteins E6 and E, clinical responses were observed in 15 of the 19 vaccinated patients, and complete regression of all lesions were seen in 9 of the 19 patients in this trial.[1]

Targeting foreign antigens thus may represent a strategy that can lead to more effective immunotherapies. These include viral epitopes as well as mutated epitopes that are also foreign to the host and therefore may represent more effective targets for these therapies than normal self-antigen.

HUMAN CANCER IMMUNOTHERAPIES

A wide variety of therapies have been evaluated in model systems and are now being developed for the treatment of patients with cancer. These include nonspecific approaches, those that involve direct immunization of patients with a variety of immunogens and approaches that involve the adoptive transfer of activated effector cells (Table 14.1). Much confusion related to the effectiveness of cancer immunotherapy has resulted from the lack of proper evaluation of the results of therapy using standard, accepted oncologic criteria such as the World Health Organization or the Response Evaluation Criteria in Solid Tumors (RECIST). Many clinical trials reported a positive use of *soft* criteria such as lymphoid infiltration or tumor necrosis that can occur in the natural course of cancer growth. Because of the delayed responses seen with some immunotherapy approaches, including tumor regression after initial tumor growth, guidelines have been published suggesting the use of an alternate set of immune-related response criteria for the evaluation of immune-based cancer treatments.[57,58] Other confusion has arisen from the use of inappropriate animal models. Although animal model systems have provided important clues that may lead to improved therapies, model systems that employ artificially introduced foreign antigens or that evaluate protection from tumor challenge do not appear to be relevant to the treatment of patients with bulky metastases. Short-term lung metastasis models involve the treatment of relatively small, nonvascularized tumors and also may not be directly relevant to the majority of tumors that are the targets of current clinical trials.

TABLE 14.1

Three Main Approaches to Cancer Immunotherapy

1. Nonspecific stimulation of immune reactions
   a) Stimulate effector cells
      IL-2 (melanoma and renal cancer)
   b) Inhibit regulatory factors
      Anti-CTLA4 (melanoma)
      Anti–PD-1 (melanoma, lung cancer)
2. Active immunization to enhance antitumor reactions (cancer vaccines)
3. Passively transfer activated immune cells with antitumor activity (adoptive immunotherapy)

Nonspecific Approaches to Cancer Immunotherapy

Progress has surged in the past 10 years in the understanding and utilization of nonspecific immune stimulation for the treatment of metastatic cancers. These agents aim to activate quiescent tumor-reactive immune cells or to remove inhibitory mechanisms to allow immunosuppressed cells to function to their full capacity. Although IL-2 and ipilimumab are currently the only immune stimulants approved by the U.S. Food and Drug Administration (FDA) for the treatment of metastatic renal cell carcinoma (IL-2) and melanoma (IL-2 and ipilimumab), new immune checkpoint inhibitors such as anti–programmed cell death 1 (anti–PD-1) have shown impressive results in recent clinical trials for patients with melanoma, renal cell cancer, and also non–small-cell lung cancer (NSCLC), and will likely be approved in the near future. As expected with nonspecific immunostimulation, systemic and bystander immune-related adverse events such as colitis has been reported with all agents in varying degrees, although most side effects are controllable and reversible if addressed aggressively and promptly by experienced clinicians. Importantly, antitumor responses seen with these immune-based modalities appear to be durable for some patients and may even be potentially curative. As with many therapies for metastatic solid tumors, preliminary trials using combination therapies have suggested better than expected response rates and survival, and confirmatory trials are in process to validate and ensure that toxicities from combining agents would not be prohibitive. Overall, patients with metastatic solid tumors may soon have wider armamentarium of off-the-shelf immunotherapy options.

Interleukin-2

Morgan et al.[59] showed that a *factor* produced in the medium from stimulated normal human blood lymphocytes can allow ex vivo growth and expansion of human T lymphocytes. The identification of this soluble T-cell growth factor (IL-2)[60,61] allowed the ability to culture T cells in vitro. IL-2 is a 15-kd glycoprotein produced in minute amounts by activated peripheral blood lymphocytes, and even with using T-cell hybridomas, minimal quantities could be purified; thus, research using IL-2 was impeded by the limited amounts of purified IL-2 available. The isolation of the cDNA clone in 1983[62] enabled the development in 1984 of recombinant IL-2,[63] which permitted the ability to mass manufacture IL-2. Although murine studies demonstrated the ability of IL-2 to mediate tumor regression,[64] early phase I clinical trials did not show any antitumor response,[65] but was instructive in showing pharmacokinetics and toxicities, which led to more effective regimens. Subsequently, IL-2 was given in higher doses (up to 720,000 IU/kg intravenously every 8 hours) in a landmark trial involving 25 patients, along with nonspecific lymphokine-activated natural killer (LAK) cells, which are non-T and non-B lymphocytes.[66] This report was the first to document the regression of advanced solid cancers (melanoma, renal cell, lung, and colon) using immunotherapy in humans.[66] A follow-up trial randomizing 181 patients to either high-dose IL-2 alone (720,000 IU/kg intravenously every 8 hours) or high-dose IL-2 and LAK cells showed that the tumor response was due to IL-2 alone and not to the nonspecific LAK cells.[67] This study also narrowed the IL-2–sensitive histologies to melanoma and renal cell cancer, which had more consistent responses.

IL-2 Therapy for Metastatic Renal Cell Cancer

Subsequent to the studies discussed previously, high-dose IL-2 was tested by additional centers and in combination with other agents for renal cell cancer. A randomized phase II trial involving 99 kidney cancer patients showed no increase in antitumor responses with the addition of interferon alfa-2b (IFNα-2b). Responses were seen for 12 (17%) of 71 patients who received high-dose IL-2 alone, with 4 complete regressions.[68] A summary report of 227 patients with metastatic renal cell cancer treated with high-dose IL-2 (defined as 600,000 IU/kg or 720,000 IU/kg given intravenously every 8 hours as tolerated up to 15 doses) from 1985 to 1996 at the Surgery Branch of the National Cancer Institute (NCI) documented a total response rate of 19%, with 10% partial and 9% complete; the longest duration of a complete response was over 10 years ongoing (134+ months).[69] Another summary report from seven phase II clinical trials from multiple institutions involving 255 patients with metastatic renal cell cancer receiving high-dose IL-2 showed the overall response rate was 14%, with 9% partial and 5% complete, and responses occurred in all sites of disease, including primary kidney tumors, bone metastases, and bulking visceral tumor burdens.[70] Although the response rates were modest, the durability of the responses was remarkable, with many responses lasting over 5 years ongoing (see Fig. 14.2). Because of the striking durability of the antitumor responses, IL-2 received FDA approval for the treatment of metastatic renal cell cancer in 1992. A follow-up report in 2000 showing the response rates of the 255 renal cell patients in the seven phase II studies to be the same, with complete responses lasting over 10 years ongoing (131+ months for the longest responder), suggesting a potential cure.[71]

To ascertain whether lower doses and/or different administration routes, which would decrease toxicity and obviate the need for inpatient hospitalization for IL-2 therapy, a trial randomizing 400 patients with metastatic renal cell cancer to either standard high-dose intravenous IL-2, low-dose intravenous IL-2 (at 72,000 IU/kg), or low-dose subcutaneous IL-2 (250,000 U/kg per dose daily Monday through Friday in the first week and then 125,000 U/kg per dose daily during the next 5 weeks).[72] Although responses were seen with all three regimens, including complete responses in the low-dose subcutaneous regimen, standard high-dose IL-2 had higher overall response rates (21%) versus low-dose intravenous IL-2 (13%; p = 0.048) and low-dose subcutaneous IL-2 (10%; p = 0.033), suggesting the superiority of the high-dose intravenous regimen.[72]

The administration of IL-2 represents the only known curative treatment for patients with metastatic renal cell cancer and should be considered as front-line therapy for suitable patients.

IL-2 Therapy for Metastatic Melanoma

Between 1985 and 1993, 270 patients with metastatic melanoma enrolled into eight clinical trials in multiple centers using high-dose IL-2 (defined as 600,000 IU/kg or 720,000 IU/kg given intravenously every 8 hours as tolerated up to 15 doses). Atkins et al.[73] reported overall response rates of 16% (43 patients), with 10% partial and 6% complete; responses occurred at all tumor sites and regardless of initial tumor burden. With median follow-up at that time of 62 months, 20 responders (47%) were still alive, with 15 surviving over 5 years.[73] A follow-up report on those patients in 2000 showed that the response rates were unchanged; with the longest response duration of >12 years ongoing, disease progression was not observed in any patient responding greater than 30 months.[74] As with renal cell cancer, the flat *tail* of the Kaplan-Meier response duration and overall survival curves (Fig. 14.3), showing the potential curative nature of the antitumor responses, was the main compelling reason the FDA approved IL-2 for the treatment of metastatic melanoma in 1998.

Research in subsequent years aimed to increase the response rates of IL-2, led by increasing interests in tumor vaccinations as melanoma-associated antigens were being characterized.[75] Pilot studies suggested that vaccinations using modified melanoma differentiation antigens such as gp100:209–217(210M) could elicit immunologic responses in nearly all patients, and when combined with high-dose IL-2, could elicit potentially higher than expected clinical antitumor responses.[75] A follow-up phase III study[76] randomized 185 patients with HLA*A0201 from 21 centers to either high-dose IL-2 or high-dose IL-2 plus gp100:209–217(210M) concurrent immunization. Although the response rates for the

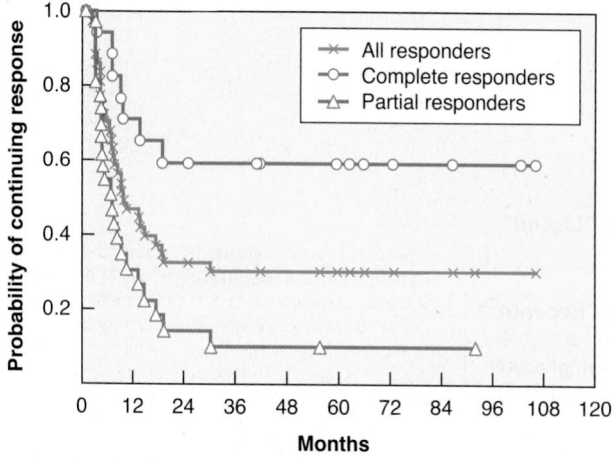

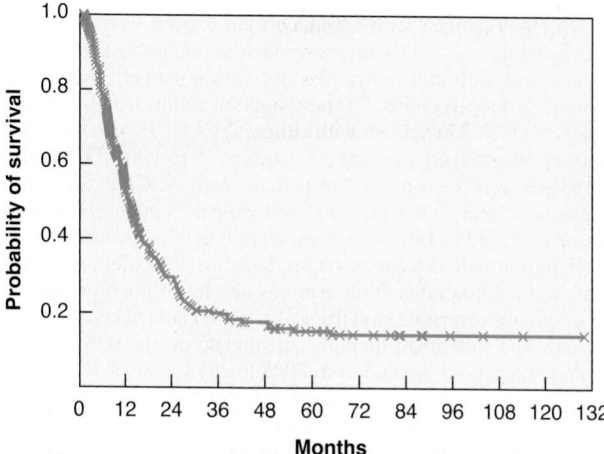

Figure 14.3 Kaplain-Meier plots of response duration (*top*) and overall survival (*bottom*) for 270 patients with metastatic melanoma who were treated with high-dose bolus IL-2 from 1985 to 1993 in eight clinical trials.[73]

IL-2 plus vaccine arm was statistically improved compared to IL-2 alone (16% versus 6%; p = 0.03), the IL-2 alone arm was notable for being much lower than in all prior studies.[76] In addition, a pilot trial of 36 melanoma patients treated high-dose IL-2 concurrently with ipilimumab (an antibody against cytotoxic T lymphocyte–associated antigen 4 discussed in the following section) gave a 25% OR rate, with 17% achieving complete response[77]; however, these data have not been further tested.

Correlative studies suggest that the total doses of IL-2 received during the first treatment course was significantly higher in patients achieving a complete response[69]; however, when limited to patients who were able to complete both cycles of the course, there was no statistical significance, suggesting that patients whose tumors progressed significantly after one cycle (and was not able to complete the second cycle of the course) accounted for some of the difference seen.[78] Responders did have a higher maximal lymphocyte count[69,78] immediately posttherapy and were more likely to develop vitiligo and thyroid dysfunction.[78] There has not been a consistent pretherapy factor that is predictive of response, although one retrospective correlative study involving 374 patients showed that patients with M1a (subcutaneous- and/or cutaneous-only disease) have a response rate of 54% compared with 12% for those with visceral M1b/c (P$_2$ <0.0001).[78]

Toxicities and Safe Administration of IL-2

High-dose IL-2 has been shown to be associated with adverse events that impact multiple organ systems.[73,79,80] The main component of

the toxicities is due to an inflammatory response mediated by the release of cytokines such as IFNγ and tumor necrosis factor alpha (TNF-α)[81] resulting in a capillary-leak syndrome[82] and decreased systemic vascular resistance, which can lead to fever, hypotension, cardiac arrhythmia, lethargy, renal insufficiency, hepatic dysfunction, body edema, pulmonary edema, and confusion; other side effects can also include nausea, diarrhea, rash, anemia, thrombocytopenia, lymphocytosis, and neutrophil chemotactic defect[83] that predispose patients to gram-positive line infections. Since the first clinical trials with IL-2 in 1984, however, much has been learned to permit its safe dosing for appropriately screened patients[82,84,85]; importantly, if patients are appropriately supported, side effects are quickly reversible once IL-2 dosing ceases.[85] Kammula et al.[86] compared the incidences of grade 3/4 toxicities between the 155 patients treated from 1985 to 1986 to 156 patients treated from 1993 through 1997 at the NCI Surgery Branch: grade 3/4 hypotension decreased from 81% to 31%, intubations from 12% to 3%, neuropsychiatric toxicities from 19% to 8%, diarrhea from 92% to 12%, line sepsis from 18% to 4%, cardiac ischemia from 3% to 0%, and mortality from 3% to 0%. In fact, no fatality occurred strictly due to IL-2 therapy since 1989.[86] Overall strategies for the safe administration of high-dose IL-2 include careful screening for appropriately selected patients with adequate cardiopulmonary reserve, having an experienced team of physicians and nurses who are cognizant of the expected toxicities of IL-2, having routine preemptive measures such as prophylactic antibiotics to prevent line infections, and aggressive and prompt management of toxicities.

Checkpoint Modulators

Anti–Cytotoxic T Lymphocyte Antigen 4

CTLA-4 is an immunosuppressive *costimulatory* receptor found on newly activated T cells (and on regulatory T cells) that binds with costimulatory ligands B7-1 and B7-2 on antigen-presenting cells.[87,88] When CTLA-4 is engaged by B7-1 or B7-2, the T cells becomes inhibited,[89,90] suggesting that CTLA-4 likely evolved as a self-protective mechanism to prevent autoimmunity (Fig. 14.4). Thus, overcoming this *checkpoint* molecule was an aim of cancer immunotherapy. After CTLA-4 blockade in murine models led to antitumor immunity,[91,92] anti–CTLA-4 antibodies were tested in clinical trials starting in 2002.

The combination of anti–CTLA-4 blocking antibodies and vaccination worked well in murine models and led to one of the early phase II studies using ipilimumab (a fully human immunoglobulin [IgG$_1$] monoclonal antibody previously called MDX-010) with two gp100 vaccines, gp100:209–217(210M) and gp100:280–288(288V), in patients with metastatic melanoma.[93] Antitumor regressions were seen (from 11% to 22% overall response rates, with up to 8% complete response rates), along with severe autoimmune toxicities such as colitis, dermatitis, and even hypophysitis,[93–95] as would be expected based on the mechanism of CTLA-4 blockade. In fact, autoimmunity adverse events appeared to correlate with response to ipilimumab.[3] The experience with these early studies led to management strategies to screen aggressively for immune-related adverse events (IRAE), such as routine screening of endocrinopathies, and to treat IRAEs promptly, including high-dose steroids if needed for severe colitis.[96,97] Overall, ipilimumab was in some ways easier to manage for the patients than IL-2 because it was an outpatient infusion given every 3 weeks; IRAEs were unpredictable, however, and can appear suddenly many weeks after receiving a dose.

In 2010, results from a landmark phase III randomized trial comparing three treatment strategies (ipilimumab alone, gp100 peptide vaccine alone, or ipilimumab plus gp100 peptide vaccine) in 676 patients with metastatic melanoma were published showing improvement in median survival in the two arms that received ipilimumab (10 months) compared to the gp100 alone arm (6 months, p <0.001), despite showing a low response rate of 7% (among 540 patients who received ipilimumab).[98] Another

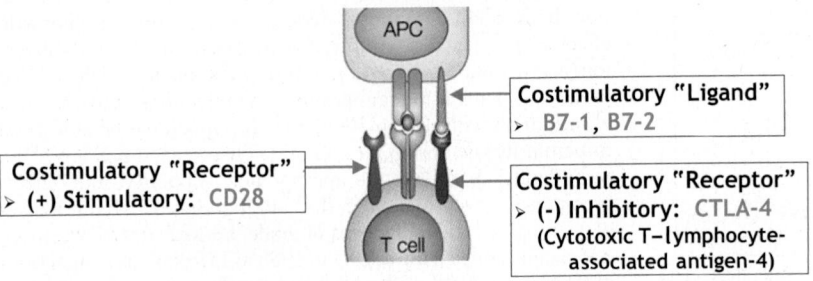

"Second Signal"

Additional signal(s) via costimulatory molecules

Figure 14.4 Mechanism of action of cytotoxic T-lymphocyte–associated antigen 4 (CTLA-4). When CD28 is engaged on the T cell, reactivity of the T cell is enhanced. When CTLA-4 is engaged on the T cell, reactivity of the T cell is inhibited. Blocking of CTLA-4 with a monoclonal antibody can elicit antitumor immunity but also autoimmunity.

phase III randomized trial comparing dacarbazine plus ipilimumab versus dacarbazine alone again showed improved survival in that arm containing dacarbazine (11.2 months versus 9.1 months; p <0.001).[99] These studies showing survival benefit led to FDA approval of ipilimumab for advanced melanoma in 2011.

The responses seen with ipilimumab appear to be durable.[100] A follow-up study of 177 patients with metastatic melanoma treated on the earliest trials at the NCI Surgery Branch using ipilimumab showed that response duration could last 99+ months ongoing.[77] In fact, 14 out of the 15 complete responders remain disease free 54+ to 99+ months ongoing, suggesting a potential cure for some patients. Interestingly, several patients who were deemed partial responders converted to complete responders several years later, because it look an average of 30 months to have all visible tumor marks on imaging scans to disappear.[77]

Ipilimumab was also tested on other solid tumors, and renal cell cancer again appears to be the only other type beside melanoma that had significant responses. Sixty-one patients with metastatic renal cell cancer were treated, and six developed a response (10%); however, 33% developed grade 3/4 IRAEs.[101] Subsequently, the availability of agents with lower toxicity profiles such as sunitinib and sorafenib prevented further enthusiasm to pursue this drug for renal cell cancer.

Another anti–CTLA-4 antibody, tremelimumab (previously called CP-675,206), has also demonstrated durable responses in melanoma patients.[102,103] A phase III randomized trial randomizing 655 patients with metastatic melanoma to either tremelimumab or physician's choice chemotherapy, however, failed to show a survival difference (despite a significantly different response duration favoring tremelimumab, 35.8 months versus 13.7 months; p = 0.0011), possibly due to crossover of chemotherapy patients enrolling into ipilimumab trials and expanded access programs.[103]

Anti–Programmed Death 1 and Anti–Programmed Death Ligand 1

PD-1 is another checkpoint modulator expressed on activated T cells. Although CTLA-4 appears to be involved in the early activation of T cells, PD-1 is involved in the later effector phase of T-cell activation and can function to prevent excessive damage to self by activated T cells in the periphery.[104,105] Interaction with its corresponding ligand, PD-L1 (B7-H1) and PD-L2 (B7-H2) leads to suppressed T-effector function. PD-L1 is expressed on hematopoietic and epithelial cells and is upregulated by cytokines such as IFNγ,[106] whereas PD-L1 is mainly on antigen-presenting cells. Given the clinical results with inhibiting the CTLA-4 checkpoint, recent efforts have focused on inhibiting the PD-1/PD-L1 and PD-1/PD-L2 interactions.

Nivolumab (previously known as BMS-936558, MDX-1106, and ONO-4538) is a fully human anti–PD-1 IgG4 monoclonal antibody that was initially tested in a phase I trial published in 2010 in which 39 patients with advanced solid cancers were treated in escalating doses.[107] Responses were seen in one patient with colon cancer, one with melanoma, and one with renal cell cancer; one patient developed colitis.[108] These hopeful results lead to a larger study in which 236 patients with either NSCLC (74 patients), melanoma (94 patients), or renal cell cancer (33 patients).[4] Objective responses were seen in 18% of patients with NSCLC, 28% with melanoma, and 27% with renal cell cancer.[4] Grade 3/4 adverse events occurred in 14% of patients, including those previously seen with ipilimumab (dermatitis, colitis, hepatitis, thyroiditis, hypophysitis, and pneumonitis). Nine patients developed pneumonitis, six of whom was reversible, and three (1%) with grade 3/4 died despite steroids and infliximab therapy.[4] An update on the status of 107 melanoma patients treated from 2008 to 2012 shows a 31% tumor response rate, with a median response duration of 2 years and a median overall survival of 16.8 months.[109]

Nivolumab was also tested in combination with ipilimumab in melanoma in either concurrent (53 patients) or sequenced (33 patients) regimens. The concurrent group experienced an overall response rate of 40%, whereas the sequenced group had a 20% response rate.[110] The concurrent group also experienced a higher rate of grade 3/4 adverse events (53%), compared to 18% in the sequenced group. Interestingly, 16 of 21 responders in the concurrent group experienced tumor reduction of 80% or greater by 12 weeks,[110] a tempo that is faster than was seen with ipilimumab.

Another anti–PD-1 developed independently, lambrolizumab (previously known as MK-3475, a humanized IgG4κ monoclonal antibody), was tested on 135 patients with metastatic melanoma.[111] The response rate was found to be 38% and was similar between those who had received ipilimumab and those who were ipilimumab naïve,[111] confirming that the antitumor response from lambrolizumab occurs via a different mechanism. Similar to nivolumab, 13% of patients developed grade 3/4 adverse events, with 4% developing pneumonitis, although none developed grade 3/4 pneumonitis.[111]

BMS-936559 is a fully human IgG4 monoclonal antibody that blocks PD-L1 ligation to both PD-1 and CD80. A phase I study was tested in 207 patients (75 with NSCLC, 55 with melanoma, 18 with colon cancer, and 17 with renal cell cancer, 17 with ovarian cancer, 14 with pancreatic cancer, 7 with gastric cancer, and 4 with breast cancer).[112] Among patients who were evaluated for response, objective responses were seen in 16% of melanoma patients, 17% of renal cell cancer patients, 10% of NSCLC patients, and 1 out of 17 ovarian cancer patients. Grade 3/4 toxicities were seen in 9% of patients.[112]

The advent of these checkpoint inhibitors brings additional treatment options to patients with selected advanced cancers, particularly those with histologies deemed previously to be outside the realm of immunotherapy such as NSCLC.[108,113] In addition, a new anti–PD-L1 (MPDL3280A) in clinical trials has also shown some efficacy in melanoma, renal cell cancer, and NSCLC in early reports.

Active Immunization Approaches to Cancer Therapy (Cancer Vaccines)

The molecular characterization of multiple cancer antigens led to a large number of clinical trials that attempted to actively immunize against these antigens with the expectation that cellular immune reactions would be generated capable of inhibiting the growth of established cancers. The results of these efforts have yet to produce significant vaccine efforts of value in the treatment of human cancer. There is a paucity of murine tumor models that suggests that active vaccine approaches can mediate the regression of established vascularized tumors; therefore, it is not surprising that these approaches have, with a few exceptions, shown little efficacy in humans. Enthusiasm about the effectiveness of cancer vaccines has often been grounded in surrogate and subjective end points, rather than reliable objective cancer regressions using standard oncologic criteria. In a review of the world literature, including 107 published cancer vaccine trials involving 2,242 patients, a 3.4% overall objective response rate was observed (Table 14.2).[114,115] In many cases, relatively soft criteria such as stable disease or the regression of individual metastases in the presence of progressive disease at other sites have been reported. A variety of immunizing vectors have been used, including tumor-derived peptides, proteins, whole tumor cells, recombinant viruses, dendritic cells, and heat-shock proteins.[116-122] Although many of these approaches can lead to the development of circulating T cells that can recognize the immunizing tumor antigen, these T cells rarely cause the inhibition of established tumors, a point that has led to much confusion in the field of tumor immunology. The generation of antitumor T cells in vivo is likely a necessary, but certainly not a sufficient criteria for the development of a clinically active immunotherapy. Often, T cells with weak avidity for tumor recognition are generated, and the tolerizing and inhibitory influences that exist in vivo must be overcome for an effective immune response to cause tumor destruction.

A prospective randomized trial of immunization with antigen-presenting cells was carried out by the Dendreon Corporation (Seattle, Washington). This trial used an antigen-presenting cell vaccine loaded with prostatic acid phosphatase linked to GM-CSF compared to placebo in men with hormone-refractory prostate cancer.[123] Of 330 patients who received the vaccine treatment,

TABLE 14.2

Experience with Therapeutic Cancer Vaccines

	Number of Trials	Number of Patients	Objective Responses
Surgery Branch, National Cancer Institute	25	541	14 (2.6%)
Published before 2005[114]	33	765	29 (4.0%)
Published 2005–2010[115]	49	936	34 (3.7%)
Total	107	2,242	77 (3.4%)

Note: Vaccines include: peptide, protein, dendritic cell, virus, plasmid DNA, and whole tumor cells.

1 objective partial response was seen. Only 8 patients experienced a PSA drop of at least 50%. There was no difference in the time to disease progression; however, the vaccine group had a median survival of 25.8 months compared to 21.7 months in the placebo group, and based on this statistically significant survival improvement, this treatment was approved by the FDA (Fig. 14.5).

Adoptive Cell Transfer Immunotherapy

Adoptive cellular immunotherapy refers to the transfer to the tumor-bearing host of immune lymphocytes with anticancer activity. The first successful administration of adoptive cell therapy (ACT) involving TIL, in combination with high-dose IL-2 was carried out at the National Cancer Institute Surgery Branch in 1988.[124] Studies that used cell transfer therapy in patients with metastatic melanoma have provided the clearest evidence of the power of the immune system to mediate the regression of advanced metastatic cancers in humans. Adoptive cell therapy has several theoretical as well as practical advantages.[125] Lymphocytes with antitumor activity can be expanded to very large numbers ex vivo for infusion into cancer patients. These cells can be tested in vitro for antitumor activity, and cells with appropriate properties such as high avidity for tumor recognition and a high proliferative potential

CANCER THERAPEUTICS

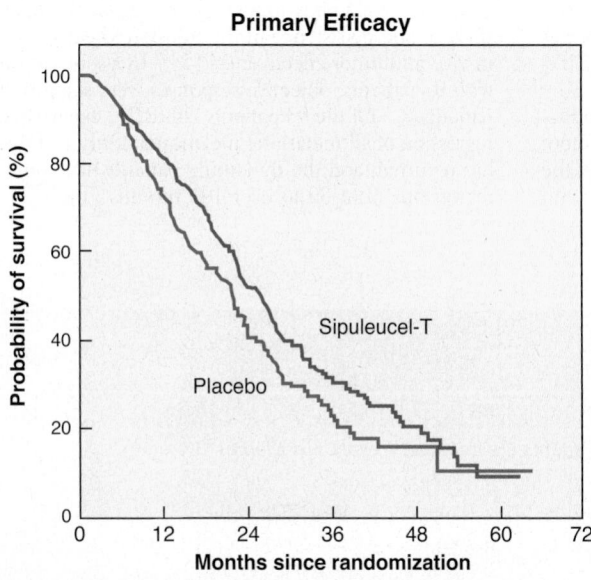

Primary Efficacy

(Y-axis: Probability of survival (%); X-axis: Months since randomization)

Sipuleucel-T
Placebo

Number at risk

Sipuleucel-T	341	274	129	49	14	1
Placebo	171	123	55	19	4	1

Figure 14.5 Kaplan-Meier estimate of the overall survival in patients with metastatic castration-resistant prostate cancer treated with Sipuleucel-T antigen–presenting cell immunotherapy. A modest but statistically significant improvement in survival was seen ($P = 0.03$).

Adoptive Transfer of Tumor Infiltrating Lymphocytes (TIL)

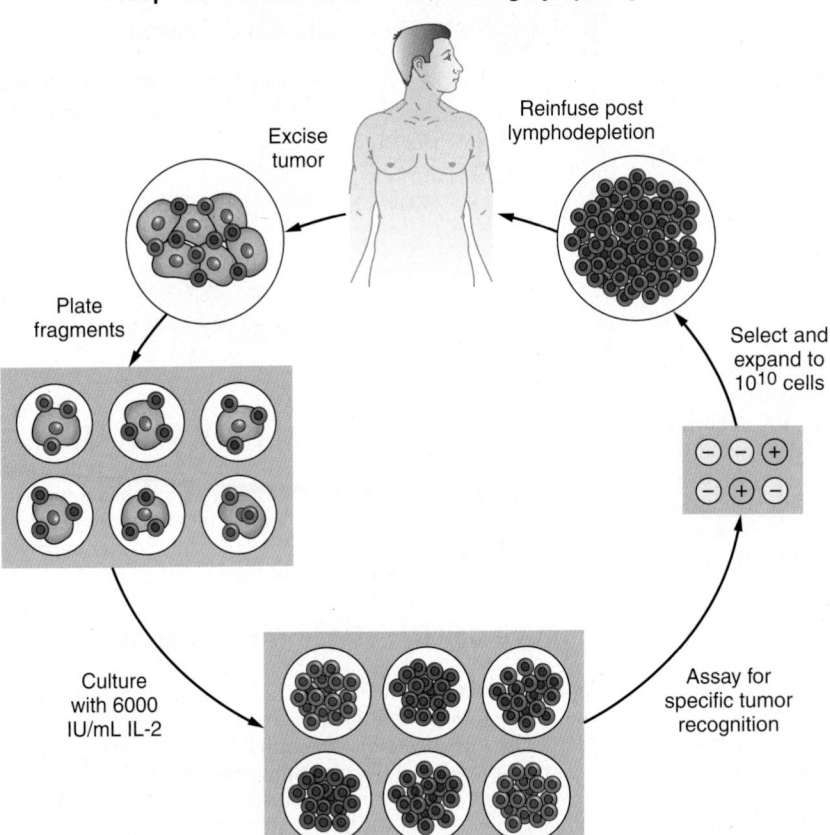

Figure 14.6 Diagram of the adoptive cell therapy of patients with metastatic melanoma. Tumors are resected and individual cultures are grown and tested for antitumor reactivity. Optimal cultures are expanded in vitro and reinfused into the autologous patient who had received a preparative lymphodepleting chemotherapy.

can be identified and selectively expanded for treatment. These cells can be activated in vitro and thus are not subjected to the tolerizing influences that exist in vivo. Perhaps, most important, the host can be manipulated prior to the transfer of the anticancer cells to provide an optimal tumor microenvironment free of in vivo suppressive factors.[125] Studies have shown that the transfer of cultured lymphocytes with antiviral activity can prevent Epstein-Barr virus (EBV) infections as well as the subsequent development of posttransplant lymphoproliferative diseases. Cultured lymphocytes have been used for the treatment of patients with established EBV-induced lymphomas.[126]

The best evidence for the ability of adoptive cell transfer to successfully treat patients with solid tumors comes from the treatment of patients with metastatic melanoma. A diagram that describes the nature of this treatment is shown in Figure 14.6. In patients with

metastatic melanoma, TILs can be obtained from resected tumor deposits and individual cultures tested to identify those with optimal anticancer activity.[124,127] These cells are then expanded ex vivo and reinfused along with IL-2, which is the requisite growth factor required for the survival and persistence of these cells. The administration of a preparative lymphodepleting chemotherapy regimen, consisting of cyclophosphamide and fludarabine with or without 2 or 12 Gy total body irradiation, could substantially enhance the survival and persistence of the transferred cells and increase their in vivo antitumor effectiveness.[128,129] In a series of three pilot trials with 93 patients, objective responses were seen in 49% to 72% of patients.[5,130] Of the 93 patients, 20 (22%) experienced a complete regression of all metastatic melanoma. Only 1 of these 20 patients has recurred, and the remaining patients have ongoing complete regressions from 80 to over 104 months (Table 14.3, Fig. 14.7).

TABLE 14.3				
Cell Transfer Therapy				
Treatment	**Total**	**PR**	**CR**	**OR**
		Number of Patients (Percentage) (Duration in Months)		
No TBI	43	16 (37%) (84, 36, 29, 28, 14, 12, 11, 7, 7, 7, 7, 4, 4, 2, 2, 2)	5 (12%) (114+, 112+, 111+, 97+, 86+)	21 (49%)
200 TBI	25	8 (32%) (14, 9, 6, 6, 5, 4, 3, 3)	5 (20%) (101+, 98+, 93+, 90+, 70+)	13 (52%)
1,200 TBI	25	8 (32%) (21, 13, 7, 6, 6, 5, 3, 2)	10 (40%) (81+, 78+, 77+, 72+, 72+, 71+, 71+, 70+, 70+, 19)	18 (72%)

Note: 20 complete responses: 19 ongoing at 70 to 114 months.

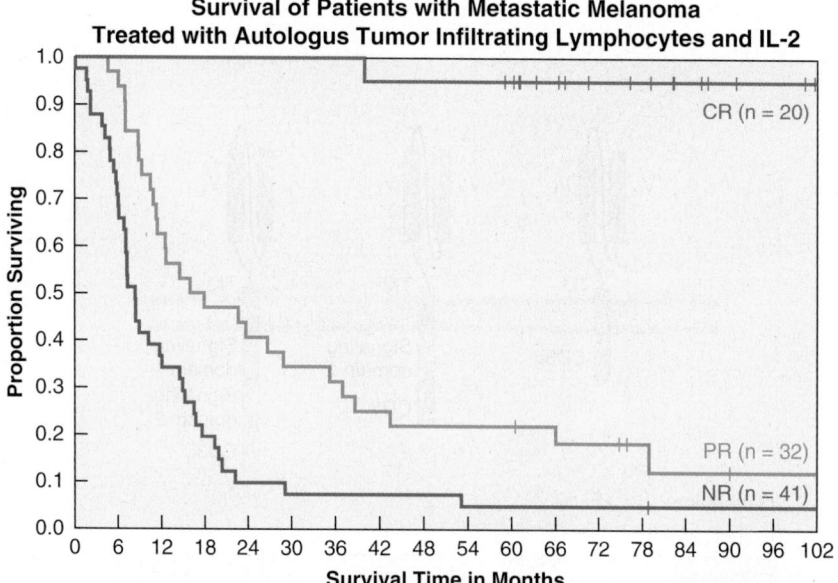

Figure 14.7 Survival curves of 93 patients treated with adoptive cell transfer using autologous TIL. The results of three consecutive trials using different preparative regimens have been combined in this analysis. Of 20 patients who achieved a complete cancer regression, only one has recurred with a median follow-up of over 8 years.[5]

The 5-year survival of these 93 patients was 29% and was similar regardless of the prior treatments that these patients had received.

Extensive genomic studies have shown that TILs that mediate complete cancer regressions recognize mutated epitopes presented by the cancer.[52] The use of exomic sequencing combined with in vitro tests of antitumor activity can be used to select for T-cell populations reactive against the cancer. This approach has now been utilized to identify T cells used to successfully treat a patient with chemotherapy-refractory cholangiocarcinoma and provides a blueprint for the application of cell transfer therapy for a variety of common epithelial cancers.[54]

The difficulty in obtaining TILs with antitumor activity from cancers other than melanoma has also led to the development of approaches using lymphocytes genetically modified using retroviral transduction to insert antitumor T-cell receptors into the normal lymphocytes of patients.[131]

Genetic Modification of Lymphocytes for Use in Adoptive Cell Therapy: Basic Principles and Applications to Solid Tumors

Efforts are in progress to genetically engineer autologous PBMCs through the introduction of exogenous high avidity receptors that specifically recognize tumor antigens (Fig. 14.8). These cells can then be expanded to large numbers in vitro and be readministered back to the patient similar to TILs in order to mediate tumor regression. The use of gene-modified cells for ACT has resulted in objective clinical responses for a variety of cancer histologies including melanoma, synovial sarcoma, and CD19-positive B-cell malignancies.[6,131–133]

There are two key requirements necessary for the use of gene-modified cells for the treatment of solid cancer. The first is the selection of an appropriate gene transfer method in order to achieve high receptor expression levels in the transferred T cells. For this discussion, we will consider both nonviral and viral-based gene delivery platforms. Generally speaking, there are two categories of nonviral gene transfer, chemical and physical. Chemical gene transfer involves the use of positively charged delivery vehicle such as calcium phosphate, cationic lipids, or polymers to form DNA complexes capable of entering a cell through endocytosis.[134] These reagents benefit from their ease of manufacture and ability to form complexes with large DNA sequences; however, low transfection efficiency of human T cells continues to be an issue.

Physical methods for gene delivery may involve direct delivery of DNA into a cell via microinjection or indirect DNA uptake via electroporation.[135] Electroporation of messenger RNA (mRNA) can achieve high levels of protein expression in cells, comparable to many of the viral-mediated gene delivery systems (gammaretroviral or lentiviral).[135,136] High-throughput electroporators should allow one to gene modify large numbers of T cells ex vivo.[137] mRNA electroporation appears to be most suited for this application, because there is significant loss of cell viability following electroporation of large amounts of DNA.[136] The electroporation of mRNA, although gaining traction as a means of redirecting T cell specificity,[137] provides for transient receptor expression because the mRNA will degrade over time. Currently, it is not clear if stable long-term receptor expression is required to mediate tumor regression. However, the main criticism of the non-viral methods described is the lack of stable gene transfer. To overcome this problem, many investigators are now using transposons such as *sleeping beauty* or *piggybac*.[138] Transposons are mobile DNA gene delivery elements encoding a gene of interest (i.e., TCR or chimeric antigen receptors [CAR]) that can randomly integrate into the genome in the presence of the transposase enzyme, thereby allowing for stable gene expression. This technology is currently being used for the ACT of CAR-modified cells targeting B-cell malignancies (see Fig. 14.8B).[139]

Viral-mediated gene delivery is currently the most common method for the genetic modification of immune cells for cancer ACT. Retroviridae is a family of RNA viruses that, upon entry into cells, undergo a process called reverse transcription whereby the viral RNA is converted into DNA as it stably integrates into the host genome. The two most common retroviral vector systems are based on the gammaretrovirus, Moloney murine leukemia virus (MLV), and the lentivirus, HIV type 1 (see Fig. 14.8B). Gammaretroviral vectors have been used in human clinical applications for over 20 years. The only reported toxicity associated with gammaretroviral engineering of human cells involved the retroviral transduction of hematopoietic stem cells for the treatment of children with severe combined immunodeficiency syndrome (X-SCID).[140] There have been no reports of clonal outgrowth following the retroviral transduction of mature T lymphocytes in adults. Highly active vectors have been generated from a variety of murine retroviruses including spleen focus forming virus (SFFV), myeloproliferative sarcoma virus (MPSV), and the murine stem cell virus (MSCV).[141–147] In most cases, these vectors are replication incompetent, but non–self-inactivating in

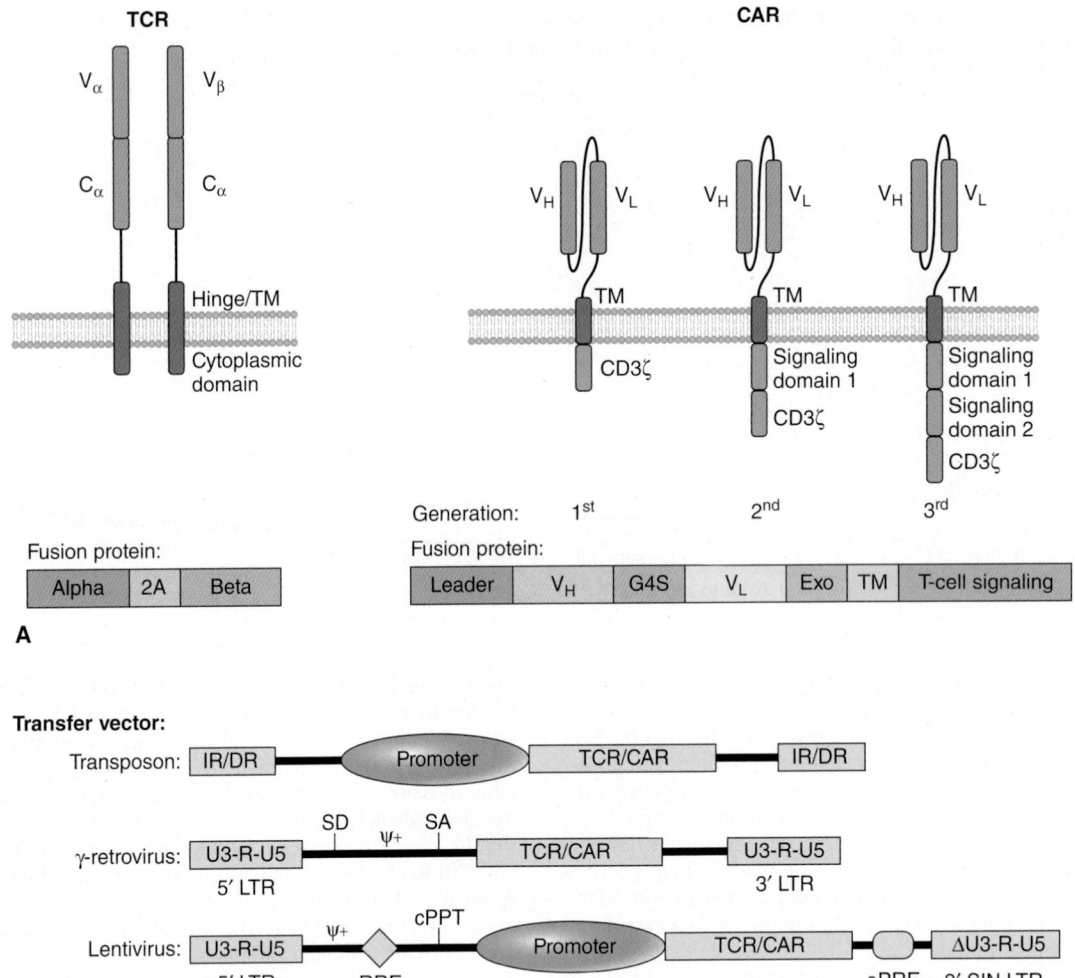

Figure 14.8 Genetic modification of T cells for the treatment of solid cancers. **(A)** In order to gene-modify T cells to confer stable tumor-specific reactivity, one can transduce T cells with an exogenous TCR derived from a naturally occurring or murine T-cell clone or a CAR derived from a tumor-specific monoclonal antibody. The TCR or CAR is synthesized as fusion proteins and inserted into the appropriate gene transfer vector. **(B)** Depending on the transfer vector selected, the T cells are then electroporated (transposon) or transduced (viral vector) to confer tumor specificity. V_α, V_β, and C_α, C_β, TCR alpha and beta chain variable and constant regions, respectively; TM, transmembrane domain; V_H and V_L, immunoglobulin variable regions; 2A and G4S, linker sequences; Exo, extracellular spacer domain; SD, splice donor; SA, splice acceptor; Ψ, packaging signal; LTR, long terminal repeat; U3, unique 3′ region; R, repeat region; U5, unique 5′ region; RRE, rev response element; cPPT, central polypurine tract; wPRE, woodchuck hepatitis virus posttranscriptional regulatory element; ΔU3, truncated unique 3′ region; SIN, self-inactivating.

that the promoter for transgene expression is derived from the viral long terminal repeat (LTR). Self-inactivating (SIN) gammaretroviral vectors have been developed that require an internal promoter to drive transgene expression. The advantage of non-SIN vectors is the ability to use a variety of retroviral packaging cell lines (PG13, Phoenix) engineered to constitutively express gag (capsid protein), pol (reverse transcriptase, integrase, and RNase H enzymes) and env (envelope protein). Transduction of these packaging lines with a non-SIN retroviral vector encoding a transgene allows for the generation of a stable packaging cell line that constitutively releases vector into the medium. This platform is easily scaled up to support large-scale vector production efforts. An alternative to the gammaretroviral vector platform is the lentiviral vector platform. There are some advantages to selecting a lentiviral vector for T-cell engineering in that one can transduce large numbers of minimally stimulated T cells,[148] transfer more complex and larger gene expression cassettes, and yield a potentially safer chromosomal integration profile as compared to gammaretroviruses. However, there has been at least one instance of clonal outgrowth

following lentiviral vector transduction of CD34+ stem cells.[149] Therefore, more data will be needed to better understand the risk of insertional mutagenesis associated with the use of lentiviral vectors. The major disadvantage with using lentiviral vectors for ACT is the lack of a robust packaging cell line, which requires transient vector production and is difficult to scale up.

The first successful application ACT involved the use of autologous T cells genetically modified with a conventional αβ TCR targeting MART-1 for the treatment of patients with melanoma.[131] The success of this approach relies on the ability to identify naturally occurring TCRs with sufficiently high avidity for the tumor antigen. For this clinical trial, a tumor-specific TCR was cloned directly from melanoma TIL. Exogenous TCR can also be generated from human PBMC following a variety of in vitro sensitization techniques or immunization of transgenic mice expressing HLA molecules. A T-cell clone expressing a low avidity TCR recognizing MART-1 was isolated and the α and β chains cloned into a gammaretroviral vector. The objective response rate from this trial was 13% (2/15).[131] In a follow-up trial with a higher avidity TCR that was cloned from the same melanoma TIL, the objective response rate increased to 30% (6/20).[150] However, patients in this trial experienced significant on-target, off-tumor toxicity with the destruction of normal melanocytes in the skin, eye, and ear. These trials showed the potential to use ACT for the treatment of solid cancers, but also highlight the importance of selecting appropriate tumor antigens to target in order to minimize normal tissue toxicities. Perhaps a better class of antigen to target for ACT would be the cancer testes antigens (CTA) that are expressed only on germ cells during fetal development and then reexpressed on cancers but not other normal tissues with the exception of the testes (see Table 14.1). Because the testes do not express class I MHC molecules, they are protected from any adverse immune response.[151] NY-ESO-1 is a CTA overexpressed on melanoma, as well as a variety of solid epithelial cancers.[152–154] A high-avidity TCR was developed targeting NY-ESO-1 and patients with metastatic melanoma or synovial cell sarcoma were treated following adoptive cell transfer using autologous lymphocytes transduced with a gammaretrovirus encoding this receptor.[6] In updated results from this trial, 8 of 17 patients (47%) with melanoma showed objective tumor responses, two of which were complete responses and ongoing at 51 and 48 months after treatment. Nine of 19 patients (47%) with synovial cell sarcoma showed objective tumor response, only one of which is complete and ongoing at 12 months. Of note, no toxicities were observed in any of these trials. Thus, targeting NY-ESO-1 and other CTAs is an attractive strategy for the application of ACT for the treatment of solid cancers (see Table 14.4 for other trials conducted at the National Cancer Institute, Surgery Branch).

Redirection of T-cell specificity using conventional TCR is constrained by HLA restriction, which limits treatment only to patients expressing a particular MHC haplotype. An alternate approach is to use CAR comprised of an monoclonal antibody single chain variable fragment (scFv) fused in frame to T-cell intracellular signaling domains capable of T-cell activation following antigen-specific binding (see Fig. 14.8A).[155] CARs, unlike conventional TCRs, are not MHC restricted but are limited by the requirement for the tumor antigen to be expressed on the cell surface. CARs can also recognize carbohydrate and lipid moieties further expanding their application. To date, there has been limited success using

CAR-based ACT for the treatment of solid cancers. In 2008, the first successful CAR trial targeting the disialoganglioside, GD2, for the treatment of neuroblastoma was reported.[156] In this trial, 4 out of 8 patients (50%) with evaluable tumor experienced tumor regression or necrosis with one complete responder. In that same year, a second CAR trial targeting CD20 on non-Hodgkin and mantle cell lymphomas was reported.[157] Of the 7 patients treated, one achieved a partial response. Much greater success has now been achieved using a CAR targeting CD19, a molecule expressed on normal B cells and virtually all B-cell lymphomas. In a trial conducted at the National Cancer Institute, Surgery Branch, Kochenderfer et al.[132] first reported that autologous T cells expressing a CAR targeting CD19 was able to mediate tumor regression in a patient with B-cell lymphoma (hematologic malignancies will be discussed in more detail elsewhere). Successfully expanding CAR-based ACT to other cancer histologies has been limited by the inability to identify suitable tumor antigens to target. At the National Cancer Institute, Surgery Branch, there are active clinical programs with CAR targeting the mutated epidermal growth factor receptor, EGFRvIII, expressed on approximately 40% of glioblastomas as well as head and neck cancers[158]; the vascular endothelial growth factor-2 receptor, VEGFR-2, expressed on tumor vasculature[159]; and mesothelin, expressed on the mesothelial lining of the pleura, peritoneum, and pericardium, but overexpressed on mesothelioma, pancreatic, and ovarian cancers.[160] These trials are currently accruing patients; however, no objective clinical responses have been observed to date. A summary of clinical trials at the National Cancer Institute, Surgery Branch using gene-modified autologous T cells for ACT are shown in Table 14.4. ACT can mediate the regression of large, established tumors in humans. Efforts to identify and specifically target novel tumor antigens are currently underway with the hope that ACT using gene-modified T cells will develop into an effective treatment for patients with a variety of solid cancers.

Genetic Modification of Lymphocytes to Treat Hematologic Malignancies

Immunologic therapies can be useful treatments for some hematologic malignancies as demonstrated by the effectiveness of mono-

TABLE 14.4

Surgery Branch, National Cancer Institute Program for the Application of Cell Transfer Therapy to a Wide Variety of Human Cancers

Receptor	Type	Cancers	Status
MART-1	TCR	Melanoma	Closed
gp100	TCR	Melanoma	Closed
NY-ESO-1	TCR	Epithelial & sarcomas	Accruing
CEA	TCR	Colorectal	Closed
CD19	CAR	Lymphomas	Accruing
VEGFR2	CAR	All cancers	Accruing
2G-1	TCR	Kidney	Accruing
IL-12	Cytokine	Adjuvant for all receptors	Accruing
MAGE-A3[a]	TCR	Epithelial	In development
EGFRvIII	CAR	Glioblastoma	Accruing
SSX-2	TCR	Epithelial	In development
Mesothelin	CAR	Pancreas & mesothelioma	Accruing
HPV16 (E6&7)	TCR	Cervical, oropharyngeal	In development

[a] MAGE-A3 TCRs; restricted by HLA-A2, A1, Cw7, DP4—covers 80% of patients.
EGFR, epidermal growth factor receptor; VEGFR2, vascular endothelial growth factor 2.

clonal antibodies in treating B-cell malignancies and the fact that allogeneic hematopoietic stem cell transplantation (alloHSCT) can cure a variety of hematologic malignancies.[161–167] The results with monoclonal antibodies and alloHSCT clearly prove that immunologic therapies have significant activity against hematologic malignancies, but monoclonal antibodies are not curative as single agents,[162,166] and alloHSCT has a substantial transplant-related mortality rate due to infections and an immunologic attack against normal tissues known as graft versus host disease (GVHD).[163,165] The proven curative potential of alloHSCT and the effectiveness of autologous T-cell transfer therapies for melanoma have encouraged the development of autologous T-cell therapies for hematologic malignancies.[125,129,163,165] Genetically engineering T cells to specifically recognize antigens expressed by malignant cells has emerged as a very promising strategy for cancer immunotherapy.[125,129,168]

T cells can be genetically engineered to express either of two types of receptors, CARs[168–171] or natural TCRs.[6,131,172] T cells expressing either a CAR or TCR gain the ability to specifically recognize an antigen.[171,172] CARs are artificial fusion proteins that incorporate antigen recognition domains and T-cell activation domains.[168,170,172] The antigen recognition domains are most often derived from monoclonal antibodies.[168,170,172] Antigen recognition by TCRs is major histocompatibility complex restricted.[125,128] In contrast to TCRs, recognition of antigens by CARs is not dependent on MHC molecules. An advantage of TCRs over CARs is that TCRs can recognize intracellular antigens, whereas CARs can only recognize cell-surface antigens.

Chimeric Antigen Receptors

CARs targeting hematopoietic antigens have been extensively studied in preclinical experiments and early-stage clinical trials.[168,170,172,173] For a protein to be a promising target for CAR-expressing T cells, it should be uniformly expressed on the malignant cells being targeted but not expressed on essential normal cells. Many cell-surface proteins with restricted normal tissue expression patterns have been identified on malignant hematologic cells, and CARs targeting many of these proteins are under development (Table 14.5).

Many factors can affect CAR T-cell therapies. The types of gene-therapy vectors encoding the DNA of the CAR could be an important factor. The types of vectors currently being used in clinical trials of CAR T cells are gammaretroviruses, lentiviruses, and transposon-based systems.[132,155,174–181] The design of the CAR fusion protein is another important factor. CAR fusion proteins include an antigen-recognition domain that is most often derived from an antibody, costimulatory domains such as CD28 and 4-1BB, and T-cell activation domains that are usually derived from the CD3z molecule.[168,170,171,182] Other factors that could impact the effectiveness of CAR T-cell therapies include the cell culture method used to prepare the cells and administration of chemotherapy or radiation therapy prior to the CAR T-cell infusions.[170,178,179] In mouse models, a profound enhancement of the antimalignancy activity of infused T cells occurs when the T-cell infusions are preceded by lymphocyte-depleting chemotherapy or radiation therapy.[183–185] Because chemotherapy can have a direct antimalignancy effect against hematologic malignancies, the administration of chemotherapy prior to infusions of T cells is a confounding factor that must always be kept in mind when interpreting the results of clinical trials of T-cell therapies.

Anti-CD19 Chimeric Antigen Receptors

CD19 is an appealing target antigen for CARs because CD19 is expressed on almost all malignant B cells, but CD19 is not expressed on normal cells except B cells.[186] The first preclinical studies of anti-CD19 CARs utilized either gammaretrovirus vectors[174] or plasmid electroporation[176] to insert genes encoding anti-CD19 CARs into human T cells. These studies and subsequent preclinical work by other groups showed that T cells expressing anti-CD19

TABLE 14.5

Hematologic Antigens Targeted by Genetically-Modified T-Cells

Antigen	Malignancy Expressing Antigen	Targeted by CAR or TCR	References
CD19	B-cell malignancies	CAR	17, 19, 21, 22, 23, 24, 25, 26, 34, 35, 55, 56
CD20	B-cell malignancies	CAR	36, 37, 38
CD22	B-cell malignancies	CAR	39, 40
CD23	B-cell malignancies	CAR	41
ROR1	B-cell malignancies	CAR	42
Kappa light chain	B-cell malignancies	CAR	43
B-cell maturation antigen (BCMA)	Multiple myeloma	CAR	44
Lewis Y antigen	Multiple myeloma and acute myeloid leukemia (AML)	CAR	45, 46
CD123	AML	CAR	47
CD30	Hodgkin lymphoma	CAR	48, 49
CD70	Hodgkin lymphoma	CAR	50
Wilms tumor-1 (WT1)	AML and acute lymphoid leukemia (ALL)	TCR	51
Aurora kinase-A	AML and chronic myeloid leukemia (CML)	TCR	52
Hyaluronan-mediated motility receptor (HMMR)	AML and ALL	TCR	53

CARs could specifically recognize and kill CD19-expressing malignant B cells in vitro and in vivo.[174–176,187] These preclinical studies compared many different CAR signaling moieties, which led most groups to utilize CARs with T-cell activation domains from the CD3z molecule and costimulatory molecules from either CD28 or 4-1BB (CD137).[165,180,182,187,188] Preclinical studies showed that lymphocyte-depleting radiation therapy administered before anti-CD19 CAR T-cell infusions was critical to the antimalignancy activity of CAR T cells.[183] The addition of lymphocyte-depleting radiation therapy prior to infusions of anti-CD19 CAR T cells increased the percentage of mice cured of lymphoma by the CAR T cells from 0% to 100%.[183] Preclinical experiments with anti-CD19 CARs have led to several early-phase clinical trials.

The first clinical trial to demonstrate in vivo activity of anti-CD19 CAR T cells in humans was conducted in the Surgery Branch of the National Cancer Institute.[132] The gammaretroviral vector used in this trial encoded a CAR with a CD28 costimulatory domain. Patients treated on this clinical trial received cyclophosphamide and fludarabine chemotherapy followed by an infusion of anti-CD19 CAR T cells and a short course of intravenous IL-2.[132,181] Clear antigen-specific activity of the anti-CD19 CAR T cells was demonstrated because blood B cells were selectively eliminated from four of the seven evaluable patients for several months.[181] The duration of B-cell depletion in these patients was much longer than the duration of B-cell depletion caused by the chemotherapy that the patients received.[132,181] This study also generated evidence of an antimalignancy effect by the anti-CD19 CAR T cells because six of seven evaluable patients with advanced B-cell malignancies obtained either complete remissions or partial remissions (Fig. 14.9).[181] One of these remissions is ongoing 45 months after treatment, and another remission is ongoing 31 months after treatment. Significant toxicity, including hypotension and neurologic toxicity, occurred during this clinical trial.[181] The severity of these toxicities correlated with the levels of serum inflammatory cytokines.[181] Except for one patient who died with influenza pneumonia, the toxicities were transient, with all toxicities resolving within 3 weeks of the anti-CD19 CAR T-cell infusions.[181]

Investigators at the Memorial Sloan Kettering Cancer Center treated nine patients with chronic lymphocytic leukemia (CLL) or acute lymphocytic leukemia (ALL) by infusing T cells that expressed a CAR with a CD28 costimulatory domain.[179] The gene therapy vector used in this work was a gammaretrovirus.[179] None of three patients treated with CAR T cells alone experienced a regression of leukemia, and CLL regressed in one of four evaluable patients treated with cyclophosphamide followed by an infusion of CAR T cells. Using the same CAR, the same group went on to treat five patients with ALL.[173] Patients received chemotherapy followed by an infusion of anti-CD19 CAR T cells. Four patients had detectable leukemia prior to their CAR T-cell infusions, and all of these patients became minimal residual disease negative after infusion of CAR T cells. Four of five patients on this trial rapidly underwent allogeneic stem cell transplantation after their CAR T-cell infusions.[173]

Investigators at the Baylor College of Medicine conducted clinical trials of anti-CD19 CAR T cells in which each patient simultaneously received infusions of two types of anti-CD19 CAR T cells.[189] One type of T cell expressed a CAR expressing a CD28 costimulatory domain. The other type of T cell was identical except that the CAR it expressed lacked a CD28 domain. Compared to the T cells lacking a CD28 moiety, the T cells expressing a CAR with a CD28 moiety had higher peak blood levels and longer in vivo persistence.[189] Patients on this trial did not receive chemotherapy, and there were no remissions of malignancy or long-term B-cell depletion.[189]

Investigators at the University of Pennsylvania reported results from three patients with CLL who were treated with chemotherapy followed by infusions of anti-CD19 CAR-expressing T cells.[133,180] The CAR used in this study was encoded by a lentiviral vector and contained a costimulatory domain from the 4-1BB molecule. Two

Before treatment

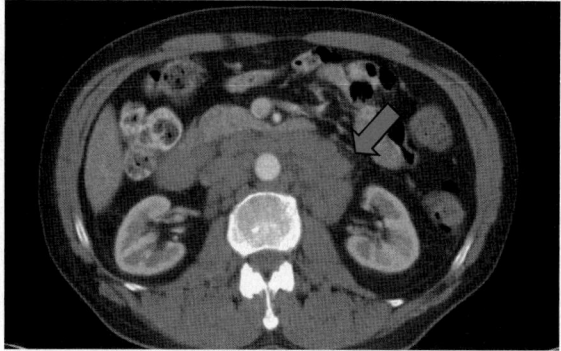

32 days after infusion

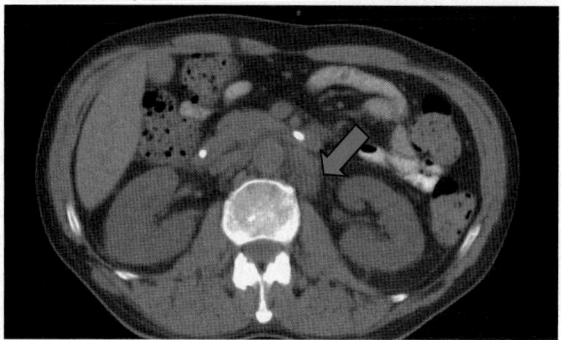

132 days after infusion

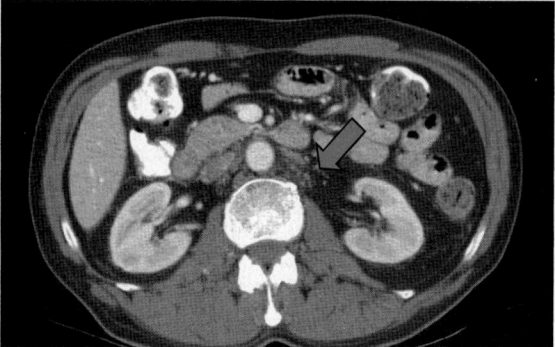

645 days after infusion

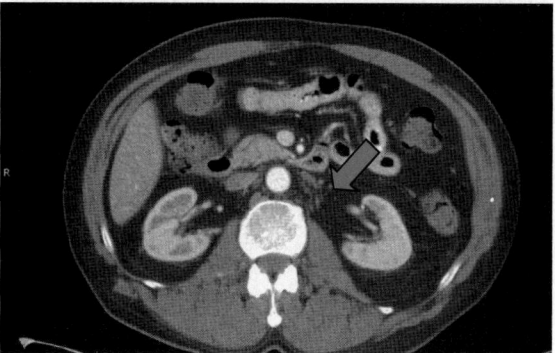

Figure 14.9 Computed tomography (CT) scans show regression of adenopathy in a patient with chronic lymphocytic leukemia (CLL) after treatment with chemotherapy followed by an infusion of autologous anti-CD19 CAR T cells. The time after the cell infusion of each CT scan is indicated. The *arrow* points to a large lymph node mass that resolved completely over time. (Reproduced from Kochenderfer JN, Rosenberg SA. Treating B-Cell cancer with T cells expressing anti-CD19 chimeric antigen receptors. *Nature Rev Clin Oncology* 2013;10:267-276, with permission.)

of the three reported patients obtained prolonged complete remissions.[180] This same CAR design was subsequently evaluated in a clinical trial enrolling patients with ALL.[190] One ALL patient obtained a prolonged complete remission but also experienced significant toxicity that was associated with elevated levels of serum cytokines.[190]

Overall, the early results with anti-CD19 CAR T cells show that this strategy holds great promise to improve the treatment of B-cell malignancies, but anti-CD19 CAR T-cell infusions are also associated with significant toxicity that is usually of short duration. Future progress will require decreasing the toxicity of anti-CD19 CAR T cells while maintaining or enhancing their antimalignancy activity. Parameters that are being studied in an effort to improve anti-CD19 CAR therapy include vector selection, CAR design, cell culture methods, and clinical application.

Chimeric Antigen Receptors and T-Cell Receptors Targeting Hematologic Antigens Other than CD19

CARs and TCRs targeting several hematologic antigens other than CD19 have been evaluated in preclinical or clinical studies. Except for CD19, the B-cell antigen CD20 has been the hematologic antigen most extensively studied as a target of CAR T cells.[191–193] Plasmid electroporation, which is not an optimal method of T-cell genetic modification, was used to transfer the anti-CD20 CAR gene to T cells in these studies. In one trial of anti-CD20 CAR T cells, patients received chemotherapy followed by infusions of T cells expressing a CAR without costimulatory domains.[192] One of seven patients obtained a partial remission that lasted 3 months. In a second trial, patients received chemotherapy followed by anti-CD20 CAR T cells expressing a CAR with both CD28 and 4-1BB costimulatory domains; in this trial, the only evaluable patient obtained a partial remission.[193]

CARs targeting other B-cell antigens including CD22,[157,194] CD23,[195] receptor tyrosine kinase–like orphan receptor-1 (ROR1),[196] and the immunoglobulin kappa light chain[197] have been evaluated in preclinical studies. CARs for treating multiple myeloma are currently being developed. B-cell maturation antigen (BCMA) is expressed on normal and malignant plasma cells, but it is not known to be expressed on other normal cells except for a small subset of mature B cells.[198] CARs targeting BCMA have undergone preclinical testing, and a clinical trial of an anti-BCMA CAR will open soon.[198] Preclinical studies have been performed on CARs targeting the Lewis Y antigen as a treatment for multiple myeloma and acute myeloid leukemia (AML),[199] and activity against AML was recently demonstrated in a phase I clinical trial of a CAR targeting the Lewis Y antigen.[200] CARs targeting the CD123 protein are undergoing preclinical testing for potential use against AML.[201] For Hodgkin lymphoma, CARs have been developed that target the CD30 protein and the CD70 protein, and anti-CD30 CARs are entering early-phase clinical trials.[202–204]

MHC-restricted TCRs targeting some antigens expressed on hematologic malignancies have undergone preclinical testing, but TCRs for treating hematologic malignancies are at a much earlier stage of development than CARs (see Table 14.1). TCRs targeting the Wilms tumor antigen-1 (WT1) are under development to treat ALL and AML.[205] Aurora kinase-A–specific TCRs and hyaluronan-mediated motility receptor (HMMR)-specific TCRs are under preclinical development as leukemia treatments.[206,207]

T-Cell Gene Therapy in the Setting of Allogeneic Hematopoietic Stem Cell Transplantation

A leading cause of death among patients undergoing alloHSCT is relapse of malignancy, and alloHSCT is often complicated by GVHD.[164,165,208] Therefore, a central goal in the field of alloHSCT is to increase the antimalignancy activity of allogeneic T cells without worsening GVHD. One way to accomplish this goal might be to genetically modify T cells to give them the ability to specifically recognize antigens expressed by malignant cells. CARs are well-suited for this task.

Two groups have recently reported promising early results treating B-cell malignancies after alloHSCT with allogeneic donor-derived T cells expressing anti-CD19 CARs.[209,210] Investigators at the National Cancer Institute treated 10 patients with B-cell malignancies that persisted despite alloHSCT and standard donor lymphocyte infusions.[209] Although patients on this trial did not receive chemotherapy before their T-cell infusions, 3 of 10 patients had objective regressions of their malignancies, and 1 patient with CLL remains in CR more than 1 year after treatment.[209] No patient developed GVHD after receiving allogeneic anti-CD19 CAR T cells on this trial.[209] Investigators at the Baylor College of Medicine reported objective antimalignancy responses in two of six patients with relapsed malignancy after infusion of donor-derived allogeneic anti-CD19 CAR T cells that were also specific for viral antigens.[210]

In an effort to improve the safety of infusions of allogeneic lymphocytes by limiting GVHD, investigators have genetically modified T cells to express *suicide genes* that cause death of the T cells containing the suicide gene when certain drugs are administered.[211–214] Suicide gene–expressing T cells are infused to treat malignancy after alloHSCT. This approach has been tested in clinical trials, and rapid abrogation of GVHD has been demonstrated.[211,213,214]

SELECTED REFERENCES

The full reference list can be accessed at lwwhealthlibrary.com/oncology.

3. Attia P, Phan GQ, Maker AV, et al. Autoimmunity correlates with tumor regression in patients with metastatic melanoma treated with anti-cytotoxic T-lymphocyte antigen-4. *J Clin Oncol* 2005;23:6043–6053.
4. Topalian SL, Hodi FS, Brahmer JR, et al. Safety, activity, and immune correlates of anti-PD-1 antibody in cancer. *N Engl J Med* 2012;366:2443–2454.
5. Rosenberg SA, Yang JC, Sherry RM, et al. Durable complete responses in heavily pretreated patients with metastatic melanoma using T-cell transfer immunotherapy. *Clin Cancer Res* 2011;17:4550–4557.
6. Robbins PF, Morgan RA, Feldman SA, et al. Tumor regression in patients with metastatic synovial sarcoma and melanoma using genetically engineered lymphocytes reactive with NY-ESO-1. *J Clin Oncol* 2011;29:917–924.
8. Van der Bruggen P, Traversari C, Chomez P, et al. A gene encoding an antigen recognized by cytolytic T lymphocytes on a human melanoma. *Science* 1991;254:1643–1647.
12. Morgan RA, Chinnasamy N, Abate-Daga D, et al. Cancer regression and neurological toxicity following anti-MAGE-A3 TCR gene therapy. *J Immunother* 2013;36:133–151.

44. Parkhurst MR, Yang JC, Langan RC, et al. T cells targeting carcinoembryonic antigen can mediate regression of metastatic colorectal cancer but induce severe transient colitis. *Mol Ther* 2011;19:620–626.
52. Robbins PF, Lu YC, El-Gamil M, et al. Mining exomic sequencing data to identify mutated antigens recognized by adoptively transferred tumor-reactive T cells. *Nat Med* 2013;19:747–752.
54. Tran E, Turcotte S, Gros A, et al. Cancer immunotherapy based on mutation-specific CD4+ T cells in a patient with epithelial cancer. *Science* 2014;344:641–645.
56. Villa LL, Costa RL, Petta CA, et al. Prophylactic quadrivalent human papillomavirus (types 6, 11, 16, and 18) L1 virus-like particle vaccine in young women: a randomised double-blind placebo-controlled multicentre phase II efficacy trial. *Lancet Oncol* 2005;6:271–278.
57. Wolchok JD, Hoos A, O'Day S, et al. Guidelines for the evaluation of immune therapy activity in solid tumors: immune-related response criteria. *Clin Cancer Res* 2009;15:7412–7420.
59. Morgan DA, Ruscetti FW, Gallo R. Selective in vitro growth of T lymphocytes from normal human bone marrows. *Science* 1976;193:1007–1008.
62. Taniguchi T, Matsui H, Fujita T. Structure and expression of a cloned cDNA for human interleukin-2. *Nature* 1983;302:305–307.

CANCER THERAPEUTICS

63. Rosenberg SA, Grimm EA, McGrogan M, et al. Biological activity of recombinant human interleukin-2 produced in *Escherichia coli*. *Science* 1984;223:1412–1414.

64. Rosenberg SA, Mule JJ, Spiess PJ, et al. Regression of established pulmonary metastases and subcutaneous tumor mediated by the systemic administration of high dose recombinant IL-2. *J Exp Med* 1985;161:1169–1188.

65. Lotze MT, Matory YL, Ettinghausen SE, et al. In vivo administration of purified human interleukin-2. II. Half life, immunologic effects and expansion of peripheral lymphoid cells in vivo with recombinant IL-2. *J Immunol* 1985;135:2865–2875.

66. Rosenberg SA, Lotze MT, Muul LM, et al. Observations on the systemic administration of autologous lymphokine-activated killer cells and recombinant interleukin-2 to patients with metastatic cancer. *N Engl J Med* 1985;313:1485–1492.

67. Rosenberg SA, Lotze MT, Yang JC, et al. Prospective randomized trial of high-dose interleukin-2 alone or in conjunction with lymphokine-activated killer cells for the treatment of patients with advanced cancer. *J Natl Cancer Inst* 1993;85:622–632.

70. Fyfe G, Fisher R, Sznol M, et al. Results of treatment of 255 patients with metastatic renal cell carcinoma who received high dose proleukin interleukin-2 therapy. *J Clin Oncol* 1995;13:688–696.

72. Yang JC, Sherry RM, Steinberg SM, et al. Randomized study of high-dose and low-dose interleukin-2 in patients with metastatic renal cancer. *J Clin Oncol* 2003;21:3127–3132.

73. Atkins MB, Lotze MT, Dutcher JP, et al. High-dose recombinant interleukin 2 therapy for patients with metastatic melanoma: analysis of 270 patients treated between 1985 and 1993. *J Clin Oncol* 1999l;17:2105–2116.

76. Schwartzentruber DJ, Lawson DH, Richards JM, et al. gp100 peptide vaccine and interleukin-2 in patients with advanced melanoma. *N Engl J Med* 2011;364:2119–2127.

77. Prieto PA, Yang JC, Sherry RM, et al. CTLA-4 blockade with ipilimumab: long-term follow-up of 177 patients with metastatic melanoma. *Clin Cancer Res* 2012;18:2039–2047.

78. Phan GQ, Attia P, Steinberg SM, et al. Factors associated with response to high-dose interleukin-2 in patients with metastatic melanoma. *J Clin Oncol* 2001;19:3477–3482.

85. Schwartzentruber DJ. Guidelines for the safe administration of high-dose interleukin-2. *J Immunother* 2001;24:287–293.

86. Kammula US, White DE, Rosenberg SA. Trends in the safety of high dose bolus interleukin-2 administration in patients with metastatic cancer. *Cancer* 1998;83:797–805.

93. Phan GQ, Yang JC, Sherry RM, et al. Cancer regression and autoimmunity induced by cytotoxic T lymphocyte-associated antigen 4 blockade in patients with metastatic melanoma. *Proc Natl Acad Sci U S A* 2003;100:8372–8377.

98. Hodi FS, O'Day SJ, McDermott DF, et al. Improved survival with ipilimumab in patients with metastatic melanoma. *N Engl J Med* 2010;363:711–723.

100. Wolchok JD, Weber JS, Maio M, et al. Four-year survival rates for patients with metastatic melanoma who received ipilimumab in phase II clinical trials. *Ann Oncol* 2013;24:2174–2180.

101. Yang JC, Hughes M, Kammula U, et al. Ipilimumab (anti-CTLA4 antibody) causes regression of metastatic renal cell cancer associated with enteritis and hypophysitis. *J Immunother* 2007;30:825–830.

107. Brahmer JR, Drake CG, Wollner I, et al. Phase I study of single-agent anti-programmed death-1 (MDX-1106) in refractory solid tumors: safety, clinical activity, pharmacodynamics, and immunologic correlates. *J Clin Oncol* 2010;28:3167–3175.

109. Topalian SL, Sznol M, McDermott DF, et al. Survival, durable tumor remission, and long-term safety in patients with advanced melanoma receiving nivolumab. *J Clin Oncol* 2014;32:1020–1030.

110. Wolchok JD, Kluger H, Callahan MK, et al. Nivolumab plus ipilimumab in advanced melanoma. *N Engl J Med* 2013;369:122–133.

112. Brahmer JR, Tykodi SS, Chow LQ, et al. Safety and activity of anti-PD-L1 antibody in patients with advanced cancer. *N Engl J Med* 2012;366:2455–2465.

114. Rosenberg SA, Yang JC, Restifo NP. Cancer immunotherapy: moving beyond current vaccines. *Nat Med* 2004;10:909–915.

115. Klebanoff CA, Acquavella N, Yu Z, et al. Therapeutic cancer vaccines: are we there yet? *Immunol Rev* 2011;239:27–44.

123. Kantoff PW, Higano CS, Shore ND, et al. Sipuleucel-T immunotherapy for castration-resistant prostate cancer. *N Engl J Med* 2010;363:422.

124. Rosenberg SA, Packard BS, Aebersold PM, et al. Use of tumor infiltrating lymphocytes and interleukin-2 in the immunotherapy of patients with metastatic melanoma. Preliminary report. *N Engl J Med* 1988;319:1676–1680.

126. Rooney CM, Smith CA, Ng CY, et al. Infusion of cytotoxic T cells for the prevention and treatment of Epstein-Barr virus-induced lymphoma in allogeneic transplant recipients. *Blood* 1998;92:1549–1555.

128. Dudley ME, Wunderlich JR, Robbins PF, et al. Cancer regression and autoimmunity in patients after clonal repopulation with anti-tumor lymphocytes. *Science* 2002;298:850–854.

130. Rosenberg SA. Cell transfer immunotherapy for metastatic solid cancer—what clinicians need to know. *Nat Rev Clin Oncol* 2011;8:577–585.

131. Morgan RA, Dudley ME, Wunderlich JR, et al. Cancer regression in patients after transfer of genetically engineered lymphocytes. *Science* 2006;314:126–129.

132. Kochenderfer JN, Wilson WH, Janik E, et al. Eradication of B-lineage cells and regression of lymphoma in a patient treated with autologous T cells genetically engineered to recognize CD19. *Blood* 2010;116:4099–4102.

133. Porter DL, Levine BL, Kalos M, et al. Chimeric antigen receptor-modified T cells in chronic lymphoid leukemia. *N Engl J Med* 2011;365:725–733.

136. Zhao Y, Zheng Z, Cohen CJ, et al. High-efficiency transfection of primary human and mouse T lymphocytes using RNA electroporation. *Mol Ther* 2006;13:151–159.

140. Singh H, Huls H, Kebriaei P, et al. A new approach to gene therapy using Sleeping Beauty to genetically modify clinical-grade T cells to target CD19. *Immunol Rev* 2014;257:181–190.

150. Johnson LA, Morgan RA, Dudley ME, et al. Gene therapy with human and mouse T-cell receptors mediates cancer regression and targets normal tissues expressing cognate antigen. *Blood* 2009;114:535–546.

155. Gross G, Waks T, Eshhar Z. Expression of immunoglobulin-T-cell receptor chimeric molecules as functional receptors with antibody-type specificity. *Proc Natl Acad Sci U S A* 1989;86:10024–10028.

156. Pule MA, Savoldo B, Myers GD, et al. Virus-specific T cells engineered to coexpress tumor-specific receptors: persistence and antitumor activity in individuals with neuroblastoma. *Nat Med* 2008;14:1264–1270.

169. Eshhar Z, Waks T, Gross G, et al. Specific activation and targeting of cytotoxic lymphocytes through chimeric single chains consisting of antibody-binding domains and the gamma or zeta subunits of the immunoglobulin and T-cell receptors. *Proc Natl Acad Sci U S A* 1993;90:720–724.

170. Kochenderfer JN, Rosenberg SA. Treating B-cell cancer with T cells expressing anti-CD19 chimeric antigen receptors. *Nat Rev Clin Oncol* 2013;10:267–276.

173. Brentjens RJ, Davila ML, Riviere I, et al. CD19-targeted T cells rapidly induce molecular remissions in adults with chemotherapy-refractory acute lymphoblastic leukemia. *Sci Transl Med* 2013;5:177ra38.

183. Kochenderfer JN, Yu Z, Frasheri D, et al. Adoptive transfer of syngeneic T cells transduced with a chimeric antigen receptor that recognizes murine CD19 can eradicate lymphoma and normal B cells. *Blood* 2010;116:3875–3886.

190. Grupp SA, Kalos M, Barrett D, et al. Chimeric antigen receptor-modified T cells for acute lymphoid leukemia. *N Engl J Med* 2013;368:1509–1518.

209. Kochenderfer JN, Dudley ME, Carpenter RO, et al. Donor-derived CD19-targeted T cells cause regression of malignancy persisting after allogeneic hematopoietic stem cell transplantation. *Blood* 2013;122:4129–4139.

213. Ciceri F, Bonini C, Stanghellini MT, et al. Infusion of suicide-gene-engineered donor lymphocytes after family haploidentical haemopoietic stem-cell transplantation for leukaemia (the TK007 trial): a non-randomised phase I-II study. *Lancet Oncol* 2009;10:489–500.

214. Di Stasi A, Tey SK, Dotti G, et al. Inducible apoptosis as a safety switch for adoptive cell therapy. *N Engl J Med* 2011;365:1673–1683.

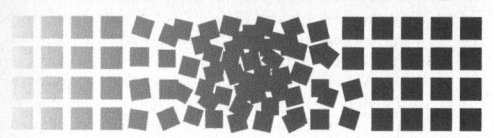

15 Pharmacokinetics and Pharmacodynamics of Anticancer Drugs

Alex Sparreboom and Sharyn D. Baker

INTRODUCTION

Drug selection and therapy considerations in oncology were originally solely based on observations of the effects produced.[1] To overcome some of the limitations of this empirical approach and to answer questions related to considerations of dose, frequency, and duration of drug treatment, it is necessary to understand the events that follow drug administration. Preclinical in vitro and in vivo studies have shown that the magnitude of antitumor response is a function of the concentration of drug,[2] and this has led to the suggestion that the therapeutic objective can be achieved by maintaining an adequate concentration at the site of action for the duration of therapy.[3] However, drugs are rarely directly administered at their sites of action. Indeed, most anticancer drugs are given intravenously or orally, and yet are expected to act in the brain, lungs, or elsewhere. Drugs must, therefore, move from the site of administration to the site of action and, moreover, distribute to all other tissues including organs that eliminate them from the body, such as the kidneys and liver. To administer drugs optimally, knowledge is needed not only of the mechanisms of drug absorption, distribution, and elimination, but also of the kinetics of these processes.[4]

The treatment of human malignancies involving drugs can be divided into two pharmacologic phases, a *pharmacokinetic* phase in which the dose, dosage form, frequency, and route of administration are related to drug level–time relationships in the body, and a *pharmacodynamic* phase in which the concentration of drug at the site(s) of action is related to the magnitude of the effect(s) produced. Once both of these phases have been defined, a dosage regimen can be designed to achieve the therapeutic objective, although additional factors need to be taken into consideration (Fig. 15.1). The clinical application of this approach allows distinctions between pharmacokinetic and pharmacodynamic causes of an unusual drug response. A basic tenet of pharmacokinetics is that the magnitude of both the desired response and toxicity are functions of the drug concentration at the site(s) of action. Accordingly, therapeutic failure results when either the concentration is too low, resulting in ineffective therapy, or is too high, producing unacceptable toxicity. Between these limits of concentrations lies a region associated with therapeutic success, the so-called *therapeutic window*.[5] Because the concentration of a drug at the site of action can rarely be measured directly, with the exception of certain hematologic malignancies, plasma or blood is commonly measured instead as a more accessible alternative.

PHARMACOKINETIC CONCEPTS

A drug's pharmacokinetic properties can be defined by two fundamental processes affecting drug behavior over time, *absorption* and *disposition*.

Absorption

Historically, most anticancer drugs have been administered intravenously; however, the use of orally administered agents is growing with the development of small-molecule targeted cancer therapeutics, such as tyrosine kinase inhibitors.[6] Moreover, drugs may also be administered regionally, for example into the pleural or peritoneal cavities,[7] the cerebrospinal fluid, or intra-arterially into a vessel leading to a cancerous tissue.[8] The process by which the unchanged drug moves from the site of administration to the site of measurement within the body is referred to as *absorption*. Loss at any site prior to the site of measurement contributes to a decrease in the apparent absorption of a drug. For an orally administered agent, this complex series of events involves disintegration of the pharmaceutical dosage form, dissolution, diffusion through gastrointestinal fluids, permeation of the gut membrane, portal circulation uptake, passage through the liver, and, finally, entry into the systemic circulation. The loss of drug as it passes for the first time through organs of elimination, such as the gastrointestinal membranes and the liver, during the absorption process is known as the *first-pass effect*.[9]

The pharmacokinetic parameter most closely associated with absorption is availability or bioavailability (F), defined as the fraction (or percent) of the administered dose that is absorbed intact. Bioavailability can be estimated by dividing the area under the plasma concentration–time curve (AUC) achieved following extravascular administration by the AUC observed after intravenous administration, and can range from 0 to 1.0 (or 0% to 100%).

Disposition

Disposition is defined as all the processes that occur subsequent to absorption of a drug; by definition, the components of disposition are *distribution* and *elimination*. Distribution is the process of reversible transfer of a drug to and from the site of measurement. Any drug that leaves the site of measurement and does not return has undergone elimination, which occurs by two processes, *excretion* and *metabolism*. Excretion is the irreversible loss of the chemically unchanged drug, whereas metabolism is the conversion of drug to another chemical species.

The extent of drug distribution can be determined by relating the concentration obtained with a known amount of drug in the body and is, in essence, a dilution space. The apparent volume into which a drug distributes in the body at equilibrium in called the volume of distribution (V_d), and may or may not correspond to an actual physiologic compartment.

The rate and extent to which a drug distributes into various tissues depend on a number of factors, including hydrophobicity, tissue permeability, tissue-binding constants, binding to serum proteins, and local organ blood flow.[10] Large apparent volumes of distribution are common for agents with high tissue binding or high lipid solubility,

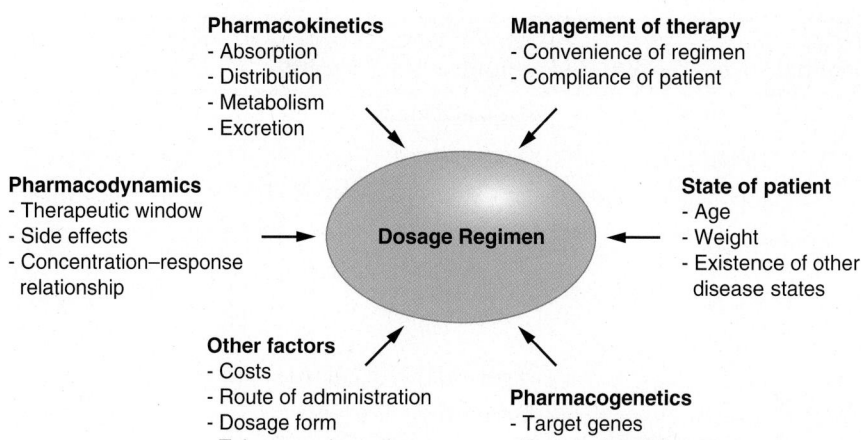

Figure 15.1 Principal determinants of dosage regimen selection for an anticancer drug

although distribution into specific body compartments may be limited by physiologic processes, such as the blood–brain barrier protecting the central nervous system[11,12] or the blood–testes barrier.[13]

Just as V_d is needed as a parameter to relate the concentration to the amount of drug in the body, there is also a need to have a parameter to relate the concentration to the rate of drug elimination, which is known as *clearance* (CL). Of all pharmacokinetic parameters, CL has the most clinical relevance because it defines the key relationship between drug dose and systemic drug exposure (AUC). Derived from V_d and CL is the parameter *elimination rate constant*, which can be regarded as the fractional rate of drug removal. It is, however, more common to refer to the half-life than to the elimination rate constant of a drug. The half-life of a drug is a useful parameter to estimate the time required to reach steady state on a multidose schedule or during a continuous intravenous drug infusion.

Dose Proportionality

When drug concentrations change in strict proportionality to the dose of drug administered, then the condition of dose proportionality (or linear pharmacokinetics) holds. If doubling the dose exactly doubles the plasma concentration or AUC, then pharmacokinetic parameters such V_d, and CL are constant and remain independent of dose and concentration.[14] By strict definition, drugs with linear pharmacokinetics are dose proportional. Dose proportionality is clinically important because it means that dose adjustments will generate predictable changes in systemic drug exposure. For drugs that lack dose proportionality, V_d and CL will demonstrate concentration or time dependence, or both, making it difficult to predict the effect of dose adjustments on drug concentration (Fig. 15.2). Factors that can contribute to a lack of dose proportional pharmacokinetics include saturable oral absorption,[15] capacity-limited distribution or protein binding,[16] and/or saturable metabolism.[17] Dose proportionality of anticancer agents is typically assessed in Phase 1 dose-escalation trials in which small groups of patients are treated at a single dose level using a parallel study design, although the statistical power of such studies to detect deviations from dose proportionality is poor. An alternative, more robust study design is a crossover study in which each patient receives a low dose, an intermediate dose, and a high dose over consecutive cycles of treatment.[18] However, such studies are relatively rare in oncology because of the required use of low, potentially ineffective doses, which may raise ethical concerns for patients.

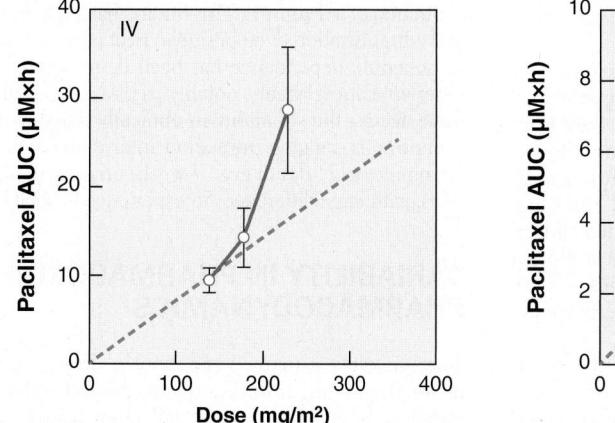
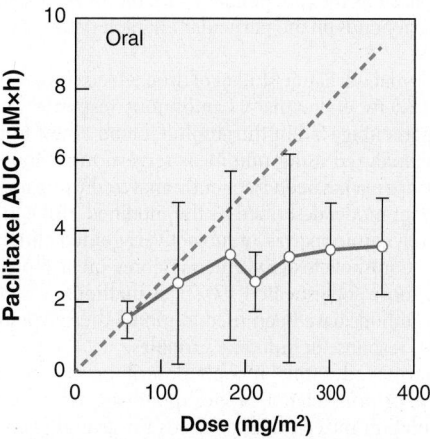

Figure 15.2 Effect of drug dose on systemic exposure to paclitaxel following intravenous (IV) or oral administration in patients with cancer. Data are expressed as mean values (symbols) and standard deviation (error bars). The *dashed line* indicates the hypothetical dose-proportional increase in the area under the plasma concentration time curve (AUC). (Data derived from van Zuylen L, Karlsson MO, Verweij J, et al. Pharmacokinetic modeling of paclitaxel encapsulation in Cremophor EL micelles. *Cancer Chemother Pharmacol* 2001;47:309–318, and Malingre MM, Terwogt JM, Beijnen JH, et al. Phase I and pharmacokinetic study of oral paclitaxel. *J Clin Oncol* 2000;18:2468–2475, respectively.)

TABLE 15.1

Examples of Systemic Exposure as a Pharmacodynamic Marker of Anticancer Drug Effects

Drug	Side Effect	Response/Survival
Carboplatin	Thrombocytopenia	Ovarian cancer
Cisplatin	Nephrotoxicity	Head and neck cancer
Cyclophosphamide	Cardiotoxicity	
Docetaxel	Neutropenia	Non–small-cell lung cancer
Doxorubicin	Neutropenia	
Epirubicin	Neutropenia	
Erlotinib	Skin rash	Non–small-cell lung and head and neck cancer
Etoposide		Non–small-cell lung cancer
5-Fluorouracil	Diarrhea, mucositis	Head and neck cancer
Imatinib		Chronic myeloid leukemia
Irinotecan	Diarrhea, neutropenia	
6-Mercaptopurine		Acute lymphoblastic leukemia
Methotrexate	Mucositis	Acute lymphoblastic leukemia
Nilotinib	Anemia, QT-interval prolongation	
Paclitaxel	Neutropenia	
Sorafenib	Hypertension, hand-foot skin reaction	Renal cell cancer
Sunitinib	Neutropenia	Renal cell cancer
Teniposide		Lymphoma

PHARMACODYNAMIC CONCEPTS

Pharmacodynamic models relate clinical drug effects with drug dose, concentration, or other pharmacokinetic parameters indicative of drug exposures (Table 15.1). In oncology, pharmacodynamic variability may account for substantial differences in clinical outcomes, even when systemic exposures are uniform. Variability in pharmacodynamic response may be heavily influenced by clinical covariates such as age, gender, prior chemotherapy, prior radiotherapy, concomitant medications, or other variables.[19] The pharmacokinetic parameters that are most often correlated with drug effects are markers of drug exposure, such as AUC. In general, the specific parameter used as the independent variable in a pharmacodynamic analysis depends on the particular characteristics of the study drug.

In oncology, pharmacodynamic studies of drug effects have most often focused on toxicity endpoints.[20] Continuous response variables, such as the percentage fall in the absolute blood count from baseline, are easily analyzed using nonlinear regression methods. Dose-limiting neutropenia has been frequently analyzed using a sigmoid maximum effect model described by the modified Hill equation. The pharmacodynamic analysis of subjectively graded clinical endpoints, such as common toxicity criteria scores on a 4-point scale, may require more sophisticated statistical methods.[21,22] Logistical regression methods have been used to model these types of categorical (ordinal) response or outcome variables.

Physiologic pharmacodynamic models describing the severity and time course of drug-related myelosuppression have been derived using population mixed-effect methods for several agents, including paclitaxel[23,24] and pemetrexed.[25] The ability of these models to predict both the severity and duration of drug-induced neutropenia substantially enhances their clinical usefulness.[26] In contrast to small-molecule therapeutics, large-molecule therapeutics such as monoclonal antibodies may not demonstrate toxicities directly related to dose levels. For these agents, a thorough understanding of the pharmacokinetic/pharmacodynamic relationships using modeling approaches may be critical for optimal dose selection.[27]

The antitumor activity of certain chemotherapeutic agents is highly schedule dependent. For such drugs, the dose fractionated over several days can produce a different antitumor response or toxicity profile compared with the same dose given over a shorter period. For example, the efficacy of etoposide in the treatment of small-cell lung cancer is markedly increased when an identical total dose of etoposide is administered by a 5-day divided-dose schedule rather than a 24-hour infusion.[28] Pharmacokinetic analysis in that study showed that both schedules produced very similar overall drug exposure (as measured by AUC), but that the divided-dose schedule produced twice the duration of exposure to an etoposide plasma concentration of >1 μg/mL. This finding has led to the use of prolonged oral administration of etoposide to treat patients with cancer.[29] Similar schedule dependence has been demonstrated for a number of other anticancer agents, notably paclitaxel[30,31] and topotecan.[32] For these agents, the variability in clinically tested treatment schedules is enormous, ranging from short intravenous infusions of less than 30 minutes to 21-day or even 7-week continuous infusion administrations, with large differences in experienced toxicity profiles.

VARIABILITY IN PHARMACOKINETICS/ PHARMACODYNAMICS

There is often a marked variation in drug handling between individual patients, resulting in variability in pharmacokinetic parameters (Fig. 15.3), which will often lead to variability in the pharmacodynamic effects of a given dose of a drug.[33] That is, an identical dose of drug may result in acceptable toxicity in one patient, and unacceptable and possibly life-threatening toxicity in another, or a clinical response in one individual and cancer progression in another. The principal underlying sources of this interindividual pharmacokinetic/pharmacodynamic variability are discussed in the following paragraphs.

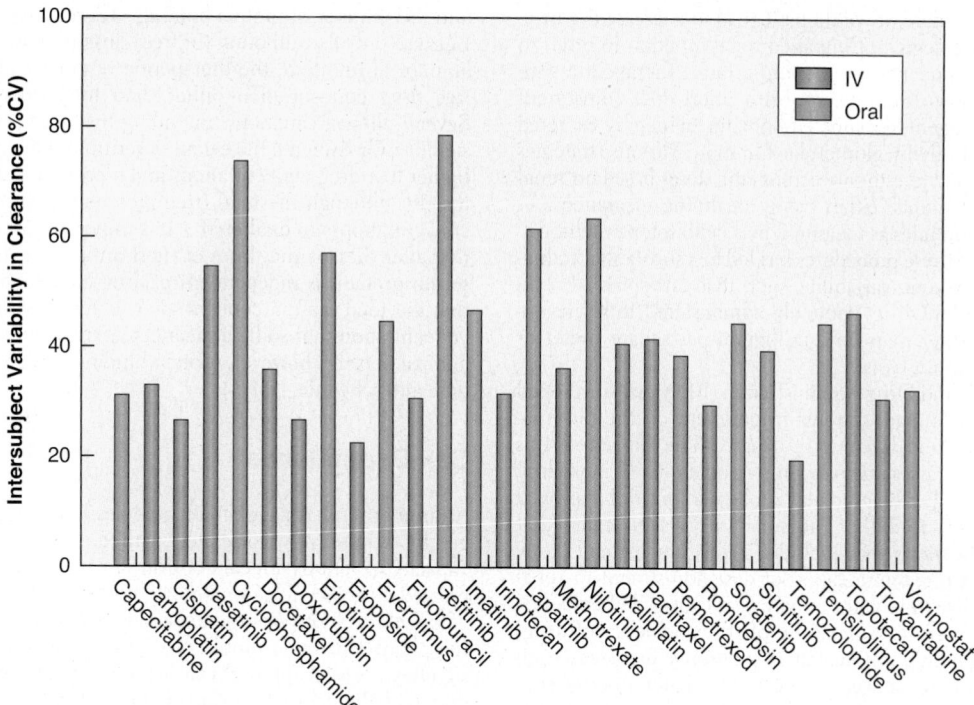

Figure 15.3 Interindividual pharmacokinetic variability of select cytotoxic agents and molecularly targeted agents expressed as a percent coefficient of variation (%CV) in apparent (oral) clearance. IV, intravenous. (Data derived from Mathijssen RH, de Jong FA, Loos WJ, et al. Flat-fixed dosing versus body surface area based dosing of anticancer drugs in adults: does it make a difference? *Oncologist* 2007;12:913–923, and publicly available prescribing information.)

Body Size and Body Composition

The traditional method of individualizing anticancer drug dosage is by using body surface area (BSA).[34] However, the usefulness of normalizing an anticancer drug dose to BSA in adults has been questioned, because, for many drugs, there is no relationship between BSA and CL.[35] Likewise, attempts to replace BSA as a size metric in dose calculation with alternate descriptors such as lean body weight, either in an average population or in individuals at the outer extremes of weight (i.e., frail, severely obese patients) have failed for many anticancer agents.[36,37] It should be pointed out that BSA is a much more important consideration in drug dose calculation for pediatric patients as compared to adults, because of the larger size range in the former population.[38] Based in part on the failure to reduce interindividual pharmacokinetic variability with the use of BSA normalization to obtain a starting dose, many of the more recently developed molecularly targeted agents are currently administered using a flat-fixed dose irrespective of an individual's BSA.[37]

Age

Changes in body composition and organ function at the extremes of age can affect both drug disposition and drug effect.[39] For example, maturational processes in infancy may alter the absorption and distribution of drugs as well as change the capacity for drug metabolism and excretion.[4] The importance of understanding the influence of age on the pharmacokinetics and pharmacodynamics of individual anticancer agents has increased steadily as treatment for the malignancies of infants,[40] adolescents,[41] and the elderly[42] has advanced. Although pediatric cancers remain rare compared with cancers in adults and the elderly population, in particular, optimizing treatment in a patient group with a high cure rate and a long expected survival becomes critical to minimize the incidence of preventable late complications while maintaining efficacy.

Pathophysiologic Changes

Effects of Disease

Pathophysiologic changes associated with particular malignancies may cause dramatic alterations in drug disposition. For example, increases in the clearance of both antipyrine and lorazepam were noted after remission induction compared with the time of diagnosis in children with acute lymphoblastic leukemia (ALL).[43] The clearance of unbound teniposide is lower in children with ALL in relapse than during first remission.[44] Because leukemic infiltration of the liver at the time of diagnosis is common, drugs metabolized by the liver may have a reduced clearance, as has been documented in preclinical models.[45]

Furthermore, in mouse models, certain tumors elicited an acute phase response that coincided with downregulation of human CYP3A4 in the liver as well as the mouse ortholog Cyp3a11.[46] The reduction of murine hepatic Cyp3a gene expression in tumor-bearing mice resulted in decreased Cyp3a protein expression and, consequently, a significant reduction in Cyp3a-mediated metabolism of midazolam. These findings support the possibility that tumor-derived inflammation may alter the pharmacokinetic and pharmacodynamic properties of CYP3A4 substrates, leading to reduced metabolism of drugs in humans.[47] This supports a possible need for disease-specific design of early clinical trials with anticancer drugs,[48] as has been recommended for docetaxel.[49]

Effects of Renal Impairment

The potential impact of pathophysiologic status on interindividual pharmacokinetic variability can be due to either the disease itself or to a dysfunction of specific organs involved in drug elimination. For example, if urinary excretion is an important elimination route for a given drug, any decrement in renal function could lead to decreased drug clearance, which may result in drug accumulation and toxicity.[50] Therefore, it would be logical to decrease the drug dose relative to the degree of impaired renal function in order to maintain plasma concentrations within a target therapeutic window. The best known example of this a priori dose adjustment of an anticancer agent remains carboplatin, which is excreted renally almost entirely by glomerular filtration. Various strategies have been developed to estimate carboplatin doses based on renal function among patients, either using creatinine clearance[51] or glomerular filtration rates as measured by a radioisotope method.[52] The application of these procedures has led to a substantial reduction in pharmacokinetic variability, such that carboplatin is currently one of the few drugs routinely administered to achieve a target exposure rather than on a milligram per square meter or milligram per kilogram basis.

The U.S. Food and Drug Administration (FDA) has developed a guidance on the impact of renal impairment on the pharmacokinetics, dosing, and labeling of drugs.[53] The impact of this guidance has been assessed following a survey of 94 new drug applications for small-molecule new molecular entities approved over the years 2003 to 2007. The survey results indicated that 41% of the applications that included renal impairment study data resulted in a recommendation of dose adjustment in renal impairment.[54] Interestingly, the survey results provided evidence that renal impairment can affect the pharmacokinetics of drugs that are predominantly eliminated by nonrenal processes such as metabolism and/or active transport. The latter finding supports the FDA recommendation to evaluate pharmacokinetic/pharmacodynamic alterations in renal impairment for those drugs that are predominantly eliminated by nonrenal processes, in addition to those that are mainly excreted unchanged by the kidneys. A striking example of a drug in the former category is imatinib, an agent that is predominantly eliminated by hepatic pathways but where predialysis renal impairment is associated with dramatically reduced drug clearance,[55] presumably due to a transporter-mediated process.[56]

Effects of Hepatic Impairment

In contrast to the predictable decline in renal clearance of drugs when glomerular filtration is impaired, it is difficult to make general predictions on the effect of impaired liver function on drug clearance. The major problem is that commonly applied criteria to establish hepatic impairment are typically not good indicators of drug-metabolizing enzyme activity and that several alternative hepatic function tests, such as indocyanine green and antipyrine, have relatively limited value in predicting anticancer drug pharmacokinetics. An alternative dynamic measure of liver function has been proposed, which is based on totaled values (scored to the World Health Organization [WHO] grading system) of serum bilirubin, alkaline phosphatase, and either alanine aminotransferase or aspartate aminotransferase to give a hepatic dysfunction score.[57] Based on pharmacokinetic studies in patients with normal and impaired hepatic function, guidelines have been proposed for dose adjustments of several agents when administered to patients with severe liver dysfunction.[58] It should be emphasized that no uniform criteria have been used in the conduct of these studies and that, ultimately, substantial advances could be made through an a priori determination of the hepatic activity of enzymes of pertinent relevance to the chemotherapeutic drug(s) of interest, as has been done for docetaxel.[59]

Effects of Serum Proteins

The binding of drugs to serum proteins, particularly those that are highly bound, may also have significant clinical implications for a therapeutic outcome.[60] Although protein binding is a major determinant of drug action, it is clearly only one of a myriad of factors that influence the disposition of anticancer drugs.[16] The extent of protein binding is a function of drug and protein concentrations, the affinity constants for the drug–protein interaction,

and the number of protein-binding sites per class of binding site. Because only the unbound (or free) drug in plasma water is available for distribution, the therapeutic response will correlate with free drug concentration rather than total drug concentration. Several clinical situations, including liver and renal disease, can significantly decrease the extent of serum binding and may lead to higher free drug concentrations and a possible risk of unexpected toxicity, although the total (free plus bound forms) plasma drug concentrations are unaltered.[61] It is important to realize, however, that after therapeutic doses of most anticancer drugs, binding to serum proteins is independent of drug concentration, suggesting that the total plasma concentration is reflective of the unbound concentration. For some anticancer agents, including etoposide[62] and paclitaxel,[63] however, protein binding is highly dependent on dose and schedule.

Sex Dependence

A number of pharmacokinetic analyses have suggested that male gender is positively correlated with the maximum elimination capacity of various anticancer drugs (e.g., paclitaxel)[8] or with increased clearance (e.g., imatinib)[64] compared with female gender. These observations have added to a growing body of evidence that the pharmacokinetic profile of various anticancer drugs exhibits significant sexual dimorphism, which is rarely considered in the design of clinical trials during oncology drug development.

Drug Interactions

Coadministration of Other Chemotherapeutic Drugs

Favorable and unfavorable interactions between drugs must be considered in developing combination regimens. These interactions may influence the effectiveness of each of the components of the combination, and typically occur when the pharmacokinetic profile of one drug is altered by the other. Such interactions are important in the design of trials evaluating drug combinations because, occasionally, the outcome of concurrent drug administration is diminished therapeutic efficacy or increased toxicity of one or more of the administered agents. Although a recent survey indicated that clinically significant pharmacokinetic interactions are relatively rare in Phase I trials of oncology drug combinations,[65] interactions appear to be more common for combinations of tyrosine kinase inhibitors with cytotoxic chemotherapeutics.[66]

Coadministration of Nonchemotherapeutic Drugs

Many prescription and over-the-counter medications have the potential to cause interactions with anticancer agents by altering their pharmacokinetic characteristics and leading to clinically significant phenotypes. Most clinically relevant drug interactions in this category are due to changes in metabolic routes related to an altered expression or function of cytochrome P450 (CYP) isozymes. This class of enzymes, particularly the CYP3A4 isoform, is responsible for the oxidation of a large proportion of currently approved anticancer drugs. Elevated CYP activity (induction), translated into a more rapid metabolic rate, may result in a decrease in plasma concentrations and to a loss of therapeutic effect. For example, anticonvulsant drugs such as phenytoin, phenobarbital, and carbamazepine can induce drug-metabolizing enzymes and thereby increase the clearance of various anticancer agents.[33]

Conversely, the suppression (inhibition) of CYP activity, for example with ketoconazole,[13,67] may trigger a rise in plasma concentrations and can lead to exaggerated toxicity commensurate with overdose. It should be borne in mind that several pharmacokinetic parameters could be altered simultaneously. Especially in the development of anticancer agents given by the oral route,

TABLE 15.2

Effect of Food on Exposure to Select Oral Anticancer Agents

Drug	Food	Effect on Drug Exposure	Manufacturer's Recommendations
Abiraterone	High-fat meal	↑ AUC 1,000%	Without food
Dasatinib	High-fat meal	↑ AUC 14%	With or without food
Erlotinib	High-fat, high-calorie breakfast	Single dose, ↑ AUC 200% Multiple dose, ↑ AUC 37%–66%	Without food[a]
Gefitinib	High-fat breakfast	↓ AUC 14%, ↓ Cmax 35%	With or without food
	High-fat breakfast	↑ AUC 32%, ↑ Cmax 35%	
Imatinib	High-fat meal	No change	With food and a large glass of water[b]
		Variability (% CV) ↓ 37%	
Lapatinib	Low-fat meal (5% fat, 500 calories)	↑ AUC 167%, ↑ Cmax 142%	Without food[c]
	High-fat meal (50% fat, 1,000 calories)	↑ AUC 325%, ↑ Cmax 203%	
Nilotinib	High-fat meal	↑ AUC 82%	Without food
Sorafenib	Moderate-fat meal (30% fat, 700 calories)	No change in bioavailability	Without food
	High-fat meal (50% fat, 900 calories)	↓ Bioavailability 29%	
Sunitinib	High-fat, high-calorie meal	↑ AUC 18%	With or without food
Everolimus	High-fat meal	↓ AUC 16%, ↓ Cmax 60%	With or without food
Vismodegib	High-fat meal	↑ AUC 74% for single dose; no effect at steady state	With or without food
Vorinostat	High-fat meal	↑ AUC 37%	With food[d]

[a] Recommended without food because the approved dose is the maximum tolerated dose.
[b] Recommended with food to reduce nausea.
[c] Recommended without food to achieve consistent drug exposure; was taken without food in clinical trials.
[d] Was taken with food in clinical trials.
AUC, area under the plasma concentration time curve; Cmax, maximum plasma concentration; CV, coefficient of variation.

oral bioavailability plays a crucial role[9]; this parameter is contingent on adequate absorption and the circumvention of intestinal and, subsequently, hepatic metabolism of the drug. It has been suggested that the prevalence of drug–drug interactions is particularly high in cancer patients receiving oral chemotherapy,[68] especially for agents that are weak bases that exhibit pH-dependent solubility.[69]

An additional consideration is related to a possible influence of food intake on the extent of drug absorption after oral administration, which can increase, decrease, or remain unchanged depending on specific physicochemical properties of the drug in question (Table 15.2). The relatively narrow therapeutic index of most of these agents means that significant inter- and intrapatient variability would predispose some individuals to excessive toxicity or, conversely, inadequate efficacy.[12]

Coadministration of Complementary and Alternative Medicine

Surveys within the past decade estimate the prevalence of complementary and alternative medicine (CAM) use in oncology patients to be as high as 87%, and in many cases the treating physician is not aware of the patients' CAM use.[70] With a larger number of participants to phase I clinical trials[71] using herbal treatments combined with allopathic therapies, the risk for herb–drug interactions is a growing concern, and there is an increasing need to understand possible adverse drug interactions in oncology at the early stages of drug development.

A number of clinically important pharmacokinetic interactions involving CAM and cancer drugs have now been recognized, although causal relationships have not always been established.[72] Most of the observed interactions point to the herbs

affecting several isoforms of the CYP family, either through inhibition or induction. In the context of chemotherapeutic drugs, St. John's wort,[73] garlic,[74] milk thistle,[75] and Echinacea[11] have been formally evaluated for their pharmacokinetic drug–interaction potential in cancer patients. However, various other herbs have the potential to significantly modulate the expression and/or activity of drug-metabolizing enzymes and drug transporters (Table 15.3), including ginkgo, ginseng, and kava.[70] Because of the high prevalence of herbal medicine use, physicians should include herb usage in their routine drug histories in order to have an opportunity to outline to individual patients which potential hazards should be taken into consideration prior to participation in a clinical trial.

Inherited Genetic Factors

The discipline of pharmacogenetics describes differences in the pharmacokinetics and pharmacodynamics of drugs as a result of inherited variation in drug metabolizing enzymes, drug transporters, and drug targets between patients.[76] These inherited variations are occasionally responsible for extensive interpatient variability in drug exposure or effects. Severe toxicity might occur in the absence of a typical metabolism of active compounds, while the therapeutic effect of a drug could be diminished in the case of an absence of activation of a prodrug, such as irinotecan.[77] The importance and detectability of polymorphisms for a given enzyme or transporter depends on the contribution of the variant gene product to pharmacologic response, the availability of alternative pathways of elimination, and the frequency of occurrence of the variant allele. Although many substrates have been identified for the known polymorphic drug metabolizing enzymes

TABLE 15.3

Effects of Common Herbal Products on Exposure to Anticancer Agents

Botanical	Concurrent Chemotherapy/Condition (Suspected Effect)
Ephedra	Avoid with all cardiovascular chemotherapy (synergistic increase in blood pressure)
Ginkgo	Caution with camptothecins, cyclophosphamide, TK inhibitors, epipodophyllotoxins, taxanes, and vinca alkaloids (CYP3A4 and CYP2C19 inhibition); discourage with alkylating agents, antitumor antibiotics, and platinum analogs (free-radical scavenging)
Ginseng	Discourage in patients with estrogen-receptor–positive breast cancer and endometrial cancer (stimulation of tumor growth)
Green tea	Discourage with erlotinib and pazopanib (CYP1A2 induction)
Japanese arrowroot	Avoid with methotrexate (ABC and OAT transporter inhibition)
St. John's wort	Avoid with all concurrent chemotherapy (CYP2B6, CYP2C9, CYP2C19, CYP2E1, CYP3A4, and ABCB1 induction)
Valerian	Caution with tamoxifen (CYP2C9 inhibition), cyclophosphamide, and teniposide (CYP2C19 inhibition)
Kava-kava	Avoid in all patients with preexisting liver disease, with evidence of hepatic injury (herb-induced hepatotoxicity), and/or in combination with hepatotoxic chemotherapy; caution with camptothecins, cyclophosphamide, TK inhibitors, epipodophyllotoxins, taxanes, and Vinca alkaloids (CYP3A4 induction)

TK, tyrosine kinase; CYP, cytochrome P450; ABC, ATP-binding cassette; OAT, organic anion transporter.

and transporters, the contribution of a genetically determined source of interindividual pharmacokinetic variability has been established for only a few cancer chemotherapeutic agents. Most of these cases involve agents for which elimination is critically dependent on a rate-limiting breakdown by a polymorphic enzyme (e.g., 6-mercaptopurine by thiopurine-S-methyltransferase; 5-fluorouracil by dihydropyrimidine dehydrogenase) or when a polymorphic enzyme is involved in the formation of a toxic metabolite (e.g., tamoxifen by CYP2D6).[78]

In addition to drug metabolism, pharmacokinetic processes are highly dependent on the interplay with drug transport in organs such as the intestines, kidneys, and liver. Genetically determined variation in drug transporter function or expression is now increasingly recognized to have a significant role as a determinant of intersubject variability in response to various commonly prescribed drugs.[79] The most extensively studied class of drug transporters are those encoded by the family of ATP-binding cassette (ABC) genes, some of which also play a role in the resistance of malignant cells to anticancer agents. Among the 48 known ABC gene products, ABCB1 (P-glycoprotein), ABCC1 (multidrug-resistance associated protein-1 [MRP1]) and its homologue ABCC2 (MRP2; cMOAT), and ABCG2 (breast cancer resistance protein [BCRP]) are known to influence the oral absorption and disposition of a wide variety of drugs.[80] As a result, the expression levels of these proteins in humans have important consequences for an individual's susceptibility to certain anticancer drug–induced side effects, interactions, and treatment efficacy, for example, in the case of genetic variation in ABCG2 in relation to gefitinib-induced diarrhea.[81]

Similar to the discoveries of functional genetic variations in drug efflux transporters of the ABC family, there have been considerable advances in the identification of inherited variants in transporters that facilitate cellular drug uptake in tissues that play an important role in drug elimination, such as the liver (Fig. 15.4). Among these, members of the organic anion-transporting polypeptides (OATP), organic anion transporters (OAT), and organic cation transporters (OCT) can mediate the cellular uptake of a large number of structurally divergent compounds.[82,83] Accordingly, functionally relevant polymorphisms in these influx transporters may contribute to interindividual and interethnic variability in drug disposition and response,[84] for example, in the case of the impact of polymorphic variants in the OCT1 gene *SLC22A1* on the survival of patients with chronic myeloid leukemia receiving treatment with imatinib.[85]

DOSE-ADAPTATION USING PHARMACOKINETIC/PHARMACODYNAMIC PRINCIPLES

Therapeutic Drug Monitoring

Prolonged infusion schedules of anticancer drugs offer a very convenient setting for dose adaptation in individual patients. At the time required to achieve steady-state concentration, it is possible to modify the infusion rate for the remainder of the treatment course if a relationship is known between this steady-state concentration and a desired pharmacodynamic endpoint. This method has been successfully used to adapt the dose during continuous infusions of 5-fluorouracil and etoposide, and for repeated oral administration of etoposide or repeated intravenous administration of cisplatin.[86] Methotrexate plasma concentrations are routinely monitored to identify patients at high risk of toxicity and to adjust leucovorin rescue in patients with delayed drug excretion. This monitoring has significantly reduced the incidence of serious toxicity, including toxic death, and in fact, has improved outcome by eliminating unacceptably low systemic exposure levels.[87] Therapeutic drug monitoring has also been applied to or is currently under investigation for several more recently developed anticancer drugs, including imatinib[88–90] and sorafenib.[91]

Feedback-Controlled Dosing

It remains to be determined how information on interindividual pharmacokinetic variability can eventually be used to devise an optimal dosage regimen of a drug for the treatment of a given disease in an individual patient. Obviously, the desired objective would be most efficiently achieved if the individual's dosage requirements could be calculated prior to administering the drug. While this ideal cannot be met completely in clinical practice, with the notable exception of carboplatin, some success may be achieved by adopting feedback-controlled dosing. In the adaptive dosage with feedback control, population-based predictive models are used initially, but allow the possibility of dosage alteration based on feedback revision. In this approach, patients are first treated with standard dose and, during treatment, pharmacokinetic information is estimated by a limited-sampling strategy and compared with that predicted from the population model with which treatment was initiated. On the basis of the comparison,

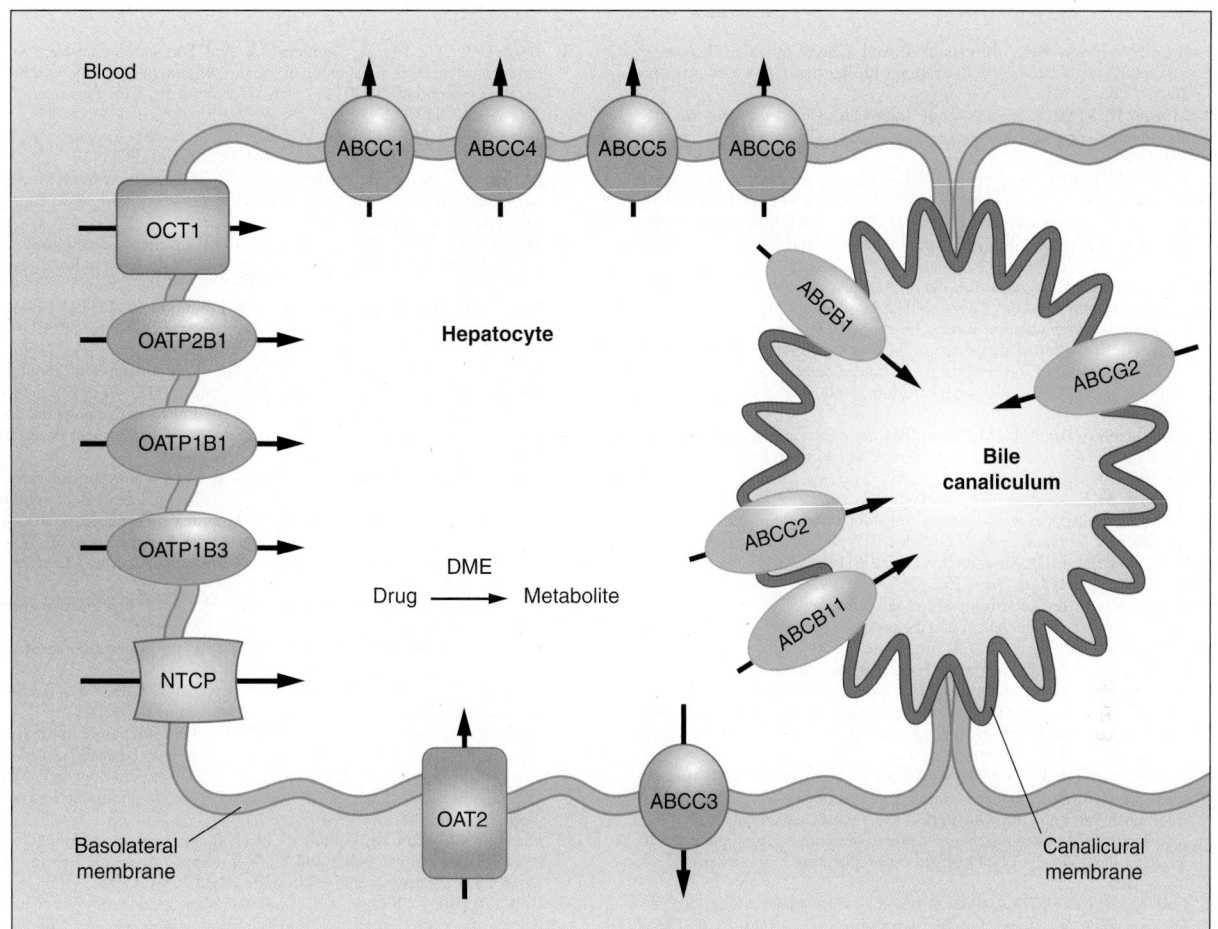

Figure 15.4 Common mechanisms for possible interactions between xenobiotics and anticancer drugs in the liver. DME, drug-metabolizing enzyme(s).

more patient-specific pharmacokinetic parameters are calculated, and dosage is adjusted accordingly to maintain the target exposure measure producing the desired pharmacodynamic effect. Despite its mathematical complexity, this approach may be the only way to deliver the desired and precise exposure of an anticancer agent.

The study of population pharmacokinetics seeks to identify the measurable factors that cause changes in the dose-concentration relationship and the extent of these alterations so that, if these are associated with clinically significant shifts in the therapeutic index, dosage can be appropriately modified in the individual patient. It is obvious that a careful collection of data during the development of drugs and subsequent analyses could be helpful to collect some essential information on the drug. Unfortunately, important information is often lost by failing to analyze this data or due to the fact that the relevant samples or data were never collected. Historically, this has resulted in the notion that tools for the identification of patient population subgroups are inadequate for most of the currently approved anticancer drugs.

However, the use of population pharmacokinetic models is increasingly studied in an attempt to accommodate as much of the pharmacokinetic variability as possible in terms of measurable characteristics. This type of analysis has been conducted for a number of clinically important anticancer drugs, including carboplatin,[92] docetaxel,[93] topotecan,[94] gefitinib,[95] and erlotinib,[96] and provided mathematical equations based on morphometric, demographic, phenotypic enzyme activity, and/or physiologic characteristics of patients, in order to predict drug clearance with an acceptable degree of precision and bias.[97]

SELECTED REFERENCES

The full reference list can be accessed at lwwhealthlibrary.com/oncology.

1. DeVita VT, Chu E. A history of cancer chemotherapy. *Cancer Res* 2008; 68:8643–8653.
2. Lieu CH, Tan AC, Leong S, et al. From bench to bedside: lessons learned in translating preclinical studies in cancer drug development. *J Natl Cancer Inst* 2013;105:1441–1456.
6. Stuurman FE, Nuijen B, Beijnen JH, et al. Oral anticancer drugs: mechanisms of low bioavailability and strategies for improvement. *Clin Pharmacokinet* 2013;52:399–414.
7. Hasovits C, Clarke S. Pharmacokinetics and pharmacodynamics of intraperitoneal cancer chemotherapeutics. *Clin Pharmacokinet* 2012;51:203–224.

9. DeMario MD, Ratain MJ. Oral chemotherapy: rationale and future directions. *J Clin Oncol* 1998;16:2557–2567.
11. Deeken JF, Loscher W. The blood-brain barrier and cancer: transporters, treatment, and Trojan horses. *Clin Cancer Res* 2007;13:1663–1674.
15. Malingre MM, Terwogt JM, Beijnen JH, et al. Phase I and pharmacokinetic study of oral paclitaxel. *J Clin Oncol* 2000;18:2468–2475.
18. van Zuylen L, Karlsson MO, Verweij J, et al. Pharmacokinetic modeling of paclitaxel encapsulation in Cremophor EL micelles. *Cancer Chemother Pharmacol* 2001;47:309–318.
19. Karlsson MO, Molnar V, Bergh J, et al. A general model for time-dissociated pharmacokinetic-pharmacodynamic relationship exemplified by paclitaxel myelosuppression. *Clin Pharmacol Ther* 1998;63:11–25.

21. Xie R, Mathijssen RH, Sparreboom A, et al. Clinical pharmacokinetics of irinotecan and its metabolites in relation with diarrhea. *Clin Pharmacol Ther* 2002;72:265–275.

24. Minami H, Sasaki Y, Saijo N, et al. Indirect-response model for the time course of leukopenia with anticancer drugs. *Clin Pharmacol Ther* 1998;64:511–521.

27. Keizer RJ, Huitema AD, Schellens JH, et al. Clinical pharmacokinetics of therapeutic monoclonal antibodies. *Clin Pharmacokinet* 2010;49:493–507.

30. Gelderblom H, Mross K, ten Tije AJ, et al. Comparative pharmacokinetics of unbound paclitaxel during 1- and 3-hour infusions. *J Clin Oncol* 2002;20:574–581.

33. Undevia SD, Gomez-Abuin G, Ratain MJ. Pharmacokinetic variability of anticancer agents. *Nat Rev Cancer* 2005;5:447–458.

34. Gurney H. Dose calculation of anticancer drugs: a review of the current practice and introduction of an alternative. *J Clin Oncol* 1996;14:2590–2611.

35. Baker SD, Verweij J, Rowinsky EK, et al. Role of body surface area in dosing of investigational anticancer agents in adults, 1991–2001. *J Natl Cancer Inst* 2002;94:1883–1888.

37. Sparreboom A, Wolff AC, Mathijssen RH, et al. Evaluation of alternate size descriptors for dose calculation of anticancer drugs in the obese. *J Clin Oncol* 2007;25:4707–4713.

38. Bartelink IH, Rademaker CM, Schobben AF, et al. Guidelines on paediatric dosing on the basis of developmental physiology and pharmacokinetic considerations. *Clin Pharmacokinet* 2006;45:1077–1097.

41. Veal GJ, Hartford CM, Stewart CF. Clinical pharmacology in the adolescent oncology patient. *J Clin Oncol* 2010;28:4790–4799.

46. Charles KA, Rivory LP, Brown SL, et al. Transcriptional repression of hepatic cytochrome P450 3A4 gene in the presence of cancer. *Clin Cancer Res* 2006;12:7492–7497.

47. Moore MM, Chua W, Charles KA, et al. Inflammation and cancer: causes and consequences. *Clin Pharmacol Ther* 2010;87:504–508.

49. Franke RM, Carducci MA, Rudek MA, et al. Castration-dependent pharmacokinetics of docetaxel in patients with prostate cancer. *J Clin Oncol* 2010;28:4562–4567.

50. Rahman A, White RM. Cytotoxic anticancer agents and renal impairment study: the challenge remains. *J Clin Oncol* 2006;24:533–536.

51. Egorin MJ, Van Echo DA, Olman EA, et al. Prospective validation of a pharmacologically based dosing scheme for the cis-diamminedichloroplatinum(II) analogue diamminecyclobutanedicarboxylatoplatinum. *Cancer Res* 1985;45:6502–6506.

52. Calvert AH, Newell DR, Gumbrell LA, et al. Carboplatin dosage: prospective evaluation of a simple formula based on renal function. *J Clin Oncol* 1989;7:1748–1756.

53. Huang SM, Temple R, Xiao S, et al. When to conduct a renal impairment study during drug development: US Food and Drug Administration perspective. *Clin Pharmacol Ther* 2009;86:475–479.

57. Twelves C, Glynne-Jones R, Cassidy J, et al. Effect of hepatic dysfunction due to liver metastases on the pharmacokinetics of capecitabine and its metabolites. *Clin Cancer Res* 1999;5:1696–1702.

59. Hooker AC, Ten Tije AJ, Carducci MA, et al. Population pharmacokinetic model for docetaxel in patients with varying degrees of liver function: incorporating cytochrome P4503A activity measurements. *Clin Pharmacol Ther* 2008;84:111–118.

61. Sparreboom A, Nooter K, Loos WJ, et al. The (ir)relevance of plasma protein binding of anticancer drugs. *Neth J Med* 2001;59:196–207.

64. Gardner ER, Burger H, van Schaik RH, et al. Association of enzyme and transporter genotypes with the pharmacokinetics of imatinib. *Clin Pharmacol Ther* 2006;80:192–201.

65. Wu K, House L, Ramirez J, et al. Evaluation of utility of pharmacokinetic studies in phase I trials of two oncology drugs. *Clin Cancer Res* 2013;19:6039–6043.

66. Hu S, Mathijssen RH, de Bruijn P, et al. Inhibition of OATP1B1 by tyrosine kinase inhibitors: in vitro-in vivo correlations. *Br J Cancer* 2014;110(4):894–898.

67. Kehrer DF, Mathijssen RH, Verweij J, et al. Modulation of irinotecan metabolism by ketoconazole. *J Clin Oncol* 2002;20:3122–3129.

68. van Leeuwen RW, Brundel DH, Neef C, et al. Prevalence of potential drug-drug interactions in cancer patients treated with oral anticancer drugs. *Br J Cancer* 2013;108:1071–1078.

69. Budha NR, Frymoyer A, Smelick GS, et al. Drug absorption interactions between oral targeted anticancer agents and PPIs: is pH-dependent solubility the Achilles heel of targeted therapy? *Clin Pharmacol Ther* 2012;92:203–213.

70. Sparreboom A, Cox MC, Acharya MR, et al. Herbal remedies in the United States: potential adverse interactions with anticancer agents. *J Clin Oncol* 2004;22:2489–2503.

76. Wheeler HE, Maitland ML, Dolan ME, et al. Cancer pharmacogenomics: strategies and challenges. *Nat Rev Genet* 2013;14:23–34.

78. Huang RS, Ratain MJ. Pharmacogenetics and pharmacogenomics of anticancer agents. *CA Cancer J Clin* 2009;59:42–55.

81. Cusatis G, Gregorc V, Li J, et al. Pharmacogenetics of ABCG2 and adverse reactions to gefitinib. *J Natl Cancer Inst* 2006;98:1739–1742.

84. Sprowl JA, Mikkelsen TS, Giovinazzo H, et al. Contribution of tumoral and host solute carriers to clinical drug response. *Drug Resist Updat* 2012;15:5–20.

87. Evans WE, Relling MV, Rodman JH, et al. Conventional compared with individualized chemotherapy for childhood acute lymphoblastic leukemia. *N Engl J Med* 1998;338:499–505.

89. Larson RA, Druker BJ, Guilhot F, et al. Imatinib pharmacokinetics and its correlation with response and safety in chronic-phase chronic myeloid leukemia: a subanalysis of the IRIS study. *Blood* 2008;111:4022–4028.

93. Bruno R, Hille D, Riva A, et al. Population pharmacokinetics/pharmacodynamics of docetaxel in phase II studies in patients with cancer. *J Clin Oncol* 1998;16:187–196.

94. Gallo JM, Laub PB, Rowinsky EK, et al. Population pharmacokinetic model for topotecan derived from phase I clinical trials. *J Clin Oncol* 2000;18:2459–2467.

95. Li J, Karlsson MO, Brahmer J, et al. CYP3A phenotyping approach to predict systemic exposure to EGFR tyrosine kinase inhibitors. *J Natl Cancer Inst* 2006;98:1714–1723.

16 Pharmacogenomics

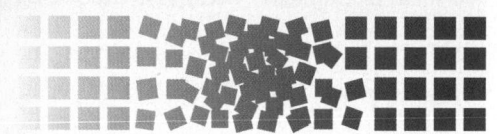

Christine M. Walko and Howard L. McLeod

INTRODUCTION

The evolution of understanding cancer biology has yielded many advances that have been translated into cancer treatment. Application of this knowledge has allowed for a shift in chemotherapeutics from traditional cytotoxic agents that worked by killing both healthy and malignant fast growing cells to chemical and biologic therapies aimed at targeting a specific gene or pathway critical to the particular cancer being treated.[1] This age of pathway-directed therapy has been made possible by the increased availability and feasibility of high throughput technology able to provide comprehensive and clinically useful molecular characterization of tumors. Translation of these efforts have resulted in improved degree to disease control for many common cancers including breast, colorectal, lung, and melanoma as well as long-term survival benefits for chronic myelogenous leukemia (CML), gastrointestinal stromal tumors (GIST), and childhood acute lymphoblastic leukemia (ALL).[2]

Pharmacogenomic-guided therapy aims the use information on DNA and RNA integrity to optimize not only the treatment choice for an individual patient, but also the dose and schedule of that treatment. The assessment of both somatic and germ-line mutations contribute to the overall individualization of cancer treatment. Somatic mutations are genetic variations found within the tumor DNA, but not DNA from the normal (germ-line) tissues, which also have functional consequences that influence disease outcomes and/or response to certain therapies. These types of mutations or biomarkers can be classified as either prognostic or predictive. Prognostic biomarkers identify subpopulations of patients with different disease courses or outcomes, independent of treatment. Predictive biomarkers identify subpopulations of patients most likely to have a response to a given therapy.[3] Germ-line mutations are heritable variations found within the individual and, in practical terms, are focused on DNA markers predictive for toxicity or therapeutic outcomes of a particular therapy as well as inheritable risk of certain cancers.[4] Pharmacogenomic mutations in the germ line provide some explanation for the interindividual and interracial variability in drug response and toxicity. For cancer chemotherapy, where cytotoxic agents are administered at doses close to their maximal tolerable dose, and therapeutic windows are relatively narrow, minor differences in individual drug handling may lead to severe toxicities. Therefore, an understanding of the sources of this variability would lead to the possibility of individualizing dosages or influencing clinical decisions that can improve patient care. Pharmacogenomics has putative utility in therapy selection, clinical study design, and as a tool to improve understanding of the pharmacology of a medication.

The term *pharmacogenetics* was initially used to define inherited differences in drug effects and typically focused on individual candidate genes. The field of pharmacogenomics now includes genomewide association studies and is used to describe genetic variations in all aspects of drug absorption, distribution, metabolism, and excretion in addition to drug targets and their downstream pathways.[5] Table 16.1 illustrates some current clinical examples of genotype-guided cancer chemotherapy. Variations in the DNA sequences encoding these proteins may take the form of deletions, insertions, repeats, frameshift mutations, nonsense mutations, and missense mutations, resulting in an inactive, truncated, unstable, or otherwise dysfunctional protein. The most common change involves single nucleotide substitutions, called single-nucleotide polymorphisms (SNP), which occur at approximately 1 per 1,000 base pairs on the human genome. Variability in toxicity or activity can also be mediated by postgenomic events, at the level of RNA, protein, or functional activity.

PHARMACOGENOMICS OF TUMOR RESPONSE

Tumor response to chemotherapy is regulated by a complex, multigenic network of genes that encompasses inherent characteristics of the tumor, differentially activated pathways of cell signaling, proliferation and DNA repair, factors that control drug delivery to the tumor cells (e.g., metabolism, transport), and cell death. These may in turn be modulated by previously administered treatment or drug exposure, which may upregulate target proteins or activate alternative pathways of drug resistance. The polygenic nature of drug response implies that a better understanding of genotype–phenotype associations would require more than the usual single-gene pharmacogenetic strategies employed to date. However, there are instances where the genomic context of a single gene within a cancer will be of high impact for specific therapeutic agents (see Table 16.1).

Pathway Directed Anticancer Therapy

One of the earliest success stories illustrating pathway-driven therapeutics is with CML. The hallmark chromosomal abnormality of this disease is the translocation of chromosomes 9 and 22 that ultimately produces the fusion gene *BCR-ABL*. This discovery in 1960 eventually led to the development of the targeted tyrosine-kinase inhibitor (TKI) imatinib and its subsequent Food and Drug Administration (FDA) approval for treatment of CML in 2001.[6] The International Randomized Study of Interferon and STI571 (IRIS) trial began enrollment in 2000 and compared imatinib with interferon and low-dose cytarabine, which was the previous standard of care for newly diagnosed patients with chronic-phase CML. All efficacy endpoints favored imatinib, including complete cytogenetic response of 76.2% with imatinib compared with 14.5% with interferon (p <0.001).[7] Overall survival (OS) after 60 months of follow-up was 89% with imatinib.[8] This example is just one of many where a once fatal disease can now be considered more akin to a chronic disease, requiring a daily medication and regular physician follow-up, similar to hypertension or diabetes. Drug development has also kept pace with these advances and now several other agents, including dasatinib, nilotinib, bosutinib, and ponatinib, have joined imatinib as treatment options for CML.

The idea of changing treatment focus from a disease-based model to a pathway-driven model is also evolving. Human epidermal

TABLE 16.1

Clinical Examples of Genotype-Guided Cancer Chemotherapy

Somatic Mutation Examples		
Drug Target	**Drug(s)**	**Malignancy**
EML4-ALK	Crizotinib	Non–small-cell lung cancer
BCR-ABL	Dasatinib, imatinib, nilotinib, bosutinib, ponatinib	Chronic myelogenous leukemia
BRAF	Vemurafenib, dabrafenib	Melanoma
Epidermal growth factor receptor (EGFR)	Erlotinib, afatinib	Non–small-cell lung cancer
HER2	Trastuzumab, lapatinib, pertuzumab, Ado-trastuzumab emtansine	Breast cancer, gastric cancer
Janus kinase 2 (JAK2)	Ruxolitinib	Myelofibrosis
Kirsten rat sarcoma viral oncogene (KRAS)	Cetuximab, panitumumab	Colorectal cancer
Rearranged during transfection (RET)	Vandetanib	Medullary thyroid cancer
Germ-Line Mutation Examples		
Gene Mutation	**Drug**	**Effect**
Cytochrome P450 (CYP) 2C19	Voriconazole	Decreased serum levels of active drug and potential decreased efficacy in patients with high enzyme levels (ultrarapid metabolizers)
CYP2D6	Tamoxifen, codeine, ondansetron	Decreased production of active metabolite and potential decreased efficacy in patients with low enzyme levels
Dihydropyrimidine dehydrogenase (DPYD)	5-Fluorouracil	Decreased elimination and increased risk of myelosuppression, diarrhea, and mucositis in patients with low enzyme levels
Glucose-6-phosphate dehydrogenase (G6PD)	Rasburicase	Risk of severe hemolysis in patients with G6PD deficiency
Thiopurine methyltransferase (TPMT)	Mercaptopurine, thioguanine, azathioprine	Decreased methylation of the active metabolite resulting decreased elimination and increased risk of neutropenia in patients with low enzyme levels
UDP-glucuronosyltransferase (UGT) 1A1	Irinotecan	Decreased glucuronidation of the active metabolite resulting decreased elimination and increased risk of neutropenia and diarrhea in patients with low enzyme levels

growth factor receptor 2 (HER2) is a transmembrane receptor tyrosine kinase that is overexpressed or amplified in up to 25% of breast cancers. Trastuzumab is a humanized monoclonal antibody directed against HER2 and demonstrated improved response rates (RR) and time to disease progression in patients with metastatic HER2 positive breast cancer and improved disease-free survival (DFS) and OS in HER2-positive breast cancer patients treated with adjuvant trastuzumab.[9] Several additional agents are now available to target the HER2 pathway and vary in their pharmacology and mechanism of action. Lapatinib is an oral TKI directed against HER2 and the epidermal growth factor receptor (EGFR), pertuzumab is a humanized monoclonal antibody that binds at a different location than trastuzumab and inhibits the dimerization and subsequent activation of HER2 signaling, and ado-trastuzumab emtansine is an antibody-drug conjugate that targets HER2-positive cells and then releases the cytotoxic antimitotic agent emtansine through liposomal degradation of the linking compound. All of these agents illustrate the progress and pharmacologic diversity of pathway-directed therapy and remain as standard of care options for HER2-positive breast cancer in either the adjuvant and/or metastatic settings.[10] HER2 expression is not limited to breast cancer, however. Though less common, HER2 expression is seen in numerous solid tumors including bladder, gastric, prostate and non–small-cell lung cancer with varying

degrees of incidence depending on the method of detection. Based on results from a large, open-label phase III randomized, international trial of 594 patients with gastric or gastroesophageal junction cancer expressing HER2 by either immunohistochemistry or gene amplification by fluorescence in situ hybridization, trastuzumab is also approved for treatment of metastatic gastric or gastroesophageal junction adenocarcinoma that expresses HER2. Patients randomized to chemotherapy in combination with trastuzumab had a median OS of 13.8 months compared with 11.1 months in the patients receiving chemotherapy alone (hazard ratio [HR], 0.74; 0.60 to 0.91, p = 0.0046).[11] Numerous examples also support that pathway-directed therapy will cross the boundaries of disease sites and that tumor genetics will become one of the biggest determining factors for treatment.

Simple expression of the drug target does not always translate into desired clinical outcomes though. Cetuximab and panitumumab are monoclonal antibodies directed against EGFR; however, it was found that colorectal cancer (CRC) patients who did not have detectable EGFR still experienced responses to these agents similar in extent to EGFR-positive patients. Kirsten rat sarcoma viral oncogene (KRAS) is a downstream effector of the EGFR pathway. Ligand binding to EGFR on the cell surface activates pathway signaling through the KRAS-RAF-mitogen-activated protein kinase (MAPK) pathway, which is thought to control cell growth, differentiation, and apoptosis.[12] Eventually it was found that CRC patients with a KRAS mutation did not derive benefit from cetuximab or panitumumab. The RR in CRC receiving either cetuximab or panitumumab who were KRAS wild type was 10% to 40% compared with near zero percent in those with KRAS mutations.[13] This finding was the result of a retrospective analysis of small group of patients and was confirmed in large, prospective trials. Additionally, it underscores the importance of tissue collection for biomarker assessment in trials with novel therapeutics. A recent clinical trial genomic analysis suggests that mutations in NRAS may also have value in predicting the utility of EGFR antibody therapy in colorectal cancer. Although the predictive value of KRAS mutation status in colorectal cancer has been well established in clinical trials, the role of KRAS in lung cancer and other malignancies is less well elucidated. Lung cancers harboring KRAS mutations have been shown to have less clinical benefit from the EGFR-targeted erlotinib in some trials, although this has not consistently been the case across all trials. Additionally, lung cancer KRAS mutation status does not appear to reproducibly predict clinical benefit from the EGFR-targeted monoclonal antibodies, as is the case in colorectal cancer.[14] Unlike the HER2 example discussed previously, the clinical application of some genetic mutations will differ between tissue of origin.

Deeper investigations and understandings of mutations driving oncogenic pathways can also elucidate mechanisms of resistance and practical therapeutic strategies for treatment and prevention. Approximately half of all cutaneous melanomas carry mutations in BRAF, with the most common being the V600E mutation. Vemurafenib is a TKI directed against mutated BRAF that demonstrated improvements in both progression-free survival (PFS) and OS when compared with the cytotoxic agent dacarbazine in previously untreated patients with metastatic melanoma carrying the BRAF V600E mutation. Vemurafenib demonstrated a 63% relative reduction in the risk of death compared with dacarbazine (p <0.001) along with a higher response rate (48% compared with 5% for dacarbazine).[15] Based on these results, vemurafenib was the first BRAF targeted TKI approved by the FDA and was soon joined by dabrafenib. Although dramatic responses to these agents have been observed, relapse almost universally occurs after a median of 6 to 8 months. Activating BRAF mutations, like V600E, result in uncontrolled activity of the MAPK pathway through activation of the downstream kinase MEK, which when phosphorylated, subsequently activates extracellular signal-regulated kinase (ERK), which ultimately translocates to the cell nucleus, resulting in cell proliferation and survival (Fig. 16.1).[16] An assessment of serial biopsies from patients treated with vemurafenib suggested numerous mechanisms for acquired resistance, including the appearance of secondary mutations in MEK.[17] This finding supports the clinical rationale for using combination therapy with a BRAF and a MEK inhibitor. The combination of dabrafenib (BRAF inhibitor) and trametinib (MEK inhibitor) was assessed in 247 metastatic melanoma patients with BRAF V600 mutations compared with dabrafenib alone. Median PFS was 9.4 months in the combination group compared with 5.8 months in the patients who received single agent therapy (HR, 0.39; 0.25 to 0.62, p <0.001). A complete or partial response was also higher in the combination therapy group (76% compared with 54%, p = 0.03). The occurrence of cutaneous squamous cell carcinoma, a known side effect of single-agent BRAF inhibitor therapy due to paradoxical activation of RAF in nonmutated cells, was also decreased in the combination therapy group (7% compared with 19%, p = 0.09), further supporting the evidence of downstream inhibition.[18] Although combination therapy does prolong the time to disease progression, resistance still occurs in patients through a variety of mechanisms. Utilization of sequential biopsies and a genetic assessment will help to inform rationale combination and sequential pathway-driven therapy trials that will ultimately aid in better understanding and mitigation of common mechanism of resistance.

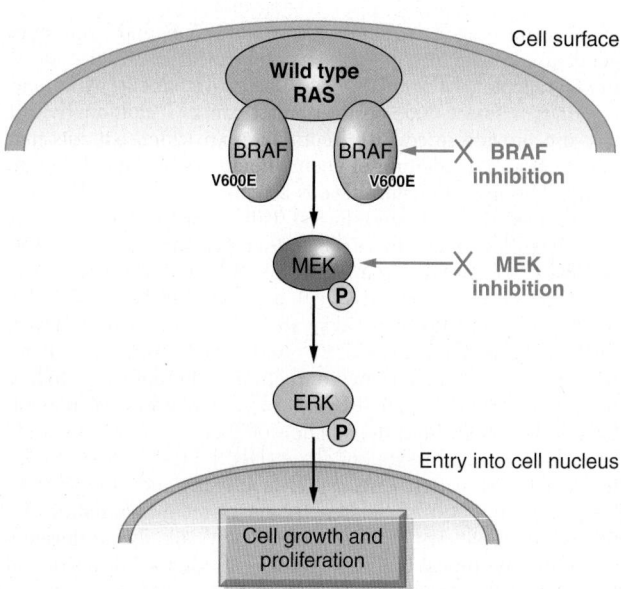

Figure 16.1 MAPK pathway in BRAF mutated melanoma. The BRAF V600E mutation results in activation of the MAPK pathway independent of growth factor binding, initially by phosphorylation (P) of MEK. MEK subsequently phosphorylates ERK. ERK then translocates to the cell nucleus and causes transcription of cellular factors, resulting in cell proliferation and survival. Because one mechanism of resistance to BRAF inhibition is through mutations in MEK, inhibition at both the upstream target of BRAF and the downstream site of MEK can prolong the clinical benefit of the BRAF inhibitor.

Although advances in basic science and drug development have translated many oncogenic driver mutations across tumor types into pathway-directed therapy, this is not the case for the majority. There are numerous examples of functionally relevant recurrent driver mutations that affect protein targets that are not currently druggable. Regardless of malignancy, one of the most commonly mutated tumor suppressors is the protein p53. Mutations can result in p53 acquiring oncogenic functions that enable proliferation, invasion, metastasis, and cell survival as well as coordinating with different proteins, such as EGFR, to enhance or inhibit its effects. However, a clinical application of p53 mutation data or directly targeting p53 has been limited, to date.[19] PIK3CA encodes a catalytic subunit of phophoinositol-3 kinase (PI3K), which includes four distinct subfamily kinases involved in regulating cell growth, motility, proliferation, and survival. Direct inhibitors of the kinase, as well as downstream targets, including AKT (protein kinase B [PKB]) and mammalian target of rapamycin (mTOR), are being assessed to target these mutations. Therapeutic challenges include understanding the complex signaling network germane to each cancer and the role of kinases in each subfamily.[20] Both the examples of p53 and PI3K illustrate the challenge of translating the multitude of somatic mutations into applications of available therapeutic agents.

Application of Genomewide Gene Expression Profiling to Guide Therapy

Single gene approaches may not reflect the overall complexity of genetic regulation of chemotherapy responses. Genomic strategies using global gene expression data are able to provide a more complete picture of the tumor through disease classification.[21] These strategies may identify subgroups of patients with early disease that need adjuvant chemotherapy, those who will not benefit from standard therapy, or help with the selection of chemotherapy from a menu of potentially active agents. Oncotype Dx is a 21-gene assay with 16 tumor-associated genes and 5 reference genes used to predict the risk of distant local recurrence in estrogen receptor (ER)-positive, HER2-negative patients with node-negative or select node-positive breast cancer. Additionally, the test also provides predictive information on which patients may benefit from the addition of chemotherapy to hormonal therapy alone. The test ultimately reports a recurrence score (RS) on a continuous scale from zero to 100. Patients with an RS <18 are considered low risk, with a 10-year distant recurrence rate (DRR) of 6.8% (95% confidence interval [CI], 4 to 9.6); RS scores of 18 to 30 are at intermediate risk, with a 10-year DRR of 14.3% (CI, 8.3 to 20.3); and RS scores ≥31 are at high risk, with a 10-year DRR of 30.5% (CI, 23.6 to 37.4).[22] Additionally, high-risk patients have the largest benefit from the addition of chemotherapy to hormonal therapy (HR, 0.26; 0.13 to 0.53), whereas low-risk patients have little benefit from the addition of chemotherapy and could consider hormonal treatment alone (HR, 1.31; 0.46 to 3.78). Intermediate risk patients are harder to classify, and clinical trials are underway to further address treatment recommendations for this group of patients.[23] These type of assays are also in development and in clinical trials for a variety of other solid tumor and hematologic malignancies.

Genetic-Guided Therapy Practical Issues in Somatic Analysis

Currently, targeted DNA capture is the most common type of somatic genetic screening and involves focusing on a few relevant candidate genes followed by deeper sequencing. These types of techniques can reveal common genes associated with a particular malignancy but also may uncover a signaling pathway that would not be obviously associated with a particular histology or tumor site. Application of a next-generation sequencing assay in 40 CRC and 24 non–small-cell lung cancer (NSCLC) tissue samples that assessed 145 cancer-relevant genes demonstrated that somatic mutations were seen in 98% of the CRC tumors and 83% of the NSCLCs (Fig. 16.2).[24] The evolution of sequencing strategies and decreasing costs has made whole genome sequencing more available in the clinical setting, and several companies offer commercially available tumor profiling services. Several limitations exist that currently restrict the broad clinical implementation of these assays, however. Although germ-line genetic assessments can be done on a peripheral blood sample or buccal swab, somatic assessments typically require biopsy tissue, which is often in limited supply and of varying quality or may not be feasible depending on the site of the cancer. Ongoing studies are assessing the

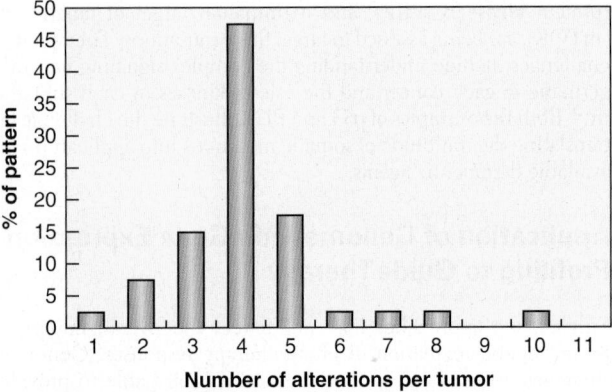

Figure 16.2 Number of alterations per tumor. Deep sequencing of 145 genes in 40 colorectal cancers found a spectrum of incidence of somatic mutations, with more than half occurring in genes that are *druggable* with medication that is either FDA approved or in late stage clinical development.

value of liquid biopsies of circulating tumor DNA.[25] Optimizing and creating uniformity in quality control of gene panel or whole-genome assessment is also needed to decrease the reporting of uncertain or erroneous identification of mutations. Once sequencing is completed, a predictive analysis is needed for the 25% to 80% of instances where variants of unknown significance are identified in genes of interest. Translation of genomic sequencing into clinical practice will require a diverse team, including pathologists, medical oncologists, surgical oncologists, information technologists, geneticists, and pharmacologists.

PHARMACOGENOMICS OF CHEMOTHERAPY DRUG TOXICITY

A drug's disposition and pharmacodynamic effects can be influenced by a number of variables, including patient age, diet, concomitant medications, and underlying disease processes. However, an individual's genetic constitution is an important regulator of variability in drug effect. Differences in drug effects are more pronounced between individuals compared to within an individual. Indeed, studies in monozygotic and dizygotic twins identified that 20% to 80% of the variation in drug disposition is mediated by inheritance.[26] Drug-metabolizing enzymes, cellular transporters, and tissue receptors are governed by genetic variation.

Advances in the treatment of most common malignancies have resulted in the availability of multiple distinct combination chemotherapy regimens with similar or equal anticancer efficacy. Therefore, differences in systemic toxicity have become a major determinant in the selection of therapy. The majority of pharmacogenomic examples affecting adverse events or efficacy from cytotoxic drugs involve hepatic metabolizing enzymes that detoxify or biotransform xenobiotics.[27,28]

Thiopurine Methyltransferase

One of the best-studied pharmacogenetic syndrome involves the metabolism of the thiopurine drugs—6-mercaptopurine (6MP), 6-thioguanine, and azathioprine—which have wide applications, including maintenance therapy for childhood ALL and adult leukemias. These prodrugs must be activated to thioguanine nucleotides in order to have antiproliferative effects. However, most of the variability in the formation of active metabolites is mediated by methylation via thiopurine methyltransferase (TPMT).[29] TPMT is a cytosolic enzyme that catalyzes S-methylation of thiopurine agents, resulting in an inactive metabolite. Erythrocyte TPMT activity has a trimodal distribution, with 90% of patients having high activity, 10% intermediate activity, and 0.3% with very low or no detectable activity. TPMT deficiency results in higher intracellular activation of 6MP to form thioguanine nucleotides, resulting in severe or fatal hematologic toxicity from standard doses of therapy.[30] The variable activity results from polymorphism in the TPMT gene, located on chromosome locus 6p22.3. Genetic variants at codon 238 (TPMT*2), codon 719 (TPMT*3C), or both codons 460 and 719 (TPMT*3A) are the most clinically significant, accounting for 95% of the patients with reduced TPMT activity.[31] Heterozygotes (one wild type and one variant allele) are common (10% of patients), and have elevated levels of active metabolites (twofold more than homozygous wild type), and required more cumulative dose reductions of 6MP for maintenance ALL chemotherapy compared to homozygous wild-type patients (Fig. 16.3).[32] Patients with a homozygous variant TPMT genotype are at a fourfold risk of severe toxicity, compared with wild-type patients.[31] TPMT genotype tests are now available commercially in a Clinical Laboratory Improvement Amendments (CLIA)-certified environment. To date, patients homozygous for TPMT variant alleles appear to tolerate 10%, and heterozygotes appear to tolerate 65% of the recommended doses of 6MP, with no apparent

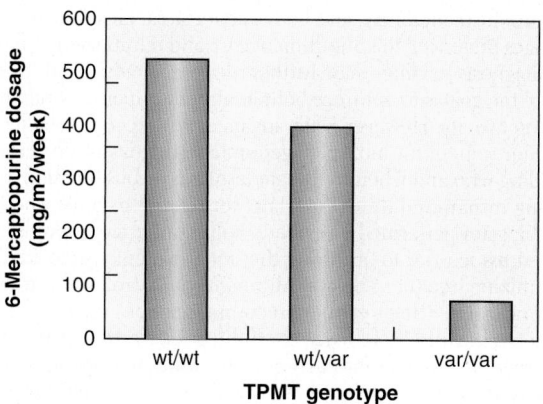

Figure 16.3 Relationship between TPMT genotype and required 6MP dose. Compared with homozygous wild-type patients, those heterozygous for a thiopurine methyltransferase (TPMT) variant allele generally require at least a 30% dose reduction in 6MP, whereas homozygous variant patients require substantial dose reductions of approximately 90% that of wild-type patients.

decrease in clinical efficacy (Fig. 16.3).[32] This has formed the basis for prospective, TPMT genotype-guided dosing of 6MP to avoid severe toxicity. Clinical Pharmacogenomics Implementation Consortium (CPIC) Guidelines recommend that homozygous wild-type patients be started at the full standard dose. Heterozygous patients should start with reduced doses at 30% to 70% of the full dose with adjustments made after 2 to 4 weeks based on myelo-suppression and disease-specific guidelines. Homozygous variant patients should start with 10% of the full dose due to the extremely high levels of the active metabolite and potential for fatal toxicity at standard doses. Adjustments should be made after 4 to 6 weeks based on myelosuppression and disease-specific guidelines.[33]

Dihydropyrimidine Dehydrogenase (DPD)

Although 5-fluorouracil (5FU) has been available for over 40 years, it remains the cornerstone of colorectal cancer chemotherapy, both in the adjuvant and metastatic settings. Additionally, the oral prodrug capecitabine ultimately undergoes activation to 5FU and is commonly used in gastrointestinal and breast malignancies. 5FU is a prodrug that is activated intracellularly to 5-fluoro-2'-deoxyuridine monophosphate (5FdUMP), which inhibits thymidylate synthase (TS), among other mechanisms of action. TS inhibition results in impaired de novo pyrimidine synthesis and suppression of DNA synthesis. Approximately 85% of a 5FU dose is catabolized by dihydropyrimidine dehydrogenase (DPD) to inactive metabolites. Therefore, DPD is a primary regulator of 5FU activity. DPD deficiency has been described, resulting in higher 5FU blood levels, greater formation of active metabolites, and severe or fatal clinical toxicity, predominately myelosuppression, mucositis, and cerebellar toxicity.[34] In theory, this toxicity could be reduced or avoided by screening for DPD activity in surrogate tissues, such as peripheral mononuclear cells. However, the technical requirements for preparation of these samples make it impractical for many practice sites. Understanding the molecular basis for DPD deficiency will provide an approach for prospective identification of patients at high risk for severe 5FU toxicity. The gene encoding DPD is composed of 23 exons, and at least 23 SNPs have been found.[35] Studies in DPD-deficient patients have identified several distinct molecular variants associated with low enzyme activity. Many of these are rare, and base substitutions, splicing defects, and frame shift mutations, have been described. The prevalent variation is the splice recognition site in intron 14 (DPYD*2A), where a G to A substitution results in the skipping of exon 14, resulting in an inactive enzyme.[36–38] This polymorphism

has been associated with severe DPD deficiency in heterozygous patients, with a homozygous genotype associated with a mental retardation syndrome. Patients with severe 5FU toxicity may harbor one or more variant alleles of DPD, and a recent study showed that 61% of cancer patients experiencing severe 5FU toxicities had decreased DPD activity in peripheral mononuclear cells, and DPYD*2A was commonly found.[39] In the patients with grade 4 neutropenia, 50% harbored at least one DPYD*2A. It is estimated that in the Caucasian population, homozygotes for the variant alleles have an incidence of 0.1% and heterozygotes occur at an incidence of 0.5% to 2%. There are additional DPD mutations that have been associated with impaired enzyme activity, including DPYD *3 and DPYD*13. CPIC guidelines recommend standard dosing for homozygous wild-type patients. Reducing the dose by at least 50% in heterozygous patients (*1/*2A) is recommended, followed by dose adjustment based on toxicity and/or pharmacokinetic testing. The use of an alternative agent is recommended in homozygous-variant patients (*2A/*2A).[34] There are many patients with severe 5FU toxicity that have normal DPD activity. This highlights that many factors, including multiple genes, are potential causes of 5FU toxicity, and there will not be one simple test to avoid this important clinical problem.

Cytochrome P450 2D6

Tamoxifen is a selective estrogen-receptor modulator used in ER-positive breast cancer in both the localized and metastatic settings. It is the drug of choice for premenopausal women and is a treatment option, along with aromatase inhibitors, for postmenopausal women. The low cost of tamoxifen also makes it a preferred therapy regardless of menopausal status in numerous countries. Tamoxifen metabolism is complex, with extensive metabolism through numerous phase I and II enzymes that produce several primary and secondary metabolites and their corresponding isomers, each possessing different antiestrogen effects.[40] The primary active metabolite is believed to be endoxifen, which is produced by the CYP3A4/5 mediated-conversion of tamoxifen to N-desmethyltamoxifen, which is then further converted to endoxifen (4-hydroxy-N-desmethyltamoxifen) via cytochrome P450 2D6 (CYP2D6). A direct relationship between endoxifen concentration and its antiestrogen effects has been demonstrated, potentially suggesting that a threshold concentration may be needed for optimal clinical effect.[41] CYP2D6 is highly polymorphic, with more than 80 allelic CYP2D6 variants described. These alleles vary in enzyme activity and prevalence with respect to race and ethnicity.[42] Based on genotype, patients can be classified by phenotype into ultrarapid metabolizers (UM; approximately 1% to 2% of patients [common alleles include *1xN, *2xN]) who carry more than two functional allele copies, extensive metabolizers (EM; 77% to 92% [e.g., *1, *2]), intermediate metabolizers (IM; 2% to 11% [e.g., *10, *17, *41]), or poor metabolizers (PM; 5% to 10% [*3, *4, *5]).[43] UM patients have the highest concentrations of endoxifen, followed by EM patients, then IM patients, and finally, PM patients have the lowest concentration. Up to a sixfold variation in endoxifen levels may be seen between homozygous PM and homozygous EM patients.[40]

The relationship between CYP2D6 genotype, endoxifen concentrations, and disease outcomes has been investigated in numerous clinical trials. One of the largest retrospective trials assessed this relationship in 1,325 women treated with adjuvant tamoxifen 20 mg daily. Approximately 46% of the patients were classified as EM, 48% were IM, and 5.9% were PM. A statistically significant increased risk of disease recurrence was seen in the IM and PM patients compared with the EM patients (HR, 1.40; 95% CI, 1.04 to 1.90 for IM; and HR 1.90, 95% CI, 1.10 to 3.28 for PM).[44] A large meta-analysis of 4,973 tamoxifen-treated patients across 12 international studies conducted by the International Tamoxifen Pharmacogenomics Consortium also supported this relationship.

CYP2D6 PM phenotypes were associated with decreased DFS (HR 1.25, 95% CI, 1.06 to 1.47, p = 0.009) when only considering the data from trials with postmenopausal women with ER-positive breast cancer who received tamoxifen 20 mg daily for 5 years.[45]

Not all trial results have been consistent, however, and dosing guidelines for genotype-guided therapy do not yet exist. Clinical trials do support the potential for genotype-guided therapy. IM patients who received an increased dose of 40 mg daily instead of the standard 20 mg were shown to have endoxifen concentrations similar to that of EM patients (p = 0.25).[46] This suggests that genotype-guided therapy with increased dose recommendations may be feasible, but additional prospective trials are needed to determine the clinical efficacy of this intervention.

CONCLUSIONS AND FUTURE DIRECTIONS

Genomic-driven cancer medicine is being translated into clinical practice through increased understanding of somatic mutations in a specific tumor that can be translated to pathway-directed therapeutics as well as germ-line mutations that affect the pharmacokinetics and pharmacodynamics of individual medications. For the practicing oncologist, knowledge of pharmacogenomics is necessary because therapeutic decisions of drug selection and dosage are being based on more molecularly and genetically defined variables than the current phenotypic information of tumor type, immunohistochemistry, and body surface area. Health-care policy changes preferring the bundling of care and reimbursement based on diagnosis coding may further drive individualized therapy where the goal is to optimize both treatment responses while minimizing toxicity. However, with advances always come challenges. Reimbursement for multiplex genomic testing is not universal, so deciding who and when to initiate testing is a consideration. Optimizing turnaround time, especially for referral patients who have had biopsies performed elsewhere, will require requesting this archived tissue prior to or during the initial patient visit to facilitate minimizing treatment delays. Although some variants have strong evidence supporting treatment recommendations, many currently do not yet. Multidisciplinary committees charged with reviewing the level of evidence for each genetic result and providing clinically actionable recommendations will be essential for translating these multigene tumor assay results into routine clinical practice. Decision tools and development of treatment guidelines will further assist with routine integration of this technology, especially for oncologists at smaller practice sites. Oncology fellowship training programs will also need to be expanded to ensure competence of new practitioners in the area of genomic-guided therapies.

Regardless of these challenges, the treatment paradigm of genomic-driven medicine and individualizing therapy has permitted the field of oncology to move beyond the limitations of nonselective cytotoxic therapy and toward the more optimal selection and dosing of oncology agents.

SELECTED REFERENCES

The full reference list can be accessed at lwwhealthlibrary.com/oncology.

1. McLeod HL. Cancer pharmacogenomics: early promise, but concerted effort needed. *Science* 2013;339:1563–1566.
2. Garraway LA. Genomics-driven oncology: framework for an emerging paradigm. *J Clin Oncol* 2013;31:1806–1814.
4. Evans WE, Relling MV. Pharmacogenomics: translating functional genomics into rational therapeutics. *Science* 1999;286:487–491.
5. Wang L, McLeod HL, Weinshilboum RM. Genomics and drug response. *N Engl J Med* 2011;364:1144–1153.
6. Druker BJ. Translation of the Philadelphia chromosome into therapy for CML. *Blood* 2008;112:4808–4817.
8. Druker BJ, Guilhot F, O'Brien SG, et al. Five-year follow-up of patients receiving imatinib for chronic myeloid leukemia. *N Engl J Med* 2006;355:2408–2417.
9. Hudis CA. Trastuzumab—mechanism of action and use in clinical practice. *N Engl J Med* 2007;357:39–51.
12. Bardelli A, Siena S. Molecular mechanisms of resistance to cetuximab and panitumumab in colorectal cancer. *J Clin Oncol* 2010;28:1254–1261.
13. Jimeno A, Messersmith WA, Hirsch FR, et al. KRAS mutations and sensitivity to epidermal growth factor receptor inhibitors in colorectal cancer: practical application of patient selection. *J Clin Oncol* 2009;27:1130–1136.
15. Chapman PB, Hauschild A, Robert C, et al. Improved survival with vemurafenib in melanoma with BRAF V600E mutation. *N Engl J Med* 2011;364:2507–2516.
17. Trunzer K, Pavlick AC, Schuchter L, et al. Pharmacodynamic effects and mechanisms of resistance to vemurafenib in patients with metastatic melanoma. *J Clin Oncol* 2013;31:1767–1774.
18. Flaherty KT, Infante JR, Daud A, et al. Combined BRAF and MEK inhibition in melanoma with BRAF V600 mutations. *N Engl J Med* 2012;367:1694–1703.
21. Ramaswamy S, Golub T. DNA microarrays in clinical oncology. *J Clin Oncol* 2002;20:1932–1941.
22. Paik S, Shak S, Tang G, et al. A multigene assay to predict recurrence of tamoxifen-treated, node-negative breast cancer. *N Engl J Med* 2004;351:2817–2826.
24. Lipson D, Capelletti M, Yelensky R, et al. Identification of new ALK and RET gene fusions from colorectal and lung cancer biopsies. *Nat Med* 2012;18:382–384.

25. Diaz LA Jr, Bardelli A. Liquid biopsies: genotyping circulating tumor DNA. *J Clin Oncol* 2014;32:579–586.
27. Evans W, Relling M. Pharmacogenomics: translating functional genomics into rational therapeutics. *Science* 1999;286:487–491.
30. McLeod H, Krynetski EY, Relling MV, et al. Genetic polymorphism of thiopurine methyltransferase and its clinical relevance for childhood acute lymphoblastic leukemia. *Leukemia* 2000;14:567–572.
33. Relling MV, Gardner EE, Sandborn WJ, et al. Clinical pharmacogenetics implementation consortium guidelines for thiopurine methyltransferase genotype and thiopurine dosing: 2013 update. *Clin Pharmacol Ther* 2013;93:324–325.
34. Caudle KE, Thorn CF, Klein TE, et al. Clinical Pharmacogenetics Implementation Consortium guidelines for dihydropyrimidine dehydrogenase genotype and fluoropyrimidine dosing. *Clin Pharmacol Ther* 2013;94:640–645.
37. Ridge S, Sludden J, Wei X, et al. Dihydropyrimidine dehydrogenase pharmacogenetics in patients with colorectal cancer. *Br J Cancer* 1998;77:497–500.
40. Mürdter TE, Schroth W, Bacchus-Gerybadze L, et al. Activity levels of tamoxifen metabolites at the estrogen receptor and the impact of genetic polymorphisms of phase I and II enzymes on their concentration levels in plasma. *Clin Pharmacol Ther* 2011;89:708–717.
41. Desta Z, Ward BA, Soukhova NV, et al. Comprehensive evaluation of tamoxifen sequential biotransformation by the human cytochrome P450 system in vitro: prominent roles for CYP3A and CYP2D6. *J Pharmacol Exp Ther* 2004;310:1062–1075.
43. Crews KR, Gaedigk A, Dunnenberger HM, et al. Clinical Pharmacogenetics Implementation Consortium (CPIC) guidelines for codeine therapy in the context of cytochrome P450 2D6 (CYP2D6) genotype. *Clin Pharmacol Ther* 2012;91:321–326.
44. Schroth W, Goetz MP, Hamann U, et al. Association between CYP2D6 polymorphisms and outcomes among women with early stage breast cancer treated with tamoxifen. *JAMA* 2009;302:1429–1436.
45. Province MA, Goetz MP, Brauch H, et al. CYP2D6 genotype and adjuvant tamoxifen: meta-analysis of heterogeneous study populations. *Clin Pharmacol Ther* 2014;95:216–227.
46. Irvin WJ Jr, Walko CM, Weck KE, et al. Genotype-guided tamoxifen dosing increases active metabolite exposure in women with reduced CYP2D6 metabolism: a multicenter study. *J Clin Oncol* 2011;29:3232–3239.

17 Alkylating Agents

Kenneth D. Tew

PERSPECTIVES

Alkylating agents were the first anticancer molecules developed, and they are still used today. After more than 50 years of use, the basic chemistry and pharmacology of this drug family is well understood and has not changed substantially. The family contains six major classes: nitrogen mustards, aziridines, alkyl sulfonates, epoxides, nitrosoureas, and triazene compounds, although a few nonstandard agents have recently been developed. Most epoxides tend to be quite nonspecific with respect to their reactivity and, as such, few have useful clinical characteristics. This chapter provides perspective on how the limited varieties of alkylating agents continue to be useful in the therapeutic management of cancer patients.

The alkylating agents are a diverse group of anticancer agents with the commonality that they react in a manner such that an electrophilic alkyl group or a substituted alkyl group can covalently bind to cellular nucleophilic sites. Electrophilicity is achieved through the formation of carbonium ion intermediates and can result in transition complexes with target molecules. Ultimately, reactions result in the formation of covalent linkages by alkylation with a broad range of nucleophilic groups, including bases in DNA, and these are believed responsible for ultimate cytotoxicity and therapeutic effect. Although the alkylating agents react with cells in all phases of the cell cycle, their efficacy and toxicity result from interference with rapidly proliferating tissues. From a historical perspective, the vesicant properties of mustard gas used during World War I were shown to be accompanied by the suppression of lymphoid and hematologic functions in experimental animals[1] and led to the development of mechlorethamine as the first alkylating agent used in the management of human cancer.[2] Subsequently, a number of related drugs have been developed, and these have roles in the treatment of a range of leukemias, lymphomas, and solid tumors. Most of the alkylating agents cause dose-limiting toxicities to the bone marrow and, to a lesser degree, the intestinal mucosa, with other organ systems also affected contingent on the individual drug, dosage, and duration of therapy. Despite the present trend toward targeted therapies, this class of "nonspecific" drugs maintains an essential role in cancer chemotherapy.

Because of the classic nature of the drug family, there have been relatively few advances in either their use or utility since publication of the previous edition of this book.

CHEMISTRY

Alkylating reactions are generally classified through their kinetic properties as S_N1 (nucleophilic substitution, first order) or S_N2 (nucleophilic substitution, second order) (Fig. 17.1). The first-order kinetics of the S_N1 reactions depend on the concentration of the original alkylating agent. The rate-limiting step is the initial formation of the reactive intermediate, and the rate is essentially independent of the concentration of the substrate. The S_N2 alkylation reaction is a bimolecular nucleophilic displacement with second-order kinetics, where the rate depends on the concentration of both alkylating agent and target nucleophile. Reactivity of electrophiles[3] suggests that the rates of alkylation of cellular nucleophiles (including thiols, phosphates, amino and imidazole groups of amino acids, and various reactive sites in nucleic acid bases) are most dependent on their potential energy states, which can be defined as "hard" or "soft," based on the polarizability of their reactive centers.[4] Although the metabolism and metabolites of nitrogen mustards and nitrosoureas differ, the active alkylating species of each is the alkyl carbonium ion (see Fig. 17.1), a highly polarized hard electrophile as a consequence of its highly positive charge density at the electrophilic center. Alkyl carbonium ions will react most readily with hard nucleophiles (possessing a highly polarized negative charge density), where the high-energy transition state (a potential energy barrier to the reaction) is most favorable. In specific terms, an active alkylating species from a nitrogen mustard will demonstrate selectivity for cellular nucleophiles in the following order: (1) oxygen in phosphate groups of RNA and DNA, (2) oxygens of purines and pyrimidines, (3) amino groups of purine bases, (4) primary and secondary amino groups of proteins, (5) sulfur atoms of methionine, and (6) thiol groups of cysteinyl residues of protein and glutathione.[3] The least favored reactions will still occur, but at much slower rates unless they are catalyzed.

Alkylation through highly reactive intermediates (e.g., mechlorethamine) would be expected to be less selective in their targets than the less reactive S_N2 reagents (e.g., busulfan). However, the therapeutic and toxic effects of alkylating agents do not correlate directly with their chemical reactivity. Clinically useful agents include drugs with S_N1 or S_N2 characteristics, and some with both.[5] These differ in their toxicity profiles and antitumor activity, but more as a consequence of differences in pharmacokinetics, lipid solubility, penetration of the central nervous system (CNS), membrane transport, metabolism and detoxification, and specific enzymatic reactions capable of repairing alkylation sites on DNA.

CLASSIFICATION

The major classes of clinically useful alkylating agents are illustrated in Table 17.1 and summarized in the following sections. Doses and schedules of the various agents are shown in Table 17.2.

Alkyl Sulfonates

Busulfan is used for the treatment of chronic myelogenous leukemia. It exhibits S_N2 alkylation kinetics and shows nucleophilic selectivity for thiol groups, suggesting that it may exert cytotoxicity through protein alkylation rather than through DNA. In contrast to the nitrogen mustards and nitrosoureas, busulfan has a greater effect on myeloid cells than lymphoid cells, thus the reason for its use against chronic myelogenous leukemia.[6]

Aziridines

Aziridines are analogs of ring-closed intermediates of nitrogen mustards and are less chemically reactive, but they have

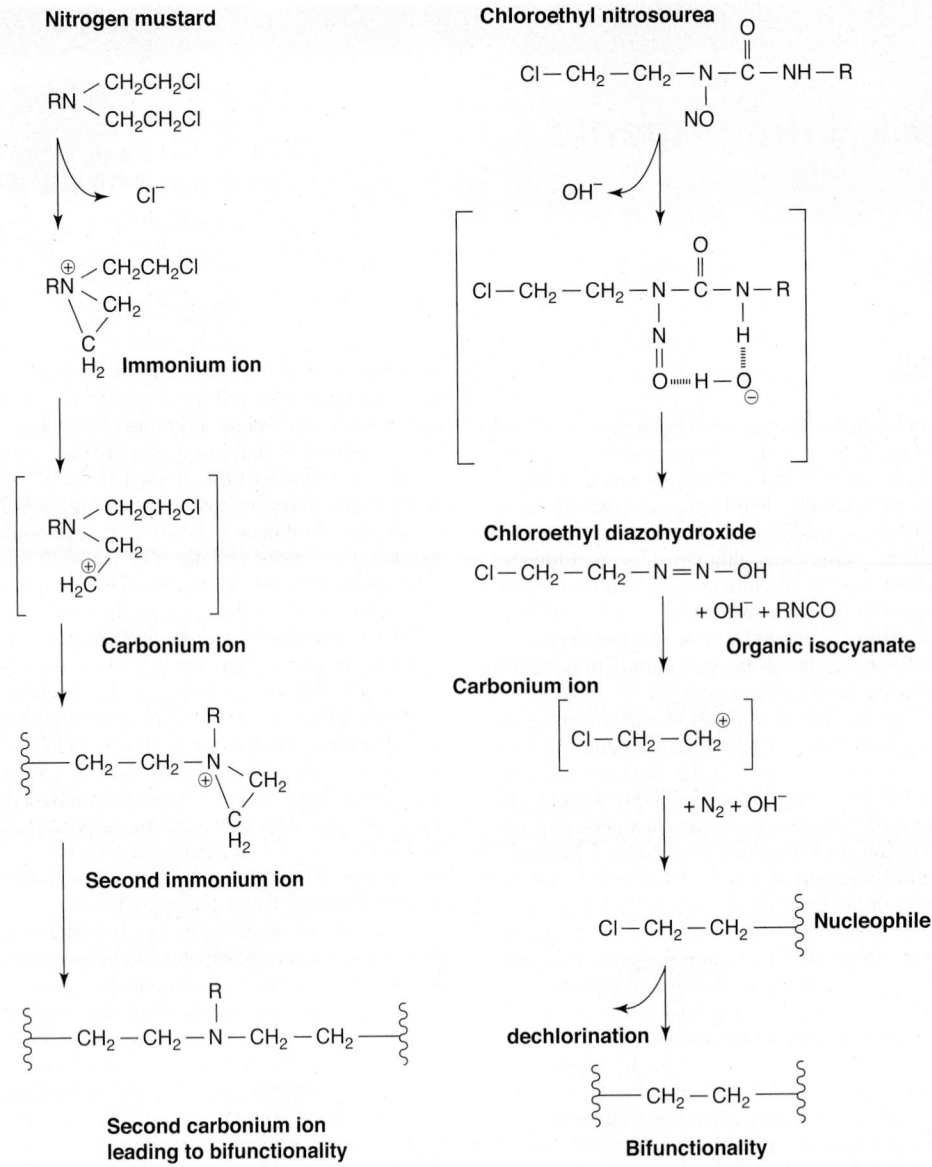

Figure 17.1 Comparative decomposition and metabolism of a typical nitrogen mustard compared to a nitrosourea. Although intermediate metabolites are distinct, the active alkylating species is a carbonium ion in each case. This electrophilic moiety reacts with target cellular nucleophiles.

equivalent therapeutic properties. Thiotepa has been used in the treatment of carcinoma of the breast, ovary, for a variety of CNS diseases, and with increasing frequency as a component of high-dose chemotherapy regimens.[7] Thiotepa and its primary desulfurated metabolite triethylenethiophosphoramide (TEPA) alkylate through aziridine ring openings, a mechanism similar to the nitrogen mustards.

Triazines

Perhaps the newest clinical development in the alkylating agent field is the emergence of temozolomide (TMZ). This agent acts as a prodrug and is an imidazotetrazine analog that undergoes spontaneous activation in solution to produce 5-(3-methyltriazen-1-yl) imidazole-4-carboxamide (MTIC), a triazine derivative. It crosses the blood–brain barrier with concentrations in the CNS approximating 30% of plasma concentrations.[8] Resistance to the methylating agent occurs quite frequently and has adversely affected the rate and durability of the clinical responses of patients. However, because of its favorable toxicity and pharmacokinetics, TMZ is

being combined with numerous other classes of anticancer drugs in an effort to improve response rates in diseases such as malignant melanomas, gliomas, brain metastasis from solid tumors, and refractory leukemias. Many of these trials are currently underway.[9]

Nitrogen Mustards

Bischloroethylamines or nitrogen mustards are extensively administered in the clinic. As an initial step in alkylation, chlorine acts as a leaving group and the β-carbon reacts with the nucleophilic nitrogen atom to form the cyclic, positively charged, reactive aziridinium moiety. Reaction of the aziridinium ring with an electron-rich nucleophile creates an initial alkylation product. The remaining chloroethyl group achieves bifunctionality through the formation of a second aziridinium. Melphalan (L-phenylalanine mustard), chlorambucil, cyclophosphamide, and ifosfamide (see Table 17.1) replaced mechlorethamine as primary therapeutic agents. These derivatives have electron-withdrawing groups substituted on the nitrogen atom, reducing the nucleophilicity of the nitrogen and rendering them less reactive, but enhancing their antitumor efficacy.

TABLE 17.1

Major Classes of Clinically Useful Alkylating Agents

Drug	Main Therapeutic Uses	Clinical Pharmacology	Major Toxicities	Notes
ALKYL SULFONATES				
Busulfan	Bone marrow transplantation, especially in chronic myelogenous leukemia	Bioavailability, 80%; protein bound, 33%; $t_{1/2}$, 2.5 h	Pulmonary fibrosis, hyperpigmentation thrombocytopenia, lowered blood platelet count and activity	Oral or parenteral; high dose causes hepatic veno-occlusive disease
ETHYLENEIMINES/METHYLMELAMINES				
Altretamine		Protein bound, 94%; $t_{1/2}$, 5–10 h	Nausea, vomiting, diarrhea, and neurotoxicity	Not widely used
Thio TEPA	Breast, ovarian, and bladder cancer; also bone marrow transplant	$t_{1/2}$, 2.5 h; urinary excretion at 24 h, 25%; substrate for CYP2B6 and CYP2C11	Myelosuppression	Nadirs of leukopenia, occur 2 wk; thrombocytopenia, 3 wk (correlates with AUC of parent drug)
NITROGEN MUSTARDS				
Mechlorethamine	Hodgkin lymphoma		Nausea, vomiting, myelosuppression	Precursor for other clinical mustards
Melphalan (L-phenylalanine mustard)	Multiple myeloma and ovarian cancer, and occasionally malignant melanoma	Bioavailability 25%–90%; $t_{1/2}$, 1.5 h; urinary excretion at 24 h, 13%; clearance, 9 mL/min/kg	Nausea, vomiting, myelosuppression	Causes less mucosal damage than others in class
Chlorambucil	Chronic lymphocytic leukemia	$t_{1/2}$, 1.5 h; urinary excretion at 24 h, 50%	Myelosuppression, gastrointestinal distress, CNS, skin reactions, hepatotoxicity	Oral
Cyclophosphamide	Variety of lymphomas, leukemias, and solid tumors	Bioavailability, >75%; protein bound, >60%; $t_{1/2}$, 3–12 h; urinary excretion at 24 h, <15%	Nausea and vomiting, bone marrow suppression, diarrhea, darkening of the skin/nails, alopecia (hair loss), lethargy, hemorrhagic cystitis	IV; primary excretion route is urine
Ifosfamide	Testicular, breast cancer; lymphoma (non-Hodgkin); soft tissue sarcoma; osteogenic sarcoma; lung, cervical, ovarian, bone cancer	$t_{1/2}$, 15 h; urinary excretion at 24 h, 15%	As for cyclophosphamide	Ifosfamide is often used in conjunction with mesna to avoid cystinuria
NITROSOUREAS				
Carmustine	Glioma, glioblastoma multiforme, medulloblastoma and astrocytoma, multiple myeloma and lymphoma (Hodgkin and non-Hodgkin)	Bioavailability, 25%; protein bound, 80%; $t_{1/2}$, 30 min	Bone marrow and pulmonary toxicities are a function of lifetime cumulative dose	Clinically, nitrosoureas do not share cross-resistance with nitrogen mustards in lymphoma treatment
Streptozotocin	Cancers of the islets of Langerhans	$t_{1/2}$, 35 min; excreted in the urine (15%), feces (<1%), and in the expired air	Nausea and vomiting; nephrotoxicity can range from transient protein urea and azotemia to permanent tubular damage; can also cause aberrations of glucose metabolism	A natural product from *Streptomyces achromogenes*
TRIAZENES				
Dacarbazine	Malignant melanoma and Hodgkin lymphoma	$t_{1/2}$, 5 h; protein bound, 5% hepatic metabolism	Nausea, vomiting, myelosuppression	IV or IM
Temozolomide	Glioblastoma; astrocytoma; metastatic melanoma	Protein bound, 15%; $t_{1/2}$, 1.8 h; clearance, 5.5 l/h/m^2	Nausea, vomiting, myelosuppression	Oral; derivative of imidazotetrazine, prodrug of dacarbazine; rapidly absorbed

$t_{1/2}$, half-life; TEPA, triethylenethiophosphoramide; AUC, area under curve; CNS, central nervous system; IV, intravenous; IM, intramuscular.

CANCER THERAPEUTICS

TABLE 17.2

Dose and Schedules of Clinically Useful Alkylating Agents

Alkylating Agent	Disease Sites and Dose Ranges Used Clinically	Notes

BCNU (Carmustine)	General antineoplastic
	150–200 mg/m^2 (IV, every 6 wks)
	Cutaneous T-cell lymphoma 200–600 mg
	  (topical solution)
	Adjunct to surgical resection of brain tumor
	  61.6 mg (implant)
		Infusion 1–2 h; in combination, dose usually reduced by
		  25%–50%
		Side effects include irritant dermatitis, telangiectasia,
		  erythema, and bone marrow suppression
		Up to 8 wafers (7.7 mg of carmustine) implanted

Busulfan	Chronic myelogenous leukemia and myeloproliferative disorders 4–8 mg (daily PO) 1.8 mg/m^2 (daily PO) Bone marrow transplant 640 mg/m^2 (daily PO)	Dispensed over 3–4 d, with cyclophosphamide

Carboplatin	Advanced ovarian cancer—monotherapy
	360 mg/m^2 (IV, every 4 wks)
	Ovarian cancer—combination
	300 mg/m^2 (IV, every 4 wks for 6 cycles)
	Ovarian cancer—IP
	200–500 mg/m^2 (IP, 2 L dialysis fluid)
	Ovarian and other sites phase 1/2 setting—
	  high-dose therapy
	800–1,600 mg/m^2 (IV)
		With cyclophosphamide
		Patients usually receive marrow transplantation or
		  peripheral stem cell support

Cisplatin	Metastatic testicular cancer:
	20 mg/m^2/d for 5 d of each cycle (IV)
	Metastatic ovarian cancer:
	75–100 mg/m^2 (IV, once every 4 wks)
	Head and neck cancer:
	100 mg/m^2 (IV)
	Bladder cancer:
	(combination prior to cystectomy)
	50–70; initiate dosing at 50
	mg/m^2 (IV, once every 3–4 wks)
	Metastatic breast cancer:
	20 mg/m^2 (IV, days 1–5 every 3 wks)
	Cervical cancer:
	70 mg/m^2 (IV, dosing cycled every 4 wks)
	Non–small-cell lung cancer:
	75 mg/m^2 (IV, every 3 wks)
	Esophageal cancer:
	75 mg/m^2 on day 1 of wks 1, 5, 8, and 11 (IV)
		With other antineoplastic agents
		With cyclophosphamide (600 mg/m^2 once every 4 wks)
		With vincristine, bleomycin, and fluorouracil
		With methotrexate and fluorouracil
		MVAC regimen (methotrexate, vinblastine, doxorubicin,
		  and cisplatin) used for cervical cancer
		Administration preceded by paclitaxel 135 mg/m^2
		  every 3 wks
		With radiation therapy

Cyclophosphamide	General antineoplastic
	1–5 mg/kg (daily PO)
	40–50 mg/kg (IV, in divided doses over 2–5 d)
	40–50 mg/kg (IV, in divided doses over 2–5 d)
	10–15 mg/kg (IV, every 7–10 d)
	10–15 mg/kg (IV, every 7–10 d)
	3–5 mg/kg (IV twice per wk)
	High-dose regimen in bone marrow transplantation
	  and for other autoimmune disorders
	200 mg/kg (IV)
	1–2.5 mg/kg (daily PO 7–14 d/mo)
		Dose used as monotherapy for patients with no
		  hematologic toxicity

Dacarbazine	General antineoplastic 2–4.5 mg/kg/d (IV) 150 mg/m^2/d (IV)	Administered for 10 d, may be repeated at 4-week intervals With other anticancer agents; treatment lasts 5 d, may be repeated every 4 wks

Etoposide	Testicular cancer
	50–100 mg/m^2/day (IV, slow infusion over
	  30–60+ min for 5 d)
	Small cell lung cancer
	35–50 mg/m^2/day (IV, slow infusion over
	  30–60+ min for 4–5 d)
		Alternatively, 100 mg/m^2/d on days 1, 3, and 5 may
		  be used; doses for combination therapy and are
		  repeated at 3- to 4-wk intervals after recovery from
		  hematologic toxicity
		Doses are for combination therapy and repeated at 3- to
		  4-wk intervals after recovery from hematologic toxicity;
		  oral dose is twice the IV, rounded to the nearest 50 mg

(continued)

TABLE 17.2

Dose and Schedules of Clinically Useful Alkylating Agents *(continued)*

Ifosfamide	General antineoplastic 1.2 g/m^2/d (IV, for 5 consecutive days)	Repeat every 3 wks
Melphalan	Multiple myeloma: 16 mg/m^2 (IV, infusion over 15–20 min) 6 mg (daily PO) Epithelial ovarian cancer: 0.2 mg/kg (daily PO)	2-week intervals for 4 doses, 4-wk intervals thereafter After 2–3 wks treatment, should be discontinued for up to 4 wks, then reinstituted at 2–4 mg/d Daily dose for a 5-d course, repeated every 4–5 wks
Streptozotocin	Pancreatic tumors 500 mg/m^2/d; 1,000 mg/m^2/d (IV; IV)	500 mg for 5 consecutive days every 6 wks, 1,000 mg is for 2 wks, followed by an increase in weekly dose not to exceed 1,500 mg/m^2/wk
Temozolomide	Brain tumors 150 mg/m^2 (daily PO)	Dose adjusted on the basis of blood counts
Thiotepa	General antineoplastic: 0.3–0.4 mg/kg (IV) Papillary carcinoma of the bladder: 60 mg/wk for 4 wks (bladder catheter) Control of serous effusions: 0.6–0.8 mg/kg (intracavitary)	Rapid administration given at 1- to 4-wk intervals 30 or 60 mL should be retained for 2 h, so the patient is usually dehydrated prior to administration of the drug

IV, intravenously; PO, by mouth; IP, intraperitoneal.

One distinguishing feature of melphalan is that an amino acid transporter responsible for uptake influences its efficacy across cell membranes.[10] Although a number of glutathione (GSH) conjugates of alkylating agents are effluxed through adenosine triphosphate–dependent membrane transporters,[11] specific uptake mechanisms are generally rare for cancer drugs. Cyclophosphamide and ifosfamide are prodrugs that require cytochrome P-450 metabolism to release active alkylating species. Cyclophosphamide continues to be the most widely used alkylating agent and has activity against a variety of tumors.[12] A cost saving with equivalent therapeutic activity was recently shown in a modified regimen of high-dose cyclophosphamide plus cyclosporine in patients with severe or very severe aplastic anemia.[13]

Nitrosoureas

The nitrosoureas form a diverse class of alkylating agents that have a distinct metabolism and pharmacology that separates them from others.[14] Under physiologic conditions, proton abstraction by a hydroxyl ion initiates spontaneous decomposition of the molecule to yield a diazonium hydroxide and an isocyanate (see Fig. 17.1). The chloroethyl carbonium ion generated is the active alkylating species. Through a subsequent dehalogenation step, a second electrophilic site imparts bifunctionality.[15] Thus, while cross-linking may occur similar to those lesions caused by nitrogen mustards, the chemistry leading to the endpoint is distinct. The isocyanate species generated are also electrophilic, showing nucleophilic selectivity toward sulfhydryl and amino groups that can inhibit a number of enzymes involved in nucleic acid synthesis and thiol balance.[16] Because carbamoylation is considered of minor importance to the therapeutic efficacy of clinically used nitrosoureas, chlorozotocin and streptozotocin were designed to undergo internal carbamoylation at the 1- or 3-OH group of the glucose ring, with the consequence that no carbamoylating species are produced.[17,18] Streptozotocin is also unusual in that most methylnitrosoureas have only modest therapeutic value. However, its lack of bone marrow toxicity and strong diabetogenic effect in animals led to its use in cancer of the pancreas (see Table 17.1).[19] The dose-limiting toxicities in humans are gastrointestinal and renal, but the drug has considerably less hematopoietic toxicity than the other nitrosoureas. Because of their lipophilicity and capacity to cross the blood–brain barrier, the chloroethylnitrosoureas

were found to be effective against intracranially inoculated murine tumors. Indeed, early preclinical studies showed that many mouse tumors were quite responsive to nitrosoureas. The same extent of efficacy was not found in humans. Subsequent analyses demonstrated that an enzyme responsible for repair of O-6-alkyl guanine (O^6-methylguanine-DNA methyltransferase [MGMT], or the Mer/Mex phenotype)[20] was expressed at low levels in mice, but at high levels in humans, a contributory factor in the reduced clinical efficacy of nitrosoureas in humans. In the 1980s, in particular, a number of new nitrosoureas were tested in patients in Europe and Japan, but none established a regular role in standard cancer treatment regimens.

MGMT promoter methylation is crucial in MGMT gene silencing and can predict a favorable outcome in glioblastoma patients receiving alkylating agents.[21] This biomarker is on the verge of entering clinical decision making and is currently used to stratify or even select glioblastoma patients for clinical trials. In other subtypes of glioma, such as anaplastic gliomas, the relevance of MGMT promoter methylation might extend beyond the prediction of chemosensitivity, and could reflect a distinct molecular profile. At this time, the standardization of MGMT assays will be critical in establishing prospective prognostic or predictive effects. In addition, eventual clinical trials will need to determine, for each subtype of glioma, the extent to which methylation patterns are predictive or prognostic and whether such assays could be incorporated into an individualized approach to clinical practice.[21]

CLINICAL PHARMACOKINETICS/PHARMACODYNAMICS

The pharmacokinetics of the alkylating agents are highly variable depending on the individual agent. Nevertheless, they are generally characterized by high reactivity and short half-lives. Although detailed studies on clinical pharmacology are available,[22] Table 17.1 summarizes some of the primary kinetic characteristics of the major clinically useful drugs. Mechlorethamine is unstable and is administered rapidly in a running intravenous infusion to avoid its rapid breakdown to inactive metabolites. In contrast, chlorambucil and cyclophosphamide are sufficiently stable to be given orally, and are rapidly and completely absorbed from the gastrointestinal tract, whereas others like melphalan have poor and variable

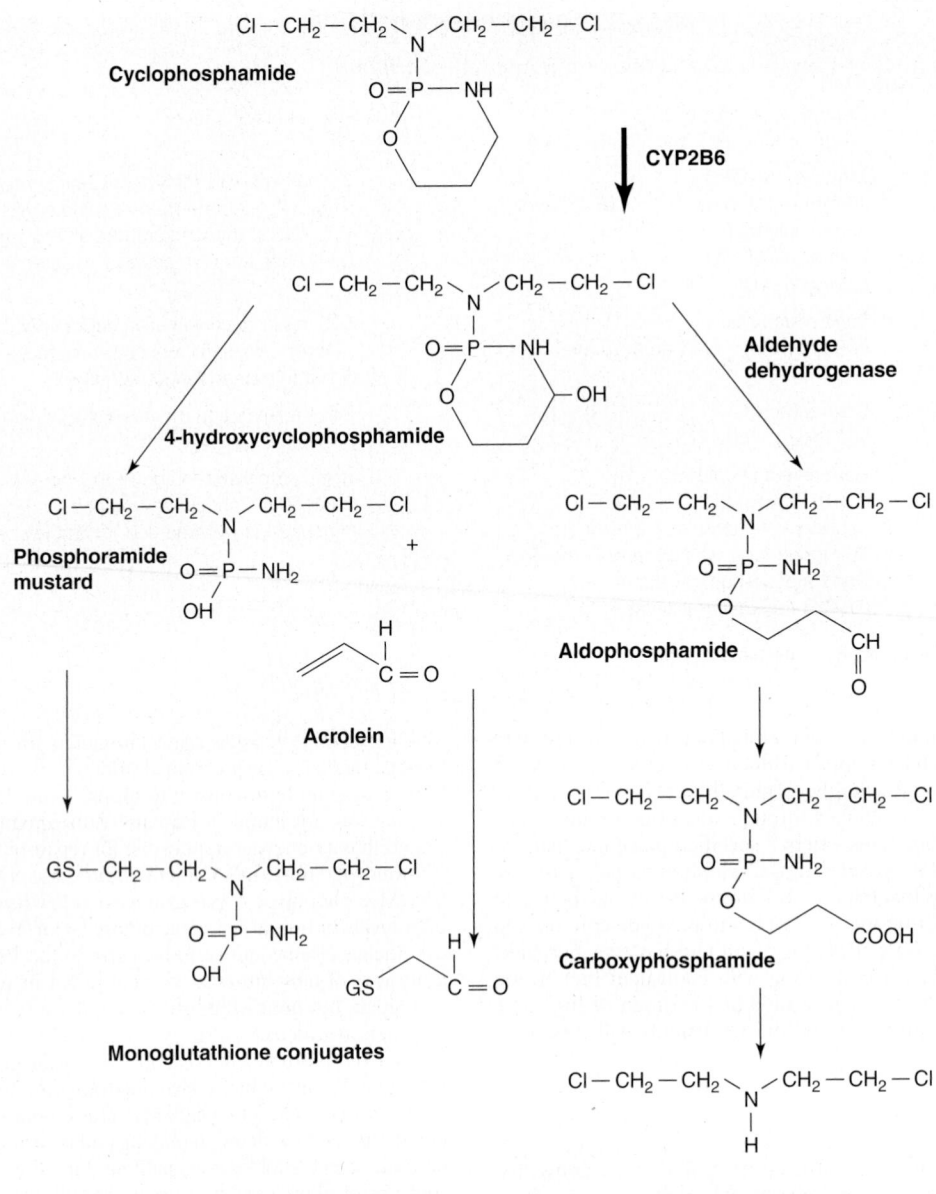

Figure 17.2 Activation and detoxification routes of metabolism for cyclophosphamide.

oral absorption. Cyclophosphamide,[23] ifosfamide, and dacarbazine are unusual in that they require activation by cytochrome P-450 in the liver before they can alkylate cellular constituents. The nitrosoureas also require activation, albeit nonenzymatic. The major route of metabolism of most alkylating agents is spontaneous hydrolysis, although many can also undergo some degree of enzymatic metabolism. This is particularly pertinent for phase II metabolic conversions where reactivity with nucleophilic thiols precedes conversion to mercapturates, with the result that most of the alkylating agents are excreted in the urine. One example of complex multistep metabolism is provided by cyclophosphamide (see Fig. 17.2). Activation by CYP2B6 is followed by the conversion of aldehyde dehydrogenase to reactive alkylating species or possible detoxification through GSH conjugation reactions. The latter is particularly important for acrolein because it is believed to contribute to the bladder toxicities associated with the drug.

The alkylating agents form covalent bonds with a number of nucleophilic groups present in proteins, RNA, and DNA (e.g., amino, carboxyl, sulfhydryl, imidazole, phosphate). Under physiologic conditions, the chloroethyl group of the nitrogen mustards undergoes cyclization, with the chloride acting as a leaving group forming an intermediate carbonium ion that attacks nucleophilic sites (see Fig. 17.1). Bifunctional alkylating agents (with two chloroethyl side chains) can undergo a subsequent cyclization to form a covalent bond with an adjacent nucleophilic group, resulting in DNA–DNA or DNA–protein cross-links. The N7 or O6 positions of guanine are particularly susceptible and may represent primary targets that determine both the cytotoxic and mutagenic consequences of therapy.[24] The nitrosoureas have a similar, but distinct, mechanism of action, spontaneously forming both alkylating and carbamoylating agents in aqueous media (see Fig. 17.1). The carbamoylating moieties are generally believed to be inconsequential to the therapeutic properties of the nitrosoureas.

THERAPEUTIC USES

The alkylating agents are frequently used in combination therapy to treat a variety of types of cancer. Perhaps the most versatile is cyclophosphamide, whereas the other alkylating agents are of more restricted clinical use. Because of early successes, many disease states are managed with drug combinations that contain several alkylating agents. Cyclophosphamide is employed to treat a variety of immune-related diseases and to purge bone marrow in autologous marrow transplant situations.[25] A general summary of the clinical uses of the primary alkylating agents is shown in Table 17.1.

TOXICITIES

The alkylating agents show significant qualitative and quantitative variability in the sites and severities of their toxicities. The primary dose-limiting toxicity is suppression of bone marrow function, with secondary limiting effects on the proliferating cells of the intestinal mucosa.

Contraindications to the use of alkylating agents would identify patients with severely depressed bone marrow function and patients with hypersensitivity to these drugs. Other listed precautions to these drugs include carcinogenic and mutagenic effects and impairment of fertility. Precaution is also advised in patients with (1) leukopenia or thrombocytopenia, (2) previous exposure to chemotherapy or radiotherapy, (3) tumor cell infiltration of the bone marrow, and (4) impaired renal or hepatic function. These drugs can also increase toxicity in adrenalectomized patients and interfere with wound healing. A brief summary of dose-limiting toxicities is shown in Table 17.1, and a narrative of each follows here.

Nausea and Vomiting

Nausea and vomiting are frequent side effects of alkylating agent therapy and are not well controlled by conventional antiemetics.[24] They are a major source of patient discomfort and a significant cause of lack of drug compliance and even discontinuation of therapy. Frequency and extent are highly variable among patients. The overall frequency of nausea and vomiting is directly proportional to the dose of alkylating agent. The onset of nausea may occur within a few minutes of the administration of the drug or may be delayed for several hours.

Bone Marrow Toxicity

Bone marrow toxicity can involve all of the blood elements, leukocytes, platelets, and red cells.[26] The extent and time course of suppression show marked interindividual fluctuation. Relative platelet sparing is a characteristic of cyclophosphamide treatment. Even at the very high doses (<200 mg/kg) of cyclophosphamide (used in preparation for bone marrow transplantation), some recovery of hematopoietic elements occurs within 21 to 28 days. This stem cell–sparing property is further reflected by the fact that cumulative damage to the bone marrow is rarely seen when cyclophosphamide is given as a single agent, and repeated high doses can be given without progressive lowering of leukocyte and platelet counts. The biochemical basis for the stem cell–sparing effect of cyclophosphamide is related to the presence of high levels of aldehyde dehydrogenase in early bone marrow progenitor cells (see Fig. 17.2). Busulfan is particularly toxic to bone marrow stem cells,[26] and treatment can lead to prolonged hypoplasia. The hematopoietic depression produced by the nitrosoureas is characteristically delayed. The onset of leukocyte and platelet depression occurs 3 to 4 weeks after drug administration and may last an additional 2 to 3 weeks.[22,26] Thrombocytopenia appears earlier and usually is more severe than leukopenia. Even if the nitrosourea is given at 6-week intervals, hematopoietic recovery may not occur between courses, and the drug dose often must be decreased when repeated courses are used.

Renal and Bladder Toxicity

Hemorrhagic cystitis is unique to the oxazaphosphorines (cyclophosphamide and ifosfamide) and may range from a mild cystitis to severe bladder damage with massive hemorrhage.[27] This toxicity is caused by the excretion of toxic metabolites (particularly acrolein) (see Fig. 17.2) in the urine, with subsequent direct irritation of the bladder mucosa. The incidence and severity can be lessened by adequate hydration and continuous irrigation of the bladder with a solution containing 2-mercaptoethane sulfonate (MESNA) and frequent bladder emptying.[26] MESNA is given in divided doses every 4 hours in dosages of 60% of those of the alkylating agent.

At high cumulative doses, all commonly used nitrosoureas can produce a dose-related renal toxicity that can result in renal failure and death.[29] In patients developing clinical evidence of toxicity, increases in serum creatinine usually appear after the completion of therapy and may be first detected up to 2 years after treatment.

Interstitial Pneumonitis and Pulmonary Fibrosis

Long-term busulfan therapy can lead to the gradual onset of fever, a nonproductive cough, and dyspnea, followed by tachypnea and cyanosis, and progressing to severe pulmonary insufficiency and death.[30] If busulfan is stopped before the onset of clinical symptoms, pulmonary function may stabilize, but if clinical symptoms are manifest, the condition may be rapidly fatal. Cyclophosphamide, bischloroethylnitrosourea, and methyl-1-(2-chloroethyl)-3-cyclohexyl-1-nitrosourea in cumulative doses exceeding 1,000 mg/m^2 may also lead to similar side effects.[31] Other alkylating agents, including melphalan, chlorambucil, and mitomycin C, can lead to pulmonary fibrosis after therapy.[32] This effect is probably caused by a direct cytotoxicity of the alkylating agent to pulmonary epithelium, resulting in alveolitis and fibrosis.

Gonadal Toxicity, Teratogenesis, and Carcinogenesis

Alkylating agents can have profound toxic effects on reproductive tissue.[33] A depletion of testicular germ (but not Sertoli) cells is accompanied by aspermia. In patients with a total absence of germ cells, an increase in plasma levels of follicle-stimulating hormone occurs. However, patients in remission and off alkylating agents for 2 to 7 years show complete spermatogenesis, indicating that testicular damage is reversible.

In women, a high incidence of amenorrhea and ovarian atrophy is associated with cyclophosphamide or melphalan therapy.[34] This seems to be age related because it developed after lower doses in older compared with younger patients, and was less likely to be reversible in the older cohort. A pathologic analysis reveals the absence of mature or primordial follicles, and endocrinology studies demonstrate decreased estrogen and progesterone levels and elevated serum follicle-stimulating hormone and luteinizing hormone levels typical of menopause.

The DNA-damaging properties of alkylating agents ensure that they are all teratogenic and carcinogenic to some degree. The administration of alkylating agents during the first trimester of pregnancy presents a definitive risk of a malformed fetus, but the administration of such drugs during the second and third trimesters does not increase the risk of fetal malformation above normal.[35]

Development of second cancer as a consequence of alkylating agent therapy has been documented. For example, a fulminant acute myeloid leukemia characterized by a preceding phase of myelodysplasia is found in some patients treated with melphalan, cyclophosphamide (which is much less leukemogenic than melphalan), chlorambucil, and the nitrosoureas.[33] This circumstance probably reflects the fact that these have been the most widely used of the alkylating agents. Also, the preponderance of patients with multiple myeloma, Hodgkin lymphoma, and carcinoma of the ovary in the reports of leukemogenesis is probably because patients with these diseases may have good responses and are often treated with alkylating agents for a number of years. The rate of occurrence of acute leukemia in patients with ovarian cancer who survive for 10 years after treatment with alkylating agents might be as high as 10%. Acute leukemia has been the most frequently described second malignancy, and it usually develops 1 to 4 years after drug exposure.[36] Other malignancies, including solid tumors, also have been reported to develop in patients treated with alkylating agents.[37]

The last four decades have yielded a significant improvement in the survival of children diagnosed with cancer (5-year survival is approximately 80%). As many as two-thirds of the survivors of childhood malignancies can experience delayed drug toxicities that may be severe or even life threatening. Such complications include impairment in growth and development, neurocognitive dysfunction, cardiopulmonary compromise, endocrine dysfunction, renal impairment, gastrointestinal dysfunction, musculoskeletal sequelae, and second cancers.[38]

Alopecia

The degree of alopecia after cyclophosphamide administration may be quite severe, especially when this drug is used in combination with vincristine sulfate or doxorubicin hydrochloride.[39] Regrowth of hair inevitably occurs after the cessation of therapy, but may be associated with a change in the color and greater curl. Use of a tourniquet or ice pack applied to the scalp during and for a short period after cyclophosphamide administration reduces the impact.

Allergic Reactions

Alkylating agents covalently bind to proteins, and these conjugates can act as haptens and produce allergic reactions.[40] An increasing number of reports of skin eruption, angioneurotic edema, urticaria, and anaphylactic reactions after the systemic administration of alkylating agents have appeared.

Immunosuppression

Alkylating agents suppress both humoral and cellular immunity in a variety of experimental systems.[41] The most immunosuppressive is cyclophosphamide, reported to cause (1) selective suppression of B-lymphocyte function, (2) depletion of B-lymphocytes, and (3) suppression of lymphocyte functions that are mediated by T cells, such as the graft-versus-host response and delayed hypersensitivity. Most intermittent antitumor regimens do not uniformly produce profound immunosuppression, and recovery is usually prompt. Sustained drug treatments can lead to severe lymphocyte depletion and profound immunosuppression and may be accompanied by an increase of viral, fungal, and protozoal infections.[41]

COMPLICATIONS WITH HIGH-DOSE ALKYLATING AGENT THERAPY

At standard doses, alkylating agents produce myelosuppression as their dose-limiting toxicity. Less severe effects on the gastrointestinal epithelium, lungs, bladder, and kidneys may become problems with long-term treatment, but rarely limit initial therapy. For this reason, and because of their steep dose response to tumor-killing curves, the alkylating agents have become a logical tool, either alone or in combination, for high-dose chemotherapy

regimens in which bone marrow toxicity is expected, and is accommodated by bone marrow transplantation, stem cell reconstitution from peripheral blood monocytes, and growth factor rescue. In this high-dose setting, toxicities that affect the gut, lungs, liver, and CNS become dose limiting and life threatening.[42] The highly lipid-soluble alkylators, especially ifosfamide, busulfan, the nitrosoureas, and thiotepa, cause CNS dysfunction, including seizures, altered mental status, cerebellar dysfunction, cranial nerve palsies, and coma.[43] High-dose ifosfamide is most frequently the cause of neurotoxicity.[44] Clinical manifestations of grade 4 neurotoxicities were reported in approximately one-fourth of those patients receiving ifosfamide. The side-chain N-linked chloroethyl moiety of ifosfamide (see Table 17.1) is more likely than the bischloroethyl group of cyclophosphamide to undergo oxidation and subsequent N-deethylation and lead to the formation of chloroacetaldehyde. High-dose busulfan is also frequently used in a variety of conditioning regimens for hematopoietic cell transplantation. In this setting, busulfan causes neurotoxicity manifesting in seizures that generally are tonic–clonic in character. Phenytoin has been the preferred drug to treat busulfan-induced seizures, although some emerging clinical data support the use of benzodiazepines, most notably clonazepam and lorazepam, to prevent busulfan-induced seizures. Moreover, the second-generation antiepileptic drug levetiracetam possesses the characteristics of optimal prophylaxis for busulfan-induced seizures.[45] At least one recent study has suggested that a polymorphism in the glutathione S-transferase A2 family may be predictive of transplant-related mortality after allogeneic stem cell transplantation,[46] perhaps indicating that a pharmacogenetic approach might be possible in this disease setting. Moreover, in a preclinical setting, a proteomic analysis identified thioredoxin as a potentially important adjuvant therapy in enhancing donor cell graft enhancement in bone marrow transplantation.[47] The possibility that this approach may benefit patients following alkylating agent–based ablation remains to be tested in a clinical setting.

Cyclophosphamide at doses exceeding 100 mg/kg during a 48-hour period (preparatory to bone marrow transplantation) can cause cardiac toxicity.[48] No evidence exists for cumulative damage to the heart after repeated moderate or low doses of the drug. Cardiac toxicity occurs with greatest frequency in patients older than 50 years or in those previously treated with anthracyclines.[48]

ALKYLATING AGENT–STEROID CONJUGATES

Adapting the rationale that steroid receptors may function to localize and concentrate attached drug species intracellularly in hormone-responsive cancers, a number of synthetic conjugates of nitrogen mustards and steroids have been developed. Of these, two made the transition into clinical use.

Prednimustine is an ester-linked conjugate of chlorambucil and prednisolone designed to function as a prodrug for chlorambucil. Release of the alkylating agent occurs after cleavage by serum esterases,[49] which can release the ester link of prednimustine, producing the hormone and active alkylating drug. The elimination phase of chlorambucil in patient plasma is significantly longer after the administration of prednimustine than after chlorambucil. Estramustine is a carbamate ester–linked conjugate of nor-nitrogen mustard and estradiol. Unlike prednimustine, the pharmacology of estramustine is governed by the presence of the carbamate group in the steroid–mustard linkage. The relative resistance of the carbamate bond to enzymatic cleavage eliminates the alkylating activity of the molecule and conveys an entirely new pharmacology.[50] The crystal structural and mechanism of action studies showed that estramustine has antimitotic activity, an activity shared by some other steroids.[51] Estramustine has found a clinical niche used in combination with other antimitotic drugs in the management of hormone refractory prostate cancer.[52]

DRUG RESISTANCE AND MODULATION

As with all drugs, intrinsic or acquired resistance to alkylating agents occurs and limits the therapeutic utility of this class of anticancer drugs.[53] A plethora of preclinical studies have characterized mechanisms by which cells develop resistance and, to a lesser degree, these have been shown to occur clinically. Because alkylating agents have a narrow therapeutic index, the emergence of resistance can have a significant impact on clinical success. Some of the factors that can contribute to the expression of resistance to alkylating agents include (1) alterations in drug uptake or transport, (2) increased repair of drug-induced nucleic acid damage, (3) failure to activate alkylating agent prodrugs, (4) increased scavenging of drug species by nonessential cellular nucleophiles, (5) increased enzymatic detoxification of drug species, and (6) altered expression of genes coding for cellular commitment to apoptosis.

RECENT DEVELOPMENTS

In the era of directed targeted therapies, the lack of specificity of alkylating agents would seem to limit the likelihood that novel drugs will be forthcoming. High toxicities, narrow therapeutic indices, and chemical instabilities are all properties that consign this drug class to the lower echelons of popularity in drug-discovery platforms. Although covalent bonding to specific target sites is one approach to direct targeting, the random electrophilic attraction toward nucleic acids and proteins is not an optimal property by today's standards. Nevertheless, the relative success of the alkylating agents in gaining therapeutic responses to diseases that are difficult to treat continues to serve as an impetus to use alkylating moieties as a means to kill cells. Some novel agents are presently in development. Cyclophosphamide and ifosfamide were prodrugs synthesized in the hope that high levels of phosphoamidase in epithelial tumors would selectively activate the drugs.[27] Other efforts to improve selectivity have centered on the synthesis of antibody–enzyme conjugates that bind to tumor-specific surface antigens. Enzymes frequently associated with the cell surface include peptidases, nitroreductases, and γ-glutamyl transpeptidase; to some degree, each has been targeted to cleave circulating alkylating prodrugs, thereby in a localized fashion releasing active alkylating species. Antibody-directed enzyme prodrug therapy is exemplified by the use of an antibody linked to the peptidase carboxypeptidase G-2, which releases an active alkylator from an inactive γ-glutamyl conjugate.[54] Linkage of the peptidase to any antibody that localizes selectively to a tumor cell membrane is a viable option. Expression of the peptidase on the cell surface then leads to prodrug activation and cell kill. Such approaches have had limited clinical impact to this time; however, their development does continue.

A further rationale for enhancing tumor-specific delivery takes advantage of the observation that glutathione-S-transferase *pi* (GSTP1-1) is preferentially expressed in a number of solid tumors and some lymphomas. In this case, the prodrug consists of an unusual alkylating agent conjugated to a substituted glutathione peptidomimetic. GSTP initiates the cleavage, thereby creating a cytotoxic alkylating species.[55] The initial canfosfamide design strategy relied on the principle that proton-abstracting sites at the active site of GST could initiate a cleavage reaction that would convert an inactive prodrug into a cytotoxic species. The presence of a histidine residue in proximity to the G binding site was integral to the removal of the sulfhydryl proton from the GSH cosubstrate, resulting in the generation of a nucleophilic sulfide anion. This moiety would be more reactive with electrophiles in the absence of GSH. Unlike other standard nitrogen mustard drugs, canfosfamide contains a tetrakis (chloroethyl) phosphorodiamidate moiety. Other compounds bearing this structure have been shown to be more cytotoxic than a similar structure with a single bis-(chloroethyl) amine group.[56]

As in other nitrogen mustards, the chlorines can act as leaving groups, thus creating aziridinium ions with electrophilic characteristics. Although the exact temporal or sequential formation of the four possible chlorine leaving events is not known, the assumption is that these species possess cytotoxic properties through their capacity to alkylate target nucleophiles, such as DNA bases. Tetrafunctionality could result in the formation of cross-links with bonding distances greater than for bifunctional agents. However, a number of caveats apply to this interpretation. For example, alkylating agents, whether mono-, bi-, or putatively tetrafunctional, generally lead to some form of myelosuppression. A number of clinical trials with canfosfamide have now been completed. These include, phase 1,[57] phase 1/2a,[58] phase 2,[59] and phase 3.[60] The phase 3 study was in platinum refractory ovarian cancer patients and proved negative for enhanced survival. Nevertheless, additional trials are still in progress.

Another targeting approach delivers the gene for a cytochrome P-450 isoenzyme to tumors by viral vector, thereby enhancing specific tumor cell activation of cyclophosphamide.[61] Because this therapy has its base in gene delivery technologies, successful development in humans will await further advances in this arena.

Laromustine is in the sulfonylhydrazine class of alkylating agents. It is presently in clinical development for the treatment of malignancies such as acute myelogenous leukemia (AML).[62] Similar to nitrosoureas, laromustine is a prodrug that yields a chloroethylating and a carbamoylating (methyl isocyanate) species. As with nitrosoureas, the cytotoxicity of laromustine is attributed primarily to the chloroethylating-mediated alkylation of DNA and subsequent interstrand cross-links.[63] The carbamoylating species can inhibit DNA repair and other cellular enzyme systems. Phase 1 trials in patients with solid tumors indicated the expected myelosuppression, although few extramedullary toxicities were observed, indicating potential efficacy in the treatment of hematologic malignancies. Phase 2 trials have been completed in patients with untreated AML, high-risk myelodysplastic syndrome, and relapsed AML. The most encouraging results have been found in patients older than 60 years with poor-risk, de novo AML for which no standard treatment exists. Laromustine is currently in phase 2/3 trials for AML and phase 2 trials for myelodysplastic syndrome and solid tumors.[64] Laromustine appears to be a promising agent in elderly patients who do not respond to or are not fit for intensive chemotherapy.

Although not a new drug, bendamustine is a unique cytotoxic agent with structural similarities to alkylating agents and antimetabolites, but it lacks cross-resistance with other established alkylating agents both in vitro and in the clinic.[65] Its mechanism of action is similar to other mustards in causing DNA intra- and interstrand cross-links. In comparison with other more commonly used alkylating agents, such as cyclophosphamide or phenylalanine mustard, more DNA double-strand breaks are formed at equitoxic dosages. Treatment with bendamustine induces a concentration-dependent apoptosis as evidenced by changes in Bcl-2 and Bax expression profiles in chronic B-cell lymphocytic leukemia.[66] DNA damage produced by bendamustine is repaired via base-excision repair mechanisms, implicating an unusual mode of action, which was recently confirmed through gene expression profiling analyses. This also provided an explanation for the lack of cross-resistance with other alkylating agents, as observed in vitro with anthracycline-resistant breast cancer and cisplatin-resistant ovarian cancer.[66,67]

Clinical studies conducted in Germany more than 30 years ago suggested activity in indolent non-Hodgkin lymphoma. Subsequent American trials showed responses in more than 70% of patients with drug refractory disease, with the implication that bendamustine may be the most effective drug in this patient population. Combinations of bendamustine and rituximab elicited response rates of 90% to 92%, with complete remission in 55% to 60% in follicular and mantle cell lymphoma. Superiority over chlorambucil in previously untreated patients with chronic lymphocytic leukemia (CLL) led to its recent approval for this disease in the United States. Bendamustine is approved in Germany for the treatment of patients with indolent non-Hodgkin lymphoma, CLL, and multiple myeloma. Activity has also been noted in patients with breast cancer and non–small-cell lung cancer.

Bendamustine has been used both as a single agent and in combination with other agents, including etoposide, fludarabine, mitoxantrone, methotrexate, prednisone, rituximab, and vincristine. A multicenter phase 2 trial in lymphomas had an overall response rate of 89%; (35% complete response and 54% partial response). In previously treated patients. the overall response rate was 76% (38% complete response and 38% partial response). The estimated median progression-free survival was 19 months.[67] In CLL patients, the drug is administered at 100 mg/m^2 intravenously over 30 minutes on days 1 and 2 of a 28-day cycle, for up to six cycles. Efficacy relative to first-line therapies other than chlorambucil has not been established. It is also indicated for the treatment of patients with indolent B-cell non-Hodgkin lymphoma that has progressed during, or within, 6 months of treatment with rituximab or rituximab-containing regimens. As with most alkylating agents, the primary dose-limiting toxicity is myelosuppression; nonhematologic toxicities were mild and included fatigue, nausea, loss of appetite, and vomiting. The optimization of dose and schedule, particularly relative to other drugs, and the management of toxicities has allowed its use in combination with a range of other chemotherapeutic agents, including prednisone, methotrexate, fludarabine, etoposide, mitoxantrone, vinca alkaloids, and rituximab. The availability of bendamustine provides another effective treatment option for patients with lymphoid malignancies, frequently reducing the side effects of the more standard cyclophosphamide, hydroxy doxorubicin, Oncovin, and prednisone (CHOP) regimen.[68] Recent approval by the U.S. Food and Drug Administration has allowed Cephalon, Inc. to market bendamustine under the trade name Treanda and, in combination with mitoxantrone and rituximab, it is now standard of care in indolent lymphomas. Trial results released in 2013 indicated that this combination more than doubled the progression-free survival in this disease[69] and there is early evidence that there may be utility in relapsed or refractory multiple myeloma.[70]

SELECTED REFERENCES

The full reference list can be accessed at lwwhealthlibrary.com/oncology.

1. Adair FE, Bagg HJ. Experimental and clinical studies on the treatment of cancer by dichlorethylsulphide (mustard gas). *Ann Surg* 1931;93(1):190–199.
6. Elson LA. Hematological effects of the alkylating agents. *Ann N Y Acad Sci* 1958;68(3):826–833.
10. Vistica DT. Cytotoxicity as an indicator for transport mechanism: evidence that murine bone marrow progenitor cells lack a high-affinity leucine carrier that transports melphalan in murine L1210 leukemia cells. *Blood* 1980;56(3):427–429.
13. Zhang F, Zhang L, Jing L, et al. (2013) High-dose cyclophosphamide compared with antithymocyte globulin for treatment of acquired severe aplastic anemia. *Exp Hematol* 2013;41:328–334.
19. Schein PS, O'Connell MJ, Blom J, et al. Clinical antitumor activity and toxicity of streptozotocin (NSC-85998). *Cancer* 1974;34(4):993–1000.
29. Schacht RG, Feiner HD, Gallo GR, et al. Nephrotoxicity of nitrosoureas. *Cancer* 1981;48(6):1328–1334.
31. Mark GJ, Lehimgar-Zadeh A, Ragsdale BD. Cyclophosphamide pneumonitis. *Thorax* 1978;33(1):89–93.
34. Miller JJ 3rd, Williams GF, Leissring JC. Multiple late complications of therapy with cyclophosphamide, including ovarian destruction. *Am J Med* 1971;50(4):530–535.
42. de Jonge ME, Huitema AD, Beijnen JH, et al. High exposures to bioactivated cyclophosphamide are related to the occurrence of veno-occlusive disease of the liver following high-dose chemotherapy. *Br J Cancer* 2006;94(9):1226–1230.
45. Eberly AL, Anderson GD, Bubalo JS, et al. Optimal prevention of seizures induced by high-dose busulfan. *Pharmacotherapy* 2008;28(12):1502–1510.
46. Bonifazi F, Storci G, Bandini G, et al. Glutathione transferase-A2 S112T polymorphism predicts survival, transplant-related mortality, busulfan and bilirubin blood levels after allogeneic stem cell transplantation. *Haematologica* 2014;99(1):172–179.
47. An N, Janech MG, Bland AM, et al. Proteomic analysis of murine bone marrow niche microenvironment identifies thioredoxin as a novel agent for radioprotection and for enhancing donor cell reconstitution. *Exp Hematol* 2013;41:944–956.
51. Punzi JS, Duax WL, Strong P, et al. Molecular conformation of estramustine and two analogues. *Mol Pharmacol* 1992;41(3):569–576.
54. Friedlos F, Davies L, Scanlon I, et al. Three new prodrugs for suicide gene therapy using carboxypeptidase G2 elicit bystander efficacy in two xenograft models. *Cancer Res* 2002;62(6):1724–1729.
58. Sequist LV, Fidias PM, Temel JS, et al. Phase 1–2a multicenter dose-ranging study of canfosfamide in combination with carboplatin and paclitaxel as first-line therapy for patients with advanced non-small cell lung cancer. *J Thorac Oncol* 2009;4(11):1389–1396.
61. Chase M, Chung RY, Chiocca EA. An oncolytic viral mutant that delivers the CYP2B1 transgene and augments cyclophosphamide chemotherapy. *Nat Biotechnol* 1998;16(5):444–448.
62. Vey N, Giles F. Laromustine (cloretazine). *Expert Opin Pharmacother* 2010;11(4):657–667.
64. Schiller GJ, O'Brien SM, Pigneux A, et al. Single-agent laromustine, a novel alkylating agent, has significant activity in older patients with previously untreated poor-risk acute myeloid leukemia. *J Clin Oncol* 2010;28(5):815–821.
69. van der Jagt R. Bendamustine for indolent non-Hodgkin lymphoma in the front-line or relapsed setting: a review of pharmacokinetics and clinical trial outcomes. *Expert Rev Hematol* 2013;6:525–537.
70. Ponisch W, Heyn S, Beck J, et al. Lenalidomide, bendamustine and prednisolone exhibits a favourable safety and efficacy profile in relapsed or refractory multiple myeloma: final results of a phase 1 clinical trial OSHO - #077. *Br J Haematol* 2013;162:202–209.

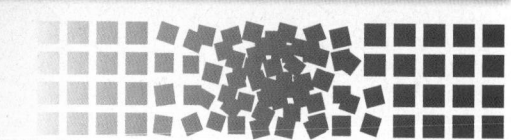

18 Platinum Analogs

Peter J. O'Dwyer and A. Hilary Calvert

INTRODUCTION

The platinum drugs represent a unique and important class of antitumor compounds. Alone or in combination with other chemotherapeutic agents, *cis*-diamminedichloroplatinum (II) (cisplatin) and its analogs have made a significant impact on the treatment of a variety of solid tumors for nearly 40 years. The unique activity and toxicity profile observed with cisplatin in early clinical trials fueled the development of platinum analogs that are less toxic and more active against a variety of tumor types, including those that have developed resistance to cisplatin. In addition to cisplatin, two other platinum complexes are currently approved for use in the United States: *cis*-diamminecyclobutanedicarboxylate platinum (II) (carboplatin) and 1,2-diaminocyclohexaneoxalato platinum (II) (oxaliplatin). Several other analogs with unique activities are in various stages of clinical development, and nedaplatin (Japan) and lobaplatin (China) are locally registered. Progress in the development of superior analogs requires a thorough understanding of the chemical, biologic, pharmacokinetic, and pharmacodynamic properties of this important class of drugs.

HISTORY

The realization that platinum complexes exhibited antitumor activity began serendipitously in a series of experiments to investigate the effect of electromagnetic radiation on the growth of bacteria, carried out by Dr. Barnett Rosenberg and colleagues beginning in 1961.[1,2] Exposure of the bacteria to an electric field resulted in a profound change in their morphology; this effect was found not to be from the electric field, but from electrolysis products produced by the platinum electrodes. An analysis of these products resulted in the identification of the cis-isomer of a platinum coordination complex as the active compound. Tests of *cis*-diamminedichloroplatinum (II) in mice bearing several model tumor types indicated that cisplatin exhibited a broad spectrum of antitumor activity. Although early clinical trials demonstrated responses in several tumor types, particularly testicular cancers, the severe renal and gastrointestinal toxicity caused by the drug nearly led to its abandonment. Work at Memorial Sloan-Kettering[3,4] showed that these effects could be ameliorated, in part, by aggressive prehydration, which rekindled interest in its clinical use. Currently, cisplatin is curative in testicular cancer and significantly prolongs survival in combination regimens for ovarian, lung, head and neck, bladder, and upper gastrointestinal (GI) cancers. Its role is being reexamined in other tumors, too, and especially breast cancer.

PLATINUM CHEMISTRY

Platinum exists primarily in either a 2+ or 4+ oxidation state. These oxidation states dictate the stereochemistry of the ligands surrounding the platinum atom. Platinum (II) compounds exhibit a square planar geometry, in which the ammine ligands (also called carrier groups) are relatively stable, whereas the opposite, more polar ligands (leaving groups) are more easily displaced and

so confer reactivity toward charged macromolecules, including DNA.[5] The stereochemistry of platinum complexes is critical to their antitumor activity as evidenced by the significantly reduced efficacy observed with *trans*-diamminedichloroplatinum (II).

In an aqueous solution, the chloride leaving groups of cisplatin are subject to mono- and diaqua substitution, particularly at chloride concentrations below 100 mmol, which characterize the intracellular environment. The administration of cisplatin in high chloride solutions (normal saline usually), therefore, contributes to stability. Intracellular formation of partially and fully aquated complexes creates the chloroaqua and hydroxoaqua cisplatin species that bind DNA.[6]

PLATINUM COMPLEXES AFTER CISPLATIN

Early in the clinical development of cisplatin, it became clear that its toxicity was a limitation to its therapeutic effectiveness, and that its activity, although striking in certain diseases, did not extend to all cancers. These observations then motivated a search for structural analogs with less toxicity and a different profile of antitumor activity. In addition, the side effects of cisplatin stimulated the development of antiemetics and other supportive care measures for use with chemotherapy. Progress in understanding the chemistry and pharmacokinetics of cisplatin has guided the development of new analogs. In general, modification of the chloride leaving groups of cisplatin results in compounds with different pharmacokinetics and reactivity towards DNA, whereas modification of the carrier ligands alters the activity of the resulting complex. The features of the more important platinum analogs that have been developed are shown in Figure 18.1.

Carboplatin

The carboplatin molecule has the same ammine carrier ligands as cisplatin. Using a murine screen for nephrotoxicity, Harrap and Calvert discovered that substituting a cyclobutanedicarboxylate moiety for the two chloride ligands of cisplatin resulted in a complex with reduced renal toxicity. This observation was translated to the clinic in the form of carboplatin, a more stable and pharmacokinetically predictable analog.[7,8] The results in humans were accurately predicted by the animal models, and marrow toxicity rather than nephrotoxicity was the principal side effect. At effective doses, carboplatin produced less nausea, vomiting, nephrotoxicity, and neurotoxicity than cisplatin. Furthermore, the myelosuppression was closely associated with the pharmacokinetics. The work of Calvert et al.[9] and Egorin and colleagues[10] showed that toxicity can be made more predictable and dose intensity less variable by dosing strategies based on the exposure. Carboplatin was shown to be indistinguishable from cisplatin in its clinical activity in all but a handful of tumor types and is the most frequently used form of platinum in current use. Cisplatin and carboplatin have almost superimposable profiles of activity in the NCI60 cell line screen, which further emphasizes the dependence of spectrum of activity on the carrier ligand.

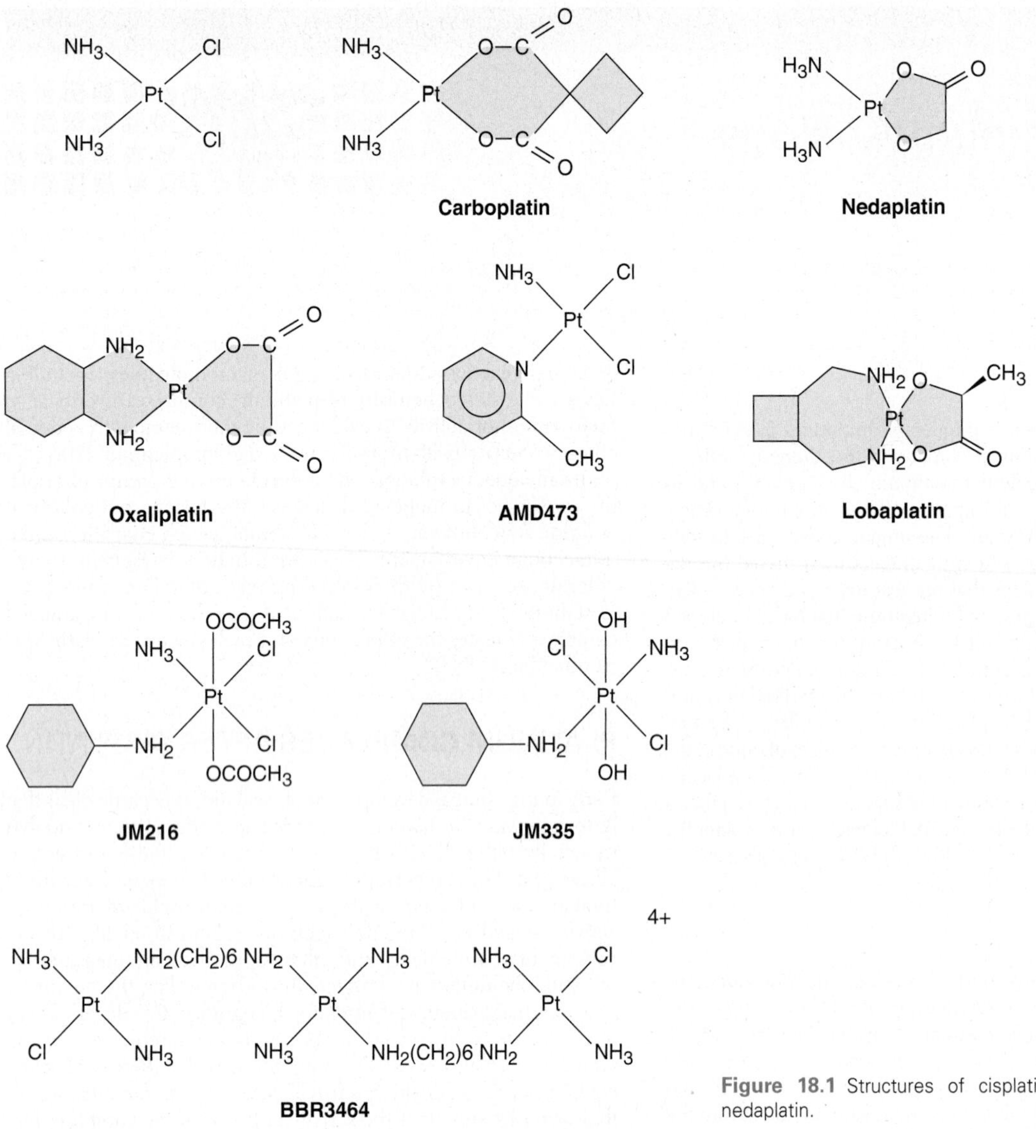

Figure 18.1 Structures of cisplatin, analogs, lobaplatin, and nedaplatin.

Oxaliplatin

Compounds with activity in cisplatin-resistant models emerged from modifications to the carrier group (see left side of the analogs in Fig. 18.1). Connors, in the late 1960s, synthesized platinum coordination compounds with varying physicochemical characteristics and found that the series that possessed a diaminocyclohexane (DACH) carrier group was active in models of cancer in vitro[11] and in vivo.[12] Subsequent studies supported the idea that DACH-based platinum complexes were non–cross-resistant with cisplatin, and DACH derivatives exhibited a unique cytotoxicity profile compared to cisplatin and carboplatin in the National Cancer Institute 60 cell line screen.[13–15] After a number of delays, a DACH analog that had been synthesized by Kidani and colleagues in the early 1970s, was developed in the clinic.[13] Oxaliplatin, a coordination compound of a DACH carrier group and an oxalato leaving group, was active in cisplatin-resistant tumor models. Like cisplatin, oxaliplatin preferentially forms adducts at the N7 position of guanine and, to a lesser extent, adenine. However, there is evidence that the three-dimensional structure of the DNA adducts and biologic response(s) they elicit are different from those of cisplatin. Oxaliplatin demonstrated activity in combination with 5-fluorouracil and leucovorin in colon cancer, a disease that is unresponsive to cisplatin. This finding validated the focus on cisplatin-resistant preclinical models to identify new active molecules. Oxaliplatin is approved for the treatment of advanced colorectal cancer, and enhances cure rates in the adjuvant setting. The therapeutic role of oxaliplatin has been found to extend to pancreatic, gastric, and esophageal cancers, in all of which it is the more active platinum derivative.

Nedaplatin and Lobaplatin

Nedaplatin is cis-diammineglycolatoplatinum, developed as a less nephrotoxic second-generation platinum analog, has been shown to be active in a range of tumors similar to that of cisplatin and carboplatin.[16] As a diammine structure, nedaplatin would fall among the cisplatin analogs analyzed in the NCI60 cell line screen,[17] and this activity is therefore anticipated. Lobaplatin is a platinum (II) complex in which the leaving group is lactic acid and the stable ammine ligand is 1,2-bis(aminomethyl)cyclobutane. In a similar way to oxaliplatin the stable ammine ligand may convey some non–cross-resistance compared to cisplatin or carboplatin. It is licensed in China for the breast cancer, small-cell lung cancer, and chronic myelogenous leukemia. It is unique among the platinum drugs for its approval for breast cancer, but there are few published clinical data and no randomized trials. It has not achieved approval in the United States or Europe.

Newer Platinum Structures

The octahedral stereochemistry adopted by platinum (IV) compounds has led investigators to speculate that they may exhibit a different spectrum of activity than that of platinum (II) drugs. Two compounds that were tested clinically without much success are ormaplatin and iproplatin. Two other platinum (IV) compounds that exhibit novel structural features, satraplatin (previously JM216) and JM335 (*trans*-ammine[cyclohexylamine]dichlorodihydroxo platinum [IV]), underwent more limited development. Satraplatin was the first orally active platinum compound, and showed some activity in lung and ovarian cancers, but despite promising activity in prostate cancer, a phase III trial was not successful.[18,19]

An approach based on the chemistry of the platinum-DNA interaction led to design and synthesis by Farrell et al.[20] of a novel class of compounds containing multiple platinum atoms (see Fig. 18.1). These bi- and trinuclear structures form adducts that span greater distances across the minor groove of DNA and have a profile of cell kill that differs from that of the small molecules. These compounds are unique in that their interaction with DNA is considerably different from that of cisplatin, particularly in the abundance of interstrand cross-links formed. Clinical development of candidate compounds is at a preliminary stage.

Efforts have been made to design novel platinum analogs that can circumvent putative cisplatin resistance mechanisms. An example is *cis*-amminedichloro(2-methylpyridine) platinum (II) (also known as *AMD473* and *ZD0473*). This compound is a sterically hindered platinum complex that was designed to have minimal reactivity with thiols and thus avoid inactivation by molecules such as glutathione.[21,22] Responses were identified with its use in the clinic, but development was curtailed based on low levels of activity. The recent description of a monofunctional platinum (II) analog, phenanthriplatin, from the lab of Lippard is potentially of great interest, based on both potency in vitro and a mechanistic profile different from existing analogs.[23] A renewed appreciation that chemotherapeutic drugs have a continuing role in managing cancer is likely to prompt additional clinical development of novel platinum structures.

MECHANISM OF ACTION

DNA Adduct Formation

DNA has long been thought to be the major therapeutic target for platinum compounds. The cytotoxic effects are determined, in part, by the structure and relative amount of DNA adducts formed. Cisplatin and its analogs react preferentially at the N7 position of guanine and adenine residues to form a variety of monofunctional and bifunctional adducts.[24] The monoadducts may form intrastrand or interstrand cross-links. The predominant lesions that are formed when platinum compounds bind DNA are d(GpG)Pt intrastrand cross-links. Cisplatin also forms interstrand cross-links between guanine residues located on opposite strands, and these account for less than 5% of the total DNA-bound platinum. The formation of adducts and cross-links has been associated with therapeutic efficacy.[25,26] These adducts may contribute to the drug's cytotoxicity because they impede certain cellular processes that require the separation of both DNA strands, such as replication and transcription. The adducts formed in the reaction between carboplatin and DNA in cultured cells are essentially the same as those of cisplatin; however, higher concentrations of carboplatin are required (20- to 40-fold for cells) to obtain equivalent total platinum-DNA adduct levels due to its slower rate of aquation.[27] Oxaliplatin intrastrand adducts form even more slowly due to a slower rate of conversion from monoadducts; however, they are formed at similar DNA sequences and regions as cisplatin adducts. At equitoxic doses, oxaliplatin forms fewer DNA adducts than

does cisplatin. This has been interpreted to mean that oxaliplatin lesions are more cytotoxic than those formed by cisplatin.

The differences observed in cytotoxicity between the diammine (e.g., cisplatin, carboplatin) and DACH platinum compounds may not depend on the type and relative amounts of the adducts formed, but on the overall three-dimensional structure of the adduct and its recognition by various cellular proteins. The major difference between them is the protrusion of the DACH moiety of oxaliplatin into the major groove of DNA, which thus produces a bulkier adduct than that of cisplatin. This bulkier, more hydrophobic adduct seems to be recognized differently by cellular proteins involved in sensing DNA damage.[28] The functional consequences are twofold: Proteins such as polymerases that recognize and participate in reactions on DNA under normal circumstances may be perturbed, whereas processes that are controlled by proteins that recognize damaged DNA may become activated (the DNA damage response). The latter group of proteins function both in the DNA repair process and in cellular signaling toward cell survival/death decisions.

DNA Interstrand Cross-Links

Although the DNA adducts are well-recognized to result in G-G interstrand cross-links, like classical alkylating agents, platinum drugs have the capacity to form intrastrand cross-links, albeit to a lesser degree. By blocking essential aspects of DNA metabolism, such as replication and transcription, intrastrand cross-links are highly cytotoxic. Recent studies have drawn attention both to the cytotoxicity of these lesions, and their differing mechanisms of repair, both replication dependent and independent.[29,30] These studies may have clinical implications in selecting patients for therapy based on the repair competence of tumors.

CELLULAR RESPONSES TO PLATINUM-INDUCED DNA DAMAGE

Multiple cellular outcomes may follow the formation of platinum-DNA adducts, including cell death by apoptosis, necrosis, or mitotic catastrophe, or cell survival by activation of various protective mechanisms including DNA repair, DNA damage signaling pathways, cell cycle arrest, and autophagy (the last may have a dual role, possibly context dependent).

Cell Fate

The cellular effects following DNA binding by platinum drugs have been analyzed. The studies of Sorenson and Eastman,[31] using DNA repair-deficient Chinese hamster ovary (CHO) cells, indicated that passage through the S phase is necessary for G2 arrest and cell death, which suggests that DNA replication on a damaged template may result in the accumulation of further damage. An aberrant mitosis was observed before apoptosis in this model.

DNA Damage Recognition

Among the initiation events that ultimately result in platinum drug–induced cell death are the binding of platinum-DNA damage recognition proteins, which then seed the accumulation of a large protein complex capable both of DNA damage signaling (as to cell cycle proteins to halt replication) and repair of the damaged DNA. Among the DNA-binding proteins are the high-mobility group proteins HMG1 and HMG2.[32–34] These proteins are capable of bending DNA as well as recognizing bent DNA structures, such as that produced by cisplatin, and different specificities for cisplatin and for oxaliplatin adducts are observed in structural studies.[35,36] Other candidate platinum-DNA damage recognition proteins include histone H1, RNA polymerase I transcription upstream binding factor (hUBF), the TATA binding protein (TBP), and proteins involved in mismatch repair (MMR). The MMR complex has been implicated in cisplatin sensitivity.[37] Studies have shown that the MSH2 and MLH1 proteins participate in the recognition of DNA adducts formed by cisplatin, but not oxaliplatin, which could contribute to differences in the cytotoxicity profiles observed between these two platinum complexes.

DNA Damage Signaling

A number of signaling events have been shown to occur after treatment of cells with platinum drugs.[38] For example, the ATM- and Rad3-related (ATR) proteins that are involved in cell-cycle checkpoint activation are activated by cisplatin. These kinases phosphorylate and activate several downstream effectors that regulate cell cycle, DNA repair, cell survival, and apoptosis, including p53, CHK2, and members of the mitogen-activated protein kinase (MAPK) pathway (extracellular signal-related kinase [ERK], c-Jun amino-terminal kinase [JNK], and p38 kinase). Recent data especially implicate signaling through the JNK pathway, and inhibition at the level of JNK seems especially relevant to platinum drug cytotoxicity in vitro and in vivo.[39,40] The pleiotropic nature of this stress response only grows, because each of these molecules subsequently controls the activity and expression of many more proteins. As a result of this complexity, acting in the context of variable genomic tumor aberrations, therapeutic strategies directed to these pathways have been slow to emerge. However, clinical trials to investigate specific inhibitors of DNA damage responses are underway and hold promise. It is also relevant to point out that these signaling pathways affect not just the tumor cell, but also may communicate to cells in the microenvironment, the responses of which may also determine the effectiveness of therapy.

IS DNA THE ONLY TARGET?

Early analyses of the action of cytotoxic drugs included a probe of whether effects on DNA were sufficient to explain drug effects. A pioneer in this field was Tritton,[41] who proposed that effects of DNA-intercalating agents on the plasma membrane could underlie the cytotoxicity of the drug. More recently, enucleated cells were shown to be susceptible to cisplatin, and a seminal paper from Voest and colleagues showed that platinum sensitivity was determined not solely by the accumulation of DNA damage in the tumor cell.[42] In analyzing the contribution of cells in the microenvironment of tumors, he showed that tumor infiltration with mesenchymal stem cells could confer drug resistance. A search for secreted factors defined platinum-induced fatty acids, metabolic products in the thromboxane synthetase, and cyclooxygenase-1 pathways as determining the effectiveness of drug therapy. A proteomic study in cisplatin-sensitive and -resistant cells confirmed the substantial effects of drug exposure on lipid metabolites and their relation to susceptibility. A current focus on therapies

directed to the microenvironment, including immunologic and anti-inflammatory interventions,[43] has the potential to expand our ability to apply platinum drugs in the clinic.

MECHANISMS OF RESISTANCE

The major limitation to the successful treatment of solid tumors with platinum-based chemotherapy is the emergence of drug-resistant tumor cells.[44] Developments in tumor biology have advanced our thinking with regard to how and when these cells emerge; heterogeneity within a tumor even at its earliest diagnosis reflects the emergence of treatment-resistant clones even in advance of selection pressure and the realization that resistance may not be specific to the DNA-damaging drug. Indeed, this may be reflected clinically in the finding that after progression on initial chemotherapy, the use of second-line therapy is usually associated with a shorter duration of response.

Currently described mechanisms of platinum drug resistance (Fig. 18.2) include reduced cellular accumulation, intracellular detoxification, repair of Pt-DNA lesions, increased damage tolerance, and the activation of cellular defense mechanisms such as autophagy. In addition, we have already alluded to exogenous influences on mechanism, as may be mediated by other cells, metabolites, of physicochemical conditions (such as hypoxia) in the tumor microenvironment. It must be acknowledged, however, that our insights are very limited as to why some tumors respond and others do not to platinum chemotherapy. As genome sequencing yields increasing and often surprising revelations about the genes that drive cancers and the complexity inherent in cancers of a single histologic type, it is likely that when associated with outcomes in large patient populations, patterns will emerge to guide selection of therapies.

Reduced Accumulation

Platinum uptake in cells occurs by simple diffusion and by carrier-mediated mechanisms. Inhibition of transport mechanisms has a marked effect on intracellular platinum accumulation, and Howell's group has shown the importance of the copper transporters CTR-1 and CTR-2 in regulating the influx of various platinum analogs in eukaryotic cells.[45,46] The contribution of these mechanisms to clinical platinum drug resistance is being explored.[47] Accumulation may also be influenced by enhanced efflux, and various transport proteins are upregulated in cell lines selected for acquired resistance, and in platinum-resistant ovarian cancers.

Inactivation

Platinum complexes are highly reactive molecules and bind rapidly to multiple cellular macromolecules. Protection from such chemicals in the environment is afforded by cellular thiols, including

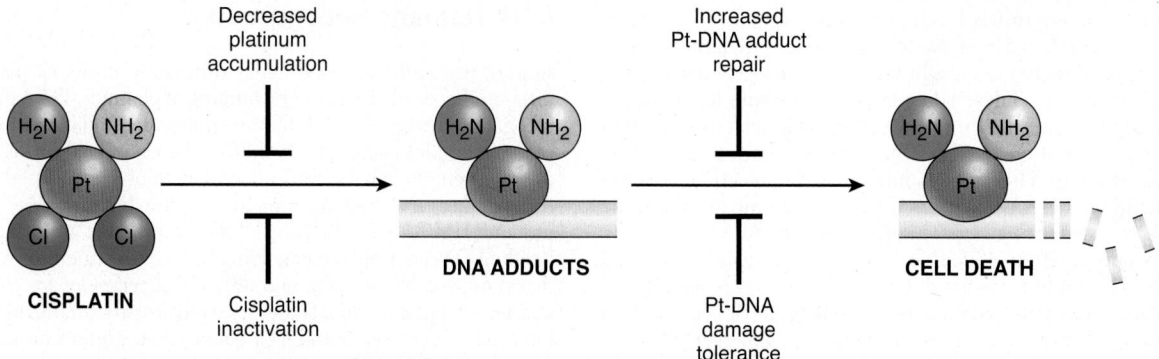

Figure 18.2 Cellular mechanisms of cisplatin resistance.

small peptides such as glutathione (GSH) and larger proteins as exemplified by metallothionein (MT). There are many reports of an association between platinum drug sensitivity and glutathione levels[48–50]; however, reducing intracellular glutathione levels with drugs such as buthionine sulfoximine has resulted in only low to modest potentiation of cisplatin sensitivity.[51] Buthionine sulfoximine was developed for clinical use, and some impact on GSH content of tumors and normal tissues was demonstrated. However, the depletion of GSH was not consistent, and ultimately, the cost of producing the active stereoisomer of the drug was judged prohibitive. Inactivation of the platinum drugs may also occur through binding to the MTs, a family of sulfhydryl-rich, low–molecular-weight proteins that participate in heavy metal binding and detoxification; however, the contribution of MT to clinical platinum drug resistance is unclear, and a therapeutic role has not emerged.

Increased DNA Repair

Once platinum-DNA adducts are formed, cells must either repair or tolerate the damage to survive. In general, the capacity to repair DNA damage seems to play a role in determining a tumor cell's sensitivity to platinum drugs and other DNA-damaging agents. For example, tumors that are unusually sensitive to cisplatin, such as testicular nonseminomatous germ cell tumors, may be deficient in their ability to repair platinum-DNA adducts.[52] The increased repair of platinum-DNA lesions in cisplatin-resistant cell lines as compared to their sensitive counterparts has been shown in several human cancer cell lines, but translation of these observations to the clinic has been difficult. The repair of platinum-DNA adducts appears to occur predominantly by nucleotide excision repair (NER), with a role for MMR under certain circumstances.[53] The molecular basis for the increased repair activity observed in cisplatin-resistant cells is not known precisely, but formation of the ERCC1/XPF protein complex may be a key step. Selvakumaran et al.[54] showed that the downregulation of ERCC-1 using an antisense approach sensitized a platinum-resistant cell line to cisplatin both in vitro and in vivo. There is substantial clinical evidence that implicates *ERCC1* expression in increased NER and cisplatin resistance, and high expression of ERCC1 has been demonstrated to confer a worse outcome after cisplatin treatment in several resistant tumors. The most extensive study of this as a marker has been in non–small-cell lung cancer, results in which were summarized and analyzed by Hubner et al.[55] In gastric cancer also, high levels of ERCC1 are associated with resistance to cisplatin treatment.[56–58] However, a recent reevaluation of discrepant results questioned the reliability of the assays of ERCC1 and their relationship to function.[59] These data suggest that there is a relationship between ERCC1 expression and treatment, but that the lag in marker development precludes implementation of a predictive assay until additional studies have been performed.

Perhaps the most striking evidence that DNA repair is a determinant of platinum drug responses is that breast and ovarian cancers occurring in BRCA1 or BRCA2 mutation carriers are particularly responsive to cisplatin or carboplatin. These cancers are also sensitive to inhibitors of poly(ADP-ribose)polymerase (PARPi), several of which are currently in clinical development. The mechanism of the sensitivity to PARPi has been elucidated. Both the BRCA1 and 2 proteins for part of the homologous recombination repair (HR) system that achieves error-free repair of double strand breaks. Carriers are heterozygous and, therefore, have normal repair function, but loss of the second allele leads to the use of error-prone backup systems and is therefore oncogenic. The cancers that arise are unable to perform HR and, therefore, are sensitive to drugs that induce single strand breaks, such as PARPi.[60,61] A mechanism of resistance to PARPi has been described, which is due to reactivation of the function of the BRCA2 leading to restoration of HR and sensitivity to PARPi.[62] This reactivation is accomplished by an intragenic deletion and the restoration of an open reading frame.

It has further been shown that such revertant cells are resistant to cisplatin as well as PARPi. Finally, recurrent cancers in BRCA2 mutation carriers, which have acquired platinum resistance, have been shown to have undergone reversion of the BRCA2 mutation.[63] This clearly shows that the HR system can be one cause of cisplatin resistance. However, not all cisplatin-resistant patients are also resistant to PARPi,[64] showing that there are multiple other causes of cis/carboplatin resistance.

Combinations of platinum drugs with PARPi are being actively pursued in patients with BRCA-related tumors and also in patients whose tumors are likely to have acquired loss of HR function (poorly differentiated serous ovarian cancer and triple negative breast cancer).

Autophagy

After platinum-DNA adduct formation, the cell detects the DNA damage and initiates signaling through multiple pathways, the effects of which include mobilization of repair proteins; arrest of the cell cycle; altered transcriptional programs; redirection of energy production and consumption; activation of cell death pathways and, simultaneously, of pathways that would counter a cell death decision, and so to permit survival. A process recently characterized to perform the last function is autophagy. Initially described as a mechanism of cell death, autophagy represents a regulated dissolution of cellular elements into a characteristic set of subcellular organelles detectable by electron microscopy and linked by a particular profile of gene expression changes.[65] Multiple stimuli precipitate these changes and have in common scarcity of nutrients that are required for survival, from oxygen and glucose withdrawal to less specific calorie deprivation, and inhibition of metabolic pathways. Autophagy is also a consequence of cytotoxic drug treatment and, more recently, has been appreciated as a means by which cells might survive the stress of cellular insults, and so become resistant to treatment.[66] Amaravadi and colleagues[67] demonstrated that autophagy reversal can sensitize tumors to cytotoxic drugs and several trials of platinum compounds along with the autophagy inhibitor hydroxychloroquine are in progress.

Increased DNA Damage Tolerance

The net result of DNA damage signaling in a sensitive tumor cell is engagement of cell death pathways, including apoptosis, and therapeutic benefit. In a resistant tumor cell, the cell survives as a consequence of one or many of these mechanisms, and this can result in platinum-DNA damage tolerance or multidrug resistance phenotype, or both. Contributors to the tolerance might include deficient DNA MMR (which could excise the adduct if NER failed), enhanced replicative bypass (which essentially ignores the adduct, allowing the cell to survive, but could contribute to the increase in mutation frequency observed in chemotherapy-treated cancers), and altered signaling through stress-related kinases such as JNK, which can both alter transcriptional programs and activate autophagy. Indeed JNK, by phosphorylating Bcl-2 or Bcl-XL, and releasing beclin-1 from inhibition, acts as a key switch to turn on autophagy. The enhanced DNA damage tolerance, in addition to permitting persistence of the cancer cell, may have an additional deleterious effect by fostering further mutagenesis within the tumor, facilitating its evolution to a more malignant phenotype.

CLINICAL PHARMACOLOGY

Pharmacokinetics

The pharmacokinetic differences observed between platinum drugs may be attributed to the structure of their leaving groups. Platinum complexes containing leaving groups that are less easily displaced exhibit reduced plasma protein binding, longer plasma half-lives, and higher rates of renal clearance. These features are

Comparative Parmacokinetics of Platinum Analogs After Bolus or Short Intravenous Infusion

	Cisplatin	Carboplatin	Oxaliplatin
$T_{1/2}\alpha$			
Total platinum	14–49 min	12–98 min	26 min
Ultrafiltrate	9–30 min	8–87 min	21 min
$T_{1/2}\beta$			
Total platinum	0.7–4.6 h	1.3–1.7 h	—
Ultrafiltrate	0.7–0.8 h	1.7–5.9 h	—
$T_{1/2}\gamma$			
Total platinum	24–127 h	8.2–40.0 h	38–47 h
Ultrafiltrate	—	—	24–27 h
Protein binding	>90%	24%–50%	85%
Urinary excretion	23%–50%	54%–82%	>50%

$T_{1/2}\alpha$, half-life of first phase; $T_{1/2}\beta$, half-life of second phase; $T_{1/2}\gamma$, half-life of terminal phase.

evident in the pharmacokinetic properties of cisplatin, carboplatin, and oxaliplatin, which are summarized in Table 18.1. Platinum drug pharmacokinetics have been reviewed.[68]

Cisplatin

After intravenous infusion, cisplatin rapidly diffuses into tissues and is covalently bound to plasma protein. More than 90% of platinum is bound to plasma protein at 4 hours after infusion. The disappearance of ultrafilterable platinum is rapid and occurs in a biphasic fashion. Half-lives of 10 to 30 minutes and 0.7 to 0.8 hours have been reported for the initial and terminal phases, respectively. Cisplatin excretion is dependent on renal function, which accounts for the majority of its elimination. The percentage of platinum excreted in the urine has been reported to be between 23% and 40% at 24 hours after infusion. Only a small percentage of the total platinum is excreted in the bile.

Carboplatin

The differences in pharmacokinetics observed between cisplatin and carboplatin depend primarily on the slower rate of conversion of carboplatin to a reactive species. Thus, the stability of carboplatin results in a low incidence of nephrotoxicity. Carboplatin diffuses rapidly into tissues after infusion; however, it is considerably more stable in plasma. Only 24% of a dose was bound to plasma protein at 4 hours after infusion. The disappearance of platinum from plasma after short intravenous infusions of carboplatin has been reported to occur in a biphasic or triphasic manner. The initial half-lives for total platinum, which vary considerably among several studies, are listed in Table 18.1. The half-lives for total platinum range from 12 to 98 minutes during the first phase ($T_{1/2}\alpha$) and from 1.3 to 1.7 hours during the second phase ($T_{1/2}\beta$). Half-lives reported for the terminal phase range from 8.2 to 40 hours. The disappearance of ultrafilterable platinum is biphasic with $T_{1/2}\alpha$ and $T_{1/2}\beta$ values ranging from 7.6 to 87 minutes and 1.7 to 5.9 hours, respectively. Carboplatin is excreted predominantly by the kidneys, and cumulative urinary excretion of platinum is 54% to 82%, most as unmodified carboplatin. The renal clearance of carboplatin is closely correlated with the glomerular filtration rate (GFR).[69] This observation enabled Calvert et al.[9] to design a carboplatin-dosing formula based on the individual patient's GFR.

Oxaliplatin

After oxaliplatin infusion, platinum accumulates into three compartments: plasma-bound platinum, ultrafilterable platinum, and platinum associated with erythrocytes. When specific and sensitive mass spectrometric techniques are used, oxaliplatin itself is undetectable in plasma, even at end infusion.[70] The active forms of the drug have not been extensively characterized. Approximately 85% of the total platinum is bound to plasma protein at 2 to 5 hours after infusion.[71] Plasma elimination of total platinum and ultrafiltrates is biphasic. The half-lives for the initial and terminal phases are 26 minutes and 38.7 hours, respectively, for total platinum and 21 minutes and 24.2 hours, respectively, for ultrafilterable platinum (see Table 18.1).[72] Thus, as with carboplatin, substantial differences between total and free platinum kinetics are not observed. As with cisplatin, a prolonged retention of oxaliplatin is observed in red blood cells. However, unlike cisplatin, oxaliplatin does not accumulate to any significant level after multiple courses of treatment.[71] This may explain why neurotoxicity associated with oxaliplatin is reversible. Oxaliplatin is eliminated predominantly by the kidneys, with more than 50% of the platinum being excreted in the urine at 48 hours.

Pharmacodynamics

Pharmacodynamics relates pharmacokinetic indices of drug exposure to biologic measures of drug effect, usually toxicity to normal tissues or tumor cell kill. Two issues to be addressed in such studies are whether the effectiveness of the drug can be enhanced and whether the toxicity can be attenuated by knowledge of the platinum pharmacokinetics in an individual. These questions are appropriate to the use of cytotoxic agents with relatively narrow therapeutic indices. Toxicity to normal tissues can be quantitated as a continuous variable when the drug causes myelosuppression. Thus, the early studies of carboplatin demonstrated a close relationship of changes in platelet counts to the area under the concentration-time curve (AUC) in the individual. The AUC was itself closely related to renal function, which was determined as creatinine clearance. Based on these observations, Egorin et al.,[10] Calvert et al.,[9] and Chatelut and colleagues[73] derived formulas based on creatinine clearance to predict either the percentage change in platelet count or a target AUC. Application of pharmacodynamically guided dosing algorithms for carboplatin has been widely adopted as a means of avoiding overdosage (by producing acceptable nadir platelet counts) and of maximizing dose intensity in the individual. There is good evidence that this approach can decrease the risk of unacceptable toxicity. Accordingly, a dosing strategy based on renal function is recommended for the use of carboplatin.

A key question is whether maximizing carboplatin exposure in an individual can measurably increase the probability of tumor regression or survival. In an analysis by Jodrell et al.,[74] carboplatin AUC was a predictor of response, thrombocytopenia, and leukopenia. The likelihood of a tumor response increased with increasing AUC up to a level of 5 to 7 mg × hour per milliliter, after which a plateau was reached. Similar results were obtained with carboplatin in combination with cyclophosphamide, and neither response rate nor survival was determined by the carboplatin AUC in a cohort of ovarian cancer patients.[75] As a result, most carboplatin recommended doses are based on an AUC in this range (for every 3 to 4 week schedules), and modifications of these are used for more frequent administration (as in combined chemoradiotherapy regimens).

The relationship of pharmacokinetics to response has been sought by investigating the cellular pharmacology of these agents.[76] The formation and repair of the platinum-DNA adducts in human cells are not easily measured. Schellens and colleagues[77,78] analyzed the pharmacokinetic and pharmacodynamic interactions of cisplatin administered as a single agent. In a series of patients with head and neck cancer, they found that cisplatin exposure (measured as the AUC) closely correlated with both the peak DNA adduct content in leukocytes and the area under the DNA-adduct time curve. These measures were important predictors of response, both individually and in logistic regression analysis. However, as an approach to determine who should or should not be treated with platinum drugs, it seems more likely that genomic analyses will provide guidance in the near future.

Pharmacogenomics

Variability in pharmacokinetics and pharmacodynamics of cyto-toxic drugs is an important determinant of therapeutic index. This interindividual variation may be attributed in part to genetic differences among patients. Targeted analyses of germ-line DNA and, increasingly, Genome-wide association studies (GWAS) approaches, have yielded genotypic features associated with results of therapy. Detoxification pathways and DNA repair have emerged as having markers attributable to response of lack of it in response to platinum drugs. Single nucleotide polymorphisms (SNP) in genes related to glutathione metabolism and in several DNA repair genes have been identified in lung cancer, breast cancer, and various GI cancers. A concern is that larger trials have not always confirmed early findings. As yet, informative SNPs that could be used to define therapeutic strategies for individual patients have not yet been defined.

FORMULATION AND ADMINISTRATION

Cisplatin (Platinol)

Cisplatin is administered in a chloride-containing solution intravenously over 0.5 to 2.0 hours. To minimize the risk of nephrotoxicity, patients are prehydrated with at least 500 mL of salt-containing fluid. Immediately before cisplatin administration, mannitol (12.5 to 25.0 g) is given parenterally to maximize urine flow. A diuretic such as furosemide may be used also, along with parenteral antiemetics. These currently include dexamethasone together with a 5-hydroxytryptamine (5-HT$_3$) antagonist. A minimum of 1 L of posthydration fluid is usually given. The intensity of hydration varies somewhat with the dose of cisplatin. High-dose cisplatin (up to 200 mg/m^2 per course) may be administered in a formulation containing 3% sodium chloride, but this method is no longer widely used. Cisplatin may also be administered regionally to increase local drug exposure and diminish side effects. Its intraperitoneal use was defined by Ozols et al.[79] and by Howell and colleagues.[80] Measured drug exposure in the peritoneal cavity is some 50-fold higher compared to levels achieved with intravenous administration. At standard dosages in ovarian cancer patients with low-volume disease, a randomized intergroup trial suggested that intraperitoneal administration is superior to intravenous cisplatin in combination with intravenous cyclophosphamide.[81] The development of combinations of carboplatin and paclitaxel has, however, superseded this technique in the treatment of ovarian cancer, and the intraperitoneal route is now infrequently used. Regional uses also include intra-arterial delivery (as for hepatic tumors, melanoma, and glioblastoma), but none have been adopted as a standard method of treatment. There is growing interest in chemoembolization for the treatment of tumors confined to the liver, and cisplatin is a component of many popular regimens.[82]

Carboplatin (Paraplatin)

Cisplatin treatment over 3 to 6 hours is burdensome for clinical resources and tiring for cancer patients. Previously given as an in-hospital treatment, it is now usually administered in the outpatient setting. The exigencies of the modern health-care environment have contributed to the expanding use of carboplatin as an alternative to cisplatin except in circumstances in which cisplatin is clearly the superior agent. Carboplatin is substantially easier to administer. Extensive hydration is not required because of the lack of nephrotoxicity at standard dosages. Carboplatin is reconstituted in chloride-free solutions (unlike cisplatin, because chloride can displace the leaving groups) and administered over 30 minutes as a rapid intravenous infusion.

Oxaliplatin (Eloxatin)

Oxaliplatin is also uncomplicated in its clinical administration. For bolus infusion, the required dose is administered in 500 mL of chloride-free diluent over a period of 2 hours. Oxaliplatin is most frequently given as a single dose every 2 weeks (85 mg/m^2) or every 3 weeks (130 mg/m^2), alone or with other active agents. It is common to pretreat patients with active antiemetics, such as a 5-HT$_3$ antagonist, but the nausea is not as severe as with cisplatin. No prehydration is required. Besides a relatively low incidence of myelosuppression, the predominant toxicity of oxaliplatin is cumulative neurotoxicity. The development of an oropharyngeal dysesthesia, often precipitated by exposure to cold, may require prolonging the duration of administration to 6 hours. On occasion, the occurrence of hypersensitivity also requires slowing the infusion.

TOXICITY

A substantial body of literature documents the side effects of platinum compounds. As noted in the section titled History, earlier in this chapter, the toxicity of cisplatin was a driving force both in the search for less toxic analogs and for more effective treatments for its side effects, especially nausea and vomiting. The toxicities associated with cisplatin, carboplatin, and oxaliplatin are described in detail in the following sections and summarized in Table 18.2. Please review the package inserts for these drugs for full prescribing information and delineation of toxic effects.

Cisplatin

The side effects associated with cisplatin (at single doses of more than 50 mg/m^2) include nausea and vomiting, nephrotoxicity, ototoxicity, neuropathy, and myelosuppression. Rare effects include visual impairment, seizures, arrhythmias, acute ischemic vascular events, glucose intolerance, and pancreatitis. The nausea and vomiting stimulated a search for new antiemetics. These effects are currently best managed with 5-HT$_3$ antagonists, usually given with a glucocorticoid, although other combinations of agents are still widely used. In the weeks after treatment, continuous antiemetic therapy may be required. Nephrotoxicity is ameliorated but not completely prevented by hydration. The renal damage to both glomeruli and tubules is cumulative, and after cisplatin treatment, serum creatinine levels are no longer a reliable guide to GFR. An acute elevation of serum creatinine level may follow a cisplatin dose, but this index returns to normal with time. Tubule damage may be reflected in a salt-losing syndrome that also resolves with time.

TABLE 18.2

Toxicity Profiles of Platinum Analogs in Clinical Use

Toxicity	Cisplatin	Carboplatin	Oxaliplatin
Myelosuppression		X	
Nephrotoxicity	X		
Neurotoxicity	X		X
Ototoxicity	X		
Nausea and vomiting	X	X	X

Ototoxicity is a cumulative and irreversible side effect of cisplatin treatment that results from damage to the inner ear. The initial audiographic manifestation is loss of high-frequency acuity (4,000 to 8,000 Hz). When acuity is affected in the range of speech, cisplatin should be discontinued under most circumstances and carboplatin substituted where appropriate. Peripheral neuropathy is also cumulative, although less common than with agents such as vinca alkaloids. This neuropathy is usually reversible, although recovery is often slow. A number of agents with the potential for protection from neuropathy have been developed, but none is yet used widely.

Carboplatin

Myelosuppression, which is not usually severe with cisplatin, is the dose-limiting toxicity of carboplatin. The drug is most toxic to the platelet precursors, but neutropenia and anemia are frequently observed. The lowest platelet counts after a single dose of carboplatin are observed 17 to 21 days later, and recovery usually occurs by day 28. The effect is dose dependent, but individuals vary widely in their susceptibility. As shown by Egorin et al.[10] and Calvert et al.,[9] the severity of platelet toxicity is best accounted for by a measure of the drug exposure in an individual, the AUC. Both groups derived pharmacologically based formulas to predict toxicity and guide carboplatin dosing. That of Calvert and colleagues targets a particular exposure to carboplatin:

$$\text{Dose (mg)} = \text{target AUC (mg} \cdot \text{min/mL)} \times \text{(GFR mL/min} + 25)$$

This formula has been widely used to individualize carboplatin dosing and permits targeting an acceptable level of toxicity. Patients who are elderly, have a poor performance status, or have a history of extensive pretreatment have a higher risk of toxicity even when dosage is calculated with these methods, but the safety of drug administration has been enhanced. In the combination of carboplatin and paclitaxel, AUC-based dosing has helped to maximize the dose intensity of carboplatin. Dosages some 30% higher than those using a dosing strategy based solely on body surface area may safely be used. A determination of whether this approach to dosing improves outcomes will require a randomized trial.

The other toxicities of carboplatin are generally milder and better tolerated than those of cisplatin. Nausea and vomiting, although frequent, are less severe, shorter in duration, and more easily controlled with standard antiemetics (i.e., prochlorperazine [Compazine]), dexamethasone, lorazepam) than that after cisplatin treatment. Renal impairment is infrequent, although alopecia is common, especially with the paclitaxel-containing combinations. Neurotoxicity is also less common than with cisplatin, although it is observed more frequently with the increasing use of high-dose regimens. Ototoxicity is also less common.

Oxaliplatin

The dose-limiting toxicity of oxaliplatin is sensory neuropathy, a characteristic of all DACH-containing platinum derivatives. This side effect takes two forms. First, a tingling of the extremities, which may also involve the perioral region, that occurs early and usually resolves within a few days. With repeated dosing, symptoms may last longer between cycles, but do not appear to be cumulative or of long duration. Laryngopharyngeal spasms and cold dysesthesias have also been reported but are not associated with significant respiratory symptoms and can be prevented by prolonging the duration of infusion. A second neuropathy, more typical of that seen with cisplatin, affects the extremities and increases with repeated doses. Definitive physiologic characterization of oxaliplatin-induced neuropathy has proven difficult in large studies. Electromyograms performed in six patients treated by Extra et al.[83] revealed an axonal sensory neuropathy, but nerve conduction velocities were unchanged. Specimens from peripheral nerve biopsies performed in this study showed decreased myelination and replacement with collagen pockets. The neurologic effects of oxaliplatin appear to be cumulative in that they become more pronounced and of greater duration with successive cycles; however, unlike those of cisplatin, they are reversible with drug cessation. In a review of 682 patient experiences, Brienza et al.[84] reported that 82% of patients who experienced grade 2 neurotoxicity or higher had their symptoms regress within 4 to 6 months. In a larger adjuvant trial, de Gramont et al.[85] reported that 12% of patients had grade 3 toxicity at the end of a 6-month treatment period and that the majority of these patients had relief, but not always complete resolution of the symptoms, by 1 year later. The persistence of the neurotoxicity has led to approaches to ameliorate it, including the use of protective agents. The use of calcium and magnesium salts intravenously before and after each infusion has been shown to be ineffective. Ototoxicity is not observed with oxaliplatin. Nausea and vomiting do occur and generally respond to 5-HT$_3$ antagonists. Myelosuppression is uncommon and is not severe with oxaliplatin as a single agent, but it is a feature of combinations including this drug. Oxaliplatin therapy is not associated with nephrotoxicity.

SELECTED REFERENCES

The full reference list can be accessed at lwwhealthlibrary.com/oncology.

2. Rosenberg B. Fundamental studies with cisplatin. *Cancer* 1985;55:2303–2316.

4. Hayes D, Cvitkovic E, Golbey R, et al. High dose cis-platinum diamine dichloride: amelioration of renal toxicity by mannitol diuresis. *Cancer* 1977;39:1372–1381.

8. Harrap K. Initiatives with platinum- and quinazoline-based antitumor molecules—Fourteenth Bruce F. Cain Memorial Award Lecture. *Cancer Res* 1995;55:2761–2768.

9. Calvert A, Newell D, Gumbrell L, et al. Carboplatin dosage: prospective evaluation of a simple formula based on renal function. *J Clin Oncol* 1989;7:1748–1756.

10. Egorin M, Echo DV, Olman E, et al. Prospective validation of a pharmacologically based dosing scheme for the cis-diamminedichloroplatinum(II) analogue diamminecyclobutanedicarboxylatoplatinum. *Cancer Res* 1985;45:6502–6506.

11. Connors T, Jones M, Ross W, et al. New platinum complexes with antitumour activity. *Chem Biol Interact* 1972;5:415–424.

13. Kidani Y, Inagaki K, Tsukagoshi S. Examination of antitumor activities of platinum complexes of 1,2-diaminocyclohexane isomers and their related complexes. *Gann* 1976;67:921–922.

16. Shimada M, Itamochi H, Kigawa J. Nedaplatin: a cisplatin derivative in cancer therapy. *Cancer Manag Res* 2013;5:67–76.

17. Fojo T, Farrell N, Ortuzar W, et al. Identification of non-cross-resistant platinum compounds with novel cytotoxicity profiles using the NCI anticancer drug screen and clustered image map visualizations. *Crit Rev Oncol Hematol* 2005;53:25–34.

20. Farrell N, Qu Y, Bierbach U, et al. Structure-activity relationships within di- and trinuclear platinum phase-I clinical anticancer agents. In: Lippert B, ed. *Cisplatin: Chemistry and Biochemistry of a Leading Anticancer Drug.* Zurich: Verlag Helvetica Chimica Acta; 1999;477–496.

23. Park GY, Wilson JJ, Song Y, et al. Phenanthriplatin, a monofunctional DNA-binding platinum anticancer drug candidate with unusual potency and cellular activity profile. *Proc Natl Acad Sci U S A* 2012;109:11987–11992.

24. Eastman A. The formation, isolation and characterization of DNA adducts produced by anticancer platinum complexes. *Pharmacol Ther* 1987;34:155–166.

26. Martens-de Kemp SR, Dalm SU, Wijnolts FM, et al. DNA-bound platinum is the major determinant of cisplatin sensitivity in head and neck squamous carcinoma cells. *PLoS One* 2013;8:e61555.

30. Zhu G, Song L, Lippard SJ. Visualizing inhibition of nucleosome mobility and transcription by cisplatin-DNA interstrand crosslinks in live mammalian cells. *Cancer Res* 2013;73:4451–4460.

31. Sorenson C, Eastman A. Mechanism of cis-diamminedichloroplatinum (II)-induced cytotoxicity: role of G2 arrest and DNA double-strand breaks. *Cancer Res* 1988;48:4484–4488.

36. Ramachandran S, Temple B, Alexandrova AN, et al. Recognition of platinum-DNA adducts by HMGB1a. *Biochemistry* 2012;51:7608–7617.

38. Kelland L. The resurgence of platinum-based cancer chemotherapy. *Nat Rev Cancer* 2007;7:573–584.

40. Vasilevskaya IA, Selvakumaran M, O'Dwyer PJ. Disruption of signaling through SEK1 and MKK7 yields differential responses in hypoxic colon cancer cells treated with oxaliplatin. *Mol Pharmacol* 2008;74:246–254.

41. Maestre N, Tritton TR, Laurent G, et al. Cell surface-directed interaction of anthracyclines leads to cytotoxicity and nuclear factor kappaB activation but not apoptosis signaling. *Cancer Res* 2001;61:2558–2561.

42. Roodhart JM, Daenen LG, Stigter EC, et al. Mesenchymal stem cells induce resistance to chemotherapy through the release of platinum-induced fatty acids. *Cancer Cell* 2011;20:370–383.

44. Galluzzi L, Senovilla L, Vitale I, et al. Molecular mechanisms of cisplatin resistance. *Oncogene* 2012;31:1869–1883.

46. Blair BG, Larson CA, Safaei R, et al. Copper transporter 2 regulates the cellular accumulation and cytotoxicity of cisplatin and carboplatin. *Clin Cancer Res* 2009;15:4312–4321.

48. Britten RA, Green JA, Broughton C, et al. The relationship between nuclear glutathione levels and resistance to melphalan in human ovarian tumour cells. *Biochem Pharmacol* 1991;41:647–649.

50. Godwin A, Meister A, O'Dwyer P, et al. High resistance to cisplatin in human ovarian cancer cell lines is associated with marked increase in glutathione synthesis. *Proc Natl Acad Sci U S A* 1992;89:3070–3074.

52. Koberle B, Grimaldi K, Sunters A, et al. DNA repair capacity and cisplatin sensitivity of human testis tumour cells. *Int J Cancer* 1997;70:551–555.

53. Martin LP, Hamilton TC, Schilder RJ. Platinum resistance: the role of DNA repair pathways. *Clin Cancer Res* 2008;14:1291–1295.

54. Selvakumaran M, Piscarcik DA, Bao R, et al. Enhanced cisplatin cytotoxicity by disturbing the nucleotide excision repair pathway in ovarian cancer cell lines. *Cancer Res* 2003;63:1311–1316.

55. Hubner RA, Riley RD, Billingham LJ, et al. Excision repair cross-complementation group 1 (ERCC1) status and lung cancer outcomes: a meta-analysis of published studies and recommendations. *PLoS One* 2011;6:e25164.

59. Friboulet L, Olaussen KA, Pignon JP, et al. ERCC1 isoform expression and DNA repair in non–small-cell lung cancer. *N Engl J Med* 2013;368:1101–1110.

60. Bryant HE, Schultz N, Thomas HD, et al. Specific killing of BRCA2-deficient tumours with inhibitors of poly(ADP-ribose) polymerase. *Nature* 2005;434:913–917.

61. Farmer H, McCabe1 N, Lord C, et al. Targeting the DNA repair defect in BRCA mutant cells as a therapeutic strategy. *Nature* 2005;434:917–921.

64. Gelmon, KA, Tischkowitz M, Mackay H, et al. Olaparib in patients with recurrent high-grade serous or poorly differentiated ovarian carcinoma or triple-negative breast cancer: a phase 2, multicentre, open-label, non-randomised study. *Lancet Oncology* 2011;12:852–861.

67. Amaravadi RK, Yu D, Lum JJ, et al. Autophagy inhibition enhances therapy-induced apoptosis in a Myc-induced model of lymphoma. *J Clin Invest* 2007;117:326–336.

68. Duffull S, Robinson B. Clinical pharmacokinetics and dose optimization of carboplatin. *Clin Pharmacokinet* 1997;33:161–183.

70. Graham MA, Lockwood GF, Greenslade D, et al. Clinical pharmacokinetics of oxaliplatin: a critical review. *Clin Cancer Res* 2000;6:1205–1218.

73. Chatelut E, Canal P, Brunner V, et al. Prediction of carboplatin clearance from standard morphological and biological patient characteristics. *J Natl Cancer Inst* 1995;87:573–580.

74. Jodrell D, Egorin M, Canetta R, et al. Relationships between carboplatin exposure and tumor response and toxicity in patients with ovarian cancer. *J Clin Oncol* 1992;10:520–528.

78. Schellens J, Ma J, Planting A, et al. Relationship between the exposure to cisplatin, DNA-adduct formation in leucocytes and tumour response in patients with solid tumours. *Br J Cancer* 1996;73:1569–1575.

81. Alberts D, Liu P, Hannigan E, et al. Intraperitoneal cisplatin plus intravenous cyclophosphamide versus intravenous cisplatin plus intravenous cyclophosphamide for stage III ovarian cancer. *N Engl J Med* 1996;335:1950–1955.

83. Extra J, Marty M, Brienza S, et al. Pharmacokinetics and safety profile of oxaliplatin. *Semin Oncol* 1998;25:13–22.

84. Brienza S, Vignoud J, Itzhaki M, et al. Oxaliplatin (L-OHP): global safety in 682 patients. *Proc Am Soc Clin Oncol* 1995;14:209.

85. André T, Boni C, Mounedji-Boudiaf L, et al. Oxaliplatin, fluorouracil, and leucovorin as adjuvant treatment for colon cancer. *N Engl J Med* 2004;350:2343–2351.

CANCER THERAPEUTICS

M. Wasif Saif and Edward Chu

ANTIFOLATES

Reduced folates play a key role in one-carbon metabolism, and they are essential for the biosynthesis of purines, thymidylate, and protein biosynthesis. Aminopterin was the first antimetabolite with documented clinical activity in the treatment of children with acute leukemia in the 1940s. This antifolate analog was subsequently replaced by methotrexate (MTX), the 4-amino, 10-methyl analog of folic acid, which remains the most widely used antifolate analog, with activity against a wide range of cancers (Table 19.1), including hematologic malignancies (acute lymphoblastic leukemia and non-Hodgkin's lymphoma) and many solid tumors (breast cancer, head and neck cancer, osteogenic sarcoma, bladder cancer, and gestational trophoblastic cancer).

Pemetrexed is a pyrrolopyrimidine, multitargeted antifolate analog that targets multiple enzymes involved in folate metabolism, including thymidylate synthase (TS), dihydrofolate reductase (DHFR), glycinamide ribonucleotide (GAR) formyltransferase, and aminoimidazole carboxamide (AICAR) formyltransferase.[1,2] This agent has broad-spectrum activity against solid tumors, including malignant mesothelioma and breast, pancreatic, head and neck, non–small-cell lung, colon, gastric, cervical, and bladder cancers.[3-5]

The third antifolate compound to have entered clinical practice is pralatrexate (10-propargyl-10-deazaaminopterin), a 10-deazaaminopterin antifolate that was rationally designed to bind with higher affinity to the reduced folate carrier (RFC)-1 transport protein, when compared with MTX, leading to enhanced membrane transport into tumor cells. It is also an improved substrate for the enzyme folylpolyglutamyl synthetase (FPGS), resulting in enhanced formation of cytotoxic polyglutamate metabolites.[6,7] When compared with MTX, this analog is a more potent inhibitor of multiple enzymes involved in folate metabolism, including TS, DHFR, and GAR and AICAR formyltransferases. This agent is presently approved for the treatment of relapsed or refractory peripheral T-cell lymphomas.[8]

Mechanism of Action

The antifolate compounds are tight-binding inhibitors of DHFR, a key enzyme in folate metabolism.[1] DHFR plays a pivotal role in maintaining the intracellular folate pools in their fully reduced form as tetrahydrofolates, and these compounds serve as one-carbon carriers required for the synthesis of thymidylate, purine nucleotides, and certain amino acids.

The cytotoxic effects of MTX, pemetrexed, and pralatrexate are mediated by their respective polyglutamate metabolites, with up to 5 to 7 glutamyl groups in a γ-peptide linkage. These polyglutamate metabolites exhibit prolonged intracellular half-lives, thereby allowing for prolonged drug action in tumor cells. Moreover, these polyglutamate metabolites are potent, direct inhibitors of several folate-dependent enzymes, including DHFR, TS, AICAR formyltransferase, and GAR formyltransferase.[1]

Mechanisms of Resistance

The development of cellular resistance to antifolates remains a major obstacle to its clinical efficacy.[9,10] In experimental systems, resistance to antifolates arises from several mechanisms, including an alteration in antifolate transport because of either a defect in the reduced folate carrier or folate receptor systems, decreased capacity to polyglutamate the antifolate parent compound through either decreased expression of FPGS or increased expression of the catabolic enzyme γ-glutamyl hydrolase, and alterations in the target enzymes DHFR and/or TS through increased expression of wild-type protein or overexpression of a mutant protein with reduced binding affinity for the antifolate. Gene amplification is a common resistance mechanism observed in various experimental systems, including tumor samples from patients. In in vitro and in vivo experimental model systems, the levels of DHFR and/or TS protein acutely increase after exposure to MTX and other antifolate compounds. This acute induction of target protein in response to drug exposure is mediated, in part, by a translational regulatory mechanism, which may represent a clinically relevant mechanism for the acute development of cellular drug resistance.

Clinical Pharmacology

The oral bioavailability of MTX is saturable and erratic at doses greater than 25 mg/m^2. MTX is completely absorbed from parenteral routes of administration, and peak serum levels are achieved within 30 to 60 minutes of administration.

The distribution of MTX into third-space fluid collections, such as pleural effusions and ascitic fluid, can substantially alter MTX pharmacokinetics. The slow release of accumulated MTX from these third spaces over time prolongs the terminal half-life of the drug, leading to potentially increased clinical toxicity. It is advisable to evacuate these fluid collections before treatment and monitor plasma drug concentrations closely.

Renal excretion is the main route of drug elimination, and this process is mediated by glomerular filtration and tubular secretion. About 80% to 90% of an administered dose is eliminated unchanged in the urine. Doses of MTX, therefore, should be reduced in proportion to reductions in creatinine clearance. Renal excretion of MTX is inhibited by probenecid, penicillins, cephalosporins, aspirin, and nonsteroidal anti-inflammatory drugs.

Pemetrexed enters the cell via the RFC system and, to a lesser extent, by the folate receptor protein. As with MTX, it undergoes polyglutamation within the cell to the pentaglutamate form, which is at least 60-fold more potent than the parent compound. This agent is mainly cleared by renal excretion, and in the setting of renal dysfunction, the terminal drug half-life is significantly prolonged to up to 20 hours. Pemetrexed, therefore, should be used with caution in patients with renal dysfunction. In addition, renal excretion is inhibited in the presence of other agents including probenecid, penicillins, cephalosporins, aspirin, and nonsteroidal anti-inflammatory drugs.

TABLE 19.1

Antimetabolites: Indications, Doses and Schedules, and Toxicities

Drug	Main Therapeutic Uses	Main Doses and Schedule	Major Toxicities
Methotrexate	Non-Hodgkin's lymphoma Primary CNS lymphoma Acute lymphoblastic leukemia Breast cancer Bladder cancer Osteogenic sarcoma Gestational trophoblastic cancer	Low dose: 10–50 mg/m² IV every 3–4 weeks Low dose weekly: 25 mg/m² IV weekly Moderate dose: 100–500 m/m² IV every 2–3 weeks High dose: 1–12 gm/m² IV over a 3- to 24-hour period every 1–3 weeks Intrathecal (IT): 10–15 mg IT 2 times weekly until CSF is clear, then weekly dose for 2–6 weeks, followed by monthly dose	Mucositis, diarrhea, myelosuppression, acute renal failure, transient elevations in serum transaminases and bilirubin, pneumonitis, neurologic toxicity
Pemetrexed	Mesothelioma Non–small-cell lung cancer	500 mg/m² IV, every 3 weeks	Myelosuppression, skin rash, mucositis, diarrhea, fatigue
Pralatrexate	Peripheral T-cell lymphoma	30 mg/m² IV, weekly for 6 weeks; cycles repeated every 7 weeks	Myelosuppression, skin rash, mucositis, diarrhea, elevation of serum transaminases and bilirubin, mild nausea/vomiting
5-Fluorouracil	Breast cancer Colorectal cancer Anal cancer Gastroesophageal cancer Hepatocellular cancer Pancreatic cancer Head and neck cancer	Bolus monthly schedule: 425–450 mg/m² IV on days 1–5 every 28 days Bolus weekly schedule: 500–600 mg/m² IV every week for 6 weeks every 8 weeks Infusion schedule: 2,400–3,000 mg/m² IV over 46 hours every 2 weeks 120-hour infusion: 1,000 mg/m²/d IV on days 1–5 every 21–28 d Protracted continuous infusion: 200–400 mg/m²/d IV	Nausea/vomiting, diarrhea, mucositis, myelosuppression, neurotoxicity, coronary artery vasospasm, conjunctivitis
Capecitabine	Breast cancer Colorectal cancer Gastroesophageal cancer Hepatocellular cancer Pancreatic cancer	Recommended dose for monotherapy is 1,250 mg/m² PO bid for 2 weeks with 1 wk rest May decrease dose of capecitabine to 850–1,000 mg/m² bid on days 1–14 to reduce risk of toxicity without compromising efficacy An alternative dosing schedule for monotherapy is 1,250–1,500 mg/m² PO bid for 1 week on and 1 week off; this schedule appears to be well tolerated, with no compromise in clinical efficacy Capecitabine should be used at lower doses (850–1,000 mg/m² bid on days 1–14) when used in combination with other cytotoxic agents, such as oxaliplatin and lapatinib	Diarrhea, hand-foot syndrome, myelosuppression, mucositis, nausea/vomiting, neurologic toxicity, coronary artery vasospasm
Cytarabine	Hodgkin's lymphoma Non-Hodgkin's lymphoma Acute myelogenous leukemia Acute lymphoblastic leukemia	Standard dose: 100 mg/m²/day IV on days 1–7 as a continuous IV infusion, in combination with an anthracycline as induction chemotherapy for acute myelogenous leukemia High-dose: 1.5–3.0 gm/m² IV q 12 hours for 3 days as a high dose, intensification regimen for acute myelogenous leukemia SC: 20 mg/m² SC for 10 days per month for 6 months, associated with IFN-α for treatment of chronic myelogenous leukemia IT: 10–30 mg IT up to 3 times weekly in the treatment of leptomeningeal carcinomatosis secondary to leukemia or lymphoma.	Nausea/vomiting, myelosuppression, cerebellar ataxia, lethargy, confusion, acute pancreatitis, drug infusion reaction, hand-foot syndrome High-dose therapy: noncardiogenic pulmonary edema, acute respiratory distress and *Streptococcus viridans* pneumonia, conjunctivitis, and keratitis
Gemcitabine	Pancreatic cancer Non–small-cell lung cancer Breast cancer Bladder cancer Hodgkin's lymphoma Ovarian cancer Soft tissue sarcoma	Pancreatic cancer: 1,000 mg/m² IV every week for 7 weeks with 1 week rest Treatment then continues weekly for 3 weeks followed by 1 week off Bladder cancer: 1,000 mg/m² IV on days 1, 8, and 15 every 28 days Non–small-cell lung cancer: 1,000-1,200 mg/m² IV on days 1 and 8 every 21 days	Nausea/vomiting, myelosuppression, flulike syndrome, elevation of serum transaminases and bilirubin, pneumonitis, infusion reaction, mild proteinuria, and rarely, hemolytic-uremic syndrome and thrombotic thrombocytopenic purpura

CANCER THERAPEUTICS

(continued)

TABLE 19.1

Antimetabolites: Indications, Doses and Schedules, and Toxicities *(continued)*

Drug	Main Therapeutic Uses	Main Doses and Schedule	Major Toxicities
6-Mercaptopurine	Acute lymphoblastic leukemia	Induction therapy: 2.5 mg/kg PO daily Maintenance therapy: 1.5–2.5 mg/kg PO daily	Myelosuppression, nausea/vomiting, mucositis and diarrhea, hepatotoxicity, immunosuppression
6-Thioguanine	Acute myelogenous leukemia Acute lymphoblastic leukemia	Induction: 100 mg/m^2 PO every 12 hours on days 1–5, usually in combination with cytarabine Maintenance: 100 mg/m^2 PO every 12 hours on days 1–5, every 4 weeks, usually in combination with other agents Single agent: 1–3 mg/kg PO daily	Myelosuppression, nausea/vomiting, mucositis and diarrhea, hepatotoxicity, immunosuppression
Fludarabine	Chronic lymphocytic leukemia Non-Hodgkin's lymphoma	25 mg/m^2 IV on days 1–5 every 28 days For oral usage, the recommended dose is 40 mg/m^2 PO on days 1–5 every 28 days	Myelosuppression, immunosuppression with increased risk of opportunistic infections, mild nausea/vomiting, hypersensitivity reaction
Cladribine	Hairy cell leukemia Chronic lymphocytic leukemia Non-Hodgkin's lymphoma	Usual dose is 0.09 mg/kg/d IV via continuous infusion for 7 days; one course is usually administered	Myelosuppression, immunosuppression, mild nausea/vomiting, fever
Clofarabine	Acute lymphoblastic leukemia	52 mg/m^2 IV daily for 5 days every 2–6 weeks	Myelosuppression nausea/vomiting, diarrhea, systemic inflammatory response syndrome, increased risk of opportunistic infections, renal toxicity

CNS, central nervous system; IV, intravenously; CSF, cerebrospinal fluid; PO, by mouth; bid, twice daily; SC, subcutaneously; IFN-α, interferon alpha.

As with other antifolate analogs, pralatrexate is transported into the cell by the RFC carrier protein and then metabolized by FPGS to form longer chain polyglutamates, with up to four additional glutamate residues attached to the parent molecule. About 34% of the parent drug is cleared in the urine during the first 24 hours after drug administration. As such, caution is advised when using pralatrexate in patients with renal dysfunction. As with MTX and pemetrexed, the concomitant administration of other agents such as probenecid, penicillins, cephalosporins, aspirin, and nonsteroidal anti-inflammatory drugs, may inhibit renal clearance.

Toxicity

The main side effects of MTX are myelosuppression and gastrointestinal (GI) toxicity, which are usually completely reversed within 14 days, unless drug-elimination mechanisms are impaired. In patients with compromised renal function, even small doses of MTX may result in serious toxicity. MTX-induced nephrotoxicity is thought to result from the intratubular precipitation of MTX and its metabolites in acidic urine. Antifolates may also exert a direct toxic effect on the renal tubules. Vigorous hydration and urinary alkalinization have greatly reduced the incidence of renal failure in patients on high-dose regimens. Acute elevations in hepatic enzyme levels and hyperbilirubinemia are often observed during high-dose therapy, but these levels usually return to normal within 10 days. Methotrexate given concomitantly with radiotherapy may increase the risk of soft tissue necrosis and osteonecrosis.

The original rationale for high-dose MTX therapy was based on the concept of selective rescue of normal tissues by the reduced folate leucovorin (LV). However, recent data suggest that high-dose MTX may also overcome resistance mechanisms caused by impaired active transport, decreased affinity of DHFR for MTX,

increased levels of DHFR resulting from gene amplification, and/or decreased polyglutamation of MTX.

The main toxicities of pemetrexed and pralatrexate include dose-limiting myelosuppression, mucositis, and skin rash, usually in the form of the hand-foot syndrome (HFS). Other toxicities include reversible transaminasemia, anorexia and fatigue syndrome, and GI toxicity. These side effects are reduced by supplementation with folic acid (350 μg orally daily) and vitamin B$_{12}$ (1,000 mg subcutaneously given at least 1 week before starting therapy, and then repeated every three cycles). To date, there is no evidence to suggest that vitamin supplementation adversely affects the clinical efficacy of pemetrexed or pralatrexate.

5-FLUOROPYRIMIDINES

The fluoropyrimidine, 5-fluorouracil (5-FU) was synthesized by Charles Heidelberger in the mid 1950s. Uracil is a normal component of RNA; as such, the rationale leading to the development of the drug was that cancer cells might be more sensitive to *decoy* molecules that mimic the natural compound than normal cells. 5-FU and its derivatives are an integral part of treatment for a broad range of solid tumors (see Table 19.1), including GI malignancies (esophageal, gastric, pancreatic, colorectal, anal, and hepatocellular cancers), breast, head and neck, and skin cancers.[11] It continues to serve as the main backbone for combination regimens used to treat metastatic colorectal cancer (mCRC) and as adjuvant therapy of early-stage colon cancer.

Mechanism of Action

5-FU enters cells via the facilitated uracil base transport mechanism and is then anabolized to various cytotoxic nucleotide forms

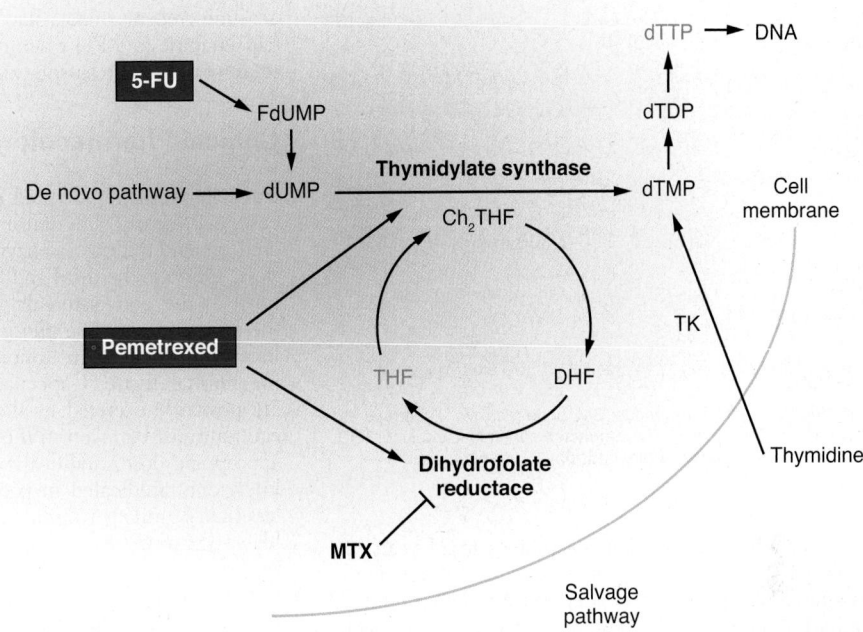

Figure 19.1 Antifolates and 5-fluorouracil (5-FU) sites of action. FdUMP, fluorodeoxyuridine monophosphate; dUMP, deoxyuridine monophosphate; dTTP, deoxythymidine triphosphate; dTDP, deoxyuridine diphosphate; dTMP, deoxythymidine monophosphate; TK, thymidine kinase; CH₂THF, 5,10-methylenetetrahydrofolate; THF, tetrahydrofolate; DHF, dihydrofolate.

by several biochemical pathways. It is thought that 5-FU exerts its cytotoxic effects through various mechanisms, including (1) the inhibition of TS, (2) incorporation into RNA, and (3) incorporation into DNA (Fig. 19.1). In addition to these mechanisms, the genotoxic stress resulting from TS inhibition may also activate programmed cell-death pathways in susceptible cells, which leads to the induction of parental DNA fragmentation.

Mechanisms of Resistance

Several resistance mechanisms to 5-FU have been identified in experimental and clinical settings. Alterations in the target enzyme TS represent the most commonly described mechanism of resistance. In vitro, in vivo, and clinical studies have documented a strong correlation between the levels of TS enzyme activity/TS protein and chemosensitivity to 5-FU. In this regard, cell lines and tumors with higher levels of TS are relatively more resistant to 5-FU. Mutations in the TS protein have been identified that lead to reduced binding affinity of the 5-FU metabolite fluorodeoxyuridine monophosphate (FdUMP) to the TS protein. Reduced expression and/or diminished activity of key activating enzymes may interfere with the formation of cytotoxic 5-FU metabolites. Decreased expression of mismatch repair enzymes, such as human mutL homolog 1 (hMLH1) and human mutS homolog 2 (hMSH2), and increased expression of the catabolic enzyme dihydropyrimidine dehydrogenase (DPD) are associated with fluoropyrimidine resistance. At this time, the relative contribution of each of these mechanisms in the development of cellular resistance to 5-FU in the actual clinical setting remains unclear.

Clinical Pharmacology

5-FU is not orally administered, given its erratic bioavailability resulting from high levels of the catabolic enzyme DPD present in the gut mucosa. After intravenous bolus doses, metabolic elimination is rapid, with a half-life of 8 to 14 minutes. More than 85% of an administered dose of 5-FU is enzymatically inactivated by DPD, the rate-limiting enzyme in the catabolism of 5-FU.

A pharmacogenetic syndrome has been identified in which partial or compete deficiency in the DPD enzyme is present in 3% to 5% and 0.1% of the general population, respectively. As DPD catalyzes the rate-limiting step in the catabolic pathway of 5-FU, a deficiency of DPD can result in a clinically dangerous increase in the anabolic products of 5-FU. Unfortunately, patients with DPD deficiency do not manifest a phenotype only until they are treated with 5-FU, and in that setting, they can develop severe GI toxicity in the form of mucositis and/or diarrhea, myelosuppression, neurologic toxicity, and in rare cases, death. In patients being treated with 5-FU or any other fluoropyrimidine, it is important to consider DPD deficiency in patients who present with excessive, severe toxicity.[12] It is now increasingly appreciated that DPD mutations are unable to account for all of the observed cases of excessive 5-FU toxicity, because up to 50% of patients who experience 5-FU toxicity will have no documented alterations in the *DPD* gene. Moreover, individuals with normal DPD enzyme activity may be diagnosed with high plasma levels of 5-FU, resulting in increased toxicity. Although DPD enzyme activity can be assayed from peripheral blood mononuclear cells in a specialized laboratory, routine phenotypic and genotypic screenings for DPD deficiency prior to 5-FU therapy are not yet available.

Biomodulation of 5-FU

Significant efforts have focused on enhancing the antitumor activity of 5-FU through biochemical modulation in which 5-FU is combined with various agents, including leucovorin, MTX, N-phosphonacetyl-L-aspartic acid, interferon-α, interferon-γ, and

TABLE 19.2

Toxicities of Different Forms of 5-FU

Route	Schedule	Dose	DLT
IV	Daily × 5, bolus	400–500 (mg/m²/d)	⇓ BM D M
IV	Weekly bolus	450–500 (mg/m²/d)	⇓ BM
IV	Daily × 5, CI	750–1,000 (mg/m²/d)	M D
IV	PCI	200–400 (mg/m²/d)	M HFS
HAI	Daily × 14–21, CI	750–1,000 (mg/m²/d)	M D
IP	32–120 hr	5 nM	M D
Oral (Xeloda)	14–21 d	2,000–2,500 (mg/m²/d)	HFS

DLT, dose limiting toxicity; IV, intravenous; BM, bone marrow; D, diarrhea; M, mucositis; CI, continuous infusion; PCI, protracted continuous infusion; HFS, hand-foot syndrome; HAI, hepatic artery infusion; IP, intraperitoneal.

a whole host of other agents.[13] For the past 20 to 25 years, the reduced folate LV has been the main biochemical modulator of 5-FU. An alternative approach has been to alter the schedule of 5-FU administration. Given the S-phase specificity of this agent, prolonged exposure of tumor cells to 5-FU would increase the fraction of cells being exposed to the drug. Overall response rates are significantly higher in patients treated with infusional schedules of 5-FU than in those treated with bolus 5-FU, and this improvement in response rate has translated into an improved progression-free survival. Moreover, the overall safety profile is improved with infusional regimens. A hybrid schedule of bolus and infusional 5-FU was originally developed in France, and this regimen has shown superior clinical activity compared with bolus 5-FU schedules. This hybrid schedule has now been simplified by using only the 46-hour infusion of 5-FU and completely eliminating the 5-FU bolus doses.

Toxicity

The spectrum of 5-FU toxicity is dose- and schedule-dependent (Table 19.2). The main side effects are diarrhea, mucositis, and myelosuppression. The dermatologic HFS is more commonly observed with infusional 5-FU therapy. Acute neurologic symptoms have also been reported, and they include somnolence, cerebellar ataxia, and upper motor signs. Treatment with 5-FU can, on rare occasions, cause coronary vasospasm, resulting in a syndrome of chest pain, cardiac enzyme elevations, and electrocardiographic changes. Cardiac toxicity seems to be related more to infusional 5-FU than bolus administration.[14]

CAPECITABINE

Capecitabine is an oral fluoropyrimidine carbamate that was rationally designed to allow for selective 5-FU activation in tumor tissue.[15] This oral agent was initially approved in anthracycline- and taxane-resistant breast cancer and subsequently approved for use in combination with docetaxel as second-line therapy in metastatic breast cancer and in combination with lapatinib, a tyrosine-kinase inhibitor of human epidermal growth factor receptor type 2 (HER2) and epidermal growth factor receptor (EGFR) in women with HER2-positive metastatic breast cancer following progression on trastuzumab-based therapy.[16] This agent is also approved by the

U.S. Food and Drug Administration (FDA) for the first-line treatment of mCRC and as adjuvant therapy for stage III colon cancer when fluoropyrimidine therapy alone is preferred.[17] In Europe and throughout much of the world, the combination of capecitabine plus oxaliplatin (XELOX) is approved for the treatment of mCRC as well as for the adjuvant therapy of stage III colon cancer.[18] In addition, recent studies have documented the noninferiority of capecitabine to 5-FU when combined with cisplatin in the treatment of metastatic gastric cancer.

Clinical Pharmacology

Capecitabine is rapidly and extensively absorbed by the gut mucosa, with nearly 80% oral bioavailability. It is inactive in its parent form and undergoes enzymatic conversion via three successive steps. Of note, the third and final step occurs in tumor tissue and involves the conversion of 5′-deoxy-5-fluorouridine to 5-FU by the enzyme thymidine phosphorylase (TP), which is expressed at much higher levels in tumors when compared with corresponding normal tissue. Capecitabine and capecitabine metabolites are primarily excreted by the kidneys, and in contrast to 5-FU, caution must be taken in the presence of renal dysfunction, with appropriate dose modification. The use of capecitabine is absolutely contraindicated in patients whose creatinine clearance is less than 30 mL per minute. The FDA and Roche have added a black box warning and strengthened the precautions section on the capecitabine label about the drug–drug interaction between warfarin and capecitabine-based chemotherapy. It is generally recommended to do weekly monitoring of the coagulation parameters (prothrombin time/international normalized ratio [PT/INR]) for all patients receiving concomitant warfarin and capecitabine, with an appropriate adjustment of warfarin dose.

Toxicity

Similar to what is observed with infusional 5-FU, the main side effects of capecitabine include diarrhea and HFS. Of note, the incidence of myelosuppression, neutropenic fever, mucositis, alopecia, and nausea/vomiting is lower with capecitabine when compared with 5-FU. Elevations in indirect serum bilirubin can be observed, but are usually transient and clinically asymptomatic. Patients in the United States appear to be unable to tolerate as high doses of capecitabine as European patients, either as monotherapy or in combination with other cytotoxic chemotherapy.[19] Although the underlying reasons for this discrepancy are not known, it may in part be related to the increased fortification of the US diet with folate and the increased focus on vitamin and folic acid supplementation.

S-1

S-1 is an oral fluoropyrimidine that consists of tegafur (FT), a prodrug of 5-FU, combined with two 5-FU biochemical modulators: 5-chloro-2,4-dihydroxypyridine (gimeracil or CDHP), a competitive inhibitor of DPD, and oteracil potassium, which inhibits phosphorylation of 5-flurouracil in the GI tract, thereby decreasing serious GI toxicities such as nausea/vomiting, mucositis, and diarrhea.[20] As with other oral agents, S-1 offers several advantages over 5-FU, including ease of administration, no risks associated with use of central venous access such as infection, thrombosis, etc., and reduced toxicities, especially neurotoxicity. Although S-1 has yet to be approved by the FDA, it has been approved for the treatment of gastric cancer, head and neck, colorectal cancer (CRC), non–small-cell lung, breast, pancreatic, and biliary tract cancers in several countries in Asia and for the treatment of advanced gastric cancer in combination with cisplatin in a large number of European countries.

Clinical Pharmacology

S-1 was designed to provide continuous 5-FU plasma exposure comparable to the intravenous (IV) infusion. FT, the 5-FU prodrug, is absorbed in the small intestine and converted to 5-FU through the liver microsomal P-450 metabolizing enzyme system (CYP2A6). Most of the 5-FU is degraded (85%) by DPD, leading to the formation of fluoro-beta-alanine (FBAL).[21] CDHP inhibits DPD, thus allowing higher concentrations of 5-FU to enter the anabolic pathway and enhance its therapeutic effect. Additionally, the inhibition of DPD leads to a decreased amount of FBAL formation, which presumably leads to reduced neurotoxicity. Oteracil is the final component of the S-1 formulation, and it inhibits orotate phosphoribosyltransferase in the GI mucosa, which prevents the formation of fluorouridine monophosphate (FUMP), thereby decreasing GI toxicity.

The maximum tolerated dose was established at 80 mg/m^2 in two divided doses for a Japanese population and 25 mg/m^2 twice a day for a Caucasian population. This interethnic variability of S-1 pharmacokinetics and pharmacodynamics has been attributed to differences in the CYP2A6 genotypes.[22] Studies have demonstrated a high frequency of allelic variants CYP2A6*4, *7, and *9 in East Asians than in Caucasians, which might be associated with reduced enzymatic activity and decreased activation of FT. On the other hand, higher FT metabolism is seen in Caucasian patients due to higher CYP2A6 activity. However, investigators have established similar 5-FU exposure between these two ethnic groups. These findings were explained by higher CDHP exposure in Asians, resulting in increased DPD inhibition and slower catabolism of 5-FU, despite having low CYP2A6 activity, whereas Caucasians had higher CYP2A6 activity but faster 5-FU clearance.

Clinical Toxicity

Clinical studies have shown that the GI toxicities associated with S-1, such as diarrhea, nausea, vomiting, and hyperbilirubinemia, are more prominent in Western patients, whereas hematologic toxicities are more prevalent in Japanese patients. The difference in safety profile cannot be explained by differences in 5-FU exposure, because pharmacokinetic studies have shown that overall drug exposures are similar. A potential explanation might involve interethnic variations in TS promoter enhancer region polymorphisms, which are more frequently seen in Asians or in Caucasians on a higher folate diet.

CYTARABINE

Cytarabine (ara-C) is a deoxycytidine nucleoside analog isolated from the sponge *Cryptotethya crypta*, and it differs from its physiologic counterpart by virtue of a stereotypic inversion of the 2'-hydroxyl group of the sugar moiety.[23] A regimen of ara-C, combined with an anthracycline and given as a 5- or 7-day continuous infusion, is considered the standard induction treatment for acute myeloid leukemia (AML). Ara-C is active against other hematologic malignancies, such as non-Hodgkin's lymphoma, chronic myelogenous leukemia, and acute lymphocytic leukemia (see Table 19.1). However, this agent has absolutely no activity against solid tumors.

Mechanism of Action

Ara-C enters cells via nucleoside transport proteins, the most important one being the equilibrative inhibitor-sensitive (ES) receptor. Once inside the cell, ara-C requires activation for its cytotoxic effects.[23,24] The first metabolic step is the conversion of ara-C to the monophosphate form ara-cytidine monophosphate (ara-CMP) by the enzyme deoxycytidine kinase (dCK) with subsequent phosphorylation to the di- and triphosphate metabolites, respectively. Ara-cytidine triphosphate (ara-CTP) is a potent inhibitor of DNA polymerases α, β, and γ, which in turn interferes with DNA chain elongation, DNA synthesis, and DNA repair. Ara-CTP is also incorporated directly into DNA and functions as a DNA chain terminator, interfering with chain elongation. Catabolism of ara-C involves two key enzymes, cytidine deaminase and deoxycytidylate deaminase. These breakdown enzymes convert ara-C and ara-CMP into the inactive metabolites, ara-uridine (ara-U) and ara-uridine monophosphate (ara-UMP), respectively. The balance between intracellular activation and degradation is critical in determining the amount of drug that is ultimately converted to ara-CTP and, thus, its subsequent cytotoxic and antitumor activity.

Mechanisms of Resistance

Several resistance mechanisms to ara-C have been described. An impaired transmembrane transport, a decreased rate of anabolism, and an increased rate of catabolism may result in the development of ara-C resistance.[23,25,26] The level of cytidine deaminase enzyme activity has been shown to correlate with clinical response in patients with AML undergoing induction chemotherapy with ara-C–containing regimens.

Clinical Pharmacology

Ara-C has poor oral bioavailability given its extensive deamination within the GI tract. Thus, ara-C is administered intravenously via continuous infusion. After administration, ara-C undergoes extensive metabolism in the liver, plasma, and peripheral tissues. Within 24 hours, up to 80% of drug is recovered in the urine as the ara-U metabolite. Ara-C crosses the blood–brain barrier when used at high doses, with cerebrospinal fluid levels between 7% and 14% of plasma levels and reaching peak levels of up to 10 μM.

Toxicity

The toxicity profile of ara-C is highly dependent on the dose and schedule of administration. Myelosuppression is dose-limiting with a standard 7-day regimen. Leukopenia and thrombocytopenia are observed most frequently, with nadirs occurring between days 7 and 14 after drug administration. GI toxicity commonly manifests as a mild-to-moderate degree of anorexia, nausea, and vomiting along with mucositis, diarrhea, and abdominal pain. In rare cases, acute pancreatitis has been observed. The ara-C syndrome has been described in pediatric patients with hematologic malignancies, usually begins within 12 hours after the start of drug infusion, and is characterized by fever, myalgia, bone pain, maculopapular rash, conjunctivitis, malaise, and occasional chest pain.

The administration of ara-C at high doses (2 to 3 g/m^2 with each dose) is associated with profound myelosuppression.[27] Severe GI toxicity in the form of mucositis and/or diarrhea is also observed. Neurologic toxicity is significantly more common with high-dose ara-C than with standard doses, and presents with seizures, cerebral and cerebellar dysfunction, and peripheral neuropathy. Clinical signs of cerebellar dysfunction occur in up to 15% of patients and include dysarthria, dysmetria, and ataxia. Change in alertness and cognitive ability, memory loss, and frontal lobe release signs reflect cerebral toxicity. Despite discontinuation of therapy, clinical recovery is incomplete in up to 30% of affected patients. Pulmonary complications may include noncardiogenic pulmonary edema, acute respiratory distress, and pneumonia, resulting from *Streptococcus viridans* infection. Other side effects associated with high-dose ara-C include conjunctivitis (often responsive to topical corticosteroids), a painful HFS, and rarely, anaphylactic reactions.

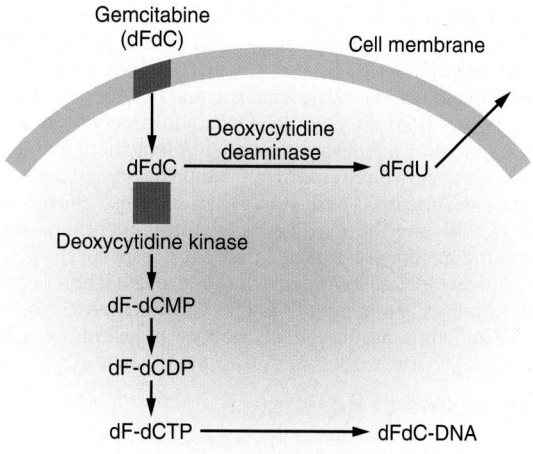

Figure 19.2 Transport and metabolism of gemcitabine. dFdC, gemcitabine; dFdU, 2',2'-difluorodeoxyuridine; dF-dCMP, gemcitabine monophosphate; dF-dCDP, gemcitabine diphosphate; dF-dCTP, gemcitabine triphosphate.

GEMCITABINE

Gemcitabine (2',2'-difluorodeoxycytidine) is a difluorinated deoxycytidine analog. Despite its similarity in structure, metabolism, and mechanism of action to ara-C, the spectrum of antitumor activity of gemcitabine is much broader.[23,28] This compound has significant clinical activity against several human solid tumors, including pancreatic, bile duct, gall bladder, small cell and non–small-cell lung, bladder, ovary, and breast cancers as well as hematologic malignancies, namely Hodgkin's and non-Hodgkin's lymphoma (see Table 19.1).

Mechanism of Action

The transport of gemcitabine into cells requires the nucleoside transporter system. Gemcitabine is inactive in its parent form and requires intracellular activation for its cytotoxic effects. The steps involved in the metabolic activation of gemcitabine are similar to those observed with ara-C, with both drugs being activated by the same enzymatic machinery to the active triphosphate metabolite (see Fig. 19.2). Gemcitabine triphosphate is then incorporated into DNA, resulting in chain termination and the inhibition of DNA synthesis and function, or the triphosphate form can directly inhibit DNA polymerases α, β, and γ, which in turn, interferes with DNA chain elongation, DNA synthesis, and DNA repair. The triphosphate metabolite is also a potent inhibitor of ribonucleotide reductase, which further mediates inhibition of DNA biosynthesis by reducing the levels of key deoxynucleotide pools.[29]

Mechanisms of Resistance

Several mechanisms of resistance to gemcitabine have been described in various preclinical experimental models.[30] Gemcitabine is a polar nucleoside analog that requires the activity of human equilibrative nucleoside transporter 1 (hENT1) to enter cells and exert its cytotoxic effects. Preclinical data in human pancreatic cancer cell lines showed that gemcitabine resistance is negatively correlated with hENT1 expression and can be induced by specific inhibitors of hENT1.[31] Clinical data also support the concept that a lack of hENT1 may be predictive of resistance to gemcitabine. CO-101, a lipid-drug conjugate of gemcitabine, was rationally designed to enter cells independently of hENT1. Unfortunately, two studies in pancreatic cancer failed to show any benefit of CO-101.

Additionally, several enzymes involved in the intracellular metabolism of gemcitabine have been implicated in the development of cellular drug resistance, including reduced expression and/or deficiency in dCK enzyme activity as well as increased expression and/or activity of the catabolic enzymes cytidine deaminase and dCMP deaminase. Recent studies have also identified a subset of CD44-positive cancer stem cells within pancreatic tumors that sustain tumor formation and growth, and are resistant to gemcitabine therapy.[33]

Clinical Pharmacology

Gemcitabine is administered via the intravenous route, typically over a 30-minute intravenous infusion, and it undergoes extensive metabolism by deamination to the catabolic metabolite, difluorodeoxyuridine (dFdU), with more than 90% of the metabolized drug being recovered in urine. Plasma clearance is about 30% lower in women and in elderly patients, and this pharmacokinetic difference may result in an increased risk of toxicity in these respective patient populations. The initial findings from pilot pharmacokinetic studies suggested that gemcitabine, when given at a fixed dose rate (FDR) intravenous infusion of 10 mg/m^2 per minute, produced the highest accumulation of active dFdCTP metabolites in peripheral blood mononuclear cells, which led to a randomized phase II trial that compared gemcitabine 1,500 mg/m^2 by FDR or 2,200 mg/m^2 of gemcitabine over 30 minutes. Although this phase II study suggested an improved overall survival with FDR, a subsequent phase III trial failed to confirm the survival advantage of gemcitabine by FDR over its conventional administration schedule.[34]

Toxicity

Gemcitabine is a relatively well-tolerated drug when used as a single agent. The main dose-limiting toxicity is myelosuppression, with neutropenia more commonly experienced than thrombocytopenia. Toxicity is schedule dependent, with longer infusions producing greater hematologic toxicity. Transient flulike symptoms, including fever, headache, arthralgias, and myalgias, occur in 45% of patients. Asthenia and transient transaminasemia may occur. Renal microangiopathy syndromes, including hemolytic-uremic syndrome and thrombotic thrombocytopenic purpura, have been reported rarely.

6-THIOPURINES

The development of the purine analogs in cancer chemotherapy began in the early 1950s with the synthesis of the thiopurines, 6-mercaptopurine (6-MP) and 6-thioguanine (6-TG). 6-MP an important role in maintenance therapy for acute lymphoblastic leukemia, whereas 6-TG is active in remission induction and in maintenance therapy for AML (see Table 19.1).

Mechanism of Action

The thiopurines, 6-MP and 6-TG, act similarly with respect to their cellular biochemistry.[34] In their respective monophosphate nucleotide forms, they inhibit enzymes involved in de novo purine synthesis and purine interconversion reactions. The triphosphate nucleotide forms can get directly incorporated into either cellular RNA or DNA, leading to the inhibition of RNA and DNA synthesis and function, respectively.

Mechanisms of Resistance

The development of cellular resistance to 6-thiopurines results from a decreased level of key cytotoxic nucleotide metabolites, either through decreased formation or increased breakdown. Resistant cells have been identified that express either complete or partial deficiency of the activating enzyme hypoxanthine-guanine phosphoribosyltransferase (HGPRT). In clinical samples derived from patients with AML, drug resistance has been associated with increased concentrations of a membrane-bound alkaline phosphatase or a conjugating enzyme, 6-thiopurine methyltransferase (TPMT), the end-result being reduced formation of cytotoxic thiopurine nucleotides. Finally, the decreased expression of mismatch repair enzymes, including hMLH1 and hMSH2, has been associated with cellular drug resistance.

Clinical Pharmacology

Oral absorption of 6-MP is highly erratic, and the relatively poor oral bioavailability is mainly related to rapid first-pass metabolism in the liver. The major route of drug elimination is via metabolism by several enzymatic pathways. 6-MP is oxidized to the inactive metabolite 6-thiouric acid by xanthine oxidase. Enhanced 6-MP toxicity may result from the concomitant administration of 6-MP and the xanthine oxidase inhibitor allopurinol. In patients receiving both 6-MP and allopurinol, the 6-MP dose must be reduced by at least 50% to 75%. 6-MP also undergoes S-methylation by the enzyme TPMT to yield 6-methylmercaptopurine.[35]

6-TG is administered orally in the treatment of AML. Its oral bioavailability is erratic, with peak plasma levels occurring 2 to 4 hours after ingestion. The catabolism of 6-TG differs from 6-MP in that it is not a direct substrate for xanthine oxidase.

TPMT enzyme activity may vary considerably among patients as a result of point mutations or loss of alleles of TPMT.[36] Approximately 0.3% of the Caucasian population expresses either a homozygous deletion or a mutation of both alleles of the *TPMT* gene. In these patients, grossly elevated thiopurine nucleotides concentrations, profound myelosuppression with pancytopenia, and extensive GI symptoms are observed after only a brief course of thiopurine treatment. An estimated 10% of patients may be at increased risk for toxicity because of heterozygous loss of the gene or a mutant allele coding for a less enzymatically active TPMT.

Toxicity

The major dose-related toxicities of the thiopurines are myelosuppression and GI toxicity in the form of nausea/vomiting, anorexia, diarrhea, and stomatitis.[37] In TPMT-deficient patients, dosage reduction to 5% to 25% of the standard dosage is necessary to prevent severe excessive toxicity. Thiopurine hepatotoxicity occurs in up to 30% of adult patients and presents mainly as cholestatic jaundice, although elevations of hepatic transaminases may also be seen. Combinations of thiopurines with other known hepatotoxic agents should be avoided, and liver function should be closely monitored. The thiopurines are also potent suppressors of cell-mediated immunity, and prolonged therapy results in an increased predisposition to bacterial and parasitic infections.

FLUDARABINE

Fludarabine (9-β-D-arabinosyl-2-fluoroadenine monophosphate, F-ara-AMP) is an active agent in the treatment of chronic lymphocytic leukemia (CLL) (see Table 19.1).[38,39] It is also active against indolent non-Hodgkin's lymphoma, prolymphocytic leukemia, cutaneous T-cell lymphoma, and Waldenström macroglobulinemia. This agent has also shown promising activity in mantle cell lymphoma. In contrast to its activity in hematologic malignancies, this compound has virtually no activity against solid tumors.

Mechanism of Action

The active cytotoxic metabolite is the triphosphate metabolite F-ara-ATP, which competes with deoxyadenosine triphosphate (dATP) for incorporation into DNA and serves as a highly effective chain terminator. In addition, F-ara-ATP directly inhibits enzymes involved in DNA replication, including DNA polymerases, DNA primase, DNA ligase I, and ribonucleotide reductase.[37] F-ara-ATP is also incorporated into RNA, causing the inhibition of RNA function, processing, and mRNA translation. In contrast to other antimetabolites, fludarabine is active against nondividing cells. In fact, the primary effect of fludarabine may result from activation of apoptosis, through an as yet ill-defined mechanisms.[39] This finding may explain the activity of fludarabine in indolent lymphoproliferative diseases with relatively low growth fractions.

Mechanisms of Resistance

The decreased expression of the activating enzyme dCK resulting in diminished intracellular formation of F-ara-AMP is one of the main resistance mechanisms identified in preclinical models.[38] A high degree of cross-resistance develops to multiple nucleoside analogs, requiring activation by dCK, including cytarabine, gemcitabine, cladribine, and clofarabine. Reduced cellular transport of drug has also been identified as a resistance mechanism.

Clinical Pharmacology

Peak concentrations of F-ara-A are reached 3 to 4 hours after intravenous administration.[40] The main route of elimination is via the kidneys, with about 25% of a given dose of drug being excreted unchanged in the urine.

Toxicity

Myelosuppression and immunosuppression are the major side effects of fludarabine as highlighted by dose-limiting and possibly cumulative lymphopenia and thrombocytopenia. Suppression of the immune system affects T-cell function more than B-cell function. Fevers, often in the setting of neutropenia, occur in 20% to 30% of patients. Lymphocyte counts, specifically CD4-positive cells, decrease rapidly after the initiation of therapy, and recovery of CD4-positive cells to normal levels may take longer than 1 year. Common opportunistic pathogens include the varicella-zoster virus, *Candida*, and *Pneumocystis carinii*. In general, patients are empirically placed on sulfamethoxazole trimethoprim prophylaxis to prevent the development of *P. carinii* infection.

CLADRIBINE

Cladribine (2-CdA) is a purine deoxyadenosine analog, and it is the drug of choice for hairy cell leukemia with activity in low-grade lymphoproliferative disorders (see Table 19.1).[41,42] Salvage treatment of patients previously treated with interferon-α or splenectomy is as effective as first-line treatment. Retreatment with cladribine results in a complete response in up to 60% of relapsing patients. In addition, this agent has promising activity in patients with CLL and non-Hodgkin's lymphoma.

Mechanism of Action

Upon entry into the cell, 2-CdA undergoes an initial conversion to cladribine-monophosphate (Cd-AMP) via the reaction catalyzed by dCK, and Cd-AMP is subsequently metabolized to the active metabolite, cladribine-triphosphate. The triphosphate metabolite competitively inhibits incorporation of the normal dATP nucleotide into DNA, a process that results in the termination of chain elongation.[43] Progressive accumulation of the triphosphate metabolite leads to an imbalance in deoxyribonucleotide pools, thereby inhibiting further DNA synthesis and repair. Finally, the triphosphate metabolite is a potent inhibitor of ribonucleotide reductase, which further facilitates the inhibition of DNA biosynthesis.

Mechanisms of Resistance

Resistance to 2-CdA has been attributed to altered intracellular drug metabolism. A reduction in the activity of dCK, the enzyme responsible for generating cytotoxic nucleotide metabolites, is a major determinant of acquired resistance. The monophosphate and triphosphate metabolites are dephosphorylated by the cytoplasmic enzyme 5'-nucleotidase. Interestingly, resistant cells derived from a patient with CLL exhibited both low levels of dCK expression and high levels of 5'-nucleotidase.

Clinical Pharmacology

2-CdA is orally bioavailable, with 50% of an administered dose orally absorbed. Approximately 50% of an administered dose of drug is cleared by the kidneys, and 20% to 35% of the drug is excreted unchanged in the urine. Of note, this nucleoside can cross the blood–brain barrier with penetration into the cerebrospinal fluid.

Toxicity

At conventional doses, myelosuppression is dose limiting. After a single course of drug, recovery from thrombocytopenia usually occurs within 2 to 4 weeks, whereas recovery from neutropenia takes place in 3 to 5 weeks. GI toxicities are generally mild, with nausea/vomiting and diarrhea. Mild-to-moderate neurotoxicity occurs in 15% of patients and is at least partly reversible with discontinuation of the drug. Immunosuppression accounts for the late morbidity observed in 2-CdA–treated patients. Lymphocyte counts, particularly CD4-positive cells, decrease within 1 to 4 weeks of drug administration and may remain depressed for several years.[44] After discontinuation of 2-CdA, a median time of up to 40 months may be required for complete recovery of normal CD4-positive counts. Although opportunistic infections occur, they do so less frequently than with fludarabine therapy. Infectious complications correlate with decreases in the CD4-positive count, and they include herpes zoster, *Candida*, *Pneumocystis*, *Pseudomonas aeruginosa*, *Listeria monocytogenes*, *Cryptococcus neoformans*, *Aspergillus*, *P. carinii*, and cytomegalovirus.

CLOFARABINE

Clofarabine is a purine deoxyadenosine nucleoside analog, and it is approved for the treatment of pediatric patients with relapsed or refractory acute lymphoblastic leukemia (see Table 19.1).[45]

Ongoing studies are exploring the benefit of clofarabine alone and in combination with other agents in less heavily pretreated patients and in the use of different dose schedules for other hematologic malignancies.[46]

Mechanism of Action

Clofarabine is inactive in its parent form and, like other purine analogs, it requires intracellular activation by dCK to form the monophosphate nucleotide, which undergoes further metabolism to the cytotoxic triphosphate metabolite. Clofarabine triphosphate is then incorporated into DNA, resulting in chain termination, and inhibition of DNA synthesis and function or the triphosphate form can directly inhibit DNA polymerases α, β, and γ, which in turn, interferes with DNA chain elongation, DNA synthesis, and DNA repair. The triphosphate metabolite is also a potent inhibitor of ribonucleotide reductase, further mediating the inhibition of DNA biosynthesis by reducing the levels of key deoxyribonucleotide pools.

Mechanisms of Resistance

Several resistance mechanisms have been identified in various preclinical systems, and they include decreased activation of the drug through the reduced expression of the anabolic enzyme deoxycytidine kinase, the decreased transport of drug into cells via the nucleoside transporter protein, and the increased expression of CTP synthetase activity resulting in increased concentrations of competing physiologic nucleotide substrate dCTP. To date, the precise resistance mechanism(s) that are relevant in the clinical setting remain to be determined.

Clinical Pharmacology

Approximately 50% to 60% of an administered dose of drug is excreted unchanged in the urine, and the terminal half-life is on the order of 5 hours. To date, the pathways for nonrenal elimination have not been well defined. Caution should be exercised in patients with abnormal renal function, and concomitant use of medications known to cause renal toxicity should be avoided during drug treatment.

Toxicity

Myelosuppression is dose limiting with neutropenia, anemia, and thrombocytopenia. The capillary leak syndrome (systemic inflammatory response syndrome) presents with tachypnea, tachycardia, pulmonary edema, and hypotension.[47] In essence, this adverse event is part of the tumor lysis syndrome and results from rapid cytoreduction of peripheral leukemic cells following treatment.[47] Other side effects may include nausea/vomiting, reversible liver dysfunction (hyperbilirubinemia and elevated serum transaminases), renal dysfunction (approximately 10%), and cardiac toxicity in the form of tachycardia and acute pump dysfunction.

REFERENCES

1. Wright DL, Anderson AC. Antifolate agents: a patent review (2006–2010). *Expert Opin Ther Pat* 2011;21:1293–1308.
2. Chattopadhyay S, Moran RG, Goldman ID. Pemetrexed: biochemical and cellular pharmacology, mechanisms, and clinical applications. *Mol Cancer Ther* 2007;6:404–417.
3. Vogelzang NJ, Rusthoven JJ, Symanowski J, et al. Phase III study of pemetrexed in combination with cisplatin versus cisplatin alone in patients with malignant pleural mesothelioma. *J Clin Oncol* 2003;21:2636–2644.
4. Kindler HL. Systemic treatments for mesothelioma: standard and novel. *Curr Treat Options Oncol* 2008;9:171–179.
5. Joerger M, Omlin A, Cerny T, et al. The role of pemetrexed in advanced non small-cell lung cancer: special focus on pharmacology and mechanism of action. *Curr Drug Targets* 2010;11:37–47.
6. Zain J, O'Connor O. Pralatrexate: basic understanding and clinical development. *Expert Opin Pharmacother* 2010;11:1705–1714.
7. Sirotnak FM, DeGraw JI, Moccio DM, et al. New folate analogs of the 10-deaza-aminopterin series. Basis for structural design and biochemical and pharmacologic properties. *Cancer Chemother Pharmacol* 1984;12:18–25.
8. O'Connor OA. Pralatrexate: an emerging new agent with activity in T-cell lymphomas. *Curr Opin Oncol* 2006;18:591–597.

9. Bertino JR, Göker E, Gorlick R, et al. Resistance mechanisms to methotrexate in tumors. *Oncologist* 1996;1:223–226.

10. Zhao R, Goldman ID. Resistance to antifolates. *Oncogene* 2003;22:7431–7457.

11. Grem JL. 5-Fluorouracil: forty-plus and still ticking. A review of its preclinical and clinical development. *Invest New Drugs* 2000;18:299–313.

12. Saif MW, Ezzeldin H, Vance K, et al. DPYD*2A mutation: the most common mutation associated with DPD deficiency. *Cancer Chemother Pharmacol* 2007;60:503–507.

13. Grem JL. Biochemical modulation of 5-FU in systemic treatment of advanced colorectal cancer. *Oncology (Williston Park)* 2001;15:13–19.

14. Saif MW, Shah MM, Shah AR. Fluoropyrimidine-associated cardiotoxicity: revisited. *Expert Opin Drug Saf* 2009;8:191–202.

15. Saif MW, Eloubeidi MA, Russo S, et al. Phase I study of capecitabine with concomitant radiotherapy for patients with locally advanced pancreatic cancer: expression analysis of genes related to outcome. *J Clin Oncol* 2005;23:8679–8687.

16. Geyer CE, Forster J, Lindquist D, et al. Lapatinib plus capecitabine for HER2-positive advanced breast cancer. *N Engl J Med* 2006;355:2733–2743.

17. Saif MW, Katirtzoglou NA, Syrigos KN. Capecitabine: an overview of the side effects and their management. *Anticancer Drugs* 2008;19:447–464.

18. Van Custem E, Verslype C, Tejpar S. Oral capecitabine: bridging the Atlantic divide in colon cancer treatment. *Semin Oncol* 2005;32:43–51.

19. Haller DG, Cassidy J, Clarke SJ, et al. Potential regional differences for the tolerability profiles of fluoropyrimidines. *J Clin Oncol* 2008;26:2118–2123.

20. Saif MW, Syrigos KN, Katirtzoglou NA. S-1: a promising new oral fluoropyrimidine derivative. *Expert Opin Investig Drugs* 2009;18:335–348.

21. Saif MW, Rosen LS, Saito K, et al. A phase I study evaluating the effect of CDHP as a component of S-1 on the pharmacokinetics of 5-fluorouracil. *Anticancer Res* 2011;31:625–632.

22. Daigo S, Takahashi Y, Fujieda M, et al. A novel mutant allele of the CYP2A6 gene (CYP2A6*11) found in a cancer patient who showed poor metabolic phenotype towards tegafur. *Pharmacogenetics* 2002;12:299–306.

23. Reiter A, Hochhaus A, Berger U, et al. AraC-based pharmacotherapy of chronic myeloid leukaemia. *Expert Opin Pharmacother* 2001;2:1129–1135.

24. Braess J, Wegendt C, Feuring-Buske M, et al. Leukemic blasts differ from normal bone marrow mononuclear cells and CD34+ hematopoietic stem cells in their metabolism of cytosine arabinoside. *Br J Haematol* 1999;105:388–393.

25. Momparler RL, Laliberte J, Eliopoulos N, et al. Transfection of murine fibroblast cells with human cytidine deaminase cDNA confers resistance to cytosine arabinoside. *Anticancer Drugs* 1996;7:266–274.

26. Cai J, Damaraju VL, Groulx N, et al. Two distinct molecular mechanisms underlying cytarabine resistance in human leukemic cells. *Cancer Res* 2008;68:2349–2357.

27. Kern W, Estey EH. High-dose cytosine arabinoside in the treatment of acute myeloid leukemia: review of three randomized trials. *Cancer* 2006;107:116–124.

28. Mini E, Nobili S, Caciagli B, et al. Cellular pharmacology of gemcitabine. *Ann Oncol* 2006;17:v7–v12.

29. Saif MW, Sellers S, Li M, et al. A phase I study of bi-weekly administration of 24-h gemcitabine followed by 24-h irinotecan in patients with solid tumors. *Cancer Chemother Pharmacol* 2007;60:871–882.

30. Bergman AM, Pinedo HM, Peters GJ. Determinants of resistance to 2′, 2′-difluorodeoxycytidine (gemcitabine). *Drug Resist Update* 2002;5:19–33.

31. Saif MW, Lee Y, Kim R. Harnessing gemcitabine metabolism: a step towards personalized medicine for pancreatic cancer. *Ther Adv Med Oncol* 2012;4:341–346.

32. Hong SP, Wen J, Bang S, et al. CD44-positive cells are responsible for gemcitabine resistance in pancreatic cancer cells. *Int J Cancer* 2009;125:2323–2331.

33. Poplin E, Feng Y, Berlin J, et al. Phase III, randomized study of gemcitabine and oxaliplatin versus gemcitabine (fixed-dose rate infusion) compared with gemcitabine (30-minute infusion) in patients with pancreatic carcinoma E6201: a trial of the Eastern Cooperative Oncology Group. *J Clin Oncol* 2009;27:3778–3785.

34. Hande KR. Purine antimetabolites. In: Chabner BA, Longo DL, eds. *Cancer Chemotherapy and Biotherapy: Principles and Practice*, 4th ed. Philadelphia: Lippincott–Raven; 2006: 212.

35. Evans WE. Pharmacogenetics of thiopurine S-methyltransferase and thiopurine therapy. *Ther Drug Monitor* 2004;26:186–191.

36. Wang L, Weinshilboum R. Thiopurine S-methyltransferase pharmacogenetics: insights, challenges, and future directions. *Oncogene* 2006;25:1629–1638.

37. Vora A, Mitchell CD, Lennard L, et al. Toxicity and efficacy of 6-thioguanine versus 6-mercaptopurine in childhood lymphoblastic leukaemia: a randomised trial. *Lancet* 2006;368:1339–1348.

38. Montillo M, Ricci F, Tedeschi A. Role of fludarabine in hematological malignancies. *Expert Rev Anticancer Ther* 2006;6:1141–1161.

39. Gandhi V, Plunkett W. Cellular and clinical pharmacology of fludarabine. *Clin Pharmacokinet* 2002;41:93–103.

40. van den Neste E, Cardoen S, Offner F, et al. Old and new insights into the mechanism of action of two nucleoside analogs active in lymphoid malignancies: fludarabine and cladribine. *Int J Oncol* 2005;27:1113–1124.

41. Gidron A, Tallman MS. 2-CdA in the treatment of hairy cell leukemia: a review of long-term follow-up. *Leuk Lymphoma* 2006;47:2301–2307.

42. Huang P, Robertson LE, Wright S, et al. High molecular weight DNA fragmentation: a critical event in nucleoside analog-induced apoptosis in leukemia cells. *Clin Cancer Res* 1995;1:1005–1013.

43. Grevz N, Saven A. Cladribine: from the bench to the bedside: focus on hairy cell leukemia. *Expert Rev Anticancer Ther* 2004;4:745–757.

44. Seto S, Carrera CJ, Kubota M, et al. Mechanism of deoxyadenosine and 2-chlorodeoxyadenosine toxicity to nondividing human lymphocytes. *J Clin Invest* 1985;75:377–383.

45. Bonate PL, Arthaud L, Cantrell WR Jr, et al. Discovery and development of clofarabine: a nucleoside analogue for treating cancer. *Nat Rev Drug Discov* 2006;5:855–863.

46. Faderi S, Gandhi V, Keating MJ, et al. The role of clofarabine in hematologic and solid malignancies: development of a next generation nucleoside analog. *Cancer* 2005;102:1985–1995.

47. Baytan B, Ozdemir O, Gunes AM, et al. Clofarabine-induced capillary leak syndrome in a child with refractory acute lymphoblastic leukemia. *J Pediatr Hematol Oncol* 2010;32:144–146.

CANCER THERAPEUTICS

20 Topoisomerase Interactive Agents

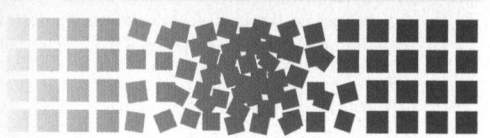

Khanh T. Do, Shivaani Kummar, James H. Doroshow, and Yves Pommier

CLASSIFICATION, BIOCHEMICAL, AND BIOLOGIC FUNCTIONS OF TOPOISOMERASES

Nucleic acids (DNA and RNA) being long polymers, topoisomerases fulfill the need for cellular DNA to be densely packaged in the cell nucleus, transcribed, replicated, and evenly distributed between daughter cells following replication without tangles. Topoisomerases are ubiquitous and essential for all organisms as they prevent and resolve DNA and RNA entanglements and resolve DNA supercoiling during transcription and replication. This chapter first summarizes the basic elements necessary to understand the mechanism of action of topoisomerases and their inhibitors. More detailed information can be found in recent reviews[1–7] and two recent books.[8,9] The second part of the chapter summarizes the use of topoisomerase inhibitors as anticancer drugs.

Classification of Topoisomerases

Human cells contain six topoisomerase genes (Table 20.1), which have been numbered historically. The commonly used abbreviations are Top1 for topoisomerases I (Top1mt being the mitochondrial topoisomerase whose gene is encoded in the cell nucleus),[10] Top2 for topoisomerases II, and Top3 for topoisomerases III. Top1 was the first eukaryotic topoisomerase discovered by Champoux and Dulbecco.[11] Topoisomerases solve DNA topologic problems by cutting the DNA backbone and religating without the assistance of any additional ligase. Top1 and Top3 act by cleaving/religating a single strand of the DNA duplex, whereas Top2 enzymes cleave and religate both strands, making a four–base pair reversible staggered cut (Fig. 20.1). It is convenient to remember that odd-numbered topoisomerases (Top1 and Top3) cleave and religate one strand, whereas the even numbered topoisomerases (Top2s) cleave and religate both strands.

Biochemical Characteristics and Cleavage Complexes of the Different Topoisomerases

The DNA cutting/relegation mechanism is common to all topoisomerases and utilizes an enzyme catalytic tyrosine residue acting as a nucleophile and becoming covalently attached to the end of the broken DNA. These catalytic intermediates are referred to as cleavage complexes (see Fig. 20.1B, E). The reverse religation reaction is carried out by the attack of the ribose hydroxyl ends toward the tyrosyl-DNA bond.

Top1 (and Top1mt) attaches to the 3′-end of the break, whereas the other topoisomerases (Top2 and Top3) have opposite polarity and covalently attach to the 5′-end of the breaks (see Table 20.1 [second column] and Fig. 20.1B, E). Topoisomerases have distinct biochemical requirements. Top1 and Top1mt are the simplest, nicking/closing, and relaxing DNA as monomers in the absence of cofactor, and even at ice temperature. Top2 enzymes, on the other hand, are the most complex topoisomerases working as dimers, requiring ATP binding and hydrolysis, and a divalent metal (Mg^{2+}) for catalysis. Top3 enzymes also require Mg^{2+} for catalysis but function as monomers without ATP requirement. Notably, the DNA substrates differ for Top3 enzymes. Whereas both Top1 and Top2 process double-stranded DNA, the Top3 substrates need to be single-stranded nucleic acids (DNA for Top3α and DNA or RNA for Top3β).[10,12,13]

Differential Topoisomerization Mechanisms: Swiveling Versus Strand Passage, DNA Versus RNA Topoisomerases

Topoisomerases use two main mechanisms to change nucleic topology. The first is by "untwisting" the DNA duplex. This mechanism is unique to Top1, which, by an enzyme-associated single-strand break, allows the broken strand to rotate around the intact strand (see Fig. 20.1B) until DNA supercoiling is dissipated. At this point, the stacking energy of adjacent DNA bases realigns the broken ends, and the 5′-hydroxyl end attacks the 3′-phosphotyrosyl end, thereby relegating the DNA. A remarkable feature of this Top1 untwisting mechanism is its extreme efficiency with a rotation speed around 6,000 rpm and relative independence from torque, thereby allowing full relaxation of DNA supercoiling.[14]

The second topologic mechanism is by "strand passage." This mechanism allows the passage of a double- or a single-stranded DNA (or RNA) through the cleavage complexes. Top2α and Top2β both act by allowing the passage of an intact DNA duplex through the DNA double-strand break generated by the enzymes. After which, Top2 religates the broken duplex. Such reactions permit DNA decatenation, unknotting, and relaxation of supercoils.[3] Top3 enzymes also act by strand passage but only pass one nucleic acid strand through the single-strand break generated by the enzymes. In the case of Top3α, the substrate is a single-stranded DNA segment (such as a double-Holliday junction), whereas in the case of Top3β, the substrate can be a single-stranded RNA segment, with Top3β acting as a RNA topoisomerase.[13,15]

TOPOISOMERASE INHIBITORS AS INTERFACIAL POISONS

Topoisomerase Inhibitors Act as Interfacial Inhibitors by Binding at the Topoisomerase–DNA Interface and Trapping Topoisomerase Cleavage Complexes

Relegation of the cleavage complexes is dependent on the structure of the ends of the broken DNA (i.e., the realignment of the broken ends). Binding the drugs at the enzyme–DNA interface misaligns the ends of the DNA and precludes relegation, resulting in the stabilization of the topoisomerase cleavage complexes (Top1cc and Top2cc). Crystal structures of drug-bound cleavage complexes have firmly established this mechanism for both Top1- and Top2-targeted drugs.[16]

TABLE 20.1

Classification of Human Topoisomerases and Topoisomerase Inhibitors

Type	Polarity	Mechanism	Genes	Proteins	Main Functions	Drugs
IB	3′-PY	Rotation/swiveling	TOP1	Top1	DNA supercoiling relaxation, replication, and transcription	Camptothecins, noncamptothecins
			TOP1MT	Top1mt		
IIA	5′-PY	Strand passage ATPase	TOP2A	Top2α	Decatenation/replication	Anthracyclines, anthracenediones, epipodophyllotoxins
			TOP2B	Top2β	Transcription	
IA	5′-PY	Strand passage	TOP3A	Top3α	DNA replication with BLM	None
			TOP3B	Top3β	RNA topoisomerase	

Top1mt, mitochondrial DNA topoisomerase; BLM, Bloom's syndrome helicare.

It is critical to understand that the cytotoxic mechanism of topoisomerase inhibitors requires the drugs to trap the topoisomerase cleavage complexes rather than block catalytic activity. This sets apart topoisomerase inhibitors from classical enzyme inhibitors such as antifolates. Indeed, knocking out Top1 renders yeast cells totally immune to camptothecin,[17,18] and reducing enzyme levels in cancer cells confers drug resistance. Conversely, in breast cancers, amplification of TOP2A, which is on the same locus as HER2, contributes to the efficacy of doxorubicin.[19] Also, cellular mutations of Top1 and Top2 that renders cells insensitive to the trapping of topoisomerase cleavage complexes produce high resistance to Top1 or Top2 inhibitors. Based on this trapping of cleavage complexes mechanism, we refer to topoisomerase inhibitors as topoisomerase cleavage complex-targeted drugs.

Top1cc-Targeted Drugs (Camptothecin and Noncamptothecin Derivatives) Kill Cancer Cells by Replication Collisions

Top1cc are cytotoxic by their conversion into DNA damage by replication and transcription fork collisions. This explains why cytotoxicity is directly related to drug exposure and why arresting DNA replication protects cells from camptothecin.[20,21] The collisions arise from the fact that the drugs, by slowing down the nicking/closing activity of Top1, uncouple the kinetics of Top1 with the polymerases and helicases, which lead polymerases to collide into Top1cc (Fig. 20.2A). Such collisions have two consequences. They generate double-strand breaks (replication and transcription runoff) and irreversible Top1–DNA adducts (see Fig. 20.2B). The replication double-strand breaks are repaired by homologous recombination, which explains the hypersensitivity of BRCA-deficient cancer cells to Top1cc-targeted drugs.[22] The Top1-covalent complexes can be removed by two pathways, the excision pathway centered around tyrosyl-DNA-phosphodiesterase 1 (TDP1)[23] and the endonuclease pathway involving 3′-flap endonucleases such as XPF-ERCC1.[24] It is also possible that drug-trapped Top1cc directly generate DNA double-strand breaks when they are within 10 base pairs on opposite strands of the DNA duplex or when they occur next to a preexisting single-strand break on the opposite strand. Finally, it is not excluded that topologic defects contribute to the cytotoxicity of Top1cc-targeted drugs (the accumulation of supercoils[25] and the formation of alternative structures such as R-loops) (see Fig. 20.2D).[26]

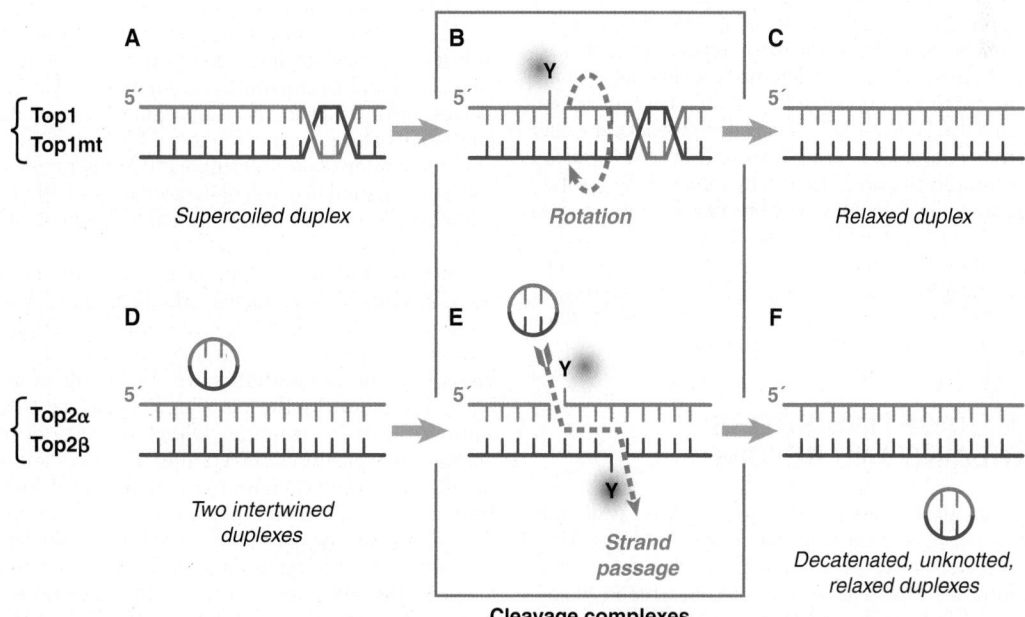

Figure 20.1 Mechanisms of action of topoisomerases. **(A–C)** Topoisomerases I (Top1 for nuclear DNA and Top1mt for mitochondrial DNA) relax supercoiled DNA **(A)** by reversibly cleaving one DNA strand, forming a covalent bond between the enzyme catalytic tyrosine and the 3′ end of the nicked DNA (the Top1 cleavage complex [Top1cc]) **(B)**. This reaction allows the swiveling of the broken strand around the intact strand. Rapid religation allows the dissociation of Top1. **(D–F)** Topoisomerases II (Top2α and Top2β) act on two DNA duplexes **(A)**. They act as homodimers, cleaving both strands and forming a covalent bond between their catalytic tyrosine and the 5′ end of the DNA break (Top2cc) **(E)**. This reaction allows the passage of the intact duplex through the Top2 homodimer (red dotted arrow) **(E)**. Top2 inhibitors trap the Top2cc and prevent the normal religation **(F)**.

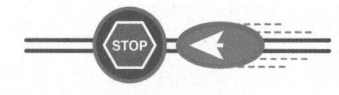

Collisions of polymerases and helicases *(green ellipse)*
with trapped Top cleavage complexes *(Stop sign)*
=> Protein-DNA complexes blocking DNA metabolism

A

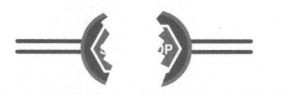

Conversion of Top1cc into DSB by replication "runoff"
=> Top1 needs to be removed by TDP1
     and /or 3'-flap endonucleases (XPF-ERCC1)
=> DSB repaired by homologous recombination
Top1cc also form DSB when on opposite strands or
opposite to a preexisting single-strand break

B

Top2cc readily form DSB when concerted cleavage
on both strands and disjunction of the homodimer

Top2cc proteolysis or mechanical disjoining

C

Topologic defects resulting from Top sequestration
in the cleavage complexes: accumulation of
=> Supercoils (Top1 and Top2) *(1)*
=> Knots (Top2) *(2)*
=> Catenanes (Top2) *(3)*

D

Figure 20.2 Mechanisms of action of topoisomerase inhibitors beyond the trapping of topoisomerase cleavage complexes. **(A)** Stalled or slow cleavage complexes lead to collisions with replication and transcription complexes. **(B)** Collisions of replication complexes with Top1cc on the leading strand for DNA synthesis generate DNA double-strand breaks by replication runoff. Top1cc can also form DNA double-strand breaks (DSBs) when they occur opposite to another Top1cc or preexisting nick. **(C)** Top2cc, which are normally held together by Top2 homodimers, can be converted to free DSBs upon Top2cc proteolysis or dimer disjunction. **(D)** Topologic defects resulting from functional topoisomerase deficiencies play a minor role in the anticancer activity of topoisomerase cleavage complex targeted drugs.

Cytotoxic Mechanisms of Top2cc-Targeted Drugs (Intercalators and Demethyl Epipodophyllotoxins)

Contrary to camptothecins, Top2 inhibitors kill cancer cells without requiring DNA replication fork collisions. Indeed, even after a 30-minute exposure, doxorubicin and other Top2cc-targeted drugs can kill over 99% of the cells, which is in vast excess of the fraction of S-phase cells in tissue culture (generally less than 50%).[27,28] The collision mechanism in the case of Top2cc-targeted drugs (see Fig. 20.2A) appears to involve transcription and proteolysis of both Top2 and RNA polymerase II.[29] Such situation would then lead to DNA double-strand breaks by disruption of the Top2 dimer interface (see Fig. 20.2C). Alternatively, the Top2 homodimer interface could be disjoined by mechanical tension (see Fig. 20.2C). Yet, it is important to bear in mind that 90% of Top2cc trapped by etoposide are not concerted and, therefore, consist in single-strand breaks,[3,30,31] which is different from doxorubicin, which traps both Top2 monomers and produces a majority of DNA double-strand breaks.[32] Finally, it is not excluded that topologic defects resulting from Top2 sequestration by the drug-induced cleavage complexes could contribute to the cytotoxicity of Top2cc-targeted drugs (see Fig. 20.2D). Such topologic defects would include persistent DNA knots and catenanes, potentially leading to chromosome breaks during mitosis.

TOPOISOMERASE I INHIBITORS: CAMPTOTHECINS AND BEYOND

Camptothecin is an alkaloid identified in the 1960s by Wall and Wani[33] in a screen of plant extracts for antineoplastic drugs. The two water-soluble derivatives of camptothecin containing the active lactone form are topotecan and irinotecan, which are approved by the U.S. Food and Drug Administration (FDA) for the treatment of several cancers. In addition, several Top1cc-targeting drugs are in clinical development, including camptothecin derivatives and formulations (including high–molecular-weight conjugates or liposomal formulations), as well as noncamptothecin compounds that exhibit greater potency or noncross resistance to irinotecan and topotecan in preclinical cancer models.[31,34–36]

Irinotecan

Irinotecan, a prodrug containing a bulky dipiperidine side chain at C-10 (Fig. 20.3), is cleaved by a carboxylesterase-converting enzyme in the liver and other tissues to generate the active metabolite, SN-38. Irinotecan is FDA approved for the treatment of colorectal cancer in the metastatic setting as first-line treatment in combination with 5-fluorouracil/leucovorin (5-FU/LV) and as a single agent in the second-line treatment of progressive colorectal cancer after 5-FU–based therapy (see Table 20.1).[37,38] Newer therapeutic uses of irinotecan include a combination with oxaliplatin and 5-FU as first-line treatment in pancreatic cancer.[39] Irinotecan is additionally used in combination with cisplatin or carboplatin in extensive-stage small-cell lung cancer[40,41] as well as refractory esophageal and gastroesophageal junction (GEJ) cancers, gastric cancer, cervical cancer, anaplastic gliomas and glioblastomas, and non–small-cell lung cancer (Table 20.2). Irinotecan is usually administered intravenously at a dose of 125 mg/m^2 for 4 weeks with a 2-week rest period in combination with bolus 5-FU/LV, 180 mg/m^2 every 2 weeks in combination with an infusion of 5-FU/LV, or 350 mg/m^2 every 3 weeks as a single agent.

Diarrhea and myelosuppression are the most common toxicities associated with irinotecan administration. Two mechanisms explain irinotecan-induced diarrhea. Acute cholinergic effects resulting in abdominal cramping and diarrhea occur within 24 hours of drug administration are the result of acetylcholinesterase inhibition by the prodrug, and can be treated with the administration of atropine. Direct mucosal cytotoxicity with diarrhea is typically observed after 24 hours and can result in significant morbidity. Symptoms are managed with loperamide. Hepatic metabolism and biliary excretion accounts for >70% of the elimination of the administered dose, with renal excretion accounting for the remainder of the dose. SN-38 is glucuronidated in the liver by UGT1A1, and deficiencies in this pathway increase the risk of diarrhea and myelosuppression. Dose reductions are recommended for patients who are homozygous for the UGT1A1*28 allele, for which an FDA-approved test for detection of the UGT1A1*28 allele in patients is available.[42,43] Additionally, dose reductions of irinotecan are recommended for patients with hepatic dysfunction, with bilirubin greater than 1.5 mg/mL.[44]

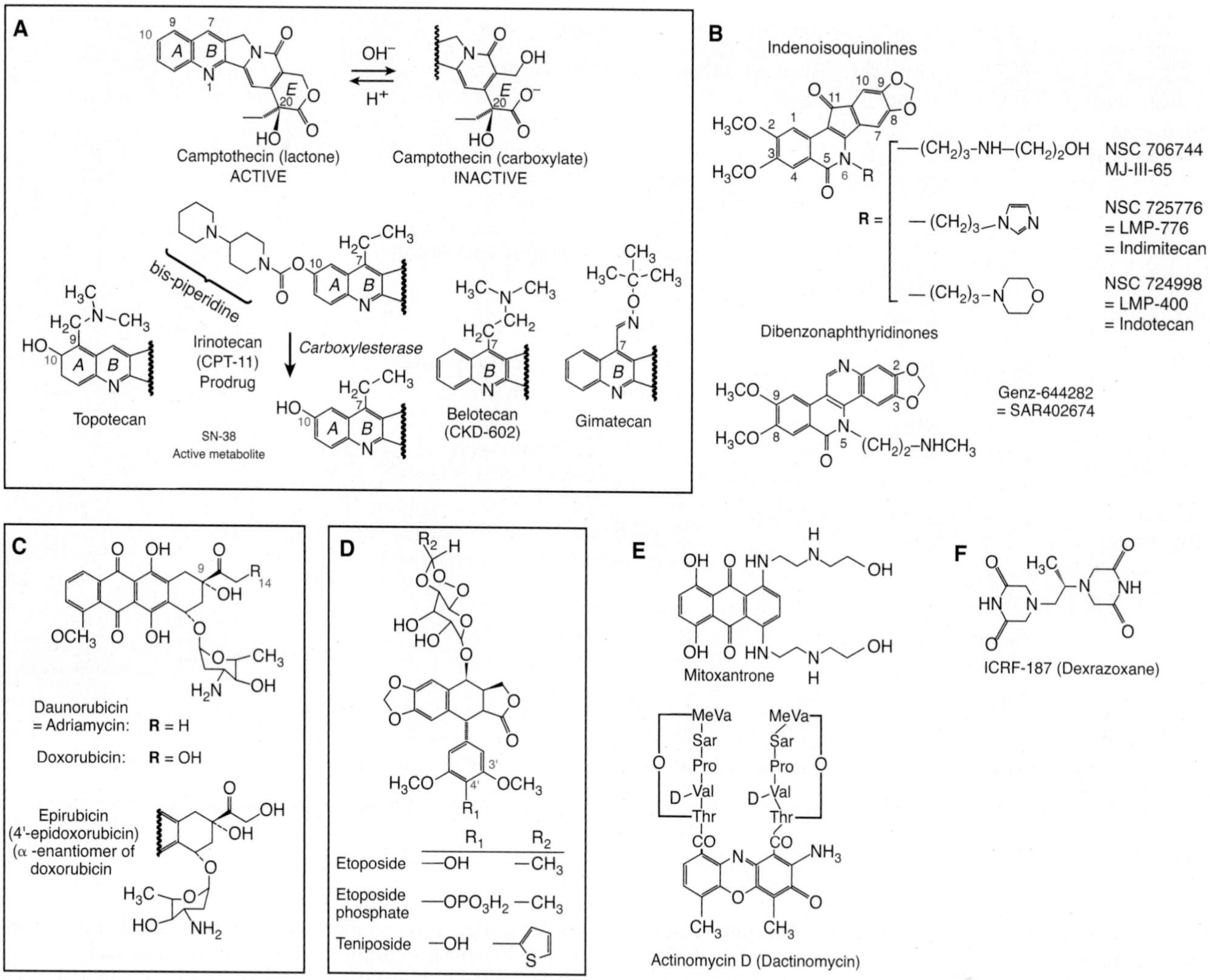

Figure 20.3 Structure of topoisomerase inhibitors. **(A)** Camptothecin derivatives are instable at physiologic pH with the formation of a carboxylate derivative within minutes. Irinotecan is a prodrug and needs to be converted to SN-38 to trap Top1cc. **(B)** Non-camptothecin derivatives in clinical trials. **(C)** Anthracycline derivatives. **(D)** Demethyl epipodophyllotoxin derivatives. **(E)** Other intercalating Top2 inhibitors acting by trapping Top2cc. **(F)** Structure of dexrazoxane, which acts as a catalytic inhibitor of Top2.

Topotecan

Topotecan contains a basic side chain at position C-9 that enhances its water solubility (see Fig. 20.3). Topotecan is approved for the treatment of ovarian cancer,[45] small-cell lung cancer,[46] and as a single agent and in combination with cisplatin for cervical cancer.[47] Additionally, it is active in acute myeloid leukemia (AML) and myelodysplastic syndrome (see Table 20.2). Topotecan is administered intravenously as a single agent at a dose of 1.5 mg/m² as a 30-minute infusion daily for 5 days, followed by a 2-week period of rest for the treatment of solid tumors or at a dose of 0.75 mg/m² as a 30-minute infusion daily for 3 days in combination with cisplatin on day 1, every 3 weeks, for the treatment of cervical cancer.

Myelosuppression is the most common dose-limiting toxicity. Extensive prior radiation or previous bone marrow–suppressive chemotherapy increases the risk of topotecan-induced myelosuppression. Other toxicities include nausea, vomiting, diarrhea, fatigue, alopecia, and transient hepatic transaminitis.

Topotecan and its metabolites are primarily cleared by the kidneys, requiring dose reduction in patients with renal dysfunction. A 50% dose reduction is recommended for patients with moderate renal impairment (creatinine clearance 20 to 39 mL per minute).

There are no formal guidelines for dose reductions in patients with hepatic dysfunction (defined as serum bilirubin >1.5 mg/dL to <10 mg/dL). Topotecan additionally penetrates the blood-brain barrier, achieving concentrations in cerebrospinal fluid that are approximately 30% that of plasma levels.[48]

Camptothecin Conjugates and Analogs

New formulations of camptothecin conjugates and analogs are currently in clinical development in an effort to improve the therapeutic index (Table 20.3). The development of camptothecin conjugates is based on the notion that the addition of a bulky conjugate would allow for a more consistent delivery system and extend the half-life of the molecule.

CRLX101, formerly IT-101, a covalent cyclodextrin-polyethylene glycol copolymer camptothecin conjugate, has plasma concentrations and area under the curve (AUC) that are approximately 100-fold higher than camptothecin, with a half-life in the range of 17 to 20 hours compared to 1.3 hours for camptothecin.[49] It has demonstrated antitumor activity in preclinical studies in irinotecan-resistant tumors with complete tumor regression in human non–small-cell lung cancer, Ewing sarcoma, and

TABLE 20.2

U.S. Food and Drug Administration–Approved Camptothecin Analogs

Irinotecan (Camptosar)	FDA approved for: Metastatic colorectal cancer	First-line therapy in combination with 5-FU/LV	Diarrhea (dose reductions are recommended for patients who are homozygous for the UGT1A1*28 allele) Myelosuppression
		Second-line therapy as a single agent	
	Category 2A[a] recommendations: Pancreatic cancer	First-line therapy in combination with oxaliplatin, 5-FU/LV	
	Extensive-stage small-cell lung cancer	First-line therapy in combination with cisplatin or carboplatin	
	Category 2B[b] recommendations: Esophageal and GEJ cancers, gastric cancer, cervical cancer, anaplastic gliomas and glioblastomas, non–small-cell lung cancer, ovarian cancer		
Topotecan (Hycamtin)	FDA approved for: Cervical cancer	Stage IVB, recurrent, or persistent carcinoma of the cervix not amenable to curative treatment with surgery and/or radiation therapy	Myelosuppression
	Ovarian cancer	After failure of initial therapy	
	Small-cell lung cancer	After failure of initial therapy	
	Class 2B recommendations: AML, MDS		

[a] Category 2A: Recommendations are based upon lower-level evidence, there is uniform National Comprehensive Cancer Network consensus that the intervention is appropriate.
[b] Category 2B: Recommendations are based upon lower-level evidence, there is National Comprehensive Cancer Network consensus that the intervention is appropriate.
MDS, myelodysplastic syndrome.

lymphoma xenograft models.[50] Preliminary data from Phase 1 studies indicate that CRLX101 is well tolerated at a dose of 15 mg/m^2 administered in a biweekly administration schedule.[51] It is currently being studied in Phase 2 studies as a single agent and in combination with chemotherapeutic agents in lung, renal cell cancer, and gynecologic malignancies.[52–54]

Etirinotecan pegol (NKTR-102), an irinotecan polymer conjugate, has a longer plasma circulation time with a lower maximum concentration of SN-38 compared with irinotecan. It was evaluated in a Phase 2 study in platinum-resistant refractory epithelial ovarian cancer at a dose of 145 mg/m^2 administered on a schedule of every 21 days; a median progression-free survival of 5.3 months and median overall survival of 11.7 months was observed.[55] Two schedules of administration, 145 mg/m^2 administered every 14 days versus every 21 days, have been tested in a Phase 2 study of NKTR-102 in patients with previously treated metastatic breast cancer.[56] Of the 70 patients evaluated in this study, 20 patients achieved an objective response (29%; 95% confidence interval [CI] 18.4 to 40.6). For both these studies, the most common adverse events

on the 21-day administration schedule were dehydration and diarrhea. Etirinotecan pegol is currently being evaluated in several phase 2 studies in lung cancer, colorectal cancer, and high-grade gliomas,[57–60] with evidence of clinical activity in refractory solid tumors. A Phase 3 trial (The BEACON Study) is underway evaluating NKTR-102 against the physicians' choice in refractory breast cancer.[61]

As an alternative to macromolecular conjugates, attempts have also been made to alter the camptothecin pentacyclic ring structure with modifications of the A and B ring (see Fig. 20.3A) in an effort to improve solubility and enhance antitumor activity. Structure–activity relationship studies have shown that substitutions at the 7, 9, and 10 positions serve to enhance the antitumor activity of camptothecin.[62] Belotecan, a novel camptothecin analog, has a water-solubilizing group at the 7 position of the B ring of camptothecin (see Fig. 20.3A). Several Phase 2 studies have evaluated belotecan in combination with carboplatin in recurrent ovarian cancer[63] and in combination with cisplatin in extensive-stage small-cell lung cancer,[64] demonstrating activity in these cancers; however, these combinations were associated with prominent hematologic toxicities. Phase 2 studies evaluating belotecan as a single agent in patients with recurrent or progressive carcinoma of the uterine cervix failed to show activity.[65] Gimatecan is a lipophilic oral camptothecin analog (see Fig. 20.3A). Pharmacokinetic studies demonstrate that gimatecan is primarily present in plasma as the lactone form (>85%), and has a long half-life of 77.1 +/− 29.6 hours, with an increase in maximum concentration (Cmax) and AUC of three- to six-fold after multiple dosing.[66] Phase 2 studies show that gimatecan has demonstrated activity in previously treated ovarian cancer, with myelosuppression as the main toxicity.[67]

Newer development of analogs have attempted to modify the E-ring through introduction of an electron-withdrawing group at

TABLE 20.3

Topoisomerase I Inhibitors in Development

Camptothecin Conjugates	Camptothecin Analogs	Noncamptothecin Agents
CRLX101	Belotecan	Indenoisoquinoline
NKTR-102	Gimatecan	Indotecan (LMP-400)
MM-398	Homocamptothecin	Indimitecan (LMP-776)
	Elomotecan	Dibenzo naphthyridine
	Diflomotecan	Genz-644282

the α position in an effort to overcome the instability of the E-ring while maintaining the binding capability of the camptothecin analog to the Top1-DNA cleavage complex. Collectively called homocamptothecin analogs, two have been tested in clinical trials and include diflomotecan[68] and elomotecan.[69] The dose-limiting toxicity in the Phase I study of elomotecan was neutropenia. A five-member E-ring derivative has also been developed and has reached a Phase 1 clinical trial.[70,71]

Noncamptothecin Topoisomerase I Inhibitors

Noncamptothecin Top1 inhibitors are in clinical development, and include indenoisoquinolines and dibenzonaphthyridines (see Fig. 20.3B). Two indenoisoquinoline derivatives are currently in clinical development, indotecan (LMP400) and indimitecan (LMP776).[72,73] Early in vitro studies show enhanced potency compared with camptothecins, and persistence of Top1 cleavage complexes.[74] Genz-644282, a dibenzonaphthyridine derivative, demonstrated enhanced antitumor activity in preclinical studies[75] and is currently being evaluated in Phase 1 clinical trials.[76]

TOPOISOMERASE II INHIBITORS: INTERCALATORS AND NONINTERCALATORS

Topoisomerase II inhibitors can be classified in two main classes: DNA intercalators, which encompass different chemical classes (Fig. 20.3C, E), and nonintercalators represented by the epipodophyllotoxin derivatives (see Fig. 20.3D). Although both act by trapping Top2 cleavage complexes (Top2cc), DNA intercalators exhibit a second effect as drug concentrations increase above low micromolar values: they block the formation of Top2cc by intercalating into DNA and destabilizing the binding of Top2 to DNA. This explains why Top2α and Top2β are trapped over a relatively narrow concentration range by anthracyclines, and why intercalators have additional effects besides trapping Top2cc, namely inhibition of a broad range of DNA processing enzymes including helicases, polymerase, and even nucleosome destabilization.

Doxorubicin

Doxorubicin and daunorubicin were the first anthracyclines discovered in the 1960s and remain among the most widely used anticancer agents over a broad spectrum of malignancies. Although doxorubicin only differs by one hydroxyl substitution on position 14 (see Fig. 20.3C), doxorubicin has a much broader anticancer activity than daunorubicin. Anthracyclines are natural products derived from *Streptomyces peucetius* variation *caesius*. They were found to target Top2 well after their clinical approval.[77] Subsequent searches for less toxic drugs and formulations led to the approval of liposomal doxorubicin, idarubicin, and epirubicin.

Anthracyclines are flat, planar molecules that are relatively hydrophobic. The quinone structure of anthracyclines (see Fig. 20.3C) enhances the catalysis of oxidation-reduction reactions, thereby promoting the generation of oxygen free radicals, which may be involved in antitumor effects as well as the cardiotoxicity associated with these drugs.[78,79] Anthracyclines are also substrates for P-glycoprotein and Mrp-1, and drug efflux is thought to be a major drug resistance determinant.[80,81]

Doxorubicin is available in a standard salt form and as a liposomal formulation. FDA-labeled indications for standard doxorubicin include acute lymphocytic leukemia (ALL), AML, chronic lymphoid leukemia, Hodgkin lymphoma, non-Hodgkin lymphoma, mantle cell lymphoma, multiple myeloma, mycosis fungoides, Kaposi sarcoma, breast cancer (adjuvant therapy and advanced), advanced prostate cancer, advanced gastric cancer, Ewing sarcoma, thyroid cancer, advanced nephroblastoma,

advanced neuroblastoma, advanced non–small-cell lung cancer, advanced ovarian cancer, advanced transitional cell bladder cancer, cervical cancer, and Langerhans cell tumors. Doxorubicin has activity in other malignancies as well, including soft tissue sarcoma, osteosarcoma, carcinoid, and liver cancer (Table 20.4). Doxorubicin is typically administered at a recommended dose of 30 to 75 mg/m² every 3 weeks intravenously.

Major acute toxicities of doxorubicin include myelosuppression, mucositis, alopecia, nausea, and vomiting. Myelosuppression is the acute dose-limiting toxicity. Other toxicities, including diarrhea, nausea, vomiting, mucositis, and alopecia, are dose and schedule related. Prophylactic antiemetics are routinely given with bolus doses of doxorubicin, and longer infusions are associated with less nausea and less cardiotoxicity. Patients should also be warned to expect their urine to redden after drug administration. Doxorubicin is a potent vesicant, and extravasation can lead to severe necrosis of skin and local tissues, requiring surgical debridement and skin grafts. Infusions via a central venous catheter are recommended. Other toxicities of doxorubicin include *radiation recall* and the risk of developing secondary leukemia. *Radiation recall* is an inflammatory reaction at sites of previous radiation and can lead to pericarditis, pleural effusion, and skin rash. Secondary leukemias are thought to be a result of balanced translocations that result from Top2 poisoning by the anthracyclines, albeit to lesser degree than other Top2 poisons, such as the epipodophyllotoxins (see the following).[82]

Anthracyclines are cleared mainly by metabolism to less active forms and by biliary excretion. Less than 10% of the administered dose is cleared by the kidneys. Dose reductions should be made in patients with elevated plasma bilirubin. Doxorubicin should be dose reduced by 50% for plasma bilirubin concentrations ranging from 1.2 to 3.0 mg/dL, by 75% for values of 3.1 to 5.0 mg/dL, and withheld for values greater than 5 mg/dL.

Liposomal Doxorubicin

Doxorubicin is also available in a polyethylene glycol (PEG)ylated liposomal form, which allows for enhancement of drug delivery. Use of liposomal doxorubicin has been associated with less cardiotoxicity even at doses exceeding 500 mg/m².[83] Additionally, liposomal doxorubicin produces less nausea and vomiting and relatively mild myelosuppression compared to doxorubicin. Unique to the liposomal formulation is the risk of hand–foot syndrome and an acute infusion reaction manifested by flushing, dyspnea, edema, fever, chills, rash, bronchospasm, and hypertension. These infusion reactions are related to the rate of infusion; therefore, the recommended administration schedule is set at an initial rate of 1 mg per minute for the first 10 to 15 minutes. The rate may be slowly increased to complete infusion over 60 minutes if no reaction occurs. Typical dosing schedules include 50 mg/m² intravenous infusion every 4 weeks for four courses in ovarian cancer, 20 mg/m² intravenous infusion every 3 weeks in AIDS-related Kaposi sarcoma, and 30 mg/m² intravenous infusion in combination with bortezomib to be given on days 1, 4, 8, and 11 every 3 weeks in multiple myeloma.

Daunorubicin

Despite its chemical similarity (see Fig. 20.3C), daunorubicin is considerably less active in solid tumors compared to doxorubicin. It is FDA approved for the treatment of ALL and AML. Daunorubicin is typically administered via intravenous push over 3 to 5 minutes at a dose of 30 to 45 mg/m² per day on 3 consecutive days in combination chemotherapy. For induction therapy for pediatric acute lymphoblastic leukemia, daunorubicin is dosed at 25 mg/m² intravenously in combination with vincristine and prednisone. In children less than 2 years of age or in those who have a body surface area less than 0.5 m², current recommendations are based on

CANCER THERAPEUTICS

TABLE 20.4

U.S. Food And Drug Administration–Approved Topoisomerase II Inhibitors in Clinical Use

Compound	Tumor Type	Clinical Indication	Major Toxicities
I. Anthracyclines			
Doxorubicin (Adriamycin)	Breast carcinoma	Adjuvant setting with axillary LN involvement following resection of primary breast cancer	Dose-dependent cardiotoxicity Myelosuppression
	ALL AML Wilms' tumor Neuroblastoma Sarcomas Ovarian cancer Transitional cell bladder cancer Thyroid cancer Gastric cancer Hodgkin lymphoma Non-Hodgkin lymphoma	In combination with other cytotoxic agents	
Pegylated liposomal doxorubicin (Doxil)	Ovarian cancer	After failure of platinum-based chemotherapy	Myelosuppression Stomatitis Hand-foot syndrome Dosage reduction recommended with hepatic dysfunction
	AIDS-related Kaposi sarcoma	After failure of prior systemic chemotherapy	
	Multiple myeloma	In combination with bortezomib	
Daunorubicin (Cerubidine)	ALL AML	Induction therapy	Dose-dependent cardiotoxicity Myelosuppression
Epirubicin (Ellence)	Breast cancer	Adjuvant therapy in patients with evidence of axillary node tumor involvement following primary resection	Dose-dependent cardiotoxicity Myelosuppression
Idarubicin (Idamycin)	AML	Induction therapy	Dose-dependent cardiotoxicity Myelosuppression
II. Anthracenediones			
Mitoxantrone (Novantrone)	Prostate cancer AML	Hormone-refractory prostate cancer	Myelosuppression
Dactinomycin (Cosmegen)	Wilms' tumor Rhabdomyosarcoma Ewing sarcoma Nonseminomatous testicular cancer Gestational trophoblastic neoplasia		Myelosuppression
III. Epipodophyllotoxins			
Etoposide (VePesid)	Small-cell lung cancer Testicular cancer	First-line in combination First-line in combination	Myelosuppression
Teniposide (Vumon)	Pediatric lymphoblastic leukemia	Refractory setting	Myelosuppression

LN, lymph node.

body mass index (1 mg/kg) rather than body surface area. A higher dose of daunorubicin at 60 mg/m^2 per day to 90 mg/m^2 per day intravenously for 3 consecutive days is currently recommended as part of the induction combination regimen for the treatment of acute myeloblastic leukemia. Daunorubicin has similar toxicities to doxorubicin, including myelosuppression, cardiac toxicity, nausea, vomiting, alopecia, and is also a vesicant. Daunorubicin is metabolized by the liver and undergoes substantial elimination by the kidneys, requiring dose reductions for both renal and hepatic dysfunction. A 50% dose reduction is recommended for either serum creatinine or bilirubin greater than 3 mg/dL, and a 25% reduction in dose for bilirubin concentrations ranging from 1.2 to 3.0 mg/dL.

Epirubicin

Epirubicin is an epimer of doxorubicin (see Fig. 20.3C) with increased lipophilicity. It is FDA approved for adjuvant therapy of breast cancer but is also used in combination for the treatment of a variety of malignancies. Epirubicin is administered intravenously at doses ranging from 60 to 120 mg/m^2 every 3 to 4 weeks. Epirubicin has a similar toxicity profile to doxorubicin but is overall better tolerated.

In addition to being converted to an enol by an aldose reductase, epirubicin has a unique steric orientation of the C-4 hydroxyl group that allows it to serve as a substrate for conjugation reactions mediated by liver glucuronosyltransferases and sulfatases. As such, dose adjustments are recommended in the setting of hepatic dysfunction. For patients with serum bilirubin of 1.2 to 3 mg/dL or aspartate aminotransferase of 2 to 4 times the upper limit of normal, a 50% dose reduction is recommended. For patients with bilirubin greater than 3 mg/dL or aspartate aminotransferase greater than 4 times the upper limit of normal, a dose reduction of 75% is recommended. Due to limited data, no specific dose recommendations are currently available for patients with renal impairment, although current recommendations are for consideration of dose adjustments in patients with serum creatinine greater than 5 mg/dL.

Idarubicin

Idarubicin is a synthetic derivative of daunorubicin, but lacks the 4-methoxy group (see Fig. 20.3C). It is FDA approved as part of combination chemotherapy regimen for AML and is also active in ALL. It is given intravenously at a dose of 12 mg/m² for 3 consecutive days, typically in combination with cytarabine. Idarubicin has similar toxicities as daunorubicin. Its primary active metabolite is idarubicinol, and elimination is mainly through the biliary system and, to a lesser extent, through renal excretion. A 50% dose reduction is recommended for serum bilirubin of 2.6 to 5 mg/dL and idarubicin should not be given if the bilirubin is greater than 5 mg/dL. Additionally, dose reductions in renal impairment are advised, but specific guidelines are not available.

Cardiac Toxicity of Anthracyclines

Anthracyclines are responsible for cardiac toxicities, and special considerations are necessary to minimize this severe side effect. Acute doxorubicin cardiotoxicity is reversible, and clinical signs include tachycardia, hypotension, electrocardiogram changes, and arrhythmias. It develops during or within days of anthracycline infusion, and its incidence can be significantly reduced by slowing doxorubicin infusion rates.

Chronic and delayed cardiotoxicity is more common and more severe because it is irreversible. Chronic cardiotoxicity with congestive heart failure peaks at 1 to 3 months but can occur even years after therapy. Myocardial damage has been shown to occur by several mechanisms. The classical mechanism is by the direct generation of reactive oxygen species (ROS) during the electron transfer from the semiquinone to quinone moieties of the anthracycline,[84] which leads to myocardial damage. ROS can also be generated by mitochondrial damage resulting from drug-mediated inactivation of the oxidative phosphorylation chain because doxorubicin accumulates not only in chromatin, but also in mitochondria.[78,79] A recent study has also related doxorubicin cardiotoxicity to the poisoning of Top2β cleavage complexes in myocardiocytes.[85] Endomyocardial biopsy is characterized by a predominant finding of multifocal areas of patchy and interstitial fibrosis (stellate scars) and occasional vacuolated myocardial cells (Adria cells). Myocyte hypertrophy and degeneration, loss of cross-striations, and the absence of myocarditis are also characteristic of this diagnosis.[86] The incidence of cardiomyopathy is related to both the cumulative dose and the schedule of administration, and predisposition to cardiac damage includes a previous history of heart disease, hypertension, radiation to the mediastinum, age greater than 65 years or younger than 4 years, prior use of anthracyclines or other cardiac toxins, and coadministration of other chemotherapy agents (e.g., paclitaxel, cyclophosphamide, or trastuzumab).[87,88] Sequential administration of paclitaxel followed by doxorubicin in breast cancer patients is associated with cardiomyopathy at total doxorubicin doses above 340 to 380 mg/m², whereas the reverse sequence of drug administration did not yield the same systemic toxicities at these doses.[89] When doxorubicin is given in a low-dose weekly regimen (10 to 20 mg/m² per week) or by slow continuous infusion over 96 hours, cumulative doses of more than 500 mg/m² can be given. Doses of epirubicin less than 1,000 mg/m² and daunorubicin

less than 550 mg/m² are considered safe. Additionally, liposomal doxorubicin is associated with less cardiac toxicity.

Cardiac function can be monitored during treatment with anthracyclines by electrocardiography, echocardiography, or radionuclide scans. Numerous studies have established the danger of embarking on anthracycline therapy in patients with underlying cardiac disease (e.g., a baseline left ventricular ejection fraction of less than 50%) and of continuing therapy after a documented decrease in the ejection fraction by more than 10% (if this decrease falls below the lower limit of normal). Because anthracycline-induced cardiotoxicity has been related to the generation of free radicals, efforts have been aimed at attenuating this effect through the targeting of redox response and reduction in oxidative stress. Dexrazoxane is a metal chelator that decreases the myocardial toxicity of doxorubicin in breast cancer patients. In two multicenter, double-blind studies, advanced breast cancer patients were randomized to chemotherapy with dexrazoxane or a placebo; dexrazoxane was shown to have a cardioprotective effect based on serial, noninvasive cardiac testing during the course of the trial and is approved for that use by the FDA.[90] Dexrazoxane chelates iron and copper, thereby interfering with the redox reactions that generate free radicals and damage myocardial lipids. Notably, dexrazoxane is also a Top2 catalytic inhibitor (see Fig. 20.3F), which potentially might minimize the therapeutic activity of anthracyclines by interfering with the trapping of Top2 cleavage complexes by anthracyclines.[2,3,91] Other agents currently in use include β-blockers and statins. A recent meta-analysis of 12 randomized controlled trials and 2 observational studies involving the use of agents to prevent the cardiotoxicity associated with anthracyclines demonstrated relatively similar efficacy regardless of which prophylactic treatment was used.[92]

Anthracenediones

Mitoxantrone (see Fig. 20.3E) is currently the only clinically approved anthracenedione. Compared to anthracyclines, mitoxantrone is less cardiotoxic owing to a decreased ability to undergo oxidation-reduction reactions and form free radicals.

Mitoxantrone is FDA approved for the treatment of advanced hormone-refractory prostate cancer[93] and AML.[94] It is typically administered intravenously at a dose of 12 to 14 mg/m² every 3 weeks in the treatment of prostate cancer, and at a dose of 12 mg/m² in combination with cytosine arabinoside for 3 days in the treatment of AML.

Toxicities are generally less severe compared to doxorubicin and include myelosuppression, nausea, vomiting, alopecia, and mucositis. Cardiac toxicity can be seen at cumulative doses greater than 160 mg/m².[95] Mitoxantrone is rapidly cleared from the plasma and is highly concentrated in tissues. The majority of the drug is eliminated in the feces, with a small amount undergoing renal excretion. Dose adjustments for hepatic dysfunction are recommended, but formal guidelines are currently not available.

Dactinomycin

Dactinomycin was the first antibiotic shown to have antitumor activity[96] and consists of a planar phenoxazone ring attached to two peptide side chains. This unique structure allows for tight intercalation into DNA between adjacent guanine–cytosine bases, leading to Top2 and Top1 poisoning and transcription inhibition.[97] Dactinomycin was one of the first drugs shown to be transported by P-glycoprotein, and represents the major mechanism of resistance.[98]

Dactinomycin is FDA approved for Ewing sarcoma,[99] gestational trophoblastic neoplasm,[100] metastatic nonseminomatous testicular cancer,[101] nephroblastoma,[102] and rhabdomyosarcoma.[103] Typically, it is administered intravenously at doses of 15 μg/kg for 5 days in combination with other chemotherapeutic agents for the treatment of nephroblastoma, rhabdomyosarcoma, and Ewing sarcoma; at does of 12 μg/kg intravenously as a single agent in the treatment of gestational trophoblastic neoplasias; and at doses of 1,000 μg/m² intravenously on day 1 as part of a combination regimen with cyclophosphamide, bleomycin, vinblastine, and cisplatin in the treatment of metastatic nonseminomatous testicular cancer. Toxicities include myelosuppression, veno-occlusive disease of the liver, nausea, vomiting, alopecia, erythema, and acne. Additionally, similar to doxorubicin, dactinomycin can cause radiation recall and severe tissue necrosis in cases of extravasation. Dactinomycin is largely excreted unchanged in the feces and urine. Guidelines for dosing in patients with impaired renal or liver function are currently not available.

Epipodophyllotoxins

Epipodophyllotoxins are glycoside derivatives of podophyllotoxin, an antimicrotubule agent extracted from the mandrake plant. Two derivatives, demethylated on the pendant ring (see R1 in Fig. 20.3D), etoposide and teniposide were shown to primarily function as Top2 poisons rather than through antimicrotubule mechanisms.[104,105] Epipodophyllotoxins poison Top2 through a mechanism distinct from that of anthracyclines and other DNA intercalators.[106] without intercalating into normal DNA in the absence of Top2. Therefore, they are "cleaner" Top2 inhibitors than the anthracyclines, anthracenediones, and dactinomycin. However, etoposide and teniposide trap Top2 cleavage complexes by base stacking in a ternary complex at the interface of the DNA and the Top2 homodimer. Mechanisms that have been implicated in resistance to etoposide include drug efflux, because epipodophyllotoxins are substrates for P-glycoprotein[107]; altered localization of Top2α; decreased cellular expression of Top2α[108]; and impaired phosphorylation of Top2.[109]

Etoposide

Etoposide (see Fig. 20.3D) is available in intravenous and oral forms. It is FDA approved for the treatment of small-cell lung cancer[110] and refractory testicular cancer.[111] It also has activity in hematologic malignancies and various solid tumors. The intravenous form is generally administered at doses of 35 to 50 mg/m² for 4 to 5 days every 3 to 4 weeks in combination therapy for small-cell lung cancer, and 50 to 100 mg/m² for 5 days every 3 to 4 weeks in combination therapy for refractory testicular cancer. The dose of oral etoposide is usually twice the intravenous dose. Oral bioavailability is highly variable due to dependence on intestinal P-glycoprotein.[112]

The dose-limiting toxicity for etoposide is myelosuppression, with white blood cell count nadirs typically occurring on days 10 to 14. Thrombocytopenia is less common than leukopenia. Additionally, mild to moderate nausea, vomiting, diarrhea, mucositis, and alopecia are associated with etoposide. Among topoisomerase inhibitors, epipodophyllotoxins have the greatest association with secondary malignancies, with etoposide having the highest risk, with an estimated 4% 6-year cumulative risk.[113] The majority of etoposide is cleared unchanged by the kidneys, and a 25% dose reduction is recommended in patients with a creatinine clearance of 15 to 50 mL per minute. A 50% dose reduction is recommended in patients with a creatinine clearance less than 15 mL per minute. Because the unbound fraction of etoposide is dependent on albumin and bilirubin concentrations, dose adjustments for hepatic dysfunction are advised, but consensus guidelines are currently not available.

Teniposide

Teniposide contains a thiophene group in place of the methyl group on the glucose moiety of etoposide (Fig. 20.3D). Teniposide is FDA approved for refractory pediatric ALL.[114,115] In pediatric ALL studies, doses ranged from 165 mg/m² intravenously in combination with cytarabine to 250 mg/m² intravenously weekly in combination with vincristine and prednisone. Similar to etoposide, the dose-limiting toxicity of teniposide is myelosuppression. Additional toxicities include mild-to-moderate nausea, vomiting, diarrhea, alopecia, and secondary leukemia. Teniposide is associated with greater frequency of hypersensitivity reactions compared to etoposide.

Teniposide is 99% bound to albumin and, as compared to etoposide, undergoes hepatic metabolism more extensively and renal clearance less extensively. No specific guidelines are currently available on dose adjustments for renal or hepatic dysfunction.

THERAPY-RELATED SECONDARY ACUTE LEUKEMIA

One of the major complications of Top2 inhibitor therapies, especially for etoposide and mitoxantrone, is acute secondary leukemia, which occurs in approximately 5% of patients. Therapy-related AMLs (t-AML) are characterized by their relatively rapid onset (they can occur only a few months after therapy) and the presence of recurrent balanced translocations involving the mixed lineage leukemia (MLL) locus on 11q23 and over 50 partner genes.[116] The molecular mechanism is likely from the disjoining of two drug-trapped Top2 cleavage complexes on different chromosomes (see Fig. 20.2C) in relationship with transcription collisions and illegitimate relegation.[117] Top2β, rather than Top2α, has been implicated in the generation of these disjoined cleavage complexes.[117,118]

FUTURE DIRECTIONS

Current challenges in the development of topoisomerase inhibitors lie in the inherent chemical instability of current and established agents. In addition to recent developments designed to enhance the stability with semisynthetic analogs and the development of novel delivery systems in an effort to achieve higher intratumoral concentrations, attention is also being focused on targeting other topoisomerase isoenzymes. Driving this trend has been the recent elucidation of the role of Top2β inhibition in the development of treatment-related cardiotoxicity and secondary AML.[86,117,118] In addition to combination chemotherapy regimens already in use, attempts have also been made for the sequential inhibition of Top1 and Top2. Based on early preclinical models suggesting synergy with sequential inhibition of Top1 and Top2,[120] phase 1 studies have evaluated the sequential administration of topotecan and etoposide in extensive-stage small-cell lung cancer and ovarian cancer, with significant myelosuppression as the dose-limiting toxicity.[121,122] Future rational drug combinations include targeting DNA repair pathways in combination with Top1 inhibition, although further characterization is needed of the specific DNA repair and stress response pathways invoked in response to DNA damage as a result of Top1 inhibition. However, one such attempt of combining topotecan with veliparib, a small molecule inhibitor of poly (ADP-ribose) polymerase, was poorly tolerated due to significant myelosuppression, thus limiting the doses of topotecan that could be safely administered.[123]

Molecular characterization of tumors to better define patient selection and the development of pharmacodynamic biomarkers to monitor the response to treatment and to optimize the combination dose and schedules is needed for the further clinical development of topoisomerase inhibitors. Validated assays have been developed to evaluate topoisomerase 1 levels and levels of plosphorylated histone H2AX (gamma-H2AX) as a marker of DNA damage response to topoisomerase inhibition,[124,125] and are being incorporated in current phase I studies of indenoisoquinolines.[72,73]

SELECTED REFERENCES

The full reference list can be accessed at lwwhealthlibrary.com/oncology.

1. Nitiss JL. DNA topoisomerase II and its growing repertoire of biological functions. *Nat Rev Cancer* 2009;9(5):327–337.
2. Nitiss JL. Targeting DNA topoisomerase II in cancer chemotherapy. *Nat Rev Cancer* 2009;9(5):338–350.
5. Wang JC. A journey in the world of DNA rings and beyond. *Annu Rev Biochem* 2009;78:31–54.
6. Wang JC. Cellular roles of DNA topoisomerases: a molecular perspective. *Nat Rev Mol Cell Biol* 2002;3(6):430–440.
16. Pommier Y, Marchand C. Interfacial inhibitors: targeting macromolecular complexes. *Nat Rev Drug Discov* 2011;11(1):25–36.
21. Hsiang YH, Lihou MG, Liu LF. Arrest of DNA replication by drug-stabilized topoisomerase I-DNA cleavable complexes as a mechanism of cell killing by camptothecin. *Cancer Res* 1989;49(18):5077–5082.
25. Koster DA, Palle K, Bot ES, et al. Antitumor drugs impede DNA uncoiling by topoisomerase I. *Nature* 2007;448(7150):213–217.
31. Pommier Y. Drugging topoisomerases: lessons and challenges. *ACS Chem Biol* 2013;8(1):82–95.
33. Wall ME, Wani MC. Camptothecin and taxol: discovery to clinic—thirteenth Bruce F. Cain Memorial Award Lecture. *Cancer Res* 1995;55:753–760.
36. Pommier Y, Cushman M. The indenoisoquinoline noncamptothecin topoisomerase I inhibitors: update and perspectives. *Mol Cancer Ther* 2009;8(5):1008–1014.
37. Douillard JY, Cunningham D, Roth AD, et al. Irinotecan combined with fluorouracil compared with fluorouracil alone as first-line treatment for metastatic colorectal cancer: a multicentre randomised trial. *Lancet* 2000;355:1041–1047.
38. Saltz LB, Cox JV, Blanke C, et al. Irinotecan plus fluorouracil and leucovorin for metastatic colorectal cancer. Irinotecan Study Group. *N Engl J Med* 2000;343:905–914.
39. Conroy T, Desseigne F, Tchou M, et al. FOLFIRINOX versus gemcitabine for metastatic pancreatic cancer. *N Engl J Med* 2011;364:1817–1825.
40. Hanna N, Bunn PA Jr, Langer C, et al. Randomized phase III trial comparing irinotecan/cisplatin with etoposide/cisplatin in patients with previously untreated extensive-stage disease small-cell lung cancer. *J Clin Oncol* 2006;24:2038–2043.
43. Innocenti F, Undevia SD, Iyer L, et al. Genetic variants in the UDP-glucuronosyltransferase 1A1 gene predict the risk of severe neutropenia of irinotecan. *J Clin Oncol* 2004;22:1382–1388.
50. Young C, Schluep T, Hwang J, et al. CRLX101 (formerly IT-101)-A novel nanopharmaceutical of camptothecin in clinical development. *Curr Bioact Compd* 2011;7:8–14.
55. Vergote IB, Garcia A, Micha J et al. Randomized multicentre phase II trial comparing two schedules of etirinotecan pegol (NKTR-102) in women with recurrent platinum-resistant/refractory epithelial ovarian cancer. *J Clin Oncol* 2013;31(32):4060–4066.
62. Basili S, Moro S. Novel camptothecin derivatives as topoisomerase I inhibitors. *Expert Opin Ther Pat* 2009;19:555–574.
66. Frapolli R, Zucchetti M, Sessa C, et al. Clinical pharmacokinetics of the new oral camptothecin gimatecan: the inter-patient variability is related to alpha1-acid glycoprotein plasma levels. *Eur J Cancer* 2010;46:505–516.
69. Trocóniz IF, Cendrós JM, Soto E, et al. Population pharmacokinetic/pharmacodynamics modeling of drug-induced adverse effects of a novel homocamptothecin analog, elomotecan (BN80927), in a Phase I dose finding study in patients with advanced solid tumors. *Cancer Chemother Pharmacol* 2012;70:239–250.

70. Takagi K, Dexheimer TS, Redon C, et al. Novel E-ring camptothecin keto analogues (S38809 and S39625) are stable, potent, and selective topoisomerase I inhibitors without being substrates of drug efflux transporters. *Mol Cancer Ther* 2007;6(12 Pt 1):3229–3238.
71. Lansiaux A, Léonce S, Kraus-Berthier L, et al. Novel stable camptothecin derivatives replacing the E-ring lactone by a ketone function are potent inhibitors of topoisomerase I and promising antitumor drugs. *Mol Pharmacol* 2007;72(2):311–319.
74. Antony S, Agama KK, Miao ZH, et al. Novel indenoisoquinolines NSC 725776 and NSC 724998 produce persistent topoisomerase I cleavage complexes and overcome multidrug resistance. *Cancer Res* 2007;67:10397–10405.
75. Kurtzberg LS, Roth S, Krumbholz R, et al. Genz-644282, a novel non-camptothecin topoisomerase I inhibitor for cancer treatment. *Clin Cancer Res* 2011;17:2777–2787.
79. Doroshow JH, Davies KJ. Redox cycling of anthracyclines by cardiac mitochondria. II. Formation of superoxide anion, hydrogen peroxide, and hydroxyl radical. *J Biol Chem* 1986;261:3068–3074.
82. Felix CA, Kolaris CP, Osheroff N. Topoisomerase II and the etiology of chromosomal translocations. *DNA Repair* 2006;5:1093–1108.
83. O'Brien ME, Wigler N, Inbar M, et al. Reduced cardiotoxicity and comparable efficacy in a phase III trial of pegylated liposomal doxorubicin HCl (CAELYX/Doxil) versus conventional doxorubicin for first-line treatment of metastatic breast cancer. *Ann Oncol* 2004;15(3):440–449.
85. Zhang S, Liu X, Bawa-Khalfe T, et al. Identification of the molecular basis of doxorubicin-induced cardiotoxicity. *Nat Med* 2012;18:1639–1642.
90. Swain SM, Whaley FS, Gerber MC, et al. Cardioprotection with dexrazoxane for doxorubicin-containing therapy in advanced breast cancer. *J Clin Oncol* 15(4):1318–1332.
92. Kalam K, Marwick TH. Role of cardioprotective therapy for prevention of cardiotoxicity with chemotherapy: a systematic review and meta-analysis. *Eur J Cancer* 2013;49:2900–2909.
93. Tannock IF, Osoba D, Stockler MR, et al. Chemotherapy with mitoxantrone plus prednisone or prednisone alone for symptomatic hormone-resistant prostate cancer: a Canadian randomized trial with palliative end points. *J Clin Oncol* 1996;14:1756–1764.
95. Shenkenberg TD, Von Hoff DD. Mitoxantrone: a new anticancer drug with significant clinical activity. *Ann Intern Med* 1986;105:67–81.
104. Chen GL, Yang L, Rowe TC, et al. Nonintercalative antitumor drugs interfere with the breakage-reunion reaction of mammalian DNA topoisomerase. *J Biol Chem* 1984;259(21):13560–13566.
106. Ross W, Rowe T, Glisson B, et al. Role of topoisomerase II in mediating epipodophyllotoxin-induced DNA cleavage. *Cancer Res* 1984;44:5857–5860.
110. Sundstrøm S, Bremnes RM, Kaasa S, et al. Cisplatin and etoposide regimen is superior to cyclophosphamide, epirubicin, and vincristine regimen in small-cell lung cancer: results from a randomized phase III trial with 5 years' follow-up. *J Clin Oncol* 2002;20:4665–4672.
111. Nichols CR, Catalano PJ, Crawford ED, et al. Randomized comparison of cisplatin and either etoposide and either bleomycin or ifosfamide in treatment of advanced disseminated germ cell tumors: an Eastern Cooperative Oncology Group, Southwest Oncology Group, and Cancer and Leukemia Group B Study. *J Clin Oncol* 1998;16:1287–1293.
113. Smith MA, Rubinstein L, Anderson JR, et al. Secondary leukemia or myelodysplastic syndrome after treatment with epipodophyllotoxins. *J Clin Oncol* 1999;17:569–577.
116. Lovett BD, Lo Nigro L, Rappaport EF, et al. Near-precise interchromosomal recombination and functional DNA topoisomerase II cleavage sites at MLL and AF-4 genomic breakpoints in treatment-related acute lymphoblastic leukemia with t(4;11) translocation. *Proc Natl Acad Sci U S A* 2001;98(17):9802–9807.

CANCER THERAPEUTICS

21 Antimicrotubule Agents

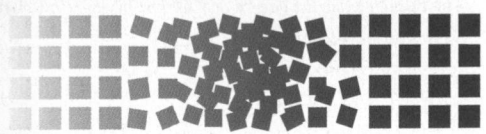

Christopher J. Hoimes and Lyndsay N. Harris

MICROTUBULES

Microtubules are vital and dynamic cytoskeletal polymers that play a critical role in cell division, signaling, vesicle transport, shape, and polarity, which make them attractive targets in anticancer regimens and drug design.[1] Microtubules are composed of 13 linear protofilaments of polymerized α/β-tubulin heterodimers arranged in parallel around a cylindrical axis and associated with regulatory proteins such as microtubule-associated proteins, tau, and motor proteins kinesin and dynein.[2] The specific biologic functions of microtubules are due to their unique polymerization dynamics. Tubulin polymerization is mediated by a nucleation-elongation mechanism. One end of the microtubules, termed the *plus end*, is kinetically more dynamic than the other end, termed the *minus end* (Fig. 21.1). Microtubule dynamics are governed by two principal processes driven by guanosine 5'-triphosphate (GTP) hydrolysis: *treadmilling* or *poleward flux* is the net growth at one end of the microtubule and the net shortening at the opposite end, and *dynamic instability*, which is a process in which the microtubule ends switch spontaneously between states of slow sustained growth and rapid depolymerization.[2] Antimicrotubule agents are tubulin-binding drugs that directly bind tubules, inhibitors of tubulin-associated scaffold kinases, or inhibitors of their associated mitotic motor proteins to, ultimately, disrupt microtubule dynamics. They are broadly classified as microtubule stabilizing or microtubule destabilizing agents according to their effects on tubulin polymerization.

TAXANES

Taxanes were the first-in-class microtubule stabilizing drugs. Ancient medicinal attempts at cardiac pharmacotherapy using material from the toxic coniferous yew tree, *Taxus* spp., were likely related to the plant's alkaloid *taxine* effect on sodium and calcium channels. Taxane compounds are the result of a drug screening of 35,000 plant extracts in 1963 that led to the identification of activity from the bark extract of the Pacific yew tree, *Taxus brevifolia*. Paclitaxel was identified as the active constituent with a report of its activity in carcinoma cell lines in 1971.[3] Motivation to identify taxanes derived from the more abundant and available needles of *Taxus baccata* led to the development of docetaxel, which is synthesized by the addition of a side chain to 10-deacetylbaccatin III, an inactive taxane precursor.[4] The taxane rings of paclitaxel and docetaxel are linked to an ester side chain attached to the C13 position of the ring, which is essential for antimicrotubule and antitumor activity. Nanoparticle albumin-bound paclitaxel (nab-paclitaxel) is a formulation that avoids the solvent related side effects of non–water-soluble paclitaxel and docetaxel. Overcoming docetaxel and paclitaxel's susceptibility to the P-glycoprotein efflux pump led to the development of cabazitaxel.[5] Cabazitaxel is synthesized by adding two methoxy groups to the 10-deacetylbaccatin III, which results in

the inhibition of the 5'-triphosphate–dependent efflux pump of P-glycoprotein.

Paclitaxel initially received regulatory approval in the United States in 1992 for the treatment of patients with ovarian cancer after failure of first-line or subsequent chemotherapy (Table 21.1).[1,4] Subsequently, it has been approved for several other indications, including advanced breast cancer after anthracycline-based regimens[6]; combination chemotherapy of lymph node–positive breast cancer in the adjuvant setting[7]; advanced ovarian cancer in combination with a platinum compound; second-line treatment of AIDS-related Kaposi sarcoma; and first-line treatment of non–small-cell lung cancer (NSCLC) in combination with cisplatin[8] (see Table 21.1). In addition to the U.S. Food and Drug Administration (FDA) on-label indications, paclitaxel is widely used for several other tumor types, such as cancers of unknown origin, bladder, esophagus, gastric, head and neck, and cervical cancers. The U.S. patent for paclitaxel expired in 2002, and a generic form of paclitaxel is now available.

Docetaxel was first approved for use in the United States in 1996 for patients with metastatic breast cancer that progressed or relapsed after anthracycline-based chemotherapy, which was later broadened to a general second-line indication (see Table 21.1).[4,6] Subsequently, it received regulatory approval in adjuvant chemotherapy of stage II breast cancer in combination with Adriamycin and cyclophosphamide (TAC)[9], and first-line treatment for locally advanced or metastatic breast cancer.[10] In addition, docetaxel has indications in nonresectable, locally advanced, or metastatic NSCLC after failure of or in combination with cisplatin therapy; metastatic castration-resistant prostate cancer in combination with prednisone[11]; first-line treatment of gastric adenocarcinoma, including gastroesophageal junction adenocarcinoma in combination with cisplatin and 5-fluorouracil (5-FU)[12]; and inoperable locally advanced squamous cell cancer of the head and neck in combination with cisplatin and 5-FU (see Table 21.1). Docetaxel came off patent in 2010 and a generic form is available.

Mechanism of Action

The unique mechanism of action for paclitaxel was initially defined by Schiff et al.[13] in 1979, who showed that it bound to the interior surface of the microtubule lumen at binding sites completely distinct from those of exchangeable GTP, colchicine, podophyllotoxin, and the vinca alkaloids.[14] The taxanes profoundly alter the tubulin dissociation rate constants at both ends of the microtubule, suppressing treadmilling and dynamic instability. Dose-dependent taxane β-tubular binding induces mitotic arrest at the G2/M transition and induces cell death. By stabilizing microtubules, they also can stall ligand-dependent intracellular trafficking, as shown in sequestration of the androgen receptor to the cytosol in metastatic prostate cancer patients treated with docetaxel, and is associated with decreased androgen-regulated gene expression, such as prostate-specific antigen (PSA).[15,16] Peripheral neuropathy is a common dose-limiting toxicity across the antimicrotubule agents and likely is a result of their direct effect on microtubules. Studies

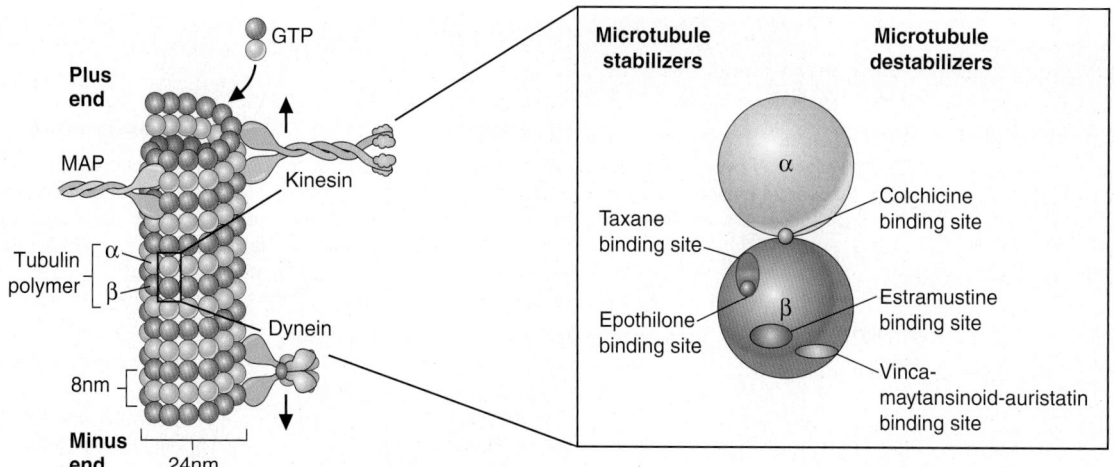

Figure 21.1 Antimicrotubule agents bind tubulin directly or inhibit its associated proteins. Taxanes and epothilones have distinct binding pockets within the same site on the interior surface of the tubule. Estramustine has a distinct site on β-tubulin, although it also directly binds microtubule-associated proteins (MAP). (Adapted from Lieberman M, Marks A. *Mark's Basic Medical Biochemistry: A Clinical Approach*. 3rd ed. Philadelphia: Lippincott Williams & Wilkins; 2009.)

have shown that they inhibit anterograde and/or retrograde fast axonal transport and can explain the demyelinating "dying back" pattern seen and the vulnerability of sensory neurons with the longest axonal projections.[17]

Recent evidence suggests that microtubule inhibitors have collateral effects during interphase that lead to cell death. For instance, paclitaxel-stabilized microtubules serve as a scaffold for the binding of the death-effector domain of pro-caspase-8, and thereby enabling a caspase-8 downstream proteolytic cascade.[18,19] This caspase-8–dependent mechanism also serves as an important basis for the understanding of the loss of function and/or low expression of the breast cancer 1, early onset gene (*BRCA1*) association with resistance to taxane therapy.[20]

Another mechanism of the anticancer effect of taxanes is currently being elaborated and is tied to the B-cell lymphoma-2 (Bcl-2) antiapoptosis family of proteins. Paclitaxel has been shown to cause the phosphorylation of Bcl-2 and the sequestration of Bak and Bim; however, this seemingly cancer-protective phosphorylation needs to be reconciled and likely correlates with Bcl-2–expression levels.[21–23] Interestingly, neutralizing Bcl-2 homology 3 (BH3) domains with compounds such as ABT-737 is synergistic with docetaxel.[24]

Clinical Pharmacology

Paclitaxel

With prolonged infusion schedules (6 and 24 hours), drug disposition is a biphasic process with values for alpha and beta half-lives averaging approximately 20 minutes and 6 hours, respectively.[4] When administered as a 3-hour infusion, the pharmacokinetics are nonlinear and may lead to unexpected toxicity with a small dose escalation, or a disproportionate decrease in drug exposure and loss of tumor response with a dose reduction. Approximately 71% of an administered dose of paclitaxel is excreted in the stool via the enterohepatic circulation over 5 days as either the parent compound or metabolites in humans. Renal clearance of paclitaxel and metabolites is minimal, accounting for 14% of the administered dose. In humans, the bulk of drug disposition is metabolized by cytochrome P-450 mixed-function oxidases—specifically, the isoenzymes CYP2C8 and CYP3A4, which metabolize paclitaxel to hydroxylated 3'p-hydroxypaclitaxel (minor) and 6α-hydroxypaclitaxel (major), as well as dihydroxylated metabolites.

Nanoparticle Albumin-Bound Paclitaxel

Nab-paclitaxel is a solvent-free colloidal suspension made by homogenizing paclitaxel with 3% to 4% albumin under high pressure to form nanoparticles of ~130 nm that disperse in plasma to ~10 nm (see Table 21.1).[25] It received regulatory approval in the United States in 2005 based on results in patients with metastatic breast cancer, and is now also approved in combination with carboplatin for first-line treatment of locally advanced or metastatic NSCLC, and in combination with gemcitabine for first-line treatment of metastatic pancreatic adenocarcinoma.[26–28] The improved responses seen with nab-paclitaxel, when compared to solvent-based paclitaxel, are not fully understood. Nab-paclitaxel likely capitalizes on several mechanisms, which include an improved pharmacokinetic profile with a larger volume of distribution and a higher maximal concentration of circulating, unbound, free drug; improved tumor accumulation by the enhanced permeability and retention (EPR) effect; and receptor-mediated transcytosis via an albumin-specific receptor (gp60) for endothelial transcytosis and binding of secreted protein acidic and rich in cysteine (SPARC) in the tumor interstitium.[29,30] In contrast to cremophor/ethanol (CrEL) solvent-based paclitaxel, nab-paclitaxel exhibits an extensive extravascular volume of distribution exceeding that of water, indicating extensive tissue and extravascular protein distribution. Some studies show that nab-paclitaxel achieves 33% higher drug concentration over CrEL-paclitaxel.[31] Additionally, the maximum concentration (Cmax), the mean plasma half-life of 15 to 18 hours, the area under curve (AUC), and the dose-independent plasma clearance correspond to linear pharmacokinetics over 80 to 300 mg/m^2.[29,32] The improved deposition of a nanoparticle, such as nab-paclitaxel in a tumor tissue, can occur passively through an EPR effect in areas of leaky vasculature, sufficient vascular pore size, and decreased lymphatic flow.[25,33] Once in the tissue, the nab-paclitaxel nanovehicle can deliver the drug locally or benefit from further receptor-mediated targeting to SPARC, which has been shown to be overexpressed, and correlates with disease progression in many tumor types.[34–38] Although preclinical models, as well as one clinical trial, have shown how nanoparticle therapy can benefit from this targeted approach,[39,40] correlative data for nab-paclitaxel is limited. The high stromal SPARC level was associated with longer survival in patients treated with nab-paclitaxel in the phase I/II study of patients with pancreatic cancer; however, this correlative analysis was not included in the phase III trial report and requires validation.[28,41]

TABLE 21.1

Antimicrotubule Agents: Dosages and Toxicities

Chemotherapeutic Agent	Dosage	Indications	Common Toxicities
Paclitaxel	135–200 mg/m^2 IV over 3 h or 135 mg/m^2 IV over 24 h every 3 wk; or 80 mg/m^2 IV over 1 h weekly	Adjuvant therapy of node-positive breast cancer; metastatic breast, ovarian, non–small-cell lung, bladder, esophagus, cervical, gastric, and head and neck cancer; AIDS-related Kaposi sarcoma; cancer of unknown origin	Myelosuppression, hypersensitivity, nausea and vomiting, alopecia, arthralgia, myalgia, peripheral neuropathy
Docetaxel	60–100 mg/m^2 IV over 1 h every 3 wk	Adjuvant therapy of node-positive breast cancer; metastatic breast, gastric, head and neck, prostate, non–small-cell lung, and ovarian cancer	Myelosuppression, hypersensitivity, edema, alopecia, nail damage, rash, diarrhea, nausea, vomiting, asthenia, neuropathy
Cabazitaxel	25 mg/m^2 IV every 3 wk over 1 h	Docetaxel-refractory metastatic castration resistant prostate cancer	Neutropenia, infections, myelosuppression, diarrhea, nausea, vomiting, constipation, abdominal pain, asthenia
Nab-paclitaxel	260 mg/m^2 IV over 30 min every 3 wk; or 125 mg/m^2 IV weekly on days 1, 8, and 15 every 28 d	Metastatic breast cancer, non–small-cell lung cancer, pancreatic cancer	Myelosuppression, nausea, vomiting, alopecia, myalgia, peripheral neuropathy
Ixabepilone	40 mg/m^2 IV over 3 h every 3 wk	Metastatic and locally advanced breast cancer	Myelosuppression, fatigue/asthenia, myalgia/arthralgia, alopecia, nausea, vomiting, stomatitis/mucositis, diarrhea, musculoskeletal pain
Vincristine	0.5–1.4 mg/m^2/wk IV (maximum 2 mg per dose); or 0.4 mg/d continuous infusion for 4 d	Lymphoma, acute leukemia, neuroblastoma, rhabdomyosarcoma, AIDS-related Kaposi sarcoma, multiple myeloma, testicular cancer	Constipation, nausea, vomiting, alopecia, diplopia, myelosuppression
Vinblastine	6 mg/m^2 IV on days 1 and 15 as part of the ABVD regimen; 0.15 mg/kg IV on days 1 and 2 as part of the PVB regimen; 3 mg/m^2 IV as part of days 2, 15, 22 MVAC regimen	Hodgkin and non-Hodgkin lymphoma; Kaposi sarcoma; breast, testicular, bladder, prostate, and renal cell cancer	Myelosuppression, constipation, alopecia, malaise, bone pain
Vinorelbine	25–30 mg/m^2 IV weekly	Non–small-cell lung, breast, cervical, and ovarian cancer	Alopecia, diarrhea, nausea, vomiting, asthenia, neuromyopathy
Estramustine	14 mg/kg PO daily in 3 or 4 divided doses	Metastatic prostate cancer	Nausea, vomiting, gynecomastia, fluid retention
Ado-trastuzumab emtansine	3.6 mg/kg IV every 3 wk	Metastatic breast cancer	Thrombocytopenia, nausea, constipation or diarrhea, peripheral neuropathy, fatigue, increased AST/ALT
Brentuximab vedotin	1.8 mg/kg every 3 wk, maximum dose 180 mg	Refractory Hodgkin lymphoma, refractory systemic anaplastic large cell lymphoma	Neutropenia, anemia, thrombocytopenia, fatigue, fever, peripheral neuropathy

ABVD, doxorubicin (Adriamycin), bleomycin, vinblastine, dacarbazine; PVB, cisplatin, vinblastine, bleomycin; MVAC, methotrexate, vinblastine, doxorubicin (Adriamycin), cisplatin; IV, intravenous; PO, by mouth; AST/ALT, aspartate amniotransferase–alanine amniotransferase.

Docetaxel

The pharmacokinetics of docetaxel on a 1-hour schedule is triexponential and linear at doses of 115 mg/m^2 or less.[4] Terminal half-lives ranging from 11.1 to 18.5 hours has been reported. The most important determinants of docetaxel clearance were the body surface area (BSA), hepatic function, and plasma α_1-acid glycoprotein concentration. Plasma protein binding is high (greater than 80%), and binding is primarily to α_1-acid glycoprotein, albumin, and lipoproteins. The hepatic cytochrome P-450 mixed-function oxidases, particularly isoforms CYP3A4 and CYP3A5, are principally involved in biotransformation. The principal pharmacokinetic determinants of toxicity, particularly neutropenia, are drug exposure and the time that plasma concentrations exceed biologically relevant concentrations. The baseline level of α_1-acid glycoprotein may be elevated as an acute phase reactant in advanced disease and is an independent predictor of response and a major objective prognostic factor of survival in patients with non–small-cell lung cancer treated with docetaxel chemotherapy.

Cabazitaxel

Cabazitaxel is a semisynthetic derivative of the natural taxoid 10-deacetylbaccatin III. It binds to and stabilizes the β-tubulin subunit, resulting in the inhibition of microtubule depolymerization and cell division, cell cycle arrest in the G_2/M phase, and the inhibition of tumor cell proliferation.[5] It is active against diverse cancer cell lines and tumor models that are sensitive and resistant to docetaxel, including prostate, mammary, melanoma, kidney, colon, pancreas, lung, gastric, and head and neck.[5] Cabazitaxel is a poor substrate for the membrane-associated, multidrug resistance P-glycoprotein efflux pump; therefore, is useful for treating docetaxel-refractory prostate cancer for which it gained FDA approval in 2010.[5] In addition, it penetrates the blood–brain barrier.[42] Pharmacokinetics of cabazitaxel is similar to docetaxel; however, cabazitaxel has a larger volume of distribution and a longer terminal half-life (mean 77.3 hours versus 11.2 hours for docetaxel).[43,44]

Tesetaxel

Tesetaxel (DJ-927, XRP6258) is a semisynthetic, orally bioavailable taxane currently in clinical trials in breast, gastric, and prostate cancer. Administration in phase I and II trials has been once per week or every 3 weeks and not associated with hypersensitivity and possibly less neurotoxicity compared to other taxanes. Dose-limiting toxicity has been neutropenia. Overall responses in phase II studies have been 50% and 38% in patients treated for first- and second-line breast cancer, respectively. A phase I/II study in advanced NSCLC showed an overall response rate of 5.6%. Tesetaxel activity is independent of P-glycoprotein expression.[45] Pharmacokinetics on a schedule of every 3 weeks have an AUC of ~1,750 ng/mL per hour, a half life of ~170 hours, and no drug interactions that have been noted.[46]

Drug Interactions

Sequence-dependent pharmacokinetic and toxicologic interactions between paclitaxel and several other chemotherapy agents have been noted. The sequence of cisplatin followed by paclitaxel (on a 24-hour schedule) induces more profound neutropenia than the reverse sequence, which is explained by a 33% reduction in the clearance of paclitaxel after cisplatin.[47] Treatment with paclitaxel on either a 3- or 24-hour schedule followed by carboplatin has been demonstrated to produce equivalent neutropenia and less thrombocytopenia as compared to carboplatin as a single agent, which is not explained by pharmacokinetic interactions. Neutropenia and mucositis are more severe when paclitaxel is administered on a 24-hour schedule before doxorubicin, compared to the reverse sequence, which is most likely due to an approximately 32% reduction in the clearance rates of doxorubicin and doxorubicinol when doxorubicin is administered after paclitaxel. Several agents that inhibit cytochrome P-450 mixed-function oxidases interfere with the metabolism of paclitaxel and docetaxel in human microsomes in vitro; however, the clinical relevance of these findings is not known.[47]

Toxicity

Paclitaxel

The micelle-forming CrEL vehicle, which is required for suspension and intravenous delivery of paclitaxel, causes its nonlinear pharmacokinetics and thereby impacts its therapeutic index. CrEL causes hypersensitivity reactions, with major reactions usually occurring within the first 10 minutes after the first treatment and resolving completely after stopping the treatment. All patients should be premedicated with steroids, diphenhydramine, and an H2 antagonist, although up to 3% will still have reactions. Those who have major reactions have been rechallenged successfully after receiving high doses of corticosteroids.

Neuropathy is the principal toxicity of paclitaxel. Paclitaxel induces a peripheral neuropathy that presents in a symmetric stocking glove distribution, at first transient and then persistent.[48] A neurologic examination reveals sensory loss, and neurophysiologic studies reveal axonal degeneration and demyelination.[48] Compared with cisplatin, a loss of deep tendon reflexes occurs less commonly; however, autonomic and motor changes can occur. Severe neurotoxicity is uncommon when paclitaxel is given alone at doses below 200 mg/m² on a 3- or 24-hour schedule every 3 weeks, or below 100 mg/m² on a continuous weekly schedule. There is no convincing evidence that any specific measure is effective at ameliorating existing manifestations or preventing the development or worsening of neurotoxicity.[48]

Neutropenia is also frequent with paclitaxel. The onset is usually on days 8 to 11, and recovery is generally complete by days 15 to 21 with an every 3 weeks dosing regimen. Neutropenia is noncumulative, and the duration of severe neutropenia—even in heavily pretreated patients—is usually brief. Severity of neutropenia is related to the duration of exposure above the biologically relevant levels of 0.05 to 0.10 μM/L, and paclitaxel's nonlinear pharmacokinetics should be considered whenever adjusting dose.[49]

The most common cardiac rhythm disturbance, a transient sinus bradycardia, can be observed in up to 30% of patients. Routine cardiac monitoring during paclitaxel therapy is not necessary but is advisable for patients who may not be able to tolerate bradyarrhythmias. Drug-related gastrointestinal effects, such as vomiting and diarrhea, are uncommon. Severe hepatotoxicity and pancreatitis have also been noted rarely. Pulmonary toxicities, including acute bilateral pneumonitis, have been reported. Extravasation of large volumes can cause moderate soft tissue injury. Paclitaxel also induces reversible alopecia of the scalp in a dose-related fashion. Nail disorders have also been reported with paclitaxel use and include ridging, nail bed pigmentation, onychorrhexis, and onycholysis. These side effects have been reported more commonly with dose-intensified paclitaxel regimens.

Recent studies have suggested a role for the adenosine triphosphatase (ATP)-binding cassette (ABC) transporter polymorphisms in the development of neuropathy and neutropenia. Sissung et al.[50] reported that patients carrying two reference alleles for the *ABCB1* (P-glycoprotein, MDR1) 3435C greater than T polymorphism had a reduced risk to develop neuropathy as compared to patients carrying at least one variant allele ($P = .09$). Data from a large controlled trial to evaluate these and other candidate polymorphisms failed to detect a significant association between genotype and outcome or toxicity for any of the genes analyzed, although the correlative studies were retrospective and the sample size was inadequate to rule out smaller differences.[51] A large randomized trial of the CALGB 40101 using an integrated genomewide associate study found two polymorphisms associated with paclitaxel-induced polyneuropathy.[52] Both are involved in nerve development and maintenance, including the hereditary peripheral neuropathy Charcot-Marie-Tooth disease gene, *FGD4*. Further studies are required to adequately assess the role of these variants in predicting toxicity from taxane therapy.

Nab-paclitaxel

Hypersensitivity reactions have not been observed during the infusion period and, therefore, steroid premedications are not necessary. The main dose-limiting toxicities are neutropenia and sensory neuropathy. In a trial comparing weekly paclitaxel 90 mg/m² to nab-paclitaxel 150 mg/m² to ixabepilone in patients with metastatic breast cancer, there was more hematologic toxicity and peripheral neuropathy in the nab-paclitaxel arm compared to the paclitaxel arm, although median progression-free survival was not significantly different at the 12-month follow-up.[53] This led to dose reductions in 45% of patients in the nab-paclitaxel arm compared with 15% for the paclitaxel arm.[53] Other toxicities include alopecia, diarrhea, nausea and vomiting, elevations in liver enzymes, arthralgia, myalgia, and asthenia.

Docetaxel

Neutropenia is the main toxicity of docetaxel.[4] When docetaxel is administered on an every 3 weeks schedule, the onset of neutropenia is usually noted on day 8, with complete resolution by days 15 to 21. Neutropenia is significantly less when low doses are administered weekly. FDA black box warnings include increased toxicity in patients with abnormal liver function and, in select NSCLC patients that received prior platinum, severe hypersensitivity reactions and severe fluid retention despite dexamethasone at-home premedication.

Hypersensitivity reactions were noted in approximately 31% of patients who received the drug without premedications in early studies.[4] Symptoms include flushing, rash, chest tightness, back pain, dyspnea, and fever or chills. Severe hypotension, bronchospasm, generalized rash, and erythema may also occur.[54] Major reactions usually occur during the first two courses and within minutes after the start of treatment. Signs and symptoms generally resolve within 15 minutes after cessation of treatment, and docetaxel can usually be reinstituted without sequelae after treatment with diphenhydramine and an H2-receptor antagonist. Docetaxel induces a unique fluid retention syndrome characterized by edema, weight gain, and third-space fluid collection. Fluid retention is cumulative and is due to increased capillary permeability. Prophylactic treatment with corticosteroids has been demonstrated to reduce the incidence of fluid retention. Aggressive and early treatment with diuretics has been successfully used to manage fluid retention. Skin toxicity may occur in as many as 50% to 75% of patients; however, premedication may reduce the overall incidence of this effect.[4] Other cutaneous effects include palmar–plantar erythrodysesthesia and onychodystrophy. Docetaxel produces neurotoxicity, which is qualitatively similar to that of paclitaxel; however, neurosensory and neuromuscular effects are generally less frequent and less severe than with paclitaxel. Mild-to-moderate peripheral neurotoxicity occurs in approximately 40% of untreated patients.[55] Asthenia has been a prominent complaint in patients who have been treated with large cumulative doses. Stomatitis appears to occur more frequently with docetaxel than with paclitaxel. Other reported toxicities of note include necrotizing enterocolitis, interstitial pneumonitis, and organizing pneumonia.[56,57]

Cabazitaxel

A phase III multi-institutional study of men with metastatic castration-resistant prostate cancer who had failed docetaxel improved overall median survival on cabazitaxel compared to mitoxantrone.[58] Cabazitaxel was approved by the FDA in June 2010 to treat metastatic castration-resistant prostate cancer in those who had received prior chemotherapy. This was despite a higher rate of adverse deaths (4.9%), a third of which were due to neutropenic sepsis. Cabazitaxel was associated with more grade 3 or 4 neutropenia (82%) than mitoxantrone (58%). Side effects reported in more than 20% of patients treated with cabazitaxel included myelosuppression, diarrhea, nausea, vomiting, constipation, abdominal pain, or asthenia. FDA black box warnings are similar to those for docetaxel.

VINCA ALKALOIDS

The vinca alkaloids have been some of the most active agents in cancer chemotherapy since their introduction 40 years ago. The naturally occurring members of the family, vinblastine (VBL) and vincristine (VCR), were isolated from the leaves of the periwinkle plant *Catharanthus roseus G. Don*. In the late 1950s, their antimitotic and, therefore, cancer chemotherapeutic potential was discovered by groups both at Eli Lilly Research Laboratories and at the University of Western Ontario, and they came into widespread use for the single-agent treatment of childhood hematologic and solid malignancies and, shortly after, for adult hematologic malignancies (see Table 21.1).[1] Their clinical efficacy in several combination therapies has led to the development of various novel semisynthetic analogs, including vinorelbine (VRL), vindesine (VDS), and vinflunine (VFL).

Mechanism of Action

In contrast to the taxanes, the vinca alkaloids depolymerize microtubules and destroy mitotic spindles.[1] At low but clinically relevant concentrations, VBL does not depolymerize spindle microtubules, yet it powerfully blocks mitosis. This has been suggested to occur as a result of the suppression of microtubule dynamics rather than microtubule depolymerization. This group of compounds binds to the β subunit of tubulin dimers at a distinct region called the vinca-binding domain. Importantly, VBL binding induces a conformational change in tubulin in connection with tubulin self-association. In mitotic spindles, the slowing of the growth and shortening or treadmilling dynamics of the microtubules block mitotic progression. Disruption of the normal mitotic spindle assembly leads to delayed cell cycle progress with chromosomes stuck at the spindle poles and unable to pass from metaphase into anaphase, which eventually induces to apoptosis. The naturally occurring vinca alkaloids VCR and VBL, the semisynthetic analog VRL, and a novel bifluorinated analog VFL have similar mechanisms of action.

Tissue and tumor sensitivities to the vinca alkaloids, which, in part, relate to differences in drug transport and accumulation, also vary. Intracellular or extracellular concentration ratios range from five- to 500-fold depending on the individual cell type, lipophilicity, tissue-specific factors such as tubulin isotype composition, and tissue-specific microtubule-associated proteins (MAP).[59–61] Although the vinca alkaloids are retained in cells for long periods of time and thus may have prolonged cellular effects, intracellular retention is markedly different among the various vinca alkaloids. For instance, VBL appears to be retained in lipophilic tissue much more than either VCR or VDS.[59] Newer theories of antimicrotubule agents' mechanism of action have emerged, suggesting that the more important target of these drugs may be the tumor vasculature, as reviewed in the next section.

Clinical Pharmacology

The vinca alkaloids are usually administered intravenously as a brief infusion, and their pharmacokinetic behavior in plasma has generally been explained by a three-compartment model. The vinca alkaloids share many pharmacokinetic properties, including large volumes of distribution, high clearance rates, and long terminal half-lives that reflect the high magnitude and avidity of drug binding in peripheral tissues. VCR has the longest terminal half-life and the lowest clearance rate; VBL has the shortest terminal half-life and the highest clearance rate; and VDS has intermediate characteristics. Although prolonged infusion schedules may avoid excessively toxic peak concentrations and increase the duration of drug exposure in plasma above biologically relevant threshold concentrations, there is little evidence to support the notion that prolonged infusions are more effective than bolus schedules. The longest half-life and lowest clearance rate of VCR may account for its greater propensity to induce neurotoxicity, but there are many other nonpharmacokinetic determinants of tissue sensitivity, as discussed in the previous section.

Vincristine

After conventional doses of VCR (1.4 mg/m^2) given as brief infusions, peak plasma levels approach 0.4 μmol. Plasma clearance is slow, and terminal half-lives that range from 23 to 85 hours have been reported. VCR is metabolized and excreted primarily by the hepatobiliary system. The nature of the VCR metabolites identified to date, as well as the results of metabolic studies in vitro, indicate that VCR metabolism is mediated principally by hepatic cytochrome P-450 CYP3A5.

Vinblastine

The clinical pharmacology of VBL is similar to that of VCR. VBL binding to plasma proteins and formed elements of blood is extensive.[62,63] Peak plasma drug concentrations are approximately 0.4 μm after rapid intravenous injections of VBL at standard doses. Distribution is rapid, and terminal half-lives range from 20 to 24 hours. Like VCR, VBL disposition is principally through the hepatobiliary system with excretion in feces (approximately 95%); however, fecal excretion of the parent compound is low, indicating that hepatic metabolism is extensive.[59]

Vinorelbine

The pharmacologic behavior of VRL is similar to that of the other vinca alkaloids, and plasma concentrations after rapid intravenous administration have been reported to decline in either a biexponential or triexponential manner.[64] After intravenous administration, there is a rapid decay of VRL concentrations followed by a much slower elimination phase (terminal half-life, 18 to 49 hours). Plasma protein binding, principally to α₁-acid glycoprotein, albumin, and lipoproteins, has been reported to range from 80% to 91%, and drug binding to platelets is extensive.[64] VRL is widely distributed, and high concentrations are found in virtually all tissues, except the central nervous system.[64] The wide distribution of VRL reflects its lipophilicity, which is among the highest of the vinca alkaloids. As with other vinca alkaloids, the liver is the principal excretory organ, and up to 80% of VRL is excreted in the feces, whereas urinary excretion represents only 16% to 30% of total drug disposition, the bulk of which is unmetabolized VRL. Studies in humans indicate that 4-O-deacetyl-VRL and 3,6-epoxy-VRL are the principal metabolites, and several minor hydroxy-VRL isomer metabolites have been identified. Although most metabolites are inactive, the deacetyl-VRL metabolite may be as active as VRL. The cytochrome P-450 CYP3A isoenzyme appears to be principally involved in biotransformation.

Vinflunine

VFL is a novel semisynthetic microtubule inhibitor with a fluorinated catharanthine moiety, which translates into lower affinity for the vinca binding site on tubulin and, therefore, different quantitative effects on microtubule dynamics.[65] The low affinity for tubulin may be responsible for its reduced clinical neurotoxicity. Despite this lower affinity, it is more active in vivo than other vinca alkaloids, and resistance develops more slowly. VFL is a new vinca and still under clinical development. Its volume of distribution is large, and has a terminal half-life of nearly 40 hours.[65] The only active metabolite is 4-O-deacetylvinflunine, which has a terminal half-life approximately 5 days longer than that of the parent compound.[65]

Drug Interactions

Methotrexate accumulation in tumor cells is enhanced in vitro by the presence of VCR or VBL, an effect mediated by a vinca alkaloid–induced blockade of drug efflux; however, the minimal concentrations of VCR required to achieve this effect occur only transiently in vivo.[66] The vinca alkaloids also inhibit the cellular influx of the epipodophyllotoxins in vitro, resulting in less cytotoxicity. However, the clinical implications of this potential interaction are unknown. L-asparaginase may reduce the hepatic clearance

of the vinca alkaloids, which may result in increased vinca-related toxicity. To minimize the possibility of this interaction, the vinca alkaloids should be given 12 to 24 hours before L-asparaginase. The combined use of mitomycin C and the vinca alkaloids has been associated with acute dyspnea and bronchospasm. The onset of these pulmonary toxicities has ranged from within minutes to hours after treatment with the vinca alkaloids, or up to 2 weeks after mitomycin C.

Treatment with the vinca alkaloids has precipitated seizures associated with subtherapeutic plasma phenytoin concentrations.[66] Reduced plasma phenytoin levels have been noted from 24 hours to 10 days after treatment with VCR and VBL. Because of the importance of the cytochrome P-450 CYP3A isoenzyme in vinca alkaloid metabolism, administration of the vinca alkaloids with erythromycin and other inhibitors of CYP3A may lead to severe toxicity.[67] Concomitantly administered drugs, such as pentobarbital and H₂-receptor antagonists, may also influence VCR clearance by modulating hepatic cytochrome P-450 metabolic processes.[66]

Toxicity

Despite close similarities in structure, the vinca alkaloids differ in their safety profiles. Neutropenia is the principal dose-limiting toxicity of VBL and VRL. Thrombocytopenia and anemia occur less commonly. The onset of neutropenia is usually day 7 to 11, with recovery by day 14 to 21, and can be potentiated by hepatic dysfunction. Gastrointestinal autonomic dysfunction, as manifested by bloating, constipation, ileus, and abdominal pain, occur most commonly with VCR or high doses of the other vinca alkaloids. Mucositis occurs more frequently with VBL than with VRL and is least common with VCR. Nausea, vomiting, diarrhea,[31,43,45] and pancreatitis[53,54] also occur to a lesser extent.

VCR principally induces neurotoxicity characterized by a peripheral, symmetric mixed sensory motor and autonomic polyneuropathy.[68,69] Toxic manifestations include constipation, abdominal cramps, paralytic ileus, urinary retention, orthostatic hypotension, and hypertension. Its primary neuropathologic effects are due to interference with axonal microtubule function. Early symmetric sensory impairment and paresthesias can progress to neuritic pain and loss of deep tendon reflexes with continued treatment, which may be followed by foot drop, wrist drop, motor dysfunction, ataxia, and paralysis. Cranial nerves are rarely affected because the uptake of VCR into the central nervous system is low. Severe neurotoxicity occurs infrequently with VBL and VDS. VRL has been shown to have a lower affinity for axonal microtubules than either VCR or VBL, which seems to be confirmed by clinical observations.[70] Mild-to-moderate peripheral neuropathy, principally characterized by sensory effects, occurs in 7% to 31% of patients, and constipation and other autonomic effects are noted in 30% of patients, whereas severe toxicity occurs in 2% to 3%.

In adults, neurotoxicity may occur after treatment with cumulative doses as little as 5 to 6 mg, and manifestations may be profound after cumulative doses of 15 to 20 mg. Patients with delayed biliary excretion or hepatic dysfunction, and those with antecedent neurologic disorders, such as Charcot-Marie-Tooth disease, hereditary and sensory neuropathy type 1, and Guillain-Barré syndrome, are predisposed to neurotoxicity.

The vinca alkaloids are potent vesicants. To decrease the risk of phlebitis, the vein should be adequately flushed after treatment. If extravasation is suspected, treatment should be discontinued, aspiration of any residual drug remaining in the tissues should be attempted, and prompt application of heat (not ice) for 1 hour four times daily for 3 to 5 days can limit tissue damage.[71] Hyaluronidase, 150 to 1,500 U (15 U/mL in 6 mL 0.9% sodium chloride solution) subcutaneously, through six clockwise injections in a circumferential manner using a 25-gauge needle (changing the needle with each new injection) into the surrounding tissues may minimize discomfort and latent cellulitis. A surgical consultation to consider early debridement is also recommended. Mild and reversible alopecia occurs in approximately 10% and 20% of patients treated with VLR and VCR, respectively. Acute cardiac ischemia, chest pains without evidence of ischemia, fever, Raynaud syndrome, hand–foot syndrome, and pulmonary and liver toxicity (transaminitis and hyperbilirubinemia) have also been reported with use of the vinca alkaloids. All of the vinca alkaloids can cause a syndrome of inappropriate secretion of antidiuretic hormone (SIADH), and patients who are receiving intensive hydration are particularly prone to severe hyponatremia secondary to SIADH.

MICROTUBULE ANTAGONISTS

Estramustine Phosphate

Estramustine is a conjugate of nor-nitrogen mustard linked to 17β-estradiol by a carbamate ester bridge. Estramustine phosphate received regulatory approval in the United States in 1981 for treating patients with castration-resistant prostate cancer (CRPC). Although the recommended daily dose of estramustine phosphate is 14 mg/kg per day, patients are usually treated in the daily dosing range of 10 to 16 mg/kg in three to four divided daily doses (see Table 21.1). Estramustine has significant activity in CRPC and had been used in combination with VBL or docetaxel. However, phase III trials in patients with CRPC showed that when combined with docetaxel, there is no added benefit to overall survival compared to docetaxel alone.[72,73]

Estramustine binds to β-tubulin at a site distinct from the colchicine and vinca alkaloid binding sites. This agent depolymerizes microtubules and microfilaments, binds to and disrupts MAPs, and inhibits cell growth at high concentrations, resulting in mitotic arrest and apoptosis in tumor cells. The selective accumulation and actions of estramustine phosphate and its metabolite, *estromus*tine, in specific tissues appear to be dependent on the expression of the estramustine-binding protein (EMBP). The disposition of estramustine is principally by rapid oxidative metabolism of the parent compound to estromustine. Estromustine concentrations in plasma are maximal within 2 to 4 hours after oral administration, and the mean elimination half-life of estromustine is 14 hours. Estromustine and estramustine are principally excreted in the feces, with only small amounts of conjugated estrone and estradiol detected in the urine (less than 1%).

In general, this agent has a manageable safety profile. Nausea and vomiting are the principal toxicities encountered. In contrast to the taxanes and the vinca alkaloids, myelosuppression is rarely clinically relevant. Common estrogenic side effects include gynecomastia, nipple tenderness, and fluid retention. Thromboembolic complications may occur in up to 10% of patients.

Epothilones

The epothilones are macrolide compounds that were initially isolated from the mycobacterium *Sorangium cellulosum*. They exert their cytotoxic effects by promoting tubulin polymerization and inducing mitotic arrest.[74] In general, the epothilones are more potent than the taxanes. In contrast to the taxanes and vinca alkaloids, overexpression of the efflux protein P-glycoprotein minimally affects the cytotoxicity of epothilones. Epothilones include the natural epothilone B (patupilone; EPO906) and several semisynthetic epothilone compounds such as aza-epothilone B (ixabepilone; BMS-247550), epothilone D (deoxyepothilone B, KOS-862), and a fully synthetic analog, sagopilone (ZK-EPO).[75]

Ixabepilone has been evaluated in several schedules using a cremophor-based formulation and is FDA approved for the treatment of patients with breast cancer.[75] It is active in breast cancer previously treated with paclitaxel or docetaxel. The principal toxicities observed include neutropenia and peripheral neuropathy,

in addition to fatigue, nausea, emesis, and diarrhea.[55,74] It also has been evaluated in other solid tumors such as ovarian, prostate, and renal cell carcinomas.[75] Epothilones are still undergoing evaluations in several clinical trials. Pharmacokinetic studies based on patupilone have shown large volume of distribution (41-fold the total body water) and low body clearance (13% of hepatic blood flow).[76] There do not appear to be active metabolites once the parent drug is hydrolyzed, which is the main elimination pathway.[76]

Maytansinoids and Auristatins: DM1, MMAE

Antibody drug conjugates (ADC) were first attempted with delivery of doxorubicin. Although tissue localization seemed promising, it became clear that the delivery of more potent chemotherapeutics was necessary.[77,78] One of the major advances for the promise of ADC came with the discovery and development of highly potent anticancer compounds such as calicheamicins, maytansinoids, and auristatins.[78] The next necessary advance was a linker that released the drug only when intended, and avoiding, or in some cases capitalizing on, in vivo proteases, oxidizing, or reducing environments. Gemtuzumab ozogamicin was the first ADC using calicheamicin, a potent DNA minor groove binder (and not a microtubule agent), approved in 2000 although withdrawn from the market in 2013 due to failed confirmatory studies. Maytansinoids and auristatins are unrelated, although are both tubulin-binding agents of the vinca binding site and inhibit tubulin polymerization.[78] They are 100- to 1,000-fold more cytotoxic that most cancer chemotherapeutics.[79]

Drug maytansinoid-1 (DM1) is the chemotherapeutic delivered using a thioether linker in the ADC ado-trastuzumab emtansine (T-DM1) that was FDA approved for patients with HER2- positive metastatic breast cancer previously treated with trastuzumab and taxane chemotherapy.[80,81] In the international phase III study, there was a 3.2-month improved progression-free survival among patients that received T-DM1 compared to those receiving standard treatment with capecitabine and lapatinib.[81] Despite a potent chemotherapeutic, the tolerability was much better in the experimental arm, which was dosed at 3.6 mg/kg intravenously every 21 days. The most common side effects in the trial were thrombocytopenia (12.8%), transient transaminitis (4.3%), as well as nausea, fatigue, myalgias, and arthralgias.[81]

Monomethyl auristatin E (MMAE) is linked to a monoclonal antibody against CD30 as an ADC (brentuximab vedotin, SGN35) and approved for refractory Hodgkin lymphoma or anaplastic large cell lymphoma. The linker is a peptide-based substrate for cathepsin-B and thereby designed to detect the lysosome/endosome compartment for drug release.[82,83] Dose-limiting toxicities include thrombocytopenia, hyperglycemia, diarrhea, and vomiting, and the most common side effects in this heavily pretreated population (including autologous stem cell transplant) includes peripheral neuropathy (42%), nausea (35%), and fatigue (34%).[84] The FDA black box warning includes contraindicated use with bleomycin due to increased pulmonary toxicity and the risk of John Cunningham (JC) virus–induced progressive multifocal leukoencephalopathy. Reports of severe pancreatitis are also emerging.[85]

MITOTIC MOTOR PROTEIN INHIBITORS

Aurora Kinase and Pololike Kinase Inhibitors

Aurora kinases are serine/threonine kinases crucial for mitosis in their recruitment of mitotic motor proteins for spindle formation. They are particularly overexpressed in high growth rate tumors. Aurora A and B kinases are expressed globally throughout all tissues, and Aurora C kinase is expressed in testes and participates in meiosis. Aurora A kinase is expressed and frequently amplified in many epithelial tumors and implicated in the microtubule-targeted agent-resistant phenotype.[86] Aurora A kinase interacts with p53, and there is evidence that p53 wild-type tumors are more sensitive to aurora A kinase inhibitors than p53 mutant tumors.[87] MLN-8237 has an IC_{50} of 1 nm for aurora A kinase and >200 nm for aurora B kinase and is in clinical development for treatment-related neuroendocrine prostate cancer.[86,88] The main dose-limiting toxicity of these agents is neutropenia. Pololike kinases (PLKs) are serine or threonine kinases crucial for cell cycle process. Overexpression of PLKs has been shown to be related to histologic grading and poor prognosis in several types of cancer. BI-2536 and ON01910 are PLK inhibitors in early clinical development.[89]

Kinesin Spindle Protein Inhibitor

Ispinesib

Kinesin spindle protein (KSP; also known as EG5) is a kinesin motor protein required to establish mitotic-spindle bipolarity.[90] Several KSP inhibitors have been evaluated in early phase clinical trials. SB-715992 (ispinesib) is a small-molecule inhibitor of KSP ATPase and has been evaluated in two different schedules.[89] The dose-limiting toxicity is neutropenia. Ispinesib was found to be inactive in phase 2 studies evaluating efficacy in patients with castration-resistant and largely docetaxel-resistant prostate cancer, advanced renal cancer, and head and neck cancer.[90–92]

MECHANISMS OF RESISTANCE TO MICROTUBULE INHIBITORS

Drug resistance is often complex and multifaceted and can involve diverse mechanisms such as (1) factors that reduce the ability of drugs to reach their cellular target (e.g., activation of detoxification pathways and decreased drug accumulation); (2) modifications in the drug target; and (3) events downstream of the target (e.g., decreased sensitivity to, or defective, apoptotic signals). Many tubulin binding agents are substrates for multidrug transporters such as P-glycoprotein and the multidrug resistance gene (*MDR1*).[93,94]

The *MDR1*-encoded gene product MDR1 (ABC subfamily B1; ABCB1) and MDR2 (ABC subfamily ABCB4) are the best-characterized ABC transporters thought to confer drug resistance to taxanes.[94,95] MDR-related taxane resistance can be reversed by many classes of drugs, including the calcium channel blockers, cyclosporin A, and antiarrhythmic agents.[94,95] However, the clinical utility of this approach has never been proven, despite several clinical trials. The role of ABC transporters in resistance to microtubule inhibitors remains to be determined.[96]

An increasing number of studies suggest that the expression of individual tubulin isotypes are altered in cells resistant to

antimicrotubule drugs and may confer drug resistance.[93,97] Inherent differences in microtubule dynamics and drug interactions have been observed with some isotypes in vitro and in vivo.[98] Several taxane-resistant mutant cell lines that have structurally altered α- and β-tubulin proteins and an impaired ability to polymerize into microtubules have also been identified.[99] Mutations of tubulin isotype genes, gene amplifications, and isotype switching have also been reported in taxane-resistant cell lines.[99] In patients, levels of class III β-tubulin have been shown to correlate with response—those with high RNA levels have poor response—and immunohistochemical stains can correlate and may be predictive.[96,100,101] As opposed to taxanes, resistance to vinca alkaloids has been associated with decreased class II β-tubulin expression.[97,98]

MAPs are important structural and regulatory components of microtubules that act in concert to remodel the microtubule network by stabilizing or destabilizing microtubules during mitosis or cytokinesis. Alterations in the activity and/or balance of stabilizing or destabilizing MAPs can profoundly affect microtubule function.[99,102] The overexpression of stathmin, a destabilizing protein, has been reported to decrease sensitivity to paclitaxel and vinblastine.[1] An analysis of predictive or prognostic factors in a large phase 3 study (National Surgical Adjuvant Breast and Bowel Project NSABP-B 28) in patients with node-positive breast cancer showed that MAP-tau, a stabilizing protein, was a prognostic factor; however, it was not predictive for benefit from paclitaxel-based chemotherapy.[1,93] In a separate randomized controlled trial in breast cancer (TAX 307), where the only variable was docetaxel, MAP-tau was also shown to be prognostic, but not predictive of taxane benefit.[103]

Additional studies have shown a correlation with *BRCA1* loss measured by gene or protein expression, or gene signatures, with resistance to taxane and sensitivity to DNA-damaging agents (such as cisplatin and anthracyclines).[104–107] *BRCA1* is a tumor-suppressor gene with DNA damage response and repair, as well as cell cycle checkpoint activation, which explains why its loss leads to enhanced cisplatin sensitivity.[20] *BRCA1* also indirectly regulates microtubule dynamics and stability and can favorably control how microtubules respond to paclitaxel treatment via their association with pro-caspase-8. The loss of *BRCA1* can lead to impaired taxane-induced activation of apoptosis due to microtubules that are more dynamic and less susceptible to taxane-induced stabilization and proximity-induced activation of caspase-8 signaling.[20]

In addition to resistance, certain tumor subtypes may be sensitive to the taxane dosing schedule. In two randomized trials of low-dose, weekly paclitaxel, the luminal breast cancer subtype was found to have a better outcome compared with the control arm. This suggests that not only the drug, but also the schedule may influence the response to therapy and that genomic approaches may reveal these insights.[108]

SELECTED REFERENCES

The full reference list can be accessed at lwwhealthlibrary.com/oncology.

1. Kavallaris M. Microtubules and resistance to tubulin-binding agents. *Nat Rev Cancer* 2010;10:194–204.
3. Wani MC, Taylor HL, Wall ME, et al. Plant antitumor agents. VI. Isolation and structure of taxol, a novel antileukemic and antitumor agent from Taxus brevifolia. *J Am Chem Soc* 1971;93:2325–2327.
5. Vrignaud P, Sémiond D, Lejeune P, et al. Preclinical antitumor activity of cabazitaxel, a semisynthetic taxane active in taxane-resistant tumors. *Clin Cancer Res* 2013;19:2973–2983.
9. Martin M, Pienkowski T, Mackey J, et al. Adjuvant docetaxel for node-positive breast cancer. *N Engl J Med* 2005;352:2302–2313.
10. Jones SE, Erban J, Overmoyer B, et al. Randomized phase III study of docetaxel compared with paclitaxel in metastatic breast cancer. *J Clin Oncol* 2005;23:5542–5551.
11. Tannock IF, de Wit R, Berry WR, et al. Docetaxel plus prednisone or mitoxantrone plus prednisone for advanced prostate cancer. *N Engl J Med* 2004;351:1502–1512.

13. Schiff PB, Fant J, Horwitz SB. Promotion of microtubule assembly in vitro by taxol. *Nature* 1979;277:665–667.
19. Komlodi-Pasztor E, Sackett D, Wilkerson J, et al. Mitosis is not a key target of microtubule agents in patient tumors. *Nat Rev Clin Oncol* 2011;8:244–250.
20. Sung M, Giannakakou P. BRCA1 regulates microtubule dynamics and taxane-induced apoptotic cell signaling. *Oncogene* 2014;33(11):1418–1428.
23. Dai H, Ding H, Meng XW, et al. Contribution of Bcl-2 phosphorylation to Bak binding and drug resistance. *Cancer Res* 2013;73(23)6998–7008.
24. Oakes SR, Vaillant F, Lim E, et al. Sensitization of BCL-2–expressing breast tumors to chemotherapy by the BH3 mimetic ABT-737. *Proc Natl Acad Sci* 2012;109:2766–2771.
25. Chauhan VP, Stylianopoulos T, Martin JD, et al. Normalization of tumour blood vessels improves the delivery of nanomedicines in a size-dependent manner. *Nat Nanotechnol* 2012;7:383–388.
26. Gradishar W, Tjulandin S, Davidson N, et al. Phase III trial of nanoparticle albumin-bound paclitaxel compared with polyethylated castor oil-based paclitaxel in women with breast cancer. *J Clin Oncol* 2005;23:7794–7803.

27. Socinski MA, Bondarenko I, Karaseva NA, et al. Weekly nab-paclitaxel in combination with carboplatin versus solvent-based paclitaxel plus carboplatin as first-line therapy in patients with advanced non–small-cell lung cancer: final results of a Phase III trial. *J Clin Oncol* 2012;30:2055–2062.

28. Von Hoff DD, Ervin T, Arena FP, et al. Increased survival in pancreatic cancer with nab-paclitaxel plus gemcitabine. *N Engl J Med* 2013;369:1691–1703.

32. Nyman DW, Campbell KJ, Hersh E, et al. Phase I and pharmacokinetics trial of ABI-007, a novel nanoparticle formulation of paclitaxel in patients with advanced nonhematologic malignancies. *J Clin Oncol* 2005;23:7785–7793.

39. Cheng CJ, Saltzman WM. Enhanced siRNA delivery into cells by exploiting the synergy between targeting ligands and cell-penetrating peptides. *Biomaterials* 2011;32:6194–6203.

40. Davis ME, Zuckerman JE, Choi CHJ, et al. Evidence of RNAi in humans from systemically administered siRNA via targeted nanoparticles. *Nature* 2010;464:1067–1070.

43. Diéras V, Lortholary A, Laurence V, et al. Cabazitaxel in patients with advanced solid tumours: results of a Phase I and pharmacokinetic study. *Eur J Cancer* 2013;49:25–34.

44. Mita AC, Denis LJ, Rowinsky EK, et al. Phase I and pharmacokinetic study of XRP6258 (RPR 116258A), a novel taxane, administered as a 1-hour infusion every 3 weeks in patients with advanced solid tumors. *Clin Cancer Res* 2009;15:723–730.

45. Yared JA, Tkaczuk KH. Update on taxane development: new analogs and new formulations. *Drug Des Devel Ther* 2012;6:371–384.

48. Kudlowitz D, Muggia F. Defining risks of taxane neuropathy: insights from randomized clinical trials. *Clin Cancer Res* 2013;19:4570–4577.

49. Henningsson A, Karlsson MO, Viganò L, et al. Mechanism-based pharmacokinetic model for paclitaxel. *J Clin Oncol* 2001;19:4065–4073.

50. Sissung T, Mross K, Steinberg S, et al. Association of ABCB1 genotypes with paclitaxel-mediated peripheral neuropathy and neutropenia. *Eur J Cancer* 2006;42:2893–2896.

53. Rugo H, Barry W, Moreno Aspitia A, et al. CALGB 40502/NCCTG N063H: Randomized phase III trial of weekly paclitaxel (P) compared to weekly nanoparticle albumin bound nab-paclitaxel (NP) or ixabepilone (Ix) with or without bevacizumab (B) as first-line therapy for locally recurrent or metastatic breast cancer (MBC). *J Clin Oncol* 2012;30.

56. Alsamarai S, Charpidou AG, Matthay RA, et al. Pneumonitis related to docetaxel: case report and review of the literature. *In Vivo* 2009;23:635–637.

58. de Bono JS, Oudard S, Ozguroglu M, et al. Prednisone plus cabazitaxel or mitoxantrone for metastatic castration-resistant prostate cancer progressing after docetaxel treatment: a randomised open-label trial. *Lancet* 2010;376:1147–1154.

62. Bender RA, Castle MC, Margileth DA, et al. The pharmacokinetics of [3H]-vincristine in man. *Clin Pharmacol Ther* 1977;22:430–435.

64. Rowinsky EK, Noe DA, Trump DL, et al. Pharmacokinetic, bioavailability, and feasibility study of oral vinorelbine in patients with solid tumors. *J Clin Oncol* 1994;12:1754–1763.

72. Petrylak D, Hussain MHA, Tangen C, et al. Docetaxel and estramustine compared with mitoxantrone and prednisone for advanced refractory prostate cancer. *N Engl J Med* 2004;351:1513–1520.

73. Tannock IF, de Wit R, Berry WR, et al. Docetaxel plus prednisone or mitoxantrone plus prednisone for advanced prostate cancer. *N Engl J Med* 2004;351:1502–1512.

74. Lee JJ, Kelly WK. Epothilones: tubulin polymerization as a novel target for prostate cancer therapy. *Nat Clin Pract Oncol* 2009;6:85–92.

76. Kelly K, Zollinger M, Lozac'h F, et al. Metabolism of patupilone in patients with advanced solid tumor malignancies. *Invest New Drugs* 2013;31:605–615.

79. Doronina SO, Toki BE, Torgov MY, et al. Development of potent monoclonal antibody auristatin conjugates for cancer therapy. *Nat Biotechnol* 2003;21:778–784.

80. Lewis Phillips GD, Li G, Dugger DL, et al. Targeting HER2-positive breast cancer with trastuzumab-DM1, an antibody–cytotoxic drug conjugate. *Cancer Res* 2008;68:9280–9290.

81. Verma S, Miles D, Gianni L, et al. Trastuzumab emtansine for HER2-positive advanced breast cancer. *N Engl J Med* 2012;367:1783–1791.

83. Younes A, Bartlett NL, Leonard JP, et al. Brentuximab vedotin (SGN-35) for relapsed CD30-positive lymphomas. *N Engl J Med* 2010;363:1812–1821.

86. Mosquera JM, Beltran H, Park K, et al. Concurrent AURKA and MYCN gene amplifications are harbingers of lethal treatment-related neuroendocrine prostate cancer. *Neoplasia* 2013;15:1–10.

94. Gottesman MM, Fojo T, Bates SE. Multidrug resistance in cancer: role of ATP-dependent transporters. *Nat Rev Cancer* 2002;2:48–58.

99. Orr GA, Verdier-Pinard P, McDaid H, et al. Mechanisms of Taxol resistance related to microtubules. *Oncogene* 2003;22:7280–7295.

100. Monzó M, Rosell R, Sánchez JJ, et al. Paclitaxel resistance in non-small-cell lung cancer associated with beta-tubulin gene mutations. *J Clin Oncol* 1999;17:1786–1793.

102. Baquero MT, Hanna JA, Neumeister V, et al. Stathmin expression and its relationship to microtubule-associated protein tau and outcome in breast cancer. *Cancer* 2012;118:4660–4669.

103. Baquero MT, Lostritto K, Gustavson MD, et al. Evaluation of prognostic and predictive value of microtubule associated protein tau in two independent cohorts. *Breast Cancer Res* 2011;13(5):R85.

106. Font A, Taron M, Gago JL, et al. BRCA1 mRNA expression and outcome to neoadjuvant cisplatin-based chemotherapy in bladder cancer. *Ann Oncol* 2011;22:139–144.

108. Martin M, Prat A, Rodriguez-Lescure A, et al. PAM50 proliferation score as a predictor of weekly paclitaxel benefit in breast cancer. *Breast Cancer Res Treat* 2013;138:457–466.

22 Kinase Inhibitors as Anticancer Drugs

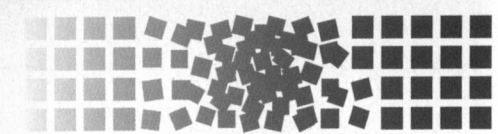

Charles L. Sawyers

INTRODUCTION

In 2001, the first tyrosine-kinase inhibitor imatinib was approved for clinical use in chronic myeloid leukemia. The spectacular success of this first-in-class agent ushered in a transformation in cancer drug discovery from efforts that were largely based on novel cytotoxic chemotherapy agents to an almost exclusive focus on molecularly targeted agents across the pharmaceutical and biotechnology industry and academia. This chapter summarizes this remarkable progress in this field over ~15 years, with the focus on the concepts underlying this paradigm shift as well as the considerable challenges that remain (Table 22.1). Readers in search of more specific details on individual drugs and their indications should consult the relevant disease-specific chapters elsewhere in this volume as well as references cited within this chapter. Readers should also note that the epidermal growth factor receptor (EGFR) and human epidermal growth factor receptor 2 (HER2) receptor tyrosine kinases covered here have also been successfully targeted by monoclonal antibodies that engage these proteins at the cell surface. These drugs, referred to as biologics rather than small molecule inhibitors, are covered in other chapters. The chapter is organized around kinase targets rather than diseases and, intentionally, has a historical flow to make certain thematic points and to illustrate the broad lessons that have been and continue to be learned through the clinical development of these exciting agents.

Perhaps the most stunning discovery from the clinical trials of the Abelson murine leukemia (ABL) kinase inhibitor imatinib was the recognition that tumor cells acquire exquisite dependence on the breakpoint cluster region protein BCR-ABL fusion oncogene, created by the Philadelphia chromosome translocation.[1] Although this may seem intuitive at first glance, consider the fact that the translocation arises in an otherwise normal hematopoietic stem cell, the survival of which is regulated by a complex array of growth factors and interactions with the bone marrow microenvironment. Although BCR-ABL clearly gives this cell a growth advantage that, over years, results in the clinical phenotype of chronic myeloid leukemia, there was no reason to expect that these cells would depend on BCR-ABL for their survival when confronted with an inhibitor. In the absence of BCR-ABL, these tumor cells could presumably rely on the marrow microenvironment, just like their normal, nontransformed neighbors. Thus, it seemed more likely that, by shutting down the driver oncogene, BCR-ABL inhibitors might halt the progression of chronic myeloid leukemia but not eliminate the preexisting tumor cells. In fact, chronic myeloid leukemia (CML) progenitors are eliminated after just a few months of anti–BCR-ABL therapy, indicating they are dependent on the driver oncogene for their survival and have "forgotten" how to return to normal. This phenomenon, subsequently documented in a variety of human malignancies, is colloquially termed *oncogene addiction*.[2] Although the molecular basis for this addiction still remains to be defined, the notion of finding an Achilles' heel for each cancer continues to captivate the cancer research community and has spawned a broad array of efforts to elucidate the molecular identity of these targets and discover relevant inhibitors.

EARLY SUCCESSES: TARGETING CANCERS WITH WELL-KNOWN KINASE MUTATIONS (BCR-ABL, KIT, HER2)

From the beginning, clinical trials of imatinib were restricted to patients with Philadelphia chromosome–positive chronic myeloid leukemia. For what seem like obvious reasons, there was never any serious discussion about treating patients with Philadelphia chromosome–negative leukemia because the assumption was that only patients with the BCR-ABL fusion gene would have a chance of responding. This was clearly a wise decision because hematologic response rates approached 90% and cytogenetic remissions were seen in nearly half of the patients in the early phase studies.[3] It was obvious that the drug worked, and imatinib was approved in record time. Unwittingly, the power of genome-based patient selection was demonstrated in the clinical development of the very first kinase inhibitor. As we will see, it took nearly a decade for this lesson to be fully learned. Today, the much larger clinical experience, with an array of different kinase inhibitors across many tumor types, has led to a much better understanding of the principles that dictate oncogene addiction that, in retrospect, were staring us in the face. Foremost among them is the notion that tumors with a somatic mutation or amplification of a kinase drug target are much more likely to be dependent on that target for survival. Hence, a patient whose tumor has such a mutation is much more likely to respond to treatment with the appropriate inhibitor. This has also led to a new paradigm at the regulatory level of drug approval requiring codevelopment of a *companion diagnostic* (a molecularly based diagnostic test that reliably identifies patients with the mutation) with the new drug.

After chronic myeloid leukemia, the next example to illustrate this principle was gastrointestinal stromal tumor (GIST), which is associated with mutations in the KIT tyrosine-kinase receptor or, more rarely, in the platelet-derived growth factor (PDGF) receptor.[4,5] Serendipitously, imatinib inhibits both KIT and the PDGF receptor; therefore, the clinical test of KIT inhibition in GIST followed quickly on the heels of the success in CML.[6] In retrospect, the rapid progress made in these two diseases was based, in part, on the fact that the driver molecular lesion (BCR-ABL or KIT mutation, respectively) is present in nearly all patients who are diagnosed with these two diseases. The molecular analysis merely confirmed the diagnosis that was made using standard clinical and histologic criteria. Consequently, clinicians could identify the patients most likely to respond based on clinical criteria rather than rely on an elaborate molecular profiling infrastructure to prescreen patients. Consequently, clinical trials evaluating kinase inhibitors in CML and GIST accrued quickly, and the therapeutic benefit became clear almost immediately.

The notion that molecular alteration of a driver kinase determines sensitivity to a cognate kinase inhibitor was further validated during the development of the dual EGFR/HER2 kinase inhibitor lapatinib. Clinical trials of this kinase inhibitor were conducted in women with advanced HER2-positive breast cancer based on earlier success in these same patients with the monoclonal antibody trastuzumab, which targets the extracellular domain of the HER2

TABLE 22.1

Kinase Inhibitors: Approved or Anticipated Approval In 2014

Target	Drug	Approved Indications	Anticipated Future Indications
ALK	Crizotinib Ceritinib	ALK mutant lung cancer	ALK mutant neuroblastoma, anaplastic lymphoma
BCR-ABL	Imatinib Dasatinib Nilotinib Bosutinib Ponatinib	Chronic myeloid leukemia Philadelphia chromosome–positive acute lymphoid leukemia T315 mutation only (ponatinib)	
BRAF	Vemurafenib Dabrafenib	BRAF mutant melanoma	Other BRAF mutant tumors
BTK	Ibrutinib	Chronic lymphocytic leukemia Mantle cell lymphoma	
EGFR	Gefitinib Erlotinib Afatinib	Lung adenocarcinoma with EGFR mutation	
HER2	Lapatinib	Her2$^+$ breast cancer	
JAK2	Ruxolitinib	JAK2 mutant myelofibrosis	
KIT	Imatinib Sunitinib	Gastrointestinal stromal tumor	
MEK	Trametinib	BRAF mutant melanoma	
PI3K delta[a]	Idelalisib	Chronic lymphocytic leukemia Indolent non-Hodgkin lymphoma	
PDGFR- α/β	Imatinib	Chronic myelomonocytic leukemia (with TEL-PDGFR-β fusion) hypereosinophilic syndrome (with PDGFR-β fusion) Dermatofibrosarcoma protuberans	
RET	Vandetanib Sorafenib Cabozantinib	Medullary thyroid cancer	
TORC1	Sirolimus (rapamycin)	Kidney cancer	
(mTOR)	Everolimus Temsirolimus	Breast cancer Tuberous sclerosis	
VEGF Receptor	Sorafenib Sunitinib Axitinib Pazopanib	Kidney cancer Hepatocellular carcinoma (sorafenib only) Pancreatic neuroendocrine tumors (sunitinib)	

[a] Approval is anticipated based on positive phase 3 data and announcement of accepted Food and Drug Administration submission by the sponsor.

kinase. Lapatinib was initially approved in combination with the cytotoxic agent capecitabine for women with resistance to trastuzumab,[7] and then was subsequently approved for frontline use in metastatic breast cancer in combination with chemotherapy or hormonal therapy, depending on estrogen receptor status. A key ingredient that enabled the clinical development of lapatinib was the routine use of HER2 gene amplification testing in the diagnosis of breast cancer, pioneered during the development of trastuzumab several years earlier. This widespread clinical practice allowed for the rapid identification of those patients most likely to benefit. If lapatinib trials had been conducted in unselected patients, the clinical signal in breast cancer would likely have been missed.

The Serendipity of Unexpected Clinical Responses: EGFR in Lung Cancer

In contrast to the logical development of imatinib and lapatinib in molecularly defined patient populations, the EGFR kinase inhibitors gefitinib and erlotinib entered the clinic without the benefit of such a focused clinical development plan. Although considerable preclinical data implicated EGFR as a cancer drug target, there was little insight into which patients were most likely to benefit. The first clue that EGFR inhibitors would have a role in lung cancer came from the recognition by several astute clinicians of remarkable responses in a small fraction of patients with lung adenocarcinoma.[8] Further studies revealed the curious clinical circumstance that those patients most likely to benefit tended to be those who never smoked, women, and those of Asian ethnicity.[9] Clearly, there was a strong clinical signal in a subgroup of patients, who could perhaps be enriched based on these clinical features, but it seemed that a unifying molecular lesion must be present. Three academic groups simultaneously converged on the answer. Mutations in the EGFR gene were detected in the 10% to 15% of patients with lung adenocarcinoma who had radiographic responses.[10–12] It may seem surprising that mutations in a gene as highly visible as EGFR and in such a prevalent cancer had not been detected earlier. But the motivation to search aggressively for EGFR mutations was not there until the clinical responses were seen. Perhaps even more surprising was the failure of the pharmaceutical company sponsors of the two most advanced compounds, gefitinib and erlotinib, to embrace this important discovery and refocus future clinical development plans on patients with EGFR mutant lung adenocarcinoma.

But that was 2004, when the prevailing approach to cancer drug development was an empiric one originally developed (with great success) for cytotoxic agents. Typically, small numbers of patients with different cancers were treated in *all comer* phase I studies (no enrichment for subgroups) with the goal of eliciting a clinical signal in at least one tumor type. A single-agent response rate of 20% to 30% in a disease-specific phase II trial would justify a randomized phase III registration trial, where the typical endpoint for drug approval is time to progression or survival. Cytotoxics were also typically evaluated in combination with existing standard of care treatment (typically approved chemotherapy agents) with the goal of increasing the response rate or enhancing the duration of response. (Note: The use of the past tense here is intentional. As we will see later in this chapter, nearly all cancer drug development today is based on selecting patients with a certain molecular profile.)

The clinical development of gefitinib and erlotinib followed the cytotoxic model. Both drugs had similarly low but convincing single-agent response rates (10% to 15%) in chemotherapy-refractory, advanced lung cancer. Indeed, gefitinib was originally granted accelerated approval by the U.S. Food and Drug Administration (FDA) in 2003 based on the impressive nature of these responses, contingent on the completion of formal phase III studies with survival endpoints.[13] The sponsors of both drugs, therefore, conducted phase III registration studies in patients with chemotherapy-refractory, advanced stage lung cancer but without prescreening patients for EGFR mutation status. (In fairness, these trials were initiated prior to the discovery of EGFR mutations in lung cancer but study amendments could have been considered.) Erlotinib was approved in 2004 on the basis of a modest survival advantage over placebo (the BR.21 trial); however, gefitinib failed to demonstrate a survival advantage in essentially the same patient population.[14,15] This difference in outcome was surprising because the two drugs have highly similar chemical structures and biologic properties. Perhaps the most important difference was drug dose. Erlotinib was given at the maximum tolerated dose, which produces a high frequency of rash and diarrhea. Both side effects are presumed *on target* consequences of EGFR inhibition because EGFR is highly expressed in skin and gastrointestinal epithelial cells. In contrast, gefitinib was dosed slightly lower to mitigate these toxicities, with the rationale that responses were clearly documented at lower doses.

In parallel with the single-agent phase III trials in chemotherapy-refractory patients, both gefitinib and erlotinib were studied as an upfront therapy for advanced lung cancer to determine if either would improve the efficacy of standard *doublet* (carboplatin/paclitaxel or gemcitabine/cisplatin) chemotherapy when all three drugs were given in combination. These trials, termed INTACT-1 and INTACT-2 (gefitinib with either gemcitabine/cisplatin or with carboplatin/paclitaxel) and TRIBUTE (erlotinib with carboplatin/paclitaxel), collectively enrolled over 3,000 patients.[16–18] Excitement in the oncology community was high based on the clear single-agent activity of both EGFR inhibitors. But, both trials were spectacular failures; neither drug showed any benefit over chemotherapy alone. The fact that EGFR mutations are present in only 10% to 15% of patients (i.e., those likely to benefit) provided a logical explanation. The clinical signal from those whose tumors had EGFR mutations was likely diluted out by all the patients whose tumors had no EGFR alterations, many of whom benefited from chemotherapy.

The convergence of the EGFR mutation discovery with these clinical trial results will be remembered as a remarkable time in the history of targeted cancer therapies, not just for the important role of these agents as lung cancer therapies, but also for missteps in deciding that the EGFR genotype should drive treatment selection. Perhaps the most egregious error came from a retrospective

analysis of tumors from patients treated on the BR.21 trial, which concluded that EGFR mutations did *not* predict for a survival advantage.[19] (EGFR gene amplification *was* associated with survival, but only in a univariate analysis.) This conclusion was concerning because less than 30% of patients on the trial had tissue available for EGFR mutation analysis, raising questions about the adequacy of the sample size. Furthermore, the EGFR mutation assay used by the authors was subsequently criticized because a significant number of the EGFR mutations reported in these patients were in residues not previously found by others, who had sequenced thousands of tumors. Many of these mutations were suspected to be an artifact of working from formalin-fixed biopsies. Fortunately, recent advances in DNA mutation detection, using massively parallel next-generation sequencing technology, have largely eliminated this concern. These new platforms are now being used in the clinical setting.

Clinical investigators in Asia, where a greater fraction of lung cancers (roughly 30%) are positive for EGFR mutations, addressed the question of whether mutations predict for clinical benefit in a prospective trial. In this study known as IPASS, gefitinib was clearly superior to standard doublet chemotherapy as frontline therapy for patients with advanced EGFR mutation–positive lung adenocarcinoma.[20] Conversely, EGFR mutation–negative patients fared much worse with gefitinib and benefited from chemotherapy. In addition, EGFR mutation–positive patients had a more favorable overall prognosis regardless of treatment, indicating that EGFR mutation is also a prognostic biomarker. The IPASS trial serves as a compelling example of a properly designed (and executed) biomarker-driven clinical trial. Although the rationale for this clinical development strategy had been demonstrated years earlier with BCR-ABL in leukemia, KIT in GIST, and HER2 in breast cancer, it was difficult to derail the empiric approach that had been used for decades in developing cytotoxic agents.

A Mix of Science and Serendipity: PDGF Receptor–Driven Leukemias and Sarcoma

The discovery of EGFR mutations in lung cancer (motivated by dramatic clinical responses in a subset of patients treated with EGFR kinase inhibitors) is the most visible example of the power of bedside-to-bench science, but it is not the only (or the first) such example from the kinase inhibitor era. Shortly after the approval of imatinib for CML in 2001, two case reports documented dramatic remissions in patients with hypereosinophilic syndrome (HES), a blood disorder characterized by prolonged elevation of eosinophil counts and subsequent organ dysfunction from eosinophil infiltration, when treated with imatinib.[21,22] Although HES resembles myeloproliferative diseases such as CML, the molecular pathogenesis of HES was completely unknown at the time. Reasoning that these clinical responses must be explained by inhibition of a driver kinase, a team of laboratory-based physician/scientists quickly searched for mutations in the three kinases known to be inhibited by imatinib (ABL, KIT, and PDGF receptor). ABL and KIT were quickly excluded, but the PDGF receptor α (PDGFR-α) gene was targeted by an interstitial deletion that fused the upstream FIP1L1 gene to PDGFR-α[23] FIP1L1-PDGFR-α is a constitutively active tyrosine kinase, analogous to BCR-ABL, and is also inhibited by imatinib. As with EGFR-mutant lung cancer, the molecular pathophysiology of HES was discovered by dissecting the mechanism of response to the drug used to treat it.

The HES/FIP1L1-PDGFR-α story serves as a nice bookend to an earlier discovery that the t(5,12) chromosome translocation, found rarely in patients with chronic myelomonocytic leukemia, creates the TEL-PDGFR-β fusion tyrosine kinase.[24] Similar to HES, treatment of patients with t(5,12) translocation-positive leukemias with imatinib has also proven successful.[25] A third example comes from dermatofibrosarcoma protuberans, a sarcoma characterized by a t(17,22) translocation that fuses the COL1A gene to the PDGFB *ligand* (not the receptor). COL1A-PDGFB is onco-genic through autocrine stimulation of the normal PDGF receptor in these tumor cells. Patients with dermatofibrosarcoma protuber-ans respond to imatinib therapy because it targets the PDGF receptor, just one step downstream from the oncogenic lesion.[26]

Exploiting the New Paradigm: Searching for Other Kinase-Driven Cancers

The benefits of serendipity notwithstanding, the growing number of examples of successful kinase inhibitor therapy in tumors with a mutation or amplification of the drug target begged for a more rational approach to drug discovery and development. In 2002, the list of human tumors known to have mutations in kinases was quite small. Due to advances in automated gene sequencing, it became possible to ask whether a much larger fraction of human cancers might also have such mutations through a brute force approach. To address this question comprehensively, one would have to se-quence all of the kinases in the genome in hundreds of samples of each tumor type. Several early pilot studies demonstrated the potential of this approach by revealing important new targets for drug development. Perhaps the most spectacular was the discovery of mutations in the BRAF kinase in over half of patients with mela-noma, as well as in a smaller fraction of colon and thyroid can-cers.[27] Another was the discovery of mutations in the JAK2 kinase in nearly all patients with polycythemia vera, as well as a significant fraction of patients with myelofibrosis and essential thrombocyto-sis.[28–30] A third example was the identification of PIK3CA muta-tions in a variety of tumors, with the greatest frequencies in breast, endometrial, and colorectal cancers.[31] PIK3CA encodes a lipid kinase that generates the second messenger phosphatidyl inositol 3-phosphate (PIP3). PIP3 activates growth and survival signaling through the AKT family of kinases as well as other downstream ef-fectors. Coupled with the well-established role of the phosphatase and tensin homolog (PTEN) lipid phosphatase in dephosphorylat-ing PIP3, the discovery of PIK3CA mutations focused tremendous attention on developing inhibitors at multiple levels of this path-way, as discussed further in the follow paragraphs.

Each of these important discoveries—BRAF, JAK2, and PIK3CA—came from relatively small efforts (less than 100 tu-mors) and generally focused on resequencing only those exons that coded for regions of kinases where mutations had been found in other kinases (typically, the juxtamembrane and kinase domains). These restricted searches were largely driven by the high cost of DNA sequencing using the Sanger method. In 2006, a compre-hensive effort to sequence all of the exons in all kinases in 100 tumors could easily exceed several million dollars. Financial sup-port for such projects could not be obtained easily through tra-ditional funding agencies because the risk/reward was considered too high. Furthermore, substantial infrastructure for sample acqui-sition, microdissection of the tumors from normal tissue, nucleic acid preparation, high throughput automated sequencing, and computational analysis of the resulting data was essential. Few in-stitutions were equipped to address these challenges. In response, the National Cancer Institute in the United States (in partnership with the National Human Genome Research Institute) and an international group known as the International Cancer Genome Consortium (ICGC) launched large-scale efforts to sequence the complete genomes of thousands of cancers. In parallel, next-generation sequencing technologies resulted in massive reduc-tions in cost, allowing a more comprehensive analysis of much larger numbers of tumors. At the time of this writing, the US effort (called The Cancer Genome Atlas [TCGA]) had reported data on 29 different tumor types (https://tcga-data.nci.nih.gov/tcga/). The international consortium has committed to sequencing 25,000 tumors representing 50 different cancer subtypes.[32] Both groups have enforced immediate release of all sequence information to the research community free of charge so that the entire scientific community can learn from the data. This policy enabled *pan can-cer* mutational analyses that give an overall view of the genomic landscape of cancer, serving as a blueprint for the community of cancer researchers and drug developers.[33,34]

Rounding Out the Treatment of Myeloproliferative Disorders: JAK2 and Myelofibrosis

Taken together with the BCR-ABL translocation in CML and FIP1L1-PDGFR-α in HES, the discovery of JAK2 mutations in polycythemia, essential thrombocytosis, and myelofibrosis pro-vided a unifying understanding of myeloproliferative disorders as diseases of abnormal kinase activation. The JAK family kinases are the primary effectors of signaling through inflammatory cytokine receptors and, therefore, had been considered compelling targets for anti-inflammatory drugs. But the JAK2 mutation discovery im-mediately shifted these efforts toward developing JAK2 inhibitors for myeloproliferative disorders. Because most patients have a com-mon JAK2 V617F mutation, these efforts could rapidly focus on screening for activity against a single genotype. Progress has been rapid. Myelofibrosis was selected as the initial indication (instead of essential thrombocytosis or polycythemia vera) because the time to registration is expected to be the shortest. Currently, ruxolitinib is approved for myelofibrosis based on shrinkage in spleen size as the primary endpoint. Clinical trials in essential thrombocytosis and polycythemia vera (versus hydroxyurea) are ongoing. Other JAK2 inhibitors are also in clinical development.

BRAF Mutant Melanoma: Several Missteps Before Finding the Right Inhibitor

As with JAK2 mutations in myeloproliferative disorders, the discov-ery of BRAF mutations in patients with melanoma launched wide-spread efforts to find potent BRAF inhibitors. One early candidate was the drug sorafenib, which had been optimized during drug discovery to inhibit RAF kinases. (Sorafenib also inhibits vascular endothelial growth factor (VEGF) receptors, which led to its ap-proval in kidney cancer, as discussed later in this chapter.) Despite the compelling molecular rationale for targeting BRAF, clinical results of sorafenib in melanoma were extremely disappointing and reduced enthusiasm for pursuing BRAF as a drug target.[35] In hindsight, this concern was completely misguided. Sorafenib dosing is limited by toxicities that preclude achieving serum lev-els in patients that potently inhibit RAF, but are sufficient to in-hibit VEGF receptors. In addition, patients were enrolled without screening for BRAF mutations in their tumors. Although the fre-quency of BRAF mutations in melanoma is high, the inclusion of patients without the BRAF mutation diluted the chance of seeing any clinical signal. In short, the clinical evaluation of sorafenib in melanoma was poorly designed to test the hypothesis that BRAF is a therapeutic target. The danger is that negative data from such clinical experiments can slow subsequent progress. It is critical to know the pharmacodynamic properties of the drug and the mo-lecular phenotype of the patients being studied when interpreting the results of a negative study.

The fact that RAF kinases are intermediate components of the well-characterized RAS/ mitogen-activated protein (MAP) kinase pathway (transducing signals from RAS to RAF to MEK to ERK) raised the possibility that tumors with BRAF mutations might re-spond to inhibitors of one of these downstream kinases (Fig. 22.1). Preclinical studies revealed that tumor cell lines with BRAF mu-tation were exquisitely sensitive to inhibitors of the downstream kinase MEK.[36] (Sorafenib, in contrast, does not show this profile of activity.[37] Thus, proper preclinical screening would have revealed the shortcomings of sorafenib as a BRAF inhibitor.) Curiously, cell lines with a mutation or amplification of EGFR or HER2, which

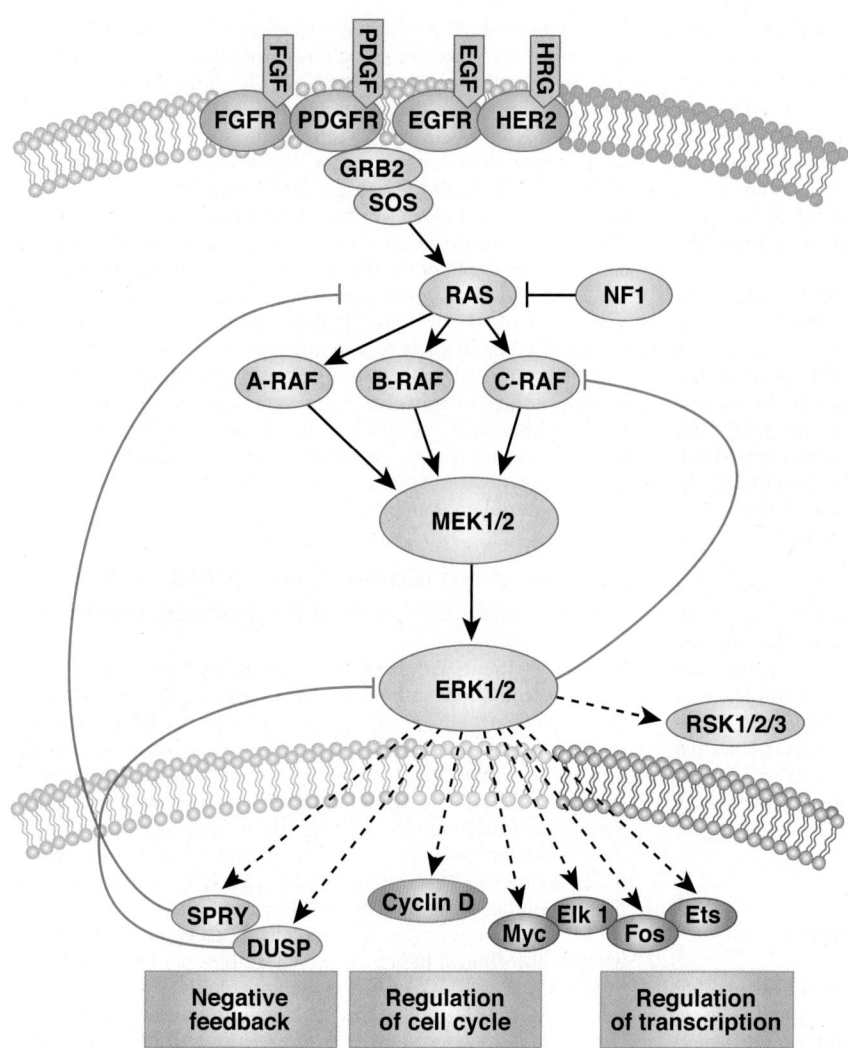

CANCER THERAPEUTICS

Figure 22.1 The RAS–RAF–MEK–ERK signaling pathway. The classical mitogen-activated protein kinase (MAPK) pathway is activated in human tumors by several mechanisms, including the binding of ligand to receptor tyrosine kinases (RTK), the mutational activation of an RTK, by loss of the tumor suppressor NF1, or by mutations in RAS, BRAF, and MEK1. Phosphorylation and, thus, activation of ERK regulates the transcription of target genes that promote cell cycle progression and tumor survival. The ERK pathway contains a classical feedback loop in which the expression of feedback elements such as SPRY and DUSP family proteins are regulated by the level of ERK activity. Loss of expression of SPRY and DUSP family members due to promoter methylation or deletion is thus permissive for persistently elevated pathway output. In the case of tumors with mutant BRAF, pathway output is enhanced by impaired upstream feedback regulation. FGF, fibroblast growth factor; HRG, heregulin; NF1, neurofibromatosis 1. (From Bernt KM, Zhu N, Sinha AU, et al. MLL-rearranged leukemia is dependent on aberrant H3K79 methylation by DOT1L. *Cancer Cell* 2011;20(1):66–78, with permission.)

function upstream in the pathway, were insensitive to MEK inhibition. Even tumor lines with RAS mutations were variably sensitive. In short, the preclinical data made a strong case that MEK inhibitors should be effective in BRAF mutant melanoma, but not in other subtypes. The reason that HER2, EGFR, and RAS mutant tumors were not sensitive to MEK inhibitors is explained, at least in part, by the existence of negative feedback loops that modulate the flux of signal transduction through MEK.[38]

In parallel with the generation of these preclinical findings, clinical trials of several MEK inhibitors were initiated. Patients with various cancers were enrolled in the early studies, but there was a strong bias to include melanoma patients. Significant efforts were made to demonstrate MEK inhibition in tumor cells by measuring the phosphorylation status of the direct downstream substrate ERK using an immunohistochemical analysis of biopsies from patients with metastatic disease. Phase I studies of the two earliest compounds in clinical development (PD325901 and AZD6244) documented reduced phospho-ERK staining at multiple dose levels in several patients for whom baseline and treatment biopsies were obtained.[39,40] (In the following, we will learn that these pharmacodynamic studies, while well intentioned, were not quantitative enough to document the magnitude of MEK inhibition in these patients.) Furthermore, clinical responses were observed in a few patients with BRAF mutant melanoma. Armed with this confidence, a randomized phase II clinical trial of AZD6244 was conducted in advanced melanoma, with the chemotherapeutic agent temozolomide (which is approved for glioblastoma) as the comparator arm. (The clinical development

of PD325901 was discontinued because of safety concerns about ocular and neurologic toxicity.) Disappointingly, patients receiving AZD6244 had no benefit in progression-free survival when compared to temozolomide-treated patients, raising further concerns about the viability of BRAF as a drug target.[41] A closer examination of the data revealed that clinical responses were, indeed, seen in patients receiving AZD6244. The fact that BRAF mutation status was not required for study entry likely diminished the clinical signal in the AZD6244 arm, a lesson learned from the EGFR inhibitor trials in lung cancer. Indeed, a different MEK inhibitor, trametinib, received FDA approval in 2013 based on activity in melanoma patients with the BRAF mutation.[42]

All doubts about BRAF as a target vanished in 2009 to 2010 when dramatic clinical responses were observed with a novel BRAF inhibitor vemurafenib (PLX4032). Like sorafenib, this compound was optimized to inhibit RAF, but with an additional focus on mutant BRAF. Vemurafenib differs dramatically from sorafenib because it potently inhibits BRAF without the additional broad range of activities that sorafenib has against other kinases like the VEGF receptor.[43] The greater selectivity of vemurafenib relative to sorafenib resulted in a much greater tolerability, such that it could be given at high doses while avoiding significant toxicity. The early days of vemurafenib clinical development were plagued by challenges in maximizing the oral bioavailability of the drug.[44] Consequently, the initial phase I clinical trial was temporarily halted to develop a novel formulation (i.e., the coingredients in the drug capsule or tablet that improve solubility and absorption through the gastrointestinal tract). Much higher serum levels were obtained in patients who received the new vemurafenib formation and, shortly thereafter, complete and partial responses were observed in about 80% of the melanoma patients with B-RAF mutant tumors. Strikingly, no activity was observed in patients whose tumors were wild type for BRAF.[45,46] The data were so compelling that vemurafenib was immediately advanced to a phase III registration trial. Similarly impressive responses in BRAF mutant melanoma patients were observed with a second potent RAF inhibitor dabrafenib,[47] providing further proof that BRAF is a important cancer target.

The vemurafenib and dabrafenib data also provide insight into why sorafenib and the early MEK inhibitor trials failed to demonstrate activity. One lesson is the critical importance of achieving adequate target inhibition. Clinical responses with vemurafenib were observed only after the drug was reformulated to achieve substantially higher serum levels. Reductions in phospho-ERK staining (as documented by immunohistochemistry) were documented in the earlier trials but, in retrospect, the assays were not sensitive enough to distinguish between modest (~50%) kinase inhibition versus more complete BRAF or MEK inhibition. Efficacy in preclinical models is significantly improved using doses that give >80% inhibition, and the human trial data suggest that this degree of pathway blockade is also required for a high clinical response rate.[46] Collectively, these experiences illustrate the critical need for quantitative pharmacodynamic assays to measure target inhibition early in clinical development. A second lesson is the importance of genotyping all patients for mutation or amplification of the relevant drug target. Not only does this ensure that a sufficient number of patients with the biomarker of interest are included in the study, but also that the results provide compelling evidence early in clinical development in support (or not) of the preclinical hypothesis.

Getting It Right: ALK and Lung Cancer

The development of the ALK inhibitor crizotinib (PF-02341066) illustrates how an unexpected signal obtained in a small number of patients can quickly shift a program in an entirely new direction with a high probability of success. The key ingredient is this story is a familiar one—a strong molecular hypothesis backed up by clinical response data in a small number of carefully selected patients. Crizotinib emerged from a drug discovery program at Pfizer that was focused on finding inhibitors of the MET receptor tyrosine kinase and entered the clinic with this target as its lead indication.[48] As we previously learned with imatinib, essentially all kinase inhibitors have activity against other targets (so called *off-target* activities), which can sometimes prove to be advantageous. Off-target activities are typically discovered by screening compounds against a large panel of kinases to establish profiles of relative selectivity against the intended target. Off-target activity, potency, and pharmaceutical properties (bioavailability, half-life) are all factors that influence the decision of which compound to advance to clinical development. The primary off-target activity of crizotinib is against the ALK tyrosine kinase.

ALK was first identified as a candidate driver oncogene in 1994 through the cloning of the t(2,5) chromosomal translocation associated with anaplastic large cell lymphoma, which creates the nucleophosmin/anaplastic lymphoma kinase (NPM-ALK) fusion gene.[49] This discovery, together with the demonstration that NPM-ALK causes lymphoma in mice, made a compelling case for ALK as a drug target in this disease. But there was limited interest in developing ALK inhibitors because this particular lymphoma subtype is rare and most commonly found in children. (Companies are generally reluctant to develop drugs solely for pediatric indications because of complexities related to dose selection and additional regulatory guidelines. Efforts to streamline this development process are underway, such as the Creating Hope Act, which provides new incentives for companies to pursue pediatric indications.) In 2007, a different ALK fusion gene called EML4-ALK was discovered in a small fraction of patients with lung adenocarcinoma, with an estimated frequency of 1% to 5%.[50] This discovery did not immediately capture the attention of drug developers, but several academic groups who had already begun testing lung cancer patients seen at their institutions for EGFR mutations simply added an EML4-ALK fusion test to the screening panel. Astute clinical investigators participating in the phase I trial of crizotinib, which was designed to include patients with a broad array of advanced cancers, were aware of the off-target ALK activity and enrolled several lung cancer patients with EML4-ALK fusions in the study. These patients had remarkably dramatic responses.[51] This serendipitous finding in a few ALK-positive patients was confirmed in a larger cohort, resulting in a strongly positive pivotal phase III study in ALK-positive lung cancer, just 2 years after the discovery of the EML4-ALK fusion.[52] Crizotinib is also being evaluated in other diseases associated with genomic alterations in ALK, including large-cell anaplastic lymphoma, neuroblastoma,[53] and inflammatory myofibroblastic sarcoma.[54]

Extending the Model to RET Mutations in Thyroid Cancer: Clinical Responses, But Why?

Subsets of patients with papillary or medullary thyroid cancer have activating mutations or translocations targeting the RET tyrosine-kinase receptor, raising the question of whether RET inhibitors might have a role in this disease.[55] Although no drugs specifically designed to inhibit RET have entered the clinic, four compounds with off-target activity against RET (vandetanib, sorafenib, motesanib, and cabozantinib) have all shown single-agent activity in thyroid cancer studies.[56-60] Vandetanib and cabozantinib are currently approved in medullary thyroid cancer based on improved progression-free survival in phase III registration trials.[61,62] Because all four compounds also inhibit VEGF receptor, it is unclear whether the clinical benefit observed in these studies is explained by inhibition of RET, VEGF receptor, or both. Unlike the crizotinib trials in ALK-positive lung cancer, enrollment in these registration studies was not restricted to patients with RET mutations. In addition to the fact that thyroid cancer patients are not routinely screened for these mutations, the primary reason for including all comers in these studies is that clinical responses are observed in a larger fraction of patients than can be accounted for based on the suspected frequency of an RET mutation. Responses in patients without RET mutation (if they occur) might be explained by mutations in other genes in the RAS-MAP kinase pathway such as BRAF or HRAS, which are found in a substantial fraction of patients and typically do not overlap with RET alterations.[55] Clearly, detailed genotype/response correlations, as demonstrated in lung cancer and melanoma, will clarify the role of these mutations in predicting the response to these drugs. Thyroid cancer is also a compelling indication for the BRAF and MEK inhibitors discussed previously in melanoma.

FLT3 Inhibitors in Acute Myeloid Leukemia: Did the Genomics Mislead Us?

Shortly after the success of imatinib, the receptor tyrosine–kinase FLT3 emerged as a compelling drug candidate based on the presence of activating mutations in about one-third of patients with acute myeloid leukemia.[63] Laboratory studies documented that FLT3 alleles bearing these mutations, which occur as internal tandem duplications (ITD) of the juxtamembrane domain or a point mutation in the kinase domain, function as driver oncogenes in mouse models, giving phenotypes analogous to BCR-ABL.[64] As with RET in thyroid cancer, no compounds had been specifically optimized to target FLT3, but several drugs with off-target FLT3 activity were redirected to acute myeloid leukemia (AML).

Disappointingly, the first three of the compounds tested (midostaurin, lestaurtinib, and sunitinib) showed only marginal single-agent activity in relapsed AML patients, even in those with FLT3 mutations.[65–67] Despite the strong molecular rationale for FLT3 as a driver lesion, questions were raised about the viability of FLT3 as a drug target. Pharmacodynamic studies showed evidence of FLT3 kinase inhibition in tumor cells, but the magnitude and duration of these effects were difficult to quantify, raising the possibility of inadequate target inhibition.[65] Indeed, the dose of all three compounds was limited by toxicities believed to be independent of FLT3. A more pessimistic interpretation was that FLT3, although presumably important for the initiation of AML, was no longer required for tumor maintenance due to the accumulation of additional driver genomic alterations. If true, even a complete FLT3 blockade with a highly selective inhibitor would be expected to fail. But this view was not supported by the fact that clinical responses were observed in the somewhat analogous situation of single-agent ABL kinase inhibitor treatment of CML in blast crisis, where BCR-ABL is just one of many additional genomic alterations that contribute to disease progression, yet complete remissions are observed in many patients.

Despite this pessimism about FLT3 as a viable drug target, several drugs are now advancing toward drug registration trials. Midostaurin, one of the early compounds that showed disappointing single-agent activity in relapsed AML, is being evaluated in a randomized phase III trial in newly diagnosed AML combined with standard induction chemotherapy. A single-arm phase II study showed higher and more durable remission rates in FLT3 mutant patients when compared to historical controls.[68] The second compound, quizartinib (AC220), is a next-generation FLT3 inhibitor with greater potency and specificity and with single-agent activity in FLT3 mutant relapsed AML—precisely the population where midostaurin and others failed.[69,70] The fact that some responder patients have relapsed with drug-resistant gatekeeper mutations in the FLT3 kinase domain provides formal proof that FLT3 is the relevant target.[71] Assuming these compounds prove successful in AML, it will be important to examine their activity in the rare cases of pediatric acute lymphoid leukemia associated with FLT3 mutation. Although the jury is still out on FLT3 inhibitors, the failure of early compounds in AML is reminiscent of the failures of early RAF and MEK inhibitors in melanoma. Collectively, these examples emphasize the importance of using optimized compounds to test a molecularly based hypothesis in patients and to focus enrollment on those patients with the relevant molecular lesion.

Kidney Cancer: Targeting the Tumor and the Host With Mammalian Target of Rapamycin and VEGF Receptor Inhibitors

A recurring theme in this chapter is the critical role of driver kinase mutations in guiding the development of kinase inhibitors. Ironically, several kinase inhibitors have been approved for kidney cancer over the past 5 years in a tumor type with no known kinase mutations. The most common molecular alteration in kidney cancer is a loss of function in the Von Hippel-Lindau (VHL) tumor suppressor gene, resulting in the activation of the hypoxia inducible factor[68] pathway.[72] As a consequence of VHL loss, which normally targets hypoxia-inducible factor (HIF) proteins for proteasomal degradation, HIF-1α and HIF-2α are constitutively active transcription factors that function as oncogenes through activation of an array of downstream target genes. Among these is the angiogenesis factor VEGF, which is secreted by HIF-expressing cells and promotes the development and maintenance of tumor neovasculature. HIF-mediated secretion of VEGF by tumor cells likely explains the highly vascular histopathology of clear cell renal carcinoma. All three currently approved angiogenesis inhibitors (the monoclonal antibody bevacizumab targeting VEGF and the kinase inhibitors sorafenib and sunitinib targeting or its receptor

VEGF receptor) have single-agent clinical activity in clear cell carcinoma.[73–75] The high specificity of bevacizumab for VEGF leaves little doubt that the activity of this drug is explained by antiangiogenic effects. In contrast, the off-target activities of sorafenib and sunitinib include several kinases expressed in kidney tumor cells, stroma, and inflammatory cells (PDGFR, RAF, RET, FLT3, and others). Interestingly, the primary effect of bevacizumab in kidney cancer is disease stabilization, whereas sorafenib and sunitinib have substantial partial response rates. This raises the question of whether the superior antitumor activity of the VEGF receptor kinase inhibitors is due to the concurrent inhibition of other kinases. However, partial responses rates with next-generation VEGF receptor inhibitors (axitinib, pazopanib, and tivozanib), all of which have greater potency and selectivity for the VEGF receptor, are similarly high, and reinforce the importance of the VEGF receptor as the critical target in kidney cancer.[76–78] Pazopanib is approved for advanced kidney cancer, whereas axitinib is approved as second-line therapy.

Two inhibitors of the mammalian target of rapamycin (mTOR) kinase (temsirolimus and everolimus) are also approved for advanced renal cell carcinoma.[79,80] Both temsirolimus and everolimus are known as rapalogs because both are chemical derivatives of the natural product sirolimus (rapamycin). Sirolimus was approved more than 10 years ago to prevent graft rejection in transplant recipients based on its immunosuppressive properties against T cells. Sirolimus also has potent antiproliferative effects against vascular endothelial cells and, on that basis, is incorporated into drug-eluting cardiac stents to prevent coronary artery restenosis following angioplasty.[81] Rapalogs differ from all the other kinase inhibitors discussed in this chapter in that they inhibit the kinase through an allosteric mechanism rather than by targeting the mTOR kinase domain. Because rapalogs also inhibit the growth of cancer cell lines from different tissues of origin, clinical trials were initiated to study their potential role as anticancer agents in a broad range of tumor types. Based on responses in a few phase I patients with different tumor types (including kidney cancer), exploratory phase II studies were conducted in several diseases. Single-agent activity of temsirolimus was observed in a phase II kidney cancer study,[82] then confirmed in a phase III registration trial.[79] The phase III everolimus trial, which was initiated after temsirolimus, was noteworthy because clinical benefit was demonstrated in patients who had progressed on the VEGF receptor inhibitors sorafenib or sunitinib.[80]

In parallel with the empirical clinical development of rapalogs, various laboratories explored the molecular basis for mTOR dependence in cancer cells. mTOR functions at the center of a complex network that integrates signals from growth factor receptors and nutrient sensors to regulate cell growth and size (Fig. 22.2). It does so, in part, by controlling the translation of various mRNAs with complex 5′ untranslated regions into protein. mTOR exists in two distinct complexes known as TOR complex 1 (TORC1) and TORC2. Rapalogs only inhibit the TORC1 complex, which is largely responsible for downstream phosphorylation of targets such as S6K1/2 and 4EBP1/2 that regulate protein translation.[83] The TORC2 complex contributes to the activation of AKT by phosphorylating the important regulatory serine residue S473 and is unaffected by rapalogs.

Two hypotheses have emerged to explain the clinical activity of rapalogs in kidney cancer. The antiproliferative activity of these compounds against endothelial cells suggests an antiangiogenic mechanism, which is consistent with the clinical activity of the VEGF receptor inhibitors. But rapalogs also inhibit the growth of kidney cancer cell lines in laboratory models where the effects on tumor angiogenesis have been eliminated. Interestingly, mRNAs for HIF1/2 are among those whose translation is impaired by rapalogs, and this effect has been implicated as the primary mechanism of rapalog activity in kidney cancer xenograft models.[84] As with the VEGF receptor inhibitors, a detailed molecular annotation of tumors from responders and nonresponders will shed light on these issues.

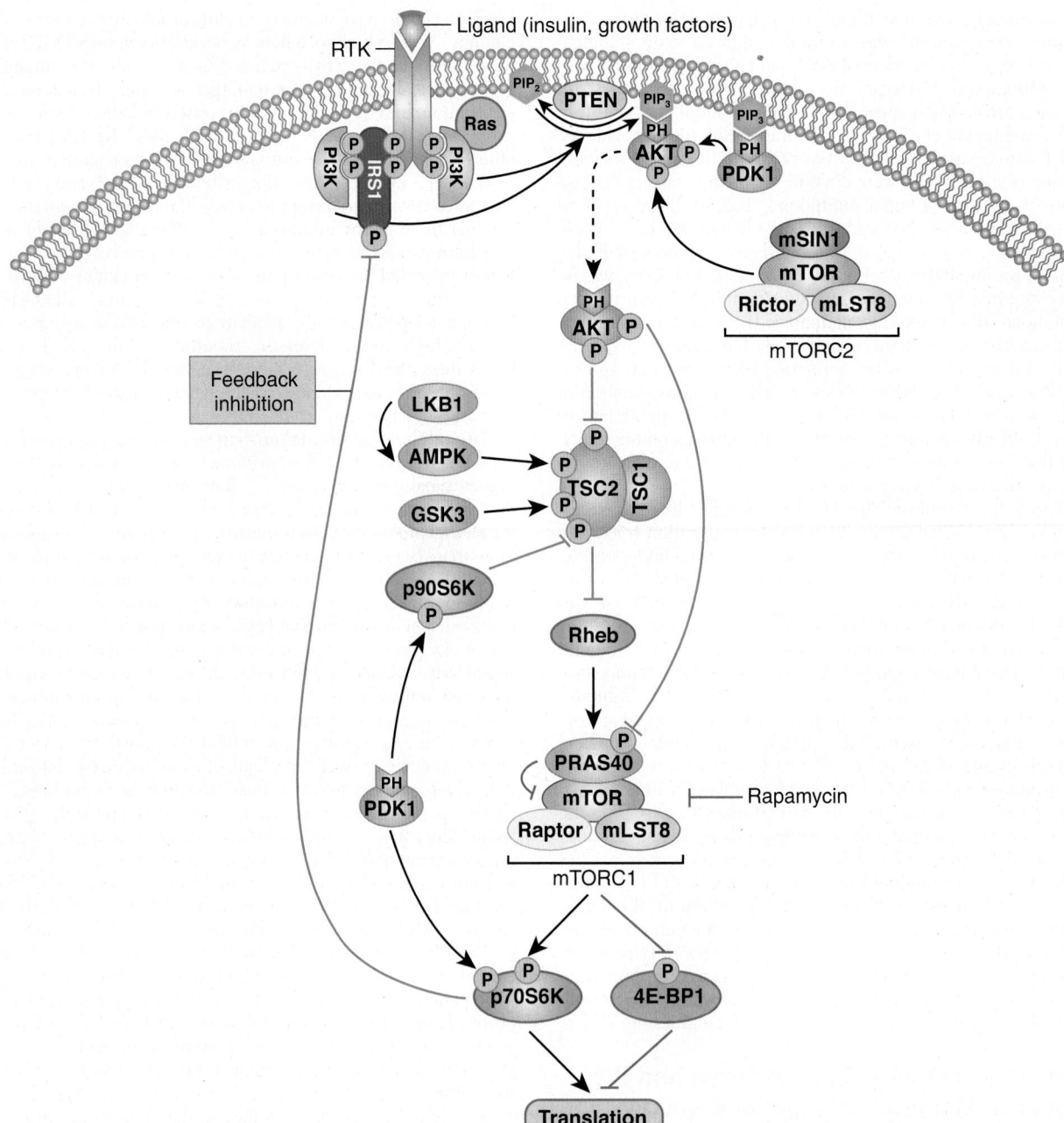

Figure 22.2 Feedback inhibition of the phosphatidylinositol 3-kinase (PI3K) pathway. Activated AKT regulates cellular growth through mammalian target of rapamycin (mTOR), a key player in protein synthesis and translation. mTOR forms part of two distinct complexes known as mTORC1, which contains mTOR, Raptor, mLST8, and PRAS40, and mTORC2, which contains mTOR, Rictor, mLST8, and mSIN1. mTORC1 is sensitive to rapamycin and controls protein synthesis and translation, at least in part, through p70S6K and eukaryotic translation initiation factor 4E–binding protein 1 (4E-BP1). AKT phosphorylates and inhibits tuberous sclerosis complex 2 (TSC2), resulting in increased mTORC1 activity. AKT also phosphorylates PRAS40, thus relieving the PRAS40 inhibitory effect on mTOR and the mTORC1 complex. mTORC2 and 3-phosphoinositide–dependent kinase (PDK1) phosphorylate AKT on Ser473 and Thr308, respectively, rendering it fully active. mTORC1-activated p70S6K can phosphorylate insulin receptor substrate 1 (IRS1), resulting in inhibition of PI3K activity. In addition, PDK1 phosphorylates and activates p70S6K and p90S6K. The latter has been shown to inhibit TSC2 activity through direct phosphorylation. Conversely, LKB1-activated AMP-activated protein kinase (AMPK) and glycogen synthase kinase 3 (GSK3) activate the TSC1/TSC2 complex through direct phosphorylation of TSC2. Thus, signals through PI3K as well as through LKB1 and AMPK converge on mTORC1. Inhibition of mTORC1 can lead to increased insulin receptor–mediated signaling, and inhibition of PDK1 may lead to activation of mTORC1 and may, paradoxically, promote tumor growth. (From Daigle SR, Olhava EJ, Therkelsen CA, et al. Selective killing of mixed lineage leukemia cells by a potent small-molecule DOT1L inhibitor. *Cancer Cell* 2011;20(1):53–65, with permission.)

Other Indications for mTOR Inhibitors: Breast Cancer and Tuberous Sclerosis Complex Mutant Cancers

Two other indications for mTOR have emerged, both based on fundamental insights from laboratory studies but from quite different angles. Preclinical studies of estrogen receptor (ER) therapy in breast cancer suggested that phosphatidylinositol 3-kinase (PI3K) pathway activation may be a mechanism of resistance and that this resistance could be prevented or overcome by combined treatment with ER-based drugs and rapalogs such as everolimus. Based on evidence that some women with progressive disease while receiving the aromatase inhibitor letrozole have clinical benefit from the addition of everolimus, randomized trials were initiated comparing everolimus + exemestane to exemestane alone (called BO-LERO-2), or everolimus + tamoxifen to tamoxifen alone (called TAMRAD). Both studies demonstrated substantial improvements in time to progression in women with metastatic breast cancer who had already failed one aromatase inhibitor,[85,86] resulting in FDA approval of the everolimus/exemestane combination. Evidence of cross-talk between the PI3K pathway and hormone receptor signaling (ER in breast cancer, androgen receptor in prostate cancer) provides a molecular rationale for the clinical benefit of combination therapy and is currently under investigation in metastatic prostate cancer.[87]

Yet another indication for rapalog therapy emerged from the genetics of children with tuberous sclerosis caused by a loss of function mutations in tuberous sclerosis complex 1 (TSC1) or TSC2, which encode the proteins hamartin and tuberin that function in the PI3K signaling pathway just upstream of mTOR. Based on laboratory studies showing that TSC1- or TSC2-deficient cells are exquisitely sensitive to rapalogs, a clinical trial was conducted in tuberous sclerosis patients with benign subependymal giant-cell astrocytomas (SEGA) that showed tumor shrinkage in 21 of 28 patients.[88] This genetic dependence on mTOR in tumors with tuberous sclerosis complex (TSC) loss has also been observed in bladder cancer. In a remarkable example of the power of comprehensive DNA sequencing to provide insight into rare clinical phenotypes, investigators examined the tumor genome of the single complete responder patient on a phase II trial of everolimus in bladder cancer and discovered somatic mutations in TSC2 as well as a second gene, NF2, that also controls mTOR activity.[89] This plus other examples of how a retrospective genomic analysis of *extraordinary responders* has led to a national effort to capture these cases, as well as prospective clinical trials of patients with the relevant tumor genotype regardless of histology (called *basket* trials).

It is unclear why rapalogs have failed in other tumor types. One explanation is the concurrence of PI3K pathway mutations with alterations in other pathways that mitigate sensitivity to rapalogs. Another possibility is the disruption of negative feedback loops regulated by mTOR that inhibit signaling from upstream receptor tyrosine kinases. Rapalogs paradoxically *increase* signaling through PI3K due to loss of this negative feedback. A primary consequence is *increased* AKT activation, which signals to an array of downstream substrates that can enhance cell proliferation and survival (other than TORC1, which remains inhibited by rapalog) (see Fig. 22.2). This problem might be overcome by combining rapalogs with an inhibitor of an upstream kinase in the feedback loop, such as HER kinases or the insulinlike growth factor receptor (IGFR), to block this undesired effect of rapalogs on PI3K activation.[90]

DIRECTLY TARGETING THE PI3K PATHWAY

Mutations or copy number alterations (e.g., amplification or deletion of oncogenes or tumor suppressor genes) in PI3K pathway genes (PIK3CA, PIK3R1, PTEN, AKT1, and others) are among the most common abnormalities in cancer. Consequently, intensive efforts at many pharmaceutical companies have been devoted to the discovery of small-molecule inhibitors targeting kinases in the PI3K pathway. Inhibitors of PI3K, AKT, and ATP-competitive (rather than allosteric) inhibitors of mTOR that target both the TORC1 and TORC2 complex are all in clinical development. Phase I clinical trials have, in general, established that the pathway can be efficiently targeted without serious toxicity other than easily manageable effects on glucose metabolism (which is anticipated based on the importance of PI3K signaling in insulin signaling). Unfortunately, there has been no evidence to date of dramatic single-agent clinical activity with any of these agents, although early results with PI3K alpha selective inhibitor BYL719 in PIK3CA mutant breast cancer appear promising.[91]

However, the first approval of a direct PI3K inhibitor in cancer is likely to come in chronic lymphocytic leukemia and in lymphoma, but not on the basis of tumor genomics. Normal and malignant B cells are dependent on PI3K delta as well as Bruton tyrosine kinase (BTK) for proliferation and survival, raising the possibility that inhibitors of these kinases might be broadly active in B-cell malignancies. Concerns about toxicity on normal B cells were alleviated, in part, by the earlier clinical success of the CD20 antibody rituximab in lymphoma, which also eliminates normal circulating B cells, but without significant clinical sequelae. The first such PI3K delta inhibitor, idelalisib, has shown impressive activity in indolent non-Hodgkin lymphoma as a single agent and in relapsed chronic lymphocytic leukemia when given in combination with rituximab. The BTK inhibitor ibrutinib, following a similar clinical development path, was recently approved as second-line therapy for chronic lymphocytic leukemia and for mantle cell lymphoma.[92,93]

COMBINATIONS OF KINASE INHIBITORS TO INDUCT RESPONSE AND PREVENT RESISTANCE

Preclinical studies indicate that combinations of kinase inhibitors are required to realize their full potential as anticancer agents. The most common rationale is to address the problem of concurrent mutations in different pathways that alleviate dependence on a single-driver oncogene. The best examples are cancers with mutations in both the RAS/MAP kinase pathway (RAS or BRAF) and the PI3K pathway (PIK3CA or PTEN). In mouse models, such doubly mutant tumors fail to respond to single-agent treatment with either an AKT inhibitor or a MEK inhibitor. However, combination treatment can give dramatic regressions.[94] Similarly, genetically engineered mice that develop KRAS-driven lung cancer respond only to combination therapy with a PI3K inhibitor and a MEK inhibitor.[95] To date, clinical trials combining different PI3K pathway and RAS/MAP kinase pathway inhibitors have been challenging due to toxicities associated with continuous, concurrent PI3K and RAS/MAP kinase pathway inhibition.

Many of the tumor types discussed in this chapter *do* respond to treatment with a single-agent kinase, but relapse despite continued inhibitor therapy. Research into the causes of "acquired" kinase inhibitor resistance has revealed two primary mechanisms: (1) novel mutations in the kinase domain of the drug target that preclude inhibition, or (2) *bypass* of the driver kinase signal by activation of a parallel kinase pathway. In both cases, the solution is combination therapy to prevent the emergence of resistance. An elegant demonstration of this approach comes from CML where resistance to imatinib is primarily caused by mutations in the BCR-ABL kinase domain.[96,97] The second-generation ABL inhibitors dasatinib and nilotinib are effective against most imatinib-resistant BCR-ABL mutants and were initially approved as single-agent therapy for imatinib-resistant CML.[98,99] Very recently, both drugs have proven superior to imatinib in the upfront treatment of CML

CANCER THERAPEUTICS

due to increased potency and fewer mechanisms of acquired resistance.[100–102] However, one BCR-ABL mutation called T315I is resistant to all three drugs. The third-generation ABL kinase inhibitor ponatinib blocks T315I and showed activity in a phase II clinical trial that included CML patients with the T315I mutation,[103] resulting in FDA approval. However, subsequent reports of severe vascular occlusive events, such as stroke and heart failure, led to withdrawal from the market, followed by approval for restricted use in T315I-mutant patients. Analogous approaches are ongoing in other diseases such as EGFR-mutant lung cancer, where acquired resistance to the frontline kinase inhibitor is also associated with mutations in the target kinase.[104,105] Promising clinical results have been reported with irreversible EGFR inhibitors such as CO-1686 and AZD9291.

The clinical development of kinase inhibitor combinations to prevent acquired resistance is relatively straightforward. Because the frontline drug is already approved, success would be determined by an improvement in response duration using the combination. The situation is more complex when two experimental compounds (e.g., a PI3K pathway inhibitor and a MEK inhibitor) are combined, neither of which shows significant single-agent activity. Older regulatory guidelines required a four-arm study that compared each single agent to the combination and to a control group in order to obtain approval of the combination. Recognizing that this design could discourage drug developers as well as patients from moving forward because it requires a large sample size, the FDA has issued new guidelines for the development of novel combinations that require a two-arm registration study comparing the combination to standard of care http://www.fda.gov/downloads/Drugs/GuidanceComplianceRegulatoryInformation/Guidances/UCM236669.pdf. A more challenging issue may be dose optimization and dose schedule that is needed to safely combine two investigational drugs. Much like the development of combination chemotherapy several decades ago, it may be important to select compounds with nonoverlapping toxicities to allow for sufficient doses of each drug to be achieved.

SPECULATIONS ON THE FUTURE ROLE OF KINASE INHIBITORS IN CANCER MEDICINE

The role of genomics in predicting a response to kinase inhibitor therapy is now irrefutable. As the number of kinase driver mutations continues to grow, the field is likely to move away from the current strategy of a *companion diagnostic* for each drug. Rather, comprehensive mutational profiling platforms that query each tumor for hundreds of potential cancer mutations are more likely to emerge as the diagnostic platform. The number of directly *actionable* mutations (meaning the presence of a mutation defines a treatment decision supported by clinical trial data) remains low, but this number will undoubtedly grow. In addition, it is becoming apparent that many patients have rare mutations (defined as rare in that histologic tumor type) but are, in theory, actionable. Because these examples are unlikely to be formally evaluated in clinical trials, many centers have opened *basket* studies (with eligibility based solely on mutation profile) to capture these cases with some reports of remarkable success.

More effort must be devoted to manipulating the dose and schedule of kinase inhibitor therapy to maximize efficacy and minimize toxicity. To date, all kinase inhibitors have been developed based on the assumption that a 24/7 coverage of the target is required for efficacy. Consequently, most compounds are optimized to have a long serum half-life (12 to 24 hours). Phase II doses are then selected based on the maximum tolerated dose determined with daily administration. But a recent clinical of the ABL inhibitor dasatinib in CML indicates that equivalent antitumor activity can be achieved with intermittent therapy.[106] By giving larger doses intermittently, higher peak drug concentrations were achieved that resulted in equivalent and possibly superior efficacy.[107] Similar results were observed in laboratory studies of EGFR inhibitors in EGFR-mutant lung cancer. Clinically robust, quantitative assays of target inhibition are needed to hasten progress in this area.

Although the focus of this chapter is kinase inhibitors, the themes developed here should apply broadly to inhibitors of other cancer targets. Inhibitors of the G-protein coupled receptor smoothened (SMO) in patients with metastatic basal cell carcinoma or medulloblastoma establish that the driver mutation hypothesis extends beyond kinase inhibitors. SMO is a component in the Hedgehog pathway, which is constitutively activated in subsets of patients with basal cell carcinoma and medulloblastoma due to mutations in the Hedgehog ligand-binding receptor Patched-1. Treatment with the SMO inhibitor vismodegib led to impressive responses in basal cell carcinoma and medulloblastoma patients whose tumors had Patched-1 mutations,[108,109] resulting in FDA approval. Other novel cancer targets are emerging from cancer genome sequencing projects. Somatic mutations in the Krebs cycle enzyme isocitrate dehydrogenase (IDH1/2) were found in subsets of patients with glioblastoma, AML, chondrosarcoma, and cholangiocarcinoma,[110–112] and the first IDH2 inhibitor has entered clinical trials in leukemia. Mutations in enzymes involved in chromatin remodeling, such as the histone methyltransferase EZH2, have been reported in lymphoma and have spurred the ongoing development of EZH2 inhibitors.[113,114] Inhibitors of another histone methyltransferase DOT1L, which is required for the maintenance of mixed lineage leukemia (MLL) fusion leukemias, are also in clinical development.[115,116] Kinase inhibitors are just the first wave of molecularly targeted drugs ushered in by our understanding of the molecular underpinnings of cancer cells. There is much more to follow.

SELECTED REFERENCES

The full reference list can be accessed at lwwhealthlibrary.com/oncology.

1. Sawyers CL. Shifting paradigms: the seeds of oncogene addiction. *Nat Med* 2009;15(10):1158–1161.
2. Weinstein IB. Cancer. Addiction to oncogenes—the Achilles heal of cancer. *Science* 2002;297(5578):63–64.
3. Druker BJ, Talpaz M, Resta DJ, et al. Efficacy and safety of a specific inhibitor of the BCR-ABL tyrosine kinase in chronic myeloid leukemia. *N Engl J Med* 2001;344(14):1031–1037.
4. Hirota S, Isozaki K, Moriyama Y, et al. Gain-of-function mutations of c-kit in human gastrointestinal stromal tumors. *Science* 1998;279(5350):577–580.
5. Heinrich MC, Corless CL, Duensing A, et al. PDGFRA activating mutations in gastrointestinal stromal tumors. *Science* 2003;299(5607):708–710.
6. Demetri GD, von Mehren M, Blanke CD, et al. Efficacy and safety of imatinib mesylate in advanced gastrointestinal stromal tumors. *N Engl J Med* 2002;347(7):472–480.
8. Kris MG, Natale RB, Herbst RS, et al. Efficacy of gefitinib, an inhibitor of the epidermal growth factor receptor tyrosine kinase, in symptomatic patients with non-small cell lung cancer: a randomized trial. *JAMA* 2003;290(16):2149–2158.
10. Paez JG, Jänne PA, Lee JC, et al. EGFR mutations in lung cancer: correlation with clinical response to gefitinib therapy. *Science* 2004;304(5676):1497–1500.
11. Lynch TJ, Bell DW, Sordella R, et al. Activating mutations in the epidermal growth factor receptor underlying responsiveness of non-small-cell lung cancer to gefitinib. *N Engl J Med* 2004;350(21):2129–2139.
12. Pao W, Miller V, Zakowski M, et al. EGF receptor gene mutations are common in lung cancers from "never smokers" and are associated with sensitivity of tumors to gefitinib and erlotinib. *Proc Natl Acad Sci U S A* 2004;101(36):13306–13311.
14. Shepherd FA, Rodrigues Pereira J, Ciuleanu T, et al. Erlotinib in previously treated non-small-cell lung cancer. *N Engl J Med* 2005;353(2):123–132.
19. Tsao MS, Sakurada A, Cutz JC, et al. Erlotinib in lung cancer - molecular and clinical predictors of outcome. *N Engl J Med* 2005;353(2):133–144.
20. Mok TS, Wu YL, Thongprasert S, et al. Gefitinib or carboplatin-paclitaxel in pulmonary adenocarcinoma. *N Engl J Med* 2009;361(10):947–957.

23. Cools J, DeAngelo DJ, Gotlib J, et al. A tyrosine kinase created by fusion of the PDGFRA and FIP1L1 genes as a therapeutic target of imatinib in idiopathic hypereosinophilic syndrome. *N Engl J Med* 2003;348(13):1201–1214.

25. Apperley JF, Gardembas M, Melo JV, et al. Response to imatinib mesylate in patients with chronic myeloproliferative diseases with rearrangements of the platelet-derived growth factor receptor beta. *N Engl J Med* 2002;347(7):481–487.

27. Davies H, Bignell GR, Cox C, et al. Mutations of the BRAF gene in human cancer. *Nature* 2002;417(6892):949–954.

28. Baxter EJ, Scott LM, Campbell PJ, et al., Acquired mutation of the tyrosine kinase JAK2 in human myeloproliferative disorders. *Lancet* 2005;365(9464):1054–1061.

29. James C, Ugo V, Le Couédic JP, et al. A unique clonal JAK2 mutation leading to constitutive signalling causes polycythaemia vera. *Nature* 2005;434(7037):1144–1148.

30. Levine RL, Wadleigh M, Cools J, et al. Activating mutation in the tyrosine kinase JAK2 in polycythemia vera, essential thrombocythemia, and myeloid metaplasia with myelofibrosis. *Cancer Cell* 2005;7(4):387–397.

31. Samuels Y, Wang Z, Bardellli A, et al. High frequency of mutations of the PIK3CA gene in human cancers. *Science* 2004;304(5670):554.

32. International Cancer Genome Consortium, Hudson TJ, Anderson W, et al. International network of cancer genome projects. *Nature* 2010;464(7291):993–998.

33. Vogelstein B, Papadopoulos N, Velculescu VE, et al. Cancer genome landscapes. *Science* 2013;339(6127):1546–1558.

34. Lawrence MS, Stojanov P, Mermel CH, et al. Discovery and saturation analysis of cancer genes across 21 tumour types. *Nature* 2014;505(7484):495–501.

35. Eisen T, Ahmad T, Flaherty KT, et al. Sorafenib in advanced melanoma: a Phase II randomised discontinuation trial analysis. *Br J Cancer* 2006;95(5):581–586.

36. Solit DB, Garraway LA, Pratilas CA, et al. BRAF mutation predicts sensitivity to MEK inhibition. *Nature* 2006;439(7074):358–362.

38. Pratilas CA, Taylor BS, Ye Q, et al. (V600E)BRAF is associated with disabled feedback inhibition of RAF-MEK signaling and elevated transcriptional output of the pathway. *Proc Natl Acad Sci U S A* 2009;106(11):4519–4524.

42. Flaherty KT, Robert C, Hersey P, et al. Improved survival with MEK inhibition in BRAF-mutated melanoma. *N Engl J Med* 2012;367(2):107–114.

45. Flaherty KT, Puzanov I, Kim KB, et al. Inhibition of mutated, activated BRAF in metastatic melanoma. *N Engl J Med* 2010;363(9):809–819.

46. Bollag G, Hirth P, Tsai J, et al. Clinical efficacy of a RAF inhibitor needs broad target blockade in BRAF-mutant melanoma. *Nature* 2010;467(7315):596–599.

47. Hauschild A, Grob JJ, Demidov LV, et al. Dabrafenib in BRAF-mutated metastatic melanoma: a multicentre, open-label, phase 3 randomised controlled trial. *Lancet* 2012;380(9839):358–365.

50. Soda M, Choi YL, Enomoto M, et al. Identification of the transforming EML4-ALK fusion gene in non-small-cell lung cancer. *Nature* 2007;448(7153):561–566.

52. Shaw AT, Kim DW, Nakagawa K, et al. Crizotinib versus chemotherapy in advanced ALK-positive lung cancer. *N Engl J Med* 2013;368(25):2385–2394.

53. Chen Y, Takita J, Choi YL, et al. Oncogenic mutations of ALK kinase in neuroblastoma. *Nature* 2008;455(7215):971–974.

63. Sawyers CL. Finding the next Gleevec: FLT3 targeted kinase inhibitor therapy for acute myeloid leukemia. *Cancer Cell* 2002;1(5):413–415.

69. Zarrinkar PP, Gunawardane RN, Cramer MD, et al. AC220 is a uniquely potent and selective inhibitor of FLT3 for the treatment of acute myeloid leukemia (AML). *Blood* 2009;114(14):2984–2992.

71. Smith CC, Wang Q, Chin CS, et al. Validation of ITD mutations in FLT3 as a therapeutic target in human acute myeloid leukaemia. *Nature* 2012;485(7397):260–263.

72. Kaelin WG Jr. The von Hippel-Lindau tumour suppressor protein: O2 sensing and cancer. *Nat Rev Cancer* 2008;8(11):865–873.

73. Yang JC, Haworth L, Sherry RM, et al. A randomized trial of bevacizumab, an anti-vascular endothelial growth factor antibody, for metastatic renal cancer. *N Engl J Med* 2003;349(5):427–434.

83. Guertin DA, Sabatini DM. Defining the role of mTOR in cancer. *Cancer Cell* 2007;12(1):9–22.

84. Thomas GV, Tran C, Mellinghoff IK, et al. Hypoxia-inducible factor determines sensitivity to inhibitors of mTOR in kidney cancer. *Nat Med* 2006;12(1):122–127.

85. Bachelot T, Bourgier C, Cropet C, et al. Randomized phase II trial of everolimus in combination with tamoxifen in patients with hormone receptor-positive, human epidermal growth factor receptor 2-negative metastatic breast cancer with prior exposure to aromatase inhibitors: a GINECO study. *J Clin Oncol* 2012;30(22):2718–2724.

86. Baselga J, Campone M, Piccart M, et al. Everolimus in postmenopausal hormone-receptor-positive advanced breast cancer. *N Engl J Med* 2012;366(6):520–529.

87. Carver BS, Chapinski C, Wongvipat J, et al. Reciprocal feedback regulation of PI3K and androgen receptor signaling in PTEN-deficient prostate cancer. *Cancer Cell* 2011;19(5):575–586.

88. Krueger DA, Care MM, Holland K, et al. Everolimus for subependymal giant-cell astrocytomas in tuberous sclerosis. *N Engl J Med* 2010;363(19):1801–1811.

89. Iyer G, Hanrahan AL, Milowsky MI, et al. Genome sequencing identifies a basis for everolimus sensitivity. *Science* 2012;338(6104):221.

90. O'Reilly KE, Rojo F, She QB, et al. mTOR inhibition induces upstream receptor tyrosine kinase signaling and activates Akt. *Cancer Res* 2006;66(3):1500–1508.

91. Gonzalez-Angulo AM, Juric D, Argilis G, et al. Safety, pharmacokinetics, and preliminary activity of the alpha-specific PI3K inhibitor BYL719: results from the first-in-human study. *J Clin Oncol* 2013;31(15 Suppl):2531.

92. Byrd JC, Furman RR, Coutre SE, et al. Targeting BTK with ibrutinib in relapsed chronic lymphocytic leukemia. *N Engl J Med* 2013;369(1):32–42.

93. Wang ML, Rule S, Martin P, et al. Targeting BTK with ibrutinib in relapsed or refractory mantle-cell lymphoma. *N Engl J Med* 2013;369(6):507–516.

95. Engelman JA, Chen L, Tan X, et al. Effective use of PI3K and MEK inhibitors to treat mutant Kras G12D and PIK3CA H1047R murine lung cancers. *Nat Med* 2008;14(12):1351–1356.

96. Gorre ME, Mohammed M, Ellwood K, et al. Clinical resistance to STI-571 cancer therapy caused by BCR-ABL gene mutation or amplification. *Science* 2001;293(5531):876–880.

97. Shah NP, Nicoll JM, Nagar B, et al. Multiple BCR-ABL kinase domain mutations confer polyclonal resistance to the tyrosine kinase inhibitor imatinib (STI571) in chronic phase and blast crisis chronic myeloid leukemia. *Cancer Cell* 2002;2(2):117–125.

98. Shah NP, Tran C, Lee FY, et al. Overriding imatinib resistance with a novel ABL kinase inhibitor. *Science* 2004;305(5682):399–401.

99. Talpaz M, Shah NP, Kantarjian H, et al. Dasatinib in imatinib-resistant Philadelphia chromosome-positive leukemias. *N Engl J Med* 2006;354(24):2531–2541.

101. Sawyers CL. Even better kinase inhibitors for chronic myeloid leukemia. *N Engl J Med* 2010;362(24):2314–2315.

104. Pao W, Miller VA, Politi KA, et al. Acquired resistance of lung adenocarcinomas to gefitinib or erlotinib is associated with a second mutation in the EGFR kinase domain. *PLoS Med* 2005;2(3):e73.

105. Antonescu CR, Besmer P, Guo T, et al. Acquired resistance to imatinib in gastrointestinal stromal tumor occurs through secondary gene mutation. *Clin Cancer Res* 2005;11(11):4182–4190.

106. Shah NP, Kantarjian HM, Kim DW, et al. Intermittent target inhibition with dasatinib 100 mg once daily preserves efficacy and improves tolerability in imatinib-resistant and -intolerant chronic-phase chronic myeloid leukemia. *J Clin Oncol* 2008;26(19):3204–3212.

107. Shah NP, Kasap C, Weier C, et al. Transient potent BCR-ABL inhibition is sufficient to commit chronic myeloid leukemia cells irreversibly to apoptosis. *Cancer Cell* 2008;14(6):485–493.

112. Ward PS, Patel J, Wise DR, et al. The common feature of leukemia-associated IDH1 and IDH2 mutations is a neomorphic enzyme activity converting alpha-ketoglutarate to 2-hydroxyglutarate. *Cancer Cell* 2010;17(3):225–234.

113. McCabe MT, Ott HM, Ganji G, et al. EZH2 inhibition as a therapeutic strategy for lymphoma with EZH2-activating mutations. *Nature* 2012;492(7427):108–112.

114. Morin RD, Johnson NA, Severson TM, et al. Somatic mutations altering EZH2 (Tyr641) in follicular and diffuse large B-cell lymphomas of germinal-center origin. *Nat Genet* 2010;42(2):181–185.

115. Bernt KM, Zhu N, Sinha AU, et al. MLL-rearranged leukemia is dependent on aberrant H3K79 methylation by DOT1L. *Cancer Cell* 2011;20(1):66–78.

116. Daigle SR, Olhava EJ, Therkelsen CA, et al. Selective killing of mixed lineage leukemia cells by a potent small-molecule DOT1L inhibitor. *Cancer Cell* 2011;20(1):53–65.

CANCER THERAPEUTICS

Histone Deacetylase Inhibitors and Demethylating Agents

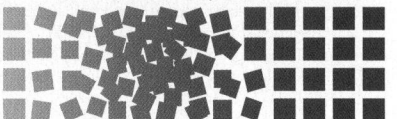

Steven D. Gore, Stephen B. Baylin, and James G. Herman

INTRODUCTION

The past decade has seen an explosive growth, especially at a genome-wide level, in our understanding of the role of chromatin in the normal regulation of gene expression and in the concept of the *epigenome*.[1-3] Concomitant with these advances has been the increasing appreciation of the role of epigenetic abnormalities in the progression of cancer[4-7] and the concept of the *cancer epigenome*. The translational consequences of this research include the possibilities for developing therapies in cancer that target epigenetic abnormalities. These are being explored in clinical trials and several have entered clinical practice.[4,5,7,8] Of these epigenetic abnormalities, the most thoroughly examined is the occurrence of abnormal cytosine guanine (CpG) promoter region DNA methylation and associated altered chromatin involving histone modifications, in the transcriptional silencing of genes, including a group of well-defined tumor suppressor genes.[4,5,7,8] However, targeting epigenetic processes to downregulate the action of overexpressed genes is also an emerging area of research.[9,10] This chapter describes the basis of epigenetic changes in cancer and discusses some of the latest approaches that target epigenetic abnormalities in cancer,[11] including those designed to induce the reexpression of silenced genes, for cancer therapy. The two approaches most mature in development are the inhibition of DNA methyltransferases, which mediate the abnormal promoter DNA methylation, and the inhibition of histone deacetylases, which remove histone modifications associated with active chromatin that alone, or in association with DNA methylation, are associated with transcriptional repression.[4,5,7,8] However, several exciting newer approaches are now in clinical trials and these will be mentioned.

Aberrant gene function and altered patterns of gene expression are key features of cancer.[4] Although genetic alterations remain the best characterized in the development and progression of cancer, increasingly it is appreciated that epigenetic abnormalities cooperate with genetic alterations in multiple ways to cause dysfunction of key regulatory pathways. Through genomic approaches to mutation discovery, there is growing recognition of the frequency of mutations in genes encoding for proteins that regulate the epigenome.[12] This chapter will outline the understanding of how each of these epigenetic alterations contribute to cancer and how derivation of therapeutic approaches may depend on understanding the biology of these changes.

EPIGENETIC ABNORMALITIES AND GENE EXPRESSION CHANGES IN CANCER

Epigenetic changes are defined as heritable alterations of gene expression patterns and cell phenotypes, which are not accompanied by changes in DNA sequence.[13] This definition clearly delineates the two key features of epigenetic regulation important for an understanding of therapies described in this chapter. Specifically, in contrast to genetic alterations (point mutations, deletions,

or translocations), epigenetic changes do not alter the coding sequence of targeted genes. Thus, reversal of epigenetic changes can potentially restore the normal function of affected genes and their encoded proteins. Second, the heritable nature of epigenetic changes—that is, the ability of a cell to pass on regulation of gene expression through DNA replication—suggests that such changes, while relatively stable, can be reversed. Thus, therapeutic reprogramming of patterns of gene expression could theoretically result in a long-term change in the cancer cell phenotype, even after the inducing drugs are removed, although to date, this has not been accomplished.

The fundamental unit that determines epigenetic states is the nucleosome that contains an octamer of histone proteins around which approximately 160 base pairs of DNA are wrapped.[13] It is the positioning of these structures, and the three-dimensional aspects of their spacing, and the regulation of this process by posttranslational modifications of the constituent histones that underpins the functions of the epigenome.[13,14]

Abnormal Gene Silencing

One key alteration in cancer, which can be associated with altered epigenetic control, is abnormal gene silencing. Normally, such silencing is fundamental and required at the level of chromatin and DNA methylation regulation for the life of multicellular eukaryotic organisms. The silencing is critical for regulating important biologic processes, including all aspects of development, differentiation, imprinting, and silencing of large chromosomal domains, including the X chromosome of female mammals.[13] For example, the diversity of structure and function of cells derived from epithelial or mesenchymal origin, ultimately differentiating into cells lining the intestine or lung or forming mature granulocytes and myocytes, result from heritable changes in gene expression that are not the result of a change in DNA sequence. Although in many species, silencing can be initiated and maintained solely by processes involving the covalent modifications of histones and other chromatin components, vertebrates utilize an additional layer of gene regulation. This process involves the only natural covalent modification of DNA in humans and is characterized by DNA cytosine methylation that occurs nearly exclusively at the fifth position of the cytosine ring in cytosines preceding guanine, the so-called CpG dinucleotide (Fig. 23.1).[13,15]

Like most biologic processes, the normal patterns of silencing can be altered, resulting in the development of disease states. Thus, activation of genes normally not expressed, or silencing of a gene that should be expressed, can contribute to the dysregulation of gene function that characterizes cancer and, when stably present, represent epigenetic alterations.[4-7] Most studies have focused on the silencing of normally expressed genes. For the purposes of understanding the rationale behind epigenetic therapy, it is important to understand the mechanisms through which such silencing occurs. Alterations in gene expression associated with epigenetic changes that give rise to a growth advantage would be expected to be selected for in the host tissue, leading to progressive dysregulated

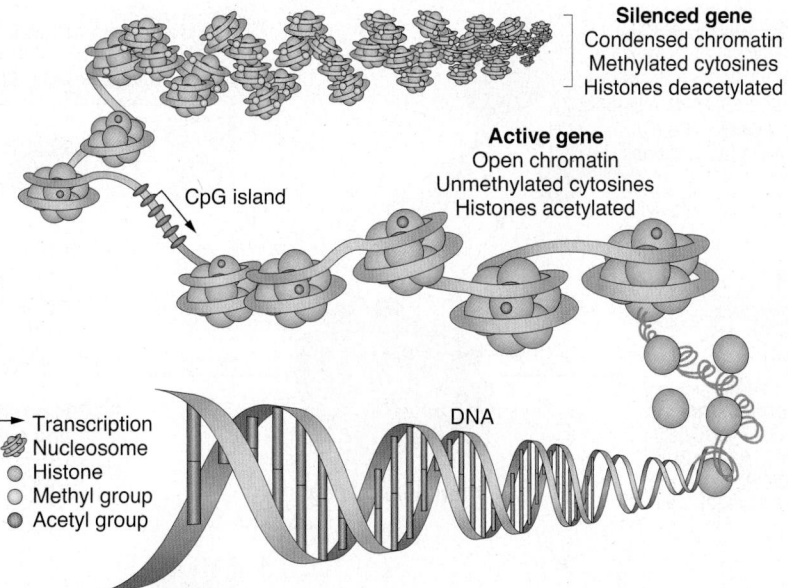

Figure 23.1 Epigenetic regulation of gene expression. In the promoter region, gene expression is controlled by a combination of DNA methylation and chromatin configuration. In normal cells, gene expression is silenced by condensing chromatin, methylating DNA, and deacetylating histones. By contrast, active genes are those with open nucleosome spacing around the transcription start site, are unmethylated, and are associated with acetylated histones. In cancer cells, CpG islands that are rich in cytosine and guanine—and are typically unmethylated to promote gene expression—can be epigenetically silenced by hypermethylation. (Redrawn with permission from Azad N, Zahnow CA, Rudin CM, et al. The future of epigenetic therapy in solid tumours—lessons from the past. *Nat Rev Clin Oncol* 2013;10:256–266.)

growth of the tumor. Such dysregulation is commonly associated with increases in promoter region DNA methylation and is associated with repressive chromatin changes.

Changes in DNA Methylation

The importance of abnormal cytosine methylation and gene silencing has been clearly established in the past 2 decades and been shown convincingly to be involved in cancer development.[4–7] The CpG dinucleotide, usually underrepresented in the genome, is clustered in the promoter regions of approximately 50% of human genes in regions termed *CpG islands*. These regions are largely protected from DNA methylation in normal cells, with the exception of genes on the inactive X chromosome and imprinted genes.[16] This protection is critical, because the methylation of promoter region CpG islands is associated with a loss of gene expression.[4–7] Abnormal de novo DNA methylation of gene promoter CpG islands is a very frequent abnormality in virtually all cancer types and is associated with a process that can serve as an alternative mechanism for loss of tumor suppressor gene function.[4–7] Although a limited number of classic tumor suppressor genes can be affected by this process, a patient's individual cancer may harbor hundreds of such genes.[4–7] Which of these latter genes are drivers of cancer, individually or in groups, versus those which are passengers reflecting only the widespread effects of a global epigenetic abnormality is a leading question in the field and the target of much research.[5,6] A clue to the importance of at least groups of the previous DNA hypermethylated genes may come from the fact that an inordinate number of them are involved in holding normal embryonic and adult stem cells in the self-renewal state and/or rendering such cells refractory to differentiation cues.[17,18] Normally, these genes are then in a poised expression state and can be induced to be activated or repressed as needed for changes in

cell state.[18] Abnormal promoter DNA methylation of such genes renders them more repressed and could be a factor in the fact that cancers inevitably exhibit cell populations with enhanced self-renewal or refractoriness to full differentiation.[18]

Recent studies have also suggested that DNA regions other than promoter CpG islands may undergo changes of DNA methylation in cancer. For example, non–CpG-rich sequences surrounding promoter CpG islands, termed CpG island shores, are abnormally methylated in cancers[19] and may be altered in stem cell populations.[20] Thus, the relative cancer specificity of changes of DNA methylation in multiple CpG regions makes reversal of these changes by targeting DNA methyltransferases, the enzymes that catalyze DNA methylation, logical for cancer therapeutics.

As a key example of the previous points, perhaps the most studied tumor suppressor gene for promoter hypermethylation is the *p16* gene, currently designated *CDKN2A*, a cyclin-dependent kinase inhibitor that functions in the regulation of the phosphorylation of the Rb protein. Hypermethylation associated with loss of expression of the *CDKN2A* gene has been found to be one of the most frequent alterations in neoplasia being common in the lung, head and neck, gliomas, colorectal, and breast carcinomas[21,22] and other cancer types. A member of the same gene family, *p15* or *CDKN2B*, also regulates Rb and is silenced in association with promoter methylation in many forms of leukemia and in the chronic myeloid neoplasm myelodysplastic syndrome (MDS).[23] These two previous changes are of much relevance for the clinical uses of epigenetic therapies discussed later.

As mentioned, many hundreds of genes may be inactivated in a single cancer by promoter methylation,[5,6,18,24] providing potential targets for gene reactivation using epigenetic therapies.[25–27] The latter represents one of the potential ways in which epigenetic therapy may be effective: Multiple genes and gene pathways, all

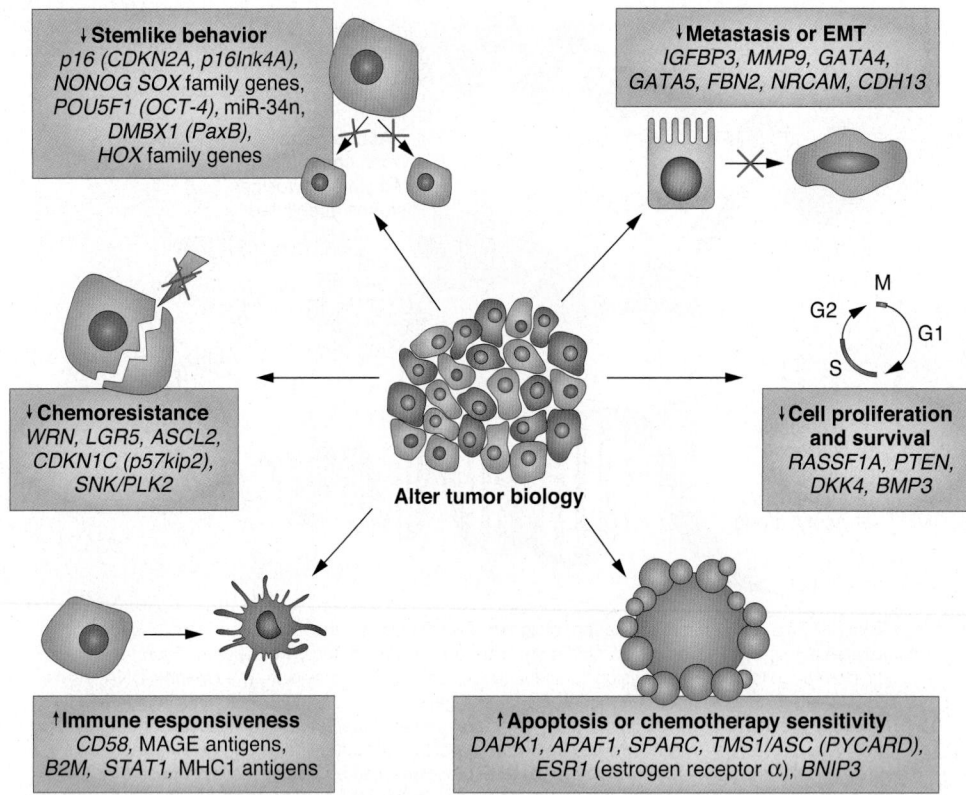

↓**Stemlike behavior**
p16 (CDKN2A, p16Ink4A),
NONOG SOX family genes,
POU5F1 (OCT-4), miR-34n,
DMBX1 (PaxB),
HOX family genes

↓**Metastasis or EMT**
IGFBP3, MMP9, GATA4,
GATA5, FBN2, NRCAM, CDH13

↓**Chemoresistance**
WRN, LGR5, ASCL2,
CDKN1C (p57kip2),
SNK/PLK2

Alter tumor biology

↓**Cell proliferation
and survival**
RASSF1A, PTEN,
DKK4, BMP3

↑**Immune responsiveness**
CD58, MAGE antigens,
B2M, STAT1, MHC1 antigens

↑**Apoptosis or chemotherapy sensitivity**
DAPK1, APAF1, SPARC, TMS1/ASC (PYCARD),
ESR1 (estrogen receptor α), *BNIP3*

Figure 23.2 Concurrent widespread changes in gene expression with epigenetic therapy. Anticancer efficacy of treatment with epigenetic-modulating agents is associated with extensive changes in gene expression that influence several biologic processes. Gene expression is increased through the direct reversal of epigenetic modifications of genomic DNA, whereas for cancer-promoting genes, gene expression is reduced by the regression of their regulatory genes. EMT, epithelial-membrane transition. (Redrawn with permission from Azad N, Zahnow CA, Rudin CM, et al. The future of epigenetic therapy in solid tumours—lessons from the past. *Nat Rev Clin Oncol* 2013;10:256–266.)

repressed by changes in DNA methylation and chromatin modification, can be reactivated by DNA methyltransferase inhibitors and histone deacetylase (HDAC) inhibitors (HDACi), thereby restoring normal cell cycle control, differentiation, and apoptotic signaling (Fig. 23.2).[8,26,28] In general, methylated CpG islands are not capable of the initiation of transcription unless the methylation signal can be overridden by alterations in factors that modulate chromatin, such as the removal of methylated cytosine-binding proteins. However, reversal of DNA methylation with secondary changes in histone modification or directed reversal of repressive histone modifications represent a target for epigenetic therapies.[8,26,28]

Most studies of DNA methylation, particularly in the study of cancer, have focused on CpG island promoter methylation. However, about 40% of human genes do not contain bona fide CpG islands in their promoters.[29] The primary focus on CpG islands has resulted from the clear demonstration that CpG-island promoter methylation permanently silences genes both physiologically and pathologically in mammalian cells. However, recent work has shown correlations between tissue-specific expression and methylation of non-CpG islands, including, for example, the maspin gene,[30] and as mentioned previously, regions near CpG islands,[19,20] suggesting that many additional genes could be regulated, either normally or abnormally, by changes in DNA methylation.

An exciting new area of DNA methylation research involves the role of this change in regulating gene enhancers: small DNA regions that regulate the expression of multiple target genes.[31–33] The presence of DNA methylation in these areas, which can reside considerable distances from the genes that are being regulated, generally works together with histone modifications to mediate a repressive state for that enhancer.[31–33] The status of enhancers is also emerging as important for cancer risk states.[34]

Chromatin in Gene Regulation

Heritable gene silencing involves the interplay between DNA methylation and histone covalent modifications. Complexes of proteins that can regulate how nucleosomes are positioned perform nucleosomal remodeling.[35–37] What was initially termed the *histone code*, with reference to how histones are modified, has emerged to be much more complex than originally envisioned. An explosion of research findings during the last several years now allows for an appreciation of how the epigenome is controlled by a complex interplay between a myriad of posttranslational histone modifications that occur on key amino acid residues of these proteins.[37] Acetylation, deacetylation, methylation, phosphorylation, and other modifications all modify chromatin structure and thereby alter gene expression.[38] Some of the enzymes that catalyze these modifications include HDACs, histone methyltransferases (HMT), and most recently, histone demethylases.[13,14,39,40] These modifications help establish heritable states at the start site of genes, but also at enhancers and other transcribed DNA regions not encoding for canonical genes. The latter areas contain noncoding RNAs (ncRNAs) and micro-RNAs (miRNAs), which play key modulatory roles for overall gene expression and protein patterns that can be altered in cancer.[41–43] Again, much research is being focused on epigenetic changes in these DNA regions, which may be important to cancer development and, potentially, to cancer management.

A link between covalent histone modifications and DNA methylation has been clearly established.[44-46] In this interaction, cytosine methylation attracts methylated DNA-binding proteins and HDACs to methylated CpG sites during chromatin compaction and gene silencing.[46,47] In addition, the DNA methylation binding protein (MBD2) interacts with the nucleosomal remodeling complex (NuRD) and directs the complex to methylated DNA.[48] This complex also binds HDACs and has recently been identified as a central player for the abnormal silencing of genes associated with promoter DNA hypermethylation in cancer.[47] Thus, the three processes of DNA cytosine methylation, histone modification, and nucleosomal remodeling are intimately linked, and alterations in these processes can result in abnormalities of gene expression in cancer-relevant genes.

Enzymes Regulating DNA Methylation and Histone Acetylation

DNA methylation involves the covalent addition of a methyl group to the 5′ position of cytosine. In mammals, three enzymes have been shown to catalyze this transfer of a methyl group from the methyl donor S-adenosylmethionine. Most of the methyltransferase activity present in differentiated cells is derived from the expression of DNMT1.[49] This enzyme is thought to be most important in maintaining DNA methylation patterns following DNA replication and thus is referred to as a maintenance methyltransferase. However, the enzyme does possess the ability to methylate previously unmethylated DNA sequences (de novo activity).[50] In contrast, the other enzymes, DNMT3a and DNMT3b, are efficient at methylating previously unmethylated DNA and thus are considered de novo methyltransferases. Each of these enzymes possesses a similar catalytic site,[51] a fact important for the inhibition of DNMT enzymes by nucleoside analogs, discussed later in this chapter.

DNA methylation is closely associated with changes in the histone modifications. As previously discussed, histone proteins are the central components of the nucleosome, and modifications of the histone tails of core histones are associated with active or repressed chromatin.[52] Although it is beyond the scope of this chapter to fully discuss the complex series of modifications to the histone tails of histone H3 and H4, a few well-characterized modifications should be mentioned that are relevant to therapies designed to target epigenetic abnormalities in cancer. In reference to currently investigated epigenetic therapies, changes in histone acetylation are of importance. Acetylation of histones H3 and H4 at key amino acids is associated with the active chromatin present at the promoters of transcribed genes, whereas the absence of histone acetylation is associated with repressed, silenced genes.[13,14,53] Histone acetyltransferases (HAT) HDACs have opposing functions to maintain the proper level of histone acetylation for gene expression.[13,14,53] HDACs specifically deacetylate the lysine residues of the histone tails, and this deacetylation is associated with condensation of nucleosome positions in what is termed a closed chromatin formation. This scenario is key to transcriptional repression. There are four classes of HDACs.[53] Class I HDACs are characterized by their similarity to the yeast Rpd3 HDAC. In humans, this class of enzymes includes HDAC1, -2, -3, and -8. These HDACs are thought to be ubiquitously expressed in tissue throughout the body. In contrast, class II HDACs are similar to yeast Hda1 and include HDAC4, -5, -6, -7, -9, and -10, and they have a greater degree of tissue specificity. Class III HDACs are similar to yeast Sir2 and are set apart from the other classes by their dependence on nicotinamide adenine dinucleotide (NAD+) as a cofactor. Finally, class IV includes HDAC11.[53]

Of the previously listed HDACs, class I and 2 HDACs have been most closely tied to gene silencing associated with abnormal promoter DNA hypermethylation.[48] These are bound to the nucleosome remodeling complex, NuRD.[48,49] Experimental decreases in NURD, after use of a DNA demethylating agent, can augment reactivation of many abnormally silenced and DNA hypermethylated genes in colon cancer cells.[48] Manipulation of these HDACs is under study in clinical trials, with and without the use of DNA methyltransferase inhibitors, and is discussed later. Another HDAC, SIRT1 in the class III of these proteins, is also involved with gene silencing.[54,55] This deacetylase has been linked to silencing of DNA hypermethylated genes, and blocking its activity can be associated with reactivation of such genes.[55]

Reversal of Layers of Gene Silencing

The interaction between DNA methylation and HDAC activity and repressive chromatin marks in maintaining aberrant silencing of hypermethylated genes in cancer has therapeutic implications for epigenetic therapies. Experimental evidence suggests that DNA methylation functions as a dominant event that stably establishes transcriptional repression. Inhibition of HDAC activity alone, by potent and specific HDACis, does not generally result in the reactivation of aberrantly silenced and densely hypermethylated genes in tumor cells.[56] In contrast, treatment with HDACis can reactivate densely silenced genes if the cells are first treated with demethylating drugs, such as 5-azacitidine.[56] The clinical implications of this observation are discussed in more detail in the following section (Table 23.1).

DNA Methyltransferase Inhibitors

Originally synthesized as cytotoxic antimetabolite drugs in the 1960s,[57] azacytosine nucleosides were recognized as inhibitors of DNA methylation in the early 1980s. The inhibitors 5-azacitidine (5AC) and 2′-deoxy-5-azacytidine induced muscle, fat, and chondrocyte differentiation in mouse embryo cells, in association with a reversal of DNA methylation.[58,59] The incorporation of azacytosine nucleosides into DNA in lieu of cytosine residues was shown to be associated with inhibition of DNMT activity.[59,60] DNMT inhibition requires the incorporation of decitabine triphosphate into DNA. The incorporated azacytosine nucleoside forms an irreversible inactive adduct with DNMT. The sequential reversal of DNA methylation then results when DNA replication proceeds in the absence of active DNMT.[61] The inhibitor 5AC must be phosphorylated and converted to decitabine diphosphate by ribonucleotide reductase before it can be activated through triphosphorylation, whereas decitabine does not require ribonucleotide reductase. The inhibitor 5AC can also be incorporated into RNA. DNMT2, a misnamed protein that is actually an RNA-specific methyltransferase,[62] becomes inhibited, leading to the depletion of methylated tRNA.[60] This may contribute to the inhibition of protein synthesis and is a potential difference between azacitidine and decitabine.[63] The previous DNA methyltransferase inhibitors not only block the catalytic activities of DNMTs, but also trigger degradation of these proteins, especially DNMTs 1 and 3B.[64-68] This latter activity is potentially important for their activities for gene reexpression because each of these two proteins, experimentally, possess transcriptional repression properties independent of their DNA methylation catalytic sites.[69,70]

The azacytosine nucleosides exhibit complex dose–response characteristics. At low concentrations (0.2 to 1 μM), the *epigenetic* activities of these drugs predominate, with dose-dependent reversal of DNA methylation[71,72] and induction of terminal differentiation in some systems.[28,71] As concentrations are increased, DNA damage and apoptosis become more prominent.[28,72] Cell lines with 30-fold resistance to the cytotoxic effects of doxifluridine,

TABLE 23.1

Small Molecules Targeting Epigenetic Abnormalities in Clinical Development

Drug	Class	Target	Dose Range	Schedule	Route of Administration
5-Azacitidine	Nucleoside	DNA methyl-transferase	30–75 mg/m²/d	Daily × 7–14 d/28 d	Subcutaneous or intravenous
2′-Deoxy-5-azacytidine	Nucleoside	DNA methyl-transferase	10–45 mg/m²/d	Daily × 3–5 d/4–6 wk	Intravenous
SG110	Nucleoside	DNA methyl-transferase	Being determined	Being determined	Subcutaneous
Valproic acid	Small chain fatty acid	Histone deacetylase (class I and II)	25–50 mg/kg/d	Daily	Oral or intravenous
Vorinostat	Hydroxamic acid	Histone deacetylase (class I and II)	400–600 mg/d	Divided doses	Oral
Entinostat	Benzamide	Histone deacetylase (class I)	2–8 mg/m²	Weekly	Oral
Belinostat	Hydroxamic acid	Histone deacetylase (class I and II)	600–1,000 mg/m²	Daily × 5/28 d	Intravenous
Romidepsin	Cyclic tetrapeptide	Histone deacetylase (class I and II)	13–18 mg/m²	Weekly	Intravenous
LBH-589	Hydroxamic acid	Histone deacetylase (class I and II)	5–11 mg/m²	Daily × 3	Intravenous
MGCD-0103	Benzamide	Histone deacetylase (class I)	40–125 mg/m²	Twice weekly	Oral
CI-994	Benzamide	Histone deacetylase (class I)	5–8 mg/m²	Daily	Oral

adriamycin, cyclophosphamide (DAC) continue to reverse methylation in response to this nucleoside, suggesting that the methylation reversing and cytotoxic activities of this compound can be separated.[73] The ability of these drugs to inhibit the cell cycle, at least in part through induction of p21$^{WAF1/CIP1}$ expression, complicates the goal of reversing DNA methylation, because the latter requires DNA replication with the azacytosine nucleoside incorporated into the DNA.

The importance of low doses of the two azacytosine nucleosides to achieve a targeted therapeutic effect has been recently explored in a series of laboratory observations. Transient exposure of both leukemia and solid tumor cells to submicromolar doses induce such cells to undergo cellular reprogramming, accompanied by decreases in ability to clone in long-term self-renewal assays and to grow as explants in immune-incompetent mice.[28] These effects occur with partial genome-wide DNA demethylation and changes in gene expression in multiple pathways potentially key for driving tumorigenesis.

The pharmacokinetic properties of the two azacytosine nucleosides are also very important to consider for their clinical use. In this regard, a major potential challenge for their usage is the fact that these drugs are highly unstable in an aqueous solution, resulting in their rapid hydrolysis and resultant inactivation.[74] In clinical practice, the drugs must be administered shortly after reconstitution. The drugs are also metabolized by cytidine deaminase,[74] leading to a short half-life in plasma. When injected subcutaneously, 5AC reaches a maximal plasma concentration at 30 minutes, with a terminal half-life of 1.5 to 2.3 hours.[75,76] At the U.S. Food and Drug Administration (FDA) approved dose of 5AC (75 mg/m² administered subcutaneously daily for 7 days), peak plasma concentrations were 3 to 5 μM, which is well within the range of DNMT inhibitory concentrations.[75,76] Intravenous (IV) administration of the same dose has led to higher peak plasma concentrations (11 μM) with a shorter half-life

(approximately 22 minutes).[75] DAC given over 1 hour IV at 15 to 20 mg/m² produced plasma concentrations of 1.1 to 1.6 μM during the infusion,[77] whereas in a phase 1 study in patients with thoracic malignancies, patients were treated with escalating doses of decitabine for 72-hour IV infusions for two 35-day cycles. The maximum tolerated total dose was 60 to 75 mg/m² with neutropenia as the dose-limiting toxicity. Steady-state plasma concentrations ranged from 25 to 40 nM, which is less than those usually used to induce expression of methylated genes in tissue culture models.[78] An oral formulation of 5AC has also been studied. The oral bioavailability of oral azacitidine ranged from 6% to 20%. Nonetheless, MDS and acute myelogenous leukemia (AML) patients receiving oral azacitidine developed clinical responses similar to patients receiving parenteral azacitidine. Oral azacitidine has also been safely administered on 14-daily and 21-daily schedules repeated monthly. The extended administration of lower daily doses may provide favorable pharmacodynamics of DNA methylation reversal given the need for ongoing cell cycling to effect methylation reversal.[79]

SGI-110 is a dinucleoside that acts as a prodrug for decitabine. This drug is being studied in myelodysplasia and AML.[80]

HISTONE DEACETYLASE INHIBITORS

The increasing recognition of the critical importance of histone modifications in regulating the transcriptional permissively of chromatin has led to intense interest in compounds that can inhibit the activity of HDAC proteins, facilitating the acetylation of lysines associated with transcriptional activation of genes. As with the DNMT inhibitors discussed previously, there are multiple, sometimes dose-dependent, effects of HDACis in preclinical studies. Some of these may truly be epigenetic, others strictly cytotoxic, and others a combination of both.[9,81–84] Some actions of HDACis may relate to altering how chromatin is central to the repair of DNA. Thus, at especially high doses, these compounds can blunt efficient repair and even induce DNA breaks.[84,85] These effects may underlie cell cycle arrest and induction of cell death as is often observed in preclinical studies of HDACis.[81–84]

Perhaps novel uses of these drugs may be inferred by results from recent studies suggesting they could be extremely powerful epigenetic therapy agents when used in proper doses, for targeted purposes, and at key time intervals. Recent studies by Settleman and colleagues[86] suggest that histone acetylation changes, and thus epigenetic mechanisms, could be a key factor for cancer therapy resistance to both targeted therapy agents and conventional chemotherapy. The mechanisms involved may involve the emergence of drug-tolerant stem-like cells.[86] In such cells, gene expression studies suggest that a protein upregulated in resistance is a histone demethylase, which diminishes a key histone modification for active transcription, H3K4methyl.[86] A very similar enzyme has been shown in other studies to be central to self-renewal of stem-like melanoma cells.[87] Key to the therapies under discussion is that, in the previous drug-resistance studies, low doses of HDACis, could reversibly reduce drug-resistant cells induced by the various anticancer drugs.[86] It is essential going forward to sort out which of these effects are dose-related off-target effects and which are desired on-target effects that can be optimized for efficacious therapy strategies.

Types of Histone Deacetylase Inhibitors

Small Chain Fatty Acids

The earliest report of the use of an HDACi to treat leukemia described the treatment of a child with refractory AML with intravenous sodium butyrate, with a concomitant clearance of peripheral blood blast cells and a decrement in bone marrow blasts.[88] No responses developed in a subsequent study of nine AML patients who were treated with intravenous butyrate.[89] Phase 1 studies of sodium phenylbutyrate (NaPB) in MDS and AML explored 7-day continuous infusions administered monthly or biweekly, and 21-day continuous infusions administered monthly.[90,91] At the maximum tolerated dose (375 mg per kilogram per day), the mean steady-state plasma concentration was 0.3 mM, within the range of HDAC inhibition.[90–92] Isolated patients developed hematologic improvement in response to NaPB.

Similar to NaPB, valproic acid (VPA) requires near millimolar concentrations to effectively inhibit HDACs. Of 18 patients with MDS or AML with trilineage dysplasia treated with VPA to target plasma concentrations of 0.3 to 0.7 mM, 6 patients developed hematologic improvement.[93] Of 20 elderly patients with AML treated with VPA, only 11 could remain in control long enough to be considered evaluable for response. Five had improvement in platelet counts.[94] VPA induced hematologic improvement in combination with all-transretinoic acid in two of eight patients treated with AML; a fluorescence in situ hybridization analysis showed definitive evidence of terminal differentiation of the malignant cells.[95] A larger study of this combination induced hematologic response in only 2 of 26 elderly patients with AML.[96] It appears unlikely that the small chain fatty acids will develop an important role in the treatment of malignancy given the availability of HDACis with vastly greater potency.

Hydroxamic Acids

The FDA approved vorinostat as the first commercially available HDACi. The approval was based on activity of this agent in cutaneous T-cell lymphoma (CTCL). Thirty-three patients with a median number of five prior systemic therapy regimens received one of three dose schedules of vorinostat in a single institution study.[97] Eight patients achieved a partial response, with a median time to response of 12 weeks and a median duration of response of 15 weeks. Overall, 45% of patients had relief of pruritus. Fatigue, diarrhea, nausea, and thrombocytopenia were common toxicities. In a multicenter phase 2 trial, 74 patients with relapsed or refractory CTCL were treated with 400 mg daily.[98] Similar to the prior study, 29% of patients responded, consisting almost entirely of partial responses. Median time to response was 56 days, and median duration of response was greater than 6 months. In phase 1 trials, responses to vorinostat have developed in other non-Hodgkin's and Hodgkin's lymphoma cases.[99] More recently, in a trial combining vorinostat with carboplatin and paclitaxel in patients with untreated, advanced, non–small-cell lung cancer (NSCLC), response rates increased significantly from 12.5% to 34%, and a trend to improved progression-free survival and overall survival was observed.[100]

Panobinostat (LBH589), a cinnamic hydroxamic acid HDACi, reduced peripheral blood blast percentage but did not induce remissions in a phase 1 trial of daily times 7 oral dosing in patients with a variety of relapsed hematologic malignancies.[101] Asymptomatic changes in electrocardiographic T waves developed in 80% of treated patients. Gastrointestinal symptoms and thrombocytopenia were common. Panobinostat has recently been approved by the FDA for the treatment of multiple myeloma.[102]

Cyclic Tetrapeptides

Romidepsin is FDA approved for the treatment of CTCL[103] and peripheral T-cell lymphoma.[104,105] Antitumor activity, including tumor lysis syndrome, was demonstrated in a phase 1 study that enrolled patients with chronic lymphocytic leukemia and AML, but no complete or partial remissions were seen.[75] The administration of romidepsin induces electrocardiographic changes, including T-wave flattening and ST-T wave depression in greater than half of the posttreatment tracings; however, no changes in serum cardiac troponin levels or left ventricular ejection fraction have been reported.[106]

Benzamides

Entinostat, formerly known as MS-275, was administered weekly times four to patients with relapsed and refractory AML in a phase 1 study. Infections, unsteady gate, and somnolence were dose-limiting toxicities. No clinical responses developed, although improvements in neutrophil counts were observed.[107] Entinostat did not increase the response rate in patients with higher risk MDS and AML with MDS-related changes when combined with azacitidine compared to azacitidine alone.[108] Most recently, however, studies NSCLC suggest that entinostat could be a valuable therapeutic agent in solid tumors when used with established therapies. When combined with the epidermal growth factor inhibitor erlotinib, in a randomized phase 2 trial for patients with recurrent advanced NSCLC, entinostat was not efficacious alone but appeared to combine with erlotinib to benefit a group of patients whose tumors contained baseline high E-cadherin levels. Overall survival in these latter patients yielded an increased survival benefit of 9.4 versus 5.4 months.[109] Finally, entinostat significantly increased survival when combined with an aromatase inhibitor in a phase 2 trial for patients with breast cancer.[110]

Pharmacodynamic Properties

The administration of oral vorinostat was associated with a transient increase in acetylation of histone H3 in peripheral blood lymphocytes, which peaked at 2 hours post dosing and reverted to baseline by 8 hours; similar changes were observed in the lymph node of a treated patient with lymphoma.[99] Treatment with vorinostat was associated with translocation of phosphorylated signal transducer and activator of transcription 3 (STAT-3) from nucleus to cytoplasm in responding patients and with reduced microvessel density.[97]

Similar changes in the acetylation of histones 2B and 3 were observed in peripheral blood cells from patients treated with LBH589.[101] Romidepsin induced acetylation of H3 and H4 in peripheral blood tumor cells within 4 hours of dosing[111]; of interest, p21$^{WAF1/CIP1}$ protein levels also increased, associated with an increase in acetylation of H4 at the p21 promoter (using chromatin immunoprecipitation). Treatment with entinostat led to increased acetylation of H3 and H4 in both peripheral blood and bone marrow. This increase was detectable within 8 hours and remained above baseline throughout the treatment cycle. Thus, this compound may provide the most prolonged inhibition of protein deacetylation of HDACis and is under current investigation.[107] Increases in p21$^{WAF1/CIP1}$ and activation of caspase 3 were also demonstrated in these samples.

EPIGENETIC THERAPY FOR HEMATOLOGIC MALIGNANCIES

DNA Methyltransferase Inhibitors

Epigenetic therapy has seen the most widespread use to date and achieved the greatest efficacy in hematologic malignancies. The therapeutic efficacy of 5AC and DAC for patients with the chronic myeloid neoplasm myelodysplasia (MDS) and AML has been well reviewed.[26,27] Their FDA approval for MDS/AML emerged only after doses were reduced, with resultant diminishing toxicities for patients. The successful development of 5AC for the treatment of MDS can be credited largely to Silverman et al.[25,112,114] in the Cancer and Leukemia Group B (CALGB). The inhibitor 5AC had successfully induced the expression of hemoglobin F in patients with sickle cell anemia.[25,112] Viewing this compound as a potential inducer of terminal differentiation, Silverman et al. conducted a series of phase 2 trials of 5AC administered as a continuous intravenous infusion or as subcutaneous injections for the treatment of MDS.[113,114] Based on significant hematologic responses, the group performed a phase 2 trial (CALGB 9221) in which patients with low- and high-risk MDS with significant hematopoietic compromise were randomly assigned to receive subcutaneous 5AC (75 mg/m^2 per day daily for 7 days, repeated on a 28-day cycle) or observation. Patients on the observation arm with progressive disease could cross over to receive 5AC. This study firmly established the ability of 5AC to induce hematologic improvement, and, less frequently, complete and partial responses.[113,115] The median time to development of AML (defined by 30% bone marrow blast cells) or death was greater in the 5AC arm by 9 months (21 versus 12 months); of note, the observation arm included patients who subsequently crossed over to 5AC treatment.

In a subsequent phase 3 trial (AZA001),[116] patients with higher risk myelodysplastic syndromes were randomly assigned one-to-one to receive 5AC (75 mg/m^2 per day for 7 days every 28 days) or conventional care (best supportive care, low-dose cytarabine, or intensive chemotherapy as selected by investigators before randomization). Three hundred fifty-eight patients were randomly assigned to receive 5AC (n = 179) or conventional care regimens (n = 179). After a median follow-up of 21.1 months (interquartile range [IQR] 15.1 to 26.9), median overall survival was 24.5 months (9.9 not reached) for the azacitidine group versus 15.0 months (5.6 to 24.1) for the conventional care group (hazard ratio [HR] 0.58; 95% confidence interval [CI], 0.43 to 0.77; p = 0.0001). At 2 years, on the basis of Kaplan-Meier estimates, 50.8% (95% CI, 42.1 to 58.8) of patients in the 5AC group were

alive compared with 26.2% (95% CI, 18.7 to 34.3) in the conventional care group (p < 0.0001). Median time to AML transformation was 17.8 months (IQR 8.6 to 36.8; 95% CI, 13.6 to 23.6) in the 5AC group compared with 11.5 months (4.9 not reached; 8.3 to 14.5) in the conventional care group (HR 0.50; 95% CI, 0.35 to 0.70; p < 0.0001). Subsequent unplanned analyses of AZA001 included an examination of elderly patients with what would now be classified as AML (blast count 20% to 30%). In these 113 patients, there remains a statistically significant improvement in survival of 24.5 months versus 16.0 months (HR 0.47; 95% CI; p = 0.0001).[117]

The early development of decitabine in MDS took place primarily in Europe under the leadership of Wijermans et al.[118,119] These investigators pursued intravenous scheduling of decitabine administered three times daily for 3 days (45 mg/m^2 per day total dose). This cycle was repeated every 6 weeks. Phase 2 studies suggested a response rate of approximately 50% in MDS patients. In a randomized trial of DAC versus observation, patients with International Prognostic Score risk categories intermediate 1 to high received the previously listed schedule of decitabine or observation. No crossover was allowed in this trial. Response rates reported were: complete response: 9%, partial response: 8%, and hematologic improvement: 13%.[120] A 10% induction death rate occurred, suggesting that this schedule of DAC may be more toxic than the CALGB schedule of 5AC (1% induction mortality). DAC has also been investigated in low-dose daily intravenous dosing[121] and in daily-times-five schedules. The latter appears convenient and well tolerated. A daily-times-five schedule (20 mg/m^2 per day) has been FDA approved[121]; 99 patients with MDS (de novo or secondary) of any French-American-British (FAB) subtype and an International Prognostic Scoring System (IPSS) score equal to or greater than 0.5 were treated, with an overall response rate of 32% (17 complete responses [CR] plus 15 marrow CRs [mCR]).[122] Among patients who improved, 82% demonstrated responses by the end of cycle two. This well-tolerated regimen allows outpatient administration and, as noted previously, provides plasma levels of decitabine that inhibit DNMTs.

The 3-day intravenous schedule of DAC has been studied in two randomized trials compared to supportive care in patients with higher risk MDS. The first trial confirmed the hematologic activity of decitabine in this patient population but failed to show an improvement in survival in the DAC-treated patients.[123] Survival was also not increased in the subsequent trial, performed by the European Organization for Research and Treatment of Cancer (EORTC).[124] The failure of the randomized decitabine trials to show a survival benefit may be partially due to study design. Both randomized trials of 5AC continued treatment until disease progression for patients who did not achieve complete remission; in fact, this meant that most patients received maintenance therapy. In contrast, both randomized trials of decitabine allowed a maximum of eight cycles of treatment. The need for maintenance therapy in patients treated with DNMT inhibitors has not been tested in prospective randomized trials. An additional difference in the conduct of the two sets of DNMT inhibitor trials involves the duration of therapy administered. The median number of cycles of treatment administered in the two randomized trials of decitabine was three, compared to nine in the azacytidine trials. This may reflect greater toxicity of the originally 3-day schedule of decitabine compared to that of the approved schedule of 5AC. Although the differences in survival may reflect differences in trial design and trial conduct, emerging data suggests that despite similarities in methylation reversal, the two drugs differ in other potentially important biologic parameters, which may contribute to clinical outcomes.[62,63,125]

Two randomized phase 3 trials have been published treating elderly AML patients (greater than 20% blasts) with decitabine, both demonstrating improvement in survival that was not statistically significant. In the European study, 233 patients received either

DAC at 15 mg/m^2 × 9 doses over 3 days on 42-day cycles or best supportive care. The patients received a median of 4 cycles (0 to 9), and the overall survival was improved in the decitabine-treated patients, but did not reach statistical significance (median overall survival [OS], 10.1 versus 8.5 months, respectively; HR, 0.88; 95% CI, 0.66 to 1.17; two-sided, log-rank p = 0.38).[126] In the M.D. Anderson Cancer Center–led multicenter trial,[127] 485 patients 65 years or older were randomly assigned to receive decitabine 20 mg/m^2 per day as a 1-hour intravenous infusion for 5 consecutive days every 4 weeks or best supportive care or low-dose cytarabine (20 mg/m^2 per day for 10 days every 4 weeks). There was a similar improvement in OS with decitabine (7.7 months; 95% CI, 6.2 to 9.2) versus the control group (5.0 months; 95% CI, 4.3 to 6.3; p = 0.108; HR, 0.85; 95% CI, 0.69 to 1.04).[127]

The azacytosine nucleosides require prolonged administration to demonstrate hematologic improvement in MDS. Median time to development of first clinical response in the CALGB studies of 5AC was three cycles; 90% of responses developed by cycle six.[114] In the phase 3 trial of decitabine, the median time to response was two cycles,[123] as also seen in the alternative regimen of decitabine.[122] It is, therefore, extremely important when treating patients with azacytosine nucleosides to commit to administering between four and six cycles of therapy before determining whether a patient is responding to treatment. Furthermore, survival benefit is seen even in patients not showing bone marrow improvement for 5AC, perhaps related to decreased transfusion requirements or delayed progression to AML.[116]

Because AML in the context of MDS is arbitrarily defined based on marrow blast count, activity of the azanucleoside analogs in AML should not be surprising. In CALGB 9221, 20 patients were reclassified upon central pathology review as meeting criteria for AML (greater than 30% blasts). Their outcomes were comparable to the overall population in the study.[115] In all three CALGB studies among patients meeting current World Health Organization (WHO) criteria for AML (greater than 20% blasts), a complete response was achieved in 9% and hematologic improvement in 26%.[114] A retrospective review of 20 patients with AML, including 8 patients with bone marrow blasts greater than 29% treated with 5AC, reported a complete remission in 4 patients, a partial response in 5, and a hematologic improvement in 3. The median duration of response was 8 months (range: 3 to 33 months).[128] DAC induced a complete hematologic response in 2 of 20 patients treated who had the blastic phase of chronic myeloid leukemia.[129] These studies suggest activity of the azacytosine nucleosides in the treatment of a subset of AML patients. Current studies do not allow for the determination of whether this subset is limited to MDS-associated AML (AML with MDS-related changes), which tends to have low white blood cell counts and have a low proliferative rate, or whether these compounds are also active for those with AML without a history of antecedent hematologic disorder. Several reports describe the sensitivity MDS and AML, characterized by abnormalities of chromosome 7 and associated with poor outcomes in response to cytarabine-based therapy to azanucleosides. In one nonrandomized retrospective study, survival of such patients following the administration of DNMT inhibitors surpassed survival in response to conventional cytotoxic chemotherapy, similar to the outcomes of AZA001.[130–132]

Although the mechanisms underlying the clinical activity of azacytosine analogs may involve reversal of gene methylation, other actions need to be considered. The administration of DAC has been shown to induce transient decrements of methylation in noncoding regions, including long interspersed nuclear element (LINE) and ALU elements.[133] Early studies that examined methylation reversal of the target gene p15^{INK4B} in response to DAC showed no correlation between methylation reversal and clinical response.[134,135] Clinical responders to DAC developed significantly higher expression of this gene following treatment, and certainly key biologic roles for this gene and its low basal expression are probable. Moreover, in one study, the clinical response was closely associated with the reversal of methylation of p15 or CDH-1 during the first cycle of treatment with 5AC followed by the HDACi NaPB.[25] In that study, it was noteworthy that the administration of 5AC prior to the addition of an HDACi was associated with the induction of histone acetylation. Although the mechanism underlying this activity is unknown, histone acetylation has been observed following DNA damage due to gamma irradiation.[136] Subsequent studies have found demethylation following treatment with either DAC or 5AC[137–140] but not consistently associated with response.[137,138,140] More work will be required to answer the important mechanistic question underpinning the clinical activity of azacytosine analogs.

Combining Inhibitors in the Treatment of Hematologic Malignancies

It is almost certain that the biggest promise of epigenetic therapy lies in strategies to combine existing and newer drugs with each other and with current chemotherapies and targeted therapies. To date, the example for existing agents is the combination of DNMT inhibitors and HDAC inhibitors based on the hypothesis from the laboratory that this paradigm leads to optimal reexpression of transcriptionally silenced genes with promoter methylation.[56,141] This in vitro treatment paradigm has led to a variety of clinical studies that have attempted to apply this concept to the treatment of hematologic malignancies. Much remains to be determined with regard to its efficacy and precisely what determines this. The first study of sequential DNMT/HDAC inhibitors administered a variety of doses of 5AC for 5 to 14 days followed by 7 days of NaPB by continuous infusion at its maximum tolerated dose to patients with MDS and AML.[25] The combination was well tolerated, and clinical responses were frequent in patients receiving 5AC at 50 mg/m^2 per day daily for 10 days and 25 mg/m^2 per day daily for 14 days, with 5 of 14 patients at those dose schedules achieving complete or partial response.

In a pilot study, 10 patients with MDS or AML were treated with 5AC at 75 mg/m^2 per day daily times seven followed by 5 days of NaPB given at 200 mg per kilogram per day as a 1- to 2-hour infusion. Three patients developed a partial response.[142]

In a similar study, investigators at the M.D. Anderson Cancer Center treated leukemic patients with decitabine (15 mg/m^2 per day IV daily times 10) and concomitant VPA at a variety of doses. Of 54 patients, 12 achieved complete remission or complete remission with incomplete platelet recovery.[143] The inhibitors 5AC, VPA, and all-transretinoic acid have been administered to patients with AML and MDS. Of 33 previously untreated patients, 14 over the age of 60 years developed a complete remission or a complete remission with inadequate platelet recovery.[144] A subsequent study of 5AC and VPA suggests increased efficacy of this combination in high-risk MDS.[145]

Entinostat has been successfully combined with azacytidine in patients with myeloid malignancies.[140] The US Leukemia Intergroup recently completed a randomized phase 2 trial of this combination compared with 5AC alone. In this study, of 149 patients, the primary endpoint of hematologic normalization was statistically similar, with 32% (95% CI, 22% to 44%) of the 5AC group reaching hematologic normalization (HN) versus 27% (95% CI, 17% to 39%) in the AZA + entinostat group. Median overall survivals were 18 months for the AZA group and 13 months for the AZA + entinostat group, but were also not statistically significant.[108] In the latter study, the administration of the combination was associated with less DNA methylation reversal compared to azacitidine monotherapy, likely due to cell cycle inhibitory effects of the HDACi. This highlights the complexity of effectively targeting epigenetic gene regulation.

It remains to be established whether combination therapies are more effective than single-agent demethylating therapies.

Epigenetically Targeted Therapy in Nonhematologic Malignancies

The efficacies that have emerged in the application of epigenetically targeted drugs to hematologic malignancies has spurred interest in using epigenetic therapy for other types of cancer. As outlined as follows, laboratory studies and clinical trials support this approach. Studies in the lab have been directed by lessons learned from therapy in hematologic malignancies, suggesting that low doses of drugs like DAC and 5AC, in the nanomolar range, may avoid excess toxicities due to off-target effects of the drugs and may maximize epigenetic effects of the agents.[28] The desired effects may require minimizing initial cellular cytotoxicity, giving tumor cells time to accrue maximal cellular reprogramming responses to the inhibition of DNMTs.[28] DAC and 5AC are effective only when they have been incorporated into DNA, after which they irreversibly inhibit DNMT catalytic activity and target these proteins for degradation.[64–68] In cell culture and mouse explants, low nanomolar doses appear to induce both human leukemic and solid tumor cells to exhibit blunting of self-renewal and tumorigenic activity of tumor stem-like cells.[28] These preclinical results suggest a key possibility that use of epigenetic therapies might inhibit these latter cell populations, which often are difficult to eradicate and are a factor in resistance to many standard cancer therapies.[146] Exhaustion of such cells over time during therapy with DAC or 5AC might explain the observation that most patients with MDS/AML take several months to reach best response.[147] Leukemic stem cells were not eliminated in one study in MDS and AML patients treated with 5AC in combination with VPA, although their frequency decreased in clinical responders.[148]

Clinical trials for common solid tumors, informed through the previous laboratory studies, have been initiated including phase 2 designs using low-dose strategies with 5AC often combined with use of histone deacetylase inhibitors. Sixty-five patients with advanced, multiply treated NSCLCs were treated with 5AC plus entinostat.[149] Only 3% of patients developed Response Evaluation Criteria (RECIST)-measureable responses; however, these two patients had durable responses, with survival of 3 to 4 years.[149] Upregulation of immunogenic pathways in NSCLC and other solid tumor cells, observed in laboratory studies, suggest a potential for sequencing DNMT inhibitors with immune checkpoint inhibitors.[150] This drug is also reported to induce antitumor responses and immune recognition in a model of pancreatic cancer.[151] Other laboratory results and emerging clinical trials also suggest the promise of combining epigenetic therapy approaches to sensitize cancers other than NSCLC to subsequent therapies. Low-dose DAC appears able to upregulate a key mediator of 5-fluorouracil (5FU) action,

uridine monophosphate (UMP) kinase, in colorectal cancer cell lines.[152] These increases correlated with a reversal of 5FU resistance. Similar to studies discussed previously, DAC plus the HDACi, trichostatin A, decreased marker identified self-renewal populations in ovarian cancer while simultaneously inducing increased sensitivity to cisplatin.[153] In advanced ovarian cancer, 5AC or DAC plus carboplatin have yielded durable responses and induced stable disease in ovarian cancer patients.[154,155] These early results are being extrapolated for verification in larger, ongoing clinical trials.

NEW APROACHES TO EPIGENETIC THERAPY

As we have outlined previously, the emerging promise for epigenetic therapy and the future of the approaches may lie in combinatorial drug strategies. Although this is already being explored with older agents, new drugs for new targets are now entering the picture.[9,11,156–158] In these efforts, several themes we have introduced in this chapter will likely dominate.

Most epigenetic therapies will not induce, when used at truly targeting doses, immediate cytotoxic effects. Therapeutic efficacy based on cellular reprogramming may require significant time to manifest. Clinical trial designs may need adaptation so that effective therapies are not discarded due to premature response evaluations. Finally, the ultimate promise for epigenetic therapy may lie with newer drugs now entering clinical trials. Outcomes with DNMT inhibitors may be improved with alternative scheduling of oral azacitidine or through prolonged pharmacokinetics of the decitabine prodrug SGI110.[79] Also, drugs targeting other proteins including BET family bromodomain proteins are generating much excitement.[9,82,156–159] BET inhibitors may interfere with localization of the oncogene C-MYC to acetylated lysines in regulatory regions of target genes.[9,82,156–159] These inhibitors are now entering clinical trials. Other promising approaches include the use of inhibitors of EZH2, the enzyme in the PcG system, which catalyzes the repressive histone mark H3K27me3.[9,82,156–159] Another clinical trial underway employs targeting of the translocation in which the protein mixed lineage leukemia (MLL) is fused with several targets, such as in infant leukemias. These translocations result in abnormal recruitment of the histone methyltransferase, DOT1L, to target genes like HOXA9.[158] This fusion induces hypermethylation of H3K79 and abnormal activation of MLL target genes.[158,160] Very selective inhibitors of DOT1L are now in clinical trials.

Epigenetically targeted therapies continue to hold great promise that reprogramming of malignant cells could alter approaches to cancer management. Strategies to merge older drugs, which we have focused on in this chapter, with the newer agents briefly discussed in this section, will underpin future trials to test this approach.

SELECTED REFERENCES

The full reference list can be accessed at lwwhealthlibrary.com/oncology.

4. Herman JG, Baylin SB. Gene silencing in cancer in association with promoter hypermethylation. *N Engl J Med* 2003;349:2042–2054.
5. Jones PA, Baylin SB. The epigenomics of cancer. *Cell* 2007;128:683–692.
7. Esteller M. Cancer epigenomics: DNA methylomes and histone-modification maps. *Nat Rev Genet* 2007;8:286–298.
8. Yoo CB, Jones PA. Epigenetic therapy of cancer: past, present and future. *Nat Rev Drug Discov* 2006;5:37–50.
14. Kouzarides T. Chromatin modifications and their function. *Cell* 2007;128: 693–705.

18. Easwaran H, Johnstone SE, Van Neste L, et al. A DNA hypermethylation module for the stem/progenitor cell signature of cancer. *Genome Res* 2012;22:837–849.
25. Gore SD, Baylin S, Sugar E, et al. Combined DNA methyltransferase and histone deacetylase inhibition in the treatment of myeloid neoplasms. *Cancer Res* 2006;66:6361–6369.
26. Azad N, Zahnow CA, Rudin CM, et al. The future of epigenetic therapy in solid tumours—lessons from the past. *Nat Rev Clin Oncol* 2013;10:256–266.
28. Tsai HC, Li H, Van Neste L, et al. Transient low doses of DNA-demethylating agents exert durable antitumor effects on hematological and epithelial tumor cells. *Cancer Cell* 2012;21:430–446.

38. Jones PA. Functions of DNA methylation: islands, start sites, gene bodies and beyond. *Nat Rev Genet* 2012;13:484–492.

39. Bannister AJ, Kouzarides T. Reversing histone methylation. *Nature* 2005; 436:1103–1106.

40. Bannister AJ, Kouzarides T. Regulation of chromatin by histone modifications. *Cell Res* 2011;21:381–395.

48. Cai Y, Geutjes EJ, de Lint K, et al. The NuRD complex cooperates with DNMTs to maintain silencing of key colorectal tumor suppressor genes. *Oncogene* 2014;33:2157–2168.

49. Bestor TH. Cloning of a mammalian DNA methyltransferase. *Gene* 1998; 74:9–12.

50. Jair KW, Bachman KE, Suzuki H, et al. De novo CpG island methylation in human cancer cells. *Cancer Res* 2006;66:682–692.

52. Jenuwein T, Allis CD. Translating the histone code. *Science* 2001;293: 1074–1080.

55. Pruitt K, Zinn RL, Ohm JE, et al. Inhibition of SIRT1 reactivates silenced cancer genes without loss of promoter DNA hypermethylation. *PLoS Genet* 2006;2:344–352.

56. Cameron EE, Bachman KE, Myohanen S, et al. Synergy of demethylation and histone deacetylase inhibition in the re-expression of genes silenced in cancer. *Nat Genet* 1999;21:103–107.

59. Jones PA, Taylor SM. Hemimethylated duplex DNAs prepared from 5-azacytidine-treated cells. *Nucleic Acids Res* 1981;9:2933–2947.

64. Kelly TK, De Carvalho DD, Jones PA. Epigenetic modifications as therapeutic targets. *Nat Biotechnol* 2010;28:1069–1078.

65. Ferguson AT, Vertino PM, Spitzner JR, et al. Role of estrogen receptor gene demethylation and DNA methyltransferase. DNA adduct formation in 5-aza-2′deoxycytidine-induced cytotoxicity in human breast cancer cells. *J Biol Chem* 1997;272:32260–32266.

66. Gabbara S, Bhagwat AS. The mechanism of inhibition of DNA (cytosine-5-)-methyltransferases by 5-azacytosine is likely to involve methyl transfer to the inhibitor. *Biochem J* 1995;307:87–92.

69. Rountree MR, Bachman KE, Baylin SB. DNMT1 binds HDAC2 and a new co-repressor, DMAP1, to form a complex at replication foci. *Nat Genet* 2000;25:269–277.

70. Bachman KE, Rountree MR, Baylin SB. Dnmt3a and Dnmt3b are transcriptional repressors that exhibit unique localization properties to heterochromatin. *J Biol Chem* 2001;276:32282–32287.

75. Gore SD, Weng LJ, Figg WD, et al. Impact of prolonged infusions of the putative differentiating agent sodium phenylbutyrate on myelodysplastic syndromes and acute myeloid leukemia. *Clin Cancer Res* 2002;8: 963–970.

CANCER THERAPEUTICS

24 Proteasome Inhibitors

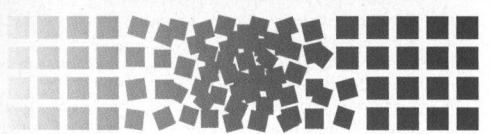

Christopher J. Kirk, Brian B. Tuch, Shirin Arastu-Kapur, and Lawrence H. Boise

BIOCHEMISTRY OF THE UBIQUITIN-PROTEASOME PATHWAY

The ubiquitin proteasome system is involved in the degradation of more than 80% of cellular proteins, including those that control cell-cycle progression, apoptosis, DNA repair, and the stress response.[1] A key step in this process is the *tagging* of proteins targeted for degradation with multiple copies of ubiquitin, a 76–amino acid protein whose primary sequence and structure is highly conserved in organisms ranging from yeasts to mammals.[2,3] Once polyubiquitinated, proteins targeted for degradation bind to the 26S proteasome, a holoenzyme composed of two 19S regulatory complexes capping a central 20S proteolytic core. The 20S core is a hollow "barrel" consisting of four stacked heptameric rings. The subunits of the rings are classified as either β subunits (outer two rings) or β subunits (inner two rings). The 19S regulatory complex consists of a lid that recognizes ubiquitinated protein substrates with high fidelity, and a base that contains six adenosine triphosphatases, unfolds protein substrates, removes the polyubiquitin tag, and threads them into the catalytic chamber of the 20S particle in an adenosine triphosphate–dependent manner.[4,5] Unlike typical proteases, the 20S proteasome in eukaryotic cells contains multiple proteolytic activities resulting in the cleavage of protein targets after many different amino acids. In most cells, the 20S core particle contains the catalytic subunits β5 (PSMB5), β1 (PSMB1), and β2 (PSMB2), accounting for chymotrypsinlike (CT-L), caspaselike (C-L), and trypsinlike (T-L) activities, respectively, each differing in their substrate preference.[6] However, in cells of hematopoietic origin, such as lymphocytes and monocytes, the proteasome catalytic subunits are encoded by homologous gene products: LMP7 (PSMB8), LMP2 (PSMB9), and MECL-1 (PSMB10).[7] These immunoproteasome subunits are also induced in nonhematopoietic cells following exposure to inflammatory cytokines such as interferon-γ (IFN-γ) and tumor necrosis factor alpha (TNF-α).[8] In the immunoproteasome, the 19S regulatory complex can be replaced with proteasome activators such as PA28, whose expression is also induced in cells following exposure to IFN-γ. Hybrid proteasomes, both for the catalytic subunits and regulatory particles, have been described.[9]

Given its key role in maintaining cellular homeostasis, the ubiquitin proteasome system appeared to be an unlikely target for pharmaceutical intervention. However, a variety of groundbreaking studies in the 1990s suggested that inhibitors of proteasome function might prove to be viable therapeutic agents.[10] Initial studies used substrate-related peptide aldehydes to investigate the proteolytic functions and specificity of the proteasome.[11] In vitro and in vivo studies with these inhibitors demonstrated their ability to induce apoptosis as well as inhibit tumor growth.[12–15] It was subsequently discovered that several natural products with antitumor activity exert their action via proteasome inhibition, providing additional rationale for the development of selective proteasome inhibitors (PIs).[16,17]

PROTEASOME INHIBITORS

Chemical Classes of Proteasome Inhibitors in Clinical Development

As of the writing of this overview, six different proteasome inhibitors comprising three distinct chemical classes have been tested in clinical trials (Table 24.1) and include: (1) dipeptide boronic acids, (2) peptide epoxy ketones, and (3) β-lactones.[18,19] Bortezomib (PS-341, Velcade), a dipeptide boronic acid, was developed by Millennium Pharmaceuticals (Cambridge, MA) and was the first PI approved for clinical use.[20] Two additional dipeptide boronic acids have entered clinical development, ixazomib/MLN 9708 (Millennium), currently in phase III studies, and delanzomib/CEP-18770 (Teva Pharmaceuticals; Frazer, PA), the clinical development of which has been halted. Carfilzomib (Onyx Pharmaceuticals; San Francisco, CA), a tetrapeptide epoxy ketone, received U.S. Food and Drug Administration (FDA) approval in 2012.[21] A second peptide epoxy ketone proteasome inhibitor, oprozomib (Onyx), entered clinical study in 2010. The third class of proteasome inhibitors, β-lactones, is represented by NPI-0052 (salinosporamide A [Marizomib]) and is currently being developed by Nereus Pharmaceuticals, Inc. (San Diego, CA). The initial approvals for both bortezomib and carfilzomib were in multiple myeloma (MM), a plasma cell neoplasm and the second most common hematologic cancer. However, the activity of PIs in other B-cell neoplasms has resulted in an expansion of the clinical utilization of this drug class.

Preclinical Activity of Proteasome Inhibitors

Each of the three classes of inhibitors has a distinct chemical mechanism of proteasome inhibition.[22] Peptide boronates form stable but reversible tetrahedral intermediates with the γ-hydroxyl (γ-OH) group of the catalytic N-terminal threonine of the proteasome active sites.[23,24] β-lactones also interact with this γ-OH, but form a completely irreversible interaction.[25] Similarly, peptide epoxy ketones form irreversible covalent adducts with the active site threonine but do so via a dual covalent adduction of γ-OH group and the free amine.[26] This interaction is highly specific for N-terminal threonine-containing hydrolases and renders peptide epoxy ketones the most selective proteasome inhibitors yet described.[27,28]

The primary targets of these PIs within the constitutive and immunoproteasomes are the CT-L subunits, β5 and LMP7, respectively. Despite accounting for less than 50% of total protein turnover by the proteasome, these subunits are essential for cell survival.[29] In MM cell lines, inhibiting both subunits (β5 and LMP7) is necessary and sufficient for tumor cell death.[30] Cytotoxicity of other tumor cell types requires the inhibition of multiple active sites beyond the CT-L activity. The combination of inhibitors specific for either the T-L or C-L activities, which have no cytotoxic activity on their own, augments the cytotoxic potential of the CT-L–specific inhibitors.[31,32]

TABLE 24.1

Proteasome Inhibitors in Clinical Development

Agent	Other Names	Drug Class	Stage of Development	Tumor Types	Route of Administration	Dose Levels	Schedule of Administration
Bortezomib	Velcade PS-341	Peptide boronate	FDA/EMEA approved	Multiple myeloma, mantle cell lymphoma	Intravenous, subcutaneous	1.3 mg/m^2	Days 1, 4, 8, & 11 (21-day cycle)
Ixazomib	MLN 9708 MLN 2238	Peptide boronate	Phase III	Multiple myeloma, AL, amyloidosis	Oral	4 mg	Once weekly (21-day cycle)
Delanzomib	CEP-18770	Peptide boronate	Phase I (discontinued)	Multiple myeloma	Intravenous	0.1–1.8 mg/m^2	Days 1, 4, 8, & 11 (21-day cycle)
Carfilzomib	Kyprolis PR-171	Peptide epoxy ketone	FDA approved, phase III	Multiple myeloma	Intravenous	20/27 mg/m^2	Days 1, 2, 8, 9, 15, & 16 (28-day cycle)
Oprozomib	ONX 0912 PR-047	Peptide epoxy ketone	Phase I/II	Multiple myeloma	Oral	150–240 mg (dose escalation ongoing)	Days 1, 2, 8, & 9 (14-day cycle) Days 1–5 (14-day cycle)
Marizomib	NPI-0052 Salinosporamide A	β-lactone	Phase II	Multiple myeloma	Intravenous	0.075–0.6 mg/m^2	Days 1, 4, 8, & 11 (21-day cycle)

EMEA, European Medicines Agency; AL, amyloid light chain.

Given its status as the first proteasome inhibitor approved for marketed use, the antitumor potential and preclinical activity of other proteasome inhibitors have generally been compared to bortezomib.[19] Carfilzomib showed equivalent antitumor activity to bortezomib in vitro against a panel of tumor cell lines under standard culture conditions but was >10-fold more potent at inducing tumor cell death when cells were exposed to drug for a 1-hour pulse, which mimics the pharmacokinetics of both compounds.[33] MLN2238 (the active agent of ixazomib) was active in the same mouse models of human tumors as bortezomib, but demonstrated greater levels of proteasome inhibition in the tumors.[34] In biochemical assays of proteasome activity, delanzomib had an identical potency and subunit activity profile to bortezomib, but in tumor cytotoxicity assays, potency relative to bortezomib was 2- to 10-fold less.[35] In addition, delanzomib appeared to be less cytotoxic than bortezomib to normal cells and had a differential effect on cytokine release in bone marrow stromal cells, suggesting a different pharmacologic activity. Oprozomib is 10-fold less potent than carfilzomib in proteasome activity assays, but showed similar antitumor activity in mouse tumor models.[36,37] Marizomib displayed greater potency against the non–CT-L active sites of the proteasome than bortezomib.[38] Interestingly, this agent synergized with bortezomib in killing tumor cells in vitro.[39] All of the second-generation inhibitors have shown activity in tumor cells made resistant to bortezomib and/or MM cells isolated from patients relapsed from bortezomib-based therapies[35,36,40–42]

The inhibition of tumor cells with proteasome inhibitors induces cell death via the induction of apoptosis through death effector caspase activation.[10] Although the mechanism underlying the induction of cell death remains to be fully elucidated, extensive research suggests a complex interplay of multiple pathways. PIs have been shown to affect the half-life of the *BH3-only* members of the Bcl-2 family, specifically BH3–interacting-domain death agonist (Bid) and Bcl-2 interacting killer (Bik).[43] Moreover the BH3-only protein NOXA is upregulated at the transcription level by PIs.[44–48] Proteasome inhibition also upregulates the expression of several key cell-cycle checkpoint proteins that include p53 (an inducer of G0/G1 cell-cycle arrest through accumulation of the cyclin-dependent kinase [CDK] inhibitor p27); the CDK inhibitor p21;

mammalian cyclins A, B, D, and E; and transcription factors E2F and Rb.[49,50] The transcription factor nuclear factor kappa B (NF-κB), an important regulator of cell survival and cytokine/growth factor production,[51] is also affected by proteasome inhibition in multiple ways. The net effect on NF-κB signaling is not consistent across various assays and cell lines, and its relative importance in the antitumor effects of PIs remains unclear. Although it is interesting to note that patients whose myeloma harbor NF-κB–activating mutations (~20%) respond better to bortezomib than those without NF-κB–activating mutations.[52–54] In MM cell lines, there is growing evidence that the major determinant of sensitivity to proteasome inhibition is the relative load of protein flux to the proteasome.[55–57] These data suggest that induction of the terminal unfolded protein response may drive cell death. Whether proteotoxic stress induced cell death reflects sensitivity to proteasome inhibitors in other tumor types remains to be determined.

Pharmacokinetics and Pharmacodynamics of Proteasome Inhibitors in Animals

Following intravenous (IV) administration to animals and humans, proteasome activity is inhibited in a dose-dependent fashion within minutes; however, PIs such as bortezomib and carfilzomib are also rapidly cleared from circulation.[55,56,58–61] Recovery of proteasome activity in animals occurs in tissues with a half-life of approximately 24 hours, mirroring the recovery time of cells exposed to sublethal concentrations of PIs in vitro and likely reflecting new protein synthesis.[33,62]

PROTEASOME INHIBITORS IN CANCER

Clinical Activity of Bortezomib

Bortezomib is typically administered on days 1, 4, 8, and 11 of a 3-week cycle either as an IV bolus or subcutaneous administration. Increasing doses of bortezomib inhibit proteasome activity in blood in a dose-dependent fashion, reaching a maximum of 74% inhibition at a dose of 1.38 mg/m^2. Daily dosing schedules in animal studies have been associated with severe toxicity and have not been attempted in humans. In clinical trials, thrombocytopenia and peripheral neuropathy (PN) were common adverse events.[20,63,64] Bortezomib has shown remarkable single-agent antitumor activity in a wide range of B-cell neoplasms, including MM, non Hodgkin lymphoma (NHL), and Waldenström macroglobulinemia (WM). In 2003, bortezomib was approved by the FDA for use as a single agent for the treatment of patients with MM following two prior therapies and who demonstrated disease progression with their most recent therapy. The primary efficacy data for this approval was derived from the SUMMIT trial in which 202 patients with heavily pretreated disease were treated with bortezomib at 1.3 mg/m^2.[65] In this trial, the overall response rate (ORR), defined as patients achieving at least a 50% reduction in serum or urine levels of the myeloma M protein, was 35%. This clinical trial was supported by the CREST trial, in which the activity of 1.3 mg/m^2 dose was determined to be superior to a dose of 1.0 mg/m^2.[66] Bortezomib is also active as a single agent in earlier stage MM patient populations. A single-agent ORR of 38%, with a 6% complete response (CR) rate, was seen in the phase III APEX study in early relapsed MM, with a time to progression (TTP) of 6.2 months and a median duration of response of 8 months.[67] In this study, the major grade 3 and 4 toxicities were PN, 12%; dysesthesia and related symptoms, 8% to 10%; anemia, 8%; diarrhea, 8%; neutropenia, 14%; and fatigue, 12%. In the frontline setting, bortezomib demonstrated a single-agent response rate of 41% (5% CR rate).[68]

Bortezomib is also approved for newly diagnosed MM in combination with velcade, melphalan and prednisone (VMP). The phase III VISTA trial evaluated VMP in patients with untreated MM who were ineligible for high-dose therapy.[69] The addition of bortezomib to the melphalan prednisone (MP) backbone significantly improved response rates in this setting with an ORR of 71% for VMP (including 30% CR) versus 35% (with only 4% CR) for MP.[52] VMP was associated with a TTP of ~24 months, compared with ~16.6 months with MP. After a 5-year follow-up, there was a 31% reduced risk of death for the VMP group versus MP-treated patients.[70]

Bortezomib has also shown promise when combined with other agents in relapsed and refractory MM patients. The combination of bortezomib with pegylated doxorubicin (Doxil, Centocor Ortho Biotech Products, L.P.; Horsham, PA) resulted in an ORR of 79% in relapsed patients, and toxicities were similar to those observed with each agent administered separately.[71] A phase III study in 646 patients with relapsed and refractory MM compared this treatment with bortezomib alone; the combination produced a 44% ORR and extended the TTP from 6 to 9.3 months.[72,73] The combination of bortezomib with revlimid, lenalidomide and dexamethasone (Rd), a standard of care in the treatment of MM, resulted in an ORR of 64% and a median duration of response of 8.7 months.[74] This activity is striking given that 53% of patients had received prior bortezomib and 75% of patients had received prior thalidomide, a closely related analog of lenalidomide. Other agents tested in combination with bortezomib include vorinostat, the anti-CS1 mAb, elotuzumab, the Hsp90 inhibitor tanespimycin, and the Akt inhibitor perifosine.[75]

Frontline combinations with bortezomib in MM patients have shown high ORRs with a notable improvement in CR rates. In longer term studies, CR rates with bortezomib-based combinations have been shown to be associated with improved clinical outcomes.[63,64] A community-based phase IIIb study evaluating bortezomib + dexamethasone (VD) versus bortezomib + thalidomide + dexamethasone (VTD) versus VMP found similar ORR (60%, 70%, and 52%, respectively) and CR rates (13%, 18%, and 15%, respectively).[63] Bortezomib + melphalan + prednisone + thalidomide (VMPT) followed by bortezomib + thalidomide (VT) maintenance resulted in a superior CR rate compared with VMP with no maintenance (34% versus 21%) and improved 2-year progression-free survival (70% versus 58.2%).[64] A protocol modification in this trial involved changing from twice weekly

to weekly bortezomib administration, which yielded similar TTP but reduced the incidence (21% versus 43%) and severity of PN (2% grade 3/4 versus 14%).[64] The bortezomib, lenalidomide, and dexamethasone combination in newly diagnosed MM resulted in a ORR of 100% in 66 patients, 29% of whom achieved a CR.[76]

Bortezomib has also shown activity in other hematologic cancers, most notably mantle cell lymphoma (MCL).[77,78] As a single agent in 155 relapsed and refractory MCL patients, bortezomib yielded an ORR of 33% (8% CR), a median duration of response of 9.2 months, and a TTP of 6.2 months.[78] Toxicities observed were similar to those seen in patients with MM and included thrombocytopenia, PN, and fatigue. When bortezomib was used to treat both newly diagnosed and refractory MCL, a response rate of 46% was observed in both populations,[77] leading to FDA approval late in 2006.

Bortezomib has been tested in a variety of solid tumors in phase I and II studies.[79] Partial responses (PR) were reported in 8% of patients with refractory non–small-cell lung cancer (NSCLC), although the TTP was 1.5 months.[80] Exacerbation of PN was common. Bortezomib was subsequently tested in combination with paclitaxel, irinotecan, and gemcitabine/carboplatin; however, results have not been encouraging. Bortezomib continues to be tested in combination with other agents in a variety of tumor types.[81,82]

Recent clinical activity and preclinical data suggest that proteasome inhibition may extend to nononcology applications. Single-agent bortezomib therapy in kidney transplant patients undergoing antibody-mediated rejection resulted in a reduction of donor-specific antibodies and improved renal function.[83] In mouse models of lupus nephritis, bortezomib resulted in a reduction of pathogenic plasma cells and the prevention of disease progression.[84] These data suggest that PIs may be useful in a wide range of B-cell–mediated diseases. However, toxicities with bortezomib, particularly PN, may prevent wider application of this particular agent.

Carfilzomib

Parallel phase I studies of carfilzomib have been conducted in patients with multiple tumor types, and two phase I dose-finding studies targeting B-cell malignancies have been completed. The first study used daily IV bolus dosing with doses up to 20 mg/m^2 for 5 consecutive days followed by 9 days of rest and resulted in substantial inhibition of proteasome activity.[85] In the second study, carfilzomib was administered daily for 2 days for 3 consecutive weeks (days 1, 2, 8, 9, 15, and 16), followed by 12 days of recovery.[86] Hematologic toxicities were the most frequent adverse events, observed along with transient, noncumulative elevations in serum creatinine, usually with increases in serum urea nitrogen and consistent with a *prerenal* etiology. New onset PN was infrequent. Among 20 evaluable patients (including bortezomib-refractory patients), 4 PRs and 1 minor response were seen. Responses were also durable, lasting more than 1 year in some cases. Although the maximum tolerated dose of carfilzomib was not established in this study, a dose of 20 mg/m^2 was initially selected for the phase II studies.

Based on the phase I studies, an open-label, single-arm, phase II study of single-agent carfilzomib in relapsed and refractory MM was initiated in 2007.[87,88] Carfilzomib was administered as an IV bolus on the twice-weekly dose schedule. Patients enrolled in the initial phase of the study (003-A0) had received a median of five prior therapies, and 78% of patients had grade 1/2 PN at entry.[87] Among 39 evaluable patients in 003-A0, 10 (26%) achieved a minor response or better, including 5 PRs, and 16 additional patients with stable disease. Based on new safety information from phase I studies, the protocol was amended and the carfilzomib dose was escalated to 27 mg/m^2 after the first cycle (003-A1).[89] In this trial, 266 patients were enrolled and all patients had previously been treated with an immunomodulatory agent (IMiD) and bortezomib and were refractory to their last therapy. An ORR of 24% with a median duration of response of 8 months was reported. Adverse events were predominantly hematopoietic (thrombocytopenia, lymphopenia, and anemia) and there was a <1% rate of grade 3 PN, despite 77% having a history of PN. Based on these findings, carfilzomib was granted conditional approval by the FDA in 2012 for the treatment of patients with relapsed and refractory myeloma who had received prior bortezomib and IMiD therapy.

The parallel PX-171-004 trial enrolled patients with relapsed MM following one to three prior treatments and who may have been refractory to one or more of these therapies.[90,91] Of the 155 patients enrolled in this trial, 120 had not received prior bortezomib-based therapy. In patients with relapsed disease, non-hematologic and hematologic toxicity profiles were similar. Despite high rates of baseline PN, reports of worsening neuropathic symptoms were infrequent (2% incidence of grade 3 and no grade 4 events). Carfilzomib demonstrated considerable activity in bortezomib-naïve patients, inducing PR or better in 46% of 54 evaluable patients at 20 mg/m^2 and 53% of patients at 27 mg/m^2.[91] The response rate in patients previously exposed to bortezomib was lower (18%).[90] Responses across groups are durable, typically 8 to 9 months.[90,91]

Based on findings in animal studies in which a 30-minute infusion of carfilzomib resulted in reduced toxicities,[61] the effect of infusional administration was tested in patients with relapsed and refractory myeloma. In a dose escalation study, PX-171-007, the MTD dose of carfilzomib was determined to be 56 mg/m^2, more than twice the dose used in the studies described previously. In a cohort of 24 patients receiving this dose and who had received a median of five prior lines of therapy (including two prior bortezomib-containing regimens), the ORR was 60%.[92] This enhanced efficacy also correlated with a greater level of inhibition of all three subunits of the immunoproteasome measured in isolated peripheral blood mononuclear cells (Lee S, et al., unpublished).[93] This same dose and infusion time is currently being explored in a phase III trial of nearly 900 patients comparing carfilzomib plus low-dose dexamethasone (Cd) to bortezomib plus low-dose dexamethasone (Vd) in MM patients with relapsed disease.

Trials of carfilzomib in combination with other agents in MM have been initiated, including a phase Ib/II safety and efficacy study of carfilzomib in combination with lenalidomide and low-dose dexamethasone (CRd) in relapsed and/or refractory MM. At the maximum planned dose, the ORR was 77% with a median duration of response of 22 months.[94] The CRd combination is now being tested in an international, multicenter, randomized, open-label phase III study in comparison with lenalidomide and low-dose dexamethasone (Rd) in approximately 780 patients with relapsed MM following one to three prior therapies. The CRd regimen has also been explored in newly diagnosed MM patients.[95] When carfilzomib is combined with Rd at a dose of 36 mg/m^2, 62% of the 53 patients treated achieved a CR. In addition, 20 of 21 patients analyzed for signs of minimal residual disease (MRD), utilizing multiparameter flow cytometry were determined to be free of MRD.

Ixazomib

Initial clinical studies of ixazomib involved dose escalation studies in patients with hematologic malignancies and explored both weekly and twice weekly dosing schedules.[96,97] Oral administration resulted in potent proteasome inhibition of ~65%. Clinical activity in patients with relapsed MM was 16%.[98] In patients with newly diagnosed MM, ixazomib plus lenalidomide and low-dose dexamethasone resulted in an ORR of 93% with 24% achieving a CR.[99] This combination is also being investigated in a phase III trial comparing this to Rd in patients with relapsed MM.

Oprozomib

Initial clinical testing of oprozomib in patients with solid tumors investigated a dosing schedule consisting of a 14-day cycle with once daily administration for 5 consecutive days.[100] In patients with relapsed and/or refractory B-cell neoplasms, two dosing schedules are being utilized: the schedule described previously and one involving 2 consecutive days of dosing repeated weekly.[101] Proteasome inhibition following the administration of oprozomib reached >80% and clinical activity was noted in patients with MM and WM. In patients receiving the 5 consecutive day schedule, 5 of 19 MM patients (26%) and 8 of 10 WM patients (80%) achieved a partial response or better. Exploration of the dose and schedule continues as a single agent and in combination with other anti-MM therapies.

Biomarkers for Proteasome Inhibitors

As described previously, PI-based therapies have proven highly effective in the treatment of MM and other B-cell neoplasms. Given that response rates in single-agent trials are generally <50%, there would be a distinct clinical benefit to identify those patients most likely to respond to proteasome inhibition prior to treatment initiation. Gene expression analysis from bone marrow–derived MM tumor cells from 169 bortezomib-treated patients and 70 dexamethasone-treated patients revealed a 100-gene signature that provided a stratification for patients likely to respond that performed better than standard staging systems.[102] However, this signature provided only a modest increase in predictive power for treatment with bortezomib versus dexamethasone. More recently, Keats et al.[54] reanalyzed this dataset based on a pathway analysis of NF-κB and the realization that TRAF3, a key regulatory of the noncanonical NF-κB pathway, is a tumor suppressor in MM cell lines. They found a dramatic enrichment for response to bortezomib in patients with low levels of TRAF3 expression. However, these data remain to be validated in a separate sample set. A transcriptomic analysis of samples derived from single-agent carfilzomib trials suggest that patients with the highest level of immunoglobulin heavy chain expression were the most sensitive to carfilzomib therapy.[103] Similar findings were noted in the expression data from bortezomib-treated patients described previously.[103] These data are supported by phenotypic data from patients progressing on bortezomib-based therapy, in which resistance to bortezomib was associated with a dedifferentiated (and lower immunoglobulin expressing) B-cell phenotype.[104] Taken together, these findings suggest that biomarkers, potentially those involving an analysis of protein load of immunoglobulin expression, may be developed to predict those patients most likely to respond to PIs.

SELECTED REFERENCES

The full reference list can be accessed at lwwhealthlibrary.com/oncology.

1. Ciechanover A. Intracellular protein degradation: from a vague idea thru the lysosome and the ubiquitin-proteasome system and onto human diseases and drug targeting. *Biochim Biophys Acta* 2012;1824:3–13.
3. Wilkinson KD. Ubiquitination and deubiquitination: targeting of proteins for degradation by the proteasome. *Semin Cell Dev Biol* 2000;11:141–148.
5. Groll M, Ditzel L, Lowe J, et al. Structure of 20S proteasome from yeast at 2.4 A resolution. *Nature* 1997;386:463–471.
8. Griffin TA, Nandi D, Cruz M, et al. Immunoproteasome assembly: cooperative incorporation of interferon gamma (IFN-gamma)-inducible subunits. *J Exp Med* 1998;187:97–104.
10. Adams J. The proteasome: a suitable antineoplastic target. *Nat Rev Cancer* 2004;4:349–360.

11. Vinitsky A, Michaud C, Powers JC, et al. Inhibition of the chymotrypsin-like activity of the pituitary multicatalytic proteinase complex. *Biochemistry* 1992;31:9421–9428.

12. Orlowski RZ, Eswara JR, Lafond-Walker A, et al. Tumor growth inhibition induced in a murine model of human Burkitt's lymphoma by a proteasome inhibitor. *Cancer Res* 1998;58:4342–4348.

16. Meng L, Mohan R, Kwok BH, et al. Epoxomicin, a potent and selective proteasome inhibitor, exhibits in vivo antiinflammatory activity. *Proc Natl Acad Sci U S A* 1999;96:10403–10408.

20. Bross PF, Kane R, Farrell AT, et al. Approval summary for bortezomib for injection in the treatment of multiple myeloma. *Clin Cancer Res* 2004;10:3954–3964.

21. Herndon TM, Deisseroth A, Kaminskas E, et al. U.S. Food and Drug Administration approval: carfilzomib for the treatment of multiple myeloma. *Clin Cancer Res* 2013;19:4559–4563.

23. Adams J, Behnke M, Chen S, et al. Potent and selective inhibitors of the proteasome: dipeptidyl boronic acids. *Bioorg Med Chem Lett* 1998;8:333–338.

27. Kisselev AF, van der Linden WA, Overkleeft HS. Proteasome inhibitors: an expanding army attacking a unique target. *Chem Biol* 2012;19:99–115.

28. Arastu-Kapur S, Anderl JL, Kraus M, et al. Nonproteasomal targets of the proteasome inhibitors bortezomib and carfilzomib: a link to clinical adverse events. *Clin Cancer Res* 2011;17:2734–2743.

30. Parlati F, Lee SJ, Aujay M, et al. Carfilzomib can induce tumor cell death through selective inhibition of the chymotrypsin-like activity of the proteasome. *Blood* 2009;114:3439–3447.

31. Britton M, Lucas MM, Downey SL, et al. Selective inhibitor of proteasome's caspase-like sites sensitizes cells to specific inhibition of chymotrypsin-like sites. *Chem Biol* 2009;16:1278–1289.

33. Demo SD, Kirk CJ, Aujay MA, et al. Antitumor activity of PR-171, a novel irreversible inhibitor of the proteasome. *Cancer Res* 2007;67:6383–6391.

34. Kupperman E, Lee EC, Cao Y, et al. Evaluation of the proteasome inhibitor MLN9708 in preclinical models of human cancer. *Cancer Res* 2010;70:1970–1980.

36. Chauhan D, Singh AV, Aujay M, et al. A novel orally active proteasome inhibitor ONX 0912 triggers in vitro and in vivo cytotoxicity in multiple myeloma. *Blood* 2010;116:4906–4915.

38. Chauhan D, Catley L, Li G, et al. A novel orally active proteasome inhibitor induces apoptosis in multiple myeloma cells with mechanisms distinct from Bortezomib. *Cancer Cell* 2005;8:407–419.

40. Chauhan D, Tian Z, Zhou B, et al. In vitro and in vivo selective antitumor activity of a novel orally bioavailable proteasome inhibitor MLN9708 against multiple myeloma cells. *Clin Cancer Res* 2011;17:5311–5321.

41. Kuhn DJ, Chen Q, Voorhees PM, et al. Potent activity of carfilzomib, a novel, irreversible inhibitor of the ubiquitin-proteasome pathway, against preclinical models of multiple myeloma. *Blood* 2007;110:3281–3290.

44. Fernandez Y, Verhaegen M, Miller TP, et al. Differential regulation of noxa in normal melanocytes and melanoma cells by proteasome inhibition: therapeutic implications. *Cancer Res* 2005;65:6294–6304.

48. Mannava S, Zhuang D, Nair JR, et al. KLF9 is a novel transcriptional regulator of bortezomib- and LBH589-induced apoptosis in multiple myeloma correlation. *Blood* 2012;119:1450–1458.

49. Koepp DM, Harper JW, Elledge SJ. How the cyclin became a cyclin: regulated proteolysis in the cell cycle. *Cell* 1999;97:431–434.

53. Chapman MA, Lawrence MS, Keats JJ, et al. Initial genome sequencing and analysis of multiple myeloma. *Nature* 2011;471:467–472.

54. Keats JJ, Fonseca R, Chesi M, et al. Promiscuous mutations activate the noncanonical NF-kappaB pathway in multiple myeloma. *Cancer Cell* 2007;12:131–144.

56. Obeng EA, Carlson LM, Gutman DM, et al. Proteasome inhibitors induce a terminal unfolded protein response in multiple myeloma cells. *Blood* 2006;107:4907–4916.

57. Shabaneh TB, Downey SL, Goddard AL, et al. Molecular basis of differential sensitivity of myeloma cells to clinically relevant bolus treatment with bortezomib. *PLoS One* 2013;8:e56132.

59. Papandreou CN, Daliani DD, Nix D, et al. Phase I trial of the proteasome inhibitor bortezomib in patients with advanced solid tumors with observations in androgen-independent prostate cancer. *J Clin Oncol* 2004;22:2108–2121.

60. Wang Z, Yang J, Kirk C, et al. Clinical pharmacokinetics, metabolism, and drug-drug interaction of carfilzomib. *Drug Metab Dispos* 2013;41:230–237.

62. Meiners S, Heyken D, Weller A, et al. Inhibition of proteasome activity induces concerted expression of proteasome genes and de novo formation of mammalian proteasomes. *J Biol Chem* 2003;278:21517–21525.

63. Lonial S, Waller EK, Richardson PG, et al. Risk factors and kinetics of thrombocytopenia associated with bortezomib for relapsed, refractory multiple myeloma. *Blood* 2005;106:3777–3784.

64. Richardson PG, Briemberg H, Jagannath S, et al. Frequency, characteristics, and reversibility of peripheral neuropathy during treatment of advanced multiple myeloma with bortezomib. *J Clin Oncol* 2006;24:3113–3120.

65. Richardson PG, Barlogie B, Berenson J, et al. A phase 2 study of bortezomib in relapsed, refractory myeloma. *N Engl J Med* 2003;348:2609–2617.

67. Richardson PG, Sonneveld P, Schuster MW, et al. Bortezomib or high-dose dexamethasone for relapsed multiple myeloma. *N Engl J Med* 2005;352:2487–2498.

69. San Miguel JF, Schlag R, Khuageva NK, et al. Bortezomib plus melphalan and prednisone for initial treatment of multiple myeloma. *N Engl J Med* 2008;359:906–917.

76. Richardson PG, Weller E, Lonial S, et al. Lenalidomide, bortezomib, and dexamethasone combination therapy in patients with newly diagnosed multiple myeloma. *Blood* 2010;116:679–686.

78. Fisher RI, Bernstein SH, Kahl BS, et al. Multicenter phase II study of bortezomib in patients with relapsed or refractory mantle cell lymphoma. *J Clin Oncol* 2006;24:4867–4874.

79. Milano A, Iaffaioli RV, Caponigro F. The proteasome: a worthwhile target for the treatment of solid tumours? *Eur J Cancer* 2007;43:1125–1133.

84. Neubert K, Meister S, Moser K, et al. The proteasome inhibitor bortezomib depletes plasma cells and protects mice with lupus-like disease from nephritis. *Nat Med* 2008;14:748–755.

88. Siegel DS, Martin T, Wang M, et al. A phase 2 study of single-agent carfilzomib (PX-171-003-A1) in patients with relapsed and refractory multiple myeloma. *Blood* 2012;120:2817–2825.

91. Vij R, Wang M, Kaufman JL, et al. An open-label, single-arm, phase 2 (PX-171-004) study of single-agent carfilzomib in bortezomib-naive patients with relapsed and/or refractory multiple myeloma. *Blood* 2012;119:5661–5670.

95. Jakubowiak AJ, Dytfeld D, Griffith KA, et al. A phase 1/2 study of carfilzomib in combination with lenalidomide and low-dose dexamethasone as a frontline treatment for multiple myeloma. *Blood* 2012;120:1801–1809.

102. Mulligan G, Mitsiades C, Bryant B, et al. Gene expression profiling and correlation with outcome in clinical trials of the proteasome inhibitor bortezomib. *Blood* 2007;109:3177–3188.

103. Loehr A, Degenhardt JD, Kwei KA, et al. Immunoglobulin expression is a major determinant of patient sensitivity to proteasome inhibitors. *Blood* 2013;122:1903.

25 Poly (ADP-ribose) Polymerase Inhibitors

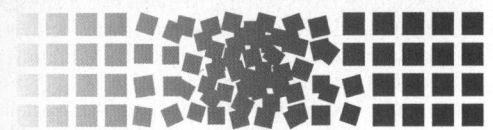

Alan Ashworth

INTRODUCTION

Cancer cells may harbor defects in DNA repair pathways leading to genomic instability. This can foster tumorigenesis but also provides a weakness that can be exploited therapeutically. Tumors with compromised ability to repair double-strand DNA breaks by homologous recombination, including those with defects in the *BRCA1* and *BRCA2* genes, are highly sensitive to blockade of the repair of DNA single-strand breaks, via the inhibition of the enzyme poly(ADP-ribose) (PARP). This provides the basis for a *synthetic lethal* approach to cancer therapy, which is showing considerable promise in the clinic.

CELLULAR DNA REPAIR PATHWAYS

DNA is continually damaged by environmental exposures and endogenous activities, such as DNA replication and cellular free-radical generation, which cause diverse lesions including base modifications, double-strand breaks (DSB), single-strand breaks (SSB), and intrastrand and interstrand cross-links.[1] These aberrations are repaired by distinct repair pathways, which are coordinated to maintain the stability and integrity of the genome. This faithful repair of DNA damage is an essential prerequisite for the maintenance of genomic integrity and cellular and organismal viability. Where one DNA strand is affected and the intact complementary strand is available as a template, the base-excision repair (BER), nucleotide-excision repair, or mismatch repair pathways are used and these pathways are highly efficient at repairing damage. DSBs, more problematic than SSBs because the complementary strand is not available as a template, are repaired by the homologous recombination (HR) or nonhomologous end-joining (NHEJ) pathways.[1]

Endogenous base damage, including SSBs, is the most common DNA aberration and it has been estimated that the average cell may repair 10,000 such lesions every day. BER is an important pathway for the repair of SSBs and involves the sensing of the lesion followed by the recruitment of a number of other proteins. PARP-1 (poly[ADP]ribose polymerase) is a critical component of the major "short-patch" BER pathway. PARP is an enzyme, discovered over 40 years ago,[2] that produces large branched chains of poly(ADP) ribose (PAR) from NAD$^+$. In humans, there are 17 members of the PARP gene family but most of these are poorly characterized.[3,4] The abundant nuclear protein PARP-1 senses and binds to DNA nicks and breaks, resulting in activation of catalytic activity causing poly(ADP)ribosylation of PARP-1 itself as well as other acceptor proteins including histones. This modification may signal the recruitment of other components of DNA repair pathways as well as modify their activity. The highly negatively charged PAR that is produced around the site of damage may also serve as an antirecombinogenic factor. In addition to the BER pathway PARP enzymes have been implicated in numerous cellular pathways.[3,4]

Two main DSB repair pathways are available within eukaryotic cells: NHEJ and HR.[5,6] HR can be further subdivided into the gene conversion (GC) and single-strand annealing (SSA) subpathways.[1]

Both GC and SSA rely on sequence homology for repair whereas NHEJ uses no, or little, homology.[2,3] NHEJ is the most important pathway for the repair of DSBs during G_0, G_1, and early S phases of the cell cycle, although it is likely active throughout the cell cycle.[7,8] This form of DSB repair usually results in changes in DNA sequence at the break site and, occasionally, in the joining of previously unlinked DNA molecules, potentially resulting in gross chromosomal rearrangements such as translocations.[9] GC uses a homologous sequence, preferably the sister chromatid, as a template to resynthesize the DNA surrounding the DSB, and therefore generally results in accurate repair of the break. Repair by GC is critically dependent on the recombinase function of RAD51 and is facilitated by a number of other proteins. SSA also involves the use of homologous sequences for the repair of DSBs, but unlike GC, SSA is RAD51-independent and involves the annealing of DNA strands formed after resection at the DSB. The detailed mechanism of SSA is still obscure but it frequently results in the loss of one of the homologous sequences and deletion of the intervening sequence.[9] SSA is a potentially important pathway of mutagenesis because a significant fraction of mammalian genomes consist of repetitive elements. GC and SSA are cell-cycle regulated and are most active in S-G_2 phases of the cell cycle.[10]

THE DEVELOPMENT OF PARP INHIBITORS

PARP inhibitors were originally developed as chemopotentiators, which are agents that enhance the effects of DNA damage—a common mechanism of action of drugs used to treat cancer. The rationale was that inhibition of the repair of chemotherapy-induced DNA damage might give greater efficacy. Early studies using relatively nonspecific PARP inhibitors such as 3-aminobenzamide, demonstrated potential synergy with alkylating agents.[11] Subsequent studies with more potent PARP inhibitors demonstrated synergy with temozolomide, an observation that was taken into a clinical trial with AG014699,[12] a PARP inhibitor developed by Pfizer. This agent is now being developed by Clovis. Although the major focus of this chapter is the use of PARP inhibitors in synthetic lethal therapeutic strategies, their use in chemopotentiation in combination with chemotherapy remains under active investigation, as described later.

BRCA1 AND *BRCA2* MUTATIONS AND DNA REPAIR

Heterozygous germline mutations in the *BRCA1* and *BRCA2* genes confer a high risk of breast (up to 85% lifetime risk) and ovarian (10% to 40%) cancer in addition to a significantly increased risk of pancreatic, prostate, and male breast cancer.[13] The genes have been classified as tumor suppressors, because the wild-type *BRCA* allele is frequently lost in tumors, a phenomenon that occurs by a variety of mechanisms. The *BRCA1* and *BRCA2* genes encode large proteins that likely function in multiple cellular pathways, including transcription, cell-cycle regulation, and the maintenance of genome integrity. However, the roles of BRCA1 and BRCA2 in DNA repair have been best documented.[14]

BRCA1- and BRCA2-deficient cells are highly sensitive to ionizing radiation and display chromosomal instability, which is likely to be a direct consequence of unrepaired DNA damage.[14] The similar genomic instability in BRCA1- and BRCA2-deficient cells and the interaction of both BRCA1 and BRCA2 with RAD51 suggested a functional link between the three proteins in the RAD51-mediated DNA damage repair process. However, although BRCA2 is directly involved in RAD51-mediated repair, affecting the choice between GC and SSA, BRCA1 acts upstream of these pathways[15]; both GC and SSA are reduced in BRCA1-deficient cells, placing BRCA1 before the branch point of GC and SSA.[15]

BRCA1 has a role in signaling DNA damage and cell-cycle checkpoint regulation,[14,15] whereas BRCA2 has a more direct role in DNA repair itself. BRCA2 is thought to promote genomic stability through a role in the error-free repair of DSBs by GC via association with RAD51. Aberrations in BRCA2-deficient cells arise at least in part by the use of the SSA pathway. NHEJ, however, is apparently unaffected in BRCA2-deficient cells.[14,15] Loss of BRCA2, therefore, results in the repair of DSBs by preferential utilization of an error-prone mechanism, which potentially explains the apparent chromosome instability associated with BRCA2 deficiency.[15]

The physical interaction between BRCA2 and RAD51 is essential for error-free DSB repair. BRCA2 is required for the localization of RAD51 to sites of DNA damage, where RAD51 forms the nucleoprotein filament required for recombination. The foci of the RAD51 protein are apparent in the nucleus after certain forms of DNA damage and these likely represent sites of repair by HR; BRCA2-deficient cells do not form RAD51 foci in response to DNA damage.[15] Two different domains within BRCA2 interact with RAD51, the eight BRC repeats in the central part of the protein and a distinct domain, TR2, at the C-terminus.[16]

PARP-1 INHIBITION AS A SYNTHETIC LETHAL THERAPEUTIC STRATEGY FOR THE TREATMENT OF BRCA-DEFICIENT CANCERS

Synthetic lethality is defined as the situation when a mutation in either of two genes individually has no effect, but combining the mutations leads to death.[17] This effect was first described and studied in genetically tractable organisms such as *Drosophila* and yeast.[17,18] This effect can arise because of a number of different gene–gene interactions. Examples include two genes in separate semiredundant or cooperating pathways, and two genes acting in the same pathway where loss of both critically affects flux through the pathway. The implication is that targeting one of these genes in a cancer where the other is defective should be selectively lethal to the tumor cells but not toxic to the normal cells. In principle, this should lead to a large therapeutic window.[19] The original suggestion that the concept of synthetic lethality could be used in the selection or development of cancer therapeutics came from Hartwell et al.,[18] and from experiments performed in yeast. Synthetic lethal screens have now been performed in a number of model organisms[20] and in human cells,[21] and these have revealed multiple potential gene–gene interactions, some of which could be exploited clinically. However, synthetic lethal therapies have not been clinically used until recently, when evidence has been provided for PARP-1 inhibition as a potential synthetic lethal approach for the treatment of BRCA-mutation–associated cancers.

PARP-1 inhibition causes failure of the repair of SSB lesions but does not affect DSB repair.[22] However, a persistent DNA SSB encountered by a DNA replication fork will cause stalling of the fork and may result in either fork collapse or the formation of a DSB.[23] Therefore, the loss of PARP-1 increases the formation of

DNA lesions that might be repaired by GC. As a loss of function of either BRCA1 or BRCA2 impairs GC,[14,15] a loss of PARP-1 function in a BRCA1- or BRCA2-defective background could result in the generation of replication-associated DNA lesions normally repaired by sister chromatid exchange. If so, this might lead to cell-cycle arrest and/or cell death. Therefore, PARP inhibitors could be selectively lethal to cells lacking functional BRCA1 or BRCA2 but might be minimally toxic to normal cells. This would indicate a synthetic lethal interaction between PARP and BRCA1 or BRCA2. Exemplifying this principle, potent inhibitors of PARP were applied to cells deficient in either BRCA1 or BRCA2. Cell survival assays showed that cell lines lacking wild-type BRCA1 or BRCA2 were extremely sensitive to these agents compared with heterozygous mutant or wild-type cells.[24,25]

To explain these observations, a model was proposed whereby persistent single-strand gaps in DNA caused by PARP inhibition when encountered by a replication fork might trigger fork arrest, collapse, and/or a DSB.[26] Alternatively, PARP-1 trapped on DNA by the inhibition of enzyme activity might also cause a fork collapse. Normally, these DSBs would be repaired by RAD51-dependent GC.[14,15] However, in the absence of BRCA1 or BRCA2, the replication fork cannot be restarted and collapses, causing persistent chromatid breaks. When repaired by the alternative error-prone DSB repair mechanisms of SSA or NHEJ, large numbers of chromatid aberrations would be induced, leading to cell lethality.[26] The idea that the defect in GC is being targeted in BRCA-deficient cells is supported by the demonstration that deficiency in other genes implicated in HR also confers sensitivity to PARP inhibitors.[27] This further suggests that this approach may be more widely applicable in the treatment of sporadic cancers with impairments of the HR pathway or BRCAness[28] (see the following).

INITIAL CLINICAL RESULTS TESTING SYNTHETIC LETHALITY OF PARP INHIBITORS AND BRCA MUTATION

Phase I studies[29] established that olaparib (AstraZeneca, London, UK; formerly KU-0059436, KuDOS Pharmaceuticals, Cambridge, UK) could be administered safely as a single agent at a dose of 400 mg twice per day. Side effects were classified as mild and were unlike those typically experienced with cytotoxic chemotherapy. Significant and durable responses were observed in patients with germ-line BRCA1 or BRCA2 mutations and breast ovary or prostate cancer. Of the 19 mutation carriers enrolled, 9 had an objective response defined by Response Evaluation Criteria in Sold Tumors (RECIST) criteria and 12 had stable disease for more than 4 months in duration. A similar magnitude of clinical responses was observed in an expanded cohort.[30] These observations are impressive because the cohort had been heavily pretreated and most were resistant to a wide range of chemotherapies.[29,30]

Phase II studies were subsequently performed in advanced breast and ovarian cancers arising in BRCA1 and BRCA2 mutation carriers.[31,32] The reported response rate was 41% in the breast study and 52% in the ovarian group; both groups had been heavily pretreated. Again, the drug was well tolerated. Another study of BRCA1/2 carriers with ovarian cancer compared olaparib with pegylated liposomal doxorubicin (PLD).[33] There was no significant difference in the response rates, but there were some differences in the patient characteristics and an unexpectedly high rate of response to PLD.

There are also reports of responses to PARP inhibitors in BRCA2 mutation carriers with prostate[34] and pancreatic[35] cancer. A number of other PARP inhibitors are in clinical development (Table 25.1), and some of these have shown efficacy in the treatment of cancers arising in BRCA1 or BRCA2 mutation carriers.[36,37]

TABLE 25.1

PARP Inhibitors in Late Stage Clinical Development

Agent	Company	Phase III Trials
Olaparib	AstraZeneca (formerly KuDOS)	BRCA-mutant ovarian cancer
Niraparib	Tesaro (formerly Merck)	Platinum sensitive ovarian cancer BRCA-mutant breast cancer
Rucaparib	Clovis (formerly Pfizer)	Platinum sensitive ovarian cancer
Veliparib	AbbVie (formerly Abbot)	Undisclosed
BMN673	BioMarin (formerly Lead)	BRCA-mutant breast cancer

Adapted from Garber, K. PARP inhibitors bounce back. *Nat Rev Drug Discov* 2013;12:725–727.

THE USE OF PARP INHIBITORS IN SPORADIC CANCERS

Germline mutations in BRCA1 or BRCA2 are relatively common in hereditary breast and ovarian cancer. However, inactivation of BRCA genes by mutation in sporadic cancers is rare, at least in breast cancer, which may seem to limit the application of PARP inhibitors to a wider range of patients. However, many tumors display features in common with BRCA-deficient tumors, including similar defects in DNA repair due to either epigenetic mutation of BRCA1, such as promoter methylation, or mutation of other components of BRCA-associated pathways.[28] This BRCA-ness may make these tumors also susceptible to PARP inhibition.[28] For example, phosphatase and tensin homolog (PTEN) mutations, which occur with a frequency estimated at 50% to 80% in sporadic tumors,[38] may cause PARP inhibitor sensitivity in preclinical models, possibly because PTEN-null cells display BRCAness phenotypes, such as the inability to efficiently repair certain forms of DNA damage.[39]

Traditional histopathologic methods and, more recently, gene expression profiling approaches have shown the phenotypic overlap between triple-negative breast cancers, basal-like breast cancers, and BRCA1 familial breast cancers.[40,41] In gene expression profiling studies, it has been observed that BRCA1 familial cancers strongly segregate with basal-like tumors and share features such as high-grade and pushing margins.[28,40,41] Although the overlap is not absolute, it leads to the hypothesis that there may be a subset of sporadic breast cancers that exhibits features of BRCAness, including deficiencies in HR and that may be susceptible to treatment with drugs such as PARP inhibitors.[26]

There have been several studies of PARP inhibitors in sporadic ovarian cancer. A study by Lederman[42] showed in a maintenance study following the response to platinum therapy a significant benefit in terms of progression-free survival (PFS) of olaparib compared to placebo. This was even more pronounced when the subgroup of BRCA mutation carriers were examined.[43] In both cases, the overall survival (OS) advantage was less than the PFS, but in the case of the BRCA mutation group, this reached statistical significance. Gelmon[44] also showed activity in sporadic ovarian cancer. In contrast, a study in sporadic triple-negative breast cancer failed to observe any benefit, although the study was small and the patients were heavily pretreated.[44]

Iniparib (initially reported as a PARP inhibitor) showed an overall survival benefit in a Phase II trial of triple-negative breast cancer in combination with gemcitabine and carboplatin compared with chemotherapy alone.[45] However, a subsequent Phase III study showed no improvement in PFS.[45] The reasons for this are uncertain, but significant questions have been raised about whether iniparib is indeed a bona fide PARP inhibitor. Therefore, it is now generally conceded that studies of iniparib have no implications for PARP inhibitors as a drug class.[46]

Which population of patients lacking a BRCA1 or BRCA2 mutation might benefit from PARP inhibitors remains unclear. This is likely to require the development of a clinical test to identify prospectively tumors with intrinsic sensitivity. Presently, most efforts are directed at developing assays of DNA repair deficiency.[47]

MECHANISMS OF RESISTANCE TO PARP INHIBITORS

Resistance to targeted therapy frequently occurs, but it was unclear how resistance might arise to a synthetic lethal therapy.[48] Potential mechanisms of resistance to PARP inhibitors have, however, been elucidated both directly in vitro, in mouse models, and in the clinic.[48] An in vitro model for resistance was developed by producing cells from the highly PARP inhibitor–sensitive BRCA2-deficient cell line CAPAN1, which carries a c.6174delT BRCA2 frameshift mutation. CAPAN1 cells cannot form damage-induced RAD51 foci, are defective for HR, and are extremely sensitive to treatment with PARP inhibitors.[49] PARP inhibitor–resistant clones were highly resistant (over 1,000-fold) to the drug and were also cross-resistant to the DNA cross-linking agent cisplatin, but not to the microtubule-stabilizing drug docetaxel. PARP inhibitors and cisplatin both exert their effects on BRCA-deficient cells by increasing the frequency of misrepaired DSBs in the absence of effective HR. Therefore, this observation indicates that the resistance of PARP inhibitor–resistant clones to PARP inhibitors might be because of restored HR. This contention was supported by the acquisition in PARP inhibitor–resistant clone cells of the ability to form RAD51 foci after PARP inhibitor treatment or exposure to irradiation.

DNA sequencing of PARP inhibitor–resistant clones revealed the unexpected presence of novel BRCA2 alleles that resulted in the elimination of the c.6174delT mutation and restoration of an open reading frame.[49] Therefore, in this case, resistance arises because of gain of function mutations in the synthetic lethal partner (BRCA2) rather than the direct drug target (PARP). Alternative mechanisms of PARP inhibitor resistance have also been described.[48] A mouse model of BRCA1-associated mammary gland cancer demonstrated the efficacy of olaparib in vivo and was used to study mechanisms of resistance.[50] Resistance seemed to be caused by the upregulation of ABCB1a/b, which encode P-glycoprotein pumps; this effect could be reversed with the P-glycoprotein inhibitor tariquidar. In addition, other alterations in DNA repair pathways have been proposed to compensate for BRCA1 deficiency resulting in PARP inhibitor deficiency.[48]

Studies of the mechanisms of resistance to PARP inhibitors in patient material are still at an early stage. Initial studies addressed the mechanism of resistance to platinum salts in BRCA mutation carriers. Cisplatin and carboplatin are part of the standard of care for the treatment of ovarian cancer, including individuals with BRCA1 or BRCA2 mutations. Platinum salts are thought to exert their BRCA-selective effects by a similar mechanism to PARP inhibitors.[15] Clinical observations suggest that BRCA mutation carriers with ovarian cancer usually respond better to these agents than patients without BRCA mutations[51,52]; however, resistance does eventually occur. To investigate this effect, BRCA1 and BRCA2 have been sequenced in tumor material from mutation carriers.[49,53] These studies revealed mutations in BRCA1 or BRCA2 that restored the open reading frame and likely contributed to platinum resistance. These observations suggest that specific mutations in BRCA1 or BRCA2 and sensitivity to therapeutics in cell lines and patients can be suppressed by intragenic deletion. Presumably, these mutations occur randomly and are then selected for by differential drug sensitivity. Therefore, the best use of these agents is likely to be earlier in the disease process when the disease burden is smaller, which will reduce the probability of resistance based on stochastic genetic reversion. Recently, similar observations of revertant *BRCA* alleles were made in two patients who became resistant after an initial response to olaparib.[54] Although preliminary, these results suggest that this mechanism is responsible for at least some of the clinical resistance observed. Doubtless, as with other targeted therapies, multiple resistance mechanisms will be implicated as further patients are studied.[48]

PROSPECTS

Currently, the treatments for cancers arising in carriers of *BRCA1* or *BRCA2* mutations are the same as those that occur sporadically matched for tumor pathology and age of onset. However, tumors in *BRCA1* or *BRCA2* mutation carriers lack wild-type *BRCA1* or *BRCA2*, but normal tissues retain a single wild-type copy of the relevant gene. This is a potentially targetable alteration that provides the basis for new mechanism-based approaches to the treatment of cancer. The biochemical difference in capacity to carry out HR between the tumor and normal tissues, in a *BRCA1* or

BRCA2 carrier, provides the rationale for this approach. Inhibiting the DNA repair protein PARP results in the generation of specific DNA lesions that require BRCA1 and BRCA2 specialized repair function(s) for their removal. Preclinical data indicate that tumors defective in wild-type BRCA1 or BRCA2 could be much more sensitive to PARP inhibition than unaffected heterozygous tissues, providing a potentially large therapeutic window. The safety and efficacy of this approach is currently being tested in clinical trials, which, if successful, may lead to registration for routine clinical use of one or more PARP inhibitors.[37]

Synthetic lethality by combinatorial targeting of DNA repair pathways may have usefulness as a therapeutic approach beyond familial cancers. The majority of solid tumors also exhibit genomic instability and aneuploidy. This suggests that pathways involved in the maintenance of genomic stability are dysfunctional in a significant proportion of neoplastic disorders.[47] Understanding which specialized DNA damage response and repair pathways are abrogated in sporadic tumor subtypes may allow for the development of therapies that target the residual repair pathways on which the cancer, but not normal tissue, is now completely dependent. These potential therapies may significantly improve response rates while causing fewer treatment-related toxicities. However, these approaches may be associated with mechanism-associated resistance, and careful consideration of their optimal use will be required.

SELECTED REFERENCES

The full reference list can be accessed at lwwhealthlibrary.com/oncology.

1. Hoeijmakers JH. Genome maintenance mechanisms for preventing cancer. *Nature* 2001;411:366–374.
2. Chambon P, Weill JD, Mandel P. Nicotinamide mononucleotide activation of new DNA-dependent polyadenylic acid synthesizing nuclear enzyme. *Biochem Biophys Res Commun* 1963;11:39–43.
11. Durkacz BW, Omidiji O, Gray DA, et al. (ADP-ribose)n participates in DNA excision repair. *Nature* 1980;283(5747):593–596.
13. Wooster R, Weber BL. Breast and ovarian cancer. *N Engl J Med* 2003;348:2339–2347.
17. Dobzhansky T. Genetics of natural populations: Xiii. Recombination and variability in populations of *Drosophila pseudoobscura*. *Genetics* 1946;31:269–290.
18. Hartwell LH, Szankasi P, Roberts CJ, et al. Integrating genetic approaches into the discovery of anticancer drugs. *Science* 1997;278:1064–1068.
19. Kaelin WG Jr. The concept of synthetic lethality in the context of anticancer therapy. *Nat Rev Cancer* 2005;5:689–698.
21. Iorns E, Lord CJ, Turner N, et al. Utilizing RNA interference to enhance cancer drug discovery. *Nat Rev Drug Discov* 2007;6:556–568.
24. Farmer H, McCabe N, Lord CJ, et al. Targeting the DNA repair defect in BRCA mutant cells as a therapeutic strategy. *Nature* 2005;434:917–921.
25. Bryant HE, Schultz N, Thomas HD, et al. Specific killing of BRCA2-deficient tumours with inhibitors of poly(ADP-ribose) polymerase. *Nature* 2005;434:913–917.
26. Ashworth A. A synthetic lethal therapeutic approach: PARP inhibitors for the treatment of cancers deficient in double-strand break repair. *J Clin Oncol* 2008;26:3785–3790.
27. McCabe N, Turner NC, Lord CJ, et al. Deficiency in the repair of DNA damage by homologous recombination and sensitivity to poly(ADP-ribose) polymerase inhibition. *Cancer Res* 2006;66:8109–8115.
28. Turner N, Tutt A, Ashworth A. Hallmarks of 'BRCAness' in sporadic cancers. *Nat Rev Cancer* 2004;4:814–819.
29. Fong PC, Boss DS, Yap TA, et al. Inhibition of poly(ADP-ribose) polymerase in tumors from BRCA mutation carriers. *N Engl J Med* 2009;361:123–134.
30. Fong PC, Yap TA, Boss DS, et al. Poly(ADP)-ribose polymerase (PARP) inhibition: frequent durable responses in BRCA carrier ovarian cancer correlating with platinum-free interval. *J Clin Oncol* 2010;28:2512–2519.
31. Audeh MW, Carmichael J, Penson RT, et al. Oral poly(ADP-ribose) polymerase inhibitor olaparib in patients with *BRCA1* or *BRCA2* mutations and recurrent ovarian cancer: a proof-of-concept trial. *Lancet* 2010;376:245–251.
32. Tutt A, Robson M, Garber JE, et al. Oral poly(ADP-ribose) polymerase inhibitor olaparib in patients with *BRCA1* or *BRCA2* mutations and advanced breast cancer: a proof-of-concept trial. *Lancet* 2010;376:235–244.
42. Ledermann J, Harter P, Gourley C, et al. Olaparib maintenance therapy in platinum-sensitive relapsed ovarian cancer. *N Engl J Med* 2012;366;1382–1392.
43. Ledermann JA, Harter P, Gourley C. Olaparib maintenance therapy in patients with platinum-sensitive relapsed serous ovarian cancer (SOC) and a BRCA mutation (BRCAm). *J Clin Oncol* 2013;31 (suppl; abstr 5505).
46. Mateo J, Ong M, Tan DS, et al. Appraising iniparib, the PARP inhibitor that never was—what must we learn? *Nat Rev Clin Oncol* 2013;10:688–696.
47. Lord CJ, Ashworth A. The DNA damage response and cancer therapy. *Nature* 2012;481:287–294.
48. Lord CJ, Ashworth A. Mechanisms of resistance to therapies targeting BRCA-mutant cancers. *Nat Med* 2013;19;1381–1388.
49. Edwards S, Brough R, Lord CJ, et al. Resistance to therapy caused by intragenic deletion in BRCA2. *Nature* 2008;451(7182):1111–1115.
53. Sakai W, Swisher EM, Karlan BY, et al. Secondary mutations as a mechanism of cisplatin resistance in BRCA2-mutated cancers. *Nature* 2008;451: 1116–1120.
54. Barber LJ, Sandhu S, Chen L, et al. Secondary mutations in BRCA2 associated with clinical resistance to a PARP inhibitor. *J Pathol* 2013;229:422–429.

26 Miscellaneous Chemotherapeutic Agents

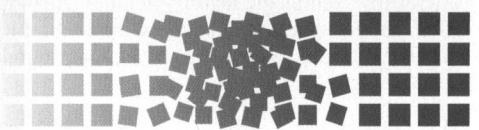

M. Sitki Copur, Scott Nicholas Gettinger, Sarah B. Goldberg, and
Hari A. Deshpande

HOMOHARRINGTONINE AND OMACETAXINE

Homoharringtonine and its congener, harringtonine, are cephalotaxine esters isolated from the evergreen tree *Cephalotaxus hainanensis*, which are distributed throughout southern and northeastern China. The two differ only by a single methylene group, but both have a similar activity against murine leukemia.[1] The primary action of homoharringtonine appears to be the inhibition of protein synthesis and chain elongation through binding to 80S ribosome in eukaryotic cells.[2] DNA effects may also be important, involving a block in progression of cells from G1 phase into S phase and from G2 phase into M phase.[3] Homoharringtonine exhibits a triphasic plasma decay with a terminal half-life of 65.3 hours and apparent volume of distribution of 2.4 L/kg.[4] In early phase I studies, homoharringtonine was administered as a 10 to 360 minute infusion daily for 10 days.[5] Dose-limiting cardiovascular toxicity with hypotension began 4 or more hours after drug administration, which was alleviated by interrupting the infusion or by fluid administration and prolonging the duration of administration. Initial clinical studies with homoharringtonine in China showed activity against acute myeloid leukemia (AML) and chronic phase chronic myeloid leukemia (CML).[6] Variable activity was observed in the initial series of phase II trials in pediatric and adult patients with acute leukemia. In early studies of homoharringtonine, a continuous intravenous (IV) infusion at 2.5 mg/m^2 per day for 10 to 14 days per month induced complete hematologic and cytogenetic responses in 72% and 31% of patients, respectively, with chronic phase CML.[7]

The greater availability of homoharringtonine led to its further testing and the development of a semisynthetic cephalotaxine ester, omacetaxine mepesuccinate.[2] The mechanism of action of omacetaxine includes inhibition of protein synthesis and is independent of direct Bcr-Abl binding. In vitro, it reduces protein levels of the Bcr-Abl oncoprotein and Mcl-1, an antiapoptotic B-cell lymphoma 2 (Bcl-2) family member. The antileukemic effect of omacetaxine is not affected by the presence of mutations in Bcr-Abl.[8] Omacetaxine is absorbed following subcutaneous administration of 1.25 mg/m^2 twice daily for 11 days with a mean half-life of 6 hours, and a volume of distribution of 141 +/−93.4 L. A phase 2 trial assessed the efficacy of omacetaxine in CML patients with T315I and tyrosine–kinase inhibitor failure. Patients received subcutaneous omacetaxine 1.25 mg/m^2 twice daily on days 1 through 14, every 28 days until hematologic response or a maximum of 6 cycles, and then days 1 through 7 every 28 days as maintenance. Complete hematologic response was achieved in 77%, with a median response duration of 9.1 months. Of patients, 23% achieved a major cytogenetic response, including a complete cytogenetic response in 16%. Hematologic toxicity included thrombocytopenia (76%), neutropenia (44%), and anemia (39%) and was typically manageable by dose reduction. Nonhematologic adverse events were mostly grade 1/2 and included infection, diarrhea, and nausea.[9]

L-ASPARAGINASE

L-Asparaginase (L-asparagine aminohydrolase, EC 3.5.1.1), which catalyzes the hydrolysis of the essential amino acid L-asparagine to L-aspartic acid and ammonia, is a naturally occurring enzyme in some microorganisms.[10,11] Although cancer cells depend on an exogenous source of L-asparagine for survival, normal cells can synthesize asparagine. In addition to the depletion of L-asparagine, it may exert its antitumor activity through a glutaminase effect, depleting essential glutamine stores and leading to the inhibition of DNA biosynthesis. It comes in three preparations, two of which are native forms purified from bacterial sources, *Escherichia coli* and *Erwinia carotovora*. A third preparation, pegylated (PEG)-L-asparaginase, is a chemically modified form of the enzyme in which native *E. coli* L-asparaginase has been covalently conjugated to polyethylene glycol.[12]

After an intramuscular (IM) injection, peak plasma levels, approximately one-half of those achieved with IV administration, are reached within 14 to 24 hours. Plasma protein binding is 30%. The pharmacokinetics vary depending on the source of the enzyme.[13] Pharmacokinetic studies in newly diagnosed children with acute lymphocytic leukemia (ALL) have shown peak serum concentrations in the range of 1 to 10 IU/mL in 24 to 48 hours of a single dose of 2,500 to 25,000 IU/m^2 of the enzyme derived from *E. coli*. After a single dose of 25,000 IU/m^2, peak serum levels are reached within 24 hours. PEG-L-asparaginase, when administered at a dose of 2,500 IU/m^2, achieves peak drug levels at 72 to 96 hours and has a significantly longer half-life (5.7 days) than the *E. coli* L-asparaginase preparation.[13] Clinical trials have demonstrated the efficacy, safety, and tolerability of PEG-L-asparaginase administered intramuscularly, subcutaneously, or intravenously as part of multiagent chemotherapy regimens in the management of newly diagnosed and relapsed pediatric and adult ALL. L-Asparaginase can antagonize antineoplastic effects of methotrexate if given concurrently or immediately before. These two drugs should be administered sequentially at least 24 hours apart. L-Asparaginase has also been shown to inhibit the metabolic clearance of vincristine and can result in increased neurotoxicity. Toxicity is less pronounced if L-asparaginase is administered after vincristine. Hypersensitivity reactions occur in up to 25% of patients as a skin rash and urticaria or serious anaphylactic reactions. The risk increases with repeat exposure, and as a single-agent use without steroids. PEG-L-asparaginase is less immunogenic than the native nonpegylated forms of the enzyme. A number of other side effects are observed that are secondary to the inhibitory effects of L-asparaginase on cellular protein synthesis. Decreased serum levels of insulin, key lipoproteins, and albumin have been reported. L-Asparaginase can cause alterations in thyroid function tests as early as 2 days after an administered dose, possibly secondary to a reduction in the serum levels of thyroxine-binding globulin. Alterations in coagulation parameters with prolonged thrombin time, prothrombin time, and partial thromboplastin time have been observed. Patients treated with L-asparaginase are at an increased risk for bleeding or thromboembolic

CANCER THERAPEUTICS

events.[14] L-Asparaginase is contraindicated in patients with a prior history of pancreatitis, because there is a 10% incidence of acute pancreatitis. Neurologic toxicity includes lethargy, confusion, agitation, hallucinations, and/or coma. In contrast to the other anticancer agents used to treat ALL, myelosuppression is rare.

BLEOMYCIN

Bleomycin is a glycopeptide antibiotic produced by the bacterium *Streptomyces verticillus*. The most active chemotherapeutical forms are bleomycin A_2 and B_2.[15] The effect of bleomycin is cell cycle specific, because its main effects are mediated in the G_2 and M phases of the cell cycle.[16] The exact mechanism for DNA strand scission has been suggested to be due to bleomycin's chelating of metal ions (primarily iron) and producing a pseudoenzyme that reacts with oxygen to produce superoxide- and hydroxide-free radicals, thus cleaving DNA. Alternatively, bleomycin may bind at specific sites in the DNA strand and induce scission by abstracting the hydrogen atom from the base, resulting in strand cleavage as the base undergoes a Criegee-type rearrangement, or bleomycin may form an alkali-labile lesion.[17] Bleomycin is used in the treatment of Hodgkin lymphoma (as a component of the ABVD and BEACOPP regimen), squamous cell carcinomas, and testicular cancer; in the treatment of plantar warts,[18] as a means of effecting pleurodesis,[19] as well as an intralesional agent with electrochemotherapy in the management of cutaneous malignancies.[20]

The oral bioavailability is poor. It must be administered via IV or IM routes. The initial distribution half-life is 10 to 20 minutes with a terminal half-life of 3 hours. Bleomycin can be administered via the intracavitary route to control malignant pleural effusions or ascites, or both. Approximately 45% to 55% of an administered intracavitary dose of bleomycin is absorbed into the systemic circulation. Elimination is primarily via the kidneys, and approximately 60% to 70% of an administered dose is excreted unchanged in the urine. Dose reductions are required if creatinine clearance is less than 25 mL per minute.

Bleomycin-induced pneumonitis, the dose-limiting toxicity of the drug, occurs in 10% of patients, and is dependent on the cumulative dose.[21] The risk increases in patients older than 70 years and in those who receive a total cumulative dose greater than 400 U. In addition, patients with an underlying lung disease, prior irradiation to the chest or mediastinum, and exposure to high concentrations of inspired oxygen are at increased risk. Increased use of granulocyte colony-stimulating factor (G-CSF) has been paralleled by an increased incidence of bleomycin-induced pulmonary toxicity. The exacerbating effects of G-CSFs seem to be associated with a marked infiltration of activated neutrophils along with the lung injury caused by the direct effects of bleomycin.[22,23] In a retrospective review, 18% of a total of 141 patients with Hodgkin lymphoma treated with a bleomycin-containing regimen developed pulmonary toxicity. G-CSF use was one of the key factors associated with the development of this complication, and omission of bleomycin had no impact on clinical outcomes.[24] Similarly the combination of brentuximab vedotin and ABVD was associated with excessive pulmonary toxicity, indicating that brentuximab vedotin and bleomycin should not be used together.[25]

Patients with bleomycin-induced pulmonary toxicity may present with cough, dyspnea, dry inspiratory crackles, and infiltrates on chest radiograph. Pulmonary function testing is the most sensitive approach to monitor patients, and pulmonary function tests should be obtained at baseline and before each cycle of therapy, with a specific focus on the carbon monoxide diffusion capacity and vital capacity. A decrease greater than 15% in either diffusion capacity of carbon monoxide or vital capacity should mandate immediate discontinuation of bleomycin. Early clinical trials and isolated case reports suggest that bleomycin-induced acute hypersensitivity reactions occur in 1% of patients with lymphoma and less than 0.5% of those with solid tumors. The reactions are mainly characterized by high-grade fever, chills, hypotension, and, in a few cases, cardiovascular collapse, which can lead to death. The exact mechanism of these reactions is unclear, but is thought to be related to the release of endogenous pyrogens from the host cells. Supportive care, including hydration, steroids, antipyretics, and antihistamines, may resolve the symptoms.

Clinicians should monitor their patients for any signs and symptoms of acute hyperpyrexic reactions during bleomycin administration. Because the onset of the reactions can occur with any dose of bleomycin and at any time, routine test dosing does not seem to predict when drug reactions may occur.[26] Mucocutaneous toxicity presents as mucositis, erythema, hyperpigmentation, induration, hyperkeratosis, and skin peeling, which may progress to ulceration, and usually develops in the 2nd and 3rd week of treatment and after a cumulative dose of 150 to 200 U of the drug. Levels of bleomycin hydrolase are relatively low in lung and skin tissue, perhaps offering an explanation as to why these normal tissues are more adversely affected by bleomycin. Myelosuppression and immunosuppression are relatively mild. In rare cases, vascular events, including myocardial infarction, stroke, and Raynaud phenomenon, have been reported.

PROCARBAZINE

Originally prepared as a monoamine oxidase inhibitor, procarbazine is a prodrug, which after oxidation of the hydrazine in the liver, undergoes a complex enzymatic and chemical breakdown to its alkylating and methylating species.[27,28] The precise mechanism of action is uncertain, but may involve damaging the DNA, RNA or transfer RNA, and the inhibition of protein synthesis. Procarbazine is a cell-cycle phase-nonspecific antineoplastic agent. This agent was initially approved by the U.S. Food and Drug Administration (FDA) in 1969 as part of the MOPP (mechlorethamine, vincristine, procarbazine, and prednisone) regimen for the treatment of Hodgkin lymphoma. Since then, it has also demonstrated clinical activity in non-Hodgkin lymphoma, cutaneous T-cell lymphoma, and brain tumors.

Procarbazine is rapidly and completely absorbed from the gastrointestinal tract. Following oral administration, peak drug levels are reached within 10 to 15 minutes. Procarbazine crosses the blood–brain barrier and rapidly equilibrates between plasma and cerebrospinal fluid after oral administration. Peak cerebrospinal fluid drug concentrations are reached within 30 to 90 minutes after drug administration. The biologic half-life of procarbazine hydrochloride in both plasma and cerebrospinal fluid is approximately 1 hour. Procarbazine is metabolized to active and inactive metabolites by chemical breakdown in an aqueous solution and the liver microsomal P-450 system. Approximately 70% of procarbazine is excreted in urine within 24 hours, and less than 5% to 10% of the drug is eliminated in an unchanged form.[29,30]

A careful food and drug history is required before starting a patient on procarbazine therapy, because there are several potential drug–drug and drug–food interactions. Patients should avoid tyramine-containing foods, such as dark beer, wine, cheese, yogurt, bananas, and smoked foods. Procarbazine produces a disulfiramlike reaction with concurrent use of alcohol. Acute hypertensive reactions may occur with coadministration of tricyclic antidepressants and sympathomimetic drugs. Concurrent use of procarbazine with antihistamines and other central nervous system (CNS) depressants can result in CNS and/or respiratory depression.

Dose-limiting toxicity is myelosuppression, more commonly thrombocytopenia, and the nadir in platelet count is generally observed at 4 weeks. Patients with glucose-6-phosphate dehydrogenase deficiency can develop hemolytic anemia while receiving procarbazine therapy. Stepwise dose increments over the first few days of drug administration may minimize gastrointestinal intolerance. On rare occasions, procarbazine may induce interstitial pneumonitis, which mandates the discontinuation of therapy. Azoospermia and infertility after treatment with MOPP can be attributed, in part, to procarbazine. Procarbazine is associated with an increased risk of secondary malignancies, especially acute leukemia.

VISMODEGIB

Vismodegib (Erivedge, GDC-0449, Genentech) is a first-in-class, small-molecule inhibitor of the Hedgehog pathway. It binds to and inhibits smoothened, a transmembrane protein that is involved in Hedgehog signaling.[31] Pharmacodynamic downmodulation in the Hedgehog pathway was shown by a 90% decrease in transcription factor Gli1 mRNA in basal-cell carcinoma biopsy specimens of patients treated for a month. One-month vismodegib treatment also significantly reduced tumor proliferation, as assessed by Ki-67 expression, but did not change apoptosis, as assessed by cleaved caspase 3. The extent of Gli1 downmodulation does not seem to correlate with pharmacokinetic levels of vismodegib in individual patients. Vismodegib is absorbed from the gastrointestinal tract, with an oral bioavailability of 32%. Food does not affect drug exposure. Elimination is mainly hepatic, with excretion in feces. The median steady-state concentration is not changed by increasing the dose from 150 mg to 270 mg, and the median time to steady state is 14 days. The half-life is estimated at 8 days after a single dose. Intermittent doses (e.g., three times per week or once per week) were associated with a decrease of 50% and 80% in effective plasma levels of unbound drug, respectively, thus reinforcing the recommended dose and schedule of 150 mg orally daily.[32] Vismodegib is approved for the treatment of adults with metastatic basal-cell carcinoma that has recurred following surgery or in those who are not candidates for surgery and who are not candidates for radiation.[33]

No dose-limiting toxic effects or grade 5 events have been observed. However, 54% of patients receiving vismodegib discontinued the medication owing to side effects, and only one out of give eligible patients was able to continue vismodegib for 18 months. Abdominal pain, fatigue, weight loss, dysgeusia, and anorexia were reasons for discontinuation of the drug. When vismodegib was withdrawn, dysgeusia and muscle cramps ceased within 1 month, and scalp and body hair started to regrow within 3 months. Other side effects reported include hyponatremia, dyspnea, muscle spasm, atrial fibrillation, aspiration, back pain, corneal abrasion, dehydration, keratitis, lymphopenia, pneumonia, urinary tract infection, and a prolonged QT interval.[34]

ADO-TRASTUZUMAB EMTANSINE

Ado-trastuzumab emtansine (T-DM1), is a HER2-targeted antibody-drug conjugate (ADC). It is a novel compound composed of trastuzumab, a stable thioether linker, and DM1. DM1, a derivative of maytansine, is a microtubule polymerization inhibitor with activity similar to that of vinca alkaloids. T-DM1 is taken up into cells after binding to HER2, allowing for cytotoxic drug delivery specifically to cells overexpressing HER2. It has a drug-to-antibody ratio of approximately 3.5:1. T-DM1 is administered intravenously every 3 weeks and has been tested in a phase I trial at doses ranging from 0.3 to 4.8 mg/kg. The maximally tolerated dose is 3.6 mg/kg, which was the dose used in further phase II–III trials. T-DM1 is metabolized by the liver, via CYP3A4/5, and has a half-life of 3.5 days.[35]

T-DM1 is approved for use in patients with metastatic HER2-positive breast cancer who have received prior trastuzumab and a taxane. This approval was based on the results of the EMILIA trial, which randomized 991 patients with HER2-positive unresectable, locally advanced or metastatic breast cancer to T-DM1 3.6 mg/kg IV every 21 days or lapatinib 1,250 mg daily plus capecitabine 1,000 mg/m² on days 1 through 14 every 21 days. All patients were previously treated with trastuzumab and a taxane. T-DM1 resulted in a progression-free survival of 9.6 months compared to 6.4 months for lapatinib plus capecitabine (hazard ratio [HR] 0.65; 95% confidence interval [CI] 0.55 to 0.77; p <0.001). The response rate and overall survival was also higher with T-DM1 compared to lapatinib plus capecitabine.[36]

Although maytansine itself is associated with significant toxicity, T-DM1 is very well tolerated overall, which is likely due to the targeted nature of the compound. Side effects from T-DM1 include thrombocytopenia, hepatotoxicity, hypersensitivity/infusion reactions, and cardiotoxicity. Nausea, fatigue, headaches, and anemia are also common. The left ventricular ejection fraction should be monitored prior to and at least every 3 months during therapy because of the potential for cardiac dysfunction.

SIROLIMUS AND TEMSIROLIMUS

Sirolimus (rapamycin) was isolated from the soil bacteria *Streptomyces hygroscopicus*, in the mid 1970s.[37] This bacterial macrolide later became the preferred immunosuppressant for kidney transplantation, because it was mildly immunosuppressive; however, in contrast to cyclosporine A, it did not enhance tumor incidence.[38] Sirolimus is the prototypic inhibitor of the mammalian target of rapamycin (mTOR), a serine/threonine protein kinase that is a highly conserved regulatory protein involved in cell-cycle progression, proliferation, and angiogenesis.[39] Signaling pathways both upstream and downstream of mTOR have been shown to be commonly dysregulated in cancer. mTOR functions through two main mechanisms, depending on the presence and activity of the mTOR-associated protein complexes, mTORC1 and mTORC2. Sirolimus and its analog compounds, temsirolimus and everolimus, form a complex with the FK-binding protein (FKBP) and inhibit activation of a subset of mTOR proteins residing within mTORC1. In contrast, mTORC2 holds mTOR in a form that is not as readily inhibited by these rapamycin analogs, and upregulation of mTORC2 may represent a mechanism by which resistance can develop to this class of compounds.

Temsirolimus (CCI-779), a novel functional ester of sirolimus, is a water-soluble dihydroxymethyl propionic acid compound that rapidly undergoes hydrolysis to sirolimus after IV administration, reaching peak concentrations within 0.5 to 2.0 hours.[40] This drug is widely distributed in tissues, and steady-state drug levels are reached in 7 to 8 days. Temsirolimus is metabolized primarily in the liver by CYP3A4 microsomal enzymes to yield sirolimus as the main metabolite. The terminal half-life of temsirolimus is 17 hours, whereas that of sirolimus is approximately 55 hours. When bound to temsirolimus, mTOR is unable to phosphorylate the key protein translation factors, such as 4E-BP1 and S6K1, leading to translational inhibition of several critical regulatory proteins involved in cell-cycle control. Several other cellular proteins involved in the regulation of angiogenesis, such as hypoxia-inducible factor-1α (HIF-1α) and vascular endothelial growth factor (VEGF), are suppressed through mTOR inhibition by temsirolimus.

Phase I studies of temsirolimus have investigated various schedules and doses, ranging from 7.5 mg to 220 mg given as weekly 30-minute infusions.[40] A phase II study in patients with cytokine-refractory renal cell cancer (RCC) investigated the efficacy and safety of three different dose levels (25 mg, 75 mg, and 250 mg, respectively) administered on a weekly schedule. This study showed promising antitumor activity for all three dose levels with no significant difference in efficacy or toxicity.[41] As a result, the 25-mg dose was eventually selected as the monotherapy dose for further study. A phase III randomized trial compared interferon, temsirolimus, and the combination of the two agents in previously untreated patients with advanced RCC who had at least three of six poor prognostic features.[42] Once-weekly IV temsirolimus, 25 mg, prolonged the median overall survival of patients with poor prognostic features by 49% from 7.3 months (95% CI, 6.1 to 8.8 months) in the interferon arm to 10.9 months (95% CI, 8.6 to 12.7 months) in the temsirolimus arm (P = .008). The temsirolimus arm also had a prolonged median progression-free survival of 5.5 months compared to 3.1 months in the interferon arm (P <.001). Moreover, temsirolimus was effective for both clear cell and non–clear cell histologies.[43,44]

Mantle cell lymphoma was the first hematologic malignancy in which mTOR inhibition was explored as a treatment strategy. The rationale for this approach was that mantle cell lymphoma is characterized by overexpression of cyclin D1, which is a cyclin whose expression appears to be tightly regulated by mTOR signaling. The early-phase clinical trials of temsirolimus showed promising activity against non-Hodgkin lymphomas, multiple myeloma, and myeloid leukemias, with some evidence of success thus far.[45]

In terms of the safety profile, the most common adverse events associated with temsirolimus were asthenia and fatigue, dry skin with acneiform skin rash, nausea/vomiting, mucositis, and anorexia. Hyperlipidemia with increased serum triglycerides and/or cholesterol as well as hyperglycemia occur in up to 90% of patients. Allergic, hypersensitivity reactions have been observed in about 10% of patients, and pulmonary toxicity, presenting as increased cough, dyspnea, fever, and pulmonary infiltrates, is a relatively rare event, occurring in less than 1% of patients. However, the risk of pulmonary toxicity increases in patients with an underlying pulmonary disease.[46]

EVEROLIMUS

Everolimus (RAD001) is an orally active hydroxyethyl ether analog of rapamycin that contains a 2-hydroxyethyl chain substitution. This molecule is significantly more water soluble than sirolimus. As with sirolimus and temsirolimus, everolimus targets mTOR by forming a complex with mTOR and FKBP, resulting in inhibition of mTOR activity. Few data are available regarding the actual differences in the ability of temsirolimus and everolimus to inhibit mTOR. One preclinical in vitro study showed that the binding of everolimus to FKBP was approximately threefold weaker than that of sirolimus.[47] In vivo studies, however, have documented similar efficacy of the two agents in terms of immunosuppressive activity as well as antitumor activity. In preclinical models, the administration of everolimus results in the inhibition of mTOR, similar to what has been observed with the other rapamycin analogs.[48] In terms of clinical pharmacology, peak drug levels are achieved within 1 to 2 hours after oral administration, and food with a high fat content reduces oral bioavailability by up to 20%. This compound is metabolized in the liver, mainly by the CYP3A4 system, and six main metabolites have been identified. In general, these metabolites are less active than the parent compound. Elimination is mainly hepatic with excretion in feces, and caution should be used in patients with moderate liver impairment (Child-Pugh class B).[49] In this setting, the daily dose of drug should be reduced to 5 mg. In patients with severe liver dysfunction (Child-Pugh class C), the use of this drug is contraindicated.

Encouraging clinical activity was initially observed in phase 1/2 trials in patients with non–small-cell lung, gastric, and esophageal cancers, sarcomas, pancreatic neuroendocrine tumors, as well as hematologic malignancies.[50–53] Presently, everolimus is indicated and approved for the treatment of adults with advanced RCC after failure with sunitinib or sorafenib; advanced hormone receptor-positive, HER2-negative breast cancer in combination with exemestane; and progressive unresectable, locally advanced, or metastatic neuroendocrine tumors of pancreatic origin (PNET).[54,55] The recommended dose of everolimus for these indications is 10 mg taken orally once daily.

The safety profile of everolimus is similar to what has been observed with temsirolimus. The most common adverse events include asthenia and fatigue, dry skin with acneiform skin rash, nausea/vomiting, mucositis, and anorexia. Hyperlipidemia with increased serum triglycerides and/or cholesterol as well as hyperglycemia occur in up to 90% of patients. Allergic, hypersensitivity reactions have been observed in about 10% of patients, and pulmonary toxicity, presenting as increased cough, dyspnea, fever, and pulmonary infiltrates, are a relatively rare event, occurring in less than 1% of patients. However, the risk of pulmonary toxicity increases in patients with an underlying pulmonary disease.

THALIDOMIDE, LENALIDOMIDE, AND POMALIDOMIDE

Thalidomide and its amino-substituted analogs, lenalidomide and pomalidomide, are small-molecule glutamic acid derivatives that possess a wide range of biologic properties, including immunomodulating, antiangiogenic, and epigenetic effects. They are classified as class I (non–phosphophodiesterase-4 inhibitory) immunomodulatory drugs (IMiDs). Although their primary mechanism of activity against malignancy is uncertain, it is believed that IMiDs exert their anticancer effects both directly on cancer cells and indirectly via effects on the tumor microenvironment and host antitumor immunity. Specific mechanisms include the inhibition of nuclear factor kappa B (NF-κB) transcriptional activity in malignant cells with a resultant decrease in the production of antiapoptotic molecules; the inhibition of surface adhesion molecule expression on both multiple myeloma cells and bone marrow stromal cells; the inhibition of the production and release of various growth factors (including vascular endothelial growth factor, basic fibroblast growth factor, tumor necrosis factor alpha, and interleukin [IL] 6) that regulate angiogenesis and tumor cell proliferation; and costimulation of IL-2 and interferon gamma (IFN-γ) release with T-helper 1 subset skewing and augmentation of cytotoxic T-cell and natural killer cell effector function.[56,57] Unlike thalidomide, both lenalidomide and pomalidomide result in cell cycle arrest and apoptosis of myeloma cells in vitro, believed in part to be related to epigenetic effects.[58] They are also more potent stimulators of IL-2 and INF-γ production and T-cell proliferation than thalidomide, and appear to additionally inhibit T-regulatory cells.[57] Clinically, lenalidomide has activity in patients with thalidomide-resistant multiple myeloma, and pomalidomide has additional activity in patients with lenalidomide-resistant disease.[59,60] Recently, the protein cereblon (cerebral protein with lon protease), a highly conserved E3 ligase, was recognized as a primary target of IMiDs teratogenic effect, and appears to be an important target of IMiD anticancer activity.[61–63] Efforts are currently under way to evaluate the expression of Cereblon as a predictive biomarker of response to IMiDs.[63] Due to the potential risk of significant teratogenicity, thalidomide, lenalidomide, and pomalidomide can only be prescribed by licensed prescribers who are registered in restricted distribution programs.

Thalidomide

Thalidomide (2-[2,6-dioxopiperidin-3-yl]-2,3-dihydro-1H-isoindole-1,3-dione; Thalomid) is a synthetic glutamic acid derivative that was initially synthesized in 1953. It was used widely in Europe between 1956 and 1962 as a sleeping aid and antiemetic for pregnant women before it was discovered to cause severe congenital malformations. Initial reports of its efficacy in multiple myeloma were published in 1999, and the 200-mg daily dose combined with pulse dexamethasone (40-mg daily dose on days 1 through 4, 9 through 12, and 17 through 20 on a 28-day schedule) was approved by the FDA in 2006 for newly diagnosed multiple myeloma. The use of thalidomide has dropped precipitously in the United States with the FDA approval of more efficacious and less toxic therapies for myeloma. Thalidomide is poorly soluble, and it is absorbed slowly from the gastrointestinal tract, reaching peak plasma concentration in 3 to 6 hours, with 55% to 66% bound to plasma proteins. The exact metabolic route and fate of thalidomide is not known. Thalidomide does not appear to be hepatically metabolized, but rather undergoes spontaneous nonenzymatic hydrolysis in plasma to multiple metabolites, with a half-life of elimination ranging from 5 to 7 hours. These metabolites are believed to be responsible for the antitumor effects of thalidomide. Less than 1% is excreted into the urine as unchanged drug.[64]

Thalidomide frequently causes drowsiness, constipation, and fatigue. Peripheral neuropathy is a common and potentially severe and irreversible side effect occurring in up to 30% of patients. Increased incidences of venous thromboembolic events, such as deep venous thrombosis and pulmonary embolus, have also been observed with thalidomide, particularly when used in combination with dexamethasone or anthracycline-based chemotherapy. Patients who are appropriate candidates may benefit from concurrent prophylactic anticoagulation or aspirin treatment.[65] Other side effects of thalidomide include rash, nausea, dizziness, orthostatic hypotension, bradycardia, and mood changes. In 2013, additional alerts were released linking thalidomide to an increased risk of developing second primary malignancies (both acute myelogenous leukemia and myelodysplastic syndrome) and arterial thromboembolic events.

Lenalidomide

Lenalidomide (3-[4-amino-1-oxo-2,3-dihydro-1H-isoindol-2-yl]piperidine-2,6-dione; Revlimid) is a thalidomide derivative that shares the immunomodulatory and antineoplastic properties of its parent compound. However, lenalidomide appears to be more potent in vitro with less nonhematologic toxicities in clinical studies. It initially received FDA approval (10-mg daily dose) in 2005 for the treatment of patients with transfusion-dependent anemia secondary to low or intermediate risk myelodysplastic syndromes associated with a deletion 5q cytogenetic abnormality, with or without additional cytogenetic abnormalities. In 2006, lenalidomide (25-mg daily dose on days 1 through 21 of a 28-day cycle) in combination with dexamethasone (40-mg daily dose on days 1 through 4, 9 through 12, and 17 through 20 on each 28-day cycle for the first four cycles, then 40 mg daily on days 1 through 4 every 28 days) was approved by the FDA for the treatment of patients with multiple myeloma who had received at least one prior therapy for multiple myeloma. In 2013, lenalidomide 25 mg daily (days 1 through 21 on repeated 28-day cycles) was additionally approved for use in refractory mantle cell lymphoma (after relapse/ progression on two lines of therapy, one of which contained bortezomid). Lenalidomide is administered orally and is rapidly absorbed from the gastrointestinal tract. Maximum plasma concentration is reached 0.625 to 1.5 hours after dosing, with approximately 30% bound to plasma proteins. The half-life of elimination is approximately 3 hours, with little information currently available concerning metabolism. Approximately 70% of an administered dose is excreted unchanged by the kidneys.[66]

Compared with thalidomide, lenalidomide is associated with less sedation, constipation, and peripheral neuropathy. However, myelosuppression in the form of neutropenia and thrombocytopenia can be dose limiting. As with thalidomide, the incidence of thromboembolic events is significant with the combination of dexamethasone and lenalidomide. A pooled analysis of 691 patients enrolled in two randomized studies reported a 12% incidence of thrombotic or thromboembolic events with the combination, compared with 4% with dexamethasone alone.[67]

Pomalidomide

Pomalidomide (4-amino-2-[2,6-dioxopiperidin-3-yl]-2,3-dihydro-1H-isoindole-1,3-dione; Pomalyst) is another thalidomide derivative designed to be more portent and less toxic than both thalidomide and lenalidomide. It is currently FDA approved (4-mg once daily dose orally on days 1 through 21 of a 28-day cycle, with or without dexamethasone) for use in patients with progressive multiple myeloma who have received at least two prior therapies, including lenalidomide and bortezomid. Pomalidomide is administered orally and is rapidly absorbed. Maximum plasma concentration is reached 2 to 3 hours after ingestion, with approximately 12% to 44% protein binding.[68] The half-life of elimination is between 7.5 and 9.5 hours. Pomalidomide is metabolized in the liver, via CYP1A2/CYP3A4 (major) and CYP2C19/CYP2D6 (minor), and excretion occurs primarily through the kidneys (73%; 2% as unchanged drug).

Like lenalidomide, pomalidomide is better tolerated than thalidomide at approved doses with less constipation, fatigue, and neuropathy.[69] The primary toxicity appreciated in myeloma trials has been myelosuppression, particularly neutropenia, which can be dose limiting. The risk of thromboembolic events is similar to that seen with thalidomide and lenalidomide. Unlike thalidomide or lenalidomide, dermatologic toxicity is rare with pomalidomide. A summary of the characteristics of the miscellaneous drugs mentioned in this chapter is provided in Table 26.1. A summary of all hematology oncology drug approvals since the last edition of the textbook can be viewed in Table 26.2.

CANCER THERAPEUTICS

TABLE 26.1

Miscellaneous Chemotherapeutic Agents

	Main Therapeutic Uses	Clinical Pharmacology	Major Toxicities	Notes
Omacetaxine	CML	Mean half-life of 6 h after subcutaneous injection	Thrombocytopenia, anemia, nausea, diarrhea	Efficacy shown in Bcr-Abl–mutated CML
L-Asparaginase	Pediatric and adult ALL	Peak concentration 7–12 h after IV administration; 30% plasma protein binding; PEG form has longer half-life of 5.7 days; antagonize effects of methotrexate if given before or concurrently	Hypersensitivity reactions, alterations in thyroid function, prolonged PT/PTT, decreased levels of vitamin K–dependent factors, acute pancreatitis	Myelosuppression is rare; hypersensitivity reaction risk increases with repeated exposure and when used as single agent; PEG form is less immunogenic
Bleomycin	Hodgkin disease, neoplastic pleural effusion, non-Hodgkin lymphoma, squamous cell carcinoma of cervix, squamous cell carcinoma of nasopharynx, squamous cell carcinoma of penis, squamous cell carcinoma of the head and neck, squamous cell carcinoma of vulva, testicular cancer	Terminal half-life of 3h; can be given intracavitary; 45%–55% of intracavitary dose absorbed systemically; elimination via kidneys if CrCl <25–35 mL/min dose reduction required	Pulmonary toxicity dose-limiting; more if age >70 y; cumulative dose >400 U; acute hypersensitivity reactions rare (1%); mucositis, erythema, hyperpigmentation	Not myelosuppressive; immunosuppressive; metabolizing enzyme; bleomycin hydrolase enzyme low in lung and skin tissue; G-CSF use seems to exacerbate pulmonary toxicity

(continued)

TABLE 26.1

Miscellaneous Chemotherapeutic Agents *(continued)*

	Main Therapeutic Uses	Clinical Pharmacology	Major Toxicities	Notes
Procarbazine	Hodgkin lymphoma	Rapid complete oral absorption; peak concentration, 10–15 min; crosses blood–brain barrier; half-life 1 h; several drug–drug and food–drug interactions; metabolized by hepatic microsomal P-450 system; 70% excreted in urine	Dose-limiting toxicity is myelosuppression, more commonly thrombocytopenia nadir at 4 wk; G-6PD–deficient patients can develop hemolytic anemia, nausea, vomiting, diarrhea, flulike symptoms, peripheral neuropathy, hypersensitivity reactions	Avoid tyramine-containing foods; disulfiramlike reaction with concurrent alcohol use; hypertensive reaction with concurrent tricyclic antidepressant use; increased risk for azoospermia/infertility and secondary malignancy
Vismodegib	Basal cell carcinoma of the skin	Oral bioavailability 32%; not affected by food	No dose limiting toxicity; abdominal pain, fatigue, weight loss, dysgeusia	Hedgehog-signaling pathway inhibitor
Ado-trastuzumabemtansine	Advanced HER2-positive breast cancer	Peak concentration near the end of infusion metabolized by CYP3A4/5; half-life, 3.5 days	Thrombocytopenia, hepatotoxicity, cardiac toxicity fatigue, nausea	Monitor cardiac function
Temsirolimus	Advanced renal cancer	Peak concentration, 0.5–2 h; widely distributed in tissues; steady-state levels reached in 7–8 d; half-life, 17 h	Asthenia, fatigue, dry skin, acneiform skin rash, mucositis, anorexia, hyperlipidemia, hyperglycemia	Efficacy shown for both clear cell and non–clear-cell histologies; efficacy in hematologic malignancies (mantle cell lymphoma, non-Hodgkin lymphoma, multiple myeloma)
Everolimus	Advanced renal cell carcinoma, breast cancer, pancreatic neuroendocrine tumor	Peak concentration, 1–2 hr; reduced bioavailability with high fat content food; metabolized by CYP3A4 system; mainly hepatic excretion	Asthenia, dry skin, nausea, vomiting, mucositis, hyperlipidemia, hyperglycemia, allergic hypersensitivity reaction, pulmonary toxicity	Contraindicated in Child-Pugh class C patients; encouraging activity in gastric, non–small-cell, lung, esophageal cancers, sarcomas; approved for organ rejection prophylaxis
Thalidomide	Multiple myeloma, erythema nodosum leprosum	Oral absorption slow; peak concentration, 3–6 h; 55%–66% bound to plasma proteins; half-life, 5–7 h; spontaneous nonenzymatic hydrolysis in plasma	Drowsiness, constipation, fatigue, skin rash, increased risk for thromboembolic complications	Pregnancy category X; may be present in semen; serious skin reactions including Stevens-Johnson syndrome
Lenalidomide	Low-to-intermediate risk myelodysplastic syndrome associated with 5q deletion, multiple myeloma	Rapid oral absorption; peak concentration, 0.6–1.5 h; half-life, 3 h; 70% excreted unchanged by kidneys	Less sedation, drowsiness, constipation than thalidomide; myelosuppression; thromboembolic events; peripheral neuropathy	Pregnancy category X; caution in patients with renal function impairment; neutropenia; thrombocytopenia may be dose limiting
Pomalidomide	Multiple myeloma who have received at least two prior therapies	Rapid oral absorption; peak concentration, 2–3 h; half-life, 7.5 h	Myelosuppression; thromboembolic events; skin toxicity rare	Better tolerated than thalidomide; effective in prior bortezomib- and lenalidomide-receiving patients

PT, prothrombin time; PTT, partial thromboplastin time; CrCl, creatinine clearance.

TABLE 26.2

U.S. Food And Drug Administration Hematology Oncology Drug Approvals 2010–2013

Drug/Manufacturer	Indication	Approval Date
Sorafenib (NEXAVAR tablets, Bayer Healthcare Pharmaceuticals Inc.)	For the treatment of locally recurrent or metastatic, progressive, differentiated thyroid carcinoma (DTC) refractory to radioactive iodine treatment.	November 22, 2013
Crizotinib (Xalkori, Pfizer, Inc.) capsules	For the treatment of patients with metastatic non–small-cell lung cancer (NSCLC) whose tumors are anaplastic lymphoma kinase (ALK) positive as detected by an FDA-approved test.	November 20, 2013
Ibrutinib (IMBRUVICA, Pharmacyclics, Inc.)	For the treatment of patients with mantle cell lymphoma (MCL) who have received at least one prior therapy.	November 13, 2013
Obinutuzumab (GAZYVA injection, for intravenous use, Genentech, Inc.; previously known as GA101)	For use in combination with chlorambucil for the treatment of patients with previously untreated chronic lymphocytic leukemia (CLL).	November 1, 2013
Pertuzumab injection (PERJETA, Genentech, Inc.)	For use in combination with trastuzumab and docetaxel for the neoadjuvant treatment of patients with HER2-positive, locally advanced, inflammatory, or early stage breast cancer (either greater than 2 cm in diameter or node positive) as part of a complete treatment regimen for early breast cancer.	September 30, 2013
Paclitaxel protein-bound particles (albumin-bound) (Abraxane for injectable suspension, Abraxis BioScience, LLC, a wholly owned subsidiary of Celgene Corporation)	In combination with gemcitabine for the first-line treatment of patients with metastatic adenocarcinoma of the pancreas.	September 6, 2013
Afatinib (Gilotrif tablets, Boehringer Ingelheim Pharmaceuticals, Inc.)	For the first-line treatment of patients with metastatic NSCLC whose tumors have epidermal growth factor receptor (EGFR) exon 19 deletions or exon 21 (L858R) substitution mutations as detected by an FDA-approved test. The safety and efficacy of afatinib have not been established in patients whose tumors have other EGFR mutations.	July 12, 2013
Denosumab (Xgeva injection, for subcutaneous use, Amgen Inc.)	For the treatment of adults and skeletally mature adolescents with a giant cell tumor of bone that is unresectable or where surgical resection is likely to result in severe morbidity.	June 13, 2013
Lenalidomide capsules (REVLIMID, Celgene Corporation)	For the treatment of patients with MCL whose disease has relapsed or progressed after two prior therapies, one of which included bortezomib.	June 5, 2013
Trametinib (MEKINIST tablet, GlaxoSmithKline, LLC)	For the treatment of patients with unresectable or metastatic melanoma with BRAF V600E or V600K mutation as detected by an FDA-approved test.	May 29, 2013
Dabrafenib (TAFINLAR capsule, GlaxoSmithKline, LLC)	For the treatment of patients with unresectable or metastatic melanoma with BRAF V600E mutation as detected by an FDA-approved test.	May 29, 2013
Radium Ra 223 dichloride (Xofigo Injection, Bayer HealthCare Pharmaceuticals Inc.)	For the treatment of patients with castration-resistant prostate cancer, symptomatic bone metastases, and no known visceral metastatic disease.	May 15, 2013
Erlotinib (Tarceva, Astellas Pharma Inc.)	For the first-line treatment of metastatic NSCLC patients whose tumors have EGFR exon 19 deletions or exon 21 (L858R) substitution mutations.	May 14, 2013
Ado-trastuzumab emtansine (KADCYLA for injection, Genentech, Inc.)	For use as a single agent for the treatment of patients with HER2-positive, metastatic breast cancer who previously received trastuzumab and a taxane, separately or in combination.	February 22, 2013
Pomalidomide (POMALYST capsules, Celgene Corporation)	For the treatment of patients with multiple myeloma who have received at least two prior therapies, including lenalidomide and bortezomib, and have demonstrated disease progression on or within 60 days of completion of the last therapy.	February 8, 2013

(continued)

TABLE 26.2

U.S. Food And Drug Administration Hematology Oncology Drug Approvals 2010–2013 *(continued)*

Drug/Manufacturer	Indication	Approval Date
Doxorubicin hydrochloride liposome injection (Sun Pharma Global FZE), a generic version of DOXIL Injection (doxorubicin hydrochloride liposome; Janssen Products, L.P.)	For the treatment of ovarian cancer in patients whose disease has progressed or recurred after platinum-based chemotherapy and for AIDS-related Kaposi sarcoma after failure of prior systemic chemotherapy or intolerance to such therapy.	February 4, 2013
Bevacizumab (Avastin, Genentech U.S., Inc.)	For use in combination with fluoropyrimidine–irinotecan- or fluoropyrimidine–oxaliplatin-based chemotherapy for the treatment of patients with metastatic colorectal cancer (mCRC) whose disease has progressed on a first-line bevacizumab-containing regimen.	January 23, 2013
Ponatinib (Iclusig tablets, ARIAD Pharmaceuticals, Inc.)	For the treatment of adult patients with chronic phase, accelerated phase, or blast phase chronic myeloid leukemia (CML) that is resistant or intolerant to prior tyrosine–kinase inhibitor (TKI) therapy or Philadelphia chromosome–positive acute lymphoblastic leukemia (Ph+ ALL) that is resistant or intolerant to prior TKI therapy.	December 17, 2012
Abiraterone acetate (Zytiga Tablets, Janssen Biotech, Inc.)	In combination with prednisone for the treatment of patients with metastatic castration-resistant prostate cancer.	December 10, 2012
Cabozantinib (COMETRIQ capsules, Exelixis, Inc.)	For the treatment of patients with progressive metastatic medullary thyroid cancer (MTC).Cabozantinib is a small molecule that inhibits the activity of multiple tyrosine kinases, including RET, MET, and VEGF receptor 2.	November 29, 2012
Omacetaxine mepesuccinate (SYNRIBO for injection, for subcutaneous use, Teva Pharmaceutical Industries Ltd.)	For the treatment of adult patients with chronic or accelerated phase CML with resistance and/or intolerance to two or more TKIs.	October 26, 2012
Paclitaxel protein-bound particles for injectable suspension, albumin-bound (ABRAXANE for injectable suspension; Abraxis Bioscience a wholly owned subsidiary of Celgene Corporation)	For use in combination with carboplatin for the initial treatment of patients with locally advanced or metastatic NSCLC who are not candidates for curative surgery or radiation therapy.	October 11, 2012
Regorafenib (Stivarga tablets, Bayer HealthCare Pharmaceuticals, Inc.)	For the treatment of patients with mCRC who have been previously treated with fluoropyrimidine-, oxaliplatin-, and irinotecan-based chemotherapy, an anti-VEGF therapy, and, if KRAS wild-type, an anti-EGFR therapy.	September 27, 2012
Bosutinib tablets (Bosulif, Pfizer, Inc.)	for the treatment of chronic, accelerated, or blast phase Ph+ CML in adult patients with resistance or intolerance to prior therapy.	September 4, 2012
Enzalutamide (XTANDI Capsules, Medivation, Inc., and Astellas Pharma US, Inc.)	For the treatment of patients with metastatic castration-resistant prostate cancer who have previously received docetaxel.	August 31, 2012
Everolimus tablets for oral suspension (Afinitor Disperz, Novartis Pharmaceuticals Corp.)	For the treatment of pediatric and adult patients with tuberous sclerosis complex (TSC) who have subependymal giant cell astrocytoma (SEGA) that requires therapeutic intervention, but that cannot be curatively resected.	August 30, 2012
Vincristine sulfate LIPOSOME injection (Marqibo, Talon Therapeutics, Inc.)	For the treatment of adult patients with Ph- ALL in second or greater relapse or whose disease has progressed following two or more antileukemia therapies.	August 9, 2012
Ziv-aflibercept injection (ZALTRAP, Sanofi U.S., Inc.)	For use in combination with 5-fluorouracil, leucovorin, irinotecan (FOLFIRI) for the treatment of patients with mCRC that is resistant to or has progressed following an oxaliplatin-containing regimen.	August 3, 2012
Everolimus tablets (Afinitor, Novartis Pharmaceuticals Corporation)	For the treatment of postmenopausal women with advanced hormone receptor–positive, HER2-negative breast cancer in combination with exemestane, after failure of treatment with letrozole or anastrozole.	July 20, 2012

(continued)

TABLE 26.2

**U.S. Food And Drug Administration Hematology Oncology Drug Approvals
2010–2013 (continued)**

Drug/Manufacturer	Indication	Approval Date
Carfilzomib injection (Kyprolis, Onyx Pharmaceuticals)	For the treatment of patients with multiple myeloma who have received at least two prior therapies, including bortezomib and an immunomodulatory agent, and have demonstrated disease progression on or within 60 days of the completion of the last therapy.	July 20, 2012
Cetuximab (Erbitux, ImClone LLC, a wholly owned subsidiary of Eli Lilly and Co.)	For use in combination with FOLFIRI for first-line treatment of patients with K-ras mutation-negative (wild-type), EGFR-expressing mCRC as determined by FDA-approved tests for this use.	July 9, 2012
Pertuzumab injection (PERJETA, Genentech, Inc.)	For use in combination with trastuzumab and docetaxel for the treatment of patients with HER2-positive metastatic breast cancer who have not received prior anti-HER2 therapy or chemotherapy for metastatic disease.	June 8, 2012
Pazopanib tablets (VOTRIENT, a registered Trademark of GlaxoSmithKline)	For the treatment of patients with advanced soft tissue sarcoma (STS) who have received prior chemotherapy.	April 26, 2012
Everolimus (Afinitor tablets, Novartis)	For the treatment of adults with renal angiomyolipoma, associated with TSC who do not require immediate surgery.	April 26, 2012
Imatinib mesylate tablets (Gleevec, Novartis Pharmaceuticals)	For the adjuvant treatment of adult patients following complete gross resection of Kit (CD117)-positive gastrointestinal stromal tumors (GIST).	January 31, 2012
Vismodegib (ERIVEDGE Capsule, Genentech, Inc.)	For the treatment of adults with metastatic basal cell carcinoma or with locally advanced basal cell carcinoma that has recurred following surgery or who are not candidates for surgery and who are not candidates for radiation.	January 30, 2012
Axitinib tablets (Inlyta, Pfizer, Inc.)	For the treatment of advanced renal cell carcinoma after failure of one prior systemic therapy.	January 27, 2012
Glucarpidase injection (Voraxaze, BTG International Inc.)	For the treatment of toxic plasma methotrexate concentrations (> 1 μmol/L) in patients with delayed methotrexate clearance due to impaired renal function.	January 17, 2012
Asparaginase *Erwinia chrysanthemi* (Erwinaze, injection, EUSA Pharma [USA], Inc.)	As a component of a multiagent chemotherapeutic regimen for the treatment of patients with ALL who have developed hypersensitivity to *E. coli*–derived asparaginase.	November 18, 2011
Ruxolitinib (Jakafi oral tablets, Incyte Corporation)	For the treatment of intermediate and high risk myelofibrosis, including primary myelofibrosis, postpolycythemia vera myelofibrosis, and postessential thrombocythemia myelofibrosis.	November 16, 2011
Cetuximab (Erbitux, ImClone LLC, a wholly-owned subsidiary of Eli Lilly and Company)	In combination with platinum-based therapy plus 5-fluorouracil (5-FU) for the first-line treatment of patients with recurrent locoregional disease and/or metastatic squamous cell carcinoma of the head and neck (SCCHN).	November 7, 2011
Eculizumab (Soliris, Alexion, Inc.)	For the treatment of pediatric and adult patients with atypical hemolytic uremic syndrome (aHUS).	September 23, 2011
Denosumab (Prolia, Amgen Inc.)	As a treatment to increase bone mass in patients at high risk for fracture receiving androgen-deprivation therapy (ADT) for nonmetastatic prostate cancer or adjuvant aromatase inhibitor (AI) therapy for breast cancer.	September 16, 2011
Crizotinib (XALKORI Capsules, Pfizer Inc.)	For the treatment of patients with locally advanced or metastatic NSCLC that is ALK-positive as detected by an FDA-approved test.	August 26, 2011

(continued)

CANCER THERAPEUTICS

TABLE 26.2

U.S. Food And Drug Administration Hematology Oncology Drug Approvals 2010–2013 (continued)

Drug/Manufacturer	Indication	Approval Date
Brentuximab vedotin (Adcetris for injection, Seattle Genetics, Inc.)	For treatment of patients with Hodgkin lymphoma after failure of autologous stem cell transplant (ASCT) or after failure of at least two prior multiagent chemotherapy regimens in patients who are not ASCT candidates and treatment of patients with systemic anaplastic large cell lymphoma (ALCL) after failure of at least one prior multiagent chemotherapy regimen.	August 19, 2011
Vemurafenib tablets (ZELBORAF, Hoffmann-La Roche Inc.)	For the treatment of patients with unresectable or metastatic melanoma with the BRAFV600E mutation as detected by an FDA-approved test.	August 17, 2011
Sunitinib (Sutent capsules, Pfizer, Inc.)	For the treatment of progressive, well-differentiated pancreatic neuroendocrine tumors (pNET) in patients with unresectable, locally advanced, or metastatic disease.	May 20, 2011
Everolimus (Afinitor tablets, Novartis Pharmaceuticals Corporation)	For the treatment of progressive PNET in patients with unresectable, locally advanced, or metastatic disease.	May 5, 2011
Abiraterone acetate (Zytiga tablets, Centocor Ortho Biotech, Inc.)	For use in combination with prednisone for the treatment of patients with metastatic castration-resistant prostate cancer (mCRPC) who have received prior chemotherapy containing docetaxel.	April 28, 2011
Vandetanib tablets (Vandetanib tablets, AstraZeneca Pharmaceuticals LP)	For the treatment of symptomatic or progressive medullary thyroid cancer in patients with unresectable, locally advanced, or metastatic disease.	April 6, 2011
Peginterferon alfa-2b (Sylatron, Schering Corporation, Kenilworth, NJ 07033)	For the treatment of patients with melanoma with microscopic or gross nodal involvement within 84 days of definitive surgical resection including complete lymphadenectomy.	March 29, 2011
Ipilimumab injection (YERVOY, Bristol-Myers Squibb Company)	For the treatment of unresectable or metastatic melanoma.	March 25, 2011
Rituximab (Rituxan, Genentech, Inc.)	For maintenance therapy in patients with previously untreated follicular, CD-20 positive, B-cell non-Hodgkin lymphoma who achieve a response to rituximab in combination with chemotherapy.	January 28, 2011
Eribulin mesylate (Halaven injection, Eisai Inc.)	For the treatment of patients with metastatic breast cancer who have previously received an anthracycline and a taxane in either the adjuvant or metastatic setting, and at least two chemotherapeutic regimens for the treatment of metastatic disease.	November 15, 2010
Everolimus (Afinitor, Novartis), an mTOR inhibitor	For patients with SEGA associated with tuberous sclerosis (TS) who require therapy but who are not candidates for surgical resection.	October 29, 2010
Dasatinib (Sprycel, Bristol-Myers Squibb)	For the treatment of newly diagnosed adult patients with Ph+ CML in chronic phase (CP-CML).	October 28, 2010
Trastuzumab (Herceptin, Genentech, Inc.)	In combination with cisplatin and a fluoropyrimidine (capecitabine or 5-FU), for the treatment of patients with HER2-overexpressing metastatic gastric or gastroesophageal (GE) junction adenocarcinoma, who have not received prior treatment for metastatic disease.	October 20, 2010
Nilotinib (Tasigna capsules, Novartis Pharmaceuticals Corporation)	For the treatment of adult patients with newly diagnosed Ph+ CP-CML.	June 17, 2010
Cabazitaxel (Jevtana injection, Sanofi-Aventis)	For use in combination with prednisone for treatment of patients with metastatic hormone-refractory prostate cancer (mHRPC) previously treated with a docetaxel-containing regimen.	June 17, 2010

SELECTED REFERENCES

The full reference list can be accessed at lwwhealthlibrary.com/oncology.

3. Baaske DM, Heinstein P. Cytotoxicity and cell cycle specificity of homoharrintonine. *Antimicrob Agents Chemother* 1977;12:298–300.

9. Jorge Cortes J, Lipton JF, Rea D, et al. Phase 2 study of subcutaneous omacetaxine mepesuccinate after TKI failure in patients with chronic-phase CML with T315I mutation. *Blood* 2012;120:2573–2580.

13. Avramis VI, Panosyan EH. Pharmacokinetic/pharmacodynamic relationships of asparaginase formulations: the past, the present and recommendations for the future. *Clin Pharmacokinet* 2005;44:367–393.

16. Chen J, Stubbe J. Bleomycins: towards better therapeutics. *Nat Rev Cancer* 2005;2:102–112.

22. Azulay E, Herigault S, Levame M, et al. Effect of granulocyte colony-stimulating factor on bleomycin-induced acute lung injury and pulmonary fibrosis. *Crit Care Med* 2003;31:1442–1448.

25. Younes A, Connors JM, Park SI et al. Brentuximab vedotin combined with ABVD or AVD for patients with newly diagnosed Hodgkin's lymphoma: a phase 1, open-label, dose-escalation study. *Lancet Oncol* 2013;14:1348–1356.

30. Preiss R, Baumann F, Regenthal R, et al. Plasma kinetics of procarbazine and azo-procarbazine in humans. *Anticancer Drugs* 2006;17:75–80.

31. Von Hoff DD, LoRusso PM, Rudin CM, et al. Inhibition of the hedgehog pathway in advanced basal-cell carcinoma. *N Engl J Med* 2009;361:1164-1172.

35. Krop IE, Beeram M, Modi S, et al. Phase I study of trastuzumab-DM1, an HER2 antibody-drug conjugate, given every 3 weeks to patients with HER2-positive metastatic breast cancer. *J Clin Oncol* 2010;28:2698–2704.

37. Sehgal SN, Baker H, Vézina C. Rapamycin (AY-22,989), a new antifungal antibiotic. II. Fermentation, isolation and characterization. *J Antibiot (Tokyo)* 1975;28:727–732.

39. Wullschleger S, Loewith R, Hall MN. TOR signaling in growth and metabolism. *Cell* 2006;124:471–484.

44. Hudes G, Carducci M, Tomczak P, et al. Temsirolimus, interferon alfa, or both for advanced renal-cell carcinoma. *N Engl J Med* 2007;356:2271–2281.

47. Schuler W, Sedrani R, Cottens S, et al. SDZ RAD, a new rapamycine derivative: pharmacological properties in vitro and in vivo. *Transplantation* 1997;64:36–42.

48. Dudkin L, Dilling MB, Cheshire PJ, et al. Biochemical correlates of mTOR inhibition by the rapamycin ester CCI-779 and tumor growth inhibition. *Clin Cancer Res* 2001;7:1758–1764.

51. Yao JC, Lombard-Bohas C, Baudin E, et al. Daily oral everolimus activity in patients with metastatic pancreatic neuroendocrine tumors after failure of cytotoxic chemotherapy: a phase II trial. *J Clin Oncol* 2010;28:69–76.

54. Yao JC, Shah MH, Ito T, et al. Everolimus for advanced pancreatic neuroendocrine tumors. *N Engl J Med* 2011;364:514–523.

55. Baselga J, Campone M, Piccart M, et al. Everolimus in postmenopausal hormone-receptor-positive advanced breast cancer. *N Engl J Med* 2012;366:520–529.

56. Shortt J, Hsu AK, Johnstone RW. Thalidomide-analogue biology: immunological, molecular and epigenetic targets in cancer therapy. *Oncogene* 2013;32:4191–4202.

57. Zhu YX, Kortuem KM, Stewart AK. Molecular mechanism of action of immune-modulatory drugs thalidomide, lenalidomide and pomalidomide in multiple myeloma. *Leuk Lymphoma* 2013;54:683–687.

61. Ito T, Ando H, Suzuki T, et al. Identification of a primary target of thalidomide teratogenicity. *Science* 2010;327:1345–1350.

62. Zhu YX, Braggio E, Shi CX, et al. Cereblon expression is required for the antimyeloma activity of lenalidomide and pomalidomide. *Blood* 2011;118:4771–4779.

65. Bennett CL, Angelotta C, Yarnold PR, et al. Thalidomide- and lenalidomide-associated thromboembolism among patients with cancer. *JAMA* 2006;296:2558–2560.

69. Lacy MQ, McCurdy AR. Pomalidomide. *Blood* 2013;122:2305–2309.

CANCER THERAPEUTICS

27 Hormonal Agents

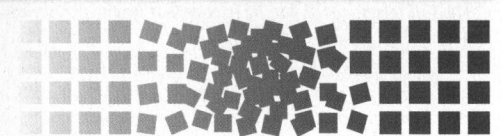

Matthew P. Goetz, Charles Erlichman, Charles L. Loprinzi, and Manish Kohli

INTRODUCTION

Hormonal agents are commonly used as a treatment of hormonally responsive cancers, such as breast, prostate, or endometrial carcinomas. Other uses for some hormonal therapies include the treatment of paraneoplastic syndromes, such as carcinoid syndrome, and symptoms caused by cancer, including anorexia. This chapter discusses the major hormonal agents for such therapy, first with an overview of their use in practice, then with more detailed pharmacologic information regarding them (Table 27.1).

SELECTIVE ESTROGEN RECEPTOR MODULATORS

Tamoxifen

Tamoxifen continues to be an important hormonal therapy for the prevention and treatment of breast cancer worldwide. The continued importance of tamoxifen is reflected in the fact that it is the only hormonal agent approved by the U.S. Food and Drug Administration (FDA) for the prevention of premenopausal breast cancer,[1] the treatment of ductal carcinoma in situ (DCIS),[2] and the treatment of surgically resected premenopausal estrogen receptor (ER)–positive breast cancer.[3]

The standard daily dose of tamoxifen is 20 mg, and the optimal duration depends on the underlying clinical setting. Although the recommended duration in the prevention and DCIS settings is 5 years, recently published prospective studies have demonstrated that for the adjuvant treatment of invasive breast cancer, a duration of 10 years (compared to 5 years) further reduced the risk of breast cancer mortality and improved overall survival.[4]

The most common toxicity from tamoxifen is hot flashes, affecting approximately 50% of treated women. These hot flashes are of varying intensity and duration. Tamoxifen-induced hot flashes appear to increase over the first 3 months of therapy and then plateau. They appear to be more prominent in women with a history of hot flashes or estrogen replacement use. Tamoxifen-induced hot flashes can be ameliorated by a number of different pharmacotherapies, including low doses of megestrol[5]; antidepressants such as venlafaxine,[6] desvenlafaxine,[7] citalopram,[8] escitalopram,[9] and paroxetine[10]; and the anticonvulsant drugs gabapentin[11] and pregabalin.[12] There is evidence that drugs that inhibit CYP2D6 (e.g., paroxetine) alter the metabolic activation of tamoxifen to endoxifen, a critical metabolite associated with in vivo tamoxifen efficacy.[13]

The estrogenic properties of tamoxifen are responsible for both beneficial and deleterious side effects. Tamoxifen increases the incidence of endometrial cancer in postmenopausal (but not premenopausal) women, with the increase in the annual incidence of endometrial cancer being approximately 2.58 (ratio of incidence rates).[14] The absolute risk depends on the duration of tamoxifen administration. For women who receive 10 years of adjuvant tamoxifen, the cumulative risk is 3.1% (mortality, 0.4%) versus 1.6% (mortality, 0.2%) for 5 years of tamoxifen.[4] The incidence of a rarer form of uterine cancer, uterine sarcoma, is also increased after tamoxifen use.[15] This form of endometrial cancer comprises approximately 15% of all uterine malignancies that develop after tamoxifen use.[15] Beneficial estrogenic effects from tamoxifen include a decrease in total cholesterol[16] and the preservation of bone density in postmenopausal women.[17] In premenopausal women, however, tamoxifen has a negative effect on bone density.[18] Although most patients do not complain of vaginal symptoms, a few complain of vaginal dryness, whereas others have increased vaginal secretions and discharge, the latter of which is an indication of the estrogenic activity of tamoxifen on the vagina. In the Arimidex, Tamoxifen, Alone or in Combination (ATAC) trial, a commonly observed tamoxifen side effect was vaginal bleeding, leading to a higher hysterectomy rate for patients randomized to tamoxifen (5%) compared to anastrozole (1%).[19] An uncommon effect from tamoxifen is retinal toxicity. This drug can also increase the risk of cataracts. However, no difference in the rate of vision-threatening ocular toxicity has been seen among prospectively treated tamoxifen patients.[20] Tamoxifen predisposes patients to thromboembolic phenomena, especially if used with concomitant chemotherapy. Depression has also been described, but the association with tamoxifen is not clear. Although liver cancers have been noted in laboratory animals, there is no established association between tamoxifen and liver cancers in humans.

Pharmacology

Tamoxifen acts by blocking estrogen stimulation of breast cancer cells, inhibiting both translocation and nuclear binding of the ER. This alters transcriptional and posttranscriptional events mediated by this receptor.[21] Tamoxifen has agonistic, partial agonistic, or antagonistic effects depending on the species, tissue, or endpoints that have been assessed. Additionally, there are marked differences between the antiproliferative properties of tamoxifen and its metabolites.[22]

Resistance to tamoxifen can be intrinsic or acquired, and the potential mechanisms for this resistance are reviewed in the following paragraphs. At each step of the signal transduction pathway with which tamoxifen or its metabolites interferes, there is the potential for an alteration in response. The most important factor appears to be the level of ER, which is highly predictive for a response to tamoxifen. Tamoxifen is ineffective in ER-negative breast cancer. Although decreased or absent expression of the progesterone receptor (PR) is associated with a worse prognosis, the relative risk reduction in tamoxifen-treated patients is the same regardless of the presence or absence of the PR.

Following binding to the ER, subsequent translocation of the tamoxifen/ER complex to the nucleus and binding to an estrogen-response element may occur. This binding prevents transcriptional activation of estrogen-responsive genes. Laboratory and clinical data have demonstrated that ER-positive breast cancers that overexpress HER2 may be less responsive to tamoxifen and

TABLE 27.1

Overview of Major Hormonal Agents Used in Cancer

Class of Drug	Individual Drug	Dose	Route of Delivery	Frequency of Delivery
Selective estrogen receptor modulator	Tamoxifen	20 mg	Oral	Once daily
	Toremifene	60 mg	Oral	Once daily
	Raloxifene	60 mg	Oral	Once daily
Aromatase inhibitor	Anastrozole	1 mg	Oral	Once daily
	Letrozole	2.5 mg	Oral	Once daily
	Exemestane	25 mg	Oral	Once daily
Estrogen receptor downregulator	Fulvestrant	500 mg	IM	Once monthly
Luteinizing hormone releasing hormone agonist	Goserelin	7.5	IM	Once monthly[a]
	Leuprolide	3.6	IM	Once monthly[a]
GnRH antagonist	Degarelix	240 mg loading dose	SC	80 mg SC monthly maintenance dose
Antiandrogen	Flutamide	250 mg	Oral	Three times daily
	Bicalutamide	50 mg	Oral	Once daily
	Nilutamide	300 mg for 30 d then 150 mg	Oral	Once daily
Cytochrome P45017 alpha inhibitors	Abiraterone Acetate	1,000 mg (four 250 mg capsules)	Oral	Once Daily
AR "super antagonists"	Enzalutamide	160–240 mg	Oral	Daily
Androgen	Fluoxymesterone	10 mg	Oral	Twice daily
Estrogen	Estradiol	10 mg	Oral	Up to three times daily
Somatostatin analog	Octreotide	Varies	SC or IV	Up to three times daily[b]
Progestational agents	Megestrol	Varies	Oral	Once daily
	Medroxyprogesterone acetate	Varies	Oral or IM	Varies

[a] Longer acting depot preparations (every 3 months) are available.
[b] Depot formulations are available.
IM, intramuscular; SC, subcutaneous; GnRH, gonadotropin-releasing hormone; CYP, cytochrome P-450; AR, androgen receptor.

to hormonal therapy in general.[23–26] In these tumors, ligand-independent activation of the ER by mitogen-activated protein kinase (MAPK) pathways may contribute to resistance.[27–29] In addition, the expression of AIB1, an estrogen-receptor coactivator, has been associated with tamoxifen resistance in patients whose breast cancers overexpress HER2.[30] In some cases, resistance may result from a decrease or loss of ER expression.[31,32] Although mutations in the ER ligand binding domain (LBD) are rare in newly diagnosed breast cancer, ER mutations are present in up to 20% of recurrent breast cancers.[33–36] These mutations lead to a conformational change in the LBD, which mimics the conformation of activated ligand-bound receptor and constitutive, ligand-independent transcriptional activity, resulting in resistance to hormonal therapy. Preclinical studies suggest that some of these mutations, although insensitive to aromatase inhibitors, retain sensitivity to higher dose selective estrogen-receptor modulators (SERM), such as endoxifen, as well as fulvestrant.[35]

The carcinogenic potential of tamoxifen has been recognized in rat studies[37–39] and in humans (endometrial cancer).[40] It has been proposed that the generation of reactive intermediates that bind covalently to macromolecules underlies the process. Such reactive intermediates have been demonstrated in vitro.[40–43] In addition, the induction of covalent DNA adducts in rat livers treated with tamoxifen has been reported.[44] Both constitutive and inducible cytochrome P-450 (CYP) enzymes have been implicated in the formation of metabolites with tamoxifen,[45,46] and the flavone-containing monooxygenase has been implicated in the formation of the N-oxide of tamoxifen. Reactive intermediates from

such metabolic steps are being evaluated for their carcinogenic potential in vitro and in vivo.

Multiple studies to evaluate tumor gene expression profiling have identified gene expression patterns or specific genes associated with resistance to tamoxifen therapy. A commonly utilized gene expression assay, Oncotype DX 21 gene assay (Genomic Health, Redwood City, California), measures the expression of genes known to be involved in estrogen signaling (e.g., ER, PR), HER2, proliferation (e.g., Ki-67), and others. In multiple different data sets, the recurrence score has been associated with a higher risk of breast cancer recurrence in patients treated with hormonal therapy (e.g., tamoxifen or aromatase inhibitors) without concomitant chemotherapy.[47–49]

The pharmacokinetics of tamoxifen is complex. The chemical structure and metabolic pathway of tamoxifen are shown in Figure 27.1. Metabolic activation of tamoxifen is associated with greater pharmacologic activity. The two most active tamoxifen metabolites are 4-hydroxytamoxifen (4-OH tamoxifen) and 4-OH-N-desmethyltamoxifen (endoxifen). A series of studies carried out to characterize endoxifen pharmacology have demonstrated that it has equivalent potency in vitro to 4-hydroxytamoxifen in ER-α and -beta (ER-β) binding,[50] for the suppression of ER-dependent human breast cancer cell line proliferation,[22,50] and in global ER-responsive gene expression.[51] A recent study suggests that endoxifen's effect on the ER may differ from 4-hydroxytamoxifen based on the observation of ER-α degradation.[52]

In women who receive tamoxifen at a dose of 20 mg per day, plasma endoxifen steady-state concentrations are generally 6 to

CANCER THERAPEUTICS

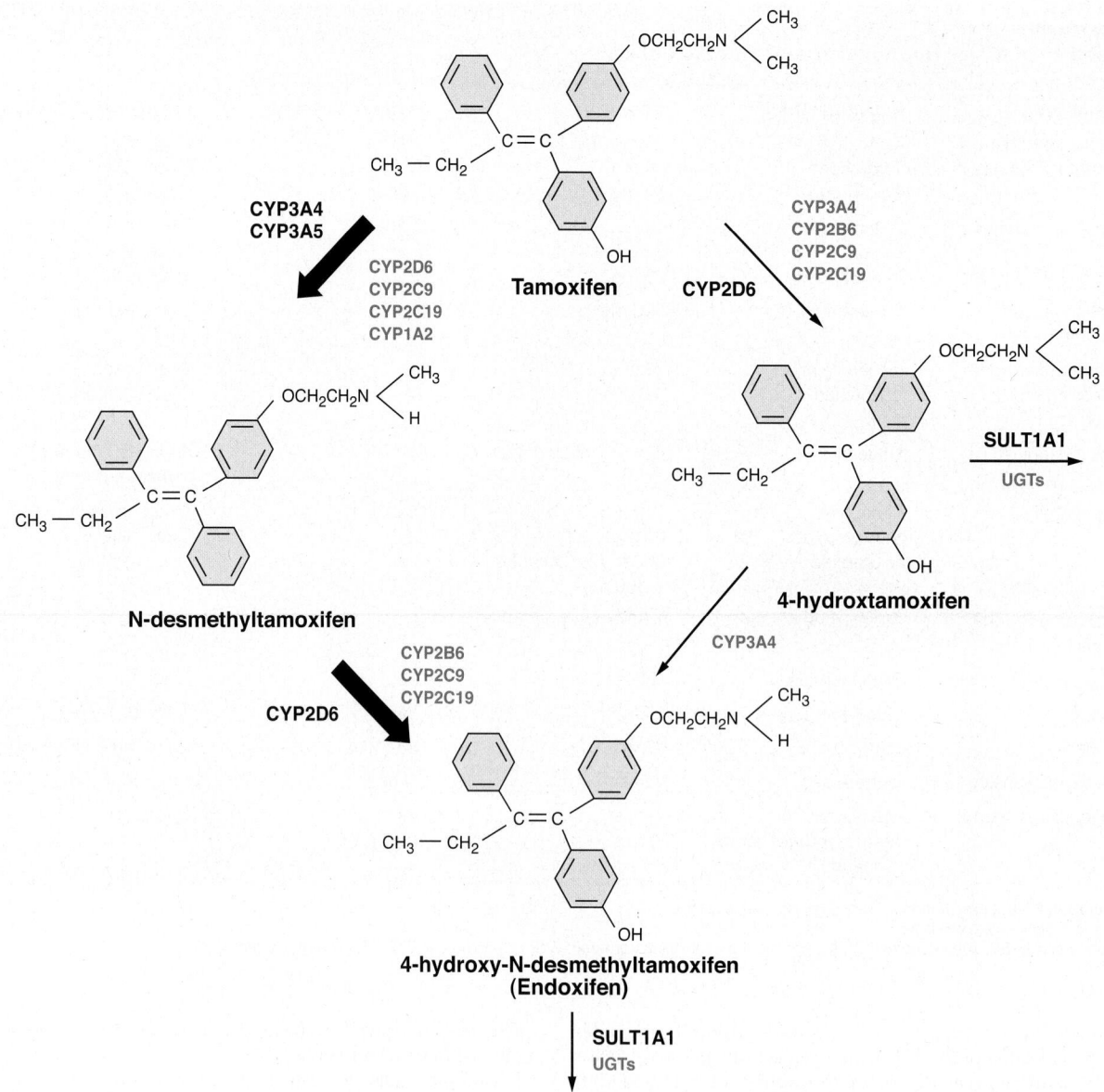

Figure 27.1 Metabolic pathway of tamoxifen biotransformation. (From Sideras K, Ingle JN, Ames MM, et al. Coprescription of tamoxifen and medications that inhibit CYP2D6. *J Clin Oncol* 2010;28:2768–2776.)

10 times higher than 4-hydroxytamoxifen.[53] Although the metabolism of tamoxifen to 4-OH-tamoxifen is catalyzed by multiple enzymes, endoxifen is formed predominantly by the CYP2D6-mediated oxidation of N-desmethyltamoxifen, the most abundant tamoxifen metabolite (see Fig. 27.1).[54] Multiple clinical studies have demonstrated that common *CYP2D6* genetic variation (leading to low or absent CYP2D6 activity) or the drug-induced inhibition of CYP2D6 significantly lowers endoxifen concentrations.[53,55] The *CYP2D6* gene is highly polymorphic, with more than 70 major alleles with four well-defined phenotypes: poor metabolizers (PM), intermediate metabolizers (IM), extensive metabolizers (EM), and ultrarapid metabolizers (UM).

The clinical studies to evaluate the association between *CYP2D6* polymorphisms and tamoxifen outcomes have yielded conflicting results. Initial[56] and follow-up data[57,58] demonstrated that CYP2D6 PM had an approximately two- to threefold higher risk of breast cancer recurrence (compared to CYP2D6 EM) and these data led an FDA special emphasis panel to recommend a tamoxifen label change to incorporate data that the *CYP2D6* genotype was an important biomarker associated with tamoxifen

efficacy.[5] However, this label change has been delayed, in part because of conflicting data from secondary analyses of 5-year tamoxifen prospective trials (ATAC,[59] BIG 1-98,[60] and ABCSG8[61]) as well as meta-analyses,[62] which demonstrate that the *CYP2D6* genotype is associated with tamoxifen efficacy when tamoxifen is administered as monotherapy for the adjuvant treatment of postmenopausal, ER-positive breast cancer. Additional support for the importance of endoxifen concentrations came from a secondary analysis of a prospective study, which demonstrated a higher risk of recurrence for women with low endoxifen concentrations.[13]

Many drugs are known to inhibit CYP2D6 activity. In tamoxifen-treated women, the coadministration of potent CYP2D6 inhibitors, such as paroxetine, converts a patient with normal CYP2D6 metabolism to a phenotypic PM.[63] Many other clinically important drugs have been reported to inhibit the CYP2D6 enzyme system, but their effects on tamoxifen metabolism have not been prospectively studied. As with the data regarding *CYP2D6* genotype, the data regarding CYP2D6 inhibitors has additionally been controversial, including two studies that reported opposite findings with regard to CYP2D6 inhibitor use and breast cancer recurrence or death.[64,65] Although the *CYP2D6* data remain controversial, we conclude that until results from prospective adjuvant studies are available, women should be counseled regarding the potential impact of the *CYP2D6* genotype on the effectiveness of adjuvant tamoxifen, and potent CYP2D6 inhibitors should be avoided. Additional caution should be used with drugs that induce CYP3A, such as rifampicin, as a these drugs have been demonstrated to substantially reduce (up to 86%) the concentrations of tamoxifen and its metabolites.[66]

Strategies to overcome low endoxifen concentrations include dose escalation of tamoxifen to 40 mg per day, which has been demonstrated to significantly increase endoxifen concentrations,[67,68] as well as the direct administration of endoxifen itself. The latter strategy is ongoing in multiple different clinical trials, and early reports suggest clinical activity in aromatase inhibitors (AI)-resistant breast cancer.[69]

Following the metabolic activation of tamoxifen, the hydroxylated metabolites undergo both glucuronidation and sulfation. Peak plasma levels of tamoxifen (maximum concentration [Cmax]) are seen 3 to 7 hours after oral administration. Assuming an oral bioavailability of 30%, the volume of distribution has been calculated to be 20 L/kg, and plasma clearance ranges from 1.2 to 5.1 L per hour.[70] The terminal half-life of tamoxifen has been reported to range between 4 and 11 days.[71,72] The elimination half-life of tamoxifen increases with successive doses, which is consistent with saturable kinetics.[71,73] The drug's distribution in tissues is extensive. Levels of the parent drug and metabolites have been reported to be higher in tissue than in plasma in animal studies.[74,75] Reports of tamoxifen concentrations 10- to 60-fold higher than plasma concentrations in the liver, lungs, brain, pancreas, skin, and bones are reported.[76,77] Elevated levels of tamoxifen with biliary obstruction have been reported.[78]

Tamoxifen has been reported to interact with warfarin,[73,79–81] digitoxin, phenytoin,[82] and medroxyprogesterone.[73] Tamoxifen-induced activation of human transcription factor pregnane X receptor (hPXR), resulting in the induction of CYP3A4, may increase the elimination of concomitantly administered CYP3A substrates,[83] such as anastrozole.[84]

Toremifene

Toremifene is an agent similar to tamoxifen. It is available in the United States for the treatment of patients with metastatic breast cancer, and is approved in other countries for the adjuvant treatment of ER-positive breast cancer. Clinical trials have demonstrated no difference in either disease-free or overall survival when toremifene was compared with tamoxifen for the treatment of ER-positive breast cancer,[85,86] and evidence exists for major cross-resistance between tamoxifen and toremifene.[87,88]

Pharmacology

Toremifene is an antiestrogen with a chemical structure that differs from that of tamoxifen by the substitution of a chlorine for a hydrogen atom that is retained when toremifene undergoes metabolism.[89] Like tamoxifen, toremifene is metabolized by CYP3A,[90] with a secondary metabolism to form hydroxylated metabolites that appear to have similar binding affinities to 4-OH tamoxifen.[89,91] The importance of these metabolites or the role of metabolism to the hydroxylated metabolites is unknown, but may play a role given the structural similarity of toremifene to tamoxifen. Although the oral bioavailability has not been defined, toremifene's oral absorption appears to be good. The time to peak plasma concentrations after oral administration ranges from 1.5 to 6.0 hours,[92] with the terminal half-lives for toremifene and one metabolite, 4-hydroxytoremifene, being 5 to 6 days.[93,94] The apparent clearance is 5.1 L per hour. The terminal half-life for the major metabolite, N-desmethyltoremifene, is 21 days.[95] The time to reach

plasma steady-state concentrations is 1 to 5 weeks. Plasma protein binding is more than 99%. As with tamoxifen, toremifene is present at higher concentrations in tissues compared to plasma with a high apparent volume of distribution (958 L). Seventy percent of the drug is excreted in feces as metabolites. Studies in patients with impaired liver function or those on anticonvulsants known to induce CYP3A have demonstrated that hepatic dysfunction decreases the clearance of toremifene and N-desmethyltoremifene,[95] whereas those patients on anticonvulsants had an increased clearance. Although toremifene appeared to be less carcinogenic than tamoxifen in preclinical models,[43,96,97] of the rates of endometrial cancer in the adjuvant studies have been similar to tamoxifen.[85]

Raloxifene

Raloxifene is an estrogen agonist and antagonist originally developed to treat osteoporosis. Large placebo-controlled randomized trials demonstrated reduced rates of osteoporosis and a reduction in new breast cancers in treated women, leading to the development of a second-generation breast cancer chemoprevention trial (National Surgical Adjuvant Breast and Bowel Project, NSAPB P2) in which raloxifene was compared with tamoxifen in high-risk postmenopausal women. In this study, tamoxifen was superior to raloxifene in terms of both invasive and noninvasive cancer events, but was associated with a higher risk of thromboembolic events and endometrial cancer.[98]

Pharmacology

Raloxifene is partially estrogenic in bone[99] and lowers cholesterol.[100] It is antiestrogenic in mammary tissue[101,102] and uterine tissue.[103]

The pharmacokinetics of raloxifene have been studied principally in postmenopausal women.[104–106] Pharmacokinetic parameters of raloxifene show considerable interindividual variation. Limited information is available on the pharmacokinetics of raloxifene in individuals with hepatic impairment, renal impairment, or both.

Raloxifene is rapidly absorbed from the gastrointestinal tract. Because raloxifene undergoes extensive first-pass glucuronidation, oral bioavailability of unchanged drug is low. Although approximately 60% of an oral dose is absorbed, the absolute bioavailability as unchanged raloxifene is only 2%. However, systemic availability of raloxifene may be greater than that indicated in bioavailability studies, because circulating glucuronide conjugates are converted back to the parent drug in various tissues.

After the oral administration of a single 120- or 150-mg dose of raloxifene hydrochloride, peak plasma concentrations of raloxifene and its glucuronide conjugates are achieved at 6 hours and 1 hour, respectively. After the oral administration of radiolabeled raloxifene, less than 1% of total circulating radiolabeled material in plasma represents the parent drug.

Results of a single-dose study in patients with liver dysfunction indicate that plasma raloxifene concentrations correlate with serum bilirubin concentrations and are 2.5 times higher than individuals with normal hepatic function. In postmenopausal women who received raloxifene in clinical trials, plasma concentrations of raloxifene and the glucuronide conjugates in those with renal impairment (i.e., estimated creatinine clearance values as low as 23 mL per minute) were similar to values in women with normal renal function.

Raloxifene and its monoglucuronide conjugates are more than 95% bound to plasma proteins. Raloxifene binds to albumin and α_1-acid glycoprotein. Raloxifene undergoes extensive first-pass metabolism to the glucuronide conjugates raloxifene 4'-glucuronide, 6-glucuronide, and 6,4'-diglucuronide. UGT1A1 and -1A8 have been found to catalyze the formation of both the 6-β-and 4'-β-glucuronides, whereas UGT1A10 formed only the 4'-β-glucuronide.[107] The metabolism of raloxifene does not appear to be mediated by CYP enzymes (such as CYP2D6), because metabolites other than glucuronide conjugates have not been identified.

The plasma elimination half-life of raloxifene at steady state averages 32.5 hours (range, 15.8 to 86.6 hours). Raloxifene is excreted principally in feces as an unabsorbed drug and via biliary elimination as glucuronide conjugates, which, subsequently, are metabolized by bacteria in the gastrointestinal tract to the parent drug. After oral administration, less than 0.2% of a raloxifene dose is excreted as the parent compound and less than 6% as glucuronide conjugates in urine.

Fulvestrant

Fulvestrant is an ER antagonist that has no known agonist activity and results in ER downregulation.[108–111] Like tamoxifen, fulvestrant competitively binds to the ER but with a higher affinity—approximately 100 times greater than that of tamoxifen,[108,112–114]—thus preventing endogenous estrogen from exerting its effect in target cells.

Results from two phase III clinical trials using the 250 mg per month dose demonstrated fulvestrant to be as effective as anastrozole in the treatment of postmenopausal women with advanced hormone receptor–positive breast cancer previously treated with antiestrogen therapy (mainly tamoxifen).[112–116] In the setting of first-line hormone-responsive metastatic breast cancer, a randomized phase III clinical trial to compare tamoxifen to fulvestrant (250 mg per month) demonstrated no differences in response or time to progression.[117] Because of pharmacology data (discussed in the following paragraphs), the 500 mg per day dose was developed. A randomized trial comparing the 250 mg per month with 500 mg per month dose demonstrated a 4-month improvement in median overall survival advantage for the higher dose.[118] For this reason, the higher dose is now the standard recommended dose.

Fulvestrant is well tolerated. The most common drug-related events (greater than 10% incidence) from the randomized phase III studies were injection-site reactions and hot flashes. Common events (1% to 10% incidence) included asthenia, headache, and gastrointestinal disturbances such as nausea, vomiting, and diarrhea, with minor gastrointestinal disturbances being the most commonly described adverse event.

Pharmacology

Fulvestrant is a steroidal molecule derived from E_2 with an alkylsulphonyl side chain in the 7-α position (Fig. 27.2). Because fulvestrant is poorly soluble and has low and unpredictable oral bioavailability, a parenteral formulation of fulvestrant was developed in an attempt to maximize delivery of the drug.[111] The intramuscular formulation provides prolonged release of the drug over several weeks. The pharmacokinetics of three different single doses of fulvestrant (50, 125, and 250 mg) have been published.[111] In this phase I/II multicenter study, postmenopausal women with primary breast cancer who were awaiting curative surgery received either fulvestrant, tamoxifen, or placebo. After single intramuscular injections of fulvestrant, the time of maximal concentration (t_{max}) ranged from 2 to 19 days, with the median being 7 days for each dose group. At the interval of 28 days, Cmin values were two- to fivefold lower than the Cmax values. For most patients in the 125- and 250-mg dose groups, significant levels of fulvestrant were still measurable 84 days after administration. Pharmacokinetic modeling of the pooled data from the 250-mg cohort was best described by a two-compartment model in which a longer terminal phase began approximately 3 weeks after administration. Because of the long time needed to reach a steady state, the 500-mg loading dose regimen was prospectively studied and determined to be superior to the 250 mg per month dose, both in terms of steady state concentrations achieved within 1 month[119] as well as progression-free and overall survival.[118]

AROMATASE INHIBITORS

At menopause, the synthesis of ovarian hormones ceases. However, estrogen continues to be converted from androgens (produced by the adrenal glands) by aromatase, an enzyme of the CYP superfamily. Aromatase is the enzyme complex responsible for the final step in estrogen synthesis via the conversion of androgens, androstenedione and testosterone, to estrogens, estrone (E_1) and E_2. This biologic pathway served as the basis for the development of the antiaromatase class of compounds. Alterations in aromatase expression have been implicated in the pathogenesis of estrogen-dependent disease, including breast cancer, endometrial cancer, and endometriosis. The importance of this enzyme is also highlighted by the fact that selective aromatase inhibitors are commonly used as first-line therapy for the treatment of postmenopausal women with estrogen-responsive breast cancer. Aminoglutethimide was the first clinically used aromatase inhibitor. When it became available, it was used to cause a *medical adrenalectomy*. Because of the lack of selectivity for aromatase and the resultant suppression of aldosterone and cortisol, aminoglutethimide is no longer recommended for treating metastatic breast cancer. Aminoglutethimide is also occasionally used to try to reverse excess hormone production by adrenocortical cancers.[120]

Aromatase (cytochrome P-450 19 [CYP19]) is encoded by the *CYP19* gene, which is highly polymorphic. Some of these variants are functionally important[121] and may have clinical significance.[122,123]

Aromatase inhibitors have been classified in a number of different ways, including first, second, and third generation; steroidal and nonsteroidal; and reversible (ionic binding) and irreversible (suicide inhibitor, covalent binding).[124] The nonsteroidal aromatase inhibitors include aminoglutethimide (first generation), rogletimide and fadrozole (second generation), and anastrozole, letrozole, and vorozole (third generation). The steroidal aromatase inhibitors include formestane (second generation) and exemestane (third generation).

Steroidal and nonsteroidal aromatase inhibitors differ in their modes of interaction with, and their inactivation of, the aromatase enzyme. Steroidal inhibitors compete with the endogenous

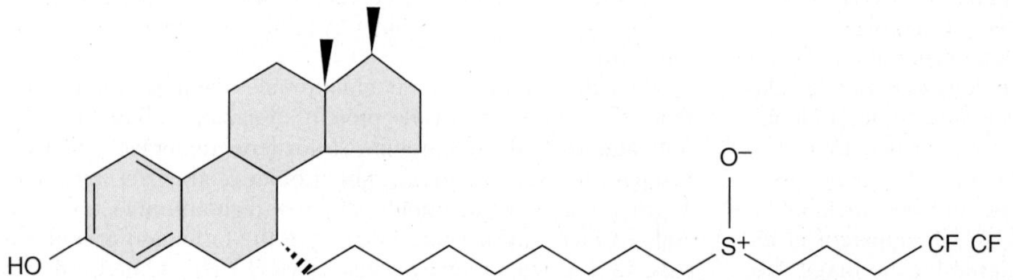

Figure 27.2 Structure of fulvestrant.

substrates, androstenedione and testosterone, for the active site of the enzyme and are processed into intermediates that bind irreversibly to the active site, causing irreversible enzyme inhibition.[19] Nonsteroidal inhibitors also compete with the endogenous substrates for access to the active site, where they then form a reversible bond to the heme iron atom so that enzyme activity can recover if the inhibitor is removed; however, inhibition is sustained whenever the inhibitor is present.[19]

Letrozole and Anastrozole

Both letrozole and anastrozole have been extensively studied in the metastatic and adjuvant settings. When compared to tamoxifen, both letrozole and anastrozole have demonstrated superior response rates and progression-free survival in the metastatic setting.[124,125] In the adjuvant setting, two trials have been performed and demonstrated superiority in terms of relapse-free survivals of both anastrozole (ATAC)[126] and letrozole (BIG 1-98).[127] Additionally, anastrozole has been studied in a sequential approach, and the sequence of tamoxifen followed by anastrozole is superior to 5 years of tamoxifen alone.[128] Anastrozole has recently been compared to placebo in women at an increased risk of developing breast cancer and was demonstrated to significantly reduce the incidence of invasive breast cancer.[129]

The side effects of both anastrozole and letrozole are similar and include arthralgias and myalgias in up to 50% of patients. Both letrozole and anastrozole are associated with a higher rate of bone fracture, compared with the tamoxifen.[130] At the present time, minimal long-term (longer than 5 years) clinical data regarding the effect of aromatase inhibitors on bones are available. When offering anastrozole for extended periods of time to patients with early breast cancer, attention to bone health is paramount, and bone density should be monitored in all patients. Prospective studies have demonstrated that bisphosphonates prevent aromatase-inhibitor–induced bone loss and a meta-analysis presented at the 2013 San Antonio Breast Cancer Symposium demonstrated that bisphosphonates reduce bone recurrences and prolong overall survival. Therefore, bisphosphonates should be considered in AI-treated patients, both in those with and without an increased risk of bone fractures.

A meta-analysis of toxicities comparing aromatase inhibitors with tamoxifen has demonstrated a 30% increase in grade 3 and 4 cardiac events with aromatase inhibitors.[131] However, prospective data demonstrate no differences in myocardial events comparing anastrozole with placebo, although an increase in hypertension was observed.[129]

No impact has been seen with anastrozole on adrenal steroidogenesis at up to 10 times the clinically recommended dose.[132] Although letrozole may decrease basal and adrenocorticotropic hormone–stimulated cortisol synthesis,[133,134] the clinical effect appears to be minimal. Aromatase inhibitors appear to have differential effects on lipids. In a study of over 900 patients with metastatic disease, anastrozole showed no marked effect on lipid profiles compared with baseline.[135] Conversely, the administration of letrozole in women with advanced breast cancer resulted in significant increases in total cholesterol and low-density lipoprotein, from baseline, after 8 and 16 weeks of therapy.[136] In the Breast International Group 1-98 trial, more women who received letrozole experienced grade 1 hypercholesterolemia compared to women who received tamoxifen.[127]

Letrozole is a nonsteroidal aromatase inhibitor with a high specificity for the inhibition of estrogen production (Fig. 27.3). Letrozole is 180 times more potent than aminoglutethimide as an inhibitor of aromatase in vitro. Aldosterone production in vitro is inhibited by concentrations 10,000 times higher than those required for inhibition of estrogen synthesis.[137,138] In a normal male volunteer study, letrozole was shown to decrease E_2 and serum E_1 levels to 10% of baseline with a single 3-mg dose. In phase I

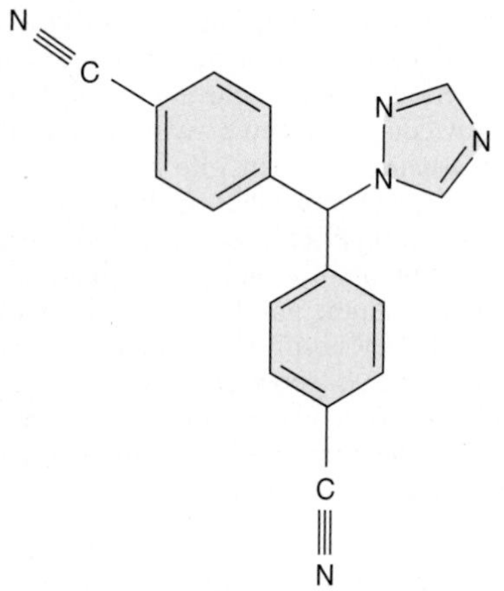

Figure 27.3 Structure of letrozole.

studies, letrozole caused a significant decline in plasma E_1 and E_2 within 24 hours of a single oral dose of 0.1 mg.[139,140] After 2 weeks of treatment, the blood levels of E_2, E_1, and estrone sulfate were suppressed 95% or more from baseline. This continued over the 12 weeks of therapy. There was no apparent alteration in plasma levels of cortisol and aldosterone with letrozole or after corticotropin stimulation.[139] In postmenopausal women with advanced breast cancer, the drug did not have any effect on follicle-stimulating hormone (FSH), luteinizing hormone (LH), thyrotropin (previously thyroid-stimulating hormone), cortisol, 17-α-hydroxyprogesterone, androstenedione, or aldosterone blood concentrations.[141,142]

Anastrozole is a nonsteroidal aromatase inhibitor that is 200-fold more potent than aminoglutethimide.[143] No effect on the adrenal glands has been detected. In human studies, the t_{max} is 2 to 3 hours after oral ingestion.[144] Elimination is primarily via hepatic metabolism, with 85% excreted by that route and only 10% excreted unchanged in urine. The main circulating metabolite is triazole after cleavage of the two rings in anastrozole by N-dealkylation. Linear pharmacokinetics have been observed in the dose range of 1 to 20 mg and do not change with repeat dosing. The terminal half-life is approximately 50 hours, and steady-state concentrations are achieved in approximately 10 days with once-a-day dosing and are three to four times higher than peak concentrations after a single dose. Plasma protein binding is approximately 40%.[145] In one study, anastrozole 1 mg and 10 mg daily, inhibited in vivo aromatization by 96.7% and 98.1%, respectively, and plasma E_1 and E_2 levels were suppressed 86.5% and 83.5%, respectively, regardless of dose.[146] Thus, 1 mg of anastrozole achieves near maximal aromatase inhibition and plasma estrogen suppression in breast cancer patients.

A recent prospective study to evaluate the pharmacokinetics of anastrozole (1 mg per day) demonstrated large interindividual variations in plasma anastrozole and anastrozole metabolite concentrations, as well as pretreatment and postdrug plasma E_1, E_2, and E_1 conjugate and estrogen precursor (androstenedione and testosterone) concentrations.[147] Further research is needed to determine the basis for the wide variability in the pharmacokinetics of anastrozole and whether these findings are clinically relevant.

Exemestane

Exemestane has a steroidal structure and is classified as a type 1 aromatase inhibitor, also known as an *aromatase inactivator*, because it irreversibly binds with and permanently inactivates the enzyme.[134] Exemestane has been compared to tamoxifen in both the metastatic and adjuvant settings. In the setting of tamoxifen-refractory metastatic breast cancer, exemestane is superior to megestrol acetate, as demonstrated in a phase III trial in which improvements in both median time to tumor progression and median survival were observed.[148] In the adjuvant setting, the international exemestane study compared 2 to 3 years of tamoxifen with 2 to 3 years of exemestane in women who had previously competed 2 to 3 years of adjuvant tamoxifen. In this trial, a switch to exemestane resulted in superior disease-free and overall survival in the hormone receptor–positive subtype. Furthermore, exemestane has been compared with the nonsteroidal agent anastrozole in the adjuvant treatment of ER-positive breast cancer, and there were no differences in disease-free or overall survival.[149] Finally, exemestane has been compared to placebo in patients at increased risk of breast cancer, and a significant reduction in the risk of developing invasive breast cancer was observed.[150]

Side Effects of Exemestane

Although preclinical studies have suggested that exemestane prevented bone loss in ovariectomized rats,[151] the Intergroup Exemestane adjuvant trial still demonstrated a higher rate of bone fracture for patients randomized to the exemestane arm and there were no differences in fracture rates comparing anastrozole with exemestane.[149] Side effects, including arthralgias and myalgias, appear to be similar to the other AIs. With regard to steroidogenesis, no impact on either cortisol or aldosterone levels was seen in a small study after the administration of exemestane for 7 days.[152] Finally, exemestane has weak androgenic properties, and its use at higher doses has been associated with steroidal-like side effects, such as weight gain and acne.[153,154] However, these side effects have not been observed with the FDA-approved dose (25 mg per day).[155]

Pharmacology

Exemestane is administered once daily by mouth, with the recommended daily dose being 25 mg. The time needed to reach maximal E_2 suppression is 7 days,[156] and its half-life is 27 hours.[157] At daily doses of 10 to 25 mg, exemestane suppresses estrogen concentrations to 6% to 15% of pretreatment levels. This activity is more pronounced than that produced by formestane and comparable to that produced by the nonsteroidal AIs, anastrozole and letrozole.[158–160] Exemestane does not appear to affect cortisol or aldosterone levels when evaluated after 7 days of treatment based on dose-ranging studies, including doses from 0.5 to 800 mg.[152] Exemestane is metabolized by CYP3A4.[134] Although drug–drug interactions have not been formally reported for exemestane, there is the potential for interactions with drugs that affect CYP3A4.[134]

GONADOTROPIN-RELEASING HORMONE ANALOGS

Gonadotropin-releasing hormone (GnRH) analogs result in a *medical orchiectomy* in men and are used as a means of providing androgen ablation for hormone-sensitive and castration refractory metastatic prostate cancer.[161] Because the initial agonist activity of GnRH analogs can cause a *tumor flare* from temporarily increased androgen levels, concomitant use of the antiandrogen flutamide or bicalutamide has been used to prevent this effect. GnRH analogs can also cause tumor regressions in hormonally responsive breast cancers[162] and have received FDA approval for the treatment of metastatic breast cancer in premenopausal women. Data suggest that these drugs may be useful as adjuvant therapy of premenopausal women with resected breast cancer.[163] The use of these drugs in combination with tamoxifen or exemestane in premenopausal women with primary breast cancer is the subject of large, ongoing, international clinical trials. The primary toxicities of GnRH analogs are secondary to the ablation of sex steroid

concentrations and include hot flashes, sweating, and nausea.[164] These symptoms can be reversed with low doses of progesterone analogs.[5] In males treated with GnRH analogs for prostate cancer, an alternate strategy of intermittent schedule of GnRH administration may result in improved tolerability and quality of life, with comparable efficacy compared with continuous GnRH analog administration in well-selected advanced prostate cancer patient cohorts.[165] However, in a recent trial comparing intermittent with continuous androgen ablation in newly diagnosed metastatic hormone sensitive prostate cancer patients, a greater risk for death from an intermittent strategy could not be conclusively ruled out although intermittent therapy resulted in small improvements in quality of life.[166]

GnRH analogs available for clinical use include goserelin[167,168] and leuprolide.[169] Both are available in depot intramuscular preparations to be given at monthly intervals. The recommended monthly dose of leuprolide is 7.5 mg and of goserelin is 3.6 mg. There are also longer acting depot preparations to be administered every 3, 4, 6, and 12 months.

Pharmacology

Analogs of the decapeptide GnRH[167,169,170] have been synthesized by modifications of position 6 in which the l-glycine has been exchanged for a d-amino acid and the C-terminal amino acid has been either replaced by an ethylamide or substituted for a modified amino acid. These changes increase the affinity of the analog for the GnRH receptor and decrease the susceptibility to enzymatic degradation. There is an amino acid structure of GnRH with the substitutions for leuprolide and goserelin. Initial administration of these compounds results in stimulation of gonadotropin release. However, prolonged administration has led to profound inhibition of the pituitary–gonadal axis.[170] Plasma E_2 and progesterone are consistently suppressed to postmenopausal or castrate levels after 2 to 4 weeks of treatment with goserelin or leuprolide.[164,171] These drugs are administered intramuscularly or subcutaneously in a parenteral sustained-release microcapsule preparation, because parenteral administration of the parent drug is otherwise associated with rapid clearance. The GnRH analogs are metabolized in the liver, kidney, hypothalamus, and pituitary gland by neutral peptidase cleavage of the peptide bond between the tyrosine in the 5 position and the amino acid in position 6 and by a postproline-cleaving enzyme that cleaves the peptide bond between proline in the 9 position and the glycine-NH₂ in the 10 position. Substitutions at the glycine 6 position and modification of the C-terminal make these analogs more resistant to this enzymatic cleavage.

Leuprolide is approximately 80 to 100 times more potent than endogenous GnRH. It induces castrate levels of testosterone in men with prostate cancer within 3 to 4 weeks of drug administration after an initial sharp increase in LH and FSH. The mechanisms of action include pituitary desensitization after a reduction in pituitary GnRH receptor binding sites and possibly a direct antitumor effect in ER-positive human breast cancer cells.[169] The depot form results in a dose rate of 210 μg per day of leuprolide. Peak concentrations of the depot form, achieved approximately 3 hours after drug administration, have been reported to range between 13.1 and 54.5 μg/L. There appears to be a linear increase in the area under the curve (AUC) for doses of 3.75, 7.5, and 15.0 mg in the depot form. The parenteral bioavailability of subcutaneously injected leuprolide is 94%. The volume of distribution ranges from 27.4 to 37.1 L. In human studies, leuprolide urinary excretion as a metabolite was the primary route of clearance.

Goserelin is approximately 100 times more potent than the naturally occurring GnRH. Like leuprolide, it causes the stimulation of LH and FSH acutely, and with subsequent administration, GnRH receptor numbers decrease, and the pituitary becomes desensitized with decreasing LH and FSH levels. Castrate levels of testosterone are achieved within 1 month. In women, goserelin inhibits ovarian androgen production, but serum levels of dehydroepiandrosterone sulfate and, to a lesser extent, androstenedione, are preserved. In vitro, goserelin has demonstrated antitumor activity in estrogen-dependent MCF7 human breast cancer cells and LNCaP2 prostate cancer cells. The drug is released at a continuous mean rate of 120 μg per day in the depot form, with peak concentrations in the range of 2 to 3 μg/L achieved. The mean volume of distribution in six patients has been reported to be 13.7 L,[172] which is consistent with extracellular fluid volume. Goserelin is principally excreted in the urine, with a mean total body clearance of 8 L per hour in patients with normal renal function. The total body clearance is reduced by approximately 75%, with renal dysfunction and the elimination half-life increased two- or threefold. However, dose adjustment for renal insufficiency does not appear to be necessary. The 5 to 10 hexapeptide and the 4 to 10 hexapeptide were detected in urine in animal studies.[173] The terminal half-life of goserelin is approximately 5 hours after subcutaneous injection. Protein binding is low, and no known drug interactions have been documented.

GONADOTROPIN-RELEASING HORMONE ANTAGONISTS

Modification to the structure of GnRH has resulted in the development of GnRH antagonist compounds that are currently being used in the treatment of prostate cancer. Abarelix was initially approved by the FDA in 2003 as the first depot-injectable GnRH antagonist, but was subsequently withdrawn in 2005. Degarelix is a synthetically modified compound with GnRH antagonist activity that was approved for use by the FDA in 2008 for the management of prostate cancer.[174] Its effect in prostate cancer treatment is to block the GnRH receptor, and thereby prevent the trigger for the production of LH, which mediates androgen synthesis. In contrast to GnRH analogs, degarelix does not cause *tumor flare* symptoms secondary to temporary increased androgen production. A large randomized clinical trial demonstrated that degarelix was associated with a rapid and sustained reduction in serum testosterone, prostate-specific antigen (PSA), FSH, and LH levels, with a loading dose of 240 mg subcutaneously, followed by a monthly maintenance dose of 80 mg[175] with comparable efficacy to leuprolide.[176] The most common side effects (greater than 10%) were hot flashes and pain at the injection site[176] when patients were provided degarelix for a 12-month period. It is unknown if degarelix will have a similar chronic side effect profile known to be associated with long-term GnRH analog use.

Pharmacology

The recommended loading dose of degarelix is 240 mg, administered as two injections of 120 mg each subcutaneously. Monthly maintenance doses of 80 mg as a 20 mg/mL solution is started 28 days after the loading dose. In an analysis of pharmacokinetic/pharmacodynamic (PK/PD) properties of degarelix in 60 healthy males, after a single subcutaneous dose, a terminal half life of 47 days was observed.[177] PK properties of degarelix have been evaluated when administered as a subcutaneous depot of drug as a gel in six different doses to 48 healthy males and when administered intravenously. Using data from several clinical trials, the rate of drug diffusion from subcutaneous administration results in detectable drug up to 60 days after a single dose compared to less than 4 days when the drug is injected intravenously.

ANTIANDROGENS

Flutamide

The antiandrogen flutamide is used in men with metastatic prostate cancer either as initial therapy, combined with GnRH analog administration, or when the metastatic prostate cancer is unresponsive, despite androgen ablation therapy. The recommended dose is 250 mg by mouth three times a day. In patients whose prostate cancer is growing despite flutamide use, stopping flutamide can sometimes cause a flutamide-withdrawal response.

The most common toxicity seen with flutamide is diarrhea, with or without abdominal discomfort. Gynecomastia, which can be tender, frequently occurs in men who are not receiving concomitant androgen ablation therapy.[178] Flutamide can rarely cause hepatotoxicity, a condition that is reversible if detected early, but this toxicity can also be fatal.[179] There is no accepted, clinically recommended testing schedule to screen for flutamide-induced hepatotoxicity other than being aware of this phenomenon and testing for liver function if hepatic symptoms develop.

Pharmacology

Flutamide is a pure antiandrogen with no intrinsic steroidal activity.[180] Flutamide's mechanism of action is as an androgen-receptor antagonist. This binding prevents dihydrotestosterone binding and subsequent translocation of the androgen-receptor complex into the nuclei of cells. Because it is a pure antiandrogen, it acts only at the cellular level. The administration of flutamide alone leads to increased LH and FSH production and a concomitant increase in plasma testosterone and E_2 levels. Plasma protein binding ranges between 94% and 96% for flutamide and between 92% and 94% for 2-hydroxyflutamide, its major metabolite. When the drug is administered three times a day, steady state levels are achieved by day 6. The elimination half-life at steady state is 7.8 hours, and 2-hydroxyflutamide achieves concentrations 50 times higher than the parent drug at steady state and has equal or greater potency than that of flutamide.[180] The elimination half-life for the metabolite is 9.6 hours. The high plasma concentrations of 2-hydroxyflutamide, as compared with flutamide, suggest that the therapeutic benefits of flutamide are mediated primarily through its active metabolite.[181]

Bicalutamide

Bicalutamide is another nonsteroidal antiandrogen that has been approved by the FDA for use in the United States. The recommended dose is one 50-mg tablet per day. One randomized trial reported that bicalutamide compared favorably with flutamide in patients with advanced prostate cancer.[182] Bicalutamide appears to be relatively well tolerated and is associated with a lower incidence of diarrhea than is flutamide.

Pharmacology

Bicalutamide has a binding affinity to the androgen receptor in the rat prostate that is four times greater than that of 2-hydroxyflutamide.[183,184] In vivo, bicalutamide caused a marked inhibition of growth of accessory sex organs in rats, with a potency 5 to 10 times greater than that of flutamide. Unlike flutamide, bicalutamide did not cause a significant increase in LH or testosterone in rats. In humans, the drug has a long plasma half-life of 5 to 7 days, so it may be administered on a weekly schedule. Pharmacokinetics of the drug showed a dose-dependent increase in mean peak plasma concentrations, and the AUC increased linearly with the dose. The half-life of bicalutamide in humans was approximately 6 days, and the drug clearance was not saturable at plasma concentrations up to 1,000 ng/mL. Daily dosing of the drug led to an approximately tenfold accumulation after 12 weeks of administration. In contrast to results in rats, serum concentrations of testosterone and LH increased significantly from baseline at all dose levels tested in humans. Whereas serum FSH concentrations remained essentially unchanged, the median serum E_2 concentrations increased significantly.[185]

Nilutamide

Nilutamide represents the third variation of an antiandrogen available for use in patients with prostate cancer. The observation of unique toxicities, night blindness, and pulmonary toxicity has limited its use.

NOVEL ANTIANDROGENS

Although testosterone depletion remains an unchallenged standard for advanced stage hormone-sensitive disease, evidence has emerged that *castration-recurrent* prostate cancer remains androgen receptor (AR) dependent and is neither *hormone refractory* nor *androgen independent*, which were commonly used terms to define the progression of advanced stage disease following androgen deprivation therapy. Recognition of AR functioning despite the paucity of circulating androgens is evidenced by the elevation of AR messenger RNA in castration-recurrent tumor tissue relative to androgen-dependent tumors and reexpression of some androgen-regulated genes during clinical castration resistance. Recently, the AR axis has been the focus of therapeutic targeting.

Abiraterone Acetate

After the failure of initial androgen manipulation with GnRH analogs and peripheral antiandrogens, prostate cancer continues to respond to a variety of second- and third-line hormonal interventions. Based on this observation, CYP17, a key enzyme in androgen and estrogen synthesis, was targeted using ketoconazole, which is a weak, reversible, and nonspecific inhibitor of CYP17 resulting in modest antitumor activity of short durability. More recently, abiraterone, a more potent (i.e., 20 times more than ketoconazole), selective, and irreversible inhibitor of CYP17, has been investigated in castration-recurrent prostate cancer, and significant objective responses have been observed.[186] Chemically, it is a 3-pyridyl steroid pregnenolone–derived compound available in an oral prodrug form of abiraterone acetate. Its main toxicity is from symptoms of mineralocorticoid excess (including hypokalemia, hypertension, and fluid overload), because continuous CYP17 blockade results in raising adrenocorticotrophic hormone (ACTH) levels that increase steroid levels upstream of CYP17, including corticosterone and deoxycorticosterone. These adverse effects are best avoided by the coadministration of steroids.

The established dose of abiraterone is 1,000 mg a day (four 250 mg tablets). Following oral administration of abiraterone acetate, the median time to maximum plasma abiraterone concentrations is 2 hours. At the dose of 1,000 mg daily, steady state values (mean ± standard deviation [SD]) of Cmax were 226 ± 178 ng/mL and of AUC were 1173 ± 690 ng.hr/mL. Abiraterone is highly bound (>99%) to the human plasma proteins, albumin and alpha-1 acid glycoprotein. The apparent steady state volume of distribution (mean ± SD) is 19,669 ± 13,358 L. No major deviation from dose proportionality was observed in the dose range of 250 mg to 1,000 mg. However, the exposure was not significantly increased when the dose was doubled from 1,000 to 2,000 mg (8% increase in mean AUC). The two main circulating metabolites of abiraterone in human plasma are abiraterone sulfate (inactive) and N-oxide abiraterone sulfate (inactive), which each account for about 43% of exposure. CYP3A4 and SULT2A1 are enzymes involved in the formation and conjugation of N-oxide abiraterone.

Enzalutamide

Enzalutamide is a new diarylthiohydantoin compound that binds AR with an affinity that is several-fold greater than the antiandrogens bicalutamide and flutamide. This class of novel AR inhibitor also disrupts the nuclear translocation of AR and impairs DNA binding to androgen response elements and the recruitment of coactivators.[187] In early clinical trials, promising results have been observed in castrate refractory and chemotherapy-resistant settings. The major metabolite of enzalutamide is N-desmethyl enzalutamide, and CYP2C8 is responsible for the formation of the active metabolite, N-desmethyl enzalutamide. Enzalutamide pharmacokinetics, in the studied dose range between 30 mg to 480 mg, exhibited a linear, two-compartmental model with first-order kinetics. In patients with mCRPC, the mean (% coefficient of variation [CV]) predose Cmin values for enzalutamide and N-desmethyl enzalutamide were 11.4 (25.9%) µg/mL and 13.0 (29.9%) µg/mL, respectively. Enzalutamide is mainly metabolized by CYP2C8 and CYP3A4. Doses ranging from 30 to 600 mg daily have been evaluated, with dose-limiting toxicities including fatigue, seizure, asthenia, anemia, and arthralgia occurring at higher dose levels. At present, enzalutamide has been approved for treating advanced castrate-recurrent prostate cancer[188] after a failure of docetaxel chemotherapy at a dose of 160 mg (four, 40 mg oral capsules). Clinical trials are ongoing to evaluate the efficacy of enzalutamide in castrate-recurrent patients who are chemotherapy naïve.

Galeterone and Orteronel

Novel CYP17 inhibitors that are more selective for 17,20-lyase over 17 α-hydroxylase are currently being developed. Orteronel (TAK-700) is an example of a highly selective 17,20 lyase, which is currently undergoing phase III clinical trials in a pre- and post-chemotherapy castrate-recurrent setting after the failure of androgen-deprivation therapy.[189] Other novel agents being developed include galeterone, which is an inhibitor of CYP 17 α-hydroxylase and C17,20 lyase. Survival mechanisms of prostate cancer cells targeted by galeterone include its binding to AR, competitive inhibition of testosterone binding, and a reduction in the quantity of AR protein within the prostate cancer cells. It can also enhance the degradation of constitutively active splice variants. Therefore, taken together, it diminishes the ability of the cells to respond to the low levels of androgenic growth signals. This agent is currently in early clinical safety and efficacy testing for advanced stage prostate cancer.

OTHER SEX STEROID THERAPIES

Fluoxymesterone

Fluoxymesterone is an androgen that has been used in women with metastatic breast cancer who have hormonally responsive cancers and who have progressed on other hormonal therapies such as tamoxifen, an aromatase inhibitor, or megestrol acetate. The usual dose is 10 mg given twice daily. Although the overall response rate is low for fluoxymesterone used in this clinical situation,[190] there are some patients who have substantial antitumor responses lasting for months or even years.

Toxicities associated with fluoxymesterone are those that would be expected with an androgen: hirsutism, male-pattern baldness, voice lowering (hoarseness), acne, enhanced libido, and erythrocytosis. Fluoxymesterone can also cause elevated liver function test results in some patients and, rarely, has been associated with hepatic neoplasms.

Pharmacology

Fluoxymesterone is a chlorinated synthetic analog of testosterone with potent androgenic and anabolic activity in humans. Limited pharmacologic information is available on this agent. Colburn,[191] using a radioimmunoassay, studied two patients after a single oral administration of a 50-mg dose. Peak serum concentrations were achieved between 1 and 3 hours after administration, with the average peak concentrations being 335 ng/mL. By 5 hours after drug administration, serum levels had declined to approximately 50% of the peak concentration. Urinary excretion of a 10-mg dose can be detected for 24 hours, and at least 6-hydroxy, 4-ene, 3-β, and 11-hydroxy metabolites of fluoxymesterone have been detected.[192]

Estrogens: Diethylstilbestrol and Estradiol

Diethylstilbestrol (DES) had been the primary hormonal therapy for postmenopausal metastatic breast cancer. Randomized comparative trials demonstrated it had a similar response rate to that of tamoxifen.[193,194] However, based on these trials, DES use was supplanted by tamoxifen, primarily because DES has more toxicity. DES is occasionally used in metastatic breast cancer patients who have hormonally sensitive cancers that have failed to respond to multiple other hormonal therapies. The usual dose in this situation is 15 mg per day, either as a single dose or as divided doses. DES was also used as androgen ablation therapy in men with metastatic prostate cancer.[195] Doses of approximately 3 mg per day result in testosterone levels that are seen in an anorchid state.

DES toxicities include nausea and vomiting, breast tenderness, and a darkening of the nipple–areolar complex. DES increases the risk of thromboembolic phenomenon, which may result in life-threatening complications. Although DES is not clinically available in the United States, similar antitumor effects and toxicities are seen with estradiol, with a target dose of 10 mg by mouth three times a day. The pharmacology of E_2 has been extensively described elsewhere.[196]

Medroxyprogesterone and Megestrol

Medroxyprogesterone and megestrol are 17-OH-progesterone derivatives differing in a double bond between C6 and C7 positions in megestrol. Historically, megestrol was used as a hormonal agent for patients with advanced breast cancer, usually at a total daily dose of 160 mg. Additionally, it is still used for the treatment of hormonally responsive metastatic endometrial cancer, at a dose of 320 mg per day. In addition, doses of 160 mg per day are occasionally used as a hormonal therapy for prostate cancer.[197] Megestrol has also been extensively evaluated for the treatment of anorexia/cachexia related to cancer or AIDS.[198–201] Various dosages ranging from 160 to 1,600 mg per day have been used. A prospective study has demonstrated a dose–response relationship with doses up to 800 mg per day.[202] Low dosages of megestrol (20 to 40 mg per day) have been shown to be an effective means of reducing hot flashes in women with breast cancer and in men who have undergone androgen ablation therapy.[5] Although megestrol had historically been commonly administered four times per day, the long terminal half-life supports once-per-day dosing.

Megestrol is a relatively well-tolerated medication, with its most prominent side effects being appetite stimulation and resultant weight gain. Although these may be beneficial effects in patients with anorexia/cachexia, they can be important problems in patients with breast and endometrial cancers. Another side effect of megestrol acetate is the marked suppression of adrenal steroid production by suppression of the pituitary–adrenal axis.[203] Although this appears to be asymptomatic in the majority of patients, reports suggest that this adrenal suppression can cause clinical problems in some patients.[204] This drug has been abruptly stopped for decades without the recognition of untoward sequelae in patients, and it seems reasonable to continue this practice. Nonetheless, if Addisonian signs or symptoms develop after drug discontinuation, corticosteroids should be administered.

Furthermore, if patients who receive megestrol have a significant infection, experience trauma, or undergo surgery, then corticosteroid coverage should be administered. There appears to be a slightly increased incidence of thromboembolic phenomena in patients receiving megestrol alone.[202] This risk appears to be higher if megestrol is administered with concomitant cytotoxic therapy.[205] There are conflicting reports regarding megestrol-causing edema.[206] If it does, the edema is generally minimal and easily handled with a mild diuretic. Megestrol may cause impotence in some men.[207] The incidence of this is controversial, although it is generally agreed that this is a reversible situation. Megestrol can cause menstrual irregularities, the most prominent of which is withdrawal menstrual bleeding within a few weeks of drug discontinuation.[5] Although nausea and vomiting have sometimes been attributed as a toxicity of this drug, there are data to demonstrate that this drug has antiemetic properties.[200,201,205] In terms of magnitude, megestrol appears to decrease both nausea and vomiting in advanced-stage cancer patients by approximately two thirds.

Medroxyprogesterone has many of the same properties, clinical uses, and toxicities as megestrol acetate. It has never been commonly used in the United States for the treatment of breast cancer but has been used more in Europe. Medroxyprogesterone is available in 2.5- and 10-mg tablets and in injectable formulations of 100 and 400 mg/L. Dosing for the treatment of metastatic breast or prostate cancer has commonly been 400 mg per week or more and 1,000 mg per week or more for metastatic endometrial cancer. Injectable or daily oral doses have been used for controlling hot flashes.

Pharmacology

The exact mechanism of antitumor effect of medroxyprogesterone and megestrol is unclear. These drugs have been reported to suppress adrenal steroid synthesis,[208] suppress ER levels,[209] alter tumor hormone metabolism,[210] enhance steroid metabolism,[211] and directly kill tumor cells.[212] In addition, progestins may influence some growth factors,[213] suppress plasma estrone sulfate formation, and, at high concentrations, inhibit P-glycoprotein.

The oral bioavailability of these progestational agents is unknown, although absorption appears to be poor for medroxyprogesterone relative to megestrol.

The terminal half-life for megestrol is approximately 14 hours,[214,215] with a t_{max} of 2 to 5 hours after oral ingestion.[216] The AUC for a single megestrol dose of 160 mg is between 2.5- and 8-fold higher than that for single-dose medroxyprogesterone at 1,000 mg with a radioactive dose of megestrol; 50% to 78% is found in the urine after oral administration, and 8% to 30% is found in the feces.

Metabolism and excretion of medroxyprogesterone have been incompletely characterized. In humans, 20% to 50% of a [^{3}H]medroxyprogesterone dose is excreted in the urine and 5% to 10% in the stool after intravenous administration.[217–219] Metabolism of medroxyprogesterone occurs via hydroxylation, reduction, demethylation, and combinations of these reactions.[220] The major urinary metabolite is a glucuronide. Less than 3% of the dose is excreted as unconjugated medroxyprogesterone in humans. Clearance of medroxyprogesterone has been reported to range between 27 and 70 L per hour.[219] The initial volume of distribution is between 4 and 8 L in humans. The mean terminal half-life is 60 hours. The t_{max} for medroxyprogesterone occurs 2 to 5 hours after oral administration. Medroxyprogesterone appears to be concentrated in the small intestine, the colon, and in adipose tissue in human autopsy studies.[221] Drug interactions of medroxyprogesterone have been reported with aminoglutethimide, which decreases plasma medroxyprogesterone levels.[222] Medroxyprogesterone may reduce the concentration of the N-desmethyltamoxifen metabolite concentration. Progestational agents also may increase plasma warfarin levels.[223] These reports are consistent with CYP3A being the site of interaction.

OTHER HORMONAL THERAPIES

Octreotide

Octreotide is a somatostatin analog that is administered for the treatment of carcinoid syndrome and other hormonal excess syndromes associated with some pancreatic islet cell cancers and acromegaly. Response rates (measured in terms of a reduction in diarrhea and flushing) are high and can last for several months to years. Occasionally, antitumor responses temporarily related to octreotide are seen with these tumors. Octreotide may be useful to alleviate 5-fluorouracil–associated diarrhea.[224–226]

Octreotide can be administered intravenously or subcutaneously. Initial doses of 50 μg are given two to three times on the first day. The dose is titrated upward, with a usual daily dose of 300 to 450 μg per day for most patients. A depot preparation is available, allowing doses to be administered at monthly intervals. Octreotide is generally well tolerated overall. It appears to cause more toxicity in acromegalic patients, with such problems as bradycardia, diarrhea, hypoglycemia, hyperglycemia, hypothyroidism, and cholelithiasis.

Pharmacology

Octreotide is an 8-amino acid synthetic analog of the 14-amino acid peptide somatostatin.[227] Octreotide has a similar high affinity for somatostatin receptors, as does its parent compound, with a concentration that inhibits the receptor by 50% in the subnanomolar range. Octreotide inhibits insulin, glucagon, pancreatic polypeptide, gastric inhibitory polypeptide, and gastrin secretion. It has a much longer duration of action than the parent compound because of its greater resistance to enzymatic degradation. Its absorption after subcutaneous administration is rapid, and bioavailability is 100% after subcutaneous injection. Peak concentrations of 4 μg/L after a 100-μg dose occur within 20 to 30 minutes of subcutaneous injection and are 20% to 40% of the corresponding intravenous injection. Both peak concentration and AUC for octreotide increase linearly with dose. The total body clearance in healthy volunteers is 9.6 L per hour. Hepatic metabolism of octreotide accounts for 30% to 40% of the drug's disposition, and 11% to 20% is excreted unchanged in the urine. The volume of distribution ranges between 18 and 30 L, and the terminal half-life is reported to be between 72 and 98 minutes. Sixty-five percent of the drug is protein bound primarily to the lipoprotein fraction.[227,228] Because of the short half-life, classic octreotide is administered subcutaneously two or three times per day.[229] A slow-release form of octreotide, designed for once-per-month administration, controls the symptoms of carcinoid syndrome at least as well as three-times-per-day octreotide.[230]

SELECTED REFERENCES

The full reference list can be accessed at lwwhealthlibrary.com/oncology.

1. Fisher B, Costantino JP, Wickerham DL, et al. Tamoxifen for the prevention of breast cancer: current status of the National Surgical Adjuvant Breast and Bowel Project P-1 study. *J Natl Cancer Inst* 2005;97:1652–1662.
2. Fisher B, Dignam J, Wolmark N, et al. Tamoxifen in treatment of intraductal breast cancer: National Surgical Adjuvant Breast and Bowel Project B-24 randomised controlled trial. *Lancet* 1999;353:1993–2000.
4. Davies C, Pan H, Godwin J, et al. Long-term effects of continuing adjuvant tamoxifen to 10 years versus stopping at 5 years after diagnosis of oestrogen receptor-positive breast cancer: ATLAS, a randomised trial. *Lancet* 2013;381:805–816.
6. Loprinzi CL, Kugler JW, Sloan JA, et al. Venlafaxine in management of hot flashes in survivors of breast cancer: a randomised controlled trial. *Lancet* 2000;356:2059–2063.
10. Stearns V, Beebe KL, Iyengar M, et al. Paroxetine controlled release in the treatment of menopausal hot flashes: a randomized controlled trial. *JAMA* 2003;289:2827–2834.
11. Pandya KJ, Morrow GR, Roscoe JA, et al. Gabapentin for hot flashes in 420 women with breast cancer: a randomised double-blind placebo-controlled trial. *Lancet* 2005;366:818–824.
12. Loprinzi CL, Qin R, Balcueva EP, et al. Phase III, randomized, double-blind, placebo-controlled evaluation of pregabalin for alleviating hot flashes, N07C1. *J Clin Oncol* 2010;28:641–647.
13. Madlensky L, Natarajan L, Tchu S, et al. Tamoxifen metabolite concentrations, CYP2D6 genotype, and breast cancer outcomes. *Clin Pharmacol Ther* 2011;89:718–725.
14. Tamoxifen for early breast cancer: an overview of the randomised trials. Early Breast Cancer Trialists' Collaborative Group. *Lancet* 1998;351:1451–1467.
15. Wickerham DL, Fisher B, Wolmark N, et al. Association of tamoxifen and uterine sarcoma. *J Clin Oncol* 2002;20:2758–2760.
16. Dewar JA, Horobin JM, Preece PE, et al. Long term effects of tamoxifen on blood lipid values in breast cancer. *BMJ* 1992;305:225–226.
17. Love RR, Mazess RB, Barden HS, et al. Effects of tamoxifen on bone mineral density in postmenopausal women with breast cancer. *N Engl J Med* 1992;326:852–856.
29. Pietras RJ, Arboleda J, Reese DM, et al. HER-2 tyrosine kinase pathway targets estrogen receptor and promotes hormone-independent growth in human breast cancer cells. *Oncogene* 1995;10:2435–2446.
30. Osborne CK, Bardou V, Hopp TA, et al. Role of the estrogen receptor coactivator AIB1 (SRC-3) and HER-2/neu in tamoxifen resistance in breast cancer. *J Natl Cancer Inst* 2003;95:353–361.
33. Zhang QX, Borg A, Wolf DM, et al. An estrogen receptor mutant with strong hormone-independent activity from a metastatic breast cancer. *Cancer Res* 1997;57:1244–1249.

34. Toy W, Shen Y, Won H, et al. ESR1 ligand-binding domain mutations in hormone-resistant breast cancer. *Nat Genet* 2013;45:1439–1445.
35. Robinson DR, Wu YM, Vats P, et al. Activating ESR1 mutations in hormone-resistant metastatic breast cancer. *Nat Genet* 2013;45:1446–1451.
36. Merenbakh-Lamin K, Ben-Baruch N, Yeheskel A, et al. D538G mutation in estrogen receptor-alpha: a novel mechanism for acquired endocrine resistance in breast cancer. *Cancer Res* 2013;73:6856–6864.
37. Fendl KC, Zimniski SJ. Role of tamoxifen in the induction of hormone-independent rat mammary tumors. *Cancer Res* 1992;52:235–237.
41. Mani C, Kupfer D. Cytochrome P-450-mediated activation and irreversible binding of the antiestrogen tamoxifen to proteins in rat and human liver: possible involvement of flavin-containing monooxygenases in tamoxifen activation. *Cancer Res* 1991;51:6052–6058.
49. Paik S, Shak S, Tang G, et al. A multigene assay to predict recurrence of tamoxifen-treated, node-negative breast cancer. *N Engl J Med* 2004;351:2817–2826.
52. Wu X, Hawse JR, Subramaniam M, et al. The tamoxifen metabolite, endoxifen, is a potent antiestrogen that targets estrogen receptor alpha for degradation in breast cancer cells. *Cancer Res* 2009;69:1722–1727.
54. Desta Z, Ward BA, Soukhova NV, et al. Comprehensive evaluation of tamoxifen sequential biotransformation by the human cytochrome P450 system in vitro: prominent roles for CYP3A and CYP2D6. *J Pharmacol Exp Ther* 2004;310:1062–1075.
55. Stearns V, Johnson MD, Rae JM, et al. Active tamoxifen metabolite plasma concentrations after coadministration of tamoxifen and the selective serotonin reuptake inhibitor paroxetine. *J Natl Cancer Inst* 2003;95:1758–1764.
56. Goetz MP, Rae JM, Suman VJ, et al. Pharmacogenetics of tamoxifen biotransformation is associated with clinical outcomes of efficacy and hot flashes. *J Clin Oncol* 2005;23:9312–9318.
58. Schroth W, Goetz MP, Hamann U, et al. Association between CYP2D6 polymorphisms and outcomes among women with early stage breast cancer treated with tamoxifen. *JAMA* 2009;302:1429–1436.
59. Rae JM, Drury S, Hayes DF, et al. CYP2D6 and UGT2B7 genotype and risk of recurrence in tamoxifen-treated breast cancer patients. *J Natl Cancer Inst* 2012;104:452–460.
60. Regan MM, Leyland-Jones B, Bouzyk M, et al. CYP2D6 genotype and tamoxifen response in postmenopausal women with endocrine-responsive breast cancer: the breast international group 1-98 trial. *J Natl Cancer Inst* 2012;104:441–451.
61. Goetz MP, Suman VJ, Hoskin TL, et al. CYP2D6 metabolism and patient outcome in the Austrian Breast and Colorectal Cancer Study Group trial (ABCSG) 8. *Clin Cancer Res* 2013;19:500–507.
62. Province MA, Goetz MP, Brauch H, et al. CYP2D6 Genotype and adjuvant tamoxifen: meta-analysis of heterogeneous study populations. *Clin Pharmacol Ther* 2014;95:216–227.

65. Kelly CM, Juurlink DN, Gomes T, et al. Selective serotonin reuptake inhibitors and breast cancer mortality in women receiving tamoxifen: a population based cohort study. *BMJ* 2010;340:c693.

67. Irvin WJ Jr., Walko CM, Weck KE, et al. Genotype-guided tamoxifen dosing increases active metabolite exposure in women with reduced CYP2D6 metabolism: a multicenter study. *J Clin Oncol* 2011;29:3232–3239.

69. Goetz MP, Suman VA, Reid JR, et al. A first-in-human phase I study of the tamoxifen (TAM) metabolite, Z-endoxifen hydrochloride (Z-Endx) in women with aromatase inhibitor (AI) refractory metastatic breast cancer (MBC) (NCT01327781). *Cancer Res* 2013;73(24 Suppl): Abstract nr PD3-4. .

70. Lien EA, Anker G, Lonning PE, et al. Decreased serum concentrations of tamoxifen and its metabolites induced by aminoglutethimide. *Cancer Res* 1990;50:5851–5857.

74. Lien EA, Solheim E, Lea OA, et al. Distribution of 4-hydroxy-N-desmethyltamoxifen and other tamoxifen metabolites in human biological fluids during tamoxifen treatment. *Cancer Res* 1989;49:2175–2183.

110. Howell A, Osborne CK, Morris C, et al. ICI 182,780 (Faslodex): development of a novel, "pure" antiestrogen. *Cancer* 2000;89:817–825.

116. Osborne CK, Pippen J, Jones SE, et al. Double-blind, randomized trial comparing the efficacy and tolerability of fulvestrant versus anastrozole in postmenopausal women with advanced breast cancer progressing on prior endocrine therapy: results of a North American trial. *J Clin Oncol* 2002;20:3386–3395.

117. Howell A, Robertson JF, Abram P, et al. Comparison of fulvestrant versus tamoxifen for the treatment of advanced breast cancer in postmenopausal women previously untreated with endocrine therapy: a multinational, double-blind, randomized trial. *J Clin Oncol* 2004;22:1605–1613.

118. Leo AD, Jerusalem G, Petruzelka L, et al. Final overall survival: fulvestrant 500 mg vs 250 mg in the randomized CONFIRM trial. *J Natl Cancer Inst* 2014;106:djt337.

121. Ma CX, Adjei AA, Salavaggione OE, et al. Human aromatase: gene resequencing and functional genomics. *Cancer Res* 2005;65:11071–11082.

124. Goss PE, Ingle JN, Martino S, et al. A randomized trial of letrozole in postmenopausal women after five years of tamoxifen therapy for early-stage breast cancer. *N Engl J Med* 2003;349:1793–1802.

126. Howell A, Cuzick J, Baum M, et al. Results of the ATAC (Arimidex, Tamoxifen, Alone or in Combination) trial after completion of 5 years' adjuvant treatment for breast cancer. *Lancet* 2005;365:60–62.

127. Thurlimann B, Keshaviah A, Coates AS, et al. A comparison of letrozole and tamoxifen in postmenopausal women with early breast cancer. *N Engl J Med* 2005;353:2747–2757.

128. Jakesz R, Jonat W, Gnant M, et al. Switching of postmenopausal women with endocrine-responsive early breast cancer to anastrozole after 2 years' adjuvant tamoxifen: combined results of ABCSG trial 8 and ARNO 95 trial. *Lancet* 2005;366:455–462.

129. Cuzick J, Sestak I, Forbes JF, et al. Anastrozole for prevention of breast cancer in high-risk postmenopausal women (IBIS-II): an international, double-blind, randomised placebo-controlled trial. *Lancet* 2014;383:1041–1048.

130. Baum M, Budzar AU, Cuzick J, et al. Anastrozole alone or in combination with tamoxifen versus tamoxifen alone for adjuvant treatment of postmenopausal women with early breast cancer: first results of the ATAC randomised trial. *Lancet* 2002;359:2131–2139.

131. Amir E, Seruga B, Nira S, et al. Toxicity of adjuvant endocrine therapy in postmenopausal breast cancer patients: a systematic review and meta-analysis. *J Natl Cancer Inst* 2011;103:1299–1309.

147. Ingle JN, Buzdar AU, Schaid DJ, et al. Variation in anastrozole metabolism and pharmacodynamics in women with early breast cancer. *Cancer Res* 2010;70:3278–3286.

149. Goss PE, Ingle JN, Pritchard KI, et al. Exemestane versus anastrozole in postmenopausal women with early breast cancer: NCIC CTG MA.27—a randomized controlled phase III trial. *J Clin Oncol* 2013;31:1398–1404.

150. Goss PE, Ingle JN, Ales-Martinez JE, et al. Exemestane for breast-cancer prevention in postmenopausal women. *N Engl J Med* 2011;364:2381–2391.

151. Goss PE, Grynpas M, Qi S, et al. The effects of exemestane on bone and lipids in the ovariectomized rat. *Breast Cancer Res Treat* 2001;69:224.

163. Kaufmann M, Jonat W, Blamey R, et al. Survival analyses from the ZEBRA study. Goserelin (Zoladex) versus CMF in premenopausal women with node-positive breast cancer. *Eur J Cancer* 2003;39:1711–1717.

166. Hussain M, Tangen CM, Berry DL, et al. Intermittent versus continuous androgen deprivation in prostate cancer. *N Engl J Med* 2013;368:1314–1325.

168. Vogelzang NJ, Chodak GW, Soloway MS, et al. Goserelin versus orchiectomy in the treatment of advanced prostate cancer: final results of a randomized trial. Zoladex Prostate Study Group. *Urology* 1995;46:220–226.

175. Van Poppel H, Tombal B, de la Rosette JJ, et al. Degarelix: a novel gonadotropin-releasing hormone (GnRH) receptor blocker—results from a 1-yr, multicentre, randomised, phase 2 dosage-finding study in the treatment of prostate cancer. *Eur Urol* 2008;54:805–813.

176. Klotz L, Boccon-Gibod L, Shore ND, et al. The efficacy and safety of degarelix: a 12-month, comparative, randomized, open-label, parallel-group phase III study in patients with prostate cancer. *BJU Int* 2008;102:1531–1538.

186. Attard G, Reid AH, A'Hern R, et al. Selective inhibition of CYP17 with abiraterone acetate is highly active in the treatment of castration-resistant prostate cancer. *J Clin Oncol* 2009;27:3742–3748.

188. Scher HI, Fizazi K, Saad F, et al. Increased survival with enzalutamide in prostate cancer after chemotherapy. *N Engl J Med* 2012;367:1187–1197.

224. Cascinu S, Fedeli A, Fedeli SL, et al. Control of chemotherapy-induced diarrhoea with octreotide in patients receiving 5-fluorouracil. *Eur J Cancer* 1992;28:482–483.

230. Rubin J, Ajani J, Schirmer W, et al. Octreotide acetate long-acting formulation versus open-label subcutaneous octreotide acetate in malignant carcinoid syndrome. *J Clin Oncol* 1999;17:600–606.

CANCER THERAPEUTICS

28 Antiangiogenesis Agents

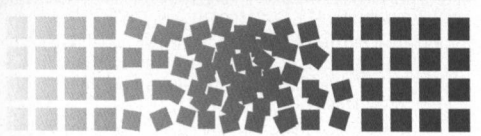

Cindy H. Chau and William Douglas Figg, Sr.

INTRODUCTION

Blood vessels are indispensable for tumor growth and metastasis, and the formation of a new network of blood vessels from the existing vasculature, termed *angiogenesis*, is one of the essential hallmarks of cancer development.[1] Indeed, it was over 70 years ago that the existence of tumor-derived factors responsible for promoting new vessel growth was postulated,[2] and that tumor growth is essentially dependent on vascular induction and the development of a neovascular supply.[3] By the late 1960s, Dr. Judah Folkman and colleagues[4] had begun the search for a tumor angiogenesis factor. In the 1971 landmark report, Folkman[5] proposed that inhibition of angiogenesis by means of holding tumors in a nonvascularized dormant state would be an effective strategy to treat human cancer, and hence laid the groundwork for the concept behind the development of *antiangiogenesis* agents. This fostered the search for angiogenic factors, regulators of angiogenesis, and antiangiogenic molecules over the next few decades and shed light on angiogenesis as an important therapeutic target for the treatment of cancer and other diseases.

A decade has passed since the regulatory approval of the first antiangiogenic drug bevacizumab, and while initial results were regarded as highly promising, clinical evidence indicated that antiangiogenic therapy also had limitations. Successful development and clinical translation of this novel class of agents depends on the complete understanding of the biology of angiogenesis and the regulatory proteins that govern this angiogenic process, topics that have been covered in greater detail in another section of this textbook. This chapter will briefly review the mechanisms underlying tumor angiogenesis followed by an in-depth discussion of antiangiogenic therapy, the modes of action of angiogenesis inhibitors, and the successes and challenges of this treatment modality.

UNDERSTANDING THE ANGIOGENIC PROCESS

Angiogenic Switch and Regulatory Proteins

Tumor development and progression depend on angiogenesis. Recruitment of new blood vessels to the tumor site is required for the delivery of nutrients and oxygen to the cancerous growths and for the removal of waste products.[6] Cancer cells promote angiogenesis at an early stage of tumorigenesis, beginning with the release of molecules that send signals to the surrounding normal host tissue and stimulate the migration of microvascular endothelial cells (EC) in the direction of the angiogenic stimulus. These angiogenic factors not only mediate EC migration, but also EC proliferation and microvessel formation in tumors undergoing the switch to the angiogenic phenotype.[7] Experimental evidence for this *angiogenic switch* was observed when hyperplastic islets in transgenic mice (RIP-Tag model) switch from small (<1 mm), white microscopic dormant tumors to red, rapidly growing tumors.[7] Dormant tumors have been discovered during autopsies of individuals who died of causes other than cancer.[8] These autopsy studies suggest that the vast majority of microscopic in

situ cancers never switch to the angiogenic phenotype during a normal lifetime. Such incipient tumors are usually not neovascularized and can remain harmless to the host for long periods of time as microscopic lesions that are in a state of dormancy.[9,10] These nonangiogenic tumors cannot expand beyond the initial microscopic size and cannot become clinically detectable, lethal tumors until they have switched to the angiogenic phenotype[11–13] through neovascularization and/or blood vessel cooption.[14] Depending on the tumor type and the environment, this switch can occur at different stages of the tumor progression pathway and ultimately depends on a net balance of positive and negative regulators. Thus, the angiogenic phenotype may result from the production of growth factors by tumor cells and/or the downregulation of negative modulators.

Changes in this angiogenic balance affecting the levels of activator and inhibitor molecules dictate whether an EC will be in a quiescent or an angiogenic state. Normally, the inhibitors predominate, thereby blocking growth. Once the balance shifts in favor of the angiogenic state, proangiogenic factors prompts the activation, growth, and division of vascular ECs, resulting in the formation of new blood vessels. Activated ECs produce and release matrix metalloproteinases (MMP) into the surrounding tissue to break down the extracellular matrix to allow the ECs to migrate and organize themselves into hollow tubes that eventually evolve into a mature network of blood vessels. Proangiogenic factors or positive regulators of angiogenesis include vascular endothelial growth factor (VEGF), basic fibroblast growth factor (PlGF), platelet-derived growth factor (PDGF), placental growth factor, transforming growth factor-β, pleiotrophins, and others.[15] Activation of the hypoxia-inducible factor 1 (HIF-1) via tumor-associated hypoxic conditions is also involved in the upregulation of several angiogenic factors.[16] The angiogenic switch also involves the downregulation of angiogenesis suppressor proteins, which include endostatin, angiostatin, thrombospondin, and others.[17,18] Most notably, however, is the link between many oncogenes and angiogenesis and the significant role oncogenes play in driving the angiogenic switch.[19,20] These proangiogenic oncogenes not only induce the expression of stimulators, but may also downregulate inhibitors of angiogenesis.[21]

Endogenous Inhibitors of Angiogenesis

The infrequency of microscopic in situ tumors that actually undergo the angiogenic switch (<1%) suggests that naturally occurring endogenous inhibitors exist in the body to defend against the angiogenic switch in pathologic conditions and to limit physiologic angiogenesis.[9] These circulating endogenous inhibitors could also prevent microscopic metastases from growing into visible tumors. Early studies by Langer et al.[22,23] demonstrated the possible existence of such inhibitors through the extraction of a functional inhibitor from cartilage, a tissue that is poorly vascularized. Since then, dozens of endogenous angiogenesis inhibitors have been identified, some of which are listed in Table 28.1.[17,18,24] Many of the endogenous inhibitors of angiogenesis that have been discovered to date are proteolytically cleaved fragments of larger proteins that are members of either the clotting/coagulation system

TABLE 28.1

Examples of Endogenous Inhibitors of Angiogenesis

Alphastatin

Angiostatin

Antithrombin III (cleaved)

Arrestin

Canstatin

Endostatin

Interferon alpha/beta (IFN-α/β)

2-Methoxyestradiol (2-ME)

Pigment epithelial-derived factor (PEDF)

Platelet factor 4 (PF-4)

Tetrahydrocortisol-S

Thrombospondin 1

Tissue inhibitor of metalloproteinase 2 (TIMP-2)

Tumstatin

Vasohibin

or members of the extracellular matrix family of glycoproteins. Endostatin is the most well-studied endogenous angiogenesis inhibitor.[25,26] Other potent endogenous angiogenesis inhibitors include thrombospondin-1[27] and tumstatin.[28] The discovery of vasohibin, an endogenous inhibitor that is selectively induced in ECs by proangiogenic stimulatory growth factors such as VEGF, demonstrated the existence of an intrinsic and EC-specific feedback inhibitor control mechanism,[29,30] whereas most endogenous inhibitors of angiogenesis are extrinsic to ECs. More recently, a second endothelium-produced negative regulator of angiogenesis has been discovered, the Dll4-Notch signaling system.[31,32] Both intrinsic factors have since been shown to control tumor angiogenesis by an autoregulatory or negative-feedback mechanism. The Dll4-Notch axis has emerged as a critical regulator of tumor angiogenesis, and inhibitors of this pathway (e.g., demcizumab, the anti-Dll4 monoclonal antibody) are currently being investigated in early phase trials of solid tumors.[33]

Perhaps the most compelling genetic evidence that endogenous inhibitors suppress pathologic angiogenesis was observed in studies using mice deficient in tumstatin, endostatin, or thrombospondin 1 (TSP-1).[34] These experiments demonstrate that normal physiologic levels of the inhibitors can retard the tumor growth and that their absence leads to enhanced angiogenesis and increased tumor growth by two- to threefold, strongly suggesting that endogenous inhibitors of angiogenesis can act as endothelium-specific tumor suppressors. The connection between a tumor suppressor protein and angiogenesis is best illustrated by the classic tumor suppressor p53. p53 inhibits angiogenesis by increasing the expression of TSP-1[35] by repressing VEGF[36] and basic fibroblast growth factor–binding protein,[37] and by degrading HIF-1,[38] which blocks the downstream induction of VEGF expression. New evidence suggests that p53 also indirectly downregulates VEGF expression via the retinoblastoma pathway in a p21-dependent manner during sustained hypoxia.[39] Furthermore, p53-mediated inhibition of angiogenesis may also occur in part via the antiangiogenic activity of endostatin and tumstatin.[40] This landmark finding clearly demonstrates that p53 not only controls cell proliferation, but can also repress tumor angiogenesis through enzymatic mobilization of these endogenous angiogenesis inhibitor proteins to prevent ECs from being recruited into the dormant, microscopic tumors, thereby preventing the switch to the angiogenic phenotype.[41] The discovery that these endogenous angiogenesis inhibitors can suppress the growth of primary tumors

raises the possibility that such inhibitors might also be able to slow tumor metastasis. Indeed, the inhibition of angiogenesis by angiostatin significantly reduced the rate of metastatic spread.

DRUG DEVELOPMENT OF ANGIOGENESIS INHIBITORS

The first angiogenesis inhibitor was reported in 1980 and involved the low-dose administration of interferon α (IFN-α).[42–44] Over the next decade, several compounds were discovered to have potent antiangiogenic activity, including protamine and platelet factor 4,[45] trahydrocortisol,[46] and the fumagillin analog TNP-470.[47] The proof of concept that targeting angiogenesis is an effective strategy for treating cancer came with the approval of the first angiogenesis inhibitor, bevacizumab, by the U.S. Food and Drug Administration (FDA). Since then, several antiangiogenic agents have received FDA approval for cancer treatment (Table 28.2), and three additional agents (pegaptanib, ranibizumab, and aflibercept) are approved for the treatment of wet age-related macular degeneration.

Rationale for Antiangiogenic Therapy

Antiangiogenic therapy stems from the fundamental concept that tumor growth, invasion, and metastasis are angiogenesis dependent; thus, blocking blood vessel recruitment to starve primary and metastatic tumors is a rational approach. The microvascular EC recruited by a tumor has become an important second target in cancer therapy. Unlike the cancer cell (the primary target of cytotoxic chemotherapy), which is genetically unstable with unpredictable mutations, the genetic stability of ECs may make them less susceptible to acquired drug resistance.[48] Moreover, ECs in the microvascular bed of a tumor may support 50 to 100 tumor cells. Coupling this amplification potential together with the lower toxicity of most angiogenesis inhibitors results in the use of antiangiogenic therapy, which should be significantly less toxic than conventional chemotherapy. However, the variable responses of antiangiogenic therapy observed in different tumor types and the fact that angiogenesis inhibitors have not delivered the benefits initially envisaged suggest that the precise mechanism of action of angiogenesis inhibitors is complex and remains incompletely understood.

Modes of Action of Antiangiogenic Agents

Various strategies for the development of antiangiogenic drugs have been investigated over the years, with these agents being classified into several different categories depending on their modes of action. Some inhibit ECs directly, whereas others inhibit the angiogenesis signaling cascade or block the ability of ECs to break down the extracellular matrix. Inhibitors may block one main angiogenic protein, two or three angiogenic proteins, or have a broad-spectrum effect by blocking a range of angiogenic regulators that can be located in both the tumor and ECs.[49] In some cases, the antiangiogenic activity is discovered as a secondary function after the drug has received regulatory approval for a different primary function. For example, bortezomib is a proteasome inhibitor that is approved for multiple myeloma and was later found to possess antiangiogenic activity via inhibiting VEGF. Some small-molecule drugs may display their antiangiogenic activity through inducing the expression of endogenous angiogenesis inhibitors such as celecoxib, a cyclooxygenase-2 (COX-2) inhibitor, which inhibits angiogenesis by increasing levels of endostatin.[25]

Some drugs possess antiangiogenic properties but with mechanisms that are not completely understood, such as thalidomide and its analogs, lenalidomide and pomalidomide, referred to as immunomodulatory drugs. Thalidomide was originally shown to inhibit angiogenesis by D'Amato et al.[50] in 1994 and this was subsequently confirmed in several different in vitro and ex vivo

TABLE 28.2

Antiangiogenic Agents that Have Received U.S. Food and Drug Administration Approval for Cancer Treatment

Drug	Class	Mechanism (Cellular Targets)	Year of Approval	Indications	Dosages
Bevacizumab (Avastin)	Anti-VEGF mAB	VEGF	2004	First- and second-line metastatic CRC	5 mg/kg IV q2wk + bolus IFL; 10 mg/kg IV q2wk + FOLFOX4
			2006	First-line NSCLC	15 mg/kg IV q3wk + carboplatin/paclitaxel
			2009	Second-line GBM	10 mg/kg IV q2wk
			2009	Metastatic RCC	10 mg/kg IV q2wk + IFN
			2013	Second-line metastatic CRC (after prior bevacizumab-containing regimen)	5 mg/kg IV q2wk or 7.5 mg/kg IV q3wk + fluoropyrimidine–irinotecan or fluoropyrimidine-oxaliplatin–based regimen
Ziv-aflibercept (Zaltrap, VEGF Trap)	Anti-VEGF mAB	VEGFA, VEGFB, PlGF1, PlGF2	2012	Metastatic CRC (after prior oxaliplatin-containing regimen)	4 mg/kg IV q2wk (1-hr infusion)
Sorafenib (Nexavar, BAY439006)	Small-molecule TKI	VEGFR2, VEGFR3, PDGFR, FLT3, c-Kit	2005	Advanced RCC	400 mg PO bid (w/o food)
			2007	Unresectable HCC	400 mg PO bid (w/o food)
			2013	RAI-refractory DTC	400 mg PO bid (w/o food)
Sunitinib (Sutent, SU11248)	Small-molecule TKI	VEGFR1, VEGFR2, VEGFR3, PDGFR, FLT3, c-Kit, RET	2006	Imatinib-resistant or -intolerant GIST	50 mg PO qd, 4 wk on/2 wk off
			2006	Advanced RCC	50 mg PO qd, 4 wk on/2 wk off
			2011	Advanced pNET	37.5 mg PO qd
Pazopanib (Votrient)	Small-molecule TKI	VEGFR1, VEGFR2, VEGFR3, PDGFR, Itk, Lck, c-Fms	2009	Advanced RCC	800 mg PO qd (w/o food)
			2012	Advanced soft tissue sarcoma	800 mg PO qd (w/o food)
Vandetanib (Caprelsa)	Small molecule TKI	RET, VEGFR, EGFR, BRK, TIE2	2011	Advanced MTC	300 mg PO qd
Axitinib (Inlyta)	Small molecule TKI	VEGFR1, VEGFR2, VEGFR3	2012	Advanced RCC (after failure of prior therapy)	5 mg PO bid
Cabozantinib (XL184, Cometriq)	Small molecule TKI	MET, VEGFR2, RET, KIT, AXL, FLT3	2012	Progressive, metastatic MTC	140 mg PO qd (w/o food)
Regorafenib (Stivarga)	Small molecule TKI	RET, VEGFR1, VEGFR2, VEGFR3, TIE2, KIT, PDGFR	2012	Previously treated metastatic CRC	160 mg PO qd × 21days (q28-day cycle)
			2013	GIST	160 mg PO qd × days 1–21 (q28-day cycle)
Temsirolimus (Torisel)	mTOR inhibitor	mTOR	2007	Advanced RCC	25 mg IV qwk (infused over 30–60 min)
Everolimus (Afinitor, RAD-001)[a]	mTOR inhibitor	mTOR	2009	Second-line advanced RCC (after VEGFR TKI failure)	10 mg PO qd
			2010	SEGA associated w/TSC	4.5 mg/m^2 PO qd
			2011	pNET	10 mg PO qd
			2012	Advanced HR+, HER2- breast cancer	10 mg PO qd
			2012	AML associated w/TSC	10 mg PO qd

[a] Afinitor Disperz (everolimus tablets for oral suspension) was approved in 2012 for children aged 1 and older who have SEGA + TSC.

mAB, monoclonal antibody; CRC, colorectal cancer; IV, intravenous; IFL, irinotecan, 5-fluorouracil, and leucovorin; FOLFOX4, 5-flourouracil, leucovorin, and oxaliplatin; NSCLC, non–small-cell lung cancer; GBM, glioblastoma multiforme; RCC, renal cell carcinoma; VEGFA, vascular endothelial growth factor A; PlGF, placental growth factor; TKI, tyrosine–kinase inhibitor; VEGFR, VEGF receptor; PDGFR, platelet-derived growth factor receptor; FLT, Fms-like tyrosine kinase; c-Kit, stem cell factor receptor; HCC, hepatocellular carcinoma; RAI, radioactive iodine; DTC, differentiated thyroid carcinoma; PO, orally; RET, glial cell line-derived neurotrophic factor receptor; pNET, pancreatic neuroendocrine tumor; GIST, gastrointestinal stromal tumor; qd, every day; Itk, interleukin-2 receptor inducible T-cell kinase; Lck, leukocyte-specific protein tyrosine kinase; c-Fms, transmembrane glycoprotein receptor tyrosine kinase; bid, twice daily; EGFR, epidermal growth factor receptor; BRK, protein tyrosine kinase 6; MTC, medullary thyroid cancer; mTOR, mammalian target of rapamycin; SEGA, subependymal giant cell astrocytoma; TSC, tuberous sclerosis complex; HR, hormone receptor; HER2, human epidermal growth factor receptor 2; AML, angiomyolipoma.

assays.[51–54] Interestingly, unlike other mechanisms of action, the antiangiogenic activity of thalidomide is believed to require enzymatic activation. The extent to which the antiangiogenic properties of thalidomide and its analogs play a role in its antimyeloma activity is not clearly understood. Several mechanisms have been proposed that involve the downregulation of cytokines in EC, the inhibition of EC proliferation, the decrease in the level of circulating ECs, or the modulation of adhesion molecules between the multiple myeloma cells and the endogenous bone marrow stromal cells, thereby decreasing the production of VEGF and interleukin 6 (IL-6).[55–59] The immunomodulatory agents are discussed in greater detail in another section of this textbook. Examples of the various types of angiogenesis inhibitors are highlighted in Table 28.3.

Drugs with antiangiogenic activity may be classified as either direct or indirect angiogenesis inhibitors. A direct angiogenesis inhibitor blocks vascular ECs from proliferating, migrating, or increasing their survival in response to proangiogenic proteins. They target the activated endothelium directly and inhibit multiple angiogenic proteins. Examples of direct angiogenesis inhibitors include many of the endogenous inhibitors of angiogenesis, such as endostatin, angiostatin, and TSP-1. Indirect angiogenesis inhibitors decrease or block expression of a tumor cell product, neutralize the tumor product itself, or block its receptor on ECs. The limitation to indirect inhibitors is that, over time, tumor cells may acquire mutations that lead to increased expression of other proangiogenic proteins that are not blocked by the indirect inhibitor. This may give the appearance of drug resistance and warrants the addition of a second antiangiogenic agent, one that would target the expression of these upregulated proangiogenic proteins. Examples of drugs that interfere with the angiogenesis-signaling pathway include the anti-VEGF monoclonal antibodies and small-molecule tyrosine–kinase inhibitors. These drugs target the major signaling pathways in tumor angiogenesis: VEGF, PDGF, and their respective receptors, as well as other growth factors and/or signaling pathways.

VEGF (also known as vascular permeability factor) is a potent proangiogenic growth factor and its expression is upregulated by most cancer cell types. It stimulates EC proliferation, migration, and survival as well as induces increased vascular permeability. The different forms of VEGF bind to transmembrane receptor tyrosine kinases (RTK) on ECs: VEGFR1 (Flt-1), VEGFR2 (KDR/Flk-1 or kinase insert domain receptor/fetal liver kinase 1), or VEGFR3 (Flt-4).[60] This results in receptor dimerization, activation, and autophosphorylation of the tyrosine–kinase domain, thereby triggering downstream signaling pathways. Other signaling molecules that may represent attractive therapeutic targets include PDGF and the angiopoietins (Ang1, Ang2). PDGF-B/PDGF receptor (R)-β plays an important role in the recruitment of pericytes and maturation of the microvasculature.[61] Ang2, which binds the Tie-2 receptor, is mostly expressed in tumor-induced neovasculature, whereby its selective inhibition results in reduced EC proliferation.[62] The angiopoietins are also involved in lymphangiogenesis, the formation of new lymphatic vessels, which plays a key role in tumor metastasis. An increased Ang2/Ang1 ratio correlates with tumor angiogenesis and poor prognosis in many cancers, thus making the angiopoietins an attractive therapeutic target. Angiopoietin inhibitors are currently under investigation in the preclinical and clinical setting.

Other strategies for targeting angiogenesis involve the tumor microenvironment. Breakdown of the extracellular matrix is required to allow ECs to migrate into surrounding tissues and proliferate into new blood vessels; thus, drugs that target MMPs, enzymes that catalyze the breakdown of the matrix, can also inhibit angiogenesis. However, clinical development of MMP inhibitors (MMPI) has yielded disappointing results.[63–66]

Integrins are cell surface adhesion molecules that play an essential role in cell–cell and cell–matrix adhesion as well as in transmitting signals important for cell migration, invasion, proliferation, and survival. The involvement of integrin in tumor angiogenesis was demonstrated in studies that show the β-4 subunit of integrin promoting endothelial migration and invasion.[67] Agents that target integrins (inhibitors of $\alpha_v\beta_3$ and $\alpha_v\beta_5$) have been evaluated as potential therapeutic options and include etaracizumab, cilengitide, and intetumumab. However, all three integrin inhibitors have proven to be largely ineffective in various early and late stage cancer trials.[68–73] In summary, the downstream effects of antiangiogenic agents, in addition to blocking angiogenesis, may involve inducing vessel regression, promoting sensitization to radiotherapy and chemotherapy by depriving ECs of VEGF's prosurvival signals, and inhibiting the recruitment of proangiogenic bone marrow–derived cells as well as reducing the self-renewal capability of cancer stem cells.[74]

CLINICAL UTILITY OF APPROVED ANTIANGIOGENIC AGENTS IN CANCER THERAPY

The following section reviews the current FDA-approved angiogenesis inhibitors (Table 28.2). These agents include: (1) the monoclonal anti-VEGF antibodies (bevacizumab and ziv-aflibercept); (2) small-molecule tyrosine–kinase inhibitors (TKI) (sorafenib, sunitinib, pazopanib, vandetanib, axitinib, cabozantinib, and regorafenib); and (3) the mammalian target of rapamycin (mTOR) inhibitors (temsirolimus and everolimus), as examples of drugs that possess antiangiogenic activity. Other approved drugs that also inhibit angiogenesis as a secondary function, such as thalidomide, are discussed in greater detail in another section of this textbook and are presented in Table 28.3.

Anti-VEGF Therapy

Bevacizumab

Bevacizumab is a recombinant humanized anti–VEGF-A monoclonal antibody that received FDA approval in February 2004 for use in combination therapy with fluorouracil-based regimens for

TABLE 28.3

Examples of Drugs that Possess Antiangiogenic Activity or Inhibit Angiogenesis as a Secondary Function

Drug	Class
Cetuximab Panitumumab Trastuzumab	EGFR/HER monoclonal antibodies
Gefitinib Erlotinib	EGFR small-molecule tyrosine–kinase receptor inhibitors
Everolimus Temsirolimus	mTOR inhibitors
Thalidomide Lenalidomide Pomalidomide	Immunomodulatory agents
Belinostat (PXD101) LBH589 Vorinostat (SAHA)	HDAC inhibitors
Celecoxib	COX-2 inhibitors
Bortezomib	Proteasome inhibitors
Zoledronic acid	Bisphosphonates
Rosiglitazone	PPAR-γ agonists
Doxycycline	Antibiotic

EGFR, epidermal growth factor receptor; mTOR, mammalian target of rapamycin HDAC, histone deacetylase; COX-2, cyclooxygenase-2; PPAR, peroxisome proliferator–activated receptor.

metastatic colorectal cancer. Bevacizumab binds VEGF and prevents the interaction of VEGF to its receptors (Flt-1 and KDR) on the surface of ECs. It is the first antiangiogenic agent clinically proven to extend survival following a large, randomized, double-blind, phase III study in which bevacizumab was administered in combination with bolus irinotecan, 5-fluorouracil, and leucovorin (IFL) as first-line therapy for metastatic colorectal cancer (CRC).[75] In 2006, its approval extended to first- or second-line treatment of patients with metastatic carcinoma of the colon or rectum. This recommendation is based on the demonstration of a statistically significant improvement in overall survival (OS) in patients receiving bevacizumab plus FOLFOX4 (5-flourouracil, leucovorin, and oxaliplatin) when compared to those receiving FOLFOX4 alone. In January 2013, it was further approved to treat mCRC for second-line treatment when used with fluoropyrimidine-based (combined with irinotecan or oxaliplatin) chemotherapy after disease progression following a first-line treatment with a bevacizumab-containing regimen based on clinical benefits observed in the randomized phase III study (ML18147).[76] Despite the benefit in the metastatic setting, the addition of bevacizumab did not improve clinical outcomes in the adjuvant setting in CRC.[77,78] In 2006, bevacizumab received an additional approval for use in combination with carboplatin and paclitaxel, and is indicated for first-line treatment of patients with unresectable, locally advanced, recurrent, or metastatic nonsquamous, non–small-cell lung cancer (NSCLC) based on the demonstration of a statistically significant improvement in OS in patients in the bevacizumab arm compared to those receiving chemotherapy alone.[79] In February 2008, the FDA granted a conditional, accelerated approval for bevacizumab to be used in combination with paclitaxel for the treatment of patients who have not received chemotherapy for metastatic human epidermal growth factor receptor 2 (HER2)-negative breast cancer. However, additional clinical trials were conducted and the new data showed only a small effect on progression free survival (PFS) without evidence of an improvement in OS or a clinical benefit to patients sufficient to outweigh the risks; thus, the FDA rescinded its approval and removed the breast cancer indication from the drug's label in November 2011.[80–82] This controversial decision continues to be debated with ongoing subgroup analyses to identify patients who would likely benefit from bevacizumab.

Bevacizumab received another accelerated approval as a single agent for patients with glioblastoma multiforme (GBM) with progressive disease following therapy in May 2009. The approval was based on the demonstration of durable objective response rates observed in two single-arm trials, AVF3708g and NCI 06-C-0064E.[83] Currently, no data have shown whether bevacizumab improves disease-related symptoms or survival in people previously treated for GBM. Moreover, phase III trials of bevacizumab in newly diagnosed GBM (RTOG 8025 and AVAglio) have shown a 3- to 4-month improvement of PFS, but no OS advantage over the standard of care.[84] The AVAglio trial improved patients' quality of life, whereas the RTOG 0825 did not and instead increased the burden of symptoms with a negative impact on cognition. Although these two studies showed that bevacizumab had a modest benefit as the initial therapy for GBM, it remained effective to treat recurrences where treatment options are limited. In July 2009, bevacizumab was approved for use in combination with IFN-α for the treatment of patients with metastatic renal cell carcinoma (RCC). Results from the AVOREN trial demonstrated a 5-month improvement in median PFS in patients treated with bevacizumab plus IFN-α-2a versus IFN-α-2a plus placebo.[85] Another phase III trial (CALGB 90206) of bevacizumab plus IFN-α versus IFN-α monotherapy was conducted in patients with previously untreated, metastatic clear cell RCC. Median PFS was 8.4 months versus 4.9 months in favor of the bevacizumab arm.[86] Both studies did not demonstrate a statistically significant advantage in OS.[87,88]

Clinical studies of bevacizumab in combination with oxaliplatin-containing and 5-fluorouracil–based regimens have shown that combination therapy is well tolerated with toxicity not being substantially greater than that of the chemotherapy alone.[89] Side effects included grade 3 hypertension, grade 1 or 2 proteinuria, a slight increase (less than two percentage points) in grade 3 or 4 bleeding, and impaired surgical wound healing in patients who underwent surgery during treatment with bevacizumab. However, potentially life-threatening events (e.g., arterial and venous thromboembolic events, gastrointestinal perforation, hemoptysis, risk of ovarian failure) have occurred in some patients, thus requiring close patient monitoring in individuals who are at greater risk of adverse events.[90] In a recent meta-analysis of RCTs, bevacizumab in combination with chemotherapy or biologic therapy, compared with chemotherapy alone, was associated with increased treatment-related mortality.[91]

Although four phase III randomized studies have demonstrated improvements in PFS for ovarian cancer (OC)—two first-line trials (GOG 218 and ICON7) and two in recurrent OC [*platinum-resistant* (AURELIA Trial) or *platinum-sensitive* (OCEANS Trial)]—the role of bevacizumab in OC remains controversial. Bevacizumab is approved for use in combination with chemotherapy in the first- and second-line treatment of advanced OC in Europe, but it is not currently licensed in the United States for this indication. Mature OS data and predictive biomarkers are key to defining the subsets of patients who will most like benefit from this therapy. More recently, a randomized, phase III trial (GOG240) has demonstrated for the first time that bevacizumab can prolong OS and PFS for women with advanced, recurrent, or persistent cervical cancer that was not curable with standard chemotherapy. At the time of writing, there are currently over 400 actively recruiting, ongoing trials investigating the clinical benefits of bevacizumab in combination with chemotherapeutic regimens or as adjuvant therapy in various stages and types of cancer (http://clinicaltrial.gov).

Ziv-aflibercept

Ziv-aflibercept (previously known as aflibercept or VEGFTrap) is a recombinant humanized fusion protein of the extracellular domains of VEGF receptor 1 (VEGFR1) and VEGFR2 with the constant region (Fc) of human immunoglobulin (Ig)G1 that binds to VEGF-A, VEGF-B, PlGF1, and PlGF2, thereby preventing these ligands from binding to and activating their cognate receptors.[92] Ziv-aflibercept has a higher VEGF-A binding affinity and more potent blockade of VEGFR1 or VEGFR2 activation than bevacizumab.[93] In tumor models, ziv-aflibercept exerts its antiangiogenic effects through regressing tumor vasculature and size, remodeling or normalizing surviving vasculature, and inhibiting ascites formation.[94] In August 2012, ziv-aflibercept received regulatory approval for use in combination with 5-fluorouracil, leucovorin, and irinotecan (FOLFIRI) for the treatment of patients with metastatic CRC that is resistant to or that has progressed following treatment with an oxaliplatin-containing regimen. Results from the pivotal phase III VELOUR trial showed that ziv-aflibercept plus FOLFIRI statistically and significantly improved PFS (median PFS, 6.90 versus 4.67 months, respectively), OS (median OS, 13.50 versus 12.06 months, respectively), and overall response rates (19% versus 11.1%, respectively) relative to placebo plus FOLFIRI.[95] Toxicities related to ziv-aflibercept were consistent with those expected from the anti-VEGF drug class. The frequency of vascular-related adverse events appeared to be higher with ziv-aflibercept than bevacizumab treatment when compared across trials. Current clinical data are insufficient to directly compare ziv-aflibercept and bevacizumab in the first- or second-line setting for metastatic CRC.

Tyrosine–Kinase Inhibitor Therapy

Sorafenib

Sorafenib is a small-molecule Raf kinase and VEGF receptor kinase (VEGFR2 and VEGFR3) inhibitor. It has been shown to exhibit broad-spectrum effects on multiple targets (PDGF receptor (PDGFR), stem cell factor (c-KIT) receptor, p38) that affect the maintenance of the tumor vasculature and angiogenesis.[96] In December 2005, the FDA granted approval for sorafenib, which is considered the first multikinase inhibitor, for the treatment of patients with advanced RCC. Safety and efficacy of sorafenib was proven in the largest randomized phase III study conducted in advanced RCC that showed prolong PFS in favor of sorafenib.[97,98] In November 2007, sorafenib was approved for the treatment of patients with unresectable hepatocellular carcinoma (HCC) based on the study results in patients with advanced HCC who had not received previous systemic treatment. Median survival and the time to radiologic progression were nearly 3 months longer for patients treated with sorafenib than for those given placebo.[99] In November 2013, sorafenib received a new indication under the FDA's priority review program for the treatment of locally recurrent or metastatic, progressive differentiated thyroid carcinoma (DTC) refractory to radioactive iodine (RAI) treatment based on positive results from the phase III DECISION trial. Treatment with sorafenib improved PFS (the primary endpoint of the trial) by 41% compared with placebo (10.8 versus 5.8 months, respectively; hazard ratio [HR], 0.587, 95% confidence interval [CI] [0.454 to 0.758]; p <0.0001).[100] The overall response rates were 12% for patients who received sorafenib versus 1% for the placebo arm. Although only about 5% to 15% of thyroid cancer patients become refractory to RAI, no standard treatments are available and, thus, sorafenib is the first agent specifically approved for RAI-resistant DTC. Sorafenib was generally well tolerated with a predictable safety profile. Common adverse events include diarrhea, rash/desquamation, fatigue, hand–foot skin reaction, alopecia, and nausea/vomiting. Grade 3/4 adverse events were 38% for sorafenib versus 28% for placebo. Sorafenib-induced hypertension occurred in patients with metastatic RCC. The treatment-related hypertension was noted to be a class effect observed not only with VEGFR inhibitors, but also with the VEGF monoclonal antibody as well.[90] No significant relationship between previously described mediators of blood pressure and the magnitude of increase was found in a study evaluating the mechanism of sorafenib-induced hypertension in patients.[101]

Sunitinib

Sunitinib (SU11248) is a small-molecule, multitargeted TKI that exhibits potent antitumor and antiangiogenic activity and inhibits VEGFR-1, -2, -3, c-KIT, PDGFR; FLT-3; colony-stimulating factor receptor type 1 receptor; and the glial cell line–derived neurotrophic factor receptor. It was rationally designed and chosen for its high bioavailability and its nanomolar-range potency against the antiangiogenic RTKs. Sunitinib received its first U.S. regulatory approval in 2006 for the treatment of gastrointestinal stromal tumor (GIST) after disease progression on, or intolerance to, imatinib and accelerated approval for the treatment of advanced RCC.[102] Sunitinib demonstrated significant efficacy (prolonged median time to progression) in imatinib-resistant or -intolerant GIST in a randomized phase III trial.[103] The accelerated approval for RCC was based on durable partial responses, with a response rate of 26% to 37%, and a median duration of response of 54 weeks from two phase II, single-arm trials of patients with cytokine-refractory RCC.[104] The accelerated approval was converted to regular approval in 2007 following confirmation of an improvement in PFS and OS in a phase III trial of sunitinib for first-line treatment of patients with treatment-naïve, metastatic RCC.[105,106] In May 2011, the drug received a new indication for the treatment of progressive, well-differentiated pancreatic neuroendocrine tumors (pNET) in patients with unresectable, locally advanced, or metastatic disease. The randomized phase III trial was discontinued early after the independent data monitoring committee observed more serious adverse events and deaths in the placebo group as well as a difference in PFS favoring sunitinib. The median PFS for patients treated with sunitinib was 10.2 months,

compared with 5.4 months for patients treated with placebo (HR, 0.427, 95% CI, 0.271 to 0.673], p <0.001).[107] Common adverse effects, including diarrhea, mucositis, asthenia, skin abnormalities, and altered taste, were more common in patients receiving sunitinib. In addition, a decrease in left ventricular ejection fraction and severe hypertension were also more commonly reported in the sunitinib arm. Grade 3 or 4 treatment-emergent adverse events were reported in 56% versus 51% of patients on sunitinib versus placebo, respectively.

Pazopanib

Pazopanib is a second-generation, multitargeted TKI that binds to VEGFR-1, -2, -3, PDGFR-α and -β, c-KIT, and several other key proteins responsible for angiogenesis, tumor growth, and cell survival. Pazopanib exhibited in vivo and in vitro activity against tumor growth, and early clinical trials demonstrated potent antitumor and antiangiogenic activity.[108] A phase III clinical trial in treatment-naïve and cytokine-pretreated patients with advanced and/or metastatic RCC showed a significant improvement in PFS and tumor response compared with placebo,[109] leading to the approval of pazopanib in the United States in October 2009. A recent, randomized phase III trial (COMPARZ) compared the efficacy and safety of pazopanib and sunitinib as first-line therapy involving patients with metastatic RCC and demonstrated that both pazopanib and sunitinib have similar efficacy, but the safety and quality-of-life profiles favor pazopanib.[110] In April 2012, pazopanib was approved for the treatment of patients with metastatic nonadipocytic soft tissue sarcoma who have received prior chemotherapy following a phase III trial that demonstrated a statistically significant improvement in PFS. The median PFS was 4.6 months for patients receiving pazopanib versus 1.6 months for the placebo arm.[111] The drug is generally well tolerated, with the most common adverse events being diarrhea, fatigue, anorexia, hypertension, and hair depigmentation, as well as laboratory abnormalities in elevated aspartate aminotransferase and alanine aminotransferase. Pazopanib has shown clinical activity in a variety of tumors, including breast cancer, thyroid cancer, HCC, and cervical cancer.[112] Ongoing phase II and III trials are further evaluating pazopanib in these malignancies.

Vandetanib

Vandetanib is an oral, small-molecule TKI that inhibits the activity of RET kinase, VEGFR, epidermal growth factor receptor (EGFR), protein tyrosine kinase 6 (BRK), TIE2, members of the ephrin (EPH) receptors kinase family, and members of the Src family of tyrosine kinases.[113] Vandetanib reduced endothelial cell migration, proliferation, survival, and angiogenesis in vitro, and it decreased tumor vessel permeability and inhibited tumor growth and metastasis in vivo. In April 2011, vandetanib received U.S. regulatory approval for the treatment of symptomatic or progressive medullary thyroid cancer (MTC) in patients with unresectable, locally advanced, or metastatic disease. Until the approval of vandetanib, no systemic therapy was approved for the treatment of unresectable MTC, making it the first molecularly targeted agent approved for this disease. Results of a randomized phase III trial of patients with unresectable, locally advanced, or metastatic MTC demonstrated statistically significant and clinically meaningful improvements in PFS for vandetanib compared with placebo (HR, 0.46; 95% CI, 0.31 to 0.69; p <0.001).[114] Common grade 3 and 4 toxicities (>5%) were diarrhea and/or colitis, hypertension and hypertensive crisis, fatigue, hypocalcemia, rash, and corrected QT interval (QTc) prolongation. Given the toxicity profile, which includes QTc prolongation and sudden death, vandetanib is only available through a restricted distribution program. Vandetanib is also the first targeted drug to show evidence of efficacy in a randomized phase II trial in patients with locally advanced or metastatic differentiated thyroid carcinoma,[115] and a phase III trial is currently underway. Early phase studies are also being conducted in solid tumors, including GIST and kidney and pancreatic cancers.

Axitinib

Axitinib is a potent and selective second-generation inhibitor of VEGFR-1, -2, and -3. The in vitro half-maximal inhibitory concentration (IC50) of axitinib is 10-fold lower for the VEGF family of receptors than for other TKIs such as pazopanib, sunitinib, or sorafenib.[116] In January 2012, axitinib received approval for the treatment of advanced RCC after the failure of one prior systemic therapy based on a phase III trial (AXIS) comparing the efficacy and safety of axitinib versus sorafenib as a second-line treatment for metastatic RCC.[117,118] The median PFS was 6.7 months with axitinib compared to 4.7 months with sorafenib (HR, 0.67; 95% CI, 0.54, 0.81; one-sided p <0.0001). This improvement in PFS was greater in the cytokine-pretreated subgroup in comparison with the sunitinib-pretreated subgroup. The most frequent adverse events with axitinib were diarrhea (all grade), hypertension (all grade), fatigue, decreased appetite, nausea, and dysphonia. Moreover, hypertension, nausea, dysphonia, and hypothyroidism were more common with axitinib, whereas palmar–plantar erythrodysesthesia, alopecia, and rash were more frequent with sorafenib. A phase III trial (AGILE) comparing axitinib with sorafenib as first-line therapy in patients with treatment-naïve metastatic RCC demonstrated no significant difference in median PFS between patients treated with axitinib or sorafenib.[119] Additionally, axitinib is being studied as a single agent as well as in combination with chemotherapy across several tumor types including HCC, NSCLC, and pancreatic and thyroid cancers.

Cabozantinib

Cabozantinib (XL184) is a small-molecule TKI with potent activity toward the MET receptor and VEGFR2, as well as a number of other receptor tyrosine kinases, including RET, KIT, AXL, and FLT-3. MET is the only known receptor for hepatocyte growth factor (HGF), and its signaling activity plays a key role in tumorigenic growth, metastasis, and therapeutic resistance. The dysregulated expression and/or activation of MET and HGF have been implicated in the development of numerous human cancers including glioma; melanoma; and hepatocellular, renal, gastric, pancreatic, prostate, ovarian, breast, and lung cancers, and is often correlated with poor prognosis.[120] Recent studies have determined that the MET pathway plays an important role in the development of resistance to VEGF pathway inhibition and that the use of VEGFR inhibitors, such as sunitinib, sorafenib, or a VEGFR2-targeting antibody, can result in the development of an aggressive tumor phenotype characterized by increased invasiveness and metastasis.[121–123] Thus, there is an advantage to targeting both the MET and VEGF pathways to disrupt angiogenesis, tumorigenesis, and cancer progression. In November 2012, cabozantinib received U.S. regulatory approval for progressive metastatic MTC based on the phase III trial that demonstrated a statistically significant PFS prolongation for the cabozantinib-treatment arm.[124] The estimated median PFS was 11.2 months for cabozantinib versus 4.0 months for placebo (HR, 0.28; 95% CI, 0.19 to 0.40; p <0.001). Manageable toxicities included diarrhea, palmar–plantar erythrodysesthesia, decreased weight and appetite, nausea, and fatigue. Cabozantinib has been effective against several solid cancers, including MTC, breast, NSCLC, melanoma, and liver cancer, and is currently being studied in clinical trials in a number of tumor types, with the most significant results observed in the reduction of bone metastatic lesions in castration-resistant prostate cancer.[125]

Regorafenib

Regorafenib is a small-molecule TKI of multiple membrane-bound and intracellular kinases including RET, VEGFR1, VEGFR2, VEGFR3, KIT, PDGFR-α, PDGFR-β, FGFR1, FGFR2, TIE2, DDR2, TrkA, Eph2A, RAF-1, BRAF, BRAFV600E, SAPK2, PTK5, and Abl pathways.[126] Regorafenib is structurally related to sorafenib and differs from the latter by the presence of a fluorine atom in the center phenyl ring, resulting in higher inhibitory potency against various proangiogenic receptors than sorafenib, including VEGFR2 and FGFR1. In September 2012, regorafenib was approved for the treatment of patients with mCRC who have been previously treated with fluoropyrimidine-, oxaliplatin-, and irinotecan-based chemotherapy, with an anti-VEGF therapy, and if KRAS wild type, with an anti-EGFR therapy. The phase III CORRECT trial that resulted in approval of the drug demonstrated a median OS of 6.4 months in the regorafenib group versus 5.0 months in the placebo group (HR, 0.77; 95% CI, 0.64 to 0.94; one-sided p = 0.0052).[127] Regorafenib is the first TKI with survival benefits in mCRC that has progressed after all standard therapies. In February 2013, it received another indication for the treatment of patients with locally advanced, unresectable, or metastatic GIST who have been previously treated with imatinib and sunitinib. This was based on positive findings of the phase III GRID trial that demonstrated a median PFS of 4.8 months for regorafenib and 0.9 months for placebo (HR, 0.27, 95% CI, 0.19 to 0.39; p <0.0001).[128] In both studies, regorafenib provided significant improvements in PFS to highly refractory patient populations who have progressed on standard treatments. The most common adverse events that were grade 3 or higher and related to regorafenib were hand–foot skin reaction, fatigue, diarrhea, hypertension, and rash or desquamation. Its clinical development as a single agent or in combination with standard chemotherapeutic agents in various malignant tumors is ongoing and includes a phase III trial in patients with HCC whose disease has progressed after treatment with sorafenib.

mTOR Inhibitors

The mTOR pathway is a central component of the PI3K/Akt signaling pathway and a regulator of many biologic processes that are essential for angiogenesis, cell proliferation, and metabolism.[129] Inhibition of the mTOR kinase prevents downstream signaling via the Akt pathway, resulting in inhibition of protein translation and cell growth. mTOR plays a key role in angiogenesis and specifically regulates the expression of HIF-1, which is upregulated by the loss of the von Hippel–Lindau gene in RCC. In May 2007, temsirolimus was approved for the treatment of advanced RCC. Efficacy and safety were demonstrated in a phase III study in previously untreated patients (n = 626) with poor risk features of metastatic RCC assigned to one of three treatment arms: IFN-α alone, temsirolimus 25 mg alone, or the combination of temsirolimus (15 mg) and IFN-α.[130] Single-agent temsirolimus was associated with a statistically significant improvement in OS when compared with IFN; the addition of temsirolimus to IFN did not improve OS. The results of the phase III INTORSECT trial compared the efficacy of temsirolimus and sorafenib in the second-line treatment of metastatic RCC after disease progression on sunitinib demonstrated that temsirolimus did not improve survival over sorafenib in the second-line setting.[131] The significant OS difference in favor of sorafenib (stratified HR, 1.31; 95% CI, 1.05 to 1.63; two-sided p = 0.01) suggested that VEGFR inhibition may be a better option than mTOR inhibitors for patients progressing on sunitinib. The most common adverse reactions that occurred were rash, asthenia, mucositis, nausea, edema, and anorexia. Rare, but serious adverse reactions associated with temsirolimus included interstitial lung disease, bowel perforation, and acute renal failure.

Everolimus (RAD001) was approved in March 2009 for patients with advanced RCC whose disease had progressed on VEGFR-targeted therapy (sunitinib or sorafenib). Efficacy was demonstrated in a phase 3 trial that study met its primary endpoint with a median PFS of 4.9 and 1.9 months in the everolimus and placebo arms, respectively (HR, 0.33; p <0.0001).[132] Everolimus is also indicated for subependymal giant cell astrocytoma (SEGA) associated with tuberous sclerosis complex (TSC), renal angiomyolipoma with TSC, progressive neuroendocrine tumors of pancreatic origin, and advanced hormone receptor-positive, HER2-negative breast cancer in combination with exemestane.[133] The most common adverse reactions were stomatitis, infections, asthenia, fatigue, cough, and diarrhea. The most common grade 3/4 adverse reactions were infections, dyspnea, fatigue, stomatitis, dehydration, pneumonitis, abdominal pain, and asthenia. Both temsirolimus and everolimus are currently being evaluated in phase I through III studies of various cancer types. By downregulating HIF-1 in the tumor cell, mTOR inhibitors may complement the effects of TKIs at the level of the EC; thus, the combination of mTOR inhibitors with other targeted agents such as bevacizumab or sorafenib/sunitinib are also being investigated.

On the Horizon: Anti-VEGFR2 Monoclonal Antibody

Ramucirumab (IMC-1121B) is a fully human IgG1 monoclonal antibody that binds with high affinity to the extracellular VEGF-binding domain of VEGFR-2. In a phase III trial (REGARD), ramucirumab monotherapy conferred a statistically significant benefit in OS and PFS compared to placebo in patients with advanced gastric or gastroesophageal junction adenocarcinoma in the second-line setting with an acceptable safety profile.[134] The survival advantage is the first to be elicited by a single-agent biologic treatment in this setting and, based on these findings, the FDA has assigned a priority review designation for ramucirumab. An ongoing phase III trial (RAINBOW) of ramucirumab in combination with chemotherapy as second-line treatment for patients with advanced gastric cancer is currently underway, and preliminary results demonstrated the trial met both its primary (OS) and secondary (PFS) endpoints. In April 2014, the U.S. FDA approved ramucirumab for use as a single agent for the treatment of patients with advanced or metastatic, gastric or gastroesophageal junction adenocarcinoma with disease progression on or after prior treatment with fluoropyrimidine- or platinum-containing chemotherapy. The recommended ramucirumab dose and schedule is 8 mg/kg administered as a 60-minute intravenous infusion every 2 weeks. The drug also marginally improved survival in the second-line treatment of NSCLC in an ongoing phase III (REVEL) trial.

COMBINATION THERAPIES

Tumor angiogenesis is a highly complex process involving multiple growth factors and their receptor signaling pathways. Based on current evidence, with a few exceptions, effective therapy will probably rely on a combinatorial approach that involves targeting multiple pathways simultaneously. However, a recent study has demonstrated that simultaneous inhibition of the VEGF and EGF pathways in combination with chemotherapy shortens rather than prolongs PFS as compared to inhibition of the VEGF pathway alone in combination with chemotherapy.[135] Whether other targeted agents exhibit beneficial effects when combined with VEGF inhibitors remains to be investigated. Moreover, a number of studies have shown that antiangiogenic agents in combination with chemotherapy or radiotherapy result in additive or synergistic effects. Several models have been proposed to explain the mechanism responsible for this potentiation, keying in on the chemosensitizing effects of antiangiogenic therapy.[136] One hypothesis is that antiangiogenic therapy may normalize the tumor vasculature, thus resulting in improved oxygenation, better blood perfusion, and consequently, improved delivery of chemotherapeutic drugs.[137] A second model suggests that chemotherapy delivered at low doses and at close, regular intervals with no extended drug-free break periods preferentially damages ECs in the tumor neovasculature.[138,139] and suppresses circulating endothelial progenitor cells.[140,141] This regimen, also called metronomic

chemotherapy, sustains antiangiogenic activity and reduces acute toxicity.[142] Thus, the efficacy of metronomic chemotherapy may increase when administered in combination with specific antiangiogenic drugs. Another model addresses the use of antiangiogenic drugs to slow down tumor cell repopulation between successive cycles of cytotoxic chemotherapy.[143] This model underscores the importance of timing and sequence in achieving the maximal therapeutic benefit from combination therapies. In fact, a preclinical study in murine tumor models demonstrated that the administration of sunitinib markedly reduced chemotherapy-induced bone marrow toxicity, suggesting that the sequential treatment regimen (delivery of antiangiogenics followed by chemotherapy) showed superior survival benefits compared with the simultaneous administration of two drugs.[144] Finally, other mechanisms that might also contribute to the synergism include angiogenesis inhibitor–induced tumor blood vessel regression, the prevention of tumor coopting of vessels from surrounding healthy tissues, and the formation of abnormal vessels in the tumor microenvironment.[145] Nevertheless, it remains a challenge to determine why bevacizumab has proved largely ineffective as a single agent, whereas VEGF RTK inhibitors have repeatedly failed in randomized phase III trials when used in combination with chemotherapy. Furthermore, an additional challenge is to determine the optimal dose and duration of antiangiogenic drugs as well as the impact of drug sequencing in combination regimens. Studies are warranted to delineate the discrepancy of bevacizumab's efficacy in the macrometastatic versus micrometastatic disease settings.[146,147]

BIOMARKERS OF ANTIANGIOGENIC THERAPY

Antiangiogenic therapy has created a need to develop effective biomarkers to assess the activity of these inhibitors. Biomarkers of tumor angiogenesis activity are important to guide clinical development of these agents and to select patients most likely to benefit from this approach. Although there are currently no validated biomarkers for clinically assessing the efficacy of or selecting patients who will respond to antiangiogenic therapies, a number of candidate markers, including tissue, imaging, and circulating biomarkers, are emerging that need to be prospectively validated.[148,149] Several avenues are currently being investigated and include tumor biopsy analysis, microvessel density, noninvasive vascular imaging modalities (positron-emission tomography, dynamic contrast-enhanced magnetic resonance imaging), and measuring circulating biomarkers (levels of angiogenic factors in serum, plasma, urine, or circulating ECs and their precursors).[150–152] Recent research efforts have focused on identifying genetic and toxicity biomarkers to predict which patients will benefit from anti-VEGF/VEGFR therapy and identify patients at risk of adverse events. The existence of VEGF single-nucleotide polymorphisms (SNP) and their association with clinical outcomes may be predictive of patient response to bevacizumab. A recent study identified a locus in VEGFR1 that correlated with increased VEGFR1 expression and poor bevacizumab treatment outcomes.[153] Moreover, a breast cancer study (E2100) reported the VEGF-2578 AA and VEGF-1154 AA genotypes predicted an improved median OS, whereas the VEGF-634 CC and VEGF-1498 TT genotypes predicted protection from grade 3/4 hypertension in the combination-treatment arm.[154] The degree of hypertension can serve as a predictive biomarker of survival in patients after bevacizumab or TKI treatment. Although an association between hypertension and anti-VEGF therapy has been described, the clinical implications of this association and the predictive value of hypertension remains to be validated prospectively. A retrospective analysis of hypertension and efficacy outcomes was conducted in seven large phase III trials (n = 6,486 patients) and, in six of seven studies, early treatment-related blood pressure increase was neither predictive of clinical benefit from bevacizumab nor prognostic for the course of the disease.[155] However, one study (AVF2107g) showed early increased blood pressure was associated with longer PFS and OS. Because genetics play a significant role in modifying the risk of hypertension,[156] it remains to be determined whether polymorphisms in the VEGF/VEGFR pathway may function as potential biomarkers to predict the association between treatment-related hypertension and response to anti-VEGF therapy, as previously implicated in the E2100 trial.[154] Other biomarkers of response include elevated VEGF and placental growth factor levels,[148,152] whereas biomarkers of resistance, including circulating basic fibroblast growth factor, stromal cell-derived factor 1α, and viable circulating endothelial cells, increased when tumors escaped treatment.[157] A first prospective biomarker study (MERiDiAN) in metastatic breast cancer is currently underway to evaluate the impact of bevacizumab in patients stratified for plasma short VEGF-A isoforms. If validated, these findings could help identify which subgroup of patients should receive antiangiogenic therapy and could lead the way to possible future tailoring of individualized antiangiogenic therapy.

RESISTANCE TO ANTIANGIOGENIC THERAPY

Despite a decade of trials with angiogenesis inhibitors, clinical experience reveals that VEGF-targeted therapy often prolongs the survival of cancer patients by only months because tumors elicit evasive resistance.[145,158] Resistance to VEGF inhibitors may be observed in late-stage tumors when tumors regrow during treatment after an initial period of growth suppression from these antiangiogenic agents. This resistance involves the reactivation of tumor angiogenesis and increased expression of other proangiogenic factors. As the disease progresses, it is possible that redundant pathways might be implicated, with VEGF being replaced by other angiogenic pathways, warranting the addition of a second angiogenesis inhibitor that would target these secondary growth factors and/or their activated receptor pathways, or the use of a multitargeted TKI antiangiogenic drug (e.g., sunitinib, sorafenib).

However, resistance to these drugs eventually occurs, implicating the existence of additional pathways mediating resistance to antiangiogenic therapies. Moreover, tumor cells bearing genetic alterations of the *p53* gene may display a lower apoptosis rate under hypoxic conditions, which might reduce their reliance on vascular supply and, therefore, their responsiveness to antiangiogenic therapy.[159] The selection and overgrowth of tumor-variant cells that are hypoxia resistant and, thus, less dependent[159] on angiogenesis and vasculature remodeling, resulting in vessel stabilization,[160] could also explain the resistance to antiangiogenic drugs. Other possible mechanisms for acquired resistance include tumor vessels becoming less sensitive to antiangiogenic agents, tumor regrowth via rebound revascularization, and vessel cooption.[161-166] Perhaps one of the most intriguing findings is that, although ECs are assumed to be genetically stable, they may under some circumstances harbor genetic abnormalities and thus acquire resistance as well.[167,168]

Recent studies report that VEGF-targeted therapies not only induce primary tumor shrinkage and inhibit tumor progression, but can also initiate mechanisms that increase malignancy to promote tumor invasiveness and metastasis.[122,123,169] These mechanisms of resistance to antiangiogenic therapy involve tumor- and host-mediated pathways and may allow for differential efficacy in different stages of disease progression.[163] Specifically, antiangiogenic drug–resistance mechanisms involve pathways mediated by the tumor, whether intrinsic or acquired in response to therapy or by the host, which is either responding directly to therapy or indirectly to tumoral cues. Taken together, antiangiogenic therapy can enhance tumor invasiveness and metastasis to facilitate and/or accelerate disease in microscopic tumors and, hence, reduce OS benefit. Understanding the mechanisms of resistance, whether intrinsic or acquired, after exposure to antiangiogenic drug treatment is essential for developing strategies that will allow for optimal exploitation of VEGF inhibitors. It is equally important to identify biomarkers of drug resistance and factors mediating this resistance because the development of reliable biomarkers can be invaluable to monitor the development of evasive resistance to angiogenesis inhibitors.

SELECTED REFERENCES

The full reference list can be accessed at lwwhealthlibrary.com/oncology.

1. Hanahan D, Weinberg RA. Hallmarks of cancer: the next generation. *Cell* 2011;144:646–674.
5. Folkman J. Tumor angiogenesis: therapeutic implications. *N Engl J Med* 1971;285:1182–1186.
7. Hanahan D, Folkman J. Patterns and emerging mechanisms of the angiogenic switch during tumorigenesis. *Cell* 1996;86:353–364.
9. Folkman J, Kalluri R. Cancer without disease. *Nature* 2004;427:787.
11. Holmgren L, O'Reilly MS, Folkman J. Dormancy of micrometastases: balanced proliferation and apoptosis in the presence of angiogenesis suppression. *Nat Med* 1995;1:149–153.
12. Naumov GN, Bender E, Zurakowski D, et al. A model of human tumor dormancy: an angiogenic switch from the nonangiogenic phenotype. *J Natl Cancer Inst* 2006;98:316–325.
13. Udagawa T, Fernandez A, Achilles EG, et al. Persistence of microscopic human cancers in mice: alterations in the angiogenic balance accompanies loss of tumor dormancy. *Faseb J* 2002;16:1361–1370.
14. Holash J, Maisonpierre PC, Compton D, et al. Vessel cooption, regression, and growth in tumors mediated by angiopoietins and VEGF. *Science* 1999;284:1994–1998.
16. Carmeliet P, Dor Y, Herbert JM, et al. Role of HIF-1alpha in hypoxia-mediated apoptosis, cell proliferation and tumour angiogenesis. *Nature* 1998;394:485–490.
19. Rak J, Yu JL. Oncogenes and tumor angiogenesis: the question of vascular "supply" and vascular "demand". *Semin Cancer Biol* 2004;14:93–104.
20. Bottos A, Bardelli A. Oncogenes and angiogenesis: a way to personalize antiangiogenic therapy? *Cell Mol Life Sci* 2013;70:4131–4140.
24. Ribatti D. Endogenous inhibitors of angiogenesis: a historical review. *Leuk Res* 2009;33:638–644.
31. Noguera-Troise I, Daly C, Papadopoulos NJ, et al. Blockade of Dll4 inhibits tumour growth by promoting non-productive angiogenesis. *Nature* 2006;444:1032–1037.
32. Ridgway J, Zhang G, Wu Y, et al. Inhibition of Dll4 signalling inhibits tumour growth by deregulating angiogenesis. *Nature* 2006;444:1083–1087.
33. Kuhnert F, Kirshner JR, Thurston G. Dll4-Notch signaling as a therapeutic target in tumor angiogenesis. *Vasc Cell* 2011;3:20.
49. Folkman J. Angiogenesis: an organizing principle for drug discovery? *Nat Rev Drug Discov* 2007;6:273–286.
60. Ferrara N, Gerber HP, LeCouter J. The biology of VEGF and its receptors. *Nat Med* 2003;9:669–676.
61. Lindahl P, Johansson BR, Leveen P, et al. Pericyte loss and microaneurysm formation in PDGF-B-deficient mice. *Science* 1997;277:242–245.
69. Desgrosellier JS, Cheresh DA. Integrins in cancer: biological implications and therapeutic opportunities. *Nat Rev Cancer* 2010;10:9–22.
74. Ellis LM, Hicklin DJ. VEGF-targeted therapy: mechanisms of anti-tumour activity. *Nat Rev Cancer* 2008;8:579–591.
75. Hurwitz H, Fehrenbacher L, Novotny W, et al. Bevacizumab plus irinotecan, fluorouracil, and leucovorin for metastatic colorectal cancer. *N Engl J Med* 2004;350:2335–2342.
79. Sandler A, Gray R, Perry MC, et al. Paclitaxel-carboplatin alone or with bevacizumab for non-small-cell lung cancer. *N Engl J Med* 2006;355:2542–2550.
90. Chen HX, Cleck JN. Adverse effects of anticancer agents that target the VEGF pathway. *Nat Rev Clin Oncol* 2009;6:465–477.
91. Ranpura V, Hapani S, Wu S. Treatment-related mortality with bevacizumab in cancer patients: a meta-analysis. *JAMA* 2011;305:487–494.
94. Gaya A, Tse V. A preclinical and clinical review of aflibercept for the management of cancer. *Cancer Treat Rev* 2012;38:484–493.
97. Escudier B, Eisen T, Stadler WM, et al. Sorafenib in advanced clear-cell renal-cell carcinoma. *N Engl J Med* 2007;356:125–134.
99. Llovet JM, Ricci S, Mazzaferro V, et al. Sorafenib in advanced hepatocellular carcinoma. *N Engl J Med* 2008;359:378–390.
101. Veronese ML, Mosenkis A, Flaherty KT, et al. Mechanisms of hypertension associated with BAY 43-9006. *J Clin Oncol* 2006;24:1363–1369.
105. Motzer RJ, Hutson TE, Tomczak P, et al. Sunitinib versus interferon alfa in metastatic renal-cell carcinoma. *N Engl J Med* 2007;356:115–124.
107. Raymond E, Dahan L, Raoul JL, et al. Sunitinib malate for the treatment of pancreatic neuroendocrine tumors. *N Engl J Med* 2011;364:501–513.
110. Motzer RJ, Hutson TE, Cella D, et al. Pazopanib versus sunitinib in metastatic renal-cell carcinoma. *N Engl J Med* 2013;369:722–731.

112. Schutz FA, Choueiri TK, Sternberg CN. Pazopanib: Clinical development of a potent anti-angiogenic drug. *Crit Rev Oncol Hematol* 2011;77:163–171.

120. Graveel CR, Tolbert D, Vande Woude GF. MET: a critical player in tumorigenesis and therapeutic target. *Cold Spring Harb Perspect Biol* 2013;5.

123. Paez-Ribes M, Allen E, Hudock J, et al. Antiangiogenic therapy elicits malignant progression of tumors to increased local invasion and distant metastasis. *Cancer Cell* 2009;15:220–231.

126. Strumberg D, Schultheis B. Regorafenib for cancer. *Expert Opin Investig Drugs* 2012;21:879–889.

130. Hudes G, Carducci M, Tomczak P, et al. Temsirolimus, interferon alfa, or both for advanced renal-cell carcinoma. *N Engl J Med* 2007;356:2271–2281.

133. Lebwohl D, Anak O, Sahmoud T, et al. Development of everolimus, a novel oral mTOR inhibitor, across a spectrum of diseases. *Ann N Y Acad Sci* 2013;1291:14–32.

136. Kerbel RS. Antiangiogenic therapy: a universal chemosensitization strategy for cancer? *Science* 2006;312:1171–1175.

137. Jain RK. Normalization of tumor vasculature: an emerging concept in antiangiogenic therapy. *Science* 2005;307:58–62.

142. Kerbel RS, Kamen BA. The anti-angiogenic basis of metronomic chemotherapy. *Nat Rev Cancer* 2004;4:423–436.

143. Hudis CA. Clinical implications of antiangiogenic therapies. *Oncology (Williston Park)* 2005;19:26–31.

145. Kerbel RS. Tumor angiogenesis. *N Engl J Med* 2008;358:2039–2049.

146. Mountzios G, Pentheroudakis G, Carmeliet P. Bevacizumab and micrometastases: Revisiting the preclinical and clinical rollercoaster. *Pharmacol Ther* 2014;141:117–124.

147. Ebos JM, Kerbel RS. Antiangiogenic therapy: impact on invasion, disease progression, and metastasis. *Nat Rev Clin Oncol* 2011;8:210–221.

148. Jain RK, Duda DG, Willett CG, et al. Biomarkers of response and resistance to antiangiogenic therapy. *Nat Rev Clin Oncol* 2009;6:327–338.

152. Lambrechts D, Lenz HJ, de Haas S, et al. Markers of response for the antiangiogenic agent bevacizumab. *J Clin Oncol* 2013;31:1219–1230.

155. Hurwitz HI, Douglas PS, Middleton JP, et al. Analysis of early hypertension and clinical outcome with bevacizumab: results from seven phase III studies. *Oncologist* 2013;18:273–280.

158. Sennino B, McDonald DM. Controlling escape from angiogenesis inhibitors. *Nat Rev Cancer* 2012;12:699–709.

161. Bergers G, Hanahan D. Modes of resistance to anti-angiogenic therapy. *Nat Rev Cancer* 2008;8:592–603.

162. Crawford Y, Ferrara N. Tumor and stromal pathways mediating refractoriness/resistance to anti-angiogenic therapies. *Trends Pharmacol Sci* 2009;30:624–630.

163. Ebos JM, Lee CR, Kerbel RS. Tumor and host-mediated pathways of resistance and disease progression in response to antiangiogenic therapy. *Clin Cancer Res* 2009;15:5020–5025.

168. Streubel B, Chott A, Huber D, et al. Lymphoma-specific genetic aberrations in microvascular endothelial cells in B-cell lymphomas. *N Engl J Med* 2004;351:250–259.

169. Loges S, Mazzone M, Hohensinner P, et al. Silencing or fueling metastasis with VEGF inhibitors: antiangiogenesis revisited. *Cancer Cell* 2009;15:167–170.

CANCER THERAPEUTICS

29 Monoclonal Antibodies

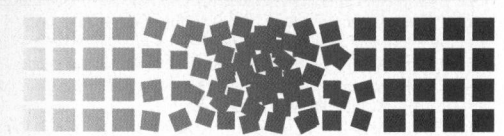

Hossein Borghaei, Matthew K. Robinson, Gregory P. Adams, and Louis M. Weiner

INTRODUCTION

Antibody-based therapeutics are important components of the cancer therapeutic armamentarium. Early antibody therapy studies attempted to explicitly target cancers based on the structural and biologic properties that distinguish neoplastic cells from their normal counterparts. The immunogenicity and inefficient effector functions of the first-generation murine monoclonal antibodies (MAb) that were evaluated in clinical trials limited their effectiveness.[1-3] Patients developed human antimouse antibody (HAMA) responses against the therapeutic agents that rapidly cleared it from the body and limited the number of times the therapy could be administered. The development of engineered chimeric, humanized, and fully human MAbs has identified a number of important and useful applications for antibody-based cancer therapy. Currently, the U.S. Food and Drug Administration (FDA) has approved 14 MAbs and MAb-conjugates for the treatment of cancer (Table 29.1) and many more are under evaluation in late-stage clinical trials.[4] Antibodies provide an important means by which to exploit the immune system by specifically recognizing and directing antitumor responses.

Antibodies are produced by B cells and arise in response to exposures to a variety of structures, termed antigens, as a result of a series of recombinations of V, D, and J germline genes. Immunoglobulin-G (IgG) molecules are most commonly employed as the working backbones of current therapeutic monoclonal antibodies, although various other isotypes of antibodies have specialized functions (e.g., IgA molecules play important roles in mucosal immunity, IgE molecules are involved in anaphylaxis). The advent of hybridoma technology by Kohler and Milstein[5] made it possible to produce large quantities of antibodies with high purity and monospecificity for a single binding region (epitope) on an antigen.

The mechanisms that antibody-based therapeutics employ to elicit antitumor effects include focusing components of the patient's immune system to attack tumor cells[6,7] and methods to alter signal transduction pathways that drive tumor progression.[8,9] Antibody-based conjugates employ the targeting specificity of antibodies to deliver toxic compounds, such as chemotherapeutics, specifically to the tumor sites.

IMMUNOGLOBULIN STRUCTURE

Structural and Functional Domains

An IgG molecule is typically divided into three domains consisting of two identical antigen-binding (Fab) domains connected to an effector or Fc domain by a flexible hinge sequence. Figure 29.1 shows the structure of an IgG molecule. IgG antibodies are comprised of two identical light chains and two identical heavy chains, with the chains joined by disulfide bonds, resulting in a bilaterally symmetrical complex. The Fab domains mediate the binding of IgG molecules to their cognate antigens and are composed of an intact light chain and half of a heavy chain. Each chain in the Fab domain is further divided into variable and constant regions, with the variable region containing hypervariable, or complementarity determining regions (CDR) in which the antigen-contact residues reside. The light and heavy chain variable regions each contain three CDRs (CDR1, CDR2, and CDR3). All six CDRs form the antigen-binding pocket and are collectively defined in immunologic terms as the idiotype of the antibody. In the majority of cases, the variable heavy chain CDR3 plays a dominant role in binding.[10]

The different isotypes of immunoglobulins are defined by the structure and function of their Fc domains. The Fc domain, composed of the CH2 and CH3 regions of the antibody's heavy chains, is the critical determinant of how an antibody mediates effector functions, transports across cellular barriers, and persists in circulation.[7,11]

MODIFIED ANTIBODY-BASED MOLECULES

Advances in antibody engineering and molecular biology have facilitated the development of many novel antibody-based structures with unique physical and pharmacokinetic properties (see Fig. 29.1). These include chimeric human-murine antibodies with human-constant regions and murine-variable regions,[12] humanized antibodies in which murine CDR sequences have been grafted into human IgG molecules, and entirely human antibodies derived from human hybridomas and, more recently, from transgenic mice expressing human immunoglobulin genes.[13] An accepted naming scheme based on "stems" was developed by the World Health Organization's International Nonproprietary Names (INN) for pharmaceuticals and is employed in the United States (Table 29.2). Engineering has also facilitated the development of antibody-based fragments. In addition to the classic, enzymatically derived Fab and F(ab')$_2$ molecules, a plethora of promising IgG-derivatives have been developed that retain antigen-binding properties of intact antibodies (see Fig. 29.1; for review see Robinson et al.[14]). The basic building block for these molecules is the 25 kDa, monovalent single-chain Fv (scFv) that is comprised of the variable domains (V$_H$ and V$_L$) of an antibody fused together with a short peptide linker. Novel, bispecific antibody-based structures can facilitate binding to two tumor antigens or bridge tumor cells with immune effector cells to focus antibody-dependent cell-mediated cytotoxicity (ADCC) or killing by T cells. An example of the former is MM-111, a bispecific gene-fused molecule composed of an anti-HER2 scFv connected to an anti-HER3 scFv via a modified form of human serum albumin.[15] Examples of the latter mechanism include small scFv-based bispecific T-cell engagers (BiTE) such as the anti-CD3/anti-CD19 molecule blinatumomab[16] and larger MAb-based antibodies such as catumaxomab, a rat/mouse anti-CD3/EpCAM bispecific MAb produced via quadroma technology.[17] Both classes of bispecifics endow selectivity and targeting properties that are not obtainable with natural antibody formats.

TABLE 29.1

FDA Approved Antibodies for the Treatment of Cancer

Generic Name (Trade Name)	Origin	Isotype (Conjugate)	Indication	Target	Initial Approval
Unconjugated MAbs					
Rituximab (Rituxan)	Chimeric	IgG1	NHL	CD20	1997
Trastuzumab (Herceptin)	Humanized	IgG1	BrCa	HER2	1998
Alemtuzumab (Campath-1H)	Humanized	IgG1	CLL	CD52	2001
Cetuximab (Erbitux)	Chimeric	IgG1	CRC, SCCHN	EGFR	2004
Bevacizumab (Avastin)	Humanized	IgG1	CRC, NSCLC, RCC, GBM	VEGF	2004
Panitumumab (Vectibix)	Human (XenoMouse)	IgG2	CRC	EGFR	2006
Ofatumumab (Arzerra)	Human (XenoMouse)	IgG1	CLL	CD20	2009
Denosumab (Prolia/Xgeva)	Human	IgG2	Metastasis-related SREs, ADT/AI-associated osteoporosis, GCT	RANKL	2010
Pertuzumab (Perjeta)	Humanized	IgG1	BrCa	HER2	2012
Immunoconjugates					
Gemtuzumab ozogamicin (Mylotarg)	Humanized	IgG4 (calicheamicin)	AML	CD33	2000[a]
Ibritumomab tiuxetan (Zevalin)	Murine	IgG1 (^{90}Y)	NHL	CD20	2002
Tositumomab (Bexxar)	Murine	IgG2A (^{131}I)	NHL	CD20	2003
Brentuximab vedotin (Adcetris)	Chimeric	IgG1 (MMAE)	HL, sALCL	CD30	2011
Ado-trastuzumab emtansine (Kadcyla)	Humanized	IgG1 (DM1)	BrCa	HER2	2013

[a] Withdrawn from the US market in June 2010.
NHL, non-Hodgkin lymphoma; BrCa, breast cancer; CLL, chronic lymphocytic leukemia; CRC, colorectal cancer; SCCHN, squamous cell carcinoma of head and neck; EGFR, epidermal growth factor receptor; NSCLC, non–small-cell lung cancer; RCC, renal cell carcinoma; GBM, glioblastoma multiforme; VEGF, vascular endothelial growth factor; SREs, skeletal-related events; ADT, androgen deprivation therapy; AI, aromatase inhibitor; GCT, giant cell tumor; RANKL, RANK ligand; AML, acute myelogenous leukemia; ^{90}Y, yttrium-90; ^{131}I, iodine-131; MMAE, Monomethyl auristatin E; HL, Hodgkin lymphoma; sALCL, systemic anaplastic large-cell lymphoma.

IgG

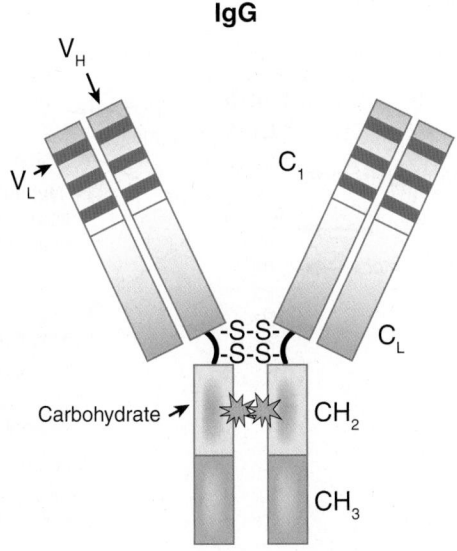

Figure 29.1 Structure of an IgG. C, constant; V, variable; H, heavy chain; L, light chain.

TABLE 29.2

Rules for Naming MAb for the Treatment of Cancer

The International Nonproprietary Names (INN) for monoclonal antibodies (MAbs) are composed of "stems" that indicate their origin, specificity, and modifications. The names include a random prefix to provide distinction from other names, a substem indicating the target specificity (-t[u]- for tumor), a substem indicating the species of origin (see the following) and a suffix (-mab), which indicates the presence of an immunoglobulin variable domain.

Substem Indication of the Species on Which the Immunoglobulin Sequence Is Based	
-o-	mouse
-xi-	chimeric
-zu-	humanized
-xizu-	chimeric/humanized
-u-	human

FACTORS REGULATING ANTIBODY-BASED TUMOR TARGETING

Antibody Size

Nonuniform distribution of systemically administered antibody is generally observed in biopsied specimens of solid tumors. Heterogeneous tumor blood supply limits uniform antibody delivery to tumors, and elevated interstitial pressures in the center of tumors oppose inward diffusion.[18] This high interstitial pressure slows the diffusion of molecules from their vascular extravasation site in a size-dependent manner.[19,20] The relatively large transport distances in the tumor interstitium also substantially increase the time required for large IgG macromolecules to reach target cells.[21]

Tumor Antigens

Access to the target antigen is undoubtedly a critical determinant of therapeutic effect of antibody-based applications. Such access is regulated by the heterogeneity of antigen expression by tumor cells. Shed antigen in the serum, tumor microenvironment, or both may saturate the antibody's binding sites and prevent binding to the cell surface. Alternatively, a rapid internalization of an antibody/antigen complex, although critical for antibody–drug conjugates (ADC), may deplete the quantity of cell surface MAb capable of initiating ADCC or cytotoxic signal transduction events. Finally, target antigens are normally *tumor associated* rather than *tumor specific*. Tumor-specific antigens are both highly desirable and rare. Typically, such antigens arise as a result of unique tumor-based genetic recombinations, such as clonal immunoglobulin idiotypes expressed on the surface of B-cell lymphomas.[22]

Antibody affinity for its target antigen has complex effects on tumor targeting. The *binding-site barrier* hypothesis postulates that antibodies with extremely high affinity for target antigen would bind irreversibly to the first antigen encountered upon entering the tumor, which would limit the diffusion of the antibody into the tumor and accumulate instead in regions surrounding the tumor vasculature.[23,24] Similarly, in tumor spheroids, the in vitro penetration of engineered antibodies is primarily limited by internalization and degradation.[25] The valence of an antibody molecule can increase the functional affinity of the antibody through an avidity effect.[26–28]

Half-Life/Clearance Rate

The concentration of intact IgG in mammalian serum is maintained at constant levels with half-lives of IgGs measured in days. This homeostasis is regulated in part by the major histocompatibility complex (MHC)-class I–related Fc receptor, FcRn (n = neonatal), a saturable, pH-dependent salvage mechanism that regulates quality and quantity of IgG in serum. This mechanism can be exploited via mutations in the Fc portion of an IgG to modulate IgGs pharmacokinetics.[29,30] Indeed, multiple strategies have been developed to increase the serum persistence of antibody-based fragments and other classes of protein therapeutics.[14,31]

Glycosylation

IgGs undergo N-linked glycosylation at the conserved Asn residue at position 297 within the C_H2 domain of the constant region. Glycosylation status of the residue has long been known to impact the ability of IgGs to bind effector ligands such as FcγR and C1q, which, in turn, affects their ability to participate in Fc-mediated functions such as ADCC and complement-dependent cytotoxicity (CDC).[32–34] The glycosylation of MAbs can be altered to increase ADCC by producing them in a cell line engineered to express β(1,4)-N-acetylglucosaminyltransferase III (GnTIII), the enzyme required to add the bisecting GlcNAc residues.[33] Defucosylation of antibody Fc domains is also associated with enhanced ADCC, and in a recently completed multicenter phase II trial of a defucosylated anti-CC chemokine receptor 4 (CCR4), MAb was associated with meaningful antitumor activity, including complete responses and enhanced progression-free survival (PFS).[35]

UNCONJUGATED ANTIBODIES

The majority of monoclonal antibodies approved for clinical use display intrinsic antitumor effects that are mediated by one or more of the following mechanisms.

Cell-Mediated Cytotoxicity

As components of the immune system, effector cells such as natural killer (NK) cells and monocytes/macrophages represent natural lines of defense against oncologically transformed cells. These effector cells express Fcγ receptors (FcγR) on their cell surfaces, which interact with the Fc domain of IgG molecules. This family is comprised of three classes (type I, II, and III) that are further divided into subclasses (IIa/IIb and IIIa/IIIb).[36] Recognition of transformed cells by immune effector cells leads to cell-mediated killing through processes such as ADCC and phagocytosis, as shown in Figure 29.2, and can be mediated by FcγRI (CD64), a high affinity receptor capable of binding to monomeric IgG, or FcγRII (CD32) and FcγRIII (CD16), which are low affinity receptors that preferentially bind multimeric complexes of IgG. Signaling through type I, IIa, and IIIa receptors results in the activation of effector cells due to associated immunoreceptor tyrosine-based activation motifs (ITAM), whereas the engagement of type IIb receptors inhibits cell activation through associated immunoreceptor tyrosine-based inhibitory motifs (ITIM).[36] Clinical results support the idea that ADCC can play a role in the efficacy of antibody-based therapies. Naturally occurring polymorphisms in FcγRs alter their affinity for human IgG1 and have been linked to clinical response.[37,38] A polymorphism in the FCGR3A gene results in either a valine or phenylalanine at position 158 of FcγRIIIa. Human IgG1 binds more strongly to FcγRIIIa-158V than FcγRIIIa-158F, and likewise to NK cells from individuals that are either homozygous for 158F or heterozygous for this polymorphism.[39] The FcγRIIIa-158v was a predictor of early response and was associated with improved PFS.

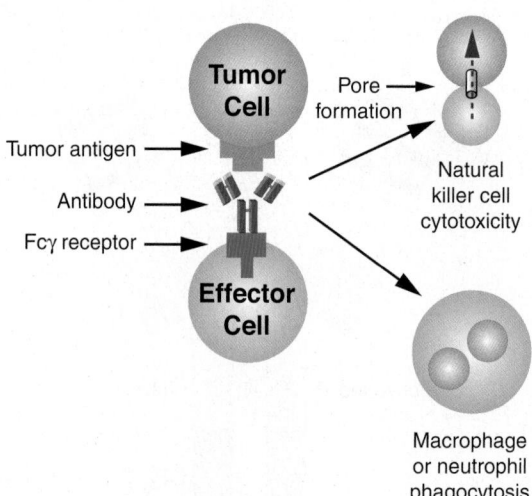

Figure 29.2 Antibody-dependent cellular cytotoxicity. The antibody engages the tumor antigen and the Fc domain binds to cellular Fc receptors to bridge effector and target cells. This bridging induces effector cell activation, resulting in natural killer cell cytotoxicity or phagocytosis by neutrophils, monocytes, or macrophages.

A second polymorphism, FcγRIIa-131H/R, did not predict early response but was an independent predictor of time to progression (TTP).[38] Taken together, these data suggest that modulating the affinity of MAbs for FcγRIIIa, FcγRIIa, or both may increase the efficacy of therapeutic MAbs.

Each class of FcγR exhibits a characteristic specificity for IgG subclasses.[40] Many groups have focused on modifying the Fc domain of IgGs to optimize the engagement of subclasses of FcγR and the induction of ADCC, based on the findings of Shields et al.,[29] who performed a series of mutagenesis experiments to map the residues required for IgG1-FcγR interaction. Antibodies such as ocrelizumab, a humanized version of rituximab, have increased binding to low affinity FcγRIIIa variants and are now in clinical trials.

An alternative to modifying the Fc region of MAbs is to create bispecific antibodies (bsAbs) that recognize both a tumor-associated antigen and a *trigger antigen* present on the surface of an immune effector cell.[43] Simultaneous engagement of both antigens can redirect the cytotoxic potential of the effector cell against the tumor.[41–43] Such antibodies are capable of eliciting effector function against tumor cell lines in vitro and in animal models. Two HER-2 directed bispecific antibodies, 2B1 and MDX-H210, have been tested in phase I clinical trials.[44,45]

Bispecific antibodies have a number of distinctive properties, including flexible choices of cytotoxic trigger molecules,[46] recruitment of effector function in the presence of excess IgG,[42] and custom tailoring of the affinity of the bsAb to match effector cell characteristics. These advantages have been facilitated by improved methods of bsAb production.[47] BiTE antibodies represent a novel class of bispecific, single-chain Fv antibodies.[48] Promising results have been seen in early phase clinical trials with at least two BiTE antibodies, one of which, blinatumomab, targets CD19/CD3.[49] Promising phase I results have also been reported in an interim analysis of an anti-EpCAM/anti-CD3 MT110 BiTE in the setting of advanced lung and gastrointestinal tumors.[50]

Complement-Dependent Cytotoxicity

In addition to cell-mediated killing (see previous), MAbs can recruit the complement cascade to kill cells via CDC. Although IgM is the most effective isotype for complement activation, it is not widely used in clinical oncology. Similar to ADCC, the human IgG subclass used to construct a therapeutic MAb dictates its ability to elicit CDC; IgG1 is extremely efficient at fixing complement, in contrast to IgG2 and IgG4.[51] Antibodies activate complement through the classical pathway, by engaging multiple C1q to trigger activation of a cascade of serum proteases, which kill the antibody-bound cells.[52,53] The anti-CD20 MAb rituximab has been found to depend in part on CDC for its in vivo efficacy.[54] Antibody engineering approaches have identified residues in the C_H2 domain of the Fc region that either suppress or enhance the ability of rituximab to bind C1q and activate CDC.[55] The ability to manipulate complement fixation through engineering approaches warrants in vivo testing to determine the impact of these changes on the efficacy and toxicity of MAbs.

ALTERING SIGNAL TRANSDUCTION

Growth factor receptors represent a well-established class of targets for therapeutic intervention. Normal signaling through these receptors often leads to mitogenic and prosurvival responses. Unregulated signaling, as seen in a number of common cancers due to receptor overexpression, promotes tumor cell growth and insensitivity to chemotherapeutic agents. Clinically relevant MAbs can modulate signaling through their target receptors to normalize cell growth rates and sensitize tumor cells to cytotoxic agents. The binding of cetuximab or panitumumab to the epidermal growth factor receptor (EGFR) physically blocks ligand binding[56] and prevents the receptor from assuming the extended conformation required for dimerization.[57] Pertuzumab binds to the dimerization domain of HER-2, thereby sterically inhibiting subsequent receptor heterodimerization with other ligand-bound family members.[58] Alternatively, signaling through growth factor receptors can be indirectly modified by MAbs that bind to activating ligands, as is seen with the anti–vascular endothelial growth factor (VEGF) MAb, bevacizumab.[59]

IMMUNOCONJUGATES

MAbs that are not capable of directly eliciting antitumor effects, either by altering signal transduction or directing immune system cells, can still be effective against tumors by delivering cytotoxic payloads. MAbs have been employed to deliver a wide variety of agents, including chemotherapy, toxins, radioisotopes, and cytokines (for review see Adams and Weiner[60]). In theory, the appropriate combination of toxic agents and MAbs could lead to a synergistic effect. For example, delivery of a therapeutic radioisotope by a MAb would be significantly enhanced if, by binding to its target antigen, the MAb also activated a signaling event that increased the target cell's sensitivity to ionizing radiation.

Catalytic toxins derived from plants catalytic toxins derived from plants (e.g., ricin) and microorganisms (e.g., Pseudomonas) represent two classes of cytotoxic agent that have been investigated for their utility in immunoconjugate strategies.[61] Although there are promising preclinical studies,[62] few successful clinical trials have been reported using this approach. In a phase I clinical trial in hairy cell leukemia patients who were resistant to cladribine, 11 of 16 patients exhibited complete remissions with minimal side effects with an anti-CD22 immunotoxin with a truncated form of *Pseudomonas exotoxin*.[63] Clinical trials with other immunotoxins have been associated with unacceptable neurotoxicity[64] and life-threatening vascular leak syndrome.[65]

Immunocytokine fusions have also been investigated as an approach to direct the patient's immune response to his or her own tumor.[66] A number of cytokines have been incorporated into antibody-based constructs, including interleukin-2 (IL-2),[67,68] interferon γ (IFN-γ),[69] tumor necrosis factor α (TFN-α),[69] VEGF,[70] and IL-12.[71]

Antibody–Drug Conjugates

The first ADC, gemtuzumab ozogamicin (Mylotarg), was approved by the FDA in 2000 for the treatment of patients with relapsed CD33-positive acute myeloid leukemia, but was voluntarily withdrawn from the US market by its manufacturer in 2010 after a confirmatory phase III trial (SWOG S0106) recommended, based on results of a planned interim analysis, that Mylotarg randomizations be terminated due to a lack of efficacy in the presence of enhanced toxicity.[72] Although two additional randomized trials[73,74] suggested that some patient populations may benefit from Mylotarg therapy, the drug remains off the market in the United States.

The majority of ADCs under development employ potent cytotoxic agents that block the polymerization of tubulin (e.g., auristatins or maytansines) or damage DNA (e.g., calicheamicins or pyrrolobenzodiazepines) by employing a variety of linkers and conjugation strategies.[75]

A variety of ADCs specific for a wide range of oncology targets are currently in clinical evaluation, with the majority of the more advanced agents being tested in the setting of diffuse malignancies.[76] The majority of these employ auristatins or maytansines as their payloads. Early observations suggest that cumulative, dose-related peripheral sensory neuropathy can result when auristatins are conjugated to an antibody via a cleavable linker, and dose-limiting thrombocytopenia can result when auristatins and maytansinoids are conjugated to the antibody via an uncleavable linker.[76,77]

Two ADCs are now approved for use in clinical practice. Ado-trastuzumab emtansine (T-DM1, Kadcyla), an ADC composed of the anti-HER2 MAb trastuzumab linked to DM1,[78] is now approved for the treatment of patients with refractory HER2/neu expressing breast cancers. The other, brentuximab vedotin (SGN-35, Adcetris), is an ADC consisting of the anti-CD30 chimeric MAb cAC10 that is linked to three to five molecules of the microtubule-disrupting agent Monomethyl auristatin E. At this point, this drug is approved for use in patients with recurrent systemic anaplastic large cell lymphoma. The clinical data associated with both of these ADCs will be discussed in subsequent sections of this chapter.

Antibodies also can be used to target liposome-encapsulated drugs[79] and other cytotoxic agents, such as antisense RNA[80] or radionuclides to tumors.

Radioimmunoconjugates

Two anti-CD20 radioimmunoconjugates have been FDA approved for radioimmunotherapy (RIT) of non-Hodgkin lymphoma (NHL). Ibritumomab (Zevalin) and tositumomab (Bexxar) are murine MAbs labeled with yttrium-90 (^{90}Y) and iodine-131 (^{131}I), respectively. Both are associated with impressive clinical efficacy.[81,82] Although these radioimmunoconjugates are effective therapeutics, cumbersome logistics surrounding their administration have significantly limited their use. Despite significant preclinical evidence supporting the use of RIT for solid malignancies, clinical results have not demonstrated consistent antitumor activity.[60]

ANTIBODIES APPROVED FOR USE IN SOLID TUMORS

Trastuzumab

Trastuzumab (Herceptin) is a humanized IgG1[83] that targets domain IV of the HER2/ErbB2 member of the EGFR/ErbB family of receptor tyrosine kinases. Gene amplification as judged by fluorescence in situ hybridization (FISH) with concomitant overexpression of HER2 protein measured by immunohistochemistry (IHC) is seen in approximately 25% of breast cancers.[84,85] HER2 amplification and overexpression is now recognized to also be a critical driver in a subset (7% to 34%) of gastric cancers.[86] Trastuzumab inhibits tumor cell growth by binding to HER2 and blocking the unregulated HER2 signaling that is associated with its high level overexpression.

Trastuzumab became the first FDA-approved monoclonal antibody for the treatment of solid tumors based on a series of studies carried out in the setting of HER2-positive metastatic breast cancer.[87,88] A subsequent phase III trial investigating trastuzumab in combination with cytotoxic chemotherapy demonstrated an improved response rate compared to chemotherapy alone, from 25.0% to 57.3% with a taxane regimen.[89]

Trastuzumab is also approved for use in the adjuvant setting based on an approximately 50% reduction in recurrence after 1 year in multiple phase III trials.[90–92] Myocardial dysfunction, seen with anthracycline therapy, was observed with increased frequency in patients receiving antibody alone[93] or with doxorubicin or epirubicin.

Recognition of HER2 as a driver in a subset of gastric cancers led to an open-label, randomized, phase III trial (ToGA) that investigated the addition of trastuzumab to standard of care chemotherapy[94] and showed increased median overall survival with higher levels of HER2 expression. A study by Gomez-Martin et al.[95] in 99 patients with metastatic gastric cancer being treated with first-line trastuzumab plus chemotherapy identified a mean HER2/CEP17 ratio of 4.7 to be an optimal cut-off to discriminate between trastuzumab-sensitive and refractory patients.

Pertuzumab

Pertuzumab (Perjeta) is a humanized IgG1 MAb that binds to domain II of HER2 and blocks ligand-dependent dimerization of HER2 with other members of the EGFR family.[96] Pertuzumab, in combination with trastuzumab and docetaxel, is approved for use as first-line therapy in HER2-positive metastatic breast cancer patients. Use of the combination is also approved for the treatment of HER2-positive, locally advanced, inflammatory, or high-risk early breast cancer (>2 cm node negative or node positive) in the neoadjuvant setting.

FDA-approval of pertuzumab was based on results of a phase III trial (CLEOPATRA) of 808 patients with locally recurrent, unresectable, or metastatic breast cancer randomized to receive trastuzumab plus docetaxel with or without the addition of pertuzumab. Inclusion of pertuzumab increased the independently assessed PFS by 6.1 months from 12.4 to 18.5 (hazard ratio [HR], 0.62 (95% confidence interval [CI], 0.51, 0.75), p <0.0001], with a trend toward improved overall survival[97] that reached statistical significance (p = 0.0008) after an additional year of follow-up.[98] The addition of pertuzumab did increase rates of grade 3 adverse events (AE), but it did not adversely affect cardiac function. Accelerated approval was granted for use of pertuzumab in combination with trastuzumab and docetaxel for the neoadjuvant treatment of high-risk early-stage breast cancer. This approval was based on results from a four-arm, open-label phase II study of 417 patients randomized to receive trastuzumab plus docetaxel, pertuzumab plus docetaxel, pertuzumab plus trastuzumab, or the triple combination. The triple combination improved the pathologic complete response (pCR) rate by 17.8% over the trastuzumab plus docetaxel arm (39.3% versus 21.5%) in the pertuzumab arm.[99] Follow-up studies to confirm a correlation between pCR and long-term clinical benefit are ongoing.

Cetuximab

Cetuximab (Erbitux) targets the EGFR. This chimeric IgG1 binds to domain III of the EGFR, with roughly a tenfold higher affinity than either EGF or transforming growth factor α (TGF-α) ligands and thereby inhibits ligand-induced activation of this tyrosine kinase receptor. Cetuximab may also function to downregulate EGFR-dependent signaling by stimulating EGFR internalization.[100] Cetuximab is approved for the treatment of colorectal cancer (CRC) and, more recently, for the treatment of squamous cell cancer of the head and neck (SCCHN).

The efficacy and safety of cetuximab against CRC was demonstrated alone and in combination with irinotecan in a phase II, multicenter, randomized, and controlled trial of 329 patients.[101] The combination of irinotecan plus cetuximab increased both the overall response and the median duration of response as compared to cetuximab alone. Additionally, patients with irinotecan refractory disease responded to treatment with the combination regimen. Recent studies in patients with colorectal cancers have indicated that patients with KRAS mutations in codon 12 or 13 should not receive anti-EGFR therapy.[101,102]

An international, multicenter, phase III trial comparing definitive radiotherapy to radiotherapy plus cetuximab in SCCHN demonstrated that EGFR blockade with radiotherapy significantly reduced the risk of locoregional failure by 32% and the risk of death by 26%. In advanced stage non–small-cell lung cancer (NSCLC) expressing EGFR, the combination of cetuximab and standard doublet chemotherapy (cisplatin plus vinorelbine) was studied in a prospective randomized phase III trial.[103] The addition of cetuximab was associated with a slight, but statistically significant, benefit in overall survival over chemotherapy alone (median overall survival 10.1 versus 11.3 months). A similar study using the carboplatin plus paclitaxel backbone in combination with cetuximab did not meet its primary endpoint of improved PFS, although cetuximab-treated patients exhibited higher objective response rates.[104] Therefore, the benefit of adding cetuximab to standard chemotherapy for patients with advanced NSCLC is unclear.

Panitumumab

Panitumumab (Vectibix) is a fully human IgG2 monoclonal antibody that binds to EGFR. Similar to cetuximab, panitumumab inhibits EGFR activation by blocking the binding of EGF and TGF-α. However, it does so by binding to EGFR with a higher affinity than cetuximab (5×10^{-11} M versus 1×10^{-10} M). As previously mentioned, the IgG2 class of antibodies does not induce activation of the immune system cell via the Fc-receptor mechanism, so panitumumab's primary action appears to be interference with EGFR–ligand interactions.

A phase III trial of 463 patients with metastatic colorectal cancer compared panitumumab plus best supportive care (BSC) to BSC alone.[105] A partial-response rate of 8% and a stable-disease rate of 28% were reported for the panitumumab arm compared with a 10% stable-disease rate in the best supportive care arm of the study. As with cetuximab, patients with metastatic colorectal cancers who have KRAS mutations in codons 12 or 13 are not routinely offered therapy with panitumumab.[106]

Bevacizumab

Bevacizumab (Avastin or rhuMAb VEGF) is a humanized monoclonal antibody targeting VEGF. VEGF is a critical determinant of tumor angiogenesis, a process that is a necessary component of tumor invasion, growth, and metastasis. VEGF expression by invasive tumors has been shown to correlate with vascularity and cellular proliferation and is prognostic for several human cancers.[107–109] Interestingly, the inhibition of VEGF signaling via bevacizumab treatment may normalize tumor vasculature, promoting a more effective delivery of chemotherapy agents.[110] Bevacizumab is approved for use as a first-line therapy for metastatic colorectal cancer and NSCLC when given in combination with appropriate cytotoxic chemotherapy regimens. Phase III clinical trials leading to the approval of bevacizumab for the treatment of colorectal cancer demonstrated improved response rates from 35% to 45% compared to fluorouracil (5-FU)–based chemotherapy alone. Enhanced response durations and improved patient survival were seen in patients treated with chemotherapy plus bevacizumab as compared to patients receiving chemotherapy alone.[111] A survival benefit was also seen in the setting of NSCLC. A randomized phase III trial (ECOG 4599) of paclitaxel and carboplatin with or without bevacizumab in patients with advanced nonsquamous NSCLC led to a significant improvement in median survival (12.5 months versus 10.2 months; p = 0.0075) for patients in the bevacizumab arm,[112] with significantly higher response rates. A higher incidence of bleeding was associated with bevacizumab (4.5% versus 0.7%). Five of 10 treatment-related deaths occurred as a result of hemoptysis, all in the bevacizumab arm.

A phase III trial randomized 722 patients with metastatic breast cancer with no prior chemotherapy for advanced disease to either paclitaxel or paclitaxel and bevacizumab.[113] PFS was significantly better in the paclitaxel plus bevacizumab arm (median, 11.8 versus 5.9 months; HR for progression, 0.60; p <0.001) with an increased response rate (36.9% versus 21.2%, p <0.001). Overall survival, however, was similar.

In contrast,[114] in a randomized phase III trial, capecitabine/bevacizumab increased response rates compared with capecitabine alone in 462 anthracycline and taxane pretreated metastatic breast cancer patients but did not meet its primary endpoint of improved PFS. Overall survival and time to deterioration in quality of life were comparable in both treatment groups.

Bevacizumab has not demonstrated activity in the adjuvant colorectal and breast cancer settings.[115,116] There was no improvement in overall survival between the two groups and the rate of invasive disease-free survival was also not significantly different between the treatment groups.

Bevacizumab is also approved for the management of recurrent glioblastomas based on results of phase II studies.[117]

Ado-Trastuzumab Emtansine

Ado-trastuzumab emtansine (T-DM1, Kadcyla) is an ADC composed of the anti-HER2 MAb trastuzumab linked to DM1, a highly potent derivative of maytansine, through a stable thioether linker.[78]

Based on two single-agent phase II trials of T-DM1[118,119] that demonstrated single-agent activity in the setting of metastatic breast cancer, two separate phase III studies were conducted. The 991 patient EMILIA trial demonstrated that T-DM1 significantly prolongs both PFS and overall survival as compared to a regimen of lapatinib plus capecitabine when used in the setting of metastatic breast cancer that had progressed after treatment with trastuzumab plus a taxane.[120] Grade 3 and worse AEs were lower in the T-DM1 arm (200, 40.8%) as compared to the lapatinib plus capecitabine arm (278, 57%). Results are still awaited from the ongoing MARIANNE trial that is assessing first-line efficacy and safety of T-DM1 alone and T-DM1 plus pertuzumab versus trastuzumab plus taxane (NCT01120184).

Denosumab

Denosumab (Xgeva) is a fully human IgG2 RANK ligand (RANKL) neutralizing antibody. Denosumab is FDA-approved for use in adults and skeletally mature adolescents who have either surgically unsalvageable giant cell tumors of the bone (GCTB) or where resection is anticipated to result in severe morbidity. Approval was based in part on two open-label, phase II trials examining subcutaneous administration of 120 mg q4 week with additional loading doses on days 8 and 15 of the first cycle.[121,122] Serious adverse events were seen in 9% of patients (n = 25). Of 187 patients, 47 (25%) exhibited partial objective responses based on modified Response Evaluation Criteria in Solid Tumors (RECIST) criteria.

Denosumab is also approved in for use in two supportive care settings based on three randomized, double-blind, placebo-controlled phase III trials evaluating its efficacy versus zoledronic acid[123–125] to reduce bone metastasis-related skeletal-related events (SRE). Based on data from two phase III trials, a second formulation and dosing schedule of denosumab is approved to increase bone mass in prostate cancer[126] and breast cancer[127] patients at high risk for bone fracture due to hormone-ablation therapies.

ANTIBODIES USED IN HEMATOLOGIC MALIGNANCIES

Rituximab

Rituximab (Rituxan) is a chimeric anti-CD20 monoclonal antibody that was the first MAb to be approved by the FDA for use in human malignancy.[128,129] Studies have shown that multiple doses can be safely administered, and in vitro studies have demonstrated multiple mechanisms by which anti-CD20 antibodies can lead to cell death.[130] Efficacy of rituximab monotherapy is well established.[131]

Rituximab has been tested in conjunction with chemotherapy based on supportive preclinical data.[132,133] The combination of rituximab with cyclophosphamide, doxorubicin, vincristine, and prednisolone (CHOP) resulted in a 95% overall response rate (55% complete response, 40% partial response) among 40 patients with low-grade or follicular B-cell non–Hodgkin lymphoma, with molecular complete remissions observed.[134] A long-term study of elderly patients with previously untreated diffuse large-cell lymphoma randomized to either CHOP chemotherapy plus rituximab (R-CHOP) or CHOP alone demonstrated a significant improvement in event-free survival, PFS, disease-free survival, and overall survival for the combination arm.[135] No significant differences in long-term toxicity were noted.

Low-grade B-cell lymphoma patients possessing the 158V/V polymorphism in FcγRIII experience superior response rates and outcomes when treated with rituximab.[37,38] These findings signify that antibody Fc domain::Fc receptor interactions underlie at least some of the clinical benefit of rituximab, and indicate a possible role for ADCC that depends on such interactions.

A combination of active agents (such as lenalidomide and thalidomide) that are also immune modulating may be additive with rituximab,[136] and perhaps synergize by increasing ADCC.[137] Cytokines such as interleukin-2 (IL-2), IL-12, or IL-15 and myeloid growth factors may also enhance therapeutic antibody activity as suggested by preclinical data demonstrating that IL-2 can promote NK cell proliferation and activation and can enhance rituximab activity[138] and clinical efficacy.[139,140] Myeloid growth factors, in combination with rituximab, may also activate ADCC.[141] Alternative approaches to induce effector cell activity by combining Toll-like receptors (TLR) agonists, such as CpG oligonucleotides, have been investigated.[142] Altering the balance of proapoptotic and antiapoptotic signals could generate more rituximab-induced cytotoxicity. BCL-2 downregulation by antisense oligonucleotides was found to enhance rituximab efficacy in preclinical testing.[143,144] However, small molecules that bind to the BH-3 domain common to many members of the BCL-2 family of proteins may be better therapeutic agents.[145–147]

Ofatumumab

The anti-CD20 ofatumumab[148] is a fully human antibody that binds an epitope on CD20 distinct from that bound by rituximab and is engineered for better complement activation, although it induces less ADCC. Ofatumumab has received regulatory approval for the treatment of patients with fludarabine-refractory chronic lymphocytic leukemia (CLL). In a recently reported, planned interim analysis that included 138 CLL patients with treatment-refractory disease or bulky (>5 cm) lymphadenopathy, treatment with ofatumumab led to an overall response rate (primary endpoint) of 47% in patients with bulky disease and 5% in patients refractory to both alemtuzumab and fludarabine.[149]

Additional humanized anti-CD20 antibodies (veltuzumab[150] and ocrelizumab) are under development.

Alemtuzumab

Alemtuzumab (Campath-1H) targets the CD52 glycopeptide, which is highly expressed on T and B lymphocytes. It has been tested as a therapeutic agent for CLL and promyelocytic leukemias, as well as other non–Hodgkin lymphomas.

Brentuximab Vedotin

Brentuximab vedotin (SGN-35, Adcetris) is an ADC consisting of the anti-CD30 chimeric MAb cAC10 that is linked to three to five molecules of the microtubule-disrupting agent Monomethyl auristatin E (MMAE). MMAE is a highly potent derivative of dolastatin. Linkage of MMAE to cAC10 occurs through a protease-cleavable linter.[151] Brentuximab vedotin is approved for treating systemic, chemotherapy-refractory anaplastic large-cell lymphomas (sALCL). It is also approved to treat patients with Hodgkin lymphoma who have progressed after an autologous stem cell transplant (ASCT). Patients ineligible for ASCT must have failed two prior multidrug chemotherapy regimens.

Brentuximab vedotin received accelerated approval in 2011 based in part on the results of two phase II trials. In a multicenter trial conducted by Pro et al.,[152] 58 patients with relapsed or refractory sALCL received brentuximab vedotin (1.8 mg per kilogram per week), and 86% of patients achieved objective response. Complete responses occurred in 57% of patients, with a median duration of 13.2 months. An additional 17 patients (29%) had partial responses. Median overall response was 12.6 months. Most common grade 3 and 4 adverse events (AE) were neutropenia (21%), thrombocytopenia (14%), and peripheral sensory neuropathy (12%). A similar trial, in Hodgkin lymphoma, was reported by Younes et al.[153] Patients (n = 102) that had failed ASCT received brentuximab vedotin on the same schedule as listed previously and were assessed for the objective response rate. In this setting, 75% of patients had objective responses, with 34% being complete remissions. The median duration of complete responses was 20.5 months, and 31 patients were progression free after a median follow-up of 1.5 years. Phase III trials to assess the known risk of neuropathy (AETHERA) and to confirm overall clinical benefit seen in the phase II trials (ECHELON-2, or ClinicalTrials.gov Identifier NCT01712490) are ongoing.

CONCLUSION

In the 35 years since Kohler and Milstein first developed the hybridoma technology that enabled antibody-based therapeutics, the field has made remarkable progress. Numerous antibody-based molecules are currently in clinical trials and many more are in development. Multiple therapeutic antibodies have a proven clinical benefit and have been licensed by the FDA. The thoughtful application of advances in cancer biology and antibody engineering suggest that this progress will continue.

SELECTED REFERENCES

The full reference list can be accessed at lwwhealthlibrary.com/oncology.

4. Reichert JM, Dhimolea E. The future of antibodies as cancer drugs. *Drug Discov Today* 2012;17:954–963.
5. Kohler G, Milstein C. Continuous cultures of fused cells secreting antibody of predefined specificity. *Nature* 1975;256:495–497.
10. Komissarov AA, Calcutt MJ, Marchbank MT, et al. Equilibrium binding studies of recombinant anti-single-stranded DNA Fab. Role of heavy chain complementarity-determining regions. *J Biol Chem* 1996;271:12241–12246.
11. Ghetie V, Popov S, Borvak J, et al. Increasing the serum persistence of an IgG fragment by random mutagenesis. *Nat Biotechnol* 1997;15:637–640.
19. Jain RK. Physiological barriers to delivery of monoclonal antibodies and other macromolecules in tumors. *Cancer Res* 1990;50:814s–819s.
29. Shields RL, Namenuk AK, Hong K, et al. High resolution mapping of the binding site on human IgG1 for Fc gamma RI, Fc gamma RII, Fc gamma RIII, and FcRn and design of IgG1 variants with improved binding to the Fc gamma R. *J Biol Chem* 2001;276:6591–6604.
31. McDonagh CF, Huhalov A, Harms BD, et al. Antitumor activity of a novel bispecific antibody that targets the ErbB2/ErbB3 oncogenic unit and inhibits heregulin-induced activation of ErbB3. *Mol Cancer Ther* 2012;11:582–593.

38. Weng WK, Levy R. Two immunoglobulin G fragment C receptor polymorphisms independently predict response to rituximab in patients with follicular lymphoma. *J Clin Oncol* 2003;21:3940–3947.
48. Mack M, Riethmuller G, Kufer P. A small bispecific antibody construct expressed as a functional single-chain molecule with high tumor cell cytotoxicity. *Proc Natl Acad Sci U S A* 1995;92:7021–7025.
49. Bargou R, Leo E, Zugmaier G, et al. Tumor regression in cancer patients by very low doses of a T cell-engaging antibody. *Science* 2008;321:974–977.
54. Di Gaetano N, Cittera E, Nota R, et al. Complement activation determines the therapeutic activity of rituximab in vivo. *J Immunol* 2003;171:1581–1587.
57. Li S, Schmitz KR, Jeffrey PD, et al. Structural basis for inhibition of the epidermal growth factor receptor by cetuximab. *Cancer Cell* 2005;7:301–311.
59. Presta LG, Chen H, O'Connor SJ, et al. Humanization of an anti-vascular endothelial growth factor monoclonal antibody for the therapy of solid tumors and other disorders. *Cancer Res* 1997;57:4593–4599.
63. Kreitman RJ, Wilson WH, Bergeron K, et al. Efficacy of the anti-CD22 recombinant immunotoxin BL22 in chemotherapy-resistant hairy-cell leukemia. *N Engl J Med* 2001;345:241–247.
66. Lode HN, Xiang R, Becker JC, et al. Immunocytokines: a promising approach to cancer immunotherapy. *Pharmacol Ther* 1998;80:277–292.

74. Castaigne S, Pautas C, Terre C, et al. Effect of gemtuzumab ozogamicin on survival of adult patients with de-novo acute myeloid leukaemia (ALFA-0701): a randomised, open-label, phase 3 study. *Lancet* 2012;379:1508–1516.

76. Lambert JM. Drug-conjugated antibodies for the treatment of cancer. *Br J Clin Pharmacol* 2013;76:248–262.

82. Witzig TE, White CA, Wiseman GA, et al. Phase I/II trial of IDEC-Y2B8 radioimmunotherapy for treatment of relapsed or refractory CD20(+) B-cell non-Hodgkin's lymphoma. *J Clin Oncol* 1999;17:3793–3803.

83. Carter P, Presta L, Gorman CM, et al. Humanization of an anti-p185HER2 antibody for human cancer therapy. *Proc Natl Acad Sci U S A* 1992;89:4285–4289.

90. Piccart-Gebhart MJ, Procter M, Leyland-Jones B, et al. Trastuzumab after adjuvant chemotherapy in HER2-positive breast cancer. *N Engl J Med* 2005;353:1659–1672.

91. Romond EH, Perez EA, Bryant J, et al. Trastuzumab plus adjuvant chemotherapy for operable HER2-positive breast cancer. *N Engl J Med* 2005;353:1673–1684.

92. Smith I, Procter M, Gelber RD, et al. 2-year follow-up of trastuzumab after adjuvant chemotherapy in HER2-positive breast cancer: a randomised controlled trial. *Lancet* 2007;369:29–36.

94. Bang YJ, Van Cutsem E, Feyereislova A, et al. Trastuzumab in combination with chemotherapy versus chemotherapy alone for treatment of HER2-positive advanced gastric or gastro-oesophageal junction cancer (ToGA): a phase 3, open-label, randomised controlled trial. *Lancet* 2010;376:687–697.

97. Baselga J, Cortes J, Kim SB, et al. Pertuzumab plus trastuzumab plus docetaxel for metastatic breast cancer. *N Engl J Med* 2012;366:109–119.

98. Swain SM, Kim SB, Cortes J, et al. Pertuzumab, trastuzumab, and docetaxel for HER2-positive metastatic breast cancer (CLEOPATRA study): overall survival results from a randomised, double-blind, placebo-controlled, phase 3 study. *Lancet Oncol* 2013;14:461–471.

101. Van Cutsem ELI, D'haens G. KRAS status and efficacy in the first-line treatment of patients with metastatic colorectal cancer (metastatic CRC) treated with FOLFIRI with or without cetuximab: The CRYSTAL experience. Abstract 2. *J Clin Oncol* 2008;26:5s.

103. Pirker R, Pereira JR, Szczesna A, et al. Cetuximab plus chemotherapy in patients with advanced non-small-cell lung cancer (FLEX): an open-label randomised phase III trial. *Lancet* 2009;373:1525–1531.

105. Gibson TB, Ranganathan A, Grothey A. Randomized phase III trial of panitumumab, a fully human anti-epidermal growth factor receptor monoclonal antibody, in metastatic colorectal cancer. *Clin Colorectal Cancer* 2006;6:29–31.

106. Amado RG, Wolf M, Peeters M, et al. Wild-type KRAS is required for panitumumab efficacy in patients with metastatic colorectal cancer. *J Clin Oncol* 2008;26:1626–1634.

111. Hurwitz H, Fehrenbacher L, Novotny W, et al. Bevacizumab plus irinotecan, fluorouracil, and leucovorin for metastatic colorectal cancer. *N Engl J Med* 2004;350:2335–2342.

112. Sandler A, Gray R, Perry MC, et al. Paclitaxel-carboplatin alone or with bevacizumab for non-small-cell lung cancer. *N Engl J Med* 2006;355:2542–2550.

113. Miller K, Wang M, Gralow J, et al. Paclitaxel plus bevacizumab versus paclitaxel alone for metastatic breast cancer. *N Engl J Med* 2007;357:2666.

120. Verma S, Miles D, Gianni L, et al. Trastuzumab emtansine for HER2-positive advanced breast cancer. *N Engl J Med* 2012;367:1783–1791.

122. Chawla S, Henshaw R, Seeger L, et al. Safety and efficacy of denosumab for adults and skeletally mature adolescents with giant cell tumour of bone: interim analysis of an open-label, parallel-group, phase 2 study. *Lancet Oncol* 2013;14:901–908.

128. Maloney D, Grillo-López A, Bodkin D, et al. IDEC-C2B8: results of a phase I multiple-dose trial in patients with relapsed non-Hodgkin's lymphoma. *J Clin Oncol* 1997;15:3266–3274.

131. Coiffier B, Haioun C, Ketterer N, et al. Rituximab (anti-CD20 monoclonal antibody) for the treatment of patients with relapsing or refractory aggressive lymphoma: a multicenter phase II study. *Blood* 1998;92:1927–1932.

135. Feugier P, Van Hoof A, Sebban C, et al. Long-term results of the R-CHOP study in the treatment of elderly patients with diffuse large B-cell lymphoma: a study by the Groupe d'Etude des Lymphomes de l'Adulte. *J Clin Oncol* 2005;23:4117–4126.

140. Khan KD, Emmanouilides C, Benson DM Jr., et al. A phase 2 study of rituximab in combination with recombinant interleukin-2 for rituximab-refractory indolent non-Hodgkin's lymphoma. *Clin Cancer Res* 2006;12:7046–7053.

149. Wierda WG, Kipps TJ, Mayer J, et al. Ofatumumab as single-agent CD20 immunotherapy in fludarabine-refractory chronic lymphocytic leukemia. *J Clin Oncol* 2010;28:1749–1755.

152. Pro B, Advani R, Brice P, et al. Brentuximab vedotin (SGN-35) in patients with relapsed or refractory systemic anaplastic large-cell lymphoma: results of a phase II study. *J Clin Oncol* 2012;30:2190–2196.

153. Younes A, Gopal AK, Smith SE, et al. Results of a pivotal phase II study of brentuximab vedotin for patients with relapsed or refractory Hodgkin's lymphoma. *J Clin Oncol* 2012;30:2183–2189.

CANCER THERAPEUTICS

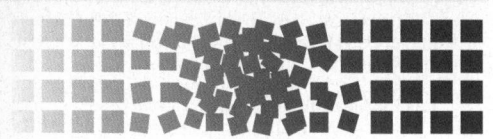

Antonio Tito Fojo and Susan E. Bates

INTRODUCTION

Approaches to response assessments have become increasingly important over the past decade as the drug development pipeline has steadily increased in volume. In 2012, an estimated 981 medicines were in development for cancer, and the number is certainly higher today.[1] The challenge is, first, how to measure the activity of an agent in the research setting, and, second, how to measure activity in the standard of care setting.

The "modern era" of drug development began in 1976 when 16 experienced oncologists treating lymphoma gathered to decide what would be considered a reliable measure of response to a therapy.[2] Each oncologist measured 12 *simulated tumor masses* employing *usual clinical methods* (i.e., calipers or rulers). A principal goal was to identify the amount of shrinkage that *could not* be ascribed to operator error and that *would not* be found if a *placebo* was administered. Moertel and Hanley recommended that *to avoid error, a 50% reduction in the product of perpendicular diameters be employed as the criterion for efficacy*.[2] It was from this beginning that our current methodologies of response assessment evolved. The important point to note is that the decision to use a 50% reduction in the product of perpendicular diameters as a measure of efficacy was made so as to reduce error and *not because it represented a value that conferred clinical benefit*.

From Calipers and Rulers in Lymphoma to the Bidimensional World Health Organization Criteria

In 1981, five years after the Moertel and Hanley report,[2] a World Health Organization (WHO) initiative developed standardized approaches for the "reporting of response, recurrence and disease-free interval."[3] The WHO criteria, like Moertel and Hanley, recommended that malignant disease be measured in two dimensions. Complete response (CR) was defined as the disappearance of all known disease, and a partial response (PR) was scored if there occurred a "50% decrease in the sum of the products of the perpendicular diameters of the multiple lesions." Thus, the 50% reduction initially chosen as an operationally optimal value became institutionalized as the threshold for declaring efficacy in the majority of cancers. This measure of efficacy was perpetuated in 2000 with the now widely used Response Evaluation Criteria in Solid Tumors (RECIST), but shifting to one dimension.[4] The authors noted "the definition of a partial response, in particular, is an arbitrary convention—there is no inherent meaning for an individual patient of a 50% decrease in overall tumor load." Nevertheless, the threshold chosen—a 30% reduction in one dimension—was comparable in volume to the 50% decrease in the sum of the products of the perpendicular diameters and thus perpetuated the 1976 standard. In spite of its arbitrary origins, the 50% reduction has held up over time. But the major impact of the WHO criteria was that it marked the beginning of a common language of response. These criteria have been revisited and refined over time, as technology

and medicine advanced. Table 30.1 compares the WHO criteria with those of RECIST 1.0 and RECIST 1.1 and three modifications of RECIST, whereas Figure 30.1 provides a visual presentation of the RECIST threshold required to qualify as response or progression.[3-9]

ASSESSING RESPONSE

RECIST 1.1

The RECIST 1.0 guidelines were updated as RECIST 1.1 in 2009, with a number of differences between the two response criteria highlighted. RECIST 1.1 preserves the same categories of response found in RECIST 1.0:

- Complete response: Complete disappearance of all disease
- Partial response: ≥30% reduction in the sum of the longest diameter of target lesions
- Stable disease: Change not meeting criteria for response or progression
- Progression: ≥20% increase in the sum of the longest diameter of target lesions

However, a decade of experience with RECIST identified several problems with the criteria, some of which could be corrected. In RECIST 1.0, minimum size varied between 1 and 2 cm depending on technique; in RECIST 1.1, a 1-cm lesion is the minimum measurable. In RECIST 1.0, 10 lesions were to be measured, 5 per organ; RECIST 1.1 reduced that to 5 lesions, 2 per organ. Response criteria in RECIST 1.0 did not address lymph nodes; in RECIST 1.1, lymph nodes decreasing to <1 cm in their short axis could constitute a complete response. Disease progression in nontarget disease was further defined to indicate that in addition to a 20% increase in target lesions over the smallest sum on study, there must be an absolute increase of 5 mm, and that an increase of a single nontarget lesion should not trump an overall disease status assessment based on target lesions.

Variations of the RECIST Criteria

The RECIST criteria have been widely used for standardizing the reporting of clinical trial results and have improved reproducibility. However, the increasing precision and codification of RECIST has led to recognition of its limitations. For example, there are unique challenges in central nervous system (CNS) disease, relating response to tumor size measurements based on contrast enhancement. Pseudoprogression refers to an increase in contrast enhancement due to a transient increase in vascular permeability after irradiation, whereas pseudoresponse is a decrease in contrast enhancement that may occur due to a reduction in vascular permeability following corticosteroids or an antiangiogenic agent such as bevacizumab.[10-12] The McDonald criteria, traditionally used in determining glioma response based

TABLE 30.1

Key Features of Response Criteria

	WHO[3]	RECIST 1.0[4]	RECIST 1.1[5]	CNS RANO Criteria[7]	RECIST Mesothelioma[8]	RECIST Immunotherapy[9]
Dimension	Uni- and bidimensional	Unidimensional	Unidimensional	Bidimensional	Unidimensional	Bidimensional
Measurable Lesion	Not defined	Longest diameter, ≥20 mm with most modalities; ≥10 mm with spiral CT	Longest diameter ≥10 mm on CT or on skin if using calipers; ≥20 mm if using CXR	Two perpendicular diameters of contrast enhancing lesions ≥10 mm	Tumor thickness perpendicular to chest wall or mediastinum, measured in two positions at three levels on transverse cuts of CT scan	Longest perpendicular diameters
Measurable Lymph Nodes	Not defined	Not defined	≥15 mm short axis	—	—	—
Disease Burden to be Assessed at Baseline	All (not specified)	Measurable target lesions up to 10 total (5 per organ); other lesions nontarget	Measurable target lesions up to 5 total (2 per organ); other lesions nontarget	Two to five lesions in patients with several lesions	Pleural disease in perpendicular diameter; nodal, subcutaneous, and other bidimensional lesions measured unidimensionally as per the RECIST criteria	5 lesions per organ, up to 10 visceral lesions and five cutaneous lesions
Sum	*Sum of the products* of bidimensional diameters or sum of linear unidimensional diameters	Sum of longest diameters of all measurable lesions	Sum of the longest diameters of target lesions with only exception use of short axis for lymph nodes	Sum of the products of perpendicular diameters of all measurable enhancing target lesions	Sum of the six measurements defines a pleural unidimensional measure	SPD with new lesions incorporated into baseline; tumor burden = $SPD_{index\ lesions}$ + $SPD_{new\ lesions}$
Complete Response	Disappearance all known disease	Disappearance all known disease	Disappearance all known disease; lymph nodes <10 mm	—	Disappearance all target lesions with no evidence of tumor elsewhere	Disappearance all lesions in two consecutive observations
Partial Response	≥50% decrease	≥30% decrease; all other no evidence of progression	≥30% decrease; all other disease, no evidence of progression	≥50% reduction; stable or decreased steroid use compared to baseline	≥30% reduction in total tumor measurement	≥50% decrease compared with baseline in two observations
Response Confirmation?	≥4 weeks apart	≥4 weeks apart	≥4 weeks apart (if response primary end point); no, if secondary endpoint	≥4 weeks apart	Repeat on two occasions ≥4 weeks apart	≥4 weeks apart

(continued)

CANCER THERAPEUTICS

TABLE 30.1

Key Features of Response Criteria *(continued)*

	WHO[3]	RECIST 1.0[4]	RECIST 1.1[5]	CNS RANO Criteria[7]	RECIST Mesothelioma[8]	RECIST Immunotherapy[9]
Progressive Disease	≥25% increase in size of one or more measurable lesions or appearance of new lesions	≥20% increase, taking as reference smallest sum in study; or appearance of new lesions	≥20% increase, with absolute increase ≥5 mm, taking as reference smallest sum in study; or appearance of new lesions	≥25%, or any new lesions	≥20% increase in the total tumor measurement over the nadir measurement, or the appearance of one or more new lesions	≥25% increase compared with nadir confirmed ≥4 weeks apart; up to five new lesions (≥5 × 5 mm) per organ incorporated into tumor burden
	Nonmeasurable disease: Estimated increase of ≥25%	Nonmeasurable disease: unequivocal progression	Nonmeasurable disease: unequivocal progression	Nonmeasurable disease: >5 mm increase in maximal diameter; ≥25% increase in SPD; or significant increase in nonenhancing lesions on same or lower dose of corticosteroids	—	New, nonmeasurable lesions (i.e., <5 × 5 mm) do not define progression
Stable Disease	Stable disease or non-PR and non-PD ≥4 weeks	Non-PR, non-PD; minimum time defined by protocol	Non-PR, non-PD; minimum time defined by protocol	—	Non-PR, non-PD	Non-irPR, non-irPD

CXR, Chest X-ray; SPD, sum of products of two largest perpendicular diameters; PD, progressive disease; irPR, immune-related partial response; irPD, immune-related progressive disease.

on two-dimensional measurements, have been recently updated as part of the Response Assessment in Neuro-Oncology (RANO) response criteria and extended to include a response assessment for metastatic CNS disease.[7,13]

Other examples where RECIST is limited include mesothelioma, gastrointestinal stromal tumors (GIST), hepatocellular cancers, among others. The pleural disease of mesothelioma increases in depth while following the pleural surface. GIST tumors may remain unchanged in size after treatment, whereas the center of the tumor mass undergoes necrosis, and progression may occur in the remaining rim.[14] Hepatocellular cancers are often treated with local–regional therapy in which the goal is tumor necrosis and treatment failure occurs in surviving viable tumor.[15] Different

strategies have emerged to quantify these diseases, including modifications of RECIST, quantifying positron-emission tomography (PET) imaging, and biomarker criteria, as will be discussed. The RECIST adaptation for mesothelioma, growing along the pleural surface, is to measure the diameter perpendicular to the chest wall or mediastinum, and to measure at three levels.[8] The adaptation for hepatocellular cancer following local therapy is measurement of the longest diameter of the tumor that shows enhancement on the arterial phase of the scan, bypassing the dense, homogeneous Lipiodol-containing necrotic area.[15]

Investigators have also observed that following immunotherapy, tumor lesions may increase in size due to the increased infiltration of T cells, even meeting criteria for RECIST-defined progressive

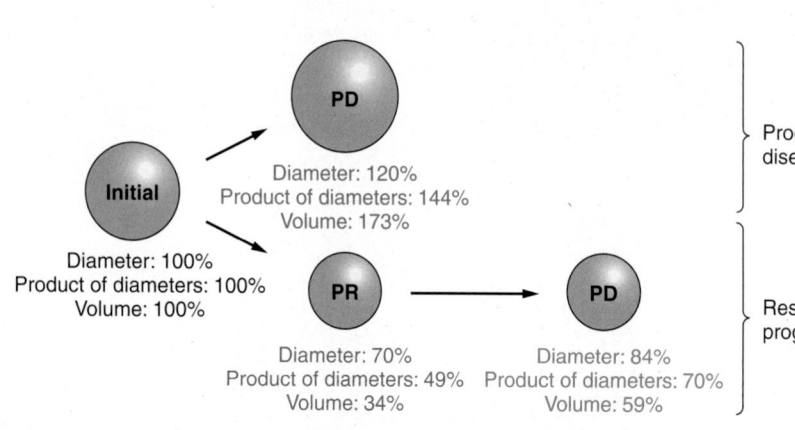

Figure 30.1 RECIST thresholds in three parameters: diameter, product of diameters, and volume. In the figure, spheres meeting RECIST criteria for progressive disease (PD) and for PR are shown with the percentage relative to the baseline calculated for each parameter. To meet the threshold for PD, the longest diameter must increase to 120%, which is equivalent to a 144% increase in the product of the perpendicular diameters and a 173% increase in the volume of a sphere. Although PR definitions are almost identical to those employed with WHO, RECIST has a higher threshold to meet PD.[6]

disease (PD). Previously radiographically undetectable lesions may appear. Departing from conventional RECIST, which defines any new lesion as PD, the immune response criteria allow the appearance of new lesions, adding them to the total tumor burden.[9] An increase in total tumor burden of >25% relative to baseline or nadir is required to define PD.

International Working Group Criteria for Lymphoma

Revised guidelines for lymphoma assessment were promulgated by the International Working Group (IWG) in 2007.[16] These guidelines incorporated 18F-fluorodeoxyglucose (FDG)-PET assessments in metabolically active lymphomas.[16] Although a CR requires the complete disappearance of detectable disease, a post-treatment residual mass is permitted if it is negative on FDG-PET and was positive at baseline. For lymphomas that are not consistently FDG avid, or if FDG avidity is unknown, a CR requires that nodes >1.5 cm before therapy regress to <1.5 cm, and nodes that were 1.1 to 1.5 cm in long axis and >1.0 cm in the short axis shrink to ≤1.0 cm in short axis. The definition of PR resembles the WHO criteria, in that a ≥50% decrease in the sum of the product of the diameters in up to six nodal masses or in hepatic or splenic nodules must be documented. Although RECIST 1.1 now includes lymph node assessment, the IWG criteria remain the assessment method typically used in lymphoma clinical trials.

ALTERNATE RESPONSE CRITERIA

The previous examples represent attempts to more accurately measure tumor burden. Evolving imaging technology enabling volumetric measurements of tumor masses may eventually resolve some of these problems, but effective therapeutic agents are required to enable validation and utilization of response assessment tools. The lack of an agent that can mediate substantial tumor shrinkage underlies the concept of *clinical benefit response* (CBR) as an endpoint in pancreatic cancer. Clinical benefit was defined as a combination of improvement in pain, performance status, and weight; the assessment of CBR supported the U.S. Food and Drug Administration (FDA) approval of gemcitabine in pancreatic cancer.[17,18] Better therapies for pancreatic cancer that result in tumor shrinkage or eradication should include and then eclipse clinical benefit.

Response criteria may be specific to a particular disease or clinical setting. Some diseases by their nature require specific strategies for response assessment.

Severity-Weighted Assessment Tool Score in Cutaneous T-Cell Lymphoma

Cutaneous T-cell lymphoma (CTCL) is a disease that can involve the entire epidermis, or comprise individual skin lesions varying widely in severity rather than size. The severity-weighted assessment tool (SWAT) assigns a factor for skin lesion severity—patch, plaque, or tumor—multiplies this factor by the percent of skin involved with each lesion type and then adds these together. This complex system formed the basis of the FDA approval of vorinostat for CTCL.[19]

Pathologic Complete Response in Breast Cancer

One unique response endpoint is the assessment of breast cancer treated in the neoadjuvant setting. The purpose of neoadjuvant therapy is to improve survival, render locally advanced cancer amenable to surgery, or to aid in breast conservation. In that setting, the absence of cancer cells in resected breast tissue has been used to define a pathologic complete response (pCR). The rate of pCR has been proposed as a surrogate endpoint for event-free survival (EFS) or overall survival (OS) to support approval of new agents or combinations of agents tested in clinical trials.[20] In a pooled analysis of 11,955 patients enrolled on 12 neoadjuvant trials, individual patients with pCR had improved EFS and OS.[21] However, at the trial level, pCR rates did not correlate with EFS or OS, a problem likely due to heterogeneity of breast cancer subtypes among the trials. Despite this, pCR rates were recently used to support the approval of pertuzumab and trastuzumab in the neoadjuvant setting.[21,22]

Computed Tomography-Based Tumor Density

One approach, often called the Choi criteria, advocates assessing tumor response in GIST, renal cell cancer, or hepatocellular cancer based on density on computed tomography (CT) scans (Table 30.2). This variation was prompted by the evident response to treatment with imatinib but with minimal tumor shrinkage.[23] The Choi criteria are still considered exploratory in GIST,[24,25] and it is too soon to know of benefits in other histologies.[26,27] Further study should determine its utility, although it will likely be confined to specific tumor types with specific drugs.

FDG-PET

Although widely used in clinical practice, FDG-PET has become part of standardized response criteria for clinical trials only in lymphoma (see Table 30.2). In solid tumors, FDG-PET can aid in the detection of new or recurrent sites of disease, and can be used as an adjunct during assessments for disease progression when using RECIST criteria.[5] Although FDG uptake is a powerful diagnostic tool and its uptake reflects a tumor's metabolic activity, it has some limitations: Some tumors have variable FDG avidity; differences can occur due to variations in patient activity, carbohydrate intake, blood glucose, and timing; and there are several benign sources of uptake, including inflammatory and postsurgical sites. Multiple methods of quantitating FDG-PET and assessing response have been proposed, but to date there is no consensus, particularly regarding the definition of a metabolic response.[28–33]

The two most widely used response criteria—the European Organisation for the Research and Treatment of Cancer (EORTC) criteria and PET Response Criteria in Solid Tumors (PERCIST) (see Table 30.2)—have been evaluated in specific disease types, but unifying FDG-PET response criteria remains a challenge in anticancer drug development.[28,30] We would note that, as shown in Figure 30.1, a 30% reduction in the diameter of a sphere—the magnitude of change required to score a response according to RECIST—represents a 65% decrease in volume. If an standardized uptake value (SUV) decrease is directly equated to a volume decrease, a reduction of 25% translates to a 10% reduction in diameter, a value that likely constitutes an insufficient response.

Serum Biomarkers of Response

The ideal response assessment method is an assay that could measure tumor quantity by a simple blood test (see Table 30.2). Circulating protein biomarkers have been identified and studied for several decades for screening, early detection of recurrent disease, determining prognosis, selecting therapy, and monitoring response to therapy. These serum tumor markers are to be distinguished from the assays determining the presence of an overexpressed or mutated molecular target. With the successful launch of therapies against such molecular targets, there has been increased interest in the assays needed to select therapy for individual patients (predictive biomarkers). The analytical and clinical validation of such assays, along with determination of their clinical utility, has created a new regulatory paradigm known as *companion diagnostics*.[34,35] This investment in the development of predictive markers for companion diagnostics has reduced the focus on protein biomarkers of treatment response relative to older literature.

As a result, there are few clinically validated biomarkers of response.[36] In addition to issues regarding sensitivity and specificity, their use and development has also been hindered by the often

CANCER THERAPEUTICS

TABLE 30.2

Alternate Response Criteria: Biomarkers

Criterion	Baseline	Response	Progression
CA-125 in ovarian cancer (GCIG criteria)[43]	CA 125 >2× ULN	CA 125 decline ≥50% confirmed at 28 days	2× nadir OR 2× ULN if normalized on therapy on two occasions 1 wk apart
PSA in prostate cancer (PSA WG1)[45,a]	PSA ≥5 ng/mL and documentation of two consecutive increases in PSA 1 wk apart	PSA decline of 50% from baseline (measured twice 3–4 wks apart)	After decrease from baseline, a 50% increase AND an increase ≥5 ng/mL, or back to baseline, whichever is lower
PSA in prostate cancer (PCWG2)[46,a]	PSA ≥2.0 ng/mL; estimate pretreatment PSA-DT: Need ≥3 values ≥4 wks apart	Report percent change from baseline (rise or fall) at 12 weeks, and separately, the maximal change (rise or fall) at any time using a waterfall plot	PSA increase ≥25% and absolute increase by ≥2 ng/mL above the nadir, confirmed by a second value ≥3 wks later (i.e., confirmed rising trend) OR PSA increase ≥25% and ≥2 ng/mL above baseline >12 wks
hCG and AFP in testicular cancer[50–51]		Decrease consistent with marker half-life: 2–3 d for hCG, 5–7 d for AFP	Rising levels usually indicate need to change therapy
Choi Criteria for CT Imaging			
Choi criteria[24–27]		≥10% decrease in tumor size OR ≥15% reduction in tumor density	An increase in tumor size ≥10% and does not meet criteria of PR by tumor attenuation on CT
FDG-PET Criteria			
EORTC criteria[29–31]	ROI should be drawn, SUV calculated	**CMR:** Complete resolution of uptake **PMR:** SUV reduction ≥25% **SMD:** SUV increase <25% and decrease <15%	**PMD:** SUV increase >25% in regions defined on baseline, or appearance of new FDG-avid lesions
PERCIST criteria[29]	SUL peak >1.5× normal liver	**CMR:** Complete resolution of uptake **PMR:** SUL reduction ≥30%	**PMD:** SUL increase >30% in regions defined on baseline, or appearance of new FDG avid lesions

[a] Guidelines for PSA assessment have evolved from those of the PSAWG1, where responses were dichotomized based on the percent decline, to those in the PCWG2 where PSA response is considered a continuous variable. Recently, emphasis has shifted to assessing PSA doubling time.
CA-125, cancer antigen 125; GCIG, Gynecologic Cancer InterGroup; ULN, upper limit of normal; PSA, prostate-specific antigen; PSAWG1, PSA Working Group 1; PCWG2, Prostate Cancer Working Group 2; PSA-DT, PSA-doubling time; hCG, human chorionic gonatropin; AFP, alpha-fetoprotein; EORTC, European Organisation for the Research and Treatment of Cancer; ROI, regions of interest; SUV, standardized uptake value; CMR, complete metabolic response; PMR, partial metabolic response; SMD, stable metabolic disease; PMD, progressive metabolic disease; PERCIST, PET response criteria in solid tumors; SUL, SUV normalized to lean body mass.

limited efficacy of therapies; response biomarkers are of little value without highly effective primary and salvage therapies. For example, a recent clinical trial indicates that in *asymptomatic patients* with ovarian cancer whose only evidence of disease progression is an isolated rising CA-125, nothing is gained by instituting treatment before there is other evidence of progression.[37,38]

■ **Cancer Antigen 125 (CA-125):** Despite recognized limitations, CA-125 is widely used. For example, the Gynecologic Cancer InterGroup (GCIG) criteria have evolved to help determine whether a patient's tumor has responded to therapy.[39–41] Response is defined as a 50% decline from an elevated baseline value, whereas progression is defined as a doubling over the nadir or the upper limit of normal.[42] In clinical practice, CA-125 levels are followed as part of standard management, but making clinical decisions on marker changes alone is not recommended.[43]

■ **Prostate-Specific Antigen (PSA):** Similar issues have confronted investigators caring for patients with prostate cancer. The PSA Working Group 1 (PCWG1) guidelines, first published in

1999, established PSA criteria, particularly for use in patients with disease that was difficult to quantify.[44] There followed a second working group (PCWG2) that recommended plotting the percent PSA change for each patient in a waterfall plot so as to avoid creating a dichotomous variable from the changes in PSA.[45] PCWG2 also recommended keeping patients on trial until evidence of a change in clinical status—either symptomatic or radiographic progression. The latter addressed concerns with patients in whom PSA changes did not reflect clinical status, particularly those with transient increases in the first 12 weeks of a new therapy.

■ **Human Chorionic Gonadotropin (hCG) and alpha fetoprotein (AFP):** Because testicular cancer is a highly curable disease with validated biomarkers, outcome assessment has focused on the rapid detection of patients whose tumors have a poor response to therapy. Because both markers have relatively short half-lives—2 to 3 days for hCG and 5 to 7 days for serum AFP—the rate of decline can be determined. Various methods have demonstrated that a rapid decline or early normalization of marker levels is indicative of a good outcome, without any one method achieving widespread acceptance.[46–48] Nonetheless, the 2010 American Society of Clinical Oncology (ASCO) guidelines on serum tumor markers concluded there was still insufficient evidence to recommend changing therapy solely on the basis of a slow marker decline.[49] Rising levels after two cycles of therapy (outside the first week of treatment when rises can be due to tumor lysis) can be considered an indication to change the treatment plan.[49,50]

Circulating Tumor Cells and Circulating Tumor DNA

Two response endpoints under recent investigation show a potential to detect the impact of therapy. One is the measurement of circulating tumor cells (CTC) in the bloodstream, enriched by one or more capture strategies, including one that has received FDA approval.[51] The number of CTCs in the blood has been shown to be prognostic, with higher levels conferring a poor prognosis, and to correlate with a response to therapy. A second approach is the determination of levels of circulating tumor DNA (ctDNA) in the blood. This is detected by quantitating the number of DNA molecules carrying a given mutation or gene rearrangement in the blood, typically detected through targeted sequencing of common mutations, or of a previously identified *mutation signature* or gene rearrangement. The amount of ctDNA appears to correlate with tumor burden, increases with stage, and in one study, was deemed more sensitive than CTC detection.[52–54] Whether these tests will ultimately prove to be more sensitive and accurate than the serum biomarkers discussed previously remains to be determined. Because targeted sequencing can be very sensitive, one concern is that false-positive ctDNA detection may occur after treatment, or intermittently in the setting of enlarging tumor masses. At the least, detection of CTCs and ctDNA is advancing our understanding of cancer biology, as studies reveal evidence of metastatic heterogeneity, clonal heterogeneity, and emergence of resistance mutations in clinical samples.

DETERMINING OUTCOME

The response measures described previously represent different approaches to quantitate tumor burden. What happens after those data are obtained varies depending on the clinical setting. In the community, less emphasis is placed on strict criteria. In the setting of a clinical trial, tumor size is measured and the response categorized. For FDA submission, these are but factors in the risk-benefit equation needed for drug approvals. The FDA conveys full approval to new agents based on true *clinical benefit* (i.e., an improvement in a *survival* endpoint or symptom relief).[55] Surrogates for clinical benefit, such as response rate, may support either regular approval or accelerated approval, depending on the setting.

Overall Response Rate, Duration of Response, and Stable Disease

Overall response rate (ORR) is the proportion of patients with a tumor size reduction of a predefined amount for a minimum time period. The FDA has generally defined ORR as the sum of PRs and CRs. Although OS remains the gold standard, ORR is often used both in drug development and in clinical practice to indicate antitumor efficacy of a given therapy. Table 30.3 summarizes the attributes and drawbacks of using ORR as a method of assessment. Using standardized definitions of response, it has been shown that ORR often correlates with OS, although ORR usually explains only a fraction of the variability of the survival

benefits.[56–58] Equally important, however, is the duration of response, a value that is measured from the time of initial response until documented tumor progression, and which assumes added importance when ORR is the endpoint for regulatory approval.

Unlike PR and CR, the FDA has generally not been willing to include *stable disease (SD)*, defined as shrinkage that qualifies as neither response nor progression, as part of the ORR, feeling it is often indicative of the underlying disease biology rather than a drug's therapeutic effect.[55,59] Nevertheless, in reporting data, investigators are increasingly using the term *CBR*, which includes CR + PR + SD and which is a misuse of the term *clinical benefit* because neither CR, PR, or SD are *objective tumor findings* that address the true *clinical benefit* of a therapy.[58,60] In the absence of standardized definitions for SD that are shown to effect meaningful changes in a clinical outcome, SD should not be used as a response endpoint. A better approach is to use nondichotomized response assessments, such as the waterfall plot or one of the kinetic analyses, discussed later.

Progression-Free Survival, Time to Progression, and Time to Treatment Failure

In cancer drug development, one usually finds ORR assessed as an indicator of activity in phase II trials, whereas randomized phase III trials rely on other endpoints such as progression-free survival (PFS) and time to progression (TTP) (see Table 30.3). Although PFS and TTP attempt to assess efficacy in close proximity to a therapy, they score outcomes differently and are not interchangeable. TTP is defined as the time from randomization to *the time of disease progression.*[55] *In TTP analyses, deaths are censored either at the time of death or at an earlier visit.* In contrast, PFS is defined from the time of randomization to the time of *disease progression or death*. Although patients who discontinue trial participation for adverse events might be censored in both analyses, patients who die while on study are censored only in the TTP analysis. Those who favor TTP argue that if a patient dies without their tumor meeting criteria for progression, one cannot accurately estimate when progression might have occurred, so the data should be censored. However, those who favor PFS argue that, in some cases, death might be an adverse effect of the therapy. High-dose therapies represent an example of why PFS might be a preferable (regulatory) endpoint. If in a given tumor there is evidence of a dose-response relationship for an active drug, then high doses may have a greater response. However, such high doses may also be responsible for a greater number of deaths. Assessing only those who survive the high dose therapy and ignoring those who die (i.e., TTP) may lead to the conclusion that the high-dose therapy is more effective. The balance sheet that includes death (i.e., PFS) would clearly demonstrate this efficacy came at too great a price.

Although many have argued that PFS and TTP should be acceptable endpoints for cancer clinical trials, in the majority of tumors there is no convincing evidence PFS is a surrogate for OS, and in those where there is some evidence, its value is arguable.[61] Table 30.3 presents the attributes and drawbacks of PFS and TTP. Note that the definition of progression is often difficult, particularly in some tumor types, and that investigator bias can influence PFS and TTP. Problems with ascertainment bias and censoring, depicted in Figure 30.2, can also impact outcomes.

Alternate endpoints include time to treatment failure (TTF), defined as a composite endpoint measuring time from randomization to discontinuation of treatment for any reason, including disease progression, treatment toxicity, and death. The FDA has not recommended TTF as a regulatory endpoint for drug approval. However, the high rates of censoring due to toxicity seen in phase III clinical trails may lead to a reassessment of this position given that most can agree that not only is efficacy important, but so too is tolerability, and TTF can capture both of these attributes.

CANCER THERAPEUTICS

TABLE 30.3

A Comparison of Important Cancer Approval Endpoints

Regulatory Evidence	Endpoints	Advantages	Disadvantages
Clinical benefit used for regular approvals	Overall survival (OS)	■ Universally accepted direct measure of clinical benefit ■ Easily measured ■ Includes treatment-related mortality that can obscure benefit in a subset ■ Precisely measured; unambiguous ■ Not dependent on assessment intervals	■ May involve larger studies ■ May require long follow-up ■ May be affected by crossover and/or sequential therapies ■ Includes noncancer deaths
	Symptom endpoints (patient-reported outcomes)	■ Patient perspective of direct clinical benefit	■ Blinding is often difficult ■ Data are frequently missing or incomplete ■ Clinical significance of small changes is unknown ■ Multiple analyses ■ Lack of validated instruments
Surrogates used for accelerated approvals or regular approvals	Disease-free survival (DFS)	■ Smaller sample size and shorter follow-up necessary compared with survival studies	■ Not statistically validated as surrogate for survival in all settings ■ Not precisely measured; subject to assessment bias, particularly in open-label studies ■ Definitions vary among studies
	Objective response rate (ORR)	■ Can be assessed in single-arm studies ■ Assessed earlier and in smaller studies compared with survival studies ■ Effect attributable to drug, not natural history	■ Not a direct measure of benefit ■ Not a comprehensive measure of drug activity ■ Only a subset of patients who benefit
	Complete response (CR)	■ Can be assessed in single-arm studies ■ Durable complete responses can represent clinical benefit ■ Assessed earlier and in smaller studies compared with survival studies ■ Definition of progressive disease (PD) identifies uniform time to end treatment and data capture	■ Not a direct measure of benefit in all cases ■ Not a comprehensive measure of drug activity ■ Small subset of patients with benefit ■ Requires prospective, consistent definition. Meaningful response durations not standardized ■ Definition of PD is arbitrary without evidence it actually represents end of benefit period
	Progression-free survival (PFS) or time to progression (TTP)[a]	■ Smaller sample size and shorter follow-up necessary compared with survival studies ■ Measurement of stable disease included ■ Not confounded by crossover or subsequent therapies ■ Generally based on objective and quantitative assessment	■ Statistically validated as surrogate for survival only in some settings ■ Not precisely measured; subject to assessment bias particularly in open-label studies ■ Definitions vary among studies; little agreement on magnitude of difference that constitutes clinical benefit ■ Requires frequent and consistent radiological or other assessments ■ Involves balanced timing of assessments among treatment arms

[a] Progression-free survival includes all deaths; time to progression censors deaths that occur before progression.
Adapted from U.S. Department of Health and Human Services, Food and Drug Administration, Center for Drug Evaluation and Research (CDER), Center for Biologics Evaluation and Research (CBER). *Guidance from Industry. Clinical Trial Endpoints for the Approval of Cancer Drugs and Biologics.* 2007. http://www.fda.gov/downloads/Drugs/.../Guidances/ucm071590.pdf.

Prespecified evaluation interval
Ideally, disease progression is reported at a prespecified evaluation interval

Ascertainment (evaluation) bias
An earlier evaluation leads to earlier scoring of progression (e.g., concern for symptoms prompt earlier evaluation)

Ascertainment (evaluation) bias
A later evaluation leads to delay in scoring progression (e.g., evaluation delayed by toxicity or treatment delays)

Censoring bias
Patient whose disease would have progressed quickly is censored early. Here censoring is "beneficial."

Censoring bias
Patient whose disease would have progressed late is censored early. Here censoring is "detrimental."

Informative censoring
Central review cannot score progression with available data. Although progression had been scored, the data is instead censored centrally. This is usually "beneficial."

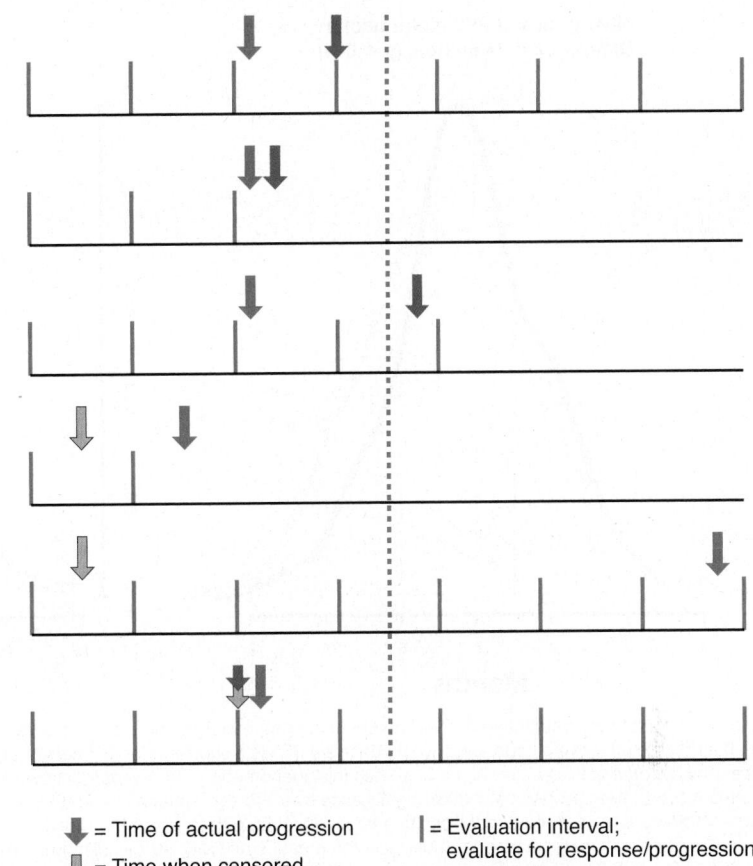

= Time of actual progression

= Time when censored

= Time progression scored

| = Evaluation interval;
    evaluate for response/progression

⋮ = Median PFS/TTP

Figure 30.2 The potential problems encountered when PFS is used as an endpoint. Ideally, as depicted at the *top,* response assessment will be conducted at a prespecified time. However, the date at which progression is scored may suffer from either ascertainment or censoring bias. Ascertainment bias can occur if either an evaluation occurs before the prespecified date or if it is delayed. For example, a clinician concerned about a patient who is not experiencing side effects and has likely been randomized to placebo may be more inclined to investigate symptoms early and document progression before the prespecified time, while delaying the evaluation of a patient randomized to the experimental arm who experiences some toxicity. Similarly, censoring—an increasing problem in randomized trials—may impact the outcome of a given study arm by either censoring patients who would experience early progression (beneficial impact) or censoring those who would have remained progression free for a long time (detrimental impact). Finally, informative censoring can occur when independent radiologic review cannot concur with an investigator's assessment of progression and censors the patient. This outcome is usually beneficial, because a patient who is very close to experiencing progression is censored. (Adapted from Villaruz LC, Socinski MA. The clinical viewpoint: definitions, limitations of RECIST, practical considerations of measurement. *Clin Cancer Res* 2013;19:2629–2636.)

Overall Survival

Defined as the time from randomization to death, OS has been considered the gold standard of clinical trial endpoints (see Table 30.3). In part, this is so because it is unambiguous and does not suffer from interpretation bias. An additional advantage of the survival endpoint is that it can balance the effect of therapies with high treatment-related mortality even if tumor control is substantially better with the new treatment. However, some worry that because patients may receive multiple lines of therapy following the clinical trial, the results may be confounded by those subsequent therapies. The latter concern is often cited as the reason why an advantage in PFS/TTP *disappears* when one looks to OS. But as a review of clinical trials confirms,[62] the magnitude of the difference does not disappear, only the statistical validity (Fig. 30.3).[63,64]

When evaluating a randomized controlled trial, it is important that the OS as well as the PFS analyses are always by intention to treat (ITT). In an ITT analysis, often described as *once randomized, always analyzed,* all patients assigned to a group at the time of randomization are analyzed regardless of what occurred subsequently.[65] An ITT analysis avoids the bias introduced by omitting dropouts and noncompliant patients that can negate randomization and overestimate clinical effectiveness.

Kaplan–Meier Plots

In a typical clinical trial, data are often presented as a Kaplan–Meier plots. In discrete time intervals, the number of patients in each group who are progression free and alive (PFS analysis) or alive (OS analysis) at the end of the interval are counted and divided by the total number of patients in that group at the beginning of the time interval. One excludes from this calculation patients censored for a reason other than progressive disease or death during the same interval. This has the advantage that it allows one to include censored patients in estimates of the probability of PFS or OS up to the point when they were censored (i.e., they are excluded only beyond the point of censoring). In most clinical trials, a fraction of patients are typically censored.

In constructing the Kaplan–Meier plot, probabilities are calculated for each interval of time. The probability of surviving

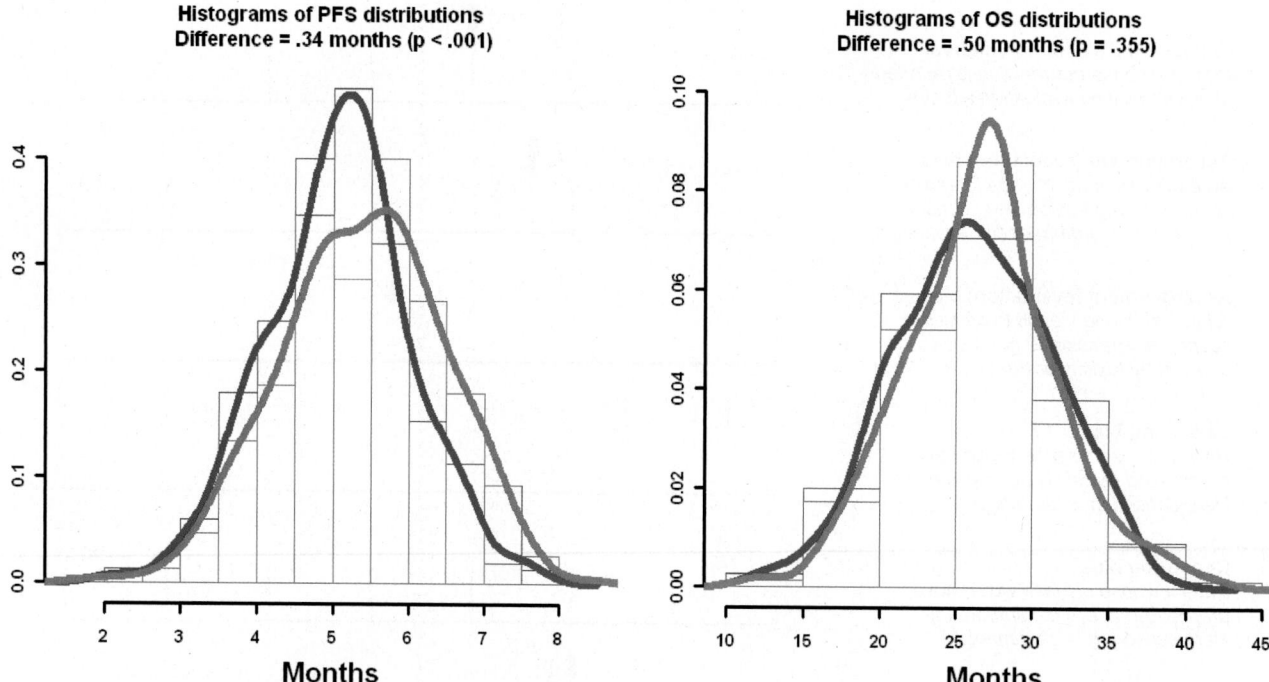

Figure 30.3 Hypothetical distribution of PFS and OS data demonstrating the *disappearance of PFS benefit*. Because chemotherapy does not exert a lasting effect on the underlying tumor biology and because PFS is a shorter interval (measured in increments, not daily as is OS) PFS differences often disappear. The *hypothetical example* shown illustrates this phenomenon. The *left panel* shows a histogram of PFS distributions with a difference of 0.34 months that nevertheless achieves statistical significance over the short interval when PFS is measured. The *right panel* depicts similar histograms for OS captured over a longer time period. Despite a larger absolute difference of 0.5 months, the OS difference does not reach statistical significance. For these hypothetical curves, random number generated data sets (with normal distribution), histograms, and density plots were generated using R version 2.11.1 (2010-05-31).[75] The differences were deliberately chosen to be small, but a similar disappearance can also occur with larger differences. As can be seen, what disappears is not the absolute benefit, but the statistical validity.

progression free or being counted as a survivor to the end of any interval of assessment is the product of the probabilities of surviving in all the preceding assessment intervals multiplied by the probability for the interval of interest. One might ask to what extent the two curves in each study differ. One measure that is of value is the median PFS or OS—a value calculated in most studies from a Kaplan–Meier plot.

Hazard Ratios

Increasingly, however, hazard ratios are cited in preference to the more traditional measures of efficacy such as the median PFS and median OS. *However, because a hazard ratio is a value that has no dimensions, it has very limited value, informing the reader only with regard to the reliability and uniformity of the data.* It does not quantify the magnitude of the benefit. A physician and, especially, a patient want to know the magnitude of the benefit (i.e., the extent to which a life will be prolonged), not what a dimensionless hazard ratio is. By definition, the *hazard ratio* is a ratio of the *hazard rates*. The hazard rate quantifies the likelihood that a patient will experience a *hazardous event* or a hazard during a defined interval of observation, and this is expressed as a rate or percent. For example, if during a given period of observation 20 of 100 patients receiving a reference or control therapy experience progression or death, their hazard rate during this interval is 0.2 (20/100). If during this same interval, only 10 of the 100 patients receiving the experimental therapy experience progression or death, their hazard rate is 0.1 (10/100). In this simple example, the hazard ratio for the interval, calculated as *the ratio of the hazard rates* is 0.5 (0.1/0.2) and indicates the likelihood of experiencing a hazardous event is reduced by 50% in the experimental arm. As commonly presented, and as this simple example illustrates, the lower the

hazard ratio, the better the experimental therapy. To determine whether the hazard ratio has statistical significance, one can (1) use a log-rank test to show that the null hypothesis that the two treatments lead to the same survival probabilities is wrong, or (2) use a parametric approach writing a regression model and fitting the data to the model so that one can establish the hazard ratio for the whole trial and its statistical significance. In many cases, the Cox proportional hazard model is used. Although the ideal hazard ratio would capture the differential benefit throughout the period of study, in practice, the extremes depicted in a Kaplan–Meier plot may not be analyzed.

Forest Plots

Interest in determining whether there is heterogeneity in a treatment effect, such that better outcomes occur in some subgroups, has led to the use of Forest plots to display treatment effects across subgroups. Although simple in concept, these plots are subject to error because subgroups are composed of smaller numbers and the confidence intervals are therefore wider than those for the entire group. The most common presentation includes a vertical line at the *no effect point* (e.g., a hazard ratio of 1.0), with symbols of varying size representing the subgroups, each with its confidence interval depicted by a line that stretches from the symbol to both sides (the symbol size is usually proportional to the size of the subgroup). If the confidence interval for a subgroup crosses the no effect point, this is commonly interpreted (not necessarily correctly) as a lack of effect in the subgroup. *The information one seeks from a Forest plot is whether the effect size for different subgroups varies significantly from the main effect, which is determined by a test for heterogeneity.*[66]

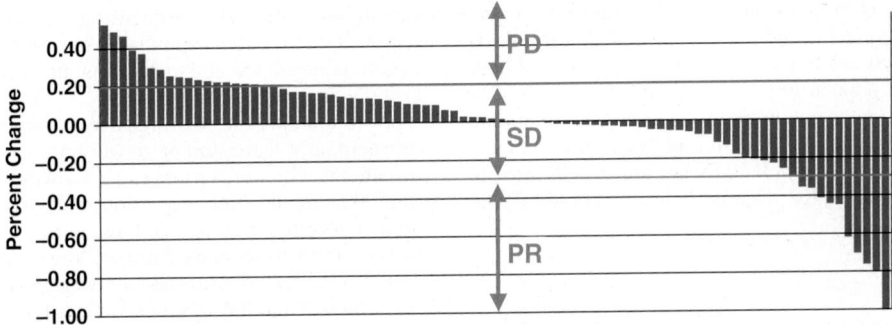

Figure 30.4 Example of a waterfall plot demonstrating for each patient the maximum benefit obtained with the study therapy. Those to the *left* represent patients whose tumors increased, and those on the *right* represent patients whose tumors regressed. The *vertical red lines* at +20% and -30% define the boundaries of stable disease according to RECIST. Ideally, all responses should be confirmed after a period of at least 4 weeks. The example shown is of patients with renal cell carcinoma treated with the microtubule targeting agent ixabepilone. (From Huang H, Menefee M, Edgerly M, et al. A phase II clinical trial of ixabepilone [Ixempra; BMS-247550; NSC 710428], an epothilone B analog, in patients with metastatic renal cell carcinoma. *Clin Cancer Res* 2010;16:1634–1641.)

Beyond Dichotomized Data

Quality of Life

The assessment of cancer patients enrolled on a clinical trial can be said to consist of two sets of endpoints: cancer outcomes and patient outcomes. Cancer outcomes measure the response of the tumor to treatment, the duration of the response, the symptom-free period, and the early recognition of relapse. In contrast, patient outcomes assess the benefit achieved with a given therapy by measuring the increase in survival and the quality of life (QOL) before and after therapy. Unfortunately, physicians tend to concentrate on cancer-related outcomes, often neglecting assessments of QOL. Although a QOL assessment in clinical settings is possible with currently available instruments, there must be continued development and refinement of these instruments. Such development must focus not only on extracting valuable information in an unbiased manner, but also and equally important, developing an instrument that is user friendly and will be completed in a high percentage of encounters.

Waterfall Plots

The arbitrary nature of the 50% cutoff set by Moertel and Hanley and its evolution to the current RECIST threshold of 30%

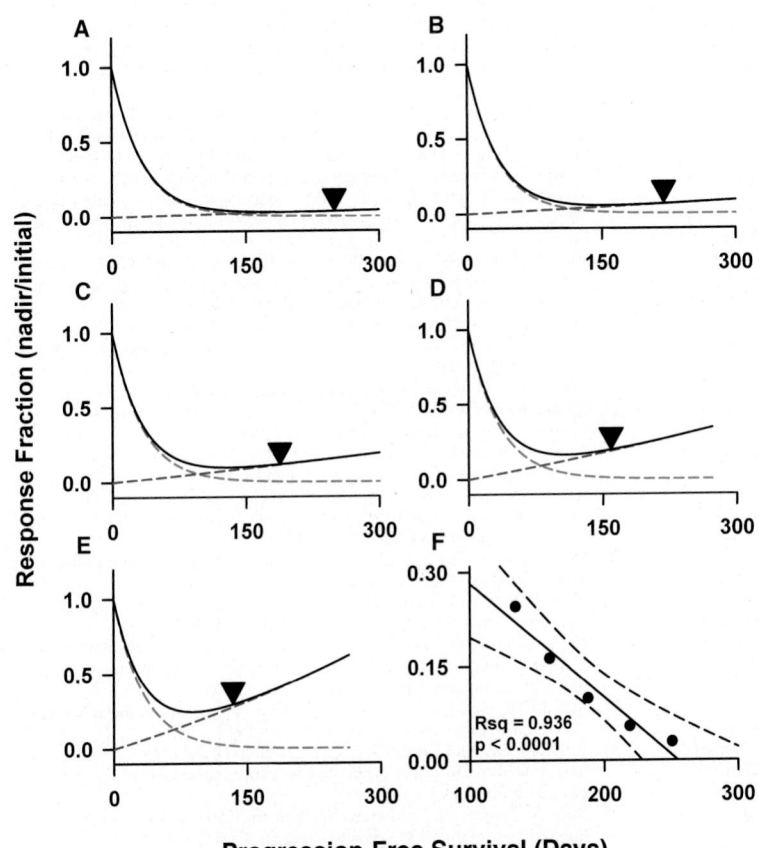

Progression-Free Survival (Days)

Figure 30.5 The effect of the growth rate constant, *g*, on two commonly reported clinical values: maximum tumor shrinkage and PFS. Tumor measurements obtained in patients can be analyzed mathematically. **(A–E)** The *black line* depicts idealized clinical data using tumor quantities measured as patients received chemotherapy. Actually, clinical measurements comprise concurrent tumor regression *(dashed red line)* and growth *(dashed blue line)* that can be described by a rate constant and a first order kinetic equation, $f(t) = exp^{(-d \cdot t)} + exp^{(g \cdot t)} - 1$, where *exp* is the base of the natural logarithm, e = 2.7182..., and *f* is the percent change in tumor measurement at time *t*, normalized to the value when treatment began. The rate constant *d* accounts for exponential decrease, whereas the rate constant *g* accounts for exponential growth occurring during treatment.[68,69] To demonstrate the correlation between the growth rate, tumor shrinkage and PFS, the *same* regression rate (*d*) has been modeled in panels *A* through *E*, whereas the growth rate constant, *g*, *increases* in each successive panel. The *black triangles* depict the point at which tumor size is 20% above the nadir (RECIST definition of PD). As the growth rate increases (i.e., faster tumor growth) from **A** to **E**, the nadir is reached sooner, and the depth of the nadir is less. **(F)** The correlation between PFS and maximum tumor shrinkage (nadir) is shown, plotting the correlation between PFS and response fraction, which is defined as the ratio of nadir to initial value.[68,69] Although idealized plots are given, the curves are based firmly on data obtained from patients enrolled on clinical trials.

reduction in the size of the maximum diameter raises valid queries as to why 30% is valuable and not 29% or 25%. On this background, waterfall plots such as the one shown in Figure 30.4 have become increasingly popular because they depict the benefit or lack thereof in all patients as a continuum of response, rather than a dichotomized response rate.[67] Waterfall plots can be generated from any quantitative assessment. If ctDNA or tumor cells prove to be as quantitative as hoped, the maximum decline could be plotted as a waterfall plot.

Growth Kinetics

Efforts to quantify tumor kinetic parameters from clinical data have been investigated in recent years. Different equations have been applied to describe the two-phase curve based on tumor size as observed in most solid tumor trials, where there is first shrinkage followed by regrowth (Fig. 30.5). These models show exponential tumor shrinkage after treatment, followed by tumor regrowth that is either exponential or linear and have been shown to correlate with OS and to discriminate effective therapies as well as individual patients within trials.[68–73] A major advantage is that more of the data are used, relative to dichotomized response assessment, and regression or growth rates can be determined even in patients who are censored in a Kaplan–Meier analysis. Equations that model both regression and growth rates confirm the clinical intuition that resistant disease is emerging even as overall tumor volume is reduced. Further, "the strategy of studying tumor growth kinetics circumvents one weakness of 'progression criteria,' which is that they inherently dichotomize a complex biological process that may be better characterized using a continuous function."[74] As shown in Figure 30.5, the response of a tumor to a therapy is exemplified by the nadir, the time to the nadir, and the time to progression or PFS, and these are all are all dependent on the growth rate.

REFERENCES

1. America's Biopharmaceutical Research Companies. *Medicines in Development for Cancer.* PhRMA Web site. http://www.phrma.org/sites/default/files/pdf/phrmamedicinesindevelopmentcancer2012.pdf.
2. Moertel CG, Hanley JA. The effect of measuring error on the results of therapeutic trials in advanced cancer. *Cancer* 1976;38:388–394.
3. Miller AB, Hoogstraten B, Staquet M, et al. Reporting results of cancer treatment. *Cancer* 1981;47:207–214.
4. Therasse P, Arbuck SG, Eisenhauer EA, et al. New guidelines to evaluate the response to treatment in solid tumors. European Organization for Research and Treatment of Cancer, National Cancer Institute of the United States, National Cancer Institute of Canada. *J Natl Cancer Inst* 2000;92:205–216.
5. Eisenhauer EA, Therasse P, Bogaerts J, et al. New response evaluation criteria in solid tumours: revised RECIST guideline (version 1.1). *Eur J Cancer* 2009;45:228–247.
6. Mazumdar M, Smith A, Schwartz LH. A statistical simulation study finds discordance between WHO criteria and RECIST guideline. *J Clin Epidemiol* 2004;57:358–365.
7. Wen PY, Macdonald DR, Reardon DA, et al. Updated response assessment criteria for high-grade gliomas: response assessment in neuro-oncology working group. *J Clin Oncol* 2010;28:1963–1972.
8. Byrne MJ, Nowak AK. Modified RECIST criteria for assessment of response in malignant pleural mesothelioma. *Ann Oncol* 2004;15:257–260.
9. Wolchok JD, Hoos A, O'Day S, et al. Guidelines for the evaluation of immune therapy activity in solid tumors: immune-related response criteria. *Clin Cancer Res* 2009;15:7412–7420.
10. Quant EC, Wen PY. Response assessment in neuro-oncology. *Curr Oncol Rep* 2011;13:50–56.
11. Hawkins-Daarud A, Rockne RC, Anderson AR, et al. Modeling tumor-associated edema in gliomas during anti-angiogenic therapy and its impact on imageable tumor. *Front Oncol* 2013;3:66.
12. Fink J, Born D, Chamberlain MC. Pseudoprogression: relevance with respect to treatment of high-grade gliomas. *Curr Treat Options Oncol* 2011;12:240–252.
13. Lin NU, Lee EQ, Aoyama H, et al. Challenges relating to solid tumour brain metastases in clinical trials, part 1: patient population, response, and progression. A report from the RANO group. *Lancet Oncol* 2013;14:e396–e406.
14. Mabille M, Vanel D, Albiter M, et al. Follow-up of hepatic and peritoneal metastases of gastrointestinal tumors (GIST) under Imatinib therapy requires different criteria of radiological evaluation (size is not everything!!!). *Eur J Radiol* 2009;69:204–208.
15. Liu L, Wang W, Chen H, et al. EASL- and mRECIST-evaluated responses to combination therapy of sorafenib with transarterial chemoembolization predict survival in patients with hepatocellular carcinoma. *Clin Cancer Res* 2014; 20:1623–1631.
16. Cheson BD, Pfistner B, Juweid ME, et al. Revised response criteria for malignant lymphoma. *J Clin Oncol* 2007;25:579–586.
17. Bernhard J, Dietrich D, Scheithauer W, et al. Clinical benefit and quality of life in patients with advanced pancreatic cancer receiving gemcitabine plus capecitabine versus gemcitabine alone: a randomized multicenter phase III clinical trial—SAKK 44/00-CECOG/PAN.1.3.001. *J Clin Oncol* 2008; 26:3695–3701.
18. Burris HA, Moore MJ, Andersen J, et al. Improvements in survival and clinical benefit with gemcitabine as first-line therapy for patients with advanced pancreas cancer: a randomized trial. *J Clin Oncol* 1997;15:2403–2413.
19. Mann BS, Johnson JR, He K, et al. Vorinostat for treatment of cutaneous manifestations of advanced primary cutaneous T-cell lymphoma. *Clin Cancer Res* 2007;13:2318–2322.
20. von Minckwitz G, Untch M, Blohmer JU, et al. Definition and impact of pathologic complete response on prognosis after neoadjuvant chemotherapy in various intrinsic breast cancer subtypes. *J Clin Oncol* 2012;30: 1796–1804.
21. Cortazar P, Zhang L, Untch M, et al. Pathological complete response and long-term clinical benefit in breast cancer: the CTNeoBC pooled analysis. *Lancet* 2014 [Epub ahead of print].
22. Bardia A, Baselga J. Neoadjuvant therapy as a platform for drug development and approval in breast cancer. *Clin Cancer Res* 2013;19:6360–6370.
23. Choi H, Charnsangavej C, Faria SC, et al. Correlation of computed tomography and positron emission tomography in patients with metastatic gastrointestinal stromal tumor treated at a single institution with imatinib mesylate: proposal of new computed tomography response criteria. *J Clin Oncol* 2007;25:1753–1759.
24. Schramm N, Englhart E, Schlemmer M, et al. Tumor response and clinical outcome in metastatic gastrointestinal stromal tumors under sunitinib therapy: comparison of RECIST, Choi and volumetric criteria. *Eur J Radiol* 2013;82:951–958.
25. Dudeck O, Zeile M, Reichardt P, et al. Comparison of RECIST and Choi criteria for computed tomographic response evaluation in patients with advanced gastrointestinal stromal tumor treated with sunitinib. *Ann Oncol* 2011;22:1828–1833.
26. Ronot M, Bouattour M, Wassermann J, et al. Alternative response criteria (Choi, European Association for the Study of the Liver, and Modified Response Evaluation Criteria in Solid Tumors [RECIST]) versus RECIST 1.1 in patients with advanced hepatocellular carcinoma treated with sorafenib. *Oncologist* 2014. http://prostatecancer.theoncologist.com/article/alternative-response-criteria-choi-european-association-study-liver-and-modified-response.
27. van der Veldt AA, Meijerink MR, van den Eertwegh AJ, et al. Choi response criteria for early prediction of clinical outcome in patients with metastatic renal cell cancer treated with sunitinib. *Br J Cancer* 2010;102:803–809.
28. Wahl RL, Jacene H, Kasamon Y, et al. From RECIST to PERCIST: evolving considerations for PET response criteria in solid tumors. *J Nucl Med* 2009;50:122S–150S.
29. Shankar LK, Hoffman JM, Bacharach S, et al. Consensus recommendations for the use of 18F-FDG PET as an indicator of therapeutic response in patients in National Cancer Institute Trials. *J Nucl Med* 2006;47:1059–1066.
30. Young H, Baum R, Cremerius U, et al. Measurement of clinical and subclinical tumour response using [18F]-fluorodeoxyglucose and positron emission tomography: review and 1999 EORTC recommendations. European Organization for Research and Treatment of Cancer (EORTC) PET Study Group. *Eur J Cancer* 1999;35:1773–1782.
31. Kramer-Marek G, Capala J. Can PET imaging facilitate optimization of cancer therapies? *Curr Pharm Des* 2012;18:2657–2669.
32. Niederkohr RD, Greenspan BS, Prior JO, et al. Reporting guidance for oncologic 18F-FDG PET/CT imaging. *J Nucl Med* 2013;54:756–761.
33. Liu Y, Litière S, de Vries EG, et al. The role of response evaluation criteria in solid tumour in anticancer treatment evaluation: results of a survey in the oncology community. *Eur J Cancer* 2014;50:260–266.
34. Rubin EH, Allen JD, Nowak JA, et al. Developing precision medicine in a global world. *Clin Cancer Res* 2014;20:1419–1427.
35. Parkinson DR, McCormack RT, Keating SM. Evidence of clinical utility: an unmet need in molecular diagnostics for cancer patients. *Clin Cancer Res* 2014;20:1428–1444.
36. Buyse M, Sargent DJ, Grothey A, et al. Biomarkers and surrogate end points—the challenge of statistical validation. *Nat Rev Clin Oncol* 2010;7:309–317.

37. Karam AK, Karlan BY. Ovarian cancer: the duplicity of CA125 measurement. *Nat Rev Clin Oncol* 2010;7:335–339.
38. Rustin GJ, van der Burg ME, Griffin CL, et al. Early versus delayed treatment of relapsed ovarian cancer (MRC OV05/EORTC 55955): a randomised trial. *Lancet* 2010;376:1155–1163.
39. Vergote I, Rustin GJ, Eisenhauer EA, et al. Re: new guidelines to evaluate the response to treatment in solid tumors [ovarian cancer]. Gynecologic Cancer Intergroup. *J Natl Cancer Inst* 2000;92:1534–1535.
40. Guppy AE, Rustin GJ. CA125 response: can it replace the traditional response criteria in ovarian cancer? *Oncologist* 2002;7:437–443.
41. Rustin GJ, Quinn M, Thigpen T, et al. Re: New guidelines to evaluate the response to treatment in solid tumors (ovarian cancer). *J Natl Cancer Inst* 2004;96:487–488.
42. Rustin GJ, Vergote I, Eisenhauer E, et al. Definitions for response and progression in ovarian cancer clinical trials incorporating RECIST 1.1 and CA 125 agreed by the Gynecological Cancer Intergroup (GCIG). *Int J Gynecol Cancer* 2011;21:419–423.
43. Eisenhauer EA. Optimal assessment of response in ovarian cancer. *Ann Oncol* 2011;22:viii49–viii51.
44. Bubley GJ, Carducci M, Dahut W, et al. Eligibility and response guidelines for phase II clinical trials in androgen-independent prostate cancer: recommendations from the Prostate-Specific Antigen Working Group. *J Clin Oncol* 1999;17:3461–3467.
45. Scher HI, Halabi S, Tannock I, et al. Design and end points of clinical trials for patients with progressive prostate cancer and castrate levels of testosterone: recommendations of the Prostate Cancer Clinical Trials Working Group. *J Clin Oncol* 2008;26:1148–1159.
46. Mazumdar M, Bajorin DF, Bacik J, et al. Predicting outcome to chemotherapy in patients with germ cell tumors: the value of the rate of decline of human chorionic gonadotrophin and alpha-fetoprotein during therapy. *J Clin Oncol* 2001;19:2534–2541.
47. Fizazi K, Culine S, Kramar A, et al. Early predicted time to normalization of tumor markers predicts outcome in poor-prognosis nonseminomatous germ cell tumors. *J Clin Oncol* 2004;22:3868–3876.
48. Toner GC. Early identification of therapeutic failure in nonseminomatous germ cell tumors by assessing serum tumor marker decline during chemotherapy: still not ready for routine clinical use. *J Clin Oncol* 2004;22:3842–3845.
49. Gilligan TD, Seidenfeld J, Basch EM, et al. American Society of Clinical Oncology Clinical Practice Guideline on uses of serum tumor markers in adult males with germ cell tumors. *J Clin Oncol* 2010;28:3388–3404.
50. Albers P, Albrecht W, Algaba F, et al. EAU guidelines on testicular cancer: 2011 update. *Eur Urol* 2011;60:304–319.
51. Yap T, Lorente D, Omlin A, et al. Circulating tumor cells: a multifunctional biomarker. *Clin Cancer Res* 2014;20:2553–2568.
52. Dawson SJ, Tsui DW, Murtaza M, et al. Analysis of circulating tumor DNA to monitor metastatic breast cancer. *N Engl J Med* 2013;368:1199–1209.
53. Punnoose EA, Atwal S, Liu W, et al. Evaluation of circulating tumor cells and circulating tumor DNA in non-small cell lung cancer: association with clinical endpoints in a phase II clinical trial of pertuzumab and erlotinib. *Clin Cancer Res* 2012;18:2391–2401.
54. Bettegowda C, Sausen M, Leary RJ, et al. Detection of circulating tumor DNA in early- and late-stage human malignancies. *Sci Transl Med* 2014;6:224ra24.
55. Pazdur R. Endpoints for assessing drug activity in clinical trials. *Oncologist* 2008;13:19–21.
56. Buyse M, Thirion P, Carlson RW, et al. Relation between tumour response to first-line chemotherapy and survival in advanced colorectal cancer: a meta-analysis. Meta-Analysis Group in Cancer. *Lancet* 2000;356:373–378.
57. Bruzzi P, Del Mastro L, Sormani MP, et al. Objective response to chemotherapy as a potential surrogate end point of survival in metastatic breast cancer patients. *J Clin Oncol* 2005;23:5117–5125.
58. Vidaurre T, Wilkerson J, Simon R, et al. Stable disease is not preferentially observed with targeted therapies and as currently defined has limited value in drug development. *Cancer J* 2009;15:366–373.
59. McKee AE, Farrell AT, Pazdur R, et al. The role of the U.S. Food and Drug Administration review process: clinical trial endpoints in oncology. *Oncologist* 2010;15:13–18.
60. Ohorodnyk P, Eisenhauer EA, Booth CM. Clinical benefit in oncology trials: is this a patient-centred or tumour-centred end-point? *Eur J Cancer* 2009;45:2249–2252.
61. Buyse M. Use of meta-analysis for the validation of surrogate endpoints and biomarkers in cancer trials. *Cancer J* 2009;15:421–425.
62. Wilkerson J, Fojo T. Progression-free survival is simply a measure of a drug's effect while administered and is not a surrogate for overall survival. *Cancer J* 2009;15:379–385.
63. Reck M, von Pawel J, Zatloukal P, et al. Overall survival with cisplatin-gemcitabine and bevacizumab or placebo as first-line therapy for nonsquamous non-small-cell lung cancer: results from a randomised phase III trial (AVAiL). *Ann Oncol* 2010;21:1804–1809.
64. Hortobagyi GN, Gomez HL, Li RK, et al. Analysis of overall survival from a phase III study of ixabepilone plus capecitabine versus capecitabine in patients with MBC resistant to anthracyclines and taxanes. *Breast Cancer Res Treat* 2010;122:409–418.
65. Hennekens C, Buring J. *Epidemiology in Medicine.* 1st ed. Boston: Little, Brown and Co.; 1987.
66. Cuzick J. Forest plots and the interpretation of subgroups. *Lancet* 2005; 365:1308.
67. Huang H, Menefee M, Edgerly M, et al. A phase II clinical trial of ixabepilone (Ixempra; BMS-247550; NSC 710428), an epothilone B analog, in patients with metastatic renal cell carcinoma. *Clin Cancer Res* 2010;16: 1634–1641.
68. Stein WD, Gulley JL, Schlom J, et al. Tumor regression and growth rates determined in five intramural NCI prostate cancer trials: the growth rate constant as an indicator of therapeutic efficacy. *Clin Cancer Res* 2011;17: 907–917.
69. Stein WD, Wilkerson J, Kim ST, et al. Analyzing the pivotal trial that compared sunitinib and IFN-α in renal cell carcinoma, using a method that assesses tumor regression and growth. *Clin Cancer Res* 2012;18:2374–2381.
70. Maitland ML, Wu K, Sharma MR, et al. Estimation of renal cell carcinoma treatment effects from disease progression modeling. *Clin Pharmacol Ther* 2013;93:345–351.
71. Claret L, Girard P, Hoff PM, et al. Model-based prediction of phase III overall survival in colorectal cancer on the basis of phase II tumor dynamics. *J Clin Oncol* 2009;27:4103–4108.
72. Claret L, Gupta M, Han K, et al. Evaluation of tumor-size response metrics to predict overall survival in Western and Chinese patients with first-line metastatic colorectal cancer. *J Clin Oncol* 2013;31:2110–2114.
73. Wang Y, Sung C, Dartois C, et al. Elucidation of relationship between tumor size and survival in non-small-cell lung cancer patients can aid early decision making in clinical drug development. *Clin Pharmacol Ther* 2009;86: 167–174.
74. Oxnard GR, Morris MJ, Hodi FS, et al. When progressive disease does not mean treatment failure: reconsidering the criteria for progression. *J Natl Cancer Inst* 2012;104:1534–1541.
75. Team RDC. R: A language and environment for statistical computing. R Foundation for Statistical Computing. Vienna, Austria: R Foundation for Statistical Computing, 2010. http://www.r-project.org.

CANCER THERAPEUTICS

PART IV

Cancer Prevention and Screening

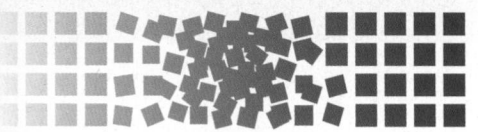

31 Tobacco Use and the Cancer Patient

Graham W. Warren, Benjamin A. Toll, Irene M. Tamí-Maury, and Ellen R. Gritz

INTRODUCTION

Tobacco is commonly described as the largest preventable cause of cancer. Over 50 years ago, tobacco was increasingly recognized as the primary cause of lung cancer, with definitive recognition for tobacco use as a causative factor in the seminal 1964 U.S. Surgeon General's Report (SGR) on Smoking and Health.[1] Recent editions of the SGR have described the widespread adverse health effects of tobacco on a spectrum of diseases, including as a causative agent for a spectrum of cancers.[2,3] Tobacco use is an addiction usually initiated in youth prior to the age of 18 and is driven by the highly addictive drug, nicotine.[4] As related to the cancer patient, considerable work has been conducted to associate tobacco use with the risk of developing cancer and how tobacco cessation can substantially reduce cancer risks. However, there is a relative paucity of effort that has been put forth to identify the effects of smoking on outcomes for cancer patients or to establish methods to help cancer patients quit smoking. Fortunately, in recent years, the importance of tobacco use by the cancer patient has been increasingly recognized as an important health behavior, including a National Cancer Institute (NCI)–sponsored conference on tobacco use in 2010, a joint sponsored NCI–American Association of Cancer Research (AACR)–sponsored workshop at the Institute of Medicine in 2012, and recent recommendations by the AACR and the American Society of Clinical Oncology (ASCO) to address tobacco use in cancer patients.[5,6] The recently released 2014 SGR now provides substantial evidence behind the effects of smoking by cancer patients with the following conclusions[7]:

1. In cancer patients and survivors, the evidence is sufficient to infer a causal relationship between cigarette smoking and adverse health outcomes. Quitting smoking improves the prognosis of cancer patients.
2. In cancer patients and survivors, the evidence is sufficient to infer a causal relationship between cigarette smoking and increased all-cause mortality and cancer-specific mortality.
3. In cancer patients and survivors, the evidence is sufficient to infer a causal relationship between cigarette smoking and increased risk for second primary cancers known to be caused by cigarette smoking, such as lung cancer.
4. In cancer patients and survivors, the evidence is suggestive but not sufficient to infer a causal relationship between cigarette smoking and the risk of recurrence, poorer response to treatment, and increased treatment-related toxicity.

The overall objective of this chapter is to discuss tobacco use by cancer patients, the clinical effects of smoking in cancer patients, methods to address tobacco use by cancer patients, and areas of needed research.

NEUROBIOLOGY OF TOBACCO DEPENDENCE

Nicotine is the primary addictive component of tobacco that increases extracellular concentrations of dopamine in the nucleus accumbens and stimulates the mesolimbic dopaminergic system,[8,9] resulting in nicotine's rewarding effect experienced by tobacco users.[10–12] Dopaminergic neurotransmission may also be involved in the assignment of incentive salience, or stimulus for a pleasure based reward, to tobacco use–related environmental cues[13,14] that may become conditioned reinforcers of tobacco use behaviors. For example, an individual who smokes while drinking their morning coffee may associate coffee, or even holding a coffee cup in their hand, with the reward from smoking. Thus, cigarette smoking is directly linked to external nontobacco-based behavioral stimuli. Activation of the nucleus accumbens has further been implicated in drug reinstatement or relapse.[15,16] Individuals who have quit tobacco use for years have restarted a tobacco habit simply by sitting next to a smoker and being exposed to secondhand smoke. Substantial work has been conducted on the addictive nature of tobacco and nicotine, and readers are referred to several comprehensive reviews on this topic.[9,12,17]

TOBACCO USE PREVALENCE AND THE EVOLUTION OF TOBACCO PRODUCTS

Much of the discussion on tobacco use epidemiology and carcinogenesis is presented in Chapter 4. In brief, the prevalence of cigarette smoking among adults in the United States decreased to 19.0% as compared with 22.8% in 2001, but it did not meet the *Healthy People 2010* objective to reduce smoking prevalence to 12%.[18,19] There have been substantial changes in the landscape of tobacco use over time as a direct consequence of cigarette-centered policies and regulations aiming to reduce the harmful effects and number of deaths caused by smoking.[20–22] Under this new landscape, novel and reemergent noncigarette tobacco products such as cigars, cigarillos, snuff, chewing tobacco, water pipes (hookahs), and other forms of tobacco consumption have been growing in demand as a consequence of aggressive and sophisticated marketing by the tobacco industry.[23] Consumption patterns have also changed due to efforts by the tobacco industry to make cigarettes appear safer, such as low tar or filtered cigarettes, and the inclusion of flavoring (menthol, vanilla, fruits, etc.).[24] Although these efforts may have changed consumption patterns, they have not reduced cancer risk. Large patient cohorts demonstrate that the introduction of low tar and filtered cigarettes actually increased risk by promoting deeper inhalation and higher rates of addiction with no reductions in cancer risk,[24,25] resulting in subsequent changes in lung cancer from centrally located squamous cell cancers to peripherally located nonsquamous cell cancers.

The relatively recent introduction of electronic cigarettes (i.e., e-cigarettes, e-cigs, nicotine vaporizers, or electronic nicotine delivery systems [ENDS]) is noteworthy. These electronic or battery-powered devices activate a heating element that vaporizes a liquid solution contained in a cartridge, and then the user inhales this vapor. Levels of nicotine as well as other chemical additives and flavors in the cartridge are uncertain and vary according to the brand.[26] Although there are no research studies that have evaluated the potential harmful effects of the use of e-cigarettes for cancer patients,[27] organizations such as the World Health Organization have already expressed concerns about the safety of these increasingly popular products.[28,29] To date, e-cigarettes have not been approved by the U.S. Food and Drug Administration (FDA) as therapeutic devices to aid in quitting smoking.[26] Readers are referred to a recent editorial on the use of e-cigarettes by cancer patients[27]; however, it will likely be several years before evidence-based health information is available.

TOBACCO USE BY THE CANCER PATIENT

The prevalence of current smoking among long-term adult cancer survivors appears to have declined in the past decade,[30] but data suggest higher rates of smoking among cancer survivors than in the general population.[30–32] These data are often biased by the fact that assessments in cancer patients may not include cancer patients who were current smokers at the time of death. As a result, estimates of smoking rates in cancer survivors may be misleading and may underestimate true tobacco use patterns for cancer patients. Furthermore, alternative tobacco products are often not assessed in cancer patients. Data from the Childhood Cancer Survivor Study and the 2009 Behavioral Risk Factor Surveillance System indicate that approximately 3% to 8% of cancer survivors use smokeless tobacco products.[33,34] Patients may be attracted to these alternative products due to less social stigma and the nonevidence-based perception that these products are healthier alternatives compared to cigarette smoking.

Continued tobacco use by cancer patients often represents a combined failure by the patient to recognize the need to stop smoking even after a cancer diagnosis and the effort by health-care providers to address tobacco use with evidence-based assessments and tobacco cessation support. Approximately 30% of all cancer patients use tobacco at the time of cancer diagnosis with higher rates in traditionally tobacco-related disease sites, such as head and neck or lung cancers, and lower rates in traditionally nontobacco-related disease sites, such as breast or prostate cancers.[35–44] However, findings from several studies indicate that cancer patients are receptive to smoking cessation interventions even as they continue to smoke.[35,38,45–50]

A cancer diagnosis can be used as a window of opportunity, or *teachable moment*, to intervene and provide assistance in the quitting process.[51] A recent study in 12,000 cancer patients, including 2,700 patients who smoked, capitalized on the teachable moment and demonstrated that less than 3% of patients who were contacted by the cessation program rejected tobacco cessation assistance.[45] However, only 1.2% of patients who received a mailed invitation participated in the program. This highlights the idea that patients may be interested in quitting, but methods such as mailed tobacco cessation information may not yield effective participation by cancer patients. Once enrolled, patients and clinicians must realize that although relapses in the general population usually occur within 1 week of cessation, relapses in cancer patients may be delayed due to cancer treatment–related variables such as surgical or other posttreatment healing.[52] Consequently, it is important to continue offering tobacco assessments and cessation support for cancer survivorship efforts.

Defining Tobacco Use by the Cancer Patient

In dealing with tobacco use by cancer patients, it is important to note that virtually all of the evidence associating tobacco with cancer treatment outcomes deals with smoking. Few studies report associations between other forms of tobacco use (e.g., smokeless, cigars, cigarillos) and outcomes in cancer patients. Furthermore, the definition of smoking across published studies varies substantially.[53] In studies of cancer patients, smoking has been defined as current (e.g., smoking after diagnosis, at diagnosis, in the weeks

before diagnosis, within the 12 months prior to diagnosis, after diagnosis, within the past 10 years), former (e.g., recent, intermediate-, or long-term quit for 1 month, 3 month, 6 month, 12 month, 2 years, 5 years, 10 years), never, quitting after diagnosis, and according to exposure (e.g., multiple pack year cutoffs, Brinkman index, years of smoking, years of smoking within a predefined period of time such as 5 years prior to diagnosis). Though the nonstandard method of addressing tobacco use in cancer patients has been observed in several reports,[54–57] there are no current standard recommendations for the definition of tobacco use by any national organization. There are four primary categories for smoking status:

1. **Never smoking** is typically defined as having smoked less than 100 cigarettes in a person's lifetime and no current cigarette use. These patients are generally considered as a reference group in many studies. Categories 2 through 4 require that a person has smoked at least 100 cigarettes in their lifetime.
2. **Former smoking** is typically defined as no current cigarette use, usually within the past year.
3. **Recent smoking** (or recent quit) is generally defined as having stopped smoking within the recent past, typically for a period of 1 week to 1 year.
4. **Current smoking** is typically defined as smoking one or more cigarettes per day every day or some days.

Ever smoking is a combination of categories 2 through 4 (i.e., former, recent, and current smokers) that has been used to report negative associations between smoking and cancer outcomes in a number of studies.[58–70] Defining smoking according to *ever* smoking status limits the ability to interpret the effects of current smoking on a clinical outcome, and nothing can be done to address a prior tobacco use history. However, defining exposure according to *current* smoking status allows for the analysis of potentially reversible effects as well as for the potential implementation of smoking cessation to prevent the adverse outcomes of smoking on cancer patients. The primary focus for the remainder of this chapter will be on *current* smoking and will include a discussion of methods to address tobacco use with the cancer patient through accurate assessments and structured tobacco cessation support.

THE CLINICAL EFFECTS OF SMOKING ON THE CANCER PATIENT

Cancer treatment is generally defined according to disease site, stage, treatment type (e.g., surgery, chemotherapy [CT], radiotherapy [RT], or biologic therapy), and primary treatment objective, such as cure or palliation. A comprehensive discussion of the effects of smoking on cancer patients is beyond the scope of a single chapter, but the 2014 SGR provides an excellent evidence base, concluding that "the evidence is sufficient to infer a causal relationship between cigarette smoking and adverse health outcomes."[7] Overall, approximately 75% to 80% of studies in the SGR demonstrated a negative association between smoking and outcome, with approximately 65% to 70% of studies demonstrating statistically significant negative associations. This chapter will provide an illustrative review of studies that demonstrate the adverse effects of tobacco across disease sites and treatment modalities (e.g., surgery, CT, RT), and effects will be discussed across the categories of *mortality, recurrence and cancer-related mortality, toxicity,* and *risk of a second primary cancer.* Evidence for the benefits of smoking cessation will also be presented within each section.

The Effect of Smoking on Overall Mortality

Substantial evidence demonstrates that current smoking by cancer patients increases the risk of overall mortality across virtually all cancer disease sites and for all treatment modalities. Currently smoking significantly increased the risk of overall mortality by between 17% to 38% as compared with never, former, and recent quit smokers in a large cohort of patients across 13 disease sites.[71] Similar but larger observations were noted in elderly current smokers from a separate cohort (hazard ratio [HR], 1.72, 95% confidence interval [CI], 1.23 to 2.42).[72] A large analysis of over 20,000 patients treated with surgery demonstrated that current smoking increased mortality by 62% in gastrointestinal cancer patients and by 50% in thoracic cancer patients with a nonsignificant trend in urologic cancer patients.[73] Several larger studies with at least 500 patients demonstrated that current smoking increases mortality in head and neck cancer,[74–77] breast cancer,[78–81] gastrointestinal cancers,[82,83] prostate cancer,[84–87] renal cancer,[88] gynecologic cancers,[89,90] and lung cancer.[91–102] Smaller studies demonstrate similar effects for hematolymphoid cancers such as leukemia and lymphoma.[103,104] Studies suggest that the effects of current smoking on mortality may be dose and time dependent, with higher risks in heavier smokers[105,106] and lesser risks in patients whose time since quitting was longer.[105]

Whereas many reports rely on retrospective chart reviews, several prospective studies demonstrate that current smoking increases mortality.[71] Browman et al.[107] was one of the first prospective studies to demonstrate that current smoking increased mortality by 2.3-fold in patients who continued to smoke during RT as compared with nonsmokers. Results from Radiation Therapy Oncology Group (RTOG) 9003 and 0129 cooperative group trials demonstrated that current smoking increased mortality in advanced head and neck cancer patients treated with RT or concurrent chemoradiotherapy (CRT),[108] with a similar effect noted in 165 cervical cancer patients treated with CRT.[109] In the randomized retinoid chemoprevention trial of 1,190 early stage head and neck cancer patients, current smoking increased mortality by 2.5-fold.[110]

Numerous studies have demonstrated that current smoking increases overall mortality as compared with former and never smokers combined.[72,75,76,101,102,107,108] The adverse effects of smoking compared with former and never smokers not only reflect the negative effects of smoking on mortality as a whole, but also demonstrate that the effects of smoking are reversible. Current smoking increased mortality risk as compared with patients who quit within the year[71] or 1 to 3 months prior to diagnosis.[111,112] Furthermore, in 284 limited-stage small-cell lung cancer patients, patients who quit smoking at or following a cancer diagnosis had a 45% reduction in mortality as compared with current smokers.[113] These studies suggest that the effects of smoking on mortality are reversible.

Collectively, these studies provide significant data associating current smoking with increased overall mortality across most disease sites, tumor stages, treatment modalities, and in both traditionally tobacco-related as well as nontobacco-related cancers. The potential significance of smoking is perhaps best exemplified by Bittner et al.,[114] who analyzed causes of death in prostate cancer patients and demonstrated that more than 90% died of causes other than prostate cancer, but that current smoking increased the risks of non–prostate cancer deaths between 3- and 5.5-fold. As a result, tobacco use and cessation may be of paramount importance to cancers with high cure rates, such as prostate cancer or breast cancer, simply because patients may be at the most risk of death from noncancer-related causes such as heart disease, pulmonary disease, or other diseases related to smoking and tobacco use.

The Effect of Smoking on Cancer Recurrence and Cancer-Related Mortality

The primary objective of cancer therapy is to cure cancer and prevent recurrence. However, smoking has been shown to increase cancer recurrence and cancer-related mortality. Across a broad spectrum of cancer patients, current smoking increased cancer mortality as compared with former and never smokers.[71] Current smoking has been shown to increase cancer mortality in patients with head and neck cancer,[108,115–118] breast cancer,[78,119]

gastrointestinal cancers,[82,120,121] prostate cancer,[41,84,122] gynecologic cancers,[89,90,106,123–125] and lung cancer.[126] Cancer recurrence, whether local or metastatic, is a key driver behind cancer-related mortality. Several studies demonstrate that current smoking increases the risk of recurrence and decreases response across multiple disease sites.[76,84,107,127,128] The effects of smoking on increasing recurrence or cancer-related mortality have also been reported in several relatively rare cancers.[120,129] In a remarkable report of patients with recurrent head and neck cancers treated with salvage surgery, continued smoking after salvage treatment continued to increase the risk of yet another recurrence by 42%.[130] The striking nature of this last study highlights the continued risks even in recurrent cancer patients and the resilience with which some cancer patients will continue to smoke.

The effects of smoking are also noted in premalignant lesions. In patients with high-grade vulvar intraepithelial neoplasia, current smoking increased the risk of persistent disease after therapy by 30-fold.[131] In a prospective trial of progesterone to treat cervical intraepithelial neoplasia (CIN), current smoking increased the risk of progression as compared with former and never smokers combined.[132] A prospective trial of 516 low-grade cervical intraepithelial neoplasia patients demonstrated that current smoking decreased response by 36%, although a similar effect was also noted in former smokers.[133]

As noted with overall mortality, several studies demonstrated that the effects of current smoking are worse than the effects of former smoking[76,86,89,109,127,134–136,137] and that the effects of smoking may be acutely reversible. Several studies also demonstrate that current smoking increases recurrence or cancer mortality, whereas former smoking has no significant effect.[41,78,82,84,85,119,122–124,138] The acutely reversible effects of smoking were shown by Browman et al.[139] who demonstrated that continued smoking increased the risk of cancer-related mortality by 23% as compared with patients who quit within 12 weeks of starting RT. In 284 colorectal cancer patients, smoking at the first postoperative visit increased the risk of cancer mortality by 2.5-fold as compared with all other patients suggesting that smoking after treatment significantly predict for adverse outcome.[121] In a notable study of over 1,400 prostate cancer patients treated with surgery, continued smoking 1 year after treatment increased the risk of recurrence 2.3-fold, but quitting smoking 1 year after treatment did not confer an increased risk of recurrence.[128] Chen et al.[138] demonstrate that patients who continue to smoke before and following a bladder cancer diagnosis have an increased risk of recurrence as compared with patients who quit in the year prior to diagnosis or within the first 3 months after diagnosis. The reversible effects of smoking on recurrence and mortality are consistent with observations on overall mortality and continue to emphasize the benefit of tobacco cessation for cancer patients who smoke at diagnosis.

The Effect of Smoking on Cancer Treatment Toxicity

Discussion of the effects of smoking on cancer treatment toxicity is highly dependent upon disease site, treatment modality (e.g., surgery, CT, RT), and timing of toxicity. Across disease sites and treatments, current smoking has been shown to increase complications from surgery,[140–149] pulmonary complications,[150,151] toxicity from RT,[117,152–156] mucositis,[157] hospitalization,[158] and vasomotor symptoms.[159] One of the largest recent studies in over 20,000 gastrointestinal, pulmonary, and urologic patients demonstrates that former or current smoking increased the risk of surgical site infection, pulmonary complications, or 30-day mortality in a site-specific manner.[73] The effects of current smoking were most significant for pulmonary complications where former smoking had a lesser or nonsignificant effect. In 13,469 lung cancer patients treated with surgery, current smoking increased the risk of postoperative death with no increased risk in former smokers.[160] Current smoking increased the risk of complications, morbidity, or reoperation following esophagectomy, pancreatectomy, or colorectal surgery.[161–163] A study of 836 prostate cancer patients treated with RT demonstrated that current smoking increased abdominal cramps, rectal urgency, diarrhea, incomplete emptying, and sudden emptying between two- and nine-fold,[164] with similar effects noted in 3,489 cervical cancer patients who smoked more than 1 pack per day (PPD).[156]

Several studies have demonstrated that the effects of smoking on cancer treatment toxicity are reversible. Stopping smoking within 3 weeks of surgery reduced wound healing complications in esophageal cancer patients treated with surgery and reconstruction.[165] In 393 T1 laryngeal cancer patients treated with RT, quitting smoking after diagnosis reduced laryngeal complications as compared with continued smoking.[152] In a large study of 7,990 lung cancer patients from the Society of Thoracic Surgeons Database, current smoking increased the risk of pulmonary complications by 80% and hospital mortality 3.5-fold.[151] However, smoking cessation for 2 weeks eliminated the risks for pulmonary complications, and cessation for 1 month eliminated risks for hospital mortality. Vaporciyan et al.[166] also showed that current smoking increased the risk of pulmonary complications 2.7-fold as compared with smoking cessation for at least 1 month prior to surgery. In a striking example of the potentially reversible effects of smoking in 205 head and neck cancer patients treated with RT,[167] 43% of smoking patients treated in the morning experienced Grade 3+ mucositis compared with 72% of smokers treated in the afternoon (p = 0.04). These data suggest that reducing smoking overnight may yield a clinical benefit in reduced toxicity. Whereas all toxicity may not be acutely reversed, these encouraging data show that patients can make clinically meaningful improvements in their health and or cancer treatment within a short time frame by quitting smoking.

The Effect of Smoking on Risk of Second Primary Cancer

Several studies have reported the effects of smoking on the risk of developing a second primary cancer. Park et al.[168] reported on over 14,000 male cancer patients and demonstrated that current smoking increased the risk of developing a second tobacco-related primary cancer twofold, with no increased risk in former smokers. A higher risk was observed in in head and neck cancer patients who smoked more than 10 cigarettes per day, with no increased risk in lighter smokers.[169] Kinoshita et al.[170] showed an 82% increased risk of developing a second primary in gastric cancer patients who are current smokers with no increased risk in former smokers. In the phase III randomized trial of isotretinoin for the prevention of a second primary tumor in 1,190 head and neck cancer patients, current smoking increased the risk of a second primary by 2.2-fold with a nonsignificant trend of 1.6-fold in former smokers.[110] Notably, 39% of patients who reported quitting within the previous year were biochemically confirmed smokers.[171] As a result, these data collectively suggest that some of the increased risk may be biased by continued smoking in patients who deny smoking by self-report.

The effects of smoking on the risk of a second primary cancer are also noted in nontobacco-related cancers and in long-term survivors. In 835 breast cancer patients, smoking increased the risk for the development of lung metastases after breast cancer by more than threefold.[172] Ford et al.[173] demonstrated that breast cancer patients who were former smokers had a threefold increased risk of developing lung cancer, but that current smokers had a 13-fold increased risk. In nearly 1,100 estrogen receptor (ER)-positive breast cancer patients, current smokers had a 1.8-fold increased risk of developing a second contralateral breast cancer, and current smokers at most recent follow-up had a 2.2-fold increased risk, but former smoking at the diagnosis or most recent follow-up had no increased risk.[174] In 2,700 5-year survivors of testicular cancer,

current smokers had a 1.8-fold increased risk of developing a second primary as compared with all other survivors.[175]

There are some studies suggesting that smoking, combined with cytotoxic therapy, may have an additive or synergistic effect on the risk of developing a second primary cancer. In 9,780 prostate cancer patients from the Cancer of the Prostate Strategic Urologic Research Endeavor (CaPSURE) study, RT increased the risk of bladder cancer by 1.6-fold, smoking increased the risk by 2.1-fold, and smoking combined with RT increased risk by 3.7-fold.[176] In ER-positive breast cancer patients, treatment with RT had no significant effect on the risk of developing a contralateral breast cancer, but RT combined with current smoking increased the risk of contralateral cancer by ninefold.[173] In a detailed analysis of Hodgkin lymphoma patients, nonheavy smokers (defined as never, former, and less than one PPD) had a second primary relative risk of between fourfold and sevenfold when treated with CT or RT as compared with patients who received no RT or CT.[177] However, heavy smokers had a sixfold increased risk in the absence of RT and CT and a 17- to 49-fold increased risk when combined with RT and/or CT. These observations suggest that smoking combined with cytotoxic cancer therapy may complement the risk of developing a second primary cancer perhaps through the promotion of mutations induced by CT and/or RT in the presence of tobacco smoke. The potential mechanisms of this effect have not been tested or defined at this time, but the mechanism of tobacco-induced carcinogenesis in prior reports[3] supports these observations.

Human Papilloma Virus, Epidermal Growth Factor Receptor, Anaplastic Lymphoma Kinase, Programmed Cell Death Protein 1, and Smoking

Data over the past decade has shown that head and neck cancers that are human papilloma virus (HPV) positive are known to have an improved prognosis as compared with HPV-negative tumors.[178] Patients who have HPV-positive tumors typically have increased p16 expression and often respond better to conventional cancer therapy, including RT and CT. Many HPV-positive patients are never smokers or have a lighter smoking history. However, smoking was an independent adverse risk factor for both overall and cancer-related mortality with a 1% increase in risk per pack-year smoked.[178] Current smoking increased cancer mortality approximately fivefold even in p16-positive patients treated with surgery.[115] Smoking also increased the risk of developing second primary cancer in both HPV-positive and HPV-negative patients.[179] As a consequence, the presence of HPV does not appear to negate the adverse effects of smoking.

A similar effect is noted in lung cancer patients with epidermal growth factor receptor (EGFR)-mutated or anaplastic lymphoma kinase (ALK)-mutated tumors. As with HPV-positive head and neck cancer patients, lung cancer patients who are light or never smokers have a higher rate of EGFR-positive tumors that may respond to biologic therapy using EGFR tyrosine–kinase inhibitors. At this time, most information regarding EGFR-based therapy for lung cancer reports on the effects of ever smoking demonstrating that ever smokers have a decreased response to EGFR therapy. Early, large, randomized trials demonstrate that Tarceva (erlotinib) and Iressa (gefitinib) provide survival and tumor control benefits specifically in never smokers.[180,181] A very similar pattern is noted for ALK-positive patients with a much higher incidence in never smokers and high response rate to the ALK kinase inhibitor crizotinib.[182] Paik et al.[183] have described the importance of driver mutations in EGFR, ALK, and KRAS demonstrating that smokers have a higher preponderance for K-ras drivers, whereas nonsmokers tend to have EGFR or ALK driver mutations. In general, patients who are smokers may be best served with conventional cancer treatments rather than these biologic therapies, but randomized controlled trials confirming this suggestion are lacking at this time.

Although there are essentially no biologic therapies that have shown to have a better response in smokers, there are exciting data presented at the 2013 European CanCer Organization (ECCO) annual conference, suggesting that anti–programmed cell death protein 1 (PD-1)–based therapies may have a better response rate in smokers.[184] These very preliminary data have yet to be replicated or expanded into randomized trials, but if expanded trials prove effective, they may represent one of the only cancer treatments that may specifically benefit smokers.

Summarizing the Clinical Effects of Smoking on the Cancer Patient

Smoking by cancer patients increases mortality, toxicity, recurrence, and the risk of a second primary cancer. There are four important conclusions, and a fifth implied conclusion, to the evidence previously presented:

1. One or more adverse effects of smoking affect all cancer disease sites.
2. One or more adverse effects of smoking affect all treatment modalities.
3. The effects of current smoking are distinct from an ever or former smoking history.
4. Several lines of evidence demonstrate that many of the effects of smoking are reversible.

Although substantial data demonstrate that smoking by cancer patients increases the risk for one or more outcomes, the largest limitations are the lack of standard tobacco use definitions, the lack of assessing tobacco use in cancer patients at follow-up, and the lack of structured tobacco cessation for cancer patients. Importantly, patients may further misrepresent tobacco use. Several studies suggest that approximately 30% of cancer patients who smoke deny tobacco use.[171,185,186] Marin et al.[187] exemplify the importance of an accurate assessment, demonstrating that patients who self-reported smoking had no significant risk associated with surgical complications; however, biochemical confirmation of smoking significantly increased the risk of surgical wound complications. This highlights the potential discrepancy between the effects of smoking based on subjective versus biochemically confirmed assessments. Due to this discrepancy, the *fifth implied conclusion* is that the adverse effects of smoking and the benefits of cessation may be more pronounced than currently reported in the literature.

ADDRESSING TOBACCO USE BY THE CANCER PATIENT

National Oncology Association Statements and Clinical Practice Guidelines

Professional societies are taking leadership roles in recognizing the need to assess patients' tobacco use and to examine the effects of tobacco use in medical treatment, including the important role of tobacco cessation. The American Medical Association (AMA) passed a resolution supporting documentation of smoking behavior in clinical trials, from trial registration through treatment, follow-up, and to end of the study or death.[188] The Oncology Nursing Society (ONS) has also advocated for assessment and cessation.[189,190] Both the AACR[5,191] and ASCO[6,192] have issued policy statements specifically addressing tobacco use in cancer patients, detailing that clinicians have a responsibility to address tobacco use, that all patients should be screened, that all patients who use tobacco should receive evidence-based tobacco cessation support, and that tobacco use should be included in clinical practice and research. These provide strong counsel to address tobacco use in the general population as well as in cancer patients.

Smoking Cessation Guidelines

Overall, the approach to tobacco cessation for the cancer patient is very similar to the approach for the general population. However, there are a few specific details that are important to consider when approaching the cancer patient who smokes. It is important to recognize that virtually all newly diagnosed cancer patients are faced with a life-changing diagnosis that will require intensive treatment approaches. Treatments, toxicity, and outcomes differ according to disease site and treatment modality. Whereas some cancer patients may have a curable cancer, others may have incurable cancer. Smoking in cancer patients is also often associated with comorbid psychiatric diseases, such as depression, that may affect dependence.[193] The urgency of cessation is also important to consider. If smoking decreases the efficacy of cancer treatment, then every effort should be made to stop tobacco use as soon as possible rather than choosing a quit date several weeks or months after a cancer diagnosis. Patients may also be burdened with a "stigma" associated with certain tobacco-related cancers,[193–197] where they may be viewed by others, or themselves, as causing their cancer due to tobacco use. As a result, the rationale and motivation for quitting tobacco use likely differs among cancer patients, but there is a consistent theme that exists. (1) All patients should be asked about tobacco use with structured assessments; (2) all patients who use tobacco or are at risk for relapse should be offered evidence-based cessation support; and 3) tobacco assessment and cessation support should occur at the time of diagnosis, during treatment, and during follow-up for all cancer patients.

Empiric treatment of tobacco use by cancer patients is fundamentally supported by Public Health Service (PHS) Guidelines that are based on evidence from tobacco cessation efforts in noncancer patients. Originally issued in 1996 and renewed in 2008, *The Clinical Practice Guideline: Treating Tobacco Use and Dependence* is a PHS-sponsored, evidence-based guideline designed to assist health-care providers in delivering and supporting effective smoking cessation treatment.[198,199] The basic recommendation states that clinicians should consistently identify, document, and treat every tobacco user seen in a health-care setting. Details of cessation support range from brief to intensive intervention, but emphasize that consistent repeated cessation support and even brief counseling are effective methods to assist patients with stopping tobacco use. It is important to note that physician-delivered interventions significantly increase long-term abstinence rates.[199] Included are newer effective medication options and strong support for counseling and the use of quit lines as effective intervention strategies. As described in the PHS Guidelines, the principal steps in conducting effective smoking cessation interventions are referred to as The 5 A's:

1. *Ask* about tobacco use for every patient.
2. *Advise* every tobacco user to quit.
3. *Assess* the willingness of patients to quit.
4. *Assist* patients with quitting through counseling and pharmacotherapy.
5. *Arrange* follow-up cessation support, preferably within the first week after the quit date.

There is a strong evidence base for these interventions as documented in the clinical practice guideline.[199]

Implementing Smoking Cessation Into Clinical Practice

An algorithm is provided to guide clinicians in implementing the five A's into clinical cancer care (Fig. 31.1).[5,45,194,199] Included in the algorithm are suggested questions that are useful to accurately assess tobacco use by cancer patients where patients can generally be divided into *current, former,* or *never* smokers. The first step (ASK) is to inquire about and document tobacco use behaviors for every

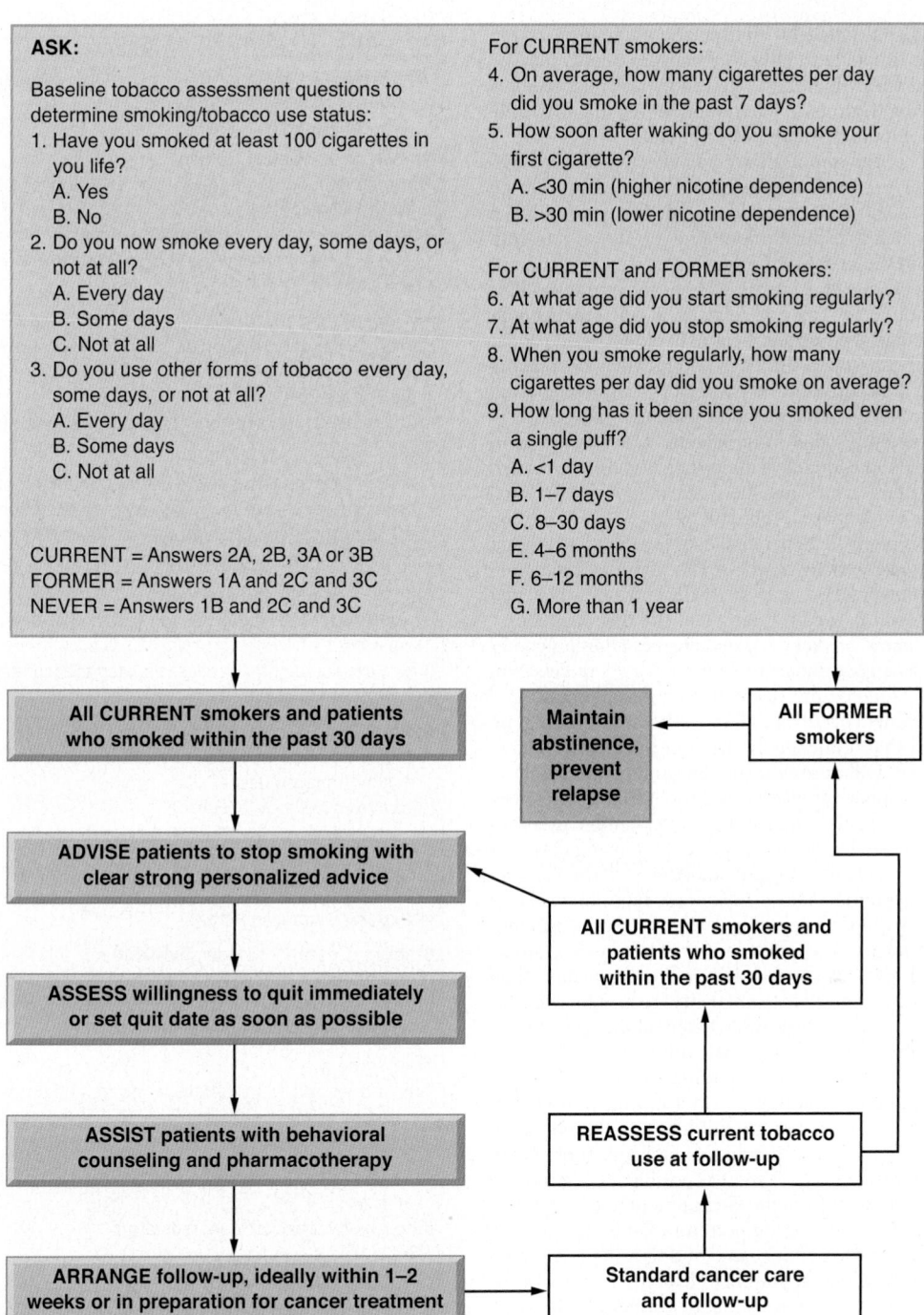

ASK:

Baseline tobacco assessment questions to determine smoking/tobacco use status:
1. Have you smoked at least 100 cigarettes in you life?
   A. Yes
   B. No
2. Do you now smoke every day, some days, or not at all?
   A. Every day
   B. Some days
   C. Not at all
3. Do you use other forms of tobacco every day, some days, or not at all?
   A. Every day
   B. Some days
   C. Not at all

CURRENT = Answers 2A, 2B, 3A or 3B
FORMER = Answers 1A and 2C and 3C
NEVER = Answers 1B and 2C and 3C

For CURRENT smokers:
4. On average, how many cigarettes per day did you smoke in the past 7 days?
5. How soon after waking do you smoke your first cigarette?
   A. <30 min (higher nicotine dependence)
   B. >30 min (lower nicotine dependence)

For CURRENT and FORMER smokers:
6. At what age did you start smoking regularly?
7. At what age did you stop smoking regularly?
8. When you smoke regularly, how many cigarettes per day did you smoke on average?
9. How long has it been since you smoked even a single puff?
   A. <1 day
   B. 1–7 days
   C. 8–30 days
   E. 4–6 months
   F. 6–12 months
   G. More than 1 year

All CURRENT smokers and patients who smoked within the past 30 days

Maintain abstinence, prevent relapse

All FORMER smokers

ADVISE patients to stop smoking with clear strong personalized advice

All CURRENT smokers and patients who smoked within the past 30 days

ASSESS willingness to quit immediately or set quit date as soon as possible

ASSIST patients with behavioral counseling and pharmacotherapy

REASSESS current tobacco use at follow-up

ARRANGE follow-up, ideally within 1–2 weeks or in preparation for cancer treatment

Standard cancer care and follow-up

Figure 31.1 This 5 A's screening and smoking cessation treatment schema for cancer patients may be integrated into clinical oncology practice.

patient at every visit including follow-up visits. Whereas a more comprehensive evaluation is necessary at the first consult, only updates to current tobacco use are needed at follow-up. Including smoking status assessments as a "vital sign" for all patients significantly increases the identification and treatment for patients.[200] Tobacco-use status stickers on paper charts or an automated reminder system for electronic records can increase compliance with tobacco assessments.[45] With the recent Meaningful Use standards that were implemented in 2011, hospitals using an electronic medical record (EMR) are essentially required to document tobacco use.[201] A recent report utilized the EMR to implement mandatory tobacco assessments in cancer patients demonstrating that just a few questions at the initial evaluation and at follow-up could yield high referral.

Less than 1% of referrals were delayed when assessments were repeated on a monthly basis rather than at every clinic visit.[45] These findings reduce the clinical burden and patient fatigue associated with repeated assessments as frequently as every day such as in patients who are treated with daily RT or CT.

At the time of this chapter release, there were no national guidelines for implementation of specific questions to assess tobacco use in cancer patients. However, Figure 31.1 provides effective questions for assessing tobacco use in cancer patients based on advice from published reports.[5,45,194,199] Current, former, and never smokers are identified in a structured manner. Patients who use tobacco within the past 30 days should have structured support to quit tobacco use, maintain abstinence, and prevent relapse.

CANCER PREVENTION AND SCREENING

Although not explicitly stated by any specific guidelines, asking about tobacco use in family members of cancer patients may be important because family members often support cancer patients during and following treatment, but continued smoking by family members can make quitting much more difficult.[202–204]

Advising is the second step in promoting effective tobacco cessation that involves giving clear, strong, and personalized advice to stop tobacco use. This advice should include the importance of quitting smoking, such as explicit information on the risks of continued smoking and the benefits of cessation for cancer treatment outcomes and overall health regardless of cancer diagnosis. This includes a discussion of how it is not "too late" to quit and that quitting will in fact benefit their cancer treatment efficacy and cancer outcome.[5] Patients can also consider the cost savings of stopping a smoking habit. Clinicians must be particularly sensitive to avoid contributing to any perceived blame for the patient's illness.[195–197,205] Clinicians must remember that most patients started smoking in adolescence and did not completely understand the risks associated with tobacco use. At the same time, the severe addiction associated with chronic tobacco use makes it difficult to stop.

The next step is *assessing* dependence and willingness to quit. Asking "How soon after waking do you smoke your first cigarette?" assesses nicotine dependence, with high dependence associated with a shorter interval between waking and the first cigarette.[206] Nicotine dependence is predictive of smoking cessation outcomes and can be used as a good indicator of the intensity of cessation treatment needed, such as the need for pharmacotherapy.[207,208] Determining the patient's motivation and interest in quitting are critical parameters that influence the types of intervention strategies to be employed. Different strategies for quitting are based on the transtheoretical model of change and motivational interviewing stance, which recognizes that unique intervention messages and strategies are needed to optimally promote smoking cessation based on a patient's readiness to quit smoking.[209,210] In the general population, recommendations encourage that clinicians set a target quit date within 30 days. However, for cancer patients, the reader is encouraged to consider an urgent need to stop smoking immediately. If patients are unable to quit immediately, then patients should be encouraged to immediately reduce tobacco use and to set a quit date as soon as possible based on the typical need to start cancer treatment in the immediate future.

Assisting patients with smoking cessation involves clinicians helping the patient design and implement a specific quit plan or broadly enhancing the motivation to quit tobacco. Promoting an effective quit strategy for cancer patients should consist of (1) setting a quit date (immediately or as soon as possible), (2) removing all tobacco-related products from the environment (e.g., cigarettes, ashtrays, lighters), (3) requesting support from family and friends, (4) discussing challenges to quitting, and (5) discussing or prescribing pharmacotherapy where appropriate. Patients should also be provided information on cessation support services (Table 31.1). In the cancer setting, patients can also be informed that smoking cessation is a critical component of cancer care over which they have complete control, thereby conferring some personal control over their cancer care.

Patients who are unwilling to quit should continue to receive repeated assessments and counseling to help motivate patients to quit smoking. These patients should be encouraged to make immediate reductions in tobacco use and work toward abstinence as soon as possible. Clinician education, reassurance, and gentle encouragement can help them to consider changing their smoking behaviors. Specific strategies include discussing the personal relevance of smoking and benefits to cessation, providing support and acknowledging the difficulty of quitting, educating patients about the positive consequences of quitting smoking, and discussing available pharmacologic methods to assist with quitting.[211] The emphasis should be placed on patient autonomy to quit. Motivational strategies for patients unwilling to quit can be employed (e.g., asking open-ended questions, providing affirmations,

TABLE 31.1

Additional Tobacco Cessation Resources for Patients and Clinicians[a]

American Association for Cancer Research
Information about the adverse effects of tobacco and advocacy for tobacco control
(http://www.aacr.org/home/public--media/science-policy--government-affairs/science-policy--government-affairs-committee/tobacco-and-cancer.aspx)

American Cancer Society
A national cancer organization providing brochures and fact sheets on the health effects of tobacco and resources for smoking cessation
(http://www.cancer.org/cancer/cancercauses/tobaccocancer/)

American Legacy Foundation
A national independent public health foundation offering programs to help people quit and resources about the health effects of tobacco use
(http://www.legacyforhealth.org/)

American Society of Clinical Oncology
Resources for tobacco cessation with an emphasis on cancer patients
(http://www.asco.org/practice-research/tobacco-cessation-and-control-resources)

Centers for Disease Control and Prevention
A collection of online resources, information, and materials about quitting tobacco use
(http://www.cdc.gov/TOBACCO/)

North American Quitline Consortium
Information on local and national cessation quitlines,
1-800-QUIT-NOW
(http://www.naquitline.org/)

Smoking Cessation Leadership Center
A collaborative dedicated to disseminating knowledge about the health effects of tobacco and assistance in cessation
(http://smokingcessationleadership.ucsf.edu/)

Smokefree.gov
Tips and resources for people trying to stop smoking
(http://smokefree.gov/)

Tobacco Free Nurses
An organization aimed at engaging nurses in tobacco cessation efforts
(http://www.tobaccofreenurses.org/)

U.S. Department of Health & Human Services, Surgeon General.gov
Tobacco use and cessation information from the Surgeon General
(http://www.surgeongeneral.gov/initiatives/tobacco/index.html)

World Health Organization
An international organization tasked with implementing and monitoring public health with a focus on tobacco control
(http://www.who.int/topics/tobacco/en/)

[a] Current as of December 2013.

reflective listening, summarizing).[198,210,212,213] Table 31.2 provides suggested methods to help clinicians promote tobacco cessation.

The final step in a clinician-delivered smoking cessation intervention involves *arranging* a follow-up contact with the patient. Ideally, cancer patients will follow an immediate quit strategy and follow-up should occur preferably within 1 to 2 weeks. However, a short-term follow-up may also benefit patients who are reluctant to quit smoking. The clinician must remember that a new cancer diagnosis is stressful and patients may rely on continued smoking to

TABLE 31.2

Select Treatment Strategies Used for Tobacco Cessation Treatments

Provide and monitor the use of nicotine replacement or other pharmacotherapy.

Provide education regarding the health effects of tobacco use and its addictive and relapsing nature.

Identify and change environmental and psychological cues for tobacco use.

Generate alternative behaviors for tobacco use.

Assist in optimization of social support for cessation efforts and address tobacco use in family members.

Prevent relapse including the identification of future high-risk situations and plans for specific behaviors in those situations.

Provide motivational interventions as needed throughout treatment.

Identify relaxation techniques such as guided imagery and progressive muscle relaxation.

Provide behavioral strategies to address depressed mood (e.g., increasing pleasurable activities).

Provide crisis intervention including appropriate referrals and emergency intervention if indicated.

Recognize and congratulate patients on success with reducing and/or quitting smoking.

relieve stress, but after absorbing the psychological effects of a new cancer diagnosis, patients may be more receptive to smoking cessation. During follow-up, clinicians should congratulate patients on successful cessation efforts, discuss accomplishments and setbacks, and assess pharmacotherapy use and problems. Patients should not be criticized for returning to smoking; rather, it is critical to create a supportive environment for patients to communicate progress, failure, and personal needs. Framing relapses as a learning experience can be helpful, and patients should be encouraged to set another quit date. Referrals to a psychologist or professionally trained smoking cessation counselor should be considered for patients with numerous unsuccessful quit attempts, comorbid depression, anxiety, additional substance abuse disorders, or inadequate social support.

Clinicians who are not well versed in tobacco cessation should realize that smoking is an extremely difficult addiction to overcome and should recognize the clinical pattern associated with cessation. As patients stop smoking, many will experience symptoms of withdrawal, including dry or sore throat, constipation, cravings to smoke, irritability, anxiety, trouble concentrating, restlessness, increased appetite, depression, and insomnia. In the first few weeks, patients may also report an increase in mucous secretions from the airways, a cough, and other upper respiratory tract symptoms. Patients and clinicians should realize that tobacco cessation requires a concerted effort, may require repeated attempts, and symptoms will not resolve immediately. Clinicians should counsel patients on a repeated basis, recognize success, and provide repeated assistance if patients relapse.

Pharmacologic Treatment for Smoking Cessation

The principles of pharmacotherapy to help patients quit smoking are fundamentally based on reducing the craving associated with nicotine withdrawal. Nicotine replacement therapy (NRT), in the form of patches, lozenges, inhalers, sprays, and gum, varenicline (Chantix), and bupropion (Zyban) are the three principal first-line pharmacotherapies recommended for use either alone or in combination according to PHS Guidelines.[199] Table 31.3 presents information on these first-line agents. Nicotine is the primary addictive substance in tobacco and NRT facilitates smoking cessation by reducing craving and withdrawal that smokers experience during abstinence. NRT also weans smokers off nicotine by providing a lower level and, in some cases, slower infusion of nicotine than smoking.[214] Strong evidence from over 100 randomized clinical trials support the use of NRT to increase the odds of quitting approximately twofold as compared with placebo.[215] Pooled analyses demonstrate that 17% of smokers receiving NRT were able to quit versus 10% with placebo after at least 6 months. Recent evidence further shows that combination therapy, or dual NRT (such as a nicotine patch and lozenge), is a very effective smoking cessation therapy that produces high quit rates.[216,217] Data suggest that activation of the nicotinic acetylcholine receptor (nAChR) may promote tumor development,[218] but evidence suggests that the negative aspects of smoking outweigh these concerns.[219,220] Furthermore, there are no clinical trials reporting negative outcomes for NRT in cancer patients as related to mortality or recurrence. Studies also demonstrate that NRT is not associated with an increased risk of carcinogenesis in the general population.[221,222] As a result, NRT should be used as a clinically proven method to help cancer patients stop smoking.

Antidepressants have been studied as non-nicotine–based pharmacotherapy in part due to depression and psychiatric disease being comorbid conditions in smokers.[223] Bupropion (Zyban) is currently the only FDA-approved antidepressant for the treatment of tobacco dependence.[199] Bupropion inhibits the reuptake of both dopamine and norepinephrine, thereby increasing dopamine and norepinephrine concentrations in the mesolimbic systems.[12,224] Bupropion also antagonizes the nAChR, thereby lowering the rewarding effects of nicotine.[225] Should an abstinent smoker relapse, bupropion may function to reduce the pleasure of cigarette smoking experienced by the smoker[226] and help to prevent further relapse. A meta-analysis found that smokers who received bupropion were twice as likely as those who received placebo to have achieved long-term abstinence at either a 6- or 12-month follow-up.[227]

Varenicline (Chantix) is a α4β2 nAChR partial agonist that produces sustained dopamine release in the mesolimbic system that received FDA approval for treating tobacco dependence in 2006. Sustained dopamine release maintains a normal systemic level of the neurotransmitter, which helps to reduce craving and withdrawal during abstinence.[228] Varenicline also antagonizes the rewarding effects of nicotine. Because varenicline attenuates the pleasure smokers experience from smoking, it may decrease motivation to smoke and protect them from relapse. One of the initially reported randomized clinical trials that compared varenicline (2 mg), bupropion (300 mg), and placebo showed that varenicline was superior to bupropion and placebo, with overall continuous abstinence rates between 10% to 23%.[229] A meta-analysis demonstrated that the 1-mg daily dose approximately doubled, whereas the 2-mg daily dose approximately tripled the likelihood of long-term abstinence at 6 months as compared to placebo.[199] As a result, the 1-mg daily dose can be considered as an alternative should the patient experience significant dose-related side effects. Several meta-analyses have shown that varenicline is superior to bupropion and placebo in the general population.[230–233]

In July 2009, the FDA issued a warning after reports that some patients attempting to quit smoking while using varenicline or bupropion experienced unusual changes in behavior, depressed mood, worsening of depression, or had thoughts of suicide. This has prompted recommendations that health-care providers elicit information about a patient's psychiatric history prior to prescribing varenicline or bupropion to closely monitor changes in mood and behavior during the course of treatment. However,

TABLE 31.3

First-Line Pharmacotherapy Agents for the Treatment of Nicotine Depedence

Agent	Dose	Mechanism	Use
Nicotine Replacement			
Transdermal (patches)	16 h or 24 h 7, 14, or 21 mg 1 patch/d	Steady state NRT to reduce craving and withdrawal	6–10 CPD: 14 mg daily × 8 wks then 7 mg daily × 2 wks >10 CPD: 21 mg daily × 6 wks, then 14 mg × 2 wks, then 7 mg × 2 wks
Gum	2 or 4 mg Max: 24 pieces/d	Short-term NRT to reduce craving and withdrawal	First cigarette >30 min after waking: 2 mg PO q1–2 hr First cigarette <30 min after waking: 4 mg PO q1–2 hr
Lozenge	2 or 4 mg Max: 20 lozenges/d	Short-term NRT to reduce craving and withdrawal	1st cigarette >30 min after waking: 2 mg PO q1–2 hr 1st cigarette <30 min after waking: 4 mg PO q1–2 hr
Nasal spray	0.5 mg/spray Max:10 sprays/hr or 80 sprays/d	Short-term NRT to reduce craving and withdrawal	1 spray/nostril q1–5 hr
Inhaler	4 mg/cartridge Max: 16 cartridges/d	Short-term NRT to reduce craving and withdrawal	1 cartridge inhaled over 20 min q1.5–6 hr
Bupropion (Zyban)	150 mg	Block nicotinic receptors and reduces reward	1 tablet daily × 3 d, then 1 tablet twice daily for 7–12 wks
Varenicline (Chantix)	0.5 or 1 mg	Dopaminergic reward and partial nicotinic receptor antagonist	0.5 mg daily × 3 d, then 0.5 mg twice daily × 3 d, then 1 mg twice daily

CPD, cigarettes per day; PO, by mouth; NRT, nicotine replacement therapy.

updated recent safety studies examining very large databases (one database of N = 119,546, one database of N = 35,800) regarding safety have shown no difference in neuropsychiatric side effects between varenicline or bupropion as compared to NRT and no increased risk of depression.[234,235] Another prospective study showed no adverse events when treating participants with current or past major depression and also showed higher abstinence rates for the varenicline group as compared to placebo at weeks 9 to 52 (20.3% versus 10.4%, p <0.001).[236] Varenicline should be considered a viable cessation pharmacotherapy for cancer patients.

The clinical practice guideline also identifies two non-nicotine–based medications—clonidine and nortriptyline—as second-line pharmacotherapies for tobacco dependence. A second-line agent is used when a smoker cannot use first-line medications due to either contraindications or lack of effectiveness. Both clonidine, an antihypertensive, and nortriptyline, a tricyclic antidepressant, have been shown to effectively assist smokers achieve abstinence.[227,237] Unfortunately, many patients who quit will eventually relapse, and rates of long-term abstinence remain low. Because smoking poses enormous health risks to individuals and their families, even a modest reduction in smoking may translate into a significant impact on public health. Clinicians should continue to encourage recalcitrant smokers to stop tobacco use and use pharmacotherapy where appropriate with repeated quit attempts.

Empirically Tested Cessation Interventions with Cancer Patients

The overwhelming majority of cessation research has been performed in the general population, but there are several studies that have been performed in cancer patients. Gritz et al.[238] conducted the first physician- or dentist-delivered randomized cessation intervention comparison in 186 newly diagnosed head and neck cancer patients. Patients were treated with either minimal advice or an enhanced intervention with trained clinicians consisting of strong personalized advice to stop smoking, a contracted quit date, tailored written materials, and booster advice sessions. No significant differences were found between treatments, but a 70.2% continuous abstinence rate was found at 12-month follow-up regardless of treatment condition, suggesting that many cancer patients can benefit from brief physician-delivered advice. A later study by Schnoll et al.,[239] comparing cognitive behavioral treatment with standardized health education advice, also failed to find significant differences in quit rates. All patients received NRT, and quit rates in both groups approached 50% at 1-month follow-up and 40% at 3-month follow-up.

Additional studies, ranging from 15 to 80 patients, examined nurse-delivered cessation interventions for a variety of cancer patients. The lowest cessation rates were found with a single session intervention: a 21% cessation rate in the intervention group versus 14% in the usual care group 6 weeks' postintervention.[240] Higher cessation rates were associated with a more intensive intervention consisting of three inpatient visits, supplementary materials, and five postdischarge follow-up contacts. Additional studies demonstrate higher cessation rates with more intensive intervention (40% to 75%) as compared with usual care (43% to 50%), suggesting more intensive interventions may yield higher cessation rates.[241–243] In general, more intense interventions appear to be more efficacious, but even brief advice is important to achieve tobacco cessation.

In a randomized trial of 432 cancer patients coordinated by the Eastern Cooperative Oncology Group (ECOG) with a physician-delivered intervention (comprised of cessation advice, optional NRT, and written materials) or usual care (unstructured advice from physicians), there were no significant intervention effects and generally low abstinence rates (12% to 15%

at 6 to 12 months).[244] However, patients with head and neck or lung cancer were significantly more likely to have quit smoking compared to patients with tumors that were not smoking related. Analyses of outcomes from the Mayo Clinic Nicotine Dependence Center found that although lung cancer patients were more likely to achieve 6-month tobacco abstinence than controls (22% versus 14%), no significant differences were observed after adjusting for covariates.[245] Garces et al.[246] also found no significant differences in abstinence rates between head and neck cancer patients and controls (33% versus 26%). However, higher abstinence rates were found for both head and neck and lung cancer patients treated within 3 months of diagnosis compared to those treated for more than 3 months after the diagnosis, emphasizing the potential importance of the *teachable moment* at the time of the cancer diagnosis.

The potential importance of addressing smoking combined with considering comorbid disease has been noted in a few studies. In a randomized head and neck cancer patients of usual care versus 9 to 11 sessions of a nurse-administered intervention consisting of cognitive-behavioral therapy and medications, targeting comorbid smoking, drinking, and depression significantly increased quit rates at 6-month follow-up for the intervention group compared to the usual control group (47% versus 31%, p <0.05).[247] In a randomized trial of 246 cancer patients treated with 9 weeks of NRT with or without bupropion, there was no significant difference with the addition of bupropion to NRT, but in patients with depressive symptoms, bupropion increased abstinence rates, lowered withdrawal, and improved quality of life.[248] Patients without depression symptoms did equally well when treated with bupropion versus transdermal nicotine and counseling alone.

Patient recruitment has been a problem noted by some studies, including 5.5 years to accrue 246 patients with telephone screening of over 7,500 potential patients.[249] A pilot trial of varenicline in thoracic oncology patients required screening 1,130 patients to accrue 49 participants randomized to a 12-week course of either varenicline or placebo paired with a behavioral counseling platform of seven sessions.[250] A randomized trial of 185 smoking cancer patients comparing the efficacy of a hospital-based standard care smoking cessation model versus standard care augmented by a behavioral tapering regimen via a handheld device before inpatient hospitalization for cancer surgery demonstrated no difference in quit rates (both 32%,).[251] However, over 29,000 patients were screened to conduct a randomized clinical trial with a smoking cancer patient population. These studies highlight the potential difficulty recruiting participants who smoke, including considerations for the importance of medical comorbidity in guiding smoking cessation treatment, patient mix (multiple tumor sites), treatment status (awaiting treatment to completed treatment), variation in stage of disease, and considering how psychiatric conditions such as depression reflect the difficulty of conducting research in the oncology setting and the importance of these variables in future studies.

Although accruing patients to intervention trials may seem discouraging, several studies demonstrate the benefit of counseling over self-help. Emmons et al.[252] conducted a randomized controlled trial in 796 young adult survivors of pediatric cancer that included six calls, tailored and targeted written materials, and optional NRT as compared with self-help. Significantly higher quit rates were found in the counseling group compared to the self-help group at all reported follow-up time points, including 12 months (15% versus 9%; p <0.01). A randomized trial of a motivational interviewing-based smoking cessation intervention in a south Australian hospital was delivered over a 3-month period, consisted of multiple contacts with a trained counselor, and provided supplementary material tailored to cancer patients with NRT.[253] The control group received brief advice to quit and generic supplementary material. Quit rates did not differ by treatment group (5% to 6% at 3-month follow-up), but the intervention group was significantly more likely to report attempts to quit smoking.

Current Tobacco Assessment and Cessation Support by Oncologists

Access to cessation support is critical to address tobacco use by cancer patients. A recent survey of 58 NCI-designated cancer centers indicated that about 80% reported a tobacco use program available to their patients and about 60% routinely offered educational materials, but less than 50% had a designated individual who provided services.[254] A recent survey of over 1,500 members of the International Association for the Study of Lung Cancer (IASLC)[255] and a parallel study of 1,197 ASCO members[256] observed that approximately 90% of physicians believe that tobacco affects outcomes, tobacco cessation should be a standard part of cancer care, and approximately 80% regularly advise patients to stop using tobacco, but only approximately 40% discuss medications or assist with quitting. Dominant perceived barriers to cessation support were patient resistance to treatment, an inability to get patients to quit, a lack of cessation resources, and a lack of clinician education. These data showed that even motivated clinicians are not regularly providing tobacco cessation support. A recent survey of 155 actively accruing cooperative group clinical trials further demonstrated that only 29% of active trials collected any tobacco use information, 4.5% collected any tobacco use information at follow-up, and none addressed tobacco cessation.[55] Few oncology meetings offer educational workshops or talks, and they are often poorly attended when they are offered.[257] Collectively, these data demonstrate that oncologists are not regularly providing cessation support and that we are not capturing tobacco use information that may be critical to understanding the effects of tobacco on cancer treatment outcomes.

More in-person talks as well as written and Web-based training should be made available, as well as new approaches that move from the traditional 5 A's model delivered by a single professional to referral systems that efficiently connect tobacco users to multiple resources for tobacco cessation.[258–260] The *ASCO Prevention Curriculum* has a chapter devoted to educating oncology healthcare professionals on the evaluation and treatment of tobacco use.[213] Innovative curricula, such as the Texas Tobacco Outreach Education Program (TOEP), are available and can facilitate program development in other states.[261] However, specialty programs in tobacco cessation treatment that are based in cancer centers and other medical centers are valuable resources that need to be further developed.

Addressing tobacco use in cancer patients may be approached in a systematic and efficient manner. A recent report highlighted the potential utility of automated tobacco assessment and smoking cessation using structured assessments in the EMR where all patients were automatically referred to a dedicated cessation program consisting of phone-based cessation support.[45] In 2,700 patients referred for cessation support, half received only a mailing and only 1% contacted the cessation program. However, in the arm with at least five phone call attempts made by the cessation service, 81% of patients were successfully contacted and only 3% refused cessation support. Furthermore, assessments implemented every 4 weeks, rather than more frequent assessments every 2 weeks, resulted in delayed cessation referrals in less than 1% of smokers. This is the first report to try and identify clinically efficient mechanisms of addressing tobacco use that may be useful in clinical practice or research that may be an effective method of increasing patient participation in cessation support, but substantial work is needed to assess who may benefit from low versus high intensity support in such a program.

Examples of Model Tobacco Treatment Programs

Several dedicated tobacco treatment programs at cancer centers have been developed. Table 31.4 contrasts the core elements of

TABLE 31.4

Attributes of Prototypical Tobacco Treatment Programs

Attribute	MDACC	RPCI	Yale	MSKCC
Tobacco assessment of all patients (EMR)	Yes	Yes	Yes	Yes
Automatic referral of all patients	Yes	Yes	No	Yes
In-person counseling	Yes	No	Yes	Yes
Telephone counseling	Yes	Yes	No	Yes
Medications prescribed	Yes	No	Yes	Yes
Biochemical confirmation (CO) testing	Yes	No	Yes	No
Free to patient	Yes	Yes	No	Yes
Third-party payment	No	No	Yes	Yes
Research studies of new treatments	Yes	Yes	Yes	Yes

MDACC, M.D. Anderson Cancer Center, Houston, TX; RPCI, Roswell Park Cancer Institute, Buffalo, NY; Yale, Yale University Hospital, Smilow Cancer Center, New Haven, CT; MSKCC, Memorial Sloan Kettering Cancer Center, New York, NY.

four active model programs at the end of 2013 (University of Texas M.D. Anderson Cancer Center, Roswell Park Cancer Institute, Yale Cancer Center, and Memorial Sloan Kettering Cancer Center), each of which employ different methods to help cancer patients quit smoking. All programs follow the evidence-based 5 A's model described previously from PHS Guidelines.[199] All programs were made available to patients at their respective medical centers and are now designed to evaluate and treat all patients who self-report current tobacco use. Importantly, not all cancer centers can treat smoking cessation in the same manner. Financing of a cessation program is critical and may include institutional funds, state funds, research funds, and third-party billing. Notably, given the broad spectrum of adverse health effects associated with smoking, cancer centers should carefully consider the potential health benefits and cost savings associated with tobacco cessation due to reductions in treatment complications and recurrence associated with smoking by cancer patients. There is no one "correct" way to create and sustain a tobacco treatment program at a cancer center, but at the very least and consistent with evidence, rigorous behavioral counseling should be provided and, if possible, medication management as well.

FUTURE CONSIDERATIONS

Research Considerations

The past several years have shown a surge in activities identifying the effects of tobacco in cancer patients and increasing awareness is being developed for cessation support at cancer centers as well as through several national organizations. There are three fundamental areas of research that need to be expanded:

1. *Evaluating the effects of tobacco use and cessation on clinical cancer outcomes.* The 2014 SGR concluded that smoking caused adverse outcomes in cancer patients,[7] but several limitations remain. Tobacco-use definitions should be standardized and implemented at diagnosis, during treatment, and follow-up. Biochemical confirmation with cotinine or exhaled carbon monoxide may improve the accuracy of tobacco assessment in at-risk groups such as current smokers who are trying to quit or patients who reported quitting in the past year.[171,185,186,262] Although smoking is the predominant form of tobacco consumption, all tobacco products should be considered. A further understanding of the effects of tobacco on the efficacy and toxicity of cancer treatment, tumor response, quality of life, survival, recurrence,

compliance, second primary, and noncancer-related comorbidity is needed. All cancer disease sites and stages are important to consider.

2. *Understanding the effects of tobacco and cessation on cancer biology.* Although not a primary focus of this chapter, tobacco and tobacco-related products increase tumor growth, angiogenesis, migration, invasion and metastasis and decrease response to conventional cancer treatments such as CT and RT. These and other areas are important to consider, including the potential effects on immune-related therapy and vaccine development. *In vivo* models of exposure and cancer response are not well developed, yet are critical to this research area. Work is also needed to assess the effect of emerging tobacco-related products such as e-cigarettes.

3. *Advance understanding of models to increase access to cessation support and increase efficacy of tobacco cessation methods for cancer patients.* This diverse area includes assessing the timing of intervention, intensity, duration, follow-up, and the potential effects of harm-reduction strategies. Cessation pharmacology requires additional consideration in combination with unique approaches to motivational and behavioral counseling in cancer patients. Significant work is needed to disseminate evidence-based cessation support and to assess the cost-effectiveness of different cessation strategies, particularly with regard to improving the cost of cancer care as a whole. Preventing relapse and evaluating the safety of transition to alternative products such as e-cigarettes is equally important and increasingly complex with the addition of new tobacco-related products. Identifying and addressing barriers to effective cessation support is also needed. As related to the cancer patient, clinicians and cessation specialists should consider how their research relates to cancer care. Taking advantage of new integrated medical management systems presents a significant opportunity to improve cessation support access as well as to develop a more effective tracking of patient outcomes.

Policy Implications and Systematic Issues

Several national and international organizations have emphasized the importance of tobacco assessments and cessation for the general population and for cancer patients that include tools to evaluate tobacco use at diagnosis, during treatment, and follow-up appointments, as well as routine support for smoking cessation.[5,6,188–191] In 2012, ASCO, with the contribution of the American Legacy Foundation, published a Tobacco Cessation Toolkit for the oncology setting.[263] This evidence-based guideline intends to help oncology providers integrate tobacco cessation strategies into their patient care. Utilization of the EMR and standardized, automated systems for more efficacious and efficient access to tobacco cessation support has also been suggested,[45] but requires participation by clinicians, institutions, insurers, and health departments. Not only should providers be aware of the need for tobacco cessation and available interventions, but health-care institutions must also build such treatment into their overall system of care. Thus, the identification of patients who smoke or use any alternative tobacco product, referral or direct treatment by providers, billing and reimbursement for treatment provided, and consistent efforts from professional oncology organizations are critically important.[257] The

tremendous public health burden from tobacco-related disability and death has not been countered by a proportional level of funding in tobacco control, cancer treatment research, or public advocacy. Researchers, clinicians, and advocates must come together to persuade policy makers to increase funding in tobacco-related research, treatment, and policy initiatives on behalf of healthy individuals and patients. A united front is critically needed in support of a common agenda that includes both increased tobacco-control efforts and additional funding for disease-related research and treatment. With clinical rationale, guidelines, and advocacy in place, the final steps in effective tobacco control and improving health outcomes are to implement these recommendations into practice.

SELECTED REFERENCES

The full reference list can be accessed at lwwhealthlibrary.com/oncology.

1. U.S. Department of Health, Education, and Welfare. *Smoking and Health: Report of the Advisory Committee to the Surgeon General of the Public Health Service.* PHS Publication No. 1103. Washington, D.C.: U.S. Department of Health, Education, and Welfare, Public Health Service, Center for Disease Control; 1964.
2. Office of the Surgeon General, Office on Smoking and Health. *The Health Consequences of Smoking. A Report of the Surgeon General.* Atlanta: Centers for Disease Control and Prevention; 2004.
3. Centers for Disease Control and Prevention, National Center for Chronic Disease Prevention and Health Promotion, Office on Smoking and Health. *How Tobacco Smoke Causes Disease: The Biology and Behavioral Basis for Smoking-Attributable Disease: A Report of the Surgeon General.* Atlanta: Centers for Disease Control and Prevention; 2010.
5. Toll BA, Brandon TH, Gritz ER, et al. Assessing tobacco use by cancer patients and facilitating cessation: an American Association for Cancer Research policy statement. *Clin Cancer Res* 2013;19:1941–1948.
6. Hanna N, Mulshine J, Wollins DS, et al. Tobacco cessation and control a decade later: American society of clinical oncology policy statement update. *J Clin Oncol* 2013;31:3147–3157.
7. U.S. Department of Health and Human Services. *The Health Consequences of Smoking—50 Years of Progress: A Report of the Surgeon General.* Atlanta: U.S. Department of Health and Human Services, Centers for Disease Control and Prevention, National Center for Chronic Disease Prevention and Health Promotion, Office on Smoking and Health; 2014.
9. Benowitz NL. Nicotine addiction. *N Engl J Med.* 2010;362:2295–2303.
24. Warren GW, Cummings KM. Tobacco and lung cancer: risks, trends, and outcomes in patients with cancer. In: *American Society of Clinical Oncology 2013 Educational Book.* 201;359–364. ASCO University Web site. http://meetinglibrary.asco.org//content/200-132. Accessed November 25, 2013.
25. Thun MJ, Carter BD, Feskanich D, et al. 50-year trends in smoking-related mortality in the United States. *N Engl J Med.* 2013;368:351–364.
27. Cummings KM, Dresler CM, Field JK, et al. E-cigarettes and cancer patients. *J Thorac Oncol* 2014;9:438–441.
36. Gritz ER. Smoking and smoking cessation in cancer patients. *Br J Addict* 1991;86:549–554.
45. Warren GW, Marshall JR, Cummings KM, et al. Automated tobacco assessment and cessation support for cancer patients. *Cancer* 2014;120:562–569.
48. Gritz ER, Nisenbaum R, Elashoff RE, et al. Smoking behavior following diagnosis in patients with stage I non-small cell lung cancer. *Cancer Causes Control* 1991;2:105–112.
55. Peters EN, Torres E, Toll BA, et al. Tobacco assessment in actively accruing National Cancer Institute Cooperative Group Program Clinical Trials. *J Clin Oncol* 2012;30:2869–2875.
56. Land SR. Methodologic barriers to addressing critical questions about tobacco and cancer prognosis. *J Clin Oncol* 2012;30:2030–2032.
57. Gritz ER, Dresler C, Sarna L. Smoking, the missing drug interaction in clinical trials: ignoring the obvious. *Cancer Epidemiol Biomarkers Prev* 2005;14:2287–2293.
71. Warren GW, Kasza K, Reid M, et al. Smoking at diagnosis and survival in cancer patients. *Int J Cancer* 2013;132:401–410.
73. Gajdos C, Hawn MT, Campagna EJ, et al. Adverse effects of smoking on postoperative outcomes in cancer patients. *Ann Surg Oncol* 2012;19:1430–1438.
80. Holmes MD, Murin S, Chen WY, et al. Smoking and survival after breast cancer diagnosis. *Int J Cancer* 2007;120:2672–2677.
84. Kenfield SA, Stampfer MJ, Chan JM, et al. Smoking and prostate cancer survival and recurrence. *JAMA* 2011;305:2548–2555.
107. Browman GP, Wong G, Hodson I, et al. Influence of cigarette smoking on the efficacy of radiation therapy in head and neck cancer. *N Engl J Med* 1993;328:159–163.
108. Gillison ML, Zhang Q, Jordan R, et al. Tobacco smoking and increased risk of death and progression for patients with p16-positive and p16-negative oropharyngeal cancer. *J Clin Oncol* 2012;30:2102–2111.

110. Khuri FR, Lee JJ, Lippman SM, et al. Randomized phase III trial of low-dose isotretinoin for prevention of second primary tumors in stage I and II head and neck cancer patients. *J Natl Cancer Inst* 2006;98:441–450.
114. Bittner N, Merrick GS, Galbreath RW, et al. Primary causes of death after permanent prostate brachytherapy. *Int J Radiat Oncol Biol Phys* 2008;72:433–440.
166. Vaporciyan AA, Merriman KW, Ece F, et al. Incidence of major pulmonary morbidity after pneumonectomy: association with timing of smoking cessation. *Ann Thorac Surg* 2002;73:420–425.
167. Bjarnason GA, Mackenzie RG, Nabid A, et al. Comparison of toxicity associated with early morning versus late afternoon radiotherapy in patients with head-and-neck cancer: a prospective randomized trial of the National Cancer Institute of Canada Clinical Trials Group (HN3). *Int J Radiat Oncol Biol Phys* 2009;73:166–172.
177. Travis LB, Gospodarowicz M, Curtis RE, et al. Lung cancer following chemotherapy and radiotherapy for Hodgkin's disease. *J Natl Cancer Inst* 2002;94:182–192.
185. Morales N, Romano M, Cummings KM, et al. Accuracy of self-reported tobacco use in newly diagnosed cancer patients. *Cancer Causes Control* 2013;24:1223–1230.
186. Warren GW, Arnold SM, Valentino JP, et al. Accuracy of self-reported tobacco assessments in a head and neck cancer treatment population. *Radiother Oncol* 2012;103:45–48.
187. Marin VP, Pytynia KB, Langstein HN, et al. Serum cotinine concentration and wound complications in head and neck reconstruction. *Plast Reconstr Surg* 2008;121:451–457.
192. American Society of Clinical Oncology. American Society of Clinical Oncology policy statement update: tobacco control—Reducing cancer incidence and saving lives. 2003. *J Clin Oncol* 2003;21:2777–2786.
193. Gritz ER, Fingeret MC, Vidrine DJ, et al. Successes and failures of the teachable moment: smoking cessation in cancer patients. *Cancer* 2006;106:17–27.
194. Gritz ER, Dresler C, Sarna L. Smoking, the missing drug interaction in clinical trials: ignoring the obvious. *Cancer Epidemiol Biomarkers Prev* 2005;14:2287–2293.
199. Fiore MC, Jaén CR, Baker TB, et al. *Treating Tobacco Use and Dependence: 2008 Update.* Rockville, MD: U.S. Department of Health and Human Services; 2008. http://www.ncbi.nlm.nih.gov/books/NBK63952/. Accessed November 25, 2013.
211. Toll BA, Rojewski AM, Duncan L, et al. "Quitting smoking will benefit your health": the evolution of clinician messaging to encourage tobacco cessation. *Clin Cancer Res* 2014;20:301–309.
213. Gritz ER, Fingeret MC, Vidrine DJ. Tobacco control in the oncology setting. In: Brawley OW, Khuri FR, Rock CL, eds. *ASCO Cancer Prevention Curriculum.* Alexandria, VA: American Society of Clinical Oncology; 2007.
218. Warren GW, Singh AK. Nicotine and lung cancer. *J Carcinog* 2013;12:1–8.
221. Jorgensen ED, Zhao H, Traganos F, et al. DNA damage response induced by exposure of human lung adenocarcinoma cells to smoke from tobacco- and nicotine-free cigarettes. *Cell Cycle* 2010;9:2170–2176.
222. Murray RP, Connett JE, Zapawa LM. Does nicotine replacement therapy cause cancer? Evidence from the Lung Health Study. *Nicotine Tob Res* 2009;11:1076–1082.
227. Hughes JR, Stead LF, Lancaster T. Antidepressants for smoking cessation. *Cochrane Database Syst Rev* 2003;(2):CD000031.
229. Jorenby DE, Hays JT, Rigotti NA, et al. Efficacy of varenicline, an alpha4beta2 nicotinic acetylcholine receptor partial agonist, vs placebo or sustained-release bupropion for smoking cessation: a randomized controlled trial. *JAMA* 2006;296:56–63.
235. Thomas KH, Martin RM, Davies NM, et al. Smoking cessation treatment and risk of depression, suicide, and self harm in the Clinical Practice Research Datalink: prospective cohort study. *BMJ* 2013;347:f5704.
236. Anthenelli RM, Morris C, Ramey TS, et al. Effects of varenicline on smoking cessation in adults with stably treated current or past major depression: a randomized trial. *Ann Intern Med* 2013;159:390–400.
238. Gritz ER, Carr CR, Rapkin D, et al. Predictors of long-term smoking cessation in head and neck cancer patients. *Cancer Epidemiol Biomarkers Prev* 1993;2:261–270.

244. Schnoll RA, Zhang B, Rue M, et al. Brief physician-initiated quit-smoking strategies for clinical oncology settings: a trial coordinated by the Eastern Cooperative Oncology Group. *J Clin Oncol* 2003;21:355–365.

248. Schnoll RA, Martinez E, Tatum KL, et al. A bupropion smoking cessation clinical trial for cancer patients. *Cancer Causes Control* 2010;21:811–820.

251. Ostroff JS, Burkhalter JE, Cinciripini PM, et al. Randomized trial of a presurgical scheduled reduced smoking intervention for patients newly diagnosed with cancer. *Health Psychol* 2013 [Epub ahead of print].

254. Goldstein AO, Ripley-Moffitt CE, Pathman DE, et al. Tobacco use treatment at the U.S. National Cancer Institute's designated Cancer Centers. *Nicotine Tob Res* 2013;15:52–58.

255. Warren GW, Marshall JR, Cummings KM, et al. Practice patterns and perceptions of thoracic oncology providers on tobacco use and cessation in cancer patients. *J Thorac Oncol* 2013;8:543–548.

256. Warren GW, Marshall JR, Cummings KM, et al. Addressing tobacco use in cancer patients: a survey of American Society of Clinical Oncology (ASCO) members. *J Oncol Pract* 2013;9:258–262.

257. Gritz ER, Sarna L, Dresler C, et al. Building a united front: aligning the agendas for tobacco control, lung cancer research, and policy. *Cancer Epidemiol Biomarkers Prev* 2007;16:859–863.

262. Society for Research on Nicotine and Tobacco Committee on Biochemical Verification. Biochemical verification of tobacco use and cessation. *Nicotine Tob Res* 2002;4:149–159.

263. American Society of Clinical Oncology. Tobacco Cessation Guide: for Oncology Providers. ASCO Web site. http://www.asco.org/sites/default/files/tobacco_cessation_guide.pdf. Accessed November 25, 2013.

32 Role of Surgery in Cancer Prevention

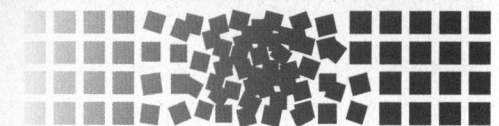

José G. Guillem, Andrew Berchuck, Jeffrey F. Moley, Jeffrey A. Norton, Sheryl G. A. Gabram-Mendola, and Vanessa W. Hui

INTRODUCTION

Since the heritable component of some cancer predispositions has been linked to mutations in specific genes, clinical interventions have been formulated for mutation carriers within affected families. The primary interventions for mutation carriers for highly penetrant syndromes, such as multiple endocrine neoplasia (MEN), familial adenomatous polyposis (FAP), hereditary nonpolyposis colorectal cancer (CRC), and hereditary breast and ovarian cancer syndromes, are primarily surgical. This chapter is divided into five sections addressing breast (S.G.A.G.), gastric (J.N.), ovarian and endometrial (A.B.), and MENs (J.F.M.) and colorectal (J.G.G., V.W.H.). For each, the clinical and genetic indications and timing of prophylactic surgery and its efficacy, when known, are provided.

Prophylactic surgery in hereditary cancer is a complex process, requiring a clear understanding of the natural history of the disease and variance of penetrance, a realistic appreciation of the potential benefit and consequence of a risk-reducing procedure in an otherwise potentially healthy individual, and the long-term sequelae of such surgical intervention, as well as the individual patient's and family's perception of surgical risk and anticipated benefit.

PATIENTS AT HIGH RISK FOR BREAST CANCER

Identification of Patients at Risk

A detailed family history is the most important tool for identifying individuals at increased risk for hereditary cancers. The US Preventive Services Task Force updated their recommendation for risk assessment, genetic counseling, and genetic testing for asymptomatic women who have not been diagnosed with a *BRCA*-related cancer. In this update, the use of a risk screening tool is highly recommended to identify appropriate patients for referral for genetic counseling.[1] The American Society of Clinical Oncology has also updated the policy on genetic and genomic testing for cancer susceptibility, and this update includes information on genetic tests of uncertain clinical utility and direct-to-consumer marketing, both of which impact the practice of oncology and preventive medicine.[2] Historically, genetic counseling and testing were offered by health-care providers. However, with the advent of direct-to-consumer marketing, individuals may obtain tests and receive results directly from a company. The American Society of Clinical Oncology still endorses pre- and posttest counseling for thorough disclosure of the impact of testing. Before any woman considers risk-reduction surgery such as bilateral mastectomy or salpingo-oophorectomy, referral to a high-risk or genetic screening program is desirable, as women often overestimate their actual breast cancer risk.[3]

The most common cancer syndromes that place women at risk for breast cancer are *BRCA1*[4] and *BRCA2*[5] gene mutations. Other less common syndromes are listed in Table 32.1.[6,7]

Following referral for genetic assessment, three groups of patients emerge.[8] The first consists of those women who have undergone genetic testing and have been found to harbor a mutated gene associated with high penetrance for breast cancer. Given that the possibility of developing breast cancer in this group may be as high as 90%, there is a role for enhanced surveillance or risk-reduction surgery. The American Cancer Society has published guidelines for magnetic resonance imaging (MRI) screening as a method for enhanced surveillance.[9] Women in this first group qualify for such screening, which can be offered annually but scheduled at 6-month intervals with screening mammography to increase the rate of identifying interval cancers. Alternatively, simultaneous screening with MRI and mammography to compare one modality with the other on an annual basis may also be offered. Another choice for this group of women is to pursue bilateral risk-reduction mastectomy with an option for immediate reconstruction. Bilateral salpingo-oophorectomy for *BRCA1* and *BRCA2* mutation carriers may also be considered, as this procedure has been shown to reduce breast cancer risk by almost 50%.[8,10] This is especially true for *BRCA2* mutation carriers, who tend to develop hormone receptor–positive breast cancers.

The second group consists of women with strong family histories suggestive of hereditary breast cancer who test negative for both the *BRCA1* and *BRCA2* mutations as well as the other described syndromes. In this group, there may not have been a family member with cancer who was tested for the mutation. Therefore, a negative test does not necessarily indicate that a woman's risk is equivalent to that of the general population.[7] There may also be an undetected mutation in such a family, indicating the possibility of higher-than-average risk for that particular woman. These women may or may not qualify for enhanced surveillance with MRI screening,[9] and accurate assessment of their risk may require the use of other risk prediction tools,[3] in addition to evaluating for the presence of lobular carcinoma in situ, atypical lobular hyperplasia, or atypical ductal hyperplasia, and determining if a more intensive surveillance regimen is necessary based on heterogeneously or extremely dense breast tissue on mammography.

The third group consists of women with a strong family history of breast cancer, who for various reasons, have chosen not to pursue genetic testing. These individuals may have other health-related problems, psychological concerns, cost issues, or they may fear perceived medical insurance discrimination. Women in all groups can be educated that with passage of the Genetic Information Nondiscrimination Act in 2008, significant advances have occurred that protect patients from discrimination by employers and health insurers.[11]

Women in the second and third groups may still qualify for bilateral risk-reduction mastectomy and immediate reconstruction. Often, women who elect this path are influenced by their family history or by witnessing breast and/or ovarian cancer deaths in close family members, giving them a significant fear of a breast or ovarian cancer diagnosis. For women in all three groups, the decision of whether to pursue risk-reducing surgery is difficult. Often, the expertise of a cancer clinical psychologist or psychiatrist

TABLE 32.1

Hereditary Carcinoma Syndromes Including Breast Cancer

Syndrome	Chromosome/Gene	Primary Carcinoma	Secondary Carcinoma	Breast Cancer Penetrance
Familial breast cancer/ovarian cancer syndrome	17g21; *BRCA1* Autosomal dominant	Breast cancer, ovarian cancer	Colon, prostate	60%–80%
Familial breast cancer/ovarian cancer syndrome	13q12; *BRCA2* Autosomal dominant	Breast cancer, ovarian cancer	Male breast cancer, endometrial, prostate, oropharyngeal, pancreatic	60%–80%
Li-Fraumeni syndrome	17p13.1 and 22q12.1; *TP53* and *CHEK2* Autosomal dominant	Soft tissue cancers (including breast)	Soft tissue sarcoma, leukemia, osteosarcoma, melanoma, colon, pancreas, adrenal syndrome, cortex, and brain tumors	50%–85% (for all types of cancers in this syndrome)
PTEN hamartoma syndrome (Cowden's)	10q23.31; *PTEN* mutation Autosomal dominant	Breast cancer	Thyroid (follicular) and endometrial carcinoma	25%–50%
Peutz-Jeghers syndrome	19p13.3; *STK11* Autosomal dominant	Gastrointestinal cancers	Esophagus, stomach, small intestine, large bowel, pancreas, lung, ovary, endometrial	29%
Diffuse gastric cancer	16q22.1; *CDH1* Autosomal dominant	Diffuse gastric cancer	Colorectal, lobular breast cancer	39% (lobular breast cancer)
Louis-Bar syndrome	11q22.3; *ATM* Autosomal recessive	Leukemia and lymphoma	Ovarian, breast, gastric, melanoma, leiomyomas, sarcomas	38% (for all types of cancers in the syndrome)

PTEN, phosphatase and tensin homolog.
Data from Lux MP, Fasching PA, Beckmann MW. Hereditary breast and ovarian cancer: review and future perspectives. *J Mol Med* 2006;84:16–28; and Shannon KM, Chittenden A. Genetic testing by cancer site: breast. *Cancer J* 2012;18:310–319.

is enlisted, as risk-reduction mastectomy involves an irreversible procedure with body image and sexual implications.[8]

Updated in 2007, the Society of Surgical Oncology published a position statement on the role of prophylactic mastectomy for patients at high risk for breast cancer, as well as those patients recently diagnosed with breast cancer who are considering contralateral prophylactic breast surgery.[12] For women at high risk, indications fall into three broad categories: presence of a mutation in *BRCA* or other susceptible genes, strong family history with no demonstrable mutation, and histologic risk factors (biopsy-proven atypical ductal hyperplasia, atypical lobular hyperplasia, or lobular carcinoma in situ especially in patients with a strong family history of breast cancer). Recommendations for patients with recently diagnosed breast cancer are similar in that they include the indications for high-risk individuals previously noted, as well as future surveillance challenges for the opposite breast (clinically and mammographically dense breast tissue or diffuse, indeterminate microcalcifications in the contralateral breast). Another important consideration is the need for symmetry in patients with large, ptotic, or disproportionately sized contralateral breasts.

Surgical Issues and Technique

In a single institution's 33-year experience,[13] the risk for breast cancer in both moderate- and high-risk groups of women based on family history was reduced by at least 89% for women who underwent bilateral prophylactic mastectomy. From a technical perspective, in this study, women either had a subcutaneous mastectomy (removal of the majority of breast tissue with sparing of the nipple–areola complex) or total mastectomy (removal of the entire breast through the nipple–areola complex). Most of the recurrences occurred in women undergoing a subcutaneous mastectomy. However, this was the most frequent procedure performed at that time and thus may have contributed to the number of increased recurrences.

Another surgical option for high-risk women is bilateral salpingo-oophorectomy. Among a cohort of women with *BRCA1* and *BRCA2* mutations, this procedure has been associated with a lower risk of mortality from both breast and ovarian cancer.[10] As an additional benefit, this procedure also decreases the risk of breast cancer in this patient population, likely through the mechanism of decreasing hormonal exposure at a younger age.

Contemporary surgical procedures for risk-reducing bilateral mastectomy include total mastectomy, skin-sparing mastectomy (preservation of the skin envelope by removal of the entire breast through a circumareolar incision around the nipple–areola complex), subcutaneous mastectomy, areola-sparing mastectomy (removal of the nipple while sparing the areola), and nipple-sparing mastectomy (removal of entire breast and nipple core tissue but preservation of nipple–areolar skin).[14] Given advances in reconstructive nipple–areolar techniques, it appears that total mastectomy with or without skin-sparing methods reduces the risk of breast cancer to the greatest extent with reasonable cosmesis. More limited and long-term follow-up data are available on areola- and nipple-sparing techniques. The potential limitations of these procedures are distortion of the nipple–areola complex and lack of sensitivity after breast tissue has been completely removed.[8]

Immediate reconstruction is offered to patients and performed in the vast majority undergoing bilateral risk-reduction mastectomy. Choices of reconstruction include a bilateral pedicled or free tissue transverse rectus abdominis muscle flap, a free bilateral deep inferior epigastric perforator flap or superficial inferior epigastric artery flap, bilateral latissimus flaps with or without implant or expanders, or bilateral implant or expander placement alone.[14] Although tissue flap transfer gives a more natural appearance and texture to the reconstructed site, individual body contour drives the ultimate plan for reconstruction. The decision about the type of reconstruction should be made by the plastic surgeon with input from the surgical oncologist, especially for the group of women with breast cancer desiring bilateral mastectomies who may require adjuvant radiation for treatment.

Although the risk reduction is dramatic for bilateral mastectomy, residual breast tissue may be left behind, especially with skin-sparing procedures. Patients should be educated that careful chest wall surveillance is recommended after such a procedure. Local recurrences after bilateral implant reconstruction are reliably detected by clinical examination. Recurrences after reconstruction with autologous tissue present most commonly on the skin 50% to 72% of the time and are detectable by physician examination.[15] Nonpalpable deeper recurrences in this setting are less common, and use of mammography image surveillance may be indicated, especially if significant breast tissue was left behind unintentionally during the bilateral mastectomy procedure. At times, an initial "screening" mammogram may be performed, if significant residual breast tissue is suspected; this should occur well after all healing has taken place to delineate the amount of visible breast tissue on imaging. This drives future decisions of whether to follow a patient with imaging. Finally, all patients should be instructed to return for clinical breast examination with the health provider if any change is noted on the reconstructed breasts, regardless of imaging plan.

Although risk-reduction bilateral mastectomy may be exceedingly beneficial for high-risk women, especially for those testing positive for *BRCA1*, *BRCA2*, or other deleterious mutations, or belonging to a family afflicted with a cancer syndrome, they are never emergent procedures. Along with risk-reduction bilateral salpingo-oophorectomy, risk-reduction bilateral mastectomy resides at the far end of the spectrum of an individual's choices.[16] These procedures should be offered only after appropriate genetic counseling and accurate assessment of a woman's actual risk for breast and ovarian cancer. An in-depth consultation with the patient and her family members is necessary prior to proceeding with an operative plan.

HEREDITARY DIFFUSE GASTRIC CANCER

Gastric cancer is the fourth most common cause of cancer worldwide and is the second leading cause of cancer mortality.[17] Although environmental agents, including *Helicobacter pylori* and diet, are the primary risk factors for this disease, approximately 10% of gastric cancers are a result of familial clustering.[18,19] Histologically, gastric cancers may be classified as either intestinal or diffuse types. The intestinal type histopathology is linked to environmental factors and advanced age. The diffuse type occurs in younger patients and is associated with a familial predisposition. Because of

a decrease in intestinal-type gastric cancers, the overall incidence of gastric cancer has declined significantly in the past 50 years. However, the incidence of diffuse gastric cancer (DGC), which is also called signet ring cell or linitis plastica, has remained stable and, by some reports, may be increasing.

Hereditary DGC (HDGC) is a genetic cancer susceptibility syndrome defined by one of the following: (1) two or more documented cases of DGC in first- or second-degree relatives, with at least one diagnosed before the age of 50; or (2) three or more cases of documented DGC in first- or second-degree relatives, independent of age of onset. The average age of onset of HDGC is 38, and the pattern of inheritance is autosomal dominant.[20] Figure 32.1 shows a pedigree with HDGC.

In 1998, inactivating germline mutations in the E-cadherin gene *CDH1* were identified in three Maori families, each with multiple cases of poorly differentiated DGC.[21] The *CDH1* mutations in these families were inherited in an autosomal dominant pattern, with incomplete but high penetrance. Onset of clinically apparent cancer was early, with the youngest affected individual dying of DGC at the age of 14.[21] Since then, germline mutations of *CDH1* have been identified in 30% to 50% of all patients with HDGC.[19,22] More than 50 mutations have been recognized across diverse ethnic backgrounds, including European, African American, Pakistani, Japanese, Korean, and others.[19] In addition to gastric cancers, germline *CDH1* mutations are associated with increased risk of lobular carcinoma of the breast, and this was the first manifestation of a *CDH1* mutation in one series.[23] *CDH1* is, to date, the only gene implicated in HDGC. Penetrance of DGC in patients carrying a *CDH1* mutation is estimated at 70% to 80%, but may be higher. The need for a systematic study of specimens is supported by recent work by Gaya et al.[24] in which initial total gastrectomy specimens were reported as negative, but detailed sectioning and analysis showed invasive carcinoma.

CDH1 is localized on chromosome 16q22.1 and encodes the calcium-dependent cell adhesion glycoprotein E-cadherin. Functionally, E-cadherin impacts maintenance of normal tissue morphology and cellular differentiation. It is hypothesized that *CDH1* acts as a tumor suppressor gene in HDGC, with loss of function leading to loss of cell adhesion and subsequently to proliferation, invasion, and metastases. Figure 32.2 shows the *CDH1* mutation for the pedigree depicted in Figure 32.1.

The germline *CDH1* mutation is most frequently a truncating mutation. Germline missense mutations are causative in a few HDGC kindreds, but are more often clinically insignificant. In vitro assays for cellular invasion and aggregation may predict the functional impact of missense mutations to aid in this distinction.[22] Within the gastric mucosa, the "second hit" leading to complete loss of E-cadherin function results from *CDH1* promoter methylation, as has been described in sporadic gastric cancer.[25]

CANCER PREVENTION AND SCREENING

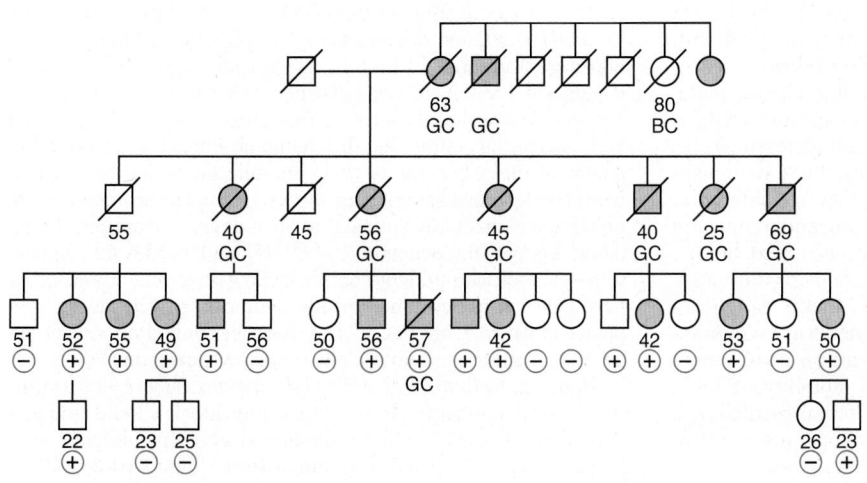

Figure 32.1 A family pedigree showing autosomal dominant inheritance of gastric cancer. Individual mutation testing results for the codon 1003 CDH1 mutation are indicated by + or −. Individuals affected with gastric cancer are *shaded*. (From Norton JA, Ham CM, Van Dam J, et al. CDH1 truncating mutations in the E-cadherin gene: an indication for total gastrectomy to treat hereditary diffuse gastric cancer. *Ann Surg* 2007;245:873.)

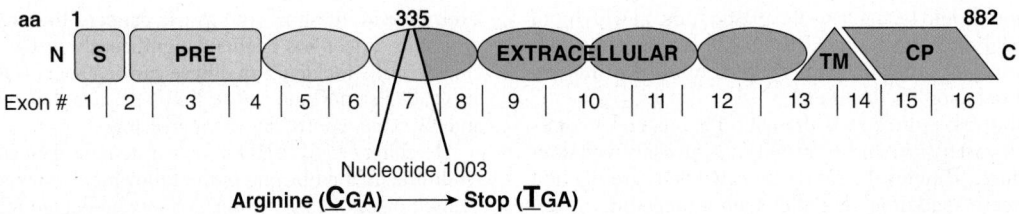

Figure 32.2 The mutation in this kindred is located in the central region of the E-cadherin gene that codes for the extracellular cadherin domains of the protein containing calcium-binding motifs important in the adhesion process. The C → T transition in exon 7 of nucleotide 1003 results in a premature stop codon (R335X), producing truncated peptides that lack the transmembrane and cytoplasmic β-catenin–binding domains essential for tight cell-cell adhesion. *Black* area indicates truncated portion of peptide. N, N-terminus; C, C-terminus; S, signal peptide; PRE, precursor sequence; TM, transmembrane domain; CP, cytoplasmic domain. (From Norton JA, Ham CM, Van Dam J, et al. CDH1 truncating mutations in the E-cadherin gene: an indication for total gastrectomy to treat hereditary diffuse gastric cancer. *Ann Surg* 2007;245:873.)

It remains unclear whether specific *CDH1* mutations are associated with distinctive phenotypic characteristics or rates of penetrance, although this may become apparent as more recurrent mutations are recognized. To date, most mutations identified have been novel and distributed throughout *CDH1*. Recognition of recurrent mutations has usually resulted from independent events; however, there is evidence for the role of founder effects in certain kindreds.[22] At present, it is also unclear whether patients with HDGC without detectable *CDH1* mutations have mutation of a different gene or merely a *CDH1* mutation that has gone unrecognized.

New recommended screening criteria for *CDH1* mutations are as follows:

1. Families with one or more cases of DGC
2. Individuals with DGC before the age of 40 years without a family history
3. Families or individuals with cases of DGC (one case below the age of 50 years) and lobular breast cancer
4. Cases where pathologists detect in situ signet ring cells or pagetoid spread of signet ring cells adjacent to diffuse type gastric cancer[15,26]

As in other familial cancer syndromes, genetic counseling should take place prior to genetic testing so that the family understands the potential impact of the results. After obtaining informed consent, a team comprising a geneticist, gastroenterologist, surgeon, and oncologist should discuss the possible outcomes of testing and the management options associated with each. Genetic testing should first be performed on a family member with HDGC or on a tissue sample if no affected relative is living. In addition to direct sequencing, multiplex ligation-dependent probe amplification is recommended to test for large genomic rearrangements. If a *CDH1* mutation is identified, asymptomatic family members may proceed with genetic testing, preferably by the age of 20.[19] If no mutation is identified in the family member with DGC, the value of testing asymptomatic relatives is low.

Among individuals found to carry a germline *CDH1* mutation, clinical screening is problematic. Histologically, DGC is characterized by multiple infiltrates of malignant signet ring cells, which may underlie normal mucosa.[27] Because these malignant foci are small in size and widely distributed, they are difficult to identify via random endoscopic biopsy. Chromoendoscopy and positron emission tomography have reportedly been used, but the clinical utility of these tools in early detection remains unproven. Lack of a sensitive screening test for HDGC makes early diagnosis extremely challenging. By the time patients are symptomatic and present for treatment, many have diffuse involvement of the stomach or linitis plastica, and rates of mortality are high. Published case reports describe patients who have presented with extensive DGC despite recent normal endoscopy and negative biopsies.[28] The 5-year survival rate for individuals who develop clinically apparent DGC is only 10%, with the majority dying before age 40.

Because of high cancer penetrance, poor outcome, and inadequacy of clinical screening tools for HDGC, prophylactic total gastrectomy is recommended as a management option for asymptomatic carriers of *CDH1* mutations.[18] Although total gastrectomy is performed with prophylactic intent in these cases, most specimens have been found to contain foci of diffuse signet ring cell cancer.[19,28,29] Foci of DGC have been identified even in patients who have undergone extensive negative screening, including high-resolution computed tomography, positron emission tomography scan, chromoendoscopy-guided biopsies, and endoscopic ultrasonography.[19] However, HGDC in asymptomatic *CDH1* carriers is usually completely resected by prophylactic gastrectomy, as pathologic analyses of resected specimens have shown only T1N0 disease.

Because these signet ring cell cancers are multifocal and distributed throughout the entire stomach, especially in the cardia,[30] prophylactic gastrectomy should include the entire stomach, and the surgeon must transect the esophagus and not the proximal stomach. Furthermore, it should be performed by a surgeon experienced in the technical aspects of the procedure and familiar with HDGC. In asymptomatic patients, lymph node metastases have not been observed; therefore, D2 lymph node resection is not necessary. The optimal timing of prophylactic gastrectomy in individuals with *CDH1* mutations is unknown, but recent consensus recommendations indicate that age 20 is reasonable.[18]

Although it is a potentially lifesaving procedure, prophylactic gastrectomy for *CDH1* mutation carries significant risks that must be considered. Overall mortality for total gastrectomy is estimated to be as high as 2% to 4%, although it is estimated to be 1% when performed prophylactically. Patients must also be aware that there is a nearly 100% risk of long-term morbidity associated with this procedure, including diarrhea, dumping, weight loss, and difficulty eating.[19] A recent study of the effects of prophylactic gastrectomy for *CDH1* mutation demonstrated that physical and mental function were normal at 12 months, but specific digestive issues were recognized. Overall, 70% had diarrhea, 63% fatigue, 81% eating discomfort, 63% reflux, 45% eating restrictions, and 44% had altered body image, suggesting that this operation impacted negatively on quality of life.[31] Because of these complications and the fact that lymph node spread has not been observed, some recommend vagus-preserving gastrectomy done either open or laparoscopically. In addition, because the penetrance of *CDH1* mutations is incomplete, some patients who undergo prophylactic gastrectomy would never have gone on to develop clinically significant gastric cancer. Prophylactic gastrectomy has, in fact, been performed on several patients reported to show no evidence of gastric cancer on pathology.[29]

Some individuals with *CDH1* mutations choose not to pursue prophylactic gastrectomy. These individuals should undergo careful surveillance, including biannual chromoendoscopy with biopsies, beginning when they are at least 10 years younger than the youngest family member with DGC was at time of diagnosis. It is recommended that any endoscopically visible lesion is targeted and that six random biopsies are taken from the following regions: antrum, transitional zone, body, fundus, and cardia. Careful white-light examination with targeted and random biopsies combined with detailed histopathology can identify early lesions and help to inform decision making with regard to gastrectomy.[32] Additionally, because women with *CDH1* mutations have a nearly 40% lifetime risk of developing lobular breast carcinoma, they should be carefully screened with annual mammography and breast MRI starting at age 35.[23] They should also do monthly self-examinations and have a breast examination by a physician every 6 months. The same surveillance recommendations are probably appropriate for HDGC families without identifiable *CDH1* mutations, although no current guidelines for this exist.

The emergence of gene-directed gastrectomy as a treatment strategy for patients with HDGC represents the culmination of a successful collaboration between molecular biologists, geneticists, oncologists, gastroenterologists, and surgeons. It is anticipated that the recognition of similar molecular markers in other familial cancer syndromes will transform the approach to the early diagnosis and treatment of a variety of tumors.

SURGICAL PROPHYLAXIS OF HEREDITARY OVARIAN AND ENDOMETRIAL CANCER

Hereditary Ovarian Cancer (*BRCA1, BRCA2*)

Inherited mutations in *BRCA1* and *BRCA2* strongly predispose women to breast cancer and to high-grade serous cancers of the ovary, fallopian tube, and peritoneum.[33,34] About two-thirds are due to *BRCA1* mutations and one-third *BRCA2* mutations, and these account for about 15% to 20% of high-grade serous cases. The lifetime risk of these gynecologic cancers increases from a baseline of 1.5% to about 15% to 25% in *BRCA2* carriers and 30% to 60% in *BRCA1* carriers.[33,34] *BRCA1/2* mutations are rare in most populations (<1 in 500 individuals); one notable exception is the Ashkenazi Jewish population, in which the carrier frequency is 1 in 40.[35] *BRCA1*-associated cases peak in the 50s and *BRCA2*-associated cancers in the 60s.[36] In addition to *BRCA1/2* mutations, germline mutations in a number of other genes in the homologous recombination DNA repair pathway confer high penetrance susceptibility to ovarian cancer (e.g., *RAD51C, RAD51D, BRIP1, PALB2*).[37] This has led to the development of more comprehensive cancer genetic testing panels that are increasingly being used to identify women who are candidates for risk-reducing salpingo-oophorectomy (RRSO).

Genetic testing for inherited high-penetrance mutations in *BRCA1/2* and other genes should be discussed with women who have a significant family history of early onset breast cancer and/or cancers of the ovary, fallopian tube, or peritoneum. Involvement of a genetic counselor prior to testing is helpful, as they have expertise in managing the inherent clinical and social issues. Most *BRCA1/2* mutations involve base deletions or insertions in the coding sequence or splice sites that encode truncated protein products that are clearly dysfunctional. Less frequently, disease-causing mutations may occur that alter a single amino acid, though most of these missense variants represent innocent polymorphisms. The clinical significance of missense mutations can sometimes be elucidated by determining whether they segregate with cancer in other family members. In addition, genomic rearrangements may occur that inactivate *BRCA1* or *BRCA2*, and identification of such alterations requires molecular testing beyond sequencing.

Penetrance of ovarian cancer is not 100% in those with clearly deleterious *BRCA1/2* mutations, but presently it is not possible to provide more precise personalized risk estimates to guide the use of RRSO. However, common variants have been discovered

in other genes that appear to affect the risk of ovarian cancer in *BRCA1/2* carriers.[38] Based on the known ovarian cancer risk–modifying loci, it has been reported that the 5% of *BRCA1* carriers at lowest risk have a lifetime risk of ≤28% of developing ovarian cancer, whereas the 5% at highest risk have a ≥63% lifetime risk. In the future, when modifier loci are more completely catalogued, more precise estimates of cancer risk may be provided to individual patients who are considering RRSO.

As about 20% of women with high-grade serous ovarian cancers have *BRCA1/2* mutations, it has been suggested that all of these women undergo genetic testing regardless of family history.[39] Mutational analysis in women with these cancers may increasingly become standard practice as the cost of genetic testing declines. Testing may also be driven by the availability of poly(ADP-ribose) polymerase inhibitor therapy for women whose cancers have germline or sporadic mutations in genes such as *BRCA1/2* and others that are involved in homologous recombination DNA repair.

RRSO is strongly recommended in women who carry *BRCA1/2* mutations because of the high mortality rate of ovarian cancer and the lack of effective screening and prevention approaches. Although screening with pelvic ultrasound and serum CA125 is generally recommended for *BRCA1/2* carriers during their 20s and 30s, it is not proven to reduce ovarian cancer mortality because even early stage high-grade cancers have a very high mortality. Oral contraceptives reduce the risk of ovarian cancer in the general population and appear to have a similar effect in *BRCA1/2* carriers, but this must be balanced against concerns regarding increased breast cancer risks.

The past practice of performing RRSO based solely on family history has been replaced by reliance on genetic testing. Clinical management of women with a strong family history in whom a deleterious germline mutation is not found, or those with variants of uncertain significance, should be resolved on a case-by-case basis. RRSO may be deemed appropriate in some cases, despite the absence of a clearly deleterious mutation. Fortunately, the risk of hereditary ovarian cancer does not rise dramatically until the mid-30s in women with *BRCA1* mutations and the 40s for women with *BRCA2* mutations.[36] As a result, most women are able to complete childbearing prior to undergoing RRSO. It is advisable for *BRCA1* carriers to undergo RRSO around age 35, as there is a 4% risk of ovarian cancer being discovered clinically or at the time of RRSO by age 40.[10] *BRCA2* carriers may choose to delay surgery into their 40s due to their lower risk of ovarian cancer, but this could diminish the protection against breast cancer that is afforded by RRSO. If a mutation carrier, particularly a *BRCA1* carrier, chooses to pursue fertility into her 40s, then she should be counseled that she is at considerable risk of developing a life-threatening cancer that is largely preventable.

Several studies have provided evidence of the efficacy of RRSO. In one early study of *BRCA1/2* carriers, RRSO reduced the rate of breast and ovarian cancer by 75% over several years of follow-up.[40] A separate study in 2002 examined outcome in 551 *BRCA1/2* carriers from various registries.[41] Among 259 women who had undergone RRSO, 6 (2.3%) were found to have stage I ovarian cancer at the time of the procedure and 2 (0.8%) subsequently developed serous peritoneal carcinoma. Among the controls, 58 (20%) women developed ovarian cancer after a mean follow-up of 8.8 years. With the exclusion of the six women whose cancers were diagnosed at surgery, RRSO reduced ovarian cancer risk by 96%. More recently, in 2014, an international registry study of over 5,783 subjects with median follow-up of 5.6 years found that RRSO reduced ovarian, tubal, and peritoneal cancer risk by 80%.[36] There was an estimated lifetime risk of primary peritoneal cancer after RRSO of about 4% for *BRCA1* carriers and 2% for *BRCA2* carriers.[36] The risk of death from all causes was reduced by 77%. A prospective cohort study noted that RRSO was associated with reduction in breast cancer–specific (hazard ratio [HR] = 0.44; 95% confidence interval [CI] = 0.26 to 0.76), ovarian cancer–specific (HR = 0.21; 95% CI = 0.06 to 0.80), and all-cause mortality (HR = 0.40; 95% CI = 0.26 to 0.61).[10]

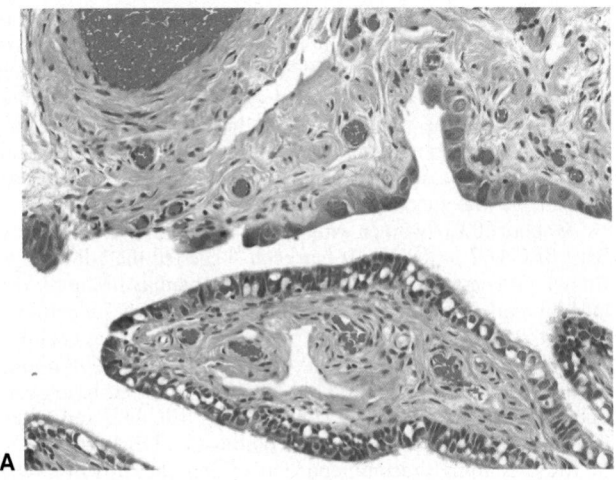 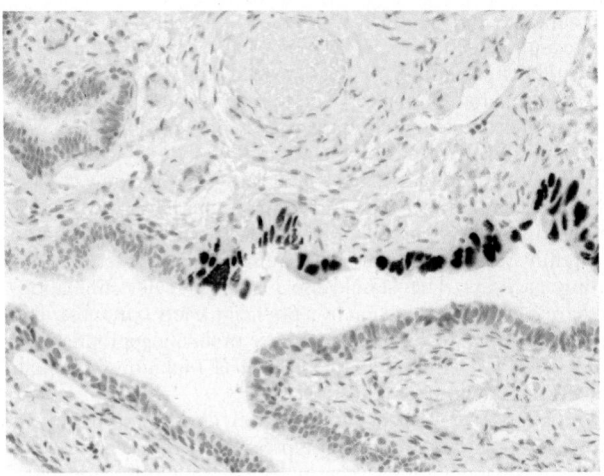

Figure 32.3 Hematoxylin and eosin **(A)** and immunohistochemical staining **(B)** demonstrating overexpression of mutant *TP53* in serous carcinoma in situ of the fallopian tube from a *BRCA1* mutation carrier who underwent risk-reducing bilateral salpingo-oophorectomy.

Removal of the ovaries, as internal organs, usually has little effect on body image and self-esteem, and most *BRCA1/2* mutation carriers elect to undergo RRSO. Insurance payers will almost always pay for RRSO in proven mutation carriers.

RRSO can be performed laparoscopically in most women, with discharge to home the same day. If a laparoscopic approach is problematic due to obesity or adhesions, the surgery can be performed through a small lower abdominal incision. Morbidity including bleeding, infection, and damage to the urinary or gastrointestinal tracts can occur, but the incidence of serious complications is very low. As the fallopian tubes and ovaries are small discrete organs, they are relatively easy to remove completely. Attention should be paid to transecting the ovarian artery and vein proximal to the ovary and tube so that remnants are not left behind. This involves opening the pelvic sidewall peritoneum, visualizing the ureter, and then isolating the ovarian blood supply. If there are adhesions between the adnexa and adjacent structures, careful dissection should be performed to ensure complete removal of the ovaries and fallopian tubes. If the uterus is not removed, care should be taken to remove the entire fallopian tube. A small portion of the tube inevitably will be left in the cornu of the uterus, but the risk of fallopian tube cancer developing in such remnants appears to be negligible.

Though there is not strong evidence that *BRCA1/2* mutations increase uterine cancer risk, many women elect to have the uterus removed as part of the surgical procedure because they have completed their family or have other gynecologic indications. Although the addition of a hysterectomy may increase operative time, blood loss, surgical complications, and hospital stay, it usually can be performed laparoscopically and serious adverse outcomes are infrequent. Furthermore, the likelihood of future exposure to tamoxifen in the context of breast cancer prevention or treatment, which increases endometrial cancer risk two- to three-fold, also argues for concomitant hysterectomy. Women who receive hormone replacement therapy after surgery will require a progestin along with estrogen to protect against the development of endometrial cancer if the uterus is not removed.

In younger women, surgical menopause after RRSO is associated with vasomotor symptoms, vaginal atrophy, decreased libido, and an accelerated onset and incidence of osteoporosis and cardiovascular disease. In premenopausal women who do not have a personal history of breast cancer, estrogen replacement can be administered to ameliorate many of the deleterious effects of premature menopause. Systemic estrogen levels are lower in oophorectomized premenopausal women taking hormone replacement than if the ovaries had been left in place. The therapeutic benefit of oophorectomy in women with breast cancer has long been

appreciated, and more recent studies support the contention that RRSO reduces the risk of breast cancer by about half in *BRCA1/2* carriers.[42] However, a meta-analysis showed that while RRSO was strongly protective against estrogen receptor–positive breast cancer (HR = 0.22), there was no protection against estrogen receptor–negative breast cancer.[42] Many carriers are identified after developing early onset breast cancer, and this group represents the most difficult in which to balance the potential risks and benefits of estrogen replacement therapy.

Early stage high-grade serous cancers and in situ lesions with *TP53* mutations have been identified in the fallopian tubes of some RRSO specimens (Fig. 32.3). This has led to a paradigm shift in which it is now thought that most high-grade serous cancers found in the ovary, fallopian tube, and peritoneum are derived from cells that originate in the tubal fimbria.[43] The frequency of occult malignancies has varied between reports, but appears to be about 3%.[43] In view of this, the pelvis and peritoneal cavity should be examined carefully. Malignant cells also have been found in peritoneal cytologic specimens, and washings of the pelvis should be obtained when performing RRSO. The pathologist should be informed of the indication for surgery and serial sections of the fallopian tubes should be performed to look for the presence of early lesions. Patients found to have occult invasive high-grade serous cancers should be treated with chemotherapy after surgery. Those with in situ lesions appear to have a good outcome without chemotherapy.[44]

Cases of peritoneal serous carcinoma indistinguishable from ovarian cancer have been observed years after RRSO, but the origin of these cancers is unclear. Some may represent recurrences of occult ovarian or tubal cancers. In this regard, retrospective examination of the ovaries and fallopian tubes sometimes has revealed primary cancers that were not originally recognized. In contrast, some of these cancers likely arise directly from fallopian tube cells that have implanted in the peritoneum and subsequently become malignant. Patients who undergo RRSO should be made aware of their residual risk of peritoneal cancer, but there is no evidence that continued surveillance using CA125 and/or ultrasound is beneficial.

HEREDITARY ENDOMETRIAL CANCER (LYNCH SYNDROME)

Although Lynch syndrome (LS, also known as hereditary nonpolyposis CRC syndrome) typically manifests as familial clustering of early onset CRC, there is also an increased incidence of several other types of cancers—most notably endometrial cancer in women.[45] About 3% of endometrial cancers are attributable to inherited mutations in the DNA mismatch repair (MMR) genes that cause LS. Most often, *MSH2* and *MLH1* are implicated, but mutations in *MSH6* and *PMS2* also occur.[45] The risk of ovarian cancer is also significantly increased in LS, but to a lesser degree than in *BRCA1/2* mutation carriers, and accounts for only about 1% of all ovarian cancers.

Cells in which one of the LS genes have been inactivated exhibit a phenomenon called microsatellite instability (MSI).[46] This occurs as DNA mismatches cause shortening or lengthening of repetitive DNA sequences and these mismatches go unrepaired. This results in generation of alleles in the cancer that contain a greater or lesser number of repeats than are present in normal cells from that individual. MSI occurs in most LS-associated colorectal and endometrial cancers.[46] However, MSI is found in about 20% of sporadic cancers that arise in these organs, and in most cases is caused by silencing of the *MLH1* gene due to promoter hypermethylation. Screening strategies for identification of MMR gene alterations in families with LS-associated cancers include analysis of tumor tissue for MSI and/or loss of DNA MMR gene expression using immunohistochemistry (IHC).[46] In cancers with MSI or loss of expression of one of the MMR genes, or in families with pedigrees suggestive of LS, these genes can be sequenced to identify disease-causing mutations, most of which cause truncated protein products.[47] Although it has been suggested that it may be cost-effective to do these tests on all endometrial cancers, this approach has not been widely adopted.[47]

The risk of a woman who carries a LS mutation developing endometrial cancer ranges from 20% to 60% in various reports.[45,48] The risk of ovarian cancer is increased to about 5% to 12%. Whereas the mean age of women with sporadic endometrial cancers is in the early 60s, cancers that arise in association with LS are often diagnosed before menopause, with the average age in the 40s. The clinical features of these endometrial cancers are similar to those of most sporadic cases (well-differentiated, endometrioid histology, early stage), and survival is about 90%. The mean age of onset of ovarian cancer in LS is in the early 40s, and the clinical features of these cancers are generally more favorable than in sporadic cases. They usually are identified at an early stage, are well- or moderately differentiated, have favorable survival, and some occur in the setting of a synchronous endometrial cancer.

Recommendations for screening and risk-reducing surgery in LS are better established for CRC than for extracolonic malignancies.[49] Transvaginal ultrasound has been proposed as a screening test for endometrial cancer (and ovarian cancer), but its efficacy is unproven.[50] Endometrial biopsy is the most sensitive means of diagnosing endometrial cancer, and it has been suggested that this should be employed periodically beginning around age 30 to 35. However, there are no published studies demonstrating that this approach prevents endometrial cancer deaths compared to simply performing a biopsy if abnormal uterine bleeding occurs.

Most experts believe that risk-reducing hysterectomy has a role in the management of some women with LS because of the high incidence of endometrial cancer. The risk of endometrial cancer is low during the prime reproductive years, and the uterus does not serve a vital function once childbearing has been completed. In view of the increased risk of ovarian cancer in LS, concomitant bilateral salpingo-oophorectomy should also be considered. One study demonstrated that there were no cases of endometrial or ovarian cancer in 61 LS carriers who underwent risk-reducing hysterectomy and bilateral salpingo-oophorectomy, while endometrial cancer occurred in 33% and ovarian cancer in 5% who retained their uterus and ovaries.[51] Despite the low risk of death from gynecologic cancers in LS, cost-effectiveness analyses of various approaches suggest that risk-reducing hysterectomy and salpingo-oophorectomy leads to both the lowest cost and the greatest increase in quality-adjusted life-years.[52] Estrogen replacement after removal of the ovaries in premenopausal women with LS is not contraindicated, as there is no evidence that this adversely affects the incidence of other cancers.

Many women with LS elect to undergo risk-reducing colectomy, which provides an opportunity to perform concomitant hysterectomy. Hysterectomy in concert with colectomy, either via laparoscopy or laparotomy, does not greatly increase operative time or surgical complications. If an endometrial biopsy has not been performed preoperatively, an intraoperative inspection of the uterine cavity and possibly frozen section should be performed to exclude the presence of cancer. If cancer is found in the uterus, surgical staging—including sampling of the regional lymph nodes—should be considered in addition to hysterectomy.[53] It is also appropriate to discuss risk-reducing hysterectomy with LS carriers who do not elect to undergo prophylactic colectomy. The operative approach (vaginal versus laparotomy versus laparoscopy) can be determined based on the presence or absence of uterine pathology (e.g., myomas), whether the patient has had prior abdominal surgery, and whether the ovaries are also to be removed.

GYNECOLOGIC CANCER RISK IN VERY RARE HEREDITARY CANCER SYNDROMES

Several very rare hereditary cancer syndromes also increase the risk of gynecologic cancers, and some of these women could potentially benefit from risk-reducing surgery to remove the ovaries and/or uterus. Peutz-Jeghers syndrome is characterized by intestinal polyps and an increased risk of colorectal and breast cancers. This rare syndrome is due to inherited mutations in the *STK11* gene. Affected women also have an increased risk of ovarian sex cord–stromal tumors with annular tubules and adenoma malignum of the cervix. Li-Fraumeni syndrome is caused by inherited mutations in the *TP53* gene, and carriers are predisposed to a number of types of cancers including sarcomas and breast cancer. The risk of ovarian cancer is increased as well, but is not a major cause of cancer in these families. Cowden syndrome is due to germline *PTEN* mutations and increases the risk of several malignancies including breast, thyroid, mucocutaneous, and endometrial cancers. Finally, small cell carcinoma of the ovary, hypercalcemic type, is due to mutations in the *SMARCA4* gene. These highly lethal ovarian cancers occur at a very young age (median 24 years) and present difficult challenges related to timing of RRSO. There are no well-accepted evidence-based guidelines for early detection and prevention of gynecologic cancers in these very rare hereditary cancer syndromes. An awareness of the risk and natural history of gynecologic cancers in these families provides a basis for counseling individual patients.

MULTIPLE ENDOCRINE NEOPLASIA TYPE 2

Gene Carriers

The MEN type 2 syndromes include MEN 2A, MEN 2B, and familial (non-MEN) medullary thyroid carcinoma (FMTC).[54–56] These are autosomal dominant inherited syndromes caused by germline mutations in the *RET* proto-oncogene. Their hallmark is the development of multifocal bilateral medullary thyroid carcinoma (MTC) associated with C-cell hyperplasia. MTCs arise from the thyroid C-cells, also called parafollicular cells. C-cells secrete the hormone calcitonin, a specific tumor marker for MTC. A slow-growing tumor in most cases, MTC causes significant morbidity and death in patients with uncontrolled local or metastatic spread. Large tumor burden is associated with diarrhea and flushing. In the MEN 2 syndromes, there is almost complete penetrance of MTC. Other features are variably expressed, with incomplete penetrance (summarized in Table 32.2).

In MEN 2A, all patients develop MTC. Approximately 42% of affected patients also develop pheochromocytomas, associated with adrenal medullary hyperplasia. Hyperparathyroidism develops in

TABLE 32.2

Clinical Features of Sporadic Medullay Thyroid Carcinoma, Multiple Endocrine Neoplasia 2A, Multiple Endocrine Neoplasia 2B, and Familial Medullary Thyroid Carcinoma

Clinical Setting	Features of MTC	Inheritance Pattern	Associated Abnormalities	Genetic Defect
Sporadic MTC	Unifocal	None	None	Somatic *RET* mutations in >20% of tumors
MEN 2A	Multifocal, bilateral	Autosomal dominant	Pheochromocytomas, hyperparathyroidism, cutaneous lichen amyloidosis, Hirshprung's disease	Germline missense mutations in extracellular cysteine codons of *RET*
MEN 2B	Multifocal, bilateral	Autosomal dominant	Pheochromocytomas, mucosal neuromas, megacolon, skeletal abnormalities	Germline missense mutation in tyrosine kinase domain of *RET*
FMTC	Multifocal, bilateral	Autosomal dominant	None	Germline missense mutations in extracellular or intracellular cysteine codons of *RET*

MTC, medullary thyroid carcinoma; MEN, multiple endocrine neoplasia; FMTC, familial medullary thyroid carcinoma.

10% to 35%. Cutaneous lichen amyloidosis and Hirschsprung's disease are infrequently associated with MEN 2A.[57–60]

MEN 2B appears to be the most aggressive form of hereditary MTC. In MEN 2B, MTC develops in all patients at a very young age (infancy). All affected individuals develop neural gangliomas, particularly in the mucosa of the digestive tract, conjunctiva, lips, and tongue; 40% to 50% develop pheochromocytomas. Patients with MEN 2B may also have megacolon, skeletal abnormalities, and markedly enlarged peripheral nerves. They do not develop hyperparathyroidism.

FMTC is characterized by development of MTC in the absence of any other endocrinopathies. MTC in these patients has a more indolent clinical course. Some individuals with FMTC may never manifest clinical evidence (i.e., symptoms or a lump in the neck), although biochemical testing and histologic evaluation of the thyroid demonstrates MTC.[55,56]

RET Genotype-Phenotype Correlations

Mutations in the *RET* proto-oncogene are responsible for MEN 2A, MEN 2B, and FMTC.[61–64] This gene encodes a transmembrane tyrosine kinase protein.[57,65] The mutations that cause the MEN 2 syndromes are activating gain-of-function mutations affecting constitutive activation of the protein. This is unusual among hereditary cancer syndromes, which are usually caused by loss-of-function mutations in the predisposition gene (e.g., familial polyposis, *BRCA1* and 2, von Hippel-Lindau, and MEN 1). More than 30 missense mutations have been described in patients affected by the MEN 2 syndromes (Fig. 32.4).

There is a relationship between the type of inherited *RET* mutation and presentation of MTC. The most virulent form is seen in patients with MEN 2B. These patients most commonly have a germline mutation in codon 918 of *RET* (ATG->ACG), although other mutations have been described (codon 883 and 922). As noted previously, MTC in MEN 2B has an extremely early age of onset (infancy). Despite its distinctive clinical appearance and associated gastrointestinal difficulties, the disease is often not detected until the patient develops a neck mass. Metastatic spread is usually present at the time of initial treatment, and calcitonin levels often remain elevated postoperatively.

MTC has a variable course in patients with MEN 2A, similar to that of sporadic MTC. Codon 634 and 618 mutations are the most common *RET* mutations associated with MEN 2A, although

mutations at other codons are also observed (see Fig. 32.4). Some patients do extremely well for many years, even with distant metastases, while others develop inanition, symptomatic liver, lung or skeletal metastases, as well as disabling diarrhea. Recurrence in the central neck, with invasion of the airway or great vessels, may cause death.

In patients with FMTC, MTC is usually indolent. These individuals most commonly have mutations of codons 609, 611, 618, 620, 768, 804, or 891, although mutations of other codons have been identified (see Fig. 32.4). Many patients with FMTC are cured by thyroidectomy alone, and even those with persistent elevation of calcitonin levels do well for many years. Occasionally, patients with FMTC survive into the seventh or eighth decade without clinical signs of disease, although pathologic examination of the thyroid will reveal MTC or C-cell hyperplasia.[66]

Risk-Reducing Thyroidectomy in *RET* Mutation Carriers

Genetic counseling and informed consent should be obtained prior to genetic testing. Specific issues that should be covered in genetic counseling sessions include explaining the patterns of heritability, likelihood of expression of different tumors, their prevention and treatment, insurability, nonpaternity, survivor guilt, and others.

It has been shown that *RET* mutation carriers may harbor foci of MTC in the thyroid gland, even when calcitonin levels are normal.[67] While the age of onset and rate of disease progression may differ, the lifetime penetrance of MTC is near 100% in carriers of *RET* mutations associated with MEN 2 syndromes. At-risk individuals who are found to have inherited a *RET* gene mutation are therefore candidates for thyroidectomy, regardless of their plasma calcitonin levels.

The best option for prevention of MTC in *RET* mutation carriers is complete surgical resection prior to malignant transformation. Prophylactic thyroidectomy prior to the development of MTC is the goal in these patients. A number of studies have demonstrated improved biochemical cure rates and/or decreased recurrence rates from early thyroidectomy, performed after positive screening by calcitonin testing or *RET* mutation testing.[68–70]

MEN 2B mutations are the highest risk level, designated level III (see Fig. 32.4).[55,71] Patients with MEN 2B have the most aggressive form of MTC, with invasive disease reported in patients <1 year of age. These patients should have preventative surgery

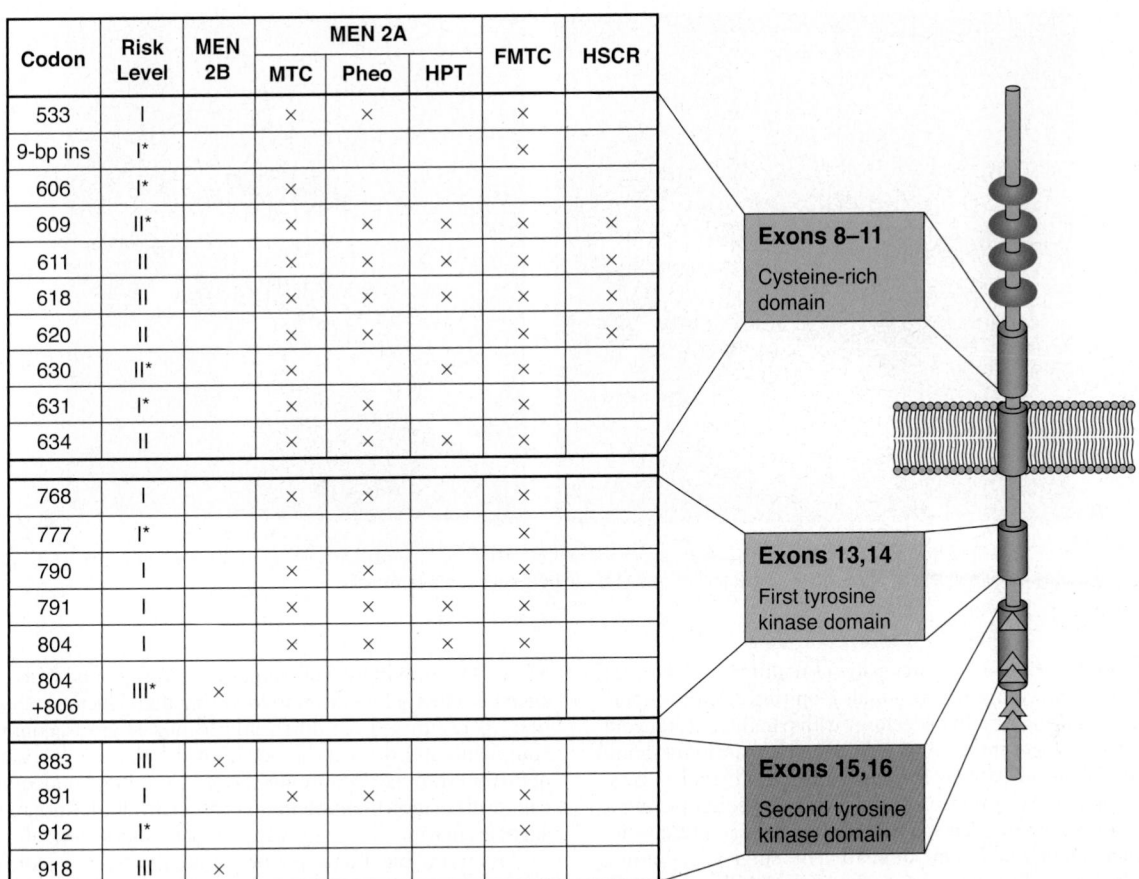

Codon	Risk Level	MEN 2B	MEN 2A			FMTC	HSCR
			MTC	Pheo	HPT		
533	I		×	×		×	
9-bp ins	I*					×	
606	I*		×				
609	II*		×	×	×	×	×
611	II		×	×	×	×	×
618	II		×	×	×	×	×
620	II		×	×		×	×
630	II*		×		×	×	
631	I*		×	×		×	
634	II		×	×	×	×	
768	I		×	×		×	
777	I*					×	
790	I		×	×		×	
791	I		×	×	×	×	
804	I		×	×	×	×	
804 +806	III*	×					
883	III	×					
891	I		×	×		×	
912	I*					×	
918	III	×					

Exons 8–11
Cysteine-rich domain

Exons 13,14
First tyrosine kinase domain

Exons 15,16
Second tyrosine kinase domain

Figure 32.4 *RET* mutation sites associated with multiple endocrine neoplasia (MEN) 2 syndromes. Codons previously reported in association with MEN-2 syndromes are listed by structural domain within the RET protein. Risk level is based on consensus guidelines or more recent clinical reports. Previously reported phenotypes for each codon are shown. MTC, medullary thyroid carcinoma; Pheo, pheochromocytoma; HPT, hyperparathyroidism; FMTC, familial medullary thyroid carcinoma; HSCR, Hirschsprung's disease. *Asterisk* indicates risk level based on recent clinical reports not available at publication of the consensus guidelines. (From Traugott AL, Moley JF. The RET protooncogene. *Cancer Treat Res* 2010;153:303–319.)

early in the first year of life, if possible. Identification and preservation of parathyroid glands can be extremely difficult in these infants, due to their small size, translucent appearance, and the presence of exuberant thymic and perithyroidal nodal tissue. These procedures should be performed by surgeons experienced in parathyroid and/or pediatric thyroid operations.

Patients with MEN 2A with mutations in codons 634, 620, 618, and 611 are also considered high risk (level II).[55,71] Patients with level II mutations should undergo a total thyroidectomy at 5 to 6 years of age. There is evidence that the risk of lymph node metastasis is very low in patients with MEN 2A under the age of 8, with normal calcitonin levels. Central lymph node dissection is associated with higher risk of hypoparathyroidism, and recurrent laryngeal nerve injury and should be reserved for patients with elevated calcitonin levels.

A larger subset of *RET* mutations, associated with MEN 2A and/or FMTC, is considered the lowest risk (level I).[55,71] These include mutations at codons 768, 790, 791, 804, and 891. For patients with low-risk level I mutations, total thyroidectomy is recommended before age 5 to 10 years. This decision, however, regarding ideal age at preventative thyroidectomy in low-risk mutation carriers, is currently being reviewed, and may be driven by additional clinical data such as the basal or stimulated serum calcitonin level.[72,73] There are no guidelines at present that address the issue of timing of surgery based on calcitonin level, and at present, pentagastrin (the primary calcitonin secretagogue used in testing) is not available in the United States. It is anticipated that within a decade, there will

be enough published data to direct timing of interventions based upon this information. As with the level II mutations, the need for central lymph node dissection should be guided by calcitonin levels and clinical features of the patient and kindred.

Until recently, some groups recommended total thyroidectomy with central neck lymph node dissection and total parathyroidectomy with autotransplantation for all *RET* mutation carriers. Recent studies and personal experience, however, have demonstrated an extremely low likelihood of nodal metastases in patients with MEN 2A or FMTC younger than 8 years of age, and in patients with a normal calcitonin level.[70] Our current strategy is to leave the parathyroid in situ in these patients, if possible.[74] Often, however, the desired complete removal of thyroid tissue results in compromise of parathyroid blood supply. In these situations, autotransplantation of devascularized parathyroid is required. We routinely remove and autotransplant the parathyroid if a central node dissection is done. In parathyroid autotransplantation, parathyroid glands are sliced into 1 mm × 3 mm fragments and autotransplanted into individual muscle pockets in the muscle of the nondominant forearm in patients with MEN 2A, or in the sternocleidomastoid muscle in patients with FMTC or MEN 2B. Patients are maintained on calcium and vitamin D supplementation for 4 to 8 weeks postoperatively.

In a recent series of thyroidectomies performed in 50 individuals with MEN 2A (identified by genetic screening), total thyroidectomy and central node dissection with parathyroidectomy and parathyroid autografting were performed in all patients (Fig. 32.5).[70]

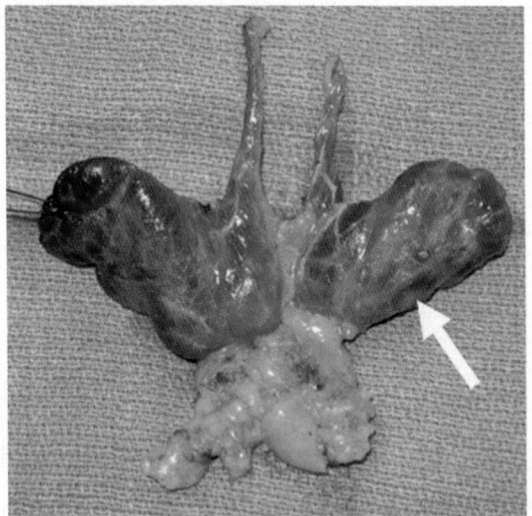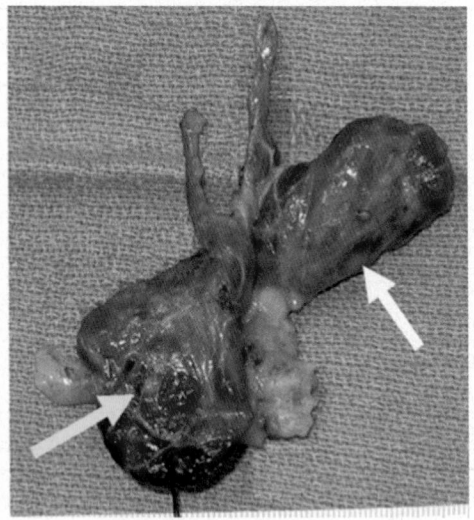

Figure 32.5 Total thyroidectomy specimen with attached central nodes from a patient with germline *RET* mutation and elevated calcitonin levels. Note small visible foci of medullary thyroid carcinoma (*arrows*).

All autografts functioned, but three patients required supplemental calcium. The percentage of individuals requiring calcium supplementation following parathyroidectomy with parathyroid autografting reportedly ranges from 0% to 18%. Parathyroidectomy should be performed in all patients showing gross parathyroid enlargement or biochemical evidence of parathyroid disease at time of surgery. The operating surgeon should have expertise in preservation of parathyroid function. It is important that the surgeon performing an operative procedure for MTC be familiar with the techniques described here. If not, the patient should be referred to a center where these procedures are routinely performed.

Some patients with MEN 2 will be found to have elevated calcitonin levels prior to thyroidectomy. This is usually associated with medullary thyroid carcinoma or C-cell hyperplasia in the gland, and may be associated with lymph node metastases. Much has been written about the correlation between preoperative calcitonin levels and extent of nodal involvement. It has been suggested that preoperative calcitonin level may guide the extent of node dissection. In a study of 300 European patients with MTC, node metastases were not identified when the preoperative basal calcitonin level was <20 pg/ml.[75] Involvement of nodal groups was correlated with basal calcitonin level as follows: ipsilateral central and lateral neck nodes (basal calcitonin >20 pg/ml), contralateral central nodes (basal calcitonin >50 pg/ml), contralateral lateral neck nodes (basal calcitonin >200 pg/ml), and mediastinal nodes (basal calcitonin >500 pg/ml). Based upon these findings, this group (who also wrote the European guidelines) recommends thyroidectomy only if basal calcitonin is <20 pg/ml, ipsilateral central and lateral neck dissection if the calcitonin is 20 to 50 pg/ml, and contralateral central neck dissection if the basal calcitonin is 50 to 200 pg/ml, with the addition of contralateral lateral neck dissection if the calcitonin is 200 to 500 pg/ml. Most experts agree that sternotomy with mediastinal neck dissection should be reserved for patients with image evidence of mediastinal disease. In contrast, most North American surgeons rely heavily upon preoperative ultrasound imaging to map the extent of nodal involvement and determine extent of surgery based upon calcitonin and imaging results.[55,74,76]

Follow-up

Following thyroidectomy, thyroid hormone replacement is required for life. Patients may need several weeks of oral calcium and vitamin D until parathyroid function recovers. Intermittent calcitonin testing may be done to monitor for persistent or recurrent MTC. The importance of regular monitoring of patients' compliance with thyroid medication following thyroidectomy should not be underestimated. Children and teenagers are frequently noncompliant, and this can be determined by routine measurement of thyroid-stimulating hormone levels. Continued noncompliance can result in growth problems. Occasionally, local human services agencies may need to be involved in particularly difficult cases.

The term "biochemical cure" is used to refer to patients with normal calcitonin levels after surgery for MTC. Complete postoperative normalization of calcitonin has been associated with decreased long-term risk of MTC recurrence, though the evidence is less clear for a survival benefit. A persistent or recurrent elevation in calcitonin indicates residual or recurrent MTC and warrants additional investigation by imaging. However, as most MTC has a fairly indolent course, patients with biochemical evidence of recurrent disease may not have corollary imaging findings for some time.

Conclusions

Identification of *RET* gene mutations in individuals at risk for developing hereditary forms of MTC has simplified management, expanding the scope of indications for surgical intervention. Patients who carry this mutation can be offered operative treatment at a very young age, hopefully before the cancer has developed or spread, and those identified as not having the mutation are spared further genetic and biochemical screening. This achievement marks a new paradigm in surgery: the indication that an operation be performed based on the results of a genetic test. As in the decision to perform any surgical procedure, meticulous preparation and detailed discussion with patient and family must precede the final recommendation. It is also important that the patient and family be involved in preoperative discussions with genetic counselors. Postoperative follow-up for compliance with thyroid medication is important, especially in children and teenagers who are still growing and developing into adults.

FAMILIAL ADENOMATOUS POLYPOSIS, *MYH*-ASSOCIATED POLUPOSIS, AND LYNCH SYNDROME

Inherited CRC syndromes with multiple adenomatous polyps include FAP, *MYH*-associated polyposis (MAP), and LS. In some cases, the diagnosis is suspected because of a striking family history

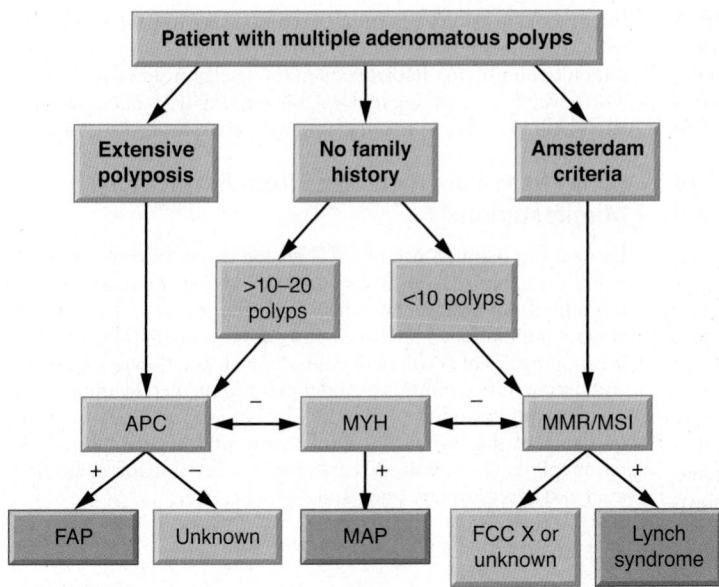

Figure 32.6 Schematic demonstrating the potential genetic workup for a patient with multiple adenomatous colorectal polyps and suspected of having an inherited colorectal cancer syndrome. APC, adenomatous polyposis coli; MMR, mismatch repair; MSI, microsatellite instability; FAP, familial adenomatous polyposis; MAP, *MYH*-associated polyposis; FCC X, familial colorectal cancer syndrome X.

of CRC, while in others, suspicion arises from a very young onset of CRC or florid polyposis.

Although adenomatous polyp burden and family history may suggest one syndrome over another, an initial negative genetic test result should be followed by further evaluation for other syndromes. For example, in clinical practice, a negative adenomatous polyposis coli (*APC*) gene test in a patient with a suspected CRC syndrome is followed by reflex testing for MAP and LS, as shown in Figure 32.6.

FAP is an autosomal dominant syndrome that accounts for <1% of the annual CRC burden, is caused by mutations in the tumor-suppressor *APC* gene. It is characterized by the presence of ≥100 adenomatous polyps in the colorectum, nearly 100% penetrance, and an inevitable risk of CRC if prophylactic colectomy is not performed.[8,77] Patients with a less severe form known as attenuated FAP (AFAP) usually present with <100 colorectal adenomas that tend to be proximally located. MAP is an autosomal recessive syndrome that often presents phenotypically as attenuated polyposis. While an estimated 2% of the general population are monoallelic carriers of a mutated base-excision-repair *MUTYH* (*MYH*) gene, biallelic germline mutations may account for 9% to 18% of patients with FAP or AFAP phenotypes who have no demonstrable *APC* mutation.[78–80]

LS accounts for 1% to 4% of all newly diagnosed CRC and is attributable to a germline mutation in one of the DNA MMR genes (*MLH1, MSH2, MSH6,* and *PMS2*).[81–83] Epigenetic silencing of the *MSH2* gene via a 3′-end deletion in *EPCAM* (*TACSTD1*), a neighbor of *MSH2* that plays a role in cell adhesion, also accounts for 20% to 25% of all suspected *MSH2* cases and 1% to 6% of LS cases overall.[84–86] LS is characterized by early age-of-onset CRC, predominance of lesions proximal to the splenic flexure, an increased rate of metachronous CRC, and a unique spectrum of benign and malignant extracolonic tumors. Lifetime risk of CRC in patients with LS may be as high as 80%.[83,87] MSI reflects a deficiency in DNA repair secondary to MMR gene mutation and is a hallmark feature of LS-associated tumors.

Variability in penetrance, phenotypic expression, and certainty of disease development mandate distinctly different surgical approaches in these three syndromes, including the type and timing of risk-reducing colon and rectal surgery.[88]

Familial Adenomatous Polyposis

Surveillance of at-risk family members should begin around age 10 to 15 years with an annual colonoscopy or flexible sigmoidoscopy.[89]

At-risk individuals who belong to families with an AFAP phenotype should undergo colonoscopic screening every 2 to 3 years starting in their late teens. Informative genetic testing is possible in families with a demonstrated *APC* mutation, and mutations are detected in most pedigrees. However, approximately 25% of patients with FAP will have a de novo *APC* mutation.[87] Severity of polyposis should be established during colonoscopy, as the timing of surgery and the risk of developing colorectal is dependent on the extent of polyp burden. Patients with mild polyposis and a correspondingly lower CRC risk can undergo surgery in their late teens. Patients with severe polyposis, a high degree of dysplasia, multiple adenomas >5 mm in size, and symptoms (bleeding, persistent diarrhea, anemia, failure to thrive, psychosocial stress, etc.) should undergo risk-reducing colorectal surgery as soon as is practical after diagnosis.[90,91] However, in carefully selected, fully asymptomatic patients who have small adenomas but a strong family history of aggressive abdominal desmoid disease, consideration can be given to delaying prophylactic colectomy, as the risk of desmoid-related complication may be greater than the risk of CRC development.

The three current surgical options for patients with FAP are total proctocolectomy (TPC) with permanent ileostomy, total colectomy with ileorectal anastomosis (IRA), and proctocolectomy with ileal pouch-anal anastomosis (IPAA). IPAA can be a double-stapled, end-of-pouch-to-anus anastomosis, which may leave behind approximately 1 cm of anal transition zone. An alternative approach, which is preferred when there is carpeting of the anal transition zone with adenomas, is to perform a mucosal stripping of the anal transition zone down to the dentate line followed by a hand-sewn per anal anastomosis of pouch to the dentate line. Selection of the optimal procedure for an individual patient is based on several factors, including characteristics of the FAP syndrome within the patient and family, differences in likely postoperative functional outcome, preoperative anal sphincter status, and patient preference.[8]

TPC with permanent ileostomy, although rarely chosen as a primary procedure, is used in patients with invasive cancer involving the sphincters or levator complex, or patients for whom an IPAA is not technically feasible (secondary to desmoid disease and foreshortening of the small bowel mesentery, making it surgically impossible to bring the ileal pouch to the anus) nor likely to lead to good function such as massive obesity or weak anal sphincters. However, TPC is occasionally chosen as a primary procedure by patients who perceive that their lifestyle would be compromised by the frequent bowel movements (five to six per day) sometimes associated with the IPAA procedure.

In addition to these issues, the key in deciding between an IPAA and an IRA is based primarily on the risk of rectal cancer development if the rectum is left in situ. The risk of rectal cancer following IRA may range from 3% to 10% at 10 years, while the risk for a secondary proctectomy for uncontrolled rectal polyposis ranges from 10% to 61% at 20 years following initial colectomy with IRA.[92–94] The magnitude of risk in an individual patient is, however, related to the overall extent of colorectal polyposis. IRA may be considered for patients with <1,000 colorectal polyps (including those with attenuated FAP) and <20 rectal adenomas, as these individuals have a relatively low risk of developing rectal cancer.[88,93] Patients with severe rectal (>20 adenomas) or colonic (>1,000 adenomas) polyposis, an adenoma >3 cm, or an adenoma with severe dysplasia should ideally undergo a risk-reducing procedure that will include a proctectomy.[90,91,93]

The risk of secondary rectal excision, due to uncontrollable rectal polyposis or rectal cancer, may be estimated by identifying the specific location of the causative APC mutation. Patients with mutations located between codons 1250 and 1464 have been shown to have a six-fold increased risk of developing rectal cancer, compared to those with mutations prior to codon 1250 or after codon 1464 (mean number of rectal polyps 42 versus 22, respectively).[8,92] Although the use of the genotype-phenotype relationship to guide patient management may be appealing,[92] it is important to recognize the variability of phenotypic expression that exists even among members of the same family. This suggests that at the current time, the choice between an IRA and an IPAA should be based primarily on clinical (rather than genetic) grounds.[90]

The risk of polyp and cancer development following primary surgery is not limited to patients undergoing IRA. In patients undergoing IPAA, neoplasia may occur at the site of ileal pouch anastomosis; the frequency appears to be greater after stapled anastomosis (28% to 31%) than after mucosectomy and hand-sewn anastomosis (10% to 14%).[95] In the case of neoplasia developing at the anal transition zone after a stapled anastomosis, transanal mucosectomy may be performed, followed by advancement of the pouch to the dentate line. Of additional concern is the development of adenomatous polyps in the ileal pouch, which occurs in approximately 45% of patients by 10-year follow-up.[96] Consequently, depending on polyp burden, lifetime endoscopic surveillance of the rectal remnant (after IRA) every 6 to 12 months or the ileal pouch (after IPAA) every 1 to 3 years is required following either procedure.[89]

Another important consideration in choosing between IPAA and IRA is postoperative bowel function and quality of life. Some studies have associated IPAA with higher frequency of both daytime and nocturnal bowel movements, higher incidence of passive incontinence and incidental soiling, and greater postoperative morbidity.[97] However, long-term follow-up demonstrates a comparable quality of life following IPAA for FAP relative to the patient's preoperative baseline.[98] Therefore, although the choice of procedure must be carefully individualized, because of the risk of rectal cancer associated with IRA, the authors favor IPAA for most patients with FAP whenever feasible. However, an IRA should be considered in specific circumstances, such as when there is mild rectal polyposis (as in AFAP), or a young patient with rectal sparing who is not interested in undergoing the multiple procedures that accompany an IPAA and diverting loop ileostomy, or a young woman interested in having children and trying to avoid the decreased fecundity associated with an IPAA procedure.[99] The use of minimally invasive techniques such as laparoscopy may reduce the risk of infertility associated with IPAA.[100,101] Though a diverting loop ileostomy should be performed in all IPAA procedures, it is not always feasible due to a number of anatomic factors such as body habitus.

Endoscopic surveillance of the rectal segment at 6- to 12-month intervals after the index surgery is recommended, with subsequent surveillance frequencies dependent on the number and size of adenomas observed.[89] Although small (<5 mm) scattered adenomas can be safely observed or removed with biopsy forceps, polyps >5 mm should be removed by snare. However, repeated fulguration and polypectomy over many years can lead to difficulty with subsequent polypectomy, reduced rectal compliance, and difficulty identifying flat cancers in the background of scar tissue. The development of severe dysplasia and/or villous adenomas not amenable to endoscopic removal is indication for proctectomy.

Long-Term Considerations from Extracolonic Manifestations

Despite the reduced risk of CRC-related death following prophylactic colectomy, patients with FAP are still at increased risk of mortality from both rectal cancer and other causes relative to the general population. The three main causes of death following IRA are progression of desmoid disease, stomach and duodenal cancer, and perioperative mortality. Additional FAP-related extraintestinal manifestations include epidermoid cysts, supernumerary teeth, osteomas of the jaw and/or skull, congenital hypertrophy of the retinal pigment epithelium, cancers of the hepatopancreatobiliary tract and genitourinary tract, and thyroid cancer.[102–104]

Desmoids

Desmoids may occur in 10% to 25% of patients with FAP.[105,106] Unlike those found in the general population, FAP-associated desmoids tend to be intra-abdominal and arise following abdominal surgery.[106,107] Although conflicting reports exist, it appears that female patients, those with extracolonic manifestations of FAP, a positive family history of desmoids, and APC mutations located at 3' of codon 1440 are at increased risk of developing desmoids.[106,108,109] These tumors often involve the small bowel mesentery as well as the retroperitoneum and are often life-threatening due to invasion or compression of adjacent viscera. Further, recurrence and morbidity rates are high following attempted resection, with recurrent disease often more aggressive than the initial desmoid. Estimated 5-year overall survival for patients with intra-abdominal desmoids causing severe symptoms such as significant pain and septic fistula/abscess, diameter >20 cm or rapidly growing, and/or need for parenteral nutrition is only 53%.[107] Therefore, desmoid resection is evaluated on an individualized case-by-case basis with surgery reserved for highly select cases.

Desmoids that involve the small bowel mesentery may preclude the formation of an IPAA secondary to foreshortening of the small bowel mesentery, especially in patients undergoing proctectomy after an initial IRA.[110] Surgery for intra-abdominal and abdominal wall desmoids should be reserved for limited disease where the likelihood of clear margins is high.

In symptomatic cases where resection of an intra-abdominal desmoid may not be feasible, intestinal bypass or ureteral stenting may be necessary to alleviate bowel or urinary obstruction secondary to mass effect. In addition to surgical intervention, several medical options with variable efficacy are available for the management of desmoid disease and include nonsteroidal anti-inflammatory drugs (e.g., sulindac), selective estrogen receptor modulators (e.g., tamoxifen), immunomodulators (e.g., imatinib, sorafenib, interferon), doxorubin-based cytotoxic chemotherapy, and radiation.

MYH-Associated Polyposis

MAP should be suspected in patients with >10 colorectal adenomas, a weak history of CRC, and no family history of FAP. The diagnosis is confirmed by *MUTYH* (*MYH*) gene testing.[80,88]

Depending on the polyp burden, the management of the colon and rectum of a patient with a biallelic *MYH* mutation can be endoscopic or surgical. If the polyp burden is limited and an endoscopic approach is pursued, colonoscopy should be performed every 1 to 3 years.[87,89] If the polyp burden is not amenable to an endoscopic approach at the time of diagnosis, then a resection is indicated. In most cases in which surgery is deemed necessary, an IRA is sufficient. However, if rectal polyposis is severe, an IPAA may be indicated. Indications for surgery following an endoscopic surveillance program include increasing polyp size or number, or worsening histology.

Extracolonic manifestations of MAP are similar to FAP and include osteomas, desmoids, congenital hypertrophy of the retinal pigment epithelium, as well as cancers of the thyroid, ovary, bladder, sebaceous gland, and breast. In addition, patients with MAP are also at a 4% lifetime risk of developing duodenal cancer and require upper endoscopies every 1 to 3 years beginning as early as ages 18 to 20 years and starting no later than ages 30 to 35 years.[87,89,111]

Lynch Syndrome

Due to the discordance associated with the term hereditary nonpolyposis colorectal cancer, the use of this term has largely been abandoned with reversion back to the eponym LS, which refers to individuals with a predisposition to CRC and other malignancies as a result of a germline MMR mutation.[112] Overall, CRC occurs in up to 80% of patients with LS by their mid-40s.[8,82] Endometrial cancer occurs in 40% to 60%, gastric cancer in 11% to 19%, urinary tract cancer in 5% to 18%, and ovarian cancer in 9% to 15% of affected individuals.[8,82,87]

The Amsterdam criteria and revised Bethesda guidelines[113] (Table 32.3) are used in clinical practice to identify patients at risk for LS who require further genetic evaluation. The Amsterdam criteria, which led to the identification of the LS-causing MMR gene mutations require that there be:

■ Three relatives (one a first-degree relative of the other two) with colorectal, endometrial, stomach, ovary, small bowel, ureteral/renal pelvis, brain, hepatobiliary, and/or sebaceous cancer;
■ In two or more successive generations;
■ With at least one case of cancer diagnosed before the age of 50;
■ And that FAP as a diagnosis is excluded.[114]

Though the Amsterdam criteria can be used clinically to identify potential patients with LS, using it alone will result in identification

of only 42% of LS mutation carriers.[115] Families meeting Amsterdam criteria but lacking an MMR mutation are referred to as having "familial colorectal cancer type X" and appear to have a lower incidence of colorectal and extracolonic cancers than those with a LS germline MMR mutation (see Fig. 32.6). Of note, they have an increased incidence of left-sided and nonmucinous microsatellite stable tumors.[77,88]

Patients with CRC who belong to pedigrees suspicious for LS should be offered screening by IHC for loss of MMR protein expression or by MSI analysis. As the sensitivity of IHC testing for loss of MMR protein expression is comparable to MSI testing, either approach can be pursued.[112] However, IHC testing is less expensive and can also identify a specific MMR protein loss, which can help target subsequent germline testing. Routine IHC testing for loss of MMR protein in individuals younger than 50 years at the time of CRC diagnosis is feasible and has led to the identification of patients with LS who might otherwise have been missed.[116,117] Patients with MSI-high tumors should undergo testing for germline MMR mutations in *MSH2, MLH1, MSH6,* and *PMS2.* Reflex IHC and/or MSI testing on all newly diagnosed CRC has been advocated by some expert groups and has been successfully implemented at some institutions.[83,112,118] However, a majority of cancer programs nationwide currently do not have a protocol for reflex testing for LS, citing lack of institutional protocols as well as fear of nonreimbursement.[119] As such, a unified move toward universal testing remains some time away. In families for which tumor tissue is not available, initial germline testing may be considered though the financial burden is not insignificant, with the cost of finding a single LS carrier measuring approximately $58,000 (compared to the $5,000 spent in finding a single LS carrier using IHC screening).[120] As in FAP, a mutation in an affected individual must be established for testing in at-risk individuals to be conclusive.

In lieu of universal testing, several predictive models such as the MMRpredict, MMRpro, and PREMM$_{1,2,6}$ have been devised in order to assess an individual's likelihood of harboring LS.[115,121,122] These models quantify an individual's risk for carrying an *MLH1, MSH2, or MSH6* germline mutation by using clinical characteristics such as age at onset of CRC and/or other LS-associated cancers, location of CRC, family history, history of synchronous or metachronous CRC, among others. A study of these predictive models demonstrated that they all performed better than the revised Bethesda guidelines in terms of identifying patients with germline mutations for LS.[123] The MMRpredict model appeared to have to be the best predictor, with a sensitivity and specificity for LS of 94% and 91%, respectively. Other validation studies, however, have not demonstrated the superiority of MMRpredict compared to the other aforementioned models.[124,125] It appears that the use of clinical characteristics in combination with MSI or MMR protein expression status in predictive models may potentially improve our ability to establish LS diagnoses in patients with CRC. However, the practicality and applicability of these tools in a clinical setting requires further assessment.

Although development of CRC in LS is not a certainty, the 80% lifetime risk, the 16% to 30% risk of metachronous CRC, and the possibly accelerated adenoma-to-carcinoma sequence mandate consideration of prophylactic surgical options.[82,87,126–129] Patients with LS who have a CRC or more than one advanced adenoma should be offered the options of prophylactic total colectomy with IRA or segmental colectomy with annual postoperative surveillance colonoscopy. Careful surveillance is also necessary after total colectomy and IRA, as the risk of high-risk adenomas and cancer in the retained rectum at a median of 104 months are 11% and 8%, respectively.[126] Although there has been no study demonstrating an improved survival for patients with LS undergoing total colectomy and IRA versus segmental colectomy, mathematical models suggest a slight survival benefit for total colectomy and IRA, especially for individuals under the age of 30.[130,131] In addition, because of increased rates of metachronous CRC development and the risk of multiple abdominal surgeries

TABLE 32.3

The Revised Bethesda Guidelines for Testing Colorectal Tumors for Microsatellite Instability

Tumors from individuals should be tested for MSI in the following situations:
1. Colorectal cancer diagnosed in a patient who is <50 y of age.
2. Presence of synchronous, metachronous colorectal, or other HNPCC-associated tumors,[a] regardless of age.
3. Colorectal cancer with the MSI-H[b] histology[c] diagnosed in a patient who is <60 y of age.[d]
4. Colorectal cancer diagnosed in one or more first-degree relatives with an HNPCC-related tumor, with one of the cancers being diagnosed under age 50 years.
5. Colorectal cancer diagnosed in two or more first- or second-degree relatives with HNPCC-related tumors, regardless of age.

MSI, microsatellite instability; HNPCC, hereditary nonpolyposis colorectal cancer; MSI-H, microsatellite instability–high.
[a] HNPCC-related tumors include colorectal, endometrial, stomach, ovarian, pancreas, ureter and renal pelvis, biliary tract, and brain (usually glioblastoma as seen in Turcot syndrome) tumors, sebaceous gland adenomas and keratoacanthomas in Muir-Torre syndrome, and carcinoma of the small bowel.
[b] MSI-H in tumors refers to changes in two or more of the five National Cancer Institute–recommended panels of microsatellite markers.
[c] Presence of tumor-infiltrating lymphocytes, Crohn's-like lymphocytic reaction, mucinous/signet ring differentiation, or medullary growth pattern.
[d] There was no consensus among the workshop participants on whether to include the age criteria in guideline 3; participants voted to keep <60 years of age in the guidelines.
From Umar A, Boland CR, Terdiman JP, et al. Revised Bethesda Guidelines for hereditary nonpolyposis colorectal cancer (Lynch syndrome) and microsatellite instability. *J Natl Cancer Inst* 2004;96:261–268.

in those undergoing a segmental resection, a total colectomy and IRA has emerged as the procedure of choice for the index cancer, with consideration for TPC in cases where a high risk of metachronous rectal cancer can be predicted.[126–128] Targeted genetic testing approaches—such as the single amplicon MSH2 A636P mutation test in Ashkenazi Jewish patients with CRC—have demonstrated how a rapid and inexpensive preoperative genetic test can help direct the extent of colon resection.[132]

LS mutation carriers with a normal colon and without a history of CRC may also be offered prophylactic colectomy in highly select situations. One rationale for this approach is the similarity of lifetime cancer risk between patients with *APC* and *MMR* gene mutations, and the fact that total abdominal colectomy with IRA produces less functional disturbance than the prophylactic procedure recommended for FAP (TPC with IPAA). However, an alternate strategy for these individuals is surveillance by colonoscopy, which is cost-effective and greatly reduces the rate of CRC development and overall mortality.[133] There is a risk of CRC development in the interval between colonoscopies, though most interval cancers tend to be early stage.[134,135] As such, given that metachronous CRC may develop in as short a duration as a median of 11.3 months,[136] the recommended interval for surveillance colonoscopies is now every 1 to 2 years.[89] While prophylactic colectomy is not routinely recommended, it may be indicated in highly select patients for whom colonoscopic surveillance is not technically possible or in those who refuse to undergo regular surveillance. A decision analysis model suggests that prophylactic subtotal colectomy at age 25 may offer a survival benefit of 1.8 years, compared with surveillance colonoscopy. The benefit of prophylactic colectomy decreases when surgery is delayed until later in life and is negligible when performed at the time of cancer development.[137] Thus, the decision between prophylactic surgery and surveillance for a gene-positive unaffected individual is based on many factors including penetrance of disease in the

family, early age-of-onset in affected family members, functional and quality-of-life considerations, and likelihood of compliance with surveillance. Table 32.4 lists some of the pros and cons of a prophylactic colectomy for germline mutation carriers for LS without a history of CRC. Patients with LS and an index rectal cancer should be offered the options of TPC with IPAA or anterior proctosigmoidectomy with primary reconstruction.[128,138] The rationale for TPC is the 10% to 15% associated risk of metachronous colon cancer in the remaining colon following the index rectal cancer. Choosing between the two procedures depends, in part, on the patient's willingness to undergo intensive surveillance of the retained proximal colon, as well as issues regarding quality of life and bowel function.

TABLE 32.4

Prophylactic Total Abdominal Colectomy and Ileorectal Anastomosis for Lynch Syndrome Patients without Cancer

Pros
- Elimination of colon cancer risk
- Elimination of need for surveillance colonoscopy
- Alleviating patient anxiety over the prospect of colon cancer development

Cons
- Persistence of risk of rectal cancer development
- Rectum still requires flexible endoscopic surveillance
- Patient anxiety of prospect of rectal cancer persists
- Possible altered bowel function
- Risk of surgery and possible associated complications

SELECTED REFERENCES

The full reference list can be accessed at lwwhealthlibrary.com/oncology.

1. Moyer VA, US Preventive Services Task Force. Risk Assessment, Genetic Counseling, and Genetic Testing for BRCA-Related Cancer in Women: U.S. Preventive Services Task Force Recommendation Statement. *Ann Intern Med* 2014;160.

2. Robson ME, Storm CD, Weitzel J, et al. American Society of Clinical Oncology policy statement update: genetic and genomic testing for cancer susceptibility. *J Clin Oncol* 2010;28:893–901.

3. Amir E, Freedman OC, Seruga B, et al. Assessing women at high risk of breast cancer: a review of risk assessment models. *J Natl Cancer Inst* 2010; 102:680–691.

8. Guillem JG, Wood WC, Moley JF, et al. ASCO/SSO review of current role of risk-reducing surgery in common hereditary cancer syndromes. *J Clin Oncol* 2006;24:4642–4660.

9. Saslow D, Boetes C, Burke W, et al. American Cancer Society guidelines for breast screening with MRI as an adjunct to mammography. *CA Cancer J Clin* 2007;57:75–89.

10. Domchek SM, Friebel TM, Singer CF, et al. Association of risk-reducing surgery in BRCA1 or BRCA2 mutation carriers with cancer risk and mortality. *JAMA* 2010;304:967–975.

11. US Equal Employment Opportunity Commission. Genetic information discrimination. http://www.eeoc.gov/laws/types/genetic.cfm. Accessed January 2, 2014.

12. Society of Surgical Oncology. Position statement on prophylactic mastectomy. http://www.surgonc.org/practice-policy/practice-management/consensus-statements/position-statement-on-prophylactic-mastectomy. Accessed February 1, 2014.

14. Eldor L, Spiegel A. Breast reconstruction after bilateral prophylactic mastectomy in women at high risk for breast cancer. *Breast J* 2009;15:S81–S89.

15. Zakhireh J, Fowble B, Esserman LJ. Application of screening principles to the reconstructed breast. *J Clin Oncol* 2010;28:173–180.

16. Gabram SG, Dougherty T, Albain KS, et al. Assessing breast cancer risk and providing treatment recommendations: immediate impact of an educational session. *Breast J* 2009;15:S39–S45.

17. Nadauld LD, Ford JM. Molecular profiling of gastric cancer: toward personalized cancer medicine. *J Clin Oncol* 2013;31:838–839.

18. Bardram L, Hansen TV, Gerdes AM, et al. Prophylactic total gastrectomy in hereditary diffuse gastric cancer: identification of two novel CDH1 gene mutations-a clinical observational study. *Fam Cancer* 2014;13:231–242.

19. Norton JA, Ham CM, Van Dam J, et al. CDH1 truncating mutations in the E-cadherin gene: an indication for total gastrectomy to treat hereditary diffuse gastric cancer. *Ann Surg* 2007;245:873–879.

21. Guilford P, Hopkins J, Harraway J, et al. E-cadherin germline mutations in familial gastric cancer. *Nature* 1998;392:402–405.

22. Kaurah P, MacMillan A, Boyd N, et al. Founder and recurrent CDH1 mutations in families with hereditary diffuse gastric cancer. *JAMA* 2007;297:2360–2372.

23. Benusiglio PR, Malka D, Rouleau E, et al. CDH1 germline mutations and the hereditary diffuse gastric and lobular breast cancer syndrome: a multicentre study. *J Med Genet* 2013;50:486–489.

25. Lee KH, Hwang D, Kang KY, et al. Frequent promoter methylation of CDH1 in non-neoplastic mucosa of sporadic diffuse gastric cancer. *Anticancer Res* 2013;33:3765–3774.

28. Huntsman DG, Carneiro F, Lewis FR, et al. Early gastric cancer in young, asymptomatic carriers of germ-line E-cadherin mutations. *N Engl J Med* 2001;344:1904–1909.

30. Rogers WM, Dobo E, Norton JA, et al. Risk-reducing total gastrectomy for germline mutations in E-cadherin (CDH1): pathologic findings with clinical implications. *Am J Surg Pathol* 2008;32:799–809.

31. Worster E, Liu X, Richardson S, et al. The impact of prophylactic total gastrectomy on health-related quality of life: a prospective cohort study. *Ann Surg* 2014;260:87–93.

32. Lim YC, di Pietro M, O'Donovan M, et al. Prospective cohort study assessing outcomes of patients from families fulfilling criteria for hereditary diffuse gastric cancer undergoing endoscopic surveillance. *Gastrointest Endosc* 2014;80:78–87.

33. Mavaddat N, Peock S, Frost D, et al. Cancer risks for BRCA1 and BRCA2 mutation carriers: results from prospective analysis of EMBRACE. *J Natl Cancer Inst* 2013;105:812–822.

34. Risch HA, McLaughlin JR, Cole DE, et al. Prevalence and penetrance of germline BRCA1 and BRCA2 mutations in a population series of 649 women with ovarian cancer. *Am J Hum Genet* 2001;68:700–710.

35. Struewing JP, Hartge P, Wacholder S, et al. The risk of cancer associated with specific mutations of BRCA1 and BRCA2 among Ashkenazi Jews. *N Engl J Med* 1997;336:1401–1408.

36. Finch AP, Lubinski J, Moller P, et al. Impact of oophorectomy on cancer incidence and mortality in women with a BRCA1 or BRCA2 mutation. *J Clin Oncol* 2014;32:1547–1553.

37. Walsh T, Casadei S, Lee MK, et al. Mutations in 12 genes for inherited ovarian, fallopian tube, and peritoneal carcinoma identified by massively parallel sequencing. *Proc Natl Acad Sci U S A* 2011;108:18032–18037.

38. Couch FJ, Wang X, McGuffog L, et al. Genome-wide association study in BRCA1 mutation carriers identifies novel loci associated with breast and ovarian cancer risk. *PLoS Genet* 2013;9:e1003212.

40. Kauff ND, Satagopan JM, Robson ME, et al. Risk-reducing salpingo-oophorectomy in women with a BRCA1 or BRCA2 mutation. *N Engl J Med* 2002;346:1609–1615.

41. Rebbeck TR, Lynch HT, Neuhausen SL, et al. Prophylactic oophorectomy in carriers of BRCA1 or BRCA2 mutations. *N Engl J Med* 2002;346:1616–1622.

44. Wethington SL, Park KJ, Soslow RA, et al. Clinical outcome of isolated serous tubal intraepithelial carcinomas (STIC). *Int J Gynecol Cancer* 2013;23:1603–1611.

45. Bonadona V, Bonaiti B, Olschwang S, et al. Cancer risks associated with germline mutations in MLH1, MSH2, and MSH6 genes in Lynch syndrome. *JAMA* 2011;305:2304–2310.

48. Watson P, Vasen HF, Mecklin JP, et al. The risk of endometrial cancer in hereditary nonpolyposis colorectal cancer. *Am J Med* 1994;96:516–520.

49. Koornstra JJ, Mourits MJ, Sijmons RH, et al. Management of extracolonic tumours in patients with Lynch syndrome. *Lancet Oncol* 2009;10:400–408.

51. Schmeler KM, Lynch HT, Chen LM, et al. Prophylactic surgery to reduce the risk of gynecologic cancers in the Lynch syndrome. *N Engl J Med* 2006;354:261–269.

54. Traugott AL, Moley JF. Multiple endocrine neoplasia type 2: clinical manifestations and management. *Cancer Treat Res* 2009;153:321–337.

55. American Thyroid Association Guidelines Task Force, Kloos RT, Eng C, et al. Medullary thyroid cancer: management guidelines of the American Thyroid Association. *Thyroid* 2009;19:565–612.

56. Wells SA Jr, Pacini F, Robinson BG, et al. Multiple endocrine neoplasia type 2 and familial medullary thyroid carcinoma: an update. *J Clin Endocrinol Metab* 2013;98:3149–3164.

57. Eng C, Clayton D, Schuffenecker I, et al. The relationship between specific RET proto-oncogene mutations and disease phenotype in multiple endocrine neoplasia type 2. International RET mutation consortium analysis. *JAMA* 1996;276:1575–1579.

70. Skinner MA, Moley JA, Dilley WG, et al. Prophylactic thyroidectomy in multiple endocrine neoplasia type 2A. *N Engl J Med* 2005;353:1105–1113.

71. Brandi ML, Gagel RF, Angeli A, et al. Guidelines for diagnosis and therapy of MEN type 1 and type 2. *J Clin Endocrinol Metab* 2001;86:5658–5671.

72. Elisei R, Romei C, Renzini G, et al. The timing of total thyroidectomy in RET gene mutation carriers could be personalized and safely planned on the basis of serum calcitonin: 18 years experience at one single center. *J Clin Endocrinol Metab* 2012;97:426–435.

74. Moley JF. Medullary thyroid carcinoma: management of lymph node metastases. *J Natl Compr Canc Netw* 2010;8:549–556.

81. Hampel H, Frankel WL, Martin E, et al. Screening for the Lynch syndrome (hereditary nonpolyposis colorectal cancer). *N Engl J Med* 2005;352:1851–1860.

83. Vasen HF, Blanco I, Aktan-Collan K, et al. Revised guidelines for the clinical management of Lynch syndrome (HNPCC): recommendations by a group of European experts. *Gut* 2013;62:812–823.

86. Rumilla K, Schowalter KV, Lindor NM, et al. Frequency of deletions of EPCAM (TACSTD1) in MSH2-associated Lynch syndrome cases. *J Mol Diagn* 2011;13:93–99.

87. Jasperson KW, Tuohy TM, Neklason DW, et al. Hereditary and familial colon cancer. *Gastroenterology* 2010;138:2044–2058.

88. Steinhagen E, Markowitz AJ, Guillem JG. How to manage a patient with multiple adenomatous polyps. *Surg Oncol Clin N Am* 2010;19:711–723.

89. National Comprehensive Cancer Network. NCCN *Clinical Practice Guidelines in Oncology: Colorectal Cancer Screening.* http://www.nccn.org/professionals/physician_gls/pdf/colorectal_screening.pdf. Accessed February 19, 2014.

90. Vasen HF, Moslein G, Alonso A, et al. Guidelines for the clinical management of familial adenomatous polyposis (FAP). *Gut* 2008;57:704–713.

91. Church J. Familial adenomatous polyposis. *Surg Oncol Clin N Am* 2009;18:585–598.

93. Sinha A, Tekkis PP, Rashid S, et al. Risk factors for secondary proctectomy in patients with familial adenomatous polyposis. *Br J Surg* 2010;97:1710–1715.

94. Koskenvuo L, Renkonen-Sinisalo L, Jarvinen HJ, et al. Risk of cancer and secondary proctectomy after colectomy and ileorectal anastomosis in familial adenomatous polyposis. *Int J Colorectal Dis* 2014;29:225–230.

97. Aziz O, Athanasiou T, Fazio VW, et al. Meta-analysis of observational studies of ileorectal versus ileal pouch-anal anastomosis for familial adenomatous polyposis. *Br J Surg* 2006;93:407–417.

101. Beyer-Berjot L, Maggiori L, Birnbaum D, et al. A total laparoscopic approach reduces the infertility rate after ileal pouch-anal anastomosis: a 2-center study. *Ann Surg* 2013;258:275–282.

102. Steinhagen E, Guillem JG, Chang G, et al. The prevalence of thyroid cancer and benign thyroid disease in patients with familial adenomatous polyposis may be higher than previously recognized. *Clin Colorectal Cancer* 2012;11:304–308.

104. Jarrar AM, Milas M, Mitchell J, et al. Screening for thyroid cancer in patients with familial adenomatous polyposis. *Ann Surg* 2011;253:515–521.

106. Nieuwenhuis MH, Lefevre JH, Bulow S, et al. Family history, surgery, and APC mutation are risk factors for desmoid tumors in familial adenomatous polyposis: an international cohort study. *Dis Colon Rectum* 2011;54:1229–1234.

107. Quintini C, Ward G, Shatnawei A, et al. Mortality of intra-abdominal desmoid tumors in patients with familial adenomatous polyposis: a single center review of 154 patients. *Ann Surg* 2012;255:511–516.

111. Nieuwenhuis MH, Vogt S, Jones N, et al. Evidence for accelerated colorectal adenoma—carcinoma progression in MUTYH-associated polyposis? *Gut* 2012;61:734–738.

112. Palomaki GE, McClain MR, Melillo S, et al. EGAPP supplementary evidence review: DNA testing strategies aimed at reducing morbidity and mortality from Lynch syndrome. *Genet Med* 2009;11:42–65.

113. Umar A, Boland CR, Terdiman JP, et al. Revised Bethesda Guidelines for hereditary nonpolyposis colorectal cancer (Lynch syndrome) and microsatellite instability. *J Natl Cancer Inst* 2004;96:261–268.

116. Lee-Kong SA, Markowitz AJ, Glogowski E, et al. Prospective immunohistochemical analysis of primary colorectal cancers for loss of mismatch repair protein expression. *Clin Colorectal Cancer* 2010;9:255–259.

117. Steinhagen E, Shia J, Markowitz AJ, et al. Systematic immunohistochemistry screening for Lynch syndrome in early age-of-onset colorectal cancer patients undergoing surgical resection. *J Am Coll Surg* 2012;214:61–67.

118. Heald B, Plesec T, Liu X, et al. Implementation of universal microsatellite instability and immunohistochemistry screening for diagnosing lynch syndrome in a large academic medical center. *J Clin Oncol* 2013;31:1336–1340.

119. Beamer LC, Grant ML, Espenschied CR, et al. Reflex immunohistochemistry and microsatellite instability testing of colorectal tumors for Lynch syndrome among US cancer programs and follow-up of abnormal results. *J Clin Oncol* 2012;30:1058–1063.

126. Kalady MF, McGannon E, Vogel JD, et al. Risk of colorectal adenoma and carcinoma after colectomy for colorectal cancer in patients meeting Amsterdam criteria. *Ann Surg* 2010;252:507–511, discussion 511–513.

127. Parry S, Win AK, Parry B, et al. Metachronous colorectal cancer risk for mismatch repair gene mutation carriers: the advantage of more extensive colon surgery. *Gut* 2011;60:950–957.

128. Kalady MF, Lipman J, McGannon E, et al. Risk of colonic neoplasia after proctectomy for rectal cancer in hereditary nonpolyposis colorectal cancer. *Ann Surg* 2012;255:1121–1125.

129. Cirillo L, Urso ED, Parrinello G, et al. High risk of rectal cancer and of metachronous colorectal cancer in probands of families fulfilling the Amsterdam criteria. *Ann Surg* 2013;257:900–904.

132. Guillem JG, Glogowski E, Moore HG, et al. Single-amplicon MSH2 A636P mutation testing in Ashkenazi Jewish patients with colorectal cancer: role in presurgical management. *Ann Surg* 2007;245:560–565.

133. Barrow P, Khan M, Lalloo F, et al. Systematic review of the impact of registration and screening on colorectal cancer incidence and mortality in familial adenomatous polyposis and Lynch syndrome. *Br J Surg* 2013;100:1719–1731.

134. Vasen HF, Abdirahman M, Brohet R, et al. One to 2-year surveillance intervals reduce risk of colorectal cancer in families with Lynch syndrome. *Gastroenterology* 2010;138:2300–2306.

138. Giardiello FM, Allen JI, Axilbund JE, et al. Guidelines on genetic evaluation and management of Lynch syndrome: a consensus statement by the US Multi-Society Task Force on Colorectal Cancer. *Dis Colon Rectum* 2014;57(8):1025–1048.

33 Cancer Risk Reducing Agents

Dean E. Brenner, Scott M. Lippman, and Susan T. Mayne

WHY CANCER PREVENTION AS A CLINICAL ONCOLOGY DISCIPLINE

Until recently, clinical oncology has been defined as a medical specialty that attempts to intervene in order to slow or reverse the final stage of the cancer process—the clonally derived, genomically damaged, invasive cell mass. Cancer is a long process, a stepwise carcinogenic progression that encompasses critical molecular events that culminate in the loss of key cellular control homeostatic functions (e.g., control of proliferation, apoptosis, invasion, angiogenesis).[1] These events occur prior to and during the morphologic changes that have historically defined neoplasia. Morphologic changes, such as subtle increases in cellular proliferation that progress to early and late precancerous lesions containing dysplastic cells, characterize the carcinogenesis process (Fig. 33.1).[1–3] Opportunities for intervention in this process can include diverse, nonpharmacologic approaches (e.g., obesity management via diet/lifestyle interventions) or pharmacologic interventions (e.g., drugs or nutrients/nonnutrient substances used as drugs) aimed at delaying or reversing the carcinogenesis process prior to or following the appearance of early morphologic changes. Cancer screening and early detection strategies (e.g., surveillance endoscopy, fecal occult blood testing, mammography) identify not only those individuals with early stage, curable malignant transformations, but also those individuals with noninvasive neoplasias who are at risk for progression to transformed invasive malignancies.

Recognizing that cancer is a continuum, oncologists are increasingly expected to be knowledgeable about a diverse array of cancer-related topics including lifestyle behaviors such as diet and exercise, risk assessment, screening, other preventive interventions, in addition to current treatments for advanced malignancy. The understanding, use, and management of interventions designed to delay or reverse the carcinogenesis process have become integral components of the this role.[4]

DEFINING CANCER RISK–REDUCING AGENTS (CHEMOPREVENTION)

Cancer risk reduction, commonly referred to as chemoprevention, is the use of a range of interventions from drugs to isolated dietary components to whole-diet modulation to block, reverse, or prevent the development of invasive cancer.[5,6] Human cancer risk reduction asserts that one can intervene at many steps in the carcinogenic process, which occurs over many years. This prolonged latency provides opportunities to intervene at many time points and at multiple events in the carcinogenic process. Successful deployment of cancer risk–reducing agent interventions requires evidence of reduced cancer-associated incidence and/or mortality.

The concept of field carcinogenesis was first described in the early 1950s as *field cancerization* in squamous cell carcinomas of the head and neck, and subsequently ascribed to many epithelial sites. The field carcinogenesis concept is that patients have a wide surface area of precancerous or cancerous tissue change that can

be detected at the gross (oral premalignant lesions, polyps), microscopic (metaplasia, dysplasia), and/or molecular (gene loss or amplification) levels. Recent molecular studies detecting profound genetic alterations in histologically normal tissue from high-risk individuals have provided strong support for the field carcinogenesis concept. The implication of the field effect is that multifocal, genetically distinct, and clonally related premalignant lesions can progress over a broad tissue region.[1] The essence of cancer risk reduction, then, is intervention within the multistep carcinogenic process and throughout a wide field.

IDENTIFYING POTENTIAL CANCER RISK–REDUCING AGENTS

Cancer risk–reducing agent identification results from the synthesis of data from population, basic, translational, and clinical sciences. Findings from all of these disciplines are combined to contribute to the identification of agents with the potential to delay or reverse the carcinogenesis process (see Fig. 33.1).

The Hanahan and Weinberg hallmarks of malignant transformation—self-sufficiency in growth signals, insensitivity to growth-inhibitory signals, evasion of apoptosis, limitless replication potential, sustained angiogenesis, and tissue invasion and metastasis[7]—reflect the loss of cellular signaling control. The molecular damage that results in transformation is triggered by a large array of genetic and environmental stressors such as chronic inflammation, oxidation, inherited genetic mutations, and exogenous environmental exposures. Many such signaling intermediates have common functions in multiple organ sites (see Fig. 33.1). The complexity and overlap of signal transduction pathways suggests that single molecular therapeutic/preventive targets may have limited effectiveness. Interventions aimed at preventing the occurrence of or overcoming the effects of molecular defects in multiple pathways or targets may be required to arrest or reverse carcinogenesis. Using the Hanahan and Weinberg hallmarks, examples of possible targets are shown in Table 33.1.

PRECLINICAL DEVELOPMENT OF CANCER RISK–REDUCING AGENTS

Similar to the development of therapeutic interventions, the assessment of efficacy and toxicity of single chemically synthesized entities, agents designed *in silico*, botanicals, nutrients/nonnutrient substances used as drugs for cancer risk–reducing agent efficacy proceeds through a translational paradigm that identifies efficacy in cell culture models, in live animal models, and in humans. Preclinical models that simulate the carcinogenesis process in target epithelia identify molecular biomarkers for modulation by interventions. These models can be used to identify potential toxicity of interventions and to assess the effect of interventions on the development and progression of preneoplasia/neoplasia.[8]

The U.S. National Cancer Institute's (NCI) PREVENT Cancer Preclinical Drug Development Program is a prime example of a

Molecular Biomarkers of Carcinogenesis

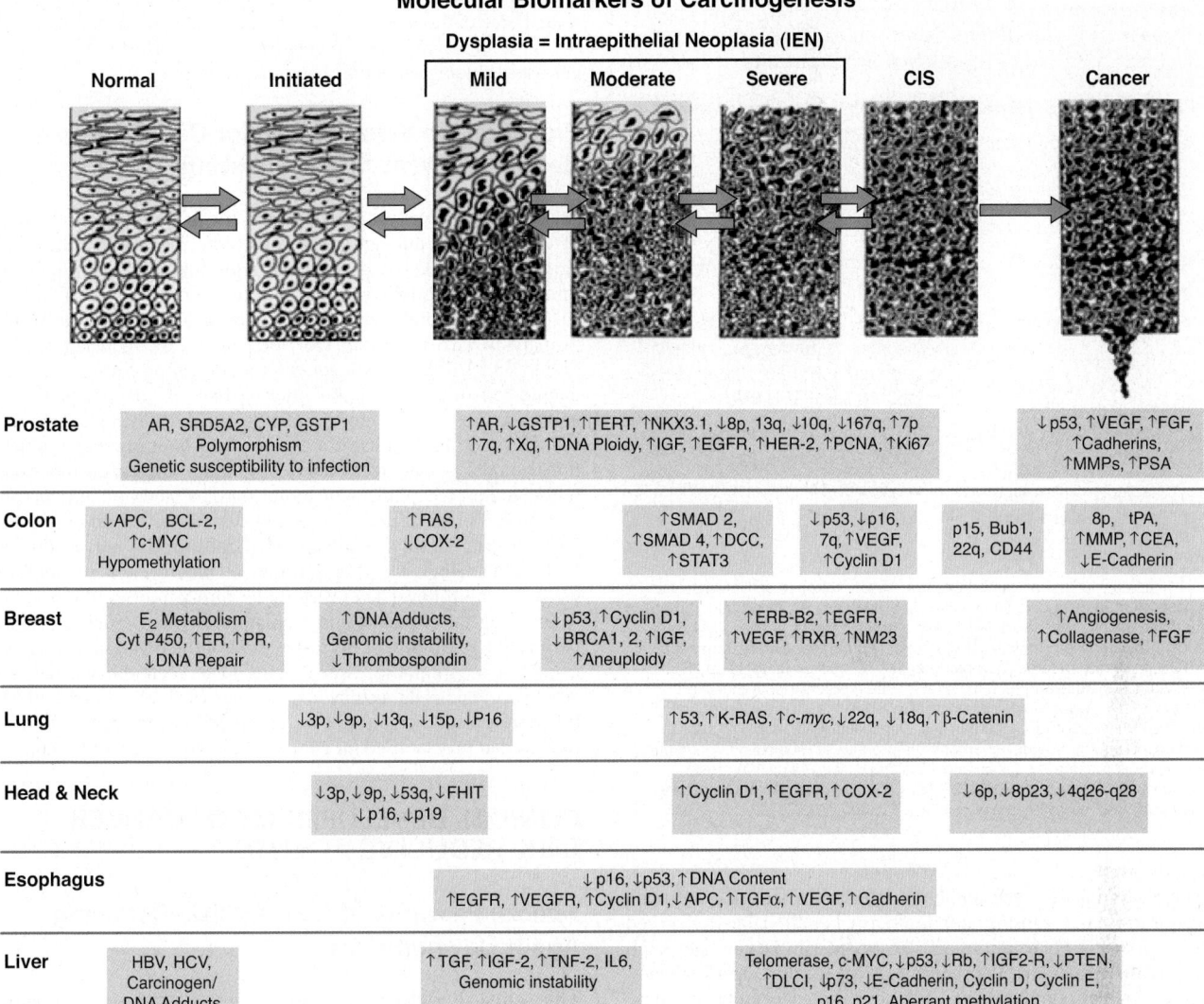

Figure 33.1 Genetic progression in major cancers. Carcinogenesis is driven by genetic progression. This progression is marked by the appearance of molecular biomarkers in distinctive patterns representing accumulating changes in gene expression and correlating with changes in histologic phenotype as cells move from normal through the early stages of clonal expansion to dysplasia and finally to early invasive, locally advanced, and metastatic cancer. The figure[257] shows candidate molecular biomarkers of genetic progression in seven target organs: the prostate,[300–302] the colon,[2] the breast,[303,304] the lung,[305–307] the head and neck,[308–311] the esophagus,[312,313] and the liver.[314] CIS, carcinoma in situ; AR, androgen receptor; CYP, cytochrome P-450; GSTP1, glutathione S transferase P1; TERT, telomerase reverse transcriptase; NKX3.1, NK 3 transcription factor related, locus 1 (prostate specific, androgren regulated); IGF, insulin-like growth factor; EGFR, epidermal growth factor receptor; HER-2, human epidermal growth factor receptor-2; PCNA, proliferating cell nuclear antigen; VEGF, vascular endothelial growth factor; FGF, fibroblast growth factor; MMP, matrix metalloproteinase; PSA, prostate-specific antigen; APC, adenomatous polyposis coli; BCL-2, B-cell lymphoma 2 gene, apoptosis control; c-MYC, v-myc avian myelocytomatosis viral oncogene homolog; COX-2, cyclooxygenase-2; SMAD, homolog of mothers against decapentaplegic + *C. Elegans* SMA protein; DCC, deleted in colon cancer gene; CEA, carcinoembryonic antigen; ER, estrogen receptor; PR, progesterone receptor; ERB-B2, Receptor tyrosine-protein kinase erbB-2, same as HER-2; RXR, retinoid X receptor; NM23, Nucleoside disphosphate kinase A; K-RAS, Kirsten rat sarcoma viral oncogene homolog; FHIT, fragile histidine triad protein; TGFα, tumor growth factor alpha; HBV, hepatitis B virus; HCV, hepatitis C virus; TNF-2, tumor necrosis factor 2; IL6, interleukin 6; PTEN, phosphatase and tensin homolog. (Figure and revised caption from Kelloff GJ, Lippman SM, Dannenberg AJ, et al. Progress in chemoprevention drug development: the promise of molecular biomarkers for prevention of intraepithelial neoplasia and cancer—a plan to move forward. *Clin Cancer Res* 2006;12:3661–3697, published with permission from the American Association for Cancer Research.)

rational strategy to select promising agents for clinical trials through a stepwise approach of preclinical in vitro testing followed by *in vivo* screening.[8–10] This system involves several phases: biochemical prescreening assays, in vitro efficacy models, in vivo short-term screening, animal efficacy testing, and preclinical toxicology testing.

Biochemical Prescreening Assays

Prescreening assays are a series of short-term, mechanistic assays developed to evaluate the ability of a test compound to modulate biochemical events presumed to be mechanistically linked to carcinogenesis.[8]

These in vitro assays are rapidly completed for potential cancer risk–reducing agents. Examples of such assays include carcinogen-DNA binding, prostaglandin synthesis inhibition, glutathione–S-transferase inhibition, and ornithine decarboxylase inhibition.

In Vitro Efficacy Models

In vitro assays test the cancer risk–reducing activity of a screened compound in four epithelial cell systems (primary rat tracheal epithelial cells, human lung tumor [A427] cells, mouse mammary organ cultures [MMOC], and human foreskin epithelial cells).

TABLE 33.1

Molecular Mechanisms Common to Transforming Cells and Potential Preventive Interventions

Characteristics of Neoplasia	Possible Molecular Targets
■ Self-sufficiency in cell growth	EGFR, platelet-derived growth factor, MAPK, PI3K
■ Insensitivity to antigrowth signals	SMADs, pRb, cyclin-dependent kinases, MYC
■ Limitless replicative potential	hTERT, pRb, p53
■ Evading apoptosis	Bcl-2, BAX, caspases, Fas, tumor necrosis factor receptor, insulin growth factor/PI3K/Akt, mTOR, p53, NF-κB, PTEN, RAS
■ Sustained angiogenesis	VEGF, basic fibroblast growth factor, integrins ($\alpha_v\beta_3$), thrombospondin-1, HIF-1α
■ Tissue invasion and metastases	MMPs, MAPK, E-cadherin

EGFR, epidermal growth factor receptor; MAPK, mitogen-activated protein kinase; PI3K, phosphoinositide 3-kinase; SMAD, drosophila protein, mothers against decapentaplegic gene and the *Elegans* protein SMA; pRb, phosphorylated Rb protein; hTERT, human telomerase reverse transcriptase; mTOR, mammalian target of rapamycin; NF-κB, nuclear factor kappa B; PTEN, phosphatase and tensin homolog; VEGF, vascular endothelial growth factor; HIF-1α, hypoxia-inducible factor-1α; MMP, Matrix metalloproteinases. Adapted from Kelloff GJ, Lippman SM, Dannenberg AJ, et al. Progress in chemoprevention drug development: the promise of molecular biomarkers for prevention of intraepithelial neoplasia and cancer—a plan to move forward. *Clin Cancer Res* 2006;12:3661–3697 and derived from Hanahan D, Weinberg RA. The hallmarks of cancer. *Cell* 2000;100:57–70.

The assays measure the ability of potential cancer risk–reducing agents to reverse transformation in normal epithelial cells exposed to carcinogens. For example, after treatment with a carcinogen such as 7,12-demethylbenz(a)anthracene, MMOCs develop lesions similar to alveolar nodules that are considered precancerous in mouse mammary glands in vivo.[11] Pretreatment of organ cultures before carcinogen exposure measures the effect of cancer risk–reducing agents in the initiation stage of carcinogenesis, whereas treatment

after carcinogen exposure measures activity during tumor promotion. Three of these assays (using rat tracheal epithelial, A427, and MMOC cells) have shown predictive values of 76% to 83% for cancer risk–reducing agent efficacy in in vivo models.[8]

Preclinical In Vivo Models for Cancer Risk–Reducing Agent Efficacy Testing

Animal models remain a crucial link in the efficacy assessment of cancer risk–reducing agents for epithelial cancer. Chemical carcinogenesis models provide the reproducible development of tumors in animals following the administration of a known chemical initiator or combination initiator/promoter and have been the primary in vivo screening tool for cancer risk–reducing agents (Table 33.2A).[12,13] Carcinogenesis models employing genetically engineered mice permit the interrogation of targeted pathways and the corresponding efficacy of cancer risk–reducing agents. Although useful for mechanistic studies, knockout or genetic mutational models create accelerated neoplastic progression that does not accurately recapitulate the more complex, stepwise, human carcinogenesis process. Recombinant alleles can be driven by the addition of drug-sensitive regulatory elements, such as tetracycline or tamoxifen analogs. The drug-sensitive regulatory elements achieve temporal control over a gene promoter through the administration of the drug that binds to the regulatory element. Such a system permits the inhibition or overexpression of the organ-specific gene using Cre recombinase, a site-specific DNA recombinase that targets DNA regions flanked by loxP sequences. Tables 33.2A and 2B list representative organ-specific chemical and transgenic mouse models that may be used for cancer risk–reducing agent testing.

CLINICAL DEVELOPMENT OF CANCER RISK–REDUCING AGENTS

Special Features of Cancer Risk–Reducing Agent Development

The clinical efficacy assessment of cancer risk–reducing agents employs phased testing (phase I to III) models used for development of drugs[14] but with crucial differences in study design and end points. Special features for the clinical development of

TABLE 33.2A

Chemical Carcinogenesis Models Used for Screening of Cancer Risk–Reducing Agents for Common Epithelial Neoplasms in Animals

Organ Site	Species	Carcinogen	End Point
Colon	Rat, mouse	Azoxymethane (AOM)	Aberrant crypts, adenomas, adenocarcinomas
Lung	Mouse	N—butyl-N-(4-hydroxybutyl)nitrosamine (NNK); benzo[a]pyrene; cigarette smoke	Adenomas, adenocarcinomas
	Hamster	Methylnitrosourea (MNU)	Squamous cell carcinomas
	Mouse	N-nitroso-tris-chloroethylurea	Squamous cell carcinomas
Breast	Rat	Dimethylbenz[a]anthracene (DMBA); MNU	Adenocarcinomas, adenomas
Prostate	Rat	MNU + testosterone	Adenocarcinomas
Bladder	Rat, mouse	N-butyl-N-(4-hydroxybutyl)nitrosamine (OH-BBN)	Transitional cell carcinoma
Pancreas	Hamster	N-nitrobis-(2-oxopropyl)amine (BOP)	Ductal carcinoma
Head and neck	Rat	4-nitroquinoline-1-oxide (4-NQO)	Tongue squamous cell carcinomas
	Mouse	DMBA	Squamous cell carcinomas
Esophagus	Rat	Dimethylbenz[a]anthracene	Squamous cell carcinomas
	Rat	Esophagogastroduodenal anastomosis + iron	Adenocarcinomas

Adapted from Steele VE, Lubet RA. The use of animal models for cancer chemoprevention drug development. *Semin Oncol* 2010;37:327–338.

TABLE 33.2B

Selected Transgenic Animal Models for Carcinogenesis Evaluation

Organ Site	Genes Targeted	End Point	References
Colon	*Apc, Lrig1, gp130, Stat3, Smad3, Wnt-β-catenin, villin, TGFBR2, Kras, Ink4a*	Adenomas and adenocarcinomas	(258, 259)
Lung	*KrasG12D, KrasG12Vgeo, PTEN, Braf*V600E, *cRaf, Egfr* L858R±T790M, *PIK3CA,* EMLA4-ALK fusion *Rb. P53*	Adenomas and adenocarcinomas Small cell	(260)
Breast	Mouse mammary tumor virus long terminal repeat promoter (MMTV) driven *BRCA1, p53, ERα,* aromatase, *TGFα, Her2/neu, wnt,* PELP-1, AIB-1	DCIS, adenocarcinomas	(261)
Prostate	Probasin promotor driving SV40 large T antigen (*TRAMP/LADY*), *c-Myc, TMPRSS-ERG, Akt, Wnt-β-catenin,* androgen receptor *Nkx3.1, FGFR1, TGF, PTEN*	Prostate intraepithelial neoplasia, neuroendocrine tumors (TRAMP); adenocarcinomas (*c-Myc, TMPRESS-ERG, Akt, Wnt,* androgen receptor) Adenocarcinomas	(262)
Pancreas	*KrasG12D* alone, *LSL-Kras, PDX-1, R26Notch, Tif1γ* Combined *PDX-1, LSL-Kras, LSL-Trp53;* combined *PDX-1, Brca2, LSL-Kras Trp53; KrasG12D* on *Mist1* locus; *PDX-1, KrasG12D+ Ink4a/Arf* or *Smad4; Ptf1a, KrasG12D, TGFBR2*	Pancreatic intraepithelial neoplasia Pancreatic adenocarcinoma	(263)

Note: Most models are mouse models. Such models will permit efficacy testing of specific pathway targets using single agent interventions, combinations, or multimechanism-based natural products.

cancer risk–reducing agents create the following challenges to be overcome: (1) the need for large therapeutic index (doses associated with potential toxicity of an intervention need to substantially exceed doses aimed at delaying or reversing transformation) for use in individuals who are asymptomatic yet may benefit from an extended (years) treatment course; (2) the long latency to malignant transformation (an assessment of effectiveness based on the reduction in cancer incidence requires studies lasting for years and involving thousands of participants); (3) adherence (once-daily dosing regimens using interventions that have sufficiently long half-lives may minimize the impact of a missed dose yet maintain the biologic impact on the physiologic target; minimal toxicity and strong psychological commitment to preventive goals also enhance adherence[15]); and (4) complex risk assessment for cancer (individuals with highly penetrant but infrequent, germ-line genetic susceptibility to breast and colon cancers[16,17] are excellent candidates for cancer risk–reducing agents and are likely to accept some toxicity for reduced cancer risk). For individuals at more modestly increased risk (e.g., long-term, current smokers; persons with a family history of cancer; women with mammographically dense breasts), quantitative risk assessment algorithms may be useful in the future to identify optimal cancer risk–reducing agents. The refinement of cancer risk calculators for breast,[18] colon,[19] and prostate cancer[20] promises to appropriately select high-risk individuals for cancer risk–reducing agents such that anticipated benefits exceed potential risks.

Biomarkers as Cancer Risk–Reducing Agent Targets and Efficacy End Points

A biomarker is a characteristic that is measured and evaluated as an indicator of normal biologic processes, pathogenic processes, or pharmacologic responses to therapeutic interventions.[21] A surrogate end point for cancer prevention assumes that a measured biologic feature will predict the presence or future development of a cancer outcome.[22] Biomarkers enable a reduction in the size and duration of an intervention trial by replacing a rare or distal end point with a more frequent, proximate end point.[23] Intraepithelial

neoplasia has served and continues to serve as a biomarker for invasive malignancy (Table 33.3). Although many advocate the use of intraepithelial neoplasia-based biomarkers as regulatory surrogate end points, others caution that intraepithelial neoplasias may not serve as sufficiently robust surrogate biomarkers for cancer incidence or mortality.[24]

In order to be useful as end points for cancer risk–reducing agent efficacy testing as regulatory end points, any biomarker must have statistical accuracy, precision, and effectiveness of results[24] that demonstrate prediction of a *hard* disease end point—cancer incidence or mortality. An independent validation data set must address defined standards of validation that minimize bias in the study design and the populations studied.[25] The biomarker must be generalizable to the specific clinical or screening population (Table 33.4).

Phases of Cancer Risk–Reducing Agent Development

Phase I cancer risk–reducing agent trials define an optimal cancer risk–reducing agent dose. An optimal cancer risk–reducing agent dose is one that is usually nontoxic, scheduled once daily, and modulates a tissue, cellular, or serum biomarker of drug activity (e.g., the dose of aspirin that inhibits prostaglandin production in a target tissue site). The definition of a maximum tolerated dose is not an essential end point of a phase I cancer risk–reducing agent trial. Higher, yet nontoxic doses may lower cancer risk–reducing agent efficacy. For example, β-carotene at high doses has pro-oxidant activity and may enhance the carcinogenesis process, whereas at low doses, it is a potent antioxidant and differentiating agent.[26]

Phase II cancer risk–reducing agent trials begin to define cancer risk–reduction efficacy. These short-term (6 months to 1 year) treatment periods gather evidence of risk reduction by assessing drug effects on tissue, cellular, or blood surrogate markers of carcinogenesis. Phase IIa trials are nonrandomized, biomarker modulation trials. Phase IIb trials are randomized, placebo-controlled trials of several hundred subjects testing, for example, whether a risk-reducing agent reduces recurrence of a previously resected intraepithelial neoplastic lesion as the primary end point. Cellular dynamic

TABLE 33.3

Common Intraepithelial Neoplasias

Epithelium	Intraepithelial Neoplasia	References
Colon and rectum	Adenoma	(264)
Lower esophagus	Barrett esophagus	(265)
Upper esophagus	Squamous dysplasia	(266, 267)
Skin: Squamous/basal cell	Actinic keratosis	(268)
Skin: Pigmented	Dysplastic nevus	(269)
Cervix	Cervical intraepithelial neoplasia	(270)
Head and neck	Leukoplakia/oral epithelial dysplasia	(271)
Prostate	Prostate intraepithelial neoplasia (PIN), intraductal carcinoma of the prostate	(272)
Lung	Bronchial dysplasia	(273)
Pancreas	Pancreatic intraepithelial neoplasia	(274)

(e.g., proliferation, apoptotic index), biochemical, or molecular (e.g., p53, cyclin D) end points may be used as secondary end points. Preoperative or *window of opportunity trials* enroll subjects for brief study periods prior to obtaining tissue by a planned resection of an invasive neoplasm. Such designs permit the exploration of biomarker modulation in the invasive neoplasm and in contiguous epithelial fields proximal and distal to the invasive neoplasm.[27]

Phase III cancer risk–reducing agent trials define reduction in a hard cancer end point such as cancer incidence or mortality. Such trials, using large, higher risk populations in a randomized, double-blinded intervention, are designed to identify a standard of preventive care for a given risk population. For example, trials of tamoxifen for the reduction of breast cancer incidence,[28,29] finasteride for the reduction of prostate cancer incidence,[30] and β-carotene for the reduction of lung cancer incidence[31] serve as examples of well-conducted, definitive phase III cancer risk–reducing agent clinical trials.

Some investigators consider randomized, controlled clinical trials with an end point sufficient for regulatory review as phase III.

TABLE 33.4

Characteristics of Biomarkers for Use as End Points in Cancer Risk–Reducing Agent Efficacy Assessment

- Variability of expression between phases of the carcinogenesis process
- Detected early in the carcinogenesis process
- Genetic progression or protein pathway based
- Target of modulation by preventive interventions
- Changes in biomarker linked to reduction in incident cancer of epithelial target
- Changes in biomarker linked to clinical benefit
- Can be quantified directly or via closely related activity such as a downstream target or upstream kinase
- Measurable in an accessible biosample (preferably urine, serum, saliva, stool, or breath)
- High throughput, technically feasible, analytical procedure with strong quality assurance/quality control procedures
- Cost-effective

Using such a definition, a clinical trial with an end point of reduction in adenoma recurrence is considered a phase III trial. Other investigators define phase III cancer risk–reducing agent trials as randomized, controlled clinical trials with a cancer incidence or mortality end point. This controversy causes confusion in the literature. For the purpose of clarity in this textbook, the latter definition of phase III trial is used—a prospective, randomized, controlled clinical trial with a cancer incidence or mortality end point. Randomized, controlled clinical trials with a surrogate biomarker end point such as an intraepithelial neoplasia (e.g., adenoma) are defined as phase IIb cancer risk–reducing agent trials.

MICRONUTRIENTS

Definition

Micronutrients comprise a large, diverse group of molecules typically ingested as part of the diet that play roles in normal human biology. This group of compounds has been investigated extensively as cancer risk–reducing agents in purified forms (i.e., supplements), as components of multiagent cocktails, and occasionally, as components of food extracts/other mixtures. Although retinoids are not micronutrients per se, they are related to retinol (vitamin A) and share certain properties with carotenoids, which are diet derived and, therefore, included along with micronutrients.

Retinoids, Carotenoids, and Antioxidant Nutrients

Overview and Mechanisms

Retinoids are the natural derivatives and synthetic analogs of vitamin A.[32] Cancer risk–reduction intervention studies have evaluated the parent compound (retinol, typically given as retinyl acetate or palmitate), naturally occurring retinoids such as all-trans–retinoic acid (ATRA) and 13-cis-retinoic acid (13cRA), and also synthetic retinoids such as etretinate and fenretinide (4-hydroxy[phenyl]retinamide [4HPR]). These agents have been of interest for cancer risk reduction for decades. Mechanistically, retinoids have been shown to modulate cellular growth and differentiation, as well as apoptosis.[32] A large body of research indicates that retinoids have activity in the promotion and progression phases of carcinogenesis, including extensive evidence of efficacy in the setting of premalignant lesions, leading to their evaluation in human Phase III trials. Nuclear retinoic acid receptors mediate many of the retinoid-signaling effects; however, retinoids interact with other signaling pathways, such as estrogen signaling in breast cancer.[33]

Carotenoids are a group of naturally occurring plant pigments, only some of which are found in appreciable levels in the human diet and human tissues, including beta-carotene, alpha-carotene, lycopene, lutein, and β-cryptoxanthin.[34] Of these, the most widely studied carotenoids for cancer risk reduction are beta-carotene and lycopene. Beta-carotene has the highest pro–vitamin A activity of the carotenoids, but alpha-carotene and β-cryptoxanthin also possess pro–vitamin A activity. Other carotenoids, such as lycopene, do not possess vitamin A activity but are known to have potent antioxidant activity, particularly with regard to singlet oxygen quenching.[35] Furthermore, eccentric cleavage products of beta-carotene,[36] as well as other non-pro–vitamin A carotenoids such as lycopene (e.g., apocarotenals, apocarotenoic acids) appear to be biologically active and may also act via retinoid-signaling pathways.[37]

Because of the known antioxidant function of carotenoids, they are often studied for risk-reducing efficacy in combination with other antioxidant nutrients, especially vitamins E and C and selenium (sometimes as a cocktail, versus placebo). Thus, we will consider this group of nutrients first, followed by other micronutrients that are thought to act via different mechanisms and/or pathways.

Epidemiology

A large body of literature indicates that people who consume greater amounts of carotenoids from foods (primarily fruits and vegetables) and people with higher serum or plasma levels of various carotenoids have a lower risk for various cancers.[38] In particular, according to the systematic review of the literature conducted by the World Cancer Research Fund/American Institute for Cancer Research,[38] foods containing carotenoids are "probably" associated with lower risks of cancers of the mouth/pharynx/larynx and lung; foods containing beta-carotene are "probably" associated with lower risks of cancers of the esophagus; and foods containing lycopene are "probably" associated with lower risks of prostate cancer. Preformed retinol intake is inconsistently associated with risks of various cancers but that, in part, likely reflects confounding, because dietary sources of preformed retinol primarily include foods of animal origin (e.g., liver, eggs, milk). Vitamin C in the diet comes primarily from the consumption of fruits and vegetables; therefore, vitamin C and carotenoids often trend together in epidemiologic findings. Vitamin E, in contrast, is found in different foods, especially nuts, seeds, and vegetable oils; intake and blood concentrations are somewhat inconsistently associated with cancer risk.[39] Selenium, being a trace mineral, is difficult to measure in the diet, but higher selenium status has been associated with a lower risk of certain cancers, although the results are not entirely consistent.[39]

Preclinical In Vivo Models

In preclinical models, retinoids induce differentiation as well as arrest proliferation[33] of various cancers, making them attractive agents for cancer risk reduction.[40] The International Agency for Research on Cancer reviewed the preclinical research involving beta-carotene, concluding that there was "sufficient" evidence of cancer preventive activity, particularly involving mouse skin tumor models and the hamster buccal pouch model.[41] Notably, there was inconsistent evidence of efficacy in respiratory tract models. Lycopene has been evaluated in numerous cell culture systems and in a variety of models of prostate carcinogenesis, including chemically induced, orthotopic implantation, transgenic, and xenotransplantation, with mixed evidence of efficacy.[42] Evidence, primarily from cell culture studies, suggests that lycopene metabolites may be at least partially responsible for anticarcinogenic activity.[37]

Clinical Trials: Retinoids, Carotenoids, and Antioxidant Nutrients

Retinoids, carotenoids, and antioxidant nutrients have been evaluated in the setting of preneoplasia/neoplasia in many different organ sites, as will be discussed. Of the many clinical trials of retinoids and carotenoids/other antioxidant nutrients, key trials with cancer incidence/recurrence as primary outcomes are tabulated (see Tables 33.5 and 33.6) and reviewed.

Clinical Efficacy in the Upper Airway

Many trials of cancer risk–reducing agents have been done in the setting of squamous cell carcinomas of the head and neck, in large part because of the substantial clinical problem of relatively high rates of recurrences and second primary tumors in curatively treated cancer patients. Early work demonstrated that high-dose 13cRA (50 to 100 mg/m² per day) produced no significant differences in disease recurrence (local, regional, or distant) but significantly lowered the rate of second primary invasive neoplasms,[43] with the benefits persisting for at least 5 years.[44] Substantial retinoid toxicity, however, including skin dryness and peeling, cheilitis, conjunctivitis, and hypertriglyceridemia, was evident in a large proportion of patients. Subsequent trials thus used lower doses of retinoids (13cRA or a synthetic retinoid, etretinate), but failed to show efficacy in reducing second primary tumor formation (Table 33.5).[45,46]

Supplemental beta-carotene has also been studied as a single agent and in combination with other agents for the prevention of second primary cancers of the mouth and throat (Table 33.6). One trial of beta-carotene alone observed no harm or benefit[47]; another observed nonsignificantly fewer second head and neck cancers but more lung cancers[48]; and a third gave beta-carotene with α-tocopherol (400 IU per day).[49] In the third trial, beta-carotene was discontinued early due to adverse findings from lung cancer prevention trials (see the following); however, after a median follow-up of 6.5 years, all-cause mortality was increased, which the authors attributed to the supplemental α-tocopherol. As will be discussed later, adverse effects of antioxidant nutrients are not limited to head and neck cancer patients; potential mechanisms for adverse effects are discussed further.

Clinical Efficacy in the Lung (Lower Airway)

Reversal of Metaplasia or Dysplasia. Active smokers and recent quitters have multiple preinvasive metaplastic and dysplastic lesions in the pulmonary tree. Most of these lesions resolve upon smoking cessation, but some remain and progress to invasive neoplasms. Unfortunately, micronutrient or retinoid interventions have not demonstrated preventive efficacy in most rigorous trials in patients with early lesions. For example, a US trial randomized 755 asbestos workers to receive beta-carotene (50 mg per day) and retinol (25,000 IU every other day) versus placebo; sputum atypia was not reduced after 5 years.[50] As another example, eligible smokers with lung metaplasia or dysplasia were randomized to 6 months of 13cRA or placebo. The extent of metaplasia decreased similarly (in approximately 50% of subjects) in both study arms.[51] Only smoking cessation was associated with a significant reduction in the metaplasia index during the 6-month intervention.

Prevention of Invasive Neoplasms. Large, phase III efficacy trials of beta-carotene plus other micronutrients for primary prevention of lung cancer have been completed, as summarized in Table 33.6. The Alpha-Tocopherol, Beta-carotene (ATBC) Trial involved 29,133 men from Finland who were heavy cigarette smokers at entry.[52] In a two-by-two factorial design, participants were randomized to receive either supplemental α-tocopherol, beta-carotene, the combination, or placebo. Unexpectedly, participants receiving beta-carotene (alone or in combination with α-tocopherol) had a statistically significant 18% increase in lung cancer incidence and an 8% increase in total mortality relative to participants receiving placebo. α-Tocopherol had no effect.

The finding of an increased incidence of lung cancer in the beta-carotene–supplemented smokers was replicated in the Carotene and Retinol Efficacy Trial (CARET), a large randomized trial of supplemental beta-carotene plus retinol versus placebo in asbestos workers and smokers.[53] This trial was terminated early, but, at the time of termination, overall lung cancer incidence was increased by 28% in the supplemented subjects and total mortality was also increased by 17%. In contrast, the Physicians' Health Study (PHS) of supplemental beta-carotene versus placebo in 22,071 male US physicians reported no significant effect—positive or negative—of 12 years of supplementation of beta-carotene on total cancer, lung cancer, or cardiovascular disease (see Table 33.6).[54] Two other trials involving supplemental beta-carotene alone (the Women's Health Study[55]) or with other antioxidant nutrients (the Medical Research Council/British Heart Foundation Heart Protection Study[56]) on overall cancer incidence also failed to observe efficacy.

Prevention of Second Primary Invasive Neoplasms. EUROSCAN was a multicenter trial employing a two-by-two factorial design to test retinyl palmitate and N-acetylcysteine (also a compound with known antioxidant activity) in preventing second primary invasive neoplasms in patients with early stage cancers

TABLE 33.5

Larger, Randomized Trials of Retinoids in Human Cancer Risk Reduction with Cancer Outcomes[a,b]

Population	Drug (Dose)	End Point	Outcomes	References
United States, prior HNSCC	13cRA (50–100 mg/m²/d)	Second primary tumor	Significant reduction in second primary tumors at 32 and 55 mos; however, substantial toxicity	(43, 44)
France, prior HNSCC	Etretinate (50/25 mg/d)	Second primary tumor	No difference	(46)
United States, prior HNSCC	13cRA (30 mg/d)	Second primary tumor	No difference	(45)
Europe, prior HNSCC, NSCLC	Vitamin A (300,000/150,000 IU/d) +/− N-acetylcysteine	Second primary tumor	No difference	(57)
United States, Prior NSCLC	13cRA (30 mg/d)	Second primary tumor	No difference, but second primary tumors were lower in nonsmokers on drug but higher in smokers on drug	(58)
Italy, prior breast cancer	4HPR (200 mg/d) No treatment	Contralateral breast cancer	Nonsignificant reduction; pre-menopausal women did better but opposite in postmenopausal women	(60)
United States, prior BCC	13cRA (10 mg/d)	Second basal cell carcinoma	No difference	(65)
United States, prior actinic keratosis	Retinol (25,000 IU/d)	Skin cancer incidence	Reduction in squamous cell carcinomas but not basal cell carcinomas	(67)
United States, prior BCC/SCC of the skin	13cRA (5–10 mg/d) Retinol (25,000 IU/d)	Second skin cancer	No significant difference for either agent	(66)
Netherlands, renal transplant patients	Acitretin (30 mg/d)	Skin cancer	Significant reduction	(64)
United States, aggressive SCC of the skin	13cRA (1 mg/kg/d) + interferon alpha	Second primary tumors and tumor recurrences	No effect	(275)
United States, prior bladder TCC	Megadose vitamins (40,000 IU retinol/d) versus RDA vitamins	Recurrence	Significant reduction in recurrence	(73)
United States, prior bladder TCC	4HPR (200 mg/d)	Recurrence	No difference	(72)

[a] Trials of retinoids that also included beta-carotene are listed under Table 33.2 only.
[b] Versus placebo unless otherwise indicated.
HNSCC, head and neck squamous cell carcinoma; NSLC, non–small-cell lung cancer; BCC, basal cell carcinoma; TCC, transitional cell carcinoma; RDA, recommended dietary allowance.

of the head and neck or lung. None of the interventions reduced second airway primary invasive neoplasms.[57] The Lung Intergroup Trial randomized patients with surgically resected lung cancer to 13cRA versus placebo and found no significant differences between the two arms in second primary tumors.[58] Notably, smoking status modified the effect of the 13cRA intervention, which was harmful in current smokers yet beneficial in former smokers.

Thus, phase III trials of both carotenoids/antioxidants and retinoids indicate that these agents overall do not reduce the risk of developing invasive lung cancers, nor do they prevent the development of second primary invasive neoplasms. However, the finding that former smokers seemed to benefit from both 13cRA[58] and beta-carotene[53] is intriguing. Mechanistic work suggests this interaction is real rather than chance (see the following), suggesting that (1) risk-reduction in smokers is especially challenging,[59] and (2) trials in former smokers may merit consideration.

Clinical Efficacy in the Breast

Moon et al.[40] first showed that fenretinide was a promising cancer risk–reducing agent for the breast, having a high therapeutic index and synergistic interaction with tamoxifen in mammary carcinogenesis model studies. This laboratory work led to a large-scale randomized trial of fenretinide (versus no treatment) for 5 years to prevent contralateral breast cancer in women aged 30 to 70 years with a history of resected early breast cancer and no prior adjuvant therapy.[60] The intervention produced no significant overall effect, although fenretinide reduced contralateral and ipsilateral breast cancer rates in premenopausal women, with an opposite (adverse) trend observed in postmenopausal women. The reduced incidence of second breast cancer in premenopausal patients persisted with longer follow-up.[61]

Retinoid X receptor (RXR)–selective retinoids are also being evaluated in preclinical and clinical studies. Ongoing work suggests that combination treatment may represent a promising new strategy to suppress both estrogen receptor–negative and estrogen receptor–positive breast tumors, and the combination of retinoids with antiestrogens may be particularly effective.[62]

Clinical Efficacy in the Skin

Retinoids have been widely studied for cancer risk–reducing efficacy in skin. Early work was done in patients who have substantial skin cancer risk either due to xeroderma pigmentosum or medication-induced immunosuppression for transplants. For example, 13cRA reduced skin cancer by 63% in patients with

TABLE 33.6

Randomized Trials of Antioxidant Nutrients in Human Cancer Risk Reduction with Cancer Outcomes[a]

Population	Drug (Dose)	End Point	Outcomes	References
United States, prior head/neck cancer	Beta-carotene (50 mg/d)	Second primary head and neck cancers	Nonsignificant reduction in second head and neck cancer, increase in lung cancer	(48)
Italy, prior head/neck cancer	Beta-carotene (75 mg/d) for 3 mos with 1 mo off	Second primary head and neck cancers	No effect on second primary tumors, nonsignificant decrease in death	(47)
Canada, prior head/neck cancer	30 mg beta-carotene/d + 400 IU vitamin E/d	Deaths	Beta-carotene discontinued, mortality increased at end of trial	(49)
Finland, male smokers	20 mg beta-carotene/d +/− 50 mg vitamin E/d	Lung cancer	Lung cancer increased with beta-carotene, no effect vitamin E	(52)
United States, smokers and asbestos workers	Beta-carotene (30 mg/d) + retinol (25,000 IU/d)	Lung cancer	Lung cancer increased with beta-carotene + vitamin A	(53)
United States, resected stage I non–small-cell lung cancer	Selenized yeast, 200 μg/d versus placebo	Second primary cancer	No effect	(276)
United States, male physicians	Beta-carotene (50 mg every other day)	Total cancer	No effect	(54)
United States, female health professionals	Beta-carotene (50 mg/ every other day)	All cancers	No effect	(55)
United Kingdom, adults at risk for coronary heart disease	20 mg beta-carotene/d + 600 mg vitamin E/d + 250 mg vitamin C/d	Total cancers	No effect	(56)
United States, prior skin cancer	50 mg beta-carotene/d	Second skin cancer	No effect	(68)
Australia	Beta-carotene (30 mg/d)	Incident squamous cell skin cancer incident basal cell skin cancer	No effect	(69)
United States, prior skin cancer	200 μg selenium/d	Second skin cancer	No effect, with longer follow-up became adverse	(70)
Linxian County, China, general population	15 mg beta-carotene/d + 30 mg vitamin E/d + 50 μg selenium/d	Stomach cancer death Esophageal cancer death	Significant decrease in stomach cancer death; no effect on esophageal cancer death	(75)
Linxian County, China, esophageal dysplasia	Multivitamin/multimineral + 15 mg beta-carotene/d	Stomach cancer death Esophageal cancer death	No effect	(78)
United States, males	200 μg selenium/d +/− 400 IU vitamin E/d	Prostate cancer incidence	No effect; with longer follow-up vitamin E became adverse	(84)
United States, male physicians II	500 mg vitamin C/d + 400 IU vitamin E every other day	Prostate cancer incidence, total cancer incidence	No effect	(86)

[a] All versus placebo.

xeroderma pigmentosum; however, severe, acute mucocutaneous toxicity with the 13cRA occurred.[63] Also, the preventive effect of the retinoid was lost after stopping retinoid therapy. In renal transplant patients, acitretin (30 mg per day) reduced the numbers of premalignant lesions, the number of patients with skin cancer, and the cumulative number of skin cancers.[64]

In lower risk populations, low-dose 13cRA (10 mg per day)[65] and retinol or 13cRA alone did not reduce the recurrence of basal or squamous cell skin cancers,[66] although retinol alone reduced squamous but not basal cell carcinomas in patients with prior actinic keratoses.[67]

Beta-carotene (50 mg per day), in a randomized trial did not reduce the recurrence of nonmelanoma skin cancers.[68] Consistent with findings in the lung, the risk was increased by 44% in current smokers randomized to beta-carotene but not in never smokers randomized to beta-carotene as compared with placebo.

Supplemental beta-carotene (30 mg per day) also did not prevent basal cell carcinoma or squamous cell carcinoma of the skin in an Australian trial.[69]

Clark et al.[70] randomized patients with a history of nonmelanoma skin cancer to 200 μg per day selenium or placebo.[70] Selenium did not reduce the incidence of second skin cancers; a further report of this trial with longer follow-up[71] indicated that there was instead a significant increase in total nonmelanoma skin cancer (hazard ratio [HR] = 1.17; 95% confidence interval [CI], 1.02 to 1.34) and squamous cell skin cancer (HR = 1.25; 95% CI, 1.03 to 1.51).

Clinical Efficacy in the Bladder

A trial of fenretinide (200 mg per day orally for 12 months) versus placebo was conducted for preventing tumor recurrence in patients with nonmuscle-invasive bladder transitional cell carcinoma after transurethral resection with or without adjuvant intravesical bacillus Calmette-Guérin; recurrence rates were similar in both groups.[72] Another trial randomized 65 patients with biopsy-confirmed transitional cell carcinoma of the bladder to a multivitamin (recommended dietary allowance [RDA] levels) alone or supplemented with 40,000 IU retinol, 100 mg pyridoxine, 2,000 mg ascorbic acid, 400 U of α-tocopherol, and 90 mg zinc.[73] The 5-year estimate of tumor recurrence was 91% in the RDA arm versus 41% in the higher-dose nutrient arm ($p = 0.0014$).

Clinical Efficacy in the Cervix

Randomized trials include four with beta-carotene (alone or with other antioxidant nutrients), and five with retinoids. Only one of these trials, involving ATRA,[74] found a significant treatment effect. This trial administered a 0.372% ATRA solution by collagen sponge in a cervical cap delivery system. There was a higher complete response rate in the ATRA group (43%) than the placebo group (27%; $p = 0.041$) among the 141 patients with moderate dysplasia; no significant differences in dysplasia regression rates between the two study arms were detected in patients with severe dysplasia. The investigators experienced substantial losses to follow-up in this patient population.

Clinical Efficacy in the Esophagus and Stomach

Certain regions of China (Huixian and Linxian) have strikingly high incidence rates of esophageal and gastric cancers. Two trials were done in Linxian County; one was a general population trial that tested the efficacy of four different nutrient combinations at inhibiting the development of esophageal and gastric cancers.[75] Those who were given the combination of beta-carotene, vitamin E, and selenium had a 13% reduction in total cancer deaths, a 4% reduction in esophageal cancer deaths, and a 21% reduction in gastric cancer deaths (see Table 33.6). None of the other nutrient combinations reduced gastric or esophageal cancer deaths significantly in this trial. The treatment benefit has been shown to persist for 10 years postintervention, with greater efficacy seen in participants under age 55 years.[76] This finding stands in contrast to most other antioxidant nutrient supplement intervention trials, suggesting that the applicability of these results for populations with adequate nutritional status and for other tumor sites may be limited.[77]

The other Linxian trial evaluated a multivitamin/multimineral preparation plus beta-carotene (15 mg per day) in residents with esophageal dysplasia.[78] There was no clear evidence of efficacy, although confidence intervals were wide.

Clinical Efficacy in the Colon/Rectum

Of the randomized trials aimed at the prevention of recurrent colorectal adenomas with micronutrients that have been completed, some used beta-carotene alone[79] or with other nonmicronutrient interventions.[80] Others evaluated beta-carotene with and without supplemental vitamins C and E.[81] None of the trials observed benefit with supplementation. A subsequent report from one trial noted that alcohol intake and cigarette smoking modified the efficacy of beta-carotene.[82] Among nonsmokers and nondrinkers, beta-carotene was associated with a significant decrease in the risk of one or more recurrent adenomas (relative risk [RR] = 0.56). Among persons who smoked and also drank more than one alcoholic drink per day, beta-carotene significantly increased the risk of recurrent adenoma (RR = 2.07).

Clinical Efficacy in the Prostate

Because oxidative stress may play a role in the etiology of prostate cancer, several antioxidant nutrients, including vitamin E, selenium, and lycopene, have been of interest for preventing prostate cancer. The largest trial to date of these nutrients is the Selenium and Vitamin E Cancer Prevention Trial (SELECT), which tested selenium and vitamin E in a two-by-two factorial design for the primary prevention of prostate cancer. Despite preliminary indications of prostate cancer risk–reducing efficacy for selenium (from a trial of selenium for skin cancer[70]) and vitamin E (from a trial of vitamin E to prevent lung cancer[83]), there was no evidence of efficacy.[84] With extended follow-up, the nonsignificant adverse effect of vitamin E became significantly adverse.[85] Negative/neutral findings also were reported for vitamins E and C and prostate and total cancer in the PHS II randomized controlled trial.[86]

The carotenoid lycopene has generated much interest with regard to prostate cancer risk, and several intervention trials have been conducted based on lycopene supplements. These studies have been small, short term, based on intermediate end points, and often lack adequate control groups. The use of a tomato sauce–based intervention is arguably a better approach to evaluate, based on animal data indicating that tomato powder (which includes lycopene along with other phytochemicals), but not lycopene alone, was effective at inhibiting prostate carcinogenesis.[87]

Mechanisms for Ineffective Retinoid and Carotenoid Cancer Risk–Reducing Activity

There are now a number of trials demonstrating that supplemental beta-carotene/retinoids given to current smokers can produce increases rather than reductions in cancer incidence. In tobacco users, beta-carotene and other carotenoids may produce oxidative carotenoid breakdown products that alter retinoid metabolism and signaling pathways, along with pro-oxidation.[88] For retinoids such as 13cRA, smoking may induce genetic and epigenetic changes in the lung that affect retinoid activity; for example, tobacco smoking can affect RAR-β expression.[58] The adverse effects of supplemental nutrients are not limited to smokers; α-tocopherol increased rather than reduced prostate cancer in SELECT (which had relatively few smokers) and selenium increased prostate cancer among men without a baseline selenium deficiency.[89] This may be a consequence of the relatively high doses used in SELECT,[77] but certainly calls into question the notion that reducing oxidative stress is a pivotal cancer risk–reduction strategy, even in nonsmokers.

It has become clear that reactive oxygen species (ROS), such as hydrogen peroxide, can act as important physiologic regulators of intracellular signaling pathways.[90,91] Data in mouse models have shown that vitamin E accelerates lung tumor growth by disrupting the ROS–p53 axis, potentially by removing oxidative damage to DNA, which can serve as a potent stimulus for p53 activation.[92] Although some of the large cancer risk–reducing trials may have failed in their primary objective, they may indirectly contribute to a clearer understanding of cancer biology, leading to the recognition that the role of oxidative stress and ROS in human disease is much more nuanced than originally hypothesized.[93]

As for the retinoids, these agents are generally too toxic to be used as single agents for risk-reducing efficacy; however, a major area of ongoing research is examining retinoids (low doses) given in combination with other agents, especially those that regulate the epigenome, such histone deacetylase (HDAC) inhibitors.[33]

Folic Acid and Other B Vitamins

Overview and Mechanisms. Folate is a water-soluble B vitamin found in foods, whereas folic acid is the synthetic form found in supplements and fortified foods. Adequate folate is critical for DNA methylation, repair, and synthesis.[94,95] The methylation status of genes can play a key role in gene silencing and gene expression, lending plausibility to the idea that folate could be a key nutrient in regulating cell growth and proliferation.

Epidemiology. Epidemiologic studies have linked low folate intake with higher risk of several cancers, most notably colorectal cancer.[96] Long-term use of multivitamin supplements, which are a major source of folate and other B vitamins, has been associated with a reduction in the risk of colon cancer in some studies, including recent (postfortification) findings.[97–99] Supporting an anticancer role of folate is that genotypes for methylene tetrahydrofolate reductase, an enzyme known to be involved in folate metabolism, predict the risk of colon cancer dependent on folate intake or status.[100] Vitamin B_6 has been less studied in relation to cancer than folate, but some epidemiologic studies suggest that vitamin B_6 may be important for colorectal cancer.[101,102] A higher risk of cancer related to deficiencies of these vitamins has been suggested for alcohol drinkers.[103]

Clinical Trials: Folic Acid and B Vitamins.

Risk-reducing efficacy for supplemental folic acid has been primarily evaluated in the setting of prevention of recurrent colorectal adenomas (i.e., in patients with prior adenomas). Of six randomized trials of folic acid, two small trials reported suggestions of benefit of folic acid supplementation.[104,105] However, benefits were not observed in two much larger trials, the Aspirin/Folate Polyp Prevention Study (AFPPS) (dose: 1 mg of folic acid daily)[106] and the United Kingdom Colorectal Adenoma Prevention (ukCAP) trial (dose: 500 μg of folic acid daily).[107] AFPPS found indications of an increased risk for advanced lesions and multiple adenomas with prolonged treatment and follow-up. A third large trial, the Nurses Health Study/Health Professionals Follow-up Study (NHS/HPFS) folic acid polyp prevention trial, showed no overall risk reduction.[108] The most recent trial, done in a Chinese population >50 years of age,[109] reported that 1 mg folic acid per day reduced sporadic colorectal adenomas when compared to no intervention (not a placebo-controlled study). One possible explanation for the discrepancy of the Chinese trial versus North American and European trials is the baseline plasma folate status. In the Chinese trial, the mean baseline folate concentration of 5 ng/mL[109] was half of the reported 10 ng/mL in a United States trial,[106] where folate fortification of the food supply occurs.

Calcium and Vitamin D

Overview and Mechanisms. There are two major forms of vitamin D: ergocalciferol (D_2) and cholecalciferol (D_3). Vitamin D_2 is absorbed through dietary sources such as fortified milk products, and D_3 is synthesized via ultraviolet (UV) B light isomerization of 7-dehydrocholestrol in the epidermis.[110] Vitamin D_3 is converted to calcitriol (1, 25-[OH]$_2$ D_3) in a two-step process requiring both hepatic and renal hydroxylation. Calcitriol binds to the vitamin D receptor, which translocates to the nucleus and binds to multiple gene promoter sites. Through this mechanism, vitamin D regulates cytoplasmic signaling pathways that impact cellular differentiation and growth through proteins such as Ras and mitogen-activated protein kinase (MAPK), protein lipase A, prostaglandins, cyclic adenosine monophosphate (AMP), protein kinase A, and phosphatidyl inositol 3 kinase.[110] 1,25(OH)$_2$D$_3$ regulates cellular proliferation and apoptosis. For example, 1,25(OH)$_2$D$_3$ can induce cleavage of caspase 3, poly (ADP-ribose) polymerase (PARP), and MAPK, leading to apoptosis. 1,25(OH)$_2$D$_3$ inhibits the expression and phosphorylation of Akt, a key regulator of cellular proliferation. The differentiation properties of 1,25(OH)$_2$D$_3$ are mediated through transcriptional activation of the CDK inhibitor p21. The effects of vitamin D on multiple signal transduction pathways operational in cancer cells are reviewed by Deeb et al.[111]

Epidemiology. Observational epidemiologic studies have shown a relatively consistent inverse association between low calcium intake, including that from supplements, and increased colorectal and colon cancer risk.[112,113] Vitamin D exposure is typically assessed by measuring 25(OH)vitamin D in plasma because exposure is derived not only from diet and supplements, but also from cutaneous synthesis following dermal exposure to UV radiation. A large number of observational studies have evaluated the association between vitamin D status and cancer risk, as systematically reviewed by the Agency for Healthcare Research and Quality (AHRQ).[114] The evidence is inconsistent for most cancer sites, with the exception of studies showing that individuals with lower blood vitamin D levels have a higher risk of colorectal cancer or adenoma. Although some observational studies have reported that higher serum vitamin D is associated with lower breast cancer risk, the association is inconsistent.[114,115] Also, there are some studies suggesting high serum vitamin D is associated with increases in certain cancers, particularly pancreatic cancer.[116]

Clinical Trials: Calcium and Vitamin D

Clinical Efficacy in the Colon. Baron et al.[117] randomized subjects with a recent history of colorectal adenomas to either calcium carbonate (1,200 mg per day of elemental calcium) or placebo. Results showed significant benefit for the calcium arm (adjusted RR = 0.81; 95% CI, 0.67 to 0.99; $p = 0.04$). In a smaller, similar study of calcium gluconolactate and carbonate (2 g elemental calcium daily), the adjusted odds ratio (OR) for adenoma recurrence was 0.66 (95% CI, 0.38 to 1.17; $p = 0.16$) for calcium treatment,[118] and while not statistically significant, it was similar to the data of Baron et al.[117]

In the largest trial of calcium and vitamin D with primary cancer end points (e.g., colon, breast), the US Women's Health Initiative (WHI) evaluated the combination of 400 IU of vitamin D per day plus 1,000 mg of calcium per day in 36,282 postmenopausal women. For colon cancer, there was no benefit observed,[119] although the mean baseline intake of calcium was already very high (more than 1,151 mg per day). With regard to vitamin D as a single agent, there was also no suggestion of benefit for colon cancer incidence in a 5-year British trial of vitamin D (100,000 IU every 4 months) that reported colon cancer incidence,[120] although this was not a primary end point.

Clinical Efficacy in the Breast. Vitamin D has received considerable attention for a possible role in the prevention of breast cancer,[121] although no trials have yet investigated vitamin D as a single agent for breast cancer risk reduction. The large WHI trial gave a combination of calcium and vitamin D, as noted previously, and there was no significant effect of this combination on breast cancer risk (HR, 0.96; 95% CI, 0.85 to 1.09).[122] Lappe et al.[123] conducted a trial that examined the relation between calcium plus vitamin D (1,100 IU per day) supplementation (versus calcium alone or placebo) in 1,179 healthy postmenopausal women in Nebraska.[123] Although fracture was the primary outcome of the trial, total cancer incidence was reportedly lower in the calcium plus vitamin D group, although the number of end points was very small (n = 50 total cancers observed during the follow-up). An ongoing randomized trial of vitamin D and omega-3 fatty acids (the VITamin D and OmegA-3 TriaL [VITAL]) among 20,000 participants is expected to provide more definitive data on a possible role of vitamin D in the prevention of breast and other cancers.[124]

Summary and Conclusion: Micronutrients

Certain agents, including the retinoids, beta-carotene, folic acid, calcium plus vitamin D, vitamin E, and selenium, have received substantial attention for a possible role in reducing the risk of cancer in humans. As reviewed herein, some of the trials have observed statistically significant reductions in the risk of the primary end point (e.g., retinoids in skin carcinogenesis models, calcium in colorectal adenomas, antioxidant nutrients in Linxian, China, for gastric cancer prevention), whereas others have observed statistically significant increases in the risk of the primary end points (beta-carotene and retinoid lung cancer prevention trials in smokers, vitamin E and prostate cancer, selenium and nonmelanoma skin cancer). Considering the completed trials, there is clear evidence against the general use of nutrient *supplements* for cancer prevention, which is the conclusion also reached by the World Cancer Research Fund/ American Institute for Cancer Research.[38] Note that there is no evidence that food sources of these nutrients increase risk.

Having noted that, there are other key themes emerging from this growing body of research. One such theme is that nutrient supplementation may be of benefit to some but not all. One such population that may benefit includes persons who are low in the nutrient of interest at baseline.[77] This was initially suggested in the Linxian Country trial (done in a micronutrient-deficient population), with growing support from subgroup analyses of several completed trials.[77] However, the hypothesis that nutrient supplementation can reduce cancer risk in subgroups selected based on inadequate nutritional status has, to date, not been formally evaluated in intervention trials.

Another consistent theme is that lifestyle factors (e.g., smoking) and genetics (polymorphisms) may determine who is most likely to benefit from supplementation. Trial data will likely be increasingly mined to identify genetic profiles associated with both better outcomes (risk prediction) and response to intervention.[125,126] Ultimately, a more personalized approach to cancer risk reduction may emerge, consistent with the movement toward a more personalized approach for cancer treatment.

Finally, nearly all of these trials initiate intervention with older adults (who are more likely to develop cancer end points during the follow-up); but, animal models suggest that the timing of exposure may likely be quite relevant. For example, folic acid may protect against initiation, but may also promote the proliferation of existing neoplasms.[127] Thus, the dose, form (food versus supplement), timing, and nutritional and lifestyle characteristics may all be relevant in affecting the efficacy of risk-reducing interventions involving nutrients and related substances. Further research, drawing upon newer tools now available through the field of nutritional genomics, will be needed to gain greater clarity on the heterogeneous biologic effects observed in nutrient-based risk reduction.

ANTI-INFLAMMATORY DRUGS

Mechanism

Nonsteroidal anti-inflammatory drugs (NSAIDs) represent a class of drugs that reduce cellular inflammation through multiple mechanisms, the most prominent of them being the modulation of eicosanoid metabolism.[128] Eicosanoids are metabolites of dietary fatty acids, primarily linoleic acid. Linoleic acid is metabolized to arachidonic acid, which is stored in the lipid membrane and, once mobilized from the membrane, further metabolized by prostaglandin-H synthases (PGHS) 1 and 2 to PGD_2, PGE_2, $PGF_{2\alpha}$, PGI_2, or thromboxane A_2 (TxA_2) by specific synthases. Leukotriene pathways involve the conversion of arachidonic acid to leukotriene A_4 by 5-lipoxygenase and subsequent hydrolysis of leukotriene A_4 to other downstream leukotrienes. Newly formed prostaglandins function primarily through binding to prostaglandin receptors (EP receptors), releasing coupled G-proteins to elicit responses in the same or neighboring cells.[129]

Prostaglandins (PG) play crucial roles in controlling cellular proliferation, apoptosis, cellular invasiveness, and angiogenesis and in modulating immunosuppression.[129] Because PGE_2 is the most abundant PG in tumors, reducing local concentrations of PGE_2 may be a pivotal cancer preventive strategy.[129]

PGHS-independent mechanisms of NSAID action may, at least in part, explain NSAID preventive efficacy.[130] A diverse group of NSAIDs inhibit apoptosis via multiple mechanisms. Among the more prominent of these mechanisms is the inhibition of cyclic guanosine monophosphate (cGMP) phosphodiesterase activity, attenuation of beta-catenin mRNA through suppressing transcription of the *CTNNB1* gene, and activation of c-Jun N-terminal kinase 1.[130] NSAIDs activate peroxisome proliferator–activated receptor (PPAR)γ, leading to increased E-cadherin

expression and reduced colony formation in vitro, while reducing PPARδ, leading to reduced resistance to apoptosis.[130] Selective cyclooxygenase 2 (COX-2) inhibitors inhibit Akt signaling and induce apoptosis of human colorectal and prostate cancer cells in vitro in a COX-2–independent manner via the inhibition of phosphoinositide-dependent kinase-1 (PDK-1). NSAIDs inhibit nuclear factor kappa B (NF-κB) at pharmacologic concentrations and key cellular proliferation signaling intermediates such as activator protein 1 (AP-1) and other intermediates of the MAPK pathway.[130] The impact of NSAIDs on carcinogenic events driven by these upstream pathways in humans as opposed to preliminary in vitro or in vivo models remains unclear.

Epidemiology

Pooled analyses of 34 controlled trials of aspirin 75 mg to 100 mg daily (69,224 participants), conducted primarily for cardiovascular disease reduction, observed reduced cancer deaths (OR, 0.63; 95% CI, 0.49 to 0.82). Most of the benefit occurred after 5 years follow-up.[131] In a pooled analysis of 150 case control and 45 cohort studies, in addition to a reduced risk of death from colorectal cancer (OR, 0.58; 95% CI, 0.44 to 0.78), chronic and frequent (once daily or more) use of aspirin also reduced the risk of death from esophageal (OR, 0.58; 95% CI, 0.44 to 0.76), gastric (OR, 0.61; 95% CI, 0.40 to 0.93), and breast (OR, 0.81; 95% CI, 0.72 to 0.93) cancers.[132] An analysis of 662,624 men and women enrolled in the American Cancer Society's Cancer Prevention Study II found that aspirin taken at least 16 times per month over a 6-year period conferred a 40% reduced risk of colorectal cancer mortality.[133] Both the 46,363 male patients of the Health Professional Study[134] and the 82,911 patients of the Nurse's Health Study[135] suggest that prolonged use (>10 years) of 325 mg of aspirin twice weekly or more reduces colorectal cancer risk (RR, 0.77; 95% CI, 0.67 to 0.88, from the Nurse's Health Study). Daily NSAID intake is associated with a 40% reduction (OR, 0.56; 95% CI, 0.43 to 0.73) in the risk of esophageal adenocarcinoma.[136]

Evidence in Preclinical In Vivo Carcinogenesis Models

NSAIDs, including aspirin, indomethacin, piroxicam, sulindac, ibuprofen, and ketoprofen, suppress colonic tumorigenesis induced chemically (1,2-dimethylhydrazine or its metabolites) or transgenically (Min^+).[137,138] The selective COX-2 inhibitors were the most efficacious colon tumorigenesis inhibitors in both chemical and transgenic rodent models.[139,140] In preclinical models, NSAIDs affect the onset and progression of cancers in the stomach, skin, breast, lung, prostate, and urinary bladder, although the evidence is more limited than for colon cancers.[141]

Clinical Trials

Key clinical trials of NSAIDs for the prevention of colorectal cancer are summarized in Table 33.7. Sulindac reduced the size and number of preexisting adenomas in patients with familial adenomatous polyposis but did not suppress the development of new adenomas,[142] whereas the selective COX-2 inhibitor, celecoxib, suppressed the development of new adenomatous polyps in patients with familial adenomatous polyposis.[143] Although these results are promising, reports of invasive neoplasms developing in familial adenomatous polyposis patients being treated with sulindac[144] raise the question of whether NSAIDs preferentially alter the formation or regression of those adenomas less likely to progress to invasive adenocarcinomas, as compared to those more likely to progress.

Randomized, double-blinded placebo controlled trials of NSAIDs as cancer risk–reducing agents for colorectal adenocarcinoma (see Table 33.7) have confirmed that aspirin suppresses

TABLE 33.7

Summary of Clinical Trials of Nonsteroidal Anti-Inflammatory Drugs as Colorectal Cancer Risk–Reducing Agents

Population	Drug (Dose), Duration	Phase	Endpoint	Outcome	References
Gene Associated					
Familial adenomatous polyposis (FAP)	Sulindac (300–400 mg/d, divided doses)	IIb	Polyp regression	Colorectal and duodenal polyps regressed in ~50%	(277, 278) (279)
Hereditary nonpolyposis colon cancer (Lynch syndrome)	Aspirin 600 mg/d, resistant starch	III	Cancer	≥2 yr, hazard ratio (HR) colon cancer 0.41; 95% CI, 0.19–0.86; all cancers Incidence rate ratio 0.37; 95% CI, 0.18–0.78; no effect of starch	(280, 281)
Sporadic Risk					
Previous adenomatous polyps, healthy subjects	Aspirin (40, 81, 325, 650 mg once per day)	I, IIa	Dose-biomarker	Aspirin dose of 81 mg daily sufficient to suppress colorectal mucosal prostaglandin E_2	(282–284)
Previous adenomatous polyps	Sulindac (300 mg), 4 mos	IIb	Polyp regression	Sulindac did not significantly decrease the number or size of polyps	(146)
Previous adenomatous polyps	Piroxicam (7.5 mg), 2 yr	IIb	Polyp recurrence	Colorectal mucosal PGE_2 reduced in piroxicam treated arm, unacceptable toxicity	(145)
Prior colorectal cancer	Aspirin (325 mg once per day), 3 yr	IIb	Polyp recurrence	Aspirin use associated with delayed development of adenomatous polyps	(285)
Previous adenomatous polyps	Aspirin (81 mg once per day or 325 mg once per day) and/or folate, 3 yr	IIb	Polyp recurrence	Low-dose aspirin reduced the recurrence of adenomatous polyps	(286)
Previous adenomatous polyps	Celecoxib and rofecoxib	IIb	Polyp recurrence	Celecoxib and rofecoxib reduced the recurrence of adenomatous polyps, unacceptable toxicity	(148–150)

CANCER PREVENTION AND SCREENING

adenoma recurrence in patients previously treated for adenomas or for cancer. Neither sulindac nor piroxicam alone suppressed adenoma formation in high-risk, sporadic populations at tolerable doses.[145,146] Sulindac, in combination with difluoromethylornithine, has potent colorectal anticarcinogenesis effects.[147] Selective COX-2 inhibitors (celecoxib, rofecoxib) reduce the recurrence of adenomas by one-third in all patients previously treated for adenomas and by one-half in patients with previously resected large (≥1 cm) adenomas,[148–150] but they are too toxic as cancer risk–reducing agents due to their cardiovascular toxicity.[151,152] Although most NSAIDs (piroxicam, indomethacin) have sufficient gastrointestinal (GI) toxicity to reduce their acceptability as cancer risk–reducing agents,[153,154] the long-term administration of low-dose aspirin in vascular prevention trials demonstrates acceptable GI toxicity.[155]

Up to 40% of individuals screened for colorectal neoplasms will have an adenomatous polyp detected and removed, yet only 10% of these lesions will progress to invasive neoplasms. To date, prospective NSAID trials of only 2 to 3 years cannot substitute for cancer incidence or mortality end points. Given the 10-year latency between adenoma formation and a cancer event, prospective trials sufficiently powered to detect colorectal cancer incidence end points are unlikely in the future.[156] Alternatively, a follow-up of patients randomized on trials of aspirin in the prevention of vascular events in the 1980s and 1990s offers secondary analysis opportunities. In a pooled analysis of three prospective vascular end point cohort studies, 20-year low-dose aspirin treatments reduced cancer deaths from all solid tumors (OR, 0.69; CI, 0.54 to 0.88) and from lung and esophageal adenocarcinomas (OR, 0.66; CI, 0.56 to 0.77).[155] Despite this, the U.S. Preventive Services Task Force (USPSTF) does not recommend the use of aspirin or NSAIDs as cancer risk–reducing agents for normal risk populations, preferring adherence to colorectal cancer screening recommendations (fecal occult blood testing and endoscopy).[153,154,157]

Minimal prospective cancer risk reduction data are available at other epithelial organ sites. Ketorolac, given as a 1% rinse solution, did not reduce the size or histology of leukoplakia lesions.[158] Celecoxib reduces the Ki67 labeling index and increases the expression of nuclear survivin without significantly changing the cytoplasmic survivin in bronchial biopsies of smokers.[159] Cancer prevention trials of aspirin as interventions for delaying progression from intraepithelial neoplasias in other epithelial sites remain ongoing for the lower esophagus.[136] No prospective, randomized trials or data are available for breast, prostate, or gynecologic cancer prevention.

EPIGENETIC TARGETING AGENTS (SELECTIVE ESTROGEN RECEPTOR MODULATORS, 5α-STEROID REDUCTASE INHIBITORS, POLYAMINE INHIBITORS)

Posttranslational pathway targets remain a fertile source of chemopreventive strategies. Phase III data support cancer risk–reduction agent efficacy of selective estrogen receptor modulators (SERM) and 5α-steroid reductase inhibitors for breast and prostate cancer prevention, respectively. Inhibitors of the polyamine pathway may be useful preventives for colorectal cancer.

Selective Estrogen Receptor Modulators

Mechanism

SERMs function as estrogen receptor (ER) agonists and antagonists depending on the SERM structure and target tissue. Predominant ERα receptors occur in the human uterus, cortical bone, and the liver; whereas predominant ERβ receptors occur in blood vessels, cancellous bone, the whole brain, and immune cells.[160,161] During carcinogenesis, the amount of ERα increases while the amount of ERβ decreases in breast tissues.[162] Ideally, a desirable SERM for cancer prevention will function as an antiestrogen in the breast and uterus, but a partial estrogen agonist in skeletal, cardiovascular, central nervous system (CNS), GI tract, and vaginal tissues. In addition, an ideal SERM will not have procoagulant effects and will not cause perimenopausal symptoms such as hot flashes.[162]

Tamoxifen. Tamoxifen is a triphenylethylene compound developed for the treatment of ER-positive breast cancer in the 1960s and 1970s.[163,164] Tamoxifen inhibits the initiation and promotion phases of breast carcinogenesis in the dimethylbenzanthracene chemical carcinogenesis model.[164,165] When tamoxifen binds to ERβ, which then binds to an AP-1 type gene promoter, it functions as an estrogen agonist. When bound to ERα, which binds to an estrogen response element (ERE) target gene promoter, tamoxifen functions as an estrogen antagonist.[162,166] Tamoxifen has estrogen antagonist effects in the human breast; partial estrogen agonist effects in bone, the cardiovascular system, and CNS; and predominant estrogen agonist effects in the uterus, liver, and vagina. The estrogen agonist effects in the liver and uterus result in tamoxifen's toxicities of thromboembolism and endometrial cancer, respectively. The clinical finding that tamoxifen reduces the incidence of contralateral second primary breast cancers during adjuvant treatment regimens catalyzed the push for its development as a cancer risk–reduction agent.[167,168]

Raloxifene. The benzothiophene structure of raloxifene confers a different tissue-specific ER-binding profile than the triphenylethylene tamoxifen. Raloxifene has greater estrogen agonist activity in bone but reduced estrogen agonist activity in the uterus. Raloxifene was studied for the treatment and prevention of osteoporosis in a large, pivotal trial (the Multiple Outcomes of Raloxifene Evaluation [MORE]) and was found to reduce the rate of vertebral fracture as compared to placebo in postmenopausal women.[169]

Lasofoxifene and Arzoxifene. Lasofoxifene and arzoxifene are third-generation SERMs developed as more potent blockers of bone resorption with the goal of reducing the risk of fractures, breast cancer, and heart disease while minimizing the SERM-induced risk of endometrial hyperplasia in postmenopausal women. Both agents proved potent in vitro and in preliminary clinical trials for bone fracture prevention.[170–173]

Selective Estrogen Receptor Modulators as Risk-Reducing Agents for Breast Cancer Prevention

Efficacy. Table 33.8 summarizes the phase III data for SERM-based breast cancer–risk reduction. In a systematic review of MEDLINE and Cochrane databases through December, 2012, the USPSTF identified seven trials of tamoxifen or raloxifene that showed a reduced incidence of invasive breast cancer by 7 to 9 cases in 1,000 women over 5 years compared to placebo.[174] Tamoxifen is more effective than raloxifene; it reduces breast cancer incidence more than raloxifene by 5 cases in 1,000 women. Both drugs reduce the incidence of ER-positive breast cancer, but neither reduces the risk of ER-negative breast cancer. Neither drug reduced breast cancer–specific or all cause mortality rates. Based on benefit–risk models, women with estimated 5-year risks of breast cancer of 3% or greater are likely to benefit from treatment.[175] Using similar

---

TABLE 33.8

Phase III, Randomized, Controlled Clinical Trials of SERMs for the Prevention of Breast Cancer

Study	Drug and Daily Dose	N =	Treatment Duration (Years)	Entry Criteria	Overall Outcome HR (95% CI)	References
NSABP P-1	Tamoxifen 20 mg Placebo	13,388	5	Gail model: 5 yr predicted risk of ≥1.66%	0.52 (0.42–0.64)	(28,287)
IBIS-I	Tamoxifen 20 mg Placebo	7,139	5	>Twofold relative risk	0.72 (0.58–0.90)	(288)
Marsden	Tamoxifen 20 mg Placebo	2,471	8	Family history	0.87 (0.63–1.21)	(289)
Italian	Tamoxifen 20 mg Placebo	5,408	5	Normal risk, hysterectomy	0.67 (0.59–0.76)	(290)
NSABP P-2 (STAR)	Raloxifene 60 mg Tamoxifen 20 mg	19,747	5	Gail model: 5 yr predicted risk of ≥1.66%	RR Raloxifene versus tamoxifen 1.02 (0.81–1.28)	(29)
MORE/CORE	Raloxifene 60 mg Placebo Raloxifene 120 mg Placebo	7,705 6,511	5	Normal risk, postmenopausal with osteoporosis	0.42 (0.29–0.60)	(291,292)
RUTH	Raloxifene 60 mg Placebo	10,101	5	Normal risk, postmenopausal with risk of coronary heart disease	0.67(0.47–0.96)	(179)
PEARL	Lasofoxifene 0.5 mg Lasofoxifene 0.25 mg Placebo	8,856	5	Normal risk, postmenopausal, with osteoporosis	0.25 mg: 0.82 (0.45–1.49) 0.5 mg: 0.21 (0.05–0.55)	(170)
GENERATIONS	Arzoxifene 20 mg Placebo	9,354	4	Normal risk, postmenopausal, with osteoporosis	0.42 (0.25–0.68)	(172)

Table and data adapted from Cuzick J, Sestak I, Bonanni B, et al. Selective oestrogen receptor modulators in prevention of breast cancer: an updated meta-analysis of individual participant data. *Lancet* 2013;381:1827–1834.

analysis methods as the USPSTF, the American Society of Clinical Oncology recommends the use of tamoxifen (20 mg per day orally for 5 years) or raloxifene (60 mg per day orally for 5 years) "in premenopausal women who are age ≥35 years with a 5-year projected absolute breast cancer risk ≥1.66% according to the NCI Breast Cancer Risk Assessment Tool (or equivalent measures), or with lobular carcinoma in situ."[176] Tamoxifen reduces the risk of in situ (preinvasive) breast neoplasms (lobular carcinoma in situ, ductal carcinoma in situ) by 50%.[177,178] The reduction during treatment persists for at least 5 years after treatment.[177,178] Raloxifene does not reduce the risk of in situ breast neoplasms.

Data from two trials designed to evaluate the safety and efficacy of lasofoxifene (PEARL)[170,171] and arzoxifene (GENERATIONS)[172,173] as bone fracture preventives have been analyzed for breast cancer–risk reduction. Their effect at reducing breast cancer incidence was captured in secondary analyses (see Table 33.8). Neither lasofoxifene nor arzoxifene have been evaluated in phase III randomized controlled breast cancer prevention trials. Arzoxifene development has been discontinued in the United States.

Toxicity Profiles. Tamoxifen causes a twofold increase in the risk of endometrial adenocarcinoma (RR, 2.13; 95% CI, 1.36 to 3.32) and is related to more benign gynecologic conditions, uterine bleeding, and surgical procedures than the placebo controls, whereas raloxifene did not increase the risk for endometrial cancer or uterine bleeding.[174] Tamoxifen causes a twofold increase in thromboembolic events (RR, 1.93; 95% CI, 1.41 to 2.64), whereas raloxifene causes a 60% increase in risk of venous thromboembolism (RR, 1.60; 95% CI, 1.15 to 2.23).[174] Raloxifene does not differ from tamoxifen in risk of fractures, other cancers, or cardiovascular events.[177] Raloxifene's lower risk of endometrial adenocarcinomas compared to tamoxifen needs to be weighed against the increased risk of stroke seen in in the MORE/CORE trials (see Table 33.8).[179] Raloxifene's effectiveness in the community may also be compromised by its poor bioavailability (2%) due to rapid phase II enzyme metabolism in the gut and liver,[180] whereas tamoxifen is more bioavailable and has active metabolites that permit a prolonged drug effect. Missed raloxifene doses may potentially compromise efficacy and prevention outcomes in widespread, community use.

Aromatase Inhibitors. In adjuvant clinical trials for breast cancer, aromatase inhibitors (anastrozole, exemestane, letrozole) given after 5 years of tamoxifen enhance the reduction of breast cancer recurrence in the contralateral breast compared to tamoxifen alone.[181] In a phase I cancer risk–reducing agent trial, letrozole reduced the Ki-67 proliferation index of breast epithelial cells aspirated from high-risk women.[182] Exemestane reduced the overall risk of ER-positive invasive breast cancer (Table 33.9). It did not reduce the risk of noninvasive breast neoplasms or ER-negative breast cancer.[183] Exemestane has no increased risk of venous thromboembolism, endometrial cancer, fracture, or cataract,[183] but losses in bone mineral density and cortical thickness of the distal tibia and radius occurred after 2 years of treatment despite calcium and vitamin D supplementation.[184] The results of the

International Breast Cancer Intervention Study II (IBIS-II), comparing anastrozole with placebo, are similar to those reported for exemestane.[185] Compared to exemestane, anastrozole decreases the incidence of ductal carcinoma in situ (DCIS), whereas exemestane does not. Neither aromatase inhibitor increased survival compared to placebo controls. The American Society of Clinical Oncology recommends exemestane for breast cancer prevention in addition to tamoxifen and raloxifene.

Use Counseling. Despite the widespread evidence of breast cancer preventive efficacy for tamoxifen and raloxifene, only 3% to 20% of eligible high-risk women agree to take tamoxifen for primary prevention.[186] The low willingness of eligible women to take tamoxifen for 5 years demonstrates the issue of risk benefit for cancer risk–reducing agents. Women with high short-term risk (5 year Gail risk of >3%)—for example, those with ER-positive atypical hyperplasia, lobular carcinoma in situ, and the majority of non–high-grade ductal carcinoma in situ lesions—have an acceptable risk to benefit ratio and are the most likely to benefit from a 5-year cancer risk–reducing agent intervention with a SERM.[175,176] The toxicity profile of aromatase inhibitors differs from SERMs. Although aromatase inhibitors may have a more favorable risk to benefit profile than SERMs, long-term outcomes and toxicity experience for aromatase inhibitor risk-reducing agent intervention are not available to date. In the National Surgical Adjuvant Breast and Bowel Project, tamoxifen-treated women with a *BRCA2* mutation but not a *BRCA1* mutation had reduced cancer incidence,[187] but subsequent data from another group have found reduced cancer risk in women with both BRCA mutations.[188] Data remain insufficient to recommend the use of SERMs for risk reduction in women with BRCA mutations.

5α-Steroid Reductase Inhibitors

Mechanism

Prostate cancers require androgens to proliferate and evade apoptosis. The primary nuclear androgen responsible for the maintenance of epithelial function is dihydrotestosterone. The testes and adrenal gland synthesize dihydrotestosterone by the conversion of testosterone by 5α-steroid reductase types 1 and 2 isozymes. Dihydrotestosterone binds to intracellular androgen receptors to form a complex that binds to DNA hormone response elements controlling cellular proliferation and apoptosis. Finasteride, a selective, competitive inhibitor of type 2 5α-steroid reductase,[189] inhibits proliferation in the transformed prostate cell. In the 3,2'-dimethyl-4-aminobiphenyl (DMAB), methylnitrosourea (MNU), and testosterone chemical carcinogenesis models in rats, finasteride reduces prostate tumor incidence by close to six-fold. Finasteride appears to be more effective in the promotion phase of prostate carcinogenesis.[190] Dutasteride inhibits both 5α-steroid reductase inhibitor[190] types 1 and 2 isoforms and has similar anticarcinogenesis activity in preclinical models to finasteride.

TABLE 33.9

Phase III, Randomized, Controlled Clinical Trials of Aromatase Inhibitors for the Prevention of Breast Cancer

Study	Drug and Daily Dose	N =	Treatment Duration (Years)	Entry Criteria	Overall Outcome HR (95% CI)	References
MAP.3	Exemestane 25 mg Placebo	4,560	5	Gail model 5 yr predicted risk of ≥2.3%	0.35 (0.18–0.70)	(183)
IBIS-II	Anastrozole 1 mg Placebo	3,851	5	RR twofold higher than general population or Tyrer-Cuzick 10-yr risk >5%	0.47 (0.32–0.68)	(185)

Phase III, Randomized, Controlled Clinical Trials of 5α-Steroid Reductase Inhibitors for the Prevention of Prostate Cancer

Study	Drug and Daily Dose	N =	Treatment Duration (Years)	Entry Criteria	Overall Outcome HR (95% CI)	References
PCPT	Finasteride 5 mg Placebo	18,880	7	Age ≥55 y, PSA ≤3 ng/mL	0.70 (0.65–0.76)	(30, 193)
REDUCE	Dutaseride 0.5 mg Placebo	6,729	4	Age 50–75 y, PSA 2.5–10.0 ng/mL, core biopsies within 6 mos	RR = 0.77 (0.70–0.85)	(192)

PSA, prostate specific antigen.

Cancer Risk–Reducing Agent Activity

Randomized, placebo-controlled cancer incidence end point risk-reducing agent clinical trials demonstrated that finasteride and dutasteride reduced the incidence of prostate cancer by approximately 22% (Table 33.10).[30,191,192] Patients who are treated with either drug yet progress to transformed neoplasms develop more tumors of a high Gleason grade (7 to 10) compared to the placebo arm (22%). After 18 years of follow-up, no significant differences in overall survival or survival after prostate cancer diagnosis were found in the finasteride-treated group compared to the placebo-treated group.[193] Sexual function side effects (e.g., erectile dysfunction, loss of libido, gynecomastia) were more common in the finasteride- or dutasteride-treated groups.[30,192]

The 5α-steroid reductase inhibitors, finasteride and dutasteride, prevent or delay carcinogenesis progression in the prostate, yet progression of high-grade lesions is unaffected. Use of finasteride for a period of 7 years reduced the incidence of prostate cancer but did not significantly affect mortality.[193] Increasing the diagnosis of low-grade prostate cancer through prostate-specific antigen (PSA) testing or intervention with a drug with a minimal toxicity profile without reducing mortality is of no benefit and "all forms of therapy cause considerable burden to the patient and to society."[193]

SIGNAL TRANSDUCTION MODIFIERS

Both cancer therapy and cancer prevention have investigated drugs that modify specific targets in signal transduction pathways. Although the emphasis in drug development has focused on cancer treatment, interventions aimed at modulating signal transduction pathways promise new approaches to interventions in the carcinogenic process. Because of the complexity of signaling systems, the inhibition of single targets may not be effective or may cause unacceptable toxicity.

Difluoromethylornithine

Mechanism

Polyamines (spermidine, spermine, and the diamine, putrescine) are required to maintain cellular growth and function.[194] In mammalian cells, polyamine inhibition by genetic mutation or pharmaceutical agents is associated with virtual cessation in cellular growth. Difluoromethylornithine (DFMO) is an enzyme-activated irreversible inhibitor of ornithine decarboxylase (which is trans-activated by the *c-MYC* oncogene and cooperates with the *RAS* oncogene in malignant transformation).[195]

Evidence in Preclinical In Vivo Carcinogenesis Models

Extensive preclinical data has found that DFMO prevents tumor promotion in a variety of systems, including skin, mammary, colon, cervical, and bladder carcinogenesis models.[194] Synergistic or additive activity with retinoids, butylated hydroxyanisole, tamoxifen, piroxicam, and fish oil has been demonstrated with low concentrations of DFMO.[194]

Clinical Trials

In phase I prevention trials, DFMO at a dose of 0.5 mg/m^2 per day reduced tissue polyamines in the colon and skin[196,197] and causes regression of cervical intraepithelial neoplasia when used topically,[198] but does not reduce tissue polyamines or other biomarkers of cellular proliferation in the human breast.[199] As a single agent, DFMO has anticarcinogenic activity for nonmelanoma skin cancers, primarily basal cell carcinoma. In combination with an NSAID (sulindac), DFMO reduced adenoma recurrences, suggesting a synergistic reduction of colorectal cancer risk (Table 33.11). Preliminary data suggest some cancer risk–reducing agent activity for the lower esophagus and the prostate (see Table 33.11).[200]

Statins

Mechanism

Statins are hydroxyl-3-methylglutaryl coenzyme A (HMG-CoA) reductase inhibitors that inhibit the conversion of HMG-CoA to mevalonate, a cholesterol precursor. The statins are a class of medications with similar structures but with variable moieties that can result in hydrophilic forms (e.g., pravastatin, rosuvastatin) and lipophilic forms (e.g., lovastatin, simvastatin, fluvastatin, atorvastatin).[201] Statins decrease the risk of cancer in preclinical studies by inhibiting *RAS*- and *RHO*-mediated cell proliferation, upregulating cell cycle inhibitors (e.g., p21 and p27), and inducing apoptosis of transformed cells and the inhibition of angiogenesis.[202]

Evidence in Preclinical In Vivo Carcinogenesis Models

Lipophilic statins delay progression of pancreatic intraepithelial neoplasias and the growth of pancreatic carcinoma xenografts. Atorvastatin alone and in combination with NSAIDs reduced colonic adenoma and adenocarcinoma incidence and multiplicity by half in rodent transgenic and chemical carcinogenesis models. Lovastatin reduced lung adenoma multiplicity but not incidence.[201]

Clinical Trials

Although several large trials of pravastatin or simvastatin on cardiovascular disease risk with cancer as secondary end points have shown no benefit for reducing cancer risk with follow-ups between 18 months to 4 years, these trials were not adequately powered to examine cancer end points.[201] Several case control studies evaluating statin effects have shown a significant association with lower risk of colorectal adenocarcinoma with odds ratios ranging from 0.53 to 0.91 for arzoxifene. A secondary analysis of a celecoxib prevention trial demonstrated no statin protection against colorectal

TABLE 33.11

Summary of Clinical Trials of Difluoromethylornithine as a Cancer Risk–Reducing Agent

Population	Dose per Day, Duration	Phase	Endpoint	Outcome	References
Low risk bladder cancer (Ta. T1. Grades 1 or 2)	1 gm versus placebo × 1 year	III	Bladder cancer recurrence	Did not prevent or delay recurrence	(293)
Prostate risk: men with family history prostate cancer, age 35–70 yr	500 mg versus placebo × 1 yr	IIb	Prostate volume, polyamines, PSA	10-fold reduction of prostate size increase over 1 yr compared to placebo, PSA reduction not significant	(294)
Nonmelanoma skin cancer	500 mg/m² versus placebo × 4–5 y	III	New nonmelanoma skin cancers	Lower rate of basal cell carcinomas per year (0.28 versus 0.40); persistent reduction in nonmelanoma skin cancers, not statistically significant	(295, 296)
Colon adenomas	DFMO: 500 mg Sulindac: 150 mg versus placebo × 3 y	IIb	Adenoma recurrence	RR for adenoma recurrence for DFMO/sulindac treatment 5 0.30 (0.18–0.49)	(147)

PSA, prostate specific antigen.

neoplasms.[203] The Women's Health Initiative (prospective longitudinal cohort of 159,319 women) found that lovastatin was associated with a lower risk of developing colorectal cancer (HR = 0.62; 95% CI, 0.39 to 0.99).[204] Prospective longitudinal studies have shown mixed results. The PHS reported statin use was inversely associated with prostate cancer (adjusted RR, 0.51),[205] whereas the Nurse's Health Study showed no association with risk of breast cancer.[206] Interventional trials to determine statin preventive efficacy for colon and breast cancer are ongoing.[201] Statins may be effective risk-reducing agents in individuals with the A/A variant of the predominant T/T genotype of rs12654264 of the HMG-CoA reductase gene.[207]

Bisphosphonates

Mechanism

Bisphosphonates are pyrophosphate analogs with a central phosphorus-carbon-phosphorus bond that resists bone degradation preventing bone loss and fractures. Second- and third-generation amino bisphosphonates (pamidronic, alendronic, risedronic, ibandronic, and zoledronic acids) inhibit farnesyl diphosphate synthase downstream of HMG-CoA reductase, leading to decreased posttranslational prenylation of GTP-binding proteins such as RAS and Rho. Amino bisphosphonates inhibit cell proliferation, angiogenesis, and cell cycle arrest while inducing apoptosis.[201]

Evidence in In Vivo Preclinical and Clinical Models

HER2-transgenic mice treated with zoledronic acid had increased tumor-free survival and overall survival. Zoledronic acid suppressed bone, lung, and liver metastases when treated prior to an injection of breast cancer cells.[201] The short-term use of bisphosphonates is associated with reduced breast cancer incidence in case control studies[208,209] and prospective cohort studies (HR = 0.68; 95% CI, 0.52 to 0.88 in a prospective cohort study).[210] Randomized trials of amino-bisphosphonates in postmenopausal women with breast cancer treated for 1 year have found a reduction of breast cancer risk in the contralateral breast (HR = 0.39; 95% CI, 0.18 to 0.88).[211] Case control data suggesting a bisphosphonate-associated reduction in colorectal cancer risk have not been confirmed by prospective cohort studies (i.e., Women's Health Initiative, Nurse's Health Study).[201]

Metformin

Mechanism

Metformin, an oral antidiabetic drug in the biguanide class, is the first-line drug of choice for the treatment of type 2 diabetes.[212] Cancers are more common in diabetics and obese individuals than their normal weight and normoglycemic counterparts, leading to the hypothesis that elevated serum insulin concentrations promote cancer risk.[213,214] Insulin and insulin-like growth factors (IGF1 and 2) stimulate cellular DNA synthesis, proliferation, and tumor growth through phosphoinositide-3 kinase (PI3K), mammalian target of rapamycin (mTOR), and the RAS-MAPK signaling pathways.[213] Metformin activates the adenosine monophosphate-activated protein kinase (AMPK) via LKB1, a protein-threonine kinase that has tumor-suppressor activity.[201] Metformin anticarcinogenesis activity appears to be broad and includes downregulation of erbB-2 and epidermal growth factor receptor (EGFR) expression, inhibiting the phosphorylation of erbB family members, IGF1R, Akt, mTOR, and STAT3 in vivo. Low doses of metformin inhibit the self-renewal/proliferation of cancer stem cells in breast, colon, and pancreatic models.[215,216]

Evidence in Preclinical In Vivo Carcinogenesis Models

Metformin reduces tobacco carcinogen–induced tumors in mice, and pancreatic premalignant and malignant tumors in hamsters.[201] However, metformin's anticarcinogenic activity appears dependent on the dose and the induced carcinogenesis process. Metformin promoted carcinogenesis in MNU-induced rat breast cancers, MMTV-Neu ER-negative breast cancers, OH-BBN induced bladder cancer, and Min+ mouse intestinal tumors using nonobese rodents.[217] Metformin cancer risk–reducing agent effects may be limited to obesity- and diabetes-associated carcinogenesis mechanisms.

Clinical Trials

Two large retrospective cohort studies have shown that metformin therapy is associated with a reduced risk of solid tumors by 25% to 30%.[201] The Women's Health Imitative observed a lower incidence of invasive breast cancer in metformin-treated women with type 2 diabetes mellitus.[218] Phase II window of opportunity randomized trials have shown reduced proliferation and increased apoptosis in resected tissue of breast cancer patients.[201]

Diet-Derived Natural Products

Mechanism

Polyphenolic phytochemicals, such as curcumin, resveratrol, epigallocatechin gallate (EGCG), genistein, and ginger, are attractive as cancer risk–reducing agents for their low toxicity and multimechanism anticarcinogenic properties. They have anti-inflammatory activity, in part through scavenging of ROS, modulation of protein kinase signal transduction pathways (e.g., STAT-3, HER2/neu, MAPK, and Akt), and downstream inhibition of eicosanoid synthesis potentially due to upstream inhibition of NF-κB and PPAR or direct blockade or inhibition of eicosanoid-metabolizing enzymes.[219–221] Curcumin, and presumably other polyphenolics, downregulate stem cell driver signaling systems Wnt, Hedgehog, and Notch with subsequent reductions of breast, pancreatic, and colonic stem cell self-renewal.[222,223]

Omega-3 fatty acids (derived from marine products) compete with omega-6 fatty acid substrates for eicosanoid-metabolizing enzymes with subsequent tissue reduction of these inflammatory mediators.[224,225] These fatty acids have other diverse anticarcinogenic mechanisms (e.g., G-protein inhibition, changes in membrane physical characteristics that alter transmembrane signaling protein dynamics) that make them attractive as cancer risk–reducing agents.[226,227]

Whole berries, black raspberries, and strawberries contain mixtures of multiple anticarcinogenic compounds such as ellagic acid, anthocyanins, and tocopherols.[228] Research-grade berries are grown in a standardized cultivation environment and assayed for key components to ensure year-to-year reproducibility despite yearly climatologic variation. Berries have potent stabilization of methylation properties in addition to the expected anti-inflammatory and antioxidative properties associated with the prominent components.[229,230]

Preclinical and Clinical Anticarcinogenesis Efficacy. Diverse diet-derived natural products have moderate-to-strong anticarcinogenic effects in both chemical and transgenic rodent carcinogenesis models (Table 33.12). Phase I clinical trials of curcumin detected little parent compound in plasma or tissues, raising the possibility of biologically active conjugates or deconjugation at the target site.[231–233] Resveratrol's plasma bioavailability exceeds that of curcumin and ginger, and partitions into human colon tissue at 10-fold concentrations compared to plasma.[219,234,235] No natural products have been studied in large prospective, cancer incidence risk–reduction trials. Using intraepithelial biomarker end points in human phase II trials, berry formulations reduce esophageal dysplasia and oral leukoplakia.[236,237] Curcumin reduces the number of colon aberrant crypt foci in human smokers.[238]

ANTI-INFECTIVES

Many infectious agents are known causes of human cancers, including the human hepatitis viruses, hepatitis B virus (HBV) and hepatitis C virus (HCV) for hepatocellular carcinoma[239]; *Helicobacter pylori* for gastric adenocarcinoma[240]; human papilloma viruses (HPV) for cervical, anal, vulva, penis, and oral cavity and pharynx carcinomas[241]; herpes virus-8 for Kaposi sarcoma[242]; Epstein-Barr virus for Burkitt and other lymphomas[243]; liver flukes for cholangiocarcinoma[244]; and schistosomes for bladder carcinoma.[245] The success of the HPV vaccine at reducing the incidence of intraepithelial neoplasia of the cervix (reviewed in Chapter 72) is one example that demonstrates the potential of immunochemoprevention for epithelial targets for which an etiologic agent can be identified.

Helicobacter pylori

Intestinal-type gastric adenocarcinoma arises through a multistep process that begins with chronic gastritis initiated by *H. pylori*, progressing through gastric mucosal atrophy, intestinal metaplasia to dysplasia, and ultimately, to adenocarcinoma.[246] *H. pylori* infects 50% of the world's population.[240] Infection occurs early in life, remains quiescent, and may be associated with chronic gastritis of variable intensity but with minimal symptoms. Although the majority of *H. pylori* organisms remain in the gastric mucous layer, 10% adhere to the gastric mucosa through adhesion *BabA*, an outer membrane protein that binds to the Lewis-B histo-blood group antigen.[240] Progression to atrophic gastritis and peptic ulcer disease (occurs in 10% to 15% of infected individuals) requires other bacterial and host cofactors.[245,246] Infection with *H. pylori* is associated with an OR of 2.7 to 6.0 for gastric cancer; *CagA* increases this risk by 20- to 40-fold. The risk of developing gastric adenocarcinoma with an *H. pylori* infection is estimated to be 1% to 3%.[245,246]

The eradication of *H. pylori* with antibiotics and anti-inflammatory agents—for example, amoxicillin, metronidazole, and bismuth subsalicylate—increases the rate of regression of nonmetaplastic gastric atrophy and intestinal metaplasia in geographically diverse regions.[247,248] A combination of a 2-week course of a proton pump inhibitor (omeprazole) and an antibiotic (amoxicillin) reduced the risk of gastric cancer in a high-risk population in China (OR = 0.61; (95% CI, 0.36 to 0.96) for 14.7 years after the treatment.[249] The sequence of giving proton pump inhibitors and antibiotic therapy does not alter the treatment outcome. In addition to contributing to gastric cancer risk, *H. pylori* infections may also contribute to pancreatic cancer risk.[250] Because *H. pylori* infections are so widespread, mass eradication campaigns in high-risk regions are being considered.[251] However, complicating this is that *H. pylori* infections have also been associated with a reduced risk of both esophageal adenocarcinoma and gastric cardia carcinoma.[252]

MULTIAGENT APPROACHES TO CANCER RISK REDUCTION

In the transition to molecularly targeted interventions, combinations of targets that logically address critical carcinogenic pathways may have greater efficacy than single agents. For example, previously demonstrated interactive signaling of EGFRs and COX-2 experiments in Min[+] mice[253] demonstrates cancer preventive synergism. Combining atorvastatin with selective or nonselective COX inhibitors enhanced the inhibition of azoxymethane-induced colon carcinogenesis in F344 rats and reduced the dose of the combined drugs required to achieve a reduction of colon carcinogenesis.[254]

DFMO plus sulindac inhibited adenoma formation in a phase IIb trial of 375 patients with a prior history of adenomas followed for 36 months (see Table 33.11).[147] Cardiovascular-adverse outcomes were higher in DFMO/sulindac-treated patients who had preexisting high baseline cardiovascular risk; however, the cardiovascular-adverse events were similar to placebo in moderate or low cardiovascular risk patients.[255] Using IGF-1 as a biomarker, Guerrieri-Gonzaga et al.[256] showed that the combination of low-dose tamoxifen with low-dose fenretinide is safe but not synergistic. As more data accumulate from in vivo models, combined drugs aimed at specific targets in coordinated signaling pathways will enter clinical biomarker-based trials. Optimal doses, toxicity, and biomarker modulation data will select those combinations useful for risk reduction trials and, ultimately, generalized use in at-risk populations.

TABLE 33.12

Selected Diet-Derived Natural Products with Cancer Risk–Reducing Activity

Nutritional Extract	Source	Mechanisms	In Vivo Anticarcinogenesis Efficacy	Human Trials	References
Curcumin ([1E,6E]-1,7-bis-[4-hydroxy-3-methoxyphenyl]-1,6-heptadiene-3,5-dione/diferuloylmethane)	Turmeric, rhizome of *Curcuma longa*	Inhibits: PGE$_2$ synthesis via direct binding to COX-2 and through inhibition of NF-κB; angiogenesis. ErbB2 transduction; PI3K-Akt transduction; Inhibits stem cell self renewal Agonist: vitamin D receptor	Colon, breast, skin	Phase I: Poor bioavailability due to biotransformation in gut, enterohepatic cycling of metabolites; Phase IIa: reduced aberrant crypt foci	(219, 238)
Resveratrol (3,5,4'-trihydroxy-trans-stilbene)	Grapes, mulberries, peanuts, and *Cassia quinquangulata* plants	Inhibits: Carcinogen activation via inhibition of phase I isozyme, eicosanoids via direct binding; NF-κB; Nrf2. Acts as a caloric restriction mimetic, activates the histone deacetylase SIRT1 and AMPK	Colorectal, breast, pancreas, skin, and prostate	Phase I: 1 g dose generated peak concentration ~2 μM, conjugates 10-fold higher; resveratrol tissue concentrations 10-fold higher than plasma; Phase IIa: Small reduction in IGF-1 and IGFBP-1	(220, 234)
Ginger (gingerols, paradols, shagaols)	Rhizome of *Zingiber officinale*	Induces apoptosis via caspase-3 mechanisms; Inhibits NF-κB activation and downstream COX-2 expression; reduces iNOS expression and ornithine decarboxylase activity	Colon, breast, skin, oral cavity, liver	Phase I: 2 g dose nontoxic; Phase IIa: Small reductions in PGE$_2$, increased Bax in upper colon crypt	(235, 297, 298)
Green tea (epigallocatechin gallate, other catechins)	Green tea extract	Inhibits: PI3K-Akt transduction, IGF-1, IGFBP-3; NK-κB; catenin reduces methylation via inhibition of DNA methyltransferase 1	Lung, prostate, skin, colorectal	Phase IIa: 500–1,000 mg/m^2 × 12 wk reduced oral premalignant lesions in 50%; Phase IIb: 2.5 g × 1 yr reduced colorectal adenoma recurrence by 50%	(221)
Omega-3 fatty acids (eicosapentaenoic acid; docosahexaenoic acid)	Fish oil	Reduction of inflammation via eicosanoid reduction; direct binding to G receptor proteins; PPAR activation; induction of anti-inflammatory lipid mediators (resolvins, protectins, maresins)	Colon, breast, prostate	Phase II: 4–7 mg/d reduced colon adenomas in familial adenomatous polyposis; ongoing trials for sporadic; extensive case control studies	(226, 299)
Berries	Black raspberries, strawberries	Reduction of methylation via inhibition of methyltransferases, re-regulated Wnt; inhibits NF-κB; inhibits cyclooxygenases; inhibits proliferation	Esophageal squamous cell, colon, skin	Phase IIb: Freeze dried strawberries reduced esophageal dysplasia; Phase IIa: Blackberry gel reduced leukoplakia	(228, 229, 236, 237)

IGFBP-1, insulin growth factor binding protein-1; iNOS, inducible isoform of nitric oxide synthase.

SELECTED REFERENCES

The full reference list can be accessed at lwwhealthlibrary.com/oncology.

4. Lippman SM, Levin B, Brenner DE, et al. Cancer prevention and the American Society of Clinical Oncology. *J Clin Oncol* 2004;22:3848–3851.

8. Steele VE, Boone CW, Lubet RA, et al. Preclinical drug development paradigms for chemopreventives. *Hematol Oncol Clin North Am* 1998;12:943–961.

22. Schatzkin A, Freedman LS, Schiffman MH, et al. Validation of intermediate end points in cancer research. *J Natl Cancer Inst* 1990;82:1746–1752.

25. Pepe MS, Feng Z, Janes H, et al. Pivotal evaluation of the accuracy of a biomarker used for classification or prediction: standards for study design. *J Natl Cancer Inst* 2008;100:1432–1438.

28. Fisher B, Costantino J, Wickerham D, et al. Tamoxifen for prevention of breast cancer: report of the National Surgical Adjuvant Breast and Bowel Project P-1 study. *J Natl Cancer Inst* 1998;90:1371–1388.

29. Vogel VG, Costantino JP, Wickerham DL, et al. Update of the National Surgical Adjuvant Breast and Bowel Project Study of Tamoxifen and Raloxifene (STAR) P-2 Trial: Preventing breast cancer. *Cancer Prev Res (Phila)* 2010;3:696–706.

30. Thompson IM, Goodman PJ, Tangen CM, et al. The influence of finasteride on the development of prostate cancer. *N Engl J Med* 2003;349:215–224.

31. Omenn G, Goodman G, Thornquist M, et al. Effects of a combination of beta carotene and vitamin A on lung cancer and cardiovascular disease. *N Engl J Med* 1996;334:1150–1155.

38. World Cancer Research Fund, American Institute for Cancer Research. *Food, Nutrition, Physical Activity, and the Prevention of Cancer: A Global Perspective*. Washington, DC: AICR; 2007.

43. Hong WK, Lippman SM, Itri LM, et al. Prevention of second primary tumors with 13cRA in squamous-cell carcinoma of the head and neck. *N Engl J Med* 1990;323:795–801.

45. Khuri FR, Lee JJ, Lippman SM, et al. Randomized phase III trial of low-dose isotretinoin for prevention of second primary tumors in stage I and II head and neck cancer patients. *J Natl Cancer Inst* 2006;98:441–450.

48. Mayne ST, Cartmel B, Baum M, et al. Randomized trial of supplemental beta-carotene to prevent second head and neck cancer. *Cancer Res* 2001;61:1457–1463.

49. Bairati I, Meyer F, Jobin E, et al. Antioxidant vitamins supplementation and mortality: a randomized trial in head and neck cancer patients. *Int J Cancer* 2006;119:2221–2224.

52. The Alpha-Tocopherol Beta Carotene Cancer Prevention Study Group. The effect of vitamin E and beta carotene on the incidence of lung cancer and other cancers in male smokers. *N Engl J Med* 1994;330:1029–1035.

57. van Zandwijk N, Dalesio O, Pastorino U, et al. EUROSCAN, a randomized trial of vitamin A and N-acetylcysteine in patients with head and neck cancer or lung cancer. For the European Organization for Research and Treatment of Cancer Head and Neck and Lung Cancer Cooperative Groups. *J Natl Cancer Inst* 2000;92:977–986.

58. Lippman SM, Lee JJ, Karp DD, et al. Randomized phase III intergroup trial of isotretinoin to prevent second primary tumors in stage I non-small-cell lung cancer. *J Natl Cancer Inst* 2001;93:605–618.

60. Veronesi U, De Palo G, Marubini E, et al. Randomized trial of fenretinide to prevent second breast malignancy in women with early breast cancer. *J Natl Cancer Inst* 1999;91:1847–1856.

62. Uray IP, Brown PH. Chemoprevention of hormone receptor-negative breast cancer: new approaches needed. *Recent Results Cancer Res* 2011;188:147–162.

63. Kraemer KH, DiGiovanna JJ, Moshell AN, et al. Prevention of skin cancer in xeroderma pigmentosum with the use of oral isotretinoin. *N Engl J Med* 1988;318:1633–1637.

65. Tangrea JA, Edwards BK, Taylor PR, et al. Long-term therapy with low-dose isotretinoin for prevention of basal cell carcinoma: a multicenter clinical trial Isotretinoin-Basal Cell Carcinoma Study Group. *J Natl Cancer Inst* 1992;84:328–332.

66. Levine N, Moon TE, Cartmel B, et al. Trial of retinol and isotretinoin in skin cancer prevention: a randomized, double-blind, controlled trial. Southwest Skin Cancer Prevention Study Group. *Cancer Epidemiol Biomarkers Prev* 1997;6:957–961.

67. Moon TE, Levine N, Cartmel B, et al. Effect of retinol in preventing squamous cell skin cancer in moderate-risk subjects: a randomized, double-blind, controlled trial. Southwest Skin Cancer Prevention Study Group. *Cancer Epidemiol Biomarkers Prev* 1997;6:949–956.

68. Greenberg ER, Baron JA, Stukel TA, et al. A clinical trial of beta carotene to prevent basal-cell and squamous-cell cancers of the skin. The Skin Cancer Prevention Study Group. *N Engl J Med* 1990;323:789–895.

69. Green A, Williams G, Neale R, et al. Daily sunscreen application and beta-carotene supplementation in prevention of basal-cell and squamous-cell carcinomas of the skin: a randomised controlled trial. *Lancet* 1999;354:723–729.

70. Clark LC, Combs GF Jr, Turnbull BW, et al. Effects of selenium supplementation for cancer prevention in patients with carcinoma of the skin. A randomized controlled trial. Nutritional Prevention of Cancer Study Group. *JAMA* 1996;276:1957–1963.

71. Duffield-Lillico AJ, Slate EH, Reid ME, et al. Nutritional Prevention of Cancer Study Group. Selenium supplementation and secondary prevention of nonmelanoma skin cancer in a randomized trial. *J Natl Cancer Inst* 2003;95:1477–1481.

74. Meyskens FL Jr, Surwit E, Moon TE, et al. Enhancement of regression of cervical intraepithelial neoplasia II (moderate dysplasia) with topically applied all-trans-retinoic acid: a randomized trial. *J Natl Cancer Inst* 1994;86:539–543.

75. Blot WJ, Li JY, Taylor PR, et al. Nutrition intervention trials in Linxian, China: supplementation with specific vitamin/mineral combinations, cancer incidence, and disease-specific mortality in the general population. *J Natl Cancer Inst* 1993;85:1483–1492.

77. Mayne ST, Ferrucci LM, Cartmel B. Lessons learned from randomized clinical trials of micronutrient supplementation for cancer prevention. *Annu Rev Nutr* 2012;32:369–390.

78. Li JY, Taylor PR, Li B, et al. Nutrition intervention trials in Linxian, China: multiple vitamin/mineral supplementation, cancer incidence, and disease-specific mortality among adults with esophageal dysplasia. *J Natl Cancer Inst* 1993;85:1492–1498.

81. Greenberg ER, Baron JA, Tosteson TD, et al. A clinical trial of antioxidant vitamins to prevent colorectal adenoma. Polyp Prevention Study Group. *N Engl J Med* 1994;331:141–147.

83. Heinonen OP, Albanes D, Virtamo J, et al. Prostate cancer and supplementation with alpha-tocopherol and beta-carotene: incidence and mortality in a controlled trial. *J Natl Cancer Inst* 1998;90:440–446.

84. Lippman SM, Klein EA, Goodman PJ, et al. Effect of selenium and vitamin E on risk of prostate cancer and other cancers: the Selenium and Vitamin E Cancer Prevention Trial (SELECT). *JAMA* 2009;301:39–51.

99. Gibson TM, Weinstein SJ, Pfeiffer RM, et al. Pre- and postfortification intake of folate and risk of colorectal cancer in a large prospective cohort study in the United States. *Am J Clin Nutr* 2011;94:1053–1062.

106. Cole BF, Baron JA, Sandler RS, et al. Folic acid for the prevention of colorectal adenomas: a randomized clinical trial. *JAMA* 2007;297:2351–2359.

107. Logan RF, Grainge MJ, Shepherd VC, et al. Aspirin and folic acid for the prevention of recurrent colorectal adenomas. *Gastroenterology* 2008;134:29–38.

108. Wu K, Platz EA, Willett WC, et al. A randomized trial on folic acid supplementation and risk of recurrent colorectal adenoma. *Am J Clin Nutr* 2009;90:1623–1631.

114. Chung M, Balk EM, Brendel M, et al. *Vitamin D and Calcium: A Systematic Review of Health Outcomes*. Evidence Report No. 183 (Prepared by the Tufts Evidence-based Practice Center). Rockville, MD: Agency for Healthcare Research and Quality; 2009.

117. Baron J, Beach M, Mandel JS, et al. Calcium supplements for the prevention of colorectal adenomas. The Calcium Polyp Prevention Study Group. *N Engl J Med* 1999;340:101–107.

119. Wactawski-Wende J, Kotchen JM, Anderson GL, et al. Calcium plus vitamin D supplementation and the risk of colorectal cancer. *N Engl J Med* 2006;354:684–696.

122. Chlebowski RT, Johnson KC, Kooperberg C, et al. Calcium plus vitamin D supplementation and the risk of breast cancer. *J Natl Cancer Inst* 2008;100:1581–1591.

132. Rothwell PM, Price JF, Fowkes FG, et al. Short-term effects of daily aspirin on cancer incidence, mortality, and non-vascular death: analysis of the time course of risks and benefits in 51 randomised controlled trials. *Lancet* 2012;379:1602–1612.

133. Thun MJ, Namboodiri MM, Heath C Jr. Aspirin use and reduced risk of fatal colon cancer. *N Engl J Med* 1991;325:1593–1596.

135. Chan AT, Giovannucci EL, Meyerhardt JA, et al. Long-term use of aspirin and nonsteroidal anti-inflammatory drugs and risk of colorectal cancer. *JAMA* 2005;294:914–923.

139. Kawamori T, Rao C, Seibert K, et al. Chemopreventive effect of celecoxib, a specific cyclooxygenase-2 inhibitor on colon carcinogenesis. *Cancer Res* 1998;58:409–412.

142. Giardiello FM, Yang VW, Hylind LM, et al. Primary chemoprevention of familial adenomatous polyposis with sulindac. *N Engl J Med* 2002;346:1054–1059.

143. Steinbach G, Lynch PM, Phillips RK. The effect of celecoxib, a cyclooxygenase-2 inhibitor, in familial adenomatous polyposis. *N Engl J Med* 2000;342:1946–1952.

147. Meyskens FL Jr, McLaren CE, Pelot D, et al. Difluoromethylornithine plus sulindac for the prevention of sporadic colorectal adenomas: a randomized placebo-controlled, double-blind trial. *Cancer Prev Res (Phila)* 2008;1:32–38.

149. Bertagnolli MM, Eagle CJ, Zauber AG, et al. Celecoxib for the prevention of sporadic colorectal adenomas. *N Engl J Med* 2006;355:873–884.

151. Bresalier RS, Sandler RS, Quan H, et al. Cardiovascular events associated with rofecoxib in a colorectal adenoma chemoprevention trial. *N Engl J Med* 2005;352:1092–1102.

156. Rothwell PM. Aspirin in prevention of sporadic colorectal cancer: current clinical evidence and overall balance of risks and benefits. *Recent Results Cancer Res* 2013;191:121–142.

157. U.S. Preventive Services Task Force. Routine aspirin or nonsteroidal anti-inflammatory drugs for the primary prevention of colorectal cancer: U.S. Preventive Services Task Force recommendation statement. *Ann Intern Med* 2007;146:361–364.

161. Kuiper GG, Carlsson B, Grandien K, et al. Comparison of the ligand binding specificity and transcript tissue distribution of estrogen receptors alpha and beta. *Endocrinology* 1997;138:863–870.

164. Jordan VC. Tamoxifen (ICI46,474) as a targeted therapy to treat and prevent breast cancer. *Br J Pharmacol* 2006;147:S269–S276.

169. Ettinger B, Black DM, Mitlak BH, et al. Reduction of vertebral fracture risk in postmenopausal women with osteoporosis treated with raloxifene: results from a 3-year randomized clinical trial. Multiple Outcomes of Raloxifene Evaluation (MORE) Investigators. *JAMA* 1999;282:637–645.

175. Moyer VA. Medications for risk reduction of primary breast cancer in women: U.S. Preventive Services Task Force recommendation statement. *Ann Intern Med* 2013;159:698-708.

176. Visvanathan K, Hurley P, Bantug E, et al. Use of pharmacologic interventions for breast cancer risk reduction: American Society of Clinical Oncology clinical practice guideline. *J Clin Oncol* 2013;31:2942–2962.

177. Vogel VG, Costantino JP, Wickerham DL, et al. Carcinoma in situ outcomes in National Surgical Adjuvant Breast and Bowel Project Breast Cancer Chemoprevention Trials. *J Natl Cancer Inst Monogr* 2010;2010:181–186.

178. Cuzick J, Sestak I, Bonanni B, et al. Selective oestrogen receptor modulators in prevention of breast cancer: an updated meta-analysis of individual participant data. *Lancet* 2013;381:1827–1834.

179. Barrett-Connor E, Mosca L, Collins P, et al. Effects of raloxifene on cardiovascular events and breast cancer in postmenopausal women. *N Engl J Med* 2006;355:125–137.

183. Goss PE, Ingle JN, Ales-Martinez JE, et al. Exemestane for breast-cancer prevention in postmenopausal women. *N Engl J Med* 2011;364:2381–2391.

185. Cuzick J, Sestak I, Forbes JF, et al. Anastrozole for prevention of breast cancer in high-risk postmenopausal women (IBIS-II): an international, double-blind, randomised placebo-controlled trial. *Lancet* 2014;383:1041–1048.

187. King MC, Wieand S, Hale K, et al. Tamoxifen and breast cancer incidence among women with inherited mutations in BRCA1 and BRCA2: National Surgical Adjuvant Breast and Bowel Project (NSABP-P1) Breast Cancer Prevention Trial. *JAMA* 2001;286:2251–2256.

192. Andriole GL, Bostwick DG, Brawley OW, et al. Effect of dutasteride on the risk of prostate cancer. *N Engl J Med* 2010;362:1192–1202.

193. Thompson IM Jr, Goodman PJ, Tangen CM, et al. Long-term survival of participants in the prostate cancer prevention trial. *N Engl J Med* 2013;369: 603–610.

198. Meyskens FL Jr, Surwit E, Moon TE, et al. Enhancement of regression of cervical intraepithelial neoplasia II (moderate dysplasia) with topically applied all-trans-retinoic acid: randomized trial. *J Natl Cancer Inst* 1994;86: 539–543.

200. Jeter JM, Alberts DS. Difluoromethylornithine: the proof is in the polyamines. *Cancer Prev Res (Phila)* 2012;5:1341–1344.

201. Gronich N, Rennert G. Beyond aspirin-cancer prevention with statins, metformin and bisphosphonates. *Nat Rev Clin Oncol* 2013;10:625–642.

203. Bertagnolli MM, Hsu M, Hawk ET, et al. Statin use and colorectal adenoma risk: results from the adenoma prevention with celecoxib trial. *Cancer Prev Res (Phila)* 2010;3:588–596.

208. Rennert G. Bisphosphonates: beyond prevention of bone metastases. *J Natl Cancer Inst* 2011;103:1728–1729.

215. Zhu P, Davis M, Blackwelder A, et al. Metformin selectively targets tumor initiating cells in erbB-2 overexpressing breast cancer models. *Cancer Prev Res (Phila)* 2014;7:199–210.

218. Chlebowski RT, McTiernan A, Wactawski-Wende J, et al. Diabetes, metformin, and breast cancer in postmenopausal women. *J Clin Oncol* 2012; 30:2844–2852.

221. Lambert JD. Does tea prevent cancer? Evidence from laboratory and human intervention studies. *Am J Clin Nutr* 2013;98:1667S–1675S.

222. Kakarala M, Brenner DE, Korkaya H, et al. Targeting breast stem cells with the cancer preventive compounds curcumin and piperine. *Breast Cancer Res Treat* 2010;122:777–785.

226. Laviano A, Rianda S, Molfino A, et al. Omega-3 fatty acids in cancer. *Curr Opin Clin Nutr Metab Care* 2013;16:156–161.

234. Gescher A, Steward WP, Brown K. Resveratrol in the management of human cancer: how strong is the clinical evidence? *Ann N Y Acad Sci* 2013;1290:12–20.

236. Stoner GD, Wang LS. Chemoprevention of esophageal squamous cell carcinoma with berries. *Top Curr Chem* 2013;329:1–20.

238. Carroll RE, Benya RV, Turgeon DK, et al. Phase IIa clinical trial of curcumin for the prevention of colorectal neoplasia. *Cancer Prev Res (Phila)* 2011;4:354–364.

249. Ma JL, Zhang L, Brown LM, et al. Fifteen-year effects of Helicobacter pylori, garlic, and vitamin treatments on gastric cancer incidence and mortality. *J Natl Cancer Inst* 2012;104:488–492.

250. Risch HA, Lu L, Kidd MS, et al. Helicobacter pylori seropositivities and risk of pancreatic carcinoma. *Cancer Epidemiol Biomarkers Prev* 2014;23:172–178.

255. Zell JA, Pelot D, Chen WP, et al. Risk of cardiovascular events in a randomized placebo-controlled, double-blind trial of difluoromethylornithine plus sulindac for the prevention of sporadic colorectal adenomas. *Cancer Prev Res (Phila)* 2009;2:209–212.

256. Guerrieri-Gonzaga A, Robertson C, Bonanni B, et al. Preliminary results on safety and activity of a randomized, double-blind, 2 × 2 trial of low-dose tamoxifen and fenretinide for breast cancer prevention in premenopausal women. *J Clin Oncol* 2006;24:129–135.

257. Kelloff GJ, Lippman SM, Dannenberg AJ, et al. Progress in chemoprevention drug development: the promise of molecular biomarkers for prevention of intraepithelial neoplasia and cancer—a plan to move forward. *Clin Cancer Res* 2006;12:3661–3697.

258. Washington MK, Powell AE, Sullivan R, et al. Pathology of rodent models of intestinal cancer: progress report and recommendations. *Gastroenterology* 2013;144:705–717.

264. Winawer SJ, Zauber AG, Ho MN, et al. Prevention of colorectal cancer by colonoscopic polypectomy. The National Polyp Study Workgroup. *N Engl J Med* 1993;329:1977–1981.

267. Taylor P, Li B, Dawsey S, et al. Prevention of esophageal cancer: the nutrition intervention trials in Linxian, China. Linxian Nutrition Intervention Trials Study Group. *Cancer Res* 1994;54:2029s–2031s.

278. Giardiello FM, Hamilton SR, Krush AJ, et al. Treatment of colonic and rectal adenomas with sulindac in familial adenomatous polyposis. *N Engl J Med* 1993;328:1313–1316.

281. Burn J, Gerdes AM, Macrae F, et al. Long-term effect of aspirin on cancer risk in carriers of hereditary colorectal cancer: an analysis from the CAPP2 randomised controlled trial. *Lancet* 2011;378:2081–2087.

282. Ruffin MT, Krishnan K, Rock CL, et al. Suppression of human colorectal mucosal prostaglandins: determining the lowest effective aspirin dose. *J Natl Cancer Inst* 1997;89:1152–1160.

286. Baron JA, Cole BF, Sandler RS, et al. A randomized trial of aspirin to prevent colorectal adenomas. *N Engl J Med* 2003;348:891–899.

288. Cuzick J, Forbes JF, Sestak I, et al. Long-term results of tamoxifen prophylaxis for breast cancer—96-month follow-up of the randomized IBIS-I trial. *J Natl Cancer Inst* 2007;99:272–282.

290. Veronesi U, Maisonneuve P, Rotmensz N, et al. Tamoxifen for the prevention of breast cancer: late results of the Italian Randomized Tamoxifen Prevention Trial among women with hysterectomy. *J Natl Cancer Inst* 2007;99:727–737.

303. Dontu G, Liu S, Wicha MS. Stem cells in mammary development and carcinogenesis: implications for prevention and treatment. *Stem Cell Rev* 2005;1:207–213.

308. Califano J, van der Riet P, Westra W, et al. Genetic progression model for head and neck cancer: implications for field cancerization. *Cancer Res* 1996; 56:2488–2492.

309. Califano J, Westra WH, Meininger G, et al. Genetic progression and clonal relationship of recurrent premalignant head and neck lesions. *Clin Cancer Res* 2000;6:347–352.

312. Barrett MT, Sanchez CA, Prevo LJ, et al. Evolution of neoplastic cell lineages in Barrett oesophagus. *Nat Genet* 1999;22:106–109.

CANCER PREVENTION AND SCREENING

Cancer Screening

Otis W. Brawley and Howard L. Parnes

INTRODUCTION

Cancer screening refers to a test or examination performed on an asymptomatic individual. The goal is not simply to find cancer at an early stage, nor is it to diagnose as many patients with cancer as possible. The goal of cancer screening is to prevent death and suffering from the disease in question through early therapeutic intervention.

The assumption that early detection improves outcomes can be traced back to the concept that cancer inexorably progresses from a small, localized, primary tumor to local–regional spread, to distant metastases and death. This linear model of disease progression predicts that early intervention would reduce cancer mortality.

Cancer screening was an element of the "periodic physical examination," as espoused by the American Medical Association in the 1920s.[1] It consisted of palpation to find a mass or enlarged lymph nodes and auscultation to find a rub or abnormal sound. Today, screening has grown to include radiologic testing, the measurement of serum markers of disease, and even molecular testing. A positive screening test leads to further diagnostic testing, which might lead to a cancer diagnosis.

The intuitive appeal of early detection accounts for the emphasis that has long been placed on screening. However, it is not widely understood that screening tests are always associated with some harm (e.g., anxiety, financial costs) and may actually cause substantial harm (e.g., invasive follow-up diagnostic or therapeutic procedures). Because screening is, by definition, done in healthy people, all early detection tests should be carefully studied and their risk–benefit ratio determined before they are adopted for widespread usage.

Screening is a public health intervention. However, some draw a distinction between screening an individual within the doctor–patient relationship and mass screening, a program aimed at screening a large population. The latter may involve advertising campaigns to encourage people to be screened for a particular cancer at a shopping mall or at a community event, such as state fair.

Screening may be either *opportunistic* (i.e., a patient sees a health-care provider who chooses to screen or not to screen) or *programmatic*. Programmatic refers to a standardized approach with algorithms for screening and follow-up as well as recall of patients for regular routine screening with quality control measures. Programmatic screening is usually more effective.

PERFORMANCE CHARACTERISTICS

The degree to which a screening test can discriminate between individuals with and without a particular disease is described by its performance characteristics. These include the a test's sensitivity, specificity, positive predictive value (PPV), and negative predictive value (NPV) (Table 34.1). It should be noted that these measures relate to the accuracy of a screening test;

they do not provide any information regarding a test's efficacy or effectiveness.

- Sensitivity is the proportion of persons designated positive by the screening test among all individuals who have the disease: true positive (TP)/(TP + false negative [FN]).
- Specificity is the proportion of persons designated negative by the screening test among all individuals who do not have the disease: true negative TN/(TN + false positive [FP]).
- Positive predictive value is the proportion of individuals with a positive screening test who have the disease: (TP)/(TP + FP).
- Negative predictive value is the proportion of individuals with a negative screening test who do not have the disease: (TN)/(TN + false negative [FN]).[2]

For a given screening test, sensitivity and specificity are inversely related. For example, as one lowers the threshold for considering a serum prostate-specific antigen (PSA) level to represent a *positive* screen, the sensitivity of the test increases and more cancers will be detected. This increased sensitivity comes at the cost of decreased specificity (i.e., more men without cancer will have *positive* screenings tests and, therefore, will be subjected to unnecessary diagnostic procedures).

Some screening tests, such as mammograms, are more subjective and operator dependent than others. For this reason, the sensitivity and specificity of screening mammography varies among radiologists. For a given radiologist, the lower his or her threshold for considering a mammogram to be suspicious, the higher the sensitivity and lower the specificity will be for them. However, mammography can have both a higher sensitivity and higher specificity in the hands of a more experienced versus a less experienced radiologist.

As opposed to sensitivity and specificity, the PPV and NPV of a screening test are dependent on disease prevalence. PPV is also highly responsive to small increases in specificity. As shown in Table 34.2, given a disease prevalence of 5 cases per 1,000 (0.005), the PPV of a hypothetical screening test increases dramatically as specificity goes from 95% to 99.9%, but only marginally as sensitivity goes from 80% to 95%. Given a disease prevalence of only 1 per 10,000 (0.0001), the PPV of the same test is poor even at high sensitivity and specificity. The positive association between breast cancer prevalence and age is the major reason why screening mammography is a better test (higher PPV) for women aged 50 to 59 than for women 40 to 49 years of age.

ASSESSING SCREENING TESTS AND OUTCOMES

Screening Test Results

Lead time bias occurs whenever screening results in an earlier diagnosis than would have occurred in the absence of screening.

TABLE 34.1

Performance Characteristics of a Screening Test

Sensitivity is the proportion designated positive by the screening test among all individuals who have the disease.

$$\frac{TP}{TP + FN}$$

Specificity is the proportion designated negative by the screening test among all those who do not have the disease.

$$\frac{TN}{TN + FP}$$

Positive predictive value is the proportion of individuals with a positive test who have the disease.

$$\frac{TP}{TP + FP}$$

Negative predictive value is the proportion of individuals with a negative test negative who do not have the disease.

$$\frac{TN}{TN + FN}$$

TP, true positive, the condition present and the test is positive; FN, false negative, the condition is present and the test is negative; FP, false positive, the condition is absent and the test is positive; TN, true negative, the condition is absent and test is negative.

Because survival is measured *from the time of diagnosis*, an earlier diagnosis, by definition, increases survival. Unless an effective intervention is available, lead time bias has no impact on the natural history of a disease and death will occur at the same time it would have in the absence of early detection (Fig. 34.1).

Length bias is a function of the biologic behavior of a cancer. Slower growing, less aggressive cancers are more likely to be detected by a screening test than faster growing cancers, which are more likely to be diagnosed due to the onset of symptoms between scheduled screenings (interval cancers). Length bias has an even greater effect on survival statistics than lead time bias (Fig. 34.2).

Overdiagnosis is an extreme form of length bias and represents pure harm. It refers to the detection of tumors, often through highly sensitive modern imaging modalities and other diagnostic tests, that fulfill the histologic criteria for malignancy

TABLE 34.2

Positive Predictive Value Given Varying Sensitivity and Specificity and Prevalence

Prevalence 0.005		Sensitivity %		
		80	90	95
Specificity %	95	7	8	9
	99	29	31	32
	99.9	80	82	83
Prevalence 0.0001		Sensitivity %		
		80	90	95
Specificity %	95	0.2	0.2	2.0
	99	0.8	0.9	0.9
	99.9	0.7	8.0	9.0

PPV improves dramatically in response to small changes in specificity. Changes in specificity influence PPV much more than changes in sensitivity. Note the influence of prevalence on PPV. Screening tests do not perform as well in populations with a low prevalence of disease.

Lead Time Bias

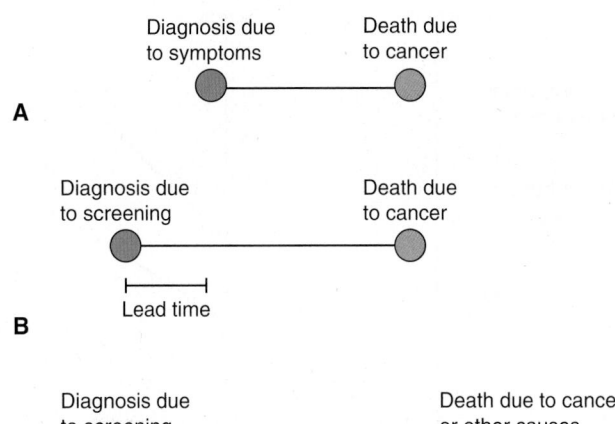

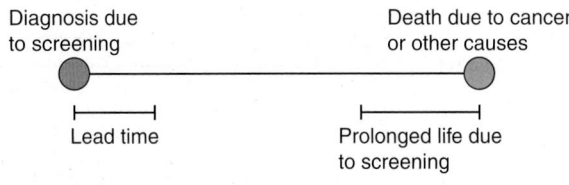

Figure 34.1 Survival is the time from cancer diagnosis to death. **(A)** Lead time bias occurs when screening results in an earlier diagnosis. Without screening, a patient is diagnosed with cancer due to symptoms. **(B)** With screening, the patient is often diagnosed earlier. When screening and treatment do not prolong life, the screened patient can have a longer survival solely due to the earlier diagnosis. The survival increase is pure lead time bias. **(C)** When screening and treatment are beneficial, the patient is diagnosed before the onset of symptoms and the patient lives beyond the point in which death would have occurred without screening.

but are not biologically destined to harm the patient (see Fig. 34.2).

There are two categories of overdiagnosis: the detection of histologically defined *cancers* not destined to metastasize or harm the patient, and the detection of cancers not destined to metastasize or cause harm *in the life span of the specific patient*. The importance of this second category is illustrated by the widespread practice in the United States of screening elderly patients with limited life expectancies, who are thus unlikely to benefit from early cancer diagnosis.

Overdiagnosis occurs with many malignancies, including lung, breast, prostate, renal cell, melanoma, and thyroid cancers.[3] Neuroblastoma provides one of the most striking examples of overdiagnosis.[4] Urine vanillylmandelic acid (VMA) testing is a highly sensitive screening test for the detection of this pediatric disease. After screening programs in Germany, Japan, and Canada showed marked increases in the incidence of this disease without a concomitant decline in mortality, it was noticed that nearby areas that did not screen had similar death rates with lower incidence.[4,5] It is now appreciated that screen-detected neuroblastomas have a very good prognosis with minimal or no treatment. Many actually regress spontaneously.

Stage shift—i.e., a cancer diagnosis at an earlier stage than would have occurred in the absence of screening—is necessary, but not sufficient, for a screening test to be effective in terms of reducing mortality. Both lead time bias and length bias contribute to this phenomenon. Although it is tempting to speculate that diagnosis at an earlier stage must confer benefit, this is not necessarily the case. For example, a substantial proportion of men treated with radical prostatectomy for what appears to be a localized prostate cancer relapse after undergoing surgery. Conversely, some men who are treated with definitive therapy would never have gone on to develop metastatic disease in the absence of treatment.

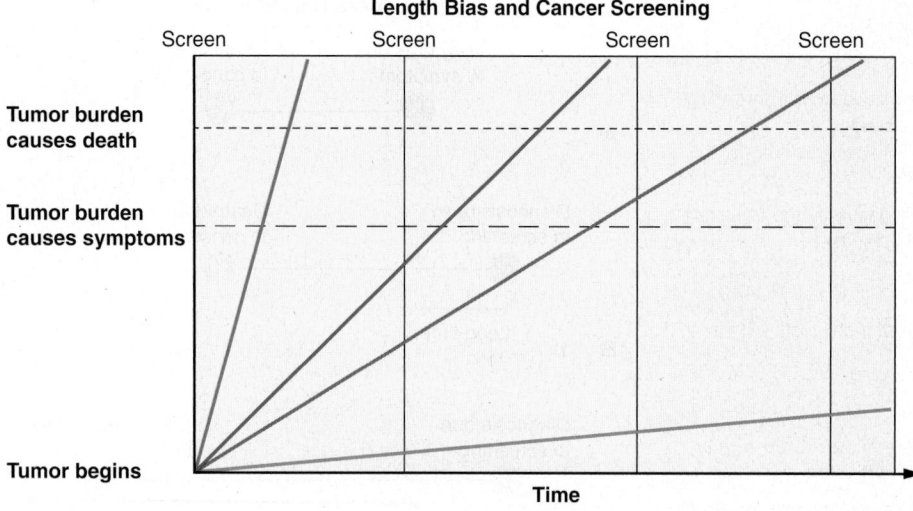

Figure 34.2 Length bias and cancer screening. The *red line* is indicative of a fast-growing tumor that is not amenable to regular screening. The *blue line* is indicative of a fast-growing tumor that can be diagnosed by screening or later by symptoms; death may possibly be prevented by treatment. The *green line* is a slower growing but potentially deadly cancer that can be detected by symptoms or several screenings and treated, possibly preventing death. The *orange line* is indicative of a very slow growing tumor that would never cause death and would never need treatment despite being screen detected. This is classic overdiagnosis.

Selection bias occurs when enrollees in a clinical study differ from the general population. In fact, people who voluntarily participate in clinical trials tend to be healthier than the general population, perhaps due to a greater interest in health and healthcare research. Screening studies tend to enroll individuals healthier than the general population. This so-called *healthy volunteer effect*[6,7] can introduce a powerful bias if not adequately controlled for by randomization procedures.

Assessing Screening Outcomes

The usual primary goal of cancer screening is to reduce mortality from the disease in question (a reduction in disease-specific mortality). Screening studies generally do not have sufficient statistical power to assess the impact of screening for a specific malignancy on overall mortality. (Lung cancer screening provides an exception to this rule; see the following.) As discussed previously, the fact that a screening test increases the percentage of people diagnosed with early stage cancer and decreases that of late stage cancer (stage shift) is not equivalent to proof of mortality reduction. Further, due to the healthy volunteer effect, case control and cohort studies cannot provide definitive evidence of mortality benefit. Prospective, randomized clinical trials are required to address this issue. In such trials, volunteers are randomized to be screened or not and are then followed longitudinally to determine if there is a difference in disease-specific or overall mortality.

A reduction in mortality rates or in the risk of death is often stated in terms of relative risk. However, this method of reporting may be misleading. It is preferable to report both the relative and absolute reduction in mortality. For example, the European Randomized Study of Screening for Prostate Cancer (ERSPC) showed that screening reduced the risk of prostate cancer death by 20%. However, this translates into only 1 prostate cancer death averted per 1,000 men screened (5 prostate cancer deaths per 1,000 men not screened versus 4 prostate cancer deaths per 1,000 men screened) and a relatively modest lifetime reduction in the absolute risk of prostate cancer death of only 0.6%, from 3.0% to 2.4%.[8]

PROBLEMS WITH RANDOMIZED TRIALS

It is important to acknowledge that even prospective, randomized trials can have serious methodologic shortcomings. For example, imbalances caused by flaws in the randomization scheme can prejudice the outcome of a trial. Other flaws include so-called *drop-in* or *contamination*, in which some participants on the control arm get the intervention. Patients on the intervention arm may also

drop out of the study. Both drop-ins and drop-outs reduce the statistical power of a clinical trial.

In the United States, it is now considered standard to obtain informed consent before randomization takes place. However, there have been several published studies that randomized participants from rosters of eligible subjects such as census lists. In these trials, informed consent was obtained after randomization and only among those randomized to the screening arm of the study. Those randomized to the control arm were not contacted, and indeed, did not know they were in a clinical trial. They were followed through national death registries. Although the study was analyzed on an intent-to-screen basis, this method can still introduce biases. For example, only patients on the intervention arm had access to the screening facility and staff for counseling and treatment if diagnosed; those in the control group were more likely to be treated in the community as opposed to high-volume centers of excellence and were less likely to be treated with surgery and more likely to be treated with hormones alone than those on the screened arm. The study arms would also tend to differ in their knowledge of the disease, which may contribute to an overestimate of the benefits of a screening test.[9]

Virtually every screening test is a balance between known harms and potential benefits. The most important risk of screening is the detection and subsequent treatment of a cancer that would never have come to clinical detection or harmed the patient in the absence of screening (i.e., overdiagnosis and overtreatment). Treatment can cause emotional and physical morbidity and even death.[10] Even when screening has a net mortality benefit, there can be considerable harm. For example, in the recent randomized trial of spiral lung computed tomography (CT) scan, approximately 27,000 current smokers and former smokers were given three annual low-dose CT scans. More than 20% had a *positive* screening CT scan, necessitating further testing. About 1,000 subsequently underwent invasive diagnostic procedures and 16 deaths were reported within 60 days of the procedure.[11] It is not known how many of these deaths were directly related to the screening.

It can be dangerous to extrapolate estimates of benefit from one population to another. In particular, studies showing that a radiographic test is beneficial to average risk individuals may not mean that it is beneficial to a population at high risk, and vice versa. For example, women at high risk for breast cancer due to an inherited mutation of a DNA repair gene may be at higher risk for radiation-induced cancer from mammographies compared to the general population; a screening test (e.g., spiral lung CT scan), shown to be efficacious in a high-risk population of heavy smokers may result in net harm if applied to a low or average risk population.

SCREENING GUIDELINES AND RECOMMENDATIONS

A number of organizations develop cancer screening recommendations or guidelines. These organizations use varying methods. The Institute of Medicine (IOM) has released two reports to establish standards for developing trustworthy clinical practice guidelines and conducting systematic evidence reviews that serve as their basis.[12,13] The U.S. Preventive Services Task Force (USPSTF) and the American Cancer Society (ACS) are two organizations that issue respected and widely used cancer guidelines (Table 34.3). Both have changed their methods to comply with the IOM standards.

The USPSTF is a panel of experts in prevention and evidence-based medicine.[14] They are primary care providers specializing in internal medicine, pediatrics, family practice, gynecology and obstetrics, nursing, and health behavior. The task force process begins by conducting an extensive structured scientific evidence review. The task force then develops recommendations for primary care clinicians and health-care systems. They adhere to some of the highest standards for recommending a screening test. They are very much concerned with the question, "Does the evidence supporting a screening test demonstrate that the benefits outweigh its harms?"

The ACS guidelines date back to the 1970s. The current process for making guidelines involves commissioning academics to do an independent systematic evidence review. A single generalist group digests the evidence review, listens to public input, and writes the guidelines. The ACS panel tries to clearly articulate the benefits, limitations, and harms associated with a screening test.[15]

BREAST CANCER

Mammographies, clinical breast examinations (CBE) by a health-care provider, and breast self-examinations (BSE) have long been advocated[16] for the early detection of breast cancer. In recent years, ultrasound, magnetic resonance imaging (MRI), and other technologies have been added to the list of proposed screening modalities.

Mammographic screening was first advocated in the 1950s. The Health Insurance Plan (HIP) Study was the first prospective, randomized clinical trial to formally assess its value in reducing death from breast cancer. In this study, started in 1963, about 61,000 women were randomized to three annual mammograms with clinical breast examination versus no screening, which was the standard practice at that time. HIP first reported that mammography reduced breast cancer mortality by 30% at about 10 years after study entry. With 18 years of follow-up, those in the screening arm had a 25% lower breast cancer mortality rate.[16]

Nine additional prospective randomized studies have been published. These studies provide the basis for the current consensus that screening women 40 to 75 years of age does reduce the relative risk of breast cancer death by 10% to 25%. The 10 studies demonstrate that the risk–benefit ratio is more favorable for women over 50 years of age. Mammography has also been shown to be operator dependent, with better performance characteristics (higher sensitivity and specificity and lower FP rates) reported by high-volume centers (Table 34.4).

It is important to note that every one of these studies has some flaws and limitations. They vary in the questions asked and their findings. The Canadian screening trial suggests mammographies and clinical breast examinations do not decrease risk of death for woman aged 40 to 49 and that mammographies add nothing to CBEs for women age 50 to 59 years.[17] On the other extreme, the Kopparberg Sweden study suggests that mammographies are associated with a 32% reduction in the risk of death for women aged 40 to 74 years.[18]

To date, no study has shown that BSEs decrease mortality. BSEs have been studied in two large randomized trials. In one, approximately 266,000 Chinese women were randomized to receive intensive BSE instruction with reinforcements and reminders compared to a control group receiving no instruction on BSE. At 10 years of follow-up, there was no difference in mortality, but the intervention arm had a significantly higher incidence of benign breast lesions diagnosed and breast biopsies preformed. In the second study, 124,000 Russian women were randomized to monthly BSEs versus no BSEs. There was no difference in mortality rates, despite the BSE group having a higher proportion of early stage tumors and a significant increase in the proportion of cancer patients surviving 15 years after diagnosis.

Ultrasonography is primarily used in the diagnostic evaluation of a breast mass identified by palpation or mammography. There is little evidence to support the use of ultrasound as an initial screening test. This modality is highly operator dependent and time consuming, with a high rate of FP findings.[19] An MRI is used for screening women at elevated breast cancer risk due to BRCA1 and BRCA2 mutations, Li-Fraumeni syndrome, Cowden disease, or a very strong family history. MRI is more sensitive but less specific than mammography, leading to a high FP rate and more unnecessary biopsies, especially among young women.[20] The impact of MRI breast screening on breast cancer mortality has not yet been determined.

Thermography, an infrared imaging technology, has some advocates as a breast cancer screening modality despite a lack of evidence from several small cohort studies.[21] Nipple aspirate cytology and ductal lavage have also been suggested as possible screening methods. Both should be considered experimental at this time.[22]

Effectiveness of Breast Cancer Screening

Breast cancer screening has been associated with a dramatic rise in breast cancer incidence. At the same time, there has been a dramatic decrease in breast cancer mortality rates. However, in the United States and Europe, incidence-by-stage data show a dramatic increase in the proportion of early stage cancers without a concomitant decrease in the incidence of regional and metastatic cancers.[23] These findings are at odds with the clinical trials data and raise questions regarding the extent to which early diagnosis is responsible for declining breast cancer mortality rates.

From 1976 to 2008, the incidence of early-stage breast cancer for American women aged 40 and older increased from 112 to 234 per 100,000. This is a rise of 122 cases per 100,000, whereas the absolute decrease in late-stage cancers was only 8 cases per 100,000 (from 102 to 94 cases per 100,000). These data raise questions regarding the magnitude of benefit, as well as the potential risks, of breast cancer screening. The discrepancy between the magnitude of the increase of early disease and the decrease of late-stage cancer and cancer mortality suggests that a proportion of invasive breast cancers diagnosed by screening represents overdiagnosis. These data suggest that overdiagnosis accounts for up to 31% of all breast cancers diagnosed by screening.[24] Others have estimated that up to 50% of breast cancers detected by screening mammography are overdiagnosed cancers. In an exhaustive review of the screening literature, a panel of experts concluded that overdiagnosis does exist and estimated it to be 11% to 19% of breast cancers diagnosed by screening.[25]

A confounding factor with regard to the mortality benefits of breast cancer screening is the improvement that has occurred in breast cancer treatment over this period of time. The effects of the advances in therapy are supported by cancer modeling studies. Indeed, the Cancer Intervention and Surveillance Modeling Network (CISNET), supported by the U.S. National Cancer Institute (NCI), has estimated that two-thirds of the observed breast cancer mortality reduction is attributable to modern therapy, rather than to screening.[26]

TABLE 34.3

Screening Recommendations for Normal-Risk Asymptomatic Subjects

Cancer Type	Test or Procedure	American Cancer Society	U.S. Preventive Services Task Force
Breast	Self-examination	Women ≥20 years: Breast self-exam is an option	"D"
	Clinical examination	Women 20–39 years: Perform every 3 years Women ≥40 years: Perform annually	Women ≥40 years: "I" (as a stand alone without mammography)
	Mammography	Women ≥40 years: Screen annually for as long as the woman is in good health	Women 40–49 years: The decision should be an individual one, and take patient context/values into account ("C") Women 50–74 years: Every 2 years ("B") Women ≥75 years: "I"
	MRI	Women >20% lifetime risk of breast cancer: Screen with MRI plus mammography annually Women 15%–20% lifetime risk of breast cancer: Discuss option of MRI plus mammography annually Women <15% lifetime risk of breast cancer: Do not screen annually with MRI	"I"
Cervical	Pap test (cytology)	Women ages 21–29 years: Screen every 3 years Women 30–65 years: Acceptable approach to screen with cytology every 3 years (see HPV test) Women <21 years: No screening Women >65 years: No screening following adequate negative prior screening Women after total hysterectomy for noncancerous causes: Do not screen	Women ages 21–65 years: Screen every 3 years ("A") Women <21 years: "D" Women >65 years, with adequate, normal prior Pap screenings: "D" Women after total hysterectomy for noncancerous causes: "D"
	HPV test	Women <30 years: Do not use HPV testing Women ages 30–65 years: Preferred approach to screen with HPV and cytology cotesting every 5 years (see Pap test) Women >65 years: No screening following adequate negative prior screening Women after total hysterectomy for noncancerous causes: Do not screen	Women ages 30–65 years: Screen in combination with cytology every 5 years if woman desires to lengthen the screening interval (see Pap test) ("A") Women <30 years: "D" Women >65 years, with adequate, normal prior Pap screenings: "D" Women after total hysterectomy for noncancerous causes: "D"
Colorectal	Sigmoidoscopy	Adults ≥50 years: Screen every 5 years Note: For all CRC screening tests, stop screening when benefits are unlikely due to life-limiting comorbidity.	Adults 50–75 years: Every 5 years in combination with high-sensitivity fecal occult blood testing (FOBT) every 3 years ("A")[a] Adults 76–85 years: "C" Adults ≥85 years: "D"
	Fecal occult blood testing (FOBT)	Adults ≥50 years: Screen every year with high sensitivity guaiac based FOBT or fecal immunochemical test (FIT) only	Adults 50–75 years: Annually, for high-sensitivity FOBT ("A") Adults 76–85 years: "C" Adults ≥85 years: "D"
	Colonoscopy	Adults ≥50 years: Screen every 10 years	Adults 50–75 years: every 10 years ("A") Adults 76–85 years: "C" Adults ≥85 years: "D"
	Fecal DNA testing	Adults ≥50 years: Screen, but interval uncertain	"I"
	Fecal immunochemical testing (FIT)	Adults ≥50 years: Screen every year	"I"
	CT colonography	Adults ≥50 years: Screen every 5 years	"I"
Lung	Complete skin examination by clinician or patient	Men and women, 55–74 years, with ≥30 pack-year smoking history, still smoking or have quit within past 15 years: Discuss benefits, limitations, and potential harms of screening. Only perform screening in facilities with the right type of CT scanner and with high expertise/specialists.	"I" ("B" draft recommendation issued for public comment in July 2013)

(continued)

TABLE 34.3

Screening Recommendations for Normal-Risk Asymptomatic Subjects *(continued)*

Cancer Type	Test or Procedure	American Cancer Society	U.S. Preventive Services Task Force
Ovary	CA-125 Transvaginal ultrasound	There is no sufficiently accurate test proven effective in the early detection of ovarian cancer. For women at high risk of ovarian cancer and/or who have unexplained, persistent symptoms, the combination of CA-125 and transvaginal ultrasound with pelvic exam may be offered.	"D" "D"
Prostate	Prostate-specific antigen (PSA)	Starting at age 50, men should talk to a doctor about the pros and cons of testing so they can decide if testing is the right choice for them. If African American or have a father or brother who had prostate cancer before age 65, men should have this talk starting at age 45. How often they are tested will depend on their PSA level.	Men, all ages: "D"
	Digital rectal examination (DRE)	As for PSA; if men decide to be tested, they should have the PSA blood test with or without a rectal exam.	No individual recommendation
Skin	Complete skin examination by clinician or patient	Self-examination monthly; clinical exam as part of routine cancer-related checkup	"I"

Note: Summary of the screening procedures recommended for the general population by the American Cancer Society and the U.S. Preventive Services Task Force. These recommendations refer to asymptomatic persons who have no risk factors for the cancer, other than age or gender.
[a] USPSTF lettered recommendations are defined as follows:
"A": The USPSTF recommends the service, because there is high certainty that the net benefit is substantial.
"B": The USPSTF recommends the service, because there is high certainty that the net benefit is moderate or moderate certainty that the net benefit is moderate to substantial.
"C": The USPSTF recommends selectively offering or providing this service to individual patients based on professional judgment and patient preferences. There is at least moderate certainty that the net benefit is small.
"D": The USPSTF recommends against the service, because there is moderate or high certainty that the service has no net benefit or that the harms outweigh the benefits.
"I": The USPSTF concludes that the current evidence is insufficient to assess the balance of benefits and harms of the service.

Questions have also been raised regarding the quality of the randomized screening trials that demonstrated the mortality benefits of mammography and clinical breast examination because these trials suffered from a variety of design flaws. In some, randomization methods were suboptimal, others reported varying numbers of participants over the years, and still others had substantial contamination (drop-ins). Perhaps more importantly, most trials were started and concluded before the widespread use of more advanced mammographic technology, before the modern era of adjuvant therapy, and before the advent of targeted therapy.

Although randomized control trials (RCT) remain the gold standard for assessing the benefits of a clinical intervention, they cannot take into account improvements in both treatment and patient awareness that occurred over time. For this reason, observational and modeling studies can provide important, complementary information.

One systematic review of 17 published population-based and cohort studies compared breast cancer mortality in groups of women aged 50 to 69 years who started breast cancer screening at different times. Although these studies are subject to methodologic limitations, only four suggested that breast cancer screening reduced the relative risk of breast cancer mortality by 33% or more and five suggested no benefit from screening. The review concluded that breast cancer screening likely reduces the risk of breast cancer death by no more than 10%.[27]

Even with these limitations, a systematic review of the data sponsored by the USPSTF concluded that regular mammography reduces breast cancer mortality in women aged 40 to 74 years.[28] The task force also concluded that the benefits of mammography are most significant in women aged 50 to 74 years.

Screening Women Age 40 to 49

Experts disagree about the utility of screening women in their forties. In the HIP Randomized Control Trial, women who entered at age 40 to 49 years had a mortality benefit at 18 years of follow-up. However, to a large extent, the mortality benefit among those aged 45 to 49 years at entry was driven by breast cancers diagnosed after they reached age 50 years.[16]

Mammography, like all screening tests, is more efficient (higher PPV) for the detection of disease in populations with higher disease prevalence (see Table 34.2). Mammography is, therefore, a better test in women age 50 to 59 years than it is among women age 40 to 49 years because the risk of breast cancer increases with age. Mammography is also less optimal in women age 40 to 49 years compared to women 50 to 59 years of age for the following reasons:

- A larger proportion have increased breast density, which can obscure lesions (lower sensitivity).
- Younger women are more likely to develop aggressive, fast-growing breast cancers that are diagnosed between regular screening visits. By definition, these *interval cancers* are not screen detected.[29]

The USPSTF meta-analysis of eight large randomized trials suggested a 15% relative reduction in mortality (relative risk [RR], 0.85; 95% confidence interval [CI], 0.75 to 0.96) from mammography screening for women aged 40 to 49 years after 11 to 20 years of follow-up. This is equivalent to a needing to invite 1,904 women to screenings over 10 years to prevent one breast cancer death. Studies, however, show that more than half of women aged 40 to 49 years screened annually over a 10-year period will have an FP mammogram necessitating further evaluation, often including biopsy. In addition, estimates of overdiagnosis in this group range from 10% to 40% of diagnosed invasive cancers.[30]

In an effort to decrease FP rates, some have suggested screening every 2 years rather than yearly. Comparing biennial with annual screening, the CISNET Model consistently shows that biennial screening of women ages 40 to 70 only marginally decreases the number of lives saved while halving the false positive rate.[29] Notably, the Swedish two-county trial, which had a planned 24-month screening interval (the actual interval was 33 months) reported one

TABLE 34.4

Randomized Controlled Trials

Study	Randomization	Sample Size	Intervention and Age at Entry	Follow-up	Finding
Health Insurance Plan, United States 1963[a,b]	Individual	60,565–60,857	MMG and CBE for 3 years Age 40–64 years	18 years	RR 0.77 (95% CI: 0.61–0.97)
Malmo, Sweden 1976[c,d]	Individual	42,283	Two-view MMG every 18–24 months × 5 Age 45–69 years	12 years	RR 0.81 (95% CI: 0.62–1.07)
Ostergotland (County E of Two-County Trial) Sweden 1977[e–g]	Geographic cluster	38,405–39,034 study 37,145–37,936 control	Three single-view MMG every 2 years women, Age 40–50 years Every 33 months women, Age 50–74	12 years	RR 0.82 (95% CI: 0.64–1.05)
Kopparberg (County W of Two-County Trial) Sweden 1977[e–g]	Geographic cluster	38,562–39,051 intervention 18,478–18,846 control	Three single-view MMG every 2 years women, Age 40–50 years Every 33 months women, Age 50–74 years	12 years	RR 0.68 (95% CI: 0.52–0.89)
Edinburgh, United Kingdom[h]	Cluster by physician practice	23,266 study 21,904 control	Initially, two-view MMG and CBE Then annual CBE with single-view MMG years 3, 5, and 7, Age 45–64 years	10 years	RR 0.84 (95% CI: 0.63–1.12)
NBSS-1, Canada 1980[i,j]	Individual	25,214 study (100% screened after entry CBE) 25,216 control	Annual two-view MMG and CBE for 4–5 years, Age 40–49 years	13 years	RR 0.97 (95% CI: 0.74–1.27)
NBSS-2, Canada 1980[i,j]	Individual	19,711 study (100% screened after entry CBE) 19,694 control	Annual two-view MMG and CBE versus CBE, Age 50–59 years	11–16 years (mean 13 years)	RR 1.02 (95% CI: 0.78–1.33)
Stockholm, Sweden 1981[k]	Cluster by birth date	40,318–38,525 intervention group 19,943–20,978 control group	Single view MMG every 28 months × 2 Age 40–64 years	8 years	RR 0.80 (95% CI: 0.53–1.22)
Gothenberg, Sweden 1982[d]	Complex	21,650 invited 29,961 control	Initial two-view MMG, then single-view MMG every 18 months × 4 Single read first three rounds, then double-read, Age 39–59 years	12–14 years	RR 0.79 (95% CI 0.58–1.08) In the evaluation phase RR 0.77 (95% CI 0.60–1.00) In follow-up phase
Age Trial[l]	Individual	160,921 (53,884 invited; 106,956 not invited)	Invited group aged 48 and younger offered annual screening by MMG (double-view first screen, then single mediolateral oblique view thereafter); 68% accepted screening on the first screen an 69% and 70% were reinvited (81% attended at least one screen) Age 39–41 years	10.7 years	RR 0.83 (95% CI: 0.66–1.04)

[a] Shapiro S, Venet W, Strax P, et al. Ten- to fourteen-year effect of screening on breast cancer mortality. *J Natl Cancer Inst* 1982;69:349–355.
[b] Shapiro S. Periodic screening for breast cancer: the HIP Randomized Controlled Trial. Health Insurance Plan. *J Natl Cancer Inst Monogr* 1997:27–30.
[c] Andersson I, Aspegren K, Janzon L, et al. Mammographic screening and mortality from breast cancer: the Malmo mammographic screening trial. *BMJ* 1988;297:943–948.
[d] Nystrom L, Rutqvist LE, Wall S, et al. Breast cancer screening with mammography: overview of Swedish randomised trials. *Lancet* 1993;341:973–978.
[e] Tabar L, Fagerberg CJ, Gad A, et al. Reduction in mortality from breast cancer after mass screening with mammography. Randomised trial from the Breast Cancer Screening Working Group of the Swedish National Board of Health and Welfare. *Lancet* 1985;1:829–832.
[f] Tabar L, Fagerberg G, Duffy SW, Day NE. The Swedish two county trial of mammographic screening for breast cancer: recent results and calculation of benefit. *J Epidemiol Community Health* 1989;43:107–114.
[g] Tabar L, Fagerberg G, Duffy SW, et al. Update of the Swedish two-county program of mammographic screening for breast cancer. *Radiol Clin North Am* 1992;30:187–210.
[h] Roberts MM, Alexander FE, Anderson TJ, et al. Edinburgh trial of screening for breast cancer: mortality at seven years. *Lancet* 1990;335:241–246.
[i] Miller AB, To T, Baines CJ, Wall C. The Canadian National Breast Screening Study-1: breast cancer mortality after 11 to 16 years of follow-up. A randomized screening trial of mammography in women age 40 to 49 years. *Ann Intern Med* 2002;137:305–312.
[j] Miller AB, Wall C, Baines CJ, et al. Twenty five year follow-up for breast cancer incidence and mortality of the Canadian National Breast Screening Study: randomised screening trial. *BMJ* 2014;348–366.
[k] Frisell J, Eklund G, Hellstrom L, et al. Randomized study of mammography screening—preliminary report on mortality in the Stockholm trial. *Breast Cancer Res Treat* 1991;18:49–56.
[l] Moss SM, Cuckle H, Evans A, et al. Effect of mammographic screening from age 40 years on breast cancer mortality at 10 years' follow-up: a randomised controlled trial. *Lancet* 2006;368:2053–2060.

of the greatest reductions in breast cancer mortality among the RCTs conducted to date.

Screening Women at High Risk

There is interest in creating risk profiles as a way of reducing the inconveniences and harms of screening. It might be possible to identify women who are at greater risk of breast cancer and refocus screening efforts on those most likely to benefit.

Risk factors for breast cancer include the following:

- Extremely dense breasts on mammography or a first-degree relative with breast cancer are each associated with at least a twofold increase in breast cancer risk
- Prior benign breast biopsy, second-degree relatives with breast cancer, or heterogeneously dense breasts each increase risk 1.5- to twofold
- Current oral contraceptive use, nulliparity, and age at first birth 30 years and older increase risk 1- to 1.5-fold.[31]

Importantly, these are risk factors for breast cancer diagnosis, not breast cancer mortality. Few studies have assessed the association between these factors and death from breast cancer; however, reproductive factors and breast density have been shown to have limited influence on breast cancer mortality.[32,33]

Genetic testing for *BRCA1* and *BRCA2* mutations and other markers of breast cancer risk has identified a group of women at high risk for breast cancer. Unfortunately, when to begin and the optimal frequency of screening have not been defined. Mammography is less sensitive at detecting breast cancers in women carrying *BRCA1* and *BRCA2* mutations, possibly because such cancers occur in younger women in whom mammography is known to be less sensitive.

MRI screening may be more sensitive than mammography in women at high risk, but specificity is lower. MRIs are associated with both an increase in FP and an increase in the detection of smaller cancers, which are more likely to be biologically indolent. The impact of MRIs on breast cancer mortality with or without concomitant use of mammographies has not been evaluated in a randomized controlled trial.

Breast Density

It is well established that mammogram sensitivity is lower in women with heterogeneously dense or very dense breasts.[29,32] However, at this time, there are no clear guidelines regarding whether or how screening algorithms should take breast density into account.

In the American College of Radiology's Imaging Network (ACRIN)/NCI 666 Trial, breast ultrasound was offered to women with increased mammographic breast density and, if either test was positive, they were referred for a breast biopsy.[34] The radiologists performing the ultrasounds were not aware of the mammographic findings. Mammography detected 7.6 cancers per 1,000 women screened; ultrasound increased the cancer detection rate to 11.8 per 1,000. However, the PPV for mammography alone was 22.6%, whereas the PPV for mammography with ultrasound was only 11.2%.

It has yet to be determined whether supplemental imaging reduces breast cancer mortality in women with increased breast density. Although it continues to be strongly advocated by some, systematic reviews have concluded that the evidence is currently insufficient to recommend for or against this approach.[35] There are also a number of barriers to supplemental imaging, including inconsistent insurance coverage, lack of availability in many communities, concerns about cost-effectiveness (particularly with regard to MRI), and the increased FP rate associated with supplemental imaging leading to unnecessary biopsies.[36]

Newer technologies may improve screening accuracy for women with dense breasts. Compared to conventional mammography, full field digital mammography (FFDM) appears to have less FPs. This could reduce the number of women needing supplemental imaging and biopsies.[37] Digital breast tomosynthesis (DBT) uses x-rays and a digital detector to generate cross-sectional images of the breasts. Data are limited, but compared to mammograms, DBT appears to offer increased sensitivity and a reduction in the recall rates.[38] Another potential supplementary imaging modality currently under investigation is three-dimensional (3-D) automated breast ultrasound, and having screening ultrasounds performed by technologists rather than radiologists.

Ductal Carcinoma In Situ

The incidence of noninvasive ductal carcinoma in situ (DCIS) has increased more than fivefold since 1970 as a direct consequence of widespread screening mammographies.[39] DCIS is a heterogeneous condition with low- and intermediate-grade lesions taking a decade or more to progress. Nevertheless, women with this diagnosis are uniformly subjected to treatment. A better understanding of this entity and an increased ability to predict its biologic behavior may enable more judicious, personalized treatment of DCIS.

There is little evidence that the early detection and aggressive treatment of low- and intermediate-grade DCIS reduces breast cancer mortality. The standard of care for all grades of DCIS is lumpectomy with radiation or mastectomy, followed by tamoxifen for 5 years. Interestingly, patterns of care studies indicate that mastectomy rates are increasing,[40] and that women are more often choosing double mastectomies for the treatment of DCIS.[41] Genomic characterization will hopefully lead to the identification of a subset of noninvasive cancers that can be treated less aggressively or even observed.

Harms

The harms and disadvantages of mammography screening include overdiagnosis, FP tests, FN tests, and the possibility of radiation-induced breast cancer.

The fact that mammography screening has increased the incidence of localized disease without a significant change in metastatic disease at the time of diagnosis suggests that there is some degree of overdiagnosis. The risk of overdiagnosis is greatest at the first screening[3] and varies with patient age, tumor type, and grade of disease.

FP screening tests lead to substantial inconvenience and anxiety in addition to unnecessary invasive biopsies with their attendant complications. In the United States, about 10% of all women screened for breast cancer are called back for additional testing, and less than half of them will be diagnosed with breast cancer.[39] The risk of a FP mammogram is greater for women under the age of 50.[37]

FN tests delay diagnosis and provide false reassurance. They are more common in younger women and in women with dense breasts.[42,43] Certain histologic subtypes are also more difficult to see on mammogram. Mucinous and lobular tumors and rapidly growing tumors tend to blend in with normal breast architecture.[44]

A typical screening mammogram provides approximately 4 mSv of radiation. It has been estimated that annual mammographies will cause up to 1 case of breast cancer per 1,000 women screened from age 40 to age 80 years. Radiation exposure at younger ages causes a greater risk of breast cancer.[45] There is also concern that ionizing radiation from mammographies might disproportionately increase the breast cancer risk for women with certain *BRCA1* or *BRCA2* mutations, because these genes are related to DNA repair.[46]

Recommendations

Women at Average Risk

The ACS and most other medical groups recommend that average risk women undergo a CBE every 3 years starting at age 20 and that women 40 years of age and over should undergo CBEs and screening mammograms annually. Women should be informed of the benefits, limitations, and harms associated with breast cancer screening. A mammography will not detect all breast cancers, and some breast cancers detected with mammographies may still have a poor prognosis. The harms associated with breast cancer screening also include the potential for FP results, causing substantial anxiety. When abnormal findings cannot be resolved with additional imaging, a biopsy is required to rule out the possibility of breast cancer. A majority of biopsies are benign. Finally, some breast cancers detected by a mammography may be biologically indolent, meaning they would not have caused a problem or have been detected in a woman's lifetime had she not undergone a mammography.

The USPSTF, the American College of Physicians, and the Canadian Task Force on the Periodic Health Examination recommend routine screening beginning at age 50 years.[30,47,48] For women aged 40 to 49 years of age, these groups advise physicians to enter into a discussion with the patient. The physician and patient should take into account individual risks and concerns before deciding to screen.[47]

An Advisory Committee on Cancer Prevention in the European Union recommends that women between the ages of 50 and 69 years be offered mammogram screening in an organized screening program with quality assurance.[49] This committee says women aged 40 to 49 years should be advised of the potential harms of screening and, if mammographic screening is offered, it should be performed with strict quality standards and double reading.

Women at High Risk

The ACS has issued guidelines for women who were known or likely carriers of a *BRCA* mutation and other rarer high-risk genetic syndromes, or at high risk for other reasons.[50] Annual screening mammographies and MRIs starting at age 30 is recommended for women:

- With a known *BRCA* mutation
- Who are untested but have a first-degree relative with a *BRCA* mutation
- Who had been treated with radiation to the chest for Hodgkin disease
- Who have an approximately 20% to 25% or greater lifetime risk of breast cancer based on specialized breast cancer risk estimation models.

COLON CANCER SCREENING

Colorectal cancer screening with the rigid sigmoidoscope dates back to the late 1960s. The desire to examine the entire colon led to the use of a barium enema and the development of fecal occult blood tests. With the development of fiber optics, flexible sigmoidoscopies and, later, colonoscopies were employed. Today, fecal occult blood testing (FOBT), stool DNA testing, flexible sigmoidoscopies, colonoscopies, and CT colonographies and, occasionally, barium enemas are all used in colorectal cancer screening. MRI colonoscopy is in development.

Screening examinations of the colon and rectum can find cancer early, but also find precancerous polyps. Randomized trials have demonstrated that endoscopic polypectomies reduce the incidence of colorectal cancer by about 20%.[51–53]

FOBT was the first colorectal screening test studied in a prospective randomized clinical trial. The Minnesota Colon Cancer Control Study randomized 46,551 adults to one of three arms: annual FOBTs, biennial screening, or usual care. A rehydrated guaiac test was used. With 13 years of follow-up, the annual screened arm had a 33% relative reduction in colorectal cancer mortality compared to the usual care group.[54] At 18 years of follow-up, the biennially screened group had a 21% reduction in colorectal cancer

mortality.[55] This study would subsequently show that stool blood testing was associated with a 20% reduction in colon cancer incidence.[51] These results were confirmed by two other randomized trials.[56,57] A reduction in colon cancer–specific mortality persisted in the Minnesota trial through 30 years of follow-up. Overall mortality was not affected.

Rehydration increases the sensitivity of FOBT at the expense of lowering specificity.[58] Indeed, rehydrated specimens have a very high FP rate. Overall, 1% to 5% of FOBTs are positive, but only 2% to 10% of those with a positive FOBT have cancer.

Fecal immunochemical tests (FIT) are stool tests that do not react to hemoglobin in dietary products. They appear to have higher sensitivity and specificity for colorectal cancer when compared to nonrehydrated FOBT tests.[59]

Fecal DNA testing is an emerging modality. These tests look for DNA sequences specific to colorectal polyps and colorectal cancer. They may have increased sensitivity and specificity compared to FOBT. Although fecal DNA tests appear to find cancer, the body of evidence on their ability to reduce colorectal cancer mortality is limited due to a lack of study. This test has been intermittently available.

Flexible sigmoidoscopies are, of course, limited to an examination of the rectum and sigmoid colon. A prospective randomized trial of once-only flexible sigmoidoscopies demonstrated a 23% reduction in colorectal cancer incidence and a 31% reduction in colorectal cancer mortality after a median 11.2 years of follow-up.[60] In the NCI's Prostate, Lung, Colorectal, and Ovarian Cancer Screening Trial (PLCO), there was a 21% reduction in colorectal cancer incidence and a 26% reduction in colorectal cancer mortality with two sigmoidoscopies done 3 to 5 years apart compared with the usual care group after a median follow-up of 11.9 years.[53] In both studies, there was no effect on proximal lesions (i.e., right and transverse colon) due to the limited reach of the scope. It is estimated that flexible sigmoidoscopies can find 60% to 80% of cancers and polyps found by colonoscopies.[61]

In two meta-analyses of five randomized controlled trials of sigmoidoscopies, there was an 18% relative reduction in colorectal cancer incidence and a 28% relative reduction in colorectal cancer mortality.[62,63] Participants ranged in age from 50 to 74 years. Follow-up ranged from 6 to 13 years.

The *colonoscopy* has become the preferred screening method of many, although there have been no prospective, randomized trials of colonoscopy screening. A positive FOBT, FIT, fecal DNA test, or sigmoidoscopy warrants a follow-up diagnostic colonoscopy. Perhaps the best support for colonoscopy screening is indirect evidence from the Minnesota Colon Cancer Control Study, which required that all participants with a positive stool blood test have diagnostic imaging of the entire colon. In the Minnesota study, more than 40% of those screened annually eventually received a colonoscopy. One can also make the argument that the sigmoidoscopy studies indirectly support the efficacy of colonoscopy screening, although it can be argued that embryologic and epidemiologic evidence indicate that the right and left colon are biologically distinct and, therefore, the mortality benefits from sigmoidoscopies do not constitute proof that a colonoscopy would similarly reduce mortality from proximal colon lesions.

In studies involving repeat colonoscopies by a second physician, 21% of all adenomas were missed, including 26% of 1 to 5 mm adenomas and 2% of adenomas 10 mm or more in length.[64] Other limitations of colonoscopies include the inconvenience of the bowel preparation and the risk of bowel perforation (about 3 out of 1,000 procedures, overall, with nearly all of the risk among patients who undergo colonoscopic polypectomies). The cost of the procedure and the limited number of physicians who can do the procedure are also of concern.

A *CT colonography* or *virtual* colonoscopy allows a physician to visually reproduce the endoscopic examination on a computer screen. A CT colonography involves the same prep as a colonoscopy, but is less invasive. It might have a higher compliance rate.

In experienced hands, the sensitivity of a CT colonography for the detection of polyps ≥6 mm appears to be comparable to that of a colonoscopy. In a meta-analysis of 30 studies, 2-D and 3-D CT colonographies performed equally well.[65]

The disadvantages of a CT colonography include the fact that it requires a colonic prep and a finding on CT requires a follow-up diagnostic colonoscopy. The rate of extracolonic findings of uncertain significance is high (~15% to 30%), and each one must be evaluated, thereby contributing to additional expense and potential morbidity. The long-term, cumulative radiation risk of repeated colonography screenings is also a concern.

Current Recommendations

The ACS, the American College of Gastroenterology, the American Gastroenterological Association, the American Society for Gastrointestinal Endoscopy, and the American College of Radiology have issued joint colorectal cancer guidelines. These groups consider FOBT, FIT, rigid and flexible sigmoidoscopies, colonoscopies, and CT colonographies to all be reasonable screening methodologies.

They recommend the following: (1) Screening modalities be chosen based on personal preference and access, and (2) average risk adults should begin colorectal cancer screening at age 50 years with *one* of the following options:

1. Annual high sensitivity FOBT or FIT
2. A flexible sigmoidoscopy every 5 years
3. A colonoscopy every 10 years
4. A double contrast barium enema every 5 years
5. A CT colonography every 5 years

No test is of unequivocal superiority. Patient preferences should be incorporated into screening in order to increase compliance. The guidelines also stress that a single screening examination is far from optimal and that patients should be in a program of regular screening.

Although some colorectal cancers are diagnosed in persons under the age of 50 years, screening persons age 40 to 49 years has low yield.[66] The guidelines also state that patients with less than a 10-year life expectancy should not be screened.

The USPSTF issued colorectal cancer screening guidelines in 2008.[67] The guidelines were based on a systematic literature review and decision models. The task force concluded that three screening strategies appear to be equivalent for adults age 50 to 75 years:

1. An annual FOBT with a sensitive test
2. A flexible sigmoidoscopy every 5 years, with a sensitive FOBT every 3 years
3. A colonoscopy every 10 years

The task force recommends that patients age 76 to 85 years be evaluated individually for screening. They found "insufficient evidence" to recommend CT colonographies or fecal DNA testing.

Patients at Increased Risk of Colorectal Cancer

Patients can have higher than average risk of colorectal cancer due to familial or hereditary factors and clinical conditions such as inflammatory bowel disease. These patients technically undergo surveillance and not screening. Nevertheless, there are few clinical studies to guide recommendations. Guidelines have been created based on professional opinion and an understanding of the biology of colorectal cancer (Table 34.5).[68]

OTHER CANCERS OF THE GASTROINTESTINAL TRACT

There are no widely accepted screening guidelines for cancers of the esophagus, stomach, pancreas, and liver. However, surveillance is advocated for some patients at high risk.

Esophageal Cancer Screening

Esophageal cancer screening has centered on endoscopic examinations for those at high risk due to chronic, severe gastroesophageal reflux disease.[69] Some physicians advocate routine endoscopic surveillance of patients with Barrett esophagus. At this time, there is no evidence that such surveillance is effective at reducing cancer mortality.

TABLE 34.5

Colon Cancer Screening Recommendations for People with Familial or Inherited Risk

Familial Risk Category	Screening Recommendation
First-degree relative[a] affected with *colorectal cancer* or an *adenomatous polyp* at age ≥60 years, or two second-degree relatives[b] affected with colorectal *cancer*	Same as average risk but starting at age 40 years
Two or more first-degree relatives with *colon cancer*, or a single first-degree relative with *colon cancer* or *adenomatous polyps* diagnosed at an age <60 years	Colonoscopy every 5 years, beginning at age 40 years or 10 years younger than the earliest diagnosis in the family, whichever comes first
One second-degree or any third-degree relative[b,c] with *colorectal cancer*	Same as average risk
Gene *carrier* or *at risk* for familial adenomatous polyposis[d]	Sigmoidoscopy annually, beginning at age 10–12 years[e]
Gene carrier or at risk for HNPCC	Colonoscopy, every 1–2 years, beginning at age 20–25 years or 10 years younger than the earliest case in the family, whichever comes first

[a] First-degree relatives include patients, siblings, and children.
[b] Second-degree relatives include grandparents, aunts, and uncles.
[c] Third-degree relatives include great-grandparents and cousins.
[d] Includes the subcategories of familial adenomatous polyposis, Gardner syndrome, some Turcot syndrome families, and attenuated adenomatous polyposis coli (AAPC).
[e] In AAPC, colonoscopy should be used instead of sigmoidoscopy because of the preponderance of proximal colonic adenomas. Colonoscopy screening in AAPC should probably begin in the late teens or early 20s.
HNPCC, hereditary nonpolyposis colon cancer.
From Winawer S, Fletcher R, Rex D, et al. Colorectal cancer screening and surveillance: clinical guidelines and rationale: update based on new evidence. *Gastroenterology* 2003;124:544–560, with permission.

Gastric Cancer Screening

Barium-meal photofluorography, serum pepsinogen, and gastric endoscopy have been proposed as screening methods for the early detection of gastric cancer. There are no randomized trials evaluating the impact of these modalities on gastric cancer mortality. Indeed, screening with barium-meal photofluorography has been studied in high-risk populations for more than 40 years without clear evidence of benefit.

Time-trend analysis and case control studies of gastric endoscopy have suggested a decrease in gastric cancer mortality among those at high risk in screened versus unscreened individuals; however, a large observational study in a high-risk population failed to demonstrate a benefit.[70,71]

Although widespread gastric screenings cannot be advocated, there may be justification for endoscopic screenings of high-risk populations. Candidates for screening might include elderly individuals with atrophic gastritis or pernicious anemia, patients who have had partial gastrectomy,[72] those with a history of sporadic adenomas, and patients with familial adenomatous polyposis or hereditary nonpolyposis colon cancer.

Pancreatic Cancer Screening

At this time, there are no data from prospective clinical trials to support a role for pancreatic cancer screening. Some patients with an extensive family history have undergone periodic CT scanning of the abdomen, but this approach has not been shown to reduce pancreatic cancer mortality. There is an ongoing search for screening biomarkers. There is a need to follow large cohorts prospectively after collecting and storing biologic samples to identify biomarkers of risk.[73]

Liver Cancer Screening

Screening for liver cancer or hepatocellular carcinoma (HCC) has focused on very high-risk individuals, such as those with cirrhosis.[54] To date, trial results are unreliable due to small study sizes and a lack of randomization.

Serum alpha-fetoprotein (AFP), a fetal-specific glycoprotein antigen, is an HCC tumor marker used in screening. It is not specific to HCC because it may be elevated in hepatitis, pregnancy, and some germ cell tumors. AFP has variable sensitivity and has not been tested in any randomized clinical trial with a mortality end point.

In one prospective, 16-year, population-based observational study, screening was done on 1,487 Alaska natives with chronic hepatis B virus (HBV) infection. The survival of those with screen-detected HCC was compared with a historical group of clinically diagnosed HCC patients.[74] With a target of AFP determination every 6 months, there was a 97% sensitivity and 95% specificity for HCC. Such high sensitivity and specificity have not been found in other studies. It is not known if AFP screening decreases HCC mortality.[75]

Hepatic ultrasound has been used as an additional method for detection of HCC. This procedure is operator dependent with variable sensitivity and specificity. Ultrasound screening is commonly used in patients with hepatitis and cirrhosis.[76,77]

Interest in CT scanning has grown due to the limitations of AFP and ultrasound. CT scans may be a more sensitive test for HCC than ultrasound or AFP.[75]

GYNECOLOGIC CANCER

Cervical Cancer Screening

Dr. George Papanicolaou first introduced the Pap smear or Pap test in the early 1940s. The test was widely adopted based on its ability to identify squamous premalignancies and malignancies (from the ectodermal cervix) and glandular dysplasia and adenocarcinomas (from the endocervix). It is, however, more sensitive at detecting squamous lesions.

The Pap test was introduced before the advent of the prospective, randomized clinical trial and, therefore, has never been so tested. However, a number of observational studies over the past 60 years support the effectiveness of this screening test.[78,79] Multiple ecologic studies have shown an inverse correlation between the introduction of Pap testing in a given country and reductions in both cervical cancer incidence and mortality.[80] Importantly, mortality reductions in these studies have been proportional to the intensity of screening. In one series, more than half of women diagnosed with cervical cancer either had never had a Pap test or had not been screened within 5 years of diagnosis.[80]

Cervical cytology has evolved over the years. The original Pap smear used an ectocervical spatula to apply a specimen ("smear") to glass slides. It later included an endocervical brush. The smear was fixed, stained, and manually examined under a microscope. That method is still used today, but a liquid-based/thin-layer system capable of being analyzed by computer is gaining in popularity.[81]

Human papillomavirus (HPV) 16 and 18 are the cause of more than 70% of cervical cancers. Thirteen other HPV subtypes are known to be associated with cervical cancer. With increasing understanding of the role of HPV in cervical disease, interest in developing tests to determine the presence of HPV DNA and RNA has grown. HPV screening can be used along with cytology (*cotesting*), in response to an abnormal cytologic test (*reflexive testing*), or as a stand-alone test. One advantage of the liquid-based/thin-layer tests over the older smears is that it makes reflexive testing easier to perform. An abnormal cytology screen can be objectively verified by testing for the presence of the HPV virus without calling the patient back.

HPV testing is especially useful because of its negative predictive value. Although a positive test for HPV infection is not diagnostic of cervical disease, a negative HPV test strongly suggests that the abnormal Pap does not represent a premalignant condition.

The utility of the HPV test is limited in younger women because one-third or more of women in their 20s have active cervical infections at any given time. The overwhelming majority of these infections and resultant dysplasia will regress and resolve within 8 to 24 months. For women over the age of 30, screening for the presence of HPV DNA or RNA appears to be superior to cytology in identifying women at risk for cervical dysplasia and cancer.[82] An HPV infection in women over the age of 30 is more likely to be persistent and clinically significant.[83] The risk of cervical cancer also increases with age, and most cervical cancer deaths occur in women over 50 years of age.

Cytologic Terminology

The terminology of the Pap smear has changed over time. The traditional cytologic categories were mild, moderate, and severe dysplasia and carcinoma in situ. *Mild* correlated with cervical intraepithelial neoplasia (CIN)1 histology on biopsy; *moderate* usually indicated CIN2; and *severe* dysplasia indicated CIN3 or carcinoma in situ.

There was some subjectivity and some overlap, especially in the area of mild and moderate dysplasia. The NCI sponsored the development of the Bethesda system in 1988. This system provides an assessment of the adequacy of the cervical specimen and a way of categorizing and describing the Pap smear findings. It more effectively and uniformly communicates cytology results from the laboratory to the patient caregiver. The Bethesda system was modified in 1991 and again in 2001.[84] Today, more than 40 international professional societies have endorsed the Bethesda system.

The Bethesda system recognizes both squamous and glandular cytologic abnormalities.

Squamous cell abnormalities include:

- Atypical squamous cells (ASC), which are categorized as either:
  - Of undetermined significance (ASC-US)
  - Cannot exclude high-grade squamous intraepithelial lesions (ASC-H)
- Low-grade squamous intraepithelial lesion (LSIL), which correlates with histologic CIN1
- High-grade squamous intraepithelial lesion (HSIL), which correlates with histologic CIN2, CIN3, and carcinoma in situ

Glandular cell abnormalities (features suggestive of adenocarcinoma) include:

- Atypical glandular cells (AGC): endocervical, endometrial, or not otherwise specified
- AGCs, favor neoplastic
- Endocervical or not otherwise specified
- Endocervical adenocarcinoma in situ (AIS)
- Adenocarcinoma

ASCs differ from normal cells but do not meet criteria for LSIL or HSIL. A small proportion of ASC-US smears are from CIN1 lesions; a smaller proportion are from CIN2 or 3. LSILs are usually due to a transient HPV infection. HSILs are more likely to be due to a persistent HPV infection and are more likely to progress to cervical cancer than LSILs.

The Lower Anogenital Squamous Terminology (LAST) project of the College of American Pathology and the American Society for Colposcopy and Cervical Pathology has proposed that histologic cervical findings be described using the same terminology as cytologic findings.[85]

Women under the age of 30 who have not received the HPV vaccine have a high incidence of HPV infection[86] and the highest prevalence of CIN. However, the overwhelming majority of these HPV infections and associated CIN will spontaneously regress.[87,88] Due to the high regression rates, cervical screening and treatment in women aged 20 to 24 years appear to have little or no impact on the incidence of invasive cervical cancer. It is estimated that about 6% of CIN1 lesions progress to CIN3, and 10% to 20% of CIN3 lesions progress to invasive cancer.[89]

The Atypical Squamous Cells of Undetermined Significance (ASCUS)-LSIL Triage Study (ALTS) evaluated women with abnormal Pap smears.[90] The investigators concluded that women with ASC-US should be tested for HPV. Those who are HPV positive should receive a colposcopy. In addition, because most women with LSIL or HSIL had an HPV infection, an immediate colposcopy and a biopsy of lesions was recommended.[91] HPV DNA testing is very sensitive for identifying CIN2 or worse pathology. Among women 30 to 69 years of age, the sensitivity of the Pap test with HPV testing was 95% compared with 55% for the Pap test alone.[92]

Performance Characteristics of Cervical Cytology

The sensitivity of cytology varies and is a function of the adequacy of the cervical specimen. It is also affected by the age of the woman and the experience of the cytologist. The addition of HPV testing increases the number of women referred for a colposcopy. Not surprisingly, sensitivity is improved by serial examinations over time versus a single screen.

Screening Recommendations

Cervical screening, like other screening tests, is associated with some degree of overdiagnosis as evidenced by the phenomenon of spontaneous regression (see previous) and, therefore, potential harm from overtreatment, such as cervical incompetence, which may reduce fertility and the ability to carry a pregnancy to term. Because dysplasia takes years to progress to cervical cancer,

increasing the screening interval can reduce overdiagnosis and excessive treatment without decreasing screening efficacy.

In 2012, the ACS, the American Society for Colposcopy and Cervical Pathology (ASCCP), and the American Society for Clinical Pathology (ASCP) issued joint screening guidelines.[93] These guidelines recommend different surveillance strategies and options based on a woman's age, screening history, risk factors, and choice of screening tests. The following are the recommendations for a woman at average risk.

- Screening for cervical cancer should begin at 21 years of age. Women aged 21 to 29 years should receive cytology screening (with either conventional cervical cytology smears or liquid-based cytology) every 3 years. HPV testing should not be performed in this age group (although it can be used to follow-up a diagnosis of ASC-US). Women under 21 years of age should not be screened regardless of their age of sexual initiation.
- For women aged 30 to 65 years, the preferred approach is to be screened every 5 years with both HPV testing and cytology (*cotesting*). It is also acceptable to continue screening every 3 years with cytology alone.
- Women should discontinue screening after age 65 years if they have had three consecutive negative cytology tests or two consecutive negative HPV test results within the 10-year period before ceasing screening, with the most recent test occurring within the last 5 years.
- Women who have undergone a hysterectomy for noncancerous conditions do not need to undergo cervical cancer screening.
- Women, regardless of age, should NOT be screened annually by any screening method.
- Women who have received HPV vaccinations should still be screened according to the previously listed schedule.

Screening in Low Resource Countries

Cytology and HPV testing is not widely available in much of the world. Cervical cancer remains a leading cause of death in many of these areas. Visual inspection of the cervix is a low-tech method of screening that is now recognized as having the potential to save thousands of lives per year. A clustered, randomized trial in India compared one-time cervical visual inspection and immediate colposcopy, biopsy, and/or cryotherapy (where indicated) versus counseling on cervical cancer deaths in women aged 30 to 59 years. After 7 years of follow-up, the age-standardized rate of death due to cervical cancer was 39.6 per 100,000 person-years in the intervention group versus 56.7 per 100,000 person-years in unscreened controls.[94,95] This was the first prospective randomized clinical trial to evaluate cervical cancer screening.

Ovarian Cancer Screening

Modalities proposed for ovarian cancer screening include the bimanual pelvic examination, serum CA-125 antigen measurement, and transvaginal ultrasound (TVU). The bimanual pelvic examination is subjective and not very reproducible, but serum CA-125 can be objectively measured. Unfortunately, CA-125 is neither sensitive nor specific. It is elevated in only about half of women with ovarian cancer and may be elevated in a number of nonmalignant diseases (e.g., diverticulosis, endometriosis, cirrhosis, normal menstruation, pregnancy, uterine fibroids).[96–98] TVU has shown poor performance in the detection of ovarian cancer in average and high-risk women.[99] There is interest in the analysis of serum proteomic patterns, but this should be considered experimental.[100,101]

The combination of CA-125 and TVU has been assessed in two large, prospective randomized trials. The U.S. trial, the Prostate Lung Colorectal and Ovarian trial (PLCO), enrolled

78,216 women of average risk age 55 to 74 years.[102,103] Participants were randomized to receive annual examinations with CA-125 (at entry and then annually for 5 years) and TVU (at entry and then annually for 3 years) (n = 39,105), or usual care (n = 39,111). Participants were followed for a maximum of 13 years, with mortality from ovarian cancer as the main study outcome. At the conclusion of the study, the number of deaths from ovarian cancer was similar in each group. There were 3.1 ovarian cancer deaths per 10,000 women years in the screened group versus 2.6 deaths per 10,000 women years in the control group (RR = 1.18; 95% CI, 0.82 to 1.71).[103]

The U.K. Collaborative Trial of Ovarian Cancer Screening (UKCTOCS) is a randomized trial assessing the efficacy of CA-125 and TVU in more than 200,000 postmenopausal women. In this trial, CA-125 is being used as a first-line test and TVU as a follow-up test using a risk of ovarian cancer algorithm (ROCA).[104] The ROCA measures changes in CA-125 over time rather than using a predefined cut point.[105] ROCA is believed to improve sensitivity for smaller tumors without measurably increasing the FP rate. A mortality assessment is expected in 2015.[106]

No organization currently recommends screening average risk women for ovarian cancer. In 2012, the USPSTF recommended against screening for ovarian cancer, concluding that there was "adequate evidence" that (1) annual screening with TVU and CA-125 does not reduce ovarian cancer mortality and (2) screening for ovarian cancer can lead to important harms, mainly surgical interventions in women without ovarian cancer.[107]

Women at High Risk for Ovarian Cancer

Although no study has shown a mortality benefit for ovarian cancer screening of high-risk individuals, a National Institutes of Health (NIH) consensus panel concluded that it was prudent for women with a known hereditary ovarian cancer syndrome, such as *BRCA1/2* mutations or HNPCC, to have annual rectovaginal pelvic examinations, CA-125 determinations, and TVU until childbearing is completed or at least until age 35 years, at which time a prophylactic bilateral oophorectomy is recommended.[108]

Endometrial Cancer Screening

There is insufficient evidence to recommend endometrial cancer screening either for women at average risk or for those at increased risk due to a history of unopposed estrogen therapy, tamoxifen therapy, late menopause, nulliparity, infertility or failure to ovulate, obesity, diabetes, or hypertension.[109] The ACS recommends that women be informed about the symptoms of endometrial cancer—in particular, vaginal bleeding and spotting—after the onset of menopause. Women should be encouraged to immediately report these symptoms to their physician.

Women at High Risk for Endometrial Cancer

Women with a suspected autosomal-dominant predisposition to colon cancer (e.g. Lynch syndrome), should consider undergoing an annual endometrial biopsy to evaluate endometrial histology, beginning at age 35 years.[110,111] This is based only on *expert opinion*, given the paucity of clinical trial data. Women should be informed about the potential benefits, harms, and limitations of testing for early endometrial cancer.

LUNG CANCER SCREENING

Lung cancer screening programs using chest radiographs (CXR) and sputum cytology began in the late 1940s.[112] An evaluation of these programs showed that screening led to the diagnosis of an increased number of cancers, an increased proportion of early stage cancers, and a larger proportion of screen-diagnosed patients surviving more than 5 years.

These findings led many to advocate for mass lung cancer screening, whereas others called for a prospective, randomized trial with a lung cancer mortality endpoint.[113] The Mayo Lung Project (MLP), which began in 1971, was such a trial. More than 9,200 male smokers were enrolled and randomized to either have sputum cytology collected and CXRs done every 4 months for 6 years or to have these same tests performed annually.

At 13 years of follow-up, there were more early stage cancers in the intensively screened arm (n = 99) than in the control arm (n = 51), but the number of advanced tumors was nearly identical (107 versus 109, respectively).[114] Despite an increase in 5-year survival (35% versus 15%) intensive screening was not associated with a reduction in lung cancer mortality (3.2 versus 3.0 deaths per 1,000 person-years, respectively).[115]

The impact of screening on cancer incidence persisted through nearly 20 years of follow-up. There were 585 lung cancers diagnosed on the intensive screening arm versus 500 on the control arm (p = 0.009) and intensive screening continued to be associated with a significant increase in disease-specific survival. However, a concomitant decrease in lung-cancer mortality did not emerge with long-term follow-up (4.4 lung cancer deaths per 1,000 person-years in the intensively screened arm versus 3.9 per 1,000 person-years in the control arm).[116] This suggests that some lung cancers diagnosed by screening would not have resulted in death had they not been detected (i.e., overdiagnosis).[116]

Two other large, randomized studies of CXR and sputum cytology were conducted in the United States during the same time period. All three studies evaluated different screening schedules rather than screening versus no screening. Paradoxically, a meta-analysis of the three studies found that more frequent screening was associated with an increase (albeit not statistically significant), rather than a decrease, in lung cancer mortality when compared with less frequent screening.[117] A study conducted in Czechoslovakia in the 1980s also failed to show a reduction in lung cancer mortality with CXR screening.[118]

More recently, the NCI conducted the PLCO trial at 10 sites across the United States. This was a prospective, randomized trial of nearly 155,000 men and women, aged 55 to 74 years. Participants were randomized to receive annual, single-view, posteroanterior CXRs for 4 years versus routine care. With 13 years of follow-up, no significant difference in lung cancer mortality was observed. A total of 1,213 lung cancer deaths occurred on the intervention arm versus 1,230 in the control group (RR, 0.99; 95% CI, 0.87 to 1.22).[119]

Low-dose computerized tomography (LDCT) is an appealing technology for lung cancer screening. It uses an average of 1.5 mSv of radiation to perform a lung scan in 15 seconds. A conventional CT scan uses 8 mSv of radiation and takes several minutes. The LDCT image is not as sharp as the conventional image, but sensitivity and specificity for the detection of lung lesions are similar.

As in the early chest radiograph trials, a number of single-arm LDCT studies reported a substantial increase in the number of early stage lung cancers diagnosed. These studies also demonstrated that 5-year survival rates were increased in screened compared to unscreened populations.

These findings led to the conduct of several randomized trials of LDCT for the early detection of lung cancer. The largest, longest, and first to report a mortality end point is the National Lung Screening Trial (NLST). In this trial, approximately 53,000 persons were randomized to receive three annual LDCT scans or single-view posteroanterior CXRs. Eligible participants were current and former smokers between 55 and 74 years of age at the time of randomization with at least a 30 pack-year smoking history; former smokers were eligible if they had quit smoking within the previous 15 years.

With a median follow-up of 6.5 years, 13% more lung cancers were diagnosed and a 20% (95% CI, 6.8 to 26.7; p = 0.004) relative reduction in lung cancer mortality was observed in the LDCT arm compared to the CXR arm.[11] This corresponds to rates of death from lung cancer of 247 and 309 per 100,000 person-years, respectively.[11] Another important finding from the NLST was a 6.7% (95% CI, 1.2 to 13.6; p = 0.02) decrease in death from any cause in the LDCT group.

NLST participants were at high risk for developing lung cancer based on their smoking history. Indeed, 25% of all participant deaths were due to lung cancer. A further analysis of the NLST shows that screening prevented the greatest number of lung cancer deaths among participants who were at the highest risk but prevented very few deaths among those at the lowest risk. These findings provide empirical support for risk-based screening.[120]

LDCT screening is clearly promising, but there are some notable caveats. The risk of a FP finding in the first screen was 21%. Overall, after three CT scans, 39.1% of participants had at least one positive screening result. Of those who screened positive, the FP rate was 96.4% in the LDCT group.[11] Positive results require additional workup, which can include conventional CT scans, a needle biopsy, bronchoscopy, mediastinoscopy, or thoracotomy. These diagnostic procedures are associated with anxiety, expense, and complications (e.g., pneumo- or hemothorax after a lung biopsy). In the LDCT study arm, there were 16 deaths within 60 days of an invasive diagnostic procedure. Of the 16 deaths, 6 ultimately did not have cancer. Although it is not known whether these deaths were directly caused by the invasive procedure, such findings do give pause. Although the radiation dose from LDCT is low, the possibility that this screening test could cause radiation-induced cancers is at least a theoretical concern. The possibility of this long-term phenomenon will have to be assessed in future analyses.

The CXR lung screening studies suggested that there is a reservoir of biologically indolent lung cancer and that a percentage of screen-detected lung cancers represent overdiagnosis. The estimated rate of overdiagnosis in the long-term follow-up of the Mayo Lung Study and the other CXR studies was 17 to 18.5%.[121] Similarly, it is estimated that 18.5% of the cancers diagnosed on the LDCT arm of the NLST represented overdiagnosis.[122]

There are estimates that widespread, high-quality screening has the potential to prevent 12,000 lung cancer deaths per year in the United States.[123] However, the NLST was performed at 33 centers specifically chosen for their expertise in the screening, diagnosis, and treatment of lung cancer. It is not known whether the widespread adoption of LDCT lung cancer screening will result in higher complication rates and a less favorable risk–benefit ratio.

Although LDCT lung cancer screening should clearly be considered for those at high risk of the disease, those at lower risk are equally likely to suffer the harms associated with screening but less likely to reap the benefits.

Following the announcement of the NLST results, the ACS, the American College of Chest Physicians (AACP), the American Society of Clinical Oncology (ASCO), and the National Comprehensive Cancer Network (NCCN) recommended that clinicians should initiate a discussion about lung cancer screening with patients who would have qualified for the trial. That is:

- Age 55 to 74 years
- At least a 30 pack-year smoking history
- Currently smoke or have quit within the past 15 years
- Relatively good health

Core elements of this discussion should include the benefits, uncertainties, and harms associated with screening for lung cancer with LDCT. Adults who choose to be screened should enter an organized screening program at an institution with expertise in LDCT screening, with access to a multidisciplinary team skilled in the evaluation, diagnosis, and treatment of abnormal lung lesions. If such a program is not available, the risks of harm due to screening may be greater than the benefits.[124,125] The guidelines recommend an annual LDCT screening with the caveat that participants in NLST had only three annual screens.

The USPSTF guidelines give LDCT a grade B recommendation, concluding that there is moderate certainty that annual screening for lung cancer with LDCT is of moderate net benefit in asymptomatic persons at high risk for lung cancer based on age, total cumulative exposure to tobacco smoke, and years since quitting.

PROSTATE CANCER SCREENING

Hugh Hampton Young first advocated the early detection of prostate cancer with a careful digital rectal examination (DRE) in 1903. Screening for prostate cancer with the DRE and serum PSA was first advocated in the mid 1980s and became commonplace by 1992. PSA screening is directly responsible for prostate cancer becoming the most common nonskin cancer in American men.

PSA is a glycoprotein produced almost exclusively by the epithelial component of the prostate gland. This protein was discovered in the late 1970s, and a serum test to measure circulating levels was developed in the early 1980s. Although PSA is prostate specific, it is not prostate cancer specific and may be elevated in a variety of conditions (e.g., benign prostatic hyperplasia, inflammation and following trauma to the gland, the presence of prostate cancer).

The PSA test has been widely advocated for prostate cancer screening because it is objective, easily measured, reproducible, noninvasive, and inexpensive. Although PSA screening increases the detection of potentially curable disease, there is substantial debate about the overall utility of the test. This is because PSA screening introduces substantial lead time and length bias as well as being associated with a high FN and FP rates and having a low positive predictive value. The prostate cancer conundrum was best summarized by the distinguished urologist, Willet Whitmore when he said, "Is cure necessary for those in whom it is possible? Is cure possible for those in whom it is necessary?"[126]

Observational studies suggest that the problem of prostate cancer overdiagnosis precedes the PSA era. In a landmark analysis with 20-year follow-up, only a small proportion of 767 men, diagnosed with localized prostate cancer in the 1970s and early 1980s and followed expectantly, died from prostate cancer: 4% to 7% of those with Gleason 2 to 4 tumors, 6% to 11% of those with Gleason 5 disease, and 18% to 30% of men with Gleason 6 cancer.[127]

Although obviously present in the pre-PSA era, overdiagnosis increased substantially after the introduction of PSA screening. This is illustrated by an examination of the prostate cancer incidence and mortality rates in Washington state and Connecticut. Due to the earlier uptake of PSA screening, the incidence of prostate cancer in Washington increased to twice that of Connecticut during the 1990s. However, mortality rates remained similar throughout the decade and, in fact, have remained similar to this day. The Surveillance, Epidemiology, and End Results (SEER) cancer registries show that, over the last 2 decades, a larger proportion of men living in western Washington have been diagnosed with prostate cancer and definitively treated, without a concomitant reduction in prostate cancer mortality compared to that of men living in Connecticut.[128]

Additional evidence of the potential for overdiagnosis comes from the unexpectedly large number of men diagnosed with prostate cancer in the Prostate Cancer Prevention Trial (PCPT). The PCPT was a prospective, randomized, placebo-controlled trial of finasteride for prostate cancer prevention. Men were screened annually during this trial, and those who had not been diagnosed with prostate cancer after 7 years on-study were asked to undergo an end-of-study prostate biopsy. Of 4,692 men on the placebo arm whose prostate cancer status had been determined by biopsy or transurethral resection (TURP), 24.4% were diagnosed with prostate cancer. Given that the lifetime risk of prostate cancer mortality in the United States is less than 3%, it is clear that many men harbor indolent prostate cancer and, therefore, are at risk of being overdiagnosed.

CANCER PREVENTION AND SCREENING

The unexpectedly high rate of positive end-of-study biopsies in men with PSA levels less than or equal to 4.0 ng/mL provided a more accurate assessment of disease prevalence and thus a more accurate assessment of PSA sensitivity than was previously possible. Of the 2,950 men on the placebo arm of the PCPT with PSA levels consistently less than or equal to 4 ng/mL who underwent end-of-study biopsies, 449 (15.2%) were diagnosed with prostate cancer. Accordingly, a PSA level <4.0 ng/mL is more likely to be a *false* negative. Because Sensitivity = True Positives / (True Positives + False Negatives), a higher FN rate means a lower sensitivity at any given PSA threshold. This has prompted some to advocate using a lower PSA threshold for recommending biopsies. However, although lowering the PSA threshold from 4.0 to 2.5 ng/mL increases the sensitivity from 24% to 42.8%, it reduces specificity from 92.7% to an unacceptably low 80%.[129]

In the PCPT, cancer was found on end-of-study biopsies at all PSA levels (e.g., including 10% of biopsies in men with PSA levels between 0.6 and 1.0 ng/mL and 6% of biopsies in men with PSA levels between 0 and 0.6 were positive), suggesting a continuum of prostate cancer risk and no cut point with simultaneously high sensitivity and high specificity. High-grade disease was also documented at all PSA levels, albeit at an overall frequency of only 2.3% of men with PSAs <4 ng/mL.[130,131]

Does Prostate Cancer Treatment Prevent Deaths?

In order for screening to work, treatment has to work. The first prospective, randomized studies showing that any prostate cancer treatment saves lives were published in the late 1990s. These studies demonstrated an overall survival benefit for the addition of long-term androgen deprivation to radiation therapy in men with locally advanced, high-risk prostate cancer.[132]

The value of surgery for localized disease was assessed by the Scandinavian Prostate Cancer Group 4 study (SPCG-4). In this trial, 695 men with clinically localized prostate cancer were prospectively randomized to receive radical prostatectomy (RP) or watchful waiting (WW). In the expectant management group, hormonal therapy was given at the time of symptomatic metastases. About 60% of those enrolled had low-grade, 23% had moderate-grade, 5% had high-grade tumors, and 12% had tumors of unknown grade. At a median follow-up of 12.8 years, the RP group had significantly lower overall (RR 0.75; p = 0.007) and prostate cancer–specific mortality (RR 0.62; p = 0.01), with 14.6% of the PR group and 20.7% of the WW group having died of prostate cancer. The number needed to treat or prevent one prostate cancer death was 15. The survival benefit associated with RP was similar before and after 9 years of follow-up and for men with low and high-risk disease. However, a subset analysis suggested that the mortality benefit of surgery was limited to men less than 65 years of age. An important limitation of this trial is that 75% of the study participants had palpable disease, only 12% had nonpalpable disease, and only 5% of the cancers had been screen detected. It is, therefore, difficult to apply these data to the US prostate cancer population, which is dominated by nonpalpable, screen-detected disease.[133]

In contrast to the SPCG-4, the Prostate Intervention versus Observation Trial (PIVOT) was conducted in the United States during the early PSA era. In this study, 731 men with screen-detected prostate cancer were randomized to receive RP or WW. Of the participants, 50% had nonpalpable disease and, using established criteria for PSA levels, grade, and tumor stage, 43% of men had low-risk, 36% had intermediate-risk, and 21% had high-risk prostate cancer. With a median follow-up of 12 years, during which time 48.4% (354 of 731) of the study participants had died, RP was associated with statistically insignificant 2.9% and 2.6% absolute reductions in overall and prostate cancer–specific mortality,

respectively. Subgroup analyses suggested mortality benefits for men with PSA values greater than 10 ng/mL and for those with intermediate- and high-risk disease.[134]

The Prospective Randomized Screening Trials

The PLCO Cancer Screening Trial was a multicenter, phase III trial conducted in the United States by the NCI. In this trial, nearly 77,000 men age 55 to 74 years were randomized to receive annual PSA testing for 6 years or usual care. At 13 years of follow-up, a nonsignificant increase in cumulative prostate cancer mortality was observed among men randomized to annual screening (RR, 1.09; 95% CI, 0.87 to 1.36).[135] The most important limitation of this trial was the high rate of PSA testing among men randomized to the control arm. This *drop-in* or *contamination* served to reduce the statistical power of the study to detect differences in outcome between the two arms. It has also been argued that, due to the high rate of PSA screening on the control arm, PLCO effectively compared regular prostate cancer screening to opportunistic screening rather than comparing screening to no screening.

The ERSPC is a multicenter trial initiated in 1991 in the Netherlands and Belgium; five additional European countries joined between 1994 and 1998.[136,137] The frequency of PSA testing was every 4 years in all countries except Sweden, in which it was every 2 years. The study results were initially reported in 2009 and updated in 2012.[136,137] Although the overall analysis of 182,160 men, aged 50 to 74, did not show a reduction in prostate cancer–specific mortality, screening was associated with a significant decrease in prostate cancer mortality in the prespecified core age group, 55 to 69 years, which included 162,243 men. After a median follow-up of 11 years, a 21% relative reduction of prostate cancer death (RR, 0.79; 95% CI, 0.68 to 0.91) was observed in this group. In absolute terms, prostate cancer mortality was reduced from 5 to 4 men per 1,000 screened and 37 men had to be diagnosed to avert one prostate cancer death. It remains to be seen whether the benefits of screening will increase with continued follow-up.

The recruitment and randomization procedures of the ERSPC differed among countries. Notably, potential participants in Finland, Sweden, and Italy were identified from population registries and underwent randomization *before* written informed consent was obtained. In some trials, men on the control arm were not aware they were in the study. Therefore, men on the intervention arm in these countries were more likely to be cared for at high-volume referral centers. This may have contributed to the higher proportion of men on the screening arm, with clinically localized cancer being treated with RPs.[138]

In a separate report on 20,000 men randomized to screening or a control group in Göteborg, Sweden, there was a 40% (95% CI, 1.50 to 1.80) risk reduction at 14 years of follow-up.[139] They reported 293 (95% CI, 177 to 799) needed to be screened and 12 needed to be diagnosed in order to prevent one prostate cancer death. Three-fourths of the men in this report and 89% of the prostate cancer deaths were included in the published ERSPC analysis. Given this, these data do not constitute independent evidence of the efficacy of prostate cancer screening.

The other site to report separately was in Finland. A total of 80,144 men were randomized to a screening or usual care arm. At 12 years after randomization, there was no statistical difference in risk of prostate cancer death (hazard ratio [HR] = 0.85; 95% CI, 0.69 to 1.04).[140] Possible explanations as to why Sweden and Finland would have such different outcomes include differences in the frequency of screening (every 2 years versus every 4 years, respectively) and the higher background rate of death from prostate cancer in the control group in the Goteborg cohort. Given that the mortality data from these two cohorts have been largely included in the ERSPC analyses, they do not provide independent evidence of the efficacy of prostate cancer screening.

The decline in prostate cancer mortality in the United States since the introduction of PSA screening 2 decades ago is often offered as evidence supporting a mortality benefit for prostate cancer screening. However, prostate cancer mortality rates have also declined in many countries that have not widely adopted screening.[141] Thus, it is likely that improvements in treatment have contributed, at least in part, to the observed decline in prostate cancer mortality. Another possible contributing factor may be the World Health Organization (WHO) algorithm for adjudicating cause of death. A change occurred just as mortality rates began to go up in the late 1970s, and WHO changed back to the older algorithm in 1991 when prostate cancer mortality began declining in many countries.[142] All of these factors, including a beneficial effect from screening, may be contributing to the declining prostate cancer mortality rates in the United States.

Screening Recommendations

The topic of prostate cancer screening tends to evoke strong emotional reactions. Although the intuitive appeal of early detection is undeniable and screening may save some lives, the magnitude of the mortality reduction is relatively small, whereas the harms associated with screening can be substantial. Whether the potential benefits outweigh the known harms is a question that each man must answer for himself based on his individual preferences.

Several professional organizations in the United States, Europe, and Canada have recently reviewed the screening data and issued screening guidelines. All acknowledge that legitimate concerns remain regarding the risk–benefit ratio of prostate cancer screening. There is also general agreement that prostate cancer screening should only be done in the context of fully informed consent and that men should know that experts do not agree as to whether the benefits of screening for this disease outweigh the harms. Most recommend against mass screening in public meeting places, malls, churches, etc.

In 2009, the American Urological Association (AUA) PSA Best Practice Statement was published, which stated, "Given the uncertainty that PSA testing results in more benefit than harm, a thoughtful and broad approach to PSA is critical. Patients need to be informed of the risks and the benefits of testing before it is undertaken. The risks of over-detection and over-treatment should be included in this discussion."[143]

In 2010, the ACS updated their guidelines, stating that the balance of benefits and harms related to prostate cancer early detection are uncertain and the existing evidence is insufficient to support a recommendation for or against the routine use of PSA screening.[144] The ACS called for discussion and shared decision making within the physician–patient relationship.

The most recent 2012 USPSTF guidelines recommend against the use of PSA screening on the basis that there is moderate certainty that the harms of PSA testing outweigh the benefits and, on that basis, recommended against PSA-based screening for all men.[14] The task force did acknowledge that some men will continue to request screening and some physicians will continue to offer it. Like the ACS and AUA, they state that screening under such circumstances should respect patient preferences.

In 2013, the AUA conducted a systematic review of over 300 studies. They recommended against screening men younger than 40 years of age, and against screening average-risk men age 40 to 54 years, most men over 70 years of age, and men with a life expectancy of less than 10 to 15 years. They recommend that screening decisions be individualized for higher risk men ages 40 to 54 years and men over 70 years of age who are in excellent health. They placed primacy on shared decision making versus physician judgments about the balance of benefits and harms at the population level.[145] Even for men aged 55 to 69 years, the AUA concluded that the quality of evidence for benefits associated with screening was moderate, whereas the quality of the evidence for harm was high. They recommended shared decision making for this group, in whom they have concluded the benefits may outweigh the harm.

SKIN CANCER SCREENING

Assessments of skin cancer screening have focused on melanoma end points with very little attention to screening for nonmelanoma skin cancer. A systematic review of skin cancer screening studies examining the available evidence through mid 2005 concluded that direct evidence of improved health outcomes associated with skin cancer screening is lacking.[146]

No randomized, clinical trial of skin cancer screening has been attempted. However, several observational studies have suggested that melanoma screening might reduce mortality. For example, a decrease in melanoma mortality did occur after a Scottish campaign to promote awareness of the signs of suspicious skin lesions and encourage early self-referral. However, uncontrolled, ecologic studies such as this provide a relatively low level of evidence, because it is not possible to determine whether the observed mortality reduction was due to screening or other factors.

More recently, the Skin Cancer Research to Provide Evidence for Effectiveness of Screening project, or SCREEN project, compared a region of Germany in which intensive skin cancer screening was performed to areas of Germany without intensive screening. Approximately 360,000 residents of the Schleswig-Holstein region aged 20 years and older participated. They chose either to be screened by a nondermatologist physician trained in skin examinations or by a dermatologist. Almost 16,000 biopsies were performed and 585 melanomas were diagnosed. Overall, 1 in 23 participants had an excisional skin biopsy and 620 persons needed to be screened to detect one melanoma. This screening effort led to a 16% and 38% increase in melanoma incidence among men and women, respectively, compared to 2 years earlier. The melanoma incidence rate returned to preprogram levels after the program ended. Of the screen-detected melanomas, 90% were less than 1 mm thick. Screening was performed in 2003 to 2004, and melanoma mortality in this region subsequently declined. In 2008, it was nearly 50% lower in both men and women compared to the rest of Germany.[147,148]

Recommendations of Experts

Skin cancer screening recommendations are based on *expert opinion*, given the absence of a randomized clinical trial data and limited observational studies. The ACS recommends monthly skin self-examinations and a yearly clinical skin examination as part of a routine cancer-related checkup.[149] The USPSTF finds insufficient evidence to recommend for or against either routine skin cancer screening of the general population by primary care providers or counseling patients to perform periodic skin self-examinations. The task force does recommend that clinicians "remain alert" for skin lesions with malignant features when performing a physical examination for other purposes, particularly in high-risk individuals. The American Academy of Dermatology recommends that persons at highest risk (i.e., those with a strong family history of melanoma and multiple atypical nevi), perform frequent self-examination and seek a professional evaluation of the skin at least once per year.[150]

High-risk individuals are persons with multiple nevi or atypical moles. There is consensus they should be educated about the need for frequent surveillance by a trained health-care provider beginning at an early age. In the United States, Australia, and Western Europe, Caucasian men age 50 years and over account for nearly half of all melanoma cases. There is some discussion that melanoma early detection efforts should be focused on this population.

REFERENCES

1. Collen MF, Dales LG, Friedman GD, et al. Multiphasic checkup evaluation study. 4. Preliminary cost benefit analysis for middle-aged men. *Prev Med* 1973;2:236–246.
2. Prorok PC, Kramer BS, Gohagan JK. Screening theory and study design: the basics. In: Kramer B, Prorok P, eds. *Cancer Screening*. New York: Marcel Dekker; 1999:29–53.
3. Welch HG, Black WC. Overdiagnosis in cancer. *J Natl Cancer Inst* 2010; 102:605–613.
4. Yamamoto K, Hayashi Y, Hanada R, et al. Mass screening and age-specific incidence of neuroblastoma in Saitama Prefecture, Japan. *J Clin Oncol* 1995;13:2033–2038.
5. Woods WG, Gao RN, Shuster JJ, et al. Screening of infants and mortality due to neuroblastoma. *N Engl J Med* 2002;346:1041–1046.
6. Friedman GD, Collen MF, Fireman BH. Multiphasic Health Checkup Evaluation: a 16-year follow-up. *J Chronic Dis* 1986;39:453–463.
7. Pinsky PF, Miller A, Kramer BS, et al. Evidence of a healthy volunteer effect in the prostate, lung, colorectal, and ovarian cancer screening trial. *Am J Epidemiol* 2007;165:874–881.
8. Boyle P, Brawley OW. Prostate cancer: current evidence weighs against population screening. *CA Cancer J Clin* 2009;59:220–224.
9. Autier P, Boyle P, Buyse M, et al. Is FOB screening really the answer for lowering mortality in colorectal cancer? *Recent Results Cancer Res* 2003;163: 254–263.
10. de Boer AG, Taskila T, Ojajarvi A, et al. Cancer survivors and unemployment: a meta-analysis and meta-regression. *JAMA* 2009;301:753–762.
11. Aberle DR, Adams AM, Berg CD, et al. Reduced lung-cancer mortality with low-dose computed tomographic screening. *N Engl J Med* 2011;365: 395–409.
12. Eden J, Levit L, Berg A, et al., eds. *Finding What Works in Health Care: Standards for Systematic Reviews*. Washington DC: The National Academies Press; 2011.
13. Graham R, Mancher M, Wolman DM, et al. Medicine CoSfDTCPGIo. Washington, DC: The National Academies; 2011.
14. Moyer VA. Screening for prostate cancer: U.S. Preventive Services Task Force recommendation statement. *Ann Intern Med* 2012;157:120–134.
15. Brawley O, Byers T, Chen A, et al. New American Cancer Society process for creating trustworthy cancer screening guidelines. *JAMA* 2011;306: 2495–2499.
16. Shapiro S. Periodic screening for breast cancer: the HIP Randomized Controlled Trial. Health Insurance Plan. *J Natl Cancer Inst Monogr* 1997:27–30.
17. Miller AB, Wall C, Baines CJ, et al. Twenty five year follow-up for breast cancer incidence and mortality of the Canadian National Breast Screening Study: randomised screening trial. *BMJ* 2014;348:g366.
18. Tabar L, Fagerberg G, Duffy SW, et al. Update of the Swedish two-county program of mammographic screening for breast cancer. *Radiol Clin North Am* 1992;30:187–210.
19. Moy L, Slanetz PJ, Moore R, et al. Specificity of mammography and US in the evaluation of a palpable abnormality: retrospective review. *Radiology* 2002;225:176–181.
20. Lord SJ, Lei W, Craft P, et al. A systematic review of the effectiveness of magnetic resonance imaging (MRI) as an addition to mammography and ultrasound in screening young women at high risk of breast cancer. *Eur J Cancer* 2007;43:1905–1917.
21. Wishart GC, Campisi M, Boswell M, et al. The accuracy of digital infrared imaging for breast cancer detection in women undergoing breast biopsy. *Eur J Surg Oncol* 2010;36:535–540.
22. Dooley WC, Ljung BM, Veronesi U, et al. Ductal lavage for detection of cellular atypia in women at high risk for breast cancer. *J Natl Cancer Inst* 2001;93:1624–1632.
23. Autier P, Boniol M, Middleton R, et al. Advanced breast cancer incidence following population-based mammographic screening. *Ann Oncol* 2011;22:1726–1735.
24. Bleyer A, Welch HG. Effect of three decades of screening mammography on breast-cancer incidence. *N Engl J Med* 2012;367:1998–2005.
25. Marmot MG, Altman DG, Cameron DA, et al. The benefits and harms of breast cancer screening: an independent review. *Br J Cancer* 2013;108:2205–2240.
26. Berry DA, Cronin KA, Plevritis SK, et al. Effect of screening and adjuvant therapy on mortality from breast cancer. *N Engl J Med* 2005;353:1784–1792.
27. Harris R, Yeatts J, Kinsinger L. Breast cancer screening for women ages 50 to 69 years a systematic review of observational evidence. *Prev Med* 2011;53:108–114.
28. Nelson HD, Tyne K, Naik A, et al. Screening for breast cancer: an update for the U.S. Preventive Services Task Force. *Ann Intern Med* 2009;151:727–737.
29. Mandelblatt JS, Cronin KA, Bailey S, et al. Effects of mammography screening under different screening schedules: model estimates of potential benefits and harms. *Ann Intern Med* 2009;151:738–747.
30. U.S. Preventive Services Task Force. Screening for breast cancer: U.S. Preventive Services Task Force recommendation statement. *Ann Intern Med* 2009;151:716–726.
31. Nelson HD, Zakher B, Cantor A, et al. Risk factors for breast cancer for women aged 40 to 49 years: a systematic review and meta-analysis. *Ann Intern Med* 2012;156:635–648.

32. Barnett GC, Shah M, Redman K, et al. Risk factors for the incidence of breast cancer: do they affect survival from the disease? *J Clin Oncol* 2008;26: 3310–3316.
33. Gierach GL, Ichikawa L, Kerlikowske K, et al. Relationship between mammographic density and breast cancer death in the Breast Cancer Surveillance Consortium. *J Natl Cancer Inst* 2012;104:1218–1227.
34. Berg WA, Blume JD, Cormack JB, et al. Combined screening with ultrasound and mammography vs mammography alone in women at elevated risk of breast cancer. *JAMA* 2008;299:2151–2163.
35. Gartlehner G, Thaler K, Chapman A, et al. Mammography in combination with breast ultrasonography versus mammography for breast cancer screening in women at average risk. *Cochrane Database Syst Rev* 2013;4:CD009632.
36. Tice JA, O'Meara ES, Weaver DL, et al. Benign breast disease, mammographic breast density, and the risk of breast cancer. *J Natl Cancer Inst* 2013;105:1043–1049.
37. Kerlikowske K, Hubbard RA, Miglioretti DL, et al. Comparative effectiveness of digital versus film-screen mammography in community practice in the United States: a cohort study. *Ann Intern Med* 2011;155:493–502.
38. Haas BM, Kalra V, Geisel J, et al. Comparison of tomosynthesis plus digital mammography and digital mammography alone for breast cancer screening. *Radiology* 2013;269:694–700.
39. Rosenberg RD, Yankaskas BC, Abraham LA, et al. Performance benchmarks for screening mammography. *Radiology* 2006;241:55–66.
40. Gomez SL, Lichtensztajn D, Kurian AW, et al. Increasing mastectomy rates for early-stage breast cancer? Population-based trends from California. *J Clin Oncol* 2010;28:e155–e157.
41. Tuttle TM, Jarosek S, Habermann EB, et al. Increasing rates of contralateral prophylactic mastectomy among patients with ductal carcinoma in situ. *J Clin Oncol* 2009;27:1362–1367.
42. Rosenberg RD, Hunt WC, Williamson MR, et al. Effects of age, breast density, ethnicity, and estrogen replacement therapy on screening mammographic sensitivity and cancer stage at diagnosis: review of 183,134 screening mammograms in Albuquerque, New Mexico. *Radiology* 1998;209:511–518.
43. Kerlikowske K, Grady D, Barclay J, et al. Effect of age, breast density, and family history on the sensitivity of first screening mammography. *JAMA* 1996;276:33–38.
44. Porter PL, El-Bastawissi AY, Mandelson MT, et al. Breast tumor characteristics as predictors of mammographic detection: comparison of interval- and screen-detected cancers. *J Natl Cancer Inst* 1999;91:2020–2028.
45. Ronckers CM, Erdmann CA, Land CE. Radiation and breast cancer: a review of current evidence. *Breast Cancer Res* 2005;7:21–32.
46. Pijpe A, Andrieu N, Easton DF, et al. Exposure to diagnostic radiation and risk of breast cancer among carriers of BRCA1/2 mutations: retrospective cohort study (GENE-RAD-RISK). *BMJ* 2012;345:e5660.
47. Qaseem A, Snow V, Sherif K, et al. Screening mammography for women 40 to 49 years of age: a clinical practice guideline from the American College of Physicians. *Ann Intern Med* 2007;146:511–515.
48. Tonelli M, Connor Gorber S, Joffres M, et al. Recommendations on screening for breast cancer in average-risk women aged 40-74 years. *CMAJ* 2011;183: 1991–2001.
49. Recommendations on cancer screening in the European Union. Advisory Committee on Cancer Prevention. *Eur J Cancer* 2000;36:1473–1478.
50. Saslow D, Boetes C, Burke W, et al. American Cancer Society guidelines for breast screening with MRI as an adjunct to mammography. *CA Cancer J Clin* 2007;57:75–89.
51. Mandel JS, Church TR, Bond JH, et al. The effect of fecal occult-blood screening on the incidence of colorectal cancer. *N Engl J Med* 2000;343: 1603–1607.
52. Nishihara R, Wu K, Lochhead P, et al. Long-term colorectal-cancer incidence and mortality after lower endoscopy. *N Engl J Med* 2013;369: 1095–1105.
53. Schoen RE, Pinsky PF, Weissfeld JL, et al. Colorectal-cancer incidence and mortality with screening flexible sigmoidoscopy. *N Engl J Med* 2012;366: 2345–2357.
54. Mandel JS, Bond JH, Church TR, et al. Reducing mortality from colorectal cancer by screening for fecal occult blood. Minnesota Colon Cancer Control Study. *N Engl J Med* 1993;328:1365–1371.
55. Mandel JS, Church TR, Ederer F, et al. Colorectal cancer mortality: effectiveness of biennial screening for fecal occult blood. *J Natl Cancer Inst* 1999;91:434–437.
56. Hardcastle JD, Chamberlain JO, Robinson MH, et al. Randomised controlled trial of faecal-occult-blood screening for colorectal cancer. *Lancet* 1996;348:1472–1477.
57. Kronborg O, Fenger C, Olsen J, et al. Randomised study of screening for colorectal cancer with faecal-occult-blood test. *Lancet* 1996;348:1467–1471.
58. Ahlquist DA, Wieand HS, Moertel CG, et al. Accuracy of fecal occult blood screening for colorectal neoplasia. A prospective study using Hemoccult and HemoQuant tests. *JAMA* 1993;269:1262–1267.
59. Levin B, Brooks D, Smith RA, et al. Emerging technologies in screening for colorectal cancer: CT colonography, immunochemical fecal occult blood tests, and stool screening using molecular markers. *CA Cancer J Clin* 2003;53:44–55.

60. Atkin WS, Edwards R, Kralj-Hans I, et al. Once-only flexible sigmoidoscopy screening in prevention of colorectal cancer: a multicentre randomised controlled trial. *Lancet* 2010;375:1624–1633.

61. Levin TR. Flexible sigmoidoscopy for colorectal cancer screening: valid approach or short-sighted? *Gastroenterol Clin North Am* 2002;31:1015–1029.

62. Littlejohn C, Hilton S, Macfarlane GJ, et al. Systematic review and meta-analysis of the evidence for flexible sigmoidoscopy as a screening method for the prevention of colorectal cancer. *Br J Surg* 2012;99:1488–1500.

63. Elmunzer BJ, Hayward RA, Schoenfeld PS, et al. Effect of flexible sigmoidoscopy-based screening on incidence and mortality of colorectal cancer: a systematic review and meta-analysis of randomized controlled trials. *PLoS Med* 2012;9:e1001352.

64. van Rijn JC, Reitsma JB, Stoker J, et al. Polyp miss rate determined by tandem colonoscopy: a systematic review. *Am J Gastroenterol* 2006;101:343–350.

65. Rosman AS, Korsten MA. Meta-analysis comparing CT colonography, air contrast barium enema, and colonoscopy. *Am J Med* 2007;120:203–210.

66. Imperiale TF, Wagner DR, Lin CY, et al. Using risk for advanced proximal colonic neoplasia to tailor endoscopic screening for colorectal cancer. *Ann Intern Med* 2003;139:959–965.

67. U.S. Preventive Services Task Force. Screening for colorectal cancer: U.S. Preventive Services Task Force recommendation statement. *Ann Intern Med* 2008;149:627–637.

68. Winawer S, Fletcher R, Rex D, et al. Colorectal cancer screening and surveillance: clinical guidelines and rationale-Update based on new evidence. *Gastroenterology* 2003;124:544–560.

69. Quintero E, Castells A, Bujanda L, et al. Colonoscopy versus fecal immunochemical testing in colorectal-cancer screening. *N Engl J Med* 2012;366:697–706.

70. Murakami R, Tsukuma H, Ubukata T, et al. Estimation of validity of mass screening program for gastric cancer in Osaka, Japan. *Cancer* 1990;65:1255–1260.

71. Kampschoer GH, Fujii A, Masuda Y. Gastric cancer detected by mass survey. Comparison between mass survey and outpatient detection. *Scand J Gastroenterol* 1989;24:813–817.

72. Stael von Holstein C, Eriksson S, Huldt B, et al. Endoscopic screening during 17 years for gastric stump carcinoma. A prospective clinical trial. *Scand J Gastroenterol* 1991;26:1020–1026.

73. Shaukat A, Mongin SJ, Geisser MS, et al. Long-term mortality after screening for colorectal cancer. *N Engl J Med* 2013;369:1106–1114.

74. McMahon BJ, Bulkow L, Harpster A, et al. Screening for hepatocellular carcinoma in Alaska natives infected with chronic hepatitis B: a 16-year population-based study. *Hepatology* 2000;32:842–846.

75. Chalasani N, Horlander JC Sr, Said A, et al. Screening for hepatocellular carcinoma in patients with advanced cirrhosis. *Am J Gastroenterol* 1999;94:2988–2993.

76. Sherman M, Peltekian KM, Lee C. Screening for hepatocellular carcinoma in chronic carriers of hepatitis B virus: incidence and prevalence of hepatocellular carcinoma in a North American urban population. *Hepatology* 1995;22:432–438.

77. Dodd GD 3rd, Miller WJ, Baron RL, et al. Detection of malignant tumors in end-stage cirrhotic livers: efficacy of sonography as a screening technique. *AJR Am J Roentgenol* 1992;159:727–733.

78. Laara E, Day NE, Hakama M. Trends in mortality from cervical cancer in the Nordic countries: association with organised screening programmes. *Lancet* 1987;1:1247–1249.

79. Christopherson WM, Lundin FE Jr, Mendez WM, et al. Cervical cancer control: a study of morbidity and mortality trends over a twenty-one-year period. *Cancer* 1976;38:1357–1366.

80. Janerich DT, Hadjimichael O, Schwartz PE, et al. The screening histories of women with invasive cervical cancer, Connecticut. *Am J Public Health* 1995;85:791–794.

81. Sawaya GF, McConnell KJ, Kulasingam SL, et al. Risk of cervical cancer associated with extending the interval between cervical-cancer screenings. *N Engl J Med* 2003;349:1501–1509.

82. Sankaranarayanan R, Nene BM, Shastri SS, et al. HPV screening for cervical cancer in rural India. *N Engl J Med* 2009;360:1385–1394.

83. Vesco KK, Whitlock EP, Eder M, et al. In: *Screening for Cervical Cancer: A Systematic Evidence Review for the US Preventive Services Task Force.* Rockville, MD: Agency for Healthcare Research and Quality; 2011.

84. Solomon D, Davey D, Kurman R, et al. The 2001 Bethesda System: terminology for reporting results of cervical cytology. *JAMA* 2002;287:2114–2119.

85. Darragh TM, Colgan TJ, Thomas Cox J, et al. The Lower Anogenital Squamous Terminology Standardization project for HPV-associated lesions: background and consensus recommendations from the College of American Pathologists and the American Society for Colposcopy and Cervical Pathology. *Int J Gynecol Pathol* 2013;32:76–115.

86. Ho GY, Bierman R, Beardsley L, et al. Natural history of cervicovaginal papillomavirus infection in young women. *N Engl J Med* 1998;338:423–428.

87. Holowaty P, Miller AB, Rohan T, et al. Natural history of dysplasia of the uterine cervix. *J Natl Cancer Inst* 1999;91:252–258.

88. Richardson H, Kelsall G, Tellier P, et al. The natural history of type-specific human papillomavirus infections in female university students. *Cancer Epidemiol Biomarkers Prev* 2003;12:485–490.

89. Melnikow J, Nuovo J, Willan AR, et al. Natural history of cervical squamous intraepithelial lesions: a meta-analysis. *Obstet Gynecol* 1998;92:727–735.

90. Cox JT, Schiffman M, Solomon D. Prospective follow-up suggests similar risk of subsequent cervical intraepithelial neoplasia grade 2 or 3 among women with cervical intraepithelial neoplasia grade 1 or negative colposcopy and directed biopsy. *Am J Obstet Gynecol* 2003;188:1406–1412.

91. Guido R, Schiffman M, Solomon D, et al. Postcolposcopy management strategies for women referred with low-grade squamous intraepithelial lesions or human papillomavirus DNA-positive atypical squamous cells of undetermined significance: a two-year prospective study. *Am J Obstet Gynecol* 2003;188:1401–1405.

92. Mayrand MH, Duarte-Franco E, Rodrigues I, et al. Human papillomavirus DNA versus Papanicolaou screening tests for cervical cancer. *N Engl J Med* 2007;357:1579–1588.

93. Saslow D, Solomon D, Lawson HW, et al. American Cancer Society, American Society for Colposcopy and Cervical Pathology, and American Society for Clinical Pathology screening guidelines for the prevention and early detection of cervical cancer. *CA Cancer J Clin* 2012;62:147–172.

94. Sankaranarayanan R, Esmy PO, Rajkumar R, et al. Effect of visual screening on cervical cancer incidence and mortality in Tamil Nadu, India: a cluster-randomised trial. *Lancet* 2007;370:398–406.

95. Szarewski A. Cervical screening by visual inspection with acetic acid. *Lancet* 2007;370:365–366.

96. Johnson CC, Kessel B, Riley TL, et al. The epidemiology of CA-125 in women without evidence of ovarian cancer in the Prostate, Lung, Colorectal and Ovarian Cancer (PLCO) Screening Trial. *Gynecol Oncol* 2008;110:383–389.

97. Duffy MJ, Bonfrer JM, Kulpa J, et al. CA125 in ovarian cancer: European Group on Tumor Markers guidelines for clinical use. *Int J Gynecol Cancer* 2005;15:679–691.

98. Moss EL, Hollingworth J, Reynolds TM. The role of CA125 in clinical practice. *J Clin Pathol* 2005;58:308–312.

99. Fishman DA, Cohen L, Blank SV, et al. The role of ultrasound evaluation in the detection of early-stage epithelial ovarian cancer. *Am J Obstet Gynecol* 2005;192:1214–1221.

100. Kobayashi E, Ueda Y, Matsuzaki S, et al. Biomarkers for screening, diagnosis, and monitoring of ovarian cancer. *Cancer Epidemiol Biomarkers Prev* 2012;21:1902–1912.

101. Ren J, Cai H, Li Y, et al. Tumor markers for early detection of ovarian cancer. *Expert Rev Mol Diagn* 2010;10:787–798.

102. Prorok PC, Andriole GL, Bresalier RS, et al. Design of the Prostate, Lung, Colorectal and Ovarian (PLCO) Cancer Screening Trial. *Control Clin Trials* 2000;21:273S–309S.

103. Buys SS, Partridge E, Black A, et al. Effect of screening on ovarian cancer mortality: the Prostate, Lung, Colorectal and Ovarian (PLCO) Cancer Screening Randomized Controlled Trial. *JAMA* 2011;305:2295–2303.

104. Menon U, Gentry-Maharaj A, Hallett R, et al. Sensitivity and specificity of multimodal and ultrasound screening for ovarian cancer, and stage distribution of detected cancers: results of the prevalence screen of the UK Collaborative Trial of Ovarian Cancer Screening (UKCTOCS). *Lancet Oncol* 2009;10:327–340.

105. Drescher CW, Shah C, Thorpe J, et al. Longitudinal screening algorithm that incorporates change over time in CA125 levels identifies ovarian cancer earlier than a single-threshold rule. *J Clin Oncol* 2013;31:387–392.

106. Sharma A, Apostolidou S, Burnell M, et al. Risk of epithelial ovarian cancer in asymptomatic women with ultrasound-detected ovarian masses: a prospective cohort study within the UK collaborative trial of ovarian cancer screening (UKCTOCS). *Ultrasound Obstet Gynecol* 2012;40:338–344.

107. Moyer VA. Screening for ovarian cancer: U.S. Preventive Services Task Force reaffirmation recommendation statement. *Ann Intern Med* 2012;157:900–904.

108. NIH consensus conference. Ovarian cancer. Screening, treatment, and follow-up. NIH Consensus Development Panel on Ovarian Cancer. *JAMA* 1995;273:491–497.

109. Smith RA, von Eschenbach AC, Wender R, et al. American Cancer Society guidelines for the early detection of cancer: update of early detection guidelines for prostate, colorectal, and endometrial cancers. Also: update 2001—testing for early lung cancer detection. *CA Cancer J Clin* 2001;51:38–75.

110. Burke W, Petersen G, Lynch P, et al. Recommendations for follow-up care of individuals with an inherited predisposition to cancer. I. Hereditary nonpolyposis colon cancer. Cancer Genetics Studies Consortium. *JAMA* 1997;277:915–919.

111. Gull B, Karlsson B, Milsom I, et al. Can ultrasound replace dilation and curettage? A longitudinal evaluation of postmenopausal bleeding and transvaginal sonographic measurement of the endometrium as predictors of endometrial cancer. *Am J Obstet Gynecol* 2003;188:401–408.

112. Scamman CL. Follow-up study of lung cancer suspects in a mass chest X-ray survey. *N Engl J Med* 1951;244:541–544.

113. Croswell JM, Ransohoff DF, Kramer BS. Principles of cancer screening: lessons from history and study design issues. *Semin Oncol* 2010;37:202–215.

114. Fontana RS, Sanderson DR, Taylor WF, et al. Early lung cancer detection: results of the initial (prevalence) radiologic and cytologic screening in the Mayo Clinic study. *Am Rev Respir Dis* 1984;130:561–565.

115. Fontana RS, Sanderson DR, Woolner LB, et al. Screening for lung cancer. A critique of the Mayo Lung Project. *Cancer* 1991;67:1155–1164.

116. Marcus PM, Bergstralh EJ, Zweig MH, et al. Extended lung cancer incidence follow-up in the Mayo Lung Project and overdiagnosis. *J Natl Cancer Inst* 2006;98:748–756.

CANCER PREVENTION AND SCREENING

117. Manser R, Wright G, Hart D, et al. Surgery for early stage non-small cell lung cancer. *Cochrane Database Syst Rev* 2005:CD004699.
118. Kubik A, Parkin DM, Khlat M, et al. Lack of benefit from semi-annual screening for cancer of the lung: follow-up report of a randomized controlled trial on a population of high-risk males in Czechoslovakia. *Int J Cancer* 1990; 45:26–33.
119. Oken MM, Hocking WG, Kvale PA, et al. Screening by chest radiograph and lung cancer mortality: the Prostate, Lung, Colorectal, and Ovarian (PLCO) randomized trial. *JAMA* 2011;306:1865–1873.
120. Kovalchik SA, Tammemagi M, Berg CD, et al. Targeting of low-dose CT screening according to the risk of lung-cancer death. *N Engl J Med* 2013; 369:245–254.
121. Kubik AK, Parkin DM, Zatloukal P. Czech Study on Lung Cancer Screening: post-trial follow-up of lung cancer deaths up to year 15 since enrollment. *Cancer* 2000;89:2363–2368.
122. Patz EF Jr, Pinsky P, Gatsonis C, et al. Overdiagnosis in low-dose computed tomography screening for lung cancer. *JAMA Intern Med* 2014;174:269–274.
123. Ma J, Ward EM, Smith R, et al. Annual number of lung cancer deaths potentially avertable by screening in the United States. *Cancer* 2013;119: 1381–1385.
124. Wender R, Fontham ET, Barrera E Jr, et al. American Cancer Society lung cancer screening guidelines. *CA Cancer J Clin* 2013;63:107–117.
125. Bach PB, Mirkin JN, Oliver TK, et al. Benefits and harms of CT screening for lung cancer: a systematic review. *JAMA* 2012;307:2418–2429.
126. Montie JE, Smith JA. Whitmoreisms: memorable quotes from Willet F. Whitmore, Jr, M.D. *Urology* 2004;63:207–209.
127. Albertsen PC, Hanley JA, Fine J. 20-year outcomes following conservative management of clinically localized prostate cancer. *JAMA* 2005;293:2095–2101.
128. Lu-Yao G, Albertsen PC, Stanford JL, et al. Screening, treatment, and prostate cancer mortality in the Seattle area and Connecticut: fifteen-year follow-up. *J Gen Intern Med* 2008;23:1809–1814.
129. Thompson IM, Chi C, Ankerst DP, et al. Effect of finasteride on the sensitivity of PSA for detecting prostate cancer. *J Natl Cancer Inst* 2006;98:1128–1133.
130. Thompson IM, Pauler DK, Goodman PJ, et al. Prevalence of prostate cancer among men with a prostate-specific antigen level < or =4.0 ng per milliliter. *N Engl J Med* 2004;350:2239–2246.
131. Thompson IM, Ankerst DP, Chi C, et al. Operating characteristics of prostate-specific antigen in men with an initial PSA level of 3.0 ng/ml or lower. *JAMA* 2005;294:66–70.
132. Widmark A, Klepp O, Solberg A, et al. Endocrine treatment, with or without radiotherapy, in locally advanced prostate cancer (SPCG-7/SFUO-3): an open randomised phase III trial. *Lancet* 2009;373:301–308.
133. Bill-Axelson A, Holmberg L, Ruutu M, et al. Radical prostatectomy versus watchful waiting in early prostate cancer. *N Engl J Med* 2011;364: 1708–1717.
134. Wilt TJ, Brawer MK, Jones KM, et al. Radical prostatectomy versus observation for localized prostate cancer. *N Engl J Med* 2012;367:203–213.
135. Andriole GL, Crawford ED, Grubb RL 3rd, et al. Prostate cancer screening in the randomized Prostate, Lung, Colorectal, and Ovarian Cancer Screening Trial: mortality results after 13 years of follow-up. *J Natl Cancer Inst* 2012;104:125–132.
136. Schroder FH, Hugosson J, Roobol MJ, et al. Screening and prostate-cancer mortality in a randomized European study. *N Engl J Med* 2009;360:1320–1328.
137. Schroder FH, Hugosson J, Roobol MJ, et al. Prostate-cancer mortality at 11 years of follow-up. *N Engl J Med* 2012;366:981–990.
138. Wolters T, Roobol MJ, Steyerberg EW, et al. The effect of study arm on prostate cancer treatment in the large screening trial ERSPC. *Int J Cancer* 2010;126:2387–2393.
139. Hugosson J, Carlsson S, Aus G, et al. Mortality results from the Goteborg randomised population-based prostate-cancer screening trial. *Lancet Oncol* 2010;11:725–732.
140. Kilpelainen TP, Tammela TL, Malila N, et al. Prostate cancer mortality in the Finnish randomized screening trial. *J Natl Cancer Inst* 2013;105: 719–725.
141. Center MM, Jemal A, Lortet-Tieulent J, et al. International variation in prostate cancer incidence and mortality rates. *Eur Urol* 2012;61:1079–1092.
142. Boyle P. Screening for prostate cancer: have you had your cholesterol measured? *BJU Int* 2003;92:191–199.
143. Greene KL, Albertsen PC, Babaian RJ, et al. Prostate specific antigen best practice statement: 2009 update. *J Urol* 2009;182:2232–2241.
144. Wolf AM, Wender RC, Etzioni RB, et al. American Cancer Society guideline for the early detection of prostate cancer: update 2010. *CA Cancer J Clin* 2010;60:70–98.
145. Carter HB. American Urological Association (AUA) guideline on prostate cancer detection: process and rationale. *BJU Int* 2013;112:543–547.
146. Wolff T, Tai E, Miller T. Screening for skin cancer: an update of the evidence for the U.S. Preventive Services Task Force. *Ann Intern Med* 2009;150: 194–198.
147. Katalinic A, Waldmann A, Weinstock MA, et al. Does skin cancer screening save lives?: an observational study comparing trends in melanoma mortality in regions with and without screening. *Cancer* 2012;118:5395–5402.
148. Breitbart EW, Waldmann A, Nolte S, et al. Systematic skin cancer screening in Northern Germany. *J Am Acad Dermatol* 2012;66:201–211.
149. Smith RA, Brooks D, Cokkinides V, et al. Cancer screening in the United States, 2013: a review of current American Cancer Society guidelines, current issues in cancer screening, and new guidance on cervical cancer screening and lung cancer screening. *CA Cancer J Clin* 2013;63:88–105.
150. U.S. Preventive Services Task Force. Screening for skin cancer: U.S. Preventive Services Task Force recommendation statement. *Ann Intern Med* 2009;150: 188–193.

35 Genetic Counseling

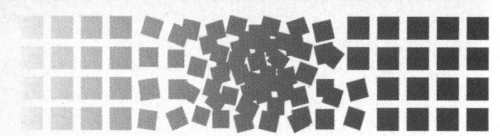

Ellen T. Matloff and Danielle C. Bonadies

INTRODUCTION

Clinically based genetic testing has evolved from an uncommon analysis ordered for the rare hereditary cancer family to a widely available tool ordered on a routine basis to assist in surgical and radiation decision making, chemoprevention, and surveillance of the patient with cancer, as well as management of the entire family. The evolution of this field has created a need for accurate cancer genetic counseling and risk assessment. Extensive coverage of this topic by the media, including Angelina Jolie's public disclosure of her *BRCA1+* status in May 2013, and widespread advertising by commercial testing laboratories have further fueled the demand for counseling and testing.

Cancer genetic counseling is a communication process between a health-care professional and an individual concerning cancer occurrence and risk in his or her family.[1] The process, which may include the entire family through a blend of genetic, medical, and psychosocial assessments and interventions, has been described as a bridge between the fields of traditional oncology and genetic counseling.[1]

The goals of this process include providing the client with an assessment of individual cancer risk, while offering the emotional support needed to understand and cope with this information. It also involves deciphering whether the cancers in a family are likely to be caused by a mutation in a cancer gene and, if so, *which one*. There are >30 hereditary cancer syndromes, many of which can be caused by mutations in different genes. Therefore, testing for these syndromes can be complicated. Advertisements by genetic testing companies bill genetic testing as a simple process that can be carried out by health-care professionals with no training in this area; however, there are many genes involved in cancer, the interpretation of the test results is often complicated, the risk of result misinterpretation is great and associated with potential liability, and the emotional and psychological ramifications for the patient and family can be powerful.[2,3] A few hours of training by a company generating a profit from the sale of these tests does not adequately prepare providers to offer their own genetic counseling and testing services.[4] Furthermore, the delegation of genetic testing responsibilities to office staff and, recently, mammography technicians, is alarming and likely presents a huge liability for these ordering physicians, their practices, and their institutions.[5,6] *Providers should proceed with caution before taking on the role of primary genetic counselor for their patients.*

Counseling about hereditary cancers differs from *traditional* genetic counseling in several ways. Clients seeking cancer genetic counseling are rarely concerned with reproductive decisions, which are often the primary focus in traditional genetic counseling, but are instead seeking information about their own and other relatives' chances of developing cancer.[1] Additionally, the risks given are not absolute but change over time as the family and personal history changes and the patient ages. The risk reduction options available are often radical (e.g., chemoprevention or prophylactic surgery), and are not appropriate for every patient at every age. The surveillance and management plan must be tailored to the patient's age, childbearing status, menopausal status, risk category, ease of screening, and personal preferences and will likely change over time with the patient. The ultimate goal of cancer genetic counseling is to help the patient reach the decision best suited to her personal situation, needs, and circumstances.

There are now a significant number of referral centers across the country specializing in cancer genetic counseling, and the numbers are growing. However, some experts insist that the only way to keep up with the overwhelming demand for counseling will be to educate more physicians and nurses in cancer genetics. The feasibility of adding another specialized and time-consuming task to the clinical burden of these professionals is questionable, particularly with average patient encounters of 19.5 and 21.6 minutes for general practitioners and gynecologists, respectively.[7,8] A more practical goal is to better educate clinicians in the area of risk assessment so that they can screen their patient populations for individuals at high risk for hereditary cancer and refer them on to comprehensive counseling and testing programs. Access to genetic counseling is no longer an issue because there are now internet, phone, and satellite-based telemedicine services available (Table 35.1), with most major health insurance companies now covering these services[9–11] and several requiring them.[12]

WHO IS A CANDIDATE FOR CANCER GENETIC COUNSELING?

Only 5% to 10% of most cancer is thought to be caused by single mutations within autosomal-dominant inherited cancer susceptibility genes.[13] The key for clinicians is to determine which patients are at greatest risk to carry a hereditary mutation. There are seven critical risk factors in hereditary cancer (Table 35.2). The first is early age of cancer onset. This risk factor, *even in the absence of a family history*, has been shown to be associated with an increased frequency of germline mutations in many types of cancers.[14] The second risk factor is the presence of the same cancer in multiple affected relatives on the same side of the pedigree. These cancers do not need to be of similar histologic type in order to be caused by a single mutation. The third risk factor is the clustering of cancers known to be caused by a single gene mutation in one family (e.g., breast/ovarian/pancreatic cancer or colon/uterine/ovarian cancers). The fourth risk factor is the occurrence of multiple primary cancers in one individual. This includes multiple primary breast or colon cancers as well as a single individual with separate cancers known to be caused by a single gene mutation (e.g., breast and ovarian cancer in a single individual). Ethnicity also plays a role in determining who is at greatest risk to carry a hereditary cancer mutation. Individuals of Jewish ancestry are at increased risk to carry three specific *BRCA1/2* mutations.[15] The presence of a cancer that presents unusually—in this case, breast cancer in a male—represents a sixth risk factor and is important even when it is the only risk factor present. Finally, the last risk factor is pathology. Certain types of cancer are overrepresented in hereditary cancer families. For example, medullary and triple negative breast

TABLE 35.1

How to Find a Genetic Counselor for Your Patient

American Board of Genetic Counselors
https://abgcmember.goamp.com/Net/ABGCWcm/Find_Counselor/ABGCWcm/PublicDir.aspx?hkey=0ad511c0-d9e9-4714-bd4b-0d73a59ee175
http://bit.ly/1kzTbk9
Directory of board-certified genetic counselors

InformedDNA
www.informeddna.com
(800) 975-4819
A nationwide network of independent genetic counselors that use telephone and internet technology to bring genetic counseling to patients and providers. Covered by many insurance companies.

National Society of Genetic Counselors
www.nsgc.org (click "Find a Counselor" button)
(312) 321-6834
For a listing of genetic counselors in your area who specialize in cancer.

National Cancer Institute Cancer Genetics Services Directory
www.cancer.gov/cancertopics/genetics/directory
(800) 4-CANCER
A free service designed to locate providers of cancer risk counseling and testing services.

cancers (where the estrogen, progesterone and Her2 receptors are all negative, often abbreviated ER-/PR-/Her2) are overrepresented in *BRCA1* families,[16,17] and the National Comprehensive Cancer Network (NCCN) BRCA testing guidelines now include individuals diagnosed with a triple negative breast cancer <age 60 years.[18] However, breast cancer patients without these pathologic findings are *not* necessarily at lower risk to carry a mutation. In contrast, patients with a borderline or mucinous ovarian carcinoma are at lower risk to carry a *BRCA1* or *BRCA2* mutation[19] and may instead

TABLE 35.2

Risk Factors that Warrant Genetic Counseling for Hereditary Cancer Syndromes

1. Early age of onset (e.g., <50 years for breast, colon, and uterine cancer)
2. Multiple family members on the same side of the pedigree with the same cancer
3. Clustering of cancers in the family known to be caused by a single gene mutation (e.g., breast/ovarian/pancreatic; colon/uterine/ovarian; colon cancer/polyps/desmoid tumors/osteomas)
4. Multiple primary cancers in one individual (e.g., breast/ovarian cancer; colon/uterine; synchronous/metachronous colon cancers; <15 gastrointestinal polyps; <5 hamartomatous or juvenile polyps)
5. Ethnicity (e.g., Jewish ancestry for breast/ovarian cancer syndrome)
6. Unusual presentation of cancer/tumor (e.g., breast cancer in a male; medullary thyroid cancer; retinoblastoma; even a sebaceous carcinoma or adenoma)
7. Pathology (e.g., triple negative [ER/PR/Her-2] breast cancer <60; medullary breast cancers are overrepresented in women with hereditary breast and ovarian cancer; a colon tumor with an abnormal microsatellite instability (MSI) or immunohistochemistry (IHC) result increases the risk for a hereditary colon cancer syndrome)

carry a mutation in a different gene. It is already well-established that medullary thyroid carcinoma, sebaceous adenoma or carcinoma, adrenocortical carcinoma before the age of 25 years, and multiple adenomatous, hamartomatous, or juvenile colon polyps are indicative of other rare hereditary cancer syndromes.[11,20] These risk factors should be viewed in the context of the entire family history, and must be weighed in proportion to the number of individuals who have not developed cancer. The risk assessment is often limited in families that are small or have few female relatives; in such families, a single risk factor may carry more weight.

A less common, but extremely important, finding is the presence of unusual physical findings or birth defects that are known to be associated with rare hereditary cancer syndromes. Examples include benign skin findings, autism, large head circumference[20,21] and thyroid disorders in Cowden syndrome, odontogenic keratocysts in Gorlin syndrome,[22] and desmoid tumors or dental abnormalities in familial adenomatous polyposis (FAP).[23] These and other findings should prompt further investigation of the patient's family history and consideration of a referral to genetic counseling.

In this chapter, the breast/ovarian cancer counseling session with a female patient will serve as a paradigm by which all other sessions may follow broadly.

COMPONENTS OF THE CANCER GENETIC COUNSELING SESSION

Precounseling Information

Before coming in for genetic counseling, the counselee should be informed about what to expect at each visit, and what information he/she should collect ahead of time. The counselee can then begin to collect medical and family history information and pathology reports that will be essential for the genetic counseling session.

Family History

An accurate family history is undoubtedly one of the most essential components of the cancer genetic counseling session. Optimally, a family history should include at least three generations; however, patients do not always have this information. For each individual affected with cancer, it is important to document the exact diagnosis, age at diagnosis, treatment strategies, and environmental exposures (i.e., occupational exposures, cigarettes, other agents).[24] The current age of the individual, laterality, and occurrence of any other cancers must also be documented. Cancer diagnoses should be confirmed with pathology reports whenever possible. A study by Love et al.[25] revealed that individuals accurately reported the primary site of cancer only 83% of the time in their first degree relatives with cancer, and 67% and 60% of the time in second and third degree relatives, respectively. It is common for patients to report a uterine cancer as an ovarian cancer, or a colon polyp as an invasive colorectal cancer. These differences, although seemingly subtle to the patient, can make a tremendous difference in risk assessment. Individuals should be asked if there are any consanguineous (inbred) relationships in the family, if any relatives were born with birth defects or mental retardation, and whether other genetic diseases run in the family (e.g., Fanconi anemia, Cowden syndrome), because these pieces of information could prove to be important in reaching a diagnosis.

The most common misconception in family history taking is that somehow a maternal family history of breast, ovarian, or uterine cancer is more significant than a paternal history. Conversely, many still believe that a paternal history of prostate cancer is more significant than a maternal history. Few cancer genes discovered thus far are located on the sex chromosomes and, therefore, both maternal and paternal history are significant and must be explored thoroughly. It has also become necessary to elicit the spouse's personal and family history of cancer. This has bearing on the cancer status of common children, but may also determine if children are at increased risk for a serious recessive genetic disease such as Fanconi anemia.[26] Children who inherit two copies of a BRCA2 mutation (one from each parent) are now known to have this serious disorder characterized by defective DNA repair and high rates of birth defects, aplastic anemia, leukemia, and solid tumors.[26] Patients should be encouraged to report changes in their family history over time (e.g., new cancer diagnoses, genetic testing results in relatives), because this may change their risk assessment and counseling.

A detailed family history should also include genetic diseases, birth defects, mental retardation, multiple miscarriages, and infant deaths. A history of certain recessive genetic diseases (e.g., ataxia telangiectasia, Fanconi anemia) can indicate that healthy family members who carry just one copy of the genetic mutation may be at increased risk to develop cancer.[26,27] Other genetic disorders, such as hereditary hemorrhagic telangiectasia, can be associated with a hereditary cancer syndrome caused by a mutation in the same gene—in this case, juvenile polyposis.[28]

Dysmorphology Screening

Congenital anomalies, benign tumors, and unusual dermatologic features occur in a large number of hereditary cancer predisposition syndromes. Examples include osteomas of the jaw in FAP, palmar pits in Gorlin syndrome, and papillomas of the lips and mucous membranes in Cowden syndrome. Obtaining an accurate past medical history of benign lesions and birth defects, and screening for such dysmorphology can greatly impact diagnosis, counseling, and testing. For example, BRCA1/2 testing is inappropriate in a patient with breast cancer who has a family history of thyroid cancer and the orocutaneous manifestations of Cowden syndrome.

Risk Assessment

Risk assessment is one of the most complicated components of the genetic counseling session. It is crucial to remember that risk assessment changes over time as the person ages and as the health statuses of their family members change. Risk assessment can be broken down into three separate components.

- What is the chance that the counselee will develop the cancer observed in his/her family (or a genetically related cancer such as ovarian cancer due to a family history of breast cancer)?
- What is the chance that the cancers in this family are caused by a single gene mutation?
- What is the chance that we can identify the gene mutation in this family with our current knowledge and laboratory techniques?

Cancer clustering in a family may be due to genetic and/or environmental factors, or may be coincidental because some cancers are very common in the general population.[29] Although inherited factors may be the primary cause of cancers in some families, in others, cancer may develop because an inherited factor increases the individual's susceptibility to environmental carcinogens. It is also possible that members of the same family may be exposed to similar environmental exposures due to shared geography or patterns in behavior and diet that may increase the risk of cancer.[30] Therefore, it is important to distinguish the difference between a familial pattern of cancer (due to environmental factors or chance) and a hereditary pattern of cancer (due to a shared genetic mutation). Emerging research is also evaluating the role and clinical utility of more common low-penetrance susceptibility genes and single nucleotide polymorphisms (SNP) that may account for a proportion of familial cancers.[31]

Several models are available to calculate the chance that a woman will develop breast cancer, including the Gail and Claus models.[32,33] Computer-based models are also available to help determine the chance that a BRCA mutation will be found in a family.[34] At first glance, many of these models appear simple and easy to use, and it may be tempting to exclusively rely on these models to assess cancer risk. However, each model has its strengths and weaknesses, and the counselor needs to understand the limitations well and know which are validated, which are considered problematic, when a model will not work on a particular patient, or when another genetic syndrome should be considered. For example, none of the existing models are able to factor in other risks that may be essential in hereditary risk calculation (e.g., a sister who was diagnosed with breast cancer after radiation treatment for Hodgkin disease).

The risk of a detectable mutation will also vary based on cancer history and the degree of relationship to an affected family member. For example, family members with early-onset breast cancer have a higher likelihood of testing positive than unaffected family members. Therefore, the risk assessment process should include a discussion of which family member is the best candidate for testing.

DNA Testing

DNA testing is now available for a variety of hereditary cancer syndromes. However, despite misrepresentation by the media, testing is feasible for only a small percentage of individuals with cancer. DNA testing offers the important advantage of presenting clients with *actual risks* instead of the empiric risks derived from risk calculation models. DNA testing can be very expensive; full sequencing and rearrangement testing of the BRCA1/2 genes currently averages $2,500, and full panel testing costs up to $7,000 per patient. Importantly, testing should begin in an affected family member whenever possible to maximize scientific accuracy. Most insurance companies now cover cancer genetic testing in families where the test is medically indicated.

One of the most crucial aspects of DNA testing is accurate result ordering and interpretation. Unfortunately, errors in ordering and interpretation are the greatest risk of genetic testing and are very common.[35] Emerging data reveal that between 30% to 50% of genetic tests are ordered inappropriately, which is problematic for patients, clinicians, and insurers.[36–38] Recent data demonstrate that many medical providers have difficulty interpreting even basic pedigrees and genetic test results.[33–35] Additional studies have demonstrated that an inaccurate interpretation of genetic testing has been shown to result in inappropriate medical management recommendations, unnecessary prophylactic surgeries, a massive waste of health-care dollars, psychosocial distress, and false reassurance for patients.[2,3]

Interpretations are becoming increasingly complicated as more tests and gene panels become available. For example, one study demonstrated that approximately 25% of high-risk families that were BRCA1 and BRCA2 negative by commercially available sequencing were found to carry a deletion or duplication in one of these genes, or a mutation in another gene.[39]

This is particularly concerning in an era in which testing companies are canvassing physicians, and now mammography technicians, and encouraging them to perform their own counseling and testing. The potential impact of test results on the patient and his/her family is great and, therefore, accurate interpretation of the results is paramount. Professional groups have recognized this and have adopted standards encouraging clinicians to refer patients to genetics experts to ensure proper ordering and interpretation of genetic tests. The U.S. Preventive Services Task Force recommends that women whose family history is suggestive of a BRCA mutation be referred for genetic counseling before being offered genetic testing.[40] The American College of Surgeons' Commission on Cancer standards include "cancer risk assessment, genetic counseling and testing services provided to patients either on site

CANCER PREVENTION AND SCREENING

or by referral, by a qualified genetics professional."[4] In an effort to reduce errors, some insurance companies are requiring genetic counseling by a certified genetic counselor before testing for hereditary breast or colon cancer syndromes.[12]

Results can fall into a few broad categories. It is important to note that a negative test result can actually be interpreted in three different ways, detailed in #2, #3, and #4, which follows.

1. Deleterious mutation "positive." When a deleterious mutation in a well-known cancer gene is discovered, the cancer risks for the patient and her family are relatively straightforward. However, with the development of multigene panels and the inclusion of many lesser known genes, the risks of detecting a mutation within a gene whose cancer risks are ill defined and medical management options unknown is much greater. Even for well-known genes, the risks are not precise and should be presented to patients as a risk range.[41,42] When a true mutation is found, it is critical to test both parents (whenever possible) to determine from which side of the family the mutation is originating, even when the answer appears obvious.

2. True negative. An individual does not carry the deleterious mutation found in her family, which ideally, has been proven to segregate with the cancer family history. In this case, the patient's cancer risks are usually reduced to the population risks.

3. Negative. A mutation was not detected, and the cancers in the family are not likely to be hereditary based on the personal and family history assessment. For example, a patient is diagnosed with breast cancer at age 38 years and comes from a large family with no other cancer diagnoses and relatives who died at old ages of other causes.

4. Uninformative. A mutation cannot be found in affected family members of a family in which the cancer pattern appears to be hereditary; there is likely an undetectable mutation within the gene, or the family carries a mutation in a different gene. If, for example, the patient developed breast cancer at age 38 years, has a father with breast cancer, and has a paternal aunt who developed breast and ovarian cancers before age 50 years, a negative test result would be almost meaningless. It would simply mean that the family has a mutation that could not be identified with our current testing methods or a mutation in another cancer gene. The entire family would be followed as high risk.

5. Variant of uncertain significance. A genetic change is identified, the significance of which is unknown. It is possible that this change is deleterious or completely benign. It may be helpful to test other *affected* family members to see if the mutation segregates with disease in the family. If it does not segregate, the variant is less likely to be significant. If it does, the variant is more likely to be significant. Other tools, including a splice site predictor, in conjunction with data on species conservation and amino acid difference scores, can also be helpful in determining the likelihood that a variant is significant. It is rarely helpful (and can be detrimental) to test *unaffected* family members for such variants. The rates of variants of uncertain significance vary greatly depending on the reporting protocols of the lab and the genes analyzed. Creation of open databases through a nationwide movement called Free the Data will likely improve variant reporting for all laboratories.

In order to pinpoint the mutation in a family, an affected individual most likely to carry the mutation should be tested first whenever possible. This is most often a person affected with the cancer in question at the earliest age. Test subjects should be selected with care, because it is possible for a person to develop sporadic cancer in a hereditary cancer family. For example, in an early-onset breast cancer family, it would not be ideal to first test a woman diagnosed with breast cancer at age 65 years because she may represent a sporadic case.

If a mutation is detected in an affected relative, other family members can be tested for the same mutation with a great degree of accuracy. Family members who do not carry the mutation found in their family are deemed true negative. Those who are found to carry the mutation in their family will have more definitive information about their risks to develop cancer. This information can be crucial in assisting patients in decision making regarding surveillance and risk reduction.

If a mutation is not identified in the affected relative, it usually means that either the cancers in the family are (1) not hereditary, or (2) caused by an undetectable mutation or a mutation in a different gene. A careful review of the family history and the risk factors will help to decipher whether interpretation 1 or 2 is more likely. Additional genetic testing may need to be ordered at this point. In cases in which the cancers appear hereditary and no mutation is found, DNA banking should be offered to the proband for a time in the future when improved testing may become available. A letter indicating exactly who in the family has access to the DNA should accompany the banked sample.

The genetic counseling result disclosure session should also include a detailed discussion of which other family members would benefit from genetic counseling and testing and referral information. This can apply not only to families who have been found to carry a deleterious mutation, but may also prove useful in other families (e.g., test a higher risk relative or determine segregation of a variant within a family).

The penetrance of mutations in cancer susceptibility genes is also difficult to interpret. Initial estimates derived from high-risk families provided very high cancer risks for *BRCA1* and *BRCA2* mutation carriers.[43] More recent studies done on populations that were not selected for family history have revealed lower penetrances.[44] Because exact penetrance rates cannot be determined for individual families at this time, and because precise genotype/phenotype correlations remain unclear, it is prudent to provide patients with a range of cancer risk and to explain that their risk probably falls somewhere within this spectrum. This can prove challenging for genes that lack published long-term data on cancer associations and risks.

Female carriers of *BRCA1* and *BRCA2* mutations have a 50% to 85% lifetime risk to develop breast cancer and between a 15% to 60% lifetime risk to develop ovarian cancer.[15,42,43] It is important to note that the classification "ovarian cancer" also includes cancer of the fallopian tubes and primary peritoneal carcinoma.[44,45] *BRCA2* carriers also have an increased lifetime risk of male breast cancer, pancreatic cancer, and possibly, melanoma.[46,47]

Options for Surveillance, Risk Reduction, and Tailored Treatment

The cancer risk counseling session is a forum to provide counselees with information, support, options, and hope. Mutation carriers can be offered: earlier and more aggressive surveillance, chemoprevention, and/or prophylactic surgery. Detailed management options for *BRCA* carriers are discussed in this chapter.

Surveillance recommendations are evolving with newer techniques and additional data. At this time, it is recommended that individuals at increased risk for breast cancer, particularly those who carry a *BRCA* mutation, have annual mammograms beginning at age 25 years, with a clinical breast exam by a breast specialist, a yearly breast magnetic resonance imaging (MRI) with a clinical breast exam by a breast specialist, and a yearly clinical breast exam by a gynecologist.[48,49] It is suggested that the mammogram and MRI be spaced out around the calendar year so that some intervention is planned every 6 months. Recent data suggest that MRI may be safer and more effective in *BRCA* carriers <40 years of age and may someday replace mammograms in this population.[50]

BRCA carriers may take a selective estrogen-receptor modulator (SERM) or aromatase inhibitor in hopes of reducing their risks of developing breast cancer. These medications have been proven effective in women at increased risk due to a positive family history of breast cancer.[51-53] There are limited data on the effectiveness of such medications in unaffected *BRCA* carriers[54-56]; however, there are some data to suggest that *BRCA* carriers taking tamoxifen as treatment for a breast cancer reduce their risk of a contralateral breast cancer.[57] Additionally, the majority of *BRCA2* carriers who develop breast cancer develop an estrogen-positive form of the disease,[58] and it is hoped that this population will respond especially well to chemoprevention. Further studies in this area are necessary before drawing conclusions about the efficacy of chemoprevention in this population. Prophylactic bilateral mastectomy reduces the risk of breast cancer by >90% in women at high-risk for the disease.[59] Before genetic testing was available, it was not uncommon for entire generations of cancer families to have at-risk tissues removed without knowing if they were *personally* at increased risk for their familial cancer. Fifty percent of unaffected individuals in hereditary cancer families will *not* carry the inherited predisposition gene and can be spared prophylactic surgery or invasive high-risk surveillance regimens. Therefore, it is clearly not appropriate to offer prophylactic surgery until a patient is referred for genetic counseling and, if possible, testing.[60]

Women who carry *BRCA1/2* mutations are also at increased risk to develop second contralateral and ipsilateral primaries of the breast.[61] These data bring into question the option of breast conserving surgery in women at high risk to develop a second primary within the same breast. For this reason, the *BRCA1/2* carrier status can have a profound impact on surgical decision making,[62] and many patients have genetic counseling and testing immediately after diagnosis and before surgery or radiation therapy. Those patients who test positive and opt for prophylactic mastectomy can often be spared radiation and the resulting side effects that can complicate reconstruction. Approximately 30% to 60% of previously irradiated patients who later opt for mastectomy with reconstruction report significant complications or unfavorable cosmetic results.[62,63]

Women who carry *BRCA1/2* mutations are also at increased risk to develop ovarian, fallopian tube, and primary peritoneal cancer, even if no one in their family has developed these cancers. Surveillance for ovarian cancer includes transvaginal ultrasounds and CA-125 testing; however, the effectiveness of such surveillance in detecting ovarian cancers at early, more treatable stages has not been proven in any population. Oral contraceptives reduce the risk of ovarian cancer in all women, including *BRCA* carriers.[64] Recent data indicate that the impact of this intervention on increasing breast cancer risk, if any, is low.[56,65] Given the difficulties in screening and in the treatment of ovarian cancer, the risk/benefit analysis likely favors the use of oral contraceptives in young carriers of *BRCA1/2* mutations[30] who are not yet ready to have their ovaries removed. Prophylactic bilateral salpingo-oophorectomy (BSO) is currently the most effective means to reduce the risk of ovarian cancer and is recommended to *BRCA1/2* carriers by the age of 35 to 40 or when childbearing is complete.[66] Specific operative and pathologic protocols have been developed for this prophylactic surgery.[67] In *BRCA1/2* carriers whose pathologies come back normal, this surgery is highly effective at reducing the subsequent risk of ovarian cancer.[68] A decision analysis, comparing various surveillance and risk-reducing options available to *BRCA* carriers, has shown an increase in life expectancy if BSO is pursued by age 40.[69] Emerging data indicate that most ovarian cancers begin in the fallopian tube, and that salpingectomy may someday be sufficient in reducing ovarian cancer risk in young women; however, more data are needed before this option is offered to patients outside of clinical trials.[70] A relatively small percentage of women who pursue BSO may develop primary peritoneal carcinoma.[44,71] There has been some debate about whether *BRCA1/2* carriers should also opt for total abdominal hysterectomy (TAH) due to the fact that small stumps of the fallopian tubes remain after BSO alone. The question of whether *BRCA* carriers are at increased risk for uterine serous papillary carcinoma (USPC) has also been raised.[72-74] If a relationship does exist between *BRCA* mutations and uterine

cancer, the risk appears to be low and not elevated over that of the general population.[75] Removing the uterus may make it possible for a *BRCA* carrier to take unopposed estrogen or tamoxifen in the future without the risk of uterine cancer, but this surgery is associated with a longer recovery time and has more side effects than does BSO alone. Each patient should be counseled about the pros and cons of each procedure and the risks associated with premature menopause before having surgery.[76]

A secondary, but important, reason for female *BRCA* carriers to consider prophylactic oophorectomy is that it also significantly reduces the risk of a subsequent breast cancer, particularly if they have this surgery before menopause.[77,78] The reduction in breast cancer risk remains even if a healthy premenopausal carrier elects to take low-dose hormone-replacement therapy (HRT) after this surgery[79] Early data suggest that tamoxifen, in addition to premenopausal oophorectomy, in *BRCA* carriers may have little additional benefit in terms of breast cancer risk reduction.[80] Research is needed in balancing quality of life issues secondary to estrogen deprivation with cancer risk reduction in these young female *BRCA1/2* carriers.

New developments are also emerging in the treatment and, possibly, the prevention of *BRCA*-related cancers. Early data revealed that breast and ovarian cancers in *BRCA* carriers were particularly sensitive to treatment with poly adenosine diphosphate (ADP)-ribose polymerases (PARP) inhibitors in combination with chemotherapy.[81,82] New trials are focusing on which chemotherapeutic regimens are most effective in mutation carriers. More data are needed on larger cohorts of patients and are currently being studies in multiple clinical trials.

Genetic counseling and testing is also available for dozens of cancer syndromes, including Lynch syndrome, von Hippel-Lindau syndrome, multiple endocrine neoplasias, and familial adenomatous polyposis. Surveillance and risk reduction for patients who are known mutation carriers for such conditions may decrease the associated morbidity and mortality of these syndromes.

Follow-up

A follow-up letter to the patient is a concrete means of documenting the information conveyed in the sessions so that the patient and his/her family members can review it over time. This letter should be sent to the patient and health-care professionals to whom the patient has granted access to this information. A follow-up phone call and/or counseling session may also be helpful, particularly in the case of a positive test result. Some programs provide patients with an annual or biannual newsletter updating them on new information in the field of cancer genetics or patient support groups. It is now recommended that patients return for follow-up counseling sessions months, or even years, after their initial consult to discuss advances in genetic testing and changes in surveillance and risk reduction options. This can be beneficial for individuals who have been found to carry a hereditary predisposition, for those in whom a syndrome/mutation is suspected but yet unidentified, and for those who are ready to move forward with genetic testing. Follow-up counseling is also recommended for patients whose life circumstances have changed (e.g., preconception, after childbearing is complete), who are preparing for prophylactic surgery, or who are ready to discuss the family genetics with their children.

ISSUES IN CANCER GENETIC COUNSELING

Psychosocial Issues

The psychosocial impact of cancer genetic counseling cannot be underestimated. Just the process of scheduling a cancer risk counseling session may be quite difficult for some individuals with a family history who are not only frightened about their own cancer risk, but also are reliving painful experiences associated with the cancer of their loved ones.[13] Counselees may be faced with an onslaught of emotions, including anger, fear of developing cancer, fear of disfigurement and dying, grief, lack of control, negative body image, and a sense of isolation.[24] Some counselees wrestle with the fear that insurance companies, employers, family members, and even future partners will react negatively to their cancer risks. For many, it is a double-edged sword as they balance their fears and apprehensions about dredging up these issues with the possibility of obtaining reassuring news and much needed information.

A person's perceived cancer risk is often dependent on many "nonmedical" variables. They may estimate that their risk is higher if they look like an affected individual, or share some of their personality traits.[24] Their perceived risks will vary depending on if their relatives were cancer survivors or died painful deaths from the disease. Many people wonder not *if* they are going to get cancer, but *when*.

The counseling session is an opportunity for individuals to express why they believe they have developed cancer, or why their family members have cancer. Some explanations may revolve around family folklore, and it is important to listen to and address these explanations rather than dismiss them.[24] In doing this, the counselor will allow the clients to alleviate their greatest fears and to give more credibility to the medical theory. Understanding a patient's perceived cancer risk is important, because that fear may *decrease* surveillance and preventive health-care behaviors.[83] For patients and families who are moving forward with DNA testing, a referral to a mental health-care professional is often very helpful. Genetic testing has an impact not only on the patient, but also on his/her children, siblings, parents, and extended relatives. This can be overwhelming for an individual and the family, and should be discussed in detail prior to testing.

To date, studies conducted in the setting of pre- and post-genetic counseling have revealed that, at least in the short term, most patients do not experience adverse psychological outcomes after receiving their test results.[84,85] In fact, preliminary data have revealed that individuals in families with known mutations who seek testing seem to fare better psychologically at 6 months than those who avoid testing.[84] Among individuals who learn they are *BRCA* mutation carriers, anxiety and distress levels appear to increase slightly after receiving their test results but returned to pre-test levels in several weeks.[86] Although these data are reassuring, it is important to recognize that genetic testing is an individual decision and will not be right for every patient or every family.

Presymptomatic Testing in Children

Presymptomatic testing in children has been widely discussed, and most concur that it is appropriate only when the onset of the condition regularly occurs in childhood or if there are useful interventions that can be applied.[87] For example, genetic testing for mutations in the *BRCA* genes and other adult-onset diseases is generally limited to individuals who are >18 years of age. The American College of Medical Genetics states that if the "medical or psychosocial benefits of a genetic test will not accrue until adulthood . . . genetic testing generally should be deferred."[88] In contrast, the DNA-based diagnosis of children and young adults at risk for hereditary medullary thyroid carcinoma (MTC) is appropriate and has improved the management of these patients.[89] DNA-based testing for MTC is virtually 100% accurate and allows at-risk family members to make informed decisions about prophylactic thyroidectomy. FAP is a disorder that occurs in childhood and in which mortality can be reduced if detection is presymptomatic.[90] Testing is clearly indicated in these instances.

Questions have been raised about the parents' right to demand testing for adult-onset diseases, and this is now happening regularly

with direct-to-consumer tests and whole exome testing of children.[91] The risks of such testing to the child, and the child's right *not* to be tested must be considered. Whenever childhood testing is not medically indicated, it is preferable that testing decisions are postponed until the children are adults and can decide for themselves whether to be tested.

Confidentiality

The level of confidentiality surrounding cancer genetic testing is paramount due to concerns of genetic discrimination. Careful consideration should be given to the confidentially of family history information, pedigrees, genetic test results, pathology reports, and the carrier status of other family members as most hospitals and clinicians transition to electronic medical records systems. The goal of electronic records is to share information about the patient with his/her entire health-care team. However, genetics is a unique specialty that involves the whole family. Patient's charts often contain Health Insurance Portability and Accountability Act (HIPAA)–protected health information and genetic test results for many other family members. This information may not be appropriate to enter into an electronic record. The unique issues of genetics services need to be considered when designing electronic medical record standards.

Confidentiality of test results *within* a family can also be of issue, because genetic counseling and testing often reveals the risk statuses of family members other than the patient. Under confidentiality codes, the patient needs to grant permission before at-risk family members can be contacted. For this reason, many programs have built in a "share information with family members" clause to their informed consent documents. It has been questioned whether or not a family member could sue a health-care professional for negligence if they were identified at high risk yet not informed.[92] Most recommendations have stated that the burden of confidentiality lies between the provider and the patient. However, more recent recommendations state that confidentiality *should* be violated if the potential harm of not notifying other family members outweighs the harm of breaking a confidence to the patient.[93] There is no patent solution for this difficult dilemma, and situations must be considered on a case-by-case basis with the assistance of the in-house legal department and ethics committee.

Insurance and Discrimination Issues

When genetic testing for cancer predisposition first became widely available, the fear of health insurance discrimination by both patients and providers was one of the most common concerns.[94,95] It appears that the risks of health insurance discrimination were overstated and that almost no discrimination by health insurers has been reported.[96] HIPAA banned the use of genetic information as a preexisting condition.[97,98] In May of 2008, Congress passed the Genetic Information Nondiscrimination Act (GINA, HR 493), which provides broad protection of an individual's genetic information against health insurance and employment discrimination.[99] In addition, the Heath Care and Education Reconciliation Act of 2010 (HR 4872) prohibits group health plans from denying insurance based on preexisting conditions and from increasing premiums based on health status.[100] Health-care providers can now more confidently reassure their patients that genetic counseling and testing will not put them at risk of losing group or individual health insurance.

More and more patients are choosing to submit their genetic counseling and/or testing charges to their health insurance companies. In the past few years, more insurance companies have agreed to pay for counseling and/or testing,[101] perhaps in light of data that show these services reduce errors related to ordering and interpreting genetic testing and that decision analyses have revealed subsequent prophylactic surgeries to be cost effective.[102] The risk of life or disability insurance discrimination, however, is more realistic. Patients should be counseled about such risks before they pursue genetic testing.

Reproductive Issues

Reproductive technology in the form of preimplantation genetic diagnosis, prenatal testing, or sperm sorting are options[103] for men and women with a hereditary cancer syndrome, but are requested by few patients for adult-onset conditions in which there are viable options for surveillance and risk reduction. Importantly, if a *BRCA2* carrier is considering having a child, it is important to assess the spouse's risk of also carrying a *BRCA2* mutation. If the spouse is of Jewish ancestry or has a personal or family history of breast, ovarian, or pancreatic cancer, *BRCA* testing should be considered and a discussion of the risk of Fanconi anemia in a child with two *BRCA2* mutations should take place.[104]

RECENT ADVANCES AND FUTURE DIRECTIONS

Cancer genetic counseling and testing were thrust into the national spotlight in the spring of 2013 when Hollywood icon Angelina Jolie publically disclosed that she was a *BRCA1* carrier. One month later the Supreme Court unanimously ruled against gene patents. Referrals for genetic testing spiked across the country and have not returned to baseline levels at most centers. Within hours of the ruling, other labs began offering less expensive and more comprehensive *BRCA* testing, dramatically changing the marketplace of genetic testing for hereditary breast cancer.

All laboratories that have entered the *BRCA* marketplace have done so by including *BRCA1* and *BRCA2* in gene panels. These panels simultaneously analyze groups of genes that contribute to increased risk for breast, colon, ovarian, uterine, and other cancers. The cost of this technology continues to decrease with some multigene panels costing just a few hundred dollars *less* than traditional *BRCA* testing (~$4,000). Some panels include only well-known genes (e.g., *p53*, *APC*, *MLH1*), although many include lesser known genes (e.g., *BRIP1*, *NBN*, *MRE11A*) for which cancer risks are ill defined and medical management options are unknown. Because testing for these genes is new to the clinical setting, it is expected to take several years to compile accurate cancer risk estimates and appropriate recommendations for surveillance and risk reduction. Furthermore, the rate of *variants of uncertain significance* will likely be more common in the lesser known genes. These changes have increased the complexity of genetic testing exponentially. In response, several state and one national insurance company have mandated genetic counseling by certified providers before they will cover cancer genetic testing. In a surprising response, the American Society of Clinical Oncology (ASCO) opposed this insurer's decision, despite more than a decade's worth of data demonstrating that the majority of physicians do not have the time or expertise to offer genetic counseling and testing([38,105-108]). The AMA will decide whether to back the ASCO resolution in June 2014.

Some companies are now offering direct-to-consumer (DTC) genetic testing via websites. The accuracy of some of these DTC genetic tests are in question, and the leading company, 23andMe, has recently come under fire by the U.S. Food and Drug Administration.[105]

Maintaining high standards for thorough genetic counseling, informed consent, and accurate result interpretation will be paramount in reducing potential risks and maximizing the benefits of genetic technology in the next century.

SELECTED REFERENCES

The full reference list can be accessed at lwwhealthlibrary.com/oncology.

3. Brierley KL, Blouch E, Cogswell W, et al. Adverse events in cancer genetic testing: medical, ethical, legal, and financial implications. *Cancer J* 2012;18:303–309.
8. Doksum T, Bernhardt BA, Holtzman NA. Does knowledge about the genetics of breast cancer differ between nongeneticist physicians who do or do not discuss or order BRCA testing? *Genet Med* 2003;5:99–105.
13. Claus E, Schildkraut J, Thompson W, et al. The genetic attributable risks of breast and ovarian cancer. *Cancer* 1996;77:2318–2324.
14. Loman N, Johannsson O, Kristoffersson U. Family history of breast and ovarian cancers and BRCA1 and BRCA2 mutations in a population-based series of early-onset breast cancer. *J Natl Cancer Inst* 2001;93:1215.
21. Pilarski R. Cowden syndrome: a critical review of the clinical literature. *J Genet Couns* 2009 Feb;18:13–27.
25. Love R, Evan A, Josten D. The accuracy of patient reports of a family history. *J Chronic Dis* 1985;38(4):289–293.
31. Stratton MR, Rahman N. The emerging landscape of breast cancer susceptibility. *Nat Genet* 2008;40:17–22.
38. Plon SE, Cooper HP, Parks B, et al. Genetic testing and cancer risk management recommendations by physicians for at-risk relatives. *Genet Med* 2011;13:148–154.
41. King MC, Marks JH, Mandell JB, et al. Breast and ovarian cancer risks due to inherited mutations in BRCA1 and BRCA2. *Science* 2003;302:643–646.
42. Antoniou A, Pharoah PD, Narod S, et al. Average risks of breast and ovarian cancer associated with BRCA1 or BRCA2 mutations detected in case Series unselected for family history: a combined analysis of 22 studies. *Am J Hum Genet* 2003;72:1117–1130.
46. van Asperen C, Brohet R, Meijers-Heijboer, et al. Cancer risks in BRCA2 families: estimates for sites other than breast and ovary. *J Med Genet* 2005;42:711–719.
47. Breast Cancer Linkage Consortium. Cancer risks in BRCA2 mutation carriers. *J Natl Cancer Inst* 1999;91:1310–1316.
48. Warner E, Plewes D, Hill K, et al. Surveillance of BRCA1 and BRCA2 mutation carriers with magnetic resonance imaging, ultrasound, mammography, and clinical breast examination. *JAMA* 2004;202:1317–1325.
49. Kriege M, Brekelmans CT, Boetes C, et al. Efficacy of MRI and mammography for breast-cancer screening in women with a familial or genetic predisposition. *N Engl J Med* 2004;29:351:427–437.

55. King M, Wieand S, Hale K. Tamoxifen and breast cancer incidence among women with inherited mutations in BRCA1 and BRCA2. *JAMA* 2001;286:2251–2256.
57. Phillips KA, Milne RL, Rookus MA, et al. Tamoxifen and risk of contralateral breast cancer for BRCA1 and BRCA2 mutation carriers. *J Clin Oncol* 2013;31:3091–3099.
59. Hartmann L, Schaid D, Woods J. Efficacy of bilateral prophylactic mastectomy in women with a family history of breast cancer. *N Engl J Med* 1999;340:77–84.
61. Turner B, Harold E, Matloff E, et al. BRCA1/BRCA2 germline mutations in locally recurrent breast cancer patients after lumpectomy and radiation therapy: Implications for breast-conserving management in patients with BRCA1/BRCA2 mutations. *J Clin Oncol* 1999;17:3017–3024.
65. Milne R, Knight J, John E, et al. Oral contraceptive use and risk of early-onset breast cancer in carriers and noncarriers of BRCA1 and BRCA2 mutations. *Cancer Epidemiol Biomarkers Prev* 2005;14:350–356.
66. Domchek S, Friebel T, Neuhausen S, et al. Mortality reduction after risk-reducing bilateral salpingo-oophorectomy in a prospective cohort of BRCA1 and BRCA2 mutation carriers. *Lancet Oncol* 2006;7:223–229.
67. Powel CB, Kenley E, Chen LM, et al. Risk-reducing salpingo-oophorectomy in BRCA mutation carriers: role of serial sectioning in the detection of occult malignancy. *J Clin Oncol* 2005;23:127–132.
77. Rebbeck T, Lynch H, Neuhausen S, et al. Prophylactic oophorectomy in carriers of BRCA1 or BRCA2 mutations. *N Engl J Med* 2002;346:1616–1622.
79. Rebbeck T, Friebel T, Wagner T, et al. Effect of short-term hormone replacement therapy on breast cancer risk reduction after bilateral prophylactic oophorectomy in BRCA1 and BRCA2 mutation carriers: the PROSE study group. *J Clin Oncol* 2005;23:7804–7810.
88. ASHG/ACMG. Points to consider: ethical, legal, and psychosocial implications of genetic testing in children and adolescents. American Society of Human Genetics Board of Directors, American College of Medical Genetics Board of Directors. *Am J Hum Genet* 1995;57:1233–1241.
99. The Genetic Information Nondiscrimination Act of 2008 (H.R. 493). Library of Congress Web site. http://thomas.loc.gov/cgi-bin/bdquery/z?d110 :h.r.00493. Accessed December 3, 2012.
108. Bellcross C, Kolor K, Goddard K, et al. Awareness and utilization of BRCA1/2 testing among U.S. primary care physicians. *Am J Prev Med* 2011;40:61–66.

CANCER PREVENTION AND SCREENING

PART V

Practice
of Oncology

36 Design and Analysis of Clinical Trials

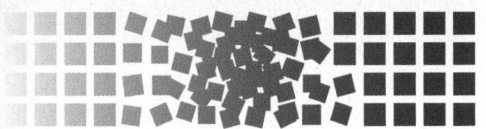

Richard M. Simon

INTRODUCTION

Clinical trials are experiments to determine the value of a treatment. There are two key components to the experimental approach. First, results rather than plausible reasoning are required to support conclusions. Second, in an experiment the treatments are assigned so that one can conclude that differences in outcome are due to differences in treatment effect. In observational studies, treatments are not assigned as part of the study, so differences in outcome between treatment groups may merely result from the fact that sicker patients received less intensive treatments. Experiments should be prospectively planned and conducted under controlled conditions to provide definitive answers to well-defined questions. Using tumor registry data to compare the survival rates of patients with prostate cancer treated with surgery to those of patients receiving radiotherapy is an example of an *observational study*, not a clinical trial. In an observational study, the investigators are passive observers. Treatment assignments, staging workup, and follow-up procedures are out of the control of the investigators, and are conducted with no considerations about the validity of the subsequent attempt at comparison. The statistical associations resulting from such studies are, consequently, a weak basis for causal inferences about relationships between the treatments administered and the outcomes observed. Surprisingly, this does not seem to be realized by the politicians and health-care administrators allocating enormous sums of money to outcomes research based on electronic medical records from general practice. In such observational studies, treatments are usually selected on the basis of subjective assessment of the prognosis of the patient, specialties of the physician, and diagnostic evaluations. Unknown patient selection factors generally are more important determinants of patient outcome than are differences between treatments. For example, Subramanian and Simon[1] found that in observational studies that developed gene expression prognostic signatures for patients with early stage nonsmall-cell lung cancer, those who received chemotherapy had poorer survivals than those who did not even after adjusting for all recorded prognostic factors.

Clinical trials require careful planning. The first result of the planning process is a written protocol. Typical subject headings for the protocol are shown in Table 36.1, and the protocol development process is discussed in more detail by Green et al.[2] The protocol should define treatment and evaluation policies for a well-defined set of patients. It also should define the specific questions to be answered by the study and should directly justify that the number of patients and the nature of the controls are adequate to answer these questions. Some clinical trials are really only guidelines for clinical management supplemented by lofty objectives with no scientific meaning and no realistic chance of providing a reliable answer to a well-defined medical question. Such studies are a disservice to the patients who are undergoing some inconvenience to contribute to the welfare of future patients.

PHASE 1 CLINICAL TRIALS

The main objectives of phase 1 trials have traditionally been to determine a dose that is appropriate for use in phase 2 and 3 trials and to determine information about the pharmacokinetics of distribution of the drug. Patients with advanced disease that is resistant to standard therapy but who have normal organ function are usually included in such trials.

Phase 1 trials are usually initiated at a low dose that is not expected to produce serious toxicity. A starting dose of one-tenth the lethal dose (expressed as milligrams per square meter of body surface area) in the most sensitive species usually is used.[3] The dose is increased for subsequent patients according to a series of preplanned steps. Dose escalation for subsequent patients occurs only after sufficient time has passed to observe acute toxic effects for patients treated at lower doses. Cohorts of three to six patients are treated at each dose level. Usually, if no dose-limiting toxicity (DLT) is seen at a given dose level, the dose is escalated for the next cohort. If the incidence of DLT is 33%, then three more patients are treated at the same level. If no further cases of DLT are seen in the additional patients, then the dose level is escalated for the next cohort. Otherwise, dose escalation stops. If the incidence of DLT is >33% at a given level, then dose escalation also stops. The phase 2 recommended dose often is taken as the highest dose for which the incidence of DLT is <33%. Usually, six or more patients are treated at the recommended dose.

The dose levels themselves are commonly based on a modified Fibonacci series. The second level is twice the starting dose, the third level is 67% greater than the second, the fourth level is 50% greater than the third, the fifth is 40% greater than the fourth, and each subsequent step is 33% greater than that preceding it. Escalating doses for subsequent courses in the same patient are generally not done, except at low doses before any DLT has been encountered.

Accelerated Titration Designs

There is no compelling scientific basis for the approach just outlined, except that experience has shown it to be safe. Traditional phase 1 trials have three limitations:

1. They sometimes expose too many patients to subtherapeutic doses of the new drug.
2. The trials may take a long time to complete.
3. They provide very limited information about interpatient variability and cumulative toxicity.

New trial designs have been developed to address these problems.[4] The *accelerated titration designs*[5] permit within-patient dose escalation and use only one patient per dose level until grade 2 or greater toxicity is seen. Doses are titrated within patients to achieve grade 2 toxicity. The analysis consists of fitting a statistical model to the full set of data that includes all grades of toxicity for all courses of a patient's treatment. The model includes parameters

TABLE 36.1

Subject Headings for a Protocol

Introduction and scientific background
Objectives
Selection of patients
Design of study (including schematic diagram)
Treatment plan
Drug information
Toxicities to be monitored and dosage modifications
Required clinical and laboratory data and study calendar
Criteria for evaluating the effect of treatment and end point
  definition
Statistical considerations
Informed consent and regulatory considerations
Data forms
References
Study chairperson, collaborating participants, addresses, and
  telephone numbers

that represent the steepness of the dose-toxicity curve, the degree of interpatient variability in the location of the dose-toxicity curve, and the degree (if any) of cumulative toxicity. All these parameters are estimated from the data.

Several variants of the accelerated titration design were studied. Design A uses conventional 40% dose steps during the initial accelerated phase, whereas designs B and C use 100% dose steps until one patient experiences DLT or two patients experience grade 2 toxicity. At that point, acceleration ceases and standard cohorts of three to six patients with 40% dose-step increments are used. These designs were compared to a control design using cohorts of three to six patients with 40% dose-step increments and no intrapatient dose escalation.

In the 20 phase 1 trials initially evaluated, only three showed any evidence of cumulative toxicity. The average number of patients required was reduced from 39.9 for the control design to 24.4, 20.7, and 21.2 for designs A, B, and C, respectively. The average number of patients who had grade 0 to 1 toxicity as their worst toxicity grade over three cycles of treatment was 23.3 for the control but only 7.9, 3.9, and 4.8 for designs A, B, and C, respectively. The average number of patients with a worst toxicity grade of 3 increased from 5.5 for the control to 6.2, 6.8, and 6.2 for designs A, B, and C, respectively. The average number of patients with a worst toxicity grade of 4 increased from 1.9 for the control to 3.0, 4.3, and 3.2 for designs A, B, and C, respectively. Accelerated titration designs appear to be effective in reducing the number of patients necessary for finding the maximum tolerated dose, for reducing the number who are undertreated, and for providing increased information. They do not necessarily reduce the length of time necessary for completion of the trial. They increase the information yield if investigators analyze the results of the trial using the model developed by Simon et al.[5] Software for fitting the model is available at http://brb.nci.nih.gov. Software for determining dose assignments and for recording the data in a spreadsheet format are also available at that website. The model of Simon et al.[5] uses actual worst grade toxicity for each course of treatment of each patient, and it enables one to determine whether there is cumulative toxicity and to estimate the variability among patients in toxic effects. The use of the accelerated titration design has been reviewed.[6,7]

Continual Reassessment Methods

O'Quigley, Pepe, and Fisher[8] used a dose-toxicity model to guide the dose escalation, as well as to determine the maximum tolerated dose. A Bayesian prior distribution is established for the steepness of the dose-toxicity curve and the distribution is updated after each patient is treated. The model is based on using only first-course treatment data and whether the patient experiences DLT. This approach is called the *continual reassessment method*. For each new patient, the model is used to determine the dose predicted to cause DLT to a specified percentage of the patients. That dose is assigned to the next patient. Many modifications of the original continual reassessment method have been subsequently proposed.[9–11]

For some tumor vaccines and molecularly targeted drugs, toxicity may not be dose limiting,[12] and the dose selected may be based on preclinical findings or on practical considerations. For some molecularly targeted drugs, preclinical studies provide a target serum concentration of the active moiety necessary to maximally inhibit the target, and drug administration can be titrated for each patient to the targeted serum concentration. This approach can be complex because it involves developing a population pharmacokinetic model relating dose to concentration as the study progresses. A simpler approach is to have separate cohorts of patients who are treated at each of several dose levels without intrapatient dose titration. A population pharmacokinetic model relating dose to concentration is fit to the data.

Ideally, a trial design should provide the smallest dose that gives maximum biologic effect. For molecularly targeted therapeutics, the biologic effect might be a measure of the degree of inhibition of the target. Because it can be very difficult to obtain tumor samples before and after treatment, biologic effect is sometimes measured in an accessible surrogate tissue, such as peripheral blood lymphocytes or skin, or by using functional imaging.[13] For therapeutic vaccines, the biologic effect might be a measure of stimulation of tumor reactive T cells.

Finding the dose that provides maximum biological effect is often not practical in a phase 1 trial, as it may require a large number of patients. For example, to have 90% power for detecting a one standard error difference in mean response between two dose levels at a one-sided 10% significance level requires 14 patients per dose level. A more limited objective is to identify a dose that is biologically active. Korn et al.[14] developed a sequential procedure for finding such a dose when the measure of biologic response is binary. During an initial accelerated phase, they treat one patient per dose level until a biologic response is seen. Then, they treat cohorts of three to six patients per dose level. With zero to one biologic responses among three patients at a dose level, they escalate to the next level. With two to three responses among three patients, they expand the cohort to six patients. With five to six biologic responses from the six patients, they declare that dose to be the biologically active level and terminate the trial. With four or fewer biologic responses at a level, they continue to escalate.

Designs have also been developed for phase zero proof of concept trials.[15,16] Patients are treated with single doses of a new drug at very low concentrations not expected to cause toxicity. This enables the investigator to obtain an early assessment of whether the molecular target of the drug is being inhibited by measuring a pharmacodynamic end point before and after drug administration. These trials require prior development of an assay for measuring the pharmacodynamic end point and an adequate database for estimating the variability of measurement for independent tissue samples of the same patient. This estimate should reflect variability of tissue sampling as well as technical variability of the assay. The approach developed depends on having a good estimate of assay variability and in having assay sufficiently reproducible to be able to reliably classify individual patients as responders or nonresponders based on the observed change in the level of the pharmacodynamic end point. The designs described by Rubinstein et al.[16] utilize a small numbers of patients for establishing whether the drug causes target inhibition in a substantial proportion of patients.

PRACTICE OF ONCOLOGY

PHASE 2 CLINICAL TRIALS

Patient Selection

Phase 2 trials have traditionally been performed separately by tumor type in patients with the least amount of prior therapy for whom no effective therapy is available. With cytotoxics, full-dose chemotherapy is often impossible in patients debilitated by prior treatment, and lack of chemotherapeutic activity in previously treated patients may not indicate lack of clinical usefulness in earlier disease. The development of molecularly targeted drugs has introduced new complexities with regard to selection and evaluation of patients for phase 3 trials. When the target of the drug is clearly known, it may be more appropriate to select patients based on target expression than based on primary site of disease. Even if target expression is not used as an eligibility criterion, the drug should be evaluated in an adequate number of patients whose tumors express the target. Consequently, it is important to have an adequate assay for the target available at the time that phase 2 development begins.

In many cases, the drug will have multiple targets; there may be several candidate assays available for each target. Expression of the target will often prove to be only part of the relevant genomic information. For example, the effectiveness of antiepidermal growth factor receptor antibodies cetuximab and pannitumumab turned out to depend on whether the tumor had an activating K-RAS mutation.[17–19]

Whereas the major objective of phase 2 trials has traditionally been to identify the primary tumor sites in which a new drug was active, a new important objective is to develop promising predictive biomarkers that identify the patients whose tumors are most (or least) likely to respond to the drug. The phase 2 development stage is also the time to select the assay(s) that will be used in the phase 3 trials of the new drug and to define the criteria that will be used to either select patients for such trials or to structure the analysis, as will be described later in this chapter.

It is often undesirable to restrict entry to phase 2 trials based on what one thinks one knows about the drug target, at least in cases where this knowledge is uncertain. It is important, however, to ensure that the activity of the drug is not missed because the phase 2 trials did not accrue enough of the right kinds of patients. The decision of whether to restrict entry based on the presumed mechanism of action will depend in part on the adverse effects of the drug.

If tumor specimens are archived for the patients entered on broad eligibility phase 2 trials, then one avoids the need to develop assays in advance for all candidate targets, but it is not possible to ensure adequate accrual for subsets of patients whose tumors are positive for the candidate markers. Pusztai, Anderson, and Hess[20] described a hybrid approach that begins with conducting a standard single-arm two-stage design for evaluating whether the overall response rate for unrestricted patients is sufficiently large. If the overall response rate is sufficient in the first stage of the standard phase 2 trial, then the second stage is completed with accrual of additional unrestricted patients. If there are too few responses overall in the first stage, then one starts a two-stage phase 2 study restricting entry to patients who are marker positive. If there are multiple markers of interest, then one restricts entry to patients positive for one of the markers and ensures that each marker has sufficient number of positive patients for evaluation. LeBlanc et al.[21] have described how multiple primary sites can be incorporated in a single phase 2 trial.

In some cases, the list of candidate targets can be narrowed using mRNA transcript expression profiling of the pretreatment specimens. By comparing pretreatment expression levels of responders to nonresponders, one can potentially prioritize targets for assay development. If one does not have a good list of candidate targets, genomewide expression profiling can be used to develop a classifier of the tumors likely to respond to the drug. Dobbin, Zhao, and Simon[22] have provided sample size guidelines for genomewide expression profiling studies and generally recommend at least 20 responders for developing a classifier. Pusztai, Anderson, and Hess[20] performed a computer simulation study to indicate that HER-2 transcript overexpression would have been missed as a predictive biomarker for treatment of advanced breast cancer with trastuzumab in whole genome expression profiling with only five responders to analyze. They recommend analysis based on candidate genes if the number of responders are very limited.

Single-Arm Phase 2 Trials

Single Agents

For most single-agent phase 2 trials, the objective is simply to determine whether the drug has activity against the tumor type in question. For this objective, response rate based on the response evaluation criteria in solid tumors guidelines may provide a satisfactory approach.[23] A variety of statistical accrual plans and sample size methods have been developed for single-arm phase 2 trials. One of the most popular approaches is the optimal two-stage design.[24] n_1 evaluable patients are entered into study in the first stage of the trial. If no more than r_1 responses are obtained among these n_1 patients, then accrual terminates and the drug is rejected as being of little interest. Otherwise, accrual continues to a total of n evaluable patients. At the end of the second stage, the drug is rejected if the observed response rate is less than or equal to r/n, where r and n are determined by the design used.

Tables 36.2 and 36.3 illustrate some of these optimized designs, and a web-based interactive computer program is available at http://linus.nci.nih.gov/brb. To select a design, the investigator specifies the target activity level of interest, p_1, and also a lower activity level, p_0, representing inadequate activity. The first row of each triplet of optimal designs provides designs with probability 0.10 of accepting drugs worse than p_0 and probability 0.10 of rejecting drugs better than p_1. Subject to these two constraints, the optimal designs minimize the average sample size. The average sample size is calculated at the lower activity level p_0 to optimize protection of patients from exposure to inactive drugs. The tables show for each design the optimal values of r_1, n_1, r, and n; the average sample size; and the probability of stopping after the first stage for a drug with activity level p_0.

These tables also show the "minimax" designs, which provide the smallest maximum sample size n that satisfies the two constraints just described. Although minimax designs have somewhat larger average sample sizes than do optimal designs, in some instances, they are preferable because the small increase in average sample size is more than compensated for by a large reduction in maximum sample size.

The designs shown in Tables 36.2 and 36.3 are two-stage designs with the potential for early stopping for lack of activity. Optimized three-stage designs have been described by Ensign et al.[25] Others have extended the design to incorporate toxicity or tumor progression information.[26–28]

Some authors have recommended use of progression-free survival instead of response[29] for evaluating molecularly targeted drugs that may be cytostatic. Single-arm phase 2 trials can be designed using Tables 36.2 and 36.3 for testing whether the proportion of patients with stable disease at a specified landmark time like 12 months after the start of treatment is greater than a specified value p_0, but that is only meaningful if the value p_0 is a stable, robust, and well-characterized stable disease rate that results from multiple large studies with control regimens. Single-arm studies using stable disease are rarely planned or analyzed with that care and hence conclusions of single-arm phase 2 trials claiming that molecularly targeted agents cause disease stabilization are often dubious.[30] Vidaurre et al.[30] have questioned, however, whether

TABLE 36.2

Simon Two-Stage Phase 2 Designs for $p_1 - p_0 = 0.20$[a]

		Optimal Design				Minimax Design			
		Reject Drug if Response Rate				Reject Drug if Response Rate			
P_0	P_1	r_1/n_1	r/n	EN (p_0)	PET (p_0)	r_1/n_1	r/n	EN (p_0)	PET (p_0)
0.05	0.25	0/9	2/24	14.5	0.63	0/13	2/20	16.4	0.51
		0/9	2/17	12.0	0.63	0/12	2/16	13.8	0.54
		0/9	3/30	16.8	0.63	0/15	3/25	20.4	0.46
0.10	0.30	1/12	5/35	19.8	0.65	1/16	4/25	20.4	0.51
		1/10	5/29	15.0	0.74	1/15	5/25	19.5	0.55
		2/18	6/36	22.5	0.71	2/22	6/23	26.2	0.62
0.20	0.40	3/17	10/37	26.0	0.55	3/19	10/36	28.2	0.46
		3/13	12/43	20.6	0.75	4/18	10/33	22.3	0.50
		4/19	15/54	30.4	0.67	5/24	13/45	31.2	0.66
0.30	0.50	7/22	17/46	29.9	0.67	7/28	15/39	35.0	0.36
		5/15	18/46	23.6	0.72	6/19	16/39	25.7	0.48
		8/24	24/63	34.7	0.73	7/24	21/53	36.6	0.56
0.40	0.60	7/18	22/46	30.2	0.56	11/28	20/41	33.8	0.55
		7/16	23/46	24.5	0.72	17/34	20/39	34.4	0.91
		11/25	32/66	36.0	0.73	12/29	27/54	38.1	0.64
0.50	0.70	11/21	26/45	29.0	0.67	11/23	23/39	31.0	0.50
		8/15	26/43	23.5	0.70	12/23	23/37	27.7	0.66
		13/24	36/61	34.0	0.73	14/27	32/53	36.1	0.65
0.60	0.80	6/11	26/38	25.4	0.47	18/27	24/35	28.5	0.82
		7/11	30/43	20.5	0.70	8/13	25/35	20.8	0.65
		12/19	37/53	29.5	0.69	15/26	32/45	35.9	0.48
0.70	0.90	6/9	22/28	17.8	0.54	11/16	20/25	20.1	0.55
		4/6	22/27	14.8	0.58	19/23	21/26	23.2	0.95
		11/15	29/36	21.2	0.70	13/18	26/32	22.7	0.67

[a] For each value of (p_0, p_1), designs are given for three sets of error probabilities (α, β). The first, second, and third rows correspond to error probability limits (0.10, 0.10), (0.05, 0.20), and (0.05, 0.10), respectively. α is the probability of accepting a drug with response probability p_0. β is the probability of rejecting a drug with response probability p_1. For each design, EN (p_0) and PET (p_0) denote the expected sample size and the probability of early termination when the true response probability is p_0.

molecularly targeted drugs are any more cytostatic than conventional chemotherapy drugs. El-Maraghi and Eisenhauer[31] have also recommended that objective response is a useful end point for screening molecularly targeted agents.

Combination Regimens

Determination whether a new drug adds anticancer activity to an active regimen is inherently comparative. In using Tables 36.2 and 36.3 to design a single-arm trial, p_0 should represent the level of activity of existing standard regimens. If this response probability is not well determined, however, because it varies among studies and varies based on patient prognostic factors, then a single-arm trial based on an assumed known p_0 may not be appropriate.

Several approaches to single-arm study design have been developed that attempt to either account for or control the variability in p_0. One approach to controlling this variability is to base the analysis of the single-arm trial on comparison to a specific set of control patients, matched for prognostic factors, and treated at the same institution as those for the new study. This can be a better approach than just using an assumed known value of p_0 as described previously, but it still assumes that adjustment for known prognostic factors is sufficient to ensure comparability. Although such historic control comparisons are not considered reliable enough to eliminate the need for phase 3 trials, if done carefully, they may provide an adequate basis for decisions about which new regimens are worthy of phase 3 evaluation.

For comparative trials of response rates using specific historic controls, the sample size should be planned using the formulas appropriate for randomized clinical trials. By inserting the number of historic controls to be used, one can compute the number of patients needed to treat on the new regimen in the single-arm phase 2 trial.[32] For binary end point data, the results of these calculations are presented in Table 36.4 for 80% power with a one-sided 10% significance level. The tabulated entries indicate that a 25 percentage-point difference can be detected with <40 new patients if there are at least 30 appropriate historic controls. The table entries indicate that detecting a 15 percentage-point difference is almost never feasible with this single-arm approach and that detecting a 20 percentage-point difference generally requires at least 50 appropriate historical controls and ≥60 new patients.

Thall and colleagues[33,34] have developed and used Bayesian methods for planning and conducting single-institution trials comparing one or more new regimens to a specific set of historic controls who received a control treatment at the same institution. The Bayesian methods provide for continual analysis of results with either tumor response or time to event end points or for joint monitoring of efficacy and toxicity. Their methods require a substantial number of patients who have been treated on protocol with an appropriate control regimen and who have been staged comparably to the patients to be treated with the new regimen.

Korn et al.[35] developed an approach for using historic control data in phase 2 multicenter trials of metastatic melanoma. They

TABLE 36.3

Simon Two-Stage Phase 2 Designs for $p_1 - p_0 = 0.15$[a]

		Optimal Design				Minimax Design			
		Reject Drug if Response Rate				Reject Drug if Response Rate			
P_0	P_1	r_1/n_1	r/n	EN (p_0)	PET (p_0)	r_1/n_1	r/n	EN (p_0)	PET (p_0)
0.05	0.20	0/12	3/37	23.5	0.54	0/18	3/32	26.4	0.40
		0/10	3/29	17.6	0.60	0/13	3/27	19.8	0.51
		1/21	4/41	26.7	0.72	1/29	4/38	32.9	0.57
0.10	0.25	2/21	7/50	31.2	0.65	2/27	6/40	33.7	0.48
		2/18	7/43	24.7	0.73	2/22	7/40	28.8	0.62
		2/21	10/66	36.8	0.65	3/31	9/55	40.0	0.62
0.20	0.35	5/27	16/63	43.6	0.54	6/33	15/58	45.5	0.50
		5/22	19/72	35.4	0.73	6/31	15/53	40.4	0.57
		8/37	22/83	51.4	0.69	8/42	21/77	58.4	0.53
0.30	0.45	9/30	29/82	51.4	0.59	16/50	25/69	56.0	0.68
		9/27	30/81	41.7	0.73	16/46	25/65	49.6	0.81
		13/40	40/110	60.8	0.70	27/77	33/88	78.5	0.86
0.40	0.55	16/38	40/88	54.5	0.67	18/45	34/73	57.2	0.56
		11/26	40/84	44.9	0.67	28/59	34/70	60.1	0.90
		19/45	49/104	64.0	0.68	24/62	45/94	78.9	0.47
0.50	0.65	18/35	47/84	53.0	0.63	19/40	41/72	58.0	0.44
		15/28	48/83	43.7	0.71	39/66	40/68	66.1	0.95
		22/42	60/105	62.3	0.68	28/57	54/93	75.0	0.50
0.60	0.75	21/34	47/71	47.1	0.65	25/43	43/64	54.4	0.46
		17/27	46/67	39.4	0.69	18/30	43/62	43.8	0.57
		21/34	64/95	55.6	0.65	48/72	57/84	73.2	0.90
0.70	0.85	14/20	45/59	36.2	0.58	15/22	40/52	36.8	0.51
		14/19	46/59	30.3	0.72	16/23	39/49	34.4	0.56
		18/25	61/79	43.4	0.66	33/44	53/68	48.5	0.81
0.80	0.95	5/7	27/31	20.8	0.42	5/7	27/31	20.8	0.42
		7/9	26/29	17.7	0.56	7/9	26/29	17.7	0.56
		16/19	37/42	24.4	0.76	31/35	35/40	35.3	0.94

[a] For each value of (p_0, p_1), designs are given for three sets of error probabilities (α, β). The first, second, and third rows correspond to error probability limits (0.10, 0.10), (0.05, 0.20), and (0.05, 0.10), respectively. α is the probability of accepting a drug with response probability p_0. β is the probability of rejecting a drug with response probability p_1. For each design, EN (p_0) and PET (p_0) denote the expected sample size and the probability of early termination when the true response probability is p_0.

reviewed 42 previous phase 2 trials in melanoma conducted by US cancer cooperative oncology groups. They found that after adjustment for performance status, sex, presence of visceral disease, and presence of brain metastases, there was little interstudy variability in survival among the arms of the phase 2 trials. Consequently, for any single-arm phase 2 trial of metastatic melanoma, one can use their results in conjunction with the prognostic makeup of the patients in the new study to synthesize a benchmark overall survival curve or a benchmark 1-year overall survival rate for use in evaluating the new regimen. They provide an example of planning a phase 2 trial using this approach that required 72 patients to have 85% to 90% power for detecting a 15 percentage-point improvement in the 1-year overall survival rate with a one-sided type 1 error of 10%. They found that this approach was less satisfactory for use with progression-free survival because interstudy variability remained substantial after adjustment for prognostic factors.

Mick, Crowley, and Carroll[36] proposed that the time to progression of a patient on a phase 2 trial be compared to the time to progression of the same patient on his/her previous trial. The ratio of these times was called a *growth modulation index*, and the agent was considered active if the index was >1.3 on average. In practice, however, follow-up intervals on various protocols are different, and there may be substantial variability and bias in computing

the ratio of progression times. As tumors grow larger, the doubling time may increase and hence in some cases the chance of false-positive findings may be inflated.[37]

Randomized Phase 2 Trials

Time to tumor progression or disease-free survival has been recommended for evaluation of single-agent phase 2 trials of drugs that may be cytostatic and for trials adding a new drug to an active regimen. Even single-agent phase 2 trials of cytotoxics have been criticized on the basis that they do not provide much evidence that the drug will be able to prolong survival when incorporated into a regimen with other active drugs. Demonstrating that the regimen incorporating the new drug prolongs progression-free survival compared to the control regimen may provide a stronger basis for conducting a phase 3 trial of the new regimen.

Simon et al.[12] suggested two key design differences between such randomized phase 2 designs and phase 3 designs. A randomized phase 2 design may use an end point that is a sensitive indicator of antitumor effect, although it may not be an acceptable phase 3 end point that directly reflects patient benefit. Such an endpoint does not need to be "validated." It is not claimed to be a valid surrogate for survival; no regulatory approval or practice standard decisions should be based on the phase 2 trials using such an intermediate

TABLE 36.4

Number of Patients to Treat in Single-Arm Phase 2 Trial Using Historic Controls and Binary End Point[a]

Proportion of Success for Historic Controls	Number of Historic Controls				
	30	40	50	75	100
0.10	94[b]	69	59	50	46
	36	32	30	28	27
	21	20	19	18	18
0.20	–	226	126	80	67
	68	49	43	36	33
	29	25	24	21	21
0.30	[c]	[c]	307	113	86
	132	69	54	41	37
	36	29	26	23	21
0.40	[c]	[c]	[c]	137	95
	267	83	59	43	37
	39	29	25	22	20
0.50	[c]	[c]	[c]	136	91
	370	80	54	38	33
	34	25	22	18	17
0.60	[c]	[c]	910	104	72
	178	56	39	28	25
	22	17	14	12	12

[a] One-sided significance level of 10% and power of 80%.
[b] First entry is number of new patients required to detect a 15 percentage-point difference. Second and third entries are for detecting 20 percentage-point and 25 percentage-point differences, respectively.
[c] Number of required new patients exceeds 1,000.

end point. The purpose of the phase 2 trial is merely to determine whether to conduct a phase 3 trial that will evaluate the new regimen with an accepted phase 3 end point The phase 2 trial may also serve to optimize the regimen that might be carried forward to phase 3 and to provide information about the best target population. The second key difference noted by Simon et al.[12] is that the type I error "alpha level" for planning and analyzing the phase 2 trial can be increased from the two-sided 5% level used for phase 3 trials. By letting this alpha level increase to a one-sided 10%, meaningful savings in number of patients required can be achieved.

How large should a randomized phase 2 design comparing a new treatment to a control regimen be? Consider, for example, a randomized phase 3 trial comparing a new regimen to a control in a patient population in which the median time to progression on the control is 6 months and the median survival is 2 years. A 25% reduction in the hazard of death amounts to a 4-month prolongation of median survival with exponential distributions. A phase 3 trial with 90% statistical power for detecting this effect at a two-sided 5% significance level would require about 510 deaths (see Table 36.7). With an average follow-up time of 2 years, 50% of the patients would have events and so the number of patients required for randomization would be just in excess of 1,000. A randomized phase 2 trial with 90% power for detecting a 33% reduction in hazard of progression corresponding to a 2-month increase in median progression-free survival at a one-sided 10% significance level would require observing 164 progression events (Table 36.5). With an average follow-up time of 2 years, >90% would have progression events and so a sample size of 180 total randomized patients would suffice. Accrual to the randomized phase 2 study could potentially be stopped early based on futility monitoring if results are not promising for the new regimen. The results in Table 36.5 show that if an imbalanced randomization is used in which two-thirds of the patients are randomized to the new treatment, the number of progression events needed increases to 185 instead of 164. So although a larger total sample size would be required, somewhat fewer patients would receive the control regimen.

The randomized phase 2 design with control regimen has also been discussed by Korn et al.[38] and by Rubinstein et al.[39] Randomized phase 2 trials can require fewer patients than phase 3 trials, but they generally require more patients than single-arm phase 2 trials. Nevertheless, they are generally necessary for evaluating time to event end points or for evaluating combination regimens. Table 36.6 shows number of patients required for randomized phase 2 trials where the primary end point is either response rate or the proportion of patients without progression by a specified landmark time.

Randomized Screening Designs

Phase 2 trials are generally viewed as a means of determining whether a particular regimen is worthy of phase 3 evaluation. They can, however, be viewed as way to screen a wide range of new regimens in order to select the most promising for phase 3 evaluation. Traditional single-arm phase 2 designs are problematic for screening when there is substantial interstudy variation in patient selection and outcome evaluation. Simon, Wittes, and Ellenberg[40] proposed the randomized phase 2 design in which multiple new regimens are randomized against each other as one way of

TABLE 36.5

Number of Total Events to Observe in Two-Arm Randomized Phase 2 Trial Based on Progression-Free Survival

Reduction in Hazard	Ratio of Medians	Equal Randomization				2:1 Randomization[a]			
		$\alpha = 0.05$[b]		$\alpha = 0.10$[b]		$\alpha = 0.05$[b]		$\alpha = 0.10$[b]	
		Power = 0.8	Power = 0.9	Power = 0.8	Power = 0.9	Power = 0.8	Power = 0.9	Power = 0.8	Power = 0.9
25%	1.33	301	417	219	319	339	469	246	358
30%	1.43	195	270	141	206	219	303	159	232
33%	1.5	155	215	113	164	175	242	127	185
40%	1.67	96	132	70	101	108	149	78	114
50%	2.0	52	72	38	55	59	81	43	62

[a] Two-thirds of patients are randomized to the new treatment group.
[b] One-sided significance level.

TABLE 36.6

Number of Patients in Each Arm of Randomized Phase 2 Trial Without Progresstion at T in Control Arm to New Treatment Arm[a]

T-mo DFS for Control Group	5% One-Sided Significance Level Increase in T-mo DFS				10% One-Sided Significance Level Increase in T-mo DFS			
	0.10	0.15	0.20	0.25	0.10	0.15	0.20	0.25
0.05	129	72	48	35	99	56	38	28
0.10	176	91	58	41	133	70	45	32
0.15	216	108	66	46	163	82	51	36
0.20	250	121	73	50	188	92	56	39
0.25	278	132	79	53	208	100	60	41
0.30	300	141	83	55	224	106	63	42
0.35	315	146	85	56	235	110	65	43
0.40	324	149	86	56	243	112	65	43

DFS, disease-free survival
[a] Eighty percent statistical power.

avoiding such interstudy variablility in prioritizing the candidate regimens.[40] This randomized design can provide more interpretable results if it also incorporates a control arm. This design is more efficient than separate randomized phase 2 trials because the control arm does not have to be replicated in all of the randomized phase 2 trials. Using the example described previously, if it takes 90 patients per arm to conduct a randomized phase 2 trial, instead of $180 \times 5 = 900$ patients to conduct randomized phase 2 trials of five new regimens, one would require only $90 \times 6 = 540$ patients, a savings of 40%. The savings in number of patients can be even more dramatic if one takes the position that the objective is not to evaluate all five new regimens, but rather to select the best one and determine whether it is worthy of phase 3 evaluation. For this selection objective, one does not require 90 patients per arm.[40] These designs have been discussed and extended by others.[41–44]

Simon et al.[12] showed that one can take advantage of the nontoxic nature of some molecularly targeted drugs to efficiently evaluate multiple regimens in the same study. They propose using a factorial design in which concurrent randomizations are made for each drugs. For example, if there are three drugs (A, B, C) being evaluated, then some patients will receive all three, some will receive pairs (AB, AC, or BC), some will receive single drugs (A, B, C), and one group will receive none of the drugs. In evaluating each drug, the time to progression for all patients receiving that drug are compared to the times for all patients not receiving that drug. The trial can be sized as if it were a single two-arm trial. The design is effective as long as there are not negative interactions among drugs. Negative interactions would result from the toxicity of one drug interfering with the full-dose administration of other drugs, which may not be a problem for many molecularly targeted drugs. The design is also useful for attempting to identify combinations that are therapeutically synergistic, a circumstance of particular importance with molecularly targeted drugs.

Rosner, Stadler, and Ratain[45] describe a "randomized discontinuation design" for phase 2 studies of therapeutically targeted drugs. All eligible patients are started on the drug and given two to four courses of treatment. Patients are then evaluated: Those with progression are removed from study, those with objective tumor response are continued on treatment, and the remaining patients are randomized to either continue or discontinue the drug. The continued and discontinued groups of randomized patients are compared with regard to time to progression. Freidlin and Simon[46] evaluated and further developed this design. It may require as large a number of patients started on treatment as a straightforward randomized phase 2 design. The advantage of the design is that because all patients start on the new regimen, accrual rate may be better with the randomized discontinuation design.

Seamless Phase 2/3 Designs

Hunsberger, Zhao, and Simon[47] developed a design for a seamless phase 2/3 design. Patients are randomized between a new regimen and control. An interim analysis is performed using a phase 2 end point such as response rate or time to progression to decide whether the results with the new treatment as sufficiently promising to continue to a phase 3 sample size. If accrual continues, then the final analysis is performed using an acceptable phase 3 end point. A similar approach was described by Goldmamn LeBlanc, and Crowley.[48] Phase 2/3 designs using Bayesian methods have been reviewed by Thall.[49] Sher and Heller[50] proposed conducting phase 3 trials with multiple experimental regimens, a control arm, and early termination of all experimental arms that are not promising. They used the statistical design of Schaid, Wieand, and Therneau[51] for time to event data. Thall, Simon, and Ellenberg[52] had studied such designs when the end point was binary. A similar approach was recommended by Parmar et al.[53] Freidlin et al.[54] have discussed statistical and practical aspects of conducting clinical trials with a control arm and multiple new treatment arms. Freidlin, McShane, and Polley[55] have also introduced a design for a randomized phase 2 design of a new drug with a candidate predictive biomarker for determining whether the drug is entirely inactive, active only in the marker positive group, or active regardless of the biomarker status. This design enables investigators to appropriately plan whether to continue biomarker development into phase 3 development.

DESIGN OF PHASE 3 CLINICAL TRIALS

Good therapeutic research requires asking important questions and getting reliable answers. The most important clinical trials are often the most difficult to conduct.[56] They may involve withholding a treatment established by tradition, transferring patient management responsibility across specialties, standardizing procedures among physicians, and sharing recognition with a large group of collaborators.

End Points

Phase 3 trials attempt to provide guidance to practicing physicians to help them make treatment decisions with their patients.

Consequently, the trials should provide reliable information concerning end points of relevance to the patients. The major end points for evaluating the effectiveness of a treatment should be direct measures of patient welfare. Survival and symptom control are two such end points. The latter is not routinely used because of the difficulty of measuring it reliably and because it may be influenced by concomitant treatments.

Although durable complete regression of metastatic disease is usually a good surrogate for prolonged survival, partial tumor shrinkage usually is not an appropriate end point for phase 3 trials. Torri et al.[57] performed a meta-analysis of the relationship between difference in response rates and difference in median survivals for randomized clinical trials of advanced ovarian carcinoma. They found that large improvements in response rates corresponded to very small improvements in median survival. Hence, use of response rate as an end point may result in giving patients increasingly intensive and toxic therapy with little or no net benefit to them. Proper validation of an end point as a surrogate for clinical benefit requires a series of randomized clinical trials in which treatment differences with regard to the candidate surrogate are related to treatment differences with regard to clinical benefit.[58–60] It is not sufficient to show that clinical outcome is related to the candidate surrogate measured on the same treatment arm as this may just reflect the known responder versus nonresponder bias.

Disease-free survival is often accepted as an important measure of clinical benefit to be used as an end point for adjuvant treatment trials. There is more controversy, however, about the use of time to progression in metastatic disease trials. The controversy relates to whether prolonged time to progression provides clinical benefit and whether it can be measured without bias. With unblinded evaluation of time to progression, there could be a reduced threshold for declaring progression for control patients so that they can cross over to the new treatment.[61] Central party blinded review of progression is often used to avoid such potential bias. Because the review is not performed in real-time, however, it can introduce additional biases of "informative censoring." Freidlin et al.[62] proposed an approach to adjusting for increased surveillance of the control group. Dodd et al.[63] proposed that central review be performed only for a subset of patients to evaluate whether local assessments were biased, not to replace local assessments.

Patient Eligibility

To ensure that the results of phase 3 trials are applicable to patients seen in the community outside of clinical research settings, the trials often involve numerous centers and extensive community participation. In order to ensure broad generalization of conclusions, most multicenter phase 3 trials have employed broad eligibility criteria. In the United Kingdom, many trials have been designed using the *uncertainty principle*, an approach that leaves much of the decision making about eligibility to the treating physician. There may be guidelines for eligibility, but the ultimate decision is made by the treating physician; if he or she is uncertain about which treatment is more appropriate for the patient, the patient is eligible.

There is a growing recognition, however, that the one of the key hallmarks of cancer is intertumor heterogeneity. Tumors that arise in the same primary site are often quite different with regard to their oncogenesis, pathophysiology, and drug sensitivity. Consequently, conducting broad eligibility clinical trials with drugs only expected to be effective for an identifiable subset of patients is often no longer an appropriate research strategy.[64–66] Particularly with molecularly targeted drugs, effectiveness is likely to be limited to a sensitive subset of tumors that may be characterized based on whether the molecular target of the drug is deregulated in the tumor. Even with cytotoxics, many patients are generally treated for each patient who benefits. The high costs of many molecularly targeted drugs make the traditional broad eligibility trial approach increasingly unsustainable.

Clinical trials can be conducted with fewer patients if patients are selected based on assays that identify the tumors likely to be sensitive to the drug in question. Simon and Maitournam[67,68] and others[69,70] have evaluated the efficiency of such targeted designs. When fewer than half of the patients "test positive" and when the new treatment has little benefit for patients who test negative, the required sample size can be dramatically reduced by restricting eligibility to patients who test positive. Simon and Zhao have made available a web-based computer program to enable investigators to compare such designs to standard broad eligibility designs (http://linus.nci.nih.gov/brb).

This targeted approach was effectively used for the development of trastuzumab in patients with metastatic breast cancer. In that case, about 450 patients whose tumors overexpressed HER-2 participated in a randomized clinical trial that provided convincing evidence that trastuzumab prolonged survival. Had the study been conducted without evaluating HER-2 expression, >8,000 patients would have been needed for similar statistical power.[67] Even had a huge study of unselected patients been conducted and given a statistically significant result, the size of the benefit would have been very small as the benefit in the 25% of patients with HER-2 overexpression would have been diluted by lack of benefit from the remaining 75%. It is questionable whether such a small benefit overall would have justified approval or use of a drug with clear and serious toxicities.

In many cases where the biologic credentials of a predictive biomarker are less compelling, one will want to include patients who are both marker positive and marker negative but to require that all patients have the marker evaluated, to size the trial so that there is adequate statistical power for evaluating treatment effect separately in the patients who are marker positive and to use a multiple testing method that ensures that the study-wise type I error level does not exceed 5%. Simon and others have described "all comers" designs of this type.[71–74] Zhao and Simon provide web-based computer programs at http://linus.nci.nih.gov/brb to facilitate use of such designs in clinical trials. Freidlin, McShane, and Korn[75] have described the use of biomarker designs in cancer clinical trials. These enrichment and all-comers designs presume that a single predictive biomarker with an analytically validated test and a threshold of positivity has been developed prior to the start of the phase 3 clinical trial. Because of the complexity of cancer biology, this is not always possible. Several adaptive designs have been developed to enable some aspects of biomarker specification to be included in the phase 3 trial while also rigorously evaluating the statistical significance of the treatment effect in the "biomarker positive" population. The "adaptive threshold design" avoids the requirement that the threshold of positivity be prespecified,[76] and the "adaptive signature design" enables multiple candidate biomarkers to be evaluated.[77,78] Hong and Simon[79] developed a run-in design that permits a pharmacodynamic, immunologic, or intermediate response end point measured after a short run-in period on the new treatment to be used as the predictive biomarker. Simon, Paik, and Hayes[80] described a prospective-retrospective approach to using archived tumor specimens for a focused re-analysis of a randomized phase 3 trial with regard to a predictive biomarker. The approach requires that archived specimens be available on most patients, and that an analysis plan focused on a single marker be developed prior to performing the blinded assays. This approach was used in establishing that a K-RAS mutation was a negative predictive biomarker for response of patients with colorectal cancer to antiepidermal growth factor receptor antibodies.

Randomization

To determine whether a new treatment cures any patients with a disease that is uniformly and rapidly fatal, history is a satisfactory control. Once we leave this setting of complete determinism, however, the definition of an adequate nonrandomized control group becomes problematic. In comparing outcomes for patients

PRACTICE OF ONCOLOGY

receiving two different treatments when the treatment assignment was not randomized, often diagnostic and staging procedures and other factors used explicitly or implicitly for selecting patients for each treatment are different. Some of these factors may be difficult to quantify but strongly prognostic. Some of the factors may be previously unsuspected as being of prognostic importance. Also, supportive care, secondary treatments, and methods of evaluation and follow-up may be different for the two treatment groups. In comparisons of a new treatment to a historic control, patients receiving the new treatment are often much more highly selected than the control group. Often, there is inadequate information to determine whether prognostic differences are present, and current known prognostic factors may not have been measured for the controls. It generally is difficult or impossible to determine whether the controls would have been eligible for the current study and in what way they represent a selection of all eligible patients.

Formation of the control group by random treatment assignment as an integral part of the planned study can avoid most of the systematic biases just mentioned. Randomization does not ensure that the study will include a representative sample of all patients with the disease, but it does help to ensure an unbiased evaluation of the relative merits of the two treatments for the types of patients entered.

It is sometimes said that randomization is unnecessary because matched historic or concurrent controls can be selected. However, matching can be done only with regard to known prognostic factors, and those factors often do not account for enough of the variation in patient outcome to assure that an unbiased historic control group can be constructed. It also is sometimes said that randomization is not effective in ensuring that the treatment groups are similar with regard to unknown prognostic factors unless the number of patients is large. This is true but reflects a misunderstanding of the purpose of randomization. Randomization does not ensure that the groups are medically equivalent, but it distributes the unknown biasing factors according to a known random distribution so that their effects can be rigorously allowed for in significance tests and confidence intervals. This is true regardless of the study size. A significance level represents the probability that differences in outcome can be the result of random fluctuations. Without a randomized treatment allocation, a "statistically significant difference" may be the result of a nonrandom difference in the distribution of unknown prognostic factors.

In many cases, there is a role for both randomized and nonrandomized trials in drug development. The nonrandomized format can in some cases be used for determining which regimens are sufficiently promising for randomized phase 3 evaluation and in clinical settings in which outcome is uniformly poor. For major questions of public health importance, unless the expected treatment effect on outcome is very large, the need for reliable answers dictates the use of randomized phase 3 trials.

Randomization of a patient should be performed after the patient has been found eligible and has consented to participate in the trial and to accept either of the randomized options. A truly random and nondecipherable randomization procedure should be used and implemented by calling a central randomization office staffed by individuals who are independent of participating physicians.

Stratification

When important prognostic factors are known for patients in a randomized trial, it is often advisable to stratify the randomization to ensure equal distribution of these factors. This is usually accomplished by preparing a separate randomization list for each stratum of patients. Each list must be balanced so that after each block of 4 to 10 patients within the stratum, the treatment groups contain equal numbers of patients. Within the blocks, the sequence of treatment assignments is random. The stratification factors must be known for each patient at the time of randomization.

It is generally best to limit stratification to those factors definitely known to have important independent effects on outcome. If two factors are closely correlated, only one needs to be included. Many clinical trialists believe that stratification is an unnecessary complication because adjustment for imbalances of known factors can be made in the analysis and has negligible effect on statistical power. Stratification may help to ensure balance for interim analyses when the sample sizes may be limited and provides the medical audience with confidence in the results, which often is not available when depending on complex adjustment methods to deal with prognostic imbalances. Stratification also is a convenient way of specifying a priori what are considered the important prognostic factors.

Many clinical trials use dynamic stratification methods. The most popular such method is that conceived by Pocock and Simon,[81] which permits effective balancing with regard to many prognostic factors. There has been some concern about the effect of adaptive stratification on analysis of treatment differences. Multiple studies, including those by Kalish and Begg,[82] have demonstrated that if the stratification factors are included in the model used for final analysis, the effect of adaptive stratification is to make the true type I error less than the nominal rate, hence the analyses are slightly conservative. Simon and Simon[83] showed that model-based analyses are not necessary to use with adaptive stratification methods. One can define a linear test statistic that reflects the treatment effect difference on the outcome adjusted for the stratification variables, and generate the null distribution of the test statistic by reapplying the adaptive stratification method. The Pocock-Simon[81] method of adaptively stratified treatment assignment is not deterministic. Consequently, one can replicate the stratified treatment assignments, holding fixed the order of patient registrations and the stratification variables of the patients, recompute the value of the test statistic for the rerandomized treatment assignment, repeat this process a thousand times, and thereby generate the null distribution of the test statistic. Consequently, although the use of adaptive stratification methods, like the use of all stratification methods, are not essential, the criticisms of their effect on final analyses are unjustified.

Sample Size

The protocol for a phase 3 trial should specify the number of patients to be accrued and the duration of follow-up after the close of accrual when the final analysis will be performed. Methods of sample size planning are usually based on the assumption that at the conclusion of the follow-up period, a statistical significance test will be performed comparing the experimental treatment to the control treatment with regard to a single primary end point. A statistical significance level of 0.05 means that if there is no true difference in treatment effectiveness, the probability of obtaining a difference in outcomes as extreme as that observed in the data is 0.05. The significance level does not represent the probability that the null hypothesis is true; it represents a probability of an observed difference, assuming that the null hypothesis is true. Conventional statistical theory ascribes no probabilities to hypotheses, only to data.

A one-sided significance level represents the probability, by chance alone, of obtaining a difference as large as and in the same direction as that actually observed. A two-sided significance level represents the probability of obtaining by chance a difference in either direction as large in absolute magnitude as that actually observed. The two-sided significance level is usually twice the one-sided significance level. Controversy exists over the appropriateness of one-sided or two-sided significance levels. Although this is a somewhat trivial issue, a two-sided significance level of 0.05 has become widely accepted as a standard level of evidence.

The probability of obtaining a statistically significant result when the treatments differ in effectiveness is called the *power* of the trial. As the sample size and extent of follow-up increases, the power increases. The power depends critically, however, on the

TABLE 36.7

Number of Events Needed for Comparing Survival Curves

Percentage Reduction in Hazard of Death	Ratio of Median Survival for Exponential Distributions	Number of Total Deaths to Observe[a]
25	1.33	508
30	1.43	330
33	1.50	257
40	1.67	162
50	2.0	88

[a] Total number of deaths in both groups to have power = 0.90 for detecting ratio of median survival. Type I error $\alpha = 0.05$ (two-sided).

size of the true difference in effectiveness of the two treatments. Generally, one sizes the trial so that the power is either 0.80 or 0.90 when the true difference in effectiveness is the smallest size that is considered medically important to detect.

Statisticians have developed useful methods for planning sample size to compare survival curves or disease-free survival curves in phase 3 trials. Table 36.7 shows the number of total events needed assuming that the *hazard ratio*—the ratio of forces of mortality for the two treatment groups—is constant over time.[84] Table 36.7 shows the total number of events that must occur in a given cohort to provide 90% power for detecting a specified reduction in the hazard for the experimental treatment relative to the control

treatment. For exponential distributions, the percentage reduction in hazard of death can be expressed as a ratio of median survivals, which is displayed in the second column of Table 36.7. When the primary end point is overall survival, the events are deaths; for disease-free survival curves, events are deaths or recurrences. The translation of the number of deaths or events required to the number of patients required depends on the actual shape of the survival distributions, the rate of accrual, and the duration of follow-up after close of accrual. Generally, however, it is best to specify the time of the final analysis as the time when the specified number of deaths or events is obtained—not in terms of absolute calendar time.

In some cases, it may be convenient to think in terms of the proportion of patients without progression or death beyond some landmark time, such as 5 years. Tables 36.8 and 36.9 provide required numbers of patients for clinical trials planned on this basis. This approach is less flexible for studies in which survival or disease-free survival is the end point, as it presumes that all patients will be followed for the landmark time as a minimum. These tables can, however, be used generally for detecting differences in a binary end point, denoted *success rate* in the tables. For comparing treatments in phase 3 trials, differences of >15 to 20 percentage-points usually are considered unrealistic. Establishing a sample size that provides good statistical power for detecting realistically expected treatment improvements is important. Many published "negative" results are actually uninterpretable because the sample sizes are too small.[85]

FACTORIAL DESIGNS

The 2^K factorial design was described in the section on randomized phase 2 trials, but it can also be used for phase 3 trials. The two-by-two factorial design is the version most often used. There are four treatment groups: one receiving neither of the two drugs

TABLE 36.8

Number of Patients in Each of Two Treatment Groups to Compare Proportions (One-Sided Test)

Smaller Success Rate	Larger Minus Smaller Success Rate									
	0.05	0.10	0.15	0.20	0.25	0.30	0.35	0.40	0.45	0.50
0.05	512[a]	172	94	62	45	35	28	23	19	16
	381[b]	129	72	48	35	27	22	18	15	13
0.10	786	236	121	76	54	40	31	25	21	17
	579	176	91	58	41	31	24	20	16	14
0.15	1,026	292	144	88	60	44	34	27	22	18
	752	216	108	66	46	34	26	21	17	14
0.20	1,231	339	163	98	66	48	36	29	23	19
	900	250	121	73	50	37	28	22	18	15
0.25	1,402	377	178	105	70	50	38	29	23	19
	1,024	278	132	79	53	38	29	23	18	15
0.30	1,539	407	189	111	73	52	38	30	23	19
	1,122	300	141	83	55	39	30	23	18	15
0.35	1,642	429	197	114	74	52	38	29	23	18
	1,196	315	146	85	56	40	30	23	18	14
0.40	1,711	441	201	115	74	52	38	29	22	17
	1,246	324	149	86	56	39	29	22	17	14
0.45	1,745	446	201	114	73	50	36	27	21	16
	1,271	327	149	85	55	38	28	21	16	13
0.50	1,745	441	197	111	70	48	34	25	19	15
	1,271	324	146	83	53	37	26	20	15	12

[a] Upper figure: significance level = 0.05, power = 0.90.
[b] Lower figure: significance level = 0.05, power = 0.80.

TABLE 36.9

Number of Patients in Each of Two Treatment Groups to Compare Proportions (Two-Sided Test)

Smaller Success Rate	Larger Minus Smaller Success Rate									
	0.05	0.10	0.15	0.20	0.25	0.30	0.35	0.40	0.45	0.50
0.05	620[a]	206	113	74	54	42	33	27	23	19
	473[b]	159	88	58	43	33	27	22	18	16
0.10	956	285	146	92	64	48	38	30	25	21
	724	218	112	71	50	38	30	24	20	17
0.15	1,250	354	174	106	73	53	41	33	26	22
	944	269	133	82	57	42	32	26	21	18
0.20	1,502	411	197	118	79	57	44	34	27	22
	1,132	313	151	91	62	45	34	27	22	18
0.25	1,712	459	216	127	84	60	45	35	28	23
	1,289	348	165	98	65	47	36	28	22	18
0.30	1,880	495	230	134	88	62	46	36	28	22
	1,414	375	175	103	68	48	36	28	22	18
0.35	2,006	522	239	138	89	63	46	35	27	22
	1,509	395	182	106	69	49	36	28	22	18
0.40	2,090	537	244	139	89	62	45	34	26	21
	1,571	407	186	107	69	48	36	27	21	17
0.45	2,132	543	244	138	88	60	44	33	25	19
	1,603	411	186	106	68	47	34	26	20	16
0.50	2,132	537	239	134	84	57	41	30	23	17
	1,603	407	182	103	65	45	32	24	18	14

[a] Upper figure: significance level = 0.05, power = 0.90.
[b] Lower figure: significance level = 0.05, power = 0.80.

A or B, one receiving A, one receiving B, and one receiving both. Although there are four treatment groups, the average effect of each treatment factor can be evaluated using all of the patients. To evaluate the effect of A, you compare outcomes for patients receiving A to outcomes for those not receiving A, ignoring B. Usually, the sample size for a two-by-two factorial trial is computed assuming that there is no interaction between the effects of the two drugs. The sample size is approximately the same as for a simple two-arm trial. The factorial design offers the possibility of answering two questions for the cost of one, but there is a risk of ambiguity in the interpretation of results.[86] For situations in which negative interactions are unlikely or in which it is unlikely that both factors will have substantial effects, the factorial design can provide a substantial improvement in the efficiency of clinical trials.

Simon and Freedman[87] developed a Bayesian method for the design and analysis of factorial trials. Their approach avoids the need to dichotomize one's assumptions that interactions either do or do not exist, and provides a flexible approach to the design and analysis of such clinical trials. The Bayesian approach also avoids a preliminary test of interaction; such tests have poor power and basing the analysis on such tests is problematic. The Bayesian model suggests that in planning a factorial trial in which interactions are unlikely but cannot be excluded, the sample size should be increased by approximately 30%, as compared to a simple two-arm clinical trial for detecting the same size of treatment effect. The 30% figure allows for a 5% prior probability of a medically important, qualitative interaction between the treatment effects.

Noninferiority Trials

Noninferiority trials often compare a standard treatment to a less invasive or more convenient therapy that is not expected to be superior to the standard treatment with regard to the primary end point.

For such trials, the secondary benefits of the new regimen, while important, is not worth reductions in effectiveness in the primary end point. Unfortunately, it is not possible to establish that the two treatments are completely equivalent with regard to the primary end point. The usual approach is to plan the trial to have high statistical power for detecting small reductions in effectiveness, and this requires a large sample size. Because failure to reject the standard null hypothesis of no treatment difference results in adoption of a new, and potentially inferior, regimen, misinterpretation of the results of noninferiority trials can result in serious problems. For the analysis of such trials, confidence intervals rather than statistical significance tests should be emphasized.[88] The confidence interval for the true difference of effectiveness gives a much clearer picture of which differences are consistent with the data. Makuch and Simon[89] and Durrleman and Simon[90] discuss this approach for planning and monitoring therapeutic equivalence trials.

Noninferiority trials are generally planned to distinguish the null hypothesis that the treatments are equivalent from the alternative that the new treatment is inferior by an amount δ. One of the key problems in designing a noninferiority trial is specification of δ. A small value of δ leads to a large trial. A large value of δ can lead to a small but meaningless trial. The reduction in effectiveness that the trial will be able to detect should be some fraction of the effectiveness of the standard treatment. For example, suppose the standard treatment is 12 months of a chemotherapy regimen that increases 5-year survival by 10 percentage-points relative to no chemotherapy and the new regimen of interest is use of the same regimen for only 6 months. If we want to have high power for detecting a reduction in effectiveness by half, then δ should represent a difference of 5 percentage-points in 5-year survival. If we want high power for detecting a reduction in effectiveness by one-quarter, then δ should represent a difference of 2.5 percentage-points in 5-year survival. An appropriate value of δ can only be determined based on a careful review of the studies that established the effectiveness of the standard treatment. If those studies do not exist or are not adequate, a noninferiority trial may not be appropriate.

Another problem in the design of noninferiority trials is the lack of internal validation of the assumption that the control treatment is actually effective for the patient population at hand. If the effectiveness of the standard treatment is highly variable among studies, there is the risk that a new regimen will be found noninferior to the standard because the standard is not effective in the current study. Consequently, noninferiority trials are only appropriate when the standard regimen is highly and reproducibly effective.

None of the conventional frequentist approaches to the design and analysis of therapeutic equivalence trials satisfactorily account for the uncertainty in estimation of the effectiveness of the standard treatment. Simon[91] developed a Bayesian approach that addresses this problem. The effectiveness of the control treatment C relative to the previous standard (P) is represented by a parameter β. Information about the effectiveness of C relative to P is summarized by a prior distribution, which is normal with mean μ_β and standard deviation σ_β. These values are obtained from a random-effects meta-analysis of the previously conducted randomized trials comparing C to P. The result of the noninferiority trial is summarized by an estimate $\hat{\delta}$ with standard error of the effectiveness of test regimen E relative to C. With some simplifying assumptions, the posterior distribution of the effectiveness of E relative to P is a normal distribution with mean $\mu_\beta + \hat{\delta}$ and variance $\sigma_\beta^2 + \sigma^2$. Simon[90] also shows how the sample size of the therapeutic equivalence trial may be planned and how the size depends critically on the strength and consistency of the evidence that the active control C is superior to P and on the size of that difference in effectiveness.

Bayesian Methods

Conventional statistical methods (i.e., *frequentist method*) regard the data collected in an experiment as being random; they test hypotheses about parameters that represent fixed but unknown treatment effects. For example, frequentist methods derive probability statements about differences in observed response rates under an assumed null hypothesis that the true response probabilities are equal. *Bayesian* statistical methods consider the parameters, as well as the data, as being random and selected from *prior distributions*. What does the assumption that the true treatment effect is a random draw from a prior distribution mean? One interpretation is that we regard the prior distribution as expressing our subjective beliefs about the value of the treatment effect based on previous experience with this treatment and other similar treatments. Such subjective prior distributions would vary among individuals based on their experience, biases, circumstances, and perhaps economic interests. Bayesian methods use Bayes' theorem to update the prior distributions of the parameters based on data from the study to produce the posterior distributions of the parameters. Using the posterior distributions, hypotheses about whether the treatments are equivalent can be tested. Consequently, Bayesian methods can derive direct probability statements about the parameters, such as "the probability that the treatment effect is 0.04." The probability statements about the parameters seem to tell us what we want to know, but the results may depend as much on our prior distributions as on the data.

Many Bayesian statisticians use "noninformative" prior distributions. For example, a noninformative prior distribution for the difference in response probabilities might be constant for all differences between −1 and +1. That noninformative prior represents the belief that huge differences are just as likely as small differences, positive differences as likely as negative differences. Consequently, methods based on apparently innocuous noninformative prior distributions may not be appropriate for real-world studies. In some cases, the treatment being evaluated can be considered "exchangeable" with other treatments that have been previously evaluated and a prior distribution can be defined based on that

previous experience. Spiegelhalter, Freedman, and Parmar[92] have suggested analysis of a clinical trial with regard to both an "enthusiastic" prior and a "skeptical" prior. The former might be held by a developer of the treatment and the later by a regulator. Robust conclusions are obtained when the data is so extensive and strong that the posterior distributions are little changed regardless of whether you use an enthusiastic or skeptical prior. Unfortunately, such robustness generally requires a very large sample size, much larger than indicated by use of standard frequentist methods. For some parameters, there may be a consensus prior distribution. For example, for evaluating cytotoxics there was generally broad consensus that large treatment-effect by patient-subset interactions were unlikely, and Simon[93] used this in a Bayesian approach to subset analysis. Generally, however, there is no meaningful prior consensus about the effect of treatment. Randomized clinical trials are done because the opinions of experts are often wrong. The subjective nature of the prior distribution is problematic for the interpretation of phase 3 clinical trials.

There are several important misconceptions about the use of Bayesian methods for clinical trials. First, some people believe that Bayesian methods provide an adequate alternative to randomized treatment assignment. In fact, however, randomization is just as important for the validity of Bayesian methods as for frequentist methods.[94] Second, some people mistakenly believe that Bayesian clinical trials require fewer patients than frequentist trials. Bayesian sample size calculations depend on the prior distribution used. Using *skeptical priors*, the sample size needed with Bayesian methods may be much larger than the conventional sample size. Third, some statisticians believe that the main impediment to use of Bayesian methods in clinical trials has been the difficulty of computing posterior distributions. The main limitation has, however, been the fact that subjectivity of analysis is problematic for phase 3 clinical trials.

Bayesian methods can be very useful for phase 1 and phase 2 trials. For such trials, the prior distribution need only be appropriate for the investigator or sponsor. For phase 3 trials, the situation is more complex. Bayesian methods are applicable to phase 3 problems in which a concensus prior is appropriate. Such priors are possible for parameters representing interaction effects,[93] for the effectiveness of active controls in noninferiority trials,[91] and for unexpected findings with multiple safety end points.[95] As indicated previously, however, subjective opinion of the investigator or sponsor should have no role in testing the primary hypothesis of whether the new treatment is better than the control for the prespecified target population. Once the basic effectiveness of the treatment is established, however, there are many other analyses that can help physicians decide how to use the new treatment. Those analyses generally cannot be answered as precisely or with as little chance of error as the testing of the primary null hypothesis. Different physicians may have varying prior beliefs about the treatment and how its effectiveness might vary among patients; Bayesian methods may be useful for physicians in determining how to implement the results in the context of the patients they see. One must recognize, however, that Bayesian models can be overfit to data like any other models and can produce poor predictions.

ANALYSIS OF PHASE 3 CLINICAL TRIALS

Intention-to-Treat Analysis

The *intention-to-treat* principle indicates that all randomized patients should be included in the primary analysis of the trial. For cancer trials, this has often been interpreted to mean all "eligible" randomized patients. Excluding patients from analysis because of treatment deviations, early death, or patient withdrawal can severely distort the results.[96–98] Often, excluded patients have poorer outcomes than do those who are not excluded. Investigators frequently rationalize that the poor outcome experienced by a patient was due to lack of compliance to treatment, but the direction of causality may be the reverse. For example, in the Coronary Drug Project, the 5-year mortality for poor adherents to the placebo regimen was 28.3%, significantly greater than the 15.1% experienced by good adherents to the placebo regimen.[99] In randomized trials, there may be poorer compliance in one treatment group than the other, or the reasons for poor compliance may differ. Excluding patients, or analyzing them separately (which is equivalent to excluding them), for reasons other than eligibility is generally considered unacceptable. The intention-to-treat analysis with all eligible randomized patients should be the primary analysis. If the conclusions of a study depend on exclusions, these conclusions are suspect. The treatment plan should be viewed as a policy to be evaluated. The treatment intended cannot be delivered uniformly to all patients, but all eligible patients should generally be evaluable in phase 3 trials.

Interim Analyses

If statistical significance tests are performed repeatedly, the probability that the difference in outcomes will be found to be statistically significant (at the 0.05 level) at some point may be considerably >5%. This probability is called the *type I error* of the analysis plan. Fleming, Green, and Harrington[100] have shown that the type I error can be as great as 26% if a statistical significance test is performed every 3 months of a 3-year trial that compares two identical treatments. Some trials are published without stating the target sample size, without indicating whether a target sample size was stated in the protocol, and without describing whether the published analysis represented a planned final analysis or was one of multiple analyses performed during the course of the trial. In such cases, one must suspect that the investigators were not aware of good statistical practices and of the dangers of informal multiple analyses.

Interim analyses can be very misleading and interfere with a physician's attempt to state honestly to the patient that there is no reliable evidence indicating that one treatment option or the other is preferable. Consequently, it has become standard in phase 3 multicenter clinical trials to have a data-monitoring committee review interim results, rather than having the monitoring done by participating physicians. This approach helps to protect patients by having interim results carefully evaluated by an experienced group of individuals and helps to protect the study from damage that ensues from misinterpretation of interim results.[101,102] Generally, interim outcome information is available to only the data-monitoring committee. The study leaders are not part of the data-monitoring committee, because they may have a perceived conflict of interest in continuing the trial. The data-monitoring committee determines when results are mature and should be released. These procedures are used only for phase 3 trials.

A number of useful statistical designs have been developed for monitoring interim results. The simplest is due to Haybittle.[103] Interim differences are discounted unless the difference is statistically significant at the two-sided $p < 0.0025$ level. If the interim differences are not significant at that level, the trial continues until its originally intended size. The final analysis is performed without regard to the interim analyses, and the type I error is almost unaffected by the monitoring. Many others have developed group-sequential methods for interim monitoring based on a prespecified number of planned interim analyses. One of the most commonly used methods is that of O'Brien and Fleming.[104] The critical p value for determining whether an interim difference should be judged statistically significant depends on the number of analyses that will be performed during the trial. For a five-stage trial—four interim analyses and one final analysis—the critical p values are shown in Table 36.10.[105] The experience of the US

cancer cooperative groups with interim analysis of phase 3 clinical trials was reviewed by Korn, Freidlin, and Mooney.[106]

Extreme treatment differences at an interim analysis are less usual in cancer clinical trials than finding that interim results do not support the hypothesis that the experimental treatment is substantially better than the control. Futility analyses are important in order to avoid exposing patients to a more toxic and debilitating new treatment E once the essential outcome of the trial is well assured.[107] Data-monitoring committees are charged with helping to make these difficult judgments. A variety of statistical approaches to "futility monitoring" have been developed.[108] Goldman, LeBlanc, and Crowley[48] have shown that futility analyses based on intermediate end points like disease-free survival can be particularly effective even in trials where the primary endpoint is survival.

The method of stochastic curtailment[109] is widely used for "futility analyses." At any interim analysis, the probability of rejecting the null hypothesis at the end of the trial is computed. This probability is calculated as being conditional on the data already obtained and on the assumption that the alternative hypothesis of superiority of the experimental treatment used initially in planning the sample size for the trial is true. If this conditional power is less than approximately 0.20, then the trial may be terminated with acceptance of the null hypothesis. The 0.20 cutoff can be raised substantially to at least 0.40 if this type of interim analysis is performed only a few times during the course of the trial. With stochastic curtailment, interim analyses need not be equally spaced, and the number of interim analyses need not be specified in advance.

Significance Levels, Hypothesis Tests, and Confidence Intervals

Medical decision making is complicated, and clinicians frequently misinterpret statistical significance tests in search of clear-cut answers from ambiguous data. A statistical significance level for comparing outcomes represents the probability of obtaining a difference as large as that actually observed if the treatments were actually of equal efficacy and differences occur merely by chance. After significance tests had been used for many years, Neyman and Pearson formalized a mathematical theory of hypothesis testing. In this theory, a study must prespecify a null hypothesis, an alternative hypothesis, and a decision rule for accepting one hypothesis and rejecting the other based on the data obtained. The theory has appealed to clinicians because it simplifies complex medical decision making by providing yes or no answers: either the difference is statistically significant or it is not. The distinction between one- and two-sided decision rules becomes crucial because a one-sided $p = 0.05$ is simply nonsignificant if a type I error of 0.05 based on a two-sided decision rule is prespecified.

TABLE 36.10				
Nominal Two-Sided Significance Levels for Early Stopping in Interim Monitoring Methods That Maintain an Overall Type I Error Level of 0.05				
Analysis Number	**Pocock[125]**	**Haybittle[103]**	**O'Brien and Fleming[104]**	**Fleming et al.[105]**
1	0.016	0.0027	0.00001	0.0051
2	0.016	0.0027	0.0013	0.0061
3	0.016	0.0027	0.008	0.0073
4	0.016	0.0027	0.023	0.0089
Final	0.016	0.049	0.041	0.0402

The concept of prespecification of hypotheses is important for medical experimentation. However, the accept–reject nomenclature of the Neyman-Pearson theory provides an oversimplified and sometimes misleading interpretation of the data. Significance levels can serve as useful aids to interpretation of results, but quibbling about whether a one-sided $p = 0.04$ is significant makes little sense. Significance levels are influenced by sample sizes, and failure to reject the null hypothesis does not mean that the treatments are equivalent. There is no simple index of truth for interpreting results. Some attempt to use the notion of statistical significance in this way, but thorough presentation, skeptical evaluation, and cautious interpretation of results always are required.

Confidence intervals are generally much more informative than are significance levels. A confidence interval for the size of the treatment difference provides a range of effects consistent with the data. The significance level tells nothing about the size of the treatment effect because it depends on the sample size. However, it is the size of the treatment effect, as communicated by a confidence interval, that should be used in weighing the costs and benefits of clinical decision making. Many so-called negative results are actually noninformative, and confidence intervals help to determine when this is the case. Simon[88] has presented a nontechnical discussion of how to calculate confidence intervals for treatment differences with the types of end points commonly used in cancer clinical trials.

Calculation of Survival Curves

Most cancer clinical trials display results by showing survival curves or disease-free survival curves. Survival curves display the probability of surviving beyond any specified time, with time shown on the horizontal axis. In disease-free survival curves, it is the time until recurrence or death that is shown. Other time-to-event distributions can be similarly represented using the same methods. The usual statistical methods are not appropriate for analyzing survival because they ignore the fact that surviving patients have a limited follow-up period after which their survivals are "censored."

The most satisfactory way of representing such data is to estimate the survival function $S(t)$. This function represents the probability of surviving more than t time units. Time t is measured from diagnosis, start of treatment, or some other meaningful time point. For randomized studies, it is best to measure time from the date of randomization. There are basically two satisfactory methods for estimating $S(t)$. The first is the life table or actuarial method[110,111] and is appropriate when the number of patients is large. The other method is the product limit method of Kaplan and Meier.[112] This method is appropriate for any number of patients, but it involves

more effort than the life table method when the number of patients is large.

The first step in the application of either method is the calculation of survival time for all patients. Survival is the duration from the chosen baseline (e.g., date of randomization) until death or date last known to be alive for patients who are not known to have died. To use the life table method, intervals for the grouping of survival times are determined. The life table, shown in Table 36.11, is then filled out. This sample life table is prepared with yearly intervals in the first column. The number of patients alive at the beginning of the interval is entered in column 2. The number who died in the interval is entered in column 4. Patients dying exactly at a time that represents a boundary between two intervals (e.g., 365 days) are considered to have died in the preceding interval (e.g., 0 to 1 year). Column 3 contains the number of patients who are lost to follow-up during the interval or who are alive with maximum follow-up duration included in the interval. These latter patients are referred to as *withdrawn alive* in the conventional life table terminology. The life table method assumes that patients lost to follow-up or withdrawn alive during the interval are at risk of death for one-half of the interval. Hence, column 5—the number alive at the start of the interval minus half the number lost or withdrawn during the interval—represents an approximate number of patients at risk of death during the interval. Column 6 gives the ratio of the number of patients who died during the interval to the number at risk during the interval. Column 7 gives the estimated probability of surviving the interval for patients alive at the start of the interval.

Column 8 should be studied carefully, because it provides the life table estimate of the survival distribution and indicates the logic behind the method. The probability of surviving >3 years after randomization, for example, equals the entry in the third row of column 8 (0.50). The logic is as follows: To survive 3 full years, the patients must survive through the first year; and given that they have survived the first year, they must survive the second year; and given that they have survived the second year, they must survive the third year. Consequently, the probability of surviving for at least 3 years is estimated by the product $p_1 \times p_2 \times p_3$ of factors in column 7. By using this product, the life table method takes maximal advantage of the mortality experience of patients with limited follow-up. The entry S_x in column 8, row x, represents the life table estimate of the probability of surviving more than x years from randomization. Computational shortcuts to observe are those for column 8 ($S_x = p_x = S_{x-1}$) and for column 2 ($l_{x+1} = l_x - w_x - d_x$).

The product limit method of Kaplan and Meier[112] is similar in concept to the life table method. With the Kaplan-Meier approach, however, the intervals are defined by the actual survival times of patients who have died. Suppose, for example, that the survivals are 3, 3, 3+, 5, 6, 8+, 8+, 10, 10, and 12+ months,

TABLE 36.11

Life-Table Method for Estimating a Survival Distribution

Years After Randomization	No. Alive at Beginning of Interval l_x	No. Lost to Follow-Up or Withdrawn Alive During Interval w_x	No. Died During Interval d_x	At Risk During Interval (Col 2 − ½Col 3)	Proportion Dying (Col 4/Col 5) q_x	Proportion Surviving (1 − Col 6) p_x	Cumulative Proportion Surviving (S_x) ($p_1 \times p_2 \times \ldots \times p_x$)
0–1	252	38	94	233	0.40	0.60	0.60
1–2	120	34	10	103	0.10	0.90	0.54
2–3	76	30	4	61	0.07	0.93	0.50
3–4	42	18	4	33	0.12	0.88	0.44
4–5	20	12	0	14	0.00	1.00	0.44
5–6	8	8	0	4	0.00	1.00	0.44

Col, column.

Kaplan-Meier Method for Estimating a Survival Distribution

Months After Randomization	No. Alive at Beginning of Interval l_x	No. Lost to Follow-Up or Withdrawn Alive During Interval w_x	No. Died During Interval d_x	Effective No. Exposed to Risk of Dying Just Before End of Interval (Col 2 − Col 3)	Proportion Dying (Col 4/Col 5) q_x	Proportion Surviving (1 − Col 6) p_x	Cumulative Proportion Surviving $(p_1 \times p_2 \times \ldots \times p_x)$ S_x
0–3	10	0	2	10	0.2	0.8	0.8
3–5	8	1	1	7	0.14	0.86	0.68
5–6	6	0	1	6	0.17	0.83	0.57
6–10	5	2	2	3	0.67	0.33	0.19

Col, column.

where a plus sign follows survivals for patients still alive. Then the intervals are 0 to 3, 3 to 5, 5 to 6, and 6 to 10 months, as shown in Table 36.12. With the Kaplan-Meier method, deaths occur only at the ends of intervals. The entry in column 5 equals $l_x - w_x$ rather than $l_x - 2w_x$ for the life table method. This is because deaths occur only at the ends of intervals here, and the number of patients at risk of death just before the interval end is $l_x - w_x$. In the entry w_x in column 3 for the Kaplan-Meier method, patients who are lost to follow- up or withdrawn alive at the end of an interval are considered not lost or withdrawn until the following interval. These differences between the Kaplan-Meier and life table methods render the former more appropriate for studies with fewer patients.

Once the values S_x have been calculated for the Kaplan-Meier method, they may be graphed with time on the horizontal axis. The graph is a step function that starts at time zero and ordinate 1.0. It drops to value S_x at time x, where x is the time at the right end of an interval. The survival curve corresponding to Table 36.12 is shown in Fig. 36.1. The tic marks are placed on the curve at 3, 8, and 12 months to represent the follow-up times of living patients. The step function can be extended horizontally out to 12 months to represent follow-up of the last patient, but the right-hand end of the curve usually is very imprecisely estimated, and concluding that a plateau exists at the level shown on the curve is often erroneous.

For any time t, the Kaplan-Meier curve is an estimator of the true unknown value of $S(t)$. The estimator is approximately normally distributed in large samples. If m patients remain alive at time x,

the standard error of the estimate can be conservatively estimated[44] as the Kaplan-Meier estimate of a survival distribution is based on the assumption that censoring is noninformative, which means that the censoring time is independent of the prognosis of the patient. Most censoring in a randomized clinical trial results from the fact that some patients are alive and still being followed at the time of analysis. This is noninformative censoring. However, if patients are lost to follow-up—if they fail to return to clinic when they are too sick to travel—then the censoring is informative and all the usual methods of survival analysis are invalidated. Consequently, it is essential to obtain follow-up information actively on *all* patients before analysis. If some patients have not been contacted for many months and their status is unknown, that information should be obtained before any analysis is performed. Examining the distribution of time since the last contact for patients not known to have died is a good way to examine the adequacy of follow-up.

The issue of informative censoring also arises in considering end points other than death. For example, one may be attempting to estimate the distribution of time until tumor recurrence in the central nervous system (CNS) in a pediatric leukemia trial. How should one handle patients whose disease recurs in the marrow without evidence of CNS recurrence? One may be tempted to censor the time to CNS recurrence of such patients at their time of marrow recurrence, but that implicitly assumes that the censoring is noninformative. Because CNS and marrow recurrence may be biologically linked, the assumption of noninformative censoring may not be valid. Other issues of informative censoring can be similarly problematic. Clearly, one should never censor patients because of lack of compliance with therapy, as this can severely bias results. More extensive discussions of statistical methods for the analysis of clinical trial data are given by Marubini and Valsecchi.[113]

Multiple Comparisons

Table 36.13 shows the probability of obtaining one statistically significant ($p < 0.05$) difference by chance alone as a function of the number of independent comparisons of two equivalent treatments. With only five comparisons, the chance of at least one false-positive conclusion is 22.6%. When the number of end points, interim analyses, and patient subsets are considered in the analysis of clinical trials, these results are disturbing.[114] The comparisons performed in clinical trials are not entirely independent, but this does not have much effect on ameliorating the problem. Fleming and Watelet[115] performed a computer simulation to determine the chance of obtaining a statistically significant treatment difference when two equivalent treatments in six subsets determined by three dichotomous variables are compared. The chance of a statistically significant difference between treatments in at least one subset was 20% at the final analysis and 39% in the final or one of the three interim analyses. Subset analysis, comparison of treatments

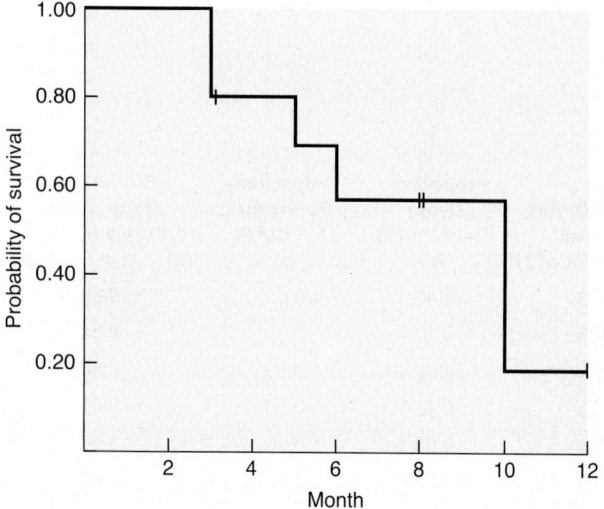

Figure 36.1 Example of estimated survival distribution.

TABLE 36.13

Probability of Obtaining at Least One Statistically Significant (P <0.05) Difference by Chance Along in Multiple Comparisons of Two Equivalent Treatments

Comparisons	Probability of at Least One "Significant" Difference (%)
1	5
2	9.7
3	14.3
4	18.5
5	22.6
10	40
20	64.1

TABLE 36.14

Summary of Guidelines for Reporting Clinical Trials[116]

- Quality control of data and response evaluations should be discussed.
- All patients registered on study should be accounted for.
- Inevaluability rate for major end points should not exceed 15%.
- No exclusions of eligible patients in comparing outcomes by treatment group.
- The sample size should be large enough to establish or conclusively rule out effects of clinically important magnitude. Confidence limits for size of treatment versus control effectiveness should be given.
- Publication should provide protocol-specified sample size and interim analysis plan as well as actual timing of analyses.
- Claims of therapeutic effectiveness should not be based on phase 2 trials.
- Generalizability of conclusions should be carefully discussed. Subset-specific claims should be justified based on prospective planning and statistical control of study-wise type I error.

with regard to multiple end points, and multiple interim analyses are common sources of erroneous conclusions. The primary end point should be defined in the protocol. Subset analyses and analyses with regard to secondary end points should be specified in advance, and statistical significance should be declared only for significance levels much defined in advance to limit the study-wise type 1 error to 5%.

Generally, it is not valid to adjust the analysis by characteristics measured after the start of treatment (e.g., compliance, dose delivered, toxicity). New approaches to subset analysis and multiple end point analysis using Bayesian methods have been described by Dixon and Simon.[93,116] Qualitative interaction tests are described by Gail and Simon.[117]

REPORTING RESULTS OF CLINICAL TRIALS

Effective reporting of results is an integral part of good research. Unfortunately, numerous reviews have indicated that the quality of reporting of clinical trial results is poor.[98,118,119] Pocock et al.[120] concluded that "overall, the reporting of clinical trials appears to be biased toward an exaggeration of treatment differences." Tannock and Murphy[98,114] have given clear illustration of how this is easily done. The guidelines summarized in Table 36.14 are adapted from those proposed by Simon and Wittes.[121]

FALSE POSITIVE REPORTS IN THE LITERATURE

Many of the positive results reported in the literature for small clinical trials are probably false positive results.[122–124] In 100 trials, suppose that there are 10 in which the experimental treatment is sufficiently better than the control such that there is a 90% chance of the difference being detected in a small or moderate-sized clinical trial. Of these 10 trials, obtaining a statistically significant difference is expected in 9. Of the remaining 90 trials, we assume that the treatments are approximately equivalent to the control. A statistically significant difference could be expected in 5% (4.5) of these. Hence, of the 13.5 (9 + 4.5) trials that yield statistically significant results, the finding is false positive in 4.5 or 33% of the cases. The 33% false discovery rate is striking but it depends on the assumption that only 10% of the trials study new treatments with large treatment effects. For large clinical trials, the size of treatment effect that can be detected with high statistical power is likely to be larger. The Eastern Cooperative Oncology Group reported that about one-third of their phase 3 clinical trials resulted in statistically significant results.[123] Assuming that most of these trials are

conducted with 90% power and a 5% statistical significance level, the false positive discovery rate is about 9%.

An additional factor to consider is that of publication bias,[125] which denotes the preference of journals to publish positive rather than negative results. A negative result may not be published at all, particularly from a small trial. If it is published, it is likely to appear in a less widely read journal than it would if the result were positive.

These observations emphasize that results in the medical literature often cannot be accepted at face value. It is important to recognize that "positive" results need confirmation, particularly positive results of small studies, before they can be believed and applied to the general population.

META-ANALYSIS

A *meta-analysis* is a quantitative summary of research on a topic. It is distinguished from the traditional literature review by its emphasis on quantifying results of individual studies and combining results across studies. Key components of this approach for therapeutics are to include only randomized clinical trials, to include all relevant randomized clinical trials that have been initiated (regardless of whether they have been published), to exclude no randomized patients from the analysis, and to assess therapeutic effectiveness based on the average results pooled across trials.[126]

Attention is restricted to randomized trials, because the bias from nonrandomized comparisons may be larger than the small to moderate therapeutic effects likely to be present. Including all relevant randomized trials that have been initiated in a geographic area (e.g., the world, or the Americas and Europe) represents an attempt to avoid publication bias. Avoiding exclusion of any randomized patients also functions to avoid bias. Assessing therapeutic effectiveness based on average pooled results is an attempt to make the evaluation on the totality of evidence rather than on extreme isolated reports. In calculating average treatment effects, a measure of difference in outcome between treatments is calculated separately for each trial. For example, an estimate of the logarithm of the hazard ratio can be computed for each trial. A weighted average of these study-specific differences is then computed, and the statistical significance of this average is evaluated. This approach to meta-analysis requires access to individual patient data for all randomized patients in each trial. It also requires collaboration of the leaders of all the relevant trials and is very labor-intensive. Nevertheless, it represents the gold standard for meta-analysis methodology.

A major issue of concern in meta-analyses is whether the individual trials are sufficiently similar to make calculation of average effects medically meaningful. If the therapeutic interventions or control treatments differ too greatly or if the patient populations are too different, the results may not be medically meaningful as a basis for making treatment decisions for individual patients. Often in cancer therapeutics, the studies will not be identical in their treatment regimens or their patient populations, but they will not be so different as to make the results meaningless. In this case, the meta-analysis may be useful for answering important questions about a class of treatments that the individual trials cannot address reliably. For example, trials evaluating adjuvant treatment of primary breast cancer often are designed to detect differences in disease-free survival, and a meta-analysis is often required to evaluate survival. Similarly, subset analysis can usually be meaningfully evaluated only in the context of a meta-analysis, because individual trials are not sized for this objective.

Meta-analysis is not an alternative to properly designed and sized randomized clinical trials. Some have suggested that one need not be concerned about computing sample size in the traditional ways, as small, randomized trials can be pooled for meta-analysis. Because most investigators would prefer to "do their own thing," this would lead to a proliferation of diverse trials of inconsequential individual size that may be too heterogeneous to permit a meaningful meta-analysis. Given that sufficient large, randomized clinical trials of very similar treatment regimens have been conducted, meta-analysis can provide supplemental information about a given class of treatments that is not available from the individual trials.

SELECTED REFERENCES

The full reference list can be accessed at lwwhealthlibrary.com/oncology.

1. Subramanian J, Simon R. Gene expression-based prognostic signatures in lung cancer: ready for clinical use? *J Natl Cancer Inst* 2010;102:464–474.
2. Green S, Benedetti J, Crowley J. *Clinical Trials in Oncology.* 2nd ed. London: Chapman & Hall/CRC; 2003.
3. Leventhal BG, Wittes RE. *Research Methods in Clinical Oncology.* New York: Raven Press; 1988.
4. Eisenhauer EA, O'Dwyer PJ, Christian M, et al. Phase I clinical trial design in cancer drug development. *J Clin Oncol* 2000;18:684–692.
5. Simon R, Freidlin B, Rubinstein L. Accelerated titration designs for phase I clinical trials in oncology. *J Natl Cancer Inst* 1997;89:1138–1147.
9. Babb J, Rogatko A, Zacks S. Cancer phase I clinical trials: efficient dose escalation with overdose control. *Stat Med* 1998;17:1103–1120.
10. Goodman SN, Zahurak ML, Piantadosi S. Some practical improvements in the continual reassessment method for phase I studies. *Stat Med* 1995;14:1149–1161.
12. Simon RM, Steinberg SM, Hamilton M, et al. Clinical trial designs for the early clinical development of therapeutic cancer vaccines. *J Clin Oncol* 2001;19:1848–1854.
15. Kummar S, Kinders R, Rubinstein L, et al. Compressing drug development timelines in oncology using phase '0' trials. *Nat Rev Cancer* 2007;7:131–139.
17. Karapetis CS, Khambata-Ford S, Jonker DJ, et al. K-ras mutations and benefit from cetuximab in advanced colorectal cancer. *N Engl J Med* 2008;359:1757–1765.
20. Pusztai L, Anderson K, Hess KR. Pharmacogenomic predictor discovery in phase II clinical trials for breast cancer. *Clin Cancer Res* 2007;13:6080–6086.
21. LeBlanc M, Rankin C, Crowley J. Multiple Histology Phase II Trials. *Clin Cancer Res* 2009;15:4256–4262.
22. Dobbin KK, Zhao Y, Simon RM. How large a training set is needed to develop a classifier for microarray data? *Clin Cancer Res* 2008;14:108–114.
23. Eisenhauer EA, Therasse P, Bogaerts J, et al. New response evaluation criteria in solid tumors: revised RECIST guideline (version 1.1). *Eur J Cancer* 2009;45:228–247.
24. Simon R. Optimal two-stage designs for phase II clinical trials. *Control Clin Trials* 1989;10:1–10.
29. Seymour L, Ivy SP, Sargent D, et al. The design of phase II clinical trials testing cancer therapeutics: consensus recommendations from the clinical trial design task force of the National Cancer Institute investigational drug steering committee. *Clin Cancer Res* 2010;16:1764–1769.
30. Vidauurre T, Wilkerson J, Simon R, et al. Stable disease is not preferentially observed with targeted therapies and as currently defined has limited value in drug development. *Cancer J* 2009;15:366–373.
31. El-Maraghi RH, Eisenhauer EA. Review of phase II trial designs used in studies of molecular targeted agents: outcomes and predictors of success in phase III. *J Clin Oncol* 2008;26:1346–1354.
34. Estey EH, Thall PF. New designs for phase 2 clinical trials. *Blood* 2003;102:442–448.
35. Korn EL, Liu PY, Lee SJ, et al. Meta-analysis of phase II cooperative group trials in metastatic stage IV melanoma to determine progression-free and overall survival benchmarks for future phase II trials. *J Clin Oncol* 2008;26:527–534.
38. Korn EL, Arbuck SG, Pluda JM, et al. Clinical trial designs for cytostatic agents: are new approaches needed? *J Clin Oncol* 2001;19:265–272.
39. Rubinstein LV, Korn EL, Freidlin B, et al. Design issues of randomized phase 2 trials and a proposal for phase 2 screening trials. *J Clin Oncol* 2005;23:7199–7206.
40. Simon R, Wittes RE, Ellenberg SS. Randomized phase II clinical trials. *Cancer Treat Rep* 1985;69:1375–1381.
45. Rosner G, Stadler W, Ratain M. Randomized discontinuation design: Application to cytostatic antineoplastic agents. *J Clin Oncol* 2002;20:4478–4484.
46. Freidlin B, Simon R. An evaluation of the randomized discontinuation design. *J Clin Oncol* 2005;23:1–5.
48. Goldman B, LeBlanc M, Crowley J. Interim futility analysis with intermediate endpoints. *Clin Trials* 2008;5:14–22.
51. Schaid DJ, Wieand S, Therneau TM. Optimal two-stage screening designs for survival comparisons. *Biometrics* 1990;77:507–513.
54. Freidlin B, Korn EL, Gray R, et al. Multi-arm clinical trials of new agents: some design considerations. *Clin Cancer Res* 2008;14:4368–4371.
55. Freidlin B, McShane LM, Polley MYC. Randomized phase II trial designs with biomarkers. *J Clin Oncol* 2012;30:3304–3309.
56. Simon R. Randomized clinical trials. Principles and obstacles. *Cancer* 1994;74:2614–2619.
57. Torri V, Simon R, Russek-Cohen E, et al. Relationship of response and survival in advanced ovarian cancer patients treated with chemotherapy. *J Natl Cancer Inst* 1992;84:407–414.
58. Buyse M, Molensberghs G, Burzykowski T, et al. The validation of surrogate endpoints in meta-analyses of randomized experiments. *Biostatistics* 2000;1:49–67.
60. Korn EL, Albert PS, McShane LM. Assessing surrogates as trial endpoints using mixed models. *Stat Med* 2004;24:163–182.
61. Fleming TR, Rothmann MD, Lu HL. Issues in using progression-free survival when evaluating oncology products. *J Clin Oncol* 2009;27:2874–2880.
62. Freidlin B, Korn EL, Hunsberger S, et al. Proposal for the use of progression-free survival in unblinded randomized trials. *J Clin Oncol* 2007;25:2122–2126.
63. Dodd LE, Korn EL, Freidlin B, et al. Blinded independent central review of progression-free survival in phase III clinical trials: important design element or unnecessary expense? *J Clin Oncol* 2008;26:3791–3796.
64. Simon R. An agenda for clinical trials: clinical trials in the genomic era. *Clin Trials* 2004;1:468–470.
65. Simon R. A roadmap for developing and validating therapeutically relevant genomic classifiers. *J Clin Oncol* 2005;23:7332–7341.
66. Simon R. New challenges for 21st century clinical trials. *Clin Trials* 2007;4:167–169.
67. Simon R, Maitournam A. Evaluating the efficiency of targeted designs for randomized clinical trials. *Clin Cancer Res* 2005;10:6759–6763.
68. Simon R, Maitournam A. Evaluating the efficiency of targeted designs for randomized clinical trials. Erratum. *Clin Cancer Res* 2006;12:3229.
69. Hoering A, LeBlanc M, Crowley J. Randomized phase III clinical trial designs for targeted agents. *Clin Cancer Res* 2008;14:4358–4367.
70. Mandrekar SJ, Sargent DJ. Clinical trial designs for predictive biomarker validation: theoretical considerations and practical challenges. *J Clin Oncol* 2009;27:4027–4034.
71. Simon R. Using genomics in clinical trial design. *Clin Cancer Res* 2008;14:5984–5993.
72. Simon RM. *Genomic Clinical Trials and Predictive Medicine.* Cambridge, UK: Cambridge University Press; 2013.
73. Karuri SW, Simon R. A two-stage Bayesian design for co-development of new drugs and companion diagnostics. *Stat Med* 2012;31:901–914.
74. Freidlin B, Sun Z, Gray R, et al. Phase III clinical trials that integrate treatment and biomarker evaluation. *J Clin Oncol* 2013;31:3158–3161.
75. Freidlin B, McShane LM, Korn EL. Randomized clinical trials with biomarkers: design issues. *J Natl Cancer Inst* 2010;102:152–160.
80. Simon RM, Paik S, Hayes DF. Use of archived specimens in evaluation of prognostic and predictive biomarkers. *J Natl Cancer Inst* 2009;101:1–7.
81. Pocock S, Simon R. Sequential treatment assignment with balancing for prognostic factors in the controlled clinical trial. *Biometrics* 1975;31:103–115.
83. Simon R, Simon N. Using randomization tests to preserve type I error with response-adaptive and covariate-adaptive randomization. *Stat Probab Lett* 2011;81:767–772.

84. Rubinstein L, Gail M, Santner T. Planning the duration of a comparative clinical trial with loss to follow-up and a period of continued observation. *J Chronic Dis* 1981;34:469–479.

88. Simon R. Confidence intervals for reporting results from clinical trials. *Ann Intern Med* 1986;105:429–435.

91. Simon R. Bayesian design and analysis of active control clinical trials. *Biometrics* 1999;55:484–487.

92. Spiegelhalter DJ, Freedman LS, Parmar MK. Bayesian approaches to randomized trials. *J R Stat Soc Series A General* 1994;157:357–387.

93. Simon R. Bayesian subset analysis: application to studying treatment-by-gender interactions. *Stat Med* 2002;21:2909–2916.

95. Simon R. Discovering the truth about tamoxifen: problems of multiplicity in the evaluation of biomedical data. *J Natl Cancer Inst* 1995;87:627–629.

96. Peto R, Pike MC, Armitage P. Design and analysis of randomized clinical trials requiring prolonged observation of each patient. II. Analysis and examples. *Br J Cancer* 1977;35:1–39.

97. Barr J, Tannock I. Analyzing the same data two ways: a demonstration model illustrate the reporting and misreporting of clinical trials. *J Clin Oncol* 1989;7:969–978.

98. Tannock I, Murphy K. Reflections on medical oncology: an appeal for better clinical trials and improved reporting of their results. *J Clin Oncol* 1983;1:66–70.

101. Ellenberg S, Fleming TR, DeMets D. *Data Monitoring Committees in Clinical Trials: A Practical Perspective*. Hoboken, NJ: Wiley; 2002.

102. Smith M, Ungerleider R, Korn E, et al. The role of independent data monitoring committees in randomized clinical trials sponsored by the National Cancer Institute. *J Clin Oncol* 1997;15:2736–2743.

103. Haybittle JL. Repeated assessment of results in clinical trials of cancer treatment. *J Radiol* 1971;44:793–797.

104. O'Brien PC, Fleming TR. A multiple testing procedure for clinical trials. *Biometrics* 1979;35:549–556.

107. Freidlin B, Korn EL. Monitoring for lack of benefit: a critical component of a randomized clinical trial. *J Clin Oncol* 2009;27:629–633.

109. Lan KKG, Simon R, Halperin M. Stochastically curtailed test in long-term clinical trials. *Commun Stat Seqen Anal* 1982;1:207–219.

112. Kaplan EI, Meier P. Nonparametric estimation from incomplete observations. *J Am Stat Assoc* 1958;53:457–481.

114. Tannock IF. False-positive results in clinical trials: multiple significance tests and the problem of unreported comparisons. *J Natl Cancer Inst* 1996;88:206–207.

115. Fleming TR, Watelet L. Approaches to monitoring clinical trials. *J Natl Cancer Inst* 1989;81:188–193.

116. Dixon DO, Simon R. Bayesian subset analysis. *Biometrics* 1991;47:871–881.

117. Gail M, Simon R. Testing for qualitative interactions between treatment effects and patient subsets. *Biometrics* 1985;41:361–372.

123. Simon R. Commentary on "Clinical trials and sample size considerations: Another perspective." *Stat Sci* 2000;15:95–110.

125. Begg CB, Berlin JA. Publication bias and dissemination of clinical research. *J Natl Cancer Inst* 1989;81:107–115.

126. Collins R, Gray R, Godwin J, et al. Avoidance of large biases and large random errors in the assessment of moderate treatment effects: the need for systematic overviews. *Stat Med* 1987;6:245–254.

37 Molecular Biology of Head and Neck Cancers

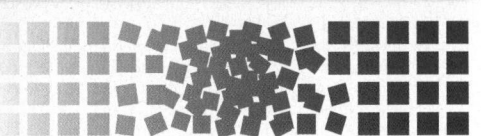

Thomas E. Carey and Mark E. P. Prince

INTRODUCTION

Incidence, Risk Factors, and Etiology

Head and neck squamous cell carcinoma (HNSCC) accounts for 90% of all malignant disease in the head and neck region of the body. With 550,000 new cases diagnosed worldwide each year, HNSCC is a major public health problem. In the United States, there are 40,000 new cases and roughly 14,000 deaths from HNSCC each year. Historically, HNSCC has been a disease of older males with heavy lifelong tobacco use, high alcohol consumption, poor diet, and bad dentition. As smoking increased among women, the male to female ratio of 5:1 observed in the 1960s declined to 3:1 in the 1990s. Most mucosal squamous cancers of the head and neck, particularly those of the oral cavity, larynx, and hypopharynx are still associated with these etiologic factors as well as other cultural habits, such as oral tobacco use, and in other countries, betel and areca nut chewing.[1,2] A small but mysterious segment of head and neck tumors arise in individuals under 40 years of age who have no known etiologic factors. In the past 10 years, we noted that at our institution, HNSCC patients under age 35 included more women than men, and during this period, four cases of tongue cancer in pregnant women were also observed.[3] The etiology of the cancers in the men and women in the young age group is unknown. A small percentage of HNSCC have a familial origin; however, when corrected for tobacco and alcohol use, most associations lose statistical significance.[4] Nevertheless, familial head and neck cancers associated with inherited defects of the CDKN2A locus causing loss of function of the cyclin-dependent kinase inhibitor p16INK4A[5] and the hMDM2 regulator p14ARF occur. Two members of a family were treated recently for HNSCC in our department. An analysis revealed that each had the same somatic CDKN2A mutation. Families with inherited mutations of cancer-related genes tend to have multiple types of malignant tumors, and second primary tumors of different histologic types.[6] In fact, CDKN2A was originally called multiple tumor suppressor gene 1 (MTS-1)[7,8] because it was so frequently mutated in multiple tumor types, including melanoma, pancreatic cancers, breast cancers, and head and neck cancers. The genes associated with an inherited predisposition to head and neck cancer include the master regulator, TP53 (Li-Fraumeni syndrome),[9] and Fanconi anemia genes, the FANC family of DNA repair genes that are also associated with the development of HNSCC.[10,11] Head and neck cancers arising in young patients and others that are independent of tobacco exposure provide a rich area for an in-depth molecular assessment to determine the underlying genetic factors.

High-Risk Human Papillomaviruses

As smoking has declined in the United States, so has the incidence of smoking-related head and neck cancer, particularly those of the oral cavity and larynx, while at the same time there has been a steady increase in tonsillar cancers.[12] Trends for head and neck cancer incidence by site in the United States and Canada indicate that oropharynx cancers have increased continuously over the past 25 years.[9,13] The oropharyngeal cancer increase began in the late 1970s and is attributed to increased rates of infection with high-risk human papillomaviruses (hrHPV) secondary to changing sexual mores that are traceable to widespread use of oral contraceptives, reduced use of condoms, and freedom to have more sexual partners, without the fear of an unwanted pregnancy. Studies in the United States, Canada, and Western Europe clearly show a trend for increasing incidence of hrHPV, notably, HPV16 in oropharyngeal cancers by year of diagnosis.[14–22] At our institution, there was a steady increase in the proportion of HPV-positive oropharynx cancer in three clinical trials done over the past decade (Table 37.1). Surveillance, Epidemiology, and End Results (SEER) data illustrate the decline in smoking-related cancers of the larynx, the increase in oropharyngeal cancer, and the remarkable decline in cervical cancer that is attributable to an early diagnosis with Pap smears, hrHPV testing, and colposcopy of cervical lesions (Fig. 37.1). In 2013, the incidence of new oropharyngeal cancer cases was expected to surpass that of cervical cancer. Unfortunately, no early detection and treatment for HPV-induced oropharynx cancer is available, but this is a rich area for investigation.

HPV is the most common sexually transmitted disease with an overall genital HPV prevalence of 42.5% in females 14 to 59 years of age as determined in the National Health and Nutrition Examination Survey (NHANES) (2003–2006).[23] In the oral cavity and oropharynx, the lymphoid-rich tissue of the tonsils is the likely reservoir of HPV. To replicate, HPV must infect the basal epithelial cell. The thin epithelium of the tonsillar crypts serves as an ideal location for the virus to infect (Fig. 37.2). HPV infection may be facilitated by concurrent inflammation within the tonsil due to other microorganisms. D'Souza et al.[24] conducted a hospital-based case control study of 100 patients with newly diagnosed oropharynx cancer to 200 noncancer patients to evaluate associations between HPV infection and oropharyngeal cancer. A high lifetime number of vaginal sex partners (≥26) and oral sex partners (≥6) was significantly associated with oropharyngeal cancer as was seropositivity for antibodies to the viral L1 protein or oral infection with any hrHPV type, most frequently HPV16. However, other high-risk HPV types are also found in roughly 10% of oropharynx tumors and in other head and neck cancer locations, notably the nasopharynx and the oral cavity; the proportion of other high-risk HPV types is much higher.[25,26] Oral and vaginal HPV infections in a series of HIV-positive and HIV-negative women revealed a significant but lower incidence of oral HPV (15%) compared to vaginal HPV (51%).[27] Oral HPV infection incidence in the general U.S. population was evaluated in the NHANES study.[28] The prevalence of oral HPV infection shows a biphasic distribution with one peak in the 30- to 34-year-old age group and a second

PRACTICE OF ONCOLOGY

TABLE 37.1

Changing HPV Involvement in Oropharynx Cancers: Over 10 Years of Study Accruals: University of Michigan Head and Neck Oncology Program

HPV Positivity by Clinical Trial and Time Period

HPV Status	UMCC 9921 1999–2001	UMCC 0221 2001–2005	UMCC 0221–like 2005–2011
HPV negative	14 (34%)	8 (10%)	6 (8%)
HPV positive	27 (66%)	75 (90%)	71 (92%)

UMCC, University of Michigan Cancer Center.

peak in the 60- to 64-year-old age group. Overall, oral HPV infection was (6.9%), with high-risk HPV types in 3.7%. Men had a higher prevalence than women (10.1% versus 3.6%), and blacks had a higher prevalence of oral HPV (10.5%) than whites (6.5%), although this difference did not reach statistical significance. It is not yet certain how oral HPV infection relates to the risk of developing HPV-induced head and neck cancer.

Fortunately, HPV-positive oropharyngeal cancers show improved response to therapy when compared to HPV-negative cancers of the same site.[29–32] Patients presenting with HPV-positive oropharyngeal cancers also tend to be younger, healthier, and have a much lower frequency of smoking and alcohol abuse.[33] However, some studies have shown that a history of smoking in patients with HPV-positive oropharynx cancer may increase the likelihood of recurrence or metastasis after treatment.[21,34] This has prompted many to consider reducing the intensity of treatment to decrease treatment-related morbidity.[35,36] In contrast to

the excellent prognosis of HPV-positive oropharynx cancers, in HPV-positive oral cancers,[37] and HPV-positive nasopharyngeal cancers,[38] the outcome may be worse than HPV-negative cancers arising in these sites.

At the University of Michigan, 80% to 90% of oropharyngeal tumors (see Table 37.1) that present are HPV positive,[21,25] and >80% of patients with HPV-positive oropharynx cancer are responders to concurrent carboplatin and taxol with intensity-modulated radiation treatment (chemoRT).[39] Critical questions for the future are to determine which patients can benefit from less intensive treatment, which patients need the intensive concurrent chemoRT treatment, and which patients need a different treatment because they fail to be cured by chemoRT. Spector et al.[40,41] showed that nodal status and, in particular, matted nodes (defined as three nodes abutting one another with loss of an intervening fat plane replaced with evidence of extracapsular spread) defines a group of patients with a greatly increased risk of distant metastasis and poor overall and disease-free survival. The molecular correlates of these highly malignant HPV-positive tumors are yet to be defined fully, but in work submitted for publication, Walline et al. have shown that integration of hrHPV into cancer-related genes is common in tumors of patients who suffer from recurrent disease and poor survival, whereas integration of the viral genome into intragenic sites was more commonly associated with good response to therapy and prolonged progression-free survival. Immune responses to HPV antigens have also been suggested to be a cause of the good response to therapy among HPV-positive oropharyngeal cancers. However, failure of a potent immune response in some cases may occur because of frequent alterations affecting the tumor necrosis factor (TNF) receptor *TRAF3*, which participates in the activation of the immune response and nuclear factor kappa B (NF-κB) signaling (TCGA Head and Neck Cancer Consortium).[42] These changes may provide a mechanism for HPV-positive tumors to

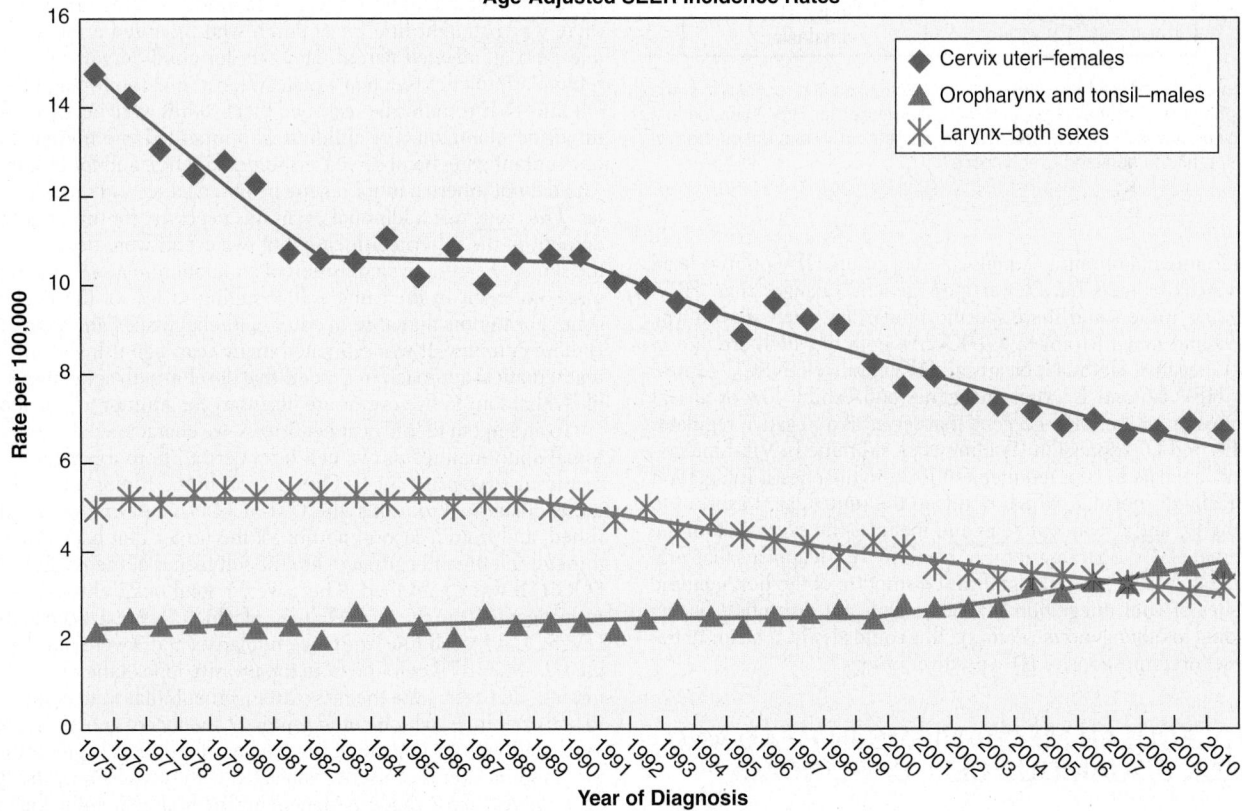

Figure 37.1 Changing incidence rates of larynx, cervix, and oropharynx cancers. Adapted by R. Meza, from Surveillance, Epidemiology, and End Results (SEER) Program Populations (1969–2011) (www.seer.cancer.gov/popdata), National Cancer Institute, Division of Cancer Control and Population Sciences (DCCPS), Surveillance Research Program, Surveillance Systems Branch, released January 2013.

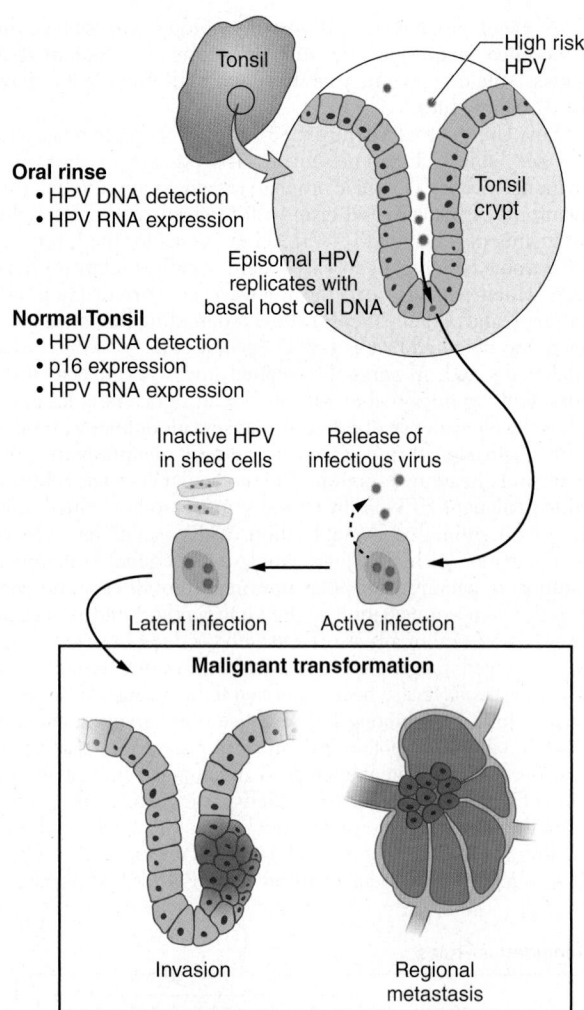

Figure 37.2 Human papillomavirus (HPV) infection and replication in the oropharynx, with the tonsil as the primary target for HPV infection and carcinogenesis. HPV detection can be carried out in oral rinses, normal tonsils, and tumors and lymph nodes.

and neck cancers and are associated with poor prognosis.[46,47] It is puzzling that only about 10% of HNSCC cases respond to treatment that targets EGFR.[48] Alternate driver pathways are suspected as an explanation for this observation. Early molecular studies of HNSCC also revealed that mutations, loss of heterozygosity, and methylation of the CDNK2A locus is very common and occurs early in HNSCC development.[49–51] Mutation and overexpression of p53 was also identified in early studies of HNSCC.[52] CyclinD1 amplification and overexpression has also been identified as an important biomarker that is associated with outcomes and responses to treatment.[53] In the landmark VA larynx trial, a biomarker analysis revealed that overexpressed p53 predicted the response to induction chemotherapy and radiation (RT).[54] Because p53 overexpression is nearly always associated with mutant p53, this suggested that tumors with wild-type p53 were less responsive to chemotherapy and RT, even though normal cells containing wild-type p53 are very sensitive to chemotherapy or RT. Thus, it was unclear why tumors with wild-type p53 were more resistant to chemotherapy and RT. Subsequent studies revealed that the combination of wild-type p53 and overexpression of Bcl-xL resulted in cisplatin resistance.[55] This suggested that Bcl-xL blocks p53-induced apoptosis, and that wild-type p53 mediates cell cycle arrest and repair mechanisms, allowing tumor cells to escape from treatment-induced damage.

In spite of our awareness of EGFR overexpression and its potential value as a target for therapy, it is still impossible to predict which head and neck cancers will respond and which will not. The same is true for many other molecular markers when only one molecular target is addressed. It is now becoming clear that it will be necessary to identify the driver pathways and target more than one cancer driver. It was postulated many years ago that a certain number of "hits" is necessary to drive a tumor. Knudsen correctly explained the tumor suppressor nature of the retinoblastoma gene by comparing the kinetics of tumor development in children with an inherited predisposition and in children who developed sporadic retinoblastoma. When time to tumor development in affected children was plotted against months from birth, there was a straight line for children who inherited a mutant allele from an affected parent. However for children with sporadic retinoblastoma the line had a plateau for several months and then fell linearly. From this he reasoned that two hits were necessary for tumor development. For children who inherited one normal and one mutant gene he observed first-order kinetics, and for children who did not inherit a mutant gene he observed second-order kinetics. Thus only one additional event was necessary for tumor development in the inherited disease, but two events were necessary in the sporadic cases, i.e. acquisition of a mutation in a cell and then a second event in the same cell, resulting in loss of the healthy gene. For tumors that arise in adult epithelial tissues, the situation is more complex. It was estimated many years ago using a similar mathematical approach in cancers that develop with aging that it is likely that four to five events are necessary for a tumor to develop.

To attempt to identify cancer drivers, we characterized chromosomal abnormalities in two cell lines derived from a patient with recurrent laryngeal cancer. One portion of the tumor was within the endolarynx. From this, the UM-SCC-17A cell line was established, and from a second portion of the tumor that had invaded through the thyroid cartilage into the soft tissues of the neck, UM-SCC-17B was established. There were a total of 22 chromosome rearrangements in the two cell lines, of which 8 were unique to the UM-SCC-17A cell line from the endolarynx and 9 were unique to the UM-SCC-17B cell line from the invasive lobe of the tumor. Of interest, however, were the five rearrangements that were common to both cell lines, which could represent the loci of genetic events associated with tumor initiation, whereas the others represent either random events or events associated with progression.[56] It will be of interest to use modern sequencing methods to identify the genetic aberrations linked to these five early chromosome rearrangements to test this hypothesis. Hahn and Weinberg tested what steps were necessary to transform normal human bronchial epithelial

evade antiviral immune responses.[42] As a group, HPV-positive head and neck cancers have fewer gross genetic changes than HPV-negative tumors and share specific similarities, such as wild-type TP53 and intact p16ink4a (CDKN2A), both of which are rare in HPV-negative HNSCC. Nearly all HPV-positive HNSCC express the HPV E6 and E7 viral oncogenes and exhibit low or absent expression of the HPV E2 gene that serves as a negative regulator of E6 and E7 expression (Walline et al. submitted). Viral integration[43] appears to be a requirement for carcinogenesis. Integration typically disrupts E2, which results in the unregulated expression of the E6 and E7 oncoproteins and includes the expression of the alternate HPV E6 transcripts E6*I and E6*II.[44] It appears that viral integration also causes a significant disruption of the host genome at sites of viral integration.[45] When significant disruption occurs leading to other genomic damage, this could also be a factor in the subset of nonresponsive HPV-positive tumors.

MOLECULAR MECHANISMS IN HEAD AND NECK SQUAMOUS CELL CARCINOMA

Early molecular studies of head and neck cancers revealed that amplification of the epidermal growth factor receptor (EGFR) gene with associated EGFR overexpression are common among head cells into tumor cells. They targeted a small but consistent set of specific pathways based on the observed abnormalities of many epithelial cancers. The necessary pathways include: ectopic expression of the catalytic unit of human telomerase, human telomerase reverse transcriptase (hTERT), to stabilize telomeres over many cell divisions; abrogation of the Rb pathway with SV40 large T oncoprotein to induce continuous cell cycle entry; inhibition of *TP53* with large T oncoprotein to facilitate cell cycle progression and to inhibit *TP53*-mediated induction of apoptosis; and introduction of the activated (oncogenic) allele of *HRAS*, to provide continuous signaling through the RAS, RAF, mitogen-activated protein kinase (MEK), extracellular signal-related kinase (ERK) kinase cascade to trigger the expression of transcription factors associated with proliferation.[57,58] This demonstration is critical to our thinking of how we will develop precision medicine for cancer because, similar to the chromosome rearrangements observed in the UM-SCC-17A and UM-SCC-17B cell lines mentioned previously, each epithelial cancer is likely to have multiple abnormalities, of which some are primary driver events and others are passenger events that have developed incidentally due to genomic destabilization. The knowledge that a limited number of events are sufficient for the conversion of a normal human epithelial cell to an immortalized, invasive tumor cell population suggests that a series of principles can be developed that control the conversion of normal to malignant behavior and that we should be able to develop strategies that will target the two or three critical pathways of an individual tumor that serve as the primary drivers of neoplastic behavior.

THE CANCER GENOME ATLAS PROJECT

Most studies have looked at individual target genes in isolation or in small combinations of genes to identify tumor driver events; however, these have largely been thwarted by the range of mechanisms that a tumor cell might acquire stochastically to become malignant. This limited our ability to assess the drivers of individual cancers and has complicated the assessment of the efficacy of pathway-targeted agents. The development of modern molecular analysis techniques has made it possible to analyze nearly all of the abnormalities in an individual tumor. Furthermore, The Cancer Genome Atlas (TCGA) project has provided us with an impressive collection of data from multiple tumors of the same types that can be used to bring us closer to developing knowledge of the types of oncogenic drivers and tumor suppressors that characterize each tumor type. By examining individual tumors in similar detail to identify the aberrant pathways, we can deduce the primary drivers and propose effective combinations of targeted therapies that can work against that individual tumor.

The Head and Neck Cancer Consortium assessed 279 previously untreated HNSCC tumors (35 of which contained HPV) for genomic alterations.[42] Sequence (exome, RNA, miRNA, some whole genome sequence), structural, epigenetic (DNA methylation), and copy number analyses as well as protein expression were carried out. The genomic gains and losses of the smoking-related HNSCC strongly resembled those in the squamous cancers of the lung[59]; however, those HNSCC tumors containing HPV had less complex genomic signatures and lacked *TP53* mutations, *HRAS*-activating mutations, and *CDKN2A* deletions and mutations, but had more frequent *PIK3CA* mutations. Also of interest was the identification of a subset of HPV-negative HNSCC that had relatively fewer *TP53* mutations and more frequent *PIK3CA* and *HRAS* mutations. Interestingly the tumors with *HRAS* mutations tended to correlate with wild-type *TP53*–containing tumors. This set was also notable for a less complex pattern of chromosome rearrangements and better survival than the other HPV-negative HNSCC tumors. In the entire HNSCC set, the most commonly mutated genes were *TP53*, *FAT1*, *CDKN2A*, *PIK3CA*, *NOTCH1*, and *MLL2*, with mutation frequencies ranging from 72% to 18%. Amplifications of receptor tyrosine kinases (RTK) were common. *EGFR* amplification was identified in 16% of tumors. Other smaller subsets of

tumors lacked EGFR amplification but contained amplification of fibroblast growth factor receptor (FGFR)1, 2, or 3. A few tumors had more than one RTK amplification, but mostly subsets could be categorized by amplification of one RTK. CyclinD1 (*CCND1*) amplification was very common, occurring in 30% of all tumors. *CCND1* amplification was observed in some tumors with RTK amplification and in a subset of tumors with *CMYC* amplification, although there was also a subset that had either *CCDN1* or *CMYC* amplification, but not both. *HRAS* mutations were found in 5%, *PIK3CA* mutations were found in 18%, *PTEN* mutations in 12%, whereas *TP53* mutations were present in 83%.

The tumor subsets defined by each of these distinct categories offers promise for better response when the correct amplified or mutated gene is targeted in those categories. Inhibitors for EGFR, FGFR, and PIK3CA are all now available and suggest that the appropriate matching of the tumor characteristics with the correct inhibitor is a fruitful area for study. Although CCND1 inhibitors are not yet available, several companies have cyclin-dependent kinase inhibitors (CDK4/6), and use of these agents is being tested in tumors with a loss of *CDKN2A* and might also be applicable in tumors with *CCND1* amplification. *NOTCH1* mutations found in 18% of HNSCC are a recently appreciated feature of a subset of HNSCC and are typically loss-of-function mutations, suggesting that *NOTCH1* is a tumor suppressor in this cancer type. In normal squamous epithelium, NOTCH1 acts to drive squamous differentiation by feeding back on the Wnt/β-catenin signaling pathway active in the proliferating basal cell. Loss of the NOTCH1 tumor suppressor function allows unopposed activity of the Wnt pathway, allowing this to become a target for therapy. Liu et al.[60] recently reported the development of a novel inhibitor of the Wnt pathway that targets Wnt secretion by inhibiting porcupine, the enzyme required for Wnt secretion. This inhibitor, LGK974, was more effective in tumor cell lines shown to have *NOTCH1* loss of function mutations, suggesting that this may be a useful agent in HNSCC tumors with NOTCH pathway abnormalities.

The next horizon for targeted agents is to find the correct combinations of targeted compounds for individual tumors. For this effort, it will be necessary to identify targets in different pathways for which effective agents exist. Such a combination might include inhibitors of RTKs, together with a CDK4/6 inhibitor or a Wnt pathway inhibitor and PIK3CA inhibitor. Many combinations are possible, and the literature will be replete with combinations of multiple targeted agents within the next few years as precision medicine approaches evolve. Rapid and comparatively inexpensive targeted or exome sequencing is now becoming available at the lab bench, with bioinformatics software and cloud computing to provide results within days. This will be an exciting era.

CANCER STEM CELLS

The isolation of highly tumorigenic subpopulations of cancer cells from solid cancers, commonly referred to as cancer stem cells (CSC), has generated a great deal of interest in the relevance of these cells to cancer progression and treatment failure. CSCs have been shown to be critical in the growth and development of primary tumors and for the development of regional and distant metastatic disease in HNSCC. CSCs are also believed to be highly resistant to conventional therapy and, therefore, likely responsible for disease recurrence and treatment failures when they occur.

CSCs were first isolated from lymphomas. A subsequent investigation of solid tumors has revealed the presence of highly tumorigenic cancer cells in essentially every solid cancer type. These highly tumorigenic cells fit the current criteria for being classified as CSCs: they are tumorigenic; they are able to reproduce the original tumor heterogeneity, including the tumorigenic and nontumorigenic cell subpopulations; and they are self-renewing. CSCs generally represent a very small subpopulation of the cancer cells. In the majority of solid tumors, they typically represent less than 10%

of the entire cancer cell population. A variety of surface markers and biologic markers have been used to isolate the CSC population from the other cancer cells in HNSCC, including CD 44, CD 133, ESA, and aldehyde dehydrogenase activity. So far, no single marker or combination of markers has proven useful for isolating CSCs from every tumor site. Additionally, none of these stem cell markers has been found to be a useful or effective target for cancer therapy.

The term *cancer stem cell* refers to the biologic behavior of the cells and not their cell of origin. Although CSCs exhibit many of the properties of normal stem cells, their cell of origin has yet to be determined. Likely, CSCs can originate from normal stem cells, early progenitor cells, and possibly more differentiated cells if they undergo the correct combination of mutations and epigenetic changes required to achieve the CSC phenotype.

Many normal stem cell genetic pathways are expressed in CSCs and are important regulators of their behavior. These genes include the transcription factors responsible for maintaining pluripotency, epithelial to mesenchymal transition, self-renewal, xenobiotic efflux, and quiescence. Embryonic stem cells are believed to be dependent on at least three critical pathways that regulate their activity: NANOG, Oct-4, and Sox-2. NANOG has been shown to inhibit differentiation, and Oct-4 is critical to self-renewal. Oct-4 and NANOG have also been recognized as important transcription factors in the reprogramming of pluripotency in adult cells. NANOG, Oct-3/4, and Sox-2 have been found to be upregulated in CSC-enriched cells derived from HNSCC grown as spheroids. Oct-4, which is known to be an important stem cell gene in epithelial stem cells, has been found to be unregulated in aldehyde dehydrogenase (ALDH)-positive HNSCC cells.[61] The overexpression of NANOG and Oct-4 has been correlated with chemotherapy resistance and the stage of cancer, suggesting that these genes play a role in treatment outcomes and in the prognosis in HNSCC.

BMI1 is a gene that is believed to be an essential stem cell–related gene that maintains the self-renewal of stem cells. To date, although *BMI1* has not been shown to be a reliable marker for CSCs in HNSCC, its potential to induce tumorigenic changes has made it an attractive target for study in CSCs. *BMI1* is expressed in CSCs from a variety of tumor types, including HNSCC, and is an important component of the polycomb complex 1, an epigenetic regulator of stem cell self-renewal and carcinogenesis.[62] Through repression of the *CDKN2A* locus and inhibition of p16Ink4A expression, *BMI1* is believed to promote cellular proliferation by blocking p16Ink4A-induced cellular senescence. *BMI1* knockdown

resulted in a significant reduction in HNSCC CSC renewal and in chemotherapy and radiation resistance.[63] Conversely, overexpression of *BMI1* in the non-CSC population of HNSCC resulted in the acquisition of self-renewal and stem cell–like properties.

Epithelial to mesenchymal transition is required to allow for cancer cell migration to occur and for the subsequent development of metastasis. Snail and Twist have been identified as critical transcription factors regulating epithelial to mesenchymal transition in stem cells and cancer cells. Increased expression of Twist has been found in both CD44-positive and ALDH-positive HNSCC, and increased Snail expression has been confirmed in ALDH HNSCC CSCs.[64] Snail expression in HNSCC CSCs has been correlated with metastasis, local recurrence, and prognosis. Increased Twist expression increases HNSCC CSC motility and loss of E-cadherin–mediated cell-to-cell contact.

Normal cells and CSCs express high levels of adenosine triphosphate (ATP)-binding cassette (ABC) transporter genes, including *ABCB1*, which encodes P-glycoprotein, and *ABCG2*. The drug-effluxing property of stem cells conferred by ABC transporters is the basis for the side-population phenotype that arises from the exclusion of the fluorescent dye Hoechst 33342 and has been used to isolate CSCs from HNSCC.[65] CSCs are likely to share many of the properties of normal stem cells that provide for a long lifespan, including resistance to drugs and toxins through the expression of ABC transporters. Therefore, tumors might have a built-in population of drug-resistant pluripotent cells—the CSCs—due to their expression of the ABC-transported genes that can survive chemotherapy and repopulate the tumor.

The Wnt/β-catenin pathway is known to be important to organogenesis and embryonic development. The major function of this pathway to is to regulate β-catenin function by its phosphorylation and proteasomal degradation. Abnormalities in the pathway can lead to β-catenin accumulation, which, in turn, results in the activation of several pathways such as cyclin D1 and CMYC, which control the G1 to S phase transition in the cell cycle. Wnt signaling is also involved in the critical cell migration process known as the epithelial–mesenchymal transition. These effects contribute to the importance of the Wnt/β-catenin in determining the CSC phenotype.

The expression of CSC genes in primary HNSCC has been found in some studies to be associated with the prognosis and response to therapy. The role of CSCs in the treatment resistance and recurrence is still being elucidated. Gaining a better understanding of the molecular pathways that regulate CSC behavior will be essential to developing therapies that target this critical population of cells.

SELECTED REFERENCES

The full reference list can be accessed at lwwhealthlibrary.com/oncology.

3. Eliassen AM, Hauff SJ, Tang AL, et al. Head and neck squamous cell carcinoma in pregnant women. *Head Neck* 2013;35:335–342.
10. Wreesmann VB, Estilo C, Eisele DW, et al. Downregulation of Fanconi anemia genes in sporadic head and neck squamous cell carcinoma. *ORL J Otorhinolaryngol Relat Spec* 2007;69:218–225.
11. van Zeeburg HJ, Snijders PJ, Wu T, et al. Clinical and molecular characteristics of squamous cell carcinomas from Fanconi anemia patients. *J Natl Cancer Inst* 2008;100:1649–1653.
13. Chaturvedi AK, Engels EA, Anderson WF, et al. Incidence trends for human papillomavirus-related and -unrelated oral squamous cell carcinomas in the United States. *J Clin Oncol* 2008;26:612–619.
14. Kreimer AR, Clifford GM, Boyle P, et al. Human papillomavirus types in head and neck squamous cell carcinomas worldwide: a systematic review. *Cancer Epidemiol Biomarkers Prev* 2005;14:467–475.
15. Gillison ML, Alemany L, Snijders PJ, et al. Human papillomavirus and diseases of the upper airway: head and neck cancer and respiratory papillomatosis. *Vaccine* 2012;30 Suppl 5:F34–F54.
16. Chaturvedi AK, Engels EA, Pfeiffer RM, et al. Human papillomavirus and rising oropharyngeal cancer incidence in the United States. *J Clin Oncol* 2011;29:4294–4301.
17. Gillison ML. Human papillomavirus-associated head and neck cancer is a distinct epidemiologic, clinical, and molecular entity. *Semin Oncol* 2004;31:744–754.
21. Maxwell JH, Kumar B, Feng FY, et al. Tobacco use in human papillomavirus-positive advanced oropharynx cancer patients related to increased risk of distant metastases and tumor recurrence. *Clin Cancer Res* 2010;16:1226–1235.
22. Worden FP, Kumar B, Lee JS, et al. Chemoselection as a strategy for organ preservation in advanced oropharynx cancer: response and survival positively associated with HPV16 copy number. *J Clin Oncol* 2008;26:3138–3146.
23. Hariri S, Unger ER, Sternberg M, et al. Prevalence of genital human papillomavirus among females in the United States, the National Health And Nutrition Examination Survey, 2003-2006. *J Infect Dis* 2011;204:566–573.
24. D'Souza G, Kreimer AR, Viscidi R, et al. Case-control study of human papillomavirus and oropharyngeal cancer. *N Engl J Med* 2007;356:1944–1956.
25. Walline HM, Komarck C, McHugh JB, et al. High-risk human papillomavirus detection in oropharyngeal, nasopharyngeal, and oral cavity cancers: comparison of multiple methods. *JAMA Otolaryngol Head Neck Surg* 2013;139:1320–1327.
26. Maxwell JH, Kumar B, Feng FY, et al. HPV-positive/p16-positive/EBV-negative nasopharyngeal carcinoma in white North Americans. *Head Neck* 2010;32:562–567.
28. Gillison ML, Broutian T, Pickard RK, et al. Prevalence of oral HPV infection in the United States, 2009–2010. *JAMA* 2012;307:693–703.
29. Fakhry C, Gillison ML. Clinical implications of human papillomavirus in head and neck cancers. *J Clin Oncol* 2006;24:2606–2611.
30. Fakhry C, Westra WH, Li S, et al. Improved survival of patients with human papillomavirus-positive head and neck squamous cell carcinoma in a prospective clinical trial. *J Natl Cancer Inst* 2008;100:261–269.

32. Worden FP, Kumar B, Lee JS, et al. Chemoselection as a strategy for organ preservation in advanced oropharynx cancer: response and survival positively associated with HPV16 copy number. *J Clin Oncol* 2008;26:3138–3146.

34. Ang KK, Harris J, Wheeler R, et al. Human papillomavirus and survival of patients with oropharyngeal cancer. *N Engl J Med* 2010;363:24–35.

35. Adelstein DJ, Ridge JA, Brizel DM, et al. Transoral resection of pharyngeal cancer: summary of a National Cancer Institute Head and Neck Cancer Steering Committee Clinical Trials Planning Meeting, November 6-7, 2011, Arlington, Virginia. *Head Neck* 2012;34:1681–1703.

36. Kimple RJ, Harari PM. Is radiation dose reduction the right answer for HPV-positive head and neck cancer? *Oral Oncol* 2013 Oct 14.

37. Duray A, Descamps G, Decaestecker C, et al. Human papillomavirus DNA strongly correlates with a poorer prognosis in oral cavity carcinoma. *Laryngoscope* 2012;122:1558–1565.

38. Stenmark MH, McHugh JB, Schipper M, et al. Nonendemic HPV-positive nasopharyngeal carcinoma: association with poor prognosis. *Int J Radiation Oncol Biol Phys* 2014;88:580–588.

41. Spector ME, Gallagher KK, Light E, et al. Matted nodes: poor prognostic marker in oropharyngeal squamous cell carcinoma independent of HPV and EGFR status. *Head Neck* 2012;34:1727–1733.

42. Hayes N, consortium T. Comprehensive genomic characterization of head and neck squamous cell carcinomas. *Nature* 2013.

47. Rubin Grandis J, Melhem MF, Gooding WE, et al. Levels of TGF-alpha and EGFR protein in head and neck squamous cell carcinoma and patient survival. *J Natl Cancer Inst* 1998;90:824–832.

48. Bonner JA, Harari PM, Giralt J, et al. Radiotherapy plus cetuximab for locoregionally advanced head and neck cancer: 5-year survival data from a phase 3 randomised trial, and relation between cetuximab-induced rash and survival. *Lancet Oncol* 2010;11:21–28.

53. Bradford CR, Kumar B, Belillile E, et al. Biomarkers in advanced larynx cancer. *Laryngoscope* 2014;124:179–187.

55. Kumar B, Cordell KG, D'Silva N, et al. Expression of p53 and Bcl-xL as predictive markers for larynx preservation in advanced laryngeal cancer. *Arch Otolaryngol Head Neck Surg* 2008;134:363–369.

57. Hahn WC, Counter CM, Lundberg AS, et al. Creation of human tumour cells with defined genetic elements. *Nature* 1999;400:464–468.

60. Liu J, Pan S, Hsieh MH, et al. Targeting Wnt-driven cancer through the inhibition of Porcupine by LGK974. *Proc Natl Acad Sci U S A* 2013;110:20224–20229.

63. Chen YC, Chang CJ, Hsu HS, et al. Inhibition of tumorigenicity and enhancement of radiochemosensitivity in head and neck squamous cell cancer-derived ALDH1-positive cells by knockdown of Bmi-1. *Oral Oncol* 2010;46:158–165.

64. Yu CC, Lo WL, Chen YW, et al. Bmi-1 regulates snail expression and promotes metastasis ability in head and neck squamous cancer-derived ALDH1 positive cells. *J Oncol* 2011;2011.

65. Clay MR, Tabor M, Owen JH, et al. Single-marker identification of head and neck squamous cell carcinoma cancer stem cells with aldehyde dehydrogenase. *Head Neck* 2010;32:1195–1201.

PRACTICE OF ONCOLOGY

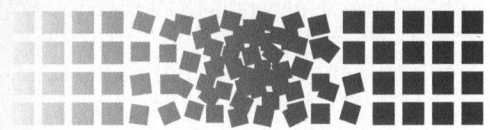

38 Cancer of the Head and Neck

William M. Mendenhall, John W. Werning, and David G. Pfister

INCIDENCE AND ETIOLOGY

The estimated number of new head and neck cancer cases (excluding skin cancer) in the United States in 2013 is 53,640; this represents 3.2% of the total new cancer cases.[1] Approximately 27% of these patients are women.[1] African Americans have a higher age-adjusted incidence than other ethnic groups. The usual time of diagnosis is after the age of 40, except for salivary gland and nasopharyngeal cancers (NPCs), which may occur in younger age groups. For many primary sites, tobacco use is associated with an increased risk. Alcohol has also been implicated as a causative factor; the effects of alcohol and tobacco may be synergistic.[2] Head and neck cancer patients have an increased risk for developing a second primary tumor (SPT), both within the head and neck and elsewhere (e.g., esophageal and lung cancers),[3] attributed to the field effect associated with tobacco and alcohol use.[4] Human papillomavirus infection (HPV; most commonly HPV-16) plays a role in the development of certain head and neck cancers, particularly those in the oropharynx.[5,6] Patients with high-risk HPV (HR-HPV)–positive head and neck cancers tend to be younger and less likely to have a strong history of tobacco and ethanol use, have a history of multiple sex partners (particularly oral-genital sex), have a better prognosis, and appear to have a lower rate of SPTs.[6–8] Prior tobacco exposure adversely affects the prognosis of HPV-related oropharynx cancers.[8,9] An increasing incidence of oral tongue squamous cell carcinoma in nonsmoking Caucasian women has been reported that does not appear to be driven by prior HPV infection, whereas the incidence of other oral cavity cancers is declining.[10] There is a long-standing association between Epstein-Barr virus (EBV) and NPC.[11] Occupational exposures are associated with the development of sinonasal tract tumors.[12]

ANATOMY AND PATHOLOGY

The anatomy pertaining to a particular primary site is described in subsequent sections. To facilitate communication, lymph nodes are organized into levels. Level I includes the submental and submandibular areas; levels II through IV include the internal jugular vein lymph nodes; level V includes the posterior triangle (Fig. 38.1).[13] Furthermore, which lymph node levels are involved is predictive of the primary site. For example, lip, oral cavity, and facial skin tumors typically spread to levels I and II initially; larynx and pharynx cancers have a predilection for spread to levels II and III.

There are no capillary lymphatics in the epithelium. The tumor must penetrate the lamina propria before lymphatic invasion can occur. One can predict the richness of the capillary network in a given head and neck site by the relative incidence of lymph node metastases at presentation. The nasopharynx and pyriform sinus have the most profuse capillary lymphatic networks. The paranasal sinuses, middle ear, and vocal cords have few or no capillary lymphatics. Muscle and fat contain few capillary lymphatics, as do bone and cartilage within the periosteum or perichondrium. There are no capillary lymphatics in the eye, and few in the orbit.

Most head and neck malignant neoplasms arise from the surface epithelium and are squamous cell carcinoma (SCC) or one of its variants, including lymphoepithelioma, spindle cell carcinoma, verrucous carcinoma, and undifferentiated carcinoma. Lymphomas and a wide variety of other malignant and benign neoplasms make up the remaining cases.[14–16]

Lymphoepithelioma is an SCC with a lymphoid stroma and occurs in the nasopharynx, tonsillar fossa, and base of tongue; it may also occur in the salivary glands. In the spindle cell variant, there is a spindle cell component that resembles sarcoma intermixed with SCC. It is generally managed like other high-grade SCCs. Verrucous carcinoma is a low-grade SCC found most often in the oral cavity, particularly on the gingiva and buccal mucosa. It usually has an indolent growth pattern and is often associated with the chronic use of snuff or chewing tobacco.

Small cell neuroendocrine carcinoma occurs rarely throughout the head and neck. Upper aerodigestive tract lymphomas almost always show a diffuse non-Hodgkin histologic pattern.

NATURAL HISTORY

Patterns of Spread

Primary Lesion

SCCs usually begin as surface lesions. Superficial tumors arising in the Waldeyer ring may be difficult to distinguish from normal lymphoid tissue. Very early surface lesions may show only erythema and a slightly elevated mucosa.

Spread is dictated by local anatomy, and thus varies by each site. Muscle invasion is common, and the tumor may spread along muscle or fascial planes a surprising distance from the palpable or visible lesion. The tumor may attach early to the periosteum or perichondrium, but bone or cartilage invasion is usually a late event. Bone and cartilage usually act as a barrier to spread; the tumor that encounters these structures will often be diverted and spread along a path of less resistance. Slow-growing gingival neoplasms may produce a smooth pressure defect of the underlying bone without bone invasion.

Tumor extension into the parapharyngeal space allows superior or inferior spread from the skull base to the low neck.

Spread inside the lumen of the sublingual, submandibular, and parotid gland ducts is uncommon. The nasolacrimal duct, however, is often invaded in ethmoid sinus and nasal carcinomas.

Perineural invasion (PNI) is observed in SCCs as well as salivary gland tumors, especially adenoid cystic carcinomas. When advanced, PNI may produce neurologic symptoms and is associated with a poorer rate of local control.[17] Tumors may track along a nerve to the skull base and central nervous system (CNS) or peripherally.

Vascular space invasion is associated with an increased risk for regional and distant metastases.

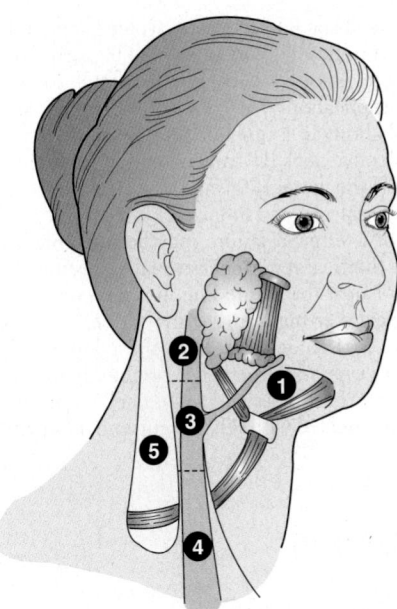

Figure 38.1 Head and neck lymph node levels.

Lymphatic Spread

The differentiation of the tumor, the size of the primary lesion, the presence of vascular space invasion, and the density of capillary lymphatics predict the risk of lymph node metastasis. Recurrent lesions have an increased risk. Histology also impacts the likelihood of lymphatic spread. Low-grade minor salivary gland tumors and sarcomas have a lower risk of lymph node metastases than SCCs arising in similar mucosal sites.

A patient may present with SCC in a cervical lymph node, and despite an extensive work-up, the site of origin may remain undetermined in approximately 50% of patients.[18] If only the neck is treated, a primary lesion may appear later, but sometimes is never found.[19]

The relative incidence of clinically positive lymph nodes on admission is determined by primary site and T stage.[20] Well-lateralized lesions spread to ipsilateral neck nodes.[21] Lesions on or near the midline, tongue base, and nasopharyngeal lesions (even when lateralized), may spread to both sides of the neck, although the risk is higher to the side occupied by the bulk of the lesion. Patients with clinically positive ipsilateral neck nodes are at risk for contralateral disease, especially if the nodes are large or multiple; obstruction of the lymphatic pathways by surgery or radiotherapy (RT) also shunts the lymphatic flow to the opposite neck.[21] When lymph node metastases appear at an unusual site, a careful search must be made for a second primary. The likelihood of retropharyngeal adenopathy is related to the presence of clinically involved lymph nodes and the primary site, and is particularly high for NPCs.[22]

Distant Spread

The risk of distant metastasis is related more to N stage and the location of involved nodes in the low neck, rather than to T stage.[23] The risk is less than 10% for N0 or N1 disease and rises to approximately 30% for N3 disease as well as N1 or N2 nodes with disease below the level of the thyroid notch. Distant metastases are found most often in the lung.[24]

DIAGNOSIS

A general medical evaluation is performed, including a thorough head and neck examination. The location and extent of

the primary tumor and any clinically positive lymph nodes is documented. Almost all patients undergo contrast enhanced computed tomography (CT) and/or magnetic resonance imaging (MRI) to further define the extent of local–regional disease. The scan(s) should be obtained prior to biopsy so that biopsy changes are not confused with the tumor. A chest radiograph is obtained to determine the presence of distant metastases and/or a synchronous primary lung cancer. Patients with N3 neck disease, as well as those with N2 disease with nodes below the level of the thyroid notch, have a 20% to 30% risk of developing distant metastases and are considered for a chest CT or positron emission tomography (PET).

Tumors amenable to transoral biopsy may be biopsied using local anesthetics in the clinic. Otherwise, direct laryngoscopy under anesthesia is performed to determine the extent of the tumor and to obtain a tissue diagnosis. Given the risk of synchronous cancers, some advocate routine triple endoscopy (i.e., laryngoscopy/pharyngoscopy, bronchoscopy, and esophagoscopy). The additional yield is low, unless diffuse mucosal abnormalities or a malignant lymph node without an identified primary site, particularly in the low neck, are present. Patients presenting with a metastatic node from an unknown primary site undergo fine-needle aspiration (FNA) of the node. An excisional biopsy is not routinely performed unless lymphoma is suspected or FNA results are equivocal. If SCC is a consideration, the excision should be done in a manner to facilitate subsequent management, including neck dissection. Occasionally, the diagnosis may be made by clinical and radiographic evaluation, and a biopsy should be avoided in situations where the treatment is definitive for RT and where obtaining a tissue sample is risky (e.g., paragangliomas, juvenile nasopharyngeal angiofibromas).[14,25]

Before the initial treatment, the patient should be evaluated by members of the team who may be involved in the initial management as well as possible salvage therapy. Head and neck surgeons, radiation oncologists, medical oncologists, diagnostic radiologists, plastic surgeons, pathologists, dentists, speech and swallowing therapists, and social workers may all play a role.

STAGING

The staging system of the American Joint Committee on Cancer (AJCC) is used.[26] In general, excisional biopsy (TX) indicates that the primary tumor cannot be assessed; T0 indicates no evidence of primary tumor; and Tis indicates carcinoma in situ. For tumors of the oral cavity and oropharynx, further staging of the primary lesion is based primarily on size criteria: 2 cm or less for T1; greater than 2 cm but no more than 4 cm for T2; greater than 4 cm for T3; and T4 tumors involve major invasion or encasement of surrounding structures (e.g., bone, carotid artery, deep musculature). For the other primary sites, further staging is less easily generalized because the anatomic extent of spread and/or functional criteria (e.g., vocal cord mobility) are used and, for certain sites, are combined with tumor size (e.g., hypopharynx, major salivary glands), and so will be given in the discussion of each respective primary site.[26] Neck staging is common to all head and neck sites, except the nasopharynx (Table 38.1).[26] Lesions may be clinically or pathologically staged. Clinical staging is more commonly used for treatment planning and the reporting of results. The format for combining T and N stages into an overall stage is depicted in Table 38.2 and is common to all sites except the nasopharynx.[26]

Stage IV represents a wide spectrum of disease. One patient may have a T1, T2, or T3 lesion with low-volume N2 neck disease and a high probability of cure (stage IVA), whereas another may have a T4b primary cancer and/or N3 neck disease and a relatively poor prognosis (stage IVB)[27]; distant metastases indicate stage IVC disease, and the treatment intent is typically palliative.

TABLE 38.1

TABLE 38.1

2010 American Joint Committee on Cancer Stages of Regional Lymph Node Involvement

NX	Regional lymph nodes cannot be assessed
N0	No regional lymph node metastasis
N1	Metastasis in a single ipsilateral lymph node, 3 cm or less in greatest dimension
N2	Metastasis in single ipsilateral lymph node, more than 3 cm but no more than 6 cm in greatest dimension; or in multiple ipsilateral lymph nodes, none more than 6 cm in greatest dimension; or in bilateral or contralateral lymph nodes, no more than 6 cm in greatest dimension
N2a	Metastasis in single ipsilateral lymph node, more than 3 cm but no more than 6 cm in greatest dimension
N2b	Metastasis in multiple ipsilateral lymph nodes, none more than 6 cm in greatest dimension
N2c	Metastasis in bilateral or contralateral lymph nodes, none more than 6 cm in greatest dimension
N3	Metastasis in a lymph node more than 6 cm in greatest dimension

Used with the permission of the American Joint Committee on Cancer (AJCC), Chicago, Illinois. The original source for this material is the *AJCC Cancer Staging Handbook*, Seventh Edition (2010) published by Springer Science and Business Media LLC, www.springerlink.com.

PRINCIPLES OF TREATMENT FOR SQUAMOUS CELL CARCINOMA

General Principles for Selection of Treatment

Surgery and RT are the only curative treatments for head and neck carcinomas. Although chemotherapy alone is not curative, it enhances the effects of RT, and thus is routinely used as part of combined modality treatment in patients with stage III or IV disease.

The advantages of surgery compared with RT, assuming similar cure rates, may include the following: (1) a limited amount of tissue is exposed to treatment, (2) the treatment time is shorter, (3) the risk

TABLE 38.2

2010 American Joint Committee on Cancer Overall Stage Grouping

Stage 0	Tis	N0	M0
Stage I	T1	N0	M0
Stage II	T2	N0	M0
Stage III	T3	N0	M0
	T1–T3	N1	M0
Stage IVA	T4a	N0–N1	M0
	T1–T4a	N2	M0
Stage IVB	Any T	N3	M0
	T4b	Any N	M0
Stage IVC	Any T	Any N	M1

Used with the permission of the American Joint Committee on Cancer (AJCC), Chicago, Illinois. The original source for this material is the *AJCC Cancer Staging Handbook*, Seventh Edition (2010) published by Springer Science and Business Media LLC, www.springerlink.com.

of immediate and late RT sequelae is avoided, and (4) RT is reserved for a head and neck SPT, which may not be as suitable for surgery.

The advantages of RT may include (1) the risk of a major postoperative complication is avoided, (2) no tissues are removed so that the probability of a functional or cosmetic defect may be reduced, (3) elective neck RT can be included with little added morbidity, and (4) the surgical salvage of RT failure is probably more likely than the salvage of a surgical failure.

Salvage of a surgical failure may be attempted by operation, RT, or both. Surgical recurrences usually develop at the resection margins, in or near the suture line. It is difficult to distinguish the normal surgical scarring from recurrent disease, and the diagnosis of recurrence is often delayed. Tumor response to RT under these circumstances is poor. Surgery, RT, or both, however, may salvage small mucosal recurrences and some neck recurrences. For bulkier recurrences treated with RT, concurrent chemotherapy is often incorporated.

MANAGEMENT

Primary Site

The management of the primary cancer will be considered separately for each anatomical site. Patients who are in poor nutritional condition may require a nasogastric (NG) tube or a percutaneous gastrostomy (PEG) before initiating RT, particularly if concomitant chemotherapy is used. Opinions vary regarding the role of prophylactic NG or PEG placement in anticipation of RT-based local toxicity in patients without significant baseline dysphagia or weight loss; a reactive strategy is preferred by many and may facilitate swallowing recovery.[28] If external-beam radiotherapy (EBRT) is selected, it may be given with either conventional once-daily fractionation, 66 to 70 Gy at 2 Gy per fraction, 5 days a week in a continuous course, or with an altered fractionation schedule. Whether an altered fractionation schedule is better than conventional fractionation depends on the altered fractionation technique that is selected. Two altered fractionation schedules shown to result in improved local–regional control rates are the University of Florida hyperfractionation and the M.D. Anderson concomitant boost techniques.[29] The results of a prospective randomized Radiation Therapy Oncology Group (RTOG) trial comparing these schedules with conventional fractionation and the Massachusetts General Hospital accelerated split-course schedule are shown in Table 38.3. Acute toxicity is increased with altered fractionation; late toxicity is comparable with conventional fractionation.[30]

Conventional EBRT techniques and/or brachytherapy will be discussed in the subsequent site-specific sections. EBRT may also be delivered with intensity-modulated radiation therapy (IMRT) to produce a more conformal dose distribution and to reduce the dose to the normal tissues.[31–33] The disadvantages of IMRT are that it is more time consuming to plan and treat the patient; the dose distribution is often less homogenous so that "hot spots" may increase the risk of late complications, the risk of a marginal miss may be increased because the fields are more conformal, the total body RT dose is higher because of increased "beam on" time and scatter irradiation, and it is more costly. Therefore, a clear reason for using IMRT versus conventional RT must be identified. The usual indication for IMRT is to reduce the dose to the contralateral parotid gland, and thus limit long-term xerostomia.[34] Another indication is to reduce the CNS dose in patients with NPC. Finally, it may be used to avoid a difficult low neck match in patients with laryngeal or hypopharyngeal cancers and a low-lying larynx. Proton therapy, which offers potential targeting and dosing advantages for selected tumors,[35] is useful for reducing the dose to the brain and the visual apparatus for patients with nasal cavity and paranasal sinus malignancies.

TABLE 38.3

Altered Fractionation: 5-Year Outcomes from the Radiation Therapy Oncology Group 90-03 Trial

Parameter	Fractionation Schedule			
	Conventional (70 Gy/35 Fx/7 wk)	Hyperfractionation (81.6 Gy/68 Fx/7 wk)	Accelerated Split Course (67.2 Gy/42 Fx/6 wk)	Accelerated Concomitant Boost (72 Gy/42 Fx/6 wk)
Number of patients	268	263	274	268
Local–regional failure	59.1%	51.2% (p = 0.037)	57.8% (p = 0.042)	51.7%
Disease-free survival	21.2%	30.7% (p = 0.013)	26.6% (p = 0.042)	28.9%
Overall survival	29.5%	37.1% (p = 0.063)	30.8%	33.5%
Cause-specific survival	42.9%	45.5%	40.9%	43.4%
Grade 3 late toxicity	25.2%	27.4%	26.8%	33.3% (p = 0.066)

Note: P values reflect comparison of the experimental arms with standard fractionation.
Fx, fractions.
From Trotti A, Fu KK, Pajak TF, et al. Long term outcomes of RTOG 90-03: a comparison of hyperfractionation and two variants of accelerated fractionation to standard fractionation radiotherapy for head and neck squamous cell carcinoma. *Int J Radiat Oncol Biol Phys* 2005;63:S70–S71.

NECK

In a classic *radical neck dissection*, the superficial and deep cervical fascia with its enclosed lymph nodes (levels I to V) is removed in continuity with the sternocleidomastoid muscle, the omohyoid muscle, the internal and external jugular veins, cranial nerve XI, and the submandibular gland. The incisions used by the surgeon will be governed largely by the primary lesion. The radical neck dissection can be *modified* to spare certain structures with the intent of decreasing morbidity and improving functional outcome without compromising disease control. There are three main types of modified radical neck dissections: type I, CN XI is spared; type II, CN XI and the internal jugular vein are spared; and type III (functional), CN XI, the internal jugular vein, and the sternocleidomastoid muscle are spared. *Selective* neck dissections are more limited and include the resection of lymph node levels that are at greatest risk for nodal metastatic spread. Examples include the lateral, posterolateral, and supraomohyoid, which include resections of lymph node levels II through IV, II through V, and I through III, respectively.

A modified or selective neck dissection is recommended for the cN0 neck, for selected clinically positive necks (mobile, 1 to 3 cm lymph nodes), and for removing residual disease after RT when there has been excellent regression of N2 or N3 disease.[36,37]

The more extensive the neck dissection, the higher the risk of complications. Complications after neck dissection include hematoma, seroma, lymphedema, wound infections and dehiscence, damage to the 7th, 10th, 11th, and 12th cranial nerves, carotid exposure, and carotid rupture. The last-mentioned complication can be minimized by covering the carotid artery with a dermal graft at the time of surgery.[36] Pain and dysfunction in the neck or shoulder may occur. Rehabilitation and anti-inflammatory medication are commonly utilized with varying benefits; acupuncture had demonstrated a benefit compared to the usual care in one randomized study.[38]

Clinically Negative Neck

The estimated incidence of subclinical disease in the regional lymphatics when the neck is cN0 is presented in Table 38.4.[39] Both RT and neck dissection are approximately 90% efficient at eradicating subclinical regional disease.[36] Alternatively, a policy of close observation may be adopted for the cN0 neck to avoid unnecessary treatment, and the neck is managed by surgery and/or RT if cervical metastases develop. The salvage rate for patients developing clinically positive lymph nodes with the primary lesion controlled is 50% to 60%.[39]

TABLE 38.4

Definition of Risk Groups for the Clinically N0 Neck

Group	Estimated Risk of Subclinical Neck Disease	T Stage	Site
I: Low risk	<20%	T1	Floor of mouth, oral tongue, retromolar trigone, gingiva, hard palate, buccal mucosa
II: Intermediate risk	20%–30%	T1	Soft palate, pharyngeal wall, supraglottic larynx, tonsil
		T2	Floor of mouth, oral tongue, retromolar trigone, gingiva, hard palate, buccal mucosa
III: High risk	>30%	T1–T4	Nasopharynx, pyriform sinus, base of tongue
		T2–T4	Soft palate, pharyngeal wall, supraglottic larynx, tonsil
		T3–T4	Floor of mouth, oral tongue, retromolar trigone, gingiva, hard palate, buccal mucosa

Reprinted with permission from Mendenhall WM, Million RR. Elective neck irradiation for squamous cell carcinoma of the head and neck: analysis of time-dose factors and causes of failure. *Int J Radiat Oncol Biol Phys* 1986;12:741–746.

PRACTICE OF ONCOLOGY

Failure of Initial Neck Treatment (596 Patients with Carcinoma of the Tonsillar Fossa, Base of Tongue, Supraglottic Larynx, or Hypopharynx at M.D. Anderson Hospital 1948–1967)

	Stage							
	N0							
Treatment	**No Treatment**	**Partial**	**Complete**	**N1**	**N2A**	**N2B**	**N3A**	**N3B**
Radiation		15%	2%	15%	27%	27%	38%	34%
Surgery	55% (16/29)	35%	7%	11%	8%	23%	42%	41%
Combined		1/5	0/6	0	0	0	23%	25%

Adapted from Barkley HT Jr, Fletcher GH, Jesse RH, et al. Management of cervical lymph node metastases in squamous cell carcinoma of the tonsillar fossa, base of tongue supraglottic larynx, and hypopharynx. *Am J Surg* 1972;124:462–467.

Elective neck irradiation (ENI) and elective neck dissection are equally effective in the management of the N0 neck, with control rates exceeding 90%.[39,40] Treatment of the entire neck is advised for primary lesions with a high rate of subclinical disease, such as the base of tongue, soft palate, supraglottis, and hypopharynx. Patients with lateralized T1 to T2 tonsillar cancers do not require elective treatment for the contralateral N0 neck[41]; T3 or T4 cancers or those with significant extension into the tongue and/or soft palate should receive bilateral neck treatment to the entire neck.

When the primary tumor is to be treated surgically, an elective neck dissection should be performed when the risk of regional lymph node metastasis is 10% to 15% or greater. Modified neck dissection has a good rate of disease control; patients who are found to have multiple positive nodes or extracapsular extension (ECE) are then referred for postoperative RT,[42] and concurrent chemotherapy is recommended in the latter circumstance.[43–46] If the primary lesion is to be treated with EBRT, ENI adds relatively little cost and modest morbidity.

Clinically Positive Neck Lymph Nodes

The rates of neck failure by N stage and treatment group reported from the M.D. Anderson Cancer Center and the University of Florida are shown in Tables 38.5 and 38.6, respectively.[40,47] In general, RT precedes surgery if the primary site is to be treated by RT or if the node was fixed. The operation precedes RT if the primary site is to be treated surgically.

Modified neck dissection is sufficient treatment for the ipsilateral neck for patients with N1 or N2A disease without ECE. RT, often combined with concurrent chemotherapy, is added for those with more advanced neck disease.[42]

When the primary lesion is to be managed by RT or chemoradiotherapy (chemoRT), then RT-based therapy alone is sufficient for patients in whom the node(s) regress completely as documented on CT obtained 4 weeks post-RT.[37,48] RT is followed by a neck dissection for patients with residual nodes that are 1.5 cm or larger, as well as those that demonstrate focal defects, enhancement, and/or calcification.[48] A PET scan done 3 months after RT is completed is an alternative to CT to assess whether there is persistent disease.[49]

McGuirt and McCabe[50] compared results of definitive surgery with and without a prior open neck biopsy and concluded the risks of neck failure, distant metastases, and complications were all increased. Ellis et al.[51] studied the results of therapy following open biopsy of a lymph node before treatment. Patients received definitive RT to the primary site and neck; a subset of patients underwent a neck dissection after RT. Open biopsy had no adverse impact on these patients compared with those who did not undergo an open biopsy.[51] Therefore, after open biopsy of the neck, RT-based therapy is recommended as the initial treatment, particularly if the primary tumor is to be managed by RT or chemoRT. Under these circumstances, no further neck treatment is needed if the neck node had been removed; if there was residual gross tumor in the neck after open biopsy, a planned neck dissection should be added depending on the results of radiologic reassessment.[48]

5-Year Rate of Neck Control According to the 1983 American Joint Committee on Cancer Stage and Treatment (459 Patients, 593 Heminecks[a])

	RT Alone		**RT + Neck Dissection**		
Stage	**No. of Heminecks**	**Control**	**No. of Heminecks**	**Control**	**Significance**
N1	215	86%	38	93%	p = 0.28
N2A	29	79%	24	68%	p = 0.60
N2B	138	70%	80	91%	p < 0.01
N3A	29	33%	40	69%	p < 0.01

Note: The University of Florida data, patients were treated October 1964 to October 1985; analysis occurred December 1988 by Eric R. Ellis, MD.
[a] Excludes 67 heminecks that received incisional or excisional biopsies before treatment.
From Mendenhall WM, Parson JT, Mancuso AA, et al. Head and neck: management of the neck. In: Perez CA, Brady LW, eds. *Principles and Practice of Radiation Oncology*, 2nd ed. Philadelphia: J.B. Lippincott Company; 1992: 790–805; and American Joint Committee on Cancer. *Manual for Staging of Cancer*. Philadelphia: J. B. Lippincott Company; 1983.

CHEMOTHERAPY

Drug therapy may be administered to prevent the development of SPTs (chemoprevention), to palliate symptoms in patients with incurable disease, to improve the odds of cure or organ preservation when combined with definitive local-regional therapy, or to decrease treatment toxicity. The first two indications are discussed here; the last two are discussed in a subsequent section.

Chemoprevention

Chemoprevention is the administration of natural or synthetic agents to reduce the risk of developing SPTs. Patients who have a head and neck SCC have an increased risk of developing an upper aerodigestive tract SPT because of exposure to carcinogens and/or genetic predisposition.[3] The risk of developing an SPT is approximately 2.7% to 4% per year[52] and may impact survival. Current data indicate the risk of SPTs is lower among patients with HR-HPV–related head and neck cancers.[6,8] Analogs of vitamin A, particularly of the retinoids, have been a particular focus of clinical investigations. At present, there is no standard role for the use of chemopreventive agents in the management of head and neck cancer.

Retinoids and beta-carotene both may cause regression of oral leukoplakia; the former appear more efficacious.[53] Lesions commonly recur after cessation of drug therapy. Chemoprevention agents do not reduce the risk of recurrence of the index cancer.

High-dose 13-*cis*-retinoic acid (100 mg/m^2 daily for 12 months) has been shown in a randomized, placebo-controlled trial to reduce the risk of SPTs in patients previously treated for stage I to IV, M0, head and neck cancer.[54] However, a large, placebo-controlled, randomized trial in 1,190 survivors of stage I and II head and neck SCC found no difference in the rate of SPTs or survival after 3 years of a low-dose schedule of this agent (30 mg per day).[55] Outcomes were better among nonsmokers and those who quit compared to smokers, emphasizing the important role of tobacco cessation as part of head and neck cancer management and strategies to decrease SPTs. Similarly, etretinate was not shown to be efficacious in decreasing SPTs.[56]

With regard to other agents, vitamin A, N-acetylcysteine, both, or neither were evaluated using a factorial design in the EUROSCAN study. No significant improvement in survival or SPTs was observed.[57] Bairati et al.[58] randomized head and neck cancer survivors to 3 years of therapy with alpha-tocopherol and beta-carotene versus placebo; the rate of SPTs was actually higher during the period of treatment, a difference that did not persist with longer follow-up. A randomized phase II, placebo-controlled trial demonstrated no significant benefit of celecoxib at 100 mg or 200 mg, both twice daily, on the control of oral premalignant lesions.[59]

Targeting the epidermal growth factor receptor (EGFR) pathway is receiving attention, because there is an association between progressive EGFR dysregulation and the transition from normal mucosa to dysplasia to SCC.[60] The concept of bioadjuvant therapy,[55] whereby drug combinations intended to reduce both the risk of SPTs and relapse from the index cancer, as well as the potential role of natural extracts are also of interest.[61]

There is no standard role for the use of HR-HPV vaccination in the prevention of head and neck cancer at this time,[62] although the impact of current vaccination programs on the incidence of head and neck cancer warrants follow-up.

Chemotherapy for Recurrent or Metastatic Disease

Single Agents

Patients with recurrent or metastatic head and neck SCCs have a median survival of 6 to 9 months, and a 1-year survival rate of 20% to 40% when treated with chemotherapy alone.[63,64] Although selected patients may derive apparent significant prolongations in survival, average survival improvements appear small at best. Morton et al.[65] reported a 2-month improvement in median survival after treatment with cisplatin, with or without bleomycin, compared to no treatment. The duration of responses is typically measured in weeks to months, not years; survival beyond 2 years is infrequent; and cures are anecdotal. Thus, the primary intent of chemotherapy in this setting is to achieve tumor regression with the hope that the potential palliative benefit and possible modest survival improvement will outweigh the side effects of treatment.

A number of drugs have been demonstrated in clinical trials to have activity in head and neck SCCs, and the list is well summarized in prior reviews.[63,64] The most commonly used include methotrexate, cisplatin, carboplatin, 5-fluorouracil, paclitaxel, and docetaxel, with reported major response rates ranging from 15% to 42%. Among other drugs with reported major response rates of 15% or greater are bleomycin, cyclophosphamide, doxorubicin, hydroxyurea, ifosfamide, irinotecan, oral uracil, ftorafur (with leucovorin), pemetrexed, vinblastine, and vinorelbine. Some of these agents (e.g., cyclophosphamide, doxorubicin, hydroxyurea) have their activity based on reported assessments in a limited number of patients from over 2 decades ago, an era when methods and criteria for response assessments may have differed from current standards. Anticipated response rates and toxicity profiles may vary based on patient selection and drug schedule. A poor performance status is associated with both lower response rates and greater potential for toxicity. The larger the amount of prior treatment also adversely affects response rates.[64]

Methotrexate is a historic standard drug used in the recurrent or metastatic disease setting. The typical standard dosing is 40 mg/m^2 intravenously weekly, with dose attenuation or increase (up to 60 mg/m^2) based on toxicity, with mucositis being a frequent reason for dose adjustment. The favorable side effect profile and convenience of administration of methotrexate make it well-suited for use in this patient population in which medical comorbidity is common, as is more advanced age. In randomized trials, higher doses increase response rates and toxicity without a significant improvement in overall survival.[66,67] Newer analogs of methotrexate (e.g., edatrexate) have not been shown to offer a therapeutic advantage in phase III trials.[68]

Cisplatin is a cornerstone drug in the modern management of head and neck cancer. Cisplatin is customarily dosed at 75 to 100 mg/m^2 intravenously every 3 to 4 weeks. The potential for renal (i.e., increase in creatinine, electrolyte abnormalities), otologic (i.e., high frequency hearing loss, tinnitus), neurologic (i.e., peripheral neuropathy), and gastrointestinal (i.e., nausea and vomiting) toxicity are widely appreciated, but these risks are manageable if patients are appropriately screened for therapy, monitored closely, and state of the art supportive care measures are applied. Further dose escalation of cisplatin has not been established to improve outcome. A randomized trial comparing 60 mg/m^2 versus 120 mg/m^2 of cisplatin failed to demonstrate a significant improvement in response or survival.[69] Carboplatin is the best studied and most commonly used platinum analog in head and neck cancer. Although generally less toxic and easier to administer than the parent drug, it is more bone marrow suppressive and may be somewhat less active. This last issue is more of a concern in the definitive treatment setting in which cure is a central endpoint, as opposed to the palliative setting, when patients often seek a less toxic alternative treatment.

Although taxanes as a class have significant activity in head and neck SCCs, hopes of clinically significant improvement in survival in the palliative setting with the introduction of these agents have yet to be realized. Neither paclitaxel or docetaxel has been demonstrated in random assignment trials to be clearly superior to methotrexate with regard to survival as an endpoint.[70] Paclitaxel dosed at 250 mg/m^2 intravenously over 24 hours with growth factor support in an Eastern Cooperative Oncology Group (ECOG) trial, yielded a major response in 12 of 30 patients (40%) including four complete responses; grade 3 or greater neutropenia occurred in 91% of patients, and there were two deaths.[71] Less cumbersome to administer and less toxic schedules are commonly used in practice (e.g., 135 to 225 mg/m² intravenously over 3 hours every 3 weeks; 80 to 100 mg/m² weekly), although their relative efficacies have not been well evaluated. A paclitaxel schedule that provides more prolonged exposure to the drug may be more efficacious,[72] although a phase II trial of 120 to 140 mg/m² over 96 hours yielded disappointing results even in treatment-naïve patients (major response rate, 13%).[65] Other toxicities besides myelosuppression include sensory neuropathy, alopecia, allergic reactions, and arrhythmia, although cardiac monitoring is not required.

Docetaxel appears less neuropathic than paclitaxel, but fluid retention and hematologic toxicity may be more problematic. A typical dose is 60 to 100 mg/m² intravenously over 1 hour. Initial studies evaluated the efficacy of the 100 mg/m² dose level, with major response rates ranging from 21% to 42%[73]; an excellent performance status is required for this higher dose. Lower doses may offer similar efficacy and better tolerance.[74] As with paclitaxel, weekly schedules are applied in practice, but the relative efficacy of weekly versus a schedule of every 3 weeks is not well-studied.

Although initial studies evaluated a bolus schedule for 5-fluorouracil, an infusional program of 1,000 mg/m² per day over 96 to 120 hours appears more efficacious in head and neck cancer.[75] Infusional 5-fluorouracil is associated with more mucositis and diarrhea than a bolus schedule, so the shorter infusion (i.e., 96 hours) is typically applied in patients who are pretreated and have received prior head and neck RT.

EGFR is highly expressed in most head and neck SCCs, and the degree of expression is inversely associated with prognosis.[76–78] As such, there has been a keen interest in drugs that target the receptor itself or steps downstream. Cetuximab, a chimeric immunoglobulin G antibody that binds the receptor, has been approved by the U.S. Food and Drug Administration for use in patients with disease refractory to platin-based therapy. As summarized in Table 38.7, the response rates in this refractory setting are similar (10% to 13%) whether cetuximab is used alone or combined with platin-based therapy; median survivals remained disappointing, ranging from 5.2 to 6.1 months.[79–82] Another EGFR antibody, zalutumumab, was compared in a randomized trial to best supportive care alone in patients with cisplatin-refractory squamous cell head and neck cancer. Among 286 entered patients, there was no significant improvement in the primary endpoint of overall survival (median 6.7 versus 5.2 months, p = 0.0648) although a significant difference was found on an exploratory post hoc analysis done 12 months after the last patient was randomized. Response rate (6.3% versus 1.1%) and progression-free survival (median 9.9 versus 8.4 weeks, p = 0.0012) were improved with zalutumumab.[83]

The small molecule tyrosine–kinase inhibitors, gefitinib and erlotinib, offer no efficacy advantage in similar refractory patients.

Major response rates and median survivals ranged from 0% to 15% and 5.9 to 8.1 months, respectively.[78,84–86] A large randomized trial (486 patients) compared gefitinib (250 or 500 mg daily) to methotrexate and demonstrated no survival improvement with either gefitinib dose.[87]

With both of these classes of agents, the development of rash was associated with clinical benefit, but this association is not fully explained by simple pharmacokinetics.[78] There is no established molecular predictor of response to these agents currently in head and neck SCC.

The successful development and approval of cetuximab in head and neck SCC highlights the potential for therapies to exploit specific molecular pathways with therapeutic effect. A number of other new agents, often with multitarget capability, are entering clinical trials. There is a good rationale for agents that target angiogenesis in head and neck SCC.[88] However, the development of bevacizumab has been cautious given the reported toxicity concerns, specifically bleeding, in patients with squamous cell lung cancer.[89] Alterations in the PI3K/Akt/mammalian target of rapamycin (mTOR) pathway are common in head and neck cancer, and activation appears independent of EGFR activation, making targeting of this pathway of great interest.[90] Cancer gene therapy, whereby genetic sequences are introduced via viral or nonviral vectors, is well-suited to head and neck tumors given the local–regional character of head and neck tumors that facilitates direct injection and the monitoring of gene expression. The tumor suppressor gene p53 has been one target, because somatic mutations of it are common in head and neck cancers, particularly among patients who have smoked cigarettes and used alcohol.[91] For example, in a phase II study of Onyx-015, a replication-competent adenovirus absent the E1B gene, major responses, including some complete regressions, occurred in 10% to 14% of treated patients.[92] In other studies, treatment with Onyx-015, or a similar virus such as H101, improved the efficacy of chemotherapy.[93,94]

Combination Therapy

Given the disappointing track record for single-agent therapy in the palliative setting, combinations of drugs have been extensively evaluated. In the early 1980s, investigators from Wayne State, building upon potential synergy between cisplatin and 5-fluororuacil, reported a major response rate of 70% with a complete response rate of 27% using a regimen of cisplatin 100 mg/m² intravenously and a 5-fluorouracil 1,000 mg/m² per day continuous infusion over 96 hours recycled every 3 weeks in patients with recurrent or disseminated disease.[95] Other investigators confirmed the significant activity of the regimen, albeit with a somewhat lower major and complete response rate on average (50% and 16%, respectively),[96] establishing it as the standard regimen to which new therapies are compared.

TABLE 38.7

Cetuximab for Recurrent or Metastatic Head and Neck Cancer: Selected Studies

Author	No. of Patients	Cancer	Chemotherapy	RR	Median PFS (Months)	Median OS (Months)
Herbst et al.[80,a]	79	SCC–POD on CDDP based	CDDP based + cetuximab	6%–20%	2.0–3.0	4.3–6.1
Baselga et al.[79,a]	96	SCC–POD on platin based	CDDP based + cetuximab	10%–11%	2.4–2.8	4.9–6.0
Trigo et al.[81]	103	SCC–POD on platin based	Cetuximab	13%	2.3	5.9
Burtness et al.[82,b]	117	SCC	CDDP	10%	2.7	8.0
		No chemo for R/M	CDDP + cetuximab	26%	4.2	9.2

[a] Range related to how POD was defined in different subgroups.
[b] Response rates were significantly different (p = 0.03): PFS (p = 0.09) and OS (p = 0.21) did not reach statistical significance.
RR, response rate; PFS, progressive-free survival; OS, overall survival; SCC, squamous cell cancer; POD, progression of disease; CDDP = cisplatin; R/M = recurrent or metastatic disease.

Despite an improvement in response rates associated with the use of combination therapies like cisplatin and 5-flurouracil, demonstrating a statistically or clinically significant improvement in survival compared to single-agent therapy has proven elusive. Table 38.8 summarizes the results of three randomized trials that compared treatment with cisplatin and infusion 5-fluorouracil to that with different single agents.[97–99] Treatment with combination chemotherapy led to a significant increase in response rate, albeit at the cost of greater toxicity. Overall survival did not significantly improve. The meta-analysis reported by Browman et al.[100] yielded similar conclusions. These data do not support the routine use of cisplatin-based combinations for patients with recurrent or metastatic SCC. Combination therapy seems most appropriate for patients with a good performance who have significant symptoms (e.g., pain) for which the higher anticipated response rate will translate into better palliation.

The activity of paclitaxel and docetaxel in head and neck cancer has fostered the development and evaluation of taxane and cisplatin combinations. Docetaxel with cisplatin is associated with a major response rate of 40% to 53%, with complete response rates approximating 6% to 18%[101,102]; a weekly schedule of paclitaxel (80 mg/m^2) and carboplatin (area under concentration [AUC] versus time curve, 2) appeared more efficacious than an every 3-week dosing (paclitaxel 175 to 200 mg/m^2 intravenously over 3 hours followed by carboplatin AUC 6) in two separate phase II studies.[103–105] ECOG compared a high-dose (200 mg/m^2) and moderate-dose (135 mg/m^2) paclitaxel, both by 24-hour infusion and followed by the same dose of cisplatin (75 mg/m^2) in a randomized study (E1393). No significant difference in response rate or survival was found between the arms.[106] Another randomized trial done under the auspices of ECOG compared standard cisplatin and 5-fluorouracil with paclitaxel 175 mg/m^2 intravenously over 3 hours and cisplatin 75 mg/m^2 (E1395).[107] Objective major response rates (27% versus 26%) and median survivals (8.7 versus 8.1 months) were no different between the arms. The reported quality of life was better on the paclitaxel arm over the first 16 weeks of treatment.[108]

Attempts have been made to improve the efficacy of combination chemotherapy through the development of a variety of triplets. The addition of interferon-alpha2b (IFN-α2b) to cisplatin and 5-fluorouracil failed to significantly improve response or survival in a randomized trial.[109] Phase II studies of a taxane with cisplatin or carboplatin and a third drug (e.g., 5-fluorouracil, ifosfamide), have yielded major response rates of 55% to 86%[110–113]; whether these regimens translate into better survival outcomes compared to a cisplatin-based doublet that may be less toxic await further evaluations.

There is great interest in the combination of standard chemotherapy with newer targeted agents. One ECOG study compared cisplatin versus cisplatin and cetuximab as first-line treatment in 123 patients. The arm including the cetuximab had a significantly higher response rate (10% versus 26%, p = 0.03), but no significant difference was found in the primary endpoint of progression-free survival (2.7 versus 4.2 months, p = 0.09) or in overall survival (8.0 versus 9.2 months, p = 0.21), although the trends favored the combination arm.[82] In a larger trial (EXTREME),[114] 442 patients were randomized to cisplatin or carboplatin and 5-fluorouracil with or without cetuximab for six cycles. Subsequent maintenance with cetuximab alone was allowed on the investigational arm, but there was no crossover to cetuximab on the standard arm. Both median progression-free (5.6 versus 3.3 months) and overall (10.1 versus 7.4 months) survivals were significantly improved on the triplet arm, at the cost of more sepsis (nine patients versus one patient; p = 0.02), grade 3 skin reactions (9%), and grade ≥3 infusion reactions. Quality of life outcomes were reported to not be significantly different between the treatment arms.[115] Tumor EGFR copy number and degree of EFGR expression were not predictive of benefit with cetuximab.[116,117] Of interest, data from Vermorken and colleagues[118] suggests that the therapeutic effect of cetuximab, when combined with chemotherapy, is mainly additive rather than synergistic. Whether allowing patients to crossover to cetuximab on the doublet arm at progression would have decreased or eliminated the observed survival difference is of interest for future research. A similar but not identically designed randomized trial evaluated cisplatin and 5-fluorouracil with or without the EGFR antibody panitumumab in 657 patients. Response rate (36% versus 25%, p = 0.0065) and median progression-free survival (5.8 versus 4.6 months, p = 0.0036) were significantly improved with the incorporation of the panitumumab, but not the primary endpoint of overall survival (11.1 versus 9.0 months, p = 0.1403). Overall survival was improved in the p16-negative subgroup (p = 0.0115).[119]

With advances in RT techniques that facilitate reirradiation with acceptable morbidity, this approach has been increasingly

TABLE 38.8

Chemotherapy for Recurrent or Metastatic Head and Neck Cancer: Selected Phase III Trials of Cisplatin/5-Fluorouracil Versus Other Options

Study	No. of Patients	Agents	Response Rates[a]	Median Survivals[b] (Months)
Jacobs et al.[98]	249	CDDP/FU	32%	5.5
		CDDP	17%	5.0
		FU	13%	6.1
Forastiere et al.[97]	277	CDDP/FU	32%	6.6
		CBDCA/FU	21%	5.0
		MTX	10%	5.6
Clavel et al.[99]	382	CDDP/MTX/BLEO/VCR	34%	8.2
		CDDP/FU	31%	6.2
		CDDP	15%	5.3
Schrijvers et al.[109]	122	CDDP/FU/IFN-α2b	38%	6.0
		CDDP/FU	47%	6.3
Gibson et al.[107]	218	CDDP/FU	27%	8.7
		CDDP/PAC	26%	8.1

[a] The following response rate differences were statistically significant at p <0.05: Jacobs et al., CDDP/FU versus both CDDP and FU; Forastiere et al., CDDP/FU versus MTX; Clavel et al., both combinations versus CDDP.
[b] All survival differences were not statistically significant.
CDDP, cisplatin; FU, 5-fluorouracil; MTX, methotrexate; CBDCA, carboplatin; BLEO, bleomycin; VCR, vincristine; IFN-α2b, interferon-alpha 2b; PAC, paclitaxel.

explored in patients with unresectable local or regional recurrence, often with integrated chemotherapy. The observed median survivals in these series are similar to those obtained in phase II trials of chemotherapy alone, but more durable responses occur in selected patients and there is a clearer plateau on the survival curve. In two larger series involving 169 and 115 patients, respectively, among patients treated with a variety of RT fractionation schedules and concurrent chemotherapy regimens, 2-year survival rates exceeded 20%.[120,121] In two sequential RTOG studies, a regimen of daily paclitaxel (20 mg/m^2) and cisplatin (15 mg/m^2) added concurrently to split-course RT (total dose 60 Gy, 1.5 Gy twice-daily fractions; granulocyte colony-stimulating factor support during off weeks) (RTOG 96-11) yielded a better 2-year survival rate than concurrent 5-fluorouracil and hydroxyurea added to the same RT schedule (RTOG 96-10) (24.9% versus 16.9%, p = 0.44).[122,123] The reported 2-year survival rates exceed the rate of 10.5%, which was observed in a subgroup of 124 patients with local disease only who had previously received RT and participated in E1393 or E1395.[124] Randomized trials comparing chemotherapy alone to reirradiation and chemotherapy are needed.

Nasopharynx Cancer

Many of the same drugs and regimens used in the treatment of head and neck SCC are also active in NPC. There are reports of a small proportion of patients with recurrent or metastatic disease being controlled long term with chemotherapy alone.[125] Available data support the use of cisplatin-based combination chemotherapy (e.g., cisplatin/5-fluorouracil; cisplatin/bleomycin/5-flurouracil +/− epirubicin), although there is a lack of randomized studies to clarify the relative efficacies and toxicities of different options. Site-specific phase II studies report major response rates of 70% or higher with regimens containing cisplatin.[126–128] In a review of the Princess Margaret Hospital experience, single-agent or noncisplatin-based combination chemotherapy was associated with a major and complete response rates of 25% and 8%, respectively, in 40 patients, whereas cisplatin-based combination therapy produced major and complete response rates of 70% and 23%, respectively, in 30 patients.[126] The substitution of carboplatin may be associated with less activity.[127]

With regard to other agents, paclitaxel as a 175 mg/m^2 3-hour infusion is active with a response rate of 22% in a series of 24 patients with undifferentiated NPCs.[128] The combination of it with carboplatin has yielded response rates consistently greater than 50%.[129–131] Gemcitabine is active in NPCs,[132,133] and combinations including it appear promising, with response rates exceeding 70%.[134,135] Capecitabine, prolonged 5-fluorouracil infusion, and cetuximab all have modest activity in the refractory setting, and no major responses were seen in one study with gefitinib.[136–139] There is keen interest in looking to exploit the association NPCs have with EBV for therapeutic purposes. Potential gene therapy approaches are discussed elsewhere.[140,141]

GENERAL PRINCIPLES OF COMBINING MODALITIES

Surgery Plus Radiation Therapy

RT may be administered preoperatively or postoperatively. An analysis of available data suggests there is no compelling difference in survival rates comparing the two sequences[42]; local–regional control may be improved with postoperative treatment.[142]

Combined modality therapy should be avoided for lesions with a high cure rate (70% or greater) by either surgery or RT alone. The increased morbidity from combined treatment is not associated with a significantly improved control rate, and many patients with local or regional failure can be salvaged by secondary procedures.

The advantages of postoperative compared with preoperative RT include less operative morbidity, more meaningful margin checks at the time of the surgery, a knowledge of tumor spread for RT planning, safe use of a higher RT dose, and no chance the patient will refuse surgery. The disadvantages of postoperative RT include the larger treatment volume necessary to cover surgical dissections, a delay in the start of RT with possible progression, and the higher dose required to accomplish the same rates of local–regional control.

Preoperative Radiation Therapy

Preoperative RT should be considered for the following situations: (1) fixed-neck nodes, (2) delayed initiation of postoperative RT by >8 weeks, (3) use of the gastric pull-up for reconstruction, and (4) open biopsy of a positive neck node.

Postoperative Radiation Therapy

Postoperative RT is considered when the risk of recurrence above the clavicles exceeds 20%. The operative procedure should be one stage and of such magnitude that RT is started no later than 6 to 8 weeks after surgery. The operation should be undertaken only if it is believed to be highly likely that all gross disease will be removed and margins will be negative.

Although no definitive randomized trials have addressed the efficacy of postoperative RT in the treatment of head and neck cancer, excellent data that has bearing on this issue is available from the Medical College of Virginia. Two groups of surgeons operated on patients with head and neck cancer: general surgical oncologists who used surgery alone and reserved RT for treatment of recurrent disease, and otolaryngologists who routinely sent patients with locally advanced disease for postoperative RT.[143] Of 441 patients, 125 were treated surgically between 1982 and 1988 and had ECE and/or positive margins, 71 were treated with surgery alone, and 54 received postoperative RT. Local control rates at 3 years after surgery alone compared with surgery and RT were: for ECE, 31% and 66% (p = 0.03); positive margins, 41% and 49% (p = 0.04); and ECE and positive margins, 0% and 68% (p = 0.001). A multivariate analysis of local control revealed that the use of postoperative RT (p = 0.0001), macroscopic ECE (p = 0.0001), and margin status (p = 0.09) were of independent significance. Cause-specific survival rates at 3 years were 41% for surgery alone and 72% for surgery and postoperative RT (p = 0.0003). A multivariate analysis of cause-specific survival showed that postoperative RT (p = 0.0001) and the number of nodes with ECE (p = 0.0001) significantly influenced this endpoint.

In another series, Lundahl et al.[144] reported on 95 patients with node-positive SCC who were treated with a neck dissection and postoperative RT at the Mayo Clinic. A matched-pair analysis was performed using a series of patients treated with surgery alone; 56 matched pairs of patients were identified. The recurrence rates in the dissected neck (relative risk [RR] = 5.82, p = 0.0002), recurrence in either side of the neck (RR = 2.21, p = 0.0052), and death from any cause (RR = 1.67, p = 0.0182) were significantly higher for patients treated with surgery alone.

Thus, it appears that postoperative RT may significantly improve both local–regional disease control and survival for patients who are at high risk for failure after surgery.

Indications for postoperative RT include close (<5 mm) or positive margins, ECE, multiple positive nodes, invasion of the soft tissues of the neck, endothelial-lined space invasion, PNI, and more than 5 mm of subglottic invasion.[42] The authors currently recommend 60 Gy in 6 weeks to 66 Gy in 6.5 weeks for patients with negative margins and fewer than three indications for RT. For patients with close (<5 mm) or positive margins, we recommend 70 Gy in 7 weeks or 74.4 Gy at 1.2 Gy twice a day. Concomitant cisplatin chemotherapy should be considered for patients with positive margins and/or ECE.[43–45]

Given the appreciation that HPV-related cancers have a better prognosis than HPV-unrelated disease, there is interest in potential deescalation of therapy with the intent of decreasing toxicity without compromise in survival.[145] Although this is an important area of future research, modification in standards of care based on the HPV status of the tumor is not recommended outside of a clinical trial at present.[146]

CHEMOTHERAPY AS PART OF CURATIVE TREATMENT

Systematically designed and randomized studies have established a role for drug therapy as part of the standard combined modality management of head and neck SCC in several settings. These include the therapy of unresectable disease, for organ preservation, and for patients with poor risk pathologic features after surgery. Chemotherapy has been shown to improve the likelihood of disease control compared to RT alone in patients with advanced disease, albeit with increased acute toxicity. In certain circumstances, response to chemotherapy has been used to triage patients to different local–regional treatments.

Chemotherapy has been integrated with surgery or RT in a variety of ways including induction, concurrent with RT, and/or maintenance. Unlike outcome studies of surgery and/or RT in which site-specific results are reported, albeit typically using a retrospective methodology, many of the trials evaluating the role of chemotherapy enrolled patients with a variety of head and neck SCCs. Even when site specific, although prospective, subsites are combined. This is less of an issue for studies evaluating therapy for NPC.[147,148] Nonetheless, important lessons have been learned from these studies, further enhanced by use of a random assignment methodology. In this section, general principles for the integration chemotherapy with local–regional treatment will be discussed with a focus on the results of randomized trials.

The Meta-Analysis of Chemotherapy on Head and Neck Cancer (MACH-NC) included 63 randomized trials published from 1965 through 1993, all of which compared local–regional treatment with or without chemotherapy.[149] Individual patient data was available on 10,741 patients. The absolute improvement in 5-year survival overall was 4% (p <0.001). However, the significant improvement appeared limited to those patients who received concomitant treatment (absolute difference of 8% at 5 years, p <0.001). Neither the difference seen at 5 years with induction (2%, p = 0.10), nor maintenance (1%, p = 0.74) chemotherapy was statistically significant.[149] In an update of this analysis, now including trials through 2000 and totaling 17,346 patients,[149] the superior efficacy of concurrent therapy was confirmed, and was greater than that seen with induction chemotherapy. Survival benefit diminished with patient age and, on subset analysis, was not significant in patients over 70 years of age.

Tumor HPV status has emerged as an important predictor of favorable treatment response and survival, particularly for patients with oropharynx cancer.[7] In ECOG 2399, the response to chemotherapy to all protocol treatment, progression free-survival, and overall survival were all improved in the HPV-positive group.[7] Subsequent analysis of RTOG 0129 demonstrated that tobacco use (>10 pack-years) and the extent of nodal disease (N2b-N3) both adversely affect the prognosis associated with HPV-positive tumors.[8]

Induction Chemotherapy

In untreated patients with local or regionally advanced M0 head and neck SCC, treatment with cisplatin-based combination chemotherapy will yield major response rates approximating 90%, with clinical complete response rates in the 30% range.[150] Enthusiasm that response rates of this magnitude should translate into

survival benefit when induction chemotherapy was combined with surgery or RT is understandable. Yet, in the original report of the MACH-NC analysis, which included 31 induction studies, all but 2 suggested no survival benefit.[149]

However, a more careful look at these and other data do provide grounds for continued interest in this approach. Many of the included studies had significant methodologic limitations by more contemporary trial standards. A subset analysis, limited to the 15 trials that used cisplatin and infusional 5-fluorouracil, suggested survival benefit (hazard ratio [HR], 0.88; 95% confidence interval [CI], 0.79 to 0.97).[149] Even in the absence of survival improvement, there seemed to be a correlation between response to chemotherapy and subsequent response to RT, which provided a basis for subsequent organ preservation initiatives.[151,152] Finally, patterns of failure were affected with less distant metastases in certain studies when induction chemotherapy was incorporated. As local–regional control improves, the rate of clinically apparent distant metastases is increasing,[153] and induction chemotherapy is, on average, better tolerated than maintenance therapy as a way to give additional systemic therapy.

The study reported originally by Paccagnella et al.[154] is illustrative of these types of trials, and provides further insights.[155] Two hundred and thirty-seven patients with stage III or IV head and neck cancer were randomized to four cycles of induction cisplatin and infusional 5-fluorouracil followed by standard local–regional treatment (i.e., surgery plus RT if resectable, RT alone if unresectable). Resectability was assessed pretreatment, not after chemotherapy, and was a stratification criteria. Overall, there was no significant difference between the arms with regard to overall survival or local–regional control, although the incidence of distant metastases was lower among patients treated with chemotherapy. On a subset analysis, however, patients with unresectable disease benefitted from the incorporation of induction chemotherapy for all outcomes, including local–regional control, distant control, and overall survival (3-year survival 24% versus 10%, p = 0.04). Among resectable patients, improvement in distant control was offset by a decrement in local–regional control with the integration of induction chemotherapy, and reported survival rates in this subgroup were similar on both treatment arms.

Historically, then, there was no established role for induction chemotherapy prior to planned surgery and postoperative RT, and a limited role only in selected settings prior to RT. However, with the incorporation of taxanes into induction regimens containing cisplatin and 5-fluororuacil, newer data suggest that the indications for induction chemotherapy may further evolve.

Three randomized trials have compared the relative efficacies of induction chemotherapy with standard cisplatin and 5-fluorouracil versus a triplet including a taxane and these same two drugs with one or both being dose adjusted.[156–158] All three studies randomized patients with advanced M0 head and neck cancer to either cisplatin and 5-fluororuacil or a triplet, followed by the same RT-based treatment. In one study, this was RT alone, whereas, in the other two, concurrent therapy with carboplatin and cisplatin, respectively, were employed. In general, the taxane-containing triplet was associated with a higher response rate to induction chemotherapy, and improved both progression-free and overall survival. More neutropenia was observed with triplet therapy but, overall, it was as well-tolerated as standard cisplatin and 5-fluorouracil.

These studies were designed to determine which induction chemotherapy was more efficacious, and provide convincing evidence that the triplet of a taxane with cisplatin and 5-flurouracil is superior to standard cisplatin and 5-fluorouracil alone as induction therapy. However, an alternative design is necessary to define the role of induction with such triplets in standard practice. For this population, as discussed in the next section, concurrent chemotherapy and RT alone without induction chemotherapy is the more established standard therapy. Randomized studies are necessary to determine whether a sequential approach using induction with a triplet followed by RT-based treatment (typically with concurrent chemotherapy), is superior to concurrent chemotherapy and RT alone such that the added duration of treatment and potential toxicity is justified.

To date, available randomized trials have failed to demonstrate a clear overall survival benefit with the incorporation of induction chemotherapy. The combination of docetaxel, cisplatin, and 5-fluorouracil has been the focus of these investigations. One study available only in abstract form was confounded by the lack of an intention to treat an analysis with unequal exclusions among treatment arms. Even with those methodologic limitations, it failed to demonstrate a significant improvement in overall survival with the incorporation of induction docetaxel, cisplatin, and 5-fluorouracil or cisplatin, and 5-fluorouracil.[159] In the PARADIGM study, 145 patients with local or regionally advanced SCC were randomized to induction docetaxel, cisplatin, and 5-fluorouracil followed by carboplatin or docetaxel concurrent with RT versus concurrent cisplatin with concomitant boost radiation. Patients could have unresectable disease or be resectable, with the intent of therapy being organ preservation. The study was closed early because of slower than expected accrual, so it was somewhat underpowered. There was no difference in overall or progression-free survival between the arms with a median follow-up of 49 months; the 3-year overall survival rates were 73% on the induction arm and 78% on the concurrent arm (p = 0.77); and the 3-year progression-free survival rates were 67% and 69%, respectively (p = 0.82). A subset analysis of the group with advanced neck disease (N2b/N2c,N3), felt to be at increased risk of distant metastases, demonstrated no advantage with the incorporation of induction chemotherapy.[160] The DECIDE trial used a similar design, but only patients with N2/N3 were eligible and, for the concurrent therapy, hydroxyurea and 5-fluorouracil was used. Among 280 patients accrued with minimum 24-months follow-up, there was no significant difference between the sequential and concurrent arms with regard to overall survival (75% versus 73%, p = 0.70) or disease-free survival (69% versus 64%, p = 0.39); the cumulative incidence of distant failure, however, was lower in the induction arm (10% versus 19%, p = 0.025).[161] Finally, in 256 enrolled patients with stage III or IVA oral cavity cancer, induction with docetaxel, cisplatin, and 5-fluorouracil prior to surgery and postoperative radiation failed to improve overall survival (p = 0.918) or disease-free survival (p = 0.897) compared to proceeding directly to surgery and postoperative radiation alone.[162]

The optimal role of induction chemotherapy is currently controversial. A review of the National Comprehensive Cancer Network (NCCN) guidelines highlights this reality, because concurrent chemoRT alone and induction followed by RT-based therapy are both listed as treatment options for certain disease scenarios.[146] Although concurrent chemoRT alone remains the standard to which new treatments are compared for local or regionally advanced disease and generally receives the higher category rating in these guidelines, induction is well-suited for certain settings in patients who are medically fit. Examples include when immediate therapy is needed in the hope of avoiding a tracheostomy or PEG, in organ preservation settings where the degree of response affects the decision to proceed with surgery versus RT-based therapy, or in patients with advanced neck disease at higher risk for distant metastases.

After induction chemotherapy, there is some controversy as to whether to proceed with RT alone or concurrent chemoRT, and if the latter, which drug to use.[156–158] Concern exists regarding the tolerance to high-dose cisplatin after cisplatin-based induction treatment. In a randomized phase II trial, concurrent cetuximab and RT was compared with high-dose cisplatin and RT after induction docetaxel, cisplatin, and 5-fluorouracil in 116 patients with advanced hypopharynx or larynx cancer. Toxicity was substantial on both arms, but treatment compliance was better with cetuximab therapy. There was no significant difference in larynx function preservation and overall survival between the arms; more local failures occurred on the cetuximab arm.[163]

Concurrent Chemotherapy and Radiation for Gross Disease

Although there are a number of ways to integrate chemotherapy with RT, available data most strongly support concurrent chemotherapy. Given proven efficacy in patients with poor prognostic and unresectable disease, more recent investigations have applied the approach in better prognostic, organ preservation, and adjuvant settings.

Concurrent chemoRT programs vary in many ways, of which the type of chemotherapy (i.e., specific agents, single, combination) and RT schedule (i.e., dose, fractionation) are the most apparent variables. In general, three main approaches can be discerned: single-agent or combination chemotherapy with continuous-course RT; combination chemotherapy with split-course RT, often with altered fractionation; and chemotherapy alternating with RT.[164] Although continuous course RT may be desirable and more attractive from a radiobiologic perspective, local toxicities may preclude it depending on the concurrent agents used. The first two approaches are the most common.

A variety of drugs and combinations have been utilized concurrently with RT. When only one drug is used, the MACH-NC indicates that the impact is largest with a platin, of which cisplatin is the predominant one studied, a conclusion shared in another meta-analysis reported by Browman and colleagues.[165] Of interest, platin plus 5-fluorouracil (HR, 0.75) offered no clear advantage compared to platin alone (HR, 0.74).[166] The results of a three-arm randomized study comparing concurrent cisplatin and RT, concurrent cisplatin, 5-fluorouracil and split-course RT (with possible resection depending on response), and definitive RT alone in patients with unresectable disease reported by Adelstein et al.,[167] in the E1392 study, are consistent with this assessment. Although daily,[168] weekly,[46,169] and every 3 week schedules of cisplatin intravenously concurrent with RT have been applied, the last schedule is the one most studied and is a widely accepted standard. If weekly dosing is used, 20 mg/m^2 weekly appears too low because it did not significantly improve overall survival or failure-free survival in one randomized study.[169] Attempts to improve the efficacy of concurrent cisplatin through intra-arterial administration[170,171] did not prove more efficacious in a randomized trial when compared to intravenously delivered cisplatin, although toxicity profiles differed.[172] In absence of a proven efficacy advantage with intra-arterial delivery, intravenous cisplatin is preferred because it is logistically easier to administer.

Most randomized trials to date have compared chemoRT to RT alone. As such, studies evaluating the efficacy of different chemoRT programs are limited. For example, for purposes of the MACH-NC analysis, "platin" included both cisplatin and carboplatin. Yet the relative efficacy of these agents, when given concurrently, is not well-studied. In one three-arm randomized study by Jeremic et al.[168] using a daily schedule for each drug with RT and a control arm of RT alone, both the cisplatin (6 mg/m^2 per day) and carboplatin (25 mg/m^2 per day) arms appeared comparable, and superior in efficacy to RT alone. However, in a randomized study reported by the Hellenic Cooperative Oncology Group using an every 3 week schedule for each drug (cisplatin 100 mg/m^2, carboplatin AUC, 6), their equivalence seemed less clear.[173] The RTOG reported a randomized phase II study comparing three different chemotherapy regimens, all delivered concurrently with 70 Gy in 2 Gy fractions: ARM 1, cisplatin 10 mg/m^2 per day and 5-fluorouracil 400 mg/m^2 per day continuous infusion for the final 10 days of treatment; ARM 2, hydroxyurea 1 g every 12 hours and 5-fluorouracil 800 mg/m^2 per day continuous infusion every other week; or ARM 3, weekly paclitaxel 30 mg/m^2 and cisplatin 20 mg/m^2. Among 231 analyzable patients, 2-year disease-free and overall survival rates were for ARM

1, 38.2% and 57.4%; for ARM 2, 48.6% and 69.4%; and for ARM 3, 51.3% and 66.6%, respectively.[174]

Because anemia may adversely affect the efficacy of RT, the integration of an appropriate hematopoietic growth factor has been investigated. In a multicenter, double-blind, randomized, placebo-controlled trial, the addition of erythropoietin 300 IU/kg three times weekly during postoperative RT was evaluated in 351 patients with head and neck SCC.[175] Although target hemoglobulin levels were reached in 82% of patients receiving erythropoietin compared to 15% receiving placebo, local–regional progression-free survival (adjusted RR, 1.62 [95% CI, 1.22 to 2.14]; p = 0.0008), local–regional progression (RR, 1.69 [CI, 1.16 to 2.47]; p = 0.007), and survival (RR, 1.39 [CI, 1.05 to 1.84]; p = 0.02) were all inferior on the erythropoietin arm. Consistent with the current FDA alert, an erythropoietin-stimulation agent is contraindicated during curative-intent RT-based therapy.[176] Transfusion then, is the preferred approach to address potential radiation resistance attributed to anemia, but a recent analysis of two randomized trials failed to demonstrate that prophylactic transfusion improved overall survival or other disease control endpoints.[177] Use of a hypoxic radiosensitizer represents another strategy to potentially address tumor hypoxia. The results of one meta-analysis were consistent with potential benefit[178]; recent randomized trials, however, have not been convincing in terms of improved disease control with such a strategy.[179,180]

An important question is whether the use of newer, more efficacious, and altered fractionated RT programs[181] obviates the benefits accrued with the addition of chemotherapy. A single institution study reported by Brizel et al.[182] compared a more aggressive RT schedule with or without concomitant 5-fluorouracil and cisplatin. Patients who underwent RT alone received 75 Gy in 60 twice-daily fractions; those who underwent concomitant chemotherapy received 70 Gy in 56 twice-daily fractions with a 7-day split. Chemotherapy consisted of two cycles of concomitant cisplatin 12 mg/m^2 per day and 5-fluorouracil 600 mg/m^2 per day each for 5 days, followed by two cycles of maintenance chemotherapy. Among the 116 patients included, chemoRT was associated with improved 3-year rates of local–regional control (70% versus 40%, p = 0.01), relapse-free survival (61% versus 41%, p = 0.08), and overall survival (55% versus 34%, p = 0.07). In another randomized study reported by Jeremic et al.,[183] the addition of daily cisplatin to hyperfractionated RT also leads to incremental benefits. The results of these studies are consistent with the MACH-NC analysis, which demonstrated significant HRs, that are consistent with benefits among patients receiving postoperative RT (HR, 0.79), conventional RT (HR, 0.83), or altered fractionated RT (HR, 0.73), suggesting a benefit for adding concomitant chemotherapy regardless of the type of RT schedule.[166]

Of note, the converse—once concurrent chemotherapy is added, does an altered fractionation RT schedule further improve outcome compared to that seen with standard fractionation—has not been established in randomized trials. Neither RTOG 0129 (standard versus concomitant boost RT both with concurrent high-dose cisplatin)[8] nor GORTEC 99-02 (accelerated RT with or without concurrent carboplatin and 5-flourouracil, standard fractionated RT with concurrent carboplatin and 5-flourouracil)[184] demonstrated improved overall survival with the incorporation of altered fractionated RT with concurrent chemotherapy versus standard fractionation with concurrent chemotherapy to justify the added logistical complexity and potential added toxicity.

For patients who are not cisplatin candidates, using a carboplatin-based program (e.g., carboplatin/5-fluorouracil)[147] or other concurrent programs that have different side effect profiles and that withstood the scrutiny of a randomized trial is recommended. There has been great interest in cetuximab and concurrent RT in this regard.[185] In a randomized study reported by Bonner et al.,[186] patients with local–regionally advanced head and neck cancer were randomized to RT alone (213 patients) or combined with weekly cetuximab dosed in a standard fashion (211 patients);

median follow-up was 54 months. The median duration of survival was 49 months after combined therapy compared with 29 months after RT alone (p = 0.03). Other than an acneiform rash and infusion reactions, grade 3 or greater complications were similar in the two groups of patients. The results of this trial have been confirmed with longer follow-ups.[186] Patients with oropharynx cancer appeared to derive the largest benefit with the integration of cetuximab, suggesting that HPV-related disease may have an improved outcome with the use of this agent; other studies, however, suggest greater activity of EGFR-directed antibody therapy in HPV-negative disease.[114,119] Randomized data comparing cetuximab and RT to other chemoRT programs are not available. One RTOG study evaluating concurrent cisplatin and RT versus cetuximab and RT in patients with HPV-related cancers is currently in progress. Investigators at Memorial-Sloan Kettering reported a phase II trial of cisplatin and cetuximab concurrent with RT in patients with local–regionally advanced head and neck SCC. Efficacy was impressive, although there were toxicity concerns.[187] The RTOG completed accrual to a large randomized trial (RTOG 0522, n = 895 evaluable patients) intended to assess the efficacy and safety of this regimen compared to concurrent cisplatin and RT. With a median follow-up of 2.4 years among surviving patients, the incorporation of cetuximab failed to significantly improve 2-year progression-free survival (63% versus 64%, p = 0.66) or overall survival (83% versus 80%, p = 0.17), but mucosal and skin toxicity were increased.[188]

Choosing among the numerous concurrent programs can be difficult. In the NCCN guidelines,[146] concurrent cisplatin with RT is the preferred choice, although several other options are listed. It is important to emphasize that concurrent chemoRT may be associated with significant toxicity; treatment-related mortality, albeit infrequent (<5% in the cooperative group setting), may occur. Morbidity from chemotherapy (dependent on the agent chosen) and RT are possible, and there are both acute (e.g., mucositis, blood count suppression) and chronic (e.g., dry mouth, swallowing dysfunction, fibrosis) toxicities. Selected studies have begun to report long-term, not just acute, toxicities.[189] Appropriate infrastructure, an experienced multidisciplinary team, and a cooperative patient are necessary to optimize both efficacy and safety.

Nasopharynx Cancer

Current practice has been particularly affected by the Intergroup Study 0099 (Table 38.9).[190] In it, 147 patients with stage III or IV NPC were randomized to definitive RT (70 Gy, 35 fractions over 7 weeks) versus cisplatin 100 mg/m^2 intravenously on days 1, 22, and 43 concurrent with the same dose of RT followed by three planned cycles of cisplatin and infusional 5-fluorouracil. Although only 63% and 53% of patients received all the planned concurrent and maintenance treatments, respectively, local–regional control, distant control, progression-free, and overall survivals were all significantly improved with chemoRT.

One of the potential limitations of the Intergroup Study was how generalizable its results would be to endemic NPCs, because 24% of patients entered in the trial had World Health Organization (WHO) type I histology. However, subsequent reports of randomized trials in which WHO types II and III predominated have similarly shown a survival advantage with concurrent cisplatin-based concurrent chemotherapy without[191–193] or with maintenance chemotherapy.[194,195]

One relatively small randomized trial (n = 206) with a median follow-up of 26.3 months, suggested that weekly carboplatin dosed at 100 mg/m^2 concurrent with RT when compared to standard high-dose cisplatin, did not yield inferior disease-free or overall survival. Both arms received adjuvant platin and 5-fluorouracil.[196] However, another randomized study involving 408 patients who received concurrent carboplatin at AUC 6 every 3 weeks after induction chemotherapy failed to demonstrate an improvement

TABLE 38.9

Selected Randomized Trials Evaluating Concurrent Chemoradiotherapy Versus Radiotherapy for Advanced Nasopharynx Cancer

Study	No. of Patients	Maintenance Chemotherapy	Treatment Arms	PFS[a,b] (p value)	OS[a] (p value)
Al-Saraff et al.[190]	147	Yes, on CDDP/RT arm	RT CDDP/RT	24% 69% (<0.001)	47% 78% (0.005)
Lin et al.[191]	284	No	RT CDDP/FU/RT	53% 72% (0.0012)	54% 72% (0.0022)
Chan et al.[198]	350	No	RT CDDP/RT	52% 60% (0.06)	59% 70% (0.049)
Wee et al.[194]	221	Yes, on CDDP/RT arm	RT CDDP/RT	53% 72% (0.0093)	65% 80% (0.0061)
Lee et al.[195]	348	Yes, on CDDP/RT arm	RT CDDP/RT	62% 72% (0.027)	78% 78% (0.97)

[a] Five-year rates for Lin et al. and Chan et al.; otherwise, 3-year rates.
[b] Disease-free rate provided for Wee et al., and failure-free rate for Lee et al.
PFS, progression-free survival; OS, overall survival; CDDP, cisplatin; FU, 5-fluorouracil; RT, radiation therapy.

in overall survival at 5 years or other disease outcomes compared to patients receiving radiation alone after the same induction regimen.[197]

Another limitation of the Intergroup Study was that it was not designed to delineate the proportional benefits of concurrent and maintenance chemotherapy. Although current NCCN guidelines recommend concurrent and maintenance chemotherapy in M0 patients with a more advanced disease based on the Intergroup experience,[146] in reviewing available data, the benefits of maintenance chemotherapy appear more controversial. As noted, other randomized studies have demonstrated a survival improvement with concurrent therapy alone.[191,198] Earlier randomized trials, summarized elsewhere, failed to demonstrate a survival benefit when either maintenance or induction chemotherapy was added to definitive RT.[199,200] Furthermore, a meta-analysis of updated individual patient data on 1,753 patients enrolled in eight randomized trials, besides confirming an absolute survival benefit of 6% at 5 years with incorporation of chemotherapy with RT (HR, 0.82, 95% CI, 0.71 to 0.91; p = 0.006), also reported a significant association between the timing of chemotherapy and overall survival (p = 0.005), with the largest benefit being attributed to concomitant therapy.[201] A recently reported randomized trial involving 508 patients with nonmetastatic, stage III to IV nasopharyngeal cancer failed to demonstrate a significant difference in 2-year failure-free survival, overall survival, local–regional failure-free survival, or distant failure-free survival after a median follow-up of 37.8 months. Of note, the direction of each of the previous endpoint comparisons favored the adjuvant arm, albeit not significantly so, with associated p values of 0.13, 0.32, 0.10, and 0.12, respectively.[202] A longer term follow-up of this trial will be of interest. Currently, the NCCN guidelines list both concurrent chemoRT followed by maintenance chemotherapy and concurrent chemoRT alone as treatment options for advanced disease, with the former having the higher category rating.[146]

Selected randomized studies have demonstrated evidence of a positive biologic effect with the use of induction chemotherapy, but no survival benefit has been documented.[200,203–205] Such promising results have engendered interest in the potential for enhanced efficacy with newer drugs and combinations. A randomized phase II trial evaluating induction with docetaxel and

cisplatin prior to concurrent cisplatin and RT was consistent with a benefit compared with concurrent cisplatin and RT alone.[200] Programs incorporating newer taxane- and cisplatin-based triplet induction regimens warrant further study.[206] There is also interest in the role of plasma EBV–DNA assays as a way to assess disease and monitor response.[199]

Organ Preservation

Organ preservation therapy is intended to control disease without compromise in survival while optimizing function or cosmesis.[207] The term implies that the tumor is potentially resectable for cure, and that the morbidity from surgery is significant. Although conservation surgical procedures can achieve the same goals, the label of organ preservation is more commonly applied to nonsurgical approaches. In that regard, the role of chemotherapy integrated with RT is best established for more advanced primary tumors. In this setting, conservation surgical procedures become less feasible, and local control rates with RT alone are lower than seen with earlier stage disease.

Total laryngectomy is one of the surgical procedures most feared by patients.[208] Thus, larynx preservation has been a central focus of many organ preservation studies, including those that established integrated chemotherapy and RT as a standard organ preservation treatment option. Studies commonly focused on patients with advanced tumors of the larynx, hypopharynx, and oropharynx (particularly the base of tongue), in whom primary surgical management would jeopardize the voice box.[209]

Initial chemoRT approaches to larynx preservation utilized induction chemotherapy. The response to initial chemotherapy was used to triage patients to either definitive RT (a partial response or better at the primary site; surgery to the primary site was reserved for salvage) or primary surgical management (lower than a partial response). The randomized and landmark Veterans Administration (VA) Larynx Preservation Study demonstrated that such an approach could be pursued in patients with advanced laryngeal cancer without compromise in survival when compared to primary treatment with surgery and RT.[151] Over 60% of patients on the chemoRT arm avoided total laryngectomy. Among

year 2, every 4 to 8 months (
thereafter. Thyroid function
if the neck was irradiated. I
x-rays or other chest imagin
cancer and to document c
imaging on outcomes is nc
with a vague recommendat
"as clinically indicated." To
purposes of lung cancer scr
ing within 6 months of thera
such as CT, MRI, and PET
to determine whether there
otherwise are not routinely
swallowing evaluations and
cated. Counseling is indic
alcohol contributed as a risl

OR

The oral cavity consists of tl
two-thirds of the tongue, th
alveolar ridges, the hard pal
The AJCC staging syste

LIP

The ratio between men ar
mately 15:1.[240] Persons wit
exposure to sunlight are mc

Anatomy

The lips are composed of tl
the external surface and muc
The transition from skin to i
The blood supply is from t
artery. The motor nerves ar
The sensory nerve to the i
CN V (V 2), and the menta

Pathology

The most common neopla
arise on the skin of the lip a
ion. Keratoacanthoma occi
mistaken grossly and histolc
Leukoplakia and CIS ai
and may precede the appea
mary lesions arising from tl
ered under the section Buc

Patterns of Spread

SCC can originate from the
may invade the adjacent si
lesions invade the adjacent
cosa, the skin and wet muc
and eventually the mental i
reported by Byers and cow
lesions, large tumor size, mi
tiated histology. Lymphatic
mandibular (IB) lymph noc
risk for lymph node metas
and is increased by high-gr
the mucosa of the lip, and I

long-term survivors, patients treated on the chemoRT arm had better emotional well-being, were less depressed, and also reported less pain.[210]

A similarly designed randomized trial in patients with pyriform sinus and aryepiglottic fold tumors reported by the European Organization for Research and Treatment of Cancer (EORTC) confirmed these findings.[152] However, a small randomized study (n = 68) limited to patients with T3 disease with a fixed cord done by the Groupe d'Etude des Tumeurs de la Tete et du Cou (GETTEC) reported that survival was superior on the primary surgery arm (84% versus 69% at 2 years, p = 0.006).[211] When the MACH-NC performed a collective analysis of the VA, EORTC, and GETTEC studies, the rate of larynx preservation among survivors was 58%. A nonsignificant (6%) decrement in survival at 5 years was seen in the chemoRT group (39% versus 45%; pooled HR, 1.19; 95% CI, 0.97 to 1.46; p = 0.10).[149]

The data reviewed in the prior section highlighting the therapeutic benefits of a concurrent chemoRT relative to an induction or RT alone approach have obvious implications for the larynx preservation setting. RTOG 91-11 was designed to assess the impacts of adding chemotherapy to RT and its timing (concurrent versus induction) with regard to achieving larynx preservation. Four hundred and ninety-seven patients with larynx cancer were randomized to one of three arms: primary RT, 70 Gy to the primary site, 50 to 70 Gy to nodes; induction chemotherapy with cisplatin and infusional 5-fluorouracil for three cycles followed by RT in responders, surgery in nonresponders; and cisplatin 100 mg/m^2 on days 1, 22, and 43 concurrent with RT. Surgical salvage was an option on all three arms. The recently updated 10-year results are summarized in Table 38.10.[148,212] As anticipated, the rate of grade 3 or 4 mucosal toxicity was highest on the concurrent arm; however, this did not translate into more significant speech or swallowing impairment at 2 years compared to the other treatment arms. Noteworthy is that, although the larynx preservation rate and local–regional control was highest and statistically superior with concurrent treatment, there was no significant difference in overall survival rates among the arms. Deaths not attributed to larynx cancer were highest in the concurrent arm (30.8%) versus 20.8% on the induction arm and 16.9% in the RT alone group, raising concern regarding the long-term morbidity of concurrent therapy. However, late effects were similar among the groups, and there were no substantial differences in speech or swallowing function reported.[212]

In another randomized larynx-preservation study, induction chemotherapy followed by RT and alternating chemotherapy and RT approaches were compared in 450 patients with advanced larynx or hypopharynx cancer. Both treatment arms used cisplatin and 5-flourouracil and allowed surgical salvage. Overall and progression-free survival rates were similar on both arms. Survival with a functional larynx in place was higher with alternating chemoRT,

although the difference was not statistically significant (median, 2.3 years versus 1.6 years; HR, 0.85; 95% CI, 0.68 to 1.06).[213]

Available randomized phase III data support a concurrent chemotherapy–RT strategy administered with organ preservation intent for patients with advanced oropharynx cancer. A phase III study from the Groupe d'Oncologie Radiothérapie Tête et Cou (GORTEC) demonstrated improved local–regional control (66% versus 42% at 3 years, p = 0.03) in patients with advanced oropharynx cancer who received concurrent chemotherapy (carboplatin and 5-fluorouracil) and RT (70 Gy) compared to RT alone.[147] A non–site-specific trial from the Cleveland Clinic, which included a high proportion of patients with advanced oropharynx cancer, yielded similar results.[214]

Although concurrent chemotherapy is the current cornerstone of organ preservation treatment of advanced disease, other paradigms deserve mention. In an Italian study, 195 patients with T2 to T4 oral cavity cancer were randomized to either primary surgical management or induction chemotherapy with cisplatin and 5-fluorouracil followed by a surgical procedure, which could be modified based on response. Overall survival was similar on both arms, but less postoperative RT was necessary (33% versus 46%) and fewer mandible resections were performed (31% versus 52%) on the chemotherapy arm.[215] As a further extension of this concept, Laccourreye and colleagues[216] have pioneered the selective observation without local–regional treatment of patients with laryngeal cancer who have a complete response to induction chemotherapy. Durable tumor control without the addition of surgery or RT has been reported in a small subset of patients with early stage tumors.[216] The University of Michigan has developed a larynx preservation program whereby the triage to RT-based treatment or surgery occurs after only one cycle of chemotherapy.[217] The intent is to improve survival and minimize morbidity through the timely selection of appropriate therapy, including referral to surgery if indicated. The implication is that induction chemotherapy has little other therapeutic benefit, and some patients who are slow to respond may be triaged unnecessarily to total laryngectomy.[218] Conversely, newer sequential strategies of induction chemotherapy followed by planned concurrent chemotherapy are looking to optimize both local–regional and distant control. Induction with more efficacious triplet chemotherapy, including a taxane combined with cisplatin and 5-fluorouracil, is already being incorporated into larynx preservation strategies with evidence of improved larynx preservation rates.[219]

Adjuvant Therapy after Surgery

The use of maintenance chemotherapy after the completion of local–regional treatment has been evaluated in several randomized trials, but with disappointing results. Suboptimal compliance

TABLE 38.10

Intergroup 91-11: Updated Results at 10 Years

RX Arms	No. of Patients	LP Rate	LRF	DMF[a]	DFS	OS
RT only	171	63.8% p <0.0012	47.2% p = 0.0015	76.0%[b]	14.8%[b]	31.2%[b]
Induction PF→RT	173	67.5% p = 0.005	48.9% p = 0.0037	83.4% p = 0.06	20.4% p = 0.06	38.8%[a] p = 0.29
Concurrent P/RT	171	81.7%[b]	65.3%[b]	83.9% p = 0.08	21.6% p = 0.04	27.5% p = 0.53

[a] Trend, p = 0.08 for induction versus concurrent arm.
[b] Comparison group.
RX, treatment; LP, larynx preservation; LRF, local-regional failure; DMF, distant metastatic failure; DFS, disease-free survival; OS, overall survival; RT. radiation therapy; PF, cisplatin/5-fluorouracil; P, cisplatin.
From Forastiere AA, Zhang Q, Weber RS, et al. Long-term results of RTOG 91-11: a comparison of three nonsurgical treatment strategies to preserve the larynx in patients with locally advanced larynx cancer. *J Clin Oncol* 2013;31:845–852.

with maintenance t
efit, because toleraı
and RT.[220] Despite
survival benefit, pat
ies, with a decrease
effect of chemothe

The results of I:
trial, 442 analyzabl
gical therapy to eit
three cycles of stan
sion followed by th
was stratified by risk
in situ (CIS) at the
features. Overall, th
vival, disease-free s
treatment arms, alt
dence of distant mo
Interestingly, on a
no significant impa
impact on survival
patients. Given the
treatment, its appli
tension. A pilot stu
current high-dose o
the adjuvant setting
improvement in lo
concurrent mitomy
concurrent with p
yielded a significaı
and survival with c

Two randomize
clarified the indica
risk adjuvant settir
similar designs.[43-4]
they had poor risk
alone (60 to 66 G
or the same RT wi
at 100 mg/m[2] ever
somewhat betweer
of two or more po
the EORTC requiı
N, N2, or N3 disea
with oral cavity or
lism.[43-45] Both stuc
local–regional con
with combined mo
into a significant ac
(p = 0.02), but on
ther study showed
addition of chemo
dition of the cispla

A subsequent a
performed to bette
benefit the most fr
Patients having evi
largest benefit fro
versely, patients ir
more positive lymp
with RT alone. Loı
consistent with thi

The EORTC a
previously untreate
al.,[225] on behalf of
the potential role o
salvage surgery. In
standard arm was
treatment significa
CI, 1.13 to 2.5], p
cantly improved ai

as the insertion of the buccinator, orbicular oris, and superior pharyngeal constrictor muscles. Behind the pterygomandibular raphe and between the medial pterygoid muscle and the ascending ramus is the pterygomandibular space, which contains the lingual and dental nerves and is related posteriorly to the deep lobe of the parotid and the parapharyngeal space. There are no minor salivary glands in the mucous membranes of the alveolar ridges.

Pathology

Most neoplasms are SCCs. Minor salivary gland tumors, usually adenoid cystic carcinomas, often occur on the posterolateral hard palate.[258] Verrucous carcinomas usually occur on the lower gingiva. Melanoma has been reported.[259]

SCC may arise within the body of the mandible or maxilla either from the odontogenic epithelium or from epithelium trapped during embryonic development. It is more frequent in the mandible than the maxilla and is most common in the molar regions. It must be distinguished from metastatic SCC and ameloblastoma.

Ameloblastoma is a rare, benign locally aggressive odontogenic tumor with an incidence of about 1% of all tumors of the maxilla and mandible; about 80% of cases occur in the mandible with the molar–ramus region most commonly involved.

Patterns of Spread

Lower Gum

SCC invades the periosteum and the adjacent buccal mucosa and floor of the mouth. Low-grade lesions tend to produce a smooth, saucerized defect before invading the mandible. Moderate to high-grade lesions invade the bone directly or through recently opened dental sockets and produce a lytic defect.

Lymphatic spread is to the level I and level II nodes. Clinically positive nodes occur in 18% to 52% of diagnoses; occult disease occurs in 17% to 19%.[20,244]

Ameloblastoma expands and destroys the bone and extends to adjacent areas by contiguous growth. Ameloblastic carcinoma, a rare malignant variant of ameloblastoma, may metastasize to regional nodes and distant sites.[260]

Upper Alveolar Ridge and Hard Palate

Most SCCs originate on the gingiva and spread secondarily to the hard palate, soft palate, buccal mucosa, and underlying bone. The maxillary antrum is invaded late unless there are recent extractions providing access. The risk for positive lymph nodes at diagnosis is 13% to 24%, and the incidence of occult disease is 22%.[20,244]

Retromolar Trigone

Carcinomas spread to the adjacent buccal mucosa, the anterior tonsillar pillar, and the maxilla. Posterior spread occurs into the pterygomandibular space and the medial pterygoid muscle. Posterolateral spread occurs into the buccinator muscle and fat pad. The first echelon lymphatics are the level I and level II nodes. The incidence of clinically positive nodes on presentation is about 30%; the risk for occult disease is 15% to 25%.

Clinical Picture

The patient with SCC may present to the dentist first with ill-fitting dentures, pain, loose teeth, or a sore that will not heal. A history of inappropriate dental extractions or root canal therapy is common. Invasion into the mandible may involve the inferior alveolar nerve and produce paresthesia of the lower lip. A background of leukoplakia is frequently present.

Retromolar trigone lesions have pain referred to the external auditory canal and preauricular area. Invasion of the pterygoid muscle produces trismus. Intra-alveolar SCC presents with a submucosal mass and dental symptoms. Roentgenograms show a lytic lesion in the mandible.

Ameloblastoma exhibits few symptoms in the early stages. Patients may notice a gradually increasing facial deformity or a loosening of teeth. An intraoral submucosal mass may be present initially; ulceration occurs as the mass increases in size. On roentgenograms, a radiolucent area is seen with the expansion of the overlying cortical plate, scalloped margins, a multilocular appearance, and/or resorption of the roots of adjacent teeth.

Minor salivary gland tumors present as a submucosal mass, enlarge slowly, and may develop a central ulceration.[261]

Differential Diagnosis

The differential diagnosis includes dental disease and underlying bony cysts or tumors.

Treatment

Selection of Treatment Modality

Lower Alveolar Ridge. The majority of lesions are managed by surgery alone or followed by postoperative RT or chemoRT. Surgery entails a marginal mandibulectomy when there is, at most, saucerization of the underlying bone. Segmental mandibulectomy and free flap reconstruction is indicated for more advanced disease.

Ameloblastoma. The treatment is surgery; however, local recurrence is a problem. Sehdev and coworkers[262] reported curettage was followed by local recurrence in 90% of mandibular ameloblastomas and in all maxillary ameloblastomas. Subsequent resection controlled 80% of the mandibular but only 40% of the maxillary tumors. The initial use of segmental mandibular resection controlled 78% (18 of 23 patients), with subsequent resection controlling those that recurred. The use of partial maxillectomy as the first treatment controlled 100% (7 of 7 patients) of maxillary ameloblastomas as opposed to only 40% when a partial maxillectomy was performed for recurrence. Limited experience with RT suggests that it may reduce the probability of progression and result in long-term local control in the occasional patient with incompletely resectable disease.[260]

Retromolar Trigone. Surgery is preferred for discrete early lesions. RT is recommended for superficial lesions involving a large surface area.[263] Advanced carcinomas are treated with surgery and postoperative RT or chemoRT

Upper Alveolar Ridge and Hard Palate. Resection alone or followed by RT or chemoRT is the usual treatment for most lesions. However, if the lesion is superficial and extensively involves the hard palate or involves a significant portion of the soft palate, then an RT-based approach should be considered for the initial therapy. If the lesion is small and discrete and there is no bone involvement, resection includes the periosteum or occasionally some underlying bone. Bone invasion requires a maxillectomy that is tailored to optimally resect the cancer. The resulting defect is usually rehabilitated with a removable prosthesis.

Irradiation Technique

Small lesions of the lower alveolar ridge and retromolar trigone may be treated by intraoral cone for all or part of their therapy. Well-lateralized lesions of the retromolar trigone and posterior alveolar ridge may be treated by either an ipsilateral mixed beam or IMRT; the latter is preferred. Parallel-opposed portals treat anterior gum lesions.

Carcinomas that involve a large surface area with little or no bone invasion may be treated by EBRT. T1 to T2 carcinomas are treated with altered fractionation; larger tumors are treated with chemoRT.

Management of Recurrence

RT failures are managed by operation. Surgical failures may be managed by surgery and postoperative RT or chemoRT[264]; Salvage procedures frequently are not attempted because of the advanced nature of the recurrence and the low chance of cure.

Results of Treatment

Mandibular Gingiva. Overholt and coworkers[265] reported 155 patients with SCCs of the lower alveolar ridge treated at M.D. Anderson between 1970 and 1990. Surgery alone was used for 131 patients; the remainder received surgery and RT. Five-year survival for patients with T1 and T2 cancers were 85% and 84%, respectively, compared with 66% and 64%, respectively, for those with T3 and T4 malignancies. Local control at 2 years was impacted by tumor size (p = 0.021) and margin status (p = 0.027), whereas 5-year cause-specific survival was influenced by tumor size (p = 0.001), margin status (p = 0.011), mandibular invasion (p ≤0.05), and the presence of lymph node metastases (p <0.001).

Retromolar Trigone. Byers and coworkers[266] reported the M.D. Anderson results for 110 previously untreated patients with SCC of the retromolar trigone treated between 1965 and 1977, with a minimum 5-year follow-up. Surgery was often selected for patients with leukoplakia, poor teeth, mandible invasion, large neck nodes, or trismus. RT was selected for poorly differentiated tumors, for mainly exophytic lesions, and lesions involving the faucial arch or soft palate or lesions having ill-defined borders, and for poor surgical risk cases. The local control rates were as follows: T1, 12 of 13 (92%); T2, 50 of 57 (88%); T3, 18 of 20 (90%); and T4, 15 of 20 (75%). Local control was similar after surgery and/or RT. The absolute 5-year survival rate was 26%.

Mendenhall and coworkers[263] reported on 99 patients with retromolar trigone SCCs treated between 1966 and 2003 with RT alone (35 patients) or combined with surgery (64 patients). The 5-year local–regional control rates after RT versus surgery and RT were for stages I through III, 51% and 87%; for stage IV, 42% and 62%; and overall, 48% and 71%, respectively. The 5-year cause-specific survival rates after RT versus surgery and RT were for stages I through III, 56% and 83%; for stage IV, 50% and 61%; and overall, 52% and 69%, respectively. A multivariate analysis revealed that the likelihood of cure was better after surgery and RT compared with definitive RT.

Hard Palate. Shibuya and coworkers[267] reported the results for 38 cases of carcinoma of the hard palate and 82 cases of carcinoma of the upper alveolar ridge treated between 1953 and 1982 in Japan. Sixty-six patients were managed initially by RT alone to the primary lesion, and 54 patients were managed by RT and surgery. The 5-year actuarial survival rate by stage was the following: for stage I, 56%; for stage II, 41%; for stage III, 32%; and for stage IV, 12%. There was no difference in survival when comparing hard palate versus upper alveolar ridge, SCC versus minor salivary gland tumors, or RT alone versus RT plus surgery as the initial therapy. The overall risk for metastatic lymph nodes was 47% for hard palate and 49% for the upper alveolar ridge. Thirty patients were recorded as having "slight bone invasion," and no metastases had a 5-year survival rate of 75% when treated by RT.

Complications of Treatment

Surgical complications include orocutaneous fistula, bone exposure, extrusion of a metal tray, and loss of graft or flap.

The complications of RT include soft tissue necrosis, bone exposure, and ORN. The risk is greatest for patients with advanced lesions of the lower gum and retromolar trigone. Huang and colleagues[268] reported the following rates of grade 3 bone and soft tissue complications in 65 patients treated for retromolar trigone carcinomas: preoperative RT, 0 of 10 patients (0%); surgery and postoperative RT, 5 of 39 patients (13%); and RT alone, 2 of 16 patients (13%).

OROPHARYNX

ANATOMY

The base of the tongue is bounded anteriorly by the circumvallate papillae, laterally by the glossotonsillar sulci, and posteriorly by the epiglottis. The vallecula is a strip of mucosa that is the transition from the base of the tongue to the epiglottis; it is considered part of the base of tongue. The musculature of the base of the tongue is contiguous with that of the oral tongue.

The tonsillar fossa is bounded anteriorly by the anterior tonsillar pillar (palatopharyngeal muscle), posteriorly by the posterior tonsillar pillar (palatopharyngeal muscle), and inferiorly by the glossotonsillar sulcus and pharyngoepiglottic fold. The pharyngeal constrictor muscle and its fascia, the mandible, and the lateral pharyngeal space bound the tonsillar region laterally. The tonsillar area is separated from the base of tongue by the glossotonsillar sulcus, which extends from the anterior tonsillar pillar to the pharyngoepiglottic fold. Beneath the mucous membrane of the sulcus are the styloglossal muscle and the stylohyoid ligament.

The soft palate is a thin, mobile muscle complex separating the nasopharynx from the oropharynx. The epithelium of the oral side of the soft palate is squamous; the epithelium of the nasopharyngeal surface is respiratory. It is contiguous laterally with the tonsillar pillars.

PATHOLOGY

SCC accounts for 95% of cancers. Lymphoepitheliomas occur in the tonsillar fossa and the base of tongue. Basaloid features suggest a HR-HPV related tumor. Lymphomas account for 5% of tonsillar and 1% to 2% of base of tongue malignancies. Minor salivary gland malignancies, plasmacytomas, and other rare tumors make up the remainder.[269,270]

PATTERNS OF SPREAD

Base of Tongue

Primary

Base of tongue SCC usually remains in the tongue unless it begins at the peripheral margin. Lateral base of tongue cancers may invade the glossotonsillar sulcus and eventually escape into the neck, because there is no effective musculature barrier at this point. Vallecular lesions spread along the mucosa to the lingual surface of the epiglottis, laterally along the pharyngoepiglottic fold, and then to the lateral pharyngeal wall and anterior wall of the pyriform sinus. Vallecular lesions frequently penetrate through the hyoepiglottic ligament to enter the preepiglottic space.

Lymphatic

The first-echelon nodes are in level II; spread is then to the level III and level IV nodes. The level Ib nodes are at risk if the tumor extends into the oral tongue or if massive upper neck disease is present. The level V nodes are involved often enough to be included in treatment plans. Approximately 75% of patients will have clinically positive neck nodes at diagnosis, and 30% will have bilateral nodes.[20] The risk of occult disease in the clinically negative neck is probably 40% to 50%.

Tonsillar Area

Anterior Tonsillar Pillar

Almost all malignancies are SCCs, and they tend to be diagnosed early when they are relatively superficial with indistinct borders. As the lesions progress, they may develop a central ulcer with a rolled margin and infiltrate the palatoglossus. The lesion may extend superiorly onto the soft palate and posterior hard palate, anterolaterally to the retromolar trigone and buccal mucosa, and inferomedially into the tongue. As these lesions advance, they eventually invade bone, extend to the skull base and nasopharynx, and invade the medial pterygoid muscle, causing trismus and temporal pain.

Tonsillar Fossa

The initial lesions tend to be exophytic with central ulceration plus an infiltrative component. As the tumor progresses, it extends into the posterior tonsillar pillar, the oropharyngeal wall, and the base of tongue. It eventually penetrates the parapharyngeal space and grows superiorly to the skull base.

Posterior Tonsillar Pillar

Posterior tonsillar pillar lesions may spread inferiorly along the palatopharyngeal muscle to its insertions into the middle pharyngeal constrictor, the pharyngoepiglottic fold, and the posterior border of the thyroid cartilage.

Lymphatic

Retromolar trigone/anterior tonsillar pillar lesions have a lower risk of clinically positive lymph nodes (45%) compared with the tonsillar fossa (76%). The distribution for the retromolar trigone/anterior tonsillar pillar on the ipsilateral side is to the jugular and level IB lymph nodes with a low risk for junctional and level V nodes. Contralateral spread is uncommon (5%) and is confined to the jugular chain. The risk of occult disease in the clinically negative neck (N0) is 10% to 15%. The incidence of positive nodes increases with T stage.

The lymph node distribution for tonsillar fossa lesions on the ipsilateral side includes the jugular, junctional, level V, and level IB lymph nodes. Contralateral spread occurs in 11% of patients and is mainly to the jugular chain lymph nodes. The risk of contralateral spread is related to invasion of the tongue near the midline of the soft palate and large ipsilateral lymph nodes that produce lymphatic obstruction. The incidence of occult disease is probably 50% to 60%.

Soft Palate

Primary

Nearly all SCCs occur on the oral side of the palate. The earliest tumors are red lesions with ill-defined borders. Spread occurs first to the tonsillar pillars and hard palate. Lateral spread may eventually penetrate the superior constrictor muscle and skull base and invade the lateral wall(s) of the nasopharynx.

Lymphatic

The spread pattern is first to the level II nodes and then to levels III and IV. Approximately 56% of patients have clinically positive nodes at presentation; 16% are bilateral.[20] The incidence of occult neck disease is approximately 20%.[271] The incidence of clinically positive nodes increases with T stage.[20]

CLINICAL PICTURE

Base of Tongue

Often, the earliest symptom is a mild sore throat or a level II neck mass. Difficulty swallowing, a nasal voice quality, and ear pain occur as the lesion enlarges. Advanced lesions fix the tongue.

Flexible fiber optic endoscopy and digital palpation are necessary for the diagnosis of early lesions of the base of tongue.

Lymphomas are usually large, mostly submucosal masses. Minor salivary gland tumors are also usually submucosal, but more discrete and firm than lymphomas.

Tonsillar Area

Anterior Tonsillar Pillar

Early symptoms include sore throat, and pain is referred to the ear. As the lesion progresses, it may cause trismus and temporal pain.

Tonsillar Fossa

An ipsilateral sore throat is common. Detection by visual examination with a tongue depressor is sufficient for most lesions. Some patients present with a node in the neck. Lymphomas tend to be large submucosal masses, but may ulcerate and appear similar to carcinomas.

Soft Palate

Patients may present with a mild sore throat that is not well localized. Advanced lesions may cause swallowing dysfunction, voice changes, regurgitation of food into the nasopharynx, trismus, temporal pain, and, rarely, CN involvement.

STAGING

The AJCC staging system is used.[26] Invasion of the deep musculature of the tongue is diagnosed if the tongue is partially fixed. Lesions that produce trismus or CN palsy are classified as T4. Pathologic staging usually results in "upstaging." Stage migration renders a meaningful comparison of outcomes between clinically and pathologically staged patients nearly impossible.

TREATMENT: BASE OF TONGUE

Selection of Treatment Modality

Surgery and RT produce similar cure rates. Because excision of the base of tongue generally causes greater disability and because of the high risk for bilateral lymphatic involvement, RT or chemoRT is usually the treatment of choice.[272]

Surgical Treatment

Patients with a low-volume T1 or early T2 cancer may be suitable for transoral laser excision and a neck dissection.[273] Transoral robotic surgery is increasingly used to facilitate resection with less morbidity. Otherwise, the surgical approach requires an incision, which splits the lip, and a mandibulotomy, which permits lateral rotation of the mandible. Suprahyoid, transhyoid, and infrahyoid approaches also can be used to resect small lesions. After the tumor has been removed, the mandibular edges are reapproximated and stabilized with a titanium reconstruction plate. Only one lingual artery may be sacrificed. A neck dissection is done in continuity with excision of the primary lesion. Removal of a large tumor requires the simultaneous removal of part of or the entire larynx.

Irradiation Technique

Parallel opposed EBRT portals encompass the primary site and bilateral cervical nodes. Interstitial brachytherapy with flexible sources, such as ^{192}Ir ribbons, may be used for part of the treatment if the lesion is relatively limited. In contrast to oral tongue cancer, there is no proven advantage in local control for interstitial boosts compared with EBRT alone.

One of the common errors in planning EBRT is a failure to recognize anterior tumor extension into the lateral floor of the mouth; this is usually appreciated on CT and/or MRI. The inferior border of the lateral portals is usually the thyroid notch unless the tumor has extended into the upper pyriform sinus or preepiglottic space.

The primary portals include the level I$_B$, II, and V nodes when the neck is N0. The superior border is approximately 2 cm above the tip of the mastoid even with clinically negative nodes to ensure coverage of the nodes near the skull base.

The bilateral lower neck nodes are always treated with a separate anterior portal. If the upper neck is clinically negative, the lower neck portals include the level 3 and 4 nodes. If the upper neck is clinically positive, the lower neck portals are more generous.

Patients are treated with 1.2 Gy per fraction twice daily to 74.4 to 76.8 Gy. An alternative is 70 Gy in 35 fractions over 30 treatment days using simultaneous integrated boost (SIB) and a concomitant boost. Most patients with a N0 neck or ipsilateral positive nodes are treated with IMRT to reduce the dose to the contralateral parotid.

Management of Recurrence

RT treatment failures are treated surgically; salvage is infrequent except for T1 and early T2 lesions. Surgical treatment failures are rarely salvaged, except for the early lesion with a discrete local recurrence. Palliative management is often preferred.

RESULTS OF TREATMENT: BASE OF TONGUE

The 5-year local control rates after definitive RT in a series of 333 patients treated at the University of Florida were for T1, 98% (n = 46); for T2, 92% (n = 125); for T3, 82% (n = 92); and for T4, 53% (n = 70).[272] The 5-year local–regional control, distant metastasis-free survival, and survival rates are depicted in Table 38.11. Severe, acute, late, and/or postoperative complications developed in 52 patients (16%).

FOLLOW-UP: BASE OF TONGUE

RT failures may present as an ulcer and must be distinguished from necrosis. Deep biopsies usually must be done under general anesthesia to obtain adequate tissue and control bleeding.

COMPLICATIONS OF TREATMENT: BASE OF TONGUE

Surgical Complications

These include an operative mortality of about 5%. Other complications include fistula, mandibular necrosis, dysphagia, aspiration pneumonia, hoarseness, trismus, and carotid rupture.

Complications of Irradiation

Bone exposure and ORN are uncommon. Mild-to-moderate soft tissue necroses occur in approximately 10% of patients, and mild-to-moderate bone exposures occur in 5% of patients treated solely by EBRT. Necroses may persist for several months and may respond to pentoxifylline. Hypoglossal nerve palsy occurs rarely.

Occasionally, patients may have difficulty swallowing due to fibrosis of the base of the tongue compounded by xerostomia. Significant aspiration is unusual. It is uncommon for a patient to develop severe swallowing disability requiring a PEG.[274]

TREATMENT: TONSILLAR AREA

Selection of Treatment Modality

The cure rates are similar after definitive RT-based treatment compared with surgery alone or combined with adjuvant RT.[275] Because morbidity is generally higher after surgery, definitive RT or chemoRT is often preferred.

Surgical Treatment

Surgery for early cancers consists of a transoral wide local excision. Transoral robotic surgery is increasingly used for surgical procedures of this site to facilitate resection with less morbidity. Larger lesions may require removal of the adjacent mandible as well as a portion of the tongue and soft palate. Depending on the size of the defect, a tongue, deltopectoral, or osteomyocutaneous flap may be required. Speech may be impaired if a significant portion of the tongue or palate has been removed.

PRACTICE OF ONCOLOGY

TABLE 38.11

Base of Tongue: 5-Year Outcomes After Radiotherapy at the University of Florida (333 Patients)

Stage	No. of Patients	Local–Regional Control	Ultimate Local–Regional Control	Distant Metastasis-Free Survival	Cause-Specific Survival	Survival
I–II	26	100%	100%	92%	91%	67%
III	58	82%	87%	90%	77%	66%
IVA	124	87%	90%	92%	84%	67%
IVB	125	58%	62%	69%	45%	33%

From Mendenhall WM, Morris CG, Amdur RJ, et al. Definitive radiotherapy for squamous cell carcinoma of the base of tongue. *Am J Clin Oncol* 2006;29:32–39.

Irradiation Technique

The portal arrangement depends on the extent of local–regional disease. If the risk for contralateral lymph node metastases is low, an ipsilateral IMRT technique is employed to reduce xerostomia.

More advanced lesions are treated with parallel opposed photon portals, usually weighted 2 to 1 or 3 to 2 to the involved side. If there are positive contralateral nodes or extension across the midline, the portals usually are equally weighted. The inferior border is placed 2 cm below the primary tumor. IMRT may be employed to irradiate both sides of the neck and reduce the dose to the contralateral parotid in patients with a N0 neck or ipsilateral positive neck nodes. The low neck is treated with a separate anterior field with a thin midline block over the larynx. Small, discrete lesions of the anterior tonsillar pillar may have part of the RT by intraoral cone.

The dose for tonsillar lesions is 74.4 to 76.8 Gy (1.2 Gy twice daily) for T1 to T3 lesions, and 76.8 Gy for T4 lesions. An alternative is 70 Gy in 35 fractions over 30 treatment days using SIB and concomitant boost.

Management of Recurrence

Surgery will salvage a good portion of T1 or T2 RT failures, but only an occasional advanced lesion is salvaged.

RESULTS OF TREATMENT: TONSILLAR AREA

The 5-year local control rates after definitive RT in a series of 503 patients treated at the University of Florida between 1964 and 2003 for cancer of the anterior tonsillar pillar versus tonsillar fossa/posterior tonsillar pillar were for T1, 70% versus 94%; for T2, 74% versus 90%; for T3, 72% versus 79%; and for T4, 57% versus 62%.[275] The local control rates are better for tonsillar fossa/posterior tonsillar pillar cancers compared with those arising in the anterior tonsillar pillar. The 5-year local–regional control, distant metastases-free survival, and survival rates are depicted in Table 38.12.[275]

COMPLICATIONS OF TREATMENT: TONSILLAR AREA

Radiation Therapy

The risk for a severe complication, usually a bone or soft tissue necrosis, requiring surgical intervention is low. The probability of a fatal complication is remote. An occasional patient, usually one treated for advanced disease, may have long-term swallowing problems. Other complications include trismus, hypoglossal

nerve entrapment, and a remote risk of an RT-induced malignancy and/or myelitis. Severe late complications occurred in 46 of 503 patients (9%).[275]

SURGICAL TREATMENT

Complications of operation include impaired swallowing, fistula, flap failure, poor wound healing, and aspiration occasionally leading to laryngectomy. The risk of severe and/or fatal complications is higher after surgery compared with RT.[275]

TREATMENT: SOFT PALATE

Selection of Treatment Modality

Although small, well-defined lesions may be excised and the neck observed, the risk of subclinical regional disease is high. Therefore, definitive RT is indicated for nearly all soft palate carcinomas; neck dissection is added as needed. Concomitant chemotherapy is indicated for patients with T3 to T4 and/or N2 to N3 disease.

Surgical Treatment

Small, discrete lesions can be managed by transoral excision and repaired by a pharyngeal flap to prevent any velopharyngeal incompetence. A tonsillectomy may also be necessary in order to obtain an adequate margin. If full-thickness resection is performed, a prosthesis is often required.

Irradiation Technique

The RT technique involves equally weighted, parallel opposed EBRT portals that include the primary lesion and the bilateral first-echelon upper neck nodes. A separate anterior portal is used to treat the low neck. If the primary lesion is discrete and the neck is clinically negative, a portion of the treatment may be given with an intraoral cone prior to EBRT.

Patients are treated with 4 to 6 MV photons to 74.4 to 76.8 Gy at 1.2 Gy per fraction, twice daily, in a continuous course. Another option is 70 Gy in 35 fractions over 30 treatment days. IMRT using the concomitant boost technique may be used to reduce the dose to one or both parotids.

Management of Recurrence

A persistent ulcer after RT is indicative of recurrent disease. Patients with a limited local recurrence after RT for a T1 or T2 lesion may be suitable for surgical salvage.

TABLE 38.12

Tonsillar Region: 5-Year Outcomes After Definitive Radiotherapy at the University of Florida (503 Patients)

Stage	No. of Patients	Local–Regional Control	Ultimate Local–Regional Control	Distant Metastasis-Free Survival	Cause-Specific Survival	Survival
I	22	66%	92%	100%	100%	54%
II	83	75%	88%	95%	86%	61%
III	95	85%	88%	97%	84%	62%
IVA	184	76%	84%	85%	73%	57%
IVB	119	58%	66%	68%	46%	33%

From Mendenhall WM, Morris CG, Amdur RJ, et al. Definitive radiotherapy for tonsillar squamous cell carcinoma. *Am J Clin Oncol* 2006;29:290–297.

RESULTS OF TREATMENT: SOFT PALATE

Chera and coworkers[276] reported on 145 patients treated with definitive RT at the University of Florida between 1963 and 2004. Local control rates at 5 years were for T1, 90%; for T2, 90%; for T3, 67%; for T4, 57%; and overall, 81%. The 5-year local–regional control and cause-specific survival rates were for stage I, 84% and 89%; for stage II, 85% and 87%; for stage III, 66% and 88%; for stage IVA, 59% and 57%; and for stage IVB, 43% and 0%, respectively.[276]

COMPLICATIONS OF TREATMENT: SOFT PALATE

Surgical Complications

Nasal speech and regurgitation of food into the nasopharynx are sequelae of full-thickness soft palate resection. A prosthesis is partially successful in correcting the functional deficit.

Complications of Irradiation

Soft-tissue necrosis is uncommon. The soft palate may become retracted following successful treatment of advanced lesions and may result in regurgitation into the nasopharynx and a slight alteration in speech. ORN requiring surgical management is rare. Severe late complications were observed in 8 of 145 patients (6%) treated with definitive RT.[276]

LARYNX

Cancer of the larynx is primarily related to cigarette smoking.[277] The effect of alcohol remains unclear, but it is probably less impactful for the larynx than for the other head and neck sites.[277]

ANATOMY

The larynx is divided anatomically into the supraglottis, glottis, and subglottis. The supraglottis consists of the epiglottis, false vocal cords, ventricles, aryepiglottic folds, and arytenoids; the arytenoids are cartilages that articulate on the cricoid. The glottis includes the true vocal cords and the anterior commissure. The subglottis is 2 cm long and extends from 5 mm below the free edge of the true vocal cords to the lower margin of cricoid cartilage.

The preepiglottic space is bounded by the epiglottis posteriorly, the hyoepiglottic ligament and vallecula superiorly, and the thyroid cartilage and thyrohyoid membrane anteriorly and laterally. It can be seen as a low-density area on a CT scan.

The supraglottis has a moderately rich capillary lymphatic plexus. The lymphatic trunks pass through the preepiglottic space and the thyrohyoid membrane to the level II nodes. A few trunks drain directly to the level III or level IV nodes. There are essentially no capillary lymphatics of the true vocal cords. The subglottis area has relatively few capillary lymphatics. The lymphatic trunks pass through the thyrocricoid membrane to the midline pretracheal (Delphian) node(s) in the region of the thyroid isthmus and/or to the level IV nodes. The subglottis also drains posteriorly through the cricotracheal membrane with some trunks going to the paratracheal (level VI) nodes, whereas others pass to the level IV nodes.

PATHOLOGY

Nearly all laryngeal cancers arise from the surface epithelium and are SCCs. Minor salivary gland tumors are rare; even rarer are soft-tissue sarcomas, lymphomas, neuroendocrine carcinomas, and plasmacytomas. Hemangiomas, chondromas, and osteochondromas are reported, but their malignant counterparts are rare.

Distinguishing between CIS and invasive SCC is often challenging because focal biopsies of the vocal cords can miss an area of microinvasion and mucosal stripping of a vocal cord lesion results in a disoriented specimen that precludes a complete evaluation of the basement membrane region. However, both CIS and microinvasive SCC are treated the same, with either endoscopic transoral laser resection or RT.

Most vocal cord SCCs are either well or moderately well differentiated. In a few cases, SCCs with a spindle cell component may be observed. Verrucous carcinoma occurs on the vocal cords in about 1% to 2% of patients with carcinoma. Supraglottic SCCs are less differentiated; verrucous cancers are rare.

PATTERNS OF SPREAD

Supraglottic Larynx

Lesions may exhibit an exophytic growth pattern with little tendency to destroy cartilage or spread to adjacent structures. Others may infiltrate and destroy cartilage and eventually amputate the tip of the epiglottis. They tend to invade the vallecula, preepiglottic space, lateral pharyngeal walls, and the remainder of the supraglottis.

False vocal cord cancers are often submucosal. Those arising from the aryepiglottic fold tend to invade the medial wall of the pyriform sinus. An inferior invasion of the vocal cords is usually a late phenomenon, and subglottic extension occurs only in advanced lesions. Lesions that extend onto or below the vocal cords are at a high risk for cartilage invasion, even if the cords are mobile.[278]

Vocal Cord

The majority of lesions begin on the free margin and upper surface of the vocal cord. About two thirds are confined to one cord, usually the anterior two thirds of the cord. Extension to the anterior commissure is frequent. As the lesion enlarges, it extends to the ventricle, false cord, vocal process of the arytenoids, and subglottis. Cancers then invade the vocal ligament and thyroarytenoid muscles, eventually reaching the thyroid cartilage where they tend to grow up or down the paraglottic space rather than invade cartilage. The conus elasticus initially acts as a barrier to subglottic extension. Advanced lesions eventually invade through the thyroid cartilage or thyrocricoid membrane to enter the neck and/or thyroid gland.

Subglottic Larynx

Subglottic cancers involve the cricoid cartilage early, and cord fixation is common.

Lymphatic

Supraglottic

Lymphatic drainage is initially to the level II nodes, and then to levels III and IV.[20] The incidence of clinically positive nodes is 55% at diagnosis; 16% are bilateral.[20] Elective neck dissection will show pathologically positive nodes in 16% to 26% of cases; observation of the neck will be followed by the appearance of positive nodes in approximately 33% of cases.

Glottic

The incidence of clinically positive nodes at diagnosis varies with T stage: T1, ≤1%; T2, ≤5%; and T3 and T4, 20% to 30%.[279] Supraglottic spread is associated with metastasis to the level II nodes. Anterior commissure and subglottic invasion is associated with level III, level IV, and Delphian node involvement.[280]

PRACTICE OF ONCOLOGY

Subglottic

Lederman[281] reported a 10% incidence of clinically positive lymph nodes on admission. Spread is primarily to the Delphian nodes and the level IV nodes.

CLINICAL PICTURE

Presenting Symptoms

Vocal Cords

Carcinoma initially causes hoarseness. Pain, dysphagia, and airway obstruction may be observed with advanced cancers.

Supraglottic Larynx

Pain on swallowing, referred to the ear by the vagus nerve and the auricular nerve of Arnold, is a frequent initial symptom. A neck mass may be the first sign of a supraglottic cancer. Late symptoms include hoarseness, weight loss, foul breath, dysphagia, and aspiration.

Physical Examination

A determination of laryngeal mobility with a laryngeal mirror or fiber optic scope frequently requires multiple examinations because the subtle distinctions between mobile, partially fixed, and fixed cords are often difficult. Preepiglottic space invasion is best appreciated on CT.

Postcricoid extension may be suspected when the laryngeal "click" disappears on physical examination. Localized pain or tenderness to palpation over the thyroid cartilage is suggestive of invasion. Advanced tumors may penetrate through the thyroid ala and be felt as a bulge on the cartilage. A CT scan may detect cartilage invasion, but irregular calcification of the cartilage, coupled with volume averaging of the CT slice, creates technical problems in appreciating early cartilage invasion.

DIFFERENTIAL DIAGNOSIS AND STAGING

The differential diagnosis includes papillomas, polyps, vocal nodules, fibromas, and granulomas. Papillomas generally occur in children and young adults, and may persist into adulthood. Vocal polyps and nodules occur at the junction of the middle and anterior one third of the true vocal cords. There is usually a history of voice abuse followed by hoarseness. Vocal cord granulomas usually occur as a result of intubation and are located on or near the posterior commissure. Endoscopic removal may be necessary if medical therapy for gastroesophageal reflux provides no improvement, although this is rare.

The staging system for the primary tumor is depicted in Table 38.13.

TABLE 38.13

2010 American Joint Committee on Cancer Staging for Laryngeal Cancer

Primary Tumor (T)	
TX	Primary tumor cannot be assessed
T0	No evidence of primary tumor
Tis	Carcinoma in situ
Supraglottis	
T1	Tumor limited to one subsite of supraglottis with normal vocal cord mobility
T2	Tumor invades mucosa of more than one adjacent subsite of supraglottis or region outside the supraglottis (e.g., mucosa of base of tongue, vallecula, medial wall of pyriform sinus) without fixation of the larynx
T3	Tumor limited to larynx with vocal cord fixation and/or invades any of the following: postcricoid area, preepiglottic tissues, paraglottic space, and/or minor thyroid cartilage erosion (e.g., inner cortex)
T4a	Tumor invades through the thyroid cartilage and/or invades tissues beyond the larynx (e.g., trachea, soft tissues of neck including deep extrinsic muscles of the tongue, strap muscles, thyroid, or esophagus)
T4b	Tumor invades prevertebral space, encases carotid artery, or invades mediastinal structures
Glottis	
T1	Tumor limited to one (T1a) or both (T1b) vocal cord(s) (may involve anterior or posterior commissure) with normal mobility
T2	Tumor extends to supraglottis and/or subglottis, and/or with impaired vocal cord mobility
T3	Tumor limited to the larynx with vocal cord fixation, and/or invades paraglottic space, and/or minor thyroid cartilage erosion (e.g., inner cortex)
T4a	Tumor invades through the thyroid cartilage and/or invades tissues beyond the larynx (e.g., trachea, soft tissues of neck including deep extrinsic muscles of the tongue, strap muscles, thyroid, esophagus)
T4b	Tumor invades prevertebral space, encases carotid artery, or invades mediastinal structures
Subglottis	
T1	Tumor limited to the subglottis
T2	Tumor extends to vocal cord(s) with normal or impaired mobility
T3	Tumor limited to larynx with vocal cord fixation
T4a	Tumor invades cricoid or thyroid cartilage and/or tissues beyond the larynx (e.g., trachea, soft tissues of neck including deep extrinsic muscles of the tongue, strap muscles, thyroid, or esophagus)
T4b	Tumor invades prevertebral space, encases carotid artery, or invades mediastinal structures

TREATMENT: VOCAL CORD CARCINOMA

Selection of Treatment Modality

Carcinoma In Situ

Vocal cord stripping may sometimes control CIS. Recurrence is frequent, and the vocal cord may become thickened and the voice hoarse with repeated stripping. We recommend RT for patients with multiple recurrences.[282]

Early Vocal Cord Lesions (T1, T2)

In most centers, RT is the initial treatment, with operation reserved for salvage of RT failures.[283] Although an open partial laryngectomy will produce comparable cure rates for selected T1 or T2 vocal cord lesions, RT is generally preferred because it is less expensive and voice quality is better. An endoscopic transoral laser resection is increasingly being used.[283] Using this technique, small midcord lesions may be treated. Voice quality depends on the extent of tissue removal and whether surgical resection involves the anterior commissure. An open partial laryngectomy or a total laryngectomy may be used as a salvage operation after RT failure.

Verrucous carcinomas are treated with a transoral laser resection or an open partial laryngectomy. Definitive RT is employed if the alternative is a total laryngectomy.

Advanced Vocal Cord Lesions (T3, T4)

Low volume cancers (≤3.5 mL) with stage III to IV disease are treated with definitive RT and concomitant chemotherapy.[284,285] Higher volume carcinomas are usually treated with a total laryngectomy, neck dissection, and postoperative RT or chemoRT.

Surgical Treatment

Stripping the cord implies transoral removal of the mucosa of the edge of the cord.

A cordectomy is an excision of the vocal cord and is usually performed via a transoral laser. The major advantages of laser excision are that it requires a day, as opposed to the 5.5 weeks that are necessary for RT, and RT may be reserved if the patient develops a second head and neck cancer.

A hemilaryngectomy is a partial laryngectomy allowing the removal of limited cord lesions with voice preservation. Restrictions include the involvement of one cord and up to 5 mm of the opposite cord, a partial fixation of one cord, and up to 9 mm of subglottic extension anteriorly and 5 mm posteriorly (to preserve the cricoid cartilage). Extension to the supraglottic or interarytenoid area is a contraindication. One arytenoid may be sacrificed; the reconstructed vocal cord must be fixed in the midline to prevent aspiration. The patient must have adequate pulmonary function. More extensive open partial laryngectomies have been described, such as the supracricoid partial laryngectomy.[286]

The last surgical alternative is a total laryngectomy with or without a neck dissection. The entire larynx is removed, the pharynx is reconstituted, and a permanent tracheostoma is created.

There are several options to accomplish voice rehabilitation after a total laryngectomy. Prosthetic devices (e.g., the Blom-Singer Voice Prosthesis) have been developed for insertion into a tracheoesophageal fistula, which permits the patient to speak without aspiration.[287] Voice rehabilitation was evaluated in 173 patients who underwent a total laryngectomy and postoperative RT at the University of Florida; 118 patients were evaluable 2 to 3 years after treatment and 69 patients were evaluated for 5 years or longer.[287] Methods of voice rehabilitation at 2 to 3 years and 5 years or more after surgery included: tracheoesophageal speech, 27% and 19%; artificial ("electric") larynx, 50% and 57%; esophageal, 1% and 3%; nonvocal, 17% and 14%; and no data, 5% and 7%, respectively.[287]

Irradiation Technique

RT for early vocal cord cancer is delivered by portals including only the primary lesion. Portals for T1 lesions extend from the thyroid notch superiorly to the inferior border of the cricoid; the posterior border depends on posterior extension of the tumor. Portals for T2 lesions are slightly larger, depending on the extent of the lesion. Patients receive 2.25 Gy per fraction once daily to 63 Gy (T1 and T2a) or 65.25 Gy (T2b).[279,288]

RT for T3 and T4 lesions include the primary lesion and the level II through IV and Delphian lymph nodes. The initial treatment is delivered at 1.2 Gy per fraction twice daily to 45.6 Gy. The portals are then reduced to include only the primary lesion; the final tumor dose is 74.4 Gy. Another option is 70 Gy in 35 fractions in over 30 treatment days. The low neck is treated through a separate anterior portal. IMRT may be useful to avoid a difficult low neck match in patients with a low-lying larynx.

Management of Recurrence

Worsening laryngeal edema suggests recurrence. Cord fixation usually implies local recurrence; fixation may rarely develop in the absence of recurrent disease.

RT failures (T1 to T2) are almost always salvaged by a cordectomy, a partial laryngectomy, or a total laryngectomy. The salvage rate for T3 lesions recurring after RT is approximately 60%.[285]

Salvage by RT-based treatment for recurrences or new tumors appearing after partial laryngectomy is about 50%. Isolated tracheostomal recurrences may be managed by RT, chemoRT, or surgery and postoperative RT-based treatment; the chance of cure is relatively low.[289] A multi-institutional surgical experience in the management of stomal recurrence was reported by Gluckman and coworkers.[289] Forty-one patients came to operation. The 2-year cause-specific survival was 24%. Patients with localized recurrences had a 5-year survival rate of 45%.

TREATMENT: SUPRAGLOTTIC LARYNX CARCINOMA

Selection of Treatment Modality

T1, T2, and low-volume (≤6 mL) T3 lesions are favorable and can be treated with definitive RT or a supraglottic laryngectomy. It is seldom necessary to combine RT and surgery for the management of the primary lesion; however, combined treatment may be indicated to control neck disease.

Patients who are candidates for a supraglottic laryngectomy must have lesions that are anatomically suitable, a resectable neck disease, and adequate pulmonary reserve to withstand aspiration. Because the likelihood of local control after RT is related to primary tumor volume, lesions >6 mL are treated with a partial laryngectomy.[290,291] The anatomic constraints include: no extension inferior to the apex of the ventricle, minimal or no involvement of the medial wall of the pyriform sinus, mobile cords, no cartilage invasion, and limited lateralized extension to the tongue base. Patients who are not candidates for the supraglottic laryngectomy are treated with RT; concomitant chemotherapy is added for those with stage III through IV disease.

When a patient presents with an early-stage primary lesion and N2B to N3 neck disease, a combined treatment is necessary to produce a high rate of neck control. Thus, the primary lesion is preferably treated with chemoRT, with neck dissection(s) added to the involved side(s) of the neck if necessary. If the patient has N1 or N2A neck disease and surgery is elected for the primary site, postoperative RT or chemoRT is only added because of unexpected findings (e.g., positive margins, multiple positive nodes, ECE). The probability of a good functional result is improved if the dose to the remaining larynx is limited to 55 Gy at 1.8 Gy per once-daily fraction. The involved neck may be boosted to a higher dose without irradiating the larynx.

Selected unfavorable T3 and T4 lesions that are mainly exophytic can be treated by chemoRT. Lesions unsuitable for RT are endophytic, high-volume cancers often associated with vocal cord fixation, which are managed by a total laryngectomy.

Surgical Treatment

Supraglottic Laryngectomy

The incision is usually an apron flap. The neck dissection is completed and left attached to the thyrohyoid membrane. The perichondrium of the larynx is elevated in continuity with the strap muscles and used to close the surgical defect. Saw cuts are made through the thyroid cartilage, and the pharynx is entered above the hyoid bone through the vallecula so the preepiglottic space is included in the specimen. The arytenoids and true vocal cords are preserved. If one arytenoid is sacrificed, the vocal cord is fixed in the midline to prevent aspiration. Suturing the perichondrium and muscle to the base of tongue closes the defect. The extended supraglottic laryngectomy may include resection of the base of tongue to the level of the circumvallate papillae as long as one lingual artery is spared.

Total Laryngectomy

The entire larynx and the preepiglottic space are resected en bloc and a permanent tracheostoma is fashioned. A portion of the thyroid gland is also removed if there is extralaryngeal or subglottic extension. The pharyngeal defect is closed, reestablishing a conduit from the pharynx into the esophagus.

Irradiation Technique

The primary lesion and both sides of the neck are included with opposed lateral portals. The inferior border of the portals depends on the inferior extent of the primary tumor; it is usually at the inferior border of the cricoid. The dose is 74.4 Gy in 62 twice-daily fractions; the lower neck nodes are irradiated through a separate anterior portal. Patients with ipsilateral positive nodes may be treated with IMRT to reduce the dose to the contralateral parotid and/or to avoid a difficult low neck match. An alternative is 70 Gy in 35 fractions over 30 treatment days.

Patients develop a sore throat, loss of taste, and moderate dryness during RT. Arytenoid edema may occur and produce the sensation of a lump in the throat. A tracheostomy is seldom necessary before the start of RT. Laryngeal edema may persist for up to a year. Neck dissection increases the degree of lymphedema; a bilateral neck dissection should be avoided, if possible.[292]

Combined Treatment Policies

If a total laryngectomy is required and the lesion is resectable, postoperative RT is preferred. The high-risk areas are usually the base of tongue and neck. The stoma is at risk when subglottic extension is present or if there is tumor in the low neck lymph nodes.

Management of Recurrence

Failures after supraglottic laryngectomy or RT frequently can be salvaged by further treatment. The salvage of recurrences that develop after total laryngectomy and adjuvant RT is uncommon.

TREATMENT: SUBGLOTTIC LARYNX CARCINOMA

Early lesions are treated with RT; advanced lesions are usually managed by a total laryngectomy and postoperative RT or chemoRT.

Results of Treatment

Vocal Cord Cancer

Surgical Results. Garcia-Serra et al.[282] reviewed 10 series containing 269 patients with CIS of the vocal cord treated with stripping; the weighted average 5-year local control and ultimate local control rates were 71.9% and 92.4%, respectively. Similarly, 10 series containing 177 patients treated with carbon dioxide laser revealed the following weighted average 5-year local control and ultimate local control rates: 82.5% and 98.1%, respectively.[282]

Thomas and coworkers[293] reported on 159 patients who underwent an open partial laryngectomy at the Mayo Clinic between 1976 and 1986. Of 159 patients, 17 had CIS; the remaining were T1 SCCs. Local recurrence developed in 11 patients (7%), and 9 eventually required a laryngectomy. Ten patients developed recurrent cancer in the neck, and distant metastases were observed in 10 patients.

A hemilaryngectomy, including the ipsilateral arytenoid, was reported by Som[294] for 130 cases of vocal cord carcinoma extending to the vocal process and face of the arytenoid. The cure rate was 74% for 104 patients with T2 lesions, and 58% for 26 patients with T3 cancers.

Foote and coworkers[295] reported on 81 patients who underwent a laryngectomy for T3 cancers at the Mayo Clinic between 1970 and 1981. Seventy-five patients underwent a total laryngectomy and six underwent a near-total laryngectomy; 53 received a neck dissection. No patient underwent adjuvant RT or chemotherapy. The 5-year rates of local–regional control, cause-specific survival, and absolute survival were 74%, 74%, and 54%, respectively.

Radiation Therapy Results. Garcia-Serra et al.[282] reviewed 22 series containing 705 patients with CIS of the vocal cord treated with RT and observed that the weighted average 5-year local control and ultimate local control rates were 87.4% and 98.4%, respectively.

The results of RT for 585 patients with T1 and T2 N0 SCC of the glottis treated by RT are presented in Table 38.14. The 5-year rates of neck control for the overall groups and for the subsets of patients who remained continuously disease free at the primary site were for T1a, 98% and 100%; for T1b, 99% and 100%; for T2a, 96% and 98%; and for T2b, 88% and 94%, respectively.[279]

The 5-year outcomes after RT alone (53 patients) versus surgery alone or combined with RT (65 patients) in a series of 118 patients with T3 fixed-cord glottic carcinomas treated at the University of Florida were for local–regional control, 62% versus 75% (p = 0.10); for ultimate local–regional control, 84% versus 82% (p = 0.95); for cause-specific survival, 75% versus 71% (p = 0.26); for overall survival, 55% versus 45% (p = 0.119); and for severe complications, 16% versus 15% (p = 0.558), respectively.[284] Hinerman et al.[296] recently updated the University of Florida experience and reported a 5-year local control rate of 63% for 87 patients with T3 fixed-cord glottic carcinomas. The likelihood of local control after RT is related to primary tumor volume and cartilage sclerosis.[297]

The probability of cure after treatment for T4 glottic carcinomas after surgery with or without adjuvant RT or definitive RT varies from 30% to 50% depending on patient selection.[296–303]

TREATMENT: SUPRAGLOTTIC LARYNX CANCER

The 5-year local control rates after definitive RT in a series of 274 patients treated between 1964 and 1998 at the University of Florida were for T1, 100% (n = 22); for T2, 86% (n = 125); for T3, 62% (n = 99); and for T4, 62% (n = 28).[304] The likelihood of local control and local control with a functional larynx is related to tumor volume; those with tumors ≤6 mL have a more favorable outcome

PRACTICE OF ONCOLOGY

TABLE 38.14

T1 to T2N0 Glottic Larynx: 5-Year Outcomes After Radiotherapy in 585 Patients

Stage	No. of Patients	Local Control	Ultimate Local Control	Local Control With Larynx Preservation	Cause-Specific Survival	Survival
T1A	253	94%	98%	95%	97%	82%
T1B	72	93%	97%	94%	99%	83%
T2A	165	80%	96%	81%	94%	76%
T2B	95	70%	93%	74%	90%	78%

Data from Chera BS, Amdur R, Morris CG, et al. T1N0 to T2N0 squamous cell carcinoma of the glottic larynx treated with definitive radiotherapy. *Int J Radiat Oncol Biol Phys* 2010;78:461–466.

than those with larger primary tumors.[291] The 5-year rates of local–regional control and cause-specific survival were for stage I, 100% and 100%; for stage II, 86% and 93%; for stage III, 64% and 81%; for stage IVA, 61% and 50%; and for stage IVB, 28% and 13%, respectively.[304] Of 274 patients, 12 (4%) experienced a severe acute or late complication, and 2 patients (1%) died as a consequence.

Lee and coworkers[305] reported on 60 patients who underwent a supraglottic laryngectomy and modified neck dissection at the M.D. Anderson Hospital between 1974 and 1987, of which 50 patients (83%) received postoperative RT. Local control was 100% and local–regional control was obtained in 56 of 60 patients (93%). The 5-year disease-free survival rate was 91%. Three of 60 patients (5%) required a complete laryngectomy for intractable aspiration.

Ambrosch and colleagues[306] reported on 48 patients treated with transoral laser resection for T1N0 (12 patients) and T2N0 (36 patients) supraglottic carcinoma. Twenty-six patients underwent a unilateral (11 patients) or bilateral (15 patients) neck dissection. Postoperative RT was administered to two patients (4%). The 5-year local control rates were 100% for pT1 cancers and 89% for pT2 malignancies. The 5-year recurrence-free survival and overall survival rates were 83% and 76%, respectively. No patient developed severe aspiration.

Complications of Treatment

Surgical Treatment

Repeated stripping of the cord may result in vocal cord fibrosis and hoarseness. Neel and coworkers[307] reported a 26% incidence of nonfatal complications for cordectomy. Immediate postoperative complications included atelectasis and pneumonia, severe subcutaneous emphysema in the neck, bleeding from the tracheotomy site or larynx, wound complications, and airway obstruction requiring a tracheotomy. Late complications included the removal of granulation tissue by a direct laryngoscopy to exclude recurrence, extrusion of cartilage, laryngeal stenosis, and obstructing laryngeal web.

The postoperative complications of hemilaryngectomy include aspiration, chondritis, wound slough, inadequate glottic closure, and anterior commissure webs.

The complication rate following supraglottic laryngectomy is about 10%, including fistula formation, aspiration, chondritis, dysphagia, dyspnea, and carotid rupture.[304]

The postoperative complications of a total laryngectomy may include perioperative death, hemorrhage, fistula, chondritis, wound breakdown, carotid rupture, dysphagia, and pharyngoesophageal stenosis.

Radiation Therapy

Soft-tissue necrosis leading to chondritis occurs in about 1% of patients. Soft-tissue and cartilage necroses mimic recurrence with hoarseness, pain, and edema; a laryngectomy may be recommended

for fear of recurrent cancer, even though biopsies show only necrosis. Chera et al.[279] recorded severe complications after definitive RT in 10 (1.7%) of 585 patients treated for T1 to T2N0 glottic SCCs.

Combined Treatment

The major late effects of combined treatment are an increased fibrosis of soft tissues, stomal stenosis, and pharyngeal stricture.

HYPOPHARYNX: PHARYNGEAL WALLS, PYRIFORM SINUS, AND POSTCRICOID PHARYNX

Both the oropharyngeal and hypopharyngeal walls will be considered together because there is no distinct difference in the presentation or treatment. The majority of hypopharyngeal lesions originate in the pyriform sinus. Postcricoid carcinomas are uncommon.

ANATOMY

The epithelium of the pharyngeal mucous membrane is squamous. The dividing point between the nasopharynx and posterior pharyngeal wall is the Passavant ridge, a muscular ring that contracts to close the nasopharynx during swallowing. Between the constrictor muscles and the prevertebral fascia covering the longitudinal prevertebral muscles is a thin layer of loose areolar tissue, the retropharyngeal space. The entire thickness of the posterior pharyngeal wall from the mucous membrane to the anterior vertebral body is no more than 1 cm in the midline. Lateral to the pharyngeal wall are the vessels, nerves, and muscles of the parapharyngeal space. The constrictor muscles are relatively thin and do not present much of an obstacle to tumor penetration. There is a variable weak spot in the lateral pharyngeal wall just below the hyoid where the middle and the inferior constrictor muscles fail to overlap. The lateral wall in this area is composed of the thin thyrohyoid membrane, which is penetrated by the vessels, nerves, and lymphatics of the laryngopharynx.

The pharyngeal walls are continuous with the cervical esophagus below; the transition to cervical esophagus is below the arytenoids (C4). The transition zone, which is 3 cm to 4 cm in length, is the postcricoid hypopharynx.

The lateral pharyngeal wall is a narrow strip of mucosa that lies behind the posterior tonsillar pillar in the oropharynx, is partially interrupted by the pharyngoepiglottic fold, and then continues into the hypopharynx, where it becomes the lateral wall of the pyriform sinus. The posterior pharyngeal wall is 4 cm to 5 cm wide and 6 cm to 7 cm in height.

The superior margin of the pyriform sinus is the pharyngoepiglottic fold and the free margin of the aryepiglottic fold. The superolateral margin of the pyriform sinus is an oblique line along the lateral pharyngeal wall opposite the aryepiglottic fold. Thus, the pyriform sinus has three walls: the anterior, lateral, and medial (there is no posterior wall). The pyriform sinus tapers inferiorly to the apex and terminates variably at a level between the superior and inferior borders of the cricoid cartilage. The superior limit of the pyriform sinus is opposite the hyoid. The thyrohyoid membrane is lateral to the upper portion of the pyriform sinus, and the thyroid cartilage, cricothyroid membrane, and cricoid cartilage are lateral to the lower portion. The internal branch of the superior laryngeal nerve, a branch of the vagus, lies under the mucous membrane on the anterolateral wall of the pyriform sinus. The auricular branch is sensory to the skin of the back of the pinna and the posterior wall of the external auditory canal.

The postcricoid pharynx is funnel shaped to direct food into the esophagus. The superior margin begins just below the arytenoids. The anterior wall lies behind the cricoid cartilage and is the posterior wall of the lower larynx. The posterior wall is a continuation of the hypopharyngeal walls. The recurrent laryngeal nerve ascends in the tracheoesophageal groove, entering the larynx posterior to the cricothyroid articulation at the junction of the hypopharynx and esophagus. Internal branches of the superior laryngeal nerve extend inferiorly anterior to the mucosa of the piriform sinuses.

PATHOLOGY

More than 95% of malignant tumors are SCCs. CIS is commonly seen at the edge of pharyngeal wall SCCs; multifocal skip areas of CIS may make it difficult to obtain clear margins if excision is done. Minor salivary gland tumors are rare.

PATTERNS OF SPREAD

Posterior Pharyngeal Wall

SCCs of the posterior wall have a tendency to remain on the posterior wall, grow up or down the wall, and infiltrate posteriorly; they seldom spread circumferentially to the lateral walls. Early lesions are red and ulcerate as they progress. The tumor may spread up the pillars, eventually reaching the palate and nasopharynx. Advanced lesions tend to terminate inferiorly at the level of the arytenoids. Direct invasion of the cervical vertebrae or skull base is uncommon.

Lateral Pharyngeal Wall

Early tumors may be well-defined exophytic lesions. As they advance, they tend to penetrate laterally through the constrictor muscle, thus entering the lateral pharyngeal space or the soft tissues of the neck.

Pyriform Sinus

Early lesions usually appear as nodular mucosal irregularities. Medial wall lesions may grow superficially along the aryepiglottic fold and arytenoids, or invade directly into the false cord and aryepiglottic fold. Medial wall lesions also extend posteriorly to the postcricoid region, cricoid cartilage, and to the opposite pyriform sinus. Extensive submucosal spread is characteristic. There is frequently an area of central ulceration. The vocal cord becomes fixed because of infiltration of the intrinsic muscles of the larynx, the cricoarytenoid joint or muscle, or less commonly, the recurrent laryngeal nerve. Spread into the cervical esophagus is a late event.

Lesions arising on the lateral wall tend toward early invasion of the posterior thyroid cartilage and the posterior superior cricoid cartilage and, eventually, invade the thyroid gland. Involvement of the pyriform sinus apex is associated with an increased risk of thyroid cartilage invasion.[308] Lesions of the lateral walls tend to spread submucosally to the posterior pharyngeal wall.

Postcricoid Pharynx

Early postcricoid lesions are rare. Lesions arising from the posterior wall tend to remain on the posterior wall. Lesions arising from the anterior wall tend to invade the posterior cricoarytenoid muscle and the cricoid and arytenoid cartilages. Advanced tumors eventually encircle the lumen.

Lymphatics

Pharyngeal Walls

The lymphatics of the pharyngeal walls terminate primarily in the jugular chain and secondarily in the level V nodes. The level II nodes are most often involved. Lindberg[20] reported 59% clinically positive nodes at diagnosis; 17% were bilateral. Retropharyngeal lymph node involvement is frequent.

Pyriform Sinus

The drainage is mainly to the jugular chain with a relatively small proportion to the level V nodes. The level II nodes are most commonly involved, but level III involvement occurs without level II metastases. At diagnosis, 75% of patients have clinically positive nodes, and at least 10% have bilateral nodes. There is no difference in the risk of lymph node metastases by T stage. The incidence of subclinical neck disease probably exceeds 50%.[309]

CLINICAL PICTURE

Tumors that are lateralized to the lateral pharyngeal wall or pyriform sinus produce a unilateral sore throat. Dysphagia, ear pain, and voice changes occur later. A neck mass may be the presenting complaint.

Lesions of the apex of the pyriform sinus or postcricoid area produce a pooling of secretions, indicating obstruction of the gullet. Arytenoid edema and an inability to see into the apex of the pyriform sinus may be observed.

STAGING

The staging system for the primary tumor is depicted in Table 38.15.

TABLE 38.15

Hypopharynx: 2010 American Joint Committee on Cancer Staging System for the Primary Tumor

T1	Tumor limited to one subsite of hypopharynx and 2 cm or less in greatest dimension
T2	Tumor invades more than one subsite of hypopharynx or an adjacent site, or measures more than 2 cm but not more than 4 cm in greatest diameter without fixation of the hemilarynx
T3	Tumor more than 4 cm in greatest dimension or with fixation of the hemilarynx or extension to esophagus
T4a	Tumor invades thyroid/cricoid cartilage, hyoid bone, thyroid gland, or central compartment soft tissue[a]
T4b	Tumor invades the prevertebral fascia, encases the carotid artery, or involves mediastinal structures

[a] Central compartment soft tissue includes the prelaryngeal strap muscles and subcutaneous fat.
Used with the permission of the American Joint Committee on Cancer (AJCC), Chicago, Illinois. The original source for this material is the *AJCC Cancer Staging Handbook*, Seventh Edition (2010) published by Springer Science and Business Media LLC, www.springerlink.com.

TREATMENT

Selection of Treatment Modality

Posterior Pharyngeal Wall

RT produces cure rates similar to those produced by surgery alone or combined with RT, and with less morbidity. Thus, almost all cancers are treated with RT.

Lateral Pharyngeal Wall

The preferred treatment is definitive RT.

Pyriform Sinus

T1 and low-volume (≤6 mL), exophytic T2 cancers with normal cord mobility can be treated either by RT or a partial laryngopharyngectomy.[310] RT is preferred because it is associated with less morbidity.

Selected high-volume endophytic T2 and T3 lesions with normal or reduced mobility may be suitable for chemoRT. The swallowing outcomes after concurrent chemoRT may be less optimal than those seen in the oropharynx and larynx.[311]

The remainders are best treated with a total laryngopharyngectomy, neck dissection, and postoperative RT or chemoRT. Patients presenting with an extensive primary lesion and extensive neck metastases are frequently offered palliative therapy.

Surgical Treatment

Posterior Pharyngeal Wall

If the lesion is high on the posterior wall, a transoral approach can be used. Lower lesions were traditionally accessed via a transhyoid approach, a lateral pharyngotomy, or a midline mandibulolabial glossotomy. More recently, transoral laser microsurgical resection has been employed to reduce the morbidity associated with open approaches, which also frequently require tracheotomy. Dissection extends deep to the tumor down to the prevertebral fascia; smaller defects heal by secondary intention without a skin graft, whereas larger defects may require a radial forearm free flap.

Pyriform Sinus

Partial Laryngopharyngectomy. A partial laryngopharyngectomy removes the false cords, epiglottis, aryepiglottic fold, and pyriform sinus; one arytenoid may be removed when necessary. The vocal cords are preserved. The following findings contraindicate a partial laryngopharyngectomy: extension to the apex of the pyriform sinus, a fixed cord, extension to contralateral arytenoid, poor pulmonary function, and large, fixed lymph nodes.

Total Laryngopharyngectomy. A total laryngopharyngectomy removes the larynx and varying amounts of the pharyngeal wall. Advanced lesions require excision of nearly the entire circumference. The pharynx is reestablished by primary closure after a partial pharyngectomy; reconstruction is accomplished with a pectoralis major myocutaneous flap or a radial forearm free flap.

Postcricoid Pharynx

A total laryngopharyngectomy with reconstruction, generally using a pectoralis major myocutaneous flap or free flap, is performed. If the lesion extends into the cervical esophagus, a gastric pull-up or jejunal free flap may be necessary.

Irradiation Technique

Posterior Pharyngeal Wall

The RT technique is opposed lateral fields to include the primary lesion and the regional nodes. Because these lesions tend to "skip" areas, the entire posterior pharyngeal wall is included initially. If the lesion extends near the arytenoids, the postcricoid pharynx, pyriform sinuses, and upper cervical esophagus are included. The retropharyngeal nodes are included even if the neck is N0. When the field is reduced at 45 Gy to avoid the spinal cord, the posterior border of the portal is placed just anterior to the spinal cord.[312] The dose is 74.4 to 76.8 Gy, at 1.2 Gy per fraction twice daily, in a continuous course. Another option is 70 Gy in 35 fractions over 30 treatment days. IMRT is useful to reduce the dose to one or both parotids. Concomitant chemotherapy should be included for stage III through IV cancers.

Pyriform Sinus

Parallel-opposed lateral portals are used to encompass the primary lesion and regional nodes on both sides. The superior border is placed 2 cm above the tip of the mastoid to cover the most superior jugular chain and the retropharyngeal lymph nodes. The posterior border encompasses the level V nodes. Clinically positive nodes behind the plane of the spinal cord require an electron boost. The anterior border is usually placed about 0.5 to 1 cm behind the anterior skin edge if it is possible to do so and adequately encompass the tumor. The inferior border is 2 cm below the inferior border of the cricoid. The remaining lower neck lymph nodes are treated through an en face portal. The doses are the same as for the posterior pharyngeal wall. IMRT is an option if the tumor can be adequately encompassed while sparing the contralateral salivary gland(s) and/or to avoid a difficult low neck match.

Combined Treatment Policies

Posterior Pharyngeal Wall

An operation should usually precede RT when a combination is selected, unless a gastric pull-up is planned.

Pyriform Sinus

Following a total laryngopharyngectomy with or without neck dissection, RT is usually recommended for indications previously outlined. RT or chemoRT is used prior to operation for patients with a large fixed node. The dose to the primary tumor ranges from 45 to 50 Gy; the fixed node(s) is boosted to 60 to 75 Gy.

Management of Recurrence

Posterior Pharyngeal Wall

Recurrence after RT may be limited to the posterior pharyngeal wall and may be suitable for surgical excision, with occasional salvage. There is frequently a persistent ulcer after RT for advanced lesions; it should be considered evidence of persistent disease if it does not heal. Surgical excision is limited posteriorly by the prevertebral fascia. RT salvage of a surgical failure is unusual.

Pyriform Sinus

The hallmark of local recurrence after RT is persistent edema, pain, and fixation of laryngeal structures. A direct laryngoscopy is required, but the biopsy may be negative. A CT and/or PET scan is often helpful for distinguishing local recurrence from necrosis. It may be necessary to recommend a total laryngopharyngectomy for salvage without a positive biopsy.

Recurrence after a total laryngopharyngectomy is usually in the soft tissues of the neck, the untreated opposite neck, the base of tongue, or stoma. Surgical failures after a partial laryngopharyngectomy for early lesions may be salvaged by a total laryngopharyngectomy. Failures after a total laryngopharyngectomy are rarely salvaged.

RESULTS OF TREATMENT

Pharyngeal Wall

The 5-year local control rates and ultimate local control rates after RT at the University of Florida for 170 patients were for T1 (n = 14), 93% and 93%; for T2 (n = 51), 84% and 91%; for T3 (n = 75), 60% and 62%; and for T4 (n = 30), 44% and 44%, respectively.[312] The 5-year local–regional control and cause-specific survival rates were for stage I, 88% and 88%; for stage II, 85% and 89%; for stage III, 49% and 44%; and for stage IV, 44% and 35%, respectively.[312]

Pyriform Sinus

The results of treatment for 80 patients with carcinoma of the pyriform sinus treated at Washington University by preoperative RT followed by a partial laryngopharyngectomy are shown in Table 38.16.[313] Seventy patients had the equivalent of AJCC T1 lesions (disease limited to the pyriform sinus), 10 patients had disease extending beyond the pyriform sinus, and none had invasion of the apex of the pyriform sinus. The cause of death was cancer in 26%, complications of treatment in 14%, and intercurrent disease in 20%. The 5-year absolute survival was 25 of 66 patients (38%) (JE Marks, Personal communication, 1979).

The results of treatment for 57 patients from the same institution who were treated by preoperative RT followed by total laryngectomy and partial pharyngectomy are depicted in Table 38.16.[313] Thirty-five patients had lesions confined to the pyriform sinus (AJCC T1) and the remainder had extension beyond the pyriform sinus (AJCC T2 to T4). The cause of death was cancer in 56% of patients, complications of treatment in 11% of patients, and intercurrent disease in 18% of patients.

The 5-year local control rates for 123 patients treated with definitive RT for T1 (23 patients) and T2 (100 patients) pyriform sinus SCCs were for T1, 85%; and for T2, 85%, respectively.[311] The 5-year rates of local–regional control and cause-specific survival were for stage I to II, 86% and 85%; for stage III, 65% and 73%; for stage IVA, 83% and 62%; and for stage IVB, 24% and 22%, respectively.[311] The 5-year distant metastasis-free survival rates were for N0, 96%; for N1, 88%; for N2, 68%; and for N3, 55%.

COMPLICATIONS OF TREATMENT

Posterior Pharyngeal Wall

Surgical Treatment Complications

Marks and coworkers[314] reported a 14% operative mortality plus major complications including pharyngocutaneous fistula (31%) and carotid rupture (14%) for patients treated with preoperative RT, 25 to 30 Gy.

Radiation Therapy Complications

Mendenhall and coworkers[312] observed 9 fatal complications (5%) in 170 patients who were treated at the University of Florida. Twenty-five patients (15%) experienced nonfatal severe complications including permanent feeding tube (17 patients), soft tissue and/or bone necrosis (7 patients), and permanent tracheostomy (1 patient).

Pyriform Sinus

Surgical Treatment Complications

The complications of a partial laryngopharyngectomy included a 12% operative mortality, fistula, aspiration, and dysphagia.[313] The complications of total laryngopharyngectomy included a treatment-related mortality of 11%, fistula, and pharyngeal stenosis.[313] The complication rate is increased by the addition of RT.

Radiation Therapy Complications

The major RT complication is laryngeal necrosis. Rabbani et al.[311] reported the following rates of moderate-to-severe complications in 123 patients: acute (2%); late (9%); and postoperative (5%).

Complications of Salvage Treatment

Attempted surgical salvage of RT failures has a significant operative morbidity and mortality; few patients are cured.

NASOPHARYNX

NPCs are uncommon in the United States. The Chinese have a high frequency; American-born second-generation Chinese maintain the risk of NPC. NPCs have been shown to have an association with elevated titers of EBV, which is independent of geography.[315] There is a 3 to 1 ratio of predominance in men. The age distribution for NPC is younger than for other head and neck sites; about 20% of patients are younger than 30 years of age.

ANATOMY

The nasopharynx is roughly cuboidal in shape. It is contiguous with the nasal cavity, inferiorly with the oropharynx, and laterally with the middle ears by way of the eustachian tubes.

The mucosa of the roof and posterior wall is often irregular because of the pharyngeal bursa, adenoids, and pharyngeal hypophysis; it tends to become smooth with age.

TABLE 38.16

Carcinoma of the Pyriform Sinus: Results of Treatment by Low Dose Radiation Therapy Plus Partial Laryngopharyngectomy or Total Laryngectomy and Partial Pharyngectomy (Washington University, St. Louis, 1964–1974)

Result	PLP (80 Patients)[a]	TLP (57 Patients)[b]
Local recurrence ± neck recurrence	14%[c]	14%
Neck recurrence ± distant metastases (primary controlled)	9%	23%
Distant metastases alone	11%	21%
5-year actuarial survival (no evidence of disease)	40%	22%

[a] T1, 70 patients; T2–T4, 10 patients (AJCC staging).
[b] T1, 35 patients; T2–T4, 22 patients (AJCC staging).
[c] Four patients salvaged.
PLP, partial laryngopharyngectomy; TLP, total laryngopharyngectomy.
Data from Marks JE, Kurnick B, Powers WE, Ogura JH. Carcinoma of the pyriform sinus: an analysis of treatment results and patterns of failure. *Cancer* 1978;41:1008–1015.

The lateral walls include the eustachian tube openings with the fossa of Rosenmüller, located behind the torus tubarius. The superolateral muscular wall of the nasopharynx is incomplete. The floor of the nasopharynx is incomplete and consists of the upper surface of the soft palate.

Lymphatics

There is an extensive submucosal lymphatic capillary plexus. The tumor spreads along three different pathways: the jugular chain, the spinal accessory chain, and the retropharyngeal pathway.[316] The lateral retropharyngeal nodes lie in the retropharyngeal space medial to the carotid artery. Directly behind the nodes are the lateral masses of C1 and C2. Inconstant lymphatic vessels may drain directly to the level III and V nodes.[13]

PATHOLOGY

Carcinomas compose about 85% and lymphomas about 10% of the malignant lesions. NPCs are classified as follows: keratinizing squamous cell carcinoma (WHO type I); nonkeratinizing carcinoma (WHO type II), and undifferentiated (WHO type III) basaloid SCC. Lymphoepithelioma is included in the WHO type II and III categories. A miscellaneous group of malignant tumors includes melanoma, plasmacytoma,[270] juvenile angiofibroma,[14] carcinosarcoma, sarcomas, nonchromaffin paragangliomas, and minor salivary gland tumors.

PATTERNS OF SPREAD

Primary

Inferior extension along the lateral pharyngeal walls and tonsillar pillars occurs in almost one third of patients. Extension into the posterior nasal cavity is frequent but is usually limited to less than 1 cm. Invasion of the posterior ethmoids, maxillary antrum, and/or orbit occurs fairly often. Skull base invasion is recognized radiographically in at least 25% of patients. The sphenoid sinus frequently is invaded. The tumor may erode through the foramen ovale, lacerum, and/or spinosum. The tumor eventually reaches the cavernous sinus and has access to CNs II to VI.

The lateral muscular wall of the nasopharynx is incomplete superiorly. The defect, termed the sinus of Morgagni, is transversed by the cartilaginous eustachian tube and the levator palatine muscle, providing access for NPCs to the lateral pharyngeal space and skull base.

Lymphatics

There is an 80% to 90% incidence of metastatic neck nodes on presentation; approximately 50% are bilateral. Low-grade SCCs produce fewer metastases (73%) than high-grade carcinomas (92%). Metastases to submental and occipital nodes may appear when there is blockage of the common lymphatic pathways either by massive neck disease or by an untimely neck dissection.

CLINICAL PICTURE

The most common presenting complaint is a painless upper neck mass. Nasal obstruction, epistaxis, sore throat, and otitis media may be observed. Facial pain may be referred from any of the three divisions of the trigeminal nerve, usually V3. Occipital or temporal headaches frequently are seen. Proptosis occurs with posterior orbital invasion. Trismus is due to the invasion of the pterygoid region.

Neurologic symptoms and signs occur in about 25% of patients. Involvement of CNs II to VI indicates extension into the cavernous sinus. CNs IX to XII and the sympathetic chain are involved in the lateral pharyngeal space.

An examination of the nasopharynx will show a lesion on the lateral wall or roof. Early lesions may be submucosal. Lymphomas tend to remain submucosal until quite large. The tumor infrequently grows very far down the posterior pharyngeal wall. The posterior tonsillar pillars may bulge into the oropharynx if an enlarged node develops in the lateral pharyngeal space. CN VI is the one most commonly involved.

STAGING

The AJCC staging system is depicted in Table 38.17.

TREATMENT

Selection of Treatment Modality

The treatment of almost all NPCs is RT-based because complete surgical resection is usually not feasible. Neck dissection is used less often in the management of neck disease because of the relatively high success rate with RT or chemoRT alone. A small adenocarcinoma or sarcoma may be excised. Juvenile angiofibromas are preferably excised because of the young age of the patient, although the tumors are quite successfully cured by RT when a complete resection is unlikely or dangerous.[14] Patients with advanced disease should receive concomitant chemotherapy.[190,192,201,317,318]

Irradiation Technique

If the tumor is thought to be limited to the nasopharynx or to have minimal soft-tissue extension, the following areas are included in the treatment volume: (1) the nasopharynx, (2) the posterior 2 cm of the nasal cavity, (3) the posterior ethmoid sinuses, (4) the entire sphenoid sinus and basioccipital bone, (5) the cavernous sinus, (6) the base of skull (7 to 8 cm width encompassing the foramen ovale, carotid canal, and foramen spinosum laterally), (7) the pterygoid fossae, (8) the posterior one third of the maxillary sinus, (9) the oropharyngeal wall to the level of the mid tonsillar fossa, (10) the retropharyngeal nodes, and (11) the neck nodes on both sides.

Extension to the skull base or involvement of CNs II to VI requires the superior border be raised to include the entire pituitary, the base of the brain in the suprasellar area, the adjacent middle cranial fossa, and the posterior portion of the anterior cranial fossa. Patients with anterior invasion into the orbit, ethmoids, or maxillary sinus require an individualized plan to produce a satisfactory dose distribution. The use of 3-dimensional CT-based treatment planning allows for the use of more conformal fields. IMRT is useful to improve coverage of the poststyloid parapharyngeal space and to reduce the dose to the parotid glands and the temporal lobes to reduce long-term morbidity. We currently treat patients to 74.4 at 1.2 Gy per fraction twice daily.

Neck Nodes. The entire neck is irradiated to the level of the clavicles. The retropharyngeal nodes are included in the treatment of the primary lesion. The upper neck nodes are included in the primary fields to the level of the thyroid notch. In the case of an N0 neck, the posterior margin is placed about 1 to 2 cm behind the posterior border of the sternocleidomastoid to encompass the high level V nodes and level 2 nodes. The portals are extended to include the submental area only if there is disease in the level IB nodes or if the patient had a neck dissection prior to RT. The lower neck is treated through an anterior portal with a shield over the larynx.

2010 American Joint Committee on Cancer Staging for Nasopharyngeal Cancer

Primary Tumor (T)

T1	Tumor confined to the nasopharynx, or tumor extends to oropharynx and/or nasal cavity without parapharyngeal extension[a]
T2	Tumor with parapharyngeal extension[a]
T3	Tumor involves bony structures of skull base and/or paranasal sinuses
T4	Tumor with intracranial extension and/or involvement of cranial nerves, hypopharynx, orbit, or with extension to the infratemporal fossa/masticator space

[a] Parapharyngeal extension denotes posterolateral infiltration of tumor.
Used with the permission of the American Joint Committee on Cancer (AJCC), Chicago, Illinois. The original source for this material is the *AJCC Cancer Staging Handbook,* Seventh Edition (2010) published by Springer Science and Business Media LLC, www.springerlink.com.

Regional Lymph Nodes (N)

NX	Regional lymph nodes cannot be assessed
N0	No regional lymph node metastasis
N1	Unilateral metastasis in lymph node(s), 6 cm or less in greatest dimension, above the supraclavicular fossa and/or unilateral or bilateral, retropharyngeal lymph nodes, 6 cm or less, in greatest dimension[a]
N2	Bilateral metastasis in cervical lymph node(s), 6 cm or less in greatest dimension, above the supraclavicular fossa[a]
N3	Metastasis in a lymph node(s),[a] >6 cm and/or to supraclavicular fossa
N3a	Greater than 6 cm in dimension
N3b	Extension to the supraclavicular fossa[b]

[a] Midline nodes are considered ipsilateral nodes.
[b] Supraclavicular zone or fossa is relevant to the staging of nasopharyngeal carcinoma and is the triangular region originally described by Ho. It is defined by three points: (1) the superior margin of the sternal end of the clavicle, (2) the superior margin of the lateral end of the clavicle, and (3) the point where the neck meets the shoulder. Note that this would include caudal portions of levels IV and VB. All cases with lymph nodes (whole or part) in the fossa are considered N3b.
Used with the permission of the American Joint Committee on Cancer (AJCC), Chicago, Illinois. The original source for this material is the *AJCC Cancer Staging Handbook*, Seventh Edition (2010) published by Springer Science and Business Media LLC, www.springerlink.com.

Stage Grouping

0	Tis	N0	M0
I	T1	N0	M0
II	T1	N1	M0
	T2	N0	M0
	T2	N1	M0
III	T1	N2	M0
	T2	N2	M0
	T3	N0	M0
	T3	N1	M0
	T3	N2	M0
IVA	T4	N0	M0
	T4	N1	M0
	T4	N2	M0
IVB	Any T	N3	M0
IVC	Any T	Any N	M1

Used with the permission of the American Joint Committee on Cancer (AJCC), Chicago, Illinois. The original source for this material is the *AJCC Cancer Staging Handbook*, Seventh Edition (2010) published by Springer Science and Business Media LLC, www.springerlink.com.

Acute Sequelae. A sore throat begins at the end of the second week of therapy and persists for 2 to 3 months after the completion of RT. A xerostomia is always present. Loss of taste and appetite is often profound; both return 1 to 6 months after completion of RT. Obstruction of the eustachian tubes may occur with secondary otitis media and hearing loss. Polyethylene tubes inserted through the eardrums to drain the middle ears can correct this condition. The obstruction often improves after a few months. Severe nausea and vomiting are uncommon.

Management of Recurrence

The majority of recurrent SCCs are diagnosed within 2 years, but lymphoepithelioma may recur many years after treatment. Headache and CN palsies usually indicate recurrence. Retreatment for local recurrences with limited RT portals and/or intracavitary brachytherapy may be rewarding, particularly if the recurrence is due to a marginal miss or low dose.[319,320]

Results of Treatment

Lee and co-workers[321] reported the following 10-year outcomes in a series of 5,037 patients treated with RT at the Queen Elizabeth Hospital, Hong Kong, between 1976 and 1985: local control, 61%; regional control, 64%; distant metastasis-free survival, 59%; and survival, 42%. Leung et al.[322] reported the following 5-year local control rates in a series of 1,070 patients: T1, 88%; T2A, 87%; T2B, 82%; T3, 69%; and T4, 69%. Chua et al.[323] evaluated 290 patients and found that primary tumor volume of more than 60 mL was associated with a lower likelihood of local control after RT. Teo and colleagues[324] evaluated a series of 903 patients treated at the Prince of Wales Hospital, Hong Kong, and observed that local control was adversely affected by advanced patient age, skull base invasion, and CN involvement. Prognostic factors associated with an increased rate of distant metastases and poor survival were male sex, skull base and CN(s) involvement, advanced neck stage, nodal fixation, and bilateral neck nodes.[324] The 5-year outcomes for 82 patients treated at the University of Florida were for local control, 78%; for regional control, 90%; for local–regional control, 76%; for distant metastasis-free survival, 80%; for cause-specific survival, 66%; and for survival, 57%.[325] Table 38.9 summarizes the results of selected randomized trials comparing chemoRT versus RT alone.

Follow-Up

The follow-up includes careful observation and laboratory testing for possible thyroid and/or pituitary hypofunction. Dental care must be closely monitored because of xerostomia.

Complications of Treatment

Primary or secondary hypopituitarism (from a hypothalamic lesion) has been reported. Brain necrosis is rare. Hypothyroidism may result from either a direct effect on the thyroid gland or an indirect effect on the pituitary. A transient CNS syndrome may appear 2 to 3 months after RT and would require several months to resolve. General weakness and extreme fatigue may be symptoms of low serum cortisol levels. Radiation myelitis of the cervical cord or brain stem is the most severe CNS complication. IMRT may be used to reduce the dose to the CNS, particularly the temporal lobes.

Trismus may occur because of fibrosis of the pterygoid muscles. Palsy of CNs IX to XII may occur several years after RT and is related to nerve entrapment in the lateral pharyngeal space. Eye complications (e.g., retrobulbar optic neuritis) may develop owing to RT of the optic nerve.[326] RT of the posterior eyeball to high doses may produce a retinopathy.[327]

NASAL VESTIBULE, NASAL CAVITY, AND PARANASAL SINUSES

Tumors of the nasal vestibule are considered separately from nasal cavity tumors because they are essentially skin cancers and have a different natural history. Primary tumors arising from the nasal cavity and paranasal sinuses are considered together because the lesions are frequently advanced when first seen and it is not always possible to determine the site of origin.

Cancer of the nasal cavity or paranasal sinuses is a relatively rare problem, with a yearly risk factor estimated at approximately one case for every 100,000 people. They occur more often in men and usually appear after the age of 40 except for minor salivary gland tumors and esthesioneuroblastomas, which may appear before the age of 20.[328] Nasal cavity and ethmoid sinus adenocarcinomas have been linked to occupations associated with wood dust, such as the furniture industry, sawmill work, and carpentry. Other occupations with dust-filled work environments, such as shoe making, baking, and the flour milling industry, also have been implicated.[72]

Carcinomas of the sphenoid and frontal sinuses are rare.

Anatomy

The nasal vestibule is the entrance to the nasal cavity. It is lined by skin in which there are numerous hair follicles and sebaceous glands. The vestibule is a three-sided, pear-shaped cavity about 1.5 cm in diameter that ends posteriorly at the limen nasi. The alar cartilages form the anterolateral wall. The medial wall is the columella, formed by the medial wing of the alar cartilage and the anterior portion of the cartilaginous septum. The floor is the maxilla.

The nasal cavity begins at the limen nasi and ends at the posterior nares, where it communicates with the nasopharynx. The lateral walls are composed of thin bony folds that project into the nasal cavity: the inferior, medial, and superior turbinates. The nasolacrimal duct enters the nasal cavity beneath the inferior turbinate. The frontal sinus and ethmoid bullae connect to the nasal cavity with openings that lie under the middle turbinate. The sphenoid sinus communicates with the nasal cavity by an opening on the anterior wall of the sinus. Approximately 20 branches of the olfactory nerves enter the nasal cavity through the cribriform plate; nerve fibers are distributed over the upper one third of the septum and the superior nasal turbinate. The epithelium is nonciliated columnar. The lower half of the nasal cavity is the respiratory portion, and the epithelium is ciliated columnar. There are numerous collections of lymphoid tissue and mucous glands beneath the epithelium.

The maxillary sinuses are single pyramidal cavities. The medial wall is the lateral wall of the nasal cavity and has one or two openings communicating with the middle meatus under the medial turbinate. The inferior wall is the hard palate. The posterolateral wall is related to the zygomatic process and the pterygomaxillary space. The superior wall is the orbital floor.

The frontal sinuses are two irregular, asymmetrical air cavities separated by a thin bony septum. They connect to the middle meatus of the nasal cavity by the frontonasal duct. They are separated from the anterior ethmoid cells by thin bony walls. The posterior wall separating the frontal sinus from the anterior cranial fossa is relatively thick.

The ethmoid sinuses consist of a number of air cells lying between the medial walls of the orbits and the lateral wall of the nasal cavity. The lateral wall is the thin porous lamina papyracea. Medially, the ethmoid air cells bulge into the lateral wall of the nasal cavity. The ethmoid cells communicate with the nasal cavity in the middle meatus. These bony walls are thin and easily traversed by the tumor. The ethmoid air cells extend far anteriorly; the lacrimal bone covers the anterior cells laterally. The midline perpendicular plate of the ethmoid separates the right and left ethmoid cells anatomically. There is no anatomic barrier between the anterior, middle, and posterior ethmoids.

The sphenoid sinus is a midline structure in the body of the sphenoid bone. The pituitary lies above, the cavernous sinuses laterally, the nasal cavity and ethmoid sinuses in front, and the nasopharynx beneath. The clivus and brain stem lie posteriorly. The pneumatization is variable and can extend into all portions of the sphenoid bone. The right and left sinuses are partially separated by an incomplete septum. The sphenoid sinus connects anteriorly with the nasal cavity in the sphenoethmoidal recess.

Lymphatics

Nasal Vestibule. The lymphatic trunks run to the level IB nodes. There is a small risk for involvement of the intercalated facial nodes just behind the commissure of the lip along the course of the facial neurovascular bundle.

Nasal Cavity and Paranasal Sinuses. The lymphatics of the nasal cavity are separated into the olfactory group and the respiratory group. According to Rouvière,[13] they do not communicate with each other. There is a connection between the lymphatic network of the olfactory region and the subarachnoid spaces, which allows some absorption of cerebrospinal fluid (CSF) into the lymphatic system. The lymphatics of the olfactory region of the nasal cavity run posteriorly to terminate in lymph nodes alongside the jugular vein at the skull base in the lateral pharyngeal space. The lymphatics of the respiratory nasal cavity terminate in the lateral retropharyngeal nodes or the level II nodes. The capillary lymphatic plexus of the nasal mucosa is probably not very profuse, judged by the relatively low incidence of metastatic nodes.

The mucosa of the paranasal sinuses has either no or very sparse capillary lymphatics.

Pathology

Benign Tumors

Inflammatory polyps, giant cell reparative granulomas, benign odontogenic tumors, and necrotizing sialometaplasia may appear in this area. Inverted papilloma is a benign, aggressive neoplasm that is associated with carcinoma in 5% to 15% of cases.[329]

Malignant Tumors

Nasal Vestibule. Almost all malignant tumors are SCCs; basal cell carcinomas and adnexal carcinomas are also reported.

Nasal Cavity and Paranasal Sinuses. SCC or one of its variants is the most common neoplasm. Minor salivary gland tumors account for about 10% to 15% of neoplasms in this region. Lymphoma and melanoma account for approximately 5% and 1% of cases, respectively. Esthesioneuroblastoma is a neuroendocrine carcinoma that originates from the olfactory mucosa. Sinonasal undifferentiated carcinoma—a more aggressive neuroendocrine malignancy—is sometimes encountered.[330] Soft tissue and bone sarcomas may occur in the nasal cavity and paranasal sinuses, including chondrosarcoma, osteosarcoma, and Ewing sarcoma.[331]

Midline lethal granuloma is a nonkiller (NK) nasal T-cell lymphoma. Unchecked, the disease is fatal. Death results from extension to the CNS, hemorrhage, sepsis, or inanition. Treatment is usually RT, which is often combined with chemotherapy.[332]

Patterns of Spread

Nasal Vestibule

Primary. Lesions of the nasal vestibule invade the alar and septal cartilages and may extend to the nasal skin. The upper lip is frequently invaded. Posterior growth into the nasal cavity is frequent.

Early cancers originating on the columella and anterior septum are often superficial lesions that ulcerate and produce a crust or scab and often present with septal perforation.

Lymphatic. Lymph node spread is usually to a solitary ipsilateral level IB node, but may be bilateral. The facial, preauricular, and submental nodes are at small risk. Wallace et al.[333] reported only 4 of 79 patients (5%) with clinically positive lymph nodes at diagnosis, but 9 patients (11%) later developed positive lymph nodes.

Nasal Cavity and Paranasal Sinuses

Nasal Cavity. The routes of spread are essentially the same for various histologies, with the exception of esthesioneuroblastoma and minor salivary gland tumors. The latter have a greater propensity for PNI.

Lesions arising in the olfactory region invade the ethmoids and the orbit, spread through the cribriform plate to the anterior cranial fossa, and spread between bone and dura. Eventually, they penetrate the dura and invade the frontal lobes. These lesions also tend to destroy the septum and may invade through the nasal bone to the skin. Lesions arising on the lateral wall of the nasal cavity invade the maxillary sinus, ethmoids, and orbit.

Esthesioneuroblastomas may show submucosal spread and may grow along olfactory nerves and penetrate through an intact dura to the frontal lobes.

The nasopharynx and sphenoid sinus are secondarily invaded in advanced lesions. The tumor may follow nerves posteriorly and superiorly toward the sphenopalatine ganglion near the skull base or along V2.

Maxillary Sinus. All walls of the sinus may be penetrated by the tumor; the pattern of spread and bone destruction is dependent on the site of origin within the sinus. Lesions arising in the anterolateral infrastructure tend to invade through the lateral inferior wall or grow through dental sockets, causing loosening of the teeth or improper seating of a denture. Ulceration follows, with the development of an oral–antral fistula. Lesions arising on the medial infrastructure readily extend into the nasal cavity.

Posterior infrastructure lesions erode through the posterolateral wall and into the infratemporal fossa and extend superiorly to the skull base. Orbital extension occurs either through the roof of the maxillary sinus, through the ethmoids and lamina papyracea, or by way of the infratemporal fossa and then through the infraorbital fissure.

Tumors arising in the suprastructure of the antrum have two general patterns of development. One group extends laterally, invades the malar bone, and produces a mass below the lateral floor of the orbit that may ulcerate through to the skin. The orbit is invaded laterally and displaces the eye superomedially. The temporal fossa is often involved, as is the zygomatic bone in advanced lesions. Suprastructure cancers that extend medially invade the nasal cavity, the ethmoid and frontal sinuses, the lacrimal apparatus, and the medial inferior orbit.

Ethmoid Sinuses. Depending on the location of the tumor, it may invade the medial orbit through the lamina papyracea, the inner canthus, and the nasal cavity. More advanced lesions invade the maxillary antrum, the nasopharynx, the sphenoid sinus, and the anterior cranial fossa.

Sphenoid Sinus. The sphenoid sinus is closely related to the CNs in the cavernous sinus: III, IV, V1, V2, and VI (Fig. 38.2). CN palsies and headaches are frequently the first clinical evidence of a sphenoid sinus tumor. A diagnosis is usually made, however, when the tumor eventually breaks through into the nasopharynx or nasal cavity where it can be seen.

Inverted Papilloma. A report of 223 cases of inverted papillomas showed the lateral nasal wall was the most commonly involved site (68%), with ethmoid and maxillary sinus involvement also being

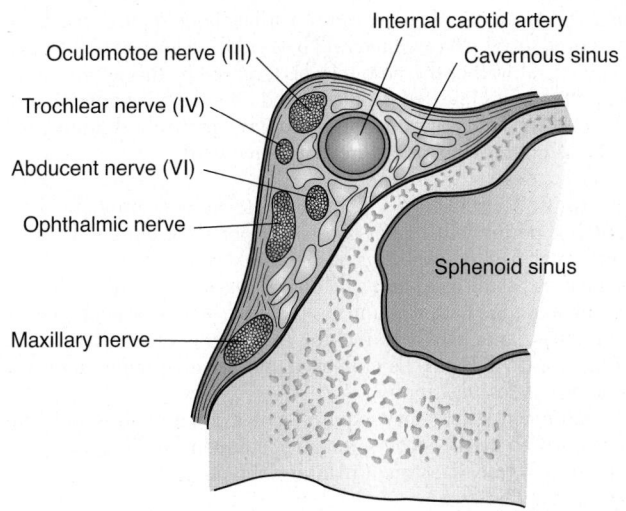

Figure 38.2 Coronal section of the cavernous sinus. (Mendenhall WM, Million RR, Mancuso AA, Stringer SP. Nasopharynx. In: Million RR, Cassisi, eds. *Management of Head and Neck Cancer: A Multidisciplinary Approach,* 2nd ed. Philadelphia: J. B. Lippincott; 1994: 606, Fig. 23-10).

common (57%), as was involvement of the septum (28%). However, ethmoid and maxillary sinus involvement without a tumor of the lateral nasal wall occurred in 4%. Intracranial extension was usually associated with a carcinoma. The tumor occurred bilaterally when there was spread through the nasal septum; multicentric sites of origin were observed.[334]

Lymphatic. The incidence of lymphatic metastases at diagnosis is 10% to 15% for nasal cavity and ethmoid sinus SCCs and probably lower for antral and sphenoid tumors. Maxillary sinus tumors that invade the oral cavity and involve the buccal mucosa, maxillary gingiva, or hard palate may spread to the level IB and level II nodes. Lesions that invade the nasal cavity or nasopharynx spread posteriorly to the parapharyngeal nodes and then to the level II nodes. The risk of cervical node involvement for esthesioneuroblastoma is approximately 20%.[328]

Clinical Picture

Nasal Vestibule

These lesions present with symptoms of a slow-growing mass with attendant crusting and occasional, minor bleeding. Septal perforation may occur.

Nasal Cavity and Paranasal Sinuses

Nasal Cavity. The earliest symptoms are a low-grade chronic infection with discharge, obstruction, and minor, intermittent bleeding. Lesions arising in the olfactory region may cause unilateral or bilateral nasal expansion of the bridge of the nose; a mass may appear near the inner canthus and eventually ulcerate. Obstruction of the nasolacrimal system may be a presenting complaint. Extension through the cribriform plate or into the ethmoid sinuses is accompanied by a frontal headache. The aberration of smell is rare. Invasion of the medial orbit produces proptosis and diplopia; a mass may be palpated in the orbit.

Maxillary Sinus. These cancers develop silently when they are confined to the sinus and produce symptoms after extension through the walls. If the tumor invades toward the oral cavity, the presenting symptoms include pain and loosening or loss of teeth. Palpation

and observation of the face may show a mass. A posterior invasion of the orbit will produce proptosis, diplopia, and conjunctival edema. Invasion of V2 in the floor of the orbit may cause paresthesia. Nasal obstruction and bleeding are common, and trismus and headaches are associated with invasion posteriorly into the pterygopalatine fossa, pterygoid muscles, infratemporal fossa, and skull base.

Cancers developing in the medial suprastructure of the antrum present with nasal symptoms of discharge or bleeding, mild infraorbital pain, an infected lacrimal sac, and displacement of the eye superolaterally with proptosis, diplopia, and conjunctival edema.

Cancer developing in the lateral suprastructure produces a mass below the lateral canthus with associated pain. The eye may be deviated medially and upward when orbital invasion occurs, producing diplopia and proptosis. The tumor may extend to the temporal fossa, producing a diffuse fullness.

Ethmoid Sinuses. Mild-to-moderate sinus pain referred to the frontal-nasal area is an early symptom. A painless mass may present near the inner canthus. Diplopia and proptosis develop with invasion of the medial orbit. Nasal discharge, epistaxis, and obstruction are frequent. Paresthesia may occur over the distribution of sensory nerves.

Staging

The AJCC staging system for the nasal cavity and paranasal sinuses is depicted in Table 38.18. Nasal vestibule tumors are staged according to the AJCC staging system for skin cancers.

Treatment

Selection of Treatment Modality

Nasal Vestibule. RT is usually the preferred treatment because of the deformity produced by excision.[333] Surgery alone is preferred for the occasional very small lesion, the removal of which will not produce cosmetic deformity or require reconstruction. A subset of patients best treated by surgery and adjuvant RT or chemoRT are those with invasion of the premaxilla.

Surgical Treatment. Excision of lesions in the nasal vestibule usually involves removal of cartilage as well as skin. Depending on the site of the lesion, the columella, the septum, or the alar cartilages will have to be removed, with a resulting cosmetic deformity that is difficult to reconstruct. If the alar cartilage has been sacrificed, either a composite graft consisting of skin and cartilage from the ear or a nasolabial flap can be used to repair the defect. If the entire external nose is resected, a prosthesis is used.

Irradiation Technique. EBRT, brachytherapy, or a combination of both may be used. EBRT is usually administered with a single anterior portal technique, which uses a combination of photons and electrons; a wax bolus ensures a homogenous dose. The dose ranges from 66 to 70 Gy at 2 Gy per fraction, once daily in a continuous course.

Interstitial brachytherapy of the nasal vestibule and nasal cavity is highly individualized and employs afterloaded ^{192}Ir needles. The implant is usually composed of two, three, or four planes of sources inserted perpendicularly through the skin surface of the external nose with crossing needles placed in the dorsum of the nose, the floor of the nasal cavity, and the upper lip. The dose varies depending on the size of the lesion.[333]

Inverted Papilloma. An inverted papilloma is treated initially by surgery. Depending on the procedure, the local recurrence rate may be fairly high, and subsequent excisions may be required. When the lesion begins to act aggressively with rapid recurrences and invasion of the sinuses, orbit, and anterior cranial fossa, it

TABLE 38.18

2010 American Joint Committee on Cancer Staging System for Nasal Cavity and Paranasal Sinus Cancers

Maxillary Sinus

TX	Primary tumor cannot be assessed
T0	No evidence of primary tumor
Tis	Carcinoma in situ
T1	Tumor limited to the maxillary sinus mucosa with no erosion or destruction of bone
T2	Tumor causing bone erosion or destruction including extension into the hard palate and/or middle nasal meatus, except extension to posterior wall of maxillary sinus and pterygoid plates
T3	Tumor invades any of the following: bone of the posterior wall of maxillary sinus, subcutaneous tissues, floor or medial wall of orbit, pterygoid fossa, ethmoid sinuses
T4a	Tumor invades anterior orbital contents, skin of cheek, pterygoid plates, infratemporal fossa, cribriform plate, sphenoid or frontal sinuses
T4b	Tumor invades any of the following: orbital apex, dura, brain, middle cranial fossa, cranial nerves other than maxillary division of trigeminal nerve (V2), nasopharynx, or clivus

Nasal Cavity and Ethmoid Sinus

TX	Primary tumor cannot be assessed
T0	No evidence of primary tumor
Tis	Carcinoma in situ
T1	Tumor restricted to any one subsite, with or without bony invasion
T2	Tumor invading two subsites in a single region or extending to involve an adjacent region within the nasoethmoid complex, with or without bony invasion
T3	Tumor extends to invade the medial wall or floor of the orbit, maxillary sinus, palate, or cribriform plate
T4a	Tumor invades any of the following: anterior orbital contents, skin of nose or cheek, minimal extension to anterior cranial fossa, pterygoid plates, sphenoid or frontal sinuses
T4b	Tumor invades any of the following: orbital apex, dura, brain, middle cranial fossa, cranial nerves other than V2, nasopharynx, or clivus

Used with the permission of the American Joint Committee on Cancer (AJCC), Chicago, Illinois. The original source for this material is the *AJCC Cancer Staging Handbook*, Seventh Edition (2010) published by Springer Science and Business Media LLC, www.springerlink.com.

should be considered a low-grade cancer and treated by a more radical removal. RT is recommended for lesions that are incompletely resected, for multiple recurrences, and for those in whom carcinoma is found.[329]

Nasal Cavity. Surgery is the preferred treatment if a gross total resection is likely; postoperative RT or chemoRT is usually indicated.[335] Definitive RT is used for incompletely resectable tumors.

Surgical Treatment. A lateral rhinotomy provides the best access for resection of lesions of the nasal cavity. Generally, reconstruction

is not necessary unless the entire cartilaginous septum has been removed, in which case there will be a saddle deformity of the nose. The lateral wall of the nose may be removed by this approach for resection of an inverted papilloma and other localized neoplasms. More advanced lesions require the removal of involved sinuses and orbit. A craniofacial procedure may be required.

Irradiation Technique. The EBRT technique emphasizes an anterior portal with one or two lateral portals. Contiguous structures such as the maxillary sinus, ethmoid sinus, medial orbit, nasopharynx, skull base, and sphenoid sinus are generally included in the initial treatment volume as required. The treatment volume is reduced after 50 Gy to include the original gross disease with a margin. IMRT may be employed and usually produces a more conformal dose distribution.

Advanced lesions may require inclusion of an entire orbit and loss of vision usually occurs, but an operation would require visual loss in any case. Treatment planning should protect the opposite eye and optic nerve.

Combined Treatment Policies

If a combined treatment is planned, we prefer surgery first. RT or chemoRT is started 4 to 6 weeks afterward. The dose is usually 60 to 65 Gy for clear margins; patients with positive margins or for a gross residual tumor after operation receive 74.4 Gy at 1.2 Gy per twice-daily fraction.

Management of Recurrence

Once the patient has had surgery or RT, it is difficult to determine the extent of recurrent disease because of changes from the previous therapy. The most common situation for salvage is RT or surgical failure that can be treated successfully by a craniofacial resection. Tumor extension to the sphenopalatine fossa with definite destruction of a pterygoid plate is a relative contraindication to craniofacial resection. CN involvement, posterior invasion near the optic chiasm, and sphenoid sinus or cavernous sinus invasion are contraindications to resection. An MRI can distinguish between exudate and a gross tumor in a sinus. The anterior wall of the sphenoid sinus may be removed, but the sinus itself cannot be completely resected. Postoperative RT should be considered whether or not margins are positive.

Maxillary Sinus

Selection of Treatment Modality. Surgery gives the best results. Early infrastructure lesions may be cured by surgery alone, but, for most other cases, RT is given postoperatively even if margins are negative. ChemoRT should be considered for a positive margin. The extension of cancer to the skull base, nasopharynx, or sphenoid sinus contraindicates excision. The pterygoid process below the foramen rotundum may be removed along with the attached pterygoid muscles, but destruction of the sphenoid bone above this point is a contraindication to operation. Procedures to resect portions of the skull base are described for special situations.

Surgical Treatment. Surgery for maxillary sinus carcinoma depends on which walls are involved. If the floor of the orbit is free of disease, then the eye and orbital rim may be left undisturbed. If, however, there is involvement through the orbital floor, then a maxillectomy with resection of the floor with or without an orbital exenteration must be performed. If the posterior wall or the pterygoid plates are involved, they too must be included in the resection. A split-thickness skin graft is used to line the cavity, and a removable dental prosthesis is then used to fill the resulting deformity in the palate. An interim prosthesis is constructed prior to surgery so it can be placed at the time of operation and act as a stent. The permanent prosthesis is constructed about 6 months after the operation.

Irradiation Technique. RT treatment planning includes the entire maxilla, the adjacent nasal cavity, the ethmoid sinus, the nasopharynx, and the pterygopalatine fossa. All or part of the orbit is included in patients with extension into or near the orbit. Target volume definition is aided by the use of treatment planning CT combined with image-fusion MRI. The prescribed dose is 74.4 Gy at 1.2 Gy per fraction twice daily for RT alone. The dose for preoperative RT varies from 50 to 60 Gy, and the dose for postoperative RT varies from 60 to 74.4 Gy.

Ethmoid Sinus

Selection of Treatment Modality. Surgery is preferred if a gross total resection is likely. Postoperative RT or chemoRT is usually indicated. Unresectable tumors are treated with chemoRT.

Surgical Treatment. Localized lesions require resection of the ethmoids with or without the ipsilateral maxilla and/or orbit. Extensive lesions require a craniofacial procedure. Endoscopic resection of selected malignant tumors involving the nasal cavity, ethmoid sinuses, and anterior skull base is being performed with increasing frequency with promising outcomes.

Irradiation Technique. RT treatment is entirely by EBRT, emphasizing treatment through an anterior field combined with one or two lateral fields. This field arrangement, weighted 2:1 or 3:1 in favor of the anterior field, provides adequate treatment of the tumor volume while avoiding excessive RT to the contralateral eye and optic nerve. Wedges are added to achieve a satisfactory dose distribution. Electrons should not be used for the anterior portal. IMRT should be considered because a more conformal dose distribution can usually be achieved.

Management of Recurrence. Recurrent disease is heralded by recurrent pain and CN palsies. Localized recurrence after surgery only may be managed by chemoRT or craniofacial resection and postoperative RT or chemoRT. RT failures may be suitable for maxillectomy or craniofacial resection.

Sphenoid Sinus

The treatment is with RT, and the technique is similar to that used for advanced NPC.

Results of Treatment

Nasal Vestibule

Goepfert and coworkers[336] reviewed the M.D. Anderson Cancer Center experience of 26 patients with nasal vestibule SCCs. The absolute 5-year survival was 78%. Ten patients were treated initially by surgery; one developed a local recurrence and was salvaged by RT. Sixteen patients were treated by RT; three developed local recurrence, and two were salvaged by an operation.

Wallace et al.[333] reviewed 71 patients treated by RT at the University of Florida for SCC of the nasal vestibule. The 5-year local control and cause-specific survival rates were for T1 to T2 (n = 43), 95% and 95%; for T4 (n = 28), 71% and no data; and overall, 86% and 91%.[333] Eight additional patients with unfavorable T4 cancers were treated with resection and adjuvant RT. All eight patients treated with surgery and RT were locally controlled; three of eight experienced severe complications.

Nasal Cavity and Ethmoid Sinus

Inverted Papilloma. Weissler and coworkers[334] reported 233 cases of inverting papilloma seen over a 35-year period. One hundred thirty-four patients had at least 1 year of follow-up. The risk of recurrence was 71% in patients who had an intranasal

procedure and 56% for those having a Caldwell-Luc approach. Patients having a lateral rhinotomy had the lowest incidence of recurrence (29%).

Weissler and coworkers[334] also reported six patients who received RT for benign inverting papilloma and nine for inverting papilloma associated with malignant disease. Twelve of the 15 patients had a complete response to RT and were free of disease for long periods of follow-up. Gomez et al.[329] reported 10 patients with advanced and/or recurrent inverting papillomas who were treated with definitive RT. Local recurrence developed in four patients (40%) at 1.5, 6.5, 12, and 13 years after treatment. Six patients remained continuously disease-free at 7, 8.5, 8.5, 9, 9, and 20.5 years after RT.

Carcinoma. Mendenhall et al.[335] reviewed 109 patients treated at the University of Florida for carcinomas of the nasal cavity (69 patients), ethmoid sinus (33 patients), sphenoid sinus (6 patients), and frontal sinus (1 patient). Fifty-six patients were treated with definitive RT, 45 with surgery and postoperative RT, and 8 with preoperative RT and surgery. The 5-year local control rates were for T1 to T3, 82%; for T4, 50%; and overall, 63%. Local control at 5 years was 43% after definitive RT and 84% after surgery and adjuvant RT (p <0.0001). A multivariate analysis revealed that both overall stage and treatment group (definitive RT versus surgery and adjuvant RT) impacted this endpoint. Cause-specific survival rates at 5 years were for stages I to III, 81%; for stage IV, 54%; and overall, 62%. A multivariate analysis of cause-specific survival revealed that T-stage, N-stage, and treatment group significantly impacted this endpoint. Of 109 patients, 31 (20%) sustained severe complications; 17 (16%) of 56 patients after definitive RT, and 14 (25%) of 53 patients after surgery and adjuvant RT.

Esthesioneuroblastoma. Elkon and coworkers[337] reviewed the literature on esthesioneuroblastoma and compiled the results of 78 cases. They concluded that either RT or surgery was sufficient treatment for early-stage disease, but that combined treatment might be advantageous for late-stage presentations. The 5-year absolute survival rate was 75% for lesions confined to the nasal cavity, 60% for those involving the nasal cavity and paranasal sinuses, and 41% for tumors extending beyond the nasal cavity and paranasal sinuses.

Monroe and coworkers[328] reported on 22 patients treated with curative intent at the University of Florida and observed the following 5-year outcomes: local control, 59%; cause-specific survival, 54%; and survival, 48%. The 5-year cause-specific survival rate was lower after definitive RT (17%) compared with craniofacial resection and postoperative RT (56%). Cervical metastases occurred in 6 of 22 patients (27%). Recurrence in the neck was observed in 4 of 9 patients, who were initially N0 and who did not receive elective neck RT compared with zero of 11 patients who were electively treated (p = 0.02).

Maxillary Sinus

Waldron and coworkers[338] reported on 110 patients treated with curative intent at the Princess Margaret Hospital with definitive RT (83 patients) or surgery and adjuvant RT (27 patients). The 5-year rates of local control and cause-specific survival were 42% and 43%, respectively. Sixty-three patients developed a local recurrence, and 25 of 63 underwent salvage surgery with a subsequent 5-year cause-specific survival of 31%.

Complications of Treatment

Surgery

Complications of a maxillectomy include failure of the split-thickness skin graft to heal, trismus, CSF leak, and hemorrhage.

PRACTICE OF ONCOLOGY

Complications of ethmoid sinus surgery include hemorrhage, meningitis, CSF leak, cellulitis and pansinusitis, brain abscess, and stroke. Complications of craniofacial resection includes meningitis, subdural abscess, CSF leak, diplopia, and hemorrhage.

Radiation Therapy

The most frequent and significant complications of RT involve the eye.[335,339,340] When only a portion of the ipsilateral eye is irradiated (the medial one third), it is possible to preserve vision in the majority of patients. When there is extensive disease in the orbit, however, the entire eye is irradiated to a high dose with almost certain loss of vision; however, these same patients would require orbital exenteration if treated by surgery. The risk for bilateral blindness can be reduced by the use of CT and MRI scans for improved treatment planning and knowledge of the tolerance of the optic nerve.

A few patients will experience a transient CNS syndrome that includes vertigo, headaches, decreased cerebration, and lethargy. This syndrome usually appears 2 to 3 months after the completion of treatment and lasts 1 to 2 months. Aseptic meningitis, chronic sinusitis, or serous otitis media can occur. High-dose RT of the nasal cavity can cause narrowing and synechiae of the nasal cavity. Douching with salt water and daily self-dilations with petrolatum-coated cotton swabs will reduce the problem. Septal perforations occur when tumor has destroyed part of the septum; these do not usually require treatment. Destruction of the nasal bone and septum by the tumor may result in cosmetic deformity. Maxillary necrosis may develop, particularly if teeth are extracted.

PARAGANGLIOMAS

Paragangliomas are an uncommon group of neoplasms that may originate anywhere glomus bodies are found. The lesions are rare before the age of 20; there is a female predominance in some series; and the lesions may occur in multiple sites in about 10% to 20% of cases, especially in patients with familial history. Carotid body tumors are associated with conditions producing chronic hypoxia, such as high-altitude habitation.

Anatomy

The normal glomus bodies in the head and neck vary from 0.1 to 0.5 mm in diameter. Tumors arising in glomus bodies (i.e., paragangliomas) arise most often from the carotid and temporal bone glomus bodies, with rare reports of tumors arising in the orbit, nasopharynx, larynx, nasal cavity, paranasal sinuses, tongue, and jaw. The temporal bone glomus bodies are not found consistently in any location. At least one half of the glomus bodies are found in the general region of the jugular fossa; the remaining are distributed along the course of the nerve of Jacobson (a branch of CN X). Approximately 20% of all temporal bone glomus bodies lie in the tympanic canaliculus, and approximately 10% are in relation to the cochlear promontory. The carotid bodies are located adjacent to the bifurcation of the common carotid. Orbital bodies are in relation to the ciliary nerve, and vagal bodies are adjacent to the ganglion nodosum of the vagus nerve.

Pathology

Paragangliomas are histologically benign tumors resembling the parent tissue and consist of nests of epithelioid cells within stroma-containing, thin-walled blood vessels and nonmyelinated nerve fibers. Although the tumor is well circumscribed, a true capsule is not seen. The criterion of malignancy is based on the development of metastases rather than the histologic appearance.

Patterns of Spread

These lesions usually grow slowly; it is usual to have a history of symptoms for a few years and, occasionally, for 20 years or longer.

Carotid Body Tumors

Carotid body tumors are usually located at the common carotid bifurcation and, as they expand, tend to displace and encircle the internal and external carotid vessels. The tumor begins in the adventitia of the artery and initially derives its blood supply from the vaso vasorum. An accessory blood supply may come from branches of the vertebral artery and the ascending cervical artery. The tumor is usually closely adherent to the wall of the carotid adjacent to the vascular pedicle, and there may be thinning of the arterial wall owing to pressure by the mass. Large masses extend toward the cervical spine, skull base, angle of the mandible, and the lateral pharyngeal space.

Temporal Bone Tumors

Glomus tympanicum lesions tend to be small when diagnosed because they produce symptoms early in their course. The tumor may involve the ossicles, the tympanic membrane, the mastoid, the external auditory canal, the semicircular canal, and the 7th, Jacobson, and Arnold nerves.

Glomus jugulare tumors invade the skull base, petrous apex, jugular vein, middle ear, and middle and posterior cranial fossae. CNs V to XII may be involved.

Lymphatic

Lymphatic metastases occur in about 5% of carotid body tumors but are very rare for temporal bone tumors. An upper neck mass may be an inferior extension of a jugular fossa or vagal tumor rather than a lymph node metastasis.

Distant Metastases

Distant metastases have rarely been reported for temporal bone tumors; carotid body tumors have a low risk for distant metastases, probably in the range of 5% or less.

Clinical Picture

Carotid Body Tumors

The most common presenting symptom is an asymptomatic, slow-growing mass in the upper neck near the carotid bifurcation. Large masses may encroach on the parapharyngeal space and produce dysphagia, pain, and CN palsies. Carotid sinus syndrome may occur because of the pressure of the mass.

On examination, the mass usually lies deep to the sternocleidomastoid muscle and is tethered to surrounding structures. Fixation occurs only in large tumors extending to the spine and skull base. Glomus vagale tumors occur more superiorly and produce a submucosal bulge in the tonsillar area.

Temporal Bone Tumors

A tumor arising in or near the middle ear presents with an insidious conductive hearing loss, pulsatile tinnitus, vertigo, and headache. Patients with lesions developing in or around the jugular fossa develop headaches, often pulsatile in nature, referred to the orbit or temple. CNs V to XII and the sympathetic nerves become affected. Lesions developing in the facial canal present with facial nerve symptoms.

A characteristic blue-red mass may be seen bulging the tympanic membrane. A mass may be appreciated in the upper neck between the mandible and mastoid. Paralysis of CNs V to XII and sympathetic nerves may occur.

Differential Diagnosis

Carotid Body Tumors

The differential diagnosis includes enlarged lymph nodes, a carotid artery aneurysm, a branchial cleft cyst, benign tumors (e.g., lipoma), and direct extension of a lateral pharyngeal wall or pyriform sinus cancer into the soft tissues of the neck.

A CT and/or MRI scan with contrast provides the diagnosis. A biopsy usually produces serious hemorrhage and is not recommended.

Temporal Bone Tumors

The differential diagnosis includes an internal carotid artery in the middle ear either as an aberrant vessel or as an aneurysm. These patients also present with hearing loss, pulsatile tinnitus, and a pulsatile mass behind the eardrum. A high jugular bulb may present as a vascular mass in the middle ear and mimic a glomus tumor. Other possibilities include an ear canal polyp, an NPC with extension to the temporal bone, acoustic neuroma, middle ear carcinoma, metastatic carcinoma, cholesteatoma, histiocytosis, chronic serous otitis, and mastoiditis.

Staging

There is no accepted staging system for paragangliomas.

Treatment

Selection of Treatment Modality

Temporal Bone Tumors. Excision is satisfactory for small lesions that can be removed without a risk of operative death or damage to normal structures. Stereotactic radiosurgery is an option for early lesions.

Early lesions of the tympanic cavity are managed successfully by excision without a loss of hearing or vestibular function. The remainder of the lesions are managed best by RT, with a very high success rate and minimal morbidity with current techniques. Partial removal of the tumor prior to RT does not improve the results and only increases the overall morbidity. Local control after RT is defined as stable disease or partial regression with no evidence of growth.

Carotid Body Tumors. Small lesions (1 to 5 cm) may be successfully removed with little risk to the patient. However, if resection of the carotid vessels is anticipated or if a large lesion is fixed or unresectable because of size, RT is the preferred initial treatment.

Surgical Treatment

Temporal Bone Tumors. Small glomus tympanicum lesions are approached through the eardrum or mastoid area and are removed. Hearing loss may occur from the operation, but if there is conductive hearing loss from the tumor, it may be correctable.

For the glomus jugulare tumors, surgery is reserved for RT failure, in which case a radical mastoidectomy or a subtotal temporal bone resection would be required. Some surgeons advocate a skull base approach.

Carotid Body Tumors. A standard neck incision is made in a skin crease at the level of the carotid bulb, and the carotid sheath and its contents are identified. The tumor is usually lying at the bifurcation of the internal and external carotid arteries, often displacing these vessels. Marked drops in blood pressure and bradycardia can be avoided by injecting the bulb area with lidocaine. Bleeding may be avoided by using the bipolar electrode before excising the mass. The mass is then removed, preserving the carotid arteries.

Preoperative embolization of feeder vessels is frequently employed to minimize intraoperative blood loss.

Irradiation Technique

RT consists of 45 Gy of 25 fractions over 5 weeks. The dose is below the tolerance of the normal tissues included in the treatment volume. Patients are treated with IMRT.

Acute RT sequelae are almost nil. The patient will have temporary hair loss in the entrance and exit areas beginning about the 3rd week. Mild nausea may occur. Late sequelae are few. The patient may develop otitis media, especially if tumor involves the middle ear.

Management of Recurrence

Patients have follow-up with annual CT or MRI scans. Recurrence after surgery usually is treated by RT. Recurrence after RT should be treated by operation if feasible; if surgery is not possible, re-RT may be considered.

Results of Treatment

Woods and coworkers[341] observed a local control rate of 89% in 71 patients with temporal bone paragangliomas who were treated surgically and followed from 1 to 22 years. Green and coworkers[342] reported a local control rate of 89% after surgery for 18 patients who had a mean follow-up of 8 years.

Hinerman et al.[25] reported on 104 patients with 121 paragangliomas who were treated with RT (115 tumors) or radiosurgery (6 tumors) and followed for a median of 8.5 years. The 10-year actuarial local control and cause-specific survival rates were 94% and 95%, respectively.

Complications of Treatment

Surgery

The major risks during operation are hemorrhage and injury to the CNs. Other complications include hemiparesis, spinal fluid leak, and hearing loss.

Irradiation

Complications include cholesteatoma and sequestrum of the mastoid and otitis media. Detectable damage to the hearing mechanism and vestibular apparatus is unlikely after 45 Gy of 25 fractions.[343]

MAJOR SALIVARY GLANDS

Tumors of the major salivary glands account for 3% to 4% of all head and neck neoplasms. The average age of patients is 55 years for malignant neoplasms, and about 40 years for benign tumors. Approximately 25% of parotid tumors and 50% of submandibular tumors are malignant.

Anatomy

The parotid gland is formed by the muscles, bones, vessels, and nerves that come in contact with the gland. The bulk of the parotid gland is superficial, extending superiorly to the zygomatic arch and anterior aspect of the external auditory canal. The anterior border does not extend beyond the opening of the parotid duct into the oral cavity opposite the second molar. Inferiorly, the gland extends between the mastoid and the angle of the mandible. The gland lies in front of and below the external auditory canal. A deep lobe extends into the parapharyngeal area, where it is in relationship to the lateral process of C1, the styloid process, and the parapharyngeal space.

The parotid gland is encompassed by fascia that is sufficient to contain most parotid infections in addition to benign tumors and low-grade malignancies. However, the fascia between the parotid gland and the conchal and tragal cartilages is thin and quickly penetrated by tumor. The fascia separating the deep lobe from the parapharyngeal space (stylomandibular fascial membrane) may be sufficiently thin to allow the tumor or infection to access the parapharyngeal space and pharynx.

The sensory nerve supply to the parotid area and part of the pinna is from the greater auricular nerve (C2 to C3). The facial nerve (VII) penetrates the parotid gland almost immediately upon leaving the stylomastoid canal and forms an extensive anatomic network within the gland and gives off branches to the muscles of expression.

The parotid gland is richly supplied from several arteries that freely anastomose and create arteriovenous bleeding during a parotidectomy. The external carotid, the internal maxillary and superficial temporal arteries, and the posterior facial vein lie deep to CN VII.

The superficial preauricular nodes lie outside the fascia of the parotid gland and immediately in front of the tragus and drain the skin of the anterior ear, temple, and upper face, including the eye and nose. They are involved most frequently by metastatic skin cancer and lymphoma, but not usually from parotid neoplasms. The preauricular nodes empty into the external jugular chain nodes, or they may communicate with the internal jugular chain nodes.

There are two nodal groups within the parotid fascia. Within the substance of the parotid gland are numerous lymph follicles and 4 to 10 small lymph nodes scattered along the posterior facial and external jugular veins. Thus, they may lie deep to CN VII. Outside the gland but within the fascia are subparotid nodes that lie in front of the tragus and between the inferior aspect of the parotid tail and the anterior border of the sternocleidomastoid muscle.

Pathology

Benign Tumors

Benign Mixed Tumors. Also called pleomorphic adenoma, these slow-growing neoplasms are surrounded by an imperfect pseudocapsule traversed by fingers of tumor. The age of appearance begins in the early 20s with a mean age of 40 years.

Papillary Cystadenoma Lymphomatosum. Also called a Warthin tumor, it is encased by a thin but complete capsule, occurs predominantly in older men, is bilateral in approximately 10% of cases, and may be multiple on one or both sides.

Benign Lymphoepithelial Lesions. Benign lymphoepithelial lesions account for about 5% of benign lesions. The tumor may be bilateral and is more common in women.

Oncocytoma. Oncocytoma is a benign, slow-growing tumor found mostly in the older age group. The encapsulated tumor has a dark appearance similar to melanoma.

Basal Cell Adenoma. The basal cell adenoma is an uncommon benign lesion, usually appearing in older people. It is cured by a simple excision. Basal cell adenoma must be distinguished from basal cell carcinoma of the skin metastatic to parotid lymph nodes.

Malignant Tumors

Low-Grade Malignancy

Acinic cell carcinoma. Acinic cell carcinomas typically are indolent low-grade neoplasms appearing in all age groups and are most common in women. Metastases occur in a small percentage of cases and cannot be predicted by the histologic picture.

Mucoepidermoid carcinoma, low grade. Most mucoepidermoid carcinomas are indolent lesions readily cured by adequate excision. They may appear in any age group and grow slowly; there is little or no capsule. They are usually well circumscribed, but they may widely infiltrate the normal gland or become fixed to skin.

High-Grade Malignancy

Mucoepidermoid carcinoma, high grade. High-grade mucoepidermoid carcinomas behave aggressively, widely infiltrating the salivary gland and producing lymph node and distant metastases. They may be difficult to distinguish from SCCs.

Adenocarcinoma, poorly differentiated carcinoma, anaplastic carcinoma, and squamous cell carcinoma. These histologies tend to appear late in life and behave aggressively. Almost all of the so-called SCCs of the parotid are metastatic from skin cancer, especially from the temple area.[344]

Malignant mixed tumor. A small percentage of benign mixed tumors may develop into a frank malignancy (carcinoma ex pleomorphic adenoma).

Adenoid cystic carcinoma. This is uncommon in the major salivary glands. Its growth rate is variable. Metastases to regional lymph nodes and distant sites occur; PNI is characteristic; and recurrences may appear many years after initial treatment.

Lymphoepithelioma (malignant lymphoepithelial lesion, "eskimoma"). Lymphoepithelioma occurs rarely in the parotid and submandibular gland. The histologic picture is that of lymphoepithelioma with varying degrees of nonmalignant lymphoid stroma.

Patterns of Spread

Benign Mixed Tumors

Benign mixed tumors of the parotid gland grow by expansion and local infiltration. Most tumors begin in the superficial lobe. Because of their slow growth, they rarely cause CN VII palsy. When incompletely excised, multiple tumor nodules develop within the tumor bed. Skin invasion may occur in recurrent lesions; bone invasion does not occur.

Malignant Tumors

Malignant neoplasms infiltrate the parotid gland, invade CN VII and the auriculotemporal nerve, and spread along nerve sheaths. The tumor may invade the adjacent skin, muscles, and bone. Deep lobe lesions invade the parapharyngeal space, the infratemporal fossa, and the skull base and compromise additional CNs.

Malignant tumors of the submandibular gland invade the gland, fix the tumor to the adjacent mandible, and invade the mylohyoid muscle and hypoglossal nerve.

Sublingual gland neoplasms usually present as a submucosal mass in the floor of the mouth. The advanced lesions show an ulcerated mass in the floor of the mouth with extension to the tongue, the mandible, and the submental soft tissues.

Lymphatic Spread

Lymph node metastases may occur from all of the malignant neoplasms. Approximately 20% to 25% of patients with malignant tumors will have clinically positive or occult metastases in lymph nodes at the time of diagnosis. Low-grade mucoepidermoid carcinoma and acinic cell adenocarcinoma have a low rate of lymph node metastasis, as do adenoid cystic cancers. The risk for lymph node metastasis increases with recurrent disease and an increased size of the primary lesion.

Clinical Picture

Parotid Gland

The majority of patients with either benign or malignant parotid tumors present with a mass. Mild, intermittent pain is occasionally present, but does not distinguish between benign and malignant tumors. Facial nerve palsy is an infrequent presenting complaint and indicates malignancy. Deep lobe tumors may produce dysphagia. Fixation or reduced mobility may occur in both benign and malignant neoplasms. Tumors presenting in the deep lobe may cause bulging of the palate and tonsil. Advanced malignant lesions may rarely affect CNs IX to XII and the sympathetic chain if the parapharyngeal space is invaded. CN V3 may be involved when tumor tracks along the auriculotemporal nerve to the skull base; pain is an associated finding.

Submandibular Gland

Both benign and malignant neoplasms present as a mass usually associated with mild pain. Nerve palsy is rarely present. The skin may be infiltrated in advanced lesions. The tumor mass usually is partially fixed to the mandible unless quite small. Loss of mobility occurs with both benign and malignant lesions.

Sublingual Gland

Sublingual gland lesions are clinically similar to floor of the mouth SCCs. They produce a mass, which is submucosal at first, that may be felt by the tongue. There is mild discomfort, if any, in the early stages.

Differential Diagnosis

Parotid Gland

Gallia and Johnson[345] reviewed 140 patients who eventually underwent a parotidectomy for diagnosis. Only 11% had malignant masses; the remainder had benign neoplasms (62%) or nonneoplastic conditions (27%). Conditions that may be confused with a parotid tumor include: (1) metastatic cancer, lymphoma, or leukemia involving parotid-area lymph nodes; (2) fatty replacement, tail of parotid; (3) chronic parotitis; (4) a Boeck sarcoid; (5) a stone in the duct; (6) cysts (branchial cleft, dermoid); (7) hypertrophy associated with diabetes; (8) hypertrophy of masseter muscle; (9) mandibular neoplasms; (10) prominent transverse process of C1; (11) penetrating foreign bodies; (12) hemangiomas/lymphangioma; and (13) a lipoma.

Submandibular Gland

The differential diagnosis of a submandibular mass includes inflammatory disease, SCC metastatic to a lymph node, and a primary neoplasm of the submandibular gland.

Gallia and Johnson[345] reviewed 110 submandibular lesions in patients who underwent biopsy. Ninety-three lesions (85%) were nonneoplastic, usually inflamed glands, and nine lesions (8%) were benign tumors. Eight patients (7%) had malignant lesions, of which three lesions were lymphoma, three were metastatic carcinoma, and two were primary submandibular gland carcinoma.

Biopsy Technique

Parotid Gland. The biopsy and definitive surgical treatment are often the same for parotid masses. Lesions lying in the superficial lobe are best biopsied by performing a superficial parotidectomy. Lesions involving both the superficial and deep lobes or just the deep lobes are "biopsied" by a total parotidectomy. An incisional

and excisional biopsy may contaminate the tumor bed, thus increasing the risk of tumor recurrence and facial nerve damage as well as increasing the extent of the definitive surgical procedure by necessitating the wide removal of the biopsy site.

An FNA cytology can be performed for diagnosis. A negative FNA does not necessarily mean that there is no tumor, therefore surgical decisions often rely heavily on clinical and radiographic findings. An FNA can be used in the inoperable or recurrent lesions when RT is the initial treatment.

Submandibular Gland. An FNA is helpful when positive for a tumor, but may delay diagnosis when falsely negative. When needle biopsy is negative, but history, physical examination, and radiographic studies suggest neoplasm, and a careful search of the head and neck area fails to reveal a primary mucosal lesion, the submandibular triangle is dissected as the biopsy procedure.

Staging

The AJCC staging system is depicted in Table 38.19.

Treatment

Selection of Treatment Modality

Parotid Gland. The initial management of resectable superficial lobe parotid masses is an en bloc superficial lobectomy. The tumor usually can be dissected free of the facial nerve. If the tumor involves the deep portion of the gland, the nerve is retracted and the deep portion excised (i.e., total parotidectomy). Skin, bone, and muscle may also be resected as needed.

Low-grade malignant neoplasms are usually managed by operation only. RT is given postoperatively for nearly all high-grade lesions. RT is advised for low-grade malignant lesions that are recurrent and those with close or positive margins on the facial nerve. Postoperative RT is advised for selected benign mixed tumors when there is microscopic residual disease after operation, and for nearly all patients after surgery for recurrent disease. RT alone is unlikely to control gross disease, and if possible, resection of any gross residual benign mixed tumor should be performed prior to RT. Inoperable malignancies are treated by definitive RT.

TABLE 38.19

2010 American Joint Committee on Cancer Staging for Major Salivary Gland Primary Tumors (T)

TX	Primary tumor cannot be assessed
T0	No evidence of primary tumor
T1	Tumor 2 cm or less in greatest dimension without extraparenchymal extension[a]
T2	Tumor more than 2 cm but not more than 4 cm in greatest dimension without extraparenchymal extension[a]
T3	Tumor more than 4 cm and/or tumor having extraparenchymal extension[a]
T4a	Tumor invades skin, mandible, ear canal, and/or facial nerve
T4b	Tumor invades skull base and/or pterygoid plates and/or encases carotid artery

[a] Extraparenchymal extension is clinical or macroscopic evidence of invasion of soft tissues. Microscopic evidence alone does not constitute extraparenchymal extension for classification purposes.
Used with the permission of the American Joint Committee on Cancer (AJCC), Chicago, Illinois. The original source for this material is the *AJCC Cancer Staging Handbook*, Seventh Edition (2010) published by Springer Science and Business Media LLC, www.springerlink.com.

Submandibular Gland. If a frozen section diagnosis shows a malignant lesion and there is no involvement of nerves, mandible, or soft tissues, submandibular triangle dissection is performed and postoperative RT is given to the submandibular bed and ipsilateral neck. If there is PNI, bone invasion, a clinically positive node, or extension to contiguous soft tissues, resection is enlarged to encompass the necessary areas. Postoperative RT is added in nearly all cases.

Surgical Treatment

Superficial Parotidectomy.
The incision is made in the preauricular crease and then curves under the earlobe posteriorly, and extends into the neck. The facial nerve is identified and the dissection is carried out between the mass and the facial nerve. Ideally, a 1-cm circumferential cuff of "normal" parotid tissue should be resected along with the tumor. However, close margins of less than 1 mm are frequently encountered because most parotid gland tumors lay close to branches of the facial nerve. In such cases, completely encapsulated tumors can frequently be resected with confidence. On the other hand, facial nerve sacrifice must be considered if the nerve branch courses directly through the tumor or when there is gross extracapsular extension into the parotid gland. The adequacy of resection is determined by frozen sections.

Total Parotidectomy.
A superficial parotidectomy is performed, the nerve is dissected free from the underlying deep lobe, and the deep lobe and tumor are removed. Occasionally, the mandible must be divided to gain access to the retromandibular portion of the deep lobe. A partial mandibulectomy is required when the mandible is invaded by tumor.

The intraparotid nodes are removed with the primary lesion. If the nodes are positive, a neck dissection is added. Neck dissection is always included for clinically positive nodes. Elective neck dissection is not done for low-grade lesions.

A radical parotidectomy implies removal of the entire parotid, the facial nerve, and other involved tissues such as skin, bone, or muscle. Part or all of CN VII must be sacrificed, and an immediate autologous nerve graft may be done. If a frozen section examination of the facial nerve is positive at the stylomastoid foramen, a mastoidectomy may be required to complete the resection. Postoperative RT is delayed for 6 weeks, and the chance of successful function is reported to be good.[346]

Radiation Therapy

The minimum treatment volume for parotid lesions includes the parotid bed and upper neck nodes. PNI indicates enlargement of the portals to cover the nerve pathways. The entire ipsilateral neck is included for high-grade lesions or for clinically positive nodes in the neck dissection specimen. The tumor dose to the primary area is 60 to 65 Gy over 6 to 7 weeks if there is no gross residual disease. Higher doses employing altered fractionation are used for patients with microscopically positive margins or gross disease.

Submandibular space EBRT portals are tailored to the extent of disease found in the surgical dissection. The entire ipsilateral neck is included. The postoperative dose is 65 to 70 Gy because the rate of recurrence, even with combined treatment, is substantial. Neutron therapy has been used in the management of unresectable salivary gland cancers.[347]

Chemotherapy for Salivary Gland Cancers

Historically, chemotherapy has been primarily used for patients with incurable disease or on prospective clinical trials. The safety and dosing of concurrent chemotherapy and RT has been established for this body region from the experience in patients with upper aerodigestive tract SCCs, and as such, this approach is sometimes applied to patients with unresectable disease or in the poor risk adjuvant setting. Available efficacy data for such an approach in this setting are limited.[348,349]

Results of Treatment

Parotid Gland

Benign Mixed Tumors. Enucleation or excision with a narrow rim of normal tissue will eventually result in a local recurrence rate of approximately 20% after 10 to 15 years of follow-up. A superficial parotidectomy will result in a recurrence rate of approximately 5%.[350] The surgical success rate for recurrent lesions depends on the number of previous operations and the size and extent of recurrence. It may be necessary to sacrifice one or several branches of CN VII and to repair the defect with a nerve graft. Postoperative RT of 66 to 70 Gy is added in selected cases in which there are close margins or microscopic residual disease, or in cases in which a subsequent recurrence would be almost impossible to manage surgically or would result in loss of the facial nerve.[351] Death because of benign mixed tumors is unlikely.

Malignant Tumors. The likelihood of cure after surgery alone for low-grade tumors is high, and adjuvant RT is usually unnecessary. The local recurrence rate for operation alone is approximately 50% to 60% for high-grade tumors.[352,353]

Garden and coworkers[354] reported 166 patients treated with surgery and postoperative RT for parotid malignancies at the M.D. Anderson Hospital between 1965 and 1989. Forty patients (24%) developed a recurrent disease that was local in 9% and regional in 6%. The histologic type did not significantly influence the likelihood of local control (p = 0.36). Twenty-five patients (15%) developed distant metastases with disease control above the clavicles. The 10- and 15-year survival rates were 60% and 52%, respectively.

Submandibular Gland

Byers and coworkers[355] reported the results of treatment for 22 malignant tumors of the submandibular gland with no prior therapy. Treatment was resection followed selectively by postoperative RT. The local control rate was 64%, and the survival rate was 50%.

Spiro[350] reported the results of surgery for 129 malignant submandibular gland carcinomas seen between 1939 and 1973. All patients had a minimum of 10 years of follow-up. Adenoid cystic carcinoma occurred in 35%, mucoepidermoid carcinoma in 29%, and malignant mixed tumor in 19%. Cervical lymph nodes were malignant in 28%. The local–regional control rate was 40%, and the cause-specific cure rate was 31% at 5 years and 22% at 10 years.

Benign tumors of the submandibular gland were resected in 106 patients, and only 2 developed a local recurrence.[350]

Chemotherapy Results

The heterogeneity and relative rarity of malignant salivary gland tumors have complicated the evaluation of systemic therapies. Prospective clinical trials are infrequent; different histologies are often combined, as are the results for major and minor salivary gland tumors. Over the last 2 decades, less than 500 patients with adenoid cystic cancer have been the subject of studies evaluating drug therapy.[356,357] Drugs like doxorubicin and 5-fluorouracil with reported activity have this claim largely based on retrospective case series, not prospective clinical trials.

Cisplatin, paclitaxel, vinorelbine, epirubicin, and mitoxantrone have major response rates in the 10% to 20% range in prospective studies in the recurrent or metastatic disease setting.[358–562] The potential importance of histology in trial design is well illustrated with the case of paclitaxel, where 3 out of 12 and 4 out of 17 patients with mucoepidermoid and adenocarcinoma responded, respectively, yet zero of 14 with adenoid cystic cancer responded.[363] Treatment with gemcitabine also did not yield any major response in patients with adenoid cystic carcinoma.[139] Cisplatin- or anthracycline-containing combinations (e.g., cyclophosphamide/doxorubicin/cisplatin; cisplatin/vinorelbine; cisplatin/5-fluorouracil, cisplatin/mitoxantrone) may increase this rate, but a major response still occurs in the minority of patients, and toxicity is increased.[356,357] The relative efficacies of single-agent versus combination chemotherapies have not been well studied. It should be emphasized that the natural history of some salivary gland cancers, of which the adenoid cystic subtype is perhaps the best example, can be quite indolent, making initial observation a prudent course.

Given these response rates, clinical trials are often an attractive option for patients, and there has been interest in the potential utility of newer targeted agents. Expression of potential molecular targets vary by pathologic subtype. For example, c-kit is commonly expressed in adenoid cystic cancer, but variably or not at all in other salivary cancer subtypes.[356] Although there have been reported responses to imatinib in case reports,[364,365] demonstrating objective responses in clinical trials where the agent has proved elusive, and so the drug remains investigational for this disease.[366,367] Data thus far for EGFR pathway and Her-2 targeted agents are limited and not compelling.[368] Of note, the androgen receptor is commonly expressed in patients with salivary duct carcinoma, and there are reports under these circumstances of response to anti-androgen therapy.[369] The oncogenic transcription factor c-myb is overexpressed in adenoid cystic cancer[370] and is informing further drug development in the disease. Dovitinib, which is designed to block fibroblast growth factor receptor (FGFR)- and vascular endothelial growth factor receptor (VEGFR)-mediated angiogenesis demonstrated activity in a phase II trial in patients with adenoid cystic cancer.[371]

Complications of Treatment

Surgery

Facial paralysis is the most important complication associated with parotid surgery. Temporary facial nerve palsy may occur due to manipulation of the nerve during operation, and function will gradually return over a few months' time. Isolated persistent weakness of the lower lip may occur due to division of the platysma muscle. Incomplete eyelid closure requires protective measures such as artificial tears, Lacri-Lube (Allergan Inc., Irvine, CA), and eye patches to prevent corneal abrasion. A variety of surgical techniques can be employed to address facial nerve deficits if functional recovery is not expected, including nerve grafting, a brow lift, gold weight implantation into the upper eyelid, lower eyelid tightening, and facial suspensory procedures. Gustatory sweating (Frey syndrome) occurs in about 10% of patients after parotidectomy and rarely requires treatment. A persistent salivary fistula is rare.

Radiation Therapy

Xerostomia is avoided by techniques that spare the contralateral salivary tissues. There may be trismus due to fibrosis of the masseter and pterygoid muscles and the temporomandibular joint. Otitis media may occur if the ear is irradiated. Localized hair loss may occur with some techniques. Osteoradionecrosis may rarely occur with high doses.

MINOR SALIVARY GLANDS

Tumors of the minor salivary gland origin are uncommon, accounting for about 2% to 3% of all malignant neoplasms of the upper aerodigestive tract. They may appear at any age, but are uncommon before age 20 and rare under age 10. They tend to occur most often in the hard palate, nasal cavity, and paranasal sinuses—areas infrequently involved by SCCs. Thus, the site of origin is related to the density of the minor salivary glands in a particular tissue.

Anatomy

Minor salivary glands are ubiquitous in the mucosa of the upper aerodigestive tract with the exception of the gingivae and the anterior portion of the hard palate, which are free of minor salivary glands. They are distributed on the undersurface of the anterior and lateral oral tongue and the base of the tongue. Aberrant salivary tissue sometimes is seen in lymph nodes, in the body of the mandible just behind the third molar teeth, and in the vestigial remnant of the nasopalatine canal in the anterior maxilla, middle ear, lower neck, sternoclavicular joint, thyroglossal duct, and other sites.

Pathology

Approximately one half of minor salivary gland tumors are malignant. The histologic varieties of malignant tumors include adenoid cystic carcinoma, mucoepidermoid carcinoma, adenocarcinoma, and malignant mixed, acinic cell, and oncocytic carcinomas. About two thirds are adenoid cystic. Mucoepidermoid carcinomas and adenocarcinomas arise predominantly in the oral cavity.

The benign tumors are pleomorphic adenomas in the great majority of cases, with a few cases of intraductal papillomas, papillary cystadenomas, basal cell adenomas, and benign oncocytomas.

Patterns of Spread

There are no minor salivary glands in the anterior half of the hard palate, so tumors arise on the posterolateral hard palate and all of the soft palate. The site of origin for floor of mouth salivary gland tumors is either the sublingual gland or a minor salivary gland.

These tumors grow by local infiltration with eventual invasion of muscle, bone, and cartilage. PNI is a common feature, particularly for adenoid cystic carcinoma. The tumor may track both centrally and peripherally along nerves, but the central spread is the more common event. Extension along nerves eventually may traverse the skull base and surface intracranially, although this spread pattern may not become manifest for several years after the original treatment. Tumor growth along a nerve may be characterized by skip areas, so that a normal nerve segment is no assurance of free margins.

The risk of positive lymph nodes is related to the site of origin and the histology. Lymph node metastases are most likely from sites with a dense capillary lymphatic network, similar to the pattern for SCC. Adenoid cystic carcinoma, low-grade mucoepidermoid carcinoma, and acinic cell carcinoma are at low risk to spread to lymph nodes; about 20% of adenoid cystic carcinomas spread to lymph nodes, but this low incidence may be related partly to their frequent site of origin in the hard palate and paranasal sinuses, areas that infrequently produce lymph node metastases. The high-grade tumors carcinomas have a 30% incidence of lymph node involvement on presentation, and eventually half will develop lymph node metastases.

Clinical Picture

The clinical picture depends on the site of origin. The signs and symptoms differ from those of SCCs arising in the same area. Many of the lesions are indolent, and the history may go back many months or even years. Because lesions develop under the epithelium, the initial lesion is a submucosal mass that is often painless until ulceration develops. PNI is expressed as pain or paresthesias. Otherwise, the clinical picture resembles that for SCCs for a given size and site. Lymph node metastases occur at predictable sites. The clinically positive nodes are usually small and mobile, but neck dissection on such a patient may show numerous small, clinically undetectable positive nodes. The same staging systems applied to SCCs may be used.

Treatment

Selection of Treatment Modality

Benign, mixed-grade tumors are managed by operation; postoperative RT sometimes is advised in cases in which margins are close or positive.[372]

The low-grade carcinoma is treated initially by an operation when feasible, but RT is sometimes used as the primary treatment for inaccessible lesions or where the functional loss would be considerable. Postoperative RT is added for close margins or for those lesions that have recurred more than once. If the patient presents after excisional biopsy of a small lesion, RT is an alternative to reexcision, particularly if the procedure would produce significant cosmetic or functional loss.

The treatment of high-grade lesions varies immensely, depending on the site of origin, stage of disease, and willingness of the patient to accept a major cosmetic or functional change subsequent to an operation. Surgery and postoperative RT are preferred; RT alone is used for unresectable cancers. There are data that support the use of neutron therapy.[347]

Surgical Treatment

Benign tumors are removed by a wide local excision that includes a cuff of normal tissue. Small, low-grade lesions with a long history of slow growth may be treated with a wide local excision including a shell of normal tissue. Large, low-grade lesions and high-grade lesions require a more radical resection. When PNI is present, it is not possible to remove all the nerves potentially involved, but the nerves that are involved should be sacrificed wherever it is reasonable to do so. As an alternative, postoperative RT may be used to cover the perineural routes of spread.

Irradiation Technique

The RT techniques and doses are similar to those for SCCs of the same anatomic site and similar tumor size, with the exception that nerve pathways must be covered for adenoid cystic carcinomas.

Subclinical PNI for adenoid cystic carcinomas must be considered to be present even if it is not seen on the biopsy or surgical sections.

Results of Treatment

Spiro and coworkers[373] reported the Memorial Sloan-Kettering Cancer Center results for 434 malignant minor salivary gland tumors, of which 90% were treated surgically. The cause-specific 5-, 10-, and 15-year cure rates were 44%, 32%, and 21%, respectively; 51% died of the original cancer. Patients with adenoid cystic carcinoma had the poorest prognosis, with about 20% surviving without recurrence. Those with adenocarcinoma had an intermediate outlook—about 35% surviving without recurrence—and mucoepidermoid carcinomas had the best control rate, with about 70% long-term cures.

Cianchetti et al.[18] reported on 140 patients treated at the University of Florida for minor salivary gland carcinomas between 1966 and 2006. The 10-year local control rate was 66%; a multivariate analysis revealed that treatment group and T-stages significantly influenced this endpoint. Patients treated with RT alone had a lower local control rate compared with those treated with surgery and RT. The 10-year outcomes were for distant metastasis-free survival, 67%; for cause-specific survival, 56%; and for overall survival, 45%.

Benign mixed tumors of minor salivary gland origin have a good prognosis. Spiro[350] reported on 81 benign tumors; 60 occurred on the palate and 13 on the lip or cheek. With a minimum follow-up of 10 years, the local recurrence rate was 6%.

Wallace et al.[374] reported on 25 patients treated with RT alone (2 patients) or combined with surgery (23 patients) for pleomorphic adenoma and followed the patients for a median of 10.5 years. Local control was obtained in 13 of 16 patients (75%) with subclinical disease and 5 of 9 patients (56%) irradiated for gross disease. The 10-year overall local control rate was 76%.

In a small randomized trial of inoperable primary or recurrent salivary gland cancers (both major and minor salivary gland cancers were allowed), neutron therapy (n = 25) improved local–regional control significantly (p = 0.009) but at the expense of more severe morbidity.[347]

SELECTED REFERENCES

The full reference list can be accessed at lwwhealthlibrary.com/oncology.

1. Siegel R, Naishadham D, Jemal A. Cancer statistics, 2013. *CA Cancer J Clin* 2013;63:11–30.
3. Erkal HS, Mendenhall WM, Amdur RJ, et al. Synchronous and metachronous squamous cell carcinomas of the head and neck mucosal sites. *J Clin Oncol* 2001;19:1358–1362.
5. Gillison ML, Koch WM, Capone RB, et al. Evidence for a causal association between human papillomavirus and a subset of head and neck cancers. *J Natl Cancer Inst* 2000;92:709–720.
6. Mendenhall WM, Logan HL. Human papillomavirus and head and neck cancer. *Am J Clin Oncol* 2009;32:535–539.
7. Licitra L, Perrone F, Bossi P, et al. High-risk human papillomavirus affects prognosis in patients with surgically treated oropharyngeal squamous cell carcinoma. *J Clin Oncol* 2006;24:5630–5636.
8. Ang KK, Harris J, Wheeler R, et al. Human papillomavirus and survival of patients with oropharyngeal cancer. *N Engl J Med* 2010;363:24–35.
9. Gillison ML, Zhang Q, Jordan R, et al. Tobacco smoking and increased risk of death and progression for patients with p16-positive and p16-negative oropharyngeal cancer. *J Clin Oncol* 2012;30:2102–2111.
10. Patel SC, Carpenter WR, Tyree S, et al. Increasing incidence of oral tongue squamous cell carcinoma in young white women, age 18 to 44 years. *J Clin Oncol* 2011;29:1488–1494.
11. Yu MC, Yuan JM. Epidemiology of nasopharyngeal carcinoma. *Semin Cancer Biol* 2002;12:421–429.
12. Luce D, Gerin M, Leclerc A, et al. Sinonasal cancer and occupational exposure to formaldehyde and other substances. *Int J Cancer* 1993;53:224–231.
13. Rouvière H. *Anatomy of the Human Lymphatic System*. Arbor, MI: Edwards Brothers; 1938.
14. McAfee WJ, Morris CG, Amdur RJ, et al. Definitive radiotherapy for juvenile nasopharyngeal angiofibroma. *Am J Clin Oncol* 2006;29:168–170.
17. Maddox WA, Urist MM. Histopathological prognostic factors of certain primary oral cavity cancers. *Oncology (Williston Park)* 1990;4:39–42.
18. Cianchetti M, Mancuso AA, Amdur RJ, et al. Diagnostic evaluation of squamous cell carcinoma metastatic to cervical lymph nodes from an unknown head and neck primary site. *Laryngoscope* 2009;119:2348–2354.
19. Erkal HS, Mendenhall WM, Amdur RJ, et al. Squamous cell carcinomas metastatic to cervical lymph nodes from an unknown head-and-neck mucosal site treated with radiation therapy alone or in combination with neck dissection. *Int J Radiat Oncol Biol Phys* 2001;50:55–63.
20. Lindberg RD. Distribution of cervical lymph node metastases from squamous cell carcinoma of the upper respiratory and digestive tracts. *Cancer* 1972;29:1446–1449.
21. Fisch U. *Lymphography of the Cervical Lymphatic System*. Philadelphia: W. B. Saunders; 1968.
22. McLaughlin MP, Mendenhall WM, Mancuso AA, et al. Retropharyngeal adenopathy as a predictor of outcome in squamous cell carcinoma of the head and neck. *Head Neck* 1995;17:190–198.
23. Al-Othman MO, Morris CG, Hinerman RW, et al. Distant metastases after definitive radiotherapy for squamous cell carcinoma of the head and neck. *Head Neck* 2003;25:629–633.
24. Merino OR, Lindberg RD, Fletcher GH. An analysis of distant metastases from squamous cell carcinoma of the upper respiratory and digestive tracts. *Cancer* 1977;40:145–151.
25. Hinerman RW, Amdur RJ, Morris CG, et al. Definitive radiotherapy in the management of paragangliomas arising in the head and neck: a 35-year experience. *Head Neck* 2008;30:1431–1438.
26. Edge SB, Byrd DR, Compton CC, eds. *AJCC Cancer Staging Handbook*. 7th ed. New York: Springer; 2010.
27. Mendenhall WM, Parsons JT, Million RR, et al. A favorable subset of AJCC stage IV squamous cell carcinoma of the head and neck. *Int J Radiat Oncol Biol Phys* 1984;10:1841–1843.

28. Koyfman SA, Adelstein DJ. Enteral feeding tubes in patients undergoing definitive chemoradiation therapy for head-and-neck cancer: a critical review. *Int J Radiat Oncol Biol Phys* 2012;84:581–589.

29. Trotti A, Fu KK, Pajak TF, et al. Long term outcomes of RTOG 90-03: A comparison of hyperfractionation and two variants of accelerated fractionation to standard fractionation radiotherapy for head and neck squamous cell carcinoma. *Int J Radiat Oncol Biol Phys* 2005;63:S70–S71.

30. Mendenhall WM, Riggs CE, Vaysberg M, et al. Altered fractionation and adjuvant chemotherapy for head and neck squamous cell carcinoma. *Head Neck* 2010;32:939–945.

31. Mendenhall WM, Amdur RJ, Palta JR. Intensity-modulated radiotherapy in the standard management of head and neck cancer: promises and pitfalls. *J Clin Oncol* 2006;24:2618–2623.

32. Mendenhall WM, Mancuso AA. Radiotherapy for head and neck cancer—is the "next level" down? *Int J Radiat Oncol Biol Phys* 2009;73:645–646.

35. Mendenhall NP, Malyapa RS, Su Z, et al. Proton therapy for head and neck cancer: rationale, potential indications, practical considerations, and current clinical evidence. *Acta Oncol* 2011;50:763–771.

36. Mendenhall WM, Villaret DB, Amdur RJ, et al. Planned neck dissection after definitive radiotherapy for squamous cell carcinoma of the head and neck. *Head Neck* 2002;24:1012–1018.

37. Yeung AR, Liauw SL, Amdur RJ, et al. Lymph node-positive head and neck cancer treated with definitive radiotherapy: can treatment response determine the extent of neck dissection? *Cancer* 2008;112:1076–1082.

38. Pfister DG, Cassileth BR, Deng GE, et al. Acupuncture for pain and dysfunction after neck dissection: results of a randomized controlled trial. *J Clin Oncol* 2010;28:2565–2570.

39. Mendenhall WM, Million RR. Elective neck irradiation for squamous cell carcinoma of the head and neck: analysis of time-dose factors and causes of failure. *Int J Radiat Oncol Biol Phys* 1986;12:741–746.

40. Barkley HT Jr., Fletcher GH, Jesse RH, et al. Management of cervical lymph node metastases in squamous cell carcinoma of the tonsillar fossa, base of tongue, supraglottic larynx, and hypopharynx. *Am J Surg* 1972;124:462–467.

41. O'Sullivan B, Warde P, Grice B, et al. The benefits and pitfalls of ipsilateral radiotherapy in carcinoma of the tonsillar region. *Int J Radiat Oncol Biol Phys* 2001;51:332–343.

43. Cooper JS, Pajak TF, Forastiere AA, et al. Postoperative concurrent radiotherapy and chemotherapy for high-risk squamous-cell carcinoma of the head and neck. *N Engl J Med* 2004;350:1937–1944.

44. Bernier J, Domenge C, Ozsahin M, et al. Postoperative irradiation with or without concomitant chemotherapy for locally advanced head and neck cancer. *N Engl J Med* 2004;350:1945–1952.

45. Cooper JS, Zhang Q, Pajak TF, et al. Long-term follow-up of the RTOG 9501/intergroup phase III trial: postoperative concurrent radiation therapy and chemotherapy in high-risk squamous-cell carcinoma of the head and neck. *Int J Radiat Oncol Biol Phys* 2012;84:1198–1205.

46. Bachaud JM, Cohen-Jonathan E, Alzieu C, et al. Combined postoperative radiotherapy and weekly cisplatin infusion for locally advanced head and neck carcinoma: final report of a randomized trial. *Int J Radiat Oncol Biol Phys* 1996;36:999–1004.

47. Mendenhall WM, Parsons JT, Mancuso AA, et al. Head and neck: management of the neck. In: Perez CA, Brady LW, eds. *Principles and Practice of Radiation Oncology*, 2nd ed. Philadelphia: J. B. Lippincott Company; 1992: 790–805.

48. Liauw SL, Mancuso AA, Amdur RJ, et al. Postradiotherapy neck dissection for lymph node-positive head and neck cancer: the use of computed tomography to manage the neck. *J Clin Oncol* 2006;24:1421–1427.

49. Ong SC, Schoder H, Lee NY, et al. Clinical utility of 18F-FDG PET/CT in assessing the neck after concurrent chemoradiotherapy for Locoregional advanced head and neck cancer. *J Nucl Med* 2008;49:532–540.

50. McGuirt WF, McCabe BF. Significance of node biopsy before definitive treatment of cervical metastatic carcinoma. *Laryngoscope* 1978;88:594–597.

51. Ellis ER, Mendenhall WM, Rao PV, et al. Incisional or excisional neck-node biopsy before definitive radiotherapy, alone or followed by neck dissection. *Head Neck* 1991;13:177–183.

54. Hong WK, Lippman SM, Itri LM, et al. Prevention of second primary tumors with isotretinoin in squamous-cell carcinoma of the head and neck. *N Engl J Med* 1990;323:795–801.

55. Khuri FR, Lee JJ, Lippman SM, et al. Randomized phase III trial of low-dose isotretinoin for prevention of second primary tumors in stage I and II head and neck cancer patients. *J Natl Cancer Inst* 2006;98:441–450.

56. Bolla M, Lefur R, Ton Van J, et al. Prevention of second primary tumours with etretinate in squamous cell carcinoma of the oral cavity and oropharynx. Results of a multicentric double-blind randomised study. *Eur J Cancer* 1994;30A:767–772.

57. van Zandwijk N, Dalesio O, Pastorino U, et al. EUROSCAN, a randomized trial of vitamin A and N-acetylcysteine in patients with head and neck cancer or lung cancer. For the European Organization for Research and Treatment of Cancer Head and Neck and Lung Cancer Cooperative Groups. *J Natl Cancer Inst* 2000;92:977–986.

58. Bairati I, Meyer F, Gelinas M, et al. A randomized trial of antioxidant vitamins to prevent second primary cancers in head and neck cancer patients. *J Natl Cancer Inst* 2005;97:481–488.

62. Haddad RI, Shin DM. Recent advances in head and neck cancer. *N Engl J Med* 2008;359:1143–1154.

66. Taylor SG 4th, McGuire WP, Hauck WW, et al. A randomized comparison of high-dose infusion methotrexate versus standard-dose weekly therapy in head and neck squamous cancer. *J Clin Oncol* 1984;2:1006–1011.

68. Schornagel JH, Verweij J, de Mulder PH, et al. Randomized phase III trial of edatrexate versus methotrexate in patients with metastatic and/or recurrent squamous cell carcinoma of the head and neck: a European Organization for Research and Treatment of Cancer Head and Neck Cancer Cooperative Group study. *J Clin Oncol* 1995;13:1649–1655.

71. Forastiere AA, Shank D, Neuberg D, et al. Final report of a phase II evaluation of paclitaxel in patients with advanced squamous cell carcinoma of the head and neck: an Eastern Cooperative Oncology Group trial (PA390). *Cancer* 1998;82:2270–2274.

79. Baselga J, Trigo JM, Bourhis J, et al. Phase II multicenter study of the antiepidermal growth factor receptor monoclonal antibody cetuximab in combination with platinum-based chemotherapy in patients with platinum-refractory metastatic and/or recurrent squamous cell carcinoma of the head and neck. *J Clin Oncol* 2005;23:5568–5577.

82. Burtness B, Goldwasser MA, Flood W, et al. Phase III randomized trial of cisplatin plus placebo compared with cisplatin plus cetuximab in metastatic/recurrent head and neck cancer: an Eastern Cooperative Oncology Group study. *J Clin Oncol* 2005;23:8646–8654.

89. Johnson DH, Fehrenbacher L, Novotny WF, et al. Randomized phase II trial comparing bevacizumab plus carboplatin and paclitaxel with carboplatin and paclitaxel alone in previously untreated locally advanced or metastatic non-small-cell lung cancer. *J Clin Oncol* 2004;22:2184–2191.

106. Forastiere AA, Leong T, Rowinsky E, et al. Phase III comparison of high-dose paclitaxel + cisplatin + granulocyte colony-stimulating factor versus low-dose paclitaxel + cisplatin in advanced head and neck cancer: Eastern Cooperative Oncology Group Study E1393. *J Clin Oncol* 2001;19:1088–1095.

107. Gibson MK, Li Y, Murphy B, et al. Randomized phase III evaluation of cisplatin plus fluorouracil versus cisplatin plus paclitaxel in advanced head and neck cancer (E1395): an intergroup trial of the Eastern Cooperative Oncology Group. *J Clin Oncol* 2005;23:3562–3567.

114. Vermorken JB, Mesia R, Rivera F, et al. Platinum-based chemotherapy plus cetuximab in head and neck cancer. *N Engl J Med* 2008;359:1116–1127.

116. Licitra L, Mesia R, Rivera F, et al. Evaluation of EGFR gene copy number as a predictive biomarker for the efficacy of cetuximab in combination with chemotherapy in the first-line treatment of recurrent and/or metastatic squamous cell carcinoma of the head and neck: EXTREME study. *Ann Oncol* 2011;22:1078–1087.

117. Licitra L, Storkel S, Kerr KM, et al. Predictive value of epidermal growth factor receptor expression for first-line chemotherapy plus cetuximab in patients with head and neck and colorectal cancer: analysis of data from the EXTREME and CRYSTAL studies. *Eur J Cancer* 2013;49:1161–1168.

118. Vermorken JB, Trigo J, Hitt R, et al. Open-label, uncontrolled, multicenter phase II study to evaluate the efficacy and toxicity of cetuximab as a single agent in patients with recurrent and/or metastatic squamous cell carcinoma of the head and neck who failed to respond to platinum-based therapy. *J Clin Oncol* 2007;25:2171–2177.

121. De Crevoisier R, Bourhis J, Domenge C, et al. Full-dose reirradiation for unresectable head and neck carcinoma: experience at the Gustave-Roussy Institute in a series of 169 patients. *J Clin Oncol* 1998;16:3556–3562.

122. Spencer SA, Harris J, Wheeler RH, et al. RTOG 96-10: reirradiation with concurrent hydroxyurea and 5-fluorouracil in patients with squamous cell cancer of the head and neck. *Int J Radiat Oncol Biol Phys* 2001;51:1299–1304.

142. Tupchong L, Scott CB, Blitzer PH, et al. Randomized study of preoperative versus postoperative radiation therapy in advanced head and neck carcinoma: long-term follow-up of RTOG study 73-03. *Int J Radiat Oncol Biol Phys* 1991;20:21–28.

143. Huang DT, Johnson CR, Schmidt-Ullrich R, et al. Postoperative radiotherapy in head and neck carcinoma with extracapsular lymph node extension and/or positive resection margins: a comparative study. *Int J Radiat Oncol Biol Phys* 1992;23:737–742.

144. Lundahl RE, Foote RL, Bonner JA, et al. Combined neck dissection and postoperative radiation therapy in the management of the high-risk neck: a matched-pair analysis. *Int J Radiat Oncol Biol Phys* 1998;40:529–534.

146. National Comprehensive Cancer Network (NCCN). Clinical Practice Guidelines in Oncology: Head and Neck Cancers. NCCN Web site. http://www.nccn.org/professionals/physician_gls/PDF/head-and-neck.pdf.Accessed October 21, 2013.

147. Calais G, Alfonsi M, Bardet E, et al. Randomized trial of radiation therapy versus concomitant chemotherapy and radiation therapy for advanced-stage oropharynx carcinoma. *J Natl Cancer Inst* 1999;91:2081–2086.

148. Forastiere AA, Goepfert H, Maor M, et al. Concurrent chemotherapy and radiotherapy for organ preservation in advanced laryngeal cancer. *N Engl J Med* 2003;349:2091–2098.

149. Pignon JP, Bourhis J, Domenge C, et al. Chemotherapy added to locoregional treatment for head and neck squamous-cell carcinoma: three meta-analyses of updated individual data. MACH-NC Collaborative Group. Meta-Analysis of Chemotherapy on Head and Neck Cancer. *Lancet* 2000;355:949–955.

PRACTICE OF ONCOLOGY

150. Adelstein DJ, Leblanc M. Does induction chemotherapy have a role in the management of locoregionally advanced squamous cell head and neck cancer? *J Clin Oncol* 2006;24:2624–2628.

151. Induction chemotherapy plus radiation compared with surgery plus radiation in patients with advanced laryngeal cancer. The Department of Veterans Affairs Laryngeal Cancer Study Group. *N Engl J Med* 1991;324:1685–1690.

152. Lefebvre JL, Chevalier D, Luboinski B, et al. Larynx preservation in pyriform sinus cancer: preliminary results of a European Organization for Research and Treatment of Cancer phase III trial. EORTC Head and Neck Cancer Cooperative Group. *J Natl Cancer Inst* 1996;88:890–899.

153. Brockstein B, Haraf DJ, Rademaker AW, et al. Patterns of failure, prognostic factors and survival in locoregionally advanced head and neck cancer treated with concomitant chemoradiotherapy: a 9-year, 337-patient, multi-institutional experience. *Ann Oncol* 2004;15:1179–1186.

158. Posner MR, Hershock DM, Blajman CR, et al. Cisplatin and fluorouracil alone or with docetaxel in head and neck cancer. *N Engl J Med* 2007;357:1705–1715.

159. Hitt R, Grau JJ, Lopez-Pousa A, et al. Final results of a randomized phase III trial comparing induction chemotherapy with cisplatin/5-FU or docetaxel/cisplatin/5-FU follow by chemoradiotherapy (CRT) versus CRT alone as first-line treatment of unresectable locally advanced head and neck cancer (LAHNC). *J Clin Oncol* 2009;27:S6009.

160. Haddad R, O'Neill A, Rabinowits G, et al. Induction chemotherapy followed by concurrent chemoradiotherapy (sequential chemoradiotherapy) versus concurrent chemoradiotherapy alone in locally advanced head and neck cancer (PARADIGM): a randomised phase 3 trial. *Lancet Oncol* 2013;14:257–264.

162. Zhong LP, Zhang CP, Ren GX, et al. Randomized phase III trial of induction chemotherapy with docetaxel, cisplatin, and fluorouracil followed by surgery versus up-front surgery in locally advanced resectable oral squamous cell carcinoma. *J Clin Oncol* 2013;31:744–751.

163. Lefebvre JL, Pointreau Y, Rolland F, et al. Induction chemotherapy followed by either chemoradiotherapy or bioradiotherapy for larynx preservation: the TREMPLIN randomized phase II study. *J Clin Oncol* 2013;31:853–859.

164. Merlano M, Benasso M, Corvo R, et al. Five-year update of a randomized trial of alternating radiotherapy and chemotherapy compared with radiotherapy alone in treatment of unresectable squamous cell carcinoma of the head and neck. *J Natl Cancer Inst* 1996;88:583–589.

166. Pignon JP, le Maitre A, Maillard E, et al. Meta-analysis of chemotherapy in head and neck cancer (MACH-NC): an update on 93 randomised trials and 17,346 patients. *Radiother Oncol* 2009;92:4–14.

167. Adelstein DJ, Li Y, Adams GL, et al. An intergroup phase III comparison of standard radiation therapy and two schedules of concurrent chemoradiotherapy in patients with unresectable squamous cell head and neck cancer. *J Clin Oncol* 2003;21:92–98.

169. Quon H, Leong T, Haselow R, et al. Phase III study of radiation therapy with or without cis-platinum in patients with unresectable squamous or undifferentiated carcinoma of the head and neck: an intergroup trial of the Eastern Cooperative Oncology Group (E2382). *Int J Radiat Oncol Biol Phys* 2011;81:719–725.

170. Robbins KT, Kumar P, Wong FS, et al. Targeted chemoradiation for advanced head and neck cancer: analysis of 213 patients. *Head Neck* 2000;22:687–693.

171. Regine WF, Valentino J, Arnold SM, et al. High-dose intra-arterial cisplatin boost with hyperfractionated radiation therapy for advanced squamous cell carcinoma of the head and neck. *J Clin Oncol* 2001;19:3333–3339.

172. Rasch CR, Hauptmann M, Schornagel J, et al. Intra-arterial versus intravenous chemoradiation for advanced head and neck cancer: Results of a randomized phase 3 trial. *Cancer* 2010;116:2159–2165.

177. Hoff CM, Lassen P, Eriksen JG, et al. Does transfusion improve the outcome for HNSCC patients treated with radiotherapy? Results from the randomized DAHANCA 5 and 7 trials. *Acta Oncol* 2011;50:1006–1014.

178. Overgaard J. Hypoxic modification of radiotherapy in squamous cell carcinoma of the head and neck—a systematic review and meta-analysis. *Radiother Oncol* 2011;100:22–32.

179. Rischin D, Peters LJ, O'Sullivan B, et al. Tirapazamine, cisplatin, and radiation versus cisplatin and radiation for advanced squamous cell carcinoma of the head and neck (TROG 02.02, HeadSTART): a phase III trial of the Trans-Tasman Radiation Oncology Group. *J Clin Oncol* 2010;28:2989–2995.

180. Janssens GO, Rademakers SE, Terhaard CH, et al. Accelerated radiotherapy with carbogen and nicotinamide for laryngeal cancer: results of a phase III randomized trial. *J Clin Oncol* 2012;30:1777–1783.

181. Bourhis J, Overgaard J, Audry H, et al. Hyperfractionated or accelerated radiotherapy in head and neck cancer: a meta-analysis. *Lancet* 2006;368:843–854.

182. Brizel DM, Albers ME, Fisher SR, et al. Hyperfractionated irradiation with or without concurrent chemotherapy for locally advanced head and neck cancer. *N Engl J Med* 1998;338:1798–1804.

184. Bourhis J, Sire C, Graff P, et al. Concomitant chemoradiotherapy versus acceleration of radiotherapy with or without concomitant chemotherapy in locally advanced head and neck carcinoma (GORTEC 99-02): an open-label phase 3 randomised trial. *Lancet Oncol* 2012;13:145–153.

185. Bonner JA, Harari PM, Giralt J, et al. Radiotherapy plus cetuximab for squamous-cell carcinoma of the head and neck. *N Engl J Med* 2006;354:567–578.

186. Bonner JA, Harari PM, Giralt J, et al. Radiotherapy plus cetuximab for locoregionally advanced head and neck cancer: 5-year survival data from a phase 3 randomised trial, and relation between cetuximab-induced rash and survival. *Lancet Oncol* 2010;11:21–28.

187. Pfister DG, Su YB, Kraus DH, et al. Concurrent cetuximab, cisplatin, and concomitant boost radiotherapy for locoregionally advanced, squamous cell head and neck cancer: a pilot phase II study of a new combined-modality paradigm. *J Clin Oncol* 2006;24:1072–1078.

188. Ang KK, Zhang QE, Rosenthal DI, et al. A randomized phase III trial (RTOG 0522) of concurrent accelerated radiation plus cisplatin with or without cetuximab for stage III-IV head and neck squamous cell carcinomas (HNC). *J Clin Oncol* 2011;29:S5500.

189. Denis F, Garaud P, Bardet E, et al. Late toxicity results of the GORTEC 94-01 randomized trial comparing radiotherapy with concomitant radiochemotherapy for advanced-stage oropharynx carcinoma: comparison of LENT/SOMA, RTOG/EORTC, and NCI-CTC scoring systems. *Int J Radiat Oncol Biol Phys* 2003;55:9–98.

190. Al-Sarraf M, LeBlanc M, Giri PG, et al. Chemoradiotherapy versus radiotherapy in patients with advanced nasopharyngeal cancer: phase III randomized Intergroup study 0099. *J Clin Oncol* 1998;16:1310–1317.

191. Lin JC, Jan JS, Hsu CY, et al. Phase III study of concurrent chemoradiotherapy versus radiotherapy alone for advanced nasopharyngeal carcinoma: positive effect on overall and progression-free survival. *J Clin Oncol* 2003;21:631–637.

192. Chan AT, Teo PM, Ngan RK, et al. Concurrent chemotherapy-radiotherapy compared with radiotherapy alone in locoregionally advanced nasopharyngeal carcinoma: progression-free survival analysis of a phase III randomized trial. *J Clin Oncol* 2002;20:2038–2044.

193. Chan AT, Hui EP, Ma BB, et al. A randomized phase II study of concurrent cisplatin-radiotherapy (RT) with or without neoadjuvant chemotherapy using docetaxel and cisplatin in advanced nasopharyngeal carcinoma (NPC) *J Clin Oncol* 2005;23:S5544.

194. Wee J, Tan EH, Tai BC, et al. Randomized trial of radiotherapy versus concurrent chemoradiotherapy followed by adjuvant chemotherapy in patients with American Joint Committee on Cancer/International Union against cancer stage III and IV nasopharyngeal cancer of the endemic variety. *J Clin Oncol* 2005;23:6730–6738.

196. Chitapanarux I, Lorvidhaya V, Kamnerdsupaphon P, et al. Chemoradiation comparing cisplatin versus carboplatin in locally advanced nasopharyngeal cancer: randomised, non-inferiority, open trial. *Eur J Cancer* 2007;43:1399–1406.

197. Huang PY, Cao KJ, Guo X, et al. A randomized trial of induction chemotherapy plus concurrent chemoradiotherapy versus induction chemotherapy plus radiotherapy for locoregionally advanced nasopharyngeal carcinoma. *Oral Oncol* 2012;48:1038–1044.

200. Chua DT, Ma J, Sham JS, et al. Long-term survival after cisplatin-based induction chemotherapy and radiotherapy for nasopharyngeal carcinoma: a pooled data analysis of two phase III trials. *J Clin Oncol* 2005;23:1118–1124.

201. Baujat B, Audry H, Bourhis J, et al. Chemotherapy in locally advanced nasopharyngeal carcinoma: an individual patient data meta-analysis of eight randomized trials and 1753 patients. *Int J Radiat Oncol Biol Phys* 2006;64:47–56.

207. Pfister DG, Laurie SA, Weinstein GS, et al. American Society of Clinical Oncology clinical practice guideline for the use of larynx-preservation strategies in the treatment of laryngeal cancer. *J Clin Oncol* 2006;24:3693–3704.

208. McNeil BJ, Weichselbaum R, Pauker SG. Speech and survival: tradeoffs between quality and quantity of life in laryngeal cancer. *N Engl J Med* 1981;305:982–987.

212. Forastiere AA, Zhang Q, Weber RS, et al. Long-term results of RTOG 91-11: a comparison of three nonsurgical treatment strategies to preserve the larynx in patients with locally advanced larynx cancer. *J Clin Oncol* 2013;31:845–852.

213. Lefebvre JL, Rolland F, Tesselaar M, et al. Phase 3 randomized trial on larynx preservation comparing sequential vs alternating chemotherapy and radiotherapy. *J Natl Cancer Inst* 2009;101:142–152.

214. Adelstein DJ, Lavertu P, Saxton JP, et al. Mature results of a phase III randomized trial comparing concurrent chemoradiotherapy with radiation therapy alone in patients with stage III and IV squamous cell carcinoma of the head and neck. *Cancer* 2000;88:876–883.

215. Licitra L, Grandi C, Guzzo M, et al. Primary chemotherapy in resectable oral cavity squamous cell cancer: a randomized controlled trial. *J Clin Oncol* 2003;21:327–333.

216. Laccourreye O, Veivers D, Hans S, et al. Chemotherapy alone with curative intent in patients with invasive squamous cell carcinoma of the pharyngolarynx classified as T1-T4N0M0 complete clinical responders. *Cancer* 2001;92:1504–1511.

217. Urba S, Wolf G, Eisbruch A, et al. Single-cycle induction chemotherapy selects patients with advanced laryngeal cancer for combined chemoradiation: a new treatment paradigm. *J Clin Oncol* 2006;24:593–598.

223. Weissberg JB, Son YH, Papac RJ, et al. Randomized clinical trial of mitomycin C as an adjunct to radiotherapy in head and neck cancer. *Int J Radiat Oncol Biol Phys* 1989;17:3–9.

224. Haffty BG, Son YH, Sasaki CT, et al. Mitomycin C as an adjunct to postoperative radiation therapy in squamous cell carcinoma of the head and neck: results from two randomized clinical trials. *Int J Radiat Oncol Biol Phys* 1993;27:241–250.

225. Janot F, de Raucourt D, Benhamou E, et al. Randomized trial of postoperative reirradiation combined with chemotherapy after salvage surgery compared with salvage surgery alone in head and neck carcinoma. *J Clin Oncol* 2008;26:5518–5523.

226. Haughey BH, Sinha P. Prognostic factors and survival unique to surgically treated p16+ oropharyngeal cancer. *Laryngoscope* 2012;122:S13–S33.
227. Daly ME, Lieskovsky Y, Pawlicki T, et al. Evaluation of patterns of failure and subjective salivary function in patients treated with intensity modulated radiotherapy for head and neck squamous cell carcinoma. *Head Neck* 2007;29:211–220.
229. Wang ZH, Yan C, Zhang ZY, et al. Impact of salivary gland dosimetry on post-IMRT recovery of saliva output and xerostomia grade for head-and-neck cancer patients treated with or without contralateral submandibular gland sparing: a longitudinal study. *Int J Radiat Oncol Biol Phys* 2011;81:1479–1487.
233. Brizel DM, Wasserman TH, Henke M, et al. Phase III randomized trial of amifostine as a radioprotector in head and neck cancer. *J Clin Oncol* 2000;18:3339–3345.
236. Trotti A, Garden A, Warde P, et al. A multinational, randomized phase III trial of iseganan HCl oral solution for reducing the severity of oral mucositis in patients receiving radiotherapy for head-and-neck malignancy. *Int J Radiat Oncol Biol Phys* 2004;58:674–681.
237. Stiff PJ, Emmanouilides C, Bensinger WI, et al. Palifermin reduces patient-reported mouth and throat soreness and improves patient functioning in the hematopoietic stem-cell transplantation setting. *J Clin Oncol* 2006;24:5186–5193.
238. Le QT, Kim HE, Schneider CJ, et al. Palifermin reduces severe mucositis in definitive chemoradiotherapy of locally advanced head and neck cancer: a randomized, placebo-controlled study. *J Clin Oncol* 2011;29:2808–2814.
239. Henke M, Alfonsi M, Foa P, et al. Palifermin decreases severe oral mucositis of patients undergoing postoperative radiochemotherapy for head and neck cancer: a randomized, placebo-controlled trial. *J Clin Oncol* 2011;29:2815–2820.
240. Fitzpatrick PJ. Cancer of the lip. *J Otolaryngol* 1984;13:32–36.
241. Byers RM, O'Brien J, Waxler J. The therapeutic and prognostic implications of nerve invasion in cancer of the lower lip. *Int J Radiat Oncol Biol Phys* 1978;4:215–217.
242. Mackay EN, Sellers AH. A statistical review of carcinoma of the lip. *Can Med Assoc J* 1964;90:670–672.
243. Mohs FE, Snow SN. Microscopically controlled surgical treatment for squamous cell carcinoma of the lower lip. *Surg Gynecol Obstet* 1985;160:37–41.
245. Chu A, Fletcher GH. Incidence and causes of failures to control by irradiation the primary lesions in squamous cell carcinomas of the anterior two-thirds of the tongue and floor of mouth. *Am J Roentgenol Radium Ther Nucl Med* 1973;117:502–508.
246. Wang CC, Biggs PJ. Technical and radiotherapeutic considerations of intra-oral cone electron beam radiation therapy for head and neck cancer. *Semin Radiat Oncol* 1992;2:171–179.
247. Rodgers LW Jr., Stringer SP, Mendenhall WM, et al. Management of squamous cell carcinoma of the floor of mouth. *Head Neck* 1993;15:16–19.
248. Pernot M, Hoffstetter S, Peiffert D, et al. Epidermoid carcinomas of the floor of mouth treated by exclusive irradiation: statistical study of a series of 207 cases. *Radiother Oncol* 1995;35:177–185.
249. Byers RM, Weber RS, Andrews T, et al. Frequency and therapeutic implications of "skip metastases" in the neck from squamous carcinoma of the oral tongue. *Head Neck* 1997;19:14–19.
250. Mendenhall WM, Van Cise WS, Bova FJ, et al. Analysis of time-dose factors in squamous cell carcinoma of the oral tongue and floor of mouth treated with radiation therapy alone. *Int J Radiat Oncol Biol Phys* 1981;7:1005–1011.
251. Mendenhall WM, Parsons JT, Stringer SP, et al. T2 oral tongue carcinoma treated with radiotherapy: analysis of local control and complications. *Radiother Oncol* 1989;16:275–281.
252. Wendt CD, Peters LJ, Delclos L, et al. Primary radiotherapy in the treatment of stage I and II oral tongue cancers: importance of the proportion of therapy delivered with interstitial therapy. *Int J Radiat Oncol Biol Phys* 1990;18:1287–1292.
253. Fein DA, Mendenhall WM, Parsons JT, et al. Carcinoma of the oral tongue: a comparison of results and complications of treatment with radiotherapy and/or surgery. *Head Neck* 1994;16:358–365.
254. Pernot M, Malissard L, Hoffstetter S, et al. The study of tumoral, radiobiological, and general health factors that influence results and complications in a series of 448 oral tongue carcinomas treated exclusively by irradiation. *Int J Radiat Oncol Biol Phys* 1994;29:673–679.
255. Chang DT, Sandow PR, Morris CG, et al. Do pre-irradiation dental extractions reduce the risk of osteoradionecrosis of the mandible? *Head Neck* 2007;29:528–536.
256. Nair MK, Sankaranarayanan R, Padmanabhan TK. Evaluation of the role of radiotherapy in the management of carcinoma of the buccal mucosa. *Cancer* 1988;61:1326–1331.
257. Diaz EM Jr., Holsinger FC, Zuniga ER, et al. Squamous cell carcinoma of the buccal mucosa: one institution's experience with 119 previously untreated patients. *Head Neck* 2003;25:267–273.
258. Mendenhall WM, Morris CG, Amdur RJ, et al. Radiotherapy alone or combined with surgery for adenoid cystic carcinoma of the head and neck. *Head Neck* 2004;26:154–162.
259. Mendenhall WM, Amdur RJ, Hinerman RW, et al. Head and neck mucosal melanoma. *Am J Clin Oncol* 2005;28:626–630.
260. Mendenhall WM, Werning JW, Fernandes R, et al. Ameloblastoma. *Am J Clin Oncol* 2007;30:645–648.
261. Cianchetti M, Sandow PS, Scarborough LD, et al. Radiation therapy for minor salivary gland carcinoma. *Laryngoscope* 2009;119:1334–1338.
262. Sehdev MK, Huvos AG, Strong EW, et al. Proceedings: Ameloblastoma of maxilla and mandible. *Cancer* 1974;33:324–333.
263. Mendenhall WM, Morris CG, Amdur RJ, et al. Retromolar trigone squamous cell carcinoma treated with radiotherapy alone or combined with surgery. *Cancer* 2005;103:2320–2325.
264. Million RR, Cassisi NJ. General principles for treatment of cancers in the head and neck: selection of treatment for the primary site and for the neck. In: Million RR, Cassisi NJ, eds. *Management of Head and Neck Cancer: A Multidisciplinary Approach*, 1st ed. Philadelphia: J. B. Lippincott Company; 1984: 43–62.
265. Overholt SM, Eicher SA, Wolf P, et al. Prognostic factors affecting outcome in lower gingival carcinoma. *Laryngoscope* 1996;106:1335–1339.
266. Byers RM, Anderson B, Schwarz EA, et al. Treatment of squamous carcinoma of the retromolar trigone. *Am J Clin Oncol* 1984;7:647–652.
267. Shibuya H, Horiuchi J, Suzuki S, et al. Oral carcinoma of the upper jaw. Results of radiation treatment. *Acta Radiol Oncol* 1984;23:331–335.
268. Huang CJ, Chao KS, Tsai J, et al. Cancer of retromolar trigone: long-term radiation therapy outcome. *Head Neck* 2001;23:758–763.
269. Mendenhall WM, Morris CG, Amdur RJ, et al. Radiotherapy alone or combined with surgery for salivary gland carcinoma. *Cancer* 2005;103:2544–2550.
270. Mendenhall WM, Mendenhall CM, Mendenhall NP. Solitary plasmacytoma of bone and soft tissues. *Am J Otolaryngol* 2003;24:395–399.
271. Lindberg RD, Barkley HT Jr., Jesse RH, et al. Evolution of the clinically negative neck in patients with squamous cell carcinoma of the faucial arch. *Am J Roentgenol Radium Ther Nucl Med* 1971;111:60–65.
272. Mendenhall WM, Morris CG, Amdur RJ, et al. Definitive radiotherapy for squamous cell carcinoma of the base of tongue. *Am J Clin Oncol* 2006;29:32–39.
273. Steiner W, Fierek O, Ambrosch P, et al. Transoral laser microsurgery for squamous cell carcinoma of the base of the tongue. *Arch Otolaryngol Head Neck Surg* 2003;129:36–43.
274. Al-Othman MO, Amdur RJ, Morris CG, et al. Does feeding tube placement predict for long-term swallowing disability after radiotherapy for head and neck cancer? *Head Neck* 2003;25:741–747.
275. Mendenhall WM, Morris CG, Amdur RJ, et al. Definitive radiotherapy for tonsillar squamous cell carcinoma. *Am J Clin Oncol* 2006;29:290–297.
276. Chera BS, Amdur RJ, Hinerman RW, et al. Definitive radiation therapy for squamous cell carcinoma of the soft palate. *Head Neck* 2008;30:1114–1119.
277. Vincent RG, Marchetta F. The relationship of the use of tobacco and alcohol to cancer of the oral cavity, pharynx or larynx. *Am J Surg* 1963;106:501–505.
278. Pillsbury HR, Kirchner JA. Clinical vs histopathologic staging in laryngeal cancer. *Arch Otolaryngol* 1979;105:157–159.
279. Chera BS, Amdur RJ, Morris CG, et al. T1N0 to T2N0 squamous cell carcinoma of the glottic larynx treated with definitive radiotherapy. *Int J Radiat Oncol Biol Phys* 2010;78:461–466.
280. Olsen KD, DeSanto LW, Pearson BW. Positive Delphian lymph node: clinical significance in laryngeal cancer. *Laryngoscope* 1987;97:1033–1037.
281. Lederman M. [The place of radiotherapy in the treatment of cancer of the larynx]. *Ann Radiol (Paris)* 1961;4:433–454.
282. Garcia-Serra A, Hinerman RW, Amdur RJ, et al. Radiotherapy for carcinoma in situ of the true vocal cords. *Head Neck* 2002;24:390–394.
283. Mendenhall WM, Werning JW, Hinerman RW, et al. Management of T1-T2 glottic carcinomas. *Cancer* 2004;100:1786–1792.
284. Mendenhall WM, Parsons JT, Stringer SP, et al. Stage T3 squamous cell carcinoma of the glottic larynx: a comparison of laryngectomy and irradiation. *Int J Radiat Oncol Biol Phys* 1992;23:725–732.
285. Mendenhall WM, Parsons JT, Mancuso AA, et al. Definitive radiotherapy for T3 squamous cell carcinoma of the glottic larynx. *J Clin Oncol* 1997;15:2394–2402.
286. Weinstein GS, El-Sawy MM, Ruiz C, et al. Laryngeal preservation with supracricoid partial laryngectomy results in improved quality of life when compared with total laryngectomy. *Laryngoscope* 2001;111:191–199.
287. Mendenhall WM, Morris CG, Stringer SP, et al. Voice rehabilitation after total laryngectomy and postoperative radiation therapy. *J Clin Oncol* 2002;20:2500–2505.
288. Yamazaki H, Nishiyama K, Tanaka E, et al. Radiotherapy for early glottic carcinoma (T1N0M0): results of prospective randomized study of radiation fraction size and overall treatment time. *Int J Radiat Oncol Biol Phys* 2006;64:77–82.
289. Gluckman JL, Hamaker RC, Schuller DE, et al. Surgical salvage for stomal recurrence: a multi-institutional experience. *Laryngoscope* 1987;97:1025–1029.
290. Mendenhall WM, Morris CG, Amdur RJ, et al. Parameters that predict local control after definitive radiotherapy for squamous cell carcinoma of the head and neck. *Head Neck* 2003;25:535–542.
291. Mancuso AA, Mukherji SK, Schmalfuss I, et al. Preradiotherapy computed tomography as a predictor of local control in supraglottic carcinoma. *J Clin Oncol* 1999;17:631–637.
292. Somerset JD, Mendenhall WM, Amdur RJ, et al. Planned postradiotherapy bilateral neck dissection for head and neck cancer. *Am J Otolaryngol* 2001;22:383–386.

PRACTICE OF ONCOLOGY

293. Thomas JV, Olsen KD, Neel HB 3rd, et al. Early glottic carcinoma treated with open laryngeal procedures. *Arch Otolaryngol Head Neck Surg* 1994;120: 264–268.

294. Som ML. Cordal cancer with extension to vocal process. *Laryngoscope* 1975; 85:1298–1307.

295. Foote RL, Olsen KD, Buskirk SJ, et al. Laryngectomy alone for T3 glottic cancer. *Head Neck* 1994;16:406–412.

296. Hinerman RW, Mendenhall WM, Morris CG, et al. T3 and T4 true vocal cord squamous carcinomas treated with external beam irradiation: a single institution's 35-year experience. *Am J Clin Oncol* 2007;30:181–185.

297. Pameijer FA, Mancuso AA, Mendenhall WM, et al. Can pretreatment computed tomography predict local control in T3 squamous cell carcinoma of the glottic larynx treated with definitive radiotherapy? *Int J Radiat Oncol Biol Phys* 1997;37:1011–1021.

298. Jesse RH. The evaluation of treatment of patients with extensive squamous cancer of the vocal cords. *Laryngoscope* 1975;85:1424–1429.

299. Ogura JH, Sessions DG, Spector GJ. Analysis of surgical therapy for epidermoid carcinoma of the laryngeal glottis. *Laryngoscope* 1975;85: 1522–1530.

300. Skolnik EM, Yee KF, Wheatley MA, et al. Carcinoma of the laryngeal glottis therapy and end results. *Laryngoscope* 1975;85:1453–1466.

301. Vermund H. Role of radiotherapy in cancer of the larynx as related to the TNM system of staging. A review. *Cancer* 1970;25:485–504.

302. Stewart JG, Jackson AW. The steepness of the dose response curve both for tumor cure and normal tissue injury. *Laryngoscope* 1975;85:1107–1111.

303. Harwood AR, Beale FA, Cummings BJ, et al. T4N0M0 glottic cancer: an analysis of dose-time volume factors. *Int J Radiat Oncol Biol Phys* 1981;7:1507–1512.

304. Hinerman RW, Mendenhall WM, Amdur RJ, et al. Carcinoma of the supraglottic larynx: treatment results with radiotherapy alone or with planned neck dissection. *Head Neck* 2002;24:456–467.

305. Lee NK, Goepfert H, Wendt CD. Supraglottic laryngectomy for intermediate-stage cancer: U.T. M.D. Anderson Cancer Center experience with combined therapy. *Laryngoscope* 1990;100:831–836.

306. Ambrosch P, Kron M, Steiner W. Carbon dioxide laser microsurgery for early supraglottic carcinoma. *Ann Otol Rhinol Laryngol* 1998;107:680–688.

307. Neel HB 3rd, Devine KD, Desanto LW. Laryngofissure and cordectomy for early cordal carcinoma: outcome in 182 patients. *Otolaryngol Head Neck Surg (1979)* 1980;88:79–84.

308. Kirchner JA. Pyriform sinus cancer: a clinical and laboratory study. *Ann Otol Rhinol Laryngol* 1975;84:793–803.

309. Ogura JH, Biller HF, Wette R. Elective neck dissection for pharyngeal and laryngeal cancers. An evaluation. *Ann Otol Rhinol Laryngol* 1971;80:646–650.

310. Pameijer FA, Mancuso AA, Mendenhall WM, et al. Evaluation of pretreatment computed tomography as a predictor of local control in T1/T2 pyriform sinus carcinoma treated with definitive radiotherapy. *Head Neck* 1998;20:159–168.

311. Rabbani A, Amdur RJ, Mancuso AA, et al. Definitive radiotherapy for T1-T2 squamous cell carcinoma of pyriform sinus. *Int J Radiat Oncol Biol Phys* 2008;72:351–355.

312. Mendenhall WM, Morris CG, Kirwan JM, et al. Definitive radiation therapy for squamous cell carcinoma of the pharyngeal wall. *Prac Radiat Oncol* 2012;2:e113–e119.

313. Marks JE, Kurnik B, Powers WE, et al. Carcinoma of the pyriform sinus. An analysis of treatment results and patterns of failure. *Cancer* 1978;41: 1008–1015.

314. Marks JE, Freeman RB, Lee F, et al. Pharyngeal wall cancer: an analysis of treatment results complications and patterns of failure. *Int J Radiat Oncol Biol Phys* 1978;4:587–593.

315. Ho JH. An epidemiologic and clinical study of nasopharyngeal carcinoma. *Int J Radiat Oncol Biol Phys* 1978;4:182–198.

316. Fletcher GH, Million RR. Malignant tumors of the nasopharynx. *Am J Roentgenol Radium Ther Nucl Med* 1965;93:44–55.

317. Chi KH, Chang YC, Guo WY, et al. A phase III study of adjuvant chemotherapy in advanced nasopharyngeal carcinoma patients. *Int J Radiat Oncol Biol Phys* 2002;52:1238–1244.

318. Chow E, Payne D, O'Sullivan B, et al. Radiotherapy alone in patients with advanced nasopharyngeal cancer: comparison with an intergroup study. Is combined modality treatment really necessary? *Radiother Oncol* 2002;63:269–274.

319. Leung TW, Tung SY, Sze WK, et al. Salvage radiation therapy for locally recurrent nasopharyngeal carcinoma. *Int J Radiat Oncol Biol Phys* 2000;48:1331–1338.

320. Mendenhall WM, Mendenhall CM, Malyapa RS, et al. Re-irradiation of head and neck carcinoma. *Am J Clin Oncol* 2008;31:393–398.

321. Lee AW, Poon YF, Foo W, et al. Retrospective analysis of 5037 patients with nasopharyngeal carcinoma treated during 1976-1985: overall survival and patterns of failure. *Int J Radiat Oncol Biol Phys* 1992;23:261–270.

322. Leung TW, Tung SY, Sze WK, et al. Treatment results of 1070 patients with nasopharyngeal carcinoma: an analysis of survival and failure patterns. *Head Neck* 2005;27:555–565.

323. Chua DT, Sham JS, Kwong DL, et al. Volumetric analysis of tumor extent in nasopharyngeal carcinoma and correlation with treatment outcome. *Int J Radiat Oncol Biol Phys* 1997;39:711–719.

324. Teo P, Yu P, Lee WY, et al. Significant prognosticators after primary radiotherapy in 903 nondisseminated nasopharyngeal carcinoma evaluated by computer tomography. *Int J Radiat Oncol Biol Phys* 1996;36:291–304.

325. Mendenhall WM, Morris CG, Hinerman RW, et al. Definitive radiotherapy for nasopharyngeal carcinoma. *Am J Clin Oncol* 2006;29:622–627.

326. Bhandare N, Monroe AT, Morris CG, et al. Does altered fractionation influence the risk of radiation-induced optic neuropathy? *Int J Radiat Oncol Biol Phys* 2005;62:1070–1077.

327. Monroe AT, Bhandare N, Morris CG, et al. Preventing radiation retinopathy with hyperfractionation. *Int J Radiat Oncol Biol Phys* 2005;61:856–864.

328. Monroe AT, Hinerman RW, Amdur RJ, et al. Radiation therapy for esthesioneuroblastoma: rationale for elective neck irradiation. *Head Neck* 2003;25: 529–534.

329. Gomez JA, Mendenhall WM, Tannehill SP, et al. Radiation therapy in inverted papillomas of the nasal cavity and paranasal sinuses. *Am J Otolaryngol* 2000;21:174–178.

330. Mendenhall WM, Mendenhall CM, Riggs CE Jr., et al. Sinonasal undifferentiated carcinoma. *Am J Clin Oncol* 2006;29:27–31.

331. Mendenhall WM, Mendenhall CM, Werning JW, et al. Adult head and neck soft tissue sarcomas. *Head Neck* 2005;27:916–922.

332. Mendenhall WM, Olivier KR, Lynch JW Jr., et al. Lethal midline granulomatosal natural killer/T-cell lymphoma. *Am J Clin Oncol* 2006;29:202–206.

333. Wallace A, Morris CG, Kirwan J, et al. Radiotherapy for squamous cell carcinoma of the nasal vestibule. *Am J Clin Oncol* 2007;30:612–616.

334. Weissler MC, Montgomery WW, Turner PA, et al. Inverted papilloma. *Ann Otol Rhinol Laryngol* 1986;95:215–221.

335. Mendenhall WM, Amdur RJ, Morris CG, et al. Carcinoma of the nasal cavity and paranasal sinuses. *Laryngoscope* 2009;119:899–906.

336. Goepfert H, Guillamondegui OM, Jesse RH, et al. Squamous cell carcinoma of nasal vestibule. *Arch Otolaryngol* 1974;100:8–10.

337. Elkon D, Hightower SI, Lim ML, et al. Esthesioneuroblastoma. *Cancer* 1979;44:1087–1094.

338. Waldron JN, O'Sullivan B, Gullane P, et al. Carcinoma of the maxillary antrum: a retrospective analysis of 110 cases. *Radiother Oncol* 2000;57: 167–173.

339. Parsons JT, Bova FJ, Fitzgerald CR, et al. Radiation retinopathy after external-beam irradiation: analysis of time-dose factors. *Int J Radiat Oncol Biol Phys* 1994;30:765–773.

340. Parsons JT, Bova FJ, Fitzgerald CR, et al. Severe dry-eye syndrome following external beam irradiation. *Int J Radiat Oncol Biol Phys* 1994;30:775–780.

341. Woods CI, Strasnick B, Jackson CG. Surgery for glomus tumors: the Otology Group experience. *Laryngoscope* 1993;103:65–70.

342. Green JD Jr., Brackmann DE, Nguyen CD, et al. Surgical management of previously untreated glomus jugulare tumors. *Laryngoscope* 1994;104:917–921.

343. Bhandare N, Antonelli PJ, Morris CG, et al. Ototoxicity after radiotherapy for head and neck tumors. *Int J Radiat Oncol Biol Phys* 2007;67:469–479.

344. Hinerman RW, Indelicato DJ, Amdur RJ, et al. Cutaneous squamous cell carcinoma metastatic to parotid-area lymph nodes. *Laryngoscope* 2008;118:1989–1996.

345. Gallia LJ, Johnson JT. The incidence of neoplastic versus inflammatory disease in major salivary gland masses diagnosed by surgery. *Laryngoscope* 1981;91:512–516.

346. Gullane PJ, Havas TJ. Facial nerve grafts: effects of postoperative irradiation. *J Otolaryngol* 1987;16:112–115.

347. Laramore GE, Krall JM, Griffin TW, et al. Neutron versus photon irradiation for unresectable salivary gland tumors: final report of an RTOG-MRC randomized clinical trial. Radiation Therapy Oncology Group. Medical Research Council. *Int J Radiat Oncol Biol Phys* 1993;27:235–240.

348. Tanvetyanon T, Qin D, Padhya T, et al. Outcomes of postoperative concurrent chemoradiotherapy for locally advanced major salivary gland carcinoma. *Arch Otolaryngol Head Neck Surg* 2009;135:687–692.

349. Guzzo M, Locati LD, Prott FJ, et al. Major and minor salivary gland tumors. *Crit Rev Oncol Hematol* 2010;74:134–148.

350. Spiro RH. Salivary neoplasms: overview of a 35-year experience with 2,807 patients. *Head Neck Surg* 1986;8:177–184.

351. Hodge CW, Morris CG, Werning JW, et al. Role of radiotherapy for pleomorphic adenoma. *Am J Clin Oncol* 2005;28:148–151.

352. Spiro RH, Huvos AG, Strong EW. Cancer of the parotid gland. A clinicopathologic study of 288 primary cases. *Am J Surg* 1975;130:452–459.

353. Woods JE, Chong GC, Beahrs OH. Experience with 1,360 primary parotid tumors. *Am J Surg* 1975;130:460–462.

354. Garden AS, el-Naggar AK, Morrison WH, et al. Postoperative radiotherapy for malignant tumors of the parotid gland. *Int J Radiat Oncol Biol Phys* 1997;37:79–85.

355. Byers RM, Jesse RH, Guillamondegui OM, et al. Malignant tumors of the submaxillary gland. *Am J Surg* 1973;126:458–463.

356. Laurie SA, Licitra L. Systemic therapy in the palliative management of advanced salivary gland cancers. *J Clin Oncol* 2006;24:2673–2678.

357. Laurie SA, Ho AL, Fury MG, et al. Systemic therapy in the management of metastatic or locally recurrent adenoid cystic carcinoma of the salivary glands: a systematic review. *Lancet Oncol* 2011;12:815–824.

358. Mattox DE, Von Hoff DD, Balcerzak SP. Southwest Oncology Group study of mitoxantrone for treatment of patients with advanced adenoid cystic carcinoma of the head and neck. *Invest New Drugs* 1990;8:105–107.

359. Vermorken JB, Verweij J, de Mulder PH, et al. Epirubicin in patients with advanced or recurrent adenoid cystic carcinoma of the head and neck: a phase II study of the EORTC Head and Neck Cancer Cooperative Group. *Ann Oncol* 1993;4:785–788.

360. Verweij J, de Mulder PH, de Graeff A, et al. Phase II study on mitoxantrone in adenoid cystic carcinomas of the head and neck. EORTC Head and Neck Cancer Cooperative Group. *Ann Oncol* 1996;7:867–869.

361. Airoldi M, Pedani F, Succo G, et al. Phase II randomized trial comparing vinorelbine versus vinorelbine plus cisplatin in patients with recurrent salivary gland malignancies. *Cancer* 2001;91:541–547.

362. Licitra L, Marchini S, Spinazze S, et al. Cisplatin in advanced salivary gland carcinoma. A phase II study of 25 patients. *Cancer* 1991;68:1874–1877.

363. Gilbert J, Li Y, Pinto HA, et al. Phase II trial of taxol in salivary gland malignancies (E1394): a trial of the Eastern Cooperative Oncology Group. *Head Neck* 2006;28:197–204.

364. Alcedo JC, Fabrega JM, Arosemena JR, et al. Imatinib mesylate as treatment for adenoid cystic carcinoma of the salivary glands: report of two successfully treated cases. *Head Neck* 2004;26:829–831.

365. Faivre S, Raymond E, Casiraghi O, et al. Imatinib mesylate can induce objective response in progressing, highly expressing KIT adenoid cystic carcinoma of the salivary glands. *J Clin Oncol* 2005;23:6271–6273.

366. Hotte SJ, Winquist EW, Lamont E, et al. Imatinib mesylate in patients with adenoid cystic cancers of the salivary glands expressing c-kit: a Princess Margaret Hospital phase II consortium study. *J Clin Oncol* 2005;23:585–590.

367. Slevin NJ, Mais KL, Bruce I, et al. Imatinib with cisplatin in recurrent and/or metastatic salivary adenoidcystic carcinoma – response assessed by FDG-PET scanning *J Clin Oncol* 2004;22:S5604.

368. Haddad R, Colevas AD, Krane JF, et al. Herceptin in patients with advanced or metastatic salivary gland carcinomas. A phase II study. *Oral Oncol* 2003;39:724–727.

369. Locati LD, Bossi B, Rinaldi GR, et al. Anti-androgen therapy in recurrent and/or metastatic salivary glands carcinoma (RSGC). Poster presented at: 2005 3rd International Symposium in Targeted Anticancer Therapies; March 3–5, 2005; Amsterdam.

370. Persson M, Andren Y, Mark J, et al. Recurrent fusion of MYB and NFIB transcription factor genes in carcinomas of the breast and head and neck. *Proc Natl Acad Sci U S A* 2009;106:18740–18744.

371. Dillon PM, Moskaluk C, Fracasso PM, et al. Phase II study of dovitinib (TKI258) in patients with progressive metastatic adenoid cystic carcinoma. *J Clin Oncol* 2013;31:S6021.

372. Mendenhall WM, Mendenhall CM, Werning JW, et al. Salivary gland pleomorphic adenoma. *Am J Clin Oncol* 2008;31:95–99.

373. Spiro RH, Koss LG, Hajdu SI, et al. Tumors of minor salivary origin. A clinicopathologic study of 492 cases. *Cancer* 1973;31:117–129.

374. Wallace AS, Morris CG, Kirwan JM, et al. Radiotherapy for pleomorphic adenoma. *Am J Otolaryngol* 2013;34:36–40.

PRACTICE OF ONCOLOGY

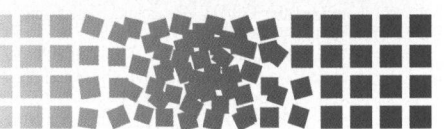

39 Rehabilitation After Treatment of Head and Neck Cancer

Douglas B. Chepeha, Teresa H. Lyden, and Marc Haxer

INTRODUCTION

Progress has been made in the past several years with survival for patients with head and neck cancer.[1] The current challenge is how to balance intensity of treatment and preserve function. Conservation surgery, radiation strategies, autogenous revascularized tissue transplantation, and treatment selection protocols continue to be used in an attempt to maintain or reestablish functional speech, voice, and swallowing in head and neck cancer patients. The ideal multidisciplinary team requires interaction among the surgical oncologists, radiation oncologists, medical oncologists, reconstructive surgeons, speech pathologists, physical therapists, occupational therapists, maxillofacial prosthodontists, dental oncologists, nutritionists, nurse oncologists, psychologists, audiologists, and social workers during pretreatment assessment and posttreatment intervention. Because radiation and chemotherapy protocols are being initiated in smaller centers, steps must be taken to ensure that the patient benefits from a multidisciplinary approach to treatment.

This chapter will focus on the rehabilitation of the *patient as a whole*. Pretreatment counseling is essential for all patients with aerodigestive tract cancer. Patients benefit from discussions regarding swallowing, voice, and speech difficulties that can result from radiation and chemotherapy regimens. Regrettably, patients who undergo radiation and chemotherapy protocols often are inadequately counseled, if at all. For rehabilitation to be effective, the patient's social, psychological, and addictive behaviors must be assessed and treated. Many of these patients have addictions to tobacco and/or alcohol at presentation and may lack social support. All these issues should be comprehensively addressed, and in so doing, the provider and the patient are often rewarded by the productive role the patient assumes for him or herself, as well as within his or her family and in the workplace.

PRETREATMENT COUNSELING

The education process begins during the initial consultation with the physician. Each team member has a specific, yet overlapping, role in preparing the patient for his or her intervention. The physicians are essential for providing information to the patient with respect to diagnosis, prognosis, and treatment options. This includes providing education to the patient on his or her specific treatment plan. Patients who are previously untreated and receive single modality treatment are going to do much better than patients who are recurrent or are going to undergo multimodality therapy. In order to design the best intervention for the patient, the physicians must also remain flexible and integrate feedback from the team. Once the plan is established, the physician team has to clearly communicate the treatment plan to the remaining members of the team so they can provide appropriate counseling.

Nursing will provide education on feeding tube and tracheotomy management. The placement of a gastrostomy or a tracheotomy tube is associated with the poorest patient-reported quality of life.[2] The patient will have little or no familiarity with these interventions; therefore, a specific explanation of the anatomy and postoperative care is important.

Preoperative counseling with the speech pathologist is another essential part of patient education and shaping expectations. The speech pathologist is often regarded by the patient as the individual who will restore communication and swallowing function posttreatment. The greatest counseling challenge for the team when working with this patient group is overcoming poor coping skills.[3] Quality of life assessments have correlated low scores in emotional well-being domains with increased *overall bother* scores.[4] The speech pathologist and other rehabilitation specialists must contend with the patient's coping mechanisms in order to facilitate rehabilitation. Speech pathologists often provide psychological counseling on an ad hoc basis, and this has shown to benefit head and neck cancer patients when compared to controls.[5] The speech pathologist must show interest in the patient's welfare, describe the expected long-term functional outcomes, and discuss the mechanics of communicative and swallowing strategies.

The patient must also be counseled on smoking and alcohol cessation. This is a central piece of the rehabilitation efforts that ideally should be handled by a cessation specialist. Smoking cessation interventions, particularly those that take into consideration alcohol intake and depression, have been shown to be efficacious for this patient population.[6] This is encouraging because smoking is highly correlated with alcohol intake and depression. An addicted patient is unlikely to be effectively rehabilitated. Therefore, the patient must understand that continuation of addictive behaviors represents the greatest risk to patient survival and future function. It is important to emphasize to the patient that there are many different ways to quit smoking. The patient should understand that alcohol is a facilitator and nicotine is a lower level carcinogen than tobacco products. Involvement of social work is important to address psychosocial and economic issues that impact cancer treatment and rehabilitation.

The use of patient volunteers who have completed treatment is an invaluable resource. They provide education and experience with regard to what one may experience during treatment, posttreatment recuperation, and long-term quality of life to patients who are preparing for treatment.

SUPPORT DURING TREATMENT AND REHABILITATION OF THE CHEMORADIATION PATIENT

Radiation alone, with concurrent chemotherapy or adjuvant after surgery, is a common treatment approach.[1] Swallowing and the voice are affected by radiation, but the effect is variable and depends on the radiation field, the radiation dose, and the concomitant chemotherapy agents. After treatment, there can be stiffness, edema, fibrosis, xerostomia, and stenosis. The severity of these effects is proportional to the aggressiveness of the treatment. To help reduce the effects of chemotherapy and radiation therapy, mobility of the aerodigestive tract should be maintained during treatment.[7] Recent, small, randomized studies support both prophylactic use of feeding gastrostomies, together with oral feeding[8] and swallow exercises during therapy,[9–11] to improve long-term swallowing and quality of life. Newer radiotherapy techniques that spare the swallowing-related structures have resulted in substantial improvements of long-term dysphagia.[12] This is facilitated by good supportive care, which includes appropriate treatment of mucositis, adequate analgesia, management of depression, maintenance of nutrition, and monitoring by the treatment team. The treatment of mucositis involves the use of mouthwash and oral care. There are many different *recipes* for mouthwashes, but the common components are an antifungal such as nystatin (Mycostatin), an antihistamine such as diphenhydramine (Benadryl), and a barrier agent such as an antacid. The approach to analgesia is a sustained release agent that covers 80% to 90% of the analgesia needs and a shorter acting agent to cover breakthrough pain. Recent efforts to identify newer agents that may reduce mucositis during radiotherapy include amifostine[13] and palifermin (keratinocyte growth factor).[14] None of these agents can yet be recommended for routine use based on the published data. To address issues relating to depression, the creation of an environment where depressive emotions or issues can be addressed is important. At present, serotonin reuptake inhibitors are the first-line antidepressants, and modafinil is added if the patient has significant symptoms of fatigue. Clonazepam is added to the antidepressant regimen if there is a significant component of anxiety or to support the withdrawal of alcohol. Transdermal testosterone is also useful for symptoms of fatigue. A free testosterone serum level should be obtained to verify that testosterone levels are low. If unable to maintain adequate nutrition orally, particularly for the patient who is receiving radiation therapy, supplemental or primary nutrition can be met via a temporary gastrostomy tube. It is important to keep the patient swallowing even if the patient is only able to take sips of liquids. If a patient is unable to swallow anything, then a nasogastric feeding tube should be inserted as a stent for the pharynx. Removal of the stent is recommended only when the lumen is patent and the patient is able to swallow again. A possible consequence of *resting* the digestive tract during chemoradiation is pharyngeal stenosis or a nonfunctional upper aerodigestive tract. If pharyngeal stenosis occurs, management is achieved through dilation in the operating room, clinic, or with a program of self-dilation.

Rehabilitation after treatment usually focuses on relief from xerostomia, maintenance of mobility of the oropharyngeal musculature, improved swallowing function (including reducing the risk of aspiration), and improvement with communication or voice. The posttreatment examination usually reveals edema, decreased sensation, and thick secretions. The thick secretions and xerostomia are managed with the regular intake of liquids. In addition, medications designed to improve salivary flow, such as pilocarpine and cevimeline, can be taken daily. Pilocarpine is indicated in the radiated patient, but a minority of patients report subjective efficacy.[15] Cevimeline is indicated for Sjögren disease but is often used off label for xerostomia, with few patients using this medication long term. Artificial saliva can be taken as a gel, spray, or a lozenge and contains methylcellulose as a lubricating agent. However, in lieu of using salivary substitutes, most patients choose to take frequent sips of water to thin secretions and keep their aerodigestive tract lubricated. The most important advance to reduce the incidence of xerostomia is intensity modulated radiation therapy (IMRT), which is a radiation delivery technique that uses selective targeting to spare salivary tissue. In cases where it is safe to spare the parotid from radiation, it has been shown that there is improved salivary flow, relief from xerostomia, and improved quality of life.[16–18] Even with better salivary flow, patients frequently need to use liquid washes to improve swallowing function by moistening dry foods and lubricating the aerodigestive tract to allow for easier bolus passage. The reduction of aspiration is facilitated by aggressive swallowing exercises[7] and the use of strategies, postures, or maneuvers. The incidence of aspiration can increase during and after treatment. Exercises are introduced focusing on improving strength, range of motion, and coordination of movement. Areas that are commonly focused on include improving mandibular, labial, and lingual range of motion and improving strength and coordination of the lips, tongue (including base of tongue), palate, posterior pharyngeal wall, and laryngeal elevation. There are several strategies that may be of benefit that include, but are not limited to, a chin tuck, an effortful swallow, supra- and supersupraglottic swallows, and the Mendelsohn maneuver.[19–21]

There are several patient factors that also affect outcome. These include continued smoking, continued alcohol consumption, gastroesophageal reflux disease, and tissue reaction to the oxidative effects of radiation. As previously mentioned, in order to facilitate optimal rehabilitation, these factors need to be addressed by the medical team as part of the patient's rehabilitation.

Posttreatment Swallowing Assessment

The team should understand which aspects of communication and swallowing functions have been compromised by treatment. Because of their training in the areas of communication and swallowing, the speech pathologist assumes a leading role in the evaluation and treatment of deficits in these areas. The site of lesion, the extent of resection, the type of reconstruction, and the use of adjunct treatment modalities will influence the extent and severity of the communication and swallowing disorder. In addition, these factors will help guide the selection of assessment tools to be used, as well as which strategies may be of benefit to the patient. In order to better understand the rehabilitation process with respect to swallowing, it may be useful to briefly review the four phases or stages of the normal swallow. The oral preparatory phase involves mastication and bolus formation. During this phase, the lips are closed anteriorly while the posterior tongue is closed against the soft palate, which keeps the bolus from prematurely spilling into the pharynx. The bolus is formed, shaped, and readied for swallowing.[22] During the oral phase, the bolus is propelled into the oropharynx as a result of the oral tongue rolling posteriorly. Once this occurs, the involuntary or pharyngeal phase of swallowing is initiated. There are multiple components to the pharyngeal phase. This phase involves palatal closure and bolus transport through the pharynx. In addition, laryngeal elevation occurs and, with this action, pharyngeal suction results along with coverage of the larynx by the base of the tongue. Glottic closure also occurs with the pharyngeal phase of the swallow and helps assist with the prevention of aspiration. Finally, relaxation of the upper esophageal sphincter facilitates the delivery of the bolus into the esophagus, and this completes the pharyngeal phase of the swallow. When the bolus enters the esophagus, this is the initiation of the esophageal phase of the swallow.[21] Any alteration of the normal aerodigestive physiology will result in compromised swallowing. Normal transit times for the oral and pharyngeal phases of the swallow are 1.5 seconds or less. These increase slightly as bolus viscosity increases.[21] Transit times for the esophageal phase of the swallow vary between 8 and 20 seconds.[21]

Swallowing can be assessed subjectively or objectively. A subjective assessment is a clinical examination that involves an evaluation of oral motor skills along with the presentation of various consistencies of foods or liquids. Observations are made with regard to oral competency, timeliness of the swallow, laryngeal elevation, and clinical signs or symptoms of aspiration. Objective measures include fiber optic endoscopic evaluation of swallowing (FEES) and videofluoroscopic swallow study (VFSS).[21,23] VFSS is performed using x-rays (cineradiography or fluoroscopy) with barium as a contrast agent to visualize swallowing movements. VFSS is an objective evaluation of swallowing function that includes all stages of the swallow during presentation of varying food consistencies. This procedure allows measured amounts of barium boluses to be followed from the lips to the stomach and, if needed, can incorporate the effects of compensatory strategies, such as postural assists or maneuvers. VFSS is ideal for patients with oropharyngeal dysphagia because it allows for an assessment of strategies and a diagnosis of aspiration severity. VFSS is expensive and time consuming. It requires at least 30 minutes to perform, involves radiation exposure, and requires both a radiologist and a speech pathologist.[21] FEES utilizes a fiber optic nasoendoscope to observe the pharyngeal and laryngeal structures directly during the pharyngeal phase of the swallow. A bolus of contrasting color is used to note premature spillage into the hypopharynx or laryngeal vestibule before the swallow initiation along with the presence of residua in the hypopharynx and laryngopharynx after a swallow. Vocal fold movement patterns can be assessed during FEES but need to be visualized independent of swallows. This examination yields minimal information relative to the oral preparatory and oral phases of the swallow. However, there are advantages to FEES, including a shorter assessment time, the avoidance of radiation, and less expensive instrumentation. The Fiber optic Endoscopic Evaluation of Swallowing with Sensory Testing (FEESST)[24] combines FEES with a technique that determines laryngopharyngeal sensory discrimination thresholds by endoscopically delivering air pulse stimuli to the mucosa.

VFSS and FEES integrate a diagnosis and intervention. During these diagnostic interventions, the food bolus size, consistency, and maneuvers are all assessed to identify the safest and most efficient method for bolus transport and clearance and to reduce or eliminate aspiration events. At the most basic level, the assessment and intervention allows the patient to continue with oral intake and minimizes aspiration. At the most sophisticated level, efficient eating can only be accomplished if the patient understands the consistencies, the bolus size, and the maneuvers that are appropriate to the speed of consumption in particular social situations. As a result, the VFSS and FEES are only as good as the knowledge and training of the speech pathologist providing the rehabilitation to this patient group. If the speech pathologist lacks this experience and training in the completion or the interpretation of either the VFSS or FEES of head and neck cancer patients, the physician must recognize and manage this situation by encouraging the patient to make the effort to go to an institution where the assessment and plan will be appropriate to the patient's needs.

Posttreatment Swallowing Rehabilitation

The speech pathologist rehabilitates swallowing disorders with use of postural assists, maneuvers, control of bolus size or rate of intake, modification of bolus consistencies, and exercises.[21,25] Postures are body positions that the patient utilizes to improve bolus control and transport. Most of the postures involve the alteration of head or body position to direct the bolus to sensate native tissue, to direct the bolus to more functional tissue, or to open the pharynx or close the larynx. Maneuvers are used to alter swallow physiology. These maneuvers are designed to improve laryngeal closure, increase the base of tongue contact with the posterior pharyngeal wall, elevate the larynx, and open the hypopharynx. Postural assists and maneuvers may be prescribed to reduce penetration (entry of the bolus into the supraglottis) and aspiration (entry of the bolus into the trachea), with the goal of achieving safe and efficient oral intake. Many patients who have been treated for advanced head and neck cancer and are in need of evaluation and rehabilitation are actively aspirating. A statistically significant correlation between aspiration detected on videofluoroscopy after chemoirradiation of head and neck cancer and the risk of subsequent aspiration pneumonia has been observed, whereas patient-reported or observer-based dysphagia were not predictive of subsequent pneumonia.[26] These findings suggest that an objective evaluation of dysphagia, such as videofluoroscopy, should be performed routinely after chemoirradiation, rather than limiting it to patients with symptoms of dysphagia. Successful rehabilitation is a reduction, not necessarily the elimination, of aspiration. Optimization of the bolus type and consistency is an art. The bolus size and type of consistencies consumed evolve during rehabilitation. Management of swallowing requires understanding of the pre- versus posttreatment physiology and the probability of improvement

during the first year following treatment. Swallowing exercises are important for strengthening, improving mobility, and improving coordination of movement. They involve both passive and active range of motion exercises. Exercises are designed to improve labial seal, mandibular movement or mouth opening, oral tongue mobility, base of tongue mobility, velopharyngeal closure, posterior pharyngeal wall strength or movement, and laryngeal elevation.

Posttreatment Speech Assessment

Speech generation involves an assessment of respiration, phonation, resonance, and articulation. For optimum phonatory function, there has to be adequate pulmonary reserve for breath support, an intact sound generator, and an intact vocal tract. Respiratory support is the driver of sound generation. Head and neck cancer patients frequently have impaired respiratory support secondary to chronic lung disease or pulmonary resection for second primary tumors. Reduced respiratory support decreases sound volume, increases vocal fatigue, and makes select consonants difficult to produce. Phonation can occur in the glottic or supraglottic larynx, the pharynx, or from an external source such as an artificial larynx. An important component of speech production is vocal resonance. If the soft palate and the lateral or posterior pharyngeal walls are not functioning properly, the voice may sound hyper- or hyponasal. Hypernasality is associated with too much sound (i.e., air leakage) into the nasopharynx during speech, whereas hyponasality is associated with inadequate nasal resonance during speech. For the sound to be shaped into intelligible speech, there must be coordination between and adequate contact of the articulators. Much of the shaping of speech occurs in the oral cavity. For articulation to be optimized, the patient has to have an intact oral sphincter, tongue tip to premaxilla contact, maxillary alveolar contact with the lateral tongue and a mobile tongue tip, obliteration of dead space within the oral cavity, and soft palate contact with the base of the tongue.

The assessment of speech after the treatment of head and neck cancer is varied depending on the site of the lesion, the treatment completed, the extent of surgical resection, and the type of reconstruction, if any. Speech deficits commonly occur in postsurgical patients but can also occur in postchemoradiation patients. Access to the surgeon's template of the surgical defect, including the involved muscles and nerves, is useful for the assessment of the postoperative patient.[27] For the assessment of resonance and velopharyngeal competence, a thorough evaluation includes an articulation assessment, an oral motor assessment, and a measurement of nasal airflow. A nasometer (Zoo Passage, Rainbow Passage, and Nasal Sentences) is used to measure nasal airflow during the recitation of standard passages. This is a relatively simple and noninvasive test. The results are compared to normative data. In addition, periodic retesting can be useful to monitor patient progress with interventions. VFSS and FEES can also be useful for the assessment of articulatory precision and velopharyngeal competency, but are better suited to the evaluation of swallowing. Articulation can be assessed by a number of survey instruments, including those that can be used for the assessment of intraoral prostheses.[28] These instruments are useful in the research setting and should be used in conjunction with the clinical examination. An interesting area of development is assessment using pressure-sensing electrode arrays. These electrodes are placed on the hard and soft palate to determine the exact location of tongue contact points during articulation. The contact points are then viewed as contrasting colored dots in a line drawing of the palate on a computer screen. This display can be used to assess and treat articulation problems particularly after tongue resection or reconstruction.

With regard to postlaryngectomy voice restoration, insufflation testing[29] is an available objective measure to assist with determining candidacy for tracheoesophageal puncture. This test provides information relative to the pressure generated within the pharyngoesophageal segment during production of structured speech tasks but has never gained widespread use among speech pathologists.

Rehabilitation of the Neck

Neck dissection is performed for the diagnosis or treatment of neck metastasis. The clinical sequelae are secondary to postoperative weakness of the trapezius muscle, which include neck stiffness, shoulder girdle weakness, and chronic pain. The extent of the neck dissection (selective versus modified), radiation, age, and weight all affect the patient's ability to rehabilitate after neck dissection.[2] Patients who undergo selective neck dissection have significantly better shoulder function than patients who undergo modified radical neck dissection with the same regional control rates.[30,31] To reduce pain and discomfort and improve mobility, passive and active range of motions have been shown to significantly improve long-term function and quality of life.[32]

Rehabilitation of the Oral Cavity

Surgery and postoperative radiation therapy remain the most common treatment approach in the oral cavity. Reconstructive surgeons must be versed in the optimization of oral function. The general approach for oral cavity reconstruction is to perform an anatomic reconstruction (Figs. 39.1 and 39.2). The goals of oral cavity reconstruction include:

- Obliteration of the oral cavity. This is achieved when all oral cavity mucosal surfaces are in contact with one another when the mouth is closed. This goal is important because it should decrease the likelihood of food getting lost in a *dead space* in the oral cavity. Additionally, it should improve the handling of secretions by bringing the revascularized free tissue transfer in contact with the remaining native mucosa.
- Maintain premaxillary contact. This is an extension of the goal of obliteration of the oral cavity. In terms of speech generation, premaxillary and palatal contact is important for maintaining the precision of articulation for a number of speech sounds. Generally, reduced precision of linguadental, alveolar, palatal, and velar sounds will occur if adequate contact is not achieved. The surgeon needs to ensure that some of the volume of the reconstructive flap is concentrated anteriorly to allow for the obliteration of the oral cavity.
- Maintain the *finger function* of the tongue. This is the ability of the tongue to sweep and clear the buccal, labial, and alveolar sulci and protrude past the coronal plane of the incisors.
- Maintain movement of secretions from the anterior to the posterior aspect of the oral cavity.
- Optimize sensation of the remaining native tissue and the revascularized free tissue transfer.

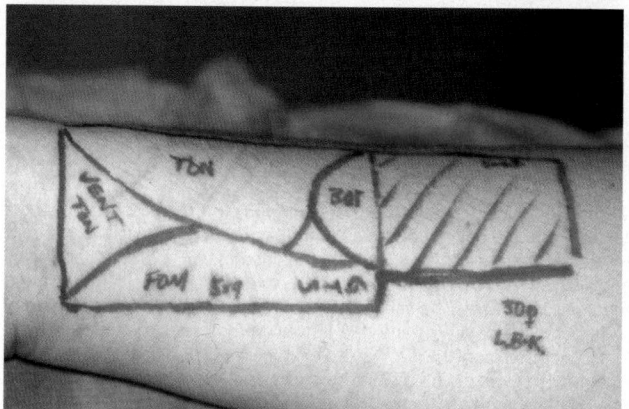

Figure 39.1 This is the preoperative *rectangle tongue* template for reconstruction of a hemiglossectomy defect. The template is marked out on the patient's forearm, will be excised, implanted, and revascularized to reconstruct the tongue.

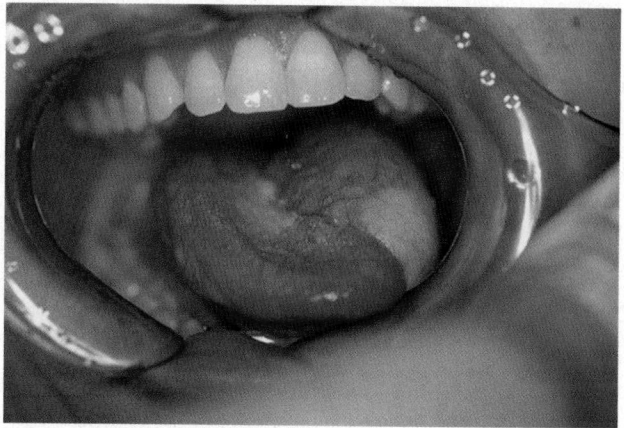

Figure 39.2 A postoperative reconstructed hemiglossectomy defect 22 months after implantation.

In general, these goals are best met with local tissue and revascularized autogenous tissue reconstruction. Traditional regional flaps, such as the pectoralis flap, are less commonly used because they are associated with higher gastrostomy tube rates.[33] There are published studies that suggest that autogenous revascularized free tissue transplantation is a disadvantage.[34] These data are not generally representative of present day reconstruction because, in this historic cohort, free flaps were used for large defects and skin grafts were used for smaller defects. The differences related more to the size of the defect than the reconstructive approach.

For oral cavity rehabilitation, the speech pathologist will perform an oral motor assessment. An assessment includes an evaluation of oral sphincter competence, the patient's ability to handle secretions, tongue to premaxillary/palatal contact, anterior–posterior movement of the tongue, location of sensate tissue, and identification of areas where food will collect (i.e., dead space). A clinical swallow examination is used to assess swallowing function with a focus on the oral phase of the swallow. The patient's ability to remove the bolus from an eating utensil (e.g., a spoon), create a labial seal, manipulate the bolus, control the bolus, and clear the bolus is assessed. The challenge for the speech pathologist is to modify the treatment plan and strategies used to compensate for the changing reconstruction during the first year of rehabilitation.

During the immediate postoperative period, the reconstruction will frequently be bulky and edematous; with radiation, the reconstruction will become smaller and the native tissue will undergo fibrosis. The objective throughout the first year is to maximize and maintain mobility of the tongue, focusing on the use of the remaining native tissue. In this patient group, use of liquid washes to add moisture and to aid in bolus passage with dry and solid consistencies should be considered the norm and not a failure of oral rehabilitation.

Maintaining the remaining native dentition is important for communication, swallowing, and for general health; therefore, including a dentist as part of the treatment team is critical. The best approach is prevention, which involves a reduction of radiation dose to the mandible when possible, the removal or restoration of carious teeth prior to treatment, regular fluoride trays before and after treatment, and the treatment of inflamed gingival tissue. Should a patient develop osteoradionecrosis, surgical excision and reconstruction is the mainstay, because hyperbaric oxygen therapy has been shown to lack efficacy in controlled clinical trials.[35]

The maxillofacial prosthodontist makes important contributions to the rehabilitation of the patient with an oral cavity defect. Dental rehabilitation with dental prostheses is important for function and cosmesis. When introducing dental prosthetics, it is important to consider the patient's ability to masticate and prevent bolus loss. The introduction of a dental prosthesis can impair bolus control by covering sensate tissue, preventing glossal–labial contact, and decreasing the functional oral opening. It is also important to ensure that the patient can perform a *tongue sweep* of the labial sulci to clear food residue, especially if a lower (mandibular) dental prosthesis is introduced. If the patient is unable to perform this maneuver, then use of a digit may be required to clear food particles while eating. Even if the patient is a good candidate for a dental prosthesis, implants may be required to assist in the retention of a lower dental prosthesis. Implants can be placed in the native mandible or in an osseous free flap for the purpose of supporting and retaining a dental prosthesis. An individual knowledgeable of the use of implants in radiated bone is important because the rate of implant failure is high and there is a risk of osteoradionecrosis.[36] Prostheses can also be useful for the rehabilitation of soft tissue deficits. For example, if the patient does not have good palatal–maxillary contact, a *palatal drop* prosthesis can be fashioned, facilitating the obliteration of dead space within the oral cavity, which allows the tongue to contact the prosthetically reconstructed palate. This may result in improved clarity of speech sounds and, therefore, overall speech intelligibility. In addition, the palatal drop prosthesis may assist in improved bolus manipulation, control, and oral transfer.

Rehabilitation After Partial Laryngeal Procedures

Both the communication and swallowing functions can be adversely affected with a partial surgical resection of the larynx. Supraglottic laryngectomy, hemilaryngectomy, and supracricoid laryngectomy all result in some degree of compromised phonatory function. Following these surgical procedures, the swallowing function is generally adversely affected in the short term, but improvement can be anticipated with the process of healing and the implementation of swallowing therapy. Postoperative dysphagia after partial laryngeal procedures is common due to a decrease in sensation and alteration of normal laryngeal anatomy. As a result, the patient is at risk for penetration and aspiration secondary to the compromise in airway protection that completion of these procedures brings about. Postoperatively, the patient will be trained on swallowing

strategies to improve laryngeal closure in an attempt to prevent aspiration. In the early stages of recovery, liquids are usually the most difficult consistency to consume due to reduced sensation in and around the laryngeal complex and incomplete laryngeal closure, thus reducing airway protection. Therefore, consumption of a modified diet (thickened liquids and purees) with or without the use of alternative means of nutrition is not uncommon until adequate airway protection can be achieved. Implementation of swallowing maneuvers, such as the supra- and supersupraglottic swallow maneuvers, are helpful in facilitating airway protection.[19–21]

Rehabilitation After Laryngectomy or Laryngopharyngectomy

After a total laryngectomy, the patient has a tracheostoma in the lower neck and a separated digestive tract. The stoma and lungs require management to prevent stomal stenosis, prevent stomal trauma, enhance humidification, and reduce tracheal crusting. There are a variety of products that prevent tracheostomal stenosis, protect the stoma from digital trauma, and enhance humidification (Fig.39.3A, B). Many of these tracheal stomal products are designed to be used with or without tracheoesophageal (TE) prostheses.

Rehabilitation of speech after a total laryngectomy has improved. Options for alaryngeal communication are TE voice, voice generated by an artificial larynx, and esophageal voice. TE voice has become the gold standard for voice rehabilitation after a total laryngectomy. The challenge with prosthetic rehabilitation is customized solutions, because one size does not fit all. There are many different types of TE voice prostheses (Fig. 39.4A, B). An experienced speech pathologist is essential for long-term patient compliance. The artificial larynx is a device that produces mechanical sound. This sound is transferred into the oral cavity via the placement of the device to the cheek or neck. Additionally, there is an option for an intraoral adapter, allowing for direct transmission of sound into the oral cavity. This device can be used short term until a patient achieves functional esophageal or TE speech. In some cases, it is used long term as the primary means of alaryngeal communication. This device can

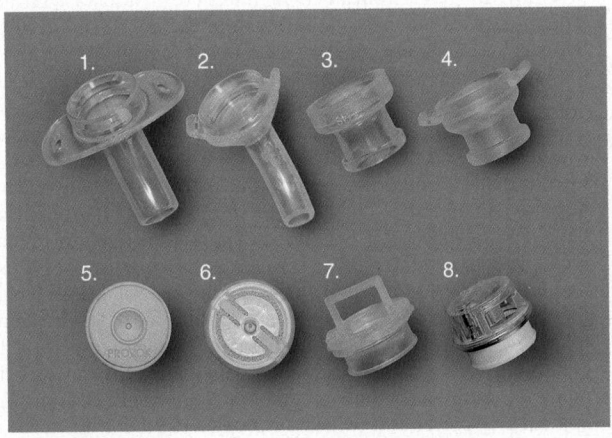 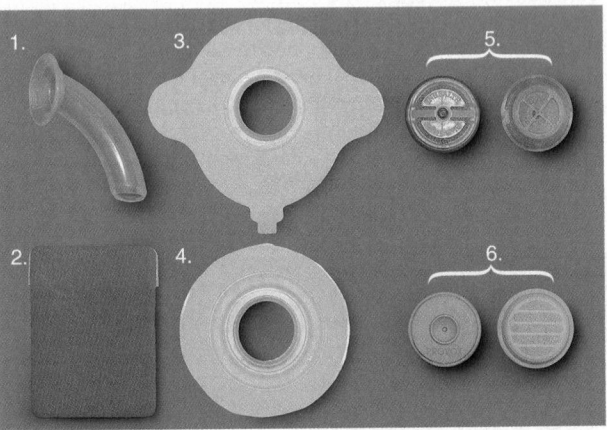

A   B

Figure 39.3 (A) Items *1* through *4* are for use in the trachea and are designed to retain the heat moisture exchange (HME) cartridge/cassette or hands-free speaking valve. Items *1* and *2* are laryngectomy tubes that are not self-retaining and are designed for use with ties. They are available in different diameters, lengths, and with or without fenestration. Items *3* and *4* are stoma buttons, are self-retaining. and are designed to be used by patients with a tracheal *lip*. If this lip of tissue is not circumferential, adequate retention is unlikely. Items *5* and *6* are examples of HME cassettes/cartridges and can be used with items *1* through *4*. Items *7* and *8* are examples of hands-free speaking valves. The valves are open during restful breathing. During tracheoesophageal (TE) sound production, the valve closes, redirecting the air through a separate device, the TE voice prosthesis. The TE prosthesis diverts air into the esophagus creating a vibratory segment so the patient can produce a voice. **(B)** Item *1* is an example of a laryngectomy tube that is used to maintain stoma patency and can be supplied with fenestrations so that it can be used with a TE voice prosthesis. Item *2* is a foam adhesive filter that is placed over the stoma and acts as a partial barrier between the trachea and environment. Items *3* and *4* are types of tracheostoma (TS) base plates. These are adhesive and attach to the peristomal skin to allow for attachment of a HME system (see items *5* and *6*) or a hands-free speaking valve. The base plates come in different shapes and adhesive strengths, but the HME attachment system is universal to facilitate the use of different brands. Items *5* and *6* are two types of HME cartridges/cassettes and must be inserted into a retention system such as a TS base plate, select laryngectomy tubes, and/or stoma buttons. The HME helps maintain the humidity and temperature of the pulmonary tract and should be worn 24 hours per day. Items *2* through *6* are single-use items and are meant to be discarded after use. Wear time of the TS baseplates can vary from several hours to several days.

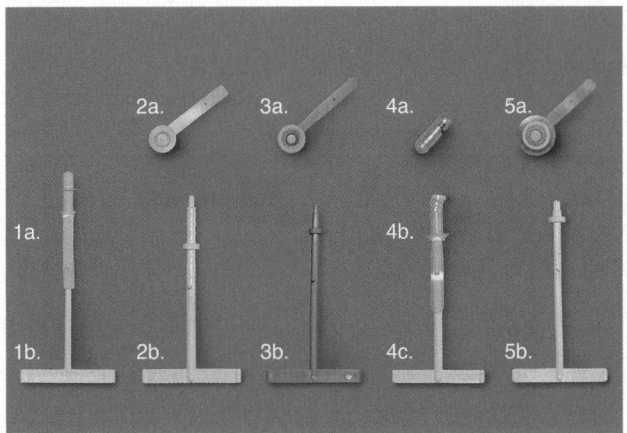

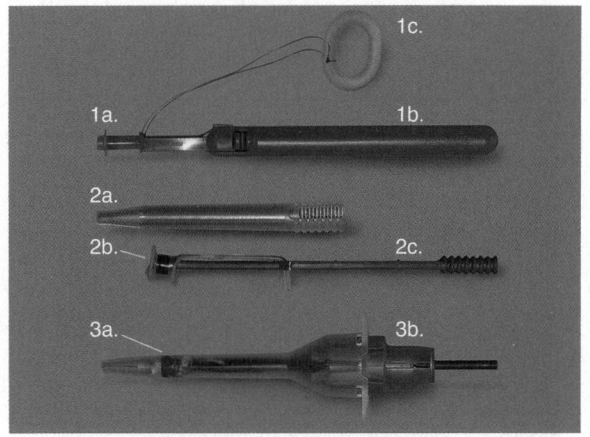

A   **B**

Figure 39.4 (A) There are many different types of tracheoesophageal (TE) prostheses. This figure is a sample of some different types. Item *1* is a duckbill voice prosthesis. Item *2a* is a low pressure voice prosthesis. These are patient changeable devices. The duckbill *(1a)* is shown attached to the insertion stick *(1b)*. Item *2a* would be attached to the insertion stick *(2b)* in the same manner. Items *3a* and *5a* are indwelling voice prostheses that are not patient changeable and are shown apart from their insertion sticks *(3b and 5b,* respectively). Item *4a* is a gel cap that has been placed on the esophageal end of an indwelling prosthesis *(4b)*, which is shown attached to the insertion stick *(4c)*. Item *5a* is an indwelling variation with large esophageal flange. This would be used in patients who experience reduced retention of their prosthesis in the TE puncture. **(B)** These are examples of TE prostheses with alternative insertion systems. Item *1a* is a patient changeable nonindwelling voice prosthesis shown on its insertion stick *(1b)*. Item *1c* is a safety washer attached to the voice prosthesis, which allows for the easy removal of the voice prosthesis in the event of accidental prosthesis dislodgement. Item *2a* is an insertion tube. The indwelling voice prosthesis *(2b)* is shown on its insertion stick *(2c)*, which is intended to be placed into the insertion tube. Item *3b* is a loaded indwelling voice prosthesis in its insertion tube. The voice prosthesis *(3a)* can be visualized on the left side of the insertion tube.

be difficult to use. Training of and practice by the patient are essential to become adept for daily communication requirements (Fig. 39.5). Another alaryngeal speech option is esophageal speech, which does not utilize devices or implants. It involves trapping air in the pharynx distal to the cricopharyngeus with a subsequent controlled release of air through the pharyngoesophageal segment to produce sound. Learning esophageal speech is time intensive and can take up to a year or longer to achieve a functional result. In some cases, fluent sound is never realized. As a result, esophageal speech is not commonly used. However, voice production with a TE voice prosthesis, in many instances, can be achieved on the day of insertion.

A wide variety of TE voice prostheses are available. Prosthesis selection is related to many factors. It is important to know that prostheses come in different diameters, lengths, amounts of valve resistance, and sizes of tracheal and esophageal retention collars.

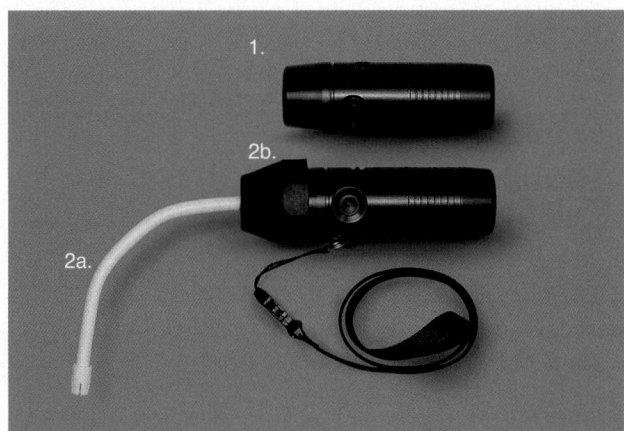

Figure 39.5 An artificial larynx. This device is a sound generator. Item *1* is shown without an attachment/attenuator and can be used with neck placement or cheek placement. When used this way, sound is directed through the neck or cheek tissue into the oral cavity. Item *2* is shown with an intraoral attenuator *(2a)* and an attachment *(2b)*. Together, the attachment and attenuator allow for the delivery of sound into the oral cavity, which can then be shaped into speech.

Additionally, there are standard prostheses and yeast-resistant prostheses. The type of voice prosthesis that is chosen will depend on the diameter, length, and integrity of the tissue that makes up the TE puncture. Candidal colonization also affects prosthesis selection. Candidal colonization of the TE prosthesis can cause accelerated deterioration and can increase the frequency of replacement. Therefore, consideration for transition to a yeast-resistant prosthesis may be indicated. There are patient-changeable and clinician-placed (i.e., indwelling) prostheses. Patient-changeable prostheses can last from less than 1 month to 3 months on average, whereas clinician-placed prosthetics can last 3 to 6 months on average. The goal is for the patient to be as independent as possible with their care. This includes daily cleaning and maintenance. The advantages of the patient-changeable prosthesis is that it is less expensive than the clinician-placed prosthesis. In addition, in the event of prosthesis failure, the patient can replace the prosthesis independently. The clinician-placed prosthesis comes with added options (e.g., antifungal, large tracheal or esophageal flanges, dual valves, weighted valves). However, the indwelling prosthesis can cost two to three times more than a patient-changeable prosthesis. Additionally, if the prosthesis fails, the time for prosthesis replacement can range from 1 to 3 days. The voice prosthesis that is selected will be based on each individual's need. In addition, social and financial factors need to be considered. Some patients have to pay for their own prosthesis out of pocket or need to travel long distances to visit the speech pathologist for replacement. Therefore, cost in combination with replacement interval and travel time has to be considered along with the clinical indication for prosthesis selection.

Voice production can be difficult for some patients even when there is a properly fitting TE prosthesis. There are several causes of aphonia following the placement of a voice prosthesis. These include posttreatment edema, spasm of the cricopharyngeus, and pharyngeal stenosis. A VFSS is utilized for the evaluation of spasm versus stenosis. If a stenosis is present, then dilation is appropriate. If there is hypertonicity of the pharyngoesophageal segment or cricopharyngeal spasm, this can be treated with botulinum toxin injection in a clinic setting or administered under fluoroscopy.

Sound production with a TE voice prosthesis requires adequate occlusion of the tracheostoma. The tracheostoma can be occluded directly with a digit, an object, a stoma filter with application of digital pressure (Fig. 39.6), or with a mechanical valve that fits over

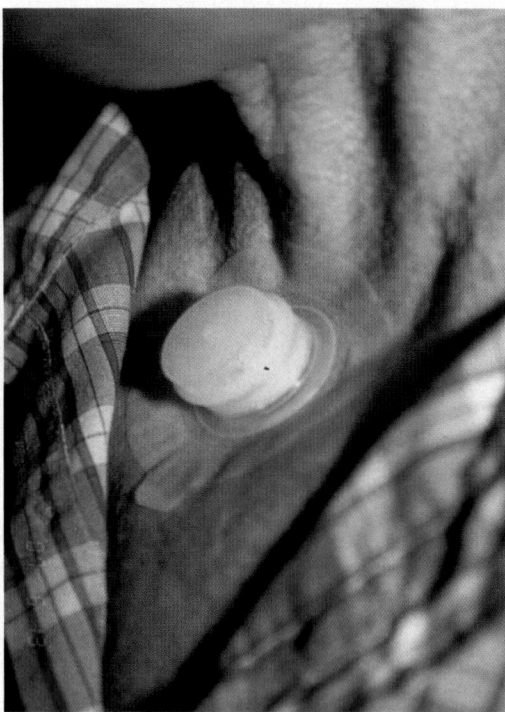

Figure 39.6 A patient with an adhesive tracheostoma baseplate heat and moisture exchange system with the cassette in position. The patient will push on the cassette for tracheoesophageal (TE) voice production.

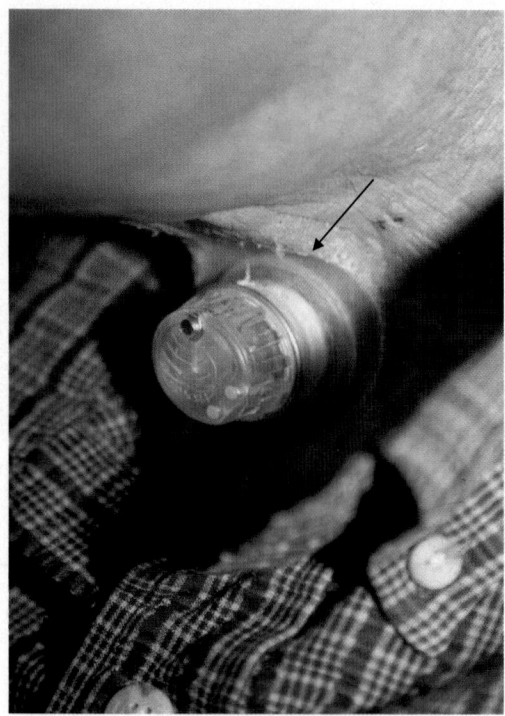

Figure 39.7 A patient with modified tracheostoma housing with hands-free speaking valve.

the stoma. A mechanical valve is considered to be *hands free* and fits into a tracheostomal housing that can be adhered to the skin adjacent to the stoma or inserted into a self-retaining tracheal button that is placed in the stoma. The hands-free devices most closely duplicate an intact larynx because the patient does not have to use a digit to occlude the stoma. Use of forced exhalation closes off the valve, shunting air through the TE prosthesis. The challenges with these devices are retention while speaking, avoiding obstruction due to secretions, and maintaining optimal respiratory support for valve closure. For effective long-term use of a tracheostomal housing used with a hands-free device, the peristomal skin must be able to withstand wound breakdown. An alternative to the adhesive tracheostomal housing is a stoma button. The button fits in the tracheostoma, and retention is facilitated by a slightly stenotic stoma and a small retention collar on the distal end of the button. For those patients who are not able to use a stoma button but who require use of a tube to maintain stoma patency, another option is a combination of the adhesive housing and the laryngectomy tube. If the retention and secretion issues can be overcome, the hands-free device is a major step forward in the rehabilitation of the head and neck cancer patient (Fig. 39.7).

Every stoma is different and, as a result, there is an endless variety of devices that assist in the retention of heat moisture exchange (HME) cassettes and hands-free devices. There are two categories of devices: peristomal, which are retained around the stoma, and intrastomal devices, which are fit into the stoma. For most patients, a peristomal base plate is fit first until adequate healing allows for an evaluation for the use of a stoma button. The tracheal stoma (TS) base plate is an adhesive-backed attachment that adheres to the peristomal skin. These can be worn daily and up to 3 days as tolerated. They come in different shapes (i.e., oval, round, oblong), types (i.e., XtraBase, Stabilibar), and varying strengths of adhesive to facilitate effective retention for the wide range of peristomal shapes. We prefer to place intrastomal devices once the patient has healed. These are frequently uncomfortable when initially fitted. These devices are called stoma buttons and can be used if there is an adequate lip at the cutaneous mucosal junction to facilitate retention. Interestingly. this creates a situation where there is a benefit to a small stoma because the stoma button can be retained effectively

and will improve the patient's overall level of comfort. Of course. this is only an option in highly supported health-care environments. The use of a stoma button will affect the placement location of the TEP. To effectively use a stoma button, the TEP needs to be placed more inferiorly so the tracheal retention collar of the stoma button does not obstruct the TE voice prosthesis. The stoma button is reused with replacement once or twice per year as needed.

There are many products available to raise the humidity level in the lungs after a laryngectomy. Generically, these items are referred to as HME systems. HME cassettes/cartridges are used to assist, in part, in the restoration of respiration lost as a result of surgery. The design varies slightly by manufacturer. Patients should be fitted as soon as the stoma is healed because these devices help to heat and increase the humidity of the air entering lungs. The result is a more comfortable patient who experiences less tracheal dryness, crusting, and less time in maintaining their stoma. As is the case with hands-free devices, they can be used with both peristomal and intrastomal devices. TE sound is generated when the HME is digitally occluded.

RESOURCES FOR REHABILITATION OF HEAD AND NECK CANCER PATIENTS

For the clinician, there are a number of useful references for the rehabilitation of head and neck cancer patients.

- Doyle PC, Keith RL. *Contemporary Considerations in the Treatment and Rehabilitation of Head and Neck Cancer.* Austin, TX: PRO-ED; 2005.
- Fried MP. *The Larynx—A Multidisciplinary Approach.* Vol. 15. Boston: Little, Brown; 1988.
- Logemann JA. *Evaluation and Treatment of Swallowing Disorders.* 2nd ed. Vol. 13. Austin, TX: PRO-ED; 1998.
- Perlman AL, Schulze-Delrieu KS. *Deglutition and Its Disorders: Anatomy, Physiology, Clinical Diagnosis, and Management.* Vol. 13. San Diego: Singular; 1997.
- Sullivan P, Guilford A. *Swallowing Intervention in Oncology.* Vol. 21. San Diego: Singular; 1999.

Many larger communities and head and neck oncology programs have or are associated with support groups. However, there are few, if any, in small rural areas. It may be helpful for a newly diagnosed head and neck cancer patient to have the opportunity to speak with a member of the support group prior to, during, and after treatment. The following include additional information about support groups:

■ Support for People with Oral and Head and Neck Cancer (SPOHNC) has a listing of support groups in the United States. In addition, it has a useful list of Web links for the head and neck cancer patient. SPOHNC can be located at www.spohnc.org, PO Box 53, Locust Valley, NY, 11560-0053, 1-800-377-0928.
■ Web Whispers is a laryngectomy online support group that provides information, has a monthly online newsletter, conducts an annual meeting, and provides loaner artificial electric larynx for members. It is located at www.webwhispers.org
■ The International Association of Laryngectomees (IAL) is an international association with educational materials, meetings, and links to medical equipment companies. IAL can be located at www.theial.com/ial.
■ Cancercare provides educational programs, counseling, information, and financial assistance. There are useful links and documents on recent cancer-related research. Patients can call

and obtain a free counseling from a social worker. It is located at www.cancercare.org. To contact telephone counseling, call 1-800-813-4673.
■ The Head and Neck Cancer Alliance has a link to a blog where patients can ask other patients about their experiences. The site is located at www.inspire.com/groups/head-and-neck-cancer-alliance/

For the patient, there is an "official" Web site for information as well as additional resources.

■ Medline Plus is a patient health information site supported by the National Library of Medicine and the National Institutes of Health. It is located at www.nlm.nih.gov/medlineplus/head-andneckcancer.html. This site is also available in Spanish.
■ Cancer.Net offers information on a variety of topics for the head and neck cancer patient. The site is located at www.cancer.net.
■ The National Cancer Institute offers information on head and neck cancer treatment, prevention, causes, and screening. The site can be accessed at www.cancer.gov/cancertopics/types/head-and-neck.
■ Brook, I. *The Laryngectomee Guide*. Washington DC: Itzhak Brook, 2013. This is a guide aimed at providing practical information that can assist laryngectomees and their caregivers. Available in print and electronically.

REFERENCES

1. Urba SG, Moon J, Giri PG, et al. Organ preservation for advanced resectable cancer of the base of tongue and hypopharynx: a Southwest Oncology Group Trial. *J Clin Oncol* 2005;23:88–95.
2. Taylor RJ, Chepeha JC, Teknos TN, et al. Development and validation of the neck dissection impairment index: a quality of life measure. *Arch Otolaryngol Head Neck Surg* 2002;128:44–49.
3. Henderson JM, Ord RA. Suicide in head and neck cancer patients. *J Oral Maxillofac Surg* 1997;55:1217–1221.
4. Terrell JE, Nanavati K, Esclamado RM, et al. Health impact of head and neck cancer. *Otolaryngol Head Neck Surg* 1999;120:852–859.
5. Hammerlid E, Persson LO, Sullivan M, et al. Quality-of-life effects of psychosocial intervention in patients with head and neck cancer. *Otolaryngol Head Neck Surg* 1999;120:507–516.
6. Duffy SA, Ronis DL, Valenstein M, et al. A tailored smoking, alcohol, and depression intervention for head and neck cancer patients. *Cancer Epidemiol Biomarkers Prev* 2006;15:2203–2208.
7. Gaziano JE. Evaluation and management of oropharyngeal dysphagia in head and neck cancer. *Cancer Control* 2002;9:400–409.
8. Silander E, Nyman J, Bove M, et al. Impact of prophylactic percutaneous endoscopic gastrostomy on malnutrition and quality of life in patients with head and neck cancer—a randomized study. *Head Neck* 2012;34:1–9.
9. Carnaby-Mann G, Crary MA, Schmalfuss I, et al. "Pharyngocise": randomized controlled trial of preventative exercises to maintain muscle structure and swallowing function during head-and-neck chemoradiotherapy. *Int J Radiat Oncol Biol Phys* 2012;83:210–219.
10. Kotz T, Federman AD, Kao J, et al. Prophylactic swallowing exercises in patients with head and neck cancer undergoing chemoradiation: a randomized trial. *Arch Otolaryngol Head Neck Surg* 2012;138:376–382.
11. Cavalot AL, Ricci E, Schindler A, et al. The importance of preoperative swallowing therapy in subtotal laryngectomies. *Otolaryngol Head Neck Surg* 2009;140:822–825.
12. Feng FY, Kim HM, Lyden TH, et al. Intensity-modulated chemoradiotherapy aiming to reduce dysphagia in patients with oropharyngeal cancer: clinical and functional results. *J Clin Oncol* 2010;28:2732–2738.
13. Eisbruch A. Amifostine in the treatment of head and neck cancer: intravenous administration, subcutaneous administration, or none of the above. *J Clin Oncol* 2011;29:119–121.
14. Le QT, Kim HE, Schneider CJ, et al. Palifermin reduces severe mucositis in definitive chemoradiotherapy of locally advanced head and neck cancer: a randomized, placebo-controlled study. *J Clin Oncol* 2011;29:2808–2814.
15. Scarantino C, LeVeque F, Swann RS, et al. Effect of pilocarpine during radiation therapy: results of RTOG 97-09, a phase III randomized study in head and neck cancer patients. *J Support Oncol* 2006;4:252–258.
16. Lin LC, Wang SC, Chen SH, et al. Efficacy of swallowing training for residents following stroke. *J Adv Nurs* 2003;44:469–478.
17. Eisbruch A, Ship JA, Dawson LA, et al. Salivary gland sparing and improved target irradiation by conformal and intensity modulated irradiation of head and neck cancer. *World J Surg* 2003;27:832–837.
18. Malouf JG, Aragon C, Henson BS, et al. Influence of parotid-sparing radiotherapy on xerostomia in head and neck cancer patients. *Cancer Detect Prev* 2003;27:305–310.
19. Fujiu M, Logemann JA. Effect of a tongue-holding maneuver on posterior pharyngeal wall movement during deglutition. *Am J Speech Lang Pathol* 1996;5:23–30.
20. Lazarus C, Logemann JA, Gibbons P. Effects of maneuvers on swallowing function in a dysphagic oral cancer patient. *Head Neck* 1993;15:419–424.
21. Logemann JA. *Evaluation and Treatment of Swallowing Disorders*. 2nd ed. Austin, TX: PRO-ED; 1998.
22. Dodds WJ, Stewart ET, Logemann JA. Physiology and radiology of the normal oral and pharyngeal phases of swallowing. *AJR Am J Roentgenol* 1990;154:953–963.
23. Murray J, Langmore SE, Ginsberg S, et al. The significance of accumulated oropharyngeal secretions and swallowing frequency in predicting aspiration. *Dysphagia* 1996;11:99–103.
24. Aviv JE, Murry T, Zschommler A, et al. Flexible endoscopic evaluation of swallowing with sensory testing: patient characteristics and analysis of safety in 1,340 consecutive examinations. *Ann Otol Rhinol Laryngol* 2005;114: 173–176.
25. Logemann JA. Role of the modified barium swallow in management of patients with dysphagia. *Otolaryngol Head Neck Surg* 1997;116:335–338.
26. Hunter KU, Schipper M, Feng FY, et al. Toxicities affecting quality of life after chemo-IMRT of oropharyngeal cancer: prospective study of patient-reported, observer-rated, and objective outcomes. *Int J Radiat Oncol Biol Phys* 2013;85:935–940.
27. Jacobson MC, Franssen E, Fliss DM, et al. Free forearm flap in oral reconstruction. Functional outcome. *Arch Otolaryngol Head Neck Surg* 1995;121:959–964.
28. Mahanna GK, Beukelman DR, Marshall JA, et al. Obturator prostheses after cancer surgery: an approach to speech outcome assessment. *J Prosthet Dent* 1998;79:310–316.
29. Lewin JS, Baugh RF, Baker SR. An objective method for prediction of tracheoesophageal speech production. *J Speech Hear Disord* 1987;52:212–217.
30. Chepeha DB, Hoff PT, Taylor RJ, et al. Selective neck dissection for the treatment of neck metastasis from squamous cell carcinoma of the head and neck. *Laryngoscope* 2002;112:434–438.
31. Chepeha DB, Taylor RJ, Chepeha JC, et al. Functional assessment using Constant's Shoulder Scale after modified radical and selective neck dissection. *Head Neck* 2002;24:432–436.
32. Salerno G, Cavaliere M, Foglia A, et al. The 11th nerve syndrome in functional neck dissection. *Laryngoscope* 2002;112:1299–1307.
33. Chepeha DB, Annich G, Pynnonen MA, et al. Pectoralis major myocutaneous flap vs revascularized free tissue transfer: complications, gastrostomy tube dependence, and hospitalization. *Arch Otolaryngol Head Neck Surg* 2004; 130:181–186.
34. Pauloski BR, Logemann JA, Colangelo LA, et al. Surgical variables affecting speech in treated patients with oral and oropharyngeal cancer. *Laryngoscope* 1998;108:908–916.
35. Annane D, Depondt J, Aubert P, et al. Hyperbaric oxygen therapy for radionecrosis of the jaw: a randomized, placebo-controlled, double-blind trial from the ORN96 study group. *J Clin Oncol* 2004;22:4893–4900.
36. Visch LL, van Waas MA, Schmitz PI, et al. A clinical evaluation of implants in irradiated oral cancer patients. *J Dent Res* 2002;81:856–859.

PRACTICE OF ONCOLOGY

40 Molecular Biology of Lung Cancer

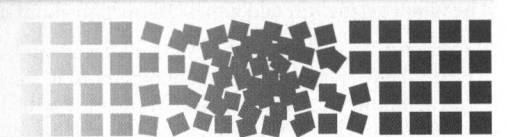

Leora Horn, Luiz Henrique de Lima Araujo, Patrick Nana-Sinkam, Gregory A. Otterson, Terence M. Williams, and David P. Carbone

INTRODUCTION

Lung cancer tumorigenesis is a multistep process of transformation from normal bronchial epithelium to overt lung cancer. Various molecular events resulting in gain or loss of function cause dysregulation of key genetic pathways involved in cellular proliferation, differentiation, apoptosis, migration, invasion, and other processes characteristic of the malignant phenotype. Mutations, including single nucleotide substitution or deletion, and translocation, deletion, or amplification of larger portions of genetic material may result from environmental factors, inherited susceptibility, or random events. Many genes are involved in tumorigenesis of both small cell lung cancer (SCLC) and non–small-cell lung cancer (NSCLC) (Table 40.1 and Fig. 40.1), but there are also unique genetic aberrations associated with each tumor type. The identification of the nature and frequency of these molecular abnormalities is necessary to determine their clinical implications (e.g., associations with smoking, histologic type, stage, survival, response to therapy), and define their clinical utility for the prevention and early diagnosis of lung cancer, and the development of therapeutic targets.

SUSCEPTIBILITY TO LUNG CANCER: GENETIC SUSCEPTIBILITY AND CARCINOGENS IN TOBACCO SMOKE

Tobacco use is the most important environmental factor associated with the development of lung cancer. Approximately 85% of lung cancer occurs in current or former smokers. Cigarette smoke contains more than 60 known carcinogens, 20 of which have been convincingly shown to cause lung tumors in laboratory animals or humans.[1] Of these, polycyclic aromatic hydrocarbons, such as benzo(a)pyrene, tobacco-specific nitrosamines, such as 4-(methylnitrosamino)-1-(3-pyridyl)-1-butanone (NNK), and aromatic amines, such as 4-aminobiphenyl, appear to have an important role in cancer causation. Nitrosamines such as NNK induce lung tumors in mice independent of the route of administration. Among the polycyclic aromatic hydrocarbons, benzo(a)pyrene is the most extensively tested and the first to be detected in tobacco smoke. Its role in cancer tumorigenesis is well described, and its diol epoxide metabolite has been implicated as a cause of mutations in the TP53 gene.[2] One of the carcinogenic effects of tobacco smoke in the lung is the formation of DNA adducts, leading to errors in DNA replication and resulting in mutations. DNA adducts have been identified in the bronchial tissue of patients with lung cancer. In current smokers, adduct levels correlate with the amount of tobacco smoke exposure.[3,4] In addition, in former smokers, the age at smoking initiation has been inversely associated with levels of DNA adducts, suggesting that the prevention of smoking in adolescence is of utmost importance in decreasing lung cancer risks.

Although tobacco use can account for the majority of lung cancers, most chronic smokers still do not develop lung cancer. Differences in inherent susceptibility may be related to variations in carcinogen metabolizing enzymes, DNA repair mechanisms, chromosome fragility, and other homeostatic mechanisms. Among genes for carcinogen-metabolizing enzymes, polymorphisms in the cytochrome P-450 genes, CYP1A1, CYP2D6, and CYP2E1, and in mu-class glutathione S-transferase (GSTM1) have received the most attention. In addition to inherent susceptibility to the carcinogenic effects of tobacco smoke, large genomewide association studies have identified lung cancer susceptibility loci at 15q25, 5p15, and 6p21.[5,6] In particular, polymorphisms in and around nicotinic cholinergic receptors at chromosome 15q25 appear to correlate with mRNA and protein expression of these receptors as well as functional changes in the calcium ion channel of the A5 nicotine receptor; these differences confer susceptibility to smoking behaviors.[7]

Researchers are optimistic that molecular epidemiology will help identify individuals at the highest risk of developing lung cancer. Such information, in addition to the smoking history, will be of great value in new lung cancer screening trials and in chemoprevention trials to identify persons at the highest risk of developing lung cancer.

MOLECULAR CHANGES IN PRENEOPLASIA

Before lung cancer is clinically recognizable, a series of morphologically distinct changes (hyperplasia, metaplasia, dysplasia, and carcinoma in situ) are thought to occur. It is believed that dysplasia and carcinoma in situ represent true preneoplastic changes. It is evident that preneoplastic cells contain several genetic abnormalities identical to some of the abnormalities found in overt lung cancer cells. For squamous cell carcinomas (SQCC), an immunohistochemical analysis has confirmed the abnormal expression of proto-oncogenes (cyclin D1) and TSGs (p53).[8] Allelotyping of precisely microdissected, preneoplastic foci of cells shows that 3p allele loss is currently the earliest known change, suggesting that one or more 3p TSGs may act as gatekeepers for lung cancer pathogenesis.[9] This is followed by 9p, 8p, and 17p allele loss and p53 mutation. Similarly, atypical alveolar hyperplasia, the potential precursor lesion of adenocarcinomas, can harbor KRAS mutations and allele losses of 3p, 9p, and 17p.[10] Other genetic alterations, such as inactivation of LKB1, whose germline mutations cause Peutz-Jeghers syndrome, have also been implicated in the development of adenocarcinoma. These observations are consistent with the multistep model of carcinogenesis and a field cancerization process, whereby the whole tissue region is repeatedly exposed to carcinogenic damage and is at risk for the development of multiple, separate foci of neoplasia.[11] Although all types of lung cancers

TABLE 40.1

Most Frequently Acquired Molecular Abnormalities in Lung Cancer

Abnormalities	Small Cell Lung Cancer	Non–Small-Cell Lung Cancer
Microsatellite instabilities	~35%	~22%
Autocrine loops	GRP/GRP receptor; SCF/KIT	TGF-α/EGFR; heregulin/HER2/neu; HGF/MET
RAS point mutation	<1%	15%–20%
EGFR mutation	<1%	<10% (West), ~40% (Asia)
EML4-ALK	0%	3%–7%
ROS1	0%	1%
RET	0%	1%
ERBB2	0%	2%–4%
PIK3CA	0%	1%–3%
FGFR	0%	20%
MYC family overexpression	15%–30%	5%–10%
P53 inactivation	~90%	~50%
RB inactivation	~90%	15%–30%
p16^{INK4A} inactivation	0%–10%	30%–70%
LKB1 inactivation	~40%–60% (IHC)	20%–40%
Frequent allelic loss	3p, 4p, 4q, 5q, 8p, 10q, 13q, 17p, 22q	3p, 6q, 8p, 9p, 13p, 17p, 19q
Telomerase activity	~100%	80%–85%
BCL2 expression	75%–95%	10%–35%

GRP, gastrin-releasing peptide; SCF, stem cell factor; TGF-α, transforming growth factor-α; EGFR, epidermal growth factor receptor; HER2, human epidermal growth factor receptor 2; HGF, hepatocyte growth factor; RB, retinoblastoma protein; IHC, immunohistochemistry.

have associated molecular abnormalities in their normal and pre-neoplastic lung epithelium, SCLC patients in particular appear to have multiple genetic alterations occurring in their histologically normal-appearing respiratory epithelium.

Molecular changes have been found not only in the lungs of patients with lung cancer, but also in the lungs of current and former smokers without lung cancer. These molecular alterations are thus important targets for use in the early detection of lung cancer and for use as surrogate biomarkers in following the efficacy of lung cancer chemoprevention. The challenge is to identify not only the prevalence and temporal sequence of molecular lesions in lung preneoplasia, but also to determine which are rate

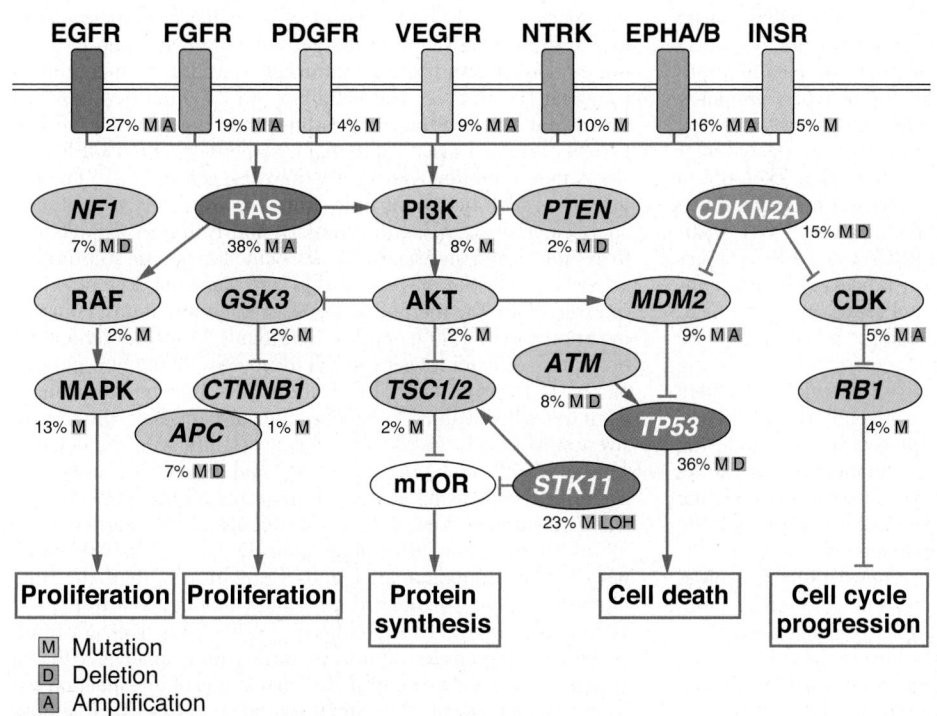

Figure 40.1 Significantly mutated pathways in lung adenocarcinomas. Genetic alterations in lung adenocarcinoma frequently occur in genes of the MAPK signaling, p53 signaling, Wnt signaling, cell cycle, and mammalian target of rapamycin (mTOR) pathways. Oncoproteins are indicated in *pink* to *red* and tumor suppressor proteins are shown in *light* to *dark blue*. The darkness of the colors is positively correlated to the percentage of tumors with genetic alterations. Frequency of genetic alterations for each of these pathway members in 188 tumors is indicated. (Reprinted by permission from Macmillan Publishers Ltd: Nature. Ding L, Getz G, Wheeler DA, et al. Somatic mutations affect key pathways in lung adenocarcinoma. *Nature* 2008;455: 1069–1075. Copyright 2007.)

PRACTICE OF ONCOLOGY

limiting and indispensable and thus represent potential candidates for intermediate biomarker monitoring and therapeutic efforts.

GENETIC AND EPIGENETIC ALTERATIONS IN LUNG CANCERS

Genomic Instability and DNA Repair Genes

Similar to other epithelial tumors, lung cancer cells typically display chromosomal instability—both numeric abnormalities (aneuploidy) of chromosomes and structural cytogenetic abnormalities.[12] Allele loss on chromosome 3p is thought to be the among the earliest genetic change occurring in both NSCLC and SCLC.[13] In addition, nonreciprocal translocations and recurrent losses involving 1p, 4p, 4q, 5q, 6p 6q, 8p, 9p, 11p, 13q, 17p, 18q, and 22q may occur, representing changes in known and potential tumor suppressor genes (TSGs).[14] Polysomes or regions of gene amplifications also occur and often involve proto-oncogenes, such as epidermal growth factor receptor (*EGFR*) and myelocytomatosis viral oncogene homolog (*MYC*).[15,16] Simple reciprocal translocations are uncommonly observed in lung cancer, although translocations that give rise to BRD4-NUT, CRCT1-MAML2, SLC34A2–ROS1, and EML4-ALK fusion proteins have been recently reported.[17–19] ALK and ROS1 translocations have been shown to drive the development and proliferation of tumors, and targeted therapy has resulted in clinical responses in patients with these abnormalities (see the following). In addition, alterations in microsatellite polymorphic repeat sequences are found in 35% of SCLC and 22% of NSCLC.[20] Most recently, a comprehensive genomic analysis of lung squamous cell cancers has revealed a high-frequency selective amplification of chromosome 3q compared to lung adenocarcinomas.[21] Furthermore, large-scale genomic profiling has established that there is a higher rate of copy number alterations, somatic rearrangements, and mutations found in squamous and adenocarcinoma lung cancers compared to other tumors.[22] For example, squamous cell lung cancers exhibit 8.1 somatic mutations per megabase (Mb) compared to other cancers where the frequency ranges from 1.0 to 3.2 mutations per megabase. These studies highlight the increased genetic complexity, genomic instability, higher mutation rate, and thus more extensive molecular heterogeneity that typifies lung cancer compared to other tumor types.

Recurring mutations in DNA repair genes are becoming increasingly recognized in multiple solid tumor types, including lung cancer. Ataxia telangiectasia mutated (ATM) plays a central role in the DNA damage response pathway that is triggered after genomic insults, including errors during replication, exposure to genotoxic drugs, or ionizing radiation, and has been identified in lung adenocarcinomas.[22–24] Alterations in other DNA repair genes have been identified, including BRCA1 and BRCA2, proteins that are both involved in the repair process of homologous recombination especially for double-strand breaks, as well as ATR, which functions in sensing and activating DNA repair in response to single-stranded DNA breaks.[22] Additionally, there is growing evidence that chromatin remodeling genes are highly mutated in lung cancer. Specifically, it has been recently shown that alterations in MLL2, MLL3, MLL4 (a group of histone-modifying genes) cluster in lung cancers, along with mutations in SMARCA4 and ARID1A (members of the SWI/SNF chromatin-remodeling complex).[21–24] Ongoing studies will serve to further evaluate the role of these putative TSGs in lung tumorigenesis.

The most powerful tumor surveillance mechanism is involved in DNA damage response and repair of errors in DNA replication.[25] The DNA glycosylase 8-oxo guanine (OGG1) specifically excises the oxidatively damaged mutagenic base 8-hydroxyguanine, which causes G:C→T:A transversions frequently found in lung cancer. Proof that OGG1 is central to this DNA repair is the evidence that lung adenocarcinoma spontaneously develops in OGG1 knockout mice and 8-hydroxyguanine accumulates in their genomes.[26,27] Individuals with low OGG activity have a greatly increased risk of developing lung cancer. Polymorphisms in other DNA repair genes including *ERCC1, XRCC1, ERCC5/XPG*, and *MGMT/AGT* have been correlated with a reduction of polyaromatic hydrocarbon DNA adduct formation as well as with lower lung cancer risks in case-control studies. Furthermore, high expression of ERCC1 is associated with decreased response to platinum-based chemotherapy, and overexpression of ERCC1 correlates with better overall prognosis in NSCLC,[28] reflecting improved repair of lethal DNA damage by platinum on the one hand, and greater DNA stability with less aggressive disease course on the other. More recent studies, however, have called into question the predictive ability of ERCC1 expression alone to predict cisplatin response, at least by immunohistochemical detection.[29] Similarly, ribonucleotide reductase M1 (RRM1) overexpression correlates with better de novo prognosis but resistance to gemcitabine.[30,31] High levels of the mismatch repair protein MSH2 have also been shown to be associated with poor survival with cisplatin, and may enhance the predictive significance of ERCC1 expression.[32] Prospective clinical trials investigating ERCC1 and RRM1 biomarker-guided therapy are currently underway.

PROTOONCOGENES, GROWTH FACTOR SIGNALING, AND GROWTH FACTOR– TARGETED THERAPIES

Advances in the understanding of lung carcinogenesis have yielded to a rapid discovery of novel driver oncogenes activated by mutations, translocations, or gene amplification. These alterations occur in genes that encode receptors or intracellular proteins crucial for cellular growth, proliferation, and survival, driving tumor formation and maintenance.

Receptor Tyrosine Kinases

EGFR is one of the most commonly mutated proto-oncogenes in lung adenocarcinoma. It is a transmembrane receptor-tyrosine kinase that is normally activated by binding with one of its ligands, members of the EGF family. EGFR-sensitizing mutations lead to constitutive activation of the tyrosine kinase and phosphorylation of downstream pathways ultimately resulting in uncontrolled proliferation, invasion, and metastasis. In 2004, investigators first noted mutations within the tyrosine-kinase domain of *EGFR* in patients who had sustained dramatic responses to the EGFR tyrosine-kinase inhibitors (TKIs), erlotinib and gefitinib.[33–35] The frequency of such mutations varies from approximately 10% of lung adenocarcinomas in North American and European populations to as high as 50% in Asia.[36–39] The leucine to arginine substitution at position 858 (L858R) in exon 21 and short in-frame deletions in exon 19 are the most common sensitizing mutations, comprising approximately 90% of cases. Sensitizing *EGFR* mutations are both prognostic for longer survival irrespective of therapy and predictive of response to EGFR TKIs.[35,39–47] Other mutations have been described within the *EGFR* gene, and for some, the responsiveness to EGFR TKI-directed therapy is similar to the deletion 19 and L858R, including the L861Q and the G719X mutations. An *EGFR* sequencing analysis of more than 1,000 patients with adenocarcinoma showed that 27 patients (2.5%) carried exon 20 insertions, representing approximately 9% of all *EGFR* mutations.[48] These mutations are found in patients who share the same phenotype as the canonical sensitivity mutations within exon 19 and 21; however, treatment with EGFR TKIs does not result in dramatic responses, and the prognosis is more analogous to that of patients with wild-type *EGFR*. A major area of investigation has been the mechanisms of acquired resistance to EGFR TKIs. Both in vitro as well as rebiopsy studies from patients who have been treated and subsequently progressed on treatment have shown two broad resistance mechanisms, secondary *EGFR* alterations and non-*EGFR bypass* mechanisms.[49] Approximately 50% of EGFR TKI resistance is due to a second site mutation, the T790M mutation occurring within exon 20.[50,51] Other, non-EGFR mechanisms of TKI resistance include *MET* amplification, *PIK3CA* mutations, and change in histology to a small cell appearance.[49] The T790M mutation is also found to be present at a very low prevalence in the germ line and appears to increase lung cancer risk independent of smoking.[52]

ERBB2 (formerly human epidermal growth factor receptor 2 [HER2]/neu) is a member of the erbB receptor family, along with *EGFR*. It is overexpressed in about 20% of NSCLCs, and amplified in 2% to 4% of cases.[53] *ERBB2* mutations have been identified in approximately 2% of NSCLCs, comprising in-frame insertions of 3 to 12 base pairs into exon 20, usually around the codon 776.[34,38,54] A meta-analysis suggested that ERBB2 overexpression is an indicator of poor survival in lung adenocarcinoma,[55] but amplification or mutations do not seem to be prognostic.[55,56] Early trials examining targeted therapies selected patients on the basis of ERBB2 overexpression and were mostly unsuccessful.[57] However, recent data suggest that trastuzumab, a recombinant humanized monoclonal antibody against ERBB2, may be active in *ERBB2*-mutant lung adenocarcinomas.[34] In addition, irreversible TKIs targeting ERBB2 are in early clinical trials.

Hepatocyte growth factor receptor (HGFR) is a receptor tyrosine kinase encoded by *MET*. MET amplification has been reported in about 2% of NSCLCs, and has been implicated in up to 20% of cases with acquired resistance to EGFR TKIs.[58] Several therapeutic strategies, including antibodies that target HGFR and anti-HGFR TKIs are under clinical evaluation in NSCLC patients, mostly aiming to prevent or overcome EGFR TKI resistance.[59–61]

Three other receptors have been nominated as potential druggable targets, especially in lung SQCC.[62,63] Insulin-like growth factor receptor 1 (IGFR1) is a tyrosine kinase receptor that activates the MAPK and PI3K/AKT/mTOR pathways, playing an important role in cancer growth and progression.[64] IGFR1 expression is higher in lung SQCC, and gene copy number has been associated with survival.[65] Despite an initial promise, phase III studies of some anti-IGFR1 agents has halted due to excess toxicities, including treatment-related deaths in the experimental arm. Fibroblast growth factor receptor 1 (FGFR1) is a member of the family of fibroblast growth factor (FGF) receptors that are dysregulated in a variety of cancers. *FGFR1* amplification has been described in approximately 20% of lung SQCCs and has been associated with cigarette smoking and worse survival.[66,67] In vitro studies showed activity with anti-FGFR inhibitors in cell lines harboring this feature, and pan-FGFR and multikinase inhibitors are in early phases of clinical investigation. Discoidin death receptor 2 (*DDR2*) is a member of the DDR family of transmembrane receptors that signals through SRC and STAT pathways. Mutations in the kinase domain have been reported in nearly 4% of lung SQCCs and were shown to yield malignant transformation in vitro.[68] Interestingly, some FDA-approved agents for chronic myelogenous leukemia seem to be active against the DDR family, including dasatinib, nilotinib, and imatinib.[69]

Translocated Genes in Lung Cancer

The anaplastic lymphoma kinase (ALK) fusion protein is an activating oncogenic driver of lung adenocarcinomas occurring in 3% to 7% of all NSCLCs.[70,71] Multiple ALK variants have been identified in lung cancer, and different ALK partners like kinesin family member 5B (KIF5B) have been described.[70,72,73] Similar to *EGFR* mutations, ALK fusions occur almost exclusively in adenocarcinomas, specifically with acinar histology, in never or former light smokers.[70,74–76] ALK fusions are not found in tumors with mutations in *EGFR* or *KRAS*, and patients appear to be of younger age compared to those with *EGFR* mutant tumors.[76] The gold standard test for *ALK* translocations is fluorescence in situ hybridization (FISH), but a variety of methods have been proposed, including immunohistochemistry, reverse transcription polymerase chain reaction (RT-PCR), and next-generation sequencing (NGS). The clinical activity of crizotinib—an oral inhibitor against c-MET, ALK, and ROS1—was impressive in early trials involving patients with the EML4-ALK translocation.[71] In a randomized phase III trial, crizotinib significantly improved progression-free survival (PFS), response rate (RR), and quality of life in comparison to second-line chemotherapy among patients with metastatic NSCLC harboring ALK translocations.[77] In a fashion analogous to that seen with EGFR TKI resistance, initial reports of resistance mechanisms include both *ALK* dependent (e.g., secondary mutations within *ALK* or amplification of the mutant *ALK* allele) and bypass tracks (e.g., the development of secondary *KRAS* and *EGFR* mutations have been described).[78–81] Importantly, several second-generation inhibitors are under clinical investigation and have shown promising activity in patients with acquired resistance to crizotinib.[82,83]

More recently, fusions involving the receptor tyrosine kinases ROS1 and RET have been described in NSCLC, each with oncogenic activity and potential utility as clinical biomarkers. ROS1 belongs to the insulin receptor family and is not normally expressed in the human lung tissue.[84] It has been demonstrated that ROS1 fusions induce autophosphorylation and downstream activation of common growth and survival pathways like mitogen-activated protein kinase (MAPK), STAT3, and PI3K/AKT. ROS1 rearrangements occur in approximately 1% to 2% of NSCLC patients, mostly in adenocarcinoma histology, younger patients, and never smokers.[85] It has been shown that selective ALK inhibitors are also active in tumors harboring *ROS1* translocations, both in vitro and in vivo.[86] RET rearrangements were only described in NSCLC in 2011, involving KIF5B as a partner.[87,88] Subsequently, CCD6, NCOA4, and TRIM33 have been described as alternative RET fusion partners.[89,90] Similar to *ALK* translocations, RET partners contain a coiled-coil domain that functions as a dimerization unit, leading to ligand-independent homodimerization of the fused protein and constitutive activation of the RET kinase activity mediated by autophosphorylation. Like ALK and ROS1, RET fusions are associated with a lack of smoking history and adenocarcinoma histology, with a frequency slightly higher than 1% in all comers.[91] Agents including cabozantinib,[90] sorafenib, sunitinib, vandetanib, and ponatinib are being evaluated in this patient population.

Intracellular Signaling

Because downstream effectors are required for intracellular transduction of incoming growth factors or receptor signals, it is not surprising that proteins important in cytoplasmic signal transduction cascades are also implicated in carcinogenesis. The *RAS* gene family—in particular, *KRAS*—can be activated by point mutations at codons 12 or 13 in exon 2 in approximately 20% to 30% of NSCLCs. *KRAS* mutations more commonly occur in patients with significant smoking history and adenocarcinoma histology.[92] Approximately 70% are G→T transversions, with the substitution of glycine by either cysteine or valine. Similar G→T transversions are observed in the mutated p53 gene, representing similar DNA damage as a result of bulky DNA adducts caused by the polycyclic hydrocarbons and nitrosamines in tobacco smoke. In a meta-analysis of 3,779 lung cancer patients, mutant *KRAS* was correlated to a worse prognosis in adenocarcinoma histology, but this link was not confirmed in a prospective study.[93] The poor prognosis has been proposed to be related to the fact that KRAS mutations rarely occur with EGFR mutations, and EGFR mutant tumors have a better prognosis than EGFR wild type. Thus, if KRAS mutations are evaluated only in EGFR wild-type tumors, the adverse prognostic effect of KRAS disappears.[94] Although the oncogenicity of aberrant *KRAS* is well established, effective agents that inhibit KRAS have not reached the clinic. Another strategy has been to target downstream effectors of RAS, like the RAF family proteins and MEK. For instance, sorafenib—a broad-spectrum kinase inhibitor including the RAF family—led to a disease control rate of 79% in the BATTLE trial[95] among patients with either KRAS or BRAF mutations. However, these findings were not confirmed in a large phase III trial.[96] The addition of selumetinib (AZD6244), a MEK1/2 inhibitor, to docetaxel significantly improved RR and PFS in a randomized, phase II trial.[97] A phase III study evaluating this combination in patients with KRAS-mutant NSCLC is ongoing. Another MEK inhibitor, trametinib (GSK1120212), also showed promising results in combination with chemotherapy in early phase I/Ib studies.[98,99] However, it is not clear whether these agents have a differential effectiveness according to the KRAS status, because similar responses have been observed in KRAS wild-type tumors.

The RAF proteins are serine/threonine kinases downstream of RAS, represented by three isoforms in mammals (ARAF, BRAF, and RAF1 [also known as CRAF]). BRAF is a known oncogene in lung adenocarcinoma, being mutated in approximately 3% of cases.[100] In contrast to melanoma, where the majority of BRAF mutations occur at valine 600 (V600E) within exon 15, V600E comprises only half of cases in lung adenocarcinoma. Interestingly, BRAF mutations are more likely to occur in former/current smokers. Dabrafenib (BRF113928)—a specific V600E BRAF inhibitor—demonstrated a promising RR of 40% in a phase II trial involving patients with lung adenocarcinoma harboring this mutation.[101] Dramatic responses have also been reported with vemurafenib, another specific inhibitor that is U.S. Food and Drug Administration (FDA)-approved for the treatment of melanoma.[102] Apart from BRAF, recurrent mutations at ARAF and RAF1 inhibitory sites were recently described in lung adenocarcinoma. Importantly, these mutations seem to be oncogenic in vitro, and may predict a response to targeted therapies, including sorafenib and MEK inhibitors.[103]

MAP2K1 (also known as MEK1) is a serine/threonine kinase downstream of RAF. In NSCLC, point mutations have been identified in 1% of cases, comprising three major nucleotide substitutions (Q56P, K57N, and D67N).[104] These mutations tend to be nonoverlapping with other drivers and induce constitutive extracellular signal-regulated kinase (ERK) phosphorylation and cell proliferation in vitro. It is still unknown if these mutations will predict clinical benefit from anti-MEK therapies.

Another frequently altered intracellular pathway in lung cancer is PI3K–AKT–mammalian target of rapamycin (mTOR). Phosphatidylinositol 3-kinases (PI3Ks) are lipid kinases that participate in regulating cell growth, proliferation, and survival. They comprise heterodimers formed by an 85-kDa regulatory subunit and a 110-kDa catalytic subunit, the latter being encoded by PIK3CA. PIK3CA mutations have been reported in several cancer types, including a frequency of 1% to 4% in lung adenocarcinoma.[105,106] However, a higher frequency of 16% was reported in the lung squamous section of The Cancer Genome Atlas (TCGA),[107] suggesting a predominance in this histologic subtype. The most common hotspots are at codons E542 and E545 in exon 9 (helical domain) and at codon H1047 in exon 20 (kinase domain). As opposed to other drivers, PIK3CA mutations often coexist with other oncogenic mutations in the case of lung adenocarcinoma and are not associated with smoking status.[108] PIK3CA mutations were shown to induce constitutive pathway activation and cell transformation in vitro[109] and have been associated with poor clinical prognosis.[110] The best strategy to target PI3K and the population to be selected is still a matter of debate.

AKT1 is downstream of PI3K and is a member of a family of serine-threonine kinases. Recurrent mutations within the plekstrin homology/lipid binding domain of AKT1 at E17K have been described in up to 1% of patients with lung adenocarcinoma.[111] This mutation causes constitutive activation of AKT and leads to cellular transformation in vitro and in vivo.[112]

Phosphatase and tensin homolog (PTEN) is a lipid/protein phosphatase that is integral to cellular processes and acts as a TSG gene by inhibiting the activity of the PI3K pathway. While germ-line mutations in PTEN lead to Cowden syndrome, somatic mutations have been found in patients with lung cancer, as well as epigenetic inactivation. PTEN mutations may be more common in smokers and those with squamous cancer, and are also seen in patients with SCLC.[113]

THE TECHNOLOGY OF GENOMIC ANALYSES OF LUNG CANCER

In recent years, technologic advances have enabled the comprehensive analyses of gene expression, copy number alterations, mutations, and other genetic perturbations across a large number of tumors.[114] In the lung cancer setting, such global approaches have led to the understanding of cancer biology and the molecular mechanisms underlying key cancer phenotypes at an unprecedented scope. More importantly, this knowledge has leveraged the identification of subsets of tumors whose biology may be affected by interventions targeted against key dysregulated genes or pathways.[115] These efforts have been increasingly applied in individual institutions or collaborative groups as will be described.

Although direct dideoxynucleotide (ddNTP) sequencing (or Sanger sequencing) has traditionally been the gold standard for the detection of recurrent point mutations in NSCLC (like EGFR), newer methodologies have been developed that are not only less dependent on the tumor fraction in the sample, but also simultaneously determine the mutational status of many genes in a single reaction. Multiplex genotyping comprises methods such as Sequenom (Sequenom, San Diego, CA) and SNaPShot (Applied Biosystems, Foster City, CA).[116,117] In an early report using these techniques from the Massachusetts General Hospital in 2009, at least one alteration was evident in 51% of 552 cases, and no overlap was observed among the main driver oncogenes.[118] More recently, the Lung Cancer Mutation Consortium (LCMC)—a collaborative group that genotyped 1,000 lung adenocarcinomas in the United States—detected genetic alterations in 54% of cases, and 97% were mutually exclusive.[119]

NGS platforms, also known as massively parallel sequencing, offer a wide range of opportunities to characterize the cancer genome for DNA, mRNA, transcription factor binding sites, microRNA (miRNA), and DNA methylation patterns.[120,121] In TCGA, 230 lung adenocarcinomas and adjacent samples were analyzed using various NGS platforms.[122] A whole-exome approach was used in all cases, whereas whole-genome sequencing was performed in 34 samples. The authors found a very high mutation rate (median 4.56 mutations per megabase), consistent with a median of 159 mutations per tumor (range, 13 to 1,339). As demonstrated in prior experiences, this was among the highest rates in TCGA projects, only behind lung SQCC and melanoma. Somatic mutations were found in known oncogenes, like KRAS, EGFR, and BRAF, as well as chromatin modifiers as ARID1A, SMARCA4, and SETD2. A number of recurrent noncanonical mutations were documented, including a MET Y1003* mutation. Lung SQCC was also explored in TCGA, including 178 pairs of tumor/normal samples from patients with stages I through IV disease.[107] A total of 48,690 nonsilent mutations were identified through whole-exome sequencing, with a mean of 360 total exonic mutations per tumor (median, 8.4 per megabase). Ten genes were considered to harbor significant mutations, including TP53, CDKN2A, PTEN, PIK3CA, KEAP1, MLL2, HLA-A, NFE2L2, NOTCH1, and RB1. Frequent alterations were present in the following pathways: CDKN2A/RB1 (cell cycle control), NFE2L2/KEAP1/CUL3 (response to oxidative stress), PI3K/AKT (apoptotic signaling), and SOX2/TP63/NOTCH1 (squamous differentiation). In addition, whole-transcriptome sequencing and microarray expression was carried out. The mRNA expression data clustered in four distinct subtypes named classical, basal, secretory, and primitive, which correlate with miRNA, methylation, somatic copy number alterations, and mutation spectrum.

As a more comprehensive insight into the lung cancer genome emerges, it becomes clear that its complex biology will require continuous efforts and more integrative analyses. For instance, it is somewhat disappointing that approximately half of lung adenocarcinomas still lack a plausible target for drug development. It comes without saying that many alterations are detected in TSGs, for which no targeted therapies are available. These observations may also serve to argue that a fraction of driver mechanisms may be mediated by epigenetic or other regulatory mechanisms, as opposed to structural genomic alterations. One approach to fill this gap is the coordinated analysis of multiple types of data from large cohorts like TCGA. For example, integrating mutational data to gene expression, miRNA, or methylation profiling could potentially determine associations with particular sets of genes. Such gene sets could be subjected to computational analyses and biochemical studies to discover the biologic and clinical significance, as well as proposing alternative therapeutic strategies. The Clinical Proteomic Tumor Analysis Consortium (CPTAC) is an ongoing program that exemplifies the integration of high-throughput cancer genomics and proteomics using samples from TCGA, as well as cell lines and xenograft models.[123]

It is also intriguing that current genomic studies rely primarily on computational approaches to identify *driver* events and distinguish them from the background of *passenger* mutations. Such analyses may be flawed not only by the relatively low sample size, but also by the filtering method on its own.[124,125] Indeed, most comprehensive genomic studies (as previously described) included a few more than a hundred samples and are not empowered to detect rare mutations. Larger efforts will be essential to achieve a larger number of cases per cancer type, as exemplified by TCGA and the International Cancer Genome Consortium. In addition, continuously improving the accuracy of analytical methods will be key to avoid false discoveries and to avoid overlooking potential targetable alterations.

EPIGENETICS/EPIGENOME

Over the last 20 years, it has become apparent that epigenetics dysregulation is nearly universal in cancers, and specifically in lung cancer. Indeed, a recent study showed that the determination of the methylation status of a four gene panel (CDKN2A, CDH13, RASSF1A, and APC) is predictive of lymph node recurrence in stage I cancers.[126] A separate study confirmed the prognostic impact of a separate panel of methylated genes.[127] Unfortunately, despite the near universal finding of hypermethylation of tumor-relevant genes and the prognostic impact of transcriptional silencing of these genes, attempts at interfering with this epigenetic program by using hypomethylating agents (usually in conjunction with histone deacetylase inhibitors) has failed to have a dramatic impact on typical tumor response criteria, although each of these trials showed tantalizing evidence of biologic effect.[128–130]

More recently, mutations within epigenetic modifying genes have been discovered in a variety of thoracic tumors. These include mutations within the SWI/SNF complex proteins SMARCA4/BRG1 and ARID1A.[24] The SWI/SNF complex is an important chromatin modeling complex that is essential in yeast and is thought to function as a tumor suppressor in many human tumors, including lung cancers. Other mutations or overexpression of other epigenetic modifiers, including histone methyltransferases, histone acetyltransferase coactivators and the histone lysine demethylase KDM2A, have been described as well.[21,131,132] Whether these mutations or overexpression of genes act as *drivers* of oncogenesis or act as passenger mutations/alterations has not yet been clarified. Furthermore, if these findings will serve as useful predictors of response to epigenetic therapy will depend on the development of well-designed prospective biomarker-driven and/or stratified trials.

TUMOR SUPPRESSOR GENES AND GROWTH SUPPRESSION

A number of TSGs have been identified that inhibit lung tumorigenesis or suppress key phenotypes in developed lung carcinomas.

Many classical tumor suppressors have been identified by decades of work examining genes involved in human-inherited cancer syndromes and elucidating their role in sporadic cancers. Germ-line mutations in some TSGs, such as LKB1/STK11, *p53*, and *RB1*, give rise to inherited tumor syndromes; however, a somatic loss of TSGs within sporadic cancers is more commonly seen, including p53, PTEN, CDKN2A (encoding both p16[INK4A] and p14[ARF]), ATM, NF1, RB1, and APC. These have all been found to be mutated or lost in lung cancer through multiple mechanisms, such as inactivating mutations, chromosomal loss, methylation, or overexpression of other proteins that inhibit the suppressive gene's expression or activity.[23,24] We discuss several of the most frequently lost TSGs in the following paragraphs.

p53 Pathway

The *p53* gene, located at chromosome 17p13, is crucial for maintaining genomic integrity in the face of cellular stress from DNA damage through gamma and ultraviolet irradiation, carcinogens, and chemotherapy. It is the most frequently mutated TSG in human malignancies, and mutations affect approximately 90% of SCLCs and >50% of NSCLCs. In NSCLCs, p53 alterations occur more frequently in SQCC (81%) than adenocarcinomas (~50%).[21,22,24] *p53* mutations have been linked to poorer prognosis retrospectively and in the TCGA Pan-Cancer analysis; however, they have not been shown to correlate with survival in a prospective randomized clinical trial.[133,134] Most p53 mutations are G→T transversions, which correlate with cigarette smoking.[2] The Li-Fraumeni syndrome of inherited germline *p53* mutation may also lead to increased susceptibility to lung cancer in adults; this risk is magnified by tobacco smoking, because carriers who smoked had a 3.16-fold higher risk for lung cancer than nonsmokers.[135] The majority of missense mutations occur in the DNA-binding domain of the protein, and five of the six most prevalently mutated sites are arginine residues that are involved with electrostatic interactions with DNA strands.[136] Missense mutations prolong the half-life of the p53 protein, leading to increased protein levels detectable with immunohistochemistry. Also, because p53 exerts its cellular actions as a tetramer, mutant forms of the protein appear to exert dominant negative effects on wild-type p53 and have also been shown to inhibit the function of p63 and p73 family members.[137]

In addition to mutational or deletional loss of p53, other regulatory components of the p53 pathway are altered in lung cancer, including the ATM gene, the p53 binding protein MDM2, and the p14[ARF] tumor suppressor. ATM and the related protein ATR are tumor-suppressive serine/threonine kinases that activate cell cycle checkpoints in response to DNA damage and, ultimately, activate and stabilize p53.[138] Although ATR and the downstream checkpoint kinases (CHEK) are mutated in less than 1% of lung adenocarcinomas, ATM has been found to have deleterious mutations in 7% of lung adenocarcinomas. These mutations were largely mutually exclusive with p53 mutations, likely indicating that mutations in both genes would have redundant effects, especially because it has been shown that gain-of-function mutations in p53 can inactivate ATM.[139,140] Conversely, the MDM2 E3 ubiquitin ligase negatively regulates p53 by binding its transcriptional activation domain, inducing its nuclear export, and by polyubiquitinating p53, marking it for proteasomal degradation.[141] Abnormal overexpression of MDM2 is found in NSCLC, where it is amplified in a significant number of tumors. MDM2 activity is inhibited by other tumor suppressor genes in the p53 pathway, including ATM and also the p14[ARF] tumor suppressor gene.[142]

When p53 is functional, it is activated by phosphorylation in response to cellular stress (e.g., DNA damage). Once activated, p53 strongly induces the expression of other tumor suppressor genes that control cell cycle checkpoints (e.g., *p21*[WAF1/CIP1]), apoptosis (*BAX*), DNA repair (*GADD45*), and angiogenesis (thrombospondin).[143] p53 activation has also been found to alter miRNA expression and maturation.[144,145] The high frequency of p53 loss across the entire spectrum of human tumors is a strong testament to its importance in inhibiting tumor development and growth. Restoring p53 activity in tumors is effective at halting their growth and could represent an effective therapy, although development of this strategy is challenging.[146] Several gene therapy clinical trials have been reported in which lung cancers are treated by an intratumoral injection introducing a wild-type *p53* gene using retroviral or adenoviral vectors.[147] Other strategies have been developed to restore p53 activity without attempting to reintroduce the entire gene into tumor cells.[148,149] The vaccination of patients with advanced cancer with a custom vaccine corresponding to their tumor's mutation in *p53* or *RAS* has demonstrated the generation of mutant oncogene–specific immune responses associated with prolonged survival.[150] A trial of p53 vaccination in SCLCs produced measurable increases in tumor-specific immune response that was associated with improved outcome and response to therapy in some patients.[151,152]

CYCLINS AND CELL CYCLE REGULATORY PATHWAYS

p16[INK4A] is a cyclin-dependent kinase (CDK) inhibitor important for the integrity of the G1 checkpoint. Loss of p16[INK4A] frees CDKs from inhibition, permitting constitutive phosphorylation of retinoblastoma (RB) protein and inactivation of its growth suppressive function. Approximately 40% of primary NSCLCs lose p16[INK4A], located on chromosome 9p21, making it the most common component of the p16[INK4A]–cyclin D1–CDK4–RB pathway to be inactivated in NSCLC. Other CDK inhibitors are also lost at a lower prevalence in NSCLC, and the RB gene is mutated or lost in a significant minority of cases.[153] In contrast, a strikingly different pattern of pathway dysregulation is observed in SCLCs, in which abnormalities in p16 are rarely observed, but RB itself is nearly always abnormal. Although p16[INK4A] point mutations in NSCLCs were observed in only 14% of tumors, homozygous deletions or aberrant promoter methylation are common mechanisms for p16[INK4A] inactivation.[20] Indeed, aberrant p16[INK4A] methylation is a frequent, early preneoplastic event in the pathogenesis of SQCC.[154] Furthermore, p16[INK4A] and p14[ARF] are alternative splice forms of RNA transcripts from the same DNA locus. p14[ARF] is also a tumor suppressor gene and functions to stabilize p53. Thus, alteration at the p16[INK4A] locus may not only abrogate p16[INK4A] function but also disrupt p53 pathway through p14[ARF].[155]

In the absence of inhibitory regulation by the CDK inhibitors, cyclins, and their catalytic partners, the CDKs phosphorylate the retinoblastoma protein, a growth-suppressive nuclear phosphoprotein located on chromosomal region 13q14. When in its active, unphosphorylated form, RB binds and inactivates proteins such as transcription factor E2F-1, preventing G1/S transition. The RB protein is absent or structurally abnormal in more than 90% of SCLCs and 15% to 30% of NSCLCs. Lung-targeted, conditional deletion of RB and p53 in mice leads to the development of SCLC that recapitulate that observed in humans.[156] Although the p16 and RB tumor-suppressive components of this pathway are frequently lost in lung cancer, the growth promoting cyclin and CDK components of the pathway are often overexpressed, and cyclin D1, cyclin E1, and CDK4 have each been shown to be amplified in a subset of lung cancers[157] and are overexpressed by immunohistochemical evaluation.

LKB1, AMPK, AND MTOR PATHWAY

LKB1 is a serine/threonine kinase that serves as a *master regulator* of several key intracellular pathways through phosphorylation of downstream regulatory kinases. Its tumor-suppressive role became apparent when it was discovered that inherited mutations in LKB1 gave rise to a rare autosomal-dominant polyposis/cancer susceptibility disease, Peutz-Jeghers syndrome.[158,159] Subsequent to this

discovery it was found that LKB1 is somatically mutated and deleted in a range of other carcinomas, most prevalently in NSCLC, where approximately 20% to 30% of adenocarcinomas exhibit LKB1 loss.[160–162] SQCCs and large cell lung carcinomas also exhibit LKB1 loss but at a lower frequency, and an immunohistochemical analysis revealed absent LKB1 expression in two-thirds of SCLCs.[163] In a mouse model, tumors rapidly develop when conditional LKB1 knockout was combined with conditional expression of oncogenic KRAS using inhaled adenovirus-expressing Cre recombinase. Additionally, whereas most other mouse models of lung tumorigenesis (e.g., oncogenic KRAS with conditional p53 deletion) cause only lung adenocarcinomas, more than half of the tumors resulting from KRAS with conditional LKB1 deletion showed squamous or mixed histology, and large cell histology was also observed.[161] LKB1 regulates a key metabolic checkpoint through its phosphorylation of the AMP-activated protein kinase AMPK. Phosphorylation of AMPK results in the suppression of tumor growth and metabolic activity by direct phosphorylation of metabolic enzymes and by activation of the tuberous sclerosis complex tumor suppressors, which block activation of the mTOR pathway.[164] In tumors that have lost LKB1, this growth-suppressive checkpoint is inactivated.[165,166] Metformin, an oral hypoglycemic drug commonly used in diabetics, activates AMPK and has been found to inhibit proliferation and colony formation in vitro.[167] Retrospective analyses demonstrate reduced incidence of cancer among diabetics treated with metformin.[168–170] In addition, metformin treatment of diabetics is associated with higher rates of complete response among neoadjuvantly treated breast cancer patients.[171] Although metformin appears to require functional LKB1 in order to effect AMPK activation, other compounds have been identified that circumvent this requirement. Thus, direct pharmacologic reactivation of the downstream tumor-suppressive functions of AMPK may be a viable therapeutic strategy for LKB1-deficient tumors. In addition to its role in regulating the AMPK metabolic checkpoint, LKB1 has many other distinct roles dependent on other downstream effector kinases, such as salt-inducible kinase, NUAK, and microtubule-affinity regulating kinase. These actions play a role in regulating a variety of cellular phenotypes important to cancer, such as cellular motility and transcriptional regulation, and LKB1 has been shown to exert profound effects in maintaining cellular polarity.[172,173] However, the relative importance of these various phenotypes in the biology of LKB1-deficient lung cancers is poorly understood.

OTHER PUTATIVE TUMOR SUPPRESSORS

Several other genes that are less well characterized than the tumor suppressor genes detailed previously have been identified as targets of recurrent mutational inactivation, chromosomal loss, and epigenetic repression in lung cancer. These candidate suppressor genes are often identified as regions of copy number loss or loss of heterozygosity (LOH) that occur in multiple tumors in large, genomewide studies of chromosomal architecture in lung cancer. Further experimentation is required to elucidate which molecular pathways and cellular phenotypes are affected and to define the functional importance of these candidates. Common regions of genomic loss surround the chromosomal regions of classical tumor suppressors CDKN2A, CDKN2B, LKB1, and RB1 (in small cell lung cancer). Other areas of recurrent loss in NSCLC occur at 9p23, 3p14.2, 3p21.3 16q23.1, 2q21.2, 4q35, 5q12.1, and 13q12.11.[157] Many of these regions are also altered in SCLC, although there are fewer data available for this tumor type. Determining the functional roles of each individual gene can be challenging. Of genes included in the regions listed previously, missense mutations have been identified in PTPRD (9p23), LRP1B (2q21.2), BLU (3p21.3), and WWOX (16q23.1).[174,175] Experimental reexpression of candidate genes has been shown to inhibit proliferation in tumor cell lines for many of these putative tumor suppressors, including PTPRD, LRP1B, WWOX (16q23.1), FHIT (3p14.2), SMARCA4 (19p13.2), PTEN (10q23), and RASSF1, FUS1, BLU, and SEMA3B (3p21.3).[176,177] However, for most of these candidates, the biologic implications of gene loss in a tumor is uncertain.

Immune Checkpoint Inhibitors

Immune checkpoint inhibitors have recently demonstrated promising results in lung cancer patients. In particular, inhibitors to cytotoxic T-lymphocyte–associated antigen 4 (CTLA-4) and programmed death 1 (PD-1) and programmed death receptor ligand 1 (PD-L1) are currently in clinical trials in both small cell and non–small-cell lung cancer patients. CTLA-4 is expressed on T cells and suppresses T-cell signaling.[178] Ipilimumab is a monoclonal antibody that inhibits CTLA-4 and is FDA approved for the treatment of melanoma. Randomized phase II trials in small cell and non–small-cell lung cancer patients demonstrated promising results when ipilimumab was combined with chemotherapy.[179,180] Randomized phase III trials in SCLCs and NSCLCs are ongoing. Antibodies that block PD-1 include nivolumab (BMS-936558) and MK3475. These agents inhibit binding of PD-1 to both its ligands, PD-L1 and PD-L2. Antibodies that block PD-L1 include MPDL3280A and MEDI-4736. These agents inhibit binding of the ligand to its receptor PD-1 and B7.1. A large phase I trial of nivolumab included 129 NSCLC patients and reported a 17.1% response rate, 1-year survival of 42%, and 2-year survival of 24%.[181,182] Based on this promising data, two randomized phase III trials in squamous and nonsquamous NSCLC patients and a single-arm phase II trial in squamous NSCLC patients have been completed with results anticipated. In patients with tumor samples available for assessment, PD-L1 expression by immunohistochemistry was associated with a response to therapy, whereas no response was observed in patients with tumors that were PD-L1 negative.[181] A phase I trial that included 85 NSCLC patients treated with MPDL3280A reported a response rate of 23%.[183] Preliminary data reported that the response rate was higher in tumors that were IHC3 positive (83%), defined as 10% of tumors staining positive for the expression of PD-L1, and in smokers. Although anti-CTLA-4 antibodies are being employed with chemotherapy in lung cancer patients, single agent data with anti-PD-1 and PD-L1 antibodies appears promising, and it is unclear if these agents should be used alone or in combination with chemotherapy or targeted therapy in lung cancer patients.

OTHER BIOLOGIC ABNORMALITIES IN LUNG CANCER

Cellular Immortality Resulting from Increased Telomerase Activity

Cellular senescence is mainly regulated by telomerase, a ribonucleoprotein enzyme responsible for maintaining telomere length by de novo synthesis of telomeres and elongation of existing telomeres. The human telomerase reverse transcriptase (hTERT) catalytic subunit is the major determinant of telomerase activity in vitro and in vivo. During normal cell division, telomere shortening leads to cell senescence and thus governs normal cell mortality. TERT maintains telomere ends via the synthesis of TTAGG nucleotide repeats. Telomerase activation is considered mandatory for tumor cells to escape senescence and contributes to immortalization and cancer pathogenesis. For example, immortalization of primary human airway epithelial cells can be achieved by the successive introduction of the simian virus SV40 early region and hTERT.[184] Malignant transformation is seen when these immortalized cells are transfected by an activated RAS oncogene. Approximately 100% of SCLCs and 80% to 85% of NSCLCs have been demonstrated to express high levels of telomerase activity.

Furthermore, hTERT gene amplification occurs in 57% of NSCLCs, suggesting that this pathway is commonly targeted in lung cancer.[185] The prognostic significance of hTERT expression or activity remains controversial, although a recent study demonstrated that the copy number of serum hTERT mRNA was independently correlated with tumor size, tumor number, presence of metastasis, likelihood of recurrence, and smoking.[186] Furthermore, elevated telomerase activity and hTERT levels have been associated with worse DFS and overall survival in patients with stage I NSCLC.[187] In preneoplastic lesions, telomerase activity or expression of its RNA component, or both, are observed in situ in lesions with the expression proportional to the severity of histology grade, supporting a temporal role for telomerase activation during lung preneoplasia.[188] Thus, telomerase activity or expression can be used as a potential biomarker to detect premalignant as well as tumor cells. For these reasons, there is much interest in developing antitelomerase drugs as new therapeutics.[189,190]

Deregulation of Apoptosis

Loss of normal apoptosis commonly occurs in many cancer types and is associated with the expansion of viable cells and the development of resistance to chemotherapy and radiation therapy. Many members of both the mitochondrial (intrinsic) and the death receptor (extrinsic) apoptotic signaling pathways are found to be abnormal in lung cancer. A member of the intrinsic pathway, the antiapoptotic gene BCL2 originally described in follicular lymphomas, is abnormally overexpressed in SCLCs (75% to 95%) and some NSCLCs (25% of SQCC and approximately 10% of adenocarcinoma) and is the prototypical member of the antiapoptotic Bcl2 family proteins.[191–193] BCL-2 expression is associated with good prognosis in NSCLCs.[194] Cytotoxicity of many chemotherapeutic agents is induced through the Bcl-2 apoptotic pathway; overexpression of Bcl-2 is associated with increased resistance to these agents.[195,196] Other prosurvival Bcl-2 family members include Bcl-xL, Bcl-w, and Mcl-1. Conversely, a number of Bcl-2 family members have proapoptotic functions, including Bim, Bak, Bax, Bad, and Puma. Given the role of Bcl-2 and other members of this family in suppressing apoptosis and in reducing the efficacy of chemotherapy and radiotherapy, considerable effort is being made to develop Bcl-2 family targeted therapeutics in combination with chemotherapy.

In the extrinsic apoptotic pathway, death receptors are members of the tumor necrosis factor (TNF)/TRAIL receptor gene superfamily that consists of more than 20 proteins with a broad range of biologic functions, including regulation of cell death and survival, differentiation, or immune regulation. The best-characterized death receptor, Fas (CD95), and its ligand, FasL, have also been implicated in lung cancer. In general, lung cancers express FasL but not the receptor. However, as T cells express Fas, one model that may help explain the resistance of lung cancer cells to immune surveillance involves the clonal deletion of immune T cells that would otherwise be directed against lung cancer antigens by this Fas–FasL interaction. Both caspase-8 and caspase-10 expression appears to be decreased in lung cancer. Homozygous deletion or methylation of the CASP8 gene has been observed in SCLC cell lines, with 79% demonstrating loss of expression, suggesting that therapies that utilize the TNF/TRAIL receptor pathway of apoptotic activation may not achieve success in SCLC due to the impaired formation of the death-inducing signaling complex (DISC).[197] Of note, TRAIL-induced apoptosis is independent of p53 gene status. Conversely, because NSCLC has high rates of p53 inactivation (but predominantly intact caspase 8 pathways) and high levels of TRAIL receptor expression, this mode of therapy may prove beneficial. Polymorphisms in the promoter region of caspase-9 have been shown to contribute to risk of lung cancer development.[198]

Another family of proteins that promote tumor survival are the inhibitors of apoptosis (IAP), which bind to and block caspase function, especially caspase-3 and -7. IAPs also inhibit apoptosis via the modulation of the transcription of nuclear factor κ B (NF-κB). In addition to X-linked inhibitor of apoptosis protein (XIAP), one of the best-known members of this class of protein is survivin. Its expression is high in the tumor but nearly nonexistent in adult normal tissue, and higher expression has been correlated with poor outcomes in NSCLCs.[199,200] The suppression of survivin has been shown to sensitize lung cancer cells to radiation, suggesting that it can be a potential target for intervention.[201] During the activation of apoptosis, another class of proteins called Smac proteins are released from the mitochondria and neutralize IAPs, by competing with caspases for the binding of IAPs. Bcl-2 family inhibitors, TRAIL receptor agonists, Smac mimetics, and IAP inhibitors are currently undergoing clinical testing as agents that sensitize lung tumor cells to chemotherapy and radiation in order to promote apoptosis.[202]

microRNAS IN LUNG CANCER DIAGNOSTICS AND THERAPY

Approximately 2 decades ago, investigators made the startling discovery that components of the human genome, previously considered to be nonfunctional, actually harbored noncoding RNAs (ncRNAs) with gene regulatory properties.[203,204] Termed microRNAs (miRNAs or miRs), these 22 nucleotide ncRNAs are now known to be highly conserved, are often localized within fragile chromosomal regions and have the capacity for gene regulation through either mRNA degradation or the inhibition of translation.[205] Given their relative short length and redundancy, it is estimated that miRNAs may regulate up to 60% of the human genome. miRNAs have been implicated as regulators of biologic processes fundamental to both the initiation and progression of cancer (differentiation, proliferation, angiogenesis).[206,207] The mechanisms of change in miRNA expression in cancers are multifactorial. First, miRNAs tend to be localized to fragile chromosomal regions. Such chromosomal regions harbor amplifications, deletions, and translocations, many of which have been described in lung cancers.[208] Thus, in some cases, patterns of miRNA deregulation may be linked to chromosomal aberrations. Changes in miRNA expression and function may also be driven by epigenetic changes, miRNA or target polymorphisms, environmental stimuli (e.g., cigarette smoke), and either tumor suppressors or oncogenes (e.g., p53).[209,210] Although the function of many miRNAs remains largely unknown, research suggests that miRNA function is both disease and cell specific.

microRNA Biogenesis

The process of miRNA biogenesis is a complex one and investigators continue to explore the mechanisms that drive miRNA production (Fig. 40.2). Initially, a long primary transcript (pri)-miRNA transcript undergoes transcription by RNA polymerase II.[211] The pri-miRNAs are then bound to the double-stranded RNA-binding domain (dsRBD) protein known as DiGeorge syndrome critical region gene 8 (DGCR8) for vertebrates.[212] Subsequently, the RNase III endonuclease termed RNASEN/Drosha converts the pri-miRNA to a smaller stem-loop ~70 nucleotide (nt) precursor miRNA (pre-miRNA). These pre-miRNAs are then transported from the nucleus to the cytoplasm using the dsRBD, Exportin 5.[213] Once in the cytoplasm, the pre-miRNA is cleaved to a mature 18 to 25 nucleotide miRNA using Dicer. The mature miRNA sequence is then loaded into the RNA-induced silencing complex (RISC) complex after which it may then form complementarity to either the 3′ or 5′ untranslated region (UTR) of a target gene to induce either RNA degradation of the inhibition of translation. It is important to recognize that investigators have now identified

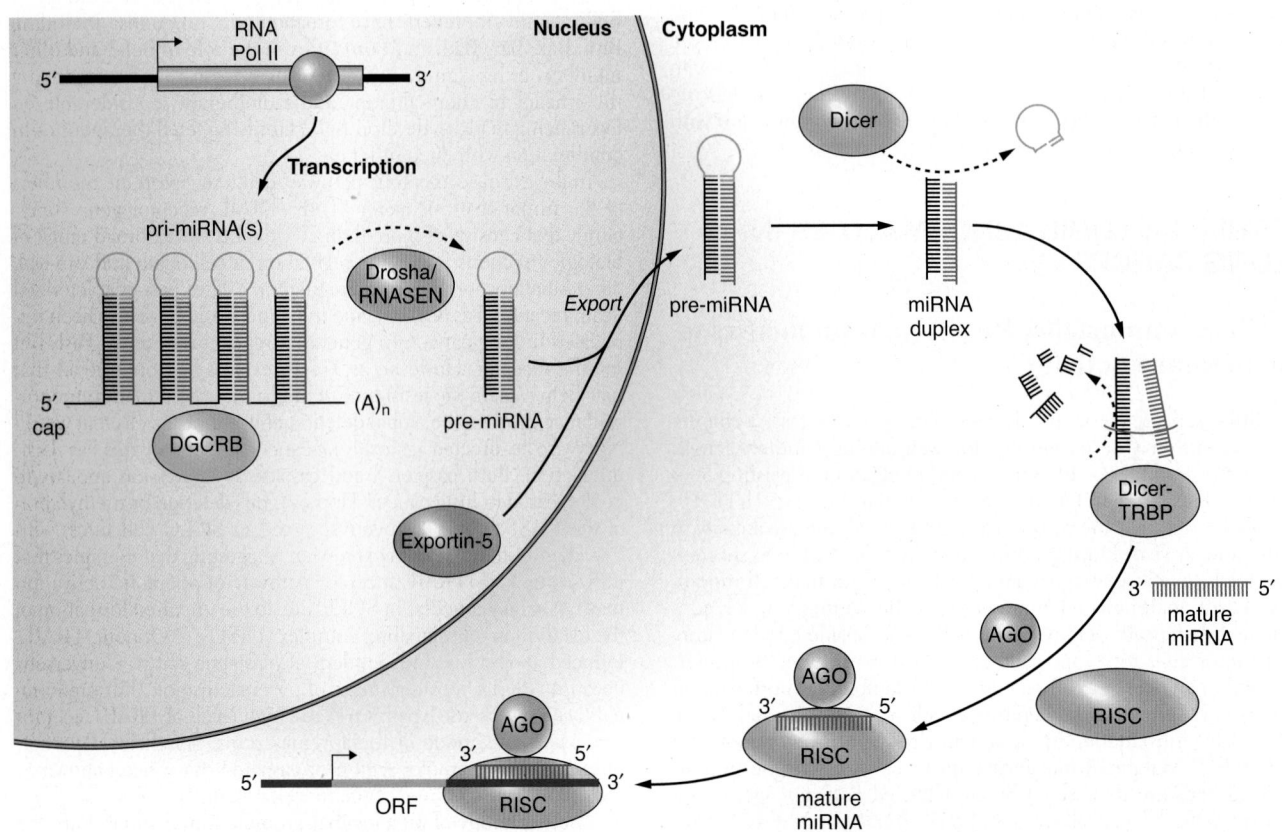

Figure 40.2 microRNA (miRNA) biogenesis.

additional mechanisms for miRNA biogenesis, suggesting that we are just beginning to understand the complexities of this process.

miRNA PROFILING IN LUNG CANCER

Early investigations in lung cancer have focused on applying high throughput platforms as a means for linking patterns of miRNA deregulation to clinical parameters. Of note, targeted the disruption of miRNA processing through the targeting of Dicer can promote lung tumorigenesis and has been associated with clinical outcome.[214] Yanaihara and colleagues[215] conducted high throughput profiling of cases of stage I adenocarcinoma of the lung. They identified over 40 miRNAs that distinguished lung tumors from adjacent uninvolved lung.[215] Of these miRNAs, decreased Let-7a-2 and increased miR-155 appeared to correlate with patient outcome. Because of that initial study, investigators have conducted multiple similar studies with the primary goals of identifying a prognostic miRNA signature[216–218] and potentially actionable miRNAs.[218]

Despite the multitude of miRNA profiling studies, investigators have yet to reach a consensus on which miRNAs confer the most accurate prognostic information. A primary reason for the lack of reproducibility is that, similar to other high throughput platforms, miRNA profiling studies are susceptible certain biases including small cohort sizes, varying platforms (array, sequencing, RT-PCR), and variability in data interpretation. In addition, most platforms are based on previously identified miRNAs. A recent study by Keller and colleagues[219] sought to use NGS to identify both previously unknown and novel mature forms of miRNAs. The authors conducted NGS on peripheral whole blood obtained from 10 patients with NSCLCs (stages 1A through IIIA) and 10 healthy control patients. They identified 32 known and 7 novel miRNAs that were significantly altered in patients with lung cancer. In addition, they identified 41 novel mature forms of previously identified precursors and 76 novel miRNAs, thus suggesting that we have yet to identify all miRNAs that may be of potential clinical and biologic relevance.

miRNAs and Mutational Status in Lung Cancer

The identification of actionable somatic mutations such as EGFR and ALK has markedly altered clinical practice in lung cancer. Few studies have correlated lung tumor mutational status with miRNA deregulation. Dacic and colleagues[220] examined EGFR-mutated, KRAS-mutated, and double-negative lung tumors for miRNA expression and identified few mutation-specific miRNAs. miR-155 was upregulated in double negative lung tumors, whereas miR-495 was upregulated only in KRAS-positive tumors and miR-25 was upregulated only in EGFR-mutated tumors. miRNAs have been implicated as drivers of both EGFR sensitivity and resistance. For example, Garofalo and colleagues[221] demonstrated that deregulation of select miRNAs miR-30b, miR-30c, miR-221/222, miR103, and miR-203 contributed to both in vitro and in vivo sensitivity of NSCLC to gefitinib.[221] Several miRNAs, including miR-128b, miR-7, and miR-145, have been validated as directly targeting EGFR.[222–224] In the case of miR-7, investigators determined both in vitro and in vivo that EGFR signaling was mediated in part by miR-7 induction in a Ras/ERK/Myc dependent manner.[225] Conversely, liposomal-mediated delivery of miR-7 has been shown to overcome EGFR resistance in T790M-mutated lung cancer cell lines.[226]

Integrating miRNAs into Clinical Decision Making in Lung Cancer

Although significant progress has been made in miRNA discovery, few miRNAs have reached clinical application in human disease; however, two recent discoveries have led to the application of miRNAs as directed therapeutics. The first involves the directed targeting of miR-122 as a therapeutic in hepatitis C, whereas the other study, which is much earlier in development, involves supplemental replacement of the tumor suppressor miRNA miR-34 in the setting of hepatocellular carcinoma or solid malignancies that have metastasized to the liver.[227,228] No such studies have reached clinical application in lung cancer; however, ongoing investigation suggests that miRNA signatures may be of value in both diagnostic and therapeutic decision making. In particular, investigators are exploring the potential for miRNA signatures in the settings of indeterminate lung nodules and early detection, histologic classification, and chemotherapeutic response, each of which can present clinical challenges. Schembri and colleagues[229] demonstrated that the human airway epithelium was susceptible to changes in miRNA expression following cigarette smoke exposure. They identified 28 miRNAs that were differentially expressed in airway epithelium from current and never smokers. One particular miRNA was miR-218, which was downregulated in smokers. Since that initial finding, studies have demonstrated downregulation of miR-218 in SQCC of the lung.[230] Few studies to date have identified a miRNA signature for solitary lung nodules.[231] The concept of integrating miRNA profiling in lung cancer early detection is an intriguing one. Using cohorts drawn from a longitudinal lung cancer screening trial, Boeri and colleagues[232] tested and identified plasma-based miRNA signatures that could predict the risk for the development of lung cancer, diagnosis, and prognosis.

Another potential area for integration for miRNA biology into the clinic is in the setting of determining chemotherapeutic response. Several studies have been conducted using miRNAs to distinguish chemosensitive from chemoresistant tumors.[34,221,233,234]

Noninvasive miRNA Detection

There have been numerous studies exploring potential noninvasive biomarkers in lung cancer. These biomarkers have included circulating DNA, transcripts, select proteins, cytokines, and angiogenic factors. Despite such exciting studies, a lack of reproducibility and a lack absence of mechanistic insight have limited the clinical impact. Recently, investigators demonstrated the utility of sputum miRNA in the early detection of lung cancer. Using a training set of 154 patients (66 with lung cancer and 68 controls) and a test set of 64 lung cancer patients and 73 smoking controls, Shen and colleagues[235] showed that sputum levels of miR-31 and miR-210 had a sensitivity of 65.2% and a specificity of 89.7% in diagnosing lung cancer. Interestingly, when combined with a computed tomography (CT) scan, the resultant specificity was higher than with a CT scan alone.[235] An independent study identified sputum miR-205, miR-210, and miR-708 as potential diagnostic biomarkers in early stage lung cancer.[236]

Investigators recognize that components of the lung tumor microenvironment, including endothelial cells, macrophages, and fibroblasts to name a few, each harbor distinct biologic programs that drive cross-talk with the primary tumor, thus fostering tumor progression. Although several mechanisms that underlie this exchange of information have been proposed and explored, there are likely to be many others. Although multiple gain of function and silencing studies have shed light on the multitude of intracellular physiologic functions of miRNAs, few have truly explored the manner by which miRNAs may carry genetic information and programming between cells and their environment. Recently, investigators have demonstrated that miRNAs may circulate both freely attached to select proteins (e.g., Ago) or lipids and packaged within extracellular vesicles (EV), including exosomes, apoptotic bodies, and microvesicles (Fig. 40.3). The concept of *packaged* miRNAs is particularly intriguing as a mechanism for the intercellular transfer of genetic material.[237] These paradigm-shifting discoveries have led to an intense investigation for novel mechanisms by which circulating miRNA may serve as mediators of intercellular communication. However, several unanswered questions remain, including defining the distribution and mechanism by which miRNAs are processed

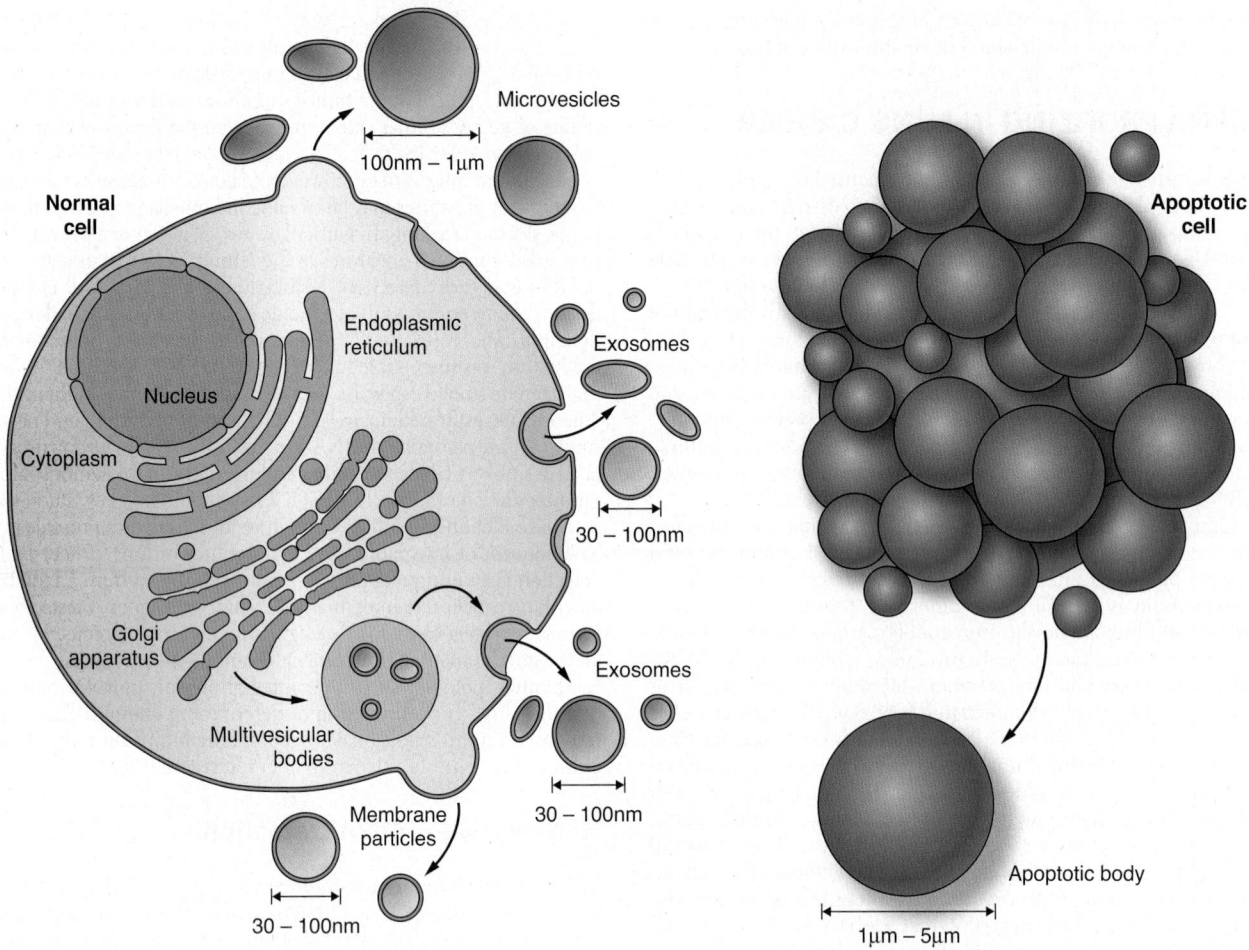

Figure 40.3 Extracellular vesicles.

for cellular release, how they are packaged into EVs versus being bound to molecules, and ultimately, their biologic function in circulation. To date, some studies suggest that the majority of circulating miRNAs are not associated with exosomes but rather are bound to select proteins.[238] Surprisingly, very few studies have examined the clinical and biologic role for extracellular miRNAs in lung cancer. Although the majority of studies to date have focused on linking global expression patterns of miRNAs in blood or other bodily fluids to clinical parameters, the reproducibility of signatures has been limited by variability in the compartment analyzed (whole blood, peripheral blood mononuclear cells [PBMC], serum, or plasma) and low cohort numbers. Identifying the *lung cancer signature* within these compartments is a major challenge.

Very few studies to date have examined for the presence of miRNAs in the circulation as either diagnostic or prognostic biomarkers in lung cancer. The earliest studies to examine miRNAs in the circulation were focused on merely providing scientific feasibility for the presence of miRNAs in the circulation. Studies have targeted whole blood, peripheral mononuclear cells, and plasma with no clearly reproducible signature.[147,148,150]

INVASION, METASTASIS, AND ANGIOGENESIS

An investigation of the molecular mechanisms of invasion and metastasis has yielded a variety of candidate genes, including cell adhesion molecules such as the cadherins, integrins, and CD44. The E-cadherin–catenin complex is critical for intercellular adhesiveness and the maintenance of normal and malignant tissue architecture. Epigenetically reduced expression of this complex in malignant disease is associated with tumor invasion, metastasis, and unfavorable prognosis in lung cancer. Another family of adhesion molecules are the integrins. α_3 Integrin has been shown to be important for normal lung development, and diminished expression correlated with a poor prognosis for patients with lung adenocarcinoma. Specific isoforms of CD44 may also be associated with lung cancer metastasis. Matrix metalloproteinases (MMP) are zinc-dependent proteases that belong to a family of endopeptidases, which degrade the extracellular matrix and basement membrane, necessary first steps in angiogenesis. The increased expression of MMPs has been strongly implicated in tumor growth, invasion, and metastasis. MMP2 and MMP9 have been associated with poorer prognosis. However, despite its established role in invasion and metastasis, many randomized phase III trials of MMP inhibitors have failed to demonstrate a survival benefit in patients with advanced lung cancer.[239] This is perhaps related to the lack of specificity of these inhibitors and recent findings that some MMPs actually inhibit tumor growth.[240] The stimuli that regulate tumor cell invasiveness are often generated or influenced by surrounding stromal or inflammatory cells and, as such, the invasive phenotype seems to be quite plastic, complex, and highly dependent on the context of the tumor microenvironment.[241]

Angiogenesis, the formation of new blood capillaries, is necessary for a tumor mass to grow beyond a few millimeters in size. The angiogenic switch results from perturbation in the balance between inducers and inhibitors, both of which are produced by tumor and host cells. Vascular endothelial growth factor (VEGF), basic fibroblast growth factor (bFGF), and angiogenic cytokines, such as interleukin-8, have all been implicated in lung cancer.[242]

Furthermore, high microvessel density (MVD) and VEGF over-expression are predictive of poor outcome. Thus, tumor angiogenesis has become a major new therapeutic target for lung cancer.[243] Clinical trials in NSCLC with bevacizumab, the humanized monoclonal antibody to VEGF, to chemotherapy prolongs PFS in phase III clinical trials, although improvements in overall survival were not always observed.[244–246]

CANCER STEM CELL HYPOTHESIS

The cancer stem cell hypothesis proposes that a self-renewing undifferentiated stem cell population comprising a small fraction of the total tumor burden gives rise to more numerous and more differentiated progeny that populate the tumor.[247] Among the characteristics reported to distinguish stemlike cells from cells constituting the bulk of tumors include the potential for supporting the continued growth of the local tumor mass, for seeding metastases throughout the body, and a resistance to cytotoxic therapies allowing the residual viable stem cells to repopulate the tumor after treatment. Because of their resistance to treatment and the potential for seeding distant metastatic disease, the study of cancer stem cells and the development of strategies effectively to eradicate all residual stem cells is of critical importance in cancer treatment.

Cancer stemlike cells can be isolated from a variety of tumor types using antibodies to unique cell surface proteins. They are capable of forming xenograft tumors at a high frequency after injection into immunocompromised mice. Empirically selected surface markers have been used to isolate putative stem cells from human breast cancer, glioblastoma multiforme, colon cancer, and other carcinomas, and these cells have a demonstrably greater potential for xenograft formation than do unselected tumor cells. The resulting tumors recapitulate the histologic appearance of the primary tumor as well as the heterogeneous expression of various surface and intracellular molecular markers.[247]

Putative lung progenitor cells have been described as cells residing at the bronchoalveolar duct junction that express both clara cell and pneumocyte markers or as lung resident cells of hematopoietic origin that express CD133.[248,249] These cells have not been conclusively shown to be lung adult stem cell populations but are intriguing and have been shown to be involved in the repair of lung tissue after injury and may be involved in cancer development. In lung tumors, CD133[250–253] and other commonly used markers of stemlike tumor cells (Hoechst dye efflux and aldehyde dehydrogenase activity)[254] have been shown to identify subsets of tumor cells that display characteristics consistent with the cancer stem cell hypothesis. CD133 has been shown to segregate with template DNA in lung cells undergoing asymmetric cell division.[255] However, conflicting reports suggest that CD133 may not define a specific subset of cells, because interconversion between CD133+ and CD133− populations is observed and CD133 expression may be associated with specific stages of cell cycle progression[256]; furthermore, some studies show no association between CD133 expression and propensity to initiate tumors.[257] The cancer stem cell hypothesis has other important grey areas as well. It is not yet certain whether a consistent developmental hierarchy would exist for every individual tumor or only in certain cases, whether lineage differentiation in a tumor can be reversible, and which basic properties should be required to define a stemlike phenotype in a given population of cells. A highly increased propensity for xenograft formation is one of the most convincing features that can be demonstrated experimentally for proposed cancer stemlike cells. However, even the reliability of this evidence is called into question by the observation that a much higher rate of tumor formation is observed when mouse tumor lines are propagated in isogenic immunocompetent mice, which raises the possibility that the xenograft initiation phenotype may be related to the ability to adapt to the tissue environment of an immunocompromised mouse, rather than a general property of enhanced tumor formation.[258]

Nevertheless, the balance of evidence from diverse tumor types favors the hypothesis that stemlike cells are present within tumors and may play a key role in certain aspects of tumor biology. Furthermore, developmental pathways that are proposed to be important in governing cancer stem cell biology may be important oncogenic drivers of proliferation and invasion for unselected tumor cell populations in certain subsets of tumors, and are important avenues of research in their own right. For instance, the activity of particular genes—achaete-scute complex homolog 1[253] and OCT4 transcription factors[251]—have been implicated in regulating this subset of lung tumor cells.

Recent studies have defined aldehyde dehydrogenase (ALDH) activity as a robust marker for lung adenocarcinoma stemlike cells.[259] ALDH-positive cells are highly tumorigenic and clonogenic as well as capable of self-renewal compared to the ALDH subpopulation. This subset and its behavior was shown to be dependent on Notch activity, specifically NOTCH3. The expression of ALDH7A1 was associated with increased risk of recurrence after surgical resection.[260]

Given the far-reaching implications of the cancer stem cell hypothesis and especially the concept that targeting developmental pathways cancer stem cells or, in particular, subsets of cancer could represent an important therapeutic strategy, these complex and exciting areas warrant further study in lung cancer.

MOLECULAR TOOLS IN THE LUNG CANCER CLINIC

Our understanding of the molecular genetic changes in lung cancer pathogenesis is advancing rapidly. Many genetic abnormalities identified in lung cancer are common to other human cancers, whereas others appear more specific to lung cancer, perhaps because of characteristics of the cells of origin and the unique nature of carcinogen exposure. Where their biochemical function is known, the proteins rendered abnormal appear to fall into several growth regulatory pathways.[261] Thus, our understanding of the fundamental workings and diverse molecular drivers of lung cancer is becoming clearer. A substantial effort has been made to translate the current scientific knowledge of these abnormalities from the bench to the bedside in order to improve patient outcomes. These approaches fall into three general categories:

- Development of early detection tools to identify primary and recurrent disease to enable effective early treatment. Because lung cancer eventually develops in only 1 of 10 cigarette smokers, the identification of persons with a genetic susceptibility to lung cancer should allow for targeting and the intensification of smoking cessation, early detection, and chemoprevention efforts. The National Lung Cancer Screening Trial (NLST)[262] randomized patients at high risk for developing lung cancer, defined as individuals between 55 and 74 years of age with a =30 pack-years history of cigarette smoking; former smokers must have quit within the previous 15 years. There was a 20% reduction in lung cancer mortality in the LDCT screened population (95% confidence interval [CI], 6.8% to 26.7%; p = 0.004). Based on this data, the U.S. Preventive Services Task Force has recommended annual CT screening for these high-risk patients. The high false-positive rate and the fact that many lung cancers arise in patients who do not meet these eligibility criteria stress the need for developing diagnostic biomarkers to aid in defining an appropriate management of CT-detected nodules and biomarkers of risk for better defining the population who would benefit from screening, including, potentially, germ line T790M.
- Development of new cancer-specific therapies based on knowledge of genetic abnormalities. These may include replacing or pharmacologically reactivating mutant tumor suppressor genes, developing new drugs targeting activated proto-oncogenes,

interfering with autocrine or paracrine growth stimulatory loops, and inhibiting angiogenesis, metastasis, and antiapoptosis. Some new therapies may be highly effective as single agents in some patients. However, it is likely that for many patients, combinations of two or more targeted or cytotoxic agents will be required to maximize clinical benefit, and determining the optimal combination of therapy for a given patient will be an additional challenge in the field.

■ Identification of prognostic and predictive biomarkers, such as the EGFR mutation and ALK-EML4, ROS1, and RET fusion

previously described that are both direct targets and predict the response and outcomes to specific therapies. Such tools will play an increasingly important role in selecting optimal treatment strategies as the number of molecularly targeted therapies expands.

These are exciting times in the molecular biology field of lung cancer, in which the science directly informs patient care and vice versa. Improved outcomes are surely to be the result, and patients can be given a degree of hope never before possible.

SELECTED REFERENCES

The full reference list can be accessed at lwwhealthlibrary.com/oncology.

6. Truong T, Hung RJ, Amos CI, et al. Replication of lung cancer susceptibility loci at chromosomes 15q25, 5p15, and 6p21: a pooled analysis from the International Lung Cancer Consortium. *J Natl Cancer Inst* 2010;102:959–971.
13. Braithwaite KL, Rabbitts PH. Multi-step evolution of lung cancer. *Sem Cancer Biol* 1999;9:255–265.
19. Soda M, Choi YL, Enomoto M, et al. Identification of the transforming EML4-ALK fusion gene in non–small-cell lung cancer. *Nature* 2007; 448:561–566.
21. Comprehensive genomic characterization of squamous cell lung cancers. *Nature* 2012;489:519–525.
22. Kandoth C, McLellan MD, Vandin F, et al. Mutational landscape and significance across 12 major cancer types. *Nature* 2013;502:333–339.
23. Ding L, Getz G, Wheeler DA, et al. Somatic mutations affect key pathways in lung adenocarcinoma. *Nature* 2008;455:1069–1075.
24. Imielinski M, Berger AH, Hammerman PS, et al. Mapping the hallmarks of lung adenocarcinoma with massively parallel sequencing. *Cell* 2012; 150:1107–1120.
29. Friboulet L, Olaussen KA, Pignon JP, et al. ERCC1 isoform expression and DNA repair in non–small-cell lung cancer. *N Engl J Med* 2013;368: 1101–1110.
30. Zheng Z, Chen T, Li X, et al. DNA synthesis and repair genes RRM1 and ERCC1 in lung cancer. *N Engl J Med* 2007;356:800–808.
33. Lynch TJ, Bell DW, Sordella R, et al. Activating mutations in the epidermal growth factor receptor underlying responsiveness of non–small-cell lung cancer to gefitinib. *N Engl J Med* 2004;350:2129–2139.
38. Shigematsu H, Takahashi T, Nomura M, et al. Somatic mutations of the HER2 kinase domain in lung adenocarcinomas. *Cancer Res* 2005;65:1642–1646.
42. Mok TS, Wu YL, Thongprasert S, et al. Gefitinib or carboplatin-paclitaxel in pulmonary adenocarcinoma. *N Engl J Med* 2009;361:947–957.
49. Sequist LV, Waltman BA, Dias-Santagata D, et al. Genotypic and histological evolution of lung cancers acquiring resistance to EGFR inhibitors. *Sci Transl Med* 2011;3:75ra26.
52. Bell DW, Gore I, Okimoto RA, et al. Inherited susceptibility to lung cancer may be associated with the T790M drug resistance mutation in EGFR. *Nat Genet* 2005;37:1315–1316.
54. Arcila ME, Chaft JE, Nafa K, et al. Prevalence, clinicopathologic associations, and molecular spectrum of ERBB2 (HER2) tyrosine kinase mutations in lung adenocarcinomas. *Clin Cancer Res* 2012;18:4910–4918.
59. Sadiq AA, Salgia R. MET as a possible target for non–small-cell lung cancer. *J Clin Oncol* 2013;31:1089–1096.
66. Weiss J, Sos ML, Seidel D, et al. Frequent and focal FGFR1 amplification associates with therapeutically tractable FGFR1 dependency in squamous cell lung cancer. *Sci Transl Med* 2010;2:62ra93.
68. Hammerman PS, Sos ML, Ramos AH, et al. Mutations in the DDR2 kinase gene identify a novel therapeutic target in squamous cell lung cancer. *Cancer Discov* 2011;1:78–89.
71. Kwak EL, Bang YJ, Camidge DR, et al. Anaplastic lymphoma kinase inhibition in non–small-cell lung cancer. *N Engl J Med* 2010;363:1693–1703.
77. Shaw AT, Kim DW, Nakagawa K, et al. Crizotinib versus chemotherapy in advanced ALK-positive lung cancer. *N Engl J Med* 2013;368:2385–2394.
79. Katayama R, Khan TM, Benes C, et al. Therapeutic strategies to overcome crizotinib resistance in non-small cell lung cancers harboring the fusion oncogene EML4-ALK. *Proc Natl Acad Sci U S A* 2011;108:7535–7540.
84. Acquaviva J, Wong R, Charest A. The multifaceted roles of the receptor tyrosine kinase ROS in development and cancer. *Biochim Biophys Acta* 2009;1795:37–52.
89. Takeuchi K, Soda M, Togashi Y, et al. RET, ROS1 and ALK fusions in lung cancer. *Nat Med* 2012;18:378–381.
94. Shepherd FA, Domerg C, Hainaut P, et al. Pooled analysis of the prognostic and predictive effects of KRAS mutation status and KRAS mutation subtype in early-stage resected non–small-cell lung cancer in four trials of adjuvant chemotherapy. *J Clin Oncol* 2013;31:2173–2181.

100. Paik PK, Arcila ME, Fara M, et al. Clinical characteristics of patients with lung adenocarcinomas harboring BRAF mutations. *J Clin Oncol* 2011; 29:2046–2051.
103. Imielinski M, Greulich H, Kaplan B, et al. Oncogenic and sorafenib-sensitivite ARAF mutations in lung adenocarcinomas. *J Clin Invest* 2014;124: 1582–1586.
104. Marks JL, Gong Y, Chitale D, et al. Novel MEK1 mutation identified by mutational analysis of epidermal growth factor receptor signaling pathway genes in lung adenocarcinoma. *Cancer Res* 2008;68:5524–5528.
105. Samuels Y, Wang Z, Bardelli A, et al. High frequency of mutations of the PIK3CA gene in human cancers. *Science* 2004;304:554.
107. Cancer Genome Atlas Research Network. Comprehensive genomic characterization of squamous cell lung cancers. *Nature* 2012;489:519–525.
111. Bleeker FE, Felicioni L, Buttitta F, et al. AKT1(E17K) in human solid tumours. *Oncogene* 2008;27:5648–5650.
115. Buettner R, Wolf J, Thomas RK. Lessons learned from lung cancer genomics: the emerging concept of individualized diagnostics and treatment. *J Clin Oncol* 2013;31:1858–1865.
116. Dias-Santagata D, Akhavanfard S, David SS, et al. Rapid targeted mutational analysis of human tumours: a clinical platform to guide personalized cancer medicine. *EMBO Mol Med* 2010;2:146–158.
117. MacConaill LE, Campbell CD, Kehoe SM, et al. Profiling critical cancer gene mutations in clinical tumor samples. *PLoS One* 2009;4:e7887.
119. Kris MG, Johnson BE, Kwiatkowski DJ, et al. Identification of driver mutations in tumor specimens from 1,000 patients with lung adenocarcinoma: The NCI's Lung cancer Mutation Consortium (LCMC). *J Clin Oncol* 2011;29:abstr CRA7506.
123. Ellis MJ, Gillette M, Carr SA, et al. Connecting genomic alterations to cancer biology with proteomics: The NCI Clinical Proteomic Tumor Analysis Consortium. *Cancer Discov* 2013;3:1108–1112.
125. Lawrence MS, Stojanov P, Polak P, et al. Mutational heterogeneity in cancer and the search for new cancer-associated genes. *Nature* 2013;499: 214–218.
140. Weir BA, Woo MS, Getz G, et al. Characterizing the cancer genome in lung adenocarcinoma. *Nature* 2007;450:893–898.
143. Menendez D, Inga A, Resnick MA. The expanding universe of p53 targets. *Nat Rev Cancer* 2009;9:724–737.
157. Beroukhim R, Mermel CH, Porter D, et al. The landscape of somatic copy-number alteration across human cancers. *Nature* 2010;463:899–905.
161. Ji H, Ramsey MR, Hayes DN, et al. LKB1 modulates lung cancer differentiation and metastasis. *Nature* 2007;448:807–810.
175. Ding L, Getz G, Wheeler DA, et al. Somatic mutations affect key pathways in lung adenocarcinoma. *Nature* 2008;455:1069–1075.
181. Topalian SL, Hodi FS, Brahmer JR, et al. Safety, activity, and immune correlates of anti-PD-1 antibody in cancer. *N Engl J Med* 2012;366: 2443–2454.
186. Miura N, Nakamura H, Sato R, et al. Clinical usefulness of serum telomerase reverse transcriptase (hTERT) mRNA and epidermal growth factor receptor (EGFR) mRNA as a novel tumor marker for lung cancer. *Cancer Sci* 2006;97:1366–1373.
192. Pezzella F, Turley H, Kuzu I, et al. bcl-2 protein in non–small-cell lung carcinoma. *N Engl J Med* 1993;329:690–694.
205. Croce CM. Causes and consequences of microRNA dysregulation in cancer. *Nat Rev Genet* 2009;10:704–714.
208. Calin GA, Croce CM. MicroRNA signatures in human cancers. *Nat Rev Cancer* 2006;6:857–866.
232. Boeri M, Verri C, Conte D, et al. MicroRNA signatures in tissues and plasma predict development and prognosis of computed tomography detected lung cancer. *Proc Natl Acad Sci U S A* 2011;108:3713–3718.
261. Bild AH, Yao G, Chang JT, et al. Oncogenic pathway signatures in human cancers as a guide to targeted therapies. *Nature* 2006;439:353–357.
262. Aberle DR, Adams AM, Berg CD, et al. Reduced lung-cancer mortality with low-dose computed tomographic screening. *N Engl J Med* 2011;365: 395–409.

41 Non-Small Cell Lung Cancer

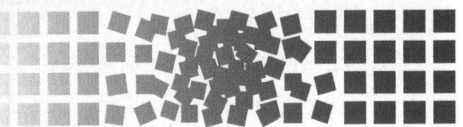

Frank C. Detterbeck, Roy H. Decker, Lynn Tanoue, and Rogerio C. Lilenbaum

INCIDENCE AND ETIOLOGY

Lung cancer is the most common cause of cancer death worldwide. The World Health Organization International Agency for Research on Cancer reported the global incidence of lung cancer at approximately 1.8 million new cases in 2012.[1] The overall ratio of mortality to incidence is high, with the 5-year survival rate in the United States still only 17%.[2] Consequently, the mortality burden is staggering, with lung cancer causing an estimated 1.59 million deaths per year around the world. Lung cancer accounts for nearly one-third of all cancer deaths in the United States and causes as many cancer deaths as the next four leading causes of cancer deaths combined (breast, colon, prostate, and pancreas).[2]

A relatively unique aspect of lung cancer is the strong association with a potentially avoidable risk factor, namely smoking. This has far-reaching psychological, social, political, and societal implications. An attitude of blame has contributed to low prioritization of lung cancer research and a lack of activism among people affected by the disease. Furthermore, this attitude and the relatively poor outcomes have promoted nihilism in both the medical and patient community about both treatment of the disease and attempts to make advances.

It is important to look beyond the simple association of lung cancer and smoking. Over half of those diagnosed with lung cancer in the United States are either never-smokers or people who quit smoking many years earlier.[3–5] Furthermore, lung cancer occurring in never-smokers is relatively common, occurring in about 20,000 individuals in the United States; this puts deaths from lung cancer in never-smokers among the top 10 causes of cancer deaths in the United States (e.g., more than cancer of the ovaries, uterus, or lymphomas).[2] This underscores that the etiology of lung cancer is complex and not well understood.

Major advances have been made in all aspects of lung cancer, from screening, to surgical, chemotherapy and radiotherapy (RT) treatment, methods of palliation, as well as the understanding of fundamental aspects of the biology of the disease. Lung cancer has become a vibrant and dynamic field, with a vast and growing literature describing advances in every facet of this disease. This makes it an impossible task to summarize the state of the art in one short chapter; it is inevitable that some areas will be missed or covered superficially, and new advances will have emerged during the course of publication. Nevertheless, this chapter is an attempt to cover the most important clinical aspects of lung cancer, which represents a major source of suffering and mortality throughout the world.

The highest incidence and mortality rates from lung cancer are observed in men in Central and Eastern Europe, Southern Europe, Eastern Asia, Micronesia, and Northern America, and in women in Northern America, Northern Europe, Australia/New Zealand, and Micronesia (Fig. 41.1). The highest estimated age-standardized lung cancer incidence rates occur in more developed regions of the world, where smoking is more prevalent (Fig. 41.2). Globally, lung cancer is still more common in men than in women, reflecting different historical and temporal exposure to tobacco smoking. The evidence does not suggest that

women are either more or less susceptible than men to the carcinogenic effects of tobacco. On a hopeful note, the incidence rates in men appear to be falling or at least stabilizing in all regions, likely reflecting the impact of successful national initiatives focused on tobacco control (Fig. 41.3). In contrast, incidence rates in women appear to be increasing in most regions or at best stabilizing in a few.

Smoking

At the turn of the 20th century, lung cancer was a rare malignancy. In an extensive autopsy review in the United States and Western Europe in 1916, Adler found that lung cancers represented <0.5% of all cancer cases.[6] Over the next several decades, a substantive increase in the incidence of lung cancer was noted; at the same time, observations of the adverse health effects of smoking were made. In 1941, Ochsner and DeBakey stated, "it is our definite conviction that the increase in the incidence of pulmonary carcinoma is due largely to the increase in smoking, particularly cigaret (*sic*) smoking."[7] Two landmark case-control studies published in 1950 by Doll and Hill[8] in the United Kingdom and Wynder and Graham[9] in the United States established a causal link between cigarette smoking and bronchogenic carcinoma. The Royal College of Physicians in the United Kingdom in 1962[10] and the Surgeon General of the United States in 1964[11] endorsed the conclusion that cigarette smoking is the major cause of lung cancer. Population trends of lung cancer incidence mirror smoking behavior, with a typical lag time of approximately 20 years (see Figs. 41.1 and 41.2). Both the number of cigarettes smoked per day and the duration of smoking correlate with lung cancer risk, with longer duration in particular being associated with a much higher risk.[12]

Cigarette smoke is a complex aerosol, with nicotine being the primary determinant of addiction and tar being the particulate residue left when nicotine and water are removed from tobacco smoke. More than 50 carcinogens in tobacco smoke have been identified, including N-nitrosoamines formed by nitrosation of nicotine during smoking, and polycyclic aromatic hydrocarbines.[13–15] The N-nitrosoamine 4-(methylnitrosamino)-1(3-pyridyl)-1-butanone is associated with DNA adduct formation and DNA mutations that result in the activation of *KRAS* oncogenes.[16,17] Both N-nitrosoamines and polycyclic aromatic hydrocarbines may be metabolically activated to become carcinogenic, or alternatively may be metabolically detoxified; the balance of these processes will determine exposure. Other carcinogens in tobacco smoke carcinogens do not require activation (e.g., benzene, vinyl chloride, or radon). The dose of carcinogen(s) received from smoking will vary with the composition of the cigarette itself, including whether a filter is present, and the intensity of inhalation. Because of regulatory mandates, cigarettes contain less nicotine and tar than in years past. However, smokers may compensate by smoking more intensively (more puffs per minute and deeper, longer inhalations) to satisfy nicotine addiction. Mentholation of cigarettes may also facilitate

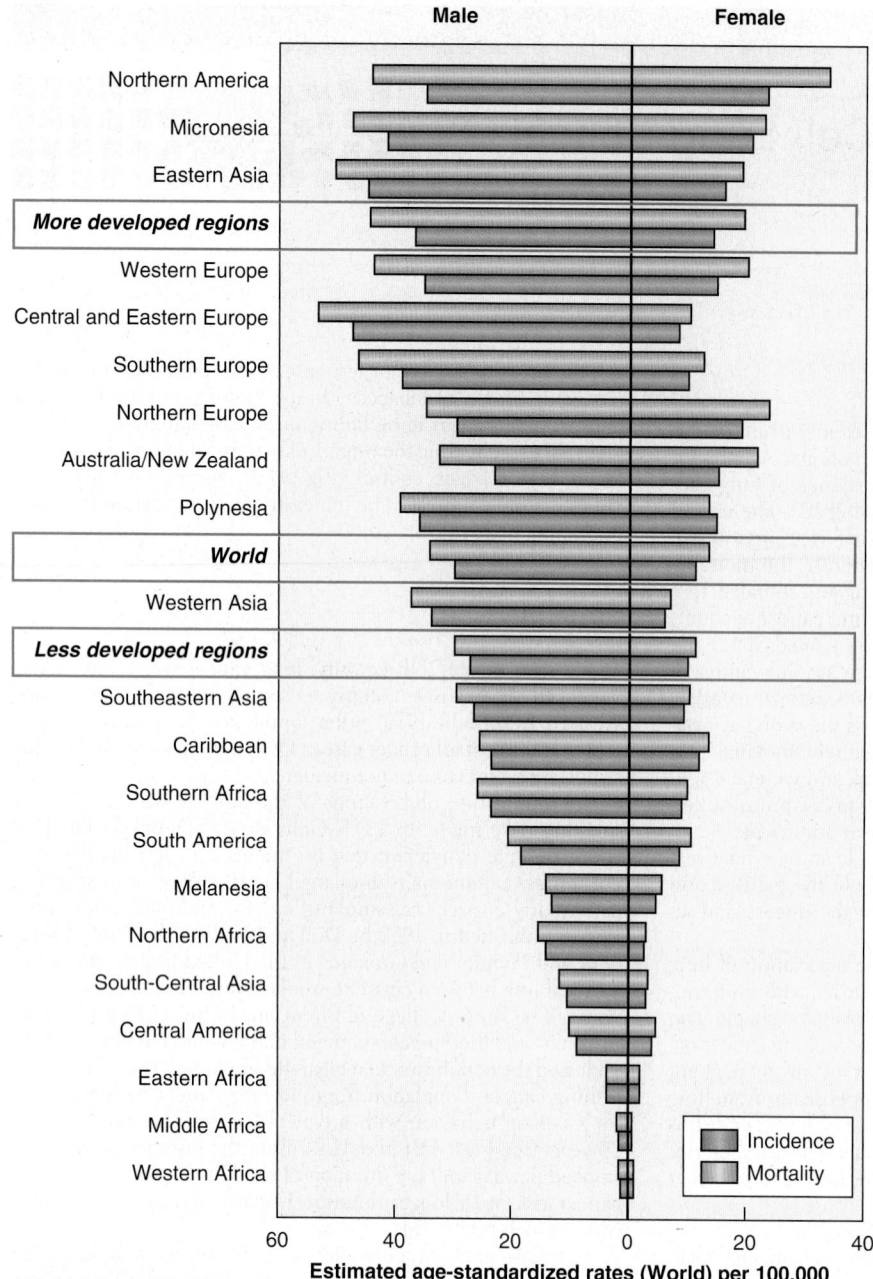

Figure 41.1 Estimated age-standardized rates of lung cancer per 100,000 population by region of the world. (Reproduced from GLOBOCAN 2012, International Agency for Research on Cancer, World Health Organization.)

more intense smoking, as it changes the aroma of the smoke and decreases the irritant effect of the smoke, thereby facilitating more intense inhalation.[18,19]

Genetic Predisposition

The cumulative lifetime risk for lifelong smokers in their eighth decade of life is approximately 16%.[20] The host factors that confer "protection" from lung cancer in the majority of individuals who smoke and never develop lung cancer, or determine increased susceptibility in those individuals who do, are not clear. An estimated 300,000 lung cancer deaths occur in nonsmokers annually in the world; in many of these cases, no specific risk or exposure can be identified.[21,22] It is widely accepted that genetic (inherited) factors as well as epigenetic (acquired) DNA changes contribute to the development of malignancy. The association of lung cancer with rare Mendelian cancer syndromes or in family aggregates supports the contribution of high-penetrance, low-frequency genes.[23,24]

Mutations in low-penetrance, high-frequency genes that encode enzymes involved in activation or detoxification of carcinogens, or enzymes involved in DNA repair, also influence lung cancer susceptibility.[25–27]

A large European case control study and meta-analysis of 41 studies demonstrated that the risk of lung cancer increased if there was a first-degree family member with lung cancer (odds ratio = 1.63) and increased further if two or more family members had lung cancer (odds ratio = 3.6).[28] The Liverpool Lung Project reported that a family history of early onset lung cancer (age <60 years) was associated with an odds ratio for lung cancer of 2.02.[29] While some polymorphisms in a few candidate genes have been identified, the broad field of host genetic factors determining lung cancer susceptibility is still poorly understood and is an area of intense investigation. We do not yet have the tools to identify which individuals might be intrinsically more likely to develop lung cancer or more vulnerable to the carcinogenic effects of cigarettes. Such knowledge eventually may help define specific populations who should be targeted for lung cancer screening.

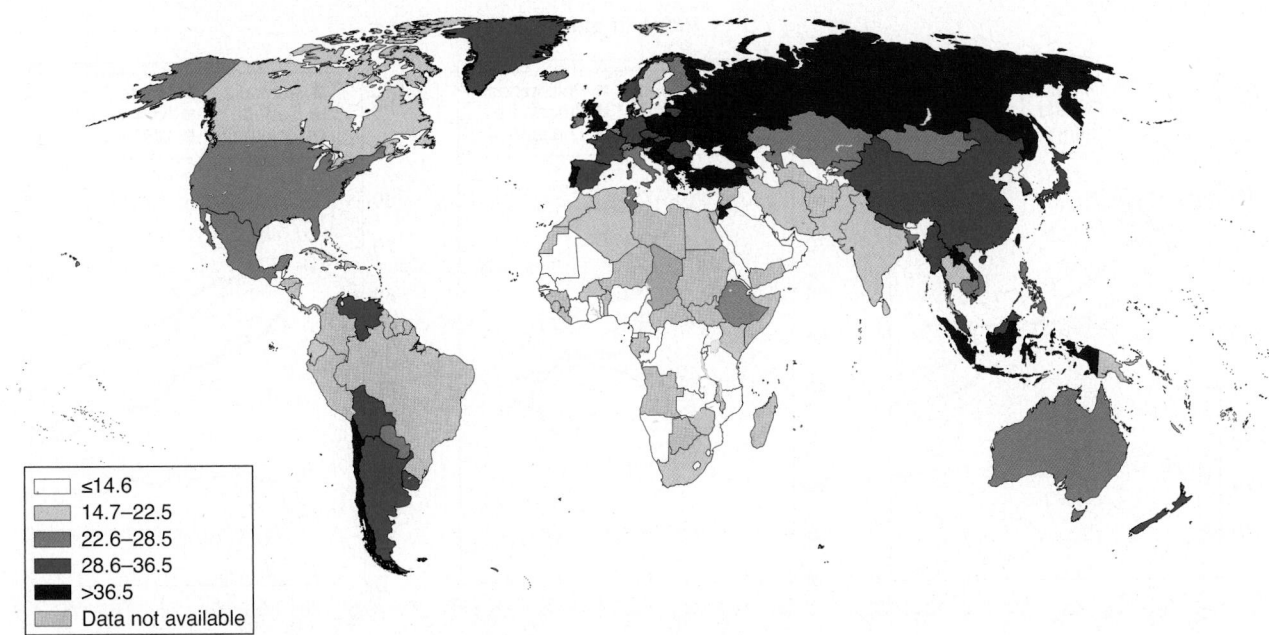

Figure 41.2 Percentage of tobacco use among adults by country in 2005. (Reproduced from GLOBOCAN 2012, International Agency for Research on Cancer, World Health Organization.)

Legend:
- ≤14.6
- 14.7–22.5
- 22.6–28.5
- 28.6–36.5
- >36.5
- Data not available

PRACTICE OF ONCOLOGY

Occupational/Environmental

Though smoking is clearly the most important modifiable risk factor, many other factors influence the development of lung cancer. It is estimated that approximately 10% of lung cancer cases are at least in part related to occupational exposures.[30] Many workplace materials have been identified as carcinogens, including, among others, arsenic, asbestos, beryllium, cadmium, chromium, nickel, radon, and vinyl chloride. Of these, asbestos is the most common, having been used widely for its insulating properties and recognized as a lung carcinogen as early as the 1940s.[31] There has been controversy as to whether asbestos exposure per se confers lung cancer risk or whether asbestosis, the associated interstitial lung disease, is required. A recent long-term follow-up of a large group of North American insulators originally studied in the early 1980s provided further data on asbestos exposure, asbestosis, and cigarette smoking.[32] In the non-smoking cohort, lung cancer risk was increased with asbestos exposure alone, and further increased if asbestosis was also present. In the smoking cohort, there was an additive risk of smoking and asbestos exposure, with a supra-additive increase in risk if both smoking and asbestosis were present. Thus it appears that while asbestosis clearly increases lung cancer risk, particularly in smokers, asbestos exposure alone also increases risk, albeit to a lesser degree.

Radon gas was first implicated as increasing lung cancer risk in workers in underground uranium mines. The awareness of radon as a carcinogen has focused attention on domestic radon gas as a common indoor pollutant.[33–36] Radon is felt to contribute to an estimated 15,000 to 20,000 lung cancer deaths in the United States annually.[36] Other indoor air pollutant carcinogens include environmental tobacco smoke and byproducts of biomass fuels used for heating and cooking. Outdoor air pollution contains carcinogens generated by fossil fuel combustion and diesel exhaust, which can be adsorbed to fine particulates small enough to be inhaled into the airways. These exposures are of particular concern in countries such as China, where indoor domestic use of coal and wood, intense urban outdoor pollution, and an epidemic of tobacco smoking are likely all contributing to an alarming rise in lung cancer incidence.

Cancer risk related to medical imaging has been an area of increasing public health concern, particularly with the escalation of use of high technology studies such as computed tomography (CT) and positron emission tomography (PET). Radiation exposure acquired in this way is cumulative, with risk extrapolated on a linear model based on known cancer risk in survivors of the atomic bomb in Japan, and after therapeutic radiation given in the past for medical diseases including tuberculosis and ankylosing spondylitis.[37–40] Based on this model, even lower cumulative doses incur some risk. Recognition of the potential harms of radiation from medical imaging makes more urgent the need to utilize these tests judiciously, develop methods to track cumulative radiation exposure to specific organs, and improve technologies that will minimize patient exposure. This need is particularly cogent anticipating implementation of lung cancer screening with low-dose chest CT scanning.

Lung cancer is typically a disease of older individuals; ironically, as overall health status improves in developing countries and those populations acquire longer life expectancy, their lung cancer risk may increase. Whether gender is a factor has been a topic of considerable debate. At present, the body of evidence does not support any significant sex-related difference in susceptibility to smoking-associated lung cancer.[41] African Americans have consistently been observed to have higher lung cancer rates as well as worse 5-year survival than Caucasian Americans.[2] In developed nations, socioeconomic factors including education and income are inversely associated with risk. Lifestyle factors, including diet and physical activity, likely influence risk. An inverse association of diets higher in fruit and vegetable (cruciferous and carotenoid-rich) consumption with lung cancer risk has been consistently described.[42,43] The evidence for physical activity is less clear, though higher levels of activity have been described as associated with lower cancer risk.[44]

The presence of underlying pulmonary disease is increasingly recognized to influence lung cancer risk. Cigarette smoking is the major etiologic factor in both lung cancer and chronic obstructive pulmonary disease (COPD). COPD per se is an independent risk factor after controlling for smoking.[45,46] The mechanism(s) by which fixed airways disease may etiologically be implicated in carcinogenesis are not defined, but potentially include mutagenesis through activation of the NF-kappaB inflammatory pathway, protease-antiprotease imbalance, or chronic inflammation itself.[47–49] The presence of interstitial lung disease has also been associated

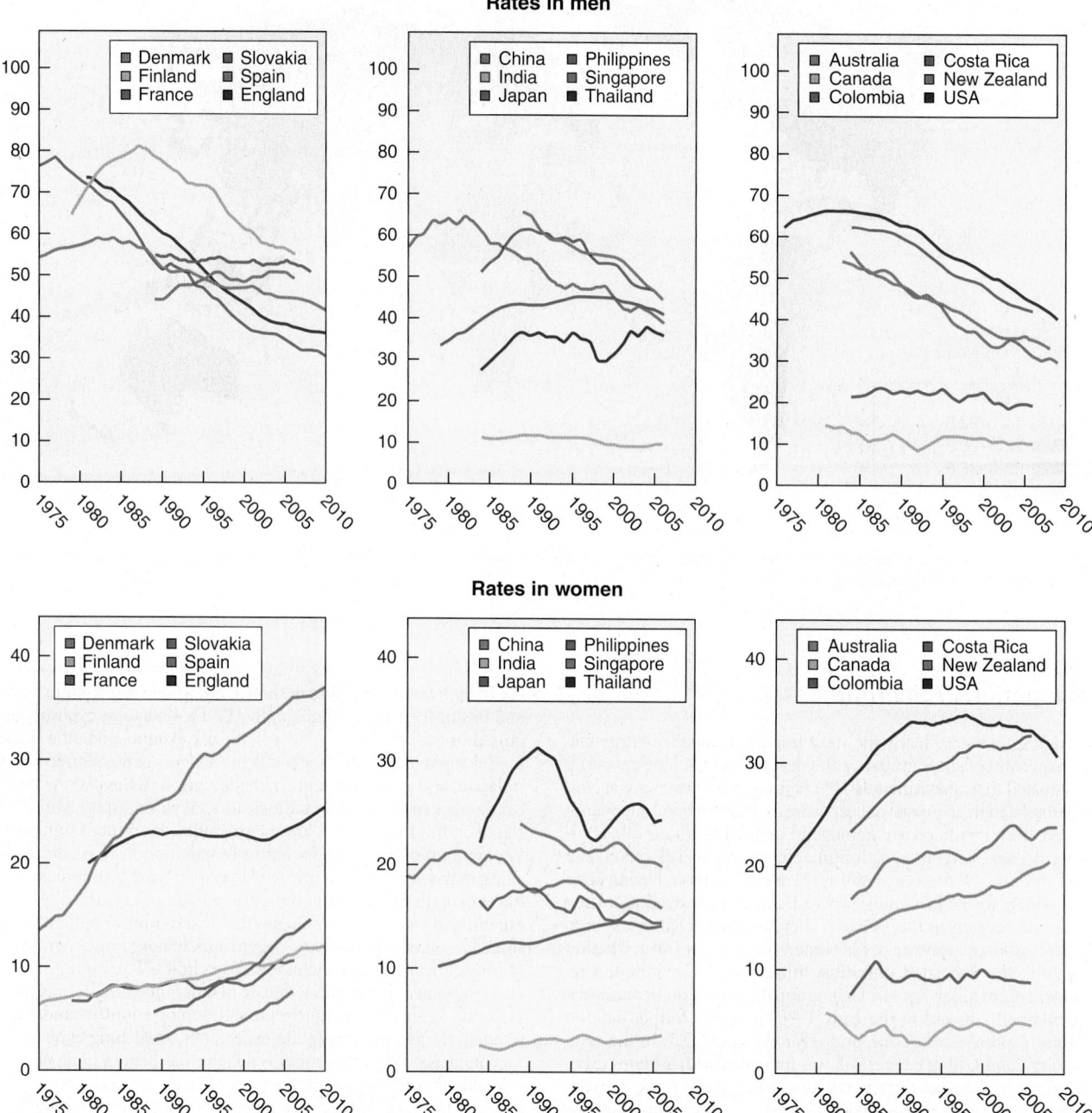

Figure 41.3 Trends in mortality from lung cancer showing the age-standardized mortality rate from lung cancer per 100,000 men (*top row*) and women (*bottom row*) in selected countries. (Reproduced from GLOBOCAN 2012. International Agency for Research on Cancer, World Health Organization.)

with an increase in lung cancer risk. In particular, patients with idiopathic pulmonary fibrosis have been reported to have an odds ratio for lung cancer of 8.25 compared to controls.[50,51] In contrast to COPD, cigarette smoking is usually not etiologically implicated in interstitial diseases, although chronic inflammation typically is felt to contribute to the pathologic process.

ANATOMY AND PATHOLOGY

Stage Classification

The stage classification for non–small-cell lung cancer (NSCLC) follows the tumor, node, metastasis (TNM) paradigm used for most solid tumors. Staging ensures a uniform standardized nomenclature to describe the anatomic extent of disease, namely the primary tumor site (T component) as well as cancer spread to nodes (N component) or distant metastatic sites (M component). The most recent (seventh edition) of the lung cancer stage classification is based on an unprecedented effort directed by the International Association for the Study of Lung Cancer (IASLC).[52–55] This involved an international database of over 100,000 patients, identified over the period 1990 to 2000 from 46 sources in 19 countries in North America, Asia, Australia, and Europe, and a sophisticated statistical analysis with extensive internal and external validation.[56] This stage classification applies to small cell and NSCLCs as well as carcinoid tumors.[57,58]

Several characteristics of the IASLC database are important to recognize in order to appropriately interpret some of the results. This was a retrospective database, with limitations in the level of details available. For example, some of the definitions of the TNM descriptors contained too few patients to allow statistical analysis of the impact of that tumor characteristic. Because the database consisted of patients diagnosed between 1990 and 2000, advances in technology (e.g., PET imaging) and treatment modalities that are routine today are not reflected. The analysis did not account for what treatment (if any) was given. In fact, there was a great deal of variation in outcomes depending on the type of source data and the geographic region. Thus, while the outcomes created a phenomenal tool to define where to draw distinctions between TNM categories and groupings, the outcomes themselves represent a global cross-section from the past with less clear relevance to specific patients today.

The definitions of the T, N, and M categories for both NSCLC and small-cell lung cancer (SCLC) are outlined in detail in Table 41.1.[59] The T, N, and M categories are then grouped to define particular stages of lung cancer (both NSCLC and SCLC), as outlined in Fig. 41.4. While ideally each stage would represent a homogeneous group of patients, this is not necessarily the case, as is evident in the range of T, N, and M combinations that comprise stage IIB or IIIA, for example. Nevertheless, the system provides a practical way of managing the complexity of a large number of T, N and M categories into a more limited number of stage groups.

TABLE 41.1

Stage Classification: T, N, M Descriptors

Category	Descriptor Definition	Subgroup[a]
T (Primary Tumor)		
T0	No primary tumor	
T1	Tumor ≤3 cm,[b] surrounded by lung or visceral pleura, not more proximal than the lobar bronchus	
T1a	Tumor ≤2 cm[b]	T1a
T1b	Tumor >2 but ≤3 cm[b]	T1b
T2	Tumor >3 but ≤7 cm[b] or tumor with any of the following[c]:	
	Invades visceral pleura, involves main bronchus ≥2 cm distal to the carina, atelectasis/obstructive pneumonia extending to hilum but not involving the entire lung	
T2a	Tumor >3 but ≤5 cm[b]	T2a
T2b	Tumor >5 but ≤7 cm[b]	T2b
T3	Tumor >7 cm[a]	$T3_{>7}$
	or directly invading chest wall, diaphragm, phrenic nerve, mediastinal pleura, parietal pericardium,	$T3_{Inv}$
	or tumor in the main bronchus <2 cm distal to the carina,[d]	$T3_{Centr}$
	or atelectasis/obstructive pneumonitis of entire lung,	
	or separate tumor nodule(s) in the same lobe	$T3_{Satell}$
T4	Tumor of any size with invasion of heart, great vessels, trachea, recurrent laryngeal nerve, esophagus, vertebral body, or carina;	$T4_{Inv}$
	or separate tumor nodule(s) in a different ipsilateral lobe	$T4_{Ipsi Nod}$
N (Regional Lymph Nodes)		
N0	No regional node metastasis	
N1	Metastasis in ipsilateral peribronchial and/or perihilar lymph nodes and intrapulmonary nodes, including involvement by direct extension	
N2	Metastasis in ipsilateral mediastinal and/or subcarinal lymph node(s)	
N3	Metastasis in contralateral mediastinal, contralateral hilar, ipsilateral, or contralateral scalene or supraclavicular lymph node(s)	
M (Distant Metastasis)		
M0	No distant metastasis	
M1a	Separate tumor nodule(s) in a contralateral lobe;	$M1a_{Contr Nod}$
	or tumor with pleural nodules or malignant pleural dissemination[e]	$M1a_{Pl Dissem}$
M1b	Distant metastasis	M1b
Special Situations		
TX, NX, MX	T, N, or M status not able to be assessed	
Tis	Focus of in situ cancer	Tis
T1[d]	Superficial spreading tumor of any size but confined to the wall of the trachea or mainstem bronchus	$T1_{SS}$

[a] These subgroup labels are not defined in the International Association for the Study of Lung Cancer publications (see Goldstraw P, Crowley J, Chansky K, et al. The IASLC Lung Cancer Staging Project: proposals for the revision of the TNM stage groupings in the forthcoming [seventh] edition of the TNM Classification of malignant tumours. *J Thorac Oncol* 2007;2:706–714; Rami-Porta R, Ball D, Crowley J, et al. The IASLC Lung Cancer Staging Project: proposals for the revision of the T descriptors in the forthcoming (seventh) edition of the TNM classification for lung cancer. *J Thorac Oncol* 2007;2:593–602; Rusch VW, Crowley J, Giroux DJ, et al. The IASLC Lung Cancer Staging Project: proposals for the revision of the N descriptors in the forthcoming seventh edition of the TNM classification for lung cancer. *J Thorac Oncol* 2007;2:603–612; Postmus PE, Brambilla E, Chansky K, et al. The IASLC Lung Cancer Staging Project: proposals for revision of the M descriptors in the forthcoming [seventh] edition of the TNM classification of lung cancer. *J Thorac Oncol* 2007;2:686–693) but are added here to facilitate a clear discussion.
[b] In greatest dimension.
[c] T2 tumors with these features are classified as T2a if ≤5 cm.
[d] The uncommon superficial spreading tumor in central airways is classified as T1.
[e] Pleural effusions are excluded that are cytologically negative, nonbloody, transudative, and clinically judged not to be due to cancer.
Reproduced with permission from the American College of Chest Physicians from Detterbeck F, Tanoue L, Boffa DJ. The new lung cancer staging system. *Chest* 2009;136:260–271.

PRACTICE OF ONCOLOGY

T/M	Subgroup	N0	N1	N2	N3
T1	T1a	Ia	IIa	IIIa	IIIb
	T1b	Ia	IIa	IIIa	IIIb
T2	T2a	Ib	IIa	IIIa	IIIb
	T2b	IIa	IIb	IIIa	IIIb
T3	T3 >7	IIb	IIIa	IIIa	IIIb
	T2 Inv	IIb	IIIa	IIIa	IIIb
	T3 Satell	IIb	IIIa	IIIa	IIIb
T4	T4 Inv	IIIa	IIIa	IIIb	IIIb
	T4 Ipsi Nod	IIIa	IIIa	IIIb	IIIb
M1	M1a Contra Nod	IV	IV	IV	IV
	M1a Pl Disem	IV	IV	IV	IV
	M1b	IV	IV	IV	IV

Figure 41.4 Stage classification: Stage groups. Inv, invasion; Satell, satellite; Ipsi Nod, ipsilateral nodule; Contra Nod, contralateral nodule; Pl Disem, pleural dissemination. (Reproduced with permission from Detterbeck F, Tanoue L, Boffa DJ. The new lung cancer staging system. *Chest* 2009;136:262.)

It is worth emphasizing what the stage classification system does and cannot accomplish. It is designed to be a consistent, stable nomenclature for the anatomic extent of disease. Although this is a major component in a patient's prognosis, the prognosis depends on many other factors, including age, comorbidities, environmental factors, and treatment factors. Particular tumor or patient factors (e.g., genetic mutations, central/peripheral lung location) may have a major impact in certain settings (e.g., a particular treatment strategy) but not in others, and at certain times during the course of the disease. Therefore, stage classification is not sufficient to capture the complexity of prognostic prediction for specific patients in specific clinical settings. Furthermore, although the anatomic extent of disease is an important component of selecting a treatment approach, this is also determined by other factors (e.g., histologic type, molecular information, patient-specific factors such as comorbidities). In addition, stage classification must remain relatively static and consistent to be useful, while treatment should continually evolve and improve. Thus, treatment must be determined by the results of clinical trials and cannot be determined merely by a stage classification nomenclature.

Histologic Classification

The histologic spectrum of lung cancer has clearly changed over the past several decades. SCLC has decreased from about 25% to <15% of all lung cancers.[60] Adenocarcinoma is now the most dominant histologic type, replacing squamous carcinoma. With the advent of more frequent CT imaging, an increased proportion of more indolent small tumors is being recognized.[61]

The histologic classification of lung cancer has become much more nuanced. In the past, the major NSCLC histologic types (adenocarcinoma, squamous cell carcinoma, and large cell carcinoma) were simply lumped together. It is critical to differentiate these because they respond differently to certain chemotherapeutic agents. Immunohistochemical stains and genetic characterization can facilitate the distinction between subtypes.[62,63] It is recognized that the vast majority of adenocarcinomas are mixed subtypes; these are now classified according to the predominant subtype with the percent of each noted in 10% increments.[63] Furthermore, the adenocarcinoma subtypes have been defined according to preinvasive, minimally invasive, and invasive groups (Table 41.2),[63] reflecting the increasingly recognized spectrum of aggressiveness of lung cancers encountered in the Western world today. Finally, bronchopulmonary carcinoid

TABLE 41.2

International Association for the Study of Lung Cancer/American Thoracic Society/European Respiratory Society Classification of Lung Adenocarcinoma in Resection Specimens

Preinvasive lesions
  Atypical adenomatous hyperplasia
  Adenocarcinoma in situ (≤3 cm, formerly BAC)
    Nonmucinous
    Mucinous
    Mixed mucinous/nonmucinous

Minimally invasive adenocarcinoma (≤3 cm lepidic predominant tumor with >5 mm invasion)
  Nonmucinous
  Mucinous
  Mixed mucinous/nonmucinous

Invasive adenocarcinoma
  Lepidic predominant (formerly nonmucinous BAC pattern, with >5 mm invasion)
  Acinar predominant
  Papillary predominant
  Micropapillary predominant
  Solid predominant with mucin production

Variants of invasive adenocarcinoma
  Invasive mucinous adenocarcinoma (formerly mucinous BAC)
  Colloid
  Fetal (low and high grade)
  Enteric

BAC, bronchioloalveolar carcinoma.
Reproduced with permission from Travis WD, Brambilla E, Noguchi M, et al. International Association for the Study of Lung Cancer/American Thoracic Society/European Respiratory Society international multidisciplinary classification of lung adenocarcinoma. *J Thorac Oncol* 2011;6:244.

and salivary gland tumors are less common types that are also included among lung cancers.[64]

Genetic Characterization

A fairly detailed understanding of cellular and genetic characteristics of cancer has emerged. A way to organize this is the concept of "hallmarks of cancer." Initially 6 hallmarks were defined; by 2011, this had increased to 10 (resisting cell death, sustaining proliferative signaling, evading growth suppressors, enabling replicative immortality, activating invasion and metastasis, inducing angiogenesis, deregulating cellular energetics, avoiding immune destruction, genome instability and mutation, tumor-promoting inflammation).[65,66] A potential 11th hallmark has recently been suggested (epigenetic or RNA deregulation).[67] The ability to identify mutations in genes that play a role in various of these mechanisms has substantiated the importance of these hallmarks as being fundamental to malignant behavior.

Genetic characterization allows better classification of lung cancers. A systematic characterization of genetic alterations in 1,255 patients with lung cancer reveals that most histologic types have a characteristic pattern of genetic alteration.[62] Large-cell lung cancer is the exception, exhibiting alterations associated with each of the other major histologic types. Using genetic characterization, the vast majority of cases initially classified simply as large-cell lung cancer could be assigned to another histologic group (e.g., adenocarcinoma, squamous carcinoma, SCLC), which was corroborated by prognostic and other similarities among the genetically grouped cohorts.[62]

Particular mutations have sparked a great deal of attention, primarily because they have led to dramatic therapeutic breakthroughs (Table 41.3). Mostly these involve driver mutations for sustained proliferative signaling. Mutations in the epidermal growth factor receptor (EGFR) gene are the best-known examples. Such driver mutations have received much attention because targeted treatment can yield dramatic results, although the overall proportion of patients with these mutations may be quite small. Particularly because identification of these genetic alterations drives the choice of treatment, some have suggested that classification based on targetable mutations may be a better way to classify lung cancers than by histologic features.

Classification by genetic alterations is thwarted by the complexity of these changes. Whole genome and whole exome sequencing of 183 lung adenocarcinomas revealed greater complexity in genetic alterations than what is seen in most other cancers.[67] Although many mutated genes were found, 15% did not have a single hallmark alteration, and almost 40% have fewer than four hallmark alterations.[67] Focusing on mutations in which a targeted therapy is available or being developed may be practical, but belies the complexity of cancer biology. Even in those instances where dramatic responses have been achieved, in most cases resistance eventually develops. Furthermore, while driver mutations can sometimes clearly play a major role in cancer growth, alterations in many of the other hallmarks of cancer are less amenable to treatment, at least at this time. Finally, the well-documented finding that some EGFR-mutated adenocarcinomas that have become resistant to treatment with a tyrosine kinase inhibitor (TKI) have been transformed into a SCLC underscores that our understanding of the fundamental nature of lung cancer is still rudimentary.

Prognostic Factors

Prediction of prognosis is fervently desired, but remains an elusive goal. Developing a system to do this is complex and must solve a number of inherent conflicts. Hence the state of affairs is that we have identified a few factors that have prognostic value (at least in some clinical settings), but it is spotty and explains only a small amount of the actual observed outcomes.

Prediction of prognosis is inherently complex.[68] There are many factors that contribute; these can be grouped roughly into environmental factors, tumor-related factors, and patient-related factors (Fig. 41.5). The prognosis is inherently linked to a specific clinical scenario and to the outcome of interest. The scenario includes treatment-related factors and timing (e.g., the prognostic significance of an EGFR mutation is different if the patient is to undergo treatment with an EGFR inhibitor, regular chemotherapy, or neither, and different prior to treatment than upon developing resistance).

There are inherent conflicts in prognostication.[68,69] We derive our knowledge from studying groups of patients with a particular characteristic, but we seek individualized prognostic prediction, tailored to a particular person. The ability to individualize is limited because we do not have sufficient detail of all of the other factors of the group to assess how well the group fits with the individual. Even if we had more and more detail, the more specific we get, the more limited the dataset available to derive the prediction becomes, and thus the greater the uncertainty about the prediction. Finally, the data we base the prediction on is inherently based on past observation, yet the prediction is for the future, and thus cannot take into account new developments that inevitably occur.

Prognostic prediction is inherently different than stage classification.[69] Stage classification is a nomenclature to describe the anatomic extent of disease. It must remain relatively static and be used in a consistent uniform manner; the classification we assign to a particular extent of tumor today must be the same as what we assign to the same extent next year or else it is a useless nomenclature. However, prognostication is inherently fluid and constantly changing as advances occur and the setting changes. Stage classification must be consistent and definitive while prognostic prediction is inherently speculative and uncertain.

TABLE 41.3

Genetic Alterations in Non–Small-Cell Lung Cancer

Genetic Alteration	Frequency	Test	Targeted Agents[a]
Nonsquamous			
KRAS mutation	25%	Sequence	None
EGFR mutation	15%	Sequence	Gefitinib, erlotinib, afatinib
ALK rearrangement	5%–7%	FISH	Crizotinib, ceritinib
ROS1 rearrangement	1%–2%	FISH	Crizotinib
HER2 (mutation only)	2%–4%	Sequence	Traztuzumab, pertuzumab, lapatinib, afatinib
BRAF mutation	2%–3%	Sequence	Vemurafenib, dabrafenib
RET rearrangement	1%–2%	FISH	Carbozantinib
MET (mutation only)	1%–2%	Sequence	None
MEK1 mutation	<1%	Sequence	None
PIK3CA mutation	1%–2%	Sequence	None
Squamous			
FGFR1 amplification	20%–25%	FISH	None
FGFR1 mutation	5%	Sequence	None
PIK3CA mutation	5%–10%	Sequence	None
DDR2 mutation	3%–5%	Sequence	Dasatinib
PTEN mutation/deletion	15%–20%	Sequence	None

FISH, fluorescence in situ hybridization.
[a] Agents listed do not all have proof of efficacy and are not all approved.

Prognostic Prediction System

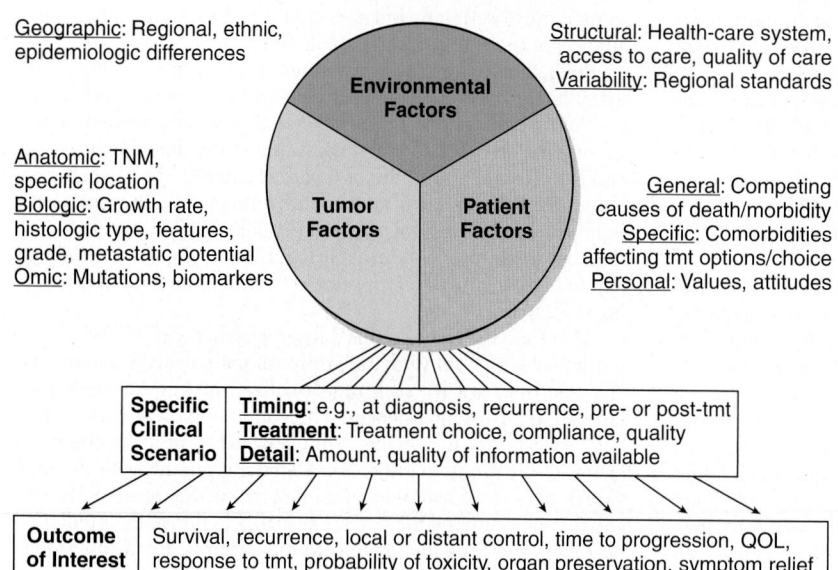

Geographic: Regional, ethnic, epidemiologic differences

Anatomic: TNM, specific location
Biologic: Growth rate, histologic type, features, grade, metastatic potential
Omic: Mutations, biomarkers

Structural: Health-care system, access to care, quality of care
Variability: Regional standards

General: Competing causes of death/morbidity
Specific: Comorbidities affecting tmt options/choice
Personal: Values, attitudes

Environmental Factors
Tumor Factors
Patient Factors

Specific Clinical Scenario	**Timing**: e.g., at diagnosis, recurrence, pre- or post-tmt
	Treatment: Treatment choice, compliance, quality
	Detail: Amount, quality of information available

| Outcome of Interest | Survival, recurrence, local or distant control, time to progression, QOL, response to tmt, probability of toxicity, organ preservation, symptom relief |

Figure 41.5 Schematic of a prognostic prediction system, taking into account environmental, patient-related, and tumor-related factors. The prediction must be specific to the clinical scenario and the outcome of interest. TNM, tumor, node, metastases; QOL, quality of life; tmt, treatment.

As part of the stage classification project, the international staging committee undertook a review of data on prognostic factors in lung cancer among surgically treated patients in the worldwide IASLC database.[70] Pathologic TNM class was most important, but age and gender also had independent prognostic significance. Histologic cell type (particularly bronchioloalveolar carcinoma [BAC]) may have some prognostic value; however, this is linked to other variables and is probably best understood when we can take into account the newer subclassification of adenocarcinoma, which was not available at the time of the analysis.[63] Many other potential factors, such as genetic features or PET intensity, were also not available for analysis. In sum, development of a prognostic model is very complex, situation specific, and constantly changing. We have only a rudimentary understanding at this point, and no overarching system of how to develop a universal prognostic prediction model.

PREVENTION AND SCREENING

Prevention

Tobacco Control

The global epidemic of lung cancer is linked most strongly to population engagement in cigarette smoking. While other modifiable risk factors (e.g., exposure to occupational or domestic carcinogens) are clearly identifiable, it is tobacco smoking that has driven the steep rises in lung cancer incidence and mortality witnessed over the last century in developed and developing nations. Primary prevention has the greatest overall potential to minimize lung cancer risk, and smoking cessation is still the most powerful intervention to diminish lung cancer risk in persons who smoke. Smoking cessation even into the seventh decade of life results in a decrease in lung cancer incidence, and so it is never too late to quit.[20,71] While smoking rates have decreased dramatically since the publication of the first surgeon general's report on the health consequences of smoking in 1964, approximately 20% of adult Americans still habitually smoke.

Important public health interventions have included stricter control of tobacco products by government regulatory agencies, limitations on cigarette advertising, particularly those geared toward children, the use of text and graphic warnings on cigarette packaging, and global initiatives to inform the public of the health hazards of smoking.[72–75]

Smoking Cessation

There are many physiologic and psychological factors that contribute to make smoking a difficult addiction to overcome. However, there have been major advances in understanding these, and solid scientific data regarding which interventions work best and in which individuals. Nicotine acts in an area of the brain associated with a sense of "safety" and "survival functions."[76] This appears to explain the paradox of difficulty in giving up smoking even when faced with a life-threatening disease that is a consequence of smoking. This struggle and the illogical nature of it, combined with the stigmatism associated with smoking, lead to feelings of shame, helplessness, and depression that further aggravate the problem.[76] It is easy to succumb to a fatalistic defense that "it is too late anyhow." However, data clearly shows that patients with lung cancer who continue to smoke approximately double their risk of dying.[76] Quitting smoking is associated with better response to treatment, better quality of life (QOL), better long-term survival, and a lower risk of second primary cancers.[76–79] Furthermore, data shows that a diagnosis of lung cancer represents a particularly opportune moment to intervene.[76]

Smoking cessation intervention should be included in the health care of any individual smoking cigarettes. It is important to use a sophisticated, evidence-based approach and an organized smoking cessation program to achieve the best results.[76] A simple recommendation to stop smoking or provision of self-help materials is largely ineffective. Several points are important. Tobacco dependence is best managed in a chronic disease model with repeated intervention over time. Intensive behavioral therapy and counseling (e.g., weekly) is of significant benefit in several randomized controlled trials (RCT). In addition, seven first-line medications reliably increase long-term smoking abstinence rates (bupropion, varenicline, nicotine patch, gum, lozenges, inhaler, and nasal spray).[76] These increase effectiveness two- or three-fold and result in abstinence rates of ~25%. Often, combinations of these may be more effective than a single intervention. These medications have been shown to be safe in most patients, including those who are about to undergo either surgery, RT, or chemotherapy. It is best to initiate the cessation interventions at the outset. Specifically, it is safe (and beneficial) for patients to stop smoking even a short time (e.g., 1 to

2 weeks) before undergoing surgery; pharmacologic interventions are safe to continue in the perioperative period as well.[76] A well-organized thoracic oncology program, therefore, should include an evidence-based smoking cessation program that is fully integrated with the diagnostic and treatment components of patient care.

Chemoprevention

The concept of chemoprevention is based on the data that lung cancer is the end result of a multistep accumulation of carcinogen-driven genetic and epigenetic changes. In theory, chemical agents might prevent these changes by a variety of proposed mechanisms, such as detoxifying carcinogens and modifying pathways that influence cell growth and behavior. Epidemiologic and animal studies had suggested that derivatives of the antioxidant vitamins A and E might be protective against lung cancer. However, large clinical trials of alpha-tocopherol and beta carotene in subjects at risk of developing lung cancer failed to demonstrate any benefit, and two studies suggested that beta carotene was actually associated with an increased incidence of lung cancer as well as cardiovascular disease.[80–83] To date, no chemopreventative intervention has been demonstrated to be of benefit for lung cancer. The focus has shifted from large RCTs to studies to better define the underlying biology and appropriate surrogate end points.[84]

Screening

At present, the majority of patients with lung cancer have advanced disease at the time of diagnosis. This preponderance of advanced disease, where prognosis is poor even with treatment, is a major contributor to the dismal overall 5-year survival rate of 18%; this contrasts starkly with breast, colon, and prostate cancers, the next three leading causes of cancer death, whose 5-year survival rates over the past several decades have increased to 90%, 65%, and nearly 100%, respectively.[2] These improved survival rates are arguably attributable at least in part to early detection resulting from widely available and broadly accepted, albeit still controversial, screening interventions.

An effective screening tool for early detection of lung cancer has been an elusive goal for decades. Several large randomized trials performed during the 1960s and 1970s evaluating lung cancer screening with chest radiography with or without sputum analysis at varying time intervals failed to demonstrate any mortality benefit,[85–89] and a Cochrane meta-analysis[90] concluded that there was no evidence to support the use of chest radiography or sputum cytology as a lung cancer screening modality. More recently, chest radiography was re-examined as a lung cancer screening tool in the Prostate, Lung, Colorectal and Ovarian trial, which enrolled 154,901 participants aged 55 to 74 years from 1993 to 2001.[91] No difference in lung cancer mortality was seen between those randomized to screening with annual chest radiography versus no screening, regardless of the degree of smoking. Together, these studies clearly demonstrate that there is no mortality benefit associated with serial chest radiography as a screening tool.

In the 1990s, intense interest was generated by the results of a number of observational studies evaluating low-dose CT (LDCT) as a lung cancer screening modality. Eventually, a number of RCTs were performed in various sites around the world. The largest of the RCTs was the National Lung Screening Trial (NLST), which included 53,454 subjects, ages 55 to 74 with at least 30 pack-years of cigarette smoking, who were either currently smoking or had quit smoking within the prior 15 years.[92] NLST subjects underwent three rounds of annual screening, randomized to either chest radiograph or LDCT. Approximately 1% of subjects had lung cancer over the duration of the trials. At a median follow-up of 6.5 years, there was a 20% relative reduction in lung cancer mortality observed in the LDCT arm (Fig. 41.6).[92] None of the other RCTs evaluating lung cancer screening with LDCT is of the scale of the NLST; in the trials in which the data has become available, the mortality benefit has been nonsignificant, and without a trend toward a benefit.[93–95] The subjects in all of these studies had smoked and were of middle to older age. A multisociety systematic review of lung cancer screening with LDCT analyzed the evidence from 8 RCTs and 13 prospective cohort studies.[96] This review found a composite significant benefit for LSCT screening, with few ensuing harms, when LDCT screening was conducted in the setting of an organized, structured program. Consistent with this, many organizations (American College of Chest Physicians [ACCP], American Cancer Society, Society of Thoracic Surgeons, American Association of Thoracic Surgery, National Comprehensive Cancer Network [NCCN], US Preventative Services Task Force) have recommended that healthy smokers or former smokers (quit <15 years ago, ≥30 pack years of smoking) age 55 to 74 years or 80 years be considered for LDCT screening.[96–101]

Teasing out further details on who to consider for screening will rely heavily on modeling studies as the effort needed for further RCTs is too great. To explore this, the Cancer Intervention and Surveillance Modeling Network developed five independent models based on a US cohort born in 1950.[102] All five models included dose-response information relating to cigarette exposure; 26 scenarios varying in age, screening frequency, and smoking exposure were modeled with respect to the percentage of cancers detected at an early stage, the number of lung cancer deaths prevented, and life-years gained were balanced against outcome measurements of harm, including the number of CT screenings

PRACTICE OF ONCOLOGY

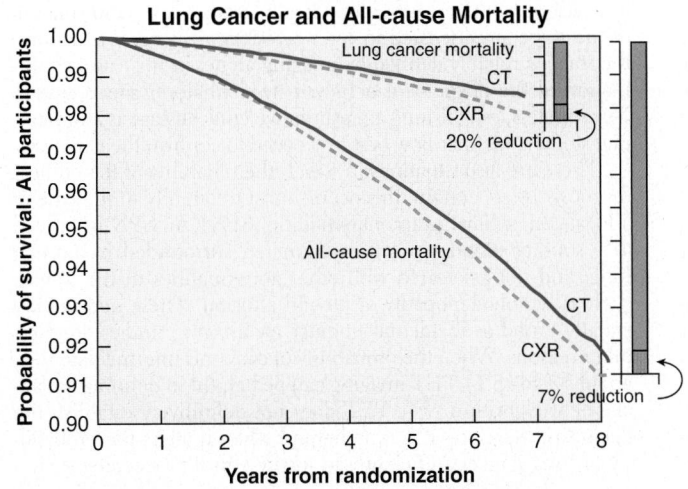

Figure 41.6 Lung cancer mortality and overall mortality reduction by computed tomography (CT) screening in the National Lung Screening Trial. CXR, chest X-ray. Data taken from Aberle D, Adams A, Berg C, et al. Reduced lung-cancer mortality with low-dose computed tomographic screening. *N Eng J Med* 2011;365:395–409.

required, the number of follow-up imaging exams, the number of overdiagnosed lung cancers, and radiation-related lung cancer deaths. Based on the models, a range of different screening scenarios are arguably valid, with different balances of benefits and harms, with the most efficient screening projected in a population similar to the NLST. On the basis of the Cancer Intervention and Surveillance Modeling Network analysis, the US Preventative Services Task Force now recommends "annual screening for lung cancer with low-dose computed tomography in adults ages 55 to 80 years who have a 30 pack-year smoking history and currently smoke or have quit within the past 15 years."[101]

There are potential downsides to screening with LDCT that must be considered in the decision to pursue screening for any population or for a given patient. The most obvious of these is the high rate (20% to 50%) of finding small nodules, which are benign and inconsequential in about 97%.[96] These findings can create unnecessary anxiety, lead to further more intense imaging with significant radiation exposure, and sometimes invasive biopsies with potential complications. In the highly organized LDCT screening studies, only 1.2% to 5.6% of subjects underwent a surgical biopsy or procedure, about 25% of these were for what turned out to be benign nodules.[97] Finally, it is clear that screening detects a higher proportion of slow-growing, less aggressive cancer, some of which may even be inconsequential.[103,104] Appropriate management of these issues that are inextricably linked to screening is essential in order to minimize harms and achieve the greatest benefits.

The complexities of the identification of the "right" population or individuals to screen, combined with the potential harms associated with LDCT screening, argue strongly that screening for lung cancer is a multifaceted process, involving much more than the simple ordering of a scan. The process for most individuals should include an individualized risk assessment for lung cancer[29,105–108]; a discussion about the potential harms of screening, including false-positive results; the potential for cumulative diagnostic radiation; and the possibility of invasive evaluation to diagnose nonmalignant disease. Smoking cessation intervention should be an integral part of this process for individuals still smoking or at risk for relapse. This process should be performed in a multidisciplinary setting. There is data to suggest that if lung cancer screening is done in an unstructured way, the ratio of benefits to harms may be significantly altered. Because implementation of lung screening is just beginning, careful consideration and monitoring is needed to see if the benefit seen in the NLST can be achieved with broader application.

DIAGNOSIS

Clinical Presentation

Approximately a quarter of patients with lung cancer are diagnosed at early stage. These patients are typically free of symptoms; their cancers are identified incidentally during evaluation of unrelated issues. While the proportion of asymptomatic early stage lung cancers may increase with the implementation of screening, at present more than half of patients have advanced lung cancer at the time of diagnosis. These patients typically come to attention because of symptoms related to the primary tumor, metastasis to distant sites, or paraneoplastic syndromes.[109]

The most common pulmonary symptoms are cough, hemoptysis, and dyspnea.[109] Cough may represent the effects of the primary tumor on the airways, with endobronchial or extrinsic airway obstruction, postobstructive atelectasis or infection, or airway inflammation with secretions. Hemoptysis may also result from airway inflammation or necrosis, but may also be related to parenchymal tumor necrosis and cavitation. Dyspnea may arise from a wide variety of tumor-related issues, including mechanical compromise of the airways, lymphangitic spread, pleural effusion, hypercoagulability with pulmonary thromboembolism, or even pericardial

effusion. Direct extension of the primary tumor to adjacent structures may cause pain from invasion of the chest wall or brachial plexus, hoarseness from impingement of the recurrent laryngeal nerve, superior vena cava (SVC) syndrome, Horner syndrome (ptosis, miosis, anhidrosis) from invasion of the sympathetic chain and stellate ganglion, or pericardial tamponade.[109]

Symptoms related to metastatic disease may be constitutional or organ related. The most common sites of NSCLC metastases are the brain, bone, liver, adrenals, and lung, though any organ can be affected. Focal neurologic symptoms, persistent headache, bony pain, or unexplained weight loss, anorexia, or fatigue should raise the suspicion for metastatic disease. Likewise, laboratory abnormalities such as anemia, liver function test abnormalities, or hypercalcemia should raise concern for distant spread.[109]

Paraneoplastic syndromes are well described with lung cancer; it is important to recognize that these syndromes are unrelated to metastatic disease and do not preclude curative intent therapy. Hyponatremia related to syndrome of inappropriate secretion of antidiuretic hormone is seen most commonly with SCLC but can occur with other malignant or benign lung processes. Hypercalcemia related to ectopic production of parathyroid hormone–related peptide is more common than hypercalcemia related to bony metastases and is most commonly associated with squamous cell carcinomas. Ectopic corticotrophin (Cushing syndrome) is usually associated with SCLC or early stage carcinoid tumors. Hypertrophic pulmonary osteoarthropathy typically manifests as symmetric and painful arthropathy of the limbs associated with characteristic findings of new periosteal bone formation of the long bones. Neurologic syndromes are less common but include the Lambert-Eaton myasthenic syndrome and encephalomyelitis-subacute sensory neuropathy, both of which are typically associated with SCLC.[109]

Diagnostic Approach

In most patients, an experienced clinician can make a clinical diagnosis of lung cancer with a high degree of reliability (>95%).[110] The main factors that contribute to this are the risk factors for development of lung cancer (e.g., age, smoking history, family history, presence of significant COPD), the clinical presentation, and the radiographic appearance of the lesion on CT (e.g., spiculated, upper lobe, node enlargement). If needed, algorithms are available that can predict the likelihood of lung cancer,[108,112–115] but the judgment of experienced clinicians is just as good.[112]

If the probability of lung cancer is high (e.g., >80%), it is generally more efficient to proceed with evaluation of the stage than confirmation of the diagnosis.[110,116,117] Frequently, this will identify a necessary procedure that will serve both to confirm the stage as well as the diagnosis. For example, biopsy of a potential solitary metastasis or of a suspicious mediastinal node can confirm both the stage and diagnosis. Those situations that require tissue confirmation of the stage are discussed in the next section. In other situations, the stage is reliably defined by imaging alone; in this case, confirmation of the diagnosis is achieved from whatever site is easiest. Nevertheless, establishing a presumptive clinical stage is an important step that defines how best to proceed to confirm the diagnosis.

There are also situations in which the reliability of the clinical diagnosis is less certain; this occurs most frequently in the case of a localized, solitary pulmonary nodule (SPN). An SPN is defined as a solitary lesion <3 cm in diameter, surrounded by normal lung, and not associated with other abnormalities in the thorax, such as lymphadenopathy or pleural effusion. These nodules are usually found as incidental findings on imaging studies done for other reasons. When the probability of cancer is intermediate (i.e., about 5% to 65%), PET imaging can be helpful in defining a management algorithm.[118,119] PET does not definitively establish the diagnosis; therefore, it is only helpful when it alters the probability of lung cancer sufficiently to justify either proceeding with a

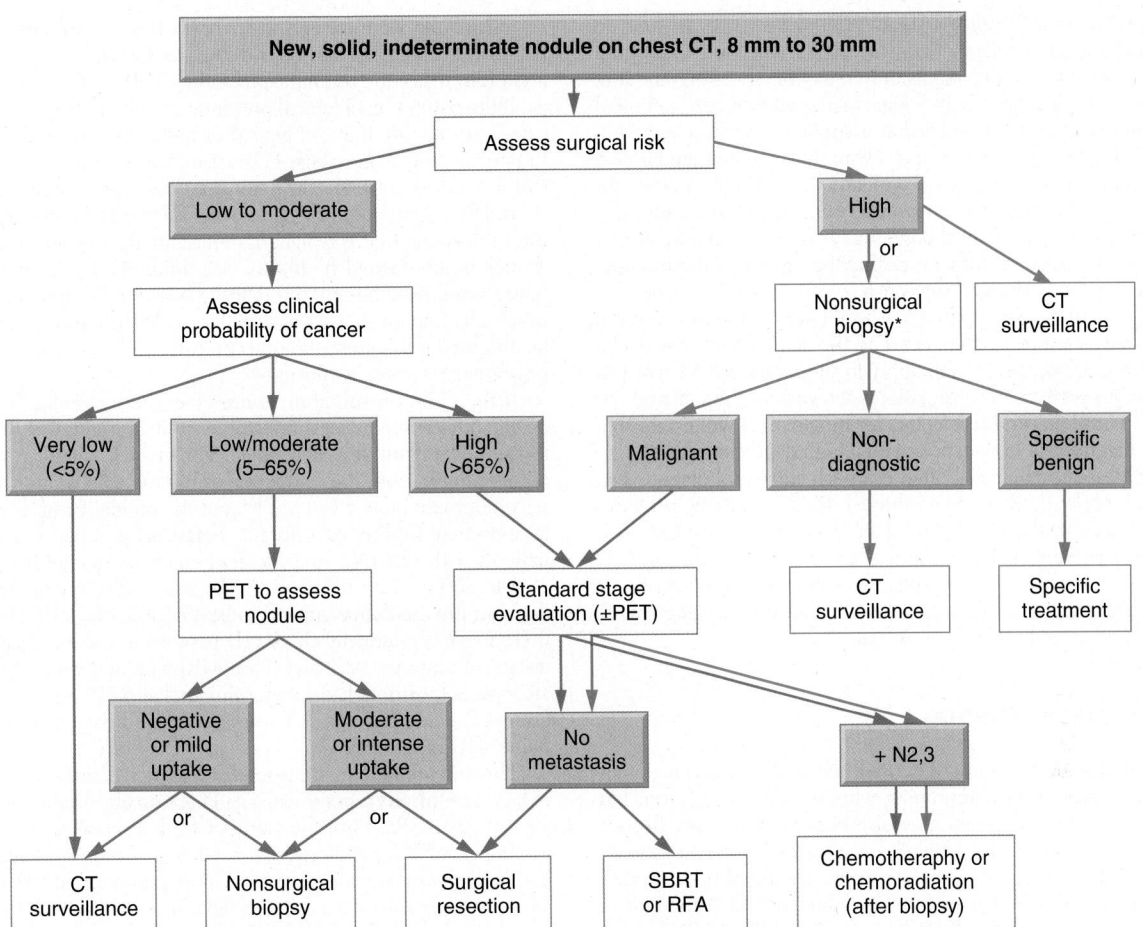

Figure 41.7 Management algorithm for individuals with solid pulmonary nodules 8 to 30 mm in diameter. *Branches* indicate steps in the algorithm following nonsurgical biopsy. *Among individuals at high risk for surgical complications, we recommend either computed tomography (CT) scan surveillance (when the clinical probability of malignancy is low to moderate) or nonsurgical biopsy (when the clinical probability of malignancy is moderate to high). PET, positron emission tomography; SBRT, stereotactic body radiotherapy; RFA, radiofrequency ablation. (Reproduced with permission from the American College of Chest Physicians Lung Cancer Guidelines, Gould MK, Donington J, Lynch W, et al. Evaluation of individuals with pulmonary nodules: when is it lung cancer? *Chest* 2013;143:e93S–120S.)

biopsy or observation. False-positive PET results may occur with any inflammatory or infectious process: tuberculosis, fungal infections, rheumatoid nodules, and sarcoidosis—when such a process is suspected, PET is generally not helpful (it does not differentiate between such a process and cancer). PET also carries a high false-negative rate with ground glass opacities (GGO), carcinoid tumors, or small lesions; in these situations, PET should also generally be avoided. Specifically, the false-negative rate of PET in a GGO is approximately 90%.[118] The false-negative rate in solid lesions <1.5 cm is ~15% and in lesions <1 cm ~30% to 50%.[118] Although the "resolution" of modern PET scanners is ~6 mm, this is a technical and not a clinical term—a lesion must have a diameter of *four times the resolution* in order to detect >90% of the 18-fluorodeoxyglucose activity that is present. This fact also explains why the detected standard uptake value of a lesion falls linearly for lesions smaller than ~2 cm, even if the actual amount of 18-fluorodeoxyglucose activity remains the same.[118,120]

A nonsurgical biopsy can be accomplished by transthoracic needle aspiration (usually guided by CT) or via bronchoscopy. This is most useful when a benign diagnosis is suspected, but this is rather uncommon.[121] In patients with a high suspicion of lung cancer, a biopsy can confirm the diagnosis, but in this situation the false-negative rate of a nonspecific diagnosis is ~20%[116]; therefore, a surgical biopsy should be pursued unless the patient is too high

risk.[119] When doing a tissue biopsy, it is crucial to obtain enough tissue for histologic and molecular characterization.[116]

To summarize, PET is most useful when there is an intermediate probability of lung cancer; PET should not be used for lesions that are <1 cm or for a GGO. A biopsy can be important in certain instances when there is doubt about the diagnosis. With a high probability of cancer, it is best to complete the stage evaluation and obtain tissue in a manner that is suited to confirm the stage as well. A detailed management approach for SPN is available for the ACCP lung cancer guidelines, as summarized in Fig. 41.7.[119]

STAGE EVALUATION

General Approach

Staging is a critical aspect of the evaluation of all patients known or suspected of having lung cancer. Clinical stage (identified by a "c" prior to the stage group) is determined by all information available before any definitive treatment. This may involve merely a simple history and physical examination, may include imaging studies, or may involve invasive biopsies or surgical procedures with sampling the primary tumor, intrathoracic lymph nodes, pleural fluid, or extrathoracic sites. Pathologic staging (identified by a "p" prior to the stage group) is determined only if surgical resection with intent to cure is performed. All patients undergo clinical staging; the subset of patients who have pathologic staging all first had a clinical stage defined that determined that a surgical resection was indicated. Pathologic staging is inherently more accurate than clinical staging; comparison of survival typically demonstrates better survival for pathologically as compared to clinically staged patients.[52] Nonetheless, it is the clinical stage that drives the initial treatment decisions, and thus it is imperative that the process of defining the clinical stage be performed rigorously.

The process of stage evaluation should begin as soon as there is a strong suspicion of lung cancer, and the data and recommendations in the rest of this section apply to such patients. As noted in the previous section, in most patients a review of the CT and the patient's symptoms and risk factors for lung cancer will establish a clinical diagnosis of lung cancer with a high degree of accuracy.[110] A thoughtful approach will often establish stage and diagnosis simultaneously and efficiently (Table 41.4). The approach to confirming the clinical diagnosis and stage is different for patients with a negative clinical evaluation and clinical stage I lesion on CT, a positive clinical evaluation suggestive of distant metastases, or those with a negative clinical evaluation but a CT suggestive of hilar or mediastinal node involvement.[110]

Extrathoracic Staging

As noted, the initial comprehensive clinical evaluation is an important first step in determining whether a primary tumor has spread. The clinical evaluation consists of a comprehensive history, physical examination, and simple laboratory testing. Constitutional symptoms, focal symptoms, abnormalities on the physical examination, or unexplained liver function abnormalities, anemia, or hypercalcemia may suggest distant metastases. Because the false-positive rate of this evaluation is around 50%, this suspicion must be confirmed. If the clinical evaluation points strongly to a particular site, further imaging or biopsy should be targeted to the observed abnormalities. For example, needle aspiration of enlarged supraclavicular nodes identified on physical examination may efficiently

establish both diagnosis and stage. If the clinical evaluation is positive but less focal, imaging for distant metastases is needed (PET and brain magnetic resonance imaging [MRI] or CT).[122]

If the patient has a typical presentation with multiple sites identified on imaging that are typical of metastases, there is no need to confirm the stage (stage IVb) histologically (although there is still a need to get tissue to document the type of cancer, which should be obtained from whatever site is easiest). However, if there is a solitary site that is typical of metastatic disease, in general this should be confirmed by biopsy (see Table 41.4). Several studies have found in such scenarios that the suspected solitary metastasis is actually benign in 10% to 50%.[123,124] Confirmation should also be obtained if the presentation is unusual or the appearance of the possible metastases is unusual.

If the clinical evaluation is negative, the incidence of finding occult distant metastases detectable by imaging varies according to the clinical intrathoracic stage. For cI by CT with a negative clinical evaluation, the incidence of finding true distant metastases is approximately 5%,[110,124–132] and the incidence of detecting a false-positive finding of a distant metastasis is actually higher. In patients with cIII (N2) the incidence of finding occult disease is 25% to 30%.[110,125,127,128,130,133–136] For stage cII, there is much less data but the incidence appears to be 15% to 20%.[110,128] Therefore, there is good reason in cII or cIII patients to pursue imaging for distant metastases: PET and brain MRI with and without contrast are optimal, although an abdominal/pelvic CT, bone scan, and brain CT with contrast is reasonable if PET is not available or brain MRI is not possible.

The value of PET imaging for the detection of distant metastases in larger cI tumors is controversial. There no clear data specifically for this group. RCTs of the value of PET in general have shown varying results depending on the clinical setting and the likelihood of metastases in the patient population included.[131,137–140] Those studies showing a benefit have included patients selected by minimal criteria (i.e., a general practitioner's suspicion of lung cancer based on a chest X-ray alone) or patients with clinical findings suggestive of metastases and little conventional imaging,[138,139] whereas those that have found no difference involved patients that had a low suspicion of metastases based on the clinical evaluation by a lung cancer specialist and who had already undergone

---

TABLE 41.4

Approach Diagnosis and Staging of Patients with Probable Lung Cancer

Clinical Scenario	Result of Clinical Evaluation	Confirmation of Extrathoracic Stage	Confirmation of Intrathoracic Stage	Confirmation of Diagnosis
NSCLC				
Peripheral cI	Neg (FN 5%)	Not needed	CT alone (FN <10%)	Surgical resection
cII, central cI	Neg (FN 5%–15%)[a]	PET	Mediastinoscopy vs. EBUS[b]	Surgical resection
cIII, discrete N2,3 enlargement	Neg (FN 30%)	PET, brain MRI	EBUS vs. mediastinoscopy[b]	Mediastinal node biopsy
cIII, diffuse infiltration	Neg (FN 30%)	PET, brain MRI	CT alone is sufficient	Easiest site[c]
cIV	Pos (FP 50%)	PET, brain MRI	not needed	Easiest site if multiple typical metastases[c] Biopsy of suspected site if solitary potential metastasis
SCLC				
Any	Any	PET, brain MRI	CT	Easiest site[c]

NSCLC Non-small cell lung cancer; cI, clinical stage I; Neg, negative; FN, false negative; CT, computed tomography; cII, clinical stage II; PET, positron emission tomography; EBUS, endobronchial ultrasound; cIII, clinical stage III; MRI, magnetic resonance imaging; cIV, clinical stage IV; Pos, positive; FP, false positive; SCLC, small-cell lung cancer;
[a] Rate not specifically defined for stage II (defined for stage I and II combined). FN rate may be up to 15%.
[b] Fine needle aspiration carries FN rate of about 30% in most series.
[c] For example, sputum, bronchoscopy, fine needle aspiration of supraclavicular node, transthoracic needle aspiration.

conventional imaging.[131,137] The ACCP and NCCN guidelines are relatively generic in recommending PET in essentially all patients with a suspected or diagnosed lung cancer, without accounting for details of the clinical stage before PET or the clinical setting (only cIa and GGO lesions are excluded from the PET recommendation by the ACCP).[110,141]

Mediastinal Staging

If there are no distant metastases, the status of the mediastinal nodes becomes critical in determining the right treatment strategy. Much information is already available from the CT scan. However, while there are situations in which it is reliable, there are also many in which it is notoriously unreliable. One can distinguish four groups of patients based on the CT findings: (A) tumors with mediastinal infiltration, meaning that discrete lymph nodes can no longer be distinguished or measured; (B) tumors with enlargement of discrete mediastinal node(s) ($\geq$1 cm in short axis diameter on an axial image); (C) normal mediastinal nodes but either N1 node enlargement or a central (hilar) tumor; and (D) peripheral tumors with no evidence of N1 or N2,3 node enlargement.[110]

In group A, clinical experience shows the false-positive rate is essentially 0; thus, invasive biopsy is not needed to confirm mediastinal involvement (Fig. 41.8). The rate of a false positive of discrete node enlargement in category B is ~40%, making invasive staging necessary. For central tumors (category C), the false-negative rate of the lack of N2,3 enlargement is ~25%, again making invasive biopsy important. In category D (peripheral tumor with no N1-3 enlargement), the false-negative rate of CT is ~10% (<10% for T1 and ~12% for T2); thus, many feel that invasive confirmation of a lack of N2,3 involvement is not needed (especially if PET is also negative; see the following), whereas some feel this rate is high enough to justify invasive biopsy.[110]

PET scanning adds information, but does not alter the indications for invasive staging significantly.[110] A positive PET in an enlarged node (group B) carries a 15% to 20% false-positive rate, whereas a negative PET in an enlarged node carries a 20% false-negative rate, making invasive biopsy necessary either way.[110] For central tumors (group C), a negative PET still has a 20% false-negative rate, and a positive PET in the mediastinum has a 20% chance of being a false positive. For a peripheral tumor with no node enlargement, a negative PET has a false-negative rate of ~3% (but a positive PET may be false positive). This data makes it clear that in groups A and D imaging can generally be considered adequate, but in groups B and C invasive biopsy is needed regardless of the PET results (unless compelling data for distant metastases is present).[110]

There are multiple techniques to invasively confirm the presence or absence of N2,3 involvement. These include traditional mediastinoscopy, video-mediastinoscopy, so-called super mediastinoscopies that involve a complete mediastinal lymphadenectomy performed as an outpatient via a cervical incision, endobronchial ultrasound (EBUS) and needle aspiration, esophageal ultrasound and needle aspiration, simple "blind" transbronchial needle aspiration, video-assisted thoracic surgery (VATS), and rarely CT-guided transthoracic needle aspiration. There are differences in which nodes are accessible, whether these procedures are applicable to multiple node sampling, and how feasible they are for sampling normal sized versus enlarged nodes (Table 41.5). The technique and thoroughness of how the procedure is done probably has a major impact on the reliability of the results.[110,142]

The choice of which invasive staging technique to use is probably best tailored to specifics of the institution and the patient. In trained hands, all can be performed with low morbidity and mortality. There is RCT data to suggest that if good quality EBUS is available, this may be the best first step in most patients.[110,143] However, the institutional availability of expertise is an important factor. In many reports, the false-negative rate of EBUS has been ~20%, although in expert hands this appears to be lower (particularly if lymphocytes are obtained). Similarly, a video-assisted lymphadenectomy via mediastinoscopy has a false-negative rate of ~2%, but is not available in most institutions. What is critical is an interest in thorough staging and experience with at least some of the various techniques available.

Confirmation of Intrathoracic Stage

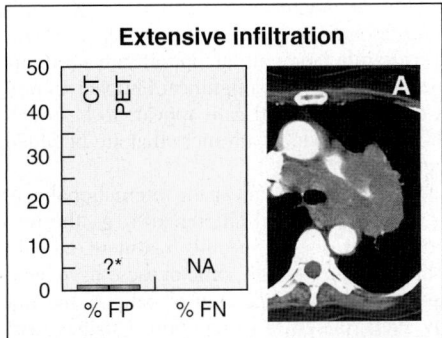

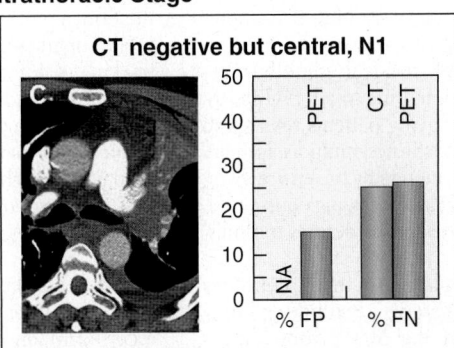

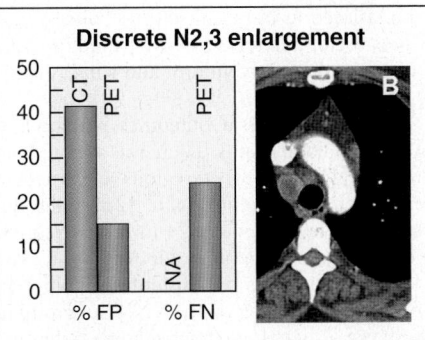

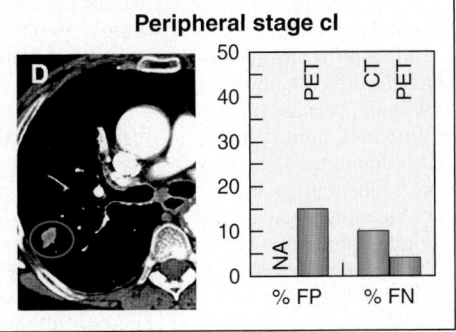

Figure 41.8 False-positive and false-negative rates for computed tomography (CT) and positron emission tomography (PET) assessment of mediastinal nodes by the American College of Chest Physicians intrathoracic radiographic (CT) classification categories. ?*, estimated, no actual data available; NA, not applicable; % FP, percent of positive test results that are false positive (= 100 − positive predictive value%); % FN, percent of negative test results that are false negative (= 100 − negative predictive value %). (Reproduced with permission from the American College of Chest Physicians Lung Cancer Guidelines, Silvestri GA, Gonazalez AV, Jantz M, et al. Methods of staging for non-small cell lung cancer: diagnosis and management of lung cancer, 3rd ed: American College of Chest Physicians evidence-based clinical practice guidelines. *Chest* 2013; 143:e211S–e250S.)

TABLE 41.5

Accessibility of Node Stations to Various Invasive Mediastinal Staging Techniques

Invasive Mediastinal Staging Technique	Accessible Lymph Node Stations
Traditional Mediastinoscopy	1, 2R, 2L, 3, 4R, 4L, anterior 7
Videomediastinoscopy	1, 2R, 2L, 3, 4R, 4L, 5, 7, 8, 10R
Anterior mediastinotomy (Chamberlain)	5, 6
Video-assisted thoracic surgery	Right-sided: R2, R4, 7, 10, 11
	Left-sided: L2, L4, 5, 6, 7, 10, 11
Transthoracic needle aspiration or biopsy	Variable; restricted to enlarged nodes
Transbronchial needle aspiration	2R, 2L, 3, 4R, 4L, 7, 10, 11
Endoscopic ultrasound with needle aspiration	4L, 5, 7, 8, 9
Endobronchial ultrasound with needle aspiration	2R, 2L, 3, 4R, 4L, 7, 10, 11, 12

MANAGEMENT BY STAGE

Overview of Lung Cancer Treatment Modalities

Structural Aspects of Patient Care

The field of lung cancer has grown to encompass a huge body of knowledge, more than what any one person can stay abreast of. Furthermore, it has become complex, with many different specialties that contribute to the evaluation and management of the patient. This makes it important to provide care in a multidisciplinary manner. The key aspect is to have a system of care delivery that is developed together with all relevant disciplines, and to have a forum for discussion so that major patient management decisions can be made with involvement of relevant specialties. It is important to provide an opportunity for different specialties to bring up points that one is unaware of, not merely to involve another specialty when one knows that they have something to offer. Unfortunately, many people think that simply having patients referred to another specialty from time to time constitutes multidisciplinary care; however, it is the system of care developed by the entire team, the ability to introduce salient points that are not being considered, and the collaborative decision making that really defines multidisciplinary care.

It is recommended and even mandated in many countries that patients with lung cancer receive care in a multidisciplinary fashion.[109,144] This is recommended by the ACCP lung cancer guidelines, based on a review of literature; specifically, the staging evaluation, the physiologic evaluation of the ability to undergo treatment, and the treatment planning should be done in a multidisciplinary setting.[144] Multidisciplinary evaluation is also recommended by the NCCN guidelines.[141] It has been difficult, however, to quantitate the impact of multidisciplinary care, because it is difficult to separate this aspect from other structural, thoroughness, and quality of care issues. A growing body of literature is showing benefits in terms of timeliness of care, more frequent use of various treatment modalities, and survival.[109,144] In the end, it may not be important to disentangle the impact of multidisciplinary care from other quality of care issues. The key point is to recognize that organization of care, which involves multiple disciplines, has a major impact on outcomes of patients with NSCLC.

There is extensive data that the care for a large proportion of patients with lung cancer is suboptimal. A study of the US National Cancer Database revealed that the proportion of patients with NSCLC and *no comorbidities* that received suboptimal care (defined as deviating from guidelines that were in place at the time) was approximately 33% for stage I, 40% for stage II, 46% for stage III, and 47% for stage IV.[145] Other studies show that there are major regional differences (more than three-fold) in the United States in the frequency of use of different treatment modalities, implying that these are not related to patient factors or what is appropriate, but likely related to regional differences in the quality of care delivery.[146,147] Several studies have shown that despite the existence of clinical guidelines for many years recommending careful mediastinal staging with biopsy confirmation, the large majority of patients are staged using CT alone (which is notoriously inaccurate).[148–150] Furthermore, such limited clinical staging was associated with dramatically worse outcomes, stage for stage (adjusted hazard ratio [HR] for death of ~1.7 to 2.3 for overall and cancer-specific survival).[148]

There is extensive evidence that structural aspects of care (e.g., case volume, specialization) have a marked effect on outcomes.[151,152] A comprehensive literature review on effect of volume/specialization in quality of cancer care concluded that "An extensive, consistent literature that supports a volume-outcome relationship was found for cancers treated with technologically-complex surgical procedures. . . . Across studies, the benefit from care at high-volume centers exceeds the benefits from breakthrough treatments."[153] In lung cancer, most of these studies have focused on surgical treatment. With very few exceptions, these studies have found lower perioperative mortality and better long-term survival in high-volume versus low-volume centers, teaching versus nonteaching facilities, and when treatment is delivered by thoracic versus general surgeons (Fig. 41.9).[151,152]

However, the relationship between volume and outcomes is not consistent on an individual institution level; there are low-volume institutions with excellent outcomes and vice versa. This suggests that volume is only a marker for other aspects of care. It is possible that low-volume centers have less availability of expertise or cutting-edge treatment interventions. However, it is much more likely that it is a marker for how organized the care delivery is. In most high-volume institutions, care will become more organized simply out of necessity. Although it has not been directly studied, there is indirect data to support that the organization of care is the critical component.[154] At any rate, developing a locally appropriate, organized, multidisciplinary process of care together with tracking of outcomes certainly represents an opportunity for many institutions, and appears likely to have a significant impact on outcomes. The impact of such organized care appears to be much greater than many treatment modality advances that are heralded as major breakthroughs.[148,155,156]

In constructing a review of lung cancer for international use, one must recognize there are regional differences (e.g., the proportion of specific cell types, use of specific treatment modalities, penetration of screening). Although some of these have been identified, their impact on the management of patients has not received much study. Nevertheless, a recognition that they exist is important. Furthermore, general conclusions and recommendations must always be tailored to the local setting. Policies may sometimes not apply because of differences in the patient population, the availability of particular interventions, and what is easily accepted in the local culture.

There are major regional differences in outcomes, perhaps best highlighted by the IASLC database results. There was a more than two-fold difference in survival rates between regions (e.g., median survival cN0 29 months versus 70 months; cN2 12 months versus 20 months for Asia versus Europe; cT1a 74 months versus 64 months, cT1b 67 months versus 46 months for Asia versus Europe, respectively).[157] The results were inconsistent, with different regions being better or worse depending on the TNM subgroup in question, although there was a slight trend toward better outcomes

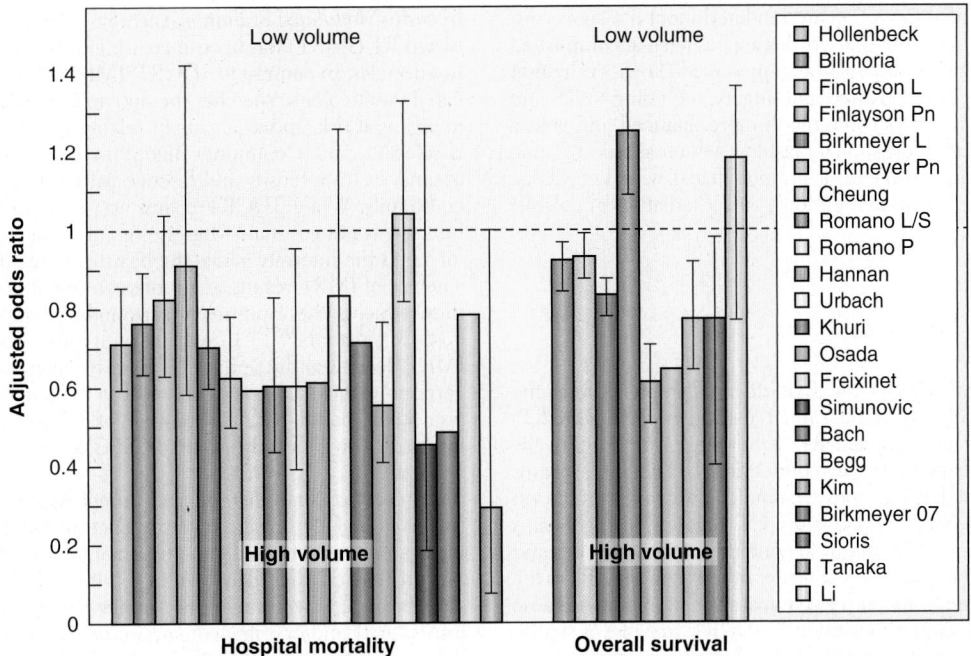

Figure 41.9 Surgical outcomes according to case volume. Perioperative mortality and long-term survival according to institutional case volume of patients undergoing surgical resection for lung cancer. (Data taken from Howington J, Blum M, Chang A, et al. Treatment of stage I and II non-small cell lung cancer: Diagnosis and management of lung cancer, 3rd ed: American College of Chest Physicians evidence-based clinical practice guidelines. *Chest* 2013;143:e278S–313S.)

in Asia.[158] It is not clear what the reasons for these differences are. It is well known that the incidence of EGFR mutation is higher in the Asian lung cancer population. There are differences in the proportion of subtypes of NSCLC. There are societal differences regarding how aggressive and which treatment modalities are generally accepted. There are differences in the availability of various technologies and treatment methods (e.g., EBUS, PET, VATS, four-dimensional RT, stereotactic body RT [SBRT], genetic testing). The impact of these differences is not clear, but it does emphasize that general recommendations need to be thoughtfully considered in light of differences as compared with the population and setting in which the data was derived.

Surgery

There have been major advances in surgical treatment of lung cancer in the past two decades, just as there have been in RT and chemotherapy. Most prominent is perhaps the use of minimally invasive resection (VATS), which makes a lung cancer resection a very different experience for the patient. The perioperative morbidity is cut in half, the hospital stay reduced to 3 to 4 days in the United States, and the return to normal functioning is dramatically quicker. This is well documented in several meta-analyses,[159–165] large-scale outcomes studies,[166–170] propensity matched studies,[168,171–182] and small randomized studies.[183–185]

While the data makes VATS the recommended treatment in the ACCP lung cancer guidelines,[151] it is used variably in different centers. Those that have embraced it perform about 80% of resections by VATS, but there remain many institutions that are not comfortable and use VATS relatively sparingly. It is likely this will change, given the amount of data supporting the VATS approach. Furthermore, robotic-assisted thoracic surgery is now being practiced at some centers. It is clear this is also a safe and effective approach. Whether there are benefits for the patient with respect to perioperative or long-term outcomes for robotic versus VATS resections is unclear.

Even open thoracotomy has changed. Smaller, muscle-sparing incisions are now commonly used. There are many newer ways of pain management that allow greater patient mobility and avoidance of complications. The management of postoperative air leaks has changed; quantitation using digital devices allows earlier chest tube removal and earlier hospital discharge.[186] Such postoperative management approaches have changed the experience for patients undergoing thoracotomy from what it typically was 20 years ago.

The value of care delivered by dedicated thoracic surgeons, who have a focused interest in noncardiac thoracic surgery and lung cancer in particular, is increasingly recognized. The ACCP lung cancer guidelines recommend that surgical care be delivered by such an individual, on the basis of a review of the literature that demonstrates better outcomes.[151] Intraoperative lymph node staging was previously often spotty; there is now a much better appreciation for the necessity to do this for both the surgeon and pathologist, and acceptance of substandard intraoperative staging is diminishing.[151]

There has also been a major advance in the ability to safely carry out extensive resections, for example involving cancers invading the thoracic inlet, vertebral column, and SVC. This makes it feasible to consider surgery as part of the treatment approach for tumors that appear to be only locally invasive. In the past, many of these tumors were simply considered unresectable; however, the modern techniques and ways of reducing morbidity make surgery a reasonable option.

The advances in surgical therapy have changed patient selection for surgery. The improved perioperative outcomes allow older and more frail patients to undergo surgery (e.g., a VATS resection or a segmentectomy).[151,166,187] Patient selection is also altered by the recognition that previous criteria had been very conservative. These had primarily defined thresholds above which there was little concern; however, they ignored the fact that risk is a continuous variable and that many patients below previous thresholds could undergo resection with quite acceptable low risk of perioperative mortality. Other previous contraindications for surgery such as a history of myocardial infarction are rendered moot if a successful intervention for the coronary artery disease has been accomplished and overall cardiac function has been preserved. Thus, evaluation of which patients can safely undergo surgery, including VATS and sublobar resection, has become much more nuanced and is best approached in a multidisciplinary fashion, which should include a dedicated thoracic surgeon, a pulmonologist with knowledge about lung cancer treatment options, and a radiation oncologist as well.

Radiation Therapy

Advances in Radiation Technique

Three-Dimensional Conformal Radiation Therapy. Before the widespread use of three-dimensional conformal RT (3DCRT) in the 1990s, the predominant RT technique for treating locally advanced lung cancer was two-dimensional. Radiation beams would be designed using bony anatomic landmarks visible on fluoroscopic imaging. 3DCRT uses CT datasets, using beams from multiple angles to conform to contoured target volumes and similarly avoid contoured normal tissue. Inherent in 3DCRT is the use of dose-volume histograms to compare the normal tissue dose among different beam arrangements. 3DCRT provides a significant advantage over two-dimensional radiation: conformal beam design and the ability to manipulate beam geometry and weighting through the planning process improves coverage of the tumor target, and decreases the dose to normal tissue. The use of CT datasets in RT planning also enables the fusion of complementary imaging modalities, such as PET or MRI.

Intensity-Modulated Radiation Therapy. The use of intensity-modulated RT (IMRT) has been increasing in frequency over the past two decades. In contrast to 3DCRT, IMRT is inverse planned. The radiation oncologist specifies the dose to tumor targets, dose limits to organs at risk, and assigns their relative priority. Beam geometry is selected, and a computer algorithm is used to determine the optimal beam intensity and fluence pattern to meet the planning constraints. While 3DCRT beams are static, in IMRT the beam intensity is not constant—the use of a dynamic multileaf collimator varies the intensity across the beam aperture during treatment. The use of IMRT results in a more conformal plan than 3DCRT, thus reducing the exposure of surrounding normal tissue to high doses of radiation.[188,189] In patients with bulky NSCLC, the use of IMRT decreased the volume of lung receiving >20 Gy by 10%, corresponding to a decrease of >10% in the calculated risk of radiation pneumonitis (RP). An example of 3DCRT and IMRT plans for a patient with locally advanced NSCLC is shown in Fig. 41.10.

Image-Guided Radiotherapy and Tumor Motion Considerations. Image-guided RT implies the presence of radiographic imaging incorporated into the radiation treatment device. Commonly used imaging devices include kilovoltage orthogonal planar imaging or cone-beam CT scanning. This allows direct visualization of the tumor target and/or critical organs immediately before treatment is delivered, while the patient is immobilized, as frequently as every treatment fraction. The use of image-guided RT allows the reduction of the expansion margin around the clinical target volume, since interfraction variations in patient positioning are reduced.[190] This can, in turn, reduce the exposure of the surrounding normal lung tissue.

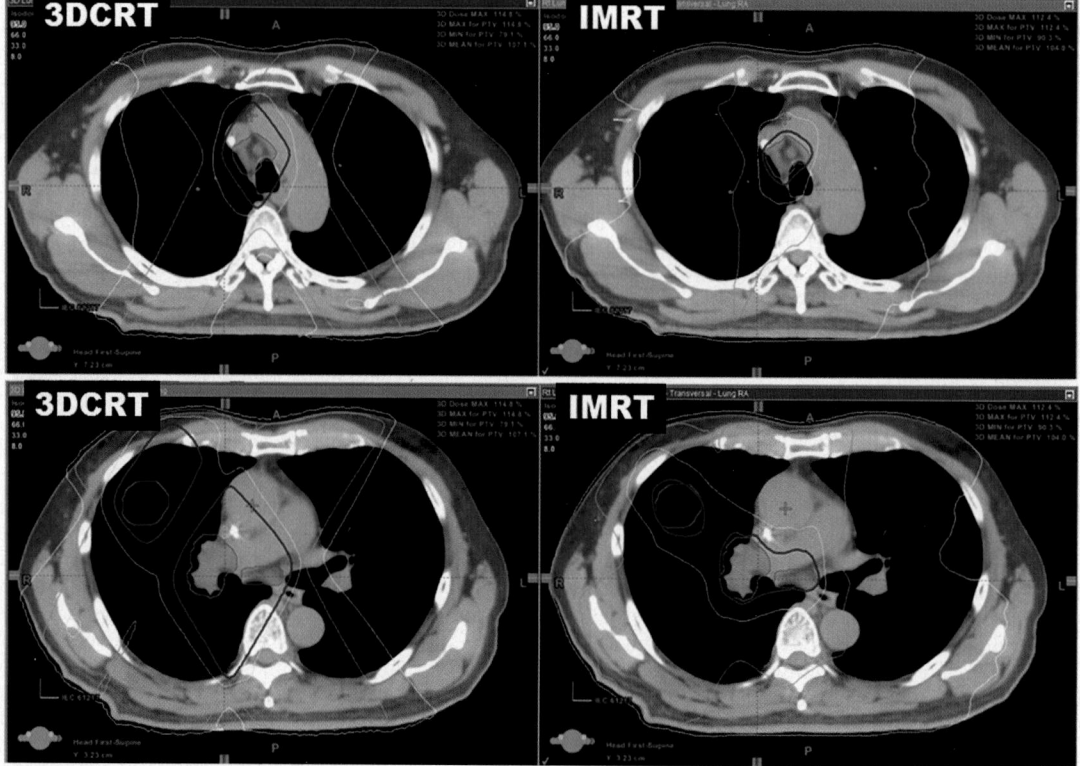

Figure 41.10. Radiation treatment plans: Comparison of two methods. A 64-year-old former smoker presented with stage IIIA non–small-cell lung cancer, with disease in the right lower lobe, hilum, and mediastinal station R4. Concurrent chemoradiation was recommended. Radiation plans were generated using three-dimensional conformal radiotherapy (3DCRT) and intensity-modulated radiotherapy (IMRT). Representative axial slices from the two plans are shown: the *top panels* compare 3DCRT (*left*) to IMRT (*right*) at the level of the aortic arch, the *bottom panels* are similarly presented for an axial level below the carina. The planning target volume is shown in *red*, isodose lines are demonstrated for 60 Gy (*dark blue*), 40 Gy (*yellow*), 20 Gy (*green*) and 5 Gy (*white*). The use of IMRT decreased the mean lung dose (16 Gy versus 13 Gy) and V20 (32% versus 23%), but increased the volume of lung receiving 5 Gy. The esophageal dose was also lower with IMRT; V30 was reduced from 41% to 23%.

A large component of the expansion margin for lung cancer is designed to allow for positional uncertainty of the tumor that corresponds with the respiratory excursion of the diaphragm. Allowing for intrafraction respiratory motion is a required part of radiation treatment planning for lung cancer, and can be accomplished in several ways. The use of four-dimensional CT scans in treatment planning allows the accurate measurement of tumor motion for an individual patient,[191] and the correlation of tumor position with an external fiducial. After the acquisition of a four-dimensional CT scan, various motion management techniques can be employed: expansion of the intended treatment volume based on the measured motion, gated treatment in which the patient is only treated during a portion of the respiratory cycle, or abdominal compression where the diaphragmatic motion is damped using external compression devices. Tumor tracking, where the radiation aperture follows tumor while it moves, is an area of growing interest.

Proton Therapy. The use of charged particle therapy such as protons is an area of active investigation in lung cancer. Protons have distinct physical characteristics that suggest they can be used to deliver thoracic radiation with a lower risk of side effects, when compared to standard photon therapy. The deposition of proton energy in tissue can be modulated by changing the beam energy, leading to much lower entry doses than photons, and an even more significant in the drop-off of the exit dose. Proton radiation beam arrangements do not need to enter and exit through lung tissue to avoid critical structures such as the spinal cord, which should decrease the risk of RP and radiation fibrosis.[192] Phase 2 trials of fractionated proton therapy with concurrent chemotherapy in locally advanced lung cancer have demonstrated excellent median survival, with relatively low toxicity.[193,194] A large cooperative group randomized trial is ongoing.

Radiation Toxicity. The risk and severity of radiation toxicity are related to the dose and volume of normal tissue that are exposed, to the presence or absence of underlying comorbidities, as well as the functional organization of the particular organ at risk. Emami et al.[195] published a comprehensive review of partial-volume organ tolerances for normal tissue that served for more than a decade as the standard source for radiation dose limits, and risk of toxicity. These parameters were based predominantly on clinical data from older, two-dimensional RT planning. Recently, a large multidisciplinary effort was undertaken, the Quantitative Analysis of Normal Tissue Effects in the Clinic, to summarize the published three-dimensional dose-volume/toxicity data in the literature, review normal tissue complication probability modeling, and provide practical guidance for organ dose limits.[196]

Radiation Pneumonitis and Pulmonary Fibrosis. Clinically significant pneumonitis occurs in somewhere between 5% and 50% of patients receiving definitive fractionated radiation for locally advanced lung cancer, and is often the dose-limiting factor in radiation planning. RP may occur during fractionated treatment or up to 18 months afterward, with a peak incidence at approximately 2 months. The most common clinical presentation is a persistent, nonproductive cough; dyspnea; low-grade fever; and fatigue. Chest X-ray or CT scan may be normal, or depending on the time course there may be GGO (within 2 to 6 months), patchy consolidation (4 to 12 months), or fibrosis (≥10 months). The earliest radiographic changes occur within the medium- to high-dose radiation volumes, though later changes may extend into unirradiated lung. Pulmonary function testing shows reduced lung volumes, tidal volumes, and diffusion capacity. A variety of dose-volume models have been evaluated as predictive metrics of RP, including threshold volumes (i.e., V_{dose}), mean lung dose (MLD), and normal tissue complication probability models. Accumulated data from the Quantitative Analysis of Normal Tissue Effects in the Clinic effort suggest that while there is gradually increasing risk with increasing

exposure, with no safe threshold dose below which the risk of RP is zero,[196] the risk of grade 2 or greater RP was <20% when the MLD was held to <20 Gy during conventional radiation fractionation. Commonly used thresholds include a V_{20} <30% to 35%, or V_5 <60%, corresponding to a risk of RP of <20%.

RP occurs less commonly after SBRT in comparison to conventionally fractionated radiation.[197] The risk of symptomatic RP does seem to follow a similar relationship to dose and volume irradiated as seen in conventionally fractionated treatment,[198] though specific dose thresholds are evolving as experience with SBRT grows. Takeda et al.[199] retrospectively examined 265 patients, and with a median follow-up of 19 months the incidence of grade 2 to 5 pneumonitis was 18.5%, 4.5%, 0%, and 0.4%, respectively. Predictors of grade 2 or higher RP on multivariate analysis included V_{20}. A large series from Indiana University examined dosimetric predictors of pneumonitis[200] in a group of 143 patients treated with SBRT. RP (grade 2 to 4) occurred in 9.4% of cases. Pneumonitis was noted in 4.3% of patients with a MLD of ≤4 Gy, compared with 17.6% of patients with MLD of >4 Gy ($p = 0.02$), and in 4.3% of patients with a V_{20} ≤4% compared with 16.4% of patients with V_{20} of ≥4% ($p = 0.03$).

RT-induced dyspnea may have several contributing causes, including not only RP but also RT to other thoracic organs at risk. Emerging evidence suggests an interaction between cardiac dose and RP,[201] and there may be additive dyspnea due to pleural and pericardial effusions, cardiomyopathy, and bronchial stenosis or bronchiectasis. Bronchial fibrosis and stenosis has been reported with radiation dose escalation beyond 70 Gy.[202]

Several patient- and treatment-related factors also impact the risk of RP, independent of dose and volume. In a large dataset derived from patients treated on Radiation Therapy Oncology Group (RTOG) trials, the risk of RP was significantly higher for tumors in the lower lung fields.[203] Older age may increase the risk of RP, and patients who continue to smoke through treatment may be at decreased risk.[196] Several chemotherapy agents that are commonly administered to patients with lung cancer concurrently are associated with an increased risk of RP, including docetaxel, gemcitabine, and particularly the commonly used carboplatin and paclitaxel combination.[204]

Glucocorticoids are commonly used to treat RP in patients who have moderate to severe symptoms, although the efficacy and appropriate starting dose and tapering schedule have not been defined in a prospective fashion. Prophylactic antibiotics or anticoagulants do not appear to effect the development of RP, although they are frequently given. Pulmonary parenchymal fibrosis is the underlying cause of long-term dyspnea after thoracic radiation, likely the result of chronic treatment-induced inflammation. No standard clinical approach has been definitively demonstrated to reverse or even slow the progression of pulmonary fibrosis, though several therapies have shown signs of activity, including pentoxifylline.[205] Amifostine is a radioprotector that has been tested in several randomized trials, with mixed results.[206,207] Captopril is an angiotensin-converting enzyme inhibitor that has been shown to reduce the development of radiation-induced fibrosis in animal models.[208]

Esophagitis and Esophageal Stenosis. Acute esophagitis is typically the dose-limiting side effect during fractionated RT for thoracic malignancies. Grade 3 or greater acute symptoms (i.e., severely altered eating/swallowing, tube feeding, parenteral nutrition, or hospitalization indicated) occurred 18% of the time, in a series of >1,000 patients undergoing chemoradiation.[204] Acute esophagitis may coexist with, and be exacerbated by, comorbid conditions such as candidiasis or reflux disease. Other factors identified as increasing the risk or severity of acute esophagitis include the use of accelerated fractionation and older patient age.[209] The use of concurrent chemotherapy is associated with an increased risk.[210] The use of concurrent bevacizumab with RT has led to case reports of fistulae.[211,212] Clinically significant late toxicity, such as stenosis or fistula formation, is less common after conventionally fractionated radiation, occurring in <5% of patients.[213,214]

Treatment of acute esophagitis is primarily supportive, frequently requiring topical agents, dietary changes, and narcotic pain medication. It is often prudent to either evaluate or treat empirically for viral or candida esophagitis. Patients may benefit from proton pump inhibitors for comorbid reflux disease, and topical agents for mucosal irritation such as sucralfate or local anesthetic agents. The ability of the radioprotectant amifostine to reduce the risk and severity of acute esophagitis has been evaluated in several prospective trials, but no benefit was noted in a large randomized, cooperative group study.[207]

Heart. For thoracic malignancies, the dose and volume of radiation to the heart and great vessels varies considerably, depending upon the anatomic distribution of the target and the treatment technique. The overall excess risk of cardiac mortality after thoracic RT is low,[215] but moderate toxicities have been reported more commonly. Acutely, this can include pericarditis, which can develop during treatment or within several months afterward. Months after radiation, there can be pericardial effusion, and over years progressive fibrosis may rarely lead to constrictive pericarditis. Ischemic changes in the cardiac muscle can manifest with a long latency and may lead clinically to congestive heart failure or ultimately a higher cardiac mortality.[216] Valvular abnormalities have been reported, presumably due to late fibrotic changes. In the great vessels, there can be accelerated atherosclerosis that worsens over years to decades, leading to an increased risk of structural damage such as aneurysm. Comorbid clinical conditions may increase the risk of RT-induced cardiac toxicity,[217] including hypertension, diabetes, obesity, and genetic predisposition. The risk of cardiac mortality from RT has been specifically demonstrated to be increased in patients over 60 years old, and by tobacco use.[218,219] There are reports that concurrent paclitaxel may also increase this risk.[220,221]

Brachial Plexus. Radiation brachial plexopathy is a rare but serious complication of fractionated radiation to conventional doses. There are case reports of early, transient neuropathy that may occur during or shortly after radiation, and may resolve spontaneously.[222] Late radiation plexopathy is more clinically significant; it manifests years after radiation to the supraclavicular area and may manifest as hypesthesia, paresthesia, and weakness of the affected arm and shoulder. It may progress to total paralysis of the affected arm, and severe pain. The dose tolerance of the brachial plexus is less defined than other thoracic organs, partly due to the difficulty in defining the plexus radiographically during radiation treatment planning. A contouring atlas has been adopted, so that more robust clinical data can be collected.[223] Late plexopathy is rare in patients who receive conventional doses of fractionated radiation.[224] For SBRT, brachial plexopathy is a more significant concern, because the biologically effective dose prescribed to the target exceeds the tolerance of the plexus.

Chemotherapy

There has been a long evolution in the treatment of NSCLC since the early editions of this textbook. It was not until the late 1980s that the benefits of chemotherapy with respect of overall survival (OS) and QOL versus supportive care were appreciated in patients with advanced disease.[225–227] In the early 1990s, a new generation of chemotherapeutic agents, used in combination with platinum analogs, consolidated the benefits of treatment and established chemotherapy.

In the mid to late 1990s, the combination of chemotherapy and RT in patients with stage III disease showed superior outcomes compared to single modality and created a new paradigm of combined modality therapy, still considered the standard to this date.[225] During the 2000s, chemotherapy was tested in the adjuvant setting

and became a new standard of care by improving the cure rates in selected patients with stage IB through IIIA disease.[228] Remarkably, over the course of two decades, or five editions of this textbook, chemotherapy has become an established treatment modality for the majority of patients with NSCLC.

The discovery of somatic mutations in a subset of lung tumors is the most significant paradigm shift in the treatment of lung cancer in the last decade. Since the initial report on EGFR,[229] the understanding that specific molecular alterations serve as oncogenic drivers, and that blockade of these pathways by specific agents can lead to robust and prolonged responses, has revolutionized the approach to patients with lung cancer. This discovery has launched the era of personalized medicine, in which patients are managed based on specific characteristics of their tumors.

The evolution of chemotherapeutic management of NSCLC has ushered in many more fundamental changes in how we think about stage IV NSCLC. At one time, it was questionable whether the treatment was worse than the disease, now this is a vibrant, successful, fast-paced field with new discoveries that challenge the ability to keep pace. There are many effective cytotoxic agents, targeted therapy, and immunotherapy, and which are used in first-, second-, and third-line settings. The treatments can be dramatically effective, and it is no longer surprising when a patient with incurable NSCLC can be successfully managed over many years. We are clearly moving toward management of stage IV NSCLC as a chronic disease.

The management of stage IV NSCLC is complex. It is not merely a question of which drug to use, but which sequence, how to plan the first course of therapy taking into account later options, and when to initiate a new treatment. Treatment is viewed less as a defined course of therapy and more as a continuum over time. The lines between treatment courses are blurred: when does a course of therapy become maintenance, when is maintenance therapy early institution of second-line treatment? More aggressive palliation of specific symptoms or conditions (brain, spine, bone metastases, airway obstruction, etc.) has far-reaching effects, including a better QOL and a more positive attitude, but also a better ability to tolerate active treatment.

The evolution of chemotherapy treatment of NSCLC has led to different end points in clinical trials. OS, once considered a hard end point, has become problematic. Because OS reflects the entire continuum of management and a combination of interventions, it is often difficult to discern what effect a particular portion of the treatment strategy has on OS. Progression-free survival (PFS) has become more prominent as it can assess a specific portion of the continuum of treatment. However, it is controversial whether and under what circumstances it is an appropriate measure.[230] More subtle measures such as toxicity and QOL are also used as primary end points. Thus, end points of clinical research have become more difficult to measure and attribute to a particular intervention. At the same time, the standards of what is considered clinically relevant and sufficient to call a trial positive has decreased.[231] The combination of these trends raises issues for clinical research moving forward.

The treatment has become much more specific; having evolved from a one-size-fits-all NSCLC approach to being histology based, and even more specifically directed to small cohorts identified by particular genetic mutations. These markers have an impact not only on response but also on susceptibility to toxicity in some cases. This radically changes the economics of treatment, research, and drug development. The specific cohorts are smaller and more difficult to identify. The need to screen a larger population to identify a few individuals can be costly and inefficient. Cost is determined not just by the cost of therapy but also cost of and ability to find the right cohort.[232–234] The dramatic response that can be seen with such targeted therapy can lead to approval of a therapy based on nonrandomized data alone, reducing the costs of drug development. However, the more limited cohort for whom it is applicable also limits the potential return. The pace of new discoveries in specific tumor subgroups creates challenges in how to conduct appropriate clinical research in a timely enough manner. New approaches to trial design, such as an adaptive Bayesian structure, may offer innovative, more flexible options than the traditional phase 1, 2, and 3 research schema.[235] There are many forces in play in the dynamic, rapidly changing field.

Preinvasive and Minimally Invasive Disease (Bronchial Intraepithelial Neoplasia, Adenocarcinoma in Situ, Ground Glass Nodules)

Bronchial intraepithelial neoplasia appears to be a precursor to central airway squamous cell carcinomas. These lesions are infrequently encountered, usually in patients with abnormal sputum cytology or during surveillance of the central airways. Although techniques have been developed (autofluorescence bronchoscopy, narrow-band imaging) that are more sensitive in detecting such lesions, it is unclear how these should be implemented.[236] Among high-risk patients who participated in a screening program, about 30% of high-grade dysplasia and 50% of carcinoma in situ lesions were observed to progress; however, the rates were highly variable among studies (with follow-up periods of ~1 to 10 years).[236] A substantial proportion of lesions regresses during follow-up. One of the problems is that there is moderate interobserver variability in the classification of such biopsies. Photodynamic therapy seems to be fairly effective at treating lesions deemed worthy of intervention, but it is not well established which lesions need intervention, as many do not progress.[236]

In 2011, a new subclassification of adenocarcinoma was introduced, covering a spectrum from atypical adenomatous hyperplasia (AAH), adenocarcinoma in situ (AIS), minimally invasive adenocarcinoma (MIA), lepidic predominant adenocarcinoma, and various types of invasive adenocarcinoma (acinar, papillary, micropapillary, etc.).[63] Although not conclusively established, this carries the implication that the earlier lesions (e.g., AAH, AIS) may be precursors to invasive adenocarcinoma. It must be emphasized that these entities can only be classified after resection (not on the basis of a limited biopsy).[63] However, there is a strong correlation between the histologic classification and the radiographic appearance, although this has not been quantitatively defined. AAH and AIS lesions generally appear as pure ground glass nodules (GGN) on CT, and MIA and lepidic predominant adenocarcinoma are often part-solid GGNs, while other types of adenocarcinoma are generally mostly solid-appearing lesions on CT. The increased use of CT has led to more frequent recognition of these lesions and creates a need to define how to manage them.

Pure GGNs are focal lesions seen incidentally on a chest CT; this is distinct from more diffuse or patchy ground glass appearance of the lung, which generally signifies benign interstitial or inflammatory lung disease. A number of studies have reported outcomes of such lesions during a period of observation of 1 to 3 years.[237] It is difficult to be precise because of slight differences in definitions and inclusion criteria and duration of follow-up. Approximately 10% to 20% of pure GGNs disappear, usually within 3 months. About 10% decrease in size, but it should be noted that approximately 20% of adenocarcinomas that were eventually resected after a period of observation were observed to have decreased in size.[237] Most remain stable, around 20% increase in size, and ~10% (range, 0% to 30%) develop a solid component.[237]

Other papers have focused on diagnoses made during observation of a GGN, which may skew the data toward the more suspicious lesions that motivated intervention. These studies have found that approximately 75% of pure GGNs are benign (and still followed), ~10% are AAH, 10% to 20% are BAC, and ~5% are adenocarcinoma.[237] It is hard to translate the older terms BAC and adenocarcinoma used in these studies into the new subclassification

of adenocarcinoma. Among studies that focused on lesions that were actually resected, ~30% of pure GGNs were benign (including AAH), the majority was BAC, and ~10% were diagnosed as adenocarcinoma. The incidence of adenocarcinoma was <5% in pure GGNs <10 mm in size, and ~25% if >10 mm.[237]

The rate of invasive cancer is substantially higher in part-solid GGNs (although these are by definition still >50% ground glass). A diagnosis of adenocarcinoma is made in ~10% during a period of observation. Of those coming to actual resection, ~30% are adenocarcinoma and most of the rest were classified as BAC; ~10% were adenocarcinoma among part-solid GGN <10 mm versus ~40% if >10 mm.[237]

Triggers for intervention are still evolving. There is a growing impression that pure GGNs may be simply observed, while a part-solid GGN usually warrants intervention, especially if the solid component has recently developed. The rate of growth should also be factored in—a lesion that has grown 2 mm in 5 years may not warrant intervention. Significant growth over the course of a year or development of a solid component should generally trigger resection.[119,237,238] Exact definition of recommendations and specific documentation of results is hampered by the short periods of follow-up in studies so far, the loose correlation between radiographic appearance and histologic results, the inability to establish a diagnosis of a preinvasive lesion before resection, and the uncertainty about the malignant potential of AAH, AIS, MIA, and even lepidic predominant adenocarcinoma.

Multiple studies suggest that a limited resection of a pure or >50% GGN results in excellent outcomes (5-year survival >95% with no recurrences).[237] One can question whether all of these lesions actually need to be resected in the first place. Nevertheless, one prospective carefully done study of limited resection found no recurrence at 5 years, but by 10 years 13% developed a staple line recurrence of a genetically apparently identical tumor, despite a reasonably wide negative margin originally.[239] The ACCP lung cancer guidelines suggest a sublobar resection for a pure GGN <2 cm with careful attention to achieving an adequate margin.[151]

Patients with GGNs often have several lesions. These lesions should be approached conceptually as independent lesions. Each lesion should be managed individually, intervening when necessary and observing other when there is no change and a low suspicion of invasive cancer.[119,237,238] There is no reason to give chemotherapy to these patients if these are independent early cancers or preinvasive lesions; chemotherapy has no role as a chemopreventative agent.

Stage I (T1,2 N0)

The standard of care for healthy patients with a clinical stage I NSCLC is surgical resection.[141,151] This is based on decades of experience showing good long-term survival rates with few recurrences after resection. Examination of the 2010-11 US National Cancer Database shows that surgery was the dominant treatment strategy (surgery in 66%, RT in 23%, and no treatment in 9%). In the US Surveillance Epidemiology and End Results (SEER)-Medicare database (i.e., patients age >65 years), the treatment given to stage cI patients in 2007 was surgery in 67%, RT in 16%, and no treatment in 18%.[240] The ACCP Lung Cancer Guideline recommends that patients with stage I NSCLC being considered for curative therapy be evaluated by a thoracic surgeon or a multidisciplinary team (even if nonsurgical therapy is being considered). Those undergoing surgery should be treated by a thoracic surgeon with a demonstrated focus on lung cancer (grade 1B).[151] There is a growing body of literature that demonstrates that outcomes are demonstrably better with specialty training and at higher volume centers (HR = 0.7 for perioperative mortality and 0.9 for long-term outcome in high-volume centers in a recent meta-analysis).[152]

Across the world, for NSCLC cases diagnosed between 1990 and 2000, staged and treated according to the local routines at the time the survival as reported by the huge IASLC database is 50% for cIa and 43% for cIb, and 73% for pIa and 58% for pIb.[52] More recent Japanese national cancer statistics demonstrate 5-year survival rates of 77% and 60% for cIa and cIb, and 84% and 66% for pIa and pIb.[241] It is important to note that only about half of the deaths within 5 years in stage I NSCLC are due to recurrences; the 5-year recurrence rate is only about 20%.[242–244] The majority (60%) of recurrences are identified within the first 2 years.[244,245] Late recurrences beyond 5 years are seen in 10% to 20% of patients, but it is unclear how many of these "recurrences" are actually new primary cancers.[246,247]

The ACCP Lung Cancer Guideline suggests that a minimally invasive (e.g., thoracoscopic [VATS] or robotically assisted) resection is preferred over an open thoracotomy for stage I NSCLC (grade 2C).[151] This is based on consistent data from small RCTs, matched case-control studies, propensity matched cohort studies, meta-analyses, and large outcomes studies, which demonstrate lower perioperative mortality, fewer complications, and shorter hospitalization as well as at least equivalent long-term stage-matched survival.[151,159,160,168,171,176,248–250] The penetration of VATS for major lung resection has been growing annually at US academic medical centers, but is performed almost exclusively by thoracic surgeons (not cardiac, general, or oncology surgeons).[251] RCTs and large database outcome studies show no difference in the ability to biopsy or resect mediastinal nodes by VATS,[159,176,183,184,252,253] although there may be a less thorough assessment of N1 nodes.[252] The ability of patients to receive adjuvant chemotherapy is improved following VATS lobectomy.[254,255]

A lobectomy remains the treatment of choice for good-risk patients with stage I NSCLC in general (ACCP Lung Cancer Guideline grade 1B).[151] This is a general conclusion, which is a different issue than asking whether an alternative resection is acceptable in patients that cannot tolerate a lobectomy, or whether there are particular cohorts for which the general statement does not apply. The recommendation for lobectomy over a more limited resection is based on better survival and lower local recurrence rates after lobectomy. Unfortunately, the data is not of high quality. This result is demonstrated by a RCT with only minor flaws,[256,257] but because it stems from the late 1980s, the relevance to the current era can be questioned. Other uncontrolled comparative studies corroborate these results, but the patients undergoing sublobar resection were clearly not the same (often not able to tolerate lobectomy or with smaller tumors). Furthermore, the sublobar resections often involved a mixture of segmentectomy and wedge resection, although segmentectomy generally results in better survival and less local recurrence than a wedge.

Specific groups that have been considered to be potentially suitable for a sublobar resection include patients with tumors <2 cm, <1 cm, pure GGO lesions, and elderly patients. For solid smaller lesions and older patients, the data is unclear; comparisons have yielded conflicting results, probably because of the inability to account for selection and confounding factors. Comparisons involving primarily wedge resection tend to show worse results, whereas those involving segmentectomy are more similar to lobectomy.[151] Two RCTs are under way to address the value of segmentectomy for solid tumors <2 cm. Increased perioperative mortality or competing causes of death such as might be present in older patients are reasonable to consider; however, clear guidance on when this tips the balance away from lobectomy is not possible from the currently available data.[151] On the other hand, there is fairly extensive data that patients with predominantly GGO lesions <2 cm consistently experience excellent 5-year outcomes after sublobar resection (predominantly segmentectomy), with the implication that it would be difficult for lobectomy to yield even better results. This led the ACCP guideline committee to recommend sublobar resection for predominantly GGO lesions <2 cm (grade 2C).[151] However, it is important to have an adequate margin, and there is data from a carefully done prospective study that segmentectomy may be associated with late recurrences (between 5 and 10 years).[239]

At the time of surgical resection, at least a systematic lymph node sampling should be performed. This involves systematically looking for and sampling a representative node from N1 and ipsilateral mediastinal node stations. Data supports that this results in more accurate staging than selective sampling.[258–261] However, there appears to be no survival benefit to a complete lymph node dissection in RCTs, at least not in clinical stage I patients.[151,260–262]

Adjuvant chemotherapy or RT is not indicated after complete resection of stage I NSCLC. Although the majority of recurrences after resection of stage I NSCLC are distant, multiple RCTs that have included stage I patients have suggested that there is no benefit to adjuvant chemotherapy.[263–265] A meta-analysis that addressed stage-specific subgroups did not find a benefit for either stage Ia or Ib.[155] An unplanned subgroup analysis in one study suggested that there may be a benefit for tumors ≥4 cm,[266] but this has not been borne out by further follow-up or other analyses. Other negative prognostic factors have been suggested (i.e., tumor differentiation, vascular invasion, histologic features), but the argument that chemotherapy will have an impact is purely speculative. The ACCP NSCLC guideline, which is more evidence based, takes the position that adjuvant chemotherapy should not be given for stage Ia or Ib with the stance that speculative arguments should not overpower RCT data.[151] The NCCN guideline, however, which is primarily consensus based, suggests considering adjuvant chemotherapy for high-risk stage Ib patients, by taking into account potential negative prognostic factors.[141] On the other hand, tegafur (an oral 5-fluorouracil agent available in Japan) has been found to improve survival in two RCTs when given orally for 2 years.[267,268]

Adjuvant RT is also not indicated after complete resection of a stage I NSCLC; in fact, the RCT data suggest it is likely to be harmful.[151,269] A more recent RCT and an outcomes analysis of the SEER database confirm this result.[270,271]

While lobectomy remains the standard of care for stage I NSCLC, there are patients who are considered poor candidates for this approach. However, poor risk for lobectomy is difficult to define. VATS resection has decreased the perioperative mortality,[272,273] data shows that lung function is reduced much less or even improved in patients with severe COPD,[272,274–276] and the majority of data mixes lobectomy and various forms of sublobar resection together (often including good-risk patients with low-risk tumors together with poor-risk patients with high-risk tumors). Furthermore, data suggest that limited pulmonary reserve correlates primarily with perioperative mortality, whereas long-term functional limitations are often due to random unpredictable events. The ACCP guideline recommends caution about undertaking lobectomy if the predicted postoperative FEV1 or predicted postoperative DLCO is <30% or <22 m on a stairclimbing test.[272] Such patients should undergo a formal exercise test and a careful multidisciplinary evaluation. While lobectomy may still be found to be appropriate, other options such as a segmentectomy, wedge, SBRT, or radiofrequency ablation (RFA) should also be considered.[272] The multidisciplinary decision making is crucial, because there are many aspects that must be taken into account (e.g., how functional the portion of lung is that contains the cancer, technical issues with doing either surgery, SBRT or RFA, and issues related to confirming the stage of the patient).

Sublobar resection undertaken as a compromise due to poor pulmonary reserve cannot be compared to sublobar resection undertaken electively because of favorable tumor characteristics. Furthermore, the outcomes for a segmentectomy cannot be compared to a wedge resection, although frequently these are combined. The available studies show that the perioperative mortality for a sublobar resection in compromised patients is around 5%, even when the resection involves a thoracotomy (not VATS).[151] The issue is one of long-term results. In the ACCP guideline review, 5-year survival after segmentectomy/wedge for stage I NSCLC in compromised patients ranged from 40% to 70%; there was a trend to worse outcomes than for lobectomy in case-matched comparisons, although the differences were not statistically significant in most studies.

The recurrence rate after sublobar resection was 0% to 18%.[151] In one of the few series to specifically compare (retrospectively) compromised patients undergoing segmentectomy versus wedge, the 5-year survival was better for segmentectomy (80% versus 48%; $p = 0.005$) and the recurrence rate was lower (16% versus 55%; $p = 0.001$).[277] In conclusion, when surgery (usually open thoracotomy) was judged to be reasonable in compromised patients, a sublobar resection could be accomplished quite safely (mortality ~5%) and the long-term outcomes were encouraging, especially for segmentectomy, which appears to be better than a wedge resection.

Nonsurgical treatment options have also emerged for compromised patients. SBRT has received the most attention. In contrast to conventionally fractionated radiation therapy, which uses small daily fractions over the course of 6 or more weeks, an SBRT treatment plan typically delivers a much higher biologically effective dose over three to five treatment visits. This requires a high degree of precision to avoid delivering the increased dose to the surrounding tissue. For lung cancer, this means highly reproducible immobilization, management of respiratory motion, and accurate localization during treatment delivery. The result is markedly higher rate of local control and survival and markedly lower toxicity when compared to conventional RT.

Because SBRT is well tolerated, does not require general anesthesia, and results in minimal damage to surrounding lung, it has been used primarily in the management of early stage lung cancers in patients who could not tolerate surgical resection of any type. In general, these appear to have been rather severely compromised patients in reported studies. The diagnosis of lung cancer was confirmed in about 75% of patients (range, 30% to 100%). In many of the studies, the cases not confirmed by biopsy were clinically diagnosed as lung cancer by a multidisciplinary tumor board on the basis of growth and/or PET activity. The lesions treated appear to have been primarily solid typical lung cancers, not indolent, ground glass tumors or screening detected cancers. The median tumor size has generally been 2 to 3 cm.

Many of the studies involving SBRT for NSCLC have reported 2-year outcomes. Survival is approximately 60% at 2 years (45% to 79%) and 40% at 5 years (24% to 50%).[151] Cancer-specific survival is approximately 75% at 2 years (50% to 90%) and 60% at 5 years (34% to 73%).[151] Disease control at the primary tumor site is approximately 90% at 2 years (83% to 100%).

Early prospective trials suggested that SBRT is associated with a higher risk of moderate to severe adverse events in a central or perihilar tumors. However, there are several published examples of safe SBRT schedules for such patients, all delivering a somewhat lower biologically effective radiation dose than that described in the RTOG 0236.[278–281] Taken together, the cumulative experience in SBRT for central lung tumors suggests that the use of more protracted fractionation, lower dose, and prioritizing normal tissue dose constraints over target volume coverage appear to reduce the risk, but there is a suggestion that this comes at the cost of somewhat lower local control. The RTOG 0813 was a phase 1/2 dose escalation study of SBRT in central tumors that has completed accrual, and the results will inform treatment of these tumors.

There is much less data for RFA, but reported OS is approximately 80% at 2 years and 30% at 5 years (20% to 61%), with a control at the primary tumor site being achieved in approximately 60% (58% to 92%). It is very difficult to compare outcomes of patients treated surgically to those treated with SBRT or RFA—the degree of comorbidity is different, the confirmation of stage and diagnosis is different, and the definition of local control outcomes are different. Randomized studies have not been able to be conducted.

In summary, it can be said that surgical resection remains the standard for stage cI NSCLC. This should involve a lobectomy with at least a systematic mediastinal node sampling and should be performed by VATS in an experienced center. Tumors that are amenable to a sublobar resection (with attention to adequate margins!) are primarily GGO lesions <2 cm; the data for small solid tumors or in elderly patients is not clear. In patients with

limited pulmonary reserve who are considered poor risk for lobectomy, segmentectomy can be accomplished safely in selected patients with good long-term outcomes. A wedge resection is probably oncologically similar to nonsurgical treatment. Although survival results appear slightly better for wedge resection than SBRT, any comparison is confounded because the patients, tumors, and workup are quite different. However, the results of such interventions appear to be good enough to justify their use and appear to be better than that of completely untreated, conventionally detected stage I NSCLC.

Stage II (T1,2 N1)

The recommended treatment for clinical stage II NSCLC without major comorbidities is surgical resection followed by adjuvant chemotherapy.[141,151] Surgery has been the mainstay of treatment for many decades; an additional benefit to adjuvant chemotherapy has been demonstrated more recently (discussed subsequently). The ACCP recommends that patients be evaluated by a thoracic surgeon with a focus on lung cancer and be discussed in a multidisciplinary forum (grade Ib).[151] This is the standard in many European countries as well.

In the IASLC database, the 5-year survival was 36% for cIIa and 25% for cIIb (representing frequent stage misclassification). Survival was 46% for pIIa and 36% for pIIb.[52] These patients were diagnosed and treated between 1990 and 2000, mostly without the availability of PET scanning and likely mostly by surgery alone. In the Japanese national database, the 5-year survival rates in 2004 were 54% and 44% for cIIa and cIIb, and 61% and 47% for pIIa and pIIb, respectively.[241] In the Lung Adjuvant Cisplatin Evaluation meta-analysis of patients receiving resection plus adjuvant chemotherapy, the 5-year survival was estimated to be 45% for stage II NSCLC.[282] In stage II NSCLC, approximately 75% of deaths are due to recurrence.[283,284]

At the time of resection, the ACCP suggests that a formal mediastinal node dissection be performed (grade 2B), because there is some data suggesting that survival may be improved.[151] Selective sampling of only abnormal-appearing nodes is clearly substandard, and does not accurately define the pathologic stage. There is no difference in the accuracy of stage definition between a systematic mediastinal node sampling and a complete mediastinal node dissection.[151,258,260] However, there is a suggestion that survival and recurrence is better after a complete node dissection from randomized and nonrandomized studies.[151,258,260,285,286] Although substandard node assessment at the time of resection has been common, it should no longer be accepted given the data and value of adjuvant chemotherapy.

Stage II NSCLC involves either hilar (N1) nodes or a central (hilar) primary tumor. Whenever possible, a sleeve resection should be performed as opposed to a pneumonectomy.[151] A sleeve resection involves resection of a portion of the bronchus to the lung with an end-to-end anastomosis of the main bronchus to that of the uninvolved lobes of the lung. The same can be done for the pulmonary artery. Although the data is retrospective and subject to potential confounding by other factors, several reviews have found lower operative mortality and complications for sleeve resection versus pneumonectomy, equivalent or better long-term survival, lower recurrence rates, and better QOL.[151,287,288]

Adjuvant chemotherapy is clearly indicated after complete resection of stage IIa,b (N1) NSCLC, and adjuvant platinum-based chemotherapy is recommended by the ACCP and NCCN clinical guidelines.[141,151] This is based on the results of several randomized trials and meta-analyses.[155] There is data suggesting that cisplatin-vinorelbine may offer the best efficacy compared with other doublets.[155,289] While a few RCTs have not been positive, they have generally had significant flaws.[151]

The benefit of adjuvant therapy rests in the use of cisplatin-based combinations.[155] Carboplatin was used in one randomized trial, exclusive to patients with stage IB disease, which did not show a statistically improvement in survival, save for a subset of patients, identified in a post hoc analysis, with tumors ≥4 cm in greatest diameter.[266] Although carboplatin may be considered an alternative for patients with an absolute contraindication to cisplatin, the majority of candidates for adjuvant chemotherapy should receive cisplatin in combination with vinorelbine, docetaxel, gemcitabine, or with pemetrexed in patients with nonsquamous histology. While the bulk of the adjuvant data is based on cisplatin-vinorelbine, other regimens have been endorsed by the National Cancer Institute. It is assumed, though not yet demonstrated, that these regimens have comparable efficacy in this setting as in more advanced stages. Four cycles of adjuvant chemotherapy are typically recommended.

There are a number of nuances to mention. While the survival benefit of adjuvant therapy is sustained in late follow-up, it is diminished and there are late intracranial failures.[263,290] The lack of benefit in some RCTs suggests that factors such as the quality of surgery, the choice of chemotherapy, and the use of RT may play an important role. Whether adjuvant chemotherapy should be used for larger primary tumors (>5 cm) without local lymph node metastasis (T2bN0M0) is unclear. The ACCP guideline does not recommend this (based on equivalent survival in JBR10 and Cancer and Leukemia Group B [CALGB] 9633),[151] but the NCCN guideline suggests this can be considered.[141]

Postoperative RT (PORT) is not recommended for completely resected NSCLC.[141,151] The PORT meta-analysis found a nonsignificant survival detriment for PORT in N1 patients.[269] However, techniques of RT have advanced from what was used in many studies included in the PORT meta-analysis, and there are nuances that may be important. A SEER analysis found slightly worse survival for stage II patients receiving adjuvant RT.[271] A subset analysis of stage II patients in the ANITA study demonstrated a 12% survival advantage of PORT in the no adjuvant chemotherapy arm, but a 16% survival disadvantage in the arm receiving adjuvant chemotherapy.[291] In the setting of a positive bronchial margin, PORT is recommended by the ACCP and NCCN, although there is very little available data addressing this.[141,151] In summary, adjuvant RT should not be used after complete resection of stage II NSCLC; while modern techniques may change this recommendation in the future, it is also possible that better adjuvant chemotherapy obviates the benefit of RT.

Preoperative chemotherapy is not recommended. This has been addressed by one RCT involving stage I-II NSCLC, although about two-thirds of the patients were stage Ib; 624 patients were randomized to either surgery alone, preoperative chemotherapy, or surgery and adjuvant chemotherapy (three cycles of paclitaxel/carboplatin).[292] There was no difference in OS or disease-free survival between any of the arms. A subgroup analysis of stage II (T3 or N1) patients found a nonsignificant trend in disease-free survival favoring preoperative chemotherapy versus surgery alone (HR = 0.88; 95% confidence interval = 0.69 to 1.12; 5-year disease-free survival 41% versus 35%; $p = 0.31$). There was no benefit to adjuvant chemotherapy versus surgery alone in this subgroup analysis (HR = 1.01; 5-year disease-free survival 37% versus 35%; $p = 0.97$). However, given the limited number of patients, no suggestive conclusions can be drawn from this experience.[292]

Locally Invasive Tumors (T3,4 N0,1)

Certain tumors are characterized by local invasiveness (or size). Although they are classified as stage IIb, IIIa or IIIb, they may be biologically different than tumors distinguished primarily by nodal involvement.

T3N0,1

T3N0M0 tumors are classified as stage IIb, whereas T3N1M0 tumors are stage IIIa.[293,294] Most commonly, this involves tumors that are locally invasive into adjacent structures, with the chest wall being the most common site. The presence or absence of pain is probably the best indicator of chest wall involvement. In patients with cT3N0M0 tumors, the ACCP and NCCN guidelines suggest imaging for potential distant metastases and invasive mediastinal staging to detect possible occult N2,3 involvement, although data defining the incidence of such involvement is not available.[141,295]

Surgical resection is the recommended therapy for T3N0,1M0 NSCLC involving the chest wall.[141,295] The 5-year survival after an en bloc complete resection is consistently 50% to 60% for T3N0M0 tumors, whereas it is <5% with no resection or an incomplete resection (even with adjuvant RT).[295] Because a discontinuous (versus en bloc) resection is associated with worse outcomes, there should be a low threshold to chest wall resection whenever there is suspicion of involvement. Several retrospective studies of completely resected patients found no difference in OS or recurrence with or without PORT[296,297] with one exception.[298] Currently, postoperative chemotherapy or RT for completely resected T3 chest wall tumors is not recommended, although the data is limited.[295]

The 5-year survival for other resected T3N0 tumors (i.e., involving the mainstem bronchus or other central T3 structures) appears to be slightly lower at about 25% to 30%.[299,300] Careful stage evaluation followed by resection is the recommended approach. There is no data that defines the role of adjuvant therapy after complete resection. Nevertheless, the NCCN guidelines recommend adjuvant chemotherapy for all T3N0,1 tumors after an R0 resection, without providing any data or details.[141] The ACCP guidelines do not address this question.

The seventh edition of the stage classification classifies tumors ≥7 cm as T3, even without invasion into adjacent structures. A few studies of large cancer databases have investigated the impact of size.[301–303] Among $T3_{\geq 7}N0$ tumors, the use of preoperative therapy was not associated with significantly better survival; negative prognostic factors were age and a size of >10 cm.[302] For $T3_{\geq 7}N1$ tumors, the best outcomes were seen after a combination of surgical resection and adjuvant chemotherapy; negative prognostic factors by multivariate analysis included a size of >10 cm and the need for pneumonectomy.[303]

Pancoast Tumors

Pancoast tumors are lung cancers that invade the structures of the thoracic inlet (i.e., the first rib, brachial plexus, subclavian vessels, or upper thoracic spine).[295,304] These tumors typically present with shoulder or arm pain; however, pain down the arm or a Horner syndrome is not required to classify a tumor as a Pancoast tumor. The key feature is the involvement of structures in a complex area that raises challenges for local treatment. There is no direct data, but given the treatment challenges it is recommended that imaging for distal metastases and invasive mediastinal staging be done routinely.[295]

The standard treatment is concurrent chemoradiation followed by resection for localized tumors.[295,305] This is based on several phase II studies that have shown better complete resection rates and lower local recurrence when compared with historical series using preoperative RT alone.[295] The chemotherapy regimen typically involves a platinum doublet (e.g., cisplatin, etoposide), and usually 45 Gy of RT is given although some recommend more.[295]

Surgical resection of Pancoast tumors has advanced, with a better understanding of the anatomy of the anterior, middle, and posterior portions of the thoracic inlet, and the advent of different surgical approaches addressing particular problems each situation presents.[304] Furthermore, techniques allowing extended resections have developed. In specialized institutions, resection and reconstruction of subclavian vessels or vertebral bodies can be accomplished safely. The long-term survival of such resections is encouraging (20% to 40%); this is usually combined with pre- or postoperative additional chemotherapy or RT.[306–311] Resection should involve a lobectomy and all involved structures; it is crucial to achieve a complete resection, and surgery should only be undertaken in an institution with the ability to carry out resection of whatever is encountered.

The outcomes of neoadjuvant chemoradiotherapy followed by resection have found an R0 resection rate of ~90% and a pathologic complete response rate of ~50%.[295] The average 5-year survival was approximately 55% (range, 37% to 84%), and the average local recurrence rate was 6%. However, it must be noted that approximately 20% of patients enrolled in these studies dropped out for various reasons, and are not included in the outcomes reported. Approximately one-third of the enrolled patients had T4 tumors, and only a few had N2,3 nodal involvement.[295] In contrast, 5-year survival of patients treated with preoperative RT and resection is ~25%, with about one-third having an incomplete resection and about two-thirds experiencing a local recurrence.

If resection cannot be accomplished, curative intent treatment with chemoradiotherapy should be considered, as suggested by ACCP and NCCN guidelines.[141,295] If palliation is the goal, RT is suggested, which is effective in relieving pain in about 75% of patients.[295]

T4N0,1

Most patients with involvement of T4 structures have involvement of N2,3 nodes; these patients should be treated with chemoradiotherapy just like patients with infiltrative stage IIIa,b (N2,3) NSCLC. However, there are a small number of patients with tumors that are locally invasive but without significant nodal involvement (T4N0,1M0). Surgical techniques have advanced significantly so that T4 structures such as the carina, SVC, aorta, and vertebral column can be resected and reconstructed relatively safely. Resection appears reasonable even when cardiopulmonary bypass is needed: in a review of all reported cases, the perioperative mortality rate was 0% and the 5-year survival was 37%.[312] However, these remain major surgical interventions and should be reserved for specialized centers. Reports from such centers demonstrate perioperative mortality rates of ~10% (lower in more recent reports), with 5-year survival rates of approximately 30%.[295] These long-term outcomes appear to be better than what is reported in series of T4 patients treated with definitive chemoradiotherapy, but this observation must be made with recognition that the resected patients are probably more highly selected.

In patients with cT4N0,1M0 tumors, a careful search for distant metastases and invasive mediastinal staging is suggested.[295] The incidence of occult N2,3 node involvement is not well documented, but many series include a substantial proportion of patients who were found to be pN2. The presence of N2,3 disease is a negative prognostic factor in many (but not all) studies.[295]

The role of preoperative chemotherapy or chemoradiotherapy is not well defined, but limited data suggest it may be of benefit.[313–315] The data generally demonstrate high rates of complete resection and good long-term survival rates after preoperative therapy. While this data cannot disentangle the effect of selection from that of treatment, it does suggest that preoperative therapy should be considered when combined with the more robust data for stage IIIa (N2) patients. demonstrating that preoperative therapy is better than primary surgical resection.[316]

Stage III (N2,3)

Stage III encompasses a large group of patients; discussion of management of these patients is aided by division into several subgroups. Although there are many ways to divide this, we find that the method used by the ACCP is simple and practical, and lends itself to clinical application.[317] We distinguish patients with "incidental N2" disease, meaning there was no reason to suspect N2 involvement preoperatively but it is nevertheless found intra- or postoperatively. The next group is patients with discrete N2,3

node involvement. Such nodes can be individually distinguished and measured, and are suspicious either due to enlargement, PET activity, or because of a central primary tumor or N1 involvement (which correlates with a ~25% chance of occult N2,3 involvement).[110] These patients are distinguished from those with infiltrative stage IIIa,b disease, in which matted nodes or tumor infiltration makes distinction/measurement of individual nodes difficult. This division can be reasonably easily defined clinically and provides a structure for discussion.

Incidental Stage IIIa (N2)

Patients in whom N2 disease is not suspected but nevertheless found post- or intraoperatively are classified as incidental N2.[317,318] It is assumed that appropriate staging for distant or mediastinal nodes has been done. If N2 is discovered intraoperatively in a patient with clinical signs pointing to possible N2 involvement (enlarged or PET-positive N1-3 nodes)—in other words an inadequately preoperatively staged patient—the ACCP suggests it is better to abort the resection and proceed first with appropriate staging.[316] The data and recommendations in the following sections only apply to patients who are incidental N2 despite appropriate preoperative stage evaluation.

Postoperative Chemotherapy. The Non-Small Cell Lung Cancer Collaborative Group[225] conducted a meta-analysis in 1995 evaluating the effect of adjuvant chemotherapy in stage I-IIIa NSCLC, including 14 trials and 4,357 patients. Five trials used alkylating agents, eight used cisplatin combinations, and three used tegafur or tegafur-uracil. There was a significant decrease in survival after treatment with alkylating agents ($p = 0.005$), no change in survival with 5-fluorouracil alone or in combination, and platinum-based chemotherapy produced an improvement in survival of 5% at 5 years ($p = 0.08$). A number of randomized trials conducted in Europe and North America since the 1995 meta-analysis have examined the efficacy of platinum-based chemotherapy after surgery. Three trials showed no significant benefit,[265,319,320] but several others showed improvement in recurrence-free survival or OS.[266,290,321–323] The Lung Adjuvant Cisplatin Evaluation meta-analysis[155] included 4,584 patients treated on the five largest platinum-based adjuvant trials (ALPI, ANITA, BLT, IALT, and JBR-10), and revealed an absolute 5-year OS benefit of 5.4%. Four of the studies included stage III disease; there were a total of 760 patients with N2 lymph nodes. Although there was no improvement in survival in stage I disease, there was a significant survival benefit in patients with stage II and III disease. There appeared to be no difference between vinorelbine, etoposide, vinca alkaloids, or other agents when combined with cisplatin.

Both the ACCP and NCCN guidelines recommend adjuvant chemotherapy for completely resected stage IIIa (N2) disease.[141,316]

Postoperative Radiotherapy. Despite appropriate preoperative staging, at times a patient will undergo surgical resection as primary therapy for presumed stage I or II disease, and mediastinal sampling at the time of surgery will be positive. For select patients, there may be a role for PORT. While the role of adjuvant chemotherapy has been relatively well defined in multiple prospective randomized trials, the indications for and benefit of PORT are subject to debate. Considerations include both the T and N stage, the status of surgical margins, and consideration of the extent and type of surgery. The variability in the extent of both surgical resection and surgical staging, both independent indicators of outcome, presents a challenge to identifying patients who might benefit from adjuvant RT.

A large retrospective SEER analysis[271] included a subset analysis of resected stage III (N2) patients (data on the margin status was not available). In this group, PORT was associated with a significant improvement in OS (27% versus 20% at 5 years). Although this retrospective analysis suffers from a lack of information about patient characteristics, how the treatment approach was selected, or details of the treatment given, it suggested lower toxicity associated with better radiation treatment techniques may have decrease the toxicity of PORT and allowed a survival benefit to emerge. A follow-up SEER study supported that treatment-related morbidity was declining as radiation techniques improved.[324] Specifically, PORT was associated with increased cardiac mortality in patients with stage II or III NSCLC between 1983 and 1988 (HR = 1.49), but not in patients treated between 1989 and 1993 (HR = 1.08; p = not significant). Similarly, a recent work stratified the randomized PORT trials by the use or nonuse of linear accelerators.[325] PORT decreased local recurrence, whether patients were treated with linear accelerators or cobalt machines. There was a survival benefit associated with PORT (an absolute increase of 13% at 5 years) when delivered with linear accelerators, but not when delivered with older cobalt units. These studies support the hypothesis that PORT delivered using modern radiation technology may be associated with a lower risk of treatment-related death than was noted in older, randomized studies, and therefore radiation-related morbidity and mortality is less likely to detract from a potential survival benefit in the modern era.

The ACCP suggests adjuvant RT when the concern about local recurrence is high.[316] The NCCN suggests that adjuvant RT sequentially after adjuvant chemotherapy may be an option, but does not specify further how to make this decision.[141]

Postoperative Chemoradiotherapy. The PORT meta-analysis and the majority of the retrospective and population-based studies of PORT examined patients that were treated before the benefit of adjuvant chemotherapy was established. In the modern era, most patients with N2 disease receive adjuvant cisplatin-based chemotherapy. The additional benefit of PORT in the setting of adjuvant chemotherapy was examined in a post hoc subset analysis of the Adjuvant Navelbine International Trialist Association (ANITA) study.[291] The trial randomized patients with stage IB to IIIA NSCLC to adjuvant cisplatin and vinorelbine, or observation. PORT was recommended, but not required or randomized, for patients with node-positive disease. Out of 840 patients, 232 received PORT. On multivariate analysis, PORT improved survival in patients with N2 disease, in both the chemotherapy and no-chemotherapy arms. Shen et al.[326] conducted a trial in completely resected stage IIIA, N2 NSCLC randomized to paclitaxel and cisplatin with or without RT. There was an improvement in local and distant relapse in the RT group, and in the subgroup of patients with two or more lymph nodes positive, there was an improvement in OS.

Single-arm prospective studies have established the efficacy and safety of PORT with concurrent chemotherapy,[327,328] and several randomized studies have evaluated PORT with or without chemotherapy. The addition of concurrent chemotherapy to PORT, compared to PORT alone, does not appear to improve local control, disease-free survival, or OS.[329–331] A comparison of sequential to concurrent chemotherapy with PORT showed increased toxicity, without an increase in OS, with concurrent therapy.[332] Together, the data suggest that when PORT and chemotherapy are recommended adjuvantly, sequential therapy provides the same benefit as concurrent with less toxicity. For patients at the highest risk of local/regional recurrence (e.g., a positive surgical margin), the value of concurrent therapy can only be extrapolated from studies demonstrating a benefit to concurrent chemoradiotherapy in patients with gross unresectable disease.

Adjuvant chemotherapy for completely resected stage IIIa (N2) disease is not recommended by either the ACCP or NCCN guidelines.[141,316]

Discrete N2 Node Involvement

Discrete N2/N3 involvement defines patients in whom individual mediastinal nodes can be identified and measured on a CT. These nodes may be enlarged on CT or normal sized but suspected by PET uptake or by other characteristics such as a central tumor or N1 node involvement.[316] The terms "resectable" and "unresectable" are specifically avoided because they are notoriously subjective and inaccurate; for example, it is consistently shown that 25% to 35% of stage IIIa (N2) patients who are selected for surgery end up with an incomplete resection.[316,317]

Such patients should undergo invasive mediastinal staging to confirm N2 or N3 involvement (the false-positive rate for discrete node enlargement on CT is ~40%, and for PET positivity it is ~15% to 20%).[110] Furthermore, such patients should undergo a careful evaluation for distant metastases, which are found in about 25% despite a negative clinical evaluation.[110] The subsequent discussion assumes that appropriate staging evaluation has been carried out; it is not acceptable to proceed to resection without thorough invasive mediastinal staging or imaging for distant metastases in patients in whom there is reasonable suspicion of N2 node involvement.[110,317] The results reported in this chapter do not apply to patients that are mismanaged (i.e., in whom clinical standards for stage evaluation prior to treatment have been ignored).

In evaluating treatment approaches for patients with discrete N2 involvement, it is best to focus on RCTs or on intent-to-treat analyses. However, the literature is replete with reported outcomes of particular cohorts of patients; these cohorts are often selected by characteristics that can only be defined in retrospect. While these studies provide data on these specific cohorts, it must be recognized that the outcomes represent not only a treatment effect but probably most predominantly the effect of selection. A common mistake is to attribute the outcomes entirely to the treatment and forget that the effect of treatment cannot be disentangled from that of selection. Another common mistake is to assume that the outcomes of patients who complete a treatment approach apply to all patients who start on this approach. The extent of attrition and its effect on outcomes is perhaps best illustrated in a comprehensive analysis of 402 preoperatively identified patients with N2 involvement who were selected for preoperative chemotherapy with planned subsequent surgery (Fig. 41.11).[333] While the 5-year survival of the patients who completed the planned approach was ~50%, this represented only about one-quarter of the original group; the 5-year survival of all patients selected for the treatment plan was only 13%. Finally, it must be emphasized that selection of a treatment approach must be based on factors that can be identified as pretreatment; the outcomes of patients according to factors that are available only in retrospect are useless to identify how to select patients for treatment.

Several RCTs have compared initial surgical resection for proven N2 versus preoperative chemotherapy.[316] These have generally found better survival in patients given preoperative therapy (average 2-year survival 40% versus 29%, 5-year survival 24% versus 17%).[316] However, most of these studies were underpowered and did not show a statistically significant difference. A 2007 Cochrane meta-analysis of stage III patients found a trend to better survival for preoperative platinum-based chemotherapy versus surgery alone (HR = 0.73; 95% confidence interval = 0.51 to 1.07; p = 0.1).[334]

Some groups have advocated that initial surgical resection is appropriate for some patients with N2 involvement. This argument is generally made citing good outcomes for cN0,1 patients with incidental N2 after resection[335]—this is not applicable to patients with N2 disease confirmed or suspected preoperatively. A few centers have published their results of preoperatively confirmed N2 patients that were selected for primary surgery: the average 5-year survival for all patients selected was 13%.[316,336–338]

In summary, the data suggests that selection of patients with good outcomes after primary surgery has not been demonstrated, and limited data suggests that outcomes are better after preoperative therapy. Neither the ACCP nor the NCCN guidelines recommend primary surgery for confirmed N2 involvement.[141,316]

However, it must be recognized that some of the data is relatively old. Techniques of mediastinal evaluation have progressed, at least in some institutions. The results of a microscopic deposit of cancer in an N2 node identified via video-assisted mediastinal

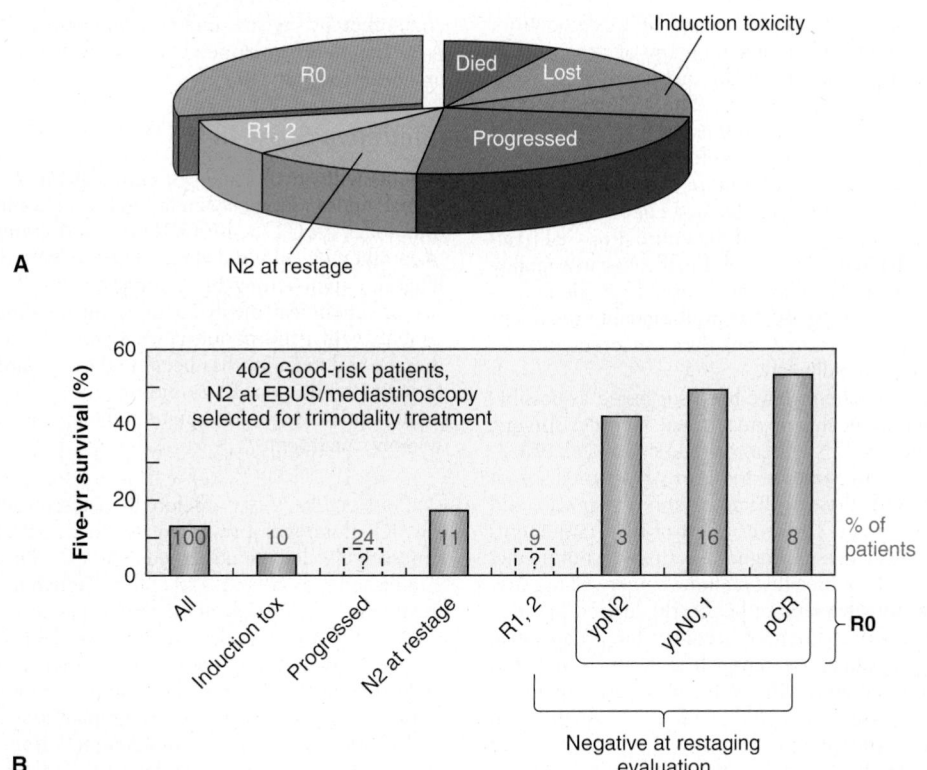

Figure 41.11 Fate of stage IIIa(N2) patients selected for neoadjuvant therapy and resection. Analysis of the fate of 402 good-risk patients, identified as having histologically proven but limited N2 involvement, who were selected as good candidates for preoperative chemotherapy followed by planned subsequent surgery. **(A)** Fate of all patients selected for this treatment approach. **(B)** Five-year survival of subgroups of patients based on subsequent outcomes and events during the planned treatment. EBUS, endobronchial ultrasound. (Data taken from Cerfolio RJ, Maniscalco L, Bryant AS. The treatment of patients with stage IIIA non-small cell lung cancer from N2 disease: who returns to the surgical arena and who survives. *Ann Thorac Surg* 2008;86:912–920.)

lymphadenectomy may not be the same as that derived from older literature. Furthermore, there appear to be regional differences, with survival being better for cN2 patients in Asia than North America or Europe.[157] However, no studies have defined how these factors can lead to appropriate selection of patients for primary surgery.

Several RCTs have compared preoperative therapy followed by surgery versus chemoradiotherapy alone.[316,339–342] These have found no significant difference, even in adequately powered studies, between these approaches, although arguably one can interpret there might be a slight trend to better survival in the surgical arms. In one larger study, a suggestion of better outcomes after treatment was completed was offset by higher treatment-related mortality in the surgical arm, particularly after pneumonectomy (Fig. 41.12).[339] However, the perioperative mortality in this study appears to have been significantly higher than in other studies.[343]

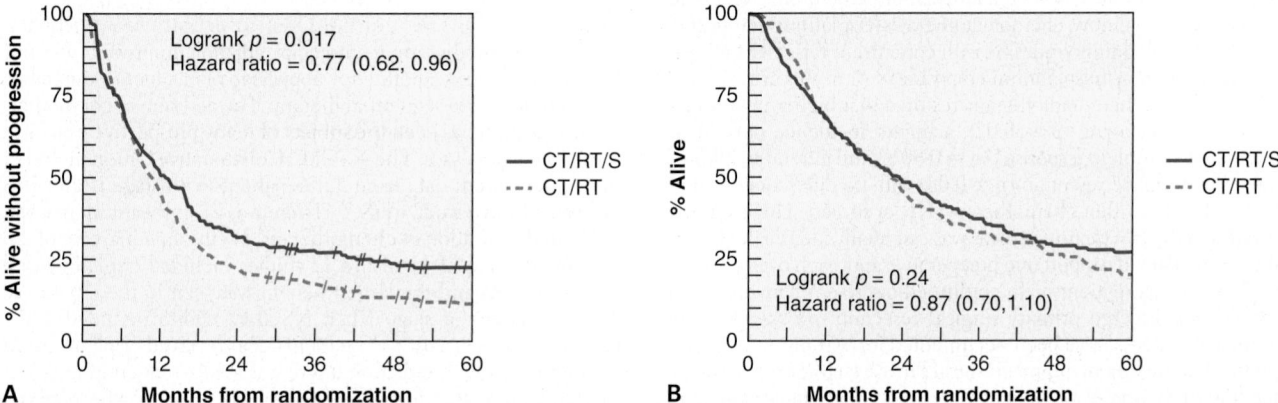

Figure 41.12 Trimodality versus bimodality treatment of stage IIIa(N2) lung cancer. Survival of patients with stage IIIA (N2) non–small-cell lung cancer treated with trimodality (CT/RT/S) versus bimodality (CT/RT) therapy from the North American Intergroup Study 0139. The initial steeper slope of the trimodality arm demonstrates the importance of the perioperative mortality rate on the overall results of trimodality therapy. **(A)** Progreesion-free survival. **(B)** Overall survival. CT/RT/S, chemotherapy and radiotherapy followed by surgery; CT/RT, chemotherapy and radiotherapy. (Reproduced with permission from Albain KS, Swann RS, Rusch VW, et al. Radiotherapy plus chemotherapy with or without surgical resection for stage III non-small-cell lung cancer: a phase III randomised controlled trial. *Lancet* 2009;374:379–386.)

Reflecting these results, both the ACCP and NCCN guidelines suggest that either definitive chemoradiotherapy or preoperative therapy followed by surgery are reasonable treatment options for patients with confirmed N2 disease.[141,316] The NCCN does not suggest how one might choose between these; the ACCP suggests that, given similar outcomes, patient preferences should factor significantly in the decision.[316] Furthermore, the ACCP suggests that the treatment strategy should be decided collectively by the multidisciplinary team of providers, and the entire proposed treatment plan should be defined at the outset. Finally, because quality of care aspects appear to play a significant role (e.g., perioperative mortality), the ACCP suggests that multimodality treatment be done at experienced centers that track their outcomes and can keep treatment-related morbidity low.

Various subgroups of patients have been suggested as possibly benefiting from a multimodality approach that includes surgery, such as those with "minimal" N2 disease, single station N2, cN0,1, younger, good surgical risk patients, those in whom mediastinal downstaging is achieved, those with radiographic response, and those requiring a lobectomy. However, most of these arguments are flawed, based on evidence of prognostic value but not predictive value for a treatment regimen that includes surgery, or because they are based on factors that cannot be clearly defined pretreatment. The best data for selection of a cohort for preoperative therapy with surgery is patients needing a lobectomy (as opposed to a pneumonectomy), although this is based on an unplanned matched-subgroup analysis in the study with an unusually high perioperative mortality after pneumonectomy.[339]

Response to preoperative therapy is often cited as a way to select patients who will benefit from resection. While this is prognostic (responders do better), there is no data that demonstrates that the better prognosis is affected whether resection is undertaken or not.[316] Furthermore, arguments that outcomes are poor in those who are not downstaged are confounded because most of the nondownstaged patients are not resected. Those that are resected despite ypN2 involvement have a 5-year survival of about 15%.[316] Finally, radiographic response by CT is notoriously inaccurate to define downstaging, and invasive methods other than a first-time mediastinoscopy are associated with high false-negative rates.[344] The data regarding survival of downstaged patients relates to the postoperative stage. Therefore, the ACCP concludes that identification of patients that are more likely to benefit from surgical resection is not possible at this time based on pretreatment characteristics.

There is also debate about the choice of preoperative therapy (chemotherapy versus chemoradiotherapy). The NCCN suggests either approach is acceptable; the ACCP does not address this issue.[141,316] This has been addressed directly in one RCT that compared preoperative chemoradiotherapy (cisplatinum/etoposide × 3, then cisplatinum/vindesine with concurrent RT of 45 Gy) versus chemotherapy (cisplatinum/etoposide × 3; in this arm, PORT was given).[345] Chemoradiotherapy resulted in a higher rate of mediastinal downstaging ($p = 0.02$), a higher incidence of a "near pathologic complete response" ($p = 0.001$), and a trend to a lower rate of incomplete resection ($p = 0.08$) with no difference in mortality related to either chemotherapy, RT, or surgery. However, the survival of the two treatment arms was essentially identical. Hence, there is no data to support one preoperative approach over another.

In summary, patients with confirmed discrete N2 involvement should not undergo primary surgical resection; no specific subgroups of patients have been documented for whom this is appropriate. The treatment approach should involve either preoperative therapy and surgery or definitive chemoradiotherapy. The outcomes of these two strategies appear to be similar, and factors such a patient preferences as well as local expertise and minimization of morbidity and mortality should play a major role in deciding upon a treatment approach. Definition of subgroups that are more likely to benefit from the inclusion of surgery is not possible from the available data; there is also no difference between preoperative

chemotherapy versus chemoradiotherapy. The treatment approach should be planned collaboratively with involvement of all of the relevant disciplines.

Infiltrative Stage III a,b

Patients with involvement of contralateral or multistation mediastinal nodes, supraclavicular nodes, or multiple clinically visible nodes on CT or PET/CT are most commonly treated with chemotherapy and radiation. This reflects not only the challenges in approaching these surgically, but the inherently higher risk of subclinical involvement of surrounding regional sites. In patients with good performance status (PS), concurrent chemotherapy and radiation has become the standard of care approach. In patients with poor PS or limiting medical comorbidities, therapeutic options include sequential therapy, RT alone, or palliative systemic treatment.

Radiotherapy Alone.
Before the widespread use of chemotherapy, RT alone was a standard treatment option for patients with unresectable, locally advanced NSCLC. The RTOG 7301 trial established the optimal dose and fractionation for single-modality treatment.[346] This study of inoperable patients randomized 375 patients to 40 Gy in 4 weeks, a split course of 40 Gy in 6 weeks, 50 Gy in 5 weeks, or 60 Gy in 6 weeks. The response rate was significantly better in the 60 Gy arm (63%), and there was parallel trend in improved OS (22% at 3 years in the high-dose arm).

In patients getting fractionated RT alone, altered fractionation and radiation dose escalation have been investigated in an effort to improve the relatively poor response and survival that is seen after standard 60 Gy. A dose escalation study conducted at the University of Michigan included 106 patients with stage I to III NSCLC, using doses from 63 to 103 Gy in daily fractions.[347] Patients were allocated to dose based on the tumor volume and risk of pneumonitis, so no optimal dose was identified, but higher dose was associated with improved control and survival. The RTOG 8311 included 840 patients in a dose escalation trial, from 60 Gy to 79.2 Gy delivered in twice-daily 1.2 Gy fractions.[348] The best OS, 29% at 2 years, was associated with 69.6 Gy twice daily. Similarly, the European Organisation for Research and Treatment of Cancer conducted a randomized phase II/III study of standard RT (60 Gy in 6 weeks) versus continuous hyperfractionated accelerated RT (CHART).[349] CHART is given in 1.5 Gy fractions, three times daily, 7 days per week, to a total dose of 54 Gy. The use of CHART was associated with improved OS (20% versus 13%), but also a higher rate of severe acute dysphagia (49% versus 19%).

Concurrent and Sequential Chemoradiotherapy.
The addition of chemotherapy to thoracic radiation improves OS, and concurrent chemoradiotherapy appears to offer superior outcomes when compared to sequential therapy. The addition of chemotherapy to radiation has been the subject of many prospective trials and several meta-analyses. The NSCLC Collaborative Group included individual patient data from 3,033 patients with stage IIIa or IIIb disease, enrolled in 22 trials.[225] There was a significant increase in OS with the addition of chemotherapy, an absolute increase of 2% at years. At total of 11 of the 22 studies included cisplatin-based chemotherapy, and the largest benefit was seen in these patients. A meta-analysis of stage IIIa,b NSCLC studies included 1,887 patients from 14 trials.[350] In patients who received cisplatin-based chemotherapy with radiation, there was a 30% reduction in 2-year mortality compared to radiation alone. In patients who received other chemotherapy, there was an 18% reduction. The preference for cisplatin-based chemotherapy was confirmed in a more recent meta-analysis, which was limited to studies that combined radiation with either cisplatin- or carboplatin-based chemotherapy.[351] They analyzed 1,764 patients from nine trials, and found an absolute improvement in OS of 4% at 2 years.

The use of concurrent, rather than sequential, chemotherapy with thoracic RT appears to improve OS, at the cost of increased acute toxicity. The RTOG 9410 was a three-arm trial: cisplatin and vindesine followed by RT (63 Gy once daily), cisplatin and vindesine with concurrent RT (63 Gy once daily), or cisplatin and etoposide concurrently with RT (69.6 Gy twice daily).[352] The median OS was significantly better in the concurrent arm with daily radiation, compared to sequential therapy (17 months versus 14.6 months), as was local control (66% versus 59%). Acute grade ≥3 toxicity was similarly higher with concurrent therapy; 48% versus 30% nonhematologic. Serious late toxicity was significantly different. The survival in the concurrent chemotherapy and twice-daily RT arm was 15.6 months, not significantly better than the control arm. This was confirmed in a trial by the West Japan Lung Cancer Group, in which patients were randomized to receive either sequential or concurrent chemotherapy.[353] The chemotherapy was cisplatin, mitomycin, and vindesine in both arms. Sequential RT was 56 Gy in 5.5 weeks; the concurrent RT was 56 Gy in 7.5 weeks with a 2-week break midcourse. The median survival was better in the concurrent arm (17 months versus 13 months). There was no difference in esophageal toxicity.

Cisplatin- and carboplatin-based are the most common chemotherapy combinations delivered concurrently with thoracic radiation, extrapolated from the superiority of such combinations in the meta-analyses of sequential treatment. The best specific combination has not yet been clearly defined. In a three-arm noninferiority trial conducted by the West Japan Lung Cancer Group, the use of concurrent weekly carboplatin (40 mg/m^2) and paclitaxel (area under the curve = 2) (CP) had comparable survival to mitomycin, vindesine, and cisplatin, and to irinotecan and carboplatin, with lower toxicity.[354] A small randomized study compared weekly carboplatin (45 mg/m^2 and area under the curve = 2, respectively) to cisplatin and etoposide (CE) delivered every 3 weeks (cisplatin 50 mg/m^2 on day 1, etoposide 50 mg/m^2 on days 1 to 5).[355] Both arms received concurrent thoracic RT to 60 Gy. The survival was superior in the CE arm (33% versus 13%). Neutropenia was more common with CE, and RP more common with carboplatin. A larger, phase 2/3 randomized study from the Chinese Academy of Medical Sciences (NCT01494558) comparing carboplatin to CE has completed enrollment and may answer this question. The use of pemetrexed in combination with platinum compounds is equally effective, and less toxic, than other combinations in patients with nonsquamous histology. The use of this combination, carboplatin (area under the curve = 5) and pemetrexed (500 mg/m^2) with thoracic RT (70 Gy), has been shown to be both safe and effective in a phase 2 study from the CALGB.[356] A large international randomized study comparing pemetrexed and cisplatin to etoposide and cisplatin with RT has been conducted but not yet reported. Attempts have been made to add targeted agents to standard chemoradiotherapy platforms in the setting of stage III disease, in an effort incorporate chemo- and radiosensitizing agents. The addition of antiangiogenics has not improved outcomes: a randomized trial adding antiangiogenic AE-941 to carboplatin and radiation failed to show an improvement in OS.[357] Similarly, a randomized trial conducted by the Eastern Cooperative Oncology Group added thalidomide to concurrent or sequential chemoradiation did not show any benefit. Bevacizumab, the monoclonal antibody to the vascular endothelial growth factor receptor has been added to chemoradiation in a phase 2 study that also incorporated an EGFR TKI and escalated radiation dose.[212] There was no improvement over standard therapy. Several phase 2 studies have incorporated the monoclonal EGFR antibody cetuximab. A randomized phase 2 study, the CALGB 30407,[356] suggested no benefit. Consistent with this, a phase 3 trial, the RTOG 0617, randomized patients getting carboplatin and thoracic RT to the addition of cetuximab. The preliminary results suggest no incremental benefit. The addition of EGFR TKIs to chemoradiation in unselected patients has been similarly disappointing; the Southwest Oncology Group S0023 randomized patients with stage III NSCLC to gefitinib or placebo after CE and RT.[358] OS was worse with gefitinib. Effort to incorporate TKIs into the treatment of stage III patients, in selected patients based on molecular profiling, are ongoing.

Induction or Adjuvant Chemotherapy with Chemoradiation. The role of adjuvant chemotherapy after definitive concurrent chemoradiation is not entirely defined and is likely dependent on the choice of concurrent systemic therapy. There are no published, randomized trials that support this specific approach with high-level evidence. The phase 3 Hoosier Oncology Group study enrolled patients receiving concurrent radiation and CE randomized to three cycles of docetaxel versus no further therapy.[359] Enrollment stopped when futility analysis determined that there would be no chance of observing a benefit; the median survival was 21.2 months after adjuvant chemotherapy and 23.3 months for observation. The continued interest in adjuvant therapy likely stems from the desire to administer more than two cycles of full-dose chemotherapy in the setting of stage III disease, consistent with that given adjuvantly after surgery. This is relevant for concurrent regimens that include two cycles of concurrent chemotherapy, but of particular interest when the concurrent regimen is weekly carboplatin, as opposed to combinations that can be delivered concurrently with radiation at full systemic dose, such as cisplatin and etoposide or cisplatin and vinorelbine.

In the induction setting, the CALGB 39081 randomized patients to two cycles of carboplatin followed by RT and weekly carboplatin, or immediate treatment with RT and weekly carboplatin.[360] In 366 enrolled patients, survival was not improved by the addition of two cycles of carboplatin before concurrent therapy. Induction therapy is not routinely employed before definitive chemoradiation but instead reserved for those patients where circumstances or disease volume precludes immediate chemoradiation.

Radiation Dose and Fractionation for Concurrent Treatment. The RTOG 7301 established 60 Gy in 6 weeks as the standard radiation for single modality therapy, and this regimen was adopted as one possible standard when combined with sequential or concurrent chemoradiotherapy. But the risk of local, in-field relapse among patients receiving definitive chemoradiation is high, between 30% and 50% depending on the length and manner of follow-up. A number of radiation dose escalation trials suggest that increasing radiation dose may improve local control and can be accomplished in at least a subset of patients. The RTOG 9311 was the first large dose escalation trial conduced with three-dimensional conformal radiation techniques. In an effort to increase the dose to the gross tumor and involved nodes, nodal regions without confirmed macroscopic or microscopic disease were not electively included. Either radiation alone or sequential chemoradiation were allowed.[327] For each patient, the lung V20 was calculated, and the maximum dose cohort was based on their predicted risk of pneumonitis. Patients were treated from 70.9 Gy to 90.3 Gy in daily 2.15-Gy fractions. Dose escalation was well tolerated up to 83.8 Gy in the lowest-risk group and 77.4 Gy in the intermediate-risk group. The follow-up study, the RTOG 0117, escalated dose in the setting of concurrent cisplatin and docetaxel.[361] The study started at 75.25 Gy in 2.15 Gy fractions and was designed to escalate by increasing the dose per fraction (and decreasing the overall treatment duration). After excess toxicity was observed at the starting dose, dose de-escalation was done, reducing to 74 Gy in 2-Gy fractions. A total of 55 patients were treated at this dose, with a median survival of 21.6 months for stage III patients. A similar, small dose escalation study in 15 stage III patients receiving weekly chemotherapy also concluded that the maximum tolerated dose was 74 Gy in two fractions[362]; the median survival was 37 months.

A series of prospective studies conducted at the University of North Carolina also evaluated escalating radiation dose from 60 Gy to 74 Gy in 2-Gy fractions, with an expansion at 74 Gy. Patients received induction and concurrent carboplatin.[363] With a median follow-up of 5 years for 62 patients, the OS at 5 years was 27%. A follow-up phase 2 study with chemoradiation to 74 Gy and erlotinib included 48 patients. The median survival was 18 months, with a 29% rate of grade 3 or 4 toxicity. The CALGB 30105 was a randomized phase 2 study that also incorporated 74 Gy into two different induction and concurrent chemotherapy schedules. The median survival was 24 months in 69 patients in the superior chemotherapy arm.[364]

Finally, the RTOG 0617 sought to determine the absolute benefit of 74 Gy, versus standard 60 Gy, with concurrent weekly carboplatin. This was a two-by-two factorial design, where patients were randomized to standard or high dose, and to standard chemotherapy or chemotherapy and cetuximab concurrently with radiation. The 74-Gy arm was closed early when futility analysis determined that there would be no benefit over 60 Gy. The result of this randomization was presented; high-dose radiation was associated with worse OS compared to standard radiation (median survival 19.5 months versus 28.7 months). There were more treatment-related deaths in the high dose arm, and a higher rate of grade 3 or greater esophagitis. Oddly, local control was worse in the high-dose arm.[365]

Altered Fractionation with Chemotherapy.

The use of standard, daily radiation fractionation is designed to balance the delivery of definitive dose to the tumor, while allowing daily repair of the surrounding normal tissue. Altered fractionation schedules take advantage of radiobiologic principles: hyperfractionation (increased number of fractions) should result in increased opportunity for normal tissue repair and a lower risk of late side effects. Accelerated radiation (shorter treatment duration) should improve local control by allowing less tumor repopulation. Hypofractionation (higher dose per fraction) is one method to achieve acceleration, typically at the cost of increased acute toxicity. SBRT is extreme hypofractionation, combined with precision targeting to reduce exposure of normal tissue. Because both hypofractionation and accelerated hyperfractionation may increase the acute side effects of radiation therapy, combining these regimens with concurrent radiosensitizing chemotherapy remains investigational.

The RTOG 9410 was a three-arm randomized trial: sequential chemoradiotherapy with 60 Gy once daily, concurrent chemoradiotherapy with 60 Gy once daily, and concurrent chemotherapy with 69.6 Gy twice daily (hyperfractionation). While the addition of concurrent chemotherapy improved survival, the hyperfractionated radiation arm was no better than daily treatment.[352] Schild et al.[366] conducted a similar phase 3 trial, comparing concurrent CE with either daily RT to 60 Gy, or twice daily RT to 60 Gy in 6 weeks. There was no difference in local control or OS.

The use of CHART improved OS when compared to daily treatment, when radiation was the sole modality, but the advantage of hyperfractionation with concurrent chemotherapy has not been similarly demonstrated. The Eastern Cooperative Oncology Group 2597 examined hyperfractionated accelerated radiation therapy with sequential chemotherapy. Patients were randomized after two cycles of carboplatin to daily radiation (64 Gy in 32 fractions) versus hyperfractionated accelerated radiation therapy (57.6 Gy three times daily over 2.5 weeks).[367] The study was closed early, partially because of the difficult logistic of three times daily treatment. Overall, 141 patients were randomized, and there was no significant difference in median survival (20.3 months versus 14.9 months favoring hyperfractionated accelerated radiation therapy).

The European Organisation for Research and Treatment of Cancer tested the use of hypofractionated RT in inoperable NSCLC.[368] Overall, 158 patients were randomized to either gemcitabine and cisplatin before RT, or low-dose daily cisplatin (6 mg/m^2) concurrent with RT. The radiation was delivered in 24 fractions of 2.75 Gy in 32 days (total 66 Gy). The combination of sequential or concurrent chemotherapy with hypofractionated radiation was well tolerated, with grade 3 esophagitis in 14% of patients in the concurrent arm. Similarly, a phase 2 trial in

49 patients with stage III disease used 60 Gy in 5 weeks with carboplatin, with a median survival of 28 months[369]; 29 of 49 patients had grade 2 or greater toxicity, and two patients died of bleeding complications.

Choice of Chemotherapy.

In the setting of stage III disease, either prior to surgical intervention (neoadjuvant therapy), or when used concurrently with RT (combined modality therapy), cisplatin-based combinations are preferred. Combinations with etoposide, vinorelbine, paclitaxel, docetaxel, and pemetrexed have all been tested in this setting. Gemcitabine is generally avoided in this context due to its potent radiosensitizing properties and potential severe complications.[370] However, unlike in adjuvant therapy, the use of carboplatin in the context of combined modality therapy for stage III disease is better documented. In particular, the use of carboplatin, administered on a weekly schedule and administered concurrently with standard thoracic RT, yielded roughly the same survival results as trials using cisplatin-based combinations.[365] In stage III disease, neither induction nor consolidation chemotherapy appears to add to concurrent treatment.[359,371] However, practitioners in the United States have been reluctant to limit treatment to two cycles of chemotherapy and tend to recommend an additional two cycles for total of four cycles.

Stage IV

Selection for Treatment

Patients with advanced NSCLC are often symptomatic and require prompt intervention. A "watch and wait" approach is generally not recommended.[372] A few selected patients who are asymptomatic at the time of the diagnosis and wish to forgo immediate treatment must be followed closely by clinical and radiographic criteria. In some circumstances, it is appropriate to administer local therapy prior to systemic therapy, such as symptomatic central nervous system disease, cord compression, painful skeletal metastases, or uncontrolled hemoptysis (discussed in more detail in the section "Specific Symptom Management"). However, chemotherapy is also an effective palliative tool and individualized judgment is recommended.

Chemotherapy is the mainstay of treatment for patients who present with stage IV disease at diagnosis or who experience recurrent disease that is not amenable to local therapy. In the 1990s and early 2000s, multiple RCTs clearly established that treatment of patients with stage IV NSCLC and good PS prolongs survival compared with basic supportive care alone.[373,374] Because this question is considered to have been clearly answered, further trials addressing this have not been conducted in the last decade.

Patients are frequently more focused on QOL and express concern that treatment with chemotherapy will negatively impact this. Multiple RCTs have evaluated this and consistently shown that treatment with chemotherapy improves QOL compared to best supportive care in good PS patients.[373,374] Chemotherapy for stage IV NSCLC is given as an outpatient; significant toxicity (grade ≥3) is uncommon. Nevertheless, QOL continues to be an important end point in studies comparing one regimen to another.

Therefore, both the ACCP and NCCN guidelines recommend that patients with stage IV NSCLC and a PS of 0,1 be treated with chemotherapy (based on level 1 evidence or a unanimous consensus, respectively).[141,374] Patients with a PS of 2 may also benefit from chemotherapy, and this is recommended by the ACCP and NCCN guidelines, but in a nuanced fashion. This patient population is addressed specifically in a subsequent section.

Recent studies have demonstrated a median survival of approximately 10 to 12 months for patients with nonsquamous histology, and 9 to 10 months for squamous carcinoma (Table 41.6).[375] The respective 1-year survival rates are 20% to 25% and 15% to 20%. These estimates are lower for patients with PS 2, regardless

TABLE 41.6

Efficacy of Chemotherapy in Advanced Non–Small-Cell Lung Cancer[a]

	ORR	PFS	MST	1-y OS
Nonsquamous				
Doublet	15%–25%	4 mo	8–10 mo	40%
Doublet + bevacizumab	25%–35%	5–6 mo	10–12mo	50%
Doublet + maintenance		5–6 mo	12–14 mo	55%–60%
Squamous				
Doublet	15%–25%	4 mo	8–10 mo	35%

ORR, objective response rate; PFS, progression-free survival; MST, median survival time; OS overall survival.
[a] Results apply to patients with performance status 0-1 and wild-type tumors.

of histology.[376] Patients with sensitizing mutations treated with targeted therapy have a more favorable outcome, as detailed in the following.

First-Line Therapy

The approach is based on the patient's histologic subtype and PS (Fig. 41.13). Patients with nonsquamous histology, regardless of PS, should have the tumor submitted for molecular analysis and, in the presence of an actionable mutation, be treated with the appropriate targeted agent. For patients with nonsquamous cancers without a mutation and for patients with squamous histology, combination chemotherapy is the standard of care for patients with PS 0-1.[141,374] Platinum-based regimens are the standard. An extensive literature has attempted to determine the "optimal platinum

analog," cisplatin or carboplatin, in advanced disease. There is a general consensus that while cisplatin may be slightly more active, particularly with respect to response rate, the impact on OS is minimal, if any, and toxicity, especially nonhematologic, is worse.[377] Carboplatin tends to be widely used in the United States, while cisplatin is still frequently utilized in Europe and Latin America. Agents that are typically combined with a platinum analog include pemetrexed (except in squamous carcinoma), paclitaxel, docetaxel, nab-paclitaxel, gemcitabine, vinorelbine, irinotecan, and etoposide (see Table 41.6). Studies have failed to demonstrate superiority of one regimen over another, and decisions regarding which agent to use are based on the toxicity profile, ease and convenience of administration, and cost.[378]

The choice of regimens tends to differ between the histologic types. Pemetrexed has no efficacy in squamous cell carcinomas and should not be used in these patients.[379] Bevacizumab, an antiangiogenesis inhibitor, has a high rate of bleeding complications in squamous cell carcinomas and should not be used in these patients.[156,380] The addition of a third cytotoxic agent does not improve outcomes and is not recommended.[381] The use of non-platinum doublets in first-line therapy is not encouraged but may be an alternative to occasional patients who have contraindications to both platinum analogs.[382]

The general standard is to administer four to six cycles of chemotherapy unless progression or toxicity prevents this.[141,374] This is administered either alone or in combination with a biologic agent (bevacizumab). The biologic agent is typically continued until disease progression (see subsequent section). In addition, administration of maintenance chemotherapy should be considered (also as discussed in a later section).

PS 2 patients have a poorer prognosis and tend to benefit less from chemotherapy.[383] However, new data have demonstrated a survival benefit for combination chemotherapy over single agent in patients with PS 2 despite higher toxicity rates.[384] This trial demonstrated a significant improvement in survival for carboplatin and pemetrexed compared to pemetrexed alone. Benefits with respect

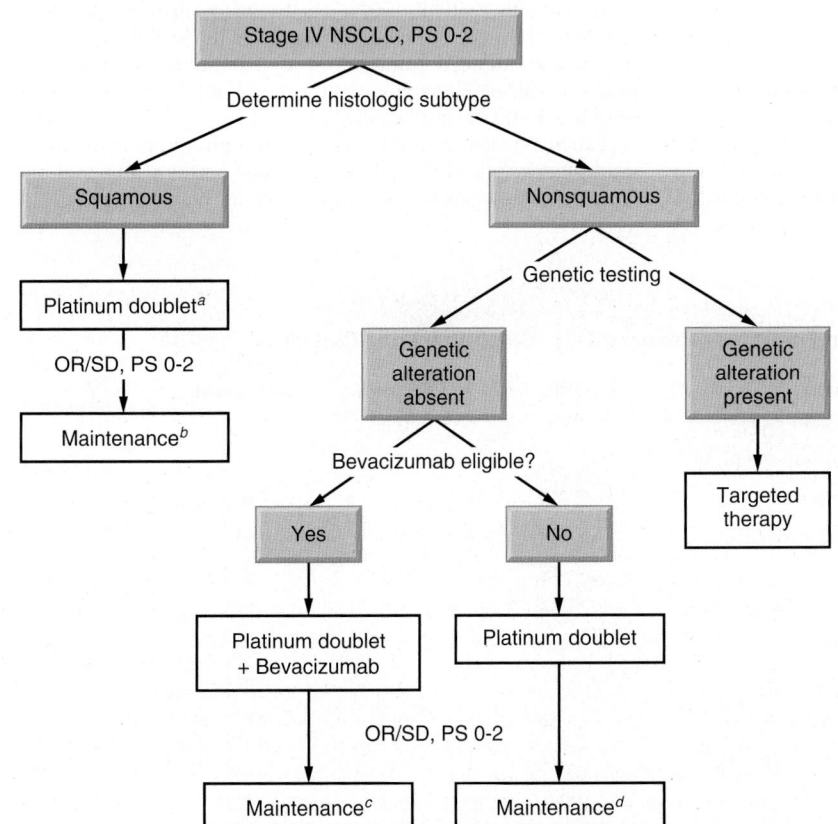

Figure 41.13 Algorithm for first-line chemotherapy management of patients with stage IV non–small-cell lung cancer (NSCLC). OR, objective response; SD, stable disease; PS, performance status.
[a] Avoid Pemetrexed
[b] Switch maintenance with Erlotinib
[c] Bevacizumab maintenance or Pemetrexed maintenance (either switch or continuation) or switch maintenance with Erlotinib
[d] Pemetrexed maintenance (either switch or continuation) or switch maintenance with Erlotinib

PRACTICE OF ONCOLOGY

to symptom reduction and QOL have also been reported in PS 2 patients.[385] Patients with PS 3 or lower are typically not candidates for chemotherapy.

Age alone is not a restriction to chemotherapy. In the past, patients aged ≥70 years were felt to be at high risk for complications and many were treated with single-agent therapy or denied active treatment altogether.[386] A robust literature published in the past decade has demonstrated that elderly patients benefit from standard combination chemotherapy compared to single agent, including a pivotal clinical trial in which the combination of carboplatin, administered weekly, was superior to single-agent therapy.[387] Toxicity, as in PS 2 patients, tends to be more severe. Carboplatin is easier to tolerate, and the use of cisplatin is discouraged in these patients. Octogenarians have been poorly represented in clinical trials, and caution is advised when applying these data to this age subset.[388]

Monoclonal Antibodies

Guidelines recommend the addition of bevacizumab, a monoclonal antibody directed against the vascular endothelial growth factor ligand, in addition to combination chemotherapy.[141,374] Bevacizumab should be continued until disease progression. This is based largely on a US RCT in which bevacizumab in combination with carboplatin led to a significant improvement in survival in patients with nonsquamous cell histology with PS 0-1.[156] However, toxicity in general and treatment-related deaths in particular were significantly higher in the bevacizumab arm, including rates of pulmonary hemorrhage, thromboembolic phenomena, and neutropenia and thrombocytopenia. A similar study conducted in Europe, using two different doses of bevacizumab in combination with cisplatin and gemcitabine, showed a significant improvement in PFS (the primary end point) but not in OS.[389]

A recent study (Pointbreak trial) compared the two most frequently used bevacizumab-containing regimens: the original carboplatin-paclitaxel-bevacizumab versus carboplatin-pemetrexed-bevacizumab developed by investigators in Chicago.[390] Both combinations were administered for four cycles followed by maintenance bevacizumab alone in the paclitaxel arm, and both pemetrexed and bevacizumab in the other arm. There was no significant difference in survival. Toxicity, while slightly different between the arms, did not seem statistically different.

These data demonstrate that bevacizumab can be used in eligible patients with advanced NSCLC in combination with chemotherapy. The benefit is modest, and toxicity can be significant. Patients with squamous cell carcinoma and hemoptysis should not receive bevacizumab, while patients on anticoagulation and with previously treated brain metastases are eligible.[391] Patients with PS 2 do not typically receive bevacizumab.

Cetuximab, a monoclonal antibody directed against the EGFR, also demonstrated a significant improvement in survival when added to cisplatin and vinorelbine in a single randomized trial.[392] However, the clinical significance of the results has been questioned and, along with other negative trials in the first- and second-line setting,[393,394] has not led to the approval of cetuximab in NSCLC. The ACCP guidelines do not recommend the addition of cetuximab to standard chemotherapy, but the NCCN guidelines suggest this is an option.[141,374] Preliminary results of a new monoclonal antibody, necitumumab, have been positive in patients with squamous cell histology, while negative in patients with adenocarcinoma.

First-Line Therapy with Targeted Agents

For patients whose tumors harbor an actionable molecular alteration, in particular EGFR-sensitizing mutations and anaplastic lymphoma kinase (ALK) rearrangement, first-line therapy with the corresponding targeted agent should be considered. Several trials have demonstrated that in patients with EGFR-mutated cancers, gefitinib, erlotinib, or afatinib yield superior response rates and longer PFS compared to standard chemotherapy, with a more favorable toxicity profile (Table 41.7).[395–399] Similarly, in patients with ALK-rearranged tumors, RCTs have confirmed the superiority of crizotinib over conventional chemotherapy.[400] However, none of the trials demonstrated a significant improvement in OS for the targeted agent compared to chemotherapy. Although this is often attributed to crossover upon progression, other explanations such as acquired resistance may also play a role.

Other trials have tested whether a combination of chemotherapy and a targeted agent is superior to either chemotherapy or the targeted agent alone in patients selected based on clinical characteristics without mutational testing.[401,402] None of these trials has demonstrated an advantage over the targeted agent, and the concurrent administration of chemotherapy and a TKI in first-line therapy is not recommended.

Importantly, patients without a known molecular alteration should not be treated with targeted agents in the first-line setting.[403] In patients who need immediate treatment and whose molecular profile is still pending, chemotherapy upfront is the best option until the results become available.

Patients treated with a targeted agent upfront are maintained until progression. At that point, depending on the nature and the tempo of the progression, options include local/ablative therapy to

---

TABLE 41.7

Chemotherapy Versus Targeted Therapy in First-Line Advanced Non–Small-Cell Lung Cancer

Target	Trial	N	Regimen	ORR (%)	PFS (mo)	MST (mo)	P
EGFR	NEJSG	228	Gefitinib	74	10.8	30.5	<0.001
			Carboplatin-paclitaxel	31	5.4	23.6	
	WJTOG	177	Gefitinib	62	9.2	36	<0.0001
			Cisplatin-docetaxel	32	6.3	39	
	Optimal	154	Erlotinib	83	13.1	22.7	<0.0001
			Carboplatin-gemcitibine	36	4.6	28.9	
	EURTAC		Erlotinib		9.7	19.3	
			Chemotherapy		5.2	19.5	
ALK	LUX Lung 3	345	Afatinib	56	6.9		0.001
			Cisplatin-pemetrexed	23	11.1		

ORR, objective response rate; PFS, progression-free survival; MST, median survival time; EGFR, epidermal growth factor receptor; NEJSG, North East Japan Study Group; WJTOG, West Japan Thoracic Oncology Group; EURTAC, EGFR mutation-positive non-small-cell lung cancer; ALK, anaplastic lymphoma kinase;

site(s) of oligoprogression and continuation of the targeted agent; change to a second generation inhibitor; and institution of chemotherapy, which can be done with or without continuation of the targeted agent.[404,405] Patients with EGFR-mutated tumors should be carefully monitored once the TKI is discontinued due to the risk of "flare," which can be severe and at times fatal.[406] It is recommended that once a change in therapy is decided, the washout period be limited to a minimum. Interestingly, patients later rechallenged with the same EGFR inhibitor often have prolonged periods of stabilization.

Maintenance Therapy

The continuation of the same combination chemotherapy regimen beyond four to six cycles yields no discernible benefit.[407–409] Assuming no evidence of progression, options at that juncture include close observation with treatment at progression or maintenance therapy. Continuation maintenance means that the nonplatinum agent used in the initial regimen is continued until disease progression. Another strategy is switch maintenance in which a new agent, one not used in the initial regimen, is initiated after the initial regimen. Both maintenance strategies have been shown to improve survival.

Continuation pemetrexed has led to an improvement in OS after four cycles of cisplatin-pemetrexed (Table 41.8).[410] A French trial also demonstrated an improvement in progression-free survival when gemcitabine was continued after four cycles of cisplatin-gemcitabine.[411] Continuation maintenance is also frequently used with bevacizumab based on the pivotal trial previously discussed,[156] despite the lack of randomized data demonstrating a benefit for maintenance versus no maintenance.

Switch maintenance therapy trials have shown a benefit for pemetrexed and erlotinib after four cycles of a platinum-based doublet (see Table 41.8).[412,413] A prior trial with docetaxel showed a progression-free survival advantage but the difference in OS, while clinically meaningful, did not reach statistical significance.[414] One criticism of these trials is that a relatively small percentage of patients randomized to the nonmaintenance arm actually received the same agent upon relapse.[415] In fact, in the Fidias trial,[414] a post hoc analysis of the patients who received this agent at the time of progression showed similar survival to those who received it as switch maintenance. This has led many thought leaders to interpret that switch maintenance is akin to early institution of second-line therapy.

Maintenance therapy must be discussed as an option rather than a universal recommendation. Several patients can be safely watched and benefit from a treatment break. On the other hand, a number of patients recur with devastating complications and miss the "window of opportunity" for second-line therapy. As of now, there are no clinical, radiographic, or biologic markers that predict outcome after first-line therapy. The ACCP and NCCN guidelines suggest maintenance pemetrexed in nonsquamous NSCLC, either as continuation maintenance if the patient is on a pemetrexed regimen, or switch maintenance if they are not.[141,374] Consideration of switch maintenance erlotinib is also suggested by both guidelines. The NCCN suggests continuation maintenance gemcitibine (category 2b), but the ACCP guideline recommends against it. However, it is clear that many factors must be considered in the decision, and clinical judgment is needed.

Second-Line Therapy

Multiple randomized trials have demonstrated that second-line therapy, with a noncross-resistant agent, leads to an improvement in survival compared to supportive care.[374] In addition, consistent improvement in QOL has been documented.[416,417] Cytotoxic agents used in this setting include docetaxel and pemetrexed.[379,418] Gemcitabine is also used in previously treated patients despite the lack of randomized data. Efficacy is similar among the chemotherapy agents, but toxicity profiles are somewhat different. EGFR TKIs have also shown benefit in this setting.[419] Erlotinib received its original approval for previously treated patients, unselected by molecular criteria, and still is used in this setting.

Recently trials have addressed whether conventional chemotherapy is preferable to erlotinib (or gefitinib where applicable) for EGFR wild-type patients in the second-line setting.[420–422] While only one trial showed an advantage with respect to OS, all trials showed a consistent trend toward better outcomes with chemotherapy. Based on these data, second-line chemotherapy is preferred for EGFR wild-type patients; erlotinib or gefitinib is usually used in these patients only after two lines of chemotherapy.

For patients whose tumors carry an EGFR mutation and who are treated with an inhibitor in the first-line setting, options at progression depend on the mechanism of resistance. The majority

PRACTICE OF ONCOLOGY

TABLE 41.8

Maintenance Chemotherapy

	Trial	Induction	Randomization	N	PFS	MST
Switch	Fidias	Cisplatin-gemcitabine	Immediate docetaxel	153	5.7	12.3
			Delayed docetaxel	156	2.7	9.7
	Ciuleanu[a]	Platinum doublet	Pemetrexed	441	4.5	15.5
			Placebo	222	2.6	10.3
	Capuzzo	Platinum doublet	Erlotinib	438	2.8	12
			Placebo	451	2.6	11
	Perol[b]	Cisplatin-gemcitabine	Erlotinib	155	2.9	11.4
			Observation	155	1.9	10.8
Continuation	Paz-Ares	Cisplatin-pemetrexed	Pemetrexed	539	4.1	13.9
			Placebo		2.8	11
	Perol[b]	Cisplatin-gemcitabine	Gemcitabine	154	3.8	12.1
			Observation	155	1.9	10.8

PFS, progression-free survival; MST, median survival time.
[a] Squamous subset.
[b] Three-arm trial: observation versus erlotinib versus gemcitabine.

of these patients have a secondary mutation, T790M, in exon 20, which shifts the affinity of the receptor preferentially to adenosine triphosphate.[423] Several new agents that target T790M are in development.[424] Other known mechanisms include conversion to a small-cell histology (usually responsive to platinum-etoposide combinations) and Her2 amplification.[405] A repeat biopsy at the time of progression is therefore advised to better guide the second-line therapy options. In addition, some patients with EGFR-mutated disease have an indolent or limited progression, including central nervous system involvement, which can be managed with local/ablative techniques, without discontinuation of the systemic therapy.[425]

Patients with ALK rearrangement also have multiple mechanisms of resistance, including de novo mutations.[426] While the same management principles apply to these patients, particularly those with indolent progression, the emergence of more specific second-generation ALK inhibitors, such as LDK 378, has become an appealing option.[427]

Third-Line Therapy

Contrary to second-line therapy, no randomized trial has shown a survival benefit for third-line therapy compared to placebo. The only agent approved for third-line therapy in the United States is erlotinib based on the same trial that led to the approval in second-line.[419] Candidates for third-line therapy were randomized to erlotinib or placebo, and those treated with the former experienced a survival benefit as well as improvement in symptom control of the same magnitude seen in second-line patients. Although no standard chemotherapy agent is formally approved for this indication, patients who have progressed on two prior lines and still maintain an acceptable PS are often treated in clinical practice with additional chemotherapy. The ACCP and NCCN guidelines recommend third-line treatment with erlotinib over basic supportive care in good PS patients.[141,374]

SPECIAL CLINICAL SITUATIONS

Oligometastases

In general, the presence of distant metastases indicates incurable disease that must be treated palliatively, usually by chemotherapy. However, a small subset of patients presents with a limited number (e.g., one to three) number of metastatic sites. This is called oligometastatic disease, and there is ample evidence that a curative intent treatment approach can be successful.

The greatest amount of data comes from patients with NSCLC and isolated brain metastases. Definitive treatment of brain metastases can be an important component of palliative-intent treatment, but in this section we focus on eradication of all known disease with intent to cure. The ACCP and NCCN guidelines recommend this be considered in NSCLC patients with isolated brain metastases.[141,295] A careful search (PET, brain MRI/CT) should be conducted to find evidence of more diffuse metastases. The number of brain metastases is not crucial as long as they can each be treated definitively.[295] Invasive mediastinal staging should be done; involvement of N2,3 nodes is considered a contraindication for curative-intent therapy.[141,295]

Treatment of patients with isolated brain metastases (T1-3N0-1M1b) generally begins with stereotactic radiosurgery or surgical resection of the brain metastases because of the devastating consequences of untreated brain lesions. Stereotactic radiosurgery and surgery for the brain metastases are complementary approaches with equivalent effectiveness; surgery is generally used with larger lesions that produce more mass effect and if the morbidity of a surgical approach is low. Curative resection of the primary lung tumor should follow the same principles dictated by the primary tumor regardless of the brain metastasis. Adjuvant chemotherapy

is then recommended, although based only on indirect data of a benefit in earlier stage patients.[141,295] There is no data regarding the sequence (i.e., after treatment of the brain metastasis, whether to resect the lung lesion followed by chemotherapy or to administer chemotherapy and then later resect the lung primary). However, given the rapid recovery in general from modern (usually VATS) lung resection, it is probably best to get this accomplished before chemotherapy in general. Both the ACCP and NCCN recommend adjuvant whole-brain RT (WBRT) as well to decrease the chance of a brain recurrence; however, the data for the benefit of WBRT (for either survival or the rate of brain recurrences) is conflicting and indirect (not specific to oligometastatic tumors and curative-intent treatment).

Outcomes of curative-intent treatment of NSCLC with isolated brain oligometastases are reasonable. The surgical mortality from both resection of the brain lesion and the lung primary is about 2% in a recent systematic review.[295] The 5-year survival is about 15% on average.[295] The outcomes are the same whether patients present with a synchronous brain metastases or a metachronous brain metastasis that is found after a previous resection of an early stage NSCLC. Prognostic factors are poorly defined; outcomes may be slightly better in patients that are younger, have good PS, and have a lower T stage of the primary tumor.

There is data supporting a similar treatment approach for patients with isolated adrenal metastases.[141,295] The staging approach and treatment strategy is similar, although the urgency of treatment of the brain metastasis missing. Usually, the adrenal metastasis is treated by surgical resection (often laparoscopic) followed in about 2 weeks by lung resection (often by VATS). Both the ACCP and NCCN recommend adjuvant chemotherapy, but this is based on extrapolation from patients with other disease stages.[141,295]

A systematic review of outcomes found an average 5-year survival of 27% with curative-intent treatment of patients with NSCLC and isolated adrenal metastases.[295] Prognostic factors have not been defined. The outcomes appear to be similar for synchronous and metachronous presentations.

Limited data is available regarding curative-intent treatment of oligometastatic disease in other distant sites. However, reported outcomes are quite good (5-year survival of 32% to 86%).[295] The observation that outcomes are better for adrenal and other sites compared with brain oligometastatic disease probably simply reflects that clinicians have been more selective in choosing patients for curative-intent treatment involving nonbrain oligometastases. A prospective trial of aggressive curative-intent treatment for nonbrain oligometastatic disease found a median survival of only 11 months; however, this trial was not very selective and included many patients with N2 disease.[428]

Second Primary Lung Cancers, Additional Nodules, and Multifocal Lung Cancer

Patients with a lung cancer and additional nodules or lesions are challenging to manage. The additional lesion may be benign, may be a synchronous second primary lung cancer, one manifestation of systemic metastases, an additional nodule of cancer, or multifocal lung cancer. Appropriate categorization is difficult because the terms and definitions are ambiguous and the usage varies over time and between centers. The ACCP lung cancer guidelines have proposed a definition of terms and a structure for classification.[158,295] This structure is based on the clinical presentation rather than pathology, which makes it applicable at the time of clinical decision making. Table 41.9 provides a summary of the approach to patients with additional lesions according to the clinical presentation. The NCCN guidelines also address these patients, but without any clarity about how to classify them.[141]

A critical step for most of these patients is evaluation by a multidisciplinary team. One must be careful; often, there is tendency

TABLE 41.9

Approach to Patients with Additional Nodule(s)

Presentation	Data Summary	Initial Evaluation	Assessment	Categorization	Management
Typical solid cancer, additional nodule on CT, no clinical signs of distant disease[a]	Large majority are benign	Multidisciplinary team[b] discussion	Judged very likely benign	Benign lesion	Treatment of primary lung cancer, observation of nodule per Fleischner guidelines
Locally advanced NSCLC, nodule(s), and clinical signs of distant disease[a]	No formal data	PET and brain MRI/CT Multidisciplinary team[b] discussion	Judged very likely stage IV	Stage IV	Stage IV treatment (i.e., chemotherapy)
			Judged unclear	Suspicious for Stage IV	Biopsy of nodule and other potential sites (N2,3 or M1b)
Typical solid cancer[c] and additional typical solid cancer[c]	~1.5% incidence	Thorough workup to rule out N2,3 or M1b Multidisciplinary team[b] discussion	Meets criteria for synchronous primaries if evaluation negative	Synchronous primaries	Manage each primary accordingly, and as patient will tolerate physiologically
Typical solid cancer and additional solid nodule	IASLC DB, but patients poorly defined, survival after resection better than for solitary M1b	Thorough workup to rule out N2,3 or M1b Multidisciplinary team[b] discussion	Judged unlikely to be synchronous second primary, but lesion suspected (or proven) malignant with same histology	Lung cancer with additional cancer nodule	Manage aggressively if T3 or T4 (consider resection), unclear if M1a (contralateral lung)
Lung cancer with GGO component and additional GGO (or semisolid) lesions	Indirect data, patients poorly defined	Multidisciplinary team[b] discussion	Fits pattern of multifocal disease	Multifocal lung cancer	Manage primary accordingly, and manage additional lesions according to guidelines for GGO

CT, computed tomography; NSCLC, non-small cell lung cancer; PET, positron emission tomography; MRI, magnetic resonance imaging; IASLC DB, International Association for the Study of Lung Cancer database; GGO, ground glass opacity.
[a] Fatigue, weight loss, anorexia, bone pain, neurologic symptoms.
[b] Team should include a chest radiologist, pulmonologist, and thoracic surgeon.
[c] Spiculated solid lesion.
Table modified from the Kozower B, Larner JM, Detterbeck FC, et al. Special treatment issues in non-small cell lung cancer: diagnosis and management of lung cancer, 3rd ed: American College of Chest Physicians evidence-based clinical practice guidelines *Chest* 2013;143:e369S–e399S.

PRACTICE OF ONCOLOGY

to be swayed by the stage classification of additional nodules (e.g., T3$_{satell}$, T4$_{ipsi\ nod}$, or M1a$_{contra\ nod}$) and forget that many if not most patients belong in other categories. The classification of T3$_{satell}$, T4$_{ipsi\ nod}$, or M1a$_{contra\ nod}$ is explicitly contraindicated when dealing with a second primary lung cancer or patients with distant metastases from lung cancer.[55] It is particularly important to remember that, in patients with a clinical and radiographic presentation consistent with early stage lung cancer and an additional subcentimeter nodule on CT, the large majority of these nodules are benign.[295,429–431] Furthermore, identification of second primary lung cancers on clinical grounds has been quite accurate (as evidenced by survival outcomes), and these have most often been of the *same* cell type. Thus, it is clinical recognition and not necessarily a biopsy result that is critical to define second primary lung cancers. Because of these and other factors, the judgment of a multidisciplinary team is important in the evaluation of patients found to have additional lesions by CT.

Second primary lung cancers occur in about 5% of resected cases (either synchronous or metachronous presentation) and at a rate of about 1.5% per patient per year after curative treatment of a NSCLC. Approximately two-thirds of second primary lung cancers have been of the same histologic type; quite consistently the outcomes of tumors classified as second primary lung cancer based on different histology versus based on other features have been the same.[295] It is reasonable to consider the radiographic appearances

in making a clinical determination of a second primary lung cancer. It has also been suggested to use molecular markers or the percentage of different subtypes of adenocarcinoma in making this determination, but this has not been extensively evaluated. All of the data available should be considered (clinical, radiographic, and pathologic) in making the determination whether a second focus of cancer is a second primary lung cancer or not.

When a synchronous second primary lung cancer is suspected, a careful search should be made for distant or mediastinal metastases as recommended by the ACCP and NCCN.[141,295] If this evaluation is negative, each primary cancer should be treated in the usual fashion for early stage cancer, provided the patient has adequate reserve. SBRT offers another treatment option. The vast majority of reported synchronous second primary lung cancers have been resected (often a limited resection); the 5-year survival after resection is approximately 25% for all and 40% if both tumors are stage pI (range, 0% to 79%).

A metachronous second primary lung cancer is best defined as a cancer with either a different histology or an interval of >4 years—in these situations, one can be fairly certain it is not a recurrence. A site of cancer of the same histologic type appearing within 2 years is most likely a metastasis, and between 2 and 4 years is a gray zone.[295] Once ~2 years have evolved, the stage of the initial NSCLC does not appear to affect the likelihood of recurrence versus new primary cancer. The judgment of a multidisciplinary team, taking all factors into account, is important in classifying the situation as a second primary lung cancer versus a recurrence.

The staging evaluation of a metachronous second primary lung cancer should generally proceed as dictated by the characteristics of the second primary tumor alone.[295] Most metachronous second primary cancers that are reported have been resected (often a limited resection); the 5-year survival after resection is approximately 30% for all and 40% for stage pI (range, 20% to 70%). No data is available regarding outcomes of unresected patients.[295]

Attention has been drawn to additional nodules ($T3_{satell}$, $T4_{ipsi\ nod}$, or $M1a_{contra\ nod}$) by the seventh edition of the lung cancer staging system.[293,294] The patients with additional nodules in the IASLC database were poorly defined, but specifically excluded those with second primary lung cancers or with distant metastases.[55] The additional nodules were probably recognized clinically in most cases (either pre- or intraoperatively) and proven pathologically to be of the same histologic type. The ACCP suggests that the additional nodule designations should be used for patients with a dominant "classic" lung cancer (i.e., solid, spiculated) and an additional solid nodule identified clinically or on pathologic examination.[158] It should be noted that most reports of patients with additional nodules of cancer have specifically excluded BAC because BAC is recognized to often present as multifocal disease. The ACCP clinically based definition effectively also excludes what was formerly called BAC pathologically from the cohort of patients classified as having additional nodules.

No additional diagnostic workup is recommended by the ACCP in patients with a secondary lesion in the same lobe ($T3_{satell}$). The data does not suggest a higher rate of occult distant or mediastinal metastases from what is predicted based on the dominant cancer, and the treatment recommendation is the same with or without an additional nodule in the same lobe (i.e., lobectomy).[295] The 5-year survival appears to be about 10% to 15% worse, stage for stage, with an additional nodule compared to the same dominant cancer without an additional nodule.[295,432] There does not appear to be a difference in survival whether there is one or several additional nodules.[295]

For additional nodules of cancer in a different lobe, the ACCP suggests a thorough search for distant disease (i.e., PET, brain MRI/CT) and invasive mediastinal staging, although direct data to support this stance is not available.[295] If there is no N2,3 or M1b disease, resection of both the dominant cancer and an ipsilateral, different lobe nodule is recommended. The reported 5-year survival for resection of such patients with ipsilateral, different lobe, additional nodules is ~20%.[295] The outcomes do appear to be better than if resection was not done. Much of the reported data comes from Asia, although there is no evidence of a geographic difference in outcomes in this cohort in the IASLC database. The survival appears to be worse if there is more than one additional ipsilateral, different lobe nodule, or with lymph node involvement.[295]

The ACCP also suggests resection of a contralateral additional nodule if thorough staging reveals no N2,3 or M1b involvement.[295] Very limited data is available on resected patients; in the IASLC database, 98% of patients were not resected, and survival was poor (5-year survival = 3%). This has been corroborated by other registry reports.[295]

Multifocal BAC was a well-recognized entity. The term BAC has been abandoned because it was used loosely in many different settings.[63] In the context of multifocal BAC, this was probably most often what would now be called a lepidic predominant invasive adenocarcinoma. The combination of abandonment of the term BAC and the seventh edition of the stage classification has left a void in how to classify multifocal lung cancer, which is still an entity that is regularly encountered. The ACCP has proposed a definition of multifocal lung cancer as multiple lesions arising from GGOs, which may develop a solid component.[158,295] This is a clinically focused definition, rather than one focused on particular pathologic findings; some of these lesions may be AAH, AIS, or MIA, but most are lepidic predominant invasive adenocarcinoma. A diffuse infiltrative pattern of disease (also called "pneumonic

type" of adenocarcinoma) is also included in the ACCP definition. For stage classification, the ACCP recommends that the T(m) designation should be used for patients with multifocal lung cancer (a designation that has been used rarely in lung cancer although it has been part of the stage classification system for more than a decade).[158,293,294]

Multifocal lung cancer appears to have a decreased propensity for nodal or systemic spread and an increased propensity for additional pulmonary foci. The ACCP lung cancer guidelines therefore suggest that for multifocal lung cancer a search for distant or mediastinal metastases (i.e., PET, invasive mediastinal staging) is not necessary unless there is clinical suspicion.[295] Additionally, the rate of recurrence after resection, which has often been a limited resection, is low. Therefore, the ACCP guidelines suggest that a limited resection be performed of any multifocal lesions that are thought to be invasive cancer.[295] Lesions that are thought not to be invasive cancer (i.e., pure GGO) should generally be followed, because most of these appear to remain stable, at least for many years.[119,151,295] Adjuvant therapy for R0 resected patients without nodal involvement is not recommended.

The published outcomes for resected patients with multifocal disease have been quite good (5-year survival of approximately 90%; range, 64% to 100%).[295]

PALLIATIVE CARE

Role of Palliative Care

A large number of patients with lung cancer will develop symptoms related to their disease. Metastases to the brain and spinal column may threaten significant neurologic compromise; airway obstruction or SVC syndrome may present urgently or with milder symptoms that progress to become severe if left untreated. And more common, less acutely severe, symptoms such as pain, dyspnea, cough, anorexia, or fatigue can significantly impact QOL, and may preclude cancer-directed therapy.[433] The importance of palliative efforts in lung cancer care was highlighted in an RCT involving 151 patients with metastatic NSCLC who received standard oncologic treatment and were randomized to receive early palliative care or not.[434] In patients who received early palliative care, there was a significant improvement in QOL and fewer depressive symptoms. Because the care mode resulted in better documentation of end-of-life preferences, patients receiving early palliative care were less likely to have aggressive resuscitation efforts and less likely to receive chemotherapy in favor of hospice care. Despite this, the authors also observed significantly improved OS (median, 11.6 months versus 8.9 months). While unexpected, this finding is consistent with prior studies that demonstrated shorter survival in patients with more severe depressed mood and worse QOL.[435] These results suggest a model for improving patient mood and QOL during cancer care, and validate the importance of the early initiation of such efforts.

Specific Symptom Management

Airway obstruction is common in patients with lung cancer, as a result of tumor mass effect, bleeding, or mucous production.[433] Therapeutic bronchoscopy is appropriate for evaluation, with interventions including mechanical disimpaction, brachytherapy, ablation, or stenting. Hemoptysis responds well to ablation with laser or electrocautery, and brachytherapy or external beam radiation may also be considered. A cough can be the direct result of malignancy, or due to secondary infection, or chemotherapy- or RT-induced pneumonitis. Evaluation and treatment for the latter etiologies should be considered, and otherwise cough suppression with opioids is appropriate. Malignant effusions, if symptomatic, respond to tunneled pleural catheters when the lung can be re-expanded. Pleurodeisis can be pursued for recurrent effusions, via talc slurry or poudrage.[433]

Pain, whether due to bone or soft tissue disease, is one of the most common symptoms of lung cancer. Nonsteroidal anti-inflammatory drugs should be prescribed to all patients, unless contraindicated, and, for those who require chronic medication, appropriate gastrointestinal prophylaxis (i.e., misprostol, H2 antagonists, or proton pump inhibitors) should be added. For those patients who have a neuropathic component to their pain, the addition of an anticonvulsant or tricyclic antidepressant improves pain control. For moderate to severe pain, morphine or an alternative narcotic is recommended.[433]

Bony metastases without pathologic fracture or significant structural weakness can be managed with short-course RT and bisphosphonates. Patients with pathologic fractures, or with focal lytic lesions that involve >50% of the cortex of weight-bearing bones, should undergo surgical fixation to prevent debilitating injury, followed by RT. Vertebral compression fractures with instability can be stabilized surgically or through augmentation procedures.

Epidural spinal cord compression (ESCC) is one of the most serious complications of metastatic cancer. The most common presenting symptom is local pain, with or without radicular component.[436,437] A bony metastatic lesion arising in the vertebral body can extend directly into the epidural space, impinging upon the spinal cord or cauda equina, or an induced vertebral compression fracture may retropulse bony fragments into the same space. Progressive pressure on the cord or nerve roots can lead to edema, ischemia, and irreversible neurologic compromise. MRI is the primary diagnostic intervention, although CT myelography may also demonstrate the characteristic impingement on the thecal sac. Additional plain films or CT imaging may be required to differentiate soft tissue extension from bony retropulsion. Corticosteroids should be administered as early as feasible. A small, single-blind randomized study of corticosteroids showed that the addition of dexamethasone to RT improved ambulation, an effect that was durable to 6 months (59% versus 33% remained ambulatory), without an effect on survival.[438] The doses administered were higher than are typically used in the modern era, 96 mg intravenously followed by 96 mg/day and tapered over 10 days. Lower doses are typically used in an effort to avoid steroid-related complications.

Surgical or augmentation procedures are indicated for ESCC when there is spinal instability or the cause of the cord impingement is bony in nature. For symptoms caused by direct tumor compression, either surgical intervention or local RT may be appropriate. Evidence suggests that neurologic compromise of short duration is more apt to be meaningfully reversed by surgery than symptoms that have been present for longer duration.[439] Patchell et al.[439] conducted a randomized trial of surgery versus RT (30 Gy in 10 fractions) in 101 patients with symptomatic ESCC, all with neurologic symptoms of <2 days duration. Patients who underwent surgery were more likely to have symptomatic relief (62% versus 19%), more likely to ambulate (84% versus 57%), and had better OS (median, 126 days versus 100 days), clearly indicating that surgery should be strongly considered in patients with ESCC, particularly those with neurologic signs and symptoms of relatively acute onset. RT as primary treatment offers reasonable palliation of pain, but is highly unlikely to restore ambulation or otherwise reverse neurologic compromise.

Lung cancer accounts for approximately half of all brain metastases. Historically, survival after diagnosis of brain metastases is poor; a median of 6 months in the most robust candidates (i.e., those of young age, good PS, and brain-only disease).[440] In patients with NSCLC, significant prognostic factors for survival in patients with brain metastases include age, PS, the presence of extracranial metastases, and the number of brain metastases.[441] The increased availability of active systemic therapy and targeted agents options has resulted in a subset of patients with brain metastases whose survival is significantly longer, increasing the importance of selecting the appropriate brain-directed therapy to maximize control and minimize potential long-term morbidity.

Brain metastases are often accompanied by significant surrounding cerebral edema, and the latter is the most common cause of symptoms such as headache, nausea, vomiting, and ataxia. Steroids with predominant glucocorticoid activity, such as dexamethasone, are commonly used to address symptomatic patients, and can partially or completely relieve symptoms in otherwise untreated patients for several weeks. There is no evidence to suggest that steroid treatment of asymptomatic patients confers any benefit. For patients with severe symptoms due to mass effect or edema that are not amenable to steroid treatment, consideration should be given to surgical decompression. Noninvasive therapies such as radiosurgery or WBRT are unlikely to acutely improve symptoms.

WBRT was the standard-of-care approach to most patients with brain metastases for several decades, since a randomized trial demonstrated a 40% improvement in OS when compared to steroid treatment and supportive care alone.[442] Because WBRT can lead to significant fatigue and somnolence in the short term, and permanent neurocognitive deficits in the late term, patients with less bulky disease or those with an expectation of more prolonged survival are frequently treated with surgery or radiosurgery in place of whole-brain treatment.

For patients with a single brain metastasis, surgery or radiosurgery, either with our without WBRT, has become the standard-of-care approach. A landmark pair of studies by Patchell et al.[443,444] established the separate roles of resection and WBRT in this setting. In the first trial, 84 patients with a solitary brain metastasis were randomized to surgical resection followed by WBRT or WBRT alone.[443] The OS was significantly longer in the surgical arm (45 weeks versus 40 weeks), reflecting the marked benefit of local therapy for patients with good PS. The use of radiosurgery in place of surgery in patients with a solitary lesion also improves OS when given in addition to WBRT in a parallel fashion.[445] The companion study from Patchell et al addressed the role of WBRT.[444] In this trial, 95 patients with a solitary metastatic lesion underwent surgery, and then were randomized to WBRT or no further therapy. The addition of WBRT significantly improved local control of the resected lesion, reduced "elsewhere" failures in the brain, but did not improve OS.[444] The significant reduction in brain recurrence seen in this study has been cited to support the routine use of WBRT after surgery or radiosurgery to a solitary brain metastasis, but the lack of any survival benefit has also been cited to suggest that active surveillance after local therapy is a reasonable approach.

Patients with one to three brain metastases may be treated with radiosurgery alone, WBRT, or both in combination. The value of radiosurgery in this population was established in the RTOG 9508,[445] in which 333 patients with one to three metastases were randomized to either WBRT alone or WBRT followed by radiosurgery. In the subset of patients with a single metastasis, the addition of radiosurgery improved OS, consistent with the Patchell trial of surgical resection in the setting of WBRT. Patients with two or three lesions who received radiosurgery in addition to WBRT had better PS at 6 months posttreatment, but no incremental survival benefit. Withholding WBRT in these patients and treating them with radiosurgery alone is predicated on avoiding the neurocognitive sequelae of WBRT. In a small randomized trial, Chang et al.[446] answered the question of whether WBRT could be avoided, randomizing patients with one to three brain metastases to either radiosurgery alone or radiosurgery and WBRT. The trial was stopped early when an interim analysis demonstrated an OS benefit to withholding WBRT. This finding was not consistent with prior surgical data and could be due to the increased opportunity to deliver subsequent chemotherapy in patients who did not have WBRT, or could be simply an anomalous finding in a relatively small study population. The clear and consistent result was that neurocognitive function was significantly better when WBRT was withheld.

In patients with poor PS or extensive extracranial disease, WBRT is appropriately the treatment of choice. In patients with more than five brain metastases, good PS, and limited extracranial disease, the role of WBRT versus stereotactic radiosurgery is ill-defined.[447] Several efforts are currently under way to determine the optimal treatment for this population.

SVC syndrome may have various neoplastic and nonneoplastic causes. Bronchogenic carcinoma is the most common cause of SVC syndrome, underlying approximately 80% of cases at diagnosis.[448] When the SVC becomes obstructed, blood returns to the heart through collateral vessels via the azygous vein or inferior vena cava. Venous collaterals dilate over weeks, compensating for the loss of SVC patency. Upper body venous pressure and resulting edema of the arm and face decrease over time, so that symptoms with sudden onset, from acute obstruction, can diminish over several weeks even without intervention. The severity of the symptoms is due not only to the degree of SVC narrowing, but also to the rapidity with which it develops. The characteristic signs include cyanosis, plethora, distention of subcutaneous veins, and edema of the head, neck, and arm. Patients may develop dyspnea and cough. In rare cases, severe and acute obstruction can result in cerebral edema or laryngeal stridor. The specific cause of SVC syndrome in a patient with known malignancy may be extrinsic compression from tumor mass or due to thrombus in the setting of hypercoagulability. Even in the case of malignant, extrinsic compression, the clinical course may be complicated by the subsequent development of a thrombus in the SVC or brachiocephalic vein, or the simultaneous tumor mass effect on the bronchi or heart.

Traditionally, SVC syndrome was viewed as a medical emergency, but accumulating experience demonstrates that the course of SVC is rarely life-threatening. In a review of 107 patients in whom intervention was withheld during evaluation, there were no serious consequences to deferring treatment until diagnosis and staging was completed.[449] The symptoms often improve without active intervention, as collateral vessels dilate.[450] Immediate intervention is warranted when symptoms are life threatening (e.g., cerebral edema leading to altered mental status, stridor,

or clinically significant hemodynamic compromise). When urgent intervention is indicated, intravascular stenting provides the most immediate relief. In the absence of life-threatening symptoms, the patient should be appropriately staged, biopsied, and the underlying malignancy treated in a manner appropriate for its stage and presentation. Patients with metastatic SCLC and SVC syndrome will likely respond to systemic therapy, which may be more appropriate than the initiation of urgent radiation. Patients with limited-stage SCLC and SVC syndrome should respond rapidly to chemoradiotherapy, or induction chemotherapy if that can be started more promptly. Patients with NSCLC and SVC syndrome are less likely to respond quickly to either chemotherapy or radiation, and so the threshold for placing an endovascular stent is somewhat lower. SVC syndrome is a poor prognostic factor in NSCLC, with a median survival from presentation of 5 months.[451]

CONCLUSION

Lung still remains by far the leading cause of cancer deaths. The blame, guilt, and nihilism that stems from the relationship of smoking to lung cancer continues to be an issue, despite a better understanding of smoking as an addiction and the fact that most patients diagnosed will have quit smoking many years earlier. However, lung cancer has become a dynamic and vibrant field. Screening is able to reduce the rate of lung cancer deaths by decreasing the proportion that is diagnosed with advanced disease. Major improvements have been made in all treatment modalities: minimally invasive surgery, better RT targeting and delivery, and a diverse array of chemotherapeutic agents and methods of palliation of many symptoms. There have also been advances in epidemiology (focusing on more than simply smoking), in imaging, in accurate definition of the stage, and on understanding some of the biologic and genetic alterations encountered. Many questions remain, but there is no question that lung cancer is a dynamic, challenging, and exciting area in which much progress is being made.

SELECTED REFERENCES

The full reference list can be accessed at lwwhealthlibrary.com/oncology.

1. GLOBOCAN 2012: Estimated Cancer Incidence, Mortality and Prevalence Worldwide in 2012. Lung Cancer [database on the Internet]. International Agency for Research on Cancer, World Health Organization. 2013 [cited January 8, 2014]. http://globocan.iarc.fr/Pages/fact_sheets_cancer.aspx.
2. Siegel R, Naishadham D, Jemal A. Cancer statistics, 2013. CA Cancer J Clin 2013;63:11–30.
20. Peto R, Darby S, Deo H, et al. Smoking, smoking cessation, and lung cancer in the UK since 1950: combination of national statistics with two case-control studies. BMJ 2000;321:323–329.
21. Samet JM, Avila-Tang E, Boffetta P, et al. Lung cancer in never smokers: clinical epidemiology and environmental risk factors. Clin Cancer Res 2009;15:5626–2645.
22. Sun S, Schiller JH, Gazdar AF. Lung cancer in never smokers—a different disease. Nat Rev Cancer 2007;7:778–790.
28. Lissowska J, Foretova L, Dabek J, et al. Family history and lung cancer risk: international multicentre case-control study in Eastern and Central Europe and meta-analyses. Cancer Causes Control 2010;21:1091–1104.
29. Cassidy A, Myles JP, van Tongeren M, et al. The LLP risk model: an individual risk prediction model for lung cancer. Br J Cancer 2008;98:270–276.
30. De Matteis S, Consonni D, Bertazzi PA. Exposure to occupational carcinogens and lung cancer risk. Evolution of epidemiological estimates of attributable fraction. Acta Biomed 2008;79:34–42.
32. Markowitz SB, Levin SM, Miller A, et al. Asbestos, asbestosis, smoking, and lung cancer. New findings from the North American insulator cohort. Am J Respir Crit Care Med 2013;188:90–96.
35. Darby S, Hill D, Auvinen A, et al. Radon in homes and risk of lung cancer: collaborative analysis of individual data from 13 European case-control studies. BMJ 2005;330:223.

41. Bain C, Feskanich D, Speizer FE, et al. Lung cancer rates in men and women with comparable histories of smoking. J Natl Cancer Inst 2004;96:826–834.
42. Gallicchio L, Boyd K, Matanoski G, et al. Carotenoids and the risk of developing lung cancer: a systematic review. Am J Clin Nutr 2008;88:372–383.
46. Turner MC, Chen Y, Krewski D, et al. Chronic obstructive pulmonary disease is associated with lung cancer mortality in a prospective study of never smokers. Am J Respir Crit Care Med 2007;176:285–290.
52. Goldstraw P, Crowley J, Chansky K, et al. The IASLC Lung Cancer Staging Project: proposals for the revision of the TNM stage groupings in the forthcoming (seventh) edition of the TNM Classification of malignant tumours. J Thorac Oncol 2007;2:706–714.
53. Rami-Porta R, Ball D, Crowley J, et al. The IASLC Lung Cancer Staging Project: proposals for the revision of the T descriptors in the forthcoming (seventh) edition of the TNM classification for lung cancer. J Thorac Oncol 2007;2:593–602.
54. Rusch VW, Crowley J, Giroux DJ, et al. The IASLC Lung Cancer Staging Project: proposals for the revision of the N descriptors in the forthcoming seventh edition of the TNM classification for lung cancer. J Thorac Oncol 2007;2:603–612.
55. Postmus PE, Brambilla E, Chansky K, et al. The IASLC Lung Cancer Staging Project: proposals for revision of the M descriptors in the forthcoming (seventh) edition of the TNM classification of lung cancer. J Thorac Oncol 2007;2:686–693.
57. Shepherd FA, Crowley J, Van Houtte P, et al. The International Association for the Study of Lung Cancer lung cancer staging project: proposals regarding the clinical staging of small cell lung cancer in the forthcoming (seventh) edition of the tumor, node, metastasis classification for lung cancer. J Thorac Oncol 2007;2:1067–1077.
58. Travis WD, Giroux DJ, Chansky K, et al. The IASLC Lung Cancer Staging Project: proposals for the inclusion of broncho-pulmonary carcinoid tumors

in the forthcoming (seventh) edition of the TNM Classification for Lung Cancer. *J Thorac Oncol* 2008;3:1213–1223.

59. Detterbeck F, Tanoue L, Boffa DJ. The new lung cancer staging system. *Chest* 2009;136:260–271.

61. Detterbeck FC. Maintaining aim at a moving target. *J Thor Oncol* 2011;6:417–422.

62. Clinical Lung Cancer Genome Project (CLCGP), Network Genomic Medicine (NGM). A genomics-based classification of human lung tumors. *Sci Transl Med* 2013;5:209ra153.

63. Travis WD, Brambilla E, Noguchi M, et al. International Association for the Study of Lung Cancer/American Thoracic Society/European Respiratory Society: international multidisciplinary classification of lung adenocarcinoma. *J Thorac Oncol* 2011;6:244–285.

64. Travis WD, Brambilla E, Muller-Hernlink HD, et al., eds. *Pathology and Genetics of Tumours of the Lung, Pleura, Thymus and Heart*. Lyon, France: IARC Press; 2004.

65. Hanahan D, Weinberg RA. Hallmarks of cancer: the next generation. *Cell* 2011;144:646–674.

67. Imielinski M, Berger AH, Hammerman PS, et al. Mapping the hallmarks of lung adenocarcinoma with massively parallel sequencing. *Cell* 2012;150:1107–1120.

70. Chansky K, Sculier J, Crowley J, et al. The International Association for the Study of Lung Cancer Staging Project: prognostic factors and pathologic TNM stage in surgically managed non-small cell lung cancer. *J Thorac Oncol* 2009;4:792–801.

76. Leone F, Evers-Casey S, Toll B, et al. Treatment of tobacco use in lung cancer: diagnosis and management of lung cancer, 3rd ed: American College of Chest Physicians evidence-based clinical practice guidelines. *Chest* 2013;143:e61S–e77S.

77. Trousse D, Barlesi F, Loundou A, et al. Synchronous multiple primary lung cancer: an increasing clinical occurrence requiring multidisciplinary management. *J Thorac Cardiovasc Surg* 2007;133:1193–1200.

81. The effect of vitamin E and beta carotene on the incidence of lung cancer and other cancers in male smokers. The Alpha-Tocopherol, Beta Carotene Cancer Prevention Study Group. *N Engl J Med* 1994;330:1029–1035.

83. Hennekens CH, Buring JE, Manson JE, et al. Lack of effect of long-term supplementation with beta carotene on the incidence of malignant neoplasms and cardiovascular disease. *N Engl J Med* 1996;334:1145–1149.

84. Szabo E, Mao JT, Lam S, et al. Chemoprevention of lung cancer: diagnosis and management of lung cancer, 3rd ed: American College of Chest Physicians evidence-based clinical practice guidelines. *Chest* 2013;143:e40S–e60S.

85. Marcus PM, Bergstralh EJ, Zweig MH, et al. Extended lung cancer incidence follow-up in the Mayo Lung Project and overdiagnosis. *J Natl Cancer Inst* 2006;98:748–756.

86. Doria-Rose VP, Marcus PM, Szabo E, et al. Randomized controlled trials of the efficacy of lung cancer screening by sputum cytology revisited: a combined mortality analysis from the Johns Hopkins Lung Project and the Memorial Sloan-Kettering Lung Study. *Cancer* 2009;115:5007–5017.

91. Oken MM, Hocking WG, Kvale PA, et al. Screening by chest radiograph and lung cancer mortality: the Prostate, Lung, Colorectal, and Ovarian (PLCO) randomized trial. *JAMA* 2011;306:1865–1873.

92. Aberle D, Adams A, Berg C, et al. Reduced lung-cancer mortality with low-dose computed romographic screening. *N Eng J Med* 2011;365:395–409.

93. Infante M, Cavuto S, Lutman FR, et al. A randomized study of lung cancer screening with spiral computed tomography. *Am J Respir Crit Care Med* 2009;180:445–453.

94. Saghir Z, Dirksen A, Ashraf H, et al. CT screening for lung cancer brings forward early disease. The randomised Danish Lung Cancer Screening Trial: status after five annual screening rounds with low-dose CT. *Thorax* 2012;67:296–301.

96. Bach PB, Mirkin JN, Oliver TK, et al. Benefits and harms of CT screening for lung cancer: a systematic review. *JAMA* 2012;307:2418–2429.

97. Detterbeck FC, Mazzone PJ, Naidich DP, et al. Screening for lung cancer: diagnosis and management of lung cancer, 3rd ed: American College of Chest Physicians evidence-based clinical practice guidelines. *Chest* 2013;143:e78S–e92S.

100. Wood D, Eapen G, Ettinger D, et al. Lung cancer screening. *J Natl Compr Canc Netw* 2011;10:240–265.

101. Moyer V, U.S. Preventive Services Task Force. Screening for lung cancer: U.S. Preventive Services Task Force recommendation statement. *Ann Intern Med* 2014;160:330–338.

102. de Koning H, Meza R, Plevritis S, et al. *Benefits and Harms of Computed Tomography Lung Cancer Screening Programs for High-Risk Populations*. AHRQ Publication No. 13-05196-EF-2. Rockville, MD: Agency for Healthcare Research and Quality; 2013.

103. Detterbeck F, Gibson C. Turning gray: the natural history of lung cancer over time. *J Thorac Oncol* 2008;3:781–792.

104. Detterbeck FC. Cancer, concepts, cohorts and complexity: avoiding oversimplification of overdiagnosis. *Thorax* 2012;67:842–845.

105. Bach PB, Gould MK. When the average applies to no one: personalized decision making about potential benefits of lung cancer screening. *Ann Intern Med* 2012;157:571–573.

106. Tammemagi MC, Katki HA, Hocking WG, et al. Selection criteria for lung-cancer screening. *N Engl J Med* 2013;368:728–736.

107. Spitz MR, Hong WK, Amos CI, et al. A risk model for prediction of lung cancer. *J Natl Cancer Inst* 2007;99:715–726.

108. Bach PB, Kattan MW, Thornquist MD, et al. Variations in lung cancer risk among smokers. *J Natl Cancer Inst* 2003;95:470–478.

109. Ost D, Yeung S, Tanoue L, et al. Clinical and organizational factors in the initial evaluation of patients with lung cancer: Diagnosis and management of lung cancer, 3rd ed: American College of Chest Physicians evidence-based clinical practice guidelines. *Chest* 2013;143:e121S.

110. Silvestri GA, Gonazalez AV, Jantz M, et al. Methods of staging for non-small cell lung cancer: diagnosis and management of lung cancer, 3rd ed: American College of Chest Physicians evidence-based clinical practice guidelines. *Chest* 2013;143:e211S–e250S.

111. Swensen SJ, Silverstein MD, Ilstrup DM, et al. The probability of malignancy in solitary pulmonary nodules: application to small radiologically indeterminate nodules. *Arch Intern Med* 1997;157:849–855.

112. Swensen SJ, Silverstein MD, Edell ES, et al. Solitary pulmonary nodules: Clinical prediction model versus physicians. *Mayo Clin Proc* 1999;74:319–329.

114. Tammemagi C, Pinsky P, Caporaso N, et al. Lung cancer risk prediction: prostate, lung, colorectal and ovarian cancer screening trial models and validation. *J Natl Cancer Inst* 2011;103:1058–1068.

115. McWilliams A, Tammemagi MC, Mayo JR, et al. Probability of cancer in pulmonary nodules detected on first screening CT. *N Engl J Med* 2013;369:910–919.

116. Rivera M, Mehta AC, Wahidi MM. Establishing the diagnosis of lung cancer: diagnosis and management of lung cancer, 3rd ed: American College of Chest Physicians evidence-based clinical practice guidelines. *Chest* 2013;143:e142S–e165S.

117. Ost DE, Niu J, S Elting L, et al. Quality gaps and comparative effectiveness in lung cancer staging and diagnosis. *Chest* 2014;145:331–345.

119. Gould MK, Donington J, Lynch W, et al. Evaluation of individuals with pulmonary nodules: when is it lung cancer? *Chest* 2013;143:e93S–e120S.

120. Vesselle H, Schmidt RA, Pugsley JM, et al. Lung cancer proliferation correlates with [F-18]fluorodeoxyglucose uptake by positron emission tomography. *Clin Cancer Res* 2000;6:3837–3844.

123. Patchell RA, Tibbs PA, Walsh JW, et al. A randomized trial of surgery in the treatment of single metastases to the brain. *N Engl J Med* 1990;322:494–500.

124. Reed C, Harpole D, Posther K, et al. Results of the American College of Surgeons Oncology Group Z0050 Trial: the utility of positron emission tomography in staging potentially operable non-small cell lung cancer. *J Thorac Cardiovasc Surg* 2003;126:1943–1951.

137. Maziak DE, Darling GE, Inculet RI, et al. Positron emission tomography in staging early lung cancer. *Ann Intern Med* 2009;151:221–228.

138. Fischer B, Lassen U, Mortensen J, et al. Preoperative staging of lung cancer with combined PET-CT. *N Engl J Med* 2009;361:32–39.

139. van Tinteren H, Hoekstra OS, Smit EF, et al. Effectiveness of positron emission tomography in the preoperative assessment of patients with suspected non-small-cell lung cancer: the PLUS multicentre randomised trial. *Lancet* 2002;359:1388–1392.

140. Herder GJ, Kramer H, Hoekstra OS, et al. Traditional versus up-front [18F] fluorodeoxyglucose-positron emission tomography staging of non-small-cell lung cancer: a Dutch cooperative randomized study. *J Clin Oncol* 2006;24:1800–1806.

141. National Comprehensive Cancer Network. Non-Small Cell Lung Cancer Version 2.2014.

142. Detterbeck F, Puchalski J, Rubinowitz A, et al. Classification of the thoroughness of mediastinal staging of lung cancer. *Chest* 2010;137:436–442.

143. Annema JT, van Meerbeeck JP, Rintoul RC, et al. Mediastinoscopy vs endosonography for mediastinal nodal staging of lung cancer. *JAMA* 2010;304:2245–2252.

144. Detterbeck FC, Lewis S, Diekemper R, et al. Executive summary: diagnosis and management of lung cancer, 3rd ed: American College of Chest Physicians evidence-based clinical practice guidelines. *Chest* 2013;143:7S–37S.

145. Little AG, Gay EG, Gaspar LE, et al. National survey of non-small cell lung cancer in the United States: epidemiology, pathology and patterns of care. *Lung Cancer* 2007;57:253–260.

148. Farjah F, Flum D, Ramsey S, et al. Multi-modality mediastinal staging for lung cancer among Medicare beneficiaries. *J Thorac Oncol* 2009;4:355–363.

149. Little AG, Rusch VW, Bonner JA, et al. Patterns of surgical care of lung cancer patients. *Ann Thorac Surg* 2005;80:2051–2056.

150. Vest M, Tanoue L, Soulos P, et al. Thoroughness of mediastinal staging in stage IIIA non-small cell lung cancer. *J Thor Oncol* 2012;7:188–195.

151. Howington J, Blum M, Chang A, et al. Treatment of stage I and II non-small cell lung cancer. *Chest* 2013;432:e278S–e313S.

152. von Meyenfeldt E, Gooiker G, van Gijn W, et al. The relationship between volume or surgeon specialty and outcome in the surgical treatment of lung cancer: a systematic review and meta-analysis. *J Thorac Oncol* 2012;7:1170–1178.

155. Pignon J-P, Tribodet H, Scagliotti GV, et al. Lung adjuvant cisplatin evaluation: a pooled analysis by the LACE Collaborative Group. *J Clin Oncol* 2008;26:3552–3559.

156. Sandler A, Gray R, Perry MC, et al. Paclitaxel-carboplatin alone or with bevacizumab for non-small-cell lung cancer. *N Engl J Med* 2006;355:2542–2550.

158. Detterbeck FC, Postmus PE, Tanoue L. The stage classification of lung cancer: diagnosis and management of lung cancer, 3rd ed: American College of Chest Physicians evidence-based clinical practice guidelines. *Chest* 2013;143:e191s–e210s.

159. Cheng D, Downey RJ, Kernstine K, et al. Video-assisted thoracic surgery in lung cancer resection: a meta-analysis and systematic review of controlled trials. *Innovations* 2007;2:261–292.

160. Yan TD, Black D, Bannon PG, et al. Systematic review and meta-analysis of randomized and nonrandomized trials on safety and efficacy of video-assisted thoracic surgery lobectomy for early-stage non-small-cell lung cancer. *J Clin Oncol* 2009;27:2553–2562.

162. Zhang Z, Zhang Y, Feng H, et al. Is video-assisted thoracic surgery lobectomy better than thoracotomy for early-stage non-small-cell lung cancer? A systematic review and meta-analysis. *Eur J Cardiothorac Surg* 2013;44:407–414.

163. Taioli E, Lee DS, Lesser M, et al. Long-term survival in video-assisted thoracoscopic lobectomy vs open lobectomy in lung-cancer patients: a meta-analysis. *Eur J Cardiothorac Surg* 2013;44:591–597.

166. Ceppa D, Kosinski A, Berry M, et al. Thoracoscopic lobectomy has increasing benefit in patients with poor pulmonary function: a Society of Thoracic Surgeons database analysis. *Ann Surg* 2012;256:487–493.

167. Farjah F, Wood DE, Mulligan MS, et al. Safety and efficacy of video-assisted versus conventional lung resection for lung cancer. *J Thorac Cardiovasc Surg* 2009;137:1415–1421.

168. Park H, Detterbeck F, Boffa D, et al. Impact of hospital volume of thoracoscopic lobectomy on primary lung cancer outcomes. *Ann Thorac Surg* 2012;93:372–379.

169. Swanson SJ, Meyers BF, Gunnarsson CL, et al. Video-assisted thoracoscopic lobectomy is less costly and morbid than open lobectomy: a retrospective multiinstitutional database analysis. *Ann Thorac Surg* 2012;93:1027–1032.

170. Licht PB, Jørgensen OD, Ladegaard L, et al. A national study of nodal upstaging after thoracoscopic versus open lobectomy for clinical stage I lung cancer. *Ann Thorac Surg* 2013;96:943–950.

172. Paul S, Sedrakyan A, Chiu YL, et al. Outcomes after lobectomy using thoracoscopy vs thoracotomy: a comparative effectiveness analysis utilizing the Nationwide Inpatient Sample database. *Eur J Cardiothorac Surg* 2013;43:813–817.

175. Su S, Scott WJ, Allen MS, et al. Patterns of survival and recurrence after surgical treatment of early stage non–small cell lung carcinoma in the ACOSOG Z0030 (ALLIANCE) trial. *J Thorac Cardiovasc Surg* 2014;147:747–753.

176. Scott WJ, Allen MS, Darling G, et al. Video-assisted thoracic surgery versus open lobectomy for lung cancer: a secondary analysis of data from the American College of Surgeons Oncology Group Z0030 randomized clinical trial. *J Thorac Cardiovasc Surg* 2010;139:976–983.

181. Jeon JH, Kang CH, Kim HS, et al. Video-assisted thoracoscopic lobectomy in non-small-cell lung cancer patients with chronic obstructive pulmonary disease is associated with lower pulmonary complications than open lobectomy: a propensity score-matched analysis. *Eur J Cardiothorac Surg* 2014;45:640–645.

182. Scott W, Matteotti R, Egleston B, et al. A comparison of perioperative outcomes of Video-Assisted Thoracic Surgical (VATS) Lobectomy with open thoracotomy and lobectomy: results of an analysis using propensity score based weighting. *Ann Surg Innov Res* 2010;4:1.

186. Pompili C, Detterbeck F, Papagiannopoulos K, et al. Multicenter international randomized comparison of objective and subjective outcomes between electronic and traditional chest drainage systems. *Ann Thorac Surg* 2014;98:490–497.

187. Cattaneo SM, Park BJ, Wilton AS, et al. Use of video-assisted thoracic surgery for lobectomy in the elderly results in fewer complications. *Ann Thorac Surg* 2008;85:231–236.

190. Grills IS, Hugo G, Kestin LL, et al. Image-guided radiotherapy via daily online cone-beam CT substantially reduces margin requirements for stereotactic lung radiotherapy. *Int J Radiat Oncol Biol Phys* 2008;70:1045–1056.

195. Emami B, Lyman J, Brown A, et al. Tolerance of normal tissue to therapeutic irradiation. *Int J Radiat Oncol Biol Phys* 1991;21:109–122.

196. Marks LB, Bentzen SM, Deasy JO, et al. Radiation dose-volume effects in the lung. *Int J Radiat Oncol Biol Phys* 2010;76:S70–S76.

197. Timmerman R, McGarry R, Yiannoutsos C, et al. Excessive toxicity when treating central tumors in a phase II study of stereotactic body radiation therapy for medically inoperable early-stage lung cancer. *J Clin Oncol* 2006;24:4833–4839.

200. Barriger RB, Forquer JA, Brabham JG, et al. A dose-volume analysis of radiation pneumonitis in non-small cell lung cancer patients treated with stereotactic body radiation therapy. *Int J Radiat Oncol Biol Phys* 2012;82:457–462.

202. Miller KL, Shafman TD, Anscher MS, et al. Bronchial stenosis: an underreported complication of high-dose external beam radiotherapy for lung cancer? *Int J Radiat Oncol Biol Phys* 2005;61:64–69.

203. Bradley JD, Hope A, El Naga I, et al. A nomogram to predict radiation pneumonitis, derived from a combined analysis of RTOG 9311 and institutional data. *Int J Radiat Oncol Biol Phys* 2007;69:985–992.

204. Palma DA, Senan S, Oberije C, et al. Predicting esophagitis after chemoradiation therapy for non-small cell lung cancer: an individual patient data meta-analysis. *Int J Radiat Oncol Biol Phys* 2013;87:690–696.

207. Movsas B, Scott C, Langer C, et al. Randomized trial of amifostine in locally advanced non-small-cell lung cancer patients receiving chemotherapy and hyperfractionated radiation: radiation therapy oncology group trial 98-01. *J Clin Oncol* 2005;23:2145–2154.

209. Turrisi AT 3rd, Kim K, Blum R, et al. Twice-daily compared with once-daily thoracic radiotherapy in limited small-cell lung cancer treated concurrently with cisplatin and etoposide. *N Engl J Med* 1999;340:265–271.

210. O'Rourke N, Roque IFM, Farre Bernado N, et al. Concurrent chemoradiotherapy in non-small cell lung cancer. *Cochrane Database Syst Rev* 2010;(6):CD002140.

214. Qiao WB, Zhao YH, Zhao YB, et al. Clinical and dosimetric factors of radiation-induced esophageal injury: radiation-induced esophageal toxicity. *World J Gastroenterol* 2005;11:2626–2629.

215. Gagliardi G, Constine LS, Moiseenko V, et al. Radiation dose-volume effects in the heart. *Int J Radiat Oncol Biol Phys* 2010;76:S77–S85.

223. Kong FM, Ritter T, Quint DJ, et al. Consideration of dose limits for organs at risk of thoracic radiotherapy: atlas for lung, proximal bronchial tree, esophagus, spinal cord, ribs, and brachial plexus. *Int J Radiat Oncol Biol Phys* 2011;81:1442–1457.

225. The Non-small Cell Lung Cancer Collaborative Group. Chemotherapy in non-small cell lung cancer: a meta-analysis using updated data on individual patients from 52 randomised clinical trials. *Br Med J* 1995;311:899–909.

228. Pignon J, Tribodet H, Scagliotti G, et al. Lung Adjuvant Cisplatin Evaluation (LACE): a pooled analysis of five randomized clinical trials including 4,584 patients. *J Clin Oncol* 2007;24:7008.

229. Lynch TJ, Bell DW, Sordella R, et al. Activating mutations in the epidermal growth factor receptor underlying responsiveness of non-small-cell lung cancer to gefitinib. *N Engl J Med* 2004;350:2129–2139.

230. Johnson DH. Setting the bar for therapeutic trials in non–small-cell lung cancer: how low can we go? *J Clin Oncol* 2014;32:1389–1391.

231. Sacher AG, Le LW, Leighl NB. Shifting patterns in the interpretation of phase III clinical trial outcomes in advanced non–small-cell lung cancer: the bar is dropping. *J Clin Oncol* 2014;32:1407–1411.

232. Atherly AJ, Camidge DR. The cost-effectiveness of screening lung cancer patients for targeted drug sensitivity markers. *Br J Cancer* 2012;106:1100–1106.

233. Djalalov S, Beca J, Hoch JS, et al. Cost effectiveness of EML4-ALK fusion testing and first-line crizotinib treatment for patients with advanced ALK-positive non-small-cell lung cancer. *J Clin Oncol* 2014;32:1012–1019.

235. Kim ES, Herbst RS, Wistuba II, et al. The BATTLE trial: personalizing therapy for lung cancer. *Cancer Discov* 2011;1:44–53.

236. Wisnievesky J, Yung RC, Mathur PN, et al. Diagnosis and treatment of bronchial intraepithelial neoplasia and early lung cancer of the central airways: diagnosis and management of lung cancer, 3rd ed: American College of Chest Physicians evidence-based clinical practice guidelines. *Chest* 2013;143:e263S–e277S.

237. Detterbeck FC, Homer RJ. Approach to the ground-glass nodule. *Clin Chest Med* 2011;32:799–810.

238. Naidich DP, Bankier AA, MacMahon H, et al. Recommendations for the management of subsolid pulmonary nodules detected at CT: a statement from the Fleischner Society. *Radiology* 2013;266:304–317.

239. Yoshida J, Ishii G, Yokose T, et al. Possible delayed cut-end recurrence after limited resection for ground-glass opacity adenocarcinoma, intraoperatively diagnosed as Noguchi Type B, in three patients. *J Thor Oncol* 2010;5:546–550.

241. Asamura H, Goya T, Koshiishi Y, et al. A Japanese Lung Cancer Registry study: prognosis of 13,010 resected lung cancers. *J Thorac Oncol* 2008;3:46–52.

246. Hubbard MO, Fu P, Margevicius S, et al. Five-year survival does not equal cure in non-small cell lung cancer: a surveillance, epidemiology, and end results-based analysis of variables affecting 10- to 18-year survival. *J Thorac Cardiovasc Surg* 2012;143:1307–1313.

251. Cooke D, Wisner D. Who performs complex noncardiac thoracic surgery in United States academic medical centers? *Ann Thorac Surg* 2012;94:1060–1064.

252. Boffa DJ, Kosinski A, Paul S, et al. Lymph node evaluation by open or video assisted approaches in 11,500 anatomic lung cancer resections. *Ann Thorac Surg* 2012;94:347–353.

253. Palade E, Passlick B, Osei-Agyemang T, et al. Video-assisted vs open mediastinal lymphadenectomy for Stage I non-small-cell lung cancer: results of a prospective randomized trial. *Eur J Cardiothorac Surg* 2013;44:244–249.

254. Petersen RP, Pham D, Burfeind WR, et al. Thoracoscopic lobectomy facilitates the delivery of chemotherapy after resection for lung cancer. *Ann Thorac Surg* 2007;83:1245–1250.

255. Jiang G, Yang F, Li X, et al. Video-assisted thoracoscopic surgery is more favorable than thoracotomy for administration of adjuvant chemotherapy after lobectomy for non-small cell lung cancer. *World J Surg Oncol* 2011;21:170.

256. Ginsberg RJ, Rubinstein LV. Randomized trial of lobectomy versus limited resection for T1 N0 non-small cell lung cancer. Lung Cancer Study Group. *Ann Thorac Surg* 1995;60:615–622, discussion 623.

259. Darling GE, Allen MS, Decker PA, et al. Number of lymph nodes harvested from a mediastinal lymphadenectomy: results of the randomized, prospective ACOSOG Z0030 trial. *Chest* 2011;139:1124–1129.

262. Allen MS, Darling GE, Pechet TT, et al. Morbidity and mortality of major pulmonary resections in patients with early-stage lung cancer: initial results of the randomized, prospective ACOSOG Z0030 trial. *Ann Thorac Surg* 2006;81:1013–1020.

263. Arriagada R, Dunant A, Pignon JP, et al. Long-term results of the international adjuvant lung cancer trial evaluating adjuvant cisplatin-based chemotherapy in resected lung cancer. *J Clin Oncol* 2010;28:35–42.

264. Scagliotti GV. The ALPI trial: the Italian/European experience with adjuvant chemotherapy in resectable non–small lung cancer. *Clin Cancer Res* 2005;11:5011s–5016s.

265. Waller D, Peake MD, Stephens RJ, et al. Chemotherapy for patients with non-small cell lung cancer: the surgical setting of the Big Lung Trial. *Eur J Cardiothorac Surg* 2004;26:173–182.

266. Strauss GM, Herndon JE II, Maddaus MA, et al. Adjuvant paclitaxel plus carboplatin compared with observation in stage IB non-small-cell lung cancer: CALGB 9633 with the Cancer and Leukemia Group B, Radiation Therapy Oncology Group, and North Central Cancer Treatment Group study groups. *J Clin Oncol* 2008;26:5043–5051.

267. Hamada C, Tanaka, F, Ohta, M, et al. Meta-analysis of postoperative adjuvant chemotherapy with tegafur-uracil in non-small-cell lung cancer. *J Clin Oncol* 2005;23:4999.

268. Wada H, Hitomi S, Teramatsu T. Adjuvant chemotherapy after complete resection in non-small-cell lung cancer. West Japan Study Group for Lung Cancer Surgery. *J Clin Oncol* 1996;14:1048–1054.

269. PORT Meta-analysis Trialists Group. Postoperative radiotherapy in non-small-cell lung cancer: systemic review and meta-analysis of individual patient data from nine randomised controlled trials. *Lancet* 1998;352:257–263.

270. Trodella L, Granone P, Valente S, et al. Adjuvant radiotherapy in non-small cell lung cancer with pathological stage I: definitive results of a phase III randomized trial. *Radiother Oncol* 2002;62:11–19.

271. Lally BE, Zelterman D, Colasanto JM, et al. Postoperative radiotherapy for stage II or III non-small-cell lung cancer using the surveillance, epidemiology, and end results database. *J Clin Oncol* 2006;24:2998–3006.

272. Brunelli A, Kim AW, Berger K, et al. Physiologic evaluation of the patient with lung cancer being considered for resectional surgery: diagnosis and management of lung cancer, 3rd ed: American College of Chest Physicians evidence-based clinical practice guidelines. *Chest* 2013;143:e166S–e190S.

274. Brunelli A, Socci L, Refai M, et al. Quality of life before and after major lung resection for lung cancer: a prospective follow-up analysis. *Ann Thorac Surg* 2007;84:410–416.

275. Bobbio A, Chetta A, Carbognani P, et al. Changes in pulmonary function test and cardio-pulmonary exercise capacity in COPD patients after lobar pulmonary resection. *Eur J Cardiothorac Surg* 2005;28:754–758.

281. Palma DA, Senan S, Haasbeek CJ, et al. Radiological and clinical pneumonitis after stereotactic lung radiotherapy: a matched analysis of three-dimensional conformal and volumetric-modulated arc therapy techniques. *Int J Radiat Oncol Biol Phys* 2011;80:506–513.

282. NSCLC Meta-analyses Collaborative Group, Arriagada R, Auperin A, et al. Adjuvant chemotherapy, with or without postoperative radiotherapy, in operable non-small-cell lung cancer: two meta-analyses of individual patient data. *Lancet* 2010;375:1267–1277.

285. Lardinois D, Suter H, Hakki H, et al. Morbidity, survival, and site of recurrence after mediastinal lymph-node dissection versus systematic sampling after cpmplete resection for non-small cell lung cancer. *Ann Thorac Surg* 2005;80:268–275.

288. Ma Z, Dong A, Fan J, et al. Does sleeve lobectomy concomitant with or without pulmonary artery reconstruction (double sleeve) have favorable results for non-small cell lung cancer compared with pneumonectomy? A meta-analysis. *Eur J Cardiothorac Surg* 2007;32:20–28.

289. Douillard J, Tribodet H, Aubert D, et al. Adjuvant cisplatin and vinorelbine for completely resected non-small cell lung cancer: subgroup analysis of the Lung Adjuvant Cisplatin Evaluation. *J Thorac Oncol* 2010;5:220–228.

290. Butts CA, Ding K, Seymour L, et al. Randomized phase III trial of vinorelbine plus cisplatin compared with observation in completely resected stage IB and II non-small-cell lung cancer: updated survival analysis of JBR-10. *J Clin Oncol* 2010;28:29–34.

291. Douillard JY, Rosell R, De Lena M, et al. Impact of postoperative radiation therapy on survival in patients with complete resection and stage I, II, or IIIA non-small-cell lung cancer treated with adjuvant chemotherapy: the Adjuvant Navelbine International Trialist Association (ANITA) randomized trial. *Int J Radiat Oncol Biol Phy* 2008;72:695–701.

292. Felip E, Rosell R, Maestre JA, et al. Preoperative chemotherapy plus surgery versus surgery plus adjuvant chemotherapy versus surgery alone in early-stage non-small-cell lung cancer. *J Clin Oncol* 2010;28:3138–3145.

293. American Joint Committee on Cancer. *AJCC Cancer Staging Manual.* 7th ed. New York, NY: Springer; 2009.

294. International Union for Cancer Control. *TNM Classification of Malignant Tumors.* 7th ed. Hoboken, NJ: Wiley-Blackwell; 2009.

295. Kozower B, Larner JM, Detterbeck FC, et al. Special treatment issues in non-small cell lung cancer: diagnosis and management of lung cancer, 3rd ed: American College of Chest Physicians evidence-based clinical practice guidelines. *Chest* 2013;143:e369S–e399S.

301. Morgensztern D, Waqar S, Subramanian J, et al. Prognostic significance of tumor size in patients with stage III non-small-cell lung cancer: a surveillance, epidemiology, and end results (SEER) survey from 1998 to 2003. *J Thorac Oncol* 2012;7:1479–1484.

303. Moreno A, Morgensztern D, Boffa D, et al. Treating stage IIIA-N1 disease: an analysis of very large, hilar lymph node positive non-small cell lung cancer using the National Cancer Data Base. *Ann Thorac Surg* 2014;97:1149–1155.

304. Detterbeck FC. Changes in the treatment of Pancoast tumors. *Ann Thorac Surg* 2003;75:1990–1997.

305. Foroulis CN, Zarogoulidis P, Darwiche K, et al. Superior sulcus (Pancoast) tumors: current evidence on diagnosis and radical treatment. *J Thorac Dis* 2013;5:S342–S358.

306. Anraku M, Waddell TK, de Perrot M, et al. Induction chemoradiotherapy facilitates radical resection of T4 non-small cell lung cancer invading the spine. *J Thorac Cardiovasc Surg* 2009;137:441–447.e1.

308. Bolton WD, Rice DC, Goodyear A, et al. Superior sulcus tumors with vertebral body involvement: a multimodality approach. *J Thorac Cardiovasc Surg* 2009;137:1379–1387.

312. Muralidaran A, Detterbeck FC, Boffa DJ, et al. Long-term survival after lung resection for NSCLC with circulatory bypass: a systematic review. *J Thorac Cardiovasc Surg* 2011;142:1137–1142.

313. Kim AW, Detterbeck FC. Surgery for T4 and N3 non-small cell lung cancer, additional pulmonary nodules and isolated distant metastases. In: Kernstine K, Reckamp K, Thomas CJ, eds. *Lung Cancer: A Multidisciplinary Approach to Diagnosis and Management.* New York, NY: Demos Medical Publishing; 2011:161–182.

315. Rusch VW, Giroux DJ, Kraut MJ, et al. Induction chemoradiation and surgical resection for superior sulcus non-small-cell lung carcinomas: long-term results of Southwest Oncology Group Trial 9416 (Intergroup Trial 0160). *J Clin Oncol* 2007;25:313–318.

316. Ramnath N, Dilling T, Harris L, et al. Treatment of stage III non-small cell lung cancer: diagnosis and management of lung cancer, 3rd ed: American College of Chest Physicians evidence-based clinical practice guidelines. *Chest* 2013;143:e314S–e340S.

317. Detterbeck F. What to do with surprise N2: intraoperative management of patients with non-small cell lung cancer. *J Thorac Oncol* 2008;3:289–302.

324. Lally BE, Detterbeck FC, Geiger AM, et al. The risk of death from heart disease in patients with nonsmall cell lung cancer who receive postoperative radiotherapy: analysis of the Surveillance, Epidemiology, and End Results database. *Cancer* 2007;110:911–917.

327. Bradley J, Graham MV, Winter K, et al. Toxicity and outcome results of RTOG 9311: a phase I-II dose-escalation study using three-dimensional conformal radiotherapy in patients with inoperable non-small-cell lung carcinoma. *Int J Radiat Oncol Biol Phys* 2005;61:318–328.

330. Pisters KM, Le Chevalier T. Adjuvant chemotherapy in completely resected non-small-cell lung cancer. *J Clin Oncol* 2005;23:3270–3278.

331. Keller SM, Adak S, Wagner H, et al. A randomized trial of postoperative adjuvant therapy in patients with completely resected stage II or IIIA non-small-cell lung cancer. Eastern Cooperative Oncology Group. *N Engl J Med* 2000;343:1217–1222.

332. Dautzenberg B, Chastang C, Arriagada R, et al. Adjuvant radiotherapy versus combined sequential chemotherapy followed by radiotherapy in the treatment of resected nonsmall cell lung carcinoma. A randomized trial of 267 patients. GETCB (Groupe d'Etude et de Traitement des Cancers Bronchiques). *Cancer* 1995;76:779–786.

333. Cerfolio RJ, Maniscalco L, Bryant AS. The treatment of patients with stage IIIA non-small cell lung cancer from N2 disease: who returns to the surgical arena and who survives. *Ann Thorac Surg* 2008;86:912–920.

334. Burdett S, Stewart L, Rydzewska L. Chemotherapy and surgery versus surgery alone in non-small cell lung cancer. *Cochrane Database Syst Rev* 2007;(3):CD006157.

335. Andre F, Grunenwald D, Pignon JP, et al. Survival of patients with resected N2 non–small-cell lung cancer: evidence for a subclassification and implications. *J Clin Oncol* 2000;18:2981–2989.

338. Vansteenkiste JF, De Leyn PR, Deneffe GJ, et al. Clinical prognostic factors in surgically treated stage IIIA-N2 non-small cell lung cancer: analysis of the literature. *Lung Cancer* 1998;19:3–13.

339. Albain KS, Swann RS, Rusch VW, et al. Radiotherapy plus chemotherapy with or without surgical resection for stage III non-small-cell lung cancer: a phase III randomised controlled trial. *Lancet* 2009;374:379–386.

342. Van Meerbeeck JP, Kramer GW, Van Schil PE, et al. Randomized controlled trial of resection versus radiotherapy after induction chemotherapy in stage IIIA-N2 non-small-cell lung cancer. *J Natl Cancer Inst* 2007;99:442–450.

344. de Cabanyes Candela S, Detterbeck F. A systematic review of restaging after induction therapy for stage IIIa lung cancer: prediction of pathologic stage. *J Thorac Oncol* 2010;5:389–398.

345. Thomas M, Rübe C, Hoffknecht P, et al. Effect of preoperative chemoradiation in addition to preoperative chemotherapy: a randomised trial in stage III non-small-cell lung cancer. *Lancet Oncol* 2008;9:636–648.

346. Perez CA, Stanley K, Rubin P, et al. A prospective randomized study of various irradiation doses and fractionation schedules in the treatment of inoperable non-oat-cell carcinoma of the lung. Preliminary report by the Radiation Therapy Oncology Group. *Cancer* 1980;45:2744–2753.

348. Cox JD, Azarnia N, Byhardt RW, et al. A randomized phase I/II trial of hyperfractionated radiation therapy with total doses of 60.0 Gy to 79.2 Gy: possible survival benefit with greater than or equal to 69.6 Gy in favorable patients with Radiation Therapy Oncology Group stage III non-small-cell lung carcinoma: report of Radiation Therapy Oncology Group 83-11. *J Clin Oncol* 1990;8:1543–1555.

349. Saunders M, Dische S, Barrett A, et al. Continuous, hyperfractionated, accelerated radiotherapy (CHART) versus conventional radiotherapy in non-small cell lung cancer: mature data from the randomised multicentre trial. CHART Steering committee. *Radiother Oncol* 1999;52:137–148.

351. Auperin A, Le Pechoux C, Pignon JP, et al. Concomitant radio-chemotherapy based on platin compounds in patients with locally advanced non-small cell lung cancer (NSCLC): a meta-analysis of individual data from 1764 patients. *Ann Oncol* 2006;17:473–483.

352. Curran WJ Jr, Paulus R, Langer CJ, et al. Sequential vs. concurrent chemoradiation for stage III non-small cell lung cancer: randomized phase III trial RTOG 9410. *J Natl Cancer Inst* 2011;103:1452–1460.

353. Furuse K, Fukuoka M, Kawahara M, et al. Phase III study of concurrent versus sequential thoracic radiotherapy in combination with mitomycin, vindesine, and cisplatin in unresectable stage III non-small-cell lung cancer. *J Clin Oncol* 1999;17:2692–2699.

354. Yamamoto N, Nakagawa K, Nishimura Y, et al. Phase III study comparing second- and third-generation regimens with concurrent thoracic radiotherapy in patients with unresectable stage III non-small-cell lung cancer: West Japan Thoracic Oncology Group WJTOG0105. *J Clin Oncol* 2010;28: 3739–3745.

356. Govindan R, Bogart J, Stinchcombe T, et al. Randomized phase II study of pemetrexed, carboplatin, and thoracic radiation with or without cetuximab in patients with locally advanced unresectable non-small-cell lung cancer: Cancer and Leukemia Group B trial 30407. *J Clin Oncol* 2011;29: 3120–3125.

357. Lu C, Lee JJ, Komaki R, et al. Chemoradiotherapy with or without AE-941 in stage III non-small cell lung cancer: a randomized phase III trial. *J Natl Cancer Inst* 2010;102:859–865.

358. Kelly K, Chansky K, Gaspar LE, et al. Phase III trial of maintenance gefitinib or placebo after concurrent chemoradiotherapy and docetaxel consolidation in inoperable stage III non-small-cell lung cancer: SWOG S0023. *J Clin Oncol* 2008;26:2450–2456.

359. Hanna N, Neubauer M, Yiannoutsos C, et al. Phase III study of cisplatin, etoposide, and concurrent chest radiation with or without consolidation docetaxel in patients with inoperable stage III non-small-cell lung cancer: the Hoosier Oncology Group and U.S. Oncology. *J Clin Oncol* 2008;26: 5755–5760.

360. Vokes EE, Herndon JE 2nd, Kelley MJ, et al. Induction chemotherapy followed by chemoradiotherapy compared with chemoradiotherapy alone for regionally advanced unresectable stage III Non-small-cell lung cancer: Cancer and Leukemia Group B. *J Clin Oncol* 2007;25:1698–1704.

361. Bradley JD, Bae K, Graham MV, et al. Primary analysis of the phase II component of a phase I/II dose intensification study using three-dimensional conformal radiation therapy and concurrent chemotherapy for patients with inoperable non-small-cell lung cancer: RTOG 0117. *J Clin Oncol* 2010;28:2475–2480.

364. Socinski MA, Blackstock AW, Bogart JA, et al. Randomized phase II trial of induction chemotherapy followed by concurrent chemotherapy and dose-escalated thoracic conformal radiotherapy (74 Gy) in stage III non-small-cell lung cancer: CALGB 30105. *J Clin Oncol* 2008;26:2457–2463.

366. Schild SE, Stella PJ, Geyer SM, et al. Phase III trial comparing chemotherapy plus once-daily or twice-daily radiotherapy in Stage III non-small-cell lung cancer. *Int J Radiat Oncol Biol Phys* 2002;54:370–378.

367. Belani CP, Wang W, Johnson DH, et al. Phase III study of the Eastern Cooperative Oncology Group (ECOG 2597): induction chemotherapy followed by either standard thoracic radiotherapy or hyperfractionated accelerated radiotherapy for patients with unresectable stage IIIA and B non-small-cell lung cancer. *J Clin Oncol* 2005;23:3760–3767.

368. Belderbos J, Uitterhoeve L, van Zandwijk N, et al. Randomised trial of sequential versus concurrent chemo-radiotherapy in patients with inoperable non-small cell lung cancer (EORTC 08972-22973). *Eur J Cancer* 2007;43:114–121.

371. Vokes EE, Herndon JE, Kelley MJ, et al. Induction chemotherapy followed by chemoradiotherapy compared wtih chemoradiotherapy alone for regionally advanced unresectable stage III Non-small-cell lung cancer: Cancer and Leukemia Group B. *J Clin Oncol* 2007;25:1698–1704.

374. Socinski MA, Evans T, Gettinger S, et al. Treatment of stage IV non-small cell lung cancer: diagnosis and management of lung cancer, 3rd ed: American College of Chest Physicians evidence-based clinical practice guidelines. *Chest* 2013;143:e341S–e368S.

375. Ellis LM, Bernstein DS, Voest EE, et al. American Society of Clinical Oncology perspective: raising the bar for clinical trials by defining clinically meaningful outcomes. *J Clin Oncol* 2014;32:1277–1280.

376. Lilenbaum RC, Herndon JE 2nd, List MA, et al. Single-agent versus combination chemotherapy in advanced non-small-cell lung cancer: the cancer and leukemia group B (study 9730). *J Clin Oncol* 2005;23:190–196.

377. Ardizzoni A, Boni L, Tiseo M, et al. Cisplatin- versus carboplatin-based chemotherapy in first-line treatment of advanced non–small-cell lung cancer: an individual patient data meta-analysis. *J Natl Cancer Inst* 2007;99:847–857.

378. Schiller JH, Harrington D, Belani CP, et al. Comparison of four chemotherapy regimens for advanced non-small-cell lung cancer. *N Engl J Med* 2002;346:92–98.

379. Hanna N, Shepherd FA, Fossella FV, et al. Randomized phase III trial of pemetrexed versus docetaxel in patients with non-small-cell lung cancer previously treated with chemotherapy. *J Clin Oncol* 2004;22:1589–1597.

380. Johnson DH, Fehrenbacher L, Novotny WF, et al. Randomized phase II trial comparing bevacizumab plus carboplatin and paclitaxel with carboplatin and paclitaxel alone in previously untreated locally advanced or metastatic non-small-cell lung cancer. *J Clin Oncol* 2004;22:2184–2191.

381. Delbaldo C, Michiels S, Syz N, et al. Benefits of adding a drug to a single-agent or a 2-agent chemotherapy regimen in advanced non-small-cell lung cancer: a meta-analysis. *JAMA* 2004;292:470–484.

382. D'Addario G, Pintilie M, Leighl NB, et al. Platinum-based versus non-platinum-based chemotherapy in advanced non-small-cell lung cancer: a meta-analysis of the published literature. *J Clin Oncol* 2005;23:2926–2936.

383. Sweeney CJ, Zhu J, Sandler AB, et al. Outcome of patients with a performance status of 2 in Eastern Cooperative Oncology Group Study E1594: a Phase II trial in patients with metastatic nonsmall cell lung carcinoma. *Cancer* 2001;92:2639–2647.

384. Zukin M, Barrios CH, Rodrigues Pereira J, et al. Randomized phase III trial of single-agent pemetrexed versus carboplatin and pemetrexed in patients with advanced non–small-cell lung cancer and Eastern Cooperative Oncology Group performance status of 2. *J Clin Oncol* 2013;31:2849–2853.

385. Hikish TF, Smith IE, O'Brien ME, et al. Clinical benefit from palliative chemotherapy in non-small-cell lung cancer extends to the elderly and those with poor prognostic factors. *Br J Cancer* 1998;78:28–33.

386. Pallis AG, Gridelli C, van Meerbeeck JP, et al. EORTC Elderly Task Force and Lung Cancer Group and International Society for Geriatric Oncology (SIOG) experts' opinion for the treatment of non-small-cell lung cancer in an elderly population. *Ann Oncol* 2010;21:692–706.

387. Quoix E, Zalcman G, Oster JP, et al. Carboplatin and weekly paclitaxel doublet chemotherapy compared with monotherapy in elderly patients with advanced non-small-cell lung cancer: IFCT-0501 randomised, phase 3 trial. *Lancet* 2011;378:1079–1088.

388. Hesketh PJ, Lilenbaum R, Chansky K, et al. Chemotherapy in patients > or = 80 with advanced non-small cell lung cancer: combined results from SWOG 0027 and LUN 6. *J Thor Oncol* 2007;2:494–498.

389. Reck M, von Pawel J, Zatloukal P, et al. Phase III trial of cisplatin plus gemcitabine with either placebo or bevacizumab as first-line therapy for nonsquamous non-small-cell lung cancer: AVAiL. *J Clin Oncol* 2009;27:1227–1234.

390. Patel JD, Socinski MA, Garon EB, et al. PointBreak: a randomized phase III study of pemetrexed plus carboplatin and bevacizumab followed by maintenance pemetrexed and bevacizumab versus paclitaxel plus carboplatin and bevacizumab followed by maintenance bevacizumab in patients with stage IIIB or IV nonsquamous non-small-cell lung cancer. *J Clin Oncol* 2013;31:4349–4357.

391. Crinò L, Dansin E, Garrido P, et al. Safety and efficacy of first-line bevacizumab-based therapy in advanced non-squamous non-small-cell lung cancer (SAiL, MO19390): a phase 4 study. *Lancet Oncol* 2010;11:733–740.

392. Pirker R, Pereira JR, Szczesna A, et al. Cetuximab plus chemotherapy in patients with advanced non-small-cell lung cancer (FLEX): an open-label randomised phase III trial. *Lancet* 2009;373:1525–1531.

393. Lynch TJ, Patel T, Dreisbach L, et al. Cetuximab and first-line taxane/carboplatin chemotherapy in advanced non-small-cell lung cancer: results of the randomized multicenter phase III trial BMS099. *J Clin Oncol* 2010;28:911–917.

394. Kim ES, Neubauer M, Cohn A, et al. Docetaxel or pemetrexed with or without cetuximab in recurrent or progressive non-small-cell lung cancer after platinum-based therapy: a phase 3, open-label, randomised trial. *Lancet Oncol* 2013;14:1326–1336.

395. Sequist LV, Yang JC-H, Yamamoto N, et al. Phase III study of afatinib or cisplatin plus pemetrexed in patients with metastatic lung adenocarcinoma with EGFR mutations. *J Clin Oncol* 2013;31:3327–3334.

396. Maemondo M, Inoue A, Kobayashi K, et al. Gefitinib or chemotherapy for non-small-cell lung cancer with mutated EGFR. *N Engl J Med* 2010;362: 2380–2388.

397. Mitsudomi T, Morita S, Yatabe Y, et al. Gefitinib versus cisplatin plus docetaxel in patients with non-small-cell lung cancer harbouring mutations of the epidermal growth factor receptor (WJTOG3405): an open label, randomised phase 3 trial. *Lancet Oncol* 2010;11:121–128.

398. Zhou C, Wu Y, Liu X, et al. Overall survival (OS) results from OPTIMAL (CTONG0802), a phase III trial of erlotinib (E) versus carboplatin plus gemcitabine (GC) as first-line treatment for Chinese patients with EGFR mutation-positive advanced non-small cell lung cancer (NSCLC) [abstract 7520]. *J Clin Oncol* 2012;30:30.

399. Rosell R, Carcereny E, Gervais R, et al. Erlotinib versus standard chemotherapy as first-line treatment for European patients with advanced EGFR mutation-positive non-small-cell lung cancer (EURTAC): a multicentre, open-label, randomised phase 3 trial. *Lancet Oncol* 2012;13:239–246.

400. Shaw AT, Kim DW, Nakagawa K, et al. Crizotinib versus chemotherapy in advanced ALK-positive lung cancer. *N Engl J Med* 2013;368:2385–2394.

401. Jänne PA, Wang X, Socinski MA, et al. Randomized phase II trial of erlotinib alone or with carboplatin and paclitaxel in patients who were never or light former smokers with advanced lung adenocarcinoma: CALGB 30406 trial. *J Clin Oncol* 2012;30:2063–2069.

402. Wu YL, Lee JS, Thongprasert S, et al. Intercalated combination of chemotherapy and erlotinib for patients with advanced stage non-small-cell lung cancer (FASTACT-2): a randomised, double-blind trial. *Lancet Oncol* 2013;14:777–786.

403. Mok TS, Wu YL, Thongprasert S, et al. Gefitinib or carboplatin-paclitaxel in pulmonary adenocarcinoma. *N Engl J Med* 2009;361:947–957.

404. Oxnard G, Arcila M, Chmielecki J, et al. New strategies in overcoming acquired resistance to epidermal growth factor receptor tyrosine kinase inhibitors in lung cancer. *Clin Cancer Res* 2011;17:5530–5537.

405. Sequist LV, Waltman BA, Dias-Santagata D, et al. Genotypic and histological evolution of lung cancers acquiring resistance to EGFR inhibitors. *Sci Transl Med* 2011;3:75ra26.

407. Socinski MA, Schell MJ, Peterman A, et al. Phase III trial comparing a defined duration of therapy versus continuous therapy followed by second-line therapy in advanced-stage IIIB/IV non-small-cell lung cancer. *J Clin Oncol* 2002;20:1335–1343.

409. Park JO, Kim SW, Ahn JS, et al. Phase III trial of two versus four additional cycles in patients who are nonprogressive after two cycles of platinum-based chemotherapy in non small-cell lung cancer. *J Clin Oncol* 2007;25:5233–5239.

410. Paz-Ares LG, de Marinis F, Dediu M, et al. PARAMOUNT: Final overall survival results of the phase III study of maintenance pemetrexed versus placebo immediately after induction treatment with pemetrexed plus cisplatin for advanced nonsquamous non-small-cell lung cancer. *J Clin Oncol* 2013;31:2895–2902.

411. Pérol M, Chouaid C, Pérol D, et al. Randomized, phase III study of gemcitabine or erlotinib maintenance therapy versus observation, with predefined second-line treatment, after cisplatin-gemcitabine induction chemotherapy in advanced non-small-cell lung cancer. *J Clin Oncol* 2012;30:3516–3524.

412. Ciuleanu T, Brodowicz T, Zielinski C, et al. Maintenance pemetrexed plus best supportive care versus placebo plus best supportive care for non-small-cell lung cancer: a randomised, double-blind, phase 3 study. *Lancet* 2009;374:1432–1440.

413. Cappuzzo F, Ciuleanu T, Stelmakh L, et al. Erlotinib as maintenance treatment in advanced non-small-cell lung cancer: a multicentre, randomised, placebo-controlled phase 3 study. *Lancet Oncol* 2010;11:521–529.

414. Fidias PM, Dakhil SR, Lyss AP, et al. Phase III study of immediate compared with delayed docetaxel after front-line therapy with gemcitabine plus carboplatin in advanced non-small-cell lung cancer. *J Clin Oncol* 2009;27:591–598.

415. Edelman M, Le Chevalier T, Soria J. Maintenance therapy and advanced non-small-cell lung cancer: a skeptic's view. *J Thor Oncol* 2012;7:1331–1336.

416. Bezjak A, Tu D, Seymour L, et al. Symptom improvement in lung cancer patients treated with erlotinib: quality of life analysis of the National Cancer Institute of Canada Clinical Trials Group Study BR.21. *J Clin Oncol* 2006;24:3831–3837.

417. Dancey J, Shepherd FA, Gralla RJ, et al. Quality of life assessment of second-line docetaxel versus best supportive care in patients with non-small-cell lung cancer previously treated with platinum-based chemotherapy: results of a prospective, randomized phase III trial. *Lung Cancer* 2004;43:183–194.

418. Shepherd FA, Dancey J, Ramlau R, et al. Prospective randomized trial of docetaxel versus best supportive care in patients with non-small-cell lung cancer previously treated with platinum-based chemotherapy. *J Clin Oncol* 2000;18:2095–2103.

419. Shepherd FA, Rodrigues Pereira J, Ciuleanu T, et al. Erlotinib in previously treated non-small-cell lung cancer. *N Engl J Med* 2005;353:123–132.

420. Ciuleanu T, Stelmakh L, Cicenas S, et al. Efficacy and safety of erlotinib versus chemotherapy in second-line treatment of patients with advanced, non-small-cell lung cancer with poor prognosis (TITAN): a randomised multicentre, open-label, phase 3 study. *Lancet Oncol* 2012;13:300–308.

421. Kim E, Hirsh V, Mok T, et al. Gefitinib versus docetaxel in previously treated non-small-cell lung cancer (INTEREST): a randomised phase III trial. *Lancet* 2008;372:1809–1818.

422. Garassino MC, Martelli O, Bettini A, et al. TAILOR: A phase III trial comparing erlotinib with docetaxel as the second-line treatment of NSCLC patients with wild-type (wt) EGFR. *J Clin Oncol* 2012;30:Abstr LBA7501.

423. Yun CH, Mengwasser KE, Toms AV, et al. The T790M mutation in EGFR kinase causes drug resistance by increasing the affinity for ATP. *Proc Natl Acad Sci U S A* 2008;105:2070–2075.

426. Gainor JF, Shaw AT. Emerging paradigms in the development of resistance to tyrosine kinase inhibitors in lung cancer. *J Clin Oncol* 2013;31:3987–3996.

427. Shaw AT, Kim DW, Mehra R, et al. Ceritinib in ALK-rearranged non–small-cell lung cancer. *N Engl J Med* 2014;370:1189–1197.

432. Port JL, Korst RJ, Lee PC, et al. Surgical resection for multifocal (T4) non-small cell lung cancer: is the T4 designation valid? *Ann Thorac Surg* 2007;83:397–400.

433. Simoff MJ, Lally B, Slade MG, et al. Symptom management in patients with lung cancer: diagnosis and management of lung cancer, 3rd ed: American College of Chest Physicians evidence-based clinical practice guidelines. *Chest* 2013;143:e455S–e497S.

434. Temel JS, Greer JA, Muzikansky A, et al. Early palliative care for patients with metastatic non-small-cell lung cancer. *N Engl J Med* 2010;363:733–742.

435. Movsas B, Moughan J, Sarna L, et al. Quality of life supersedes the classic prognosticators for long-term survival in locally advanced non-small-cell lung cancer: an analysis of RTOG 9801. *J Clin Oncol* 2009;27:5816–5822.

438. Sorensen S, Helweg-Larsen S, Mouridsen H, et al. Effect of high-dose dexamethasone in carcinomatous metastatic spinal cord compression treated with radiotherapy: a randomised trial. *Eur J Cancer* 1994;30a:22–27.

439. Patchell RA, Tibbs PA, Regine WF, et al. Direct decompressive surgical resection in the treatment of spinal cord compression caused by metastatic cancer: a randomised trial. *Lancet* 2005;366:643–648.

444. Patchell RA, Tibbs PA, Regine WF, et al. Postoperative radiotherapy in the treatment of single metastases to the brain: a randomized trial. *JAMA* 1998;280:1485–1489.

445. Andrews DW, Scott CB, Sperduto PW, et al. Whole brain radiation therapy with or without stereotactic radiosurgery boost for patients with one to three brain metastases: phase III results of the RTOG 9508 randomised trial. *Lancet* 2004;363:1665–1672.

446. Chang EL, Wefel JS, Hess KR, et al. Neurocognition in patients with brain metastases treated with radiosurgery or radiosurgery plus whole-brain irradiation: a randomised controlled trial. *Lancet Oncol* 2009;10:1037–1044.

447. Tsao MN, Rades D, Wirth A, et al. Radiotherapeutic and surgical management for newly diagnosed brain metastasis(es): an American Society for Radiation Oncology evidence-based guideline. *Pract Radiat Oncol* 2012;2:210–225.

448. Wilson LD, Detterbeck FC, Yahalom J. Clinical practice. Superior vena cava syndrome with malignant causes. *N Engl J Med* 2007;356:1862–1869.

450. Yu JB, Wilson LD, Detterbeck FC. Superior vena cava syndrome—a proposed classification system and algorithm for management. *J Thorac Oncol* 2008;3:811–814.

PRACTICE OF ONCOLOGY

42 Small Cell and Neuroendocrine Tumors of the Lung

M. Catherine Pietanza, Lee M. Krug, Abraham J. Wu, Mark G. Kris, Charles M. Rudin, and William D. Travis

SMALL CELL LUNG CANCER

Incidence and Etiology

Although the incidence of small cell lung cancer (SCLC) is declining, it remains a worldwide public health problem. The Surveillance, Epidemiologic, and End Results (SEER) database reports the proportion of SCLC cases among all lung cancers in the United States decreased from 17% to 13% in the past 30 years (Fig. 42.1),[1] whereas the age-adjusted rates per 100,000 decreased from 10.65 in 1990 to 6.74 in 2010.[2] Among the predicted 228,190 lung cancer cases in the United States in 2013,[3] an estimated 29,665 cases of SCLC were diagnosed.

Only 2% to 3% of patients with this malignancy are never smokers[4,5]; thus, as tobacco exposure causes SCLC in over 97% of cases, its incidence rates mirror smoking patterns. Peak cigarette consumption occurred in the 1960s, but declined following the Surgeon General's report linking smoking to cancer and the subsequent ban on tobacco advertising on television.[6] The percentage of men who smoke decreased from 50% in 1965 to 21.6% in 2011, which is a much greater proportional reduction than in women, who went from a rate of 32% to 16.5% during the same time period.[6,7] Correspondingly, the incidence of SCLC in men peaked in 1984 and since has been trending steadily down, whereas in women, the incidence peaked later and only has declined slightly.[8] The gender gap has narrowed such that currently about half of the patients diagnosed with SCLC are women (see Fig. 42.1).

Anatomy and Pathology

Neuroendocrine tumors of the lung encompass a spectrum of tumors, including low-grade typical carcinoid, intermediate-grade atypical carcinoid, high-grade large cell neuroendocrine carcinoma (LCNEC), and SCLC.[9] Because of their shared neuroendocrine properties, these tumors have common morphologic, ultrastructural, immunohistochemical, and molecular features. Despite this, there are also important differences in clinical, epidemiologic, histologic, and molecular characteristics.

SCLC is readily diagnosed on small specimens such as bronchoscopic biopsies, fine-needle aspirates, core biopsies, and cytology. The diagnosis of SCLC is based primarily on light microscopy (Fig. 42.2A): dense sheets of small cells with scant cytoplasm, finely granular nuclear chromatin, inconspicuous or absent nucleoli, and frequent mitoses. Necrosis is common and frequently shows large areas. The tumor cells usually measure less than the diameter of three small resting lymphocytes. They are round to be fusiform in shape and have scant cytoplasm. The nuclear chromatin is finely granular and nucleoli are inconspicuous or absent.[9–11] The mitotic rate is characteristically high, averaging 60 to 80 per 2 mm². Crush artifact is a frequent finding in small transbronchial or mediastinal biopsy specimens and can make pathologic interpretation difficult. The tumor cells of SCLC also have a tendency to show a streaming artifact. This can also occur with non–small-cell lung cancer (NSCLC), lymphoma, and chronic inflammation. In surgically resected specimens where the tumor cells achieve better fixation, the cells of SCLC appear larger than in small biopsies.[10,12] When a component of NSCLC, including adenocarcinoma, squamous cell carcinoma, large cell carcinoma, spindle cell carcinoma, and giant cell carcinoma, is present, the term *combined SCLC* is used with mention of the specific histology of the non–small-cell component.[9,10] In resected specimens, combined SCLC may occur in up to 28% of cases.[10] To diagnose combined SCLC and large cell carcinoma, the large cell carcinoma component must comprise at least 10% of the overall tumor.[9,10]

The following immunohistochemical stains are helpful in difficult cases. A pancytokeratin antibody such as AE1/AE3 is useful to confirm if the tumor is a carcinoma. Neuroendocrine differentiation can be demonstrated using a panel of markers such as CD56, chromogranin, and synaptophysin. However, up to 10% of SCLCs may be negative for all neuroendocrine markers.[13] A high proliferation rate of 80% to 100% should be seen with Ki-67. Thyroid transcription factor-1 (TTF-1) is positive in 70% to 80% of small cell carcinomas.[14–16] Notably, TTF-1 can be positive in extrapulmonary small cell carcinomas, so it is not useful in determining the primary site of small cell carcinomas.[17]

Genetics

SCLC has been characterized by frequent inactivating mutations in the critical tumor suppressor genes *TP53* (75% to 90%)[18] and *RB1* (60% to 90%).[19,20] A mouse model with conditional inactivation of these two tumor suppressors in the lung generates lung tumors histologically and biologically similar to human SCLC.[21]

Recent reports including exome, transcriptome, and limited whole genome sequencing have provided insights into the fuller landscape of genetic alterations in SCLC.[22,23] In addition to confirming *TP53* and *RB1* inactivation, these studies define other alterations of interest in SCLC, with potential therapeutic implications. One consistent finding from both reports was an exceptionally high degree of genomic alteration in this tumor type, including mutations, insertions, deletions, large scale copy number alterations, and gross inter- and intrachromosomal rearrangements. *MYC* family member alterations, including gene amplification of *MYC*, *MYCN*, and *MYCL1*, as well as a recurrent gene fusion involving *MYCL1*, are frequent in SCLC and may represent important drivers of SCLC oncogenesis. The tumor suppressor phosphatase and tensin homolog (*PTEN*) appears to be inactivated in approximately 10% of SCLC, and mutations of other factors in the same signaling pathway were also identified. Other alterations implicated as potential drivers in subsets of SCLC include amplification of the tyrosine kinase *FGFR1* (in 6% of cases) and of the developmental regulator and transcription factor *SOX2* (in up to 27% of cases). The therapeutic implications of the large majority of

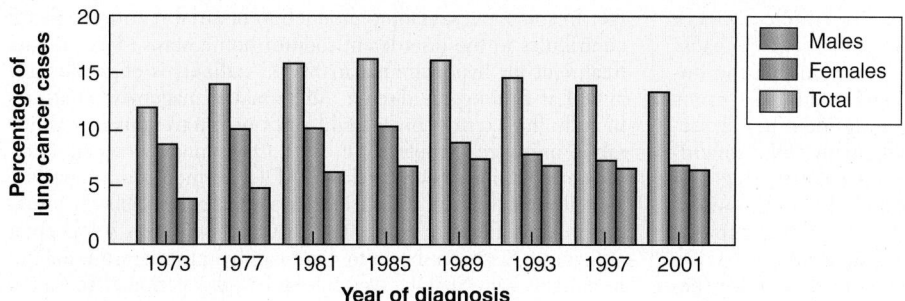

Figure 42.1 Patients diagnosed with small cell lung cancer as a percentage of all lung cancer cases and the breakdown by gender.

the genetic alterations documented to date in SCLC have not been defined.

Several reports have described the rare phenomenon of transformation to SCLC as a mechanism of acquired resistance to epidermal growth factor receptor (EGFR) tyrosine-kinase inhibitors (TKI) in patients initially treated for *EGFR*-mutant lung adenocarcinomas.[4] Of those cases with acquired resistance to EGFR TKIs, 3% to 14% will undergo SCLC transformation. Importantly, pure SCLC lack *EGFR* mutations and *ALK* rearrangements, even in those patients with this malignancy who are never smokers.[4,24] However, in the rare cases of SCLC transformation as a mechanism of acquired resistance to EGFR TKIs, there is persistence of the original *EGFR* mutation in the tumors confirmed on biopsy. In all cases where SCLC has been documented as a mechanism of

acquired resistance to EGFR TKIs, the original tumor was a pure adenocarcinoma prior to EGFR TKI treatment, and the transformation was validated by histologic examination and confirmed by expression of neuroendocrine markers.

Screening

Screening computed tomography (CT) scans detect NSCLCs at an earlier stage compared to chest x-ray (CXR), or no screening, and can decrease lung cancer–specific mortality in heavy smokers.[25] However, the natural history of SCLC is characterized by rapid tumor growth and early metastatic spread. As such, the diagnosis of SCLC in an asymptomatic patient is rare.

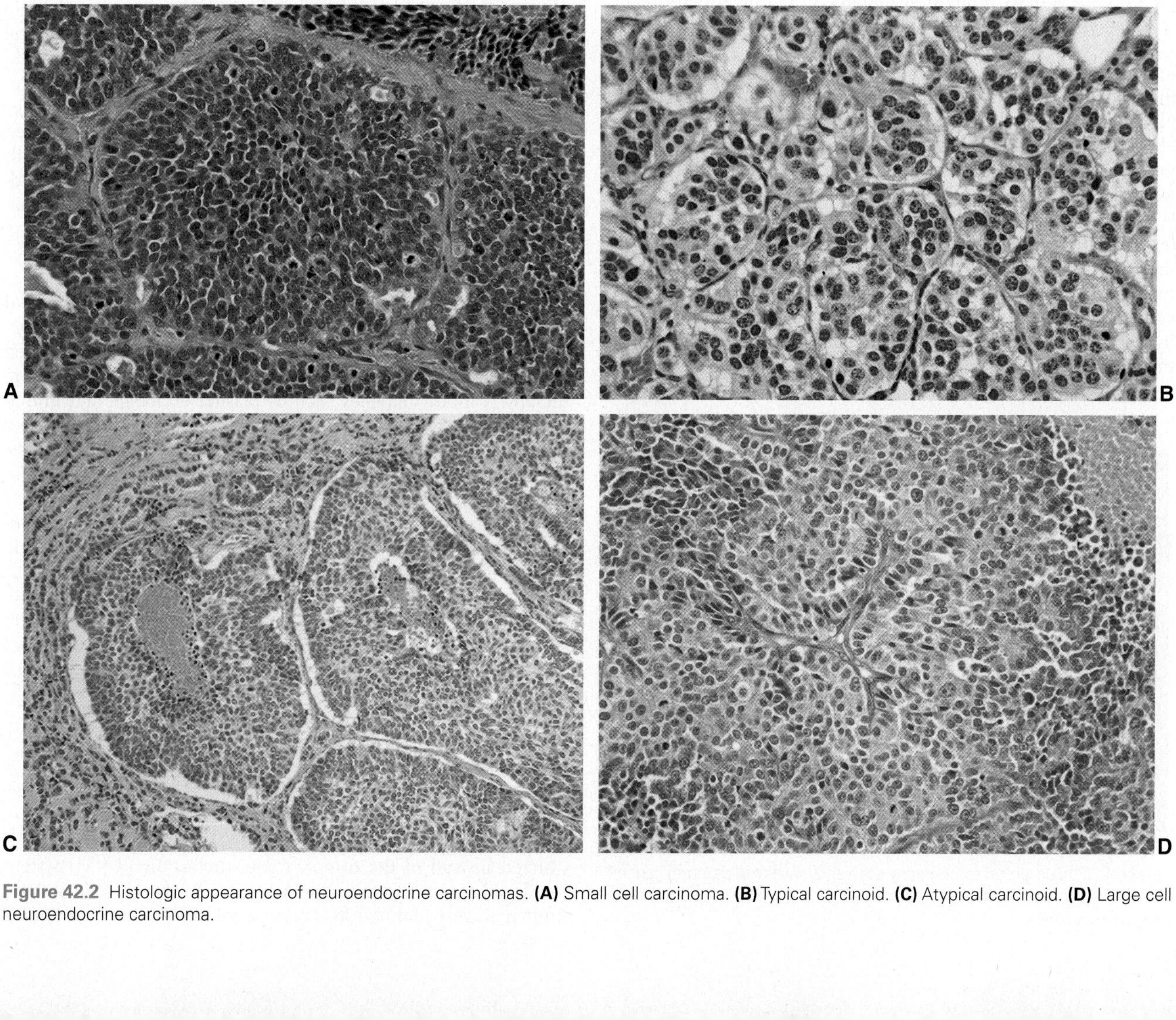

Figure 42.2 Histologic appearance of neuroendocrine carcinomas. **(A)** Small cell carcinoma. **(B)** Typical carcinoid. **(C)** Atypical carcinoid. **(D)** Large cell neuroendocrine carcinoma.

PRACTICE OF ONCOLOGY

The National Lung Screening Trial (NLST) enrolled 53,454 Americans age 55 to 74 years with a history of at least 30 pack-years of cigarette smoking, and randomly assigned them to undergo three annual screenings with either low-dose CT scans (LDCT) or standard CXR. LDCT screening identified a preponderance of adenocarcinomas, including many with bronchioloalveolar subtype. SCLCs were not detected at early stages by either LDCT or CXR in the NLST. Although the study demonstrated a reduction in lung-cancer specific mortality compared to CXR, the similar rates and patterns of detection of SCLC make it unlikely that LDCT screening will reduce mortality specific to SCLC. Therefore, screening for SCLC by any method is not recommended.[25]

Diagnosis

Presenting symptoms in patients with SCLC can be constitutional, pulmonary, the result of extrathoracic spread, or due to paraneoplastic disorders.[26,27] In one series in which patient-reported symptoms were recorded using the Lung Cancer Symptom Scale, fatigue was the most common, symptom with decreased physical activity, cough, dyspnea, decreased appetite, weight loss, and pain occurring sometime in the course of the illness in the majority of patients.[27] Hemoptysis was noted in 14% in the same series.[27] The primary tumor often presents as a large central mass invading or compressing the mediastinum. Superior vena cava obstruction is present at diagnosis in 10% of patients with SCLC (Fig. 42.3),[28] and in these cases, the symptoms are often worsened by associated thrombosis in the compromised blood vessel. Chest imaging typically shows hilar and mediastinal adenopathy. Rarely, SCLC presents as a solitary pulmonary nodule.[29,30] No more than 2% of SCLC present as a superior sulcus tumor.[31]

Most patients with SCLC have metastases at diagnosis. Bone involvement is usually characterized by osteolytic lesions, often in the absence of bone pain, or elevations in the serum alkaline phosphatase.[32] Osteoblastic bone metastases do occur in some patients. Hepatic and adrenal lesions are typically asymptomatic. Brain metastases can be detected in at least 18% of patients at diagnosis,[33] which are often asymptomatic.

Paraneoplastic syndromes are common in SCLC and differ from those observed with NSCLC. SCLC accounts for approximately 75% of the tumors associated with the syndrome of inappropriate antidiuretic hormone (SIADH). Although serum concentrations of antidiuretic hormone are elevated in the majority of those with SCLC, only approximately 10% of patients fulfill the criteria of SIADH, and symptoms are present in no more than

5%. In some cases, ectopic production of atrial natriuretic factor contributes to the disorder in sodium homeostasis. The primary treatment for hyponatremia in SCLC patients is chemotherapy aimed at treating the disease. Additional management strategies include fluid restriction in mild cases or intravenous hypertonic saline in severe, symptomatic cases. Older pharmacologic interventions that have been used in SIADH, include demeclocycline and lithium, both of which induce nephrogenic diabetes insipidus.[34] More recently, tolvaptan, an oral vasopressin V2-receptor antagonist, has been shown to significantly improve serum sodium in patients with SIADH over a 4- and 30-day period.[35] Tolvaptan therapy should be initiated while patients are in the hospital to allow monitoring of the therapeutic response. Increased serum levels of adrenocorticotropic hormone can be detected in up to 50% of patients with lung cancer, but Cushing syndrome develops in only 5% of patients with SCLC. Low serum sodium is an adverse prognostic factor,[36] and patients with Cushing syndrome have a very limited survival.[37] The primary treatment of Cushing syndrome in SCLC patients is chemotherapy, although agents such as ketoconazole and mitotane have been used.[38] Hypercalcemia is rare in SCLC.

Paraneoplastic neurologic disorders seen in patients with SCLC include sensory, sensorimotor, and autoimmune neuropathies and encephalomyelitis.[39] These syndromes are thought to occur through autoimmune mechanisms, and antinuclear antibodies that bind to SCLC and to neuronal tissues have been identified. Symptoms may precede the diagnosis by many months and are often the presenting complaint. They may also be the initial sign of relapse from remission. An aggressive search may be required to discover small tumor nodules causing profound neurologic syndromes. Subacute peripheral sensory neuropathy associated with the anti-Hu antibody may be the most frequent paraneoplastic neurologic disorder seen in those with SCLC. Less common is the Lambert-Eaton syndrome, characterized by proximal muscle weakness that improves with continued use, hyporeflexia, and dysautonomia. Classic electromyographic findings confirm the diagnosis. The cause is related to autoantibody impairment of voltage-gated calcium channels. Rarer neurologic disorders seen in patients with SCLC include cerebellar degeneration or retinopathy. Two studies conflicted when evaluating whether the presence of paraneoplastic antibodies have prognostic implications[40,41]; the utilization of different techniques to measure antibody levels may account for the discrepant results.[42]

In contrast to the endocrine syndromes, for which successful treatment of the tumor effectively controls the symptoms, the occurrence and severity of the neurologic symptoms is unrelated to tumor bulk and usually does not resolve with antineoplastic therapy. Various therapies such as plasma exchange and immunosuppressive therapy with agents such as corticosteroids, cyclophosphamide, and tacrolimus have been tried, but generally offer little benefit. In patients with Lambert-Eaton syndrome, two randomized placebo-controlled trials of 3,4 diaminopyridine, which blocks potassium channel efflux from nerve terminals, demonstrated that treatment with this agent increases compound muscle action potentials and significantly improves muscle strength.[43] In a randomized trial with a crossover design, intravenous immunoglobulin also improved limb strength as measured by myometry over placebo in 10 patients with Lambert-Eaton syndrome.[43] However, the benefit was short lived and began to dissipate after just 8 weeks.

Staging

A simple two-stage system, introduced by the Veterans' Administration Lung Study Group (VALSG), has historically been utilized instead of the tumor, node, metastasis (TNM) system employed for most other cancer types.[44] In the VALSG system, limited stage is defined as disease confined to one hemithorax

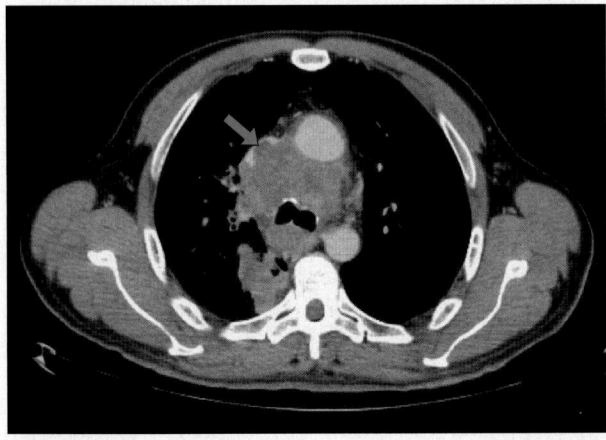

Figure 42.3 Computed tomography scan showing small cell lung cancer with an infiltrative mediastinal mass causing compression of the superior vena cava (*arrow*).

that can be "encompassed" in a "tolerable" radiation field. These patients currently are treated with a combined modality approach. All other patients are considered to have extensive-stage disease. At presentation, approximately two-thirds of patients with SCLC have extensive disease and one-third have limited-stage disease.[1]

In the VALSG staging system, the appropriate classification of ipsilateral pleural effusion, supraclavicular lymphadenopathy (ipsilateral or contralateral), or contralateral mediastinal lymphadenopathy as either limited or extensive stage remains controversial. Some large series have not found a survival difference between patients with an isolated ipsilateral pleural effusion and other patients with limited SCLC.[45] However, analyses of two large cooperative group databases, which included over 4,000 patients, showed that the survival of individuals with an isolated effusion was similar to that of patients with extensive disease.[46,47] In clinical practice, it is assumed that an effusion is malignant unless three criteria are met: the fluid is transudative, nonhemorrhagic, and cytologically negative on repeated examinations. Patients with a malignant effusion are appropriate to exclude from a combined modality treatment because hemithoracic radiotherapy to encompass the entirety of the pleura is impractical.

The presence of supraclavicular lymphadenopathy commonly is associated with extensive disease but, when encountered in patients with otherwise limited disease (5% of cases), carries a trend toward poorer survival.[47] Contralateral mediastinal involvement also is usually classified as limited-stage disease. However, two studies that evaluated twice-a-day radiation regimens excluded patients with contralateral hilar disease to reduce the normal lung volume irradiated and the risk for toxicity.[48,49]

For patients who appear to have limited-stage SCLC, some additional tests may be appropriate to confirm this assessment. Unilateral iliac crest bone marrow aspiration and biopsy are still a routine part of staging for many oncologists and should be performed in limited-stage patients with elevations of serum lactate dehydrogenase (LDH)[50,51] and evidence of myelophthisis (nucleated red blood cells, leukopenia, or thrombocytopenia) on the peripheral blood smear. If there is evidence of a pleural effusion, a thoracentesis or thoracoscopy may help confirm that the effusion is nonbloody, transudative, and cytologically negative. Effusions too small to permit image-guided sampling should not be considered in staging.[52] Osseous abnormalities seen on positron-emission tomography (PET) or bone scan require confirmation with magnetic resonance imaging (MRI), CT scan, or biopsy if they represent the only disease site that makes a patient extensive stage.

For the American Joint Committee on Cancer (AJCC) seventh edition, the use of a TNM staging system for SCLC has been revisited. To establish the accuracy of outcomes based on stage, cases of completely resected SCLC were staged using the same definitions as used for NSCLC.[53] The use of pathologic stage was necessary to accurately stage the patients used for this analysis. More favorable outcomes of patients have been reported in patients previously classified as *very limited* disease (i.e., no evidence of mediastinal metastases by CT or mediastinoscopy) treated with chemotherapy and radiation, as compared with other patients with limited-stage disease.[54–56] The use of the TNM system is best applied for cases of early stage disease and may have less relevance for the majority of patients presenting with metastatic disease.

Clinical and Serologic Predictive and Prognostic Factors

Multivariable analyses suggest that performance status is a strong and reproducible predictive and prognostic factor.[47,57,58] Poorer performance status can additionally identify individuals at higher risk for treatment-related complications. Several other clinical

parameters have been proposed. Female gender has been associated with improved response and survival in patients with SCLC.[47,57,58] Older age (variably defined) has not been identified as an adverse prognostic factor in patients with SCLC in most[59–62] but not all[36,46,47] series. Older age has been associated with decreased performance status and more comorbid illnesses and often results in compromised chemotherapy dose intensity,[63,64] which may partially explain its prognostic implications. Certain metastatic sites, such as the liver,[65–67] the brain,[66,68] bone marrow,[67] and bone,[68] as well as the total number of metastatic sites involved,[47] have been found to be of prognostic significance for patients with extensive-stage disease. Paraneoplastic Cushing syndrome has been correlated with a poor response to therapy and short survival.[37] Continued use of tobacco during combined modality therapy was identified as an adverse prognostic factor in a group of 186 patients with limited disease.[69] Elevation of serum LDH is found in 33% to 57% of all patients with SCLC and up to 85% of patients with extensive-stage disease and is a strong prognostic and predictive factor.[46,57,65,66,68,70–72] Serum LDH elevation is associated with the presence of bone marrow involvement.[50] Although many other serum markers have been proposed to have prognostic significance, including neuron-specific enolase,[61,66] chromogranin, and precursors of gastrin-releasing peptide,[73,74] none have been strong and reliable enough to warrant general use. Carcinoembryonic antigen (CEA) has been found to predict outcome in SCLC in multiple series.[57,75,76]

Management by Stage

General Recommendations for Initial Management

Once the pathologic diagnosis of SCLC is confirmed, a complete history and physical examination is the next step. Special attention should be paid to the cigarette smoking history. If a patient is a current smoker, he or she should be advised to quit immediately in the strongest terms and offered the most aggressive smoking cessation intervention available.[69] If the patient is a never smoker, the pathologic diagnosis of SCLC should be reviewed as only 2% to 3% of never smokers develop SCLC.[4,5] The National Comprehensive Cancer Network (NCCN) has compiled consensus guidelines for the initial evaluation of individuals with SCLC.[52] A complete blood cell count (CBC) with platelet count, electrolytes, calcium, creatinine, blood urea nitrogen (BUN), liver function tests, and LDH are recommended. All patients should undergo a contrast-enhanced CT scan of the chest, a gadolinium-enhanced MRI of the head, and whole-body PET or a bone scan. A PET scan can identify sites of metastases undetected by other modalities[77–79] and can replace the bone scan.[80]

All fit patients (Karnofsky performance status greater than 60% or Eastern Cooperative Oncology Group [ECOG] performance status 0, 1, or 2) should initially receive combination chemotherapy with etoposide plus either cisplatin or carboplatin for four to six cycles (Fig. 42.4).[52] Supportive data, specifics of chemotherapy regimens, duration of therapy, and alternatives for patients with contraindications or special needs are discussed in the sections that follow. Patients with limited-stage disease should receive the chemotherapy concurrently with twice-daily thoracic irradiation beginning with the first, second, or third cycle.[49,81,82] Patients who achieve a response to chemotherapy should receive prophylactic whole-brain radiotherapy at the conclusion of chemotherapy or chemoradiotherapy.[83] There is no routine recommendation for the treatment of patients who have a Karnofsky performance status of 50% or less or ECOG performance status 3 or 4. Because the toxicity of all treatment worsens and effectiveness lessens in patients with a low performance status, clinicians must carefully evaluate the agent(s) used and the appropriateness and goals of therapy individually. For many patients in this low performance status group, supportive care only and referral to hospice are the best options.

Treatment Paradigm for Small Cell Lung Cancer

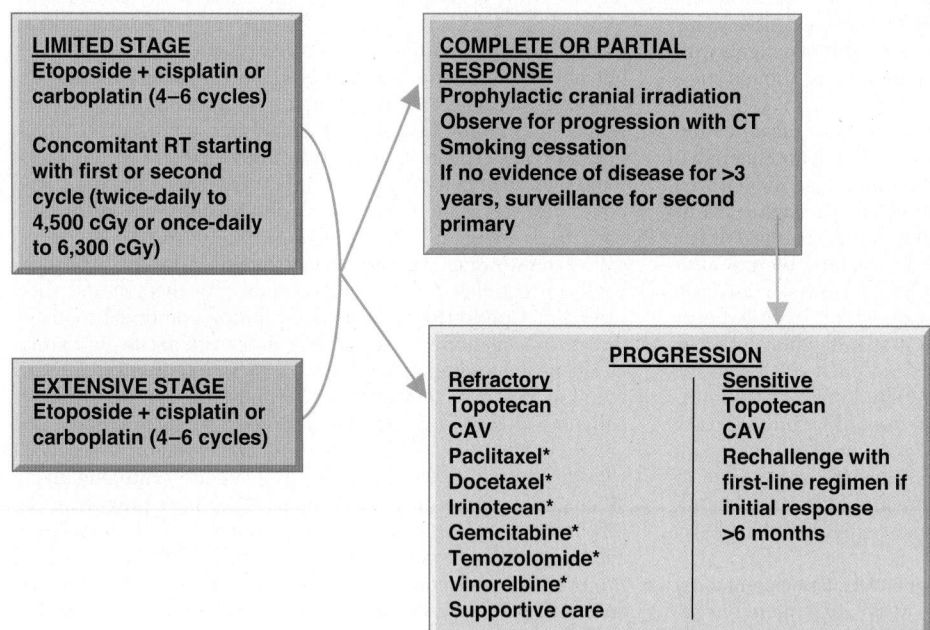

Figure 42.4 General treatment paradigm for small cell lung cancer. *Single agents evaluated in phase II trials with activity in SCLC.

Chemotherapy

Evolution of Chemotherapy Regimens. The sensitivity of SCLC to chemotherapy agents was recognized about 50 years ago, and the primary role of systemic treatment in SCLC was established early on. Alkylating agents, anthracyclines, vinca alkaloids, and antifolates all showed single-agent efficacy. In the 1980s, the epipodophyllotoxin, etoposide, and the platinum analogs, cisplatin and carboplatin, were introduced, and their activity ranged from 40% to 60% in previously untreated patients.[84] Since then, numerous other chemotherapeutic agents have demonstrated activity in SCLC, but aside from the camptothecins, the drugs identified in the 1970s and 1980s remain the backbone of therapy. Ultimately, randomized trials of combinations demonstrated superior activity to single agents.[85,86]

Livingston et al.[87] developed the cyclophosphamide, doxorubicin, vincristine (CAV) combination, and reported on 358 patients who received this combination followed sequentially by thoracic and brain irradiation. For patients with extensive disease, the complete response rate was 14%, the overall response rate was 57%, and the median survival was 26 weeks. For patients with limited disease, the rates were 41%, 75%, and 52 weeks, respectively. With these data, CAV became the standard chemotherapy regimen.

With the identification of etoposide as perhaps the most active agent, several modifications of the CAV regimen that included etoposide were tested. A randomized trial showed greater response duration and survival with cyclophosphamide, doxorubicin, and etoposide (CAE) compared with CAV.[88] Hong et al.[89] compared intensive cyclophosphamide and vincristine (CV) (with the dose of cyclophosphamide increased from 1,000 to 2,000 mg/m^2) to CAV and to cyclophosphamide, etoposide, and vincristine (CEV) and reported that patients treated with CV had a shorter survival and experienced more myelosuppression than those treated on the other two arms. Five randomized trials have evaluated the addition of etoposide (CAVE) to the CAV regimen.[90–94] In the three studies in which the doses of CAV were equivalent in each arm,[90–92] a better response rate was evident in the arm that contained etoposide, in at least some patient subsets, with increased hematologic toxicity, although a nonstatistical improvement in survival was seen in only one study.[90] Two studies intensified components of this regimen in the CAV arm compared to the CAVE arm,[93] leading to equivalent myelotoxicity, response rates, and survival.

The etoposide/cisplatin (EP) regimen was tested in SCLC cases because this combination produced synergistic activity in preclinical systems. In addition, both agents could be given at full doses because of less myelosuppression with cisplatin. The first report by Sierocki et al.[95] at Memorial Sloan-Kettering Cancer Center in 1979 demonstrated the activity of this combination in SCLC. Subsequent studies by Evans et al.[96,97] reported response rates of 55% in patients previously treated with CAV and 86% in newly diagnosed patients. Einhorn et al.[98] reported that two cycles of consolidation with EP, when added to the treatment of patients with limited disease who were responding to six cycles of CAV, produced longer survival than with CAV only. Three randomized trials have compared EP to cyclophosphamide, vincristine, and an anthracycline.[99–101] Less myelosuppression occurred with EP, and, if given with radiation, patients experienced less esophagitis and interstitial pneumonitis. Furthermore, the largest trial showed that EP produced a better median (15 months versus 10 months) and 5-year (10% versus 3%) survival for patients with limited disease.[101] Retrospective analyses and meta-analyses also support the superiority of cisplatin- or carboplatin-containing chemotherapy for SCLC.[102–104] As a result, EP is now the standard first-line chemotherapy regimen for SCLC (Table 42.1).

Carboplatin has been substituted for cisplatin in SCLC chemotherapy regimens in an effort to decrease nonhematologic toxicities. Randomized trials comparing cisplatin and carboplatin suggest that they may have similar efficacy. The Hellenic Cooperative Oncology Group randomized 147 patients with either limited or extensive disease to receive etoposide 100 mg/m^2 days 1 to 3, and cisplatin 100 mg/m^2 or carboplatin 300 mg/m^2.[105] Concurrent radiation also was administered to responding patients starting with the third cycle. Response and survival were similar in the two arms. Nausea, vomiting, nephrotoxicity, and neurotoxicity were significantly lower in the patients who received carboplatin, as was grade 4 leukopenia. However, the sample size of this study is inadequate to confirm equivalent efficacy. A meta-analysis that evaluated individual subject data from four randomized trials with a total of 663 patients found that median overall survival (OS), median progression-free survival (PFS), and response rates were similar in the cisplatin and carboplatin arms. Although hematologic toxicities were higher in those patients that receive carboplatin, nonhematologic toxicities were increased in those that receive cisplatin.[106] Based on these data, etoposide and carboplatin can

TABLE 42.1

Randomized Clinical Trials Comparing Etoposide and Cisplatin to Other Chemotherapy Regimens

Study (Ref.)	Stage	Treatment Arm	No. of Patients	Overall Response Rate (%)	Median Survival (months)	1-Year Survival (%)	2-Year Survival (%)
Fukuoka, et al.[99]	Limited and extensive	EP	97	78	9.9	NR	12
		CAV	97	55	9.9	NR	10
		CAV/EP alternating	94	76	11.8 ($p = 0.056$)	NR	21
Roth, et al.[100]	Extensive	EP	159	61	8.6	NR	NR
		CAV	156	51	8.3	NR	NR
		CAV/EP alternating	162	59	8.1	NR	NR
Sundstrom, et al.[101]	Limited and extensive	EP	218	NR	10.2 ($p = 0.0004$)	NR	14
		Cyclophosphate, epirubicin, vincristine	218	NR	7.8	NR	6
Skarlos, et al.[105]	Limited and extensive	EP	71	69	12.5	NR	NR
		Etoposide/carboplatin	72	78	11.8	NR	NR
Noda, et al.[108]	Extensive	EP	77	52	9.4	58	20
		Irinotecan/cisplatin	77	65	12.8 ($p = 0.002$)	38	5
Hanna, et al.[425]	Extensive	EP	110	44	10.2	35	8
		Irinotecan/cisplatin	221	48	9.3	35	8
Lara, et al.[109]	Extensive	EP	327	57	9.1	34	NR
		Irinotecan/cisplatin	324	60	9.9	41	NR
Eckardt, et al.[115]	Extensive	EP	395	69	9.4	31	NR
		Oral topotecan/cisplatin	389	63	9.2	31	NR
Miyamoto, et al.[130]	Limited and extensive	EP	45	78	12.8	53	15
		Ifosfamide with EP	47	74	13.0	62	17
Loehrer, et al.[131]	Extensive	EP	84	67	7.3	27	5
		Ifosfamide with EP	87	73	9.1 ($p = 0.045$)	36	13
Mavroudis, et al.[135]	Limited and extensive	EP	71	48	10.5	37	NR
		Paclitaxel with EP	62	50	9.5	38	NR
Niell, et al.[136]	Extensive	EP	282	68	9.9	37	8
		Paclitaxel with EP	283	75	10.6	38	11

EP, etoposide and cisplatin; CAV, cyclophosphamide, doxorubicin, and vincristine; NR, not reported.

be considered an appropriate first-line regimen, particularly in patients who cannot tolerate cisplatin.

More recently, platinum combinations with topotecan and irinotecan have emerged as potential regimens for initial therapy. Irinotecan was shown to have single-agent efficacy in Japanese studies.[107] The Japan Clinical Oncology Group compared cisplatin and irinotecan to EP as initial treatment in extensive disease.[108] The study was terminated after 154 of the planned 230 patients were enrolled because median (12.8 months versus 9.4 months) and 2-year (19.5% versus 5.2%) survival were significantly better in the group treated with cisplatin and irinotecan. Significant diarrhea occurred only in the irinotecan group, and myelosuppression was the most common toxicity in both groups and more frequent with EP. Two confirmatory studies were subsequently launched in the United States. In the first trial, the irinotecan/cisplatin schedule was modified in an effort to decrease toxicity, leading to equivalent response rates (48% for irinotecan/cisplatin versus 44% for EP), median time to progression (4 versus 5 months), and median OS (9 versus 10 months).[425] The Southwest Oncology Group (SWOG) compared these two regimens with the same dose and schedule used in the Japanese trial and also showed, in a well-powered study, that outcomes are equivalent with the two regimens in Caucasian patients.[109] High response rates have been reported in several trials using irinotecan and carboplatin with varied dosing schedules.[110,111] A phase III trial comparing that regimen with etoposide/cisplatin showed improved survival, but

the median survival of 7 months in the control arm, which used oral etoposide, was lower than expected.[112] Many hypothesize that population-based polymorphisms in uridine 5′-diphospho (UDP)-glucuronosyltransferase (UGT1A1), the enzyme responsible for detoxifying SN-38, the active metabolite of irinotecan, may account for differences in toxicity and efficacy between Japanese and Americans.[113] The regimen of topotecan plus cisplatin also has undergone phase II and III testing.[114,115] Eckardt et al.[115] reported the results of a randomized trial including 784 patients in which patients received oral topotecan (1.7 mg/m^2 per day for 5 days) plus cisplatin, or standard etoposide and cisplatin. The response rates, median survival, and 1-year survival were identical. Severe neutropenia occurred more often with EP, but oral topotecan and cisplatin caused more anemia and thrombocytopenia.

Strategies to Improve Outcomes with Chemotherapy Regimens

Alternating Cycles of Combination Chemotherapy Regimens. The recognition of clonal heterogeneity within a tumor and the intolerability of treatment regimens that included more than four drugs due to overlapping toxicity led to trials of alternating chemotherapy combinations. The somatic mutation model developed by Goldie et al.[116] predicted that the best probability of cure was achieved by the earliest possible introduction and the most rapid alternation of all active agents. If two equally effective non–cross-resistant regimens were available, the model predicted that alternating between regimens every other cycle would be more effective than alternating after every three cycles or giving one regimen continuously for five cycles before switching to the second regimen.

Many randomized clinical trials have tested the concept of alternating multidrug combinations.[100,117–121] The fact that the EP regimen was effective in patients who had progressed after cyclophosphamide-based chemotherapy suggested that these drug combinations were non–cross-resistant.[122] With this in mind, the National Cancer Institute of Canada conducted a study in which 289 patients were randomized to CAV or CAV alternating with EP.[119] Chemotherapy was given for a total of six cycles. The response rate (65% versus 47%), PFS, and median survival time (10 months versus 8 months) favored the patients who had received alternating therapy. The authors postulated that these findings could be the result of the inclusion of a more active regimen (i.e., EP) within the alternating arm, an advantage due to greater drug diversity with five effective drugs rather than three, or support of the Goldie et al. concept. A Japanese study compared CAV to EP to alternating CAV/EP in 288 patients with limited or extensive stage disease.[99] Patients with limited disease received four cycles of chemotherapy followed by thoracic irradiation and were found to have improved survival with the alternating regimen compared with CAV ($p = 0.058$) or EP ($p = 0.032$). No differences in survival were noted in the patients with extensive disease. Roth et al.[100] evaluated 437 patients with extensive disease in a randomized trial comparing EP for four cycles, CAV for six cycles, or CAV alternating with EP for a total of six cycles. Although a slight improvement occurred in PFS ($p = 0.052$) with the alternating regimen, there was no difference in response rate or OS among the treatment arms. The patients whose tumors did not respond to CAV and were crossed over to EP were twice as likely to benefit as individuals who initially received EP and were crossed over to CAV, although these differences were not significant (28% versus 14% for induction responders who relapsed and 15% versus 8% for patients with primary resistance). The modest activity seen when refractory patients were crossed over from one of these regimens to the other suggests that the CAV and EP combinations are not entirely cross-resistant, which works against a primary assumption of the Goldie et al. hypothesis. Taking all of these studies together, alternating regimens appears to have slight or no benefit over initial treatment with EP alone.

Additional studies have evaluated alternating chemotherapy introduced after achieving a response to an induction regimen.[123–125] The National Cancer Institute of Canada designed a randomized trial in which 300 patients with limited disease received either CAV for three cycles followed by EP for three cycles or CAV alternating with EP for a total of six cycles.[126] Response rates, time to treatment failure, or survival did not differ. Wolf et al.[123] randomized 321 patients to treatment with ifosfamide plus etoposide given until a response plateau, followed by CAV or ifosfamide plus etoposide alternating with CAV. A total of six cycles of chemotherapy were delivered in each arm. No difference in outcome was noted.

Studies also have evaluated alternating more intensive regimens. For example, a German multicenter trial demonstrated that an alternating eight-drug regimen was superior to CAV.[127] Two other European trials testing three drugs regimens alternating with four drug regimens found no survival advantage to that approach.[120,128] Again, the median survival times observed in these studies were no different from those that used EP alone.[99,100]

Addition of a Third Chemotherapeutic Agent to Etoposide Plus Cisplatin. All efforts to add a third drug to the standard EP regimen have resulted in more toxicity with little or no improvement in survival. The three-drug regimen of etoposide, ifosfamide, and cisplatin (VIP), developed initially for refractory germ cell tumors, also has been evaluated in SCLC.[129] In randomized trials comparing VIP to EP, one study, which included patients with limited and extensive disease, found no difference in survival between the two treatment groups,[130] whereas another, which was larger and enrolled only patients with extensive disease, identified a significant difference in median survival (9 months versus 7 months) and 2-year survival rates (13% versus 5%).[131] In both studies, myelosuppression was more severe in the ifosfamide-containing arm. Single-arm studies substituting carboplatin for cisplatin in ifosfamide, carboplatin, and etoposide (ICE) have shown impressive response rates, yet cumulative myelosuppression.[132,133] A large trial comparing ICE plus a midcycle dose of vincristine to other standard therapy demonstrated an improvement in the median and 1-year survival rates.[134] However, an increased rate of septicemia was noted with ifosfamide, carboplatin, and etoposide-vincristine (ICE-V) (15% versus 7% in the control arm).

Studies that added paclitaxel to EP reach the same conclusion: enhanced toxicity with similar efficacy. Two studies that compared EP to EP plus paclitaxel showed that the addition of the third drug increased toxicity, as well as treatment-related mortality, without improving survival.[135,136] A German study that added paclitaxel to etoposide and carboplatin demonstrated a significantly better median survival (13 months versus 12 months) and 3-year survival (17% versus 9%) only in patients with limited disease as compared to treatment with etoposide, carboplatin, and vincristine.[137]

Maintenance Therapy. A large number of randomized studies have examined whether maintenance chemotherapy prolongs survival in SCLC.[117,138–148] Three studies that randomized patients in complete remission after induction therapy to maintenance treatment or observation identified improved survival with the prolonged treatment program in some patient groups.[117,141,144] The Cancer and Leukemia Group B (CALGB) randomized 258 patients to one of four chemotherapy regimens, and 57 patients in complete remission underwent a second randomization to maintenance therapy or observation. Among the 46 patients with limited disease who proceeded to the second randomization, the median survival was improved with maintenance chemotherapy (17 months versus 7 months).[144] However, the initial regimens used in this study might be considered inferior to currently used treatments. In a second study, patients treated with six cycles of CAV and in complete remission were randomized to six additional cycles of the same chemotherapy or observation.[141] For the patients with extensive disease, the median survival was improved by approximately 4 months with maintenance treatment. In an ECOG trial, patients were randomized to CAV alternating with another three-drug combination or CAV alone and, subsequently, those in complete remission after six to eight cycles of induction underwent a second randomization to maintenance treatment or observation.[117] Patients assigned to CAV and maintenance therapy had a longer PFS and OS ($p = 0.09$) than patients who received only CAV with no maintenance. In contrast, for the patients who received the six-drug regimen, those who were given no maintenance survived longer than the patients who received maintenance treatment. These studies suggest that there may be patients—perhaps those with particularly chemotherapy-sensitive disease—who derive a benefit from maintenance. In unselected patients, however, clinical trials that have evaluated treatment programs that extend beyond six cycles of chemotherapy have not demonstrated an advantage in survival.

The Medical Research Council randomized 265 patients who had responded to six cycles of induction chemotherapy to an additional six cycles of maintenance or observation.[138] Overall, there was no difference in survival between patients treated with 6 or 12 cycles of chemotherapy, although for patients in complete remission at the time of randomization, a subset analysis suggested that maintenance provides a survival benefit. Three other large studies that randomized patients responding to 5 or 6 cycles of induction to a total of 12 cycles of chemotherapy or observation found no difference in outcome.[142,143,146] Another study that randomized patients with limited disease from the start of chemotherapy to a total of 6 or 12 cycles identified inferior survival in the arm treated with the longer course of therapy.[140]

Other studies have evaluated whether four cycles of chemotherapy are adequate.[139,145,149] Spiro et al.[149] designed a study that included a double randomization at diagnosis. Patients received four or eight cycles of CEV and on relapse were given additional chemotherapy or supportive care. Of the four treatment arms, patients who received four cycles of chemotherapy and only supportive care at relapse had a significantly inferior median survival of 30 weeks. Four cycles of treatment were found to be adequate, provided that chemotherapy was offered to patients appropriate for additional therapy at relapse. Two additional studies evaluated four cycles of induction with longer treatment programs. A European trial randomized patients with limited and extensive disease who responded to four cycles of EP to CAV for up to 10 additional cycles or to observation with no survival differences, although the study had limited power due to small sample size.[139] ECOG enrolled 402 eligible patients with extensive-stage disease into a trial that delivered four cycles of EP followed by a randomization of patients with at least stable disease to four additional cycles of topotecan or to observation.[145] Although maintenance therapy increased the time before documentation of disease progression, there was no difference in OS.

Two recent meta-analyses have been conducted evaluating maintenance chemotherapy showing small improvements in survival and an increase in toxicity.[150,151] Bozcuk and colleagues[150] reported an improved 1- and 2-year survival by 9% and 4%, respectively. Although Rossi et al.[151] showed a significant OS benefit (hazard ratio [HR], 0.89, 95% confidence interval [CI], 0.81 to 0.92; $p = 0.02$) for maintenance treatment, this improvement was projected to an additional 2 weeks.[151] Further, there was a high heterogeneity among the included trials.

In summary, four to six cycles of chemotherapy appear to be optimal in the management of limited and extensive SCLC. After the completion of this initial treatment, patients should be monitored closely and then offered further chemotherapy at the time of progression. Both the NCCN and the European Society of Medical Oncology Guidelines support this approach.[52,152]

Dose Intensification. In experimental models, numerous chemotherapy drugs display log-linear or near linear dose-response curves,[153] and high-dose chemotherapy has proven effective at treating hematologic diseases. It seemed reasonable to test the hypothesis that more intensive chemotherapy could improve outcomes in SCLC. Methods used have included the use of higher chemotherapy doses without or with hematopoietic growth factor support, shortened cycle length, or extreme dose intensification with marrow or peripheral blood stem cell support.

Several investigators evaluated whether increasing the dose of drugs beyond the usual dose improves survival.[154–159] Three randomized trials comparing standard versus high-dose CAV[156,158] or EP[157] found no difference in response rates or median survival. No hematopoietic growth factors were used in these three trials, and, as such, myelosuppression and infections were significantly more severe in the high-dose arms. A randomized trial that did utilize granulocyte-macrophage colony-stimulating factor (GM-CSF) with dose escalation found that excess toxicity actually resulted in lower drug delivery and poorer response and survival rates in the dose-intense arm.[159] Only a French study with 105 limited-stage patients demonstrated improvements in PFS at 2 years (28% versus 8%) and OS (43% versus 26%) with the administration of higher drug doses.[154] Few oncologists have embraced this approach.

A number of studies have evaluated whether shortening the interval between chemotherapy cycles improves survival. A multicenter study randomized 300 patients, mostly with limited-stage disease, to six cycles of ICE-V delivered every 4 weeks or every 3 weeks.[160] In a second randomization, patients were given GM-CSF or placebo after each chemotherapy cycle. The delivered dose intensity was increased by 26% in the group receiving chemotherapy every 3 weeks compared to those treated every 4 weeks. The median survival (443 days versus 351 days) and the

2-year survival rate (33% versus 18%) were better in the intensified arm ($p = 0.0014$). GM-CSF did not reduce the incidence or the duration of febrile neutropenia, and there was no difference in survival between the patients who received GM-CSF or placebo. In a subsequent study, ICE given every 4 weeks was compared to ICE given every 2 weeks with support of GM-CSF, and autologous blood collected before the cycle was reinfused 24 hours after the chemotherapy.[161] Although the median delivered dose intensity was increased by 82% without significant increased toxicity, no survival benefit was identified. Two studies compared treatment with cyclophosphamide, doxorubicin, and etoposide given either every 3 weeks, or every 2 weeks with GM-CSF support.[162,163] The larger trial,[163] which also included a higher percentage of limited-stage patients, showed an improvement in complete response rate and OS, but the other trial did not. No fewer than four randomized trials have shown that intensive multidrug weekly regimens are no better, yet significantly more toxic than standard regimens.[164–167]

Numerous reports cite the use of high-dose chemotherapy with autologous bone marrow or stem cell rescue for treating SCLC.[168–186] These studies have included small numbers of highly selected patients.[161,182,183,187–189] Survival has not been shown to be better than conventional treatment. As in other chemosensitive solid tumors like breast cancer, high-dose chemotherapy with stem cell support does not appear to have a role in SCLC.

Treatment After Relapse Following Initial Therapy. The strongest predictor of outcome for patients with relapsed SCLC is the duration of remission. As such, patients are distinguished as having *sensitive* or *refractory* disease. The term *sensitive* implies an appropriate response to initial therapy that is maintained for 3 months or more. These patients have a higher likelihood of response to any additional chemotherapy; although, at best, it is approximately half that expected in the first-line setting. Survival from the start of a second regimen averages around 6 months. Patients with *refractory* disease either had no response to initial therapy or progressed within 3 months after completing treatment. Their chance of response to additional therapy is less than 10%, and their median survival from the start of a second regimen is 4 months.

The only approved agent in relapsed disease is topotecan. Ardizzoni et al.[190] reported a phase II trial in which topotecan, administered at a dose of 1.5 mg/m² daily for 5 days, yielded a response rate of 38% in sensitive patients and 6% in refractory patients. Median survival from the start of second-line therapy was 7 and 5 months, respectively. A randomized trial compared topotecan, administered at that same dose and schedule, to CAV in patients who relapsed at least 2 months after initial therapy.[191] The response rates for topotecan (24%) and for CAV (18%) were similar. The median survival was 6 months in both arms. Symptom improvement was better with topotecan for four of the eight symptoms queried, and as such, the U.S. Food and Drug Administration approved intravenous topotecan for sensitive relapsed SCLC. Oral topotecan has also undergone extensive testing in patients with relapsed SCLC. In a randomized phase II study, oral topotecan at a dose of 2.3 mg/m² daily for 5 days was comparable to intravenous topotecan 1.5 mg/m² daily for 5 days with regard to response rate (23% versus 15%), median survival (32 weeks versus 25 weeks), and symptom control.[192] Subsequently, the Medical Research Council showed that oral topotecan improved survival in relapsed sensitive and refractory SCLC over best supportive care alone (26 versus 14 weeks, respectively).[193] Oral topotecan led to a response rate of 7%, with a slower deterioration of quality of life and symptomatology. Another phase III study randomized 309 SCLC patients who had relapsed ≥90 days after first-line therapy to receive oral topotecan or intravenous topotecan.[194] The overall response rate and median survival time were 18.3% and 33 weeks, respectively, for patients who received oral topotecan compared to 21.9% and 35 weeks, respectively, for those who received intravenous topotecan. Although oral topotecan was associated with a lower incidence of grade 4 neutropenia, diarrhea occurred more often in this group of patients. Oral topotecan also has received regulatory approval for second-line therapy of SCLC.

Amrubicin, a third-generation synthetic 9-amino-anthracycline with diverse molecular effects including DNA intercalation, inhibition of topoisomerase II, and stabilization of topoisomerase IIa cleavable complexes, has been studied extensively and has received approval in Japan for SCLC treatment.[195] A randomized phase II trial conducted there showed higher response rates and PFS compared with topotecan.[196] Two North American phase II trials of amrubicin showed encouraging results.[197,198] In patients with refractory SCLC, the overall response rate for single-agent amrubicin was found to be 21%, with median PFS and OS of 3.2 and 6 months, respectively. Subsequently, 76 patients with sensitive SCLC were randomized in a 2:1 fashion to receive amrubicin or topotecan. Amrubicin treatment resulted in a significantly higher response rate than topotecan (44% versus 15%, $p = 0.021$), which led to improved PFS (4.5 versus 3.3 months) and OS (9.2 versus 7.6 months).[198] Despite phase II activity, preliminary results of the phase III study, which compared amrubicin to topotecan, were disappointing.[199] Although the activity of amrubicin was apparent, there was no statistically significant difference in OS observed between the two arms. The trend favored amrubicin (HR, 0.82; 95% CI, 0.68 to 0.99; $p = 0.036$), especially in the subgroup of patients with primary refractory disease (HR, 0.77; 95% CI, 0.59 to 1.0; $p = 0.047$). Although lower hematologic adverse events were noted in the amrubicin arm, these patients had a higher incidence of infections. The role of amrubicin for the treatment of patients with relapsed SCLC remains to be defined.

Temozolomide is an oral alkylating agent that crosses the blood–brain barrier. A phase II clinical trial of temozolomide in 64 patients with relapsed sensitive or refractory SCLC has been performed.[200] Temozolomide therapy was well tolerated and associated with an overall response rate of 20% in this patient population, with a 23% response rate in the sensitive group (n = 48) and a 13% response rate in the refractory cohort (n = 16). Responses also were noted in patients receiving temozolomide as third-line treatment and in those with brain metastases.[200] There is an ongoing multicenter phase II study comparing temozolomide and veliparib (a poly [ADP-ribose] polymerase [PARP] inhibitor) versus temozolomide and placebo in patients with relapsed sensitive and refractory SCLC (ClinicalTrials.gov identifier: NCT01638546).

Multiple trials have been conducted using other agents in this patient population. A list of single agents and their activity in relapsed SCLC is found in Table 42.2, many of which also have been tested in combination studies. In summary, the optimal drug or combination of drugs in relapsed SCLC has not been established. Single-agent topotecan or CAV are appropriate for patients with sensitive relapse. These regimens also could be used for patients with refractory SCLC, although the response rates are lower. Agents evaluated in phase II trials with activity in SCLC can be considered. For patients with relapse 6 months or more after initial therapy, rechallenging with the same regimen as used in first-line treatment is also a consideration.[52]

Immunotherapy and Other Targeted Therapies

In light of the therapeutic plateau achieved with current chemotherapy, investigators have studied a wide range of novel therapies in the hopes of improving outcomes (Table 42.3).

Receptor Tyrosine Kinases and Growth Factors. Small molecule kinase inhibitors are now established therapies for several diseases, but as yet, have not proven efficacious in SCLC. c-Kit protein expression has been reported in 28% to 93% of SCLC tumors.[201] In vitro studies support the role of c-kit and its ligand, stem cell factor (SCF), on SCLC autocrine and paracrine growth stimulation,[202] and imatinib has demonstrated growth inhibition

of multiple SCLC cell lines.[203] Nonetheless, three phase II studies in SCLC failed to demonstrate a single radiologic response to imatinib, even when enrollment was restricted to patients with tumors expressing c-kit protein by immunohistochemistry.[201,204,205]

The PI3K/AKT/mammalian target of rapamycin (mTOR) signal pathway is defective in SCLC: SCLC cells possess a constitutively active PI3K[206] and harbor PI3K and PTEN mutations[22,23,207]; phosphorylated AKT is present in 70% of tumors in SCLC patients[208]; and protein expression of mTOR, S6K1, and phosphorylated 4EBP1 are elevated in SCLC cells compared to type II epithelial cells.[209] Such alterations lead to growth, survival, and chemotherapy resistance in SCLC. Temsirolimus—the small molecule inhibitor of mTOR—was evaluated in an ECOG trial in which patients were randomized after initial chemotherapy to maintenance therapy with either high-dose or low-dose temsirolimus.[210] Although the PFS (1.8 months versus 2.5 months) and OS were better for the high dose arm (6.5 months versus 9.0 months), these results were no better than those observed in the previous ECOG trial of topotecan maintenance therapy,[145] suggesting no added benefit from temsirolimus. Similarly, a phase II trial of everolimus in relapsed SCLC did not demonstrate antitumor activity for this agent.[211]

The insulinlike growth factor receptor (IGF-1R), a member of the insulin receptor subclass of receptor tyrosine kinase, is activated by the ligands IGF-1 and IGF-2 and signals mitogenic and antiapoptotic signaling pathways contributing to cellular transformation and malignant growth.[208] IGF-1R and its ligand, IGF-1, are expressed at increased levels in SCLC.[208] The IGF-1R activates the PI3K-AKT pathway in SCLC, playing a role in the development and growth of the disease, as well as resistance to chemotherapy.[208] Therefore, targeted inhibition of IGF-1R represents an attractive approach to enhancing chemotherapeutic efficacy and inhibiting tumor recurrence in patients with SCLC. Yet, the ECOG 1508 phase II study evaluating the monoclonal antibody, cixutumumab, together with cisplatin and etoposide in a randomized trial, failed to show an improvement in PFS with IGF-1R inhibition.[212]

Developmental Pathways: The Hedgehog Pathway. The Hedgehog pathway is essential in early lung development and has a role in regulating stem cell maintenance and differentiation.[213] Hedgehog signaling may play a significant role in the development and proliferation of SCLC, which is a relatively undifferentiated airway epithelial tumor that may recapitulate aspects of early lung development.[214,215] In vitro and in vivo studies have demonstrated that Hedgehog antagonists can inhibit SCLC and, when administered following chemotherapy, such inhibition may delay or prevent the recurrence of residual disease.[215] The ECOG 1508 phase II randomized trial in patients with extensive stage disease included an arm evaluating the addition of vismodegib, a Hedgehog inhibitor, to cisplatin and etoposide, which unfortunately, did not lead to an improvement in PFS.[212]

Nonreceptor Oncogenes: Bcl-2 Genes. The antiapoptotic gene product, bcl-2 protein, is expressed in 80% to 90% of SCLC tumor samples and, as such, is a potential therapeutic target.[216,217] Oblimersen (G3139) is an antisense oligonucleotide that suppresses bcl-2 expression. The CALGB conducted a series of studies with oblimersen in combination with chemotherapy for SCLC.[218,219] In a randomized phase II study of etoposide/carboplatin with or without oblimersen, survival was inferior in the patients receiving oblimersen (HR for OS, 2.13; $p = 0.02$).[220] Insufficient suppression of bcl-2 by this agent may explain its lack of efficacy. Navitoclax, a selective high-affinity small molecule inhibitor of bcl-2 and bcl-x_L (another antiapoptotic protein of the Bcl-2 family), resulted in dramatic tumor responses in SCLC cell line xenograft tumors as a single agent and enhanced the efficacy of standard cytotoxic agents against SCLC models.[221–227] Yet, a recent phase II study of navitoclax demonstrated limited activity in patients

TABLE 42.2

Activity of Single Agent Chemotherapy in Relapsed Small Cell Lung Cancer

Drug (Ref.)	Dose/Schedule	N	Sensitive/Refractory	Response Rate (%)	Median Survival (mo)
Topotecan (IV)[190]	1.5 mg/m^2 daily × 5 days	45	Sensitive	38	6.9
		47	Refractory	6	4.7
Topotecan (IV)[191]	1.5 mg/m^2 daily × 5 days	107	Sensitive (60 days)	24	6.0
Topotecan (IV)[192]	1.5 mg/m^2 daily × 5 days	54	Sensitive	15	5.8
Topotecan (oral)[192]	2.3 mg/m^2 daily × 5 days	52	Sensitive	23	7.5
Topotecan (oral)[193]	2.3 mg/m^2 daily × 5 days	71	Sensitive + refractory	7	6.0
		30	Sensitive	3	
		41	Refractory	10	
Topotecan (IV)[194]	1.5mg/m^2 daily × 5 days	151	Sensitive	22	8.8
Topotecan (oral)[194]	2.3 mg/m^2 daily × 5 days	153	Sensitive	18	8.0
Irinotecan[107]	100 mg/m^2 weekly	16	Sensitive[a]	47	6.2
Paclitaxel[426]	175 mg/m^2 every 3 wks	24	Refractory	29	3.0
Docetaxel[427]	100 mg/m^2 every 3 wks	34	Not specified[b]	25	NR
Gemcitabine[428]	1,000 mg/m^2 d1, 8, 15 every 4 wks	46	Both	12	7.1
Gemcitabine[429]	1,250 mg/m^2 d1, 8 every 3 wks	27	Both	0	6.4
Gemcitabine[430]	1,000 mg/m^2 d1, 8, 15 every 4 wks	38	Refractory	13	4.0
Vinorelbine[431]	25 mg/m^2 weekly	24	Both	13	5.0
Vinorelbine[432]	30 mg/m^2 weekly	26	Sensitive	16	NR
Amrubicin[433]	40 mg/m^2 daily × 3 every 3 wks	44	Sensitive	52	10.3
		16	Refractory	50	11.6
Amrubicin[434]	40 mg/m^2 daily × 3 every 3 wks	75	Refractory	21	6.0
Amrubicin[198]	40 mg/m^2 daily × 3 every 3 wks	50	Sensitive	44%	9.2
Amrubicin[199]	40 mg/m^2 daily × 3 every 3 wks	225	Sensitive	31% (both sensitive	9.2
		199	Refractory	& refractory)	6.2
Picoplatin[435]	120–150 mg/m^2 every 3 wks	24	Sensitive	8	8.1
		13	Refractory	15	6.2
Picoplatin[436]	150 mg/m^2 every 3 wks	6	Sensitive	4	6.1
		27	Resistant[c]	(all three groups)	(all three groups)
		44	Refractory[d]		
Picoplatin[437]	150 mg/m^2 every 3 wks	268	Relapsed disease[e]	4	4.7
Temozolomide[200]	75 mg/m^2 daily for 21 out of 28 days	48	Sensitive	23	6.0
		16	Refractory	13	5.6

[a] All but one patient had a chemotherapy-free interval of >90 days.
[b] Previously untreated patients also included.
[c] Defined as patients that relapsed within 90 days of the end of first-line platinum-containing chemotherapy.
[d] Defined as patients that did not have a response to first-line platinum-containing chemotherapy.
[e] Defined as those patients with relapse <6 months of completing first-line platinum-based chemotherapy.
IV, intravenous; NR, not reported; N, number of patients.

with recurrent and progressive SCLC.[228] Results of a completed phase I trial of navitoclax with first-line combination chemotherapy for SCLC are not yet available (ClinicalTrials.gov identifier: NCT00878449). A third agent, obatoclax mesylate, which is a small-molecule BH3-mimetic that exhibits binding affinity for a range of bcl-2 family members, has been evaluated in various clinical scenarios. A phase II trial of obatoclax mesylate added to topotecan did not exceed the historic response rate seen in topotecan alone in patients with relapsed SCLC.[229] The phase II randomized study of carboplatin and etoposide with or without obatoclax followed by maintenance obatoclax in patients with newly diagnosed extensive stage SCLC failed to meet its primary endpoint of improved response rate for those receiving obatoclax, although there was a trend for improved PFS (6 versus 5.4 months, $p = 0.084$) and OS (10.6 versus 9.9 months, $p = 0.052$).[230]

Angiogenesis Inhibitors. Angiogenesis inhibitors have entered into standard clinical practice for numerous malignancies, and they are being tested in SCLC as well. Two phase III trials that tested thalidomide as maintenance therapy after first-line chemotherapy showed no significant effect on OS.[231,232] Likewise, vandetanib, an oral TKI of vascular endothelial growth factor receptor 2 (VEGFR-2) and EGFR, failed to improve PFS in a randomized phase II maintenance trial.[233] In all of these cases, toxicity was significantly greater in the treatment arms. Similarly, sorafenib (inhibitor of RAF; VEGFR-2,-3; platelet-derived growth factor receptor alpha [PDGFRα]) and cediranib (inhibitor of VEGFR-1, -2, -3; PDGFRβ; c-KIT) showed minimal activity for relapsed disease when evaluated as single agents, although cediranib demonstrated a promising PFS of 8 months when administered with cisplatin and etoposide in a phase I study.[234–236]

PRACTICE OF ONCOLOGY

TABLE 42.3

Immunotherapies and Other Targeted Agents That Have Undergone Testing in Small Cell Lung Cancer

Agent (Ref.)	Mechanism of Action	Study Design	Result
Interferon-alfa[438–441]	Immunomodulator	Phase III (multiple)	Two studies with improved survival in limited-stage patients, two studies with no survival benefit
Interferon-gamma[442, 443]	Immunomodulator	Phase III (multiple)	No improvement in survival
Interleukin-2[444]	Immunomodulator	Phase II	21% response rate but excessive toxicity
Warfarin[445,446]	Anticoagulant	Randomized phase II Randomized phase III	Significant improvement in PFS and OS Warfarin added to chemotherapy significantly improved response rates, and nonsignificant improvement in PFS and OS
Aspirin (1 g/d)[447]	Anticoagulant	Randomized phase II	Aspirin added to chemotherapy did not improve survival
Subcutaneous unfractionated heparin[448]	Anticoagulant	Randomized phase II	Heparin added to chemotherapy during first 5 weeks of treatment led to significantly improved response rates and PFS, as well as OS in limited stage disease
Ipilimumab[245]	Humanized anti-CTLA4 antibody	Randomized phase II	Improved immune-related PFS when administered with carboplatin/paclitaxel in phased dosing schedule in chemo-naïve extensive stage SCLC
Marimastat[449]	Matrix metalloproteinase inhibitor	Phase III	No improvement in PFS or OS
Tanomastat[450]	Matrix metalloproteinase inhibitor	Phase III	No improvement in PFS or OS
Imatinib[201,204,205]	c-Kit tyrosine kinase inhibitor	Phase II (multiple)	No responses
Temsirolimus[210]	mTOR inhibitor	Randomized phase II	Improved survival at higher dose but no improvement in outcome compared with prior trials
Everolimus[211]	mTOR inhibitor	Phase II	Limited antitumor activity in relapsed SCLC
Tipifarnib[451]	Farnesyl transferase inhibitor	Phase II	No responses
Cixutumumab[212]	Monoclonal IGF-1R antibody	Randomized phase II	No improvement in PFS when added to cisplatin/etoposide in chemo-naïve extensive stage SCLC
Vismodegib[212]	Hedgehog pathway inhibitor	Randomized phase II	No improvement in PFS when added to cisplatin/etoposide in chemo-naïve extensive stage SCLC
Oblimersen[220]	Bcl-2 antisense	Randomized phase II	No improvement in response rate
Navitoclax[228]	Bcl-2 and bcl-x_L inhibitor	Phase II	Limited activity in recurrent and progressive disease
Obatoclax mesylate[229,230]	BH3-mimetic exhibits binding affinity for bcl-2 family members, including bcl-2, bcl-XL, and mcl-1	Phase II Randomized phase II	No increased response rate when added to topotecan in relapsed SCLC Trend toward improved response rate, PFS and OS in chemo-naïve extensive stage SCLC
Bortezomib[452]	Proteosome inhibitor	Phase II	One response in refractory patient (2% overall response rate)
BEC-2 + Bacille Calmette-Guerin (BCG) adjuvant[453]	Ganglioside (GD3) anti-idiotype vaccine	Phase III	No improvement in PFS or OS
Thalidomide[231,232]	Multiple immunomodulatory effects, also inhibits VEGF	Phase III Phase III	Improved survival from 8.7 to 11.7 months but not significant (HR, 0.74; $p = 0.16$) No improvement in any parameters
Vandetanib[233]	Tyrosine kinase inhibitor of VEGFR-2 and EGFR	Randomized phase II	No improvement in PFS
Sorafenib[234]	RAF, VEGFR-2, VEGFR-3, PDGFRα inhibitor	Phase II	5% response rate in relapsed disease

(continued)

TABLE 42.3

Immunotherapies and Other Targeted Agents That Have Undergone Testing in Small Cell Lung Cancer (continued)

Agent (Ref.)	Mechanism of Action	Study Design	Result
Cediranib[235,236]	VEGFR-1, VEGFR-2, VEGFR-3, PDGFRβ, c-KIT inhibitor	Phase II	Minimal activity as a single agent in relapsed disease
		Phase I	8-month PFS with cisplatin and etoposide
Bevacizumab[238-241]	Monoclonal antibody to VEGF	Phase II (multiple)	No increased risk of hemorrhage
			Favorable survival compared with historical control
		Randomized phase II	Improved PFS for bevacizumab, but not in OS

PFS, progression-free survival; OS, overall survival; mTOR, mammalian target of rapamycin; VEGF, vascular endothelial growth factor; PDGFR, platelet-derived growth factor receptor.

Sunitinib, which is known to inhibit VEGFR-1, -2, -3; PDGFRα; PDGFRβ; c-KIT; and FLT3, was evaluated in a phase II trial as maintenance treatment after chemotherapy in patients with untreated extensive-stage SCLC (CALGB 30504).[237] After receiving four to six cycles of etoposide with cisplatin or carboplatin, patients were randomized to sunitinib or placebo until progression of disease. Patients in the placebo arm could cross over to receive sunitinib at the time of progression. The study met its primary endpoint of PFS after chemotherapy from the time of randomization (3.77 versus 2.3 months for sunitinib and placebo, respectively; HR, 1.53; 90% CI, 1.03 to 2.27; $p = 0.037$). Further, there was evidence of single-agent activity for sunitinib as maintenance therapy and at crossover, as well as a trend toward improvement in survival.[237]

Multiple phase II studies adding the VEGF monoclonal antibody, bevacizumab, to chemotherapy have not shown any increased risk of pulmonary hemorrhage in this cohort of patients who commonly have central tumors and have yielded favorable survival rates when compared to historical controls.[238-240] A randomized phase II study evaluated cisplatin or carboplatin plus etoposide with or without bevacizumab, for four cycles followed by single-agent bevacizumab or placebo until progression or unacceptable toxicity in patients with untreated extensive stage SCLC.[241] Median PFS was higher in the bevacizumab group than in the placebo group (5.5 versus 4.4 months; HR, 0.53; 95% CI, 0.32 to 0.86); however, there was no difference observed in OS, but a trend that favored placebo was noted (9.4 versus 10.9 months for bevacizumab and placebo groups, respectively; HR, 1.16; 95% CI, 0.66 to 2.04). Although no new or unexpected safety signals for bevacizumab were observed, the trend toward worse OS calls future prospects of bevacizumab into question unless a biomarker for benefit is discovered to select patients for this therapy.

Antigen-Independent Immunotherapy: Ipilimumab. Ipilimumab, a humanized immunoglobulin (Ig)G1 monoclonal antibody against cytotoxic T-lymphocyte antigen-4 (CTLA-4), has been approved for the treatment of patients with metastatic melanoma.[242] By blocking the inhibitory signal provided by CTLA-4, this class of antibodies can prolong the activation and proliferation of tumor-directed cytotoxic T cells, thus promoting an antitumor immune response.[243] A randomized, double-blind, three arm phase II trial in patients with untreated stage IIIB/IV NSCLC or extensive stage SCLC was performed to evaluate the efficacy and safety of paclitaxel and carboplatin with or without ipilimumab given on two dosing schedules.[244] Among the 130 patients with SCLC, the phased dosing schedule, in which ipilimumab was started in cycle three of paclitaxel and carboplatin, appeared to improve immune-related PFS (median 6.4 months for the phased ipilimumab arm versus 5.3 months for the control arm ($p = 0.03$)), immune-related best overall response rate (71% [95% CI, 55 to 84] versus 53% [95% CI, 38 to 68]) and OS (median 12.9 months versus 9.9 months [p = 0.13]), compared to paclitaxel and carboplatin, whereas the concurrent regimen did not lead to improved outcomes.[245] Ipilimumab did not potentiate the toxicities of the chemotherapy, but was associated with moderate immune-related adverse events.[245] Given these favorable results, a randomized, multicenter, double-blind phase III trial comparing the efficacy of platinum/etoposide with or without ipilimumab in patients with newly diagnosed extensive stage disease SCLC, with OS as the primary endpoint, has been conducted and the results are forthcoming. (ClinicalTrials.gov identifier: NCT01450761).

As seen previously, distinct pathways contribute to the pathogenesis of SCLC, leading to its unique biology and clinical features. The therapeutic strategies employed previously to target the basic molecular and cellular changes in SCLC have not led to significant changes in the management and outcomes of the disease, thus far. However, continued, rational, target-based approaches ultimately should lead to improved survival of patients with SCLC.

Radiation

Role of Radiotherapy in Limited Disease. Despite being exquisitely chemo- and radioresponsive, neither modality alone controls all aspects of disease. The CALGB trial of the late 1980s demonstrated that 90% of patients treated with chemotherapy alone failed locally.[246] The meta-analysis of Pignon and Arriagada[247] provided more data to mandate thoracic radiotherapy, but a number of treatment issues remained to be determined, including sequencing of radiation with chemotherapy, early versus late radiotherapy, altered fractionation, and prophylactic cranial irradiation.

Concurrent combined modality therapy is the standard treatment for SCLC patients with limited-stage disease.[52] It requires close coordination between medical and radiation oncologists. A combined modality treatment approach requires patients with an excellent performance status. Single-modality therapy may be appropriate for those who are debilitated or have serious comorbidities. If the patient's condition improves sufficiently after the initial chemotherapy or radiotherapy, subsequent treatment with the other modality may be considered. Although gains in radiotherapy delivery and integration with PET imaging have been made, disease failure in local, distant, and sanctuary sites continue to be substantial clinical challenges.

Sequencing of Radiation with Chemotherapy. Concurrent therapy is the delivery of chemotherapy and radiation therapy throughout the same time period. Sequential therapy is the delivery of one modality only after the completion of the other, often requiring a delay to allow for adequate recovery from the initial modality. A 1992 meta-analysis evaluated trials in which

PRACTICE OF ONCOLOGY

more than 2,100 patients with limited-stage SCLC were randomized to receive chemotherapy alone or with chest irradiation.[248] Patients given combined modality therapy had a 14% reduction in death rate and an absolute 5.4% improvement in 3-year survival compared with those who received chemotherapy alone. Both differences were highly significant. A second and independent meta-analysis reached similar conclusions.[249]

The trials included in the meta-analysis used cyclophosphamide- and doxorubicin-based chemotherapy, which is excessively toxic when given with concurrent thoracic radiotherapy. Therefore, individual trials used strategies such as sequential or interdigitated chemoradiation and used different chemotherapy regimens during the concurrent phases. However, the current standard chemotherapy regimen of cisplatin and etoposide can be used safely with concurrent radiotherapy.

Thoracic Radiation Dose and Fractionation. Due to the radioresponsiveness of SCLC, modest doses of radiation from 45 to 50 Gy have been used. However, with modest-dose radiation therapy there is a high rate of local failure. For example, in the Intergroup trial, the control arm of 45 Gy given once daily had a 75% rate of intrathoracic relapse.[250] Therefore, higher radiation doses or intensification (i.e., acceleration) appear necessary to improve local control. A retrospective review from Massachusetts General Hospital suggested that there may be continued dose response beyond 50 Gy.[251] The maximum tolerated dose of concurrent thoracic chemoradiation seems to be 45 to 51 Gy with a twice-daily approach and 70 Gy daily.[252] However, the advent of highly conformal radiotherapy techniques, such as intensity-modulated radiation therapy (IMRT) and the shift away from targeting clinically uninvolved nodal stations, may lead to tolerance of higher radiation doses, as discussed in the following paragraphs.

CALGB-39808 determined that 70 Gy delivered with daily fractions of 2 Gy with concurrent chemotherapy is feasible in the cooperative group setting and was associated with a median survival of 22.4 months and acceptable rates of esophagitis and pneumonitis.[253] Other CALGB trials also have used 70 Gy of thoracic irradiation with concurrent chemotherapy.[254] Once-daily fractionation is more familiar for radiation oncologists and typically is more convenient for patients, although it should be noted that some patients prefer the decreased overall treatment duration with a twice-daily schedule.

SCLC appears to be an ideal neoplasm for twice-daily treatment in that it has a high growth fraction, short cell cycle time, and small-to-absent shoulder on the in vitro cell survival curve, which may allow for a reduction in long-term pulmonary toxicity while maintaining antitumor efficacy.[255] Pilot studies in the late 1980s combining etoposide and platinum with twice-daily chest radiation were promising, with median survivals greater than 2 years and, in most series, low rates of pneumonitis.[250,256,257] An Intergroup study randomized 417 patients with limited-stage SCLC receiving 45 Gy in either daily fractions of 1.8 Gy or twice-daily fractions of 1.5 Gy, both given concurrently with the first of four cycles of EP.[49] Although fractionation is the obvious variable, the overall duration of radiotherapy varied as well (3 weeks versus 5 weeks), and longer treatment times may exert selective pressure on the emergence of resistant clones. The target volume included the primary tumor, bilateral mediastinal nodes, and the ipsilateral hilum, excluding uninvolved supraclavicular nodes. Local failure was reduced from 52% to 36% with the twice-daily schedule ($p = 0.06$). Of interest, only 6% of patients with twice-daily radiation failed in both local and distant sites, compared to 23% with daily treatment ($p = 0.01$). More importantly, although statistically significant differences in survival were not seen at 2 years,[257] by 5 years the survival was 16% with once-daily treatment, compared to 26% with a twice-daily schedule ($p = 0.04$).[49] All patients who achieved less than complete response were scored as local failures, but some of those treated with the accelerated scheme who achieved only a partial response survived, as well as those with a complete response,

implying that the local failure rate was overestimated by imaging on that arm. There was a higher frequency of grade 3 esophagitis with twice-daily treatment, but overall long-term morbidities were not significantly different between the two arms.

A North Central Cancer Treatment Group trial attempted to reduce morbidity of twice-daily radiation by inserting a 2.5-week pause between two courses of 24 Gy each (therefore, the overall course was longer than the standard duration).[48,258] After three cycles of induction chemotherapy, fit and responding patients were randomized to receive either the 48 Gy split-course regimen, or 54 Gy in a once daily regimen in 6 weeks.[258] The 20% rate of 5-year survival was less than the benchmark 26% from the Intergroup trial. However, a follow-up trial used a higher dose of twice-daily radiation (total 60 Gy) with a 2-week treatment break and reported a favorable 5-year survival of 24%.[259]

A phase I trial conducted by the Radiation Therapy and Oncology Group (RTOG) and CALGB evaluated the use of 70 Gy delivered in daily fractionation or 45 Gy given in twice-a-day fractionation.[260] Although it was intended to establish the maximum-tolerated doses (MTD) of irinotecan given with cisplatin and thoracic radiation, it also was the first trial to evaluate 70 Gy delivered at cycle one. Of the 15 patients treated to 70 Gy, 2 had dose-limiting toxicities (diarrhea, esophagitis, and cardiovascular complications).

RTOG-9712 was a phase I trial to establish the MTD of radiation therapy with delayed accelerated hyperfractionation.[261] With this technique, a large field encompassing the gross tumor and mediastinum was treated to 45 Gy. A smaller field that encompassed only the gross tumor was treated as a second daily 1.8 Gy treatment for the last 3 to 11 days. The MTD was found to be 61.2 Gy with this regimen, which subsequently was evaluated in RTOG-0239, a phase II trial.[262] It reported a 2-year OS of 37%, short of the predicted survival of 60%. However, the regimen demonstrated an excellent local control of 73%.

Currently, a randomized phase III trial is being conducted by the RTOG and CALGB to evaluate three fractionation schemes: 45 Gy in 1.5-Gy twice-daily fractions (standard), 70 Gy in 2-Gy fractions (Arm B), and 61.2 Gy with delayed accelerated hyperfractionation (Arm C). In the first part of this trial, toxicity was to be assessed and the less toxic of Arms B and C was to be compared head to head with the standard arm. Although no clear difference in toxicity was observed between Arms B and C, the delayed accelerated hyperfractionation arm has been dropped due to slow accrual, and the study is continuing as a two-arm trial. A separate Phase III randomized trial is also evaluating once versus twice-daily radiotherapy with concurrent chemoradiotherapy in Europe, comparing 66 Gy in daily 2-Gy fractions against the same control arm of 45 Gy in twice-daily 1.5-Gy fractions. Until results from these trials are available, twice-daily fractionation as established by the Intergroup trial remains the reference regimen for fit patients. However, it should be noted that the logistical and toxicity obstacles with twice-daily treatment apparently are substantial, because a recent survey of practice patterns indicated that fewer than a quarter of limited-stage SCLC patients receive twice-daily treatment in the United States.[263]

Early Versus Late Radiotherapy. Randomized trials have yielded conflicting results on whether concurrent irradiation is best given early or late in the chemotherapy program. There have been multiple meta-analyses of the timing of thoracic irradiation.[264–268] One meta-analysis[265] reviewed seven randomized trials with a total of 1,524 patients that addressed the timing of radiotherapy relative to chemotherapy. Early radiation therapy was defined as beginning before 9 weeks after the initiation of chemotherapy and before the third cycle of chemotherapy. Late radiation therapy began 9 weeks or more after the initiation of chemotherapy or after the beginning of the third cycle. They reported a small but statistically significant improvement in 2-year survival for patients receiving early radiation therapy. A greater benefit was observed in patients receiving hyperfractionated radiation. Another meta-analysis[269] evaluated four randomized trials consisting of 1,056 patients to determine whether the time from the start of chemotherapy until the end of radiotherapy (SER) was a predictor of survival. They found that there was a significantly higher 5-year survival rate in the treatment arms with a shorter SER. In addition, a low SER was associated with a higher incidence of severe esophagitis. This suggests that an important factor in the treatment of SCLC involves counteracting accelerated repopulation that occurs after treatment with chemotherapy. However, definitive evidence that early integration of radiotherapy leads to improved survival remains elusive. A recent randomized trial from Korea assigned patients to receive radiotherapy (albeit a nonstandard regimen of 52.5 Gy) with either the first or third cycle of chemotherapy with cisplatin or etoposide. There was no difference in survival or local control, but rather an increase in febrile neutropenia with early radiotherapy, suggesting that later integration of radiotherapy was preferable.[82]

In clinical practice, it is often prudent to initiate chemotherapy immediately in these patients who are typically highly symptomatic and not delay treatment until radiation treatment planning is complete. Starting radiotherapy with the second cycle of chemotherapy is more readily achievable and should preserve the potential gains in efficacy obtained with early integration of radiotherapy with chemotherapy.

Radiation Therapy Treatment Volumes and Technique. An early randomized trial by SWOG showed no difference in recurrence rate whether pre- or postchemotherapy imaging was used to determine radiation therapy treatment fields.[270] Of course, if early radiation therapy is used, then there is no postchemotherapy treatment volume. The Intergroup trial[49] included gross disease, the bilateral mediastinum, and the ipsilateral hilum in the treatment field. The uninvolved supraclavicular area was excluded. RTOG-9712[261] allowed for the treatment of the uninvolved supraclavicular area in the setting of apical tumors. A small phase II trial suggested that there may be increased elective nodal failure in the supraclavicular area if it is excluded from the treatment field.[271] Consultants from the International Atomic Energy Agency reviewed available literature in 2008 and found little evidence to guide the use of elective nodal irradiation.[272] However, a number of prospective and retrospective experiences have since been published and increasingly suggest that involved-field radiation therapy is not associated with an excessive rate of local–regional failure, particularly in an era of routine PET staging. A Dutch phase II trial of concurrent chemoradiation limited radiotherapy (RT) fields to the primary tumor and clinically involved lymph nodes and reported a relatively low local failure rate of 16%.[273]

Utilizing PET to guide the design of limited radiotherapy fields appears to reduce the probability of elective nodal failure due to the improved sensitivity of PET to detect nodal disease compared to CT alone. A follow-up trial from the same group that found a worrisome rate of elective nodal failure when utilizing involved-field RT in CT-staged patients showed that the rate of isolated nodal failure was only 3% with PET staging, compared to 11% without.[274] A retrospective experience from the M.D. Anderson Cancer Center similarly showed a low rate of isolated elective nodal failure in a PET-staged cohort of patients who were treated with IMRT, a technique that gives lower incidental radiation doses to untargeted lymph node regions and, therefore, would theoretically increase the risk of elective nodal failure.[275] Overall, these and other recent publications suggest that with modern staging and treatment techniques, the omission of elective nodal irradiation does not lead to an excessive rate of isolated nodal failure.[276–278] Neither of the ongoing trials of daily versus twice-daily thoracic radiotherapy employ elective nodal irradiation in any of the trial arms (with the exception of mandatory coverage of hilar lymph nodes in the CALGB trial), indicating that the omission of elective nodal irradiation is increasingly considered within the standard of care for PET-staged patients.

In addition to the omission of elective nodal irradiation, another area of investigation in radiation technique is the implementation of more highly conformal delivery methods, such as IMRT or proton therapy. These techniques allow for significantly greater control of the location of radiation dose, particularly of incidental radiation dose outside of the target volume. Although this would seem to be an unequivocal advantage, theoretic concerns have persisted regarding the sensitivity of these techniques to respiratory organ motion, and the possibility that decreasing the incidental dose outside of the target volume might increase rates of regional or nodal failure. Investigators from the M.D. Anderson Cancer Center retrospectively compared outcomes with patients receiving standard three-dimensional (3D)-conformal radiation therapy and IMRT, and found no significant difference in OS or DFS.[279] Proton therapy, which reduces the dose outside of the target volume more fully than is possible with any form of photon radiotherapy, has not yet been widely used in SCLC, with only one small report published so far.[280] However, if the phase III trials demonstrate an advantage to higher dose radiotherapy, then IMRT and photon therapy are likely to gain in importance, because highly conformal techniques are often required to achieve high target doses while respecting dose limits to critical normal structures.

Toxicity of Radiation Therapy. The addition of chest irradiation has increased myelosuppressive, pulmonary, and esophageal complications of treatment, particularly with concurrent cyclophosphamide-based regimens.[281–283] Esophagitis is a difficult toxicity to compare because trials often use unique grading systems. However, most trials with concurrent chemoradiation with a cisplatin-based regimen report a 10% to 25% rate of severe esophagitis.[284] A retrospective review revealed that various radiation dosimetric parameters, such as mean esophageal dose and volume of esophagus receiving 15 Gy, were associated with a higher incidence of grade 3 or worse esophagitis in patients receiving twice-daily radiation.[285] More recently, a large individual patient data meta-analysis of esophagitis after concurrent thoracic chemoradiotherapy indicated that the best predictor of esophagitis was the volume of esophagus receiving greater than or equal to 60 Gy, with the highest risk seen when 17% or more of the esophagus was exposed to such doses.[286]

Radiation pneumonitis (RP) has not been as well studied in SCLC as it has in NSCLC, most likely due to the fact that most trials have used a moderate dose of radiation therapy, below which high rates of RP rarely are seen. Recent trials report a RP rate of approximately 10%.[253,287] This is lower than some of the trials reported in the 1980s and 1990s, probably due to improved radiation therapy techniques and better distinction between pneumonitis and other etiologies of respiratory distress, such as infection or tumor recurrence. The volume of lung receiving 20 Gy (V20) is a standard parameter used to predict lung toxicity in patients with NSCLC. A recent collaborative effort to define consensus dose limits for RP recommended that the V20 be kept below 30% to 35% in order to keep the risk of pneumonitis less than 20%.[288] It has been shown to have value in patients receiving concurrent accelerated hyperfractionated treatment for SCLC as well, with a V20 less than 25% associated with a lower rate of RP.[289]

Role of Chest Irradiation in Extensive Disease. Reviews of the historical literature indicated that the addition of chest irradiation plus chemotherapy for patients who have extensive-stage SCLC may improve local control in the thorax, but without change in survival.[290,291] Successive large studies by the SWOG also confirmed a benefit on local control but not survival.[118,292] Because patients with extensive disease generally achieve complete response rates of only 20% to 25% with current chemotherapy regimens and frequently relapse in distant metastatic sites, it is unsurprising that the routine application of additional local therapy did not have a clear impact on survival. Several clinical trials have randomized patients with extensive disease to chemotherapy alone or in combination with irradiation to the chest disease, as well as to some or all sites of overt distant metastases.[292–295] Although most of these did not show survival advantages with the addition of radiotherapy, it is notable that the most recent trial did.[293] In this trial, patients with at least a partial response to chemotherapy at the primary site and a complete response in distant sites were randomized to receive thoracic radiation with additional chemotherapy, or chemotherapy alone. Thoracic radiotherapy was associated with significantly better survival and a trend toward better local control. A recent, small phase II trial of consolidative thoracic radiation suggested that rates of symptomatic recurrence in the chest were low with this strategy and may, therefore, have an important quality of life benefit irrespective of any survival benefit.[296] Preliminary results from the Dutch phase III trial randomizing extensive stage SCLC patients who have had a response to four to six cycles of chemotherapy to thoracic radiation therapy or no thoracic radiation therapy has found a survival benefit at two years but not at one year, which was the primary endpoint.[297] The RTOG is conducting a randomized trial in which patients with extensive-stage disease and four or fewer metastatic lesions (excluding the central nervous system [CNS]) receive prophylactic cranial irradiation and consolidative RT to the thorax and all metastatic sites, or prophylactic cranial irradiation (PCI) alone. Although the routine use of consolidative thoracic radiation cannot yet be justified, the improved local control, attendant impact on symptomatic progression, and possible survival benefit make it a reasonable consideration in patients with significant responses to initial chemotherapy.

Prophylactic Cranial Irradiation. Brain metastases are detected in at least 18% of SCLC patients at diagnosis[33] and eventually are diagnosed in another 20% to 25%, with an increasing likelihood seen with lengthening survival.[298,299] An actuarial analysis reveals a probability of brain metastases ranging from 50% to 80% in patients who survive 2 years.[298,230] At postmortem examination, they are found in up to 65% of patients.[301] Because these metastases are sometimes the sole site of clinical relapse and are frequently clinically disabling, PCI has been recommended by many,[302] but not all,[303] authorities. The rationale is essentially an extrapolation from original strategies used in acute lymphocytic leukemia of childhood.

A large number of early prospective randomized trials assessed the benefit of PCI given at or within a few months of diagnosis.[144,304–307] When these trials were considered together, PCI reduced the frequency of clinically detectable brain metastases from 24% to 6%. However, no significant impact of PCI on survival was seen in any of those studies. Retrospective analyses suggested that virtually all benefit with PCI was confined to patients who achieved a complete remission from their initial treatment.[300] In an actuarial analysis, partial responders or nonresponders have similar risks of recurrence in the brain regardless of whether PCI was administered. This is not surprising because persistent systemic cancer could readily metastasize to the CNS after the completion of PCI.

In a meta-analysis of almost 1,000 patients in seven trials between 1977 and 1995, patients were evaluated with and without PCI after initially obtaining a complete response.[308] PCI doses ranged from 24 to 40 Gy in most patients. The meta-analysis suggested that a significant gain in survival with PCI, with 3-year survival figures increasing from 15% to almost 21%. PCI significantly decreased the probability of brain metastases and increased the likelihood of disease-free survival. Higher doses appeared to have no impact on survival, although seemed to have an increasing effect of preventing brain metastases. A trend also was seen toward a decreased risk of brain metastases when PCI was administered earlier. The meta-analysis was not able to assess the impact of PCI on cognitive function, because most of the studies did not include thorough neurocognitive assessments. Two studies that assessed baseline neuropsychological function before treatment demonstrated that many patients appear to have abnormalities of cognitive function as initial manifestations of their cancer, even when brain metastases were not detected and before any treatment.[309,310]

An Intergroup trial evaluated standard-dose versus higher dose PCI after complete response for limited-stage disease.[311] Seven hundred twenty patients were randomized to either 25 Gy in 10 fractions or 36 Gy delivered in 18 daily fractions of 2 Gy or 24 twice-daily fractions of 1.5 Gy. There was no significant difference in incidences of brain metastases between the standard-dose group and the high-dose group. The OS was significantly was worse in the higher dose group, although this was due to extracranial disease progression rather than toxicity. The reason for this counterintuitive result remains unclear. This study further established 2,500 cGy in 10 fractions as the standard dose of PCI for limited-stage patients, although some practitioners use a regimen of 3,000 cGy in 15 fractions, which should have similar biologic efficacy.

A recent EORTC randomized trial demonstrated a survival benefit with PCI in patients with extensive-stage SCLC who had had a response to chemotherapy.[83] The use of PCI significantly improved the rate of 1-year freedom from symptomatic brain metastases from 14.6% to 40.4% and the 1-year survival from 13.3% to 27.1% in the 286 randomized patients. Various fractionation schemes were used, but the most common ones were 20 Gy in five fractions and 30 Gy in 10 fractions. A common criticism of this trial is its lack of mandatory pretreatment brain imaging to rule out clinically occult brain metastases, raising the question of whether the observed survival benefit was due to treatment of patients who already had detectable brain metastases. In an era of routine and regular imaging of the brain with sensitive MRI examinations, it has been suggested that the actual rate of developing brain metastases in thoroughly staged extensive-stage patients is relatively low, which may attenuate the potential benefit of routine PCI in this cohort. Nevertheless, the results of the EORTC trial established PCI as a standard consideration for all extensive-stage patients achieving a response to initial therapy.

A major concern with recommending PCI is the significant risk of toxicity associated with it. It is evident that some long-term survivors have neurologic and intellectual impairment as well as abnormalities on CT scan that may be related to PCI.[312,313] In one study, CT scan and CNS abnormalities were significantly more frequent in patients who had received PCI or therapeutic brain irradiation than in those who had not.[314] These findings were especially disturbing because complete responders are at greater risk for possible complications. Many deficits on neuropsychological testing have been unsuspected on casual examination, but a few patients have obvious major impairments. CT scan abnormalities continue to worsen for several years after treatment has ended, although the abnormalities may eventually stabilize.[315] Neurologic abnormalities were most prominent in one series of patients who were given PCI concurrently with high-dose chemotherapy or in individual radiation fractions of 4 Gy.[312] Some authorities suggest that PCI should be administered only in standard fractions of 2 Gy after the completion of chemotherapy.[250]

After PCI, neuropsychological and imaging abnormalities may or may not be due to PCI. Chemotherapy, paraneoplastic syndromes, micrometastases, and chronic cigarette and alcohol abuse may be important contributors. In one study that evaluated cognitive function in patients before and after chemoradiation but before PCI, deficits were discovered in verbal memory, frontal lobe function, and motor coordination within both groups of patients.[118] A similar, more recent study indicated that 47% of SCLC patients had impaired cognitive function before PCI, and that PCI was not associated with persistent declines in cognitive function.[316] The administration of methotrexate, procarbazine, and lomustine has decreased over the past 15 years; these particular agents have been incriminated in neuropsychological dysfunction. One of the studies included in the meta-analysis had almost 300 patients who were randomized to receive PCI after having achieved a complete remission to initial treatment.[304] There were no obvious differences in the neuropsychological function between the two groups, but only 33 patients underwent a complete reassessment at 18 months. Inasmuch as neuropsychological abnormalities possibly due to PCI progress over time, these data are insufficient to exclude radiation-associated cognitive damage, but they are nonetheless relevant.

A recent decision analysis suggests that for patients who have had a complete response to initial therapy, PCI offers a better quality-adjusted life expectancy, even if a mild to moderate neurotoxicity rate was assumed.[317] If PCI is not administered concurrently with chemotherapy, radiation-induced permeability alterations that allow more of the chemotherapeutic agent into the brain parenchyma should be obviated. The authors' guidelines for PCI, after a thorough discussion with the patient of potential risks and benefits, are as follows: (1) PCI is typically recommended as soon as a partial or complete response to induction therapy has been confirmed, and after acute toxicities have resolved, which is typically 2 to 4 weeks after completion of all chemotherapy. Note that in the EORTC trial of PCI for extensive-stage patients, PCI was given 4 to 6 weeks after chemotherapy. (2) The standard fractionation of 2500 cGy in 10 fractions is recommended for all patients in whom PCI is deemed appropriate, with a consideration of 2000 cGy in five fractions for extensive-stage patients for whom, due to borderline performance status or significant logistical impediments, shortening overall treatment time is felt to be important.

Role of Chemotherapy and Radiation Therapy to the Neuraxis. For overt metastatic lesions within the CNS, doses of 3 Gy daily to a dose of 30 Gy typically is used. Overt intracranial metastases appear to be more difficult to sterilize than intrathoracic disease.[318] Due to the propensity for SCLC patients to develop multifocal brain metastases, stereotactic treatment for brain metastases is typically not appropriate because the risk of brain relapse beyond the treated lesion would be unacceptably high. However, in the context of prior whole brain radiation or prophylactic cranial irradiation, stereotactic treatment may be considered as a salvage option.[319]

Chemotherapy also is a therapeutic option for brain metastases, perhaps because the blood–brain barrier is disrupted in the setting of macroscopic metastatic disease. Small series of patients in whom brain metastases were present at diagnosis have been treated with standard chemotherapy regimens without radiation, and the majority have demonstrated clinical and radiographic improvement.[320] Chemotherapy also has been used at the time of relapse, and response rates of 33% to 43% have been reported.[320–322] In previously treated patients, the response to chemotherapy in the brain appears to be comparable to the response rates in other organs, and it is not dissimilar from the activity of irradiation, which in one series produced a partial response rate of 50%; the median survival was 4.7 months in a series of 22 patients.[323] In the phase II trial evaluating temozolomide in patients with relapsed or refractory SCLC, patients with progressive brain metastases that had received prior cranial irradiation demonstrated an intracranial response to the agent.[200] Thus, although brain irradiation remains the standard for patients who have not been previously irradiated, chemotherapy is a reasonable option for those in whom recurrent disease develops after prior brain radiation, particularly if active systemic disease is also present.

Surgery

Even before the advent of combination chemotherapy for SCLC, the poor outcomes in various case series clearly indicated that surgery is not advisable as a sole treatment modality in this disease.[324–327]

Given that SCLC patients generally present with bulky unresectable disease, studies evaluating surgery are limited. In some cases, patients who undergo thoracotomy for an abnormal pulmonary nodule are unexpectedly diagnosed with SCLC.[55] About 4% of solitary pulmonary nodules are diagnosed as SCLC.[29,30] In these cases, a complete surgical resection should be performed and the patient should be referred for adjuvant therapy. Based on current recommendations, patients with N0 disease should then receive adjuvant chemotherapy, whereas patients with nodal involvement should receive chemotherapy and mediastinal radiation.[52]

Nodal status and primary tumor (T) status have significant effects on the survival of patients who have undergone resection. Angeletti et al.[328] and Shepherd et al.[329] reported increased survival

of node-negative compared to N1 and N2 patients after surgical resection and postoperative chemotherapy, whereas Macchiarini et al.[330] found a decrease in 5-year survival with increasing T category in surgically resected patients without nodal metastases. Rea et al.[331] reported that 51 stage I or II SCLC patients resected and given chemotherapy after resection had 5-year survival rates of 52% (stage I) and 30% (stage II). In the review by Lucchi et al.,[332] stage I or II resected SCLC patients who underwent postoperative chemotherapy had 5-year survival rates of 47% and 15%, respectively. Stage III patients from this series who underwent surgery followed by adjuvant therapy had a 5-year survival of 14%. The largest experience examining the role of surgery followed by adjuvant therapy in SCLC was a cooperative group trial conducted by the International Society of Chemotherapy Lung Cancer Study Group.[54] Four-year survival rates for completely resected, pathologically staged SCLC patients with N0 (n = 69), N1 (n = 58), and N2 (n = 36) who received postoperative therapy were 60%, 36%, and 33%, respectively. Based on these studies, most authorities believe that surgery may have a role as part of a multimodality approach, but only for patients with stage I disease.[52] A mediastinoscopy should be performed in all patients who are being considered for resection of known SCLCs. In a large series from the University of Toronto, surgery followed by chemotherapy had the same outcome as treatment in the reverse order.[329]

Surgical resection also has been studied as a way of reducing the risk of local recurrence in patients with limited disease after the completion of chemoradiation. Although most patients with SCLC succumb to metastatic disease, local recurrence occurs in 35% to 50%.[49] Furthermore, tumors may have a mixed histology such that residual NSCLC remains after treatment of the more chemosensitive SCLC component. Of 38 cases resected after chemoradiation in a University of Toronto study, 29 had pure SCLC but 4 were pure NSCLC, 2 had a mixed histology, and 3 had no residual tumor.[333] Several groups have reported the feasibility of this approach, although notably in these prospective studies, only about half of the cases were resectable and pneumonectomies were frequently required.[305–307] One randomized trial attempted to address the question of whether surgical resection of persistent local disease adds any benefit to the usual approach of chemoradiation for limited-stage patients.[334] The Lung Cancer Study Group enrolled 328 patients who were first treated with CAV for five cycles. Fit patients with at least a partial response were then randomized to surgical resection or not. All patients were then intended to receive thoracic and prophylactic cranial irradiation. As with the previously reported studies, only a fraction of the patients were eligible for surgery after induction therapy; only 146 patients were randomized, and this diminished the power of the statistical analysis. Nonetheless, no differences in OS or even in local control rates were noted between the two groups. NSCLC or mixed NSCLC/SCLC comprised 11% of the resected specimens. These data suggest that surgical resection of residual disease in limited-stage SCLC does not improve outcomes. The use of surgery for patients with SCLC should be restricted to patients with stage I tumors.

Palliative Care

Survivorship Issues

Although minor advances have transpired over the past 3 decades, there has been no dramatic change in outcomes for SCLC since the introduction of EP chemotherapy in the late 1970s, with median survival improving only by 2 months from 7 to 9 months between 1972 and 1990.[335] Although this therapy significantly changes the natural history of SCLC, and the use of twice-daily concomitant radiotherapy and prophylactic cranial irradiation adds incremental benefit in patients with limited disease, the number of persons cured remains small. Few patients with extensive disease attain long-term survival. Patients are at greatest risk of dying from SCLC during the first 24 months after diagnosis. This risk declines between years 2 and 3 and is further reduced beyond year 3. In the SEER program database, OS at 2, 3, and 5 years was 12%, 7%, and 5%, respectively.[336]

Excessive mortality in long-term survivors is due primarily to the development of second primary tumors, mainly NSCLC, and other illnesses associated with cigarette smoking.[67,337–340] Late relapse can occur in approximately 10% of patients at 5 years.[341] Overall, the relative risk of a second primary tumor in patients who survive beyond 2 years is increased 3.5-fold. The second lung cancer risk is increased 13-fold among those who received chest irradiation.[337] Because most of the second primary tumors are NSCLC or other malignancies of the upper aerodigestive tract, it is likely that field cancerization due to tobacco exposure has occurred.[337,338] The risk of a second primary tumor increases significantly over time and with continued smoking. Treatment with alkylating agents further magnifies this risk.[337] For example, the risk of a second lung cancer in patients who continue to smoke was approximately fourfold more than those who stopped before the diagnosis of SCLC and twofold greater in patients who received chest irradiation compared to nonirradiated patients. The cumulative risk of a second lung cancer was 32% at 12 years and continued to increase beyond that time point. Secondary leukemias have been seen as well.[339,340] Patients successfully treated for SCLC constitute an extraordinarily high-risk group for second malignancies and require close surveillance. The cigarette smoking status of every long-term survivor of SCLC should be assessed at every visit. Aggressive smoking cessation efforts should be marshaled for any patient who expresses an interest in quitting. In addition, this population should be considered for studies evaluating new surveillance technologies and chemoprevention.

Long-term survivors are also at increased risk for non–cancer-related problems, including complications of treatment (e.g., pulmonary fibrosis in patients receiving thoracic irradiation, neurologic impairment both as a consequence of treatment with cranial irradiation and paraneoplastic effects of SCLC, and the acceleration of coronary artery disease following thoracic irradiation) as well as tobacco-related illnesses like heart disease, stroke, and chronic obstructive pulmonary disease. In a French study of patients surviving beyond 30 months, treatment-related sequelae included neurologic impairment in 13% of the patients, pulmonary fibrosis in 18%, and cardiac disorders in 10%.[342] A return to work was possible in 40% of these patients and was not influenced by the presence of late treatment-related complications. In a Danish analysis of patients surviving 5 years or more, there was a sixfold increased risk of death from noncancer causes, particularly cardiovascular and pulmonary diseases.[343] Physicians who care for survivors of SCLC should aggressively implement all strategies to reduce cardiovascular disease. These patients should be considered high risk and managed like any other high-risk individual.

TYPICAL AND ATYPICAL CARCINOID TUMORS

Incidence and Etiology

Although over 60% of carcinoid tumors originate in the gastrointestinal system, about 25% of all carcinoids have a pulmonary origin, representing the second most common involved site.[344] Pulmonary carcinoids comprise about 2% of all primary lung tumors.[345] Over the past 30 years, the age-adjusted incidence rate in pulmonary carcinoids has significantly increased, which may represent the improvement in classification of these tumors, as well as the rise of imaging techniques.[344] There is a higher incidence of pulmonary carcinoids in women compared to men and whites compared to blacks.[346,347]

Atypical carcinoids, which have a higher likelihood of metastatic spread or relapse after surgery, are distinguished from the typical carcinoids, which have a more favorable prognosis. Ten percent

to 30% of pulmonary carcinoids are atypical.[348–350] Patients with typical carcinoids are approximately 10 years younger than those with atypical carcinoids, which occur in the 6th decade of life.[347,351] Carcinoids are not clearly caused by smoking like SCLC and LCNEC, although some series suggest that a higher percentage of patients with atypical carcinoid smoke as compared to patients with typical carcinoid tumors.[347,348,352] Pulmonary carcinoids occur rarely in association with multiple endocrine neoplasia type 1 (MEN-1) syndrome. Some sporadic pulmonary carcinoid tumors demonstrate inactivation of the *MEN-1* gene located on chromosome 11q13.[353]

Anatomy and Pathology

All carcinoids are malignant. Typical carcinoids are low grade and atypical carcinoids are intermediate grade. Although carcinoid tumors can be diagnosed by small biopsies or cytology, it is difficult to separate a typical from an atypical carcinoid. This distinction usually requires a surgical biopsy or resection specimen. The histologic appearance of typical and atypical carcinoids is similar with a uniform population of tumor cells arranged in organoid nests with a moderate amount of cytoplasm with an eosinophilic hue (see Fig. 42.2B,C). The finely granular nuclear chromatin frequently has a salt-and-pepper appearance. There are a wide variety of histologic patterns in these tumors, including spindle cell, oncocytic, glandular, follicular, clear cell, and melanocytic. Stromal ossification can occur as well. Atypical carcinoids show increased mitoses (see Fig. 42.2C) with 2 to 10 mitoses per 2 mm^2 or necrosis that is typically punctate.[354] Mitotic activity is the most important way to distinguish typical from atypical carcinoid. The most useful immunohistochemical neuroendocrine markers are chromogranin, synaptophysin, and CD56. If the mitotic count is 11 or more mitoses per 2 mm^2 (10 high power fields), a diagnosis of LCNEC or SCLC is favored over atypical carcinoid.[354,355] In small specimens where mitotic figures are difficult to demonstrate, it may be helpful to use Ki-67 staining because most typical carcinoids show less than 5% staining, atypical carcinoids are usually 10% to 30%, and most LCNECs or SCLCs usually have a very high proliferation index of 80% to 100%.[356]

Nodular neuroendocrine proliferations 0.5 cm or larger are called *carcinoid tumors*. Smaller proliferations are called *tumorlets*, which are separated from carcinoid tumors by size, but with identical morphology of cells. Tumorlets usually are incidental histologic findings of no clinical significance, although they can be seen in interstitial or airway inflammatory and fibrosing conditions. A very rare condition called *diffuse idiopathic pulmonary neuroendocrine cell hyperplasia* (DIPNECH) is regarded as a preinvasive condition for pulmonary carcinoids. Patients with DIPNECH have widespread neuroendocrine cell hyperplasia and tumorlets in their airways and can develop multiple carcinoid tumors.[357]

Screening

Screening for pulmonary carcinoids is not useful. They represent a very small percentage of all lung malignancies and have an indolent natural history. In one study, atypical carcinoid was diagnosed in only 2 of 31,567 (0.006%) asymptomatic patients undergoing baseline lung cancer screening CT scans.[358]

Diagnosis

Two-thirds of carcinoids develop in the major bronchi. As a result, the most common presenting symptoms include obstructive pneumonia, pleuritic pain, atelectasis, dyspnea, and cough.[348,359] Hemoptysis may occur in 10% to 20% of patients. Up to 30% of patients with pulmonary carcinoid tumors are asymptomatic at presentation. In contrast to carcinoids of gastrointestinal origin, carcinoid syndrome (facial flushing, diarrhea, wheezing) is rare in pulmonary carcinoids, occurring in only about 2% of cases.[348,359] Cushing syndrome due to ectopic corticotropin production has been reported in approximately 2% of pulmonary carcinoids.[360] A rare manifestation of pulmonary carcinoids is acromegaly due to the ectopic production of growth hormone–releasing hormone (GHRH), yet these tumors are the most common cause of extrapituitary secretion of GHRH.[361]

The initial workup proceeds in a similar fashion as with other lung tumors, but once a diagnosis of carcinoid is confirmed, more specific radiologic and serologic evaluations for these neuroendocrine tumors may be employed. A biopsy of the central tumors can be easily obtained by bronchoscopy. A biopsy of peripheral lesions by fine needle can be performed, but a definitive diagnosis may be difficult to ascertain in small cytology samples. In addition to routine chest imaging with CT scans, nuclear medicine studies are helpful adjuncts for staging (Fig. 42.5). Due to the overexpression of somatostatin receptors, immunoscintigraphy by somatostatin analogs such as octreotide is widely used. In one series, the sensitivity and specificity was 90% and 83%, respectively.[362] In patients with somatostatin receptor–positive pulmonary carcinoids, octreotide scans have been found to be useful for follow-up and in the detection of recurrent disease, as well as for guiding treatment options.[363] Fluorine-18 (18F) fluorodeoxyglucose (FDG)-PET scanning may be less accurate because these indolent tumors generally have a low standard uptake value (SUV),[364] but some still advocate its potential

use.[365] Recent series have shown that 18F-FDG–PET is useful for the assessment of intermediate- and high-grade neuroendocrine tumors and may have prognostic value.[366,367] Elevated chromogranin A levels have been measured in serum or plasma, although they have been found to be lower in pulmonary carcinoids compared to gastroenteropancreatic endocrine tumors.[368,369] In the setting of advanced or metastatic disease, chromogranin A levels can be useful to follow disease activity.[369] Urinary 5-hydroxyindoleacetic acid (5-HIAA) may be elevated in patients with carcinoid syndrome.

Staging

Pulmonary carcinoid tumors are staged according to the TNM classification used for NSCLC in the AJCC seventh edition. The International Association for the Study of Lung Cancer (IASLC) proposed and approved this in 2009 when it was determined that the TNM staging system was helpful in predicting the prognosis for pulmonary carcinoids.[370] Applying this staging system to cases in the National Cancer Institute SEER registry and cases submitted to the IASLC database, it was determined that 5-year OS for patients with stage I was 93%, stage II was 74% to 85%, stage III was 67% to 75%, and stage IV was 57%.[370] Survival is significantly better for

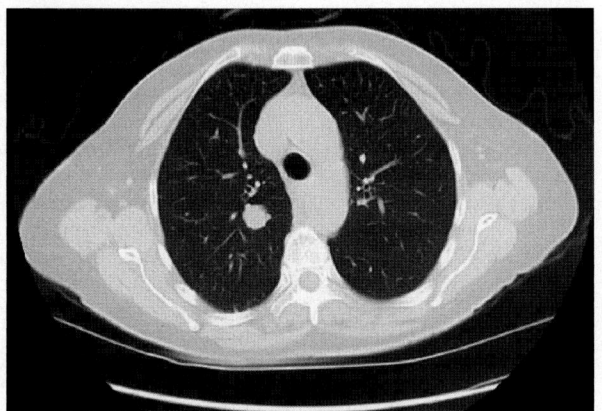
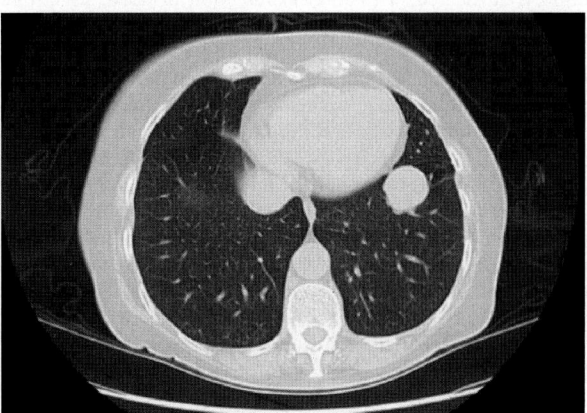
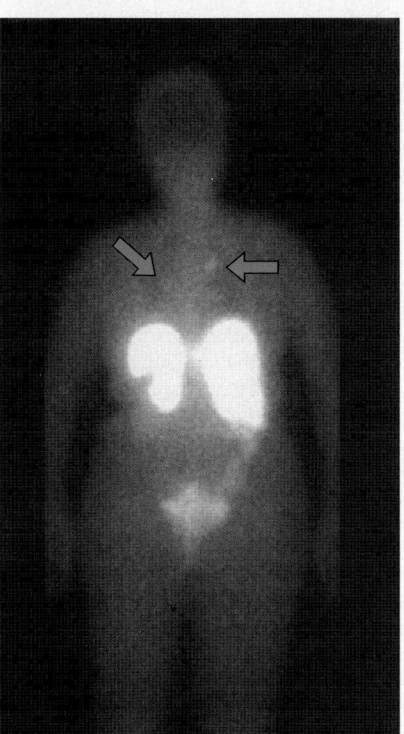

Figure 42.5 (A) Computed tomography scan and **(B)** associated octreotide scan of a patient with bilateral typical carcinoid.

typical carcinoid than for atypical carcinoid. Five-year and 10-year survival rates have been reported at 87% and 87%, respectively, for typical carcinoids, whereas they were 56% and 35%, respectively, for atypical carcinoids.[353] Predictors of survival include stage, tumor size, higher mitotic rates (i.e., atypical subtype), and age greater than 60.[347,352,370] Importantly, patients with multiple nodules have a very favorable prognosis, likely reflected by the fact that these individuals tend to have the underlying preinvasive lesion, diffuse idiopathic pulmonary neuroendocrine cell hyperplasia.[370]

Management by Stage

Stages I, II, and III

Surgery is the primary treatment modality and the only curative option for patients with pulmonary carcinoids. Because carcinoids often present centrally, a pneumonectomy or bilobectomy is frequent, but most patients undergo a lobectomy.[345,352] For patients with favorable prognostic features, such as typical histology and the absence of lymph node involvement, a more limited resection has been proposed.[359,371] Patients with atypical carcinoids should be resected using the same principles guiding surgery for NSCLC.[372]

Because mediastinal lymph node metastases occur in patients with pulmonary carcinoids, complete mediastinal lymph node dissection is advocated, with surgical resection of nodal metastases when feasible.[351,373–377] Multiple series have found decreased incidences of local recurrence[351,375] and improved survival when a complete mediastinal lymph node dissection is performed.[350,373]

Adjuvant chemotherapy after surgical resection for patients with typical carcinoid with or without regional lymph node metastases (stages I, II, and III) is not recommended,[378] because the risk of recurrence has been shown to be low: In a series of 291 resected typical carcinoids, only 3% of patients suffered recurrence.[351,379] Similarly, following surgical resection, patients with stage I atypical carcinoid are followed expectantly. However, because systemic recurrence occurs more frequently in patients with atypical carcinoid with N1 or N2 involvement (stages II and III), documented to be as high as 26% in a surgical series,[379] adjuvant chemotherapy after surgical resection has been advocated by some,[378] but it is unknown whether this is beneficial. There is no defined adjuvant regimen for atypical carcinoid, yet due to similarities with SCLC, etoposide with cisplatin or carboplatin is generally used.[378]

The use of radiation therapy for carcinoid tumors is most similar to its pattern of use in NSCLCs. For tumors that are resectable, adjuvant radiation therapy is typically recommended in situations of residual disease (R1 resection) and mediastinal lymphadenopathy (N2 disease). The use of adjuvant radiation therapy for nodal disease is probably of greater utility in the more aggressive atypical carcinoid.[378] In patients with unresectable disease, radiation therapy can be used after induction chemotherapy or concurrently.[380] Doses of 60 Gy are typical. Carcinoid tumors are less responsive to radiation therapy than SCLC.[381]

Stage IV

Data regarding the efficacy of chemotherapy specifically in pulmonary carcinoid (as opposed to gastrointestinal carcinoids) are lacking, because this tumor type has not been studied independently of other neuroendocrine tumors and occasionally has been omitted from such trials. Many of the studies have used older classification systems for carcinoids and different criteria for response. Various chemotherapeutic agents have been used, including doxorubicin, 5-fluorouracil, dacarbazine, cisplatin, carboplatin, etoposide, streptozocin, and interferon-alpha.[368,382] Yet, in general, carcinoid tumors have no significant therapies that consistently induce regression.

Octreotide has been used in the treatment of these tumors. Retrospective reviews, including small numbers of patients with pulmonary carcinoids, have reported on the use of somatostatin analogs with improvement in carcinoid syndrome symptoms, as well as prolonged disease control and survival, with very few individuals achieving a tumor response.[383,384,385] These results are similar to the experience with octreotide in gastrointestinal carcinoids.[386] Notably, the recent PROMID study showed that long-acting–release octreotide acetate significantly prolonged time to tumor progression compared with placebo in patients with newly diagnosed functionally active or inactive well-differentiated midgut neuroendocrine tumors (14.3 versus 6 months; HR, 0.34; 95% CI, 0.20 to 0.59; p = 0.000072). However, there was no improvement in OS.[387] Although some studies evaluating peptide receptor radionuclide therapy with radiolabeled somatostatin analogs in patients resistant to octreotide have included bronchial carcinoids, the number of patients with this histology is small thus far to generate any meaningful conclusions. However, such agents have been found to have reasonable response rates and outcomes in patients with pancreatic neuroendocrine tumors and gastrointestinal carcinoids.[388]

Regimens typically used for SCLC often are recommended.[378,389] However, typical carcinoids and atypical carcinoids are clearly less chemosensitive than SCLCs. In two small series that included 26 patients in total treated with chemotherapy (mostly etoposide and cisplatin), the response rate was about 20%.[368,380] EP was administered to 18 patients with foregut-origin carcinoids (lung and thymus) who had progressed after first- or second-line treatment in a prospective study. Radiographic response was noted in 2 of the 5 patients with atypical carcinoid (40%) and in 5 of the 13 with typical carcinoid (39%). The median response duration was 9 months (range, 6 to 30 months).[390] Similarly, etoposide with cisplatin or carboplatin was administered to 17 pulmonary carcinoid patients, with a 23.5% radiologic response (2 patients each with atypical and typical carcinoid) and median PFS of 7 months.[385]

Newer agents are being studied actively in neuroendocrine carcinoma. Temozolomide, a nonclassical oral alkylating agent, has been evaluated either alone or in combination with other agents. Thirteen patients with pulmonary carcinoids (10 typical, 3 atypical) were included in a retrospective study using single-agent temozolomide. Four of these patients (31%) had a partial response to treatment (3 typical, 1 atypical), and 62% derived clinical benefit (response or stable disease) with temozolomide.[391] In a larger retrospective study of 31 patients that included both typical and atypical pulmonary carcinoids, a partial response to treatment was noted in 3 patients (14%), whereas stable disease was observed in 11 patients (52%); median PFS and OS were 5.3 months and 23.2 months, respectively.[392] Eighteen patients with carcinoid and pancreatic neuroendocrine tumors metastatic to the liver that received capecitabine and temozolomide, were evaluated for response and outcome.[393] The overall response rate was 61%, and three of the four carcinoid patients attained clinical benefit (complete response, n = 1; partial response, n = 1, stable disease, n = 1). From the time of liver metastases, median PFS and OS were 14 months (range, 4 to 18 months) and 83 months (range, 18.5 to 140 months) for this combination, respectively. These results suggest that the regimen of capecitabine and temozolomide is active and may prolong survival in this malignancy.[393] In contrast, in two prospective trials that included patients with carcinoid tumors, a 7% response rate was noted using temozolomide with thalidomide and no response was observed using temozolomide and bevacizumab.[394,395] However, because some studies have shown promising results for temozolomide, either alone or in combination with other agents in metastatic pulmonary carcinoids, larger prospective studies should be developed.

The mTOR pathway, which regulates cell growth, proliferation, and metabolism, has been implicated in the pathogenesis of neuroendocrine tumors.[396] To determine if the addition of everolimus improved PFS, the randomized, placebo-controlled phase III study of everolimus plus octreotide long-acting repeatable (LAR) (RADIANT-2) included 429 patients with low-grade or intermediate-grade carcinoids, of which 44 were of pulmonary histology.[396] Median PFS was 16.4 months (95% CI, 13.7 to 21.2 months) for the group receiving the combination of everolimus and octreotide LAR compared to 11.3 months (95% CI, 8.4 to 14.6 months) in the octreotide LAR–only group (HR, 0.77; 95% CI, 0.59 to 1.0, $p = 0.026$); thus achieving the primary endpoint of the study. For the 44 bronchial carcinoid patients, median PFS was 13.6 and 5.6 months in the everolimus plus octreotide LAR group versus octreotide LAR–only group, respectively.[396] Currently, we are awaiting results from the randomized, double-blind, phase III study of everolimus versus placebo in patients with advanced neuroendocrine tumors of gastrointestinal (GI) or lung origin only (RADIANT-4) (ClinicalTrials.gov identifier: NCT01524783). Well-differentiated carcinoid tumors are highly vascularized and extensively express VEGF, Hypoxia inducible factor 1-alpha, and microvessel density.[397] As such, angiogenesis inhibitors have been investigated in this disease. In a phase II study, in low- to intermediate-grade neuroendocrine tumors, patients were randomized to receive either bevacizumab or pegylated interferon-alfa-2b (IFNα–2b). Only four patients with pulmonary carcinoids were included in this trial, where an 18% partial response rate was observed in the bevacizumab group compared with no responses in the pegylated IFNα–2b arm.[398] Fourteen patients with foregut carcinoids of the lung and stomach were included in a phase II study using sunitinib, a multitargeted oral TKI. The overall response rate for patients with carcinoid tumors was only 2.4% with a median time tumor progression of 10.2 months.[399] In contrast, in pancreatic neuroendocrine carcinoma, the randomized phase III trial of sunitinib versus placebo, demonstrated a significant improvement in PFS (11.4 versus 5.5 months, respectively; HR, 0.42; 95% CI, 0.26 to 0.66; $p <0.001$).[400]

In patients with liver metastases, hepatic artery embolization, with or without intra-arterial chemotherapy has been associated with responses and improved outcomes in carcinoid patients.[401] Nine patients with pulmonary carcinoids who developed liver metastases underwent hepatic artery chemoembolization in a recently reported single institution retrospective review. Prolonged stable disease lasting up to 19 months was noted in eight of these patients, with three achieving a partial response.[385] A newer embolization method, utilizing injectable particles conjugated to yttrium-90, permits the delivery of internal radiation into hepatic arteries that supply carcinoid liver metastases.[397] Because randomized trials in embolization methods are lacking and some do experience treatment-related toxicities, patients must be selected carefully for these procedures.

In the approach to metastatic carcinoid tumors, many advocate using somatostatin analogs as first-line treatment in patients with well-differentiated tumors with little tumor bulk in the setting of a positive octreotide scan[363,383] and chemotherapy for those with more rapidly progressing tumors or those who have progressed on less toxic treatments.[402,403] Additional prospective, randomized studies are needed for both traditional cytotoxic and molecularly targeted agents in this disease, because early results are promising. Palliative radiation therapy can be used for symptomatic lesions.[381]

LARGE CELL NEUROENDOCRINE CARCINOMA

Incidence and Etiology

LCNEC of the lung was first described in 1991 as a form of high-grade non–small-cell neuroendocrine carcinoma.[404] LCNEC accounts for about 3% of surgically resected lung cancers.[405] In previously reported series, LCNEC patients have a median age of 62 years (range, 33 to 87 years) and the vast majority of patients are male cigarette smokers.[347,405]

Anatomy and Pathology

In the 2004 World Health Organization (WHO) classification, LCNEC is classified as a variant of large cell carcinoma.[9,405,406] There are four ways that neuroendocrine differentiation can be manifest within large cell carcinomas: (1) If both neuroendocrine

morphology by light microscopy as well as neuroendocrine differentiation by immunohistochemistry or electron microscopy are seen, the tumor is classified as LCNEC; (2) if there is no neuroendocrine morphology by light microscopy and neuroendocrine differentiation is seen by immunohistochemistry or electron microscopy, the tumor is classified as large cell carcinoma with neuroendocrine differentiation (LCC-NED); (3) if the tumor lacks both neuroendocrine morphology by light microscopy and neuroendocrine differentiation by immunohistochemistry or electron microscopy, it is classified as a classic large cell carcinoma; and (4) if the neuroendocrine morphology (LCNEM) has neuroendocrine morphology but lacks neuroendocrine differentiation by electron microscopy or immunohistochemistry, it is classified as large cell carcinoma.[9,405,406] Little is known about the latter category.

LCNEC are diagnosed based on the following criteria (Fig. 42.2D): (1) neuroendocrine morphology with organoid nesting, palisading, or rosettelike structures; (2) high mitotic rate greater than 10 mitoses per 2 mm^2 (average 60 to 80 mitoses per 2 mm^2); (3) non–small-cell cytologic features, including large cell size, low nuclear or cytoplasmic ratio, nucleoli, or vesicular chromatin; and (4) neuroendocrine differentiation by immunohistochemistry (chromogranin, CD56, or synaptophysin) or electron microscopy.[9,354] The tumor grows in organoid nests with peripheral palisading and rosettelike structures. The tumor cells have abundant cytoplasm, prominent nucleoli, and frequent mitoses.

When LCNEC has components of adenocarcinoma, squamous cell carcinoma, giant cell carcinoma, or spindle cell carcinoma, it is called combined LCNEC and the specific components present should be mentioned.[9,354] Adenocarcinoma is the histologic type found most often in combined LCNEC. When SCLC is combined with LCNEC, the tumor becomes a combined SCLC, and LCNEC and should be regarded as a SCLC.

LCNEC will be positive for pancytokeratin and at least one neuroendocrine marker such as chromogranin, CD56, or synaptophysin. TTF-1 will be positive in 60% to 80% of cases. There is a very high proliferation index with 80% to 100% positive tumor cells.[405,407] When the differential diagnosis of basaloid carcinoma is a consideration, diffuse strong staining for p63 or p40 would favor this diagnosis over LCNEC.[15]

It is difficult to make the diagnosis of LCNEC on small biopsies or cytology because the characteristic neuroendocrine morphologic pattern and neuroendocrine differentiation by immunohistochemistry are difficult to demonstrate in minute pieces of tissue.[405,407] Therefore, in the vast majority of cases, a definite diagnosis of LCNEC will require a surgical biopsy. Separation of LCNEC from SCLC requires consideration of multiple histologic features such as cell size, nucleoli, chromatin pattern, and nuclear to cytoplasmic ratio, rather than a single criterion. Artifacts such as those introduced by frozen sections or poor quality hematoxylin and eosin-stained sections, can distort cellular morphology, resulting in confusion with SCLC.[11,405,407]

Screening

Clinically, LCNEC is characterized by similar behavior to SCLC, with rapid tumor growth and early metastatic spread.[347] Further, LCNEC represents a small percentage of all lung malignancies. In one study, LCNEC was diagnosed in only 15 of 31,567 (0.05%) asymptomatic patients undergoing baseline lung cancer screening CT scans.[358] Therefore, screening for LCNEC is not useful.

Diagnosis

In patients with LCNEC, presenting symptoms mimic those of SCLC and other NSCLC. For example, in one series of 83 patients, the main symptoms were hemoptysis (30%), chest pain (22%), dyspnea (16%), cough (16%), and weight loss (13%); only 4% of patients were asymptomatic.[408] Ectopic hormone production and paraneoplastic syndromes are typically absent.[347]

LCNEC generally present as peripheral tumors. When centrally located, endobronchial growth and obstructive pneumonia can be found.[409] On CT scan, these tumors are often well defined and lobulated, without air bronchograms or calcifications; spiculated margins are less commonly observed.[409,410] Inhomogeneous enhancement is found in larger diameter (33 mm or larger) tumors secondary to necrosis.[409] LCNEC typically have homogenously high FDG uptake on PET scans, which is helpful in locating extrathoracic metastases.[410] A definitive diagnosis may be difficult to determine in small specimens or by cytology, as indicated previously[405,407]; thus, a surgical biopsy is often needed in LCNEC.

Staging

The TNM classification used for NSCLC in the AJCC seventh edition is used for the staging of LCNEC.

Survival for LCNEC is poor and appears to be significantly worse than that of nonneuroendocrine NSCLC.[411] In a series of 335 pathologic stage IA NSCLCs comprising 259 adenocarcinomas, 65 squamous cell carcinomas, and 11 large cell neuroendocrine carcinomas, the histology of LCNEC was found to have a significant adverse prognostic impact and was predictive of poorer overall survival.[411] Asamura et al.[347] found that the survival curve of LCNEC can be superimposed on that for SCLC, with no difference in survival stage for stage between the two, confirming the findings of multiple other series. Reported overall 5-year survival after surgical resection of LCNEC ranges between 15% and 57%,[405] indicating that the recurrence rate after surgery is high. Data from different series reveal that the 5-year survival rate ranges between 33% to 62% in stage I patients, 18% to 75% in stage II patients, 8% to 45% in stage III patients, and 0% in stage IV patients.[347,408,411–413] Factors significantly related to survival among clinicopathologic parameters are tumor stage and size (less than 3 cm versus 3 cm or greater),[406] as well as male gender.[414]

Management by Stage

Patients with LCNEC are managed as if they have NSCLC with the same treatment algorithm stage for stage. The controversy in LCNEC centers on the choice of chemotherapy. Based on the neuroendocrine features, should LCNEC be treated with the same chemotherapy regimens used for SCLC? Certainly the aggressive natural history and propensity to metastasize are similar to SCLC, yet LCNEC clearly does not demonstrate the same chemosensitivity. Published reports about LCNEC are not instructive because essentially all are small, retrospective series with a focus on patients who underwent surgery. Details regarding chemotherapy treatment, such as the agents used or the response rates, are generally not provided.

Stages I, II, and III

For patients with early stage LCNECs, resection is recommended. The modalities of choice are either lobectomy or pneumonectomy, with systematic nodal dissection.[415] After careful mediastinal lymph node sampling, patients without lymph node metastases seem to experience improved survival.[415]

Given the aggressive nature of LCNEC, surgery alone is not sufficient for its treatment. Several small, retrospective studies have attempted to discern the role of neoadjuvant or adjuvant chemotherapy in LCNEC. In this setting, the use of SCLC-based regimens is supported. A Japanese group compiled data on 16 patients who received postoperative chemotherapy and 57 who did not.[413] For all patients, the 5-year survival was 62% for stage I, 18% for stage II, and 17% for stage III. The authors noted that the 5-year survival for the five patients with stage I disease who received adjuvant chemotherapy was 100%, whereas it was 51% for the 23 patients who did not. Postoperative chemotherapy did not affect survival for other stages.[413] In a retrospective review of 100 patients

with resected LCNEC evaluating the use of perioperative chemotherapy,[414] there was no association observed between OS and receipt of neoadjuvant (n = 22) or adjuvant (n = 20) platinum-based regimens (OS at 5 years was 50% for no therapy versus 45% for those that received chemotherapy, p adjusted for propensity score = 0.18). However, when the analysis was restricted to patients with completely resected advanced stage IB-IIIA disease, the receipt of platinum-based chemotherapy in either the induction and/or the adjuvant setting was marginally associated with improved median OS: 2 years (95% CI, 1 to 5.3 years) in the no platinum chemotherapy group, compared to 7.4 years (95% CI, 2.5 to not reached) in the platinum chemotherapy group (p adjusted for propensity score = 0.052).[414] In a retrospective analysis of 144 surgical LCNEC cases, Veronesi et al.[412] showed that although perioperative chemotherapy only led to a trend toward improved survival in stage I patients, a statistically significant survival benefit was found across all stages compared to surgery alone (p = 0.04). In a retrospective review of 45 surgically resected patients with LCNEC, patients who did not receive chemotherapy after surgery were more likely to die than patients who underwent surgery plus chemotherapy (n = 23) (HR, 9.472; 95% CI, 1.050 to 85.478; p = 0.0457).[416] An improvement in OS was found in 23 of 63 patients who received perioperative platinum-based chemotherapy compared to those who underwent surgery alone (74.4% versus 32.3%, respectively; p = 0.042).[417] A multivariate analysis utilizing age, gender, pathologic stage, surgical procedure, and perioperative chemotherapy revealed that those patients who underwent surgery with chemotherapy had a significantly better prognosis than those who underwent surgery alone (HR, 0.323; 95% CI, 0.112 to 0.934, p = 0.0371).[417]

As stated, SCLC-based regimens in the adjuvant treatment of LCNEC is supported, in particular. Iyoda et al.[418] performed a prospective analysis on 15 LCNEC patients who received adjuvant chemotherapy with EP and compared outcomes to a historic cohort of LCNEC patients treated without platinum-based adjuvant therapy. Prolonged survival was noted for the patients that received at least two cycles of SCLC-based regimens; the 5-year overall survival rates were 88.9% and 47.4% in the adjuvant chemotherapy group and in the control group, respectively. Further, those receiving platinum-based adjuvant chemotherapy were noted to have a significantly lower rate of tumor recurrence when compared to patients receiving non–platinum-based adjuvant chemotherapy or no adjuvant chemotherapy.[419] Finally, in an Italian retrospective series of 83 LCNEC cases, the 13 patients who received SCLC-based regimens had significantly better survival than the 15 patients who received drug combinations used in NSCLC (median survival, 42 months versus 11 months, respectively; p <0.0001). The best prognosis was noted in stage I LCNEC patients who received SCLC-based adjuvant chemotherapy. In univariate and multivariate analyses, the administration of adjuvant chemotherapy with cisplatin or carboplatin plus etoposide was the most important variable correlating with survival.[408] The interpretation of these reports is limited by their retrospective nature and the small sample size. However, these data, along with the known poor natural history and the routine use of adjuvant chemotherapy for SCLC and NSCLC, suggest that postoperative treatment with etoposide and cisplatin is appropriate in patients with completely resected LCNEC, including patients with stage I disease.

Data regarding the use of radiation therapy in this disease are sparse, but its role in the adjuvant setting is likely similar to that in NSCLC. As per the NCCN guidelines, definitive radiation therapy is recommended for patients who are unable to undergo surgical resection.[420]

Stage IV

The optimal chemotherapeutic regimen in relapsed or stage IV disease is not defined, although treatment with platinum-based regimens is advocated. Several studies have shown that the response rate of LCNEC to cisplatin-based chemotherapy is comparable to SCLC. A retrospective series of 20 patients with advanced LCNEC (stage IIIA, 3; stage IIIB, 6; stage IV, 6; postoperative recurrence, 5) treated with platinum-based therapy showed a response rate of 50% (complete response, 1; partial response, 9).[421] Interestingly, the response rate for chemotherapy-naïve patients (64%) was better than those patients who were previously treated (17%).[421] Rossi et al.[408] showed that in metastatic disease, the 12 patients who received SCLC-based chemotherapy had a significantly better median survival than the 15 patients who received common NSCLC regimens (51 versus 21 months, respectively; p <0.001). Only the patients who received SCLC-based chemotherapy had a complete or partial response. In another retrospective review of 45 patients with pathologically confirmed LCNEC receiving first-line chemotherapy, response rates and outcomes were compared between those that received SCLC (n = 11) and NSCLC (n = 34) regimens. Those treated with SCLC regimens had nonsignificant higher response rates and median PFS and OS compared to patients in the NSCLC chemotherapy group (73% versus 50%, p = 0.19; 6.1 versus 4.9 months, respectively, p = 0.41; 16.5 versus 9.2 months, respectively, p =0.10).[422]

Two single arm, multicenter phase II studies have been performed in patients with newly diagnosed stage IV LCNEC, each of which had the response rate as the primary endpoint.[423,424] In Japan, 44 patients were enrolled to receive cisplatin and irinotecan every 4 weeks. After careful pathologic review, 30 patients had confirmed LCNEC, whereas 10 actually were reclassified as SCLC. Comparing the two groups, the response rate for this regimen was 47% and 80% for patients with LCNEC and SCLC, respectively (p = 0.082). The median PFS and OS were higher in the SCLC group compared to the LCNEC group, 6.2 months versus 5.8 months (p = 0.382), and 17.3 months versus 12.6 months (p = 0.047), respectively.[423] In the multicenter French study, 42 patients were enrolled to receive EP every 21 days. Here, the LCNEC pathology was confirmed in 29 patients, the response rate of which was 34%. In the analysis confined to the patients with confirmed LCNEC, the median PFS was 5 months and the median OS was 8 months, which was not significantly different than the group with other confirmed diagnoses (SCLC, 9; NSCLC, 1; and atypical carcinoid, 1).[424]

As can be seen, information regarding the treatment of LCNEC has been derived from small studies and suggests that these cancers should be treated as SCLC, although the response rates are lower and outcomes are inferior. Larger, randomized prospective studies are needed to determine the optimal treatment regimen for this disease.

SELECTED REFERENCES

The full reference list can be accessed at lwwhealthlibrary.com/oncology.

1. Govindan R, Page N, Morgensztern D, et al. Changing epidemiology of small-cell lung cancer in the United States over the last 30 years: analysis of the surveillance, epidemiologic, and end results database. *J Clin Oncol* 2006;24:4539–4544.
4. Varghese A, Zakowski MF, Yu HA, et al. Small-cell lung cancers in patients who never smoked cigarettes. *J Thorac Oncol* 2014:9:892–896.
9. Travis WD, Brambilla E, Muller-Hermelink HK, et al. *Pathology and Genetics: Tumours of the Lung, Pleura, Thymus and Heart.* Lyon: International Agency for Research on Cancer; 2004.
10. Nicholson SA, Beasley MB, Brambilla E, et al. Small cell lung carcinoma (SCLC): a clinicopathologic study of 100 cases with surgical specimens. *Am J Surg Pathol* 2002;26:1184–1197.
11. Travis WD. Update on small cell carcinoma and its differentiation from squamous cell carcinoma and other non-small cell carcinomas. *Mod Pathol* 2012;25:S18–S30.
22. Peifer M, Fernandez-Cuesta L, Sos ML, et al. Integrative genome analyses identify key somatic driver mutations of small-cell lung cancer. *Nat Geneti* 2012;44:1104–1110.
23. Rudin CM, Durinck S, Stawiski EW, et al. Comprehensive genomic analysis identifies SOX2 as a frequently amplified gene in small-cell lung cancer. *Nat Genet* 2012;44:1111–1116.
25. Aberle DR, Adams AM, Berg CD, et al. Reduced lung-cancer mortality with low-dose computed tomographic screening. *N Engl J Med* 2011;365:395–409.
26. Chute CG, Greenberg ER, Baron J, et al. Presenting conditions of 1539 population-based lung cancer patients by cell type and stage in New Hampshire and Vermont. *Cancer* 1985;56:2107–2111.
35. Verbalis JG, Adler S, Schrier RW, et al. Efficacy and safety of oral tolvaptan therapy in patients with the syndrome of inappropriate antidiuretic hormone secretion. *Eur J Endocrinol* 2011;164:725–732.
39. Darnell RB, Posner JB. Paraneoplastic syndromes involving the nervous system. *N Engl J Med* 2003;349:1543–1554.
44. Zelen M. Keynote address on biostatistics and data retrieval. *Cancer Chemother Rep [3]* 1973;4:31–42.
46. Albain KS, Crowley JJ, LeBlanc M, et al. Determinants of improved outcome in small-cell lung cancer: an analysis of the 2,580-patient Southwest Oncology Group data base. *J Clin Oncol* 1990;8:1563–1574.
49. Turrisi AT 3rd, Kim K, Blum R, et al. Twice-daily compared with once-daily thoracic radiotherapy in limited small-cell lung cancer treated concurrently with cisplatin and etoposide. *N Engl J Med* 1999;340:265–271.
50. Doll DC. Serum lactate dehydrogenase and bone marrow involvement in small-cell carcinoma of the lung. *N Engl J Med* 1985;312:1262.
51. Van den Brande P, Demedts M. Serum lactate dehydrogenase in small-cell lung cancer. *N Engl J Med* 1989;320:61.
52. Kalemkerian GP, Akerley W, Bogner P, et al. Small cell lung cancer. *J Natl Compr Canc Netw* 2013;11:78–98.
53. Vallieres E, Shepherd FA, Crowley J, et al. The IASLC Lung Cancer Staging Project: proposals regarding the relevance of TNM in the pathologic staging of small cell lung cancer in the forthcoming (seventh) edition of the TNM classification for lung cancer. *J Thorac Oncol* 2009;4:1049–1059.
54. Karrer K, Ulsperger E. Surgery for cure followed by chemotherapy in small cell carcinoma of the lung. For the ISC-Lung Cancer Study Group. *Acta Oncol* 1995;34:899–906.
59. Yuen AR, Zou G, Turrisi AT, et al. Similar outcome of elderly patients in intergroup trial 0096: Cisplatin, etoposide, and thoracic radiotherapy administered once or twice daily in limited stage small cell lung carcinoma. *Cancer* 2000;89:1953–1960.
67. Lassen U, Osterlind K, Hansen M, et al. Long-term survival in small-cell lung cancer: posttreatment characteristics in patients surviving 5 to 18+ years—an analysis of 1,714 consecutive patients. *J Clin Oncol* 1995;13:1215–1220.
71. Quoix E, Purohit A, Faller-Beau M, et al. Comparative prognostic value of lactate dehydrogenase and neuron-specific enolase in small-cell lung cancer patients treated with platinum-based chemotherapy. *Lung Cancer* 2000;30:127–134.
76. Sculier JP, Feld R, Evans WK, et al. Carcinoembryonic antigen: a useful prognostic marker in small-cell lung cancer. *J Clin Oncol* 1985;3: 1349–1354.
77. Bradley JD, Dehdashti F, Mintun MA, et al. Positron emission tomography in limited-stage small-cell lung cancer: a prospective study. *J Clin Oncol* 2004;22:3248–3254.
80. Cheran SK, Herndon JE 2nd, Patz EF Jr. Comparison of whole-body FDG-PET to bone scan for detection of bone metastases in patients with a new diagnosis of lung cancer. *Lung Cancer* 2004;44:317–325.
82. Park K, Sun J-M, Kim S-W, et al. Phase III trial of concurrent thoracic radiotherapy with either the first cycle or the third cycle of cisplatin and etoposide chemotherapy to determine the optimal timing of thoracic radiotherapy for limited-disease small cell lung cancer. *J Clin Oncol* 2012;30: abstract 7004.
83. Slotman B, Faivre-Finn C, Kramer G, et al. Prophylactic cranial irradiation in extensive small-cell lung cancer. *N Engl J Med* 2007;357:664–672.
92. Jett JR, Everson L, Therneau TM, et al. Treatment of limited-stage small-cell lung cancer with cyclophosphamide, doxorubicin, and vincristine with or without etoposide: a randomized trial of the North Central Cancer Treatment Group. *J Clin Oncol* 1990;8:33–38.
99. Fukuoka M, Furuse K, Saijo N, et al. Randomized trial of cyclophosphamide, doxorubicin, and vincristine versus cisplatin and etoposide versus alternation of these regimens in small-cell lung cancer. *J Natl Cancer Inst* 1991;83: 855–861.
100. Roth BJ, Johnson DH, Einhorn LH, et al. Randomized study of cyclophosphamide, doxorubicin, and vincristine versus etoposide and cisplatin versus alternation of these two regimens in extensive small-cell lung cancer: a phase III trial of the Southeastern Cancer Study Group. *J Clin Oncol* 1992;10: 282–291.
101. Sundstrom S, Bremnes RM, Kaasa S, et al. Cisplatin and etoposide regimen is superior to cyclophosphamide, epirubicin, and vincristine regimen in small-cell lung cancer: results from a randomized phase III trial with 5 years' follow-up. *J Clin Oncol* 2002;20:4665–4672.

PRACTICE OF ONCOLOGY

102. Chute JP, Venzon DJ, Hankins L, et al. Outcome of patients with small-cell lung cancer during 20 years of clinical research at the US National Cancer Institute. *Mayo Clin Proc* 1997;72:901–912.

105. Skarlos DV, Samantas E, Kosmidis P, et al. Randomized comparison of etoposide-cisplatin vs. etoposide-carboplatin and irradiation in small-cell lung cancer. A Hellenic Co-operative Oncology Group study. *Ann Oncol* 1994;5:601–607.

106. Rossi A, Di Maio M, Chiodini P, et al. Carboplatin- or cisplatin-based chemotherapy in first-line treatment of small-cell lung cancer: the COCIS meta-analysis of individual patient data. *J Clin Oncol* 2012;30:1692–1698.

108. Noda K, Nishiwaki Y, Kawahara M, et al. Irinotecan plus cisplatin compared with etoposide plus cisplatin for extensive small-cell lung cancer. *N Engl J Med* 2002;346:85–91.

109. Lara PN Jr, Natale R, Crowley J, et al. Phase III trial of irinotecan/cisplatin compared with etoposide/cisplatin in extensive-stage small-cell lung cancer: clinical and pharmacogenomic results from SWOG S0124. *J Clin Oncol* 2009;27:2530–2535.

115. Eckardt JR, von Pawel J, Papai Z, et al. Open-label, multicenter, randomized, phase III study comparing oral topotecan/cisplatin versus etoposide/cisplatin as treatment for chemotherapy-naive patients with extensive-disease small-cell lung cancer. *J Clin Oncol* 2006;24:2044–2051.

117. Ettinger DS, Finkelstein DM, Abeloff MD, et al. A randomized comparison of standard chemotherapy versus alternating chemotherapy and maintenance versus no maintenance therapy for extensive-stage small-cell lung cancer: a phase III study of the Eastern Cooperative Oncology Group. *J Clin Oncol* 1990;8:230–240.

129. Loehrer PJ Sr, Rynard S, Ansari R, et al. Etoposide, ifosfamide, and cisplatin in extensive small cell lung cancer. *Cancer* 1992;69:669–673.

136. Niell HB, Herndon JE 2nd, Miller AA, et al. Randomized phase III intergroup trial of etoposide and cisplatin with or without paclitaxel and granulocyte colony-stimulating factor in patients with extensive-stage small-cell lung cancer: Cancer and Leukemia Group B Trial 9732. *J Clin Oncol* 2005;23:3752–3759.

142. Giaccone G, Dalesio O, McVie GJ, et al. Maintenance chemotherapy in small-cell lung cancer: long-term results of a randomized trial. European Organization for Research and Treatment of Cancer Lung Cancer Cooperative Group. *J Clin Oncol* 1993;11:1230–1240.

143. Lebeau B, Chastang C, Allard P, et al. Six vs twelve cycles for complete responders to chemotherapy in small cell lung cancer: definitive results of a randomized clinical trial. The "Petites Cellules" Group. *Eur Respir J* 1992;5:286–290.

145. Schiller JH, Adak S, Cella D, et al. Topotecan versus observation after cisplatin plus etoposide in extensive-stage small-cell lung cancer: E7593—a phase III trial of the Eastern Cooperative Oncology Group. *J Clin Oncol* 2001;19:2114–2122.

154. Arriagada R, Le Chevalier T, Pignon JP, et al. Initial chemotherapeutic doses and survival in patients with limited small-cell lung cancer. *N Engl J Med* 1993;329:1848–1852.

157. Ihde DC, Mulshine JL, Kramer BS, et al. Prospective randomized comparison of high-dose and standard-dose etoposide and cisplatin chemotherapy in patients with extensive-stage small-cell lung cancer. *J Clin Oncol* 1994;12:2022–2034.

167. Murray N, Livingston RB, Shepherd FA, et al. Randomized study of CODE versus alternating CAV/EP for extensive-stage small-cell lung cancer: an Intergroup Study of the National Cancer Institute of Canada Clinical Trials Group and the Southwest Oncology Group. *J Clin Oncol* 1999;17:2300–2308.

183. Humblet Y, Symann M, Bosly A, et al. Late intensification chemotherapy with autologous bone marrow transplantation in selected small-cell carcinoma of the lung: a randomized study. *J Clin Oncol* 1987;5:1864–1873.

191. von Pawel J, Schiller JH, Shepherd FA, et al. Topotecan versus cyclophosphamide, doxorubicin, and vincristine for the treatment of recurrent small-cell lung cancer. *J Clin Oncol* 1999;17:658–667.

193. O'Brien ME, Ciuleanu TE, Tsekov H, et al. Phase III trial comparing supportive care alone with supportive care with oral topotecan in patients with relapsed small-cell lung cancer. *J Clin Oncol* 2006;24:5441–5447.

194. Eckardt JR, von Pawel J, Pujol JL, et al. Phase III study of oral compared with intravenous topotecan as second-line therapy in small-cell lung cancer. *J Clin Oncol* 2007;25:2086–2092.

196. Inoue A, Sugawara S, Yamazaki K, et al. Randomized phase II trial comparing amrubicin with topotecan in patients with previously treated small-cell lung cancer: North Japan Lung Cancer Study Group Trial 0402. *J Clin Oncol* 2008;26:5401–5406.

199. Jotte R, Von Pawel J, Spigel DR, et al. Randomized phase III trial of amrubicin versus topotecan as second-line treatment for small cell lung cancer. *J Clin Oncol* 2011;29:abstract 7000.

200. Pietanza MC, Kadota K, Huberman K, et al. Phase II trial of temozolomide in patients with relapsed sensitive or refractory small cell lung cancer, with assessment of methylguanine-DNA methyltransferase as a potential biomarker. *Clin Cancer Res* 2012;18:1138–1145.

201. Krug LM, Crapanzano JP, Azzoli CG, et al. Imatinib mesylate lacks activity in small cell lung carcinoma expressing c-kit protein: a phase II clinical trial. *Cancer* 2005;103:2128–2131.

220. Rudin CM, Salgia R, Wang X, et al. Randomized phase II Study of carboplatin and etoposide with or without the bcl-2 antisense oligonucleotide oblimersen for extensive-stage small-cell lung cancer: CALGB 30103. *J Clin Oncol* 2008;26:870–876.

228. Rudin CM, Hann CL, Garon EB, et al. Phase II study of single-agent navitoclax (ABT-263) and biomarker correlates in patients with relapsed small cell lung cancer. *Clin Cancer Res* 2012;18:3163–3169.

230. Langer CJ, Albert I, Kovacs P, et al. A randomized phase II study of carboplatin and etoposide with or without pan-BCL-2 antagonist obatoclax in extensive-stage small cell lung cancer. *J Clin Oncol* 2011;29: abstract 7001.

237. Ready N, Pang H, Gu L, et al. Chemotherapy with or without maintenance sunitinib for untreated extensive-stage small cell lung cancer: a randomized, placebo controlled phase II study CALGB 30504 (ALLIANCE). *J Clin Oncol* 2013;31:abstract 7506.

241. Spigel DR, Townley PM, Waterhouse DM, et al. Randomized phase II study of bevacizumab in combination with chemotherapy in previously untreated extensive-stage small cell lung cancer: results from the SALUTE trial. *J Clin Oncol* 2011;29:2215–2222.

245. Reck M, Bondarenko I, Luft A, et al. Ipilimumab in combination with paclitaxel and carboplatin as first-line therapy in extensive-disease-small-cell lung cancer: results from a randomized, double-blind, multicenter phase 2 trial. *Ann Oncol* 2013;24:75–83.

246. Perry MC, Eaton WL, Propert KJ, et al. Chemotherapy with or without radiation therapy in limited small-cell carcinoma of the lung. *N Engl J Med* 1987;316:912–918.

248. Pignon JP, Arriagada R, Ihde DC, et al. A meta-analysis of thoracic radiotherapy for small-cell lung cancer. *N Engl J Med* 1992;327:1618–1624.

253. Bogart JA, Herndon JE 2nd, Lyss AP, et al. 70 Gy thoracic radiotherapy is feasible concurrent with chemotherapy for limited-stage small-cell lung cancer: analysis of Cancer and Leukemia Group B study 39808. *Int J Radiat Oncol Biol Phys* 2004;59:460–468.

258. Schild SE, Bonner JA, Shanahan TG, et al. Long-term results of a phase III trial comparing once-daily radiotherapy with twice-daily radiotherapy in limited-stage small-cell lung cancer. *Int J Radiat Oncol Biol Phys* 2004;59:943–951.

262. Komaki R, Paulus R, Ettinger DS, et al. Phase II study of accelerated high-dose radiotherapy with concurrent chemotherapy for patients with limited small-cell lung cancer: Radiation Therapy Oncology Group protocol 0239. *Int J Radiat Oncol Biol Phys* 2012;83:e531–e536.

264. Spiro SG, James LE, Rudd RM, et al. Early compared with late radiotherapy in combined modality treatment for limited disease small-cell lung cancer: a London Lung Cancer Group multicenter randomized clinical trial and meta-analysis. *J Clin Oncol* 2006;24:3823–3830.

265. Fried DB, Morris DE, Poole C, et al. Systematic review evaluating the timing of thoracic radiation therapy in combined modality therapy for limited-stage small-cell lung cancer. *J Clin Oncol* 2004;22:4837–4845.

271. De Ruysscher D, Bremer RH, Koppe F, et al. Omission of elective node irradiation on basis of CT-scans in patients with limited disease small lung cancer: a phase II trial. *Radiother Oncol* 2006;80:307–312.

275. Shirvani SM, Komaki R, Heymach JV, et al. Positron emission tomography/computed tomography-guided intensity-modulated radiotherapy for limited-stage small-cell lung cancer. *Int J Radiat Oncol Biol Phys* 2012;82: e91–e97.

279. Shirvani SM, Juloori A, Allen PK, et al. Comparison of 2 common radiation therapy techniques for definitive treatment of small cell lung cancer. *Int J Radiat Oncol Biol Phys* 2013;87:139–147.

334. Lad T, Piantadosi S, Thomas P, et al. A prospective randomized trial to determine the benefit of surgical resection of residual disease following response of small cell lung cancer to combination chemotherapy. *Chest* 1994;106: 320S–323S.

347. Asamura H, Kameya T, Matsuno Y, et al. Neuroendocrine neoplasms of the lung: a prognostic spectrum. *J Clin Oncol* 2006;24:70–76.

348. Fink G, Krelbaum T, Yellin A, et al. Pulmonary carcinoid: presentation, diagnosis, and outcome in 142 cases in Israel and review of 640 cases from the literature. *Chest* 2001;119:1647–1651.

351. Thomas CF Jr, Tazelaar HD, Jett JR. Typical and atypical pulmonary carcinoids : outcome in patients presenting with regional lymph node involvement. *Chest* 2001;119:1143–1150.

352. McCaughan BC, Martini N, Bains MS. Bronchial carcinoids. Review of 124 cases. *J Thorac Cardiovasc Surg* 1985;89:8–17.

363. Granberg D, Sundin A, Janson ET, et al. Octreoscan in patients with bronchial carcinoid tumours. *Clin Endocrinol (Oxf)* 2003;59:793–799.

370. Travis WD, Giroux DJ, Chansky K, et al. The IASLC Lung Cancer Staging Project: proposals for the inclusion of broncho-pulmonary carcinoid tumors in the forthcoming (seventh) edition of the TNM Classification for Lung Cancer. *J Thorac Oncol* 2008;3:1213–1223.

373. Garcia-Yuste M, Matilla JM, Cueto A, et al. Typical and atypical carcinoid tumors: analysis of the experience of the Spanish Multi-centric Study of Neuroendocrine Tumors of the Lung. *Eur J Cardiothorac Surg* 2007;31:192–197.

379. Lou F, Sarkaria I, Pietanza C, et al. Recurrence of pulmonary carcinoid tumors after resection: implications for postoperative surveillance. *Ann Thorac Surg* 2013;96:1156–1162.

391. Ekeblad S, Sundin A, Janson ET, et al. Temozolomide as monotherapy is effective in treatment of advanced malignant neuroendocrine tumors. *Clin Cancer Res* 2007;13:2986–2991.

393. Fine RL, Gulati AP, Krantz BA, et al. Capecitabine and temozolomide (CAPTEM) for metastatic, well-differentiated neuroendocrine cancers: The Pancreas Center at Columbia University experience. *Cancer Chemother Pharmacol* 2013;71:663–670.

396. Pavel ME, Hainsworth JD, Baudin E, et al. Everolimus plus octreotide long-acting repeatable for the treatment of advanced neuroendocrine tumours associated with carcinoid syndrome (RADIANT-2): a randomised, placebo-controlled, phase 3 study. *Lancet* 2011; 378:2005–2012.

400. Raymond E, Dahan L, Raoul JL, et al. Sunitinib malate for the treatment of pancreatic neuroendocrine tumors. *N Engl J Med* 2011;364:501–513.

405. Travis WD, Krug LM, Rusch V, et al. Large Cell Neuroendocrine Carcinoma. *Textbook of Uncommon Cancer*. Chichester, England: John Wiley & Sons, Ltd.; 2006: 298–306.

412. Veronesi G, Morandi U, Alloisio M, et al. Large cell neuroendocrine carcinoma of the lung: a retrospective analysis of 144 surgical cases. *Lung Cancer* 2006;53:111–115.

413. Iyoda A, Hiroshima K, Toyozaki T, et al. Adjuvant chemotherapy for large cell carcinoma with neuroendocrine features. *Cancer* 2001;92:1108–1112.

414. Sarkaria IS, Iyoda A, Roh MS, et al. Neoadjuvant and adjuvant chemotherapy in resected pulmonary large cell neuroendocrine carcinomas: a single institution experience. *Ann Thorac Surg* 2011;92:1180–1186.

415. Zacharias J, Nicholson AG, Ladas GP, et al. Large cell neuroendocrine carcinoma and large cell carcinomas with neuroendocrine morphology of the lung: prognosis after complete resection and systematic nodal dissection. *Ann Thorac Surg* 2003;75:348–352.

423. Niho S, Kenmotsu H, Sekine I, et al. Combination chemotherapy with irinotecan and cisplatin for large-cell neuroendocrine carcinoma of the lung: a multicenter phase II study. *J Thorac Oncol* 2013;8:980–984.

424. Le Treut J, Sault MC, Lena H, et al. Multicentre phase II study of cisplatin-etoposide chemotherapy for advanced large-cell neuroendocrine lung carcinoma: the GFPC 0302 study. *Ann Oncol* 2013;24:1548–1552.

425. Hanna N, Bunn PA Jr, Langer C, et al. Randomized phase III trial comparing irinotecan/cisplatin with etoposide/cisplatin in patients with previously untreated extensive-stage disease small-cell lung cancer. *J Clin Oncol* 2006;24:2038–2043.

437. Ciuleanu T, Samarzjia M, Demidchik Y, et al. Randomized phase III study (SPEAR) of picoplatin plus best supportive care or best supportive care alone in patients with SCLC refractory or progressive within 6 months after first-line platinum-based chemotherapy. *J Clin Oncol* 2010;28:abstract 7002.

PRACTICE OF ONCOLOGY

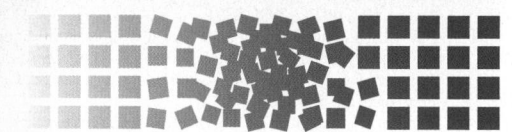

43 Neoplasms of the Mediastinum

Robert B. Cameron, Patrick J. Loehrer, and Percy P. Lee

THYMIC NEOPLASMS

Incidence and Etiology

Thymic neoplasms, predominantly thymomas, constitute 30% and 15% of anterior mediastinal masses in adults and children, respectively. Surveillance, Epidemiology, and End Results (SEER) data suggest that 15 thymomas occur in every 100,000 person-years, are more common in males and Pacific Islanders, and increase in frequency into the 8th decade of life.[1] Other studies document an incidence as low as 0.15 to 0.32 per 100,000 persons. No specific etiology or risk factors are known, but a well-known association with myasthenia gravis (MG) does exist. Thymic carcinoma is a rare, aggressive thymic neoplasm that has a particularly poor prognosis and infrequently is associated with MG or other paraneoplastic syndromes.[2] Like thymoma, it is an epithelial tumor, but unlike thymoma it exhibits malignant cytologic features. Although it is unclear if thymoma and thymic carcinoma share a common cell of origin because molecular markers are unique for each, both most often are located in the anterior mediastinum, although other sites have been reported.[3] Suster and Rosai[4] reported on 60 patients with thymic carcinoma ranging in age from 10 to 76 years and with a slight male predominance. Nearly 70% of patients had symptoms of cough, chest pain, or superior vena cava syndrome. Extensive local invasion and distant metastases are more common than in thymomas.

Anatomy and Pathology

The thymus is an incompletely understood lymphatic organ functioning in T-lymphocyte maturation. It is composed of thymocytes, lymphocytes, and an epithelial stroma. Although lymphomas, carcinoid tumors, and germ-cell tumors all may arise within the thymus, only thymomas, thymic carcinomas, and thymolipomas arise from true thymic elements.[5,6] The thymus develops from a paired epithelial anlage in the ventral portion of the third pharyngeal pouch and is closely associated with the developing parathyroid glands.[7] The thymic epithelial stromal cells are likely derived from both ectodermal and endodermal components.[8] During weeks 7 and 8 of development, the thymus elongates and descends caudally and ventromedially into the anterior mediastinum. Lymphoid cells arrive during week 9 and are separated from the perivascular spaces by a flat epithelial cell layer that creates the blood–thymus barrier. Maturation and differentiation occurs in this antigen-free environment and, during the 4th fetal month, lymphocytes begin to circulate to peripheral lymphoid tissue.[8] Six subtypes of epithelial cells have been identified in the mature thymus.[8] Four exist primarily in the cortical region and two in the medullary region. Type 6 cells form Hassall corpuscles that are characteristic of the thymus. These cells have an ectodermal origin and are displaced into the thymic medulla, where they hypertrophy, form tonofilaments, and finally appear as concentric cells without nuclei.[7,8]

At maturity, the thymus gland is an irregular, lobulated organ. It attains its greatest relative weight at birth, but its absolute weight increases to 30 to 40 g by puberty. During adulthood, it slowly involutes and is replaced by adipose tissue. Ectopic thymic tissue has been found to be widely distributed throughout the mediastinum and neck, particularly the aortopulmonary window and retrocarinal area, and often is indistinguishable from mediastinal fat.[9] This ectopic tissue is the likely explanation for thymomas outside the anterior mediastinum and possibly for failure in some cases of a simple thymectomy to improve MG.

THYMOMA

Ninety percent of thymomas occur in the anterior mediastinum and the remainder arise in the neck or other areas of the mediastinum, including, rarely, the heart.[10] The normal contour of the thymus is biconcave or flat. The diseased thymus gland displays a more convex margin. Thymomas grossly are lobulated, firm, tan-pink to gray tumors that may contain cystic spaces, calcification, or hemorrhage. They may be encapsulated, adherent to surrounding structures, or frankly invasive. Microscopically, thymomas arise from thymic epithelial cells, although thymocytes or lymphocytes may predominate histologically. True thymomas contain cytologically bland cells and should be distinguished from thymic carcinomas, which have malignant cytologic characteristics. Originally, in 1976, Rosai and Levine[11] proposed that thymomas be divided into three types: lymphocytic, epithelial, or mixed (lymphoepithelial). In 1985, Marino and Muller-Hermelink[12] proposed a histologic classification system determined by the thymic site of origin—that is, cortical thymomas, medullary thymomas, and mixed thymomas—which were later subdivided further.[13,14] To unify the pathology of thymic neoplasms[15–17] the World Health Organization (WHO) adopted a new classification system for thymic neoplasms (Table 43.1).[17] WHO type A and B2 tumors are more likely to present with locoregional disease, compared with WHO type B3 and C tumors.[18,19]

Although Suster and Moran[20] have proposed a simpler classification schema that separates thymic tumors into three categories of thymic carcinoma: well-differentiated (WHO types A, AB, B1, and B2), moderately differentiated (WHO type B3), and poorly differentiated (WHO type C), the full WHO classification system remains more broadly accepted.

Currently, the terms *noninvasive* and *invasive* thymoma are preferred over *benign* and *malignant* designations. Noninvasive thymomas have an intact capsule, are mobile, and are easily resected, although they can be adherent to adjacent organs. In contrast, invasive thymomas invade surrounding structures and should be removed with en bloc resection of involved structures despite a benign cytologic appearance. Metastatic disease may occur in both noninvasive and invasive thymomas and is most commonly seen as pleural implants or pulmonary nodules. Metastases to extrathoracic sites, such as the liver, brain, bone, and kidney, rarely occur.[21]

In 1981, Masaoka et al.[22] developed a surgical staging system, shown in Table 43.2. An update of this series of 273 patients confirmed that both WHO histology and clinical staging were independently predictive of 20-year survival.[23] The Groupe

TABLE 43.1

World Health Organization Classification System for Thymic Epithelial Tumors

Tumor Type	Cells	Clinicopathologic Classification	Histologic Terminology
A	Spindle or oval	Benign thymoma	Medullary
B B1 B2 B3	Epithelioid or dendritic	Category I malignant thymoma	Cortical; organoid Lymphocyte rich; predominately cortical Cortical Well-differentiated thymic carcinoma
AB		Benign thymoma	Mixed
C		Category II malignant thymoma	Nonorganotypic; thymic carcinoma, epidermoid keratinizing and nonkeratinizing carcinoma, lymphoepitheliomalike carcinoma, sarcomatoid carcinoma, clear-cell carcinoma, basaloid carcinoma, mucoepidermoid carcinoma, undifferentiated carcinoma

From Patterson GA. Thymomas. *Semin Thorac Cardiovasc Surg* 1992;4:39–44 with permission.

d'Etudes des Tumeurs Thymiques (GETT) has another surgically oriented staging system.[24] The Istituto Nazionale Tumori system combines the Masaoka classifications in three distinct stage groupings (locally restricted, locally advanced, and systemic disease) and may better encompass all WHO subtypes.[25] Although the Masaoka staging system[26] and a tumor-node-metastasis (TNM) classification system[27] (Table 43.3) also have been used in staging thymic carcinoma, their utility is largely unproven.

THYMIC CARCINOMA

The histologic classification of thymic carcinoma was proposed by Levine and Rosai[28] and revised by Suster and Rosai.[4] Tumors are classified broadly as low or high grade. Low-grade tumors include squamous cell carcinoma, mucoepidermoid carcinoma, and basaloid carcinoma. High-grade neoplasms include lymphoepitheliomalike carcinoma and small-cell, undifferentiated, sarcomatoid, and clear-cell carcinomas.[4,26,29,30] Although the histologic classification of thymic carcinomas was designed to be descriptive, correlations with prognosis have been made. For instance, low-grade tumors may have

a more favorable clinical course (median survival rates of 25.4 months to more than 6.6 years) when compared with higher grade malignancies (median survival of only 11.3 months to 15.0 months).[4,26]

Molecular profiling of rare solid tumors, such as thymic neoplasms, has taken place over the past decade.[31] Emerging analyses do suggest that mutations in genes of the epidermal growth factor receptor (EGFR) and KIT pathways have documented a progressive increase in observed genomic aberrations from WHO subtype A thymoma to WHO subtype C thymic carcinoma.[32]

Diagnosis

A meticulous history and physical examination, along with serologic and imaging studies, usually suggests the diagnosis. Although most anterior mediastinal masses are thymic malignancies, other etiologies also exist (Table 43.4). An improved pathologic analysis of image-guided percutaneous core needle biopsy specimens makes surgical biopsy rarely necessary.

Symptoms and Signs

Approximately 40% of mediastinal masses are asymptomatic and discovered incidentally on routine chest imaging.[1] The remaining 60% have symptoms related to either compression or direct invasion of adjacent mediastinal structures or to paraneoplastic syndromes. Asymptomatic patients are more likely to have benign lesions, whereas symptomatic patients more often harbor malignancies. Davis et al.[33] found that 85% of patients with a malignancy were symptomatic, but only 46% of patients with benign neoplasms had identifiable complaints. The most common symptoms are chest pain, cough, and dyspnea. Superior vena cava syndrome, Horner syndrome, hoarseness, and neurologic deficits are less common and often signal a malignancy.[33] Systemic syndromes associated with mediastinal neoplasms are shown in Tables 43.4 and 43.5.

Associated Systemic Syndromes

A myriad of associated systemic disorders may be identified in 71% of patients with thymomas, including autoimmune diseases (MG, systemic lupus erythematosus, polymyositis, myocarditis, Sjögren syndrome, ulcerative colitis, Hashimoto thyroiditis, rheumatoid arthritis, sarcoidosis, and scleroderma), endocrine disorders (hyperthyroidism, hyperparathyroidism, stiff-person syndrome, Addison disease, and panhypopituitarism), blood disorders (red cell aplasia, hypogammaglobulinemia, T-cell deficiency syndrome, erythrocytosis, pancytopenia, megakaryocytopenia, T-cell lymphocytosis, and pernicious anemia), neuromuscular syndromes (myotonic dystrophy,

TABLE 43.2

Thymoma Staging System of Masaoka

Stage	Description	5-/10-year Survival (%)
I	Macroscopically completely encapsulated and microscopically no capsular invasion	96/67
II	1. Macroscopic invasion into surrounding fatty tissue or mediastinal pleura, or 2. Microscopic invasion into capsule	86/60
III	Macroscopic invasion into neighboring organs (pericardium, great vessels, lung)	69/58
IV	a. Pleural or pericardial dissemination, or b. Lymphogenous or hematogenous metastasis	50/0

Adapted from Masaoka A, Monden Y, Nakahara K, Tanioka T. Follow-up study of thymomas with special reference to their clinical stages. *Cancer* 1981;48:2485–2492.

TABLE 43.3

Istituto Nazionale Tumori Tumor-Node-Metastatis (TNM)–Based Staging System

TNM	Description
T1	No capsular invasion
T2	Microscopic invasion into the capsule, or extracapsular involvement limited to the surrounding fatty tissue or normal thymus
T3	Direct invasion into the mediastinal pleura and/or anterior pericardium
T4	Direct invasion into neighboring organs, such as the sternum, great vessels, and lungs; implants to the mediastinal pleura or pericardium, only if anterior to phrenic nerves
N0	No lymph nodes metastasis
N1	Metastasis to anterior mediastinal lymph nodes
N2	Metastasis to intrathoracic lymph nodes other than anterior mediastinal
N3	Metastasis to prescalene or supraclavicular nodes
M0	No hematogenous metastasis
M1a	Implants to the pericardium or mediastinal pleura beyond the sites defined in the T4 category
M1b	Hematogenous metastasis to other sites, or involvement of lymph nodal stations other than those described in the N categories

Stage Grouping	Description
I	Locally restricted disease
	T1–2 N0 M0
II	Locally advanced disease
	T3–4 N0 M0
	Any T N1–2 M0
III	Systemic
	Any T N3 M0
	Any T any N M1

Classification Description of Residual Disease	
R0	No residual tumor
R1	Microscopic residual tumor
R2a	Local macroscopic residual tumor after reductive resection (more than 80% of the tumor)
R2b	Other features of residual tumor

Adapted from Shimizu J, Hayashi Y, Monita K, et al. Primary thymic carcinoma: a clinicopathological and immunohistochemical study. *J Surg Oncol* 1994;56:159–164.

TABLE 43.4

Systemic Syndromes Associated with Mediastinal Neoplasms

Tumor	Syndrome
Thymoma	Acute pericarditis, Addison disease, agranulocytosis, alopecia areata, Cushing syndrome, hemolytic anemia, hypogammaglobulinemia, limbic encephalopathy, myasthenia gravis, myocarditis, nephrotic syndrome, panhypopituitarism, pernicious anemia, polymyositis, pure red cell aplasia, rheumatoid arthritis, sarcoidosis, scleroderma, sensorimotor radiculopathy, stiff-person syndrome, thyroiditis, ulcerative colitis
Hodgkin lymphoma	Alcohol-induced pain, Pel-Ebstein fever
Neurofibroma	von Recklinghausen disease, osteoarthritis
Thymic carcinoid	Multiple endocrine neoplasia
Neuroblastoma	Opsomyoclonus, erythrocyte abnormalities
Neurilemoma	Peptic ulcer

PRACTICE OF ONCOLOGY

TABLE 43.5

Systemic Manifestations of Hormone Production by Mediastinal Neoplasms

Symptoms	Hormone	Tumor
Hypertension	Catecholamines	Pheochromocytoma, chemodectoma, neuroblastoma, ganglioneuroma
Hypercalcemia	Parathyroid hormone	Parathyroid adenoma
Thyrotoxicosis	Thyroxine	Thyroid
Cushing syndrome	ACTH	Carcinoid tumor
Gynecomastia	HCG	Germ cell tumor
Hypoglycemia	? Insulin	Mesenchymal tumors
Diarrhea	VIP	Ganglioneuroma, neuroblastoma, neurofibroma

ACTH, adrenocorticotropic hormone; HCG, human chorionic gonadotropin; VIP, vasoactive intestinal polypeptide.

myositis, and Eaton-Lambert syndrome), as well as other disorders (hypertrophic osteoarthropathy, nephrotic syndrome, minimal change nephropathy, pemphigus, and chronic mucocutaneous candidiasis).[34] Symptoms of one or more of these disorders may lead to the original discovery of the mediastinal tumor.

Myasthenia Gravis

MG is the most common autoimmune disorder associated with thymoma, occurring in 30% to 50% of patients.[35] Younger women and older men usually are affected, with a female-to-male ratio of 2:1. Myasthenia is a disorder of neuromuscular transmission. The temporal association is variable and a prolonged interval between the diagnosis of MG and the development of a visible thymic tumor can occur.[36] Symptoms (e.g., diplopia, ptosis, dysphagia, fatigue) begin insidiously and result from the production of antibodies to the postsynaptic nicotinic acetylcholine receptor at the myoneural junction. Ocular symptoms are the most frequent initial complaint, eventually progressing to generalized weakness in 80% of cases. The role of the thymus in MG remains unclear, but autosensitization of T lymphocytes to acetylcholine-receptor proteins or an unknown action of thymic hormones remains possible.[37] The altered microenvironment may adversely impact the output of T-regulatory (Treg) cells, thus altering autoimmune homeostasis.[38] Pathologic thymic changes are noted in 70% of MG patients, with lymphoid hyperplasia predominating and thymomas seen only in 15% of patients.[37]

The treatment of MG involves the use of anticholinesterase mimetic agents (i.e., pyridostigmine bromide [Mestinon]). In severe cases, plasmapheresis may be required to remove high antibody titers. Thymectomy has become an increasingly accepted procedure in the treatment of MG, although the indications, timing, and surgical approach remain controversial.[39] Some improvement in MG symptoms frequently occurs after a thymectomy, but complete remission rates vary from 7% to 63%.[39] Patients with thymomas do not respond as well to a thymectomy as MG patients without thymomas. Age 54 years and older and a symptom duration of less than 1 year are associated with poor outcomes[40]; however, MG does not necessarily portend a poor outcome.[41]

Red Cell Aplasia

Pure red cell aplasia, an autoimmune disorder, occurs in 5% of patients with thymomas.[42] Of patients with red cell aplasia, 30% to 50% have associated thymomas. Affected patients are older than 40 years of age in 96% of cases. A bone marrow examination reveals an absence of erythroid precursors and, in 30% of cases, a poorly understood associated decrease in platelet and leukocyte numbers. A thymectomy has produced remission in up to 38% of patients. For patients with recurrent disease, octreotide and prednisone were effective in case reports.[42,43]

Hypogammaglobulinemia

Hypogammaglobulinemia is seen in 5% to 10% of patients with thymoma (Good syndrome), and 10% of patients with hypogammaglobulinemia have been shown to have thymoma. Recurrent sinusitis is a common associated symptom in such patients. Defects in both cellular and humoral immunity have been described, and many patients also have red cell hypoplasia.[44] Thymectomy has not proven beneficial in this disorder.

Radiographic Imaging Studies

Imaging studies initially localize mediastinal neoplasms.[45] The posteroanterior and lateral chest radiographs define the location, size, density, and calcification of a mass, which helps focus the initial diagnostic testing; however, an intravenous contrast-enhanced spiral computed tomography (CT) scan remains the best imaging modality to accurately assess the nature of the lesion (cystic versus solid), detect fat and calcium, determine the relationship to surrounding anatomic structures, and, in some instances, predict invasiveness of the tumors.[46,47]

Recent advances in electrocardiogram-gating and real-time magnetic resonance imaging (MRI) and angiography have dramatically increased the usefulness of this modality in the evaluation of mediastinal masses. Not only is it superior to CT in defining vascular involvement, but an MRI scan can also detect subtle differences in tumor contour, capsule clarity, and intratumoral signal (low), which correlate with the WHO classification of thymomas.[48]

Recently, the usefulness of positron emission tomography (PET) scans in the evaluation of thymic tumors has expanded significantly. In a study of 51 patients, Benveniste et al. suggested that 18-fluorodeoxyglucose (18F-FDG) uptake by PET/CT scans was higher in thymic carcinoma than thymomas. Additionally, higher *focal* 18F-FDG uptake correlated with B3 thymomas, and greater 18F-FDG avid tumor volume predicted higher stage tumors.[49] In a contemporary study of 47 patients, Lococo et al. demonstrated that maximum standardized uptake values (SUV_{max}) and SUV_{max}/tumor size index, as determined by PET/CT, not only distinguished thymomas from thymic carcinomas, but also both parameters correlated with WHO malignancy grade and SUV_{max} predicted Masaoka stage.[50] On serial PET/CT imaging, decreased 18F-FDG uptake in 56 patients with stage III/IV thymic epithelial malignancies treated after only 6 weeks of chemotherapy was shown by Thomas et al.[51] to correlate with longer progression-free survival (11.5 versus 4.6 months; p = 0.044) and a trend toward longer overall survival (31.8 versus 18.4 months; p = 0.14).

Serology and Chemistry

Many germ-cell neoplasms release chemical markers into the serum that may be measured to confirm a diagnosis, evaluate the response to therapy, and monitor for tumor recurrence. Lactate dehydrogenase, α-fetoprotein (AFP), and human chorionic gonadotropin-β (β-hCG) are common tumor markers that should be obtained in male patients with anterior mediastinal masses. Also, adrenocorticotropic hormone, thyroid hormone, and parathormone may help differentiate certain mediastinal masses (see Table 43.4).

Invasive Diagnostic Tests

An accurate histologic diagnosis is essential for appropriate treatment of nearly all mediastinal neoplasms. Although some patients may still require open surgical biopsies, CT- or ultrasound-guided percutaneous needle biopsy is now standard in the initial evaluation of mediastinal masses.[10] Although fine-needle specimens may distinguish carcinomas from benign pathology, core biopsies are necessary for most mediastinal neoplasms, especially lymphoma and thymoma. Recent series report diagnostic yields for percutaneous needle biopsy in excess of 90%.[52] Complications include simple pneumothorax (25%), hemoptysis (7% to 15%), and pneumothorax, requiring chest tube placement (5%).[52] In some circumstances, fine-needle aspiration of posterior and middle mediastinal tumors can be performed endoscopically using transesophageal ultrasonography.[53]

Surgical procedures occasionally are still required in the diagnosis of mediastinal tumors. A mediastinoscopy is a relatively simple procedure with a diagnostic accuracy of more than 90% for biopsies of the upper middle and, in some surgeons' hands, the anterior and posterior mediastinum.[54] Anterior parasternal mediastinotomy (Chamberlain procedure) yields a diagnosis in 95% of anterior mediastinal masses and may be accomplished under local anesthesia.[54,55] A thoracoscopy is a minimally invasive procedure that provides a diagnostic accuracy of nearly 100% in most areas of the mediastinum.[54] Currently, thoracotomy rarely is necessary solely as a diagnostic procedure.

Management by Stage

Thymomas, albeit slow growing, should be considered potentially malignant neoplasms. Surgery, radiation, and chemotherapy all may play a role in their management.[41,56] Few prospective, well-designed clinical trials in the management of thymomas have been conducted, particularly evaluating the role of surgery and radiotherapy; however, the newly formed International Thymic Malignancy Interest Group is planning cohort studies to help guide diagnostic and therapeutic interventions.[57]

Masaoka Stage I/II Thymoma

Complete surgical resection is the mainstay of therapy for stage I/II thymomas and is the most important predictor of long-term survival.[58–61] Although a median sternotomy with a vertical or submammary skin incision is most commonly used, bilateral anterolateral thoracotomies with transverse sternotomy, or the *clam-shell procedure*, is useful with advanced or laterally displaced large tumors. Recently, the use of minimally invasive surgery in stage I and II thymomas has expanded dramatically. One study comparing 76 thoracoscopic thymectomies to 44 transsternal resections reported a shorter hospital stay with the thoracoscopies.[62] Similarly, two reports of robotic-assisted surgery, including a multicenter European study, were associated with less blood loss, fewer complications, and a shorter hospital stay, as well as similar operative times and short-term outcomes compared to sternotomies.[63,64] Although randomized, prospective clinical trials are still lacking, it is highly likely that minimally invasive surgery in the hands of experienced

surgeons can produce identical oncologic outcomes with less morbidity than open surgery, as has been shown in other thoracic tumors, such as lung and esophageal cancers.

During any surgery, a careful assessment of areas of possible invasion and adherence should be made. Extended total thymectomy, including all tissue anterior to the pericardium from the diaphragm to the neck and laterally from one phrenic nerve to the other, including en bloc pericardium, phrenic nerve, chest wall, lung, and diaphragmatic resection (with reconstruction) in up to two-thirds of cases in order to achieve an R0 resection is recommended in all good performance status patients.[41,58–60] Operative mortality is less than 3% in experienced centers.[41]

In the past, ionizing radiation has been used to treat various stages of thymomas. Furthermore, modern imaging, three-dimensional treatment planning, and delivery techniques have allowed thoracic radiotherapy to be prescribed in a safer fashion than noted in the past century. Radiation therapy is delivered in doses ranging from 30 to 60 Gy in 1.8- to 2.0-Gy fractions for 3 to 6 weeks.[58,65,66] There are suggestions of a dose–response relationship with local control in some patients, albeit from retrospective data, although it is not clear that doses exceeding 60 Gy offer any consistent advantage[67,68]; however, completely resected and microscopic residual disease can be well controlled with only 40 to 45 Gy.[61,69] Emerging data suggest that certain histologic subtypes (WHO type B1 and B2) are more likely to respond to radiotherapy compared to others subtypes (WHO type B3), suggesting that the response is limited to the lymphocytic and not the epithelial cell component of the tumors.[41,70–72] Gating techniques to minimize respiratory variation and intensity-modulated radiation therapy are new techniques that can minimize the dose heterogeneity, increase total dose and fraction size, and minimize toxicity.[69,73,75]

Masaoka Stage III/IV Thymoma

The role of subtotal surgical resection, or *debulking* surgery, in stage III and IV disease remains highly controversial.[76] Several studies have documented improved 5-year survival rates after subtotal resection compared to a biopsy alone.[58,61] Another study suggested no survival advantage to *debulking* surgery followed by radiation when compared with radiation alone, and a more recent report reached the opposite conclusion.[76] The use of surgery in recurrent disease remains to be defined.

Radiation therapy may be beneficial in selected patients with locally advanced disease.[61,65,67,77] Large variations in the amount of tumor treated, radiation delivered, and tumor biology, however, make interpretation of these results difficult.[61,67,78,79]

Cytotoxic chemotherapy has been used with increasing frequency in the treatment of invasive thymomas.[80] Both single-agent and combination therapy have demonstrated activity in the adjuvant and neoadjuvant settings. Doxorubicin, cisplatin, ifosfamide, corticosteroids, and cyclophosphamide all have been used as single-agent therapies.[81] The most active agents are cisplatin, doxorubicin, ifosfamide, and corticosteroids; however, only a few single agents, such as cisplatin, ifosfamide, pemetrexed, gefitinib, and imatinib, have undergone formal phase II trials.

A number of molecular targets have been identified in thymic tissue.[83] Overexpression of the EGFR has been found in more than two thirds of patients, mostly WHO B2 and 3 subtypes.[84–86] The overexpression of *c-kit* is common in thymic carcinoma, although *c-kit* mutations are less frequent.[85,87,88]

Thymic Carcinoma

The optimal treatment of thymic carcinoma remains undefined, but currently, a multimodality approach, including surgical resection, postoperative radiation, and chemotherapy, is recommended.[89] Initial surgical resection followed by radiation has been used in most studies.[4,26,27,29,90] Complete resection should be attempted, but often is not possible.[26,91] One analysis noted a 9.5-month median survival after resection and postoperative photon-beam radiation therapy,[90] with a trend toward improved survival in other studies.[4,26,29] Chemotherapy with cisplatin-based regimens similar to those used with thymomas have produced variable responses in a small number of patients.[4,26,29] Combinations of doxorubicin, cyclophosphamide, and cisplatin also have generated partial responses, as has the combination of 5-fluorouracil and leucovorin in recurrent disease. Use of neoadjuvant chemotherapy has been reported in a small number of patients.[89,92]

Results of Treatment

Thymoma

In nearly 700 patients in the SEER database treated between 1973 and 1998, advanced disease was associated with decreasing survival.[42] According to various retrospective series, the 5- and 10-year survival rates for stage I, III, and IV tumors are reported to be 89% to 95% and 78% to 90%; 70% to 80% and 21% to 80%; and 50% to 60% and 30% to 40%, respectively.[58,93] Ten-year disease-free survival rates of 74%, 71%, 50%, and 29% also have been reported for stage I, II, III, and IV disease, respectively.[58] Long-term results from an experienced Indiana University group has yielded a 66% 1-year overall survival.[41] Although Maggi et al.[58] reported a 10% overall recurrence rate in 241 patients, less than 5% of noninvasive thymomas and 20% of invasive thymomas were noted to recur. A large Japanese multi-institutional experience with 1,320 patients reported 5-year survival rates of 100%, 98.4%, 88.7%, 70.6%, and 52.8% for Masaoka stages I, II, III, IVa, and IVb, respectively.[59] Although MG once was considered an adverse prognostic factor, this is no longer the case because of improved perioperative care, and in fact, MG actually may be associated with an improved survival owing to earlier tumor detection.[41,94] Complete surgical resection of thymomas is associated with an 82% overall 7-year survival rate, whereas survival with incomplete resection is 71%, and with biopsy is only 26%.[58] Survival after a complete tumor resection has been similar in patients with noninvasive and invasive thymomas in several studies.[59,60] Patients with MG and thymoma have a 56% to 78% 10-year survival rate and a 3% recurrence rate with 4.8% (1.7% since 1980) operative mortality after an extended thymectomy.[61,95] Rarely, a syndrome of myasthenia crisis may occur following surgery and may lead to increased perioperative morbidity.[95]

Although the data on whether outcomes are related to WHO subtype is inconclusive,[41,71,72] it may be that when coupled with other factors such as completeness of resection, the WHO subtype may be prognostic in some patients.[96]

For example, in stage I thymomas, adjuvant radiotherapy has been administered but has not improved on the excellent results with surgery alone (more than 80% 10-year survival rate).[58,61] In stage II and III invasive disease, adjuvant radiation can decrease recurrence rates after complete surgical resection from 28% to 5%.[67] In addition, Pollack et al.[65] reported an increase in 5-year disease-free survival for stage II to IVa from 18% to 62% with the addition of adjuvant radiation, despite a 50% infield relapse rate in patients recurring with prior radiation. Stage II patients with cortical tumors[97,98] and invasion of pleura or the pericardium are most likely to benefit from postoperative radiation.[77] Preoperative radiotherapy for extensive tumors has been reported in limited studies that suggest a decreased tumor burden and potential for tumor seeding at the time of surgery, although multivariate analyses suggested that chemotherapy may have played a role.[58,61] Data suggest that not all Masaoka stage II patients may necessarily require postoperative radiotherapy (PORT).[56,101] Indeed, a review of SEER registry data from 1975 to 2003 demonstrated a worse cancer-specific survival for patients with resected, localized thymoma who received PORT compared to those without (91% versus 98%; p = 0.03). For patients with regional disease, PORT had a slight but nonstatistically significant difference (91% versus 86%; p = 0.12).[102] The absence of statistically significant therapeutic efficacy for PORT, despite

the suggestion of a lower local recurrence rate (i.e., 0% versus 8%) again has been confirmed in two recent studies.[102]

Masaoka Stage III/IV Thymoma

The role of subtotal surgical resection or *debulking* surgery in stage III and IV disease remains highly controversial.[76] Several studies have documented 5-year survival rates from 60% to 75% after subtotal resection and 24% to 40% after biopsy alone.[58,61] Although one study did suggest no survival advantage to debulking followed by radiation when compared with radiation alone, another more recent experience reached the opposite conclusion.[76] The use of surgery in recurrent disease remains to be defined. Maggi et al.[58] reported a 71% 5-year survival rate in 12 surgery patients and a 41% survival rate in 11 patients treated with radiation and chemotherapy alone. Prolonged tumor-free survival also was reported by Kirschner[74] in 23 patients. However, Urgesi et al.[78] noted a 74% 5-year survival rate in 11 patients undergoing surgery and radiation, compared with 65% in 10 patients treated with radiation alone (not statistically different). In 71 patients with thymoma (WHO types A and B3) with stage I to IVA disease, 53 (75.3%) patients are alive and free of disease, with 6 additional patients alive with disease with a mean follow-up of 66 months.[41]

Radiation therapy may be beneficial in selected patients with locally advanced disease.[61,63,65,68,77] Radiotherapy after incomplete surgical resection produces local control rates of 35% to 74% and 5-year survival rates ranging from 50% to 70% for stage III and 20% to 50% for stage IVa tumors.[61,66,67] In addition, Ciernik et al.[67] and others[78] have reported similar survival rates (87% 5-year and 70% 7-year) in patients treated with radiation alone compared with partial surgical resection and adjuvant radiation in small numbers of stage III and IV patients and patients with intrathoracic recurrences. Weksler et al.[105] reviewed SEER data on 322 patients with stage III thymoma who received postoperative adjuvant radiation and found that by multivariate analysis, disease-specific survival was improved (p = 0.049) but overall survival was not. However, large variations in the amount of tumor treated, radiation delivered, and tumor biology in particular make interpretation of these results difficult at best.[61,67,78,79]

Cytotoxic chemotherapy has been used with increasing frequency in the treatment of invasive thymomas.[80] Both single-agent and combination therapy have demonstrated activity in the adjuvant and neoadjuvant settings. The most commonly used active agents are cisplatin and doxorubicin; however, only a few single agents, such as cisplatin, ifosfamide, pemetrexed, gefitinib, and imatinib, have undergone formal phase II trials.[80] Cisplatin at doses of 100 mg/m² has produced complete responses lasting up to 30 months, but lower doses (50 mg/m²) have associated response rates of only 10%.[81] In 13 earlier patients, ifosfamide (with mesna) was given at a single dose of 7.5 g/m² or as a continuous infusion of 1.5 g/m² per day for 5 days every 3 weeks and resulted in five (38.7%) complete and one (7.7%) partial responses.[106] Varying regimens of corticosteroids have shown effectiveness in the treatment of all histologic subtypes of thymoma (with and without myasthenia), with a 77% overall response rate in limited numbers of patients.[82,107,108] Corticosteroids also have been effective for patients unsuccessful with chemotherapy[82]; however, the actual impact may only be on the lymphocytic and not the malignant epithelial component of the tumor.

Combination chemotherapy regimens have shown higher response rates and have been used in both neoadjuvant and metastatic settings in the treatment of advanced invasive, metastatic, and recurrent thymoma. Cisplatin plus doxorubicin-containing regimens appear to be the most active. Fornasiero et al.[93] reported a 43% complete and 91.8% overall response rate with a median survival of 15 months in 37 previously untreated patients with stage III or IV invasive thymoma treated with monthly (median, 5 months) cisplatin, 50 mg/m² on day 1; doxorubicin, 40 mg/m² on day 1; vincristine, 0.6 mg/m² on day 3; and cyclophosphamide, 700 mg/m² on day 4. Loehrer et al.[109] documented 10% complete and 50% overall response rates with a median survival of 37.7 months in 29 patients with metastatic or locally progressive recurrent thymoma treated with cisplatin, 50 mg/m^2; doxorubicin, 50 mg/m^2; and cyclophosphamide, 500 mg/m^2, given every 3 weeks for a maximum of eight cycles after radiotherapy. Park et al.[110] retrospectively described 35% complete and 64% overall response rates with a median survival of 67 months in responding and 17 months in nonresponding patients in 17 patients with invasive stage II and IV thymoma initially treated after relapse with cyclophosphamide, doxorubicin, and cisplatin, with or without prednisone. The European Organisation for Research and Treatment of Cancer noted 31% complete and 56% overall response rates with a median survival of 4.3 years in a small study of 16 patients with advanced thymoma treated with cisplatin and etoposide.[111] The addition of ifosfamide to cisplatin and etoposide had a lower than anticipated response rate (approximately 32%) in patients with thymoma and thymic carcinoma in a prospective Eastern Cooperative Oncology Group (ECOG) trial of 28 patients.[90]

ECOG also conducted a prospective trial in patients with thymoma (n = 25) and thymic carcinoma (n = 21) who were treated with carboplatin plus paclitaxel, with a 33% objective response rate for the former group and 24% for the latter.[112] In total, these data suggest higher objective response rates achieved with anthracycline-based regimens.

Combined Modality Approaches

The use of neoadjuvant (induction or preoperative) chemotherapy has been evaluated as part of a multimodality approach to stage III and IV thymoma. Six combined reports document 31% complete and 89% overall response rates in 61 total patients treated with a variety of neoadjuvant chemotherapy regimens (80% cisplatin based).[113] Twenty-two patients (36%) underwent surgery, with 11 (18%) achieving a complete resection (all treated with cisplatin). Nineteen patients were treated with radiotherapy, but only five patients had disease-free survivals exceeding 5 years. Rea et al.[114] reported 43% complete and 100% overall response rates with median and 3-year survival rates of 66 months and 70%, respectively, in 16 stage III and IVa patients treated initially with cisplatin, doxorubicin, vincristine, and cyclophosphamide, followed by surgery. At surgery, 69% were completely resected and the other 31% received postoperative radiation. A recent report from the Amsterdam team noted a 50% objective response rate using the Response Evaluation Criteria in Solid Tumors (RECIST) criteria in 16 patients with locally advanced tumors.[111] Macchiarini et al.[115] reported similar findings. Recently, the Japan Clinical Oncology Group reported a phase II trial (JCOG 9606) that treated 23 patients with unresectable stage III thymoma with 9 weeks of chemotherapy, including cisplatin 25 mg/m^2 on weeks 1 through 9; vincristine 1 mg/m^2 on weeks 1, 2, 4, 6, and 8; and doxorubicin 40 mg/m^2 and etoposide 80 mg/m^2 CODE on days 1 through 3 of weeks 1, 3, 5, 7, and 9.[116] Twelve patients (57%) completed the planned 9-week therapy without mortality. Of 21 eligible patients, zero, 13 (62%), and 7 achieved a complete response, partial response, and stable disease, respectively. Subsequently, 13 (62%) underwent thoracotomies, with 9 (39%) undergoing complete R0 resection and postoperative radiotherapy (48 or 60 Gy in completely or incompletely resected disease, respectively). Progression-free survival at 2 and 5 years was 80% and 43%, respectively, and overall survival at 5 and 8 years was 85% and 69%, respectively. Survival was not improved by surgical resection. Finally, 25% complete (3 patients) and 92% overall response rates (11 patients) with an 83% 7-year disease-free survival rate (10 patients) were reported in only 12 patients at the M.D. Anderson Cancer Center who received cisplatin, doxorubicin, cyclophosphamide, and prednisone induction chemotherapy followed by surgical resection (80% complete) and adjuvant radiotherapy for locally advanced (unresectable) thymoma.[117] The degree of chemotherapy-induced tumor necrosis correlated with Ki-67 expression.

Using two to four cycles of cisplatin, doxorubicin, and cyclophosphamide chemotherapy and sequential radiotherapy (54 Gy), a multi-institutional prospective trial demonstrated a 22% complete and 70% overall response rate. Also noted was a median survival of 93 months and a Kaplan-Meier 5-year failure-free survival rate of 54.3% in 23 patients with stage III (22/23) unresectable thymoma (GETT stage IIIA/IIIB), stage IV (1/23) thymoma, and thymic carcinoma (2/23).[118] Approximately 25% of these patients also had MG. Although these results compare favorably with those obtained with neoadjuvant therapy followed by surgical resection and radiation, further data are required. In summary, postoperative (adjuvant) chemotherapy cannot be recommended based on these data.[41]

Molecularly Targeted Therapy

Molecular profiles of thymic epithelial malignancies have shown some differences between thymoma and thymic carcinoma, but overall, clinically relevant findings are inconsistent.[119] For example, EGFR often is overexpressed in thymic epithelial malignancies, but activating mutations are rare.[119–125] However, with rare case reports of radiographic responses to cetuximab in advanced thymoma,[122,123] a combined-modality phase II trial in locally advanced or recurrent but resectable stage II and IVA patients is now underway (NCT01025089). Other trials with gefitinib as a single agent and erlotinib plus bevacizumab in previously treated patients had minimal activity. Tyrosine–kinase inhibitors also have been investigated. Despite an initial reported brief thymic carcinoma response to imatinib, two subsequent trials in 20 thymic carcinoma patients failed to find any activity.[124] Some antitumor activity has been reported in thymic malignancies with dasatinib, an oral, multitargeted kinase inhibitor of *Bcr-Abl* and *src* kinases; ephrin receptor kinases; platelet-derived growth factor receptor; c-kit; and with sunitinib, another multikinase inhibitor.[125] A phase II sunitinib study in patients with previously treated thymic malignancies is underway (NCT01621568). The histone deacetylase inhibitor, belinostat, has demonstrated a promising 65% control rate (response rate = 5%) in a 41 patient phase II study and currently is being tested in combination with first-line chemotherapy (NCT01100944).[126] Thymus-specific targeted therapy, specifically with somatostatin analogs, has shown promise in small clinical trials.[84] Although the mechanism of action is unclear, inhibition of the insulinlike growth factor or EGFR pathways are possible. Response rates were seen in more than one third (37%) of patients with tumors that were resistant to cytotoxic chemotherapy with octreotide plus prednisone.[84] The median and progression-free survival of 15 months and 14 months, respectively, is encouraging. In thymoma patients with positive radionuclide octreotide scans, 12.5% of the patients demonstrated a partial response to octreotide alone, which increased to 32% with the addition of prednisone.[84]

Thymic Carcinoma

The prognosis of thymic carcinoma is poor because of early metastatic involvement of mediastinal, cervical, and axillary lymph nodes; the pleura; the lungs; the brain; bone; and the liver.[4,92,128] The overall survival rate at 5 years is approximately 35%.[4,26] The recently reported Japanese experience noted a 88.2%, 51.7%, and 37.6% 5-year survival in patients with stages I/II, III, and IV, respectively.[59] Improved survival has been correlated with encapsulated tumors, lobular growth pattern, low mitotic activity, early-stage tumors, low histologic grade, lymphoepitheliomalike histology, and complete surgical resection.[4,87,91,108] Furthermore, in multivariate analysis of SEER data, Masaoka stage and ethnicity emerge as significant determinants of survival in thymic carcinoma patients undergoing complete resection.[108] In addition, patients with stage IVa disease appear to benefit more from treatment than those with more disseminated disease (stage IVb).[88]

THYMIC CARCINOID

Thymic carcinoid tumors are rare, male-predominant tumors that are associated with Cushing syndrome, multiple endocrine neoplasia, and, rarely, carcinoid syndrome.[129–136] Thymic neuroendocrine tumors may be differentiated from similar pulmonary tumors by their different PAX 8 (32% versus 8%) and thyroid transcription factor 1 (TTF-1) (8% versus 76%) staining characteristics.[136] Complete surgical resection with adjuvant radiotherapy for incompletely resected tumors is recommended.[130–133] Chemotherapy rarely has been used.[137,138] Although a 5-year survival rate of 60% has been reported with complete surgical resection,[131] long-term survival is generally poor and is correlated with the extent of disease and the degree of tumor differentiation.[139]

THYMOLIPOMA

Thymolipomas are rare soft, lobulated, and encapsulated benign neoplasms of the anterior mediastinum, which are composed of mature adipose and thymic tissue and account for 1% to 5% of thymic neoplasms.[140] They are also known as *lipothymomas*, *mediastinal lipomas with thymic remnants*, and *thymolipomatous hamartomas*.[140,141] A review of 27 patients noted an equal gender distribution and a mean age of 27 years.[141] Approximately 50% of patients presented with symptoms of vague chest pain, dyspnea, and tachypnea. Others have reported an association with MG, red cell aplasia, hypogammaglobulinemia, lichen planus, and Graves disease in adult patients, but less often than with thymoma.[140,142–144] They often attain a large size before becoming symptomatic[145] and frequently are found in the anterior–inferior mediastinum "draped along the diaphragm" and connected to the thymus by a small pedicle, conforming to the shape of the cardiac and mediastinal structures.[141] Microscopically, more than 50% consists of adipose tissue with the remainder being thymic tissue, often with calcified Hassall corpuscles.[141] Malignant transformation does not occur. Treatment is a complete resection.[145]

GERM CELL TUMORS

Incidence and Etiology

Mediastinal germ-cell (MGC) neoplasms account for only 2% to 5% of all germinal tumors but constitute 50% to 70% of all extragonadal tumors.[146] Most commonly seen in the anterior mediastinum, they account for 10% to 15% of all primary mediastinal tumors. MGC tumors are most commonly diagnosed in the third decade of life, but patients as old as 60 years of age have been reported. The incidence is equal in all ethnicities. Benign teratomas are the most common MGC tumor, accounting for 70% of the MGC tumors in children and 60% of those in adults. They can occur at any age, but most commonly occur between 20 and 40 years of age. Primary pure mediastinal seminomas account for roughly 35% of malignant MGC tumors and principally arise in men aged 20 to 40 years.[147] Although benign germ-cell tumors have no sex predilection, 90% of adult malignant germ-cell tumors occur in men, with a mean age of 29. Both benign and malignant extragonadal pediatric germ-cell tumors occur with equal sex distribution.

Anatomy and Pathology

Extragonadal germ-cell tumors arise along the body's midline from the cranium (pineal gland) to the presacral area, corresponding to the embryologic urogenital ridge, presumably from aberrantly migrated germ cells.[146] MGC tumors are broadly classified as benign or malignant. Benign tumors include mature teratomas and mixed teratomas with an immature component of less than 50%. Malignant germ-cell tumors are divided into seminomas (dysgerminomas) and nonseminomatous tumors. In addition, MGC tumors have a propensity to develop a component of non–germ-cell malignancy (e.g., rhabdomyosarcoma, adenocarcinoma, permeative neuroectodermal tumor), which can become the predominant histology.

Teratomas

Teratomas contain elements from all three germ-cell layers, with a predominance of the ectodermal component in most tumors, including the skin, hair, sweat glands, sebaceous glands, and teeth. The mesoderm is represented by fat, smooth muscle, bone, and cartilage. Respiratory and intestinal epithelium are often seen as the endodermal component. Teratomas may be solid or cystic in appearance and are often referred to as *dermoid cysts* if unilocular. The majority of mediastinal teratomas are composed of mature ectodermal, mesodermal, and endodermal elements and exhibit a benign course. Immature teratomas, which phenotypically appear as malignant ectodermal, mesodermal, or endodermal tumors, behave aggressively and generally are not responsive to therapy.

Seminomas

Seminomas uncommonly may exist in a pure form, but any elevation of serum AFP levels indicates the presence of at least a small element of nonseminomatous tumor.

Nonseminomatous Tumors

Mediastinal nonseminomatous germ-cell tumors are most commonly found in the anterior mediastinum and appear grossly as invasive, lobulated masses with a thin capsule. Nonseminomatous tumors include embryonal carcinomas, choriocarcinomas, yolk sac tumors, and immature teratomas.[148] They may occur in pure form, but in approximately one third of cases, multiple cell types are present. Other malignant components, including adenocarcinoma, squamous cell carcinoma, small cell undifferentiated carcinoma, neuroblastoma, rhabdomyosarcoma, or other sarcomas, may be present or even predominate, as usually occurs in immature teratomas.[146] Other synchronous hematologic malignancies, such as acute myeloid leukemia, acute nonlymphocytic leukemia, erythroleukemia, myelodysplastic syndrome, malignant histiocytosis, thrombocytosis, and most interestingly, acute megakaryocytic leukemia, also have been reported and may antedate the discovery of the germ-cell tumor. Karyotypic abnormalities, particularly the 47XXY pattern of Klinefelter syndrome, have been found in up to 20% of patients.[149] Of patients, 85% to 95% have systemic disease at the time of diagnosis. Common metastatic sites include the lungs, pleura, lymph nodes, the liver, and, less commonly, bone.[147]

Diagnosis

Many patients with benign tumors, including 50% of teratomas, are asymptomatic; however, 90% to 100% of patients with malignant tumors have symptoms of chest pain, dyspnea, cough, fever, or complaints from compression or invasion of adjacent mediastinal structures.[149,150] Seminomas typically grow slowly and metastasize later than their nonseminomatous counterparts, and they may reach a large size by the time of diagnosis with 20% to 30% remaining asymptomatic until discovered.[147] Symptoms are usually related to their affects on the surrounding mediastinal structures. Pulmonary and other intrathoracic metastases are present in 60% to 70% of patients, whereas extrathoracic metastases usually involve bone.[147]

The determination of serum tumor markers is important in the diagnosis and follow-up of MGC tumors. Immunoassays for serum β-hCG and AFP should be obtained in all patients who have suspicious mediastinal masses. The elevation of β-hCG and AFP confirm a malignant tumor, and AFP (60% to 80%), β-hCG (30% to 50%), or both are elevated in 80% to 85% of nonseminomatous germ-cell tumors.[150] Patients with pure seminoma may have low levels of β-hCG, but AFP is not detected unless a nonseminomatous component also exists. Patients with benign teratomas have normal markers. Isochromosome 12p is diagnostic of undifferentiated germ-cell malignancies even in the absence of elevated serum markers.

PRACTICE OF ONCOLOGY

MGC tumors typically are detected by standard chest radiographs, which are abnormal in 95% of cases. Most masses are noted in the anterior mediastinum, but 3% to 8% of tumors arise within the posterior mediastinum.[149] Chest CT scans demonstrate large inhomogeneous masses containing areas of hemorrhage and necrosis and also define the extent of disease, the relationship to surrounding structures, and the presence of cystic areas and calcification within the tumor. In teratomas, sonographic patterns may improve the diagnostic accuracy of CT scans alone.[151] Abdominal imaging should be performed to assess for liver metastases. Careful examination of the testes, including a testicular ultrasound, should always be performed; however, a blind testicular biopsy or orchiectomy in patients with normal physical and ultrasound findings is not indicated because an isolated anterior mediastinal mass without retroperitoneal adenopathy is not consistent with a primary testicular tumor.[146] The diagnosis of nonseminomatous germ-cell tumors in young males with anterior mediastinal masses and elevated serum tumor markers (AFP and β-hCG) may be made without a tissue biopsy, and treatment may be initated.[152] If a tissue confirmation is necessary, a core needle biopsy with cytologic staining for tumor markers usually is adequate. Rarely, an open biopsy via an anterior mediastinotomy approach is necessary.[152]

Management by Histology

MGC tumors are not formally staged according to the American Joint Committee on Cancer (AJCC) staging system but can be characterized as localized, locally advanced, and metastatic. Due to the lack of a staging system, these tumors will be discussed by histologic subtype.

Teratoma

Treatment of a mature mediastinal teratoma consists of complete surgical resection, which results in excellent long-term cure rates.[148] The tumor may be adherent to surrounding structures, necessitating resection of the pericardium, pleura, or the lung. Radiotherapy and chemotherapy play no role in the management of this tumor. For teratomas with a malignant component (immature) in patients over 15 years of age, adjuvant cisplatin-based combination chemotherapy (four cycles of cisplatin, etoposide, and bleomycin or vinblastine, ifosfamide, and cisplatin) is recommended. Neoadjuvant chemotherapy may be considered if the tumor is not completely resectable.[148]

Seminoma

The treatment of mediastinal seminoma has evolved since the early 1970s. Seminomas are extremely radiosensitive tumors, and for many years, high-dose mediastinal radiation was used as the definitive therapy, resulting in long-term survival rates of 60% to 80%.[152] Radiation therapy in the extragonadal seminoma, including recommendations for mediastinal and bilateral supraclavicular fields as well as for doses of 35 to 45 Gy was reviewed by Hainsworth.[147]

Mediastinal seminoma, however, often presents as a bulky, extensive, and locally invasive disease, requiring large radiotherapy portals that would result in excessive irradiation of surrounding the normal lung, heart, and other structures. Additionally, 20% to 40% of irradiated patients fail at distant sites.[147] Currently, due to these limitations, only an isolated mediastinal seminoma with minimal disease is managed with radiotherapy alone. Instead, the use of cisplatin-based combination chemotherapy, which was previously used only in advanced gonadal seminoma, is now used as first-line therapy. Lemarie et al.[150] reported that 12 of 13 patients treated experienced complete remission, with only 2 subsequent recurrences. Bokemeyer et al.[153] reported an international analysis of 51 patients with mediastinal seminoma. Chemotherapy was primarily cisplatin based (45, 88%), but carboplatin was also used (3, 5.9%) and had a lower objective response rate (80% versus 93%). In this study, patients were treated with chemotherapy (38, 74.5%),

chemotherapy and radiation (10, 19.6%), or radiation alone (3, 5.9%). The progression-free survival and overall survival were 77% and 88%, respectively. Patients with extrathoracic metastases (6, 11.8%) had a worse prognosis. In a collective review of 52 patients by Hainsworth,[147] 14 patients had received prior radiation therapy, but all underwent chemotherapy with cisplatin and various combinations of cyclophosphamide, vinblastine, bleomycin, or etoposide. Complete responses to treatment were noted in 85% of patients, with 83% disease-free long-term survival.

Pure mediastinal seminoma, even with visceral metastases, falls into the intermediate-risk category of the new International Staging System for Germ Cell Tumors, and all patients should be treated with curative intent. Locally advanced and bulky disease should be treated initially with cisplatin-based combination chemotherapy, which is most often four cycles of cisplatin and etoposide with or without supradiaphragmatic radiotherapy. Patients with distant metastases should undergo chemotherapy alone as the initial treatment. Salvage chemotherapy (vinblastine, ifosfamide, and cisplatin) may be required for persistent or recurrent disease.[154]

Despite a recent report of 76.9% long-term survival patients using primary surgical resection followed by adjuvant therapy,[155] most authors believe that surgery does not play a role in the definitive treatment of a seminoma.[152] In addition, surgical debulking of large tumors has not been shown to be of benefit in improving local control or survival.[147]

The management of patients with residual radiographic abnormalities after chemotherapy is controversial. Studies have shown that the residual mass is a dense scirrhous reaction or fibrosis in 85% to 90% of patients, and the presence of a viable seminoma is rare. Others have shown a 25% incidence of residual viable seminoma in these patients treated with chemotherapy followed by resection of residual masses larger than 3 cm.[155] Close observation without surgery is recommended for residual masses after chemotherapy unless the mass enlarges.[147,152] An evaluation with PET scans is superior to CT alone in seminoma patients with a sensitivity and specificity of 80% and 100%, respectively, versus 73% and 73% for CT alone. There were no false-positive scans in lesions larger than 3 cm, and all 11 lesions greater than 3 cm with a residual tumor were PET avid, making this a useful modality to avoid unnecessary surgery and empiric radiation therapy.[147,152]

Nonseminomatous Germ-Cell Tumors

The mainstay of treatment of nonseminomatous germ-cell tumors is cisplatin-based chemotherapy, which is identical to that of gonadal nonseminomatous germ-cell tumors and is discussed more completely in Chapter 70. Overall complete remission rates of 40% to 64% were obtained in most series.[147,148,150,153] In an international review of 287 patients, responses were noted in 178 (64%), and the progression-free and overall survival were 62% and 45%, respectively.[153] Patients with relapsing mediastinal nonseminomatous germ-cell tumors do extraordinarily poorly even with salvage therapy, such as vinblastine, ifosfamide, and cisplatin,[154] with only 9 of 79 patients (11%) becoming disease free in one study.[153] Surgical resection of the residual disease despite persistently elevated tumor markers has been reported by several authors to be beneficial.[155–157]

Prognosis

Immature teratomas are potentially malignant tumors, and their prognosis is influenced by the anatomic site of the tumor, the patient's age, and the fraction of the tumor that is immature.[148] In patients younger than 15 years, immature teratomas behave similarly to their mature counterparts. In older patients, they may behave as highly malignant tumors. Nonseminomatous MGC tumors carry a poorer prognosis than either pure extragonadal seminomas or their gonadal nonseminomatous counterparts. All primary mediastinal nonseminomatous germ-cell tumors fall into the poor-risk category of the International Germ Cell Consensus Classification.[158]

SELECTED REFERENCES

The full reference list can be accessed at lwwhealthlibrary.com/oncology.

1. Engels EA, Pfeiffer RM. Malignant thymoma in the United States: demographic patterns in incidence and associations with subsequent malignancies. *Int J Cancer* 2003;105:546–551.
5. Tomaszek S, Wigle DA, Keshavjee S, et al. Thymomas: review of current clinical practice. *Ann Thorac Surg* 2009;87:1973–1980.
19. Detterbeck FC. Clinical value of the WHO classification system of thymoma. *Ann Thorac Surg* 2006;81:2328–2334.
20. Suster S, Moran CA. Thymoma classification: current status and future trends. *Am J Clin Pathol* 2006;125:542–554.
23. Okumura M, Ohta M, Tateyama H, et al. The World Health Organization Histologic Classification System reflects oncologic behavior of thymoma. *Cancer* 2002;94:624–632.
24. Gamondes JP, Balawi A, Greenland T, et al. Seventeen years of surgical treatment of thymoma: factors influencing survival. *Eur J Cardiothorac Surg* 1991;5:124–131.
26. Hsu CP, Chan CY, Chen CL, et al. Thymic carcinoma: ten years' experience in twenty patients. *J Thorac Cardiovasc Surg* 1994;107:615–620.
32. Girard N, Shen R, Guo T, et al. Comprehensive genomic analysis reveals clinically relevant molecular distinctions between thymic carcinomas and thymomas. *Clin Cancer Res* 2009;15:6790–6799.
35. Rinadi TP, Batocchi AP, Evoli A, et al. Thymic lesions and myasthenia gravis: diagnosis based on mediastinal imaging and pathological findings. *Acta Radiol* 2002;43:380–384.
38. Ströbel P, Preisshofen T, Helmreich M, et al. Pathomechanisms of paraneoplastic myasthenia gravis. *Clin Dev Immunol* 2003;10:7–12.
41. Okereke IC, Kesler KA, Morad MH, et al. Prognostic indicators after surgery for thymoma. *Ann Thorac Surg* 2010;89:1071–1077.
46. Bogot NR, Quint LE. Imaging of thymic disorders. *Cancer Imaging* 2005;5:139–149.
48. Inoue A, Tomiyama N, Fujimoto K, et al. MR imaging of thymic epithelial tumors: correlation with World Health Organization classification. *Radiat Med* 2006;24:171–181.
49. Benveniste MF, Moran CA, Mawlawi O, et al. FDG PET-CT aids in the preoperative assessment of patients with newly diagnosed thymic epithelial malignancies. *J Thorac Oncol* 2013;8:502–510.
50. Lococo F, Cesario A, Okami J, et al. Role of combined (18)F-FDG-PET/CT for predicting theWHO malignancy grade of thymic epithelial tumors: A multicenter analysis. *Lung Cancer* 2013;82:245–251.
51. Thomas A, Mena E, Kurdziel K, et al. 18F-fluorodeoxyglucose positron emission tomography in the management of patients with thymic epithelial tumors. *Clin Cancer Res* 2013;19:1487–1493.
56. Falkson CB, Bezjak A, Darling G, et al. The management of thymoma: a systematic review and practice guideline. *J Thorac Oncol* 2009;4:911–919.
57. Detterbeck F, Giaccone G, Loehrer P, et al. International thymic malignancy interest group. *J Thorac Oncol* 2010;5:1–2.
58. Maggi G, Casadio C, Cavallo A, et al. Thymoma: results of 241 operated cases. *Ann Thorac Surg* 1991;51:152–156.
59. Kondo K, Monden Y. Therapy for thymic epithelial tumors: a clinical study of 1,320 patients from Japan. *Ann Thorac Surg* 2003;76:878–884.
61. Cowen D, Mornex RF, Bachelot T, et al. Thymoma: results of a multicentric retrospective series of 149 non-metastatic irradiated patients and review of the literature. *Radiother Oncol* 1995;34:9–16.
62. Liu TJ, Lin MW, Hsieh MS, et al. Video-assisted thoracoscopic surgical thymectomy to treat early thymoma: a comparison with the conventional transsternal approach. *Ann Surg Oncol* 204;21:322–328
63. Marulli G, Rea F, Melfi F, et al. Robot-aided thoracoscopic thymectomy for early-stage thymoma: a multicenter European study. *J Thorac Cardiovasc Surg* 2012;144:1125–1130.
64. Weksler B, Tavares J, Newhook TE, et al. Robot-assisted thymectomy is superior to transsternal thymectomy. *Surg Endosc* 2012;26:261–266.
68. Zhu G, He S, Fu X, et al. Radiotherapy and prognostic factors for thymoma: a retrospective study of 175 patients. *Int J Radiat Oncol Biol Phys* 2004;60:1113–1119.
71. Wright CD, Wain JC, Wong DR, et al. Predictors of recurrence in thymic tumors: importance of invasion, World Health Organization histology, and size. *J Thorac Cardiovasc Surg* 2005;130:1413–1421.
72. D'Angelillo RM, Trodella L, Ramella S, et al. Novel prognostic groups in thymic epithelial tumors: assessment of risk and therapeutic strategy selection. *Int J Radiat Oncol Biol Phys* 2008;71:420–427.
79. Mornex F, Resbeut M, Richard P, et al. Radiotherapy and chemotherapy for invasive thymomas: a multicentric retrospective review of 90 cases. *Int J Radiat Oncol Biol Phys* 1995;32:651–659.
80. Schmitt J, Loehrer PJ. The role of chemotherapy in advanced thymoma. *J Thorac Oncol* 2010;5:357–360.
83. Hammond-Thelin LA, Thomas CR Jr. Systemic therapeutic options in thymic malignancies: a glimpse of hope. *Rev Recent Clin Trials* 2007;2:191–205.
84. Loehrer PJ Sr, Wang W, Johnson DH, et al. Octreotide alone or with prednisone in patients with advanced thymoma and thymic carcinoma: an Eastern Cooperative Oncology Group phase II trial. *J Clin Oncol* 2004;22:293–299.
89. Magois E, Guigay J, Blancard PS, et al. Multimodal treatment of thymic carcinoma: report of nine cases. *Lung Cancer* 2008;59:126–132.
95. Fang W, Chen W, Chen G, et al. Surgical management of thymic epithelial tumors: a retrospective review of 204 cases. *Ann Thorac Surg* 2005;80:2002–2007.
101. Korst RJ, Kansler AL, Christos PJ, et al. Adjuvant radiotherapy for thymic epithelial tumors: a systematic review and meta-analysis. *Ann Thorac Surg* 2009;87:1641–1647.
104. Berman AT, Litzky L, Livolsi V, et al. Adjuvant radiotherapy for completely resected stage 2 thymoma. *Cancer* 2011;117:3502–3508.
105. Weksler B, Shende M, Nason KS, et al. The role of adjuvant radiation therapy for resected stage III thymoma: a population-based study. *Ann Thorac Surg* 2012;93:1822–1828.
112. Lemma GL, Lee JW, Aisner SC, et al. Phase II study of carboplatin and paclitaxel in advanced thymoma and thymic carcinoma. *J Clin Oncol* 2011;29:2060–2065.
116. Kunitoh H, Tamura T, Shibata T, et al. A phase II trial of dose-dense chemotherapy followed by surgical resection and/or thoracic radiotherapy in locally advanced thymoma: report of a Japan Clinical Oncology Group trial (JCOG 9606). *Br J Cancer* 2010;103:6–11.
118. Papadopoulos KP, Thomas CR Jr. Current chemotherapy options for thymic epithelial neoplasms. *Expert Opinion Pharmacother* 2005;6:1169–1177.
119. Girard N, Shen R, Guo T, et al. Comprehensive genomic analysis reveals clinically relevant molecular distinctions between thymic carcinomas and thymomas. *Clin Cancer Res* 2009;15:6790–6799.
121. Suzuki E, Sasaki H, Kawano O, et al. Expression and mutation statuses of epidermal growth factor receptor in thymic epithelial tumors. *Jpn J Clin Oncol* 2006;36:351–356.
157. Kesler KA, Einhorn LH. Multimodality treatment of germ cell tumors of the mediastinum.*Thorac Surg Clin* 2009;19:63–69.

PRACTICE OF ONCOLOGY

44 Molecular Biology of the Esophagus and Stomach

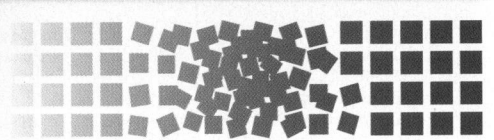

Anil K. Rustgi

INTRODUCTION

This chapter will deal with the molecular biology of esophageal and gastric cancers. The reader is referred to Chapters 45 and 46 for detailed information about the epidemiology, etiology, pathology, clinical manifestations, diagnosis, and therapy of esophageal and gastric cancers. There are several key aspects in the elucidation of the genetic basis of esophageal and gastric cancers through molecular biology approaches. These include, but are not limited to, new insights into underlying pathogenesis, possibilities for risk stratification and prognosis, correlations with traditional pathology classification schemes, the development of new diagnostics, and potential applications in molecular imaging and therapy. In considering the genetic underpinnings of esophageal and gastric cancers, critical appraisal is required of oncogenes, tumor suppressor genes, and DNA mismatch repair genes as they modulate, either positively or negatively, growth factor receptor–mediating signaling cascades, transcription of target genes, and cell-cycle progression. These molecular networks conspire to influence cellular behaviors, such as proliferation, differentiation, apoptosis, senescence, and response to stress and injury. The exquisite equilibrium that is the signature of normal cellular homeostasis is perturbed in uncontrolled cell growth, resulting in the eventual evolution of premalignant stages and malignant transformation. However, the time required for malignant transformation varies, depending on cellular- and tissue-specific context, and is affected by environmental factors.

The salient features of tumorigenesis and the acquisition of the malignant phenotype that are required, as described by Hanahan and Weinberg,[1] include growth signal autonomy, the ability to surmount antigrowth signals, the evasion of apoptosis, unlimited replicative ability, angiogenesis, and invasion and metastatic potential. More recently, the role of inflammation in carcinogenesis has gained much attention.

MOLECULAR BIOLOGY OF ESOPHAGEAL CANCER

The vast majority of esophageal cancers are of two subtypes: esophageal squamous cell cancer (ESCC) and esophageal adenocarcinoma (EAC). ESCC is preceded by squamous dysplasia, whereas EAC is preceded by a Barrett esophagus (BE) or an incomplete intestinal metaplasia of the normal squamous epithelium of the esophagus (Fig. 44.1). A BE undergoes transition from low-grade and high-grade dysplasia before progressing into EAC. ESCC and EAC have common and divergent genetic features as manifest by alterations in canonical oncogenes and tumor suppressor genes in somatic cells of tumors (Table 44.1). However, inherited predisposition to ESCC is rare, as described in *tylosis palmaris et*

plantaris. Although the gene mutation for tylosis has remained elusive, the region of allelic deletion is on chromosome 17p.[2] Similarly, there is no classic syndrome that distinguishes familial BE or familial EAC. That being said, studies continue to analyze families with BE in an effort to identify relevant genes or single-nucleotide polymorphisms. It is estimated that about 7% of patients with BE may have a family history. In a model-free linkage analysis of concordant-affected and discordant sibling pairs with BE/EAC, and tested independently prospectively in BE/EAC patients (and ancestry-matched controls), three genes—*MSR1, ASCC1*, and *CTHRC1*—were associated with BE/EAC.[3] An initial genome-wide association study (GWAS) revealed that common variants at chromosome 16q24.1 (the closest gene is *FOXF1*, which may be involved in esophageal organogenesis) and major histocompatibility complex (MHC) locus (chromosome 6p21) are associated with BE.[4] Subsequently, another GWAS revealed new susceptibility loci in BE/EAC in the following chromosomes and genes: chromosome 19p13-*CRTC1* (encoding cAMP repsonse element binding protein [CREB]-regulated transcription coactivator) gene; chromosome 9q22-*BARX1* gene, which is a transcription factor important in esophageal and gastric organogenesis; and chromosome 3p14-near the *FOXP1* gene, which regulates esophageal development).[5]

Epidermal Growth Factor Receptor

The epidermal growth factor receptor (EGFR) family of receptor tyrosine kinases stimulates a number of signal transduction cascades (e.g., *Ras/Raf/MEK/ERK, PI3K/AKT*) that regulate diverse cellular processes, such as proliferation, differentiation, survival, migration, and adhesion. These signaling pathways are important in normal cellular homeostasis, but aberrant activation of the EGFR members is crucial in esophageal carcinogenesis. This family of receptors comprises EGFR (also referred to as *erbB1, erbB2, erbB3*, and *erbB4*). The receptors have the ability to homo- or heterodimerize on engagement with one of several ligands: transforming growth factor α (TGF-α), EGF, amphiregulin, heparin-binding EGF-like growth factor, betacellulin, and epiregulin. The tyrosine phosphorylation of homo- or heterodimers of EGFRs creates docking sites for signaling proteins or adapter proteins. EGFR is commonly overexpressed in early-stage esophageal cancer, and overexpression correlates with a poor prognosis.[6–9] EGFR overexpression is typically due to increased engagement with ligands and decreased turnover. However, the mutation of a tyrosine residue in the cytoplasmic domain is rare. Increased expression of TGF-α and EGF has been detected in BE, EAC, and ESCC.[10–14] EGFR overexpression may predict a poor response to chemoradiotherapy[15,16] and is associated with decreased survival in patients with squamous cell carcinoma.[15] Furthermore, EGFR overexpression was associated with recurrent disease and diminished overall survival in patients undergoing an esophagectomy for ESCC.[16,17]

Normal esophagus ⟶ Squamous dysplasia ⟶ Squamous cell cancer

Normal esophagus ⟶ Intestinal metaplasia ⟶ Low-grade dysplasia ⟶ High-grade dysplasia ⟶ Adenocarcinoma

Figure 44.1 Progression of stages in esophageal squamous cell cancer and esophageal adenocarcinoma.

Cyclin D1 and p16INK4a

Cyclins, cyclin-dependent kinases (CDK), and cyclin-dependent kinase inhibitors (CDKi [such as p15, p16, p21, and p27]) regulate the mammalian cell cycle. During the G1 phase, the cyclin D1 oncogene complexes with either CDK4 or CDK6 to phosphorylate the retinoblastoma (pRb) tumor suppressor protein and, in so doing, relieves the negative regulatory effect of pRb, allowing the E2F family of transcription factors to propel the cell cycle toward the G1/S phase transition.[18] Toward the late G1 phase, cyclin E complexes with CDKs to phosphorylate p107, which is related to pRb, and liberates more E2F members to navigate the cell cycle into S phase. As with EGFR, cyclin D1 overexpression is found in premalignant lesions, such as esophageal squamous dysplasia or BE, and the majority of early-stage ESCC or EAC.[19,20] Additionally, cyclin D1 overexpression correlates with poor outcomes and survival as well as poor response to chemotherapy.[21,22]

Although cyclin D1 overexpression accounts for cyclin D1 dysregulation, other mechanisms include mutations in cyclin D1 and mutations in Fbx4, which is the E3 ligase for cyclin D1, thereby preventing degradation of cyclin D1 in the cytoplasm and reimportation into the nucleus, where it exerts its oncogenic effects.[23]

In a similar vein, *p16INK4a* is an early genetic alteration, via promoter hypermethylation, point mutation, or allelic deletion, in BE and EAC, but interestingly, is a late event in ESCC. Loss of heterozygosity of 9p21, the locus for both p16 and p15, has been demonstrated with high frequency in both dysplastic Barrett epithelium and Barrett adenocarcinoma (90% and more than 80% of cases, respectively).[24,25] Promoter hypermethylation, which prevents tumor suppressor function by blocking transcription, has been documented and correlates with the degree of dysplasia in BE. It is present in up to 75% of specimens with high-grade dysplasia and is found in almost 50% of patients with adenocarcinoma of the esophagus.[24,26] Point mutations of p16 in ESCC have been found, and promoter hypermethylation has been noted in up to 50% of these tumors.[27,28] An *Rb* gene mutation is not found in either type of esophageal neoplasm, but allelic loss of 13q, where the locus of the *Rb* gene resides, is found in up to 50% of patients with Barrett adenocarcinoma and squamous cell carcinoma.[29] This can correlate with diminished or loss of pRb protein in BE with dysplasia, EAC, and ESCC.[30]

TABLE 44.1

Common Molecular Genetic Alterations Observed in Esophageal and Gastric Cancers

Oncogenes

Epidermal growth factor receptor (*EGFR*)

Cyclin D1

Tumor Suppressor Genes

P16INK4a

TP53

E-cadherin

p120 catenin

DNA Mismatch Repair Genes (*hMLH1, hMSH2*)

Mismatch repair instability

TP53 Tumor Suppressor Gene

TP53 is the most commonly known mutated gene in human cancer.[31–33] *TP53* is a tumor suppressor that interrupts the G1 phase to evaluate and permit the repair of damaged DNA, which may arise from environmental exposure (e.g., irradiation, ultraviolet light) or cellular stress.[34] In the face of irreparable damage, *p53* induces apoptosis. The *p53* transcription factor binds DNA to activate or suppress a large repertoire of target genes.[35] *TP53* mutations induce the loss of cell-cycle checkpoints and promote genomic instability. The majority of *TP53* mutations occur in the DNA-binding region, and more than 80% of them are missense mutations resulting in loss of wild-type *p53* function.[36] Wild-type TP*p53* has a short half-life and is difficult to detect by immunohistochemistry; a mutation in *p53* results in the stabilization of the protein and allows for easier detection by immunohistochemistry.

The detection of the mutated p53 protein by immunohistochemistry has been demonstrated with increasing frequency during histologic progression from BE (5%) through dysplasia (65% to 75%) to frank adenocarcinoma (up to 90%).[37–39] Thus, the *p53* mutation or loss of heterozygosity appears early in BE and EAC. Both mutant p53 protein detected by immunohistochemistry and specific *p53* gene mutations detected by genomic sequencing have been identified in 40% to 75% of patients with ESCC.[40–42] The presence of a *p53* point mutation correlates with a response to induction chemoradiotherapy and predicted survival after esophagectomy in patients with either ESCC or EAC.[43]

Telomerase Activation

The maintenance of telomere length allows DNA replication to be sustained indefinitely. The aberrant expression of telomerase has been observed in most esophageal cancers examined to date.[43] Morales et al.[44] observed increased telomerase expression in 100% of adenocarcinoma and BE cases with high-grade dysplasia. Telomerase activation is important, but alternative mechanisms to maintain the length of telomeres may operate in these cancers as well.[45]

Tumor Invasion and Metastasis

The loss of cell–cell adhesion can lead to both invasion and metastases. Alterations in expression of E-cadherin, a cell–cell adhesion molecule, or its associated catenins (e.g., p120 catenin or p120ctn) disrupt cell–cell interactions, which results in the potential for tumor progression.[46] Reduced expression of E-cadherin has been correlated with progression from BE, to dysplasia, and finally to adenocarcinoma, and is also observed in ESCC.[47,48]

Models of Esphageal Squamous Cell Cancer and Esophageal Adenocarcinoma

Advances in the diagnosis and therapy of esophageal neoplasms will ultimately be fostered through cell lines, xenotransplantation mouse models, surgically based rodent models, and genetically engineered mouse models. There is a vast array of cell lines established from primary and metastatic human esophageal cancers that allow the perturbation of gene expression to gauge effects on cellular behavior. Recently, organotypic (three-dimensional) cell culture models, which mimic human tissue, have revealed that the combination of EGFR and mutant *p53* results in the transformation of human esophageal epithelial cells immortalized with human telomerase reverse transcriptase (hTERT).[49]

In transgenic mice in which cyclin D1 is targeted to the esophagus, esophagi reveal evidence of dysplasia that evolves into squamous cell cancer on crossbreeding the mice with *p53* loss.[50] More recently, the conditional knockout of p120ctn in the esophagi of mice results in invasive ESCC.[51] Rodents have also been treated with nitrosamines to yield esophageal papillomas and ESCC.[52]

A classic rodent model involves a total gastrectomy followed by an esophagojejunostomy.[53] This creates a milieu whereby the esophagus is exposed to high concentrations of bile (*nonacid reflux*) with the development of BE and EAC. Recently, two genetically engineered mouse models have changed our views of BE and EAC. The targeted expression of the interleukin-1β, a cytokine, to the mouse esophagi, results in esophageal and gastroesophageal inflammation, the development of BE, and long latency to EAC.[54] However, the time for EAC development is hastened by adding bile acid to drinking water consumed by the mice or by crossbreeding these mice with mice null for the *p16INK4a* allele.[54] Another model involves the global knockout of p63, which is important in squamous stem cells and progenitor cells, revealing Barrett-like cells in the postnatal period when the mice die from other causes.[55] In each of these two models, the cells that give rise to the Barrett cells or Barrettlike cells migrate from the gastric–squamous forestomach junction to the junction–distal esophagus.[54,55]

Functional Genomics

The underlying fate switch between ESCC and EAC may also be influenced by the expression and function of *lineage*-specific transcriptional factors as demonstrated through functional genomics. To that end, SOX2, found to be part of an amplicon on chromosome 3q26.33 in human ESCC, fosters growth of these cancers. This may have implications in the therapy of human ESCC.[56] Similarly, GATA6, a known transcriptional factor, has been reported to be overexpressed in EAC.[57] Exome and whole-genome sequencing of EAC has revealed >20 genes that are mutated significantly, some of which include newly identified chromatin-modifying factors.[58]

MOLECULAR BIOLOGY OF GASTRIC CANCER

The most common type of gastric cancer is adenocarcinoma, of which there are two subtypes: intestinal and diffuse. They are distinguished by different anatomic locations within the stomach, variable clinical outcomes, and different pathogenesis. The intestinal type of sporadic gastric adenocarcinoma has a hallmark progression from normal gastric epithelium, to chronic atrophic gastritis (typically due to *Helicobacter pylori* infection), to intestinal metaplasia (which has some overlapping but also different features than intestinal metaplasia of BE), to dysplasia, to cancer (Fig. 44.2). Diffuse-type gastric adenocarcinoma is even more invasive and aggressive in its behavior, has overlap with lobular-type breast cancer, and may be highlighted by E-cadherin loss.

Inherited Susceptibility

Case-control studies have observed consistent—up to threefold—increases in risk for gastric cancer among relatives of patients with gastric cancer.[59,60] Studies of monozygotic twins have even shown a slight trend toward increased concordance of gastric cancers compared with dizygotic twins.[61,62] Large families with an autosomal dominant, highly penetrant inherited predisposition for the development of gastric cancer are rare. However, early-onset diffuse gastric cancers have been described and linked to the *E-cadherin/CDH1* locus on chromosome 16q and associated with mutations in this gene.[63] This seminal finding has been confirmed in other studies with gastric cancers at a relatively high (67% to 83%) penetrant rate.[64–67] Thus, E-cadherin mutation testing should be considered in the appropriate clinical setting. In fact, prophylactic gastrectomy should be strongly considered in families with germ-line E-cadherin mutation even without gross mucosal abnormalities by endoscopic examination of the stomach.[68] Recently, germ-line alpha-catenin mutations have been described as well in these families.[69]

Lynch syndrome, or hereditary nonpolyposis colon cancer, involves germ-line mutations of DNA mismatch repair genes.[70] Gastric adenocarcinoma may be observed in some families with Lynch syndrome. Gastric cancers have also been noted to occur in patients with familial adenomatous polyposis and Peutz-Jeghers syndrome.[70]

Role of *Helicobacter pylori* Infection and Other Host–Environmental Factors

As a commensal organism, *H. pylori* infection is widely prevalent throughout the world. Despite its classification by the World Health Organization as a class I carcinogen, infection with *H. pylori* does not typically lead to gastric cancer. This underscores the importance of other factors, such as virulence, environmental factors, and host factors, as well as genetic polymorphisms (e.g., interleukin-1β, a potent inhibitor of acid secretion).[71] The blood group A phenotype has been reported to be associated with gastric cancers.[72,73] *H. pylori* may adhere to the Lewis blood group antigen, indicating a factor for increased risk for gastric cancer.[74] Small variant alleles of a mucin gene, *Muc1*, were found to be associated with gastric cancer patients when compared with a blood donor control population.[75] Epstein-Barr virus infection has been noted in a certain type of gastric carcinoma (lymphoepithelioid type), although the importance of this is unclear.[76]

Molecular Genetic Alterations

In contrast to ESCC, EAC, pancreatic cancer, and colon cancer, in which certain oncogenes and tumor suppressor genes are altered with high frequency, such degree of alteration is not observed in sporadic gastric cancers. A reasonably prevalent alteration is microsatellite instability, the result of changes in DNA mismatch repair genes (see Table 44.1). Microsatellite instability and associated alterations of the *TGF-β II receptor, IGFRII, BAX, E2F-4, hMSH3,* and *hMSH6* genes are found in a subset of gastric carcinomas.[77–81] Microsatellite instability has been found in 13% to 44% of sporadic gastric carcinomas.[82] A high degree of microsatellite instability occurs in gastric cancers of the intestinal type, reduced involvement of lymph nodes, enhanced lymphoid infiltration, and better prognosis.[83] This is reminiscent of colon cancers associated with Lynch syndrome.

The *p53* tumor suppressor gene is consistently altered in most gastric cancers.[84] In a study of the promoter region of p16 in gastric cancers, a significant number (41%) exhibited CpG island methylation.[85] Many cases with hypermethylation of promoter regions displayed the phenotype with a high degree of microsatellite instability and multiple sites of methylation, including the *hMLH1* promoter region.[86]

E-cadherin may be down-regulated in gastric carcinogenesis by a point mutation, allelic deletion, or promoter methylation.[87,88]

Normal gastric mucosa⟶ chronic atrophic gastritis ⟶ Intestinal metaplasia ⟶ Low-grade dysplasia ⟶ High-grade dysplasia ⟶ Adenocarcinoma

Figure 44.2 Progression of stages in intestinal-type gastric adenocarcinoma.

In addition, during the epithelial–mesenchymal transition, E-cadherin transcription can be silenced by transcriptional factors such as Snail and Slug. However, it is not clear if the epithelial–mesenchymal transition is an important process in gastric carcinogenesis, as is believed to be the case, for example, in breast cancer.

Alterations in a number of other oncogenes and tumor suppressor genes have been described in a very small subset of gastric cancers by polymerase chain reaction–based or immunohistochemical analysis, but the variability in methods and lack of uniformity in quality control make these observations less compelling. Current efforts in deep sequencing of gastric adenocarcinomas through the Cancer Genome Tumor Atlas (CGTA) consortium should reveal new insights in the near future.

Models of Gastric Cancer

Genetically engineered mouse models of gastric cancer have emerged in rapid fashion in recent years, indicating that activated Wnt signaling and induced downstream effectors, *p53* inactivation, *APC* gene inactivation, *Smad4* gene inactivation, and gastrin are critical factors.[89–92] Gastric cancers in these protean mouse models are facilitated by concomitant infection with *Helicobacter*.[93–96] Furthermore, the recruitment of bone marrow stem cells may augment the effects of *Helicobacter* infection during gastric carcinogenesis.[96] Recently, it has been demonstrated that overexpression of interleukin-1β in mice results in gastric inflammation and cancer, with concomitant recruitment of immature myeloid cells (also referred to as *myeloid-derived suppressor cells*).[97]

SELECTED REFERENCES

The full reference list can be accessed at lwwhealthlibrary.com/oncology.

1. Hanahan D, Weinberg RA. The hallmarks of cancer. *Cell* 2011;144: 646–674.
3. Orloff M, Peterson C, He X, et al. Germline mutations in MSR1, ASCC1, and CTHRC1 in patients with Barrett esophagus and esophageal adenocarcinoma. *JAMA* 2011;306:410–419.
4. Su Z, Gay LJ, Strange A, et al. Common variants at the MHC locus and at chromosome 16q24.1 predispose to Barrett's esophagus. *Nat Genet* 2012;44: 1131–1136.
5. Levine DM, Ek WE, Zhang R, et al. A genome-wide association study identifies new susceptibility loci for esophageal adenocarcinoma and Barrett's esophagus. *Nat Genet* 2013;45:1487–1493.
23. Barbash O, Zamfirova P, Lin DI, et al. Mutations in Fbx4 inhibit dimerization of the SCF(Fbx4) ligase and contribute to cyclin D1 overexpression in human cancer. *Cancer Cell* 2008;14(1):68–78.
32. Vogelstein B, Kinzler KW. Cancer genes and the pathways they control. *Nat Med* 2004;10:789–799.
45. Opitz OG, Suliman Y, Hahn WC, et al. Cyclin D1 overexpression and p53 inactivation immortalize primary oral keratinocytes by a telomerase-independent mechanism. *J Clin Invest* 2001;108(5):725–732.
49. Okawa T, Michaylira CZ, Kalabis J, et al. The functional interplay between EGFR overexpression, hTERT activation, and p53 mutation in esophageal epithelial cells with activation of stromal fibroblasts induces tumor development, invasion, and differentiation. *Genes Dev* 2007;21: 2788–2803.
50. Opitz OG, Harada H, Suliman Y, et al. A mouse model of human oral-esophageal cancer. *J Clin Invest* 2002;110:761–769.
51. Stairs DB, Bayne LJ, Rhoades B, et al. Deletion of p120-catenin results in a tumor microenvironment with inflammation and cancer that establishes it as a tumor suppressor gene. *Cancer Cell* 2011;19:470–483.
54. Quante M, Bhagat G, Abrams JA, et al. Bile acid and inflammation activate gastric cardia stem cells in a mouse model of Barrett-like metaplasia. *Cancer Cell* 2012;21:36–51.
55. Wang X, Ouyang H, Yamamoto Y, et al. Residual embryonic cells as precursors of a Barrett's-like metaplasia. *Cell* 2011;145:1023–1035.
56. Bass AJ, Watanabe H, Mermel CH, et al. SOX2 is an amplified lineage-survival oncogene in lung and esophageal squamous cell carcinomas. *Nat Genet* 2009;41:1238–1242.
57. Lin L, Bass AJ, Lockwood WW, et al. Activation of GATA binding protein 6 (GATA6) sustains oncogenic lineage-survival in esophageal adenocarcinoma. *Proc Natl Acad Sci USA* 2012;109:4251–4256.
58. Dulak AM, Stojanov P, Peng S, et al. Exome and whole-genome sequencing of esophageal adenocarcinoma identifies recurrent driver events and mutational complexity. *Nat Genet* 2013;45:478–486.
67. Pharoah PD, Caldas C. Incidence of gastric cancer and breast cancer in CDH1 (E-cadherin) mutation carriers from hereditary diffuse gastric cancer families. *Gastroenterology* 2001;121:1348–1353.
69. Majewski IJ, Kluijt I, Cats A, et al. An α-E-catenin (CTNNA1) mutation in hereditary diffuse gastric cancer. *J Pathol* 2013;229:621–629.
71. El Omar EM, Rabkin CS, Gammon MD, et al. Increased risk of non-cardiac gastric cancer associated with proinflammatory cytokine gene polymorphisms. *Gastroenterology* 2003;124:1193–1201.
82. Seruca R, Santos NR, David L, et al. Sporadic gastric carcinomas with microsatellite instability display a particular clinicopathologic profile. *Int J Cancer* 1995;64:32–36.
88. Grady WM, Willis J, Guilford PJ, et al. Methylation of the CDH1 promoter as the second genetic hit in hereditary diffuse gastric cancer. *Nat Genet* 2000;26:16–17.
89. Taketo MM. Wnt signaling and gastrointestinal tumorigenesis in mouse models. *Oncogene* 2006;25:7522–7530.
91. Teng Y, Sun AN, Pan XC, et al. Synergistic function of Smad4 and PTEN in suppressing forestomach squamous cell carcinoma in the mouse. *Cancer Res* 2006;66:6972–6981.
93. Wang TC, Dangler CA, Chen D, et al. Synergistic interaction between hypergastrinemia and *Helicobacter* infection in a mouse model of gastric cancer. *Gastroenterology* 2000;118:36–47.
96. Houghton J, Stoicov C, Nomura S, et al. Gastric cancer originating from bone marrow-derived cells. *Science* 2004;306:1568–1571.
97. Tu S, Bhagat G, Cui G, et al. Overexpression of interleukin-1beta induces gastric inflammation and cancer and mobilizes myeloid-derived suppressor cells in mice. *Cancer Cell* 2008;14:408–419.

PRACTICE OF ONCOLOGY

45 Cancer of the Esophagus

Mitchell C. Posner, Bruce D. Minsky, and David H. Ilson

INTRODUCTION

Esophageal cancer is unique among the gastrointestinal tract malignancies because it embodies two distinct histopathologic types: squamous cell carcinoma and adenocarcinoma. Which type of cancer occurs in a given patient or predominates in a given geographic area depends on many variables, including individual lifestyle, socioeconomic pressures, and environmental factors. In recent decades, the United States, along with many other Western countries, has witnessed a profound increase in incidence rates of adenocarcinoma, whereas squamous cell carcinoma continues to predominate worldwide. Although it would seem appropriate to individualize treatment of these tumors, in the past, they have often been managed as a single entity. Although present-day therapeutic interventions have begun to have an impact, with statistically significant improvement in survival over the most recent 3 successive decades, cancer of the esophagus remains a highly lethal disease as evidenced by the case fatality rate of 90%. However, a more thorough understanding of the initiating events, the molecular biologic basis, and treatment successes and failures has begun to spawn a new era of therapy aimed at targeting both adenocarcinoma and squamous cell carcinoma of the esophagus.

EPIDEMIOLOGY

The epidemiology of esophageal cancer is defined by its substantial variability as a function of histologic type, geographic area, gender, race, and ethnic background.[1] Because of the recent increase in incidence rates of adenocarcinoma, especially in the Western hemisphere, epidemiologic studies are now distinguishing between histologic types when reporting results, whereas in the past, incidence rates of esophageal cancer reflected only squamous cell carcinoma. This remains true in high-incidence areas where published rates are not obtained from population-based tumor registries. These high-incidence areas include Turkey, northern Iran, southern republics of the former Soviet Union, and northern China, where incidence rates exceed 100 per 100,000 person-years. Incidence rates of squamous cell carcinoma may vary 200-fold between different populations in the same geographic area because of unique cultural practices. The highest incidence rates for males (more than 15 per 100,000 person-years) reported from population-based tumor registries were in Calvados, France; Hong Kong; and Miyagi, Japan; and the highest rates for females (more than 5 per 100,000 person-years) were in Bombay, India; Shanghai, China; and Scotland.[2]

Esophageal cancer is relatively uncommon in the United States, and the lifetime risk of being diagnosed with the disease remains less than 1%.[3] It was estimated that 17,990 new cases would be identified in 2013, with 15,210 patients expected to die of the disease.[4] Age-adjusted incidence rates are essentially equivalent among African American and Caucasian men (Fig. 45.1), although the predominant histologic type in African American men is squamous cell carcinoma. The incidence rates for African American men peaked in the early 1980s, and since then they

have shown a marked decline to the current rate of approximately 7 per 100,000 person-years.[3] Incidence rates among Caucasian men increased up until the year 2000, reflecting the marked increase in the incidence of adenocarcinoma of the esophagus of more than 400% in the past 2 decades, but now have stabilized between 7 and 8 per 100,000 person-years.[3] Although the incidence of esophageal cancer in Caucasian females (1.6 per 100,000) is lower than that in Caucasian males, rates of adenocarcinoma have increased in women by more than 300% during the past 20 years. Similar trends have been noted in Western European countries. This trend of increased incidence of adenocarcinoma of the esophagus has paralleled the upward trend in rates of both gastroesophageal reflux disease and obesity.

A steady decline in esophageal cancer mortality has been noted since the mid-1980s in the non-Caucasian U.S. population, whereas a marked increase in mortality was noted among Caucasian men and women during the same period (Fig. 45.2).[3] The mortality rates among men are markedly higher than women, regardless of race. Although survival rates for all esophageal cancer patients are uniformly dismal, regardless of race or gender, 5-year relative survival rates have significantly improved since the 1970s (5% if diagnosed in 1975 to 1977 versus 19% if diagnosed in 2003 to 2009) based on Surveillance, Epidemiology, and End Results (SEER) population-based tumor registry reporting.[3] There is no survival difference related to cell type (squamous cell carcinoma versus adenocarcinoma).

ETIOLOGIC FACTORS AND PREDISPOSING CONDITIONS

Squamous cell carcinoma and adenocarcinoma of the esophagus share some risk factors, whereas other risk factors are specific to one histologic type or the other.

Tobacco and Alcohol Use

Tobacco and alcohol use are considered the major contributing factors in the development of esophageal cancer worldwide. It is estimated that up to 90% of the risk of squamous cell carcinoma of the esophagus in Western Europe and North America can be attributed to tobacco and alcohol use.[5] Population-based studies demonstrate that tobacco and alcohol use are independent risk factors, and their effects are multiplicative, as evidenced by the association of the highest risk of developing esophageal cancer with heavy use of both agents. Approximately 65% and 57% of squamous cell carcinomas of the esophagus have been attributed to smoking tobacco for longer than 6 months in Caucasian and African American men, respectively, in the United States.[6] There appears to be a dose–response effect related to the duration and intensity of smoking, and, importantly, there is an impressive (up to 50%) reduction in the risk of developing squamous cell carcinoma of the esophagus for those who quit smoking and an inverse relationship between risk and the length of time since cessation of

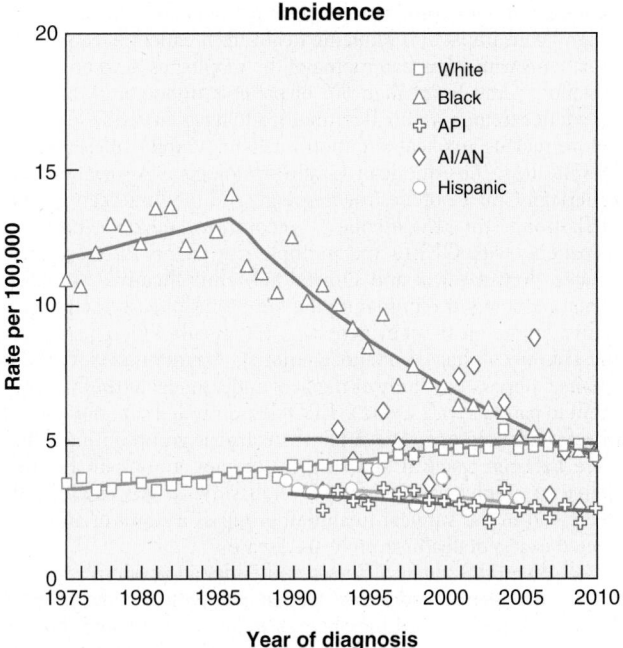

Figure 45.1 Surveillance, Epidemiology and End Results (SEER) age-adjusted esophageal cancer incidence rates in the United States. API, Asian/Pacific Islanders; AI/AN, American Indians/Alaska Natives.

tobacco use.[7] Cigarette smoking in adenocarcinoma of the esophagus leads to a twofold increase in risk for heavy smokers (more than one pack per day).[7,8] Quitting smoking does not appear to decrease the risk of adenocarcinoma, which remains elevated for decades after smoking cessation.[7,8] This suggests that tobacco carcinogens may affect carcinogenesis early on in esophageal adenocarcinoma, and, therefore, the decline in prevalence of smoking in the United States has not had an impact on the risk for the disease. Consistent with this hypothesis, cigarette smoking was recently identified as

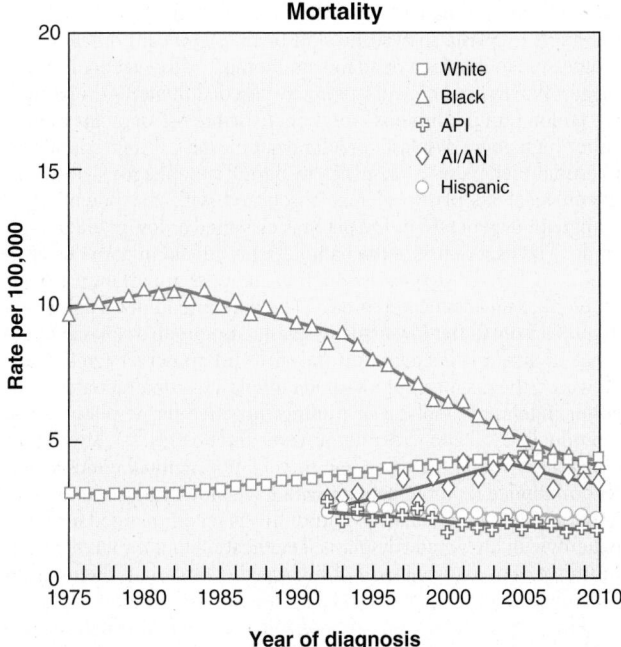

Figure 45.2 Surveillance, Epidemiology and End Results (SEER) age-adjusted esophageal cancer mortality rates in the United States. API, Asian/Pacific Islanders; AI/AN, American Indians/Alaska Natives.

a risk factor for the development of Barrett's esophagus. Specifically, when analyzing data from five case-control studies involving 1,059 patients with Barrett's esophagus, 1,332 patients with gastroesophageal reflux disease (GERD), and 1,143 population-based controls, patients with Barrett's esophagus were significantly more likely to have ever smoked than either control cohort (odds ratio [OR] = 1.67 versus population-based controls; OR = 1.61 versus GERD controls). Furthermore, increasing the pack-years of smoking increased the risk of Barrett's esophagus.[9]

Alcohol is a major contributing factor in the increased risk of esophageal squamous cell carcinoma in Western countries, likely accounting for 80% of squamous cell carcinoma of the esophagus in men in the United States.[6] A dose–response relationship exists between the amount of alcohol ingested and the risk of developing squamous cell carcinoma.[10,11] In most studies, the most commonly consumed beverage in a specific geographic region is the one most frequently associated with increased risk.[1] Although specific carcinogens may be present in a variety of alcoholic beverages, in all likelihood, it is alcohol itself—either as a mechanical irritant, promoter of dietary deficiency, or contributor to susceptibility to other carcinogens—that leads to carcinogenesis. Large population-based case-control studies in both the United States and Australia revealed no relationship between alcohol intake and risk of esophageal adenocarcinoma.[12]

Diet and Nutrition

For both squamous cell carcinoma and adenocarcinoma of the esophagus, case-control studies provide evidence of a protective effect of a diet enriched with fruits and vegetables, especially those eaten raw.[7,13] These food groups contain a number of micronutrients and dietary components such as vitamins A, C, and E; selenium; carotenoids; and fiber, which may prevent carcinogenesis. Deficiencies of the aforementioned nutrients and dietary components (in particular, selenium), have been associated with an increased risk of esophageal squamous cell carcinoma in some parts of the world.[14] Consumption of hot beverages has been suggested as a risk factor for esophageal cancer in South America.[15] More recently, a diet enriched with "animal products and related components" was significantly associated with the development of esophageal carcinoma (OR = 1.64; 95% confidence interval [CI], 1.06 to 2.55), whereas diets high in "vitamins and fiber" and "other polyunsaturated fatty acids and vitamin D" were protective of developing esophageal carcinoma (OR = 0.50 and 0.48, respectively).[16]

Socioeconomic Status

Low socioeconomic status as defined by income, education, or occupation is associated with an increased risk for esophageal squamous cell carcinoma and, to a lesser degree, for adenocarcinoma.[8,17] In the United States, it is estimated that 39% and 69% of squamous cell carcinomas of the esophagus in Caucasian men and African American men, respectively, are related to low annual income.[6] A number of occupational and industrial hazards, including exposure to perchloroethylene (e.g., dry cleaners, metal polishers), combustion products, and fossil fuels (e.g., chimney sweeps, printers, gas station attendants, asphalt and metal workers), silica and metal dust, and asbestos, as well as viral exposure via meat packing and slaughtering, have been suggested as possible risk factors for squamous cell carcinoma but not adenocarcinoma of the esophagus.[2]

Obesity

The prevalence of obesity in the United States markedly increased from 12.8% in the early 1960s to almost 23% between 1988 and 1994.[18] This upward trend parallels that seen for incidence rates of esophageal adenocarcinoma. Increased body mass index (BMI) is a risk factor for adenocarcinoma of the esophagus, and individuals with the highest BMI have up to a sevenfold greater risk of esophageal cancer than those with a low body mass index.[7,19–21] The mechanism by which obesity contributes to an increased risk of esophageal adenocarcinoma is uncertain, although the linkage between obesity and GERD is presumed to be a chief, but not the sole, factor. Recent reports suggest that the presence of abdominal/ intra-abdominal or central obesity rather than BMI itself may increase the risk of Barrett's esophagus and, subsequently, esophageal adenocarcinoma.[22–24] Because of the influence of nutritional and socioeconomic factors, the risk of squamous cell carcinoma of the esophagus increases with decreasing BMI.

Gastroesophageal Reflux Disease

GERD has been implicated as one of the strongest risk factors for the development of adenocarcinoma of the esophagus.[25,26] Chronic reflux is associated with Barrett's esophagus, the premalignant precursor of esophageal adenocarcinoma. Population-based case-control studies that examined the relationship between symptomatic reflux and risk of adenocarcinoma of the esophagus have demonstrated that increased frequency, severity, and chronicity of reflux symptoms are associated with a 2- to 16-fold increased risk of adenocarcinoma of the esophagus, regardless of the presence of Barrett's esophagus.[25,26] Trends in incidence rates of GERD during the past 3 decades parallel the time trends of increasing incidence of adenocarcinoma in the United States.

Helicobacter pylori Infection

Infection with *Helicobacter pylori*, and particularly with cagA+ strains, is inversely associated with the risk of adenocarcinoma of the esophagus.[27,28] The mechanism of action is unclear, although an *H. pylori* infection can result in chronic atrophic gastritis, leading to decreased acid production and potentially reducing the development of Barrett's esophagus. Although infection by *H. pylori* cagA+ strains by itself may not increase the risk of squamous cell carcinoma, the concurrent presence of gastric atrophy and *H. pylori* infection has been reported to significantly increase the risk of squamous cell carcinoma.[29] Atrophic gastritis may promote bacterial overgrowth, leading to intragastric nitrosation, with the production of nitrosamines increasing the risk of esophageal squamous cell carcinoma.

Barrett's Esophagus

Barrett's esophagus is defined by the presence of intestinal metaplasia (mucin-producing goblet cells) in columnar cell–lined epithelium that replaces the normal squamous epithelium of the distal esophagus.[30–32] The appearance at endoscopy of salmon-colored columnar epithelium extending about the gastroesophageal junction contrasts with the pale, pink-colored normal squamous epithelium of the esophagus. Although other types of mucosa (gastric, fundic, or junctional type) have been identified in Barrett's esophagus, specialized intestinal metaplasia confirmed by histologic examination of biopsy specimens is required for the diagnosis of Barrett's esophagus. The absolute risk to develop adenocarcinoma in a year, once thought to be 1 in 100, is now estimated to be 0.12% to 0.33%.[33–36] Regardless of this revised absolute risk, Barrett's esophagus remains the single most important risk factor for developing esophageal adenocarcinoma, with a relative risk of 11.3 (95% CI, 8.8 to 14.4), implying that patients with Barrett's esophagus are 11-fold more likely to develop esophageal adenocarcinoma than individuals without Barrett's esophagus. Patients with short- and long-segment Barrett's esophagus are at risk of developing dysplasia and subsequently adenocarcinoma.[37]

The prevalence of Barrett's esophagus in the general population undergoing endoscopy is approximately 1.5%[38]; for those with reflux symptoms, the presence of Barrett's esophagus is 2.3%, and in those without reflux symptoms, it is 1.2%. The utility of screening patients with symptomatic reflux is unproven and unlikely to have a significant impact on reducing death from cancer because 40% of patients with adenocarcinoma of the esophagus have no history of reflux,[25] and fewer than 5% of patients undergoing resection for adenocarcinoma were documented to have Barrett's esophagus before seeking medical attention for their symptomatic cancer.[39] Despite this, the American Gastroenterological Association, the American College of Gastroenterology, and the American Society of Gastrointestinal Endoscopy[40–42] recommend selective screening of patients with GERD and multiple risk factors for esophageal cancer. Both medical and surgical antireflux therapies are effective at reducing or eliminating the symptoms of gastroesophageal reflux, but no clear-cut evidence exists that either therapy reduces the risk of esophageal adenocarcinoma. A randomized Veterans Affairs Cooperative Study of medical and surgical antireflux treatment in patients with severe GERD demonstrated superior control of reflux symptoms in the surgical treatment group but no difference between medical and surgical therapy groups in the incidence of esophageal cancer.[43] Overall survival was significantly decreased in the surgical treatment group as a result of an unexpected excess of deaths from heart disease.

All three U.S. medical societies mentioned previously recommend surveillance endoscopy for patients with the diagnosis of Barrett's esophagus, and the grade of dysplasia determines the endoscopy interval.[40–42] Uncontrolled studies suggest that adenocarcinomas identified by surveillance methods are detected at an earlier stage and are associated with a more favorable outcome after an esophagectomy.[44–46] However, the efficacy of surveillance endoscopy is unclear, and there are no convincing data demonstrating that surveillance prevents cancer or improves life expectancy.[47–49] Macdonald et al.[49] followed 143 patients with Barrett's esophagus for an average of 4.4 years with surveillance endoscopy and identified only one patient with asymptomatic esophageal adenocarcinoma. Similar findings were reported by O'Connor et al.[47] These studies suggest that routine surveillance of patients with Barrett's esophagus is unlikely to alter the natural history of this disease due to the low incidence of adenocarcinoma. Some authors suggest that surgical antireflux therapy causes regression of metaplastic epithelium or interrupts progression from Barrett's esophagus to low-grade and high-grade dysplasia,[50,51] but convincing evidence is lacking. A prospective, randomized trial of medical treatment versus open Nissen fundoplication in patients with Barrett's esophagus with or without low-grade dysplasia showed no statistically significant difference in progression to dysplasia or adenocarcinoma.[52] Observational studies suggest that the use of acid suppressive medial therapy—in particular, proton pump inhibitors—may decrease the risk of progression to either high-grade dysplasia or adenocarcinoma.[53] Progression from intestinal metaplasia to dysplasia in Barrett's esophagus signifies an unequivocal neoplastic change associated with the potential for malignant degeneration. Dysplasia is classified as low grade or high grade. The experience of the pathologist is crucial in correctly diagnosing high-grade dysplasia, which is the most important predictor for esophageal adenocarcinoma.[54] The differentiation of high-grade dysplasia from either low-grade dysplasia, indefinite dysplasia, or absence of dysplasia is straightforward (85% interobserver agreement). However, the diagnosis of low-grade dysplasia as differentiated from either indefinite dysplasia or findings negative for dysplasia is less reproducible (50% to 75% interobserver agreement).[55,56] Any degree of dysplasia warrants endoscopic surveillance. Annual endoscopy is recommended for those patients with low-grade dysplasia, and more frequent screening (i.e., every 3 months) is recommended for those patients with high-grade dysplasia if eradication therapy has not been instituted. The management of high-grade dysplasia is discussed in Treatment of Premalignant and T1 Disease, later in this chapter.

The proposed stepwise carcinogenic sequence in which specialized intestinal metaplasia proceeds to low-grade dysplasia, high-grade dysplasia, and frank carcinoma suggests a potential opportunity for chemoprevention to disrupt the succession to cancer. Buttar et al.,[57] recognizing that carcinogenesis in Barrett's esophagus is associated with the increased expression of cyclooxygenase-2 (COX-2), examined the effect of COX-2 inhibitors on the development of Barrett's esophagus and adenocarcinoma in a preclinical model. Both selective and nonselective COX-2 inhibitors were effective at inhibiting Barrett's esophagus–related adenocarcinoma. A meta-analysis of two cohort and seven case-control studies comprising 1,813 cancer cases demonstrated a protective association between aspirin or nonsteroidal anti-inflammatory drugs (NSAID) and esophageal cancer.[58] These findings suggest that NSAIDs may act as potential chemopreventive agents. A small, phase IIb randomized placebo-controlled trial of celecoxib in 100 patients with Barrett's esophagus and low- or high-grade dysplasia failed to demonstrate a protective effect against progression of Barrett's dysplasia to adenocarcinoma.[59] The ongoing ASPECT trial in the United Kingdom, a phase III randomized study of aspirin and esomeprazole chemoprevention in Barrett's metaplasia, is evaluating the effect of high- and low-dose esomeprazole, with and without low-dose aspirin, on the progression of Barrett's esophagus to high-grade dysplasia or cancer. More than 2,500 patients have been enrolled in this chemoprevention trial with a planned follow-up of at least 8 years.

Tylosis

Tylosis (focal nonepidermolytic palmoplantar keratoderma) is a rare disease inherited in an autosomal-dominant manner that is characterized by hyperkeratosis of the palms and soles and esophageal papillomas. Patients with this condition exhibit abnormal maturation of squamous cells and inflammation within the esophagus and are at extremely high risk of developing esophageal cancer.[60,61] The tylosis esophageal cancer (*TOC*) gene has been mapped to 17q25 by linkage analysis of pedigrees.[62] The *TOC* gene is also frequently deleted in sporadic human esophageal cancers.[63,64] Envoplakin, which encodes a protein component of desmosomes that is expressed in esophageal keratinocytes, has been mapped to the *TOC* region[61]; however, no tylosis-specific mutations involving this gene have been observed.[65]

Plummer–Vinson/Paterson–Kelly Syndrome

Plummer–Vinson syndrome, also known as Paterson–Kelly syndrome, is characterized by iron-deficiency anemia, glossitis, cheilitis, brittle fingernails, splenomegaly, and esophageal webs. Approximately 10% of individuals with Plummer–Vinson/Paterson–Kelly syndrome develop hypopharyngeal or esophageal epidermoid carcinomas.[66] The mechanisms by which these tumors arise have not been fully defined, although nutritional deficiencies as well as chronic mucosal irritation from retained food particles at the level of the webs may contribute to the pathogenesis of these neoplasms.[67]

Caustic Injury

Squamous cell carcinomas may arise in lye strictures, often developing 40 to 50 years after a caustic injury.[68] The majority of these cancers are located in the middle third of the esophagus. The pathogenesis of these neoplasms may be similar to that implicated in esophageal cancers arising in patients with Plummer–Vinson/Paterson–Kelly syndrome. These cancers are often diagnosed late because chronic dysphagia and pain caused by the lye strictures obscure symptoms of esophageal cancer.

Achalasia

Achalasia is an idiopathic esophageal motility disorder characterized by increased basal pressure in the lower esophageal sphincter, incomplete relaxation of this sphincter after deglutition, and aperistalsis of the body of the esophagus. A 16- to 30-fold increase in esophageal squamous cancer risk has been noted in achalasia

patients.[69,70] In a retrospective analysis, Aggestrup et al.[71] observed the development of esophageal carcinomas in 10 of 147 patients undergoing an esophagomyotomy for achalasia. These neoplasms are believed to result from prolonged irritation from retained food in the midesophagus and arise an average of 17 years after the onset of achalasia. The chronic dysphagia and pain attributable to megaesophagus contributes to their late diagnosis in achalasia patients.[72]

Human Papillomavirus Infection

Human papillomavirus (HPV) infection may contribute to the pathogenesis of esophageal squamous cell cancer in high-incidence areas in Asia and South Africa.[73] This oncogenic virus encodes two proteins (E6 and E7) that sequester the *Rb* and *p53* tumor suppressor gene products. Using polymerase chain reaction techniques, de Villiers et al.[74] detected HPV DNA sequences in 17% of esophageal squamous cell cancers in patients from China. In an additional study using similar techniques, Lavergne and de Villiers[75] identified a broad spectrum of HPV in approximately one-third of esophageal cancer specimens obtained from patients living in high-incidence areas in China and South Africa. Shibagaki et al.[76] detected HPV sequences in 15 of 72 (21%) esophageal cancer specimens obtained from Japanese patients. In contrast, neither evidence of HPV infection nor HPV DNA sequences have been observed in cancers arising in low-incidence areas.[77–80]

Prior Aerodigestive Tract Malignancy

Patients with upper aerodigestive tract cancers develop second primary cancers at a rate of approximately 4% per year.[81] Nearly 10% of secondary neoplasms arising in patients with prior histories of oropharyngeal of lung carcinoma arise in the esophagus.[82–84] Interestingly, *p53* mutational analysis of multiple primary cancers of the aerodigestive tract in 17 patients demonstrated complete discordance of the *p53* genotype between separate primary tumors from the same patient, which suggests that *p53* is not functioning as a tumor susceptibility gene in this setting.[85]

Comparative Genomics

Cancers of the esophagus and stomach are heterogenous and are noted to have genomic instability, as measured by greater somatic copy number alterations when compared with lower gastrointestinal tract tumors.[86] For esophageal and gastroesophageal junction (GEJ) adenocarcinomas, amplification of certain genes rather than gene mutations may be more important drivers of oncogenesis, including targetable kinases such as epidermal growth factor receptor (EGFR), ERBB2, fibroblast growth factor receptor (FGFR)1 and 2, and MET. The most commonly affected genes by mutation include TP53 and CDKN2A.[87] A recent study reported the results of whole-exome sequencing of esophageal adenocarcinoma and esophageal squamous cell carcinoma, and identified notable differences that support the different epidemiology and risk factors for these two distinct diseases.[88] In addition to mutations in TP53, investigators identified NOTCH1 as an important gene in esophageal squamous cell carcinoma development. Also of note, the investigators found conserved mutations in matched samples of Barrett's esophagus and esophageal adenocarcinoma, supporting the progressive molecular pathogenesis of esophageal adenocarcinoma.[88]

APPLIED ANATOMY AND HISTOLOGY

Anatomy

The esophagus bridges three anatomic compartments: the neck, the thorax, and the abdomen (Fig. 45.3). The esophagus extends from the cricopharyngeus muscle at the level of the cricoid

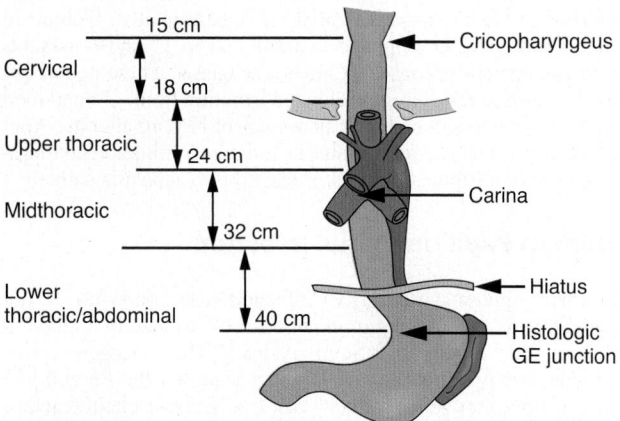

Figure 45.3 Anatomy of the esophagus with landmarks and recorded distance from the incisors used to divide the esophagus into topographic compartments. GE, gastroesophageal.

cartilage to the gastroesophageal junction.[89] The borders of the cervical esophagus span from the cricopharyngeus to the thoracic inlet (approximately 18 cm from the incisors). The remainder of the esophagus is commonly divided into thirds, with the upper third extending from the thoracic inlet to the carina (approximately 24 cm from the incisors), the middle third extending from the carina to the inferior pulmonary veins (32 cm from the incisors), and the distal esophagus traversing the remaining distance into the abdomen to the GEJ (40 cm from the incisors). Squamous cell carcinoma of the esophagus is the predominant histology in the cervical esophagus and upper and middle thirds (above the pulmonary vein) of the thoracic esophagus, whereas adenocarcinoma predominates in the distal esophagus.

Adenocarcinomas of the GEJ present a unique challenge because appropriate management of these tumors as either esophageal or gastric cancers has been uncertain. Siewert et al.[81] have offered a classification system based on demographics, histopathologic variables, and patterns of lymphatic spread that provides clarity, is well established, and has been generally accepted worldwide (Fig. 45.4). In this classification scheme, type I tumors are considered adenocarcinomas of the distal esophagus and type II and III lesions are classified as gastric cancers (cardia and subcardia). This classification system allows for a tailored and consistent surgical approach to these tumors as well as consistency in reporting outcome results associated with therapeutic interventions. However, it should be noted that in the most recent guidelines established by the American Joint Committee on Cancer, GEJ tumors are included under the esophageal cancer staging classification.[90]

The pattern of lymphatic drainage of the esophagus influences the choice of surgical approach, based on tumor location in the esophagus (Fig. 45.5). Tumors of the cervical and upper third of the thoracic esophagus drain to cervical and superior mediastinal lymph nodes. Tumors of the middle third of the esophagus drain both cephalad and caudad with lymph nodes at risk in the paratracheal, hilar, subcarinal, periesophageal, and pericardial nodal basins. Lesions in the distal esophagus primarily drain to lymph nodes in the lower mediastinum and celiac axis region. Because of the extensive lymphatic network within the wall of the esophagus, skip metastases for upper third lesions have been noted in celiac axis nodal basins, and likewise, cervical lymph node metastases have been noted in as many as 30% of patients with distal esophageal lesions. Some surgeons recommend a more radical oncologic procedure, a combined transthoracic and abdominal approach for lesions of the middle and distal esophagus,[91,92] and others recommend a three-field (cervical, mediastinal, and abdominal) lymphadenectomy for all tumors of the middle through distal esophagus.[93,94] However, lymph node metastases are initially limited in an overwhelming majority of patients to regional lymph nodes. Lymph node involvement in lymphatic basins distant from the primary tumor are rarely identified unless metastases to regional lymph nodes have already occurred,[95] which suggests the potential of sentinel lymph node sampling to direct surgical dissection.[96]

Histology

Squamous cell carcinomas account for approximately 40% of esophageal malignancies diagnosed in the United States and the majority of cases arising in high-incidence areas throughout the world.[97] Approximately 60% of these neoplasms are located in the middle third of the esophagus, whereas 30% and 10% arise in the distal third and proximal third of the intrathoracic esophagus, respectively. These tumors are associated with contiguous or noncontiguous carcinoma in situ as well as widespread submucosal lymphatic dissemination.

Adenocarcinomas frequently arise in the context of Barrett's esophagus; because of this, these tumors occur in the distal third of the esophagus. No significant survival differences have been noted in adenocarcinoma patients compared with individuals with squamous cell cancers.

Rarer cancers of the esophagus include squamous cell carcinoma with sarcomatous features, adenoid cystic, and mucoepidermoid carcinomas. These neoplasms are indistinguishable clinically and prognostically from the more common types of esophageal carcinoma.

Small cell carcinomas account for approximately 1% of esophageal malignancies and arise from argyrophilic cells in the basal

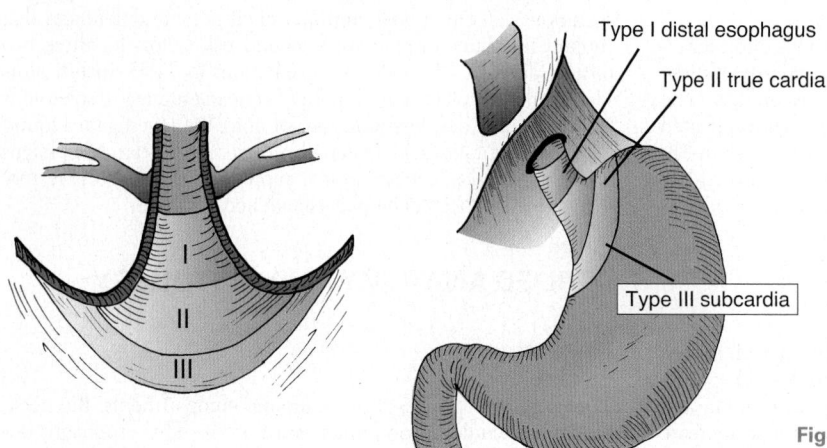

Figure 45.4 Anatomic classification of gastroesophageal junction tumors.

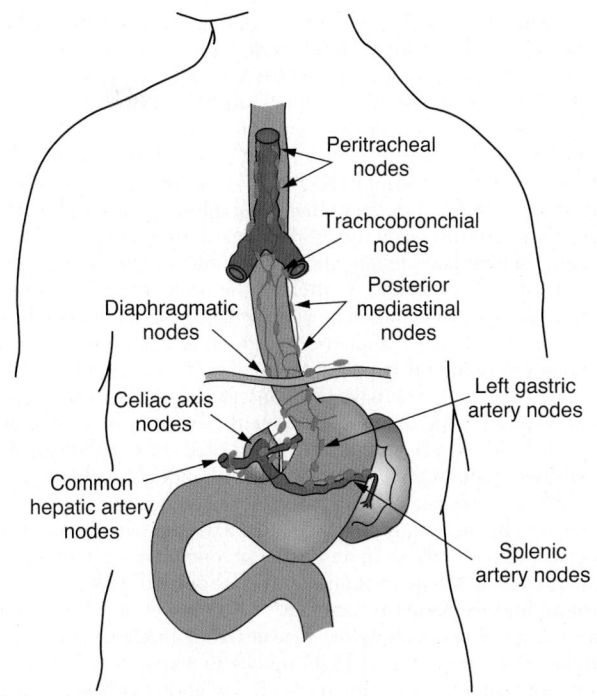

Figure 45.5 Lymphatic drainage of the esophagus with anatomically defined lymph node basins.

Peritracheal nodes

Trachcobronchial nodes

Posterior mediastinal nodes

Diaphragmatic nodes

Celiac axis nodes

Common hepatic artery nodes

Left gastric artery nodes

Splenic artery nodes

layer of the squamous epithelium. These neoplasms are usually located in the middle or lower third of the esophagus and may be associated with an ectopic production of a variety of hormones, including parathormone, secretin, granulocyte colony-stimulation factor, and gastrin-releasing peptide; individuals with these cancers often present with systemic disease.[98–100] Recent series have reported patients with locally advanced disease treated with systemic chemotherapy in combination with either radiation therapy, surgery, or both, with some patients achieving long-term disease-free survival.[101]

Leiomyosarcoma is the most common mesenchymal tumor that affects the esophagus, still accounting for less than 1% of esophageal malignancies. These neoplasms are lower third tumors presenting as bulky masses with hemorrhaging and necrosis. Malignant lymphoma and Hodgkin lymphoma rarely involve the esophagus and is usually secondary to extension from other sites. Patients with AIDS may exhibit Kaposi sarcoma involving the esophagus. Malignant melanoma involving the esophagus is exceedingly rare and presents as a bulky polypoid intraesophageal tumor of varying color depending on melanin production.

NATURAL HISTORY AND PATTERNS OF FAILURE

At presentation, the overwhelming majority of patients have locally or regionally advanced or disseminated cancer, irrespective of histologic type.[4,102] The lack of a serosal envelope and the rich submucosal lymphatic network of the esophagus lead to extensive local infiltration and lymph node involvement. Evidence suggests that occult micrometastases are invariably present, and recurrence patterns confirm that distant failure is a significant and universally fatal component of relapse.[103–107] Bone marrow samples obtained during rib resections performed at an esophagectomy revealed disseminated tumor cells in up to 90% of patients sampled.[108,109] The lung, liver, and bone are the most common sites of distant disease, with depth of tumor invasion and lymph node involvement predictive of tumor dissemination.[89,103,104]

Median survival after esophagectomy for patients with localized disease is 15 to 18 months with a 5-year overall survival rate of 20% to 25%. Patterns of failure after an esophagectomy suggest that both the location of tumor and histologic type may influence the distribution of recurrence. In patients with cancers of the upper and middle thirds of the esophagus, which are predominately squamous cell carcinomas, local–regional recurrence predominates over distant recurrence, whereas in patients with lesions of the lower third, where adenocarcinomas are more frequently located, distant recurrence is more common.[103,104] Only a very small percentage of patients (fewer than 5%) develop a clinically evident recurrence at cervical sites.[95]

The addition of chemotherapy, radiotherapy, or chemoradiation to surgery alters patterns of failure, although reported results are not consistent. Preoperative radiotherapy and preoperative chemoradiation may reduce the rate of local–regional recurrence but have no obvious effect on the rate of distant metastases.[107–111] In two prospective randomized trials recently updated with a long-term follow-up of preoperative chemotherapy plus surgery versus surgery alone that reported patterns of failure, one study showed a slight but not statistically significant decrease in distant relapse with chemotherapy,[105,112] whereas the other demonstrated equivalent distant recurrence rates in both the preoperative chemotherapy and surgery-alone arms.[106,113] Treatment failure patterns after definitive chemoradiation without surgical resection reveal that the concurrent administration of chemotherapy and radiotherapy provides better local control than radiotherapy alone, and that the administration of chemotherapy may reduce systemic recurrence; however, the long-term follow-up of both randomized and nonrandomized patients treated with primary chemoradiation failed to indicate a clear reduction in distant disease recurrence compared with radiation therapy alone.[114] Although the addition of surgery further reduces local failure from 45% to 32%,[115] it does not diminish the systemic recurrence and, in fact, may enhance it by allowing patients to manifest distant disease because they do not succumb to local–regional failure.[116,117] These patterns of relapse suggest that any further improvement in overall outcome for patients with esophageal cancer will be achieved through advances in systemic therapy.

CLINICAL PRESENTATION

The most noticeable symptoms are dysphagia and weight loss. Dysphagia signifies locally advanced disease or distant metastases, or both. Patients describe progressive dysphagia, with initial difficulty in swallowing solids, then liquids. Control of this single symptom impacts most on the patient's quality of life. Patients with squamous cell carcinoma of the esophagus more often have a history of tobacco or alcohol abuse, or both. Weight loss is seen in approximately 90% of patients with squamous cell carcinoma. Patients with adenocarcinoma of the esophagus tend to be Caucasian males from middle to upper socioeconomic classes who are overweight, have a symptomatic gastroesophageal reflux, and have been treated with antireflux therapy.

Approximately 20% of patients experience odynophagia (painful swallowing). Additional presenting symptoms include dull retrosternal pain, bone pain secondary to bone metastases, and cough or hoarseness secondary to paratracheal nodal or recurrent laryngeal nerve involvement. These types of symptoms suggest unresectable locally advanced disease or metastases. Unusual presentations are pneumonia secondary to tracheoesophageal fistula or exsanguinating hemorrhage due to aortic invasion.

DIAGNOSTIC STUDIES AND PRETREATMENT STAGING

Patients with symptoms of dysphagia should undergo an upper endoscopy and a biopsy to establish a tissue diagnosis. Biopsies or cytologic brushings have a diagnostic accuracy approaching 100%.[118,119]

A targeted biopsy can be enhanced by the use of chromoendoscopy techniques using vital dyes, including indigo carmine, Lugol iodine solution, methylene blue, and toluidine blue.[120,121] Autofluorescence imaging and narrow band imaging are emerging endoscopic techniques that allow for a detailed inspection of mucosa.[122–125]

A focused history taking should elicit information on predisposing factors for esophageal cancer, including tobacco use, alcohol use, symptomatic reflux, a diagnosis of Barrett's esophagus, and history of head and neck or thoracic malignancy. Prior surgery on the stomach or colon may influence the choice of reconstructive conduit to restore alimentary continuity at the time of an esophagectomy. Findings on history and physical examination that would prompt further diagnostic testing include hoarseness, cervical or supraclavicular lymphadenopathy, pleural effusion, or new onset of bone pain.

A chest radiography and a liquid oral contrast examination of the esophagus and stomach have been replaced by a computed tomography (CT) scan and a flexible endoscopy. An esophagogastroscopy allows for a precise evaluation of the extent of esophageal and gastric involvement and can precisely measure the distance of the tumor from the incisors to appropriately categorize the tumor's location. An upper endoscopy also allows for the identification of "skip" lesions or second primaries as well as indicates the presence and extent of Barrett's esophagus. A bronchoscopy should be reserved for those patients with tumors of the middle and upper esophagus to rule out invasion of the membranous trachea and possible tracheoesophageal fistula, although an endoscopic ultrasound is now the procedure of choice to identify these unusual manifestations.

Pretreatment staging procedures establish the depth of esophageal wall penetration, regional lymph nodes, and the presence of distant metastases so that patients can be guided to appropriate treatment. A CT scan of the chest and abdomen is mandatory. A recent single institution review of 201 CT scans in 99 patients undergoing staging for esophageal cancer indicated that imaging of the pelvis did not contribute added staging information, and it may not need to be routinely performed.[126] CT scans are highly accurate (approaching 100%) at detecting liver or lung metastases and suggesting peritoneal carcinomatosis (e.g., ascites, omental infiltration, peritoneal tumor studding).[127–129] Accuracy for detecting aortic involvement or tracheobronchial invasion exceeds 90%.[128,130,131] A CT scan is inaccurate in determining T stage and N stage.[127,128,130,132–134] The accuracy of endoscopic ultrasonography (EUS) in determining both T and N stage is a function of its ability to clearly delineate the multiple layers of the esophageal wall[135,136] and its use of multiple criteria, including shape, border pattern, echogenicity, and size, to determine lymph node involvement.[137,138] EUS is superior to CT scans in both T and N staging of esophageal cancer.[139,140] The overall accuracy for T staging is approximately 85%, and for N staging it is approximately 75%.[141] The accuracy of determining lymph node involvement has been increased to 85% to 100% with the use of linear-array EUS with a channel that allows for passage of a needle to perform tissue aspiration for cytology.[134,142,143] EUS is highly operator dependent and is limited in its ability to define relatively superficial lesions as either T1 or T2.[141,144,145] This distinction is critical to allow for the use of minimal resection techniques for T1 lesions and to avoid preoperative chemoradiation for T1 and T2 tumors. Miniprobe high-frequency (20 MHz) sonographic catheters that can be passed through the working channel of the standard endoscope are now being used and provide improved accuracy.[146,148] A new generation of endoscopes that are thin caliber may traverse almost all obstructing lesions, allowing for an EUS assessment.[148] The accuracy of EUS in assessing a response to induction chemoradiation is severely limited, and its use frequently leads to overstaging because the fibrotic changes induced by treatment mimic residual tumor,[149,150] although recent data may indicate some utility for posttherapy EUS.[151]

The fluorine-18 (^{18}F) fluorodeoxyglucose (FDG) positron emission tomography (PET) scan is being widely applied in the management of esophageal cancer. The accuracy of FDG-PET scans in assessing regional lymph nodes falls somewhere between the low and high accuracy of CT scans and EUS, respectively.[152,153] In the detection of distant metastases, an FDG-PET scan is superior to CT, with a sensitivity, specificity, and accuracy all in the range of 80% to 90%.[153,154] PET scans, in combination with CT (PET-CT fusion or hybrid FDG-PET/CT) scans, further improves specificity and accuracy of noninvasive staging.[155] This leads to the detection of unsuspected metastatic disease (upstaging) in 15% of patients, which leads to alteration of the intended treatment plan in at least 20% of patients. Currently, the utility of PET to detect distant disease not identified by other imaging modalities confirms a role for PET that is complementary to other staging procedures, although it should not supplant them.

FDG-PET may also have value in evaluating response to chemotherapy and radiotherapy. Weber et al.[156] demonstrated that decreased FDG uptake significantly correlated with pathologically confirmed response in patients treated with induction chemotherapy before esophagectomy for esophageal adenocarcinoma. A prospective validation study confirmed that a decrease in the standard uptake value of 35% or more during preoperative chemotherapy may predict histologic response and is associated with improved survival and decreased recurrence.[157] Brucher et al.,[158] from the same institution, Technische Universitat Munchen, showed a similar result of decreased FDG uptake in responders compared with nonresponders in patients with squamous cell carcinoma of the esophagus treated with preoperative chemoradiation. The MUNICON trial from the group led by Lordick et al.[159] examined PET scan response during induction chemotherapy in 110 patients with adenocarcinoma of the GEJ. PET scan nonresponders (54 patients) assessed after 2 weeks of induction chemotherapy were referred for immediate surgery rather than continuing with the full 3-month course of preoperative chemotherapy. Survival in these patients (median, 26 months) was comparable to nonresponding patients in a preceding trial (median, 18 months) who continued the full 3 months of chemotherapy prior to surgery, indicating that discontinuation of an ineffective therapy and referral for earlier surgery did not compromise outcome. Survival, however, was inferior in the PET-nonresponding patients compared with the PET responders. Although PET response may identify patients in whom ineffective preoperative therapy should be discontinued, whether or not referral of such patients for alternative chemotherapy, or chemoradiation, is warranted remains to be established. The MUNICON II trial explored whether PET scan nonresponders could have their outcome improved by further treatment with salvage neoadjuvant chemoradiotherapy consisting of single-agent cisplatin combined with 3,000 cGy of radiation therapy followed by surgery. When comparing PET scan nonresponders from MUNICON II treated with additional chemoradiation to nonresponders from the MUNICON trial, the R0 resection rate was not improved and there was no difference in either time to progression or overall survival across trials.[160] The small sample size and the utilization of suboptimal chemotherapy and radiotherapy dosing on the PET scan nonresponder arm make this trial difficult to interpret. One series of patients treated with induction chemotherapy, followed with serial PET scans, identified some patients who progressed on induction chemotherapy. Several of these patients achieved durable disease control, including pathologic complete response, when changed to an alternative chemotherapy during radiation therapy, suggesting that salvage with alternative treatment may be possible.[161] Although pathologic responses on this trial were seen in virtually only early PET scan responding patients, other trials have not shown a clear correlation with early response seen on PET scan during induction chemotherapy with subsequent pathologic response to chemoradiotherapy.[161] Two recent systematic reviews of the current available literature that addressed the evaluation of tumor response by PET scan to neoadjuvant therapy concluded that, although PET scans are the best imaging modality available to assess response, the current data

CALGB 80803 Schema

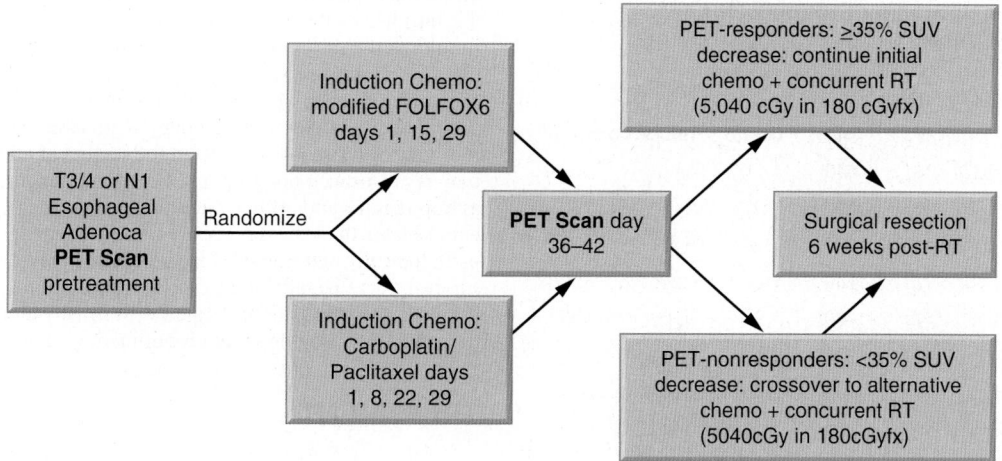

Figure 45.6 Alliance Intergroup randomized phase II trial (CALGB 80803) in resectable adenocarcinoma of the esophagus. SUV, standard update value; RT, radiation therapy.

do not support recommending the routine use of PET scans to guide therapeutic decisions.[162,163] The ALLIANCE Cooperative Group is currently prospectively evaluating the use of PET scans to direct preoperative chemoradiotherapy. Accrual is ongoing to a randomized phase II trial (CALGB 80803) designed to answer the question of whether nonresponders to induction preoperative chemotherapy subsequently treated with a nonoverlapping chemoradiotherapy regimen prior to surgery improves outcome (Fig 45.6).

Minimally invasive surgical techniques (laparoscopy, thoracoscopy, or both) are being used for the staging of both local–regional and distant disease. Performing laparoscopy as the initial procedure at the time of a planned esophagectomy adds little in the way of time and cost to the procedure and allows for the detection of unsuspected distant metastases, which spares the morbidity of laparotomy in 10% to 15% of cases.[164,165] Although studies suggest improved pretreatment staging with minimally invasive surgical approaches,[166–168] such approaches have not been embraced because of the morbidity, length of hospital stay, and cost associated with what is considered an additional procedure.

A study comparing the health-care costs and efficacy of staging procedures, including CT scans, EUS fine-needle aspirations (FNA), PET scans, and thoracoscopies or laparoscopies reported that CT scans plus EUS FNAs were the least expensive and offered the most quality-adjusted life-years on average than all the other strategies. PET scans plus EUS FNAs were somewhat more effective but also more expensive.[169]

PATHOLOGIC STAGING

The most recent guidelines established by the American Joint Committee on Cancer (AJCC) for the staging of esophageal cancer are outlined in Tables 45.1 and 45.2.[90] Changes between the current (seventh edition) and immediate past staging guidelines are highlighted. The tumor location is now defined by the position of the proximal edge of the tumor and is designated as upper, middle, or lower esophagus. Esophagogastric junction tumors are now included in the esophageal cancer staging schema. The primary tumor (T) stage is based on depth of tumor invasion into and through the wall of the esophagus. T stage is now listed as high-grade dysplasia that includes all noninvasive neoplastic epithelium, which was formerly called carcinoma in situ. T1 tumors are now subclassified as T1a (the tumor invades the lamina propria or muscularis mucosae) and T1b (the tumor invades the submucosa). T4 tumors that invade adjacent structures are now subclassified as

PRACTICE OF ONCOLOGY

TABLE 45.1

Tumor (T), Node (N), Metastasis (M) Staging System for Esophageal Cancer

Primary Tumor (T)

TX	Primary tumor cannot be assessed
T0	No evidence of primary tumor
Tis	High grade dysplasia[a]
T1	Tumor invades lumina propria, muscularis mucosae, or submucosa
T1a	Tumor invades lamina propria or muscularis mucosae
T1b	Tumor invades submucosa
T2	Tumor invades muscularis propria
T3	Tumor invades adventitia
T4	Tumor invades adjacent structures
T4a	Resectable tumor invading pleura, pericardium, or diaphragm
T4b	Unresectable tumor invading other adjacent structures, such as aorta, vertebral body, trachea, etc.

Regional Lymph Nodes (N)

NX	Regional lymph nodes cannot be assessed
N0	No regional lymph node metastasis
N1	Regional lymph node metastasis involving 1 to 2 nodes
N2	Regional lymph node metastases involving 3 to 6 nodes
N3	Regional lymph node metastases involving 7 or more nodes

Distant Metastasis (M)

M0	No distant metastasis (no pathologic M0; use clinic M to complete stage group)
M1	Distant metastasis

[a] High-grade dysplasia includes all noninvasive neoplastic epithelium that was formerly called carcinoma in situ, a diagnosis that is no longer used for columnar mucosae anywhere in the gastrointestinal tract.
Used with permission of the American Joint Committee on Cancer (AJCC), Chicago, Illinois. The original source for this material is the *AJCC Cancer Staging Manual*, Seventh Edition (2010) published by Springer Science and Business Media LLC, www.springer.com, page 109.

TABLE 45.2

Classification of Staging Groupings for Esophageal Cancer

Squamous Cell Carcinoma[a]

Group	T	N	M	Grade	Tumor Location[b]
0	Tis (HGD)	N0	M0	1	Any
IA	T1	N0	M0	1, X	Any
IB	T1	N0	M0	2–3	Any
	T2–3	N0	M0	1, X	Lower, X
IIA	T2–3	N0	M0	1, X	Upper, middle
	T2–3	N0	M0	2–3	Lower, X
IIB	T2–3	N0	M0	2–3	Upper, middle
	T1–2	N1	M0	Any	Any
IIIA	T1–2	N2	M0	Any	Any
	T3	N1	M0	Any	Any
	T4a	N0	M0	Any	Any
IIIB	T3	N2	M0	Any	Any
IIIC	T4a	N1–2	M0	Any	Any
	T4b	Any	M0	Any	Any
	Any	N3	M0	Any	Any
IV	Any	Any	M1	Any	Any

Adenocarcinoma

Group	T	N	M	Grade
0	Tis (HGD)	N0	M0	1, X
IA	T1	N0	M0	1–2, X
IB	T1	N0	M0	3
	T2	N0	M0	1–2, X
IIA	T2	N0	M0	3
IIB	T3	N0	M0	Any
	T1–2	N1	M0	Any
IIIA	T1–2	N2	M0	Any
	T3	N1	M0	Any
	T4a	N0	M0	Any
IIIB	T3	N2	M0	Any
IIIC	T4a	N1–2	M0	Any
	T4b	Any	M0	Any
	Any	N3	M0	Any
IV	Any	Any	M1	Any
Stage unknown				

[a] Or mixed histology including a squamous component, or not otherwise specified.
[b] Location of the primary cancer site is defined by the position of the upper (proximal) edge of the tumor in the esophagus.
Used with permission of the American Joint Committee on Cancer (AJCC), Chicago, Illinois. The original source for this material is the *AJCC Cancer Staging Manual*, Seventh Edition (2010) published by Springer Science and Business Media LLC, www.springer.com, page 109.

T4a (a resectable tumor invading the pleura, pericardium, or diaphragm) and T4b (an unresectable tumor). The nodal (N) stage is determined by the presence of involved regional lymph nodes and is now subclassified according to the number of regional lymph nodes involved. The subclassification of metastasis (M) based on distant lymph node involvement (e.g., celiac node metastases for distal esophageal tumors) is no longer used. An analysis of 336

esophageal cancer patients who underwent resection alone recommended that the AJCC system be revised to take into account the number of involved lymph nodes, and that 18 lymph nodes should be the minimum harvested to provide for an accurate staging.[170] The current AJCC guidelines do not specify the number of lymph nodes to be removed, but instead suggest that the surgeon resect as many lymph nodes as possible while minimizing morbidity. Future refinements in the staging of esophageal cancer may result from incorporation of computational modalities such as nomograms and artificial neural networks that may predict outcome better than the TNM-based staging systems.[171] Successive pathologically determined stage groups are predictive of length of survival.[89,102] Overall survival for adenocarcinoma and squamous cell carcinoma in patients treated with surgery alone, as staged by the new AJCC staging system is outlined in Figure 45.7.[172]

TREATMENT

The paucity of appropriately designed studies to scientifically determine the most effective therapeutic strategy in esophageal cancer fuels an ongoing debate and undermines the potential for achieving consensus. Although there is no disagreement that esophageal resection prevents progression from high-grade dysplasia to invasive carcinoma and is curative for T1 lesions limited to the mucosa, the morbidity and mortality associated with esophagectomy has created appropriate enthusiasm for alternative approaches such as mucosal ablation and endoscopic resection. Surgery has always been considered the most effective way of ensuring both local–regional control and long-term survival for patients with tumors invading into or beyond the submucosa with or without lymph node involvement. Some investigators suggest that extending the limits of resection will further improve an outcome. However, surgery alone or any other single modality fails in most patients, which has led oncologists to embrace chemoradiation and some to question the necessity for surgical intervention. Chemoradiation with or without resection is the most common therapeutic regimen offered to patients with locally advanced (stage II or III) esophageal carcinoma in the United States and its use has increased dramatically in the past decade.[102,173]

Treatment of Premalignant and T1 Disease (Localized to the Mucosa Only)

High-grade dysplasia in Barrett's esophagus is the most powerful predictor of subsequent invasive adenocarcinoma and is associated with a per-year cancer incidence of 6%, thereby warranting therapeutic intervention. The rationale for esophagectomy is that resection completely eradicates the mucosa at risk, which prevents progression to invasive carcinoma. This is supported by older surgical series reporting previously unidentified invasive cancer, which was present in up to 40% of resected specimens.[174–177] The argument against esophagectomies is that most patients with high-grade dysplasia do not develop invasive carcinoma in their lifetimes and, in the era of endoscopic resection, that early cancers can be effectively addressed without an esophagectomy. Those supporting endoscopic methods, ranging from surveillance to mucosal ablative and resection techniques, argue that this allows for the identification of patients with an early invasive lesion that is readily amenable to cure or elimination of the mucosa at risk, thus preventing progression. Indeed, patients with superficial invasive tumors confined to the mucosa, and those with T1a disease in particular, have little or no risk of lymph node metastases[178,179] and are considered candidates for endoscopic therapies.

Surveillance

Endoscopic surveillance is based on the assumptions that the majority of patients will not progress to invasive carcinoma[180] and

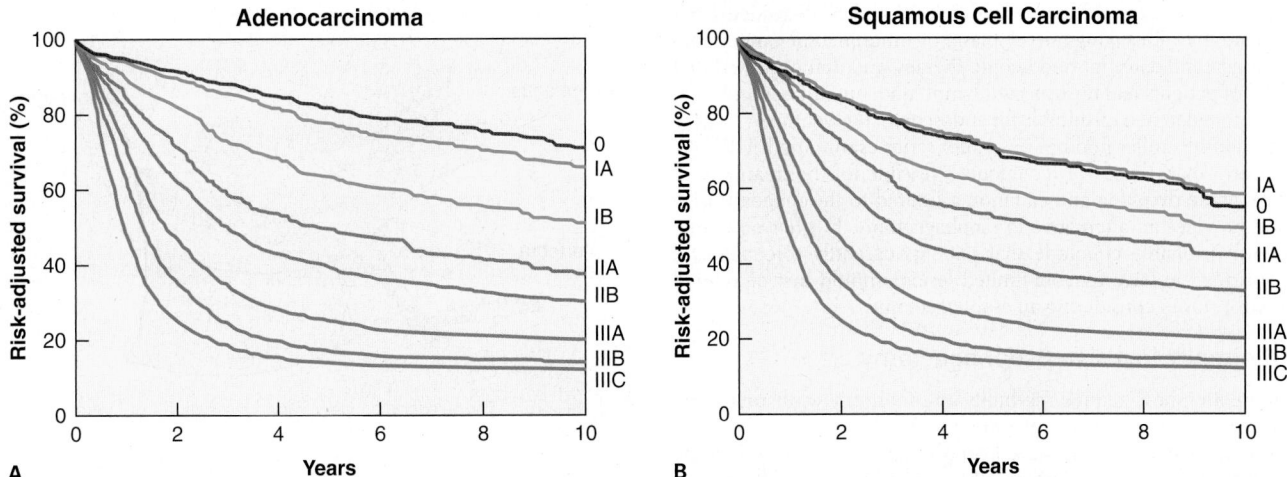

Figure 45.7 Risk-adjusted survival for **(A)** adenocarcinoma and **(B)** squamous cell carcinoma of the esophagus according to stage groups based on the seventh edition of the American Joint Commission on Cancer staging system.

that actual cancers detected by surveillance are at an earlier stage and are therefore curable.[181] Studies demonstrating that patients with Barrett's esophagus–associated adenocarcinomas detected by surveillance have an earlier stage of disease and have better survival than those detected at an initial endoscopy provide supportive evidence for surveillance.[44–46,174] Critics counter this argument with reports identifying invasive adenocarcinoma in up to 45% of esophagectomy specimens from patients with a diagnosis of high-grade dysplasia.[175–177] Proponents of surveillance management argue that these patients were not on an endoscopic surveillance program with strict biopsy criteria, and that strict pathologic criteria of invasive disease (submucosal invasion or beyond) were not utilized.[182]

Proposed guidelines for surveillance include serial endoscopy at 3- to 6-month intervals with multiple four-quadrant biopsies at 1- to 2-cm intervals.[33] The downside of endoscopic vigilance is that in a certain percentage of patients, invasive cancer goes undetected and the patients will not be candidates for potentially curative treatment.[183–185] This must be weighed against the morbidity and mortality of an esophagectomy. It is important to note that the extent of high-grade dysplasia does not predict the presence of occult adenocarcinoma identified at an esophagectomy and, therefore, cannot necessarily be applied to a subjective quantification of disease.[186]

Ablative Methods

The mechanism of action of all mucosal ablative techniques, including photodynamic therapy (PDT), laser ablation, multipolar electrocoagulation, argon plasma coagulation, and radiofrequency ablation, is destruction of the mucosal layer. The premise for managing high-grade dysplasia with endoscopic ablative therapy is that mucosal injury in an acid-controlled environment via proton-pump inhibitors eliminates the premalignant mucosa and resurfaces the esophageal lining with regenerated squamous epithelium.[181]

PDT involves the administration of an inactive photosensitizing agent that, when exposed to light of the proper wavelength, results in oxygen radical production and tissue destruction. Results of a phase III multicenter study that randomized 208 patients on a two to one basis to either PDT plus omeprazole or omeprazole alone demonstrated improved eradication of high-grade dysplasia in the PDT arm (77% versus 39%; p <0.0001) at a 24-month follow-up.[187] A marked reduction in the occurrence of adenocarcinoma was noted in the PDT-treated group (13% versus 28%); however, the results emphasize the risk of development of invasive cancer in a relatively short follow-up interval of 24 months.

These results highlight the limitations of PDT, and due to the complexity of treatment and inconvenience of exposure to photosensitizing agents, PDT has fallen out of favor. Limited experience with thermal ablation for high-grade dysplasia has been reported. Small series of either laser ablation[188–189] or argon plasma coagulation[190,191] of high-grade dysplasia suggest that high-grade dysplasia can be eradicated; however, the follow-up period in these studies was short, and invasive carcinoma has subsequently been documented. Radiofrequency ablation is now considered the preferred ablation technique. A randomized trial in 127 patients with Barrett's esophagus and either low- or high-grade dysplasia assigned patients to either a sham endoscopic procedure or to treatment with radiofrequency ablation.[192] Patients assigned to receive radiofrequency ablation were treated with a circumferential ablation device employing an inflatable cylindrical balloon, bringing electrodes into contact with the esophageal lining, with four applications performed per session, and up to four sessions performed over 9 months. At 12 months, a complete eradication of metaplasia occurred in 77.4% of the radiofrequency ablation patients compared to 2.3% in the control group. Although the development of cancer in either group was uncommon, progression to cancer in the ablation group was significantly less in the control group. More long-term follow-up beyond the 12 months in this trial as well as other confirmatory studies are required.

Endoscopic Mucosal Resection

Endoscopic mucosal resection (EMR) is now considered an essential diagnostic, staging, and therapeutic option available for patients with either high-grade dysplasia or superficial esophageal cancers (T1a). The EMR technique either involves a submucosal injection of fluid to lift and separate the lesion from the underlying muscular layer or the use of suction to trap the lesion into a cylinder, which allows for a full resection and tissue retrieval with a snare or endoscopic knife for appropriate histologic examination. Ell et al.[193] prospectively examined the utility of endoscopic resection in 100 consecutive patients with low-risk adenocarcinoma (no ulceration, mucosal lesion, no vascular or lymphatic invasion, less than 20 mm, and not poorly differentiated). Complete local remission was achieved in 99 of 100 patients; at a median follow-up of 33 months, 11% of patients developed recurrent or metachronous carcinomas, all successfully treated with repeat endoscopic resection. The calculated 5-year survival rate was 98% and no patient died of esophageal cancer. In a previous study from the same group,[194] the complete remission rate in patients with less favorable lesions was 59%, which emphasizes the need to adhere to strict criteria to optimize disease eradication.

A report examining the value of EUS and EUS-guided FNA in patients with high-grade dysplasia or intramucosal cancer considered candidates for endoscopic therapy and demonstrated that 20% of patients had unsuspected lymph node metastases and were therefore deemed unsuitable for endoscopic intervention.[195] These results and similar findings in smaller series examining EMR[196,197] confirm that use of this technique is feasible for the treatment of high-grade dysplasia and carcinoma limited to the mucosa (T1a) and provides an alternative to esophagectomy. Furthermore, one could justifiably conclude that patients carefully screened and confirmed to have mucosa-limited lesions should first be offered EMR prior to considering an esophagectomy.[198,199]

Minimally Invasive Esophagectomy

In an attempt to reduce morbidity and mortality while achieving an equivalent oncologic outcome, minimally invasive techniques for esophageal resection have been designed and continue to be investigated. A variety of minimally invasive approaches have been used for esophagectomies, including laparoscopic, thoracoscopic, combined laparoscopic and thoracoscopic, and hand-assisted techniques and robotic assisted.[200–204] These techniques have been described and are similar in conduct to open procedures of transthoracic and transhiatal esophagectomy (detailed in Surgical Resection) except for the nuances of the minimally invasive approach (Figs. 45.8 and 45.9). These procedures have been applied to the treatment of all stages of potentially resectable esophageal cancer, but until oncologic equivalency to open techniques is confirmed, it would seem to be most applicable in the management of premalignant and early-stage disease.

By far the largest single-institution experience with minimally invasive esophagectomies (MIE) has been reported by Luketich et al.,[205] which included 1,011 consecutive patients, the vast majority (95%) of whom had malignant disease. Approximately equivalent numbers of patients underwent either a three-incision MIE or, more recently, an Ivor Lewis MIE. The median intensive care unit stay was 2 days, the median length of hospital stay was 8 days, 30-day perioperative mortality was 1.7%, and the R0 resection rate was 98%. Median follow-up was only 20 months, and stage-specific

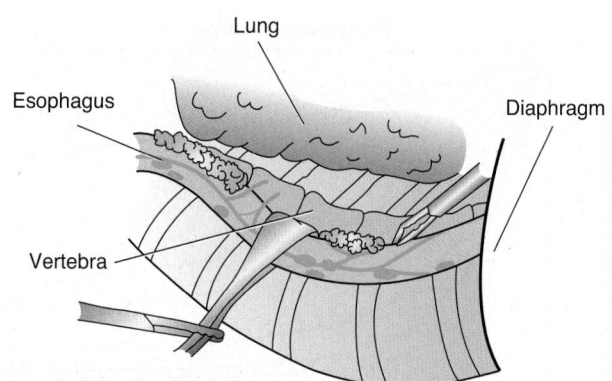

Figure 45.9 Thoracoscopic view and dissection of intrathoracic esophagus.

survival was similar to that reported in a series with open esophagectomies. This group concluded that MIEs are safe and an appropriate surgical approach in experienced hands. The same group reported their experience with 100 consecutive patients with T1 esophageal cancer who underwent esophagectomy, 80% of which were performed via a minimally invasive approach. The 30-day mortality was 0% and a R0 resection was achieved in 99%. N1 disease was present in 21% of patients, the majority of whom (90%) had T1b lesions with submucosal invasion. At a median follow-up of 5.5 years, 5-year overall survival was 62% and 3-year disease-free survival was 80%. The authors concluded that esophagectomies remain the standard of care for patients with T1 esophageal cancer.[206] The results following minimally invasive esophagectomies reported by this group at the University of Pittsburgh are both promising and impressive, but whether they are reproducible in other institutions and therefore more broadly applicable need to be determined through further study.[207,208] The first, multicenter, randomized controlled trial of MIEs versus open esophagectomies recently reported its short-term results. Patients (n = 115) were randomly assigned to MIEs or open esophagectomies with the primary endpoint of postoperative pulmonary infection within 2 weeks of surgery. MIEs were associated with a statistically significant reduction in pulmonary infections and in length of stay. There was no difference detected in either 30-day or in-hospital mortality, and postoperative complication rates were similar. Patients randomized to the MIE arm had statistically significant longer operative times and decreased operative blood loss. Long-term oncologic outcomes are pending, but R0 resection rates and lymph node retrieval were equivalent between minimally invasive and open approaches.[209]

Nonresection or Ablative Therapy

There is limited experience with the use of radiation or chemoradiation in the curative setting for patients with cT1N0 disease. Sai et al.[210] from Kyoto University treated 34 patients who were either medically inoperable or refused surgery with either external beam alone (64 Gy) or external beam (52 Gy) plus 8 to 12 Gy with brachytherapy. With a median follow-up of 61 months, 5-year results were 59% survival, 68% local relapse-free survival, and 80% cause-specific survival. Treating a similar population of 63 patients with chemoradiation plus brachytherapy, Yamada et al.[211] reported 66% survival, 64% disease-free survival, and 76% cause-specific survival at 5 years. In a recent cohort study of patients with clinical stage T1bN0 esophageal squamous cell carcinoma of the thoracic esophagus, nearly 20% of patients in the surgery cohort of 102 patients had nodal involvement on pathologic inspection. Patients who received definitive chemoradiotherapy (n = 71) had a higher risk of disease recurrence. Local recurrence in the definitive chemoradiotherapy cohort could be controlled by salvage esophagectomy

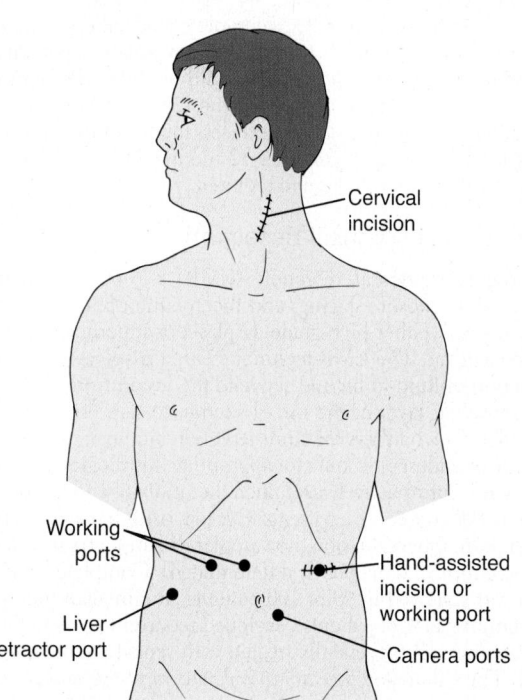

Figure 45.8 Abdominal port sites and incisions used for minimally invasive esophagectomy.

30% of the time, with the remaining ultimately dying of progressive esophageal adenocarcinoma.[212] These data highlight the importance of patient selection in the decision process for local–regional therapy for early stage esophageal carcinoma.

Treatment of Localized Disease

Surgery has traditionally been the treatment of choice for patients with localized, resectable carcinoma of the esophagus and continues to be a component of a more comprehensive approach to esophageal cancer in a substantial number of patients. Failure of surgery alone to significantly alter the natural history of esophageal cancer has resulted in considerable and appropriate enthusiasm for multimodality therapy approaches. The shift toward multimodal treatment is not only theoretically sound, but is also supported by results from phase III randomized trials. Recent trials, unlike their predecessors, which were statistically underpowered and often came to conflicting conclusions about the worth of preoperative therapeutic regimens (radiation, chemotherapy, or chemoradiation), consistently demonstrate benefit to neoadjuvant therapy compared to surgery alone. Results from clinical trials have also brought into question the role of surgery in a multimodal approach to treatment of esophageal cancer, with studies (almost exclusively in squamous cell cancer) suggesting the absence of a survival benefit for the addition of surgery after chemoradiation, despite improved local disease control. Most clinicians and investigators consider some form of combined modality treatment that includes surgery to be the standard of care for localized, resectable esophageal cancer.

Surgical Resection

Decisions regarding surgical technique are routinely based on personal bias, comfort level of the surgeon, and a subjective view of tumor biology because solid evidence from scientifically designed trials is nonexistent. Studies that used health services–linked databases have demonstrated a statistically significant association between performance of surgery in hospitals designated as high-volume esophagectomy institutions with lower complication and mortality rates.[214–217] A study from the Netherlands noted a significant reduction in postoperative morbidity, decrease in length of stay, reduction in in-hospital mortality, and improved 2-year survival following centralization of esophageal resections in high volume units when compared to before the centralization project was introduced.[218] Importantly, the strength of the inverse volume–outcome relationship for esophagectomy has significantly increased over time (2008 to 2009 versus 2000 to 2001) with the adjusted odds ratio of mortality in very low volume hospitals increasing substantially compared to that of very high volume hospitals.[219]

Transhiatal Esophagectomy. The transhiatal route for esophageal resection has gained favor, especially among surgeons in the United States, concurrent with the rising incidence of adenocarcinoma of the distal esophagus, which is readily approachable and effectively dissected through the diaphragmatic hiatus (Table 45.3). The technique is as follows.[220,221] It is prudent to initially perform laparoscopic exploration to rule out disseminated disease and, if it is confirmed, to abort the intended resection before exposing the patient to the risks of laparotomy. Through a midline incision, the stomach is mobilized by dividing all vascular attachments while preserving the right gastroepiploic and right gastric vessels on whose pedicle the reconstructive conduit will be based. The duodenum is fully mobilized via a Kocher maneuver and a pyloric drainage procedure is performed, which has been demonstrated in prospective randomized trials to reduce gastric stasis and minimize pulmonary complications such as aspiration.[222,223] Cautery division of the diaphragmatic crus allows for wide access to the mediastinum and dissection under direct vision of the middle and lower third of the esophagus. A left cervical incision provides

TABLE 45.3

Conventional Approaches to Esophageal Resection for Cancer

Transhiatal
- Laparotomy and cervical approach
- Peritumoral or two-field lymph node dissection
- En bloc resection feasible for distal esophageal tumors
- Cervical anastomosis

Transthoracic
- Ivor Lewis
  - Right thoracotomy and laparotomy
  - Peritumoral or two-field lymph node dissection
  - En bloc resection feasible for middle/distal thoracic tumors
- McKeown or "three hole"
  - Right thoracotomy, laparotomy, cervical approach
  - Peritumoral, two-field or three-field lymph node dissection
  - En bloc resection feasible for mid- or distal thoracic tumors
  - Cervical anastomosis
- Left thoracotomy
  - Left thoracotomy with or without cervical approach
  - Peritumoral lymph nodes dissection
  - Intrathoracic or cervical anastomosis
- Left thoracoabdominal
  - Left thoracoabdominal approach
  - Peritumoral or two-field lymph node dissection
  - Intrathoracic anastomosis

exposure to the cervical esophagus, and circumferential dissection of the cervical esophagus is carried down to below the thoracic inlet to the upper thoracic esophagus, with care to avoid injury to the recurrent laryngeal nerve. The remainder of the dissection at the level of and superior to the carina is completed by blunt dissection through the esophageal hiatus.

The cervical esophagus is then divided, the stomach and attached intrathoracic esophagus are delivered through the abdominal wound, and a gastric tube, which will serve as the reconstructive conduit, is fashioned using multiple applications of a linear stapling device. The gastric tube is then transposed through the posterior mediastinum to the cervical wound, where a cervical esophagogastric anastomosis is performed. The stomach is considered by most surgeons as the replacement conduit of choice for the resected esophagus. A segment of colon, usually based on the ascending branch of the inferior mesenteric artery, is an effective esophageal substitute if for any reason the stomach is deemed unsuitable for reconstruction or if it is the surgeon's preference. Although the original intent of this approach was not to perform a methodical lymph node dissection, a standard two-field lymphadenectomy (abdominal and lower mediastinal) can readily be achieved, and for that matter, if the surgeon is so inclined, a radical en bloc resection can be performed, as described by Bumm et al.[224]

The stated advantages attributed to the transhiatal approach to esophagectomy include avoidance of a thoracotomy incision, which thereby minimizes pain and subsequent postoperative pulmonary complications; elimination of the lethal complications of mediastinitis associated with an intrathoracic anastomotic leak; and a shorter duration of operation, which results in decreased morbidity and mortality.[221] Limitations and disadvantages of transhiatal esophagectomy include poor visualization of upper and middle thoracic esophageal tumors, increased anastomotic leak rate with subsequent stricture formation, the possibility of chylothorax, and the possibility of recurrent laryngeal nerve injury. The largest experience with transhiatal esophagectomy was reported by Orringer et al.[225] and included 1,525 patients with esophageal

TABLE 45.4

TABLE 45.4

Results of Transhiatal Esophagectomy for Esophageal Cancer

Study (Ref.)	Year	No. of Patients (n)	Histologic Type	Perioperative Mortality (%)	5-Year Survival (%)
Gelfand et al.[227]	1992	160	A	0.9	21
Gertsch et al.[229]	1993	100	A/S	3	23
Vigneswaran et al.[228]	1993	131	A/S	2.3	21
Dudhat and Shinde[231]	1998	80	S	7.5	37
Orringer et al.[226]	1999	800	A/S	4.5	23
Bolton and Teng[230]	2002	124	A/S	1.6	27.3

A, adenocarcinoma; S, squamous cell carcinoma.

cancer, 79% of whom had adenocarcinoma and 21% of whom had squamous cell carcinoma. Tumors were located in the lower third of the esophagus in 82% and in the middle or upper third in 18%. In-hospital mortality was 3%. The most common complications were anastomotic leak (12%) and recurrent laryngeal nerve palsy (4.5%). Leak of a cervical esophageal gastric anastomosis was handled simply, in most patients with opening of the cervical wound, followed by local wound care. Hoarseness from recurrent laryngeal nerve injury resolved spontaneously in 99% of cases. Overall 5-year survival was 29%, and stage-specific 5-year survival was 65% for stage I, 28% for stage II, 29% for stage IIB, and 11% for stage III. These results reflect those reported from other surgical series of transhiatal esophagectomy (Table 45.4).[226–231]

Transthoracic Esophagectomy. The transthoracic esophagectomy has been the most common surgical approach used to resect carcinomas of the esophagus and is the standard procedure against which all other techniques are measured (see Table 45.3). Although a left thoracotomy provides adequate exposure to tumors of the distal esophagus, a right thoracotomy affords access to upper, middle, and distal esophageal lesions and is the preferred route for transthoracic exposure. A right thoracotomy combined with an upper midline laparotomy (Ivor Lewis esophagectomy) is the technique most commonly used for esophageal resection and is briefly described here.[221] The abdominal portion of the procedure duplicates that of the transhiatal approach previously detailed and includes mobilization of the stomach and distal esophagus, upper abdominal lymphadenectomy, pyloromyotomy, and placement of a feeding jejunostomy before abdominal wound closure and repositioning for the thoracic component of the procedure. A muscle-sparing right lateral thoracotomy is performed through the fifth or sixth intercostal space. The azygos vein is divided, the mediastinal pleura incised, the intrathoracic esophagus mobilized, and a mediastinal lymph node dissection performed.

After division of the proximal esophagus in the chest to ensure an adequate margin, the GEJ and stomach are pulled into the thoracic cavity. The stomach is then divided with a linear stapler, the specimen is removed, and an esophagogastric anastomosis is performed. An alternative approach has been described in which the right thoracotomy is the initial stage of the procedure followed by repositioning of the patient supine for an abdominal and left cervical incision to achieve a cervical esophagogastric anastomosis.[232,233] Initial experience with a minimally invasive Ivor Lewis esophagectomy has also been reported.[234]

The transthoracic approach provides direct visualization and exposure of the intrathoracic esophagus, facilitating a wider dissection to achieve a more adequate radial margin around the primary tumor and more thorough lymph node dissection, which theoretically results in a more sound cancer operation. In patients with significant comorbid conditions, the combined effects of an abdominal and thoracic incision may compromise cardiorespiratory function. An intrathoracic anastomotic leak can lead to mediastinitis, sepsis, and death. In addition, esophagitis in the nonresected thoracic esophagus may occur secondary to bile reflux. The three-incision (cervical, thoracic, and abdominal) modification of the procedure effectively eliminates the potential for complications associated with an intrathoracic esophagogastric anastomosis.

Numerous authors have reported results of transthoracic esophagectomy; however, most, if not all, of these reports include patients who were resected via other surgical approaches and underwent a more extended lymphadenectomy (Table 45.5).[235–240] Both overall and stage-specific 5-year survival rates were similar to those seen with a transhiatal esophagectomy. The most reliable data may be derived from prospective randomized trials in which there is a surgery-alone control arm. In only one of those trials[240] was a transthoracic approach the only surgical procedure allowed. In that trial, median survival time on the surgery alone arm was 18.6 months and 5-year survival rate was 26%.

TABLE 45.5

Results of Transthoracic Esophagectomy for Esophageal Cancer

Study (Ref.)	Year	No. of Patients (n)	Histologic Type	Perioperative Mortality (%)	5-Year Survival (%)
Wang et al.[238]	1992	368	S	6.5	7.6
Lieberman et al.[239]	1995	258	A/S	5	27
Adam et al.[237]	1996	597	A/S	6.9	16.3
Sharpe and Moghissi[235]	1996	562	A/S	9	18
Bosset et al.[240]	1997	139	S	3.6	26
Ellis[236]	1999	455	A/S	3.3	24.7

A, adenocarcinoma; S, squamous cell carcinoma.

Transhiatal Versus Transthoracic Esophagectomy. The controversy regarding the optimal surgical approach for esophageal cancer remains unresolved. Two large meta-analyses have compared transhiatal esophagectomy with transthoracic esophagectomy based on collective reviews of numerous individual studies.[241,242] Both reports include studies that compared transhiatal with transthoracic esophagectomies, studies of transhiatal esophagectomies only, and studies of transthoracic esophagectomies only. Rindani et al.[241] reviewed 5,483 patients from 44 series published between 1986 and 1996. Perioperative mortality was significantly higher in the transthoracic esophagectomy group than in the transhiatal group (9.5% versus 6.3%), whereas overall perioperative complications were not significantly different. Transhiatal esophagectomies resulted in a higher incidence of anastomotic leak, anastomotic stricture, and recurrent laryngeal nerve injury. Overall 5-year survival was similar: 24% for transhiatal esophagectomies and 26% for transthoracic esophagectomies. Hulscher et al.[242] performed a collective review of 50 studies performed between 1990 and 1999 yielding 7,527 patients. Postoperative mortality was significantly greater in the transthoracic group than in transhiatal group (9.2% versus 5.7%). Transthoracic esophagectomies were associated with a significantly higher risk of pulmonary complications (18.7% versus 12.7%), whereas patients treated with a transhiatal esophagectomy had a higher anastomotic leak rate (13.6% versus 7.2%). Five-year survival was not significantly different, with a 23% 5-year survival for transthoracic and a 21.7% 5-year survival with transhiatal esophagectomies. A third meta-analysis of over 50 comparative studies with a total of 5,905 patients included studies published up to 2010 and also included the largest randomized controlled trial. In-hospital or 30-day mortality was significantly higher in the transthoracic group (10.6% versus 7.2%) as was pulmonary complications and length of stay (4 days greater). Anastomotic leak (16.9% versus 10.6%), anastomotic stricture and vocal cord paralysis was significantly higher in the transhiatal group. Five-year overall survival was not statistically different between the transthoracic (26.6%) and transhiatal (25.8%) groups.[243] A prospective database based on the Veterans Administration National Surgical Quality Improvement Program analyzed perioperative outcome in 945 patients: 562 who underwent transthoracic esophagectomy and 383 who underwent resection through a transhiatal approach.[244] There was no difference in overall mortality (10% for transthoracic approach versus 9.9% for transhiatal approach) or morbidity (47% for transthoracic versus 49% for transhiatal). A large population-based study evaluated transhiatal and transthoracic esophagectomies through the SEER Medicare-linked database from 1992 to 2002.[245] A lower operative mortality was found after transhiatal esophagectomies (6.7% versus 13.1%). Although observed 5-year survival was higher after a transhiatal esophagectomy, after adjusting for stage, patient, and provider factors, no significant 5-year survival difference was found.

Four phase III trials have prospectively examined the outcomes for patients randomly assigned to undergo either a transhiatal or a transthoracic esophagectomy.[246–249] No definitive conclusions can be drawn from three of these trials because of the extremely small sample size. The trial in the Netherlands, however, deserves special attention. Hulscher et al.[249] randomly assigned 220 patients with middle or distal esophageal carcinoma to undergo either a transhiatal esophagectomy or a transthoracic esophagectomy. The transthoracic group underwent a systematic mediastinal and upper abdominal lymph node dissection. Although the number of lymph nodes retrieved was significantly higher in the transthoracic group (31 versus 16; $p < 0.001$), there was no difference in the radicality of the two procedures with equivalent R0, R1, and R2 resections. Postoperative pulmonary complications, ventilatory time, intensive care unit stay, and hospital stay were significantly higher in those patients assigned to the transthoracic group. Despite the higher perioperative morbidity, there was no statistically significant increase in in-hospital mortality (4% versus 2% for transthoracic versus transhiatal esophagectomy, respectively; $p = 0.45$).

At a median follow-up of 4.7 years, there were no significant differences between the transhiatal and transthoracic esophagectomy groups with respect to median disease-free interval (1.4 years versus 1.7 years) and median overall survival time (1.8 years versus 2.0 years), respectively. Likewise, no significant differences were noted in local–regional recurrence, distant recurrence, and combined local–regional and distant recurrence for patients randomly allocated to the transthoracic or transhiatal esophagectomy arm. The investigators point out that a trend toward improved disease-free survival (39% versus 27%) and overall survival (39% versus 29%) at 5 years favored the transthoracic approach group. However, a recent update on this study that provided complete 5-year survival data demonstrated that survival was equivalent in patients randomized to either a transhiatal (34%) or transthoracic (36%) resection.[250]

Either the transhiatal or transthoracic procedure can be performed with acceptable morbidity and mortality in experienced hands and, with either technique, the outcome is remarkably similar.

Extended Esophagectomy. In an attempt to improve on the dismal results reflected in high local recurrence rates and poor overall survival with standard transhiatal and transthoracic esophagectomy techniques, some surgeons have examined extending the limits of resection to accomplish a more effective primary tumor excision and lymph node dissection. Two concepts guide the intent of these more extended resections: en bloc resection of the primary tumor with its adjacent surrounding tissue and systematic lymph node dissection, encompassing either two (mediastinal and abdominal) or three (cervical, mediastinal, and abdominal) lymph node basins (Fig. 45.10). Although some investigators have focused and reported separately on en bloc esophagectomies and extended lymphadenectomies, most of the techniques described encompass both components of this "radical" approach. An en bloc esophagectomy involves the resection of middle and lower esophageal tumors with an envelope of adjacent tissue that includes the mediastinal pleura laterally, the pericardium anteriorly, and the azygos vein and thoracic duct posterolaterally with the surrounding periesophageal tissue and lymph nodes. For tumors traversing the esophageal hiatus, a cuff of diaphragm is resected. In addition to a thorough mediastinal lymph node dissection extending from the tracheal bifurcation to the esophageal hiatus, an upper abdominal lymph node dissection incorporating lymph nodes along the portal vein, common hepatic artery, celiac trunk, left gastric artery, and splenic artery is included to achieve a two-field lymph node dissection.[251] A three-field lymph node dissection extends the lymphadenectomy to the superior mediastinum, including nodes along the course of the right and left recurrent laryngeal nerves, and, through a separate collar incision in the neck, completes the dissection with removal of the lower cervical nodes, including the deep external and lateral cervical lymph node basins.[96,97]

Most of the series that examine the utility of extended esophagectomies are retrospective and involve a single institution. Hagen et al.[91] reported on 100 consecutively treated patients who had undergone an en bloc esophagectomy with two-field lymphadenectomies; none of the patients received additional preoperative or postoperative chemotherapy or radiotherapy. The perioperative mortality was 6%, with the most common complications being pneumonia (19%), subphrenic abscess (13%), respiratory failure (9%), anastomotic leak (10%), and empyema (7%). Local recurrence was detected in only one patient and overall actuarial 5-year survival was 52%. Patients with stage III lesions had a 25% actuarial 5-year survival. Altorki et al.[92] reviewed the results for 128 patients who underwent an esophagectomy at a single institution; 61% received an en bloc esophagectomy and the remainder underwent a standard esophageal resection. Approximately 40% of those undergoing the more extended resection had a three-field lymphadenectomy; the others had a systematic two-field lymphadenectomy. The in-hospital mortality for the en bloc resection

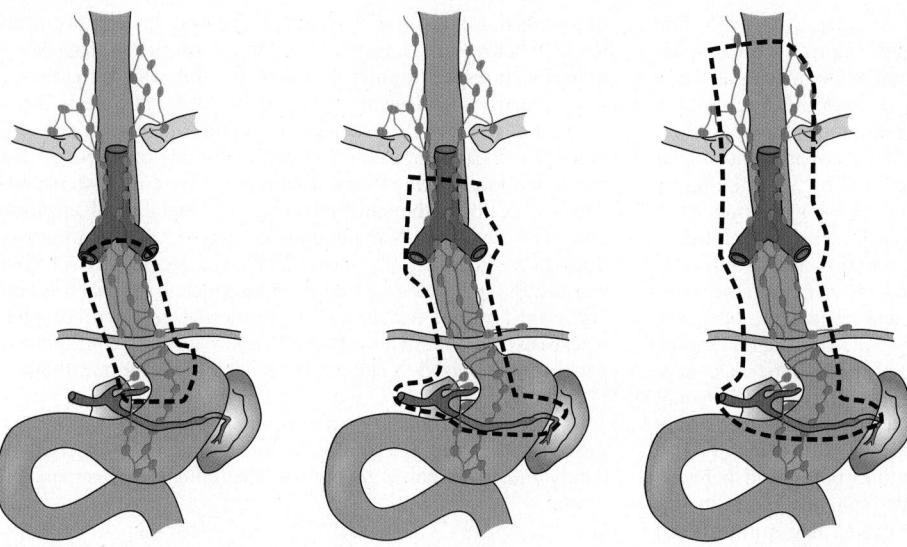

Figure 45.10 *Left to right:* Standard, two-field, and three-field lymphadenectomy.

group was 5.1%, similar to that for those undergoing a standard resection. The most common postoperative complications in the extended resection group were respiratory events (24%) and anastomotic leak (12.8%), but no significant differences were noted in comparison to the standard resection group. Four-year survival for the en bloc group was 41.5% overall and 34.5% for stage III patients, with both of these survival figures markedly better than those for the standard resection group. However, both of the studies described here are single-institution, retrospective analyses for which the results, at least in part, if not completely, can be attributed to selection bias and enhanced staging, leading to stage migration. It is interesting to note that similar results have been achieved without a thoracotomy using a transhiatal approach as described earlier in Transhiatal Esophagectomy.[224]

A group at Cornell University also separately examined 80 patients who underwent an esophagectomy with a three-field lymphadenectomy.[94] Overall 30-day mortality was 5%, with 31% of patients developing major postoperative complications, including the need for reintubation (16%), anastomotic leak (11%), and recurrent laryngeal nerve injury (9%). Overall 5-year survival was 51%. Cervical lymph node metastases were identified in 36% of patients, and the 5-year survival rate for those with positive cervical lymph nodes was 25%. Lerut et al.[252] reported on 174 patients, equally divided between squamous cell and adenocarcinoma histology, who underwent a three-field lymphadenectomy. Hospital mortality was only 1.2%, with an overall mortality of 58%. Five-year survival for stage III patients was 36.8%. Twenty-three percent of patients with adenocarcinoma and 25% of those with squamous cell carcinoma had positive cervical nodes. Five-year survival for patients with positive cervical lymph nodes was 27% and 12%, respectively, for squamous cell and adenocarcinoma histology. The authors suggest that a three-field lymphadenectomy may have a role in patients with squamous cell carcinoma, but this remains investigational for patients with adenocarcinoma. These results, although impressive, may also reflect both selection bias and stage migration. In addition, the expertise required to perform these technically demanding procedures effectively limits their application to specialized centers only and a fraction of the patients who might benefit from these procedures if an actual advantage were proven.

The Hulscher trial, discussed previously, which also employed an en bloc resection of the esophagus, compared to transhiatal esophagectomies, failed to improve outcome.[250] A small study by Nishihira et al.[253] of 62 patients showed an improved, but not statistically significant, survival advantage for extended lymphadenectomies (66.2% versus 48%; $p = 0.19$). Patients in this study were also randomly assigned to receive either chemoradiation or

chemotherapy alone after surgery, confounding the interpretation of the results.

The body of evidence confirms that extended resections improve staging and may enhance local–regional control; however, there are no reliable data confirming a survival benefit for these procedures.

Adjuvant Therapy

Preoperative Chemotherapy. Nearly three-fourths of patients newly diagnosed with esophageal cancer present with locally advanced (stage IIB or III) disease. The poor survival rate achieved with surgery alone, and given the patterns of both local and systemic disease recurrence, has provided the impetus for the evaluation of preoperative (induction) chemotherapy in patients with resectable esophageal cancer.

The benefits of induction chemotherapy include the potential downstaging of the disease to facilitate surgical resection, improvement in local control, relief of dysphagia in patients responding to induction chemotherapy, and the potential eradication of micrometastatic disease. An esophagectomy after induction therapy enables a comprehensive pathologic assessment of treatment response, which may be important in selecting patients for postoperative adjuvant therapy. The disadvantages of preoperative chemotherapy include the potential development of chemotherapy resistance and the delay in definitive treatment with the risk of further spread of the disease. These are important concerns because approximately 50% of patients do not respond to current chemotherapeutic regimens. Further compromise of the patient's already marginal nutritional status due to a delay in local disease control is also of concern when surgery is not the initial treatment.

Trials evaluating the use of induction chemotherapy followed by surgery for the treatment of esophageal cancer have been under way since the late 1970s. This strategy was evaluated in parallel with studies of concurrent chemoradiation followed by surgery or chemoradiation as definitive therapy. Early trials used cisplatin and bleomycin-based chemotherapy.[254–257] Use of cisplatin and 5-fluorouracil (5-FU)[258–262] led to the initiation of randomized trials in the 1980s. For lesions of squamous histology, the response rate to two or three cycles of cisplatin (100 mg/m² on day 1) and 5-FU (1,000 mg/m² per day for 96 or 120 hours) every 3 weeks ranged between 42% and 66%, with a 0% to 10% pathologically confirmed complete-response rate; curative resection rates were between 40% and 80%, and median survival was from 18 to 28 months.[258–262] Lesions were staged with a barium esophagogram and CT scan initially and then again before surgery to assess the response to induction therapy.

TABLE 45.6

Randomized Trials of Preoperative Chemotherapy

Study (Ref.)	Treatment	No. of Patients (n)	Histologic Type	Median Survival (months)	3- or 5-Year Survival (%)
Nygaard et al.[263]	Preop C/B	50	S		3 yr: 3
	Surgery	41			3 yr: 9
Roth et al.[264]	Preop C/VDS/B and adjuvant C/VDS	19	S	9	5 yr: 25
	Surgery	20		9	5 yr: 5
Schlag[265]	Preop C/5-FU	34	S	10	NS
	Surgery	41		10	NS
Boonstra et al.[269]	Preop C/etoposide	86	S	16	5 yr: 26
	Surgery	85		12	5 yr: 17
Kelsen et al. (Intergroup 0013)[105,112]	Preop C/5-FU and adjuvant C/5-FU	213	S/A	15	3 yr: 26
	Surgery	227		16	3 yr: 23
Allum et al.[106,113]	Preop C/5-FU	400	S/A	16.8	5 yr: 23
	Surgery	402	A	13.3	5 yr: 17
Cunningham et al.[266]	Preop/postop ECF	250	A	24	5 yr: 36
	Surgery	253	A	20	5 yr: 23
Ychou et al.[267]	Preop/postop CF	113	A	—	5 yr: 38
	Surgery	111	A	—	5 yr: 24
Schuhmacher et al.[268]	Preop CF	72	A	65	—
	Surgery	72	A	53	—

Preop, preoperative; C, cisplatin; B, bleomycin; VDS, vindesine; S, squamous cell carcinoma; A, adenocarcinoma; ECF, epirubicin/cisplatin; 5-FU, 5-fluorouracil; postop, postoperative.

Nine randomized trials evaluating the use of preoperative chemotherapy in esophageal cancer patients are summarized in Table 45.6.[105,106,263–269] Four of the trials enrolled only patients with squamous cell carcinoma,[263–265,267–269] whereas half to two-thirds of patients enrolled in the two more recent and largest trials (U.S. Intergroup and Medical Research Council) had adenocarcinoma of the esophagus, GEJ, or cardia.[105,106] Another large randomized trial treated mostly gastric cancer, although one-fourth of patients enrolled had adenocarcinoma of the distal esophagus or GEJ.[266] Two recent small European trials treated only adenocarcinoma of the esophagus and stomach with half or more of patients having esophageal or GEJ adenocarcinoma.[267,268]

No improvement in survival was noted in three small trials enrolling fewer than 100 patients each, with the small sample size making study interpretation difficult.[263–266] Boonstra et al.[269] reported a survival advantage for preoperative chemotherapy in the final report of a study initially published in abstract form back in 1997. This study, enrolling 171 patients with squamous cell carcinoma, differed from other trials by requiring a response assessment after two courses of preoperative chemotherapy. Patients showing no response underwent immediate surgery, whereas patients showing a response received two more courses of chemotherapy before surgery. The regimen consisted of cisplatin (80 mg/m² on day 1) and etoposide (100 mg/m² intravenously on days 1 to 2 and 200 mg/m² orally on days 3 to 5). Median overall survival in the surgery arm was 12 months compared to 16 months for surgery plus chemotherapy. Fewer patients went on to surgery after preoperative chemotherapy (89%) compared to patients undergoing immediate surgery (97%). Rates of R0 resection favored the chemotherapy arm, but the difference was nonsignificant ($p = 0.09$). Overall survival was superior with preoperative chemotherapy (hazard ratio [HR], 0.71; $p = 0.03$) with the 5-year survival for chemotherapy plus surgery 26% compared to 17% for surgery alone.

The U.S. Intergroup mounted a large, potentially definitive trial, INT-0113. A total of 467 patients with resectable esophageal cancer were randomly assigned to one of two treatment groups: (1) three cycles of cisplatin and 5-FU followed by surgery and then, for those patients whose resection was curative (R0), two additional cycles of cisplatin and 5-FU as adjuvant treatment; or (2) immediate surgery.[105] In contrast to other trials, a barium esophagogram was the only test required to assess clinical response to preoperative chemotherapy. Thus, it is not surprising that only a 19% response rate was reported. Survival and pattern of failure were the major study end points. No differences were observed between the surgery control group and the preoperative cisplatin and 5-FU group in terms of curative resection rate (59% versus 62%), treatment mortality (6% versus 7%), overall median survival (16.1 months versus 14.9 months), or 3-year survival (26% versus 23%) (Fig. 45.11). Furthermore, the median survival of patients who had a curative resection was the same in both treatment groups (27.4 months versus 25.0 months). The pattern of failure was also similar for the two treatment groups (local recurrence 31% versus 32%, and distant recurrence of 50% versus 41% in the surgery-alone group compared to those receiving induction chemotherapy followed by surgery, respectively). Tumor histologic type did not influence response to treatment. A recent update of the trial reported no late benefit for preoperative chemotherapy.[112] The importance of achieving an R0 resection in the updated analysis was emphasized, with these patients achieving long-term survival, whereas patients with an R1 resection treated only with surgery all died of recurrent disease. The only patients with R1 resection achieving long-term survival were those receiving protocol-permitted postoperative chemoradiotherapy: Among 34 patients treated with surgery alone with R1 resection, 18 received postoperative chemoradiotherapy and 9 (21%) achieved long-term survival. These results indicated that R1 resection patients may be salvaged with postoperative chemoradiotherapy.

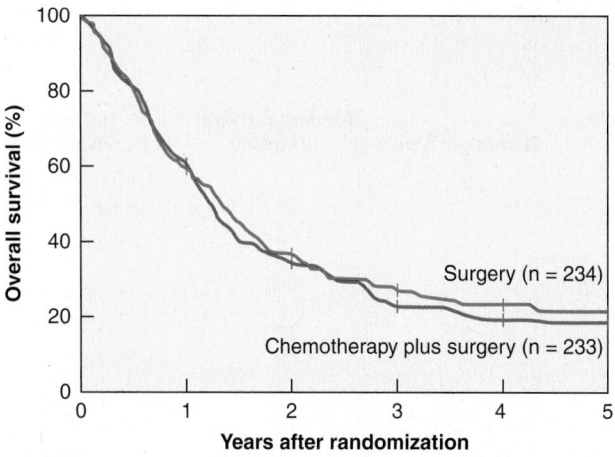

Figure 45.11 Overall survival US Intergroup trial INT-0113 comparing patients randomized to preoperative chemotherapy versus surgery alone.

Although no improvement in survival was demonstrated for preoperative chemotherapy on INT-0113, the trial importantly provides a contemporary surgical experience in the treatment of esophageal squamous carcinoma and adenocarcinoma. Important outcomes in this trial include a postoperative death rate well below 10%, the lack of difference in survival for lesions of different histologic types, and the fact that an R0 curative resection (regardless of treatment) conferred a median survival time of more than 2 years.

In contrast to the results of the 467-patient U.S. Intergroup trial, the Medical Research Council (MRC) Oesophageal Cancer Working Group demonstrated a statistically significant 9% improvement in 2-year survival rate (43% versus 34%) (Fig. 45.12) with preoperative cisplatin and 5-FU.[106] A total of 802 patients, 31% with squamous lesions and 69% with adenocarcinoma or lesions of undifferentiated histologic type, were enrolled. Patients were randomly assigned either to receive two courses of cisplatin (80 mg/m²) and 5-FU (1,000 mg/m² per day, continuous infusion for 4 days) 3 weeks apart followed by surgery or to undergo immediate surgery. The curative resection (R0) rate (60% versus 54%) and the percentage of randomly assigned patients undergoing surgery (92% versus 97%) were similar for the two treatment groups, although the improvement in curative resection rate did reach statistical significance. Patients receiving preoperative chemotherapy had improved median survival (16.8 months versus 13.3 months) and 2-year survival rate (43% versus 34%) (Fig. 45.12). Overall survival was significantly improved with preoperative chemotherapy

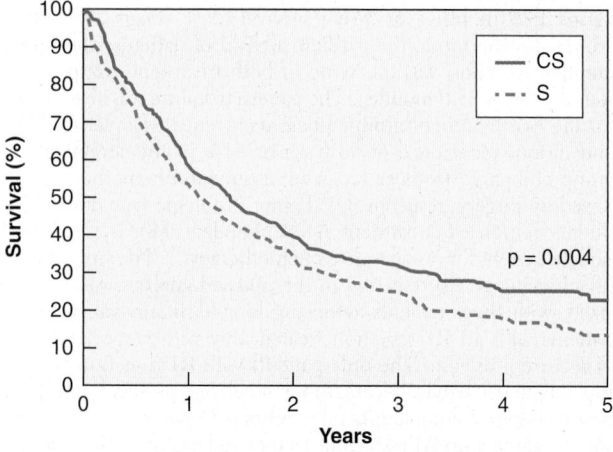

Figure 45.12 Overall survival Medical Research Council (MRC) Oesophageal Cancer Working Group trial comparing patients randomized to preoperative chemotherapy (CS) versus surgery alone (S).

($p = 0.004$; HR, 0.79; 95% CI, 0.67 to 0.93). The estimated reduction in risk of death was 21%. The postoperative mortality rate was 10% in both treatment groups. Pathologic complete responses were rare and were reported in 4% of patients undergoing preoperative chemotherapy. These authors recently reported an update of this trial at a median follow-up of 6 years.[113] Although a survival benefit was maintained in the preoperative chemotherapy arm, it had diminished to only 6% at 5 years (23.0% for preoperative therapy versus 17.1% for surgery; HR, 0.84; $p = 0.03$). There was no difference in pattern of failure—in particular, the development of distant metastatic disease—in the chemotherapy surgery versus surgery alone group, with the authors attributing the survival improvement with preoperative chemotherapy to the enhancement of rate of curative resection. The modest survival improvement with preoperative chemotherapy in this trial update is consistent with a 4.3% survival benefit observed in a recent meta-analysis of preoperative chemotherapy reported in abstract form, in which updated survival data from individual trials were obtained in over 2,000 patients in nine studies.[270]

There is no clear explanation for the discrepancy in survival outcome for the INT and MRC trials, whereas survival of the surgery control groups was essentially the same. The MRC study had the advantage of a larger sample size and greater power to observe a small difference. A greater proportion of patients who received chemotherapy underwent surgery in the MRC study, 92% compared with 80% in the INT trial. Although a microscopically complete resection (R0) was performed in similar proportions in the two trials, the MRC trial indicated a higher rate of R0 resection with preoperative chemotherapy compared to surgery alone. The duration of preoperative chemotherapy in the MRC trial was shorter and may have lessened the risk to patients of disease progression during induction therapy.

Positive results of another recent trial of perioperative chemotherapy in gastric and distal esophagus or GEJ cancer have been reported. In a trial by Cunningham et al.,[266] 503 patients were assigned to three cycles of preoperative and three cycles of postoperative epirubicin/cisplatin/5-FU or surgery alone. Preoperative chemotherapy resulted in significant improvement in patient survival, with a 6-month improvement in progression-free survival, a 4-month improvement in median survival, and a 13% improvement in 5-year overall survival (23% to 36%), all of which are statistically significant. Despite the survival improvement with pre- and postoperative chemotherapy, there was no improvement in the rate of curative resection in patients treated with preoperative chemotherapy compared with surgery alone (66% to 69%), and there were no cases of pathologic complete response to preoperative chemotherapy. Downstaging was also observed with preoperative chemotherapy, with a shift to earlier T and N stage tumors with preoperative chemotherapy compared to surgery alone. Because 26% of patients on this trial had tumors in the GEJ and lower esophagus, the results may apply to locally advanced esophageal cancer. The median follow-up was 47 months in the surgery-alone arm and 49 months in the chemotherapy arm.

Two recent studies from Europe also came to conflicting results for any benefit for preoperative chemotherapy. Ychou and colleagues[267] randomized 234 patients with esophageal, GEJ, or gastric adenocarcinoma to immediate surgery or to perioperative chemotherapy with cisplatin and fluorouracil. Rates of R0 resections were improved with preoperative chemotherapy to 84% compared to 74% for surgery alone ($p = 0.04$). At a median follow-up of 5.7 years, preoperative chemotherapy improved 5-year survival from 24% to 38%. On the other hand, Schuhmacher and colleagues[268] for the European Organisation for Research and Treatment of Cancer (EORTC) reported a negative trial of 144 patients with GEJ junction or gastric adenocarcinoma randomized to surgery alone or to two 48-day cycles of infusional fluorouracil and cisplatin.[268] In contrast to all earlier studies reported, this trial performed modern presurgical staging including endoscopic ultrasound, CT scan, and laparoscopic staging, and only endoscopic stage T3 to T4 tumors were eligible. The R0 resection was improved from 67% for surgery to 82% for preoperative chemotherapy ($p = 0.036$). At a median follow-up of 4.4 years, median survival was 65 months for the chemotherapy arm versus 63 months for surgery alone (HR, 0.84; $p = 0.466$) and 2-year overall survival was equivalent (70% for surgery alone, and 73% for the chemotherapy arm). Both arms had higher than expected median survival.

Despite the inconsistency of these outcomes, preoperative cisplatin and 5-FU is now the standard of care for resectable esophageal cancers—in particular, adenocarcinoma of the esophagus and GEJ—in the United Kingdom and in much of Europe, whereas this approach has not been generally accepted for esophageal cancer in the United States.

Preoperative Radiation Therapy. The high rate of local failure after esophagectomies engendered interest in the use of radiation therapy in conjunction with surgery. The incidence of local failure in the surgical control arms of randomized trials of preoperative radiation therapy reported by Mei et al.[271] and Gignoux et al.[272] was 12% and 67%, respectively. The local failure rate in the surgical control arm of the randomized trial of postoperative radiation therapy conducted by Teniere et al.[273] was 35% for patients with negative local–regional lymph nodes and 38% for patients with positive local–regional lymph nodes. The surgical control arm of INT-0113 provides a modern, more relevant baseline for the results of surgery alone. As discussed in Preoperative Chemotherapy, there was a 31% local failure rate in patients undergoing an R0 resection and a total local failure rate (including the additional 30% of patients with persistent disease) of 61%. Six randomized trials of preoperative radiation therapy for patients with clinically resectable disease have been reported.[263,271,272,274–276] Overall, preoperative radiation therapy did not increase the resectability rate, and only two series reported local failure rates. Although Mei et al.[271] reported no difference in local failure, Gignoux et al.[272] observed a significantly lower local failure rate in patients who received preoperative radiation therapy than in those treated with surgery alone (46% versus 67%, respectively).

Two trials have reported an improvement in survival. In the series of Nygaard et al.,[263] patients who received preoperative radiation therapy (with or without chemotherapy) had a significant improvement in overall 3-year survival (18% versus 5%; $p = 0.009$). The 48 patients who received preoperative radiation therapy without chemotherapy had a 20% 3-year survival rate; however, this did not reach statistical significance. This was not a pure radiation study, and the benefit may have been partly because of the chemotherapy. A similar improvement in survival was reported by Huang et al.[276] (46% versus 25%). A meta-analysis from the Oesophageal Cancer Collaborative Group also showed no clear evidence of a survival advantage with preoperative radiation therapy.[110]

Design flaws in these trials include the failure to use conventional doses of radiation therapy, the use of split-course radiation therapy, and failure to allow an adequate interval (4 to 8 weeks) between the completion of radiation therapy and surgery. The only study that allows an analysis of the effect of radiation fractionation is a randomized trial performed in France involving patients with squamous cell carcinomas who received chemoradiation using continuous-course versus split-course radiation.[277] The 95 patients who received a continuous-course regimen had a significantly higher local control rate (57% versus 29%) and 2-year event-free survival rate (33% versus 23%), and a borderline, significantly higher 2-year survival rate (37% versus 23%). Because it is less effective than continuous-course therapy, split-course radiation therapy is not recommended.

In summary, because only two of the six series have reported local failure rates, it is difficult to draw firm conclusions regarding the influence of preoperative radiation therapy on local control. Nonrandomized trials[278,279] also reported no survival benefit. Based on the available data from randomized trials, preoperative radiation therapy does not appear to significantly decrease local failure rate or improve survival in esophageal cancer patients.

Preoperative Chemoradiation. The rationale for trimodal therapy—chemoradiation followed by surgery—is based on the pattern of both local and distant failure associated with surgery alone or chemoradiation without surgery, which are the two treatment options established as standards of care based on data from randomized controlled trials. The results for patients randomly assigned to the surgery control arm of the INT-0113 trial revealed a 61% rate of failure in controlling local disease.[105] Similarly, the two Intergroup trials (RTOG-85-01 and INT-0123) that evaluated nonsurgical treatment (concurrent cisplatin and 5-FU, and radiotherapy), which are discussed in greater detail later in this chapter, showed unacceptably high rates of local failure (44% to 53%).[280,281] Most of the agents active against esophageal cancer (i.e., 5-FU, cisplatin, carboplatin, mitomycin C, paclitaxel, irinotecan, docetaxel, capecitabine, and oxaliplatin) are known to enhance radiosensitivity in cancer cells. Chemotherapy in conjunction with radiotherapy may both sensitize radiation therapy to improve local control as well as impact a reduction on systemic disease recurrence. Treatment with chemoradiation followed by an esophagectomy has the potential to: (1) downstage the disease, (2) increase the rate of complete resection with negative circumferential margins, and (3) eradicate occult micrometastatic disease.

Nonrandomized Trials. Most trials have used 5-FU and cisplatin-based chemotherapy combined with radiation therapy[111,282–301] although more recent trials incorporate paclitaxel, docetaxel, oxaliplatin, or irinotecan in two- or three-drug combination regimens.[101,302–314]

Since the initial trials by Leichman et al.[315] and the Southwest Oncology Group (SWOG-8037),[282] results of many phase II single-institution or multicenter trials of preoperative chemoradiation have been published.[316] Most trials used cisplatin (75 to 100 mg/m^2) and 5-FU (1,000 mg/m^2 per day continuous infusion for 4 or 5 days) with concurrent radiotherapy followed by surgery in 4 to 8 weeks. In most series, the pathologic complete-response rate (based on total number treated) was approximately 25%. The highest pathologic complete-response rates have been reported in trials treating mainly squamous cancers, and as more modern series predominantly treat adenocarcinoma, pathologic complete-response rates are consistently lower. Intensive chemoradiation regimens using hyperfractionated radiotherapy were evaluated by Forastiere et al.,[284,285] Raoul et al.,[295] and Adelstein et al.[292] Some of these regimens achieved higher pathologically determined complete-response rates and survival rates, usually with corresponding increases in acute toxicity. However, no clear advantage to altered fractionation schedules has been shown. The total dose of radiotherapy with concurrent chemotherapy varied from 30 Gy in earlier series up to 60 Gy, followed by surgery. Pathologic complete-response rates are uniformly in the 15% to 20% range with lower doses of radiation,[282,286,297,298] whereas total doses exceeding 50 Gy are associated with increased toxicity and perioperative complications.[296] Doses of 44 to 50 Gy using standard fractionation and concurrent therapy with cisplatin plus 5-FU generally result in pathologic complete-response rates of 25% to 40%[111,284, 286,287,290,292,295,299] and acceptable toxicity with postoperative mortality rates well below 10%. As will be discussed later, the CROSS randomized trial of preoperative chemoradiation used 41.4 Gy and achieved a significant survival benefit with neoadjuvant therapy.[317]

Most trials use conventional fractionation and doses of radiotherapy (45.0 to 50.4 Gy) with concurrent chemotherapy. In addition to overall outcome, some investigators have sought to determine whether preoperative endoscopy with biopsy can accurately assess response to treatment and whether achievement of pathologically confirmed complete response after chemoradiation improves overall survival. Bates et al.[287] reported a 65% 3-year survival rate in patients who achieved a pathologic confirmed complete response, compared with a 25% survival rate in those who did not. In 106 of 262 (41%) patients who achieved a pathologic complete response with preoperative chemoradiation, the 5-year survival was 52% compared with 38% in partial responders ($p < 0.001$) and 19% in nonresponders ($p < 0.001$).[301]

In other trials with long-term follow-up, investigators observed 5-year survival rates of 60% to 67% and 27% to 32% for those with pathologic complete response and those with residual disease after induction therapy, respectively.[111,284] In addition, the fact that long-term survival was observed in approximately 30% of patients with a residual tumor in the resected specimen suggests that surgery is an important component following chemoradiation.

At present, no methods short of surgical resection can accurately determine which patients will be found to have no residual tumor in the resected esophageal specimen after chemoradiation. Bates et al.[287] noted a 41% false-negative rate with preoperative endoscopy and biopsy. Sarkaria et al.[318] reported the correlation of postchemoradiotherapy endoscopy findings and surgical pathologic findings in 156 patients with esophageal cancer. Although 76% had a biopsy-negative endoscopy after preoperative therapy, only 31% of these patients were found to be pathologic complete responders at subsequent surgery. Chedella et al.[319] reported the results of 284 patients who received preoperative chemoradiation at M.D. Anderson Cancer Center, and at 5 to 6 weeks posttreatment, underwent restaging with endoscopy, biopsy, and PET-CT scan. The 24% of patients who achieved a pathologic complete response (pCR) had a higher median survival compared to those who did not achieve a pCR (95 versus 55 months).[319] Of note, only 31% of patients who achieved a clinical complete response were found to have a pCR.

Yang et al.[320] made similar observations about the accuracy of posttherapy biopsy. Jones et al.[321] reported that CT scans had a sensitivity of 65%, a specificity of 33%, a positive predictive value of 58%, and a negative predictive value of 41% in evaluating pathologic response after preoperative chemoradiation in esophageal cancer patients. Many studies show that EUS performed after chemoradiation is also a poor predictor of complete response because of the inability to distinguish postirradiation fibrosis and inflammation from residual tumor. Reported staging accuracy is below 50%.[323–324]

To further pursue the selective surgical approach as a treatment modality, it will be critical to establish the definition of an adequate response. However, the ability to predict a pCR prior to surgery is variable. A multivariate analysis by Gaca and colleagues[325] reported that posttreatment nodal status ($p = 0.03$), but not the degree of primary tumor response, predicted disease-free survival. Fields et al.[326] reviewed 714 patients treated at Memorial Sloan Kettering Cancer Center (MSKCC) and reported that there was a significant improvement in 5-year survival in the 60 patients who achieved a pCR compared with the 549 who did not (55% versus 35%; $p = 0.036$).[326]

The value of FDG-PET scans for restaging after chemoradiation remains to be established. Several studies of esophageal cancer patients show that an early decrease in FDG uptake after chemotherapy can predict clinical response.[156,327,328] In addition, multiple studies have evaluated the ability of FDG-PET scans to predict a pCR following chemoradiation.[328–332] Flamen et al.[328] evaluated the predictive value of PET scans after chemoradiation in patients receiving preoperative treatment. The sensitivity and positive predictive value of PET scans for identifying a pathologically determined complete response were 67% and 50%, respectively. Both false-positive PET findings (residual FDG activity in an area of intense inflammatory activity on histopathologic analysis) and false-negative findings occurred at the primary tumor site. Vallbohmer et al.[329] treated 119 patients with preoperative chemoradiation (cisplatin, 5-FU, and 36 Gy) and reported a nonsignificant association between major responders and FDG-PET results ($p = 0.056$). However, there was no clear standardized uptake value threshold that predicted a response.

Possible reasons for discrepant findings include the inflammatory effect of chemoradiation as well as a lack of standardization of FDG-PET protocols and techniques and definitions of a pathologic response.

Few studies have reported a long-term follow-up to determine actual survival rates at 5 years. Rates range from 25% reported by Bedenne et al.[297] for a series of 96 patients with squamous cell esophageal cancer to as high as 39% reported by Meredith et al.[301]

Taken together, data from nonrandomized trials accumulated during nearly 3 decades suggest an approximate 5% to 10% improvement in survival compared with historical surgery controls. However, substantially greater improvement in survival is seen in patients who are downstaged to pathologically confirmed complete response or minimal residual disease.

Patterns of failure after chemoradiation and resection are influenced by histologic type, with a greater likelihood of local recurrence for patients with squamous cell carcinoma of the esophagus and predominantly distant recurrence for those with adenocarcinoma of the distal esophagus, GEJ, and cardia. In a literature review of trials of preoperative chemoradiation published between 1980 and 2000, Geh et al.[316] found that the overall risk of relapse was 46%, but that the majority of relapses, 80%, were at distant sites; local–regional recurrence alone constituted only 9% of treatment failures. These cumulative data correspond with individual reports from other major centers[111,287,292,294] and suggest that preoperative chemoradiation followed by surgery leads to better local–regional control than does surgery alone or chemoradiation without surgery.

Newer regimens employing various combinations of 5-FU, cisplatin or oxaliplatin, taxanes, and irinotecan with radiotherapy report pathologic complete-response rates similar to those for previous cisplatin and 5-FU plus radiotherapy preoperative regimens, and rates of survival are also similar.

Meluch et al.[306] reported mature trial results for a combination of carboplatin, 5-FU, and paclitaxel plus concurrent radiotherapy. Among a total of 123 patients, the pathologic complete-response rate was 38%, and after a median follow-up of 45 months, the 3-year survival rate was 41%. Grade 3 or 4 leukopenia (73% of patients), esophagitis (43%), and hospitalization (57%) suggest that this regimen added toxicity without providing incremental improvement in survival. Toxicity on trials of paclitaxel and cisplatin on a once-weekly schedule, with conventional dose fractionation of radiation therapy, have reported lesser degrees of esophagitis.[303,308,333] McCurdy et al.[334] from the M.D. Anderson Cancer Center reported that the addition of taxanes to chemoradiation increased both the FDG-PET scan–determined pulmonary metabolic response and the radiation pneumonitis response compared with non–taxane-containing regimens. Weekly carboplatin combined with weekly paclitaxel and concurrent radiotherapy also appeared to have a favorable toxicity profile in a recent phase II trial treating 54 patients with adenocarcinoma and squamous cell carcinoma of the esophagus, and this regimen formed the basis of the recent Dutch CROSS Trial, which will be discussed.[310,317] The rate of pathologic complete response was 25%. Rates of grade 3 and 4 neutropenia (15%) and esophagitis (8%) were relatively low, but were in agreement with other trials employing a weekly paclitaxel and platinum drug chemotherapy regimen.

Swisher et al.,[308] Ajani et al.,[309] Bains et al.,[307] Ilson et al.,[101] and Rivera et al.[314] have published pilot experiences in the administration of induction chemotherapy before chemoradiotherapy and then surgery as a strategy to increase pathologically determined complete-response rate and to reduce distant failure. Some trials of induction chemotherapy have noted significant relief of patients' dysphagia and the rare need to place feeding tubes for nutritional support in patients.[101,307] The RTOG-0113 performed a phase II randomized trial comparing paclitaxel and 5-FU to paclitaxel and cisplatin plus radiation therapy.[312] Both arms were associated with significant toxicity, and the study did not meet its 1-year survival end point.

In summary, some of these newer regimens appear to be more toxic than cisplatin and 5-FU plus radiotherapy, whereas others suggest a potentially more favorable toxicity profile; the pathologic complete-response rates and survival estimates show no consistent benefit, but longer follow-up is needed. The interpretation of survival rates from these studies must be done cautiously, given the likelihood of stage migration due to the incorporation of EUS and PET scans into routine staging evaluation. Roof et al.[300] reported a single-institution experience of 177 patients treated with either cisplatin, 5-FU, or paclitaxel in combination with cisplatin, 5-FU, and radiation therapy as preoperative treatment in esophageal cancer. The 3-year overall survival was similar for the 5-FU/cisplatin–treated patients (39%) compared with those receiving paclitaxel in combination with 5-FU/cisplatin (42%). Pathologic complete-response rates were also comparable for two-drug (42%) compared with three-drug therapy (37%). In two sequential trials from Urba et al.[335,336] that evaluated two-drug paclitaxel cisplatin therapy plus radiation in one trial, and three-drug 5-FU, cisplatin, and paclitaxel plus radiation in another trial, there was also no difference in pathologic complete-response rates (17% to 19%). These rates of pathologic complete response were significantly lower than other trials reporting pathologic complete-response rates of 37% to 38% for three-drug therapy.[300]

The Eastern Cooperative Oncology Group (ECOG) reported response and survival[337] outcomes in a randomized phase II trial testing two of these combinations (E1201), limited to patients with resectable adenocarcinoma of the distal esophagus, GEJ, and cardia. The two preoperative treatments tested were (1) paclitaxel (50 mg/m^2, 1-hour infusion) followed by cisplatin (30 mg/m^2) on days 1, 8, 15, 22, 29, and concurrent radiotherapy (45 Gy); and (2) cisplatin (30 mg/m^2) followed by irinotecan (65 mg/m^2) on days 1, 8, 22, 29, and concurrent radiotherapy (45 Gy). Patients in each arm proceeded to esophagectomy followed by three cycles of adjuvant paclitaxel and cisplatin (arm 1) or cisplatin and irinotecan (arm 2). Staging with esophageal EUS was an eligibility requirement. A preliminary report indicated comparable rates of pathologic complete response for the two regimens of 15% to 16%,

with the lower than expected pathologic complete-response rate likely partly due to the exclusive treatment of adenocarcinoma on this trial.[338] The median survival on the paclitaxel arm was 20.9 months, and 34.9 months on the irinotecan arm (difference nonsignificant). Although the results are comparable to other modern phase II trials in esophageal adenocarcinoma, neither regimen appeared superior to more conventional 5-FU and cisplatin-based therapy.

Randomized Trials. Randomized trials comparing preoperative chemoradiation with surgery alone in patients with clinically resectable disease are listed in Table 45.7.[107,114,240,317,339–344] The series of Le Prise et al.[345] is not included because patients received sequential rather than concurrent chemotherapy and radiotherapy. Most trials combined cisplatin and 5-FU[339–341] or single-agent cisplatin[240] with concurrent radiotherapy.

The Bosset et al.[240] trial was limited to patients with stage I or II squamous cell carcinoma based on a previously defined CT scan staging system, whereas the trials of Urba et al.,[107] Burmeister et al.,[341] Tepper et al.,[342] and van Hagen et al.[317] treated adenocarcinoma and squamous cell carcinoma, and the trial of Walsh et al.[339,340] was designed for locally advanced, resectable adenocarcinoma. A significant difference in the median and 3-year survival rates was observed in the Walsh, Tepper, and Van Hagen et al. trials. It is noteworthy that the pathologically determined complete-response rate was consistent for all studies, 25% to 28%, with the exception of the Burmeister et al. trial, which indicated a statistically significant lower pathologic complete-response rate for adenocarcinoma (9%) compared to squamous cell carcinoma (27%). Van Hagen et al. reported a pathologic complete response rate of 24% for adenocarcinoma and 49% for squamous cell carcinoma. Comparable rates of 3-year survival for patients in each of the investigational treatment groups (30% to 40%) was also observed. Higher 5-year survival rates, however, were reported on the Tepper et al. trial (39%) and the Van Hagen et al. trial (47%).

Urba et al.[107] at the University of Michigan randomly assigned 100 patients (75 with adenocarcinoma, 25 with squamous cell

PRACTICE OF ONCOLOGY

TABLE 45.7

Results of Preoperative Chemoradiation for Esophageal Cancer: Randomized Trials

Study (Ref.)	No. of Patients (n)	Histology	Chemotherapy	RT (Gy)	R0 Resection (%)	Pathologic Complete Response (%)	Median Survival (months)	Overall Survival 3-, and 5-Year Overall Survival (%)
Bosset et al.[240]	282	S	C + RT + surgery	37	78	26	19	5 yr: 26
			Surgery		68		19	5 yr: 26
Walsh et al.[339]	113	A	CF + RT + surgery	40	NS	25	16	3 yr: 32
					NS	—	11	3 yr: 6
Urba et al.[107]	100	S/A	CF + RT + surgery	45	90	28	18	3 yr: 30
			Surgery		90	—	17	3 yr: 16
Burmeister et al.[341]	256	S/A	CF + RT + Surgery	35	80	9 (A) 27 (S)	22	NS
			Surgery	44	59	—	19	NS
Tepper et al.[342]	56	S/A	CF + RT + surgery	50.4	NS	40	54	5 yr: 39
			Surgery		NS	—	22	5 yr: 16
Van Hagen et al.[317]	366	S/A	CaP + RT + surgery	41.4	92	24 (A) 49 (S)	49	3 yr: 58 5 yr: 47
			Surgery		69	—	24	3 yr: 50 5 yr: 34
Lee et al.[343]	102	S	CF + RT + surgery		NS	49	28	3 yr: 46
			Surgery		NS	—	27	3 yr: 46

S, squamous cell carcinoma; C, cisplatin; RT, radiation therapy; A, adenocarcinoma; NS, not stated; Ca, carboplatin; P, paclitaxel.

carcinoma) to receive (1) preoperative cisplatin (20 mg/m^2 on days 1 to 5 and 17 to 21), vinblastine (1 mg/m^2 on days 1 to 4 and 17 to 20), 5-FU (300 mg/m^2 per 24 hours on days 1 to 21), and concurrent radiotherapy (1.5 Gy twice a day to 45 Gy), followed on day 42 by a transhiatal esophagectomy, or (2) immediate surgery. A survival analysis after a median follow-up of 8.2 years for surviving patients revealed a nonsignificant improvement favoring preoperative chemoradiation (3-year survival, 30% versus 16%; $p = 0.15$). A significant decrease in local–regional recurrence as a component of first failure was observed (19% recurrence rate for the combined treatment group versus 42% for the group undergoing immediate surgery; $p = 0.02$). However, there was no difference in the rates of distant metastases, 60% and 65%, respectively. Although overall survival rates were not significantly different, there was a 31% lower risk of death, after adjustment for other prognostic factors, for patients randomly assigned to receive trimodal therapy, which suggests a possible benefit and the need for a trial adequately powered to detect a smaller survival difference. Consistent with phase II trial data, patients who achieved a pathologically confirmed complete response had better survival outcomes, with a median survival time of 50 months and 3-year survival rate of 64%, compared to those with residual disease in the resected specimen, who had a median survival time of 12 months and a 3-year survival rate of 19%. The low statistical power of this trial may have failed to detect a potential modest survival benefit for chemoradiation compared to surgery alone.

In their series, Walsh et al.[339] reported a significant survival advantage for patients receiving preoperative chemoradiation. A total of 113 patients with adenocarcinoma of the esophagus, GEJ, and cardia were randomly assigned to receive (1) two cycles (weeks 1 and 6) of 5-FU (15 mg/kg per 24 hours on days 1 to 5), cisplatin (75 mg/m^2 on day 7), plus concurrent radiotherapy (2.67 Gy per day to 40 Gy) followed by esophagectomy; or (2) immediate surgery alone. Chemoradiation was well tolerated. The incidence of acute toxicity of grade 3 or higher was 15%. The operative mortality was 9% in the multimodality treatment arm compared with 4% in the surgery control arm. After a median follow-up of surviving patients of 18 months, a significant improvement in both median survival time (16 months versus 11 months; $p = 0.01$) and 3-year survival rate (32% versus 6%; $p = 0.01$) was observed in patients who received preoperative therapy compared with those treated with surgery alone. A major criticism of this trial was the low 3-year survival rate (6%) in the surgical control arm. This probably reflects a patient population with more advanced disease than in those enrolled in the other two trials. CT scan staging was not required. More than 80% of patients had lymph node metastases.[340]

A third randomized trial of preoperative chemoradiation was reported by Bosset et al.[240] of the EORTC. A total of 282 patients with clinically resectable (early stage I and II) squamous cell carcinoma were randomly assigned to undergo either preoperative chemoradiation or surgery alone. The preoperative regimen consisted of five daily fractions of 3.7 Gy each followed by a 2-week rest and another 3.7 Gy for 5 days. Chemotherapy was limited to cisplatin, 80 mg/m^2, 0 to 2 days before starting each 5 days of radiotherapy. Rates of curative resection were significantly higher in patients undergoing preoperative chemoradiation (81%) compared with immediate surgery (69%). After a median follow-up of 55 months, patients who received preoperative chemoradiation had a significantly better 3-year disease-free survival rate (40% versus 28%) and local disease-free survival (relative risk [RR], 0.6), yet had no improvement in median survival time (19 months) or overall 3-year survival (36%) compared with patients treated with surgery alone. However, this chemoradiation regimen was unconventional in design; not only was the radiation split course and delivered with unusually high doses per fraction, but the doses of chemotherapy would not be considered adequate for systemic therapy. The threefold higher postoperative mortality in the combined modality arm (12%) compared with the surgery-alone arm (4%) may have undercut any potential overall survival benefit for chemoradiation.

The trial reported by Burmeister et al.[341] treated 256 patients with adenocarcinoma and squamous cell carcinoma with either surgery alone, or preoperative cisplatin, 5-FU, and radiation followed by surgery. The combined modality arm received one cycle of 5-FU dosed at 800 mg/m^2 per day during a 4-day continuous infusion in combination with cisplatin 80 mg/m^2 on day 1, plus concurrent radiotherapy (2.33 Gy per day to 35 Gy) followed by esophagectomy. Chemoradiation was well tolerated, with the most common toxicities grade 3 or 4 esophagitis (16%) or nausea and vomiting (5%). There was no difference in surgical complications in either treatment group, with an overall operative mortality of 5%. After a median follow-up of 65 months, no significant difference was seen in either median overall survival time (22 months versus 19 months with surgery alone) or 3-year survival rate. The chemoradiation group had a higher rate or curative resection (80%) compared with the surgery-alone arm (59%). Pathologic complete responses were significantly less common in adenocarcinoma (9%) compared with squamous cell carcinoma (27%). A univariate analysis indicated that patients with squamous cell cancer had significantly better progression-free and overall survival when treated with preoperative chemoradiation. The low rate of pathologic complete responses in patients with adenocarcinoma on this trial raises concern about the adequacy of chemotherapy delivered (one cycle) during radiotherapy.

A similar trial was reported by Lee et al.[343] from Korea. A total of 102 patients with squamous cell cancer were randomized to surgery alone versus preoperative therapy with 45.6 Gy (1.2 Gy twice a day) plus 5-FU/cisplatin. There was no difference in median survival (28 months versus 27 months).

The sixth randomized trial by Tepper et al.[342] reported the results of an Intergroup trial led by the Cancer and Leukemia Group B (CALGB-9781), in which patients were randomly assigned to receive either (1) immediate surgery or (2) two cycles of cisplatin, 5-FU, and concurrent radiotherapy (total dose, 50.4 Gy) followed by surgery. This trial, activated in July 1998 and projected to enroll 475 patients, was terminated early because of failure to meet accrual targets. However, follow-up was available in 56 patients ultimately randomized and treated on protocol. With a median follow-up of 6 years, 5-year survival was significantly improved with the addition of preoperative chemoradiation (39% versus 16%; $p = 0.005$). Interpretation of this trial is confounded by the small number of patients treated.

The most contemporary trial recently reported by Van Hagen et al., the CROSS Trial,[317] has for many practitioners established a new standard or care for preoperative chemoradiotherapy. This study randomized 366 patients with squamous cell carcinoma or adenocarcinoma of the esophagus or GEJ to treatment with (1) preoperative carboplatin at an area under the curve of 2 mg/mL per minute and paclitaxel 50 mg/m^2 once weekly for 5 weeks, and concurrent radiotherapy (1.8 Gy daily to 41.4 Gy in 23 fractions, followed by transthoracic esophagectomy or transhiatal esophagectomy for GEJ cancers, or (2) immediate surgery. Unlike earlier trials, this more modern trial staged all patients by endoscopic ultrasound and CT scan, and patients were required to have either node-positive or T2-3Nany disease. The majority of patients treated had adenocarcinoma (75%), and most tumors involved the distal third of the esophagus (58%). The majority of patients were node positive (65%), and slightly more patients on the chemoradiotherapy arm had T3 tumors (84%) compared to the surgery-alone arm (78%). At a median follow-up of 45 months, the trial showed a significant survival benefit (Fig 45.13) for chemoradiotherapy added to surgery, with a median survival increased from 24 to 49 months (HR, 0.0657; $p = 0.003$), and improvement in 2- and 5-year overall survival (67% and 47% versus 50% and 34%; HR, 0.665). The rate of R0 resection was significantly improved on the chemoradiotherapy arm (95% compared

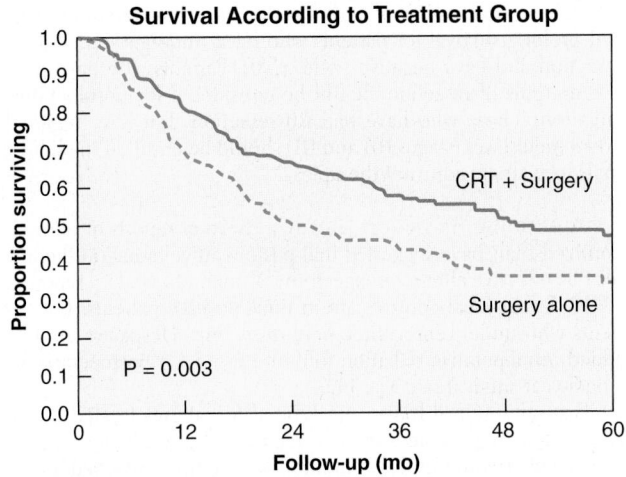

Survival According to Treatment Group

Figure 45.13 Overall survival CROSS trial comparing patients randomized to preoperative chemoradiotherapy (CRT + surgery) versus surgery alone.

to 69%; $p < 0.001$). Pathologic complete responses were seen in 24% of adenocarcinomas and 49% of squamous cancers. Survival benefits were significant for both histologies, but with an even greater benefit for squamous cancers (HR, 0.453) compared to adenocarcinomas (HR, 0.741). Therapy was well tolerated with grade 3 or 4 hematologic toxicity seen in 7% patients, and grade 3 or 4 nonhematologic toxicity seen in less than 13%. There was no difference in either operative morbidity or mortality, and mortality was below 4% in each arm, which is considered consistent and appropriate with modern day surgical outcomes in high-volume centers. Many investigators feel that this well-conducted chemoradiotherapy trial using a well-tolerated, relatively easy to administer therapeutic regimen established a new standard of care for squamous cell carcinomas and adenocarcinomas of the distal esophagus or GEJ.

Some additional insight may be obtained from a small trial reported by Stahl et al.,[344] a multicenter phase III trial directly comparing preoperative chemotherapy to combined chemoradiotherapy followed by surgery in patients with GEJ adenocarcinoma. The trial did not meet accrual goals and randomized only 119 eligible patients with Siewert I to III GEJ adenocarcinoma. The strength of the trial was the rigorous pretherapy staging, including EUS and laparoscopy, and the balance in treatment arms by clinical stage. Patients were assigned to (1) 2.5 cycles of a 6-week schedule of weekly 5-FU 2 g/m², 24-hour infusion and leucovorin 500 mg/m², 2-hour infusion plus biweekly cisplatin 50 mg/m², or (2) two cycles of the same regimen, followed by 3 weeks of radiotherapy given in 15 fractions at a dose of 2 Gy combined with cisplatin 50 mg/m² on day 1 and 8 and etoposide 80 mg/m² on days 3 to 5. The primary end point was 3-year overall survival. Comparable numbers of patients had an R0 resection after chemotherapy (69.5%) compared to chemoradiotherapy (72%). More patients on the chemoradiotherapy arm achieved a pathologic complete response (15.6%) compared to the chemotherapy arm (2.0%), and more patients were node negative (64.4% compared to 36.7%, respectively). Three-year survival trended superior in the chemoradiotherapy group (47.4%) compared to the chemotherapy group (27.7%; $p = 0.07$), and freedom from local tumor progression also favored the chemoradiotherapy group (76.5% versus 59%; $p = 0.06$). More in-hospital deaths occurred in the chemoradiotherapy arm (10.2% versus 3.8%; not statistically significant). The authors concluded that preoperative chemoradiotherapy could be considered a standard of care based on the favorable comparison to preoperative chemotherapy alone.

The accumulated experience from phase II and III trials indicates the following concerning chemoradiation using cisplatin and infusional 5-FU–based therapy followed by an esophagectomy:

- In approximately two-thirds of patients, the disease is downstaged.
- A survival advantage exists for patients experiencing downstaging to pathologically confirmed complete response or minimal residual disease status.
- Surgery appears to be an important component of treatment to eliminate persistent disease after chemoradiation, especially for adenocarcinoma. Of this group, 20% to 30% will be long-term survivors. The higher rates of pathologic complete response for squamous cancers make an argument for primary chemoradiotherapy without surgery, and this issue will be reviewed in the Radiation Therapy section.
- Local–regional control is improved, whereas distant failure is frequent and is the major cause of death.
- Rates of curative resection may be improved with preoperative chemoradiation.

Controversy continues about the optimal management of adenocarcinoma of the distal esophagus or GEJ, in particular the relative merits of preoperative chemotherapy versus combined chemoradiotherapy followed by surgery. Two ongoing randomized trials may shed light on this debate once completed. One trial, the CRITICS trial being run in the Netherlands and Sweden (NCT00407186), assigns patients with adenocarcinoma of the distal esophagus, GEJ, and stomach to all receive pre- and postoperative chemotherapy in addition to surgery; patients are randomized postoperatively to continue to receive either chemotherapy alone, or to chemotherapy combined with postoperative radiotherapy. Another trial, TOPGEAR (NCT01924819), being run by the Australasian Gasto-Intestinal Trials Group (AGITG) will treat patients with esophageal, GEJ, or gastric cancers with perioperative chemotherapy, with patients randomized to receive combined radiation therapy with preoperative chemotherapy or to preoperative chemotherapy alone.

Meta-analyses lend support to the inclusion of chemotherapy and radiation therapy as part of surgical management. Two studies evaluated in a combined analysis randomized trials predominantly of preoperative chemotherapy[346] and preoperative chemotherapy and radiation therapy compared to surgery alone.[347] These studies pooled the results of 11 to 25 randomized trials treating between 2,300 and nearly 4,200 patients. Preoperative chemotherapy improved 2-year survival by 5.1% to 6.3% for preoperative chemotherapy alone, and preoperative combined chemoradiation improved 2-year survival by 8.7%. Because of the toxicity and ongoing controversy about the benefit associated with preoperative combined chemoradiation, the priority should be given to enrolling patients in clinical trials.

Targeted Agents

Limited studies have evaluated the combination of a targeted agent with either definitive, nonoperative chemoradiotherapy, or preoperative chemoradiotherapy. Two pilot trials combining the vascular endothelial growth factor (VEGF) ligand-targeted agent, bevacizumab, added to chemoradiotherapy failed to improve outcome compared to historical controls.[313,348] The EGFR-targeted agent cetuximab was combined with definitive chemoradiotherapy in two recently reported trials. First is the SCOPE-1 trial where 258 patients with stages I through III cancer (25% adenocarcinoma) were randomized to 50 Gy/capecitabine/cisplatin ± cetuximab without planned surgery.[349] The trial was stopped early since it met its futility rules. Patient who received cetuximab had inferior 2-year survival (41% versus 56%) and higher nonheme grade 3+ acute toxicity (79% versus 63%). The second is the recently completed RTOG 0436 trial in which patients with nonoperable esophageal cancer were randomized to 50.4

Gy/paclitaxel ± cetuximab, reported only in abstract form.[350] On this nonoperative trial, of the 328 patients, the majority had adenocarcinoma. There was no difference in outcome with the addition of cetuximab to chemoradiotherapy, with no increase in rates on endoscopic clinical complete response, and no differences in overall survival and no impact on either adenocarcinoma of squamous cell carcinoma histology. These negative results add to the accumulating literature, also discussed in the section on metastatic disease, that currently available EGFR-targeted therapies are ineffective in esophageal cancer. A phase I/II trial combining the HER2-targeted agent trastuzumab with chemoradiotherapy[351] in esophageal cancer led to a randomized phase III trial in esophageal adenocarcinoma being conducted by RTOG (NCT01196390). Patients with esophageal or GEJ adenocarcinoma whose tumors test HER2 positive are randomized to chemoradiotherapy with weekly carboplatin AUCS 2 and paclitaxel 50 mg/m^2 for six doses combined with 50.4 Gy of radiotherapy followed by surgery, with or without the addition of trastuzumab during chemoradiotherapy and as a surgical adjuvant therapy for 1 year after surgery. As will be reviewed in the section covering advanced disease, with the exception of trastuzumab, suitable targets as well as active targeted agents remain to be established in the combined modality treatment of esophageal cancer.

Postoperative Chemotherapy. Administering chemotherapy after surgery to patients who have already received chemotherapy or chemoradiation preoperatively has not been easily achieved in phase II[257,258,299] and phase III trials.[105,264] This is exemplified by the INT-0113 trial, in which only 38% of patients who were candidates for adjuvant cisplatin and 5-FU therapy received the two planned courses.[105]

In Japan, surgery includes the removal of the primary lesion plus extended dissection of lymph nodes in the mediastinum, neck, and abdomen. The Japanese Oncology Group has evaluated postoperative chemotherapy in a series of randomized trials.[352–355] One study of 205 patients who had undergone resection compared observation with two courses of adjuvant cisplatin and vindesine.[354] Median follow-up was 59 months, and the 5-year survival rate was 45% in the control arm and 48% in the adjuvant treatment arm, which indicated no survival benefit from this chemotherapy regimen.

A second trial of adjuvant chemotherapy in 242 patients had the same study design, except that the chemotherapy was cisplatin and 5-FU administered for two courses after curative resection.[353,355] At a median follow-up of 40.4 months, no differences were observed in the 5-year survival estimates (51% versus 61% for adjuvant chemotherapy; $p = 0.3$). The estimated 5-year disease-free survival rate was improved with chemotherapy (58% for the chemotherapy versus 46% for observation; $p = 0.05$). Disease-free survival for node-negative patients was 77% in the surgery-alone group versus 82% in the adjuvant treatment group ($p = 0.3$), and for node-positive patients 35% in the surgery-alone group versus 53% in the adjuvant treatment group ($p = 0.06$). These data suggest that adjuvant chemotherapy may benefit node-positive patients, but this was an unplanned subset analysis on this trial. The ECOG completed a phase II trial (E8296) to evaluate adjuvant therapy consisting of cisplatin (75 mg/m^2) and paclitaxel (175 mg/m^2 during 3 hours) every 3 weeks for four courses in 55 patients with completely resected, T3, or node-positive adenocarcinoma of the esophagus, GEJ, or cardia.[356] The majority (89%) had lymph node involvement. The majority of these (84%) were able to complete all four cycles of chemotherapy. The 2-year survival rate was 60%, which compared favorably with results for contemporary historical controls.[105]

In summary, the available data for postoperative adjuvant chemotherapy suggest a possible prolongation of survival for patients who have had a potentially curative (R0) resection and have lymph node–positive (N1) disease. There are no data to indicate or suggest that the administration of postoperative adjuvant chemotherapy will prolong survival for patients who have undergone a curative resection and have negative nodes (N0). Patients who have positive margins of resection should be considered for postoperative radiation. Those who have had R0 resections but have regional nodal metastases (stages IIB and III) should be enrolled in clinical trials to evaluate adjuvant therapies.

Postoperative Radiation Therapy. Several reports of nonrandomized trials have suggested that postoperative radiation therapy may be effective after esophagectomy. Yamamoto et al.[357] reported a 94% 2-year local control rate in node-positive patients. For patients who underwent a three-field dissection, Hosokawa et al.[358] added intraoperative radiation followed by 45 Gy postoperatively. The 5-year survival rate was 34%.

Two randomized trials were limited to patients treated in the adjuvant setting. Teniere et al.[273] reported the results for 221 patients with squamous cell carcinoma randomly assigned to receive either surgery alone or postoperative radiation therapy (45 to 55 Gy at 1.8 Gy per fraction). Postoperative radiation therapy was found to have no significant impact on survival. In the series of Fok et al.,[359] patients with both squamous cell carcinomas and adenocarcinomas receiving either curative or palliative resections were evaluated; although the total dose of radiation therapy was conventional, the dose per fraction (3.5 Gy) was unconventional. No significant decrease in local failure or distant failure or improvement in the median survival time was achieved with the addition of postoperative radiation therapy.

Postoperative Chemoradiation. The only randomized trial of postoperative chemoradiation is the Intergroup trial INT-0116.[360] Although the goal of this trial was to examine the role of postoperative adjuvant chemoradiation in gastric cancer, 20% of patients had adenocarcinoma of the GEJ. Eligible patients included those with stage IB, II, IIIA, IIIB, or IV nonmetastatic adenocarcinoma of the stomach or GEJ after curative resection. Patients were randomly assigned to receive either observation alone or postoperative chemoradiation consisting of four monthly cycles of bolus 5-FU and leucovorin plus 45 Gy concurrent radiation with cycle two. A total of 603 patients were registered. Pretreatment characteristics were similar in both arms, and most patients had locally advanced disease. Approximately two-thirds of the patients had pT3 or pT4 tumors and approximately 85% had positive local–regional nodes.

Patients randomly assigned to receive postoperative chemoradiation had a significant decrease in local failure as the first site of failure (19% versus 29%) and an increase in median survival (36 months versus 27 months), 3-year relapse-free survival (48% versus 31%), and overall survival (50% versus 41%; $p = 0.005$). Although 17% of patients could not complete all therapy as planned, there was only one treatment-related death. With a median follow-up of 10 years, the improvement in survival with postoperative chemoradiation remains statistically significant.[360] An analysis of the impact of HER2 status in the INT-0116 trial revealed that HER2-negative patients had a survival benefit from chemoradiation whereas patients who underwent surgery only did not.[361]

The other role for postoperative radiation therapy is in cases of positive surgical margins. Based on the RTOG-85-01 trial, patients selected for treatment with postoperative radiation should receive chemoradiation.[280,362,363]

Definitive Chemoradiation

Although definitive chemoradiation is a treatment option for patients with localized resectable esophageal carcinoma, especially those with cervical esophageal squamous cell carcinoma or those not considered ideal resection candidates, this therapeutic approach is discussed in detail in Chemoradiation in the next section.

Treatment of Locally Advanced Disease

Radiation Therapy

The 1996 to 1999 patterns of care study examined 414 patients who received radiation therapy as part of definitive or adjuvant management at 59 institutions.[364] Overall, 51% had adenocarcinoma and 49% had squamous cell carcinoma. With a median follow-up of 8 months, a multivariate analysis revealed that patients who received chemoradiation followed by surgery had a significant decrease in local–regional recurrence (HR, 0.40; p <0.0001) and survival (HR, 0.32; p = 0.001) compared with those who did not undergo surgery. A similar significant decrease in local–regional recurrence (HR, 1.36; p = 0.01) and survival (HR, 1.32; p <0.03) was seen in those patients who received their care at large radiation oncology centers (treating 500 or more new cancer patients per year) compared with small centers (treating fewer than 500 new cancer patients per year). In a similar patterns of care study of 767 patients treated in Japan from 1998 to 2001, 220 (29%) received preoperative or postoperative radiation, or both, with or without chemotherapy.[365]

The effect of histologic type (adenocarcinoma versus squamous cell carcinoma) is unclear. Most series suggest that squamous cell cancers have a higher response rate compared with adenocarcinomas; however, no clear difference in outcome was found. The National Cancer Institute Intergroup has randomized trials that stratify patients by lesion histologic type. Until these data are available, the impact of histologic type cannot be adequately assessed, and it is reasonable to treat both types of lesions in a similar fashion.

Primary Nonsurgical Therapy. Primary therapy for esophageal cancer is either surgical or nonsurgical. The patient population selected for treatment with each modality is usually different. For several reasons, this results in a selection bias against nonsurgical therapy. Patients with unfavorable prognostic features are more commonly selected for treatment with nonsurgical therapy. These features include medical contraindications and primary unresectable or actual metastatic disease. Surgical series report results based on pathologic stage, whereas nonsurgical series report results based on clinical stage. Pathologic staging has the advantage of excluding some patients with metastatic disease not identified during clinical staging. Because some patients treated without surgery are approached in a palliative rather than a curative fashion, the intensity of chemotherapy and the doses and techniques of radiation therapy used may be suboptimal.

The difficulty of accurately staging esophageal cancer preoperatively is discussed in Diagnostic Studies and Pretreatment Staging, earlier in this chapter. The efficacy of FDG-PET scans as a complement to CT scans and EUS must be emphasized. Undetected metastatic disease was identified by PET scans in 15% of patients in the series by Flamen et al.[328] and in 20% of patients in the series by Downey et al.[327]

Radiation Therapy Alone. Many series have reported results of external-beam radiation therapy alone. Most include patients with unfavorable features such as clinical T4 disease and multiple positive lymph nodes. For example, in the series of De-Ren,[366] 184 of the 678 patients had stage IV disease. Overall, the 5-year survival rate for patients treated with conventional doses of radiation therapy alone is 0% to 10%.[362,366,367] The use of radiation therapy as a potentially curative modality requires doses of at least 50 Gy at 1.8 to 2.0 Gy per fraction. Shi et al.[368] reported a 33% 5-year survival rate with the use of late-course accelerated fractionation to a total dose of 68.4 Gy. However, in the radiation-therapy–alone arm of the RTOG-85-01 trial in which patients received 64 Gy at 2 Gy per day with modern techniques, all patients were dead of their disease by 3 years.[280,363]

Collectively, these data indicate that radiation therapy alone should be reserved for palliation or for patients who are medically unable to receive chemotherapy. As is discussed in the following section, the results of chemoradiation are more favorable, and it remains the standard of care.

Definitive Chemoradiation

Conventional Approaches

Comparison of Definitive Chemoradiation and Surgery. There are many single-arm, nonrandomized trials of chemoradiation alone, and they have included patients with disease at a variety of stages.[335–338] Few series examine patients with T1 or T2 disease.[369,370] In the series reported by Coia et al.,[369] patients received 5-FU and mitomycin C concurrently with 60 Gy of radiation therapy. When results for clinical stage I and II disease are combined, the local failure rate was 25%, the 5-year actuarial local relapse-free survival was 70%, and the 5-year actuarial survival was 30%.

Six randomized trials compared radiation therapy alone with chemoradiation.[114,263,280,371–375] Of these six trials, five used suboptimal doses of radiation and three used inadequate doses of systemic chemotherapy, and some studies used sequential chemotherapy and radiotherapy rather than concurrent therapy. For example, in the series of Araujo et al.,[375] patients received only one cycle of 5-FU, mitomycin C, and bleomycin. The EORTC trial used subcutaneous methotrexate.[371] In the Scandinavian trial reported by Nygaard et al.,[263] patients received low doses of chemotherapy (cisplatin, 20 mg/m^2, and bleomycin, 10 mg/m^2, for a maximum of two cycles). An analysis of pooled data from these trials reported a significant local control and survival benefit at 1 year for chemoradiation compared with radiation therapy alone.[376] Chemoradiation was associated with a significant increase in adverse effects, including life-threatening toxicities.

In the ECOG EST-1282 trial,[374] patients who received chemoradiation had a significantly increased median survival compared with those who received radiation alone (15 months versus 9 months; p = 0.04) but experienced no improvement in 5-year survival (9% versus 7%). However, this was not a pure nonsurgical trial because approximately 50% of patients in each arm underwent surgery after receiving 40 Gy of radiation. Furthermore, this decision depended on the individual investigator's preference. The operative mortality was 17%. Finally, the Pretoria trial reported by Slabber et al.,[373] which was limited to a total of 70 patients with T3 squamous cell cancers, used a low-dose (40 Gy) split-course radiation schedule.

The only trial that was designed to deliver adequate doses of systemic chemotherapy with concurrent radiation therapy was the RTOG-85-01 trial reported by Herskovic et al.,[280] and updated by Al-Sarraf et al.[372] This Intergroup trial primarily included patients with squamous cell carcinoma. Patients received four cycles of 5-FU (1,000 mg/m^2 per 24 hour × 4 days) and cisplatin (75 mg/m^2 on day 1). Radiation therapy (50 Gy at 2 Gy per day) was given concurrently with day 1 of chemotherapy. Curiously, cycles three and four of chemotherapy were delivered every 3 weeks (weeks 8 and 11) rather than every 4 weeks (weeks 9 and 13). This intensification may explain, in part, why only 50% of the patients finished all four cycles of the chemotherapy. The control arm was given radiation therapy alone, albeit at a higher dose (64 Gy) than the chemoradiation arm.

Patients who received chemoradiation had a significant improvement in median survival (14 months versus 9 months) and 5-year survival (27% versus 0%; p <0.0001).[344] There was a clear plateau in the survival curve. Minimum follow-up was 5 years, and the 8-year survival was 22%.[114,375] The histologic type did not significantly influence the results: 21% of patients with squamous cell carcinomas (n = 107) were alive at 5 years compared with 13% of patients with adenocarcinoma (n = 23) (p was not significant). Although African Americans had larger primary tumors, all of which were squamous cell cancers, there was no difference in their survival compared with that of Caucasians.[377] The incidence of local failure as the first site of failure (defined as local persistence or recurrence) was also decreased in the chemoradiation arm (47% versus 65%). The protocol was closed early because of the positive results; however, after this early closure, an additional 69 eligible patients were treated with the same chemoradiation regimen. In this nonrandomized combined modality group, the 5-year survival was 14% and local failure was 52%.

Chemoradiation not only improves the results compared with radiation alone but also is associated with a higher incidence of toxicity. In the 1997 report of the RTOG-85-01 trial, patients who received chemoradiation had a higher incidence of acute grade 3 toxicity (44% versus 25%) and acute grade 4 toxicity (20% versus 3%) compared with those who received radiation therapy alone. Including the one treatment-related death (2%), the incidence of total acute grade 3+ toxicity was 66%.[372] The 1999 report examined late toxicity. The incidence of late grade 3+ toxicity was similar in the chemoradiation arm and in the radiation-alone arm (29% versus 23%).[114] However, grade 4+ toxicity remained higher in the combined modality arm (10% versus 2%). Interestingly, the nonrandomized chemoradiation group experienced a similar incidence of late grade 3+ toxicity (28%) but a lower incidence of grade 4 toxicity (4%), and there were no treatment-related deaths.

Based on the positive results from the RTOG-85-01 trial, the conventional nonsurgical treatment for esophageal carcinoma is chemoradiation. Notwithstanding, the local failure rate in the RTOG-85-01 chemoradiation arm was 45%, and there is room for improvement. Therefore, new approaches, such as intensification of chemoradiation and escalation of the radiation dose, have been developed in an attempt to help improve these results.

Randomized Trials. Although there are a number of trials comparing preoperative chemoradiation with surgery alone, there are only two trials that directly compare nonoperative treatment with surgery. One randomized trial compared surgery with radiation alone[378] and one compared surgery with chemoradiation.[379] Both series have small numbers of patients, limited follow-up, and neither report a difference in survival.

Nonrandomized Trials. The positive results of RTOG-85-01, demonstrating a 27% 5-year survival rate for patients treated with definitive chemoradiation compared with no 5-year survival after treatment with radiotherapy alone, is a major advance. This treatment option has influenced the selection of patients for nonsurgical management because it provides an alternative for restoring swallowing function in patients with locally advanced disease for whom resection would likely be palliative.

For patients with earlier-stage disease that appears resectable, definitive chemoradiation may also be appropriate treatment; however, prospective trials comparing this approach with surgery, stratified by stage, have not been performed. Nonetheless, nonrandomized comparisons of contemporary series suggest that the nonsurgical approach offers a survival rate that is the same or better than that achievable with surgery alone. For example, the median survival time and 5-year survival rate were 14 months and 27%, respectively, in the chemoradiation arm of RTOG-85-01, and 20 months and 20%, respectively, in INT-0122.[380] In comparison, the median survival in the surgical control arm of the Dutch trial reported by Kok et al.[269] was 11 months, and the median survival time and 5-year survival rate in the surgical control arm of INT-0113 were 16 months and 20%, respectively. Likewise, the local failure rates were similar. The incidence of local failure (local recurrence plus local persistence of disease) as the first site of failure was 45% in RTOG-85-01 and 39% in INT-0122. If all patients, including patients failing to undergo surgery or patients having an R2 resection are included, the local failure as the first site of failure was 61% on the surgical trial INT-0113, which is actually higher than the 45% reported on RTOG-85-01. The treatment-related mortality rates were also similar (2% in RTOG-85-01, 9% in INT-0122, and 6% in INT-0113).

In summary, the local failure, survival, and treatment-related mortality rates for nonsurgical and surgical therapies are similar. Although the results are comparable, it is clear that both the nonsurgical and surgical approaches have limited success.

Necessity for Surgery After Chemoradiation. Two randomized trials examine whether surgery is necessary after chemoradiation. In the Fédération Francaise de Cancérologie Digestive (FFCD) 9102 trial, 444 patients with clinically resectable T3-4N0-1M0 squamous cell or adenocarcinoma of the esophagus received initial chemoradiation.[116] Patients initially received two cycles of 5-FU, cisplatin, and concurrent radiation (either 46 Gy at 2 Gy per day or split course 15 Gy weeks 1 and 3). The 259 patients who had at least a partial response were then randomized to surgery versus additional chemoradiation, which included three cycles of 5-FU, cisplatin, and concurrent radiation (either 20 Gy at 2 Gy per day or split course 15 Gy). Two-year local control was 66% in the surgery arm versus 57% in the chemoradiation-alone arm. There was no significant difference in 2-year survival (34% versus 40%; $p = 0.44$) or median survival (17.7 months versus 19.3 months) in patients who underwent surgery versus additional chemoradiation. These data suggest that patients who initially respond to chemoradiation should complete chemoradiation rather than stop and undergo surgery. Using the Spitzer index, there was no difference in global quality of life; however, a significantly greater decrease in quality of life was observed in the surgery arm during the postoperative period (7.52 versus 8.45; $p < 0.01$, respectively).[381] A separate analysis revealed that compared with split course radiation, patients who received standard course radiation had improved 2-year local relapse-free survival rates (77% versus 57%; $p = 0.002$) but no significant difference in overall survival (37% versus 31%).[382]

The German Oesophageal Cancer Study Group compared preoperative chemoradiation followed by surgery versus chemoradiation alone.[117] In this trial, 172 eligible patients age 70 years or more with uT3-4N0-1M0 squamous cell cancers of the esophagus were randomized to preoperative therapy (three cycles of 5-FU, leucovorin, etoposide, and cisplatin, followed by concurrent etoposide, cisplatin, plus 40 Gy) followed by surgery versus chemoradiation alone (the same chemotherapy but the radiation dose was increased to 60 to 65 Gy with or without brachytherapy). The pathologic complete response (pCR) rate was 33%. Despite a decrease in 2-year local failure (36% versus 58%; $p = 0.003$), there was no significant difference in 3-year survival (31% versus 24%) for those who were randomized to preoperative chemoradiation followed by surgery versus chemoradiation alone.

The current standard of care is to perform esophagectomy following chemoradiation in patients that can tolerate this approach. However, it is known that a subset of patients will have a complete response to chemoradiation. Further, patients with pCR have improved survival. Data from both Berger et al.[383] and Rohatgi et al.[384] suggest that patients who achieve a pCR had an improvement in survival compared to those who do not (5-year: 48% versus 15%, and median: 133 months versus 34 months, respectively). In these patients, surgical resection may not be necessary and has led to the concept of *selective* surgery after preoperative chemoradiation.

Swisher et al.[385] reported a retrospective analysis of patients who underwent a salvage compared with a planned esophagectomy at the M.D. Anderson Cancer Center from 1987 to 2000. The operative mortality was higher in those who underwent salvage versus planned surgery (15% versus 6%), but there was no difference in survival (25%). Because only 13 patients were identified who had salvage, the results need to be interpreted with caution. This approach formed the basis of a phase II Radiation Therapy Oncology Group (RTOG) trial (RTOG 0246), which prospectively examined the approach of preoperative paclitaxel/CDDP and 50.4 Gy followed by selective surgery in patients with either residual disease or recurrent disease in the absence of distant metastasis. In this trial of 43 patients with locally advanced disease, 21 patients required surgical resection after chemoradiation due to residual

(17 patients) or recurrent (3 patients) disease and one patient by choice.[386] This approach led to a 1-year overall survival of 71% and was closed early because it did not meet the predetermined survival rate of 78%.

Tumor Markers and Predictors of Response to Chemoradiation. It would be helpful to predict which tumors have a higher likelihood of responding to radiation or chemoradiation. Geh et al.[316] performed a systematic review to identify factors associated with a higher rate of pCR in patients receiving preoperative chemoradiation. The analysis was limited to the 26 trials meeting four criteria: (1) at least 20 patients treated, (2) a single chemoradiation regimen was delivered, (3) 5-FU, cisplatin, or mitomycin C–based chemotherapy was used, and (4) there was information on patient numbers, age, resection, and pCR rates. Overall, the pCR rate was 24% and the probability of pCR increased with increasing radiation dose ($p = 0.006$) and the use of a 5-FU-based ($p = 0.003$) or cisplatin-based ($p = 0.018$) regimen. In contrast, increased radiation treatment time ($p = 0.035$) and median age ($p = 0.019$) both decreased the chance of a pCR.

Data from both Berger et al.[383] and Rohatgi et al.[384] suggest that patients who achieve a pCR had an improvement in survival compared with those who do not (5-year, 48% versus 15%, and median, 133 months versus 34 months, respectively). However, the ability to predict a pCR prior to surgery is variable, as discussed earlier. A multivariate analysis by Gaca et al.[387] reported that posttreatment nodal status ($p = 0.03$), but not the degree of primary tumor response, predicted disease-free survival. Studies have linked tumor lymphocytic infiltration as well as the apoptotic index with response to chemoradiation.[388] Additional studies have linked a large number of proteins and genes involved in a wide array of signaling cascades with response to chemoradiation. Examples include alterations in diverse signaling cascades involving PI3 kinase, p53, EGFR, and hypoxia-inducible factor 1 alpha (HIF-1a).[389–394] Unfortunately, the vast majority of these studies lack validation and the specificity required to be used clinically. One recent study generated a micro-RNA signature to predict pCR from tumors in 52 patients treated uniformly with chemoradiation.[395] This signature was then validated in a separate cohort of 72 patients treated similarly. When combined with clinical stage, the area under the curve (AUC) for pathologic complete response (pCR) was 0.77 ($p = 2 \times 10^{-41}$).

Posttreatment imaging does not consistently identify the response. An ultrasound following chemoradiation does not accurately predict a pCR.[396] In contrast, Blackstock et al.[397] reported that the percentage of decrease in standard uptake value measured by 18F-FDG-PET predicted response, and Brucher et al.[398] found that it correlated with survival. McLoughlin et al.[399] treated 81 patients with preoperative chemoradiation and reported that FDG-PET scans were able to predict a pathologic complete response with 62% sensitivity, 44% specificity, and 56% accuracy.

The predictive ability of molecular markers has been examined. In 38 patients with squamous cell carcinoma who received chemoradiation with or without surgery, tumors without *p53* expression and tumors with weak *Bcl-X$_L$* expression showed a higher response to chemotherapy (56% and 53%, respectively) than tumors positive for *p53* or with strong *Bcl-X$_L$* expression (30% and 32%, respectively; *p* not significant).[400] After preoperative chemoradiation, patients with *p53*-negative tumors had a significantly better mean survival than those with *p53*-positive tumors (31 months versus 11 months; $p = 0.0378$). By multivariate analysis, Pomp et al.[401] found that overexpression of p53 resulted in a decrease in the survival in 69 patients with squamous cell carcinoma or adenocarcinoma treated with radiation alone. In one study, there was a correlation between decreasing levels of four phospholipids and increasing T stage and grade.[402]

Understanding the mechanism of radioresistance through the identification and targeting of molecular pathways by serum protein profiling[403] and the identification of genes involved in apoptosis,[404] activated transcription factor nuclear factor κB (NF-κB),[392]

and microvascular density[405] may offer new opportunities for therapeutic advances.

Intensification of Chemoradiation. The phase II Intergroup trial 0122 (ECOG-PE289/RTOG-90-12) was designed to intensify treatment in the RTOG-85-01 combined modality arm.[381] Both the chemotherapy and radiation therapy in INT-0122 were intensified by 20%.[406] The median survival time was 20 months and the 5-year actuarial survival rate was 20%. Similar toxicities were reported by Ishikura et al.[407] for 139 patients with squamous cell cancers treated with 5-FU, cisplatin, and 60 Gy of radiation. However, the higher radiation dose (64.8 Gy) in INT-0122 was tolerated and compared with the 50.4 Gy of radiation in the Intergroup trial INT-0123, discussed as follows.

A potential advantage of neoadjuvant chemotherapy is the early identification of those patients who may or may not respond to the chemotherapeutic regimen being delivered concurrently with chemoradiation. Ilson et al.[101] have shown that the change in standard update value (SUV) on FDG-PET scan was able to predict which patients showed a response to the full course of chemotherapy followed by chemoradiotherapy. Weider and associates[408] reported similar findings in 38 patients with squamous cell cancers. As discussed previously, the use of an early PET scan during induction chemotherapy to direct subsequent chemotherapy during combined chemoradiotherapy is the subject of an ongoing Alliance Trial.

Amini et al.[409] performed a retrospective review of 141 patients who achieved an initial clinical complete response (cCR) after chemoradiation. By a multivariate analysis, the initial SUV of >10 and poorly differentiated tumors had a significantly higher incidence of in-field failure.[409]

Intensification of the Radiation Dose. Another approach to the dose intensification of chemoradiation is increasing the radiation dose above 50.4 Gy. There are two methods by which to increase the radiation dose to the esophagus: brachytherapy and external-beam radiation therapy.

Brachytherapy. Intraluminal brachytherapy allows for the escalation of the dose to the primary tumor while protecting the surrounding dose-limiting structures such as the lung, heart, and spinal cord.[410] A radioactive source is placed intraluminally via bronchoscopy or a nasogastric tube. Brachytherapy has been used both as primary therapy (usually palliative)[411,412] and as a boost after external-beam radiation therapy or chemoradiation.[413–415] It can be delivered by high-dose rate or low-dose rate.[416] Although there are technical and radiobiologic differences between the two dose rates, there are no clear therapeutic advantages for either.

Series that combine brachytherapy with external-beam radiation therapy or chemoradiation report results similar to those for conventional chemoradiation. Yorozu et al.[415] reported a local failure rate of 57% and a 5-year actuarial survival of 28% in 46 patients with stage T2-3N0-1M0 disease. Even for a more favorable subset of patients with clinical T1 to T2 disease, Yorozu et al.[417] reported a local failure rate of 44% and a 5-year survival of 26%. In the series by Pasquier et al.,[414] local failure was 23% and 5-year survival was 36%. In an updated series by Ishikawa et al.,[418] 59 patients with submucosal esophageal cancer received external-beam therapy followed by brachytherapy in 36 patients with either low-dose rate caesium-137 (^{137}Cs) (17 patients) or high-dose rate iridium-192 (^{192}Ir) (19 patients). Patients selected to receive a brachytherapy boost had a significantly higher 5-year cause specific survival (86% versus 62%; $p = 0.04$).

In the RTOG-92-07 trial, 75 patients with squamous cell cancers (92%) or adenocarcinomas (8%) of the thoracic esophagus received the RTOG-85-01 combined modality regimen (5-FU, cisplatin, and 50 Gy of radiation) followed by a boost during cycle three of chemotherapy with either low-dose rate or high-dose rate intraluminal brachytherapy.[419] Because of low accrual, the low-dose rate option was discontinued and the analysis was limited to patients who received the high-dose rate treatment. High-dose rate brachytherapy was delivered in weekly fractions of 5 Gy during weeks 8, 9, and 10. After the development of several fistulas, the fraction delivered at week 10 was discontinued. Although the complete-response rate was 73%, the rate of local failure was 27%. Rates of acute toxicity were 58% for grade 3, 26% for grade 4, and 8% for grade 5 (treatment-related death). The cumulative incidence of fistula was 18% per year and the crude incidence was 14%. Of the six treatment-related fistulas, three were fatal. Given the significant toxicity, this treatment approach should be used with caution.[420] Based on these and other data, the American Brachytherapy Society has developed guidelines for esophageal brachytherapy.[421–423]

External-Beam Therapy: 2D and 3D Techniques. Because almost all patients in both the INT-0122 trial who started radiation therapy were able to complete the full dose (64.8 Gy), this higher dose of radiation was used in the experimental arm of the Intergroup esophageal trial INT-0123 (RTOG-94-05).[281] In this trial, patients with either squamous cell carcinoma or adenocarcinoma who were selected for nonsurgical treatment were randomly assigned to receive a slightly modified RTOG-85-01 combined modality regimen with 50.4 Gy of radiation versus the same chemotherapy with 64.8 Gy of radiation.

The modifications to the original RTOG-85-01 chemoradiation arm includes (1) using 1.8-Gy fractions to 50.4 Gy rather than 2-Gy fractions to 50 Gy; (2) treating with 5-cm proximal and distal margins for 50.4 Gy rather than treating the whole esophagus for the first 30 Gy followed by a cone down with 5-cm margins to 50 Gy; (3) cycle three of 5-FU and cisplatin did not begin until 4 weeks after the completion of radiation therapy rather than 3 weeks after; and (4) cycles three and four of chemotherapy were delivered every 4 weeks rather than every 3 weeks.

INT-0123 was closed to accrual in 1999 with 218 patients after an interim analysis revealed that it was unlikely that the high-dose arm would achieve superior survival compared with the standard-dose arm: There was no significant difference in median survival time (13.0 months versus 18.1 months) or 2-year survival rate (31% versus 40%) between the high-dose and standard-dose arms.[281] Although 11 treatment-related deaths occurred in the high-dose arm compared with 2 in the standard-dose arm, 7 of the 11 deaths occurred in patients who had received 50.4 Gy or less.

Although the crude incidence of local failure or persistence of local disease (or both) was lower in the high-dose arm than in the standard-dose arm (50% versus 55%), as was the incidence of distant failure (9% versus 16%), these were not significant. Although retrospective data from the M.D. Anderson Cancer Center suggest a positive correlation between radiation dose and local–regional control,[422] the results of the INT-0123 trial maintain the standard dose of 50.4 Gy.

The modifications to the original RTOG-85-01 chemoradiation arm outlined earlier did not adversely affect the local control or survival rate in the control arm of INT-0123. Therefore, the radiation doses and field design used in the control arm of INT-0123 should be used.

Radiation can be intensified not only by increasing the total dose, but also by using accelerated fractionation or hyperfractionation. This approach has revealed modest results. Zaho and colleagues[424] treated 201 patients with squamous cell cancer using 41.4 Gy followed by late-course accelerated hyperfractionation to 68.4 Gy. The results were similar to RTOG 85-01 (38% local failure and 26% 5-year survival). Choi and colleagues[425] treated 46 patients with 5-FU/cisplatin and twice per day radiation using a concurrent boost technique and reported a 37% 5-year survival. Additionally, Lee et al.[343] reported on a trial of 102 patients with locally advanced disease, limited to squamous cell carcinoma, randomized to surgery alone versus preoperative therapy with 45.6 Gy (1.2 Gy twice per day) plus 5-FU/cisplatin. There was no difference in median survival (28 versus 27 months). Thus, although these approaches appear to be reasonable, there appears to be a significant increase in acute toxicity without any clear therapeutic benefit.

Dose Escalation: Intensity Modulated Radiation Therapy and Protons. A criticism of many dose escalation trials in the definitive management of locally advanced esophageal cancer is the use of conventional two-dimensional (2D) and three-dimensional (3D) radiation techniques. Trials using newer techniques such as intensity-modulated radiation therapy (IMRT) and protons may be able to deliver higher doses of radiation with a more tolerable toxicity profile. Multiple dosimetric studies comparing standard 3D-conformal radiotherapy and IMRT, generally have found improved sparing of the heart, lung, or both using either static field or arc-based IMRT.[426–435] This has led multiple clinical centers to begin the routine use of IMRT in this disease. A retrospective analysis of these data does not suggest an inferior outcome and may provide decreased toxicity versus non-IMRT treatment techniques.[436–438] Investigators at the M.D. Anderson Cancer Center reported the results of 676 patients with locally advanced disease treated with either IMRT (263 patients) or 3D conformal radiation therapy (3DCRT) (413 patients).[436] On a multivariate analysis, IMRT was associated with improved survival ($p = 0.004$), but not cancer-specific survival ($p = 0.86$). The survival difference between 3DCRT and IMRT was thought to be due to a higher level of cardiac deaths ($p = 0.05$) and unexplained deaths ($p = 0.003$) in the 3DCRT patients, suggesting that decreased cardiac dose may have a direct impact on patient outcome. Although this and other comparisons between 3DCRT and IMRT are retrospective, a randomized trial is unlikely, thus the available data may represent the best comparison.

Another theoretical advantage of IMRT is the possibility of dose escalation. With the use of IMRT, a simultaneous integrated boost (SIB) may be performed while maintaining commonly used lung and heart dosimetric constraints. Retrospective data from Zhang and colleagues[422] suggest a positive correlation between radiation dose and local–regional control. This has led to a phase I studying examining this approach in locally advanced disease. However, at this point, based on results of the INT-0123 trial, the standard dose of external beam radiation remains 50.4 Gy.

New Chemoradiation Regimens. Because 75% to 80% of patients die of metastatic disease, advances in systemic therapies are necessary for a further improvement of results. The most widely used chemotherapeutic regimen to be combined with radiation for the treatment of esophageal cancer is 5-FU and cisplatin. A number of new cytotoxic and targeted regimens are being evaluated in both the preoperative and nonoperative setting. These are discussed previously in the section on preoperative chemoradiation regimens.

Palliation of Esophageal Cancer with Radiation Therapy

Palliation of Dysphagia and Bleeding. Many of the series examining dysphagia are retrospective, and most do not use objective criteria to define and assess dysphagia. Some do not report the number of patients presenting with dysphagia or the percentage who receive palliative treatment until the time of death. Furthermore, few series carefully examine other variables that may influence the results, such as histologic type, stage, and location of the primary tumor.

Options for palliation include stents, feeding tubes, chemotherapy, and external-beam radiation therapy or brachytherapy (or both). The selection of the technique is variable and commonly is based on physician preference. In a randomized trial from the Dutch SIREC Study Group of stent versus one 12-Gy fraction of brachytherapy, dysphagia, as measured by a variety of quality-of-life scales, improved more rapidly after stent placement; however, long-term relief was superior after brachytherapy.[412] Median survivals were similar (145 days versus 155 days).

Patients for whom stents fail are commonly treated with palliative radiation. Li et al.[439] reported that the presence of a metal stent increases the radiation dose 5% to 10% at a 0.5-cm depth in the esophageal wall. Therefore, the radiation dose should be decreased by 5% to 10% when a metal stent is in the radiation field. Nishimura et al.[440] reported a high-grade 3+ complication rate in 47 patients who underwent stent placement before or during radiation treatment and recommend that stent placement be delayed until radiation therapy has failed.

As seen in Table 45.8, series have examined the palliative benefits of either radiation alone[371,441–444] or chemoradiation.[406,443,445–450] Overall, external-beam radiation therapy alone provides palliation of dysphagia in 70% to 80% of patients.

The most comprehensive and carefully performed analysis of swallowing function in patients receiving chemoradiation is by Coia et al.[450] Using a swallowing score modified from O'Rourke et al.,[451] they analyzed 102 patients treated with three 5-FU–based combined modality regimens. Before the start of therapy, 95% of patients had some degree of dysphagia. Within 2 weeks after the start of treatment, 45% had improvement in dysphagia, and by the completion of the 6-week therapy, 83% had improvement. Overall, 88% experienced an improvement in dysphagia. The median time to improvement was 4 weeks (range, 1 to 21 weeks), and all but two patients could swallow at least soft or solid foods. Harvey et al.[446] treated 106 patients and reported that 78% had improvement of at least one grade in their dysphagia score; 51% maintained swallowing improvement until the time of last follow-up.

Intraluminal brachytherapy is also an effective, albeit a more limited method, achieving palliation of dysphagia in 35% to 80% of patients and a median survival of 5 months. A major limitation of brachytherapy is the effective treatment distance. The primary isotope is [192]-Ir, which is usually prescribed to treat to a distance of 1 cm from the source. Any portion of the tumor that is more than 1 cm from the source will receive a suboptimal radiation dose, confirmed by pathologic analysis of surgical specimens.[452] Given its limited effective range, brachytherapy is usually not as successful as external-beam radiation therapy in treating the entire tumor volume. However, in a randomized trial, there was no difference in local control or survival with high-dose–rate brachytherapy as opposed to external-beam radiation therapy.[452]

If a patient requires rapid palliation (within a few days), alternative approaches such as laser treatment or stent placement are recommended. Although external-beam radiation with or without chemotherapy takes at least 2 weeks to produce palliation, once palliation is achieved it is more durable than that provided by the other palliative modalities because external-beam radiation treats the problem (the gross tumor mass), not just the symptom. If external-beam radiation is not possible, then intraluminal brachytherapy should be considered because it is an effective modality for decreasing symptoms such as dysphagia and bleeding. Chemotherapy by itself may also substantially relieve dysphagia when used as an initial treatment of metastatic disease.

Treatment in the Setting of Tracheoesophageal Fistula

The presence of a malignant tracheoesophageal fistula usually results in poor survival, although occasionally, patients may survive for a prolonged period. Historically, radiation therapy was believed to be contraindicated for these patients for fear of exacerbating the fistula as the tumor responded. More recently, there have been reports to the contrary. In a Mayo Clinic series, 10 patients with malignant tracheoesophageal fistulas received 30 to 66 Gy external-beam radiation, and the median survival time was 5 months.[453] A series from Japan that treated 24 patients with fistulization to the airway reported ultimate closure of the fistula after chemoradiotherapy in 17 patients, with time to closure ranging from 6 to 280 days.[454]

TABLE 45.8

Palliation of Dysphagia with Radiation Therapy with or without Chemotherapy

Study (Ref.)	No. of Patients	Palliation of Dysphagia[a]	
		At the End of Treatment (%)	Duration
Radiation Therapy Alone			
Wara et al.[441]	103	89	6-mo average
Petrovich et al.[442]	133	87	34% = 6 mo 18% = 3 mo 35% = 3 mo
Roussel et al.[371]	69	70	—
Caspers et al.[444]	127	71	54% until death
Whittington et al.[443]	25	—	5% at 9 mo
Chemoradiation			
Coia et al.[450]	102	88	67%–100% until death
Seitz et al.[445]	35	100[b]	—
Whittington et al.[443]	26	—	87% 3-y actuarial
Algan et al.[447]	8	100	—
Gill et al.[448]	71	60	—
Urba et al.[449]	27	—	59% until death
Izquierdo et al.[406]	25	64	Median, 5 mo
Harvey et al.[446]	106	78	51% until lost follow-up

[a] See text for definition and number of patients presenting with dysphagia.
[b] Patients had dilation or neodymium yttrium-aluminum garnet laser treatment at the start of therapy.

Although the experience is very limited, the data suggest that radiation treatment does not necessarily increase the severity of a malignant tracheoesophageal fistula and it can be administered safely. It is unclear if radiation treatment improves outcome.

Acute and Long-Term Toxicity of Radiation Therapy.
The toxicity of radiation therapy is a function of what the total dose is, what technique is used, and whether the patient has received chemotherapy. Essentially all patients experience lethargy and esophagitis commencing 2 to 3 weeks after the start of radiation therapy; these symptoms usually resolve 1 to 2 weeks after completion of therapy.

The most carefully documented acute toxicity data for patients who receive radiation therapy alone (without chemotherapy) are from the control arm of RTOG-85-01 in which patients received radiation therapy alone to a dose of 64 Gy.[280,372] The incidence of acute grade 3 toxicity was 25% and the incidence of acute grade 4 toxicity was 3%. The incidence of long-term grade 3+ toxicity and long-term grade 4+ toxicity was 23% and 2%, respectively. Radiation therapy can produce esophageal strictures, as can surgery. The total incidence of stricture (benign plus malignant) in patients receiving radiation therapy alone or radiation combined with chemotherapy is 20% to 40% in a modern series and up to 60% in historical series,[455] with up to 50% malignant, associated with recurrence. The incidence of stricture is lower in series in which careful radiation techniques were used. Coia et al.[450] examined a subset of 25 patients who experienced local control and survived at least 1 year. The incidence of benign stricture was 12%. Radiation toxicity is related to dose–volume effects.[456]

One series examined the functional outcomes of benign and malignant strictures.[451] Patients received 45 to 56 Gy and 53% received some form of chemotherapy. Of the 24 patients (30%) who developed a benign stricture, 71% were able to tolerate a full or soft diet and required dilation, with a median interval between dilations of 5 months. Even in the subset of patients who develop a benign stricture, dilation is effective in the majority of patients. In contrast, in the 28% of patients who developed a malignant stricture, dilation was unsuccessful and esophageal intubation was required.

The high incidence of fistula reported in the RTOG-92-07 trial of chemoradiation plus intraluminal brachytherapy (18% actuarial, 14% crude) has not been seen in series using radiation therapy or chemoradiation. The incidence of other long-term grade 3+ toxicities such as pneumonitis or pericarditis is 5%.

The effect of radiation on pulmonary function was examined by Gergel et al.[457] Patients received 39.6 Gy with anterior–posterior fields followed by radiation with oblique fields to a total dose of 50.4 Gy, plus concurrent chemotherapy with oxaliplatin and 5-FU. Results of pulmonary function tests administered before and a median of 16 days after radiation revealed significant declines in diffusing capacity for carbon monoxide and total lung capacity. Investigators at the M.D. Anderson Cancer Center performed retrospective treatment-planning studies on 10 patients and found that IMRT reduced the dose volume of exposed normal lung but had no clinically meaningful differences on the irradiated volumes of spinal cord, heart, liver, or total body integral doses.[426] The impact of respiratory and organ movement on defining target volumes is being investigated.[458,459]

The issue of treatment-related deaths in patients who receive chemoradiation is complex. Although the incidence was only 2% in RTOG-85-01, subsequent trials have reported a higher treatment-related mortality rate (i.e., 9% in INT-0122 and 8% in RTOG-92-07). These mortality rates are lower than the 10% to 15% incidence reported in historical surgical series, although only slightly higher than the 6% reported in the surgical control arm of INT-0113.[105] It is interesting to note that, as the mortality rate with surgery has decreased, there has been a corresponding increase in the treatment-related mortality rate reported in the nonoperative trials. As previously discussed in Primary Nonsurgical Therapy,

this may be partly related to bias in selecting patients to be treated with the nonoperative approach.

Radiation Field Design and Treatment Techniques.
Just as expert surgical skills are required for a successful esophagectomy, radiation field design for esophageal cancer requires careful planning. Historically, the standard radiation dose, based on INT-0123, for patients selected for chemoradiation is 50.4 Gy at 1.8 Gy per fraction. However, recent data from the CROSS trial suggest that 41.4 Gy in the same fractionation may be sufficient to treat in the preoperative setting. As previously described, some investigators have performed dose escalation; however, based on INT-0113, dose escalation above 50.4 Gy should not be performed off protocol. Additionally, radiation should be delivered without treatment breaks, as randomized data from France reveal a higher local control (57% versus 29%) and 2-year survival rate (37% versus 23%) with continuous course compared with split course radiation.[382]

The radiation field should include the primary tumor with 5 cm superior and inferior margins and 2 cm lateral margins. The primary local–regional lymph nodes should receive the same dose. For cervical (proximal) primary tumors (defined as at or proximal to the carina), the treatment volume includes the bilateral supraclavicular nodes, and for GEJ (distal) primaries, the celiac axis nodes should be included.

Treatment Modality.
At many centers, the standard of care in radiotherapy for locally advanced esophageal cancer is 3D conformal radiotherapy using a beam arrangement optimized via CT scan–based planning. However, as mentioned previously, many clinicians have used IMRT with a possible benefit with regard to toxicity and no apparent compromise in oncologic outcome.[436] A comparison of three techniques is shown in Figure 45.14. If IMRT is to be used, careful attention should be given to target delineation. In addition, particularly in the case of distal/GEJ tumors, 4D CT or other forms of motion management should be considered.

Recently, proton radiotherapy has become more available as a treatment modality. By virtue of its physical characteristics, proton radiotherapy is thought to decrease dose to critical structures, in large part by minimizing the low-dose "bath" often seen with IMRT. This is to some degree shown in dosimetric studies, with V5, V10, and V20 to the lung and heart with protons compared to IMRT (see Fig. 45.14). Several studies have examined patient outcome after treating with proton radiotherapy. Sugahara and colleagues[460] examined outcomes in 46 patients with squamous cell carcinoma treated with protons with or without photons to a median total dose of 76 Gy.[460] The 5-year local control rate was for T1: 83%, for T2 through 4: 29%, and for survival T1: 55% and for T2 through 4: 13%. Koyama[461] reported mean actuarial survival rates of 60% for patients with superficial and 39% for those with advanced disease treated to mean total doses of 78 to 81 Gy. The incidence of esophageal ulcer was 67%. In the United States, Lin and colleagues[462] retrospectively reviewed 62 patients treated with proton radiotherapy for locally advanced disease. Overall, 47% were treated with surgical resection following chemoradiation, with a pCR rate in these patients of 28%. In this series, two patients (3.2%) developed symptomatic pneumonitis and an additional two patients died due to treatment-related factors. Proton therapy remains experimental and is currently being evaluated in a randomized trial.

Target Delineation.
Although CT scans can identify adjacent organs and structures, it may be limited in defining the extent of the primary tumor. Leong and colleagues[463] have demonstrated that the addition of PET/CT scan information for treatment planning improved the identification of the gross tumor volume (GTV). The GTV based on CT scan information alone excluded PET-avid disease in 11 of 16 patients (69%), 5 of whom would have resulted in a geographic miss of gross tumor. Thus, in many centers, it is

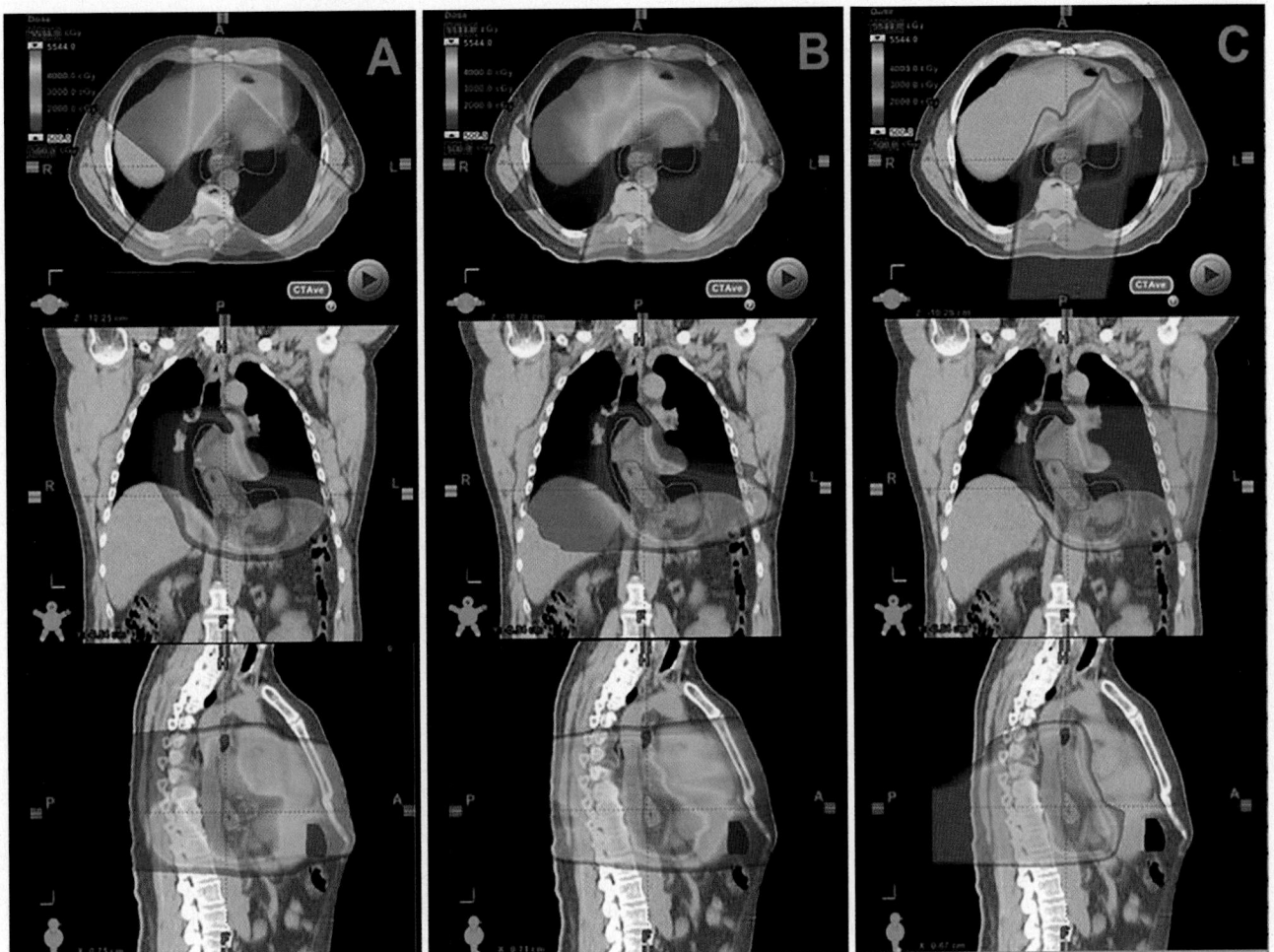

Figure 45.14 Comparative radiation treatment plans. **(A)** 3D-CRT, **(B)** IMRT, and **(C)** proton beam comparison between treatment modalities. In this selected case, both IMRT and protons provide improved lung and cardiac sparing compared to 3D-CRT. Proton beam decreases liver dose compared to other modalities. (Modified from Zhang Z, Liao Z, Jin J, et al. Dose response relationship in locoregional control for patients with stage II–III esophageal cancer treated with concurrent chemotherapy and radiotherapy. *Int J Radiat Oncol Biol Phys* 2005;61:656–664.)

customary to obtain pretreatment FDG-PET scans, not only to identify patients with occult metastatic disease, but also to assist in target delineation. Conversely, MRI has also been suggested to delineate esophageal tumors, although initial studies showed limited benefit in tumor or positive lymph node delineation.[464] Thus, the use of MRI in this context remains experimental. Thus, the current recommendation for target delineation includes using contrasted CT and EGD/EUS findings, as well as FDG-PET.

Limiting Toxicity of Chemoradiation. Depending on the location of the primary tumor, there are a number of sensitive organs that will be in the radiation field. Specifically, the most well-studied organs at risk in the context of treating esophageal cancer include the lungs and heart. Radiation pneumonitis is clearly linked to the dose and volume of lung treated. Various single dosimetric parameters have been proposed to estimate the probability of developing radiation pneumonitis after radiotherapy.[428,465–469] Investigators from the Netherlands compared different normal tissue complication probability (NTCP) models to predict radiation pneumonitis.[468] Using the observed incidence of radiation pneumonitis among breast cancer, malignant lymphoma, and inoperable non–small-cell lung cancer (NSCLC) patients, they found that the underlying local dose-effect relation for radiation pneumonitis was linear. This was better represented by the mean lung dose (MLD) model, rather than a step function model represented by a threshold dose such as V20. In their patient population, the MLD

was the most accurate predictor for the incidence of radiation pneumonitis. Willner and colleagues[466] performed an analysis of pneumonitis risk from dose volume histogram (DVH) parameters among patients treated with 3D conformal radiotherapy.[466] Their data indicated that it is reasonable to disperse the dose outside the target volume over large areas in order to reduce the volumes of lung receiving >40 Gy. They found that reducing the high-dose volume reduces the pneumonitis rate more than a corresponding reduction in the low-dose regions of the DVH. Additionally, Konski and colleagues[470] were able to correlate cardiac toxicity to dosimetric and patient factors. Specifically they recommended a threshold of V20, V30, and V40 below 70%, 65%, and 60%, respectively, to decrease symptomatic cardiac toxicity. In general, practice a MLD <20 Gy is standard. Cardiac dose constraints are not as clearly defined, but a V30 <35% is reasonable.

In the palliative setting, there are a variety of radiation-treatment regimens.[471] The goal is rapid palliation of symptoms and the most common approach is to treat anteroposteriorly and posteroanteriorly, including the primary tumor with 2-cm margins, in 10 3-Gy fractions to a total dose of 30 Gy.

Treatment of Metastatic Disease

A variety of single-agent and combination chemotherapy regimens have been evaluated in patients with recurrent or metastatic carcinoma of the esophagus. Phase II clinical trials in this population have identified drugs with activity that have been integrated into combined modality regimens for the treatment of earlier stage disease. Standard criteria for evaluating treatment response require that serial measurement of disease be possible. For the esophageal cancer patient with metastatic disease to distant organ sites or lymph nodes, treatment response can be reliably assessed using spiral CT scans or MRI. The serial tumor measurement for response assessments in patients with disease limited to the esophagus is less reliable. An endoscopy with brushings and biopsy may be performed to confirm a clinically determined complete response; however, a biopsy is subject to sampling error, and biopsy findings are not a reliable indicator of complete histologic resolution of disease. Whole-body FDG-PET performed before and during or after chemotherapy may be a valuable noninvasive method of predicting tumor response and a favorable treatment outcome. Several studies have shown that a reduction in tumor FDG uptake (median decrease in standardized uptake value) correlates with response and longer survival.[154,158,327] Until the mid-1990s, the accumulated experience with chemotherapy was almost entirely in patients with squamous cell tumors. With the rising incidence of adenocarcinoma of the distal esophagus, GEJ, and cardia in the United States and Western industrialized countries, patients with this histologic type now make up more than half of referrals for chemotherapy. Most trials of new agents and combined modality regimens now include patients with both tumor types. Modern chemotherapy trials in advanced disease also treat gastric adenocarcinoma in concert with adenocarcinoma of the GEJ and distal esophagus, and some trials also include squamous esophageal cancer.

Single-Agent Chemotherapy

Studies of single-agent chemotherapy for esophageal cancer are summarized here. Response data for many of the older drugs have come from broad phase I and II trials conducted in the 1970s and 1980s, which included small numbers of esophageal cancer patients.[472–481] Bleomycin, 5-FU, mitomycin, and cisplatin have been used most frequently because of their single-agent activity and additive or synergistic effects with radiation. Because of the potential for pulmonary toxicity, bleomycin is no longer included in combination regimens, having been replaced by 5-FU. Similarly, mitomycin is used less often because of its toxicity profile, which includes hemolytic–uremic syndrome and cumulative myelosuppression.

Seven trials examined the use of cisplatin for single-agent therapy in esophageal cancer patients,[479,482–487] six of which used dosages ranging from 50 to 120 mg/m^2 every 3 to 4 weeks. The cumulative response rate in patients with metastatic or recurrent disease was 21%. Vinorelbine is a semisynthetic vinca alkaloid that has less neurotoxicity than vincristine and vinblastine. Phase II trials in metastatic squamous cell cancer of the esophagus report response rates of 20% to 25% using weekly or biweekly dosing schedules.[488,489] In a subsequent trial, Conroy et al.[490] evaluated the doublet of vinorelbine and cisplatin. A total of 71 patients with metastatic squamous cell cancer were treated, and a 34% response rate was observed. Vinorelbine was evaluated in a phase II trial in 29 patients with adenocarcinoma of the esophagus who had failed prior chemotherapy, with minor activity (7% response rate) observed.[491]

The taxane paclitaxel has been tested in both adenocarcinoma and squamous cell carcinoma of the esophagus. Paclitaxel promotes the stabilization of microtubules and is a cycle-specific agent affecting cells in the G2/M phase. Paclitaxel also enhances radiation effects and may be both concentration and schedule dependent.[492] Three trials of single-agent paclitaxel have been reported. One used the maximum tolerable dose of 250 mg/m^2, derived from initial phase I trials using a 24-hour infusion schedule.[493] The overall response rate was 32% (34% in 33 patients with adenocarcinoma, and 28% in 18 patients with squamous cell

carcinoma). The second trial tested a regimen of 140 mg/m^2 infused during 96 hours in patients previously treated using a shorter infusion schedule of paclitaxel-containing combination chemotherapy.[494] No responses were observed. The third trial evaluated single-agent paclitaxel administered by a weekly 1-hour infusion at a dose of 80 mg/m^2 in a large multicenter phase 2 setting.[495] A modest response rate of 15% was observed in 65 patients without prior chemotherapy treatment (16% in the 50 patients treated with adenocarcinoma and 13% in the 15 patients treated with squamous cell carcinoma). Limited activity (5%) was seen in patients with prior chemotherapy. Despite the low response rate, the median survival was 274 days, and toxicity, including hematologic toxicity, was minimal.

Docetaxel was evaluated at a dose of 100 mg/m^2, every 3 weeks in a combined esophageal and gastric cancer trial treating 33 patients with gastric cancer and 8 patients with esophageal adenocarcinoma.[496] Two of the eight patients (25%) with esophageal adenocarcinoma had a major response. Overall, grade 4 neutropenia occurred in 88% of patients and neutropenic fever in 46%. A larger trial of docetaxel 75 mg/m^2 in 22 patients with esophageal adenocarcinoma reported a response rate of 18% in chemotherapy-naïve patients and no responses in previously treated patients.[496] Febrile neutropenia occurred in 32% of patients. A recent trial of 70 mg/m^2 every 3 weeks in 49 patients with squamous cell carcinoma reported a 20% response rate.[497] Eighty-eight percent of patients had grade 3 or 4 neutropenia and 18% had febrile neutropenia.

Drugs that have been adequately tested in squamous cell cancer of the esophagus and have response rates less than 5% are the methotrexate analog dichloromethotrexate[498] and trimetrexate,[499,500] and etoposide,[501,502] ifosfamide,[503,504] and carboplatin.[505,506] A more contemporary study of etoposide in untreated patients with squamous cell carcinoma reported a response rate of 19% (5 of 26 patients).[507] Carboplatin has been studied in both adenocarcinoma and squamous cell carcinoma, and, in contrast to the activity of a single agent, responses to carboplatin were observed in only 3 of 59 chemotherapy-naïve patients. Therefore, substitution of single-agent carboplatin for cisplatin is not recommended when treating patients with either adenocarcinomas or squamous cell carcinomas of the esophagus. Nonetheless, carboplatin combination regimens used as part of combination chemotherapy, in chemoradiation (as previously discussed) and in metastatic disease regimens (discussed later), appear to have comparable activity to cisplatin-based therapy.

Topotecan and gemcitabine have been separately evaluated in both histologic tumor types and have been shown to be inactive.[508–510] The topoisomerase II inhibitor irinotecan has been evaluated in two phase II trials in adenocarcinoma of the stomach and GEJ, with a response rate of 15% observed.[511,512]

Combined-Agent Chemotherapy

Older trials (before the mid-1990s) and those in Europe were almost exclusively limited to patients with squamous cell carcinoma. Because esophageal cancer is a relatively uncommon malignancy, many studies include a heterogeneous population of treatment-naïve patients with locally advanced intrathoracic disease as well as patients with recurrent or metastatic disease. Not only is there variation in the patient population, but more recent trials usually limit eligibility to patients with no prior chemotherapy and performance status of 0 or 1. Thus, in the absence of comparative trials, newer regimens may appear more effective.

Most series consist of small numbers of patients; therefore, the 95% CIs are large and nearly all responses are partial. On average, the duration of response ranges from 3 to 6 months.

Trials conducted in the 1980s testing three-drug regimens such as cisplatin, bleomycin, and vindesine[255,513] and cisplatin and mitoguazone combined with vindesine[514] or vinblastine[515] yielded response rates of 30% to 40% in patients with squamous cell carcinoma. Toxicity was primarily moderate myelosuppression. Bleomycin and

TABLE 45.9

Randomized Phase II–III Chemotherapy Trials In Esophageal and GE Junction Cancers

Regimen	Patients (N)	Histologic Type	Response Rate (%)	Overall Survival	Reference
C + 5-FU vs C	88	S	35 19	28 wks 33 wks	483
ECF vs FAMTX	274	A	45 21	8.9 mos 5.7 mos	517
ECF vs MCF	690	A/S	42 44	9.4 mos 8.7 mos	518
ECF vs ECX vs EOF vs EOX	1002	A/S	41 46 42 48	9.9 mos 9.9 mos 9.3 mos 11.2 mos	520
5-FU + O vs 5-FU + C	220	A	35 25	10.7 mos 8.8 mos	521
5-FU + C vs Cape + C	316	A	32 46	9.3 mos 10.5 mos	522
5-FU + C vs S-1 + C	1,053	A	32 29	7.9 mos 8.6 mos	524
CF vs DCF	445	A	26 36	8.6 mos 9.2 mos	525
5-FU + O +/− D	143	A	49 28	17.3 mos 14.5 mos	526
5-FU + C vs 5-FU + Irino	333	A	26 32	8.7 mos 9.0 mos	549

C, cisplatin; S, squamous cell carcinoma; ECF, epirubicin/cisplatin; FAMTX, 5-FU/doxorubicin/methotrexate; A, adenocarcinoma; EOX, epirubicin/cisplatin or oxaliplatin/5-FU or capecitabine; O, oxaliplatin; Cape, capecitabine; D, docetaxel; Irino, irinotecan.

mitoguazone were subsequently replaced by 5-FU to reduce toxicity and to take advantage of its synergistic activity with cisplatin.

The two-drug combination of cisplatin (100 mg/m^2 on day 1) and 5-FU (1,000 mg/m^2 per day continuous infusion for 96 to 120 hours) has been the standard regimen for 2 decades to treat patients with either squamous cell carcinoma or adenocarcinoma. A 35% response rate was observed in patients with metastatic, recurrent, or locally advanced incurable squamous cell cancer of the esophagus.[483] Higher response rates (in the 40% to 60% range) were reported in trials administering two or three cycles of cisplatin and 5-FU as induction therapy before surgery. The difference in response rates may be related to better performance status, better nutrition, and smaller volume disease in the surgical candidates. Despite the common use in the oncology community of the combination of 5-FU and cisplatin for the treatment of esophageal carcinoma, only one trial conducted by the EORTC has directly addressed the issue of the comparative efficacy of single-agent cisplatin and the combination of 5-FU and cisplatin (Table 45.9).[483] Patients with locally advanced or metastatic squamous cell carcinoma were randomly assigned to receive either cisplatin (100 mg/m^2) plus continuous-infusion 5-FU (1,000 mg/m^2 per day, days 1 to 5) or to cisplatin (100 mg/m^2) alone, with both regimens repeated every 3 weeks. The cisplatin/5-FU arm had a higher response rate (35%) and better median survival (33 weeks) than the cisplatin arm (19% and 28 weeks, respectively), but these findings were not statistically significant. Cisplatin/5-FU was also more toxic, with 16% treatment-related deaths for the combination.

Cisplatin in combination with tegafur uracil (UFT), an oral 5-FU pro-drug combining tegafur with uracil, an inhibitor of the enzyme dihydropyrimidine dehydrogenase that degrades 5-FU,

has also been evaluated in esophageal cancer. A response rate of 46% was reported.[516]

Recent phase III trials have compared the addition of a third agent to cisplatin/5-FU versus cisplatin/5-FU alone. The Royal Marsden group developed the ECF regimen, a combination of epirubicin (50 mg/m^2) and cisplatin (60 mg/m^2) every 3 weeks in combination with daily protracted continuous infusion 5-FU (200 mg/m^2 per day) in gastric cancer. The ECF regimen was compared in a phase III trial in gastric and GEJ adenocarcinoma with a bolus regimen of 5-FU, doxorubicin, and methotrexate (FAMTX) (see Table 45.9).[517] The ECF regimen resulted in a superior response rate (45% versus 21%), failure-free survival (7.4 months versus 3.4 months), and median survival (8.9 months versus 5.7 months) in comparison with FAMTX. The ECF regimen had a tolerable toxicity profile, with less than 10% rates of grade 3 or 4 diarrhea or stomatitis. A more recent trial treating nearly 600 patients with advanced esophageal squamous and adenocarcinoma and gastric adenocarcinoma compared the ECF regimen with a similar regimen substituting mitomycin (7 mg/m^2 every 6 weeks) for epirubicin (see Table 45.9).[518] This trial validated the previously reported response rate and median survival for the ECF regimen (42%, 9.4 months), but the response rate and median survival observed for the mitomycin combination regimen (44%, 8.7 months) were identical to those of ECF. Given that there was no difference in efficacy for the epirubicin- versus mitomycin-containing arms, this study raises the question of whether or not the addition of a third agent makes a difference in outcome when combined with cisplatin and protracted infusion 5-FU. Of the 533 patients enrolled in this trial, 40 had squamous cell carcinoma of the esophagus and the remainder had adenocarcinoma (125, esophagus; 125, gastroesophageal junction; 243, stomach). There was a significantly higher response rate among patients with GEJ cancers than among those with distal gastric cancers (48% versus 37%).

Oxaliplatin, as a potential substitute for cisplatin, and oral capecitabine, as a substitute for 5-FU, have been explored in phase II trails[519] and, more recently, phase III randomized trials in esophageal and gastric adenocarcinoma (see Table 45.9). Cunningham et al.[520] reported results of a 1,000 patient phase III trial in esophageal squamous cell and adenocarcinoma and gastric cancer, evaluating the frontline use of oxaliplatin or capecitabine. This trial compared conventional ECF with the substitution of capecitabine for infusional 5-FU, and oxaliplatin for cisplatin. The trial employed a two-by-two design, with the control arm ECF, and the experimental arms including capecitabine (625 mg/m^2 twice daily) substituted for infusional 5-FU; oxaliplatin (130 mg/m^2) substituted for cisplatin; and a fourth arm with a substitution of both capecitabine and oxaliplatin. Capecitabine was found to be noninferior to 5-FU, and oxaliplatin noninferior to cisplatin, with comparable rates of antitumor response and progression-free survival across the four treatment arms. A toxicity analysis favored oxaliplatin over cisplatin for neutropenia, alopecia, renal toxicity, and thromboembolism. In a planned comparison of ECF to EOX (epirubicin, oxaliplatin, capecitabine), median survival was superior for EOX (11.2 months versus 9.9 months; HR, 0.80; $p = 0.02$). A second phase III trial from the German AIO group compared infusional 5-FU (24-hour infusion) plus leucovorin combined with either oxaliplatin (85 mg/m^2) or cisplatin (50 mg/m^2) once every 2 weeks in 220 patients with metastatic gastroesophageal adenocarcinoma.[521] Like the Cunningham et al. trial, oxaliplatin was found to be noninferior to cisplatin. Oxaliplatin caused significantly less nausea and vomiting, fatigue, renal toxicity, and thromboembolism. Remarkable on both arms of this trial was the relatively low level of grade 3 or 4 toxicities in all categories, running less than 10% to 15%, which was likely due to the 2 weekly schedule of chemotherapy mimicking colorectallike cancer scheduling of chemotherapy. Response rates (24.5% to 34.8%), progression-free (3.9 months versus 5.8 months), and overall survival (8.8 months versus 10.7 months) were comparable between the two treatment arms, although all end points trended higher on the oxaliplatin arm. Lastly, a third phase III trial reported by Kang et al.[522] compared capecitabine (1,000 mg/m^2) twice a day for 14 days to 5-FU (800 mg/m^2 per day continuous infusion) for 5 days, cycled every 3 weeks with cisplatin (80 mg/m^2). Like the Cunningham et al. trial, capecitabine was found to be noninferior to 5-FU. Rates of toxicity on the treatment arms were similar, as were measures of progression-free (5.0 months versus 5.6 months) and overall survival (9.3 months versus 10.5 months). Based on the results of these three phase III trials, the substitution of oxaliplatin for cisplatin, or capecitabine for 5-FU, seems justified. The two-drug regimens in the Al-Batran et al.[521] and Kang et al.[522] trials had favorable toxicity profiles and efficacy compared to the three drug regimens of Cunningham et al., and whether or not epirubicin is required as part of therapy in metastatic disease is unclear.

An alternative oral 5-FU agent, S-1, combines the 5-FU prodrug tegafur with a bowel protectant (oteracil) and an inhibitor of dihydropyrimidine dehydrogenase (gimeracil). A phase III trial conducted in Japan evaluated S-1 40 to 60 mg twice a day for 3 weeks as a single agent, versus S-1 plus cisplatin (60 mg/m^2), cycled once every 5 weeks, in advanced gastric cancer. S-1 plus cisplatin was superior to S-1 alone, with improved rates of response (54% versus 31%), progression-free (6 months versus 4 months), and overall survival (13 months versus 11 months).[523] Based on encouraging data for S-1, a phase III superiority trial comparing S-1 50 mg/m^2 in two daily divided doses for 21 days was compared to infusional 5-FU 1,000 mg/m^2 per day for 5 days, cycled every 28 days (see Table 45.9).[524] Both arms were combined with cisplatin, with a lower dose of cisplatin combined with S-1 (75 mg/m^2) compared to the 5-FU arm (100 mg/m^2). A lower dose of S-1 than that used in the Japanese trials was mandated due to greater toxicity for S-1 reported in Western patients in prior phase I and II trials. The trial failed to demonstrate superiority for the S-1 arm, with

equivalent rates of overall survival (7.9 months versus 8.6 months). The S-1 arm had less toxicity than 5-FU, but the lesser cisplatin dose likely accounted for much of the toxicity differences between the treatment arms. Whether S-1 will be adopted in practice in Western countries has yet to be established.

The addition of docetaxel as a third agent added to 5-FU and cisplatin has also recently been reported in a phase III trial of GEJ and gastric cancer (see Table 45.9). 5-FU dosed at 1,000 mg/m^2 by continuous infusion during 5 days combined with cisplatin (100 mg/m^2) was compared with cisplatin (75 mg/m^2), 5-FU (750 mg/m^2) by continuous infusion during 5 days, and docetaxel (75 mg/m^2) in 445 patients with metastatic gastric or GEJ adenocarcinoma.[525] Docetaxel resulted in a higher response rate and time to progression (36%, 5.6 months) compared with 5-FU and cisplatin (26%, 3.7 months), but only a marginal median survival improvement (0.6 months) was noted for three-drug therapy. Toxicity was substantial in both treatment arms, including hematologic and gastrointestinal toxicity, with 80% of patients receiving the three-drug combination experiencing grade 3 or 4 neutropenia. The recent trials of 5-FU infusion combination chemotherapy indicate improved therapy tolerance and potentially enhanced antitumor activity, employing either a once every 2 week or a more protracted infusion of 5-FU as in the ECF regimen. The addition of a third agent, including epirubicin or docetaxel, to 5-FU and cisplatin may modestly increase response rates and survival, but, in the case of docetaxel combination therapy, may result in substantial therapy-related toxicity. The use of relatively high and relatively toxic doses of cisplatin (75 to 100 mg/m^2) is also called into question, given data from the British phase III ECF trials that indicate potential better therapy tolerance for 60 mg/m^2 without evident compromising of treatment efficacy. The tolerance of a three-drug regimen may also be influenced by patient age. In a phase III trial targeting 143 patients with esophagogastric cancer 65 years or older, Al-Batran and colleagues[526] compared a regimen of biweekly infusional 5-FU and oxaliplatin with or without the addition of docetaxel (see Table 45.9). A higher response rate was reported for triplet therapy with no impact on overall survival, and resulted in much higher rates of toxicity and an actual detriment in quality of life measures compared to two-drug therapy.

Five trials using interferon-α_{2a} (IFN-α_{2a}) as a biomodulator of 5-FU suggested possible benefit.[527–531] These phase 2 trials combined IFN-α_{2a} with 5-FU and with cisplatin combined with continuous-infusion 5-FU, with response rates reported ranging from 27% to 50%, with a suggestion of higher response rates seen in squamous cell carcinoma. Etoposide and cisplatin with or without 5-FU have also undergone a phase II evaluation.[532–534] Combination regimens that include paclitaxel have been evaluated in esophageal cancer patients. In three phase II trials of paclitaxel and cisplatin, response rates ranged from 43% to 50%; activity was comparable in both histologic tumor types, often with severe hematologic toxicity.[535–537] A phase I trial of weekly carboplatin dosed from an area under the curve of 2 to 5 combined with a 1-hour infusion of paclitaxel, 100 mg/m^2, in 40 patients with advanced esophageal and GEJ cancer had an overall response rate of 54%.[538]

The three-drug combination of paclitaxel (175 mg/m^2, 3-hour infusion), combined with cisplatin (20 mg/m^2 daily days 1–5) and 5-FU (1,000 mg/m^2 per day continuous infusion $\times$ 120 hours) was evaluated in a multicenter 60 patient trial.[539] A 48% response rate was reported (56% in patients with squamous cell cancer and 46% in patients with adenocarcinoma). Toxicity resulted in unplanned hospitalizations for 48% of patients.

Although the dose and schedule of paclitaxel in combination with other active drugs varies among phase II trials, shorter infusion schedules of paclitaxel, in particular the weekly 1-hour schedule, result in less myelotoxicity.

Other regimens of interest include those containing irinotecan. First reported was the doublet of irinotecan and cisplatin administered in low dose on a weekly schedule.[540] In vitro studies demonstrated sequence-dependent synergy for cisplatin followed by irinotecan, which prevents the removal of cisplatin-induced DNA interstrand cross-links. Two trials yielded encouraging results (51% to

57% response) with a regimen of cisplatin (30 mg/m^2) followed by irinotecan (65 mg/m^2) administered weekly for 4 weeks, repeated every 6 weeks in adenocarcinoma and squamous cancer.[540,541] Dysphagia and global quality of life were improved in the majority of patients in one of these trials.[540] In both studies, toxicity consisted of myelosuppression, diarrhea, and fatigue. Irinotecan 50 mg/m^2 combined with weekly cisplatin 25 mg/m^2 and docetaxel 30 mg/m^2, days 1 and 8 every 21 days, was studied in a phase II trial in 39 patients with esophagogastric cancer.[542] An encouraging response rate of 54% was observed, with tolerable rates of grade 3 and 4 neutropenia (21%) and diarrhea (26%). However, a recent randomized phase II trial reported only in abstract form compared the chemotherapy regimens FOLFOX, irinotecan and cisplatin, and ECF, all combined with the EGFR-targeted agent cetuximab (Table 45.10).[543] The FOLFOX and ECF arms had similar response rates and overall survival, and the toxicity analysis favored the FOLFOX arm, and has led to further questioning of the contribution of epirubicin to a two-drug combination of oxaliplatin and a fluorinated pyrimidine. Notable, however, was the inferior performance of the irinotecan–cisplatin arm, which had the lowest rates of response and overall survival.

Recent studies exploring non–cisplatin-containing combination regimens have employed the taxanes and irinotecan. Although these trials have indicated encouraging response rates in the phase II setting, substantial hematologic and diarrheal toxicities of these regimens may not offer an advantage over the older cisplatin-containing regimens.[544–548] Docetaxel has been evaluated in combination with irinotecan in four recent phase II trials. Two trials evaluated irinotecan doses of 100 to 160 mg/m^2 and docetaxel doses of 50 to 60 mg/m^2 administered once every 3 weeks. Two trials evaluated the day 1 and day 8 schedule of irinotecan (50 to 55 mg/m^2) and docetaxel (25 to 35 mg/m^2) cycled every 3 weeks. Response rates range from 13 to 30 hematologic toxicity, which exceeded 50% in patients treated on the schedule of once every 3 weeks, seemed to be less using the day 1 and day 8 schedule compared with the once every 3 weeks schedule.

A phase III comparison of cisplatin and infusional 5-FU to the combination of irinotecan and infusional 5-FU was recently reported in advanced esophagogastric cancer (see Table 45.9).[549] Response rates (25.8% to 31.8%) and progression-free (4.2 months versus 5.0 months), and overall survival (8.7 months versus 9.0 months) were comparable for the two regimens. Toxicity favored the irinotecan 5-FU arm. Data from this trial and the oxaliplatin-based studies conducted in Europe have led to greater utilization of both irinotecan and oxaliplatin in combination with infusional 5-FU for the treatment of advanced esophagogastric cancer at European centers.

Docetaxel and either vinorelbine or capecitabine were evaluated in phase II trials in squamous cell carcinoma[550,551] with response rates of 46% to 60%. In summary, recent trials of combination regimens that include paclitaxel or irinotecan appear to have comparable response rates to previous regimens; however, the duration of response remains brief. In addition, the toxicities recorded in some of these phase II single-institution experiences have been excessive.

Targeted Agents

Phase III trials of targeted agents studied alone or in combination with chemotherapy are outlined in Table 45.10. Validation of the activity of a growth factor receptor–targeted agent, trastuzumab, was recently achieved in esophagogastric cancer (see Table 45.10).[552] Over 3,800 patients with gastric or GEJ adenocarcinoma were screened for overexpression of the HER2 receptor by fluorescence in situ hybridization (FISH) and immunohistochemistry; 22.1% tested positive. Five hundred ninety-four patients were ultimately randomized to chemotherapy alone with (1) capecitabine 1,000 mg/m^2 twice a day for 14 days or (2) infusional 5-FU 800 mg/m^2 per day for 5 days, combined with cisplatin 80 mg/m^2 on day 1, cycled every 3 weeks, or to chemotherapy plus trastuzumab 6 mg/kg once every 3 weeks. The majority of patients received capecitabine plus cisplatin as the chemotherapy regimen. All end points were improved with the addition of trastuzumab to chemotherapy, including antitumor response (47.3% versus 34.5%), progression-free survival (6.7 months versus 5.5 months), and overall survival (13.8 months versus 11.1 months) (HR, 0.74; $p = 0.0046$). Toxicity was comparable for the two

TABLE 45.10

Phase II–III Randomized Trials of Targeted Agents

Regimen	Patients (N)	Histologic Type	Response Rate (%)	Overall Survival (months)	Reference
Cape-C +/− trastuzumab	584	A	47 / 35	13.8 / 11.1	552
FOLFOX vs Irino-C vs ECF + cetuximab	210	A/S	54 / 46 / 58	12.4 / 8.9 / 11.5	561
EOX +/− panitumumab	553	A	46 / 42	8.8 / 11.3	562
Cape-C +/− cetuximab	904	A	29 / 29	10 / 10	563
5-FU–C +/− cetuximab	62	S	19 / 13	9.5 / 5.5	564
Cape-C +/− bevacizumab	774	A	46 / 37	12.1 / 10.1	566
Ramucirumab vs placebo	355	A	3 / 3	5.2 / 3.8	567
Everolimus vs placebo	656	A	4 / 2	5.4 / 4.3	568

Cape, capecitabine; C, cisplatin; A, adenocarcinoma; FOLFOX, 5-FU + oxaliplatin; Irino-C, irinotecan-cisplatin; ECF, epirubicin/cisplatin; S, squamous cell carcinoma; EOX, epirubicin/cisplatin or oxaliplatin/5-FU or capecitabine.

treatment arms, with no significant cardiotoxicity from trastuzumab other than an asymptomatic, less than 10% drop in left ventricular ejection fraction, which was slightly higher on the trastuzumab arm compared to chemotherapy alone (4.6% versus 1.1%). Based on these results, the inclusion of trastuzumab in the first-line treatment of HER2+ metastatic esophagogastric cancer should now be considered. Based on these data and pilot data combining trastuzumab with chemoradiotherapy in esophageal cancer RTOG has undertaken a phase III trial (RTOG-1010) comparing preoperative chemoradiotherapy with carboplatin and paclitaxel with or without trastuzumab in locally advanced adenocarcinoma of the esophagus and GEJ, as discussed previously.

In patients with localized esophageal adenocarcinoma, HER2+ disease was associated with a significantly lower tumor grade, earlier stage of disease with fewer malignant lymph nodes, and the presence of Barrett's esophagus. These features of HER2+ localized esophageal cancer led to an independent improvement in disease-specific survival (HR, 0.54; 95% CI, 0.35 to 0.84) and overall survival ($p = 0.0022$), suggesting that HER2+ is a favorable prognostic feature in localized esophageal adenocarcinoma.[553]

With evidence for effectiveness of agents targeting the EGFR in NSCLC (including receptor-associated tyrosine-kinase inhibitors) and in colorectal cancer (including monoclonal antibodies blocking the binding of the EGFR ligand), recent phase II trials have evaluated EGFR-targeted agents in esophageal squamous cell and adenocarcinoma. A recent phase II trial of the EGFR tyrosine-kinase inhibitor gefitinib failed to indicate activity for esophageal adenocarcinoma, but limited activity was observed in squamous cell cancer.[554] A second trial indicated some limited activity for adenocarcinoma,[555] but in both trials, most patients experienced early disease progression. A phase II trial of the EGFR tyrosine-kinase inhibitor erlotinib reported a 9% response rate in 44 patients with adenocarcinoma of the GEJ.[556] With these mixed phase II trial results, a recent negative trial for an EGFR tyrosine-kinase inhibitor was reported only in abstract form by Dutton et al.[557] The trial compared best supportive care to treatment with gefitinib in patients with esophageal and GEJ adenocarcinomas progressing on conventional chemotherapy. In this large trial, no difference in overall survival could be demonstrated for gefitinib compared to supportive care alone.

Monoclonal antibodies targeting the EGFR, including cetuximab and panitumumab, have proceeded to phase III trial investigation combined with chemotherapy, based on promising data from phase II trials.[558–560] The randomized phase II trial conducted by the CALGB and ECOG evaluated three modern chemotherapy regimens combined with cetuximab in the first-line treatment of esophageal and GEJ cancer (see Table 45.10),[561] and was discussed previously. The regimens used were weekly irinotecan–cisplatin, ECF, and FOLFOX (5-FU, leucovorin, and oxaliplatin). The trial indicated comparable response rates, progression-free survival, and overall survival for the FOLFOX and ECF plus cetuximab arms, whereas the irinotecan–cisplatin arm was inferior. The final results of this study may not contribute much to the debate about EGFR-targeted agents, because two large phase III trials of these agents combined with chemotherapy failed to improve outcomes. Waddell and colleagues[562] reported results of the REAL-3 trial in esophagogastric cancer, comparing patient treatment with EOX with or without the EGFR antibody panitumumab (see Table 45.10).[562] In the 553 patients treated, although response rates for treatment with or without panitumumab were similar, overall survival was significantly inferior on the panitumumab arm (11.3 versus 8.8 months) and progression-free survival trended inferior for panitumumab (7.4 versus 6.0 months). Toxicity rates were higher on the panitumumab arm, and the chemotherapy starting doses were lower with panitumumab than on the chemotherapy alone arm. Prognostic biomarkers studied on the trial included *KRAS* mutation, *PIK3CA* kinase mutation, and loss of phosphatase and tensin homolog (PTEN). These markers were affected in a tiny minority of patients, and no clear biomarker has emerged from this trial. The potential deleterious effect of adding an EGFR anti-

body to the treatment of esophagogastric cancer was also seen in a recent chemoradiotherapy trial, discussed earlier, in which adding cetuximab to definitive chemoradiotherapy in esophageal cancer also appeared to worsen outcomes.[349] A second negative trial for EGFR-targeted antibodies in advanced disease was reported by Lordick et al. (see Table 45.10).[563] The 904 patients with esophagogastric cancer were randomized to treatment with capecitabine and cisplatin with or without cetuximab. Progression-free survival and overall survival also trended inferior on the cetuximab arm (progression-free survival, 5.6 versus 4.4 months; overall survival, 10.7 versus 9.4 months), and response rates were identical (29%). In contrast to these negative trials, Lorenzen et al.[564] reported results of a small phase II trial in advanced squamous cancer of the esophagus comparing 5-FU–cisplatin with or without cetuximab (see Table 45.10). Outcomes were poor on both arms of the trial; however, response rates and overall survivals were improved on the cetuximab arm (19% versus 13%; 9.5 months versus 5.5 months). A larger phase III trial in squamous cancer of the esophagus is now ongoing (NCT01627379) to evaluate panitumumab combined with 5-FU and cisplatin. RTOG-0436, adding cetuximab to primary chemoradiotherapy in locally advanced esophageal cancer,[350] was discussed earlier, and was also a negative trial for the addition of EGFR-targeted therapy.

Another growth factor receptor pathway under active investigation is the vascular endothelial growth factor (VEGF) receptor pathway, based on trials that demonstrate improved effectiveness for chemotherapy in colorectal cancer when combined with the anti–VEGF-A ligand monoclonal antibody bevacizumab. A recent phase II trial combined bevacizumab at a dose of 15 mg/kg every 3 weeks in combination with a day 1 and day 8 schedule of irinotecan (65 mg/m^2) and cisplatin (30 mg/m^2).[565] The multicenter trial treated 47 patients treated with metastatic adenocarcinoma of the GEJ and more distal gastric cancer. An encouraging response rate of 65% was observed, with a suggestion of improvement in time to tumor progression (8.9 months) compared with historical controls. A phase III trial combining bevacizumab with either 5-FU or capecitabine plus cisplatin in 774 patients with esophagogastric adenocarcinoma was recently reported by Ohtsu and colleagues (see Table 45.10).[566] Despite improvements in progression-free survival (5.3 to 6.7 months) and response rate (37% to 46%), a trend toward improvement in overall survival did not reach statistical significance (10.1 to 12.1 months; HR, 0.87; $p = 0.1002$). Another VEGF-targeted agent, ramucirumab, which blocks ligand binding to the receptor VEGF2, indicated a positive effectiveness in refractory esophagogastric cancer compared to placebo.[567] Fuchs and colleagues[567] randomized 355 patients progressing on 5-FU or platinum-based chemotherapy to best supportive care plus placebo versus best supportive care plus ramucirumab administered once every 2 weeks. Although no significant antitumor responses were seen, overall survival was significantly improved with ramucirumab (3.8 to 5.2 months) and toxicity was limited to a slight increase in hypertension. Results for studies of the combination of ramucirumab with chemotherapy in first- or second-line treatment are pending publication. The positive results for ramucirumab have led to a resurgent interest in the study of VEGF-targeted agents in esophageal cancer.

Finally, a recent large, placebo-controlled trial in chemotherapy refractory esophagogastric cancer compared placebo to the mammalian target of rapamycin (mTOR)–targeted agent everolimus in 656 patients (see Table 45.10).[568] Although progression-free survival was slightly improved with everolimus, there was no improvement in overall survival (5.4 months for everolimus versus 4.3 months for placebo).

STAGE-DIRECTED TREATMENT RECOMMENDATIONS

Although level I evidence is lacking to support ironclad recommendations regarding the most effective treatment of patients grouped by stage in many clinical situations, reasonable trial-generated information exists to suggest appropriate therapeutic interventions for patients grouped under broad staging categories.

Resection remains the standard by which all other treatment options must be measured for patients with high-grade dysplasia in the setting of Barrett's esophagus or T1 disease limited to the mucosa, with the caveat that esophagectomy-associated mortality must be extremely low. EMR may be considered an appropriate first step in addressing patients with mucosa-limited lesions. Intensive long-term endoscopic surveillance for patients with Barrett's esophagus–associated high-grade dysplasia is necessary to limit both cancer- and treatment-related mortality.

An esophagectomy is an appropriate method for treating patients with stage I, II, and III disease. Alternatively, definitive chemoradiation is a therapeutic option for patients with stage II and III disease, especially those who are not considered surgical candidates or who have squamous cell carcinoma at or above the carina. The high rate of persistent or recurrent local–regional disease after definitive chemoradiation suggests that additional local therapy in the form of surgery may be necessary and beneficial. This potential benefit may be realized only if perioperative mortality is minimized. Preoperative chemoradiation has been proven to be more effective than surgery alone, and is now appropriately embraced by US oncologists for patients with resectable stage IIB and III esophageal cancers. Defining more effective regimens must continue to be the focus of well-designed clinical trials. Postoperative chemoradiation should be reserved for patients with resected adenocarcinoma of the GEJ. Preoperative chemotherapy is an accepted standard of care in the United Kingdom but is still considered investigational in the United States. All patients with unresectable or stage IV disease are ideally suited for clinical trials exploring novel therapeutic agents and approaches.

SELECTED REFERENCES

The full reference list can be accessed at lwwhealthlibrary.com/oncology.

3. Howlader N, Noone AM, Krapcho M, et al. (eds). SEER Cancer Statistics Review, 1975–2010. Bethesda, MD: National Cancer Institute. SEER Web site. http://seer.cancer.gov/csr/1975_2010/. April 2013.

4. Siegel R, Naishadham D, Jemal A. Cancer Statistics, 2013. *CA Cancer J Clin* 2013;63:11–30.

9. Cook MB, Shaheen NJ, Anderson LA, et al. Cigarette smoking increases risk of Barrett's esophagus: an analysis of the Barrett's and Esophageal Adenocarcinoma Consortium. *Gastroenterology* 2012;142:744–753.

16. Bravi F, Edefonti V, Randi G, et al. Dietary patterns and the risk of esophageal cancer. *Ann Oncol* 2012;23:765–770.

22. Edelstein ZR, Farrow DC, Bonner MP, et al. Central adiposity and risk of Barrett's esophagus. *Gastroenterology* 2007;133:403–411.

24. Lagergren J. Influence of obesity on the risk of esophageal disorders. *Nat Rev Gastroenterol Hepatol* 2011;8:340–347.

25. Lagergren J, Bergstrom R, Lindgren A, et al. Symptomatic gastroesophageal reflux as a risk factor for esophageal adenocarcinoma. *N Engl J Med* 1999;340:825–831.

26. Chow WH, Finkle WD, McLaughlin JK, et al. The relation of gastroesophageal reflux disease and its treatment to adenocarcinomas of the esophagus and gastric cardia. *JAMA* 1995;274:474–477.

27. Islami F, Kamangar F. *Helicobacter pylori* and esophageal cancer risk: a meta-analysis. *Cancer Prev Res (Phila)* 2008;1:329–338.

31. Spechler SJ. Clinical practice. Barrett's esophagus. *N Engl J Med* 2002;346:836–842.

33. Spechler SJ. Barrett esophagus and risk of esophageal cancer: a clinical review. *JAMA* 2013;310:627–636.

35. Bhat S, Coleman HG, Yousef F, et al. Risk of malignant progression in Barrett's esophagus patients: results from a large population-based study. *J Natl Cancer Inst* 2011;103:1049–1057.

36. Hvid-Jensen F, Pedersen L, Drewes AM, et al. Incidence of adenocarcinoma among patients with Barrett's esophagus. *N Engl J Med* 2011;365:1375–1383.

40. Spechler SJ, Sharma P, Souza RF, et al. American Gastroenterological Association. American Gastroenterological Association medical position statement on the management of Barrett's esophagus. *Gastroenterology* 2011;140:1084–1091.

41. Katz PO, Gerson LB, Vela MF. Guidelines for the diagnosis and management of gastroesophageal reflux disease. *Am J Gastroenterol* 2013;108:308–328.

42. Evans JA, Early DS, Fukami N, et al. Standards of Practice Committee of the American Society for Gastrointestinal Endoscopy. The role of endoscopy in Barrett's esophagus and other premalignant conditions of the esophagus. *Gastrointest Endosc* 2012;76:1087–1094.

43. Spechler SJ, Lee E, Ahnen D, et al. Long-term outcome of medical and surgical therapies for gastroesophageal reflux disease: follow-up of a randomized controlled trial. *JAMA* 2001;285:2331–2338.

46. Ferguson MK, Durkin A. Long-term survival after esophagectomy for Barrett's adenocarcinoma in endoscopically surveyed and nonsurveyed patients. *J Gastrointest Surg* 2002;6:29–35.

52. Faybush EM, Sampliner RE. Randomized trials in the treatment of Barrett's esophagus. *Dis Esophagus* 2005;18:291–297.

53. Singh S, Garg SK, Singh PP, et al. Acid-suppressive medications and risk of oesophageal adenocarcinoma in patients with Barrett's oesophagus: a systematic review and meta-analysis. *Gut* 2013;Nov 12 [Epub ahead of print].

54. Haggitt RC. Barrett's esophagus, dysplasia, and adenocarcinoma. *Hum Pathol* 1994;25:982–993.

59. Heath E, Canto MI, Piantadosi S, et al. Secondary chemoprevention of Barrett's esophagus with celecoxib: results of a randomized trial. *J Natl Cancer Inst* 2007;99:545–557.

81. Siewert JR, Feith M, Werner M, et al. Adenocarcinoma of the esophagogastric junction. Results of surgical therapy based on anatomic-topographic classification in 1,002 consecutive patients. *Ann Surg* 2000;232:353–361.

86. Dulak AM, Schumacher SE, van Lieshout J, et al. Gastrointestinal adenocarcinomas of the esophagus, stomach, and colon exhibit distinct patterns of genome instability and oncogenesis. *Cancer Res* 2012;72:4383–4393.

87. Dulak AM, Stojanov P, Peng S, et al. Exome and whole genome sequencing of esophageal adenocarcinoma identifies recurrent driver events and mutational complexity. *Nat Genet* 2013;5:478–486.

88. Agrawal N, Jiao Y, Bettegowda C, et al. Comparative genomic analysis of esophageal adenocarcinoma and squamous cell carcinoma. *Cancer Discov* 2012;2:899–905.

90. Edge SB, Byrd DR, Compton CC, et al. American Joint Commission on Cancer. *AJCC Cancer Staging Manual*. 7th ed. New York: Springer-Verlag; 2009.

101. Ilson DH, Minsky BD, Ku GY, et al. Phase 2 trial of induction and concurrent chemoradiotherapy with weekly irinotecan and cisplatin followed by surgery for esophageal cancer. *Cancer* 2012;118:2820–2827.

105. Kelsen DP, Ginsberg R, Pajak RF, et al. Chemotherapy followed by surgery compared with surgery alone for localized esophageal cancer. *N Engl J Med* 1998;339:1979–1984.

106. Medical Research Council Oesophageal Cancer Working Group. Surgical resection with or without preoperative chemotherapy in oesophageal cancer: a randomised controlled trial. *Lancet* 2002;359:1727–1733.

107. Urba SG, Orringer MB, Turrisi A, et al. Randomized trial of preoperative chemoradiation versus surgery alone in patients with locoregional esophageal carcinoma. *J Clin Oncol* 2001;19:305–313.

110. Arnott SJ, Duncan W, Gignoux M, et al. Preoperative radiotherapy in esophageal carcinoma: a meta-analysis using individual patient data (Oesophageal Cancer Collaborative Group). *Int J Radiat Oncol Biol Phys* 1998;41:579–583.

112. Kelsen DP, Winter KA, Gunderson LL, et al. Long-term results of RTOG Trial 8911 (USA Intergroup 113): a random assignment trial comparison of chemotherapy followed by surgery compared with surgery alone for esophageal cancer. *J Clin Oncol* 2007;25:3719–3725.

113. Allum WH, Stenning SP, Bancewicz J, et al. Long term results of a randomized trial of surgery with or without preoperative chemotherapy in esophageal cancer. *J Clin Oncol* 2009;27:5062–5067.

114. Cooper JS, Guo MD, Herskovic A, et al. Chemoradiotherapy of locally advanced esophageal cancer: long-term follow-up of a prospective randomized trial (RTOG 85-01). Radiation Therapy Oncology Group. *JAMA* 1999;281:1623–1627.

116. Bedenne L, Michel P, Bouche O, et al. Chemoradiation followed by surgery compared to chemoradiation alone in squamous cancer of the esophagus: FFCD 9102. *J Clin Oncol* 2007;25:1160–1168.

117. Stahl M, Stuschke M, Lehmann N, et al. Chemoradiation with and without surgery in patients with locally advanced squamous cell cancer of the esophagus. *J Clin Oncol* 2005;23:2310–2317.

151. Jost C, Binek J, Schuller JC, et al. Endosonographic radial tumor thickness after neoadjuvant chemoradiation therapy to predict response and survival in patients with locally advanced esophageal cancer: a prospective multicenter phase II study. Swiss Group for Clinical Cancer Research (SAKK 75/02). *Gastrointest Endosc* 2010;7:1114.

152. Flamen P, van Cutsem E, Lerut T, et al. The utility of positron emission tomography with 18F-fluorodeoxyglucose (FDG-PET) to predict the pathologic response and survival of esophageal cancer after preoperative chemoradiation therapy (CRT). *Proc Am Soc Clin Oncol* 2001;20:127a.

157. Ott K, Weber WA, Lordick F, et al. Metabolic imaging predicts response, survival, and recurrence in adenocarcinomas of the esophagogastric junction. *J Clin Oncol* 2006;24:4692–4698.

PRACTICE OF ONCOLOGY

159. Lordick F, Ott K, Krause BJ, et al. PET to assess early metabolic response and to guide treatment of adenocarcinoma of the oesophagogastric junction: the MUNICON phase II trial. *Lancet Oncol* 2007;8:797–805.

160. zum Büschenfelde CM, Herrmann K, Schuster T, et al. 18F-FDG PET-guided salvage neoadjuvant radiochemotherapy of adenocarcinoma of the esophagogastric junction: the MUNICON II trial. *J Nucl Med* 2011;52:1189–1196.

161. Klaeser B, Nitzsche E, Schuller JC, et al. Limited predictive value of FDG-PET for response assessment in the preoperative treatment of esophageal cancer: results of a prospective mutli-center trial (SAKK 75/01). *Onkologie* 2009;32:724–730.

162. Rebollo Aguirre AC, Ramos-Font C, Villegas Portero R, et al. 18F-fluorode-oxiglucose positron emission tomography for the evaluation of neoadjuvant therapy response in esophageal cancer: systematic review of the literature. *Ann Surg* 2009;250:247–254.

163. Kwee R. Prediction of tumor response to neoadjuvant therapy in patients with esophageal cancer with the use of 18F FDG PET: a systematic review. *Radiology* 2010;254:707–717.

170. Rizk N, Venkatraman E, Park B, et al. The prognostic importance of the number of involved lymph nodes in esophageal cancer: implications for revisions of the American Joint Committee on Cancer staging system. *J Thorac Cardiovasc Surg* 2005;132:1374–1381.

172. Rice TW, Rusch VW, Ishwaran H, et al. Cancer of the esophagus and esophagogastric junction: data-driven staging for the seventh edition of the American Joint Committee on Cancer/International Union Against Cancer Cancer Staging Manuals. Worldwide Esophageal Cancer Collaboration. *Cancer* 2010;116:3763–3773.

173. Merkow RP, Bilimoria KY, McCarter MD. Use of multimodality neoadjuvant therapy for esophageal cancer in the United States: assessment of 987 hospitals. *Ann Surg Oncol.* 2012;19:357–364.

178. Stein HJ, Feith M, Brucher BL, et al. Early esophageal cancer: pattern of lymphatic spread and prognostic factors for long-term survival after surgical resection. *Ann Surg* 2005;242:566–573.

179. Dunbar KB, Spechler SJ. The risk of lymph-node metastases in patients with high-grade dysplasia or intramucosal carcinoma in Barrett's esophagus: a systematic review. *Am J Gastroenterol* 2012;107:850–862.

180. Rastogi A, Puli S, El-Serag HB, et al. Incidence of esophageal adenocarcinoma in patients with Barrett's esophagus and high-grade dysplasia: a meta-analysis. *Gastrointest Endosc* 2008;67:394–398.

182. Konda VJ, Ross AS, Ferguson MK. Is the risk of concomitant invasive esophageal cancer in high-grade dysplasia in Barrett's esophagus overestimated? *Clin Gastroenterol Hepatol* 2008;6:159–164.

186. Dar MS, Goldblum JR, Rice TW, et al. Can extent of high grade dysplasia in Barrett's oesophagus predict the presence of adenocarcinoma at oesophagectomy? *Gut* 2003;52:486–489.

187. Overholt BF, Lightdale CJ, Wang KK, et al. Photodynamic therapy with porfimer sodium for ablation of high-grade dysplasia in Barrett's esophagus: international, partially blinded, randomized phase III trial. *Gastrointest Endosc* 2005;62:488–498.

192. Shaheen NJ, Sharma P, Overholt BF, et al. Radiofrequency ablation in Barrett's esophagus and dysplasia. *N Engl J Med* 2009;360:2277–2288.

193. Ell C, May A, Pech O, et al. Curative endoscopic resection of early esophageal adenocarciomas (Barrett's cancer). *Gastrointest Endosc* 2007;65:3–10.

198. Chennat J, Konda V, Ross AS, et al. Complete Barrett's eradication endoscopic mucosal resection: an effective treatment modality for high-grade dysplasia and intramucosal carcinoma—an American single-center experience. *Am J Gastroenterol* 2009;104:2684–2692.

199. Bennett C, Vakil N, Bergman J, et al. Consensus statements for management of Barrett's dysplasia and early-stage esophageal adenocarcinoma, based on a Delphi process. *Gastroenterology* 2012;143:336–346.

204. Dunn DH, Johnson EM, Morphew JA, et al. Robot-assisted transhiatal esophagectomy: a 3-year single-center experience. *Dis Esophagus* 2013;26:159–166.

205. Luketich JD, Pennathur A, Awais O. Outcomes after minimally invasive esophagectomy: review of over 1000 patients. *Ann Surg* 2012;256:95–103.

206. Pennathur A, Farkas A, Krasinskas AM, et al. Esophagectomy for T1 esophageal cancer: outcomes in 100 patients and implications for endoscopic therapy. *Ann Thorac Surg* 2009;87:1048–1054.

208. Wu PC, Posner MC. The role of surgery in the management of oesophageal cancer. *Lancet Oncol* 2003;4:481–488.

209. Biere SS, van Berge Henegouwen MI, Maas KW, et al. Minimally invasive versus open oesophagectomy for patients with oesophageal cancer: a multicentre, open-label, randomised controlled trial. *Lancet* 2012;379:1887–1892.

215. Birkmeyer JD, Siewers AE, Finlayson EV, et al. Hospital volume and surgical mortality in the United tates. *N Engl J Med* 2002;346:1128–1137.

218. Wouters MW, Karin-Kos H, le Cessie S, et al. Centralization of esophageal cancer surgery: does it improve clinical outcomes? *Ann Surg Oncol* 2009;16:1789–1798.

219. Reames BN, Ghaferi AA, Birkmeyer JD, et al. Hospital Volume and Operative Mortality in the Modern Era. *Ann Surg* 2013 Dec 23 [Epub Ahead of Print].

220. Posner MC. Techniques of esophageal resection. In: Posner MC, Vokes EE, Weichselbaum RR, eds. *Cancer of the Upper Gastrointestinal Tract.* Hamilton, Ontario: BC Decker; 2002:1.

225. Orringer MB, Marshall B, Chang AC, et al. Two thousand transhiatal esophagectomies: changing trends, lessons learned. *Ann Surg* 2007;246:363–372.

232. McKeown KC. Total three-stage oesophagectomy for cancer of the oesophagus. *Br J Surg* 1976;63:259–262.

234. Bizekis C, Kent MS, Luketich JD, et al. Initial experience with minimally invasive Ivor Lewis esophagectomy. *Ann Thorac Surg* 2006;82:402–406.

240. Bosset JF, Gignoux M, Triboulet JP, et al. Chemoradiotherapy followed by surgery compared with surgery alone in squamous cell cancer of the esophagus. *N Engl J Med* 1997;337:161–167.

242. Hulscher JB, Tijssen JG, Obertop H, et al. Transthoracic versus transhiatal resection for carcinoma of the esophagus: a meta-analysis. *Ann Thorac Surg* 2001;72:306–313.

243. Boshier PR, Anderson O, Hanna GB. Transthoracic versus transhiatal esophagectomy for the treatment of esophagogastric cancer: a meta-analysis. *Ann Surg* 2011;254:894–906.

245. Chang AC, Ji J, Birkmeyer NJ, et al. Outcomes after transhiatal and transthoracic esophagectomy for cancer. *Ann Thorac Surg* 2008;85:424–429.

249. Hulscher JB, van Sandick JW, deBoer AG, et al. Extended transthoracic resection compared with limited transhiatal resection for adenocarcinoma of the esophagus. *N Engl J Med* 2002;347:1662–1669.

250. Omloo JM, Lagarde SM, Hulscher JB, et al. Extended transthoracic resection compared with limited transhiatal resection for adenocarcinoma of the mid/distal esophagus: five-year survival of randomized clinical trial. *Ann Surg* 2007;246:992–1000.

252. Lerut T, Nafteux P, Moons J, et al. Three-field lymphadenectomy for carcinoma of the esophagus and gastroesophageal junction in 174 R0 resections: impact on staging, disease-free survival, and outcome: a plea for adaptation of TNM classification in upper-half esophageal carcinoma. *Ann Surg* 2004;240:962–972.

266. Cunningham D, Allum W, Stenning SP, et al. Perioperative chemotherapy versus surgery alone for resectable gastroesophageal cancer. *N Engl J Med* 2006;355:11–20.

267. Ychou M, Boige V, Pignon JP, et al. Perioperative chemotherapy compared with surgery alone for resectable gastroesophageal adenocarcinoma: an FNLCC and FFCF multicenter phase III trial. *J Clin Oncol* 2011;29:1715–1721.

268. Schuhmacher C, Gretschel S, Lordick F, et al. Neoadjuvant chemotherapy compared with surgery alone for locally advanced cancer of the stomach and cardia: European Organization for Research and Treatment of Cancer randomized Trial 40954. *J Clin Oncol* 2010;28:5210–5218.

269. Boonstra JJ, Kok TC, Wijnjoven BPL, et al. Chemotherapy followed by surgery versus surgery alone in patients with resectable oesophageal squamous cell carcinoma: long-term results of a randomized trial. *BMC Cancer* 2011;11:181.

270. Thirion PG, Michiels S, LeMaitre A, et al. Individual patient data based meta analysis assessing preoperative chemotherapy in resectable oesophageal cancer. *J Clin Oncol* 2007;25:4512.

273. Teniere P, Hay JM, Fingerhut A, et al. Postoperative radiation therapy does not increase survival after curative resection for squamous cell carcinoma of the middle and lower esophagus as shown by a multicenter controlled trial. French University Association for Surgical Research. *Surg Gynecol Obstet* 1991;173:123.

280. Herskovic A, Martz K, Al-Sarraf M, et al. Combined chemotherapy and radiotherapy compared with radiotherapy alone in patients with cancer of the esophagus. *N Engl J Med* 1992;326:1593–1598.

281. Minsky B, Pajak T, Ginsberg RJ, et al. INT 0123 (Radiation Therapy Oncology Group 94–05) phase III trial of combined-modality therapy for esophageal cancer: high-dose versus standard-dose radiation therapy. *J Clin Oncol* 2002;20:1167–1174.

284. Forastiere A, Orringer MB, Perez-Tamayo C, et al. Preoperative chemoradiation followed by transhiatal esophagectomy for carcinoma of the esophagus: final report. *J Clin Oncol* 1993;11:1118–1123.

301. Meredith K, Weber J, Turaga K, et al. Pathologic response after neoadjuvant therapy is the major determinant of survival in patients with esophageal cancer. *Ann Surg Oncol* 2010;17:1159–1167.

302. Leichman LP, Goldman BH, Bohanes PO, et al. S0356: A phase II clinical and a prospective molecular trial with oxaliplatin, fluorouracil, and external-beam radiation therapy before surgery for patients with esophageal adenocarcinoma. *J Clin Oncol* 2011;29:4555–4560.

317. Van Hagen P, Hulshof MC, van Lanschot JJ, et al. Preoperative chemoradiotherapy for esophageal or junctional cancer. *N Engl J Med* 2012;366:2074–2084.

318. Sarkaria IS, Rizk NP, Bains MS, et al. Post-treatment endoscopic biopsy is a poor predictor of pathologic response in patients undergoing chemoradiation therapy for esophageal cancer. *Ann Surg* 2009;249:764–767.

319. Chedella NKS, Suzuki A, Xiao L, et al. Association between clinical complete response and pathological complete response after preoperative chemoradiation in patients with gastroesophageal cancer: analysis in a large cohort. *Ann Oncol* 2013;24:1262.

320. Yang Q, Cleary KR, Yao JC, et al. Significance of post-chemoradiation biopsy in predicting residual esophageal carcinoma in the surgical specimen. *Dis Esophagus* 2004;14:38–43.

326. Fields RC, Strong VE, Gonen M, et al. Recurrence and survival after pathologic complete response to preoperative therapy followed by surgery for gastric or gastroesophageal adenocarcinoma. *Br J Cancer* 2011;104:1840–1847.

327. Downey RJ, Akhurst T, Ilson D, et al. Whole body 18FDG-PET and the response of esophageal cancer to induction therapy: results of a prospective trial. *J Clin Oncol* 2003;21:428–432.

328. Flamen P, Van Cutsem E, Lerut A, et al. Positron emission tomography for assessment of the response to induction radiochemotherapy in locally advanced oesophageal cancer. *Ann Oncol* 2002;13:361–368.

329. Vallböhmer D, Holscher AH, Dietleiin M, et al. [18F] fluorodeoxyglucose-positron emission tomography for the assessment of histologic response and prognosis after completion of neoadjuvant chemoradiation in esophageal cancer. *Ann Surg* 2009;250:888–894.

330. Klayton T, Li T, Yu JQ, et al. The role of qualitative and quantitative analysis of F18-FDG positron emission tomography in predicting pathologic response following chemoradiotherapy in patients with esophageal carcinoma. *J Gastrointest Surg* 2012;43:612–618.

332. Monjazeb AM, Riedlinger G, Aklilu M, et al. Outcomes of patients with esophageal cancer staged with [18F] fluorodeoxyglucose positron emission tomography (FDG-PET): can postradiochemotherapy FDG-PED predict the utility of resection? *J Clin Oncol* 2010;28:4714–4721.

334. McCurdy M, McAleer MF, Wei W, et al. Induction and concurrent taxanes enhance both the pulmonary metabolic response and the radiation pneumonitis response in patients with esophagus cancer. *Int J Radiat Oncol Biol Phys* 2010;76:816–823.

337. Kleinberg L, Powell ME, Forastiere AA, et al. Survival outcome of E1201: an Eastern Cooperative Oncology Group randomized phase II trial of neoadjuvant preoperative paclitaxel/cisplatin/radiotherapy or irinotecan/cisplatin/radiotherapy in endoscopy with ultrasound stage esophageal adenocarcinoma. *J Clin Oncol* 2008;26:4532.

338. Kleinberg LR, Eapen S, Hamilton S, et al. E1201: an Eastern Cooperative Oncology Group (ECOG) randomized phase II trial to measure response rate and toxicity of preoperative combined modality paclitaxel/cisplatin/RT or irinotecan/cisplatin/RT in adenocarcinoma of the esophagus. *Int J Rad Oncol Biol Phys* 2006;66:s173.

339. Walsh TN, Noonan N, Hollywood D, et al. A comparison of multimodal therapy and surgery for esophageal adenocarcinoma. *N Engl J Med* 1996;335:462–467.

341. Burmeister BH, Smithers BM, Gebski V, et al. Surgery alone versus chemoradiotherapy followed by surgery for resectable cancer of the oesophagus: a randomised controlled phase III trial. *Lancet Oncol* 2005;6:659–668.

342. Tepper J, Krasna MJ, Niedzwiecki D, et al. Phase III trial of trimodality therapy with cisplatin, fluorouracil, radiotherapy, and surgery compared with surgery alone for esophageal cancer: CALGB 9781. *J Clin Oncol* 2008;26:1086–1092.

344. Stahl M, Walz MK, Stuschke M, et al. Phase III comparison of preoperative chemotherapy compared with chemoradiotherapy in patients with locally advanced adenocarcinoma of the esophagogastric junction. *J Clin Oncol* 2009;27:851–856.

345. Le Prise E, Etienne PL, Meunier B, et al. A randomized study of chemotherapy, radiation therapy, and surgery versus surgery for localized squamous cell carcinoma of the esophagus. *Cancer* 1994;73:1779–1784.

346. Kaklamanos IG, Walker GR, Ferry K, et al. Neoadjuvant treatment for resectable cancer of the esophagus and gastroesophageal junction: a meta-analysis of randomized clinical trials. *Ann Surg Oncol* 2003;10:754–761.

347. Sjoquist KM, Burmeister BH, Smithers BM, et al. Survival after neoadjuvant chemotherapy or chemoradiotherapy for resectable oesophageal carcinoma: an updated meta-analysis. *Lancet Oncol* 2011;12:681–692.

349. Crosby T, Hurt CN, Falk S, et al. Chemoradiotherapy with or without cetuximab in patients with oesophageal cancer (SCOPE-1): a multicenter, phase 2/3 randomized trial. *Lancet Oncol* 2013;14:627–637.

360. MacDonald J, Benedetti J, Smalley S, et al. Chemoradiation of resected gastric cancer: a 10-year follow-up of the phase III trial INT 0116 (SWOG 9008). *Proc Am Soc Clin Oncol* 2009;27:205s.

361. Gordon MA, Gundacker HM, Benedetti J, et al. Assessment of HER2 gene amplification in adenocarcinomas of the stomach or gastroesophageal junction in the INT-0116/SWOG9008 clinical trial. *Ann Oncol* 2013;24:1754–1761.

363. al-Sarraf M, Martz K, Herskovic A, et al. Superiority of chemo-radiotherapy (CT-RT) vs radiotherapy (RT) in patients with esophageal cancer. Final report of an Intergroup randomized and confirmed study. *Proc Am Soc Clin Oncol* 1996;15:abst 206.

364. Suntharalingam M, Moughan J, Cola LR, et al. Outcome results of the 1996–1999 patterns of care survey of the national practice for patients receiving radiation therapy for carcinoma of the esophagus. *J Clin Oncol* 2005;23:2325–2331.

372. al-Sarraf M, Martz K, Herskovic A, et al. Progress report of combined chemo-radiotherapy versus radiotherapy alone in patients with esophageal cancer: an Intergroup study. *J Clin Oncol* 1997;15:277–284.

376. Wong RK, Malthaner RA, Zuraw L, et al. Combined modality radiotherapy and chemotherapy in nonsurgical management of localized carcinoma of the esophagus: a practice guideline. *Int J Radiat Oncol Biol Phys* 2003;55:930–942.

378. Yu J, Ren R, Sun X, et al. A randomized clinical study of surgery versus radiotherapy in the treatment of resectable esophageal cancer. *Proc Am Soc Clin Oncol* 2006;24:181s.

379. Chiu PWY, Chan ACW, Leung SF, et al. Multicenter prospective randomized trial comparing standard esophagectomy with chemoradiotherapy for treatment of squamous esophageal cancer: early results from the Chinese University Research Group for Esophageal Cancer (CURE). *J Gastrointest Surg* 2005;9:794.

382. Crehange G, Maingon P, Peignaux K, et al. Phase III trial of protracted compared with split-course chemoradiation for esophageal cancer: Federation Francophone de Cancerologie Digestive 9102. *J Clin Oncol* 2007;25:4895–4901.

385. Swisher SG, Hofsetter W, Wu TT, et al. Proposed revision of the esophageal cancer staging system to accommodate pathologic response (pP) following preoperative chemoradiation (CRT). *Ann Surg* 2005;241:810–817.

386. Swisher SG, Winter KA, Komaki RU, et al. A phase II study of a paclitaxel-based chemoradiation regimen with selective surgical salvage for resectable locoregionally advanced esophageal cancer: initial reporting of RTOG 0246. *Int J Radiat Oncol Biol Phys* 2012;82:1967–1972.

395. Skinner HD, Xu E, Lee JH, et al. A validated miRNA expression profile for response to neoadjuvant therapy in esophageal cancer. *Proc ASCO* 2013;31:4078(abstr).

398. Brucher BL, Becker K, Lordick F, et al. The clinical impact of histopathologic response assessment by residual tumor cell quantification in esophageal squamous cell carcinomas. *Cancer* 2006;106:2119–2127.

399. McLoughlin J, Melis M, Siegel E, et al. Are patients with esophageal cancer who become PET negative after neoadjuvant chemoradiation free of cancer. *J Am Coll Surg* 2008;206:879–886.

412. Homs MY, Essink-Bot ML, Borsboom GJ, et al. Quality of life after palliative treatment for oesophageal carcinoma—a prospective comparison between stent placement and single dose chemotherapy. *Eur J Cancer* 2004;40:1862–1871.

418. Ishikawa H, Nonaka T, Sakurai H, et al. Usefulness of intraluminal brachytherapy combined with external beam radiation therapy for submucosal esophageal cancer: long-term follow-up results. *Int J Rad Oncol Biol Phys* 2010;76:452–459.

419. Gaspar LE, Qian C, Kocha WI, et al. A phase I/II study of external beam radiation, brachytherapy and concurrent chemotherapy in localized cancer of the esophagus (RTOG 92–07): preliminary toxicity report. *Int J Radiat Oncol Biol Phys* 1997;37:593–599.

421. Gaspar LE, Nag S. Herskovic A, et al. American Brachytherapy Society (ABS) consensus guidelines for brachytherapy of esophageal cancer. *Int J Radiat Oncol Biol Phys* 1997;38:127–132.

428. Kole TP, Aghayere O, Kwah J, et al. Comparison of heart and coronary artery doses associated with intensity-modulated radiotherapy versus three-dimensional conformal radiotherapy for distal esophageal cancer. *Int J Radiat Oncol Biol Phys* 2012;83:1580–1586.

429. Yin L, Wu H, Gong J, et al. Volumetric-modulated arc therapy vs. c-IMRT in esophageal cancer: a treatment planning comparison. *World J Gastroenterol* 2012;18:5266–5275.

436. Lin SH, Wang L, Myles B, et al. Propensity score-based comparison of long-term outcomes with 3-dimensional conformal radiotherapy vs. intensity-modulated radiotherapy for esophageal cancer. *Int J Radiat Oncol Biol Phys* 2012;84:1078–1085.

440. Nishimura Y, Nagata K, Katano S, et al. Severe complications in advanced esophageal cancer treated with radiotherapy after intubation of esophageal stents: a questionnaire survey of the Japanese Society for Esophageal Diseases. *Int J Radiat Oncol Biol Phys* 2003;56:1327.

450. Coia LR, Soffen EM, Schultheiss TE, et al. Swallowing function in patients with esophageal cancer treated with concurrent radiation and chemotherapy. *Cancer* 1993;71:281–286.

452. Sur M, Sur R, Cooper K, et al. Morphologic alterations in esophageal squamous cell carcinoma after preoperative high dose rate intraluminal brachytherapy. *Cancer* 1996;77:2200–2205.

455. Minsky BD. The adjuvant treatment of esophageal cancer. *Sem Radiat Oncol* 1994;4:165–169.

462. Lin SH, Komaki R, Liao Z, et al. Proton beam therapy and concurrent chemotherapy for esophageal cancer. *Int J Radiat Oncol Biol Phys* 2012;83:e345–e351.

470. Konski A, Li T, Christensen M, et al. Symptomatic cardiac toxicity is predicted by dosimetric and patient factors rather than changes in 18F-FDG PET determination of myocardial activity after chemoradiotherapy for esophageal cancer. *Radiother Oncol* 2012;104:72–77.

471. Rueth NM, Shaw D, D'Cunha J, et al. Esophageal stenting and radiotherapy: a multimodal approach for the palliation of symptomatic malignant dysphagia. *Ann Surg Oncol* 2012;19:4223–4228.

483. Bleiberg H, Conroy T, Paillot B, et al. Randomised phase II study of cisplatin and 5-fluorouracil (5-FU) versus cisplatin alone in advanced squamous cell oesophageal cancer. *Eur J Cancer* 1997;33:1216–1220.

517. Webb A, Cunningham D, Scarffe JH, et al. Randomized trial comparing epirubicin, cisplatin, and fluorouracil versus fluorouracil, doxorubicin, and methotrexate in advanced esophagogastric cancer. *J Clin Oncol* 1997;15:261–267.

518. Ross P, Nicholson M, Cunningham D, et al. Prospective randomized trial comparing mitomycin, cisplatin, and protracted venous-infusion fluorouracil (PVI 5-FU) with epirubicin, cisplatin, and PVI 5-FU in advanced esophagogastric cancer. *J Clin Oncol* 2002;20:1996.

520. Cunningham D, Starling N, Rao S, et al. Capecitabine and oxaliplatin for advanced esophagogastric cancer. *N Engl J Med* 2008;358:36–46.

521. Al-Batran S, Hartmann J, Probst S, et al. Phase III trial in metastatic gastroesophageal adenocarcinoma with fluorouracil, leucovorin plus either oxaliplatin or cisplatin: a study of the Arbeitsgemeinschaft Internistische Onkologie. *J Clin Oncol* 2008;26:1435–1442.

522. Kang YK, Kang KW, Shin DB, et al. Capecitabine/cisplatin versus 5-fluorouracil/cisplatin as first-line therapy in patients with advanced gastric cancer: a randomized phase III noninferiority trial. *Ann Oncol* 2009;20:666–673.

523. Koizumi W, Narahara H, Hara T, et al. S-1 plus cisplatin versus S-1 alone for first line treatment of advanced gastric cancer (SPIRITS Trial): a phase III trial. *Lancet Oncol* 2008;9:215–221.

524. Ajani JR, Correa A, Walsh G, et al. Multicenter phase III comparison of cisplatin/S-1 with cisplatin/infusional fluorouracil in advanced gastric or gastroesophageal adenocarcinoma study: the FLAGS Trial. *J Clin Oncol* 2010;28:1547–1553.

525. Van Cutsem E, Moiseyenko VM, Tjulandin S, et al. Phase III study of docetaxel and cisplatin plus fluorouracil compared with cisplatin and fluorouracil as first-line therapy for advanced gastric cancer: a report of the V325 study group. *J Clin Oncol* 2006;24:4991–4997.

526. Al-Batran SE, Pauligk C, Homann N, et al. The feasibility of triple-drug chemotherapy combination in older adult patients with esophagogastric cancer: a randomized trial of the Abreitsgemeinschaft Internistische Onkologie (FLOT65+). *Eur J Cancer* 2013;49:835–842.

540. Ilson DH, Saltz L, Enzinger P, et al. Phase II trial of weekly irinotecan plus cisplatin in advanced esophageal cancer. *J Clin Oncol* 1999;17:3270–3275.

541. Ajani JA, Baker J, Pisters PW, et al. CPT-11 plus cisplatin in patients with advanced, untreated gastric or gastroesophageal junction carcinoma: results of a phase II study. *Cancer* 2002;94:641–646.

542. Enzinger PC, Ryan D, Clark J, et al. Weekly docetaxel, cisplatin, and irinotecan (TPC): results of a multicenter phase II trial in patients with metastatic esophagogastric cancer. *Ann Oncol* 2009;20:475–480.

543. Enzinger PC, Burtness BA, Hollis DR, et al. CALGB 80403 / ECOG 1206: Randomized phase II study of standard chemotherapy plus cetuximab for metastatic esophageal cancer. *J Clin Oncol* 2010;28:15S.

549. Dank M, Zaluski J, Barone C, et al. Randomized phase III study comparing irinotecan combined with 5-fluorouracil and folinic acid to cisplatin combined with 5-fluorouracil in chemotherapy naive patients with advanced adenocarcinoma of the stomach or esophagogastric junction. *Ann Oncol* 2008;19:1450–1457.

552. Bang YJ, Van Cutsem E, Fevereislova A, et al. Trastuzumab in combination with chemotherapy versus chemotherapy alone for treatment of HER2-positive advanced gastric or gastroesophageal junction cancer (ToGA): a phase 3, open-label, randomized controlled trial. *Lancet* 2010;376:687–697.

553. Yoon HH, Shi Q, Sukov WR, et al. Association of HER2/ErbB2 expression and gene amplification with pathologic features and prognosis in esophageal adenocarcinomas. *Clin Cancer Res* 2012;18:546–554.

557. Dutton SJ, Blazeby JM, Petty RD, et al. Patient-reported outcomes from a phase III muticenter, randomized double-blind, placebo-controlled trial of gefitinib versus placebo in esophageal cancer progressing after chemotherapy: Cancer Oesophagus Gefitinib (COG). *J Clin Oncol* 2012;30:S34.

558. Pinto C, DiFabio F, Siena S, et al. Phase II study of cetuximab in combination with FOLFIRI in patients with untreated advanced gastric or gastroesophageal junction adenocarcinoma. *Ann Oncol* 2006;18:510–517.

559. Lorenzen S, Schuster T, Porschen R, et al. Cetuximab plus cisplatin 5-fluorouracil versus cisplatin 5-fluorouracil alone in first line metastatic squamous cell carcinoma of the esophagus: a randomized phase II trial. *Ann Oncol* 2009;20:1667–1673.

560. Lordick F, Luber B, Lorenzen S, et al. Cetuximab plus oxaliplatin/leucovorin/5-fluorouracil in first line metastatic gastric cancer: a phase II study. *Br J Cancer* 2010;102:500–505.

561. Enzinger PC, Burtness BA, Hollis DR, et al. CALGB 80403/ECOG 1206: Randomized phase II study of standard chemotherapy plus cetuximab for metastatic esophageal cancer. *J Clin Oncol* 2010;28:15S.

562. Waddell T, Cunningham D, Gonzalez D, et al. Epirubicin, oxaliplatin, and capecitabine with or without panitumumab for patients with previously untreated esophagogastric cancer (REAL-3): a randomized, open-label phase 3 trial. *Lancet Oncol* 2013;14:481.

563. Lordick F, Kang YK, Chung HC, et al. Capecitabine and cisplatin with or without cetuximab for patients with previously untreated gastric cancer (EXPAND): a randomized, open-label phase 3 trial. *Lancet Oncol* 2013;14:490–499.

564. Lorenzen S, Schuster T, Porschen R, et al. Cetuximab plus cisplatin-5-fluorouracil versus cisplatin-5-fluorouracil alone in first-line metastatic squamous cell carcinoma of the esophagus: a randomized phase II study of the Arbeitsgemeinschaft Internistische Onkologie. *Ann Oncol* 2009;20:1667–1673.

566. Ohtsu A, Shah MA, van Cutsem E, et al. Bevacizumab in combination with chemotherapy as first-line therapy in advanced gastric cancer: a randomized, double-blind, placebo-controlled phase III study. *J Clin Oncol* 2011;29:3968–3976.

567. Fuchs CS, Tomasek J, Yang CJ, et al. Ramucirumab monotherapy for previously treated advanced gastric or gastro-esophageal junction adenocarcinoma (REGARD): an international, randomized, multicenter, placebo-controlled, phase 3 trial. *Lancet* 2014;383:31–39.

568. Ohtsu A, Ajani JA, Bai YX, et al. Everolimus in previously treated, advanced gastric cancer: results of the randomized, double-blind, phase III GRANITE-1 Study. *J Clin Oncol* 2013;31:3935–3943.

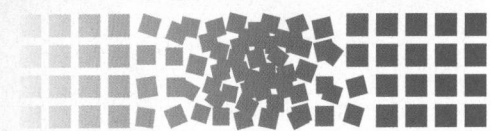

46 Cancer of the Stomach

Itzhak Avital, Alexander Stojadinovic, Peter W. T. Pisters, David P. Kelsen, and Christopher G. Willett

INTRODUCTION

Adenocarcinoma of the stomach was the leading cause of cancer-related death worldwide through most of the 20th century. It now ranks second only to lung cancer, and an estimated 870,000 new cases are diagnosed annually, and 650,000 deaths (10% of all cancer deaths) worldwide.[1] In 2011, the epidemiologic data on cancer of the stomach was updated. It now ranks fourth after lung cancer, breast cancer, and colorectal cancer. An estimated 989,600 new cases are diagnosed annually, with 738,000 deaths (10% of all cancer deaths) worldwide.[2] In the West, the incidence of gastric cancer has decreased, potentially because of changes in diet, food preparation, and other environmental factors. The declining incidence has been dramatic in the United States, where this disease ranked sixth as a cause of cancer-related death during the period of 2000 to 2005.[3] It is estimated that in 2009, 21,130 new gastric cancer cases were diagnosed in the United States, with approximately 10,600 deaths.[3] Data was updated for 2014 where an estimated 22,220 new cases will be diagnosed in the United States, with approximately 10,990 deaths.[4] Prognosis remains poor except in a few countries. The explanations for this finding are multifactorial. The lack of defined risk factors, disease-specific symptoms, and the low incidence of gastric cancer has contributed to the late stage at diagnosis seen in most Western countries. In Japan, where gastric cancer is endemic, more patients are diagnosed at an early stage, which is reflected in higher overall survival (OS) rates.

The decline in incidence has been limited to noncardia gastric cancers.[5] The number of newly diagnosed cases of proximal gastric and esophagogastric junction (EGJ) adenocarcinomas has increased six-fold since the mid-1980s.[6] These proximal tumors are thought to be biologically more aggressive and more complex to treat. The only chance of cure is complete surgical resection. However, even after what is believed to be a "curative" gastrectomy, disease recurs in the majority of patients. Efforts to improve these poor results have focused on developing effective pre- and postoperative systemic and regional adjuvant therapies. This chapter details the state-of-the-art regarding the origins, screening, diagnosis, treatment, and palliation of this significant worldwide health problem.

ANATOMIC CONSIDERATIONS

The stomach begins at the gastroesophageal junction and ends at the pylorus (Fig. 46.1). Cancers arising from the proximal greater curvature may directly involve the splenic hilum and tail of pancreas, whereas more distal tumors may invade the transverse colon. Proximal cancers may extend into the diaphragm, spleen, or the left lateral segment of the liver. A recent study reported on the potential benefits and harms of complete resection even when the tumor invades adjacent abdominal visceral structures (pT4b).[7] In this large multicenter cohort series of 2,208 patients who underwent curative intent resection, 206 patients had pT4b tumors and 112 underwent resection of adjacent organs as part of en bloc gastric cancer resection. The overall 5-year survival rate for this group of patients was 27.2%, suggesting that patients do have a chance at long-term survival if their tumor can be removed en bloc with involved adjacent organs, thereby supporting the role of multivisceral resection if required and technically feasible.[7]

The blood supply to the stomach is extensive and is based on vessels arising from the celiac axis (see Fig. 46.1). The right gastric artery arises from the hepatic artery proper (50% to 68%), left hepatic artery (29% to 40%), or from the common hepatic artery (3.2%). The left gastric artery originates from the celiac axis directly (90%) and may arise from the common hepatic artery (2%), splenic artery (4%), or aorta or from the superior mesenteric artery (3%). Both right and left gastric arteries course along the lesser curvature. Along the greater curvature are the right gastroepiploic artery, which originates from the gastroduodenal artery at the inferior border of the proximal duodenum (rarely from the superior mesenteric artery), and the left gastroepiploic artery (highly variable artery), branching from the distal (72%), inferior, middle splenic artery laterally. The short gastric arteries (vasa brevia, five to seven separate vessels) arise directly from the splenic artery or the left gastroepiploic artery. The posterior (dorsal) gastric artery (17% to 68%) may arise from the splenic artery to supply the distal esophagus, cardia, and fundus. The preservation of any of these vessels in the course of a subtotal gastrectomy for carcinoma is not necessary, and the most proximal few centimeters of remaining stomach are well supplied by collateral flow from the lower segmental esophageal arterial arcade. The rich submucosal blood supply of the stomach is an important factor in its ability to heal rapidly and produce a low incidence of anastomotic disruption following radical gastric resection. The venous drainage of the stomach tends to parallel the arterial supply. The venous efflux ultimately passes through the portal venous system, and this is reflected in the fact that the liver is the primary site for distant metastatic spread.

The lymphatic drainage of the stomach is extensive, and distinct anatomic groups of perigastric lymph nodes have been defined according to their relationship to the stomach and its blood supply. There are six perigastric lymph node groups. In the first echelon (stations 1 through 6) are the right and left pericardial nodes (stations 1 and 2). Along the lesser curvature are the lesser curvature nodes (station 3) and the suprapyloric nodes (station 5). Along the greater curvature, the gastroepiploic nodes or greater curvature nodes (station 4), and the subpyloric nodes (station 6). In the second echelon (stations 7 through 12) are the nodes along named arteries, which include the left gastric, common hepatic, celiac, splenic hilum, splenic artery, and hepatoduodenal lymphatics (stations 7 through 12, respectively), which drain into the celiac and periaortic lymphatics. The third echelon (stations 13 through 16) contains the posterior to pancreatic head, superior mesenteric artery, middle colic artery, and para-aortic lymphatics (stations 13 through 16, respectively). Proximally are the lower esophageal lymph nodes; extensive spread of gastric cancer along the intrathoracic lymph channels may be manifested clinically by a metastatic lymph node in the left supraclavicular fossa (Virchow's node) or left axilla (Irish's node). Tumor spread to the lymphatics in the hepatoduodenal ligament can extend along the falciform ligament and result in subcutaneous periumbilical tumor deposits (Sister Mary Joseph's nodes).

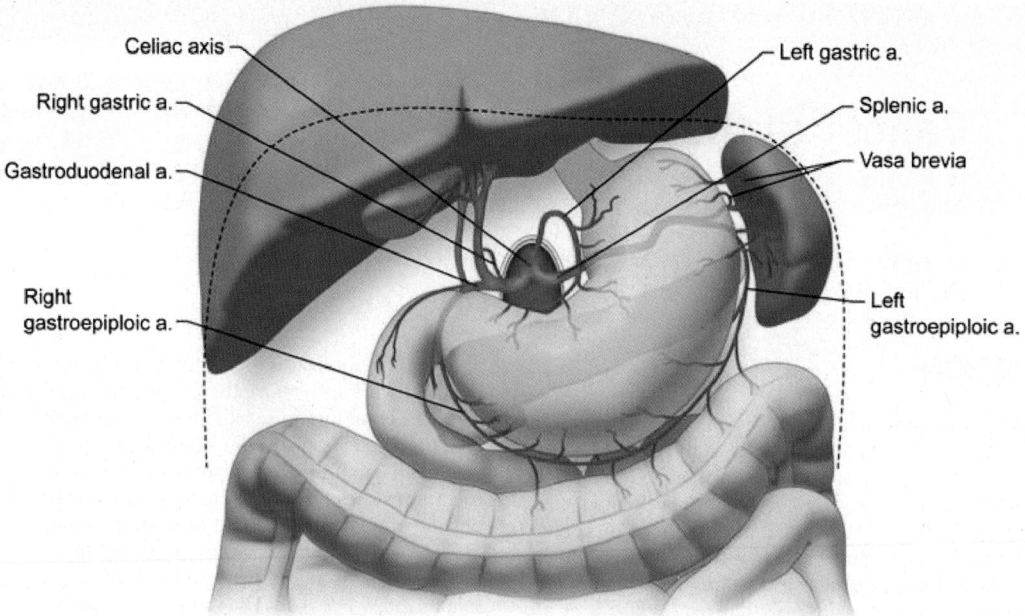

Figure 46.1 Blood supply to the stomach and anatomic relationships of the stomach with other adjacent organs likely to be involved by direct extension of a T4 gastric tumor.

PATHOLOGY AND TUMOR BIOLOGY

Approximately 95% of all gastric cancers are adenocarcinomas. The term *gastric cancer* refers to adenocarcinoma of the stomach. Other malignant tumors are rare and include squamous cell carcinoma, adenoacanthoma, carcinoid tumors, small cell carcinoma, mucinous carcinoma, hepatoid adenocarcinoma, oncocytic (parietal gland) carcinoma, sarcomatoid carcinoma, lymphoepithelioma-like carcinoma, adenocarcinoma with rhabdoid features, gastric carcinoma with osteoclastlike giant cells, neuroendocrine tumor, gastrointestinal stromal tumor, or leiomyosarcoma.[8] Although no normal lymphoid tissue is found in the gastric mucosa, the stomach is the most common site for lymphomas of the gastrointestinal tract. The increased awareness of association between mucosa-associated lymphoid tissue lymphomas and *Helicobacter pylori* may explain, in part, the rise in incidence,[9] although the incidence of mucoas-associated lymphoid tissue gastric lymphomas is decreasing likely because of effective treatment against *H. pylori*.[10]

In terms of pathogenesis, two new concepts are worth mentioning: bone marrow participation in gastric carcinogenesis and gastric cancer stem cells. It has been hypothesized that the gastric epithelial cells acquiring abnormal phenotype (resembling intestinal epithelium) originate from gastric stem cells localized to the only cell replication zone of the gastric glands (i.e., the isthmus). However, Houghton et al.,[11] Stoicov et al.,[12,13] and Li et al.[14] demonstrated in a rodent model of *Helicobacter*-induced gastric cancer that the entire cancer mass was derived from cells originating in the bone marrow. This interesting phenomenon was observed by other authors studying solid cancers in patients receiving bone marrow transplantation.[15] Recent evidence proposes the existence of cancer stem cells or stemlike cancer cells in various cancers. Although controversial, cancer stem cells are defined as cancer cells with the exclusive ability to initiate tumors, metastasize, and self-renew tumors. In gastric cancer, several investigators suggested the existence of gastric cancer stem cells (i.e., CD44+) and side population cells.[16,17] These cells showed relative resistance to chemotherapy and radiation, and exclusive ability to initiate tumors. These important observations might lead to novel approaches to the diagnosis and treatment of gastric cancer in the next decade.

HISTOPATHOLOGY

Several staging schemas have been proposed based on the morphologic features of gastric tumors. The Borrmann classification divides gastric cancer into five types depending on macroscopic appearance. Type I represents polypoid or fungating cancers, type II encompasses ulcerating lesions surrounded by elevated borders, type III represents ulcerated lesions infiltrating the gastric wall, type IV includes diffusely infiltrating tumors, and type V gastric cancers are unclassifiable cancers.[18] The gross morphologic appearance of gastric cancer and the degree of histologic differentiation are not independent prognostic variables. Ming[19] has proposed a histomorphologic staging system that divides gastric cancer into either a prognostically favorable expansive type or a poor prognosis infiltrating type. Based on an analysis of 171 gastric cancers, the expansive-type tumors were uniformly polypoid or superficial on gross appearance, whereas the infiltrative tumors were almost always diffuse. Grossly ulcerated lesions were divided between the expansive or infiltrative forms. Broder's classification of gastric cancer grades tumors histologically from 1 (well-differentiated) to 4 (anaplastic). Bearzi and Ranaldi[20] have correlated the degree of histologic differentiation with the gross appearance of 41 primary gastric cancers seen on endoscopy. Ninety percent of protruding or superficial cancers were well differentiated (Broder's grade 1), whereas almost half of all ulcerated tumors were poorly differentiated or diffusely infiltrating (Broder's grades 3 and 4).

The most widely used classification of gastric cancer is by Laurén.[21] It divides gastric cancers into either intestinal or diffuse forms. This classification scheme, based on tumor histology, characterizes two varieties of gastric adenocarcinomas that manifest distinctively different pathology, epidemiology, genetics, and etiologies. The intestinal variety represents a differentiated cancer with a tendency to form glands similar to other sites in the gastrointestinal tract, but in particular the colon type; hence the intestinal type. In contrast, the diffuse form exhibits very little cell cohesion with a predilection for extensive submucosal spread and early metastases. Although the diffuse-type cancers are associated with a worse outcome than the intestinal type, this finding is not independent of tumor, node, and metastasis (TNM) stage. The molecular pathogenesis of these two distinct forms of gastric cancer is also different. Although the intestinal type represents

H. pylori–initiated multistep progression with less defined progressive genetic alterations, the diffuse type main carcinogenic event is loss of expression of E-cadherin (*CDH1* gene). E-cadherin is a molecule involved in cell-to-cell adhesion; loss of its expression leads to noncohesive growth, hence the diffuse type. In tumors that display both intestinal and diffuse phenotypes, the *CDH1* mutation and loss of E-cadherin function are observed only within the diffuse phenotype.[22]

PATTERNS OF SPREAD

Carcinomas of the stomach can spread by local extension to involve adjacent structures and can develop lymphatic metastases, peritoneal metastases, and distant metastases. These extensions can occur by the local invasive properties of the tumor, lymphatic spread, or hematogenous dissemination. The initial growth of the tumor occurs by penetration into the gastric wall, extension through the wall, within the wall longitudinally,[23] and subsequent involvement of an increasing percentage of the stomach. The two modes of local extension that can have major therapeutic implications are tumor penetration through the gastric serosa, where the risk of tumor invasion of adjacent structures or peritoneal spread is increased, and lymphatic involvement. Zinninger[24] has evaluated spread within the gastric wall and has found a wide variation in its extent. Tumor spread is often through the intramural lymphatics or in the subserosal layers.[23] Local extension can also occur into the esophagus or the duodenum.[25] Duodenal extension is rare (0.5% to 1.8% of all resected cases),[26] portrays poor prognosis, and is principally through the muscular layer by direct infiltration and through the subserosal lymphatics, but is not generally to any great extent.[27] Extension into the esophagus occurs primarily through the submucosal lymphatics.[28]

Local extension does not occur solely by radial intramural spread but also by deep invasion through the wall to adjacent structures[23] (omentum, spleen, adrenal gland, diaphragm, liver, pancreas, or colon). Many studies report that 60% to 90% of patients had primary tumors penetrating the serosa or invading adjacent organs and that at least 50% had lymphatic metastases. In the largest series reporting on 10,783 patients with gastric cancer from Korea, 57% of the patients had lymph node metastasis, and the average number of involved lymph nodes was five.[29,30] Of the 1,577 primary gastric cancer cases admitted to Memorial Sloan Kettering Cancer Center (MSKCC) between July 1, 1985, and June 30, 1998, 60% of the 1,221 resected cases had evidence of serosal penetration and 68% had positive nodes. Lymph node metastases were found in 18% of pT1 lesions, and 60% of pT2 lesions after R0 resection in 941 patients. The highest incidence of lymphatic metastasis was seen in tumors diffusely involving the entire stomach. Tumors located at the gastroesophageal junction also had a high incidence relative to other sites.[31]

The pattern of nodal metastases also varies depending on the location of the primary site. In a study, reporting on 1,137 patients with early gastric cancer (EGC), tumors located in the upper, middle, and lower third of the stomach had 12%, 10%, and 8% nodal involvement, respectively. The most common nodal station metastases for the upper, middle, and lower third of the stomach were stations 3 (lesser curvature), 3/4/7 (lesser/greater curvature/left gastric artery), and 3/4/6 (lesser/greater curvature/infrapyloric), respectively.[32] Earlier studies that included more advanced gastric cancers showed that the left gastric artery nodes were at increased risk for nodal metastases independent of tumor location.[32,33]

Gastric cancer recurs in multiple sites, locoregionally and systemically. Patterns of failure are variable. These differences are likely related to the patient cohorts evaluated, the time at which failure was determined, and the method of determination of failure patterns. Recent series from the MSKCC and Korea do shed light on modern patterns of failure.[31,34] In the report from MSKCC, recurrence patterns of 1,038 patients who underwent

R0 gastrectomy with D2 lymphadenectomy (61%) were analyzed; complete data on recurrence were available in 367 (74%) of 496 patients who experienced recurrence. The locoregional area was involved in 199 (54%) patients. Distant sites were involved in 188 (51%) patients, and peritoneal recurrence was detected in 108 (29%) patients. More than one site of recurrence was detected: distal, peritoneal, and locoregional recurrences in 9 (2.5%); locoregional and peritoneal in 34 (9.3%); locoregional and distant in 61 (16.6%); and distant and peritoneal in 15 (4.1%) patients. On multivariate analysis, peritoneal recurrence was associated with female gender, advanced T stage, and distal and diffuse type tumors; locoregional recurrence was associated with proximal location, early T stage, and intestinal type tumors. In the study from Korea, recurrence patterns were analyzed in 2,038 patients who were treated with potentially curative gastrectomy.[34] Of 508 patients who developed recurrence, 33% involved locoregional sites, 44% were peritoneal, and 38% were distant. At time of presentation, 35% of patients presented with distant metastasis, with 4% to 14% having liver metastases.[35,36]

CLINICAL PRESENTATION AND PRETREATMENT EVALUATION

Signs and Symptoms

Because of the vague, nonspecific symptoms that characterize gastric cancer, many patients are diagnosed with advanced-stage disease. Patients may have a combination of signs and symptoms such as weight loss (22% to 61%)[37]; anorexia (5% to 40%); fatigue, epigastric discomfort, or pain (62% to 91%); and postprandial fullness, heart burn, indigestion, nausea, and vomiting (6% to 40%). None of these unequivocally indicates gastric cancer. In addition, patients may be asymptomatic (4% to 17%).[38] Weight loss and abdominal pain are the most common presenting symptoms at initial encounter.[39–41] Weight loss is a common symptom, and its clinical significance should not be underestimated. Dewys et al.[42] found that in 179 patients with advanced gastric cancer, >80% of patients had a >10% decrease in body weight before diagnosis. Furthermore, patients with weight loss had a significantly shorter survival than did those without weight loss.[40]

In some patients, symptoms may suggest the presence of a lesion at a specific location. Up to 25% of the patients have history/symptoms of peptic ulcer disease.[39] A history of dysphagia or pseudoachalasia may indicate the presence of a tumor in the cardia with extension through the gastroesophageal junction.[43] Early satiety is an infrequent symptom of gastric cancer but is indicative of a diffusely infiltrative tumor that has resulted in loss of distensibility of the gastric wall. Delayed satiety and vomiting may indicate pyloric involvement. Significant gastrointestinal bleeding is uncommon with gastric cancer; however, hematemesis does occur in approximately 10% to 15% of patients, and anemia in 1% to 12% of patients. Signs and symptoms at presentation are often related to spread of disease. Ascites, jaundice, or a palpable mass indicate incurable disease.[40] The transverse colon is a potential site of malignant fistulization and obstruction from a gastric primary tumor. Diffuse peritoneal spread of disease frequently produces other sites of intestinal obstruction. A large ovarian mass (Krukenberg's tumor) or a large peritoneal implant in the pelvis (Blumer's shelf), which can produce symptoms of rectal obstruction, may be palpable on pelvic or rectal examination.[37,44] Nodular metastases in the subcutaneous tissue around the umbilicus (Sister Mary Joseph's node) or in peripheral lymph nodes such as in the supraclavicular area (Virchow's node) or axillary region (Irish's node) represent areas in which a tissue diagnosis can be established with minimal morbidity.[45] There is no symptom complex that occurs early in the evolution of gastric cancer that can identify individuals for further diagnostic measures. However, alarming symptoms (dysphagia, weight loss, and palpable abdominal mass) are independently associated with survival; increased number and the specific symptom is associated with mortality.[40,41]

Screening

A list of risk factors associated with gastric cancer is outlined in Table 46.1. These factors might be use for risk stratification in screening programs. Mass screening programs for gastric cancer have been most successful in high-risk areas, especially in Japan.[46] A variety of screening tests have been studied in Japanese patients, with a sensitivity and specificity of approximately 90%.[40] Screening typically includes serology for *H. pylori*, the use of double-contrast barium radiographs, or upper endoscopy with risk stratification (OLGA staging system for gastric cancer risk[46,47]).

Ohata et al.[48] reported on 4,655 asymptomatic patients with an average age of 50 years old who were followed for 7.7 years. Atrophic gastritis was identified using pepsinogen and *H. pylori* testing: 2,341 (52%) were *H. pylori*–positive with nonatrophic gastritis, 967 (21%) were *H. pylori*–negative without atrophic gastritis, 1,316 (28%) were *H. pylori*–positive with atrophic gastritis,

---

TABLE 46.1

Factors Associated with Increased Risk of Developing Stomach Cancer

Acquired Factors
- Nutritional
  - High salt consumption
  - High nitrate consumption
  - Low dietary vitamin A and C
  - Poor food preparation (smoked, salt cured)
  - Lack of refrigeration
  - Poor drinking water (well water)
- Occupational
  - Rubber workers
  - Coal workers
- Cigarette smoking
- *Helicobacter pylori* infection
- Epstein-Barr virus
- Radiation exposure
- Prior gastric surgery for benign gastric ulcer disease
- Prior treatment for mucosa-associated lymphoid tissue lymphoma

Genetic Factors
- Type A blood
- Pernicious anemia
- Family history without known genetic factors (first-degree relative with gastric cancer)
- Hereditary diffuse gastric cancer (*CDH1* mutation)
- Familial gastric cancer
- Hereditary nonpolyposis colon cancer
- Familial adenomatous polyposis
- Li-Fraumeni syndrome
- *BRCA1* and *BRAC2*
- Precursor lesions
  - Adenomatous gastric polyps
  - Chronic atrophic gastritis
  - Dysplasia
  - Intestinal metaplasia
  - Menetrier disease
- Ethnicity (in the United States, gastric cancer is more common among Asian/Pacific Islanders, Hispanics and African Americans)
- Obesity (the strength of this link is not clear)

---

and 31 (0.7%) had severe atrophic gastritis. The rates of gastric cancer development per population per year were 107/100,000 for *H. pylori*–positive with nonatrophic gastritis, 0/100,000 for *H. pylori*–negative without atrophic gastritis, 238/100,000 for *H. pylori*–positive with atrophic gastritis, and 871/100,000 for severe atrophic gastritis. Thus the number of endoscopies needed to detect one cancer was 1/1,000, 0/1,000, 1/410, and 1/114, respectively. Similar data were reported on 6,985 patients by Watabe et al.[49] Surveillance in endemic populations is clinically important because EGC has a very high cure rate with surgical treatment. However, the fact that gastric cancer remains one of the top causes of death in Japan indicates the limitations of a mass-screening program when the entire population at risk is not effectively screened. However, more recent studies indicate that for surveillance programs to be effective and feasible from an economical perspective, they should be instituted only in high-risk populations (>20/100,000 incidence of disease) and include the following components: detection and eradication of *H. pylori*, serum pepsinogen (pepsinogen I/II ratio), endoscopy with biopsy, and risk stratification before and after *H. pylori* eradication using a system such as the OLGA staging system for gastric cancer risk. Such programs are expected to avoid long-term repeated screening of approximately 70% of the population who are at low risk of developing gastric cancer.[46,50–52] A US study found that screening and eradication of *H. pylori* in Japanese Americans is cost-effective in preventing gastric cancer.[53] These findings were confirmed by two studies from the United Kingdom.[54,55]

PRETREATMENT STAGING

Tumor Markers

Most gastric cancers have at least one elevated tumor marker, but some benign gastric diseases show elevated serum tumor markers as well. Tumor markers in gastric cancer continue to have limited diagnostic usefulness, with their role more informative in follow-up after primary treatment. The most commonly used markers are serum carcinoembryonic antigen (CEA), cancer antigen (CA) 19-9, CA 50, and CA 72-4. There is wide variation in the reported serum levels of these markers; positive CEA and CA 19-9 levels varied from 8% to 58% and 4% to 65%, respectively. Overall, the sensitivity of each serum tumor marker alone as a diagnostic marker of gastric cancer is low. However, when the levels are elevated, it does usually correlate with stage of disease. Combining CEA with other markers, such as CA 19-9, CA 72-4, or CA 50, can increase sensitivity compared with CEA alone.[56–62]

In a large study evaluating serum CEA, α-fetoprotein, human chronic gonadotropin-β, CA 19-9, CA 125, as well as tissue staining for *HER2* in gastric cancer patients, only human chronic gonadotropin-β level >4 IU/L and a CA 125 level ≥350 U/mL had prognostic significance. Elevated serum tumor marker levels in gastric cancer before chemotherapy may reflect not just tumor burden but also biology of disease.

Endoscopy

Endoscopy is the best method to diagnose gastric cancer as it visualizes the gastric mucosa and allows biopsy for a histologic diagnosis. Chromoendoscopy helps identify mucosal abnormalities through topical mucosal stains. Magnification endoscopy is used to magnify standard endoscopic fields by 1.5- to 150-fold. Narrow band imaging affords enhanced visualization of the mucosal microvasculature. Confocal laser endomicroscopy permits in vivo, three-dimensional microscopy including subsurface structures with diagnostic accuracy, sensitivity, and specificity of 97%, 90%, and 99.5%, respectively.[63–65]

Endoscopic ultrasound (EUS) is a tool for preoperative staging and selection for neoadjuvant therapy. It is used to assess the T and N stage of primary tumors. A study of 225 patients from MSKCC found that the concordance between EUS and pathology was lower than expected. The accuracy for individual T and N stage were 57% and 50%, respectively. However, the combined assessment of N stage and serosal invasion identified 77% of the patients at risk of disease-related death after curative resection.[66] Other investigators compared the accuracy of EUS with that of multidetector computed tomography (MDCT) and magnetic resonance imaging (MRI) and found that the overall accuracy was 65% to 92% (EUS), 77% to 89% (MDCT), and 71% to 83% (MRI) for T stage, and 55% to 66% (EUS), 32% to 77% (MDCT) for N stage, respectively. The corresponding sensitivity and specificity for serosal involvement were 78% to 100% (EUS), 83% to 100% (MDCT), and 89% to 93% (MRI) for T stage, and 68% to 100% (EUS), 80% to 97% (MDCT), and 91% to 100% (MRI) for N stage, respectively.[65,67]

Computed Tomography

Once gastric cancer is suspected, a triphasic CT with oral and intravenous contrast of the abdomen, chest, and pelvis is imperative. In a study of 790 patients who underwent MDCT prior to surgery, the overall accuracy in determining T stage was 74% (T1 46%, T2 53%, T3 86%, and T4 86%), and for N staging it was 75% (N0 76%, N1 69%, and N2 80%). The sensitivity, specificity, and accuracy for lymph node metastasis were 86%, 76%, and 82%, respectively.[68] MDCT with thin-sliced multiplanar reconstruction (MPR) and water filling is increasingly used. The accuracy rate for advanced gastric cancer was 96% and for EGC it was 41%. An improvement on axial CT and MPR-MDCT was the addition of staging with three-dimensional MPR-MDCT. The detection rate for MPR with virtual gastroscopy was 98%. MPR-MDCT with combined water and air distention is superior to conventional axial imaging.[69]

Magnetic Resonance Imaging

MRI is not used routinely in preoperative staging of gastric cancer. Several studies have demonstrated that CT and MRI are comparable in terms of accuracy and understaging.[70,71] However, MRI is a useful modality to further characterize liver lesions identified on preoperative CT staging workup.

Positron Emission Tomography

Whole-body 2-[18F]-fluoro-2-deoxyglucose (FDG) positron emission tomography (PET) is being applied increasingly in the evaluation of gastrointestinal malignancies. In gastric cancer, approximately half of the primary tumors are FDG-negative; the diffuse (signet cell) subtype was most likely to be non-FDG avid, likely because of decreased expression of the glucose transporter-1 (Glut-1).[72] In patients with non-FDG–avid primary tumor, FDG-PET/CT is not useful.[72–76] PET/CT was tested as a tool to predict response to neoadjuvant chemotherapy. Ott et al.[77] reported 90% 2-year survival in patients with PET-defined response (<35% decrease standardized uptake value [SUV]) versus 25% for patients not responding to PET. PET response could be detected as early as 14 days. At least 60% of the patients were PET-nonresponding patients and thus could have been spared further chemotherapy. Authors of the MUNICON trial reported on patients who were PET nonresponders by day 14 after cisplatin and fluorouracil (5-FU) (CF) neoadjuvant chemotherapy, and subsequently were sent for surgery, and patients who were PET responders and continued 3 months of neoadjuvant therapy before surgery. The PET-responding patients had a survival benefit (hazard ratio [HR] = 2.13; p <0.15). In PET-nonresponding patients, stopping the chemotherapy did not affect long-term survival.[78] Recent

studies, including one large meta-analysis, showed that in terms of diagnostic accuracy and lymph node staging EUS, MDCT, MRI, and PET/CT are comparable modalities. There were no significant differences between mean sensitivities and specificities.[79,80] Even in patients whose tumors were FDG-avid, FDG-PET/CT scans did not identify occult peritoneal disease (0 of 18), but did identify extraperitoneal M1 disease in nine patients with bone ($n = 2$), liver ($n = 4$), and retroperitoneal lymph node ($n = 3$) involvement. In patients with FDG-avid tumors, PET may be useful in detecting metastatic disease and follow-up for recurrence. Interestingly, the presence of Glut-1– and FDG-avid gastric cancers may be associated with decreased OS.[72] The role of PET/CT in the primary staging of gastric cancer remains to be established; its role might be better defined in advanced disease.

In a prospective study of 113 patients who were clinically staged as locally advanced but nonmetastatic gastric cancer (T3-T4, Nx or N+, M0), investigators found that FDG-PET/CT did identify occult metastatic disease in about 10% of patients. In this study, FDG-PET/CT did not identify occult peritoneal disease, suggesting a necessary role for laparoscopy in preoperative staging of locally advanced gastric cancer. A cost evaluation was also performed, and it suggested that if FDG-PET/CT is included as part of the staging algorithm, that would result in an estimated cost savings of approximately $13,000 US dollars per patient.[81]

Staging Laparoscopy and Peritoneal Cytology

Staging laparoscopy with peritoneal lavage should be an integral part of the pretreatment staging evaluation of patients believed to have localized gastric cancer. Current noninvasive modalities used in preoperative staging of gastric cancer have sensitivities significantly lower than 100%, particularly in cases of low-volume peritoneal carcinomatosis.[82–84] Current CT techniques cannot consistently identify low-volume macroscopic metastases that are ≤5 mm in size. Laparoscopy directly inspects the peritoneal and visceral surfaces for detection of CT-occult, small-volume metastases. Staging laparoscopy also allows for assessment of peritoneal cytology and laparoscopic ultrasound. Laparoscopic staging is done to spare nontherapeutic operations and for potential stratification in various trials.[85]

The rate of detection of CT-occult M1 disease by laparoscopy depends on the quality of CT scanning and interpretation.[86] Muntean et al.[87] reported on 98 patients with primary gastric cancer: 45 underwent staging laparoscopy with subsequent surgery and 53 went directly to surgery. An unnecessary laparotomy was avoided in 38% of the patients. The overall sensitivity and specificity were 89% and 100%, respectively. Nonetheless, even high-quality MDCT is insufficiently sensitive for detection of low-volume extragastric disease and thus CT, EUS, and laparoscopy are complementary staging studies.[88,89]

The value of peritoneal cytology as a preoperative staging tool in patients with gastric cancer who are potential candidates for curative resection by EUS and CT has been examined by several investigators. Bentrem et al.[90] reported on 371 patients who underwent R0 resection, 6.5% of whom had positive cytology after staging laparoscopy. Median survival of patients with positive cytology was 14.8 versus 98.5 months for patients with negative cytology findings (p <0.001). Positive cytology predicted death from gastric cancer (relative risk = 2.7; p <0.001) and is tantamount to M1 disease. Several groups confirmed these findings and concluded that staging laparoscopy with peritoneal cytology can change the management of gastric cancer in 6.5% to 52% of patients.[83,91–94]

Laparoscopy can be performed as a separate staging procedure prior to definitive treatment planning or immediately prior to planned laparotomy for gastrectomy. When performed as a separate procedure, laparoscopy has the disadvantage of the additional risks and expense of a second general anesthetic. However, separate procedure laparoscopy allows the additional staging information including cytology acquired at laparoscopy to be reviewed and discussed with the patient and in multidisciplinary treatment group prior to definitive treatment planning. Laparoscopic ultrasound (LUS) and "extended laparoscopy" are techniques that may increase the diagnostic yield of laparoscopy. Preliminary results reveal conflicting data on the added benefit of LUS and extended laparoscopy.[95–97] Further prospective studies will be required to evaluate the cost-benefit relationship of LUS and extended laparoscopy in the routine or selective workup of patients with gastric cancer.

Although laparoscopic staging is thought to detect CT-occult metastatic disease in approximately 40% of patients and spares nontherapeutic operations in approximately one-third of patients with gastric cancer, one needs to remember that tumor biology, not staging, will eventually guide outcomes. Clearly, not all patients benefit from preoperative laparoscopic staging; therefore, future studies should address the issue of selective laparoscopy based on noninvasive staging (i.e., patients with T1 tumors). Staging laparoscopy with or without cytology should be considered only if therapy will be altered consequent to information obtained by laparoscopy.[82]

STAGING, CLASSIFICATION, AND PROGNOSIS

For patients with surgically treated gastric adenocarcinoma, both pathologic staging (American Joint Committee on Cancer [AJCC]/International Union Against Cancer [UICC] or Japanese system) and classification of the completeness of resection (R classification) should be done. Although not formal components of the stage grouping, the AJCC recommends collection of additional prognostic factors: tumor location, serum CEA and CA 19.9, and histopathologic grade and type.[98]

American Joint Committee on Cancer/International Union Against Cancer Tumor, Node, Metastasis Staging

The AJCC/UICC TNM staging system for gastric cancer is outlined in Table 46.2.[98] The AJCC/UICC stage-stratified survival rates of 10,601 patients treated by surgical resection from the Surveillance, Epidemiology, and End Results program 1973 to 2005 public-use file diagnosed in years 1991 to 2000 are shown in Fig. 46.2. Several definitions in the most recent version of the AJCC (2010) differ from the previous version (2002). Tumors arising at the EGJ including Siewert type I or arising in the stomach ≤5 cm from the EGJ and crossing into the EJG including Siewert types II and III are staged using the TNM system for esophageal adenocarcinoma. Gastric tumors lying ≤5 cm from the EGJ but that do not cross the EGJ into the esophagus are staged as gastric cancer.[98]

In the AJCC/UICC staging system, tumor (T) stage is determined by depth of tumor invasion into the gastric wall and extension into adjacent structures (Fig. 46.3). The relationship between T stage, the overall stage, and survival is well defined (see Fig. 46.2). Nodal stage (N) is based on the number of involved lymph nodes, a criterion that may predict outcome more accurately than the location of involved lymph nodes.[99,100] Tumors with 1 to 2 involved nodes are classified as pN1, 3 to 6 involved nodes are classified as pN2, and those with 7 or more involved nodes are classified as pN3 (N3a has 7 to 15 nodes and N3b has ≥16 nodes). The use of numerical thresholds for nodal classification has gained increasing acceptance, although the extent of lymphadenectomy and rigor of pathologic assessment may affect results.[101,102] The nodal numerical threshold approach is based on observations that

TABLE 46.2

American Joint Committee on Cancer Staging of Gastric Cancer 2010: Definition of Tumor, Nodes, Metastasis

Primary Tumor (T)

TX	Primary tumor cannot be assessed
T0	No evidence of primary tumor
Tis	Carcinoma in situ: intraepithelial tumor without invasion of the lamina propria
T1	Tumor invades lamina propria, muscularis mucosae, or submucosa
T1a	Tumor invades lamina propria or muscularis mucosae
T1b	Tumor invades submucosa
T2	Tumor invades muscularis propria
T3	Tumor penetrates subserosal connective tissue without invasion of visceral peritoneum or adjacent structures
T4	Tumor invades serosa (visceral peritoneum) or adjacent structures
T4a	Tumor invades serosa (visceral peritoneum)
T4b	Tumor invades adjacent structures

Regional Lymph Nodes (N)

NX	Regional lymph node(s) cannot be assessed
N0	No regional lymph node metastasis
N1	Metastasis in 1 to 2 regional lymph nodes
N2	Metastasis in 3 to 6 regional lymph nodes
N3	Metastases in more than 7 regional lymph nodes
N3a	Metastasis in 7–15 regional nodes
N3b	Metastasis in 16 or more regional nodes

Distant Metastasis (M)

MX	Presence of distant metastasis cannot be assessed
M0	No distant metastasis
M1	Distant metastasis

Stage Grouping

O	Tis	N0	M0
IA	T1	N0	M0
IB	T2	N0	M0
	T1	N1	M0
IIA	T3	N0	M0
	T2	N1	M0
	T1	N2	M0
IIB	T4a	N0	M0
	T3	N1	M0
	T2	N2	M0
	T1	N3	M0
IIIA	T4a	N1	M0
	T3	N2	M0
	T2	N3	M0
IIIB	T4b	N0	M0
	T4b	N1	M0
	T4a	N2	M0
	T3	N3	M0
IIIC	T4b	N2	M0
	T4b	N3	M0
	T4a	N3	M0
IV	Any T	Any N	M1

Used with the permission of the American Joint Committee on Cancer (AJCC), Chicago, Illiois. The original source for this material is the AJCC Cancer Staging Manual, Seventh Edition (2010) published by Springer Science and Business Media LLC, www.springer.com, page 123.

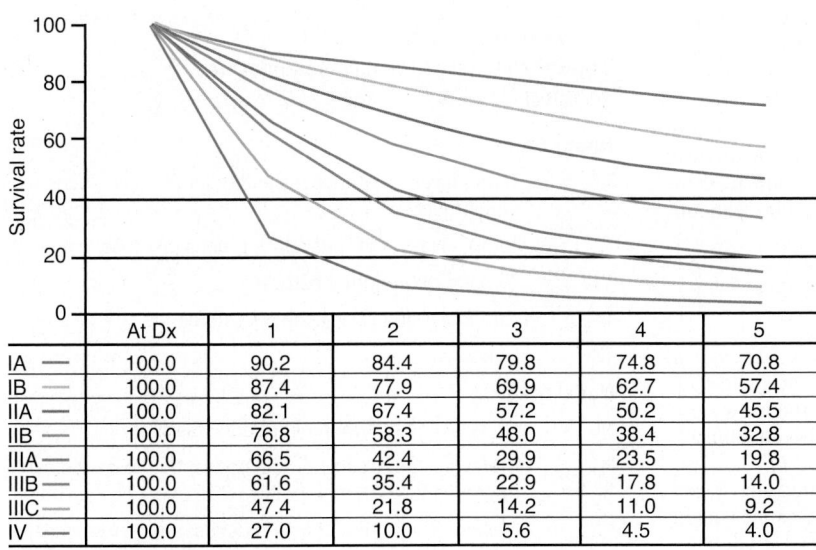

	At Dx	1	2	3	4	5
IA —	100.0	90.2	84.4	79.8	74.8	70.8
IB —	100.0	87.4	77.9	69.9	62.7	57.4
IIA —	100.0	82.1	67.4	57.2	50.2	45.5
IIB —	100.0	76.8	58.3	48.0	38.4	32.8
IIIA —	100.0	66.5	42.4	29.9	23.5	19.8
IIIB —	100.0	61.6	35.4	22.9	17.8	14.0
IIIC —	100.0	47.4	21.8	14.2	11.0	9.2
IV —	100.0	27.0	10.0	5.6	4.5	4.0

Figure 46.2 Disease-specific survival by American Joint Committee on Cancer stage grouping. *Numbers* beneath x-axis indicate patients at risk. (From Crew KD, Neugut AI. Epidemiology of gastric cancer. *World J Gastroenterol* 2006;12:354, with permission.)

survival decreases as the number of metastatic lymph nodes increases,[103,104] and that survival significantly decreases at three or more involved[103] lymph nodes and again at seven or more involved lymph nodes.[30,105]

Given the reliance on numerical thresholds for nodal staging, it is extremely important that adequate number of lymph nodes are retrieved surgically and examined pathologically. However, recent reports document poor compliance with AJCC staging primarily because the number of lymph nodes removed and/or examined (≤15) was insufficient.[104,106] Positive peritoneal cytology is classified as M1. Ratio-based lymph node classification (number of positive nodes over number of total nodes resected and evaluated) is an alternative to the threshold-based system currently utilized by the AJCC/UICC staging systems. It may minimize the confounding effects of regional variations in the extent of lymphadenectomy and pathologic evaluation on lymph node staging and thereby

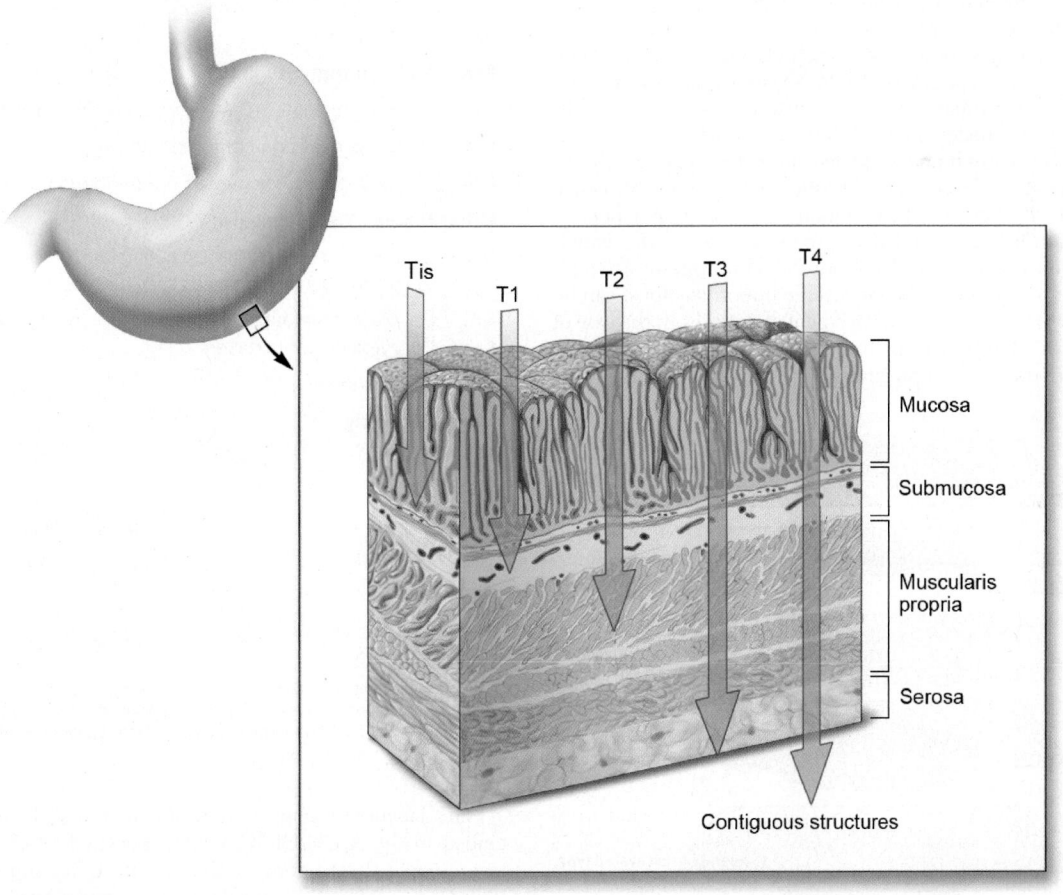

Figure 46.3 Definition of American Joint Committee on Cancer/International Union Against Cancer T stage based on depth of penetration of the gastric wall.

reduce stage migration.[107–109] Sun et al.[108] evaluated the ratio between metastatic and examined lymph nodes (RML) in a group of 2,159 patients who underwent curative gastrectomy. The anatomic location, number of positive lymph nodes (AJCC/UICC), and RML were analyzed for staging accuracy and relationship to survival. RML was an independent prognostic factor for survival and reduced stage migration. These findings were confirmed by several investigators reporting on approximately 2,000 patients treated by R0 gastrectomy.[107,109–112]

Japanese Staging System

The most recent *Japanese Classification for Gastric Carcinoma* was published in 1998.[113–116] The Japanese classification and staging system is more detailed than the AJCC/UICC staging system and places more emphasis on the distinction between clinical, surgical, pathologic, and "final" staging (prefixes "c," "s," "p," and "f," respectively). For example, a surgically treated and staged patient with locally advanced, nonmetastatic gastric cancer might be staged as pT3, pN2, sH0, sM0, stage f-IIIB (where H0 denotes no hepatic metastases and the "f" prefix denotes final clinicopathologic stage). The Japanese classification system also includes a classification system for EGC (Fig. 46.4).

In the combined superficial types, the type occupying the largest area should be described first, followed by the next type (e.g., IIc + III). Type 0I and type 0IIa are distinguished as follows: type 0I, the lesion has a thickness of more than twice that of the normal mucosa; type 0IIa, the lesion has a thickness up to twice that of the normal mucosa.

Similar to the AJCC/UICC staging system, primary tumor (T) stage in the Japanese system is based on the depth of invasion and extension to adjacent structures, as outlined in Table 46.3.[117] However, the assignment of lymph node (N) stage involves much more rigorous pathologic assessment than is required for AJCC/UICC staging. The Japanese system extensively classifies 18 lymph node regions into four N categories (N0 to N3) depending on their relationship to the primary tumor and anatomic location.[118] Most perigastric lymph nodes (nodal stations 1 through 6) are considered group N1. Lymph nodes situated along the proximal left gastric artery (station 7), common hepatic artery (station 8), celiac axis (station 9), splenic artery (station 11), and proper hepatic artery (station 12) are defined as group N2. Para-aortic lymph nodes (station 16) are defined as group N3. However, some lymph nodes, even perigastric nodes for specific tumor locations, can be regarded as M1 disease (i.e., involvement of station 2 in the case of antral tumors). This is because their involvement in antral tumors is rare and portrays a poor prognosis.[117]

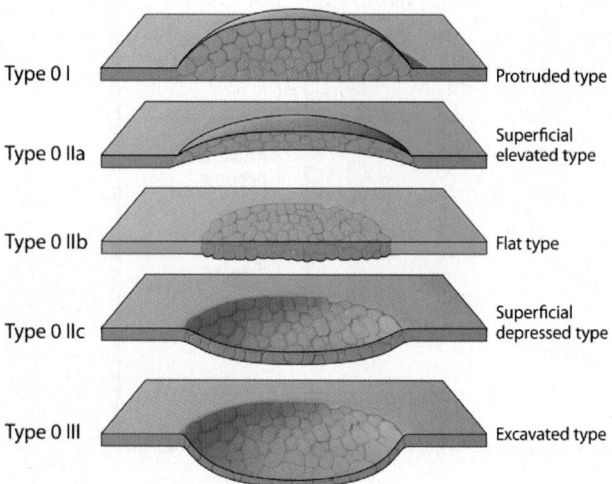

Figure 46.4 Japanese classification system for early gastric cancer.

Type 0 I — Protruded type

Type 0 IIa — Superficial elevated type

Type 0 IIb — Flat type

Type 0 IIc — Superficial depressed type

Type 0 III — Excavated type

TABLE 46.3

Japanese Gastric Cancer Association Staging System

Tumor Stage

T1	Tumor invasion of mucosa and/or muscularis mucosa or submucosa
T2	Tumor invasion of muscularis propria or subserosa
T3	Tumor penetration of serosal
T4	Tumor invasion of adjacent structures
TX	Unknown

Nodal Stage

N0	No evidence of lymph node metastasis
N1	Metastasis to group 1 lymph nodes, but no metastasis to groups 2 to 3 lymph nodes
N2	Metastasis to group 2 lymph nodes, but no metastasis to group 3 lymph nodes
N3	Metastasis to group 3 lymph nodes
NX	Unknown

Hepatic Metastasis Stage (H)

H0	No liver metastasis
H1	Liver metastasis
HX	Unknown

Peritoneal Metastasis Stage (P)

P0	No peritoneal metastasis
P1	Peritoneal metastasis
PX	Unknown

Peritoneal Cytology Stage (CY)

CY0	Benign/indeterminate cells on peritoneal cytology[a]
CY1	Cancer cells on peritoneal cytology
CYX	Peritoneal cytology was not performed

Other Distant Metastasis (M)

M0	No other distant metastases (although peritoneal, liver, or cytologic metastases may be present)
M1	Distant metastases other than the peritoneal, liver, or cytologic metastases
MX	Unknown

Stage Grouping

	N0	N1	N2	N3
T1	IA	IB	II	
T2	IB	II	IIIA	
T3	II	IIIA	IIIB	IV
T4	IIIA	IIIB		
H1, P1, CY1, M1				

[a] Cytology believed to be "suspicious for malignancy" should be classified as CY0.
Adapted from Japanese Gastric Cancer Association. Japanese Classification of Gastric Carcinoma - 2nd English Edition. *Gastric Cancer* 1998;1:10.

The Japanese staging system also includes elements not included in the AJCC/UICC system (see Table 46.3). These are macroscopic descriptions of the tumor (EGC subtype or Borrmann type for more advanced tumors), extent of peritoneal metastases (classified as P0-1), extent of hepatic metastases (H0-1), and peritoneal cytology findings (CY0-1). Recent comparison of the

Japanese and AJCC/UICC staging systems in 731 patients suggests that both are comparable.[119] However, older studies suggest that the AJCC/UICC system more accurately estimates prognosis.[101]

Classification of Esophagogastric Junction Cancers

EGJ cancers (i.e., tumors with a definitive component involving the EGJ) are no longer classified by the AJCC as gastric cancers per se. They are briefly reviewed here for historical reasons. Siewert and Stein[120] classified adenocarcinomas of the EGJ (Siewert classification) into three distinct clinical entities that arise within 5 cm of the EGJ: type I arises in the distal esophagus and may infiltrate the EGJ from above, type II arises in the cardia or the EGJ, and type III arises in the subcardial stomach and may infiltrate the EGJ from below. The assignment of tumors to one of these subtypes is based on morphology and the anatomic location of the epicenter of the tumor. The Siewert classification has important therapeutic implications.[121] The lymphatic drainage routes differ for type I versus types II and III lesions. The lymphatic pathways from the lower esophagus pass both cephalad and caudad. In contrast, the lymphatic drainage from the cardia and subcardial regions is caudad. Thus, the Siewert classification provides a practical means for choosing among surgical options. For type I tumors, esophagectomy is required, whereas types II and III tumors can be treated by transabdominal gastrectomy.[121,122]

Resection Classification

The R classification system indicates the amount of residual disease left after tumor resection.[123] R0 indicates no gross or microscopic residual disease, R1 indicates microscopic residual disease (positive margins), and R2 signifies gross residual disease. The R classification has implications for individual patient care and clinical research. Results of clinical trials that include surgery should include information on R status. Readers should be aware of the dual use of the "R" terminology in the gastric cancer literature. Prior to 1995, the Japanese staging and treatment vernacular included an "R level," which described the extent of lymphadenectomy. The latter is now classified by "D" (for dissection) level.

GASTRIC CANCER NOMOGRAMS: PREDICTING INDIVIDUAL PATIENT PROGNOSIS AFTER POTENTIALLY CURATIVE RESECTION

Kattan et al.[103] have developed a nomogram for predicting individual patient 5-year disease-specific survival using established prognostic factors derived from a population of 1,039 patients with gastric cancer treated by R0 surgical resection without neoadjuvant therapy at a single institution (nomograms@mskcc.org). Clinicopathologic factors incorporated in the nomogram include age and gender, primary tumor site, Laurén classification, numbers of positive and negative lymph nodes resected, and depth of invasion. This nomogram was subsequently validated by several authors. Peeters et al.[124] found that the nomogram prognosticates better then the AJCC staging system. Novotny et al.[125] validated the nomogram in 862 patients from Germany and the Netherlands; Strong et al.[126] compared outcomes using the nomogram in 711 patients from the United States and 1,646 patients from Korea. This tool may be useful for individual patient counseling regarding the use of adjuvant therapy, follow-up scheduling, and clinical trial eligibility assessment, and is available for personal handheld computer devices at www.nomograms.org.

Recently, a large retrospective cohort study of 1,273 patients who underwent resection revealed that having a positive family history of gastric cancer (defined as a self-reported history of cancer in first-degree relatives) was associated with significant reduction in disease-free survival (DFS; $p = 0.012$), relapse-free survival ($p = 0.006$), and OS ($p = 0.005$) when compared with those who did not have a family history of gastric cancer. The improvement in outcomes was more pronounced among patients with stage III or IV gastric cancer, with significant adjusted HRs for DFS (HR = 0.49; 95% confidence interval [CI] = 0.29 to 0.84), relapse-free survival (HR = 0.47; 95% CI = 0.30 to 0.87), and OS (HR = 0.47; 95% CI = 0.26 to 0.84), respectively.[127]

TREATMENT OF LOCALIZED DISEASE

Stage I Disease (Early Gastric Cancer)

Classification of Early Gastric Cancer and Risk for Nodal Metastases

The Japanese Research Society for Gastric Cancer has classified EGCs based on endoscopic criteria first established for the description of T1 tumors. The current classification system is used for both in situ and invasive tumors and categorizes tumors based on endoscopic findings as follows: protruded, type 0I; superficial elevated, type 0IIa; flat, type 0IIb; superficial depressed, type 0IIc; and excavated, type 0III (see Fig. 46.4). The English language version of the Japanese EGC classification contains excellent color photos of these subtypes.[128] This classification system is important in describing patients treated by newer gastric-sparing approaches for EGC, such as endoscopic mucosal resection (EMR).[114–116,129] The risk for lymph node metastasis is important when evaluating treatment options for patients with EGC. The frequency and anatomic distribution of nodal disease are related to the depth of tumor invasion. In a Japanese series of >5,000 patients who underwent gastrectomy with lymph node dissection for EGC, none of the 1,230 patients with well-differentiated intramucosal tumors <3 cm in diameter (regardless of ulceration) had lymph node metastases.[130] None of the 929 patients with EGC without ulceration had nodal metastases, irrespective of tumor size. In contrast, in the subset of >2,000 patients with tumors that invaded the submucosa, the frequencies of lymph node involvement for tumors ≤1.0 cm, 1.1 to 2.0 cm, 2.1 to 3.0 cm, and >3.0 cm were 7.9%, 13.3%, 15.6%, and 23.3%, respectively. Thus, once tumors penetrate into the submucosa, the risk for nodal metastasis increases with tumor size.[131–137] The estimates of the frequency of nodal disease in EGC are based on conventional light-microscopic histologic assessment. However, the use of more sensitive techniques such as serial sectioning of individual lymph nodes, immunohistochemistry, or reverse transcriptase-polymerase chain reaction may increase the frequency of detection of occult micrometastatic disease.[138] The clinical significance of micrometastasis remains unknown.

Endoscopic Mucosal Resection

A subset of patients with EGC can undergo an R0 resection without lymphadenectomy or gastrectomy. The Japanese have popularized EMR for EGC. This approach involves the submucosal injection of fluid to elevate the lesion and facilitate complete mucosal resection under endoscopic guidance. Most centers reporting significant experience with EMR are in Japan. There is less experience with EMR in Western countries. Only patients with tumors that have extremely low metastatic potential should be offered EMR. These are generally well-differentiated, superficial type IIa or IIc lesions, <3 cm in diameter, and located in an easily manipulated area. Tumors invading the submucosa are at increased risk for metastasizing to lymph nodes and are not usually considered candidates for EMR.

Recently, Bennett et al.[139] reviewed the available data reporting on EMR for EGC. No randomized controlled trial (RCT) reported on EMR. The indications for EMR are well-differentiated lesions, size ≤20 mm in elevated type, ≤10 mm in depressed type, no ulceration, and limited to the mucosa.[140] The incidence of lymph node metastases for such lesions is approximately 1%. Complete resection of selected EGCs can be accomplished in a majority of cases (73.4% to 98%).[139,141,142]

Two retrospective reports indicated that EMR can reduce the risk of local residual tumor, and repeat EMR is an effective option.[143,144] Recurrence after EMR varies with type of EGC. Ida et al.[145] reported on 412 patients: 8 of 199 (4.0%) had recurrence of lesions size 20 to 40 mm; 5 patients were retreated by EMR and 3 underwent open surgery; and none had lymph node metastases. Patients (0/305) with lesions ≤20 mm did not have recurrence. Complication rates associated with EMR are low. Bleeding and perforation are reported in 0% to 20.5% and 0% to 5.2 % of patients, respectively.[141,146–149] The reported morbidity and mortality rates in patients undergoing open surgery ($n = 256$) versus EMR ($n = 56$) were 0.8% and 7.8% versus 0% and 16%, repsectively.[139,150]

Fukase et al.[151,152] reported on the long-term outcomes of patients undergoing open surgery ($n = 116$) versus EMR ($n = 59$). For patients age 65 year or under, the 5- and 10-year survival rates were 100% and 91.7% versus 92.8% and 92.8%, with open surgery and EMR, respectively. For patients older than 65 years of age, the 5- and 10-year survival rates were 100% and 75% versus 80.8% and 80.8%, respectively. The differences were not statistically significant. Similar results were reported by Park et al.[153] and Kim et al.[154]

There are emerging variations of EMR techniques, including the cap suction and cut versus a ligating device. As outcome studies accumulate demonstrating favorable survival, EMR is emerging as the definitive management of selected EGCs and is not just reserved for patients in whom gastrectomy cannot be considered. However, RCTs are needed to establish an outcome advantage over open surgery.[140,155–165]

Limited Surgical Resection

Given the low rate of nodal involvement for patients with EGC, limited resection may be a reasonable alternative to gastrectomy for some patients. There are no well-accepted pretreatment criteria for selection of patients for limited resection. Based on available pathology studies, patients with small (<3 cm) intramucosal tumors and those with nonulcerated intramucosal tumors of any size may be candidates for EMR or limited resection. Surgical options for these patients may include gastrotomy with local excision. This procedure should be performed with full-thickness mural excision (to allow accurate pathologic assessment of T status) and is often aided by intraoperative gastroscopy for tumor localization. Formal lymph node dissection is not required in these patients.

Gastrectomy

Gastrectomy with lymph node dissection should be considered for patients with EGC who cannot be treated with EMR or limited surgical resection, and/or patients who have intramucosal tumors with poor histologic differentiation, or size >3 cm, or who have tumor penetration into the submucosa or beyond. Gastrectomy with lymph node dissection allows for adequate pathologic staging and local therapy for these patients at increased risk of nodal metastasis. Dissection of level I lymph nodes is a reasonable minimum standard at this time for higher risk EGCs. The roles for nodal "sampling" without formal node dissection (D0 dissection) and sentinel lymph node (SLN) mapping and biopsy in the treatment of EGC remain undefined at this time.

Stage II and Stage III Disease

Surgery

Surgical resection of the primary tumor and regional lymph nodes is the cornerstone of treatment for patients with localized gastric cancer. However, for stage II and III disease, surgery is necessary but often not sufficient for cure. The general therapeutic goal is to achieve a microscopically complete resection (R0). A complete discussion of all the technical details of gastric resection and reconstruction is beyond the scope of this chapter. However, specific surgical issues of oncologic significance are addressed here, including the extent of gastrectomy, extent of regional lymph node dissection, and role of partial pancreatectomy and splenectomy. Additional technical details can be found in surgical atlases and the section "Technical Treatment-Related Issues."

Extent of Resection for Mid- and Distal Gastric Cancers. The extent of gastrectomy required for satisfactory primary tumor treatment depends primarily on the gross and microscopic status of surgical margins. For most clinical situations, a 5-cm grossly negative margin around the tumor and microscopically negative surgical margin (R0) are the treatment goals. When gastrectomy is performed with curative intent, frozen-section assessment of proximal and distal resection margins should be used intraoperatively to improve the likelihood that an R0 resection has been attained. Three relatively small prospective RCTs have compared total gastrectomy with partial (subtotal) gastrectomy for distal gastric cancer.[166–168] Overall morbidity, mortality, and oncologic outcome were comparable in each of these RCTs. When the general oncologic goal of an R0 resection can be achieved by a gastric-preserving approach, partial gastrectomy is preferred over total gastrectomy. This is particularly relevant for distal gastric cancers, for which a gastric-preserving R0 approach may minimize the risks of specific sequelae of total gastrectomy such as early satiety, weight loss, and the need for vitamin B_{12} supplementation.

Extent of Resection for Proximal Gastric Cancer. There are many choices for surgical management of adenocarcinomas arising at the EGJ or in the proximal stomach (Siewert types II and III). Many abdominal surgeons have advocated transabdominal approaches with resection of the lower esophagus and proximal stomach or total gastrectomy. Surgeons trained in thoracic surgery have frequently advocated a combined abdominal and thoracic procedure (often termed *esophagogastrectomy*) with an intrathoracic or cervical anastomosis between the proximal esophagus and the distal stomach, or a procedure termed *transhiatal (or blunt) esophagectomy* (THE), which involves resection of the esophagus and EGJ with mediastinal dissection performed in a blunt fashion through the esophageal hiatus of the diaphragm. When THE is performed for adenocarcinoma of the EGJ, gastrointestinal continuity is restored by low cervical anastomosis of the stomach (usually advanced through the esophageal bed in the posterior mediastinum) to the cervical esophagus. Selection among the options has been dependent primarily on individual surgeon training and experience.

The optimal surgical procedure for patients with localized tumors of the EGJ and proximal stomach is a matter of considerable debate. A recently completed Dutch RCT compared transthoracic esophagogastrectomy (TTEG, with abdominal and thoracic incisions) with THE in 220 patients with adenocarcinoma of the esophagus and EGJ.[169] Although this trial was designed for patients with esophageal cancer, 40 (18%) of the patients had adenocarcinomas of the EGJ (Siewert type II), and the operations evaluated are among those considered for patients with Siewert type II or III cancers. Perioperative morbidity was higher after THE, but there was no significant difference in in-hospital mortality compared with TTEG. Although median overall, disease-free, and quality-adjusted survival did not differ significantly between the groups, there was a trend toward improved OS at 5 years with TTEG. These results are judged equivocal, and there is currently no consensus on the optimal surgical approach for patients with Siewert type II tumors.[170] Until longer follow-up of the Dutch trial is available and/or additional RCTs are performed, the surgical approach to these patients will continue to be individualized and determined by a constellation of factors including surgeon factors (training and experience), patient factors (age, comorbid conditions, and functional status), and tumor factors (pretreatment T and N stage).

Extent of Lymphadenectomy.

There has been intense debate surrounding the extent of lymphadenectomy. It involves at least two important issues: (1) adequate staging in terms of the number of lymph nodes resected surgically and examined pathologically, and (2) adequate therapy (i.e., do some forms of lymphadenectomy result in better outcomes?).[171–182]

Single-institution reports suggest that the number of pathologically positive lymph nodes is of prognostic significance,[100,102,180,183–185] and that removal and pathologic analysis of at least 15 lymph nodes is required for adequate pathologic staging.[99,186] Indeed, the current AJCC staging system accounts for these issues and therefore requires analysis of ≥16 lymph nodes to assign a pathologic N stage.[187] The possible therapeutic benefit of extended lymph node dissection D2 versus D1 dissection has been the focus of six RCTs, which are summarized in Table 46.4.[167,188–193] These trials were performed because retrospective and prospective nonrandomized evidence suggested that extended lymph node dissection may be associated with improved long-term survival.[194] The RCTs tested the hypothesis that removal of additional pathologically positive lymph nodes (not generally removed as part of a standard lymph node dissection) improves survival. The larger RCTs attempted to follow what are referred to as the "Japanese rules" for lymph node classification and dissection that govern the extent of nodal dissection required based on anatomic location of the primary tumor.[195] Using these Japanese definitions, the RCTs compared limited lymphadenectomy of the perigastric lymph nodes (D1 dissection) to en bloc removal of second-echelon lymph nodes (D2 dissection). At least two of the completed trials are underpowered for their primary end point, OS.[167,188] The trials from the Medical Research Council (MRC) of the United Kingdom[189] and the Dutch Gastric Cancer Group[190] have received the most attention and discussion.

The MRC trial registered 737 patients with gastric adenocarcinoma; 337 (46%) patients were ineligible by staging laparotomy because of advanced disease, and 400 (54%) patients were randomized at the time of laparotomy to undergo D1 (200) or D2 (200) lymph node dissection. Postoperative morbidity was significantly greater in the D2 group (46% versus 28%; p <0.001), and in-hospital mortality rates were also significantly higher in the D2 group than in the D1 group (13% versus 6%, p <0.04).[189] The most frequent postoperative complications were related to anastomotic leakage (D2 26% versus D1 11%), cardiac complications (8% versus 2%), and respiratory complications (8% versus 5%). The excess morbidity and mortality seen in the D2 group were thought to be related to the routine use of distal (left) pancreatectomy and splenectomy. Partial pancreatectomy and splenectomy were performed to maximize clearance of lymph nodes at the splenic hilum, primarily for patients with proximal tumors; however, many surgeons now believe that adequate lymph node dissection can be performed with pancreas- and spleen-preserving techniques. Long-term follow-up analysis of patients in the MRC trial demonstrated comparable 5-year OS rates of 35% and 33% in the D1 and D2 dissection groups, respectively. Survival based on death from gastric cancer as the event was also similar in the D1 and D2 groups (HR = 1.05; 95% CI = 0.79 to 1.39), as was recurrence-free survival (HR = 1.03; 95% CI = 0.82 to 1.29). The authors concluded that classic Japanese-style D2 lymphadenectomy (with partial pancreatectomy and splenectomy) offered no survival advantage over D1 lymphadenectomy.

The Dutch Gastric Cancer Group conducted a larger RCT with optimal surgical quality control comparing D1 to D2 lymph node dissection for patients with gastric adenocarcinoma that was updated in 2010 after 15-year follow-up.[196] Between 1989 and July 1993, 1,078 patients were entered, of whom 996 patients were eligible; 711 patients were randomized to D1 dissection (n = 380) or

D2 dissection (n = 331). To maximize surgical quality control, all operations were monitored.[197] Initially, this oversight was done by a Japanese surgeon who trained a group of Dutch surgeons, who in turn acted as supervisors during surgery at 80 participating centers. Notwithstanding the extraordinary efforts to ensure quality control of the two types of lymph node dissection, both noncompliance (not removing all lymph node stations) and contamination (removing more than was indicated) occurred, thus blurring the distinction between the two operations and confounding the interpretation of the oncologic end points.[196,198] The postoperative morbidity rate was higher in the D2 group (43% versus 25%; p <0.001), the reoperation rate was also higher at 18% (59/331) versus 8% (30/380), and the mortality rate was also significantly higher in the D2 group (10% versus 4%; p = 0.004). Patients treated with D2 dissection also required a longer hospitalization.[199] As in the MRC trial, partial pancreatectomy and splenectomy were performed en passant in the D2 group. Five-year survival rates were similar in the two groups: 45% for the D1 group and 47% for the D2 group (95% CI for the difference = −9.6% to 5.6%). The subset of patients who had R0 resections, excluding those who died postoperatively, had cumulative risks of relapse at 5 years of 43% with D1 dissection and 37% with D2 dissection (95% CI for the difference = −2.4% to 14.4%).

The Dutch investigators concluded that there was no role for the routine use of D2 lymph node dissection in patients with gastric cancer. At 15-year follow-up, 174/711 (25%) patients were alive, all but one without recurrence. The OS was 21% (82/711) and 29% (92 patients) for the D1 and D2 groups, respectively (p = 0.34). Interestingly, gastric cancer–specific death was higher in the D1 group 48% (182/380) versus 37% (123/331). Local recurrence was higher in the D1 group 22% (82/380) versus 12% (40/331), and regional recurrence 19% (73/380) versus 13% (43/331). The authors concluded that after 15 years of follow-up, D2 lymphadenectomy is associated with lower locoregional recurrence and gastric cancer–specific death rates than D1 lymphadenectomy. D2 resection is also associated with higher postoperative mortality, morbidity, and reoperation rates. Examining the results after 15-year follow-up and given the data regarding gastric cancer–specific mortality, local recurrence, and regional recurrence, the authors revised their original conclusion: "Because spleen-preserving D2 resection is safer in high-volume centers, it is the recommended surgical approach for patients with potentially curable gastric cancer."[196]

Degiuli et al.[191] reported on the Italian Gastric Cancer Study Group experience with a prospective randomized trial comparing pancreas-sparing D1 versus D2. There were 76 patients randomized to undergo D1 and 86 D2 resections. Complication rates were higher in the D2 group: 16.3% versus 10.5%. Postoperative mortality was higher in the D1 group: 1.3% versus 0% in the D2 group. Thus far, no survival data are available. The authors concluded that, in experienced hands, the morbidity and mortality can be as low as shown by Japanese surgeons.

Wu et al.[192] reported on a randomized trial comparing D1 versus D3 dissections.[199] There were no operative deaths, and morbidity was only 12%. At median follow-up of 94.5 months, D3 showed better overall 5-year survival of 59.5% (95% CI = 50.3 to 68.7) versus 53.6% (95% CI = 44.2 to 63.0; p = 0.041), and a trend toward better DFS at 5 years: 40.3% versus 50.6% (p = 0.197). Only 13% had pancreas or splenic resection as compared with 23% in the Dutch trial. The authors concluded that D3 as compared to D1 offers survival benefit. As far as the authors of this chapter understand, this is the first RCT to demonstrate survival advantage for more extensive lymphadenectomy (D3). As such, it requires careful examination. Roggin and Posner[200] have critically reviewed the work by Wu et al.[192] One controversial element of this trial was the use of OS versus gastric cancer–specific survival; 17/111 (15%) of the reported deaths were not related to tumor recurrence, resulting in very small survival benefit.

Interpretation of the existing level 1 evidence is encumbered by a number of issues that have been discussed in detail elsewhere.[171,172] The primary concerns relate to whether (1) the increased operative

TABLE 46.4

Prospective Randomized Trials Comparing D1 Versus D2 and D3 Resection for Potentially Curable Gastric Carcinoma

Study (Ref.)	Extent of Lymphadenectomy		
	D1	D2	*P* Value
Groote Schuur Hospital, Cape Town, 1988[188]			
Number of patients	22	21	—
Length of operation (h)	1.7 ± 0.6	2.33 ± 0.7	<0.005
Transfusions (units/group)	4	25	<0.05
Postoperative stay (d)	9.3 ± 4.7	13.9 ± 9.7	<0.05
5-y overall survival (log rank test)	0.69	0.67	NS
Prince of Wales Hospital, Hong Kong, 1994[167]			
Number of patients	25	29	—
Length of operation (h)	140	260	<0.05
Operative blood loss (ml)	300	600	<0.05
Postoperative stay	8	16	<0.05
Median survival (d)	1,511	922	<0.05
Medical Research Council Trial, United Kingdom, 1999[189,193]			
Number of patients	200	200	—
Operative mortality (%)	6.5	13	<0.04
Postoperative complications (%)	28	46	<0.001
5-y overall survival (%)	35	3	NS
Dutch Gastric Cancer Trial, The Netherlands, 1999 (2009, 15-y F/U update)[190,196]			
Number of patients	380	331	—
Operative mortality rate (%)	4	10	0.004
Postoperative complications (%)	25	43	<0.001
Postoperative stay (d)	18	25	<0.001
5-y overall survival (%)	45	47	NS
11-y F/U overall survival (%)	30	35	0.53
11-y F/U survival (perioperative death excluded)	32	39	0.10
15y F/U overall survival	21	29	0.34
15y F/U gastric cancer–specific death	48	37	0.01
Italian Gastric Cancer Study Group, 2004[191]			
Number of patients	76	86	—
Operative mortality rate (%)	1.3	0	NS
Postoperative complication (%)	10.5	16.3	0.29
Postoperative stay (d)	12	12	NS
5-y overall survival	NS	NS	NS
Yang-Ming University, Taiwan, 2006[192]			
Number of patients	110	111, D3	
Operative mortality rate (%)	0	0	
Postoperative complication (%)	10.1	17.1	0.012
Postoperative stay (d)	15	19.6	0.001
5-y overall survival	53.6	59.5	0.041

NS, not stated; F/U, follow-up.

mortality associated with protocol-mandated partial pancreatectomy and splenectomy for patients with proximal tumors undergoing D2 dissection prevented identification of a potential therapeutic impact of extended lymph node dissection, and (2) the phenomena of noncompliance and contamination led to homogenization of the operative procedures to such an extent that the fundamental hypothesis was not tested. Owing to these interpretation issues, the question of a possible therapeutic benefit of D2 dissection remains unsettled.

Many Japanese gastric surgeons have considered the caveats associated with the MRC and Dutch trials and believe that, notwithstanding inherent patient selection and stage migration biases,[171,196,198,201,202] the existing retrospective data provide sufficient proof of a clinical benefit of D2 dissection. On this basis, D2 dissection has been adopted as the standard of care for patients with localized, higher-risk gastric cancer in many centers in Japan and some specialized centers in the West.[203] The Japanese Clinical Oncology Group (JCOG-9501) has investigated an even more aggressive surgical approach in an RCT evaluating standard D2 versus D2-plus (para-aortic node dissection [PAND]) in the management of completely resected (R0) T2–4 gastric cancer.[204,205] Between July 1995 and April 2001, 523 patients from 25 institutions were registered. Patients were randomized intraoperatively to undergo D2 lymphadenectomy alone (263 patients) or D2 lymphadenectomy plus PAND (260 patients). The primary end point was OS. Postoperative morbidity was higher in the PAND group (28% versus. 21%; $p = 0.07$), and mortality was similar at 0.8% in each group. Five-year OS for patients undergoing PAND was 70.3% versus 69.2% (HR = 1.03; $p = 0.85$). There was no significant difference in recurrence-free survival. The authors concluded that, as compared to D2 lymphadenectomy, PAND when added to D2 lymphadenectomy does not improve survival rates.

Another Japanese study compared D2 with extended PAND (D4).[206] This trial randomized patients to undergo gastrectomy with D2 ($n = 135$) or D4 ($n = 134$) lymphadenectomy. The 5-year survival rates were 52.6% versus 55%, respectively ($p = 0.8$). The authors concluded that prophylactic D4 dissection is not recommended. In an RCT, a Western group from Poland investigated D2 dissection versus extended D2 dissection defined according to the Japanese Gastric Cancer Association classification.[207] They randomized 275 patients with gastric cancer to gastrectomy with D2 ($n = 141$) versus D2 + lymphadenectomy ($n = 134$). The overall postoperative morbidity and mortality were similar and did not differ statistically. Survival data are not available at this time.[207] Thus, the limits of radical surgery have been reached in Japan and the pendulum has swung back toward D2 dissection in clinical settings in which this can be safely performed.[201]

In summary, lymph nodes should be considered as indicators that the gate was opened rather than as the gate keepers for cure.[208] None of the prospective RCT trials executed in the West demonstrated survival advantage for more extensive lymphadenectomy. However, none of these studies were powered enough to detect single-digit difference in 5-year OS. Several non-a priori planned subgroup analyses were done and showed some survival advantage for certain subgroups. These analyses cannot be used to form evidence-based medicine, but should be used to form hypotheses for further RCT studies. In high-volume specialty centers, spleen- and pancreas-preserving D2 dissection is performed safely, and can potentially result in decreased gastric cancer–specific mortality based on 15 years of follow-up from the Dutch study (D2 37% versus 48%; $p = 0.01$).[196]

A recently published RCT from the multicenter Italian Gastric Cancer Study Group compared D1 to D2 lymphadenectomy for gastric adenocarcinoma with primary outcome of OS over median follow-up of 8.8 years.[209] There was no significant difference in OS (5-year OS = 66.5% versus 64.2%), operative morbidity (12% versus 17.9%), and mortality (3% versus 2.2%) in patients undergoing D1 and D2 gastrectomy; however, subgroup analysis suggested a trend toward improved disease-specific survival with

D2 gastrectomy in patients with advanced T-stage (pT2-4) and node-positive disease (5-year disease-specific survival: D1 versus D2 = 38% versus 59%; $p = 0.055$).

A systematic review and meta-analysis of eight RCTs encompassing over 2,000 patients (D1, $n = 1,042$; D2, $n = 1,002$) evaluated the safety and efficacy of extended lymphadenectomy in gastric cancer.[210] A significant increase in operative morbidity and mortality was evident in patients undergoing extended D2 lymphadenectomy, with a trend in decreased disease-specific mortality in those having spleen- and pancreas-preserving gastrectomy. Longer-term survival is required to ascertain oncologically relevant outcome benefit with D2 gastrectomy.

Partial Pancreatectomy and Splenectomy Resect or Preserve? Partial (left, distal) pancreatectomy and splenectomy have been performed as part of D2 lymph node dissection to remove the lymph nodes along the splenic artery (station 11) and lymph nodes within the splenic hilum (station 12), primarily for patients with tumors located in the proximal and midstomach. Indeed, partial pancreatectomy and splenectomy were required for patients with proximal tumors in the D2 arm of the Dutch and MRC RCTs but were required only for direct tumor extension in the D1 arm. In the Dutch and MRC D1 versus D2 randomized trials, splenectomy was associated with increased risk of surgical complications and operative mortality. In addition, a multivariate analysis suggested that splenectomy is associated with inferior long-term survival. The frequent performance of splenectomy (e.g., 30% of patients in the D2 arm versus 3% in the D1 arms of the Dutch trial) in the patient undergoing extended D2 lymphadenectomy, with its associated adverse effects on both short- and long-term mortality, confounds the interpretation of the Dutch and MRC RCTs. Thus, the hypothesis that spleen- and pancreas-preserving D2 lymph node dissection improves survival remains unproven. There is an evolving consensus that splenectomy should be performed only in cases with intraoperative evidence of direct tumor extension into the spleen, or its hilar vasculature, or when the primary tumor is located in the proximal stomach along the greater curvature.[211] Partial pancreatectomy should be performed only in cases of direct tumor extension to the pancreas.

Recent reports have described pancreas- and spleen-preserving forms of D2 dissection.[212–218] This organ-preserving modification of classic D2 dissection allows for dissection of some station 11 and 12 lymph nodes without the potential adverse effects of pancreatectomy and/or splenectomy. In a small single-institution RCT recently reported from Chile, Csendes et al.[219] randomized 187 patients with localized proximal gastric adenocarcinoma to treatment by total gastrectomy with D2 lymph node dissection plus splenectomy or total gastrectomy with D2 lymphadenectomy alone. Operative mortality was similar in both groups (splenectomy group, 3%; control group, 4%). However, septic complication rates were higher in the splenectomy arm than in the control arm ($p < 0.04$). There was no difference in 5-year OS between study groups, although it is not clear that the trial was designed with survival as the primary end point. Other investigators confirmed these findings.[218,220,221]

The JCOG is conducting a multi-institutional RCT (JCOG 0110-MF) comparing D2 dissection with and without splenectomy for patients diagnosed with proximal gastric cancer.[222] The hypothesis to be tested is that 5-year OS of patients treated by extended D2 dissection *without* splenectomy is 5% less than that of patients treated by D2 dissection *with* splenectomy. With a planned accrual of 500 patients, this design will provide 70% power to reject the null hypothesis when 5-year OS is 3% greater following splenic preservation compared with splenectomy.[222] The results of this trial will better define the short- and long-term effects of splenectomy for patients with proximal gastric cancers undergoing extended lymphadenectomy.

In an effort to reduce operative morbidity and mortality without compromising oncologic outcome in patients undergoing extended lymphadenectomy for gastric adenocarcinoma, eight clinical trials have compared laparoscopic to open gastrectomy with D2 lymph node dissection. A meta-analysis was conducted of these eight trials, which enrolled nearly 1,500 patients with gastric cancer to assess the feasibility and safety of laparoscopic total gastrectomy with D2 lymphadenectomy compared to the same operation done in the standard open manner.[223] The laparoscopic technique was associated with significantly longer operative time, less operative blood loss, fewer analgesic requirements, earlier return of bowel function, shorter hospital stay, and reduced operative morbidity (relative risk = 0.70; 95% CI = 0.50 to 0.98; $p = 0.035$). The total number of lymph nodes removed surgically and analyzed pathologically as well as operative mortality was not significantly different between groups. Further well-designed clinical RCTs are warranted to define the role of laparoscopic gastrectomy and extended lymphadenectomy for gastric adenocarcinoma. (A more detailed discussion follows in the section titled "Minimally Invasive Surgery for Gastric Resection.")

Laparoscopy clearly has a role in the complete staging of disease in patients with gastric adenocarcinoma and the detection of radiologically occult macroscopic, or microscopic peritoneal cytology positive-only metastasis. Laparoscopy and peritoneal cytology are important for accurate staging and the detection of occult metastatic disease. This methodology adds value to modern imaging techniques, for positive microscopic peritoneal cytology-only disease is tantamount to macroscopic M1 disease in terms of oncologic outcome.

A recent international multidisciplinary expert panel created statements to define processes of care relevant to the perioperative management of patient with gastric cancer.[224] Ten processes were deemed essential to maintaining quality of care:

1. CT of the abdomen and pelvis is part of preoperative staging.
2. PET scans are not routinely indicated.
3. Adjuvant therapy should be considered.
4. Clinical trials should be conducted and patients considered for participation.
5. Treatment decision making should involve a multidisciplinary team.
6. Hospitals must have sufficient systems in place to support the care of patients with gastric cancer.
7. Sixteen or more lymph nodes should be resected and staged pathologically.
8. Surgery should only be performed to palliate major symptoms in the setting of metastatic disease.
9. Surgeons experienced in the treatment of gastric cancer should be performing the operations.
10. These surgeons should also have advanced laparoscopic surgery experience for laparoscopic gastric resection.

These processes were deemed to be of indeterminate necessity for maintaining quality of care:

1. Diagnostic laparoscopy before treatment
2. Multidisciplinary approach to patients with linitis plastica
3. Genetic testing for diffuse gastric cancer, family history, or age <45 years at time of diagnosis
4. Endoscopic removal of select T1aN0 lesions
5. D2 lymphadenectomy in curative intent cases
6. D1 lymphadenectomy for EGC or patients with comorbidities
7. Frozen section analysis of gastric resection margins
8. Nonemergent cases performed in a hospital with a volume of >15 gastric cancer resections per year
9. By a surgeon who performs more than six gastric resections per year

Individualized Assessments of Lymph Node Involvement. Recent attention has focused on methods of individual assessment of risk of lymphatic spread. These techniques offer the possibility of tailoring surgical therapy for an individual patient based on clinico-

pathologic risk assessment of the primary tumor and/or preoperative or intraoperative identification of SLNs, or primary draining lymph nodes. At present, at least three approaches to individual nodal risk assessment have been evaluated: computer modeling, preoperative endoscopic peritumoral injection, and SLN biopsy.

Preoperative Computer Modeling of Individual Patient Nodal Involvement. Kampschoer et al.[225] have developed a computer program to estimate the probability of spread to specific nodal regions for an individual patient using his or her pretreatment clinicopathologic data. The program incorporated data on tumor size, depth of infiltration, primary tumor location, grade, type, and macroscopic appearance of primary tumors from 2,000 patients with surgically resected gastric cancers treated at the National Cancer Center of Tokyo. The data set used for matching individual patient data is continuously updated and now includes >8,000 patients. This computer model has been validated in non-Japanese patients in Germany[226] and Italy.[227] In the United States, Hundahl et al.[228] retrospectively applied this computer model to evaluate the surgical treatment of patients entered into the intergroup trial of adjuvant 5-FU–based chemoradiation. The Kampschoer et al.[225] program was used to estimate the likelihood of disease in undissected regional node stations, defining the sum of these estimates as the Maruyama index of unresected disease. Fifty-four percent of participating patients underwent D0 lymphadenectomy. The median index was 70 (range = 0 to 429). In contrast to D level, the Maruyama index proved to be an independent prognostic factor of survival, even with adjustment for the potentially linked variables of T stage and number of positive nodes. More recent and smaller studies confirmed these findings.[229–231]

Preoperative Endoscopic Peritumoral Injection. The hypothesis that peritumoral injection of compounds designed to optimize lymph node dissection improves lymph node clearance was addressed in a small RCT evaluating preoperative endoscopic vital dye staining with CH40 prior to D2 dissection. The frequency of positive lymph nodes in patients injected with CH40 before D2 dissection was greater than that observed in patients treated by D2 dissection alone.[232] This approach optimized the yield of lymph node dissection presumably by directing surgeons to include specific lymph nodes in the dissection that might have otherwise been left in situ and/or by directing pathologists to examine specific areas of the lymphadenectomy specimens. Further prospective studies of this approach are required to confirm the feasibility of this technique and to assess its impact on intraoperative decision making regarding the extent of lymphadenectomy and accuracy of specimen dissection and nodal retrieval in anatomic pathology.

Sentinel Lymph Node Biopsy. The goal of SLN biopsy is to identify the node or nodes believed to be the first peritumoral lymph nodes in the orderly spread of gastric adenocarcinoma from the primary site to the regional lymph nodes. Sampling of this lymph node(s) may allow for prediction of the nodal status of the entire lymph node basin, possibly obviating extended nodal dissection and its attendant morbidity in patients found to have a negative SLN. Recent pilot studies have evaluated the feasibility, sensitivity, and specificity of SLN biopsy for patients with gastric cancer.[233–242] These pilot studies demonstrated that SLN identification is feasible in approximately 95% of patients. However, most patients with gastric cancer have multiple "sentinel" nodes, with mean numbers of SLNs per patient ranging from 2.6 to 6.3. The aggregate experience to date suggests that among patients with pathologically involved lymph nodes, SLN results in false-negative assessment of pathologic regional nodal status in 11% to 60% of patients. Thus, the preliminary data available suggest that SLN biopsy cannot reliably replace lymph node dissection as a means of accurately staging regional nodal basins in gastric adenocarcinoma.[243–247]

In a large study of nearly 400 patients, the ability and accuracy of SLNs was examined in a prospective, multicenter phase 2 study.[248] Patients with early T stage gastric cancer (cT1 or cT2, tumor <4 cm) were evaluated with SLN mapping, followed by gastrectomy and D2 dissection. The SLN mapping technique identified 57 patients who had nodal involvement, of which 53 had true positive SLNs, resulting in 99% accuracy. Though further validation is needed, these results are quite encouraging.

The JCOG multicenter trial (JCOG-0302) assessed the feasibility and accuracy of indocyanine green (ICG) SLN mapping at time of surgery prior to gastrectomy and lymphadenectomy for EGC (T1).[249] Single sections of ICG-stained SLNs were examined intraoperatively using frozen section with hematoxylin and eosin stain. The primary study end point was the proportion of false-negative SLNs. Study accrual was halted after 440 of the planned 1,550 patients were enrolled when the proportion of false negatives was found to be unexpectedly and unacceptably high (46%). The authors appropriately concluded that SLN mapping and biopsy using ICG and intraoperative single nodal frozen section evaluation using hematoxylin and eosin staining is inappropriate for clinical use in EGC.

Volume-Outcome Relationships for Gastrectomy. Recent studies have established a clear relationship between institutional gastrectomy volume and perioperative mortality rates—the so-called volume-outcome relationship. The recent analysis of a national database by Birkmeyer et al.[250–252] of 31,854 patients who underwent gastrectomy between 1994 and 1999 demonstrated an inverse relationship between institutional gastrectomy volume and operative mortality rates. The odds ratio for gastrectomy-related death was lowest among patients treated within hospitals in the highest gastrectomy volume quintile (odds ratio = 0.72; 95% CI = 0.63 to 0.83). A separate analysis evaluating surrogate end points for morbidity demonstrated that gastrectomy at high-volume centers was associated with the shortest duration of hospital stay and the lowest readmission rates.[253–256] Similar findings were noted by Hannan et al.[257] in an analysis of the New York State Department of Health's administrative database. Their analysis of 3,711 patients who underwent gastrectomy between 1994 and 1997 included adjustments for covariates such as age, demographic variables, organ metastasis, socioeconomic status, and comorbidities. Patients who had a gastrectomy at hospitals in the highest-volume quartile had an absolute risk-adjusted mortality rate that was 7.1% (p <0.0001) lower than those treated at hospitals in the lowest-volume quartile, although the overall mortality rate for gastrectomy was only 6.2%.

These studies demonstrate that the risk-adjusted mortality rates for gastrectomy are significantly lower when gastrectomy is performed by high-volume providers.[258–261] It is likely that the variations in gastrectomy-related mortality rates relate in part to surgeon training and their patient age-volume[262–264] and experience with the procedure. Data on gastrectomy volume obtained from general surgeons undergoing recertification after a minimum of 7 years in practice demonstrate that the mean number of gastric resections performed by recertifying general surgeons in the United States is only 1.4 per year.[265] Thus, given the data supporting a relationship between hospital and provider volumes and the morbidity and mortality rate of gastric resection, there are reasons to consider regionalization of the surgical treatment of gastric cancers.

Outcome in Japan Versus Western Countries. Stage-stratified survival rates for gastric adenocarcinoma are higher in Japan than in most Western countries. The reasons for this are complex, are incompletely understood, and cannot be fully addressed within the context of a chapter covering all aspects of gastric cancers.

Important differences in the epidemiology of gastric cancer may contribute to observed differences in outcome in Japan versus Western countries. First, the better-prognosis intestinal-type (Laurén classification)[266] tumors are seen more commonly in Japan, whereas the diffuse-type cancers (poorer prognosis) are more frequent in Western series. These regional differences in the frequencies of intestinal and diffuse cancers are believed to be related to the higher incidence of *H. pylori* infection and atrophic gastritis in Japan. Second, poorer-prognosis proximal gastric cancers are less frequent in Japan.[267–269] Indeed, the progressive increase in proximal gastric cancers observed in the West has not been observed in Japanese populations.

Regional differences in the diagnostic criteria for EGC also may contribute to regional differences in observed outcome. In Japan, gastric carcinoma is diagnosed based on its structural and cytologic features without consideration of invasion of the lamina propria. In contrast, Western pathologists consider invasion of the lamina propria to be an essential element of the diagnosis of carcinoma.[270–274] As a consequence, unequivocally neoplastic noninvasive lesions are classified as carcinoma in Japan, but as dysplasia by Western pathologists.[270] To overcome these differences, the Padvova,[275] Vienna,[276] and Revised Vienna[276] classifications have recently been proposed. However, until there is worldwide consensus and implementation of uniform diagnostic criteria for EGC, comparative assessments of the outcome of patients with EGC treated in Japan and Western countries should acknowledge the selection bias associated with different diagnostic criteria.

Stage migration is a well-documented factor contributing to the stage-specific differences in outcome between Japanese and Western patients.[277] Stage migration arises because there is widespread use of extensive D2 or D3 lymphadenectomy combined with rigorous pathologic assessment of the lymphadenectomy specimen in Japan. More accurate stage assignment of Japanese patients leads to secondary stage migration—improvement in stage-specific survival without improvement in OS. The frequency and impact of stage migration were quantified by the Dutch Gastric Cancer Group in their RCT comparing D1 and D2 lymph node dissection.[190,278] Stage migration occurred in 30% of patients in the D2 group, and the stage-specific decreases in survival rates attributable to stage migration were 3% for AJCC/UICC stage I disease, 8% for stage II, 6% for stage III, and 12% for stage IIIB, with the more accurately staged D2 group having higher survival rates.[278]

In addition to regional differences in epidemiology, diagnostic criteria for EGC, and stage migration, other factors may contribute to the observed differences in stage-stratified survival. Such factors may include genetic, environmental, and biologic differences between Japanese and Western patients and tumors. These factors have been less well studied, but were addressed in a comprehensive review by Davis and Sano.[279]

Outcome in Korea Versus Western Countries. A separate evaluation was performed comparing gastric cancer survival following curative intent resection in Korea versus the United States.[126] This study compared two independent, single-institution prospectively maintained databases from 1995 to 2005: one from MSKCC (n = 711 curatively resected patients who did not receive neoadjuvant therapy) and another from St. Mary's Hospital in Seoul, South Korea (n = 1,646 patients, also curatively resected without receiving preoperative therapy). All patients had a D2 dissection and adequate nodal staging. There were notable differences in the two cohorts: patients from the United States were more likely to have proximal tumors and more advanced stage compared with patients resected in Korea. However, when controlling for all known risk factors, stage for stage, patients from Korea still had better OS (HR = 1.3; 95% CI = 1.0 to 1.7; p = 0.05). These data cannot exclude differences in underlying cancer biology as a potential explanation for the observed differences in survival in gastric cancer between patients treated in Korea versus those treated in the United States.

Minimally Invasive Surgery for Gastric Resection

The utilization of laparoscopy in gastric surgery has been increasing over the past decade. There are a plethora of non-RCTs reporting on laparoscopic distal gastrectomy, total gastrectomy, and D2 dissection, and practically every open procedure has been tested using laparoscopy. We will review here the available data from published RCTs. There are no RCTs reporting on total gastrectomies.[280] None of the current RCTs reporting on laparoscopy in gastric cancer are of sufficient quality and magnitude to be considered "practice changing." Huscher et al.[281,282] reported on the largest RCT testing laparoscopic ($n = 29$) versus open ($n = 30$) subtotal gastrectomy for distal gastric cancer. After 5 years of follow-up, overall morbidity and mortality were equivalent. Laparoscopic resection resulted in less blood loss, shorter hospital stay, longer operative time, and earlier resumption of oral intake; these were reported by other authors as well.[283,284] There was no difference in the number of lymph nodes harvested. Overall 5-year and DFS did not differ significantly. The authors concluded that laparoscopic subtotal gastrectomy is feasible and has similar short- and long-term outcomes as open surgery.

Kim et al.[285] reported on laparoscopy-assisted distal gastrectomy (LADG) versus open distal gastrectomy (ODG) for early gastric cancer. This trial was designed to test the 5-year survival utilizing noninferiority design. The interim analysis showed less blood loss ($p < 0.001$), reduced amount of analgesic used ($p < 0.019$), shorter hospital stay ($p < 0.0001$), fewer number of lymph nodes harvested in the LADG arm ($p < 0.05$), and improved short-term quality of life (QOL) parameters on global health ($p < 0.0001$). The authors concluded that comparison of LADG with ODG resulted in improved QOL outcomes in patients followed up to 3 months. The authors have now reported long-term follow-up data.[286] In this study, the authors evaluated 2,976 patients who were treated with either laparoscopic gastrectomy (1,477 patients) or open gastrectomy (1,499 patients) between April 1998 and December 2005. With a median follow-up of 70.8 months, there was no difference in survival between the two resection methodologies, with the exception that for stage IA gastric cancer, laparoscopic gastrectomy had a improved survival (95.3% 5-year survival) versus open gastrectomy (90.3% 5-year survival) ($p < 0.001$).[286] Recently, Ohtani et al.[287] performed meta-analysis of RCT that compared LADG versus ODG for EGC. Their report confirmed the results from Kim et al.[286] and Lee and Han.[288]

A recent update and meta-analysis analyzed data on 784 patients enrolled in eight RCTs[289] comparing laparoscopy-assisted to open gastrectomy for resectable gastric cancer. Despite the fact that operative time was significantly prolonged in the laparoscopy group and that analgesic use, operative blood loss, nodal yield, morbidity (overall and anastomotic), and mortality were *no* different when compared with open gastrectomy, there were a number of clinically important benefits observed in those undergoing minimally invasive surgery. Pulmonary morbidity (odds ratio = 0.43; 95% CI = 0.20 to 0.93; $p = 0.03$), duration of postoperative ileus (missing data = −0.23; 95% CI = −0.41 to −0.05), and hospital stay (missing data = −1.72; 95% CI = −3.40 to 0.04) were significantly reduced in the laparoscopy-assisted gastrectomy group. The survival benefit of minimally invasive surgery in resectable gastric cancer has yet to be definitively demonstrated.[289]

Laparoscopy is another tool in the armamentarium of the surgical oncologist. The question is not whether it can be done laparoscopically, certainly it can; the question is whether it should be done in patients with gastric adenocarcinoma. Recently, a meta-analysis of six clinical trials (658 patients) compared laparoscopic versus open gastrectomy for distal EGC.[290] In this analysis, the authors noted significant reductions in postoperative complications and length of hospital stay in the laparoscopic group, whereas the open gastrectomy group had less operating time and a greater number of lymph nodes harvested. There were no notable differences in the time to return of bowel function, incidence of wound infection, postoperative abscess formation, or anastomotic leak or pulmonary complications, suggesting that there may be some advantages of the laparoscopic approach. The oncologic equivalence, however, has not been adequately tested. Whether the energy, time, and capital invested in developing laparoscopic surgery for gastric

cancer is worth it is the relevant question particularly in an era of skyrocketing medical costs. Certainly, beyond the short term there seems to be no advantage of laparoscopic surgery in gastric cancer. In view of the reported morbidity and mortality in specialty centers, the advantage gained by laparoscopic gastric resection over the first few days underlines the question of whether we should invest more in innovative therapies to eradicate gastric cancer than the simple technical aspects of noninvasive extirpative surgery.

A large prospective random assignment study from Korea is underway in which 1,415 patients with EGC (pT1-2 N0) are randomly assigned to receive either open or laparoscopic distal gastrectomy.[291] Final results of this expected "definitive" phase 3 study are expected to be available in September 2015. A similar large phase 3 study for stage IA and stage IB gastric cancer was initiated in Japan in March 2010. This study randomizes 920 patients from 33 institutions, with the primary end point of OS.[292] Together, it is anticipated that these two pivotal studies will definitively define the role of laparoscopic-assisted gastrectomy in EGC.

Adjuvant Therapy

Patients with EGCs (e.g., patients with AJCC stage I and some stage II) have a good chance of cure with surgery alone. However, the Japanese S-1 adjuvant study indicates that the prognosis for even stage II tumors can be improved with systemic chemotherapy.

Adjuvant therapy indicates administration of a treatment following a potential curative resection of the primary tumor and regional lymph nodes. Therapy after resections that leave microscopic or gross disease are not adjuvant treatment, but rather therapy for known disease, which is palliative in nature. Neoadjuvant chemotherapy involves the use of systemic treatment before potentially curative surgery.

There are several theoretical reasons for beginning adjuvant therapy soon after operation (perioperative chemotherapy). Studies have shown a rapid increase in cell growth of metastases after a primary tumor has been removed related to a decline in certain circulating factors, which serve to inhibit angiogenesis or other cell-cycle promotors, once the primary tumor is removed. Perioperative or neoadjuvant chemotherapy has been studied because the ability to perform a R0 resection in gastric cancer is difficult. In addition, a substantial number of patients undergoing gastrectomy have prolonged recovery. Neoadjuvant chemotherapy has a dual goal: allowing a higher rate of R0 resections and treatment of micrometastatic disease early in the course of treatment.

Adjuvant Systemic Therapy. The results of selected recent RCTs comparing adjuvant chemotherapy with surgery alone are summarized in Table 46.5. Japanese investigators studied S-1, an oral fluoropyrimidine, in a group of 1,059 patients (stages II to IIIB). S-1 was given for 12 months (4 weeks on/2 weeks off). A total of 529 patients received S-1 plus operation and 530 patients underwent operation only. The 3-year OS was 80.1% and 70.1%, respectively (HR = 0.68).[293]

The 5-year survival update was recently reported and demonstrated a sustained benefit in 5-year OS of 71.7% with adjuvant S-1 versus 61.1% with surgery alone (HR = 0.669; 95% CI = 0.540 to 0.828).[294] In addition, another Asian study from Korea reported the results of adjuvant capecitabine and oxaliplatin.[295] In this study, patients were required to have a D2 resection, and those with stage II-IIIB were then randomly assigned to receive 6 months (eight cycles) of capecitabine/oxaliplatin or observation. This was a large study, in which 520 patients were randomly assigned to receive adjuvant chemotherapy and 515 to surgery alone. The study met its primary endpoint of 3-year DFS (74% [95% CI = 69 to 79] with chemotherapy versus 59% [53% to 64%] with surgery alone; $p < 0.0001$). In contradistinction to the positive results using S-1, and the MAGIC and ACCORD 07 trials described later, Di Costanzo et al.[296] did not find a benefit to the use of cisplatin, epirubicin, leucovorin, and 5-FU as adjuvant therapy.

TABLE 46.5

Adjuvant Therapy for Gastric Cancer: Phase 3 Trials

Study (Ref.)	No. of Patients	Three-y DFS (%)	Overall 5-y Survival (%)	HR
S-1[293]				
Surgery	530	60	70	
Adjuvant	529	72	80	0.38
INT-116[339]				
Surgery	275	31	41	1.35
Adjuvant	281	48	50	
GOIRC[296]				
Surgery	128	42[a]	49	0.90
Adjuvant	130	43[a]	48	
MAGIC[327]				
Surgery	253	25	23	0.75
Neoadjuvant	250	38	36	
ACCORD-07[318]				
Surgery	111	25	21	0.69
Neoadjuvant	113	40	34	

DFS, disease-free survival; HR, hazard ratio; INT, Intergroup Trial; GOIRC, Gruppo Oncologico Italiano di Ricerca Clinica; MAGIC, Medical Research Council Adjuvant Gastric Infusional Chemotherapy; ACCORD, the French Action Clinique Coordonnées en Cancérologie Digestive.
[a] Five-year DFS.

Several meta-analyses of adjuvant chemotherapy in gastric cancer have been reported. Recently, Buyse et al.[297] reported a meta-analysis that included individual patient data; 16 trials involving 3,710 patients were available for analysis. They found an OS benefit in favor of adjuvant chemotherapy (HR = 0.83; 95% CI = 0.76 to 0.91; p <0.0001). The absolute benefit was 6.3% at 5 years. The GASTRIC group conducted a meta-analysis; as of 2010, individual patient data for 17 trials involving 3,838 patients were available for analysis. They found an OS benefit in favor of adjuvant chemotherapy (HR = 0.82; 95% CI = 0.75 to 0.90; p >0.001). The absolute benefit was 5.9% at 5 years.[298] Shown in Table 46.5 are the results of recent trials in which adjuvant chemotherapy plus potentially curative resection was studied. The five most recent trials indicate that adjuvant therapy decreases the risk of recurrence by approximately 10%.[299] The use of systemic therapy plus potentially curative resection is considered a standard of care for patients with locally advanced gastric cancers. The most effective regimen to use, whether or not it is best to give therapy perioperatively, and the role of postoperative radiation *plus* systemic therapy are the focus of ongoing clinical research trials.

Adjuvant Intraperitoneal Chemotherapy. Peritoneal recurrence is a common pattern of failure for patients with gastric cancer, even after curative resection.[31,298] The median survival time of patients with peritoneal recurrence is 3 to 6 months. The rationale is based on the observation that drug concentrations within the peritoneal cavity are much higher than those achievable by intravenous or oral drug adminsitration. The data are a mixture of retrospective reviews, pilot phase 2 trials, and several small phase 3 trials. No definitive conclusions can yet be drawn regarding the effectiveness of intraperitoneal postoperative chemotherapy in this setting.

There are several modes of administering intraperitoneal chemotherapy: hyperthermic intraoperative peritoneal chemotherapy (HIPEC), normothermic intraoperative chemotherapy (NIIC) given at the conclusion of the operation, early postoperative intraperitoneal (normothermic) chemotherapy (EPIC), or delayed postoperative intraperitoneal (normothermic) chemotherapy. The theoretical advantage of intraoperative treatment is better drug distribution and the ability to use hyperthermia (HIPEC) to enhance microscopic tumor cytotoxicity. Most trials in gastric cancer have used either 5-FU or floxuridine, mitomycin C, or cisplatin for intraperitoneal chemotherapy.[300–309] Yan et al.[310] performed a meta-analysis of the RCTs reporting on adjuvant intraperitoneal chemotherapy for patients undergoing curative gastric resection; 10 trials involving 1,474 patients were included. A total of 775 patients had resection alone, and 873 patients had resection plus intraperitoneal treatment. A significant improvement in survival was associated with HIPEC (HR = 0.6; 95% CI = 0.43 to 0.83; p = 0.002) or HIPEC plus EPIC (HR = 0.45; 95% CI = 0.29 to 0.68; p = 0.0002). There was only a trend toward survival benefit with NIIC (p = 0.06), but this was not significant with either EPIC alone or delayed postoperative intraperitoneal (normothermic) chemotherapy. The authors concluded that HIPEC with or without EPIC after curative gastric resection is associated with modest improvement in survival and increased complication rate.

Recently, Kang et al.[311] reported on 640 patients with serosal-positive gastric cancer who underwent resection and were then randomized to receive intravenous mitomycin-C (20 mg/m^2) at 3 to 6 weeks after surgery and oral doxifluridine (460 to 600 mg/m^2 per day) starting 4 weeks after the administration of mitomycin-C and continuing for 3 months, or to receive intraoperative intraperitoneal cisplatin (100 mg), intravenous mitomycin-C (15 mg/m^2) on postoperative day 1, followed by oral doxifluridine for 12 months, and six monthly intravenous cisplatin (60 mg/m^2). Results indicated potential improvement in progression-free survival (PFS) and OS for the intraperitoneal cisplatin therapy arm. Kuramoto et al.[312] reported in a retrospective fashion that extensive intraperitoneal lavage performed with 10 L of normal saline after curative resection and before NIIC is superior to surgery alone or to surgery plus NIIC.

Immunochemotherapy

The use of adjuvant immunostimulants given in combination with cytotoxic chemotherapy (immunchemotherapy) has been studied primarily in Asia. The detailed results of these trials have been discussed in the previous edition of this textbook. Although the data available suggest that immunochemotherapy may be valuable, larger and adequately powered clinical trials are necessary to evaluate the clinical utility and efficacy this approach.

Perioperative and Neoadjuvant Chemotherapy. Perioperative (pre- and postoperative) or neoadjuvant chemotherapy is an attractive concept in gastric cancer because many patients have locally advanced tumors at diagnosis, particularly in Western countries. There are two goals of perioperative treatment: to increase the likelihood of an R0 resection, and treat micrometastatic disease early. After gastric resection, many patients have a prolonged recovery, delaying initiation of adjuvant therapy. Phase 2 trials involving either purely preoperative or perioperative treatment demonstrated that there was no increase in anticipated surgical morbidity or mortality when compared to controls.[313,314] Brenner et al.[314] reported on patients with locally advanced, high-risk gastric cancer who received preoperative CF followed by intraperitoneal chemotherapy after resection. At 43 months of follow-up, 39.5% of patients were still alive. Evaluating efficacy at the primary site is difficult in gastric cancer. Kelsen et al.[315] compared EUS with pathologic stage in assessing objective regression after neoadjuvant chemotherapy. They found that even though EUS was an accurate test in previously untreated patients following administration of chemotherapy, after chemotherapy and prior to surgery, EUS was inaccurate in measuring the depth of invasion (T stage) or lymph node involvement.

FDG-PET scan as a predictive marker of response to preoperative chemotherapy has been studied in patients with gastric cancer. Ott et al.[77] reported on 44 patients with locally advanced gastric cancer who underwent PET scans prior to and after receiving chemotherapy. A decreased SUV was able to differentiate between patients who responded pathologically to treatment and those who did not.[315] These data suggest that functional imaging may eventually prove to be a useful predictive marker for efficacy. Studies in which systemic therapy is changed on the basis of an early PET scan are now under way. As previously noted, for patients with gastric cancer, approximately 20% to 25% of patients will not have an informative PET scan, so this technique cannot be used as a predictive marker for these patients.

FDG-PET and PET/CT scan are being evaluated in Japan as a potentially useful modality for the purpose of gastric cancer. A recently published trial from the National Center for Global Health and Medicine in Tokyo studied over 150,000 asymptomatic patients as part of it FDG-PET screening.[316] With a sensitivity and positive predictive value of 38% and 34%, respectively, the authors appropriately concluded that gastric endoscopy should be included as part of screening programs in order to increase rate of gastric cancer detection.[316]

After phase 2 studies demonstrated safety and suggested efficacy, several perioperative chemotherapy phase 3 trials were conducted (see Table 46.5). English investigators led by Cunningham et al.[317] reported the final results of a well-designed, random assignment study comparing surgery alone with surgery and perioperative chemotherapy in patients with gastroesophageal junction and gastric cancers (the MAGIC trial). All patients had potentially resectable disease prior to entrance into the study. Patients assigned to perioperative chemotherapy were treated with the epirubicin–cisplatin–5-FU (ECF) regimen. Chemotherapy was given both before and after surgery. A total of 503 patients were entered into the study; three-quarters had gastric cancer and one-quarter had gastroesophageal junction or lower esophageal adenocarcinomas. The ECF chemotherapy was well tolerated, with no increase in surgical morbidity or mortality. There was a shift to an earlier stage overall in patients receiving perioperative chemotherapy, as well as an improved R0 resection rate. With a median follow-up of 4 years, there was a significant improvement in both disease-free and OS for patients receiving perioperative chemotherapy: 5-year survival rate was 36% for those receiving perioperative chemotherapy and 23% for those receiving surgery alone (HR = 0.75; 95% CI = 0.6 to 0.9; p = 0.009). The authors concluded that ECF perioperative chemotherapy improves outcome for patients with resectable gastric cancer without increasing operative morbidity or mortality. This important trial was a well-designed, adequately powered study demonstrating an advantage of systemic treatment plus surgery when compared with operation alone.

More recently, French investigators reported the results of a similar trial (ACCORD 07-FFCD 9703) using CF prior to surgery versus surgery alone.[318] Approximately half the patients receiving preoperative chemotherapy also received postoperative treatment using the same regimen. The results were similar to those of the MAGIC trial, with 5-year OS being 24% for those undergoing operation alone versus 30% for those who received perioperative chemotherapy. There was a similar improvement in DFS. The results of the ACCORD 07 trial support the results of the MAGIC study.

Summary for Neoadjuvant Chemotherapy. The results of the MAGIC and ACCORD 07 trials have shown that systemic chemotherapy regimens that are only modestly effective in palliating patients with advanced disease can have a small but clinically meaningful effect on survival when given in the perioperative setting. New and potentially effective cytotoxic agents as well as new biologic agents are now being introduced in the treatment of patients with gastric malignancy. Studies involving perioperative chemotherapy using these agents are now in the advanced planning stage. The results of the perioperative chemotherapy, MAGIC and

ACCORD 07, trials and of postoperative S-1, and Intergroup Trial (INT 0116) chemoradiation studies support the use of systemic therapy as an important component of the treatment plan for patients with locally advanced gastric cancers. The best strategy to pursue—that is, whether to give systemic therapy first followed by operation or to proceed directly to operation followed by systemic treatment plus or minus radiation given after surgery—has yet to be determined.

Given that the role of neoadjuvant chemotherapy in gastric cancer remains controversial, a systematic review and meta-analysis of six RCTs (aggregate n = 781) was conducted to gain insights about the potential benefit of neoadjuvant chemotherapy followed by surgery as compared to surgery alone.[319] Outcomes analyzed in this meta-analysis were OS, rate of R0 resection, downstaging effect of neoadjuvant chemotherapy, operative morbidity, and mortality. No significant difference were evident when comparing neoadjuvant chemotherapy and surgery to surgery alone for these outcome variables; odds ratios were as follows for OS 1.16 (0.85 to 1.58; p = 0.36), R0 resection 1.24 (0.78 to 1.96; p = 0.36), operative morbidity 1.25 (0.75 to 2.09; p = 0.39), and mortality 3.60 (0.59 to 22.45; p = 0.17).

Adjuvant Radiation and Chemoradiation Therapy. The recognition of the high rates of local and regional failure following surgery in patterns of failure analyses has served as the basis for clinical trials assessing the value of radiation therapy with and without chemotherapy as an adjuvant treatment in gastric cancer. Although these studies have all addressed the important question of whether clinical outcome is enhanced by adjuvant radiation therapy, there has been marked variability in radiation dose and schedule, sequence with surgery (preoperatively, intraoperatively, or postoperatively), and the use of concurrent and maintenance chemotherapy. These differences in study design may explain in part the conflicting results observed in phase 3 studies.

Two randomized phase 3 trials have studied the use of external beam radiation therapy (EBRT) alone with surgery.[320–322] Although both studies used similar radiation dose and schedule, sequence with surgery differed. In the British Stomach Cancer Group study, 436 patients were randomized to surgery alone, postoperative radiation therapy (45 to 50 Gy in 25 to 28 fractions), or cytotoxic chemotherapy with mitomycin, doxorubicin, and 5-FU.[320,321] The 5-year survival for surgery alone was 20%, for surgery plus radiation therapy 12%, and for surgery plus chemotherapy 19%. In this study, no survival advantage was observed for patients who received postoperative EBRT, although there was an apparent improvement in local control, demonstrating that local disease could be affected by adjuvant radiation therapy. Locoregional failure was documented in only 15 of 153 (10%) in the radiation arm versus 39 of 145 (27%) in the surgery-alone arm, and 26 of 138 (19%) in the mitomycin, doxorubicin, and 5-FU group. Interpretation of these results is complicated by the inclusion of 171 patients undergoing resection with gross or microscopic residual carcinoma. These patients would not be candidates for current gastric surgical adjuvant trials in the United States. In addition, approximately one-third of patients randomized to receive adjuvant treatment did not receive the assigned therapy. Of 153 patients randomized to the postoperative radiation arm, only 104 (68%) received a dose of 40.5 Gy or more, and 36 (24%) received none.

In contrast, the results of a phase 3 study from Beijing demonstrated a survival benefit for patients with gastric cardia carcinoma receiving preoperative radiation and surgery versus surgery alone.[322] In this study, 370 patients with gastric cardia carcinoma were randomized to 40 Gy in 20 fractions over 4 weeks of preoperative irradiation and surgery or surgery alone. The 5-year survival rates of preoperative radiation and surgery and the surgery-alone group were 30% and 20%, respectively (10-year, 20% and 13%, respectively; p = 0.009). Further, both local and regional nodal control was improved in patients undergoing preoperative radiation and surgery (61% and 61%, respectively) versus surgery

(48% and 45%, respectively) only. Morbidity and mortality rates were not increased in patients receiving preoperative therapy.[323]

As the price role of adjuvant radiation in resectable gastric cancer remains controversial, an updated systematic review and meta-analysis of 13 RCTs[324] was conducted to gain insights about the potential benefit of adjuvant (including neoadjuvant) radiation and surgery versus surgery alone for resectable gastric cancer.[323] Outcomes analyzed in this meta-analysis were OS, and DFS. Postoperative radiation was associated with a significant improvement in both OS (HR = 0.78; 95% CI = 0.70 to 0.86; p <0.001) and DFS (HR = 0.71; 95% CI = 0.63 to 0.80; p <0.001). Similar improvement in OS (HR = 0.83; 95% CI = 0.67 to 1.03; p = 0.087) and DFS (HR = 0.77; 95% CI = 0.91 to 0.65; p = 0.002) was observed in five RCTs comparing surgery + adjuvant chemoradiation to surgery + adjuvant chemotherapy for resectable gastric cancer. This meta-analysis suggests that radiation following gastrectomy translates to ∼20% DFS and OS benefit.

An alternative approach to postoperative or preoperative radiation is intraoperative radiation therapy (IORT).[325] The advantage of this technique is the ability to deliver a single large fraction (10 to 35 Gy) of radiation to the tumor or tumor bed while excluding or protecting surrounding normal tissue from the high-dose field. This approach permits high-dose radiation with minimal normal tissue treatment. Two randomized trials have examined the efficacy of IORT in combination with surgery for patients with gastric carcinoma.[326,327] Abe et al.[326] from Kyoto University performed a randomized trial of 211 patients with gastric cancer comparing surgery alone with surgery and IORT (28 to 35 Gy). For patients with tumor confined to the gastric wall (stage I), 5-year survival rates were similar for IORT and for resection alone. However, patients with Japanese stages II to IV disease who received IORT in conjunction with resection showed improved survival over patients who underwent resection without radiation. Among patients with stage IV disease (who usually had local residual disease after maximal resection), there were no 5-year survivors who received surgery alone; however, 15% of the patients who received IORT were alive at 5 years. The experience with IORT in gastric cancer at Kyoto University suggested that IORT may be beneficial in the treatment of locally advanced carcinoma of the stomach.

To further evaluate this approach, Sindelar et al.[327] at the National Cancer Institute conducted a prospective RCT comparing surgical resection and IORT with conventional therapy in gastric carcinoma. Patients in the experimental group underwent gastrectomy, and IORT was administered to the gastric bed (20 Gy). Patients in the control group underwent resection and postoperative EBRT to the upper abdomen (50 Gy in 25 fractions) for advanced-stage cancers extending beyond the gastric wall. Of the 100 patients screened for the study, 60 were randomized and underwent exploratory surgery. Nineteen patients were excluded intraoperatively because of unresectability or metastases, leaving 41 patients in the study. The median survival for patients with tumors of all stages was 25 months for the IORT group and 21 months for the control group (p = NS). Locoregional disease relapse occurred in 7 of 16 IORT patients (44%), and in 23 of 25 patients (92%) control patients (p <0.001). Complication rates were similar between IORT and control patients. Although IORT was not associated with a significant advantage over conventional therapy in terms of OS, IORT did significantly improve locoregional disease control. Based on these results, the use of IORT in gastric cancer remains investigational.

Because of the promising results in the early studies of combined-modality therapy for locally advanced (unresectable) or subtotally resected gastric cancer, investigators also have studied this combination of surgery and radiation in resectable gastric carcinoma. A small study from South Africa randomized 66 patients with resected gastric cancer (T (1–3), N (1–2), M0) to low-dose postoperative radiation (20 Gy in eight fractions over 10 days) and 5-FU, or to no further therapy after surgery.[328] No difference in survival was observed between the patients undergoing surgery and adjuvant

therapy and those undergoing surgery alone. Given the subtherapeutic doses of radiation used in this study, it is difficult to draw any definitive conclusions as to the efficacy of adjuvant radiation therapy and 5-FU. In 1984, Moertel et al.[329] reported the results of a prospective randomized trial conducted at the Mayo Clinic with 62 patients with poor prognosis, but completely resected gastric cancers who were randomized to either surgery alone or surgery followed by radiation (37.5 Gy in 24 fractions over 4 to 5 weeks) with concurrent 5-FU. A nonstratified, prerandomization scheme was used with a 2:3 ratio favoring treatment. Ten of the thirty-nine patients refused further therapy and were observed. When analyzed by intent to treat, the adjuvant arm had statistically significant improvement in both relapse-free survival and OS (overall 5-year survival 23% versus 4%; p <0.05). When patient outcome was compared with actual treatment received (29 adjuvant treatment, 33 surgery alone), 5-year survival continued to favor the adjuvant group (20% versus 12%), but the differences were not statistically significant in view of the small patient numbers. The 10 patients who refused assignment to adjuvant treatment had more favorable prognostic findings than the other two groups of patients. When the two groups with equally poor prognostic factors were compared, the 5-year OS was 20% versus 4%, with an advantage to those receiving adjuvant radiation and 5-FU treatment. When analyzed by treatment delivered, locoregional relapse was decreased with adjuvant treatments (54% with surgery alone versus 39% with irradiation and 5-FU).

The Intergroup Trial (INT 0116) randomized patients to receive surgery alone or surgery plus postoperative 5-FU–based chemotherapy and radiation.[330] The trial included patients with stages IB–IVA nonmetastatic adenocarcinoma of the stomach or GEJ. After en bloc resection, 556 patients were randomized to either observation alone or postoperative combined-modality therapy consisting of one monthly 5-day cycle of 5-FU and leucovorin, followed by 45 Gy in 25 fractions plus concurrent 5-FU and leucovorin (4 days in week 1, 3 days in week 5) followed by two monthly 5-day cycles of 5-FU and leucovorin. Nodal metastases were present in 85% of the cases. With 5 years of median follow-up, 3-year relapse-free survival was 48% for adjuvant treatment and 31% for observation (p = 0.001); 3-year OS was 50% for treatment and 41% for observation (p = 0.005). The median OS in the surgery-only group was 27 months, compared with 36 months in the chemoradiotherapy group; the HR for death was 1.35 (95% CI = 1.09 to 1.66; p = 0.005). The hazard ratio for relapse in the surgery-only group as compared with the chemoradiotherapy group was 1.52 (95% CI = 1.23 to 1.86; p <0.001). The median duration of relapse-free survival was 30 months in the chemoradiotherapy group and 19 months in the surgery-only group. Patterns of failure were based on the site of first relapse only and were categorized as local, regional, or distant. Local recurrence occurred in 29% of the patients who relapsed in the surgery-only group and 19% of those who relapsed in the chemoradiotherapy group. Regional relapse, typically abdominal carcinomatosis, was reported in 72% of those who relapsed in the surgery-only group and 65% of those who relapsed in the chemoradiotherapy group. Extra-abdominal distant metastases were diagnosed in 18% of those who relapsed in the surgery-only group and 33% of those who relapsed in the chemoradiotherapy group. Treatment was tolerable, with three (1%) toxic deaths. Grade 3 and 4 toxicity occurred in 41% and 32% of cases, respectively. The results of this large study demonstrate a clear survival advantage for the use of postoperative chemoradiation and strongly support the integration of postoperative chemoradiation into the routine care of patients with curatively resected high-risk carcinoma of the stomach and GEJ.

The US Gastrointestinal Intergroup has recently completed a second randomized prospective trial (Cancer and Leukemia Group B 80101) in patients with completely resected high-risk gastric cancer, comparing two chemotherapy regimens given before and after 5-FU–based chemoradiation. This study examines the use of one cycle of postoperative ECF (epirubicin 50 mg/m², cisplatin 60 mg/m², and continuous infusion 5-FU 200 mg/m² per day for 21 days) followed by radiation therapy with concurrent continuous infusion 5-FU (200 mg/m^2 per day) and two additional cycles of ECF. This is compared with one cycle of postoperative 5-FU and leucovorin followed by concurrent continuous infusion 5-FU (200 mg/m^2 per day) and two additional cycles of 5-FU and leucovorin. This study was recently reported in abstract form and failed to demonstrate a survival advantage of the addition of ECF therapy to standard 5-FU and leucovorin.[331]

To address the important question of the value of postoperative radiation following D2 resection, a Korean phase 3 study comparing postoperative cisplatin/capecitabine (XP) versus postoperative XP with capecitabine and radiation was reported.[332] In this study, 458 patients were enrolled, with 228 randomly assigned to receive adjuvant chemotherapy (XP for six cycles) and 230 patients assigned to receive adjuvant chemoradiation (XPx2 → capecitabine and radiation → XPx2). Although the primary end point of improved 3-year DFS was not met ($p = 0.862$), in the subset of patients with node-positive gastric cancer ($n = 396$), adjuvant chemoradiotherapy was associated with a superior DFS (HR = 0.6865; 95% CI = 0.4735 to 0.9952; $p = 0.471$). Based on these intriguing data, the investigators have initiated a confirmatory study limited to patients with lymph node–positive resected gastric cancer (ARTIST-II).

To address the role of adjuvant chemoradiation in light of the MAGIC trial, the Dutch Colorectal Cancer Group has initiated the CRITICS trial. This study is a phase 3 prospective randomized trial that investigates whether chemoradiotherapy (45 Gy in 5 weeks with daily cisplatin and capecitabine) after preoperative chemotherapy (3 × epirubicin, cisplatin, and capecitabine) and adequate (D1+) gastrectomy leads to improved survival in comparison with postoperative chemotherapy alone (3 × epirubicin, cisplatin, and capecitabine). Further evaluating the role of adjuvant radiation therapy, a Korean phase 3 trial (the ARTIST study) is randomizing patients undergoing D2 gastrectomy to adjuvant cisplatin and capecitabine, with or without radiation therapy.

Although no phase 3 trials have tested the value of preoperative radiation plus chemotherapy for patients with gastric cancer, two phase 2 trials for patients with esophagus cancer have included either lesions of the gastric cardia or the EGJ.[333,334] In both trials, the trimodality study arm demonstrated an improvement in OS when compared with the control arm of surgery alone. The series by Walsh et al.[333] (adenocarcinoma of the esophagus or gastric cardia) demonstrated a median survival of 16 months versus 11 months, and 3-year survival of 32% versus 6% ($p = 0.01$), with the statistically significant advantage to trimodality treatment. The US GI Intergroup phase 3 trial (adenocarcinoma or squamous cell of esophagus or EGJ), which closed prematurely because of low accrual, reported a median survival of 54 months versus 22 months, and 5-year survival of 39% versus 16% ($p = 0.008$), with a significant advantage associated with the trimodality arm.[334] In addition, a recent phase 3 randomized German trial compared preoperative chemotherapy alone (5-FU, leucovorin, and cisplatin) versus the same regimen followed by low-dose radiation therapy (30 Gy) with concurrent cisplatin and etoposide in patients with adenocarcinoma of the lower esophagus or gastric cardia. Although the trial was closed early because of poor accrual (126 patients), patients receiving radiation therapy had significantly higher pathologic complete response rates (2% versus 16%; $p = 0.03$) and trend toward improved survival (3-year survival 47% versus 28%; $p = 0.07$).[335]

Preoperative chemoradiation data for patients with gastric cancer exclusively is limited to phase 2 studies from single institutions and cooperative groups. The MD Anderson Cancer Center has reported a study in which 33 patients completed a preoperative protocol that started with induction chemotherapy of 5-FU, leucovorin, and cisplatin, followed by 45 Gy of radiation therapy in 25 fractions over 5 weeks with concurrent infusional 5-FU. In 28 patients (85%), a gastrectomy was performed and D2 lymph node dissection was attempted. Pathologic complete and partial responses were found in 64% of all operated patients. These patients showed a significant longer median survival of 64 months in

comparison with 13 months in patients with tumors that showed no pathologic response to preoperative chemoradiation.[336] In a study from the same institution, 41 patients with operable gastric cancer received two cycles of continuous 5-FU, paclitaxel, and cisplatin followed by 45 Gy of radiation therapy with concurrent 5-FU and paclitaxel. An R0 resection was achieved in 78% of patients; pathologic complete response was seen in 25% and pathologic partial response in 15% of patients. Pathologic response, R0 resection, and postoperative T and N stage correlated with overall and DFS.[337]

The Radiation Therapy Oncology Group (RTOG 9904) reported the results of a phase 2 study of 49 patients undergoing induction 5-FU, leucovorin, and cisplatin followed by concurrent radiation therapy, and infusional 5-FU and paclitaxel. Resection was attempted 5 to 6 weeks after chemoradiation. The pathologic complete response and R0 resection rates were 26% and 77%, respectively. At 1 year, more patients with tumors exhibiting a pathologic complete response (89%) were alive than patients with tumors having less favorable pathologic treatment response (66%). Grade 4 toxicity occurred in 21% of patients. These data appear to support a phase 3 study evaluating preoperative radiation therapy and chemotherapy versus postoperative radiation therapy and chemotherapy.[338]

TECHNICAL TREATMENT-RELATED ISSUES

Surgery

Surgery begins with careful laparoscopic staging and examination. Inspection for the presence of ascites, hepatic metastases, peritoneal seeding, disease in the pelvis (such as a "drop" metastasis), or ovarian involvement should be performed. Once distant metastases have been ruled out, depending on the location of the lesion, a bilateral subcostal incision or a midline abdominal incision can be used to gain adequate exposure to the upper abdomen. The stomach should be inspected to assess the location and extent of the primary tumor. The size and location of the primary tumor dictate the extent of gastric resection. A D2 lymphadenectomy sparing the spleen and pancreas can be done safely, and provides an excellent surgical specimen for pathologic staging, but this procedure should only be performed by or with an experienced surgeon.

The D2 subtotal gastrectomy commences with mobilization of the greater omentum from the transverse colon. After the omentum is mobilized, the anterior peritoneal leaf of the transverse mesocolon is incised along the lower border of the colon, and a plane is developed down to the head of the pancreas. The infrapyloric lymph nodes are dissected and the origin of the right gastroepiploic artery and vein are ligated. With a combination of blunt and sharp dissection, the plane of dissection continues on to the anterior surface of the pancreas, extending to the level of the common hepatic and splenic arteries. This maneuver can be tedious, but it theoretically provides additional protection against serosal spread of tumor to the local peritoneal surface. The right gastric artery is ligated. At this point, the duodenum is divided distal to the pylorus. The stomach and omentum are then reflected cephalad. The gastrohepatic ligament is divided close to the liver up to the gastroesophageal junction. Dissection is then continued along the hepatic artery toward the celiac axis. Once near the celiac axis, the lymph node–bearing tissue is dissected until the left gastric artery is visualized and can be divided at its celiac origin. The proximal peritoneal attachments of the stomach and distal esophagus can then be incised, and the proximal extent of resection is defined. For tumors of the mid- and proximal stomach, dissection of the lymph nodes along the splenic artery and splenic hilum is important. This technique is not indicated for antral tumors, given the low rate of splenic hilar nodal metastases seen with tumors in this anatomical location. The stomach is then divided 5 cm proximal to the tumor, which dictates the extent of gastric resection. Despite the fact that the entire blood supply of the stomach has been interrupted, a cuff of proximal stomach invariably shows good vascularization from the feeding distal esophageal arcade. When feasible, most surgeons prefer to anastomose jejunum to stomach rather than to esophagus because of the technical ease and excellent healing seen with gastrojejunal anastomosis. Reconstruction using a variety of techniques has been described and is a matter of personal choice.

Antibiotics Prophylaxis

One RCT ($n = 501$) tested single-dose cefazolin or ampicillin-sulbactam 30 minutes before surgery versus multiple dose regimen for 3 days postoperatively. There were no differences in surgical site infections or complication.[280,339]

Nasogastric Drainage After Gastrectomy

The Italian Total Gastrectomy Study Group reported on the largest RCT comparing total gastrectomy with Roux-en-Y with and without nasogastric tube ($n = 237$). There were no differences in overall morbidity, leak rate, hospital stay, and time to diet.[340] Other authors confirmed that nasogastric tube is not necessary after gastrectomy.[341–343]

Intraperitoneal Drains After Gastrectomy

As with other pathologies, two RCTs concluded that drains after gastrectomy are generally not indicated, and in certain situations can increase significantly operative morbidity.[344,345]

Reconstruction After Gastrectomy

Iivonen et al.[346] compared Roux-en-Y with and without pouch. They randomized 48 patients and found significantly less dumping syndrome and early satiety but with no differences at 15 months of follow-up. Fein et al.[347] reported on 138 patients randomized in a similar fashion; they found similar QOL at 1 year but significantly improved QOL at 3-, 4-, and 5-year follow-up. It seems that reconstruction with pouch has long-term advantages and may be recommended as the standard reconstruction.[280]

Radiation Treatment

Technique of Radiation Therapy

Idealized portals generated from patterns of failure data should be modified on the basis of the individual patient's initial extent of disease.[348,349] Based on the likely sites of locoregional failure, the gastric/tumor bed, anastomosis and gastric remnant, and regional lymphatics should be included in most patients undergoing post-gastrectomy radiation.[350–353] Major nodal chains at risk include the lesser and greater curvature; celiac axis; pancreaticoduodenal, splenic, supra-pancreatic, and porta hepatis groups; and, in some, para-aortic to the level of mid-L3.

The relative risk of nodal metastases at a specific nodal location depends on both the site of origin of the primary tumor, and other factors including width and depth of invasion of the gastric wall.[349] Tumors that originate in the proximal portion of the stomach and the GEJ have a higher propensity of spread to nodes in the mediastinum and pericardial region, but a lower likelihood of involvement of nodes in the region of the gastric antrum, periduodenal area, and porta hepatis. Tumors that originate in the body of the stomach can spread to all nodal sites, but have the highest likelihood of spreading to nodes along the greater and lesser curvature near the location of the primary tumor mass. Tumors that originate in the distal stomach, in the region of the gastric antrum, have a high likelihood of spread to the periduodenal, peripancreatic, and porta hepatis nodes, whereas they have a lower likelihood of spread

to the nodes near the cardia of the stomach, the periesophageal and mediastinal nodes, or to the splenic hilar nodes. Any tumor originating in the stomach has a high propensity of spread to nodes along the greater and lesser curvature, although they are most likely to spread to those sites in close anatomic proximity to the primary tumor mass. Guidelines for defining the clinical target volume for postoperative irradiation fields have been developed based on location and extent of the primary tumor (T stage), and location and extent of known nodal involvement (N stage).[349] In general, for patients with node-positive disease, there should be wide coverage of tumor bed, remaining stomach, resection margins, and nodal drainage regions. For node-negative disease, if there is a good surgical resection with pathologic evaluation of at least 15 nodes, and there are wide surgical margins proximal and distal to the primary tumor (at least 5 cm), treatment of the nodal beds is optional. Treatment of the remaining stomach should depend on a balance of the likely normal tissue morbidity and the perceived risk of local relapse in the residual stomach.

Although parallel-opposed anteroposterior/posteroanterior (AP/PA) fields are a practical arrangement for tumor bed and nodal irradiation, three-dimensional multifield techniques should be used if they can improve long-term tolerance of normal tissues. Tightly contoured fields should be designed to spare as much normal tissue as possible. Over the past decade, a shift has occurred toward more sophisticated treatment techniques that use multiple and often noncoplanar beams including three-dimensional and intensity-modulated radiation therapy. Attention has also been placed on accurate three-dimensional target delineated fields based on CT anatomy rather than only two-dimensional field design. In addition to refinements in radiation therapy target definition based on CT planning, technologic advances including study of and solutions for variability in target and normal organ location during a treatment course (day to day interfraction variability) and actual treatment delivered (intrafraction variability caused by respiration) have been undertaken. Interfraction variability in stomach location can be substantial, particularly among patients treated with neoadjuvant chemoradiation because of daily variations in gastric filling. Because of this, patients should generally be treated with an empty stomach. Intrafraction changes in target shape (deformation) and location are asymmetric and mainly from respiratory motion. Movement, particularly in the cranial-caudad dimension, frequently exceeds 1 to 1.5 cm. Image guidance, four-dimensional treatment planning, and respiratory gating have been developed to address these challenges.

More routine use of multiple field techniques should be considered when preoperative imaging exists to allow accurate reconstruction of target volumes. Single-institution data suggest that multiple field arrangements may produce less toxicity.[354] Although AP/PA fields can be weighted anteriorly to keep the spinal cord dose at acceptable levels using only parallel-opposed techniques, a four-field technique, if feasible, can spare spinal cord radiation exposure, with improved dose homogeneity. Dependent on the posterior extent of the gastric fundus, either oblique or more routine lateral portals can be used to deliver a 10- to 20-Gy component of irradiation to spare the spinal cord or kidney. When lateral fields are used, liver and kidney tolerance limits the use of lateral fields to ≤20 Gy. With the wide availability of three-dimensional treatment-planning systems, it may be possible to target more accurately the high-risk volume, and to use unconventional field arrangements to produce superior dose distributions. To accomplish this without marginal misses, it will be necessary to both carefully define and encompass the various target volumes, given that the use of oblique or noncoplanar beams could potentially exclude target volumes that would be included in AP/PA fields or nonoblique four-field techniques (AP/PA and laterals). In most patients, a portion of both kidneys are within the treatment field, but at least two-thirds to three-fourths of one kidney should be excluded beyond a dose of 20 Gy. For proximal gastric lesions, ≥50% of the left kidney is commonly within the irradiation portal, and the right kidney must be appropriately spared. For distal lesions with narrow or positive duodenal margins, a similar amount of right kidney often is included, and every effort must be taken to spare the left kidney from irradiation in order to maintain function. Late renal sequelae have not been encountered with these techniques, assuming normal renal function bilaterally.[355–357]

With proximal gastric lesions or lesions at the EGJ, a 3- to 5-cm margin of distal esophagus should be included. If the lesion extends through the entire gastric wall, a major portion of the left hemidiaphragm should be included. In these circumstances, blocking can decrease the volume of irradiated heart.

TREATMENT OF ADVANCED DISEASE (STAGE IV)

Treatment of Advanced Gastric Cancer: Palliative Systemic Chemotherapy

Chemotherapy Versus Best Supportive Care

The modest activity and substantial toxicity of cytotoxic chemotherapy has raised the question, Does palliative systemic therapy with available agents have clinical utility? That is, there was controversy as to whether a meaningful advantage is attained by early initiation of systemic therapy as opposed to providing best supportive care. Although this is a difficult hypothesis to test because of patient and physician preferences and biases, several random assignment trials were performed in the 1990s in patients with advanced incurable gastric cancer addressing this issue.

Wagner et al.[358] performed a meta-analysis for the Cochrane collaboration. They included three random assignment trials involving a total of 184 patients in whom the study design was to initiate systemic chemotherapy plus best supportive care or to provide best supportive care alone. Median survival and OS were evaluated (Table 46.6). Patients receiving chemotherapy as part of their treatment had better OS than those receiving best supportive care only, with an overall HR of 0.39 (95% CI = 0.28 to 0.52). The median survival was improved from 4.3 months for best supportive care to approximately 11 months for chemotherapy. Note that

the median survival for patients receiving chemotherapy is consistent with several more recent trials. There was also a modest improvement in time to progression (TTP; 7 months for patients receiving chemotherapy versus 2.5 months for patients receiving best supportive care). Wagner et al.[358] concluded that the evidence supporting initiating chemotherapy for patients with advanced incurable gastric cancer was convincing.

In a fourth trial, QOL was assessed. The average quality-adjusted survival for patients undergoing chemotherapy was superior to patients receiving best supportive care (6 months versus 12 months). Importantly, in those best supportive care trials that reported 2-year survival (≥24 months), only patients undergoing chemotherapy survived for that period of time. The 2-year survival rate was 5% to 14% for patients receiving combination chemotherapy versus 0% for patients receiving best supportive care. More recently, the preliminary results of a small study testing the use of single-agent chemotherapy versus best supportive care in patients who have already received chemotherapy were reported. Previously treated patients were randomly assigned to best supportive care or to single-agent irinotecan plus best supportive care. Although the study was initially powered to require 120 patients, accrual to this type of trial was difficult and a total of only 40 patients were eventually randomized. There was a modest improvement in OS, with median survival for those receiving irinotecan of 123 days, and median survival for those with best supportive care 73 days (HR = 2.85).[359] These results are in concert with the earlier studies in previously untreated patients and indicate that systemic therapy has a modest but real and clinically meaningful effect on outcome. Many cytotoxic agents have been studied in patients with advanced gastric cancer; when used as single agents, modest activity has been identified for drugs from five different classes. More recently, targeted therapy has been tested. The following section summarizes the data for the use of systemic cytotoxic chemotherapy when given with palliative intent. An extensive discussion of older agents can be found in prior editions of this textbook.

Single-Agent Chemotherapy

For most drugs, a variety of doses and schedules have been studied. In the absence of comparative trials using the same agent with different doses and schedules, superiority of one regimen over the other cannot be assessed. Table 46.7 gives a listing of agents that have demonstrated at least modest activity in the treatment of gastric cancer and which are routinely employed as part of standard practice options. Drugs with little or no activity, especially if they were evaluated prior to 2000, are not included in this table.

5-FU is the parent fluorinated pyrimidine that has been the most extensively studied single agent in gastric cancer. An antimetabolite, the drug has been used in a variety of schedules and doses in various epithelial malignancies of gastrointestinal origin. One method involved the use of rapid intravenous injections on a weekly basis, or daily for 5 consecutive days. In gastric cancer, continuous infusion 5-FU has been used more recently. During the 1990s, in several studies, 5-FU was the control arm of a random assignment trial or was studied as a single agent (with leucovorin) in a prospective phase 2 trial. This allowed an assessment using more modern criteria of activity. The studies from the 1990s suggest overall response rates of 10% to 20%, with a median duration of response, or TTP, of approximately 4 months. As is the case in other diseases, the major toxicities reported in gastric cancer for 5-FU are mucositis, diarrhea, or mild myelosuppression. Because continuous intravenous infusion schedules can be cumbersome, oral analogues of 5-FU have been studied in gastric cancer. Three oral drugs of this class have undergone study in gastric cancer. These are tegafur and uracil (UFT), S-1 (tegafur and two modulators, 5-chloro-2,4-dihydroxypyridine and potassium oxonate), and capecitabine (Xeloda, Hoffmann-La Roche, Basel, Switzerland). The data for these agents are also shown in Table 46.7. S-1 has been most extensively studied in Japan. Although a response rate to

TABLE 46.6

Chemotherapy for Advanced Gastric Cancer: Treatment Versus Best Supportive Care

Regimen	No. of Patients	Median Survival (mo)	Survival Rate (%) 1y	Survival Rate (%) 2y
FAMTX	30	10	40	6
BSC	10	3	10	0
FEMTX	17	12	—	—
BSC	19	3	—	—
ETOPLF	10	10	—	—
BSC	8	4	—	—
ELF	52	10.2	34.6	9.6
BSC	51	5	7.8	0
Irinotecan	21	123[a]	—	—
BSC	19	73[a]	—	—

F, fluorouracil; A, doxorubicin; MTX, methotrexate; BSC, best supportive care; E, epirubicin; ETOP, etoposide; L, leucovorin.
[a] Median survival in days.
Modified from Wils J. The treatment of advanced gastric cancer. *Semin Oncol* 1996;23:397.

TABLE 46.7

Activity of Selected Single Agents in Advanced Gastric Cancer

Drug	Response Rate (%)
Fluorinated Pyrimidines	
5-Fluorouracil	21
UFT	28
S-1	49
Capecitabine	26
Antibiotics	
Doxorubicin hydrochloride	17
Epirubicin hydrochloride	19
Heavy Metals	
Cisplatin	19
Taxanes	
Paclitaxel	17
Docetaxel	19
Camptothecans	
Irinotecan hydrochloride	23

UFT, tegafur and uracil; S-1, tegafur and two modulators, 5-chloro-2, 4-dihydroxypyridine and potassium oxonate.
From van De Velde CJH, Kelsen D, Minsky B. Gastric cancer: clinical management. In: Kelsen D, Daly JM, Kern SE, et al., eds. *Principles and Practice of Gastrointestinal Oncology.* 2nd ed. Philadelphia: Lippincott Williams & Wilkins; 2008, with permission.

single-agent S-1 of 44% to 54% was reported in Japanese patients, the response rate among European patients was substantially lower. Like capecitabine, S-1 is now undergoing study in combination with other agents, particularly cisplatin. UFT combines tegafur and uracil. In gastric cancer, a response rate of 28% was seen in Japanese patients. In a small European study, Okines et al.[360] reported the results of a European Organisation for Research and Treatment of Cancer (EORTC) study combining UFT and leucovorin. A 16% response rate was seen in a group of 23 patients. Capecitabine has been tested in fewer single-agent studies in gastric cancer. The data available suggest similar activity as seen with other oral fluorinated pyrimidines. Capecitabine has recently been extensively studied in combination with cisplatin or oxaliplatin (see "The REAL-2 Trial").

Platinum compounds are an important part of the treatment of gastric cancer. The parent analogue, cisplatin, was studied in the 1980s. In both previously treated and untreated patients, a response rate of approximately 15% was reported. The major toxicities for cisplatin are nausea and vomiting, peripheral neuropathy, ototoxicity, and nephropathy. The development of efficacious antiemetics has significantly improved control of nausea and vomiting. An analogue of cisplatin, carboplatin, has been less well studied in gastric cancer; it appears to have less activity in this disease, as compared to other epithelial malignancies. Most recently, oxaliplatin, a diamino cyclohexane extensively used in the treatment of colorectal cancer, was included as part of combination chemotherapy for gastric cancer. The data for combination therapy, including oxaliplatin and data from the REAL-2 trial, are shown later.

A third class of cytotoxic agents with activity in gastric cancer is the taxanes. Both paclitaxel and docetaxel have been studied as single agents in gastroesophageal cancers. Docetaxel has been more extensively studied than paclitaxel. De Cosimo et al.[361] reviewed trials in which docetaxel was used as single agent. Patients may have received prior treatment, and 262 patients were evaluable for

response. The overall response rate was 19%. The major toxicities were neutropenia, alopecia, and edema. Allergic reactions were seen in about 25% of patients. The most common dosing schedule for docetaxel is 100 mg/m^2 every 3 weeks. When reported, the median TTP while on docetaxel therapy was 6 months. A schedule using lower doses given once weekly has also been studied with similar activity. On the basis of a large randomized study comparing CF to docetaxel-cisplatin–5-FU (DCF), docetaxel was approved by the US Food and Drug Administration for the treatment of advanced gastric cancer. Paclitaxel has also been studied in gastric cancer, although in smaller numbers of patients, and has a similar degree of cytotoxic activity.

A fourth class of active agent is represented by irinotecan. It has been studied both as a single agent and in combination with other cytotoxic agents. When used alone, response rates of 15% to 25% have been reported in both previously treated and untreated patients with advanced gastric cancer. Wagner et al.[358] reviewed the data for combinations, including irinotecan versus multidrug combinations not including irinotecan. They concluded that irinotecan-containing multidrug chemotherapy combinations had a modest survival benefit, which was not statistically significant, when compared with regimens not including irinotecan. The major toxicities of irinotecan are myelosuppression and diarrhea.

Anthracyclines also have activity in gastric cancer. Single-agent data from the 1960s and 1970s show a response rate for doxorubicin of 17%, and for epirubicin a similar response rate of approximately 19%. The anthracyclines have undergone more extensive study in combination chemotherapy for advanced gastric cancer.

Single-Agent Versus Combination Chemotherapy

The potential advantage of giving combination chemotherapy versus single-agent chemotherapy has been evaluated by Wagner et al.[358] in an update of their original Cochrane review. They found that combination chemotherapy had a significant survival advantage when compared to single-agent chemotherapy (HR = 0.82; 95% CI = 0.74 to 0.90). The difference in average median survival, however, was modest: 8.3 months for combination chemotherapy versus 6.7 months for single-agent chemotherapy. In the updated analysis, a test for heterogeneity was not statistically significant; they concluded that this indicated that the results of the different studies were consistent. A secondary analysis for response rate and for TTP also favored combination chemotherapy. Not surprisingly, toxicity is higher when several agents are given together, although this was not statistically significant. Treatment-related mortality was only slightly higher (1.5%) for patients receiving combination chemotherapy versus 1.1% when single-agent chemotherapy was used.

They also evaluated the role of several different combinations of cytotoxic agents, including anthracyclines as part of combination chemotherapy. In this analysis, three studies with a total of 500 patients were included. Wagner et al.[358] found that including anthracyclines in a CF combination had a modest survival advantage over CF alone (HR = 0.77; 95% CI = 0.62 to 0.95). A similar advantage to anthracyclines in combination was found when 5-FU–anthracycline combinations without cisplatin were studied. In contrast to anthracyclines, there was a more modest, albeit not statistically significant, benefit for irinotecan-containing combinations. Once again, there was a modest improvement in OS for docetaxel-containing regimens, but this did not reach statistical significance. The response rate as a secondary objective was 36% for docetaxel-containing regimens versus 31% for nondocetaxel-containing regimens (not statistically significant). Oral fluoropyrimidines when compared to intravenous fluoropyrimidine therapy also showed no significant difference in median OS. The meta-analysis is in concert with the results of the REAL-2 trial, which indicated noninferiority for oral capecitabine when compared to intravenous 5-FU. Similarly, oxaliplatin regimens were compared to cisplatin-containing regimens with modest superiority to oxaliplatin.

In summary, there are five classes of cytotoxic chemotherapy agents in which single agents have modest activity in gastric cancer. The response rates range from 10% to 25%, and the median duration of response is relatively short (4 to 6 months). As a result of the single-agent trials, 5-FU or capecitabine (or other oral fluoropyrimidines), cisplatin or oxaliplatin, docetaxel, and less commonly, paclitaxel, epirubicin, and irinotecan are the major components of conventional combination cytotoxic systemic chemotherapy regimens.

Like other malignancies, multidrug regimens using agents that have single-agent activity have been extensively studied in gastric cancer. This section will focus on phase 3 random assignment trials. For some combinations, only phase 2 data are available. The recent Cochrane review summarizing a comparison of different regimens including three-drug versus two-drug combinations has already been discussed.[358]

Cisplatin-Fluorouracil. One of the most widely used combination chemotherapy regimens in upper gastrointestinal tract malignancies, including gastric cancer, is the two-drug combination of CF. Although this regimen has been used for several decades, with a variety of doses and schedules employed, since 2000, several phase 3 random assignment trials have been performed in which CF was the control arm. This allowed an opportunity for an evaluation of the efficacy of this combination, in patients with advanced incurable gastric cancer, both in terms of response rate, PFS, and OS, using currently accepted criteria for efficacy and toxicity of treatment. Table 46.8 shows the data from six studies in which CF was the control arm.[362] The doses of cisplatin used were 80 to 100 mg/m^2 per course. 5-FU was given as a continuous 24-hour infusion from days 1 through 5 at a dose of 800 to 1,000 mg/m^2 per day. Cycles were usually given on an every 28-day basis. Efficacy outcomes were consistent across these trials. Response rates, PFS, and OS were quite similar. Major objective tumor regression was reported in 20% to 30% of patients; complete clinical remission was very uncommon, however. The median TTP or PFS, depending on the study, ranged from 3.7 months to 4.1 months, with median survival ranging from 7.2 months to 8.6 months. Two-year survival was between 7% and 10%. CF was compared to a variety of other agents in these trials.

Vanhoefer et al.,[363] reporting for EORTC, compared CF to methotrexate, 5-FU, and doxorubicin (FAMTX); a third group of patients received etoposide, leucovorin, and 5-FU combination. There was no significant difference in outcome among the three arms. A Japanese study (JC 09205) also had three systemic therapy arms.[364] 5-FU was compared to CF, and to a third arm of uracil/tegafur plus mitomycin. In this study, there was no advantage for the two-drug combination of CF over 5-FU alone. The final results of the TAX315 trial have recently been published.[365] The details of this study are described later. An advantage was seen for the DCF arm. The CF control arm results were similar to those seen in the earlier trials previously described. The two-drug combination of 5-FU plus irinotecan was compared to CF by Dank et al.[366] CF was equivalent to irinotecan plus 5-FU. Kang et al.[367] reported the results of the RCT comparison between CF versus cisplatin-capecitabine. This study was designed as a noninferiority trial with the hypothesis that capecitabine-cisplatin was not inferior to CF. The end point was PFS. The dose of cisplatin was slightly lower than in the studies described earlier (80 mg/m^2). However, therapy was given on every-3-week basis; 316 patients were treated. The median PFS was 5 months for CF; median survival was 9.3 months. Ajani et al.[368] reported the results of the FLAGS trial, which is described in more detail later. In this study involving 1,029 eligible patients, the control arm of CF had a median OS of 7.9 months.

In summary, the random assignment trials discussed previously indicate consistent data for efficacy (and toxicity) for the two-drug combination CF. The Japanese study raises the question as to whether there is a substantial clinical advantage to CF over

---

TABLE 46.8

Combination Chemotherapy in Advanced Gastric Cancer: Cisplatin-Fluorouracil-Containing Regimens Used as the Control Arm in Random Assignment Trials

Study (Ref.)	Drug	Dose (mg/ml)	Schedule (d)	No. of Patients	RR (%)	Median TTP/ PFS (mo)	Median Survival (mo)	Two-y Survival (%)
EORTC[363]	C	100	1	127	20	4.1	7.2	~10
	F	1,000	1–5					
JCOG[364]	C	20	1–5	105	36	7.3	3.9	7
	F	800	1–5					
Dank et al.[366]	C	100	1	163	26	4.2	8.7	~10
	F	1,000	1–5					
TAX325[365]	C	100	1	224	25	3.7	8.6	9
	F	1,000	1–5					
FLAGS[368]	C	100	1	508	32	5.5	7.9	~10
	F	1,000	1–5					
Kang et al.[367]	C	80	1	156	32	5.5	9.3	~10
	F	800	1–5					
REAL-2[360,362,374]	E	50	1	289	41	6.2	9.9	~15
	C	60	1					
	F	200	Daily					

RR, recovery rate; TTP, time to progression; PFS, progression-free survival; EORTC, European Organisation for Research and Treatment of Cancer; C, cisplatin; F, fluorouracil; JCOG, Japan Clinical Oncology Group; E, epirubicin; FLAGS, Cisplatin/S-1 With Cisplatin/Infusional Fluorouracil in Advanced Gastric or Gastroesophageal Adenocarcinoma Study; REAL, Randomized Trial of EOC +/− Panitumumab for Advanced and Locally Advanced Esophagogastric Cancer.
Modified from van De Velde CJH, Kelsen D, Minsky B. Gastric cancer: clinical management. In: Kelsen D, Daly JM, Kern SE, et al., eds. *Principles and Practice of Gastrointestinal Oncology*. 2nd ed. Philadelphia: Lippincott Williams & Wilkins; 2008, with permission.

5-FU alone, but the meta-analysis performed by Wagner et al.[358] supports the use of combination over single-agent chemotherapy. Although still commonly used as a conventional standard of practice palliative treatment, the recent demonstration of modest superiority when docetaxel is added to CF (assuming that a more well-tolerated regimen using the three agents can be developed) as well as the noncomparative data using ECF, which is discussed later, suggest that CF may not be the most effective option for therapy in patients with advanced gastric cancer. The slight advantage in longer-term survival (2-year survival) in the TAX325 and in the irinotecan–5-FU–leucovorin (FOLFIRI) studies of 15% to 20%, as compared to 15% to 20% for ECF, suggests that at least some patients may have longer-term survival with newer regimens.

Although type and incidence of treatment-related toxicity is consistent across most CF trials and is generally tolerable, it can be severe on occasion. For example, in the EORTC trial, grade 3 or 4 neutropenia was seen in approximately one-third of patients; one-quarter of patients had grade 3 or 4 nausea or vomiting. Similarly, in the more recent TAX325 trial, overall grade 3 or 4 toxicity was seen in 75% of patients receiving CF; in the FLAGS trial, treatment-related mortality occurred in 4.9% of patients receiving CF. Some toxicity may be ameliorated by improved supportive care. For example, newer antiemetics such as aprepitant should improve control of severe nausea and vomiting. More widespread use of supportive cytokine agents may decrease the incidence of neutropenic fever. Nonetheless, it should be recognized that CF, using the doses and schedules described previously, is associated with substantial toxicity in some patients.

The use of oral fluoropyrimidines in place of intravenous 5-FU has been studied in several phase 3 trials, including that of Kang et al.[367] described earlier, the REAL-2 trial, and the FLAGS trial comparing CF to cisplatin–S-1. In FLAGS trial, 1,029 patients received either cisplatin 100 mg/m^2 and 5-FU 1,000 mg/m^2 as a continuous 5-day infusion or a slightly lower dose of cisplatin plus oral S-1.[368] Median OS was 8.6 months for patients receiving cisplatin plus S-1 versus 7.9 months in the CF arm, with less toxicity for the cisplatin–S-1 combination. These three trials indicate that oral fluoropyrimidine when given with a platinum compound is not inferior to intravenous 5-FU plus cisplatin.

Docetaxel, Cisplatin, and Fluorouracil. Van Cutsem et al.[365] have reported the final results of a large-scale random assignment trial comparing the DCF combination to CF (the TAX325 trial). Previously untreated patients with advanced gastric cancer received either DCF (221 analyzable patients) or CF using the doses and schedules previously described (224 patients). The primary end point of the study was TTP and was powered to detect an increase in median TTP from 4 to 6 months. The two arms of the study were well balanced for prognostic factors, including weight loss, performance status, and extent of disease. The median TTP was 3.7 months for patients receiving CF and 5.6 months for those receiving DCF (HR = 1.47; p = 0.0004). As a secondary end point, survival was also modestly increased from 8.6 months for CF to 9.2 months for DCF. The 2-year survival rate, however, was increased greater than two-fold in the DCF treatment arm (2-year OS: 8.8% for CF and 18.4% for DCF). Another measure of efficacy favoring DCF was tumor response to treatment (37% for DCF and 25% for CF). Although this study indicated an advantage to the three-drug combination of DCF, toxicity was also increased and was very substantial. Eighty-one percent of all patients receiving DCF had at least one grade 3 or 4 nonhematologic toxicity, as well as substantially more hematologic toxicity. Of the patients receiving CF, 14% had neutropenic fever, as did 30% of patients receiving DCF. However, there was no difference in the treatment-related mortality rate for the two arms. This study led to the recent approval of docetaxel by the US Food and Drug Administration for the treatment of gastric cancer when given in association with CF.

Like epirubicin, docetaxel, when added to CF, has a modest improvement in efficacy. The very substantial toxicity seen with the DCF regimen, however, has led to concerns regarding its general use. A number of studies have been performed using modifications of DCF to develop a more tolerable regimen. Several strategies have been pursued, most of which involve using somewhat lower doses of docetaxel and 5-FU, or modifications in the schedule as to duration of 5-FU infusion or timing of the cisplatin dose. The preliminary results of a phase 2 trial comparing one of these modified DCF regimes to the original DCF schedule indicate that modifications of the treatment schedule may decrease toxicity while maintaining treatment efficacy.[369]

Irinotecan Plus Fluorouracil-Leucovorin. A three-drug combination of FOLFIRI has been studied extensively in metastatic colorectal cancer. A random-assignment phase 2 study comparing FOLFIRI with cisplatin-irinotecan indicated a potential advantage for the FOLFIRI-type regimen.[370] Therefore, a definitive phase 3 trial was performed with CF as the control arm.[366] A total of 170 patients received irinotecan–5-FU) and 163 received CF. The primary end point was TTP. The analysis allowed for a noninferiority comparison between the two arms. The study was reasonably well balanced for the usual prognostic indicators; approximately 20% of patients had EGJ tumors. There was no significant difference in the major objective response rate (32% for irinotecan–5-FU and 26% for CF) nor in median TTP (5 months for irinotecan–5-FU and 4.2 months for CF). Overall median survival was also similar between groups (9 months for irinotecan–5-FU and 8.7 months for CF). Time to treatment failure was 4 months versus 3.4 months for irinotecan–5-FU and CF, respectively (p = 0.018). Irinotecan–5-FU was better in terms of toxic deaths (0.6% versus 3%), discontinuation for toxicity (10% versus 22%), neutropenia, thrombocytopenia, and stomatitis but not diarrhea than CF. The investigator's final conclusion was that irinotecan–5-FU was not inferior to CF and was somewhat less toxic.

Epirubicin, Cisplatin, and Fluorouracil. English investigators have extensively studied the three-drug combination ECF. Two random-assignment phase 3 trials have compared the ECF with a noncisplatin-containing combination (FAMTX) or with a mitomycin-cisplatin–5-FU (MCF) combination.[371] In the first study, ECF was more effective than FAMTX both in terms of response rate and median OS (8.7 months versus 6.1 months). Two-year survival was also superior for the ECF combination (14% versus 5%). In the second study, Ross et al.[371] compared ECF with MCF. In this larger study, 574 patients were treated. The primary end point was 1-year survival. The overall objective response rates were similar between the two arms (ECF 50% and MCF 55%). Toxicity was tolerable, although myelosuppression was greater for the experimental MCF arm. There was a slightly improved median duration of survival for ECF (9.4 months versus 8.7 months) and for 1-year survival (40% for ECF and 32% for MCF). There was no significant difference in 2-year survival, which was approximately 15% for both arms. Several studies have demonstrated that a small percentage of patients with advanced unresectable gastric cancer actually survive 2 years. Data for the ECF regimen as the control arm of the REAL-2 trial are discussed later.

Cisplatin Plus Irinotecan. Cisplatin is a commonly used agent in gastric cancer, and irinotecan has been combined with this drug as well as with other agents. In single-arm phase 2 studies, response rates were encouraging and toxicity was tolerable with irinotecan-cisplatin. This observation led to a somewhat larger random-assignment phase 2 trial comparing irinotecan-cisplatin with the irinotecan–5-FU regimen previously described.[370] Sixty-two patients received irinotecan–5-FU and 61 received irinotecan-cisplatin. The dose schedule used for the irinotecan-cisplatin arm was higher than that from earlier irinotecan-cisplatin regimens. In this study, the response rate was higher for irinotecan–5-FU than for irinotecan-cisplatin, as was the TTP. Although irinotecan-cisplatin in the dose and schedule used in the random-assignment phase 2 trial previously described was less effective than irinote-can–5-FU, other investigators have pursued this regimen using different schedules. These studies have been performed in patients with esophageal, gastroesophageal, and gastric cancers. One irinotecan-cisplatin regimen was used with bevacizumab.[372]

Fluorouracil-Leucovorin-Oxaliplatin. As is the case for irinotecan-containing regimens, oxaliplatin plus 5-FU is a standard practice option for patients with both metastatic and locally advanced colon cancer. In part because of this data, 5-FU–leucovorin-oxaliplatin (FOLFOX) regimens have also been studied in gastric cancer. The toxicity spectrum is similar to that seen in patients with colorectal cancer, with the dose-limiting toxicity of peripheral neuropathy (oxaliplatin). Myelosuppression, mucositis, and diarrhea typical for 5-FU regimens were noted as well. Several FOLFOX phase 2 studies have now been reported in gastric cancer. Overall response rates of approximately 50% were observed, with median TTP of 5 to 6 months and median OS ranging from 10 to 12 months.[373]

The REAL-2 Trial

Partly on the basis of these studies, a phase 3 trial comparing an oxaliplatin-based regimen with cisplatin-containing combinations was performed. Cunningham et al.[374] in the REAL-2 trial studied 1,002 patients who were randomized to one of four treatment groups: a control arm of ECF and three investigational arms. The central question in this study was: Can capecitabine be substituted for 5-FU and/or oxaliplatin substituted for cisplatin. The four arms were ECF, epirubicin-oxaliplatin–5-FU, epirubicin-cisplatin-capecitabine, and epirubicin-oxaliplatin-capecitabine (EOX). The four regimens are shown in Table 46.9. Patients were stratified for performance status and extent of disease. The primary end point was in OS. The study was powered to show noninferiority for capecitabine compared with 5-FU and oxaliplatin compared with cisplatin. There were approximately 250 patients per arm. The study design was a two-by-two comparison. A total of 40% of patients had primary gastric cancer, and the remainder had either EGJ or esophageal cancers, with 10% of patients having squamous cell cancer of the esophagus. There was no difference in median OS between the arms (ECF 9.9 months, epirubicin-oxaliplatin–5-FU 9.3 months, epirubicin-cisplatin-capecitabine 9.9 months, and EOX 11.2 months). The 1-year OS was also similar and ranged from 38% to 47%, the best outcome evident with EOX and the lowest with the control arm of ECF. The authors concluded the oxaliplatin could be substituted for cisplatin, and capecitabine could be substituted for 5-FU in the palliative setting.

Al-Batran et al.[375] reported the results of a trial comparing a FOLFOX regimen with 5-FU–leucovorin-cisplatin (FLP). A modified FOLFOX-6 schedule was used for the experimental arm. The FLP regimen used slightly lower doses of 5-FU and cisplatin (50 mg/m^2) every 2 weeks. The study was powered for superiority of FOLFOX over FLP. A total of 220 patients were randomized between the two arms. There was no significant difference in TTP ($p = 0.08$) and OS (10.7 fluorouracil 2,600 mg/m^2 via 24-hour infusion, leucovorin 200 mg/m^2, and oxaliplatin 85 mg/m^2 [FLO] every 2 weeks versus 8.8 [FLP] months). Although this study did not demonstrate superiority for oxaliplatin-containing regimens, it does support the results of the REAL-2 study for noninferiority comparing oxaliplatin and cisplatin. The FOLFOX regimen was slightly less toxic.

Finally, Kang et al.[367] compared XP with CF. A total of 160 patients received XP and 156 patients received CF. The XP arm was not inferior, with a median PFS of 5.6 months versus 5 months for CF. OS was 10.5 months versus 9.3 months for XP versus CF (HR = 0.85; 95% CI = 0.64 to 1.13; $p = 0.008$ versus noninferiority margin of 1.25). The authors concluded that XP can be considered an effective alternative to CF.

It is of note that FOLFOX, FOLFIRI, and capecitabine-containing regimens are widely used in colorectal cancer. In metastatic colorectal cancer, the median TTP using these regimens is approximately 7 to 8 months and the median survival (even without the use of bevacizumab) is 20 to 24 months. The 1-year survival for patients with stage IV unresectable colon cancer is approximately 70%, and, using these regimens, 2-year survival approaches 40%. As shown earlier, the same regimens used in patients with gastric or EGJ tumors result in substantially shorter times to progression and significantly shorter median survivals. There are more classes of active cytotoxic agents with demonstrated activity in EGJ than there are for colorectal cancer. In upper gastrointestinal tract malignancies, oxaliplatin, cisplatin, 5-FU, irinotecan, capecitabine, taxane, and anthracyclines have at least modest single-agent activity, whereas the taxanes and anthracyclines are not active in colorectal cancer. These differences in efficacy outcomes suggest biologic differences between these malignancies, despite the histologic similarities (e.g., "intestinal-type" gastric cancers).

As is the case for other solid epithelieal malignancies, an important area of investigation is the development of better preclinical models, such as murine models, and the identification of predictive and prognostic biomarkers, which may well be different between gastrointestinal tumors arising in the upper and lower gastrointestinal tract. On the other hand, using targeted therapies, predictive markers may be the same in different cancers; for example, overexpression or amplification of *HER2* is a predictive marker for the use of the monoclonal antibody trastuzumab in both breast and now gastric cancers. It is also possible that the use of another cytotoxic treatment regimen (second-line treatment) after progression of disease on the first treatment regimen in gastroesophageal cancers would lead to a similar outcome as seen in colorectal cancers. For example, in the REAL-2 trial, only 15% of patients received additional therapy at the time of progression of disease. The irinotecan versus best supportive care study described previously suggests that at least some patients will have a modest survival benefit to second-line treatment.

TABLE 46.9

REAL-2 Regimens

Drug	Dose (mg/m^2)	Day(s)	Week(s)[a]
ECF			
Epirubicin	50 mg/m^2 IV	1	Every 3 wk
Cisplatin	60 mg/m^2 IV	1	
PVI 5-FU	200 mg/m^2/d[b]	1	
EOF			
Epirubicin	50 mg/m^2 IV	1	Every 3 wk
Oxaliplatin	130 mg/m^2 IV	1	
PVI 5-FU	200 mg/m^2/d[b]	1	
ECX			
Epirubicin	50 mg/m^2 IV	1	Every 3 wk
Cisplatin	60 mg/m^2 IV	1	
Capecitabine	625 mg/m^2/BID	1	
EOX			
Epirubicin	50 mg/m^2 IV	1	Every 3 wk
Oxaliplatin	130 mg/m^2 IV	1	
Capecitabine	625 mg/m^2/BID	1	

REAL, Randomized Trial of EOC +/− Panitumumab for Advanced and Locally Advanced Esophagogastric Cancer; ECF, epirubicin-cisplatin-fluorouracil; PVI, protracted venous-infusion; 5-FU, 5-fluorouracil; EOF, epirubicin-oxaliplatin-5-FU; IV, intravenously; ECX, epirubicin-cisplatin-capecitabine; BID, twice a day; EOX, epirubicin-oxaliplatin-capecitabine.
[a] Planned treatment duration 24 weeks (eight cycles).
[b] PVI 5-FU delivered by central venous access catheter.
Modified from Cunningham D, Okines AF, Ashley S, et al. Capecitabine and oxaliplatin for advanced esophagogastric cancer. *N Engl J Med* 2008;358:36.

Second-Line Therapy

Despite numerous chemotherapy options, the majority of patients who progress on first-line therapy are currently not treated with second-line chemotherapy in the West. In several series, only 20% to 50% of patients received second-line treatment.[376,377] Patients with gastric cancer often have numerous comorbidities and complications of their malignancy (i.e., failure to thrive with significant protein-calorie losses, peritoneal carcinomatosis with limited bowel function) that preclude the safe administration of second-line therapy. Alternatively, as many as 70% of patients from Japan and other parts of Asia receive second-line therapy. Recently, there have been two random assignment studies that demonstrate the benefits of second-line therapy.[378,379]

In one study, previously treated patients were randomly assigned to best supportive care or to single-agent irinotecan plus best supportive care. Although the study was initially powered to require 120 patients, accrual to this type of trial was difficult and a total of only 40 patients were eventually randomized. Despite the small sample size, the investigators observed a significant improvement in the HR for death (HR = 0.48) with the administration of irinotecan ($p = 0.012$).[359] In a more recent and larger Korean study, 201 patients were randomized to second-line chemotherapy (either irinotecan or docetaxel) after progression on CF therapy. These investigators confirm an improvement in median OS with chemotherapy from 3.8 months with best supportive care alone to 5.1 months with the addition of chemotherapy.[379] Together, these studies definitely establish that patients with metastatic gastric cancer who have maintained their performance status should be considered for second-line palliative chemotherapy as a standard of practice.

A random assignment study was conducted in patients with advanced gastric cancer comparing paclitaxel and irinotecan in the refractory setting.[380] In this study, 223 patients were randomly assigned to either cytotoxic drug, with no difference in OS observed (median OS 9.5 months with paclitaxel and 8.4 months with irinotecan; HR = 1.13; $p = 0.38$).

Targeted Therapy

The Epidermal Growth Factor Receptor Superfamily: Monoclonal Antibodies

Trastuzumab. Overexpression or amplification of *HER2* (*EGFR2*) occurs in approximately 20% of patients with gastric cancer; it varies with the subtype. A phase 3 study of trastuzumab plus chemotherapy versus chemotherapy alone was performed in patients with gastric cancer overexpressing *HER2*. The preliminary results of the ToGA trial have been recently reported.[381] Among 3,807 patients, 594 patients had *HER2*-positive gastric cancer. They were randomized to receive either CF or XP given every 3 weeks for six cycles, or the same chemotherapy plus trastuzumab. The median OS was 13.5 months for patients receiving trastuzumab plus chemotherapy versus 11.1 months for those receiving chemotherapy alone (HR = 0.74; $p = 0.0048$). The response rate was 47% for patients receiving trastuzumab plus chemotherapy versus 35% for those receiving chemotherapy alone. There was no significant difference in toxicity between treatment arms. Trastuzumab has been approved in Europe for *HER2*-positive gastric cancer. The ToGA trial used a *HER2* scoring system similar to that used in breast cancer. *HER2* was more likely to be positive in patients with EGJ tumors than in more distal tumors (33% versus 20%); patients with diffuse gastric cancer were much less likely to have an *HER2*-positive (6%) tumor.[382]

Cetuximab and Panitumumab. Cetuximab is an antibody against epidermal growth factor receptors. In a trial combining cetuximab plus weekly infusions of oxaliplatin and 5-FU, and DL-folinic acid, 46 patients with advanced gastric cancer were treated.

Toxicity was tolerable; the response rate was 56%; however, OS was 9.5 months. K-Ras mutations were rare.[383]

The Epidermal Growth Factor Receptor Superfamily: Tyrosine Kinase Inhibitors

Lapatinib. Lapatinib is the first dual inhibitor of HER1 (EGFR1) and HER2 (EGFR2). Two phase 2 trials have evaluated lapatinib monotherapy in patients with advanced gastric cancer. In one study, 3 of 46 patients had partial responses. In the second study, 21 patients with EGJ adenocarcinomas were treated without objective responses.

Gefitnib and Erlotinib. Both are epidermal growth factor receptor tyrosine kinase inhibitors. In a large study, a 9% response rate was seen for EGJ tumors versus no responses among patients with gastric cancer; other studies have failed to demonstrate activity even in EGJ tumors.

The Vascular Endothelial Growth Factor Superfamily: Monoclonal Antibodies

Bevacizumab. Bevacizumab is a humanized monoclonal antibody that binds the vascular endothelial growth factor ligand (VEGF-A). In gastric cancer, Shah et al.[372] reported on combining cisplatin plus irinotecan with bevacizumab (phase 2). Among 47 patients, the median TTP was 9.9 months. A second phase 2 study evaluating bevacizumab with DCF also showed promising activity, with median PFS of 12 months and median OS of 17 months.[384] This trial demonstrated potential efficacy with acceptable toxicity; follow-up phase 2 trials also demonstrated acceptable toxicity.[385] The AVAGAST multinational phase 3 trial comparing bevacizumab plus CP versus CP alone has now completed accrual.[386,387] Results have been reported.[388]

In this phase 3 study, 774 patients were randomly assigned to XP ($n = 387$) or XP/bevacizumab ($n = 387$). The study did not meet the primary end point of improving OS (12.1 months with XP/bevaciuamb versus 10.1 months with XP; $p = 0.1002$), but did demonstrate improvement in PFS (6.7 months versus 5.3 months; $p = 0.0037$) and overall response rates (46.0% versus 37.4%; $p = 0.0315$) with XP/bevacizumab versus XP alone, respectively.[386,387] In this study, there was distinct geographic variation in which patients enrolled from Asia appeared not to have significant benefit from the addition of bevacizumab. These results support the concept of significant worldwide disease heterogeneity.

A biomarker evaluation was prospectively performed from the AVAGAST study, in which plasma samples were available from 92% of the study population and tissue samples were available from 94% of the study population.[389] In this analysis, baseline plasma VEGF-A levels and tumor neuropilin-1 expression were identified as potential predictors of bevacizumab efficacy. Specifically, patients with high baseline plasma VEGF-A appeared to benefit from bevacizumab therapy (HR = 0.72; 95% CI = 0.57 to 0.93), and similarly, patients with low baseline expression of neuropilin-1 also showed a trend toward improved OS with bevacizumab (HR = 0.75; 95% CI = 0.59 to 0.97). These data, if validated, may provide important insights pertaining to the geographic heterogeneity observed with this international phase 3 study, and importantly, may identify a population of patients for whom bevacizumab would have substantial efficacy when combined with chemotherapy.

The Vascular Endothelial Growth Factor Superfamily: Tyrosine Kinase Inhibitors

Sunitinib. Sunitinib is an oral inhibitor of VEGF receptor [VEGFR]-1, -2, -3, and PDGFR-α, -β, and c-kit. Bang et al.[389] reported on a phase 2 trial of sunitinib as second-line treatment for advanced gastric cancer. Response rate, PFS, and OS were 2 of 72 patients, 11.1 weeks, and 47.7 weeks, respectively. Sorafenib is another multityrosine kinase inhibitor (VEGFR-2, -3; platelet-derived growth factor receptor–β; Flt-3; Raf-1; and c-kit). The ECOG5203, a phase 2 trial investigating docetaxel plus cisplatin plus sorafenib in gastric cancer, suggested clinical efficacy (response rate = 39%; PFS = 5.8 months; OS = 15.9 months).[390]

Recently, a random assignment phase 2 study of apatinib, a tyrosine kinase inhibitor that selectively inhibits VEGFR2, appears to be active in advanced gastric cancer.[391] In this study, 144 patients were randomly assigned to placebo or two different doses of apatinib. Patients assigned to apatinib had a statistically significant improved OS (4.83 and 4.27 months in the apatinib arms versus 2.5 months in the placebo; $p = 0.0017$), with nine patients demonstrating a radiographic partial response.

In addition, a second study has demonstrated efficacy of VEGFR2 inhibition as monotherapy in gastric cancer. Ramucirumab (IMC-1121B) is a fully human IgG1 monoclonal antibody targeting VEGFR-2. The Regard study was a placebo-controlled, double blind, phase 3 international trial conducted in the second-line setting in patients with metastatic gastric or EGJ adenocarcinoma. Median OS was 5.2 months for ramucirumab and 3.8 months for placebo (HR = 0.776; 95% CI = 0.603 to 0.998; $p = 0.0473$). The significance of this study is that it provides a proof-of-principal that antiangiogenic therapy does have activity in gastroesophageal malignancies. The Regard study supports the concept that subtypes of gastric cancer exist and may be differentially sensitive to antiangiogenic therapy.[392]

Inhibition of Mammalian Target of Rapamycin (Protein Kinase)

Everolimus. An oral inhibitor of the mammalian target of rapamycin has shown activity against gastric cancer in preclinical phase 1 studies.[393,394] Doi et al.[394] reported on a phase 2 trial testing everolimus in metastatic gastric cancer. In 53 patients, the disease control rate (complete response rate plus partial response plus stable disease) was 56%, and the median PFS and OS were 2.7 and 10.1 months, respectively. Based on these encouraging results, a phase 3 study was performed comparing everolimus to best supportive care.[395] In this study, 656 patients were randomized in a 2:1 fashion to everolimus versus placebo. Median OS was similar in both arms, 5.4 months versus 3.2 months (HR = 0.9; 95% CI = 0.75 to 1.08; $p = 0.12$).

In summary, new agents targeting dysregulated cancer pathways are now undergoing study in gastric cancer. At the present time, trastuzumab remains the only drug of this type that has demonstrated efficacy, in combination with cytotoxic chemotherapy, in gastric cancer.

Predictive Markers and Early Assessment of Response in Gastric and Gastroesophageal Tumors

The recognition that several different classes of cytotoxic anticancer agents and targeted pathway agents have activity in subgroups of patients suggests the possibility that predictive markers or a gene signature might allow "customized" precision cancer care that will spare patients from unnecessary toxicity from ineffective therapy, such as testing for *HER2* identifies patients who could benefit from trastuzumab. Molecular markers that might indicate resistance or sensitivity to CF are reviewed elsewhere in this book.[396] Ooi et al.[396] and other investigators[397–399] have used gene expression arrays to identify pathways and gene signatures to predicting clinical prognosis. Ott et al.[77] reported that a drop in SUV of 35% after neoadjuvant chemotherapy was associated with significant pathologic response to systemic treatment. Similar findings were reported by Shah et al.[400] and Weber.[401] Overall, PET may allow early identification of patients responding to systemic therapy.

SURGERY IN TREATMENT OF METASTATIC GASTRIC CANCER

Given the recent improvements in systemic therapy for gastric cancer, the question whether resection of limited metastases from gastric cancer can provide survival benefit remains unanswered. To ask this question in a scientific manner, the surgery branch of the National Institutes of Health/National Cancer Institute is currently accruing patients to a prospective RCT comparing gastrectomy, metastasectomy plus systemic therapy, versus systemic therapy alone (the GYMSSA Trial, clinicaltrials.gov no. NCT00941655).[402]

The GYMSSA trial randomized patients with metastatic gastric cancer to gastrectomy, cytoreductive surgery (CRS)/HIPEC plus Folfoxiri (GYMS arm) versus Folfoxiri alone (SA arm) to study OS. All patients underwent comprehensive staging including laparoscopy. To date, the study accrued 16 evaluable patients. Seven of nine patients in the multimodality GYMS arm achieved complete cytoreduction, with median follow-up of 23 months. Median OS was 12 months in the GYMS arm and 10.2 months in the SA arm; 1- and 2-year OS was 44% and 22% versus 0% and 0%, respectively. Two patients in the GYMS arm lived beyond 23 months, and one up to 12 months. No patient in the SA arm lived longer than 12 months.

Kerkar et al.[401,402] reviewed the published data reporting on liver resection for gastric cancer; 19 studies reported on 436 patients. The majority of the patients had synchronous isolated liver gastric metastases. Overall, the 1-, 3-, and 5-year survival rates were 62%, 30%, and 27%, respectively; 13% (48/358) were alive at 5 years, and in studies with >10 years of follow-up, 4% (48/358) survived for >10 years.[402]

Standard of care for patients with pulmonary gastric metastases is chemotherapy with a median survival of 6 months.[403] Kemp et al.[403] reviewed the published data reporting on lung resections for gastric cancer; 21 studies reported on 43 patients. Eighty-two percent of patients (34/43) had a solitary lesion. At a median follow-up of 23 months, 15 of 43 (35%) patients had no evidence of disease. The overall 5-year survival was 33%.

Gastric carcinomatosis occurs in 5% to 50% of patients undergoing surgery with curative intent.[404–410] The median survival for such patients is 1.5 months to 3.1 months.[404,411–413] Overall data are limited; however, several investigators reported on CRS plus HIPEC for gastric carcinomatosis; the median OS ranged from 6 to 21 months, and 5-year survival ranged from 6% to 16% with operative mortality of 2% to 7% mortality. In patients with optimal cytoreduction-CCR-0/1 (no macroscopic or disease <5 mm), the 5-year survival was 16% to 30%. Complete cytoreduction was possible in only 44% to 51% of the patients.[309,414–418] In 2008, the Fifth International Workshop on Peritoneal Surface Malignancy indicated that peritonectomy, intraoperative, and early postoperative HIPEC potentially can be a powerful therapy against gastric cancer peritoneal carcinomatosis.[419–424]

Bidirectional chemotherapy utilizing intraperitoneal and systemic induction chemotherapy prior to CRS and HIPEC has been studied (retrospectively) in patients with peritoneal carcinomatosis of gastric origin undergoing treatment in a specialized peritoneal surface malignancy unit in Japan. A recent study of 194 patients with gastric carcinomatosis treated initially and responsive (response rate 78%) to intraperitoneal docetaxel (20 mg/m^2) and cisplatin (30 mg/m^2) followed by four cycles of oral S-1 (60 mg/m^2), followed by CRS/HIPEC reported median OS of 16 months and 1-, 2-, and 5-year survival of 66%, 32%, and 11%, respectively.[425] Operative morbidity and moratlty were 24% and 4%, respectively. Response to bidirectional intraperitoneal and systemic chemotherapy, low tumor burden (peritoneal cancer index ≤6) and completeness of cytoreduction (CCR0/1) were independently associated with improved OS on multivariate analysis.

Surgery for Palliation

Because survival for patients with advanced gastric cancer is poor, any proposed operation could have a good chance of providing sustained symptomatic relief while minimizing the attendant morbidity and need for prolonged hospitalization. Ekbom and Gleysteen[426] have reviewed the results of palliative resection versus intestinal bypass (gastrojejunostomy) in 75 patients with advanced gastric cancer. The most frequent symptoms for which patients underwent operation included pain, hemorrhage, nausea, dysphasia, or obstruction. Operative mortality was 25% for gastrojejunostomy, 20% for palliative partial or subtotal gastrectomy, and 27% for total or proximal palliative gastrectomy. The most common and often fatal complication was anastomotic leak. After gastrojejunostomy, 80% of patients had relief of symptoms for a mean of 5.9 months compared with palliative resection, which provided relief of symptoms in 88% of patients for a mean of 14.6 months. Although the duration of palliation was significantly longer after resection (p <0.01), the selection criteria for resection versus bypass were not controlled, and some bias against performing a palliative resection in high-risk patients with more advanced disease may have occurred. Meijer et al.[427] also reported on a retrospective analysis of 51 patients undergoing either palliative intestinal bypass or resection. In 20 of 26 patients (77%) undergoing resection, palliation was considered moderate to good with a mean survival of 9.5 months. After gastroenterostomy, some palliation was noted in 8 of 25 patients (30%), and survival was 4.2 months. Butler et al.[428] have presented the results of total gastrectomy for palliation in 27 patients with advanced gastric cancer. Operative mortality was only 4%, whereas morbidity occurred in 48% of patients. Median survival was 15 months, with a survival rate of 38% at 2 years. This substantial survival rate at 2 years reflects that, although all patients were symptomatic before surgery, only half had stage IV disease. Patients with linitis plastica present a very difficult therapeutic challenge. Resection may provide palliation of symptoms; however, survival after total gastrectomy is exceedingly poor, ranging from 3 months to 1 year.

Bozzetti et al.[429,430] have reviewed the outcomes of 246 patients with advanced gastric cancer who underwent simple exploratory laparotomy alone, gastrointestinal bypass, or palliative resection at the National Cancer Institute of Milan. When survival was compared in patients with similar type and extent of disease, a consistent trend was seen for improved median OS with palliative resection in patients with local spread (4 months versus 8 months) and distant spread of disease (3 months versus 8 months). Boddie et al.[431] have reported similar results in 45 patients undergoing palliative resection at the MD Anderson Cancer Center for advanced gastric cancer. Operative mortality for resection was 22%. In 21 patients who had undergone a palliative bypass procedure, OS was significantly shorter than for those undergoing palliative gastric resection (p <0.01).

In select patients with symptomatic advanced gastric cancer, resection of the primary disease appears to provide symptomatic relief with acceptable morbidity and mortality, even in the presence of macroscopic residual disease.

RADIATION FOR PALLIATION

To date, no studies have evaluated the use of radiation therapy in patients with locally recurrent or metastatic carcinoma of the stomach. Its use is likely to be limited to palliation of symptoms such as bleeding or controlling pain secondary to local tumor infiltration. Although minimal data are available, radiation therapy seems to be anecdotally effective in controlling bleeding, as is true in other primary tumor sites. Pain from local tumor invasion can also be palliated with radiation. On rare occasions, a case may arise of a patient with a focal local recurrence without metastases who would be amenable to relatively high-dose radiation therapy in order to try to prolong quality-adjusted survival or in whom radiation therapy would be given as an adjuvant to surgical resection. At present, however, no data support such an approach.

SELECTED REFERENCES

The full reference list can be accessed at lwwhealthlibrary.com/oncology.

5. Anderson WF, Fraumeni FJ, Rosenberg PS, et al. Age-specific trends in incidence of noncardia gastric cancer in US adults. *JAMA* 2010;303:1723–1728.
21. Laurén P. The two histological main types of gastric carcinoma: diffuse and so-called intestinal-type carcinoma: an attempt at a histo-clinical classification. *Acta Pathol Microbiol Scand* 1965;64:31–49.
47. Rugge M, Kim JG, Mahachai V, et al. OLGA gastritis staging in young adults and country-specific gastric cancer risk. *Int J Surg Pathol* 2008;16:150–154.
66. Bentrem D, Gerdes H, Tang L, et al. Clinical correlation of endoscopic ultrasonography with pathologic stage and outcome in patients undergoing curative resection for gastric cancer. *Ann Surg Oncol* 2007;14:1853–1859.
77. Ott K, Fink U, Becker K, et al. Prediction of response to preoperative chemotherapy in gastric carcinoma by metabolic imaging: results of a prospective trial. *J Clin Oncol* 2003;21:4604–4610.
78. Lordick F, Ott K, Krause BJ, et al. PET to assess early metabolic response and to guide treatment of adenocarcinoma of the oesophagogastric junction: the MUNICON phase II trial. *Lancet Oncol* 2007;8:797–805.
83. Conlon KC. Staging laparoscopy for gastric cancer. *Ann Ital Chir* 2001;72:33–37.
98. Edge SB, Compton CC. The American Joint Committee on Cancer: the 7th edition of the AJCC Cancer Staging Manual and the future of TNM. *Ann Surg Oncol* 2010;17:1471–1474.
99. Karpeh MS, Leon L, Klimstra D, et al. Lymph node staging in gastric cancer: is location more important than number? An analysis of 1,038 patients. *Ann Surg* 2000;232:362–371.
100. Smith DD, Schwarz RR, Schwarz RE. Impact of total lymph node count on staging and survival after gastrectomy for gastric cancer: data from a large US-population database. *J Clin Oncol* 2005;23:7114–7124.
103. Kattan MW, Karpeh MS, Mazumdar M, et al. Postoperative nomogram for disease-specific survival after an R0 resection for gastric carcinoma. *J Clin Oncol* 2003;21:3647–3650.
114. Kurihara M, Aiko T. The new Japanese classification of gastric carcinoma: revised explanation of "response assessment of chemotherapy and radiotherapy for gastric carcinoma." *Gastric Cancer* 2001;4:9–13.

120. Siewert JR, Stein HJ. Classification of adenocarcinoma of the oesophagogastric junction. *Br J Surg* 1998;85:1457–1459.
139. Bennett C, Wang Y, Pan T. Endoscopic mucosal resection for early gastric cancer. *Cochrane Database Syst Rev* 2009;(4):CD004276.
167. Robertson CS, Chung SC, Woods SD, et al. A prospective randomized trial comparing R1 subtotal gastrectomy with R3 total gastrectomy for antral cancer. *Ann Surg* 1994;220:176–182.
168. Bozzetti F, Marubini E, Bonfanti G, et al. Subtotal versus total gastrectomy for gastric cancer: five-year survival rates in a multicenter randomized Italian trial. Italian Gastrointestinal Tumor Study Group. *Ann Surg* 1999;230:170–178.
169. Hulscher JB, van Sandick JW, de Boer AG, et al. Extended transthoracic resection compared with limited transhiatal resection for adenocarcinoma of the esophagus. *N Engl J Med* 2002;347:1662–1669.
172. Kodera Y, Schwarz RE, Nakao A. Extended lymph node dissection in gastric carcinoma: where do we stand after the Dutch and British randomized trials? *J Am Coll Surg* 2002;195:855–864.
188. Dent DM, Madden MV, Price SK. Randomized comparison of R1 and R2 gastrectomy for gastric carcinoma. *Br J Surg* 1988;75:110–112.
189. Cuschieri A, Weeden S, Fielding J, et al. Patient survival after D1 and D2 resections for gastric cancer: long-term results of the MRC randomized surgical trial. Surgical Co-operative Group. *Br J Cancer* 1999;79:1522–1530.
190. Bonenkamp JJ, Hermans J, Sasako M, et al. Extended lymph-node dissection for gastric cancer. *N Engl J Med* 1999;340:908–914.
191. Degiuli M, Sasako M, Calgaro M, et al. Morbidity and mortality after D1 and D2 gastrectomy for cancer: interim analysis of the Italian Gastric Cancer Study Group (IGCSG) randomised surgical trial. *Eur J Surg Oncol* 2004;30:303–308.
192. Wu CW, Hsiung CA, Lo SS, et al. Nodal dissection for patients with gastric cancer: a randomised controlled trial. *Lancet Oncol* 2006;7:309–315.
196. Songun I, Putter H, Kranenbarg EM, et al. Surgical treatment of gastric cancer: 15-year follow-up results of the randomised nationwide Dutch D1D2 trial. *Lancet Oncol* 2010;11:439–449.
197. Bonenkamp JJ, Hermans J, Sasako M, et al. Quality control of lymph node dissection in the Dutch randomized trial of D1 and D2 lymph node dissection for gastric cancer. *Gastric Cancer* 1998;1:152–159.

PRACTICE OF ONCOLOGY

199. Bonenkamp JJ, Songun I, Hermans J, et al. Randomised comparison of morbidity after D1 and D2 dissection for gastric cancer in 996 Dutch patients. *Lancet* 1995;345:745–748.

201. Chen XZ, Hu JK, Zhou ZG, et al. Meta-analysis of effectiveness and safety of D2 plus para-aortic lymphadenectomy for resectable gastric cancer. *J Am Coll Surg* 2010;210:100–105.

203. Brennan MF. Lymph-node dissection for gastric cancer. *N Engl J Med* 1999;340:956–958.

206. Yonemura Y, Wu CC, Fukushima N, et al. Randomized clinical trial of D2 and extended paraaortic lymphadenectomy in patients with gastric cancer. *Int J Clin Oncol* 2008;13:132–137.

213. Doglietto GB, Pacelli F, Caprino P, et al. Pancreas-preserving total gastrectomy for gastric cancer. *Arch Surg* 2000;135:89–94.

217. Yao XX, Yan C, Yan M, et al. [A comparative study on the efficacy of spleen-preserving modified D2 radical gastrectomy and D2 radical gastrectomy with splenectomy]. *Zhonghua Wei Chang Wai Ke Za Zhi* 2010;13:111–114.

228. Hundahl SA, Macdonald JS, Benedetti J, et al. Surgical treatment variation in a prospective, randomized trial of chemoradiotherapy in gastric cancer: the effect of undertreatment. *Ann Surg Oncol* 2002;9:278–286.

293. Sakuramoto S, Sasako M, Yamaguchi T, et al. Adjuvant chemotherapy for gastric cancer with S-1, an oral fluoropyrimidine. *N Engl J Med* 2007;357:1810–1820.

296. Di Costanzo F, Gasperoni S, Manzione L, et al. Adjuvant chemotherapy in completely resected gastric cancer: a randomized phase III trial conducted by GOIRC. *J Natl Cancer Inst* 2008;100:388–398.

297. Buyse ME, Pignon J. Meta-analyses of randomized trials assessing the interest of postoperative adjuvant chemotherapy and prognsotic factors in gastric cancer. *J Clin Oncol* 2009;27:4539.

299. GASTRIC (Global Advanced/Adjuvant Stomach Tumor Research International Collaboration) Group, Paoletti X, Oba K, et al. Benefit of adjuvant chemotherapy for resectable gastric cancer: a meta-analysis. *JAMA* 2010;303:1729–1737.

313. Kelsen D, Karpeh M, Schwartz G, et al. Neoadjuvant therapy of high-risk gastric cancer: a phase II trial of preoperative FAMTX and postoperative intraperitoneal fluorouracil-cisplatin plus intravenous fluorouracil. *J Clin Oncol* 1996;14:1818–1828.

314. Brenner B, Shah MA, Karpeh MS, et al. A phase II trial of neoadjuvant cisplatin-fluorouracil followed by postoperative intraperitoneal floxuridine-leucovorin in patients with locally advanced gastric cancer. *Ann Oncol* 2006;17:1404–1411.

315. Downey RJ, Akhurst T, Ilson D, et al. Whole body 18FDG-PET and the response of esophageal cancer to induction therapy: results of a prospective trial. *J Clin Oncol* 2003;21:428–432.

320. Allum WH, Hallissey MT, Ward LC, et al. A controlled, prospective, randomised trial of adjuvant chemotherapy or radiotherapy in resectable gastric cancer: interim report. British Stomach Cancer Group. *Br J Cancer* 1989;60:739–744.

321. Hallissey MT, Dunn JA, Ward LC, et al. The second British Stomach Cancer Group trial of adjuvant radiotherapy or chemotherapy in resectable gastric cancer: five-year follow-up. *Lancet* 1994;343:1309–1312.

322. Zhang ZX, Gu XZ, Yin WB, et al. Randomized clinical trial on the combination of preoperative irradiation and surgery in the treatment of adenocarcinoma of gastric cardia (AGC)—report on 370 patients. *Int J Radiat Oncol Biol Phys* 1998;42:929–934.

325. Gunderson L, Willet G, Harrisson B, et al., eds. *Intraoperative Irradiation: Techniques and Results.* Totowa, NJ: Humana Press; 1999.

326. Abe M, Takahashi M, Ono K, et al. Japan gastric trials in intraoperative radiation therapy. *Int J Radiat Oncol Biol Phys* 1988;15:1431–1433.

327. Sindelar WF, Kinsella TJ, Tepper JE, et al. Randomized trial of intraoperative radiotherapy in carcinoma of the stomach. *Am J Surg* 1993;165:178–186, discussion 186–187.

330. Macdonald JS, Smalley SR, Benedetti J, et al. Chemoradiotherapy after surgery compared with surgery alone for adenocarcinoma of the stomach or gastroesophageal junction. *N Engl J Med* 2001;345:725–730.

333. Walsh TN, Noonan N, Hollywood D, et al. A comparison of multimodal therapy and surgery for esophageal adenocarcinoma. *N Engl J Med* 1996;335:462–467.

334. Tepper J, Krasna MJ, Niedzwiecki D, et al. Phase III trial of trimodality therapy with cisplatin, fluorouracil, radiotherapy, and surgery compared with surgery alone for esophageal cancer: CALGB 9781. *J Clin Oncol* 2008;26:1086–1092.

358. Wagner AD, Unverzagt S, Grothe W, et al. Chemotherapy for advanced cancer. *Cochrane Database Syst Rev* 2010;(3):CD004064.

359. Thuss-Patience PC, Kretzschmar A, Deist T, et al. Irinotecan versus best supportive care as second-line therapy in gastric cancer: a randomized phase III study of the Arbeitsgemeinschaft Internistische Onkologie (AIO). *J Clin Oncol* 2009;27:Abstr 4540.

360. Okines AF, Norman AR, McCloud P, et al. Meta-analysis of the REAL-2 and ML17032 trials: evaluating capecitabine-based combination chemotherapy and infused 5-fluorouracil-based combination chemotherapy for the treatment of advanced oesophago-gastric cancer. *Ann Oncol* 2009;20:1529–1534.

361. Di Cosimo S, Ferretti G, Fazio N, et al. Docetaxel in advanced gastric cancer—review of the main clinical trials. *Acta Oncol* 2003;42:693–700.

363. Vanhoefer U, Rougier P, Wilke H, et al. Final results of a randomized phase III trial of sequential high-dose methotrexate, fluorouracil, and doxorubicin versus etoposide, leucovorin, and fluorouracil versus infusional fluorouracil and cisplatin in advanced gastric cancer: a trial of the European Organization for Research and Treatment of Cancer Gastrointestinal Tract Cancer Cooperative Group. *J Clin Oncol* 2000;18:2648–2657.

364. Ohtsu A, Shimada Y, Shirao K, et al. Randomized phase III trial of fluorouracil alone versus fluorouracil plus cisplatin versus uracil and tegafur plus mitomycin in patients with unresectable, advanced gastric cancer: the Japan Clinical Oncology Group Study (JCOG9205). *J Clin Oncol* 2003;21:54–59.

365. Van Cutsem E, Moiseyenko VM, Tjulandin S, et al. Phase III study of docetaxel and cisplatin plus fluorouracil compared with cisplatin and fluorouracil as first-line therapy for advanced gastric cancer: a report of the V325 Study Group. *J Clin Oncol* 2006;24:4991–4997.

366. Dank M, Zaluski J, Barone C, et al. Randomized phase III study comparing irinotecan combined with 5-fluorouracil and folinic acid to cisplatin combined with 5-fluorouracil in chemotherapy naive patients with advanced adenocarcinoma of the stomach or esophagogastric junction. *Ann Oncol* 2008;19:1450–1457.

367. Kang YK, Kang WK, Shin DB, et al. Capecitabine/cisplatin versus 5-fluorouracil/cisplatin as first-line therapy in patients with advanced gastric cancer: a randomised phase III noninferiority trial. *Ann Oncol* 2009;20:666–673.

369. Shah MA, Stoller R, Shibata S, et al. Random assignment multicenter phase II study of modified docetaxel, sisplatin, flourouracil (mDCF) versus DCF with growth factor support (GCSF) in metastatic gastroesophageal adenocarcinoma (GE). *J Clin Oncol* 2010;28:Abstr 4014.

370. Pozzo C, Barone C, Szanto J, et al. Irinotecan in combination with 5-fluorouracil and folinic acid or with cisplatin in patients with advanced gastric or esophageal-gastric junction adenocarcinoma: results of a randomized phase II study. *Ann Oncol* 2004;15:1773–1781.

371. Ross P, Nicolson M, Cunningham D, et al. Prospective randomized trial comparing mitomycin, cisplatin, and protracted venous-infusion fluorouracil (PVI 5-FU) with epirubicin, cisplatin, and PVI 5-FU in advanced esophagogastric cancer. *J Clin Oncol* 2002;20:1996–2004.

372. Shah MA, Ramanathan RK, Ilson DH, et al. Multicenter phase II study of irinotecan, cisplatin, and bevacizumab in patients with metastatic gastric or gastroesophageal junction adenocarcinoma. *J Clin Oncol* 2006;24:5201–5206.

373. Nardi M, Azzarello D, Maisano R, et al. FOLFOX-4 regimen as first-line chemotherapy in elderly patients with advanced gastric cancer: a safety study. *J Chemother* 2007;19:85–89.

374. Cunningham D, Okines AF, Ashley S, et al. Capecitabine and oxaliplatin for advanced esophagogastric cancer. *N Engl J Med* 2008;358:36–46.

375. Al-Batran SE, Hartmann JT, Probst S, et al. Phase III trial in metastatic gastroesophageal adenocarcinoma with fluorouracil, leucovorin plus either oxaliplatin or cisplatin: a study of the Arbeitsgemeinschaft Internistische Onkologie. *J Clin Oncol* 2008;26:1435–1442.

381. Van Cutsam E, Kang Y, Chung H, et al. Efficacy results from the ToGA trial: a phase III study of trastuzumab added to standard chemotherapy (CT) in first-line human epidermal growth factor receptor 2 (HER2)-positive advanced cancer (GC). *J Clin Oncol* 2009;27:Abstr LBA450.

382. Bang Y, Chung H, Sawaki A, et al. HER2-positivity rates in advanced gastric cancer (GC): results from a large international phase III trial. *J Clin Oncol* 2008;26:Abstr 4526.

383. Lordick F, Luber B, Lorenzen S, et al. Cetuximab plus oxaliplatin/leucovorin/5-fluorouracil in first-line metastatic gastric cancer: a phase II study of the Arbeitsgemeinschaft Internistische Onkologie (AIO). *Br J Cancer* 2010;102:500–505.

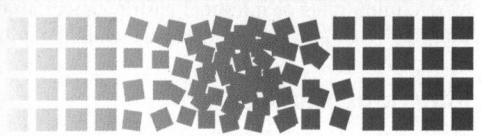

47 Genetic Testing in Stomach Cancer

Nicki Chun and James M. Ford

INTRODUCTION

Gastric cancer encompasses a heterogeneous collection of etiologic and histologic subtypes associated with a variety of known and unknown environmental and genetic factors. It is a global public health concern, accounting for 700,000 annual deaths worldwide, and currently ranks as the fourth leading cause of cancer mortality, with a 5-year survival of only 20%. The incidence and prevalence of gastric cancer vary widely, with Asian/Pacific regions bearing the highest rates of disease.

Recent and rapid advances in molecular genetics have provided an understanding of the cause for many inherited cancer syndromes, offering possibilities for individual genetic testing, family counseling, and preventive approaches. For most cancer syndromes, however, not every individual tested is found to have inherited a germ-line mutation in a candidate gene, suggesting additional uncharacterized alterations in other genes that result in similar outcomes. Nevertheless, the ability to genetically define many individuals and families with inherited cancer syndromes allows for a multidisciplinary approach to their management, often including the consideration of surgical and medical preventive measures. Without question, such complex management and decision making should be centered in the high-risk cancer genetics clinic, where physicians, genetic counselors, and other health professionals jointly consider optimal management for patients and families at high risk for developing cancer.

Approximately 3% to 5% of gastric cancers are associated with a hereditary predisposition, including a variety of Mendelian genetic conditions and complex genetic traits. Identifying those gastric cancers associated with an inherited cancer risk syndrome is the purview of cancer genetics clinics. The keystone to any cancer genetics evaluation is a complete, three-generation family history. Pedigree analyses suggesting an inherited gastric cancer risk include familiar features such as multiple affected relatives tracking along one branch of the family in an autosomal-dominant pattern, young ages at onset, and additional associated malignancies related to an identified syndrome. It is imperative to document the histology of the gastric tumors and other familial cancers because this is the initial node in the decision tree of an inherited gastric cancer syndrome differential. Finally, there are clinical criteria for recognized gastric cancer syndromes published by expert consensus panels that assist genetic practitioners in assessing both the likelihood of identifying an underlying germ-line DNA mutation and guide management in the absence of a molecular confirmation. Herein, we review the literature regarding incidence, recurrence risks, and defined gastric cancer genetic syndromes to assist in providing genetic counseling for families affected by gastric cancer.

HISTOLOGIC DEFINITIONS AND DESCRIPTIONS

Gastric cancer has traditionally been subtyped pathologically according to Lauren's[1] classification published in 1965 and revised by Carneiro et al.[2] in 1995. The four histologic categories include: (1) glandular/intestinal, (2) border foveal hyperplasia, (3) mixed intestinal/diffuse, and (4) solid/undifferentiated.

More clinically relevant, the majority of gastric cancers can be subdivided into intestinal type or diffuse type. Diffuse tumors exhibit isolated cells that typically develop below the mucosal lining and often spread and thicken until the stomach appears hardened into the morphologic designation called *linitis plastica*. Diffuse gastric tumors frequently feature *signet ring cells*, named for the marginalization of the nucleus to the cell periphery due to high mucin content. Intestinal-type gastric tumors more often present as solid masses with atrophic gastritis and intestinal metaplasia at the periphery. The intestinal subtype is seen more commonly in older patients, whereas the diffuse type affects younger patients and has a more aggressive clinical course. The relative proportions of gastric cancer subtypes worldwide are 74% intestinal versus 16% diffuse and 10% other,[3] although diffuse gastric cancer is becoming relatively more common in Western countries. The importance of distinguishing these two main histopathologic types of gastric cancer is highlighted by finding specific genetic changes associated with the different types. For the purposes of genetic counseling, E-cadherin (*CDH1*) mutations are found exclusively in the diffuse type.[4–8] Whereas intestinal-type hereditary gastric cancer families have been identified clinically, no genetic associations have yet been discovered.

As individual molecular profiling of solid tumors becomes more common in the future, we expect classification systems will evolve based on tumor biology more than histology. Advances in deciphering the mechanisms of gene alterations that lead to gastric cancer include gene mutation, amplification, deletion, and epigenetic methylation.[9] For example, two recent studies have performed whole-exome sequencing of human gastric tumors and identified a number of known (e.g., *p53*, *PTEN*, *PIK3CA*), but also previously unreported somatic gene mutations and pathway alterations. Both found *ARID1A* inactivating gene mutations in the majority of microsatellite-instable tumors, a member of the SWI-SNF chromatin remodeling family.[10,11] However, whether any of these somatic gene alterations are found to confer cancer risk when mutated in the germ line remains to be determined.

ETIOLOGY

Analogous to other common cancers, a host of factors are implicated as causes of gastric cancer. Widely diverse geographical disparities suggest both environmental and genetic contributions. Furthermore, a strong association with endemic *Helicobacter pylori* carrier rates implicates infection as a major risk factor. There are likely to be a host of factors contributing to the development of most gastric cancers.

Environmental Risk Factors

Geographic variations in gastric cancer rates have prompted investigations of shared diet and lifestyle variables. Gastric cancer is correlated with the chronic ingestion of pickled vegetables, salted fish, excessive dietary salt, smoked meats, and with smoking.[12–16]

Fruits and vegetables may have a protective effect. The influence of environmental factors as causes of gastric cancer is highlighted by declining rates of intestinal gastric cancer among immigrants from high-incident countries to low-incident countries.

Infectious Risk Factors

H. pylori infection is endemic in the Asian–Pacific basin.[17] Transmission routinely occurs through family contacts in childhood and leads to atrophic gastritis.[18,19] As evidenced by high indigenous infection rates, *H. pylori* is insufficient to singularly cause gastric cancer, suggesting complex interactions between virus and host genetic backgrounds. However, *H. pylori* species are consistently implicated as a major risk factor primarily associated with intestinal-type gastric cancer. Studies in a variety of high- and low-risk populations have found odds ratios ranging from 2.56 to 6 for noncardia gastric cancer.[20]

The Epstein-Barr virus has recently been implicated in about 10% of gastric carcinoma worldwide, or an estimated 80,000 cases annually. Epstein-Barr virus–associated gastric cancer shows some distinct clinicopathologic characteristics, such as male predominance, predisposition to the proximal stomach, and a high proportion in diffuse-type gastric carcinomas. Mechanistically, Epstein-Barr virus gastric tumors display epigenetic promoter methylation of many cancer-related genes, causing downregulation of their expression.[21]

Genetics

Five to 10% of gastric cancer is associated with strong familial clustering and attributable to genetic factors. Shared environmental factors account for the majority of familial clustering of the intestinal type; however, approximately 5% of the total gastric cancer burden is thought to be due to germ-line mutations in genes causing highly penetrant, autosomal-dominant gastric cancer risk of both intestinal and diffuse subtypes. We review the definitions of hereditary gastric cancer families and recognize genetic syndromes associated with increased gastric cancer risk.

EPIDEMIOLOGY OF GASTRIC CANCER

Gastric cancer is now the fourth most common malignancy worldwide, with rates having fallen steadily since 1975 when global statistics were first compared. The incidence and prevalence of gastric cancer vary widely among world populations. High-risk countries (reported incidence × 100,000 per year) include Korea (41.4), China (41.3), Japan (31.1), Portugal (34.4), and Colombia (20.3). Intermediate-risk countries include Malaysia, Singapore, and Taiwan (11 to 19, respectively), whereas low-risk areas include Thailand (8), Northern Europe (5.6), Australia (5.4), India (5.3), and North America (4.3). More than 70% of cases occur in developing countries, and men have roughly twice the risk of women.[22] In 2008, estimates of gastric cancer burden in the United States were 21,500 cases (13,190 men and 8,310 women) and 10,880 deaths.[23] The median age at diagnosis for gastric cancer is 71 years, and 5-year survival is approximately 25%.[24] Only 24% of stomach cancers are localized at the time of diagnosis, 30% have lymph node involvement, and another 30% have metastatic disease. Survival rates are predictably higher for those with localized disease, with corresponding 5-year survival rates of 60%.

The worldwide decline in the incidence of gastric cancer has been attributed to modifications in diet, improved food storage and preservation, and decreased *H. pylori* infection. Fresh fruit and vegetable consumption, refrigeration, decreased urban crowding, and improved living conditions have reduced *H. pylori* exposure and carrier rates. By contrast, the incidence of diffuse-type gastric cancer is stable, and in North America, it may even be increasing.[16,25–27]

TABLE 47.1
Clinical Criteria for CDH1 Testing Defined by the 2010 International Gastric Cancer Linkage Consortium

1. Two gastric cancer cases in the family: one confirmed diffuse type and one diagnosed at the age of <50 y
2. Three confirmed diffuse gastric cancers in first- or second-degree relatives independent of age
3. Diffuse gastric cancer diagnosed at age <40 y (no additional family history needed)
4. Personal or family history (first- or second-degree) of diffuse gastric cancer and lobular breast cancer, one diagnosed at age <50 y

From Fitzgerald RC, Hardwick R, Huntsman D, et al. Hereditary diffuse gastric cancer: Updated consensus guidelines for clinical management and directions for future research. *J Med Genet* 2010;47:436–444.

Familial Gastric Cancer

Shared environmental factors, such as diet and *H. pylori* infection, account for the majority of familial clustering of the intestinal type of gastric cancer, with no known causative germ-line variants. However, few nongenetic risks for diffuse gastric cancer have been identified, supporting a larger role for hereditary factors. Approximately 5% of the total gastric cancer burden is thought to be due to germ-line mutations in genes causing a highly penetrant, autosomal-dominant predisposition. The International Gastric Cancer Linkage Consortium (IGCLC) has redefined genetic classification of familial intestinal gastric cancer to reflect the background incidence rate in a population (Table 47.1).

Thus, countries with high incidence of intestinal-type gastric cancer (China, Korea, Japan, Portugal) use criteria analogous to the Amsterdam criteria invoked for Lynch syndrome:

- At least three relatives with intestinal gastric cancer, one a first-degree relative of the other two
- At least two successive generations affected, and
- Gastric cancer diagnosed before the age of 50 years in at least one individual

In countries with a low incidence of intestinal-type gastric cancer (United States, United Kingdom):

- At least two first-/second-degree relatives affected by intestinal gastric cancer, one diagnosed before the age of 50 years, or
- Three or more relatives with intestinal gastric cancer at any age

Familial intestinal gastric cancer families are similarly prevalent as familial diffuse gastric cancer families, yet a germ-line genetic defect underlying the disease remains to be identified.[28] Hemminki et al.[29] reported Swedish data on all available types of cancer in first-degree relatives by both parent and sibling probands. The relative risks (RR) for gastric cancer were greater than 3 for siblings with any relative with gastric cancer and greater than 5 when a sibling was younger than 50 years. Shin et al.[30] assessed 428 gastric cancer subjects and 368 controls in Korea for the risk of gastric cancer in first-degree relatives and found an RR of 2.85 with one first-degree relative and greater than 5 in a first-degree relative with *H. pylori* and a positive family history. Therefore, in the high-incident countries of Japan and Taiwan, population screening for gastric cancer has greatly enhanced early detection, leading to 5-year survival rates of greater than 90%.[31]

Hereditary Diffuse Gastric Cancer

In 1999, the first IGCLC defined hereditary diffuse gastric cancer (HDGC) as families with (1) two cases diffuse gastric cancer in first-/second-degree relatives with one younger than 50 years, and

(2) three cases diffuse gastric cancer at any age.[32] The first clear evidence for a gastric cancer susceptibility genetic locus was the identification in 1998 of a germ-line inactivating mutation in the gene encoding for E-cadherin (CDH1) in a large, five-generation Maori family from New Zealand with 25 kindred with early-onset diffuse gastric cancer.[33] The age at diagnosis of gastric cancer ranged upward from 14 years, with the majority occurring in individuals younger than 40 years. The pattern of inheritance of gastric cancer was consistent with an autosomal-dominant susceptibility gene with incomplete penetrance. Similar reports of CDH1 mutations in widely diverse HDGC cohorts from Asia, Europe, and North America followed soon thereafter.[34–39] Germ-line CDH1 mutations have been found to be associated with approximately 30% of families with HDGC, with a lifetime risk for gastric cancer of greater than 80%, and up to 60% risk for female carriers developing lobular breast cancer.[40] To date, CDH1 is the only gene implicated in HDGC. Worldwide, about 100 CDH1 mutation–positive families have been reported.[41]

E-cadherin Mutations and Gastric Cancer

The E-cadherin gene coding sequence gives rise to a mature protein consisting of three major domains, a large extracellular domain (exons 4 to 13), smaller transmembranes (exons 13 to 14), and cytoplasmic domains (exons 14 to 16). As in other autosomal-dominant cancer predisposing genes, only one CDH1 allele is mutated in the germ line, and the majority of genetic changes lead to truncation of the protein, with mutations distributed throughout the gene's 2.6 kb of coding sequence and 16 exons without any apparent hotspots. Somatic CDH1 mutations have been identified in about half of sporadic diffuse gastric cancers, but occur rarely in intestinal gastric cancer. CDH1 encodes the calcium-dependent cell-adhesion glycoprotein E-cadherin. E-cadherin is a transmembrane protein that connects to the actin cytoskeleton through a complex with catenin proteins.[5,42] Functionally, E-cadherin impacts the maintenance of normal tissue morphology and cellular differentiation. With regard to HDGC, it is believed that CDH1 acts as a tumor suppressor gene, with the mutation of CDH1 leading to a loss of cell adhesion, proliferation, invasion, and metastasis.[43]

Genetic Testing for HDGC

At the second meeting of the IGCLC in 2010, HDGC guidelines[44] were extended to recommend CDH1 genetic testing to families with the following:

- Cases of gastric cancer in which one case is histopathologically confirmed as diffuse and younger than 50 years
- Families with both lobular breast cancer and diffuse gastric cancer, with one diagnosed younger than 50 years
- Probands diagnosed with diffuse gastric cancer younger than 40 years, with no family history of gastric cancer

Using the initial IGCLC criteria for HDGC, CDH1 mutation testing yielded a detection rate of 30% to 50%.[45] Interestingly, a pattern began to emerge of lower CDH1 mutation rates among HDGC families in high gastric cancer incidence populations and higher rates in low-incident countries.[46,47] Other reports suggest that the rate of CDH1 mutations in isolated cases of diffuse gastric cancer younger than 35 years is similar in both low- and high-risk countries, hovering at around 20%.[48]

Approximately 50% to 70% of clinically diagnosed HDGC families have no identifiable genetic mutation. Multiple candidate loci have been investigated without identifying causative mutations that would account for the large number of non-CDH1 HDGC families.[49–51] Huntsman's group has published a report of multiplex ligation-dependent probe amplification-based exon duplication/deletion studies performed on 93 non-CDH1 families

and found 6.5% carried large genomic deletions, bringing the detection rate up to 45.6% in their cohort of 160 families.[52]

As CDH1 mutation families were identified, data on these families provided the foundation for genetic counseling information. Initially, the cumulative risk of gastric cancer by the age of 80 years in HDGC families was initially estimated as 67% for men and 83% for women. The age at onset shows marked variation between and within families. The median age at onset in the 30 Maori CDH1 mutation carriers who developed gastric cancer was 32 years, which was significantly younger than the median age of 43 years in individuals with gastric cancer from other ethnicities.[53] More recent reports of the lifetime risks of diffuse gastric cancer suggest greater than 80% in both men and women by the age of 80 years.[48,54]

The lifetime risk for lobular breast cancer among female CDH1 carriers, originally estimated to be in the range of 20% to 40%, now approaches 60%, with an average age of 53 years at the time of diagnosis.[36,54,55] Of note, CDH1 mutations have been seen in up to 50% of sporadic lobular breast cancer. Pathologic similarities between diffuse gastric and lobular breast carcinomas such as high mucin content with associated signet ring features and loss of E-cadherin on immunohistochemistry hint at a common molecular mechanism.[56,57] To evaluate the CDH1 carrier rate in women with lobular breast cancer without a family history of diffuse gastric cancer, a multicenter study of 318 women with lobular-type breast cancer diagnosed before the age of 45 years and known to be BRCA1/2-negative were sequenced for CDH1 mutations. Only four possibly pathogenic mutations were identified for a rate of 1.3%, suggesting CDH1 is a rare cause of early lobular cancer without associated gastric cancer family history.[58]

Signet ring colon cancer has been reported in two families with germ-line CDH1, but no screening guidelines have been suggested.[45,59] Nonsyndromic cleft lip and/or palate was reported in seven individuals from three families in the Netherlands and in four individuals from two families in France. There is speculation that defects in the cell-adhesion role of E-cadherin may contribute to this developmental anomaly, although no association can be drawn from these scant case reports.[40,60]

Like other familial cancer syndromes with an autosomal-dominant inheritance pattern, high penetrance for heterozygotes, and significant mortality unless diagnosed early, genetic counseling and testing should occur early, and a comprehensive screening plan should be developed, as well as the consideration of prophylactic surgery. Pretest and posttest genetic counseling should be provided to individuals from HDGC kindred who are undergoing genetic testing for germ-line CDH1 mutations. Because cases of gastric cancer in HDGC families have been reported in individuals as young as 14 years, HDGC may be considered one of the sets of hereditary cancer syndromes, such as MEN 2–associated medullary thyroid cancer, Li–Fraumeni syndrome (LFS), and familial adenomatous polyposis (FAP), in which genetic testing is potentially clinically useful in children.

SCREENING AND MANAGEMENT OF CANCER RISK IN HDGC

Diagnosing gastric cancer in its early stages provides the best chance for curative resection but is a difficult task. Symptoms due to gastric cancer are generally nonspecific and do not appear until the disease is more advanced. The survival of early gastric cancer (e.g., not beyond the mucosa or submucosa) is much better than advanced lesions, so identifying these lesions at the earliest of stages is imperative for optimal survival. Endoscopy is generally considered to be the best method to screen for gastric cancer, but diagnosing diffuse gastric carcinoma is most difficult, because these lesions tend not to form a grossly visible exophytic mass, but rather spread submucosally as single cells or clustered islands of cells. Improved chromoendoscopic-aided methods for directed

PRACTICE OF ONCOLOGY

biopsies to diagnose these early diffuse lesions may prove beneficial, but so far all approaches at screening, including computed tomography and positron emission tomography imaging, have proven disappointing.[61]

Given the inadequacy of clinical screening in HDGC, prophylactic total gastrectomy is offered to carriers of germ-line *CDH1* mutations.[62,63] In every published series of this approach, nearly all specimens contain multiple foci of intramucosal diffuse signet ring cell cancer. Currently, there is information available from 96 total gastrectomies in the setting of HDGC,[44] approximately three-quarters of which were performed in asymptomatic *CDH1* carriers following negative screening endoscopy and biopsies. Only three cases did not show evidence for early invasive carcinoma, and in two of these, tiny foci of in situ signet ring cell carcinoma were observed.[44] Although malignant foci are generally localized to the proximal one-third of the stomach,[64] lesions may be distributed throughout the entire stomach, necessitating a total gastrectomy for comprehensive prevention. The optimal timing of prophylactic gastrectomy is unknown but is generally recommended when the unaffected carrier is 5 years younger than the youngest family member who has developed clinical symptoms of HDGC. Clinical management and screening strategies remain uncertain for families who meet criteria for HDGC but are negative for *CDH1* mutations or variants of unknown significance, although a screening endoscopy is often suggested.

The impact and long-term outcomes of prophylactic gastrectomy on carriers' lifestyle and health are significant, particularly because 20% to 30% of carriers may never develop invasive gastric cancer. Certainly, all patients experience some level of morbidity, including diarrhea, weight loss, and difficulty eating. Mortality due to this indication for a gastrectomy has not been reported. Early evidence suggests that women can successfully carry healthy pregnancies after a gastrectomy.[65] Most importantly, to date, there have been no reports of gastric cancer recurrence in a member of an HDGC family after a prophylactic total gastrectomy.

Women with HDGC also exhibit up to 60% lifetime risk for developing breast cancer, primarily of the lobular type, and as more women are prevented from developing diffuse gastric cancer, breast cancer screening is of great relevance. The correct approach to screening for lobular breast cancer in women with HDGC is not known, but is based on approaches used in other hereditary breast cancer susceptibility syndromes. Although prophylactic mastectomies have been shown to effectively prevent the development of breast cancer and result in improved long-term survival in *BRCA1/2* mutation carriers, such an approach remains completely investigational for women in HDGC families. The prognosis of lobular cancers that develop in HDGC patients is currently unknown, and given the relatively late onset compared with breast cancers in *BRCA1/2* carriers, prophylactic mastectomies may not be appropriate. Therefore, standard screening recommendations include annual breast magnetic resonance imaging (MRI) and mammogram starting at the age of 35 years.[66,67] An open question is whether chemoprevention with tamoxifen may benefit women with HDGC, given its role in reducing breast cancer risk in half in women at elevated risk because of age, family history, or history of biopsy-proven lobular carcinoma in situ.[68]

In summary, individuals from HDGC families with inherited germ-line mutations in the *CDH1* gene face up to an 80% likelihood of developing gastric cancer and, for women, an additional 60% chance of developing lobular breast cancer during their lifetime, with significant risk beginning at relatively young ages. Such levels of overall cancer risk are similar to that of developing breast or colon cancer for carriers of *BRCA1* or 2 gene mutations, or mismatch repair gene mutations, respectively. Therefore, rigorous surveillance and the consideration of prophylactic surgery are important for the management of these individuals. At the very least, a regular endoscopic examination with a random biopsy of the stomach should be performed every 6 to 12 months, probably starting 10 years earlier than the youngest affected patient in the

family, or by the age of 25 years. Because mucosal abnormalities tend to occur late in diffuse gastric cancer and delay the endoscopic diagnosis, a prophylactic gastrectomy should be seriously considered as a means of preventing gastric carcinoma, although it clearly comes with high morbidity. It is somewhat less clear as to the correct approach for the screening and prevention of lobular breast cancer in women with HDGC. Adherence to standard recommendations for screening mammographies for breast cancer should be followed. The consideration of investigative approaches to screening with MRI and chemoprevention with tamoxifen or other agents are appropriate. The decision to perform a prophylactic gastrectomy should be balanced with age-based risk, based on age-specific penetrance data, as well as many other personal factors. Therefore, it is essential that patients carrying the gene have the opportunity for extensive counseling, discussion, and reflection with knowledgeable clinicians, geneticists, and counselors before making the decision to proceed.

OTHER HEREDITARY CANCER SUSCEPTIBILITY SYNDROMES WITH INCREASED GASTRIC CANCER RISK

Lynch Syndrome

The seminal report of a family with dominantly inherited colon and gastrointestinal (GI) cancers in 1979 by Lynch and Lynch[69] began decades of defining and refining this hereditary syndrome. Lynch syndrome is caused by a germ-line mutation in a mismatch DNA repair gene (*MLH1*, *MSH2*, *MSH6*, *PMS2*, or *EPCAM*) and is thus associated with tumors exhibiting microsatellite instability (MSI). It is estimated that 2% to 4% of all diagnosed colorectal cancers[70] and 2% to 5% of all diagnosed endometrial cancers[71] are due to Lynch syndrome. With a frequency estimated at 1 in 440 in the United States,[72] it is similar to the BRCA carriage rate. The lifetime risks for Lynch syndrome–associated cancers are highest for colorectal cancer at 52% to 82% (mean age at diagnosis, 44 to 61 years), followed by an endometrial cancer risk of 25% to 60% in women (mean age at diagnosis, 48 to 62 years), a 6% to 13% risk for gastric cancer (mean age at diagnosis, 56 years), and 4% to 12% for ovarian cancer (mean age at diagnosis, 42.5 years).[70–78]

Lynch syndrome–associated gastric cancers predominantly show intestinal histology (more than 90% of the cases). This correlation echoes the strong association between MSI tumor phenotype and intestinal gastric cancer. The International Collaborative Group on hereditary nonpolyposis colorectal cancer (HNPCC) developed the original Amsterdam Criteria in 1991. Revisions followed, with Bethesda criteria outlined in 1997 and revisions in 2004 with the inclusion of extracolonic tumor risks, including gastric cancer.[79,80]

MSI screening by molecular and/or immunohistochemistry for the four common Lynch protein products (MSH2, MSH6, MLH1, and PMS2) should be considered in families who meet the Bethesda criteria. Because 15% of all gastric tumors exhibit MSI histology, the majority of these have acquired this mutator phenotype through sporadic mutations, and further germ-line testing of individuals with MSI-positive tumors is necessary to confirm a molecular diagnosis of Lynch syndrome.

Hereditary Breast Ovarian Cancer Syndrome

Hereditary breast and ovarian cancer due to germ-line *BRCA1* and *BRCA2* mutations is perhaps the most well-defined and recognized inherited cancer syndrome. With a prevalence of 1 in 300 to 400 in most populations and up to 1 in 40 in selected groups with founder mutations (most notably those with Ashkenazi Jewish ancestry), it represents the most common of the hereditary disorders due to high-risk mutations. Carriers face a five- to six-fold increased risk of generally early-onset breast cancer and 10- to 20-fold increased risk for ovarian, fallopian, and primary peritoneal malignancies. Male carriers have a recognized increased risk for prostate cancer and male breast cancer. *BRCA1* and *BRCA2* have been implicated in multiple cellular functions but serve primary roles as tumor suppressor genes recruited to maintain genomic stability through DNA double-strand break repair. Following the cloning of the *BRCA1* and *BRCA2* genes in 1994 and 1995,[81,82] the Breast Cancer Linkage Consortium convened to pool data and generate a body of clinical information to assist in the counseling and management of BRCA carriers, resulting in a seminal publication outlining the spectrum of *BRCA* mutation–associated cancer risks. In 173 breast–ovarian cancer families with *BRCA2* mutations from 20 centers in Europe and North America, the RR of gastric cancer was 2.59 (95% confidence interval [CI], 1.46 to 4.61).[83] Carriers of the 6174 delT *BRCA2* Ashkenazi Jewish founder mutation in Israel found gastric cancer to be the most common malignancy after breast and ovarian. Conversely, 5.7% of patients with gastric cancer in Israel were found to carry this *BRCA2* mutation[84]; 20.7% of a Polish cohort of families with both gastric and breast malignancies were attributable to mutations in *BRCA2*. A *BRCA2* mutation was also found in 23.5% of women with ovarian cancer and a family history of stomach cancer in this population.[85,86]

Several studies have implicated *BRCA1* mutations as a risk factor for gastric cancer. A large Swedish population-based study published in 1999 involving 150 malignant tumors from 1,145 relatives in *BRCA1* found an RR of 5.86 (95% CI, 1.60 to 15.01) and observed that gastric cancer diagnosed before the age of 70 years was twice as common in carrier families compared with the general population. They did not observe the same risk with *BRCA2*.[87,88]

Brose et al.[89] observed the highest RR for gastric cancer (6.9) in 147 families with *BRCA1* mutations in Pennsylvania. Risch et al.[90] also observed an RR of 6.2 in first-degree relatives of 39 *BRCA1* mutation carrier families and, to a lesser extent, in 21 *BRCA2* families in Ontario, Canada.

More recently, a meta-analysis of more than 30 studies of tumor risk in *BRCA1* and *BRCA2* carriers found an RR of 1.69 (95% CI, 1.21 to 2.38) for gastric cancer, the highest risk after breast, ovarian, and prostate, followed closely by pancreatic cancer, with an RR of 1.62 (1.31 to 2.00).[91] No pathology details were included in these studies, and it is unknown if one of the histologic subtypes of gastric cancer predominates in BRCA-associated tumors.

Familial Adenomatous Polyposis

FAP is a rare colon cancer syndrome associated with the striking presentation of early-onset multiple colonic adenomas and, in classic form, a near-complete certainty of early colon cancer without prophylactic surgical intervention. Incidence estimates for FAP range from 1 in 10,000 to 20,000, and almost one-third of those diagnosed carry a de novo mutation, making family history unreliable for ascertainment of many cases. Extracolonic findings include upper GI adenomas, fundic gland polyps, and desmoids tumors. A wide spectrum of extracolonic tumors can occur, including relatively rare cancers such as hepatoblastomas, duodenal adenocarcinomas, and adrenal, pancreatic, thyroid, biliary tract, and brain tumors. Additional diagnostic aids can include the finding of congenital hypertrophy of the retinal pigment epithelium, supernumerary teeth, osteomas, cutaneous lipomas, and cysts.

It is estimated that the lifetime risk for upper GI cancer in FAP is approximately 4% to 12%, of which only 0.5% to 2% are gastric cancers, although this risk has been reported as 7- to 10-fold higher in Asia.[75,92,93] Approximately 50% of individuals with FAP have gastric fundus polyps, and 10% have adenomas of the stomach. Although gastric fundus polyps are unlikely to have malignancy potential, gastric adenomas can occasionally develop into invasive

disease.[94] Prophylactic gastrectomies are even discussed for diffuse fundic gland polyps showing high-grade dysplasia or large polyps.[95] Attenuated FAP is a muted form of classic FAP characterized by fewer than 100 colonic adenoma, a later median age and lower overall risk of colon cancer, and a high proportion of fundic gland polyps, suggesting a measurable risk for gastric cancer.[96–99]

Li–Fraumeni Syndrome

LFS is a devastating cancer syndrome with an extremely high risk for a multitude of tumor types. The most common malignancies are early-onset breast cancers and sarcomas, followed by brain tumors, leukemia, lung cancer, and then gastric cancer.[100] Four families were originally described by Drs. Li and Fraumeni[101] in 1969. The risk of an initial primary cancer is 50% by the age of 30 years and 90% by the age of 70 years,[102] with sex-specific differences in lifetime cancer risk of 73% in males and close to 100% in females primarily accounted for by an excessively high breast cancer risk.[103] There are high risks for multiple primary cancers, with 60% of carriers developing a second tumor and 4% developing a third malignancy.[104] Previously thought to be extraordinarily rare with an incidence of 1 in 50,000 to 100,000, recently relaxed testing criteria suggest the actual carrier rate may be several times higher. Of individuals who meet classic LFS clinical criteria, 70% are found to carry a *TP53* germ-line mutation. The de novo mutation rate is now estimated at 7% to 20%.[105] A negative family history can no longer exclude the consideration of LFS, and clinical criteria have been updated to recommend P53 testing for single cases of adrenal cortical carcinoma, choroid plexus carcinoma, and breast cancer under the age of 30 years.

Although not one of the hallmark tumors of LFS, the International Agency for Research on Cancer database reports that gastric cancer is frequency seen in up to 2.8% of LFS families.[106] Somatic *TP53* alterations are associated with both the intestinal and diffuse forms of gastric cancer in equal frequency. However, *TP53* constitutional mutations are very rarely documented in the overall gastric cancer mutational spectrum. Among 62 TP53 mutant LFS families seen at the Dana-Farber Cancer Institute in Boston and the National Cancer Institute, gastric cancer was diagnosed in 4.9% of affected members.[107] The mean and median ages at gastric cancer diagnosis were 43 and 36 years, respectively (range, 24 to 74 years), compared with the median age of 71 years in the general population based on Surveillance Epidemiology and End Results (SEER) data. Five families (8.1%) reported two or more cases of gastric cancer. A pathology review of the available tumors revealed both intestinal and diffuse histologies. A study of 180 families with LFS in the Netherlands found a concordant rate of gastric cancer among carriers with an RR of 2.6 (95% CI, 0.5 to 7.7).[108]

Peutz–Jeghers Syndrome

Peutz–Jeghers syndrome (PJS) is a rare inherited disorder of GI hamartomas, polyposis, and, most strikingly, early development of pigmented lesions on the lips, oral mucosa, and fingers. Incidence rates are estimated in the range of 1 in 25,000 to 250,000. Initially described by Peutz[109] in 1921 and subsequently by Jeghers et al.[110] in 1949, PJS is characterized by both hamartomatous and adenomatous polyposis throughout the GI tract and a high predisposition to GI malignancies. The clinical diagnosis of PJS is made on the basis of histologically confirmed hamartomatous polyps and two of the following: (1) positive family history, (2) hyperpigmentation of the digits and mucosa of the external genitalia, and (3) small bowel polyposis.[111] The mucocutaneous hyperpigmentation characteristically occurs on the buccal mucosa or near the eyes, nose, mouth, axilla, or fingertips. Typically noticeable by the age of 5 years, they frequently fade by puberty. Classic pigmented lesions in a first-degree relative of a diagnosed individual are sufficient to meet criteria for PJS.

Inherited Cancer Syndromes with Associated Gastric Cancer Risks

Cancer Syndrome	Gene	Frequency	Gastric Cancer Risk (%)	Reference
HDGC	CDH1	Vary rare	>801	Fitzgerald et al.[44]
Hereditary breast/ovarian cancer	BRCA1/2	1/40–1/400	2.6–5.5	Brose et al.[89]
Lynch syndrome	MLH1, MSH2, MSH6, PMS2, Epcam	1/440	6–13	Chen et al.,[72] Watson et al.[77]
Li–Fraumeni syndrome	P53	1/5,000	2.8	Gonzalez et al.[105]
FAP	APC	1/10–20,000	0.5–2.0	Garrean et al.[92]
Juvenile polyposis	SMAD4, BMPR1A	1/16–100,000	21	Howe et al.[121]
PJS	STK11	1/25–250,000	29	Giardiello et al.,[113] van Lier et al.[114]

Chronic GI bleeds, anemia, and recurrent obstruction due to intussusception are frequent complications and often require surgical intervention. Among GI cancers, gastric cancer was found to be the third most frequent tumor in PJS, after small intestine and colorectal carcinoma. The cumulative cancer risk is 47% at the age of 65 years.[112] RRs reported for colon, stomach, and small intestine neoplasms have been as high as 84, 213, and over 500, respectively.[113] Increased risk is also present for other GI cancers (e.g., pancreatic, esophageal), as well as neoplasms outside the GI tract (lung, breast, ovarian, and endometrial). Other tumors associated with PJS are benign ovarian tumors called sex cord tumors with annular tubules, calcifying Sertoli tumors of the testes, and adenoma malignum of the cervix.

A Dutch team reviewed 20 PJS cohort studies and 1 meta-analysis published between 1975 and 2007 with a total of 1,644 patients.[114,115] They found the cumulative lifetime risks of GI cancers of 38% to 66%, and for all cancers, a lifetime risk range of 37% to 93%. Specifically, the gastric cancer risks were 29%, the third most common malignancy after colorectal and breast cancers. Understandably, this prompted a call for screening upper endoscopies every 2 to 5 years starting at the age of 20 years, whereas others suggested initiating endoscopies at the age of 8 years with addition of colonoscopies at the age of 20 years and breast screening at the age of 25 years.

STK11/LKB1 is the only gene identified to cause PJS, and mutations are found in 70% of those who meet clinical criteria.[116] Of affected individuals, 50% have a family history of PJS, and 50% may represent de novo mutations, although the penetrance of PJS has yet to be confirmed. The absence of a mutation in STK11 does not preclude a diagnosis of PJS in individuals meeting the clinical diagnostic criteria.

Juvenile Polyposis Syndrome

Juvenile polyposis syndrome (JPS) is another very rare, hereditary cancer syndrome with a broadly defined incidence rate between 1 in 16,000 and 1 in 100,000.[117–120] The diagnosis is based on the presence of multiple hamartomatous polyps with a distinct morphology termed juvenile, although JPS is not restricted to development in childhood. Solitary juvenile polyps occur in 1% to 2% of the general population.

The diagnosis of JPS requires more than five juvenile polyps in the colorectum, multiple juvenile polyps throughout the GI tract, or a number of juvenile polyps in an individual with a known family history of juvenile polyps. There is wide interfamilial and intrafamilial variability in number and distribution of polyps. Juvenile polyps are commonly benign, but the risk of malignant transformation is present. Larger polyps have been noted to contain adenomatous regions, resulting in a high lifetime risk of colorectal cancer approaching 20% by the age of 35 years and 68% by the age of 60 years. Gastric cancer has been found in 21% of JPS patients affected with gastric polyps, and increased incidence of pancreatic and small bowel cancers has also been reported (Table 47.2).[121]

Approximately 75% of JPS cases are familial, and 25% of JPS cases appear to be de novo. Two genes have been implicated as the cause of JPS in 40% of affected individuals: SMAD4 (or MADH4) and BMPR1A, with an approximate equal frequency.[121,122] The majority of JPS cases are due to as yet unidentified gene(s). Mutations in SMAD4 are also associated with hereditary hemorrhagic telangiectasia (HHT), also known as Osler–Weber–Rendu syndrome. HHT is associated with visceral bleeding, telangiectasias, or arteriovenous malformations. Currently, 15% to 22% of SMAD4 mutation carriers are suspected of having combined JPS/HHT.[123]

Surveillance recommendations for screening individuals with JPS include monitoring for rectal bleeding, anemia, and GI symptoms from infancy and additional complete blood counts, upper endoscopies, and colonoscopies at the age of 15 years, or when symptoms are present. An endoscopy is repeated every 1 to 3 years, depending on polyp load. In families with SMAD4 mutations, HHT surveillance begins in early childhood.

CONCLUSIONS

Hereditary gastric cancer is a relatively unusual disease. Given the very poor prognosis for most gastric cancer patients once diagnosed, every effort should be made to identify lesions early when they are still curable. Genetic testing for gastric cancer susceptibility allows for the identification of families with elevated risk for this and other tumors and the development of rational surveillance strategies for early detection. Unfortunately, reliable screening tools for gastric cancer are not available, and prophylactic surgical gastrectomies have proven beneficial in certain autosomal-dominant, high-penetrance genetic syndromes, including HDGC caused by germ-line CDH1 mutations. Genetic testing for other gastric cancer risk genes may also be warranted, as reviewed here. Major goals for clinical cancer genetics include identifying additional risk alleles to explain cancer susceptibility in families without known germ-line variants and to develop more robust tools for clinical screening for gastric cancer in high-risk individuals. Finally, the advent of whole genome sequencing of germ-line DNA and tumor genomes will lead to the rapid identification of novel variants and risk alleles of various penetrance. A challenge for the next generation of cancer genetics professionals will be the interpretation of multiple rare variants found in personal genomes and integration with schemes for the prevention and early detection of gastric cancer.

REFERENCES

1. Lauren P. The two histological main types of gastric carcinoma: diffuse and so-called intestinal-type carcinoma. An attempt at a histo-clinical classification. *Acta Pathol Microbiol Scand* 1965;64:31–49.
2. Carneiro F, Seixas M, Sobrinho-Simoes M. New elements for an updated classification of the carcinomas of the stomach. *Pathol Res Pract* 1995;191:571–584.
3. Wu H, Rusiecki JA, Zhu K, et al. Stomach carcinoma incidence patterns in the United States by histologic type and anatomic site. *Cancer Epidemiol Biomarkers Prev* 2009;18:1945–1952.
4. Machado JC, Soares P, Carneiro F, et al. E-cadherin gene mutations provide a genetic basis for the phenotypic divergence of mixed gastric carcinomas. *Lab Invest* 1999;79:459–465.
5. Becker KF, Atkinson MJ, Reich U, et al. E-cadherin gene mutations provide clues to diffuse type gastric carcinomas. *Cancer Res* 1994;54:3845–3852.
6. Tamura G, Sakata K, Nishizuka S, et al. Inactivation of the E-cadherin gene in primary gastric carcinomas and gastric carcinoma cell lines. *Jpn J Cancer Res* 1996;87:1153–1159.
7. Muta H, Noguchi M, Kanai Y, et al. E-cadherin gene mutations in signet ring cell carcinoma of the stomach. *Jpn J Cancer Res* 1996;87:843–848.
8. Carneiro F, Santos L, David L, et al. T (Thomsen-Friedenreich) antigen and other simple mucin-type carbohydrate antigens in precursor lesions of gastric carcinoma. *Histopathology* 1994;24:105–113.
9. Jang BG, Kim WH. Molecular pathology of gastric carcinoma. *Pathobiology* 2011;78:302–310.
10. Wang K, Kan J, Yuen ST, et al. Exome sequencing identifies frequent mutation of ARID1A in molecular subtypes of gastric cancer. *Nat Genet* 2011;43:1219–1223.
11. Zang ZJ, Cutcutache I, Poon SL, et al. Exome sequencing of gastric adenocarcinoma identifies recurrent somatic mutations in cell adhesion and chromatin remodeling genes. *Nat Genet* 2012;44:570–574.
12. Pedrazzani C, Corso G, Velho S, et al. Evidence of tumor microsatellite instability in gastric cancer with familial aggregation. *Fam Cancer* 2009;8:215–220.
13. Palli D, Russo A, Ottini L, et al. Red meat, family history, and increased risk of gastric cancer with microsatellite instability. *Cancer Res* 2001;61:5415–5419.
14. Buermeyer AB, Deschenes SM, Baker SM, et al. Mammalian DNA mismatch repair. *Annu Rev Genet* 1999;33:533–564.
15. La Torre G, Chiaradia G, Gianfagna F, et al. Smoking status and gastric cancer risk: an updated meta-analysis of case-control studies published in the past ten years. *Tumori* 2009;95:13–22.
16. McMichael AJ, McCall MG, Hartshorne JM, et al. Patterns of gastro-intestinal cancer in European migrants to Australia: The role of dietary change. *Int J Cancer* 1980;25:431–437.
17. Nomura A, Stemmermann GN, Chyou PH, et al. *Helicobacter pylori* infection and gastric carcinoma among Japanese Americans in Hawaii. *N Engl J Med* 1991;325:1132–1136.
18. Parsonnet J, Friedman GD, Vandersteen DP, et al. Helicobacter pylori infection and the risk of gastric carcinoma. *N Engl J Med* 1991;325:1127–1131.
19. Helicobacter and Cancer Collaborative Group. Gastric cancer and *Helicobacter pylori*: a combined analysis of 12 case control studies nested within prospective cohorts. *Gut* 2001;49:347–353.
20. Cavaleiro-Pinto M, Peleteiro B, Lunet N, et al. Helicobacter pylori infection and gastric cardia cancer: Systematic review and meta-analysis. *Cancer Causes Control* 2011;22:375–387.
21. Chen JN, He D, Tang F, et al. Epstein-Barr virus–associated gastric carcinoma: A newly defined entity. *J Clin Gastroenterol* 2010;46:262–271.
22. Ferlay J, Shin HR, Bray F, et al. Estimates of worldwide burden of cancer in 2008: GLOBOCAN 2008. *Int J Cancer* 2008;127:2893–2917.
23. Jemal A, Siegel R, Ward E, et al. Cancer statistics, 2008. *CA Cancer J Clin* 2008;58:71–96.
24. Correa P. Is gastric cancer preventable? *Gut* 2004;53:1217–1219.
25. Henson DE, Dittus C, Younes M, et al. Differential trends in the intestinal and diffuse types of gastric carcinoma in the United States, 1973–2000: Increase in the signet ring cell type. *Arch Pathol Lab Med* 2004;128:765–770.
26. Roosendaal R, Kuipers EJ, Buitenwerf J, et al. Helicobacter pylori and the birth cohort effect: Evidence of a continuous decrease of infection rates in childhood. *Am J Gastroenterol* 1997;92:1480–1482.
27. Borch K, Jonsson B, Tarpila E, et al. Changing pattern of histological type, location, stage and outcome of surgical treatment of gastric carcinoma. *Br J Surg* 2000;87:618–626.
28. Oliveira C, Seruca R, Carneiro F. Genetics, pathology, and clinics of familial gastric cancer. *Int J Surg Pathol* 2006;14:21–33.
29. Hemminki K, Li X, Czene K. Swedish empiric risks: familial risk of cancer: data for clinical counseling and cancer genetics. *Int J Cancer* 2004;108:109–114.
30. Shin CM, Kim N, Yang HJ, et al. Stomach cancer risk in gastric cancer relatives: Interaction between Helicobacter pylori infection and family history of gastric cancer for the risk of stomach cancer. *J Clin Gastroenterol* 2010;44:e34–e39.
31. Yokota T, Kunii Y, Teshima S, et al. Significant prognostic factors in patients with early gastric cancer. *Int Surg* 2000;85:286–290.
32. Caldas C, Carneiro F, Lynch HT, et al. Familial gastric cancer: Overview and guidelines for management. *J Med Genet* 1999;36:873–880.
33. Guilford P, Hopkins J, Harraway J, et al. E-cadherin germline mutations in familial gastric cancer. *Nature* 1998;392:402–405.
34. Gayther SA, Gorringe KL, Ramus SJ, et al. Identification of germ-line E-cadherin mutations in gastric cancer families of European origin. *Cancer Res* 1998;58:4086–4089.
35. Guilford PJ, Hopkins JB, Grady WM, et al. E-cadherin germline mutations define an inherited cancer syndrome dominated by diffuse gastric cancer. *Hum Mutat* 1999;14:249–255.
36. Keller G, Vogelsang H, Becker I, et al. Diffuse type gastric and lobular breast carcinoma in a familial gastric cancer patient with an E-cadherin germline mutation. *Am J Pathol* 1999;155:337–342.
37. Richards FM, McKee SA, Rajpar MH, et al. Germline E-cadherin gene (CDH1) mutations predispose to familial gastric cancer and colorectal cancer. *Hum Mol Genet* 1999;8:607–610.
38. Shinmura K, Kohno T, Takahashi M, et al. Familial gastric cancer: Clinico-pathological characteristics, RER phenotype and germline p53 and E-cadherin mutations. *Carcinogenesis* 1999;20:1127–1131.
39. Yoon KA, Ku JL, Yang HK, et al. Germline mutations of E-cadherin gene in Korean familial gastric cancer patients. *J Hum Genet* 1999;44:177–180.
40. Kluijt I, Siemerink EJ, Ausems MG, et al. CDH1-related hereditary diffuse gastric cancer syndrome: Clinical variations and implications for counseling. *Int J Cancer* 2012;131:367–376.
41. Guilford P, Humar B, Blair V. Hereditary diffuse gastric cancer: Translation of CDH1 germline mutations into clinical practice. *Gastric Cancer* 2010;13:1–10.
42. Grunwald GB. The structural and functional analysis of cadherin calcium-dependent cell adhesion molecules. *Curr Opin Cell Biol* 1993;5:797–805.
43. Birchmeier W. E-cadherin as a tumor (invasion) suppressor gene. *Bioessays* 1995;17:97–99.
44. Fitzgerald RC, Hardwick R, Huntsman D, et al. Hereditary diffuse gastric cancer: updated consensus guidelines for clinical management and directions for future research. *J Med Genet* 2010;47:436–444.
45. Brooks-Wilson AR, Kaurah P, Suriano G, et al. Germline E-cadherin mutations in hereditary diffuse gastric cancer: assessment of 42 new families and review of genetic screening criteria. *J Med Genet* 2004;41:508–517.
46. Oliveira C, de Bruin J, Nabais S, et al. Intragenic deletion of CDH1 as the inactivating mechanism of the wild-type allele in an HDGC tumour. *Oncogene* 2004;23:2236–2240.
47. Suriano G, Yew S, Ferreira P, et al. Characterization of a recurrent germ line mutation of the E-cadherin gene: Implications for genetic testing and clinical management. *Clin Cancer Res* 2005;11:5401–5409.
48. Oliveira C, Sousa S, Pinheiro H, et al. Quantification of epigenetic and genetic 2nd hits in CDH1 during hereditary diffuse gastric cancer syndrome progression. *Gastroenterology* 2009;136:2137–2148.
49. Keller G, Vogelsang H, Becker I, et al. Germline mutations of the E-cadherin (CDH1) and TP53 genes, rather than of RUNX3 and HPP1, contribute to genetic predisposition in German gastric cancer patients. *J Med Genet* 2004;41:e89.
50. Kim IJ, Park JH, Kang HC, et al. A novel germline mutation in the MET extracellular domain in a Korean patient with the diffuse type of familial gastric cancer. *J Med Genet* 2003;40:e97.
51. Oliveira C, Ferreira P, Nabais S, et al. E-cadherin (CDH1) and p53 rather than SMAD4 and caspase-10 germline mutations contribute to genetic predisposition in Portuguese gastric cancer patients. *Eur J Cancer* 2004;40:1897–1903.
52. Oliveira C, Senz J, Kaurah P, et al. Germline CDH1 deletions in hereditary diffuse gastric cancer families. *Hum Mol Genet* 2009;18:1545–1555.
53. Pharoah PD, Guilford P, Caldas C. Incidence of gastric cancer and breast cancer in CDH1 (E-cadherin) mutation carriers from hereditary diffuse gastric cancer families. *Gastroenterology* 2001;121:1348–1353.
54. Kaurah P, MacMillan A, Boyd N, et al. Founder and recurrent CDH1 mutations in families with hereditary diffuse gastric cancer. *JAMA* 2007;297:2360–2372.
55. Schrader KA, Masciari S, Boyd N, et al. Hereditary diffuse gastric cancer: association with lobular breast cancer. *Fam Cancer* 2008;7:73–82.
56. Berx G, Becker KF, Hofler H, et al. Mutations of the human E-cadherin (CDH1) gene. *Hum Mutat* 1998;12:226–237.
57. Berx G, Cleton-Jansen AM, Strumane K, et al. E-cadherin is inactivated in a majority of invasive human lobular breast cancers by truncation mutations throughout its extracellular domain. *Oncogene* 1996;13:1919–1925.
58. Schrader KA, Masciari S, Boyd N, et al. Germline mutations in CDH1 are infrequent in women with early-onset or familial lobular breast cancers. *J Med Genet* 2011;48:64–68.
59. Oliveira C, Bordin MC, Grehan N, et al. Screening E-cadherin in gastric cancer families reveals germline mutations only in hereditary diffuse gastric cancer kindred. *Hum Mutat* 2002;19:510–517.
60. Frebourg T, Oliveira C, Hochain P, et al. Cleft lip/palate and CDH1/E-cadherin mutations in families with hereditary diffuse gastric cancer. *J Med Genet* 2006;43:138–142.
61. Cisco RM, Ford JM, Norton JA. Hereditary diffuse gastric cancer: Implications of genetic testing for screening and prophylactic surgery. *Cancer* 2008;113:1850–1856.

PRACTICE OF ONCOLOGY

62. Huntsman DG, Carneiro F, Lewis FR, et al. Early gastric cancer in young, asymptomatic carriers of germ-line E-cadherin mutations. *N Engl J Med* 2001;344:1904–1909.

63. Norton J, Ham C, Van Dam J, et al. CDH1 truncating mutations in the E-cadherin gene: An indication for total gastrectomy to treat hereditary diffuse gastric cancer. *Ann Surg* 2007;45:873–879.

64. Rogers W, Dobo E, Norton J, et al. Risk-reducing total gastrectomy for germ-line mutations in E-cadherin (CDH1): pathologic findings with clinical implications. *Am J Surg Pathol* 2008;32:799–809.

65. Kaurah P, Fitzgerald R, Dwerryhouse S, et al. Pregnancy after prophylactic total gastrectomy. *Fam Cancer* 2010;9:331–334.

66. Saslow D, Boetes C, Burke W, et al. American Cancer Society guidelines for breast screening with MRI as an adjunct to mammography. *CA Cancer J Clin* 2007;57:75–89.

67. Daly M, Axilbund J, Buys S, et al. Genetic/familial high-risk assessment: breast and ovarian. *J Natl Compr Cancer Netw* 2010;8:562–594.

68. Wolmark N, Dunn BK. The role of tamoxifen in breast cancer prevention: Issues sparked by the NSABP Breast Cancer Prevention Trial (P-1). *Ann N Y Acad Sci* 2001;949:99–108.

69. Lynch HT, Lynch PM. The cancer-family syndrome: a pragmatic basis for syndrome identification. *Dis Colon Rectum* 1979;22:106–110.

70. Palomaki GE, McClain MR, Melillo S, et al. EGAPP supplementary evidence review: DNA testing strategies aimed at reducing morbidity and mortality from Lynch syndrome. *Genet Med* 2009;11:42–65.

71. Meyer LA, Broaddus RR, Lu KH. Endometrial cancer and Lynch syndrome: clinical and pathologic considerations. *Cancer Control* 2009;16:14–22.

72. Chen S, Wang W, Lee S, et al. Prediction of germline mutations and cancer risk in the Lynch syndrome. *JAMA* 2006;296:1479–1487.

73. Aarnio M, Salovaara R, Aaltonen LA, et al. Features of gastric cancer in hereditary non-polyposis colorectal cancer syndrome. *Int J Cancer* 1997;74:551–555.

74. Aarnio M, Sankila R, Pukkala E, et al. Cancer risk in mutation carriers of DNA-mismatch-repair genes. *Int J Cancer* 1999;81:214–218.

75. Park YJ, Shin KH, Park JG. Risk of gastric cancer in hereditary nonpolyposis colorectal cancer in Korea. *Clin Cancer Res* 2000;6:2994–2998.

76. Vasen HF, Wijnen JT, Menko FH, et al. Cancer risk in families with hereditary nonpolyposis colorectal cancer diagnosed by mutation analysis. *Gastroenterology* 1996;110:1020–1027.

77. Watson P, Vasen HF, Mecklin JP, et al. The risk of extra-colonic, extra-endometrial cancer in the Lynch syndrome. *Int J Cancer* 2008;123:444–449.

78. Gylling A, Abdel-Rahman WM, Juhola M, et al. Is gastric cancer part of the tumour spectrum of hereditary non-polyposis colorectal cancer? A molecular genetic study. *Gut* 2007;56:926–933.

79. Rodriguez-Bigas MA, Boland CR, Hamilton SR, et al. A National Cancer Institute Workshop on hereditary nonpolyposis colorectal cancer syndrome: meeting highlights and Bethesda guidelines. *J Natl Cancer Inst* 1997;89:1758–1762.

80. Umar A, Boland CR, Terdiman JP, et al. Revised Bethesda guidelines for hereditary nonpolyposis colorectal cancer (Lynch syndrome) and microsatellite instability. *J Natl Cancer Inst* 2004;96:261–268.

81. Miki Y, Swensen J, Shattuck-Eidens D, et al. A strong candidate for the breast and ovarian cancer susceptibility gene BRCA1. *Science* 1994;266:66–71.

82. Wooster R, Bignell G, Lancaster J, et al. Identification of the breast cancer susceptibility gene BRCA2. *Nature* 1995;378:789–792.

83. The Breast Cancer Linkage Consortium. Cancer risks in BRCA2 mutation carriers. *J Natl Cancer Inst* 1999;91:1310–1316.

84. Figer A, Irmin L, Geva R, et al. The rate of the 6174delT founder Jewish mutation in BRCA2 in patients with non-colonic gastrointestinal tract tumours in Israel. *Br J Cancer* 2001;84:478–481.

85. Jakubowska A, Nej K, Huzarski T, et al. BRCA2 gene mutations in families with aggregations of breast and stomach cancers. *Br J Cancer* 2002;87:888–891.

86. Jakubowska A, Scott R, Menkiszak J, et al. A high frequency of BRCA2 gene mutations in Polish families with ovarian and stomach cancer. *Eur J Hum Genet* 2003;11:955–958.

87. Johannsson O, Loman N, Moller T, et al. Incidence of malignant tumours in relatives of BRCA1 and BRCA2 germline mutation carriers. *Eur J Cancer* 1999;35:1248–1257.

88. Lorenzo B, Hemminki K. Risk of cancer at sites other than the breast in Swedish families eligible for BRCA1 or BRCA2 mutation testing. *Ann Oncol* 2004;15:1834–1841.

89. Brose MS, Rebbeck TR, Calzone KA, et al. Cancer risk estimates for BRCA1 mutation carriers identified in a risk evaluation program. *J Natl Cancer Inst* 2002;94:1365–1372.

90. Risch H, McLaughlin J, Cole D, et al. Prevalence and penetrance of germline BRCA1 and BRCA2 mutations in a population series of 649 women with ovarian cancer. *Am J Hum Genet* 2001;68:700–710.

91. Friedenson B. BRCA1 and BRCA2 pathways and the risk of cancers other than breast or ovarian. *MedGenMed* 2005;7:60.

92. Garrean S, Hering J, Saied A, et al. Gastric adenocarcinoma arising from fundic gland polyps in a patient with familial adenomatous polyposis syndrome. *Am Surg* 2008;74:79–83.

93. Offerhaus GJ, Giardiello FM, Krush AJ, et al. The risk of upper gastrointestinal cancer in familial adenomatous polyposis. *Gastroenterology* 1992;102:1980–1982.

94. Burt RW. Gastric fundic gland polyps. *Gastroenterology* 2003;125:1462–1469.

95. Lynch HT, Snyder C, Davies JM, et al. FAP, gastric cancer, and genetic counseling featuring children and young adults: A family study and review. *Fam Cancer* 2010;9:581–588.

96. Lynch HT, Smyrk T, McGinn T, et al. Attenuated familial adenomatous polyposis (AFAP). A phenotypically and genotypically distinctive variant of FAP. *Cancer* 1995;76:2427–2433.

97. Abraham SC, Nobukawa B, Giardiello FM, et al. Fundic gland polyps in familial adenomatous polyposis: neoplasms with frequent somatic adenomatous polyposis coli gene alterations. *Am J Pathol* 2000;157:747–754.

98. Bianchi LK, Burke CA, Bennett AE, et al. Fundic gland polyp dysplasia is common in familial adenomatous polyposis. *Clin Gastroenterol Hepatol* 2008;6:180–185.

99. Dunn K, Chey W, Gibbs J. Total gastrectomy for gastric dysplasia in a patient with attenuated familial adenomatous polyposis syndrome. *J Clin Oncol* 2008;26:3641–3642.

100. Olivier M, Goldgar DE, Sodha N, et al. Li-Fraumeni and related syndromes: correlation between tumor type, family structure, and TP53 genotype. *Cancer Res* 2003;63:6643–6650.

101. Li F, Fraumeni JJ. Soft-tissue sarcomas, breast cancer, and other neoplasms. A familial syndrome? *Ann Intern Med* 1969;71:747–752.

102. Malkin D, Li F, Strong L, et al. Germ line p53 mutations in a familial syndrome of breast cancer, sarcomas, and other neoplasms. *Science* 1990;250:1233–1238.

103. Wu CC, Shete S, Amos CI, et al. Joint effects of germ-line p53 mutation and sex on cancer risk in Li-Fraumeni syndrome. *Cancer Res* 2006;66:8287–8292.

104. Hisada M, Garber J, Fung C, et al. Multiple primary cancers in families with Li-Fraumeni syndrome. *J Natl Cancer Inst* 1998;90:606–611.

105. Gonzalez K, Buzin C, Noltner K, et al. High frequency of de novo mutations in Li-Fraumeni syndrome. *J Med Genet* 2009;46:689–693.

106. Corso G, Pedrazzani C, Marrelli D, et al. Familial gastric cancer and Li-Fraumeni syndrome. *Eur J Cancer Care (Engl)* 2010;19:377–381.

107. Masciari S, Dewanwala A, Stoffel EM, et al. Gastric cancer in individuals with Li-Fraumeni syndrome. *Genet Med* 2011;13:651–657.

108. Ruijs MW, Verhoef S, Rookus MA, et al. TP53 germline mutation testing in 180 families suspected of Li-Fraumeni syndrome: Mutation detection rate and relative frequency of cancers in different familial phenotypes. *J Med Genet* 2010;47:421–428.

109. Peutz J. Very remarkable case of familial polyposis of mucous membrane of intestinal tract and nasopharynx accompanied by peculiar pigmentations of skin and mucous membrane. *Nederl Maandschr Geneesk* 1921;10:134–146.

110. Jeghers H, Mc KV, Katz KH. Generalized intestinal polyposis and melanin spots of the oral mucosa, lips and digits; a syndrome of diagnostic significance. *N Engl J Med* 1949;241:1031–1036.

111. Giardiello FM, Welsh SB, Hamilton SR, et al. Increased risk of cancer in the Peutz-Jeghers syndrome. *N Engl J Med* 1987;316:1511–1514.

112. Lim W, Olschwang S, Keller JJ, et al. Relative frequency and morphology of cancers in STK11 mutation carriers. *Gastroenterology* 2004;126:1788–1794.

113. Giardiello F, Brensinger J, Tersmette A, et al. Very high risk of cancer in familial Peutz-Jeghers syndrome. *Gastroenterology* 2000;119:1447–1453.

114. van Lier MG, Wagner A, Mathus-Vliegen EM, et al. High cancer risk in Peutz-Jeghers syndrome: A systematic review and surveillance recommendations. *Am J Gastroenterol* 2010;105:1258–1264.

115. van Lier MG, Westerman AM, Wagner A, et al. High cancer risk and increased mortality in patients with Peutz-Jeghers syndrome. *Gut* 2011;60:141–147.

116. Gruber SB, Entius MM, Petersen GM, et al. Pathogenesis of adenocarcinoma in Peutz-Jeghers syndrome. *Cancer Res* 1998;58:5267–5270.

117. Allen BA, Terdiman JP. Hereditary polyposis syndromes and hereditary non-polyposis colorectal cancer. *Best Pract Res Clin Gastroenterol* 2003;17:237–258.

118. Finan MC, Ray MK. Gastrointestinal polyposis syndromes. *Dermatol Clin* 1989;7:419–434.

119. Lindor NM, Greene MH. The concise handbook of family cancer syndromes. Mayo Familial Cancer Program. *J Natl Cancer Inst* 1998;90:1039–1071.

120. Utsunomiya J, Gocho H, Miyanaga T, et al. Peutz-Jeghers syndrome: its natural course and management. *Johns Hopkins Med J* 1975;136:71–82.

121. Howe JR, Sayed MG, Ahmed AF, et al. The prevalence of MADH4 and BMPR1A mutations in juvenile polyposis and absence of BMPR2, BMPR1B, and ACVR1 mutations. *J Med Gene* 2004;41:484–491.

122. Sayed MG, Ahmed AF, Ringold JR, et al. Germline SMAD4 or BMPR1A mutations and phenotype of juvenile polyposis. *Ann Surg Oncol* 2002;9:901–906.

123. Gallione C, Richards J, Letteboer T, et al. SMAD4 mutations found in unselected HHT patients. *J Med Genet* 2006;43:793–797.

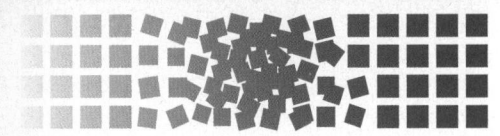
48 Molecular Biology of Pancreas Cancer

Scott E. Kern and Ralph H. Hruban

INTRODUCTION

Pancreatic cancer is a genetic disease. This perspective is supported by reproducible patterns of genetic mutations that accumulate during pancreatic tumorigenesis. These patterns indicate the operation of a selective process favoring the emergence of specific constellations of genetic changes. According to this genetic theory, most pancreatic cancers share a common foundation of genetic mutations disrupting specific cellular regulatory controls. These shared abnormalities are responsible for the processes of cancer growth, invasion, and metastasis in individual patients.

Four categories of mutated genes play a role in the pancreatic tumorigenesis: oncogenes, tumor-suppressor genes, genome-maintenance genes, and tissue-maintenance genes (summarized in Table 48.1). Some of these mutations are germline (i.e., they are transmitted within a family), whereas somatic mutations, acquired during life, contribute to tumorigenesis within a tissue but are not passed to offspring.

The most common cancer type of pancreatic cancer is pancreatic ductal adenocarcinoma (PDA). PDA is the primary focus of clinical and molecular research and is thus highlighted in this chapter. Other clinically and molecularly distinct forms of cancer occur in the pancreas and must be distinguished from PDA; they are discussed here in lesser detail.

In recent years, techniques were developed to sequence all of the genes of individual cancers. Whole-exome sequencing of PDAs revealed an average of 63 somatic mutations per tumor.[1] Most of these mutations undoubtedly are nonfunctional *passenger* mutations, each mutated at a low frequency and not contributing to tumorigenesis. Indeed, most passenger mutations might arise as tissues age before tumorigenesis even begins.[2] Smoking is associated with a doubling of the risk for pancreatic cancer, and remarkably, it is also associated with a 40% increase of the prevalence of low-frequency mutations in the cancers.[3] Only a subset of the mutations in PDA, however, are responsible for *driving* the neoplastic process in the ducts; only they are discussed further here. Modeling of a comprehensive study mapping gene mutations in multiple regions of primary PDAs and their metastases indicated a general timeline of tumorigenesis, invasion, and metastasis. According to this model, about a decade of time passes between the first driver mutation initiating the precursor neoplasm and the emergence of the first cell having the genotype of the invasive cancer; metastatic ability is acquired after another 5 years, and with patient death following about 2 years later.[4]

Telomere abnormalities and manifestations of chromosome instability are the most common alterations in pancreatic neoplasia. Four genes are mutated in most PDAs: the *KRAS*, *p16/CDKN2A*, *TP53*, and *SMAD4/DPC4* genes. Other recurrent genetic abnormalities are seen at a lower frequency, including internal deletions of exons of *FAM190A/CCSER1*; mutations in the genes *BRCA2*, *PALB2*, *FANCC*, *FANCG*, *FBXW7*, *BAX*, and *RB1*, in the transforming growth factor beta (TGF-β) receptors *TGFBR1* and *TGFBR2*, in the activin receptors *ACVR1B* and *ACVR2*, in various chromatin-remodeling genes such as *ARID1A*, in the genes *MKK4*, *STK11*, *MLL3*, *ATM*, *GUCY2F*, *NTRK3*, and *EGFR*, and in cationic trypsinogen; alterations in the mitochondrial genome; amplifications; various chromosomal deletions; inactivation of DNA mismatch-repair genes; and rarely, the maintenance of the Epstein-Barr virus genome as an episome. Irregular sizes and numbers of centrosomes were observed in 85% of pancreatic cancers and some adenomas, but in no tissues of chronic pancreatitis or normal pancreas.[5]

Knowing the genes that are mutated in a cancer can have direct clinical impact. For example, some patients develop pancreatic cancer because of an inherited mutation, and these patients and their families could benefit from genetic counseling.[6–9] A distinct morphologic subtype of pancreatic cancer, the medullary cancer, can suggest such an inherited mutation.[10,11] Another example of clinical impact includes the analysis of the genetic alterations in precursors to invasive pancreatic neoplasia, which indicated that most carcinomas arise by a process of progressive intraductal tumorigenesis, suggesting that these intraductal lesions might be detected and treated before a patient develops an invasive cancer.[12] Epigenetic changes in DNA methylation and in gene expression are also highly specific for the cancerous cells and can serve as markers of disease.

COMMON MOLECULAR CHANGES

Telomere shortening is an early and prevalent genetic change identified in the pancreatic precursor lesions.[13] Telomere shortening experimentally predisposes cells to chromosome fusion (translocations) and the missegregation of genetic material during mitosis.[14] Later in tumorigenesis, the telomerase is often reactivated,[15,16] moderating the telomere erosive process while permitting continued chromosomal instability.[17]

The *KRAS* gene mediates signals from growth factor receptors and other signaling inputs (Fig. 48.1). The mutations present in most pancreatic cancers convert the normal Kras protein (a protooncogene) to an oncogene, causing the protein to become overactive in transmitting growth factor–initiated signals.[18] *KRAS* is mutated in over 90% of conventional pancreatic ductal carcinomas.[19] Among the first genetic changes in the ducts is a *KRAS* gene mutation (see Table 48.1),[20,21] and recent evidence from advanced gene sequencing techniques indicates that their prevalence in early lesions is higher than was previously thought.[22]

As one of the most commonly mutated genes in pancreatic cancer, the Ras protein is an attractive target for the development of gene-specific therapies, and an understanding of the normal biology of the Ras protein should help in the development of these Ras-targeted therapies. Ras proteins require an attachment to the plasma membrane for activity. For many proteins, including Ras, a hydrophobic prenyl group is essential for the attachment. Either farnesyl (15-carbon) or geranylgeranyl (20-carbon) makes a covalent thioether linkage at a cysteine residue located near the C-terminal end of Ras proteins, termed the CAAX motif. Working mostly in artificial legacy models of the *HRAS* oncogene (rather than the more widely available but experimentally less tractable natural *KRAS*-mutant cancer cell lines), the farnesylation reaction

TABLE 48.1

Genetic Profile of Pancreatic Ductal Carcinoma

Gene	Gene Locations	Frequency in Cancers (%)	Timing During Tumorigenesis[a]	Mutation Origin
Oncogenes				
KRAS	12p	95	Early–Mid	Som.
BRAF	7q	4		Som.
AKT2	19q	10–20		Som.
GUCY2F	Xq	3		Som.
NTRK3	15q	1		Som.
EGFR	7p	1		Som.
EBV genome		<1		
Tumor-Suppressors/Genome-Maintenance Genes				
CDKN2A/p16	9p	>90	Mid–Late	Som. > Germ.
TP53	17p	75	Late	Som.
SMAD4	18q	55	Late	Som.
BRCA2 and PALB2	13q/16p	5	Late	Germ. > Som.
FANCC and FANCG	9q/9p	3		Germ. or Som.
CCSER1/FAM10A	4q	4[c]		Som.
MAP2K4	17p	4		Som.
LKB1/STK11	19p	4		Som. > Germ.
ACVR1B	12q	2		Som.
TGFBR1[b]	9q	1		Som.[c]
MSI⁻/TGFBR2[b]	3p	1		Som.[c]
MSI⁺/TGFBR2	3p	4		Som. > Germ.[d]
ACVR2	2q	4		Som. > Germ.[d]
BAX	19q	4		Som. > Germ.[d]
MLH1	3p	4		Som. > Germ.[d]
FBXW7/Cyclin E deregulated	4q	6		Som.[e]
ATM	11q	<1[f]		Germ.
Tissue-Maintenance Genes				
PRSS1	7q	<1[f]	Prior	Germ.

[a] Stage of appearance of the genetic changes during the intraductal precursor phase of the neoplasm, where known. For BRCA2, most mutations are inherited, but the loss of the second allele is reported only in a single advanced pancreatic intraepithelial neoplasia.
[b] Few homozygous deletions of the TGFBR1 gene and the TGFBR2 gene have been identified in non-MSI (microsatellite instability) pancreatic cancers.
[c] The prevalence of exonic transcript deletions is much higher than the prevalence of homozygously deleted exons given here.
[d] In MSI+ tumors, the mismatch repair defect is usually somatic in origin; the TGFBR2, ACVR2, and BAX alterations are somatic.
[e] A single example of homozygous mutation of the FBXW7 gene is reported in a series having a 6% prevalence of cyclin E overexpression. To date, cyclin E amplification is reported only in cell lines.
[f] The prevalence of mutations in severely affected families is higher than the prevelance among unselected cancers given here.
Som., (prevalence of) somatic mutation or methylation; Germ., (prevalence of) germline mutation.

was readily inhibited by various means; in these models, the Ras protein was rendered inactive and was often accompanied by cytotoxicity limited to the mutant cells.

Although many types of compounds capable of blocking the farnesyltransferase enzyme were developed as drugs, they have not been successful anticancer agents. Reasons are many. Although the Hras protein is linked predominantly through farnesyl groups, the Kras protein can be alternately prenylated by geranylgeranyl linkages. The latter is thought to be critical for a wider number of cellular proteins, and for fear of excessive toxicity, geranylgeranyl linkages have not usually been considered as an attractive drug target. The Kras protein may bind more tightly than Hras to the farnesyltransferase enzyme, necessitating higher drug concentrations.[18]

Additionally, the artificial models usually employed the engineered overexpression of the Ras protein, a situation in which the unattached Ras proteins would serve as a dominant-negative inhibitor, binding the essential interacting proteins and sequestering them in the cytoplasm to ensure the inactivation of the many downstream Ras pathways. Such a concentration-driven mechanism would presumably not occur under the normal levels of Ras proteins present in human cancers.[23] Indeed, it is proposed that the limited efficacy of farnesyltransferase inhibitors (FTI) observed in some experimental models and in clinical trials may be attributable to a cellular target not yet identified.[24] Attention has turned to compounds that target the downstream mediators, such as Raf and Mek protein kinase inhibitors.

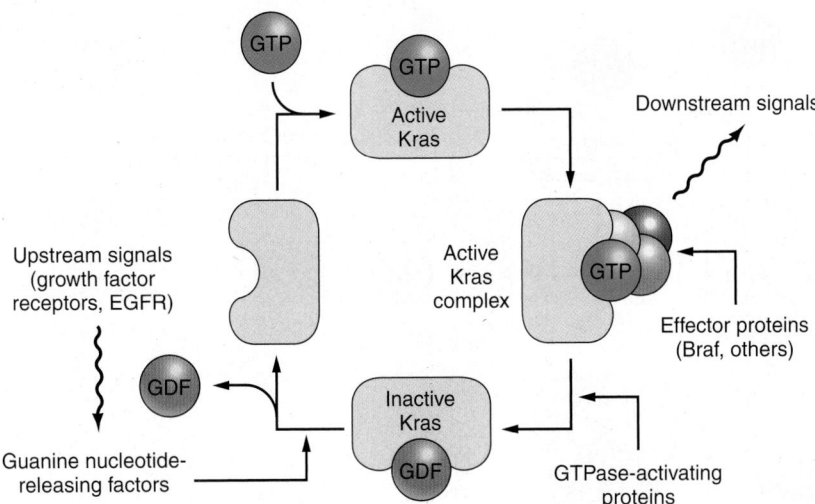

Figure 48.1 The KRAS pathway. KRAS normally integrates and regulates signals arising in the growth factor receptors that are passed to KRAS using the Grb2 and the Sos1 nucleotide exchange factor. The active GTP-bound form of KRAS recruits effector proteins such as Raf1 and Braf, in turn stimulating the downstream mitogen-activated protein kinases, such as MEK and ERK, and activating certain transcription factors. The EGF receptor can be overexpressed and occasionally mutated to provide inappropriately strong upstream signals, and the BRAF protein can be activated by point mutation, but more often in pancreatic cancer, the Kras protein is mutated. These latter mutations impair the GTPase-activating protein (GAP)–stimulated reaction that normally returns KRAS to the inactive state.

The Smad pathway mediates signals initiated upon the binding of the extracellular proteins TGF-β, activin, and bone morphogenic proteins to their receptors (Fig. 48.2). These signals are transmitted to the nucleus by proteins of the Smad family of related genes, including *SMAD4 (DPC4)*.[25] Once in the nucleus, Smad protein complexes bind specific recognition sites on DNA and cause the transcription of certain genes.[26] Mutations in the *SMAD4* gene are found in nearly half of pancreatic carcinomas, including homozygous deletions or intragenic mutations combined with loss of heterozygosity (LOH).[27] Other Smad genes are also occasionally mutated in pancreatic cancer.[1] Also, homozygous deletions and mutation/LOH affecting the TGF-β receptor genes are seen in a few pancreatic cancers.[28] A more common abnormality, in pancreatic as well as in other tumor types, is the underexpression of TGF-β receptors, which may render cells resistant to the normal suppressive effects of the TGF-β ligand.[29]

The *p16/RB1* pathway is a key control of the cell division cycle (Fig. 48.3). The retinoblastoma protein (Rb1) is a transcriptional regulator and regulates the entry of cells into S phase. A complex of cyclin D and a cyclin-dependent kinase (Cdk4 and Cdk6) phosphorylates and thereby regulates Rb1. The p16 protein is a Cdk-inhibitor that binds Cdk4 and Cdk6.[30–32] Virtually all pancreatic carcinomas suffer a loss of *p16* gene function through homozygous deletions, a mutation combined with LOH, or promoter

methylation of the *p16/CDKN2A* gene associated with a lack of gene expression.[33,34] In addition, inherited mutations of the *p16/CDKN2A* gene cause a familial melanoma/pancreatic cancer syndrome known as familial atypical multiple mole melanoma (FAMMM).[35–39] Only rare pancreatic cancers have an inactivating mutation of the *RB1* gene.[40]

The protein product of the *TP53* gene, Tp53, binds to specific sites of DNA and activates the transcription of certain genes that control the cell division cycle and apoptosis.[41,42] The Tp53 protein, normally a short-lived protein, becomes phosphorylated and stabilized after DNA damage and other cellular stresses (Fig. 48.4). In about 75% of pancreatic cancers, the *TP53* gene has point mutations that inhibit the ability of p53 to bind DNA or, occasionally, other types of inactivating mutation.[43–45]

Most human carcinomas have chromosomal instability (CIN), which produces changes in chromosomal copy numbers or aneuploidy.[46] Most pancreatic cancers have complex karyotypes, including deletions of whole chromosomes and subchromosomal regions.[47–49] CIN is the process that causes most of the tumor deletions (i.e., LOH).[50] A few percent of pancreatic carcinomas, however, do not have significant gross or numerical chromosomal changes and instead have a different form of genetic instability; they have defects in DNA mismatch repair, producing high mutation rates at sites of simple repetitive sequences (microsatellites), termed microsatellite instability (MSI).[10,11,51–54] The pattern of

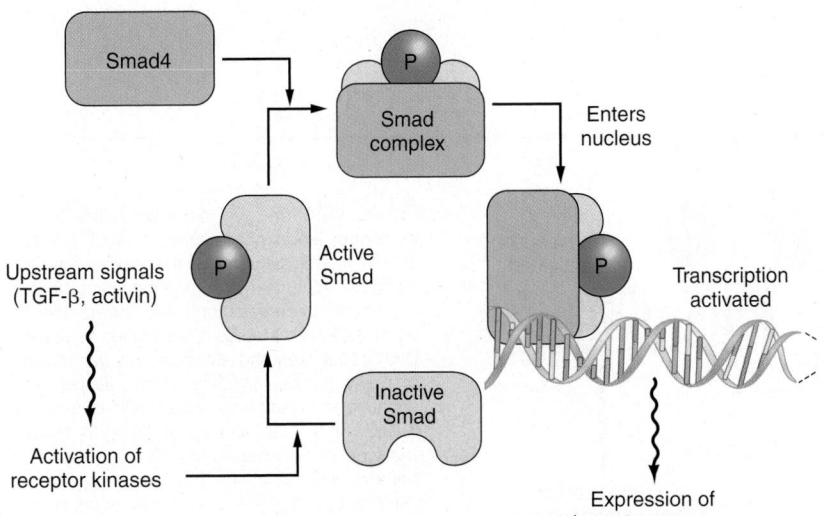

Figure 48.2 The TGF-β/Activin/Smad pathway. Dimeric kinase receptors of the TGF-β superfamily respond to extracellular ligands, causing phosphorylation of one or more of the receptor-associated Smad proteins and leading them to complex with the unphosphorylated common Smad, Smad4. This complex binds to specific DNA sequences and works with other transcription factors to stimulate gene expression. Mutations in pancreatic cancer can inactivate either partner of the dimeric receptors that respond to extracellular TGF-β or activin. More commonly, however, mutations and large deletions in the SMAD4 gene destabilize its protein product or ablate gene expression.

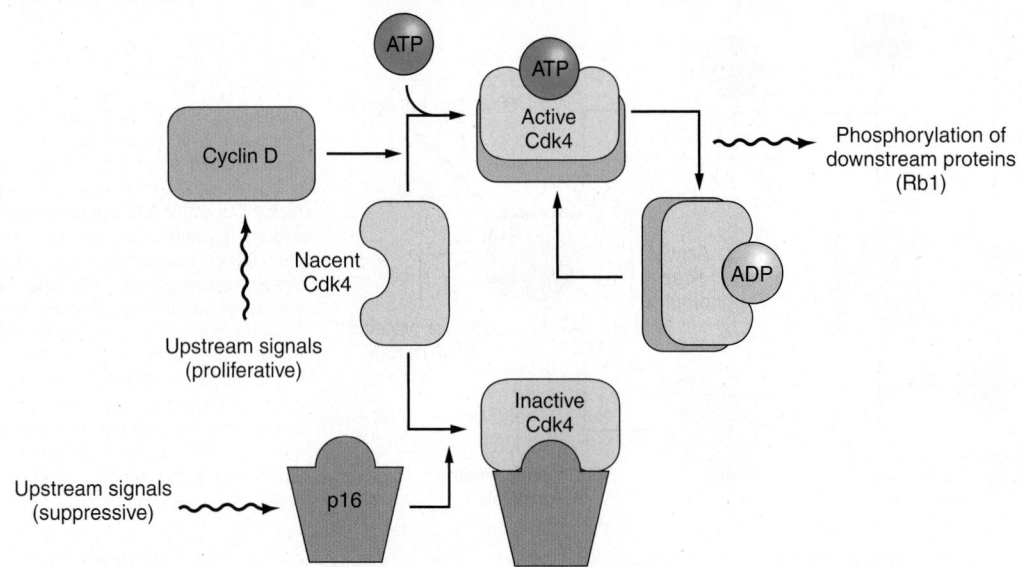

Figure 48.3 The p16/RB1 pathway. p16 binds to, inhibits, and thereby controls the availability of the cyclin-dependent kinases Cdk4 and Cdk6 (not shown). When activated by binding to cyclin D, these kinases phosphorylate and thereby inactivate the Rb1 tumor-suppressor protein. The activity of p16 is controlled in a complex manner, through changes in gene expression and by displacement reactions involving other similar kinase inhibitor proteins. p16 mutations and deletions are nearly ubiquitous in pancreatic cancer, resulting in dysregulation of these cyclin-dependent kinases that regulate the cell division cycle.

genetic damage in these carcinomas differs considerably from the pattern in carcinomas with CIN. The type II TGF-β and activin receptors (*TGFBR2*) and (*ACVR2*), as well as the *BAX* gene, have a repetitive sequence within their protein-coding regions, and biallelic inactivating mutations of these sequences are seen in many MSI pancreatic cancers.[28,54–57]

There are also alterations in pancreatic carcinomas, some probably being important to tumorigenesis, that are not attributed to genetic mutations. These include the expression of telomerase,[15,16] the underexpression of TGF-β receptors,[29] and the overexpression of the growth-stimulating Her-2/neu cell surface receptor[58–61] and growth factor-related proteins.[62] Some of these activities are proposed to be attractive as therapeutic targets, although supportive clinical evidence is not yet available. Pancreatic carcinomas also have reproducible alterations in gene expression, such as overexpression of the proteins mesothelin and prostate stem cell antigen (PSCA), that currently can serve as diagnostic aids in the histopathologic interpretation of biopsies and surgical resections.[57–59]

The epigenetic patterns of gene hypermethylation and various patterns of overexpression of RNA transcripts and proteins in pancreatic cancers are considered promising for developing additional diagnostic markers for the analysis of pancreatic secretions and for noninvasive diagnostic screening.[63]

Genetic patterns are also found among other diagnostic categories of pancreatic neoplasia. The precursor lesions of PDAs, termed pancreatic intraepithelial neoplasia (PanIN), in their most advanced grade closely resemble the genetic patterns of the conventional invasive PDAs. However, the lesions other than the PDAs, including the intraductal papillary mucinous neoplasms (IPMN), the mucinous cyctic neoplasms (MCNs), acinar cell carcinomas, well-differentiated neuroendocrine tumors, pancreatoblastomas, and solid pseudopapillary neoplasms (SPNs), diverge significantly from the patterns of PanINs and typical invasive PDAs. These differences could be used in the future for differential diagnosis of lesions upon biopsy.

Cystic neoplasms such as IPMNs, serous cystadenomas (SCAs), MCNs, and SPNs appear to have relatively few mutant genes in

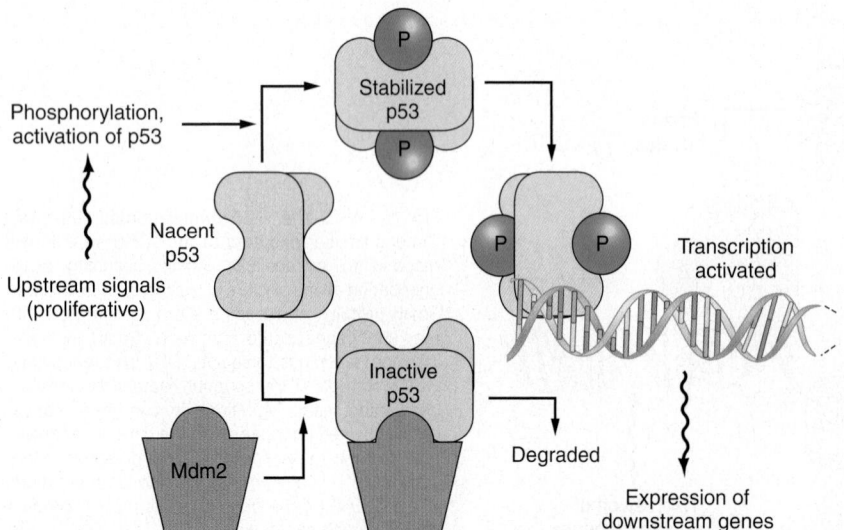

Figure 48.4 The p53 pathway. Many modes of control affect p53 activity, one of which is shown in the diagram. Stresses such as DNA damage result in the phosphorylation of p53, preventing its degradation by an Mdm2-directed pathway. When stabilized, p53 binds to specific DNA sequences and activates the transcription of many genes, including Mdm2 as part of a negative feedback loop. When p53 is mutated, it fails to bind effectively to DNA to activate transcription. Because Mdm2 then lacks its transcriptional stimulus from p53, mutant but inactive p53 proteins are usually expressed at very high levels.

each tumor, yet the genes involved are remarkably distinct.[64–66] Mutations in *GNAS* or *KRAS* were found in 96% of IPMNs; those in *RNF43* were present in many IPMNs and MCNs; those in *CTNNB1* were ubiquitous among the SPNs; and those in *VHL* affected half of the SCAs. *GNAS* mutations were found in collected pancreatic secretions samples of two thirds of familial and sporadic cases of IPMNs, but not in controls, and their presence predicted subsequent emergence or increasing size of detected cysts.[67] *PIK3CA* mutations are present in some IPMNs and the colloid carcinomas that can derive from them.[68] *CTNNB1* (beta-catenin) mutations are present in virtually all solid-pseudopapillary neoplasms[69] and pancreatoblastomas.[70] These genetic data suggested utilities in detection, diagnostic classification, and prognostication when clinically managing pancreatic cysts.

Mutations of *MEN1* and either the *DAXX* or *ATRX* genes are found in most well-differentiated pancreatic neuroendocrine tumors (PanNET).[71,72] Nearly two thirds of these tumors (a subset uniformly harboring *DAXX* or *ATRX* mutations) were found to have abnormal telomeres, indicating an active process termed alternative lengthening of telomeres (ALT). ALT is distinct from the typical activation of telomerase implicated in most types of cancer.[73] The distinguishing patterns of mutations also firmly establish that high-grade small- and large-cell neuroendocrine carcinomas of the pancreas, despite having histologic similarities with well-differentiated PanNETs, arise through different tumorigenic mechanisms.[74]

Lower-Frequency Genetic Changes

The causative genes of *Fanconi anemia* play a role in human tumorigenesis. The *BRCA2* gene represents Fanconi complementation group D1 and is thought to aid DNA strand repair.[75] Because of this function, it is perhaps best to categorize *BRCA2* as a genome-maintenance gene rather than a conventional tumor-suppressor. As many as 7% of apparently *sporadic* pancreatic cancers (more, in instances of familial aggregation) harbor an inactivating intragenic inherited mutation of one copy of the *BRCA2* gene, accompanied by LOH.[1,2,66] The *PALB2* gene represents Fanconi group N, and its protein product functions by binding the Brca2 protein.[76] Three percent of familial pancreatic cancers harbored a germ-line inactivating mutation of *PALB2*, and in a tumor studied in depth, the other copy was inactivated by a somatic mutation.[1,77,78] The *FANCC* and *FANCG* genes have somatic or germ-line mutations in some pancreatic cancer patients, again with loss of the wild-type allele in the cancer.[79] The known hypersensitivity of Fanconi cells to interstrand DNA cross-linking agents, such as cisplatin, melphalan, and mitomycin C, suggested that pancreatic cancers with Fanconi pathway genetic defects would be especially susceptible to treatment with such agents.[80–83] Occasional complete remissions of pancreatic cancer have been reported with therapies that included DNA cross-linkers,[84–88] and there are recent reports of prolonged responses using such agents in patients having *BRCA2* mutations.[89,90] Cells made experimentally deficient for Fanconi genes are also hypersensitive to certain nongenotoxic compounds,[91] and patients that have *BRCA2*-mutant cancers other than pancreatic cancer are reported to respond to therapeutic drug inhibition of the poly (ADP-ribose) polymerase enzyme, which normally becomes activated to facilitate DNA-strand repair.[92] These opportunities are being explored in clinical trials.

A genomic mutational pattern (a *signature*) typical of cancers having *BRCA1* or *BRCA2* inactivation is reported in about 12% of pancreatic cancers.[93] This pattern involves nucleotide substitutions of broad diversity and indicates that the functions of BRCA genes extend to repair mechanisms not yet well explored. Among natural compounds tested, *BRCA2*- and *PALB2*-null cancers seem most hypersensitive to the toxicity of acetaldehyde,[94] a requisite metabolite of alcohol and a natural food constituent. Acetaldehyde creates deoxynucleotide adducts, but the mutagenic effects of acetaldehyde in carriers of *BRCA2* and *PALB2* mutations are not yet explored with focused epidemiologic studies. Remarkably, *BRCA1* gene mutations were not found in unselected pancreatic cancers or pancreatic cancer families.[95] Nonetheless, pancreatic cancers do occur in carriers of *BRCA1*-inactivating mutations.[96,97] In these persons, the relatively high rate of LOH affecting the other *BRCA1* copy indicates that a loss of *BRCA1* function likely fosters tumorigenesis in these patients.[96]

A hotspot of genomic homozygous deletions affects the *FAM190A* gene, producing deletions of internal exons and typically resulting in in-frame deletions of the protein-coding sequence.[98,99] In addition to these genomic mutations, more than a third of PDAs have similar in-frame deletions affecting the *FAM190A* transcripts and/or defective expression of the Fam190a protein, but yet without an identifiable genomic mutation.[99,100] Fam190a functions in mitosis and in ensuring mononuclear daughter cells after the abscission (separation) phase of cell division.[100] Fam190a abnormalities thus might contribute to chromosomal instability during tumorigenesis.

The *mitochondrial genome* is mutated in a majority of pancreatic cancers.[101–103] These mutations most likely represent genetic drift, and perhaps do not directly contribute to the process of tumorigenesis.[103] Such mutations, however, could potentially serve as a diagnostic target due to the large number of copies of the mitochondrial genome in human carcinoma cells.[102,103]

Genes encoding components of the SWI/SNF chromatin-remodeling complex, including *ARID1A*, *ARID1B*, and *PBRM1*, are each occasionally mutated in PDA, in total affecting nearly a third of these tumors.[104,105]

The *MAP2K4* (*MKK4*) gene participates in a stress-activated protein kinase pathway.[81,82] It is stimulated by various influences, including chemotherapy, and its downstream effects include apoptosis and cellular differentiation. The *MKK4* gene is inactivated by homozygous deletions or mutation coupled with LOH in about 4% of pancreatic cancers.[106,107] The experimental loss of one or both copies of the *MKK4* gene in cancer cells reduced Jun kinase activation and its expression. Such gene dose-dependent effects could rationalize the high rate of loss of chromosomal arm 17p, affecting 90% of pancreatic cancers and more than half of the *TP53* wild-type cancers.[108]

Germ-line mutations of the *STK11* (*LKB1*) gene, a serine-threonine kinase, are responsible for Peutz-Jeghers syndrome (PJS).[109,110] PJS was anecdotally associated with pancreatic cancer.[111] A follow-up study examined lifetime risk, finding nearly a third of PJS patients to have developed pancreatic cancer.[112] Sporadic pancreatic cancers, independent of PJS, also can lose the gene by homozygous deletion or by somatic mutation/LOH in about 4% of cases.[113]

Kinase oncogenes are mutated at low frequency, including the *GUCY2F*, *EGFR*, and *NTRK3* genes.[91,92] This class of mutations is important in that these mutations can be targeted with antikinase drugs.[93]

Gene amplification also occurs in pancreatic cancer. Amplified regions include the *AKT2* gene within an amplicon on chromosome 19q, which involves about 10% to 20% of cases studied.[94–96] About 6% of pancreatic cancers overexpress the oncogene *CCNE1* (cyclin E). Two mechanisms have been demonstrated, cyclin E gene amplification and the genetic inactivation of the *FBXW7* (*AGO*) gene, which normally serves to degrade cyclin E during the normal phases of the cell division cycle.[7,114]

The patterns of *chromosomal deletion* in pancreatic cancer are complex. In one study, from 1.5% to 32% of all tested loci in the PDAs of different patients had a deletion.[115] For most lost regions, we know of no particular tumor-suppressor genes targeted by the deletions. Conversely, in some regions known to harbor tumor-suppressor genes, the known mutated genes do not justify the high observed prevalence rates of LOH unless gene dose-dependent effects are postulated.[108] Individual homozygous deletions are found at some additional genetic locations, again without a definitive target gene yet identified for most of these events.[98]

Defects in DNA mismatch repair (microsatellite instability, MSI) are seen in a small minority of pancreatic cancers. These cancers typically have a medullary histologic phenotype[10] and mutations of the type II TGF-β (*TGFBR2*) and activin (*ACVR2*) receptor genes.[28,55,56] They can also have mutations of the pro-apoptotic *BAX* gene[54] and of the growth factor pathway mediator *BRAF* gene (affecting the same pathway, presumably, as mutations of the *KRAS* gene).[10,11,54,114] The MSI tumors do not have the propensity for large chromosomal alterations and gross aneuploidy.[17,116] In a study of four cases of pancreatic cancers having MSI, all lacked expression of the Mlh1 protein.[11] Not all cancers with a medullary phenotype have MSI. Yet, medullary pancreatic carcinomas as a whole have a number of clinical and genetic differences as compared to those with conventional histologic appearance; the carcinomas have pushing rather than infiltrative borders, the *KRAS* gene often is wild type, and there is often a family history of malignancy.[5,6,47] A reported case of Epstein-Barr virus (EBV)–associated pancreatic cancer[11] had a medullary phenotype with heavy lymphocytic infiltration. Due to its distinctive features, it is advisable to separately designate the medullary category in the reporting of all clinical, genetic, and pathologic studies of pancreatic cancer.

Inherited or somatic inactivating mutations in the *ATM* gene accompany the loss of the wild-type allele of the cancers, indicating another tumor-suppressor gene for PDAs.[117,118]

Inherited mutations of the *cationic trypsinogen (PRSS1)* gene prevent the inactivation of prematurely activated trypsin within the ducts, causing a familial form of severe, early-onset acute pancreatitis.[119] Some affected kindred have a cumulative risk of pancreatic cancer that approaches 40% by the time the affected individuals reach 60 years of age.[120] This cancer diathesis falls in a unique category of cancer susceptibility, in that the predisposition emanates from genetic alterations of a tissue-maintenance gene, one that is not an oncogene, a tumor-suppressor gene, or a genome-maintenance gene.

In summary, pancreatic cancer is fundamentally a genetic disease. An understanding of the genes altered in pancreatic cancer has led to a better understanding of the familial aggregation of pancreatic cancer, which in turn, it is hoped, will lead to effective gene-specific targeted therapies for this deadly form of cancer.

SELECTED REFERENCES

The full reference list can be accessed at lwwhealthlibrary.com/oncology.

1. Jones S, Zhang X, Parsons DW, et al. Core signaling pathways in human pancreatic cancers revealed by global genomic analyses. *Science* 2008; 321:1801–1806.
4. Yachida S, Jones S, Bozic I, et al. Distant metastasis occurs late during the genetic evolution of pancreatic cancer. *Nature* 2010;467:1114–1117.
6. Goggins M, Schutte M, Lu J, et al. Germline BRCA2 gene mutations in patients with apparently sporadic pancreatic carcinomas. *Cancer Res* 1996; 56:5360–5364.
11. Wilentz RE, Goggins M, Redston M, et al. Genetic, immunohistochemical, and clinical features of medullary carcinomas of the pancreas: a newly described and characterized entity. *Am J Pathol* 2000;156:1641–1651.
12. Hruban RH, Wilentz R, Kern SE. Genetic progression in the pancreatic ducts. *Am J Pathol* 2000;156:1821–1825.
15. Hiyama E, Kodama T, Shinbara K, et al. Telomerase activity is detected in pancreatic cancer but not in benign tumors. *Cancer Res* 1997;57:326–331.
18. Cox AD, Der CJ. Ras family signaling: therapeutic targeting. *Cancer Biol Ther* 2002;1:599–606.
20. Caldas C, Hahn SA, Hruban RH, et al. Detection of K-ras mutations in the stool of patients with pancreatic adenocarcinoma and pancreatic ductal hyperplasia. *Cancer Res* 1994;54:3568–3573.
21. Klimstra DS, Longnecker DS. K-ras mutations in pancreatic ductal proliferative lesions. *Am J Pathol* 1994;145:1547–1550.
27. Hahn SA, Schutte M, Hoque ATMS, et al. DPC4, a candidate tumor-suppressor gene at 18q21.1. *Science* 1996;271:350–353.
28. Goggins M, Shekher M, Turnacioglu K, et al. Genetic alterations of the TGF beta receptor genes in pancreatic and biliary adenocarcinomas. *Cancer Res* 1998;58:5329–5332.
29. Baldwin RL, Friess H, Yokoyama M, et al. Attenuated ALK5 receptor expression in human pancreatic cancer: correlation with resistance to growth inhibition. *Int J Cancer* 1996;67:283–288.
33. Caldas C, Hahn SA, da Costa LT, et al. Frequent somatic mutations and homozygous deletions of the p16 (MTS1) gene in pancreatic adenocarcinoma. *Nat Genet* 1994;8:27–31.
35. Goldstein AM, Fraser MC, Struewing JP, et al. Increased risk of pancreatic cancer in melanoma-prone kindreds with p16INK4 mutations. *N Engl J Med* 1995;333:970–974.
37. Whelan AJ, Bartsch D, Goodfellow PJ. Brief report: a familial syndrome of pancreatic cancer and melanoma with a mutation in the CDKN2 tumor-suppressor gene. *N Engl J Med* 1995;333:975–977.

41. Kern SE, Kinzler KW, Bruskin A, et al. Identification of p53 as a sequence-specific DNA-binding protein. *Science* 1991;252:1708–1711.
50. Hahn SA, Seymour AB, Hoque ATMS, et al. Allelotype of pancreatic adenocarcinoma using a xenograft model. *Cancer Res* 1995;55:4670–4675.
62. Preis M, Korc M. Signaling pathways in pancreatic cancer. *Crit Rev Eukaryot Gene Expr* 2011;21:115–129.
65. Wu J, Jiao Y, Dal Molin M, et al. Whole-exome sequencing of neoplastic cysts of the pancreas reveals recurrent mutations in components of ubiquitin-dependent pathways. *Proc Natl Acad Sci U S A* 2011;108:21188–21193.
66. Wu J, Matthaei H, Maitra A, et al. Recurrent GNAS mutations define an unexpected pathway for pancreatic cyst development. *Sci Transl Med* 2011;3:92ra66.
72. Jiao Y, Shi C, Edil BH, et al. DAXX/ATRX, MEN1, and mTOR pathway genes are frequently altered in pancreatic neuroendocrine tumors. *Science* 2011;331:1199–1203.
77. Jones S, Hruban RH, Kamiyama M, et al. Exomic sequencing identifies PALB2 as a pancreatic cancer susceptibility gene. *Science* 2009;324:217.
79. van der Heijden MS, Yeo CJ, Hruban RH, et al. Fanconi anemia gene mutations in young-onset pancreatic cancer. *Cancer Res* 2003;63:2585–2588.
94. Ghosh S, Sur S, Yerram SR, et al. Hypersensitivities for acetaldehyde and other agents among cancer cells null for clinically-relevant Fanconi anemia genes. *Am J Pathol* 2014;184:260–270.
99. Scrimieri F, Calhoun ES, Patel K, et al. FAM190A rearrangements provide a multitude of individualized tumor signatures and neo-antigens in cancer. *Oncotarget* 2011;2:69–75.
105. Shain AH, Giacomini CP, Matsukuma K, et al. Convergent structural alterations define SWItch/Sucrose NonFermentable (SWI/SNF) chromatin remodeler as a central tumor suppressive complex in pancreatic cancer. *Proc Natl Acad Sci U S A* 2012;109:E252–E259.
107. Teng DH-F, Perry III WL, Hogan JK, et al. Human mitogen-activated protein kinase kinase 4 as a candidate tumor suppressor. *Cancer Res* 1997;57:4177–4182.
111. Giardiello FM, Welsh SB, Hamilton SR, et al. Increased risk of cancer in the Peutz-Jeghers syndrome. *N Engl J Med* 1987;316:1511–1514.
117. Roberts NJ, Jiao Y, Yu J, et al. ATM mutations in patients with hereditary pancreatic cancer. *Cancer Discov* 2012;2:41–46.
119. Whitcomb DC, Gorry MC, Preston RA, et al. Hereditary pancreatitis is caused by a mutation in the cationic trypsinogen gene. *Nature Genet* 1996; 14:141–145.

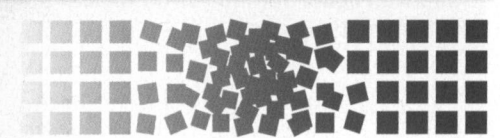
49 Cancer of the Pancreas

Jordan M. Winter, Jonathan R. Brody, Ross A. Abrams, Nancy L. Lewis, and Charles J. Yeo

INTRODUCTION

Pancreatic ductal adenocarcinoma (PDA) is the 12th most common cancer in the United States, but the 4th most frequent cause of cancer-related death.[1] There are 44,000 new cases of PDA each year in the United States and 38,000 deaths.[2] Although the death rates of most common cancers have declined over the past 80 years, the death rates for PDA have remained flat to slightly increased.[1] Based on demographic, incidence, and survival projections, PDA death rates are expected to eclipse death rates from breast and colon cancer within the next decade, and become the 2nd most deadly cancer. In short, PDA remains a deadly disease and is currently only curable in a minority of patients with localized and resectable disease.

Disease-specific survival has not changed significantly in the past 4 decades, regardless of disease stage. Patients with metastatic disease continue to have a 5-year survival of 2% or less.[1,3,4] A recent single-institution, retrospective analysis of patients with resected PDA revealed similar overall survivals in the 2000s and the 1980s.[5] The similarity in overall survival over time is not at all surprising considering the relatively modest advances in chemotherapy during this time. Although targeted and immunotherapies are now routinely used to treat certain other cancer types, personalized medicines with novel biologic therapies have not yet been successful for PDA.

This chapter provides a comprehensive overview of the pathobiology and management of pancreatic cancer, focusing on PDA. The less common types of pancreatic cancer (e.g., pancreatic neuroendocrine tumors and pancreatic cysts) will be discussed briefly. Current management strategies are placed in an historical context, and the latest understanding of the genetics and molecular biology of pancreatic cancer is reviewed. The management of PDA requires a multidisciplinary approach that involves surgeons, medical oncologists, radiation oncologists, radiologists, gastroenterologists, palliative medicine specialists, nurses, nutritionists, and many others. Herein, the roles of surgery, chemotherapy, and radiation will be emphasized. As much as possible, treatment strategies are framed in the context of the American Joint Committee on Cancer (AJCC) 7th edition staging scheme.[6]

STAGING

Pancreatic cancer is staged according to the AJCC, 7th edition, TNM staging system (Table 49.1).[6] Presented survival data are based on 1998 data.[7] T-stage is defined as follows: Tis is carcinoma in situ (pancreatic intraepithelial neoplasia [PanIN-3]); T1 is 2 cm or less and confined to the pancreas; T2 is greater than 2 cm and confined to the pancreas; T3 extends beyond the pancreas; and T4 invades visceral vessels, rendering the tumor unresectable. N-stage is defined as follows: N0 reflects no regional lymph node metastases; and N1 reflects regional lymph node metastases. M-stage is defined as follows: M0 reflects no distant metastases; and M1 reflects distant metastases.

EPIDEMIOLOGY

Like most cancers, PDA develops as a result of acquired genetic defects over many years, and therefore, most often occurs in the elderly. The median age at onset is 71 years, and nearly 74% of patients are diagnosed between the ages of 55 and 84. Only 12% of patients are diagnosed under 55, and 14% after the age of 84. The age-adjusted incidence rate in the United States is 12 out of 100,000, and the lifetime risk of developing PDA is 1.5%, or 1 in 67. African Americans have a slightly increased risk compared to Caucasians.[8]

Genetic Risk Factors

The greatest risk factor for pancreatic cancer is a strong family history. Approximately 10% of all pancreatic cancers are familial, defined as a family history involving at least two affected first-degree relatives (FDR) (e.g., parents, offspring, and siblings).[9] The lifetime risk is 40% (32-fold) for patients with three or more affected FDRs, 10% for patients with two FDRs (6.4-fold), and 6% for patients with 1 FDR (4.6-fold).[10] Some of the genetic defects underlying familial pancreatic cancer have been discovered, but known genetic defects only account for 10% to 15% of all familial cases.[11] Specific genetic abnormalities are discussed in greater detail in the Pathology and Biology section.

Environmental Risk Factors: Tobacco, Occupational Hazards, and Alcohol Consumption

Many environmental risk factors have been formally evaluated via meta-analyses performed by the Pancreatic Cancer Case Control Consortium (PanC4, http://panc4.org/index.html). Smoking tobacco is the best characterized environmental risk factor for PDA. A large meta-analysis of 83 studies calculated a relative risk increase at 1.74 for active smokers (this is substantially less than having even a single FDR).[12] Importantly, the risk decreases for former smokers, and returns to baseline after 20 years of smoking cessation.[12] These results were confirmed by the PanC4 consortium, which also noted that the number of daily cigarettes is directly proportional to the risk of developing PDA.[13] Not surprising, high-risk individuals with a family history who also smoke carry twice the risk, compared to similar patients who do not smoke.[14,15] Cigars are also associated with an increased risk for PDA, whereas smokeless tobacco is not.[16] The impact of environmental tobacco smoke (i.e., second-hand smoke) on long-term risk is unclear.[17,18] Among the many carcinogens in tobacco products, N-nitrosamines and the polycyclic aromatic hydrocarbons (PAH) are suspected to be the greatest culprits.[19]

With regard to occupational risk hazards, chlorinated hydrocarbons and PAHs have been most consistently found to correlate with PDA, and to increase relative risk by a comparable degree

TABLE 49.1

American Joint Committee on Cancer Staging for Pancreatic Cancer

Stage	T	N	M	Median Survival, All Patients (Months)	Median Survival, Resected Patients (Months)
0	Tis	N0	M0	N/A	N/A
1A	T1	N0	M0	10.0	24.1
1B	T2	N0	M0	9.1	20.6
IIA	T3	N0	M0	8.1	15.4
IIB	T1	N1	M0	9.7	12.7
	T2	N1	M0		
	T3	N1	M0		
III	T4	Any N	M0	7.7	10.6
IV	Any T	Any N	M1	2.5	4.5
Total				4.4	12.6

Modified from Bilimoria KY, Bentrem DJ, Ko CY, et al. Validation of the 6th edition AJCC Pancreatic Cancer Staging System: report from the National Cancer Database. *Cancer* 2007; 110:738–744.

as smoking.[20] The former compound type is associated with dry cleaning and metal work, and, with the latter, exposure occurs with metalwork and aluminum production. According to the PanC4 consortium, mild or moderate alcohol consumption does not predispose one to PDA, whereas heavy alcohol consumption ($\geq$9 drinks per day) is associated with an odds ratio (OR) of 1.6.[21]

Medical Risk Factors: Pancreatitis, Diabetes, and Obesity

Like smoking, chronic pancreatitis is a well-accepted risk factor for PDA, with an OR of 2.7 for patients with over 2 years of disease. The OR skyrockets for patients with less than 2 years of chronic pancreatitis (13.6), in large part because the pancreatitis in these patients represents a presenting symptom of PDA, as oppose to a contributing cause.[22] A preponderance of the evidence from over a dozen studies suggests that obesity is a mild contributing risk factor for PDA (OR 1 to 1.5). Proposed mechanistic links include hormonal (e.g., insulin and insulin-like growth factor 1 [IGF-1]) and inflammatory influences on pancreatic cells, as well as increased carcinogen exposure related to food consumption.[23] Although a link between type II diabetes mellitus (DM) and pancreatic cancer has been extensively studied, a causal association has not been clearly established. Two meta-analyses have been performed that examined more than 30 studies performed over 4 decades. Type II DM is associated with a twofold risk increase for PDA. Patients with long-standing DM (>5 years) have a mildly increased risk compared to patients without DM, suggesting that the disease may indeed contribute to tumorigenesis. Similar to obesity, increased levels of insulin and IGF-1 have been implicated. As with chronic pancreatitis, the highest risk for PDA is clearly in patients with recent onset of DM (<5 years, and particularly within 1 year), suggesting that DM is principally a manifestation of PDA, as opposed to a true risk factor in these patients.[24,25]

PATHOLOGY AND BIOLOGY

The normal pancreas contains two epithelial cell types: exocrine and endocrine cells. Most of the pancreas is comprised of exocrine cells, which line an organized ductal network. Acinar cells line the smallest ducts; they synthesize and secrete digestive enzymes. Larger ducts are lined by intercalated duct cells, and secrete bicarbonate and water. Ultimately, the ducts converge into the main pancreatic duct, which drains into the duodenum. The endocrine component makes up just 1% of the pancreas, and consists of islets of Langerhans. These hormone-producing cell clusters are primarily involved with glucose homeostasis. The principal endocrine cell types include the A (alpha), B (beta), and D (delta) cells, which synthesize glucagon, insulin, and somatostatin, respectively. The different cell types are believed to give rise to the different variants of pancreatic neoplasms.

Pancreatic cancer refers to a heterogeneous group of malignant pathologies that originate in the pancreas, and nearly all are epithelial in origin. They are categorized by their gross appearance (solid or cystic), as well as the predominant cell differentiation pattern (ductal, acinar, or endocrine). Primary pancreatic mesenchymal (e.g., sarcomas) and lymphoid neoplasms are exceptionally rare, and will not be reviewed here. Dozens of different epithelial pancreatic neoplasms have been described, but over 85% are the conventional pancreatic (tubular) ductal adenocarcinomas, and more than 98% of cancers fit into one of the following additional diagnoses: solid types, which include pancreatic endocrine neoplasms, acinar cell carcinomas, and pancreatoblastomas; and cystic types, which include mucinous cystic neoplasms, intraductal papillary mucinous neoplasms, and solid-pseudopapillary neoplasms. These diagnoses are typically made based on microscopic appearance, but a diagnosis may be confirmed with immunolabeling of specific proteins. Uncommon variants of ductal adenocarcinoma that are rarely encountered will not be reviewed. These include adenosquamous carcinoma, colloid noncystic adenocarcinoma, hepatoid carcinoma, signet ring carcinoma, medullary carcinoma, and undifferentiated carcinoma. The classification and nomenclature of pancreatic epithelial neoplasms has been reviewed by Klimstra, Pitman, and Hruban.[26]

EXOCRINE PANCREATIC CANCERS

Pancreatic Ductal Adenocarcinoma

Although the molecular mechanisms that underlie aggressive PDA biology remain poorly understood, there are certain features of PDA that are unique or defining, and will be highlighted in this section on pathobiology as well as in the Future Directions and Challenges section at the end of the chapter. These include molecular heterogeneity, a tendency for perineural invasion, remarkable tolerance to nutrient deprivation, and abundant stroma.

PDA Pathology

PDAs appear as ill-defined, sclerotic, yellow-white masses on gross inspection. The edges are poorly defined and infiltrative. Histologically, they are characterized by perineural invasion in almost all cases (much more frequently than in other common adenocarcinomas like colon and breast). Microscopic vessel and lymphatic invasion are common, and tumor necrosis is frequently present. Even in localized and resected cases, PDAs are rarely encountered at the T1 stage nor are they well differentiated, which drives home the fact that PDA is seldom diagnosed *early* in the life span of the tumor, at a *curable* stage.[27] On light microscopy, the cells typically form infiltrative gland-forming structures, separated from each other by a tenacious desmoplastic reaction. Lymph node spread is present in the majority of resection specimens with localized disease. Immunohistochemical markers typically seen include cytokeratins (e.g., 7, 8, 13, 18, 19), CA19-9, B72.3, CA-125, and DUPAN-2. The nonneoplastic desmoplastic (stromal) component comprises more than 70% of the tumor mass (a higher proportion than other common solid tumors), and is commonly referred to as

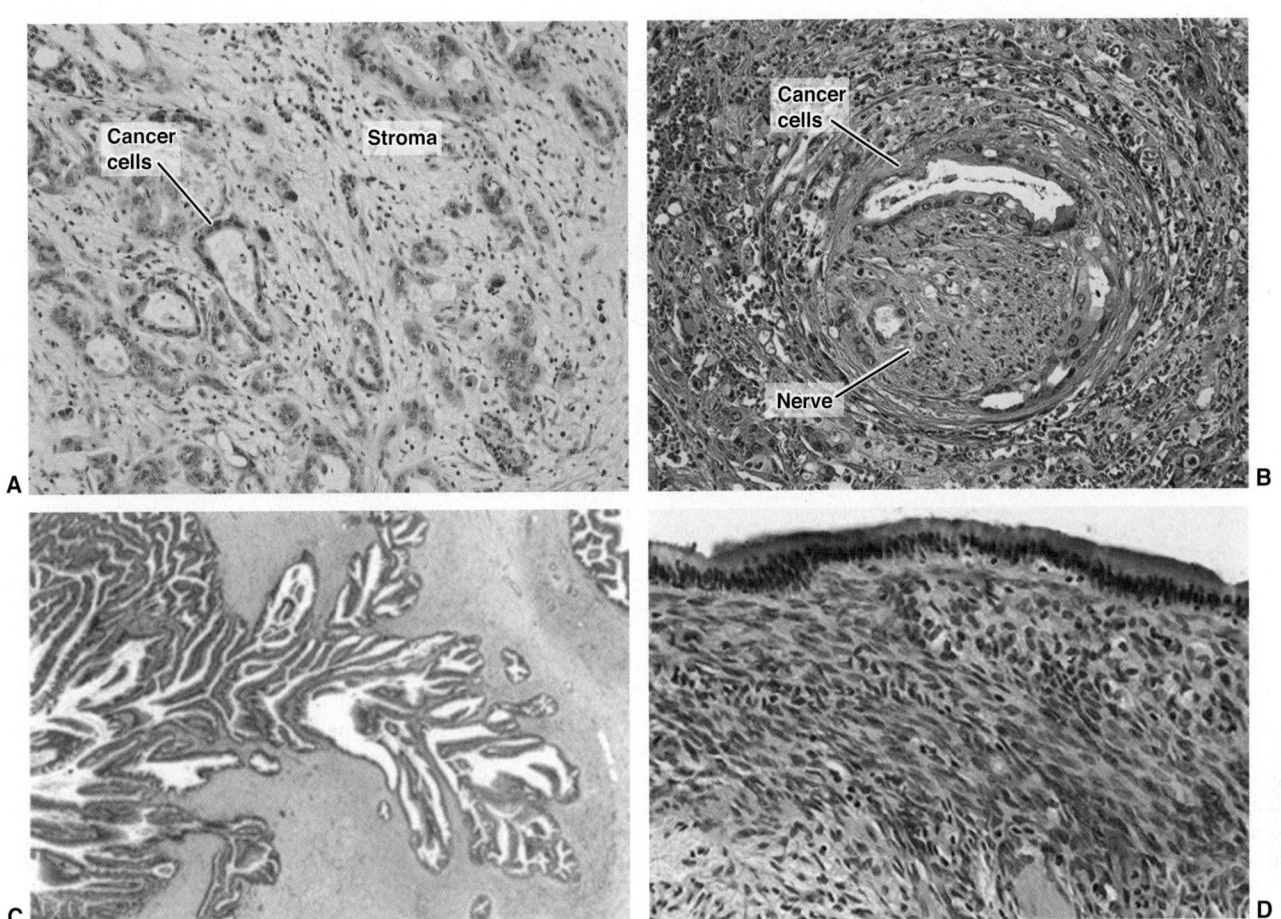

Figure 49.1 High-power photographs of PDA. **(A)** PDA containing dense stroma. **(B)** PDA with perineural invasion. **(C)** Intraductal papillary mucinous neoplasms. **(D)** Mucinous cystic neoplasms.

the tumor microenvironment (TME). The stroma consists of an extracellular matrix and numerous cell types, including inflammatory cells, pancreatic stellate cells, endothelial cells, nerve cells, fibroblasts, and myofibroblasts. The stroma is hypovascular with a low vessel density and high interstitial fluid pressure, resulting in a poorly perfused epithelial compartment, and the characteristic *hypodense* appearance on cross-sectional imaging obtained with intravenous contrast. Classic histologic features of PDA are depicted in Figure 49.1.[28]

The stroma creates a barrier to effective drug delivery[29] and is believed to contribute to the overall virulence of the tumor. Sophisticated mathematical modeling reveals that austere conditions in the TME impose profound selection pressures on cancer cells, leading to the generation and dominance of aggressive cancer subclones.[30] These subclones are chemoresistant and well adapted to survive extreme conditions present in the TME. Not surprisingly, PDA cells are more resistant to nutrient deprivation than most aggressive cancer types.[31] There is now a concerted effort to develop strategies to target the tumor microenvironment in PDA (see Future Directions and Challenges).

PDA development follows an adenoma to carcinoma sequence, similar to previous descriptions for colon cancer.[32] Precursor lesions are referred to as PanIN lesions (pancreatic intraepithelial neoplasia), and are graded from PanIN-1 to PanIn-3. Early PanIN lesions are common (present 20% of individuals at autopsy[33]) and most do not progress to PDA in an individual's lifetime. PanIN-1A lesions are tall columnar cells with abundant mucin; PanIN-1B lesions are similar but have a papillary appearance. PanIN-2 lesions have nuclear abnormalities. PanIN-3 lesions were formerly called carcinoma in situ; they exhibit true cribriforming, budding cells

into lumen, loss of nuclear polarity, and mitoses. PanIN-3 lesions are found in roughly 2% of autopsy specimens from individuals who died from nonpancreatic diseases (Fig. 49.2).[33] The similar lifetime risk of PDA suggests that a high proportion of PanIN-3 lesions develop into clinically significant cancer. Future effective early detection strategies would ideally discover and treat PanIN-3 lesions.[28]

PDA Genetics

Unlike breast and other cancers, PDA cannot be subgrouped by molecular characteristics at the present time to guide therapy or to inform prognosis. However, whole-exome sequencing of numerous PDAs were performed and provided unprecedented insight into the genetics of PDA.[34,35] High throughput sequencing data emphasize the molecular complexity of PDA. Out of 24 PDA genomes, 1,327 different genes (~7% of coding genes) were found to have at least one somatic mutation, and 148 different genes had at least two mutations (0.7%).[35] There were an average of 60 genetic alterations per tumor, and each PDA had a unique genetic fingerprint. Unfortunately, sequencing studies did not identify any novel high frequency mutated *cancer genes* as promising therapeutic targets. A more practical approach to *personalized therapy* is to group the genetically altered genes into 12 core signaling pathways (e.g., apoptosis, DNA damage, and 10 others), as proposed by Jones et al.[35] These pathways are universally dysregulated and therefore may be more realistic therapeutic targets than single genes.[35] A separate study found that axon guidance genes were also mutated at a higher rate than what was expected by chance, although the functional importance of these neuron-related genes in cancer is still unknown.[34]

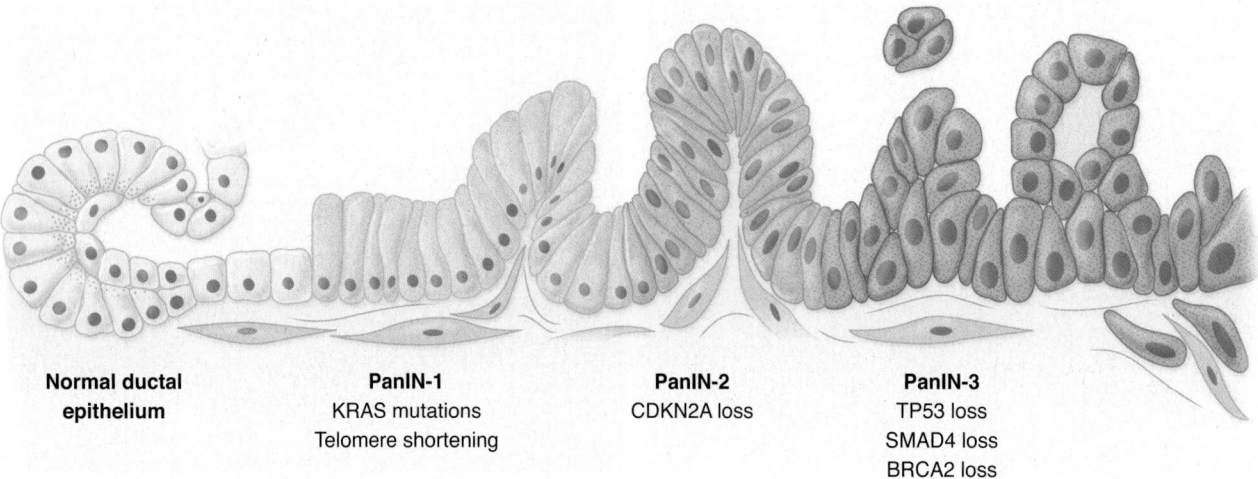

Normal ductal epithelium	PanIN-1	PanIN-2	PanIN-3
	KRAS mutations	CDKN2A loss	TP53 loss
	Telomere shortening		SMAD4 loss
			BRCA2 loss

Figure 49.2 PanIN sequence with observed molecular changes. (From Maitra A, Hruban RH. Pancreatic cancer. *Annu Rev Pathol* 2008;3:157–188.)

A genetically altered gene may be categorized as an oncogene (with gain-of-function mutations), a tumor suppressor gene (loss-of-function), or a genome maintenance gene (loss-of-function). For the latter two gene types, both copies of the gene are typically inactivated; one allele is lost by somatic mutation and the other by chromosomal or allelic loss (loss of heterozygosity [LOH]). Oncogenic Kras is altered in more than 90% of PDAs, and is usually an early event in tumorigenesis.[28,35,36] Somatic Kras mutations mostly occur in codon 12, and rarely occur in codons 13 and 61.[37] The sequence alterations inactivate GTPase function, leaving GTP continuously engaged and the oncogene constitutively activated. Activated Kras positively regulates multiple signaling pathways, including the BRAF/mitogen-activated protein kinase (MAPK) pathway (proliferation), phosphatidylinositol 3-kinase (PI3K)/mammalian target of rapamycin (mTOR) (cell growth and survival), and Phospholipase C (PLC)/Protein kinase C (PKC)/Ca^{++} (calcium and second messenger signaling).[38] To date, attempts to pharmacologically inhibit Kras have been unsuccessful.[39] However, because of its early development in nearly all PDAs, the importance of this molecule will continue to preoccupy pancreatic researchers in hopes of finding an effective targeted therapy with a large therapeutic window (see Future Directions section).

The remaining *high frequency* mutated pancreatic cancer genes are tumor suppressor genes. The pattern of frequent allelic loss mutations in PDA due to chromosome instability (losses are more common than gains[40]), promotes a fertile environment of genetic experimentation that favors loss of function mutations. Allelotype mapping reveals that genetic loss ranges from 17% to 80% of the genome in a given PDA.[41] Allelic loss is nonrandom across the PDA genome; LOH *hot spots* (areas where genetic loss most commonly occurs) harbor the most important tumor suppressors genes in PDA: CDKN2A (9p), TP53 (19p), and SMAD4 (18q).

CDKN2A (p16) is inactivated in roughly 95% of PDAs, either through homozygous deletion (deletion of both alleles), somatic mutation combined with LOH (deletion of one allele), or promoter hypermethylation. Inactivation of the gene abrogates the RB1-mediated G1/S checkpoint in the cell cycle (which allows unchecked inhibition of RB1 by CDK4), promoting cell cycle progression and cancer cell proliferation.[42,43] TP53 mutations combined with LOH also occur in the majority of PDAs (~75%).[44] TP53 is a critical component of the DNA damage response. In the face of a cytotoxic stress, TP53 induces cell cycle arrest (at G1 or G2 of the cell cycle), allowing cells to repair their DNA prior to DNA synthesis or mitosis. Thus, TP53 loss contributes to chromosome instability and aneuploidy observed in PDA.[45] TP53 has been targeted experimentally by reactivating the mutant isoform[46] or by targeting the G2/M checkpoint with WEE1 inhibitors

(TP53-deficient tumors are particularly dependent on the G2/M checkpoint).[47] SMAD4/DPC4 is inactivated in roughly half of PDAs through either homozygous deletion or mutation combined with LOH.[48,49] SMAD4 is part of the transforming growth factor β (TGFβ) receptor pathway, and like the other two aforementioned tumor suppressor genes, regulates the cell cycle at the G1/S checkpoint.[28] Interestingly, preservation of SMAD4 protein expression is associated with a local predominant progression pattern in PDA, which could be used to guide patient selection for radiotherapy.[49]

A group of genome maintenance genes (BRCA2, PALB2, FANCC, FANCG) involved in the Fanconi anemia DNA repair pathway (mutated in <10% of PDAs) are particularly intriguing because tumors deficient in this pathway are highly susceptible to DNA damaging agents and poly(ADP-ribose) polymerase (PARP) inhibitor therapy.[28] Mutations in these genes are often present in the germline, and will be discussed further in the section on genetic syndromes associated with pancreatic cancer.

Analyses of laser capture microdissected pancreatic tissues have elucidated the chronologic sequence of major genetic changes in pancreatic tumorigenesis. Telomere shortening and *Kras* mutations are believed to be the earliest events (PanIN-1)[50,51]; *p16* loss occurs at the PanIN-2 stage[52]; and TP53, SMAD4, and BRCA2 inactivation occur later during the PanIN-3 stage (see Fig. 49.2).[53,54] Major chromosome instability, characterized by large-scale allelic copy number changes, is rarely observed in PanIN lesions, and is principally limited to LOH *hot spots*.[55–57]

Iacobuzio-Donahue and colleagues[49] recently launched into pioneering work by extending the molecular progression model of pancreatic cancer to the most advanced stages of disease, through a rapid autopsy program in which primary tumors and paired metastases were sequenced and compared. The investigators distinguished *founder mutations* (those that arise early in tumorigenesis and are present throughout a tumor; about two-thirds of mutations) from *progressor mutations* (mutated in subclonal populations of cells, and absent in the parental clones; about one-third of mutations).[58] Interestingly, progressor mutations that existed throughout a metastatic deposit were also identified in certain microdissected foci in the primary tumor, but not throughout the primary. This finding demonstrated that parent clones giving rise to specific metastases can actually be defined and mapped in the primary tumor. Although previous sequencing studies highlighted intertumoral heterogeneity, this study was the first to identify intratumoral genetic heterogeneity in PDAs, with profound implications on therapy.

Roughly 10% of PDAs are familial, and only 10% of the familial subgroup are associated with a previously defined genetic syndrome.[59] Table 49.2 summarizes those familial syndromes and

TABLE 49.2

Familial Disorders Linked to Predisposition to Pancreatic Ductal Adenocarcinoma

Disease	Gene/Pathway	Lifetime Risk
Inherited pancreatitis	SPINK1/PRSS1	40%
Peutz-Jeghers syndrome	LKB1	30%
Familial atypical multiple mole melanoma (FAMMM)	CDKN2A	15%
Hereditary breast and ovarian cancer	BRCA2	5%
Familial breast cancer	PALB2	?
Ataxia telangiectasia	ATM	?
Familial (>3 FDRs)	Unknown	40%
Familial (2 FDRs)	Unknown	10%
Familial (1 FDRs)	Unknown	6%

FDR, first-degree relative.

genetic defects that have been identified in pancreatic cancer kindreds. Hereditary breast and ovarian cancer is the most common familial syndrome, and the Peutz-Jeghers syndrome confers the highest lifetime risk. Importantly, several of the familial syndromes are associated with defects in DNA repair pathways (BRCA2, PALB2), which likely render tumors particularly susceptible to therapy with DNA damaging agents (e.g., mitomycin C, platinum agents) and PARP inhibitors.[11] Other genetic predisposition alterations, such as single nucleotide polymorphisms (SNP) likely play a role in cancer risk, but remain to be fully characterized. Ongoing whole-exome sequencing efforts in familial patients will almost certainly uncover additional genetic abnormalities that predispose individuals to PDA.

There are currently no universal guidelines or proven strategies for screening high-risk individuals. The Cancer of the Pancreas Screening (CAPS) project has been the principal mechanism to study this patient population and generate recommendations. In one CAPS study, 225 asymptomatic, high-risk individuals were screened with magnetic resonance imaging (MRI), computed tomography (CT) scans, or endoscopic ultrasound (EUS) and the results were interpreted in a blinded fashion. An abnormality was identified in 92 patients (42%), and 5 were recommended to undergo a pancreatectomy (2%). High-grade dysplasia was present in three out of the five specimens.[60] These data highlight that while successes are possible, the general yield of screening programs, even in this high-risk group, is relatively low.

Recently, a 49 member multidisciplinary panel made the following recommendations (with varying degrees of agreement amongst panelists): candidates for screening include FDRs of individuals with familial pancreatic cancer (at least two FDRs); patients with Peutz-Jeghers syndrome; and p16, BRCA2, and HNPCC mutation carriers with one affected FDR. There was also consensus that EUS and MRI were the preferred surveillance strategies. Routine surveillance should be performed annually, and suspicious solid masses should be further evaluated by CT scanning. Screening should begin around 50 years of age.[61]

Other Aspects of PDA Biology

Genetically engineered mouse models (GEMM) of PDA have provided a valuable research tool to study PDA biology.[62] The workhorse of pancreatic cancer research in this area has been the conditional Kras model, where pancreas-specific promoters are exploited to target oncogenic Kras expression exclusively to the pancreas. Kras mutant mice develop pancreatic precursor lesions (e.g., PanIN lesions). Compound mutant mice with an additional genetic abnormality (e.g., mutant TP53 or CDKN2A) develop invasive and metastatic PDA, simulating human PDA. Similarly, Kras mutant mice with induced pancreatitis also develop invasive PDA. Genetic variations have also been generated that recapitulate pancreatic cystic tumors (SMAD4 loss or TGFα overexpression). The contributions of these models have been immeasurable. For instance, cell lineage tracing experiments in GEMMs reveal that PDA likely originates from acinar or centroacinar cells, as opposed to ductal cells (i.e., acinar-to-ductal metaplasia). GEMMs are enabling the development of molecular and bioimaging assays to detect late PanIN and early invasive lesions. Because GEMMs develop tumors with a robust stroma compartment, therapeutic strategies targeting the stroma can be tested. Early results suggest that this strategy enhances therapeutic efficacy of standard cytotoxic therapy. Finally, these models can be used to test and refine chemoprevention strategies before moving to humans.

Cancer genetics (e.g., mutations) have been prioritized over the last few decades in PDA cancer research, in large part because of the reproducibility of the findings and because the genetic model of tumorigenesis is straightforward and accepted. However, it is now clear that other molecular changes are also paramount for PDA development and maintenance. These include epigenetic abnormalities (methylation and histone modification), transcriptional regulation, and posttranscriptional regulation (microRNAs and RNA binding proteins).[28]

Less Common Pancreatic Cancers

Acinar Cell Carcinoma

Acinar cell carcinomas may have a slightly better prognosis (median survival of 33 months) than conventional PDA. The presentation is similar, except that patients may occasionally develop a paraneoplastic syndrome related to lipase hypersecretion, leading to subcutaneous fat necrosis and polyarthralgia. Microscopically, tumors grow in a trabecular pattern with minimal intervening stroma. Immunohistochemical confirmation is made with positive labeling for pancreatic enzymes (e.g., lipase, trypsin, chymotrypsin, amylase).[63] Cystic variants have been reported as well, and described as acinar cystadenoma or cystadenocarcinoma.[26] Twice the number of somatic mutations per tumor is present (~130 per tumor) compared to PDA, and allelic loss is comparable (27% fractional loss). Whole-exome sequencing did not reveal a consistent genetic pattern; no gene was mutated in more than 30% of cancers, and mutant genes previously identified in diverse pancreatic tumor types (e.g., TP53, SMAD4, RNF43, MEN1, GNAS) and nonpancreatic tumors (e.g., BRAF, PTEN, RB1, APC) were identified. Additionally, some mutant familial genes were identified (e.g., ATM, BRCA2, PALB2), suggesting that this tumor may arise in a familial pattern.[64] Interestingly, no Kras mutations were identified.

Pancreatoblastoma

Pancreatoblastoma is the most common pancreatic malignancy in children and usually occurs in the first 8 years of life. These tumors have been associated with the Beckwith-Wiedmann and familial adenomatous polyposis syndromes. Elevated levels of serum α-fetoprotein and hormones have been described. Cures are often achievable with resection in children, although one-third of patients present with metastatic disease. Cases have been reported in adults as well, with survival after resection that is comparable to conventional PDA.[65] Microscopically, these tumors contain acinar cells, but other cell types (e.g., neuroendocrine, ductal) are often present. Pancreatoblastomas have been whole-exome sequenced in only two adult cases.[64] These tumors acquire relatively few mutations (~15 per tumor), and SMAD4 and CTNNB1 are typical. Kras mutations have not been reported.

Intraductal Papillary Mucinous Neoplasms

Intraductal papillary mucinous neoplasms (IPMN) are mucin-producing cystic neoplasms that arise from (and therefore communicate with) pancreatic ducts.[66] Similar to PanIN lesions, they follow a progression pattern: low-grade dysplasia, moderate-grade dysplasia, high-grade dysplasia, and frank invasive carcinoma. Benign IPMNs are subgrouped according to their papillary appearance on microscopy (see Fig. 49.1), with each type associated with a particular mucin expression pattern: intestinal (MUC5AC, MUC2), gastric-foveolar (MUC5AC, MUC6), pancreatobiliary (MUC5AC, MUC1), and intraductal oncocytic neoplasm (MUC1, MUC6). Clinically, IPMNs are classified as involving the side-branch ducts or the main-pancreatic duct, with some tumors involving both of these. IPMNs are the most common pancreatic cystic neoplasms and with increased usage of high-resolution cross-sectional imaging, are believed to develop in roughly 1% to 5% of the general population.[67] Although all benign IPMNs are technically *premalignant*, there is a wide range of malignant potential amongst encountered cysts. For instance, main duct IPMNs harbor associated cancers 40% of the time, whereas small side-branched IPMNs without any concerning radiographic features have a cancer risk closer to 5% or less.[68] Thus, there has been considerable effort to try to determine which IPMNs harbor invasive cancer or are at highest risk for malignant transformation and warrant resection. The Sendai guidelines recommend resection for IPMNs that are either symptomatic, >3 cm in diameter, contain solid components (e.g., mural nodules), have malignant cells on cytology, or involve the main pancreatic duct.[68] Invasive cancer associated with IPMNs are most commonly either tubular (conventional PDA) or colloid subtypes. The former is typically more aggressive and develops from pancreatobiliary IPMNs, whereas the latter usually develops from intestinal subtypes. Although IPMN-associated cancers have a more favorable prognosis than conventional PDA, this has been attributed to the lower stage at diagnosis; when matched stage for stage, the two pancreatic cancer types are associated with similar outcomes.[69] Moreover, a recent multi-institution analysis of IPMNs with small foci of invasion (all <2 cm invasive component) indicates a significant recurrence risk (~20%) regardless of the size of the invasive component (Jordan M. Winter, MD, unpublished, July 2014).

Whole-exome sequencing of IPMN lesions revealed roughly half the number of mutations (~27 per tumor) compared to PDA. There was a high incidence of RNF43 mutations, which is a tumor suppressor with E3 ubiquitin ligase activity (involved in protein degradation).[70] Additionally, Kras and GNAS mutations occurred with high frequency.

Mucinous Cystic Neoplasms

Mucinous cystic neoplasms (MCN) are typically large cysts lined by tall, columnar epithelium (see Fig. 49.1). Benign MCNs are categorized similar to IPMNs from low- to high-grade dysplasia, and roughly one-third of cases harbor invasive cancer. Additionally, RNF43 and Kras mutations are frequently present (as with IPMNs). Distinguishing features of MCNs (from IPMNs) include a large predominance in woman, the cysts are typically localized on the left side of the pancreas, ovarian stroma underlying the epithelial component is pathognomonic (even in men), there is no communication with the pancreatic duct, and GNAS mutations have not been identified.[26,70]

Solid-Pseudopapillary Neoplasms

Solid-pseudopapillary neoplasms (SPNs) solid and cystic tumors are eponymously referred to as Hamoudi or Franz tumors. They typically occur in young women and may arise throughout the gland. Histologically, they consist of noncohesive polygonal cells that form solid masses, but develop cystic components over time with frequent intracystic hemorrhage. The tumors are considered low-grade malignancies, with a 10% risk of lymph node spread in resected specimens, and a 95% lifetime recurrence-free survival rate after resection.[71] SPNs develop fewer than five somatic mutations per tumor, but virtually all SPNs harbor CTNNB1 (β-catenin) mutations. This molecular abnormality is believed to contribute to the poor cohesion between cells apparent on microscopy (wild type β-catenin interacts with E-cadherin at cell–cell junctions).

ENDOCRINE PANCREATIC CANCERS

The classification of pancreatic neuroendocrine tumors (PNET) has been challenging based on the heterogenous biology of this tumor type. Recent staging systems have been adopted based on size and lymph node metastases, with different versions in the United States (AJCC 7th ed. 2010, same as exocrine pancreatic cancer) and Europe (European Neuroendocrine Tumor Society [ENETS]).[72] The ENETS system also considers biologic parameters and has simplified the World Health Organization classification according to the following scheme: G1 (well differentiated, <2 mitoses per 10 High power field (HPF), <3% KI67 index); G2 (well differentiated, intermediate grade: 2 to 20 mitoses per 10 HPF, 3% to 20% KI67 index); and G3 (high grade or poorly differentiated: >20 mitoses per 10 HPF, >20% KI67 index).[73] Typically, G1 tumors are considered benign and cured with resection, whereas G2 tumors are considered malignant. However, the distinction (benign versus malignant) is not always clear. Older studies observed that half of PNETs were nonfunctional and half were functional due to the presence of measurable hormones in serum.[74] The balance has shifted dramatically toward nonfunctional tumors being more common, in large part due to small, incidentally discovered PNETs identified on cross-sectional imaging obtained for nonpancreatic reasons.

Pancreatic neuroendocrine cancers have an incidence of roughly 0.2 out of 100,000 (versus 12 out of 100,00 for PDAs), yet autopsy studies show that small PNETs are very common (~10% of deceased individuals).[75] They comprise roughly 5% of all resected pancreatic cancers (on par with IPMN associated cancers).[27] PNETs are typically well demarcated and hypervascular. Therefore, they focally enhance on the arterial phase in imaging studies with intravenous contrast. Microscopically, neoplastic cells are arranged in a nested fashion with a high density of intratumoral microvessels (in contrast to PDA). The majority of well-differentiated PNETs have an indolent course and are cured with surgery alone. Even patients with metastatic disease have a 5-year survival around 50%.[72] Insulinomas are the most common functional PNETs (30% to 45%) and symptoms are associated with excessive endogenous insulin production (Whipple triad: documented hypoglycemia, symptoms of hypoglycemia, improved symptoms with correction of hypoglycemia).[76] Gastrinomas comprise roughly 20% of functional PNETs, and cause peptic ulcer disease and diarrhea from hypergastrinemia. Less common functional PNETs include glucagonomas (associated with glucose intolerance and migratory necrolytic erythema), VIPomas (watery diarrhea), and somatostatinomas (steatorrhea, diabetes mellitus, and gallstones). Familial syndromes associated with the development of PNETs include multiple endocrine neoplasia 1 (MEN1 gene), von Hippel-Lindau disease (VHL), neurofibromatosis (NF1), and tuberous sclerosis (TSC1 or TSC2).

The genetic landscape of PNETs has now been defined through whole-exome sequencing.[77] Compared to PDAs, there are fewer somatic mutations per tumor (~16). Kras mutations have not been observed. Commonly mutated genes included MEN1 (44% of PNETs), chromatin remodeling genes (43%: DAXX and ATRX), and mTOR pathway genes (15%: phosphatase and tensin homolog [PTEN], PIK3CA, and TSC2). This latter gene group likely renders many PNETs vulnerable to systemic targeted therapy using mTOR inhibitors. Although surgery is the principal therapy for local disease, treatment options have greatly expanded for advanced disease, and include local liver-directed therapies (radiofrequency ablation), regional liver-directed therapies (bland, chemo, and radioembolization), and systemic therapies (cytotoxic drugs, targeted agents, somatostatin analogs including radio-labeled drugs). The complex management of PNETs is discussed in other reviews on the subject.[78]

STAGE I AND II: LOCALIZED PANCREATIC DUCTAL ADENOCARCINOMA

Anatomy

The evaluation and treatment of localized pancreatic cancer requires a strong understanding of the anatomy of the pancreas and nearby structures. The pancreas is an elongated gland in the retroperitoneum that crosses the midline at the L2 spinal level (Fig. 49.3). It is bounded anteriorly by the stomach and posteriorly by the inferior vena cava, aorta, left adrenal gland, and left kidney. The descriptive anatomy of the gland is grossly separated into four components. The head is the right-most portion, and sits within the duodenal C-loop. It includes parenchyma to the right of the superior mesenteric vessels and contains the uncinate process, which projects inferomedially, extending to the right lateral border of the superior mesenteric artery. The common bile duct runs within (or rarely just posterior) to the pancreatic head and enters the duodenum at the ampulla of Vater with the main pancreatic duct. Moving leftward, the neck of the pancreas lies anterior to the superior mesenteric vein–portal vein axis. The superior mesenteric vessels run posterior to the pancreatic neck, and course inferiorly across the anterior border of the third portion of the duodenum. The body of the pancreas extends to the left of the superior mesenteric vessels. The gland transitions distally into the pancreatic tail anterior to the left kidney, and courses toward the splenic hilum.

Presentation

The most common presenting symptoms associated with PDA located in the right side of the pancreas (head, neck, or uncinate process) include jaundice (75%), weight loss (50%), abdominal pain (40%), or nausea (10%).[27] Jaundice occurs as a result of obstruction of the common bile duct and is often associated with pruritus. Other symptoms or findings associated with an obstructed bile duct include acholic stools and tea-colored urine. An obstructed pancreatic duct may induce acute pancreatitis and result in exocrine insufficiency associated with steatorrhea. Patients with left-sided PDAs (body or tail) typically experience abdominal pain, back pain, and nausea. New onset DM (within 1 year of diagnosis) occurs in roughly 10% of patients with PDA, based on our own institutional experience and others (unpublished).[79]

PRACTICE OF ONCOLOGY

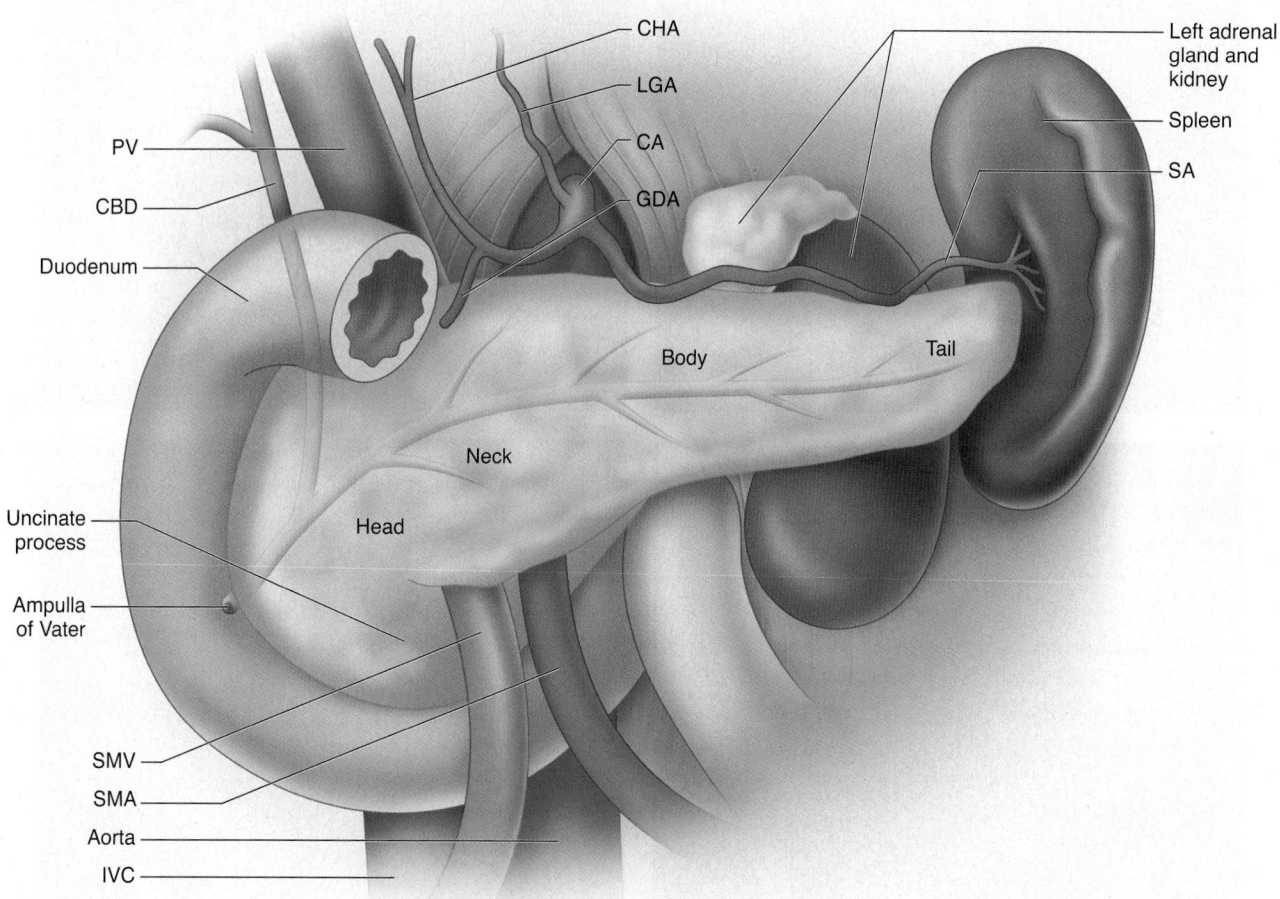

Figure 49.3 Pancreatic and peripancreatic anatomy. CBD, common bile duct; PV, portal vein; CHA, common hepatic artery; LGA, left gastric artery; CA, celiac axis; GDA, gastroduodenal artery; SA, splenic artery; SMV, superior mesenteric vein; SMA, superior mesenteric artery; IVC, inferior vena cava. (Courtesy of Jennifer Brumbaugh, Department of Surgery, Thomas Jefferson University.)

Evaluation and Assessing Resectability

Although periampullary cancer (adenocarcinoma of the pancreas, ampulla of Vater, bile duct, or periampullary duodenum) should be considered in any patient who presents with a conjugated hyperbilirubinemia, the likelihood is highest in older patients (e.g., >55 years). In individuals with an expected pancreatic cancer, a thorough history and physical should be performed, followed by appropriate imaging for staging and to assess resectability. Critical findings on physical exam include scleral icterus, jaundice, and lymphadenopathy (e.g., Sister Mary Joseph or Virchow nodes). A chest x-ray or chest CT scan is performed to assess for pulmonary metastases and as a baseline study. Either a high-quality MRI or CT scan of the abdomen is performed to evaluate the pancreas and measure the extent of disease. We typically prefer CT for its superior resolution and detailed depiction of the relevant vasculature. Water is administered as oral contrast, and nonionic intravenous contrast is rapidly injected. Slices are captured at 1-mm intervals from the diaphragm to the iliac crests at three different times or phases: early arterial, late arterial, and venous. Multiplanar reformatting and three-dimensional (3D) surface rendering is performed during the early arterial and venous phases (Fig. 49.4).[80] Positron-emission tomography (PET)/CT scans do

not add much additional value and are not routinely performed in the initial assessment for resectability.

Resection is attempted if (1) patients are medically fit for a pancreatectomy, (2) there is no evidence of metastases, and (3) patients are believed to have *resectable* disease. Resectability is ultimately decided by the operating surgeon, but general guidelines have been proposed and are based on the likelihood of achieving a complete, margin-negative resection.[81,82] Resectability equates to a high probability of an R_0 resection; borderline resectability equates to a likely result of an R_1 resection (positive microscopic margins); and unresectable (or locally advanced) PDA is likely to result in R_2 resection (residual macroscopic disease). Resectable lesions do not invade the superior mesenteric artery (SMA), celiac axis (CA), common hepatic artery (CHA), or superior mesenteric–portal vein axis (SMV-PV). In contrast, locally advanced lesions encase (i.e., >180° invasion) any of the previously mentioned arteries or occlude the SMV-PV such that no reconstructive options remain. Borderline resectable lesions involve the visceral vessels to a lesser extent; they can abut the visceral arteries (<180° invasion), distort the visceral veins, or even occlude the SMV-PV, but with venous reconstruction still technically feasible (Table 49.3).[83] Most pancreatic surgeons offer patients with resectable lesions an attempt at resection (although some centers advocate neoadjuvant treatment prior to resection even for resectable lesions[84]). Patients with locally advanced lesions are recommended

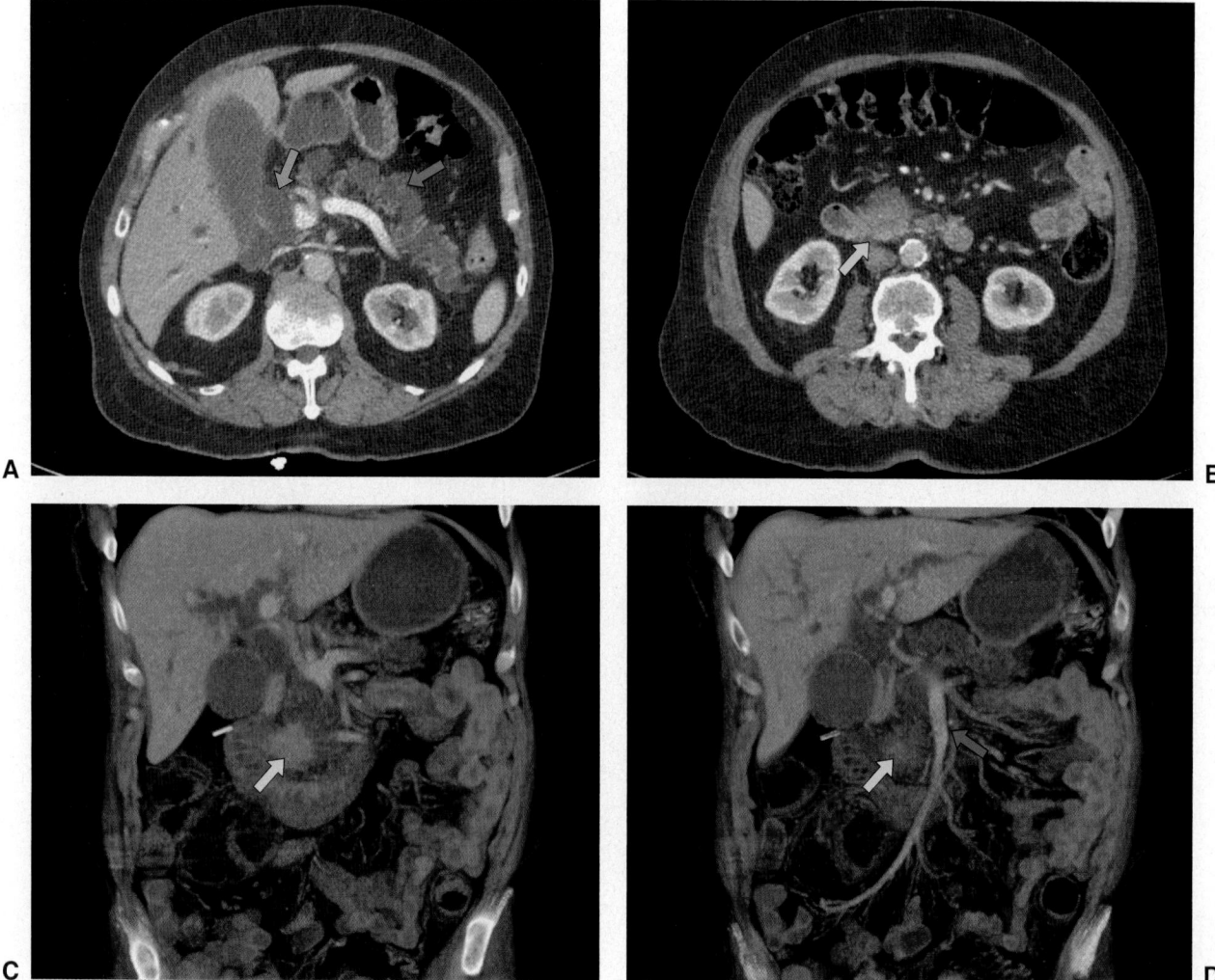

Figure 49.4 Slices from a triphasic CT scan in a patient with resectable pancreatic cancer. **(A)** Late arterial phase. Double duct sign with dilated common bile and pancreatic ducts, and an atrophic pancreatic body. **(B)** Mass. **(C)** Coronal reconstructions, venous phase, with the mass apparent, and **(D)** clearly away from the superior mesenteric–portal vein axis (SMV/PV) axis. *Yellow arrow* = PDA; *green arrow* = common bile duct; *red arrow* = pancreatic duct; and *blue arrow* = SMV. (Courtesy of Jennifer Brumbaugh, Department of Surgery, Thomas Jefferson University.)

TABLE 49.3

Criteria for Reseectability

Vessel	Resectable R_0 Resection Likely	Borderline Resectable R_1 Resection Likely	Locally Advanced R_2 Resection Likely
SMA	No abutment	Tumor abutment	Tumor encasement
Celiac axis/ hepatic artery	No abutment	Tumor abutment	Tumor encasement
SMV–PV	Abutment may be present but no vein distortion	Vein Distortion or short-segment occlusion with suitable vessel above and below	Occluded and no technical option for reconstruction

Note: R_0 = gross total resection; histologically <u>negative</u> margins.
R_1 resection = gross total resection; one or more histologically <u>positive</u> margins.
R_2 resection = subtotal resection, visible tumor unresected.
Abutment is ≤180° vessel circumference; encasement is >180° vessel circumference.
SMA, superior mesenteric artery; SMV–PV, superior mesenteric vein–portal vein.
Modified from Varadhachary GR, Tamm EP, Abbruzzese JL, et al. Borderline resectable pancreatic cancer: definitions, management, and role of preoperative therapy. *Ann Surg Oncol* 2006;13:1035–1046.

to undergo palliative treatment without the intent to cure. Considerable debate remains for borderline PDAs; resection may be offered, but increasingly, neoadjuvant treatment is recommended for even abutment or narrowing of the SMV-PV.[81] Neoadjuvant chemotherapy (± radiation) can facilitate resection, and may improve the likelihood of a complete resection with negative margins, even in the absence of a radiographic response.[85]

Obtaining a tissue diagnosis is not essential for all cases. Indications include instances when (1) neoadjuvant treatment is advised or (2) the pretest probability of an alternative diagnosis is considerable (e.g., suspicion for benign causes of pancreatitis, medically managed neoplasms such as lymphoma, or a benign stricture). In these instances, an EUS with fine-needle aspiration (FNA) biopsy is an effective method for obtaining tissue and has an accuracy in excess of 90%.[86] When the diagnosis is clear based on imaging and history, it is appropriate to proceed to attempted resection without a preoperative tissue diagnosis. Similarly, placement of an endoscopic biliary stent is frequently performed in jaundiced patients preoperatively, but is essential in only selected cases. A multicenter prospective and randomized trial compared routine preoperative biliary drainage with delayed resection to early surgery without stenting in jaundiced patients with pancreatic cancer. Serious complications were increased nearly twofold in the routine biliary drainage group (74% versus 39%; p <0.001), suggesting that biliary decompression be reserved for jaundiced patients unable to undergo resection in a short-time frame (1 to 2 weeks).[86] A pancreaticoduodenectomy is safely performed, even when the total bilirubin is markedly elevated. Patients, who are otherwise healthy, with normal renal function and clotting parameters will usually tolerate a safely performed pancreaticoduodenectomy with a total bilirubin as high as 20 mg/dL.

Surgery

Technical aspects of a pancreatectomy are detailed elsewhere and are well beyond the scope of this chapter, hence will only be reviewed briefly here. For right-sided pancreatic cancers, a pancreaticoduodenectomy (PD) is performed. The specimen includes the gallbladder, duodenum, head of the pancreas (the pancreatic transection typically is at the level of the neck), proximal jejunum, and distal common bile duct. The most proximal retained jejunum is brought up into the right upper quadrant, and three anastomoses to the pancreas remnant, common hepatic duct, and proximal duodenum (or stomach) are performed (Fig. 49.5A). A distal pancreatectomy for PDA involves resection of the pancreatic body and tail, with an en bloc splenectomy performed to ensure a proper lymphadenectomy. The transected surface of the

pancreatic remnant is closed with suture (Fig. 49.5B) or staples. A central pancreatectomy or local excision for a PDA is seldom if ever performed for PDA due to inadequate lymph node harvest.

A minimally invasive pancreatectomy using laparoscopy or a robotic-assisted approach may be safely performed. Although a minimally invasive approach is more common for benign and premalignant lesions, a presumed diagnosis of PDA is not a contraindication.[87] A meta-analysis comparing open versus laparoscopic distal pancreatectomies for PDA revealed similar oncologic and pathologic outcomes in the two groups. Patients undergoing laparoscopy had a shorter postoperative stay by 4 days, less blood loss, and fewer surgical site infections.[88] Importantly, studies comparing the two techniques have not been prospective and randomized, and are, therefore, all subject to selection bias, with the more difficult resections falling into the open group. Although most high-volume pancreatic centers offer minimally invasive left-sided resections, laparoscopic PD is more technically challenging, and only a handful of centers have a significant experience.[89] These centers report comparable outcomes with minimally invasive versus open pancreatic surgery in their own experience, although an advantage of laparoscopic PD has not yet been proven in a prospective and randomized study.

International Study Group of Pancreatic Surgery Contributions

Surgically related mortality after PD has improved dramatically over the last 3 decades, and is lower than 5% at most high volume centers.[27] However, morbidity remains high (~40%). The most common complications include pancreatic leak (20%), delayed gastric emptying (15%), and wound infection (10%). Bile and duodenal leaks occur in roughly 3% and 1% of patients, respectively.[27] The greatest limitation to studies focused on pancreatectomy-related complications has been a lack of standard definitions across institutions, making comparisons between institutions' reports difficult. The formation of an International Study Group of Pancreatic Surgery (ISGPS) to address this issue has been a great advance in pancreatic surgery–related outcomes research. The group has published consensus criteria and definitions for complication grading on the following pancreatic-specific morbidities: postoperative pancreatic fistula (leak),[90] delayed gastric emptying,[91] and postpancreatectomy hemorrhage.[92] In addition, the group established concrete guidelines on reporting features and management of the pancreatic remnant/anastomosis (e.g., duct size, gland texture, mobilization distance, type of anastomosis, suture used, use of stent).[93] Definitions of postpancreatectomy-related mortality, bile leak,[94] and wound infection also vary in the literature, and

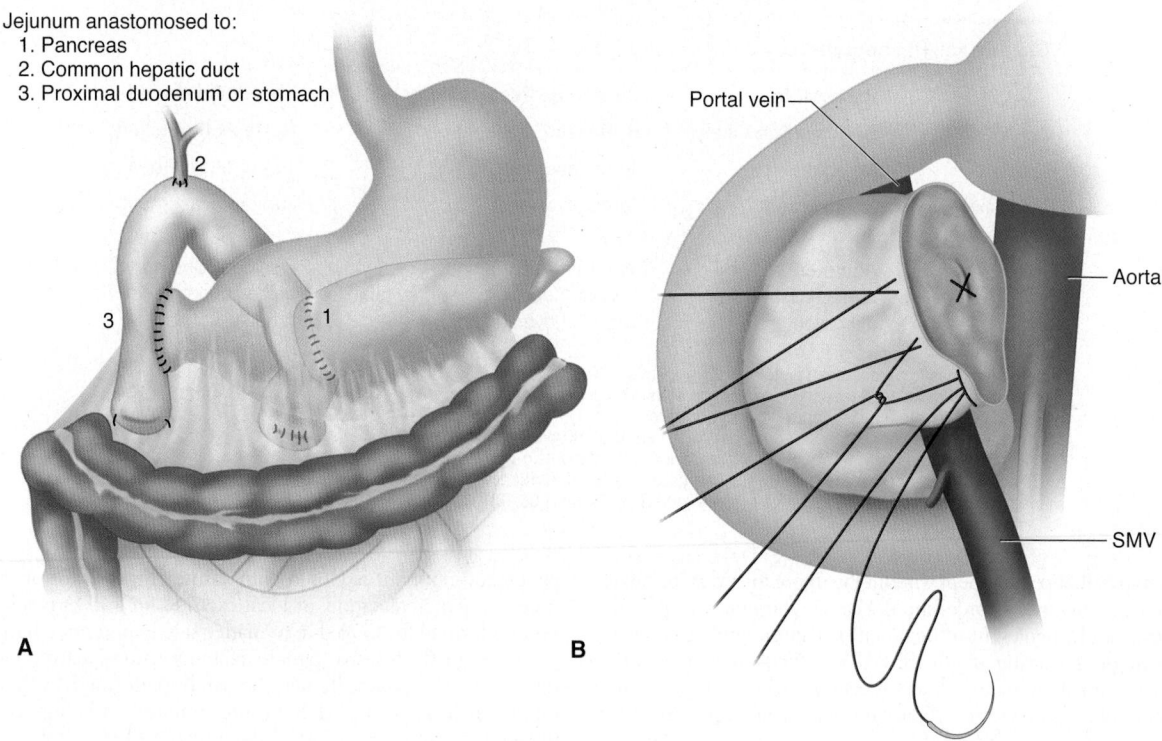

Jejunum anastomosed to:
1. Pancreas
2. Common hepatic duct
3. Proximal duodenum or stomach

A

B

Figure 49.5 (A) Standard reconstruction after a pancreaticoduodenectomy, with an end-to-side pancreaticojejunostomy, an end-to-side hepatic jejunostomy, and a retro-colic and end-to-side duodenojejunostomy. **(B)** Suture closure of the pancreatic remnant after distal pancreatectomy.

a strategy to standardize terms and complication grading for these outcomes would enhance the surgical literature.

Surgical Trials

There have been numerous prospective and randomized surgical trials that have shaped the surgical management of PDA. A trial unique to PDA, compared to other common cancers, is a study demonstrating superiority of resection over best nonoperative therapy for the management of resectable disease.[95] A total of 42 patients in Japan with resectable PDA were randomized to either standard pancreatectomy without adjuvant treatment or to chemoradiation alone (50.4 Gy with continuous fluorouracil [5-FU] at 200 mg/m^2 per day) without surgery. Randomization occurred at laparotomy and patients randomized to chemoradiation had only an open biopsy and abdominal closure. The only multivariate predictor of survival in the study was the treatment group (hazard ratio [HR] = 0.4; p = 0.02), with the group undergoing resecting having superior survival (median overall survival (OS), 13 versus 9 months).

Pancreaticoduodenectomy

A comprehensive list of surgical trials in patients undergoing pancreaticoduodenectomy is provided in Table 49.4. Regarding technical aspects of the operation, one of the more studied questions compares pylorus preserving pancreaticoduodenectomy (PPPD) to distal gastrectomy plus pancreaticoduodenectomy (classic PD).[96–102] Karanicolas et al.[97] performed a meta-analysis of six randomized trials including 574 patients. PPPD was associated with a reduced operative time by more than 1 hour (p <0.001), less blood loss (284 mL; p <0.001), and fewer blood transfusions. There was a nonsignificant trend toward improved mortality in the same direction (0.4; p = 0.09). There was not a significant difference in delayed gastric emptying. Multiple randomized studies have also

examined the location of the enteroenterostomy (antecolic versus retrocolic), and no significant differences were observed.[103–107]

A postoperative pancreatic fistula (POPF) remains the most challenging complication after PD. Clinically significant leaks (e.g., requiring treatment intervention) occur in roughly 10% of cases. Risk factors include soft pancreatic texture, a fatty pancreas, a small pancreatic duct, high intraoperative blood loss, and a high postoperative serum amylase level.[108,109] Numerous randomized trials have attempted to reduce the pancreatic leak rate, although few have succeeded. Ineffective interventions include fibrin glue,[110,111] octreotide,[112–119] and internal pancreatic stenting.[27] Mixed results have been reported with pancreaticogastrostomy (versus standard pancreaticojejunostomy).[120–126] The pancreaticojejunostomy *technique* was recently examined, comparing a two-layered invagination technique with interrupted outer stitches and a continuous inner layer, against a duct-to-mucosa technique. The pancreatic leak rate was more than twofold higher with the latter approach (7% grade B/C versus 17%; p = 0.03).[127] A binding pancreaticojejunostomy (versus invagination) is a second technique shown to have a decreased pancreatic leak rate. With this technique, an end-to-end pancreaticojejunostomy is performed; 3 cm of the pancreatic remnant is mobilized and telescoped within the jejunum. No leaks were observed in 106 patients in the latter group, although these data have not yet been replicated.[128] Interestingly, there now have been three randomized trials showing a lower pancreatic leak rate associated with external pancreatic duct stenting (the pancreatic duct stent is brought out through the bowel and skin as a drain),[129–131] whereas a fourth study revealed no benefit.[132] In the past, trials using somatostatin or its analogs have had mixed outcomes in lowering pancreatic leak rates. Recently, a phase III trial using pasireotide (SOM230, a potent somatostatin analog) was completed at Memorial Sloan-Kettering Cancer Center, and revealed a statistically significant lower pancreatic leak rate in patients receiving subcutaneous injections of the study drug

TABLE 49.4

Randomized Surgical Trials with Pancreaticoduodenectomy

Author	Year	Trial	Result
Doi[95]	2008	Surgery vs. chemoradiation for PDA	↑ Survival with surgery
Riall[137]	2005	PD vs. PD with lymphadenectomy	= Survival
Pedrazzoli[136]	1998	PD vs. PD with lymphadenectomy	= Survival
Farnell[135]	2005	PD vs. PD with lymphadenectomy	= Survival
Brennan[138]	1994	Preoperative TPN vs. none	↑ Morbidity with TPN
Ke[133]	2013	Roux-en-Y PJ vs. standard	↓ Grade B POPF with Roux-en-Y
Fischer[281]	2010	Hemodilution vs. standard intraoperative IVF	↑ POPF with hemodilution
Uemura[282]	2008	Ulinastatin vs. placebo	↓ Pancreatitis with ulinastatin
Jo[283]	2006	Glutamine supplement vs. none	= Morbidity
Conlon[139]	2001	Drain vs. no drain	= Complications and mortality
Bassi[284]	2010	Late vs. early drain removal	↑ Complications with late
Van Buren[140]	2013	Drain vs. no drain	↑ Mortality with drain
Van der Gaag[86]	2010	Preoperative biliary drainage vs. none	↑ Morbidity with drainage
Poon[130]	2007	External MPD stent vs. no stent	↓ POPF with external stent
Kuroki[285]	2011	External MPD stent vs. no stent	= POPF
Pessaux[129]	2011	External MPD stent vs. no stent	↓ POPF with external stent
Motoi[131]	2012	External MPD stent vs. no stent	↓ POPF with external stent
Kamoda[286]	2008	External MPD stent vs. internal stent	= POPF
Tani[287]	2010	External MPD stent vs. internal stent	= POPF
Winter[27]	2006	Internal MPD stent vs. no stent	= POPF
Yeo[126]	1995	PG vs. PJ	= POPF
Arnaud[121]	1999	PG vs. PJ	↓ POPF with PG
Takano[125]	2000	PG vs. PJ	↓ POPF with PG
Duffas[123]	2005	PG vs. PJ	= POPF
Bassi[122]	2005	PG vs. PJ	= POPF
Fernandez-Cruz[124]	2008	PG vs. PJ	↓ POPF with PG
Klempa[119]	1991	Octreotide vs. none	= POPF
Beguiristain[113]	1995	Octreotide vs. none	= POPF
Yeo[112]	2000	Octreotide vs. placebo	= POPF
Gouillat[115]	2001	Octreotide vs. placebo	= POPF
Shan[117]	2003	Octreotide vs. none	= POPF
Kollmar[116]	2008	Octreotide vs. placebo	= POPF
Fernandez-Cruz[114]	2013	Octreotide vs. placebo	= POPF
Wang[118]	2013	Octreotide vs. placebo	= POPF
Allen[a]	2013	SOM230 vs. placebo	↓ POPF with SOM230
Reissman[288]	1995	MPD duct ligation vs. PJ	↑ POPF with ligation
Tran[289]	2002	MPD duct ligation vs. PJ	= POPF
Lillemoe[110]	2004	Fibrin glue to PJ vs. none	= POPF
Martin[111]	2013	Fibrin glue to PJ vs. none	= POPF
Bassi[290]	2003	Invagination PJ vs. duct-to-mucosa	= POPF
Berger[127]	2009	Invagination PJ vs. duct-to-mucosa	↓ POPF with invagination
Peng[128]	2007	Binding PJ vs. invagination	↓ POPF with binding PJ
Yeo[291]	1993	Erythromycin vs. placebo	↓ DGE with erythromycin
Tani[107]	2006	Antecolic vs. retrocolic DJ	↓ DGE with antecolic DJ
Gangavatiker[104]	2011	Antecolic vs. retrocolic DJ	= DGE

(continued)

Randomized Surgical Trials with Pancreaticoduodenectomy *(continued)*

Author	Year	Trial	Result
Imamura[103]	2013	Antecolic vs. retrocolic DJ	= DGE
Tamandl[106]	2013	Antecolic vs. retrocolic DJ	= DGE
Eshuis[105]	2014	Antecolic vs. retrocolic DJ	= DGE
Paquet[99]	1998	PPPD vs. classic	= DGE
Bloechle[96]	1999	PPPD vs. classic	= DGE
Wenger[102]	1999	PPPD vs. classic	= Morbidity
Tran[101]	2004	PPPD vs. classic	= DGE
Lin[98]	2005	PPPD vs. classic	↑ DGE with PPPD
Seiler[107]	2005	PPPD vs. classic	= DGE

Note: Shading pattern highlights similar trials.
[a] Personal communication with senior author.
TPN, total parenteral nutrition; PJ, pancreaticojejunostomy; POPF, postoperative pancreatic fistula; IVF, intravenous fluid; MPD, main pancreatic duct; PG, pancreaticogastrostomy; DJ, duodenojejunostomy; DGE, delayed gastric emptying; PPPD, pylorus preserving pancreaticoduodenectomy.

(Peter J. Allen, email communication, January 2014). Roux-en-Y reconstruction performed to isolate the pancreaticojejunostomy (PJ) from the other two anastomoses did not decrease the overall leak rate, but the proportion of clinically significant leaks was substantially reduced (74% versus 29% of all leaks; p = 0.01).[133]

In addition to these important technical trials relevant to the management of right-sided pancreatic neoplasms, other studies have informed the management of patients undergoing PD. A group of studies established that a radical retroperitoneal lymphadenectomy does not confer improved cancer-specific survival (four randomized trials).[134–137] Additionally, routine adjuvant parenteral nutrition has proven to be detrimental.[138] A previous single-institution randomized trial suggested that routine nondrainage after a pancreatic resection is safe,[139] whereas a recent multi-institution and randomized study revealed a much higher mortality rate in patients without drains,[140] leaving this issue unresolved.

Distal Pancreatectomy

A distal pancreatectomy and splenectomy for left-sided PDA is a simpler operation than pancreaticoduodenectomy, yet also carries significant risk. POPF is the principal morbidity associated with distal pancreatectomy. Clinically significant leaks occur in roughly 10% of cases. In 10% to 20% of cases, a leak is appreciable as amylase-rich fluid in surgical drains, but does not add morbidity. There are now roughly a half-dozen randomized clinical trials examining the effect of pancreatic stump management on POPF, ranging from staplers to mattress sutures. In summary, no positive interventions have been discovered. The DISPACT trial was the largest of these trials. This European multi-institution study analyzed 352 patients, and compared stapled and hand-sewn closures. The pancreatic leak rate was roughly 30% in both groups (p = 0.56).[141] Fibrin sealant and falciform ligament patches have also been tested, with no observed benefit.[142, 143] Interestingly, ultrasonic dissection of the pancreas with ligation of all visualized ducts in nonfibrotic glands was associated with improved pancreatic leak rates compared to conventional division and suturing (n = 58, 4% versus 26%, p = 0.02). Roughly 20 4-0 silk ligatures were used per neck transection in the ultrasonic dissection group, and transection took 10 extra minutes, on average.[144]

Palliative Surgery

There have been five randomized trials directly comparing hepaticojejunostomy with endoscopic or percutaneous biliary decompression for patients with malignant periampullary obstruction.[145]

A meta-analysis revealed that OS is the same between the groups, although total hospital days after randomization was twofold more in the stenting group, principally related to recurrent biliary obstruction requiring intervention. The authors recommend that for patients projected to live more than 6 months, a surgical biliary (as well as gastric bypass) be considered. Two separate randomized studies have demonstrated that prophylactic gastrojejunostomy in nonobstructed patients decreased the absolute risk of subsequent gastric outlet obstruction by roughly 20%, but did not affect OS.[146,147] Finally, there is evidence that celiac neurolysis with alcohol injected at laparotomy in patients with unresectable disease improves quality of life and OS.[148]

Operative and Surgical Pathology Reporting

Just as the ISGPS has sought to standardize complication reporting, there have been efforts to standardize operative and pathology reporting to facilitate collaboration between institutions, establish a minimum standard of quality, and provide consistency to the literature. With regard to the operative dictation, a description of the clinical stage (relationship to mesenteric vessels and evidence of metastatic disease) is important. Specific mention of the liver, peritoneum, and small intestines is necessary. Blood loss and the need for transfusion are recorded. The surgical technique used to dissect the uncinate process should be described, as well as the management of the SMA and SMV (e.g., were they skeletonized? resected? the method of visceral vessel repair?). The anastomotic techniques need to be described. The important elements of the pancreaticojejunostomy have been addressed by the ISGPS, as mentioned previously.[93] If a frozen section analysis was performed, the results should be stated. Similarly, any gross residual disease must be reported.[149]

Standards for pathology reporting have been established by the College of American Pathologists, and protocols are available at the Web site (http://www.cap.org/apps/cap.portal). On the pathology review, tumor site (e.g., head, uncinate, body, tail), maximum tumor diameter (in centimeters), histologic type or subtype, and histologic grade (well, moderate, or poor) are provided. Extension into extrapancreatic tissue is described. Margins are assessed (e.g., involvement or distance), including the uncinate, pancreatic neck, common bile duct, and duodenum. The distance to the margin (in millimeters) from the tumor should be stated. The posterior pancreatic surface margin is also reported, although this is not a transected or surgical margin. Microscopic invasion of the lymphatics, small vessels, and nerves are indicated. The TNM stage and the component elements are provided according to the

AJCC 7th edition staging system. A minimum of 12 lymph nodes should be evaluated. Treatment effect is described if the patient has received neoadjuvant therapy.

Assessing Prognosis

Although PDA is widely viewed as an aggressive cancer, like other common cancers, tumors display a wide range of biology. The median survival after resection for PDA is around 18 months in large series[27]; roughly 20% of patients survive more than 5 years, and a comparable number suffer cancer-specific mortality within just 1 year of surgery.[5] There would be substantial value in accurately predicting patients' cancer-specific outcome; at the present time, there are no reliable tests to predict prognosis. The most frequently considered adverse prognostic factors include conventional pathologic features (lymph node metastases, poor differentiation, tumor size >3cm, and positive resection margins). The approximate proportions of resected PDAs that fulfill each criterion are 75%, 40%, 50%, and 40%, respectively.[27] It must be remembered that each of these individual prognostic factors are weak predictors of outcome, with multivariate Cox proportional hazards ratios only around 1.5. Winter et al.,[162] studied 137 patients who underwent resection for PDA and died within 1 year from their disease or survived more than 30 months (patients with intermediate survival were excluded). Adverse pathologic features were frequently present in long-term survivors; for instance, 65% of patients in the long survivor group had lymph node metastases in the resected specimen. Conversely, lymph node metastases were not detected in 17% of the short survivor group, yet they still recurred early after resection and succumbed to their disease.

Perhaps the most robust prognostic marker routinely used in patients with localized and resectable PDA is the *postoperative* CA 19-9 level. CA 19-9 is a high–molecular-weight glycolipid that is a sialylated derivative of the Lewis a antigen (normally expressed by epithelial cells and absorbed onto the surface of erythrocytes). The oligosaccharide epitope is also present on mucins secreted by pancreatic cancer cells and detectable in the serum. A markedly elevated *preoperative* CA 19-9 level has some prognostic value (on par with conventional pathologic features). *Preoperative* CA 19-9 has also been used by some surgeons as a predictor of unresectable disease when the lesion appears resectable on imaging. Roughly 30% of patients with serum values above 300 U/mL were found to have a contraindication to resection on staging laparoscopy.[150] However, preoperative CA 19-9 is particularly limited in patients with biliary obstruction because the antigen is falsely elevated in this setting.[151–153] In addition, the sensitivity suffers because 5% to 10% of the population are unable to express CA 19-9 due to Lewis antigen variability (related to the presence or absence of a fucosyltransferase).[154–156] As noted previously, CA 19-9 is most informative after resection when biliary obstruction is no longer a confounding variable and there has been macroscopic clearance of the disease. In a landmark ad hoc analysis of the Radiation Therapy Oncology Group (RTOG) 9704 adjuvant trial, an elevated postoperative CA 19-9 level (≥180 U/mL, drawn 1 to 2 months after resection) was associated with a multivariate proportional HR of 3.6.[154] Interestingly, Lewis antigen-negative individuals (who cannot express elevated serum CA 19-9) had the same survival as patients with low CA 19-9 levels for unclear reasons.

Patterns of Failure

Although OS after resection for PDA is roughly 18 months,[27] patients typically recur by 1 year,[159] indicating a short survival time once a recurrence is detected (comparable in survival to patients with metastatic disease). Recurrences have been reported in virtually every organ site, but most commonly occur in the retroperitoneum (57%), liver (51%), peritoneum (35%), and lung (15%). Interestingly, lung recurrences are typically delayed, and rarely

occur early after resection. A study of recurrence patterns out of Memorial Sloan-Kettering revealed that 12% of resected patients developed a local-only recurrence pattern; 33% had metastatic disease only and 46% had both local and metastatic disease (recurrence status was unknown in the remaining patients).[160]

Identifying biomarkers to predict patterns of recurrence could help select the patients who are most likely to benefit from intensive local therapy (radiation). The most intriguing biomarker to date in this area of research has been SMAD4. A study of pancreatic adenocarcinomas from an autopsy series (n = 65) revealed that a local predominant pattern was associated with intact SMAD4 expression (7 of 9 cases), whereas a disseminated pattern was associated with absent SMAD4 expression (16 of 22 cases).[49] This pattern was confirmed in tissue samples of patients from a phase II trial of locally advanced PDA.[161] Out of 15 patients with SMAD4-positive tumors, 11 had progression in a local-predominant pattern. In contrast, 10 of 14 patients with absent SMAD4 had significant distant spread. These studies suggest that patients having tumors with intact SMAD4 are most likely to benefit from radiation, whereas those patients with absent SMAD4 should only receive systemic therapy. However, a study of resected PDA samples revealed that resection alters the natural history of PDA recurrence, such that SMAD4 status is no longer predictive of recurrence pattern in this setting.[160] Other biomarkers[162] were examined as part of that study, and MUC1 expression was associated with a metastatic recurrence pattern. In a multivariate analysis, lymph node spread was the only variable (including the tested biomarkers) associated with pattern of failure. Patients without regional lymph node metastases had an increased risk of a local-only recurrence, typically in a relatively delayed fashion.[160] These data highlight that some patients would likely benefit from intensified local therapy, whereas others are best suited to receive systemic therapy only. Future studies are needed to define a personalized approach.

Adjuvant Therapy

According to the National Comprehensive Cancer Network (NCCN) guidelines, adjuvant chemotherapy is recommended for patients who recover well from pancreatic resection. Acceptable strategies include chemotherapy alone (gemcitabine, 5-FU, or capecitabine monotherapy), or chemoradiation plus chemotherapy (gemcitabine or 5-FU monotherapy, either given before or after chemoradiation).[157] Unfortunately, these regimens all consist of single-agent therapy with minimally effective agents. A meta-analysis of five randomized adjuvant trials including 951 patients concluded that adjuvant therapy provides a 3-month median survival advantage, and a 3% absolute improvement in 5-year survival. To put these findings in perspective, patients typically require a 6-month course of adjuvant treatment to achieve a 3-month survival.[158] Although these figures may appear unappealing to many patients, the reality is more complex; many patients receive no benefit at all, and may even be harmed with treatment, whereas a subset of patients receive a robust and durable survival benefit with these adjuvant treatments. Identifying which patients are most likely to experience a survival benefit is as important as discovering superior treatment regimens.

Adjuvant Trials

There have been eight prospective and randomized adjuvant trials that have shaped current treatment recommendations, including: five European trials, two in the United States, and one in Japan (Table 49.5).[163–170] Out of these eight trials, only four were considered positive with respect to the planned primary end point (one in the United States and three in Europe).[164,165,168,169] The continent where these trials were performed has played an important factor in defining the standard of care adjuvant treatment strategy around the world; chemoradiation is commonly performed in addition to chemotherapy in the United States, whereas chemotherapy

TABLE 49.5

Prospective and Randomized Adjuvant Trials for Pancreatic Cancer

Trial	Year	N	Randomization	OS (Months)	P
GITSG[168]	1985	43	Bolus 5-FU/4,000 cGy vs. observation	**20 vs. 11**	**0.04**
Bakkevold[169a]	1993	61	AMF vs. observation	**23 vs. 11**	**0.04**
EORTC[163a]	1999	218	Continuous 5-FU/4,000 cGy vs. observation	21.6 vs. 19.2	0.5
ESPAC-1[165]	2004	289	Bolus 5-FU vs. observation (2 × 2 design)	**20.1 vs. 15.5**	**0.009**
Japan[167]	2006	89	5-FU/cisplatin vs. observation	12.5 vs. 15.8	0.9
ESPAC-3[166]	2010	1088	Gemcitabine vs. 5-FU	23.6 vs. 23.0	0.4
RTOG 9704[170]	2011	451	Gemcitabine + ChemoXRT vs. 5-FU + ChemoXRT	18.7 vs. 17.3	0.9
CONKO-001[164]	2013	368	Gemcitabine vs. observation	**22.8 vs. 20.2**	**0.01**

Note: Statistically significant findings in bold (p <0.05).
[a] Included all periampullary cancers.
OS, overall survival; AMF, adriamycin, mitomycin C, 5-FU; ChemoXRT, Chemoradiation.

(without radiation) is the standard in Europe. The principal adjuvant trials will briefly be reviewed, emphasizing the strengths and weaknesses of the studies.

The Gastrointestinal Tumor Study Group (GITSG) trial was the first of the adjuvant trials and was a small phase III trial (by today's standards, n = 49 patients treated between 1974 and 1982) performed in the United States. Patients in the experimental arm received 40 Gy (split course with 20 Gy in each course, and a 2-week break in the middle). Bolus 5-FU was administered weekly for 2 years as maintenance therapy (500 mg/m^2), but was given daily for the first 3 days of each radiation course. The treatment arm was compared to an observation only arm, and the chemoradiation group had superior survival (20 versus 11 months; p = 0.04). The study has been criticized for its small sample size. Furthermore, it is not known whether the observed benefit was attributable to chemoradiation, to maintenance chemotherapy, or to both. Nevertheless, this landmark study established a role for adjuvant chemoradiation as an acceptable treatment for resected PDA in the United States.

Two small trials (in Norway[169] and Japan[167]) were performed over the last 15 years that provided equivocal results for chemotherapy alone, compared to surgery only. In the Norwegian trial, authored by Bakkevold et al.,[169] 61 patients with periampullary cancer (only 47 with PDA) were randomized to receive doxorubicin, mitomycin C, and 5-FU (six cycles), or observation. Patients receiving adjuvant chemotherapy had an improved median survival (23 versus 11 months; p = 0.04), but 2-year survival was similar (43% versus 32%; p = 0.1). In the Japanese trial, 89 patients were randomized to just two cycles (separated by 4 to 8 weeks) of 5-FU (500 mg/m^2 as a continuous infusion over 5 days) plus cisplatin (80 mg/m^2 on day 1 of each cycle), versus observation. OS was similar in the two groups (12.5 versus 15.8, respectively; p = 0.9).

The European Organization for Research and Treatment of Cancer (EORTC) trial was Europe's response to the GITSG trial and proved to be the largest adjuvant trial for PDA at that time.[163] A total of 218 patients with either PDA or other periampullary cancer were randomized to chemoradiation or observation. The treatment arm received split-course radiation for 40 Gy (as with GITSG). However, 5-FU was given as a continuous infusion (as opposed to bolus) on days 1 through 5 of each radiation course (for a total of 125 mg/m^2). No maintenance chemotherapy was administered. OS was 21.6 months with treatment and 19.2 months with observation (p = 0.5).

The European Study Group for Pancreatic Cancer (ESPAC-1) was the next large randomized adjuvant trial.[165] A total of 289 patients were randomized to a 2×2 design, with one of the four groups receiving no treatment. Treatment groups included (1) chemoradiation (40 Gy split-course radiation with bolus 5-FU at 500 mg/m^2 on days 1 through 3 of radiation, as with GITSG)

followed by chemotherapy (bolus leucovorin at 20 mg/m^2 and 5-FU at 425 mg/m^2 daily for 5 days, every 28 days for six cycles); (2) adjuvant chemotherapy only (without chemoradiation) as previously defined for group 1; (3) chemoradiation only (without chemotherapy) as previously defined for group 1; and (4) no treatment. The two groups receiving chemotherapy (groups 1 and 2) had superior survival as compared to those who did not (20.1 versus 15.5 months; p = 0.009). When chemoradiation was analyzed separately, the OS were 15.9 months with the two chemoradiation groups (groups 1 and 3) and 17.9 months without chemoradiation (groups 2 and 4; p = 0.05). When patients who received chemotherapy only were excluded from the no chemoradiation group (leaving just patients in the observation group), there was still a strong trend toward improved survival without chemoradiation. The results have been widely questioned because of the complex study design and because patients apparently received suboptimal radiation therapy (split course, no central quality of radiation control, 9% protocol violation, a very high [62%] local failure rate compared to recent trials). Although this study established chemotherapy alone as an acceptable standard of care in Europe and other parts of the world, oncologists in North America remain largely divided on the role of chemoradiation.

The Charité Onkologie (CONKO-001) trial primarily took place in German centers between 1998 and 2004,[159] with updated results recently reported.[164] The trial was an appropriate follow-up to ESPAC-1, which was interpreted in Europe as evidence in favor of adjuvant chemotherapy (without chemoradiation). Moreover, only 5-FU–based adjuvant chemotherapy had been tested up to that point, whereas the superiority of gemcitabine over 5-FU had been established for patients with advanced PDA (discussed in the Stage IV: Metastatic Disease section).[171] A total of 368 patients were randomized to receive six cycles of gemcitabine (4-week cycles) at a weekly dose of 1,000 mg/m^2 every 3 weeks with a 1 week break versus observation alone. Chemoradiation was not included in the treatment arm. The initial report reached its primary end point of disease-free survival (13.4 versus 6.9 months; p <0.001), but OS was not significantly different.[159] However, the updated analysis demonstrated improved OS with gemcitabine (22.8 versus 20.2 months; p = 0.01).[164] The small absolute difference in survival could be explained, in part, by the fact that 38% of patients did not receive the planned dose of gemcitabine and 13% did not receive at least one full cycle. In addition, most patients in the control arm received palliative chemotherapy once a recurrence was detected. Grade 3 through 4 toxicities were extremely rare in the treatment arm (no specific toxicity occurred in more than 3% of patients in the gemcitabine group). Although the median survival advantage is modest, it should be emphasized that the 5-year survival advantage was 10% (20.7% versus 10.2%; p <0.05) and the 10-year survival advantage was 5% (12.2% versus 7.7%).

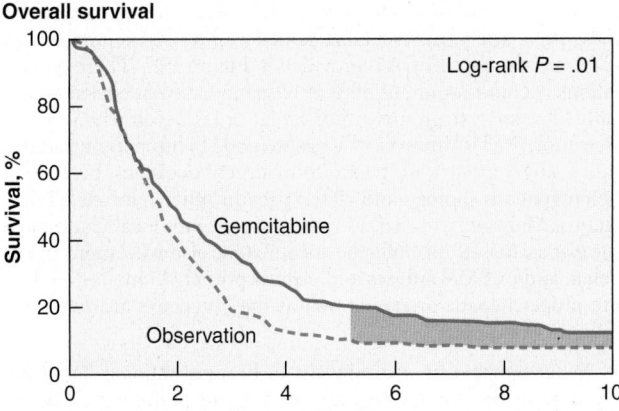

Figure 49.6 Improved long-term survival with gemcitabine monotherapy, in the CONKO-001 trial. The *highlighted area* represents patients who likely had a substantial benefit from gemcitabine monotherapy. (Modified from Oettle H, Neuhaus P, Hochhaus A, et al. Adjuvant chemotherapy with gemcitabine and long-term outcomes among patients with resected pancreatic cancer: the CONKO-001 randomized trial. *JAMA* 2013;310: 1473–1481.)

These data provide very strong evidence that, in a small subset of patients (i.e., 1 in 10), gemcitabine monotherapy is highly effective (Fig. 49.6). The opportunity to achieve long-term survival due to gemcitabine (albeit uncommon) is an important consideration for patients contemplating adjuvant treatment, despite the meager improvement in median survival.

The European ESPAC-3 trial is the largest adjuvant trial to date, and directly compared chemotherapy with gemcitabine (1,000 mg/m^2 over 30 minutes weekly, 3 out of 4 weeks) versus 5-FU (bolus folinic acid at 20 mg/m^2 plus bolus 5-FU at 425 mg/m^2 on days 1 to 5, every 28 days for six cycles as administered in ESPAC-1). As with CONKO-001, no adjuvant chemoradiation was given. Median OS were 23.6 and 23.0 months, respectively (p = 0.4), demonstrating equivalence between the two agents. However, this study did not change the emerging paradigm of frontline gemcitabine monotherapy at most centers, because toxicity was less with gemcitabine (14% serious adverse events with 5-FU versus 7.5% with gemcitabine; p <0.001). The increased toxicity due to 5-FU was primarily related to increased stomatitis and diarrhea.

Finally, RTOG 9704 was the second United States adjuvant trial, completed in 2002[172] and updated in 2011.[170] The trial's treatment arms paralleled the ESPAC-3 study (5-FU versus gemcitabine), except patients in both treatment groups received 5-FU–based chemoradiation in the middle of their adjuvant chemotherapy course. Total treatment duration in both groups was 6 months, and the study question related to chemotherapy (5-FU versus gemcitabine), and not the role of chemoradiation. A total of 451 patients were randomized to chemotherapy with 5-FU at 250 mg/m^2 per day given as a continuous infusion (different from ESPAC-3) or gemcitabine 1,000 mg/m^2 given weekly. Patients received one chemotherapy cycle prior to chemoradiation (3 weeks) and 12 additional weeks afterwards (two cycles of 5-FU consisting of 4 weeks on and 2 weeks off; three cycles of gemcitabine with 3 weeks on and 1 week off). Chemoradiation was given to all study patients as 50.4 Gy with continuous infusion 5-FU (250 mg/m^2 per day), and prospective quality assurance was performed. The primary end points of the study were OS for the whole cohort and for pancreatic head cancers. For all patients, OS was similar in the gemcitabine and 5-FU arms (18.5 versus 16.4 months; p = 0.5). In patients with pancreatic head tumors (86% of the total study population), those receiving gemcitabine had a trend toward superior survival in the multivariate analysis (20.5 versus 17.1 months; p = 0.08). The site of first relapse was recorded in this study, and was distant in roughly

70% of patients, and local–regional in 30% (a low figure relative to the local recurrence rate reported in ESPAC-1). Subsequent sites of recurrence were not reported. The RTOG-9704 study had several additional informative findings. Patients treated at centers that did not meet the quality assurance standards had inferior outcomes.[173] As previously described, postoperative CA 19-9 was identified as an important prognostic variable and should be considered in planning future adjuvant trials.[154] Finally, the inferior outcomes in patients with PDA of the left side of the pancreas raises questions about whether this group should be included in adjuvant trials with chemoradiation.

Future Questions and Ongoing Adjuvant Trials

Based on these trials, 6 months of adjuvant therapy is clearly supported as the standard of care for patients with resected PDA. Whether adjuvant chemoradiation is important remains an unanswered question, and is the subject of an ongoing randomized trial in the United States (RTOG 0848, NCT01013649). The study compares the impact of chemotherapy alone to chemotherapy plus chemoradiation. Patients in the radiation arm will receive 28 fractions of 1.8 Gy (50.4 Gy total, either 3-D conformal or intensity-modulated radiotherapy) and either capecitabine (825 mg/m^2 twice daily) or 5-FU (250 mg/m^2 per day as a continuous infusion for the duration of radiation) as a radiosensitizer. Unlike the RTOG 9704 trial, chemoradiation is administered after five cycles of gemcitabine-based chemotherapy have been completed. This trial design reflects an emerging trend in many centers toward deferring chemoradiation until after chemotherapy is completed in order to maximize systemic control early on and to spare patients who recur early at distant sites the cost and morbidity of radiation. The next ESPAC trial (ESPAC-4, ISRCTN96397434) is evaluating the role of doublet therapy (gemcitabine plus capecitabine versus gemcitabine alone) in the adjuvant setting. It is worth pointing out that this regimen did not improve OS in advanced pancreatic cancer (see the Stage IV: Metastatic Disease section).[174] CONKO-005 (DRKS00000247) is testing the addition of erlotinib to the standard-of-care gemcitabine (versus gemcitabine alone) based on a small, but statistically significant improvement in survival in the metastatic setting.[175,176] As discussed later in detail, two regimens, (1) gemcitabine plus nab-paclitaxel and (2) FOLFIRINOX, were recently shown to be superior to gemcitabine in the metastatic setting.[177,178] In light of these encouraging results, there are plans to test both regimens in the adjuvant setting (NCT01964430 and NCT01526135, respectively), using a similar control arm in both studies (gemcitabine monotherapy). Finally, the role of neoadjuvant chemotherapy in patients with resectable disease is not known. There are selected centers that routinely treat patients with resectable disease with neoadjuvant therapy,[54] and the NCCN guidelines recommend that such an approach be conducted as part of a clinical trial. In one of the largest series, from the M.D. Anderson Cancer Center,[84] outcomes are favorable (34 months) for patients who ultimately make it to pancreatic resection. The median survival of the entire cohort (22.7 months) in an intent-to-treat analysis is similar to historical controls with localized disease (see Table 49.5). Proponents argue that a neoadjuvant approach allows for an objective assessment of treatment response, early treatment of microscopic metastases, and an additional 3 to 6 months to monitor disease biology before committing to an operation with substantial risk. It is likely that as adjuvant treatment improves, more centers will move to a neoadjuvant paradigm, similar to the treatment of other upper gastrointestinal cancers.

Surveillance Postresection

The current NCCN guidelines recommend that patient follow-up after resection should include visits every 3 to 6 months for 2 years, and then annually. Surveillance CT scans and serial tumor markers (CA 19-9 at minimum) should be assessed, along with a history and physical exam. These recommendations are not based on Level 1 evidence, but rather expert consensus.[179] In practice, surveillance patterns range widely from close follow-up with CT imaging and CA 19-9 levels every 3 months, to no routine surveillance at all.[180] Poor outcomes after recurrence (roughly 6 to 12 months in the adjuvant trials discussed previously), and a lack of proven benefit for salvage chemotherapy, argue against close surveillance. However, as the number of second-line agents with activity against PDA increases, so will the opportunity to prolong survival with early detection of recurrence and intervention. It should be noted that a rise in CA 19-9 often precedes radiographic evidence of recurrence by 3 to 12 months.[181] However, initiating chemotherapy based on changes in tumor marker levels alone is not currently recommended (although widely practiced), due to the risk of false positive and false negative results.[153,154]

There are a few reports that support the benefit of close surveillance and early intervention. One study, presented in abstract form, described 139 patients who underwent resection for PDA. All patients were advised to have CT scan and CA 19-9 surveillance every 3 months in the first year, every 6 months in the 2nd year, and annually thereafter. The patients were retrospectively analyzed in three groups: those who followed the recommendations, those who underwent surveillance but with less frequency than recommended, and those who did not follow up. Survivals in the three groups were 16.6, 15.7, and 8.7 months, respectively. The authors concluded that close follow-up is advisable. Notably, the proportions of patients who received adjuvant treatment in each group were not reported.

Selected patients may even benefit from a metastasectomy. Pulmonary metastases (as compared to liver or peritoneal metastases) typically occur in a delayed fashion after surgery.[160] Therefore, the biology and natural history of patients who develop isolated pulmonary metastases may represent a unique subgroup where resection of these lesions is beneficial. The Johns Hopkins group identified 31 patients with isolated lung metastases at a median of 34 months post pancreatectomy. A total of 9 had the lung lesion resected, and these patients survived an additional 19 months (range 5 to 29 months) after the intervention.[182]

STAGE III: LOCALLY ADVANCED DISEASE

AJCC Staging Versus "Intent of Management"–Based Staging

In the current (7th) edition of AJCC staging for pancreatic adenocarcinoma, stage III cancers are T_4, N_{any} M_0 malignancies, with T_4

defined as a "tumor [that] involves the celiac axis or the superior mesenteric artery (unresectable primary tumor)." A representative CT scan of stage III PDA is provided in Figure 49.7. These presentations account for about 30% of all pancreatic cancers and typically have an average survival of 1 year or less, even when treated (see Table 49.1). However, it is problematic to lump these patients into a single group with regard to treatment decisions, because of heterogeneous biology and differences in other relevant clinical factors. Management decisions for patients with locally advanced tumors are based on both the local extent of involvement of the celiac and/or SMA arteries and critical primary branches, such as the proper hepatic artery, as well as the clinician's answer to the following questions:

1. What therapeutic goal appears to be most rational based not only on the tumor staging, but also on performance status, weight loss, and significant comorbid illnesses? Along these lines, is the treatment potentially curative? Is minimal or moderate antineoplastic intensity more appropriate? Or is treatment supportive and purely palliative?
2. What is the level of treatment intensity that this patient would be able to accept and withstand psychologically and emotionally in addition to physiologically?
3. What are the support structures surrounding this patient, and are they up to the challenges that will be incurred by the management selected?

Pragmatically, stage III clinical presentations have been divided into *borderline resectable* and *clearly unresectable* (introduced previously in the section Stage I, II: Localized Disease, Evaluation and Assessing Resectability), with the conceptual distinction being the probability of safely and successfully resecting the tumor without antecedent chemotherapy or chemoradiotherapy.

Basic Management Considerations

The initial evaluation of patients with presumed pancreatic adenocarcinoma will be the same whether the patient ultimately is demonstrated to have a resectable, borderline resectable, or locally unresectable disease at presentation. This component of management has been addressed previously in the chapter (see Stage I, II: Localized Disease, Presentation and Evaluation and Assessing Resectability). For patients treated initially with chemotherapy or chemoradiation, several additional management considerations need to be considered (also relevant for patients with resectable disease who are to receive neoadjuvant treatment).

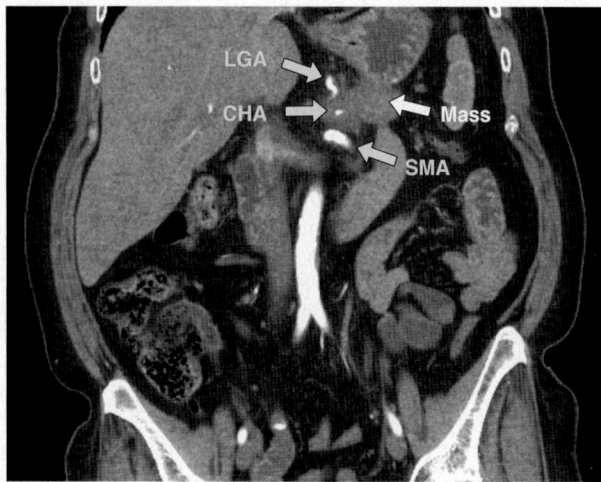
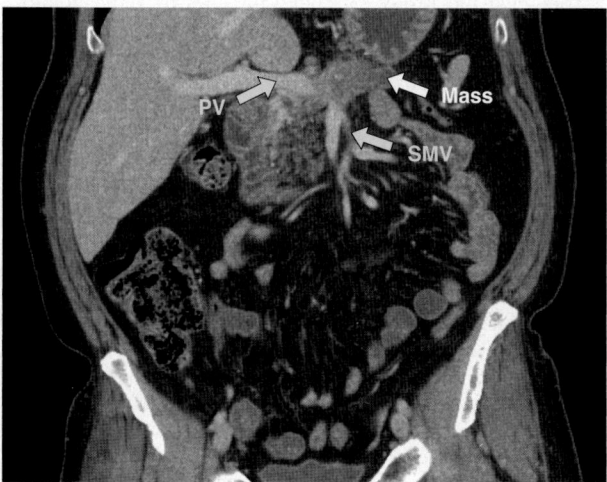

Figure 49.7 CT scans of a locally advanced, stage III PDA in the pancreatic body. Coronal images. **(A)** The arterial phase. Visceral arteries named are left gastric artery (LGA), common hepatic artery (CHA), and superior mesenteric artery (SMA). The CHA is encased. **(B)** The venous phase. The portal splenic confluence is completely occluded.

Patients generally require histologic confirmation of a pancreatic cancer diagnosis prior to treatment. Additionally, relief of obstructive jaundice and duodenal obstruction is necessary when present. These interventions will be concurrent with other basic assessments and interventions such as nutritional optimization, treatment of dehydration and electrolyte abnormalities, pain management, and attention to depression if present. It is important to emphasize that multidisciplinary teams with focused, management experience for gastrointestinal (GI) malignancies of the upper abdomen achieve the best results, and include expertise in pathology, chemotherapeutic, radiotherapeutics, surgical management, interventional radiology, and endoscopy, as mentioned in the opening of the chapter.[183]

Local–Regional Unresectable Disease

Impact of Prognostic Factors in the Management of Locally Unresectable Patients

Patients with locally advanced, or stage III, PDA have an average OS between 7 and 12 months (Table 49.6). Several patient-specific factors have been adversely associated with outcome in this context, including anemia, poor performance status, elevated CA 19-9, and elevated Charlson Comorbidity Score. In addition, use and response to systemic chemotherapy as the initial treatment, prior to chemoradiotherapy, appears to favorably predict (and possibly impact) survival.[184–187]

Evolution of Management for Local–Regional Unresectable Disease

The early, practice defining, randomized experiences have been reviewed in many prior publications and textbooks,[188] and key ones are highlighted in Table 49.6. It is important to remember how dated some studies are with respect to patient selection and evaluation, chemotherapy selection, and radiation planning and delivery (typically delivered as 2-D nonconformal, split course, low-dose therapy). Nevertheless, these papers established proof of principle for treatment feasibility with acceptable toxicity, and the value of 5-FU–based radiosensitization in this context.

From the mid 1990s through the first decade of the current century, there have been a series of important lessons learned in the management of locally advanced pancreatic cancer. Acceptable chemoradiation strategies integrating insights gained from past studies are summarized in Table 49.7. There is a biologic basis for needing both improved local control and improved systemic control to optimize results.

Improved local control in pancreatic cancer has been strongly suggested by the autopsy studies by Iacobuzio-Donahue et al.,[49] previously described (see the Stage I, II: Localized Disease, Adjuvant Therapy section), and validated in patients with locally advanced disease.[161] Investigators observed that patients with tumors having intact SMAD4 expression were more likely to have locally destructive tumors and a lower burden of metastatic disease than patients with tumors showing SMAD4 loss. Recently, Oshima et al.[189] found that abnormal TP53 expression (either absence or

TABLE 49.6

Selected Locally Advanced Pancreatic Ductal Adenocarcinoma Randomized Trials

Year	Study Name	Patient Number	Radiation (Gy)	Chemotherapy	Median Survival (Months)
1980[292]	SWOG	33	60	MeC, 5-FU, SMF	8.8
		29	60	MeC, 5-FU, testolactone	6.9
1981[293]	GITSG	83	60	5-FU	**9.4**
		86	40	5-FU	**9.8**
		25	60	None	5.3
1985[192]	ECOG	37	40	5-FU	8.3
		34	None	5-FU	8.2
1985[294]	GITSG	73	60	5-FU	8.5
		70	40	Doxorubicin	7.6
1988[190]	GITSG	22	54	5-FU, SMF	**9.7**
		21	None	SMF	7.4
1994[295]	Mayo Clinic	44	50–60	5-FU	7.8
		43	50–60	Hycanthone	7.8
2005[296]	ECOG	62	60	None	8.4
		64	60	5-FU, MMC	7.1
2008[191]	FFCD/SFRO	59	60	Gemcitabine	8.6
		60	None	Gemcitabine	**13**
2011[193]	ECOG	34	50	Gemcitabine	**11.1**
		37	None	Gemcitabine	**9.2**
2013[207]	SCALOP	38	50, Gemcitabine	Gemcitabine, Capecitabine	**15.2**
		36	50, Capecitabine	Gemcitabine, Capecitabine	**13.4**

Note: Statistically significant findings are in bold (p <0.05).
MeC, Methyl-CCNU; SMF, streptozotocin, mitomycin C, 5-FU.

PRACTICE OF ONCOLOGY

TABLE 49.7

Recommended Radiation Treatment Volumes in Commonly Used Chemoradiation Regimens for Localized Pancreatic Cancer

Chemotherapy Choice	Chemotherapy Dose and Schedule	Radiation Dose and Schedule	No Arterial Involvement or Abutment with Likely Resectability (T3 or T4)	Extensive Arterial Involvement with Uncertain Resectability or Arterial Encasement/Unresectable (T4)
Gemcitabine	400–500 mg/m^2 weekly	50.4 Gy over 5.5 wks (good PS) or 30 Gy over 2 wks (poor PS)	GTV only	GTV only
	1 g/m^2 weekly	36 Gy over 3 wks	GTV only	GTV only
	40 mg/m^2 twice weekly	50.4 Gy over 5.5 wks	GTV + ENI	GTV only
Capecitabine	800–825 mg/m^2 twice per day on days of radiation	50.4 Gy over 5.5 wks (good PS) or 30 Gy over 2 wks (poor PS)	GTV + ENI	GTV only
PVI 5-FU	225 mg/m^2 daily or 300 mg/m^2 on days of radiation	50.4 Gy over 5.5 wks (good PS) or 30 Gy over 2 wks (poor PS)	GTV + ENI	GTV only

PS, performance status; GTV, gross tumor volume; ENI, elective nodal irradiation; PVI, protracted venous infusion.
Modified from Royal RE, Wolfe RA, Crane CH. Cancer of the pancreas. In: DeVita VT Jr, Lawrence TS, Rosenberg SA, eds. *DeVita, Hellman, and Rosenberg's Cancer: Principles & Practice of Oncology*. 9th ed. Philadelphia: Lippincott Williams & Wilkins; 2011.

nuclear accumulation) was associated with a local–regional recurrence pattern in patients with resected PDA, whereas CDKN2A loss was associated with widespread metastases.[189] Similar to an aforementioned study by Winter et al.,[160] SMAD4 expression was not associated with pattern of failure in this patient cohort following resection.[189]

Past studies suggest that the controversy of using chemotherapy alone versus chemoradiotherapy should be reframed to acknowledge that there might be potential roles of each. There have been several randomized trials comparing chemotherapy to chemotherapy plus chemoradiation,[190–193] with mixed results (each appear in Table 49.6). An older ECOG study published in 1985 (with the aforementioned limitations) compared weekly 5-FU against the same chemotherapy treatment preceded by 40 Gy radiation (combined with 5-FU) and found no difference in survival. The multi-institution French Fédération Francophone de Cancérologie Digestive-Société Française de Radiothérapie Oncologie (FFCD/SFRO) study found decreased survival in patients receiving 60 Gy radiation concomitantly with 5-FU and cisplatin, and followed with maintenance gemcitabine, compared to gemcitabine alone (8.6 versus 13 months). The chemoradiation regimen used in this trial has been criticized as being particularly toxic (more on this in the following).[191] The LAP-07 trial with gemcitabine or gemcitabine plus erlotinib for four cycles, followed by either chemoradiotherapy or additional chemotherapy (two cycles), failed to show any difference in survival between the two arms. About one-third of patients had progressed by the time of the second randomization. The trial results, although final, have only been reported in abstract form.[194] However, a GITSG study from 1988 comparing 5-FU and radiation followed by streptozotocin, mitomycin C, and 5-FU chemotherapy to the same chemotherapy alone showed an improved median survival (9.7 versus 7.4 months) with multimodality therapy.[190] Most recently, ECOG 4201 from 2011 suggested that locally advanced patients randomly assigned to receive chemoradiotherapy with gemcitabine followed by five cycles of gemcitabine alone did better than patients receiving gemcitabine without radiotherapy (11.1 versus 9.2 months; p = 0.016).[193] It is noted that this trial was closed, with only 71 patients accrued and analyzed, a potential criticism of the results. Other nonrandomized studies suggesting benefit to using a combination of modalities, rather than one modality, include the recently reported Massachusetts General Hospital experience (improved survival with chemotherapy plus chemoradiation versus chemoradiation alone, HR = 0.46; p <0.001),[184] and a German study in which treatment decisions were assigned from tumor board discussions

(chemoradiotherapy plus chemoradiation, median survival 13.0 months versus 8.0 months without additional chemotherapy).[195] On further analysis, the authors could not find prognostic factor variation between to the two groups to explain this difference.

Gemcitabine has been found to be marginally superior to 5-FU in the metastatic setting.[171] The drug also has marginal efficacy as a single-agent adjuvant therapy after resection for PDA.[164] There is some suggestion that it may be better than 5-FU in the adjuvant setting, when chemoradiation is included,[170] although there is no such trend in a European trial comparing these agents without chemoradiation.[166,170] Thus, there has been interest in exploring gemcitabine as a radiation sensitizer; indeed, the drug is potent in this role based on preclinical and clinical data.[196] Investigators from the M.D. Anderson Cancer Center, the University of Michigan, and other sites explored the use of gemcitabine with radiotherapy in various contexts, with the following observations: Radiotherapy fields designed to cover gross tumor and at risk nodal basins cannot safely be targeted with concurrent gemcitabine unless the gemcitabine dose is reduced from the chemotherapy-only level of 1,000 mg/m^2 to 300 to 600 mg/m^2. Additionally, the daily fraction size should not exceed 1.8 Gy when targeting expanded fields with draining lymph nodes. If the desire is to administer full-dose gemcitabine (1,000 mg/m^2) weekly with higher radiation doses (e.g., 2.4 Gy fractions), then radiotherapy must be limited to gross tumor only with tight margins, and special attention must be given toward inadvertent targeting organs such as the duodenum, stomach, and small bowel. Subsequent studies have demonstrated that respecting these guidelines allows for acceptable toxicity, especially when combined with appropriate supportive care measures, treatment planning that accounts for target and organ movement with respiration, and intensity modulated planning and delivery aimed at minimizing doses to sensitive critical organs.[196–200]

The work of Ben Joseph et al.[197] at the University of Michigan validates this approach. Investigators conducted a phase I/II dose escalating study of radiotherapy dose over 25 fractions (totaling 50 to 60 Gy) in 50 patients, all deemed to have locally advanced PDA (not borderline resectable). The maximal tolerated dose was 55 Gy (2.2 Gy per fraction) in combination with fixed-dose rate gemcitabine (1,000 mg/m^2). Patients had a median survival of 14.8 months and 24% (12 of 50 patients, a very high rate compared to previous studies[161,191,201,202]) underwent resection (10 R$_0$ and 2 R$_1$). Among resected patients, the median survival was 32 months. A meta-analysis of three randomized trials and one comparative retrospective study (including 229 patients) revealed a small but significant survival advantage with gemcitabine-based chemoradiation (at 12 months: HR, 1.5; p = 0.03), over 5-FU–based treatment, although toxicity was higher.[203]

Technologic advances combined with greater understanding of the mechanisms and impact of acute radiation toxicity have improved the safety profile of treatment. Excessive acute toxicity quickly results when the radiation fractional dose increases, the total dose increases, the field sizes are too large for the degree of drug sensitization or intensity, or radiation is delivered without careful consideration of limiting dose volume to the stomach, duodenum, small bowel, or other critical organs. There is increasing consensus that such toxicity can be associated with symptoms, increased costs, and decreased survival.[191,200]

Capecitabine is an appealing alternative to 5-FU or gemcitabine as a radiosensitizer. Capecitabine is a prodrug of 5-FU with near-complete oral bioavailability. It is converted to its active form through a three-step process, with the last step occurring more reliably within tumor cells than in nonmalignant cells, due to higher thymidine phosphorylase levels. Thus, systemic levels of active 5-FU are actually decreased with capecitabine, theoretically widening the therapeutic window of the drug. Aside from hand–foot syndrome associated with capecitabine, clinical trials reproducibly demonstrate an improved safety profile. The efficacy of capecitabine is comparable to 5-FU, at least in studies of other cancer types that directly compare them.[204] Importantly, oral dosing obviates the need for semipermanent venous access and the attendant risks of thrombosis and infection. Nonrandomized data demonstrate that capecitabine (typically administered at a daily dose of around 1,600 mg/m^2) has comparable efficacy to continuous infusion 5-FU, and an improved toxicity profile, as a radiosensitizer in patients with locally advanced PDA receiving intensity-modulated radiation therapy (IMRT).[205,206] Finally, the recently published SCALOP I randomized trial in patients with locally advanced PDA, has suggested mildly increased efficacy (OS 15.2 versus 13.4 months; p = 0.01) and decreased toxicity of capecitabine with irradiation, as compared to gemcitabine. In this study, sensitized radiation was administered after four cycles of gemcitabine and capecitabine chemotherapy (randomization was performed after three cycles).[207] Note that the chemosensitizing dose of gemcitabine (300 mg/m^2) was lower than the fixed-dose rate levels successfully used in the abovementioned Ben Josef study.[197]

A final lesson from previous studies of chemoradiation for locally advanced pancreatic adenocarcinoma demonstrate that induction chemotherapy prior to chemoradiation has advantages. Nevertheless, chemotherapy, chemoradiation, or both have been studied and are acceptable approaches for locally advanced PDA. There are no level 1 data conclusively supporting one approach over the other. However, several studies provide a meaningful rationale for beginning with induction chemotherapy. Roughly two-thirds of patients with locally advanced PDA develop systemic metastases during treatment. Some of these individuals are less likely to benefit from radiation, and the costs and side effects of local radiation therapy may be avoided.[208] An ad hoc analysis of a prospective, nonrandomized study (GERCOR), revealed that patients with locally advanced PDA who received consolidation chemoradiation after induction chemotherapy had improved survival, as compared to those who had chemotherapy alone (15.0 versus 11.7 months; p <0.001).[208] This has been validated by other retrospective data.[209] The SCALOP trial, as previously described, showed that sequenced chemoradiation after chemotherapy achieves very good results with locally advanced PDA.[207] The GERCOR LAP-07, described previously, warrants additional mention here, because no benefit was observed with chemoradiation (50.4 Gy plus capecitabine) after chemotherapy (gemcitabine plus erlotinib or gemcitabine alone), as compared to additional chemotherapy (n = 269; OS, 15.2 versus 16.4 months; p = 0.8).[194]

Along these lines, certain multidrug combinations with higher response rates for advanced PDA than gemcitabine monotherapy (see the Stage IV: Metastatic Disease section) are also promising regimens for locally advanced PDA. FOLFIRINOX (5-FU, oxaliplatin, leucovorin, and irinotecan) has a response rate of 27% in the locally advanced setting,[210] which rivals the best results with multimodality therapy.[197,207] Planned and ongoing trials with FOLFIRINOX, as well as with nab-paclitaxel plus gemcitabine (with or without radiation), will help establish the role of these treatments for locally advanced PDA.

Management of Borderline Resectable Patients

Current NCCN guidelines for borderline resectable patients favor neoadjuvant therapy over directly going to surgery, while acknowledging the validity of both approaches and the absence of phase III data to definitively answer the issue.[157] A meta-analysis of 182 patients from 10 prospective trials of borderline resectable patients included seven studies reporting on the impact of chemoradiation (with or without chemotherapy) and three on chemotherapy alone.[211] At restaging following neoadjuvant therapy, 16% of patients responded to treatment, 69% had stable disease, and 19% showed progression. The median survival for the cohort was 22.0 months, and treatment-related grade 3 to 4 toxicity was observed in 32% of patients. Surgical exploration was performed in 69% of patients, and 80% of surgically explored patients were resected. Moreover, 83% of resected specimens had microscopically negative resection margins. Among resected patients, 61% were alive at 1 year, and 44% were alive at 2 years. The median survival in this highly selected and favorable group was 22.0 months.

Although the survival of patients with borderline PDA after neoadjuvant treatment and resection is comparable to patients with resectable PDA,[27] these data should be interpreted with a few points of caution. First, the study was underpowered and not designed to determine the best neoadjuvant regimen; thus, treatment choice is largely dependent on institutional preferences. Second, resected patients represent 56% of the total cohort, and are enriched for patients with tumors that have favorable biology. In these nonrandomized studies, it is possible that intrinsic biologic factors were more important determinants of survival than neoadjuvant treatment. Notably, nonresected patients with borderline PDA have a survival around 1 year, which is similar to patients with locally advanced disease.[212] Finally, roughly 40% of patients with potentially resectable tumors do not undergo resection when a neoadjuvant approach is used. Whether unresected patients suffered a missed opportunity for resection (and therefore for long-term survival) or were spared ineffective surgery is unknown. Most likely, the answer lies somewhere in the middle.

EMERGING ROLE OF STEREOTACTIC BODY RADIOTHERAPY

SBRT is hypofractionated (one to five fractions) radiotherapy given in doses that, in aggregate, do not exceed 50 to 60 Gy per course. Single fraction courses are usually in the dose range of 20 to 25 Gy. The number of fractions and dose per fraction is determined by tumor size and radiation tolerance of the involved and/or adjacent organs. To be safe, these large-dose fractions are given with extra attention to immobilization, controlling for respiratory movement, image guidance, and dose shaping around critical structures. The risk of severe or lethal normal organ damage is substantial in the absence of proper attention to all required, relevant considerations. In pancreatic applications, the primary dose-limiting structure is the duodenum, followed by the stomach, remaining small bowel, and other adjacent organs/structures. This approach has been applied with and without chemotherapy in a variety of pancreatic contexts, including locally unresectable, borderline resectable, locally recurrent, and as an adjuvant management boost after conventional radiotherapy.[213–215] These studies demonstrated feasibility and acceptable toxicity in experienced hands, although the exact role of this modality remains to be defined.

STAGE IV: METASTATIC DISEASE

Approximately 50% of patients with PDA will be diagnosed with distant metastatic (stage IV) disease at the time of presentation.[1] Prognosis is dismal, with a median OS of less than 6 months and an estimated 2-year survival of only 2%.[3,7] Chemotherapy in this setting improves survival by just a few additional months. Therefore, the goals of therapy in this patient population are to prolong survival, as well as to palliate symptoms.

Gemcitabine as a Gold-Standard Therapy for Metastatic Pancreatic Adenocarcinoma

5-FU was the principal treatment option for metastatic pancreatic cancer through the 1990s, although response rates were under 20% and median survival was just 6 months.[216] Other agents or combinations of drugs failed to show any improvement over 5-FU monotherapy until a landmark study in 1997 by Burris et al.[171] demonstrating the superiority of gemcitabine for advanced PDA. Since that study, gemcitabine has become the single most important pancreatic cancer therapy, and the standard treatment arm in at least 19 phase III studies (Table 49.8).

Gemcitabine (difluorodeoxycytidine [dFdC]) is a nucleoside analog of deoxycytidine, and it is administered as a prodrug. Upon entry into the cell, gemcitabine is phosphorylated by deoxycytidine kinase (DCK) to a monophosphate form (dFdCMP). Similar to the association between thymidine phosphorylase and the prodrug capecitabine, elevated DCK levels in tumor cells (compared to normal tissues)[217] enhance the therapeutic window of gemcitabine. dFdCMP is then phosphorylated into active diphosphate (dFdCDP) and triphosphate (dFdCTP) forms. The active metabolites incorporate into DNA and inhibit chain elongation. Moreover, they deplete nucleotide pools by competitively inhibiting ribonucleotide reductase.[218]

In the 1997 Burris trial, 126 patients with advanced pancreas cancer were randomized to either of two arms: (1) gemcitabine 1,000 mg/m^2 weekly for 7 weeks followed by 1 week of rest, then 3 doses per week every 4 weeks thereafter, or (2) bolus 5-FU 600 mg/m^2 once per week.[171] Patients primarily had metastatic disease, although 26% had locally advanced disease. Treatment in both arms was generally well tolerated. Grade 3 through 4 hematologic toxicities were higher with gemcitabine, including neutropenia (25.9% versus 4.9%), thrombocytopenia (9.7% versus 0%) and anemia (9.7% versus 0%). Grade 3 through 4 nausea was also more frequent in the gemcitabine arm (9.5% versus 4.8%). Clinical benefit, based on pain score, performance status, and weight, was noted in 23.8% of patients in the gemcitabine arm versus only 4.8% in the 5-FU arm (p = 0.0022). The survival advantage with gemcitabine was just over 5 weeks, with median OS of 5.65 and 4.41 months, respectively (p = 0.0025). Survival at 12 months was 18% in the gemcitabine arm versus 2% in the 5-FU arm. Partial tumor responses were observed in 5% of patients in the gemcitabine group, and stable disease was observed in 39%. In contrast, no partial tumor responses were observed with 5-FU, and only 19% of patients experienced stable disease. As a result, gemcitabine was approved by the U.S. Food and Drug Administration (FDA) in 1997 for first-line treatment for locally advanced unresectable or metastatic pancreas cancer.

Two studies have focused on modifying the dosing and infusion rates of gemcitabine in order to increase the concentration of intracellular, activated gemcitabine. Tempero et al.[219] compared two

---

TABLE 49.8

Phase III Studies of Gemcitabine + Drug "X", Compared to Gemcitabine

Author	Year	N	Drug "X"	Gemcitabine OS (Months)	Combination OS (Months)	P Value
Collucci[223]	2002	107	Cisplatin	5.0	7.5	0.43
Berlin[199]	2002	327	5-FU	5.4	6.7	0.09
Bramhall[229]	2002	239	Marimastat	5.8	5.98	0.95
Rocha Lima[227]	2004	360	Irinotecan	6.6	6.3	0.79
Richards[297]	2004	565	Pemetrexed	6.3	6.2	0.85
Van Cutsem[233]	2004	688	Tipifarnib	6.5	6.9	0.75
Louvet[226]	2005	300	Oxaliplatin	7.1	9.0	0.13
Herrmann[174]	2005	319	Capecitabine	7.3	8.4	0.31
Heinemann[225]	2006	192	Cisplatin	6.0	7.5	0.15
Stathopoulous[228]	2006	130	Irinotecan	6.5	6.4	0.97
Abou-Alfa[221]	2006	349	Exatecan	6.2	6.7	0.52
Moore[175]	2007	569	Erlotinib	6.2	5.9	**0.04**
Poplin[220]	2009	574	Oxaliplatin	4.9	5.7	0.10
Cunningham[224]	2009	533	Capecitabine	6.2	7.1	0.08
Philip[232]	2010	745	Cetuximab	5.9	6.3	0.23
Kindler[231]	2010	602	Bevacizumab	5.9	5.8	0.95
Kindler[230]	2011	632	Axitinib	8.3	8.5	0.54
Conroy[177]	2011	342	FOLFIRINOX[a]	6.8	11.1	**<0.001**
Von Hoff[178]	2013	861	Nab-paclitaxel	6.7	8.5	**<0.001**

Note: Statistically significant findings are in bold (p <0.05).
[a] The experimental arm was FOLFIRINOX alone; all other experimental arms listed in this table include a drugs in combination with gemcitabine.

different dose-intense regimens (compared to the Burris regimen) in a randomized phase II study. A total of 92 patients were randomized to either *standard* 30 minute infusion at a dose of 2,200 mg/m^2 versus 1,500 mg/m^2 over 150 minutes at a fixed-dose rate (FDR) of 10 mg/m^2 per minute.[219] All patients had locally advanced (8%) or metastatic pancreatic cancer (92%). Although there was no difference in the primary end point (i.e., time to treatment failure), patients in the standard arm had a median OS of 5 months, whereas those in the FDR had a median survival of 8 months (p = 0.013). Pharmacokinetic analyses showed a twofold increase in the intracellular (peripheral mononuclear cells) concentration of gemcitabine triphosphate with FDR gemcitabine, even though the total dose given was 30% less. Consistent with these data, grade 3 to 4 hematologic toxicity was also greater with FDR gemcitabine. Subsequently, the Eastern Cooperative Oncology Group (ECOG) conducted a three-arm phase III study (E6201) comparing gemcitabine (1,000 mg/m^2) plus oxaliplatin (100 mg/m^2) every 2 weeks versus a weekly 30-minute infusion of gemcitabine (1,000 mg/m^2) versus weekly FDR gemcitabine (1,500 mg/m^2 as previous).[220] A total of 832 patients were enrolled. The study confirmed an increase in OS for the FDR arm compared to the 30-minute infusion of gemcitabine arm (6.2 months versus 4.9 months; p = 0.04). However, the OS benefit actually did not meet the prespecified criteria for significance (a 33% decrease in survival). In addition, patients experienced greater toxicities with grade 3 to 4 neutropenia and thrombocytopenia in the FDR gemcitabine arm, consistent with the earlier phase II trial. Of note, there was no survival advantage with the combination of gemcitabine and oxaliplatin. Based on these data, the fixed-dose rate of gemcitabine can be considered a reasonable alternative to the standard 30-minute gemcitabine infusion, albeit with greater toxicity.

A Decade of Failed Attempts to Move Beyond Gemcitabine Monotherapy

In addition to oxaliplatin, there have been numerous attempts over the past decade to augment the therapeutic benefit of gemcitabine in patients with advanced disease, using additional therapeutic agents in combination with gemcitabine (see Table 49.8). Conventional cytotoxic agents that have been tested include cisplatin, oxaliplatin, 5-FU, capecitabine, irinotecan, and exatecan. Despite promising phase II data, the aforementioned doublets all failed to show any benefit over gemcitabine monotherapy.[174,220–228] In addition, novel targeted or biologic therapies have been tested in combination with gemcitabine, including marimastat (metalloproteinase inhibitor), tipifarnib (a farnesyltransferase inhibitor, targeting Kras signaling), cetuximab (epidermal growth factor receptor [EGFR] inhibitor), bevacizumab (angiogenesis inhibitor), and axitinib (multitarget tyrosine kinase inhibitor).[229–233] In general, the addition of these agents to gemcitabine failed to markedly change OS.

A few of the biologic agents warrant special mention based on the promise of therapeutic efficacy in other cancer types or in early phase clinical trial data in the treatment of advanced PDA. EGFR is expressed in 60% of PDAs,[162] and amplification or high polysomy at the EGFR locus is identified in half of the affected patients.[234] Moreover, targeting EGFR is effective in certain nonpancreatic cancers (e.g., lung, colorectal, head and neck). Therefore, there is a strong therapeutic rationale for targeting EGFR in the treatment of PDA. Cetuximab is a monoclonal antibody with affinity for EGFR, which was tested in a small phase II study in patients with advanced pancreatic cancer as a combination therapy with gemcitabine.[235] In the 41 patients with EGFR-positive tumors, the median OS was 7.1 months with a 1-year OS of 31.7%, suggesting a potential benefit when compared to historical controls.[171] However, in the large and definitive phase III trial conducted by the Southwest Oncology Group (SWOG S0205),[232] this combination failed to improve the outcome of patients when compared

to gemcitabine alone. A total of 745 patients were accrued, with median survivals of 6.3 (combination) and 5.9 months, respectively (p = 0.23). Objective response rates and progression-free survival were also similar between the two groups.

Angiogenesis has proven to be a worthy target in the solid tumor arena, and prior successes served as the impetus for the Cancer and Leukemia Group B (CALGB 80303) double-blind, placebo-controlled randomized phase III trial comparing gemcitabine plus bevacizumab versus gemcitabine alone.[231] A total of 602 treatment-naïve patients with advanced pancreatic cancer were accrued. The median OS were 5.8 and 5.9 months, respectively (p = 0.95). Again, response rates and progression-free survival were similar. Axitinib is another antiangiogenic factor, and a potent inhibitor of vascular endothelial growth factor receptor (VEGFR)1, 2, and 3. A randomized phase II trial with 103 patients demonstrated a nonsignificant improvement in OS; this prompted a larger phase III trial comparing gemcitabine 1,000 mg/m^2 on days 1, 8, and 15 every 28 days plus axitinib 5 to 10 mg orally daily, or gemcitabine plus placebo.[230] There were 632 patients in the trial, which closed at an interim analysis when the futility boundary was crossed. Median OS was 8.5 months in the gemcitabine/axitinib arm and 8.3 months in the gemcitabine/placebo arm.

Two recently published meta-analyses examined the numerous randomized controlled clinical trials of gemcitabine-based combination therapy in aggregate. These studies included more than 8,000 patients enrolled in over 25 trials.[236,237] Despite the fact that virtually all of these studies were negative independently, both meta-analyses found a small survival benefit (OR >0.9 with p <0.05) with combination therapy, although toxicity was higher. Although these findings do not justify routine use of the examined regimens, they suggest that a small subset of patients (~10% to 20%) do receive a benefit and affirm that further work to identify the best candidates for specific combination therapies is warranted.

Modest Breakthroughs in the Treatment of Advanced Pancreatic Cancer

Two additional treatments have been approved for the treatment of advanced PDA by the FDA: erlotinib and nab-paclitaxel. The former drug is an oral tyrosine kinase inhibitor of the EGFR that was approved in 2005 for use in combination with gemcitabine for locally advanced unresectable or metastatic pancreatic cancer.[175] The National Cancer Institute of Canada Clinical Trials Group (NCIC-CTG) conducted a large international phase III double-blind randomized trial of 569 patients with advanced or metastatic pancreatic adenocarcinoma, comparing gemcitabine intravenous (IV) 1,000 mg/m^2 weekly × 7 weeks followed by 1 week of rest, then weekly × 3 every 4 weeks plus erlotinib 100 mg or 150 mg per day orally versus gemcitabine plus placebo. Toxicities, including diarrhea and the typical acneiform rash associated with EGFR inhibitors, were slightly worse in the erlotinib arm. Nevertheless, these toxicities were mostly grade 1 to 2 and easily manageable. The gemcitabine/erlotinib arm experienced an improved median OS (6.24 months versus 5.91 month), with 1-year OS of 23% and 17%, respectively. Based on this study, combination gemcitabine and erlotinib became a standard of care in the first-line treatment of locally advanced or metastatic pancreas cancer in patients with a reasonably good performance status at many centers. Enthusiasm for the combination has certainly been tempered by the fact that the survival benefit amounted to just 10 days with the combination therapy. Moreover, erlotinib adds roughly $10,000 per month to the cost of treatment.[238] With that said, gemcitabine/erlotinib is clearly a more effective treatment for a subgroup of 5% to 10% of patients than gemcitabine monotherapy, and identifying predictive markers to select these individuals would be a significant advance and a step towards personalized treatment for pancreatic cancer. Notably, individuals who experienced a skin rash had improved disease control (p = 0.05) and improved survival

(Cox regression HR = 0.37; p = 0.04). Kras mutation status was tested based on prior data that wild-type Kras in colorectal cancers is predictive of response to anti-EGR therapy.[239] Unfortunately, no such correlation was found, although the study was underpowered, in large part because nearly all PDAs harbor Kras mutations.[234]

Building on the modest success of the gemcitabine/erlotinib doublet, Van Cutsem et al.[240] evaluated the same combination with or without bevacizumab in a randomized phase III study (published prior to the negative phase III gemcitabine/bevacizumab study).[240] Six hundred and seven patients were randomized to receive gemcitabine 1,000 mg/m² per week × 7 weeks over 8 weeks and × 3 every 4 weeks for subsequent cycles plus erlotinib 100 mg per day and bevacizumab 5 mg/kg every 2 weeks, or gemcitabine/erlotinib plus placebo. The median OS were 7.1 months for the bevacizumab arm and 6.0 months for the control arm (p = 0.2). Of note, there was an improvement in progression-free survival with the experimental treatment (4.6 versus 3.6 months; p = 0.0002). Grade 3 through 5 adverse events were comparable. Although the primary end point of OS was not met, there was an apparent favorable trend across all end points, providing a modicum of optimism that the gateway towards improved outcomes was opening, if ever so slightly.

Nab-paclitaxel was approved by the FDA in September 2013 as a second agent indicated for combination therapy with gemcitabine. Paclitaxel binds with high affinity to microtubules, thereby stabilizing tubule polymerization and inhibiting cell mitosis. Nab-Paclitaxel is bound to albumin, resulting in improved pharmokinetic efficiency and higher intratumoral drug levels, compared to the standard solvent-based paclitaxel formulation (standard paclitaxel pharmokinetics is otherwise limited by the hydrophobic nature of the molecule).[241] The exact mechanism of improved nab-paclitaxel delivery is not completely understood, but evidence points to protein–protein interactions between albumin and receptors that mediate transport (e.g., gp60) or that enhance drug targeting in the stroma (secreted protein, acidic, cysteine-rich [SPARC]).[242] Interestingly, a recent study of drug pharmokinetics in a genetically engineered SPARC-null mouse demonstrated that intratumoral nab-paclitaxel levels were not dependent on SPARC expression and that the drug does not target the stroma in this model.[243]

In an early phase I/II study, gemcitabine 1,000 mg/m² with nab-paclitaxel 125 mg/m² weekly × 3 every 28 days, resulted in tumor shrinkage in 48% of patients (substantially higher than the 5% rate previously seen with gemcitabine alone[171]) and a median OS of 12.2 months (more than twice the survival with gemcitabine).[244] With these promising results, a large international phase III study was conducted, randomizing 861 patients with advanced PDA to receive either gemcitabine/nab-paclitaxel or gemcitabine alone.[178] The MPACT study met its primary end point (Fig. 49.8), with a

Overall survival

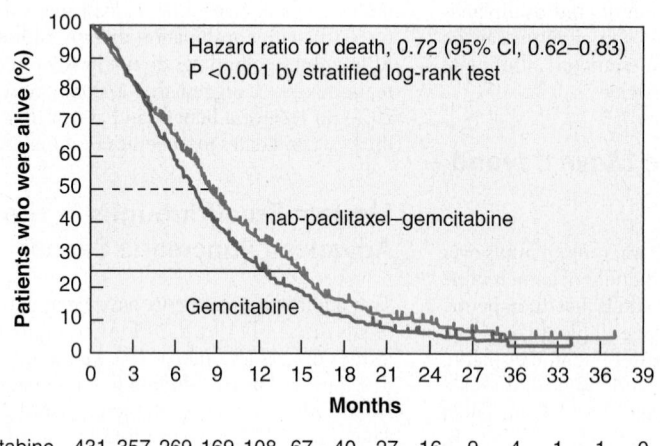

No. at risk												
nab-Paclitaxel–Gemcitabine	431	357	269	169	108	67	40	27	16	9	4	1	1	0
Gemcitabine	430	340	220	124	69	40	26	15	7	3	1	0	0	0

A

Progression-free survival, according to independent review

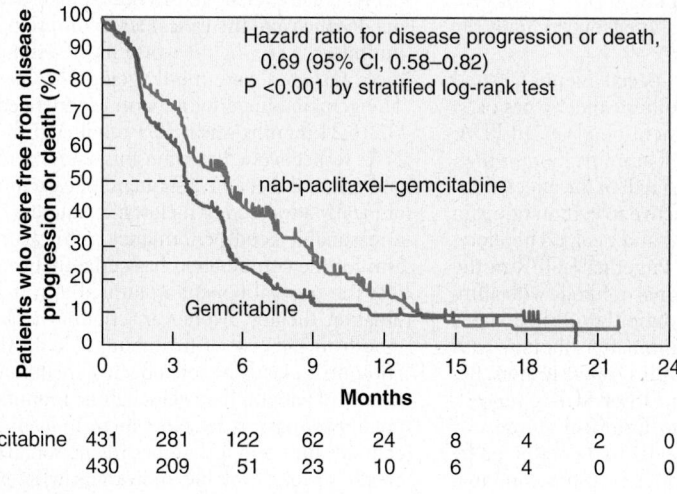

No. at risk								
nab-Paclitaxel–Gemcitabine	431	281	122	62	24	8	4	2	0
Gemcitabine	430	209	51	23	10	6	4	0	0

B

Figure 49.8 Kaplan–Meier curves for survival and progression-free survival for nab-paclitaxel versus gemcitabine. CI, confidence interval. (From Von Hoff DD, Ervin T, Arena FP, et al. Increased survival in pancreatic cancer with nab-paclitaxel plus gemcitabine. *N Engl J Med* 2013;369:1691–1703.)

median OS of 8.5 months in the gemcitabine/nab-paclitaxel arm and 6.7 months in the gemcitabine group (p <0.001). Progression-free survivals were 5.5 and 3.7 months, respectively (p <0.001). The 1-year OS were 35% versus 22%, and the 2-year OS were 9% versus 4%, respectively. Patients receiving combination therapy had a higher response rate as well (23% versus 7%; p <0.001). Grade 3 or higher toxicities that were more common in the nab-paclitaxel arm included neutropenia (38% versus 27%), fatigue (17% versus 7%), and neuropathy (17% versus 1%). Given the results of this trial, gemcitabine combined with nab-paclitaxel has eclipsed gemcitabine plus erlotinib as a standard of care in the first-line treatment of advanced, unresectable, or metastatic pancreatic adenocarcinoma. Importantly, the cost of adding nab-paclitaxel is not trivial ($8,000 per month).

Although gemcitabine has served as the principal backbone for pancreatic cancer therapy in most clinical trials, including patients with advanced PDA, studies were also being conducted on a combination of other drugs with proven success in colorectal cancer, including FOLFIRINOX. In 2003, the results of a phase I study were reported, which included 34 evaluable patients in total, and 6 with advanced pancreatic cancer. Two of the patients with pancreatic cancer experienced an objective response, with one complete responder.[245] These observations spawned a single-arm phase II trial in 47 chemotherapy-naïve patients with advanced pancreatic

cancer.[210] In the 46 evaluable patients, the overall response rate was 26%, with a 4% complete response rate. Median time to progression was 8.2 months and the median OS was 10 months. A randomized phase II trial was initiated, comparing the regimen to gemcitabine. Promising results in 88 patients were presented at the American Society of Clinical Oncology (ASCO) 2007 conference (response rate of 38.7% versus 11.7%), and the study continued on as the large, randomized phase III PRODIGE 4/ACCORD 11 study.[246]

The PRODIGE 4/ACCORD 11 study randomized 342 patients with a performance status of ECOG 0-1 to receive FOLFIRINOX (oxaliplatin 85 mg/m², irinotecan 180 mg/m², leucovorin 400 mg/m², and 5-FU 400 mg/m² IV bolus followed by 5-FU 2,400 mg/m² as a 46- hour continuous infusion every 2 weeks) versus gemcitabine 1,000 mg/m² weekly × 7 weeks followed by 1 week of rest, then 3 times per weekly × 3 every 4 weeks.[177] The primary end point was overall survival OS (Fig. 49.9). The FOLFIRINOX group had a median OS of 11.1 months compared to 6.8 months in the gemcitabine alone arm (p <0.001). Median progression-free survivals were 6.4 months and 3.3 months (p <0.001), respectively. Objective response rates were 31.6% versus 9.4% (p <0.001), and disease control rates (response + disease stability) were 70.2% and 50.9%, respectively. The FOLFIRINOX regimen resulted in substantially more toxicity, including higher grade 3 and 4 neutropenia (45% versus 21%), febrile neutropenia (5.4%

PRACTICE OF ONCOLOGY

Overall survival

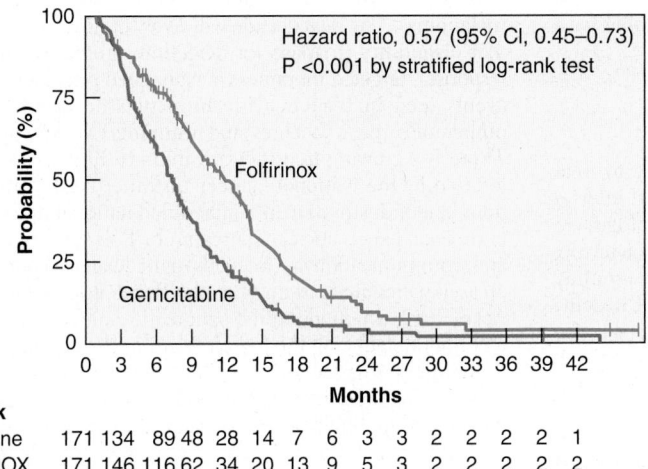

No. at risk

Gemcitabine	171	134	89	48	28	14	7	6	3	3	2	2	2	2	1
FOLFIRINOX	171	146	116	62	34	20	13	9	5	3	2	2	2	2	2

A

Progression-free survival

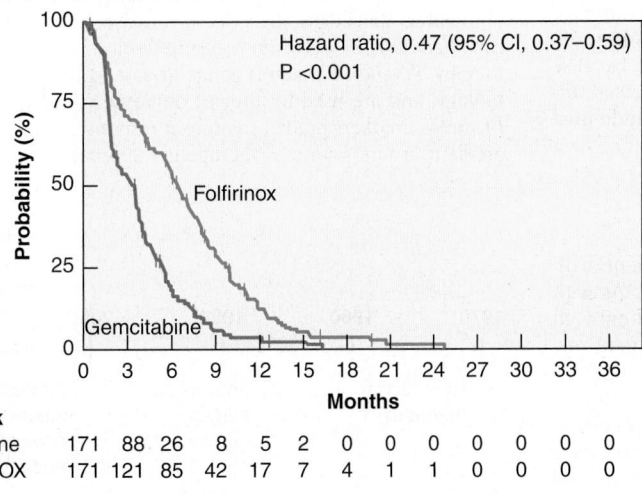

No. at risk

Gemcitabine	171	88	26	8	5	2	0	0	0	0	0	0	0
FOLFIRINOX	171	121	85	42	17	7	4	1	1	0	0	0	0

Figure 49.9 Kaplan–Meier curves for survival and progression-free survival for FOLIRINOX. (From Conroy T, Desseigne F, Ychou M, et al. FOLFIRINOX versus gemcitabine for metastatic pancreatic cancer. *N Engl J Med* 2011;364:1817–1825.)

B

versus 1.2%), thrombocytopenia (9.1% versus 3.6%), diarrhea (12.7% versus 1.8%), and sensory neuropathy (9% versus 0%). Despite these significant side effects, only 31% of patients in the FOLFIRINOX group had a definitive degradation in quality of life (QoL), as compared to 66% in the gemcitabine group. The time to definitive deterioration (based on the EORTC QoL questionnaire) was also significantly longer for the FOLFIRINOX group in the areas of global health status; physical, cognitive, and social functioning; and multiple symptom domains (e.g., fatigue and pain).[247]

Finally, a recently reported phase III trial in Japan compared gemcitabine alone (standard dosing) versus S-1 alone (80 to 120 mg per day for 28 days every 42 days) versus the combination of gemcitabine (1,000 mg/m^2 × 2 every 21 days) plus S-1 (60 to 100 mg per day for 14 days every 21 days). S-1 is an oral fluoropyrimidine derivative available in Japan with activity against PDA. A total of 832 patients with locally advanced or metastatic PDA were included in the analysis. OS were 8.8, 9.7, and 10.1 months (p = 0.15 for combination therapy compared to gemcitabine alone), respectively. Objective responses were higher with S-1 monotherapy (21%) and combination therapy (29%), than gemcitabine alone (13%). Gemcitabine was associated with more hematologic toxicities compared to S-1, whereas S-1 was associated with more diarrhea.[248] Combination therapy was the most toxic regimen.

Taken together, these trials establish gemcitabine alone, S-1 (in Japan), gemcitabine plus nab-paclitaxel, gemcitabine plus erlotinib, and FOLFIRINOX as the current standard of care treatments for metastatic pancreatic cancer. The latter regimen is recommended for patients with excellent performance status (ECOG 0 or 1), whereas the other regimens are applicable for a broader patient population (ECOG 0–2).

Monitoring Treatment Response

In the current era, with multiple active drugs available to treat PDA, patients increasingly have second-line options after a first-line therapy fails. Therefore, it is important for oncologists to closely monitor patients for signs of progression. Patients typically have weekly laboratory testing, and are seen biweekly or monthly by medical oncologists who assess for signs of treatment toxicity. With regard to treatment response, patients undergo repeat imaging (CT scans or magnetic resonance imaging [MRI]) every 8 weeks and responses are assessed by Response Evaluation Criteria in Solid Tumors (RECIST) criteria. CA 19-9 levels are serially drawn every 8 weeks. A falling CA 19-9 level in response to treatment is associated with improved survival, with the greatest decreases being associated with the best outcomes.[249–253] CEA and CA-125 are not FDA-approved biomarkers for PDA, and have far less accuracy then CA 19-9. Nevertheless, they may be helpful to monitor response to therapy, particularly in patients who do not express CA 19-9 due to Lewis antigen polymorphism variability. In the face of rising tumor markers and tumor progression, oncologists should pay close attention to performance status, because patients with an ECOG status of 2 or greater have an expected survival around 2 months and are not likely to benefit from additional chemotherapy.[231]

Symptom Palliation

Although extending survival is a primary objective in patients with PDA, the palliation of symptoms is equally important. As with other aspects of care, palliative-focused therapy in the patient with PDA requires a multidisciplinary team approach. Treatment recommendations are often based on the etiology of the symptoms, which may be multifactorial. Contributing factors include the metabolic burden of the tumor, treatment toxicity, or mechanical obstruction from the tumor. Optimization of nutritional intake is paramount and could be exacerbated by cancer cachexia and pancreatic insufficiency. Aggressive pain management frequently

requires minimally invasive interventions such as celiac plexus neurolysis (endoscopic or percutaneous), in addition to systemic narcotics. Active surveillance and prompt treatment of thromboembolic events, biliary obstruction, and gastric outlet obstruction are critical. Psychosocial issues for the patient and family must be addressed. Often, the extent of symptoms and deterioration in performance status precludes additional antitumor-directed therapy. Even with expert care, there is a 1% to 4% mortality rate related to treatment.[177,178] Therefore, oncologists need to have frank discussions with patients and family members about best supportive care (e.g., no chemotherapy or radiation) when appropriate.

FUTURE DIRECTIONS AND CHALLENGES

The timeline of pancreatic cancer therapy can be summarized as follows (Fig. 49.10): Through the 1970s, no effective therapies existed; between 1980 and 2000, surgical outcomes markedly improved, permitting safe treatment of early stage PDA at high volume centers; between 2000 and the present, modest improvements in chemotherapy and radiation have improved outcomes and the safety profile of these treatments. Over the same time span, there have been dramatic advances in the genetic and molecular understanding of pancreatic cancer development and survival, although this new knowledge has not yet translated into improved patient outcomes. It is becoming more apparent, however, that the field is on the cusp of substantial breakthroughs, similar to those experienced recently in many other cancer types (e.g., breast, colon, melanoma). The next decade will likely produce improved molecular diagnostics (markers for detection, prognosis, and treatment response), targeted therapies (personalized oncology), antistromal agents used in tandem with antineoplastic agents, and immunotherapies (e.g., vaccines and immune checkpoint inhibitors). There is a growing trend toward multi-institutional collaboration fostered by the National Cancer Institute (NCI), private foundations, and industry, as well as scheduled national meetings focused entirely on pancreatic cancer research. This surge in collaboration and communication between thought leaders, coupled with increased national attention (e.g., the Recalcitrant Cancer Research Act of 2012, which identified pancreatic cancer as a high priority), will undoubtedly jolt the field forward in the coming years.

In this closing section, we will broadly discuss some of the most encouraging areas of research, address some of the greatest challenges, and highlight areas that warrant investigative pursuit.

Biomarkers: Diagnostic, Prognostic, and Predictive

Biomarkers can be separated into three categories. *Diagnostic* biomarkers detect the presence of disease. They are relevant for *early detection*, as well as to measure disease burden in response to therapy. *Prognostic* markers gauge disease aggressiveness or tumor biology, and are used to forecast outcome or recurrence pattern. *Predictive* markers predict treatment response, and are the key ingredient to a personalized therapeutic approach.

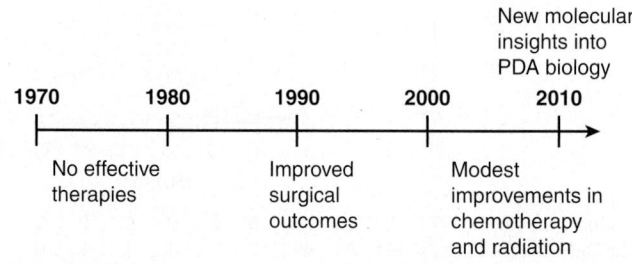

Figure 49.10 Timeline of advances in PDA-related therapy and science.

Effective early detection of PDA could have the greatest impact on PDA-specific outcomes, but may also be the least likely to come to fruition. Such a test would need to identify premalignant lesions that are at very high risk of developing into an invasive lesion (PanIN-3). Genetically engineered mouse data suggest that tumor dissemination can still occur even at the premalignant stage[254]; nevertheless, it is still believed (albeit unproven) that treatment of PanIN-3 lesions would be curative for most patients. Moreover, PanIN-3 (i.e., carcinoma in situ) lesions are likely far enough along in the tumor progression sequence that the risk of overtreatment would not outweigh the potential benefit of treatment (including surgical intervention).[33,255]

There are several challenges associated with early detection research. First, most diagnostic biomarker research to date merely distinguishes invasive PDA (in resected patients) from normal controls. This research largely misses the point, because the index lesions are not *curable* precursor lesions. Most individuals with *localized* invasive cancer already harbor occult metastases. Presently, only 6% of resected PDAs (and <1% of all PDAs) are diagnosed at stage I, and the resection of PanIN-3 disease in the absence of invasive carcinoma is exceedingly rare.[27,256] Second, current CT scanning technology fails to reliably detect PDAs below 2 cm, because PDAs are poorly demarcated and are hypodense compared to normal pancreata.[80] Curable lesions (i.e., PanIN-3 lesions) are likely one-quarter the size of this lower limit.[224] Third, the sensitivity required for effective screening tests is much higher than commonly appreciated. Pannala et al.[79] calculated that an early detection biomarker with 99% sensitivity and specificity would detect all PDAs in the general population, but would also result in a 1% false positive rate due to the relatively low prevalence of PDA (false positives outnumbering true positives by an astounding 25:1). Restricting early detection tests to *high-risk* individuals would improve the positive predictive value, but of course end up missing sporadic PDAs, which comprise the large majority of cases. Finally, serum based tests have a low pretest probability of detecting molecular analytes derived from *noninvasive* lesions that do not have access to the circulatory system. As an illustration of this point, we recently prepared plasma from fresh phlebotomy draws in patients with PDA, and performed a Kras mutation screen using a high-sensitivity commercial mutation detection assay (BEAMing, which detects mutant genes in a background of wild-type DNA at ratios >1:10,000).[257] Mutations were detected at low rates even in patients with high invasive disease burden: two out of nine patients with metastatic disease and zero out of three with localized disease (Jordan M. Winter, unpublished observation). With improved high-throughput instrumentation and bioinformatics strategies available, researchers are now better equipped to interrogate analytes beyond DNA (e.g., metabolome, transcriptome, proteome) in search of a molecular beacon of early PDA. National tissue banking programs, such as the NCI-sponsored Early Detection Research Network, are critical to this pursuit.

There are currently no effective prognostic panels for PDA, akin to the validated Oncotype Dx panels for breast, colon, and prostate cancers. Limitations are primarily due to relatively low tissue availability and to a tighter survival distribution necessitating even higher sample numbers for analyses. Nevertheless, the technology currently exists (e.g., gene expression arrays or Nanostring multiplex gene expression analyses [Seattle, WA]) to develop prognostic panels for PDA. Improved prognostics could identify patients who harbor particularly aggressive tumors that may appear resectable by imaging, yet are best managed with neoadjuvant chemotherapy to treat occult metastases and perhaps avoid ineffective surgery.

There has been some intriguing work in this area. Stratford et al.[258] used fresh frozen tumors from 15 resected PDAs and 15 metastatic PDAs (from autopsies) to identify a gene expression signature using cDNA microarrays associated with metastatic disease. The researchers then tested the derived signature in two separate cohorts of patients with resected disease and found that the panel predicted poor survival. The gene signature has not yet been validated by a separate group.[258] In a separate study, protein expression patterns of 13 putative PDA biomarkers were examined in a large cohort of short- and long-term survivors after resection. The investigators found that MUC1 and mesothelin (MSLN) expression were far more predictive of early cancer-specific death than conventional pathologic features. Again, these findings require validation.[162]

There are no proven predictive markers for standard pancreatic cancer therapies. Data from the phase II gemcitabine/nab-paclitaxel study suggested that stromal SPARC expression is associated with improved outcome.[244] Data from the more recent phase III study are forthcoming. No predictive markers of gemcitabine have been consistently validated in samples from randomized trials. Human equilibrative nucleoside transporter 1 (hENT1) is a nucleoside transporter involved in gemcitabine uptake. Increased expression was associated with improved survival in patients receiving gemcitabine in the RTOG 9704 study,[259] but no association was observed in a randomized study comparing gemcitabine and an hENT1-independent gemcitabine derivative.[260] Brody et al. have identified the RNA binding protein, HuR, as a candidate predictive marker of gemcitabine efficacy in two retrospective institutional cohorts.[261,262] HuR regulates and stabilizes DCK, which phosphorylates and activates gemcitabine. Investigators are currently evaluating samples from the adjuvant ESPAC3 trial (gemcitabine versus 5-FU) to validate this finding. Finally, our group at Thomas Jefferson recently observed that DCK expression was associated with improved survival in patients receiving 5-FU chemotherapy in the RTOG 9704 trial. This finding was recapitulated in cell lines (unpublished).

Targeted Therapy

As a result of whole-exome sequencing, the vast majority of genes mutated in PDA with high frequency are now known. Unfortunately, no novel high frequency *druggable* targets were identified. Many mutated genes can be categorized within core signaling pathway (12 were initially described),[35] and there have growing efforts to try to develop therapies targeting these pathways (as opposed to a specific genetically altered gene). In addition, there has been a redoubling of efforts to target Kras, as a result of the empty genetic search for promising new targets. As stated, Kras is mutated in virtually every PDA, as well as most cells within each PDA. Although attempts to inhibit Kras have eluded researchers thus far, numerous innovative approaches are currently under investigation. These include developing novel compounds to directly bind and inhibit RAS through rational drug design; developing drugs that restore GTP hydrolytic function in mutant RAS; interference with RAS posttranslational modification (e.g., prenylation, proteolytic processing, carboxyl methylation); inhibition of RAS expression (e.g., RNA interference); inhibition of downstream RAS signaling (e.g., Raf-MEK-ERK and PI3K pathways); and identifying pathways that are required for survival in Kras mutant cells (synthetic lethal approach). As evidence of the importance that the NCI has placed on this research, the NCI recently announced an initiative focused on targeting Kras, and plans to divert $10 million annually to support the program (http://frederick.cancer.gov/News/RASCancerGeneticsInitiative.aspx).

Heterogeneity as an Obstacle to Targeted Therapy

PDAs exhibit tremendous molecular heterogeneity, both between and within tumors. The genetic fingerprint of each tumor is unique: each with a different set of mutated genes and chromosome copy number changes.[35,41] Yachida et al.[255] revealed that

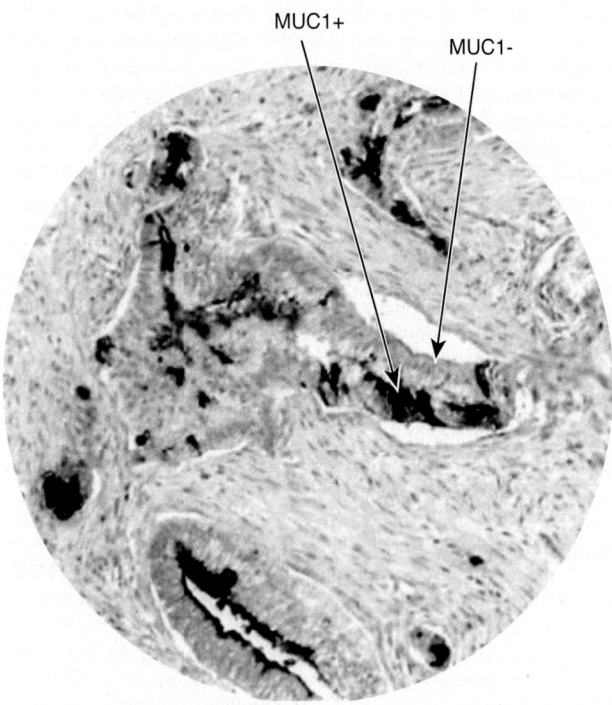

Figure 49.11 MUC1 expression in a pancreatic cancer. A focus of invasive cancer reveals areas of positive (+) and negative (−) MUC1 expression *(arrows)*.

genetic abnormalities differ across a given pancreatic tumor, with genetically distinct foci in the primary, that give rise to clonal populations in metastatic deposits. An immunohistochemical survey of pancreatic cancer biomarkers illustrates the diversity in protein expression.[162] For instance, MUC1 is absent in 15% of PDAs, but is diffusely expressed (>75% of neoplastic cells) in 30%. Even a single focus of PDA containing both MUC1-positive and MUC1-negative cells illustrates biologic variation within a given tumor (Fig. 49.11). Keeping with this pattern, metabolic gradients exist in tumors due to the proximity of neoplastic cells to patent blood vessels as well as due to the dynamic nature of the tumor microenvironment. Microecologic niches result,[263] which are reflected in the varied expression patterns of metabolic enzymes across tumor sites (e.g., primary and metastases) in patients with PDA.[264] Basic cell cycle dynamics drive proteomic changes in a single cell over time, even in the most stable circumstances. PDA heterogeneity is, therefore, a certainty, yet has emerged as the unaddressed truth, as the cancer field pursues a *personalized* approach to cancer therapy. Single molecule targeting is likely to fail because of PDA heterogeneity. An example from another cancer type is illustrative. Extreme heterogeneity, based on the expression pattern of the estrogen receptor, was observed in a human ovarian cancer prior to treatment. After treatment, the expression pattern was dramatically altered in the same tumor sample, when only chemoresistant clones survived.[265] A multitargeted approach may be necessary, similar to the standard treatment strategy against HIV. Therapeutic strategies that are significantly more *tunable* than conventional medicinal pharmacology may also be useful, such as nanoparticle-delivered gene therapy.[266]

Targeting the Stroma

Over 70% of a PDA is comprised of stroma, and a worse outcome was observed in patients with tumors exhibiting a higher stromal content.[267] The hypovascular stroma is viewed as an obstacle to drug delivery, and explains why gemcitabine is potent against xenografts (with low stromal content), but ineffective in autochthonous genetically engineered mouse models of PDA.[268] Stromal depletion in KPC mice (mice with conditional and pancreatic-specific expression of mutant Kras and TP53) with a Hedgehog pathway inhibitor improved gemcitabine delivery to tumors and decreased tumor burden. The same effects were observed in a separate study that used a drug targeting the extracellular matrix protein, hyaluronic acid.[269] Thus, targeting the tumor stroma is a promising strategy to improve the efficacy of conventional pancreatic cancer treatments and is a high research priority.

Metabolism

There is a growing appreciation and understanding of the malignant metabolic phenotype, although Otto Warburg first observed fundamental metabolic differences between cancer and normal cells nearly 100 years ago. The proliferative demands of pancreatic cancer cells, along with the adaptive requirements for survival in an austere tumor microenvironment (characterized by an abundant, yet nutrient-deprived stroma), require complex mechanisms to reprogram metabolic pathways.[270] In fact, PDA cells are particularly tolerant to nutrient deprivation compared to other cancers.[31] Recently, mutant Kras was found to alter metabolic pathways, leading to increased glycolysis,[271] altered amino acid metabolism through noncanonical enzyme pathways,[272] and macropinocytosis of protein as an additional fuel source.[273] Metabolic reprogramming through posttranscriptional regulation of metabolic enzymes by a stress response RNA-binding protein was found to be an independent survival mechanism of PDA cells under nutrient deprivation.[274] A better understanding of PDA metabolism will likely expose metabolic dependencies as important therapeutic targets.

Immunotherapy

Immunotherapy was the 2013 Science Breakthrough of the Year,[275] as a result of multiple new therapies for nonpancreatic malignancies (especially melanoma). Many of the treatments work by targeting immunologic checkpoints (i.e., immunosuppressive pathways induced by cancer cells). Inhibition of these molecules with antibodies unleashes the body's immune system against the tumor in some patients.[276,277] T-cell adoptive therapy is another emerging immunotherapy with successes in nonpancreatic cancers, where T cells from patients are genetically engineered ex vivo to target the patient's own tumor.[278] Thus, there is an urgent need to understand how these strategies can be used or modified to treat pancreatic cancer.

There are immunotherapies that have had some preclinical and early clinical trial success against pancreatic cancer. CD40 is a molecule on the surface of tumor-associated macrophages that stimulates T-cell–dependent antitumor immunity. In a recent phase I study, patients with treatment-naïve advanced PDA were treated with gemcitabine and a monoclonal antibody that binds and stimulates CD40. There was a 19% response rate and biologic indicators of a strong immune response (e.g., increased cytokine levels).[279] A pancreatic cancer vaccine (algenpantucel-L, NewLink Genetics Corporation, Ames, IA) has also been developed in which pancreatic cancer cell lines are genetically engineered to express an immunogenic nonhuman epitope. The vaccine is delivered intradermally, and was given to 70 patients as part of a phase II study, along with gemcitabine and chemoradiation (similar to the RTOG 9704 regimen). The 12-month OS of patients who received the vaccine and conventional adjuvant treatment was 86%, which compared favorably with historical controls.[280] Vaccine-related toxicity was minimal. A phase III adjuvant trial was recently completed in North America, and the results are pending.

CONCLUSION

Improvements in pancreatic cancer treatment over the past 2 decades include safer surgical management, safer radiation treatment, and modest but notable improvements in systemic treatments. With modern chemotherapy, roughly half of patients experience temporary disease control. Nevertheless, the disease is still lethal in most patients and survival beyond 2 years is a rare event. For those of us who routinely treat this disease, progress cannot come soon enough. However, advances are imminent, and there is reason for optimism. The Pancreatic Cancer Action Network has publicized its desire to dramatically improve patient outcomes by the year 2020, and the scientific community is rallying to the charge.

SELECTED REFERENCES

The full reference list can be accessed at lwwhealthlibrary.com/oncology.

1. Siegel R, Naishadham D, Jemal A. Cancer statistics, 2013. *CA Cancer J Clin* 2013;63:11–30.
5. Winter JM, Brennan MF, Tang LH, et al. Survival after resection of pancreatic adenocarcinoma: results from a single institution over three decades. *Ann Surg Oncol* 2012;19:169–175.
6. Edge SE, Byrd DR. *AJCC Cancer Staging Manual.* New York: Springer; 2009.
7. Bilimoria KY, Bentrem DJ, Ko CY, et al. Validation of the 6th edition AJCC Pancreatic Cancer Staging System: report from the National Cancer Database. *Cancer* 2007;110:738–744.
8. National Cancer Institute. SEER Stat Fact Sheets: Pancreas Cancer. http://seer.cancer.gov/statfacts/html/pancreas.html.
11. Klein AP. Genetic susceptibility to pancreatic cancer. *Mol Carcinog* 2012;51:14–24.
13. Bosetti C, Lucenteforte E, Silverman DT, et al. Cigarette smoking and pancreatic cancer: an analysis from the International Pancreatic Cancer Case-Control Consortium (Panc4). *Ann Oncol* 2012;23:1880–1888.
20. Andreotti G, Silverman DT. Occupational risk factors and pancreatic cancer: a review of recent findings. *Mol Carcinog* 2012;51:98–108.
21. Lucenteforte E, La Vecchia C, Silverman D, et al. Alcohol consumption and pancreatic cancer: a pooled analysis in the International Pancreatic Cancer Case-Control Consortium (PanC4). *Ann Oncol* 2012;23:374–382.
22. Duell EJ, Lucenteforte E, Olson SH, et al. Pancreatitis and pancreatic cancer risk: a pooled analysis in the International Pancreatic Cancer Case-Control Consortium (PanC4). *Ann Oncol* 2012;23:2964–2970.
23. Bracci PM. Obesity and pancreatic cancer: overview of epidemiologic evidence and biologic mechanisms. *Mol Carcinog* 2012;51:53–63.
24. Huxley R, Ansary-Moghaddam A, Berrington de Gonzalez A, et al. Type-II diabetes and pancreatic cancer: a meta-analysis of 36 studies. *Br J Cancer* 2005;92:2076–2083.
25. Ben Q, Xu M, Ning X, et al. Diabetes mellitus and risk of pancreatic cancer: A meta-analysis of cohort studies. *Eur J Cancer* 2011;47:1928–1937.
26. Klimstra DS, Pitman MB, Hruban RH. An algorithmic approach to the diagnosis of pancreatic neoplasms. *Arch Pathol Lab Med* 2009;133:454–464.
27. Winter JM, Cameron JL, Campbell KA, et al. 1423 pancreaticoduodenectomies for pancreatic cancer: A single-institution experience. *J Gastrointest Surg* 2006;10:1199–1210.
28. Winter JM, Maitra A, Yeo CJ. Genetics and pathology of pancreatic cancer. *HPB (Oxford)* 2006;8:324–336.
29. Neesse A, Michl P, Frese KK, et al. Stromal biology and therapy in pancreatic cancer. *Gut* 2011;60:861–868.
30. Anderson AR, Weaver AM, Cummings PT, et al. Tumor morphology and phenotypic evolution driven by selective pressure from the microenvironment. *Cell* 2006;127:905–915.
31. Izuishi K, Kato K, Ogura T, et al. Remarkable tolerance of tumor cells to nutrient deprivation: possible new biochemical target for cancer therapy. *Cancer Res* 2000;60:6201–6207.
34. Biankin AV, Waddell N, Kassahn KS, et al. Pancreatic cancer genomes reveal aberrations in axon guidance pathway genes. *Nature* 2012;491:399–405.
35. Jones S, Zhang X, Parsons DW, et al. Core signaling pathways in human pancreatic cancers revealed by global genomic analyses. *Science* 2008;321:1801–1806.
41. Calhoun ES, Hucl T, Gallmeier E, et al. Identifying allelic loss and homozygous deletions in pancreatic cancer without matched normals using high-density single-nucleotide polymorphism arrays. *Cancer Res* 2006;66:7920–7928.
49. Iacobuzio-Donahue CA, Fu B, Yachida S, et al. DPC4 gene status of the primary carcinoma correlates with patterns of failure in patients with pancreatic cancer. *J Clin Oncol* 2009;27:1806–1813.
55. Baumgart M, Werther M, Bockholt A, et al. Genomic instability at both the base pair level and the chromosomal level is detectable in earliest PanIN lesions in tissues of chronic pancreatitis. *Pancreas* 2010;39:1093–1103.
56. Hong SM, Vincent A, Kanda M, et al. Genome-wide somatic copy number alterations in low-grade PanINs and IPMNs from individuals with a family history of pancreatic cancer. *Clin Cancer Res* 2012;18:4303–4312.
60. Canto MI, Hruban RH, Fishman EK, et al. Frequent detection of pancreatic lesions in asymptomatic high-risk individuals. *Gastroenterology* 2012;142:796–804.
61. Canto MI, Harinck F, Hruban RH, et al. International Cancer of the Pancreas Screening (CAPS) Consortium summit on the management of patients with increased risk for familial pancreatic cancer. *Gut* 2013;62:339–347.
62. Perez-Mancera PA, Guerra C, Barbacid M, et al. What we have learned about pancreatic cancer from mouse models. *Gastroenterology* 2012;142:1079–1092.
64. Jiao Y, Yonescu R, Offerhaus GJ, et al. Whole exome sequencing of pancreatic neoplasms with acinar differentiation. *J Pathol* 2014;232:428–435.
66. Shi C, Hruban RH. Intraductal papillary mucinous neoplasm. *Hum Pathol* 2012;43:1–16.
70. Wu J, Jiao Y, Dal Molin M, et al. Whole-exome sequencing of neoplastic cysts of the pancreas reveals recurrent mutations in components of ubiquitin-dependent pathways. *Proc Natl Acad Sci U S A* 2011;108:21188–21193.
77. Jiao Y, Shi C, Edil BH, et al. DAXX/ATRX, MEN1, and mTOR pathway genes are frequently altered in pancreatic neuroendocrine tumors. *Science* 2011;331:1199–1203.
78. Falconi M, Bartsch DK, Eriksson B, et al. ENETS Consensus Guidelines for the management of patients with digestive neuroendocrine neoplasms of the digestive system: well-differentiated pancreatic non-functioning tumors. *Neuroendocrinology* 2012;95:120–134.
79. Pannala R, Basu A, Petersen GM, et al. New-onset diabetes: a potential clue to the early diagnosis of pancreatic cancer. *Lancet Oncol* 2009;10:88–95.
81. Callery MP, Chang KJ, Fishman EK, et al. Pretreatment assessment of resectable and borderline resectable pancreatic cancer: expert consensus statement. *Ann Surg Oncol* 2009;16:1727–1733.
82. Evans DB, Erickson BA, Ritch P. Borderline resectable pancreatic cancer: definitions and the importance of multimodality therapy. *Ann Surg Oncol* 2010;17:2803–2805.
83. Varadhachary GR, Tamm EP, Abbruzzese JL, et al. Borderline resectable pancreatic cancer: definitions, management, and role of preoperative therapy. *Ann Surg Oncol* 2006;13:1035–1046.
84. Evans DB, Varadhachary GR, Crane CH, et al. Preoperative gemcitabine-based chemoradiation for patients with resectable adenocarcinoma of the pancreatic head. *J Clin Oncol* 2008;26:3496–3502.
85. Katz MH, Fleming JB, Bhosale P, et al. Response of borderline resectable pancreatic cancer to neoadjuvant therapy is not reflected by radiographic indicators. *Cancer* 2012;118:5749–5756.
86. van der Gaag NA, Rauws EA, van Eijck CH, et al. Preoperative biliary drainage for cancer of the head of the pancreas. *N Engl J Med* 2010;362:129–137.
87. Kooby DA, Hawkins WG, Schmidt CM, et al. A multicenter analysis of distal pancreatectomy for adenocarcinoma: is laparoscopic resection appropriate? *J Am Coll Surg* 2010;210:779–785.
90. Bassi C, Dervenis C, Butturini G, et al. Postoperative pancreatic fistula: an international study group (ISGPF) definition. *Surgery* 2005;138:8–13.
95. Doi R, Imamura M, Hosotani R, et al. Surgery versus radiochemotherapy for resectable locally invasive pancreatic cancer: final results of a randomized multi-institutional trial. *Surg Today* 2008;38:1021–1028.
97. Karanicolas PJ, Davies E, Kunz R, et al. The pylorus: take it or leave it? Systematic review and meta-analysis of pylorus-preserving versus standard whipple pancreaticoduodenectomy for pancreatic or periampullary cancer. *Ann Surg Oncol* 2007;14:1825–1834.
141. Diener MK, Seiler CM, Rossion I, et al. Efficacy of stapler versus hand-sewn closure after distal pancreatectomy (DISPACT): a randomised, controlled multicentre trial. *Lancet* 2011;377:1514–1522.
151. Barton JG, Bois JP, Sarr MG, et al. Predictive and prognostic value of CA 19-9 in resected pancreatic adenocarcinoma. *J Gastrointest Surg* 2009;13:2050–2058.
154. Berger AC, Garcia M Jr, Hoffman JP, et al. Postresection CA 19-9 predicts overall survival in patients with pancreatic cancer treated with adjuvant chemoradiation: a prospective validation by RTOG 9704. *J Clin Oncol* 2008;26:5918–5922.
158. Boeck S, Ankerst DP, Heinemann V. The role of adjuvant chemotherapy for patients with resected pancreatic cancer: systematic review of randomized controlled trials and meta-analysis. *Oncology* 2007;72:314–321.
159. Oettle H, Post S, Neuhaus P, et al. Adjuvant chemotherapy with gemcitabine vs observation in patients undergoing curative-intent resection of pancreatic cancer: a randomized controlled trial. *JAMA* 2007;297:267–277.
160. Winter JM, Tang LH, Klimstra DS, et al. Failure patterns in resected pancreas adenocarcinoma: lack of predicted benefit to smad4 expression. *Ann Surg* 2013;258:331–335.

PRACTICE OF ONCOLOGY

161. Crane CH, Varadhachary GR, Yordy JS, et al. Phase II trial of cetuximab, gemcitabine, and oxaliplatin followed by chemoradiation with cetuximab for locally advanced (T4) pancreatic adenocarcinoma: correlation of Smad4(Dpc4) immunostaining with pattern of disease progression. *J Clin Oncol* 2011;29:3037–3043.

162. Winter JM, Tang LH, Klimstra DS, et al. A novel survival-based tissue microarray of pancreatic cancer validates MUC1 and mesothelin as biomarkers. *PLoS One* 2012;7:e40157.

163. Smeenk HG, van Eijck CH, Hop WC, et al. Long-term survival and metastatic pattern of pancreatic and periampullary cancer after adjuvant chemoradiation or observation: long-term results of EORTC trial 40891. *Ann Surg* 2007;246:734–740.

164. Oettle H, Neuhaus P, Hochhaus A, et al. Adjuvant chemotherapy with gemcitabine and long-term outcomes among patients with resected pancreatic cancer: the CONKO-001 randomized trial. *JAMA* 2013;310:1473–1481.

165. Neoptolemos JP, Stocken DD, Friess H, et al. A randomized trial of chemoradiotherapy and chemotherapy after resection of pancreatic cancer. *N Engl J Med* 2004;350:1200–1210.

166. Neoptolemos JP, Stocken DD, Bassi C, et al. Adjuvant chemotherapy with fluorouracil plus folinic acid vs gemcitabine following pancreatic cancer resection: a randomized controlled trial. *JAMA* 2010;304:1073–1081.

167. Kosuge T, Kiuchi T, Mukai K, et al. A multicenter randomized controlled trial to evaluate the effect of adjuvant cisplatin and 5-fluorouracil therapy after curative resection in cases of pancreatic cancer. *Jpn J Clin Oncol* 2006;36:159–165.

168. Kalser MH, Ellenberg SS. Pancreatic cancer. Adjuvant combined radiation and chemotherapy following curative resection. *Arch Surg* 1985;120:899–903.

169. Bakkevold KE, Arnesjo B, Dahl O, et al. Adjuvant combination chemotherapy (AMF) following radical resection of carcinoma of the pancreas and papilla of Vater—results of a controlled, prospective, randomised multicentre study. *Eur J Cancer* 1993;29A:698–703.

170. Regine WF, Winter KA, Abrams R, et al. Fluorouracil-based chemoradiation with either gemcitabine or fluorouracil chemotherapy after resection of pancreatic adenocarcinoma: 5-year analysis of the U.S. Intergroup/RTOG 9704 phase III trial. *Ann Surg Oncol* 2011;18:1319–1326.

171. Burris HA 3rd, Moore MJ, Andersen J, et al. Improvements in survival and clinical benefit with gemcitabine as first-line therapy for patients with advanced pancreas cancer: a randomized trial. *J Clin Oncol* 1997;15:2403–2413.

175. Moore MJ, Goldstein D, Hamm J, et al. Erlotinib plus gemcitabine compared with gemcitabine alone in patients with advanced pancreatic cancer: a phase III trial of the National Cancer Institute of Canada Clinical Trials Group. *J Clin Oncol* 2007;25:1960–1966.

177. Conroy T, Desseigne F, Ychou M, et al. FOLFIRINOX versus gemcitabine for metastatic pancreatic cancer. *N Engl J Med* 2011;364:1817–1825.

178. Von Hoff DD, Ervin T, Arena FP, et al. Increased survival in pancreatic cancer with nab-paclitaxel plus gemcitabine. *N Engl J Med* 2013;369:1691–1703.

179. O'Reilly EM, Lowery MA. Postresection surveillance for pancreatic cancer performance status, imaging, and serum markers. *Cancer J* 2012;18:609–613.

180. Sheffield KM, Crowell KT, Lin YL, et al. Surveillance of pancreatic cancer patients after surgical resection. *Ann Surg Oncol* 2012;19:1670–1677.

182. Arnaoutakis GJ, Rangachari D, Laheru DA, et al. Pulmonary resection for isolated pancreatic adenocarcinoma metastasis: an analysis of outcomes and survival. *J Gastrointest Surg* 2011;15:1611–1617.

190. Treatment of locally unresectable carcinoma of the pancreas: comparison of combined-modality therapy (chemotherapy plus radiotherapy) to chemotherapy alone. Gastrointestinal Tumor Study Group. *J Natl Cancer Inst* 1988;80:751–755.

191. Chauffert B, Mornex F, Bonnetain F, et al. Phase III trial comparing intensive induction chemoradiotherapy (60 Gy, infusional 5-FU and intermittent cisplatin) followed by maintenance gemcitabine with gemcitabine alone for locally advanced unresectable pancreatic cancer. Definitive results of the 2000-01 FFCD/SFRO study. *Ann Oncol* 2008;19:1592–1599.

192. Klaassen DJ, MacIntyre JM, Catton GE, et al. Treatment of locally unresectable cancer of the stomach and pancreas: a randomized comparison of 5-fluorouracil alone with radiation plus concurrent and maintenance 5-fluorouracil—an Eastern Cooperative Oncology Group study. *J Clin Oncol* 1985;3:373–378.

193. Loehrer PJ, Sr., Feng Y, Cardenes H, et al. Gemcitabine alone versus gemcitabine plus radiotherapy in patients with locally advanced pancreatic cancer: an Eastern Cooperative Oncology Group trial. *J Clin Oncol* 2011;29:4105–4112.

194. Hammel P, Florence H, Van Lathem J, et al. Comparison of chemoradiotherapy (CRT) and chemotherapy (CT) in patients with a locally advanced pancreatic cancer (LAPC) controlled after 4 months of gemcitabine with or without erlotinib: Final results of the international phase III LAP 07 study. *J Clin Oncol* 2013;31:suppl; abstr LBA4003.

197. Ben-Josef E, Schipper M, Francis IR, et al. A phase I/II trial of intensity modulated radiation (IMRT) dose escalation with concurrent fixed-dose rate gemcitabine (FDR-G) in patients with unresectable pancreatic cancer. *Int J Radiat Oncol Biol Phys* 2012;84:1166–1171.

207. Mukherjee S, Hurt CN, Bridgewater J, et al. Gemcitabine-based or capecitabine-based chemoradiotherapy for locally advanced pancreatic cancer (SCALOP): a multicentre, randomised, phase 2 trial. *Lancet Oncol* 2013;14:317–326.

210. Conroy T, Paillot B, Francois E, et al. Irinotecan plus oxaliplatin and leucovorin-modulated fluorouracil in advanced pancreatic cancer—a Groupe Tumeurs Digestives of the Federation Nationale des Centres de Lutte Contre le Cancer study. *J Clin Oncol* 2005;23:1228–1236.

211. Festa V, Andriulli A, Valvano MR, et al. Neoadjuvant chemo-radiotherapy for patients with borderline resectable pancreatic cancer: a meta-analytical evaluation of prospective studies. *JOP* 2013;14:618–625.

214. Rwigema JC, Parikh SD, Heron DE, et al. Stereotactic body radiotherapy in the treatment of advanced adenocarcinoma of the pancreas. *Am J Clin Oncol* 2011;34:63–69.

218. Mini E, Nobili S, Caciagli B, et al. Cellular pharmacology of gemcitabine. *Ann Oncol* 2006;17 Suppl 5:v7–v12.

219. Tempero M, Plunkett W, Ruiz Van Haperen V, et al. Randomized phase II comparison of dose-intense gemcitabine: thirty-minute infusion and fixed dose rate infusion in patients with pancreatic adenocarcinoma. *J Clin Oncol* 2003;21:3402–3408.

220. Poplin E, Feng Y, Berlin J, et al. Phase III, randomized study of gemcitabine and oxaliplatin versus gemcitabine (fixed-dose rate infusion) compared with gemcitabine (30-minute infusion) in patients with pancreatic carcinoma E6201: a trial of the Eastern Cooperative Oncology Group. *J Clin Oncol* 2009;27:3778–3785.

230. Kindler HL, Ioka T, Richel DJ, et al. Axitinib plus gemcitabine versus placebo plus gemcitabine in patients with advanced pancreatic adenocarcinoma: a double-blind randomised phase 3 study. *Lancet Oncol* 2011;12:256–262.

231. Kindler HL, Niedzwiecki D, Hollis D, et al. Gemcitabine plus bevacizumab compared with gemcitabine plus placebo in patients with advanced pancreatic cancer: phase III trial of the Cancer and Leukemia Group B (CALGB 80303). *J Clin Oncol* 2010;28:3617–3622.

232. Philip PA, Benedetti J, Corless CL, et al. Phase III study comparing gemcitabine plus cetuximab versus gemcitabine in patients with advanced pancreatic adenocarcinoma: Southwest Oncology Group-directed intergroup trial S0205. *J Clin Oncol* 2010;28:3605–3610.

235. Xiong HQ, Rosenberg A, LoBuglio A, et al. Cetuximab, a monoclonal antibody targeting the epidermal growth factor receptor, in combination with gemcitabine for advanced pancreatic cancer: a multicenter phase II Trial. *J Clin Oncol* 2004;22:2610–2616.

236. Ciliberto D, Botta C, Correale P, et al. Role of gemcitabine-based combination therapy in the management of advanced pancreatic cancer: a meta-analysis of randomised trials. *Eur J Cancer* 2013;49:593–603.

240. Van Cutsem E, Vervenne WL, Bennouna J, et al. Phase III trial of bevacizumab in combination with gemcitabine and erlotinib in patients with metastatic pancreatic cancer. *J Clin Oncol* 2009;27:2231–2237.

244. Von Hoff DD, Ramanathan RK, Borad MJ, et al. Gemcitabine plus nab-paclitaxel is an active regimen in patients with advanced pancreatic cancer: a phase I/II trial. *J Clin Oncol* 2011;29:4548–4554.

248. Ueno H, Ioka T, Ikeda M, et al. Randomized phase III study of gemcitabine plus S-1, S-1 alone, or gemcitabine alone in patients with locally advanced and metastatic pancreatic cancer in Japan and Taiwan: GEST study. *J Clin Oncol* 2013;31:1640–1648.

255. Yachida S, Jones S, Bozic I, et al. Distant metastasis occurs late during the genetic evolution of pancreatic cancer. *Nature* 2010;467:1114–1117.

292. McCracken JD, Ray P, Heilbrun LK, et al. 5-Fluorouracil, methyl-CCNU, and radiotherapy with or without testolactone for localized adenocarcinoma of the exocrine pancreas: a Southwest Oncology Group Study. *Cancer* 1980;46:1518–1522.

293. Moertel CG, Frytak S, Hahn RG, et al. Therapy of locally unresectable pancreatic carcinoma: a randomized comparison of high dose (6000 rads) radiation alone, moderate dose radiation (4000 rads + 5-fluorouracil), and high dose radiation + 5-fluorouracil: The Gastrointestinal Tumor Study Group. *Cancer* 1981;48:1705–1710.

294. Radiation therapy combined with Adriamycin or 5-fluorouracil for the treatment of locally unresectable pancreatic carcinoma. Gastrointestinal Tumor Study Group. *Cancer* 1985;56:2563–2568.

295. Earle JD, Foley JF, Wieand HS, et al. Evaluation of external-beam radiation therapy plus 5-fluorouracil (5-FU) versus external-beam radiation therapy plus hycanthone (HYC) in confined, unresectable pancreatic cancer. *Int J Radiat Oncol Biol Phys* 1994;28:207–211.

296. Cohen SJ, Dobelbower R, Jr., Lipsitz S, et al. A randomized phase III study of radiotherapy alone or with 5-fluorouracil and mitomycin-C in patients with locally advanced adenocarcinoma of the pancreas: Eastern Cooperative Oncology Group study E8282. *Int J Radiat Oncol Biol Phys* 2005;62:1345–1350.

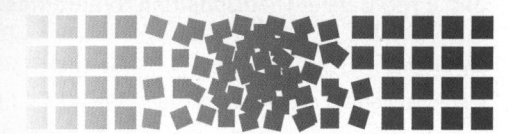

Jennifer E. Axilbund and Elizabeth L. Wiley

INTRODUCTION

It is estimated that 5% to 10% of pancreatic cancer (adenocarcinoma) is familial,[1,2] and individuals with a family history of pancreatic cancer are at a greater risk of developing pancreatic cancer themselves.[3] Although there is evidence of a major pancreatic cancer susceptibility gene,[4] it remains elusive. Therefore, the majority of families with multiple cases of pancreatic cancer do not have an identifiable causative gene or syndrome, making risk assessment and counseling challenging. However, a subset of pancreatic cancer is attributable to known inherited cancer predisposition syndromes (Table 50.1).

SELECTED GENES THAT MAY CAUSE PANCREATIC CANCER

BRCA2

The BRCA2 gene is associated with hereditary breast and ovarian cancer syndrome, and often presents as premenopausal breast cancer, ovarian cancer, and/or male breast cancer. The Breast Cancer Linkage Consortium[5] reported a 3.5-fold (95% confidence interval [CI], 1.9 to 6.6) increased risk of pancreatic cancer in BRCA2 gene mutation carriers. Subsequent studies in the United Kingdom and the Netherlands showed a relative risk of 4.1 and 5.9, respectively.[6,7] In a United States–based study, 10.9% (17 out of 156) of families with a BRCA2 mutation reported a family history of pancreatic cancer. The median ages at diagnosis for males and females were 67 and 59 years, respectively, which differed statistically from the Surveillance, Epidemiology and End Results (SEER) database (70 years old for males and 74 years old for females; $p = 0.011$).[8] Although genotype–phenotype data remain sparse, the BRCA2 K3326X variant was found in 5.6% (8 out of 144) of familial pancreatic cancer patients compared with 1.2% (3 out of 250) of those with sporadic pancreatic cancer (odds ratio [OR], 4.84; 95% CI, 1.27 to 18.55; $p <0.01$).[9]

Approximately 17% of pancreatic cancer patients who have at least two additional relatives with pancreatic cancer carry deleterious mutations in the BRCA2 gene.[10] Estimates for the prevalence of BRCA2 mutations with two first-degree relatives with pancreatic cancer are 6% to 12%,[11,12] and BRCA2 mutations also explain a portion of apparently sporadic pancreatic cancers.[13] However, prevalence varies between populations. Out of 145 Ashkenazi Jews with pancreatic cancer, 6 (4.1%) were found to have a deleterious BRCA2 mutation when compared with cancer-free controls (OR, 3.85; 95% CI, 2.1 to 10.8; $p = 0.007$), although no differences were noted in age at diagnosis or clinical pathologic features.[14] An earlier, smaller study found a deleterious BRCA2 mutation in 3 (13%) of 23 Ashkenazi Jews with pancreatic cancer, unselected for family history.[15] Among Ashkenazi Jewish probands with breast cancer who reported a family history of pancreatic cancer, 7.6% (16 out of 211) had a BRCA2 mutation.[16] By comparison, no BRCA2 mutations were found in studies of pancreatic cancer in Korea or Italy.[17,18]

BRCA1

Similar to BRCA2, mutations in BRCA1 are associated with a markedly increased risk for premenopausal breast cancer and ovarian cancer. The Breast Cancer Linkage Consortium reported a 2.26-fold (95% CI, 1.26 to 4.06) increased risk of pancreatic cancer in families with a BRCA1 mutation,[19] and Brose et al.[20] estimated a threefold higher lifetime risk. However, more recently, in the United Kingdom, Moran et al.[6] found no elevation in pancreatic cancer risk in 268 families with a known BRCA1 mutation. A United States–based study reported that 11% (24 out of 219) of their families with a BRCA1 mutation had at least one individual with pancreatic cancer, with median ages at diagnosis of 59 years for males and 68 years for females. Again, this was significantly younger than reported in the SEER database ($p = 0.0014$).[8] Al-Sukhni et al.[21] molecularly evaluated pancreatic tumors from seven known BRCA1 mutation carriers and found a loss of heterozygosity of BRCA1 in five (71%), with confirmed loss of the wild-type allele in three of the five compared with only one (11%) of nine sporadic controls. This suggests that BRCA1 germ-line mutations do, in fact, predispose some individuals to pancreatic cancers.

Familial breast cancer registries in the United States and Israel have evaluated the mutation status of families that reported pancreatic cancer in addition to breast cancer and ovarian cancer. In the US study of 19 families with breast, ovarian, and pancreatic cancer, 15 carried a deleterious mutation in BRCA1 and 4 in BRCA2,[22] whereas the Israeli study reported an equal number of BRCA1 and BRCA2 families.[23]

Another study, specifically of Ashkenazi Jewish families, reported a BRCA1 mutation in 7% of probands with breast cancer who also had a family history of pancreatic cancer,[16] which was, again, equal to the prevalence of BRCA2 mutations. Thus, within the Ashkenazi Jewish population, BRCA1 and BRCA2 mutations may contribute more equally to risk in families with both breast and pancreatic cancer. However, these studies all examined cohorts of families selected because of clustering of breast and/or ovarian cancer with pancreatic cancer. When families were selected on the basis of familial pancreatic cancer alone, BRCA1 mutations were less prevalent. None of the sixty-six families with three or more cases of pancreatic cancer had a deleterious BRCA1 mutation, including those who also reported a family history of breast and/or ovarian cancer.[24] An evaluation of Ashkenazi Jewish patients ascertained on the basis of pancreatic cancer alone showed a 1.3% (2 out of 145) prevalence of BRCA1 mutations.[14] Therefore, BRCA1 may explain a small subset of families showing a clustering of pancreatic cancer with breast and/or ovarian cancer, but is unlikely to explain most families with site-specific pancreatic cancer.

PALB2

PALB2 (partner and localizer of BRCA2) was recognized as the FANCN gene in 2007, and biallelic mutation carriers develop

TABLE 50.1

Inherited Cancer Predisposition Syndromes that Increase the Risk for Pancreatic Cancer

Syndrome	Gene(s)	Risk of Pancreatic Cancer	Predominant Features
Hereditary breast and ovarian cancer	BRCA1	RR, 2.26–3	Malignancies: Breast (particularly premenopausal), ovary, male breast, prostate
	BRCA2	RR, 3.5–5.9	Malignancies: Breast (particularly premenopausal), ovary, male breast, prostate, melanoma (cutaneous and ocular)
Familial atypical multiple mole and melanoma	CDKN2A	RR, 7.4–47.8	Malignancies: Melanoma (often multiple and early onset) Other: Dysplastic nevi
Hereditary pancreatitis	PRSS1	SIR, 57	Other: Chronic pancreatitis
Hereditary nonpolyposis colorectal cancer (Lynch syndrome)	MLH1 MSH2 MSH6 PMS2 EPCAM	SIR, 0–8.6	Malignancies: Colorectum, endometrium, ovary, stomach, small bowel, urinary tract (ureter, renal pelvis), biliary, brain (glioblastoma), skin (sebaceous)
PJS	STK11	SIR, 132	Malignancies: Colorectum, small bowel, stomach, breast, gynecologic Other: Melanin pigmentation (mucocutaneous), small-bowel intussusception

SIR, standardized incidence ratio.

Fanconi anemia.[25,26] Monoallelic mutation carriers were shown to be at an increased risk for breast cancer (relative risk [RR], 2.3; 95% CI, 1.4 to 3.9).[27] The prevalence of PALB2 mutations among familial breast cancer cases is low across ethnicities; PALB2 mutations are relatively nonexistent in breast cancers in the Irish and Icelandic populations and are found in approximately 1% of Italians, African Americans, Chinese, and Spanish breast cancer families, and in 2% of young South African breast cancer patients.[28–35] An analysis of 1,144 US familial breast cancer cases found a PALB2 mutation in 3.4% (33 out of 972) of non-Ashkenazi Jews and none (0 out of 172) of Ashkenazi Jews. The estimated risk for breast cancer was 2.3-fold by the age of 55 years (95% CI, 1.5 to 4.2) and 3.4-fold by the age of 85 years (95% CI, 2.4 to 5.9). There was also a fourfold risk for male breast cancer ($p = 0.0003$) and a sixfold risk for pancreatic cancer ($p = 0.002$).[36] Among French Canadian women with bilateral breast cancer, a PALB2 mutation was found in 0.9% (5 out of 559) compared with none of the 565 women with unilateral breast cancer ($p = 0.04$), and first-degree relatives of PALB2 mutation carriers had a 5.3-fold risk for breast cancer (95% CI, 1.8 to 13.2).[37]

PALB2 founder mutations have been identified in several populations, including the c.2323C>T (Q775X) mutation in French Canadians.[38] Another example is the Finnish founder mutation c.1592delT. This mutation was found in 2.7% (3 out of 113) of familial breast and/or breast/ovarian cancer families compared with 0.2% (6 out of 2,501) of controls (OR, 11.3; 95% CI, 1.8 to 57.8; $p = 0.005$).[39] One percent (18 out of 1,918) of breast cancer cases unselected for family history also had this founder mutation. The hazard ratio for breast cancer was estimated at 6.1 (95% CI, 2.2 to 17.2; $p = 0.01$), with a penetrance of 40% by the age of 70 years.[40]

PALB2 has not been shown to be a significant contributor to familial clustering of other cancers, including melanoma, ovarian cancer, and prostate cancer,[41–43] but has been identified in familial pancreatic cancer kindreds. Specifically, Jones et al.[44] identified a PALB2 mutation in a familial pancreatic

cancer proband, and subsequently found PALB2 mutations in 3 out of 96 additional families, suggesting that 3% to 4% of familial pancreatic cancer may be attributed to this gene. Other populations have found lower mutation frequencies, ranging from absent in the Dutch (0 out of 31) to 3.7% (3 out of 81) in Germans.[45,46] When ascertained on the basis of co-occurrence of breast and pancreatic cancer in the same individual or family, prevalence varied, again, from absent in the Dutch (0 out of 45) and United States–based studies (0 out of 77) to 4.8% (3 out of 62) in Italians.[42,47,48]

CDKN2A

The p16 transcript of the CDKN2A gene is an important cell cycle regulator. Germ-line mutations in the CDKN2A gene predispose individuals to multiple early-onset melanomas. Somatic CDKN2A mutations are also frequently identified in pancreatic adenocarcinomas and precursor lesions, indicating a role for this gene in pancreatic cancer development and progression.[49–51]

The risk of pancreatic cancer with CDKN2A mutations varies based on genotype. In a study of 22 families with the Dutch founder mutation, p16-Leiden, which is a 19–base-pair deletion in exon 2, the relative risk of pancreatic cancer was 47.8 (95% CI, 28.4 to 74.7).[52] The age-related risks have been shown to be less than 1%, 4%, 5%, 12%, and 17% by ages 40, 50, 60, 70, and 75 years, respectively.[53] Regarding other mutations, the Genes, Environment and Melanoma Study assessed relative risks for nonmelanoma cancers in 429 first-degree relatives of 65 melanoma patients with a CDKN2A mutation. Five pancreatic cancers were reported compared with 41 pancreatic cancers among 23,452 first-degree relatives of 3,537 noncarriers, for a relative risk of 7.4 (95% CI, 2.3 to 18.7; $p = 0.002$).[54] A United States–based study estimated penetrance to be 58% by the age of 80 years (95% CI, 8% to 86%) and noted a hazard ratio of 25.8 ($p = 2.1 \times 102^{13}$) in those who ever smoked cigarettes.[55]

Mutation prevalence in pancreatic cancer families varies by population. In an Italian study, 5.7% of 225 consecutive patients with pancreatic cancer had an identified *CDKN2A* mutation.[56] The predominant mutations were the E27X and G101W founder mutations, although others were also represented. Of 16 patients classified as having familial pancreatic cancer, 5 (31%) carried *CDKN2A* mutations, leading the authors to conclude that this gene may account for a sizeable subset of Italian familial pancreatic families. By comparison, no *CDKN2A* mutations were found in 51 Polish pancreatic cancer patients diagnosed at younger than 50 years.[57] Similarly, an analysis of 94 German pancreatic cancer patients who had at least one other first-degree relative with pancreatic cancer revealed no *CDKN2A* mutations.[58] However, two of five families with at least one pancreatic cancer and at least one melanoma had an identified mutation.[59] Similarly, a Canadian study found a *CDKN2A* mutation in 2 of 14 families with both pancreatic cancer and melanoma.[60] Finally, a United States–based study found 9 *CDKN2A* mutations in an unselected series of 1,537 pancreatic cancer cases (0.6%). The prevalence increased to 3.3% and 5.3% for those who reported a first-degree relative with pancreatic cancer or melanoma, respectively.[55] Thus, in the majority of populations, the co-occurrence of melanoma appears to be a significant indicator of an underlying *CDKN2A* mutation.

SELECTED SYNDROMES THAT INCREASE THE RISK OF PANCREATIC CANCER

Hereditary Nonpolyposis Colorectal Cancer

Hereditary nonpolyposis colorectal cancer (HNPCC), also referred to as Lynch syndrome, is the most common form of hereditary colon cancer, and it accounts for 2% to 5% of colorectal cancers. In addition to a high lifetime risk for colorectal cancer, affected individuals are at an increased risk for multiple other cancers. HNPCC results from mutations in mismatch repair (MMR) genes, and colon cancers that arise in Lynch syndrome typically demonstrate microsatellite instability (MSI). Four percent of all pancreatic adenocarcinomas demonstrate MSI.[61] Yamamoto et al.[62] assessed tumor characteristics in three *MLH1* mutation carriers with both colon and pancreatic cancer, and found that both tumor types had similar properties, including high MSI, loss of MLH1 protein expression, wild-type KRAS and p53, and poor differentiation. These findings support an inherited basis for the development of both types of cancer.[62]

Pancreatic cancer has been described in HNPCC kindreds as early as 1985, although data regarding the risk of pancreatic cancer in HNPCC have varied.[63–68] Barrow et al.[64] studied 121 families with known MMR mutations; 2 of 282 extracolonic cancers were pancreatic, leading to a 0.4% cumulative lifetime risk for pancreatic cancer (95% CI, 0% to 0.8%). By comparison, Geary et al.[65] studied 130 families with MMR mutations and found 22 cases of pancreatic cancer, half of which were in confirmed or obligate carriers. Pancreatic cancer in these families was seven times more common than expected, and the familial relative risk was 3.8 ($p = 0.02$). In addition, these tumors were 15 times more common in individuals younger than 60 years, suggesting an earlier average age at diagnosis as compared with the general population.[65] Another United States–based study of HNPCC families found the lifetime risk for pancreatic cancer to be 1.31% by the age of 50 years (95% CI, 0.31% to 2.32%) and 3.68% by the age of 70 years (95% CI, 1.45% to 5.88%). These risks are higher than those from the SEER data of 0.04% and 0.52% at ages 50 and 70 years, respectively.[66]

Regarding the prevalence of HNPCC in pancreatic cancer, Gargiulo et al.[69] assessed 135 pancreatic cancer patients. Nineteen of these patients had a family history that was suggestive of HNPCC, and of the 11 patients whose DNA was available for analysis, only one deleterious MMR mutation was found. Thus, MMR mutations presumably account for only a small proportion of pancreatic cancer patients.

Hereditary Pancreatitis

Hereditary pancreatitis (HP) is a rare form of chronic pancreatitis. Several genes have been linked to chronic pancreatitis, including *SPINK1*, *CTFR*, and *CTRC*, but the *PRSS1* gene on chromosome 7q35 accounts for the majority of hereditary cases. *PRSS1* mutations are inherited in an autosomal-dominant fashion and have an 80% penetrance for pancreatitis. Affected individuals begin experiencing symptoms of pancreatic pain and acute pancreatitis early in life. Several studies have shown an increase in pancreatic cancer risk associated with HP, and cumulative lifetime risk estimates range from 18.8% to 53.5%.[70–72] Lowenfels et al.[71] observed an increased risk associated with paternal inheritance. Tobacco use in patients with HP has been shown to increase the risk for pancreatic cancer twofold (95% CI, 0.7 to 6.1), pancreatic and HP patients who smoke developed cancer 20 years earlier than did their nonsmoking counterparts.[73]

Peutz–Jeghers Syndrome

Peutz–Jeghers syndrome (PJS) is an autosomal-dominant condition characterized by mucocutaneous pigmentation and hamartomatous polyps of the gastrointestinal tract. PJS is caused by mutations on the *STK11* (*LKB1*) gene. The lifetime risk to develop any cancer has been estimated to be as high as 93%,[74] with no sex difference in cancer risk noted.[74,75] Risk for pancreatic cancer in PJS is estimated to be 8% to 36% by the age of 70 years.[74–76] Grützmann et al.[77] analyzed 39 individuals with familial pancreatic cancer, and none were found to carry mutations in *STK11*. In 2011, Schneider et al.[58] confirmed these findings in their study of 94 familial pancreatic cancer kindreds. Therefore, although *STK11* mutations confer a high lifetime risk for pancreatic cancer in individuals with PJS, germ-line *STK11* mutations are not thought to account for hereditary pancreatic cancer.

EMPIRIC RISK COUNSELING AND MANAGEMENT

Having a first-degree relative with apparently sporadic pancreatic cancer has a moderate effect on risk (OR, 1.76; 95% CI, 1.19 to 2.61).[78] In familial pancreatic cancer kindreds (defined as a family with a pair of affected first-degree relatives), the risk of pancreatic cancer increases with the number of affected first-degree relatives (Table 50.2).[3] These findings suggest that high-penetrance genes may be causing the clustering of pancreatic cancer in families with two or three pancreatic cancer cases. Thus, individuals with multiple affected first-degree relatives are at an appreciably increased risk for pancreatic cancer and may be candidates for increased surveillance.

TABLE 50.2

Risk of Pancreatic Cancer in Familial Pancreatic Cancer Kindreds Based on Number of Affected First-Degree Relatives

Number of Affected FDRs	SIR (95% CI)
1	4.5 (0.54–16.3)
2	6.4 (1.8–16.4)
3	32 (10.4–74.7)

FDR, first-degree relatives; SIR, standardized incidence ratio.

PRACTICE OF ONCOLOGY

Ideally, high-risk patients would be able to undergo noninvasive, inexpensive pancreatic cancer screening; however, to date, a highly sensitive and specific method for pancreas surveillance has not been recognized. Screening of high-risk patients with endoscopic ultrasound, magnetic resonance imaging, and/or magnetic resonance cholangiopancreatogram has been shown to be effective at identifying early neoplasms, both benign and malignant.[79–82] However, it is unknown if these methods actually prevent pancreatic cancer or improve overall survival by detecting presymptomatic disease. In addition, there is great interest in developing a biomarker for premalignant or early-stage disease, although none, including CA19-9, have been proven effective.[83] Thus, whenever possible, it is recommended that high-risk patients undergo pancreatic screening through a research study.

REFERENCES

1. Lynch HT, Smyrk T, Kern SE, et al. Familial pancreatic cancer: A review. *Semin Oncol* 1996;23:251–275.
2. Klein AP, Hruban RH, Brune KA, et al. Familial pancreatic cancer. *Cancer J* 2001;7:266–273.
3. Klein AP, Brune KA, Petersen GM, et al. Prospective risk of pancreatic cancer in familial pancreatic cancer kindreds. *Cancer Res* 2004;64:2634–2638.
4. Klein AP, Beaty TH, Bailey-Wilson JE, et al. Evidence for a major gene influencing risk of pancreatic cancer. *Genet Epidemiol* 2002;23:133–149.
5. The Breast Cancer Linkage Consortium. Cancer risks in BRCA2 mutation carriers. *J Natl Cancer Inst* 1999;91:1310–1316.
6. Moran A, O'Hara C, Khan S, et al. Risk of cancer other than breast or ovarian in individuals with BRCA1 and BRCA2 mutations. *Fam Cancer* 2012;11:235–242.
7. van Asperen CJ, Brohet RM, Meijers-Heijboer EJ, et al. Cancer risks in BRCA2 families: Estimates for sites other than breast and ovary. *J Med Genet* 2005;42:711–719.
8. Kim DH, Crawford B, Ziegler J, et al. Prevalence and characteristics of pancreatic cancer in families with BRCA1 and BRCA2 mutations. *Fam Cancer* 2009;8:153–158.
9. Martin ST, Matsubayashi H, Rogers CD, et al. Increased prevalence of the BRCA2 polymorphic stop codon K3326X among individuals with familial pancreatic cancer. *Oncogene* 2005;24:3652–3656.
10. Murphy KM, Brune KA, Griffin C, et al. Evaluation of candidate genes MAP2K4, MADH4, ACVR1B, and BRCA2 in familial pancreatic cancer: Deleterious BRCA2 mutations in 17%. *Cancer Res* 2002;62:3789–3793.
11. Hahn SA, Greenhalf B, Ellis I, et al. BRCA2 germline mutations in familial pancreatic carcinoma. *J Natl Cancer Inst* 2003;95:214–221.
12. Couch FJ, Johnson MR, Rabe KG, et al. The prevalence of BRCA2 mutations in familial pancreatic cancer. *Cancer Epidemiol Biomarkers Prev* 2007;16:342–346.
13. Goggins M, Schutte M, Lu J, et al. Germline BRCA2 gene mutations in patients with apparently sporadic pancreatic carcinomas. *Cancer Res* 1996;56:5360–5364.
14. Ferrone CR, Levine DA, Tang LH, et al. BRCA germline mutations in Jewish patients with pancreatic adenocarcinoma. *J Clin Oncol* 2009;27:433–438.
15. Figer A, Irmin L, Geva R, et al. The rate of the 6174delT founder Jewish mutation in BRCA2 in patients with non-colonic gastrointestinal tract tumours in Israel. *Br J Cancer* 2001;84:478–481.
16. Stadler ZK, Salo-Mullen E, Patil SM, et al. Prevalence of BRCA1 and BRCA2 mutations in Ashkenazi Jewish families with breast and pancreatic cancer. *Cancer* 2012;118:493–499.
17. Cho JH, Bang S, Park SW, et al. BRCA2 mutations as a universal risk factor for pancreatic cancer has a limited role in Korean ethnic group. *Pancreas* 2008;36:337–340.
18. Ghiorzo P, Pensotti V, Fornarini G, et al. Contribution of germline mutations in the BRCA and PALB2 genes to pancreatic cancer in Italy. *Fam Cancer* 2012;11:41–47.
19. Thompson D, Easton DF. Cancer incidence in BRCA1 mutation carriers. *J Natl Cancer Inst* 2002;94:1358–1365.
20. Brose MS, Rebbeck TR, Calzone KA, et al. Cancer risk estimates for BRCA1 mutation carriers identified in a risk evaluation program. *J Natl Cancer Inst* 2002;94:1365–1372.
21. Al-Sukhni W, Rothenmund H, Borgida AE, et al. Germline BRCA1 mutations predispose to pancreatic adenocarcinoma. *Hum Genet* 2008;124:271–278.
22. Lynch HT, Deters CA, Snyder CL, et al. BRCA1 and pancreatic cancer: pedigree findings and their causal relationships. *Cancer Genet Cytogenet* 2005;158:119–125.
23. Danes BS, Lynch HT. A familial aggregation of pancreatic cancer. An in vitro study. *JAMA* 1982;247:2798–2802.
24. Axilbund JE, Argani P, Kamiyama M, et al. Absence of germline BRCA1 mutations in familial pancreatic cancer patients. *Cancer Biol Ther* 2009;8:131–135.
25. Reid S, Schindler D, Hanenberg H, et al. Biallelic mutations in PALB2 cause Fanconi anemia subtype FA-N and predispose to childhood cancer. *Nat Genet* 2007;39:162–164.
26. Xia B, Dorsman JC, Ameziane N, et al. Fanconi anemia is associated with a defect in the BRCA2 partner PALB2. *Nat Genet* 2007;39:159–161.
27. Rahman N, Seal S, Thompson D, et al. PALB2, which encodes a BRCA2-interacting protein, is a breast cancer susceptibility gene. *Nat Genet* 2007;39:165–167.
28. McInerney NM, Miller N, Rowan A, et al. Evaluation of variants in the CHEK2, BRIP1 and PALB2 genes in an Irish breast cancer cohort. *Breast Cancer Res Treat* 2010;121:203–210.
29. Gunnarsson H, Arason A, Gillanders EM, et al. Evidence against PALB2 involvement in Icelandic breast cancer susceptibility. *J Negat Results Biomed* 2008;7:5.
30. Papi L, Putignano AL, Congregati C, et al. A PALB2 germline mutation associated with hereditary breast cancer in Italy. *Fam Cancer* 2010;9:181–185.
31. Ding YC, Steele L, Chu LH, et al. Germline mutations in PALB2 in African-American breast cancer cases. *Breast Cancer Res Treat* 2011;126:227–230.
32. Zheng Y, Zhang J, Niu Q, et al. Novel germline PALB2 truncating mutations in African American breast cancer patients. *Cancer* 2012;118:1362–1370.
33. Cao AY, Huang J, Hu Z, et al. The prevalence of PALB2 germline mutations in BRCA1/BRCA2 negative Chinese women with early onset breast cancer or affected relatives. *Breast Cancer Res Treat* 2009;114:457–462.
34. Blanco A, de la Hoya M, Balmaña J, et al. Detection of a large rearrangement in PALB2 in Spanish breast cancer families with male breast cancer. *Breast Cancer Res Treat* 2012;132:307–315.
35. Sluiter M, Mew S, van Rensburg EJ. PALB2 sequence variants in young South African breast cancer patients. *Fam Cancer* 2009;8:347–353.
36. Casadei S, Norquist BM, Walsh T, et al. Contribution of inherited mutations in the BRCA2-interacting protein PALB2 to familial breast cancer. *Cancer Res* 2011;71:2222–2229.
37. Tischkowitz M, Capanu M, Sabbaghian N, et al. Rare germline mutations in PALB2 and breast cancer risk: A population-based study. *Hum Mutat* 2012;33:674–680.
38. Foulkes WD, Ghadirian P, Akbari MR, et al. Identification of a novel truncating PALB2 mutation and analysis of its contribution to early-onset breast cancer in French-Canadian women. *Breast Cancer Res* 2007;9:R83.
39. Erkko H, Xia B, Nikkilä J, et al. A recurrent mutation in PALB2 in Finnish cancer families. *Nature* 2007;446:316–319.
40. Erkko H, Dowty JG, Nikkilä J, et al. Penetrance analysis of the PALB2c.1592delT founder mutation. *Clin Cancer Res* 2008;14:4667–4671.
41. Sabbaghian N, Kyle R, Hao A, et al. Mutation analysis of the PALB2 cancer predisposition gene in familial melanoma. *Fam Cancer* 2011;10:315–317.
42. Adank MA, van Mil SE, Gille JJ, et al. PALB2 analysis in BRCA2-like families. *Breast Cancer Res Treat* 2011;127:357–362.
43. Tischkowitz M, Sabbaghian N, Ray AM, et al. Analysis of the gene coding for the BRCA2-interacting protein PALB2 in hereditary prostate cancer. *Prostate* 2008;68:675–678.
44. Jones S, Hruban RH, Kamiyama M, et al. Exomic sequencing identifies PALB2 as a pancreatic cancer susceptibility gene. *Science* 2009;324:217.
45. Harinck F, Kluijt I, van Mil SE, et al. Routine testing for PALB2 mutations in familial pancreatic cancer families and breast cancer families with pancreatic cancer is not indicated. *Eur J Hum Genet* 2012;20:577–579.
46. Slater EP, Langer P, Niemczyk E, et al. PALB2 mutations in European familial pancreatic cancer families. *Clin Genet* 2010;78:490–494.
47. Stadler ZK, Salo-Mullen E, Sabbaghian N, et al. Germline PALB2 mutation analysis in breast-pancreas cancer families. *J Med Genet* 2011;48:523–525.
48. Peterlongo P, Catucci I, Pasquini G, et al. PALB2 germline mutations in familial breast cancer cases with personal and family history of pancreatic cancer. *Breast Cancer Res Treat* 2011;126:825–828.
49. Kanda M, Matthaei H, Wu J, et al. Presence of somatic mutations in most early-stage pancreatic intraepithelial neoplasia. *Gastroenterology* 2012;142:730–733.
50. Remmers N, Bailey JM, Mohr AM, et al. Molecular pathology of early pancreatic cancer. *Cancer Biomark* 2011;9:421–440.
51. Bartsch D, Shevlin DW, Tung WS, et al. Frequent mutations of CDKN2 in primary pancreatic adenocarcinomas. *Genes Chromosomes Cancer* 1995;14:189–195.
52. de Snoo FA, Bishop DT, Bergman W, et al. Increased risk of cancer other than melanoma in CDKN2A founder mutation (p16-Leiden)-positive melanoma families. *Clin Cancer Res* 2008;14:7151–7157.
53. Vasen HF, Gruis NA, Frants RR, et al. Risk of developing pancreatic cancer in families with familial atypical multiple mole melanoma associated with a specific 19 deletion of p16 (p16-Leiden). *Int J Cancer* 2000;87:809–811.
54. Mukherjee B, Delancey JO, Raskin L, et al. Risk of non-melanoma cancers in first-degree relatives of CDKN2A mutation carriers. *J Natl Cancer Inst* 2012;104:953–956.

55. McWilliams RR, Wieben ED, Rabe KG, et al. Prevalence of CDKN2A mutations in pancreatic cancer patients: Implications for genetic counseling. *Eur J Hum Genet* 2011;19:472–478.
56. Ghiorzo P, Fornarini G, Sciallero S, et al. CDKN2A is the main susceptibility gene in Italian pancreatic cancer families. *J Med Genet* 2012;49:164–170.
57. Debniak T, van de Wetering T, Scott R, et al. Low prevalence of CDKN2A/ARF mutations among early-onset cancers of breast, pancreas and malignant melanoma in Poland. *Eur J Cancer Prev* 2008;17:389–391.
58. Schneider R, Slater EP, Sina M, et al. German national case collection for familial pancreatic cancer (FaPaCa): ten years experience. *Fam Cancer* 2011; 10:323–330.
59. Bartsch DK, Sina-Frey M, Lang S, et al. CDKN2A germline mutations in familial pancreatic cancer. *Ann Surg* 2002;236:730–737.
60. Lal G, Liu L, Hogg D, et al. Patients with both pancreatic adenocarcinoma and melanoma may harbor germline CDKN2A mutations. *Genes Chromosomes Cancer* 2000;27:358–361.
61. Goggins M, Offerhaus GJ, Hilgers W, et al. Pancreatic adenocarcinomas with DNA replication errors (RER⁺) are associated with wild-type K-ras and characteristic histopathology. Poor differentiation, a syncytial growth pattern, and pushing borders suggest RER⁺. *Am J Pathol* 1998;152:1501–1507.
62. Yamamoto H, Itoh F, Nakamura H, et al. Genetic and clinical features of human pancreatic ductal adenocarcinomas with widespread microsatellite instability. *Cancer Res* 2001;61:3136–3144.
63. Lynch HT, Voorhees GJ, Lanspa SJ, et al. Pancreatic carcinoma and hereditary nonpolyposis colorectal cancer: a family study. *Br J Cancer* 1985;52:271–273.
64. Barrow E, Robinson L, Alduaij W, et al. Cumulative lifetime incidence of extracolonic cancers in Lynch syndrome: A report of 121 families with proven mutations. *Clin Genet* 2009;75:141–149.
65. Geary J, Sasieni P, Houlston R, et al. Gene-related cancer spectrum in families with hereditary non-polyposis colorectal cancer (HNPCC). *Fam Cancer* 2008;7:163–172.
66. Kastrinos F, Mukherjee B, Tayob N, et al. Risk of pancreatic cancer in families with Lynch syndrome. *JAMA* 2009;302:1790–1795.
67. Aarnio M, Sankila R, Pukkala E, et al. Cancer risk in mutation carriers of DNA-mismatch-repair genes. *Int J Cancer* 1999;81:214–218.
68. Vasen HF, Offerhaus GJ, den Hartog Jager FH, et al. The tumor spectrum in hereditary non-polyposis colorectal cancer: a study of 24 kindreds in the Netherlands. *Int J Cancer* 1990;46:31–34.
69. Gargiulo S, Torrini M, Ollila S, et al. Germline MLH1 and MSH2 mutations in Italian pancreatic cancer patients with suspected Lynch syndrome. *Fam Cancer* 2009;8:547–553.
70. Howes N, Lerch MM, Greenhalf W, et al. Clinical and genetic characteristics of hereditary pancreatitis in Europe. *Clin Gastroenterol Hepatol* 2004;2:252–261.
71. Lowenfels AB, Maisonneuve P, Di Magno EP, et al. Hereditary pancreatitis and the risk of pancreatic cancer. International Hereditary Pancreatitis Study Group. *J Natl Cancer Inst* 1997;89:442–446.
72. Rebours V, Boutron-Ruault MC, Schnee MF, et al. Risk of pancreatic adenocarcinoma in patients with hereditary pancreatitis: a national exhaustive series. *Am J Gastroenterol* 2008;103:111–119.
73. Lowenfels AB, Maisonneuve P, Whitcomb DC, et al. Cigarette smoking as a risk factor for pancreatic cancer in patients with hereditary pancreatitis. *JAMA* 2001;286:169–170.
74. Giardiello FM, Brensinger JD, Tersmette AC, et al. Very high risk of cancer in familial Peutz–Jeghers syndrome. *Gastroenterology* 2000;119:1447–1453.
75. Lim W, Olschwang S, Keller JJ, et al. Relative frequency and morphology of cancers in STK11 mutation carriers. *Gastroenterology* 2004;126:1788–1794.
76. Hearle N, Schumacher V, Menko FH, et al. Frequency and spectrum of cancers in the Peutz–Jeghers syndrome. *Clin Cancer Res* 2006;12:3209–3215.
77. Grützmann R, McFaul C, Bartsch DK, et al. No evidence for germline mutations of the LKB1/STK11 gene in familial pancreatic carcinoma. *Cancer Lett* 2004;214:63–68.
78. Jacobs EJ, Chanock SJ, Fuchs CS, et al. Family history of cancer and risk of pancreatic cancer: A pooled analysis from the Pancreatic Cancer Cohort Consortium (PanScan). *Int J Cancer* 2010;127:1421–1428.
79. Canto MI, Hruban RH, Fishman EK, et al. Frequent detection of pancreatic lesions in asymptomatic high-risk individuals. *Gastroenterology* 2012;142:796–804.
80. Ludwig E, Olson SH, Bayuga S, et al. Feasibility and yield of screening in relatives from familial pancreatic cancer families. *Am J Gastroenterol* 2011;106:946–954.
81. Verna EC, Hwang C, Stevens PD, et al. Pancreatic cancer screening in a prospective cohort of high-risk patients: A comprehensive strategy of imaging and genetics. *Clin Cancer Res* 2010;16:5028–5037.
82. Langer P, Kann PH, Fendrich V, et al. Five years of prospective screening of high-risk individuals from families with familial pancreatic cancer. *Gut* 2009;58:1410–1418.
83. Goggins M. Markers of pancreatic cancer: working toward early detection. *Clin Cancer Res* 2011;17:635–637.

PRACTICE OF ONCOLOGY

51 Molecular Biology of Liver Cancer

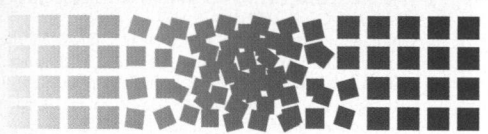

Jens U. Marquardt and Snorri S. Thorgeirsson

INTRODUCTION

Hepatocellular carcinoma (HCC) is the fifth most common cancer in men and the seventh most common cancer in women worldwide, accounting for at least 600,000 deaths annually.[1] Although rates in traditionally high-incidence regions such as southeast Asia and sub-Sahara Africa has stabilized and slowly declined due to generalized vaccination programs, the incidence and mortality rates of HCC have doubled in the United States and Europe in the past 4 decades and are predicted to continue rising.[2] Several confounding factors (e.g., immigration from high-incidence countries) contribute to these high numbers in the western world, and HCC is currently among the fastest growing causes of cancer related deaths in the United States. Small HCCs can be cured by resection and/or liver transplantation. However, at the time of diagnosis, less than 20% of patients are eligible for these treatment options.[3] These observations make it clear that liver cancer is a major health problem in the United States and Europe and highlight the critical need for both improved understanding and treatment options of this deadly disease.

The major etiologic agents responsible for chronic liver disease, cirrhosis, and ultimately, HCC are known and well characterized (e.g., hepatitis B virus [HBV], hepatitis C virus [HCV], ethanol abuse). Other etiologic factors include nonalcoholic fatty liver disease (NAFLD) and other metabolic disorders that have become particularly relevant in Western countries due to a sharp increase in prevalence and a high number of HCCs without underlying cirrhosis.[4]

Over the last decades, molecular mechanisms of liver diseases that are associated with increased risk of HCC as well as several cellular alterations that precede HCC have been identified.[5,6] Research into the molecular pathogenesis of HCC is currently focused on the interrelationship of abnormal genomics, epigenomics, proteomics, and downstream alterations in molecular signaling pathways. The primary goal of this research is to integrate the new data with clinicopathologic features of HCC in order to uncover new diagnostic tools, improve treatment options, and implement effective prevention strategies.[7]

The recent introduction of next-generation whole genomic technologies permits simultaneously detection of the expression of tens of thousands of genes in small samples from normal and diseased tissues.[8] High-throughput microarray-based technologies and the recent advent of next-generation whole genome DNA sequencing offer a unique opportunity to define the descriptive characteristics (i.e., phenotype) of a biologic system in terms of the genomic readout (e.g., gene expression, coding mutations, insertions and deletions in DNA, splicing variants, copy number variations, chromosomal translocations). Integrated analyses and the interpretation of biologic systems has caused a paradigm shift in biologic research, from the classic reductionism to systems biology.[9] Fundamental to the systems approach is the hypothesis that disease processes are driven by aberrant regulatory networks of genes and proteins that differ from the normal counterparts. The application of multiparametric measurements promises to transform current approaches of diagnosis and therapy, providing the foundation for predictive and preventive personalized medicine.[10]

In this chapter we discuss both the molecular hallmarks of hepatocarcinogenesis in the context of next-generation high-throughput genomic technologies, and the implications for clinical and translational efforts.

GENETIC ALTERATIONS IN LIVER CANCER

During the last decade, a detailed map of the structural variation in the human cancer genome has been generated.[11] This map reveals that tumor development is the consequence of intragenic mutations in approximately 140 genes belonging to 12 signaling pathways regulating three core cellular processes—cell fate, cell survival, and genome maintenance—that can promote or "drive" tumorigenesis in the majority of human cancers.[11] Hepatocarcinogenesis can, therefore, be considered a multistep process that is orchestrated by a sequence of epigenetic and genetic alterations leading to disruption in these core processes by the activation or inhibition of key downstream signaling such as p53, WNT, β-catenin, MYC, the ErbB family, as well as chromatin modifications.[11]

Structural variation and chromosomal aberrations in tumors are traditionally regarded as evidence of gene deregulation and genome instability, and may facilitate the identification of crucial genes and regulatory pathways that are perturbed in diseases.[12] Large, genomewide association studies (GWAS) recently identified liver disease–specific susceptibility loci, including in HCC.[13,14] Most of these studies employed powerful high-throughput microarray technology for single nucleotide polymorphism (SNP) genotyping and array-based comparative genomic hybridization (aCGH). These technologies enable a high-throughput analysis of DNA copy number and yield comprehensive information for determining the molecular pathogenesis of human HCC.

A meta-analysis of aCGH studies of chromosome aberrations in human HCC shows that specific chromosomal gains and losses correlate with etiology and histologic grade.[15] In HCC, the most frequent amplifications of genomic material involve 1q (57.1%), 8q (46.6%), 6p (22.3%), and 17q (22.2%), whereas losses are most common in 8p (38%), 16q (35.9%), 4q (34.3%), 17p (32.1%), and 13q (26.2%). Deletions of 4q, 16q, 13q, and 8p correlate with HBV infection and a lack of HCV infection. Chromosomes 13q and 4q are significantly underrepresented in poorly differentiated HCC, and gains of 1q correlate with other high-frequency alterations.[16] Amplifications and deletions often occur on chromosome arms at sites of oncogenes (e.g., MYC on 8q24) and tumor suppressor genes (e.g., RB1 on 13q14), as well as at several loci that contain genes with known and/or suspected oncogenic functions (e.g., FZD3, WISP1, SIAH-1, and AXIN2), all of which modulate the WNT signaling pathway. In these meta-analyses, etiology and poor differentiation of HCC correlated with specific genomic alterations. In preneoplastic dysplastic nodules (DN), amplifications are most frequent in 1q and 8q, whereas deletions occur in 8p, 17p, 5p, 13q, 14q, and 16q.[16] A gain of 1q appears to be an early event that develops in DN, possibly predisposing affected cells to acquire additional chromosomal aberrations.

A comprehensive collection of common aberrations from both human and rodent HCC is provided in the OncoDB.HCC database (http://oncodb.hcc.ibms.sinica.edu.tw).[17] This database provides a useful, validated, and graphic integration of published data derived from loss of heterozygosity (LOH) analyses, aCGH, gene expression microarrays, as well as proteomics, which is publically assessable for the validation of possible molecular targets.

Recently, a systematic strategy to identify potential driver genes by integrating whole genome copy number data with gene expression profiles of HCC patients was introduced.[18] Using regional pattern recognition approaches, the authors discovered the most probable copy number–dependent regions and 50 potential driver genes. At each step of the process, the functional relevance of the selected genes was evaluated by estimating the prognostic significance of the selected genes. Further validation using small interference RNA-mediated knockdown experiments showed proof-of-principle evidence for the potential driver roles of the genes in HCC progression (i.e., *NCSTN*, *SCRIB*). In addition, the systemic prediction of drug responses using the Connectivity Map,[19] a compendium of functional connections between drugs and genes, implicated the association of the 50 genes with specific signaling molecules associated with hepatocarcinogenesis (*mTOR*, *AMPK*, and *EGFR*). It was concluded that the application of an unbiased and integrative analysis of multidimensional genomic data sets can effectively screen for potential driver genes and provide novel mechanistic and clinical insight into the pathobiology of HCC.

In a similar approach, a recent study used an integrative approach combining information from high-resolution aCGH and gene expression profiling with clinical data from HCC patients to identify copy-number variations (CNV) in HCC with functional relevance for tumor progression.[20] The investigation was restricted to genes that showed (1) recurrent CNVs, (2) correlation of the CNVs and the transcriptome, and (3) a selective association to patients' outcomes to distinguish "drivers" from passengers. The authors were able to demonstrate significant differences in CNVs between patients with good and poor outcome and generated a 10-gene signature as a molecular predictor of patient survival and validated the signature in several independent cohorts. Both these studies elegantly illustrate the power of multilayer integrative analyses to identify the functional significance of genomic alterations in human HCC.

EPIGENETIC ALTERATIONS IN LIVER CANCER

Epigenetic alterations such as DNA methylation are important factors in tumor development for many cancers.[21] Changes in DNA methylation patterns are believed to be early events in hepatocarcinogenesis, preceding allelic imbalances and ultimately leading to cancer progression, thereby adding considerable complexity to the pathogenesis of liver cancer.[22]

Global hypomethylation and promoter hypermethylation in certain cancer-related genes are known drivers of hepatocarcinogenesis with an association to biologic behavior and prognosis.[23] Methylation patterns can further be used to classify patients according to different etiological factors (e.g. HBV, HCV, alcohol).[24,25] Moreover, in addition to changes in global methylation patterns, distinct methylation patterns strongly correlate with clinical characteristics of HCC patients.[23] Methylation patterns in a 807 cancer-related gene panel could successfully separate primary HCC samples according to their biologic subtype.[26] Consistent with previous studies, patients with progenitor cell origin displayed the worst clinical outcome.[27] The confirmation of a multistep, epigenetic-driven sequence of molecular alteration in hepatocarcinogenesis could further be demonstrated in HBV-related liver cancers. A stepwise hypermethylation of CpG islands of nine well-

described genes was seen from cirrhotic nodules over dysplastic nodules (low and high grade) to early carcinoma (eHCC) and, finally, progressed HCC (pHCC).[28]

More recently, integrative genome-wide methylation analyses have been applied to 71 human HCC patients.[29] The methylation data were combined with those from a microarray analysis of gene reexpression in four hepatoma cell lines following their exposure to DNA methylation inhibitors. A total of 13 candidate tumor suppressor genes were identified using this approach and, subsequently, *SMPD3* and *NEFH* were functionally validated as tumor suppressor genes in HCC. The authors could further show that *SMPD3* not only affects tumor aggressiveness, but also that reduced levels are an independent prognostic factor for early recurrence of HCC.

Although genetic changes in chromatin modulators are among the most common alterations in HCC (see the following), the role of epigenetic alterations beyond DNA methylation such as modification of histones (e.g., acetylation, methylation, phosphorylation, ubiquitylation, SUMOylation) are not well studied in HCC.[30] The fact that modifications of both repressing (e.g., H3 lysine 27 and histone H3 Lysine 9) and activating histone marks (e.g., H3 lysines 4) have a significant impact on the expression of critical genes associated with hepatocarcinogenesis highlight the need for whole genomic approaches such as chromatin immunoprecipitation with microarray technology (ChIP-chip) and ChIP sequencing (ChIP-seq) to address the role of these changes in a more global perspective.[31]

MicroRNAs are epigenetically active, small RNAs that are critically involved to regulate protein expression.[32] Distinct MicroRNA expression patterns contribute to the definition of the cellular phenotype, including the regulation of proliferation, cell signaling, and apoptosis. Not surprisingly, the aberrant expression of microRNAs is associated with cancer initiation, propagation, and progression. Several microRNAs are frequently deregulated in HCC and associated with certain clinicopathologic features.[33] Several studies have demonstrated that microRNAs play an essential role in HCC progression by directly contributing to cell proliferation, apoptosis, and metastasis of HCC as well as by targeting a large number of critical protein-coding genes involved in hepatocarciongenesis.[34] The profiling of microRNA expression by microarray revealed subclasses associated with clinicopathologic features as well as mutations in several oncogenic pathways such as β-catenin and *HNF1A*.[35] Furthermore, microRNA profiling of 89 HCC samples using a ligation-mediated amplification method revealed three distinct clusters HCCs reflecting the clinical behavior of the tumors as well as identifying the microRNAs family mir-517 with increased tumorigenicity of HCC cells.[36]

Ji and colleagues[37] confirmed the therapeutic potential of microRNA-based treatment modalities in HCC. The authors demonstrated that miR-26 levels are associated with a response to adjuvant therapy with interferon α (IFN-α) and, more recently, developed a simple and reliable companion diagnostic (MIR26-DX) to select HCC patients for adjuvant IFN-α therapy as a first step to successfully translate information from large scale analyses into the clinics.[38]

MUTATIONAL LANDSCAPE OF GENETIC ALTERATIONS IN HCC: THE NEXT GENERATION

Sophisticated next-generation sequencing (NGS) technologies are now applied in cancer research for complete and cost-efficient analyses of cancer genomes at a single nucleotide resolution and have advanced into valuable tools in translational medicine.[12] The implementation of NGS to solid tumors like HCC is challenging because the proportion of normal cells or the stromal composition within a given sample contributes to the genomic signature and, therefore, may require additional coverage (i.e., read depth). Also, HCCs often arise in the background of a chronically diseased liver with underlying cirrhosis, fibrosis, or HBV or HCV infection, which may complicate the tumor/normal variant discovery when compared to the peritumoral liver tissue or even blood.[39] Therefore, the number of studies where NGS technologies—in particular, whole exome sequencing—have been applied to investigate HCC is, so far, limited and only conducted on a few patients.[40] However, all the studies revealed that the landscape of molecular alterations in HCC is relatively broad, with the number of mutations found ranging from 5 to 121 mutations per tumor. Thus, due to the genetic heterogeneity, a rather complex interaction of multiple mutations in the development of a singular HCC has to be assumed.[41–44] Although no clear oncogenic addiction has been demonstrated, a high number of mutations in p53 and Wnt/β-catenin signaling were detected (Fig. 51.1). Thus, results from in-depth analyses strengthen existing evidence that p53 and Wnt/β-catenin signaling are among the most common molecular changes involved in HCC development. Another interesting finding is the high frequency of genetic alteration in genes involved in chromatin remodeling. Overall, 16% to 24% of HCCs showed genetic alterations in these pathways, thereby suggesting a causative association with hepatocyte transformation and highlighting recent evidence for the key role of epigenetics in hepatocarcinogenesis.[45]

Two recent studies on whole exome/genome sequencing of 87 and 88 human HCCs as well as matched normal tissue[46,47] con-

firmed the previous studies that β-catenin (10% and 15.9%) and TP53 (18% and 35.2%) are the most frequently mutated oncogene and tumor suppressor, respectively, in HCC.[46,47] The study by Kan et al.[47] also detected several drugable mutations, including activating mutations of Janus kinase 1 (9.1%), which might provide an option for novel individualized therapeutic interventions. Interestingly, Nault et al.,[48] using traditional Sanger sequencing, identified somatic mutations activating telomerase reverse transcriptase as both the earliest and the most frequent mutations in human preneoplastic lesions (25%) as well as hepatocellular carcinomas (59%) and is associated with activating *CTNNB1* mutations.[48]

Compared to whole-genome sequencing, the application of RNA sequencing in liver cancer is currently limited to three studies. One study investigated the transcriptomes of 10 matched HBV-related HCC cases, identifying a total of 1,378 differentially expressed genes with a specific enrichment of chromosome location on 8q21.3 to 24.3.[49] Another study investigated three paired nontumor and tumor specimens demonstrating that *ADAR1*-mediated *AZIN1* RNA editing is linked to tumor initiation and development in liver cancer.[50]

Sequential molecular alterations during human hepatocarcinogenesis from dysplastic lesions to eHCC and, ultimately, pHCC are not clearly defined. This lack of information represents a major challenge in the clinical management of patients at risk. Although recent results associating MYC activation with early stages of malignant conversion into HCC, detailed molecular sequences that drive premalignant lesions into pHCC still remain

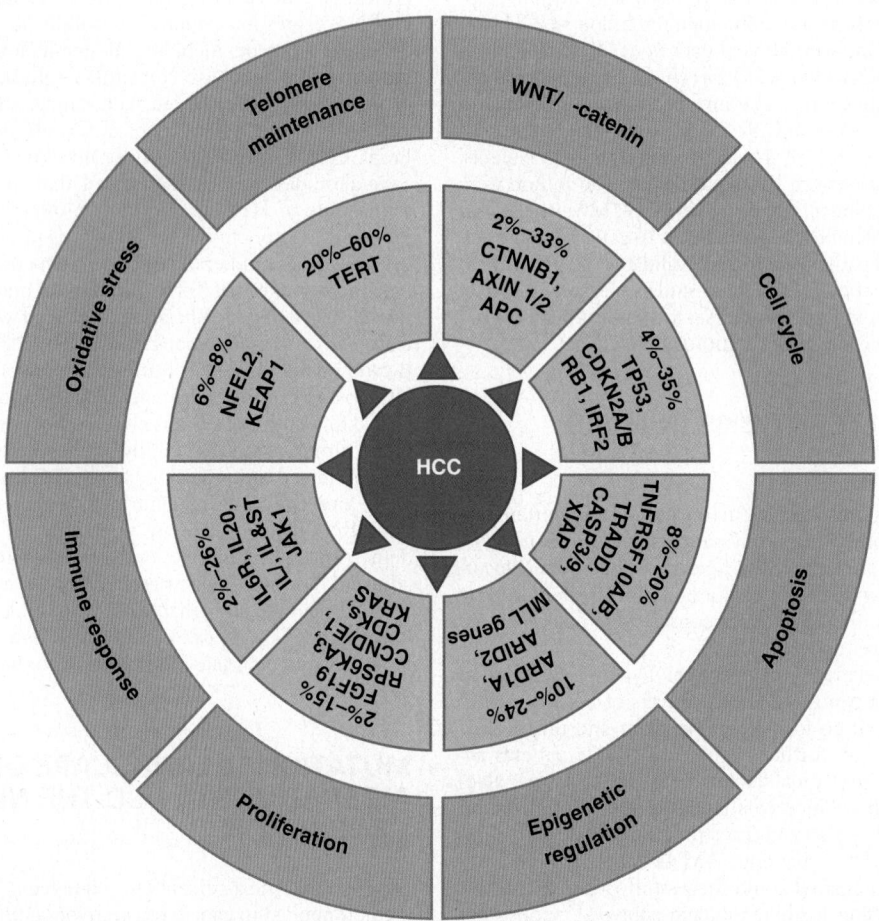

Figure 51.1 Major oncogenic pathways and genetic landscape in hepatocellular carcinoma (HCC). The scheme shows the major disrupted pathways in HCC patients (*outer circle*). The *inner circle* emphasizes the frequency of genetic alterations within the corresponding pathways and their putative contribution to hepatocarcinogenesis. Frequencies are based on results from recent whole genomic studies.[41–44] Representative members of each pathway most frequently altered in HCC are also shown.

to be clarified.[51] In the third study, integrative transcriptome sequencing to the tumor-free surrounding liver (n = 7), low-grade (n = 4) and high-grade dysplastic lesions (n = 9), eHCC (n = 5), and pHCC (n = 3) from eight HCC patients with HBV infections was applied.[52] The results of the study indicate that molecular profiles of dysplastic lesions and eHCC are quite uniform. In contrast, a sharp increase in heterogeneity on both mRNA and DNA levels is observed in progressed HCC. These molecular alterations result in massive deregulation of key oncogenic molecules such as transforming growth factor beta 1 (TGF-β1), MYC, PI3K/AKT, and suggest that activation of prognostically adverse signaling pathways is a late event during hepatocarcinogenesis (Fig. 51.2).

THE MICROENVIRONMENT OF LIVER CANCER

HCC develops on the basis of chronic liver disease and, in more than 80% of the cases, with preexisting liver cirrhosis. For a complete understanding of the molecular mechanisms of hepatocarcinogenesis, the underlying liver disease leading to a chronically altered inflamed liver microenvironment has to be appreciated.[53] Recent research efforts have focused on the identification of key factors that contribute to the disruption of the liver microenvironment and the generation of an adverse niche(s) that promotes hepatocarcinogenesis. Among the most prominent factors involved in the so called inflammation-fibrosis-cancer axis is the nuclear factor kappa B (NF-κB) pathway.[54] The dominant role of this pathway for hepatocarcinogenesis is well documented.[54] However, the absence of NF-κB by genetic loss of the NF-κB master regulator *NEMO* significantly enhanced liver cancer development in a mouse model, indicating that inhibition of NF-κB may not only exert beneficial effects, but also may negatively impact hepatocyte viability, especially when NF-κB inhibition is pronounced.[55]

The importance of the microenvironment is further highlighted in a recent study demonstrating that transplantation of hepatic progenitor cells gave rise to cancer only when introduced into a liver with chronic damage and compensatory proliferation.[56] Interestingly, similar to observations made in human hepatocarcinogenesis, the cells resembling these progenitor cells quiescently resided within dysplastic lesions for several months before the appearance of HCC. During this time, the progenitor cells acquired autocrine interleukin (IL)-6 signaling that stimulated in vivo growth and malignant progression, which might be a general mechanism of progenitor cell–induced HCC.

However, the microenvironment does not only contribute to tumor initiation. Although gene-expression profiles of tumor tissue failed to yield a significant association with survival, a 186-gene signature generated from the surrounding nontumoral liver tissue was highly correlated with outcomes in a cohort of more than 300

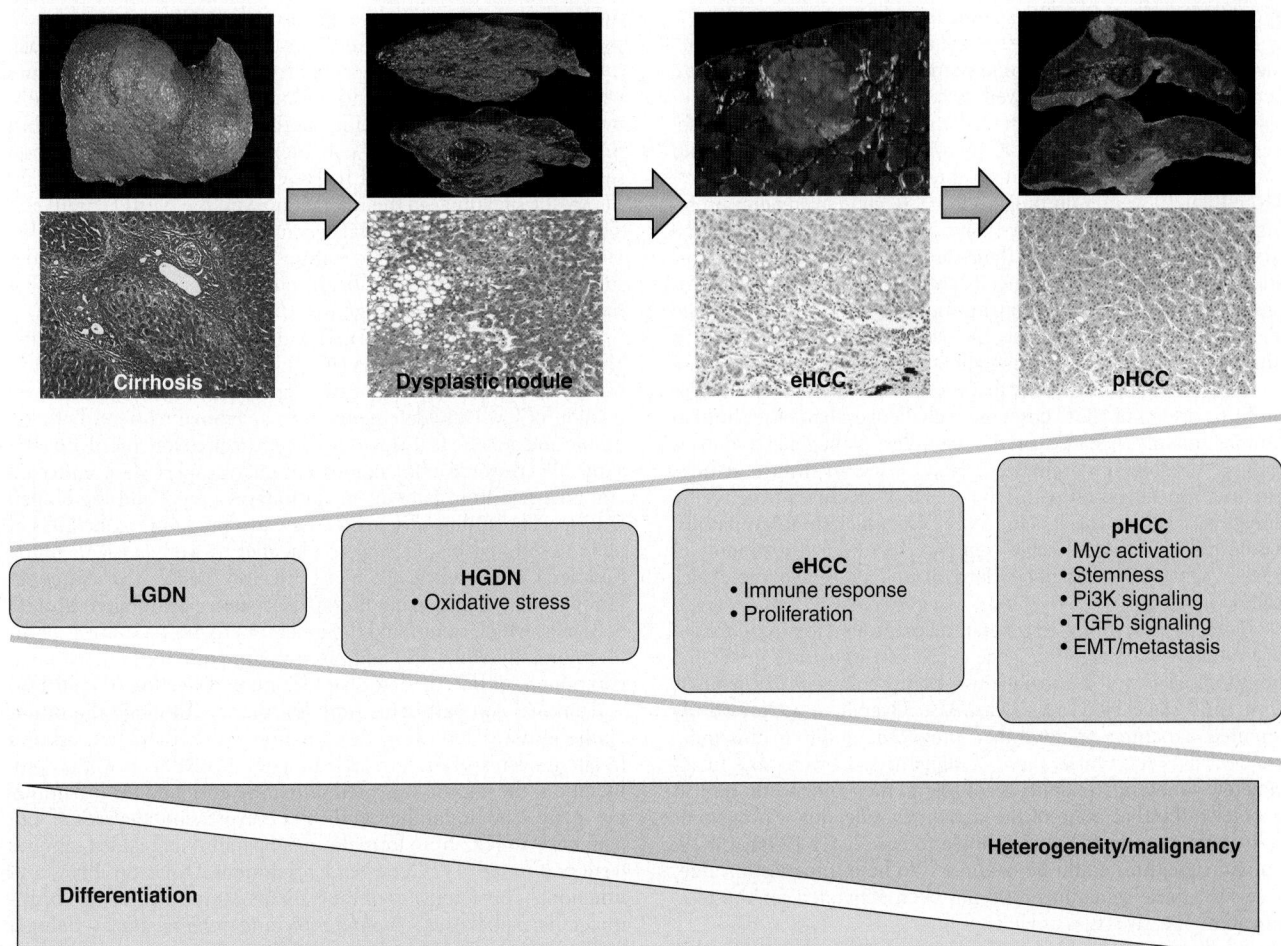

Figure 51.2 Sequential evolution of liver cancer. The current concept considers hepatocarcinogenesis as a multistep process that develops on the basis of a chronically altered microenvironment (i.e., cirrhosis) and progresses from dysplastic nodules (high grade and low grade) over early HCC to progressed HCC *(upper panels)*. On the molecular level, the different stages are characterized by progressive activation of signaling pathways related to oxidative stress, immune response, and proliferation *(middle panel)*. However, the activation of prognostically adverse signaling occurs late during the evolution of liver cancer. During this process, a progressive loss of differentiation with a concomitant acquisition of malignant and invasive properties is observed *(lower panel)*. LGDN, low-grade dysplastic nodule; HGDN, high-grade dysplastic nodule; EMT, epithelial-mesenchymal transition.

HCC patients.[57] Consistently, this poor-prognosis signature contained gene sets associated with inflammation, such as IFN signaling, NF-κB, and tumor necrosis factor α (TNF-α). Further, a gene set enrichment analysis showed that the downstream targets of IL-6 were strongly associated with the poor-prognosis signature, again confirming the importance of this signaling for hepatocarcinogenesis.

Together, these studies demonstrate the complexity of molecular mechanisms influencing the development and progression of liver cancer that are exerted by epigenetic and genetic alterations and a cross-talk between microenvironment and damaged hepatocytes and/or cancer cells, respectively.

CLASSIFICATION AND PROGNOSTIC PREDICTION OF HEPATOCELLULAR CARCINOMA

The application of microarray technologies to characterize tumors on the basis of global gene expression has had a significant impact on both basic and clinical oncology.[10] The goal of tumor microarray studies generally includes the discovery of subsets of tumors (class discovery), which enables diagnostic classification (class comparison), a prediction of clinical outcome (class prediction), and mechanistic analysis. Verification and validation of the primary results are essential for the discovery of oncogenic pathways and the identification of therapeutic targets.[8]

The goal of all staging systems is to separate patients into homogeneous prognostic groups to permit the selection of the most appropriate surveillance as well as to find a specific therapy for each subtype. Although much work has been devoted to establishing prognostic models for HCC by using clinical information and pathologic classification, many issues still remain unresolved.[58] More than 20 studies on prognostic HCC gene expression profiling, as well as several reviews, have appeared during the last 10 years.[4] However, results from these studies are quite heterogeneous and, besides disruption in general cancer-related processes such as proliferation, apoptosis, neoangiogenesis as well as prometastatic and proinflammatory gene sets, the overall similarity was low, thus limiting a successful implementation into clinical practice. A potential explanation is the fact that the interpretation of molecular profiling studies of HCC poses more challenges than other human tumors, mainly because of the complex pathogenesis of this cancer.[59] As already emphasized, HCC arises in diverse settings ranging from infection with HBV or HCV to chronic metabolic diseases as varied as diabetes, NAFLD, and hemochromatosis. These different disease stages represent complex assortments of genetic and epigenetic aberrations as well as altered molecular pathways.[39,60]

A recent study aimed to generate a composite prognostic model by evaluating 22 prognostic gene expression signatures generated from tumors as well as cirrhotic tissues in a cohort of 287 patients with early stage HCC (BCLC 0/A).[61] Overall, most previously reported signatures retained their prognostic ability in this independent data set. Out of these 22 signatures, 17 were able to adequately subclassify patients according to their prognostic trait. It is noteworthy that none of the signatures reflecting a progenitor cell origin (i.e., EpCAM, hepatoblastoma-C2, CK19-rat, CK19-human signature) could be confirmed to be of prognostic value. However, these signatures have not been generated for the classification of early stages of HCC.

Another important finding of this study was the observation that gene expression profiles obtained from paired biopsies from the center and periphery of the same tumor in 15 tumor specimens showed a high (>80%) transcriptomic concordance. Although these observation provide at least some evidence for stability of gene expression signatures in paired biopsies and suggests a low influence of sampling error, more in-depth analyses are needed to better define the intratumoral genetic heterogeneity of HCC that is likely to contribute to the high tumor recurrence and chemoresistance of the disease.[62,63]

Nault et al.[64] aimed to identifying a robust molecular signature to accurately predict the clinical outcome of HCC patients who underwent curative surgical resection. They identified a panel of five genes (TAF9, RAMP3, HN1, KRT19, and RAN) in a training cohort of 314 HCC patients with a strong prognostic relevance and further validated this panel in two independent validation cohorts with different HCC etiologies.[64] The five-genes panel was associated with disease-specific survival both in the training and in the validation cohort, and was found to be significantly more accurate in predicting the patients' prognosis (i.e., survival and recurrence) when compared to known gene expression signatures. Due to the simplicity of the panel and its reproducibility in different technologies (i.e., gene expression microarray and real-time reverse-transcription polymerase chain reaction [qRT-PCR]), the work by Nault et al. has a high potential for implementation into the clinical management of HCC. In particular, the score may be helpful to stratify patients at high risk for relapse and tumor-related death before the decision of liver resection or transplantation is made. However, independent validation of this prognostic algorithm by different groups and independent cohorts is needed before the panel can be used for clinical decision making.

Two independent studies provide evidence that the oncofetal marker SALL4 could be an attractive therapeutic target in HCC with progenitor cell origin.[65,66] High SALL4 expression was significantly associated with overall survival of patients in large independent cohorts. Further, and consistent with its oncofetal role, SALL4 overexpressing tumors shared similar molecular profiles with fetal progenitor cells and stemness-associated HCC. Finally, by using RNAi and a specific inhibitory 12-AA peptide against SALL4, the authors could convincingly show that SALL4 possessed therapeutic potential in HCC by interacting with PTEN/PI3K-AKT signaling via the interaction with the NuRD complex.[67] These studies confirm several recent observations indicating that HCCs harboring phenotypic features of stem/progenitor cells constitute a subclass of therapeutically challenged cancer patients that have a particularly poor prognosis.[27,68,69]

Contrary to HCCs, the molecular pathology of intrahepatic cholangiocellular carcinoma (ICC) is less well investigated. Most of the studies on cholangiocarcinogenesis focused on the investigation of few candidate genes.[70] In a seminal work on both genomic and genetic features of ICC gene expression, profiles of 104 surgically resected cholangiocarcinoma samples were collected and analyzed from patients in Australia, Europe, and the United States.[71] The authors discovered new two prognostic subclasses of patients defined by a 238-gene classifier as well as KRAS mutations and increased levels of EGFR and HER2, and concomitantly validated promising therapeutic strategies in different ICC cell lines, which resembled the different prognostic subtypes. Furthermore, this study also addressed the importance of the stromal component of ICC by laser capture microdissection of epithelial and stromal compartments from 23 tumors. Although the tumor epithelium was defined by deregulation of the HER2 network and frequent overexpression of EGFR, c-MET, pRPS6 as well as proliferation, the stroma was predominantly enriched for inflammatory gene sets. In another study, gene expression analyses of 149 patients with ICC from formalin-fixed paraffin-embedded samples were performed.[72] A Gene Set Enrichment Analysis (GSEA) and functional characteristics of the patients again revealed two broad molecular subclasses—*proliferation* and *inflammation*—defined by the differential expression of 1,565 significant genes. The proliferation class was associated with aggressive tumor biology as well as a poor prognosis and was characterized by molecular enrichment of oncogenic pathways (e.g., RAS/RAF/MAPK, VEGF, and PDGF). The inflammation class displayed a better prognosis and enrichment of immune-related signaling, in particular IL-10 and signal transducer and activator of transcription 3 (STAT3) signaling. Furthermore, a subgroup of ICCs in the proliferation class shared features of several previously published prognostic HCC signatures with a possible progenitor cell origin, which supported the hypothesis that these tumors may be derived from a common origin or precursor cell(s). This hypothesis is supported by recent work by Woo et al.,[73] which applied an integrative oncogenomic approach to address the clinical and functional implications of the overlapping phenotype of combined hepatocellular cholangiocarcinoma (CHC), a histopathologic intermediate between HCC and cholangiocellular carcinoma (CC).

CONCLUSION AND PERSPECTIVE

Next-generation technologies, in particular gene expression microarrays and, more recently, next-generation sequencing, have provided an extraordinary opportunity for integrative analyses of the cancer (epi-) genome as well as transcriptome. Array-based gene expression profiling not only has advanced our understanding of cancer biology, but also has begun to influence decision making in clinical oncology, which may ultimately allow for the development of more effective therapies. The power of gene expression profiling of HCC can be further enhanced by cross-comparison analyses of multiple gene expression data sets from human HCC and the rich database of HCC in animal models.[74,75] The success of these new analytical approaches, comparative and/or integrative functional genomics, suggests that integration of independent data sets will enhance our ability to identify robust predictive markers. Despite the success of these approaches in preclinical translational studies, the clinical application of gene expression profiling is still immature. Although current signatures accurately classify HCCs according to their natural biology, they are unable to predict the response to currently used therapies.[59] Furthermore, HCC with progenitor cell features display a particular aggressive behavior, which might indicate that tumor heterogeneity and resulting chemoresistance might be generated in molecularly plastic cancer stem cells (CSCs).[76] Because CSCs by definition are a rare subpopulation of cells, their molecular profile might be diluted by the bulk of tumor cells, which further hampers therapeutic progress.[77] However, based on the exciting results of recent studies and the advent of NGS technologies that offer unprecedented depths and resolution, it seems reasonable to predict that the genomic technologies will play an increasingly important role in clinical oncology. The immediate focus undoubtedly will be on incorporating these whole-genomic technologies into clinical trials. To achieve this ambitious goal, systematic and standardized collections of tissue specimens from HCC patients (e.g., mandatory biopsies) for subsequent prospective molecular analyses are urgently needed to ultimately improve the diagnosis and treatment of liver cancer patients.

SELECTED REFERENCES

The full reference list can be accessed at lwwhealthlibrary.com/oncology.

2. El-Serag HB. Hepatocellular carcinoma. *N Engl J Med* 2011;365:1118–1127.
3. Bruix J, Sherman M, American Association for the Study of Liver D. Management of hepatocellular carcinoma: an update. *Hepatology* 2011;53:1020–1022.
4. Marquardt JU, Galle PR, Teufel A. Molecular diagnosis and therapy of hepatocellular carcinoma (HCC): an emerging field for advanced technologies. *J Hepatol* 2012;56:267–275.
6. Thorgeirsson SS, Grisham JW. Molecular pathogenesis of human hepatocellular carcinoma. *Nature Genet* 2002;31:339–346.
8. Quackenbush J. Microarray analysis and tumor classification. *N Engl J Med* 2006;354:2463–2472.
11. Vogelstein B, Papadopoulos N, Velculescu VE, et al. Cancer genome landscapes. *Science* 2013;339:1546–1558.
15. Moinzadeh P, Breuhahn K, Stutzer H, et al. Chromosome alterations in human hepatocellular carcinomas correlate with aetiology and histological grade—results of an explorative CGH meta-analysis. *Br J Cancer* 2005;92:935–941.
18. Woo HG, Park ES, Lee JS, et al. Identification of potential driver genes in human liver carcinoma by genomewide screening. *Cancer Res* 2009;69:4059–4066.
22. Feinberg AP, Ohlsson R, Henikoff S. The epigenetic progenitor origin of human cancer. *Nat Rev Genet* 2006;7:21–33.
23. Calvisi DF, Ladu S, Gorden A, et al. Mechanistic and prognostic significance of aberrant methylation in the molecular pathogenesis of human hepatocellular carcinoma. *J Clin Invest* 2007;117:2713–2722.
27. Lee JS, Heo J, Libbrecht L, et al. A novel prognostic subtype of human hepatocellular carcinoma derived from hepatic progenitor cells. *Nat Med* 2006;12:410–416.
29. Revill K, Wang T, Lachenmayer A, et al. Genome-wide methylation analysis and epigenetic unmasking identify tumor suppressor genes in hepatocellular carcinoma. *Gastroenterology* 2013;145:1424–1435.e1–25.
30. Esteller M. Epigenetics in cancer. *N Engl J Med* 2008;358:1148–1159.
32. Lujambio A, Lowe SW. The microcosmos of cancer. *Nature* 2012;482:347–355.
36. Toffanin S, Hoshida Y, Lachenmayer A, et al. MicroRNA-based classification of hepatocellular carcinoma and oncogenic role of miR-517a. *Gastroenterology* 2011;140:1618–1628.e16.
37. Ji J, Shi J, Budhu A, et al. MicroRNA expression, survival, and response to interferon in liver cancer. *N Engl J Med* 2009;361:1437–1447.
41. Fujimoto A, Totoki Y, Abe T, et al. Whole-genome sequencing of liver cancers identifies etiological influences on mutation patterns and recurrent mutations in chromatin regulators. *Nat Genet* 2012;44:760–764.
42. Guichard C, Amaddeo G, Imbeaud S, et al. Integrated analysis of somatic mutations and focal copy-number changes identifies key genes and pathways in hepatocellular carcinoma. *Nat Genet* 2012;44:694–698.

43. Li M, Zhao H, Zhang X, et al. Inactivating mutations of the chromatin remodeling gene ARID2 in hepatocellular carcinoma. *Nat Genet* 2011;43:828–829.
44. Totoki Y, Tatsuno K, Yamamoto S, et al. High-resolution characterization of a hepatocellular carcinoma genome. *Nat Genet* 2011;43:464–469.
46. Cleary SP, Jeck WR, Zhao X, et al. Identification of driver genes in hepatocellular carcinoma by exome sequencing. *Hepatology* 2013;58:1693–1702.
47. Kan Z, Zheng H, Liu X, et al. Whole-genome sequencing identifies recurrent mutations in hepatocellular carcinoma. *Genome Res* 2013;23:1422–1433.
48. Nault JC, Mallet M, Pilati C, et al. High frequency of telomerase reverse-transcriptase promoter somatic mutations in hepatocellular carcinoma and preneoplastic lesions. *Nat Commun* 2013;4:2218.
52. Marquardt JU, Seo D, Andersen JB, et al. Sequential transcriptome analysis of human liver cancer indicates late stage acquisition of malignant traits. *J Hepatol* 2014;60:346–353.
54. Karin M. Nuclear factor-kappaB in cancer development and progression. *Nature* 2006;441:431–436.
56. He G, Dhar D, Nakagawa H, et al. Identification of liver cancer progenitors whose malignant progression depends on autocrine IL-6 signaling. *Cell* 2013;155:384–396.
57. Hoshida Y, Villanueva A, Kobayashi M, et al. Gene expression in fixed tissues and outcome in hepatocellular carcinoma. *N Engl J Med.* 2008;359:1995–2004.
58. Thorgeirsson SS. Genomic decoding of hepatocellular carcinoma. *Gastroenterology* 2006;131:1344–1346.
60. Farazi PA, DePinho RA. Hepatocellular carcinoma pathogenesis: from genes to environment. *Nat Rev Cancer* 2006;6:674–687.
61. Villanueva A, Hoshida Y, Battiston C, et al. Combining clinical, pathology, and gene expression data to predict recurrence of hepatocellular carcinoma. *Gastroenterology* 2011;140:1501–1512.e2.
64. Nault JC, De Reynies A, Villanueva A, et al. A hepatocellular carcinoma 5-gene score associated with survival of patients after liver resection. *Gastroenterology* 2013;145:176–187.
66. Yong KJ, Gao C, Lim JS, et al. Oncofetal gene SALL4 in aggressive hepatocellular carcinoma. *N Engl J Med* 2013;368:2266–2276.
71. Andersen JB, Spee B, Blechacz BR, et al. Genomic and genetic characterization of cholangiocarcinoma identifies therapeutic targets for tyrosine kinase inhibitors. *Gastroenterology* 2012;142:1021–1031.e15.
72. Sia D, Hoshida Y, Villanueva A, et al. Integrative molecular analysis of intrahepatic cholangiocarcinoma reveals 2 classes that have different outcomes. *Gastroenterology* 2013;144:829–840.
76. Marquardt JU, Thorgeirsson SS. Stem cells in hepatocarcinogenesis: evidence from genomic data. *Semin Liver Dis* 2010;30:26–34.

PRACTICE OF ONCOLOGY

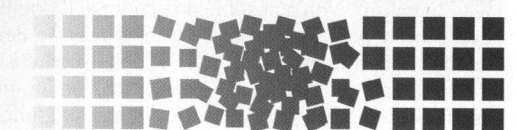

52 Cancer of the Liver

Yuman Fong, Damian E. Dupuy, Mary Feng, and Ghassan Abou-Alfa

INTRODUCTION

Primary cancers of the liver represent the fifth most common malignancy worldwide and the second most common cause of death from cancer. This is due the relationship of hepatocellular carcinoma to chronic hepatitis B virus (HBV) and hepatitis C virus (HCV) infections.[1] The prognosis of untreated hepatocellular carcinoma (HCC) has a dismal prognosis, with a 5-year survival rate below 10%.[2] The combination of cancer and chronic liver disease add significant complexity to treatment. The great progress in understanding the natural history, pathogenesis, and tumor biology of HCC has resulted in effective treatment options. For localized HCC, surgical resection and orthotopic liver transplantation (OLT) are the gold standard therapies. Formidable radiologic directed local and regional therapies, radiation therapy, and systemic therapies now round out a full arsenal of treatments even for disseminated disease. There have also been marked advances in therapies for hepatitis[3] and in care of the associated liver parenchymal disease. However, this optimism may be negated by the continued lack of a true breakthrough in screening and early detection, and the continued rising incidence of HCC globally.

EPIDEMIOLOGY

The annual number of worldwide liver cancer cases (748,300) closely resembles the number of deaths (695,900). Long-term survival rates are 3% to 5% in most cancer registries. In the United States, approximately 30,640 new tumors of the liver and intrahepatic bile ducts are diagnosed each year, with 21,670 deaths estimated annually.[1] HCC is 2.3 times more common in men than in women, and this difference is consistent globally. Androgen and androgen receptor (AR) have long been implicated in this male-dominance feature.[4] In the United States, rates of HCC are two times higher in Asians than African Americans, which are two times higher than those in Caucasians. There has been a significant overall increase in the incidence of HCC in the United States during the past 25 years.[5] This parallels the increase in HCV infection, the increase in immigrants from HBV-endemic countries, and an increase in nonalcoholic fatty liver disease. The widespread utilization of HBV vaccination is leading to a decrease in liver cancer in some areas. A dramatic demonstration of this is available from Taiwan, where an HBV vaccine was introduced in 1984, and a reduction of liver cancer was observed in children from 0.54 per 100,000 to 0.2 per 100,000 during a 16-year period.[6]

ETIOLOGIC FACTORS

Viral Hepatitis and Hepatocellular Carcinoma

The variable geographic incidence of liver cancer[7] reflects the variable geographic incidence in HCV and HBV infections, which account for 75% of the world's cases. Both case control studies and cohort studies have shown a strong association between chronic hepatitis B carriage rates and increased incidence of HCC. Beasley et al.[8] followed Taiwanese male postal carriers who were hepatitis B surface antigen (HBsAg)-positive and found an annual HCC incidence of 495 per 100,000. This represented a 98-fold greater risk than observed in HBsAg-negative individuals. By evaluating apparently asymptomatic HBsAg-positive blood donors at American Red Cross centers, a relative risk of 12.7 was noted for liver cancer compared with HBsAg-negative individuals. A multivariate analysis has been used to determine *risk scores* for the development of HCC.[9] Factors predictive of HCC include male gender, advanced age, specific promoter mutations, the presence of cirrhosis, and higher viremia levels. If validated, this may improve patient selection for surveillance.

The exact mechanism by which HBV infection causes HCC is not known.[10,11] Some have postulated that the effect of HBV on hepatic carcinogenesis is indirect, through the process of inflammation, regeneration, and fibrosis associated with chronic hepatitis and cirrhosis. Consistent with this hypothesis, 70% of cases of HBV-related HCC occur in association with cirrhosis. It is well known that cirrhosis of all causes may result in HCC.

There is evidence that the effect may be a direct viral effect. HBV DNA may become integrated within the chromosomes of infected hepatocytes, and in some HCCs, this integration of viral genetic material may occur in a critical location within the cellular genome. For example, integration of HBV DNA has been observed within the retinoic acid receptor alpha gene and within the human cyclin A gene, both of which play crucial roles in cellular growth. However, in most cases, the HBV DNA integration appears to be random. The hepatitis B x gene (*HBx*) product has been implicated in causing HCC because it is a transcriptional activator of various cellular genes associated with growth control. *HBx* has been found to interact with *p53*, interfering with its function as a tumor suppressor.

HCV is an RNA virus without a DNA intermediate form, and therefore, cannot integrate into hepatocyte DNA. In contrast to HBV, HCV is more likely to lead to chronic infection (10% versus 60% to 80%), and cirrhosis (20-fold increase).[12] The typical interval between HCV-associated transfusion and subsequent HCC is only about 30 years (compared with 40 to 50 years for HBV). The state of the liver also differs in that HCV-associated HCC patients tend to have more frequent and more advanced cirrhosis. In HBV-associated HCC, only half the patients have cirrhosis. The risk of developing HCC in a patient with HCV-related cirrhosis is 5% per year versus 0.5% per year for HBV-related cirrhosis.

There have been extensive efforts to establish the molecular pathways involved in the pathogenesis of HCC.[13,14] Some of the abnormalities that are commonly found in HCC include (1) cell-cycle dysregulation associated with somatic mutations or loss of heterozygosity in *TP53*, silencing of *CDKN2A* or *RB1*, or *CCND1* overexpression; (2) increased angiogenesis accompanied by overexpression or amplification of *VEGF*, *PDGF*, and *ANGPT2*; (3) evasion of apoptosis as a result of activation of survival signals such as nuclear factor kappa B (NF-κB); and (4) reactivation of *TERT*.

There is emerging evidence of the importance of microRNAs and epigenetic alterations such as hypermethylation in the pathogenesis of HCC. MicroRNA-155 (miR-155) levels were significantly increased in patients infected with HCV, and overexpression of miR-155 was associated with nuclear accumulation of beta-catenin by increased Wnt signaling, thereby implicating this pathway in HCV-associated hepatocellular carcinogenesis.[15]

Alcohol-Induced Hepatocarcinogenesis

There is a strong association between alcoholic cirrhosis and the development of HCC. By itself, chronic alcohol consumption has carcinogenic effects. Thus, chronic alcohol intake is known to lead to oxidative stress in the liver, inflammation, and cirrhosis. Ethanol is metabolized by alcohol dehydrogenases and cytochrome P-450, producing acetaldehyde and reactive oxygen species. Acetaldehyde binds directly to proteins and DNA. It damages mitochondria, initiating apoptosis. P-450 metabolism leads to reactive oxygen species, which lead to lipid consumption peroxidation, protein oxidation, and DNA adducts.[16] Alcohol leads to monocyte activation and inflammatory cytokine production. Oxidative stress has been demonstrated in alcoholic cirrhosis through increased isoprostane, a marker of lipid peroxidation.[17] Oxidative stress promotes the development of fibrosis and cirrhosis, creating a permissive HCC microenvironment. Oxidative stress may also lead to decreased Signal Transducers and Activators of Transcription 1 (STAT1)-directed activation of interferon gamma (IFNγ) signaling with consequent hepatocyte damage.[18]

Nonalcoholic Fatty Liver Disease

HCC has been linked to nonalcoholic fatty liver disease (NAFLD). NAFLD is present in 30% of the general adult population, in 90% of morbidly obese adults (body mass index [BMI] $\geq$40 kg/m^2), and in close to 74% of those with diabetes.[19–21] The risk of HCC due to NAFLD appears to be less than that of chronic hepatitis C. A recent US study reported a 2.6% yearly cumulative incidence of HCC in NAFLD and 4% in HCV cirrhosis.[22] Similarly, a prospective 5-year study from Japan reported a rate of HCC of 11.3% among patients with NAFLD cirrhosis compared to 30.5% among those with HCV-associated cirrhosis.[23] A recent study from Germany identified nonalcoholic steatohepatitis (NASH) as the most common etiology of HCC (24%), surpassing chronic hepatitis C (23.3%), chronic hepatitis B (19.3%), and alcoholic liver disease (12.7%).[24]

Diabetes and obesity have been established as independent risk factors for HCC, and that association holds true in the setting of NAFLD and associated NASH.[25,26] However, there is also increasing evidence suggesting that NAFLD contributes to noncirrhotic HCC, and that HCC can develop in patients with metabolic syndrome and NAFLD in the absence of NASH and fibrosis.[27]

Other Etiologic Considerations

In addition to alcoholic cirrhosis and viral hepatitis, several underlying conditions have been found to be associated with an increased risk for the development of HCC (Table 52.1). These include autoimmune chronic active hepatitis, cryptogenic cirrhosis, and metabolic diseases. Metabolic diseases include hemochromatosis (iron accumulation), Wilson disease (copper accumulation), α$_1$-antitrypsin deficiency, tyrosinemia, porphyria cutanea tarda, glycogenesis types 1 and 3, citrullinemia, and orotic acid urea. In children, congenital cholestatic syndrome (Alagille syndrome) is associated with a familial type of HCC.

Chemical Carcinogens

Probably the best-studied and most potent ubiquitous natural chemical carcinogen is a product of the *Aspergillus* fungus,

TABLE 52.1

Conditions Associated with Human Hepatocellular Carcinoma

Condition	Risk
Cirrhosis	
Hepatitis B virus	High
Hepatitis C virus	High
Alcohol	High
Autoimmune chronic active hepatitis	High
Cryptogenic cirrhosis	High
Cirrhosis due to nonalcoholic fatty liver disease	High
Primary biliary cirrhosis	Low
Hereditary hemochromatosis	High
α$_1$-Antitrypsin deficiency	High
Wilson disease	Low
Metabolic Diseases (without Cirrhosis)	
Hereditary tyrosinemia	High
α$_1$-Antitrypsin deficiency	Moderate
Ataxia telangiectasia	Moderate
Types 1 and 3 glycogen storage disease	Moderate
Galactosemia	Moderate
Citrullinemia	Moderate
Hereditary hemorrhagic telangiectasia	Moderate
Porphyria cutanea tarda	Moderate
Orotic aciduria	Moderate
Alagille syndrome (congenital cholestatic syndrome)	Moderate
Environmental	
Thorotrast	Moderate
Androgenic steroids	Moderate
Cigarette smoking	Low to moderate
Aflatoxin	Moderate

called aflatoxin B$_1$.[28] *Aspergillus flavus* mold and aflatoxin product can be found in a variety of stored grains, particularly in hot, humid parts of the world, where grains such as rice are stored in unrefrigerated conditions. In the months following the monsoons in Southeast Asia, most village-based grains can be seen to be covered by a white layer of aflatoxin that is consumed with the grain. Data on aflatoxin contamination of foodstuffs correlate well with incidence rates of HCC in Africa and to some extent in China.

There is considerable literature on the hepatocarcinogenicity of anabolic steroids as well as the induction of benign adenomas by estrogens.[29] Although estrogens are capable of causing HCC in rodents, an epidemiologic association in humans has never been clearly shown. In an industrial society, a large number of environmental pollutants, particularly pesticides and insecticides, are known rodent hepatic carcinogens. In a recent case-control study, cumulative lifetime tobacco use of more than 11,000 packs and Asian ethnicity were independent predictors of HCC development amongst a cohort of patients with chronic liver disease, including HCV.[30]

STAGING

Multiple clinical staging systems for hepatic tumors have been described. The most widely used is the American Joint Committee on Cancer/tumor-node-metastasis (AJCC/TNM) (Table 52.2).[31] Adverse prognostic features include large size, multiple tumors, vascular invasion, and lymph node spread. Macroscopic or microscopic vascular invasions, in particular, have profound effects on prognosis. Stage III disease contains a mixture of lymph node–positive and –negative tumors. Stage III patients with positive lymph node or stage IV disease have a poor prognosis, and few patients survive 1 year.

The prognosis in patients with HCC is very much influenced by the presence and severity of underlying liver disease as well. The Child-Pugh scoring system is the most commonly used tool for assessing cirrhosis (see Table 52.2).[32] It encompasses five parameters—bilirubin, albumin, prothrombin time, clinical ascites, and clinical encephalopathy—each of which is scored from one to three depending on severity. The key limitation of the Child-Pugh scoring system is its lack of any parameters pertaining to the cancer itself. Despite that, it remains incorporated into many HCC clinical trials as a tool to measure the extent of liver disease in the study populations, and thus, its use may not fade away any time soon. However, this main limitation of the Child-Pugh scoring system has been overcome by other scoring systems. Among those, the first to be established is the Okuda staging system. The

TABLE 52.2A

Staging for Liver Function and Cancer: American Joint Commission on Cancer Staging for Hepatocellular Cancer

T	TX	Primary tumor cannot be assessed		
	T0	No evidence of primary tumor		
	T1	Solitary tumor without vascular invasion		
	T2	Solitary tumor with vascular invasion, or multiple tumors no more than 5 cm		
	T3a	Multiple tumors more than 5 cm		
	T3b	Tumor involving a major branch of the portal or hepatic vein(s)		
	T4	Tumor(s) with direct invasion of adjacent organs other than the gallbladder or with perforation of visceral peritoneum		
N	NX	Regional lymph nodes cannot be assessed		
	N0	No regional lymph node metastasis		
	N1	Regional lymph node metastasis		
M	MX	Distant metastasis cannot be assessed		
	M0	No distant metastasis		
	M1	Distant metastasis		
Stage Grouping				
I	T1	N0	M0	
II	T2	N0	M0	
IIIA	T3a	N0	M0	
IIIB	T3b	N0	M0	
IIIC	T4	N0	M0	
IVA	Any T	N1	M0	
IVB	Any T	Any N	M1	

Edge SB, Byrd DR, Compton CC, et al., eds. *The American Joint Committee on Cancer: AJCC Cancer Staging Manual*, 7th ed. New York:Springer;2010:197.

TABLE 52.2B

Child-Pugh Grading of Cirrhosis[a]

Measurement	1 Point	2 Points	3 Points
Bilirubin (mg/dL)	1–1.9	2–2.9	>2.9
Prolongation of PT	1–3	4–6	>6
Albumin (g/dL)	>3.5	2.8–3.4	<2.8
Ascites	None	Mild	Moderate/severe
Encephalopathy	None	Grade 1 or 2	Grade 3 or 4

[a] Grade A = 5–6 points; grade B = 7–9 points; grade C = 10–15 points.
PT, prothrombin time.

Cancer of the Liver Italian Program (CLIP) score was defined and studied prospectively in patients with HCC mainly caused by HCV.[33,34] The CLIP score consists of the Child-Pugh score parameters combined with a subjective assessment of tumor in the liver, the presence or absence of portal vein thrombosis, and the alpha-fetoprotein (AFP) level. The addition of vascular endothelial growth factor levels to the CLIP parameters (V-CLIP) has been shown to provide a significantly more precise prognosis, but has yet to be prospectively validated.[35] The Chinese University Prognostic Index (CUPI) scoring system was developed in patients with mainly HBV-related HCC.[36] The CUPI parameters are bilirubin, ascites, AFP, alkaline phosphatase, the tumor extent (AJCC/TNM 5th edition), and clinical symptoms at presentation. A French system called the Groupe d'Etude et de Traitement du Carcinoma Hepatocellulaire (GETCH) staging system consists of bilirubin, Karnofsky performance score, AFP, alkaline phosphatase, and portal vein thrombosis.[37] Another scoring system that is mainly used in Japan is the Japan Integrated Staging (JIS) score.[38]

Another commonly used scoring system is the Barcelona Clinic Liver Cancer (BCLC) classification system.[39] The BCLC couples prognosis with treatment assignment and has been validated prospectively.[40] However, it has been shown to be less valuable in the setting of more advanced disease, defined as BCLC category C.[41,42] In retrospective analyses of patients with advanced-stage HCC seen by medical oncologists, the CLIP scoring system was noted to be the most informative regarding the outcome of this specific patient population.

DIAGNOSIS

The tests used to diagnose HCC include radiologic studies and pathologic diagnosis with biopsy. Core biopsies are most preferred because of the tissue architecture given by this technique. For patients suspected of having portal vein involvement, a core biopsy of the portal vein may be performed.[43] Morphologic features, such as stromal invasion, help distinguish high-grade dysplastic nodules from HCC.[44]

The American Association for the Study of Liver Diseases (AASLD),[45] and the European Association for the Study of the Liver (EASL)[46] have outlined noninvasive criteria for the diagnosis of HCC. EASL recommends that lesions that are greater than 2 cm with characteristic radiologic features of arterial hyperenhancement on two different imaging modalities, or on one imaging modality alongside with a serum AFP of 400 ng/dL or more, are diagnostic of HCC, and no biopsy is needed. The AASLD added venous washout as a requisite radiologic feature. Detection of a lesion larger than 2 cm that exhibits both arterial hyperenhancement and venous washout in a single imaging modality concomitant with an AFP >200 ng/mL is sufficient to diagnose HCC.[47] Bialecki et al.[48] found a sensitivity and specificity of 89.1% and 100%, respectively, for liver biopsy compared to 64.9% and 62.8%, respectively, for the noninvasive EASL criteria. The fear of biopsy-related hemorrhage is dissuaded by a 0.4% rate, and tumor seeding occurs at a low rate of 1.6%. When seeding does occur, it can be treated by local resection and is seldom a cause of morbidity and mortality.[49,50]

TREATMENT OF HEPATOCELLULAR CARCINOMA

Many treatment options for HCC are available (Table 52.3). Resection and liver transplantation represent the potentially curative options with the longest track record. For small tumors, ablation and radiotherapy (RT) are quite effective and may be curative.

Surgical Resection for Hepatocellular Carcinoma

Patient Selection

Liver resection is the preferred treatment for the noncirrhotic patient with HCC. These patients generally have normal liver function, no portal hypertension, and can tolerate major liver resections with acceptable morbidity and low mortality. The selection of noncirrhotic patients with HCC for resection is as for other malignant lesions. Resection should be considered for patients where a complete resection of tumor is possible while preserving greater than 30% functional liver. If the potential remnant liver volume may be less than 30%, portal vein embolization is now a well-accepted preoperative preparatory method for increasing the potential remnant liver volume and safety of the resection.[51]

For cirrhotic patients, the primary determinant of outcome and selection of therapy is the degree of hepatic dysfunction and portal hypertension. Traditionally, only compensated cirrhotics

---

TABLE 52.3

Treatment Options for Hepatocellular Carcinoma

- Surgery
  - Partial hepatectomy
  - Liver transplantation
- Local ablative therapies
  - Cryosurgery
  - Microwave ablation
  - Ethanol injection
  - Acetic acid injection
  - Radiofrequency ablation
- Regional therapies: hepatic artery transcatheter treatments
  - Transarterial chemotherapy
  - Transarterial embolization
  - Transarterial chemoembolization
  - Transarterial yttrium-90 microspheres
  - Transarterial ^{131}I-lipiodol
  - Proton or carbon ion therapy
  - Conformal radiation therapy
  - Stereotactic radiation therapy
  - Palliative low-dose radiation therapy
- Systemic therapies
  - Chemotherapy
  - Targeted therapy (sorafenib)[a]
  - Immunotherapy
  - Hormonal therapy
- Supportive care

[a] Sorafenib is the only systemic therapy with level 1 evidence, proving a survival benefit.

(Child-Turcotte-Pugh class A) were candidates for hepatic resection, whereas patients with significant hepatic functional dysfunction (Child class B or C) are generally not selected for resection because of poor outcome.[51] Portal hypertension can be indirectly assessed clinically by the presence of splenomegaly, esophagogastric varices, and thrombocytopenia (platelet count <100.000/mm^3) or directly determined by hepatic venous wedge pressures ($\geq$10 mmHg). With recent advances in perioperative care, there is growing evidence that liver resection for HCC in well-selected patients with mild portal hypertension is safe and can achieve a comparable outcome as in patients without portal hypertension.[52,53]

The future remnant liver mass is another important factor to be considered in cirrhotic patients before resection. A too small remnant liver volume is associated with an increased risk for postresectional liver failure.[54] There is a general consensus that the critical remnant liver volume in cirrhotic patients is 50%,[55] and portal vein embolization should be considered if the future remnant liver volume is expected to be below 50%.[56–59] Some investigators have even attempted to sequential employ transarterial chemoembolization (TACE) to control the tumor or portal vein embolization (PVE) to increase residual liver volume, followed by definitive surgical resection.[56,57] The sequential use of TACE and PVE results in more efficient hypertrophy of the future remnant liver compared to PVE alone.[51]

In other parts of the world, dynamic liver function tests are also employed for the assessment of suitability for liver resection. These include the indocyanine green (ICG) test and technetium-99m diethylenetriaminepentaacetic acid-galactosyl human serum albumin (technetium-99m galactosyl human serum albumin [99mTc-GSA] scintigraphy).[51,55] An ICG retention rate of less than 14% proved to be a safe indicator for major hepatectomy in cirrhotic patients, whereas retention rates above 20% are considered a contraindication for major hepatectomy.[60–62]

Patient medical comorbidities considered are similar to an assessment for any major surgery. Some studies have reported age and gender to be independent risk factors for poor outcome after resection of HCC.[63] Other studies indicate that advanced age is more a surrogate for medical fitness, and that, with careful patient selection, elderly patients benefit as much from resection as younger patients.[64] Comorbidities as represented by American Society of Anesthesia (ASA) grade have been shown to correlate with survival.[65]

Outcomes of Resection and Prognostic Factors

With improving patient selection and perioperative care, the outcome of hepatic resection for HCC has been continuously improved during the past 2 decades. Many large series of the past 10 years show that resection is associated with a perioperative mortality rate of less than 7%, and patients achieve an overall survival rate of 30% to 50% (Table 52.4).[65–75] Many major centers are recently reporting operative mortalities less than 2%,[68,70,74] even in cirrhotic patients.

Tumor factors most important for outcome are TNM staging at presentation, macro- and microvascular invasion, and the number of tumors. Large HCC has a propensity for vascular invasion and growth of tumor intraluminally. This is associated with intrahepatic satellite metastases via the portal venous system and is frequently associated with small satellite tumors. Intraluminal spread through the hepatic veins leads to pulmonary metastases.

One surgical factor prognostic for outcome is surgical margins. There is no clear margin size that has been universally agreed upon, but there is consensus on importance of an R0 resection.[76] Most surgeons prefer at least a 1-cm margin. In one 225 patient study, a 1-cm margin was associated with a 77% 3-year survival versus 21% for those with less than a 1-cm margin.[72] It must be noted that in a randomized controlled trial, a 2-cm margin was associated with a decrease in recurrence as well as improved survival.[77] Studies have demonstrated improved outcome for anatomic versus nonanatomic resections for HCC.[78] In a series of 210 patients, 5-year survival rates were 66% for anatomic versus 35% in

TABLE 52.4

Results of Surgical Resection for Hepatocellular Carcinoma

First Author	Year Published	Number of Patients	Cirrhosis	Minor Resections[a]	Mortality	5-Year Overall Survival Rate
Zhou[66]	2001	2,366	—	72%	2.7%	50%
Kanematsu[68]	2002	303	55%	76%	1.6%	51%
Belghiti[67]	2002	328	50%	—	6.4%	37%
Wayne[69]	2002	249	73%	73%	6.1%	41%
Ercolani[65]	2003	224	100%	—	—	42%
Wu[70]	2005	426	100%	55%	1.6%	46%–61%[b]
Capussotti[71]	2005	216	100%	24%	8.3%	34%
Hasegawa[72]	2005	210	39%	—	0.0%	35%–66%[b]
Nathan[73]	2009	788	—	—	—	39%
Yang[74]	2009	481	77%	—	1.7%	20%–48%[b]
Wang[75]	2010	438	—	—	7.5%	43%

Note: Selected series with more than 200 patients over the past decade. Areas marked by a dash are not defined.
[a] Minor resections are defined as ≤ segmentectomy.
[b] Range of 5-year overall survival among different subgroups.

nonanatomic resections.[72] For small solitary tumors, anatomic resections seem to be less important.[79] Choice of margin and the anatomic approach for cancer clearance must be weighed against better perioperative outcome for limited parenchymal resection in cirrhotic patients.

Liver Transplantation for Hepatocellular Carcinoma

Patient Selection

Theoretically, liver transplantation is the ideal therapy for HCC in cirrhotic patients because it treats both the cancer as well as the underlying parenchymal disease. However, early experience with transplants produced dismal results. Bismuth et al.[80] was one of the first groups to consider that, in advanced disease, the likelihood of systemic disease was so high that recurrence rates, and therefore long-term outcomes, were unacceptably poor. They demonstrated that patients with limited disease (uninodular or binodular <3 cm tumors) had much better outcomes with transplant than resection (83% 5-year survival versus 18%).[80]

The landmark works of Mazzaferro et al.[81] have defined the most commonly used criteria for the selection of patients with HCC for transplantation. In their paper they defined the Milan criteria for transplantation as a single tumor less than 5 cm or three or fewer tumors all individually less than 3 cm (Fig. 52.1). Using these criteria for selection, patients transplanted had a very favorable outcome, including a 4-year actuarial survival rate of 85% and a recurrence-free survival rate of 92%. The suitability of these criteria for the selection of patients for transplant has been confirmed by numerous studies (Table 52.5).[81–94]

The excellent outcomes of HCC patients within the Milan criteria led many to explore more expansive and inclusive criteria.[90] The most accepted of the expanded criteria is that from the University of California San Francisco (UCSF) group. They reported excellent results after transplant for solitary tumor ≤6.5 cm, three or fewer nodules with the largest ≤4.5 cm, and total tumor diameter ≤8 cm (see Fig. 52.1). The UCSF criteria was associated with a survival of 90% and 75% at 1 and 5 years, respectively.[90,95]

The largest experience to date using transplantation for HCC was reported from the University of California, Los Angeles

(UCLA).[96] In this study of 467 transplants performed for HCC, the overall 1-, 3-, and 5-year survivals were 82%, 65%, and 52%, respectively. Transplanted patients with tumors beyond the UCSF criteria had a survival below 50%.

Living Donor Liver Transplant

Because of the shortage of cadaveric livers, living donor liver transplant (LDLT) has become an increasingly utilized modality for the treatment of patients with decompensated cirrhosis. In many Asian countries, where prevalence of HCC is high, living related transplants are the most common liver transplants performed. Survival

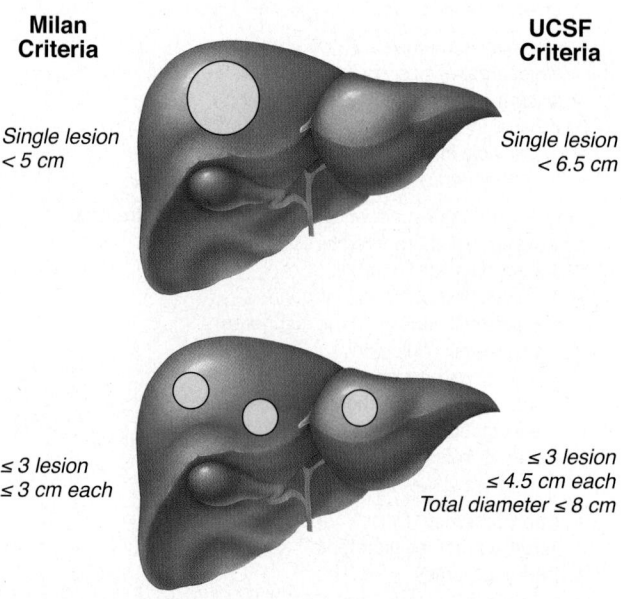

Milan Criteria
Single lesion <5 cm
≤ 3 lesion
≤ 3 cm each

UCSF Criteria
Single lesion <6.5 cm
≤ 3 lesion
≤ 4.5 cm each
Total diameter ≤ 8 cm

Figure 52.1 Milan (single lesion ≤5 cm, or no more than 3 lesions ≤3 cm) and University of California, San Francisco (UCSF) criteria (single lesion ≤6.5 cm, or no more than 3 lesions ≤4.5 cm and a total diameter of 8 cm) for patients with HCC and who are undergoing liver transplantation.

PRACTICE OF ONCOLOGY

TABLE 52.5

Results of Liver Transplantation for Early Hepatocellular Carcinoma

Study	Number of Patients	Tumor Number and Size	Neoadjuvant Therapy	Survival (%)[a]
Mazzaferro et al., 2009[81]	444	1 ≤5 cm; 3 ≤3 cm	None	73
	1,112	Beyond Milan criteria	None	54
Pelletier et al., 2009[85]	2,790	1≤5 cm; 3 ≤3 cm	None	61
	346	Beyond Milan criteria	None	32
Herrero et al., 2008[86]	47	1 ≤5 cm; 3 ≤3 cm	None	70
	26	Beyond Milan criteria	None	73
Onaca et al., 2007[87]	631	1 ≤5 cm; 3 ≤3 cm	None	62 (5 y RFS)
	575	Beyond Milan criteria	None	43 (5 y RFS)
Decaens et al., 2006[88]	279	1 ≤5 cm; 3 ≤3 cm	None	60
	44	UCSF criteria	None	46
	145	Beyond UCSF criteria	None	35
Bigourdan et al., 2003[89]	17	1 ≤5 cm; 3 ≤3 cm	TACE	71
Yao et al., 2001[90]	46	1 ≤5 cm; 3 ≤3 cm	TACE/ETOH	72
Tamura et al., 2001[91]	56	<5 cm	± TACE	71
Regalia et al., 2001[92]	122	1 ≤5 cm; 3 ≤3 cm	TACE	80
Jonas et al., 2001[93]	120	1 ≤5 cm; 3 ≤3 cm	None	71
Llovet et al., 1998[94]	58	<5 cm	None	74
Mazzaferro et al., 1996[81]	48	1 ≤5 cm; 3 ≤3 cm	TACE	75 (4 y)

[a] All are 5-year survivals, except where noted.
RFS, recurrence-free survival; ETOH, alcohol.

outcomes for all patients undergoing LDLT are comparable to the results with deceased donors (Table 52.6).[97–102] The disadvantage is clearly the risk to the living donor, with morbidity as high as 40% and a 0.5% mortality. The greatest concern is that LDLT may encourage transplants for patients with unfavorable biology (outside of the established Milan or UCSF criteria) and pose unjustified risk to two lives, including the healthy individual.

Multimodality Management While Awaiting Transplant

To qualify for the wait list, a biopsy or one of the following criteria must be fulfilled: AFP >200 mg/mL, arteriogram confirming the tumor or arterial enhancement followed by portal venous washout on computed tomography (CT) scans or magnetic resonance imaging (MRI), or a history of local–regional treatment. Patients should be assessed radiologically for number and size of tumors, to rule out extrahepatic disease and vascular involvement. Patients with tumors less than 2 cm in size or patients who do not qualify for the Milan criteria can be listed for transplant, but they will receive no additional priority points for the tumor. The tumor should

be assessed every 3 months by CT scans or MRI to rule out progression of disease beyond the established criteria.

To reduce the likelihood of tumor progression while on the wait list, many local treatments are used, including TACE, percutaneous radiofrequency ablation (RFA), or percutaneous ethanol injection (PEI). TACE involves selective embolization of the arterial feeding vessels for the hepatoma with occlusive particles with or without admixed chemotherapeutic agents. TACE limits wait list dropout, decreases posttransplant recurrence, and can downstage HCC that is beyond transplant criteria.[103] A dropout rate of 14% was found in a series of patients treated with TACE as bridge to transplant, which compared very favorably to a dropout rate of 38% for an untreated group of patients reported by the Barcelona Liver Cancer study group.[104,105]

For small, solitary tumor, PEI[106] or RFA can be effective treatment options for use as a bridge to transplant. In a series of 52 patients treated with RFA, the dropout rate was 6% at 12 months due to tumor progression with a 3-year disease-free survival of 76% for the 41 patients eventually transplanted.[107] Mazzaferro et al.[108] reported no dropout for their patients treated with RFA as bridge to transplant, with a 3-year survival of 83%.

TABLE 52.6

Results of Living Donor Liver Transplantation for Hepatocellular Carcinoma with Patient Selection Based on the Milan Criteria

Study	Patients Meeting Milan Criteria		Patients Exceeding Milan Criteria	
	Number	3-Year Survival (%)	Number	3-Year Survival (%)
Todo et al., 2004[99]	137	80	172	60
Hwang et al., 2005[100]	151	91	62	62
Takada et al., 2006[101]	49	68	44	59
Sugawara et al., 2007[102]	68	79	10	60

ADJUVANT AND NEOADJUVANT THERAPY

Adjuvant Therapy

A recent report of a randomized trial of adjuvant IFNα-2b described an improved 5-year survival in patients with stage III/IVA tumor from 24% to 68% ($p = 0.038$).[109] In a separate, larger study, IFNα-2b therapy was not associated with reducing postoperative recurrence in a population at risk for viral hepatitis–induced hepatocellular carcinoma. In this study of 268 patients, the median recurrence-free survival was 42.2 and 48.6 months with observation and IFNα-2b therapy, respectively (p = 0.828).[110]

Another approach that has been evaluated is intrahepatic ^{131}I-lipiodol. In a randomized study of 43 patients, adjuvant ^{131}I-lipiodol administered via the hepatic artery was compared with observation after resection of HCC. There was an improvement in median disease-free survival noted in favor of the ^{131}I-lipiodol arm (57.2 versus 13.6 months; $p = 0.037$).[111] However, a long-term follow-up of this trial at 10 years failed to show the same survival advantage.[112]

The best-studied systemic adjuvant therapy so far is acyclic retinoid, which was evaluated against placebo following surgical resection in 89 patients.[113] Patients who received acyclic retinoid had a recurrence rate of 27% compared with 49% for patients who received placebo ($p = 0.04$) after a median follow-up period of 38 months. The prevention of second primary HCC was more marked after a median follow-up of 62 months ($p = 0.002$, log rank test), but the difference in survival rates did not reach significance until after 6 years, with an estimated 6-year survival of 74% versus 46%, respectively ($p = 0.04$).[114]

Sorafenib, which will be discussed at length in the Systemic Therapy section, was also studied in the adjuvant setting. In a pilot study of 31 patients with HCC who had undergone curative resection and were at high risk of recurrence, sorafenib prolonged the time to recurrence (21.5 versus 13.4 months; $p = 0.006$) and significantly lowered recurrence rate (29.4% versus 70.7%; $p = 0.006$).[115] A currently fully accrued yet not reported phase III trial (STORM) randomized patients to adjuvant sorafenib versus placebo after surgery, radiofrequency ablation, or percutaneous alcohol injection with a primary end point of recurrence-free survival (Clinical Trial: NCT00692770). A phase II randomized, placebo-controlled study evaluating whether adjuvant sorafenib can prevent recurrence of HCC in high-risk orthotopic liver transplant recipients is currently enrolling (Clinical Trial: NCT01624285).

Neoadjuvant Therapy

Two randomized controlled trials and seven nonrandomized trials have evaluated preoperative transarterial chemotherapy. No clear advantage in disease-free or overall survival was found in these studies.[116–118] Postoperative transarterial chemotherapy has been examined in four randomized controlled trials and three nonrandomized controlled trials. A meta-analysis of these trials revealed a significant improvement in disease-free and overall survival.[117] The regimens consisted of Lipiodol and chemotherapy agents, including doxorubicin, mitomycin, and cisplatin. An analysis of postoperative adjuvant systemic chemotherapy trials demonstrated no consistent advantage in terms of disease-free or overall survival.[113,119–122]

A combination regimen of systemic therapy that has been studied extensively in advanced HCC provided input for its potential use in the neoadjuvant setting. PIAF (cisplatin, IFNα-2b, doxorubicin, and 5-fluorouracil) have shown in a phase II study a response rate of 26% with a median survival of approximately 9 months.[123] Of the 13 patients (26%) who had a partial response, 9 underwent surgery and 4 (9%) achieved a complete pathologic response to chemotherapy. These results illustrated that chemotherapy for HCC is effective in selected patients and suggest the possible use of PIAF as neoadjuvant therapy for medically fit patients with good liver function in whom cytoreduction might permit future resectability. The potential for cure would justify the risk of the significant toxicity profile of PIAF.

Choice of Resection, Ablation, or Transplantation

Although liver resection versus liver transplantation as primary therapy for patients with small HCC and adequate hepatic reserve is hotly debated, in most cases resection and OLT are complementary and not competing therapies. A number of studies report comparable overall survival rates for primary resection and primary OLT for transplantable HCC (Table 52.7).[89,124–134]

Patients with limited disease have potentially curative treatment options. There is general consensus that in patients with no underlying liver dysfunction, limited disease should be resected because this gives the best chance of cure without an ongoing need of immunosuppression dictated by transplantation. The outcomes of resection are quite good, with 5-year survivals of 30% to 50% (see Table 52.4).

For patients with end-stage liver disease (ESLD) and limited HCC, OLT is currently the best treatment modality. However, OLT can only be offered only to a small proportion of patients due to donor organ shortage. Therefore, liver resection remains the most important surgical therapy in patients with HCC and well-preserved liver function (Child class A).[51] Using resection as first-line therapy with salvage transplantation saved for recurrence is a common approach, especially for geographic regions with a high incidence of HCC and a low liver donation rate.[135,136] Resection can, therefore, be used as bridge therapy before OLT to control the tumor burden in patients who fulfill the Milan[81] or UCSF[90] criteria. In a study from a large Asian transplant center, the majority of patients (79%) who developed tumor recurrence after resection of small HCC were still eligible for salvage transplantation.[137] Primary resection also allows the opportunity to pathologically assess the tumor and adjacent liver tissue.[136] Pathologic prognostic factors such as micro- or macrovascular invasion, satellitosis, or occult tumors can be used as selection criteria for salvage liver transplantation in the case of recurrent tumor disease.

Patients with large HCC beyond the Milan or UCSF criteria have a less favorable outcome than those with small HCC.[81,90] Patients in the United States outside the accepted criteria can be transplanted based on the physiologic Model for End-Stage Liver Disease (MELD) score but do not receive any exception points for HCC. In an analysis of 94 patients with HCC exceeding the Milan criteria, results of resection was compared to OLT.[138] The overall survival rate was 66% for both groups even though the mean tumor size was 10 cm for the resection group and 6.4 cm for the OLT group. The results suggest that resection and OLT in patients with HCC beyond the Milan criteria have similar outcomes. A proposed algorithm of care from the Barcelona Clinic is shown in Figure 52.2.

Ablative Therapy For Localized Hepatocellular Cancer

Chemical Ablation

Chemicals destroy tumor tissue by direct dehydration of the cytoplasm, protein denaturation, and consequent coagulation necrosis as well as from indirect ischemia from vascular thrombosis from endothelial damage.[139,140] The direct instillation of chemicals such as absolute ethanol or acetic acid has been long studied for the treatment of HCC.[141–143] Chemical ablation is very inexpensive and, therefore, it is more widely used in developing countries with a high incidence of HCC. Intratumoral instillation of acetic acid for the treatment of HCC compares favorably

TABLE 52.7

Recent Studies Comparing Long-Term Outcome of Patients with Hepatocellular Carcinoma Treated Primarily with Resection (and Salvage Transplantation) or Primary Liver Transplantation

First Author	Year Published	Primary Therapy	Sample Size	5-Year Overall Survival Rate (%)	5-Year Disease-Free Survival Rate (%)
Lee[127]	2010	Transplantation	78	68	75[a]
		Resection	130	52	50
Facciuto[128b]	2009	Transplantation	119	62	—
		Resection	60	61	—
Del Gaudio[129]	2008	Transplantation	147	58	54
		Resection	80	66	41
Shah[130]	2007	Transplantation	140	64	78[a]
		Resection	121	56	60
Poon[131]	2007	Transplantation	85	44	—
		Resection	228	60	—
Margarit[126]	2005	Transplantation	36	50	64[a]
		Resection	37	78	39
Bigourdan[89]	2003	Transplantation	17	71	80[a]
		Resection	20	36	40[a]
Adam[132]	2003	Transplantation	195	61[b]	58[a]
		Resection	98	50	18
Belghiti[133]	2003	Transplantation	70	—	59
		Resection	18	—	61
Figueras[134]	2000	Transplantation	85	60	60[a]
		Resection	35	51	31

[a] Significant difference as reported in the original study.
[b] Fourth-year survival rates are reported for patients meeting the Milan criteria.
Adapted from Rahbari NN, Mehrabi A, Mollberg NM, et al. Hepatocellular carcinoma: current management and perspectives for the future. *Ann Surg* 2011;253:453–469, Table 3, with permission from Lippincott Williams & Wilkins.

with that of ethanol treatment.[144,145] Moderate quality evidence supports that RFA is superior to chemical ablation for the treatment of HCC.[146] Chemical ablation requires multiple applications, and thus, thermal ablation has largely replaced chemical ablation in many cases. In certain anatomic locations, such as adjacent to the major biliary tree or gallbladder, the combination of thermal ablation and ethanol ablation has shown some benefit.[147,148]

Radiofrequency Ablation

RFA is currently the most widely used ablative technique for the treatment of liver malignancies. The term *radiofrequency* applies to all electromagnetic energy sources with frequencies less than 30 MHz, although most clinically available devices function in the 375 to 500 kHz range. The technique for thermal ablation in the liver by using RFA was first described in animal liver models in 1990[149,150] and was later reported in a patient in 1995.[151]

In this technique, the RF electrode is placed into the tumor with imaging guidance. The electrode is coupled to an RF generator and is grounded by means of a grounding pad or pads applied to the thighs. The RF generator produces a voltage between the active electrode (applicator) and the reference electrode (grounding pad), establishing electric field lines that oscillate with the alternating current. This oscillating electric field causes electron collisions with the adjacent molecules closest to the applicator, inducing frictional heating.[152] Tissue heating to temperatures greater than 60°C leads to immediate cell death. Thus, for any given RFA procedure, the application of energy from the applicator is maximized to create a zone of tissue necrosis that encompasses the tumor and a margin of normal parenchyma.[153] The volume of ablation achieved is based

on the energy balance between heat conduction of the local RF energy applied and heat convection from the circulating blood and extracellular fluid.

In the United States, there are three commercially available percutaneous RFA systems (Fig. 52.3). Two of the systems (Boston Scientific/RadioTherapeutics and RITA Medical Systems) use a deployable RF array electrode that consists of 4 to 16 small wires (tines) deployed through a 14- to 17-G needle. Because the tines of the Boston Scientific device (LeVeen electrode) curve back toward the handle (see Fig. 52.3), the array is initially deployed in the deep portion of the tumor. In contrast, the RITA electrode tines course forward and laterally so the probe is deployed on the near surface of the tumor. The LeVeen electrode measures impedance only, and treatment time depends on repeated increases in impedance during active heating, which is a measure of tissue desiccation indicative of adequate thermocoagulation. With the RITA system, temperature readings are obtained throughout the ablation cycle from multiple peripheral thermocouples. The RITA system also has perfusion electrodes (see Fig. 52.3) that introduce small amounts of saline into the tissue to enhance the distribution of tissue heating. The third RF system (Cool-tip; Covidien) utilizes a single or triple "cluster" perfusion electrode (three single electrodes spaced 5 mm apart; see Fig. 52.3), the tip of which is positioned in the deepest part of the tumor.

Cold saline or water is pumped internally within the shaft of the electrode to keep its tip cooler than the adjacent heated tissue, thus reducing charring, which in turn helps the thermal conduction to occur at a greater distance from its source. The single or cluster RF electrode contains a thermocouple embedded in its tip, which is used to measure intratumoral temperature. A switching controller can be used with the Covidien system, allowing the placement of up to three separate single electrodes spaced 1.5 to

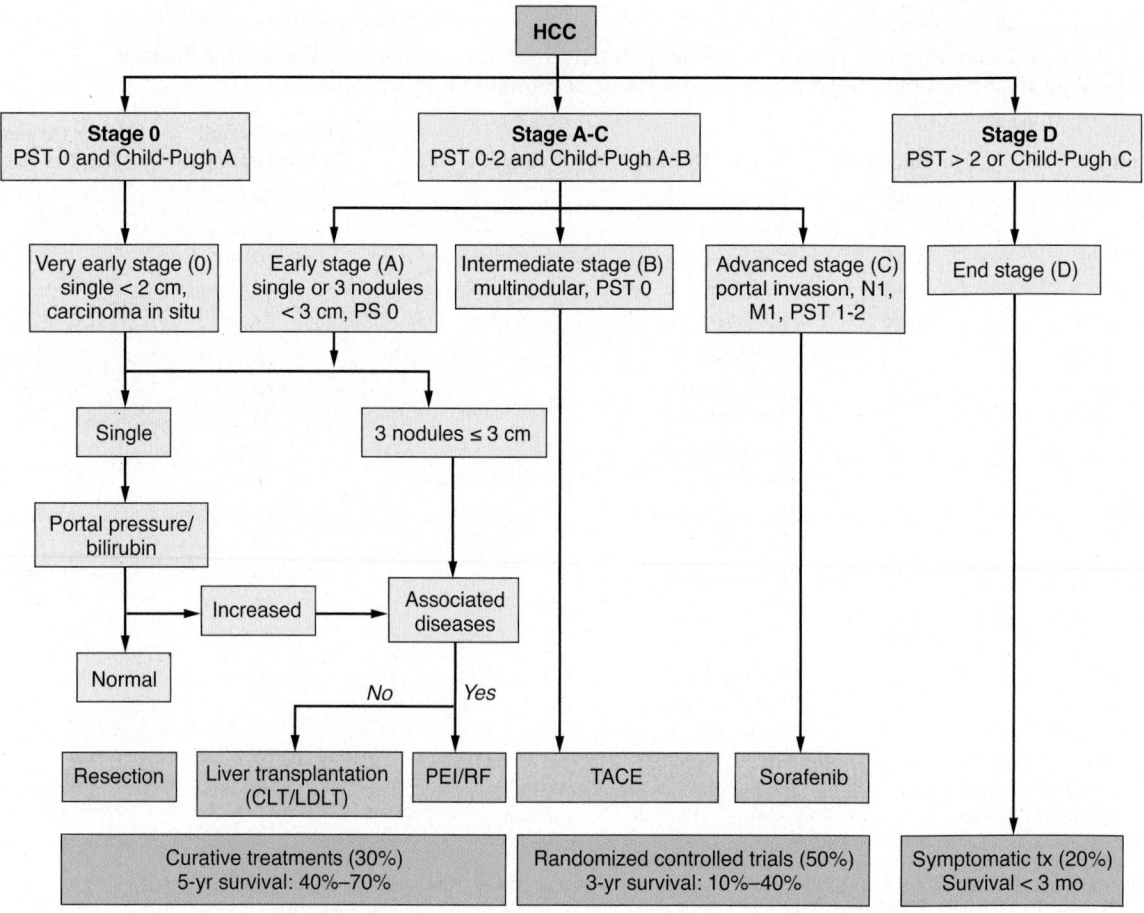

Figure 52.2 Strategy for staging and treatment assignment for patients with HCC according to the BCLC staging system. PST, performance status; CLT, cadaveric liver transplantation; tx, treatment.

2.5 cm apart, thus increasing the duty cycle of the generator to enable the creation of a greater volume of tissue thermocoagulation in a single application, as compared with three separate ablations that might be required with a single electrode. Most of the thermal ablation data regarding the treatment of liver tumors has been reported with RFA.[154–156]

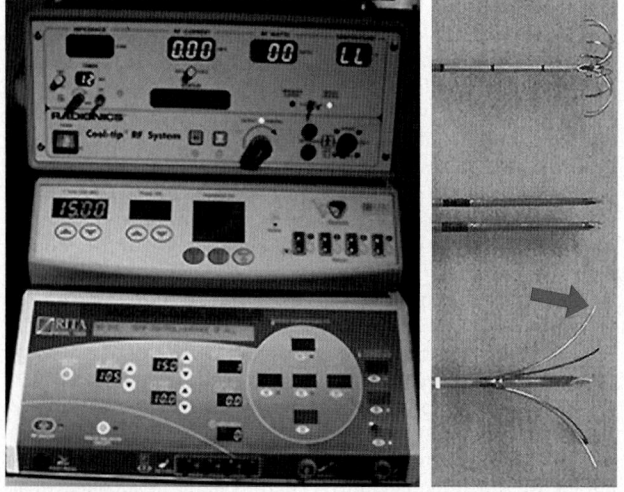

Figure 52.3 Radiofrequency ablation equipment currently available in the United States. The three most popular generators *(left)* and needle designs *(right)* are shown.

Microwave Ablation

Like RFA, microwave ablation (MWA) uses electromagnetic waves to produce heating. Unlike RFA, the MW energy is not an electrical current and is in a much higher frequency range that extends from 300 MHz to 300 GHz. The broader deposition of MW energy creates a much larger zone of active heating. MW applicators available for clinical use generally operate in the 900 to 2,450 MHz range.[157] Microwave tissue heating occurs because of the induction of kinetic energy in surrounding water molecules. Because of their electron configuration, water molecules have highly polar properties and function as small electric dipoles, with the negative charges preferentially localized around the oxygen nucleus. The rapidly alternating electric field of the MW antenna causes water molecules to spin rapidly in an attempt to align with electromagnetic charges of opposite polarity. These spinning water molecules interact with neighboring tissues, transferring a portion of their kinetic energy. Because temperature is merely a proxy measurement of molecular kinetic energy, this energy transfer results in local tissue hyperthermia.

Currently, there are six MWA systems that are commercially available in the United States and Europe.[158] These systems use either a 915-MHz generator (Evident, Covidien; MicrothermX, BSD Medical, Salt Lake City, UT; Avecure, MedWaves, San Diego, CA) or a 2,450-MHz generator (Certus 140, NeuWave Medical, Madison, WI; Amica, Hospital Service, Rome, Italy; Acculis MTA, Microsulis Medical, Hampshire, England) and straight antennae with varying active tips 0.6 to 4.0 cm in length. Perfusion of the antenna shaft is required for five of the six systems, with either room-temperature fluid or carbon dioxide to reduce conductive heating of the nonactive portion of the antenna, thus preventing damage to the skin and tissues proximal to the active tip. A single applicator is used with a single generator in four of the systems. Two have the ability to power up to three antennae with a single generator and treat large tumors (Fig. 52.4). Because most of the microwave systems have only recently received U.S. Food and Drug Administration approval, there are no published data at this time on the differences between systems in clinical safety or effectiveness. Similar safety and efficacy results for the treatment of metastatic colorectal liver metastases have been reported.[159] Perceived advantages of MW over RF energy include a greater heating profile and less severe heat sink effects.[160] Less heat sink effects may reduce local recurrences, and the larger resultant ablative volume when using the synergistic effect of multiple applicators simultaneously will allow a faster treatment time when compared to RFA.[161,162] Large trials evaluating safety show a similar safety profile compared with RF.[163] In Asia, MWA technology has been used for the treatment of liver tumors for a long period of time, and their extensive experience has created the development of appropriate treatment guidelines.[163]

Outcomes of Ablations

To date, the literature is replete with retrospective, single and multicenter cohorts with very few randomized controlled or cooperative group trials evaluating the benefits of liver ablation.

Regardless, many institutions around the world perform liver ablation for primary and metastatic liver tumors given its relative safety, low cost, and low toxicity. Many factors affect the success of thermal ablation treatment for liver malignancies, some of which include: tumor size, proximity to blood vessels, operator experience, the presence of underlying liver disease, extrahepatic disease in patients with secondary liver malignancies, overall patient health, and implementation alongside synergistic therapies in a collegial, multidisciplinary treatment clinic. The ever present argument for surgery as first-line treatment in these patients would be to properly stage the patient because preoperative imaging can underestimate the extent of liver and extrahepatic disease.[164] Of course, not all patients are fit for surgery, and ablation is an attractive minimally invasive option for older and frailer patients. Tumors adjacent to larger (>3 mm) blood vessels may be undertreated due to the thermal sink effect.[165] Proper device selection to effectively eradicate tumors adjacent to vessels should be improved, in theory, with hotter energy sources such as MWA compared to RFA.[166] A novel, largely, nonthermal electrical ablation technology called irreversible electroporation that is purported to be unaffected by thermal sink effects may play a role in treating tumors adjacent to blood vessels and critical structures, but there are no mature data at this time.[167]

With a myriad of thermal ablation devices available to hepatic surgeons, hepatologists, and interventional radiologists, studies

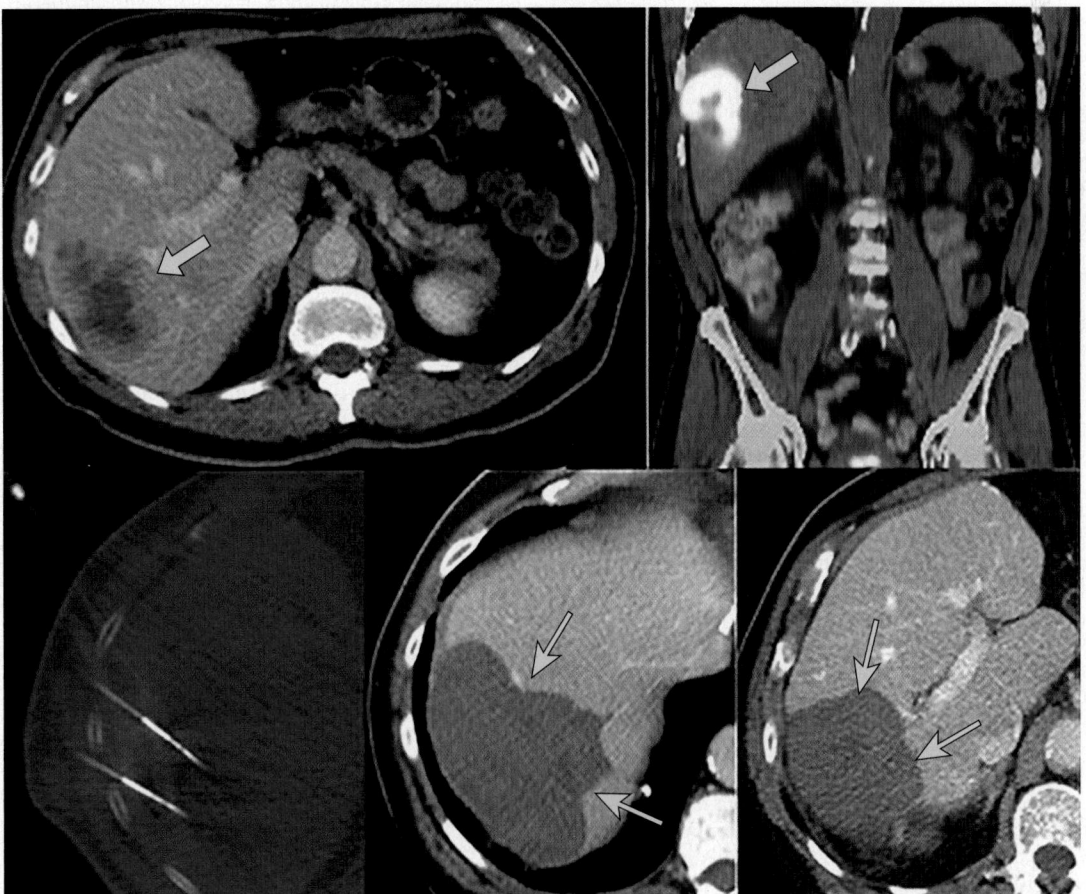

Figure 52.4 A 73-year-old man with previously resected colorectal metastatic disease in the left lobe of the liver who recurred in the right lobe despite 5-flourouracil, oxaliplatin, leukovorin (FOLFOX) chemotherapy. An axial contrast enhanced CT scan and coronal fludeoxyglucose–positron-emission tomography (FDG-PET) CT scan *(top panel)* show a large heterogeneous colorectal cancer (CRC) metastasis in the right lobe. The patient refused additional chemotherapy and ablation was offered as palliative therapy. Given the size of the mass, microwave ablation was performed with multiple antennas under CT guidance *(bottom left)*. The patient responded to the treatment extremely well, and a current 20-month follow-up contrast enhanced CT scan *(bottom right)* shows a large coagulation defect *(small arrows)* without evidence of recurrence in the liver.

have shown that it is incumbent upon these operators to gain experience with a particular device before optimal results can be expected.[164,168] This can be difficult not only in low patient volume ablation practices, but also in general given the rapid technologic changes that occur in this arena whereby a newer technology is perceived to be an improvement over an existing technology prior to rigorous scientific study. The presence of underlying cirrhosis will affect treatment options and outcomes in patients presenting with HCC. In general, HCC patients with Child-Pugh class C cirrhosis who are not on a liver transplant list and do not undergo liver-directed therapies have a median survival of less than 4 months. Therefore, treatment with thermal ablation is unlikely going to affect long-term survival.[169] In patients with Child-Pugh class A cirrhosis, data suggest thermal ablation can rival surgery when tumors are solitary and smaller (<5 cm) and less in number (< three tumors each under 3 cm).[170] However, for patients who are healthier with a normal performance status, surgical resection may provide better long-term survival compared to RFA.[171] It makes clinical sense that in patients with limited extrahepatic disease, liver-directed therapy could improve outcomes, although the outcomes themselves may be as much due to underlying tumor biology and not necessarily the treatment.[154,155] Given the complexity of any given patient with hepatic malignancy, it is important to first and foremost apply any treatment or treatments under the supervision of a team of experts whose primary goal is to provide the most cost-effective, comprehensive treatment based on evidenced-based medicine when available alongside patient centered outcomes.

Liver Resection Versus Ablative Therapy for Hepatocellular Carcinoma

With recent improvements in imaging that allows for the early diagnosis of cancer and facile guidance for interventional therapies, ablative modalities such as RFA are increasingly accepted as effective treatment for small tumors. Ablative techniques are less invasive and have the promise of being better tolerated than resections or transplantation. In retrospective studies, data suggest that for small HCCs (≤2 to 3 cm), RFAs result in similar outcomes as resections.[172–174]

Recently, four randomized trials comparing RFA and hepatic resection have been reported (Table 52.8).[175–178] Two of them, Chen et al. and Huang et al., compared tumors fulfilling the Milan tumor criteria for transplantation. Chen et al.[175] compared resection to RFA for tumors less than 5 cm in size. The 1-, 3- and 4-year survivals were 93%, 73% and 64%, respectively, for resection, and 96%, 71%, and 68%, respectively, for RFA. The authors concluded that RFA was as effective as surgical resection in the treatment of solitary HCCs ≤5 cm in terms of overall and disease-free survival after 4 years with no significant difference in outcome between the two groups on follow-up. Huang et al.[177] concluded that surgical resections have better outcomes than RFAs. This conclusion was based on a recurrence rate at 5 years of 63% in the RFA group and 41% in the resection group. However, it must be pointed out that more patients in the resected group had tumors less than 3 cm in size. In addition, the overall survival was not statistically different between the two treatment groups.

Feng et al.[178] and Liang et al.[176] confirmed the similar efficacy of RFA to resection in tumors <4 cm. Both groups found RFA and resection to have similar overall survival in a follow-up period after 3 years. It appears that for small HCCs, particularly in patients with cirrhosis, RFA can produce similar cancer outcomes with much lower morbidity. Figure 52.5 illustrates a recommended algorithm of care for small HCCs.

Embolic Therapies for Regional Disease

For patients with multifocal liver-predominant disease who are not candidates for resection or transplantation, transcatheter ablative methods have emerged as the most commonly used treatment worldwide. These techniques rely on the dual blood supply of the liver: arterial and portal venous. The portal vein provides over 75% of the blood flow to the hepatic parenchyma, whereas the hepatic artery is the primary nutrient supply of tumors. Selectively delivering agents transarterially targets the tumor while sparing the liver.

There are currently three main categories of percutaneously administered transcatheter intra-arterial therapies: TACE, bland hepatic artery embolization (HAE), and radioembolization (RAE). The usual chemotherapeutic agents used are mitomycin C, doxorubicin, and aclarubicin. The majority of the effects of embolic therapies derive from tumor ischemia produced by occlusion of the arterial vessels. Thus, bland embolizations (without chemotherapy), even with a nonpermanent agent such as Gelfoam, can produce a high likelihood of tumor killing. RAE involves the administration of yttrium-90 (a pure β emitter) that can be loaded in glass or resin microspheres intra-arterially.[179] This is really not an embolization, in that the goal is not occlusion of the arterial inflow, but more brachytherapy. RAE will be further discussed.

Patient Selection

Performance status, underlying liver disease, and degree of portal hypertension are important patient selection criteria. Although minimally invasive, following embolization, patients commonly experience a postembolization syndrome of pain, fever, and nausea that may last for several days to a few weeks. It often takes 4 to 6 weeks to recover to baseline performance status.

Although embolization in patients with normal liver, or well-compensated cirrhosis, has a low risk of liver failure, the risk of further compromising liver function and hastening death in poorly compensated cirrhosis is significant. This is because a basis of TACE is that the portal blood flow will protect the noncancerous liver from the treatment agents and ischemia. Thus, portal vein occlusion is considered a contraindication to both TACE[180] and HAE because of the risk of liver failure. Ascites, which is an indication of severe portal hypertension, or measured reversal of portal blood flow is a relative contraindication.

Results of Treatment

It has always been apparent that embolic therapies can result in a high rate of tumor response (>50%). Excellent results (level IIa evidence) following chemoembolization have also been reported from Japan in 8510 patients treated between 1994 and 2001, with 1-, 3-, and 5-year survival of 82%, 47%, and 26%, respectively.[29] With well-designed trials, there is also now level I evidence of a survival benefit to conventional TACE as demonstrated in randomized trials published by Llovett et al.,[181] Lo et al.,[182] and Becker et al.[183] In the trial by Lo et al.,[182] patients were randomized to TACE (cisplatin + Lipiodol + Gelfoam) versus control (no treatment). The 2-year survival was 31% for TACE versus 11% for controls. In the trial by Llovet et al.,[181] patients randomized to TACE (doxorubicin + Lipiodol + Gelfoam) had a 2-year survival of 63% versus 27% for control. In the study from Becker et al.,[183] TACE (mitomycin C [MMC] + Lipiodol + Gelfoam) + PEI resulted in a 39% 2-year survival compared to 18% for TACE. What seems clear from these data is that arterial embolotherapy is an effective method of treating HCC and can prolong the patient's survival. Comparable, or better, survival results have been demonstrated with bland embolization.[119]

Radiation Therapy for Hepatocellular Carcinoma

Radiation therapy for liver tumors was historically limited by hepatic toxicity but, with improved imaging, treatment planning, and treatment delivery, it now is an excellent option, particularly for patients with unresectable tumors or who are medical inoperable.

TABLE 52.8

Randomized Controlled Trials of Hepatic Resection Versus RF Ablations for HCC Reported After 2000

Author/Year Country	Treatment	Number	Age	Tumor Number	Characteristics Diameter	Disease-Free Survival (%)				Overall Survival (%)				p
						1 Year	3 Years	4 Years	5 Years	1 Year	3 Years	4 Years	5 Years	
Chen (2006)[175]	RES	90	49±11	1	≤5 cm	87	69	46	—	93	73	64	—	NS
	RFA	71	52±11	1	≤5 cm	86	64	52	—	96	71	68	—	
Liang (2008)[176a]	RES	44	49±12	≤3	≤5 cm	—	—	—	—	79	45	31	28	0.8
	RFA	66	55±11	≤3	≤5 cm	—	—	—	—	77	49	40	40	
Huang (2010)[177]	RES	115	56 ±13	≤3	≤5 cm (77%)	85	61	—	51	98	92	76	76	NS
	RFA	115	57 ±14	≤3	≤5 cm (73%)	82	46	—	29	87	70	—	55	
Feng (2012)[178]	RES	84	47(18–76)	≤2	≤4 cm	91	61	—	—	96	75	—	—	0.3
	RFA	84	51(24–83)	≤2	≤4 cm	86	50	—	—	93	67	—	—	

[a]Treatments for recurrent disease.

RES, resected patients; DFS, disease-free survival; OS, overall survival; NS, not significant.

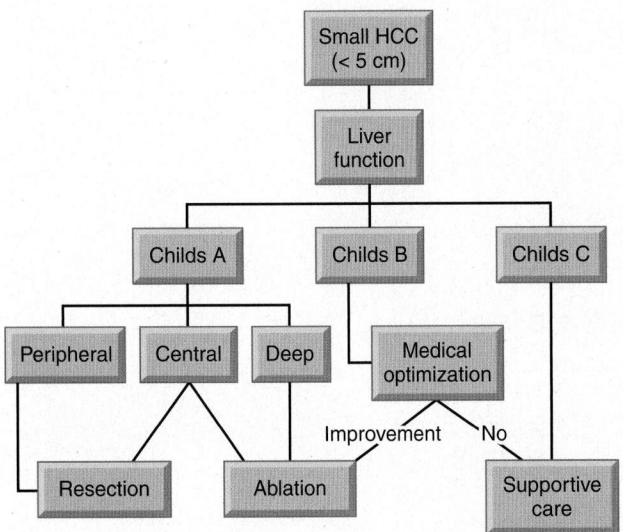

Figure 52.5 The treatment algorithm for a small HCC.

Tumors not likely to be effectively treated by radiofrequency ablation due to size over 3 cm or proximity to the diaphragm, large vessel, or gallbladder are also good candidates for RT. With proper care, tumors near gastrointestinal (GI) structures can also be treated. Side effects are typically minimal, and commonly include mild fatigue, and less commonly include nausea, mild radiation dermatitis, pain associated with tumor edema, or worsening liver dysfunction. Radiation can be delivered using external beam or brachytherapy. Patients with metastases to the bone, brain, adrenals, or other locations can be effectively palliated with RT, as can patients with pain from large primary tumors.[184]

External Beam Radiotherapy

Fractionated Treatment

Because the liver is one of the most radiosensitive organs in the body, treatment planning and delivery must be done carefully to maximize dose to the tumor and to minimize dose to the normal liver. The primary toxicity of concern is radiation-induced liver disease (RILD), which can be categorized as classic and nonclassic. Classic RILD is a constellation of anicteric ascites, hepatomegaly, and elevated liver enzymes (particularly alkaline phosphatase), which typically occurs within 4 months of therapy and is a type of veno-occlusive disease, similar to that which can be seen after high-dose chemotherapy conditioning for bone marrow transplantation.[185] Nonclassic RILD, a recently coined classification, can occur in patients with hepatitis and cirrhosis, and is characterized by jaundice and markedly elevated serum transaminases (>5 times the upper limit of normal) within 3 months of completion of therapy. This is thought to represent direct hepatocyte rather than endothelial injury.[186] RILD is typically self-limited, but can be serious, even leading to mortality. It is managed symptomatically, using diuretics and paracentesis. Even low doses to the whole liver of 25 Gy in 10 fractions or 32 Gy in 1.5 Gy per fraction twice daily are associated with a more than 5% risk of radiation-induced liver disease, particularly for patients with cirrhosis and already compromised liver function. Other toxicities that can occur include gastric or duodenal bleeding,[187] although both of these risks can be minimized using careful treatment planning, image guidance, and treatment delivery. It is important to consider factors including cirrhosis, prior liver-directed therapies, and hepatitis B and C, which add to the dose and volume models for the prediction of RILD. ICG is also used in Asia as a pretreatment assessment for the safety

of RT, similar to its use for the safety of liver resection.[188,189] In the United States, the University of Michigan has pioneered its use to measure individual tolerance to radiation, which can be quite variable. Even some patients with good pretreatment liver function can experience rapid decline, so customizing treatment is crucial.[190]

At the University of Michigan, investigators created the normal-tissue complication probability (NTCP) model that quantitatively described the relationship between radiation dose and liver volumes and the probability of developing RILD.[191] Dose was customized per patient to give an anticipated risk of 5% to 15%. Due to the variety of tumor and liver sizes and geometries, prescribed doses ranged from 40 to 90 Gy. Patients who received 75 Gy or more had a higher median survival of 24 versus 15 months. Progression-free survival was also improved with higher doses.[192–195] A prospective phase II trial from France treated patients to 66 Gy in 2 Gy fractions, with a response rate of 92%.[196] The largest published experiences are from Asia, which has a very high incidence of HCC. In a multicenter retrospective patterns-of-care study among 10 institutions in Korea, 398 patients with HCC were described. Of those, 70% were Child class A, 54% had tumors >5 cm, and 40% had portal vein thrombosis. Nearly all had received prior treatment, mostly TACE. In this series, higher dose (biologic effective dose over 53 Gy) also correlated with better survival.[197] Other groups have combined TACE and RT, with various schedules, although mostly using RT to treat residual disease. In a Korean study of 73 patients with incomplete response to TACE, 38 received RT, whereas the rest received additional TACE. Patients who received radiation had a higher 2-year survival of 37% versus 14% (p = 0.001).[198,199]

Another use for RT is to treat tumor thrombus in the portal vein, with the goals of decreasing portal pressure and allowing the safe delivery of embolic therapies. The largest series from Taiwan reports a 25% response rate. Compared with a dismal 1-year survival of 9% for nonresponders, responders had a better survival of 21% for those still not eligible for definitive therapies, and 29% for those who ultimately had additional therapy.[200]

Other crucial components of a liver RT program not always available for standard RT include adequate imaging with arterial and portal venous phase imaging with CT scans and MRI for tumor delineation, motion assessment, and management tools four-dimensional computed tomography (4D-CT) scan, treatment gating), and precise image guidance (cone beam CT scan) on the treatment machine. Because liver tumors move with respiration, accurate assessment and management of this will aid in proper tumor targeting and normal tissue avoidance. Some common methods include forced breath hold for tumor immobilization and 4D-CT scans to assess and help account for motion.[201,202] Fiducials can also be placed within or near the tumor percutaneously prior to treatment planning, with daily alignment on the treatment machine, because external anatomy is a poor surrogate for internal anatomy and tumor location.

Stereotactic Body Radiotherapy

Stereotactic body radiotherapy (SBRT) is a relatively new method of delivering high-dose, high-precision therapy in just a few treatments, rather than spread out daily over a course of several weeks. With high doses per fraction, the biologic effect is much more than with the same total dose delivered in a standard fractionated course, up to the equivalent to 80 to 150 Gy in 2-Gy fractions (see Fig. 52.5). This technique was pioneered by Blomgren et al.,[203] who treated 20 liver tumors, including 8 HCCs in the 1990s. Since then, the literature has mostly been populated by small retrospective studies. A few prospective studies have been quite informative. Mendez-Romero et al.[204] initially started treating patients with a schedule of 25 Gy in five fractions, but after two patients experienced local failure, the dose was raised to 30 Gy in three fractions for the rest of the study. The 1-year local control was 75%, with all failures in the low-dose group. One Child-Pugh class B patient experienced grade 5 nonclassic RILD, leading the authors to advise others to be very cautious with similar patients.[204] The next and largest studies were a phase I and II trial from Princess Margaret Hospital.[205,206] Of 41 initial patients, 31 had HCC. Patients were treated with a six-fraction course of SBRT delivered over 2 weeks, with the dose individualized based on the University of Michigan NTCP model, escalated from 5% to 20%. The median dose was 36 Gy (range, 24 to 54 Gy) and the median tumor volume was 173 mL (range, 9 to 1,913 mL). Even for these relatively large tumors, approximately 50% had a response to treatment, and 42% had stable disease. Median survival was 12 months. No patients developed classic RILD, although 26% had grade 3 elevation of liver enzymes and 16% had a decline from Child class A to B within 3 months after treatment. Recently, the results from the full 102 patients from both the phase I and II portions of the trial were reported.[206] Of the patients, 93% had underlying liver disease, 52% had received prior therapy, and 55% had tumor vascular thrombosis. The 1-year local control was excellent, at 87%. However, 30% of patients had grade 3 or higher toxicity, some of which possibly contributed to mortality. This illustrates the tenuous balance between treatment safety and efficacy and the need for improved predictive models of safety for individual patients.

Another phase I study reported 100% local control after 36 to 48 Gy in three to five fractions. Similar to what was seen in the Mendez-Romero study, patients with Child-Pugh class B liver failure were prone to liver toxicity.[207] Truly, these patients need extra attention and consideration. Many larger retrospective studies have confirmed these smaller prospective results.[208–210]

Charged particles, including protons and carbon ions, are being investigated for treatment of HCC. These have the advantage of lower entrance and minimal exit dose, due to a difference in dose deposition properties. In a Japanese retrospective review, 162 patients were treated with 72 Gy in 16 fractions using protons with a 5-year local control and survival of 87% and 24%, respectively. There were no grade 3 or higher toxicities.[211] In a phase II proton study, 51 patients received 66 Gy in 10 fractions. The 5-year local control and survival rates were 88% and 39%, respectively. There were no cases of RILD, although 26% had a decline in liver function.[212] Currently, carbon-ion therapy is only available in a few centers worldwide. In Japan, 24 patients were treated on a phase I/II dose-escalation study. Twenty-four patients received from 50 to 80 Gy in 15 fractions, with local control and survival similar to other reports, at 81% and 25%, respectively.[213] Despite the technologic imperative that newer is better, charged particles are not the miracle treatment some may assume. The high-dose treatment region cannot be shaped as conformally as with standard photon radiotherapy (SBRT and intensity modulated radiotherapy [IMRT]), and image guidance is currently rudimentary, therefore, ensuring the accuracy of treatment is difficult. However, because the liver is extremely sensitive to radiation, reducing the moderate and low-dose regions could potentially aid in protecting the normal liver and allowing for escalation of tumor dose. The next few years should yield exciting developments.

Brachytherapy

In contrast to other tumor sites such as prostate, gynecologic, and breast, liver brachytherapy typically involves an injection of a radioisotope for regional therapy, rather than interstitial or intracavitary therapy, although small experiences in interstitial therapy have been reported.[214,215] Radioembolization, like chemoembolization, takes advantage of the liver's dual blood supply and the arterial enhancement of HCC. Rather than chemotherapy and embolic material, radioisotopes linked to either glass (TheraSphere, Nordion, Canada) or resin (SIRTeX Medical, Inc., Lane Cove, New South Wales, Australia) microspheres are injected into the hepatic artery (HA). This outpatient treatment is typically delivered through

either the right or the left HA, although with favorable anatomy, it can be delivered more selectively. Whole liver treatment is usually reserved for metastases rather than HCC due to the risk of liver injury. The most common isotope is yttrium-90, a pure beta emitter, with an effective path length of 5 mm and a half-life of 65 hours. Ninety percent of the energy is deposited within 5 mm of the sphere, therefore, side effects are quite localized. The dose to the individual tumors is not well characterized, but is prescribed to 80 to 150 Gy, depending on liver function, to the entire treated portion of the liver, assuming equal distribution and based on pretreatment angiography. Side effects are typically quite tolerable and consist of mild nausea, pain, and fatigue. Rare complications could include hepatobiliary dysfunction, radiation pneumonitis, and GI ulceration. Risk factors associated with early mortality include an infiltrative tumor, a tumor encompassing over 50% to 70% of the liver, albumin <3 g/dL, bilirubin >2 mg/dL, and lung dose >30 Gy.[216] With proper patient selection, this procedure is relatively safe. Although both RAE and chemoembolization can deliver regional therapy, which is particularly useful for multifocal HCC, it is currently unclear which treatment may be preferred for which patients. No randomized trials comparing these two modalities have been completed; however, a retrospective comparison suggests that RAE may have a longer time to progression with reduced toxicity and similar overall survival.[179] In general, response rates are 30% to 50%, with a time to progression of 6 to 16 months depending on stage and portal vein thrombus.[217,218] Treatment may be repeated.[219]

Toxicities

RT is typically very well tolerated. Mild fatigue can be attributed both to the treatment itself and to the travel related to multiple appointments for the treatment. Mild nausea can be prevented by premedicating with an antiemetic. Radiation dermatitis is highly unusual due to the extremely conformal distribution of radiation dose. Occasionally, the treatment of large tumors can cause a pain flare due to local edema. These acute effects typically resolve within a few weeks after treatment. Late effects could include RILD, as discussed previously, in addition to GI ulceration and renal dysfunction, although these risks can be avoided by minimizing the dose to these structures to below acceptable levels.[187]

Systemic Therapy for Hepatocellular Carcinoma

First-Line Single-Agent Therapies

A large number of controlled and uncontrolled clinical studies have been performed with most of the major classes of cancer chemotherapy, given intravenously as single agent or in combination. However, these systemic therapies, and other chemotherapy combinations studied, have had no proven benefits on survival in HCC.[220] Many other nonchemotherapeutic agents have also been tried without definitive success, including luteinizing hormone-releasing hormone agonists, tamoxifen, IFN, Sandostatin, megestrol, vitamin K, thalidomide, interleukin-2, ^{131}I-lipiodol, and ^{131}I-ferritin.

Given the vascular nature of HCC and that vascular endothelial growth factor (VEGF) promotes HCC development and metastasis, antiangiogenic agents have been studied extensively in the setting of advanced HCC. Increased levels of VEGF have been observed and have been associated with inferior survival.[221]

Sorafenib a multi–tyrosine kinase inhibitor with antiangiogenic effects are thought to be mediated by the blockade of VEGFR-2/-3, platelet-derived growth factor receptor (PDGFR)-β, and other receptor tyrosine kinases.[222] The clinical efficacy of sorafenib in HCC was first reported in a multicenter phase II study of 137 patients with systemic treatment-naïve, inoperable HCC and varying hepatic reserve (72% Child-Pugh class A, 28% Child-Pugh class B) received the agent, with a primary end point of evaluating response by World Health Organization (WHO) criteria.[223] Although only

2.2% of the study population achieved a confirmed objective response by WHO criteria, 42% of the study population had extended disease control. There was a median overall survival of 9.2 months, which was encouraging when compared to historical controls. Subsequently, the Sorafenib Hepatocellular Carcinoma Assessment Randomized Protocol (SHARP) trial enrolled 602 patients with advanced HCC, Child-Pugh class A, and who had not received prior systemic therapy.[224] The majority of the study population was recruited from the Western Hemisphere. Patients were randomly assigned to receive sorafenib at 400 mg orally twice a day (N = 299) or best supportive care (N = 303). The coprimary end points of the study were overall survival and time to symptomatic progression. Median overall survival was 10.7 months in the sorafenib arm versus 7.9 months in the placebo arm (hazard ratio [HR] = 0.69; 95% confidence interval [CI], 0.55 to 0.87). A predefined subset analysis indicated that the survival benefit of sorafenib was independent of performance status and disease burden.

Parallel to the SHARP trial, the Asia-Pacific study assessed the efficacy and tolerability of sorafenib in comparison with best supportive care in the patients with advanced HCC geographically localized to Asia.[225] As expected and in contrast to the SHARP trial, the Asia-Pacific study was enriched with patients with HBV-related HCC (73% of the total study population). The trial confirmed that sorafenib, when compared to best supportive care, was tolerable and led to a statistically significant improvement in disease control, time to radiographic progression, and overall survival. However, the magnitude of the overall survival benefit on the Asia-Pacific study was not as substantial as observed on the SHARP study—the median overall survival was only 6.5 and 4.2 months for patients receiving sorafenib and placebo, respectively. The inclusion of patients who were more ill prior to beginning therapy than those patients on the SHARP study might explain this difference. Another postulate is that the observed differential outcomes on the two trials were due to differing treatment patterns between Asia and Western countries. Intense local–regional therapies might be more common in Asia, thus leading to the selection of patients on the Asia-Pacific study who are presenting later in the course of their disease. The inclusion criteria for the Asia-Pacific study, however, do not necessarily support this assertion. Alternatively, specific viral etiologic factors might affect prognosis and influence the responsiveness of liver cancer to sorafenib.

In an unplanned subset analysis of the SHARP study, patients with HBV-related HCC who were treated with sorafenib had a modest prolongation in median overall survival over placebo (9.7 versus 6.1 months).[226] However, HCV-related HCC patients treated with sorafenib appeared to derive a more substantial survival improvement over placebo (14.0 versus 7.4 months). A retrospective analysis of the initial phase II study of sorafenib observed similar etiologic-dependent trends in survival. Patients who were infected with HCV lived longer (N = 13, 12.4 months) than did patients infected with HBV (N = 33, 7.3 months; p = 0.29). The recently reported phase III study of first-line sunitinib indicates that there may in fact be differential outcomes relative to disease cause and ethnic origin, with median overall survival for HCV-associated HCC ranging from 18.3 months for patients with living outside of Asia to 7.9 months for patients living in Asia.[227] Etiologic-dependent genomic differences in HCC might explain improved outcomes to sorafenib in patients with HCV-related HCC. *CTNNB1* mutations are more commonly observed in HCV-related HCC but not in HBV-related HCC and are associated with a specific WNT gene expression profile.[228] Sorafenib can modulate this gene signature, interfere with WNT signaling output, and lead to HCC growth suppression in preclinical models. Etiologic-dependent differences in outcome might also be explained by HCV core protein-induced upregulation of the sorafenib target CRAF, among other kinases.[229] Finally, in vitro data suggest that sorafenib can directly inhibit HCV viral replication, although the clinical importance of this observation is debatable.[230] Although more exploration is certainly required, it should be emphasized that the utility of sorafenib

is not undercut by this observation, and it remains an effective and life prolonging therapy for HCC, irrespective of etiologic factor.

Several other small receptor tyrosine kinase inhibitors have been studied. Thus far, emerging results have been disappointing with the major phase III studies of antiangiogenic therapy failing to improve upon sorafenib in the first-line setting. Sunitinib, an inhibitor of vascular endothelial growth factor receptor (VEGFR)-1/-2 with greater potency than sorafenib, plus an inhibitor of PDGFR-α/β, c-KIT, FLT3, RET, and other kinases, has been studied in three phase II studies with three different dosing schedules of the agent as a treatment for advanced HCC.[231–233] A subsequent randomized phase III study of sunitinib, dosed continuously, versus sorafenib in patients with advanced HCC and Child Pugh class A liver function was initiated and rapidly enrolled 530 patients on the sunitinib arm and 544 on the sorafenib arm.[227] The study, powered to test the dual hypotheses of noninferiority and superiority with regard to overall survival, was halted by an independent data monitoring committee due to futility and safety concerns. The median overall survival for the sunitinib arm was 7.9 versus 10.2 months for the sorafenib arm (HR, 1.30; one-sided p = 0.9990; two-sided p = 0.0014).

Brivanib, a dual inhibitor of VEGFR and fibroblast growth factor receptor (FGFR), demonstrated modest antitumor activity in both treatment-naïve and in those patients who had failed prior antiangiogenic therapy in two separate phase II studies.[234,235] Based on these data, a large randomized phase III study compared brivanib to sorafenib in patients with systemic treatment-naïve, advanced HCC.[236] This noninferiority trial did not meet its primary end point; median overall survival with brivanib treatment was 9.5 months versus 9.9 months with sorafenib (HR, 1.06; 95% CI, 0.93 to 1.22; p = 0.3730).

Linifanib, a selective inhibitor of VEGFR and PDGFR, also failed to improve upon the modest survival advantage of sorafenib despite early encouraging efficacy data.[237] A large multicenter, randomized, phase III study of sorafenib versus linifanib as a first-line therapy for advanced HCC, failed to meet both prespecified end points of superiority and noninferiority. The median overall survival for linifanib was 9.1 months versus 9.8 months for sorafenib (HR = 1.046; 95%, CI 0.896 to 1.221).

Over 20 separate clinical trials have assessed or are assessing bevacizumab, a monoclonal antibody directed against VEGF, in patients with advanced HCC. Evaluated regimens include monotherapy and combination therapy with chemotherapy, targeted agents, and embolization procedures. In general, completed studies have reported higher response rates than those observed with other tyrosine kinase inhibitors; however, adverse events such as arterial/venous thrombotic events and variceal hemorrhage (some fatal) are more common. A phase II study in advanced HCC with extrahepatic disease found a 14% overall response rate with bevacizumab monotherapy.[238] It has not moved to later stage trials due to concerns regarding bleeding.

First-Line Combination Therapies

The addition of cytotoxic chemotherapy or targeted therapy to bevacizumab may augment antitumor activity. Response proportions with various cytotoxic combinations range from 9% to 20%, with disease control rates reportedly as high as 78%.[239–241] Bevacizumab and erlotinib may offer enhanced antitumor activity with a response rate of 24% and favorable patient outcomes with a median overall survival of 13.7 months.[242] A multicenter, randomized phase II trial of bevacizumab combined with erlotinib (Clinical Trial: NCT00881751) versus sorafenib monotherapy is ongoing. Similarly, the SEARCH trial confirmed that the addition of erlotinib to sorafenib provided no benefit in HCC. In this randomized, placebo-controlled, double-blind, phase III study the combination of sorafenib and erlotinib were compared to sorafenib alone in the first-line setting in 720 patients with advanced HCC. There was no statistically significant difference between study arms with regard to the primary end point of overall survival (combination 9.5 months, sorafenib 8.5 months; HR = 0.93; 95%, CI 0.78 to 1.11).

In the attempt to improve upon the modest results observed with sorafenib, investigators have proposed combination strategies with cytotoxic chemotherapy and novel biologic agents. Prior to the approval of sorafenib, doxorubicin was evaluated as monotherapy or in combination with sorafenib in a randomized, double-blind, phase II study.[243] The trial enrolled 96 patients with treatment-naïve advanced HCC and Child-Pugh class A liver function. The primary end point of the study was time to progression. In a planned exploratory analysis, both time to progression, as determined by independent review, and progression-free survival were increased by approximately 4 months, and the median overall survival doubled in favor of combined therapy (13.7 versus 6.5 months; p = 0.006). Cardiac toxicity was notable, with a higher proportion of patients on the combination experiencing left ventricular systolic dysfunction (19% versus 2%). Although the majority of such cases were asymptomatic, the median cumulative doxorubicin dose was limited to 165 mg/m^2. The dramatic increase in survival over placebo was striking; however, the lack of sorafenib as a comparator arm limits the interpretation of the trial. Doxorubicin may contribute little to outcome. The observed benefit in the doxorubicin–sorafenib group may be due to the effects of sorafenib alone. Alternatively, the combination may be synergistic. Inhibition of the mitogen-activated protein kinase (MAPK) pathway by sorafenib may restore chemosensitivity by enhancing proapoptotic pathways and dampening multidrug resistance (MDR) pathways. Anthracycline-induced cytotoxicity is mediated by the proapoptotic kinase ASK1.[244] Growth factor–induced MAPK activation, via FGF, has been shown to abrogate ASK1 activity. Blockade of the RAF kinases by sorafenib might, therefore, augment the antitumor activity of doxorubicin. Furthermore, MAPK activation leads to the induction of the MDR-1 pump.[245] Sorafenib decreases ATP-binding cassette/MDR protein gene expression, thereby restoring HCC sensitivity to doxorubicin in vitro.[246] A randomized phase III study of sorafenib versus sorafenib and doxorubicin in the first-line setting is currently underway (Clinical Trial: NCT01015833). A phase II study of doxorubicin plus sorafenib in second-line setting after sorafenib failure is currently underway (Clinical Trial: NCT01840592).

Gemcitabine and oxaliplatin (GEMOX) therapy has established efficacy in HCC,[247] and there is reason to believe that addition of sorafenib to gemcitabine might offer synergistic antitumor effects.[246] The GEMOX–sorafenib versus sorafenib was recently tested in a randomized phase II study (GONEXT).[248] The trial enrolled 95 patients with advanced HCC. The primary end point was 4-month progression-free survival of greater than or equal to 50%. The combination of GEMOX plus sorafenib resulted in a 4-month progression-free survival rate of 61% compared to 54% in the sorafenib monotherapy group. The combination was feasible, and efficacy data were encouraging (overall response rate [ORR] 16%, DCR 77%).

Second-Line Therapies

The interest in developing novel agents for advanced HCC and the positive outlook on improved outcome led to a rapidly evolving field studying second-line therapies, with already several phase III clinical trials reported, still on-going, or planned.

Overexpression of c-MET and its ligand hepatocyte growth factor (HGF) occur in up to 80% of human HCC tumors.[249] Transgenic mice that overexpress MET in hepatocytes developed HCC, and inactivation of this transgene leads to tumor regression, mediated by apoptosis and growth suppression.[250] Blocking MET with several different multitargeted tyrosine kinase inhibitors small molecules induce in vitro HCC growth suppression, cell-cycle arrest, and decreased viability as well as growth suppression and survival prolongation in vivo.[251] Based on these data, several MET inhibitors are already being studied in the setting of advanced HCC. Tivantinib, a selective MET receptor tyrosine kinase inhibitor, was

evaluated at two doses in a randomized, placebo-controlled phase II in advanced HCC patients who had progressed after first-line therapy.[252] This study reported a statistically significant difference in outcomes between high-MET expressing tumors in favor of tivantinib. For patients with high MET-expressing tumors (defined as ≥50% 3 to 4+ expression), tivantinib therapy resulted in a median time to progression of 2.7 months in comparisons to 1.4 months for placebo (HR, 0.43; 95% CI, 0.19 to 0.97) and a median overall survival of 7.2 months versus 3.8 months for placebo (HR, 0.38, 0.18 to 0.81). Importantly, no such differences between the agent and placebo were observed in low-MET expression tumors. This strongly suggests that MET expression is a predictive biomarker for MET-directed targeted therapy in HCC. Additionally, in patients on the placebo arm, high tumoral MET expression was associated with an improved overall survival when compared with low tumoral MET expression (3.8 months versus 9 months; HR, 2.94; 95% CI, 1.16 to 7.43). This observation indicates that MET expression may also be prognostic in this disease. Given these data, tivantinib is being compared with placebo in a double-blind, randomized phase III study in patients with advanced HCC and high-MET expressing tumors in the second-line setting (Clinical Trial: NCT01755767). Cabozantinib, an inhibitor of MET and VEGFR-2, has also shown promising efficacy data in a cohort of 41 patients with advanced HCC.[253] In 78% of patients, tumor regression was observed by Response Evaluation Criteria in Solid Tumors (RECIST) with a 5% confirmed partial response rate. Median progression-free survival for the cohort was estimated at 4.2 months, and median overall survival 15.1 months. A phase III study of cabozantinib versus placebo in patients with advanced HCC in the second-line setting is underway (Clinical Trial: NCT01908426). A different view on the biology of met inhibition differs between those two studies, where the tivantinib approach is to treat only patients with met-positive tumors defined as ≥50% 3 to 4+ expression, whereas the cabozantinib study will take all comers, arguing that it is not known yet how much met positivity is needed, if at all, considering the multikinase nature of both drugs.

The mammalian target of rapamycin (mTOR) pathway plays a critical role in hepatocarcinogenesis, and in xenograft mouse models, blockade of this pathway results in HCC growth suppression—but not regression or cellular apoptosis—and in lengthening of survival.[254] These observations, as well as retrospective data indicating enhanced survival among patients receiving sirolimus immunosuppression following liver transplantation for HCC, led to the development of a phase I/II study of everolimus established that 10 mg daily was a safe dose.[255] The phase II portion, a two-stage efficacy design, did not meet its prespecified boundary for expansion to the second stage. Of 25 evaluable patients, 1 (4%) had a partial response and 10 (40%) had stable disease. Median time to progression was 3.9 months and median overall survival was 8.4 months. Nonetheless, everolimus was investigated in the second-line setting after sorafenib failure in the phase III, randomized, placebo-controlled EVOLVE-1 study (Clinical Trial: NCT01035229) that was recently reported as negative.

A randomized phase III study of brivanib after progression of disease on sorafenib versus best supportive care also failed to meet its primary end point of improved overall survival.[256] Among 395 randomized patients, 87% had disease progression while on sorafenib, median overall survival was 9.4 months in the brivanib group versus 8.2 months in the placebo group (HR, 0.89; 95.8% CI, 0.69 to 1.15; p = 0.3307). This study's importance lies in defining what may be the true and current median survival of patients with advanced HCC, preserved liver function, and who have failed at least one prior line of therapy. The median survival of such population seems to be better than anticipated and may be reflective of the involvement of multidisciplines, ensuring better management of patients with advanced HCC. A selection bias, of course, could not be ruled out in the brivanib study as portal invasion and/or thrombosis was noted in 12% of placebo patients versus 25% on the brivanib arm.[256]

Ramucirumab, a monoclonal antibody blocking VEGFR-2, was recently assessed in a phase II study comprised of 43 patients with systemic treatment-naïve advanced HCC.[257] The median progression-free survival was 4 months and the median survival was 12 months. Based on these data, a randomized phase III study of ramucirumab versus best supportive care in the second-line setting is ongoing (Clinical Trial: NCT01140347).

The biosynthesis of the nonessential amino acid arginine occurs as part of the urea cycle and is dependent upon the enzymes argininosuccinate synthetase and argininosuccinate lyase. Messenger RNA encoding argininosuccinate synthetase is not present in subsets of hepatocellular carcinomas; therefore, arginine must be extracted from the circulation.[258] Pegylated arginine deiminase (ADI-PEG 20) is an arginine-degrading enzyme isolated from *Mycoplasma* that is formulated with polyethylene glycol (molecular weight: 20 kDa). In preclinical models, ADI-PEG 20 decreases HCC cell viability at low nanomolar concentrations, reduces serum arginine levels to undetectable levels, and prolongs survival in HCC xenograft mouse models. A phase I/II study demonstrated an excellent safety profile in a patient population comprised with a high burden of disease and impaired hepatic function.[259] The most common events were injection site reactions and isolated lab abnormalities, such as elevated fibrinogen. Of 19 patients evaluable, 2 (10.5%) had a complete response, 7 (36.8%) had a partial response, and 7 (36.8%) had stable disease. The duration of response ranged from 37 to more than 680 days. A subsequent study reported a disease control rate of 63.1%, a 2.6% objective response rate, and a median overall survival of 11.4 months.[260] This exclusively European patient population was composed predominantly of HCV-associated (79%) HCC confined to the liver (84%) with otherwise excellent hepatic function (81%). In contrast, Yang and colleagues[261] tested the agent in a heavily pretreated Asian population with HBV-associated (69%) extrahepatic (58%) hepatocellular carcinoma. In this study, no objective responses were noted and the median overall survival was 7.3 months. Currently, a double-blind placebo-controlled study of ADI-PEG 20 after prior systemic therapy is ongoing (Clinical Trial: NCT01287585).

Systemic Treatments for Patients with Advanced Liver Cirrhosis

Both the SHARP and Asia-Pacific studies were limited to patients with unresectable or metastatic HCC who also had preserved liver function. The benefit of sorafenib in patients with Child-Pugh class B and C has not been established. Sorafenib's safety in patients who are not Child-Pugh class A is of concern. A subgroup analysis of the phase II sorafenib study reported higher rates of hepatic decompensation, represented by worse hyperbilirubinemia, encephalopathy, and ascites in Child-Pugh class B compared to Child-Pugh class A patients.[262] Patients in this subgroup had a shorter treatment duration as well as shorter survival in Child-Pugh class B (3.2 months) versus Child-Pugh class A patients (9.5 months). In a Japanese study, there were no differences in the incidence of adverse events between Child-Pugh class A and B groups, despite a geometric means of area under the curve (AUC_{0-12}) and maximum serum concentration (Cmax) at steady state that were slightly lower in patients with Child-Pugh class B cirrhosis compared with Child-Pugh class A.[263] Similar findings have been reported from the phase IV study of sorafenib known as GIDEON.[264] Child-Pugh class B and C patients were treated for a shorter duration, had a shorter median survival on sorafenib, and were more likely to develop hepatic and serious drug-related adverse events. A phase I study of sorafenib pharmacokinetics in patients with hepatic dysfunction helped establish some guidance on the use of sorafenib among patients with advanced Child-Pugh score.[265] For a serum bilirubin ≤1.5 × upper limit of normal (ULN), sorafenib at the full dose of 400 mg twice daily can be given, whereas for a bilirubin 1.6 to 3 × ULN, half that dose should be considered. For albumin <2.5 mg/dL, no more than 200 mg once daily should be given. There was no safe dose identified for patients with a bilirubin >3 × ULN. Other antiangiogenic therapies have shown to be detrimental in cirrhotics (Fig. 52.6).[237]

TREATMENT OF OTHER PRIMARY LIVER TUMORS

Fibrolamellar Hepatocellular Carcinoma

Fibrolamellar HCC is a rare primary liver cancer that differs significantly from the usual HCC. Fibrolamellar HCC occurs in a much younger age group (peak incidence, 3rd decade), is usually not associated with cirrhosis or viral hepatitis, and affects males and females equally. Additionally, a much higher percentage (>15%) of patients with fibrolamellar HCC presents with positive lymph nodes than normal variant HCC.

Whether the diagnosis of fibrolamellar HCC portends a more favorable outcome after surgical treatment remains controversial.[266–269] Resection is the first-line of therapy. For those patients in whom the tumor is thought to be unresectable, liver transplantation provides an effective alternative. Pinna et al.[269] described 13 patients with fibrolamellar HCC who received transplantation between 1968 and 1995 and reported 1-, 3-, and 5-year patient survival rates of approximately 90%, 75%, and 38%, respectively.[269] Given that most patients transplanted presented as young patients with advanced disease, this is not an unacceptable survival rate. El-Gazzaz et al.[270] reported similar survival rates. Contrary to what was previously reported, in a large 95 patient retrospective analysis, with 50% presented with stage IV disease, median survival was limited to 6.7 years. Factors significantly associated with poor survival were female sex, advanced stage, lymph node metastases, macrovascular invasion, and unresectable disease.[271]

There is a great need for new, effective systemic therapies for advanced fibrolamellar HCC. A study is underway evaluating everolimus plus estrogen deprivation with leuprolide and letrozole for unresectable fibrolamellar HCC (Clinical Trial: NCT01642186).

Hepatoblastoma

Hepatoblastoma is the most common primary cancer of the liver occurring in childhood. The annual incidence of hepatoblastoma ranges from 0.5 to 1.5 cases per million children, with a peak incidence occurring within the first 2 years of life.[272] Hepatoblastoma is highly sensitive to chemotherapy, which often renders unresectable tumors resectable. Surgical resection is considered the first line of therapy. However, for those tumors that cannot be converted to resectable lesions but without distant metastasis, most can be rescued with liver transplantation. Survival rates for these children after liver transplantation is excellent, with 1-, 3-, and 5-year survivals reported at 92%, 92%, and 83%, respectively.[272]

Epithelioid Hemangioendothelioma

Epithelioid hemangioendothelioma is a very rare tumor of vascular origin that can originate in the liver; it occurs predominantly in females. The tumor is often confused with other more aggressive cancers, particularly cholangiocarcinoma, angiosarcoma, and HCC. The clinical course of epithelioid hemangioendothelioma is quite variable. In the review by Makhlouf et al.,[273] 137 cases were described, and survival ranged from 4 months to 28 years. Of interest, one patient who received no treatment survived for 27 years without evidence of metastasis. Surgical resection is considered to be the treatment of choice. However, in multifocal disease, a short observation may be reasonable to help decide between observation, ablation, resection, or transplant as the course of action. The presence of metastatic disease does not seem to influence survival and should not be considered an absolute contraindication to either surgical resection or transplantation.

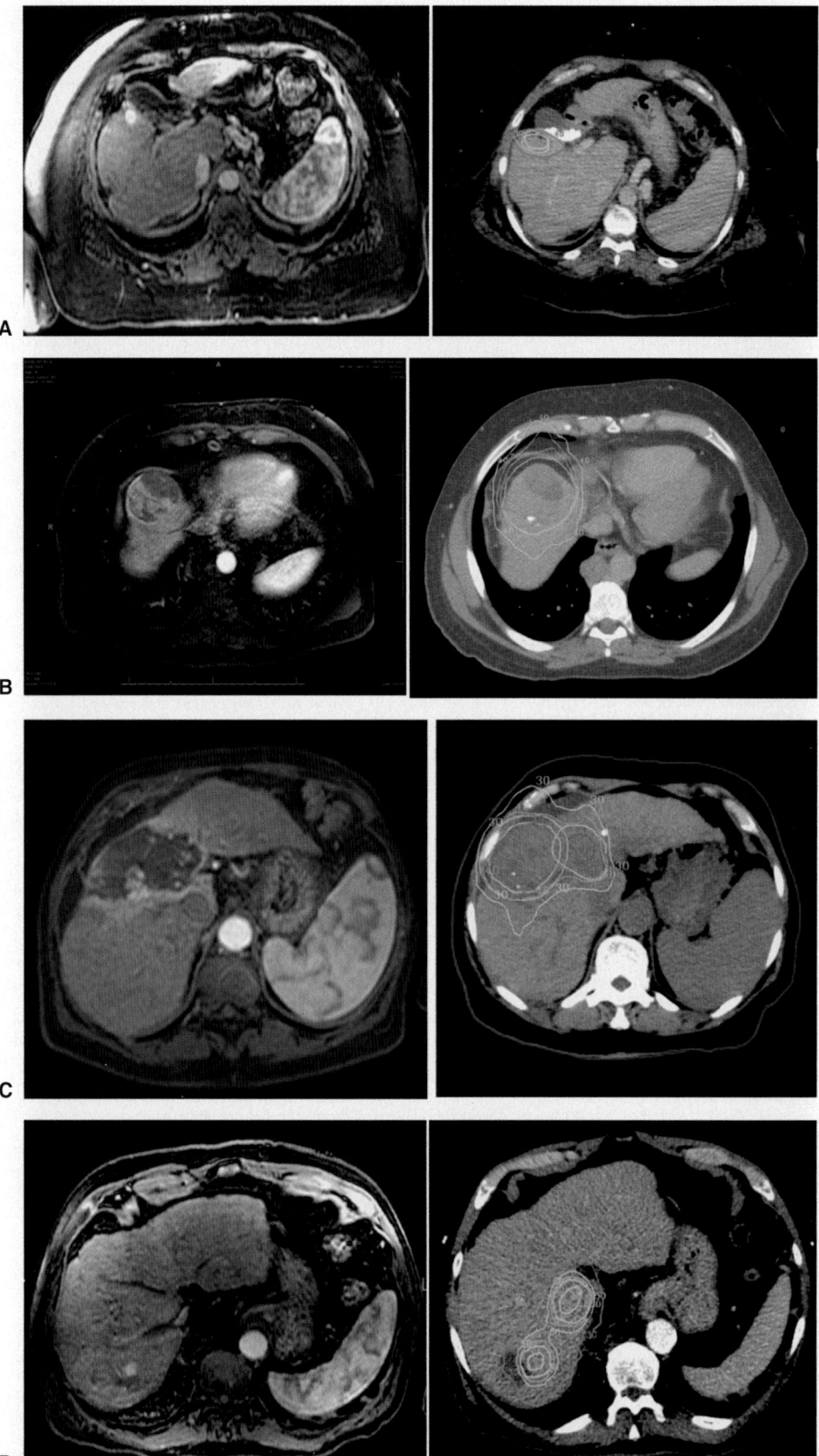

Figure 52.6 An SBRT can be used to treat single **(A, B)** or multiple **(C, D)** tumors in three to five high-dose, highly focused treatments. Planning is typically performed by fusing MRI images **(A, C)** with a planning CT scan **(B, D)** for accurate targeting. Special attention must be given to minimizing radiation dose to the remaining liver, particularly for patients with preexisting liver dysfunction.

SELECTED REFERENCES

The full reference list can be accessed at lwwhealthlibrary.com/oncology.

2. Llovet JM, Bustamante J, Castells A, et al. Natural history of untreated non-surgical hepatocellular carcinoma: rationale for the design and evaluation of therapeutic trials. *Hepatology* 1999;29:62–67.

6. Chang MH, Chen TH, Hsu HM, et al. Prevention of hepatocellular carcinoma by universal vaccination against hepatitis B virus: the effect and problems. *Clin Cancer Res* 2005;11:7953–7957.

8. Beasley RP, Hwang LY, Lin CC, et al. Hepatocellular carcinoma and hepatitis B virus. A prospective study of 22,707 men in Taiwan. *Lancet* 1981;2:1129–1133.

9. Yuen MF, Tanaka Y, Fong DY, et al. Independent risk factors and predictive score for the development of hepatocellular carcinoma in chronic hepatitis B. *J Hepatol* 2009;50:80–88.

10. Blum HE, Moradpour D. Viral pathogenesis of hepatocellular carcinoma. *J Gastroenterol Hepatol* 2002;17:S413–S420.

13. Hoshida Y, Toffanin S, Lachenmayer A, et al. Molecular classification and novel targets in hepatocellular carcinoma: recent advancements. *Semin Liver Dis* 2010;30:35–51.

14. Villanueva A, Newell P, Chiang DY, et al. Genomics and signaling pathways in hepatocellular carcinoma. *Semin Liver Dis* 2007;27:55–76.

21. Williams CD, Stengel J, Asike MI, et al. Prevalence of nonalcoholic fatty liver disease and nonalcoholic steatohepatitis among a largely middle-aged population utilizing ultrasound and liver biopsy: a prospective study. *Gastroenterology* 2011;140:124–131.

22. Ascha MS, Hanouneh IA, Lopez R, et al. The incidence and risk factors of hepatocellular carcinoma in patients with nonalcoholic steatohepatitis. *Hepatology* 2010;51:1972–1978.

26. Regimbeau JM, Colombat M, Mognol P, et al. Obesity and diabetes as a risk factor for hepatocellular carcinoma. *Liver Transpl* 2004;10:S69–S73.

34. Prospective validation of the CLIP score: a new prognostic system for patients with cirrhosis and hepatocellular carcinoma. The Cancer of the Liver Italian Program (CLIP) Investigators. *Hepatology* 2000;31:840–845.

39. Llovet JM, Bru C, Bruix J. Prognosis of hepatocellular carcinoma: the BCLC staging classification. *Semin Liver Dis* 1999;19:329–338.

45. Bruix J, Sherman M. Management of hepatocellular carcinoma: an update. *Hepatology* 2011;53:1020–1022.

51. Clavien PA, Petrowsky H, DeOliveira ML, et al. Strategies for safer liver surgery and partial liver transplantation. *N Engl J Med* 2007;356:1545–1559.

60. Fan ST, Lo CM, Liu CL, et al. Hepatectomy for hepatocellular carcinoma: toward zero hospital deaths. *Ann Surg* 1999;229:322–330.

67. Belghiti J, Regimbeau JM, Durand F, et al. Resection of hepatocellular carcinoma: a European experience on 328 cases. *Hepatogastroenterology* 2002;49:41–46.

74. Yang LY, Fang F, Ou DP, et al. Solitary large hepatocellular carcinoma: a specific subtype of hepatocellular carcinoma with good outcome after hepatic resection. *Ann Surg* 2009;249:118–123.

75. Wang J, Xu LB, Liu C, et al. Prognostic factors and outcome of 438 Chinese patients with hepatocellular carcinoma underwent partial hepatectomy in a single center. *World J Surg* 2010;34:2434–2441.

81. Mazzaferro V, Regalia E, Doci R, et al. Liver transplantation for the treatment of small hepatocellular carcinomas in patients with cirrhosis. *N Engl J Med* 1996;334:693–699.

83. Hemming AW, Cattral MS, Reed AI, et al. Liver transplantation for hepatocellular carcinoma. *Ann Surg* 2001;233:652–659.

84. Mazzaferro V, Llovet JM, Miceli R, et al. Predicting survival after liver transplantation in patients with hepatocellular carcinoma beyond the Milan criteria: a retrospective, exploratory analysis. *Lancet Oncol* 2009;10:35–43.

89. Bigourdan JM, Jaeck D, Meyer N, et al. Small hepatocellular carcinoma in Child A cirrhotic patients: hepatic resection versus transplantation. *Liver Transpl* 2003;9:513–520.

93. Jonas S, Herrmann M, Rayes N, et al. Survival after liver transplantation for hepatocellular carcinoma in cirrhosis according to the underlying liver disease. *Transplant Proc* 2001;33:3444–3445.

96. Duffy JP, Vardanian A, Benjamin E, et al. Liver transplantation criteria for hepatocellular carcinoma should be expanded: a 22-year experience with 467 patients at UCLA. *Ann Surg* 2007;246:502–509.

108. Mazzaferro V, Battiston C, Perrone S, et al. Radiofrequency ablation of small hepatocellular carcinoma in cirrhotic patients awaiting liver transplantation: a prospective study. *Ann Surg* 2004;240:900–909.

110. Chen LT, Chen MF, Li LA, et al. Long-term results of a randomized, observation-controlled, phase III trial of adjuvant interferon Alfa-2b in hepatocellular carcinoma after curative resection. *Ann Surg* 2012;255:8–17.

113. Muto Y, Moriwaki H, Ninomiya M, et al. Prevention of second primary tumors by an acyclic retinoid, polyprenoic acid, in patients with hepatocellular carcinoma. Hepatoma Prevention Study Group. *N Engl J Med* 1996;334:1561–1567.

121. Mazzaferro V, Romito R, Schiavo M, et al. Prevention of hepatocellular carcinoma recurrence with alpha-interferon after liver resection in HCV cirrhosis. *Hepatology* 2006;44:1543–1554.

124. Cherqui D, Laurent A, Mocellin N, et al. Liver resection for transplantable hepatocellular carcinoma: long-term survival and role of secondary liver transplantation. *Ann Surg* 2009;250:738–746.

131. Poon RT, Fan ST, Lo CM, et al. Difference in tumor invasiveness in cirrhotic patients with hepatocellular carcinoma fulfilling the Milan criteria treated by resection and transplantation: impact on long-term survival. *Ann Surg* 2007;245:51–58.

132. Adam R, Azoulay D, Castaing D, et al. Liver resection as a bridge to transplantation for hepatocellular carcinoma on cirrhosis: a reasonable strategy? *Ann Surg* 2003;238:508–518.

133. Belghiti J, Cortes A, Abdalla EK, et al. Resection prior to liver transplantation for hepatocellular carcinoma. *Ann Surg* 2003;238:885–892.

155. Gillams AR, Lees WR. Five-year survival in 309 patients with colorectal liver metastases treated with radiofrequency ablation. *Eur Radiol* 2009;19:1206–1213.

167. Kingham TP, Karkar AM, D'Angelica MI, et al. Ablation of perivascular hepatic malignant tumors with irreversible electroporation. *J Am Coll Surg* 2012;215:379–387.

175. Chen MS, Li JQ, Zheng Y, et al. A prospective randomized trial comparing percutaneous local ablative therapy and partial hepatectomy for small hepatocellular carcinoma. *Ann Surg* 2006;243:321–328.

176. Liang HH, Chen MS, Peng ZW, et al. Percutaneous radiofrequency ablation versus repeat hepatectomy for recurrent hepatocellular carcinoma: a retrospective study. *Ann Surg Oncol* 2008;15:3484–3493.

177. Huang J, Yan L, Cheng Z, et al. A randomized trial comparing radiofrequency ablation and surgical resection for HCC conforming to the Milan criteria. *Ann Surg* 2010;252:903–912.

178. Feng K, Yan J, Li X, et al. A randomized controlled trial of radiofrequency ablation and surgical resection in the treatment of small hepatocellular carcinoma. *J Hepatol* 2012;57:794–802.

179. Salem R, Lewandowski RJ, Kulik L, et al. Radioembolization results in longer time-to-progression and reduced toxicity compared with chemoembolization in patients with hepatocellular carcinoma. *Gastroenterology* 2011;140:497–507.

181. Llovet JM, Real MI, Montana X, et al. Arterial embolisation or chemoembolisation versus symptomatic treatment in patients with unresectable hepatocellular carcinoma: a randomised controlled trial. *Lancet* 2002;359:1734–1739.

184. Soliman H, Ringash J, Jiang H, et al. Phase II trial of palliative radiotherapy for hepatocellular carcinoma and liver metastases. *J Clin Oncol* 2013;31:3980–3986.

193. Ben-Josef E, Normolle D, Ensminger WD, et al. Phase II trial of high-dose conformal radiation therapy with concurrent hepatic artery floxuridine for unresectable intrahepatic malignancies. *J Clin Oncol* 2005;23:8739–8747.

198. Shim SJ, Seong J, Han KH, et al. Local radiotherapy as a complement to incomplete transcatheter arterial chemoembolization in locally advanced hepatocellular carcinoma. *Liver Int* 2005;25:1189–1196.

205. Tse RV, Hawkins M, Lockwood G, et al. Phase I study of individualized stereotactic body radiotherapy for hepatocellular carcinoma and intrahepatic cholangiocarcinoma. *J Clin Oncol* 2008;26:657–664.

209. Sanuki N, Takeda A, Oku Y, et al. Stereotactic body radiotherapy for small hepatocellular carcinoma: a retrospective outcome analysis in 185 patients. *Acta Oncol* 2014;53:399–404.

210. Bibault JE, Dewas S, Vautravers-Dewas C, et al. Stereotactic body radiation therapy for hepatocellular carcinoma: prognostic factors of local control, overall survival, and toxicity. *PLoS One* 2013;8:e77472.

217. Salem R, Lewandowski RJ, Atassi B, et al. Treatment of unresectable hepatocellular carcinoma with use of 90Y microspheres (TheraSphere): safety, tumor response, and survival. *J Vasc Interv Radiol* 2005;16:1627–1639.

223. Abou-Alfa GK, Schwartz L, Ricci S, et al. Phase II study of sorafenib in patients with advanced hepatocellular carcinoma. *J Clin Oncol* 2006;24:4293–4300.

226. Bruix J, Raoul JL, Sherman M, et al. Efficacy and safety of sorafenib in patients with advanced hepatocellular carcinoma: subanalyses of a phase III trial. *J Hepatol* 2012;57:821–829.

236. Johnson PJ, Qin S, Park JW, et al. Brivanib versus sorafenib as first-line therapy in patients with unresectable, advanced hepatocellular carcinoma: results from the randomized phase III BRISK-FL study. *J Clin Oncol* 2013;31:3517–3524.

243. Abou-Alfa GK, Johnson P, Knox JJ, et al. Doxorubicin plus sorafenib vs doxorubicin alone in patients with advanced hepatocellular carcinoma: a randomized trial. *JAMA* 2010;304:2154–2160.

256. Llovet JM, Decaens T, Raoul JL, et al. Brivanib in patients with advanced hepatocellular carcinoma who were intolerant to sorafenib or for whom sorafenib failed: results from the randomized phase III BRISK-PS study. *J Clin Oncol* 2013;31:3509–3516.

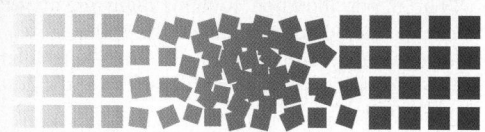

53 Cancer of the Biliary Tree

Tushar Patel and Mitesh J. Borad

INTRODUCTION

The biliary tract or the biliary drainage system includes the intra- and extrahepatic bile ducts and the gallbladder. Cancers associated with the biliary tract may be associated with biliary tract epithelia along the entire biliary tract from the intrahepatic ductules to the ampulla of Vater.

Cholangiocarcinomas are cancers of the biliary tract that are associated with the intrahepatic or extrahepatic bile ducts. The term *cholangiocarcinoma* encompasses three distinct tumor types that vary in their risk factors, presentation, natural history, and management.[1,2] Intrahepatic cholangiocarcinomas (iCCA) arise from the intrahepatic biliary tract beyond the second order ducts. Distal extrahepatic cholangiocarcinomas (dCCA) arise from the common hepatic duct extending up to the junction with the cystic duct up to the papilla. Perihilar cholangiocarcinomas (pCCA) arise from the second order ductal division within the liver and the large extracellular ducts up to the confluence with the cystic duct. In addition to cholangiocarcinomas, cancers such as gallbladder cancer and some ampullary cancers also arise from the biliary tract.

The presentation, diagnosis, and management of intrahepatic, perihilar, and distal cholangiocarcinomas and of gallbladder cancer are separately described in this chapter.

Periampullary tumors can arise from biliary as well as pancreatic, duodenal, or ampullary tissues. The presentation, evaluation, and management of periampullary tumors of biliary tract origin are identical to those of any of the other types of periampullary tumors, namely pancreatic, duodenal, or ampullary tumors. In most instances, the distinction between the tissue type of origin is obscure or may only be made on a histopathologic examination. These cancers will not be described in this chapter.

As a group, cancers of the biliary tract are rare. They are often diagnosed at an advanced stage and are associated with a poor prognosis. Management of these patients requires a multidisciplinary approach by a team with experience in their management and which includes hepatobiliary surgeons, hepatologists, gastroenterologists, diagnostic and interventional radiologists, pathologists, medical oncologists, and radiation oncologists. If the relevant and necessary expertise is not available locally, an early referral to experienced centers should be considered.

ANATOMY OF THE BILIARY TRACT

The biliary tract consists of the intrahepatic and extrahepatic bile ducts and is responsible for transporting bile from the liver to the intestine. Development of bile ducts requires complex intercellular interactions and signaling. Notch signaling is a critical determinant of both biliary differentiation and morphogenesis leading to the formation of normal bile ducts. Activation of Notch in liver progenitor cells results in differentiation to biliary ductal cells, whereas activation of Notch signaling in the hepatic lobule promotes ectopic biliary differentiation and duct formation. Experimentally enforced Notch signaling in adult murine hepatocytes causes them to reprogram to a biliary phenotype and can result in cholangiocarcinoma formation.

Within the liver, bile ducts along with branches of the hepatic artery and portal vein constitute the portal triad, which is directed to each lobule of the liver. The adult liver is divided into eight segments delineated by blood supply and venous drainage. These segments delineate and guide the resections of the liver. The main left hepatic duct exits the liver at the base of the umbilical fissure, and the main right hepatic duct exits the liver between segments V and VI. The caudate lobe drains directly into the left main hepatic duct via numerous small branches.

The confluence of the right and left hepatic ducts occurs in the hilum. The porta hepatis consists of the bile duct, the portal vein, and the hepatic artery, from right to left. At the hilum, the portal vein is posterior; the right hepatic artery generally passes between the common bile duct and the portal vein; and the cystic artery passes anterior to the bile duct. The proximity of the portal vein and hepatic artery to the bile duct in the hilum leads to early vessel involvement or occlusion from pCCA, which affects the options for surgical resection. Arterial anomalies are common, and if not recognized, could lead to inadvertent injury during dissection within the porta hepatis.

The cystic duct may enter the common duct near the confluence of the right and left ducts, or distally near the duodenum. It may also enter the right hepatic duct. The distal bile duct travels posterior within the head of the pancreas and then joins the pancreatic duct in a common channel leading to the ampulla of Vater.

The lymph node drainage of the bile ducts involves the superior pancreaticoduodenal, retroportal, or proper hepatic nodes first, then the peripancreatic, celiac, and interaortocaval lymph nodes.[3] Lymph nodes in the porta hepatis may be difficult to remove because of attached venous branches from the portal vein or fixation of tumor-involved lymph nodes to the bile duct, portal vein, hepatic artery, or the head of the pancreas. However, a multi-institutional cohort study reported that the presence of lymph node metastases significantly and adversely affected patient survival (hazard ratio [HR], 2.21; p <0.001), and may explain the survival benefit of a lymphadenectomy for iCCA.

The location of the primary tumor within the gallbladder and the proximity of the portal vein, hepatic artery, and bile duct are all important factors in the surgical management of this tumor. The gallbladder is attached to segments IVb and V of the liver, and these segments may be involved early in tumors of the fundus and body of the gallbladder. The gallbladder has a thin mucosal wall, a narrow lamina propria, and only a single muscle layer. Once this is penetrated, the tumor can access major lymphatic and vascular channels leading to early lymphatic and hematogenous spread. Tumors of the infundibulum or cystic duct can also obstruct the common bile duct and may involve the portal vein.

The lymphatic drainage of the gallbladder first involves cystic and pericholedochal nodes, before extending to nodes posterior to the pancreas, portal vein, and common hepatic artery. Finally, the flow reaches the interaortocaval, celiac, and superior mesenteric artery lymph nodes. Node-bearing adipose tissue posterior to the head of the pancreas and portal vein may be involved early, whereas drainage to the hilum does not occur.[4] Direct connections may exist from the pericholedochal nodes to

PRACTICE OF ONCOLOGY

the interaortocaval nodes, limiting the ability to control disease spread with a regional lymph node dissection.

The upper abdomen contains many organs with relative low tolerance to radiation, such as the spinal cord, kidneys, liver, stomach, duodenum, and small bowel. The tolerance of these at-risk organs poses significant limitations to the dose used in radiation therapy.

CHOLANGIOCARCINOMA

Nomenclature of Cholangiocarcinoma

The nomenclature used for cholangiocarcinomas has evolved over time and has been variably applied. As an example, epidemiological reports have either included perihilar tumors with iCCA or as extrahepatic tumors with dCCA. In addition, iCCA have long been reported along with other primary tumors of the liver. Because of the failure to recognize the different tumor types, the true incidence, prevalence, and natural history are not well established. The relative distribution of tumors within the biliary tract is also unclear. pCCA are the most common type of cholangiocarcinoma (CCA) worldwide. In one study, only 8% of cholangiocarcinomas seen were iCCA.[5] However, these data are not supported by clinical observations in practice and do not accurately reflect disease distribution because they are from a single center series and influenced by referral patterns.[5] The seventh edition of 2010 American Joint Committee on Cancer (AJCC) staging system classifies each of type of cancer of the biliary tract as separate entities with distinct staging and biologic properties.[6]

Classification of all of these diverse cancers as a single group of biliary tract cancers has resulted in a lack of recognition of their distinctive clinical behavior, nature, and management. The individual risk factors and specific molecular pathogenesis of iCCA, pCCA, or dCCA are also not well understood. Likewise, a lack of distinction between these cancers in therapeutic clinical trials has limited progress in identifying useful and optimal therapies for the individual types of cancers. Most clinical studies have included all types of biliary tract cancers, including gallbladder cancer and ampullary cancer, and have reported results in an aggregate fashion. Although specific etiologic and molecular differences are now becoming recognized, an improved understanding will emerge only once these distinctive cancer types are recognized as separate cancers in future population-based reports, patient-based studies, or laboratory investigations.

Etiology of Cholangiocarcinoma

Risk Factors

Although these cancers often occur sporadically without any identifiable risk factors, there are some well-defined risk factors. These include infections, conditions resulting in chronic biliary tract inflammation, drug/toxins, or congenital causes.[1,7–11] Because the individual risk factors for the different types of cholangiocarcinoma have not yet been delineated, we will review common risk factors associated with these cancers in this section. Where tumor specific risk factors are known, they will be discussed in the relevant sections.

Infestation with *Opisthorchis viverrini* and *Clonorchis sinensis* results in chronic inflammation of the bile duct, and are associated with CCAs. These two parasitic liver flukes are classified as group 1 carcinogens by the International Agency for Research on Cancer.[12] These liver flukes are highly prevalent in certain geographic regions such as Southeast Asia and, in particular, in Northeast Thailand. The geographic restriction of liver flukes has resulted in a highly variable disease prevalence in different parts of the world varying from 87 per 100,000 in Thailand to 1 to 2

per 100,000 in the United States.[13] Liver fluke infection with *O. viverrini* or *C. sinensis* species is associated with ingestion of raw fish containing the larva of liver flukes. Infestation is reversible with treatment with praziquantel. The degree of infestation as measured by stool egg count is related to the risk for CCA. Liver fluke infestation is associated with intrahepatic stones as well as with elevated nitrates, and animal and human studies suggest that N-nitroso compounds may be involved in carcinogenesis. The diagnosis of cancer is often difficult and delayed. Once cancer develops, the prognosis is similar to that of CCA in patients that do not have a fluke infestation.

Other infectious diseases that have been associated with CCA include HIV, and chronic hepatitis B virus (HBV) and hepatitis C virus (HCV) infections.[14] A recent meta-analysis of case-control studies reported an increased risk of iCCA in patients with HBV and HCV infection.[15,16] There appear to be regional differences in the risk of chronic hepatitis associated iCCA, although these are not well characterized.

Inflammatory conditions are less common, but their prevalence is more widely distributed. Primary sclerosing cholangitis (PSC) is an autoimmune condition affecting the biliary tract and characterized by inflammation within the biliary tract and subsequent development of diffuse multifocal biliary ductal strictures. CCA can occur in 5% to 10% of patients with PSC[17] and occurs more frequently in patients with chronic ulcerative colitis than in the general population.[18] A high incidence of CCA occurs in patients with coexisting PSC and ulcerative colitis.[19] Up to 50% of patients with PSC with CCA have this diagnosed within a year of their initial diagnosis with PSC.[20] The presence of underlying liver dysfunction resulting from biliary tract disease complicates surgery or chemotherapy.[21]

Chronic calculi of the intrahepatic and extrahepatic bile ducts (hepatolithiasis) outside the gallbladder is rare, but predisposes one to cancer formation. In Southeast Asia, chronic portal bacteremia and portal phlebitis are associated with intrahepatic pigmented stones, and subsequently, increased risk of cholangiocarcinoma. Cancers may develop even after stone removal, potentially related to stasis and cholangitis related to fibrosis induced by stone disease.[22]

An anomalous pancreatic–biliary duct junction may lead to a chronic inflammatory state in the bile duct via reflux of pancreatic juice into the biliary tree. This has been associated with an increased risk of CCA.[23]

Biliary tract cystic diseases are associated with an increased risk of malignancy, which can arise in noncystic portions of the biliary tract. Tumors can occur in patients with untreated choledochal cyst disease.[24,25] A choledochal cyst is a rare condition, manifest by congenital cystic dilatation(s) of the bile ducts. Bile stasis in the cysts leads to chronic inflammation of the duct. Of patients with choledochal cysts, 10% to 20% will develop CCA if left untreated or managed with surgical drainage alone.[26] Early excision of the choledochal cyst has been proposed to reduce the risk of CCA. Caroli disease is a rare variant of choledochal cysts that results in intrahepatic ductal dilatation and an increased risk of developing CCA.[27]

Recent epidemiologic studies indicate that occupational exposure to asbestos or to certain volatile compounds used in the printing industry such as 1,2-dichloropropane may also increase the risk of cancer.[28,29] Exposure to dioxin has also been implicated, although the data are not conclusive. Other potential carcinogens include radionuclides, radon, and nitrosamines.[30] Thorotrast (thorium dioxide) is a vascular contrast agent that is associated with an increased risk of cancer, but has not been used since the 1940s.[31] The risks associated with cigarette smoking are not well quantified.[15,30]

Recently, liver cirrhosis has been identified as a risk factor for iCCA.[15] Consistent with this observation, risk factors for cirrhosis, such as chronic hepatitis C, chronic hepatitis B, and alcohol, are also associated with a higher risk for iCCA.[15,32,33] Because these are also dominant risk factors for hepatocellular cancers, these observations suggest potential common risk mechanisms of tumorigenesis in liver epithelia.

Molecular Pathogenesis of Cholangiocarcinomas

The mechanism and events responsible for neoplastic transformation in the biliary tract are not well understood. It is postulated that chronic inflammation and infection in biliary epithelia and their interactions with other stromal cells' active inflammatory signaling such as those involving interleukin-6 (IL-6), inducible nitric oxide synthase (iNOS), and cyclooxygenase 2 (COX-2).[34] These result in a proliferative stimulus to epithelial cells involving epidermal growth factor receptor (EGFR), RAS/mitogen-activated protein kinase (MAPK), IL-6, or MET signaling. Malignant transformation occurs in the setting of genetic alterations and epigenetic changes on this background, and results in the deregulation of several signaling pathways that can enhance malignant cell growth, apoptosis, and tumor cell behavior. Tumors may arise from malignant transformation of biliary epithelial cells, progenitor cell populations, or transdifferentiation of hepatocytes.

Several genetic and epigenetic alterations and deregulated signaling pathways have been identified.[35] In PSC, inflammation results in the activation of the nuclear factor κB (NF-κB) signaling and increased tumor necrosis factor alpha (TNF-α) and IL-6. IL-6 is an important contributor to cholangiocarcinogenesis and has been associated with several molecular events such as alterations in EGFR, p38, and p42/44 MAPK and altered let-7 microRNAs.[34] Alterations in hepatocyte growth factor/MET signaling and in the EGFR family with overexpression of EGFR and HER-2/neu have been identified. Autocrine growth loops have been identified, involving hepatocellular growth factor (HGF)/MET and IL-6/glycoprotein 130 (gp130).[36] Alterations in the glycosylation of mucins (MUC proteins) and sialosyl-Tn antigen may be relevant, although their contribution in not well defined.[37]

Genetic alterations that have been identified, including activating mutations of KRAS, loss of TP53, mutations in IDH2 and IDH1, and rarely, alterations in BRAF, NRAS, and PI3K.[35,38–40] Tissue-specific activation of the K-ras G12D mutation in genetically engineered mice results in invasive iCCA, which is augmented by the addition of a loss in p53.[41] Mutations of Her-2/neu and c-MET have also been reported.[42] The genetic mutations observed may vary with type of tumor. Thus, IDH1/2 mutations are not seen with pCCA or dCCA, but may occur in up to 25% of iCCA, whereas K-ras mutations are more common in the former.[43,44]

Notch signaling is a complex, evolutionarily conserved pathway that is needed for normal bile duct development. Notch and several of its downstream targets SOX9, sex determining region Y-box 9, and hepatocyte nuclear factor 1β, may be involved in CCA pathogenesis. SOX9 is strongly expressed in intrahepatic bile ducts. Loss of SOX9 in CCA is associated with higher tumor grade and stage, and is an independent adverse prognostic factor for survival.[45] Nuclear colocalization of deltalike ligand 4 (DLL4) with Notch receptor 1 or 3 was associated with nodal metastases, less histologic differentiation, and worse survival of extrahepatic CCA and gallbladder cancer.

In addition to genetic changes, epigenetic changes resulting from alterations in promoter methylation of tumor suppressor genes such as SOCS-3, RASSF1A, p14ARF, and p16^{INK4A} as well as changes in some microRNAs such as miR-21 and miR-200c have been described.[35] Genomic studies have started to identify distinct subgroups of iCCA on patterns of gene expression, but these need to be validated and their clinical applications defined.[35,46–48]

Although the specific molecular pathogenesis of pCCA tumors is unknown, it is postulated that tumorigenesis results from a similar sequence of events to that described previously with the additional contribution of cholestasis. The reasons for the predilection of these tumors to occur in the hilar region are not clear. Morphologically and genetically, pCCA more closely resemble extrahepatic dCCA than iCCA. The pathogenesis of pCCA and dCCA is presumed to be similar to that described for iCCA, with an additional contribution of cholestasis. Some of these tumors may originate from progenitor cell populations in the submucous glands, and in tumors that have maintained differentiation, mucin production may be prominent. A subtype of iCCA may arise from a progenitor cell within the liver that results in tumors with histologic and genetic features of mixed hepatocellular carcinoma–cholangiocellular carcinoma.

A sequence of progression from normal mucosa to adenomatous hyperplasia, dysplasia, carcinoma in situ, and then invasive cancer similar to that described for other mucosal cancers may also occur in the biliary tract. Two precursor lesions are identified: biliary intraepithelial carcinoma neoplasia, which is more common, and intraductal papillary neoplasm of the bile duct.[38]

Pathology of Cholangiocarcinomas

Gross Morphology

The gross morphology can be exophytic, (nodular) mass forming, intraductal, or periductal infiltrating (or sclerosing). Mass-forming and periductal infiltrating (or both combined) are the most common types encountered. iCCAs are more likely to be nodular and mass forming, whereas pCCAs and dCCAs are more likely to be sclerosing, although not exclusively so. The sclerosing type is associated with an intense desmoplastic reaction and often manifest as diffuse thickening of the ducts without a defined mass. The nodular type tends to result in a mass lesion and usually arises within the liver. Intraductal tumors are less common and can encompass a range of lesions from preneoplastic to invasive carcinomas. In some patients, dCCAs may present only as a thickened bile duct wall involved in a dense fibrous scar. Polypoid or papillary cancers have the best prognosis. Papillary cancers represent a low-grade adenocarcinoma that is represented by a polypoid mass filling the lumen of the bile duct, with minimal invasion and no desmoplastic reaction.[49]

Histology

More than 90% of tumors are epithelial adenocarcinomas.[50] Other variants include well-differentiated, pleomorphic, giant cell, adenosquamous, oat cell, and colloid carcinomas. Other types, such as squamous cell carcinomas, sarcomas, small cell cancer, and lymphomas account for less than 5%. Sclerosing tumors are characterized by an extensive fibrous stroma with interspersed tumor cells. Papillary tumors may have papillary fronds with extension into the bile duct lumen, and may produce extracellular mucin. Nodular mass-forming tumors may vary with appearances akin to sclerosing type or with tubular pattern. Satellites are common and may result from spread along the bile ducts or from vascular invasion and intrahepatic metastatic spread. Regional lymph node metastases and perineural invasion are common with pCCAs and dCCAs. Distant metastases can occur, but are unusual.[51]

Intrahepatic Cholangiocarcinoma

Incidence and Etiology

iCCAs are cancers of the biliary tract that arise from intrahepatic bile ducts beyond the second order ductal system within the liver. They are the second most common primary epithelial malignancy of the liver, but are uncommon cancers in the United States. The incidence and mortality from iCCAs have been reported to be increasing in the United States and in many other countries.[52,53] The incidence of these cancers increases with age, with the majority of patients aged 65 years or older. Patients with defined risk factors such as PSC or choledochal cysts tend to develop tumors at a younger age. These tumors are slightly more common in men. There are racial and ethnic variations prevalent, with the highest prevalence among Hispanics in the United States (1.22 per 100,000) and the lowest among African Americans (0.3 per 100,000).[54]

Diagnosis

Patients with iCCAs may be asymptomatic, with the initial presentation being a mass lesion within the liver. When symptoms occur, these may include nonspecific right upper quadrant pain, or weight loss. In contrast to pCCAs or dCCAs where obstructive jaundice occurs early, jaundice occurs late with iCCAs and usually indicates extensive disease.[55] Occasionally, a centrally located iCCA may present with jaundice due to extrinsic compression of the main ducts. Other presentations are rare, and include mucobilia or a tumor embolizing into the extrahepatic bile ducts, resulting in pain, jaundice, or even pancreatitis.[56]

The diagnosis of iCCA involves demonstrating a mass lesion within the liver using abdominal computed tomography (CT) or magnetic resonance imaging (MRI).[57] On CT scan, the lesion is usually of low attenuation with only mild enhancement seen with contrast.[58] On a T1-weighted MRI, iCCAs are usually of low intensity, but may have high intensity on T2-weighted images. Centripetal filling in after gadolinium administration may be observed on MRI. Ductal dilation is often present peripheral to the tumor. Local vascular invasion is often seen by CT scan, MRI, or angiography.[59,60]

The differential diagnosis includes hepatocellular cancer (HCC) or metastatic cancer from other primary tumors. Cirrhosis is a risk factor for both iCCAs and HCCs. Imaging findings are often used to diagnose liver masses as HCCs without obtaining a biopsy. Characteristic imaging features of iCCAs that may be helpful in distinguishing these tumors from HCCs are slow uptake of contrast, particularly in highly desmoplastic tumors, and a peripheral rim of enhancement. A liver biopsy should be considered for a diagnosis if the tumor is inoperable due to extensive spread or if other lesions such as focal nodular hyperplasia are strongly suspected. Otherwise, in potentially resectable cases, further staging studies, including a laparoscopy, would be considered.

Grossly, iCCAs may be well or poorly demarcated, single, or multiple. Mucin production, fibrosis between the acini of tumor tissue, and a more overtly glandular pattern are the main differentiating characteristics from HCC.

Immunohistochemical staining for specific cytokeratins may also be helpful. Unlike HCCs, some cholangiocarcinomas stain positively for CA19-9 or carcinoembryonic antigen (CEA), or αvβ6 integrin, but not for hepatocyte antigen.[61] It may be difficult to distinguish iCCA from a liver metastasis of extrahepatic origin if a cytological analysis shows adenocarcinoma. Cytokeratin 7 or cytokeratin 20 may be helpful to establish a biliary origin. Cytokeratin 20 expression is focal and rare in iCCAs in contrast to being diffuse and common in colorectal cancer metastases.[62] If a primary site cannot be identified, a diagnosis of iCCA should be presumed.

Staging

The tumor-node-metastasis (TNM) system devised by the AJCC should be used for staging these cancers.[6] The seventh edition (2010) separated the staging of iCCAs from that of hepatocellular cancer, as well as from perihilar or distal CCAs. Table 53.1 shows the staging system for iCCAs.

Management

Most treatment information has been derived from small series gathered over several years, with variable definitions of disease used and, therefore, the best approaches to treatment are not clarified. Consensus guidelines have been proposed for management.[63,64]

TABLE 53.1

American Joint Committee on Cancer TNM Staging for Intrahepatic Cholangiocarcinoma

Primary Tumor (T)

TX	Primary tumor cannot be assessed
T0	No evidence of primary tumor
Tis	Carcinoma in situ (intraductal tumor)
T1	Solitary tumor without vascular invasion
T2a	Solitary tumor with vascular invasion
T2b	Multiple tumors, with or without vascular invasion
T3	Tumor perforating the visceral peritoneum or involving the local extrahepatic structures by direct invasion
T4	Tumor with periductal invasion; the pathologic definition of periductal invasion is the finding of a longitudinal growth pattern along the intrahepatic bile ducts on both gross and microscopic examination

Regional Lymph Nodes (N)

NX	Regional lymph nodes cannot be assessed
N0	No regional lymph node metastasis
N1	Regional lymph node metastasis present

Distant Metastasis (M)

M0	No distant metastasis
M1	Distant metastasis present

Anatomic Stage/Prognostic Groups

Stage 0	Tis	N0	M0
Stage I	T1	N0	M0
Stage II	T2	N0	M0
Stage III	T3	N0	M0
Stage IVA	T4	N0	M0
	Any T	N1	M0
Stage IVB	Any T	Any N	M1

Used with the permission of the American Joint Committee on Cancer (AJCC), Chicago, Illinois. The original source for this material is the *AJCC Cancer Staging Manual*, Seventh Edition (2010) published by Springer Science and Business Media LLC, www.springerlink.com, page 203.

An algorithm for the management of these cancers is shown in Figure 53.1.

Surgery. Indications for resectability are not well described. The goal is to resect the tumor with an adequate margin of normal tissue, and to obtain microscopically free resection margins, while retaining enough liver tissue behind for the patient to have adequate liver function after surgery. The resection may vary from nonanatomic resections to segmental anatomic resections. Intrahepatic metastases tend to occur as multiple satellites, and although their presence impacts prognosis, it should not define resectability. However, for widespread hepatic metastases, curative resection is unlikely, and other forms of therapy should be considered. The presence of underlying advanced cirrhosis with portal hypertension may preclude surgical resection. Extrahepatic spread portends a poor prognosis, and carcinomatosis should be considered a contraindication to resection. A staging laparoscopy can help define respectability prior to a full laparotomy and is recommended.[65]

Outcomes after surgical resection for iCCAs have been reported in small series in the literature. The resectability rate ranges from 32% to 90%. The mortality of resection is slightly higher than se-

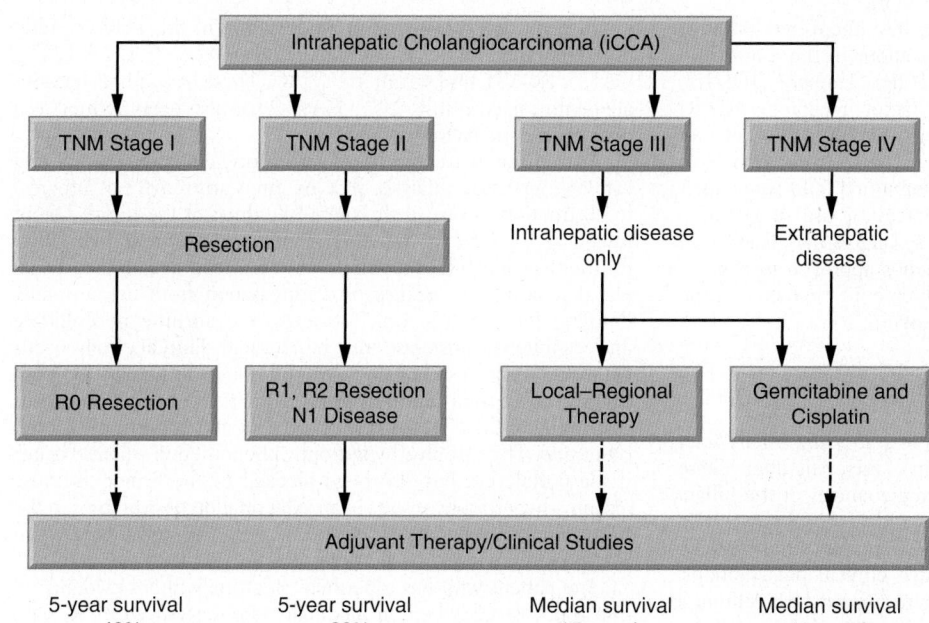

Figure 53.1 Algorithm for the management of intrahepatic cholangiocarcinoma.

ries of hepatic resection for other indications, but is generally less than 10%. Lymph node metastases, positive margin status, and vascular invasion were reported as significant prognostic factors in an analysis of 449 patients.[66] Other prognostic factors include satellite metastases, nodal metastases, tumor size, and a CA19-9 level greater than 1,000. Although rare, intrahepatic intraductal papillary tumors have an excellent prognosis if completely resected.[67,68]

The median survival after surgical resection is ~36 months. The 5-year survival rate with a curative R0 resection is ~60%, but curative resections are possible only in about 30% of patients. There is high risk of tumor recurrence both locally with intrahepatic metastases as well as with extrahepatic disease. However, there are no established guidelines for surveillance and follow-up after surgical resection for iCCAs. As a guide, surveillance could consist of laboratory tests of liver function and CA19-9 and radiologic evaluations every 3 months for the first 2 years after surgery and every 6 months thereafter for the first 5 years could be considered and modified based on the perceived risk. The role and utility of surveillance has not been formally established. Surgery is generally not indicated for recurrent CCAs.

Liver Transplantation. The outcomes from liver transplantation for iCCAs, unlike those for hilar CCAs have been disappointing, with a 5-year survival rate of 29% in data from the European Liver Transplant Registry.[69] As a result of these poor outcomes, liver transplantation is not generally offered for this indication.

Local–Regional Therapies. Local–regional therapy for unresectable iCCAs include transarterial chemoembolization (TACE), transarterial radioembolization (TARE), radiofrequency ablation (RFA), or microwave ablation. They may be used for palliation and local control in persons with a good performance status. A median survival time of 20 months with TACE and 43.7 months with TARE have been reported in case series. For tumors smaller than 3 cm, RFA resulted in a median survival time of 38.5 months. Most tumors present with a large bulky tumor precluding complete ablation, and there is a potential risk of biliary complications arising from bile duct damage.

Chemotherapy. Based on pivotal data from the UK-ABC-02 study, gemcitabine in combination with cisplatin has been established as the standard of care for patients with biliary cancers.[70] Gemcitabine was dosed at 1000 mg/m^2 in combination with cisplatin at 25 mg/m^2, with both agents given intravenously on days 1 and 8 every 21 days for a maximum of 6 months. The study was conducted using a phase II/III design and enrolled 410 patients across centers in the United Kingdom. Stratification was done based on the extent of disease (locally advanced versus metastatic), primary tumor site (intrahepatic/extrahepatic bile ducts, ampullary, gallbladder), performance status (Eastern Cooperative Oncology Group [ECOG] score 0, 1, or 2), prior therapy (yes/no), and recruiting center. The median overall survival in the gemcitabine/cisplatin group was 11.7 months compared to 8.1 months in the gemcitabine only group (p <0.001; 95% CI, 9.5 to 14.3) with a hazard ratio of 0.64 (95% CI, 0.52 to 0.80). Efficacy was evident across a range of endpoints, including progression-free survival (8 months versus 5 months; HR, 0.63; p <0.001) and response rate (26.1% versus 15.5%). Prespecified subgroups described earlier all derived clinical benefit. Only 17.6% (72 of 410) patients went on to receive second-line therapy. The role of subsequent lines of therapy with regard to survival benefit remains to be defined, but fluoropyrimidine-based regimens have demonstrated preliminary evidence of efficacy in studies with small numbers of patients with cholangiocarcinoma/gallbladder cancer,[71,72] and should be investigated in larger, controlled studies. Of patients, 58.8% (241 of 410) had involvement of the bile ducts in this study; 19.5% (80 of 410) had intrahepatic disease; 17.8% (73 of 410) had intrahepatic involvement; and 13.9% (57 of 410) had hilar disease. Survival benefit was most prominent in the intrahepatic group on a subgroup analysis (HR, 0.57; 95% CI, 0.34 to 0.94). The subgroup analyses were not powered to demonstrate benefit within each subgroup and, as such, should be viewed as hypothesis generating. Response rate was 19% versus 11.7% in the subgroup comprising both biliary and ampullary cancers.

At a conceptual level, there is support for the consideration of combined modality chemoradiation therapy for patients with unresectable disease using gemcitabine- or fluoropyrimidine-based strategies, and efficacy has been observed in small studies.[73,74] However, definitive data through controlled trials remains unavailable and, as such, this remains an area of active investigation, particularly from the standpoint of patient selection and advantages over chemotherapy alone.

The advent of molecular profiling has uncovered putative therapeutic targets, which include aberrations in the *Akt–PI3K–mammalian target of rapamycin* (*mTOR*), Fanconi, *IDH1/2*, *ERBB–MEK*, and fibroblast growth factor receptor (*FGFR*) pathways.[43,75,76] Fusions in fused in glioblastoma–repressor of silencing 1 (*FIG–ROS1*) and various *FGFR2* fusions such as *FGFR2–BICC* and others have been identified, and more such events will be identified with the increasing use of genomic sequencing studies. The pursuit of these targets may lead to an eventual individualized and heterogeneous approach to patients with both refractory and untreated disease in lieu of empiric approaches such as gemcitabine and cisplatin.

Perihilar Cholangiocarcinoma

pCCAs are cancers that arise from the extrahepatic biliary tract from the second order ducts to the origin of the cystic duct. These cancers are amongst the commonest malignancies of the biliary tract encountered in many parts of the world.

pCCAs should be distinguished from nonhilar, distal extracellular tumors because of their distinctive clinical presentations, natural history, staging, and management approaches. Although distinctive molecular and pathologic differences have yet to be determined, and the pathogenesis of these tumors may be similar, dCCAs are far less common than pCCAs and have better treatment outcomes. The reason for the predilection of pCCAs to predominantly arise at the liver hilum is not known.

Tumors that cause ductal obstruction at the hilar region are occasionally referred to as Klatskin tumors. However, the series reported in the classical paper by Klatskin included both intrahepatic and extrahepatic cancers, and was reported in an era in which the biliary tract was inaccessible to noninvasive preoperative imaging.[77] Thus, use of the term *Klatskin tumor* to describe pCCAs is inaccurate, confusing, and best avoided.

Diagnosis

Patients with early-stage cancers are often asymptomatic. Most patients present with painless jaundice and its clinical sequelae of dark urine, light stool, and pruritus. Nonspecific gastrointestinal symptoms such as anorexia and nausea, as well as mild weight loss and fatigue are not unusual. Most patients will present with painless obstructive jaundice, associated with pruritus, abdominal pain, weight loss (30% to 50%), and fever in about 20%.[78] The other clinical presentation of pCCAs are indistinguishable from other malignancies causing large bile ductal obstruction such as dCCAs or pancreatic cancer. Obstruction of the bile duct and biliary stasis may lead to bacterial colonization and cholangitis, particularly in patients with biliary stones. Patients with cholangitis can present with high fever, pain, nausea, vomiting, and rigors.

Serum biochemical tests will reveal the evidence of cholestasis with elevations in bilirubin, alkaline phosphatase, and γ-glutamyltransferase. Serum aminotransferase levels may be normal or mildly elevated in the early stages. Serum CEA and CA19-9 levels are the most commonly elevated serum tumor markers. CA19-9 has limited value because levels can be elevated in benign biliary tract disease, cholangitis, or cholestasis. CA19-9 levels above 100 U/mL were found to be 89% sensitive and 86% specific for the diagnosis of malignancy in patients with PSC.[79,80] CEA levels also have a low predictive value for cancer and are not helpful for a diagnosis.[79,81] Both CA19-9 and CEA levels may be elevated in bile specimens in the presence of cancer.[82] A combined index of CA19-9 and CEA has been proposed, with studies showing mixed results in predicting cancer. The presence of cholangitis or hepatolithiasis can cause elevations of tumor markers, and these tests should be repeated after symptoms have resolved. CA19-9 is a carbohydrate cell–surface antigen related to Lewis blood group antigens. Patients with a negative Lewis blood group antigen (representing 10% of the population) cannot synthesize

CA19-9 and will not manifest an elevation in this marker. Additional potential markers for CCA include CA242, CA72-4, CA50, CA125, RCAS1, and serum *MUC5AC*. These have all been evaluated with mixed results.[80,83–87] CA19-9 has also been defined as a poor prognostic factor in CCA.[88]

A diagnosis is usually based on history, cholangiography and cytology, or tissue analysis. pCCAs often arise and can progress to obstruction of one of the main bile ducts at the hilum before involving the other main duct. Unilateral obstruction of either the right or left bile duct alone may not lead to jaundice or an elevated bilirubin because of compensation from the normally draining lobe of the liver. However, the alkaline phosphatase and γ-glutamyltransferase may be elevated. Jaundice may occur when the tumor extends down the bile ducts to involve the confluence of the right and left ducts. Unilateral obstruction results in atrophy of the affected side of the liver and hypertrophy of the other side. This atrophy–hypertrophy phenomenon will also occur if the portal vein has also been blocked by the tumor. Because atrophy–hypertrophy results in an axial rotation of structures in the hepatoduodenal ligament, its effects need to be considered when interpreting imaging studies or in planning hepatic resections.[89]

Any patient who has a perihilar stricture, without evidence of ductal disease elsewhere in the biliary tree suggestive of PSC, and who has not had previous biliary surgery that might have resulted in stricture, is considered to have pCCA. The diagnosis and evaluation of these tumors depends on the available diagnostic technologies and expertise. The goals are to (1) ascertain the nature and extent of obstruction, (2) obtain tissue for diagnosis if possible, and (3) stage the tumor to determine spread and metastasis to guide therapy. An abdominal ultrasound will confirm the presence of a biliary obstruction. Additional testing with either a CT or MRI/magnetic resonance cholangiopancreatography (MRCP) is needed to identify the potential and for staging if a malignancy is suspected. The accuracy of CT and MRI/MRCP for the prediction of the extent of ductal involvement ranges from 84% to 91%; for hepatic arterial invasion, it ranges from 83% to 93%; for portal vein invasion, from 86% to 98%, and for lymph node metastasis, from 74% to 84%.[90–92]

Biliary tract imaging (cholangiography) with cytology is used to establish the diagnosis. Tissue biopsies can be obtained under fluoroscopic guidance, or using cholangioscopy during endoscopic retrograde cholangiopancreatography (ERCP). A cholangioscopy may allow for direct visualization, but often provides a lower amount of tissue for analysis.[93–96] In one study, direct visualization for biliary strictures using a miniendoscope identified malignancy in 11 of 20 patients and resulted in modification of diagnosis of biliary stricture in 20 of 29 patients.[97]

Peroral cholangioscopy using the spyglass system may also be associated with a higher rate of cholangitis. Confocal laser endomicroscopy is an emerging technique that may be helpful. Specific criteria (Miami criteria) for the diagnosis of a malignancy within a stricture using this technique have been proposed, but need to be further validated, and the specificity needs to be improved.[98] An endoscopic ultrasound (EUS) with fine-needle aspiration (FNA) may also be helpful for a diagnosis or to predict unresectability by detecting nodal spread. An intraductal ultrasound performed using an ultrasound probe passed into the common bile duct increased the accuracy of ERCP from 58% to 90%.[99]

pCCAs are less accessible than other distal CCAs for sampling. The highly desmoplastic nature of these tumors further limits the amount of cellular material that may be obtained for a cytologic analysis. As a result, establishing a tissue diagnosis of pCCA is extremely difficult. The diagnostic sensitivity of tissue or cytology examination remains poor. Indeed, benign disease has been noted in about 10% of surgical resections performed for presumed pCCAs.[100–102] A positive diagnosis with brush cytology ranges from 44% to 80%,[103–105] with pooled data from over 800 CCA patients reporting a sensitivity of 42%, a specificity of 98%, and a positive predictive value (PPV) of 98% among patients with confirmed cancer.[103] A brush cytology is diagnostic and very useful when positive, but of little value when negative. In a study of 74 patients with pancreaticobiliary strictures, the sensitivity and specificity of brush cytology were 56% and 100%, respectively, and the positive predictive value was 100%.[106] Intraductal tissue biopsies also have a low diagnostic yield with a pooled sensitivity of 56%, a specificity of 97%, and a PPV of 97%. The use of multiple sampling techniques should be considered to improve the diagnostic yield of sampling.

Mucobilia on ERCP is an uncommon finding that is highly suggestive of a papillary CCA. Papillary tumors could be either intrahepatic or extrahepatic. FNA is also useful if a mass can be seen on ultrasound examination or on CT scan.

Staging

Disease staging in pCCA requires an assessment of the extent of ductal involvement as well as the extent of involvement of the liver parenchyma, lymph nodes, and vasculature and distant metastases.[107] The TNM system (Table 53.2) does not help to define surgical resectability and, therefore, may not adequately predict outcome.[51] A classification for hilar tumors was introduced and modified by Bismuth.[108] This classification is based on the level of ductal involvement by the tumor, and provides a guide as to the extent of surgical resection that may be required for tumor eradication. However, it is not a true staging system and has low accuracy.[109] A registry of pCCA has been initiated to collect data that may serve as a resource to guide the development of meaningful future staging classifications.[110]

Management

A suggested approach to the management of pCCA is presented in Figure 53.2. The local extent of the disease along the biliary tree can be determined by direct or imaging-defined cholangiography—either ERCP, magnetic resonance cholangiography MRCP or percutaneous transhepatic cholangiography (PTC). However, the extent of disease may not be appreciated because of tumor spread along the wall of the bile duct without lumenal compromise. PTC or MRCP may be more useful than ERCP in establishing the upper extent of disease. MRCP is less invasive, but may need to be supplemented with direct cholangiography at times. Vascular invasion has been assessed by MRI/MR angiography, angiography, or Doppler ultrasound. An MRI is useful to assess liver invasion or vascular involvement not clearly identified on CT scans. CT scans or MR angiography are replacing the need for an invasive angiography to assess vascular involvement. Color-flow Doppler ultrasound is very dependent on the operator, but can be effective at evaluating portal vein involvement and, in some cases, hepatic artery involvement.[111] Positron-emission tomography (PET)/CT scans, intraductal ultrasound (US), and EUS have all been used for staging. EUS with FNA may also be helpful for a diagnosis by detecting distal lymph node involvement. A staging laparoscopy with or without ultrasound can identify tumor spread beyond that detected on cholangiography, vascular encasement, or lymph node involvement.

Liver Transplantation. Liver transplantation has emerged as a viable option for the treatment of early stage, unresectable pCCA in highly selected patients.[112] For patients with tumors that are unresectable, a complete hepatectomy with liver transplantation may provide the only chance for a cure. The presence of extrahepatic nodal disease or metastases is a contraindication to transplant. In carefully selected patients, a multimodality approach combining preoperative chemoradiation, staging laparoscopy, and orthotopic liver transplantation has resulted in overall 5-year survival rates of up to 82%. A study of the combined experience of several centers showed an overall survival of 53% on an intention-to-treat analysis, with a 65% recurrence-free survival after 5 years.[112] It should be noted that these data reflect results obtained with a highly selected group of patients.

The availability of adequate organs for transplantation has limited the use of liver transplantation as a treatment modal-

TABLE 53.2

American Joint Committee on Cancer TNM Staging System for Perihilar Cholangiocarcinoma

Primary Tumor (T)

TX	Primary tumor cannot be assessed
T0	No evidence of primary tumor
Tis	Carcinoma in situ
T1	Tumor confined to the bile duct, with extension up to the muscle layer or fibrous tissue
T2a	Tumor invades beyond the wall of the bile duct to surrounding adipose tissue
T2b	Tumor invades adjacent hepatic parenchyma
T3	Tumor invades unilateral branches of the portal vein or hepatic artery
T4	Tumor invades main portal vein or its branches bilaterally, or the common hepatic artery, or the second-order biliary radicals bilaterally, or unilateral second-order biliary radicals with contralateral portal vein or hepatic artery involvement

Regional Lymph Nodes (N)

NX	Regional lymph nodes cannot be assessed
N0	No regional lymph node metastasis
N1	Regional lymph node metastasis (including nodes along the cystic duct, common bile duct, hepatic artery, and portal vein)
N2	Metastasis to periaortic, pericaval, superior mesenteric artery, and/or celiac artery lymph nodes

Distant Metastasis (M)

M0	No distant metastasis
M1	Distant metastasis

Anatomic Stage/Prognostic Groups

Stage 0	Tis	N0	M0
Stage I	T1	N0	M0
Stage II	T2a-b	N0	M0
Stage IIIA	T3	N0	M0
Stage IIIB	T1–3	N1	M0
Stage IVA	T4	N0–1	M0
Stage IVB	Any T	N2	M0
	Any T	Any N	M1

Used with the permission of the American Joint Committee on Cancer (AJCC), Chicago, Illinois. The original source for this material is the *AJCC Cancer Staging Manual*, Seventh Edition (2010) published by Springer Science and Business Media LLC, www.springerlink.com, page 221.

ity for pCCA. The use of living donor liver transplantation may overcome some of the limitations of organ availability for this indication because 5-year survival after living donor living transplantation (LDLT) was 69% compared with 63% after deceased donor transplantation. The outcomes are better in patients with pCCAs arising in the setting of PSC, with a 72% 5-year survival compared with 51% in non-PSC patients. Furthermore, patients with pCCAs undergoing neoadjuvant chemoradiation and liver transplantation have a quality of life that is similar to those for patients undergoing transplantation for other indications.[113] If liver transplantation is being considered as a treatment option, FNA of the hilar lesion by EUS should be avoided because of the risk of tumor seeding.

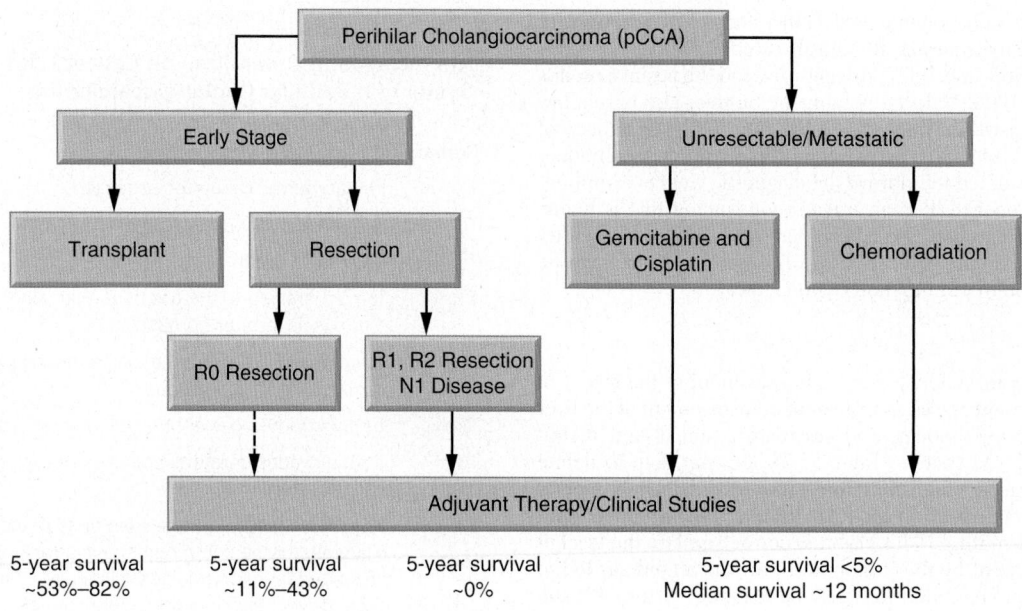

Figure 53.2 Algorithm for the management of perihilar cholangiocarcinoma.

In early reports, EBRT and bolus fluorouracil (5-FU), followed by brachytherapy, 5-FU, and liver transplantation, was used.[114,115] Out of 28 patients, 11 were excluded because of metastatic disease found at the time of exploratory surgery. The rest underwent liver transplantation with an identifiable tumor noted on explant in 10 patients; 2 patients had recurrence after 40 months and 54 months, respectively; and 2 died of non–cancer-related causes. The median duration of follow-up was 41.8 months (range, 2.8 to 105.5 months); the 5-year actuarial survival rate for those transplanted was 87%. A follow-up protocol added a intrabiliary brachytherapy using iridium seeds after external beam radiation therapy (EBRT) and maintenance therapy with capecitabine until transplantation.[115] Out of 56 enrolled patients, 28 received a transplant. The actuarial 1- and 5-year survivals were 88% and 82%, respectively, after transplantation. A similar protocol that combined neoadjuvant brachytherapy and infusional 5-FU followed by transplantation was reported, with 5 of 17 patients (29%) achieving long-term disease-free survival.[93] Other small series have demonstrated 3-year survival rates from 0% to 53%.[116]

Earlier studies of liver transplantation for patients with all types of CCA in unselected patients showed very poor results. Meyer et al.[117] reported the results of liver transplantation for cholangiocarcinoma in 207 patients collected by the Cincinnati Transplant Tumor Registry. Fifty-one percent had recurrence, with a median time of recurrence of 9.7 months, and the median time between recurrence and death being 2 months. In a series of 7 patients undergoing liver-related transplant for CCA, 6 were alive after a median follow-up of 20 months. Recurrences were noted in all patients in this series with iCCA.[118]

Surgery. Surgical resection is complex and associated with mortality and morbidity. The results of surgical resection for pCCA have been reported in many retrospective single-institution surgical series. The goals of surgical resection are to remove the tumor with negative resection margins. An en bloc resection of at least one lobe of the liver, the extrahepatic bile duct, and a complete periportal lymphadenectomy may be required.

The preoperative assessment serves to define the extent of resection that may be required. There is a role for preoperative biliary drainage in some, but not all patients. This could be performed either percutaneously or endoscopically with stenting or placement of a nasobiliary tube. Biliary drainage can alleviate symptoms in patients with severe obstructive jaundice, renal dysfunction, or pruritus.[119] However, preoperative decompression can increase complications during or after surgery.[120–123] Cholangitis may occur following bacterial colonization of bile and stenting may induce fibrosis, making it difficult to delineate the extent of tumor.[120] Five randomized trials and a meta-analysis have not demonstrated a benefit, although retrospective studies suggest a disadvantage to preoperative stenting.[124] It may be appropriate if a hemihepatectomy for CCA is planned in a jaundiced patient or if a pancreaticoduodenectomy is to be done in a patient with long-standing or severe jaundice. Other preoperative preparations include correcting a vitamin K deficiency and bowel preparation. The use of MRCP to guide decision making toward surgical resection may avoid the need for more invasive cholangiography and stenting.

Excision of the bile ducts may be possible up to the first order branches of the right and left bile ducts. If the tumor extends beyond this on one side, a partial hepatectomy may be needed, and a Roux-en-Y reconstruction performed. The contralateral preserved bile duct should be transected at the level of the first segmental branch to maximize the chance of a negative margin. If the resection is extended beyond the first order branches, a main drainage channel may need to be fashioned by suturing the individual segmental or sectoral ducts together. A caudate lobe resection is often routinely performed because invasion of the caudate ducts may occur. Several early branches of the left hepatic duct drain the caudate lobe and can be involved with the tumor involving the left main hepatic duct. Indeed, 46% of pCCAs microscopically involve the caudate lobe.[125,126]

Surgery is indicated in the absence of distant metastases where a preoperative workup suggests that an R0 resection is feasible. Bilateral biliary involvement to the point that all four sectional ducts are involved precludes curative resection.[127] Other indicators of unresectability include bilateral intrahepatic bile duct spread, involvement of the main trunk of the portal vein, involvement of both branches of the portal vein or bilateral involvement of the hepatic artery and portal vein, or a combination of vascular involvement on one side of the liver with extensive bile duct involvement on the other side.[89] With vascular replacement, it may be possible to resect some tumors previously considered unresectable.

A periportal lymphadenopathy is not a contraindication, and resection with microscopic positive margins (R1) determined after resection can provide significant palliation. A lymphadenectomy should include all soft tissue in the porta hepatis, excluding the portal vein and hepatic artery. The common hepatic artery nodes, the celiac artery nodes, the peripancreatic nodes, and the interaortocaval lymph nodes should be assessed because dissection may be indicated. Adequate staging may require sampling of at least seven nodes.[128]

Resectable disease is present in approximately one-third of patients with suspected pCCA. In a series from 2001 to 2008, of 118 patients referred for surgery, 51% were resectable and 41% underwent R0 resection.[129] Operative mortality averaged about 8%[130]; 5-year survival rates after resection have ranged from 10% to 35%. The results of surgical resection highly depend on whether negative resection margins are achieved.[107,131–135] Frozen sections are used to evaluate tumor margins at the time of surgery and to guide the extent of resection. However, the desmoplastic nature of these tumors and fibroinflammatory changes related to the presence of a biliary stent, often restricts an accurate determination of the presence of a tumor in frozen sections.

When negative margins are obtained, median survival of patients with a tumor-free margin is ~3.4 years with a 5-year survival rate from 11% to 43%. However, when margins are positive, median survival is 1 to 1.2 years and 5-year survival is almost zero.[107,132,135,136] With positive microscopic margins, there were no 5-year survivors in one study.[137] Other negative prognostic variables include tumor stage, nodal disease, tumor grade, bilirubin concentration, serum albumin level, postoperative sepsis, and absence of mucobilia.[119,135,136,138,139] Recurrences most commonly occur locally at the resection bed or within the retroperitoneal lymph nodes. Distant metastases occur in one-third of cases, most commonly within the lung, mediastinum, liver, or peritoneum. Improved outcomes seen in more recent series may reflect increasing use of routine liver resections.

There are no established guidelines for surveillance and follow-up after surgical resection. There is high risk of recurrence, with peritoneal spread, hepatic metastases, local extrahepatic recurrence, and distant metastases (most commonly lung). Laboratory and radiologic evaluations every 3 months for the first 2 years after surgery and at longer 6-month intervals thereafter could be considered based on the perceived risk. The role of CA19-9 as a surveillance indicator is not established, but persistently rising levels may precede radiologic evidence of recurrence. The role of CT scans or MRI for surveillance and detection of tumor recurrence has not been evaluated in clinical trials. MRIs may be preferable to CT scans for surveillance because of the ability to concomitantly visualize the biliary tract. In a recent study, PET/CT scans demonstrated a higher positive predictive value compared to CT scans alone (94% versus 78%) for nodal metastases and a higher sensitivity (95% versus 63%) for distant metastases.[140] Surgery is generally not indicated for recurrent CCA. Close surveillance and early diagnosis of recurrences may allow for eligibility for clinical trials.

Adjuvant Therapy. There is a lack of conclusive data regarding the efficacy of adjuvant radiation therapy or chemoradiation therapy for patients who have a gross residual tumor, a tumor involving the resection margins, or regional lymph nodes involved with a tumor after undergoing resection with curative intent. The reported series have been small with the potential for selection bias, and there are no randomized trials that support any particular adjuvant approaches as standard. There is a need to explore and effectively evaluate new regimens for adjuvant therapy in these patients. It is recommended that patients are enrolled in clinical trials to define the role of adjuvant therapy. Similarly, there is a paucity of data upon which to base decisions on the use of adjuvant chemotherapy. In a randomized study, mitomycin C and 5-FU were compared with observation alone in a study of 508 patients with resected pancreaticobiliary cancers that included 139 patients with bile duct cancers.[141] No apparent differences in overall or 5-year disease-free survival were noted. A phase III study comparing adjuvant capecitabine versus observation

alone in surgically resected patients has completed enrollment in the United Kingdom and outcomes data are eagerly awaited (NCT00363584). The primary endpoint of this study is 2-year overall survival. An analogous phase III study using gemcitabine in combination with oxaliplatin versus observation alone is underway in France with disease-free survival as the primary endpoint (NCT01313377). Data from these two pivotal studies will help define the role of adjuvant therapy more definitively. In the interim, the recommendation for patients is to participate in clinical trials whenever feasible.

Palliative Care. For unresectable tumors, palliation may be performed by percutaneous or endoscopic stent placement or by surgical bypass.

Stent Placement. The goal is to drain the most functional lobe of the liver with a stent that traverses the malignant obstruction and allows for internal drainage. Percutaneous biliary drainage is more appropriate for the drainage of intrahepatic ducts and may be required for access to these ducts. Both internal and external biliary drainage are possible. Both plastic and metallic stents may be used, with one study reporting a longer survival and lower complication rates with the latter.[142] Biliary catheters may exit the skin and remain capped. This allows for irrigation and provides easy access for cholangiography and stent changes as needed. However, percutaneous draining catheters may decrease quality of life. An attempt should be made to enable the drainage of greater than 50% of more of the liver volume, irrespective of whether one or more stents are used or one or more segments are drained. Imaging-based volumetric assessments may be useful to determine whether drainage will be adequate. A guided approach using MRCP may be beneficial to routine bilateral stenting. If bilateral stents are placed, they may be used side by side or by contralateral stenting through the mesh of the first stent (stent in stent). Plastic stents typically clog within 2 to 6 months, whereas metal stents last longer, up to 8 to 10 months. Endoscopic metallic stenting should be performed by an experienced biliary endoscopist. Catheter tract recurrence is a rare complication of PTC-placed stents, and was reported in 6 of 441 patients (2.6%) who underwent percutaneous biliary drainage for pCCAs.[143] Patients with catheter tract recurrence had a lower survival than those without recurrence (17.5 months versus 23.0 months; $p = 0.089$).

Surgery. Surgical approaches have not been shown to be superior to percutaneous or endoscopic biliary drainage. A surgical bypass may avoid the need for long-term biliary tube placement, and its associated morbidity, such as cholangitis, occlusion, and need for frequent replacement. The disadvantage of surgical bypass for palliation is the morbidity associated with the procedure when there is limited overall life expectancy. If advanced unresectable disease is encountered at the time of a laparotomy for presumed resectable tumors, a bypass could be performed for palliation to avoid the need for another procedure. A surgical bypass for pCCA involving a bypass to intraparenchymal ducts using a defunctionalized limb of jejunum can be technically challenging but quite effective for palliation. A surgical biliary enteric bypass to segment III (Bismuth–Corlette cholangiojejunostomy), where the bile duct is accessed through the liver parenchyma anteriorly avoids the hilar region that may be involved with the tumor.[144] A bypass to right-sided ducts may be challenging.[145,146] The right lobe could be drained by a bypass to the anterior sectoral bile duct. Surgical implantation of large-bore tubes through the tumor has been used in the past but is rarely employed now.

Photodynamic Therapy. Photodynamic therapy with stenting has shown to improve survival, reduce cholestasis, and improve quality of life compared to stenting alone in a randomized study.[147–149] In a small, multicentered, randomized controlled trial of 39 patients, patients who received photodynamic therapy with biliary stenting survived 493 days compared with 98 days for those treated with stenting alone.[142] In a recently published meta-analysis of 6 studies, 170 patients received photodynamic therapy and were compared with 157 who had biliary stenting alone.[150] There were statistical improvements in patient survival and performance status, and a trend in the decline of serum bilirubin was significantly improved and the risk of biliary sepsis was similar (15%). These data also suggest a possible role for photodynamic therapy in these patients.

Radiation Therapy. There are very few data regarding the efficacy of the use of radiation therapy either alone or in combination with other techniques for advanced stage disease, either unresectable or resected with gross residual tumor. Most of the reported series are small and no randomized comparisons exist. Long-term survivors have been rarely described.

External-beam irradiation was successful in clearing jaundice in 10 of 11 patients in a recent report; no other decompressive measures were used.[151] Brachytherapy has been applied through percutaneous tubes, with a median survival of 23 months.[152] The combination of surgery and radiotherapy was reported to provide a median survival of 14 months in unresectable or recurrent disease.[153] However, other series have reported no benefit with radiation.[154] Stereotactic body radiotherapy (SBRT) may have some efficacy but has the potential for severe toxicity. In a study of 27 patients (26 with pCCA and 1 with iCCA), of whom 18 were treated on a prospective phase II trial and received 45 Gy in three fractions over 5 to 8 days,[155] the median overall survival was 10.6 months and the local control at 1 year was 84% with a median follow-up of 5.4 years. Six patients had severe duodenal or pyloric ulceration, and three patients developed duodenal stenosis. Interestingly, no such toxicity was observed in another group of 13 patients with Klatskin tumors.[156] Eight of these received 48 Gy in four fractions and the others received a range of doses (32 to 56 Gy in 3 to 4 Gy per fraction), and median survival was 33.5 months.

No formal comparative studies have been performed, although the median survival of 1 year observed with radiation therapy appears to be superior to 3 months with chemotherapy or 6 months with best supportive care alone.

Other Approaches. Endobiliary radiofrequency ablation may potentially provide benefits that are similar to the use of photodynamic therapy for palliation of malignant ductal obstruction, but the experience with this has been limited.[157] EUS-guided biliary drainage through a transgastric approach is technically feasible, but has high complication rates, such as bile leakage and peritonitis (20%) even in experienced hands.[158–162]

Systemic Therapy. As described earlier, based on the UK-ABC-02 data, gemcitabine and cisplatin should be regarded as the standard of care for patients with perihilar cholangiocarcinoma with unresectable disease. Although fluoropyrimidine-based therapies have shown evidence of preliminary efficacy, the role of subsequent lines of systemic chemotherapy remains to be definitively defined. Similarly, molecular profiling of these cancers may eventually result in a paradigm shift, allowing for the individualized treatment of patients based on single-agent/combination therapy based on perturbation of aberrant pathways.

Distal Cholangiocarcinoma

dCCAs are cancers arising from the extrahepatic common hepatic duct between the junction of the cystic duct and the papilla, but not involving either the cystic duct or the ampulla of Vater.

There is heterogeneity of cancers that arise from the extrahepatic bile duct. Other cancers that arise from the extrahepatic ducts but are considered separately from dCCAs include tumors

at the liver hilum or cystic duct. Cancers arising at the hilum are considered separately as pCCAs, whereas those arising within the cystic duct are considered along with other gallbladder cancers.

Diagnosis

The typical presentation of dCCAs is with obstructive jaundice. In the case of tumors arising below the insertion of the cystic duct, the gallbladder may be palpable. The presentation is similar to that of pCCAs or cancers arising from the head of the pancreas. Patients may present with jaundice associated with pruritus, weight loss, fever, and occasionally, with abdominal pain. Cholangitis may occur, but is rare as a presenting symptom in the absence of prior interventions directed toward the biliary tract such as cannulation or stent placement. Bile is sterile, but can serve as a medium for bacterial growth and can become contaminated with instrumentation. Patients with cholangitis may present with fever, abdominal pain, nausea, vomiting, and rigors. Bacteremia with biliary tract flora such as *Escherichia coli*, Klebsiella, Proteus, *Pseudomonas aeruginosa*, Serratia, Streptococcus, and Enterobacter may be present.

The presence of obstructive jaundice is an indication for further diagnostic testing to evaluate for malignant obstruction resulting from tumors of the bile ducts.

Laboratory tests suggest extrahepatic biliary obstruction with elevations in serum bilirubin, alkaline phosphatase, and γ-glutamyltransferase levels. Transaminase levels may be elevated, but typically to a lesser level.

Tumor markers may not be very helpful. CA19-9 has low accuracy for diagnosis because the levels may be increased in the presence of pancreatic cancer, or in the presence of cholangitis or biliary obstruction from other causes. In patients with PSC, a cutoff of 100 IU has a sensitivity of 89% and specificity of 86% for CCA in PSC.[163] The King's College group index that incorporates both CEA and CA19-9 values has attained similar sensitivities for cancer arising in patients with PSC.[164] Bile CEA levels are reportedly elevated in CCA, but not in benign diseases, other than intrahepatic stones.[138]

Evaluation involves abdominal US, and body imaging with CT scans or MRI, as well as biliary tract imaging with ERCP. US is cheap, noninvasive, and is the best initial test for the detection of biliary stones or for ductal dilation that can occur with long-standing obstruction. Abdominal imaging with either a CT scan or MRI should be obtained for the patient with painless jaundice in whom malignancy is suspected. The advantage of MRI is that an MRCP could also be performed at the same time. Although a CT scan can identify mass lesions, an ERCP or MRCP may be needed to evaluate for the site and nature of biliary obstruction if no mass lesions are noted.

In patients without PSC and with no visible mass lesions, the presence of a single stricture by ERCP indicates a malignancy. In patients with PSC, a malignancy may be associated with the deterioration of clinical status and liver function tests. However, dCCAs may also present in these patients without any change in liver biochemistries. There are no data to determine the efficacy, timing, or effectiveness of screening and surveillance for a malignancy in patients with PSC, although this is often done in clinical practice using CT scans or an MRI/MRCP, with CA19-9.[164] The diagnosis of malignancy in patients who have a biliary tract stricture can be very difficult. Because of the dense associated stroma, well-differentiated cancers with little invasion are difficult to differentiate from the bile duct that has a fibrotic scar or stricture from PSC or other prior biliary injury. The presence of malignant-appearing cells within nerve sheaths (perineural invasion) is an important diagnostic criterion of malignancy that is not present in a benign stricturing disease such as PSC.

The differential diagnosis includes any cause of painless obstructive jaundice such as choledocholithiasis, pCCA, or pancreatic cancer. As with pCCA, dCCAs must be differentiated from benign fibroinflammatory strictures such as from immunoglobulin (Ig) G4 cholangiopathy or sclerosing cholangitis.[165] The former can occur in the extrahepatic and intrahepatic ducts and is diagnosed by an elevated IgG4 in the serum, or by an increased number of IgG4-positive cells in tissue samples. The failure to consider these diagnoses may lead to inappropriate therapies, such as long-term stenting or hepatic resection, and these strictures may respond to corticosteroids.

Cancers of the lower bile ducts may not be readily distinguished from ampullary, duodenal, or pancreatic cancers. Although all of these cancers present in a similar manner to dCCA, establishing a diagnosis is helpful because dCCAs are less likely to metastasize widely and may have a more favorable outcome with aggressive treatment.

Staging

The AJCC's TNM system may be used for staging dCCAs (Table 53.3).[6] Prior TNM staging systems did not consider separate staging systems for extrahepatic bile duct tumors. However, the seventh edition (2010) separated the staging of dCCAs from that of pCCAs. In order to determine resectability of the tumor, staging is necessary to identify the extent of tumor spread and the relationship to portal vein and superior mesenteric artery. EUS with FNA may be useful in determining the extent of tumor spread and involvement of local lymph nodes.[166] Although PET scanning for staging has been proposed, the benefit has not yet been shown.[167] A staging laparoscopy with or without US may enable the direct visualization of the peritoneal surfaces for metastatic implants, as well as detect vascular or nodal invasion, any of which would preclude resection for cure.[127,168,169]

Management

An approach to the evaluation and management of the patient with suspected dCCA is presented in Figure 53.3.

Biliary Decompression. If the distal ducts are dilated and extending into the lower common bile duct, therapeutic decompression by ERCP or percutaneous stenting could be performed at the time of the initial evaluation. We recommend obtaining brushings at ERCP even if no masses have been seen on abdominal imaging studies.

Surgery. Surgical resection can be considered for locally confined dCCA without major vascular involvement or distant metastases. An intraoperative assessment with the help of the pathologist

PRACTICE OF ONCOLOGY

TABLE 53.3

American Joint Committee on Cancer TNM Staging System for Distal Cholangiocarcinoma

Primary Tumor (T)

TX	Primary tumor cannot be assessed
T0	No evidence of primary tumor
Tis	Carcinoma in situ
T1	Tumor confined to the bile duct histologically
T2	Tumor invades beyond the wall of the bile duct
T3	Tumor invades the gallbladder, pancreas, duodenum, or other adjacent organs without involvement of the celiac axis, or the superior mesenteric artery
T4	Tumor involves the celiac axis, or the superior mesenteric artery

Regional Lymph Nodes (N)

NX	Regional lymph nodes cannot be assessed
N0	No regional lymph node metastasis
N1	Regional lymph node metastasis

Distant Metastasis (M)

M0	No distant metastasis
M1	Distant metastasis

Anatomic Stage/Prognostic Groups

Stage 0	Tis	N0	M0
Stage IA	T1	N0	M0
Stage IB	T2	N0	M0
Stage IIA	T3	N0	M0
Stage IIB	T1	N1	M0
	T2	N1	M0
	T3	N1	M0
Stage III	T4	Any N	M0
Stage IV	Any T	Any N	M1

Used with the permission of the American Joint Committee on Cancer (AJCC), Chicago, Illinois. The original source for this material is the *AJCC Cancer Staging Manual*, Seventh Edition (2010) published by Springer Science and Business Media LLC, www.springerlink.com, page 229.

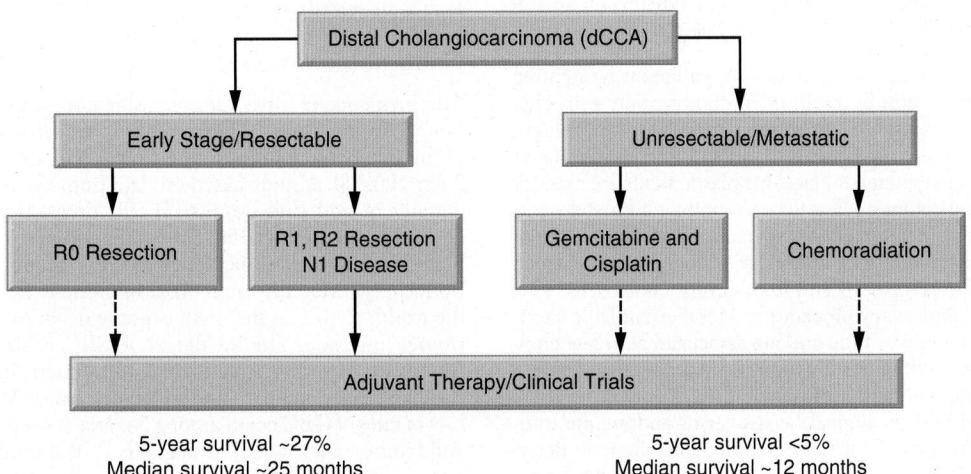

Figure 53.3 Algorithm for the management of distal cholangiocarcinoma.

must dictate the extent of resection. For localized dCCAs, a pancreaticoduodenectomy with resection of the extrahepatic bile duct to the level of the confluence may be required. Although dCCAs often involve the intrapancreatic portion of the common hepatic duct, on rare occasions the tumor may be confined to a small region of the duct and removed by an extrahepatic bile duct resection without a pancreaticoduodenectomy. The peripancreatic and periportal lymph nodes should be removed and examined, along with the interaortocaval lymph nodes, if necessary.

Although the incidence of dCCAs is lower than that of pCCAs, the resectability rate of dCCAs is much higher than that of pCCAs, which may contribute to improved outcomes. A pancreaticoduodenectomy with distal bile duct resection has a reasonable chance of providing a margin-negative resection for dCCAs. There is considerable morbidity and a mortality rate from 2% to 10%. Morbidity can arise from biliary fistulas in about 2% of patients or a fistula from the pancreatic–jejunal anastomosis in 5% to 10% of patients. Although many patients require pancreatic enzyme replacement after this procedure, few develop diabetes. Short-term outcomes and/or quality of life are similar between the pylorus-preserving and standard types of pancreaticoduodenectomy.[170,171] Extensive en bloc–combined hepatic and pancreatic resections could be considered in the rare circumstance that there is extensive involvement of the entire bile duct without any evidence of distant spread. The morbidity of such extensive surgery is very high, and the overall prognosis is poor.[126] The 5-year survival rates after an R0 resection is 27%, with a median survival time of 25 months. The expected 5-year survival is between 23% and 50%. Prognostic factors for poor survival include high p53 expression, nodal metastases, positive margins, pancreatic invasion, and perineural invasion.[172,173]

There are no established guidelines for surveillance and follow-up after surgical resection. Laboratory and radiologic surveillance modalities and intervals will be determined on perceived risk on an individual basis. Tumor recurrence may occur locally within the peritoneum or local nodes or with distant metastases.

Adjuvant Therapy. Postoperative adjuvant radiotherapy can be administered by intraoperative radiotherapy (IORT), EBRT, intrabiliary brachytherapy, or a combination of modalities. EBRT is widely available, noninvasive, and can deliver a homogeneous dose to a large volume. In most series, EBRT has been used to deliver a dose of 40 to 50 Gy (at 1.80 Gy per day) to the tumor bed and draining lymph node basin. In some series, a smaller volume (i.e., a boost) was treated with additional EBRT, intraluminal brachytherapy, or IORT to a total dose of 60 Gy or more. Most commonly, radiotherapy is administered in a continuous course during 5 to 6 weeks. However, the role of radiotherapy from an efficacy standpoint remains to be definitively ascertained. Similarly, as described earlier, the role of chemotherapy remains an area of active investigation in patients with biliary cancers.

Palliative Care. For unresectable dCCA, palliation by stenting for biliary decompression by itself, or in combination with chemotherapy may be considered. Plastic or metal stent placement can be performed at the time of ERCP or PTC, and an internal or external drainage. In general, replaceable plastic stents are used for those with a life expectancy of less than 6 months, and metal stents are used for those with a longer life expectancy, based on results of a randomized controlled trial.[174] Plastic stents need to be replaced every 3 months for best results and to minimize cholangitis. This requires repeated endoscopy procedures. Metal expandable stents remain patent for a longer time and are associated with less cholangitis, but they cannot be readily removed. Tumor advancement may lead to a complete stent occlusion.

A randomized trial of surgical bypass versus endoscopic intubation favored the latter.[175] Unresectability can often be determined preoperatively, but if unresectability is determined only at the time of an open exploration, a palliative bypass for biliary

decompression and jejunal bypass may be performed. A surgical bypass to the common bile duct does involve the morbidity associated with laparotomy and bowel anastomosis. A laparoscopic bypass of a distal bile duct obstruction can be performed,[145] usually with a cholecystojejunostomy. This will be unsuccessful if the common bile duct at the level of the cystic duct is involved with the tumor.

The efficacy of radiation therapy for advanced unresectable disease has never been evaluated in prospective randomized trials. Radiation therapy can result in biliary tract and intestinal complications. The available data is based on small retrospective reviews with heterogeneous patient populations that have been treated with a wide variety of modalities and techniques. As described earlier, based on the UK-ABC-02 data, gemcitabine and cisplatin should be regarded as the standard of care for patients with dCCA. Although fluoropyrimidine-based therapies have shown evidence of preliminary efficacy, the role of subsequent lines of systemic chemotherapy remains to be definitively defined. Similarly, molecular profiling of these cancers may eventually result in a paradigm shift, allowing for individualized treatment of patients based on single-agent/combination therapy predicated on the perturbation of aberrant pathways.

GALLBLADDER CANCER

Incidence and Etiology

Gallbladder cancers (GBC) are cancers that arise from the gallbladder mucosa. GBC is the fifth most common malignancy of the gastrointestinal tract. The incidence of GBC correlates with the prevalence of cholelithiasis. Patients who have gallstones for longer than 40 years have a significantly higher incidence of GBC than those who have had gallstones for a shorter time. It has been postulated that 1% of patients aged 65 years or more with gallstones would develop GBC, and this may reflect the duration of stone disease.[176] GBC affects women three to four times more often than men and is more common in Caucasians than in African Americans. The incidence of GBC increases with age, with the greatest incidence in persons aged 65 or more. However, there have been isolated reports of GBC diagnosed in children.[177–179] Mortality trends have been variable. Germany and the Netherlands have relatively high mortality rates from GBC, but have shown declines in most age groups. Sweden, France, and Bulgaria show steady upward trends. In Japan, the incidence increased through the 1980s but has stabilized in recent years.[180] GBC incidence in the United States, Britain, and Canada has stabilized or declined. These changes have occurred coincident with the rise in the number of laparoscopic cholecystectomies.[181]

Geographic Variation

The incidence of GBC varies considerably with geographic location.[224] In the United States, GBC is the most common cancer of the biliary tract, but is a rare cancer with an incidence of 1 to 2 per 100,000. A study based on data from the Surveillance, Epidemiology, and End Results (SEER) program reported an incidence of 1.2 cases per 100,000 population per year in the United States.[182] The highest incidence of GBC occurs in Chileans and Bolivians.[183] Mortality from GBC in Chile is 5.2%, the highest in the world.[184] GBC is the main cause of death from cancer among women in Chile. The incidence of GBC is also high in Native American, Hispanic American, Latin American, Japanese, and Zimbabwean women,[185] and in Americans of Mexican origin.[186] Lower rates of GBC occur among Nigerians, New Zealand Maoris, and Chinese natives and immigrants.[185] Within the United States and the United Kingdom, urban areas show higher incidences than rural regions. It has been suggested that lower socioeconomic status may lead to delayed access to cholecystectomy, which may increase GBC rates.[187]

Ethnicity

There are considerable ethnic differences in the incidence of GBC. In contrast to the general population, the incidence of GBC is much higher in Native Americans in the Southwest United States and in Mexican Americans. In Mexico, the highest incidence of GBC is in *mestizos* (i.e., people of mixed ancestry). The incidence of GBC in Spain, Cuba, and Puerto Rico is low, suggesting that the geographic and ethnic variations noted in GBC incidence in North and South America may be related to Native American rather than Spanish heritage. In Bolivia, differences are related to tribal origin.[185]

Risk Factors

Established risk factors include gallstone disease, bile composition, calcification of the gallbladder wall, congenital biliary cysts or ductal anatomy, some infections, environmental carcinogens, and drugs. Some of the noted geographic differences may reflect genetic differences. Although gallstone disease is associated with GBC, the mechanisms predisposing to this increased risk are not known. Cholecystolithiasis is present in 70% to 90% of patients with GBC, and the incidence of GBC in patients with cholecystolithiasis ranges from 0.5% to 3%.[188] The risk of GBC was increased in a prospective cohort study of patients with gallstones, although the incidence (9 per 10,000 per person-years), and the absolute number of cases of GBC (5 of 2,583 people) in this population was low.[189] The duration of gallstone disease, the patient age, the size of gallstones, and possible carcinogenic effects of gallstones, such as from the chemical composition or bacteria within the stones, may be important; although, in one study patients with cancers did not have larger stones, nor were their stones of higher cholesterol content.[190,191]

Although familial clusters of GBC have been reported, an inherited predisposition has not been found in large series.[192] A recent cohort study from Sweden found an association among first-degree relatives, specifically among parents (relative risk [RR], 5.1; 95% confidence interval [CI], 2.4 to 9.3) or offspring (RR, 4.1; 95% CI, 2.0 to 7.6).[235] Genetic variants in DNA repair pathways may be involved in gallbladder carcinogenesis.[193]

There is a high incidence of GBC in patients with an anomalous pancreatic–biliary duct junction (APBJ), and this risk is independent of the presence of gallstones. Studies from Japan have linked APBJ to other biliary tract cancers as well as GBC.[194] About 2% of Japanese patients examined had APBJ, with about 75% of these cases associated with a choledochal cyst and duct dilation. The rest were noted to have normal caliber bile ducts.[194,195] Patients with APBJ get cancer at a younger age than patients with sporadic GBC. Children with APBJ frequently have epithelial hyperplasia of the gallbladder.[196]

GBC has been associated with partial or complete calcification of the gallbladder wall (porcelain gallbladder). The association is controversial, with some studies reporting an incidence up to 25%, and other studies disputing the association.[197,198]

Salmonella typhi carriage has been associated with GBC. Typhoid carriers may also suffer chronic inflammation of the gallbladder and have a sixfold higher risk of gallbladder cancer.[199] *Helicobacter bilis* and *Helicobacter pylori* have been identified in bile specimens and have been demonstrated to increase the risk of carcinoma by about sixfold.[200,201]

Exposure to toxic environmental factors in the automotive, rubber, textile, and metal industries have been associated with GBC.[183,190,202] Chemicals implicated in gallbladder carcinogenesis include methyldopa, oral contraceptives, isoniazid.[203–205]

An elevated body mass index has been associated with GBC. Although many cohort studies have identified obesity as a risk factor for GBC, this parallels the risk for gallstone disease. Other rare associations with gallbladder cancer include previous gastric surgery, inflammatory bowel disease, and polyposis coli.

Pathology

Sixty percent of GBCs occur in the fundus, 30% occur in the body, and 10% occur in the neck of the gallbladder. Tumors that arise in the neck and the Hartman pouch may infiltrate the cystic and common bile duct, making them clinically and radiographically indistinguishable from pCCAs. They may be isolated tumors or involve the gallbladder through intramural spread analogous to linitis plastica of the stomach. Gallbladder cancer can spread early by direct extension into the liver and other adjacent organs. This cancer also has a propensity to seed and grow in the peritoneal cavity, and along needle biopsy sites and in laparoscopic port sites. At autopsy, GBC patients have a 91% to 94% incidence of lymphatic metastasis, 65% to 82% have an incidence of hematogenous metastasis, and 60% have an incidence of peritoneal spread.[206,207] Hematogenous metastasis tends to be from invasion into small veins that extend directly from the gallbladder into the portal venous system, leading to hepatic metastases in segments IV and V of the liver. There is a high propensity for intra-abdominal recurrence after resection, with distant metastasis occurring late in the course. The only common extra-abdominal site of metastasis is the lung. It is rare, however, to have metastasis to the lung in the absence of advanced local–regional disease.

GBC can be categorized into infiltrative, nodular, and papillary forms. The infiltrative tumors are the most common form and cause thickening and induration of the gallbladder wall, sometimes extending to involve the entire gallbladder. These tumors spread in a subserosal plane. Tumor seeding into the peritoneal cavity can occur if the subserosal plane is violated during and the presence of the tumor is not recognized at the time of cholecystectomy. Advanced tumors can invade the liver and can result in a thick wall of tumor encasing the gallbladder. Nodular or massforming GBCs can show early invasion through the gallbladder wall into the liver or neighboring structures. Despite this invasiveness, it may be easier to control surgically than the infiltrative form, where the margins are less defined. Papillary carcinomas exhibit a polypoid or cauliflowerlike appearance and fill the lumen of the gallbladder with only minimal invasion of the gallbladder wall. The prognosis of these tumor is better than other forms of GBC.

Most malignant neoplasms of the gallbladder are adenocarcinomas. Primary malignant mesenchymal tumors of the gallbladder have been described, including embryonal rhabdomyosarcoma, leiomyosarcoma, malignant fibrous histiocytoma, angiosarcoma, and Kaposi sarcoma. Other primary rare tumors of the gallbladder include carcinosarcomas, carcinoids, lymphomas, and melanomas. In addition, the gallbladder can be involved with metastatic cancers from numerous sites. Many tumors exhibit more than one histologic pattern. The only histologic type with clear prognostic significance is the papillary adenocarcinoma, which has a markedly improved survival compared with all other histologic types. There is also evidence to suggest that oat cell carcinomas, adenosquamous tumors, and carcinosarcomas have a poorer survival rate.[208]

Gallstones are found in more than 75% of all patients with GBC. In the presence of gallstones, chronic mucosal irritation predisposes one to malignant transformation. Cholesterol stones are the most common type associated with GBC. Bile from high endemic areas is more mutagenic than that from low endemic areas.[209] Although the chemical composition of stones or bile may be related to the development of cancer, there are no conclusive data linking biliary bile acids to GBC. A potential mechanism of carcinogenesis may involve the excretion of dietary or chemical metabolites within bile, with bile acids acting as cocarcinogens. Experimentally, GBC was induced by the carcinogen dimethylnitrosamine in 68% of hamsters with cholesterol pellets inserted into the gallbladder compared to 6% of controls fed the carcinogen alone.[210] Calcification is the end stage of a long-standing inflammatory process, and calcification of the gallbladder (porcelain gallbladder) is associated with cancer in 10% to 25% of cases. Despite this association, the incidence of GBC in patients with gallstones is only 0.3% to 3%.

Cancers arising from gallbladder mucosa behave similar to other adenocarcinomas of the gastrointestinal tract. Premalignant to invasive malignant changes can be found; metastatic spread occurs by lymphatic and vascular routes; the diagnosis is often delayed; and survival is related to the stage. Interestingly, at the population level, mortality is also inversely related to cholecystectomy rates.[211] GBC originates as mucosal lesions and, as growth progresses, the tumor invades the wall of the gallbladder. The lack of a well-defined muscularis leads to early entry of invasive GBC into the perimuscular connective tissue. Lymphatic, neural, and hematogenous invasions occur earlier with GBC than with other cancers of the gut.

Adenocarcinomas progress from metaplasia–dysplasia to carcinoma in situ to cancer. Chronic inflammation may play a role in the development of premalignant lesions.[212] Two types of metaplasia—intestinal and squamous—have been found in patients with GBC. The relation of intestinal metaplasia to the subsequent development of GBC has not been determined. Squamous metaplasia, in which squamous epithelium replaces the normal gallbladder epithelium, is a rare premalignant lesion associated with squamous cell cancer of the gallbladder. Cholecystitis follicularis, a rare type of inflammation, has been reported in a few cases of GBC, but its premalignant potential is unclear.[212] Progression from dysplasia to carcinoma in situ to invasive cancer in the gallbladder epithelium can take about 15 years.[213] Dysplastic changes are found in adjacent mucosa in most GBCs. Gallbladder adenomas are rarely encountered or associated with dysplasia.

Several mutations have been reported in GBCs. K-ras and p53 mutations are common.[186,214] Mutant *p53* is found in 92% of invasive carcinomas, 86% of carcinoma in situ, and 28% of dysplastic epithelium, but not in adenomas.[215] K-ras mutations are identified in 39% of GBCs.[216] Data on the expression of ras and myc are conflicting. In one study, b-RAF mutations were evident in 33% of GBCs.[217] The *erbB2* oncoprotein is overexpressed in some patients with GBC, and transgenic mice that express *erbB2* in the gallbladder epithelium develop GBC. Activated *EGFR* and *c-MET* may occur.[218,219] The fragile histidine triad (*FHIT*) gene is a candidate tumor suppressor gene in GBCs.[220] Epigenetic inactivation of *SEMA3B* and *FHIT* occurs in some GBCs.[221]

The malignant potential of APBJ is quite high and this anatomic variant is associated with premalignant histologic changes of epithelial hyperplasia with a papillary or villous appearance. The nonmalignant areas of the gallbladder of patients with APBJ-associated GBC show increased hyperplastic changes in the gallbladder mucosa compared with patients with sporadic GBCs.[222] In a cat model, side-to-side biliary–pancreatic anastomosis produced hyperplastic changes in the gallbladder within 6 months.[223] Although K-ras mutations are not commonly observed in lesions associated with gallstones, they are frequently identified in dysplastic lesions associated with APBJ. The differences in presentation, morphology, and molecular changes indicate that there are at least two distinct pathways to gallbladder carcinogenesis associated with either stone disease or with APBJ.[224]

Prevention

The low incidence of GBCs in some countries may be related to the rate of cholecystectomy performed for gallstone disease. However, the prevention of GBCs is not considered as a sole indication to perform cholecystectomy in patients who have asymptomatic gallstones. The incidence of gallbladder cancer is low compared with the incidence of gallstones in the population.

In certain high-risk conditions involving abnormalities within the gallbladder wall, a prophylactic cholecystectomy could be considered. A calcified or *porcelain* gallbladder is an indication

for cholecystectomy in the asymptomatic patient, because up to 25% of cases will be associated with gallbladder cancer. Patients with pancreaticobiliary maljunction and a normal-sized bile duct may benefit from a prophylactic cholecystectomy.[225] A study of northern Indian women reported a benefit of prophylactic cholecystectomy.[226] A serum CA19-9 evaluation and bile cytology may be helpful in making a preoperative diagnosis of cancer. A laparoscopic cholecystectomy could be reserved for those with normal markers and negative cytology. For those highly suspicious of cancer, the laparoscopic approach is not reasonable because of the risk for inadvertent seeding of the peritoneal cavity.

Diagnosis

Patients with gallbladder cancer are often asymptomatic. When symptoms occur, they may be similar to biliary colic or chronic cholecystitis, and are nonspeciifc. In contrast to biliary colic, patients with GBCs may have diffuse abdominal pain of a more constant nature. As a result of the low index of suspicion, patients with gallbladder cancer present with symptoms at an advanced stage of disease, or as incidental findings at the time of imaging or cholecystectomy for unrelated reasons. Recent weight loss and persistent right upper quadrant pain should raise the suspicion of GBCs in elderly patients over 70 years of age.

In early stage disease, symptoms can mimic those of cholelithiasis and cholecystitis or they may be related to associated cholelithiasis. Pain may be dull and aching, colicky, sharp, constant, or intermittent, with radiation to the back and associated with nausea, vomiting, and anorexia. At more advanced stages, jaundice, weight loss, hepatomegaly, a palpable mass, or ascites may develop. Jaundice can result from the obstruction of extrahepatic bile ducts by direct tumor growth or from metastatic disease. Jaundice is a poor prognostic sign, and 85% of patients with jaundice have unresectable tumors.[188] Mirizzi syndrome, in which compression of the common hepatic duct results from an impacted stone in the gallbladder neck, can be a presentation of GBC. Rarely, duodenal or colonic obstruction, cholecystoenteric fistula, or evidence of extraabdominal metastases such as palpable mass, ascites, or paraneoplastic syndromes such as acanthosis nigricans may occur. These indicate an advanced malignancy and unresectable disease.

Tumor spread can involve the liver and the extrahepatic biliary tree by direct spread. Liver metastases without full-thickness invasion of the gallbladder wall occurs in less than 10% of cases. Lymph node metastasis to the cystic, pericholedochal, peripancreatic, and celiac nodes occurs early, and are present at the time of diagnosis in more than half of patients. Direct invasion of the duodenum or colon, intraperitoneal spread, Krukenberg tumors (i.e., ovarian metastases), and hematogenous dissemination can also occur.[3]

Laboratory findings lack specificity and are not diagnostic. Patients may have increased alkaline phosphatase and bilirubin levels as a result of ductal obstruction in advanced cases. Serum CEA or CA19-9 may be elevated, but these tumor markers are not diagnostic. A CA19-9 level above 20 U/mL has a 79% sensitivity and a 79% specificity for the diagnosis of GBCs. A CEA greater than 4 ng/mL is 93% specific for GBCs, but sensitivity is only 50% for detecting cancer. CA125 has also been reported to be a reasonable marker for gallbladder cancer in some small studies.[227]

An ultrasound is the usual initial diagnostic study whenever gall bladder or biliary tract disease is suspected. Findings on ultrasonography of the gallbladder that are suggestive, but not diagnostic, of GBCs include thickening of the wall, a lumenal mass, calcification, or a mass lesion. A comparison between patients with unsuspected GBCs and those with benign gallbladder disease found that a solitary stone or displaced stone, or an intralumenal or invasive mass were more commonly associated with cancer.[228] On ultrasonography, a discontinuous gallbladder mucosa, echogenic mucosa, and submucosal echolucency were significantly more common in GBC than in benign gallbladder disease. A polypoid mass was present in 27% and a gallbladder-replacing or invasive mass was present in 50% of cases of GBC examined.[228]

Mucosal thickening should be viewed with suspicion. US will detect polyps that may represent nonmalignant lesions such as adenomas, papillomas, or cholesterolosis in addition to GBCs. An invasive cancer is more likely in polyps greater than 1 cm in diameter. The accuracy of US for staging disease extent or spread is low (38% in one study).[229] EUS is useful for a further diagnosis of polyps or gallbladder wall thickening. EUS has a higher sensitivity (92% versus 54%) and specificity (88% versus 54%) for GBC than US. It can also enable FNA of any suspicious masses or aspiration of bile for cytology. If a tumor is present, EUS can be useful for staging by assessing tumor wall invasion or distant nodal spread.

Abdominal CT scans or MRI can identify intraluminal polyps, gallbladder wall thickening, mass lesions, hepatic involvement, nodal enlargement, or other distant spread. CT scanning will reveal a mass partially obliterating the gallbladder lumen, a polypoidal mass, or diffuse wall thickening. However, only one-third of pathologically positive nodes are identified preoperatively by CT scan. The use of MRI for the diagnostic workup of GBC can be helpful. MRCP may provide more detailed information than can be provided by US or CT scan.[230] MRI may be helpful in determining vascular invasion and nodal involvement. There is almost no role for cholangiography using ERCP or PTC, although these may occasionally be needed to plan the extent of surgical resection by determining the extent of ductal involvement or spread.[231]

Fluorodeoxyglucose (FDG)-PET scanning has low sensitivity for extrahepatic disease. However, PET scanning may identify a disease that has not been radiologically apparent and resulted in a change in stage and treatment in 17% to 23% of cases with presumed localized resectable disease in one study.[65] For suspicious lesions on US, PET scanning has been reported to have a sensitivity of 0.80 and a specificity of 0.82, a positive predictive value of 0.67, and a negative predictive value of 0.90.[232]

The need for tissue biopsy before definitive exploration and resection of a mass that is suspicious for GBC is controversial because of the risks of the tumor seeding into the peritoneal cavity or abdominal wound. Bile cytology may avoid these and should be performed whenever any patient suspected of having GBC who undergoes ERCP or PTC. The diagnostic accuracy of combined ERCP and bile cytology is 50% for gallbladder cancers. The sensitivity of bile cytology alone for the diagnosis of GBC has been reported between 50% and 73%.[233] If referral for surgical management is being considered, a diagnosis based on bile cytology or percutaneous FNA cytology would be preferable to operative or laparoscopic biopsy.

Percutaneous FNA or core needle biopsy are indicated for unresectable masses. The risk of tumor seeding within the needle tract is greater with the latter. EUS-directed FNA for gallbladder lesions is associated with a 80% sensitivity and 100% specificity.[234] Percutaneous FNA has an 88% accuracy for gallbladder cancers with a negligible false-positive rate.[233] EUS may be useful to distinguish between inflammatory nodes and metastatic disease during an evaluation of periportal and peripancreatic adenopathy. A staging laparoscopy to determine the extent of spread may be helpful for some patients.[127,169]

Survival of patients with GBC is related to stage and histologic type of cancer. Lymph node involvement is rare in stage T1 tumors[235,236]; that is, lymph node involvement almost never occurs until the muscularis has been penetrated. After that, lymph node involvement is common, occurring in about 50% of stage II patients and in 70% to 80% of patients in stage III and IV. There is a close correlation between lymph node involvement and prognosis. Most long-term survivors are patients with well-differentiated tumors that were minimally invasive. These are usually found incidentally at or immediately after cholecystectomy.

GBCs may be identified incidentally at the time of cholecystectomy; the incidence ranges from 0.3% to 1%. If this occurs during a laparoscopic procedure, the potential for port-site

implantation should be considered,[237,238] and the gallbladder is extracted in a plastic bag. Implantation can arise due to physical contact between the tumor and port site tissues during extraction, or can be related to positive-pressure pneumoperitoneum.[239] The tissue surrounding the trocar ports is excised because seeding may have occurred. Early reoperation may be necessary if the tumor is discovered on later pathologic examination, or with uncertainty about residual tumor. Stage I gallbladder carcinomas with clear resection margins may not require further surgical treatment.

Gallbladder polyps may be malignant but are rarely so when they are smaller than 1 cm in diameter. In a series of patients with gallbladder polyps, none were malignant if less than 1 cm in diameter, but 23% of polyps larger than 1 cm were malignant.[240] In another series, 88% of polyps larger than 1 cm in diameter were malignant, and polyps larger than 1.8 cm were more likely to contain a more advanced stage of cancer.[241] FNA is an accurate way of distinguishing between polyps due to cholesterolosis and neoplastic polyps,[233] especially for polyps that are larger than 1 cm in diameter[242]; however, it is much less accurate in determining whether a neoplastic polyp is an adenoma or carcinoma.[242] Doppler US imaging of blood flow within a neoplastic polyp may also be useful in distinguishing these lesions from benign polyps.

Staging

Several staging systems have been described for GBC. These systems incorporate clinical and pathologic characteristics with prognostic significance. These include the modified Nevin system, the Japanese Biliary Surgical Society system, and the AJCC TNM staging system.[6,235,243] The use of these different staging systems makes it difficult to compare the treatment results of different series in the literature. The AJCC TNM staging system should be used for the standardization of reporting across studies so as to enable a comparison of treatment results. This staging system is shown in Table 53.4. Stage 1 includes tumors that invade the lamina propria or muscle layer. Tumors can arise in the Rokitansky–Aschoff sinuses and are considered stage I in a subserosal position. Tumors with invasion into the perimuscular connective tissue are considered stage II, and liver invasion is stage III. Extensive nodal metastasis to periaortic, pericaval, superior mesenteric artery, or celiac artery is now considered stage IVA. Patients with distant metastasis are considered stage IVB. GBCs undergo histopathologic grading from G1 (well differentiated) to G4 (undifferentiated). Although the grade does not factor into staging, it has prognostic significance, with high-grade tumors having a worse prognosis.

Management

Most studies of treatment approaches for GBC are from small case series or are heterogenous studies that include other biliary tract cancers. As a result, the optimal approaches to surgery or palliative therapy with chemoradiation are unknown. The stage of the disease determines the treatment approach and prognosis.[235] The diagnosis of GBC usually occurs at advanced stages TNM III or IV, and most patients in advanced stages are not resectable.[244,245] A suggested management scheme is outlined in Figure 53.4.

Surgery. Surgery is the only potentially curative option for GBCs. Absolute contraindications to surgery include distant metastases, vascular involvement, or nodal spread beyond the hepatoduodenal ligament. When GBC is suspected, an open cholecystectomy is preferable to laparoscopic excision to minimize the potential impact of tumor implantation due to gallbladder perforation and bile spillage that are more frequent with the latter. An extraserosal cholecystectomy excises the gallbladder on a deeper plane than a standard cholecystectomy, so that the gallbladder and all connective tissue down to actual liver tissue are removed. The extent of resection will depend on the extent of disease spread. For T1 lesions where the tumor has not penetrated the muscularis mucosa and margins are negative, cholecystectomy is sufficient and can

TABLE 53.4

American Joint Committee on Cancer TNM Staging of Gallbladder Cancer

Primary Tumor (T)

TX	Primary tumor cannot be assessed
T0	No evidence of primary tumor
Tis	Carcinoma in situ
T1	Tumor invades lamina propria or muscular layer
T1a	Tumor invades lamina propria
T1b	Tumor invades muscular layer
T2	Tumor invades perimuscular connective tissue; no extension beyond serosa or into liver
T3	Tumor perforates the serosa (visceral peritoneum) and/or directly invades the liver and/or one other adjacent organ or structure, such as the stomach, duodenum, colon, pancreas, omentum, or extrahepatic bile ducts
T4	Tumor invades main portal vein or hepatic artery or invades two or more extrahepatic organs or structures

Regional Lymph Nodes (N)

NX	Regional lymph nodes cannot be assessed
N0	No regional lymph node metastasis
N1	Metastases to nodes along the cystic duct, common bile duct, hepatic artery, and/or portal vein
N2	Metastases to periaortic, pericaval, superior mesenteric artery, and/or celiac artery lymph nodes

Distant Metastasis (M)

M0	No distant metastasis
M1	Distant metastasis

Anatomic Stage/Prognostic Groups

Stage 0	Tis	N0	M0
Stage I	T1	N0	M0
Stage II	T2	N0	M0
Stage IIIA	T3	N0	M0
Stage IIIB	T1–3	N1	M0
Stage IVA	T4	N0–1	M0
Stage IVB	Any T	N2	M0
	Any T	Any N	M1

Used with the permission of the American Joint Committee on Cancer (AJCC), Chicago, Illinois. The original source for this material is the *AJCC Cancer Staging Manual*, Seventh Edition (2010) published by Springer Science and Business Media LLC, www.springerlink.com, page 213–214.

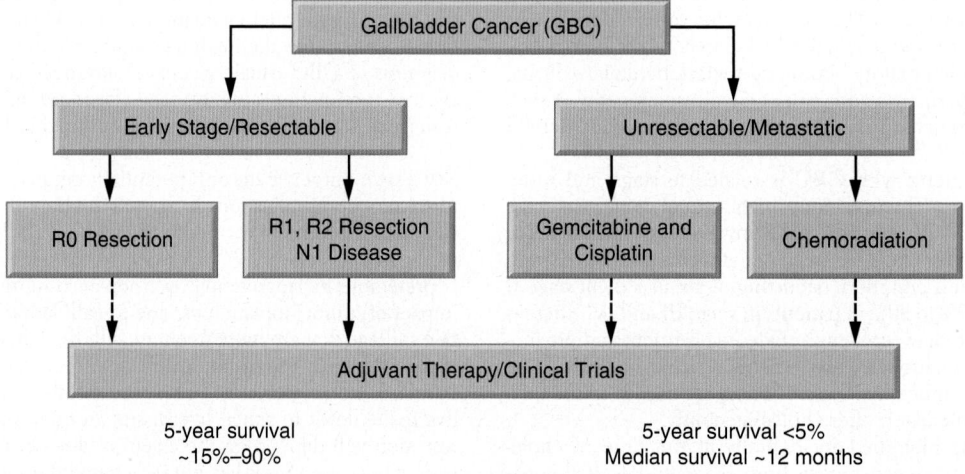

Figure 53.4 Algorithm for the management of gallbladder carcinoma.

be curative. Direct tumor growth into the liver or duodenum or colon is not a contraindication to surgery, but the extent of spread will guide the extent of resection for these T2 to T4 lesions. Thus, wedge resection of the liver, portal lymph node dissection, and extrahepatic bile duct resection, or even a pancreaticoduodenectomy may be needed in addition to a cholecystectomy. If there is obvious penetration to the serosal layer on the deep surface of the gallbladder, or if margins are positive, or the muscularis has been penetrated, resection of at least liver segments IVb and V, and a lymph node dissection are performed. If the cystic duct resection margin is positive, then, in addition, the extrahepatic bile duct is excised to clear margins. A more extensive liver resection may be required if the tumor has penetrated further into the liver. If negative resection margins are achieved, 5-year survival rates range from 90% in stage I disease, 80% in stage II, 40% in stage III, and 15% in stage IV. Lymph node involvement portends a worse prognosis than local hepatic invasion alone.[243,245] A pancreaticoduodenectomy may be considered for T2 to T4 disease, but the results remain poor in advanced stages.[246]

Randomized studies did not show a benefit of preoperative biliary decompression for jaundiced patients.[247–249] However, these studies were performed in an era in which surgical intervention mostly involved palliative bypass of the biliary tree, and the potential benefits of preoperative decompression prior to either pancreaticoduodenectomy or liver resection are not defined.

Adjuvant Therapy. GBC has a high risk of systemic spread and local–regional failure and adjuvant chemotherapy and radiotherapy are recommended by most cancer centers.

As with other biliary tract cancers, published reports on adjuvant radiotherapy or chemoradiation therapy after a resection for gallbladder cancer consist of retrospective reviews that vary in the type of radiation treatment (e.g., EBRT, brachytherapy, or IORT) and the extent of surgical resection (complete or incomplete). As a result, they cannot provide adequate evidence upon which a standard treatment recommendation could be based.

A median survival of approximately 2 years has been reported for patients receiving adjuvant therapy.

In a study of 21 patients who received postoperative adjunct EBRT with 5-FU, EBRT was applied to a median dose of 54 Gy in fractions of 1.8 to 2.0 Gy per day, with one patient also receiving 15 Gy of IORT after EBRT, the median survival rates were 0.6, 1.4, and 15.1 years, and 2-year local control rates were 0%, 80%, and 88% for patients with gross residual tumor, microscopic residual tumor, and no residual disease, respectively.[250] For six patients who received more than 54 Gy, the 3-year local control rate was 100% compared with 65% for 15 patients who received less than 54 Gy. In a randomized trial comparing mitomycin C and 5-FU with observation alone that enrolled 140 patients with gallbladder cancers, a significantly better 5-year survival was seen with chemotherapy, but these differences were not apparent when an intent-to-treat analysis was performed.[141]

Chemotherapy. Although the role of chemotherapy given in the adjuvant setting has not been defined definitively, given the poor outcomes for patients with resected disease, it remains an area of active investigation. As described earlier, data from pivotal phase III studies using gemcitabine- or fluoropyrimidine-based

regimens is eagerly awaited. New approaches beyond the currently available chemotherapeutic agents are needed for these cancers to achieve any improvements in survival. Understanding the molecular and genomic contributors to this cancer may enable more focused therapy in the future.

Palliative Care. Advanced GBC has a 1-year survival rate of less than 5%. Although the resection of gross disease may provide palliation and, in some instances, a chance for cure, it may not always be possible. Patients with advanced disease should be considered for clinical trials. The aggressive nature and dismal prognosis of advanced unresectable cancer should be considered when deciding on palliative management. The goals of palliative treatment are to prevent biliary and bowel obstruction and to relieve pain.

Stenting. If biliary obstruction is present, percutaneous stenting for relief of obstruction can be performed by percutaneous or endoscopic approaches similar to that for other cancers such as dCCAs and pCCAs.

Surgery. Surgical bypass is not usually warranted because of the poor expected survival. The resection of hematogenous metastasis or of distant nodal disease is not justified.

Chemotherapy. In the UK-ABC-02 study described earlier, 36.3% (149 of 410) of the patients had advanced gallbladder cancer. The response rate was 37.7% versus 21.4%. Median overall survival and progression-free survival differences were not reported separately, but the survival benefit did demonstrate significance on a subgroup analysis in patients with gallbladder cancer (HR, 0.63; 95% CI, 0.42 to 0.89). As such, the standard of care in patients with advanced GBC is also regarded to be gemcitabine in combination with cisplatin. As described previously, although fluoropyrimidine-based therapies have shown evidence of preliminary efficacy, the role of subsequent lines of systemic chemotherapy remains to be definitively defined. Akin to CCA, therapeutic strategies based on genomic profiling of tumors will also be an area of critical study to best define approaches that can be more individualized in nature.

Regional Therapy. Regional therapy is possible for gallbladder cancer. In one study, a 48% overall response rate and a prolongation of median survival from 5 to 14 months compared with historical controls was reported with intra-arterial mitomycin C.[251]

Radiation Therapy. EBRT may be considered for symptomatic patients. The limited data available suggest that tumor control is rarely possible, although some GBCs may be radiosensitive and spread is mainly by local–regional growth.[252,253] However, radiation therapy may be considered for palliation of jaundice in some cases, or used in multimodality approaches combining EBRT with a 5FU-based treatment. The latter approach is supported by consensus guidelines from the European Society of Medical Oncology and the National Comprehensive Cancer Network.[254] Although the benefit of EBRT is minimal, with a median survival of only 6 to 8 months, it does appear to be well tolerated and may improve symptoms and prolong survival in selected patients.

SELECTED REFERENCES

The full reference list can be accessed at lwwhealthlibrary.com/oncology.

1. Patel T. Cholangiocarcinoma—controversies and challenges. *Nat Rev Gastroenterol Hepatol* 2011;8:189–200.
2. Razumilava N, Gores GJ. Classification, diagnosis, and management of cholangiocarcinoma. *Clin Gastroenterol Hepatol* 2013;11:13–21.
5. DeOliveira ML, Cunningham SC, Cameron JL, et al. Cholangiocarcinoma: thirty-one-year experience with 564 patients at a single institution. *Ann Surg* 2007;245:755–762.
6. Edge SB, Compton CC. The American Joint Committee on Cancer: the 7th edition of the AJCC cancer staging manual and the future of TNM. *Ann Surg Oncol* 2010;17:1471–1474.

8. Tyson GL, El-Serag HB. Risk factors for cholangiocarcinoma. *Hepatology* 2011;54:173–184.

11. Welzel TM, Graubard BI, El-Serag HB, et al. Risk factors for intrahepatic and extrahepatic cholangiocarcinoma in the United States: a population-based case-control study. *Clin Gastroenterol Hepatol* 2007;5:1221–1228.

15. Palmer WC, Patel T. Are common factors involved in the pathogenesis of primary liver cancers? A meta-analysis of risk factors for intrahepatic cholangiocarcinoma. *J Hepatol* 2012;57:69–76.

17. Broome U, Olsson R, Loof L, et al. Natural history and prognostic factors in 305 Swedish patients with primary sclerosing cholangitis. *Gut* 1996;38:610–615.

23. Hasumi A, Matsui H, Sugioka A, et al. Precancerous conditions of biliary tract cancer in patients with pancreaticobiliary maljunction: reappraisal of nationwide survey in Japan. *J Hepatobiliary Pancreat Surg* 2000;7:551–555.

25. Flanigan DP. Biliary carcinoma associated with biliary cysts. *Cancer* 1977;40:880–883.

27. Taylor AC, Palmer KR. Caroli's disease. *Eur J Gastroenterol Hepatol* 1998;10:105–108.

29. Kumagai S, Kurumatani N, Arimoto A, et al. Cholangiocarcinoma among offset colour proof-printing workers exposed to 1,2-dichloropropane and/or dichloromethane. *Occup Environ Med* 2013;70:508–510.

32. Shaib YH, El-Serag HB, Davila JA, et al. Risk factors of intrahepatic cholangiocarcinoma in the United States: a case-control study. *Gastroenterology* 2005;128:620–626.

35. Sia D, Tovar V, Moeini A, et al. Intrahepatic cholangiocarcinoma: pathogenesis and rationale for molecular therapies. *Oncogene* 2013;32:4861–4870.

38. Hezel AF, Deshpande V, Zhu AX. Genetics of biliary tract cancers and emerging targeted therapies. *J Clin Oncol* 2010;28:3531–3540.

41. O'Dell MR, Huang JL, Whitney-Miller CL, et al. Kras(G12D) and p53 mutation cause primary intrahepatic cholangiocarcinoma. *Cancer Res* 2012;72:1557–1567.

42. Aishima SI, Taguchi KI, Sugimachi K, et al. c-erbB-2 and c-MET expression relates to cholangiocarcinogenesis and progression of intrahepatic cholangiocarcinoma. *Histopathology* 2002;40:269–278.

43. Borger DR, Tanabe KK, Fan KC, et al. Frequent mutation of isocitrate dehydrogenase (IDH)1 and IDH2 in cholangiocarcinoma identified through broad-based tumor genotyping. *Oncologist* 2012;17:72–79.

44. Voss JS, Holtegaard LM, Kerr SE, et al. Molecular profiling of cholangiocarcinoma shows potential for targeted therapy treatment decisions. *Hum Pathol* 2013;44:1216–1222.

46. Sia D, Hoshida Y, Villanueva A, et al. Integrative molecular analysis of intrahepatic cholangiocarcinoma reveals 2 classes that have different outcomes. *Gastroenterology* 2013;144:829–840.

47. Andersen JB, Spee B, Blechacz BR, et al. Genomic and genetic characterization of cholangiocarcinoma identifies therapeutic targets for tyrosine kinase inhibitors. *Gastroenterology* 2012;142:1021–1031.

48. Andersen JB, Thorgeirsson SS. Genetic profiling of intrahepatic cholangiocarcinoma. *Curr Opin Gastroenterol* 2012;28:266–272.

50. Lim JH. Cholangiocarcinoma: morphologic classification according to growth pattern and imaging findings. *AJR Am J Roentgenol* 2003;181:819–827.

51. Burke EC, Jarnagin WR, Hochwald SN, et al. Hilar Cholangiocarcinoma: patterns of spread, the importance of hepatic resection for curative operation, and a presurgical clinical staging system. *Ann Surg* 1998;228:385–394.

52. Patel T. Increasing incidence and mortality of primary intrahepatic cholangiocarcinoma in the United States. *Hepatology* 2001;33:1353–1357.

53. Patel T. Worldwide trends in mortality from biliary tract malignancies. *BMC Cancer* 2002;2:10.

54. McLean L, Patel T. Racial and ethnic variations in the epidemiology of intrahepatic cholangiocarcinoma in the United States. *Liver Int* 2006;26:1047–1053.

57. Choi BI, Han JK, Shin YM, et al. Peripheral cholangiocarcinoma: comparison of MRI with CT. *Abdom Imaging* 1995;20:357–360.

59. Soyer P, Bluemke DA, Sibert A, et al. MR imaging of intrahepatic cholangiocarcinoma. *Abdom Imaging* 1995;20:126–130.

62. Rullier A, Le Bail B, Fawaz R, et al. Cytokeratin 7 and 20 expression in cholangiocarcinomas varies along the biliary tract but still differs from that in colorectal carcinoma metastasis. *Am J Surg Pathol* 2000;24:870–876.

66. Ribero D, Pinna AD, Guglielmi A, et al. Surgical Approach for long-term survival of patients with intrahepatic cholangiocarcinoma: a multi-institutional analysis of 434 patients. *Arch Surg* 2012;147:1107–1113.

70. Valle J, Wasan H, Palmer DH, et al. Cisplatin plus gemcitabine versus gemcitabine for biliary tract cancer. *N Engl J Med* 2010;362:1273–1281.

71. Lee S, Oh SY, Kim BG, et al. Second-line treatment with a combination of continuous 5-fluorouracil, doxorubicin, and mitomycin-C (conti-FAM) in gemcitabine-pretreated pancreatic and biliary tract cancer. *Am J Clin Oncol* 2009;32:348–352.

72. Moretto R, Raimondo L, De Stefano A, et al. FOLFIRI in patients with locally advanced or metastatic pancreatic or biliary tract carcinoma: a monoinstitutional experience. *Anticancer Drugs* 2013;24:980–985.

75. Arai Y, Totoki Y, Hosoda F, et al. FGFR2 tyrosine kinase fusions define a unique molecular subtype of cholangiocarcinoma. *Hepatology* 2014;59:1427–1434.

76. Wu YM, Su F, Kalyana-Sundaram S, et al. Identification of targetable FGFR gene fusions in diverse cancers. *Cancer Discov* 2013;3:636–647.

80. Hultcrantz R, Olsson R, Danielsson A, et al. A 3-year prospective study on serum tumor markers used for detecting cholangiocarcinoma in patients with primary sclerosing cholangitis. *J Hepatol* 1999;30:669–673.

82. Chen CY, Shiesh SC, Tsao HC, et al. The assessment of biliary CA 125, CA 19-9 and CEA in diagnosing cholangiocarcinoma—the influence of sampling time and hepatolithiasis. *Hepatogastroenterology* 2002;49:616–620.

85. Nehls O, Gregor M, Klump B. Serum and bile markers for cholangiocarcinoma. *Semin Liver Dis* 2004;24:139–154.

87. Wongkham S, Sheehan JK, Boonla C, et al. Serum MUC5AC mucin as a potential marker for cholangiocarcinoma. *Cancer Lett* 2003;195:93–99.

88. Hatzaras I, Schmidt C, Muscarella P, et al. Elevated CA 19-9 portends poor prognosis in patients undergoing resection of biliary malignancies. *HPB (Oxford)* 2010;12:134–138.

90. Masselli G, Gualdi G. Hilar cholangiocarcinoma: MRI/MRCP in staging and treatment planning. *Abdom Imaging* 2008;33:444–451.

91. Masselli G, Manfredi R, Vecchioli A, et al. MR imaging and MR cholangiopancreatography in the preoperative evaluation of hilar cholangiocarcinoma: correlation with surgical and pathologic findings. *Eur Radiol* 2008;18:2213–2221.

93. Chen YK, Parsi MA, Binmoeller KF, et al. Single-operator cholangioscopy in patients requiring evaluation of bile duct disease or therapy of biliary stones (with videos). *Gastrointest Endosc* 2011;74:805–814.

95. Shah RJ, Langer DA, Antillon MR, et al. Cholangioscopy and cholangioscopic forceps biopsy in patients with indeterminate pancreaticobiliary pathology. *Clin Gastroenterol Hepatol* 2006;4:219–225.

100. Verbeek PC, van Leeuwen DJ, de Wit LT, et al. Benign fibrosing disease at the hepatic confluence mimicking Klatskin tumors. *Surgery* 1992;112:866–871.

103. de Bellis M, Sherman S, Fogel EL, et al. Tissue sampling at ERCP in suspected malignant biliary strictures (Part 2). *Gastrointest Endosc* 2002;56:720–730.

106. Ferrari Junior AP, Lichtenstein DR, Slivka A, et al. Brush cytology during ERCP for the diagnosis of biliary and pancreatic malignancies. *Gastrointest Endosc* 1994;40:140–145.

107. Jarnagin WR, Fong Y, DeMatteo RP, et al. Staging, resectability, and outcome in 225 patients with hilar cholangiocarcinoma. *Ann Surg* 2001;234:507–517.

108. Bismuth H, Nakache R, Diamond T. Management strategies in resection for hilar cholangiocarcinoma. *Ann Surg* 1992;215:31–38.

110. Deoliveira ML, Schulick RD, Nimura Y, et al. New staging system and a registry for perihilar cholangiocarcinoma. *Hepatology* 2011;53:1363–1371.

111. Neumaier CE, Bertolotto M, Perrone R, et al. Staging of hilar cholangiocarcinoma with ultrasound. *J Clin Ultrasound* 1995;23:173–178.

112. Darwish Murad S, Kim WR, Harnois DM, et al. Efficacy of neoadjuvant chemoradiation, Followed by liver transplantation, for perihilar cholangiocarcinoma at 12 US centers. *Gastroenterology* 2012;143:88–98.

113. Murad SD, Heimbach JK, Gores GJ, et al. Excellent quality of life after liver transplantation for patients with perihilar cholangiocarcinoma who have undergone neoadjuvant chemoradiation. *Liver Transpl* 2013;19:521–528.

115. Heimbach JK, Haddock MG, Alberts SR, et al. Transplantation for hilar cholangiocarcinoma. *Liver Transpl* 2004;10:S65–S68.

116. Shimoda M, Farmer DG, Colquhoun SD, et al. Liver transplantation for cholangiocellular carcinoma: analysis of a single-center experience and review of the literature. *Liver Transpl* 2001;7:1023–1033.

119. Lillemoe KD, Cameron JL. Surgery for hilar cholangiocarcinoma: the Johns Hopkins approach. *J Hepatobiliary Pancreat Surg* 2000;7:115–121.

120. Hochwald SN, Burke EC, Jarnagin WR, et al. Association of preoperative biliary stenting with increased postoperative infectious complications in proximal cholangiocarcinoma. *Arch Surg* 1999;134:261–266.

123. Liu F, Li Y, Wei Y, et al. Preoperative biliary drainage before resection for hilar cholangiocarcinoma: whether or not? A systematic review. *Dig Dis Sci* 2011;56:663–672.

124. Sewnath ME, Karsten TM, Prins MH, et al. A meta-analysis on the efficacy of preoperative biliary drainage for tumors causing obstructive jaundice. *Ann Surg* 2002;236:17–27.

126. Nimura Y, Kamiya J, Kondo S, et al. Aggressive preoperative management and extended surgery for hilar cholangiocarcinoma: Nagoya experience. *J Hepatobiliary Pancreat Surg* 2000;7:155–162.

128. Ito K, Ito H, Allen PJ, et al. Adequate lymph node assessment for extrahepatic bile duct adenocarcinoma. *Ann Surg* 2010;251:675–681.

131. Bengmark S, Ekberg H, Evander A, et al. Major liver resection for hilar cholangiocarcinoma. *Ann Surg* 1988;207:120–125.

132. Washburn WK, Lewis WD, Jenkins RL. Aggressive surgical resection for cholangiocarcinoma. *Arch Surg* 1995;130:270–276.

134. Iwasaki Y, Okamura T, Ozaki A, et al. Surgical treatment for carcinoma at the confluence of the major hepatic ducts. *Surg Gynecol Obstet* 1986;162:457–464.

136. Nagorney DM, Donohue JH, Farnell MB, et al. Outcomes after curative resections of cholangiocarcinoma. *Arch Surg* 1993;128:871–877.

137. Otani K, Chijiiwa K, Kai M, et al. Outcome of surgical treatment of hilar cholangiocarcinoma. *J Gastrointest Surg* 2008;12:1033–1040.

138. Nakeeb A, Pitt HA, Sohn TA, et al. Cholangiocarcinoma. A spectrum of intrahepatic, perihilar, and distal tumors. *Ann Surg* 1996;224:463–473.

139. Klempnauer J, Ridder GJ, von Wasielewski R, et al. Resectional surgery of hilar cholangiocarcinoma: a multivariate analysis of prognostic factors. *J Clin Oncol* 1997;15:947–954.
140. Lee SW, Kim HJ, Park JH, et al. Clinical usefulness of 18F-FDG PET-CT for patients with gallbladder cancer and cholangiocarcinoma. *J Gastroenterol* 2010;45:560–566.
141. Takada T, Amano H, Yasuda H, et al. Is postoperative adjuvant chemotherapy useful for gallbladder carcinoma? A phase III multicenter prospective randomized controlled trial in patients with resected pancreaticobiliary carcinoma. *Cancer* 2002;95:1685–1695.
142. Hii MW, Gibson RN, Speer AG, et al. Role of radiology in the treatment of malignant hilar biliary strictures 2: 10 years of single-institution experience with percutaneous treatment. *Australas Radiol* 2003;47:393–403.
144. Jarnagin WR, Burke E, Powers C, et al. Intrahepatic biliary enteric bypass provides effective palliation in selected patients with malignant obstruction at the hepatic duct confluence. *Am J Surg* 1998;175:453–460.
145. Witzigmann H, Lang H, Lauer H. Guidelines for palliative surgery of cholangiocarcinoma. *HPB (Oxford)* 2008;10:154–160.
147. Ortner ME, Caca K, Berr F, et al. Successful photodynamic therapy for nonresectable cholangiocarcinoma: a randomized prospective study. *Gastroenterology* 2003;125:1355–1363.
150. Leggett CL, Gorospe EC, Murad MH, et al. Photodynamic therapy for unresectable cholangiocarcinoma: a comparative effectiveness systematic review and meta-analyses. *Photodiagnosis Photodyn Ther* 2012;9:189–195.
151. Ohnishi H, Asada M, Shichijo Y, et al. External radiotherapy for biliary decompression of hilar cholangiocarcinoma. *Hepatogastroenterology* 1995;42:265–268.
152. Leung J, Guiney M, Das R. Intraluminal brachytherapy in bile duct carcinomas. *Aust N Z J Surg* 1996;66:74–77.
155. Kopek N, Holt MI, Hansen AT, et al. Stereotactic body radiotherapy for unresectable cholangiocarcinoma. *Radiother Oncol* 2010;94:47–52.
157. Steel AW, Postgate AJ, Khorsandi S, et al. Endoscopically applied radiofrequency ablation appears to be safe in the treatment of malignant biliary obstruction. *Gastrointest Endosc* 2011;73:149–153.
159. Yamao K, Bhatia V, Mizuno N, et al. EUS-guided choledochoduodenostomy for palliative biliary drainage in patients with malignant biliary obstruction: results of long-term follow-up. *Endoscopy* 2008;40:340–342.
163. Nichols JC, Gores GJ, LaRusso NF, et al. Diagnostic role of serum CA 19-9 for cholangiocarcinoma in patients with primary sclerosing cholangitis. *Mayo Clin Proc* 1993;68:874–879.
164. Ramage JK, Donaghy A, Farrant JM, et al. Serum tumor markers for the diagnosis of cholangiocarcinoma in primary sclerosing cholangitis. *Gastroenterology* 1995;108:865–869.
166. Tio TL, Cheng J, Wijers OB, et al. Endosonographic TNM staging of extrahepatic bile duct cancer: comparison with pathological staging. *Gastroenterology* 1991;100:1351–1361.
167. Kluge R, Schmidt F, Caca K, et al. Positron emission tomography with [(18)F]fluoro-2-deoxy-D-glucose for diagnosis and staging of bile duct cancer. *Hepatology* 2001;33:1029–1035.
174. Prat F, Chapat O, Ducot B, et al. A randomized trial of endoscopic drainage methods for inoperable malignant strictures of the common bile duct. *Gastrointest Endosc* 1998;47:1–7.
175. Smith AC, Dowsett JF, Russell RC, et al. Randomised trial of endoscopic stenting versus surgical bypass in malignant low bileduct obstruction. *Lancet* 1994;344:1655–1660.
180. Randi G, Franceschi S, La Vecchia C. Gallbladder cancer worldwide: geographical distribution and risk factors. *Int J Cancer* 2006;118:1591–1602.
183. Strom BL, Soloway RD, Rios-Dalenz JL, et al. Risk factors for gallbladder cancer. An international collaborative case-control study. *Cancer* 1995;76:1747–1756.
186. Lazcano-Ponce EC, Miquel JF, Munoz N, et al. Epidemiology and molecular pathology of gallbladder cancer. *CA Cancer J Clin* 2001;51:349–364.
189. Maringhini A, Moreau JA, Melton LJ 3rd, et al. Gallstones, gallbladder cancer, and other gastrointestinal malignancies. An epidemiologic study in Rochester, Minnesota. *Ann Intern Med* 1987;107:30–35.
190. Strom BL, Soloway RD, Rios-Dalenz J, et al. Biochemical epidemiology of gallbladder cancer. *Hepatology* 1996;23:1402–1411.
194. Chijiiwa K, Kimura H, Tanaka M. Malignant potential of the gallbladder in patients with anomalous pancreaticobiliary ductal junction. The difference in risk between patients with and without choledochal cyst. *Int Surg* 1995;80:61–64.
200. Matsukura N, Yokomuro S, Yamada S, et al. Association between Helicobacter bilis in bile and biliary tract malignancies: H. bilis in bile from Japanese and Thai patients with benign and malignant diseases in the biliary tract. *Jpn J Cancer Res* 2002;93:842–847.
207. Perpetuo MD, Valdivieso M, Heilbrun LK, et al. Natural history study of gallbladder cancer: a review of 36 years experience at M. D. Anderson Hospital and Tumor Institute. *Cancer* 1978;42:330–335.
211. Diehl AK, Beral V. Cholecystectomy and changing mortality from gallbladder cancer. *Lancet* 1981;2:187–189.
214. Itoi T, Watanabe H, Ajioka Y, et al. APC, K-ras codon 12 mutations and p53 gene expression in carcinoma and adenoma of the gall-bladder suggest two genetic pathways in gall-bladder carcinogenesis. *Pathol Int* 1996;46:333–340.
217. Saetta AA, Papanastasiou P, Michalopoulos NV, et al. Mutational analysis of BRAF in gallbladder carcinomas in association with K-ras and p53 mutations and microsatellite instability. *Virchows Arch* 2004;445:179–182.
219. Nakazawa K, Dobashi Y, Suzuki S, et al. Amplification and overexpression of c-erbB-2, epidermal growth factor receptor, and c-MET in biliary tract cancers. *J Pathol* 2005;206:356–365.
222. Hanada K, Itoh M, Fujii K, et al. K-ras and p53 mutations in stage I gallbladder carcinoma with an anomalous junction of the pancreaticobiliary duct. *Cancer* 1996;77:452–458.
227. Shukla VK, Gurubachan, Sharma D, et al. Diagnostic value of serum CA242, CA 19-9, CA 15-3 and CA 125 in patients with carcinoma of the gallbladder. *Trop Gastroenterol* 2006;27:160–165.
232. Rodriguez-Fernandez A, Gomez-Rio M, Medina-Benitez A, et al. Application of modern imaging methods in diagnosis of gallbladder cancer. *J Surg Oncol* 2006;93:650–664.
234. Meara RS, Jhala D, Eloubeidi MA, et al. Endoscopic ultrasound-guided FNA biopsy of bile duct and gallbladder: analysis of 53 cases. *Cytopathology* 2006;17:42–49.
236. Tsukada K, Hatakeyama K, Kurosaki I, et al. Outcome of radical surgery for carcinoma of the gallbladder according to the TNM stage. *Surgery* 1996;120:816–821.
242. Wu SS, Lin KC, Soon MS, et al. Ultrasound-guided percutaneous transhepatic fine needle aspiration cytology study of gallbladder polypoid lesions. *Am J Gastroenterol* 1996;91:1591–1594.
245. Ruckert JC, Ruckert RI, Gellert K, et al. Surgery for carcinoma of the gallbladder. *Hepatogastroenterology* 1996;43:527–533.
247. Hatfield AR, Tobias R, Terblanche J, et al. Preoperative external biliary drainage in obstructive jaundice. A prospective controlled clinical trial. *Lancet* 1982;2:896–899.
250. Kresl JJ, Schild SE, Henning GT, et al. Adjuvant external beam radiation therapy with concurrent chemotherapy in the management of gallbladder carcinoma. *Int J Radiat Oncol Biol Phys* 2002;52:167–175.
253. Todoroki T, Iwasaki Y, Orii K, et al. Resection combined with intraoperative radiation therapy (IORT) for stage IV (TNM) gallbladder carcinoma. *World J Surg* 1991;15:357–366.
254. Eckel F, Brunner T, Jelic S, Grp EGW. Biliary cancer: ESMO Clinical Practice Guidelines for diagnosis, treatment and follow-up. *Ann Oncol* 2011;22:vi40–vi44.

PRACTICE OF ONCOLOGY

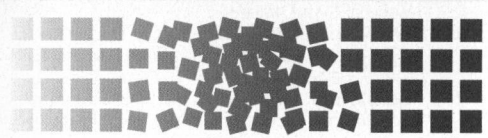

54 Cancer of the Small Bowel

Ronald S. Chamberlain, Krishnaraj Mahendraraj, and Syed Ammer Shah

SMALL BOWEL CANCER

Although the small intestine comprises 75% of the length and 90% of the total absorptive surface of the gastrointestinal tract, less than 3% of gastrointestinal malignancies occur in the small bowel.[1] Small bowel cancers (SBC) are 40- to 60-times less common than colorectal cancer. The rarity of SBCs makes them difficult to diagnose, especially considering their varied clinical presentation. With an increasing incidence and advanced stage at diagnosis, it has become even more important to understand the pathology of these rare but deadly cancers.

Epidemiology

SBC accounts for ~3% of all the gastrointestinal cancers with an equal male to female ratio and a median age of 66 years. The American Cancer Society estimates there will be 9,160 new cases of SBCs in 2014, with 1,210 deaths.[2,3] This number represents a steady increase in the incidence of SBCs from ~6,100 new cases per year in the 1980s based on information derived from the Surveillance, Epidemiology, and End Results (SEER) database registries.[1–5,8]

There are more than 40 SBC histologic subtypes, with 93% of them comprised of four major types: carcinoid (37.4%), adenocarcinoma (36.9%), lymphoma (17.3%), and gastrointestinal stromal tumors (8.4%).[6] Historically, adenocarcinoma had a higher incidence than carcinoid tumors, but this has changed over the past decade.[5–8] In terms of the location, ~50% of SBC occur in the duodenum, where adenocarcinoma predominates, followed by the jejunum (30%) and ileum, where lymphoma is more common proximally, and carcinoid tumors distally. There is an increased incidence of SBC among colon cancer patients and the reverse is true also, suggesting a similar causal mechanism rather than a surveillance bias or the carcinogenic effects treating the index primary.[6,9,10]

Pathogenesis and Risk Factors

Proposed risk factors for the predisposition to small bowel neoplasms are varied, although it is notable that 64% of small bowel tumors are malignant. Proposed factors that have been associated with SBC include:

1. Advanced age: SBCs occur predominantly in the elderly with a mean age of ~66 years.
2. Specific inheritable syndromes predisposing to SBC[11–32]:
   - *Familial adenomatosis polyposis (FAP) syndromes.* FAP is an autosomal-dominant disorder attributable to a mutation in the adenomatosis polyposis coli (APC) gene and characterized by the development of hundreds or thousands of polyps throughout the gastrointestinal tract, but predominately in the large bowel. FAP patients have a 100% lifetime risk of developing colorectal cancer, and this has led to a clearly defined role for total colectomy or proctocolectomy to prevent cancer development. FAP patients also inherit a 4% to 12% lifetime risk of developing adenocarcinoma of the duodenum or periampullary region, which is 300 times that of the general population, necessitating screening esophagogastroduodenoscopy (EGD) as part of the work-up.[11–18]
   - *Hereditary nonpolyposis colon cancer (HNPCC).* HNPCC, also known as Lynch syndrome, is a hereditary condition that results from a germ-line mutation in DNA mismatch repair genes, primarily *MSH2* and *MLH1*. This mutation predisposes one not only to an 80% lifetime risk of colorectal cancer, but also to an increased risk of endometrial, gastric, ovarian, urinary, small bowel, biliary, and skin cancers.[19,20] HNPCC patients have a SBC lifetime risk of 1% to 4%, or a 100-fold greater risk than the general population, which also tends to present 10 to 20 years earlier.[20] SBC may be the initial presentation of HNPCC in a small cohort of patients, and some clinicians recommend small bowel surveillance for this group.[20–25]
   - *Peutz-Jeghers syndrome (PJS).* PJS is an autosomal-dominant disorder characterized by benign hamartomatous polyps in the intestine along with melanocytic macules on the lips and oral mucosa. PJS is due to a mutation in the *STK11 (LKB1)* tumor suppressor gene, which results in a significant increased inherited risk for multiple cancer types, with the highest risk involving the gastrointestinal tract. By the age of 70 years, the cumulative gastrointestinal (GI) cancer risk is approximately 57% (colon cancer followed by SBC), which represents a 15-fold increased risk compared to the general population.[27,28]
   - *MUTYH-associated polyposis (MAP).* First described in 2002, the *MUTYH* gene encodes for DNA glycosylase, which is involved in oxidative DNA damage repair and belongs to the family of DNA mismatch repair genes. Mutations in this gene result in heritable predisposition to GI cancers, including SBC in an autosomal-recessive fashion. Mutations of this gene results in G to T transversions, usually involving the *APC* and *KRAS* gene, thus predisposing individuals to cancer development.[29,30]
   - *Cystic fibrosis.* A marginally increased risk of SBC has been documented in cystic fibrosis patients.[31]
3. *Inflammatory bowel disease.* Although only 2% of Crohn disease (CD) patients will develop a small bowel malignancy (typically an adenocarcinoma associated with >10 years of disease and involving the distal small bowel), this represents a 10- to 60-times higher risk than the general population.[33–35] Specifically, SBCs in CD occur more commonly in men, in the distal ileal location, are more common in small bowel bypass loops and in strictures, and in patients with exposure to asbestos or other carcinogens such as halogenated aromatic compounds.[36] A meta-analysis identified a 33.2 relative risk (95% confidence interval [CI], 15.9 to 60.9) of developing small bowel cancer among CD patients.[37–39]

4. *Celiac disease or sprue (CS).* CS is an autoimmune disorder characterized by villous atrophy, crypt hyperplasia, and increased intraepithelial lymphocytes caused by a reaction to the wheat protein gliadin in the presence of specific pairs of allelic variants in two HLA *DQ2/DQ8* genes. CS is associated with an increased risk of *enteropathy-associated T-cell lymphoma* (EATL), which can occur in up to 39% of patients with severe or refractory CS (RCS). The overall prevalence of RCS is low (0.6% to 1.5%). RCS can be subclassified into RCS type 1, which is characterized by increased but nonclonal expansion of intraepithelial lymphocytes (IEL), or RCS type 2, which displays clonal expansion of IELs that evolve into EATL in 60% to 80% of such patients within 5 years.[40–42]

5. *Immunosuppression.* Iatrogenic (therapeutic) or posttransplant immunosuppression is a generalized dysregulator of homeostasis and predisposes certain patients to both lymphomas and sarcomas. Small bowel lymphomas that develop in these patients are predominantly B-cell as opposed to T-cell lymphomas. Posttransplant lymphoproliferative disorders (PTLD) that occur develop primarily post–Epstein Barr viral infection and are typically B-cell lymphomas.

6. *Other malignancies.* The patient with other primary malignancies may also be at increased risk for SBCs. This includes patients with prior colorectal, pancreas, periampullary, uterine, ovarian, prostrate, thyroid, skin, and soft tissue tumors.[9,10,43] In fact, 30% to 40% of patients with SBCs have a synchronous malignancy, which may be associated with the primary pathologic entity or may reflect shared genetic or environmental risk factors.

7. *Modifiable risk factors.* Modifiable risk factors implicated in SBCs include alcohol use and obesity. In a recent large Asian study involving over 500,000 patients with a 10.6-year follow-up, a higher body mass index (>27.5 kg/m^2) and alcohol use (>400 g of ethanol per week) were associated with increased SBC risk. Notably, smoking is not associated with an increased risk of developing SBC.[44–46] Abstinence, weight loss, and dietary modifications (including adhering to a gluten-free diet in those with celiac disease) have been suggested to reduce the risk of SBCs.

Clinical Features

SBC presents in a variety of ways and is more likely to be symptomatic early in the disease course compared to benign tumors.[47,48] The most common presenting symptoms are abdominal pain (45% to 76%), nausea and vomiting (16% to 52%), weight loss (28% to 45%), fatigue and anemia (15% to 30%), and gastrointestinal bleeding (7% to 23%).[49–52] The most common clinical sign

of pallor is seen in ~40% of patients. Up to 77% of SBCs present acutely with either small bowel obstruction or perforation, particularly adenocarcinomas.[47] Patients with familial or genetic predisposition to SBCs present, on average, 10 years earlier compared to sporadic cases.[52–56]

In comparing different SBC histologies, adenocarcinoma is most often associated with abdominal pain and obstruction, whereas sarcomas and lymphomas are more often associated with bleeding and perforation, respectively. Adenocarcinomas are frequently found in the duodenum, carcinoid tumors affect the ileum and sarcomas, and lymphomas are found throughout the entire small bowel.

Diagnosis

The diagnosis of SBC is often delayed as a result of its rarity and nonspecific presentation. The mean duration of symptoms prior to an accurate SBC diagnosis ranges from 8 to 12 months.[48–51] A high index of clinical suspicion is imperative if the diagnosis is to be made early. In many instances, a preoperative diagnosis is not established because patients present emergently with hemorrhage, perforation, or obstruction. No single diagnostic test has sufficient sensitivity or specificity to be considered a gold standard.[141–167]

Conventional abdominal radiographs have a limited, nonspecific role in the diagnosis of SBCs. Plain abdominal radiographs are helpful when an obstruction exists, but even then accuracy is only 50% to 60%. A single or double contrast small bowel follow through (SBFT) is well suited for examination of luminal abnormalities and mucosal abnormalities, but is time consuming and associated with an accuracy ranging from 33% to 60%.[78–82] Small bowel enteroclysis may improve this accuracy to 90%.[57] A major limitation of both SBFT and enteroclysis is their inability to evaluate extraluminal pathology, which is circumvented by cross-sectional imaging, such as computed tomography (CT) scans and magnetic resonance imaging (MRI). CT- and MRI-based enteroclysis has improved the sensitivity and specificity of small bowel tumor detection compared to conventional enteroclysis.[58–60]

In clinical practice, a CT scan of the abdomen with oral and intravenous contrast is the most common diagnostic test utilized in the acute and chronic setting. Pathognomonic CT signs that differentiate between types of small bowel lesions have been well described. Adenocarcinoma appears as a discrete tumor mass with annular narrowing, abrupt concentric or irregular "overhanging edges," or as an ulcerative lesion. Lesions in the duodenum are typically intraluminal polyps, whereas more distal polypoid lesions present with intussusception and a characteristic "target sign" (Figs. 54.1 and 54.2).[61]

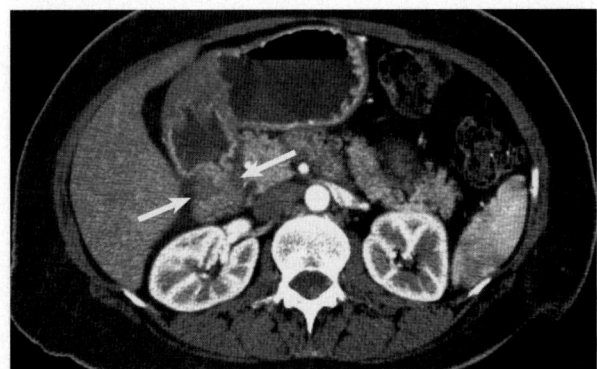
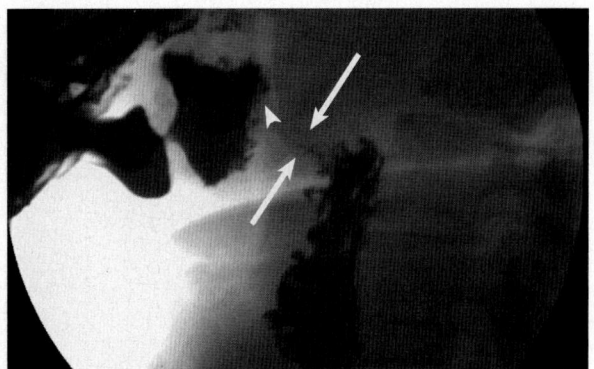

Figure 54.1 Moderately differentiated primary small bowel adenocarcinoma. **(A)** The contrast-enhanced axial computed tomography image shows an annular soft tissue lesion (*arrows*) in the duodenum, resulting in circumferential luminal narrowing and wall thickening. **(B)** A lateral image from subsequent upper gastrointestinal series shows the annular "apple-core" lesion, resulting in advanced narrowing of the duodenal lumen (*arrows*). Note the compressed, overhanging edges (*arrowhead*) of the small bowel at the margin of the mass.

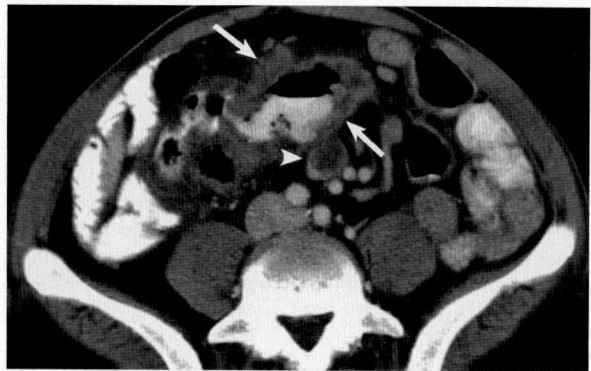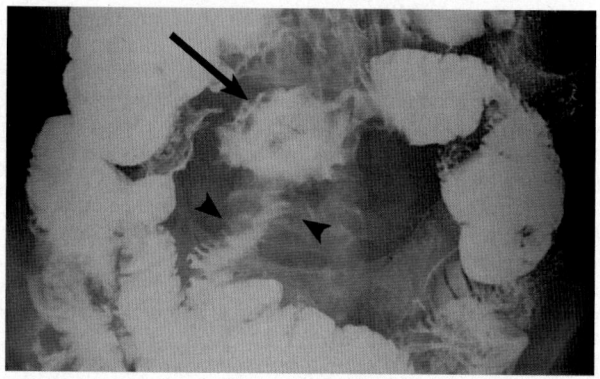

Figure 54.2 A small bowel intussusception due to primary small bowel adenocarcinoma. **(A)** A contrast-enhanced axial computed tomography image shows a small bowel target sign consistent with intussusception; the intussusceptum (*arrowhead*) telescopes into the intussuscipiens (*arrow*). The lead point for the intussusceptions was a primary small bowel carcinoma. **(B)** An image from small bowel follow through shows the "coiled spring" appearance of the intussusceptum (arrowhead) as it telescopes into the intussuscipiens (arrow).

Carcinoid tumors appear as hyperintense luminal masses due to increased vascularity. The tumors typically have intense desmoplastic reaction in response to biochemical products produced by the tumor that results in puckering of the adjacent mesentery, giving a characteristic stellate pattern on the CT scan not necessarily reflecting mesenteric invasion (Fig. 54.3).

Small bowel lymphomas present as circumferential mural thickening with low homogeneous attenuation and a characteristic aneurysmal dilatation in which the involved segment shows cavitary dilatation with a nodular, irregular luminal contour and peripheral bowel wall thickening (Fig. 54.4).[62] Sarcomas appear as homogeneous, well-circumscribed, hypervascular masses on CT (Fig. 54.5).[63–65]

The MRI has a defined niche in the assessment of early small bowel lesions given its improved soft tissue delineation and it may be pivotal in detecting early small bowel pathology (Table 54.1).[66–70] Somatostatin receptor scans (octreoscan) and metaiodobenzylguanidine (MIBG) scans may be helpful in localizing and diagnosing of small bowel carcinoid tumors. Octreoscan employs a ^{111}In-diethylenetriaminepentaacetic acid analog that targets somatostatin receptors. Over 90% of carcinoid tumors express somatostatin receptors, and this test has a sensitivity of 80% to 100%. Octreoscans may also provide a functional map of the tumor for anticipated radiolabelled immunotherapy-targeted therapy depending on the stage of the disease.[71]

Positron emission tomography (PET)/CT scans are useful in the initial diagnosis and in disease staging for small bowel adenocarcinomas (SBA), lymphomas, and gastrointestinal stromal tumor (GIST).[72,74] Fludeoxyglucose ([18]FDG)-PET has a limited role in the diagnosis and staging of carcinoid tumors because they are not [18]FDG avid; however, it may play important role in ascertaining treatment response and detecting disease recurrence.[72–74]

Two notable advances are double-balloon enteroscopy, or push enteroscopy, and video capsule endoscopy (VCE), which were both introduced in 2001. Double-balloon enteroscopy is a technically challenging procedure that permits the evaluation of the entire small bowel and tissue sampling, which is not possible with VCE. Double-balloon enteroscopy most commonly detects symptomatic lesions, including areas of ulceration, stenosis, and GI bleeds, with a sensitivity of 74% to 81%.[75–83] VCE is effective at identifying 50% of new SBC lesions and 87% of all lesions, with a relatively low miss rate of 10%.[84–93]

ADENOCARCINOMA

Adenocarcinoma of the small bowel is the second most common histologic SBC subtype, comprising 36.9% of cases.[94] The annual incidence is estimated at 7.3 case per million worldwide. In the United States, 3,050 new cases of SBA are anticipated in 2013.[94,95] Patients with SBA usually present between the 6th and 8th decade of life, with earlier presentations in patients with genetic, autoimmune, or inflammatory conditions (Table 54.2).

SBAs display a slight predominance for men, with age-adjusted incidence rates highest among African Americans (14.1 per 10[6]) followed by Caucasians (7.7 per 10[6]), Hispanics (6.2 per 10[6]), and

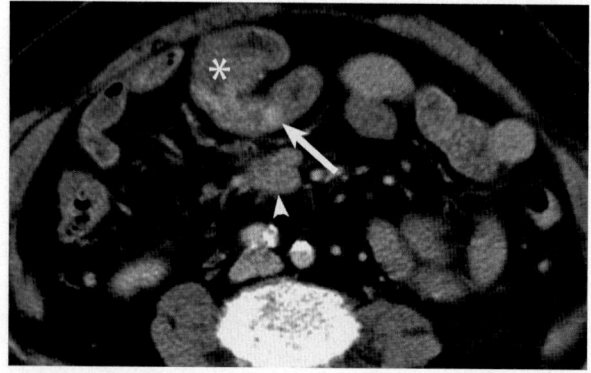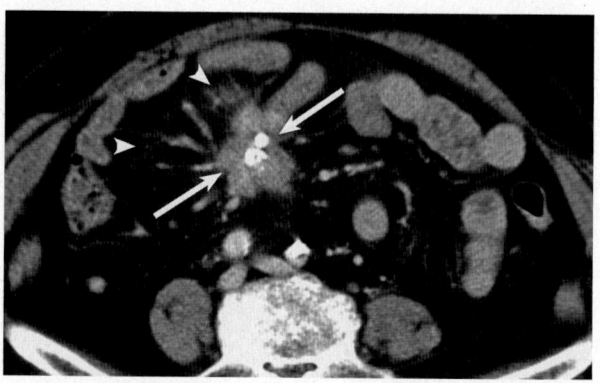

Figure 54.3 Primary ileal carcinoid. **(A)** A contrast-enhanced computed tomography (CT) shows a tethered and thickened segment of ileum (*asterisk*) containing a small submucosal enhancing lesion (*arrow*), consistent with primary carcinoid. Note partially imaged metastasis (*arrowhead*) in the adjacent mesentery. **(B)** A more inferior CT image shows a stellate mesenteric carcinoid metastasis (*arrows*) with central calcification and desmoplastic reaction (*arrowheads*) in the adjacent fat.

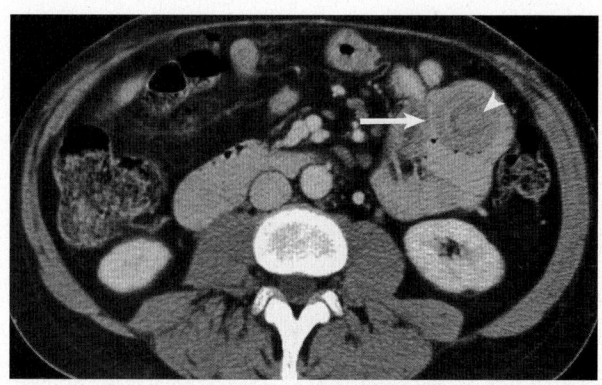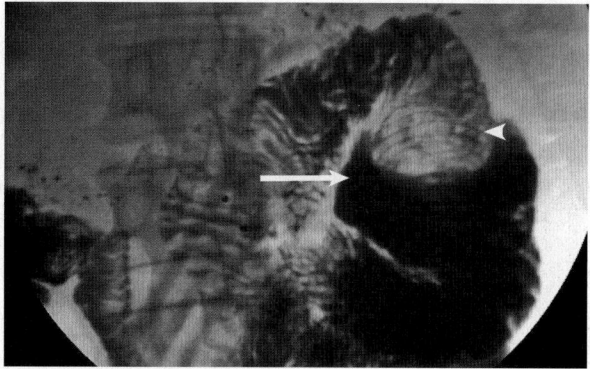

Figure 54.4 Primary small bowel lymphoma. **(A)** A contrast-enhanced computed tomography (CT) image shows aneurysmal luminal dilatation and extensive wall thickening of a segment of small bowel (*arrows*). Note enlarged adjacent mesenteric node (*arrowhead*). **(B)** A radiograph from the small bowel follow through shows a small bowel segment with luminal dilatation (*arrow*) and extensive mural thickening and irregularity (*arrowheads*) corresponding to the diseased segment on the CT.

Asian/Pacific Islanders (5.5 per 10^6). Adenocarcinoma incidence decreases distally in the small bowel, with the highest incidence in the duodenum (50% to 5%), followed by the jejunum (16%) and ileum (13%). Most SBA patients present at an advanced stage (American Joint Committee on Cancer [AJCC] stage III or greater) resulting in a poor overall 5-year disease-free survival (of about 30%) and mean survival (20 months).[50] Outcomes are worse for duodenal tumors (28% 5-year survival) compared to jejunal and ileal lesions (38% 5-year survival).

Etiology

SBA shares several etiologic features with colorectal cancers (CRC), leading to the adoption of similar treatment strategies, although they are biologically distinct diseases. The most obvious similarity between SBA and CRC is a common etiopathogenic pathways because both cancers are more common in patients with FAP, HNPCC, and inflammatory bowel disease. Available data imply a similar adenoma to carcinoma sequence in both SBA and CRC. As with CRC, the risk of progression is associated with the size of the adenoma (8.3% for lesions <1 cm and 30% for lesions >1 cm) and histology (14.3 % for tubular, 23.1% for tubulovillous, and 36% for villous).[96–99] A number of molecular similarities and dissimilarities between these two cancers have also been reported. In a recent genomic hybridization study looking at GI cancers, SBA was more similar to CRC than to stomach cancer.[100] In addition, *HER2* oncogene amplification is low in SBA similar to CRC in contrast to gastric cancer.[97,98,101,102] Microsatellite instability (MSI) and loss of mismatch repair proteins is present in 18% to 35% of SBAs versus 15% of CRCs.[77–79] Approximately 50% of the SBA cases reflect sporadic methylation of the *MLH1* gene with a relatively high incidence of MSI and MLH1 methylation in CD associated SBA (67% to 73%).[106–117]

Staging and Prognosis

The AJCC staging system for SBA is depicted in Table 54.3. Given the nonspecific initial presentation of SBAs, 32% of patients present with stage IV disease, 27% present with stage III, 30% present with stage II, and 10% present with stage I.[102] Less than 50% of SBA patients are curative surgical candidates. Survival by stage is 63% for stage I, 48% for stage II, 32% for stage III, and about 4% for stage IV.[102] Multivariate regression analyses identified age over 55 years, males, African Americans, T4 tumor, lymph node involvement and ratio, duodenal followed by ileal primary, poor differentiation, metastatic disease, and positive margins as associated with a poor prognosis.[94,102,120–122] Recent investigations into molecular determinants have also identified the CpG island methylator phenotype (CIMP) status, E-cadherin loss, and aberrant β-catenin expression as also associated with a worse prognosis.[106,118]

Management

The site of the disease, the stage at presentation, the available expertise, patient comorbidities, and patient performance status are all important considerations in determining the optimal management for individual SBA patients.

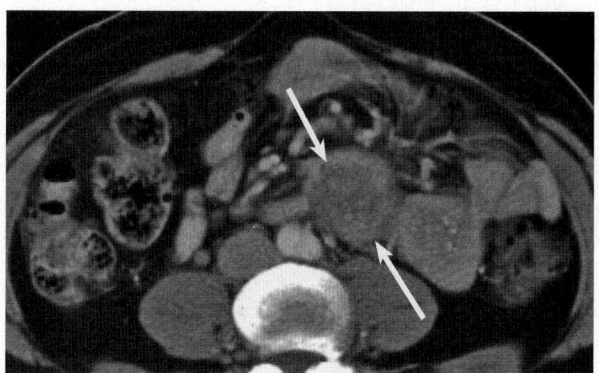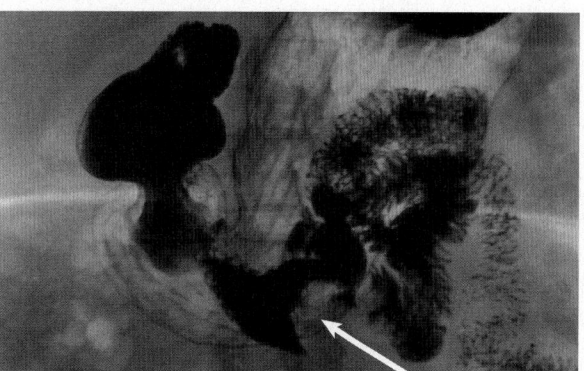

Figure 54.5 A gastrointestinal stromal tumor of the small bowel. **(A)** A contrast-enhanced computed tomography image shows a solid, heterogeneously enhancing mass (*arrows*) arising from the submucosa of the third portion of the duodenum. **(B)** An image from upper gastrointestinal series shows a filling defect (*arrow*) in the third portion of the duodenum due to the submucosal gastrointestinal stromal tumor.

TABLE 54.1

Risk Factors and Predisposing Conditions in the Development of Small Bowel Cancer

Risk Factor	Lifetime Risk	Small Bowel Cancer Type
Genetic		
FAP (2%–5%)	2%–5%	Periampullary adenocarcinoma, duodenal/jejunal adenocarcinoma,
HNPCC	1%–4%	adenocarcinoma, Gardner syndrome, desmoid duodenal adenocarcinoma,
Peutz-Jeghers syndrome	15-fold	gastrointestinal cancers
MUTYH-associated polyposis	4%	
Cystic fibrosis		
Autoimmune/Inflammatory		
Crohn disease	(>10 yr) 2%	Ileal adenocarcinoma, jejunal lymphoma/ adenocarcinoma, celiac disease immunosuppressive lymphoma, posttransplant lymphoproliferative disorder, neurofibromatosis, paragangliomas

Malignant Conditions
Colorectal, prostate, pancreas, uterine, skin and soft tissue tumors

Benign Conditions
Cholecystectomy, peptic ulcer disease

Other Conditions
Male gender, African American, advanced age, high-fat diet, obesity, alcohol

TABLE 54.2

Magnetic Resonance Findings of Common Small Bowel Neoplasms

Tumor Type	Growth Pattern	Margins	Secondary Intestinal Findings	Type of Lymphatic and Mesenteric Spread	MRI Findings
Adenocarcinoma	Short annular lesion with intraluminal growth, predominantly in duodenum	Irregular margins	Stenotic lesion with proximal obstruction	Local–regional metastases	Isointense to muscle on T1, heterogeneous signal on T2, hypovascular after Gd
Lymphoma	Long segmental infiltrating lesion	Smooth regular contours with preservation of the perivisceral fat plane	Aneurysmal dilatation without obstruction	Bulky retroperitoneal metastases	Isointense to muscle on T1, heterogeneous signal on T2, moderate enhancement after Gd
GIST	Intramural submucosal mass with extraserosal extension	Smooth lobulated contours	Aneurysmal dilatation, stenosis or obstruction usually absent	Peritoneal metastatic nodules, adenopathy rare	Inhomogeneous lesions, isointense on T1, mildly hyperintense on T2, peripheral enhancement in large lesions
Carcinoid	Focal asymmetric predominantly in ileum	Irregular margins; mesenteric stranding and kinking of the involved segment	Intermittent obstruction possible proximal to the kinked loop	Hypervascular mesenteric metastases with spiculated margins and local adenopathy with calcification	Isointense to muscle on T1, heterogeneous hyperintense on T2, hypervascular on Gd

Gd, gadolinium.
Adapted from Crusco F, Giovagnoni A, et al. Malignant small bowel neoplasms: spectrum of disease on MR imaging. *Radiol Med* 2010;115:1279–1291.

TABLE 54.3

American Joint Committee on Cancer Staging of Small Intestinal Cancer

Primary Tumor	
Tx	Primary tumor cannot be assessed
T0	No evidence of primary tumor
Tis	*Carcinoma in situ*
T1a	Tumor invades lamina propria
T1b	Tumor invades submucosa[a]
T2	Tumor invades muscularis propria
T3	Tumor invades through the muscularis propria into the subserosa or into the nonperitonealized perimuscular tissue (mesentery or retroperitoneum) with extension ≤2 cm[a]
T4	Tumor perforates the visceral peritoneum or directly invades other organs or structures (includes other loops of small intestine, mesentery, or retroperitoneum >2 cm, and abdominal wall by way of serosa; for duodenum only, invasion of pancreas or bile duct)

Regional Lymph Nodes	
Nx	Regional lymph nodes cannot be assessed
N0	No regional lymph node metastasis
N1	Metastasis in 1–3 regional lymph nodes
N2	Metastases in ≥4 regional lymph nodes

Distant Metastasis	
M0	No distant metastasis
M1	Distant metastasis

Anatomic Stage/Prognostic Group			
Stage	*T*	*N*	*M*
0	Tis	N0	M0
I	T1	N0	M0
	T2	N0	M0
IIA	T3	N0	M0
IIB	T4	N0	M0
IIIA	Any T	N1	M0
IIIB	Any T	N2	M0
IV	Any T	Any N	Any M

[a] The nonperitonealized perimuscular tissue is, for the jejunum and ileum, part of the mesentery. For the duodenum in areas where serosa is lacking, it is part of the interface with the pancreas.
Used with the permission of the American Joint Committee on Cancer (AJCC), Chicago, Illinois. The original source for this material is the *AJCC Cancer Staging Manual*, Seventh Edition (2010) published by Springer Science and Business Media LLC, www.springerlink.com, page 129.

Surgery for Local–Regional Disease

Surgery is the treatment for local–regional confined SBAs.[50] The 5-year survival of resected versus unresected patients is 54% versus 0%.[122] The optimal surgical treatment depends on the location of the primary tumor, with duodenal adenocarcinomas managed by either a pancreaticoduodenectomy or segmental resection. Both procedures are equivalent with regard to long-term survival, with segmental resection associated with less postoperative morbidity and length of hospitalization.[122–125] Jejunal and ileal adenocarcinomas are treated with oncologic-appropriate segmental resection. A right hemicolectomy is the appropriate oncologic approach to tumors near the ileocecal valve.

Adjuvant Therapy

Recurrence in SBAs is predominantly distant and rarely local–regional (86% versus 18%, respectively).[50] Although duodenal SBAs have a higher incidence of local failure, distant recurrence still predominates (59% versus 19%, respectively, and combined, 22%).[94,126,127] Most treatment strategies are based on fluorouracil (5-FU) or, more recently, 5-FU/oxaliplatin–based regimens. Overman et al.[129] reported adjuvant therapy improved disease-free survival (hazard ration [HR], 0.23, 95% CI, 0.06 to 0.89, p = 0.03), but not overall survival (HR, 0.48, 95% CI, 0.13 to 1.74, p = 0.26) in patients receiving adjuvant chemotherapy (5-FU or platinum based).[129] Multiple retrospective studies have demonstrated a mixed response for adjuvant chemotherapy in SBAs.[49,50,128–130]

The role of hyperthermic intraperitoneal chemotherapy (HIPEC) in the treatment of SBCs has been investigated in four small trials involving a total of 30 patients with peritoneal carcinomatosis. These patients underwent HIPEC followed by adjuvant chemotherapy, with a reported mean overall survival of 22.2 months compared to 12 months on conventional treatment strategies. The results are encouraging, but the numbers are too small to draw any robust conclusions.[140]

Treatment for Metastatic Disease

Limited randomized controlled trials defining a role for chemotherapy versus best supportive care (BSC) in patients with advanced SBAs have been performed. Multiple retrospective studies have demonstrated a small survival advantage for palliative chemotherapy approaches compared to BSC alone (Table 54.4).[49,50,131–136]

Although there are *no* randomized trials comparing different regimens, a number of SBA clinical trials are currently accruing in an effort to more precisely define the role of chemotherapy in advanced SBA. The role of surgery for all advanced/metastatic SBC is purely palliative. Specific patients might benefit from an intestinal bypass to maintain an enteral means of nutrition and an improved quality of life.[120,137–139]

CARCINOID TUMORS

Carcinoid tumors are slow growing neoplasms that arise from the neuroendocrine cells of Kulchitsky. Of these cells, 75% occur in the gastrointestinal tract (44.7% in the small bowel and 19.6% in the rectum), followed by the lung, bronchus, and rarely the liver, pancreas, or gonads. Given the fourfold increase in the incidence of carcinoids that has occurred over the past 2 decades, carcinoids are now the most common SBC (36.9%) according to the National Cancer Database.[167,168]

Clinical Presentation and Prognosis

Of small bowel carcinoids, 44.7% occur in the small bowel, and over 50% of these are found in the ileum.[168] Carcinoid tumors are most common in the 7th decade of life (mean age, 66 years), in males (52.4%), and in Caucasians (80.4%). Most carcinoids present in an advanced stage (75%) as a result of a significant delay and difficulty in diagnosis. Despite the advanced stage, most carcinoids follow an indolent course, with an overall 5-year survival ranging from 52% to 77%.[170–174] Tumors over 10 mm and those with a transmural depth of invasion are the primary risk factors for local–regional progression and metastasis.[175]

TABLE 54.4

Current Clinical Trials for Advanced Small Bowel Adenocarcinoma

Identifier	Phase	Tumor Type	N	Therapy Line	Agent
NCT00354887	II	Small bowel adenocarcinoma and ampullary	30	1st	CAPOX + bevacizumab
NCT00433550	II	Small bowel adenocarcinoma	33	1st	CAPOX + irinotecan
NCT01202409	II	Small bowel adenocarcinoma and ampullary	20	1st	CAPOX + panitumumab (KRAS wild type)
NCT00987766	1b	Duodenal + ampullary	22	1st	GEMOX + erlotinib
NCT01730586	II	Small bowel adenocarcinoma	10	>2nd	Nab-paclitaxel

CAPOX, capecitabine + oxaliplatin, GEMOX, gemcitabine + oxaliplatin, Nab-paclitaxel, nano-article albumin-bound paclitaxel.
Adapted from Raghav K, Overman MJ. Small bowel adenocarcinoma—existing evidence and evolving paradigms. *Nat Rev Clin Oncol* 2013;10:534–544.

Carcinoid Syndrome

Carcinoid syndrome is an array of symptoms that occurs in patients with carcinoid tumors of the bronchus or metastatic to the liver. Symptoms of carcinoid syndrome include diarrhea, cutaneous flushing, and wheezing. These symptoms are precipitated by stress, alcohol intake, and certain physical activities, and are secondary to the systemic release of several tumor-derived factors, including serotonin, dopamine, tachykinins, histamine, and prostaglandins, all of which are metabolized by the liver. Up to 80% of patients with small bowel carcinoids develop carcinoid syndrome, and it is the presenting complaint in 10% to 17% of patients. The mainstay of treatment for carcinoid syndrome is somatostatin, which prevents the secretion of hormones by binding to a specific receptor on the tumor surface.[192,193] Although octreotide is effective in most patients, interferon α (IFN-α) may benefit patients who do not respond to octreotide alone.[187] The antihistamine cyproheptadine has also been used successfully for refractory carcinoid symptoms.[188]

Management

Surgery for Local–Regional Disease

An oncologic segmental resection of the tumor is the preferred treatment for localized small bowel carcinoids.[176] Five-year survival after resection of localized disease ranges between 50% and 85%. Of small bowel carcinoids, 29% are associated with other noncarcinoid neoplasms, necessitating a thorough inspection of the entire bowel at surgery. Appendiceal carcinoids smaller than 2 cm can be treated with a simple appendectomy, whereas larger tumors require a right hemicolectomy. Pretreatment with octreotide prior to anesthetic induction is recommended because surgical intervention/manipulation can precipitate a carcinoid crisis.[177–180]

Surgery for Metastatic Disease

The liver is the most common site of carcinoid metastasis. Liver resection along with primary tumor resection is recommended for resectable metastatic disease. More radical surgical debulking or cytoreductive surgery has been used for patients with extensive bilobar liver disease, liver failure, or extensive metastatic disease to provide prolonged disease-free survival. Several studies have shown that liver resection can improve the 5-year survival rate from 36% to 61% compared to historic controls.[181–183] Although long-term data are lacking, percutaneous or laparoscopic local ablative techniques such as radiofrequency, microwave, or cryoablation represent alternative cytoreductive modalities for the treatment of metastatic carcinoid tumors. Cytoreductive strategies not only prolong survival, but are also associated with a decrease in octreotide doses required to control carcinoid symptoms. A number of retrospective series have demonstrated that surgical resection is superior to systemic therapy with regard to both overall survival and symptom management.[184]

Hepatic Artery Embolization

Transcatheter hepatic arterial embolization (HAE) with or without chemotherapy has been utilized extensively for both symptom control and as a definitive treatment for unresectable carcinoid liver metastasis.[185] HAE may be performed with gel foam, polyvinyl alcohol, or microspheres. The addition of chemotherapy allows for the delivery of much higher intratumoral concentrations than can be achieved with systemic therapy. Known complications include transient or fulminant liver failure, liver abscesses, and postembolization syndrome (fever, abdominal pain, leukocytosis, elevations in liver function tests).[185]

Systemic Chemotherapy

Several chemotherapeutics have been studied extensively in the management of carcinoid metastases, including 5-FU, streptozotocin, and doxorubicin. All have yielded modest response rates of ~20%. In addition, IFN-α has been purported to achieve tumor stabilization in 20% to 40% of cases, and octreotide has been shown to prevent the progression of metastatic carcinoids in several small case series.[186–190] Tyrosine–kinase inhibitors like imatinib or sunitinib can induce a delay in tumor cell growth in preclinical studies and disease stability in 83% of patients treated over a 1-year period. In a recent phase II study, bevacizumab, a monoclonal antibody that targets vascular endothelial growth factor (VEGF), was shown to stabilize disease in 95% of patients when combined with octreotide compared to 68% stabilization when octreotide was combined with IFN-α.[191,218,219]

Palliative Surgery

The decision to perform palliative resection for disseminated carcinoid tumors should carefully balance the surgical risks and perceived patient benefits. Orthotopic liver transplantation for patients with unresectable liver-only disease remains investigational and is currently performed by only a small number of transplant centers.

SMALL BOWEL LYMPHOMA

Lymphoma is the third most common SBC, comprising 10% to 20% of cases. Of such cases, 20% to 40% are extranodal lymphomas, which arise within a solid organ, and ~50% of extranodal lymphomas are GI lymphomas.[194–198] Of GI lymphomas, 75% are located in the stomach, followed by the small bowel, colon, and other organs such as the pancreas and the liver. GI lymphomas have a peak incidence in the 7th decade of life, with a male to female ratio of 1.5:1. The incidence of small bowel lymphomas has increased in the United States over the last 2 decades, correlating with an increase in lymphomas among immunocompromised patients. Increased immigration from the Middle East—where primary intestinal lymphoma constitutes the most common primary extranodal disease—may also account for some of the increase in small bowel lymphomas. Additional risk factors include Crohn disease and prior radiation exposure.

Staging and Prognosis

The most important prognostic indicator for intestinal lymphoma is tumor spread. Most GI lymphomas are of the non-Hodgkin type and are staged based on the Ann Arbor staging system: stage I disease is limited to a single site; stage II tumors are confined to below the diaphragm and are separated into two subgroups, namely those with regional (stage II 1E) and distant (stage II 2E) lymph node involvement; stage III has involvement of organs on both sides of the diaphragm; and stage IV represents widespread dissemination, including the liver and the spleen. Primary intestinal lymphomas can be differentiated from secondary lymphomas by the absence of superficial and mediastinal lymphadenopathies on work-up, if there is no evidence of disease on both peripheral blood smears and bone marrow biopsies, if the disease is localized to a specific small bowel segment and regional draining mesenteric lymph nodes only, and if there is no evidence of hepatic or splenic involvement (except via direct extension from the primary tumor).

Variants

Mucosal-Associated Lymphoid Tissue Lymphoma

Marginal zone B-cell lymphomas (MALT) are the most common primary gastrointestinal lymphomas. They occur more commonly in the stomach, followed by the small bowel (most commonly, the ileocecal region), the colon, and the esophagus. MALTs occur predominately in men and peak in the 6th decade of life. They present as unifocal, ulcerated overhanging lesions, characterized by cellular heterogeneity and bearing close resemblance to normal gut-associated lymphoid tissue (Peyer patch and mesenteric nodal tissue). Nonneoplastic reactive lymphoid follicles surrounded by centrocytes are characteristic, with the neoplastic focus occupying the marginal zone or intrafollicular region. These tumor cells express elevated levels of immunoglobulin (Ig)M and B-cell–associated antigens (including CD19, CD20, CD22, and CD79a). Most tumors are CD5, CD10, and CD23 negative and CD43 variable. MALT lymphomas are not associated with *Bcl-2* or *Bcl-1* rearrangements.

MALT lymphomas may be associated with chronic inflammatory conditions, including autoimmune disorders such as Sjögren syndrome and Hashimoto thyroiditis. The majority of patients present with stage I or II disease. Therapy is multimodal and includes surgical resection and/or chemoradiation therapy, with small bowel lymphomas having a better prognosis than gastric tumors. Some studies suggest that MALT tumors may be antigen driven, especially by *Campylobacter jejuni* and *Helicobacter pylori*. Regression has been reported with eradication of *H. pylori* infection using antibiotics.[194]

Diffuse Large B-Cell Lymphoma

The second most common small bowel lymphoma is diffuse large B-cell lymphoma (DLBCL), also known as large cell immunoblastic, large-cleaved follicular center cell, centroblastic D immunoblastic cell, or diffuse mixed lymphocytic and histiocytic cell. DLBCL occurs more frequently in men, with a median age of 54 to 61 years, and primarily involves the ileocecal region. DLBCLs present as unifocal ulcerated lesions, composed of diffuse large B cells with large nuclei that are twice the size of a normal lymphocyte. Tumor cells are CD19, CD20, CD22, and CD79a positive. *Bcl-2 gene* mutation is present in approximately 30% of the cases. Immunosuppression is an important risk factor for DLBCL. Surgery is the mainstay of treatment for localized disease, followed by adjuvant radiation or chemotherapy.[195] Overall 5-year survival is between 50% and 70% with multimodality therapy.[196]

Burkitt Lymphoma

Burkitt lymphoma of the small bowel accounts for <5% of all small bowel lymphomas. It can occur endemically or sporadically and is highly aggressive. The endemic subtype is seen predominantly in Central Africa; it affects children with a peak incidence at 8 years of age, is associated with Epstein-Barr virus (EBV) infection, and involves the GI tract in only 20% to 30% of cases. Conversely, sporadic Burkitt lymphoma occurs more commonly in Westernized countries, affects a broader age group, is not associated with EBV infections and commonly affects the GI tract (ileocecal region). Clinically, they can mimic appendicitis by presenting as large masses. Microscopically, cells are monomorphic medium-sized cells with round nuclei and an abundant basophilic cytoplasm. It is a rapidly growing tumor with short doubling time; the high rate of proliferation gives it a *starry sky* pattern due to the numerous macrophages that have ingested apoptotic tumor cells. Treatment primarily consists of chemotherapy, usually vincristine, cyclophosphamide, doxorubicin, and methotrexate.[197]

Mantle Cell Lymphoma

Mantle cell lymphoma (MCL) is a rare primary GI lymphoma that follows either an indolent or very aggressive course. MCL commonly affects men (ratio, 4:1) in their 6th or 7th decades of life and has a predilection for the small bowel and colon. Macroscopically, MCLs appear as multiple, whitish polypoid lesions that share morphologic features with nodal lymphomas. CD5+ B cells are located within the mantle zone that surrounds the germinal centers. Four histologic subtypes have been described: nodular, diffuse, mantle zone, and blastic. The blastic type has the worst prognosis, whereas the nodular and diffuse types have the best prognosis. MCLs have been associated with t(11:14) (q13; q32) chromosomal translocation, causing overexpression of cyclin D1. The vast majority of MCLs present in stage IV disease.

T-Cell Lymphoma

T-cell lymphomas (TCL) of the small bowel are less common than their B-cell counterparts, accounting for approximately 15% of all small bowel lymphomas. TCLs affect men and women equally and most commonly arise in the jejunum or the proximal ileum. TCLs may remain localized; however, dissemination is common. They typically present as large circumferential ulcers, in the absence of large masses, with associated mesenteric lymphadenopathy. As with other types of lymphomas, obstruction and perforation are common presentations. Microscopically, transmural replacement of the intestinal wall by highly pleomorphic lymphoid cells may be seen. A large number of surrounding intraepithelial lymphocytes may also show cellular atypia. Tumor cells stain positive for CD3, CD7, CD8, and CD103 and negative for CD4. Small bowel TCLs are known as EATLs due to their association with long-standing enteropathies, primarily celiac disease. EATL is described in approximately 5% to 10% of all patients with celiac disease, and the relative risk of developing a lymphoma in this setting is 25- to 100-fold higher than normal patients. Prognosis is generally poor, with a 5-year survival rate of 10%.[198]

GASTROINTESTINAL STROMAL TUMORS

GIST tumors arise from the intestinal cells of Cajal and are characterized by the presence of a gain-of-function c-kit (CD117) mutation. The c-kit protein codes for a tyrosine–kinase receptor involved in cellular proliferation, apoptosis, and differentiation.

Epidemiology and Genetics

GISTS are the most common mesenchymal tumor of the small bowel, despite comprising only 0.5% to 1% of all GI tumors. There are between 4,500 to 6,000 GISTs per year in the United States, with the stomach being the most common site.[199–204] Incidence rates are equal in both genders and peak between 50 and 60 years of age. Small bowel GISTs are most commonly found in the jejunum, followed by the ileum, and the duodenum and typically present with pain, intussusception, or bleeding. Approximately 80% to 90% of all GIST tumors contain a c-kit mutation (CD117), whereas the remainder have a mutation in another tyrosine–kinase receptor gene or platelet-derived growth factor (PDGF) receptor alpha. It is now recognized that a vast majority of tumors previously identified as leiomyomas and leiomyosarcomas were actually CD117+ GIST. The molecular discoveries have allowed for the development of the specific c-kit tyrosine–kinase inhibitor imatinib (Gleevec), a drug initially designed to treat chronic myelogenous leukemia.

Prognosis and Behavior

All GISTs have the potential for malignancy, and approximately 50% of resected patients will have disease recurrence within 5 years. Of GISTs, 30% to 50% are clinically malignant. Most GISTs have a c-kit gain-of-function mutation, allowing for the prediction of clinical behavior and recurrence risk stratification.[205–208] Tumors larger than 2 cm have a higher risk of recurrence and metastasis. This risk increases significantly for tumors larger than 3 cm to 5 cm. The mitotic rate has also been studied, and GISTs with five or more mitoses per 50 high-powered field (HPF) have a worse prognosis, whereas mitotic rates higher than 10 per 50 HPF predicts high recurrence and metastatic rates regardless of tumor size or location, with 5-year survival rates ~25%. The tumor site also plays an important role in prognosis, with jejunal and ileal GISTs displaying more malignant behavior compared to duodenal, rectal, or gastric GISTs.

Management

Surgery

R0 surgical resection is the mainstay therapy for all GISTs. Extensive resection of the surrounding uninvolved tissue has not been shown to improve outcomes. A routine lymphadenectomy is not indicated because GISTs rarely metastasize to regional lymph nodes. Intraoperative tumor rupture and spillage has been linked to carcinomatosis, necessitating a meticulous surgical technique. The peritoneum and liver are the main sites of metastasis and recurrence, and both should be inspected during surgical exploration.[209–212]

Adjuvant Therapy

Adjuvant imatinib therapy improves recurrence-free survival after complete surgical resection of localized disease. The ACOSOG Z9001 trial was a randomized phase III double-blinded, placebo-controlled multicenter trial where 713 patients were assigned to receive either 400 mg of imatinib or placebo daily for 1 year after complete resection of a c-kit–positive, 3 cm (or more) GIST. One-year progression-free survival was 98% in the imatinib arm and 83% in the placebo arm.[213]

Similar results were found in the Z9000 trial, a phase II, intergroup trial led by the American College of Surgeons Oncology Group, in which 106 patients who had undergone complete surgical resection of GIST were prescribed imatinib 400 mg per day for 1 year followed by serial radiologic evaluation. At 7.7 years of follow-up, the patients receiving imatinib had 1-, 3-, and 5-year overall survival rates of 99%, 97%, and 83%, respectively,

compared to a 5-year overall survival rate of 35% for historic controls. Progression-free survival for 1, 3, and 5 years was 96%, 60%, and 40%, respectively.[214]

In patients in whom the initial complete surgical resection is not possible, the use of imatinib therapy has resulted in a significant prolongation of survival, with 80% of patients achieving a 5-year overall survival versus 9 months' survival with no therapy.[215] Neoadjuvant imatinib is also effective at reducing large tumor burdens and may facilitate margin-negative, organ-sparing resections.[216,217] Regorafenib is another novel multitargeted kinase inhibitor being used in GIST management that inhibits the Ras/Raf/Mek pathways as well as VEGF receptor 2 (VEGFR2) signaling.[219]

OTHER MESENCHYMAL TUMORS

Leiomyomas and Leiomyosarcomas

Small bowel leiomyomas and leiomyosarcomas arise from the muscularis propria and muscularis mucosa. They have a varied presentation, primarily involving tumor ulceration and bleeding as the tumor enlarges. Because tumor growth is initially localized and primarily extraluminal, obstruction does not occur until very late in the disease course.[223] Leiomyosarcomas stain positive for desmin and actin and are negative for CD117 (c-kit and CD34). Metastasis is via hematologic routes and is mainly to the liver and peritoneum. About one third of patients have metastasis at the time of diagnosis, and prognosis is very poor.[228–231]

Desmoid Tumors

Frequently confused with GISTs, these spindle cell tumors originate from musculoaponeurotic structures throughout the body and are histologically defined by fibroblastic proliferation and the formation of bundles of spindle cells around blood vessels in a dense hypocellular fibrous stroma. Desmoids occur with higher frequency in patients with FAP and Gardner syndrome.[234] Few mitotic figures are seen, and necrosis is usually absent. Desmoids stain for vimentin, smooth muscle actin, and nuclear beta catenin. Although desmoids tumors are benign with no potential for metastasis, they tend to be locally aggressive and recur even after complete resection.[238] Treatment is surgical resection with a wide margin to ensure negative microscopic margins; however, this may be difficult due to the anatomic location and the involvement of vital structures. Other treatment modalities include chemotherapy (methotrexate and vinblastine, doxorubicin), radiation therapy, nonsteroidal anti-inflammatory agents, and antiestrogens (tamoxifen).[235–237]

Inflammatory Fibroid Polyps

These benign lesions are uncommonly seen in the small bowel. They are typically submucosal and consist of a mixture of small granulation tissue–like vessels, spindle cells, and inflammatory cells. They can stain positively for CD34; however, they do not stain for CD117 with the exception of very small areas of stroma within these tumors.[232,233]

Schwannomas

Although relatively rare in the small bowel, schwannomas of the GI tract are often found in the stomach, colon, and esophagus. They are benign lesions, and present as rubbery yellowish trabeculated tumors characterized by lymph node aggregates around their periphery with nuclear palisading Verocay bodies and hyalinized vessels similar to schwannomas found elsewhere in the body. Schwannomas stain strongly for S100 and glial fibrillary acidic protein, but are CD117, CD 34, and smooth muscle actin negative.[224,225]

Inflammatory and Myofibroblastic Tumors

Inflammatory mesenchymal tumors typically present as solid white masses with infiltrative margins. Although their precise etiology is uncertain, several authors have suggested that they are benign reactions to infectious processes, although local recurrence has been reported. These tumors rarely behave in a malignant fashion and are histologically composed of spindle cells admixed with lymphocytes and plasma cells. Unlike GIST, they stain negatively for CD117 and CD 34, but positive for desmin, muscle-specific actin, and cytokeratin.[226,227]

METASTATIC CANCER TO THE SMALL BOWEL

Metastatic tumors to the small intestine are 2.5 times more common than are primary SBCs. Metastatic spread to the small intestine from distant primary sites is more frequent than to any other site in the GI tract. The main routes by which secondary neoplasms reach the small bowel is primary dependent and includes direct extension (for colonic, pancreatic, and gastric cancers), intraperitoneal spread (ovarian cancer), and lympho- or hematogenous embolization (melanoma, and lung and breast cancers).

Epidemiology

Melanoma is the most common cancer to metastasize to the small bowel, with up to 4.4% of all melanoma patients demonstrating small bowel metastases. Malignant melanoma is the primary tumor in 50% to 70% of all small bowel metastases, with the terminal ileum being the most often affected site.[220–223] Primary melanomas of the intestine are extremely rare, with few case reports found in the literature.[239]

Clinically, small bowel metastases can present with obstruction, perforation, intussusception, malabsorption, and/or GI bleeding. Obstruction is commonly seen in association with metastatic lobular breast carcinoma. A wide array of nonspecific symptoms may also be present, including abdominal discomfort, distension, and diarrhea. Typical features of intestinal metastases include intestinal wall thickening, submucosal spread, and ulcers. Melanomas and sarcomas may appear as nodules or polyps. Metastases are typically located deep within the submucosa or the muscularis propria of the small bowel, with little involvement of the mucosa.[221–223]

Intestinal metastases usually represent at a late stage of the disease, during which other sites of hematogenous metastases are also frequently found. However, the prognosis for patients with small bowel metastasis varies widely according to the primary tumor type and patient-specific factors. Metastatic melanomas or renal carcinomas with isolated metastasis to the small bowel may be associated with prolonged survival after resection. Other more common primary tumors that metastasize to the small bowel are uterus, cervix, colon, lung, and breast tumors.

Management

The management of small bowel metastatic disease is defined by the primary tumor of origin. Isolated small bowel metastasis warrants segmental resection to prevent bowel obstruction, to maintain nutrition, or as part of a debulking procedure (e.g., ovarian, appendiceal). Most often, systemic therapy is the modality of choice for advanced/diffuse small bowel involvement. A diffuse disease may rarely warrant debulking or treatment with HIPEC on established protocols.

SELECTED REFERENCES

The full reference list can be accessed at lwwhealthlibrary.com/oncology.

2. Siegel R, Ma J, Zou Z, et al. Cancer statistics, 2014. *CA Cancer J Clin* 2014;64:9–29.
8. Chow JS, Chen CC, Ahsan H, et al. A population-based study of the incidence of malignant small bowel tumours: SEER, 1973-1990. *Int J Epidemiol* 1996;25:722–728.
9. Neugut AI, Santos J. The association between cancers of the small and large bowel. *Cancer Epidemiol Biomarkers Prev* 1993;2:551–553.
10. Scelo G, Anderson A et al. Associations between small intestine cancer and other primary cancers: An international population-based study. *Int J Cancer* 2006;118:189–196.
11. Schiessling S, Kihm M, Ganschow P, et al. Desmoid tumour biology in patients with familial adenomatous polyposis coli. *Br J Surg* 2013;100:694–703.
27. Hearle N, Schumacher V, Menko FH, et al. Frequency and spectrum of cancers in the Peutz-Jeghers syndrome. *Clin Cancer Res* 2006;12:3209–3215.
29. Yamaguchi S, Ogata H, Katsumata D, et al. MUTYH-associated colorectal cancer and adenomatous polyposis. *Surg Today* 2014;44:593–600.
31. Maisonneuve P, Marshall BC, Knapp EA, et al. Cancer risk in cystic fibrosis: a 20-year nationwide study from the United States. *J Natl Cancer Inst* 2013;105:122–129.
38. Hemminki K, Li X, Sundquist J, et al. Cancer risks in ulcerative colitis patients. *Int J Cancer* 2008;123:1417–1421.
46. Boffetta P, Hazelton WD, Chen Y, et al. Body mass, tobacco smoking, alcohol drinking and risk of cancer of the small intestine—a pooled analysis of over 500,000 subjects in the Asia Cohort Consortium. *Ann Oncol* 2012;23:1894–1898.
47. Neugut AI, Jacobson JS, Suh S, et al. The epidemiology of cancer of the small bowel. *Cancer Epidemiol Biomarkers Prev* 1998;7:243–251.
49. Halfdanarson TR, McWilliams RR, Donohue JH, et al. A single-institution experience with 491 cases of small bowel adenocarcinoma. *Am J Surg* 2010;199:797–803.
50. Dabaja BS, Suki D, Pro B, et al. Adenocarcinoma of the small bowel: presentation, prognostic factors, and outcome of 217 patients. *Cancer* 2004;101:518–526.
54. Negri E, Bosetti C, Vecchia C, et al. Risk factors for adenocarcinoma of the small intestine. *Int J Cancer* 1999;82:171–174.
61. Gore RM, Mehta UK, Newmark GM, et al. Diagnosis and staging of small bowel tumours. *Cancer Imaging* 2006;6:209–212.
63. Levy AD, Remotti HE, Thompson WM, et al. Gastrointestinal stromal tumors: radiologic features with pathologic correlation. *Radiographics* 2003;23:283–304.
69. Van Weyenberg SJ, Van Waesberghe JH, Ell C, et al. Enteroscopy and its relationship to radiological small bowel imaging. *Gastrointest Endosc Clin N Am* 2009;19:389–407.
74. Cronin CG, Scott J, McDermott S, et al. Utility of PET/CT in the evaluation of small bowel pathology. *Br J Radiol* 2012;85:1211–1221.
76. Kita H, Yamamoto H, Yano T, et al. Double balloon endoscopy in two hundred fifty cases for the diagnosis and treatment of small intestinal disorders. *Inflammopharmacology* 2007;15:74–77.
94. Bilimoria KY, Bentrem DJ, Wayne DJ, et al. Small bowel cancer in United States: changes in epidemiology, treatment and survival over the last 20 years. *Ann Surg* 2009;249:63–71.
97. Pan SY, Morrison H. Epidemiology of cancer of the small intestine. *World J Gastrointest Oncol* 2011;3:33–42.
98. Raghav K, Overman MJ. Small bowel adenocarcinomas-existing evidence and evolving paradigms. *Nat Rev Clin Oncol* 2013;10:534–544.
102. Overman MJ, Hu CY, Kopetz S, et al. A population-based comparison of adenocarcinoma of large and small intestine: insights into a rare disease. *Ann Surg Oncol* 2012;19:1439–1445.
106. Lee HJ, Lee OJ, Jang KT, et al. Combined loss of E-cadherin and aberrant β-catenin protein expression correlates with poor prognosis for small intestinal adenocarcinomas. *Am J Clin Pathol* 2013;139:167–176.
111. Bläker H, Aulmann S, Helmchen B, et al. Loss of SMAD4 function in small intestinal adenocarcinoma: comparison of genetic and immunohistochemical findings. *Pathol Res Pract* 2004;200:1–7.
118. Fu T, Pappou EP, Guzzetta AA, et al. CpG island methylator phenotype-positive tumours in the absence of MLH1 methylation constitute a distinct subset of duodenal adenocarcinomas and are associated with poor prognosis. *Clin Cancer Res* 2012;18:4743–4752.
120. Howe JR, Karnell LH, Menck HR, et al. American College of Surgeons Commission on Cancer and the American Cancer Society. Adenocarcinoma of the small bowel: review of national cancer database 1985-1995. *Cancer* 1999;86:2693–2706.
130. Kelsey CR, Nelson JW, Willett CG, et al. Duodenal adenocarcinoma: patterns of failure after resection and the role of chemoradiotherapy. *Int J Radiat Oncol Biol Phys* 2007;69:1436–1441.

132. Koo DH, Yun SC, Hong YS, et al. Systemic chemotherapy for treatment of advanced small bowel adenocarcinoma with prognostic factor analysis: retrospective study. *BMC Cancer* 2011;11:205.

136. Zaanan A, Gauthier M, Malka D, et al. Second-line chemotherapy with fluorouracil, leucovorin, and irinotecan (FOLFIRI regimen) in patients with advanced small bowel adenocarcinoma after failure of first-line platinum-based chemotherapy: a multicentre AGEO study. *Cancer* 2011;117:1422–1428.

168. Modlin IM, Lye KD, Kidd M. A 5-decade analysis of 13,715 carcinoid tumors. *Cancer* 2003;97:934–959.

169. Maggard MA, O'Connell JB, Ko CY. Updated population-based review of carcinoid tumors. *Ann Surg* 2004;240:117–122.

174. Soga J. Early-stage carcinoids of the gastrointestinal tract: an analysis of 1914 reported cases. *Cancer* 2005;103:1587–1595.

184. Osborne DA, Zervos EE, Strosberg J, et al. Improved outcome with cytoreduction versus embolization for symptomatic hepatic metastases of carcinoid and neuroendocrine tumors. *Ann Surg Oncol* 2006;13:572–581.

185. Gupta S, Yao JC, Ahrar K, et al. Hepatic artery embolization and chemoembolization for treatment of patients with metastatic carcinoid tumors: the M.D. Anderson experience. *Cancer J* 2003;9:261–267.

187. Tiensuu Janson EM, Ahlström H, Andersson T, et al. Octreotide and interferon alfa: a new combination for the treatment of malignant carcinoid tumours. *Eur J Cancer* 1992;28:1647–1650.

188. Moertel CG, Kvols LK, Rubin J. A study of cyproheptadine in the treatment of metastatic carcinoid tumor and the malignant carcinoid syndrome. *Cancer* 1991;67:33–36.

195. Fischbach W, Dragosics B, Kolve-Goebeler ME, et al. Primary gastric B-cell lymphoma: results of a prospective multicenter study. The German-Austrian Gastrointestinal Lymphoma Study Group. *Gastroenterology* 2000;119:1191–1202.

197. Blum KA, Lozanski G, Byrd JC. Adult Burkitt leukemia and lymphoma. *Blood* 2004;104:3009–3020.

198. Al-Toma A, Verbeek WH, Hadithi M, et al. Survival in refractory coeliac disease and enteropathy associated T cell lymphoma: retrospective evaluation of single centre experience. *Gut* 2007;56:1373–1378.

212. Nguyen SQ, Divino CM, Wang JL, et al. Laparoscopic management of gastrointestinal stromal tumors. *Surg Endosc* 2006;20:713–716.

213. Dematteo RP, Ballman KV, Antonescu CR, et al. Adjuvant imatinib mesylate after resection of localised, primary gastrointestinal stromal tumour: a randomised, double-blind, placebo-controlled trial. *Lancet* 2009;373: 1097–1104.

214. DeMatteo RP, Ballman KV, Antonescu CR, et al. Long-term results of adjuvant imatinib mesylate in localized, high-risk, primary gastrointestinal stromal tumor: ACOSOG Z9000 (Alliance) Intergroup phase 2 trial. *Ann Surg* 2013;258:422–429.

218. Yao JC, Shah MH, Ito T, et al. Everolimus for advanced pancreatic neuroendocrine tumors. *N Engl J Med* 2011;364:514–523.

219. Raymond E, Dahan L, Raoul JL, et al. Sunitinib malate for the treatment of pancreatic neuroendocrine tumors. *N Engl J Med* 2011;364:501–513.

221. Bender GN, Maglinte DD, McLarney JH, et al. Malignant melanoma: patterns of metastasis to the small bowel, reliability of imaging studies, and clinical relevance. *Am J Gastroenterol* 2001;96:2392–2400.

225. Levy AD, Quiles AM, Miettinen M, et al. Gastrointestinal schwannomas: CT features with clinicopathologic correlation. *Am J Roentgenol* 2005;184: 797–802.

226. Kovach SJ, Fischer AC, Katzman PJ, et al. Inflammatory myofibroblastic tumors. *J Surg Oncol* 2006;94:385–391.

237. de Camargo VP, Keohan ML, D'Adamo DR, et al. Clinical outcomes of systemic therapy for patients with deep fibromatosis (desmoid tumor). *Cancer* 2010;116:2258–2265.

239. Sachs DL, Lowe L, Chang AE, et al. Do primary small intestinal melanomas exist? Report of a case. *J Am Acad Dermatol* 1999;41:1042–1044.

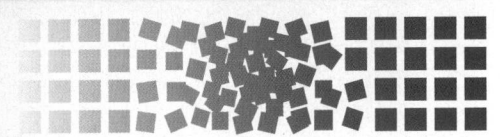

55 Gastrointestinal Stromal Tumor

Paolo G. Casali, Angelo Paolo Dei Tos, and Alessandro Gronchi

PRACTICE OF ONCOLOGY

INTRODUCTION

Gastrointestinal stromal tumors (GIST) are mesenchymal neoplasms of the gastrointestinal tract, whose tumor cell's normal counterpart is the interstitial cell of Cajal. This serves as a *pacemaker* of gastrointestinal motility, providing an interface between autonomic nerve stimulation and the muscle layer of the gastrointestinal wall.[1] GISTs are rare cancers, which were defined as a distinct disease in the 1990s, having been classified within smooth muscle neoplasms for decades from their first description in the 1960s.[2,3] Coincidentally, in 2000, they became targetable by new tyrosine-kinase inhibitors (TKI), given the role played by KIT and platelet-derived growth factor receptor alpha (PDGFRA) in their pathogenesis.[4–7] As of today, GISTs serve as an advanced model displaying both potentials and limits of currently available molecularly targeted agents in medical oncology of solid cancers.

From the clinical point of view, surgery is the mainstay treatment when GISTs are localized, and adjuvant therapy is used depending on their risk of relapse. Apparently, adjuvant therapy with TKIs is mainly able to delay relapse, if due to occur, rather than to avoid it. In the advanced disease, TKIs have substantially improved the prognosis of KIT-mutated GISTs and have become standard treatment. They face the major limiting factor of secondary resistance, which affects most patients and is marked by genetic heterogeneity. A minority of GISTs do not harbor mutations to either KIT or PDGFRA genes and, therefore, are called *wild type* (WT). They are less amenable to available TKIs, although their natural history tends to be less aggressive. Their variegated nature adds to the complexity of GISTs as a whole.

In brief, GISTs are more complex than initially believed, whereas targeted therapy has substantially improved their prognosis but is challenged by its apparent inability to eradicate the disease (even minimum residual disease), and by the heterogeneity of the secondary resistance it often gives rise to in the advanced setting. Intense translational and clinical research is underway. All this and the rarity of the disease strongly suggest to refer GIST patients to institutions or networks specializing in their treatment and study.

INCIDENCE AND ETIOLOGY

GISTs are rare cancers. Their crude incidence is suggested to be approximately 1.5 out of 100,000 per year (roughly 5,000 new cases in the United States yearly), with the limitations deriving from the fact that only recently were they identified as a clinicopathologic entity.[8,9] However, there are a number of small GISTs that are clinically meaningless and generally go undetected. In addition, microscopic GISTs (micro-GIST) might be found incidentally in as many as 10% to 25% of stomachs.[10,11] The reasons why the vast majority do not give rise to clinically overt diseases are not known, especially considering the fact that most of them harbor the same mutations to KIT and PDGFRA of fully developed diseases, which implies that alterations of these proto-oncogenes are not solely the pathogenetic drivers of GISTs.[12] Thus, the incidence of histologic GISTs may be much higher than that of clinical cases, which remains low. Prevalence is low as well, although roughly half of clinical GISTs are cured by surgery, and the median survival of advanced GISTs has improved with the use of TKIs and is likely still improving.

GISTs can occur at any age, with a median occurrence at 60 to 65 years. A small minority of GISTs affect children and adolescents: most of them are WT for KIT and PDGFRA and may take place within selected syndromes. In general, GISTs are slightly more incident in males than females. Succinate dehydrogenase (SDH)-deficient WT GISTs typically occur in young females.

No specific causes are known, although the pathogenesis of KIT- and PDGFRA-mutated GISTs has been elucidated in essence. There are some predisposing conditions for WT GISTs, which include the Carney triad (marked by GIST, pulmonary chondromas, and extra-adrenal paragangliomas), the hereditary Carney-Stratakis syndrome (marked by GIST and familial paragangliomas), and type 1 neurofibromatosis (NF-1).[13–15] Hereditary syndromes driven by germ-line mutations to KIT or PDGFRA are very rare but well recognized.[16,17]

ANATOMY AND PATHOLOGY

More than half of GIST cases arise from the stomach, one-fourth from the small bowel, roughly 5% from the rectum, and a small minority from the esophagus.[7] Some GISTs have been labeled as *extragastrointestinal*, apparently arising from the mesentery, omentum, and retroperitoneum; however, it remains unknown whether these are lesions detached from their gastrointestinal origin and/or are metastases from an unknown primary tumor.

Morphologically, GISTs can be made up of spindle cells (in more than two-thirds of cases), epithelioid cells, or both (Fig. 55.1 A,B).[18] Epithelioid-cell GISTs are more common in the stomach and include those that are PDGFRA mutated. Aside from this, there are no major clinical implications in the microscopic aspect of lesions. Importantly, there are no pathologic clues to make a distinction between malignant GISTs and others whose clinical behavior is actually benign. Thus, many GISTs behave as benign diseases as a matter of fact, but this cannot be forecast histologically or molecularly. It follows that all GISTs are currently considered malignant neoplasms, although with a highly variable risk of distant relapse, which is negligible in a significant proportion of them. This is the reason why risk classification systems are generally used in the clinic as prognosticators, being based today on a pathologic factor (i.e., the mitotic count) and two clinical variables (tumor size and tumor site).[19–24]

Immunohistochemically, the hallmark of most GISTs is their positivity for KIT (CD117) and DOG-1 (Fig. 55.2 A,B).[25–27] A low proportion of GISTs are CD117 negative, which is typical of PDGFRA-mutated GISTs, but immunohistochemical status does not reflect the mutational status with regard to KIT and PDGFRA, per se, so that it has no concrete predictive value for sensitivity to TKIs. Thus, CD117 has only a meaning in the pathologic differential diagnosis. Given their morphology, GISTs must be differentiated

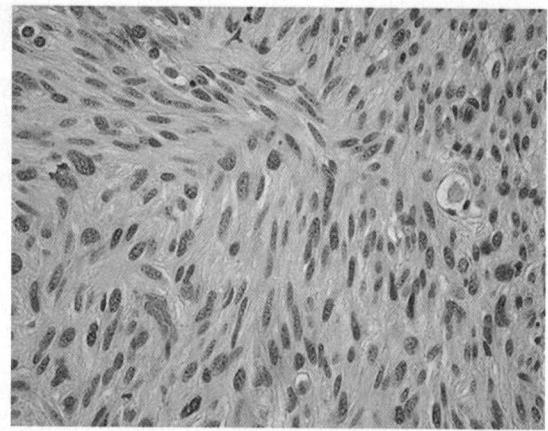
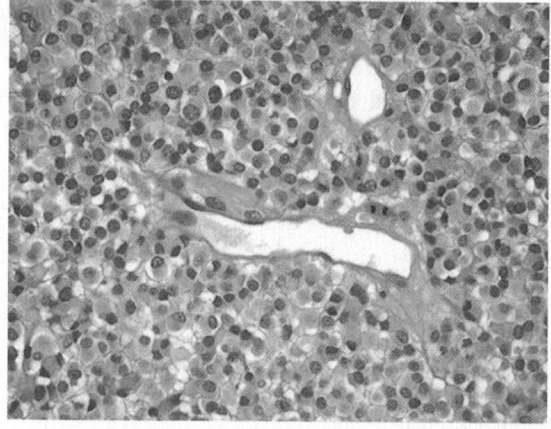

Figure 55.1 **(A)** Spindle-cell GIST. **(B)** Epithelioid-cell GIST.

from other soft tissue tumors of the gastrointestinal wall, including those of smooth muscle and neural origin and desmoid-type fibromatosis, endocrine tumors, melanocytic tumors, lymphomas, etc. Desmin is rarely positive, as opposed to vimentin and CD34. A negative stain for SDHB identifies the subgroup of SDH-deficient WT GISTs.[28,29]

Molecularly, GIST have become a relatively heterogeneous and complex group of lesions.[30] Gain-of-function mutations of the oncogenes located on chromosome 4 (4q12) coding for the type III receptor tyrosine kinases KIT and PDGFRA can be found in approximately 80% of GISTs.[5,6,31] Pathogenetically, they are the drivers of the disease and, therapeutically, underlie the efficacy of currently used TKIs. They are mutually exclusive and result in the constitutive activation of either KIT or PDGFRA, which normally are autoinhibited, being activated by the binding of their respective ligands (i.e., stem-cell factor [Steel factor] and platelet-derived growth factor A). The activation of the receptor binds two molecules of KIT or PDGFRA (dimerization), giving rise to downstream oncogenic signaling, which for both KIT and PDGFRA involves the RAS/MAPK and the PI3K/AKT/mammalian target of rapamycin (mTOR) pathways (Fig. 55.3). Mutations can be deletions, insertions, and missense mutations. They affect: exon 11 of the KIT oncogene, encoding for the juxtamembrane domain of the KIT receptor, in slightly less than 70% of GISTs; exon 9 of KIT, encoding for the extracellular domain of the receptor, in less than 10%; exon 13 and 17 of KIT, encoding for the intracellular ATP-binding pocket and activation loop domains, respectively, in a small minority of GISTs. Approximately 10% of GIST have mutations homologous to these, which affect PDGFRA (i.e., exon 12, 14, and 18 of the oncogene, with 70% being represented by the

exon 18 D842V mutation). The latter is known for its wide lack of sensitivity to available TKIs, along with a few other rare exon 18 mutations, whereas the deletion of codons 842 to 845 is sensitive. Possibly because of their similarity with different kinds of normal interstitial cell of Cajal, some tumor cell mutations correlate with elective primary sites of origin. In particular, exon 9 mutations of KIT are preferably found in the small bowel, and PDGFRA mutations are found in the stomach.

Approximately 10% to 15% of GISTs are WT for KIT and PDGFRA. They make up a family of tumor subsets with different pathogenetic backgrounds and, to some extent, different natural histories (see Fig. 55.3). Their classification is evolving.[5,6,31] In essence, as of today, one may identify: (1) SDH-deficient GISTs; (2) neurofibromatosis (NF)-1–related GISTs; or (3) others, including those with the BRAF V600E mutation. In fact, half of WT GISTs are marked by alterations involving the SDH complex, which is crucial for the Krebs cycle and mitochondrial respiratory cell function. Immunohistochemically, these GIST are negative to SDHB staining. A group of them includes *pediatric* GISTs and can be associated with the Carney triad.[13] In fact, these GISTs tend to arise in children and young adults of the female sex, are gastric and multifocal, can metastasize to lymph nodes, have a rather indolent evolution. When the Carney triad is fully expressed, it includes GISTs, pulmonary chondromas, and paragangliomas. Given the absence of mutations to the SDH complex, a posttranscriptional defect leading to dysfunctions of the SDH complex may be in place. These GISTs are SDHA positive. On the other hand, a group of SDH-deficient GISTs carries germ-line mutations of the SDHA, SDHB, or SDHC units of the SDH complex[32,33] and may be related to the Carney-Stratakis syndrome.[14] This is marked by

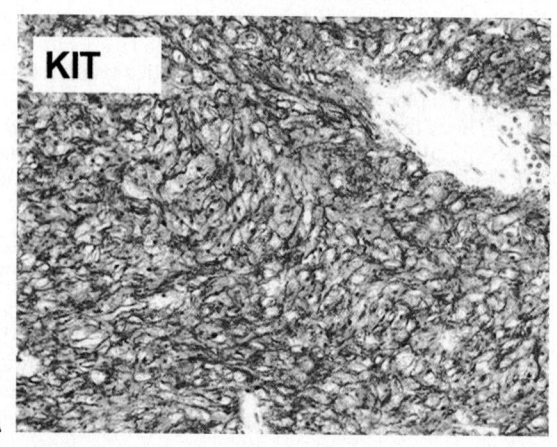
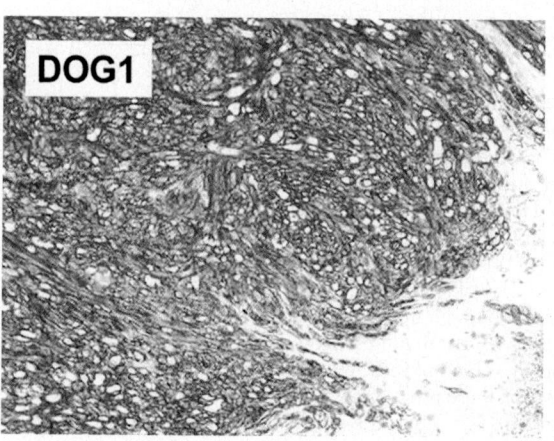

Figure 55.2 Immunostaining for KIT (CD117) and DOG1.

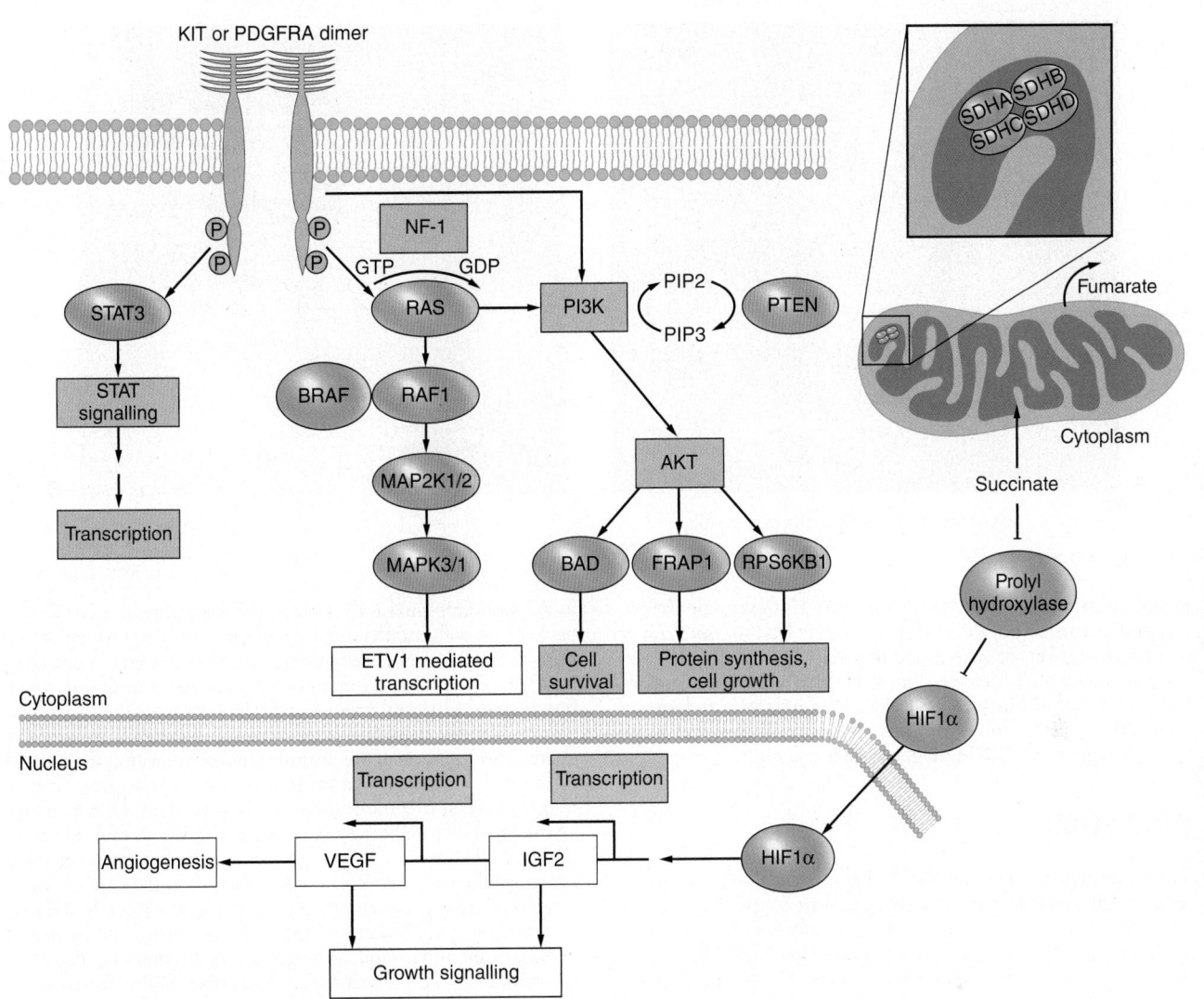

Figure 55.3 Signaling in KIT/PDGFRA-mutated and WT GIST. (From Joensuu H, Hohenberger P, Corless CL. Gastrointestinal stromal tumour. *Lancet* 2013;382:973–983.)

GIST and paragangliomas. Immunohistochemically, GISTs with SDHA mutations are negative to SDHA staining. The median age of these patients is somewhat higher and the female to male predominance is lower, but the course of disease is indolent as well. Then, WT SDHB-positive GISTs can occur in the context of NF-1, and their pathogenetic mechanism is supposed to be the absence of neurofibromin (i.e., the product of the NF-1 gene), which is mutated.[34,35] This may lead to increased activity of the RAS pathway. GISTs related to NF-1 are typically multicentric as well, and have a rather indolent course, but arise from the small bowel. Of course, NF-1 may coexist with a non–NF-1-related GISTs. Finally, the remaining SDHB-positive GISTs are probably a basket of different conditions: some were reported to have the V600E mutation of BRAF[36,37] or, more rarely, HRAS, NRAS, and PIK3 mutations.[5] All this makes the so-called WT GISTs a variegated family of tumors, which can now be identified not only through a negative definition (i.e., by the lack of KIT and PDGFRA mutations), but through immunohistochemical or cytogenetic markers, pointing to specific subsets with different natural histories.

A very rare subset of familial GISTs does exist, being marked by mutations of KIT or PDGFRA affecting the germ line.[16,17] They parallel mutations found in sporadic GISTs and lead to the multicentric and multifocal occurrence of GISTs. The behavior of these GISTs is variable (i.e., it is often indolent but some lesions turn out to become aggressive). Hyperplasia of interstitial cells of Cajal can be found, which may entail altered motility of the gastrointestinal tract. Urticaria pigmentosa and other alterations of skin pigmentation may complete the syndrome.

It is then clear how important genotyping has become for GIST patients. In fact, genotyping has an obvious predictive value, which is crucial for all patients who are candidates for medical therapy, whether in the advanced or in the adjuvant setting. In addition, genotyping has prognostic implications, at least given the peculiar natural history of WT GISTs. Finally, genotyping confirms the pathologic diagnosis in KIT/PDGFRA-mutated GIST, or leads to further pathologic and molecular assessments in WT GISTs. Thus, although there are subsets of GISTs with such a low risk of relapse as not to make them candidates for any medical therapy, a mutational analysis is currently felt as a companion to virtually any pathologic diagnosis of GISTs.

SCREENING

GISTs are rare cancers. Therefore, population-based screening policies are unforeseeable. As for all rare cancers, the clinical aim should be a timely diagnosis in the individual patient with symptoms and/or signs of disease. A difficulty thereof is the anatomical tendency of GIST lesions to grow outwards from the gastrointestinal wall, so that they may go undetected for long

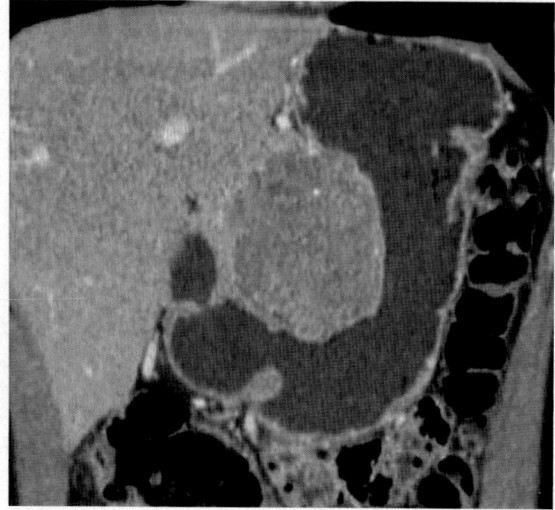
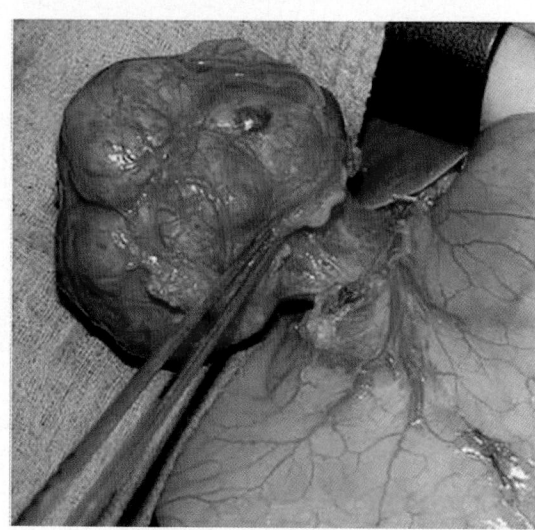

Figure 55.4 GIST growing outward of the gastric wall.

periods even when endoscopically explored. However, endoscopic procedures carried out for other reasons may lead to some risk of *overdiagnosis*, even in such a rare disease, when small gastric lesions are incidentally detected. Some of them will be benign entities, and others will be GISTs unlikely to ever grow as to become clinically relevant. Only a minority of them will turn out to be clinically aggressive GISTs caught in their making.

DIAGNOSIS

The outward growth of many GISTs (Fig. 55.4) within the gastrointestinal wall is one of the reasons why several are diagnosed relatively late, either as major abdominal masses or as causes of gastrointestinal bleeding, hemoperitoneum, perforations (Fig. 55.5). Therefore, as many as one-fourth of GISTs are diagnosed in a clinical emergency, often leading to surgical explorations resulting in the unexpected finding of the disease. One-fourth of GISTs are discovered incidentally during diagnostic assessments (whether an endoscopic procedure, ultrasound, or computed tomography [CT] scan) done for other reasons. The remaining are diagnosed because of symptoms of compression from an abdominal mass, or chronic anemia, fatigue, and the like. Therefore, GISTs should be included in the differential diagnosis of abdominal masses. When their pertinence

to the gastrointestinal wall is clear, the possibility of a GIST may be obvious, with a differential diagnosis mainly against epithelial tumors, small bowel endocrine tumors, lymphomas, paragangliomas, etc. Otherwise, retroperitoneal sarcomas and desmoid-type fibromatosis, germ cell tumors, and lymphomas are the main alternatives. Notably, when this is the clinical presentation, surgery is of choice only for some of the possible alternatives within the clinical differential diagnosis. In addition, preoperative treatments may be resorted to even in some of the surgical indications. On top of this, an intraoperative pathologic differential diagnosis is prohibitive. In principle, therefore, a diagnostic core needle biopsy is suggested by many, allowing pathologic diagnosis and, in the case of GIST, a mutational analysis, prior to any surgical exploration. In the case of gastric or rectal lesions, a biopsy can be carried out by means of endoscopic ultrasound, although, for gastric tumors, the risk of perforation should be factored in depending on the presentation. A CT/ultrasound-guided percutaneous biopsy is the other option, apparently with a negligible risk of dissemination if done at a center of expertise, again factoring in the clinical presentation.[38] There may remain some cases in which the difficulty of an endoscopic or percutaneous biopsy and the easiness of a surgical exploration would suggest the latter. In general, however, a biopsy prior to any therapeutic planning can minimize the number of abdominal masses undergoing futile surgery.

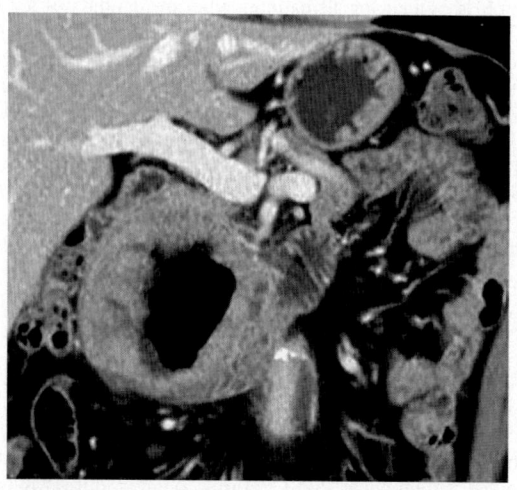
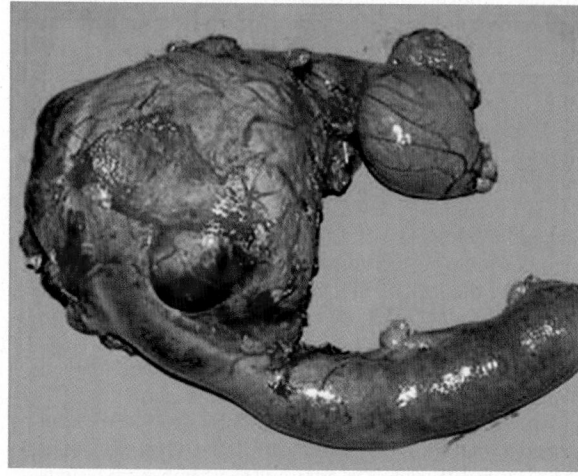

Figure 55.5 Duodenal GIST with an intratumoral perforation.

Follow-ups after potentially eradicating surgery is aimed at picking up relapses at an early stage. Local relapses are infrequent and tend to develop outwards from the gastrointestinal wall: therefore, an endoscopy is generally not used as a routine follow-up procedure. A CT scan is the most sensitive exam to pick up peritoneal and liver metastases and is recommended. It can be replaced by magnetic resonance imaging (MRI), while ultrasound is much less sensitive on the peritoneum. The maximum risk interval averages 2 to 3 years after surgery or, if an adjuvant therapy was done, after its completion. Long-term relapses are unlikely, although they are occasionally observed, especially in GISTs with a low mitotic rates. All this helps drive rational follow-up policies for potentially cured patients, though there is a lack of any empirical evidence of their effectiveness.[39]

STAGING

Conventional stage classification is seldom used.[40] Clinicians mainly distinguish localized from metastatic disease and, if the disease is localized and amenable to complete surgery, quantify the risk of relapse.[20,22,24]

Current risk classification systems are based on the combination of mitotic count, tumor size, and site of origin. Indeed, the mitotic count is the main prognostic factor, proportionally correlating to the risk of relapse. Its downside has turned out to be its possibly low reproducibility rate, but clearly this can be higher if the pathologist is aware of its importance in driving treatment choices. Tumor size is the next prognostic factor. On one side, it singles out very small gastric lesions (<2 cm), which may undergo watchful surveillance if incidentally discovered endoscopically. On the other, it highlights lesions in excess of 5 to 10 cm, which have a worse prognosis. With regard to the primary site, gastric lesions have a better prognosis than small bowel and rectal GISTs. Thus, the combination of these three factors allows one to forecast a risk of relapse by using tools such as the Armed Forces Institute of Pathology (AFIP) risk classification, the Memorial Sloan Kettering Cancer Center (MSKCC) nomogram, or the contour maps. The contour maps have the advantage of treating both the mitotic rate and tumor size as continuous variables as they are, so that the accuracy is increased especially for intermediate-risk cases (Fig. 55.6). Also, reproducibility issues become less crucial by factoring mitotic count as a continuous variable. In addition, contour maps segregate the prognosis

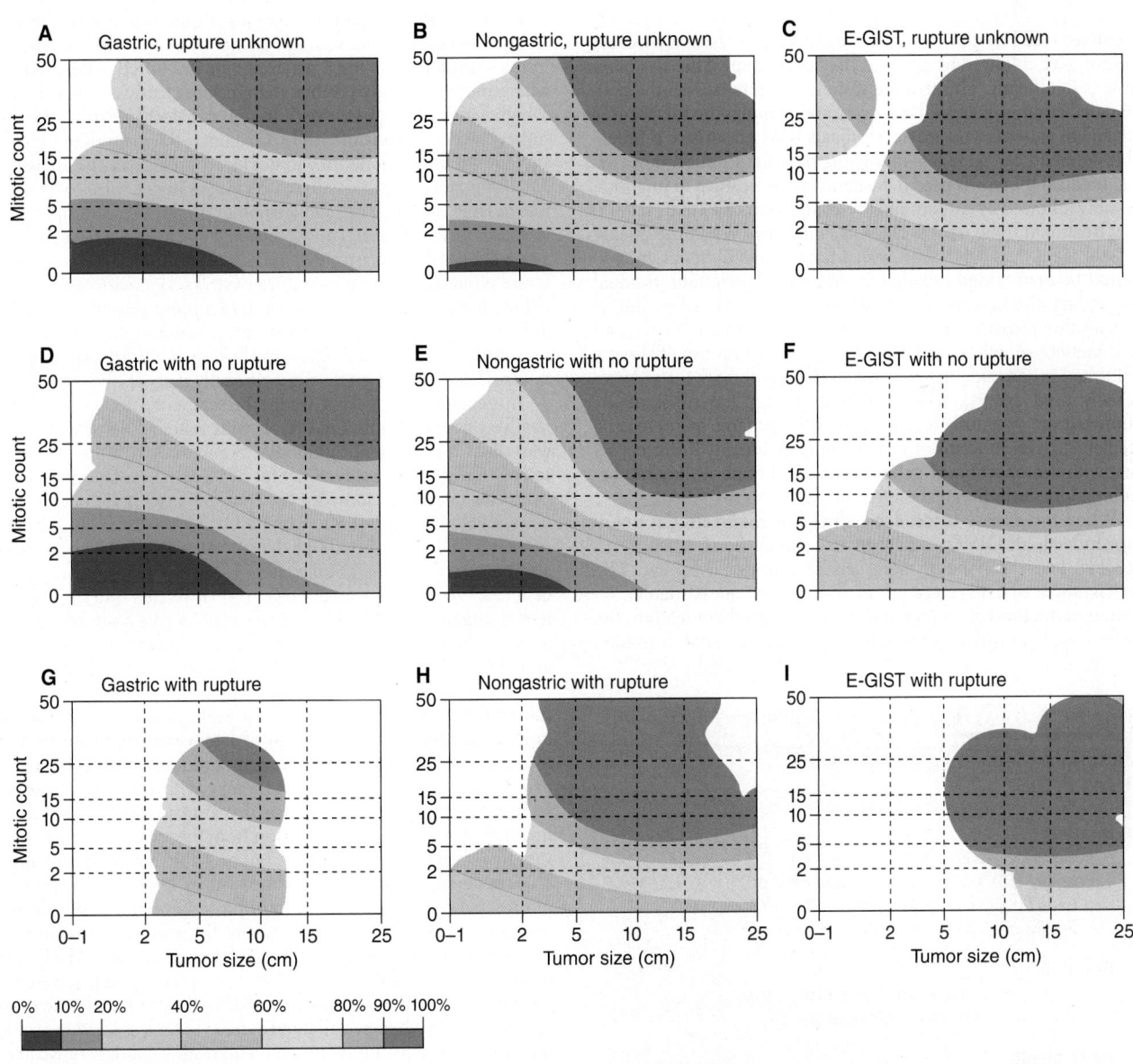

Figure 55.6 Contour prognostic maps in localized GISTs. (From Joensuu H, Vehtari A, Riihimäki J, et al. Risk of gastrointestinal stromal tumour recurrence after surgery: an analysis of pooled population-based cohorts. *Lancet Oncol* 2012;13:265–274.)

PRACTICE OF ONCOLOGY

of lesions that underwent tumor rupture, which is a highly adverse prognostic factor in diseases anatomically facing the peritoneum.[41]

The natural history of advanced GISTs is marked by their potential extension to the peritoneum and/or the liver. Thus, a CT scan is the staging procedure of choice to rule out metastatic disease. Lung metastases are rare, with the possible exception of rectal GISTs, although a chest CT scan is generally used to extend a staging workup to lungs and the mediastinum. Bone metastases are possible, but they are usually confined to the very advanced stages of disease, so that the skeleton is not routinely assessed in the lack of symptoms.[42] Other sites of distant metastases are exceedingly rare. Lymph node regional metastases are not typical of GISTs, as for mesenchymal tumors in general, with the remarkable exception of WT GISTs occurring in children and/or within syndromes. In addition, all *syndromic* GISTs may be multifocal and multicentric.[43,44] This is not tantamount to metastatic spread, being rather a marker of their inherent natural history. All these features of the natural history of GISTs drive staging procedures, in addition to the potential for other syndromic correlates, depending on the presentation.

MANAGEMENT BY STAGE

Localized GISTs with no evidence of distant metastases are treated with surgery, followed by adjuvant medical therapy if the risk of relapse is significant. This treatment strategy capitalizes on the consolidated curative potential of surgery and prolongs the relapse-free interval of patients who are not eradicated. When surgery is unfeasible or could be made less mutilating or easier through downsizing, medical therapy is used if the genotype is sensitive to imatinib, possibly followed by surgery and the completion of a medical adjuvant treatment if the risk of relapse is significant. When the disease is metastatic, medical therapy with TKIs is standard treatment and should be maintained indefinitely. Surgery of metastatic residual responding disease can be used when reasonably feasible, but its added value prognostically is unproven. When imatinib fails and/or is ineffective, other available TKIs and judicious use of surgery of limited progression are resorted to (see Table 55.1 for conventionally used agents). This treatment strategy has substantially improved the prognosis of advanced GIST patients by increasing median survival in terms of years if compared to any historical series, with a proportion of patients, limited though it may be, becoming long-term progression-free survivors.

When the disease is localized, surgery is the treatment mainstay. Indeed, all GISTs ≥2 cm in size should be resected when possible, because none of them can be considered *benign*. The management of GISTs <2 cm in size is more questionable.[45–47] Although the low risk of progression of GISTs <2 cm leads to the recommendation of a conservative approach, a reliable mitotic index cannot be determined by biopsy or fine-needle aspiration (FNA), thus preventing the identification of those at higher risk. Therefore, both observation and resection for GISTs 1 to 2 cm can be considered, and the risks and benefits of one versus the other should be discussed with the patient. The endoscopic resection of small gastric GISTs could be an option in these presentations. Risks of perforation may be low, although the decision is made on a case-by-case basis. Regardless of their size, any small GIST that is symptomatic (e.g., bleeding from erosions through the mucosa) or increases in size on serial follow-up should be resected.

A laparotomic or laparoscopic/laparoscopy-assisted resection of primary GISTs should be performed following standard oncologic principles. On laparotomy/laparoscopy, the abdomen should be thoroughly explored to identify and remove any previously undetected peritoneal metastatic deposits.[48–51] Although primary GISTs may demonstrate inflammatory adhesions to surrounding organs, true invasion is not frequent. The goal of surgery is R0 excision. A macroscopically complete resection with negative or positive microscopic margins (R0 or R1 resection, respectively) is associated with a better prognosis than a macroscopically incomplete excision (R2 excision).[52,53] Available series have not clearly shown that R1 surgery is associated with a definitely higher risk of local failure, so that the decision whether to reexcise a lesion already operated on with microscopically positive margins is doubtful, aside from the fact that sometimes a reexcision may not be technically foreseeable in the gastrointestinal tract. An exception are GIST of the rectum, where microscopically positive margins are clearly associated with a higher risk of local failure.[54] In general, local relapse after R0 surgery is very unlikely in GISTs. Of course, the margins of a big lesion toward the peritoneum will not be covered by any clean tissue, and this may well be the main reason for the high peritoneal relapse rate of large tumors even after complete surgery. Tumor rupture or violation of the tumor capsule during surgery are associated with a very high risk of recurrence, and therefore should be avoided.[41] Some clinicians approach ruptured GISTs as already metastatic, although there may be different kinds of *rupture*, possibly leading to different risk levels. A lymphadenectomy is not routinely required, because lymph nodes are rarely involved (in adult patients) and are thus resected only when they are clinically suspect.

In general, surgery is a wedge or segmental resection of the involved gastric or intestinal tract, with margins that can be less wide than for an adenocarcinoma. Sometimes, a more extensive resection (e.g., total gastrectomy for a large proximal gastric GIST, pancreaticoduodenectomy for a periampullary GIST, or abdominoperineal resection for a low rectal GIST) is needed. In the rare syndromic GIST (either SDH deficient or NF-1 related), tumors are often multifocal and confined either to the stomach (SDH-deficient GIST) or the small bowel (NF-1–related GIST). The extent of surgery should be decided on a case-by-case basis, taking into account the risk of recurrence, the lack of benefit from currently available TKIs, and the actual behavior of the underlying disease.[55]

Adjuvant medical therapy with imatinib was demonstrated to substantially improve relapse-free intervals, although with a trend to lose the benefit in a time span of 1 to 3 years from the end of therapy.[56–58] This was shown through randomized trials that compared 1 and 2 years of adjuvant therapy with imatinib versus no adjuvant therapy, and 3 years versus 1 year of adjuvant therapy with imatinib. As of today, the suggestion from these studies is that adjuvant therapy with TKIs can delay, but probably not avoid, a relapse, if this is due to occur. This correlated with a survival improvement in one trial[57] and with a trend to improvement of a potential surrogate for survival in another,[58] where the surrogate was survival free from changing the original tirosine kinase inhibitor (TKI)—in practice, survival without secondary resistance. In fact, secondary resistance is the limiting factor of TKIs in the advanced setting, so that an adjuvant therapy will be beneficial as long as it either avoids recurrences or at least prolongs freedom from secondary resistance, but by no means shortens it. Thus, the risk of any detrimental effect was ruled out for adjuvant therapy durations up to 3 years. In this

---

TABLE 55.1

Standard Medical Agents Currently Used in GIST

◼ **Imatinib**
- 400 mg by mouth daily
- Possibly 800 mg by mouth daily, in case of:
  ○ Exon 9 KIT-mutated GIST
  ○ Progression on imatinib 400 mg

◼ **Sunitinib**
- 50 mg by mouth daily for 4 wks every 6 wks
- 37.5 mg by mouth daily continuously

◼ **Regorafenib**
- 160 mg by mouth daily for 3 wks every 4 wks

sense, going beyond 3 years would seem logical, given the tendency to lose the benefit after 1 to 3 years from stopping adjuvant therapy, but such a policy should be validated by clinical trials ruling out any adverse effect on secondary resistance. Results from clinical studies on longer durations of adjuvant therapy are therefore expected. Currently, adjuvant therapy is recommended for 3 years and is reserved for patients with a significant risk of relapse, as long as the benefit in absolute terms will be higher as the risk increases, as is the case with all adjuvant therapies. In a sense, the lack of a tangible impact on the long-term relapse rate encourages one to exclude relatively low-risk patients, which is, to some extent, at odds with what is done with adjuvant cytotoxic chemotherapy in some solid cancers. This said, the magnitude of risk that is worth an adjuvant therapy with imatinib for 3 years may well be subject to a shared decision making with the individual patient, and, as a matter of fact, is generally placed above 30% to 50%. Logically, a benefit can be expected for patients whose genotype is potentially sensitive to imatinib.[59] In practice, this leads to the selection of all patients with a KIT-mutated GIST or a PDGFRA-mutated sensitive GIST (with the exception of the D842V exon 18 mutation and the few others which are insensitive in vitro and in vivo to imatinib). Given the benefit shown with the use of a double dose of imatinib (800 mg daily) for advanced GIST patients with an exon 9 KIT-mutated GIST,[60] such a dosage can be selected for them, although there is a lack of any formal demonstration in the adjuvant setting. WT GISTs are much less sensitive to imatinib, and adjuvant studies

are lacking with other TKIs, which may be potentially more active. Even more importantly, the natural history of WT GISTs is often less aggressive. These are the reasons why many clinicians currently do not select WT GISTs patients for any adjuvant treatment.

Given the extensive use of adjuvant therapy with imatinib in the high-risk populations and the activity of the drug, several recent multi-institutional retrospective series have questioned the need for extensive resections such as pancreaticoduodenectomy, abdominal perineal resection, or total/proximal gastrectomy, when tumor downsizing can be likely achieved with a preoperative medical treatment. In practice, preoperative imatinib can shrink gastric, periampullary, or rectal GISTs to such an extent as to allow more limited excisions (wedge gastrectomy, excision of periampullary lesions, transanal/perineal resection of rectal GISTs, respectively), and imatinib can then be continued postoperatively to complete the *adjuvant* treatment (Fig. 55.7). Thus, if extensive surgery is required for complete tumor removal, preoperative imatinib should be considered.[61–64] In addition to this, there are some big abdominal masses that may be felt by the surgeon as implying a significant risk of tumor rupture during surgery, which can be treated with preoperative imatinib. Because downsizing is the clinical end point in these cases, the duration of pre-operative medical therapy is generally 6 to 12 months, which corresponds to the time interval when the maximum degree of tumor shrinkage was shown to occur in studies on advanced GISTs.[65] In addition, mutational status is important in order to select patients likely to respond to imatinib,

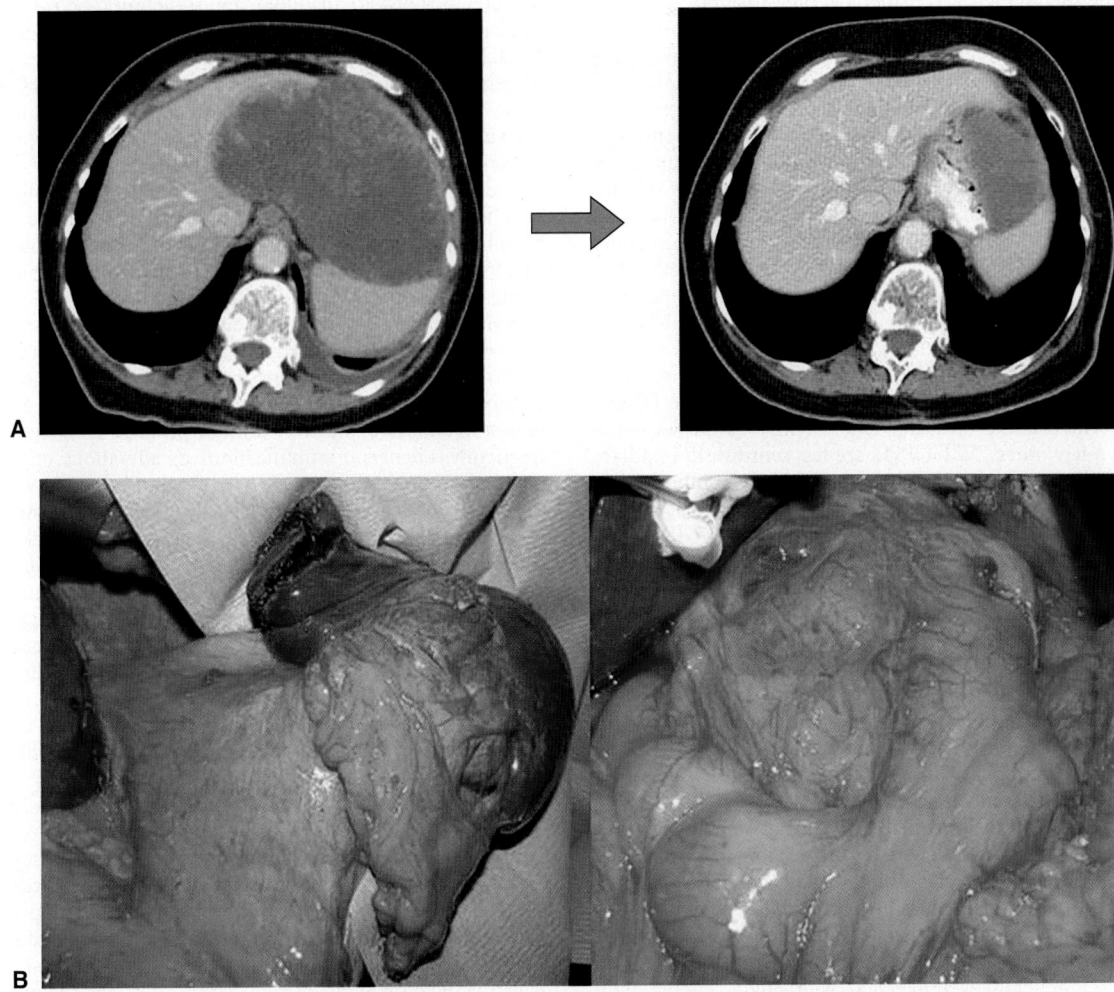

Figure 55.7 (A) Tumor shrinkage of a gastric primary GIST after 12 months of preoperative imatinib, **(B)** allowing for a sleeve gastrectomy plus splenectomy and liver resection with preservation of most of the stomach after resection.

and tumor response should be monitored closely. Positron-emission tomography (PET) scans are a resource, because they can demonstrate tumor responsiveness in a matter of weeks.

Syndromic GISTs can present with multifocal and/or multicentric disease, which may imply delicate surgical decisions. Thus, in WT GISTs, such as those occurring in children and young adults or in NF-1 patients, one should take into account the indolent behavior of many lesions and the possible presence of hyperplasia of the interstitial cells of Cajal on one side, and the possibility that single lesions may be aggressive on the other. Surgery should judiciously factor in all this. In addition, the relative lack of sensitivity of WT GISTs to available TKIs may suggest to resort to surgery more liberally than is currently done with KIT-mutated GISTs.

With regard to the highly rare syndromes of familial GISTs from germ-line mutations of KIT or PDGFRA, treatment is challenging and may involve resorting to surgery and/or TKIs depending on the behavior and extent of clinically relevant lesions.

When the disease is metastatic or locally advanced, medical therapy is the best choice and is currently based on imatinib continued indefinitely.[66–69] However, given the limiting factor of secondary resistance, some clinicians prefer to surgically resect some highly localized first distant relapses, thus delaying the start of imatinib to a subsequent relapse. It is unproven whether this approach may delay progression, its rationale being to delay the onset of time to secondary resistance by delaying the onset of any use of TKIs. Theoretically, the downside may be starting medical therapy with a higher tumor burden, which was shown to be related to a shorter time to secondary resistance to imatinib.

In fact, initial tumor burden is virtually the only prognostic factor in the metastatic GIST patient starting imatinib.[70] On the other hand, although above 80% overall, the probability of response is strictly correlated with the mutational status, which is, therefore, the main predictive factor.[71–73] KIT-mutated GIST are responsive in most cases, including the most frequent genotype, marked by mutations of exon 11. This applies also to patients who underwent adjuvant imatinib and who did not experience tumor relapse during the adjuvant period, so that these patients are currently approached the same way as those who have not been already exposed to imatinib. The standard daily dosage of imatinib is 400 mg. However, there are data derived from retrospective subgroup analyses that suggest progression-free survival is better with doses higher than 400 mg (i.e., 800 mg daily) for exon 9 KIT-mutated GIST patients.[60] Thus, many institutions treat these patients with 800 mg. PDGFRA-mutated GIST patients can be sensitive to imatinib as well, with the remarkable exception of the D842V mutation, which is the most frequent amongst PDGFRA mutations, and a few others. WT GISTs are less sensitive to imatinib, which may, however, be active in some patients. Sunitinib is an alternative option, because it was shown to have some activity in WT GISTs.[74] Generally, the clinical decision in WT GISTs, and of course PDGFRA D842–mutated patients, takes into account the natural history of these subtypes, which is often less aggressive than in KIT-mutated GISTs. Thus, surgical options, including ablations, may be resorted to when the relapse is limited. However, in sensitive genotypes medical therapy is an option even when surgery is feasible, and any decision on surgery is usually delayed to when the tumor response has been established. This allows for the possibility of being certain about a patient's responsiveness to a medical therapy that will need to be prolonged indefinitely because the disease is metastatic.

In fact, a discontinuation trial showed that stopping therapy after 1, 3, or 5 years is followed by progression in a matter of months.[75] It is true that reestablishing therapy generally leads to a new response, but its quality may be inferior to the previous one.[76] In any case, intervals to progression would be remarkably short, and an untenable *stop-and-go* treatment policy would be the result.

Imatinib is generally well tolerated, with fatigue, edema, mild diarrhea, and anemia as frequent complaints, along with less frequent toxicities, such as neutropenia, skin rash, and others.[67–69]

Clinical wisdom needs to be exercised in order to maintain dose intensity vis-à-vis side effects.[77] The number of patients truly intolerant to imatinib should be exceedingly low.

Secondary resistance is the limiting factor of imatinib, with a median time to the event averaging 2 years in the frontline advanced setting. One cannot rule out that current patients, who are generally put on therapy with lower tumor burdens, may show improved progression-free survival intervals over the earliest series. More importantly, the range of time to secondary resistance is wide, with a limited proportion of patients, averaging 10%, who become long-term progression-free survivors. Currently, there are no known prognostic factors for long-term progression-free survivorship, excluding the mutational status, which affects tumor response to imatinib, and tumor burden at the onset of imatinib therapy, which affects the duration of response. The group of long-term progression-free survivors may thus represent either just the "tail" of a curve driven by the stochastic mechanisms of secondary resistance, or the result of specific genomic profiles, still to be elucidated.

In an attempt to download tumor burden, thus potentially prolonging time to secondary resistance, surgery of residual responding disease has been resorted to in many institutions, and its results were retrospectively, but not prospectively, evaluated, with the exception of an underpowered randomized prospective study in patients who had only peritoneal disease.[78–83] These case series analyses showed a better prognosis for patients undergoing surgery, but a selection bias may well explain the results. Prospective trials have not been successful; therefore, the decision whether to surgically excise metastatic lesions responding to imatinib is currently left to a shared decision making with the patient in conditions of uncertainty. Of course, clinical presentations are manifold, and sometimes the easiness of the surgical resection is the main factor leading to the decision, and vice versa. In general, many institutions currently avoid resorting to major surgery for responding metastases. In any case, only patients amenable to complete resection of all lesions should be candidates for this kind of surgery. In this sense, surgery may be less often indicated in peritoneal compared to liver metastases, because the former are frequently underestimated by available imaging modalities and the selection of completely clearable tumors is less feasible. However, the clinician must be aware that imatinib needs to be continued after surgery, even if surgery was complete. In fact, some patients enrolled in the discontinuation trial of imatinib had had a complete excision of their metastatic lesions.[74] In addition, surgery of metastatic GISTs was never proved to be eradicating in the pre-imatinib era.[84]

Progression during therapy with imatinib is often due to secondary resistance, which essentially is marked by the occurrence of new mutations to the same primarily mutated oncogene, or, less frequently, oncogene amplifications or alterations of alternative pathways.[5] It is left to elucidate whether these secondary mutations should be biologically viewed as developing de novo. Secondary mutations entail such consequences as to lower the binding capacity of the KIT or PDGFRA receptor for imatinib and/or to circumvent its inhibiting action by escape mechanisms.[85] It was demonstrated that secondary resistance can be heterogeneous, so that more mutations can be detected in different lesions, or even within the same lesion.[86,87] Of course, this is a major limiting factor for second-line agents targeting KIT or PDGFRA. Secondary mutations in KIT-mutated GISTs are relatively limited in number, affecting exons 13 and 14, which encode the ATP-binding pocket, or exons 17 and 18, which encode the activation loop. Many resistant PDGFRA-mutated GISTs acquire the D842V mutation, which encodes for the activation loop of the receptor.

Clinically, the progression may be *limited* in a substantial proportion of cases. This means that progression is radiologically evident only in one or a few lesions, with the others still progressing. A typical clinical pattern is the *nodule within the nodule* (i.e., a small hyperdensity within a responding hypodense lesion on CT scan).[88] Given the scope of activity of further-line therapies, many clinicians now tend to treat limited progression conservatively from the medical point of view, resorting to selected surgical or ablative procedures to get rid of the progressing component of the disease, while continuing imatinib for the remaining. This might delay the moment when the first TKI is switched to a second-line one. Though this policy is not based on prospective clinical studies, it makes sense in the economy of advanced GISTs following the introduction of TKIs. Clearly this does not apply to *generalized* progressions.

Radiologic progression should be confirmed, taking into account the peculiarities of tumor response patterns in GISTs undergoing TKIs. Furthermore, before attributing progression on frontline imatinib to molecular secondary resistance, one should rule out any lack of patient compliance with therapy, which may often go unnoticed and even be underappreciated by the patient. Another mechanism leading to resistance can lie in changes of the pharmacokinetics of the drug. There is evidence that pharmacokinetics can undergo variations with time, in addition to being variable across individuals.[89] This has led to the evaluation of the importance of maintaining target plasma levels of imatinib.[90] There are limitations to the standardization of such assessments, and available data pointing to a correlation with progression-free survival are retrospective in nature. Thus, at the moment, we lack any convincing formal demonstration that pharmacokinetics is a factor able to personalize medical therapy (i.e., to drive changes in drug dosages in the lack of evident progression). However, available evidence also suggests that it can well be a variable with many orally administered targeted agents. At least, plasma levels may be assessed in the single patient: in case of clinical progression, to rule out that a major pharmacokinetic issue does exist at that stage; in case of unexpected side effects; and in case of comedications potentially able to interfere with the drug metabolism.

In the case of clinical progression with imatinib 400 mg daily, an option widely used is to increase the dose to 800 mg daily. This proved temporarily successful in a limited proportion of patients crossing over to the higher dose in randomized trials that compared 400 mg with 800 mg as frontline therapy for advanced GISTs.[91] When valuing this benefit, one should probably discount patients who had an exon 9 mutation and who started with 400 mg, and possibly some patients failing to comply with therapy, whereas other patients may have benefited due to the correction of pharmacokinetics problems.

Standard second-line therapy is sunitinib, which is a TKI inhibiting KIT and PDGFRA but also displaying antiangiogenic activity by the inhibition of vascular endothelial growth factor receptor (VEGFR)1, 2, and 3. It was shown to be effective at increasing progression-free survival by 5 months in a randomized trial versus placebo in patients failing (or intolerant) to imatinib.[92] Its molecular profile is such as to include activity on exon 9 KIT mutations as well as on secondary mutations of regions coding for the ATP-binding pocket, thus potentially covering mutations which are, respectively, less affected or not affected by imatinib.[93] What limits the potential of molecular prediction in further-line therapies of GISTs is basically the heterogeneity that often underlies secondary resistance, so that the presence of a secondary mutation is unlikely to be alone, although potentially sensitive to available agents. However, the activity of sunitinib against some secondary mutations and probably its antiangiogenic activity underlie its clinical efficacy after failing to imatinib. Its tolerability profile is less favorable, with fatigue and hand–foot syndrome as its main side effects, variable though they may be across patients. Although the clinical trial evaluated a regimen of sunitinib given 50 mg daily for 4 weeks, with a 2-week rest, a continuous regimen with a daily dose of 37.5 mg can be used as well.[94]

Regorafenib, another TKI with activity on KIT and PDGFRA as well as VEGFR1, 2, and 3, and thus with antiangiogenic properties, is standard third-line therapy for advanced GIST patients. In fact, it was shown to be effective as a third-line therapy in patients failing both imatinib and sunitinib, by providing a median advantage of 4 months of progression-free survival over placebo in a randomized clinical trial.[95] Its tolerability profile is close to sunitinib,

with hand–foot syndrome, hypertension, fatigue, and diarrhea as main side effects.[96]

An observation made in this trial was the persistence of some activity when therapy was carried on beyond progression.[97] In other words, a subset of patients, although arbitrarily selected by investigators on clinical grounds, went on with therapy beyond their first progression, achieving a second progression-free interval that approximated the previous one. This would suggest that a subset of progressing patients have a disease that might be slowed down by continuing the TKI in spite of the progression. This observation likely applies to all TKIs, at least in selected patients, and is worth testing prospectively by developing criteria to single out those patients who are more likely to benefit. In general, this parallels the clinical feeling that stopping any kind of TKI may accelerate tumor progression, even when resistance to that TKI has been established. Indeed, a criticism that was made to placebo-controlled trials on new TKIs in GIST is the lack of any tyrosine kinase inhibition in the control group, possibly worsening its outcome in comparison to what could happen by continuing the TKI already in use or by rechallenging the disease with a TKI used earlier.

In fact, in anecdotal cases and also in a small randomized clinical trial, it was shown that rechallenging a progressing GIST patient with TKIs used at an earlier stage can be beneficial, at least temporarily.[98] In other words, reestablishing imatinib in patients who underwent the drug as frontline therapy and then switched to others results in a benefit in terms of progression-free survival that is not far from what is achievable with further-line agents. One may speculate that there is a process of reexpansion of tumor clones that were sensitive to imatinib and might have been narrowed by the selective pressure of the drug, as long as resistant clones were emerging.

Following third-line therapy, there is no standard option at the moment, aside from rechallenge, and clearly patients are eligible for clinical studies on new agents. New drugs investigated in currently ongoing trials include other TKIs targeting KIT and PDGFRA; agents targeting downstream pathways (e.g., PI3K/AKT); agents targeting heat shock proteins, given their chaperone function for KIT and PDGFRA; among others. Clearly, agents with a mechanism of action other than imatinib, sunitinib, and regorafenib try to address the limiting factor of the heterogeneous nature of secondary resistance. Combinations of agents with different mechanisms of action are tried as well, although their added toxicity may be prohibitive even when they are reasonably well tolerated as single drugs. Future directions might try to exploit molecular diagnostics such as the *liquid biopsy* (i.e., the assessment of secondary mutations on circulating DNA shed by tumor cells). The sensitivity of this technique for primary and secondary mutations of GISTs has been demonstrated.[99] Thus, it looks promising for the future, to allow a degree of molecular personalization of therapy, whether following secondary resistance or before it establishes clinically, as a means to avoid or delay its occurrence. Combinations or rotations of TKIs might be tested, rationally driven by liquid biopsies. This could exploit the peculiarities of resistance seen with TKIs in GISTs. In fact, the efficacy of treatment beyond progression and of rechallenge suggests that sensitive and resistant clones may fluctuate within the tumor load, depending on the selective pressure they are exposed to. This would be consistent with the model of a *liquid resistance*, which, clinically, could be exploited by employing new strategies as from the upfront approach with TKIs.

A methodologic issue in the medical therapy of GISTs with all TKIs lies in the peculiar patterns displayed by tumor response as compared to those observed with standard cytotoxic chemotherapy of solid cancers and lymphomas.[100,101] These patterns of tumor response are marked by the possible lack of tumor shrinkage in the face of substantial changes in tumor tissue and tumor metabolic activity. Although most observations derive from imatinib in frontline therapy, in essence, they regard all TKIs, the main difference being possibly the weakness of tumor response to further-line therapies, so that some of these aspects may look less clear cut in the further-line therapy setting as opposed to the frontline. Under these patterns of tumor response, first of all, in the presence of symptoms, a subjective response may take place very early. In a matter of days, if not hours, after starting an effective TKI, a symptomatic patient may well feel a clear degree of subjective improvement. As far as imaging is concerned, this is paralleled by metabolic response as assessed through a fludeoxyglucose (FDG)-PET scan.[102] A positive PET scan may turn negative in a few days. Of course, this does not correspond to the disappearance of the tumor lesion, but rather be the consequence of the metabolic *switch off* that the tumor undergoes when an effective TKI targets its cells. The reverse is true as well, so that any stop of therapy rapidly entails a *switch on* of functional imaging. Again, this does not correspond to clinical progression, which would follow only for longer interruptions of therapy. This should be taken into account when assessing functional tumor response, because, for instance, any lack of compliance with therapy in the days the exam is made might affect metabolic response as detected through PET scanning. For example, metabolic switch on was observed by PET scans performed during the 2 weeks off of therapy with sunitinib. In principle, this adds to the feeling that TKIs need to be maintained in order to preserve tumor response, in the context of a *clinically cytostatic* effect. It goes without saying that when a PET scan has become negative, the tumor lesion will not be visible to functional imaging, so that a CT scan, MRI, or ultrasounds need to be used in order to appreciate the evolution of tumor lesions. The radiologic response, as assessed through CT scans and MRI, is marked by tumor shrinkage and/or changes in tumor tissue. Tumor shrinkage may well appear very early, but, in some cases, it is lacking in the early phases of treatment, or even later on, so that tumor lesions look unchanged dimensionally. Sometimes tumor size may even increase. In these cases, however, if a response is in place, the radiologic aspect will show substantial changes to the tumor tissue. On a CT scan, this means a decrease in density of responding lesions, with decreased contrast enhancement. On an MRI, it entails an hypointense signaling on T1-weighted images and hyperintense on T2-weighted images, and decreased contrast enhancement. These changes are substantial in GIST patients undergoing frontline therapy with imatinib, so that recording tumor response is generally unchallenging for the clinician, provided tumor shrinkage is not the only criterion. Signs of nondimensional response may prove less obvious when the tumor response is less clear cut, as with further-line therapy with TKIs. Functional imaging may help, although it is exposed to the same limitations as well if the response is less striking. However, when the response is overt, the main shortfalls of nondimensional tumor response assessments lie in the difficulty to standardize reproducible (i.e., reliable) instruments, as is needed in clinical trials. In this sense, Response Evaluation Criteria in Solid Tumors (RECIST) criteria for tumor response assessment are based on the measurement on one diameter of selected target lesions and, thus, have a good record of reproducibility.[103] However, their *validity* is, by definition, unsatisfactory in the presence of a nondimensional response. Choi criteria were worked out in GISTs to accommodate these patterns of response, by factoring tumor hypodensity on CT scans in addition to a decrease in size.[104] Their validity in predicting progression-free survival was demonstrated and compared favorably with RECIST criteria, while paralleling functional imaging with PET scanning. Then, aside from the need to use easily reproducible instruments in the research setting, for the clinician the message coming from the GIST model is simple, inasmuch as it points to the existence of nondimensional patterns of tumor response, which can be easily highlighted through CT scans and MRI on one side and through functional imaging with PET scan on the other. One should be aware that the meaning of a radiologic response through CT scans or MRI is deeply different from metabolic response assessed through a PET scan. In fact, a PET

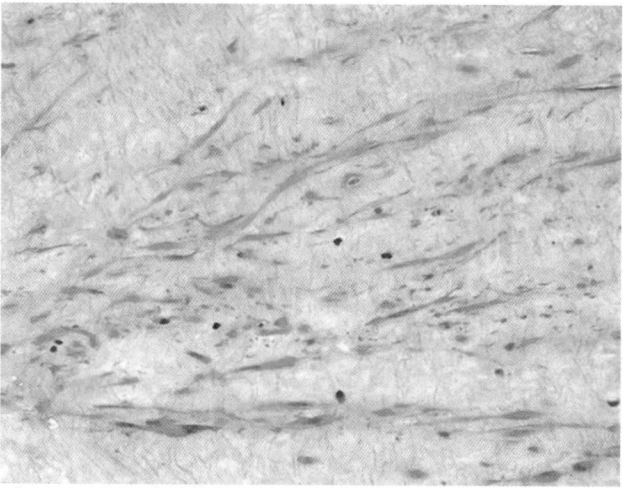

Figure 55.8 Pathologic tumor response of a GIST lesion following therapy with imatinib.

scan measures the biological effect of a TKI on the tumor cells very early, but does not necessarily imply any anatomical change in the tumor. On the contrary, CT scans and MRI detect actual changes in the tumor tissue, which correspond to pathologic signs of tumor response. These were found to take shape in terms of a myxoid degeneration widely affecting responding tumor lesions, with signs of apoptosis (Fig. 55.8). A variable proportion of vital cells may be detected, especially to the periphery of lesions (pointing in principle to the prospects of regrowth in case of discontinuation of the TKI). In this sense, a nondimensional tumor response does not mean just *absence of progression*; indeed, it is all about an actual pathologic response, with major changes to the tumor tissue. Of course, all tumor changes one can see when a tumor response is in place have their counterparts when the tumor progresses. Thus, increased tumor density and contrast enhancement on a CT scan will mark tumor progression, with or without an increase in tumor size. This may well affect just a portion of the tumor lesions, such as its periphery or a small part (as is the case with the *nodule within the nodule*). In brief, the quality of the tumor tissue should be observed, in addition to its size, in order to detect both response and progression in GISTs undergoing a TKI. Whatever the response pattern, whether dimensional or not, a tumor response on a CT scan or MRI says that the tumor is undergoing pathologic changes that clearly correlate with the prognosis. In fact, both dimensional and nondimensional tumor responses have clearly correlated with improved outcome in clinical trials, as opposed to progression. Only secondary resistance, or treatment interruption, will terminate a dimensional or nondimensional tumor response, with radiological signs that, as said, will be dimensional or nondimensional as well.

PALLIATIVE CARE

The natural history of GISTs that are not cured by initial surgery is dominated by abdominal spread involving the liver and the peritoneum. Liver failure as well as intestinal and urinary obstructions are thus the main palliative challenges. This may well carry the need of palliative surgery in selected patients. Extra-abdominal metastases are occasionally seen, mainly to the bone, and can require palliative irradiation. A systemic sign such as fatigue may add to asthenia induced by anemia as well as directly by TKIs. In fact, the existence of three lines of standard medical therapy, the potentials of rechallenge, and the availability of many agents of interest, either within clinical studies or among TKIs developed for other diseases, lead to treating many GIST patients with molecularly targeted therapy even in the very advanced stages of disease. In this sense, the usual palliative challenges of abdominal malignancies meet the new palliative challenges posed by the use of TKIs, which revolutionized the field of the disease.

Indeed, all phases of treatment of GIST are currently a model for the medical oncology of new molecularly targeted agents. The model continues to shed light on their potentials in solid cancers as well as on their current limitations. It also demonstrates how clinical methodology is deeply affected by these agents, not only for medical oncologists, but for all members of the multidisciplinary cancer team, from surgeons to palliative physicians. Interestingly, the model of GISTs shows how a multidisciplinary approach remains crucial in solid cancers, in all phases of disease, and in the era of molecularly targeted therapies, too.

SELECTED REFERENCES

The full reference list can be accessed at lwwhealthlibrary.com/oncology.

1. Kindblom L-G, Remotti HE, Aldenborg F, et al. Gastrointestinal pacemaker cell tumor (GIPACT): gastrointestinal stromal tumors show phenotypic characteristics of the interstitial cell of Cajal. *Am J Pathol* 1998;152:1259–1269.
4. Hirota S, Isozaki K, Moriyama Y, et al. Gain of function mutations of c.kit in human gastrointestinal stroma tumors. *Science* 1998;279:577–580.
5. Corless CL. Gastrointestinal stromal tumors: what do we know now? *Mod Pathol* 2014;27:S1–S16.
6. Barnett CM, Corless CL, Heinrich MC. Gastrointestinal stromal tumors: molecular markers and genetic subtypes. *Hematol Oncol Clin North Am* 2013;27:871–888.
7. Joensuu H, Hohenberger P, Corless CL. Gastrointestinal stromal tumour. *Lancet* 2013;382:973–983.
8. Nilsson B, Bumming P, Meis-Kindblom JM, et al. Gastrointestinal stromal tumors: the incidence, prevalence clinical course, and prognostication in the pre-imatinib mesylate era – a populationbased stady in western Sweden. *Cancer* 2005;103:821–829.
10. Agaimy A, Wunsch PH, Hofstaedter F, et al. Minute gastric sclerosing stromal tumors (GIST tumorlet) are common in adults and frequently show c-kit mutations. *Am J Surg Pathol* 2007;31:113–120.
11. Kawanowa K, Sakuma Y, Sakurai S, et al. High incidence of microscopic gastrointestinal stromal tumors in the stomach. *Hum Pathol* 2006;37:1527–1535.
12. Rossi S, Gasparotto D, Toffolatti L, et al. Molecular and clinicopathologic characterization of gastrointestinal stromal tumors (GISTs) of small size. *Am J Surg Pathol* 2010;34:1480–1491.
13. Carney JA. Gastric stromal sarcoma, pulmonary chondroma, and extraadrenal paraganglioma (Carney Triad): natural history, adrenocortical component, and possible familial occurrence. *Mayo Clin Proc* 1999;74:543–552.
14. Stratakis CA, Carney JA. The triad of paragangliomas, gastric stromal tumors and pulmonary chondromas (Carney triad) and the dyad of paragangliomas and gastric stromal sarcomas (Carney–Stratakis syndrome): molecular genetics and clinical implications. *J Intern Med* 2009;266:43–52.
16. Li FP, Fletcher JA, Heinrich MC, et al. Familial gastrointestinal stromal tumor syndrome: phenotypic and molecular features in a kindred. *J Clin Oncol* 2005;23:2735–2743.
17. Postow MA, Robson ME. Inherited gastrointestinal stromal tumor syndromes: mutations, clinical features, and therapeutic implications. *Clin Sarcoma Res* 2012;2:16.
18. Miettinen MM, Corless CL, Debiec-Rychter M, et al. Gastrointestinal stromal tumors. In: Fletcher CDM, Bridge JA, Hogendoorn PCW, Mertens F, eds. Lyon, France: IARC; 2013: 164–167.
20. Miettinen M, Lasota J. Gastrointestinal stromal tumors: pathology and prognosis at different sites. *Semin Diagn Pathol* 2006;23:70–83.
24. Joensuu H, Vehtari A, Riihimäki J, et al. Risk of gastrointestinal stromal tumour recurrence after surgery: an analysis of pooled population-based cohorts. *Lancet Oncol* 2012;13:265–274.
28. Doyle LA, Nelson D, Heinrich MC, et al. Loss of succinate dehydrogenase subunit B (SDHB) expression is limited to a distinctive subset of gastric wild-type gastrointestinal stromal tumours: a comprehensive genotype-phenotype correlation study. *Histopathology* 2012;61:801–809.
29. Wagner AJ, Remillard SP, Zhang YX, et al. Loss of expression of SDHA predicts SDHA mutations in gastrointestinal stromal tumors. *Mod Pathol* 2013;26:289–294.
30. Ricci R, Dei Tos AP, Rindi G. GISTogram: a graphic presentation of the growing GIST complexity. *Virchows Arch* 2013;463:481–487.
31. Nannini M, Biasco G, Astolfi A, et al. An overview on molecular biology of KIT/PDGFRA wild type (WT) gastrointestinal stromal tumours (GIST). *J Med Genet* 2013;50:653–661.
32. Janeway KA, Kim SY, Lodish M, et al. Defects in succinate dehydrogenase in gastrointestinal stromal tumors lacking KIT and PDGFRA mutations. *Proc Natl Acad Sci U S A* 2011;108:314–318.
33. Miettinen M, Killian JK, Wang ZF, et al. Immunohistochemical loss of succinate dehydrogenase subunit A (SDHA) in gastrointestinal stromal tumors (GISTs) signals SDHA germline mutation. *Am J Surg Pathol* 2013;37:234–240.
35. Maertens O, Prenen H, Debiec-Rychter M, et al. Molecular pathogenesis of multiple gastrointestinal stromal tumors in NF1 patients. *Hum Mol Genet* 2006;15:1015–1023.

36. Agaram NP, Wong GC, Guo T, et al. Novel V600E BRAF mutations in imatinib-naive and imatinib-resistant gastrointestinal stromal tumors. *Genes Chromosomes Cancer* 2008;47:853–859.
38. Eriksson M, Reichardt P, Sundby Hall K, et al. Needle biopsy through the abdominal wall for the diagnosis of GIST – Does it pose any risk for tumor cell seeding and recurrence? Presented at: 2012 Connective Tissue Oncology Society Meeting; November 17, 2012; Prague.
39. Plumb AA, Kochhar R, Leahy M, et al. Patterns of recurrence of gastrointestinal stromal tumour (GIST) following complete resection: implications for follow-up. *Clin Radiol* 2013;68:770–775.
40. Edge S, Byrd DR, Compton CC, eds. *AJCC Cancer Staging Manual*. 7th ed. New York: Springer; 2010.
41. Hohenberger P, Ronellenfitsch U, Oladeji O, et al. Pattern of recurrence in patients with ruptured primary gastrointestinal stromal tumour. *Br J Surg* 2010;97:1854–1859.
44. Kim SY, Janeway K, Pappo A. Pediatric and wild-type gastrointestinal stromal tumor: new therapeutic approaches. *Curr Opin Oncol* 2010;22:347–350.
47. Lim YJ, Son HJ, Lee JS, et al. Clinical course of subepithelial lesions detected on upper gastrointestinal endoscopy. *World J Gastroenterol* 2010;16:439–444.
50. Ohtani H, Maeda K, Noda E, et al. Meta-analysis of laparoscopic and open surgery for gastric gastrointestinal stromal tumor. *Anticancer Res* 2013;33:5031–5041.
52. DeMatteo RP, Lewis JJ, Leung D, et al. Two hundred gastrointestinal stromal tumors: recurrence patterns and prognostic factors for survival. *Ann Surg* 2000;231:51–58.
53. McCarter MD, Antonescu CR, Ballman KV, et al. Microscopically positive margins for primary gastrointestinal stromal tumors: analysis of risk factors and tumor recurrence. *J Am Coll Surg* 2012;215:53–59.
55. Mussi C, Schildhaus HU, Gronchi A, et al. Therapeutic consequences from molecular biology for gastrointestinal stromal tumor patients affected by neurofibromatosis type 1. *Clin Cancer Res* 2008;14:4550–4555.
56. Dematteo RP, Ballman KV, Antonescu CR, et al. Adjuvant imatinib mesylate after resection of localised, primary gastrointestinal stromal tumour: a randomised, double-blind, placebo-controlled trial. *Lancet* 2009;373:1097–1104.
57. Joensuu H, Eriksson M, Sundby Hall K, et al. One vs three years of adjuvant imatinib for operable gastrointestinal stromal tumor: a randomized trial. *JAMA* 2012a;307:1265–1272.
58. Casali PG, Le Cesne A, Poveda Velasco A, et al. Imatinib failure-free survival (IFS) in patients with localized gastrointestinal stromal tumors (GIST) treated with adjuvant imatinib (IM): The EORTC/AGITG/FSG/GEIS/ISG randomized controlled phase III trial. *J Clin Oncol* 2013;31:abstr 10500.
60. Gastrointestinal Stromal Tumor Meta-Analysis Group (MetaGIST). Comparison of two doses of imatinib for the treatment of unresectable or metastatic gastrointestinal stromal tumors: a meta-analysis of 1,640 patients. *J Clin Oncol* 2010;28:1247–1253.
61. Fiore M, Palassini E, Fumagalli E, et al. Preoperative imatinib mesylate for unresectable or locally advanced primary gastrointestinal stromal tumors (GIST). *Eur J Surg Oncol* 2009;35:739–745.
62. Rutkowski P, Gronchi A, Hohenberger P, et al. Neoadjuvant imatinib in locally advanced gastrointestinal stromal tumors (GIST): the EORTC STBSG experience. *Ann Surg Oncol* 2013;20:2937–2943.
64. Wang D, Zhang Q, Blanke CD, et al. Phase II trial of neoadjuvant/adjuvant imatinib mesylate for advanced primary and metastatic/recurrent operable gastrointestinal stromal tumors: long-term follow-up results of Radiation Therapy Oncology Group 0132. *Ann Surg Oncol* 2012;19:1074–1080.
66. Joensuu H, Roberts PJ, Sarlomo-Rikala M, et al. Effect of the tyrosine kinase inhibitor STI571 in a patient with a metastatic gastrointestinal stromal tumor. *N Engl J Med* 2001;344:1052–1056.
67. Blanke CD, Demetri GD, von Mehren M, et al. Long-term results from a randomized phase II trial of standard- versus higher-dose imatinib mesylate for patients with unresectable or metastatic gastrointestinal stromal tumors expressing KIT. *J Clin Oncol* 2008;26:620–625.
68. Verweij J, Casali PG, Zalcberg J, et al. Progression-free survival in gastrointestinal stromal tumours with high-dose imatinib: randomised trial. *Lancet* 2004;364:1127–1134.
69. Blanke CD, Rankin C, Demetri GD et al. Phase III randomized, intergroup trial assessing imatinib mesylate at two dose levels in patients with unresectable or metastatic gastrointestinal stromal tumors expressing the kit receptor tyrosine kinase: S0033. *J Clin Oncol* 2008;26:626–632.

PRACTICE OF ONCOLOGY

70. Van Glabbeke M, Verweij J, Casali PG, et al. Initial and late resistance to imatinib in advanced gastrointestinal stromal tumors are predicted by different prognostic factors: a European Organisation for Research and Treatment of Cancer-Italian Sarcoma Group-Australasian Gastrointestinal Trials Group study. *J Clin Oncol* 2005;23:5795–5804.

71. Heinrich MC, Owzar K, Corless CL, et al. Correlation of kinase genotype and clinical outcome in the North American Intergroup Phase III Trial of imatinib mesylate for treatment of advanced gastrointestinal stromal tumor: CALGB 150105 Study by Cancer and Leukemia Group B and Southwest Oncology Group. *J Clin Oncol* 2008;26:5360–5367.

74. Janeway KA, Albritton KH, Van Den Abbeele AD, et al. Sunitinib treatment in pediatric patients with advanced GIST following failure of imatinib. *Pediatr Blood Cancer* 2009;52:767–771.

75. Le Cesne A, Ray-Coquard I, Bui BN, et al. French Sarcoma Group. Discontinuation of imatinib in patients with advanced gastrointestinal stromal tumours after 3 years of treatment: an open-label multicentre randomised phase 3 trial. *Lancet Oncol* 2010;11:942–949.

76. Patrikidou A, Chabaud S, Ray-Coquard I, et al. Influence of imatinib interruption and rechallenge on the residual disease in patients with advanced GIST: results of the BFR14 prospective French Sarcoma Group randomised, phase III trial. *Ann Oncol* 2013;24:1087–1093.

77. Joensuu H, Trent JC, Reichardt P. Practical management of tyrosine kinase inhibitor-associated side effects in GIST. *Cancer Treat Rev* 2011;37:75–88.

78. DeMatteo RP, Maki RG, Singer S, et al. Results of tyrosine kinase inhibitor therapy followed by surgical resection for metastatic gastrointestinal stromal tumor. *Ann Surg* 2007;245:347–352.

80. Raut CP, Wang Q, Manola J, et al. Cytoreductive surgery in patients with metastatic gastrointestinal stromal tumor treated with sunitinib malate. *Ann Surg Oncol* 2010;17:407–415.

81. Mussi C, Ronellenfitsch U, Jakob J, et al. Post-imatinib surgery in advanced/metastatic GIST: is it worthwhile in all patients? *Ann Oncol* 2010;21:403–408.

82. Wang D, Zhang Q, Blanke CD, et al. Phase II trial of neoadjuvant/adjuvant imatinib mesylate for advanced primary and metastatic/recurrent operable gastrointestinal stromal tumors: long-term follow-up results of Radiation Therapy Oncology Group 0132. *Ann Surg Oncol* 2012;19:1074–1080.

85. Wang WL, Conley A, Reynoso D, et al. Mechanisms of resistance to imatinib and sunitinib in gastrointestinal stromal tumor. *Cancer Chemother Pharmacol* 2011;67:S15–S24.

86. Liegl B, Kepten I, Le C, et al. Heterogeneity of kinase inhibitor resistance mechanisms in GIST. *J Pathol* 2008;216:64–74.

89. Judson I, Ma P, Peng B, et al. Imatinib pharmacokinetics in patients with gastrointestinal stromal tumour: a retrospective population pharmacokinetic study over time. EORTC Soft Tissue and Bone Sarcoma Group. *Cancer Chemother Pharmacol* 2005;55:379–386.

90. Demetri GD, Wang Y, Wehrle E, et al. Imatinib plasma levels are correlated with clinical benefit in patients with unresectable/metastatic gastrointestinal stromal tumors. *J Clin Oncol* 2009;27:3141–3147.

91. Zalcberg JR, Verweij J, Casali PG, et al. EORTC Soft Tissue and Bone Sarcoma Group, the Italian Sarcoma Group; Australasian Gastrointestinal Trials Group. Outcome of patients with advanced gastro-intestinal stromal tumours crossing over to a daily imatinib dose of 800 mg after progression on 400 mg. *Eur J Cancer* 2005;41:1751–1757.

92. Demetri GD, van Oosterom AT, Garrett CR, et al. Efficacy and safety of sunitinib in patients with advanced gastrointestinal stromal tumour after failure of imatinib: a randomised controlled trial. *Lancet* 2006;368:1329–1338.

93. Heinrich MC, Maki RG, Corless CL, et al. Primary and secondary kinase genotypes correlate with the biological and clinical activity of sunitinib in imatinib-resistant gastrointestinal stromal tumor. *J Clin Oncol* 2008;26:5352–5359.

94. George S, Blay JY, Casali PG, et al. Clinical evaluation of continuous daily dosing of sunitinib malate in patients with advanced gastrointestinal stromal tumour after imatinib failure. *Eur J Cancer* 2009;45:1959–1968.

95. Demetri GD, Reichardt P, Kang YK, et al. Efficacy and safety of regorafenib for advanced gastrointestinal stromal tumours after failure of imatinib and sunitinib (GRID): an international, multicentre, randomised, placebo-controlled, phase 3 trial. *Lancet* 2013;381:295–302.

96. De Wit M, Boers-Doets CB, Saettini A, et al. Prevention and management of adverse events related to regorafenib. *Support Care Cancer* 2014;22:837–846

97. Casali PG, Reichardt P, Kang Y, et al. Clinical benefit with regorafenib across subgroups and post-progression in patients with advanced gastrointestinal stromal tumor (GIST) after progression on imatinib (IM) and sunitinib (SU): phase 3 GRID trial update. *Ann Oncol* 2012;23:ix478.

98. Kang YK, Ryu MH, Yoo C, et al. Resumption of imatinib to control metastatic or unresectable gastrointestinal stromal tumours after failure of imatinib and sunitinib (RIGHT): a randomised, placebo-controlled, phase 3 trial. *Lancet Oncol* 2013;14:1175–1182.

99. Demetri GD, Jeffers M, Reichardt P, et al. Mutational analysis of plasma DNA from patients (pts) in the phase III GRID study of regorafenib (REG) versus placebo (PL) in tyrosine kinase inhibitor (TKI)-refractory GIST: correlating genotype with clinical outcomes. *J Clin Oncol* 2013;31:abstr 10503.

102. Van den Abbeele AD. The lessons of GIST—PET and PET/CT: a new paradigm for imaging. *Oncologist* 2008;13:8–13.

104. Choi H, Charnsangavej C, Faria SC, et al. Correlation of computed tomography and positron emission tomography in patients with metastatic gastrointestinal stromal tumor treated at a single institution with imatinib mesylate: proposal of new computed tomography response criteria. *J Clin Oncol* 2007;25:1753–1759.

56 Molecular Biology of Colorectal Cancer

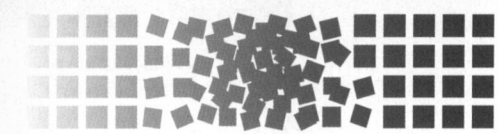

Ramesh A. Shivdasani

INTRODUCTION

The cumulative lifetime risk of developing colorectal cancer (CRC) in the United States is about 6% (www.cancer.gov/statistics) and increases about fourfold in persons with a family history of CRC. Fewer than 5% of cases, however, occur in patients with inherited predisposition syndromes. Most CRCs are therefore considered sporadic, although 20% to 30% of cases might have a familial basis despite the absence of a known germ-line defect, and genomewide association (GWA) studies reveal at least 20 alleles that elevate the risk of developing CRCs. Characteristic somatic mutations, DNA repair defects, chromosomal instability, and epigenetic alterations promote the disease. Predisposing conditions and somatic mutations profoundly inform the molecular understanding of CRCs and serve as a paradigm for the genetic basis of cancer.

MULTISTEP MODELS OF COLORECTAL TUMORIGENESIS

The genetic basis of CRC is best appreciated in light of the adenoma–carcinoma sequence. CRCs invariably arise within benign precursor polyps that show epithelial overgrowth, dysplasia, abnormal differentiation, and, sometimes, foci of tissue invasion. Pedunculated polyps are the most significant precursor lesions, with those larger than 1 cm harboring about a 15% risk of progressing to carcinoma over 10 years; endoscopic removal of these adenomas reduces CRC incidence and mortality.[1] The prevalence of polyps in the United States, estimated at up to 50% by age 70,[2] dwarfs the 6% lifetime risk of CRCs because few adenomas progress to invasive cancer and the successive aberrations that promote invasion and malignancy take 1 to 3 decades to accumulate.[3]

Nonclassical adenomas, such as hyperplastic polyps, were previously thought to have little potential to spawn invasive CRCs, but two serrated precursor lesion forms are now recognized.[4] Serrated adenomas with cytologic dysplasia occasionally evolve into common CRCs with chromosomal instability and *KRAS* mutation, whereas sessile serrated adenomas that lack dysplasia can spawn CRCs with microsatellite instability (MSI-hi), *BRAF* mutation, and abundant CpG island methylation.[5,6] About 8% of sporadic CRCs originate in such lesions, retain a serrated epithelium with characteristic nuclear morphology, and carry a relatively poor prognosis.

Although cancer progression has both genetic (somatic mutations) and epigenetic (unrelated to altered DNA sequence) underpinnings, we presently know more about the former than the latter. Alterations in several classes of genes drive tumors: oncogenes; tumor suppressors, including genes that repair damaged DNA; and those that help control other genes (epigenetic modifiers). Selected mutations appear at high frequencies in different tumor types and stages, allowing for the assignment of typical sequences (Fig. 56.1), although mutational order can vary and most tumors do not carry every alteration. These mutations support the idea of cancer as a multifaceted disease that breaches natural checks on cell survival, growth, and invasion.[7] Few specific mutations correlate strongly

with particular histologic features or patient survival and most affect multiple cellular functions. Particular genotypes do, however, define CRC subtypes and response to certain therapies. MSI-hi tumors typically arise in the ascending colon and carry a good prognosis; adjuvant 5-fluorouracil provides little benefit in stage II cases of this variety. *KRAS* or *BRAF* mutations, together accounting for about half of all cases, limit response to epidermal growth factor receptor (EGFR) antibodies[8,9] and are contraindications for this treatment. The prognostic and predictive value of other molecular features will become clearer as new therapies enter the clinic. Meanwhile, specific mutations reveal normal controls on colonic cells, possibly guiding future prevention strategies and key signaling pathways for rational drug development.

Global Events in Colorectal Cancer

CRCs acquire genetic instability in stereotypic ways that favor the accumulation of hundreds to thousands of somatic aberrations (see Fig. 56.1). About 80% of tumors display widespread chromosomal gains, losses, and translocations—phenomena that lead to gene amplifications, rearrangements, and deletions.[10] These tumors carry, on average, below 100 somatic nonsynonymous point mutations. Chromosomal segregation defects may account for chromosomal instability (CIN), as the segregation factor *Bub1* illustrates in mice,[11] but few specific gene defects are implicated confidently. Beyond weak associations with structural changes on chromosomes 8 and 18,[12] specific cytogenetic features barely influence disease patterns or patient outcomes.

About 15% of CRCs appear globally euploid but carry thousands of point mutations and small deletions or insertions near nucleotide repeat tracts—the defect designated as MSI-hi.[13] Features and the molecular determinants of disease progression in MSI[+] adenomas differ from those associated with CIN; for example, *BRAF V600E* mutations are more common in MSI[+] precursor adenomas than in other types.[14] Because hypermutability, whether associated with CIN or MSI, results in many changes that are inconsequential or even detrimental to tumors, the mere presence of a mutation does not signify a pathogenic role. Therefore, two features are used to distinguish *driver* from *passenger* mutations: appearance in a high fraction of tumor specimens, and ideally, the experimental demonstration of its contribution to a malignant property.

Epigenetic mechanisms may be as significant as mutations in cancer but are less well understood. Various covalent histone modifications and methylation of cytosine residues in DNA represent prominent modes of gene regulation,[15] the latter being far better characterized in CRCs than the former. 5'-CpG-3' dinucleotide pairs are particular targets for methylation in localized areas of high CpG content in promoters, where methylation silences adjacent genes. CRCs show 8% to 15% lower total DNA methylation than normal tissue,[16] even in colorectal adenomas.[17] Reduced pericentromeric methylation might decrease the fidelity of chromosomal segregation and altered methylation or loss of imprinting at the *IGF2* locus increase CRC risk,[18] suggesting broad effects of global hypomethylation on cell growth. However,

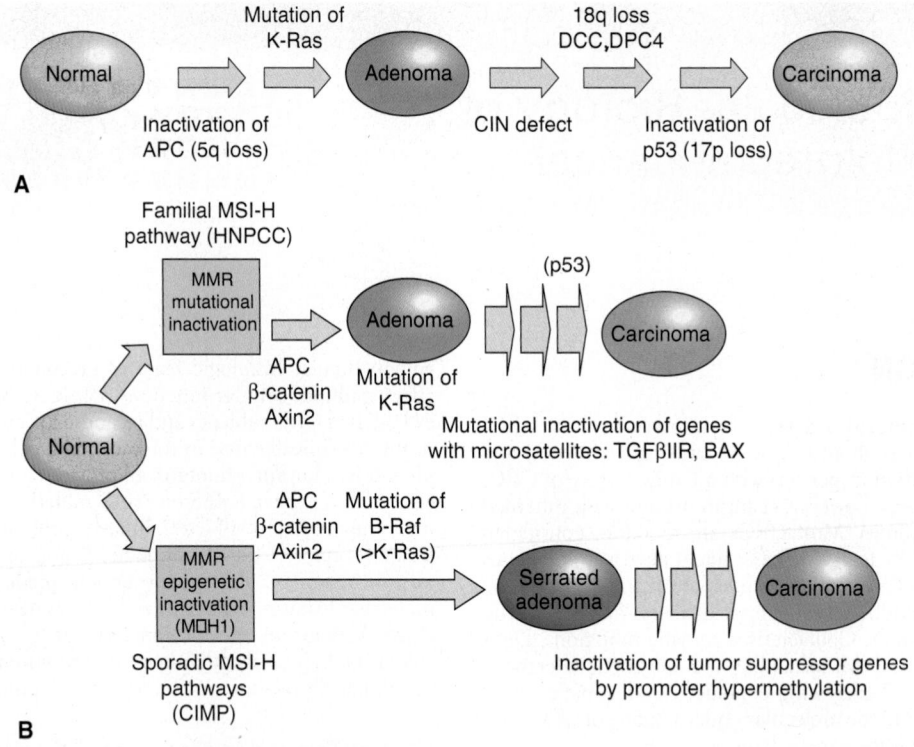

Figure 56.1 Genetic pathways to colorectal carcinoma. All colorectal cancers (CRCs) arise within benign adenomatous precursors, fueled by mutations that serially enhance malignant behavior. Mutations that activate the Wnt signaling pathway seem to be necessary initiating events, after which two possible courses contribute to the accumulation of additional mutations. **(A)** Chromosomal instability is a feature of up to 80% of CRCs and is commonly associated with activating KRAS point mutations and loss of regions that encompass *P53* and other tumor suppressors on 18q and 17p, often but not necessarily in that order. **(B)** About 20% of CRCs are euploid but defective in DNA mismatch repair (MMR), resulting in high microsatellite instability (MSI-hi). MMR defects may develop sporadically, associated with CpG island methylation (CIMP), or as a result of familial predisposition in hereditary nonpolyposis colorectal cancer (HNPCC). Mutations accumulate in the *KRAS* or *BRAF* oncogenes, *p53* tumor suppressor, and in microsatellite-containing genes vulnerable to MMR defects, such as *TGFβIIR*. Epigenetic inactivation of the MMR gene *MLH1* and activating *BRAF* point mutations are especially common in serrated adenomas, which progress, in part, through the silencing of tumor suppressor genes by promoter hypermethylation. Progression from adenoma to CRC takes years to decades, a process that accelerates in the presence of MMR defects. CIN, chromosomal instability.

its precise significance is unclear because some animals show increased tumor susceptibility with global hypomethylation,[19] whereas *Apc*Min mice lacking or overexpressing the de novo DNA methyltransferase DNMT3B show reduced or accelerated progression of small adenomas, respectively.[20,21]

Against a backdrop of genomewide *hypo*methylation, a distinct subset of CRCs shows coordinate *hyper*methylation of many CpG-rich promoters, conferring the CpG island methylator phenotype (CIMP), with transcriptional attenuation of tumor suppressor genes such as *HIC1* and Wnt-inhibiting *SFRPs*.[22,23] Whole-genome methylation analyses have confirmed the existence of this once controversial entity[24] and features that distinguish it from *KRAS*-mutant CIN disease—origin in sessile serrated adenomas; strong association with *BRAF*-mutant, right-sided MSI-hi tumors with *MLH1* gene methylation;[25] and distinctive gene expression patterns.[26]

Although the features cited previously, especially MMR and CIMP, overlap to some degree, CRCs seem to fall into three general categories: (1) traditional, (2) alternative, and (3) serrated, which are characterized by CIN, DNA mismatch repair, and CIMP, respectively (see Fig. 56.1). The Cancer Genome Atlas (TCGA) Network classified CRCs into nonhypermutated (generally CIN+) and hypermutated (encompassing MMR and CIMP) categories.[26] Other variations on the classical adenoma–carcinoma sequence are also recognized. A 10-fold elevated risk of CRC in patients with long-standing ulcerative colitis (UC)[27] likely reflects

heightened mutation in a setting of ongoing mucosal injury and repair. UC-associated CRCs often arise within flat adenomatous plaques and nonadenomatous areas of dysplasia. Compared to sporadic cases, *TP53* mutations occur earlier in the cancer sequence,[28] *APC* inactivation is less frequent, and methylation of the *p16*INK4a tumor suppressor gene is more common.[29]

INHERITED SYNDROMES OF INCREASED CANCER RISK HIGHLIGHT EARLY EVENTS AND CRITICAL PATHWAYS IN COLORECTAL TUMORIGENESIS

Two uncommon but highly penetrant Mendelian syndromes, familial adenomatous polyposis (FAP) and hereditary nonpolyposis colorectal cancer (HNPCC), together account for almost 5% of cases. *MYH*-associated polyposis (MAP), polymerase proofreading-associated polyposis (PPAP), familial juvenile polyposis (FJP), Peutz-Jeghers syndrome (PJS), and Cowden disease, each occurring in fewer than 1 in 200,000 births, also elevate the risk of CRCs (Table 56.1). Knowledge about the genes responsible for these inherited disorders allows for accurate molecular diagnosis, risk assessment, and targeted prevention in affected families. It also profoundly informs understanding of the considerably larger proportion of sporadic cases.

TABLE 56.1

Genetics of Inherited Colorectal Tumor Syndromes

Syndrome	Features Commonly Seen in Affected Individuals	Gene Defect
Syndromes with Adenomatous Polyps		
Familial adenomatous polyposis (FAP)	Multiple adenomas (>100) and colorectal carcinomas; duodenal polyps and carcinomas; gastric fundus polyps; congenital hypertrophy of retinal epithelium	*APC* (>90%)
– Gardner syndrome	Same as FAP, with desmoid tumors and mandibular osteomas	*APC*
– Turcot syndrome	Polyposis and CRC with brain tumors (medulloblastoma, glioblastoma)	*APC, MLH1*
Attenuated adenomatous polyposis coli (AAPC)	Less than 100 polyps, although marked variation in polyp number (from ~5 to >1,000 polyps) seen in mutation carriers within a single family	*APC* (5′ mutations)
Hereditary nonpolyposis colorectal cancer (HNPCC)	CRC with modest polyposis; high risk of endometrial cancer; some risk of ovarian, gastric, urothelial, hepatobiliary, and brain cancers	*MSH2, MLH1, MSH6* (together >90%), *PMS2* (about 5%)
MYH-associated polyposis (MAP)	Multiple gastrointestinal polyps, autosomal recessive	*MYH*
Polymerase proofreading-associated polyposis (PPAP)	Large adenomas, early-onset CRC, elevated risk of endometrial cancer only	*POLE* or *POLD1*
Syndromes with Atypical Polyps		
Peutz-Jeghers syndrome (PJS)	Hamartomatous polyps throughout the gastrointestinal (GI) tract; mucocutaneous pigmentation; estimated 9- to 13-fold increased risk of GI and non-GI cancers	*STK11* (30%–70%)
Cowden disease	Multiple hamartomas involving breast, thyroid, skin, brain, and GI tract; increased risk of breast, uterus, thyroid, and some GI cancers	*PTEN* (85%)
Juvenile polyposis syndrome	Multiple hamartomas in youth, predominantly in colon and stomach; variable increase in colorectal and stomach cancer risk; facial changes	*BMPR1A* (25%), *SMAD4* (15%), *ENG*
Hereditary mixed polyposis (HMPS)	Polyps of highly heterogeneous form and size, a few of which progress to CRC; confined to rare Ashkenazi Jewish kindreds; only CRC risk is elevated	*GREM1* (imputed)

Familial Adenomatous Polyposis and the Central Importance of Wnt Signaling

FAP is an autosomal-dominant monogenic disorder that underlies about 0.5% of all CRCs. Individuals develop hundreds to thousands of colonic polyps by their early 20s, and the lifetime risk of CRC approaches 100% at a median age of 39. Extraintestinal manifestations include (1) duodenal and gastric adenomas; (2) congenital hypertrophy of the retinal pigmented epithelium; (3) osteomas and mesenteric desmoid tumors in the Gardner syndrome variant[30]; (4) brain tumors in the Turcot syndrome variant[31]; and rarely, (5) cutaneous cysts, thyroid tumors, or adrenal adenomas. Although most of these extraintestinal features are benign, rare patients develop hepatoblastoma or thyroid cancer. Reflecting similar homeostatic mechanisms in the small and large bowel epithelia, a 5% to 10% risk of periampullary adenocarcinoma mandates endoscopic monitoring of the duodenum after prophylactic colectomy.[32]

The gene responsible for FAP, *adenomatous polyposis coli* (APC), encodes a 300 kDa protein. Germ-line mutations occur throughout the locus, clustering in the 5′ half and exon 15,[33] mostly introducing premature truncations. A few mutations correlate with phenotypic severity or specific extraintestinal manifestations, but identical mutations can produce different features. Mutations clustered in the extreme 5′ or 3′ ends of APC exons lead to the variant attenuated APC, with few polyps or CRCs developing late in life.[34] The I1307K allele, present in Ashkenazi Jews,

barely doubles the lifetime risk of CRC over the background and does not affect APC protein function but replaces an $(A)_3T(A)_4$ coding sequence with an $(A)_8$ tract that is occasionally targeted for nearby truncating mutations.[35] The identification of specific APC mutations in probands allows for a reliable testing of family members. Minimal recommendations for carriers include screening colonoscopy annually after age 10, gastroduodenoscopy after age 25, and treatment with nonsteroidal anti-inflammatory drugs to reduce CRC risk.[36] A prophylactic colectomy is highly recommended, with continued vigilance over the rectal stump and other at-risk tissues.

The larger significance of the APC gene derives from its somatic inactivation in about 80% of sporadic CRCs and adenomas,[37] including tiny polyps without dysplasia. APC inactivation is a rate-limiting step in the development of most polyps, and knowledge of its cellular functions supports this gatekeeper role. Attesting to the tumor suppressor function, CRCs that arise sporadically or in FAP show loss of heterozygosity and biallelic APC inactivation, with one copy usually lost by deletion. Because APC encodes several functional domains, truncated mutant proteins might interfere with various cellular activities. Disruption of its role in chromosome segregation might, for example, contribute to CIN.[38] However, attention on APC rightly centers on its control of the Wnt signaling pathway. About half the sporadic CRCs with intact APC function carry activating point mutations in CTNNB1,[39,40] which encodes β-catenin, a transcriptional effector of Wnt signaling; many of the rest carry fusions of genes that encode R-spondin cofactors.[41] Moreover, acute APC loss in mice produces intestinal defects identical to those observed upon Wnt pathway activation.[42] APC mutations are uncommon in sporadic cancers outside the intestine.

Wnts are secreted glycoprotein morphogens with diverse developmental and homeostatic functions, and, especially in the intestine, their role is intimately tied to that of R-spondins.[43,44] In the absence of Wnt ligands, cells use a complex containing APC, AXIN2, and other cytosolic proteins to promote casein kinase I- and glycogen synthase kinase (GSK)-3β-mediated phosphorylation of conserved serine and threonine residues at the N-terminus of β-catenin; this phosphorylation targets β-catenin for ubiquitin-mediated proteasomal degradation. The binding of Wnt ligands to a surface complex containing a FRIZZLED protein and the obligate coreceptor LRP5/6 inhibits the APC-AXIN2 destruction complex and stabilizes a pool of cytosolic β-catenin (Fig. 56.2), distinct from the abundant cellular stores that attach to E-cadherin on the inner cell surface. Accumulated β-catenin translocates to the cell nucleus, where it coactivates genes bound by sequence-specific transcription factors of the T-cell factor (TCF) family. Of the four proteins in this family, TCF4 is especially important in normal bowel epithelium and CRCs[39,45] and nuclear β-catenin is necessary to activate target genes.[46]

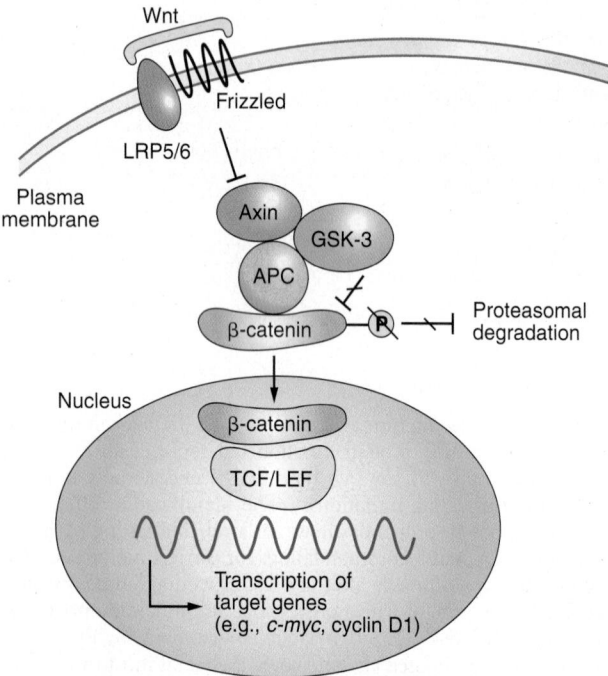

Figure 56.2 Outline of Wnt signaling, the key driver pathway in colorectal cancer. Members of the Wnt family of glycoprotein morphogens bind the cell surface coreceptors Frizzled and LRP5/6. In the absence of Wnt binding, normal cells use a complex containing APC, Axin, and other cytoplasmic proteins to promote GSK-3β–mediated phosphorylation of the β-catenin N-terminus, which targets β-catenin for proteasomal degradation (from Clevers H. Wnt/β-catenin signaling in development and disease. *Cell* 2006;127:469). Binding of a Wnt ligand to Frizzled and its obligate coreceptor LRP5/6 antagonizes the APC/Axin destruction complex, stabilizing β-catenin (CTNNB1), which moves into the nucleus and coactivates genes through T-cell factor/lymphoid enhancer factor (TCF/LEF) transcription factors. Either of the two principal gatekeeper events in colorectal cancer, inactivating *APC* or activating *CTNNB1* mutations, results in constitutive, Wnt-independent stabilization of β-catenin and unregulated activation of the cognate transcriptional program. Wnt signaling in the intestine is normally confined to crypt progenitors, and its aberrant activation by *APC* or *CTNNB1* mutations confers a permanent cryptlike state that favors cell replication.

CTNNB1 mutations in CRC invariably target residues for N-terminal phosphorylation and the mutant protein hence, resists degradation. Thus, both alternative gatekeeper lesions in CRC, inactivating *APC* or activating *CTNNB1* mutations, result in constitutive, Wnt ligand-independent stabilization of β-catenin. *R-SPONDIN* genes are translocated in up to 10% of cases, all with wild-type *APC* and *CTNNB1*,[41] and the gene fusions are probably pathogenic because they potentiate Wnt signaling. *TCF4* (also known as *TCF7L2*) mutations are surprisingly common,[26] but their roles and effects are unclear, as is the functional significance of rare *AXIN2* mutations in MSI[+] cases[47] and of *TCF3* or *TCF4* gene fusions in microsatellite stability (MSS) cases.[48]

Normal intestinal crypt stem and progenitor cells require Wnt signaling to proliferate, and *APC* or *CTNNB1* mutation-induced loss of this ligand dependence liberates cells from a potent regulatory restraint. Accordingly, the Wnt-dependent transcriptional program in CRC cell lines overlaps significantly with that in intestinal crypts.[49] Cycling crypt base cells that express the surface marker LGR5 are especially vulnerable to Wnt-induced transformation in mice, suggesting that CRC arises from stem cells and not from mature descendants.[50] Laboratory evidence suggests that even advanced CRCs remain dependent on constitutive Wnt pathway activity.[49] The TCF4–β-catenin complex controls hundreds of candidate genes,[49,51] but the individual significance of most target genes is unclear. A*pc* mutant mice lacking CD44 and selected other Wnt-pathway targets develop fewer adenomas,[52] but *MYC* seems especially vital because its absence in mouse intestines completely abrogates effects of acute APC loss.[53,54]

Hereditary Nonpolyposis Colorectal Cancer and the Role of DNA Mismatch Repair

HNPCC, or Lynch syndrome, an autosomal-dominant disorder that confers about 70% lifetime risk of developing CRCs, usually before age 50, is estimated to account for 2% to 4% of all cases. Affected individuals do not lack colonic polyps (nearly all CRCs, syndromic or sporadic, arise within benign precursors), but develop many fewer polyps than patients with FAP, a condition that must be excluded to satisfy diagnostic criteria for HNPCC (Table 56.2).[55] Cancers tend to develop in the ascending colon and patients are also predisposed to develop tumors of the endometrium (35% to 50% lifetime risk), ovary and upper urothelium (7% to 8% risk), stomach, small intestine, biliary tract, and brain—a spectrum reflected in the revised Amsterdam II criteria (see Table 56.2).[56] Cancers in HNPCC show pronounced variation in the lengths of microsatellite DNA sequences, and MSI at two or more among a panel of five mono- and dinucleotide tracts (BAT26, BAT25, D5S346, D2S123, and D17S250) confers the MSI-hi designation. CRCs harboring CIN represent a distinct class and show MSS or, in a small fraction, instability of unclear significance at just one of the five test regions (MSI-lo).

HNPCC results from germ-line mutations in any of several genes that enable DNA mismatch repair (MMR), a proofreading process that corrects base-pair mismatches and short insertions and deletions in the normal course of DNA replication. MMR in mammalian cells is mediated by homologs of bacterial and yeast repair proteins, MutS homologs (MSH) 1 through 6, MutL homologs (MLH) 1 through 3, PMS1, and PMS2. Both MLH1 and PMS2 are recruited to sites of DNA mismatch as a MutLα complex and in turn recruit MSH2-MSH6 (MutSβ) or MSH2-MSH3 (MutSβ) heterodimers to sites of 1-bp or 2- to 4-bp errors, respectively. These proteins efficiently excise the strand that carries the mismatch and resynthesize and ligate the repaired DNA. Germ-line mutations in *MSH2*, *MLH1*, *MSH6*, and *PMS2* together explain about 95% of kindreds,[57–59] including a subset with germ-line loss of the stop codon of *TACSTD1*, which results in silencing of its 3′ neighbor *MSH2* by hypermethylation.[60,61]

PRACTICE OF ONCOLOGY

TABLE 56.2

Criteria for Clinical Diagnosis of Hereditary Nonpolyposis Colorectal Cancer

A. Revised Amsterdam Criteria (Clinical Diagnosis)
1. Three or more family members with histologically verified HNPCC-related cancers, one of whom is a first-degree relative of the other two
2. Two successive affected generations
3. One or more of the HNPCC-related cancers (see C, which follows) diagnosed before age 50
4. Exclusion of familial adenomatous polyposis (FAP)

B. Revised Bethesda Guidelines (Criteria to Prompt Microsatellite Instability Testing of Tumors)
1. Diagnosis of CRC before age 50
2. Synchronous or metachronous presence of CRC or other HNPCC-associated cancer
3. CRC diagnosed before age 60 with histopathologic features associated with MSI-hi
4. CRC in at least one first-degree relative with an HNPCC-related tumor, with one of the cancers diagnosed before age 50
5. CRC in two or more first-degree relatives with HNPCC-related tumors, regardless of age

C. Spectrum of Sites for HNPCC-related Cancers
Colon and rectum, endometrium, stomach, ovary, pancreas, ureter and renal pelvis, biliary tract, small intestine, brain, sebaceous gland adenomas, and keratoacanthomas

MSI-hi colon cancers typically show exophytic growth, lymphoid infiltrates, mucinous signet-ring differentiation, and a medullary growth pattern; Bethesda guidelines (see Table 56.2) combine clinical and phenotypic features to facilitate a diagnosis of HNPCC.[62] When these criteria are met, tumor DNA should be tested either for MSI in a simple, polymerase chain reaction (PCR)-based assay or by immunohistochemistry for the absence of the commonly implicated MLH1, MSH2, and MSH6 proteins.[63] Because Bethesda guidelines might miss up to a quarter of cases, experts now recommend testing all colon cancers arising in patients under 70 years.[64,65] Coupled with thorough personal and family histories, positive results should prompt DNA testing for *MLH1, MSH2, MSH6,* or *PMS2* mutations.[66] The identification of mutant alleles and carriers allows for the targeting of cost-effective screening and interventions that are proven to reduce mortality[65] (e.g., preventive colonoscopy screening every 1 to 2 years, starting around 30 years of age; family counseling; aspirin therapy). Carriers should consider prophylactic subtotal colectomy, hysterectomy, and oophorectomy; females should at least have an annual endometrial evaluation soon after age 30.

In incipient cancers, random events first disrupt function of the wild-type allele of a mutant MMR gene and the resulting *mutator phenotype* promotes DNA replication errors at rates 10^2 to 10^3 times higher than the background.[13,57] Consequently, adenomas progress into carcinomas over 3 to 5 years instead of 2 or more decades.[67] Paradoxically, the prognosis for patients with MSI-hi CRCs is better than for those with sporadic MSS disease, perhaps because many resulting somatic mutations place tumors at a disadvantage. Both of the most commonly inactivated genes, *ACVR2A* and *TGFBR2*, encode receptors for specific ligands of the transforming growth factor beta (TGF-β) family and contain vulnerable mononucleotide tracts in their coding sequences.[26,68] TGF-β inhibits the proliferation of intestinal epithelial cells, and biallelic *TGFBR2* inactivation is detected in over 90% of MSI-hi and 15% of MSS, sporadic CRCs.[69] Other genes mutated in familial MSI-hi colon tumors encode the proapoptotic genes *CASP5* and *BAX*[70]; transcription factor genes, including *TCF4*[71]; and the epidermal growth factor receptor (EGFR)[72]; but *KRAS* and, especially, *BRAF* mutations are rare. CRC pathogenesis requires deregulated APC–β-catenin gatekeeper function irrespective of MMR status.[73]

MSI-hi is observed in 12% to 15% of sporadic cases of CRC,[74] often in older patients with early-stage disease. Such tumors seem to arise from sessile serrated adenomas in the ascending colon and do not reflect unrecognized germ-line mutation or somatic disruption of a known MMR gene.[75] Rather, most but not all cases reflect *MLH1* gene inactivation by biallelic promoter hypermethylation and show activating *BRAF* mutations and CIMP.[76–78]

MYH-Associated Polyposis and Polymerase Proofreading-Associated Polyposis

Germ-line mutations in *MYH*, a homolog of the *Escherichia coli* base excision-repair gene *MutY* cause MAP, a recessively inherited syndrome of multiple adenomas and CRC.[79] CRC develops later in life than in FAP, polyp numbers vary widely, and extracolonic tumors are less frequent than in HNPCC (see Table 56.1). Because MYH is a DNA glycosylase that helps repair oxidative DNA damage, tumors are not associated with MSI but with somatic G:C to T:A mutations, including in the *APC* gene. Two alleles, *Y165C* and *G382D*, account for most cases, and CRCs develop in homozygotes or compound heterozygotes, with no risk elevation in monoallelic carriers.[80] Surveillance recommendations are the same as in HNPCC.

Rare kindreds with a dominantly inherited high risk of CRC carry particular germ-line defects in *POLE* and *POLD1*, which encode the proofreading exonuclease activities of the leading- and lagging-strand DNA polymerases ε and δ, respectively.[81] Clinical findings of large adenomas and early-onset CRCs resemble those in HNPCC or MAP, including elevated endometrial cancer risk in women with mutant *POLD1*. Tumors carry thousands of mutations, but stable microsatellite tracts reveal a third familial *mutator* mechanism in CRCs. Hypermutation in the absence of MSI accounts for about 3% of sporadic CRCs, nearly all of which have a somatic *POLE* exonuclease domain and also *APC* mutations.[26] *POLE* and *POLD1* are nonclassical tumor suppressors because, instead of deletion or truncation, specific missense mutations affect proofreading function, and the wild-type allele is usually retained. Until further characterization of PPAP leads to formal surveillance recommendations, it is prudent to adopt those developed for HNPCC.

Familial Juvenile Polyposis and the Peutz-Jeghers, Hereditary Mixed Polyposis, and Cowden Syndromes

Patients with FJP develop premalignant hamartomatous polyps in the stomach or the small or large intestine by adolescence[82,83] and may give a revealing family history, although a significant minority represent the first case in their families. Germ-line mutations in genes encoding the bone morphogenetic protein (BMP) receptor *BMPR1A*, the accessory TGF-β receptor endoglin, *ENG*, or the *SMAD4* signal transducer emphasize the role of TGF-β signaling in disease pathogenesis (see Table 56.1).[84,85] Indeed, sporadic CRCs are often insensitive to the growth inhibitory effects of TGF-β and loss of BMP function in mice expands stem and progenitor cells, leading to polyposis or ectopic crypts.[86–88] Not all patients carry these mutations, indicating that additional genes remain undiscovered. Notably, a conditional *Smad4* deletion from mouse intestinal cells does not affect growth, whereas selective loss in T lymphocytes causes intestinal mucosal thickening and polyps.[89] These findings confound simple interpretations of TGF-β function and implicate stromal inflammation in intestinal tumorigenesis.

Patients with PJS also develop benign tumors that contain differentiated but disorganized cells (hamartomas), mainly in the small intestine but also in the colon or stomach, sometimes leading to hemorrhage or intussusception. PJS shows autosomal-dominant inheritance and is associated with macular lesions on the skin and buccal mucosa; bladder and bronchial polyps; and a propensity to develop a range of cancers, including those of the lung, breast, and female reproductive organs (see Table 56.1). The lifetime risk for all cancers exceeds 90%, the incidence of small intestine, stomach, and pancreas cancers is 50 to 500 times higher than the general population, and CRC risk is elevated nearly 100-fold.[90] Serine–threonine kinase 11 (STK11, also known as LKB1), the implicated tumor suppressor gene,[91] acts at the nexus of diverse cellular pathways and functions. Its principal activity, exerted through the adenosine monophosphate (AMP)-activated protein kinase AMPK, seems to be in linking nutrient and energy utilization to controls over cellular structure, particularly cell polarity.[92] STK11 also modulates the Rheb-GDP:Rheb-GTP cycle and downstream activities of the tuberous sclerosis gene TSC2 and the mammalian target of rapamycin (mTOR),[93] key regulators of protein synthesis and cell growth. The roles of STK11 in cell polarity and metabolism are busy areas of research, likely to hold vital clues into CRC pathogenesis and rational therapy.

Confined to rare Ashkenazi Jewish kindreds descended from a single founder, patients with HMPS develop polyps of several diverse morphologies and CRCs but no other cancers.[94] A 40-kb duplication upstream of GREM1 seems to activate a distant enhancer of this BMP antagonist gene, driving ectopic and high expression in the colonic epithelium.[95] The resulting increased crypt cell turnover likely accelerates the accumulation of oncogenic mutations. GREM1 is also the locus of a CRC risk allele identified at 15q13.3 in a GWA study.[96]

Cowden disease encompasses diverse mucosal lesions, specific cutaneous lesions (facial trichilemmomas and acral verrucous papules), and breast fibroadenomas, neurofibromas, lipomas, and meningiomas.[97] The syndrome results from germ-line mutations in PTEN, a tumor suppressor gene encoding the phosphatase and tensin homolog deleted on chromosome 10,[98] and the second most frequently mutated gene in cancers after TP53. The lipid phosphatase PTEN dephosphorylates key phosphoinositide (PI) signaling molecules[99] and accordingly regulates intracellular growth signaling negatively through PI-3 kinase and its downstream effectors AKT and mTOR. The CRC risk in Cowden syndrome is modest, and PTEN mutations are rare in sporadic cases, but protein immunostaining is lost in about 40% of CRCs, often as a result of promoter hypermethylation,[100] thus highlighting its tumor suppressor role.

Significance of Inherited Syndromes of Elevated Colorectal Cancer Risk

Following a clinical diagnosis of the previous Mendelian syndromes, patients and family members should be tested for pertinent germ-line mutations, receive genetic counseling, and enter programs for cancer prevention and screening. The corresponding molecular defects profoundly inform an understanding of sporadic CRCs, in particular, revealing the seminal role of Wnt signaling and early, rate-limiting effects of APC inactivation or CTNNB1 activation. Similarly, STK11 and PTEN loss in inherited and sporadic CRCs shed light on crucial molecular pathways, whereas HNPCC and PPAP help classify the disease and reveal the significance of features such as MSI, which is present in 12% to 15% of sporadic cases. Even in the absence of a recognized predisposition syndrome, individuals with a history of CRC in a first-degree relative are up to 4 times more likely to develop CRC than those without a family history. Specific environmental factors that compound the risk of developing CRCs are complex and insufficiently characterized, but include obesity, excessive consumption of red meat, physical inactivity, and vitamin D deficiency.[101] Because many of

these factors converge on insulin signaling, some experts propose that insulin and insulinlike growth factors play a seminal role in CRCs.[102] However, three of every four CRCs arise in individuals lacking a well-defined risk factor, and it is unknown to what extent particular genotypes confer sensitivity to environmental variables.

The cancer spectrum in HNPCC or PPAP and the particular predilection for CRC remain unexplained. Colonic, endometrial, and selected other epithelia may be especially sensitive to the kind of mutations that occur in the setting of defective DNA mismatch and base-excision repair, loss of wild-type tumor suppressor alleles may occur more readily in these tissues, or they may lack repair safeguards that protect other cell types.

Insights from Genomewide Association Studies

The quarter or more of sporadic CRC cases with a familial component[103,104] probably have diverse molecular etiologies, with low risk conferred by some common genetic variants and interaction of individual risk alleles with other genes and with environmental factors. Large multinational GWA studies have interrogated thousands of genomes and, to date, have uncovered statistical association of CRC risk with at least 20 distinct loci, including those linked to single nucleotide polymorphisms (SNPs) rs6983267 at 8q24.21, rs4939827 on 18q21, and rs3802842 at 11q23 (Table 56.3). The frequency of risk alleles ranges from less than 10% to half or more of the human population and each one elevates CRC risk no more than 7% to 25% above the background in persons with the nonrisk allele.[105,106] Even if homozygosity at some loci and additive effects compound this risk, allele frequencies are such that the cumulative risk rises no more than 50% to 250% over the background. As a result, the total effect of all identified risk variants explains, at most, 5% to 7% of cases with a family history; it is not presently feasible to predict an individual's precise risk or modify screening recommendations on the basis of known genotypes. Nevertheless, the identification of risk loci is a crucial advance for an eventually thorough understanding of disease determinants.

The specific causal significance of most of these DNA sequence variants is unclear and many localize far from coding genes, with growing evidence that they correspond to regulatory regions for control of nearby genes. This implies that an altered expression of the linked genes either transforms normal colonocytes at low frequency or, more likely, influences the oncogenic potential of other events. Particularly strong association occurs with the SNP rs6983267 at 8q24.21, which lies in a gene desert near low-risk susceptibility alleles for breast and prostate cancers. Molecular studies indicate that each culpable region acts as a tissue-specific enhancer controlling the nearest gene, CMYC,[107–109] thereby modulating disease risk.[110] Attesting to the role of TGF-β signaling in colonic epithelial homeostasis, risk alleles on chromosomes 18q21 and 14q22 are linked to SMAD7 and BMP4, respectively.[111,112] Some genes near risk variants are not expressed in the colonic mucosa, suggesting a role for extraepithelial genetic effects from stromal or immune cells. In summary, at least 20 common polymorphisms elevate CRC risk modestly and with sufficiently low penetrance that effect detection requires large population-based analyses. The pathophysiologic functions of these loci will likely inform future prevention and screening strategies and help determine how risk alleles interact with environmental factors.

ONCOGENE AND TUMOR SUPPRESSOR GENE MUTATIONS IN COLORECTAL CANCER PROGRESSION

Building on the foundation of lost gatekeeper functions in Wnt signaling, somatic mutations in oncogenes and tumor suppressor

TABLE 56.3

Single Nucleotide Polymorphisms Conferring Increased Risk of Colorectal Cancer

Chromosomal Location	Imputed SNP (Risk Allele)	Nearest Gene	Risk Allele Frequency in Controls	Odds Ratio, 95% CI	P Value
18q21.1	rs4939827 (T)	SMAD7	0.53	1.16–1.24	8×10^{-28}
8q23.3	rs16892766 (C)	EIF3H	0.07	1.20–1.34	3×10^{-18}
8q24.21	rs6983267 (G)	MYC	0.49	1.16–1.39	1×10^{-14}
10p14	rs10795668 (A)		0.48	1.10–1.16	3×10^{-13}
6p21	rs1321311 (A)	CDKN1A	0.25	1.07–1.13	1×10^{-10}
20p12.3	rs961253 (A)		0.36	1.08–1.16	2×10^{-10}
11q13.4	rs3824999 (C)	POLD3	0.51	1.05–1.10	4×10^{-10}
11q23.1	rs3802842 (C)	C11orf93	0.29	1.08–1.15	6×10^{-10}
Xp22.2	rs5934683 (T)	SHROOM2	0.38	1.04–1.10	7×10^{-10}
14q22.2	rs4444235 (C)	BMP4	0.46	1.08–1.15	8×10^{-10}
19q13.11	rs10411210 (C)	RHPN2	0.90	1.10–1.20	5×10^{-9}
16q22.1	rs9929218 (G)	CDH1	0.29	1.06–1.12	1×10^{-8}
15q13.3	rs4779584 (T)	GREM1	0.19	1.14–1.34	5×10^{-7}
1q41	rs6691170 (T)		0.35	1.13	
20q13.33	rs4925386 (C)	LAMA5	0.68	1.11	
12q13.3	rs11169552 (C)		0.72	1.12	
3q26.2	rs10936599 (C)	MYNN	0.76	1.07	

CI, confidence interval.

genes cumulatively confer malignant properties. The particular spectrum of recurring mutations in CRC provides a framework to decipher the oncogenic signaling circuits and develop rational targeted drugs (Table 56.4). The high collective frequency of recurrent KRAS, BRAF, and PIK3CA mutations places EGFR and downstream extracellular signal-regulated kinase (ERK, also known as mitogen-activated protein kinase [MAPK]) signaling at the center of research and therapeutic efforts.

The *KRAS, BRAF,* and *PIK3CA* Oncogenes

Ras-family G-proteins transduce growth factor signals and are aberrantly activated in a wide variety of cancers. KRAS is mutated in about 40% of CRCs[113] and NRAS in another 5% to 8% of cases. Mutations in both genes cluster in codons 12 or 13, and less frequently at codon 61. KRAS mutations appear even in lesions of low malignant potential, such as aberrant crypt foci lacking dysplasia,[114] and certainly in small polyps, although their frequency increases with lesion size.[115] A KRAS mutation is not required to initiate adenomas, but contributes to disease progression when combined with other genetic alterations, and specific interference with mutant KRAS in CRC cells and xenografts impedes cell growth.[116,117] Among the many different growth factor receptor signals that KRAS transduces in diverse cells, its activity in the colonic epithelium and CRC is particularly related to EGFR signaling, which is important for two reasons. First, inasmuch as Wnt and EGFR signaling drive normal gut epithelial turnover, CRC appears to subvert tissue-specific homeostatic circuits. Second, because a KRAS mutation introduces intracellular defects that lock EGFR signaling in the "on" state, EGFR antibodies are ineffective in this subset of CRCs[8] and targeted therapies will need to interfere further downstream in the signaling pathway.

Because KRAS acts early in transducing signals from EGFR and other receptor tyrosine kinases, KRAS mutations can potentially deregulate several effector pathways for cell survival, proliferation, invasion, and metastasis (Fig. 56.3). Constitutive phosphorylation of ERKs accompanies KRAS mutation, reflecting the activation of the ERK/MAPK pathway.[118] KRAS-mediated growth factor signaling recruits RAF kinases to the plasma membrane and triggers MEK1 and MEK2 kinases to activate ERK1 and ERK2, which in turn phosphorylate proteins that control the G_1–S cell cycle transition, among other substrates.[119] Although other, non–KRAS-mediated growth factor pathways also activate the MAPK cascade, signaling in CRC is most often deregulated through activating mutations in KRAS or BRAF. BRAF is mutated in about 10% of CRCs, especially those associated with MSI and CIMP.[120,121] The most common BRAF mutation in CRCs, melanoma, and selected other cancers, V600E, affects a residue within the activation loop of the kinase domain and constitutively activates kinase function, probably by several hundred-fold and acting as a phosphomimetic.[122] Like mutant KRAS, activated BRAF also phosphorylates ERKs, lifting intrinsic restraints on cell growth. Indeed, KRAS, NRAS, and BRAF mutations are mutually exclusive in CRCs,[26,120] highlighting their actions in a common cellular pathway and reflecting alternative routes to the same end.

Several features of BRAF-mutant CRCs are noteworthy. First, the defect confers a worse prognosis than KRAS mutations in advanced disease,[9,123] which indicates distinctive molecular or cellular features. Second, the BRAF mutation is a hallmark of nonfamilial MSI-hi CRC and occurs early in the natural history of sessile serrated adenomas.[121] Third, whereas forced Kras activation in the mouse intestine has a modest independent consequence,[124,125] BrafV600E expression rapidly induces persistent generalized hyperplasia with a high penetrance of crypt dysplasia, serrated morphology, and MSI-hi invasive cancers that show Wnt pathway activation.[126] Fourth, tumors mutant for either KRAS or BRAF intrinsically resist treatment with EGFR antibodies.[9,123] Fifth, BRAFV600E mutant melanomas initially respond to selective,

Recurrent Somatic Gene Mutations in Human Colorectal Cancers

Gene	Frequency	CRC Class	Known Cellular or Oncogenic Function
Oncogenes			
KRAS	35%–40%	CIN	RTK signaling
PIK3CA	18%–20%	Mostly CIN	RTK signaling
BRAF	7%–15%	MSI-hi, CIMP	RTK signaling
NRAS	9%	CIN	RTK signaling
ERBB3	~8%	CIN	RTK signaling
CTNNB1	~5%	All	Wnt pathway activation
Tumor Suppressor Genes			
APC	85%	All	Wnt pathway inactivation
TP53	50%	CIN predominant	Stress, hypoxia response; DNA replication
SMAD4	10%	CIN	
FBXW7	10%	CIN	
SOX9	5%	CIN	Wnt-dependent ISC function
ACVR2A		MSI-hi	Wnt pathway activity
TGFBR2		MSI-hi	TGF-β signaling
MSH3		MSI-hi	DNA mismatch repair
MSH6		MSI-hi	DNA mismatch repair
POLE		Hypermutated (non-MSI)	DNA polymerase ε
Epigenetic Modifier Genes (Roles Are Emerging)			
ARID1A		MSI-hi	Chromatin remodeling
SIN3A			Transcriptional repression
SMARCA5			Chromatin remodeling
NCOR1			Transcriptional repression
JARID2			Histone modification
TET1, 2, 3			DNA demethylation

RTK, receptor tyrosine kinase; ISC, intestinal stem cell.

ATP-competitive BRAF inhibitors such as vemurafenib and take months to manifest secondary resistance,[127] whereas *BRAF*V600E mutant CRCs are intrinsically resistant and barely respond to the same agents. This is because BRAF inhibition in CRC quickly induces feedback EGFR signaling through KRAS and CRAF, restoring stimuli for cell replication (melanoma cells hardly express EGFR and therefore avoid this feedback activation).[128,129] Because BRAF inhibition renders cells newly sensitive to direct antagonism of EGFR, a combined antagonism of BRAF and EGFR signaling may be beneficial.

KRAS signals are transduced not only through ERKs, but also through phosphatidylinositol (PI) 3-kinase (PI3K),[118,130] which phosphorylates the intracellular lipid PI-4,5-bisphosphate at the three position, triggering a cascade that promotes cell survival and growth.[131] Up to 20% of CRCs carry activating mutations in *PIK3CA*, the gene encoding the catalytic p110 subunit of PI3K. Mutations cluster in exons 9 and 20 and seem to arise late in the adenoma–carcinoma sequence, possibly coincident with invasion[132]; many fewer CRCs carry related *PIK3R1* mutations. Cellular PI3K activity is countered by the product of the *PTEN* gene, which is inactivated (usually by deletion) in another 10% of cases. Although both PI3K and BRAF act downstream of KRAS, only *BRAF* and *KRAS* mutations are mutually exclusive; up to one-fifth of *KRAS*-mutant CRCs also have *PIK3CA* mutations, implying that these oncogenes are not trivially redundant. One reason could

be that mutant KRAS activates PI3K signaling inefficiently.[133] More likely, oncogenic signaling pathways are less strictly linear than is convenient to depict. Indeed, seemingly parallel streams of KRAS signaling through RAF–MEK and PI3K (see Fig. 56.3) interact extensively with one another and both streams feed into the mTOR, which coordinates cell growth with nutrient responses.[134] Lastly, insulinlike growth factor 2 (IGF2) is overexpressed in at least 15% of CRCs as a result of focal gene amplifications, loss of imprinting, and other mechanisms.[26] Overexpression of *IGF2* and its downstream effector IRS2 is mutually exclusive with *PIK3CA* mutations and *PTEN* deletions, strongly implying that the underlying genetic aberrations represent alternative means to disrupt the same signaling circuit.

MYC, CDK8, and Control of Cell Growth and Metabolism

Although the *MYC* and *CDK8* oncogenes are rarely mutated in CRC, considerable gene amplification is seen in at least 10% of cases, with moderate increases in copy number and expression in up to 25% of cases.[26,135] Aberrant *MYC* gene regulation likely explains the significant GWA studies risk allele rs6983267 and MYC expression is not only a prominent outcome of Wnt signaling,[49] but may account for the bulk of the tumor effect in *Apc*-mutant

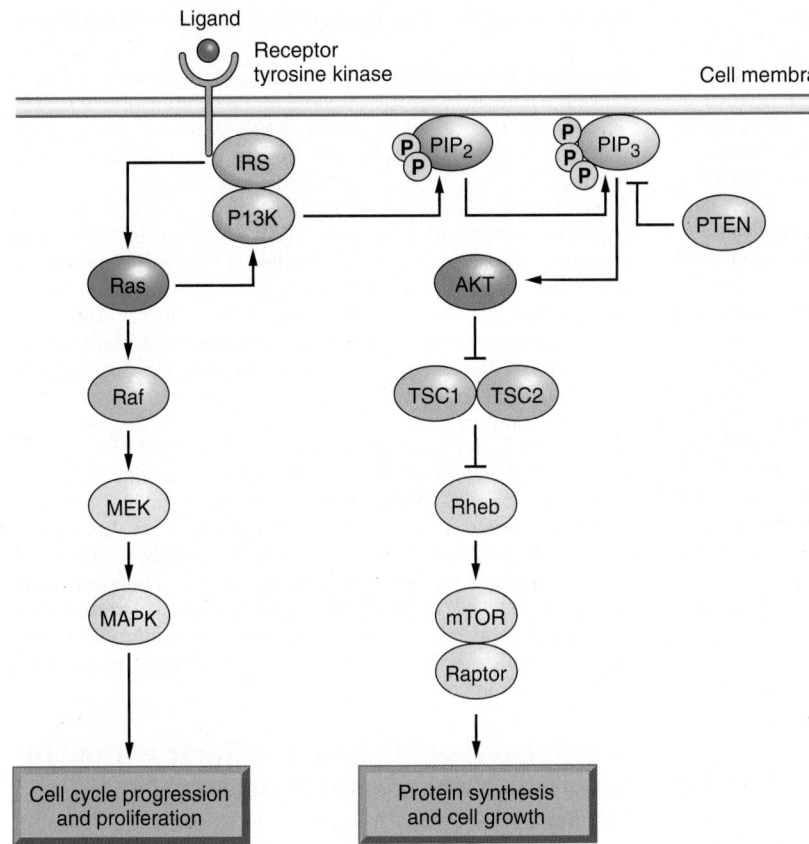

Ligand

Receptor tyrosine kinase

Cell membrane

IRS

P13K

Ras

Raf

MEK

MAPK

Cell cycle progression and proliferation

PIP₂

PIP₃

PTEN

AKT

TSC1 TSC2

Rheb

mTOR

Raptor

Protein synthesis and cell growth

Figure 56.3 Signaling pathways, oncogenic mutations, and therapeutic opportunities in CRC. It is instructive to consider common genetic alterations in CRC in light of a common canonical outline of signaling through receptor tyrosine kinases, among which the EGFR is a prime example. *KRAS*, the oncogene mutated in up to 40% of CRCs, signals receptor activation through RAF proteins (including BRAF, which is mutated in 5% to 8% of CRCs) and phosphatidylinositol 3-kinase (PI3K), whose catalytic PIK3CA subunit is mutated in 15% to 20% of CRCs. These transducers in turn activate the intracellular mitogen-activated protein kinase and AKT or mTOR pathways, respectively. Hence, common mutations confer growth factor independence on cells, resulting in dysregulated proliferation, protein synthesis, and metabolism. They also represent promising targets for therapeutic interference with aberrantly activated signaling cascades.

mouse intestines.[54] CDK8, a cyclin-dependent kinase component of the Mediator complex, couples transcription factors to the basal transcriptional machinery and hence resembles MYC in regulating thousands of genes, including those necessary for cellular metabolism, proliferation, and self-renewal. CDK8 activity in CRC is particularly associated with β-catenin.[135] Indeed, although *APC*, *CTNNB1*, and probably *RSPO* mutations kick start colonic adenomas, additional genetic events in CRC potentiate Wnt activity. Disrupting this seminally important pathway and/or its downstream effector MYC may therefore be imperative in CRC therapy, but poses formidable challenges, in part because that requires interfering with protein–protein interactions downstream of conventional druggable nodes.[136]

TP53 and Other Tumor Suppressors

The allelic loss of chromosome 17p is observed in three of every four CRCs but <10% of adenomatous polyps.[115] The remaining *TP53* allele is inactivated in most tumors with 17p loss of heterozygosity (LOH), most often at codons 175, 245, 248, 273, or 282.[137] *TP53* mutations, found in half of all CRCs and LOH of 17p thus appear to arise late in the transition from adenoma to carcinoma, possibly facilitating progression. Cells with an intact *TP53* function undergo cell cycle arrest and apoptosis when faced with stress from DNA damage, hypoxia, reduced nutrient access, or aneuploidy. *TP53* loss may allow cells to overcome these barriers to tumor survival and progression, but confers no specific disease features in CRCs.

LOH of chromosome 18q, which is rare in small to midsize adenomas, is observed in >60% of CRCs and nearly all liver metastases from MSS tumors.[138] This sequence implicates loss of resident genes in disease progression, but 18q LOH does not by itself confer a poor prognosis.[139] The minimal common region of LOH contains two candidate tumor suppressor genes[140]: *SMAD4* (*DPC4*) in about one-third of cases and *DCC* (deleted in

colorectal cancer, a receptor for Netrin axonal guidance proteins) in the rest. *SMAD4/DPC4* and *SMAD2* are positive and negative regulators of TGF-β signaling, respectively, and closely linked on 18q. Somatic *SMAD4* mutations are present in 10% to 15% of CRCs with LOH, and germ-line mutations are noted in some FJP kindreds[141]; *SMAD2* and *DCC* are rarely mutated in CRC,[142] but *DCC* mRNA and protein are lost in >50% of cases.[143] Together, these findings suggest a complex, multifactorial basis for the selection of 18q LOH in CRC.

FBXW7 (F-box and WD40 repeat domain containing 7), another gene frequently inactivated in CRCs, encodes a receptor subunit of Skp, Cullin, F-box-containing (SCF)-E3 ubiquitin ligase complexes, which target multiple regulators of cell growth, such as MYC and JUN transcription factors, for degradation. Monoallelic missense mutations tend to cluster in arginine residues within a β-propeller domain that recognizes specific substrates, including NOTCH, JUN, DEK, and TGIF1 in intestinal cells.[144,145]

THE MUTATIONAL LANDSCAPE OF COLORECTAL CANCER

Early analyses of protein-coding genes in a few CRCs produced average estimates of 81 mutations per tumor and spawned the useful idea that the mutational landscape of CRC contains few mountains (genes such as *APC*, *KRAS*, *TP53*, and *PIK3CA*, with frequent mutations) or hills (less frequent but functional mutations [e.g., *BRAF*^V600E]).[146] Although many additional events are individually infrequent and may contribute to neoplasia sporadically or represent *passenger* mutations, they tend to congregate in genes that control cell adhesion, signaling, DNA topology, and the cell cycle.[147] In general, CRCs show a genomewide bias toward C:G to T:A transitions at 5′-CpG-3′ sites and a lower frequency of mutations in 5′-TpC-3′ dinucleotides than observed, for example, in breast cancer.[146] Such findings may eventually link specific environmental factors to characteristic mutational spectra. Moreover, an average of 17 genes are deleted or amplified to 12 or more copies per CRC cell,[148] and the oncogenes *ERBB2, MYC, KRAS, MYB, IGF2, CCND1,* and *CDK8* are in aggregate amplified or overexpressed in most cases, usually together with neighboring genes. Nearly half the copy number alterations—28 amplifications and 22 deletions, including 15 recurrent changes encompassing <12 genes—identified in one study[149] also appear in other cancers. CRCs thus reflect the perturbation of selected pathways of replicative and tissue homeostasis, some in common with most cancers and others restricted to CRCs.

Detailed data from two genome-scale studies of nearly 300 CRCs and matched normal tissue corroborate these general observations and provide reliable catalogs of genetic alterations.[26,41] These comprehensive efforts revealed *RSPO* gene fusions and up to 10% incidence of monoallelic missense mutations in *SOX9,* a transcription factor target of Wnt signaling that is highly expressed and active in intestinal crypt stem and progenitor cells.[150] Additionally, MSI-hi tumors showed frequent mutations in the *ARID1A* chromatin remodeling factor gene, which may affect a broad swath of other genes. An updated, partial list of recurrent genetic alterations in CRC (see Table 56.4) indicates that few new mutations fall in genes that appeal to the pharmaceutical industry, such as tyrosine or serine/threonine kinases.

Prognostic and Predictive Value of Molecular Properties and Tumor Genotypes

These specific genetic alterations might confer particular clinical behaviors, prognoses, or drug responses. Mutational, chromosome structural, and gene expression profiles are virtually identical in colonic and rectal adenocarcinomas. Aneuploidy and tetraploidy confer a worse prognosis than MSI-hi status in early-stage disease,[151] and the benefits of adjuvant 5-fluorouracil therapy may be restricted to patients with MSS tumors.[152,153] Because nearly all CRCs have a constitutive Wnt pathway activity, this element alone has limited prognostic value and outcomes seem unaffected by whether *APC* or *CTNNB1* mutations stimulate the pathway. The presence of *KRAS* or *BRAF* mutations and possibly also *PIK3CA* mutation or loss of PTEN expression predicts a lack of response to EGFR monoclonal antibodies.[8,154] These are important observations because they direct treatment decisions and because, unlike leukemias or breast cancer, CRCs had previously resisted subgrouping on the basis of specific gene alterations. For example, mutations in the two most frequently affected oncogenes, *KRAS* or *PIK3CA,* seem not to impact survival in stage III or stage IV disease treated with chemotherapy,[9,155] although they will likely predict responses to new agents that target MEK or PI3 kinase signaling, respectively. Patients with metastatic *BRAF*-mutant CRC have especially low survival and respond poorly to current chemotherapy regimens, including adjuvant fluoropyrimidines in stage III disease.[9,156]

AN INTEGRATED MODEL FOR COLORECTAL CANCER INITIATION AND PROGRESSION

Intensive molecular investigation has informed our understanding of CRC for more than 2 decades, with crucial independent contributions from delineation of the adenoma–carcinoma sequence, uncommon familial syndromes, the Wnt–Rspo–β-catenin pathway, and EGFR signaling through the KRAS–BRAF–ERK and PIK3CA–AKT–mTOR pathways. Together with whole-genome analyses of CRC and refined investigation of intestinal crypt biology in animals, a large corpus of knowledge now permits a coherent model of disease initiation and advance.

Animal Models of Colorectal Cancer Genetics

Similar intestinal cell properties and genetics in humans and mice make the laboratory mouse valuable in the investigation of CRCs. The *multiple intestinal neoplasia* (*Min*) strain has a truncating mutation in *Apc* and phenocopies human FAP with respect to intestinal adenomas,[157] although tumors form mainly in the small bowel. *Apc^Min* mice are a cornerstone for the genetic analysis of intestinal polyps and deregulated Wnt signaling, but other *Apc* mutants also have value. A *D716* allele increases the number of adenomas, all with loss of the wild-type copy,[158] whereas a larger fraction of *Apc^1638N* adenomas appear in the colon[159]; *Apc^Pirc* rats carry a stop codon at position 1137 and more than half the tumors arise in the colon.[160] Deletion of the N-terminal degradation domain of murine β-catenin also stabilizes the protein and induces widespread intestinal polyposis.[161] Expression of activated *Kras* alleles in the intestinal epithelium of otherwise intact mice barely affects cell signaling or proliferation, but similar to human CRCs, expression on *Apc* mutant backgrounds expands progenitor cell numbers and hastens adenoma progression.[124,125] In contrast, activated *Braf* induces crypt hyperplasia, followed by invasive cancers with deregulated Wnt and ERK signaling.[126] The inactivation of murine genes for DNA MMR[162] leads to more lymphomas than intestinal tumors, with some mutants showing neither but revealing roles in meiosis; MMR is nevertheless necessary for protecting cells from mutation and malignancy.

Integrated Insights from the Study of Human Colorectal Cancers and Mouse Intestinal Crypts

Animal studies strongly suggest that CRCs originate in resident intestinal epithelial stem cells.[50] These cells, characterized mainly in the mouse small bowel, replicate frequently and neutral drift ensures that each normal crypt contains a monoclonal population of five to eight functional stem cells.[163,164] Gatekeeper mutations in *APC* or *CTNNB1* in one such cell induce constitutive Wnt pathway activity; the attendant growth advantage allows this mutant stem cell to dominate that crypt and eventually take hold as a monoclonal population. Notably, the outcome of this stochastic process is not inevitable: Neutral drift permits either wild-type or *APC*-mutant cells to replace each other quite rapidly, but a selective advantage in the latter gives them a demonstrable edge over their wild-type siblings.[165] Once a mutant stem cell clone is established, with no competing wild-type cells remaining in that crypt, it can flourish indefinitely and accumulate mutations as they occur, by chance or by virtue of a hypermutable state, so long as a mutation is not lethal or severely detrimental. Again, the outcome is not inevitable: Few polyps advance into carcinomas and others may even regress. Eventually, various combinations of mutations that co-opt existing signaling circuits confer invasive properties on a fraction of adenomas. Indeed, the bulk of observed mutations represent alternative means to dysregulate the same few pathways—Wnt, EGFR, TGF-β, IGF2, and PI3K—that control normal colonic cell turnover. Therefore, although specific genes, such as *BRAF* and *PIK3CA,* represent obvious targets for molecular therapy, it may be more useful in the long run to consider CRCs with broad respect to the pathways in which commonly mutated genes operate.

SUMMARY

The adenoma–carcinoma sequence represents the overt pathologic manifestation of sequential genetic alterations that promote cell growth, survival, and invasion. Molecular genetic studies have revealed crucial underlying mutations and the contribution of specific defects toward CRC pathogenesis. Colonic adenomas begin with deregulated Wnt signaling and this pathway's functions in intestinal crypt homeostasis lead us to interpret cancer in relation to pools of normal tissue stem cells. MSI-hi distinguishes CRCs that arise in the setting of HNPCC and about 15% of sporadic cases from the larger fraction of cases with CIN, leading to a molecular classification into at least three disease subgroups with distinctive features, natural histories, and treatment considerations. Somatic mutations associated with tumor progression involve a small selection of signaling and homeostatic pathways, revealing candidate therapeutic targets. Further work on the biologic functions of inherited and somatic mutations will help design novel, rational, and targeted therapies. Much also remains unknown about how environmental factors impinge on the implicated key pathways to modulate CRC risk and about specific interventions to prevent a cancer whose incidence and lethality in developed countries is second only to lung cancer.

SELECTED REFERENCES

The full reference list can be accessed at lwwhealthlibrary.com/oncology.

3. Jones S, Chen WD, Parmigiani G, et al. Comparative lesion sequencing provides insights into tumor evolution. *Proc Natl Acad Sci USA* 2008;105:4283–4288.
5. Noffsinger AE. Serrated polyps and colorectal cancer: new pathway to malignancy. *Annu Rev Pathol* 2009;4:343–364.
8. Van Cutsem E, Köhne CH, Hitre E, et al. Cetuximab and chemotherapy as initial treatment for metastatic colorectal cancer. *N Engl J Med* 2009;360:1408–1417.
13. Ionov Y, Peinado MA, Malkhosyan S, et al. Ubiquitous somatic mutations in simple repeated sequences reveal a new mechanism for colonic carcinogenesis. *Nature* 1993;363:558–561.
14. Spring KJ, Zhao ZZ, Karamatic R, et al. High prevalence of sessile serrated adenomas with BRAF mutations: a prospective study of patients undergoing colonoscopy. *Gastroenterology* 2006;131:1400–1407.
16. Goelz SE, Vogelstein B, Hamilton SR, et al. Hypomethylation of DNA from benign and malignant human colon neoplasms. *Science* 1985;228:187–190.
22. Toyota M, Ahuja N, Ohe-Toyota M, et al. CpG island methylator phenotype in colorectal cancer. *Proc Natl Acad Sci U S A* 1999;96:8681–8686.
26. Cancer Genome Atlas Network. Comprehensive molecular characterization of human colon and rectal cancer. *Nature* 2012;487:330–337.
37. Powell SM, Zilz N, Beazer-Barclay Y, et al. APC mutations occur early during colorectal tumorigenesis. *Nature* 1992;359:235–237.
41. Seshagiri S, Stawiski EW, Durinck S, et al. Recurrent R-spondin fusions in colon cancer. *Nature* 2012;488:660–664.
42. Sansom OJ, Reed KR, Hayes AJ, et al. Loss of Apc in vivo immediately perturbs Wnt signaling, differentiation, and migration. *Genes Dev* 2004;18:1385–1390.
46. Roose J, Clevers H. TCF transcription factors: molecular switches in carcinogenesis. *Biochim Biophys Acta* 1999;1424:M23–M37.
49. van de Wetering M, Sancho E, Verweij C, et al. The beta-catenin/TCF-4 complex imposes a crypt progenitor phenotype on colorectal cancer cells. *Cell* 2002;111:241–250.
50. Barker N, Ridgway RA, van Es JH, et al. Crypt stem cells as the cells-of-origin of intestinal cancer. *Nature* 2009;457:608–611.
54. Sansom OJ, Meniel VS, Muncan V, et al. Myc deletion rescues Apc deficiency in the small intestine. *Nature* 2007;446:676–679.
55. Vasen HF, Watson P, Mecklin JP, et al. New clinical criteria for hereditary nonpolyposis colorectal cancer (HNPCC, Lynch syndrome) proposed by the International Collaborative group on HNPCC. *Gastroenterology* 1999;116:1453–1456.
57. Fishel R, Kolodner RD. Identification of mismatch repair genes and their role in the development of cancer. *Curr Opin Genet Dev* 1995;5:382–395.
59. Liu T, Yan H, Kuismanen S, et al. The role of hPMS1 and hPMS2 in predisposing to colorectal cancer. *Cancer Res* 2001;61:7798–7802.
65. Vasen HF, Blanco I, Aktan-Collan K, et al. Revised guidelines for the clinical management of Lynch syndrome (HNPCC): recommendations by a group of European experts. *Gut* 2013;62:812–823.
68. Markowitz S, Wang J, Myeroff L, et al. Inactivation of the type II TGF-beta receptor in colon cancer cells with microsatellite instability. *Science* 1995;268:1336–1338.
76. Cunningham JM, Christensen ER, Tester DJ, et al. Hypermethylation of the hMLH1 promoter in colon cancer with microsatellite instability. *Cancer Res* 1998;58:3455–3460.
79. Sieber OM, Lipton L, Crabtree M, et al. Multiple colorectal adenomas, classic adenomatous polyposis, and germ-line mutations in MYH. *N Engl J Med* 2003;348:791–799.
81. Palles C, Cazier JB, Howarth KM, et al. Germline mutations affecting the proofreading domains of POLE and POLD1 predispose to colorectal adenomas and carcinomas. *Nat Genet* 2013;45:136–144.
84. Howe JR, Sayed MG, Ahmed AF, et al. The prevalence of MADH4 and BMPR1A mutations in juvenile polyposis and absence of BMPR2, BMPR1B, and ACVR1 mutations. *J Med Genet* 2004;41:484–491.
85. Sweet K, Willis J, Zhou XP, et al. Molecular classification of patients with unexplained hamartomatous and hyperplastic polyposis. *J Am Med Assoc* 2005;294:2465–2473.
91. Hemminki A, Markie D, Tomlinson I, et al. A serine/threonine kinase gene defective in Peutz-Jeghers syndrome. *Nature* 1998;391:184–187.
93. Shaw RJ, Bardeesy N, Manning BD, et al. The LKB1 tumor suppressor negatively regulates mTOR signaling. *Cancer Cell* 2004;6:91–99.
98. Liaw D, Marsh DJ, Li J, et al. Germline mutations of the PTEN gene in Cowden disease, an inherited breast and thyroid cancer syndrome. *Nat Genet* 1997;16:64–67.
105. Tomlinson I, Webb E, Carvajal-Carmona L, et al. A genome-wide association scan of tag SNPs identifies a susceptibility variant for colorectal cancer at 8q24.21. *Nat Genet* 2007;39:984–988.
106. Tenesa A, Farrington SM, Prendergast JG, et al. Genome-wide association scan identifies a colorectal cancer susceptibility locus on 11q23 and replicates risk loci at 8q24 and 18q21. *Nat Genet* 2008;40:631–637.
107. Pomerantz MM, Ahmadiyeh N, Jia L, et al. The 8q24 cancer risk variant rs6983267 shows long-range interaction with MYC in colorectal cancer. *Nat Genet* 2009;41:882–884.
108. Tuupanen S, Turunen M, Lehtonen R, et al. The common colorectal cancer predisposition SNP rs6983267 at chromosome 8q24 confers potential to enhanced Wnt signaling. *Nat Genet* 2009;41:885–890.
113. Bos JL, Fearon ER, Hamilton SR, et al. Prevalence of ras gene mutations in human colorectal cancers. *Nature* 1987;327:293–297.
114. Pretlow TP. Aberrant crypt foci and K-ras mutations: earliest recognized players or innocent bystanders in colon carcinogenesis? *Gastroenterology* 1995;108:600–603.
115. Vogelstein B, Fearon ER, Hamilton SR, et al. Genetic alterations during colorectal-tumor development. *N Engl J Med* 1988;319:525–532.
118. Ebi H, Corcoran RB, Singh A, et al. Receptor tyrosine kinases exert dominant control over PI3K signaling in human KRAS mutant colorectal cancers. *J Clin Invest* 2011;121:4311–4321.
119. Downward J. Targeting RAS signalling pathways in cancer therapy. *Nat Rev Cancer* 2003;3:11–22.
120. Rajagopalan H, Bardelli A, Lengauer C, et al. Tumorigenesis: RAF/RAS oncogenes and mismatch-repair status. *Nature* 2002;418:934.
122. Davies H, Bignell GR, Cox C, et al. Mutations of the BRAF gene in human cancer. *Nature* 2002;417:949–954.
124. Sansom OJ, Meniel V, Wilkins JA, et al. Loss of Apc allows phenotypic manifestation of the transforming properties of an endogenous K-ras oncogene in vivo. *Proc Natl Acad Sci U S A* 2006;103:14122–14127.
126. Rad R, Cadinanos J, Rad L, et al. A genetic progression model of Braf(V600E)-induced intestinal tumorigenesis reveals targets for therapeutic intervention. *Cancer Cell* 2013;24:15–29.
128. Corcoran RB, Ebi H, Turke AB, et al. EGFR-mediated re-activation of MAPK signaling contributes to insensitivity of BRAF mutant colorectal cancers to RAF inhibition with vemurafenib. *Cancer Discov* 2012;2:227–235.
129. Prahallad A, Sun C, Huang S, et al. Unresponsiveness of colon cancer to BRAF(V600E) inhibition through feedback activation of EGFR. *Nature* 2012;483:100–103.
130. Gupta S, Ramjaun AR, Haiko P, et al. Binding of ras to phosphoinositide 3-kinase p110alpha is required for ras-driven tumorigenesis in mice. *Cell* 2007;129:957–968.
134. Shaw RJ, Cantley LC. Ras, PI(3)K and mTOR signalling controls tumour cell growth. *Nature* 2006;441:424–430.
146. Sjoblom T, Jones S, Wood LS, et al. The consensus coding sequences of human breast and colorectal cancers. *Science* 2006;314:268–274.
157. Moser AR, Pitot HC, Dove WF. A dominant mutation that predisposes to multiple intestinal neoplasia in the mouse. *Science* 1990;247:322–324.
161. Harada N, Tamai Y, Ishikawa T, et al. Intestinal polyposis in mice with a dominant stable mutation of the beta-catenin gene. *EMBO J* 1999;18:5931–5942.
163. Lopez-Garcia C, Klein AM, Simons BD, et al. Intestinal stem cell replacement follows a pattern of neutral drift. *Science* 2010;330:822–825.
164. Snippert HJ, van der Flier LG, Sato T, et al. Intestinal crypt homeostasis results from neutral competition between symmetrically dividing Lgr5 stem cells. *Cell* 2010;143:134–144.
165. Vermeulen L, Morrissey E, van der Heijden M, et al. Defining stem cell dynamics in models of intestinal tumor initiation. *Science* 2013;342:995–998.

PRACTICE OF ONCOLOGY

57 Cancer of the Colon

Steven K. Libutti, Leonard B. Saltz, Christopher G. Willett, and Rebecca A. Levine

INTRODUCTION

A more thorough understanding of the molecular basis for this disease, coupled with the development of new therapeutic approaches, has dramatically altered the way in which patients with colorectal cancer (CRC) are managed. This chapter and the one that follows will provide an up-to-date description of the current state of the science and outline a multidisciplinary approach to the patient with colon or rectal cancer.

EPIDEMIOLOGY

Incidence and Mortality

Globally, nearly 1,200,000 new CRC cases are believed to occur, which accounts for approximately 10% of all incident cancers, and mortality from CRC is estimated at nearly 609,000.[1] In 2010, there were an estimated 141,570 new cases of CRC and 51,370 deaths in the United States.[2] As such, CRC accounts for nearly 10% of cancer mortality in the United States. Prevalence estimates reveal that in unscreened individuals age 50 years or older, there is a 0.5% to 2.0% chance of harboring an invasive CRC, a 1.0% to 1.6% chance of an in situ carcinoma, a 7% to 10% chance of a large (≥1 cm) adenoma, and a 25% to 40% chance of an adenoma of any size.[3]

Age impacts CRC incidence greater than any other demographic factor. To that end, sporadic CRC increases dramatically above the age of 45 to 50 years for all groups. In almost all countries, age-standardized incidence rates are less for women than for men. Although CRC incidence has been steadily decreasing in the United States and Canada, the incidence is rapidly increasing in Japan, Korea, and China.[1] In the United States from 2002 to 2006, the age-standardized incidence rates per 100,000 population were 59.0 for men and 43.6 for women when combined for all races.[2] Recognizing that decreases in age-standardized CRC incidence and mortality rates are apparent in the United States over the past 10 to 15 years, such trends may be counterbalanced by prolonged longevity.

While the incidence of CRC in the United States has decreased overall, presumably due to aggressive screening of the population over age 50, there has been a dramatic increase in younger patients. A new study using data from the Surveillance Epidemiology and End Results (SEER) program found a rising incidence of CRC over the last 20 years in patients aged 20 to 49. The most pronounced growth was in the age group 40 to 44 where colon and rectal cancer increased 56% and 94%, respectively. Based on these findings and the fact that CRC in younger patients tends to be more advanced, the authors recommend lowering the age for average risk screening by 10 years.[4,5]

Geographic Variation

The incidence rate for Alaskan Natives exceeds 70 per 100,000,[6] while that for Gambia and Algeria is <2 per 100,000.[7] Generally speaking, CRC incidence and mortality rates are the greatest in developed Western nations.[1,7] The reader is referred to the most recent detailed incidence and mortality rates in different countries over time according to gender, ethnicity, and anatomic site as established by the National Cancer Institute on their website.

As mentioned, there appears to be a recent decrease in age-standardized CRC incidence and mortality rates within the United States. From 1999 to 2006, CRC incidence and mortality both decreased.[2] Furthermore, 5-year survival improved. These trends are apparent regardless of gender, race, or ethnic group, except for Native Americans. Although at an initial glance one might invoke alterations in dietary and lifestyle factors, or the utilization of chemopreventive agents, it is clear that enhanced use of colonoscopy with polypectomy represents a significant reason for the improvements in trends in some areas.[8]

Emigration Patterns in Population Groups

Seminal studies have revealed that migrants from low-incident areas to high-incident areas assume the incidence of the host country within one generation.[9–12] For example, for Chinese who immigrate to the United States, higher CRC rates have been ascribed to greater meat consumption and diminished physical activity in contrast to controls within their original country.[10] These and other studies underscore the importance of environmental exposure in CRC incidence and provide a platform for attention to dietary and lifestyle modification as preventive measures.

Race and Ethnicity

Although dietary and lifestyle factors are of paramount importance in low-incident regions of the world, especially Asia and Africa, nonetheless there are certain trends along racial or ethnic lines. For example, an inherited adenomatosis polyposis coli (APC) gene mutation, I1307K, confers a higher risk of CRC within certain Ashkenazi Jewish families that is not apparent in other ethnic groups.[13,14] Inherited mutations in the DNA mismatch repair genes may be more common among African Americans,[15] in part accounting for anatomic variation in colon cancers among races in the United States,[16,17] an area that is receiving much attention in epidemiology- and biology-based research.

One recent study extracted data from the Adjuvant Colon Cancer ENdpoinTs (ACCENT) collaborative group database to analyze time-to-event end points for black and white patients participating in 12 randomized controlled adjuvant phase 3 trials of resected stage II and III colon cancer. In this cohort of 14,611 patients—controlling for sex, stage, age, and treatment type—both overall 5-year survival rates and 3-year recurrence-free survival rates were significantly worse for black patients (68.2% versus 72.8% and 68.4% versus 72.1%, respectively). However, recurrence-free interval was similar, arguing against a differential response to the adjuvant therapy itself. The authors concluded that poorer outcomes were more likely related to confounding factors not measured such as toxicity, comorbid conditions, and racial disparities in care for recurrent disease.[18]

Socioeconomic Factors

Generally, cancer incidence and mortality rates have been higher in economically advantaged countries.[19,20] This may be related to consumption of a high fat and high red meat diet, lack of physical activity with resulting obesity, and variations in mortality causes over a longitudinal period of time.

Anatomic Shift

Classically, colon cancer was believed to be a disease of the left or distal colon. However, the incidence of right-sided or proximal colon cancer has been increasing in North America[17,21] and Europe.[22] Similar trends have been observed in Asian countries.[23] This anatomic shift is likely multifactorial: (1) due to increased longevity; (2) as a response to luminal procarcinogens and carcinogens, which can vary between different sites of the colon and rectum; and (3) because of genetic factors, which can preferentially involve defects in mismatch repair genes with resulting microsatellite instability (MSI) in proximal colon cancers and chromosomal instability pathway predominant in left-sided colon and rectal cancers. These developments in anatomic variation will necessarily impact considerably on screening procedures, response to chemoprevention, response to chemotherapy, and, ultimately, disease-specific survival.[24–26]

ETIOLOGY: GENETIC AND ENVIRONMENTAL RISK FACTORS

Inherited Predisposition

Family history confers an increased lifetime risk of CRC, but that enhanced risk varies depending on the nature of the family history (Table 57.1). Familial factors contribute importantly to the risk of sporadic CRC, depending upon the involvement of first- or second-degree relatives and the age of onset of CRC. Involvement of at least one first-degree relative with CRC serves to double the risk of CRC.[27] There is further enhancement of the risk if a case is affected prior to the age of 60. Similarly, the likelihood of harboring premalignant adenomas or CRC is increased in first-degree

TABLE 57.1

Etiology of Colon Cancer: Environmental Factors

Increased Incidence	Decreased Incidence
High-caloric diet	High-fiber diet??
High red meat consumption	Antioxidant vitamins
Overcooked red meat??	Fresh fruit/vegetables
High saturated fats	Nonsteroidal anti-inflammatories
Excess alcohol consumption	Coffee
Cigarette smoking	High calcium
Sedentary lifestyle	High Magnesium
Obesity	Bisphosphonates
Diabetes	

relatives of persons with CRC.[28,29] The National Polyp Study reveals compelling data; the relative risk (RR) for parents and siblings of patients with adenomas compared to spousal controls was 1.8, which increased to 2.6 if the proband was younger than age 60 at adenoma detection.[30]

Provocative assessments of population groups suggest a dominantly inherited susceptibility to colorectal adenomas and cancer, which may account for the majority of sporadic CRC, but this may have variable inheritance based on the degree of exposure to environmental factors.[31] What are these susceptibility factors? The answer has yet to emerge. Nonetheless, genetic polymorphisms may be of paramount importance, such as in glutathione-s-transferase,[32] ethylene tetrahydrofolate reductase,[33,34] and N-acetyltransferases, especially NAT1 and NAT2.[35] In fact, genetic polymorphisms can vary among different racial and ethnic groups, which may provide clues to the geographic variation of CRC as well.

Environmental Factors

Seminal studies have underscored the importance of environmental factors as contributing to the pathogenesis of CRC. One has to take population-based studies into the context of methodologies employed, lead-time bias, time-lag issues, definition of surrogate and true end points, and the role of susceptibility factors.

One such population-based study recently evaluated risk factors for CRC from the Women's Health Initiative, a comprehensive prospectively collected database of 150,912 postmenopausal women, in which 1,210 developed colon cancer and 282 developed rectal cancer. Eleven risk factors were independently associated with colon cancer, some which have little or no previous support in the literature (age, waist girth, use of hormone therapy at baseline [protective], years smoked, arthritis [protective presumably due to medications used], relatives with CRC, lower hematocrit levels, fatigue, diabetes, less use of sleep medication, and cholecystectomy). Three of these factors were also significantly associated with an increased risk of rectal cancer (age, waist girth, and not taking hormone therapy).[36]

Diet

Total Calories

Obesity and total caloric intake are independent risk factors for CRC as revealed by cohort and case-control studies.[37,38] Increased body mass may result in a two-fold increase in CRC risk, with a strong association in men with colon but not rectal cancer. Weight gains during early to middle adulthood have also recently been linked with increased risk of colon but not rectal cancer. This relationship too seems more prominent in men than women in a large prospective study.[39]

Meat, Fat, and Protein

Ingestion of red meat but not white meat is associated with an increased CRC risk,[40,41] and as such, per capita consumption of red meat is a potent independent risk factor. Whether the total abstinence from red meat leads to a decreased CRC incidence has not been clarified, as there are studies with opposing results.[42] Also unclear is whether the type of red meat or the degree of processing or cooking method make any difference. While Probst-Hensch et al.[43] found fried, barbecued, and processed meats to be associated with CRC risk, especially for rectal cancer, with odds ratio (OR) of 6, follow-up reports do not consistently support these claims. In the population-based Norwegian Women and Cancer cohort including 84,538 participants, highly processed meat intake (especially sausage) was associated with increased CRC risk but meat cooking methods and total meat intake were not.[44]

A second study of 53,988 participants reported no difference with processed meat intake either. The authors did find that cancer risk was associated with different meat subtypes (i.e., animal of origin) which varied by tumor location—specifically, colon cancer risk was significantly elevated in the setting of high lamb intake (incidence rate ratio = 1.07) and rectal cancer risk was affected by pork (incidence rate ratio = 1.18).[45] However, McCullough et al.[46] recently reported a positive association in patients with nonmetastatic CRC between red and processed meat consumption before cancer diagnosis with higher risk of death after definitive surgery.

Coffee

Coffee contains numerous bioactive compounds that may modulate cancer risk but previous epidemiologic studies investigating its role in CRC have yielded ambiguous results. In a recent meta-analysis of 41 studies (25,965 patients), Li et al.[47] found a significant inverse association from case-control data for CRC (OR = 0.85) and colon cancer (OR = 0.79), but not rectal cancer. This was particularly true among females and in Europe.[47] Stronger evidence comes from the National Institutes of Health–AARP Diet and Health Study, a large prospective US cohort including 489,706 members. In this report, both caffeinated and decaffeinated coffee drinkers had a decreased risk of colon cancer, particularly of proximal tumors (hazard ratio [HR] for more than six cups a day = 0.62), and decaffeinated coffee drinkers also had a decreased risk of rectal cancer. While known confounders such as smoking and red meat consumption were adjusted for, further investigation is warranted to confirm and clarify this association.[48]

Fiber

Classically, a high-fiber diet was associated with a low incidence of CRC in Africa,[49] with numerous studies substantiating this premise.[50] Protection was believed to be afforded from wheat bran, fruit, and vegetables.[41] A high-fiber diet was believed to dilute fecal carcinogens, decrease colon transit time, and generate a favorable luminal environment. The European Prospective Investigation into Cancer and Nutrition is an ongoing multicenter prospective cohort study, which was one of the largest and most influential studies to initially report an inverse association between dietary fiber and CRC. More long-term data, with a mean follow-up of 11 years and a near three-fold increase in CRC cases, further supports this claim while providing a more precise estimation by fiber food source as well. After multivariable adjustments, total dietary fiber was found to be inversely associated with both colon and rectal cancers (HR per 10 g/day increased in fiber = 0.87), and this did not differ by age, sex, lifestyle, or other dietary factors.[51] However, other large, well-controlled studies show no inverse relationship between CRC and fiber intake.[52] In a study of nearly 90,000 women from ages 34 to 59 who were followed for 16 years, no protective effect was noted between fiber and incidence of either adenomatous polyp or CRC.[52] This was further corroborated by two large randomized controlled trials that evaluated high-fiber diets for moderate duration and discovered a lack of effect on the number, size, and histology of polyps found on colonoscopy.[53,54] At this point, therefore, it is unclear whether dietary fiber plays any substantial role in the risk of developing CRC.

Vegetables and Fruit

A protective effect of vegetables and fruits against CRC is generally believed to be true.[40] This has been observed with raw, green, and cruciferous vegetables. Whether certain agents such as antioxidant vitamins (E, C, and A), folate, thioethers, terpenes, and plant phenols may translate into effective chemopreventive strategies requires further investigation, although the data for folate intake are sound.[55]

Taking this nutritional data a step further, Bamia et al.[56] recently evaluated the impact of the Mediterranean diet on CRC risk in a large European cohort. This diet, introduced in the 1960s as "health-protecting," includes a high intake of vegetables, fruits, nuts, fish, cereals, and legumes with moderate alcohol consumption and low consumption of dairy and meat. The authors found an 8% to 11% decreased CRC risk when comparing patients with the highest to lowest diet adherence rates (HR = 0.89). The association was strongest for women and colon tumors.[56]

Other dietary factors under recent investigation include calcium, magnesium, and vitamin D. Calcium has been historically implicated as having a protective effect, perhaps due to its ability to bind injurious bile acids with reduction of colonic epithelial proliferation.[57] This is supported through cell culture models. However, population-based studies are not definitive.

A recent meta-analysis evaluating the influence of magnesium intake demonstrated a modest risk reduction, with pooled RRs of 0.81 for colon cancer and 0.94 for rectal cancer. This association persisted even after results were adjusted for calcium intake in six of the analyzed studies.[58]

Vitamin D has been shown to inhibit cell proliferation and increase apoptosis in vitro, and its deficiency is considered an important risk factor for many types of solid cancers. In a meta-analysis of 18 prospective studies, vitamin D intake and blood 25 (OH)D levels were found to be inversely associated with the risk of CRC as well (RR = 0.79 and 0.62 for colon cancer, respectively; RR = 0.78 and 0.61 for rectal cancer, respectively). While this report offers only preliminary observational data, larger randomized trials for vitamin D supplementation are warranted[59] and would be needed before routine vitamin D supplementation could be recommended for the purpose of CRC prevention. It is noteworthy that the Institute of Medicine, while supporting vitamn D supplementation to maintain bone health, found the evidence insufficient to support vitamin D as being protective against colorectal or any other cancer.[60]

Lifestyle

Physical inactivity has been associated with CRC risk, for colon more than rectal cancer. A sedentary lifestyle may account for an increased CRC risk, although the mechanism is unclear. Data suggest that physical activity after the diagnosis of stages I to III colon cancer may reduce the risk of cancer-related and overall mortality, and that the amount of aerobic exercise correlates with a reduced risk of recurrence following resection of stage III colon cancer.[61] More recently, positive associations have been established between increased amounts of recreational physical activity before and after CRC diagnosis and lower mortality.[62]

Most studies of alcohol have demonstrated at most a minimally positive effect. Associations are strongest between alcohol consumption in men and risk of rectal cancer. Perhaps interference with folate metabolism through acetaldehyde is responsible.[63]

Prolonged cigarette smoking is associated with the risk of CRC.[40] Cigarette smoking for >20 pack-years was associated with large adenoma risk and >35 pack-years with cancer risk. To examine the impact of smoking cessation on the attenuation of this risk, Gong et al.[64] conducted a pooled analysis of eight studies, including 6,796 CRC cases and 7,770 controls. The authors found that former smokers also remained at increased risk for up to 25 years after quitting. However, this varied substantially by cancer subsite with risk declining immediately for proximal colon and rectal cases but not until 20 years after smoking cessation for distal colon tumors.[64]

Diabetes

Type 2 diabetes has previously been implicated in the development of CRC, but it has been difficult to separate this association from other confounding lifestyle factors such as smoking and obesity.

Two recent meta-analyses provide further evidence that this condition is in fact a significant indepent risk factor. Yuhara et al.[65] identified 14 studies, most of which controlled for smoking, obesity, and physical exercise, and demonstrated that diabetes was associated with increased risk of both colon and rectal cancer (RR = 1.38 and RR = 1.20, respectively).[65] A second report, analyzing 24 studies, found a similar association (RR = 1.26) with even higher risk for those patients on insulin therapy (RR = 1.61).[66]

Drugs

Nonsteroidal Anti-Inflammatory Drugs

Population-based studies strongly support inverse associations between use of aspirin and other nonsteroidal anti-inflammatory drugs (NSAID) and the incidences of both CRC and adenomas.[67–69] As a result, NSAIDs and selective cyclooxygenase 2 (COX-2) inhibitors have been investigated intensively in hereditary and sporadic CRC.

Long-term results have just been reported from the CAPP2 study, the first double-blind randomized controlled trial of aspirin chemoprevention with cancer as the primary end point. In this study, 861 carriers of Lynch syndrome were randomly assigned to aspirin or placebo. With a mean follow-up of 55.7 months, the authors report a significantly decreased incidence of CRC in the treatment group as well as a trend toward reduction in extracolonic Lynch syndrome–associated cancers. Importantly, there was no significant difference in adverse events such as gastrointestinal (GI) bleeding, ulcers, or anemia during the intervention period. These data provide strong rationale for the routine use of aspirin chemoprevention in Lynch syndrome and establish a foundation for further study in sporadic neoplasia. In a combined analysis of four large randomized trials of lower-dose aspirin (75 to 300 mg/day) involving 14,033 patients, aspirin taken for 5 years or more was associated with a reduced 20-year incidence and mortality due to CRC (absolute reduction = 1.76%; 95% confidence interval [CI] = 0.61 to 2.91; p = 0.001). Reduction was largely confined to right-sided tumors.[70] In addition to generalized chemoprevention, the question of asprin and other NSAIDs in patients with a diagnosis of CRC has been addressed. Liao et al.[71] have reported evidence that suggests that aspirin therapy after CRC diagnosis may be beneficial to those patients whose tumors have a PIK3CA mutation, but not in those with wild-type PIK3CA.[71] However, PIK3CA mutation status had no impact on the influence of the COX-2 inhibitor rofecoxib on cancer recurrence.[72]

Bisphosphonates

In addition to being one of the most commonly used medications for osteoporosis, bisphosphonates have been shown to have various antiproliferative, antiangiogenic, proapoptotic, and antiadhesive effects in preclinical studies. Practical impact on malignant disease, however, has been inconsistent. Singh et al.[73] performed a recent meta-analysis demonstrating a statistically significant 17% reduction in CRC incidence with bisphosphonate use. This finding was observed independently for both proximal and distal colon cancers as well as rectal cancers, highlighting another potential pathway for chemoprevention.[73]

Biomarkers

In an effort to improve screening protocols and advance understanding of colorectal carcinogenesis, investigators are focusing on a variety of biomarkers for increased risk as well.

Toriola et al.[74] evaluated the role of C-reactive protein and serum amyloid A, two common inflammatory mediators, in the Women's Health Initiative Observational Study. With over 900 case-control pairs for each marker, the authors found that elevated concentrations of both C-reactive protein and serum amyloid A conferred significantly increased risk of colon cancer (OR = 1.50, p = 0.006). This is not surprising given the role inflammation plays in colorectal carcinogenesis as well as the new promising data surrounding NSAID chemoprevention.[74]

Leptin, a peptide hormone produced by adipocytes, is also thought to contribute to CRC pathogenesis. A recent prospective analysis found that soluble leptin receptor levels, which may regulate leptin function, was strongly inversely associated with both CRC and colon cancer risk (RR = 0.55 and RR = 0.42, respectively). This finding was independent of leptin levels and other circulating biomarkers.[75] Chi et al.[76] performed a similar investigation of insulin-like growth factor peptides, also implicated in CRC carcinogenesis, and found that high levels of insulin-like growth factor I and insulin-like growth factor II significantly increased cancer risk (OR = 1.25 and OR = 1.52, respectively).[76] Along these lines, high circulating levels of C-peptide, a direct marker of hyperinsulinemia, may also be a predictive factor for increased CRC risk, as indicated in a recent meta-analysis.[77]

Human Papillomavirus

While human papillomavirus is well-established as the critical pathogenic force behind cervical and anogenital cancer, its role in colorectal malignancy is less clear. An association between the two was first reported in 1990 and since then, a growing number of studies have detected the virus in colon adenocarcinoma specimens. In the first meta-analysis to address this topic (including 16 articles and 1,436 patients), Damin, Ziegelmann, and Damin[78] not only reported a high prevalence of human papillomavirus (31.9%) in affected patients, but also found a strong correlation between human papillomavirus positivity and increased CRC risk (OR = 10.04; 95% CI = 3.7 to 27.5). These results may indicate an alternative pathway of colorectal carcinogenesis that could have vast implications for treatment and prevention.[78]

FAMILIAL COLORECTAL CANCER

Familial Adenomatous Polyposis

Familial adenomatous polyposis (FAP) constitutes 1% of all CRC incidence (Table 57.2). Hallmark features include hundreds to thousands of colonic polyps that develop in patients in their teens to 30s, and if the colon is not surgically removed, 100% of patients progress to CRC. Extracolonic manifestations include benign conditions—congenital hypertrophy of the retinal pigment epithelium, mandibular osteomas, supernumerary teeth, epidermal cysts, adrenal cortical adenomas, desmoid tumors (although these tumors may lead to obstruction)—and malignant conditions—thyroid tumors, gastric small intestinal polyps with a 5% to 10% risk of duodenal or ampullary adenocarcinoma, and brain tumors.[79] The brain tumors may be of two types—glioblastoma multiforme or medulloblastoma—and the particular association of brain tumors and colonic polyposis is called Turcot syndrome.[80] The colonic polyps in Turcot syndrome are fewer and larger than in classic FAP. An attenuated form of FAP harbors up to 100 colonic polyps and has a predisposition to colorectal cancer in patients when they are in their 50s or 60s.[81]

FAP is an autosomally dominant disorder with nearly 100% penetrance. However, about 30% of patients have de novo mutations and are without an ostensible family history. Based on karyotypic analysis that reveals an interstitial deletion on human chromosome 5q and subsequent genetic linkage analysis to 5q21, the gene responsible for FAP was identified as *APC*. Patients with FAP inherit a mutated copy of the *APC* gene, thereby predisposing them to early onset polyposis. During life, patients with FAP acquire inactivation of the remaining *APC* gene copy, which accelerates the progression to CRC. Interesting genotypic-phenotypic

TABLE 57.2

Familial and Nonfamilial Causes of Colorectal Cancer

Syndromes with Adenomatous Polyps

APC gene mutations (1%):
- Familial adenomatous polyposis
- Attenuated APC
- Turcot syndrome (two-thirds of families)

MMR gene mutations (3%):
- Hereditary nonpolyposis colorectal cancer types I and II
- Muir-Torre syndrome
- Turcot syndrome (one-third of families)

Syndromes with hamartomatous polyps (<1%)

Peutz-Jeghers (*LKB1*)

Juvenile polyposis (*SMAD4, PTEN*)

Cowden (*PTEN*)

Bannayan-Ruvalcaba-Riley

Mixed polyposis

Other Familial Causes (up to 20%–25%)

Family history of adenomatous polyps (*MYH*)

Family history of colon cancer:
- Risk more than three times greater if two first-degree relatives or one first-degree relative <50 y with colon cancer
- Risk two times greater if second-degree relative affected

Familial colon-breast cancer

Nonfamilial Causes

Personal history of adenomatous polyps

Personal history of colorectal cancer

Inflammatory bowel disease (ulcerative colitis, Crohn's colitis)
- Radiation colitis
- Ureterosigmoidostomy
- Acromegaly
- Cronkhite-Canada syndrome

TABLE 57.3

Criteria for Identifying At-Risk Individuals for Mismatch Repair Deficiency (High Microsatellite Instability)

Amsterdam I Criteria

At least three relatives with colorectal cancer

One relative should be a first-degree relative of the other two

At least two successive generations should be affected

At least one colorectal cancer case before age 50

FAP should be excluded

Tumors should be verified histopathologically

Amsterdam II Criteria

At least three relatives with HNPCC-associated cancer (colorectal, endometrial, small bowel, ureter, or renal pelvis)

At least two successive generations should be affected

At least one case before age 50

FAP should be excluded

Tumors should be verified histopathologically

Bethesda Criteria (for Identification of Patients with Colorectal Tumor who Should Undergo Testing for MSI)

Cancer in families that meet Amsterdam criteria

Two HNPCC-related cancers, including colorectal or extracolonic

Colorectal cancer and a first degree relative with colorectal cancer and/or HNPCC-related extracolonic cancer and/or colorectal adenoma: one cancer before age 45 and adenoma before age 40

Colorectal cancer or endometrial cancer before age 45

Right-sided colorectal cancer with an undifferentiated pattern on histopathology before age 45

Signet-ring cell type colorectal cancer before age 45

Adenoma before age 40

FAP, familial adenomatous polyposis; HNPCC, hereditary nonpolyposis colorectal cancer; MSI, microsatellite instability.

---

associations exist between the location of the *APC* gene mutation and certain clinical manifestations, such as congenital hypertrophy of the retinal pigment epithelium, desmoid tumors, and classic FAP versus attenuated FAP.

The *APC* gene comprises 15 exons and encodes a protein of nearly 2,850 amino acids (310 kDa). Nearly all germline mutations in the *APC* gene lead to a truncated protein, which can be detected through molecular diagnostic assays that can be integrated into genetic counseling and genetic testing of affected patients and at-risk family members.[82,83] The functions of the APC protein and the interrelated pathways and regulatory molecules will be discussed later.

Hereditary Nonpolyposis Colorectal Cancer

Hereditary nonpolyposis CRC (HNPCC) accounts for about 3% of all CRCs. Salient features include up to 100 colonic polyps (hence the term nonpolyposis), preferentially, albeit not exclusively, in the right or proximal colon.[84] There is an accelerated rate of progression to CRC in these diminutive, at times flat, polyps with mean age of onset of CRC being 43 years. This is designated HNPCC type I. HNPCC type II is distinguished by extracolonic tumors that originate in the stomach, small bowel, bile duct, renal pelvis, ureter, bladder, uterus and ovary, skin, and perhaps the pancreas.

The lifetime risk of CRC in HNPCC is 80%, up to 50% to 60% for endometrial cancer, and 1% to 13% for all other cancers.[84,85] Of note, a variant of HNPCC involves skin tumors and is designated as Muir-Torre syndrome. HNPCC is defined classically by the modified Amsterdam criteria (Table 57.3).

HNPCC is an autosomally dominant disorder with about 80% penetrance. Genetic and biochemical approaches led to the discovery of the involvement of human DNA mismatch repair genes in HNPCC. Recognized as the human orthologues of mismatch repair genes described in bacteria and yeast, human mismatch repair genes encode enzymes that repair errors during DNA replication that may occur spontaneously or upon exposure to an exogenous agent (e.g., ultraviolet light, chemical carcinogen). Mutations in one of these mismatch repair genes results in MSI, which creates a milieu of somatic mutations of target genes—TGF-β2 receptor, *bax*, *IGF* type I receptor, among others—in HNPCC-associated tumors.[86] About 60% of germline mutations in HNPCC are found in either the *hMLH1* gene or the *hMSH2* gene, but mutations in other members of this family—*hMSH6, hPMS1, hPMS2*—are rare, thereby indicating that other genes are involved but have yet to be discovered. Genetic testing is not facile for HNPCC as it is for FAP, but it involves sequencing both the *hMLH1* and *hMSH2* genes (Table 57.4). If a germline mutation is found, then the remaining at-risk family members can be genetically screened.

TABLE 57.4

Genetic Testing in Inherited Colorectal Cancer

FAP	APC protein truncating testing (preferred). If APC mutation found, screen for mutation in family. Less desirable alternatives: gene sequencing, linkage testing.
HNPCC	MSI testing in tumor.[a] If MSI present, proceed to sequencing of both *hMLH1* and *hMSH2* genes. If mutation found, screen for mutation in family.

FAP, familial adenomatous polyposis; APC, adenomatosis polyposis coli; HNPCC, hereditary nonpolyposis colorectal cancer; MSI, microsatellite instability.
[a] Immunohistochemistry may be an option.

MSI testing and hMLH1/hMSH2 immunohistochemistry (IHC) can be performed on tumor specimens as a possible prelude to genetic testing.

Hamartomatous Polyposis Syndromes

Hamartomatous polyposis syndromes are rare syndromes, mostly affecting the pediatric and adolescent population, and represent <1% of CRCs annually. Peutz-Jeghers syndrome involves large but few colonic and small bowel polyps that can manifest by GI bleeding or obstruction and an increased risk of CRC. The polyps are distinguished by a smooth muscle band in the submucosa. Hallmark clinical features on physical examination include freckles on the hands, around the lips, in the buccal mucosa, and periorbitally. Associated characteristics include sinus, bronchial, and bladder polyps, and about 5% to 10% of patients have sex cord tumors. Patients can also develop lung and pancreatic adenocarcinomas. The gene responsible for this syndrome is *LKB1*, a serine threonine kinase.

Juvenile polyposis have overlapping clinical manifestations with Peutz-Jeghers, but the polyps tend to be confined to the colon, although cases of gastric and small bowel polyps have been described and there is an increased risk of CRC. Extracolonic manifestations are not prevalent. This is a polygenic disease, involving germline mutations in *PTEN*, *SMAD4*, *BMPR1*, or other genes yet to be identified.

Cowden syndrome harbors hamartomatous polyps anywhere in the GI tract, and surprisingly, there is no increased risk of CRC. However, about 10% of patients will have thyroid tumors and nearly 50% of patients have breast tumors. Germline *PTEN* mutations have been reported.

It is estimated that about 20% to 30% of CRCs are compatible with an inherited predisposition, independent of known syndromes.[87] The identification of other responsible genes will have great clinical impact. Intensive approaches are being pursued through sibling-pair studies and other familial studies. As previously mentioned, patients may be predisposed to an increased risk of adenomatous polyps as well in the context of a family history of sporadic adenomatous polyps.

ANATOMY OF THE COLON

The colon and rectum make up the segment of the digestive system commonly referred to as the large bowel. Defined as the portion of intestine from the ileocecal valve to the anus, the large bowel is approximately 150 cm in length. It is divided into five segments defined by its vascular supply and by its extraperitoneal or retroperitoneal location: the cecum (with appendix) and ascending colon, the transverse colon, the descending colon, the sigmoid colon, and the rectum. The anatomy of the rectum will be discussed in detail in the chapter on rectal cancer. The large bowel has a muscular wall and can be distinguished from the small intestine by its increased diameter, the presence of haustra, appendices epiploicae, and tenia coli. The tenia consist of condensations of longitudinal muscle fibers starting near the base of the appendix and continuing throughout the abdominal colon to form a continuous longitudinal muscle coat in the upper rectum. Haustra are outpouchings of bowel wall separated by folds that give a classic appearance on radiography or barium enema.

The right colon is made up of the cecum (with appendix) and ascending colon. It is anterior to the right kidney and the duodenum. Its vascular supply is from branches of the superior mesenteric artery (SMA). The SMA divides into the middle colic artery and the trunk of the SMA. The middle colic artery immediately forms two to three large arcades in the transverse mesocolon. The SMA ileocolic arterial branches then extend from the SMA. The right colic artery arises as a separate branch from the SMA in 10.7% of cases.[88] The ileocolic artery gives off a right colic artery to the upper ascending colon and forms an anastomosis with branches from the middle colic artery. The ileal branch of the ileocolic artery gives off branches to the distal small bowel and cecum, whereas the colic branch supplies the ascending colon. An anastomosis occurs between the distal SMA and the ileal branch of the ileocolic artery at the junction of the terminal ileum and cecum. The right colon is a retroperitoneal structure.

The transverse colon is supplied by branches of the middle colic artery. It is the first portion of the colon considered to be intraperitoneal, and its length can vary. Its boundaries are defined by the hepatic flexure on the right and the splenic flexure on the left. Both of these points are fixed. The hepatic flexure abuts the gallbladder fossa, while the splenic flexure lies anterior to the splenic hilum and the tail of the pancreas. The descending colon is where the colon once again becomes a retroperitoneal structure, and it is defined as the segment of colon from the splenic flexure to the sigmoid colon. The descending colon is the first segment of the left side of the colon and receives its blood supply from the inferior mesenteric artery. The inferior mesenteric artery arises from the aorta and gives off the left colic artery. It also gives off three to four sigmoidal arteries, which supply the intraperitoneal sigmoid colon. The anastomosis between the vessels of the middle colic artery and those of the left colic artery and right colic artery is known as the marginal artery of Drummond. The arcade, which effectively connects the left and right circulations, is known as the arc of Riolan. The arterial supply to the colon is depicted in Fig. 57.1.

The venous and lymphatic drainage of the colon parallels the arterial supply, and all three vessels course and divide within the colonic mesocolon (Fig. 57.2). The mesocolon therefore contains the regional lymph nodes (LN) for the segment of colon it supplies and drains. The efferent lymphatic channels pass from the submucosa to the intramuscular and subserosal plexus of the bowel to the first tier of LNs lying adjacent to the large intestine and known as *epicolic nodes*.[89] *Paracolic nodes* lie on the marginal vessels along the mesenteric side of the colon and are frequently involved in metastases. *Intermediate nodes* are found along the major arterial branches of the SMA and inferior mesenteric artery in the mesocolon. The *principal nodes* are found around the origin of these vessels from the aorta, and they drain into retroperitoneal nodes. The drainage of the superior and inferior mesenteric veins, which drain the ascending, transverse, descending, and sigmoid colon, is to the portal vein. The rectum is drained by rectal tributaries to the vena cava.

The extent of resection of the colon is defined by the vascular supply and by the need to take the regional draining LNs.[90,91] A careful understanding of the colonic anatomy, structure, location, and vascular supply is therefore critical in order to perform a safe and effective cancer operation. The segmental resections important for removal of lesions in various locations within the colon will be described in greater detail in later sections.

PRACTICE OF ONCOLOGY

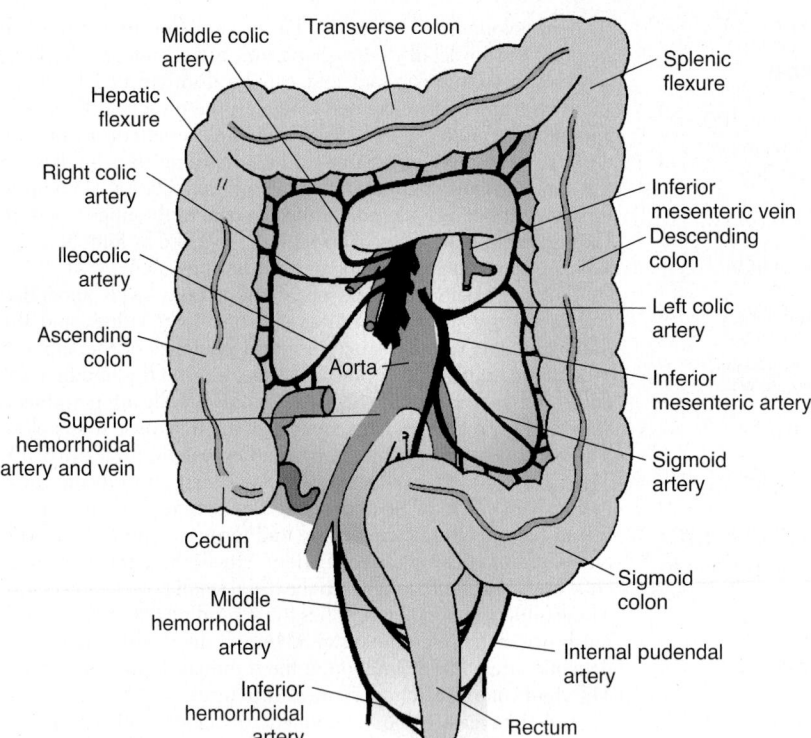

Figure 57.1 The anatomy of the colon with particular emphasis on the vascular supply.

DIAGNOSIS OF COLORECTAL CANCER

Symptoms associated with CRC include lower GI bleeding, change in bowel habits, abdominal pain, weight loss, change in appetite, and weakness, and in particular, obstructive symptoms

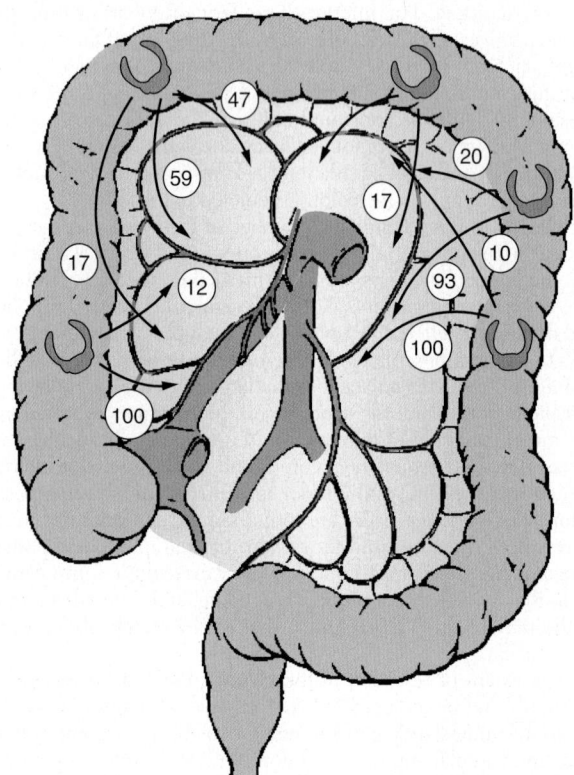

Figure 57.2 The lymphatic drainage of lesions in various anatomic locations throughout the colon.

are alarming.[92] However, apart from obstructive symptoms, other symptoms do not necessarily correlate with stage of disease or portend a particular diagnosis.[93]

Physical examination may reveal a palpable mass, bright blood per rectum (usually left-sided colon cancers or rectal cancer) or melena (right-sided colon cancers), or lesser degrees of bleeding (hemoccult-positive stool). Adenopathy, hepatomegaly, jaundice, or even pulmonary signs may be present with metastatic disease. Obstruction by colon cancer is usually in the sigmoid or left colon, with resulting abdominal distention and constipation, whereas right-sided colon cancers may be more insidious in nature. Complications of CRC include acute GI bleeding, acute obstruction, perforation, and metastasis with impairment of distant organ function.

Laboratory values may reflect iron-deficiency anemia, electrolyte derangements, and liver function abnormalities. The carcinoembryonic antigen (CEA) may be elevated and is most helpful to monitor postoperatively, if reduced to normal as a result of surgery.[94]

Evaluation should include complete history, family history, physical examination, laboratory tests, colonoscopy, and pan-body computed tomography (CT) scan.[95] For rectal cancer, additional imaging techniques, such as magnetic resonance imaging or endoscopic ultrasound, are utilized to further characterize the primary tumor prior to therapy (see Chapter 60). Upon completion of diagnosis and staging for both colon and rectal tumors, it is essential to incorporate the expertise from medical, radiation, and surgical oncologists in order to formulate and implement an optimal treatment plan.

With the advent of molecular biologic techniques, attention has been drawn to stool-based tools and new blood-based tests. Technology now exists to extract genomic DNA or protein from stool and assay for evidence of genetic alterations.[96,97] Large-scale validation studies are in progress, one of which has just been published, describing an automated multitarget sDNA assay (fecal immunochemical testing) with a 90% specificity and 98% sensitivity for the detection of CRC, as well 83% sensitivity for advanced adenoma with high-grade dysplasia.[98] In addition, Epi proColon (Epigenomics AG, Berlin, Germany), a blood-based test, was shown to be noninferior to fecal immunochemical testing in preliminary results from a multicenter double blind comparative study (press release from Epigenomics AG, December 4, 2012). One particularly attractive pathway for stool-based diagnostics would be able to stratify patients as high, moderate, or low risk for CRC and thus influence screening modalities and frequency of screening. In a complementary fashion, functional genomics are being applied to pair-wise comparisons of normal colon and CRCs to sample the entire human genome of nearly 30,000 genes to discover those genes, known and novel, that may be upregulated or downregulated and possibly linked to detection, prognosis, and therapy.

SCREENING FOR COLORECTAL CANCER

Debate is vigorous as to the best approaches for screening, and multiple factors influence that decision: simplicity and rapidity so as to enhance patient compliance, benefit to risk ratio, sensitivity, specificity, cost-effectiveness, and other economic factors. To that end, currently, optical colonoscopy likely offers the most effective approach when one considers all of these factors.

The average-risk patient is defined as a man or woman above the age of 50 without personal or family history of adenomatous polyps or CRC and absence of any occult or acute GI bleeding. Screening recommendations or guidelines for average-risk and high-risk individuals are presented in Table 57.5.

Optical colonoscopy is currently the most sensitive method for screening. Advantages include direct visualization, with the ability to remove polyps (with rate-limiting factors of size and anatomic location) and to obtain biopsies. Disadvantages involve the preparation, invasive nature of the procedure, and potential side effects that include perforation (although this is <1%).

The digital rectal examination should be part of the general physical examination. Anorectal masses may be palpated. Flexible sigmoidoscopy does not require conscious sedation and hemodynamic monitoring, and will typically allow visualization of the rectum, sigmoid colon, and descending colon to the splenic flexure. Flexible sigmoidoscopy should not be considered as a single screening measure but requires coupling with barium enema. Barium enema allows visualization of the entire colon, and experience is necessary to ensure proper visualization of the rectum. Barium enema affords advantages of ease of preparation, lack of conscious sedation and hemodynamic monitoring, and ability to visualize polyps and masses. However, small polyps may be missed. Furthermore, if a luminal polyp or mass is identified, then colonoscopy will be necessary for polypectomy or biopsies.

New noninvasive technologies, such as CT and magnetic resonance colonography, are receiving increased attention in clinical studies, which demonstrate overall feasibility, as well as some advantages.[99]

Two meta-analyses published in 2011 provide strong support for the implementation of CT colonography as a viable alternative to optical colonoscopy in both average and high-risk populations.

TABLE 57.5

Recommendations for Colorectal Cancer Screening in Average-Risk and Increased-Risk Patients from the Gastrointestinal Consortium Panel

Average-Risk Patient (Different Options)
1. FOBT: Offer yearly screening with FOBT using a guaiac-based test with dietary restriction or an immunochemical test without dietary restriction. Two samples from each of three consecutive stools should be examined without rehydration. Patients with a positive test on any specimen should be followed up with colonoscopy.
2. Flexible sigmoidoscopy: Offer flexible sigmoidoscopy every 5 y.
3. FOBT plus flexible sigmoidoscopy: Offer screening with FOBT every year combined with flexible sigmoidoscopy every 5 y. When both tests are performed, the FOBT should be done first.
4. Colonoscopy: Offer every 10 y.
5. DCBE: Offer every 5 y.

Increased Risk for Colorectal Cancer
1. Family history of colorectal cancer or polyps. People with a first-degree relative (parent, sibling, or child) with colon cancer or adenomatous polyp diagnosed at age <60 y or two first-degree relatives diagnosed with colorectal cancer at any age should be advised to have screening colonoscopy starting at age 40 y or 10 y younger than the earliest diagnosis in the family, whichever comes first, and repeated every 5 y.
2. FAP: Flexible sigmoidoscopy to start at ages 10 to 12 y. Genetic testing (for FAP, upper endoscopy with side-viewing scope) should be done every 1 to 3 y.
3. HNPCC: Colonoscopy every 1 to 2 y starting at ages 20 to 25 y or 10 y younger than the earliest case in the family, whichever comes first. Genetic testing (for HNPCC, consideration should be given to screening for uterine and ovarian cancer with hysteroscopy and transvaginal ultrasound, the frequency of which varies within centers).
4. Personal history of adenomatous polyps
   A. If one or more polyps that are malignant or large and sessile or colonoscopy is incomplete, then follow-up colonoscopy should be in the short term.
   B. If three of more polyps, follow-up colonoscopy in 3 y.
   C. If one or two polyps (<1 cm), follow-up colonoscopy in 5 y (or more).
5. Personal history of colorectal cancer
   A. Colonoscopy is incomplete at time of diagnosis of colorectal cancer due to obstruction, then repeat colonoscopy 6 mo after surgical resection.
   B. Colonoscopy is complete at time of diagnosis of colorectal cancer, then repeat colonoscopy in 3 y, and if that is normal, then repeat every 5 y.
6. Inflammatory bowel disease (ulcerative colitis, Crohn's colitis). Surveillance colonoscopy is recommended.

FOBT, fecal occult blood testing; DCBE, double-contrast barium enema; FAP, familial adenomatous polyposis; HNPCC, hereditary nonpolyposis colorectal cancer. From Rex DK, Johnson DA, Lieberman DA, et al. Colorectal cancer prevention 2000: screening recommendations of the American College of Gastroenterology. American College of Gastroenterology. *Am J Gastroenterol* 2000;95:868–877; Winawer S, Fletcher R, Rex D, et al. Colorectal cancer screening and surveillance: clinical guidelines and rationale-Update based on new evidence. *Gastroenterology* 2003;124:544–560.

In a review of 4,086 asymptomatic patients, de Haan et al.,[100] estimates sensitivities of 82.9% and 87.9% and specificities of 91.4% and 97.6% for adenomas ≥6 mm and ≥10mm, respectively.

In a complementary analysis looking exclusively at cancer detection, Pickhardt et al.[101] concludes that CT colonography is not only clinically equivalent to colonoscopy but perhaps even more suitable for initial investigation given consistently high sensitivity (96.1%) without heterogeneity across 49 studies, and 11,151 patients, despite wide variation in technique.

Other reports suggest advantages in long-term costs and patient compliance, although these issues remain controversial.[102,103]

Lastly, CT colonography may also offer improvements in preoperative staging as one study found this technique to be highly predictive of T3-4 tumors. Whether this information will prove as clinically relevant in colon cancer as it is for the rectum remains to be seen.[104]

STAGING AND PROGNOSIS OF COLORECTAL CANCER

This discussion will focus primarily on those prognostic and predictive indicators that are best supported by available data and are appropriate for use and consideration in current practice. The reader should remain aware of the potential for rapid changes and advances in this area, however.

Staging

Although many factors have been identified that have an impact on recurrence and survival, none exceeds stage in terms of prognostic significance.[105] Staging of CRC should be done using the current TNM (tumor, node, metastasis) classification of the American Joint Committee on Cancer (AJCC)/International Union Against Cancer (UICC) staging system (Table 57.6).[106] Other systems should be regarded as of historical significance only and must be comprehended solely for the purposes of understanding the studies that were performed and reported in the past using these older classifications.

TABLE 57.6

Tumor (T) Node (N) Metastasis (M) Classification of Colorectal Cancer

Stage	T	N	M
0	Tis	N0	M0
I	T1	N0	M0
	T2	N0	M0
IIA	T3	N0	M0
IIB	T4a	N0	M0
IIC	T4b	N0	M0
IIIA	T1-T2	N1-N2a	M0
IIIB	T3-T4a	N1	M0
	T2-T3	N2a	M0
	T1-T2	N2b	M0
IIIC	T4a	N2a	M0
	T3-T4a	N2b	M0
	T4b	N1-N2	M0
IVA	T any	N any	M1a
IVB	T any	N any	M1b

Used with the permission of the American Joint Committee on Cancer (AJCC), Chicago, Illinois. The original source for this material is the *AJCC Cancer Staging Manual*, Seventh Edition (2010) published by Springer Science and Business Media LLC, www.springer.com, page 144.

The Dukes Classification and Its Modifications

In the 1930s, Cuthbert Dukes, a Scottish pathologist working predominantly on a classification scheme for rectal cancer, developed the classification system that bears his name. The system, and the several modifications to it made by Dukes and others, is at this time of historical interest only, and the reader is referred to chapters in earlier editions of this book for further details.

Tumor, Node, Metastasis Classification

The current AJCC/UICC staging system for CRC is now the only classification system that should be used.[106] The TNM system classifies colorectal tumors on the basis of the invasiveness (not size) of the primary (T stage), the number (not size or location) of local-regional LNs containing metastatic cancer (N stage), and the presence or absence of distant metastatic disease (M stage) (see Table 57.6).

T Stage. A designation of Tx refers to the inability to describe the extent of tumor invasion due to incomplete information. In situ adenocarcinoma (Tis) includes cancers confined to the glandular basement membrane or lamina propria. The terms *high-grade dysplasia* and *severe dysplasia* are synonymous with in situ carcinoma and are also classified as Tis. T1 tumors invade into but not through the submucosa. T2 tumors invade into but not through the muscularis propria, and T3 tumors invade through the muscularis propria into the subserosa or into nonperitonealized pericolic or perirectal tissue. T4 tumors perforate the visceral peritoneum (T4a) or invade other named organs or structures (T4b). Tumors invading other colorectal segments by way of the serosa (i.e., carcinoma of the cecum invading the sigmoid) are classified as T4b. A tumor that is adherent to other structures or organs macroscopically is classified clinically as T4b; however, if the microscopic examination of the adhesions is negative, then the pathologic classification is pT3. The V and L substaging should be used to identify the presence or absence of vascular or lymphatic invasion. The "p" prefix denotes pathologic (rather than clinical) assessment, and the "y" prefix is attached to those tumors that are being reported after neoadjuvant (presurgical) treatment. For example, the pathologic T stage of a tumor showing only penetration into the submucosa after preoperative therapy would be ypT1. Recurrent tumors are reported with an "r" prefix (rpT3).

N Stage. Because of the prognostic significance associated with increased numbers of LNs inspected (see the following discussion), the current TNM classification scheme calls for at least 12 LNs to be analyzed, and both the number of nodes that are positive for tumor and the total number of nodes inspected should be reported. The term Nx is applied if no description of LN involvement is possible because of incomplete information. A pN0 designation may be made even if fewer than the recommended number of nodes are present; however, the prognostic significance of this pN0 designation is weaker. N0 denotes that all nodes examined are negative. N1a includes tumors with metastasis in one regional LN. N1b refers to involvement of two or three nearby LNs. N1c defines the presence of cancer cells found in areas of fat near LNs, but not in the LNs themselves. N2a indicates metastasis in four to six regional LNs. N2b denotes involvement of greater than seven nodes. Metastatic nodules or foci found in the pericolic, perirectal, or adjacent mesentery without evidence of residual LN tissue are regarded as being equivalent to a regional node metastasis and are counted accordingly.

Stage I disease is defined as T1-2N0 in a patient without distant metastases (M0). Stage II disease is defined as T3-4N0M0. The T-stage carries prognostic significance for stage II, and therefore T3N0 is classified as IIA, and T4a-bN0 is classified as IIB and IIC, respectively.

Node positivity in the absence of M1 disease defines stage III CRC. Recently, the prognostic significance of tumor invasiveness (T stage) has been reincorporated into the assessment of risk in stage III patients. In an exhaustive review of over 50,000 patients, Greene et al.[107] demonstrated the prognostic significance of T stage within node-positive patients. Within the N1 category T stage was found to be highly prognostic, with T1-2 patients fairing significantly better than T3-4. Within the N2 population, the prognosis was worse than either subgroup of N1 patients, with T stage no longer carrying prognostic significance. Thus T stage is prognostic in patients with N0 and N1 but not N2 disease. The current TNM staging system takes these findings into account and now stratifies stage III patients into IIIA (T1-2N1), IIIB (T3-4N1), and IIIC (T any, N2). Stages IIIA, B, and C are highly prognostic for survival.

M Stage. Patients are designated M0 if no evidence of distant metastases is present. Identification of distant metastases denotes a classification of M1. Involvement of the external iliac, common iliac, para-aortic, supraclavicular, or other nonregional LNs is classified as distant metastatic (M1) disease. The M1 category is subdivided into M1a, defined as spread of tumor to one distant organ or set of distant LNs, and M1b, where spread has occurred to more than one distant organ or sets of LNs or spread has occurred to the peritoneum. Although the TNM staging system is regarded as the most comprehensive tool for prognostic and predictive purposes, a major criticism of the last two revisions is that survival of stage IIIA patients continues to be superior to stage IIB. This disparity, which is actually more pronounced in the seventh edition of AJCC manual, has been attributed to inadequate LN assessment and understaging. However, a recent review of SEER data showed this problem persists even in a subset analysis of patients with >12 LNs, highlighting the need for additional refinement and perhaps the incorporation of nonanatomic prognostic factors.[108]

Residual Tumor (R Stage) at Margins of Resection. Tumors that are completely resected with histologically negative margins are classified as R0. Tumors with a complete gross resection but with microscopically positive margins are classified as R1, the positive margin indicating that at least microscopic tumor remains in the patient. Patients who have incomplete resections with grossly positive margins are classified as having had an R2 resection. The R0, R1, and R2 designations carry strong prognostic implications.

Identification of the proximal and distal margins of resection is relatively straightforward, and definitions of these margins are well understood. A more complex and often misunderstood (as well as underreported) margin of resection is the circumferential radial margin (CRM). All three margins (proximal, distal, and CRM) should be specifically commented upon in the pathology report, as all three have prognostic significance.

The CRM is, by definition, a surgically dissected surface. It is defined as the cut retroperitoneal or perineal soft tissue margin closest to the deepest penetration of tumor. It is considered positive if tumor is present microscopically (R1) or macroscopically (R2) on a *cut* radial or lateral aspect of the surgical specimen. For the ascending colon, descending colon, and upper rectum, which are incompletely encased by peritoneum, the CRM is created by dissection of the retroperitoneal aspect of the bowel. In the case of the lower rectum, which is not encased by peritoneum, the CRM is created by sharp dissection of the mesorectum.

A tumor simply penetrating into pericolonic or perirectal fat does not necessarily constitute a positive CRM, but rather is simply a description of a T3 primary. A tumor that involves a peritonealized surface of the bowel and not a surgically cut surface does not constitute a positive CRM, but rather constitutes a T4a primary. If, however, the cut surface at the deepest penetration of the tumor is positive, then the CRM is positive and the resection is staged R1 (microscopic) or R2 (macroscopic). A positive CRM is highly predictive of local recurrence and should prompt consideration of adjuvant treatment.

Prognosis

Histologic Grade

Although histologic grade has been shown to have prognostic significance, there is significant subjectivity involved in scoring of this variable, and no one set of criteria for determination of grade are universally accepted.[105] The majority of staging systems divide tumors into grade 1 (well differentiated), grade 2 (moderately differentiated), grade 3 (poorly differentiated), and grade 4 (undifferentiated). Many studies collapse this into low grade (well to moderately differentiated) and high grade (poorly differentiated or undifferentiated). Greene et al.[107] demonstrated that this two-tiered split has important prognostic significance.

College of American Pathologists Consensus Statement. The College of American Pathologists (CAP) has published an expert panel consensus statement outlining their interpretation of the validity and usefulness of a large number of putatively prognostic and predictive factors in CRC.[109] Variables were categorized as belonging to categories I through IV. Category I was defined as those factors proven to be of prognostic import based on evidence from multiple, statistically robust, published trials and generally used in patient management. Category IIA included factors intensively studied biologically or clinically and repeatedly shown to have prognostic value for outcome or predictive value for therapy that is of sufficient import to be included in the pathology report, but that remains to be validated in statistically robust studies. Category IIB included factors shown to be promising in multiple studies but lacking sufficient data for inclusion in category I or IIA. Category III included factors felt to be not yet sufficiently studied to determine their prognostic value, and category IV included those factors that are adequately studied to have convincingly shown no prognostic significance. A number of these factors are discussed in further detail in the following.

The T, N, and M categories of the current AJCC/UICC staging system were all classified as category I. Other category I inclusions were blood or lymphatic vessel invasion and residual tumor following surgery with curative intent (the R category). Although not assessed pathologically, an elevation of the preoperative CEA level was also felt to merit category I inclusion. Factors in category IIA included tumor grade, radial margin status (for resection of specimens with nonperitonealized surfaces), and residual tumor in the resection specimen following neoadjuvant therapy. Factors in category IIB (many of which are discussed in further detail in the following) included histologic type, histologic features associated with MSI (i.e., host lymphoid response to tumor and medullary or mucinous histologic type), high degree of MSI (MSI-H), loss of heterozygosity (LOH) of 18q (DCC [deleted in colon cancer] gene loss), and tumor border configuration (infiltrating versus pushing border). Factors grouped in category III included DNA content, all other molecular markers except for LOH of 18q/DCC and MSI-H, perineural invasion, microvessel density, tumor cell–associated proteins or carbohydrates, peritumoral fibrosis, peritumoral inflammatory response, focal neuroendocrine differentiation, nuclear organizing regions, and proliferation. Those factors in category IV (proven to be of no significance) included tumor size and gross tumor configuration.

Total Number of Lymph Nodes

It has been well established that an adequate number of LNs must be sampled before a patient can be considered node negative, and careful pathologic technique has been demonstrated to be crucial to adequate nodal interpretation. Failure to adequately dissect and display the mesentery will lead to underreporting and understaging.[110,111] It should be noted that an insufficient number of LNs reported could be due to a suboptimal nodal dissection at operation, a less than thorough search for nodes by the pathologist, or some combination of the two. Additional patient- and tumor-related factors may also affect LN count independent of pathologist or surgeon. Belt et al.[112] found a significant association between MSI phenotype and high LN yield in both stage II and III colon cancers, with the strongest effect in the latter group. The authors postulate that this may be due to a more prominent lymphocytic antitumor response known to be exhibited by MSI-H cancers.[112] Another report suggests that low body mass index is associated with increased LN yield, although it did not affect relapse-free or overall survival in stage III cancers. Proximal tumor location, well- or moderately differentiated histology, and stage IIIC cancer were also significant variables for adequate LN recovery.[113] Finally, a multivariate analysis of two large prospective US cohort databases (121,701 women and 51,529 men) demonstrated that specimen length, tumor size, ascending tumor location, T3N0M0 stage, and year of diagnosis were positively associated with negative node count (p <0.002). Mutation of KRAS was borderline significant and requires further study. The authors recommend that these variables be taken into account when judging adequacy of LN harvest and devising individualized treatment plans in the future.[114] An analysis was reported on outcome versus nodal sampling in the patients who participated in an Intergroup trial (INT-0089), a large four-arm trial of different 5-fluorouracil (5-FU)–based adjuvant chemotherapies in patients with colon cancer. Multivariate analyses were performed on the node-positive (2,768 patients) and node-negative (648 patients) groups separately. The median number of LNs reported in the assessable patients on this trial was 11 (range, 1 to 87). Survival (overall, cancer-specific, and disease-free [DFS]) was found to decrease with an increasing number of involved LNs (p = 0.0001 for all three survival end points). However, after controlling for the number of involved nodes, survival increased with the total number of nodes (positive plus negative) reported (p = 0.0001 for overall survival, cancer-specific survival, and DFS). Even in patients who were node negative, overall survival (p = 0.0005) and cancer-specific survival (p = 0.007) were significantly increased as the number of reported LNs increased.

In a different secondary analysis of the Intergroup trial (INT-0089), a mathematical model was created to estimate the probability of a true node-negative result on the basis of the number of LNs examined in a subset of patients who had at least 10 LNs reported in their resection specimen.[115] A total of 1,585 patients with stage III or high-risk stage II colon cancer were evaluated. This model concluded that when 18 nodes are examined, there is a <25% probability of true node negativity in T1 and T2 tumors. However, examination of <10 LNs was needed in T3 and T4 tumors to achieve the same probability. The overall conclusions of this analysis were that a very significant proportion of patients are understaged, and that such understaging could have important implications for decisions regarding adjuvant therapy and for overall prognosis.

The CAP consensus statement suggests that a minimum of 12 to 15 LNs should be examined in order to determine node negativity.[109] Availability of fewer nodes should therefore be regarded as a relative high-risk factor in terms of prognosis and should be factored into decisions regarding adjuvant therapy. Further support for this recommendation comes from a newly published Danish cohort study that indicates that the advantage of larger LN harvest extends beyond more accurate staging. In addition to improved outcomes for node-negative patients, the authors found a significant increase in overall survival for stage III patients with >12 LNs removed as well (58.6% versus 45.2% for <12 LNs), despite a higher prevalence of N2 disease in this group. This may be related to better surgical technique or an underlying benefit of wider lymphadenectomy in general. LN ratio was also shown to be an important independent prognostic indicator and, in fact, superior to N-stage in predicting survival for stage III patients. This finding is consistent with a number of previous reports, many of which have advocated for incorporation of this parameter into the AJCC staging system.[116–120]

Microscopic Nodal Metastases

The advent of improved pathologic techniques and sensitive methods such as IHC or polymerase chain reaction may have an impact on the number of positive LNs detected and may have important prognostic significance.[121,122] However, the prognostic value of these positive LNs, which otherwise would not be detected, remains controversial. In a recent review of 16 studies with survival data, Sirop et al.[123] found only 8 papers that reported definitely poorer outcomes, whereas the remainder were either equivocal in their conclusions or demonstrated no influence on outcome at all. Jeffers et al.[124] evaluated LNs from 77 patients who were found to have negative LNs by routine examination with immunocytochemical staining for cytokeratin AE1:AE3. Nineteen patients (25%) were found to have immunohistochemical evidence of micrometastases; however, there was no difference in survival between the microscopically positive and negative patients. A larger trial by Faerden et al.,[125] on the other hand, did demonstrate adverse prognostic impact. In this study, 39 of 126 patients with stage I/II colon cancer were noted to have micrometastases or isolated tumor cells (MM/ITC+) on IHC staining. Prospective median 5-year follow-up of MM/ITC+ compared to MM/ITC- patients revealed recurrence rates of 23% versus 7% (p = 0.010) and 5-year DFS of 75% versus 93% (p = 0.012), respectively.[125] If micrometastases are reported, the methodology by which they are detected should be specified, as it is likely that differences in reliability and reproducibility of different techniques will emerge. Although the actual TNM staging is not altered by the presence of micrometastases, many clinicians choose to regard the presence of such a finding as a poor prognostic variable in their consideration of adjuvant treatment.

Sentinel Node Analysis

Sentinel node analysis is an approach that has received attention in the management of cutaneous melanoma and breast cancer.[126,127] This technique has been proposed as a means of increasing the yield and the diagnostic information for colon cancer.[91,92] The technique for sentinel node mapping and biopsy for colon cancer has been described by Saha et al.[128] Unlike sentinel node approaches for melanoma and breast, where the goal is to potentially limit the extent of an unnecessary formal dissection of a node basin, the goal of the sentinel node in colon cancer is to focus the pathologic analysis on fewer nodes so a more extensive study can be performed. The same extent of node dissection is performed regardless of the sentinel node procedure. The initial studies of sentinel node biopsy demonstrated it was technically feasible, with accuracy rates >80% and upstaging in 15.4% of patients according to a recent prospective trial.[129–131] In addition, Saha et al.[132] suggest that sentinel LN mapping may not just improve staging accuracy but influence the extent of nodal dissection as well. In this study, sentinel LN mapping detected aberrant lymphatic drainage in 22%, which in turn led to a change in operation (i.e., more extensive resection). In two patients, the aberrant sentinel nodes were the only positive nodes identified.[132] However, not all subsequent studies have shown positive results. False-negative rates as high as 60% have been reported, and some studies have failed to demonstrate any change in the stage determination of the lesion.[133] Based on the available data, two conclusions can be reached. First, from a technical standpoint, sentinel node dissection at the time of a colon resection can be performed and the sentinel node accurately identified. Second, the utility of this technique has not yet been established and further large-scale trials are required to establish its role in the staging of patients with CRC.

Blood or Lymphatic Vessel Invasion

Although there have been conflicting reports in the literature, the CAP consensus statement gave blood and lymphatic vessel invasion category I status, indicating that the preponderance of evidence strongly supports the reliability of these findings as indicators of poorer prognosis.[109] Unfortunately, considerable heterogeneity exists in the methodology for examining and reporting of vessel involvement. The finding of vessel involvement increases with the number of sections examined, and differentiation of postcapillary venules from lymphatics is often not possible. These aspects can make interpretation of some older data on this topic potentially problematic. Current recommendations are that at least three blocks of tumor (optimally five or more) each have a single section examined using hematoxylin and eosin stain to look for tumor invasion of vessels. Vessels not definitively interpreted as venules or lymphatics should be reported as angiolymphatic vessels.

Histologic Type

Several histologic types of CRC carry specific independent prognostic significance. Signet ring carcinomas are characterized by >50% of cells demonstrating the "signet ring" morphology in which intracellular mucin accumulation displaces the nuclei and cytoplasm toward the cellular periphery. This histology carries an adverse prognosis.[134,135] The prognostic significance of the finding of mucinous (>50% mucinous) carcinoma remains controversial. Although some reports list mucinous type as an adverse histology, this has not been consistently demonstrated. Most findings of adverse prognosis with mucinous histology are based on univariate analyses. The one finding in a multivariate analysis of a poor prognostic outcome with mucinous tumors was based on a study of tumors presenting with obstruction, a presentation that is in itself high risk. Some reports have lumped mucinous and signet cell tumors together and found this to be a negative prognostic factor; however, this may simply reflect the negative impact of the signet cell tumors, and its meaning regarding the risk of a mucinous histology is unclear. Small cell (extrapulmonary oat cell) tumors are high-grade neuroendocrine tumors with clearly adverse prognostic features. The prognostic significance of focal neuroendocrine differentiation is, however, unclear (CAP category III). Most data indicate that extensive neuroendocrine differentiation is associated with a poorer prognosis.[136] Medullary carcinoma is a subtype characterized by an absence of glands and distinctive growth pattern that previously would have been classified as undifferentiated. It is typically infiltrated with lymphocytes. This histologic subtype is tightly associated with MSI-H and carries a more favorable prognosis.[137] Histologic types other than signet ring, small cell, and medullary carcinomas are routinely designated in the pathology report; however, the majority of these other histologic types carry no established independent prognostic significance.

Microsatellite Instability

As discussed earlier in this chapter, there are two distinct mutational pathways that can give rise to CRC: the MSI pathway or the chromosomal instability pathway. Microsatellites are sections of DNA in which a short sequence of nucleotides (most commonly a dinucleotide) is repeated multiple times.[138] MSI is a situation in which a microsatellite has gained or lost repeat units and so has undergone a change in length, resulting in frame shift mutations or base-pair substitutions. Approximately 15% of CRCs display these mutations. This form of genetic destabilization is typically associated with defective DNA mismatch repair function. Studies of HNPCC tumor specimens demonstrated mutations in mismatch repair genes such as *MLH1* and *MSH2*. These genes encode proteins that repair nucleotide mismatches. The phenotype of tumors with this defect is termed the MSI-H–instability phenotype.

The majority (approximately 85%) of patients with CRC have cancers characteristic of the chromosomal instability pathway, typically having genetic alterations involving LOH, chromosomal amplifications, and chromosomal translocations. These are known as the microsatellite-stable (MSS) tumors. MSI-H tumors have a number of different features relative to low MSI (MSI-L)

or MSS colorectal tumors.[139,140] MSI-L and MSS tumors tend to behave and present similarly. MSI-H tumors are more frequently right-sided, high grade, and mucinous type.[24,141] They are characteristically associated with increased peritumoral lymphocytic infiltration and are characteristically diploid, whereas MSS tumors are more likely to be aneuploid.[142,143] MSI-H CRCs are more likely to have a larger primary at the time of diagnosis but are more likely to be node negative. Patients with MSI-H CRCs have a better long-term prognosis than stage-matched patients with cancers exhibiting MSS.[144]

Watanabe et al.[145] evaluated MSI status as well as allelic loss from chromosomes 18q, 17b, and 8p, as well as cellular levels of p53 and p21$^{wafl/c1p1}$ proteins as potential prognostic markers. Tumors were analyzed from 460 stage III and high-risk stage II patients who had been treated with 5-FU–based adjuvant therapy. A total of 62 of 298 tumors evaluated for MSI status (21%) were found to be MSI-H. Of the MSI-H tumors, 38 (61%) had a mutation of the gene for type II receptor of transforming growth factor (TGF)-β1. In this analysis, MSI-H was a favorable prognostic indicator for 5-year DFS ($p = 0.02$) and trended toward being a favorable independent prognostic indicator, but did not reach statistical significance for overall survival ($p = 0.20$). However, the 5-year survival among patients with MSI-H was 74% in the presence of a mutated gene for the type II receptor of TGF-β1 and 46% in patients whose tumors lacked this mutation (RR = 2.90; 95% CI = 1.14 to 7.34; $p = 0.04$). MSI-H cells are relatively resistant to 5-FU in vitro.[146] All of the patients in Watanabe et al.'s[145] analysis received 5-FU–based chemotherapy. The TGF-β1 pathway inhibits tumor proliferation by causing a late G_1 cell cycle arrest. Therefore, a mutated and presumably nonfunctional *TGF-β1* gene could favor increased proliferation, which would be anticipated to confer increased susceptibility to cytotoxic chemotherapy. A recent evaluation of the prognostic significance of MSI in the N0147 adjuvant trial[147] demonstrated a more nuanced result. When looking at the colon overall, MSI was not found to be predictive. However, when divided by side, MSI was found to carry a favorable prognosis for right-sided colon lesions, but was a negative prognostic factor in left-sided colon lesions. The reasons for this difference is not clear; however, the different embryologic origins of the left and right colon may play a role in these observations.

BRAF

BRAF mutation, present in 10% to 20% of CRCs, is linked to a subset of MSI-H tumors that are sporadic and generally have poorer prognosis. Ogino et al.[148] confirmed this relationship in comparative analysis of 506 stage III patients enrolled in the Cancer and Leukemia Group B (CALGB) 89803 trial. BRAF-mutated patients had significantly worse overall survival (HR = 1.66) compared to wild-type, a finding that was most pronounced in the setting of MSS.[148] In a follow-up study, Lochhead et al.[149] also identified combined BRAF/MSI status as a powerful prognosticator and recommends stratification of all patients into poor (MSS/BRAF mutant), intermediate (MSS/BRAF wild-type), and favorable (MSI-H/BRAF wild-type) groups in order better inform treatment strategies. Douillard et al.[150] confirmed BRAF mutation to be a poor prognostic factor in patients with stage IV disease as well.

Allelic Loss of 18q (*DCC* Gene Loss)

Allelic LOH that involves chromosome 18q occurs in half or more of all CRCs. Allelic loss of 18q typically involves the *DCC* gene; however, other genes in this region, such as Smad2 and Smad4, may also be relevant to CRC development. DCC expression is greatly reduced or absent in many colorectal carcinomas, and loss of DCC is associated with metastasis and an adverse prognosis.[151] The specific product of the DCC gene has been shown to be the netrin-1 receptor. In the nonpathologic state, this receptor guides the migration of neuronal axons. DCC induces apoptosis in the absence of netrin-1 binding. DCC is cleaved by caspase, and mutation of the site at

TABLE 57.7

Loss of Heterozygosity (Allelic Loss) at 18q and Prognosis in Patients with Stage III Colon Cancer

Allelic Status of 18q	No. of Patients	Five-Y Survival (%)	P Value
No loss	112	69	0.005
Loss	109	50	

From Watanabe T, Wu TT, Catalano PJ, et al. Molecular predictors of survival after adjuvant chemotherapy for colon cancer. *N Engl J Med* 2001;344: 1196–1206.

which caspase 3 cleaves DCC suppresses the proapoptotic effect of DCC completely. Binding of netrin-1 to DCC blocks apoptosis.[152] Loss of DCC as a result of allelic loss in 18q could therefore be anticipated to impair apoptosis, thereby resulting in greater resistance to chemotherapy. This hypothesized mechanism of action of 18q LOH is attractive; however, it should be emphasized that it is not at all clear to what extent DCC is the active moiety in the setting of 18q allelic loss. Watanabe et al.[145] evaluated allelic loss from chromosome 18q as a potential prognostic indicator in archived specimens of tumors from patients who were treated in one of two national Intergroup adjuvant trials (INT 0035 or INT 0089). MSI status was also evaluated, as were 17p, 8p, and cellular levels of p53 and p21$^{waf1/c1p1}$ proteins. Tumors were analyzed from 460 stage III and high-risk stage II patients who had been treated with 5-FU–based adjuvant therapy. Allelic loss of 18q was present in 155 of 319 cancers (49%). Allelic loss in 18q was highly prognostically significant in this analysis (Table 57.7). In the stage III patients with allelic loss of 18q, 5-year overall survival was 50%, while in those with retained 18q alleles, 5-year survival was 69% ($p = 0.005$). Other markers evaluated in this analysis were not shown to be prognostically significant.

Host Lymphoid Response

Lymphocytic infiltration has been identified as a favorable prognostic indicator. Whether this is a truly independent predictor of outcome is not clear, however, as this finding is tightly associated with MSI-H, a favorable prognostic factor. Along these lines, the prognostic value of neutrophil-to-lymphocyte ratio has also been recently evaluated. Chiang et al.[153] found that elevated preoperative neutrophil-to-lymphocyte ratio (>3) was associated with significantly worse DFS in stage I to III colon but not rectal cancers on multivariate analysis. In another study, neutrophil-to-lymphocyte ratio (>5) was also found to be an independent risk factor for recurrence. While the direct impact of this parameter is difficult to explain, the authors of the first study postulate that it may represent a measure of innate-to-adaptive immunity under stress with relative lymphopenia, as a marker of depressed cell-mediated immunity, conferring survival disadvantage.[153,154]

Tumor Border Configuration

The configuration of the tumor border (infiltrating versus pushing border) has been shown to have independent prognostic significance. An infiltrating border, characterized by an irregular, infiltrating pattern at the tumor edge (also known as focal dedifferentiation or tumor budding), has been shown in multivariate analyses to portend a poorer prognosis than tumors with smooth, pushing borders.

Carcinoembryonic Antigen

An elevated preoperative CEA is a poor prognostic factor for cancer recurrence. Although there is variability in the available data regarding the level that denotes a prognostic cutoff, a preoperative CEA level >5 ng/ml is considered a category I poor prognostic indicator

by the CAP consensus panel.[109] Patients in whom the elevated CEA fails to normalize after a potentially curative operation are at particularly high risk. Several authors have presented evidence that indicates that CEA is an independent prognostic factor. In a report of 572 patients who underwent curative resection for node-negative colon cancer, the preoperative CEA level and the stage of disease predicted survival by both univariate and multivariate analyses.[155] Given the prognostic significance of the preoperative CEA, it is reasonable to recommend that all patients who undergo operation for CRC have a serum CEA drawn prior to operation.

No other serum markers have been demonstrated to be reliably prognostic or predictive in CRC. Cancer antigen (CA) 19-9, a factor that has become widely used for pancreas cancer, has no role at this time in the routine management of CRC.

Obstruction and Perforation

Carcinoma of the colon that is complicated by obstruction or perforation has been recognized as having a poorer prognosis. Data obtained from 1,021 patients with Dukes stage B and C CRC, who were entered into randomized clinical trials of the National Surgical Adjuvant Breast and Bowel Project (NSABP) showed that the presence of bowel obstruction strongly influenced the outcome. The effect of bowel obstruction was more pronounced when the obstruction was located in the right colon. The larger-sized tumor needed to block the ascending colon completely might allow a longer time for these tumors to grow and spread when compared with tumors located in the descending colon.

A review of the Massachusetts General Hospital records compared patients who presented with obstruction or perforation with a control group who underwent curative resection. The actuarial 5-year survival rate seen in patients who presented with obstruction was 31%, in contrast to 59% in historical controls. For patients with localized perforation, the 5-year actuarial survival rate was 44%. The Gastrointestinal Tumor Study Group (GITSG) multivariate analysis concluded that obstruction was an important indicator of prognosis, independent of Dukes stage. Bowel perforation was a poor prognostic factor only for DFS.

Category III Factors

Multiple factors, while of investigational interest, are at this time not appropriate for routine clinical use and have so been designated as category III (defined as not sufficiently studied to prove their prognostic value) by the CAP consensus panel. These include DNA content, or ploidy, and proliferation indices. Also included in category III are all molecular markers other than MSI and 18q deletions, such as thymidylate synthase (TS), dihydropyrimidine dehydrogenase (DPD), and p53 mutational status. Perineural invasion, microvessel density, tumor cell–associated proteins or carbohydrates, peritumoral fibrosis, peritumoral inflammatory response, and focal neuroendocrine differentiation are also category III. The area of molecular prognostic markers is one of particular activity, however, and it is anticipated that clinical trials that are now ongoing will shed light on these important areas.

Perineural Invasion

The ability of CRCs to invade perineural spaces as far as 10 cm from the primary tumor has long been described. Early reports suggest an increased disease recurrence rate and worse 5-year survival. Multivariate analyses have failed to show the prognostic significance of this finding. The CAP consensus panel classified perineural invasion as category III (insufficient evidence of determine prognostic significance).

Tumor Size and Configuration

Studies have consistently shown that both the size and configuration of the primary tumor in CRC do not carry prognostic significance (CAP category IV). In a review of 391 patients, the mean diameter of Dukes stage B2 tumors was actually greater than the mean diameter of stage C2 tumors (p <0.001) and D tumors (p <0.05). The size of the primary tumor showed no relationship to 5-year adjusted survival. These results were confirmed by the NSABP experience.[156] Tumor configuration is described as exophytic (fungating), endophytic (ulcerative), diffusely infiltrative (linitis plastica), or annular. The vast majority of studies have failed to show any of these configurations to have consistent independent prognostic significance. Linitis plastica has been related to a poor prognosis; however, this may be due to the signet cell and other high-grade features of the tumors that are typically associated with this morphology.

Hemorrhage or Rectal Bleeding

It has been speculated that tumors that present with bleeding might be found earlier and therefore might be associated with a better prognosis. This has not been confirmed by data. In the GITSG multivariate analysis, the presence of melena or rectal bleeding showed a trend as a prognostic factor for prolonged survival but failed to reach statistical significance (p = 0.08). One large study found bleeding to be a favorable prognostic indicator on univariate analysis; however, this finding disappeared on multivariate analysis. Bleeding at presentation does not appear to carry any significance.

Primary Tumor Location

Large retrospective reviews of data from the NSABP suggest that right-sided colon cancers carry a worse prognosis than left-sided ones. However, poorer prognosis for patients with disease in the left colon has also been reported. Several investigators report no difference based on the location of the primary tumor. The large GITSG colon cancer experience showed that tumor location (left, right, and rectosigmoid or sigmoid) was of low prognostic value. A recent analysis of SEER-Medicare data by Weiss et al.[157] provides additionally ambiguous results. Of 53,801 patients, 67% had right-sided colon cancer and were more likely to be older, women, and diagnosed with more advanced stage and with more poorly differentiated tumors. However, on multivariate analysis, there was no significant difference in mortality for all stages combined or for stage I. Compared to left-sided lesions, right-sided cancers were associated with a lower mortality within the stage II subgroup (HR = 0.92; p = 0.001) but higher mortality within stage III (HR = 1.12; p = 0.001). Critics of this report point out that a less aggressive treatment approach was likely employed in this older study population, as at least 40% of stage III cases did not receive adjuvant therapy and nearly half underwent inadequate LN harvest. Regardless, these results further dispel the notion of a straightforward relationship between tumor location and mortality.[157]

Body Mass Index

While obesity is known to be a risk factor for the development of colon cancer, the prognostic impact of body mass index on long-term outcomes is controversial. In a cohort study conducted within a large randomized trial of 3,759 patients with high-risk stage II or III colon cancer (INT-0089), obese women had significantly worse overall mortality (HR = 1.34; 95% CI = 1.07 to 1.67); however, this finding was not apparent in men.[158] Sinicrope et al.[159] found the opposite gender correlation using the ACCENT database, a pooled resource of 25,291 participants in national and international adjuvant chemotherapy trials. On multivariate analysis, with a median follow-up of 7.8 years, obese and underweight men, but not women, had significantly poorer survival compared to overweight and normal weight patients.[159] And in another prospective cohort of 913 patients with stage II and III colon cancer, Alipour et al.[160] found no association between obesity (as measured by either body mass index or body surface area) and oncologic outcomes. Evidently, this topic warrants further study before any conclusions can be drawn.[160]

Diabetes Mellitus

The influence of diabetes mellitus on outcome is also unclear. In the INT-0089 cohort, diabetes conferred a strong disadvantage with affected patients experiencing a significantly worse DFS (48% versus 59%; p <0.0001), overall survival (57% versus 66%; p <0.0001), and recurrence-free survival (56% versus 64%; p = 0.012) at 5 years. Median survival for diabetics was 6 years, whereas for nondiabetics it was 11.3 years.[158] Other reports, however, have generated less consistent results. Among 2,278 subjects from the Cancer Prevention Study-II Nutrition Cohort, patients with CRC and type 2 diabetes were at higher risk of all-cause mortality (ACM; RR = 1.53), but only those without insulin use were at higher risk for CRC-specific mortality. These results are in line with previous evidence that hyperinsulinemia (as in poorly controlled diabetes) plays an important role in tumorigenesis and metastasis of CRC.[161] Another population-based study did not find any such an association in 6,974 patients with colon cancer. Disease-specific mortality was only significantly increased for patients with rectal cancer (n = 3,888, 10% of whom were diabetic; HR = 1.30). While hyperinsulinemia is again implicated, the authors call for additional study to clarify specific pathways responsible for these rectum-specific findings.[162]

Gender

Female sex has generally been considered a favorable prognostic factor, but data is limited and inconclusive. In the first study to examine the impact of gender in the era of oxaliplatin-based therapy, Cheung et al.[163] performed a prospectively planned, pooled analysis of 33,345 patients participating in the ACCENT database of randomized trials. The authors found a significant but very modest survival advantage for women with early stage disease that persisted across all ages, stages, and types of adjuvant therapy. Sex was not a predictive factor for treatment efficacy, however, suggesting that chemotherapy regimens should be not be altered based on this parameter.[163]

Smoking

As discussed earlier, prolonged cigarette smoking appears to be a moderate risk factor for CRC with continued effect even after smoking cessation. Increasing evidence indicates that this association differs not just by tumor site but also by molecular features, such as the presence of MSI-H and BRAF mutations, which cumulatively seem to confer the strongest risk. Impact on survival has now also been reported in a recent study analyzing data from a large multicenter randomized adjuvant chemotherapy trial (N0147). The authors found that smokers experienced significantly shorter 3-year DFS (74% versus 70%; HR = 1.21) that was most evident in BRAF wild-type and KRAS-mutated tumors.[164]

Blood Transfusions

Considerable controversy has surrounded the question of an association between perioperative blood transfusions and the recurrence rate of CRC. Some investigators have reported worse DFS in patients who require transfusions. By multivariate analysis in a large prospective study, however, no negative influence of transfusion on survival could be detected, and it does not appear that perioperative blood transfusions carry negative prognostic value. A retrospective analysis evaluating 1,051 patients treated with curative surgery for stage II or III colorectal adenocarcinoma at the Mayo Clinic demonstrated that the use of blood components probably had no impact on disease recurrence, and the documented adverse impact of transfusions is more likely due to other variables or to the underlying illness necessitating the transfusion.[165]

Oncogenes and Molecular Markers

Oncogenes and molecular markers are discussed extensively in another chapter. At present, none of the markers under investigation has achieved adequate validity to permit routine clinical use. However, the study of molecular markers continues to progress and continues to advance the understanding of the development and treatment of CRC. TS continues to be a major area of investigation. Data are conflicting on its prognostic significance; however, preliminary studies suggest that high TS levels may be predictive for resistance to 5-FU–based therapies.[166] At present, there is no role for TS determinations in routine clinical practice. The p53 gene located on chromosome 17p is a well-known tumor suppressor gene. The abnormal p53 appears to be a late phenomenon in colorectal carcinogenesis. This mutation may allow the growing tumor with multiple genetic alterations to evade cell cycle arrest and apoptosis. In a retrospective review of 141 patients with resected stage II and III colon carcinoma, a p53 mutation increased the risk of death by 2.82 times in patients with stage II disease and by 2.39 times in patients with stage III colon carcinoma. The Southwest Oncology Group assessed the prognostic value of p53 in 66 patients with stage II and 163 stage III colon cancer. p53 expression was found in 63% of cancers and was associated with favorable survival in stage III but not stage II disease. Seven-year survival with stage III disease was 56% with p53 expression versus 43% with no p53 expression ($p = 0.012$).[167] Overall, the data are conflicting on the utility of p53 as a prognostic variable, and it does not have a use at this time in standard practice.

Epidermal growth factor receptor (EGFR) is an important molecular target for antibody-based therapy in various cancer types and is ubiquitous in colonic tissue. The prognostic impact of this biomarker was recently addressed in a meta-analysis demonstrating worse postoperative survival in patients with high compared to low EGFR expression (HR = 2.34).[168]

Genetic Polymorphisms

Extensive preliminary work is indicating that genetic polymorphisms can potentially have important predictive implications in terms of both efficacy and toxicity with chemotherapy. For example, the UGT1A1 polymorphism has been correlated with CPT-11 toxicity, and TS and XRCC1 polymorphisms may predict efficacy for oxaliplatin or 5-FU combinations.[169] Although a commercial assay is currently available for measurement of UGT1A1 polymorphisms, it is not, at this time, clear how, or if, this assay should be used in routine practice. Currently, there are no specific guidelines for dose modifications on the basis of UGT1A1 polymorphism, and the 7/7 mutation, associated with higher toxicity, has also been associated with greater antitumor activity. These approaches will require considerable more validation and exploration before they can be considered for standard management.[170]

APPROACHES TO SURGICAL RESECTION OF COLON CANCER

The management of colon cancer is best understood as a multimodality approach tailored to the stage of disease. However, there are certain basic tenets of surgical management for the resection of the primary lesion that can be applied across various pathologic stages. Therefore, in order to provide a clear description of these techniques, they will first be described based on the type of surgical resection. These procedures will then be referred to throughout the discussion of stage-specific treatment.

Colonoscopic Resection of Polyps

Many lesions of the colon are first detected during endoscopic procedures. These lesions can range from small hyperplastic polyps to large fungating invasive carcinomas. The appearance of these lesions often indicates their relative potential for malignancy. However, the only definitive way to make a diagnosis is through a pathologic examination of the tissue. Therefore, the goal of a colonoscopic biopsy or resection is to, whenever feasible, remove the lesion in its entirety and preserve a tissue architecture in order to achieve both a therapeutic resection and an accurate pathologic diagnosis. Various techniques can be employed for the removal of lesions in the colon depending on their size and location. Biopsy forceps and snares are the two most commonly employed instruments used during a colonoscopy. These devices are fashioned from flexible coated wires that can conform to the shape of the colonoscope and can also conduct electrical current in order to achieve coagulation and hemostasis.

Bleeding and perforation, while uncommon, are seen at an increased frequency during a therapeutic as opposed to a diagnostic colonoscopy.[171,172] Small polypoid lesions (up to 5 to 8 mm) that are found during the course of a colonoscopic examination can often be removed in their entirety along with a small amount of normal mucosa using a biopsy forceps. Bleeding is usually minimal but can be controlled by electrocautery if persistent. Larger well-pedunculated polyps can often be removed using a technique employing a snare and electrocautery. The snare is placed over the polypoid lesion and cinched down at the base of the polyp. Once tightened, an electrical current is applied and the polyp is resected. If the lesions are too large to be retrieved through the working port of the colonoscope, they can be held in place with a snare just beyond the tip of the colonoscope where they can be kept in view and withdrawn with the scope from the patient. It is important, when sending these specimens to pathology, to properly orient the polyp so as to indicate the base where the resection took place as well as the other positions of the lesion. This will allow the pathologist to provide important information as to the margin status for the resection. Carcinoma in situ as well as stage I invasive carcinomas found in a well-pedunculated polyp can be treated with colonoscopic resection, as described previously, and no further surgical management is needed as long as there is a negative margin >2 mm and the tumor is well-differentiated without lymphovascular invasion or extension of malignant cells beyond the stalk (Haggitt levels 1 to 3).[173] If these criteria are not met, further therapy is required. It is for this reason that it is often helpful to mark the site of the polyp resection with an agent that will leave a "tattoo" to guide additional intervention.

Larger lesions with a broad base or sessile lesions are best biopsied to make a diagnosis rather than resected using the colonoscope. The risk of perforation or inadequate resection margins is greatly increased with broad-based and sessile lesions. Multiple biopsies should be taken in order to determine whether the lesion harbors an invasive cancer, and further resection decisions are made based on the pathologic findings. In cases where there is low suspicion for malignancy, an endoscopic mucosal or submucosal resection may be attempted, usually by a gastroenterologist with advanced interventional endoscopic expertise. However, if such a lesion is left behind, it is of critical importance to note the position of the lesion in order that it might be more easily found if a subsequent procedure is required. In addition to determining the depth of insertion of the scope, which can be highly inaccurate with flexible instruments, other landmarks including the appendiceal orifice or ileocecal valve in the cecum and the liver/splenic shadows at the flexures should be noted. The most important step however is to properly mark the polyp site with 1 ml of tattoo injected submucosally in each of four quadrants for definitive intra- and extraluminal recognition at a later date.[174]

For lesions that cannot be resected through the scope or are found to be invasive carcinomas that are sessile or broad based, a variety of surgical resections can be employed depending on the position of the lesion and its T stage. It is important to keep in mind, however, that the formal staging of the lesion does not occur until after the resection is completed; therefore, if there is any suspicion of an invasive carcinoma being present, a definitive oncologic resection should be performed.[175]

Bowel Preparation

An important part of the preoperative regimen for a colon resection is the proper cleansing of the bowel in order to reduce the risk of postoperative complications as well as to allow for easier visualization during the procedure, particularly with the laparascopic approach. A variety of regimens have been described, and there are many that have demonstrated efficacy.[176,177] Although there are several choices described in the literature, the basic components of a bowel preparation are a mechanical cleansing of the bowel using a cathartic or volume-displacing agent and appropriate antibiotic prophylaxis.[178,179] Recently, some studies have suggested that mechanical bowel preparation may be unnecessary; however, this remains controversial.[180,181]

For rectal and low sigmoid tumors, a number of surgeons also perform distal rectal washout prior to resection, with the professed intention of eliminating exfoliated intraluminal cancer cells that may increase local recurrence risk. There has been little evidence to support this theory, and washout has not been routinely recommended as standard practice. However, a recent meta-analysis of nine studies and 5,395 patients is the first to demonstrate a significant benefit to this maneuver with a nearly two-fold reduction in local recurrence rates (5.79% versus 10.05%; $p < 0.00001$). While the lack of randomized controlled trials limits the strength of this data, the authors conclude that distal washout should be reconsidered in all patients given the minimal cost, time, and risk it entails.[182]

Anatomic Resection

For invasive carcinomas of the colon, stages I through III, the surgical approach will be dictated by the size and location of lesions in the colon.[183,184] The location will determine what region of bowel is removed, and the extent of its resection is dictated by its vascular and lymphatic supply.

Resection of the Right Colon

Lesions in the cecum and ascending colon are managed with a right hemicolectomy (Fig. 57.3A,B). The right colon is mobilized from the retroperitoneum by incising its retroperitoneal attachments, taking care to avoid injury to the ureter, inferior vena cava, duodenum, and gonadal vessels. The colon is mobilized from the ileum to the transverse colon, taking care at the hepatic flexure not to injure the gallbladder or duodenum. The ileocolic, right colic, and right branch of middle colic vessels are then ligated and divided. A proximal ligation in order to allow for the removal of colonic mesentery along with LNs is performed for staging purposes. Once the vascular supply is divided and the intervening mesenteric tissue ligated and divided, attention can be addressed to the resection of the colonic tissue.

There are a variety of techniques for dividing the colon. This can be done between clamps using scalpel or using a variety of stapling devices. One method would be to use a linear GI anastigmatic stapler. After making a small hole just below the colonic wall though the mesentery at the point chosen for resection, the stapler can be positioned across the colon and fired, thus dividing the tissue. This is then repeated across the ileum just proximal to the ileocecal valve. Once divided, all remaining mesenteric tissue is carefully ligated and divided, and the colonic specimen can be removed. Although a no-touch "technique" has been advocated in the past, studies have demonstrated that this has no influence on recurrence or seeding of distant disease.[185] Once the right colon has been removed, intestinal continuity can be re-established by creating an anastomosis between the terminal ileum and the remaining transverse colon using either a hand-sewn or stapled technique.

Resection of the Transverse Colon

For lesions located in the transverse colon, a variety of approaches can be undertaken. Those lesions that are proximal and

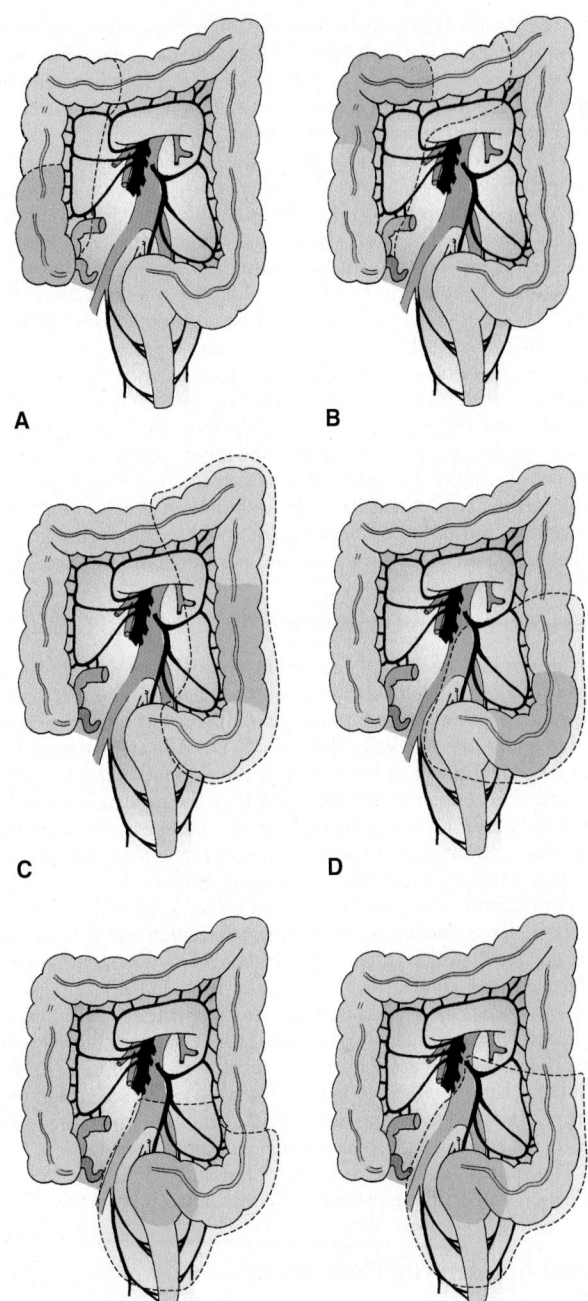

Figure 57.3 **(A)** Surgical resection for a cecal or ascending colon cancer. **(B)** Surgical resection for a cancer at the hepatic flexure. **(C)** Surgical resection for a descending colon cancer. **(D)** Preferred surgical procedure for cancer of the middle and proximal sigmoid colon. In poor-risk patients, the inferior mesenteric artery and the left colic artery may be preserved. **(E)** Surgical resection for cancer of the rectosigmoid. **(F)** A more radical surgical resection for cancer of the rectosigmoid.

near the hepatic flexure can be resected with an extended right hemicolectomy. This extension should encompass up to and include the middle colic vessel. The advantage of such a resection over a true transverse colectomy is that the anastomosis performed to restore intestinal continuity involves an anastomosis between the ileum and the remaining colon. Due to the improved blood supply delivered by the small bowel mesentery, there is a decreased risk of an anastomotic leak in an ileocolic as opposed to a colocolic anastomosis.[175] Likewise, a lesion in the distal transverse colon can be resected with an extended left hemicolectomy, which

PRACTICE OF ONCOLOGY

will be described in more detail in the following section. For those lesions that are in the midportion of the transverse colon, however, a transverse colectomy can be performed. This procedure requires mobilization of the right colon in order to allow this tissue to be brought over for an anastomosis following the resection.

The omentum is divided from the greater curvature of the stomach up to and including its attachments at the splenic helium. The omentum can often be a source of micrometastatic disease and therefore its resection at the time a transverse colectomy is indicated. After dividing the omentum and mobilizing the right and transverse colon up to and including the splenic flexure, the middle colic artery is ligated at its trunk and smaller vessels from the right and left colic artery branches can be ligated and divided as required. A linear stapler can once again be used to divide the colonic tissue, and then the mobilized right colon can be anastomosed to the descending colon in an end-to-end fashion using a hand-sewn anastomosis or using a side-to-side stapled technique. Depending on the size of the transverse colon, however, it is often safer and easier to resect the right and transverse colon and connect the ileum to the descending colon. This allows enough colonic reserve for water absorption and normal bowel movements.

Resection of the Descending and Sigmoid Colon

For lesions in the proximal descending colon, the splenic flexure is mobilized and the left colic artery can be ligated and divided with the portion of colon removed by mobilizing the splenic flexure and dividing the omentum (Fig. 57.3C,D). The transverse colon can be brought over to the region of the sigmoid colon for anastomosis. For lesions in the midportion of the descending colon, a left hemicolectomy can be performed, taking care to ligate the left colic vessel along with some sigmoidal branches and taking an adequate portion of mesentery for staging purposes.

For lesions that involve the sigmoid colon, a sigmoid colectomy can be performed with margins of resection on either side of the lesion. The descending colon is mobilized (together with the splenic flexure as needed) and connected to the rectum using either a hand-sewn anastomosis or stapling device. The mesentery can be divided either at the level of the sigmoidal branches with preservation of the left colic artery or at the origin of the inferior mesenteric pedicle (Fig. 57.3E,F). While the latter approach is preferred by some to achieve greater mobilization and higher lymph node counts, neither this nor a more extensive left hemicolectomy has resulted in improved survival.

The approaches to the resection of lesions below the peritoneal reflection will be discussed in the chapter on rectal cancer.

Total Abdominal Colectomy

For patients with ulcerative colitis or familial polyposis syndrome who either have evidence of invasive carcinoma or are at significant risk for the development of invasive carcinoma, a total abdominal colectomy may be required. This can be performed by mobilization of the right colon, transverse colon along the omentum, taking the omentum as part of the resection, the hepatic and splenic flexures, as well as the complete mobilization of the descending colon down to the peritoneal reflection. Ligation of the ileocolic, right colic, middle colic, left colic, and sigmoid branches will allow for removal of the colon down to the peritoneal reflection. For ulcerative colitis and familial polyposis syndromes without evidence of carcinoma below the peritoneal reflection, the operation can be terminated at this point with ileorectal anastomoses and careful surveillance of the remaining rectum via proctoscopy. However, in order to remove all tissue at risk for further lesions, a total protocolectomy is often advocated.[186,187] Although this procedure can be performed as an abdominal perineal resection with a permanent end ileostomy, most surgeons now advocate one of many continent pull-through procedures in order to preserve fecal continence in a patient population that is often very young. Such

procedures provide very good control of continence and a relatively normal lifestyle.[188]

SURGICAL MANAGEMENT OF COMPLICATIONS FROM PRIMARY COLON CANCER

Patients with primary lesions of the colon can present with obstruction, bleeding, and perforation. The surgical management of these patients can be complex, requiring intraoperative decisions tailored to the situation encountered. Blood per rectum can be one of the most frightening experiences for patient and physician alike. Bleeding from a CRC can occur anywhere from the cecum to the distal rectum. Although bleeding can be temporized with endoscopic fulguration and the patient supported with transfusion, definitive management of the lesion with either surgery or radiation therapy will ultimately be required. Other maneuvers such as angiographic embolization may provide only a temporary solution. Fortunately, life-threatening hemorrhage due to a colon cancer primary is a rare occurrence. More often, these lesions lead to a chronic blood loss, resulting in anemia.

Colonic obstruction due to a primary tumor is not uncommon. Obstructing colon lesions present several important issues. First, the acute obstruction must be managed. Ideally, an exploration with resection of the tumor and primary anastomosis with or without a diversion is ideal. However, given the fact that the operation will be performed on unprepared bowel and the patient's physical condition may be less than optimal, resection without an anastomosis and an end colostomy should be considered. In some instances, the obstructing lesion may present significant technical hurdles for resection in the setting of an acutely dehydrated and ill patient. In these circumstances, a decompression maneuver that can be performed rapidly and with minimal morbidity such as a transverse loop colostomy or a colostomy and mucous fistula can be performed to temporize the situation and allow the patient to be prepared and resuscitated adequately for a definitive resection at a second exploration.

Bypass operations should be reserved only for the most extreme circumstances as complications following these procedures due to repeat obstructions and leakage with abdominal sepsis are not insignificant.

Another option is to place an endoscopic stent either for temporary decompression or for definitive palliation of unresectable lesions. Multiple studies over the past 10 years have demonstrated the feasibility and safety of this maneuver in selected patients.[189–194] As a bridge to surgery, stenting can provide a minimally invasive means for converting an emergency situation into an elective one, allowing time for resuscitation, bowel prep, and adjuvant therapies. In a small randomized, controlled trial from 2009, Cheung et al.[195] reported additional advantages including significantly reduced rates of perioperative morbidity and stoma creation.

While short-term data seem to support the use of self-expanding metallic stents (SEMS) as a bridge to surgery, other reports as well long-term results from a recent comparative trial do not.[196,197] Sabbagh et al.[198] performed a head-to-head, intention-to-treat analysis of 87 patients undergoing either stenting or emergency surgery, using a propensity score to correct for selection bias. Overall survival at 3 and 5 years was significantly better in the surgery group (66% versus 44%, $p = 0.015$, and 62% versus 25%, $p = 0.0003$, respectively) and remained superior even when patients with perforation and metastatic disease were excluded (74% versus 51%, $p = 0.02$, and 67% versus 30%, $p = 0.001$, respectively). Five-year cancer-specific mortality was significantly higher in the SEMS group (48% versus 21%, $p = 0.02$) and there were trends toward worse 5-year DFS and increased recurrence as well as mean time to recurrence. Based on these findings, the authors have markedly changed their management of left-sided malignant obstruction, now reserving SEMS strictly for palliative indications and patients with high postoperative mortality risk.[198]

Laparoscopic Colon Resection

Since its introduction to the field of general surgery for gallbladder resection, the use of laparoscopic surgery has found increasing applications.[199] Laparoscopic surgery has become a particularly important addition to the armamentarium of the surgical oncologist. The use of laparoscopy for the staging of the extent of disease for peritoneal malignancies, pancreatic cancer, colon cancer, and gastric cancer is now widely accepted.[200–202] Laparoscopic resection has also found a niche for the removal of adrenal tumors, the spleen, and distal pancreas.[203,204] The use of laparoscopic approaches for the resection of malignant lesions in the colon is now becoming more common.

With the increasing application of laparoscopic techniques to colon cancer surgery, concerns ranging from inadequacy of resection margins, inadequacy of LN sampling, and the potential seeding of port sites with malignant cells have been raised.[205–207] Although these concerns are important, there are several potential advantages for laparoscopic approaches to the surgical management of colon cancer. Issues regarding length of incision, patient recovery time, and return to bowel function are often cited as justification for a laparoscopic approach. However, just as important are the technical advantages of surgery utilizing laparoscopic systems. The improved visualization due to magnification provided by video laparoscopy allows much more intricate and careful dissections in the deep pelvis, which could potentially reduce postoperative morbidity from low anterior resections that utilize a mesorectal excision technique. The ability to carefully trace vessels in the mesentery under magnification could improve the ability to perform high ligations in order to retrieve a greater number of LNs for sampling.

The technical difficulties faced during laparoscopic resection of the colon relate, in general, to the size of the specimen being removed and the need to perform an anastomosis. Each of these can be overcome through careful placement of incisions for specimen removal as well as a judicious use of stapling devices in order to perform both intracorporeal as well as a combination of intracorporeal and extracorporeal anastomotic techniques. A number of studies have examined the relative risks and benefits of the laparoscopic resection of colon cancer.[205,208–210] A prospective random assignment trial conducted by Clinical Outcomes of Surgical Therapy Study Group examined both the oncologic outcomes with respect to DFS and overall survival as well as the impact of laparoscopic versus open surgery on patient recovery, pain management, and time to return of bowel function. An initial report on quality of life showed only a modest short-term benefit for laparoscopic resection versus a conventional open procedure,[211] but the overall results of the trial with respect to oncologic outcomes demonstrated equivalence between the laparoscopic and open approach.[212]

Long-term follow-up from the corresponding UK randomized study (CLASICC Trial Group), which was similarly designed to compare laparoscopic to conventional surgery for colon and rectal cancer, and that initially reported noninferiority results in 2007, lends further support to the laparoscopic approach. With a median follow-up of 62.9 (range, 22.9 to 92.8) months, the authors found no statistically significant differences in overall survival (82.7% versus 78.3%), DFS (77% versus 89.5%), or local recurrence.[213,214]

Over a period of 10 years, the group from the Colon and Rectal Clinic of Orlando, Florida, performed a prospective nonrandomized study comparing laparoscopic to open resection for colorectal carcinoma. Laparoscopic resection was offered selectively in the absence of a large mass, invasion into the abdominal wall or adjacent organs, or if the patient did not have multiple prior operations.[205] All laparoscopic resections were performed with curative intent, and 20% of the patients whose procedures were converted to open resection were included in the laparoscopic resection group based

on an intention-to-treat model. The study measured oncologic outcomes and compared them with a computerized case-matched open resection group, using case-matching variables consisting of age, gender, site of primary tumor (colon versus rectum), and TNM stage. The group who received laparoscopic resection was followed prospectively and the data were updated on a regular basis. Follow-up of these patients consisted of a combination of office visits, telephone calls, and a review of the US Social Security Death Index Database. There were 172 patients in each group, and the groups were well matched for age, TMM stage, prior chemo- or radiation therapy, and site of the primary tumor (colon versus rectum).

Thirty-day mortality was 1.2% in the laparoscopic resection group and 2.4% in the open resection group; however, this difference was not statistically significant. The local recurrence rate of the laparoscopic group was 3.5% compared to a local recurrence rate in the open group of 2.9%. The stage-for-stage overall 5-year survival rate between the two groups was similar, and the conclusion of the authors, while acknowledging drawbacks based on the nonrandomized nature of the study, was that there was no significant difference in outcomes between using laparoscopic approaches versus an open approach in the management of primary colon and rectal tumors. There was, however, no formal cost analysis in this study, and, therefore, although oncologic outcomes were no different between the two groups, it is impossible to determine whether one group was superior to the other with respect to other outcomes.

A case-matched comparison of clinical and financial outcomes following laparoscopic and open colorectal surgery has been performed.[206] The group at the Cleveland Clinic studied patients from a prospective database who had undergone laparoscopic or open colectomy and were matched for age, gender, and disease-related groupings. A group of 150 patients undergoing laparoscopic colectomy was compared to a matched group of patients undergoing open colectomy. There was no difference found between the two groups for diagnosis, complications, or 30-day readmission rate. Although operating room costs were significantly higher after laparoscopic colectomy, this was offset by a decrease in the length of hospital stay with an overall significant reduction in total costs. This is attributed mainly to a lower cost for pharmacy, laboratory, and ward nursing expenses.

The ultimate role of laparoscopic resection in the management of CRC has yet to be determined. The studies discussed have shed some light on the relative risks and benefits as well as costs of these two procedures. The questions will remain, however, if the procedures are equivalent and whether deviating from the accepted gold standard of open resection for the management of CRC will be warranted. Longer follow-up will hopefully assist in this assessment.

In the meantime, exploration of other minimally invasive approaches to resection is ongoing. Early studies report the feasibility and safety of single port surgery, or "SILC" (single-incision laparoscopic colectomy), as well as equivalent oncologic outcomes at 2 years, and robotic colectomy has also been performed although its greatest potential is thought to lie with rectal dissection.[215–221] Natural orifice surgery is another area of interest with data accumulating on transvaginal specimen extraction as well as a pure transrectal approach.[222–224] Whether any of these novel modalities will offer real advantages (other than cosmesis) to offset the significant drawbacks of increased technical difficulty, operating time, and cost remains to be seen.

POLYPS AND STAGE I COLON CANCER

The management of polyps and stage I colon cancer is through surgical resection. Most cancer in polyps is not diagnosed until after the polypectomy is performed. Therefore, with respect to pedunculated lesions, care should be taken to resect the stalk completely, down to its base. Invasive early stage I cancers found in a polyp managed by polypectomy do not require further resection if there is a negative margin >2 mm and the tumor is well-differentiated without lymphovascular invasion or extension of malignant cells beyond the stalk (Haggitt levels 1 to 3).[173,225] Sessile lesions that are biopsied and shown to harbor an invasive cancer should be managed with a segmental colon resection. Large polypoid lesions may also require a segmental resection.

Because the stage of the lesion will not be determined until after the resection, all colon cancer lesions managed with a segmental resection should be approached the same way. The type of resection will be dictated by the location of the lesion, as has been described. Following a complete resection of a stage I lesion, no further adjuvant therapy is required. Patients managed in this way can expect a 5-year survival of over 95%.[225] Those that recur are most likely improperly classified stage II or III lesions.

STAGE II AND STAGE III COLON CANCER

Adjuvant Chemotherapy Considerations

The earliest clinical trials of adjuvant chemotherapy in colon cancer were conducted in the 1950s, utilizing the limited arsenal of anticancer agents that were available at that time. Many of these agents are now known to have no meaningful activity in metastatic CRC, and thus would not be studied in the adjuvant setting today.

The adjuvant trials of the 1950s through the mid-1980s tended to be small by current standards. Based perhaps on an unrealistically optimistic expectation of what magnitude of benefit might be achieved from the use of available chemotherapies, the size of the trials did not allow evaluation of more modest clinical benefits. A large meta-analysis of controlled randomized trials of adjuvant therapy published through 1986 indicated a nonsignificant trend toward an overall survival benefit, with a mortality OR of 0.83 in favor of therapy (95% CI = 0.70 to 0.98).[226] This sobering analysis suggested that substantially larger trials would be needed to detect the modest advantages that available chemotherapies might afford.

Large-Scale Randomized Trials

The large-scale 5-FU trials have been well summarized previously, and the reader who is interested in the details is referred to subject-relevant chapters in the previous edition of this book.[227] The outcome of numerous trials performed largely in the 1990s can be briefly summarized as follows. Trials comparing 5-FU–based therapy to surgery only demonstrated a clear benefit in terms of 5-year DFS (essentially, an increased cure rate) for stage III patients who received chemotherapy.[228,229] Six months of chemotherapy was sufficient, and no further benefit was provided by extending treatment to either nine or twelve months. Levamisole, an agent initially thought to be active, was, in fact inactive, and high-dose leucovorin did not confer superior efficacy over low-dose leucovorin, so comparisons of various 5-FU/leucovorin schedules did not demonstrate clear superiority of one schedule over the other in terms of efficacy. However, the Mayo Clinic daily times five schedule was substantially more toxic than either weekly bolus of biweekly infusion schedules. Alfa interferon conferred substantial toxicity and provided no benefit.[230–234]

Oral Fluoropyrimidine Therapies

Oral administration of 5-FU proved to be problematic secondary to erratic bioavailability. This was likely due in large part to variable effects of DPD, the rate-limiting enzyme in catabolism of 5-FU, on the first pass clearance of oral 5-FU by the liver. Two oral 5-FU prodrugs, capecitabine and uracil/tegafur (UFT), have demonstrated efficacy in metastatic disease that is comparable to the Mayo Clinic schedule of parenteral 5-FU/leucovorin. Both of these agents have now been studied in the adjuvant setting in comparison to the now defunct Mayo Clinic 5-FU schedule. In a study designed to assess for noninferiority in 3-year DFS, Twelves et al.[235] randomly assigned 1,987 patients with resected stage III colon cancer to receive either oral capecitabine (1,004 patients) or Mayo Clinic bolus 5-FU plus leucovorin (983 patients). Each treatment was planned for 24 weeks. DFS in the capecitabine group was at least equivalent to that in the 5-FU/leucovorin group (in the intention-to-treat analysis [p <0.001] for the comparison of the upper limit of the HR with the noninferiority margin of 1.20), and capecitabine resulted in significantly fewer adverse events than Mayo Clinic bolus 5-FU/leucovorin (p <0.001). Overall, this trial demonstrates that capecitabine is a reasonable alternative to intravenous 5-FU/leucovorin in the adjuvant treatment of colon cancer in reliable, motivated patients who are able to comply with a complex schedule of oral medication. However, as discussed in the following, while possibly appropriate for some stage II patients, 5-FU/leucovorin alone is no longer the standard postsurgical adjuvant treatment for stage III colon cancer. As such, the role of single-agent capecitabine in the adjuvant management of resected colon cancer remains limited at this time. Data supporting its use with concurrent intravenous oxaliplatin are discussed subsequently.

The NSABP C-06 trial assessed the use of oral UFT plus oral leucovorin in the treatment of stage II and III colon cancer.[236] A total of 1,608 patients with stage II (47%) and stage III (53%) colon cancer were randomly assigned to receive either oral UFT with leucovorin or intravenous 5-FU with leucovorin. With a median follow-up of 62.3 months, there were no significant differences in DFS or overall survival between the treatment groups. Toxicity and primary quality of life end points were similar in the two groups. As such, similar to the situation with capecitabine, the combination of oral UFT with leucovorin is an acceptable alternative to parenteral 5-FU/leucovorin; however, use of fluoropyrimidine plus leucovorin alone is no longer routine standard practice (see the following) in the adjuvant treatment of at least stage III disease. Furthermore, UFT is not commercially available in the United States.

Combination Adjuvant Therapies

Clinical trials in the metastatic setting have established the antitumor activity of combinations of agents, including irinotecan, oxaliplatin, bevacizumab, cetuximab, and panitumumab (see discussion of treatment of metastatic disease for more details). Although it had been assumed that activity in the metastatic setting would translate into an increased cure rate in the adjuvant setting, this assumption has turned out to be overly simplistic and often untrue. Of the agents listed previously, only the addition of oxaliplatin to fluoropyrimidines has resulted in benefit in the adjuvant setting.

Oxaliplatin

Oxaliplatin plus biweekly infusional 5-FU/leucovorin was first evaluated in the adjuvant setting in the Multicenter International Study of Oxaliplatin/5-Fluorouracil/Leucovorin in the Adjuvant Treatment of Colon Cancer (MOSAIC) trial.[237] The results of this trial are summarized in Table 57.8. A total of 2,246 stage II and III patients were randomized to the LV5FU2 regimen, a biweekly infusional and bolus 5-FU/leucovorin regimen that has been demonstrated to have comparable efficacy to the Mayo Clinic daily times five bolus schedule in the adjuvant setting, or to the FOLFOX-4 regimen, which is LV5FU2 plus oxaliplatin on day 1.[230] For the combined stage II and III study population, the 5-year DFS rates were 73.3% and 67.4% in the FOLFOX-4 and LV5FU2 groups, respectively (HR = 0.80; 95% CI = 0.68 to 0.93; p = 0.003).[237] Six-year overall survival rates were statistically significantly improved by 2.5% (78.5% versus 76.0% in the FOLFOX-4

TABLE 57.8

Results of The Mosaic Trial: Biweekly Infusional Fluorouracil/Leucovorin Versus 5-Fluorouracil/Leucovorin Plus Oxaliplatin in Patients with Stage II and III Colon Cancer

	FOLFOX (%)	5FULV2 (%)	P Value
Five-y disease-free survival (stage II+III)	73.3	67.4	0.003
Six-y overall survival (stage II+III)	78.5	76.0	0.046
Six-y overall survival (stage III only)	72.9	68.7	0.023
Six-y overall survival (stage II only)	85	83.3	0.65
Grade 3–4 neutropenia	41	5	
Grade 3–4 diarrhea	11	7	
Grade 3 neuropathy	12	0	
Grade 2 neuropathy	32	0	

FOLFOX, fluorouracil/leucovorin plus oxaliplatin; 5FULV2, fluorouracil/leucovorin.

and LV5FU2 groups, respectively; HR = 0.84; 95% CI = 0.71 to 1.00; $p = 0.046$). For the stage III population, the 6-year overall survival rates were improved by 4.2% (72.9% versus 68.7%, respectively; HR = 0.80; 95% CI = 0.65 to 0.97; $p = 0.023$), whereas for the stage II population, the addition of oxaliplatin conferred no survival benefit (6-year survival 85.0% and 83.3%, respectively; $p = 0.65$). A more recent update showed that even amongst the stage II patients with high-risk factors, an improved outcome with the addition of oxaliplatin was not evident. While toxicity was regarded as manageable, the FOLFOX-4 regimen resulted in 41% grade 3 or 4 neutropenia versus 5% in the control arm, and 11% grade 3 or 4 diarrhea versus 7%. All-cause mortality in the first 60 days was 0.5% in each arm. Peripheral sensory neuropathy, a toxicity not present in the LV5FU2 control arm, was a frequent occurrence on the FOLFOX-4 arm. Grade 2 neuropathy was reported in 32% of the patients, and grade 3 occurred in 12%. In some cases, the duration of the neuropathy was substantial. One year after completion of therapy, 30% of patients still experienced some grade of neuropathy (0.8% grade 2 and 1.3% grade 3). Four years after completion of therapy, 15.4% still had some degree of neuropathy, and 0.7% still had grade 3 neuropathy. It is reasonable to assume that the toxicity still present at 4 years out from the last treatment is essentially permanent.

Oxaliplatin has also been combined with a weekly bolus 5-FU regimen in an adjuvant trial. The NSABP C-07 trial studied the FLOX regimen of oxaliplatin given on weeks 1, 3, and 5 plus weekly bolus 5-FU/leucovorin on weeks 1 through 6, repeated at 8-week cycles, versus the standard weekly Roswell Park regimen of 5-FU/leucovorin.[238] A total of 2,409 patients were randomized to FLOX or to 5-FU/leucovorin. A total of 29% of patients had stage II disease and 71% had stage III. With a median follow-up of 8 years, FLOX showed a superior DFS, with 69.4% versus 64.2% alive and free of disease at five years (HR = 0.82; 95% CI = 0.72 to 0.93; $p = 0.002$). However, the overall survival difference was not statistically significantly different between the two arms. Treatment-related deaths were 1.3% versus 1.1% in the FLOX and 5-FU/leucovorin arms, respectively. Grade 2 or higher neurotoxicity was reported in 30.4% of patients on the FLOX arm versus 3.6% on 5-FU/leucovorin. Grade 3 diarrhea was 38.1% and 32.4% in the two arms, respectively, reflecting the higher incidence of serious diarrhea with the weekly bolus 5-FU regimen. Kidwell et al.[239] published long-term data regarding the persistent neurotoxic side effects of oxaliplatin beyond 4 years from this same NSABP C-07 trial, and found that there was a statistically but not clinically significant increase in total neurotoxicity for those who received the agent, with initial differences between the two groups dissipating by 7 years. However specific symptoms of numbness and tingling in the hands and feet did remain substantially elevated over time.[239]

Another recent study examined the effect of diabetes and other comorbidities on oxaliplatin-induced neuropathy. With symptoms identified in 65% of patients, hypertension, smoking, and diabetes were associated with higher trends although not statistically significant differences in severe neuropathy. Additionally, patients with diabetes developed oxaliplatin-induced neuropathy at a significantly lower cumulative dose, highlighting the importance of tailoring patient-specific regimens to minimize toxicity.[240]

In an exploratory analysis, however, the authors noted significant age-related differences in response to oxaliplatin, finding statistically improved overall survival in patients <70 years old, whereas older patients actually fared worse with increased grade 4-5 toxicity (OR = 1.59) and a 4.7% decrease in 5-year overall survival.

This age-treatment interaction has also been supported by a 2012 pooled analysis of 5,489 patients >75 years old from four large data sets that demonstrated minimal benefit of oxaliplatin in this group.[241] Moreover, post hoc analysis of MOSAIC data as well as revised findings from the ACCENT study (which initially showed no age-related difference) further indicate the limited clinical utility of this agent in older patients.[241,242] Taking all this into account, the 2013 National Comprehensive Cancer Network (NCCN) guidelines now recommend individualizing the decision to add oxaliplatin to adjuvant regimens in the elderly.[243]

More recently, a 1,866-patient study comparing capecitabine plus oxaliplatin (Cape/Ox) with bolus 5-FU/leucovorin in the adjuvant treatment of stage III colon cancer has been reported.[244] The Cape/Ox regimen had a statistically significant DFS advantage over 5-FU/leucovorin, with 66.1% of patients alive and disease-free at 5 years with Cape/Ox versus 59.8% with 5-FU/leucovorin. The difference between arms in overall survival at 5 years favored the Cape/Ox arm by 3.4%; however, this difference did not reach statistical significance at the time of this analysis ($p = 0.15$). The efficacy results of the FOLFOX and Cape/Ox studies appear more similar than different at this point in time and appear to justify interchangeability of these regimens in the adjuvant setting. Data for FLOX regimens appear to show higher rates of serious or life-threatening diarrhea, and the lack of a statistically significant survival benefit at 6 years is notable. The higher degree of severe and life-threatening diarrhea seen with FLOX would appear to be a potential reason for favoring FOLFOX or Cape/Ox over FLOX, although in the absence of a head-to-head comparison, the relative safety and efficacy when comparing one or these regimens to the other is impossible to know with certainty. The Cape/Ox regimen is a reasonable consideration only in highly reliable, motivated patients who can be expected to comply with taking multiple pills of capecitabine orally (typically three to five pills, twice daily) for 2 weeks on, 1 week off, in the setting of concurrent emetogenic intravenous chemotherapy.

Irinotecan

Based on improved overall survival in the first- and second-line metastatic settings, it was widely assumed that irinotecan would be beneficial to patients in the adjuvant setting.[245–247] This assumption has turned out to be incorrect, however, and the results of the adjuvant trials with this agent underscore the importance of both performing trials in the adjuvant setting and waiting for the results of those trials before adopting changes in practice.

The CALGB studied the weekly schedule of irinotecan plus bolus 5-FU and leucovorin (IFL). Early safety analysis of this trial identified an alarming elevation in early mortality for the experimental arm on this trial, with 18 deaths within the first 4 months of treatment on the IFL arm versus 6 deaths within the same time period on the control arm ($p = 0.008$).[248] At a median follow-up of 2.1 years in each arm, futility boundaries for both DFS and overall survival had been crossed; thus, the final result of this trial is that the addition of irinotecan provided no benefit, while increasing toxicity, including lethal toxicity.[249]

Results of adding irinotecan to biweekly infusional 5-FU/leucovorin (LV5FU2 versus FOLFIRI) were also negative. In the ACCORD 02 trial, 400 patients with high-risk stage III disease (defined as four or more positive nodes or perforated or obstructed primary tumors) were randomly assigned to LV5FU2 versus FOLFIRI. In this high-risk population, there was no benefit seen in the FOLFIRI group, and in fact the study trended insignificantly in favor of the nonirinotecan-containing arm (3-year DFS 60% for LV5FU2 versus 51% for FOLFIRI).[250]

A second, larger trial of LV5FU2 versus FOLFIRI was conducted by the PETACC-3 investigators.[251] The prespecified primary efficacy analysis of this trial was based on 2,094 patients with stage III disease. At a median follow-up of 6.5 years, there was no statistically significant difference in the 5-year DFS (56.7% versus 54.3% for FOLFIRI versus LV5FU2, respectively; $p = 0.1$) or in 5-year overall survival (73.6% versus 71.3%, respectively; $p = 0.94$). FOLFIRI was associated with an increased incidence of grade 3 or 4 GI events and neutropenia.

Taken together, the results of these three trials to evaluate irinotecan in the adjuvant setting clearly establish that despite having substantial activity in the metastatic setting, irinotecan has no meaningful activity, and no role, in the adjuvant treatment of colon cancer. Of interest, an analysis from the CALGB trial suggested that patients with MSI-H showed a benefit from inclusion of irinotecan in their adjuvant treatment; however, a similar, substantially larger analysis from the PETACC-3 trial contradicted this and showed no benefit from adding irinotecan in patients with MSI-H.[252,253]

Bevacizumab

As detailed subsequently, bevacizumab has demonstrated the ability to favorably augment standard chemotherapy for metastatic disease and has become a part of standard management in that arena. This led to evaluation of this agent in the adjuvant setting. In the NSABP C-08 trial, 2,672 patients, 25% with stage II and 755 with stage III colon cancer, were randomized to receive modified FOLFOX-6, either alone or with bevacizumab.[254] A design imbalance that could have been problematic had this been a positive trial, the FOLFOX was given for 6 months in each arm, while the bevacizumab was given both with the FOLFOX and then for an additional 6 months, for a total of 1 year of bevacizumab. This was, however, a fully negative trial, so the issues regarding the design of the trial are moot. With a median follow-up of 5 years, the addition of bevacizumab to FOLFOX did not improve either the DFS or the overall survival. DFS was 77.9% versus 75.1% ($p = 0.35$) for the study overall, and DFS was 73.5% versus 71.7% ($p = 0.55$) for the

stage III patients. Five-year overall survival was 82.5% versus 80.7% ($p = 0.56$) for the entire study, and 78.7% versus 77.6% for the stage III patients. There was a separation between the curves at the 1-year mark; however, this began to diminish a few months later and was all but absent by year 3. This finding suggests that bevacizumab did delay progression of micrometastases in some patients, but only for as long as it was continued. Bevacizumab did not contribute to the eradication of micrometastases and thus did not improve the cure rate in the adjuvant setting. Although some might choose to interpret these data to suggest that if bevacizumab were continued indefinitely, an improved survival *might* be seen, the long-term consequences of lifelong suppression of vascular endothelial growth factor (VEGF), as well as the psychological, social, and economic considerations involved, render such an approach inappropriate, especially considering that only a very small percentage of patients so treated would actually have the potential to benefit, if there is a benefit. Another trial, termed the AVANT trial, also explored the use of bevacizumab in the adjuvant treatment of stage III colon cancer, and also found no benefit.[255] This study randomized 3,451 patients, 2,876 of whom had stage III disease, to FOLFOX4, FOLFOX4 plus bevacizumab, or Cape/Ox plus bevacizumab. The bevacizumab-containing arms did not achieve a statistically significant improvement in DFS. After a minimum of 60 months follow-up, overall survival data suggested a possible detriment with the addition of bevacizumab, as the survival in the two bevacizumab-containing arms trended toward inferior to the FOLFOX-alone control arm; however, these differences did not reach statistical significance.

Thus, the available evidence suggests that bevacizumab is not beneficial in the treatment of colon cancer in the adjuvant setting, and might, in fact, be harmful. Until and unless data to the contrary emerge, bevacizumab should not be used in the adjuvant treatment of stage II and III colon cancer.

Cetuximab

As outlined in detail in the following, cetuximab has demonstrated clinical activity in metastatic CRC, prompting investigation of its usefulness in the adjuvant setting. Intergroup trial N0147 randomized patients with stage III colon cancer to modified FOLFOX-6 with or without cetuximab.[256] Once investigators became aware that the study included only patients whose tumors lacked mutations in the KRAS gene (see the following), the study was modified to obtain KRAS genotyping on all patients and to only enroll those with wild-type KRAS. Despite this selection, this large, adequately powered, randomized phase 3 trial showed no benefit for the addition of cetuximab to FOLFOX in the adjuvant treatment of patients with KRAS–wild-type stage III colon cancer. DFS and overall survival curves trended insignificantly in favor of the FOLFOX-alone control arm, and the addition of cetuximab was overtly harmful in patients >70 years of age. Cetuximab should therefore not be used in the treatment of stage III colon cancer.

Panitumumab

Panitumumab, like cetuximab, is a monoclonal antibody that blocks ligand binding to the EGFR. Although no investigations have been reported to evaluate panitumumab in the adjuvant setting, results in the metastatic setting suggest that panitumumab and cetuximab are extremely similar in terms of target, mechanism of action, mechanisms of resistance, and clinical activity. It is therefore extremely unlikely that these agents would differ in the adjuvant setting, and statements regarding cetuximab in this setting may be reasonably applied to panitumumab.

TREATMENT OF STAGE II PATIENTS

The optimal management of patients with stage II colon cancer remains undefined. Although the role of adjuvant therapy in patients with stage II colon cancer has not been firmly established, it is interesting to see what practice patterns have been emerging. Using the SEER-Medicare linked database, Schrag et al.[257] identified 3,151 patients age 65 to 75 with resected stage II colon cancer and no adverse prognostic features. Using Medicare billing records, they identified those patients who did or did not receive chemotherapy within 3 months of operation. Their review identified that 27% of patients received chemotherapy during the 3-month postoperative period. Younger age, white race, unfavorable tumor grade, and low comorbidity were associated with a greater likelihood of receiving treatment. The 5-year survival was 75% for untreated patients and 78% for those patients who received therapy in this nonrandomized comparison. After adjusting for known between-group differences, the HR for survival associated with adjuvant treatment was 0.91 (95% CI = 0.77 to 1.09). Thus, despite the lack of proven benefit, a substantial percentage of Medicare beneficiaries have received adjuvant chemotherapy for stage II disease.

Because stage II patients as a group have a relatively favorable prognosis, benefits from treatment could only be expected if either a highly efficacious therapy were used or if extremely large trials were done to detect very subtle differences. The International Multicentre Pooled Analysis of B2 Colon Cancer Trials meta-analysis provides one of the largest samples of stage II patients.[258] A total of 1,016 stage II patients were randomized between 5-FU/leucovorin and surgery alone. The surgery-only arm had a long-term overall survival rate of 81% versus 83% for those stage II patients who received adjuvant 5-FU/leucovorin. This absolute difference of 2% closely approached, but did not reach, statistical significance.

More recently, published studies have not generated any consensus on this topic. In a large retrospective, population-based analysis of 3,716 patients undergoing surgery for stage II disease with or without adjuvant chemotherapy, there was a statistically significant survival advantage for the adjuvant group (12 years versus 9.2 years). However, this is not a randomized trial, and patients receiving chemotherapy were more likely to be younger, with left-sided lesions and a higher LN yield, all of which are now known to be favorable prognostic factors. As such, it is difficult to draw conclusions from this study.[259] Another study that evaluated data from 24,847 patients, 75% of whom had one or more prognostic features, found no survival benefit from an adjuvant regimen.[260] Finally, Wu et al.[261] performed a systematic review of 12 randomized controlled trials including both colon and rectal cancers that suggested some improvement in 5-year overall survival and DFS for both tumor sites as well as a significant reduction in recurrence risk for stage II colon cancers. While the review has substantial flaws that limit interpretation of these results, it does indicate that larger, higher-quality trials are warranted.[261] One such study underway is the SACURA trial, a multicenter, randomized phase 3 study designed to evaluate the superiority of a 1-year adjuvant regimen compared to observation in stage II colon cancer. Investigators will seek to identify "high-risk factors of recurrence/death" as well as predictors of efficacy and toxicity in the adjuvant arm. End points include DFS, overall survival, and recurrence-free survival as well as the incidence and severity of adverse events. Results from this trial will hopefully facilitate a definitive therapeutic strategy for stage II colon cancers moving forward.[262]

Several prognostic indicators have been identified that correlate with a higher risk for subsequent failure in stage II patients. These include obstruction or perforation of the bowel wall as well as other less-established risk factors, such as elevated preoperative or postoperative CEA, poorly differentiated histology, and tumors not demonstrating high levels of MSI, or an 18q deletion in colorectal tumors, which may correlate with a poor prognosis.[145,263–265] Additionally cited poor prognostic factors include macroscopically infiltrating-type tumors, high serum CA 19-9 levels, extensive venous invasion, male gender, age >50 years old, and <12 dissected LNs.[266] It appears that stage II patients with one or more of these risk factors have a poorer prognosis, one closer to patients with stage III disease. Whether adjuvant chemotherapy can provide similar benefits in these patients as it does in stage III

patients remains a matter of conjecture, and in the absence of definitive data, definitive recommendations on this topic cannot be made at this time. In fully informed high-risk stage II patients, it is reasonable to consider adjuvant treatment. All reports form the MOSAIC trial have shown no benefit for the addition of oxaliplatin to 5-FU/leuvocorin in terms of overall survival of stage II patients. Uniquivocally, stage II patients lacking high-risk factors have not been shown to benefit from oxliplatin, and considering the short- and long-term toxicities of this agent, oxaliplatin should not be used in the management of good-risk stage II patients. A recent update of the outcomes for stage II patients on the MOSAIC trial demonstrates no benefit to use of oxaliplatin, even in patients on the trial with one or more high-risk factors.[242] Whereas patients with exceptionally poor risk stage II tumors may still seem reasonable for consideration of oxaliplatin-containing regimens, these negative data suggest that routine use of oxaliplatin in most patients with stage II colon cancer is unlikely to be appropriate.

Impact of Microsatellite Instability on Treatment in Stage II and III Colon Cancer

Ribic et al.[267] investigated the usefulness of MSI status as a predictor of benefit from 5-FU–based adjuvant chemotherapy in 570 stage II and III patients from five randomized trials in which no treatment control arm was used. MSI-H was exhibited in 95 patients (16.7%), MSI-L in 60 patients (10.5%), and MSS in 415 patients (72.8%). In the 287 patients who did not receive adjuvant chemotherapy, those with tumors exhibiting MSI-H had superior 5-year survival compared to patients with MSI-L or MSS tumors (HR = 0.31; $p = 0.004$). In the population of patients who received adjuvant chemotherapy, there was no difference in survival between the patients with MSI-H and patients without MSI-H ($p = 0.8$). In the patients with MSI-L or MSS tumors, chemotherapy resulted in improved survival versus no chemotherapy (HR = 0.72; $p = 0.04$). However, 5-FU/leuvocorin did not improve survival in the patients with MSI-H tumors (Table 57.9).

5-FU/leuvocorin was associated with improved outcome in both stage II and III patients with MSS or MSI-L, with an HR of 0.67 (95% CI = 0.39 to 1.15) in stage II patients and 0.69 (95% CI = 0.47 to 1.01) in patients with stage III cancer. In contrast, in patients with MSI-H tumors, treatment did not improve survival,

TABLE 57.9

Microsatellite Instability Versus Outcome with 5-Fluorouracil-Based Adjuvant Chemotherapy

	No. of Patients	Five-Y Disease-Free Survival (%)	P Value
All Patients			
Adjuvant chemotherapy	285	70	0.06
No adjuvant chemotherapy	287	62	
Patients with MSI-L/MSS			
Adjuvant chemotherapy	230	70	0.01
No adjuvant chemotherapy	245	59	
Patients with MSI-H			
Adjuvant chemotherapy	53	69	0.11
No adjuvant chemotherapy	42	83	

MSI-L, low level of microsatellite instability; MSS, microsatellite stable; MSI-H, high level of microsatellite instability.
From Ribic CM, Sargent DJ, Moore MJ, et al. Tumor microsatellite-instability status as a predictor of benefit from fluorouracil-based adjuvant chemotherapy for colon cancer. *N Engl J Med* 2003;349:247–257.

and in fact was associated with a trend toward worse outcome for both stage II (HR for death = 3.28; 95% CI = 0.86 to 12.48) and stage III cancers (HR = 1.42; 95% CI = 0.36 to 5.56). Of note, an analysis of MSI status from the NSABP failed to corroborate the results of the Ribic et al.[267] study, and the authors concluded that in their trial there was no interaction between MSI status and treatment effect, and that their data do not support the use of MSI-H as a predictive marker for chemotherapy benefit.[268] However, an updated expansion on the data from the Ribic et al.[267] report appears to corroborate the original findings, leading the authors of that study to suggest that MSI determinations should be performed on all stage II patients, and that stage II patients with MSI-H should not be treated with fluoropyrimidines alone.[269] The Eastern Cooperative Oncology Group I is leading a trial (ECOG 5202) in which patients with MSI-H and absence of LOH in chromosome 18q are being selected for observation, on the hypothesis that these patients will have a highly favorable prognosis with observation alone, whereas others are being assigned to FOLFOX chemotherapy and randomized to with or without bevacizumab. This trial has accrued and data are pending at the time of this writing.

An analysis of data indicate that patients with MSI-H stage III tumors, while having a more favorable prognosis than MSS tumors, do nevertheless achieve benefit from, and in the absence of contraindications, should receive, 5-FU–based adjuvant therapy.[270] This recommendation is further supported when considering oxaliplatin-based chemotherapy in stage III disease. This would be reasonable to expect, as platinum-DNA adducts are not removed by the mismatch repair enzymes that are deficient in MSI tumors. A more recent analysis of MSI impact in stage III disease in the N0147 trial suggested a more complex and nuanced impact, with MSI-H tumors having a favorable prognostic impact when arising in the right side of the colon, but actually having a negative prognostic impact when occurring in the left colon.[147] The reasons for this difference remain unclear; however, the different embryologic origins of the left and right colon, and the resultant different venous drainges, may contribute to this.

The incidence of MSI has more recently been shown to vary with stage of disease presentation, with 22% of stage II patients, 12% of stage III, and only 3.5% of stage IV patients found to exhibit MSI, consistent with the data that MSI-H is a favorable *prognostic* factor. Data from the PETACC-3 trial suggest that it is a strong prognostic factor in stage II disease; however, it was less so in stage III.[271–273]

Other Molecular Markers

As the majority of stage II, and even stage III, patients do not benefit from adjuvant therapy, it would be highly desirable to be able to identify those patients who are both at risk for recurrent disease (i.e., harbor micrometastases) and those whose micrometastases are sensitive to, and will be eradicated by, a particular chemotherapy. At present there are no such validated markers, with the possible exception of MSI, as discussed previously. KRAS mutations have no prognostic value in the adjuvant setting, and as there is no role for use of anti-EGFR agents in the adjuvant setting, the expense of genotyping patients with less than stage IV disease is difficult to justify.[273,274] BRAF mutations appear to be prognostic of poorer overall survival in stage II disease that is not MSI-H; however, this appears to be regardless of therapy, and so again it provides no information to inform treatment decision making.[273] At present, no molecular test has been validated as useful for making adjuvant treatment decisions, and none should be utilized outside of a clinical trial. More recently, a genetic profiling assay utilizing 21-gene signature analysis has become available.[271] This assay has been shown to provide risk stratification with stage II patients who are classified as having from 8% to 22% chance of recurrence. However, there was no interaction with treatment, meaning that the test is prognostic, identifying relatively lower or higher risk

individuals, but it provided no guidance on whom to treat. Thus, despite the interesting data outlined in the following, it would appear to be of little value in decision making at this time.

Despite this limitation, research efforts have been increasingly focused on developing and refining such gene signatures over the past few years, with three that stand out presently, promising to improve and possibly replace current risk stratification models.[275] Unfortunately, none of these approaches are able to predict who will or will not benefit from adjuvant chemotherapy. While these prognostic scores may be of scientific interest, at present they are not recommended for routine clinical use in NCCN guidelines, as they appear to offer little if any guidance in terms of treatment decisions.

The Oncotype DX Recurrence Score, which is the only externally validated assay available for commercial use, is based on a 12-gene signature that separates 3-year recurrence risk into low, intermediate, and high (12%, 18%, 22%, respectively), independent of clinicopathologic features, and with enhanced accuracy. It has been shown to be highly prognostic in stage II and III patients receiving 5-FU/leucovorin, and enables better discrimination of absolute oxaliplatin benefit as a function of risk. A recent analysis of long-term costs and outcomes in "average-risk" stage II colon cancers (T3, MSS) concluded that this signature, when applied appropriately, could potentially reduce adjuvant chemotherapy use by 17% with increased quality-adjusted life expectancy of 0.035 years and cost-savings of $2,971 per patient.[276]

Another interesting signature, ColoPrint (Agendia Inc. USA, Irvine, CA), is an 18-gene prognostic classifier developed on fresh-frozen tumor tissue to identify 5-year metastasis-free survival. Separating patients into two risk categories, this assay is particularly precise in identifying low-risk stage II cases that be managed without chemotherapy irrespective of MSI status. It also appears to better classify high-risk patients than clinicopathologic factors alone. While the signature has been validated twice in retrospective trials, it is not yet available for commercial use. A large prospective clinical validation study is under way (PARSC: Prospective Analysis of Risk Stratification by ColoPrint) that may better clarify the role of ColoPrint specifically in the management of stage II disease.[277]

Colorectal Cancer DSA (Almac Diagnostics, Craigavon, Unite Kingdom) is the most recently reported signature, based on 634 genes, developed to identify stage II patients at higher risk of recurrence (HR = 2.53) and cancer-related death (HR = 2.21) at 5 years. It has been shown to perform independently of known prognostic factors. While this assay is also not available for commercial use at the time of this writing, a prospective validation trial in stage II patients is being planned.[278]

The lack of clear direction on the matter of treatment of good-risk stage II patients is reflected in a current consensus statement, which, while not recommending therapy for all stage II patients, does recommend a medical oncology consultation for the purpose of discussing the pros and cons of chemotherapy for all stage II patients.[279]

TREATMENT OPTIONS FOR STAGE III PATIENTS

It is clear that in the absence of medical or psychiatric contraindications, patients with node-positive colon cancer should receive postoperative chemotherapy. At the very least, a 5-FU–based regimen would appear to be appropriate, and approximately 6 months of therapy would be supported by the majority of trials. The daily times five Mayo Clinic schedule or a variant has been shown to be more toxic than other 5-FU/leucovorin schedules; therefore, daily times five schedules should not be used. Oral capecitabine or oral UFT/leucovorin are acceptable alternatives if a fluoropyrimidine-only approach is selected. At this time, the data for incorporation of oxaliplatin into the routine adjuvant treatment of colon cancer appears compelling, and the FOLFOX schedule is now the most widely used adjuvant therapy. FLOX is an acceptable alternative; however, nonrandomized comparisons suggest that FLOX may carry a higher risk of serious diarrhea than FOLFOX. Cape/Ox is also an acceptable alternative in appropriately motivated and reliable patients. Although the pivotal adjuvant study was done with FOLFOX-4, in practice this regimen is rarely used, and the modified FOLFOX-6 regimen, which has been the basis for all FOLFOX-based National Cancer Institute Intergroup adjuvant and metastatic trials, is routinely used due to its greater convenience. The risk of peripheral neuropathy and the possibility of long-term neuropathy must be considered in the selection of therapy. At the time of this writing, FOLFOX or Cape/Ox are the regimens of choice in treatment of all patients with stage III colon cancer in the absense of specific contraindications. The long-term morbidity of oxaliplatin treatment has become more appreciated; however, it is anticipated that risk stratification strategies may become available in the near future to identify those patients who are likely to benefit from oxaliplatin treatment.

Irinotecan-based regimens should not be used in the adjuvant setting, as randomized data have shown increased toxicity and no long-term benefit. Bevacizumab, cetuximab, and panitumumab should also not be used in the adjuvant setting, as they add toxicity and expense, and do not add benefit.

Timing of Treatment

Traditionally, adjuvant chemotherapy is commenced within 8 weeks of surgery. However, this time frame is somewhat arbitrary, based largely on what has been mandated in clinical trials. A 2010 meta-analysis pooled data from 13,158 patients with stage II or III disease and concluded that delaying treatment beyond this interval was associated with interior survival (RR = 1.20).[280] However, these data are retrospective, nonrandomized, and fail to adequately consider the collateral implications of whatever medical and surgical conditions might have contributed to the delay in start of therapy. As such, these findings should be regarded as hypothesis-generating only, and certainly not definitive. Another study that included only stage III cancers found no such clear correlation. Secondary analysis did demonstrate a trend toward poorer outcomes after 8 weeks, particularly in younger patients (<66 years) as well as significantly inferior survival for patients beginning chemotherapy after 9 and 10 weeks (HR of death = 1.68 and 1.67, respectively).[281]

Investigational Adjuvant Approaches

Portal Vein Infusion

The NSABP C-02 trial randomized 1,158 patients with Dukes A, B, or C colon cancers to either a 7-day portal vein infusion of 5-FU (600 mg/m² per day) or to surgery alone.[282] A modest, albeit statistically significant, advantage in DFS (74% versus 64% at 4 years) was demonstrated for the group who received intraportal chemotherapy; however, no difference was seen in the incidence of hepatic recurrences.

Similar findings were reported from a 533 patient trial performed by the Swiss Group for Clinical Cancer Research.[283,284] In this trial, intraportal chemotherapy included 10 mg/m² mitomycin C by 2-hour infusion followed by a 7-day infusion of 5-FU at a dose of 500 mg/m² per day. The 5-year DFS and overall survival were modestly improved in the intraportal treatment versus surgery-only groups (57% versus 48%, and 66% versus 55%, respectively).

Subsequently, a large meta-analysis of intraportal chemotherapy trials involving over 4,000 patients in 10 randomized studies revealed only a 4% improvement in 5-year overall survival for the patients who received portal infusion. At present, intraportal adjuvant chemotherapy has not been accepted as routine practice and remains limited to clinical investigations.

Intraperitoneal Chemotherapy

A small, single-arm study explored the feasibility of immediate postoperative intraperitoneal floxuridine and leucovorin plus systemic 5-FU and levamisole.[285] A randomized trial of 241 stage II and III patients compared intraperitoneal plus systemic 5-FU/leucovorin to systemic 5-FU/levamisole.[286] With 4 years' median follow-up, no benefit was seen for the stage II patients. Among the 196 eligible patients with stage III disease, however, a 43% reduction in mortality was seen. This small trial is encouraging but would require further corroboration before being accepted into standard practice.

Hyperthermic intraperitoneal chemotherapy has been explored as a possible means of providing a benefit in patients at high risk for developing peritoneal metastases. Sammartino et al.[287] explored this hypothesis in a small case control study of patients with T3/4 lesions and mucinous or signet ring cell histology who underwent either standard resection or extended surgery (including omentectomy, bilateral adnexectomy, hepatic round ligament resection, and appendectomy) followed by hyperthermic intraperitoneal chemotherapy. The experimental group experienced statistically significantly decreased rates of peritoneal recurrence (4% versus 22%) as well as improved DFS (36.8 months versus 21.9 months; p <0.01). Large randomized trials would be necessary, however, before nonresearch use of this highly aggressive and potentially toxic treatment strategy could be considered.[287]

Vaccines

Vaccination strategies endeavor to stimulate the patient's immune system to recognize and eradicate the patient's tumor cells. An ideal immunologic target molecule would be a highly antigenic epitope that is always expressed on the tumor and never expressed on normal tissue. Such an ideal target has yet to be identified; however, a number of approaches have been explored.

CEA is a commonly expressed antigen in colorectal carcinomas. Unfortunately, CEA does not appear to be particularly immunogenic. Several approaches have been pursued in an attempt to increase immune recognition of CEA. Thus, a number of avenues of investigation are being pursued; however, at this time the use of vaccine therapy for treatment of resected colon cancer remains highly investigational.

One tumor-associated antigen that may be a more promising candidate is the MUC1 glycoprotein, which is abnormally expressed on neoplastic cells in a hypoglycosylated form that induces humoral and cellular response. A vaccine based on this antigen was found to be highly immunogenic in the premalignant setting, inducing long-term memory responses and no significant toxicity when administered to patients with advanced colonic adenomas. Subsequent studies will determine whether these results translate into meaningful clinical outcomes.[288]

Active Specific Immunotherapy

Irradiated cancer cells maintain their immunogenicity; however, they are unable to proliferate. Active specific immunotherapy is a maneuver in which patients are immunized with a preparation of their own irradiated tumor cells plus an immunostimulant such as bacillus Calmette-Guérin. This technique has been explored for some time now as a potential adjuvant immunotherapy for CRC. Overall, trials have failed to show a benefit for the use of active specific immunotherapy in the management of colon cancer, and its use should remain limited to investigational settings.

Preoperative Chemotherapy

Investigators are currently exploring the role of preoperative chemotherapy in the management of nonmetastatic disease. A pilot phase of the first randomized trial to address this topic (FOxTROT) has recently been completed, demonstrating the feasibility and safety of this approach in locally advanced, operable colon cancer. The 150 patients who underwent meticulous radiologic staging were randomly assigned to receive 6 weeks of preoperative oxaliplatin/5-FU/l-folinic acid followed by surgery and 18 weeks of postoperative chemotherapy or upfront resection followed by

24 weeks of treatment. There were no significant differences in postoperative morbidity between the two groups. While a small proportion of the patients receiving preoperative therapy had apparent progression during the time between staging and surgery, there were no tumor-related complications during this interval. Overall, preoperative therapy resulted in significant downstaging, including reductions in apical node involvement and incomplete resections as well as two pathologic complete responses. Whether these results will translate into improved survival and potentially change the accepted pathway for management of nonmetastatic disease remains to be seen. A larger phase 3 trial now under way will hopefully shed light on this issue in the near future.[289]

FOLLOW-UP AFTER MANAGEMENT OF COLON CANCER WITH CURATIVE INTENT

Follow-up after definitive management has two primary goals. First, patients with a history of CRC are at higher risk than the general population for a second colon cancer primary.[290,291] A colonoscopic screening may benefit in the early detection of a second primary malignancy or detection of a benign polyp, which can then be resected, potentially preventing the development of an invasive cancer.

Second, surveillance may increase the chance of identifying local regional or distant recurrence that is potentially curable by surgery. It should be noted that it is this detection of potentially curable recurrent or second primary disease that justifies routine postoperative surveillance. To date, there are no compelling data that indicate that early detection of unresectable asymptomatic metastatic disease is of benefit to the patient. In other words, if recurrent disease is unresectable and therefore incurable, there is no urgency to identify it; there is no compelling evidence that the early initiation of palliative chemotherapy is of benefit in the asymptomatic, incurable patient. Although the choice of follow-up routine and which studies to include in that follow-up have been the subject of much debate in the colon cancer literature,[292-295] subsequent analyses have shown that most interventions that have been considered are not value-added and not appropriate for routine use. The American Society of Clinical Oncology (ASCO) has recently updated its guidelines for postsurgical follow-up.[296] These recommendations are for physical examination and blood CEA monitoring every 3 to 6 months for the first 3 years, and every 6 months for years 4 and 5. CT scans of the chest and abdomen are recommended once a year for the first 3 years. Positron emission tomography (PET) scans are specifically not recommended for routine screening and surveillance. NCCN guidelines differ only slightly in that they recommend annual CT scanning for up to 5 years and include CT scans of the pelvis. Colonoscopy is recommended at 1 year after resection (or 3 to 6 months after resection if a complete colonoscopy was not performed prior to surgery) and then 3 years later, and then every 5 years. CT scans

and CEA monitoring should not be continued beyond 5 years. Of note, older studies advocating routine monitoring of complete blood count, liver function studies, lactate dehydrogenase, chest X-rays, and fecal occult blood monitoring have not been supported by subsequent data, and none of these are recommended for routine monitoring of patients at this time. The role of CEA measurement in patients following definitive management of CRC has been controversial.[94,297,298] ASCO carefully reviewed its utility in an additional panel guided in 1996.[299] Their recommendation for CEA monitoring then, which was confirmed in the surveillance guideline panel review, was postoperative serum CEA testing to be performed every 3 months in patients with stage II or III disease for up to 3 years after diagnosis. An elevated CEA level, if confirmed by retesting, warranted further evaluation for metastatic disease.

This further workup of an elevated CEA typically consists of a colonoscopy and a CT scan of the chest, abdomen, and pelvis. If these studies are negative, the clinician is faced with a dilemma. The question of what to do in the face of a rising serum CEA level in the absence of imageable disease by conventional imaging modalities is one that has been addressed in clinical trials.[300-305] Strategies to image CEA expression might improve upon the detection capability of standard imaging studies. Several studies were performed using immunoscintigraphy with an antibody directed against CEA or Tag72, a CEA-like glycoprotein (CEA scan and OncoScint [Cytogen Corp, Lonza Biologics, Princeton, NJ] scan, respectively).[306-308] The results of these studies using antibody-directed immunoscintigraphy were variable, and at this time, CEA scintigraphy is no longer considered standard care. In an older study, in order to more directly address this clinical dilemma, a prospective study was performed comparing CEA immunoscintigraphy to PET using 18-fluorodeoxyglucose (FDG) and blind "second look" laparotomy.[303]

In this study patients with a rising CEA level without imageable disease by CT scan of the chest, abdomen, and pelvis as well as colonoscopy and abdominal ultrasound were enrolled along with patients with a single site of otherwise resectable disease. All patients had a CEA scan performed as well as a PET scan with FDG. All patients who failed to demonstrate evidence of disease outside of the abdominal cavity went on to have an exploratory laparotomy by a surgeon who had no knowledge of the CEA or the FDG scan results. A second surgeon participated in the remainder of the exploration after thoroughly reviewing all studies including the nuclear medicine scans. Twenty-eight patients were studied in this fashion, and the trial demonstrated that PET scan with FDG was far superior to CEA scans in detecting recurrence; roughly 30% of the patients on the study potentially benefited by having recurrent disease treated at the time of surgery (Fig. 57.4).

Based on these findings, it appears that serum CEA surveillance following definitive management of a primary CRC is a reasonable surveillance technique. If the CEA level is elevated on repeat testing, imaging studies should be performed consisting of CT scans and a through evaluation of the colon with colonoscopy

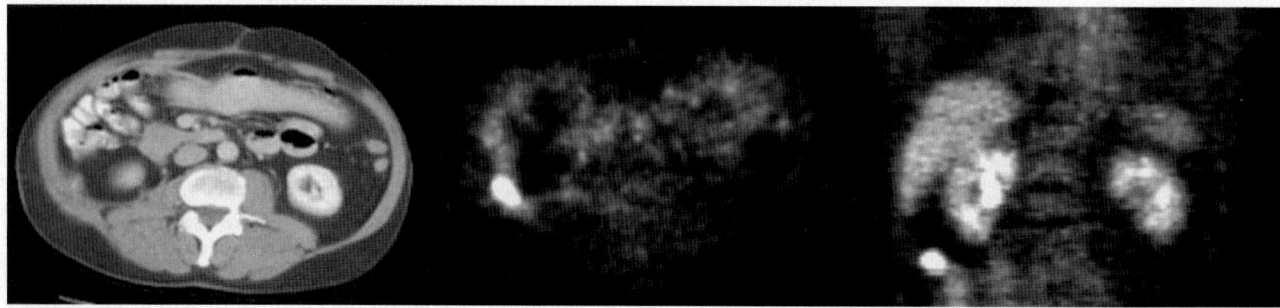

Figure 57.4 From left to right, the *first panel* depicts a contrast-enhanced computed tomography scan image of a patient with a rising carcinoembryonic antigen following a definitive resection of a right colon cancer. The *middle and far panels* show the same region imaged with fluorodeoxyglucose position emission tomography. (From Libutti SK, Alexander HR Jr, Choyke P, et al. A prospective study of 2-[18F] fluoro-2-deoxy-D-glucose/positron emission tomography scan, 99mTc-labeled arcitumomab [CEA-scan], and blind second-look laparotomy for detecting colon cancer recurrence in patients with increasing carcinoembryonic antigen levels. *Ann Surg Oncol* 2001;8:779.)

performed as well. If no recurrence or second primary is detected, watchful waiting and repeat of CT imaging at approximately 3-month intervals versus a PET scan with FDG can be considered. If disease is discovered, it should be managed as indicated. If no disease is detected, then continued surveillance is warranted with repeat CEA levels and CT or magnetic resonance imaging at intervals.[303,309]

The role of physical examination has also been evaluated.[310] The ASCO panel noted that no formal examination of the contribution of physician's history and physical examination to help outcomes of CRC has been performed. However, data from the larger studies of surveillance showed that 80% of recurrences were found by CEA testing, whereas only 20% were found by routine history and physical examination done at the same time.[311] This has been confirmed by other studies.[312,313] Although no direct effects were shown on history or physical examination about the impact and detection or outcome in the surveillance period, a physician–patient encounter provides a vital link for other studies that may influence outcome. Therefore, while not in itself substantiated by the data in the literature, it is felt that routine postresection visits be performed every 3 to 6 months for the first 3 years following resection and every 6 months during years 4 and 5.

The role of liver function tests as a means for detecting colorectal recurrence has also been carefully evaluated. No studies that were reviewed by the ASCO panel demonstrated any benefit for the routine use of liver function test measurements in the post-surveillance period.[310,314] In fact, studies suggest that other routine blood tests such as CEA detected recurrence far earlier than liver function test abnormalities.[94] Therefore, the 2005 ASCO consensus panel did not recommend the routine use of liver function test measurements in the postresection surveillance period.

Routine fecal occult blood testing, routine complete blood counts, and routine chest X-rays were all not thought to be of benefit in postoperative surveillance. Although the panel was not in uniform agreement with respect to chest X-ray, it was thought that all three of these modalities should be reserved for the evaluation of the patient with evidence of recurrence such as a rising CEA level or a positive endoscopy. Each of these modalities in and of itself was not found to be useful.

The panel recommended that annual CT of the chest and abdomen (with pelvis for rectal cancer) be performed for 3 years in those patients at higher risk for recurrence who could be candidates for curative-intent surgery of a recurrence. With respect to colonoscopy and flexible proctosigmoidoscopy, the panel, after reviewing the literature, recommended that all patients have a colonoscopy for the pre- or perioperative documentation of the cancer and to ascertain that the remainder of the colon is free from polyps. Further, the panel agreed that the data were sufficient to recommend colonoscopy at 3 years to detect new cancers and polyps and then every 5 years if normal. However, they did not recommend routine annual colonoscopy as follow-up following definitive management of patients with CRC. Further, the panel concluded that colonoscopy was superior to flexible proctosigmoidoscopy and therefore should be performed as previously discussed for patients following both colon and rectal cancer surgery. Other studies have also supported the routine use of colonoscopic examination following definitive management of CRC.[315,316]

A meta-analysis and systematic review of randomized trials to address the impact of close postoperative surveillance on overall survival following definitive management of CRC was also performed by Renehan et al.[317] A total of five randomized trials that met their inclusion criteria were reviewed, representing 1,342 patients. For four of the studies, intensive follow-up consisted of blood work including serum CEA, colonoscopy, physical examination, abdominal ultrasound, and CT scans. In one study, no CEA measurements or CT scans were performed. Follow-up in the intensive arm was performed every 3 months for 2 years and then every 6 months thereafter up to 5 years, with yearly CT scans and endoscopy. All five studies had a control arm subjected to a less aggressive follow-up regimen, which varied from study to study

ranging from no specific follow-up to interval laboratory tests and plain X-rays or ultrasound. They found that there was an absolute reduction in mortality of 9% to 13% by employing an aggressive follow-up regimen, consisting of serum CEA measurements and CT scans. Two studies in particular showed the greatest impact on survival.

In summary, a rational postoperative surveillance program would include CEA measurements every 3 to 6 months and a yearly CT scan of the chest, abdomen, and pelvis (for rectal cancer) for the first 3 years. Colonoscopy can be performed every 3 to 5 years following the resection. At the time of CEA measurements, a physician encounter should be scheduled where a discussion of patient symptoms and a physical examination can be performed. If a rising serum CEA is detected on two consecutive measurements in the absence of imageable disease by CT scan, a PET scan with FDG can be considered. Lesions found on colonoscopy should be managed appropriately either with colonoscopic resection or surgical management. These surveillance guidelines should allow for the early detection of either resectable recurrence or second primary lesions and therefore the potential to impact patient outcome.

SURGICAL MANAGEMENT OF STAGE IV DISEASE

For a select group of patients with metastatic CRC, complete surgical resection of stage IV disease (discussed in detail in Chapter 60) may be an option and may provide a long-term survival advantage. This is especially true with respect to metastatic sites in the liver and lung. Resection of locoregional recurrence can also benefit the patient with respect to local control and overall outcome. Numerous regional approaches have also been explored for the treatment of stage IV colon cancer depending on the organ or body cavity involved. Organ-specific infusional therapy, isolated or continuous perfusion therapy, radiofrequency ablation or cryotherapy, surgical debulking, and radiation are all technical approaches that have been performed. Many of these regional strategies as well as surgical metastasectomy will be discussed in separate chapters and therefore will not be specifically addressed here.

MANAGEMENT OF UNRESECTABLE METASTATIC DISEASE

Unresectable metastatic CRC is generally not curable with current technology. Management centers around palliation and control of symptoms, control of tumor growth, and attempts to lengthen progression-free and overall survival. Given the palliative nature of such treatments, extreme care must be taken to adequately assess each individual's potential for both benefit and harm from chemotherapy. Care must also be taken with surgical interventions as well. Quality-of-life issues must be frankly and objectively discussed with patients and their caregivers so that informed decisions can be made and expectations can be contained within a realistic framework. The issue of whether patients presenting with unresectable stage IV disease should have their primary tumors resected has been the matter of some debate. Although such resections had been routinely performed in the past, more recent data suggest that such interventions are not required, and may in fact be counterproductive. Temple et al.[318] reviewed the linked SEER-Medicare databases and found that of 9,011 elderly patients presenting with synchronous stage IV disease, that 72% had undergone resection of the primary, and that the 30-day mortality for these resections was 10%. In a retrospective review, Poultsides et al.[319] demonstrated that 93% of 233 patients never required surgical intervention on their primary tumors. More recently, the NSABP C-10 trial prospectively addressed this question, treating

90 patients with unresectable stage IV disease and intact, asymptomatic primary tumors with initial medical management with FOLFOX-6 plus bevacizumab. Twelve patients (14%) experienced major morbidity due to the intact primary tumor. This study met its prespecified end points for acceptability of intial nonoperative management, and the investigators concluded that good performance status patients with asymptomatic primaries can be spared initial noncurative resection of their primaries.[320]

Surgical intervention can be a very effective method of palliation and is often indicated in cases of impending obstruction, perforation, bleeding, or pain. However, it can also be associated with high postoperative morbidity and mortality. Stillwell et al.[321] identifies several adverse prognostic factors that can guide clinicians considering surgical palliation versus other less aggressive maneuvers. In a retrospective analysis of 379 patients who underwent palliative resection, elderly ($\geq$70 years) patients with advanced local disease or extrahepatic metastases were at greatest risk for postoperative mortality. Other independently associated factors included emergency operation and medical complications. Advanced nodal disease (N2) and poor tumor differentiation were significant predictors of decreased long-term survival.[321]

The chemotherapy options available and the developmental work that supports their utility are outlined subsequently. It is of paramount importance to keep in mind that virtually all of the clinical trials done in patients with metastatic disease were performed by design on patients who are in good overall general medical condition. Entry criteria for most trials require a favorable performance status and acceptable bone marrow, renal, and hepatic function, and they often specify evidence of reasonable nutritional intake.

It is not reasonable to extrapolate the results of these trials to patients who do not conform to these entry criteria. The likelihood of benefit in a poor performance status patient is substantially diminished, and the likelihood of a serious adverse event is greatly increased. Patients with hepatic or renal dysfunction may be particularly prone to additional toxicity if the drug is cleared or metabolized by these organs. Patients with marginal nutritional intake may have their nutritional deficiencies further exacerbated by drugs that produce nausea or anorexia, and patients with partial or complete bowel obstruction or other causes of prolonged GI transit time may have increased toxicity from those drugs that undergo an enterohepatic recirculation.

Thus, chemotherapy for patients with incurable metastatic disease should be approached with appropriate caution. Good performance status in well-motivated patients with good bone marrow reserve and good organ function portend a significant potential for substantial benefits from chemotherapy and should be strongly considered for aggressive therapy. Patients with poor performance status and significant comorbidities should be considered for either less aggressive therapies or for supportive care only.

Fluorouracil

Virtually the entire history of chemotherapy for CRC has revolved around the use of 5-FU. Developed by Heidelberger et al.[322] and patented in 1957, it is a source of frustration and humility for investigators working to move beyond it that over 50 years later this agent remains at the very core of most chemotherapeutic approaches to CRC.

5-FU must be metabolized before it can exert cytotoxic activity. The details of 5-FU metabolism are covered in a separate chapter. The history of investigations of 5-FU in CRC treatment has been well summarized in previous editions of this book.[227] 5-FU remained the only drug available to treat CRC for almost four decades, during which time numerous agents were studied for their ability to "biomodulate" 5-FU. Of these, only leucovorin remains in use today, and it is debatable whether this reduced folate truly contributes to the efficacy of 5-FU. Most studies that evaluate the same dose of 5-FU with or without leucovorin find that both activity and toxicity are increased in the leucovorin arm, whereas studies that evaluate single-agent 5-FU versus an equitoxic schedule of a lower dose of 5-FU plus leucovorin find equivalent activity. Nevertheless, use of leucovorin persists in most standard regimens today. Data comparing bolus versus infusional schedules of 5-FU show a slight benefit for infusions. These infusional schedules achieved widespread acceptance in Europe sooner than in the United States. It was not until the advent of combination schedules of 5-FU plus other active agents that the benefits of infusional schedules, especially in terms of improved toxicity, asserted themselves in North American practice. A selection of commonly used 5-FU regimens is outlined in Table 57.10.[323–325]

TABLE 57.10

Commonly Used 5-Fluorouracil Regimens[a]

Name of Regimen	Author (Ref.)	Schedule (All Agents Administered Intravenously)
Roswell Park	Haller et al., 1998[231]	LV 500 mg/m^2 over 2 hr; 5-FU 500 mg/m^2 by bolus 1 hr into LV infusion. Treatments given weekly for 6 consecutive wk, repeated every 8 wk.
Low-dose weekly LV	Jager et al., 1996[323]	LV 20 mg/m^2 over 5–15 min, followed by bolus 5-FU 500 mg/m^2; treatments given weekly for 6 consecutive wk, repeated every 8 wk.
Protracted venous infusion	Lokich et al., 1989[324]	5-FU 300 mg/m^2/d by continuous infusion.
AIO (weekly 24-hr infusion)	Kohne et al., 1998[325]	LV 500 mg/m^2 over 2 hr, followed by 5-FU 2,600 mg/m^2 over 24 hr, repeated weekly.
LV5FU2	de Gramont et al., 1997[341]	LV 200 mg/m^2 over 2 hr days 1 and 2, followed by bolus 5-FU 400 mg/m^2/day 1 and 2, followed by 5-FU 600 mg/m^2 over 22 hr days 1 and 2; cycle repeated every 14 d.
Simplified LV5FU2	Adapted from Andre et al., 1999[333]	LV 400 mg/m^2 over 2 hr, followed by bolus 5-FU 400 mg/m^2, followed by 5-FU 1,200 mg/m^2/d times 2 d (2,400 mg/m^2 over 46–48 hr); cycles repeated every 14 d.

LV, leucovorin; 5-FU, 5-fluorouracil; AIO, Arbeitsgemeinschaft Internistische Onkologie (Oncology Working Group, Germany).
[a] Doses listed are recommended starting doses for good performance status patients with normal renal, hepatic, and bone marrow function. Individual dose adjustments may be required.

Capecitabine

Capecitabine is a 5-FU precursor that is administered orally. It is absorbed intact through the gut and then activated by a series of enzymatic alterations. Some data suggest that thymidine phosphorylase levels are higher in tumor than in normal tissue. This could, in theory, provide a degree of preferential intratumoral activation; however, clinical trials do not appear to support a substantially better therapeutic index than 5-FU.[326] Phase 2 studies demonstrate that this agent has substantial activity in CRC, with an acceptable toxicity profile.[327] Because the addition of leucovorin did not appear to show any benefit, clinical development went forward without additional biomodulation. Phase 3 randomized clinical trials, performed both in the United States and Europe, have now shown that this orally administered agent is at least as effective as intravenous 5-FU/leucovorin, and the side effect profile of capecitabine is superior to the daily times five Mayo Clinic schedule of 5-FU/leucovorin.[328,329] However, as this bolus daily times five schedule is now known to be unacceptably toxic and is not used anymore, the relevance of the toxicity comparison is questionable. Head-to-head studies of modern infusional 5-FU/leucovorin regimens versus capecitabine have never been done; however, a reasonable extrapolation from available data would suggest that these two approaches are extremely similar in efficacy and tolerability. The dose used in these pivotal trials was 1,250 mg/m^2 given twice daily for 14 days followed by a 7-day rest. The major side effects of capecitabine appear to be palmar-plantar erythrodysesthesia, commonly called hand-foot syndrome, and to a lesser extent diarrhea. The hand-foot toxicity is frequently a dose-limiting side effect, and although the approved starting dose is 1,250 mg/m^2 twice daily, this dose is based on trials conducted mainly in Europe. For unclear reasons, possibly related to higher serum folate levels, American patients tolerate capecitabine less well than European patients, and clinicians in the United States often choose to initiate therapy at a lower dose and escalate if little or no toxicity is seen.

Irinotecan

Irinotecan (CPT-11) is a semisynthetic derivative of camptothecin, a plant alkaloid extracted from the wood of the Asian tree *Camptotheca acuminate*.[330] CPT-11 possesses a bulky dipiperidino side chain linked to the camptothecin molecule via a carboxyl-ester bond. This side chain provides solubility but greatly decreases anticancer activity. Carboxylesterase, a ubiquitous enzyme with primary activity in the liver and gut, cleaves the carboxyl-ester bond to form the more active metabolite 7-ethyl-10-hydroxycamptothecin (SN-38).[331] SN-38 is as much as 1,000-fold more potent in inhibiting topoisomerase I than irinotecan and is thus the predominant active form of the drug. CPT-11 is often considered to be a prodrug for SN-38; however, this concept may be a bit too simplistic, as achieved CPT-11 concentrations may be several logs higher than those of SN-38.

Camptothecin, CPT-11, and SN-38 function as inhibitors of topoisomerase I (topo I). Topo I is a nuclear enzyme that aids in DNA uncoiling for replication and transcription. When topo I binds to DNA, it causes a reversible single-stranded break in the DNA, allowing the intact strand to pass through the break to relieve torsional stress on the coiled helix, and then reseals the break. CPT-11 and SN-38 stabilize these single-stranded breaks. Although the stabilized breaks do not cause irreversible damage, the collision of replication forks with open single-stranded breaks results in double-stranded breaks, leading to lethal DNA fragmentation. The early development of irinotecan and its single-agent schedules have been well documented in earlier editions of this textbook.[227]

CPT-11 in First-Line Combination Regimens

Numerous phase 1 combinations of 5-FU, usually with leucovorin, plus CPT-11, were tried. Saltz et al.[332] reported a phase 1 trial built on the weekly CPT-11 schedule that had been selected for phase 1 development in North America. A low dose of weekly leucovorin was utilized in order to reduce the potential for 5-FU/leucovorin–induced diarrhea. The phase 1 trial showed that the full single-agent dose of 125 mg/m^2 of CPT-11 could be given with 500 mg/m^2 of 5-FU and 20 mg/m^2 leucovorin, with all drugs given weekly for 4 consecutive weeks followed by a 2-week break. This and other CPT-11/5-FU/leucovorin regimens are summarized in Table 57.11. This combination of IFL was compared to the Mayo Clinic schedule of 5-FU/leucovorin in a multicenter, multinational phase 3 trial.[247] For regulatory reasons, a single-agent CPT-11 arm was included as well. The IFL arm was found to be superior to Mayo Clinic 5-FU/leucovorin in terms of response rate, time to tumor progression, and overall survival. The CPT-11–alone arm appeared to be comparable in efficacy to the 5-FU/leucovorin arm. The overall incidence of severe toxicity was similar in all arms of this trial. More serious diarrhea and vomiting were seen with IFL, while more neutropenia, neutropenic fever, and stomatitis were seen with 5-FU/leucovorin. Treatment-related deaths occurred in 1% of patients in each arm of this trial. Although this IFL schedule represented a step forward over the Mayo Clinic 5-FU/leucovorin schedule, neither of these are recommended for current use. As outlined in the following, the infusional 5-FU schedules have a superior safety and efficacy profile and are preferred for use, especially in combination regimens.

TABLE 57.11

Commonly Used Irinotecan/5-Fluorouracil Combination Regimens^a

Name of Regimen	Author (Ref.)	Schedule (All Agents Administered Intravenously)
FOLFIRI	Douillard et al., 2000[246]	Irinotecan 180 mg/m^2 over 2 hr; LV 200 mg/m^2 concurrently with irinotecan (can be given in same line through "Y" connector); followed by 5-FU bolus 400 mg/m^2, followed by 5-FU 600 mg/m^2 infusion over 22 hr. Irinotecan given day 1 only. All other meds given days 1 and 2. Cycle repeated every 14 d.
FOLFIRI (simplified)	Andre et al., 1999[333]	Irinotecan 180 mg/m^2 over 90 min; LV 400 mg/m^2 concurrently with irinotecan (can be given in same line through "Y" connector); followed by 5-FU bolus 400 mg/m^2, followed by 5-FU 1,200 mg/m^2/d times 2 d (2,400 mg/m^2 infusion over 46–48 hr). Cycle repeated every 14 d.
FUFIRI	Douillard et al., 2000[246]	Irinotecan 80 mg/m^2, then LV 500 mg/m^2, followed by 5-FU 2,300 mg/m^2; all drugs given weekly for 6 wk, repeated every 7 wk.

FOLFIRI, irinotecan, 5-FU, LV; LV, leucovorin; 5-FU, 5-fluorouracil; FUFIRI, 5-FU, LV.
^{a} Doses listed are recommended starting doses for good performance status patients with normal renal, hepatic, and bone marrow function. Individual dose adjustments may be required.

In Europe, a parallel study to investigate the benefit of adding irinotecan to a 5-FU–based schedule was undertaken.[246] Two high-dose intermittent infusional schedules were developed. In France, a biweekly treatment for 2 consecutive days was explored, while German investigators, building on their experience with weekly 24-hour high-dose infusions of 5-FU, combined CPT-11 with this schedule. A randomized phase 3 trial was performed in which a participating center chose which of these two schedules would be used, and then the patients were randomized to that 5-FU/leucovorin schedule plus or minus CPT-11. Again, response rate, progression-free survival, and overall survival were superior in the CPT-11–containing arm of the trial. Of note, only the cohort treated with the biweekly schedule demonstrated a statistically superior survival over the 5-FU/leucovorin control arm, and the biweekly combination schedule is the only one registered for use in the United States.

More recently, the biweekly schedule of LV5FU2 plus irinotecan has been studied with a simplified LV5FU2 infusion schedule.[333] This schedule, known as FOLFIRI (FOL for folinic acid, F for 5-FU, and IRI for irinotecan), was initially studied as a salvage regimen; however, this has now gained widespread acceptance as a first-line treatment option, based on the data discussed subsequently.

The BICC-C (Bolus, Infusional, or Capecitabine with Camptosar-Celecoxib) trial is the only trial to directly compare weekly bolus IFL to FOLFIRI.[334] This trial utilized a modified bolus IFL schedule, giving treatment on days 1 and 8, repeated on a 3-week cycle. This modified IFL was compared to FOLFIRI as well as to capecitabine/irinotecan. The first phase of this trial (430 patients) confirmed the superior safety and efficacy of FOLFIRI over IFL (median progression-free survival 7.6 months for FOLFIRI versus 5.8 months; $p = 0.007$) and over capecitabine/irinotecan (progression-free survival 5.7 months; $p = 0.003$). The trial was halted when bevacizumab (see the following) became commercially available, and a second phase randomized 117 patients to modified IFL plus bevacizumab versus FOLFIRI plus bevacizumab (capecitabine/irinotecan was dropped from the second phase of this trial). This second phase showed a significant overall survival advantage for FOLFIRI/bevacizumab over modified IFL/bevacizumab ($p = 0.002$). The BICC-C trial also had a second randomization of all patients to celecoxib versus placebo. Celecoxib was found to provide no benefit in terms of either safety or efficacy and does not appear to have a role as part of standard chemotherapy of this disease.

Oxaliplatin

Oxaliplatin (1,2-diaminocyclohexane (trans-l) oxalatoplatinum) is a third-generation platinum compound of the diaminocyclohexane family. Initial single-agent phase 1 studies established that oxaliplatin could be safely administered, with evidence of clinical activity.[335,336] No significant nephrotoxicity was seen. Nausea and vomiting, minimal leucopenia, and rare thrombocytopenia were observed. Extra et al.[335] were the first to describe in detail the most notable toxicity encountered with oxaliplatin: neurotoxicity. This neurotoxicity manifested as paresthesias and dysesthesias of the hands, feet, perioral region, and throat. Pharyngolaryngeal dysesthesia, a sensation of choking without overt airway blockage, was described as well. These neurologic toxicities were induced or worsened by exposure to cold. Early single-agent explorations with oxaliplatin have been well outlined in the prior edition of this textbook.[337]

Oxaliplatin/5-Fluorouracil/Leucovorin Combination Trials

Based on a series of phase 2 trials by Levi et al., Giachetti et al.[338] from the same group reported a phase 3 trial of chronomodulated 5-FU/leucovorin alone or with oxaliplatin.[338–340] Two hundred patients were randomly assigned to receive a 5-day course every 3 weeks of chronomodulated 5-FU and leucovorin (700 and 300 mg/m² per day, respectively; peak delivery rate at 4 a.m.) with or without oxaliplatin on the first day of each course (125 mg/m², as a 6-hour infusion). The group who received oxaliplatin had a superior response rate (53% versus 16%; $p < 0.001$). Progression-free survival was also superior, just reaching statistical significance (8.7 months versus 7.4 months; $p = 0.048$). There were no differences in median overall survival (19.4 months and 19.9 months, respectively). Survival outcomes in this trial are somewhat difficult to interpret as extensive use of resection of metastatic disease was applied in both arms.

Most of the combination 5-FU/leucovorin/oxaliplatin trials have used flat (nonchronomodulated) administration of agents and have centered on variants of the FOLFOX regimen. The acronym FOLFOX (FOL for folinic acid [leucovorin], F for fluorouracil, OX for oxaliplatin) refers to a series of combinations of these agents. These are biweekly (every other week) regimens using 2 days of infusional 5-FU on a 14-day cycle (LV5FU2).[341] The FOLFOX-1, -2, and -3 regimens employed various alterations in dosing of each oxaliplatin, 5-FU, and leucovorin.[342,343] They are of historical interest, but were never evaluated in randomized trials. FOLFOX-3 and FOLFOX-4 were reported in a combined series to have a response rate of 21% in a population of patients who had progressed on the same 5-FU/leucovorin schedule without oxaliplatin.[342] The FOLFOX-4 regimen had a modestly higher response rate and lower toxicity than FOLFOX-3 (which used higher doses of 5-FU and leucovorin), and FOLFOX-4 appeared to be better tolerated. The more commonly used oxaliplatin/5-FU/ leucovorin combinations are outlined in Table 57.12.[344,345]

A randomized phase 3 trial was undertaken to evaluate FOLFOX-4 versus the LV5FU2 schedule in patients with previously untreated metastatic CRC (essentially a trial of LV5FU2 with or without oxaliplatin).[346] Patients treated with FOLFOX-4 had a statistically significantly superior outcome in terms of response rate (51% versus 22%; $p = 0.001$) and progression-free survival (9 months versus 6.2 months; $p = 0.0003$). The FOLFOX arm had a 1.5-month improvement in median overall survival; however, this did not reach statistical significance (16.2 months versus 14.7 months; $p = 0.12$). The number of patients experiencing grade 3 or 4 neutropenia was increased with FOLFOX-4 over 340 (42% versus 5% of patients). Grade 3 or 4 diarrhea (12% versus 5%) was also increased in the FOLFOX arm. Neurotoxicity, virtually absent in the LV5FU2 arm, was frequent in the FOLFOX arm, with 18% of patients experiencing grade 3 neurosensory toxicity.

The FOLFOX-4 regimen has also been evaluated in a multicenter randomized trial in second-line therapy following failure of first-line IFL chemotherapy.[347] Patients were randomly assigned to one of three arms: FOLFOX-4, LV5FU2, or single-agent oxaliplatin. Response rates were 10% for FOLFOX, 0% for LV5FU2, and 1% for oxaliplatin alone ($p < 0.0001$ for FOLFOX versus LV5FU2). Time to tumor progression was also superior for FOLFOX-4 (4.6 months) versus LV5FU2 (2.7 months) and oxaliplatin alone (1.6 months). These data confirm initial clinical impressions that oxaliplatin/5-FU combinations have superior activity to single-agent oxaliplatin, even in 5-FU–refractory disease. FOLFOX-4 has activity in IFL-refractory disease; however, single-agent oxaliplatin essentially does not.

Further modifications have been made to the FOLFOX schedule. FOLFOX-5 was designed with an increased dose of oxaliplatin to 100 mg/m² every 14 days; however, this regimen was never tested in clinical trials. FOLFOX-6 utilized this 100 mg/m² oxaliplatin dose with a simplified 5-FU/leucovorin schedule.[348] Oxaliplatin 100 mg/m² is given over 2 hours, with leucovorin 400 mg/m² given concurrently via a "T" connector. These are then followed by a 400 mg/m² bolus of 5-FU, and then a 46-hour infusion of 5-FU at 2,400 to 3,000 mg/m². More recently, the FOLFOX-7 regimen has been reported, utilizing a 130 mg/m² dose of oxaliplatin

TABLE 57.12

Selected Commonly Used Oxaliplatin/5-Fluorouracil Combination Regimens[a]

Name of Regimen	Author (Ref.)	Schedule (All Agents Administered Intravenously)
FOLFOX-4	de Gramont et al., 2000[346]	Oxaliplatin 85 mg/m^2 over 2 hr; LV 200 mg/m^2 concurrently with oxaliplatin (can be given in same line through "Y" connector); followed by 5-FU bolus 400 mg/m^2, followed by 5-FU 600 mg/m^2 infusion over 22 hr. Oxaliplatin given day 1 only. All other meds given days 1 and 2. Cycle repeated every 14 d.
FOLFOX-6	Tournigand et al., 2004[349]	Oxaliplatin 100 mg/m^2 over 2 hr; LV 400 mg/m^2 concurrently with oxaliplatin (can be given in same line through "Y" connector); followed by 5-FU bolus 400 mg/m^2, followed by 5-FU 1,200 mg/m^2/d times 2 d (2,400 mg/m^2 infusion over 46–48 hr). Cycle repeated every 14 d.
Modified FOLFOX-6	Widely used in current phase 3 trials, Wolmark et al. 2009[344]	Oxaliplatin 85 mg/m^2 over 2 hr; LV 400 mg/m^2 concurrently with oxaliplatin (can be given in same line through "Y" connector); followed by 5-FU bolus 400 mg/m^2, followed by 5-FU 1,200 mg/m^2/d times 2 d (2,400 mg/m^2 infusion over 46–48 hr). Cycle repeated every 14 d.
FUFOX	Grothey et al., 2002[345]	Oxaliplatin 50 mg/m^2 over 2 hr, followed by LV 500 mg/m^2, followed by 5-FU 2,000 mg/m^2 over 24 hr, weekly for 5 wk, repeated every 6 wk.

FOLFOX, folinic acid, 5-FU, oxaliplatin; LV, leucovorin; 5-FU, 5-fluorouracil; FUFOX, 5-FU, folinic acid.
[a] Doses listed are recommended starting doses for good performance status patients with normal renal, hepatic, and bone marrow function. Individual dose adjustments may be required.

every 14 days. The simplified leucovorin/5-FU administration of FOLFOX-6 is maintained, with deletion of the bolus 5-FU. Oxaliplatin is discontinued after 3 months, with planned reintroduction after 12 weeks or sooner if clinical progression occurs.[349] This rationale appears promising, both for treatment of metastatic disease and for potential use in the adjuvant setting. Given the similar response rates after 12 weeks, it would appear that the increased dose of oxaliplatin in FOLFOX-7 is unnecessary. A reasonable approach to standard use of FOLFOX in the metastatic setting is to use a modified FOLFOX-6, with 85 mg/m^2 of oxaliplatin and simplified LV5FU2 at a dose of 2,400 mg/m^2 over 46 to 48 hours (1,200 mg/m^2 per day for 2 consecutive days). As discussed in the following, the OPTIMOX trial data support cessation of oxaliplatin after 12 weeks and reintroduction of the oxaliplatin at a later date upon disease progression. It had been previously hypothesized that administration of high doses of calcium and magnesium with

oxaliplatin would be protective against neurotoxicity, but a definitive trial has now demonstrated that this is not the case.[350]

Comparisons of Oxaliplatin- and Irinotecan-Based Combinations

With both oxaliplatin- and irinotecan-based regimens showing encouraging activity, the question of which agent to use first was addressed by a number of investigators. Tournigand et al.[349] reported a phase 3 trial of FOLFOX-6 versus FOLFIRI. This trial utilized identical simplified LV5FU2 schedules, with the only variable being oxaliplatin or irinotecan. All patients were planned to crossover to the other regimen at time of progression, and the primary end point was time to tumor progression after *both* chemotherapy regimens. Results are shown in Table 57.13. Although the study is somewhat underpowered at a total of 226 patients, the

TABLE 57.13

Comparison of First-Line Use of Irinotecan Versus Oxaliplatin in Conjunction with the Same Simplified Biweekly Infusional 5-Fluorouracil/Leucovorin Schedule

	FOLFIRI (*n* = 109 Patients Treated)	FOLFOX-6 (*n* = 111 Patients Treated)	*P* Value
Major objective response rate (partial plus complete responses)	56%	54%	0.68
Time to tumor progression (on first-line regimen)	8.5 mo	8.1 mo	0.65
Time to tumor progression (after first- and second-line regimen)	14.4 mo	11.5 mo	0.65
Overall survival (from initial randomization)	20.4 mo	21.5 mo	0.9
Two-yr overall survival	41%	45%	
Grade 3–4 neutropenia	25%	44%	
Neutropenic fever	6%	1%	
Grade 3–4 diarrhea	14%	11%	
Neuropathy (grade 3)	0%	34%	
Alopecia (grade 2)	24%	9%	

FOLFIRI, irinotecan, 5-fluorouracil, leucovorin; FOLFOX, folinic acid, 5- fluorouracil, oxaliplatin.
From Tournigand C, Andre T, Achille E, et al. FOLFIRI followed by FOLFOX6 or the reverse sequence in advanced colorectal cancer: a randomized GERCOR study. *J Clin Oncol* 2004;22:229–237.

results show a striking consistency between regimens, suggesting that use of either FOLFOX-6 or FOLFIRI in first-line treatment is acceptable. A somewhat larger trial of 360 patients randomized to FOLFOX-4 versus the equivalent FOLFIRI schedule, utilizing the same LV5FU2 dose and schedule in each arm, again shows comparable efficacy data, with differing and predictable toxicity profiles.[351]

The North Central Cancer Treatment Group–led US Intergroup study N9741, a complex and important trial that underwent many iterations before its completion, initially opened as a four-arm trial comparing the Mayo Clinic 5-FU/leucovorin control arm to three different CPT-11/5-FU/leucovorin regimens: weekly bolus IFL as reported by Saltz et al.,[247] a "Mayo II" schedule of CPT-11 on day 1 and bolus 5-FU/low-dose leucovorin on days 2 to 5, or the biweekly infusional schedule of LV5FU2 plus CPT-11 as reported by Douillard et al.[246] and Goldberg.[352] After accruing a small number of patients, the trial was closed to incorporate three oxaliplatin-containing arms: FOLFOX-4, IROX (a once every 3 weeks combination of irinotecan and oxaliplatin, without 5-FU), and a modified Mayo Clinic schedule of bolus 5-FU plus low-dose leucovorin days 1 through 5, with oxaliplatin given on day 1. The infusional LV5FU2 plus CPT-11 arm was dropped. This created a six-arm trial. In March 2000, the trial was again halted, based on presentation of evidence that the combination of CPT-11/5-FU/leucovorin, using either bolus or infusional schedules, was superior to 5-FU/leucovorin. The Mayo Clinic control arm of N9741 was now dropped, and weekly bolus IFL became the control arm. At the same time, ongoing real-time monitoring of fatal toxicities identified unacceptably high rates of treatment-related mortality in the oxaliplatin plus Mayo Clinic 5-FU/leucovorin and in the CPT-11 plus 5-FU/leucovorin arms. These schedules were also dropped from the trial and from further development, leaving a three-arm trial of CPT-11 plus bolus 5-FU/leucovorin (IFL), oxaliplatin plus infusional LV5FU2 (FOLFOX-4), and oxaliplatin plus CPT-11 (IROX).

The trial was stopped a third time in April 2001, when monitoring of the trial indicated what appeared to be a higher than expected early mortality in the IFL control arm.[248] This observation, however, was based on utilization of a new metric, the 60-day ACM. This metric records death from *any* cause within 60 days of initial therapy. The 60-day ACM of the IFL arm was initially noted to be 4.5%. Because this was a new metric, however, there were no readily available historical controls; no one had ready access to data to say what the 60-day ACM had been in previous trials, either with IFL or with 5-FU/leucovorin regimens. The 4.5% ACM was therefore compared to the previously reported death rate for the IFL regimen, which was 0.9%. However, the previously reported death rate was the treatment-related death rate, the percentage of deaths judged by the investigators to have been caused by treatment, not all deaths within 60 days of starting therapy. Of further concern to the safety monitoring committee, however, the experimental arms (FOLFOX-4 and IROX) each showed 60-day ACMs of 1.8% (compared to 4.5% for the IFL control arm). This information was difficult to put into context, however, because the efficacy of the two experimental arms had not yet been established.

In fact, the 60-day ACM on the original phase 3 trial of IFL (subsequently calculated after N9741 was halted) was 6.7%, and the 60-day ACM for the Mayo Clinic control arm of that trial was found to be 7.3%. Although the 7.3% 60-day ACM appeared subjectively to be unusually high, no historical baseline data on 60-day ACM in 5-FU–based regimens were readily available. To help interpret these data, an analysis was undertaken to determine the 60-day ACM in multiple large-scale randomized trials that had used 5-FU/leucovorin schedules over the prior decade. This analysis confirmed that 60-day ACM regularly was encountered at a rate of 5% to 8% in the treatment of metastatic CRC.[353] Thus the 60-day ACM for the IFL regimen was actually *lower* on N9741 than in previous trials and was *lower* than what had been seen consistently with 5-FU/leucovorin regimens alone. In the final analysis of N9741, the 60-day ACM seen in the IFL, FOLFOX-4, and IROX arms were 4.5%, 2.6%, and 2.7%, respectively, and these differences were not statistically significant.

The efficacy results of N9741, however, were statistically significant and showed superior outcome for the patients randomized to FOLFOX-4, as compared to those randomized to either IFL or IROX, in terms of response rate, time to tumor progression, and overall survival (Table 57.14).[354] Toxicity for FOLFOX-4 was also superior for virtually all parameters, except of course neurotoxicity. The results of the IROX arm did not statistically significantly differ from those of the IFL arm in terms of toxicity, response, or time to tumor progression; however, survival was borderline statistically significantly better in the IROX arm than the IFL arm ($p = 0.04$).

TABLE 57.14

Results of Intergroup Trial N9741: Irinitecan Plus Bolus 5-Fluorouracil/Leucovorin, Oxaliplatin Plus Infusional 5-Fluorouracil/Leucovorin, and Irinotecan Plus Oxaliplatin in First-Line Treatment of Patients with Metastatic Colorectal Cancer

	IFL (*n* = 264)	FOLFOX-4 (*n* = 267)	IROX (*n* = 264)	*P* Value (IFL vs. FOLFOX)
Major objective response rate (partial plus complete responses)	31%	45%	35%	0.03
Time to tumor progression	6.9 mo	8.7 mo	6.5 mo	0.001
Overall survival	15.0 mo	19.5 mo	17.4 mo	0.0001
Received second-line therapy with active drug not included in first-line regimen	24% (oxaliplatin)	60% (irinotecan)	50% (fluorouracil)	Not given
Grade 3–4 neutropenia	40%	50%	36%	0.35
Neutropenic fever	15%	4%	11%	0.001
Grade 3–4 diarrhea	28%	12%	24%	0.001
Grade 3–4 nausea	16%	6%	19%	0.001
Grade 3 neuropathy	3%	18%	7%	0.001
60-d all cause mortality	4.5%	2.6%	2.7%	Not significant

IFL, 5-fluorouracil, leucovorin; FOLFOX4, oxaliplatin plus infusional 5-fluorouracil/leucovorin; IROX, irinotecan plus oxaliplatin
From Goldberg RM, Sargent DJ, Morton RF, et al. A randomized controlled trial of fluorouracil plus leucovorin, irinotecan, and oxaliplatin combinations in patients with previously untreated metastatic colorectal cancer. *J Clin Oncol* 2004;22:23–30.

Taken together, where do these trials leave us in terms of first-line use of oxaliplatin- and irinotecan-based regimens? Data from trial N9741 indicate that FOLFOX-4 is superior to IFL in both response rate and time to tumor progression. Overall survival was superior in the FOLFOX-4 arm versus IFL as well; however, interpretation of the survival results of N9741 is somewhat complicated due to imbalances between arms in availability of effective second-line therapy. Second-line CPT-11 was available to all patients who had received FOLFOX-4. Oxaliplatin, however, was not commercially available in the United States during the course of N9741. To what degree this imbalance in second-line therapy may have influenced the survival result is unknown. Also, as IFL contains bolus 5-FU, while FOLFOX-4 contains infusional leucovorin/5-FU2, it is difficult to isolate the irinotecan versus oxaliplatin component from the 5-FU bolus versus 5-FU infusion component.

Two other trials indicate that the FOLFOX and FOLFIRI regimens have similar safety and efficacy, with differing toxicity profiles.[349,351] Thus, FOLFOX has comparable efficacy to FOLFIRI, whereas FOLFOX has a superior response rate, time to tumor progression, and possibly some degree of survival benefit over IFL. Toxicity with irinotecan-based regimens shows a higher degree of alopecia. Diarrhea and neutropenia are increased on the bolus 5-FU schedule but are similar between FOLFOX and FOLFIRI. Oxaliplatin-based regimens, however, have neurotoxicity, absent from the irinotecan-based regimens, which can be problematic in some patients. It would therefore seem reasonable at this time to favor the use of a high-dose intermittent infusional 5-FU/leucovorin schedule plus either oxaliplatin (i.e., FOLFOX) or CPT-11 (i.e., FOLFIRI). Data do not support continued routine use of the bolus IFL schedule, nor are there randomized data to support the routine use of a bolus 5-FU/leucovorin schedule with oxaliplatin in the metastatic setting. Routine use of IROX is also not supported by the currently available body of data.

Whether to use an irinotecan-based or oxaliplatin-based combination in first-line treatment of good performance status patients can be considered a matter of patient preference, and discussion of the differing toxicity profiles is appropriate to help individuals decide. It is hoped that in the near-term future molecular prognostic indicators and pharmacogenomics will provide useful guidance for the individualization of therapies, but such approaches remain investigational at this time.

The only oxaliplatin schedule registered for use in the United States is FOLFOX-4; however, the modified FOLFOX-6 would appear at this time to be a very reasonable schedule for routine clinical use when the decision is made to use an oxaliplatin/5-FU combination.

The recognition of neurotoxicity as a major limitation of the FOLFOX regimens led to the investigation of optimization of oxaliplatin (the OPTIMOX study).[355] In this trial, patients were randomly assigned to receive either standard FOLFOX-4 until progression or 12 weeks of FOLFOX-7, followed by planned cessation of oxaliplatin and continuation of the LV5FU2. As designed, the study called for a reintroduction of oxaliplatin after 6 months of LV5FU2, although this actually occurred in the minority of patients and outcomes were superior in those patients in whom reintroduction of oxaliplatin occurred.[356] The primary end point was duration of disease control, the time from initiation of treatment until either progression through all agents (including failure after reintroduction of oxaliplatin if this was done), or death. Duration of disease control as well as progression-free survival and overall survival were not statistically significantly different between the two arms. As anticipated, toxicity, including neurotoxicity, was substantially reduced in the OPTIMOX arm. This OPTIMOX strategy of planned interruption of oxaliplatin can be considered a standard care option in metastatic disease. It is important to discuss plans for such planned interruptions with patients at the beginning of therapy so that they will not be surprised or alarmed at the removal of one of the drugs.

Although a regimen of oxaliplatin, weekly bolus 5-FU, and low-dose weekly leucovorin (bFOL) appeared promising in an initial phase 2 trial, two sequential randomized phase 2 trials, known as TREE-1 and TREE-2, suggest modestly inferior activity for the bFOL schedule compared with FOLFOX or Cape/Ox.[357,358] Thus, in the metastatic setting, oxaliplatin with bolus 5-FU schedules is therefore not recommended for routine use.

Use of planned sequential administration of FOLFOX and FOLFIRI has also been proposed, both in terms of pretreatment for potentially resectable patients with liver metastases and in terms of adjuvant treatment of earlier stage disease. Several groups are also exploring the use of "triple therapy" with oxaliplatin, CPT-11, and 5-FU/leucovorin (FOLFOXIRI). A randomized phase 3 trial conducted in Italy reported that FOLFOXIRI is tolerable and offers a modest survival benefit over FOLFIRI. These trials utilized higher doses of 5-FU than are likely to be tolerable by American patients, and use of this combination has not gained widespread acceptance.[359]

As discussed previously, a trial comparing FOLFIRI to capecitabine/irinotecan suggested inferior outcome for the capecitabine-containing regimen.[334] However, a large randomized trial has now compared Cape/Ox versus FOLFOX. The study also had a two-by-two randomization to with or without bevacizumab (discussed subsequently). This trial demonstrated the Cape/Ox regimen to be noninferior to FOLFOX, and each had acceptable toxicity, indicating that Cape/Ox is an acceptable alternative to FOLFOX.[360] It should be noted that the Cape/Ox regimen requires a motivated, reliable patient who will be able to take multiple pills of oral medication on a complex schedule, even in the setting of potentially emetogenic oxaliplatin.

Duration of Therapy

Controversy continues to exist regarding the optimal duration of chemotherapy for palliation of metastatic disease. Traditional practice for many years had been to continue chemotherapy until either unacceptable toxicity, clinical deterioration, or disease progression. When efficacy of treatment was more limited, with the duration of therapy typically limited to a small number of months, the issue of treatment breaks did not seem relevant. Now, with patients typically living multiple years with metastatic CRC and with some treatments maintaining control for more extended periods of time, the need for patients to have breaks (often referred to as "treatment holidays" or "chemotherapy-free intervals" [CFI]) is greater, and there is considerable interest in using these approaches. Both physically and psychologically, many patients appear to both need and derive benefit from these treatment interruptions.

The concept of noncontinuous chemotherapy has been investigated for some time now. Maughan et al.[361] conducted a randomized trial of continuous versus interrupted treatment in 354 patients who were responding or who had stable disease after receiving 12 weeks of either 5-FU– or raltitrexed-based chemotherapy. Patients were randomized to either continue chemotherapy until progression or to stop chemotherapy after the first 12 weeks, followed by a planned restarting on the same chemotherapy at the time of progression. At randomization, 41% of patients had achieved a major objective response and 59% had stable disease. There was no evidence of a difference in overall survival, the primary end point, between the two groups, with an HR of 0.87 ($p = 0.23$, favoring the intermittent arm).

More recently, the idea of planned early cessation of all chemotherapy was investigated in the OPTIMOX-2 trial.[362] A total of 202 patients with previously untreated metastatic CRC were treated. All patients received six cycles of modified FOLFOX-7 followed by either continued LV5FU2 until progression, or a complete cessation of all chemotherapy (a CFI). Patients on both arms were planned to receive retreatment with FOLFOX following tumor progression. The results of this study did not support the use of this planned, early interruption in therapy, as the median duration of disease control, progression-free survival, and overall survival were all inferior in the arm with the early planned CFI. This should not be misconstrued as evidence that CFIs are contraindicated, but rather that early planned CFIs for all patients is not an appropriate strategy. The authors suggest that this study indicates there are no pretreatment parameters that can identify a priori those patients who can successfully benefit from a CFI. Thus, specific decisions regarding use and timing of CFIs cannot be made in advance of starting treatment; rather, clinical judgment must be exercised in deciding on treatment interruptions for CFIs in responding patients after a favorable response. In a retrospective review of 822 patients in the two OPTIMOX studies, after excluding those patients who had early progression within the first 3 months of treatment as well as those who underwent complete gross resection of metastatic disease within 3 months of stopping chemotherapy, Perez-Staub et al.[363] noted that there was no indication of a detriment in survival when comparing those patients who took a CFI versus those who did not. In fact, in this retrospective, nonrandomized analysis, the median survival was 37.5 months in patients who had a CFI versus 21.2 months in matched patients who did not have a CFI. Of note, median overall survival of patients who stopped chemotherapy earlier than 3 months was 24 months, whereas it was 42 months when a CFI was taken between 3 and 9 months into therapy, and 44 months when a CFI was taken later than 9 months into chemotherapy. These studies were accomplished prior to the use of bevacizumab. Some clinicians have advocated the continuation of bevacizumab during CFIs. Such an approach is not supported by data, and given the absence of activity of single-agent bevacizumab in CRC, use of single-agent bevacizumab during otherwise CFIs is not recommended at this time.

Other investigators specifically addressed the question of whether rechallenge with 5-FU after a planned treatment interruption could produce a response. A pooled analysis was conducted on 613 patients involved in three randomized trials of first-line 5-FU–based therapy.[364] All patients had a planned maximum treatment period of 6 months. Patients with responding or stable disease at the end of that period were observed off treatment with a plan for retreatment at the time of disease progression. Median time to rechallenge was 11.7 months. Seventeen percent of patients had an objective response to rechallenging. Median survival for the group was 14.8 months. These nonrandomized data indicate that patients have a meaningful response rate at time of reinstitution of chemotherapy.

A similar approach was explored in patients who received second-line irinotecan therapy.[365] A total of 333 patients entered into a trial to receive 24 weeks of irinotecan. Patients who remained in the study at the end of that time were to be randomized to either continue treatment or to stop therapy. Of the 333 patients, most came off the study due to progression or toxicity before reaching the 24-week mark. Fifty-five patients with responding or stable disease agreed to randomization. Although the numbers available for comparison were small, there were no differences between the arms in progression-free survival or overall survival, nor were there differences in quality-of-life scores.

Overall, there appears to be no compelling evidence that continuation of chemotherapy indefinitely is necessary for optimal control of metastatic disease. The option of discontinuation of therapy after a reasonable period of time appears to be an appropriate consideration in standard practice.

Combination versus Single-Agent Chemotherapy

Given that combination regimens are invariably associated with more toxicity than single agents, the question of the need for universal upfront use of these combinations was investigated. The CAIRO (CApecitabine, IRinotecan, Oxaliplatin) trial randomized 820 patients to sequential versus concurrent therapies (Table 57.15).[566] In the sequential arm, first-line therapy was single-agent capecitabine. Upon failure, single-agent irinotecan was used, and then third-line therapy was Cape/Ox (since single-agent oxaliplatin is essentially inactive in 5-FU–refractory CRC). The combination arm used Cape/Ox as first-line therapy and capecitabine and irinotecan as second-line therapy. The primary end point, median overall survival, was not statistically significantly different between the two arms (17.4 months for combination versus 16.3 months for the sequential arm; $p = 0.33$). Dose-limiting toxicity (grade 3 or 4) was not significantly different between the two groups; in fact, grade 3 hand-foot syndrome was somewhat more common in the sequential arm (13% versus 7%; $p = 0.004$).

Similar findings were reported in the FOCUS study.[367] In this trial, a total of 2,135 patients were randomized to one of three arms. Arm A was sequential therapy, with initial treatment given with 5-FU on the leucovorin/5-FU2 (biweekly infusional) schedule until progression, at which point second-line therapy was given with single-agent irinotecan. Arm B also gave biweekly LV5FU2 until failure, and then LV5FU2 was continued with the addition of either oxaliplatin or irinotecan (this was a second randomization within this arm). Thus, second-line therapy was a change from biweekly LV5FU2 to either FOLFOX or FOLFIRI in this arm. In arm C, patients began with combination chemotherapy, and within this arm were randomized to either FOLFOX or FOLFIRI. The primary end point, median overall survival, for arm A was 13.9 months. For arm B, survival was 15.0 months for irinotecan and 15.2 months for oxaliplatin. Arm C had a median overall survival of 16.7 months for the FOLFIRI patients and 15.4 months for those treated with FOLFOX. Only the difference between arm A and the irinotecan arm of arm C reached statistical significance ($p = 0.01$). Arm B (initial LV5FU2 followed by FOLFOX or FOLIRI) was noninferior to arm C (initial FOLFOX or FOLIRI) (HR = 1.06; 90% CI = 0.97 to 1.17).

Taken together, the CAIRO and FOCUS trials provide a strong argument that not all patients with unresectable metastatic disease require exposure to the toxicity of combination therapy, and

TABLE 57.15

Sequential Versus Combination Chemotherapy with Capecitabine, Irinotecan, and Oxaliplatin in Advanced Colorectal Cancer: Efficacy End Points

	Overall Survival	One-Yr Survival	Progression-Free Survival (First Line)	Response Rate
Sequential Cape, then Iri, then Cape/Ox (n = 401)	16.3 mo	64%	5.8 m	20%
Combination Cape/Iri, then Cape/Ox (n = 402)	17.4 mo	67%	7.8 m	41%
P value	0.33	0.38	0.0002	0.0001

Cape, capecitabine; Iri, irinotecan; Ox, oxaliplatin.
From Koopman M, Antonini NF, Douma J, et al. Sequential versus combination chemotherapy with capecitabine, irinotecan, and oxaliplatin in advanced colorectal cancer (CAIRO): a phase III randomised controlled trial. *Lancet* 2007;370:135–142.

TABLE 57.16A

Efficacy Outcomes, First-Line Treatment of Metastatic Colorectal Cancer: Irinotecan Plus Bolus 5-Fluorouracil/Leucovorin Plus Placebo Versus 5-Fluorouracil/Leucovorin Plus Bevacizumab

Regimen	No. of Patients	Response Rate	Progression-Free Survival	Overall Survival
IFL + placebo	411	34.8%	6.2 mo	15.6 mo
IFL + bevacizumab	402	44.8% $p = 0.004$	10.6 mo $p < 0.001$	20.3 mo $p < 0.001$

IFL, 5-fluorouracil, leucovorin.

that initial use of fluorinated pyrimidine alone in patients with previously untreated metastatic CRC is a treatment alternative that needs to be carefully considered.

Bevacizumab

Bevacizumab is a humanized monoclonal antibody that binds to VEGF, thereby substantially reducing the amount of circulating ligand and thus preventing receptor activation.[368,369] The first trial of bevacizumab in CRC was a modest-sized, three-arm, randomized phase 2 trial in which a total of 104 patients were randomly assigned to either one of two different doses levels of bevacizumab (5 mg/kg or 10 mg/kg) plus weekly 5-FU/leucovorin or to 5-FU/leucovorin alone.[370] The response rate, time to tumor progression, and overall survival were superior in the 5-FU/leucovorin with 5 mg/kg bevacizumab arm. Despite the small size and limited statistical power of this study, this result would served as the basis for design of the pivotal phase 3 trial of bevacizumab in CRC.

The initial design of the phase 3 pivotal trial was a comparison between 5-FU/leucovorin plus placebo to 5-FU/leucovorin plus 5 mg/kg of bevacizumab. However, as the randomized phase 2 trial, discussed previously, was nearing completion, the randomized phase 3 trial was reported, which demonstrated a modest but statistically significant survival advantage for the IFL regimen (irinotecan plus weekly bolus 5-FU/leucovorin) compared with 5-FU/leucovorin alone.[247] As a result of this trial, the IFL regimen was then felt to be the appropriate control arm for subsequent phase 3 trials. There were no safety data at the time, however, on the combination of bevacizumab plus IFL. As a result of this, a three-arm trial was designed that contained (1) 5-FU/leucovorin/bevacizumab, (2) IFL/bevacizumab, and (3) IFL/placebo (the control arm).[371] The design included a preplanned analysis of safety on all arms when enrollment reached 100 patients per arm, with a further plan to close the 5-FU/leucovorin/bevacizumab arm at that time if the safety data indicated acceptable tolerability and safety of the IFL/bevacizumab arm.

In the final efficacy analysis, the IFL/bevacizumab cohort experienced superior outcome compared to the IFL/placebo group in response rate (45% versus 35%; $p <0.003$), progression-free survival (10.6 months versus 6.2 months; $p <0.00001$), and overall survival (20.3 months versus 15.6 months; $p = 0.00003$) (Table 57.16A).

It should be noted that no crossover to second-line bevacizumab in the IFL/placebo control arm was allowed in this trial.

In order to better understand the effects of bevacizumab in conjunction with 5-FU/leucovorin, Kabbinavar et al.[372] combined the data from three separate modest-sized trials to create a more robust data set. In this combined analysis of 5-FU/leucovorin with or without bevacizumab, there was a statistically significant survival advantage for the patients who received bevacizumab. Given the favorable aspects of the biweekly infusional LV5FU2 schedule used in the FOCUS trial, the LV5FU2 schedule would seem most appropriate for combination with bevacizumab.[373] At the same time as the pivotal front-line study was accruing, the Eastern Cooperative Oncology Group (ECOG) also performed a trial (ECOG-3200) to evaluate the use of bevacizumab in the second-line setting.[374] This trial randomized patients who had failed irinotecan and 5-FU but were naive to bevacizumab, to one of three arms: bevacizumab/FOLFOX, FOLFOX alone, or bevacizumab. The investigators chose to investigate a 10 mg/kg bevacizumab dose. Overall, a modest but statistically significant improvement in median overall survival was demonstrated for FOLFOX-4 with bevacizumab versus FOLFOX-4 alone (12.5 months versus 10.7 months; $p = 0.0024$), and grade 3 or 4 toxicities were not increased. The bevacizumab-alone arm had substantially inferior progression-free survival and an investigator-adjudicated response rate of 3%, suggesting that single-agent bevacizumab does not have meaningful activity in CRC and should not be used. It is important to note that this trial was performed *exclusively* in patients who had *not* received bevacizumab in the first-line setting. This trial provides no data on whether use of bevacizumab with a second-line regimen after progression on a first-line bevacizumab-containing regimen is efficacious.

Although it was performed in second-line patients, the ECOG-3200 trial was the first trial to provide safety data for the combination of bevacizumab plus FOLFOX. As a result of this, even before front-line data were available, bevacizumab plus FOLFOX had become widely accepted as a front-line option in the United States for metastatic CRC. More recently, the NO16966 trial directly addressed the question of front-line bevacizumab plus oxaliplatin-based therapy (Table 57.16B).[375] In this trial, 1,400 patients with previously untreated CRC were randomly assigned to

TABLE 57.16B

Efficacy Outcomes, First-Line Treatment of Metastatic Colorectal Cancer: Capeox/Folfox Plus Placebo Versus Capeox/Folfox Plus Bevacizumab

Regimen	No. of Patients	Response Rate	Progression-Free Survival	Overall Survival
CapeOx/FOLFOX + placebo	701	49%	8.0 mo	19.9 mo
CapeOx/FOLFOX + bevacizumab	699	47% $p = 0.31$	9.4 mo $p = 0.0023$	21.3 mo $p = 0.078$

CapeOx, capecitabine, oxaliplatin; FOLFOX, fluorouracil, leucovorin, oxaliplatin.
From Saltz LB, Clarke S, Diaz-Rubio E, et al. Bevacizumab in combination with oxaliplatin-based chemotherapy as first-line therapy in metastatic colorectal cancer: a randomized phase III study. *J Clin Oncol* 2008;26:2013–2019.

either FOLFOX-4 or Cape/Ox and then to either placebo or bevacizumab, in a two-by-two randomization. Although the study did show a statistically significant progression-free survival advantage for the addition of bevacizumab (9.4 months versus 8.0 months for chemotherapy with bevacizumab versus chemotherapy with placebo, respectively; HR = 0.83; p = 0.003), this difference was more modest than the 4.4-month progression-free survival difference seen in the initial bevacizumab with IFL front-line trial. Overall survival improvement with bevacizumab approached, but did not reach, statistical significance (21.3 months versus 19.9 months; HR = 0.89; p = 0.077) Also, in the NO16966 trial, the addition of bevacizumab to front-line oxaliplatin-based chemotherapy did not confer any response benefit. It is noteworthy that the majority of patients on this trial discontinued treatment, presumably due to nonbevacizumab-related toxicity issues, before progression. This may have diminished the impact of bevacizumab on survival and progression-free survival but would not have impacted the response rate.

Toxicity

In terms of toxicity, grade 3 hypertension was higher in the bevacizumab/IFL arm than in the placebo/IFL arm (11% versus 2%) in the IFL/bevacizumab study.[371] Hypertension is now widely recognized as a common side effect of bevacizumab, and monitoring for and treatment of hypertension with antihypertensive medications is a routine part of bevacizumab management. Incidences of overall thromboembolic events and proteinuria were not statistically different between the two arms. However, two rare but extremely serious toxicities were encountered with increased frequency in the bevacizumab-containing arm: GI perforations and arterial thrombotic events.

The GI perforations were a group of events that included a perforated gastric ulcer, small bowel perforations, and free air under the diaphragm without identified sources. Although these were somewhat heterogeneous in nature, it was noted that six such events occurred on the bevacizumab-containing arm (one fatal) compared with none on the chemotherapy-alone arm. No clear risk factors for these perforations could be identified from this trial. Interestingly, GI perforations were not frequent occurrences in large cooperative group trials in patients with lung cancer or breast cancer; however, an unusually high GI perforation rate has recently halted accrual on a trial of bevacizumab in patients with ovarian cancer. These ovarian observations illustrate an important aspect about GI perforations in association with bevacizumab: there is not an association between the presence of an intact primary tumor in the colon and a GI perforation. Concerns have been expressed by some clinicians about the possibility of needing to remove an asymptomatic primary colorectal tumor in a patient with synchronous stage IV disease before using bevacizumab out of an unsubstantiated fear that the primary will put the patient at risk for perforation. At present, there are no data to support this assumption, and surgery for an asymptomatic primary tumor in a stage IV patient is not routinely indicated, regardless of whether there are plans to use a bevacizumab-containing chemotherapy regimen.[319]

The other rare but very serious identified increased risk with bevacizumab-containing treatment was that of arterial thrombotic events. Initially, no clear indication of this risk was detected in the pivotal phase 3 trial. However, in a combined analysis of several trials, an important observation was made. Here again, multiple events were combined into one metric. Thus, cerebral vascular accidents, myocardial infarctions, transient ischemic attacks, and angina were combined to create the metric of arterial thrombotic events. The observed incidence of these events was 2.5% in the nonbevacizumab-containing control arms versus 5.0% in the bevacizumab-containing experimental arms. It was noted that patients who had histories of cardiovascular or atherosclerotic disease appeared to be at greater risk for increased bevacizumab-related arterial thrombotic complications. In addition, a further

analysis of these events suggested that the risk was essentially linear over time, indicating that the risk of a new arterial thrombotic event was the same in earlier versus later months of exposure.[376]

Another complication of bevacizumab that has been rarely described in the literature is fistula formation. Ganapathi et al.[377] reports a 4.1% incidence of this problem in a review of 222 patients with metastatic CRC. Two-thirds were perineal or anal with the remainder colovesicular, occuring an average of 3.9 months after initiation of treatment. Cessation of bevacizumab led to fistula healing in nearly all cases; however, three patients required fecal diversion. The authors suggest that this complication has been underreported thus far and stress the importance of early recognition.[377]

Bevacizumab Beyond Progression

Prior studies had demonstrated the activity of bevacizumab when added to first-line chemotherapy, and the ECOG 3200 trial had shown that bevacizumab added to second-line chemotherapy in bevacizumab-naïve patients. Until recently, however, data were lacking regarding the question of continuation of bevacizumab with second-line therapy after progression of disease through a first-line, bevacizumab-containing regimen. This question has now been addressed by the TML trial.[378] In this trial, 820 patients who had progressed through a first-line, bevacizumab-containing regimen were assigned to a noncross-resistant chemotherapy regimen (irinotecan plus fluoropirymidine if previously treated with oxliplatin or oxaliplatin-fluoropyrimidine if previously treated with irinotecan) and then randomized to receive bevacizumab with this second-line chemotherapy or not. The arm receiving bevacizumab showed a modest but statistically significant survival benefit of 1.4 months (overall survival of 11.2 months versus 9.8 months; HR = 0.81; 95% CI = 0.69 to 0.94; p = 0.0062). Grade 3 to 5 bleeding or hemorrhage (8 [2%] versus 1 [1%]), GI perforation (7 [2%] versus 3 [1%]), and venous thromboembolisms (19 [5%] versus 12 [3%]) were more common in the bevacizumab plus chemotherapy group than in the chemotherapy-alone group.

Aflibercept

Aflibercept is a fusion molecule containing the binding domains of VEGF receptors 1 and 2 bound to the human immunoglobulin (Ig) G Fc fragment, forming a VEGF trap molecule. Aflibercept binds all human VEGF A isoforms, VEGF B, and placental growth factor with greater affinity than the native receptors for these ligands. Aflibercept has been evaluated in the large scale phase 3 VELOUR trial, in which 1,226 patients who had progressed on a first-line oxaliplatin-containing regimen were randomized to receive second-line FOLFIRI plus aflibercept 4 mg/kg versus FOLFIRI plus placebo. All treatments were given every 2 weeks. Thirty percent of patients had received prior bevacizumab with their first-line treatment regimen, while the remainder were naïve to anti-VEGF therapy. The group receiving aflibercept achieved a modest, but statistically significant overall survival benefit of 1.4 months (13.50 months versus 12.06 months; HR = 0.817; 95% CI = 0.713 to 0.937; p = 0.0032).[379] PFS was also statistically significantly improved from 4.67 months to 6.9 months with the addition of aflibercept (p <0.0001). Reponse rate was improved from 11.1% to 19.8%.

The findings of the VELOUR and TML trials show striking similarities to one another. Each utilized an anti-VEGF strategy in second-line treatment in conjunction with active chemotherapy, and each shows a 1.4-month survival benefit. Given these findings, use of either with second-line FOLFIRI (if second-line FOLFIRI is deemed appropriate) would seem reasonable. Aflibercept has not demonstrated benefit in conjunction with oxaliplatin-based regimens at the time of this writing, and so use of aflibercept with oxaliplatin-based chemotherapy is not recommended. Furthermore, a change from FOLFIRI-aflibercept to

FOLFIRI-bevacizumab (or vice versa) is not supported by current data, nor is use of either aflibercept or bevacizumab as a single agent. As such, aflibercept presents an option for second-line therapy in conjunction with FOLFIRI, but does not create a new line of therapy in the continuum of treatment.

Regorafenib

Regorafenib is a small molecule multitargeted tyrosine kinase inhibitor. It is closely related to its parent compound, sorafenib, and differs only by the addition of a fluorine atom. After phase 1 trials identified preliminary evidence of activity in patients with refractory CRC, a large phase 3 trial of regorafenib versus placebo was undertaken.[380] A total of 760 patients, all with ECOG grade 0 or 1 performance status, who had progressed through all standard therapies, were randomized 2:1 to received regorafenib 160 mg orally daily versus placebo. The regorafenib group achieved a modest but statistically significant overall survival benefit of 1.4 months (6.4 months versus 5.0 months; HR = 0.77; 95% CI = 0.64 to 0.94; $p = 0.0052$). Response was essentially nonevident, with a response rate of 1% in the regorafenib arm. Grade 3 hand-foot syndrome (17%) and grade 3 fatigue (10%) were the most common toxicities encountered on the regorafenib arm. Regorafenib monotherapy can be considered as a standard care option for good performance status patients who have progressed through standard therapies. Studies assessing the use of regorafenib in earlier lines of therapy and in combination with cytotoxic agents are in progress at the time of this writing.

Cetuximab and Panitumumab

The EGFR, also called HER-1, is a transmembrane glycoprotein receptor. When the external binding domain of the EGFR binds specific ligands, such as epidermal growth factor or TGF-α, receptor dimerization occurs (either homodimerization with another EGFR or heterodimerization with another member of the EGFR family). This in turn stimulates phosphorylation of the tyrosine kinases on the intracellular domain of the receptor, which initiates a signaling cascade, which ultimately regulates cell proliferation, migration, adhesion, differentiation, and survival.[381–383] Cetuximab (c-mab), is a chimeric IgG$_1$ monoclonal antibody that recognizes and binds to the extracellular domain of the EGFR. Panitumumab (p-mab) is a fully human IgG$_2$ monoclonal antibody that also targets the EGFR. Binding of either c-mab or p-mab to this receptor does not cause receptor activation, but rather results in a steric interference with the ligand binding site.[384]

Preclinical models of cetuximab, or its murine precursor, demonstrated more substantial activity when given in combination with cytotoxic chemotherapy. Based on these observations, and on a single anecdotal report of a major response to cetuximab plus irinotecan in a young woman with irinotecan-refractory CRC, a multicenter phase 2 trial was initiated. This trial, reported in abstract form only, was conducted in patients who were determined by their treating investigator to have progressed on irinotecan.[385] Patients were treated with cetuximab at a dose of 400 mg/m^2 loading dose week 1 over 2 hours, followed by weekly 250 mg/m^2 over 1 hour. Irinotecan was given on the same dose and schedule as had previously failed. Irinotecan dose reductions made previously, prior to study entry, were maintained upon initiation of the study treatment.

One hundred twenty patients with irinotecan-refractory CRC were identified and enrolled. In addition, in a parallel portion of the trial, 28 patients with clinically and radiographically stable disease after receiving a minimum of 3 months of irinotecan therapy were also enrolled and treated by the addition of cetuximab to their ongoing irinotecan therapy. The response outcome of this "stable disease cohort" was not reported; only those patients who were felt to be irinotecan refractory were included in the initial report. As reported by an independent response assessment committee, 22.5% of irinotecan-refractory patients achieved a major objective response. The irinotecan-related toxicity was relatively mild in this population, at least in part because many patients had already had irinotecan dose modifications made prior to starting on this trial. Of the side effects specifically attributable to cetuximab, 3% of patients developed an allergic, anaphylactoid reaction requiring discontinuation of cetuximab therapy, and 75% of patients experienced a skin rash (12% grade 3), a rash now recognized to be characteristic of all EGFR inhibitors. This rash superficially resembles acne, leading to its initial description as an acneiform rash. However, microscopically this is not acne, and topical acne medications are ineffective in its management. An interesting observation from this trial, which has since been corroborated in multiple trials, is that the presence and severity of the rash appeared to be associated with response in this study.

The results seen in the phase 2 cetuximab plus irinotecan combination trial raised the question, both from a scientific and from a regulatory perspective, of the activity of single-agent cetuximab in irinotecan-refractory CRC. A small phase 2 trial was therefore quickly designed and accrued. In this trial, 5 of 57 patients (9%) achieved a partial response confirmed by an independent radiologic review.[386]

Based on the preliminary results of the initial phase 2 cetuximab plus irinotecan study, described previously, a subsequent larger trial, ultimately reported by Cunningham et al.,[245] was designed to provide confirmatory evidence of the activity of cetuximab in CRC (Table 57.17). This large, randomized phase 2 trial in patients with irinotecan-refractory CRC, which has become known as the BOND trial, compared cetuximab plus irinotecan to cetuximab monotherapy. A total of 329 patients were randomized in a two-to-one schema. The response rates of 22.9% for cetuximab plus irinotecan and 10.8% for cetuximab alone were virtually identical to the response rates that had been reported previously in the two US phase 2 trials, confirming the activity of this agent in CRC. Time to tumor progression in the Cunningham et al.[245] study was

PRACTICE OF ONCOLOGY

TABLE 57.17

Efficacy Outcomes: Cetuximab Plus Irinotecan Versus Cetuximab Alone in Irinotecan-Refractory Colorectal Cancer

	No. of Patients	Response Rate (95% CI)	Disease Control (95% CI)	Median TTP (mo)	Median OS (mo) (95% CI)
Cetuximab	111	11% (6%–18%)	32% (24%–42%)	1.5	6.9 (5.6–9.1)
Cetuximab + irinotecan	218	23% (18%–29)[a]	56% (49%–62%)[b]	4.1[c]	8.6 (7.6–9.6)

CI, confidence interval; TTP, time to progression; OS, overall survival.
[a] $p = 0.0074$.
[b] $p = 0.0001$.
[c] $p < 0.0001$.
From Cunningham D, Humblet Y, Siena S, et al. Cetuximab monotherapy and cetuximab plus irinotecan in irinotecan-refractory metastatic colorectal cancer. *N Engl J Med* 2004;351:337–345.

4.1 months for the combination versus 1.5 months for single-agent cetuximab. Survival in the two arms was not significantly different; however, the study was neither designed nor powered to address the issue of a survival advantage for cetuximab, and cetuximab was given to all patients on both arms of the study.

A National Cancer Institute Canada phase 3 trial compared cetuximab plus best supportive care to best supportive care alone in 572 patients who had exhausted standard treatment options.[387] The median overall survival was improved by 1.5 months (from 4.6 months to 6.1 months) in the cetuximab group compared to supportive care alone. Partial responses occurred in 23 patients (8.0%) in the cetuximab group versus none in the supportive care group ($p <0.001$).

Similar results were reported with panitumumab. As seen with single-agent cetuximab, phase 2 evaluations of panitumumab in patients with CRC indicate approximately a 10% response rate, with over 90% of patients experiencing some degree of acneiform-like rash.[388,389] The fully human nature of this antibody appears to reduce the likelihood of anaphylactoid infusion reactions, with only 1 of the 148 patients treated after experiencing a dose-limiting allergic reaction. A randomized trial of panitumumab versus best supportive care in the salvage setting demonstrated a modest (8 weeks versus 7.3 weeks) but highly statistically significant improvement in median progression-free survival for single-agent panitumumab over best supportive care (HR = 0.54; $p <0.000000001$). Response rate to p-mab was 10%. There was no difference in overall survival; however, there was extensive postprogression crossover, which obscures this end point.[390]

KRAS and Other Determinants of Anti–Epidermal Growth Factor Receptor Resistance

Perhaps the most important development in the use of anti-EGFR agents over the past several years has been the recognition that these agents only have the potential to be beneficial to patients whose tumors have nonmutated, or wild-type, KRAS gene. KRAS is a signal transduction protein that is a critical intermediate in transmission of growth and survival signals from the EGFR to the nucleus. Mutations in exon 2 of the gene that encodes for the KRAS protein lead to constitutive activation of this signaling pathway, which renders blocking of the EGFR-binding site on the surface useless. Several small retrospective series identified KRAS mutations as being incompatible with responses to cetuximab.[391,392] Subsequently, Amado et al.[393] demonstrated that the activity of panitumumab in the registration study referenced previously was limited to those patients with wild-type KRAS. In this trial, 92% of patients had tissue available for KRAS genotyping, and 43% of tumors were found to harbor a mutation in codons 12 or 13 in exon 2 of KRAS. The objective response rate to single-agent panitumumab was 17% in KRAS wild-type tumors and 0% in those tumors that had a KRAS

mutation. The progression-free survival in the patients with KRAS wild-type tumor who received panitumumab was 12.3 weeks versus 7.3 weeks for best supportive care. In patients with KRAS-mutated tumors, there was no difference in progression-free survival with panitumumab versus best supportive care. Again, overall survival in this trial could not be interpreted due to extensive postprogression crossover.

Similarly, analysis of the National Cancer Institute Canada study, discussed previously, demonstrated that activity of cetuximab as a single agent in chemotherapy-refractory disease was limited to the KRAS wild-type patients only (Table 57.18).[394] Approximately 70% of patients in this trial had tissue available for KRAS genotyping, and 42% were found to have mutated KRAS. Those with mutated KRAS showed no evidence of clinical benefit from cetuximab, while patients whose tumors had wild-type K-ras showed a 4.7-month improvement in median overall survival with cetuximab versus best supportive care (9.5 months versus 4.8 months; HR for death = 0.55; 95% CI = 0.41 to 0.74; $p <0.001$). In the control group who received best supportive care, KRAS mutation status had no impact on median overall survival ($p = 0.97$). Although some data have suggested that tumors with KRAS exon 2, codon 13 mutatuions might still garner some benefit from first-line treatment with cetuximab or panitumumab,[395] subsequent data have refuted this, and any KRAS exon 2 mutation remains a firm contraindication to treatment with an EGFR inhibitor. (More recently, a retrospective analysis suggested that in addition to exon 2 KRAS mutations, tumors with mutated BRAF, NRAS, or PIK3CA were significantly associated with a low response rate to cetuximab or panitumumab.[396]) The question of the impact of other KRAS mutations outside of exon 2 has been further addressed, as has the impact of NRAS mutations. Data strongly suggest that the presence of any KRAS or NRAS mutation confers resistance to cetuximab and panitumumab, and that these agents should not be used in patients whose tumors harbor any of these mutations.[150] The role of BRAF genotyping remians less definitive. While an unpreplanned retrospective subset analysis of a combination of two first-line trials suggests some possible contribution of cetuximab in patients with BRAF-mutated tumors, most published datasets of patients treated in the nonfirst-line setting show essentially no activity for cetuximab or panaitumumab in patients with BRAF-mutated tumors.

Genotyping for KRAS mutation status should now be regarded as standard practice in all patients with stage IV disease, and cetuximab and panitumumab should only be considered in patients with nonmutated KRAS.[397] Importantly, using a matched set of resected metastases and primary tumors from 84 patients, Vakiani et al.[398] demonstrated near-complete concordance between primary and metastasis for RAS, BRAF, and PIK3CA. Therefore, genotyping of the primary tumor is sufficient and patients do not need to be subjected to a biopsy of a metastatic site for the purposes of tissue genotyping.

It is prudent to obtain KRAS genotyping at the time that stage IV disease is diagnosed, not necessarily because the information is needed for first-line therapy, as only a minority of patients will be

TABLE 57.18

Cetuximab Versus Best Supportive Care in Metastatic Chemotherapy-Refractory Colorectal Cancer

	Overall Survival		Progression-Free Survival		Response Rate	
	KRAS Wt	KRAS Mut	KRAS Wt	KRAS Mut	KRAS Wt	KRAS Mut
Cetux	9.5 mo	4.5 mo	3.7 mo	1.8 mo	12.8%	1.2%
BSC	4.8 mo	4.6 mo	1.9 mo	1.8 mo	0%	0%
P value	0.001	0.89	0.001	0.96	NR	NR

Wt, wild type; Mut, mutant; Cetux, cetuximab; BSC, best supportive care; NR, not reported.
From Karapetis CS, Khambata-Ford S, Jonker DJ, et al. K-ras mutations and benefit from cetuximab in advanced colorectal cancer. *N Engl J Med* 2008;359: 1757–1765.

appropriate for first-line anti-EGFR therapy, but because whether a patient can consider the use of cetuximab or panitumumab in the course of multiple lines of therapy is easier to both determine and to deal with early on when there are multiple options, rather than waiting until all other options are exhausted. At present, there is no role for determining KRAS status in stage I, II, or III disease, as there is no basis for use of EGFR agents in other than stage IV.

Preliminary data suggests that KRAS status might play a role in oxaliplatin sensitivity as well. In vitro analysis, published by Lin et al.[399] demonstrated that this mutation caused downregulation of ERCC1 (excision repair cross-complementation group 1), which led to enhanced oxaliplatin sensitivity. Overexpression of ERCC1 has been shown previously to be associated with resistance to platinum-based therapy in a number of cancers. Improved understanding of this pathway may prove critical toward defining new targets for KRAS-mutant CRC treatment.[399]

Cetuximab or Panitumumab in First-Line Therapy

A 1,200-patient study of FOLFIRI with or without cetuximab, known at the CRYSTAL trial, has been reported.[400] The primary end point of the trial, progression-free survival, was statistically significantly improved with the addition of cetuximab, albeit by only 0.9 month, or 27 days. When the study was analyzed in terms of KRAS genotype, those patients with mutated KRAS showed no benefit, while those with wild-type KRAS showed a progression-free survival improvement of 1.2 months, or 37 days, but also a median overall survival improvement from 20.0 months to 23.5 months (HR = 0.796; p = 0.0093).[401] Response rates were also statistically significantly higher (57.3% versus 39.7%) in the cetuximab arm for the KRAS wild-type tumors. Skin rash and diarrhea were increased in the cetuximab arm. As has been noted in virtually all trials of anti-EGFR agents, there was a strong correlation between severity of skin rash and clinical benefit, with progression-free survival advantage being limited to those patients with grade 2 or 3 skin rash. BRAF was confirmed as a poor prognostic factor but was not predictive of response to cetuximab in this trial. The numbers of BRAF-mutated tumors limit the power to detect a predictive role of BRAF in this trial, however.

FOLFOX with or without cetuximab had been initially investigated in a randomized phase 2 trial in which the primary end point was response rate.[402] A total of 337 patients were treated. The overall response rate was improved by the addition of cetuximab from 36% to 46%, a result that did not achieve statistical significance (p = 0.64). For the KRAS wild-type patients, however, the result was more robust, with an improvement from 37% to 61% (p = 0.011). Progression-free survival was very modestly, albeit statistically significantly improved in the KRAS wild-type patients by a median of 15 days; however, progression-free survival was statistically significantly *worse* in the cetuximab arm in those patients whose tumors had mutated KRAS.

However, several larger phase 3 trials have cast considerable doubt on the role of cetuximab in conjunction with oxaliplatin-based therapy. In the Medical Research Council COIN trial, 1,603 patients with previously untreated metastatic CRC were treated with oxaliplatin plus a fluoropyrimidine (either the FOLFOX or Cape/Ox regimen) and randomized to receive cetuximab in addition or not. In the patients with KRAS wild-type tumors (367 with cetuximab plus oxaliplatin-containing chemotherapy and 362 with oxaliplatin-containing chemotherapy alone), there was no improvement in overall survival (17.9 months versus 17 months; HR = 1.04; p = 0.67) or in progression-free survival (8.6 months versus 8.6 months in the two arms). Overall response rate increased from 57% to 64% with the addition of cetuximab (p = 0.049). The data from this trial do not support use of cetuximab with front-line oxaliplatin-based chemotherapy. Outcomes were worse with the addition of cetuximab to capecitabine plus oxaliplatin, and the use of that combination is specifically not recommended.[403] In addition, the Nordic VII trial investigated the addition of cetuximab to the Nordic FLOX regimen of oxaliplatin, bolus 5-FU and leucovorin in a 571-patient phase 3 trial.[404]

Patients were randomized to one of three arms: Nordic FLOX given continuously, cetuximab plus Nordic FLOX given continuously, or cetuximab plus Nordic FLOX given intermittently. There were no statistically significant differences in the median progression-free survival between the three arms (7.9 months, 8.3 months, and 7.3 months, respectively). Overall survival also showed no difference between the three arms (20.4 months, 19.7 months, and 20.3 months, respectively). Even in patients with KRAS wild-type tumors, cetuximab did not provide demonstrable benefit.

Taken in the aggregate, the data do not lend substantial support to the use of cetuximab with oxaliplatin-based chemotherapy. Curiously, however, the results with panitumumab are somewhat different. In a phase 3 trial of FOLFOX with or without panitumumab (6 mg/kg every 14 days), 1,183 patients were randomized, of whom 60% had wild-type KRAS.[405] Progression-free survival was modestly but statistically significantly improved with panitumumab in the KRAS wild-type patients (9.6 months versus 8 months; p = 0.02), and response rate was increased from 48% to 55%. However, as was seen with cetuximab, in the patients with KRAS-mutated tumors, the addition of panitumumab resulted in a statistically significant *worsening* of median progression-free survival from 8.8 months in the control arm to 7.3 months in the panitumumab-containing arm. In an updated analysis focusing on KRAS wild-type patients only, as statistically significant survival benefit was seen with the addition of panitumumab in this cohort.[150] The addition of panitumumab resulted in increased skin rash, diarrhea, and hypomagnesemia.

Also reported in abstract form is a phase 3 trial of second-line FOLFIRI with or without panitumumab.[406] Despite this being a second-line study, patients had an excellent performance status (ECOG 0 or 1 in 94% of patients). KRAS mutations were present in 45% of patients. For the patients with KRAS wild-type tumors, the progression-free survival was statistically significantly improved in the panitumumab-containing arm (5.9 months versus 3.9 months; p = 0.004), and response rate was improved as well (35% versus 10%). Overall survival differences in favor of the panitumumab arm (14.5 months versus 12.5 months) did not reach statistical significance (p = 0.1). There were no differences in efficacy outcomes with the addition of panitumumab in the patients with KRAS-mutated tumors. Again, skin rash, diarrhea, and hypomagnesemia were increased in the panitumumab arm.

More recently the long-awaited initial results of the NCI cooperative group 80405 study have been reported in abstract form. In this trial, patients with previously untreated metastatic colorectal cancer with wild-type KRAS were enrolled. Patients were assigned to receive either FOLFOX or FOLFIRI per physician preference, and then randomized to receive either cetuximab or bevacizumab. There was no difference in overall survival, the primary study endpoint, between the cetuximab and bevacizumab arms (29.0 months vs 29.9 months, p = 0.34).[407]

Toxicities of Anti–Epidermal Growth Factor Receptor Monoclonal Antibodies

The primary toxicity of cetuximab and panitumumab is an acne-like rash, which is seen to some degree in from 75% to 100% of patients treated. This rash is not acne, and it is accompanied by skin dryness and paronychial cracking. Other than moisturizers, which are recommended, no topical agents have been shown to be of benefit in the treatment of this rash. Drying agents and retinoids, such as are used in the treatment of acne, are contraindicated. Anecdotal reports of benefit for topical steroids or antibiotics do not have supportive randomized data, and as the natural history of the rash is to wax and wane, interpretation of these anecdotal reports is problematic. There are data suggesting that prophylactic use of oral antibiotics may somewhat mitigate the severity of the rash.[408] Importantly, it has been well established that there is a clear correlation between severity of skin rash and favorable outcome with

EGFR agents.[409] The mechanism of this correlation has not yet been determined; however, it is clear that benefit from these agents is virtually confined to those patients who experience a grade 2 or 3 skin rash. A severe rash does not guarantee a response or clinical benefit; however, absence of a rash after the first month of therapy is virtually incompatible with clinical benefit from these agents. This is an important point to consider, especially in consideration of front-line use; only those patients with a very substantial rash stand a chance of benefit.

Hypersensitivity reactions, which are anaphylactoid in nature and are completely separate and distinct from the skin rash toxicity discussed previously, occur in approximately 3% of patients with cetuximab and <1% of patients with panitumumab. Almost all of these reactions are first-dose events. Dramatic regional differences in the frequency of these reactions have been noted, with serious hypersensitivity reactions to cetuximab noted in up to 20% of patients in North Carolina and Tennessee, while the serious hypersensitivity reaction rate in the northeastern United States is <1%.[410] Subsequently, it has been demonstrated that there is a high prevalence of cetuximab-specific IgE in Tennessee, suggesting cross-reactivity with an environmental allergen.[411] Panitumumab does not appear to exhibit this marked regional variation in incidence of hypersensitivity reaction, and would be the clearly preferred agent over cetuximab in these areas of high incidence of cetuximab hypersensitivity.

It should be noted that the incidence of skin rash appears to be quite similar between cetuximab and panitumumab, as does the degree of clinical activity. Thus, outside of the areas that see high frequency of cetuximab hypersensitivity reactions, there appears to be little reason to favor one agent over the other. Case reports and anecdotal evidence suggest that patients who experience hypersensitivity to cetuximab do typically tolerate panitumumab. There is no basis, however, for using one of these agents after clinical failure on the other.

Another more recently recognized toxicity of anti-EGFR therapy is hypomagnesemia.[412] This result is due to hypermagnesemia, presumably promoted by EGFR antagonism in the loop of Henle. Regular monitoring of serum magnesium levels, and intravenous magnesium supplementation, when indicated, should be practiced routinely with anti-EGFR therapies. Oral magnesium is unlikely to provide adequate supplementation, as diarrhea from this is often dose-limiting.

Cetuximab and Panitumumab in Epidermal Growth Factor Receptor–Negative Patients

From the outset of clinical development, the assumption was made that quantitative EGFR expression would be predictive of the activity, or lack thereof, of an anti-EGFR antibody, and that an absence of demonstrable EGFR expression would therefore preclude clinical activity of cetuximab or panitumumab. For this reason, all early trials with these agents required that the patient's tumor shows EGFR positivity by IHC as a criterion for study eligibility. This assumption, that EGFR expression would be predictive, has never been supported by clinical or preclinical data and has been refuted by all clinical data that have addressed the issue. All of the reported cetuximab trials to date, the earlier ones of which excluded EGFR-negative patients altogether, have demonstrated absolutely no correlation between the intensity of the EGFR expression and clinical response.[245,385] Additionally, the results of a small cohort of nine patients who were EGFR-negative and treated with cetuximab were reported in abstract form.[413] Two major objective responses were reported by the investigators, one of which was confirmed as a major response by third-party review and one of which was not.

On the basis of the lack of correlation between EGFR staining intensity and response, as well as the small data set outlined previously, a decision was made at Memorial Sloan Kettering Cancer Center in New York that patients with EGFR-negative CRC

would not be excluded from standard off-protocol treatment with cetuximab simply on the basis of EGFR status. Subsequently, a retrospective review was conducted using the computerized pharmacy records to identify all patients who had received non-research cetuximab-based therapy at Memorial Sloan Kettering Cancer Center in the first 3 months of cetuximab's commercial availability. This review identified 16 patients with irinotecan-refractory, EGFR-negative CRC who had been treated. Fourteen of these patients had received cetuximab in combination with irinotecan and two had received cetuximab alone. Of the 16, four patients experienced major objective (response rate = 25%; 95% CI = 4% to 46%), demonstrating that the hypothesis that a negative EGFR stain would preclude the possibility of response to cetuximab is false.[414] A similar lack of correlation of EGFR staining and activity with panitumumab has also more recently been reported.[415]

Because current EGFR IHC techniques have no predictive value, these techniques have no role in current management of CRC. The exclusion of a patient from cetuximab-based or panitumumab-based therapy solely on the basis of EGFR IHC is not appropriate. Likewise, no patient, with CRC or otherwise, should be given an anti-EGFR treatment solely on the basis of a high EGFR IHC expression.

Bevacizumab Plus Anti–Epidermal Growth Factor Receptor Agents

Given the reported activity of both bevacizumab and cetuximab, investigators logically became interested in the idea of concurrent use of these agents. Both some limited preclinical data, as well as mechanistic understandings of potential interaction between anti-EGFR and anti-VEGF pathways, supported the concept. As will be discussed subsequently, this concept serves as yet another example of perfectly logical, well-thought out assumptions supported by preliminary clinical evidence that turned out to be incorrect when subjected to the appropriately rigorous test of an adequately powered clinical trial.

The first study to attempt to administer bevacizumab and cetuximab concurrently was a small randomized phase 2 study of bevacizumab added to cetuximab alone or to cetuximab plus irinotecan in patients with irinotecan-refractory CRC.[416] This was a feasibility trial to assess the safety of concurrent administration of these agents and to look for preliminary evidence of efficacy. The study concluded that coadministration of these two monoclonal antibodies together was feasible, and that the preliminary data were encouraging. It should be noted, however, that this was a small feasibility trial with 41 and 40 patients, respectively, reported in each arm. Furthermore, this study was conducted in patients who were naive to both cetuximab and bevacizumab. As most patients now receive bevacizumab with their first-line regimen, the results in the bevacizumab-naive population might not necessarily have a bearing on current practice today. A small follow-up trial in patients with prior progression on a front-line bevacizumab-containing regimen showed far less activity, with 3 of 33 patients (9%) achieving a partial response and a median time to tumor progression of 3.9 months.[417] These small trials were designed to serve as the safety pilots for large-scale front-line studies that combined bevacizumab plus cetuximab with front-line chemotherapy. Two such studies have now been reported, with alarming results, which highlights the dangers of jumping to conclusions prior to the availability of mature, definitive data.

The CAIRO-2 study randomized 755 patients with previously untreated metastatic CRC to Cape/Ox-bevacizumab with or without concurrent cetuximab (Table 57.19A).[418] Not only was there not a benefit to the addition of cetuximab, but the group receiving cetuximab actually had a worse median progression-free survival of 9.4 months, compared to 10.7 months in the Cape/Ox-bevacizumab–alone arm ($p = 0.01$). Response rates were identical

TABLE 57.19A

Capecitabine, Oxaliplatin, and Bevacizumab with or without Cetuximab in Metastatic Colorectal Cancer

Overall	Median Progression-Free Survival	Median Response	Objective Survival Rates
COB (n = 332)	20.3 mo	10.7 mo	50%
COB plus cetux (n = 317)	19.4 mo	9.4 mo	52.7%
P value	0.16	0.01	0.49

COB, capecitabine, oxaliplatin, bevacizumab; cetux, cetuximab.
From Tol J, Koopman M, Cats A, et al. Chemotherapy, bevacizumab, and cetuximab in metastatic colorectal cancer. *N Engl J Med* 2009;360:563–572.

(44%) in the two arms. Furthermore, quality-of-life scores were lower in the cetuximab-containing arm. Overall survival was not statistically significantly different between the two groups. Even for the wild-type KRAS patients, there was no benefit in progression-free survival with the addition of cetuximab. As might now be anticipated (Table 57.19B), within the cetuximab-containing arm, patients whose tumors had mutated KRAS had statistically significantly decreased progression-free survival compared to those with wild-type KRAS tumors (8.1 months versus 10.5 months; $p = 0.04$). However, for the patients with KRAS mutations, those who received cetuximab also had a worse outcome than those on the noncetuximab-containing control arm (progression-free survival 8.1 months versus 12.5 months, $p = 0.003$; overall survival 17.2 months versus 24.9 months, $p = 0.03$).

Another study that investigated the use of combined bevacizumab plus anti-EGFR monoclonal antibody was the Panitumumab in Advanced Colon Cancer Evaluation (PACCE) trial.[419] This trial used FOLFOX-bevacizumab (823 patients) or FOLFIRI-bevacizumab (230 patients) and randomized them with or without concurrent panitumumab. Again, the result of adding the anti-EGFR to chemotherapy plus bevacizumab was not only not beneficial, but was actually detrimental. The median progression-free survival for the overall study was 10.0 months versus 11.4 months for the panitumumab-containing versus chemotherapy-bevacizumab–alone arm. The median overall survival was decreased by 5.1 months, from 24.5 months in the control arm to 19.4 months in the panitumumab arm. Toxicity, including not only skin rash but also diarrhea, infections, and pulmonary embolisms, was more frequent in the panitumumab-containing arm, and worse outcomes were seen in the panitumumab-containing arm regardless of KRAS mutation status.

Clearly, the concurrent use of anti-EGFR monoclonal antibodies, bevacizumab, and cytotoxic chemotherapy, despite supportive encouraging preliminary data, is not an acceptable treatment strategy. The reasons for this unanticipated negative interaction remain unknown at this time.

Oral Epidermal Growth Factor Receptor, Vascular Endothelial Growth Factor, and Cyclooxygenase-2 Inhibitors

The limited experiences with the oral EGFR tyrosine kinase inhibitors gefitinib (ZD1839) and erlotinib (OSI-774) in CRC have been essentially negative, and at present there is no role for these agents in this disease.[420,421] This is consistent with the findings that the activating mutation seen in lung cancer required for anti-EGFR tyrosine kinase activity does not appear to occur in CRC.

Oral VEGF tyrosine kinase inhibitors, with the exception of regorafenib noted previously, have been similarly disappointing. Sunitinib showed essentially no activity as a single agent in chemotherapy-refractory disease, and front-line trials of chemotherapy with or without sunitinib, as well as chemotherapy with or without sorafenib, have now been closed early by their respective data monitoring committees for futility.[422] Two large, randomized trials of FOLFOX with or without the investigational VEGF tyrosine kinase inhibitor PTK-787 have also been reported as negative trials.

Cyclooxygenase-2 Inhibitors. Cyclooxygenase-2 (COX-2) catalyzes the synthesis of prostaglandins in the inflammatory response process. COX-2 has been frequently shown to be upregulated in malignant and premalignant tissues. COX-2 expression has been correlated with increased invasiveness, resistance to apoptosis, and increased angiogenesis.[423] The science behind COX-2 inhibition appeared so compelling that many clinicians had chosen to add drugs such as celecoxib or rofecoxib (now withdrawn from the market for safety reasons) in the absence of efficacy data with the assumption that "it couldn't hurt." Evidence that use of either NSAIDs or selective COX-2 inhibitors has a beneficial role in the treatment of CRC is lacking. The large randomized BICC-C trial showed no benefit whatsoever for the use of celecoxib in terms of either safety or efficacy.[334] In the absence of any emerging data to the contrary, routine use of COX-2 inhibitors with chemotherapy is not recommended.

The role of aspirin as an adjuvant agent is also of particular interest, especially after a recent case-control study suggested that

TABLE 57.19B

Impact of KRAS Mutation Status on Addition of Cetuximab to Capecitabine, Oxaliplatin, and Bevacizumab

	Overall Survival COB + COB cetux	Progression-Free Survival COB + COB cetux
KRAS wild-type	22.4 mo 21.8 mo (p = 0.64)	10.6 mo 10.5 mo (p = 0.30)
KRAS mutated	24.9 mo 17.2 mo (p = 0.03)	12.5 mo 8.1 mo (p = 0.003)

COB, capecitabine, oxaliplatin-bevacizumab; cetux, cetuximab.
From Tol J, Koopman M, Cats A, et al. Chemotherapy, bevacizumab, and cetuximab in metastatic colorectal cancer. *N Engl J Med* 2009;360:563–572.

initiation of this medication after diagnosis reduced overall CRC specific mortality (HR = 0.53; 95% CI = 0.33 to 0.86).[424] The ASCOLT study is the first randomized, placebo-controlled trial designed to investigate this question in patients with stage III-IV and high-risk stage II disease. End points will include DFS and overall survival with anticipated follow-up of 5 years.[425]

In the meantime, a large observational study of 4,481 patients lends further support to the potential therapeutic benefits of aspirin in CRC. The authors report a 23% decrease in disease-specific mortality for patients who took aspirin for any length of time after diagnosis compared to nonaspirin users as well as a 30% lower disease-specific mortality for those who took aspirin for 9 months after diagnosis. A survival benefit was also found for prediagnosis users, although this was less pronounced at 12%.[426]

Other Novel Agents

The number of agents that are undergoing early evaluation in CRC is too large to allow a complete discussion of these in this chapter. Many are variations on the currently available agents and are unlikely to substantially move the field if successful in gaining approval. At present, no new agent with a unique mechanism of action has been identified as having meaningful activity in CRC. Furthermore, all of these at this point are of research interest only and do not have a role in standard treatment of CRC at this time.

MOLECULAR PREDICTIVE MARKERS

With the availability now of a number of active agents, the ability to prospectively select a particular drug or drug combination that would have an increased likelihood of efficacy or a decreased likelihood of toxicity would be clinically useful. Such means of rational selection do not yet exist.

One avenue of investigation has been the elucidation of markers of resistance to 5-FU based on knowledge of its metabolic pathways. Studies have indicated that high levels of either TS, DPD,[427] or thymidine phosphorylase, as measured in a tumor specimen by reverse transcription–polymerase chain reaction, predict for failure to respond to an infusional 5-FU regimen.[166,428,429] These observations are intriguing but are insufficient to exclude the use of 5-FU in a particular patient, and they need to be validated in large-scale prospective trials before being applied to routine practice. There is, at this time, no role for the use of these markers in standard practice. Others have investigated genomic analysis as an indicator of response or toxicity.[170,430] Although these approaches appear promising, they are not yet validated and should not be considered as part of standard care.

A recently reported mechanism of resistance thought to be independent of other mutations or MSI involves the tumor suppressor gene TFAP2E (transcription factor AP-2 epsilon) and its downstream target DKK4(dickkopf homolog 4 protein). In an analysis of 220 patients with CRC, Ebert et al.[431] found that hypermethylation of TFAP2E led to decreased protein expression and was significantly associated with nonresponse to 5-FU–based chemotherapy, whereas hypomethylation yielded a six-fold higher likelihood of response. Moreover, TFAP2E hypermethylation in vitro led to overexpression of DKK4, which was in turn associated with increased chemoresistance to 5-FU but not irinotecan and oxaliplatin. The authors suggest that future studies focus on specific targeting of DKK4 to overcome this pathway of chemoresistance.[431]

SELECTED REFERENCES

The full reference list can be accessed at lwwhealthlibrary.com/oncology.

1. Jemal A, Center MM, DeSantis C, et al. Global patterns of cancer incidence and mortality rates and trends. *Cancer Epidemiol Biomarkers Prev* 2010;19:1893–1907.
2. Jemal A, Siegel R, Xu J, et al. Cancer statistics, 2010. *CA Cancer J Clin* 2010;60:277–300.
3. Lieberman DA, Weiss DG, Bond JH, et al. Use of colonoscopy to screen asymptomatic adults for colorectal cancer. Veterans Affairs Cooperative Study Group 380. *N Engl J Med* 2000;343:162–168.
4. Davis DM, Marcet JE, Frattini JC, et al. Is it time to lower the recommended screening age for colorectal cancer? *J Am Coll Surg* 2011;213:352–361.
7. Parkin DM, Pisani P, Ferlay J. Global cancer statistics. *CA Cancer J Clin* 1999;49:33–64, 1.
8. Nelson RL, Persky V, Turyk M. Determination of factors responsible for the declining incidence of colorectal cancer. *Dis Colon Rectum* 1999;42:741–752.
13. Laken SJ, Petersen GM, Gruber SB, et al. Familial colorectal cancer in Ashkenazim due to a hypermutable tract in APC. *Nat Genet* 1997;17:79–83.
15. Weber TK, Chin HM, Rodriguez-Bigas M, et al. Novel hMLH1 and hMSH2 germline mutations in African Americans with colorectal cancer. *JAMA* 1999;281:2316–2320.
18. Yothers G, Sargent DJ, Wolmark N, et al. Outcomes among black patients with stage II and III colon cancer receiving chemotherapy: an analysis of ACCENT adjuvant trials. *J Natl Cancer Inst* 2011;103:1498–1506.
20. Wilmink AB. Overview of the epidemiology of colorectal cancer. *Dis Colon Rectum* 1997;40:483–493.
21. Obrand DI, Gordon PH. Continued change in the distribution of colorectal carcinoma. *Br J Surg* 1998;85:246–248.
24. Thibodeau SN, French AJ, Cunningham JM, et al. Microsatellite instability in colorectal cancer: different mutator phenotypes and the principal involvement of hMLH1. *Cancer Res* 1998;58:1713–1718.
25. Fink D, Nebel S, Norris PS, et al. The effect of different chemotherapeutic agents on the enrichment of DNA mismatch repair-deficient tumour cells. *Br J Cancer* 1998;77:703–708.
27. Fuchs CS, Giovannucci EL, Colditz GA, et al. A prospective study of family history and the risk of colorectal cancer. *N Engl J Med* 1994;331:1669–1674.
29. Guillem JG, Forde KA, Treat MR, et al. Colonoscopic screening for neoplasms in asymptomatic first-degree relatives of colon cancer patients. A controlled, prospective study. *Dis Colon Rectum* 1992;35:523–529.

30. Winawer SJ, Zauber AG, Gerdes H, et al. Risk of colorectal cancer in the families of patients with adenomatous polyps. National Polyp Study Workgroup. *N Engl J Med* 1996;334:82–87.
31. Ponz de Leon M, Scapoli C, Zanghieri G, et al. Genetic transmission of colorectal cancer: exploratory data analysis from a population based registry. *J Med Genet* 1992;29:531–538.
36. Hartz A, He T, Ross JJ. Risk factors for colon cancer in 150,912 postmenopausal women. *Cancer Causes Control* 2012;23:1599–1605.
39. Renehan AG, Flood A, Adams KF, et al. Body mass index at different adult ages, weight change, and colorectal cancer risk in the National Institutes of Health-AARP Cohort. *Am J Epidemiol* 2012;176:1130–1140.
40. Potter JD. Colorectal cancer: molecules and populations. *J Natl Cancer Inst* 1999;91:916–932.
41. Willett WC, Stampfer MJ, Colditz GA, et al. Relation of meat, fat, and fiber intake to the risk of colon cancer in a prospective study among women. *N Engl J Med* 1990;323:1664–1672.
44. Parr CL, Hjartaker A, Lund E, et al. Meat intake, cooking methods and risk of proximal colon, distal colon and rectal cancer: the Norwegian Women and Cancer (NOWAC) cohort study. *Int J Cancer* 2013;133:1153–1163.
46. McCullough ML, Gapstur SM, Shah R, et al. Association between red and processed meat intake and mortality among colorectal cancer survivors. *J Clin Oncol* 2013;31:2773–2782.
48. Sinha R, Cross AJ, Daniel CR, et al. Caffeinated and decaffeinated coffee and tea intakes and risk of colorectal cancer in a large prospective study. *Am J Clin Nutr* 2012;96:374–381.
49. Burkitt DP. Epidemiology of cancer of the colon and rectum. 1971. *Dis Colon Rectum* 1993;36:1071–1082.
51. Murphy N, Norat T, Ferrari P, et al. Dietary fibre intake and risks of cancers of the colon and rectum in the European prospective investigation into cancer and nutrition (EPIC). *PLoS One* 2012;7:e39361.
53. Schatzkin A, Lanza E, Corle D, et al. Lack of effect of a low-fat, high-fiber diet on the recurrence of colorectal adenomas. Polyp Prevention Trial Study Group. *N Engl J Med* 2000;342:1149–1155.
54. Alberts DS, Martinez ME, Roe DJ, et al. Lack of effect of a high-fiber cereal supplement on the recurrence of colorectal adenomas. Phoenix Colon Cancer Prevention Physicians' Network. *N Engl J Med* 2000;342:1156–1162.
55. Wargovich MJ. New dietary anticarcinogens and prevention of gastrointestinal cancer. *Dis Colon Rectum* 1988;31:72–75.
56. Bamia C, Lajiou P, Buckland G, et al. Mediterranean diet and colorectal cancer risk: results from a European cohort. *Eur J Epidemiol* 2013;28:317–328.

57. Bostick RM, Fosdick L, Wood JR, et al. Calcium and colorectal epithelial cell proliferation in sporadic adenoma patients: a randomized, double-blinded, placebo-controlled clinical trial. *J Natl Cancer Inst* 1995;87:1307–1315.

58. Chen GC, Pang Z, Liu QF. Magnesium intake and risk of colorectal cancer: a meta-analysis of prospective studies. *Eur J Clin Nutr* 2012;66:1182–1186.

59. Ma Y, Zhang P, Wang F, et al. Association between vitamin D and risk of colorectal cancer: a systematic review of prospective studies. *J Clin Oncol* 2011;29:3775–3782.

62. Campbell PT, Patel AV, Newton CC, et al. Associations of recreational physical activity and leisure time spent sitting with colorectal cancer survival. *J Clin Oncol* 2013;31:876–885.

64. Gong J, Hutter C, Baron JA, et al. A pooled analysis of smoking and colorectal cancer: timing of exposure and interactions with environmental factors. *Cancer Epidemiol Biomarkers Prev* 2012;21:1974–1985.

66. Deng L, Gui Z, Zhao L, et al. Diabetes mellitus and the incidence of colorectal cancer: an updated systematic review and meta-analysis. *Dig Dis Sci* 2012;57:1576–1585.

68. Thun MJ, Namboodiri MM, Heath CW Jr. Aspirin use and reduced risk of fatal colon cancer. *N Engl J Med* 1991;325:1593–1596.

69. Rosenberg L, Louik C, Shapiro S. Nonsteroidal antiinflammatory drug use and reduced risk of large bowel carcinoma. *Cancer* 1998;82:2326–2333.

70. Rothwell PM, Wilson M, Elwin CE, et al. Long-term effect of aspirin on colorectal cancer incidence and mortality: 20-year follow-up of five randomised trials. *Lancet* 2010;376:1741–1750.

71. Liao X, Lochhead P, Nishihara R, et al. Aspirin use, tumor PIK3CA mutation, and colorectal-cancer survival. *N Engl J Med* 2012;367:1596–1606.

73. Singh S, Singh AG, Murad MH, et al. Bisphosphonates are associated with reduced risk of colorectal cancer: a systematic review and meta-analysis. *Clin Gastroenterol Hepatol* 2013;11:232–239.e1.

74. Toriola AT, Cheng TY, Neuhouser ML, et al. Biomarkers of inflammation are associated with colorectal cancer risk in women but are not suitable as early detection markers. *Int J Cancer* 2013;132:2648–2658.

78. Damin DC, Ziegelmann PK, Damin AP. Human papillomavirus infection and colorectal cancer risk: a meta-analysis. *Colorectal Dis* 2013;15:e420–428.

79. Rustgi AK. Hereditary gastrointestinal polyposis and nonpolyposis syndromes. *N Engl J Med* 1994;331:1694–1702.

82. Powell SM, Petersen GM, Krush AJ, et al. Molecular diagnosis of familial adenomatous polyposis. *N Engl J Med* 1993;329:1982–1987.

84. Chung DC, Rustgi AK. The hereditary nonpolyposis colorectal cancer syndrome: genetics and clinical implications. *Ann Intern Med* 2003;138:560–570.

87. Burt RW. Familial risk and colorectal cancer. *Gastroenterol Clin North Am* 1996;25:793–803.

88. Garcia-Ruiz A, Milsom JW, Ludwig KA, et al. Right colonic arterial anatomy. Implications for laparoscopic surgery. *Dis Colon Rectum* 1996;39:906–911.

90. Colquhoun PH, Wexner SD. Surgical management of colon cancer. *Curr Gastroenterol Rep* 2002;4:414–419.

93. Majumdar SR, Fletcher RH, Evans AT. How does colorectal cancer present? Symptoms, duration, and clues to location. *Am J Gastroenterol* 1999;94:3039–3045.

94. Rocklin MS, Senagore AJ, Talbott TM. Role of carcinoembryonic antigen and liver function tests in the detection of recurrent colorectal carcinoma. *Dis Colon Rectum* 1991;34:794–797.

95. Stotland BR, Siegelman ES, Morris JB, et al. Preoperative and postoperative imaging for colorectal cancer. *Hematol Oncol Clin North Am* 1997;11:635–654.

98. Lidgard GP, Domanico MJ, Bruinsma JJ, et al. Clinical performance of an automated stool DNA assay for detection of colorectal neoplasia. *Clin Gastroenterol Hepatol* 2013;11:1313–1318.

99. Pickhardt PJ, Choi JR, Hwang I, et al. Computed tomographic virtual colonoscopy to screen for colorectal neoplasia in asymptomatic adults. *N Engl J Med* 2003;349:2191–2200.

103. Boone D, Halligan S, Taylor SA. Evidence review and status update on computed tomography colonography. *Curr Gastroenterol Rep* 2011;13:486–494.

105. Compton CC. Surgical pathology of colorectal cancer. In Saltz LB, ed. *Colorectal Cancer: Multimodality Management*. Totowa, NJ: Humana Press; 2002:247–265.

106. Edge SB, ed. *AJCC Cancer Staging Manual*. Vol. 7. Berlin: Springer; 2010.

107. Greene FL, Stewart AK, Norton HJ. A new TNM staging strategy for node-positive (stage III) rectal cancer: An analysis of 5,988 patients. In *Thirty-Ninth Annual Meeting of the ASCO*. Chicago, IL: American Society of Clinical Oncology; 2003.

109. Compton CC, Fielding LP, Burgart LJ, et al. Prognostic factors in colorectal cancer. College of American Pathologists Consensus Statement 1999. *Arch Pathol Lab Med* 2000;124:979–994.

110. Ratto C, Sofo L, Ippoliti M, et al. Accurate lymph-node detection in colorectal specimens resected for cancer is of prognostic significance. *Dis Colon Rectum* 1999;42:143–154, discussion 154–158.

114. Morikawa T, Tanaka N, Kuchiba A, et al. Predictors of lymph node count in colorectal cancer resections: data from US nationwide prospective cohort studies. *Arch Surg* 2012;147:715–723.

115. Joseph NE, Sigurdson ER, Hanson AL, et al. Accuracy of determining nodal negativity in colorectal cancer on the basis of the number of nodes retrieved on resection. *Ann Surg Oncol* 2003;10:213–218.

119. Hong KD, Lee SI, Moon HY. Lymph node ratio as determined by the 7th edition of the American Joint Committee on Cancer staging system predicts survival in stage III colon cancer. *J Surg Oncol* 2011;103:406–410.

120. Gao P, Song YX, Wang ZN, et al. Integrated ratio of metastatic to examined lymph nodes and number of metastatic lymph nodes into the AJCC staging system for colon cancer. *PLoS One* 2012;7:e35021.

121. Liefers GJ, Cleton-Jansen AM, van de Velde CJ, et al. Micrometastases and survival in stage II colorectal cancer. *N Engl J Med* 1998;339:223–228.

125. Faerden AE, Sjo OH, Bukholm IR, et al. Lymph node micrometastases and isolated tumor cells influence survival in stage I and II colon cancer. *Dis Colon Rectum* 2011;54:200–206.

128. Saha S, Wiese D, Badin J, et al. Technical details of sentinel lymph node mapping in colorectal cancer and its impact on staging. *Ann Surg Oncol* 2000;7:120–124.

131. Viehl CT, Guller U, Cecini R, et al. Sentinel lymph node procedure leads to upstaging of patients with resectable colon cancer: results of the Swiss prospective, multicenter study sentinel lymph node procedure in colon cancer. *Ann Surg Oncol* 2012;19:1959–1965.

132. Saha S, Johnston J, Korant A, et al. Aberrant drainage of sentinel lymph nodes in colon cancer and its impact on staging and extent of operation. *Am J Surg* 2013;205:302–305, discussion 305–306.

134. Cusack JC, Giacco GG, Cleary K, et al. Survival factors in 186 patients younger than 40 years old with colorectal adenocarcinoma. *J Am Coll Surg* 1996;183:105–112.

138. de la Chapelle A. Microsatellite instability. *N Engl J Med* 2003;349:209–210.

139. Boland CR, Thibodeau SN, Hamilton SR, et al. A National Cancer Institute Workshop on Microsatellite Instability for cancer detection and familial predisposition: development of international criteria for the determination of microsatellite instability in colorectal cancer. *Cancer Res* 1998;58:5248–5257.

141. Thibodeau SN, Bren G, Schaid D. Microsatellite instability in cancer of the proximal colon. *Science* 1993;260:816–819.

144. Gryfe R, Kim H, Hsieh ET, et al. Tumor microsatellite instability and clinical outcome in young patients with colorectal cancer. *N Engl J Med* 2000;342:69–77.

145. Watanabe T, Wu TT, Catalano PJ, et al. Molecular predictors of survival after adjuvant chemotherapy for colon cancer. *N Engl J Med* 2001;344:1196–1206.

147. Sinicrope FA, Mahoney MR, Smyrk TC, et al. Prognostic impact of deficient DNA mismatch repair in patients with stage III colon cancer from a randomized trial of FOLFOX-based adjuvant chemotherapy. *J Clin Oncol* 2013;31:3664–3672.

148. Ogino S, Shima K, Meyerhardt JA, et al. Predictive and prognostic roles of BRAF mutation in stage III colon cancer: results from intergroup trial CALGB 89803. *Clin Cancer Res* 2012;18:890–900.

150. Douillard JY, Oliner KS, Siena S, et al. Panitumumab–FOLFOX4 treatment and RAS mutations in colorectal cancer. *N Engl J Med* 2013;369:1023–1034.

151. Fearon E, Cho KR, Nigro JM, et al. Identification of a chromosome 18q gene that is altered in colorectal cancers. *Science* 1990;247:49–56.

155. Harrison LE, Guillem JG, Paty P, et al. Preoperative carcinoembryonic antigen predicts outcomes in node-negative colon cancer patients: a multivariate analysis of 572 patients. *J Am Coll Surg* 1997;185:55–59.

156. Wolmark N, Fisher B, Wieand HS. The prognostic value of the modifications of the Dukes' C class of colorectal cancer. An analysis of the NSABP clinical trials. *Ann Surg* 1986;203:115–122.

157. Weiss JM, Pfau PR, O'Connor ES, et al. Mortality by stage for right- versus left-sided colon cancer: analysis of surveillance, epidemiology, and end results—Medicare data. *J Clin Oncol* 2011;29:4401–4409.

159. Sinicrope FA, Foster NR, Yothers G, et al. Body mass index at diagnosis and survival among colon cancer patients enrolled in clinical trials of adjuvant chemotherapy. *Cancer* 2013;119:1528–1536.

161. Dehal AN, Newton CC, Jacobs EJ, et al. Impact of diabetes mellitus and insulin use on survival after colorectal cancer diagnosis: the Cancer Prevention Study-II Nutrition Cohort. *J Clin Oncol* 2012;30:53–59.

164. Phipps AI, Shi Q, Newcomb PA, et al. Associations between cigarette smoking status and colon cancer prognosis among participants in North Central Cancer Treatment Group Phase III Trial N0147. *J Clin Oncol* 2013;31:2016–2023.

166. Leichman CG, Lens HJ, Leichman L, et al. Quantitation of intratumoral thymidylate synthase expression predicts for disseminated colorectal cancer response and resistance to protracted-infusion fluorouracil and weekly leucovorin. *J Clin Oncol* 1997;15:3223–3229.

173. National Comprehensive Cancer Network Guidelines for Colon Cancer, Version 3.2011, www.nccn.org.

174. Huang EH, Forde KA. Surgical implications of colonoscopy. *Semin Laparosc Surg* 2003;10:13–18.

175. Libutti SK, Forde KA. Surgical considerations III: bowel anastomosis. In Cohen A, Weaver S, eds. *Cancer of the Colon, Rectum and Anus*. New York, NY: McGraw Hill; 1995:445–456.

176. Guenaga KF, Matos D, Castro AA, et al. Mechanical bowel preparation for elective colorectal surgery. *Cochrane Database Syst Rev* 2003;(2):CD001544.

180. Ram E, Sherman Y, Weil R, et al. Is mechanical bowel preparation mandatory for elective colon surgery? A prospective randomized study. *Arch Surg* 2005;140:285–288.

PRACTICE OF ONCOLOGY

183. Benson AB 3rd, Choti MA, Cohen AM, et al. NCCN Practice Guidelines for Colorectal Cancer. *Oncology (Williston Park)* 2000;14:203–212.

184. McGinnis LS. Surgical treatment options for colorectal cancer. *Cancer* 1994; 74:2147–2150.

189. Khot UP, Lang AW, Murali K, et al. Systematic review of the efficacy and safety of colorectal stents. *Br J Surg* 2002;89:1096–1102.

192. Lee HJ, Hong SP, Cheon JH, et al. Long-term outcome of palliative therapy for malignant colorectal obstruction in patients with unresectable metastatic colorectal cancers: endoscopic stenting versus surgery. *Gastrointest Endosc* 2011;73:535–542.

194. White SI, Abdool SI, Frenkiel B, et al. Management of malignant left-sided large bowel obstruction: a comparison between colonic stents and surgery. *ANZ J Surg* 2011;81:257–260.

195. Cheung HY, Chung CC, Tsang WW, et al. Endolaparoscopic approach vs conventional open surgery in the treatment of obstructing left-sided colon cancer: a randomized controlled trial. *Arch Surg* 2009;144:1127–1132.

197. van Hooft JE, Bemelman WA, Oldenburg B, et al. Colonic stenting versus emergency surgery for acute left-sided malignant colonic obstruction: a multicentre randomised trial. *Lancet Oncol* 2011;12:344–352.

198. Sabbagh C, Brower F, Diouf M, et al. Is stenting as "a bridge to surgery" an oncologically safe strategy for the management of acute, left-sided, malignant, colonic obstruction? A comparative study with a propensity score analysis. *Ann Surg* 2013;258:107–115.

201. Hartley JE, Monson JR. The role of laparoscopy in the multimodality treatment of colorectal cancer. *Surg Clin North Am* 2002;82:1019–1033.

205. Patankar SK, Larach SW, Ferrara A, et al. Prospective comparison of laparoscopic vs. open resections for colorectal adenocarcinoma over a ten-year period. *Dis Colon Rectum* 2003;46:601–611.

212. Clinical Outcomes of Surgical Therapy Study Group. A comparison of laparoscopically assisted and open colectomy for colon cancer. *N Engl J Med* 2004;350:2050–2059.

214. Green BL, Marshall HC, Collinson F, et al. Long-term follow-up of the Medical Research Council CLASICC trial of conventional versus laparoscopically assisted resection in colorectal cancer. *Br J Surg* 2013;100:75–82.

217. Katsuno G, Fukunaga M, Nagakari K, et al. Single-incision laparoscopic colectomy for colon cancer: early experience with 31 cases. *Dis Colon Rectum* 2011;54:705–710.

219. Yun JA, Yun SH, Park YA, et al. Single-incision laparoscopic right colectomy compared with conventional laparoscopy for malignancy: assessment of perioperative and short-term oncologic outcomes. *Surg Endosc* 2013;27: 2122–2130.

220. deSouza AL, Prasad LM, Park JJ, et al. Robotic assistance in right hemicolectomy: is there a role? *Dis Colon Rectum* 2010;53:1000–1006.

221. Luca F, Ghezzi TL, Valvo M, et al. Surgical and pathological outcomes after right hemicolectomy: case-matched study comparing robotic and open surgery. *Int J Med Robot* 2011 [ePub ahead of print].

223. Park JS, Choi GS, Kim HJ, et al. Natural orifice specimen extraction versus conventional laparoscopically assisted right hemicolectomy. *Br J Surg* 2011;98:710–715.

225. Nivatvongs S. Surgical management of early colorectal cancer. *World J Surg* 2000;24:1052–1055.

228. Efficacy of adjuvant fluorouracil and folinic acid in colon cancer. International Multicentre Pooled Analysis of Colon Cancer Trials (IMPACT) investigators. *Lancet* 1995;345:939–944.

229. Wolmark N, Fisher B, Rockette H, et al. Postoperative adjuvant chemotherapy or BCG for colon cancer: results from NSABP protocol C0-1. *J Natl Cancer Inst* 1988;80:30–36.

233. Comparison of flourouracil with additional levamisole, higher-dose folinic acid, or both, as adjuvant chemotherapy for colorectal cancer: a randomised trial. QUASAR Collaborative Group. *Lancet* 2000;355:1588–1596.

234. O'Connell MJ, Laurie JA, Kahn M, et al. Prospectively randomized trial of postoperative adjuvant chemotherapy in patients with high-risk colon cancer. *J Clin Oncol* 1998;16:295–300.

235. Twelves C, Wong A, Nowacki MP, et al. Capecitabine as adjuvant treatment for stage III colon cancer. *N Engl J Med* 2005;352:2696–2704.

236. Lembersky BC, Wieand HS, Petrelli NJ, et al. Oral uracil and tegafur plus leucovorin compared with intravenous fluorouracil and leucovorin in stage II and III carcinoma of the colon: results from National Surgical Adjuvant Breast and Bowel Project Protocol C-06. *J Clin Oncol* 2006;24:2059–2064.

237. Andre T, Boni C, Navarro M, et al. Improved overall survival with oxaliplatin, fluorouracil, and leucovorin as adjuvant treatment in stage II or III colon cancer in the MOSAIC trial. *J Clin Oncol* 2009;27:3109–3116.

239. Kidwell KM, Yothers G, Ganz PA, et al. Long-term neurotoxicity effects of oxaliplatin added to fluorouracil and leucovorin as adjuvant therapy for colon cancer: results from National Surgical Adjuvant Breast and Bowel Project trials C-07 and LTS-01. *Cancer* 2012;118:5614–5622.

241. McCleary NJ, Meyerhardt JA, Green E, et al. Impact of age on the efficacy of newer adjuvant therapies in patients with stage II/III colon cancer: findings from the ACCENT database. *J Clin Oncol* 2013;31:2600–2606.

242. Tournigand C, Andre T, Bonnetain F, et al. Adjuvant therapy with fluorouracil and oxaliplatin in stage II and elderly patients (between ages 70 and 75 years) with colon cancer: subgroup analyses of the Multicenter International Study of Oxaliplatin, Fluorouracil, and Leucovorin in the Adjuvant Treatment of Colon Cancer trial. *J Clin Oncol* 2012;30:3353–3360.

243. Benson AB 3rd, Bekali-Saab T, Chan E, et al. Localized colon cancer, version 3.2013: featured updates to the NCCN Guidelines. *J Natl Compr Canc Netw* 2013;11:519–528.

244. Haller DG, Tabernero J, Maroun J, et al. Capecitabine plus oxaliplatin compared with fluorouracil and folinic acid as adjuvant therapy for stage III colon cancer. *J Clin Oncol* 2011;29:1465–1471.

245. Cunningham D, Humblet Y, Siena S, et al. Cetuximab monotherapy and cetuximab plus irinotecan in irinotecan-refractory metastatic colorectal cancer. *N Engl J Med* 2004;351:337–345.

246. Douillard JY, Cunnungham D, Roth AD, et al. Irinotecan combined with fluorouracil compared with fluorouracil alone as first-line treatment for metastatic colorectal cancer: a multicentre randomised trial. *Lancet* 2000;355: 1041–1047.

247. Saltz LB, Cox JV, Blanke C, et al. Irinotecan plus fluorouracil and leucovorin for metastatic colorectal cancer. Irinotecan Study Group. *N Engl J Med* 2000;343:905–914.

249. Saltz LB, Niedzwiecki D, Hollis D, et al. Irinotecan fluorouracil plus leucovorin is not superior to fluorouracil plus leucovorin alone as adjuvant treatment for stage III colon cancer: results of CALGB 89803. *J Clin Oncol* 2007;25:3456–3461.

253. Bertagnolli MM, Niedzwiecki D, Compton CC, et al. Microsatellite instability predicts improved response to adjuvant therapy with irinotecan, fluorouracil, and leucovorin in stage III colon cancer: Cancer and Leukemia Group B Protocol 89803. *J Clin Oncol* 2009;27:1814–1821.

254. Allegra CJ, Yothers G, O'Connell MJ, et al. Bevacizumab in stage II-III colon cancer: 5-year update of the National Surgical Adjuvant Breast and Bowel Project C-08 trial. *J Clin Oncol* 2013;31:359–364.

255. de Gramont A, Van Cutsem E, Schmoll HJ, et al. Bevacizumab plus oxaliplatin-based chemotherapy as adjuvant treatment for colon cancer (AVANT): a phase 3 randomised controlled trial. *Lancet Oncol* 2012;13:1225–1233.

256. Alberts SR, Sargent DJ, Nair S, et al. Effect of oxaliplatin, fluorouracil, and leucovorin with or without cetuximab on survival among patients with resected stage iii colon cancer: a randomized trial. *JAMA* 2012;307:1383–1393.

258. Efficacy of adjuvant fluorouracil and folinic acid in B2 colon cancer. International Multicentre Pooled Analysis of B2 Colon Cancer Trials (IMPACT B2) Investigators. *J Clin Oncol* 1999;17:1356–1363.

262. Ishiguro M, Mochizuki H, Tomita N, et al. Study protocol of the SACURA trial: a randomized phase III trial of efficacy and safety of UFT as adjuvant chemotherapy for stage II colon cancer. *BMC Cancer* 2012;12:281.

266. Sato H, Maeda K, Sugihara K, et al. High-risk stage II colon cancer after curative resection. *J Surg Oncol* 2011;104:45–52.

267. Ribic CM, Sargent DJ, Moore MJ, et al. Tumor microsatellite-instability status as a predictor of benefit from fluorouracil-based adjuvant chemotherapy for colon cancer. *N Engl J Med* 2003;349:247–257.

269. Sargent DJ, Marsoni S, Thibodeau SN, et al. Confirmation of deficient mismatch repair (dMMR) as a predictive marker for lack of benefit from 5-FU based chemotherapy in stage II and III colon cancer (CC): A pooled molecular reanalysis of randomized chemotherapy trials. *J Clin Oncol* 2008;26:4008.

270. Sinicrope FA, Foster NR, Thibodeau SN, et al. DNA mismatch repair status and colon cancer recurrence and survival in clinical trials of 5-fluorouracil-based adjuvant therapy. *J Natl Cancer Inst* 2011;103:863–875.

273. Roth AD, Tejpar S, Delorenzi M, et al. Prognostic role of KRAS and BRAF in stage II and III resected colon cancer: results of the translational study on the PETACC-3, EORTC 40993, SAKK 60-00 trial. *J Clin Oncol* 2010;28: 466–474.

275. Sharif S, O'Connell MJ. Gene signatures in stage II colon cancer: a clinical review. *Curr Colorectal Cancer Rep* 2012;8:225–231.

279. Benson AB 3rd, Schrag D, Somerfield MR, et al. American Society of Clinical Oncology recommendations on adjuvant chemotherapy for stage II colon cancer. *J Clin Oncol* 2004;22:3408–3419.

283. Long term results of single course of adjuvant intraportal chemotherapy for colorectal cancer. Swiss Group for Clinical Cancer Research (SAKK). *Lancet* 1995;345:349–352.

286. Scheithauer W, Kornek GV, Marczell A, et al. Combined intravenous and intraperitoneal chemotherapy with fluorouracil + leucovorin vs fluorouracil + levamisole for adjuvant therapy of resected colon carcinoma. *Br J Cancer* 1998;77:1349–1354.

287. Sammartino P, Sibio S, Biacchi D, et al. Prevention of Peritoneal Metastases from Colon Cancer in High-Risk Patients: Preliminary Results of Surgery plus Prophylactic HIPEC. *Gastroenterol Res Pract* 2012;2012:141585.

289. Foxtrot Collaborative Group. Feasibility of preoperative chemotherapy for locally advanced, operable colon cancer: the pilot phase of a randomised controlled trial. *Lancet Oncol* 2012;13:1152–1160.

291. Burt RW. Colon cancer screening. *Gastroenterology* 2000;119:837–853.

292. Mandel JS, Bond JH, Church TR, et al. Reducing mortality from colorectal cancer by screening for fecal occult blood. Minnesota Colon Cancer Control Study. *N Engl J Med* 1993;328:1365–1371.

296. Meyerhardt JA, Mangu PB, Flynn PJ, et al. Follow-up care, surveillance protocol, and secondary prevention measures for survivors of colorectal cancer: American Society of Clinical Oncology clinical practice guideline endorsement. *J Clin Oncol* 2013;31:4465–4470.

299. Clinical practice guidelines for the use of tumor markers in breast and colorectal cancer. Adopted on May 17, 1996 by the American Society of Clinical Oncology. *J Clin Oncol* 1996;14:2843–2877.

303. Libutti SK, Alexander HR Jr, Choyke P, et al. A prospective study of 2-[18F] fluoro-2-deoxy-D-glucose/positron emission tomography scan, 99mTc-labeled arcitumomab (CEA-scan), and blind second-look laparotomy for detecting colon cancer recurrence in patients with increasing carcinoembryonic antigen levels. *Ann Surg Oncol* 2001;8:779–786.

310. Desch CE, Benson AB 3rd, Somerfield MR, et al. Colorectal cancer surveillance: 2005 update of an American Society of Clinical Oncology practice guideline. *J Clin Oncol* 2005;23:8512–8519.

313. Ohlsson B, Breland U, Ekberg H, et al. Follow-up after curative surgery for colorectal carcinoma. Randomized comparison with no follow-up. *Dis Colon Rectum* 1995;38:619–626.

315. Inadomi JM, Sonnenberg A. The impact of colorectal cancer screening on life expectancy. *Gastrointest Endosc* 2000;51:517–522.

317. Renehan AG, Egger M, Saunders MP, et al. Impact on survival of intensive follow up after curative resection for colorectal cancer: systematic review and meta-analysis of randomised trials. *BMJ* 2002;324:813.

319. Poultsides GA, Servais EL, Saltz LB, et al. Outcome of primary tumor in patients with synchronous stage IV colorectal cancer receiving combination chemotherapy without surgery as initial treatment. *J Clin Oncol* 2009; 27:3379–3384.

320. McCahill LE, Yothers G, Sharif S, et al. Primary mFOLFOX6 plus bevacizumab without resection of the primary tumor for patients presenting with surgically unresectable metastatic colon cancer and an intact asymptomatic colon cancer: definitive analysis of NSABP trial C-10. *J Clin Oncol* 2012;30:3223–3228.

321. Stillwell AP, Buettner PG, Siu SK, et al. Predictors of postoperative mortality, morbidity, and long-term survival after palliative resection in patients with colorectal cancer. *Dis Colon Rectum* 2011;54:535–544.

322. Heidelberger C, Chaudhuri NK, Danneberg P, et al. Fluorinated pyrimidines, a new class of tumor inhibitory compounds. *Nature* 1957;179:663–666.

323. Jager E, Heike M, Bernhard H, et al. Weekly high-dose leucovorin versus low-dose leucovorin combined with fluorouracil in advanced colorectal cancer: results of a randomized mulitcenter trial. *J Clin Oncol* 1996;14:2274–2279.

324. Lokich JJ, Ahlgren JD, Gullo JJ, et al. A prospective randomized comparison of continuous infusion fluorouracil with a conventional bolus schedule in metastatic colorectal carcinoma: a Mid-Atlantic Oncology Program Study. *J Clin Oncol* 1989;7:425–432.

329. Van Cutsem E, Twelves C, Cassidy J, et al. Oral capecitabine compared with intravenous fluorouracil plus leucovorin in patients with metastatic colorectal cancer: results of a large phase III study. *J Clin Oncol* 2001;19:4097–4106.

330. Pizzolato JF, Saltz LB. The camptothecins. *Lancet* 2003;361:2235–2242.

333. Andre T, Louvet C, Maindrault-Goebel F, et al. CPT-11 (irinotecan) addition to bimonthly, high-dose leucovorin and bolus and continuous-infusion 5-fluorouracil (FOLFIRI) for pretreated metastatic colorectal cancer. GERCOR. *Eur J Cancer* 1999;35:1343–1347.

334. Fuchs CS, Marshall J, Mitchell E, et al. Randomized, controlled trial of irinotecan plus infusional, bolus, or oral fluoropyrimidines in first-line treatment of metastatic colorectal cancer: results from the BICC-C Study. *J Clin Oncol* 2007;25:4779–4786.

335. Extra JM, Espie M, Calvo F, et al. Phase I study of oxaliplatin in patients with advanced cancer. *Cancer Chemother Pharmacol* 1990;25:299–303.

336. Raymond E, Chaney SG, Taamma A, et al. Oxaliplatin: a review of preclinical and clinical studies. *Ann Oncol* 1998;9:1053–1071.

338. Giacchetti S, Perpoint B, Zidani R, et al. Phase III multicenter randomized trial of oxaliplatin added to chronomodulated fluorouracil-leucovorin as first-line treatment of metastatic colorectal cancer. *J Clin Oncol* 2000;18:136–147.

342. Andre T, Bensmaine MA, Louvet C, et al. Multicenter phase II study of bimonthly high-dose leucovorin, fluorouracil infusion, and oxaliplatin for metastatic colorectal cancer resistant to the same leucovorin and fluorouracil regimen. *J Clin Oncol* 1999;17:3560–3568.

344. Wolmark N, Yothers G, O'Connell MJ, et al. A phase III trial comparing mFOLFOX6 to mFOLFOX6 plus bevacizumab in stage II or III carcinoma of the colon: Results of NSABP Protocol C-08. *J Clin Oncol* 2009;27:Abstr LBA4.

347. Rothenberg ML, Oza AM, Bigelow RH, et al. Superiority of oxaliplatin and fluorouracil-leucovorin compared with either therapy alone in patients with progressive colorectal cancer after irinotecan and fluorouracil-leucovorin: interim results of a phase III trial. *J Clin Oncol* 2003;21:2059–2069.

349. Tournigand C, Andre T, Achille E, et al. FOLFIRI followed by FOLFOX6 or the reverse sequence in advanced colorectal cancer: a randomized GERCOR study. *J Clin Oncol* 2004;22:229–237.

352. Goldberg RM. N9741: a phase III study comparing irinotecan to oxaliplatin-containing regimens in advanced colorectal cancer. *Clin Colorectal Cancer* 2002;2:81.

354. Goldberg RM, Sargent DJ, Morton RF, et al. A randomized controlled trial of fluorouracil plus leucovorin, irinotecan, and oxaliplatin combinations in patients with previously untreated metastatic colorectal cancer. *J Clin Oncol* 2004;22:23–30.

355. Tournigand C, Cervantes A, Figer A, et al. OPTIMOX1: a randomized study of FOLFOX4 or FOLFOX7 with oxaliplatin in a stop-and-Go fashion in advanced colorectal cancer—a GERCOR study. *J Clin Oncol* 2006;24:394–400.

360. Cassidy J, Clarke S, Diaz-Rubio E, et al. Randomized phase III study of capecitabine plus oxaliplatin compared with fluorouracil/folinic acid plus oxaliplatin as first-line therapy for metastatic colorectal cancer. *J Clin Oncol* 2008;26:2006–2012.

361. Maughan TS, James RD, Kerr DJ, et al. Comparison of intermittent and continuous palliative chemotherapy for advanced colorectal cancer: a multicentre randomised trial. *Lancet* 2003;361:457–464.

362. Chibaudel B, Maindrault-Goebel F, Lledo G, et al. Can chemotherapy be discontinued in unresectable metastatic colorectal cancer? The GERCOR OPTIMOX2 Study. *J Clin Oncol* 2009;27:5727–5733.

363. Perez-Staub N, Chibaudel B, Figer A, et al. Who can benefit from chemotherapy holidays after first-line therapy for advanced colorectal cancer? A GERCOR study. *J Clin Oncol* 2008;26:Abstr 4037.

366. Koopman M, Antonini NF, Douma J, et al. Sequential versus combination chemotherapy with capecitabine, irinotecan, and oxaliplatin in advanced colorectal cancer (CAIRO): a phase III randomised controlled trial. *Lancet* 2007;370:135–142.

367. Seymour MT, Maughan TS, Ledermann JA, et al. Different strategies of sequential and combination chemotherapy for patients with poor prognosis advanced colorectal cancer (MRC FOCUS): a randomised controlled trial. *Lancet* 2007;370:143–152.

368. Ferrara N, Hillan KJ, Gerber HP, et al. Discovery and development of bevacizumab, an anti-VEGF antibody for treating cancer. *Nat Rev Drug Discov* 2004;3:391–400.

371. Hurwitz H, Fehrenbacher L, Novotny W, et al. Bevacizumab plus irinotecan, fluorouracil, and leucovorin for metastatic colorectal cancer. *N Engl J Med* 2004;350:2335–2342.

374. Giantonio BJ, Catalano PJ, Meropol NJ, et al. Bevacizumab in combination with oxaliplatin, fluorouracil, and leucovorin (FOLFOX4) for previously treated metastatic colorectal cancer: results from the Eastern Cooperative Oncology Group Study E3200. *J Clin Oncol* 2007;25:1539–1544.

375. Saltz LB, Clarke S, Diaz-Rubio E, et al. Bevacizumab in combination with oxaliplatin-based chemotherapy as first-line therapy in metastatic colorectal cancer: a randomized phase III study. *J Clin Oncol* 2008;26:2013–2019.

376. Skillings JA, Johnson DH, Miller K, et al. Arterial thromboembolic events (ATEs) in a pooled analysis of 5 randomized, controlled trials (RCTs) of bevacizumab (BV) with chemotherapy. *J Clin Oncol* 2005;23:3019.

378. Bennouna J, Sastre J, Arnold D, et al. Continuation of bevacizumab after first progression in metastatic colorectal cancer (ML18147): a randomised phase 3 trial. *Lancet Oncol* 2013;14:29–37.

379. Van Cutsem E, Tabernero J, Lakomy R, et al. Addition of aflibercept to fluorouracil, leucovorin, and irinotecan improves survival in a phase III randomized trial in patients with metastatic colorectal cancer previously treated with an oxaliplatin-based regimen. *J Clin Oncol* 2012;30:3499–3506.

380. Grothey A, Van Cutsem E, Sobrero A, et al. Regorafenib monotherapy for previously treated metastatic colorectal cancer (CORRECT): an international, multicentre, randomised, placebo-controlled, phase 3 trial. *Lancet* 2013;381:303–312.

381. Ciardiello F, Tortora G. A novel approach in the treatment of cancer: targeting the epidermal growth factor receptor. *Clin Cancer Res* 2001;7:2958–2970.

384. Thomas SM, Grandis JR. Pharmacokinetic and pharmacodynamic properties of EGFR inhibitors under clinical investigation. *Cancer Treat Rev* 2004;30:255–268.

386. Saltz LB, Meropol NJ, Poehrer PJ Sr, et al. Phase II trial of cetuximab in patients with refractory colorectal cancer that expresses the epidermal growth factor receptor. *J Clin Oncol* 2004;22:1201–1208.

387. Jonker DJ, O'Callaghan CJ, Karapetis CS, et al. Cetuximab for the treatment of colorectal cancer. *N Engl J Med* 2007;357:2040–2048.

390. Van Cutsem E, Peeters M, Siena S, et al. Open-label phase III trial of panitumumab plus best supportive care compared with best supportive care alone in patients with chemotherapy-refractory metastatic colorectal cancer. *J Clin Oncol* 2007;25:1658–1664.

393. Amado RG, Wolf M, Peeters M, et al. Wild-type KRAS is required for panitumumab efficacy in patients with metastatic colorectal cancer. *J Clin Oncol* 2008;26:1626–1634.

394. Karapetis CS, Khambata-Ford S, Jonker DJ, et al. K-ras mutations and benefit from cetuximab in advanced colorectal cancer. *N Engl J Med* 2008;359:1757–1765.

397. Allegra CJ, Jessup JM, Somerfield MR, et al. American Society of Clinical Oncology provisional clinical opinion: testing for KRAS gene mutations in patients with metastatic colorectal carcinoma to predict response to anti-epidermal growth factor receptor monoclonal antibody therapy. *J Clin Oncol* 2009;27:2091–2096.

398. Vakiani E, Janakiraman M, Shen R, et al. Comparative genomic analysis of primary versus metastatic colorectal carcinomas. *J Clin Oncol* 2012;30:2956–2962.

399. Lin YL, Liau JY, Yu SC, et al. KRAS mutation is a predictor of oxaliplatin sensitivity in colon cancer cells. *PLoS One* 2012;7:e50701.

400. Van Cutsem E, Kohne CH, Hitre E, et al. Cetuximab and chemotherapy as initial treatment for metastatic colorectal cancer. *N Engl J Med* 2009;360:1408–1417.

401. Van Cutsem E, Kohne CH, Lang I, et al. Cetuximab plus irinotecan, fluorouracil, and leucovorin as first-line treatment for metastatic colorectal cancer: updated analysis of overall survival according to tumor KRAS and BRAF mutation status. *J Clin Oncol* 2011;29:2011–2019.

403. Maughan TS, Adams RA, Smith CG, et al. Addition of cetuximab to oxaliplatin-based first-line combination chemotherapy for treatment of advanced colorectal cancer: results of the randomised phase 3 MRC COIN trial. *Lancet* 2011;377:2103–2114.

404. Tveit KM, Guren T, Glimelius B, et al. Phase III trial of cetuximab with continuous or intermittent fluorouracil, leucovorin, and oxaliplatin (Nordic FLOX) versus FLOX alone in first-line treatment of metastatic colorectal cancer: the NORDIC-VII study. *J Clin Oncol* 2012;30:1755–1762.

405. Douillard JY, Siena S, Cassidy J, et al. Randomized, phase III trial of panitumumab with infusional fluorouracil, leucovorin, and oxaliplatin (FOLFOX4) versus FOLFOX4 alone as first-line treatment in patients with previously untreated metastatic colorectal cancer: the PRIME study. *J Clin Oncol* 2010;28:4697–4705.

409. Perez-Soler R, Saltz L. Cutaneous adverse effects with HER1/EGFR-targeted agents: is there a silver lining? *J Clin Oncol* 2005;23:5235–5246.

411. Chung CH, Mirakhur B, Chan E, et al. Cetuximab-induced anaphylaxis and IgE specific for galactose-alpha-1,3-galactose. *N Engl J Med* 2008;358:1109–1117.

412. Schrag D, Chung KY, Flombaum C, et al. Cetuximab therapy and symptomatic hypomagnesemia. *J Natl Cancer Inst* 2005;97:1221–1224.

414. Chung KY, Shia J, Kemeny NE, et al. Cetuximab shows activity in colorectal cancer patients with tumors that do not express the epidermal growth factor receptor by immunohistochemistry. *J Clin Oncol* 2005;23:1803–1810.

418. Tol J, Koopman M, Cats A, et al. Chemotherapy, bevacizumab, and cetuximab in metastatic colorectal cancer. *N Engl J Med* 2009;360:563–572.

419. Hecht JR, Mitchell E, Chidiac T, et al. A randomized phase IIIB trial of chemotherapy, bevacizumab, and panitumumab compared with chemotherapy and bevacizumab alone for metastatic colorectal cancer. *J Clin Oncol* 2009;27:672–680.

423. Blanke CD. Celecoxib with chemotherapy in colorectal cancer. *Oncology (Huntingt)* 2002;16:17–21.

424. Chan AT, Ogino S, Fuchs CS. Aspirin use and survival after diagnosis of colorectal cancer. *JAMA* 2009;302:649–658.

425. Ali R, Toh HC, Chia WK, et al. The utility of Aspirin in Dukes C and High Risk Dukes B Colorectal cancer—the ASCOLT study: study protocol for a randomized controlled trial. *Trials* 2011;12:261.

426. Bastiaannet E, Sampieri K, Dekkers OM, et al. Use of aspirin postdiagnosis improves survival for colon cancer patients. *Br J Cancer* 2012;106:1564–1570.

430. Iqbal S, Lenz HJ. Targeted therapy and pharmacogenomic programs. *Cancer* 2003;97:2076–2082.

431. Ebert MP, Tanzer M, Balluff B, et al. TFAP2E-DKK4 and chemoresistance in colorectal cancer. *N Engl J Med* 2012;366:44–53.

58 Genetic Testing in Colon Cancer (Polyposis Syndromes)

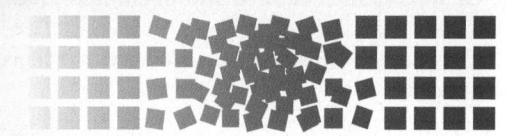

Kory W. Jasperson

INTRODUCTION

Hereditary colonic polyposis conditions account for less than 1% of all colorectal cancers (CRC). Accurate classification of these conditions is imperative, given their distinct cancer risks, management strategies, and consequent risk to relatives. However, overlapping features and atypical or attenuated presentations make diagnosis difficult in some cases. Determining the histologic types of colorectal polyps identified is especially useful in guiding diagnostic strategies. Adenomatous polyps are the predominant lesion in familial adenomatous polyposis (FAP), attenuated FAP (AFAP), and *MUTYH* (MutY human homolog)–associated polyposis (MAP), whereas hamartomatous polyps are the primary gastrointestinal lesion in Peutz–Jeghers syndrome (PJS), juvenile polyposis syndrome (JPS), and Cowden syndrome (CS). Extracolonic features, which are highlighted for each syndrome in Tables 58.1 to 58.3 are also important clues in the diagnostic workup. Genetic testing is now available for these conditions and, in most cases, allows for a precise diagnosis.

ADENOMATOUS POLYPOSIS

Familial Adenomatous Polyposis and Attenuated Familial Adenomatous Polyposis

Of all of the colonic polyposis conditions, FAP is both the most common and the best characterized. FAP is caused by germ-line mutations in the adenomatous polyposis coli (*APC*) gene and is estimated to occur in about 1 in 10,000 individuals. With the classic presentation of FAP, hundreds to thousands of adenomatous polyps occur by the age of 20 to 40 years.[1] The attenuated or less severe colonic phenotype associated with AFAP may mimic sporadic colon polyps and cancer, or other known syndromes, such as MAP. This creates diagnostic difficulties when evaluating an individual with moderate adenomatous polyposis. Other conditions linked to germ-line *APC* mutations include Gardner syndrome (with association of colonic polyposis and osteomas, epidermoid cysts, fibromas, and/or desmoid tumors) and Turcot syndrome (with association of colonic polyposis and medulloblastomas).[2] However, it is now believed that the features associated with Gardner syndrome and Turcot syndrome are the result of variable expressivity of *APC* mutations as opposed to being distinct clinical entities.

Colon Phenotype

Although adenomatous polyps associated with FAP have a similar malignancy rate as those that develop in the general population, the sheer number of polyps present in FAP results in nearly a 100% lifetime risk of CRC in untreated individuals. In FAP, colorectal polyps begin to develop on average around the age of 16 years.[1] The mean age at CRC onset is 39 years, with 7% developing CRC by 21 years and 95% before the age of 50 years.[3]

In AFAP, the lifetime risk of CRC is approximately 70% with an average age at onset in the 50s.[4] The colonic phenotype of AFAP is quite variable, even within the same family. Colonoscopies in 120 mutation-positive individuals within the same family revealed that 37% had less than 10 adenomatous colon polyps (average age, 36 years; range, 16 to 67 years), 28% had 10 to 50 polyps (average age, 39 years; range, 21 to 76 years), and 35% had greater than 50 polyps (average age, 48 years; range, 27 to 49 years).[4] In addition, the total number of polyps per individual ranged from zero to 470.[4]

Extracolonic Features

The most common extracolonic finding in individuals with FAP and AFAP is upper gastrointestinal tract polyps. Although the colonic phenotype in AFAP is less severe than in FAP, the upper gastrointestinal phenotype is comparable. Adenomatous polyps of the duodenum (20% to 100%) and the periampullary region (at least 50%) are common.[5,6] The relative risk of duodenal or periampullary carcinoma in FAP is estimated to be 100 to 330 times greater than the general population, although the absolute risk is only around 5%.[5] The majority of FAP- and AFAP-associated small-bowel carcinomas arise in the duodenum.

Fundic gland polyps are found in most cases of FAP/AFAP and often number in the hundreds.[7] Unlike polyps in the colon or small bowel, fundic gland polyps are a type of hamartoma. They are typically small (1 to 5 mm), sessile, and usually asymptomatic and are located in the fundus and body of the stomach.[7] Adenomatous polyps of the stomach are occasionally found in FAP and AFAP.[8] Gastric cancers arising from fundic gland polyps have been reported in FAP, although most are believed to arise from adenomatous polyps.[8] Individuals with FAP have an 800-fold increased risk for desmoid tumors (aggressive fibromatoses), with a lifetime risk of 10% to 30%.[9–11] Risk factors for desmoid tumors in FAP include a family history of desmoid tumors, *APC* mutations 3′ to codon 1,399 (genotype–phenotype correlation), female sex, and previous abdominal surgery.[10] Although desmoid tumors do not metastasize, they can be locally invasive, aggressive, and difficult to treat, resulting in significant morbidity and the second leading cause of mortality in FAP.[12]

The phenotypic spectrum of germ-line *APC* mutations also includes other benign findings such as osteomas, epidermoid cysts, fibromas, dental abnormalities, and congenital hypertrophy of the retinal pigment epithelium (CHRPE). In addition, there are increased risks for other cancers, including those of the pancreas, thyroid, bile duct, brain (typically medulloblastoma), and liver (specifically hepatoblastoma).[6]

Management

Without treatment, CRC is inevitable in FAP. However, with early screening and polypectomies, in addition to prophylactic colectomies after polyps become too difficult to manage endoscopically, most CRCs can be prevented in AFAP and FAP. In FAP, annual

TABLE 58.1

Characteristic Features and Recommendations: Adenomatous Polyposis Conditions

Lifetime Cancer Risks	Management Recommendations	Nonmalignant Features
FAP (*APC*)		
Colorectum (100%)	Annual colonoscopy/sigmoidoscopy by 10–12 y until colectomy	100–1,000s of colorectal adenomas
Duodenum (5%)	Upper endoscopy every 1–4 y by 25–30 y	Fundic gland polyposis
Stomach (≤1%)		Duodenal polyposis
Thyroid (1%–2%)	Annual physical examination	CHRPE, epidermoid cysts, osteomas
Pancreas (1%–2%)		Dental abnormalities
Hepatoblastoma (1%–2%)		Desmoid tumors
Medulloblastoma (<1%)		
AFAP (*APC*)		
Colorectum (70%)	Colonoscopy every 1–2 y by 18–20 y	10–100 colonic adenomas (range, 0–100s)
Duodenum (5%)	Upper endoscopy every 1–4 y by 25–30 y	Fundic gland polyposis
Stomach (≤1%)		Duodenal polyposis
Thyroid (1%–2%)	Annual physical examination	Other nonmalignant features are uncommon
Pancreas (1%–2%)		
MAP (biallelic *MUTYH*)		
Colorectum (80%)	Colonoscopy every 3 y by 25–30 y	10–100 colonic adenomas (range, 0–100s)
Duodenum (4%)	Upper endoscopy every 3–5 y by 30–35 y	Multiple hyperplastic and sessile serrated polyps possible
		Duodenal adenomatous polyposis

Data derived from National Comprehensive Cancer Network. NCCN Guidelines and Clinical Resources Web site. Colorectal Cancer Screening, Version 1.2012. 2012. http://www.nccn.org. Accessed April 3, 2012.

colonoscopies or flexible sigmoidoscopies are recommended starting around the age of 10 years.[13] In AFAP, screening begins in the late teenage years, and colonoscopies, rather than sigmoidoscopies, are necessary because of proximally located polyps.[13] Colectomies can sometimes be avoided in AFAP, which is not the case for individuals with FAP. After polyps become too numerous (usually >20 to 30 polyps) to manage endoscopically or when adenomas with advanced histology are identified, a prophylactic colectomy is advised.[13] A proctocolectomy with an ileal pouch anal anastomosis is the standard surgery in FAP, whereas a total colectomy with ileorectal anastomosis is often the preferred approach with AFAP or in FAP cases with limited rectal involvement.[13,14] Continued screening of the remaining rectum or ileal pouch is still necessary.[13]

Recently, it has been shown that duodenal cancer detected through surveillance improves survival compared with individuals presenting because of symptoms.[15] The National Comprehensive Cancer Network (NCCN) currently recommends the consideration of an esophagogastroduodenoscopy (EGD) with a side-viewing examination beginning around the age of 25 years for duodenal cancer surveillance.[13] The extent of duodenal polyps, as defined by the Spigelman staging criteria, is used to determine the EGD follow-up interval.[13] Additional considerations for the management in individuals with germ-line *APC* mutations are outlined and updated annually by the NCCN (www.nccn.org).

Genetic Testing and Counseling

A clinical diagnosis of FAP is considered when at least 100 colorectal adenomatous polyps are detected by the 2nd or 3rd decade of life.[6] Genetic testing of *APC* is still recommended to clarify extracolonic cancer risks and to help determine FAP status in relatives.

Genetic testing has also been shown to be cost-effective,[16] although it is unlikely to change colon management for cases with extensive adenomatous polyposis.

Given the phenotypic variability, a consensus as to what constitutes a diagnosis of AFAP has not been reached. The NCCN currently recommends that individuals with greater than 10 cumulative colorectal adenomas be referred for genetic counseling and the consideration of genetic testing.[13] The identification of an *APC* mutation in these less severe polyp cases confirms a diagnosis of AFAP. It is also noteworthy that individuals with 100 or more adenomatous polyps may have AFAP if polyp development occurs at a later age (typically after 40 years).

Differentiating among FAP, AFAP, and other colonic polyposis conditions is not always straightforward. Family history, which is consistent with an autosomal-dominant mode of inheritance, is suggestive of FAP/AFAP and increases the likelihood of finding an *APC* mutation.[6] However, 10% to 30% of probands with germ-line *APC* mutations are de novo (new mutation) cases, and consequently, their parents are unaffected.[6,17] In addition, it is not uncommon for individuals with AFAP to have less than 10 cumulative adenomatous polyps.[4] In patients with fewer polyps, it is not clear whether genetic testing should be performed.[13] However, it is important that these individuals be closely followed up, and if multiple adenomas continue to develop, genetic testing should be reconsidered.

Unlike what is found in some of the other conditions described in this review, hyperplastic or hamartomatous colon polyps are not known to be associated with FAP/AFAP. Therefore, if multiple hyperplastic or hamartomatous colon polyps are found in an individual, a genetic testing of *APC* is unlikely to be informative. Other features associated with *APC* mutations that may assist with making a diagnosis of AFAP or FAP include fundic gland polyposis, duodenal adenomatous polyps, osteomas, CHRPE, desmoid tumors, and hepatoblastoma.[6]

MUTYH-Associated Polyposis

As the name implies, MAP is a colonic polyposis condition caused by germ-line mutations in the *MUTYH* gene. Contrary to the other conditions described in this review, MAP is inherited in an autosomal-recessive pattern. In 2002, Al-Tassan et al.[18] were the first to describe a family with biallelic (homozygous or compound heterozygous) mutations in *MUTYH*, which is part of the base excision repair system. In this family, three siblings had CRC and/ or multiple colorectal adenomas, but no detectable mutations in *APC*.[18] All three of the affected siblings were found to have compound heterozygous mutations in *MUTYH*, whereas the other four unaffected siblings did not.[18]

It is now widely accepted that MAP is associated with a significant increased risk for multiple colorectal adenomas and cancer. Whether monoallelic *MUTYH* carriers have a modest increase in risk of CRC is debatable.[19] Monoallelic mutations in *MUTYH* are found in 1% to 2% of the general population, whereas biallelic mutations account for less than 1% of all CRCs.[20]

Colonic Phenotype

There are a number of similarities between the colonic phenotype of MAP and AFAP, including the average number, proximal distribution, and young age at onset of adenomas and cancers.[4,19] *MUTYH*-associated polyposis is associated with a 28-fold increased risk of CRC, with a penetrance of 19% by the age of 50 years, 43% by 60 years, and 80% by 70 years.[19,21] Although the risk of CRC has been reported to be as high as 100%,[22] the actual penetrance is likely to be incomplete and similar to that of AFAP. The total number of polyps in MAP is also highly variable, with some individuals developing CRC without polyps, whereas others have more than 500 colorectal polyps.[23] Typically, affected individuals have between 10 and 100 polyps.[23]

Adenomas are the predominant polyp type seen not only in AFAP and FAP, but also in MAP. Unlike individuals with germ-line *APC* mutations, serrated polyps are common in MAP. Serrated polyps include hyperplastic polyps, sessile serrated polyps (also referred to as sessile serrated adenomas), and traditional serrated adenomas.[24] Boparai et al.[25] evaluated 17 individuals with MAP and found that almost one-half (47%) had hyperplastic and/or sessile serrated polyps. In addition, three met the criteria for hyperplastic polyposis, now known as serrated polyposis. The World Health Organization diagnostic criteria for serrated polyposis include an individual with any of the following: (1) at least five serrated polyps proximal to the sigmoid colon with at least two larger than 10 mm; (2) greater than 20 serrated polyps of any size, but distributed through the colon; and (3) any number of serrated polyps proximal to the sigmoid colon in an individual with a first-degree relative with serrated polyposis.[24] Interestingly, Chow et al.[26] also identified biallelic *MUTYH* mutations in 1 (~3%) of 38 cases meeting hyperplastic polyposis/serrated polyposis criteria. Another family involving three brothers with biallelic *MUTYH* mutations has recently been reported, further highlighting this variability in phenotype. Their history included one with CRC at the age of 48 years but had no additional polyps, another was 38 years old and reportedly met criteria for serrated polyposis but had only two confirmed adenomas, and the other brother was 46 years old and had four hyperplastic polyps removed.[27] Currently, the etiology of serrated polyposis is largely unknown; however, there is growing evidence that the base excision repair pathway may be involved in a minority of these cases.

Boparai et al.[25] also compared the frequency of *KRAS* mutations and G:C to T:A transversions in hyperplastic or sessile serrated polyps in individuals with MAP to controls. In MAP, 51 (70%) of 73 serrated polyps had *KRAS* mutations, and 48 (94%) of these 51 had G:C to T:A transversions, whereas in the control group, only 7 (17%) of 41 serrated polyps had *KRAS* mutations, and 2 (29%) of 7 had G:C to T:A transversions.[25] These findings support an association between MAP and serrated polyps.

Extracolonic Features

A number of extracolonic findings have been reported in individuals with MAP.[23] However, it is still unclear whether most of these manifestations are chance occurrences or due to an underlying defective *MUTYH*. In a study of 276 individuals with MAP, only two developed duodenal cancer.[22] However, compared with the general population, the risk of duodenal cancer was significantly elevated, with a standard incidence ratio of 129 and an estimated lifetime risk of 4%.[22] Although the lifetime risk of duodenal cancer is similar between MAP and FAP/AFAP (4% and 5%), gastric and duodenal polyps are far less common in MAP. Of 150 individuals with MAP who underwent an EGD, 11% had gastric polyps, whereas 17% had duodenal polyps.[22]

Extraintestinal malignancies have also been reported in MAP,[22] although the data supporting an association are conflicting.[28,29] Desmoid tumors, thyroid and brain cancer, CHRPE, osteomas, and epidermoid cysts are rarely seen in MAP.[23]

Genetic Counseling and Testing

Since the first reported family with biallelic *MUTYH* mutations was described in 2002, more than 500 individuals with MAP have been confirmed.[23] As was the case with this first MAP family, genetic testing strategies to evaluate for *MUTYH* are typically targeted toward individuals with multiple colorectal adenomas. However, there are many other factors that can influence genetic testing approaches for *MUTYH* and *APC* mutations. Family history; age at polyp onset; types, location, and total number of polyps; CRC history (including age at onset and location); ethnicity; and extracolonic features are just some of the factors that influence genetic testing strategies and detection rates. The purpose of this review was not to present every scenario and strategy for *MUTYH* and *APC* genetic testing, but instead to outline some key concepts and considerations when multiple adenomas are detected.

Given the inheritance pattern of MAP, it is uncommon for more than one generation to be affected; however, a family history of CRC in more than one generation does not exclude MAP. Consanguinity (sharing a common ancestor) is seen in some MAP families and is an important element to evaluate for when taking a history. Siblings of affected individuals have a one in four chance (25%) of having MAP, whereas parents and children are obligate carriers. Therefore, when there is clear evidence of recessive inheritance in a family (more than one sibling affected in a family, but no one else), genetic testing should start with *MUTYH*. *APC* should still be evaluated in these families if no *MUTYH* mutations are identified, because germ-line mosaicism can result in more than one affected sibling with FAP and unaffected parents.[30] To clarify risk to offspring, spouses of individuals with MAP should also be offered *MUTYH* genetic testing. This strategy has been shown to be cost-effective.[31]

Generally, germ-line *APC* mutations are more common than biallelic *MUTYH* mutations; therefore, unless there is clear evidence for recessive inheritance in a family, *APC* genetic testing typically precedes *MUTYH* analysis. There are two common mutations in *MUTYH* that are found in the majority of affected individuals: Y179C and G396D (previously known as Y165C and G382D). These hotspot mutations were found in the original MAP family.[18] According to Nielsen et al.,[23] a review up to 2009 revealed more than 100 distinct *MUTYH* mutations. In individuals with Northern European ancestry and MAP, at least one of the two hotspot mutations are found in 90% of cases.[23,32] Testing specifically for the hotspot mutations, followed by full *MUTYH* sequencing only if one of these mutations is found, is often performed. In other populations, the scope of *MUTYH* mutations is less well understood, and therefore, full gene sequencing of *MUTYH* is often performed in individuals of non–Northern European ancestry. Similar to *APC*, genetic testing of *MUTYH* is considered when greater than 10 adenomas are documented.[13,23] The detection rates of biallelic *MUTYH* mutations

PRACTICE OF ONCOLOGY

in individuals with 10 to 100 and 100 to 1,000 polyps are 28% and 14%, respectively.[23] Given the growing evidence that hyperplastic and sessile serrated polyps are associated with MAP, these polyps should also be included in the total polyp count when considering when to test someone for *MUTYH* mutations. Individuals with FAP/AFAP are not known to develop numerous serrated polyps; therefore, genetic testing of *APC* in someone with multiple serrated polyps is unlikely to be informative. The NCCN guidelines do not currently recommend genetic testing of *MUTYH* in individuals with multiple serrated polyps and no adenomas.[13]

It is not unusual for individuals with MAP or AFAP to present with early-onset CRC and few to no polyps.[4,33] However, a consensus as to whether genetic testing of *APC* or *MUTYH* should be performed in these cases has not yet been reached.[13,23]

Management

Colonoscopy screening starting at around the age of 25 years is recommended for individuals with MAP.[13] The frequency of screening depends on polyp burden. As is the case with AFAP and FAP, colectomy is advised when polyps become endoscopically uncontrollable. EGDs should be considered in the 30s and, if duodenal adenomas are found, managed the same as in AFAP and FAP.[13] Currently, the evidence does not support increased CRC screening in monoallelic *MUTYH* carriers.

HAMARTOMATOUS POLYPOSIS

Peutz–Jeghers Syndrome

PJS is an autosomal dominant condition caused by mutations in the *STK11/LKB1* gene. It is estimated to occur in 1 in 50,000 to 200,000 births.[34] The two most characteristic manifestations of PJS are the distinct gastrointestinal-type hamartomas, called Peutz–Jeghers polyps, and the mucocutaneous melanin pigmentation. Both of these features are included in the diagnostic criteria for PJS (Table 58.2). Although it is not 100% penetrant and can fade with time, mucocutaneous hyperpigmentation in PJS typically presents in childhood. By the age of 20 years, 50% of individuals present with small-bowel obstruction, intussusception, and/or bleeding due to small-bowel polyps.[35] The polyps in PJS can also number in the hundreds and are most often found in the small intestine, followed by the colon and the stomach.[34]

The cancer risks associated with PJS are more significant after the age of 30 years, although earlier-onset malignancies do occur. In the largest study to date of 419 individuals with PJS, the risk of developing any cancer was 2% by the age of 20 years, 5% by 30 years, 17% by 40 years, 31% by 50 years, 60% by 60 years, and 85% by 70 years.[36] Gastrointestinal tract cancers had the highest cumulative risk. The specific cancer risks associated with PJS are outlined in Table 58.3.

Juvenile Polyposis Syndrome

JPS is an autosomal-dominant condition caused by germ-line mutations in *SMAD4* or *BMPR1A* genes, with an incidence of 0.6 to 1 in 100,000 and a de novo rate of 25% to 50%.[37,38] Juvenile polyps are the hallmark lesion in JPS.[38] They are most commonly found in the colorectum and can number in the hundreds, although the carpeting of polyps is not usually seen in JPS like it is in FAP.[38] Of note, solitary juvenile polyps can occur in children without JPS (see Table 58.2). Hematochezia is the most common presenting symptom and, similar to PJS, intussusception and obstruction are common. The highest risk of cancer (see Table 58.3) in JPS is CRC. Gastric cancers typically occur only in the setting of gastric polyposis, which is more commonly present in individuals with

TABLE 58.2

Testing and Diagnostic Criteria for Peutz–Jeghers Syndrome, Juvenile Polyposis Syndrome, and Cowden Syndrome

PJS

A clinical diagnosis of PJS is considered when any of the following are met:
(1) ≥3 histologically confirmed Peutz–Jeghers polyps
(2) Any number of Peutz–Jeghers polyps and a family history of PJS
(3) Characteristic, prominent, mucocutaneous pigmentation and a family history of PJS
(4) ≥1 Peutz–Jeghers polyp and characteristic, prominent, mucocutaneous pigmentation

JPS

A clinical diagnosis of JPS is considered when any of the following are met:
(1) 3–5 juvenile polyps of the colorectum
(2) Juvenile polyps throughout the gastrointestinal tract
(3) ≥1 juvenile polyp in an individual with a family history of JPS

CS[a]

Genetic testing for CS is considered in individuals meeting any of the following criteria:
(1) Adult onset Lhermitte–Duclos disease
(2) Autism spectrum disorder and macrocephaly
(3) ≥2 major criteria (one must be macrocephaly)
(4) ≥3 major criteria without macrocephaly
(5) Bannayan–Riley–Ruvalcaba syndrome
(6) One major and ≥3 minor criteria
(7) ≥2 biopsy-proven trichilemmomas
(8) ≥4 minor criteria

Major Criteria	Minor Criteria
Multiple gastrointestinal (GI) hamartomas/ganglioneuromas	A single GI hamartoma/ganglioneuroma
Nonmedullary thyroid cancer	Thyroid adenoma or multinodular goiter
Breast cancer	Fibrocystic disease of the breast
Endometrial cancer	Mental retardation (i.e., IQ ≤75)
Mucocutaneous lesions	Autism spectrum disorder
One biopsy proven trichilemmoma	Fibromas
Multiple palmoplantar keratoses	Renal cell carcinoma
Multiple cutaneous facial papules	Uterine fibroids
Macular pigmentation of glans penis	Lipomas
Multifocal/extensive oral mucosal papillomatosis	
Macrocephaly (megalocephaly) (at least 97th percentile)	

IQ, intelligence quotient.
[a] Data derived from: National Comprehensive Cancer Network. NCCN Guidelines and Clinical Resources Web site. Colorectal Cancer Screening, Version 1.2012. 2012. http://www.nccn.org. Accessed April 3, 2012.

TABLE 58.3

Characteristic Features and Recommendations: Peutz–Jeghers Syndrome and Juvenile Polyposis Syndrome

Lifetime Cancer Risks	Management Recommendations	Nonmalignant Features
PJS (*STK11*)		
Breast (54%)	Annual mammogram and breast magnetic resonance imaging by age 25 y	Mucocutaneous pigmentation
Colon (39%)	Colonoscopy every 2–3 y by age 25 y	
Pancreas (11%–36%)	CA19-9 and magnetic resonance cholangiopancreatography and/or endoscopic ultrasound every 1–2 y	Peutz–Jeghers polyps
Stomach (29%)	Upper endoscopy by 25–30 y; consider small-bowel visualization (computed tomography [CT] enterography, small-bowel enteroclysis) by 8–10 y	
Small bowel (13%)		
Ovary[a] (21%)	Annual pelvic examination and Pap smear	
Uterine/cervix[b] (11%)		
Lung (15%)	No specific recommendations	
Testicle[c] (<1%)	Annual testicular examination	
JPS (*SMAD4* and *BMPR1A*)		
Colon (40%–50%)	Colonoscopy by age 15 y repeating annually if polyps are present and every 2–3 y if no polyps	Juvenile polyps Features of hereditary hemorrhagic telangiectasia
Stomach (21% if gastric polyps are present)	Upper endoscopy by age 15 y repeating annually if polyps are present and every 2–3 y if no polyps	Congenital defects

[a] Sex cord tumor with annular tubules.
[b] Adenoma malignum.
[c] Sertoli cell tumor.
Data derived from: National Comprehensive Cancer Network. NCCN Guidelines and Clinical Resources Web site. Colorectal Cancer Screening, Version 1.2012. 2012. http://www.nccn.org. Accessed April 3, 2012.

PRACTICE OF ONCOLOGY

mutations in *SMAD4* than in *BMPR1A*.[37] JPS occurring in infancy (also known as juvenile polyposis of infancy) is often fatal, but rare. Hereditary hemorrhagic telangiectasia symptoms, such as arteriovenous malformations, telangiectasia, and epistaxis, occur in some individuals with mutations in *SMAD4*, but not *BMPR1A*.[37]

Cowden Syndrome

CS, which is part of the phosphatase and tensin homolog (PTEN) hamartoma tumor syndrome, occurs in about 1 in 200,000 to 1 in 250,000 individuals and is caused by germ-line mutations in the *PTEN* gene.[39] It is a multisystem disorder associated with characteristic mucocutaneous features, macrocephaly, and a variety of cancers and gastrointestinal manifestations.[39] Although other malignancies may be seen in CS, the primary cancers associated with CS include breast (25% to 50%), nonmedullary thyroid (3% to 10%), and endometrial (5% to 10%).[39] A recent study estimated that the lifetime risk for these cancers in *PTEN* mutation carriers was 85%, 35%, and 28%, respectively.[40] However, these risks are likely overestimates, because Tan et al.[40] failed to accurately account for ascertainment bias in their study.

Gastrointestinal polyps are one of the most common features in CS.[41] Polyps develop throughout the gastrointestinal tract, from the esophagus to the rectum, and numerous polyps or diffuse polyposis can be seen.[41] Multiple, white flat plaques in the esophagus, called glycogenic acanthosis, also occur in the setting of CS. In a large study of 127 individuals with *PTEN* mutations, 39 underwent at least 1 EGD, and 8 (~23%) had glycogenic acanthosis, 26 (~67%) had duodenal and/or gastric polyps, and only 2 (5%) had fundic gland polyps.[41] Of the 67 individuals who underwent

at least 1 colonoscopy, 62 (~93%) had colonic polyps, and 16 met criteria for hyperplastic polyposis.[41] Although hamartomas predominate, a variety of other colon polyps also develop, including adenomatous, hyperplastic, sessile serrated, ganglioneuromatous, inflammatory, lymphoid, and lipomatous. Of all of the mutation carriers in this large study, nine (7%) were diagnosed with CRC.[41]

Peutz–Jeghers Syndrome, Juvenile Polyposis Syndrome, and Cowden Syndrome: Genetic Counseling and Testing

Hamartomatous polyps consist of an overgrowth of cells native to the tissue in which they occur. They are rare, account for a minority of all colon polyps, and can be a red flag for an underlying cancer predisposition syndrome. When hamartomatous polyps are found in an individual, the differential diagnosis depends, in part, on the histologic type, total number, and age at onset of the polyps. Hamartomas can often be misdiagnosed as other polyp types, and therefore, review by a gastrointestinal pathologist should be considered.[42] When hamartomatous colonic polyps are identified, EGD and a thorough physical examination may identify extracolonic manifestations leading to a precise diagnosis. A detailed family history is also imperative. Diagnostic criteria for JPS and PJS are summarized in Table 58.2. Guidelines for genetic testing of CS, which are quite extensive and include a number of extraintestinal features, are also included in Table 58.2. Given the complexity of genetic testing for CS, the NCCN updates their guidelines annually.[13] Management considerations are reviewed for PJS and JPS in Table 58.3 and are also updated annually by the NCCN.[13]

CONCLUSIONS

There are numerous presentations that may warrant genetic testing for hereditary colonic polyposis conditions. Simplified guidelines for referral for genetic counseling include individuals with any of the following: (1) greater than 10 colonic adenomas, (2) three or more hamartomatous polyps, or (3) at least one Peutz–Jeghers polyp. Other manifestations in these individuals may help target

genetic testing to a specific condition. Once the genetic cause has been identified in an affected individual, predictive testing in at-risk relatives is critical. Family members who test negative can be spared the increased surveillance and risk-reducing procedures that are warranted for family members who test positive. It is important that health-care providers involved in the care of patients with hereditary colonic polyposis conditions stay updated with management guidelines because recommendations are constantly evolving.

REFERENCES

1. Petersen GM, Slack J, Nakamura Y. Screening guidelines and premorbid diagnosis of familial adenomatous polyposis using linkage. *Gastroenterology* 1991;100:1658–1664.
2. Foulkes WD. A tale of four syndromes: familial adenomatous polyposis, Gardner syndrome, attenuated APC and Turcot syndrome. *QJM* 1995;88:853–863.
3. Jasperson KW, Tuohy TM, Neklason DW, et al. Hereditary and familial colon cancer. *Gastroenterology* 2010;138:2044–2058.
4. Burt RW, Leppert MF, Slattery ML, et al. Genetic testing and phenotype in a large kindred with attenuated familial adenomatous polyposis. *Gastroenterology* 2004;127:444–451.
5. Gallagher MC, Phillips RK, Bulow S. Surveillance and management of upper gastrointestinal disease in familial adenomatous polyposis. *Fam Cancer* 2006;5:263–273.
6. Jasperson KW, Burt RW. APC-associated polyposis conditions. In: Pagon RA, Bird TD, Dolan CR, et al., eds. *Gene Reviews*. Seattle: University of Washington; 1993.
7. Burt RW. Gastric fundic gland polyps. *Gastroenterology* 2003;125:1462–1469.
8. Garrean S, Hering J, Saied A, et al. Gastric adenocarcinoma arising from fundic gland polyps in a patient with familial adenomatous polyposis syndrome. *Am Surg* 2008;74:79–83.
9. Nieuwenhuis MH, Casparie M, Mathus-Vliegen LM, et al. A nation-wide study comparing sporadic and familial adenomatous polyposis-related desmoid-type fibromatoses. *Int J Cancer* 2011;129:256–261.
10. Nieuwenhuis MH, Lefevre JH, Bulow S, et al. Family history, surgery, and APC mutation are risk factors for desmoid tumors in familial adenomatous polyposis: an international cohort study. *Dis Colon Rectum* 2011;54:1229–1234.
11. Sinha A, Tekkis PP, Gibbons DC, et al. Risk factors predicting desmoid occurrence in patients with familial adenomatous polyposis: a meta-analysis. *Colorectal Dis* 2011;13:1222–1229.
12. Nieuwenhuis MH, Mathus-Vliegen EM, Baeten CG, et al. Evaluation of management of desmoid tumours associated with familial adenomatous polyposis in Dutch patients. *Br J Cancer* 2011;104:37–42.
13. Colon Cancer, Version 1.2015. Clinical Practice Guidelines in Oncology (NCCN Guidelines). National Comprehensive Cancer Network. http://www.nccn.org. Accessed September 3, 2014.
14. Guillem JG, Wood WC, Moley JF, et al. ASCO/SSO review of current role of risk-reducing surgery in common hereditary cancer syndromes. *J Clin Oncol* 2006;24:4642–4660.
15. Bulow S, Christensen IJ, Hojen H, et al. Duodenal surveillance improves the prognosis after duodenal cancer in familial adenomatous polyposis. *Colorectal Dis* 2011;14:947–952.
16. Cromwell DM, Moore RD, Brensinger JD, et al. Cost analysis of alternative approaches to colorectal screening in familial adenomatous polyposis. *Gastroenterology* 1998;114:893–901.
17. Hes FJ, Nielsen M, Bik EC, et al. Somatic APC mosaicism: An underestimated cause of polyposis coli. *Gut* 2008;57:71–76.
18. Al-Tassan N, Chmiel NH, Maynard J, et al. Inherited variants of MYH associated with somatic G:C-->T:A mutations in colorectal tumors. *Nat Genet* 2002;30:227–232.
19. Lubbe SJ, Di Bernardo MC, Chandler IP, et al. Clinical implications of the colorectal cancer risk associated with MUTYH mutation. *J Clin Oncol* 2009;27:3975–3980.
20. Cleary SP, Cotterchio M, Jenkins MA, et al. Germline MutY human homologue mutations and colorectal cancer: a multisite case-control study. *Gastroenterology* 2009;136:1251–1260.
21. Jenkins MA, Croitoru ME, Monga N, et al. Risk of colorectal cancer in monoallelic and biallelic carriers of MYH mutations: a population-based case-family study. *Cancer Epidemiol Biomarkers Prev* 2006;15:312–314.
22. Vogt S, Jones N, Christian D, et al. Expanded extracolonic tumor spectrum in MUTYH-associated polyposis. *Gastroenterology* 2009;137:1976–1985, e1–e10.
23. Nielsen M, Morreau H, Vasen HF, et al. MUTYH-associated polyposis (MAP). *Crit Rev Oncol Hematol* 2011;79:1–16.
24. Snover DC, Ahnen DJ, Burt RW, et al. Serrated polyps of the colon and rectum and serrated polyposis. In: Bosman FT, Carneiro F, Hruban RH, et al., eds. *WHO Classification of Tumours of the Digestive System*. 4th ed. Lyon, France: IARC; 2010:160–165.
25. Boparai KS, Dekker E, Van Eeden S, et al. Hyperplastic polyps and sessile serrated adenomas as a phenotypic expression of MYH-associated polyposis. *Gastroenterology* 2008;135:2014–2018.
26. Chow E, Lipton L, Lynch E, et al. Hyperplastic polyposis syndrome: Phenotypic presentations and the role of MBD4 and MYH. *Gastroenterology* 2006;131:30–39.
27. Zorcolo L, Fantola G, Balestrino L, et al. MUTYH-associated colon disease: Adenomatous polyposis is only one of the possible phenotypes. A family report and literature review. *Tumori* 2011;97:676–680.
28. Out AA, Wasielewski M, Huijts PE, et al. MUTYH gene variants and breast cancer in a Dutch case-control study. *Breast Cancer Res Treat* 2012;134:219–227.
29. Santonocito C, Paradisi A, Capizzi R, et al. Common genetic variants of MUTYH are not associated with cutaneous malignant melanoma: Application of molecular screening by means of high-resolution melting technique in a pilot case-control study. *Int J Biol Markers* 2011;26:37–42.
30. Schwab AL, Tuohy TM, Condie M, et al. Gonadal mosaicism and familial adenomatous polyposis. *Fam Cancer* 2008;7:173–177.
31. Nielsen M, Hes FJ, Vasen HF, et al. Cost-utility analysis of genetic screening in families of patients with germline MUTYH mutations. *BMC Med Genet* 2007;8:42.
32. Goodenberger M, Lindor NM. Lynch syndrome and MYH-associated polyposis: Review and testing strategy. *J Clin Gastroenterol* 2011;45:488–500.
33. Wang L, Baudhuin LM, Boardman LA, et al. MYH mutations in patients with attenuated and classic polyposis and with young-onset colorectal cancer without polyps. *Gastroenterology* 2004; 127:9–16.
34. Offerhaus GJA, Billaud M, Gruber SB. Peutz–Jeghers syndrome. In: Bosman FT, Carneiro F, Hruban RH, et al., eds. *WHO Classification of Tumours of the Digestive System*. 4th ed. Lyon, France: IARC; 2010:160–165.
35. Latchford AR, Phillips RK. Gastrointestinal polyps and cancer in Peutz–Jeghers syndrome: clinical aspects. *Fam Cancer* 2011;10:455–461.
36. Hearle N, Schumacher V, Menko FH, et al. Frequency and spectrum of cancers in the Peutz–Jeghers syndrome. *Clin Cancer Res* 2006;12:3209–3215.
37. Gammon A, Jasperson K, Kohlmann W, et al. Hamartomatous polyposis syndromes. *Best Pract Res Clin Gastroenterol* 2009;23:219–231.
38. Offerhaus GJ, Howe JR. Juvenile polyposis. In: Bosman FT, Carneiro F, Hruban RH, et al., eds. *WHO Classification of Tumours of the Digestive System*. 4th ed. Lyon, France: IARC; 2010:166–167.
39. Pilarski R. Cowden syndrome: a critical review of the clinical literature. *J Genet Couns* 2009;18:13–27.
40. Tan MH, Mester JL, Ngeow J, et al. Lifetime cancer risks in individuals with germline PTEN mutations. *Clin Cancer Res* 2012;18:400–407.
41. Heald B, Mester J, Rybicki L, et al. Frequent gastrointestinal polyps and colorectal adenocarcinomas in a prospective series of PTEN mutation carriers. *Gastroenterology* 2010;139:1927–1933.
42. Sweet K, Willis J, Zhou XP, et al. Molecular classification of patients with unexplained hamartomatous and hyperplastic polyposis. *JAMA* 2005;294:2465–2473.

59 Genetic Testing in Colon Cancer (Nonpolyposis Syndromes)

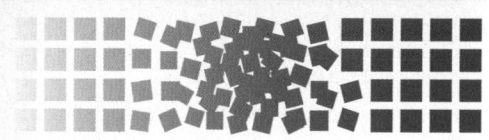

Leigha Senter-Jamieson

INTRODUCTION

Approximately 5% to 10% of colorectal cancers (CRC) are hereditary and are often categorized by the presence or absence of polyposis as a predominant feature. Lynch syndrome (LS), also sometimes referred to as hereditary nonpolyposis CRC, is the most common form of hereditary CRC, accounting for approximately 2.2%[1] of population-based CRCs diagnosed in the United States. LS also accounts for 2.3%[2] of all newly diagnosed endometrial cancers (EC), and individuals with LS also have an increased risk of developing other cancers, including cancers of the ovary, stomach, small bowel, urothelium, and biliary tract.[3] Given these increased cancer risks, cancer screening recommendations for individuals with LS differ significantly from general population screening recommendations with a goal of reducing the cancer risk and burden to the extent possible.

Mutations in one of four mismatch repair genes (*MLH1*, *MSH2*, *MSH6*, and *PMS2*) cause LS, and clinical genetic testing is available for all of them. Unlike most other hereditary cancer syndromes, however, clinical testing for LS typically begins with microsatellite instability (MSI) testing and/or immunohistochemical (IHC) staining of tumor tissue before germ-line genetic testing. This difference in testing approach, although not always possible, allows for targeted genetic analysis and, in most cases, reduced cost. Here, we review key considerations in genetic counseling for LS.

Cancer Risks

CRCs and ECs are the two most common LS-associated malignancies, and there have been several calculations of lifetime cancer risks reported in the literature. Differences in ascertainment and testing approaches have led not only to a wealth of data, but also to a wide range of risk estimates for consideration by clinicians and patients. Consistently, studies have found that the lifetime CRC risk for men with LS is higher than the risk for women with LS. The lifetime CRC risk for males is 27% to 92%, whereas the risk for females is 22% to 68%.[4,5] The most recent large study of carriers of *MLH1*, *MSH2*, and *MSH6* mutations estimated lifetime CRC risks for males and females to be 38% and 31%, respectively.[6] The average age at CRC diagnosis tends to be younger in LS (estimated 45 to 59 years) than that in the general population.[6,7] The lifetime risk of EC for women with LS based on recent data is estimated to be 33% to 39%.[6,8] Individuals with LS who have already been diagnosed with CRC also have an increased risk (10-year risk of 16%) of developing a second primary CRC.[9]

In addition to sex differences in LS-associated cancer risks, there appear to be some differences in gene-specific–associated cancer risks, as well. *MLH1* and *MSH2* seem to be associated with a higher overall cancer risk than risks associated with *MSH6* or *PMS2*.[10,11] A variable expression of phenotype both within and among families with LS is common. Therefore, as a general rule, management of families with LS (discussed later) should always take into account the family history.

Malignancies of the ovary, stomach, small bowel, urothelium, and biliary tract are also seen with greater frequency in individuals with LS when compared with the general population. Although cumulative risk estimates of these less common tumor types have been published, they are usually based on fewer cases than studies focused on CRCs and ECs, and have typically shown a lifetime cancer risk of less than 10%.[3] There have also been reports of LS-associated pancreatic and breast cancers, but the data have been inconsistent. A recent prospective study showed an increased risk of developing both tumor types when comparing carriers of *MMR* gene mutations to their unaffected relatives.[12] Additional data are necessary, however, to determine whether screening recommendations should change based on these reported risks. Some individuals with LS also have a predisposition to developing sebaceous lesions and keratoacanthomas of the skin. When an individual has one of these lesions in addition to a visceral organ malignancy, they have a variant of LS called Muir–Torre syndrome.[13] Some recent studies suggest that these skin lesions are more common in LS than originally thought and that sebaceous tumors of the skin should be considered part of the typical LS spectrum.[14] Another variant of LS characterized by the presence of glioblastomas is called Turcot syndrome. Turcot syndrome is more commonly caused by mutations in the *APC* gene but has been described in individuals with mismatch repair (MMR) deficiency, as well.[15]

CLINICAL CLASSIFICATION: AMSTERDAM CRITERIA AND BETHESDA GUIDELINES

In 1991, the International Collaborative Group on Hereditary Non-Polyposis CRC wrote the Amsterdam I criteria[16] and revised them in 1999 (Amsterdam II criteria)[17] to clinically classify families as having LS (Table 59.1). The Amsterdam criteria rely heavily on extensive family history and do not take into account the full spectrum of possible LS-associated tumors. The less stringent Bethesda guidelines (written in 1997 and revised in 2004)[18,19] (Table 59.2) were written to include these less common LS-associated tumors as well as pathologic features that are common in LS-associated CRCs. Unlike the Amsterdam criteria, which were meant to diagnose LS based on familial criteria, the Bethesda guidelines were meant to determine who should have tumor screenings for LS and relied less on family history. It has been repeatedly shown, however, that these clinical classification systems do not reliably predict LS in all patient populations, particularly for those populations outside the cancer genetics clinics dedicated to high-risk patients.[1,20]

TUMOR SCREENING

Microsatellites are pieces of DNA sequence where a single nucleotide or group of nucleotides is repeated multiple times. In general, the number of repeated nucleotide sequences should remain the same within a person's cells, but when this number of repeats

TABLE 59.1

Revised Amsterdam Criteria

≥3 relatives with colorectal, endometrial, small bowel, ureter, and/or renal pelvis cancer AND
One of these relatives is a first-degree relative[a] of the other two AND
≥2 successive generations are affected AND
At least one diagnosis is at the age of <50 y
Familial adenomatous polyposis is excluded
Tumors should be verified pathologically/histologically

[a] First-degree relative: parent, sibling, or child.
From Vasen HF, Watson P, Mecklin JP, et al. New clinical criteria for hereditary nonpolyposis colorectal cancer (HNPCC, Lynch syndrome) proposed by the International Collaborative group on HNPCC. *Gastroenterology* 1999;116:1453–1456.

TABLE 59.3

Genetic Testing Strategies Based on IHC Pattern

Absence MLH1 and PMS2	*MLH1* methylation and/or *BRAF* testing[a] OR *MLH1* germ-line testing[b] ■ If negative, consider *PMS2* germ-line testing[20]
Absence PMS2 only	*PMS2* germ-line testing ■ If negative consider *MLH1* germ-line testing[21]
Absence MSH2 and MSH6	*MSH2* germ-line testing ■ If negative, *TACSTD1* deletion testing ■ If negative, *MSH6* germline testing
Absence MSH6 only	*MSH6* germ-line testing ■ If negative, consider *MSH2* germ-line testing

[a] If personal/family history highly suggestive of LS, it is appropriate to forgo *MLH1* methylation/*BRAF* testing.
[b] Unless otherwise noted, "germ-line testing" here refers to sequencing/large rearrangement testing.

differs in one or two alleles, MSI is present.[21] In the case of LS, five microsatellite markers are used as the standard with which to measure MSI, and a tumor is considered to have a high level of MSI (MSI-H) if at least 40% of the markers are unstable.[22] Nearly all LS-associated tumors display MSI, but the presence of MSI is not diagnostic of LS, given that approximately 10% to 15% of all CRCs, in general, also display MSI.[23,24] MSI testing, however, can be used as a screening tool to help identify individuals for whom germ-line genetic testing for mutations in *MLH1*, *MSH2*, *MSH6*, and/or *PMS2* is indicated. A clinical diagnosis of LS can be made if a person has an MSI-H CRC and meets the Amsterdam II criteria (see Table 59.1).

Immunohistochemistry can be used to determine the presence or absence of MMR proteins in a tumor specimen and is another available screening test for LS. The absence of one or more MMR proteins in tumor tissue indicates dysfunction of the corresponding *MMR* gene, but additional analyses are required to determine if the dysfunction is germ line or somatic in nature. The benefit of performing IHC staining over MSI testing is that results from IHC staining can direct the approach to genetic testing. For instance, if a patient has CRC that demonstrates an absence of MSH2 and MSH6 proteins, testing for MSH2 with procession to testing for MSH6 if the MSH2 test results are negative is recommended. In

the context of this IHC result, it is generally not necessary to test for mutations in *MLH1* and/or *PMS2*. Strategies for genetic testing based on IHC results are included in Table 59.3.[25,26] In comparing tumor screening strategies, using MSI and IHC staining together will identify the majority of LS cases. Because the sensitivity of either test is not 100%, using either test alone will leave 5% to 10% of LS cases undetected.[27,28]

Epigenetic events unrelated to LS can cause a tumor to demonstrate MSI and an absence of MLH1 and PMS2 proteins upon IHC staining. These results can often be attributed to hypermethylation of the *MLH1* promoter and/or a somatic *BRAF* mutation (V600E). Several studies have shown that the V600E *BRAF* mutations are not associated with LS, and there have been very few exceptions.[11,29] Both of these tests can be performed on CRC tissue to help determine whether germ-line genetic testing should be pursued, further streamlining the genetic testing process, but this should be interpreted in the context of clinical familial presentation because sensitivities and specificities for these tests are not 100%. It is important to note that it is possible but rare to have inherited *MLH1* promoter hypermethylation.[30]

Similar approaches to screening EC with MSI and/or IHC staining are appropriate. However, because somatic *BRAF* mutations are uncommon in ECs, *BRAF* testing is not an appropriate test for ECs that are MSI-H and/or MLH1- and PMS2-protein deficient.[31] There are less data to support MSI and/or IHC testing using other LS-associated tumor tissue, but many reports suggest that it is at least feasible in the absence of additional testing options.[32]

In 2009, the Evaluation of Genomic Application in Practice and Prevention Working Group recommended that individuals with newly diagnosed CRCs be offered genetic testing for LS. Although the Evaluation of Genomic Application in Practice and Prevention Working Group did not specify the best approach for genetic testing, performing a tumor analysis with IHC staining allows for more targeted genetic testing and was considered to be an acceptable strategy.[33] In addition, multiple reports have shown that tumor screening with IHC staining is a cost-effective strategy for identifying LS in the CRC patient population.[34,35] Ladabaum et al.[35] compared the differences among multiple testing strategies with regard to effect of life-years, cancer morbidity and mortality, and cost. They concluded that IHC staining with inclusion of *BRAF* gene testing if the MLH1 protein was absent was the preferred method of identifying LS among CRC patients.[35] The effectiveness of screening for LS in these reports has been dependent on the ability to test family members of the initially diagnosed

TABLE 59.2

Revised Bethesda Guidelines

Individuals with CRC should be tested for MSI if they have any of the following:
■ CRC at the age of <50 y
■ Synchronous CRC (>1 CRC at the same time) or metachronous CRC (>1 CRC diagnosed at different times) or other LS-associated tumors[a]
■ CRC with MSI-H histology (tumor-infiltrating lymphocytes, Crohnlike lymphocytic reaction, mucinous or signet-ring differentiation, medullary growth pattern) in a patient aged <60 y
■ CRC or LS-associated tumor[a] diagnosed at the age of <50 y in FDR
■ CRC or LS-associated tumor[a] in 2 FDR and/or SDR at any age

[a] CRC, EC, stomach, small bowel, ovary, pancreas, ureter and renal pelvis, biliary tract, brain tumor, sebaceous adenomas, keratoacanthomas.
FDR, first-degree relative (parent, sibling, child); SDR, second-degree relative (grandparent, aunt, uncle, grandchild).
From Umar A, Boland CR, Terdiman JP, et al. Revised Bethesda guidelines for hereditary nonpolyposis colorectal cancer (Lynch syndrome) and microsatellite instability. *J Natl Cancer Inst* 2004;96:261–268.

LS patient; therefore, genetic counseling and dissemination of information to relatives of probands are crucial for an effective diagnosis and the prevention of cancer.

GENETIC TESTING

In many situations, as mentioned previously, tumor screening tests are performed before germ-line genetic testing, but there are situations where this is not possible or desired (e.g., sufficient tumor tissue is unavailable, all individuals affected with cancer in a family are deceased). In the absence of IHC results to direct genetic testing, germ-line testing is typically done in a stepwise fashion beginning with *MLH1* and *MSH2*, which account for 32% and 38% of mutations, respectively.[9] If no mutations are identified, testing for mutations in *MSH6* and *PMS2* is indicated. Mutations in these two genes are less common and account for 14% and 15% of LS, respectively.[9] It is important for testing to include sequencing as well as an analysis of deletions and duplications because all mutation types have been reported in the *MMR* genes.

Recently, deletions in *TACSTD1* (also known as *EPCAM*), which is not an *MMR* gene, have been reported to cause an inactivation of *MSH2* and a lack of expression of the MSH2 protein when IHC staining is performed. Therefore, testing for deletions in *TACSTD1* is indicated when the MSH2 protein is absent on IHC staining, but no germ-line *MSHS2* mutation has been identified.[36]

GENETIC COUNSELING FOR LYNCH SYNDROME

Inherited in an autosomal dominant manner, first-degree relatives of individuals with LS have a 50% chance of having inherited the syndrome as well, making the communication of these risks to family members of patients with LS very important. Data have shown that compliance with the screening recommendations, as follows, is effective at reducing the risk of dying of cancer in individuals with LS, and this should be communicated to at-risk families. A large study of *MMR* mutation carriers in Finland found that despite the increased risks of CRCs and ECs, cancer mortality was not increased when individuals followed the intensive screening protocol and/or opted to have prophylactic surgery.[37]

MANAGEMENT OF LYNCH SYNDROME

Individuals with LS require personalized management planning with the goal of reducing their cancer risks. Although many groups have put forth screening recommendations in the literature, the LS surveillance and screening recommendations from the National Comprehensive Cancer Network, which are updated annually, are commonly used in clinical practice. Based on these current recommendations, individuals with LS should have colonoscopy every 1 to 2 years beginning at the age of 20 to 25 years or 2 to 5 years earlier than the youngest CRC in the family if diagnosed before the age of 25 years. (A colonoscopy may be recommended to start at the age of 30 years in families with *MSH6* and *PMS2* mutations if the CRC age at onset in the family is not younger than the age of 30 years given the reduced penetrance with these genes.) Given that there is no clear evidence to support screening for endometrial and/or ovarian cancers, women with LS are recommended to consider a prophylactic hysterectomy and a bilateral salpingo-oophorectomy upon completion of childbearing. Some clinicians may find endometrial sampling, transvaginal ultrasound, and CA-125 serum screening to be helpful; however, these tools should be used at their discretion. To screen for gastric and small-bowel cancers, individuals with LS should consider an esophagogastroduodenoscopy with an extended duodenoscopy and a capsule endoscopy every 2 to 3 years beginning at the age of 30 to 35 years. An annual urinalysis beginning at the age of 25 to 30 years can be used to screen for urothelial cancers, and an annual physical examination to assess for symptoms of central nervous system tumors is reasonable.[38]

A 2011 study by Burn et al.[39] showed through a randomized trial with postintervention double-blind follow-up that daily use of 600 mg of aspirin for a minimum of 25 months reduced the risk of CRCs by almost 60% in individuals with LS. Like other studies of aspirin use on cancer risk, cumulative use seemed to make a difference in the study because a reduced risk became evident over time. The optimum dose and duration of use of aspirin in individuals with LS still need to be established, but based on this evidence, many clinicians are considering aspirin therapy as chemoprevention in this population.

ACKNOWLEDGMENT

The author thanks Kory Jasperson for his review of the manuscript.

REFERENCES

1. Hampel H, Frankel WL, Martin E, et al. Screening for the Lynch syndrome (hereditary nonpolyposis colorectal cancer). *N Engl J Med* 2005;352:1851–1860.
2. Hampel H, Panescu J, Lockman J, et al. Comment on: Screening for Lynch syndrome (hereditary nonpolyposis colorectal cancer) among endometrial cancer patients. *Cancer Res* 2007;67:9603.
3. Barrow E, Robinson L, Alduaij W, et al. Cumulative lifetime incidence of extracolonic cancers in Lynch syndrome: a report of 121 families with proven mutations. *Clin Genet* 2009;75:141–149.
4. Vasen HF, Wijnen JT, Menko FH, et al. Cancer risk in families with hereditary nonpolyposis colorectal cancer diagnosed by mutation analysis. *Gastroenterology* 1996;110:1020–1027.
5. Quehenberger F, Vasen HF, van Houwelingen HC. Risk of colorectal and endometrial cancer for carriers of mutations of the hMLH1 and hMSH2 gene: correction for ascertainment. *J Med Genet* 2005;42:491–496.
6. Bonadona V, Bonaiti B, Olschwang S, et al. Cancer risks associated with germline mutations in MLH1, MSH2, and MSH6 genes in Lynch syndrome. *JAMA* 2011;305:2304–2310.
7. Hampel H, Stephens JA, Pukkala E, et al. Cancer risk in hereditary nonpolyposis colorectal cancer syndrome: Later age of onset. *Gastroenterology* 2005;129:415–421.
8. Stoffel E, Mukherjee B, Raymond VM, et al. Calculation of risk of colorectal and endometrial cancer among patients with Lynch syndrome. *Gastroenterology* 2009;137:1621–1627.
9. Palomaki GE, McClain MR, Melillo S, et al. EGAPP supplementary evidence review: DNA testing strategies aimed at reducing morbidity and mortality from Lynch syndrome. *Genet Med* 2009;11:42–65.
10. Baglietto L, Lindor NM, Dowty JG, et al. Risks of Lynch syndrome cancers for MSH6 mutation carriers. *J Natl Cancer Inst* 2010;102:193–201.
11. Senter L, Clendenning M, Sotamaa K, et al. The clinical phenotype of Lynch syndrome due to germ-line PMS2 mutations. *Gastroenterology* 2008;135:419–428.
12. Win AK, Young JP, Lindor NM, et al. Colorectal and other cancer risks for carriers and noncarriers from families with a DNA mismatch repair gene mutation: a prospective cohort study. *J Clin Oncol* 2012;30:958–964.
13. Lynch HT, Lynch PM, Pester J, et al. The cancer family syndrome. Rare cutaneous phenotypic linkage of Torre's syndrome. *Arch Intern Med* 1981;141:607–611.
14. South CD, Hampel H, Comeras I, et al. The frequency of Muir-Torre syndrome among Lynch syndrome families. *J Natl Cancer Inst* 2008;100:277–281.
15. Hamilton SR, Liu B, Parsons RE, et al. The molecular basis of Turcot's syndrome. *N Engl J Med* 1995;332:839–847.
16. Vasen HF, Mecklin JP, Khan PM, et al. The International Collaborative Group on Hereditary Non-Polyposis Colorectal Cancer (ICG-HNPCC). *Dis Colon Rectum* 1991;34:424–425.
17. Vasen HF, Watson P, Mecklin JP, et al. New clinical criteria for hereditary nonpolyposis colorectal cancer (HNPCC, Lynch syndrome) proposed by the International Collaborative group on HNPCC. *Gastroenterology* 1999;116:1453–1456.

18. Rodriguez-Bigas MA, Boland CR, Hamilton SR, et al. A National Cancer Institute workshop on hereditary nonpolyposis colorectal cancer syndrome: meeting highlights and Bethesda guidelines. *J Natl Cancer Inst* 1997; 89:1758–1762.

19. Umar A, Boland CR, Terdiman JP, et al. Revised Bethesda guidelines for hereditary nonpolyposis colorectal cancer (Lynch syndrome) and microsatellite instability. *J Natl Cancer Inst* 2004;96:261–268.

20. Morrison J, Bronner M, Leach BH, et al. Lynch syndrome screening in newly diagnosed colorectal cancer in general pathology practice: from the revised Bethesda guidelines to a universal approach. *Scand J Gastroenterol* 2012;46:1340–1348.

21. de la Chapelle A, Hampel H. Clinical relevance of microsatellite instability in colorectal cancer. *J Clin Oncol* 2010;28:3380–3387.

22. Boland CR, Thibodeau SN, Hamilton SR, et al. A National Cancer Institute Workshop on Microsatellite Instability for cancer detection and familial predisposition: development of international criteria for the determination of microsatellite instability in colorectal cancer. *Cancer Res* 1998;58:5248–5257.

23. Hampel H, Frankel WL, Martin E, et al. Feasibility of screening for Lynch syndrome among patients with colorectal cancer. *J Clin Oncol* 2008;26:5783–5788.

24. Samowitz WS, Curtin K, Lin HH, et al. The colon cancer burden of genetically defined hereditary nonpolyposis colon cancer. *Gastroenterology* 2001;121:830–838.

25. Niessen RC, Kleibeuker JH, Westers H, et al. PMS2 involvement in patients suspected of Lynch syndrome. *Genes Chromosomes Cancer* 2009;48:322–329.

26. Zighelboim I, Powell MA, Babb SA, et al. Epitope-positive truncating MLH1 mutation and loss of PMS2: Implications for IHC-directed genetic testing for Lynch syndrome. *Fam Cancer* 2009;8:501–504.

27. Lindor NM, Burgart LJ, Leontovich O, et al. Immunohistochemistry versus microsatellite instability testing in phenotyping colorectal tumors. *J Clin Oncol* 2002;20:1043–1048.

28. Ruszkiewicz A, Bennett G, Moore J, et al. Correlation of mismatch repair genes immunohistochemistry and microsatellite instability status in HNPCC-associated tumours. *Pathology* 2002;34:541–547.

29. Loughrey MB, Waring PM, Tan A, et al. Incorporation of somatic BRAF mutation testing into an algorithm for the investigation of hereditary nonpolyposis colorectal cancer. *Fam Cancer* 2007;6:301–310.

30. Hitchins MP, Ward RL. Constitutional (germline) MLH1 epimutation as an aetiological mechanism for hereditary non-polyposis colorectal cancer. *J Med Genet* 2009;46:793–802.

31. Mutch DG, Powell MA, Mallon MA, et al. RAS/RAF mutation and defective DNA mismatch repair in endometrial cancers. *Am J Obstet Gynecol* 2004;190:935–942.

32. Weissman SM, Bellcross C, Bittner CC, et al. Genetic counseling considerations in the evaluation of families for Lynch syndrome—a review. *J Genet Couns* 2011;20:5–19.

33. Evaluation of Genomic Applications in Practice and Prevention (EGAPP) Working Group. Recommendations from the EGAPP Working Group: Genetic testing strategies in newly diagnosed individuals with colorectal cancer aimed at reducing morbidity and mortality from Lynch syndrome in relatives. *Genet Med* 2009;11:35–41.

34. Mvundura M, Grosse SD, Hampel H, et al. The cost-effectiveness of genetic testing strategies for Lynch syndrome among newly diagnosed patients with colorectal cancer. *Genet Med* 2010;12:93–104.

35. Ladabaum U, Wang G, Terdiman J, et al. Strategies to identify the Lynch syndrome among patients with colorectal cancer: A cost-effectiveness analysis. *Ann Intern Med* 2011;155:69–79.

36. Niessen RC, Hofstra RM, Westers H, et al. Germline hypermethylation of MLH1 and EPCAM deletions are a frequent cause of Lynch syndrome. *Genes Chromosomes Cancer* 2009;48:737–744.

37. Jarvinen HJ, Renkonen-Sinisalo L, Aktan-Collan K, et al. Ten years after mutation testing for Lynch syndrome: cancer incidence and outcome in mutation-positive and mutation-negative family members. *J Clin Oncol* 2009;27:4793–4797.

38. National Comprehensive Cancer Network. NCCN Guidelines & Clinical Resources. NCCN Guidelines for Detection, Prevention, and Risk Reduction [v.1.2012]. 2012. http://www.nccn.org/professionals/physician_gls/recently_updated.asp

39. Burn J, Gerdes AM, Macrae F, et al. Long-term effect of aspirin on cancer risk in carriers of hereditary colorectal cancer: an analysis from the CAPP2 randomised controlled trial. *Lancet* 2011;378:2081–2087.

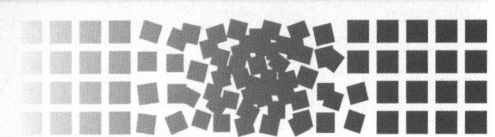

60 Cancer of the Rectum

Steven K. Libutti, Christopher G. Willett, Leonard B. Saltz,
and Rebecca A. Levine

INTRODUCTION

Information concerning epidemiology and systemic approaches to the management of both colon and rectal cancer was given in another chapter in this book. This chapter will focus on issues unique to rectal cancer with an emphasis on radiation, combined modality therapy, and sphincter-preserving surgery.

ANATOMY

The anatomy of the rectum can be very confusing as there are differing definitions of the relevant landmarks. In the upper portion of the rectum, there are changes both in the musculature of the large bowel and in the relationship to the peritoneal covering that roughly coincide. In the lower portion of the rectum, the mucosal changes occur at roughly the same location as the anal sphincter.

The anatomy of the rectum is usually divided into three portions (Fig. 60.1). The lower rectum is the area approximately from 3 to 6 cm from the anal verge. The midrectum goes from 5 to 6, to 8 to 10 cm, and the upper rectum extends approximately from 8 to 10, to 12 to 15 cm from the anal verge, although the retroperitoneal portion of the large bowel often reaches its upper limit approximately 12 cm from the anal verge. In some patients, especially elderly women, the peritonealized portion of the large bowel can be located much lower than these definitions. The determination of the location of the boundary between rectum and sigmoid colon is important in defining adjuvant therapy, with the rectum usually being operationally defined as that area of the large bowel that is at least partially retroperitoneal.

Externally, the upper extent of the rectum can be identified where the tenia spread to form a longitudinal coat of muscle. The upper third of the rectum is surrounded by peritoneum on its anterior and lateral surfaces but is retroperitoneal posteriorly without any serosal covering. At the rectovesical or rectouterine pouch, the rectum becomes completely extra-/retroperitoneal. The rectum follows the curve of the sacrum in its lower two-thirds. It enters the anal canal at the level of the levator ani. The anorectal ring is at the level of the puborectalis sling portion of the levator muscles.

The location of a rectal tumor is most commonly indicated by the distance between the anal verge, dentate (pectinate or mucocutaneous) line, or anorectal ring and the lower edge of the tumor. These points of reference are all different for different individuals. Also, these measurements differ depending on the method of measurement. This can be important clinically, as the measurement from a flexible endoscopy can substantially overestimate the distance to the tumor from the anal verge or other landmark. The distance from the anal sphincter musculature is clinically of more importance than the distance from the anal verge, as it has implications for the ability to perform sphincter-sparing surgery. The lack of a peritoneal covering over most of the rectum is a major reason for the higher risk of local failure after primary surgical management of rectal cancer compared to colon cancer. The

mesorectum is usually used as the structure to define the extent of a total mesorectal excision (TME), with most of the perirectal fatty tissue and perirectal lymph nodes (LN) contained within its boundaries.

Lymphatic Drainage

The lymphatic drainage of the upper rectum follows the course of the superior hemorrhoidal artery toward the inferior mesenteric artery. Lymph nodes that are above the midrectum and therefore drain along the superior hemorrhoidal artery are often part of the mesentery that is removed during resections of the intraperitoneal portion of the colon. Lesions that arise in the rectum below approximately 6 cm are in a region of the rectum that is drained by lymphatics that follow the middle hemorrhoidal artery. Nodes involved from a cancer in this region can include the internal iliac nodes and the nodes of the obturator fossa. These regions deserve particular attention during the resection and irradiation of lesions in this location. When lesions occur below the dentate line, the lymphatic drainage is via the inguinal nodes and external iliac chain, which has major therapeutic implications, especially for the radiation fields. The corollary of this high risk of inguinal node involvement for the very low-lying tumors is that tumors located above the dentate line are at low risk of inguinal node involvement, and these nodes as well as the external iliacs do not need to be treated.

Bowel Function

Fecal continence is maintained through the function of both the sphincter mechanism and the preservation of the normal pelvic floor musculature, which creates a neorectal angle or rectal sling. The pelvic floor is composed of the levator ani muscles, which separate the pelvis from the perineum and ischiorectal fossa. The urethra, vagina, and anus pass through the levator muscles.

Preservation of fecal continence during surgery for rectal cancer is therefore dependent on a thorough understanding of the anatomic relationships of the musculature and the sphincter mechanism. Maintenance of the sphincter apparatus without preservation of the muscular angles will not have the desired result. These anatomic constraints, especially with respect to lateral margins, make the use of adjuvant chemotherapy and radiation therapy critical to a successful surgical outcome. This is true from both an oncologic as well as a bowel function perspective.

Autonomic Nerves

The preservation of both bladder and sexual function depends on the surgeon's understanding of the autonomic nerve supply to the pelvic organs.[1,2] The hypogastric plexus is formed from the sympathetic trunks as they converge over the sacral promontory. These sympathetic nerves are found beneath the pelvic peritoneum

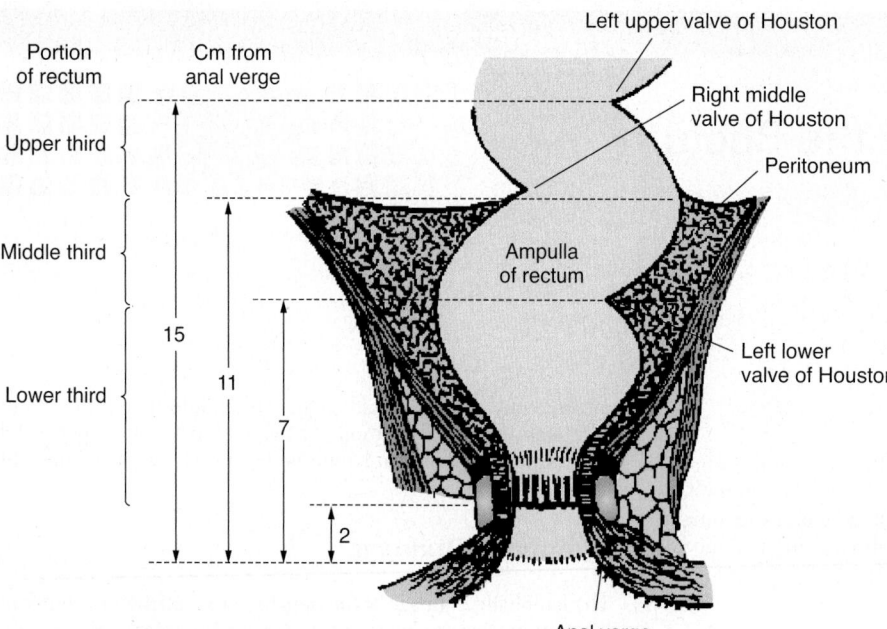

Figure 60.1 Division of the rectum into upper, middle, and lower thirds.

along the lateral pelvic sidewalls lateral to the mesorectum. The second, third, and fourth sacral nerve roots give rise to parasympathetic fibers to the pelvic viscera. The parasympathetic fibers proceed laterally as the nervi erigentes to join the sympathetic fibers at the site of the pelvic plexus that is just lateral and somewhat anterior to the tips of the seminal vesicle in men.[1,2] In order to preserve these structures and, therefore, sexual and bladder function, a sharp rather than a blunt technique should be used to dissect the mesorectum.[3–6]

STAGING

Standard clinicopathologic staging is the best indicator of prognosis for patients with rectal cancer. For rectal cancer, it is increasingly common to use clinical staging as the basis for the decision to initiate neoadjuvant chemoradiation therapy. Therefore, the accuracy of that initial staging is critically important, both for management and for prognosis. There have been a large number of studies that have evaluated other prognostic markers, including pathologic, socioeconomic, and molecular, as described more fully in Chapter 57. However, even though many of these appear to have prognostic value, there are none that are commonly used to define management. This is related to the large number of tests that could be used, the lack of standardization of these tests, as well as the lack of knowledge as to how to incorporate them into the patient management scheme. The molecular marker that has engendered the most interest is the deletion of 18q.[7] These markers have been fully reviewed elsewhere.[8,9]

The staging system that should be used in the evaluation of patients with rectal cancer is the American Joint Committee on Cancer/International Union Against Cancer TNM (tumor, node, metastases) staging system (fully described in Chapter 57), which has been recently revised to subcategorize patients with stage III (node-positive) tumors. The Dukes staging system or its multiple modifications has been used for many years, but provides less information than the TNM system and should not be used. There have been gradual changes in the TNM system that primarily reflect the stage grouping rather than the system itself. The other systems should be acknowledged for their historical interest and for initially defining many of the high-risk factors for this disease.

Patients now often have both a clinical (preoperative) stage, which may define the need for neoadjuvant therapy, and a pathologic (postoperative) stage. Initial therapy with chemoradiation can produce substantial downstaging (approximately 15% of patients will have a pathologic complete response, and as many as 40% in those with more favorable tumors). While some believe that the degree of response to neoadjuvant therapy should alter subsequent treatment, and this is in fact an area of active investigation (see later discussion), the current standard of care dictates that all surgical planning and adjuvant therapy be determined based on the initial clinical stage regardless of tumor response. This guideline is based in part on the idea that a good tumor response locally to chemoradiation does not translate into reduced risk of having micrometastatic disease, and thus does not lessen the need for adjuvant postoperative chemotherapy. Whether this will continue to be true in the face of newer data and more aggressive neoadjuvant regimens remains to be seen. Numerous studies have indicated that tumor response to neoadjuvant therapy is an important predictor of multiple oncologic end points for patients completing the full course of multimodal therapy. Patients with pathologic complete response in particular demonstrate excellent long-term results, with local recurrence rates as low as 0.7%, and significantly improved disease-free survival (DFS) and overall survival (OS) compared to nonresponders at 5 years (odds ratio [OR] = 3.28 and OR = 4.33, respectively).[10–12] It is unclear at this time whether such a favorable outcome can be maintained should the course of treatment be altered based on postneoadjuvant reassessment.

Although it is not standard practice to alter treatment based on local response to neoadjuvant therapy, preoperative restaging prior to surgery may still be valuable not only as a prognostic predictor but also for detecting interval metastatic progression. Multiple studies recommend repeating serum carcinoembryonic antigen (CEA) levels, for example, between chemoradiation and surgery as this value as well as the pre- to posttreatment ratio may be more important in predicting survival than the initial measurement.[13–15] In addition, Ayez et al.[16] advocate restaging with chest and abdominal computed tomography (CT), as this changed management in 12% of their patients, and spared 8% from undergoing noncurative rectal surgery, due to new findings of progressive metastatic disease.[16]

The major change that has occurred in the newest version of the staging system is the acknowledgment that both the T stage and the N stage have independent prognostic importance for local control, DFS, and OS.[17,18] Thus, for patients with N0 and N1 tumors viewed separately, the extent of the primary tumor in the rectum is of additional prognostic importance. Patients with T1-2N1 tumors have a relatively favorable prognosis and an outcome superior to that of other stage III patients. In fact, patients with T3N0M0 disease (stage II) have outcomes slightly inferior to those with T1-2N1M0, demonstrating the independent prognostic importance of T stage. These distinctions may allow future decisions to be more individualized as to the adjuvant therapy required.

Although at one level staging is very straightforward, the actuality of proper staging is much more difficult as it relies on multiple quality control issues that can mislead the clinician regarding proper therapy. For instance, it has been well demonstrated that for patients with colon and rectal cancer who are pathologically staged as N0, the prognosis is markedly improved for those in whom more than 12 to 14 nodes were identified by the pathologist compared with those in whom fewer nodes were identified.[19] This could be a surgical issue (fewer nodes were removed) or a pathologist issue (fewer nodes were identified), but it suggests that many patients were inappropriately understaged, which could result in inappropriate therapy. Others have shown that staging accuracy continues to improve as the pathologist recovers more nodes, with accuracy leveling off at approximately 12 to 20 nodes recovered.[20,21] (See discussion in Chapter 57). In rectal cancer, however, N staging presents a particular challenge as there are often fewer LNs in the specimen and preoperative radiotherapy is thought to reduce that number even further.[22–24] In fact, one recent report suggests that LN harvests <12 in pretreated specimens may be a marker of high tumor response and improved rather than compromised oncologic outcome. In this study of 237 patients, local recurrence rates were significantly higher in the LN >12 group as compared to those with "inadequate" LN retrieval (11% versus 0%; $p = 0.004$).[25] As with colon cancer, the percentage of positive nodes is likely of greater prognostic importance than total LN number (M. Meyers, 2007, personal communication).[26–28] The same issue relates to T-stage determination. If the pathologist does not look carefully for evidence of extension of tumor through the muscularis propria, the patient can be understaged, resulting in inappropriate treatment. Close or positive circumferential margins are a poor prognostic factor, which can only be found if the pathologist assiduously evaluates the radial margins.[29,30]

The standard staging procedure for rectal cancer entails a history, physical examination, complete blood cell count, liver and renal function studies, as well as CEA evaluation. The routine laboratory studies are quite insensitive to the presence of metastatic disease, but they are usually ordered as a screen of organ function prior to surgery or chemoradiation therapy. High CEA levels are associated with poorer survival (see Chapter 57) and give an indication as to whether follow-up CEA determinations are likely to be useful. A careful rectal examination by an experienced examiner is an essential part of the pretherapy evaluation in determining distance of the tumor from the anal verge or from the dentate line, involvement of the anal sphincter, amount of circumferential involvement, clinical fixation, sphincter tone, and so forth, and has not been replaced by imaging studies or endoscopy. Colonoscopy or barium enema to evaluate the remainder of the large bowel is essential (if the patient is not obstructed) to rule out synchronous tumors or the presence of polyposis syndromes.

Local staging is completed with one of two imaging modalities, endorectal ultrasound (EUS) or pelvic magnetic resonance imaging (MRI). Each provides similar overall accuracy in T and N determination, and each has its advantages as well as drawbacks. The decision of which to use generally depends on local institutional expertise and resource availability.

EUS defines five interface layers of the rectal wall: mucosa, muscularis mucosa, submucosa, muscularis propria, and perirectal fat, as shown in Figure 60.2. Rectal tumors are generally hypoechoic and disrupt the interfaces depending on the level of tumor extension. The accuracy of EUS depends heavily on the experience and skill of the operator. In experienced hands, EUS has an overall accuracy rate for T stage of 75% to 95% with an

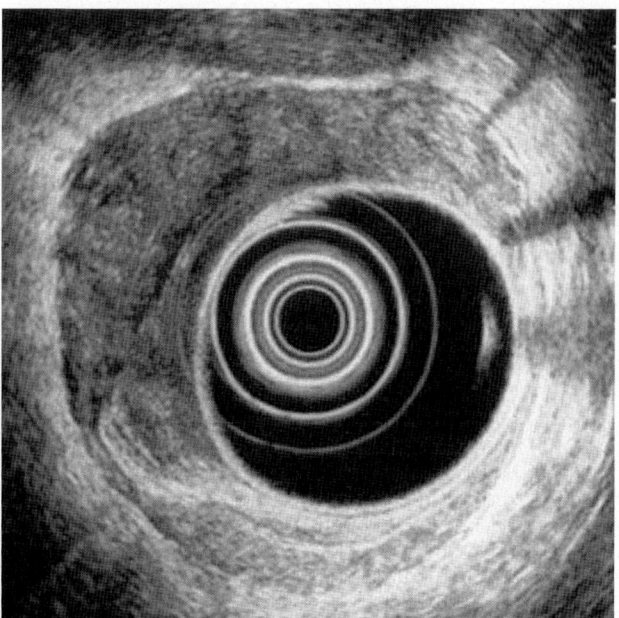

Figure 60.2 Endorectal ultrasound of a T3 tumor of the rectum, extension through the muscularis propria, and into perirectal fat.

overstaging of approximately 10% to 20% in T2 disease because of an inability to distinguish a desmoplastic response and postbiopsy changes from local tumor invasion, and approximately a 10% rate of understaging because of an inability to detect microscopic tumor extension.[31–33]

EUS is less accurate in determining N stage than for T stage, with an overall accuracy rate of 62% to 83%.[31,32] Understaging occurs because many nodal metastases from rectal cancer are small, even micrometastatic, and not easily detected by EUS. In addition, some nodes are located beyond the range of the ultrasound transducer and thus cannot be seen during the procedure. Overstaging is often related to an inflammatory response, perhaps secondary to previous biopsy or manipulation. EUS is not accurate for determining tumor regression after preoperative radiation and chemotherapy, as inflammatory changes and scarring can persist in the rectal wall or in perirectal soft tissue and may not reflect persisting tumor. Newer ultrasound techniques, such as three-dimensional ultrasound, are being explored but have not yet made it into standard practice.

Endorectal coil MRI allows discernment of the layers of the bowel wall and is similar in accuracy to EUS. Thin-section pelvic MRI with a surface coil also allows one to visualize the mesorectal fascia and thus to predict the likely distance of the surgical resection margin when performing a TME. The MERCURY Study Group confirmed this key advantage of MRI in their landmark 2005 multicenter trial, where specificity for predicting clear margins in 408 patients with varying stages of rectal cancer was 92%.[34] Although there has been great interest in this technique since then, followup studies still show a disappointing overall accuracy for T and N staging, which fails to surpass EUS in experienced hands. In one study of 96 patients who had MRI followed by TME, of 22 patients classified as having T2 disease on MRI, 3 had T1 and 6 had T3 tumors. Of 61 patients classified as having T3 disease on MRI, 8 had T2 tumors and 2 had T4. Thus, 6 of 22 (27%) patients who might have benefited from preoperative therapy for T3 disease would not have received that therapy. Eight of sixty-one patients (13%) would have received preoperative treatment inappropriately based on the MRI T stage.[35] For nodal status, 8 of 33 MRI-positive nodes were clinically negative, and 7 of 57 MRI-negative nodes were pathologically positive.[36] The presence of nodal disease identified by

MRI is also primarily determined by size, so the accuracy is similar to that of CT (<80%), although defining node positivity based on irregular border or mixed signal intensity could help improve sensitivity and specificity.[35]

While the accuracy of MRI in determining T and N stage is imperfect, newer studies have focused on other radiographic features that may prove more relevant to prognosis and treatment planning than the traditional American Joint Committee on Cancer classification. In addition to defining the circumferential resection margin (CRM) of a low rectal cancer, high-resolution MRI can be used to predict tumor regression grade (TRG) after neoadjuvant therapy. TRG in the surgical specimen is a measure of response to preoperative chemoradiation and has been shown to correlate strongly with OS and DFS. In the first prospective study to address MRI-predicted TRG, Shihab et al.[37] found this too was significantly associated with long-term outcomes. A prognostic role was also demonstrated for pretreatment MRI, specifically in the characterization of tumor invasion into the pelvic floor muscles. Based on these results, the authors postulate that MRI-defined factors may be extraordinarily useful for modifying treatment in both the pre- and postneoadjuvant settings.[37] Patel et al.[38] offer a similar conclusion in their subgroup analysis from the original MERCURY study, which likewise found MRI-predicted TRG and CRM to be significant prognostic markers.

Two studies have taken this issue a step further by investigating exactly how MRI parameters can and should alter therapy. In another extension of the MERCURY trial, Taylor et al.[39] identified patients with "good prognosis" MRI (as defined by predicted negative CRM, absence of extramural venous invasion, and T2/T3a/T3b regardless of N stage) and referred them directly for TME resection without chemoradiation. Survival and recurrence outcomes were highly favorable, suggesting that early MRI can improve patient stratification for more selective and appropriate targeting of preoperative therapy.[39] In the postneoadjuvant setting, MRI can be used to identify poor responders who may require alternative treatments or more radical resection such as the extralevator abdominoperineal approach described by Shihab et al.[40]

Finally, pelvic MRI may also help predict which patients are at increased risk for distant synchronous metastases and would therefore benefit from more extensive pretreatment imaging such as positron emission tomography (PET)/CT or liver MRI. Hunter et al.[41] found that adverse features demonstrated on pelvic MRI (extramural venous invasion, extramural spread of >5 mm or T4, involved CRM or intersphincteric plane for low tumors) were significantly associated with a higher incidence of distant metastases (OR = 6.0; p <0.001). The authors recommend using MRI-based risk stratification to identify patients who may benefit not only from more meticulous staging but also from more aggressive treatment regimens.[41]

M staging for rectal cancer is determined in the same way as colon cancer: with a baseline CT scan to evaluate the chest, abdomen, and pelvis.[42] There has been much debate about the relative value of CT versus MRI or PET, particularly in assessing the liver, without any clear resolution. This decision depends heavily on the institutional expertise and the equipment available.

CT has an overall sensitivity of 70% to 85%, which might be improved with multidetector-improved CT technology, although the data do not yet prove that contention.[43] MRI is superior in characterizing liver lesions and distinguishing cysts and hemangiomas from tumor, especially with the use of enhancement with gadolinium or other agents.[44] PET with [18F]fluorodeoxyglucose shows promise as the most sensitive study for the detection of metastatic disease in the liver and especially in abdominal LNs for which CT and MRI are relatively insensitive. In addition, a meta-analysis of whole-body PET showed a sensitivity of 97% and a specificity of 76% in evaluating for recurrent colorectal cancer.[45] However, PET is not standardly used in preoperative staging, or recommended by National Comprehensive Cancer Network guidelines, and the incremental gain from routine PET scan appears to be small.[46]

A 2013 study has re-emphasized this point, reporting that preoperative PET/CT had no impact on disease management in 96.8% of enrolled patients and advocating against its routine use for primary staging.[47] PET is probably most valuable in restaging patients with recurrence or suspected recurrence to detect additional metastatic sites prior to attempted resection of metastatic disease.

SURGERY

The surgical management of primary rectal cancer presents unique problems for the surgeon based in large part on the anatomic constraints of the pelvis. The primary goal of achieving a complete oncologic resection must be balanced with the desire for optimal nerve and sphincter preservation, which can be quite challenging in such a confined space.

Stage I

The treatment of early-stage rectal cancer can be confusing as there are many approaches that can be used, and patient selection is critical to outcome. In addition, the risk of nerve injury and damage to the anal sphincter is substantial for low-lying tumors and must be taken into consideration, along with the desire not to have a permanent colostomy for early-stage disease. Thus, the options for these patients are primarily those of local therapies without abdominal surgery, abdominal resection of the rectum with anastomosis and retention of the anal sphincter, and abdominal-perineal resection. The last two options are discussed in detail in "Stages II and III Rectal Cancer."

Small early-stage lesions of the rectum that are diagnosed on physical examination or by colonoscopy/proctoscopy can often be managed with local resection. Local resection can be performed colonoscopically (as described in the Chapter 57), or lesions can be removed via a transanal excision with the patient positioned in a prone or lithotomy position. Appropriate retractors can provide visualization, and resection should extend into the perirectal fat with a surrounding margin of normal tissue.[48] For selected T1 and T2 lesions without evidence of nodal disease, transanal excision often provides an adequate resection of the primary tumor mass and can spare the patient the morbidity of a more extensive rectal resection. However, it does not stage the nodal drainage areas and therefore cannot provide as complete staging and management of the tumor as a definitive resection. In the effort to minimize the risk of locoregional failure, criteria for local excision have been established: the tumor must be within 8 to 10 cm of the anal verge, be well or moderately well differentiated, encompass <40% of the circumference of the bowel wall, and contain no evidence of lymphovascular invasion on biopsy. For T2 lesions, local resection should be followed by adjuvant chemoradiation. While these criteria are not strongly evidence-based (and are evolving along with surgical technology), a growing body of literature supports this approach particularly for T1 lesions. In a review of 677 T1 and T2 cancers after TME, Saraste et al.[49] identified three significant risk factors for LN invasion (and hence relative contraindications for local excision): T2 stage (OR = 2.0), poor differentiation (OR = 6.5), and vascular infiltration (OR = 3.4) with likelihood of LN positivity ranging from 6% to 78% depending on how many were found. Further support for these criteria comes from a study of 25 high-risk T1 rectal cancers, half of which were treated by transanal excision only (due to comorbidities or patient refusal to undergo resection) and the remainder with immediate conventional reoperation after local excision. Local recurrence was significantly higher in patients undergoing local excision only (50% versus 7.7%, mean follow-up 62 months), and there was a trend toward decreased 5-year survival (63% versus 89%). There were no differences in age, gender, or tumor characteristics between the two groups.[50] On the other hand, for low-risk T1 lesions in the prospective phase 2 Cancer and Leukemia Group B study, local excision alone was associated with low recurrence and good survival rates that remained durable with long-term follow-up. For T2 lesions, however, even with adjuvant therapy, the role of local excision is less clear, as Saraste et al.[49] would predict, these were associated with higher recurrence rates.[51] Whether the addition of neoadjuvant therapy might be helpful is a focus of multiple investigations. The American College of Surgeons Oncology Group has published preliminary results from its recently completed phase 2 trial of neoadjuvant capecitabine, oxaliplatin, and radiation therapy followed by local excision for ultrasound T2 tumors (ACOSOG Protocol Z6041).[52] The authors report that 49 of 77 patients were downstaged and 44% achieved a complete pathologic response (pCR). There was one positive margin and one patient with a positive node. Rates of treatment-related toxicity and perioperative complications were high, however, requiring dose reduction and potentially compromising response. Follow-up trials are planned to improve upon the therapeutic ratio of this approach and better evaluate long-term efficacy.[53] More long-term results are reported from another prospective trial that supports the role of local excision following neoadjuvant therapy in selected T2N0 lesions with favorable features. Lezoche et al.[54] randomized 100 patients to either endoluminal resection or to laparoscopic or open TME, following neoadjuvant chemoradiation. Downstaging and pCR rates were similar in both groups, occurring in 51% and 28% of patients, respectively. With a mean follow-up of 9.6 years, oncologic outcomes were also essentially equivalent—with similar local recurrence rates and incidence of distant metastases (8% versus 6% and 4% versus 4%, respectively) and no difference in DFS.[54]

Performing a good transanal excision requires substantial technical expertise as the surgeon must retain control over the primary tumor and obtain adequate mucosal margins as well as deep resection into the perirectal fat. Once removed, the tumor must be well laid out for the pathologist so that all relevant margins can be properly evaluated. There is some experience using preoperative radiation therapy and chemotherapy for small lesions, but care must be taken to have the site of the primary tumor well marked with a tattoo if this approach is taken, as excellent regression could make identification of the primary site difficult.

Newer techniques for transanal excision, including transanal endoscopic microsurgery (TEMS) and transanal minimally invasive surgery, have recently gained popularity based on improved visualization of the lesion. TEMS makes use of a standard laparoscopic light source and monitoring system combined with specialized instruments and scopes. The technique allows for videoscopic magnification and the placement of instruments through an operating sigmoidoscope. TEMS and its counterpart transanal minimally invasive surgery, which uses the more basic single port laparoscopic technology, may be applied, in general, to the same patients who are candidates for traditional transanal resection. However, these methods are most useful for excising more proximal lesions that are beyond the reach of standard surgical instruments and too large for removal through a colonoscope. Preliminary data supports the role of TEMS in both benign and early-stage malignant lesions with improved margin negativity and DFS compared to transanal resection for T1 and T2 lesions in a recent report.[55] Another meta-analysis found significant reductions in morbidity and mortality compared to conventional surgery and equivalent 5-year survival rates for T1 tumors.[56] Studies that include T2 lesions and selective use of adjuvant therapy have demonstrated 5-year OS and cancer-specific survivals over 90%, with recurrence rates between 4% to 9%.[57,58] Moreover, the TEMS procedure fairs quite favorably with respect to long-term quality of life and functional outcome as most defecatory parameters return to baseline by 5 years, according to prospective data.[59] Other reports are less encouraging with recurrence rates following TEMS resection as high as 30%,[60] and therefore close endoscopic surveillance is recommended.

Stages II and III Rectal Cancer

The primary treatment of patients with stages II and III rectal cancer (T3-4 and/or node-positive) is surgical. However, in contrast to the treatment of patients with stage I disease, there is a strong body of information to suggest that combined modality therapy with radiation therapy and chemotherapy should be used in conjunction with surgical resection. This conclusion is based on both patterns of failure data, which demonstrate a substantial incidence of local, regional, as well as distant disease failure, and the fact that this incidence of tumor recurrence at all sites is decreased with the use of trimodality therapy.

The desire when performing a resection for rectal cancer is to preserve intestinal continuity and the sphincter mechanism whenever possible while still maximizing tumor control. Therefore, careful preoperative screening is crucial in the determination of the location of the lesion and its depth of invasion. As previously described, it is convenient to think of the rectum as divided into thirds for the purposes of the evaluation and preoperative determination of the surgical approach for resection. The upper third of the rectum is often considered the region of large intestine from the sacral prominence to the peritoneal reflection. These lesions are in almost all cases managed with a low anterior resection in much the same way as a sigmoid colon cancer (see Chapter 57). An adequate 1- to 2-cm distal mucosal margin can be achieved for these lesions well above the sphincter mechanism, and intestinal continuity can be restored using either a hand-sewn technique or a circular stapling device inserted through the rectum.[61,62]

Tumors in the middle and lower thirds of the rectum can be considered as lying entirely below the peritoneal reflection. The resection of these tumors can be challenging because of the confines of the pelvic skeletal structure, and the ability to perform a resection with an adequate distal margin is significantly influenced by the size of the lesion. Nevertheless, tumors of the middle third of the rectum in most cases can be safely resected with a low anterior resection, with restoration of intestinal continuity and preservation of a continent sphincter apparatus.

Lesions in the distal third of the rectum, defined as those within 6 cm of the anal verge, can present the greatest challenge to the surgeon with respect to sphincter preservation. This is often influenced by the extent of lateral invasion of the lesion into the muscles of the sphincter apparatus and how close distally the tumor is to the musculature of the anal canal. The abdominal perineal resection (APR) has historically been considered the standard treatment for patients with rectal cancers located within 6 cm of the anal verge. This procedure requires a transabdominal as well as a transperineal approach with removal of the entire rectum and sphincter complex. A permanent end colostomy is created and the perineal wound either closed primarily or left to granulate in after closure of the musculature.

Although an APR is associated with a relatively low rate of local recurrence, it is not without the obvious problems of the need for a permanent colostomy and loss of intestinal continuity and sphincter function. Therefore, intense interest has been focused on developing approaches to the resection of tumors in the distal third of the rectum that would both avoid local regional recurrence and preserve intestinal continuity and sphincter continence.

Traditionally, tumors within 1 to 2 cm of the dentate line—that is, those that can be removed with at least a 1-cm distal margin—have been considered candidates for sphincter preservation and restoration of intestinal continuity via a coloanal anastomosis, which is commonly protected by a diverting loop ileostomy that can be reversed in 6 to 12 weeks.[63,64] Newer data suggest that when TME and preoperative radiotherapy are routinely employed, even smaller margins are acceptable without oncologic compromise, as long as they are microscopically negative.[65] In fact, one of the advantages of neoadjuvant therapy is thought to be an increase in sphincter-sparing procedures due to reduction in tumor bulk, which would normally preclude identification of this slight but critical margin.[63,66] A recent systematic literature review identified seven studies addressing this topic, most of which implemented pre- or postoperative radiotherapy, and three of which reported results related to a margin of <5 mm. There were no statistically significant differences in local recurrence rates regardless of margin status. This data contributes to the growing evidence that a 1 cm (or even 5 mm) margin may be unnecessary and, more importantly, that strategies employed solely to achieve this margin (such as an APR or intersphincteric resection [ISR] for distal T1 lesions) may in fact be unnecessary as well.[67]

While controversial in the United States, ISR has been described extensively abroad as a method involving at least partial resection of the internal sphincter designed to improve margin status without sacrificing sphincter function.[68] Recently, a large systematic review addressed the efficacy of this approach, identifying 14 (mostly retrospective) studies with 1,289 patients who underwent both open and laparoscopic ISR. Median follow-up was 56 (range, 1 to 227) months. Overall oncologic outcomes did not appear to be compromised with R0 resection achieved in 97% and a mean local recurrence rate of 6.7% (range, 0% to 23%). In addition, mean 5-year OS and DFS rates were 86.3% and 78.6%, respectively. Functional outcomes, however, were widely variable with only 51.2% of patients reporting "perfect continence," while an average of 29.1% experienced fecal soiling, 23.8% incontinence to flatus, and 18.6% complained of urgency.[69]

It has been postulated that neoadjuvant chemoradiation, while improving locoregional control and rates of margin-negative resection, has a deleterious effect on long-term functional outcomes, particularly after surgery for ultralow tumors. However, a recent multivariate analysis did not support this in ISR cases, finding the only significant predictors of continence were distance of the tumor from the anal ring and distance of the anastomosis from the anal verge. There was also no difference with age or extent of internal sphincter resection.[70] Another report did find significant functional differences when comparing partial ISR (resection above the dentate line), subtotal ISR (resection at the dentate line), and total ISR (resection from the intersphincteric groove). Patients with more extensive sphincter resection had higher fecal incontinence scores, more frequent nocturnal leakage, and more problems with discrimination. In addition, manometric studies at 12 months showed greater reductions in mean resting pressure. Overall though, quality of life was maintained in the majority of patients and function improved over time in both studies.[71]

Chemoradiation should be used preoperatively when performing sphincter-preserving resections for T3 or T4 rectal lesions or for any node-positive disease stages II or III. There is some evidence that preoperative radiation results in less morbidity than postoperative radiation therapy when a coloanal anastomosis is planned. In a study of 109 patients treated with a low anterior resection and a straight coloanal anastomosis, those receiving preoperative radiation therapy had a lower incidence of adverse effects on anal function than those receiving postoperative radiation.[72] The authors attributed this to sparing of the neorectum from these effects. Relative benefits and outcomes for preoperative chemoradiation versus postoperative chemoradiation will be discussed in detail in following sections.

Total Mesorectal Resection

The goal of the resection of rectal tumors is the removal of the tumor with an adequate margin as well as removal of draining LNs and lymphatics to properly stage the tumor and to reduce the risk of recurrence and spread. For lesions in the intraperitoneal colon, the lymphatics and vascular supply are found in the mesentery associated with that region of bowel.

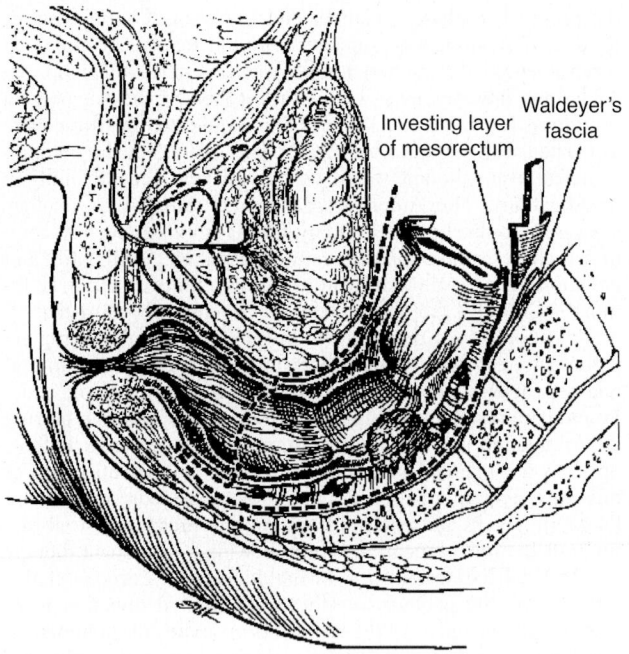

Figure 60.3 Total mesorectal excision.

In the rectum, the mesorectum is the structure that contains the blood supply and lymphatics for the upper, middle, and lower rectum. Most involved LNs for rectal cancers are found within the mesorectum, with T1 lesions associated with positive LNs in 5.7% of cases, T2 lesions having positive LNs in 20% of cases, and T3 and T4 lesions having positive LNs in 65% and 78% of cases, respectively.[73]

The anatomy and approach to mesorectal excision is depicted in Figure 60.3. This operation involves a sharp dissection occurring in an avascular plane between the fascia propria of the rectum and the presacral membrane, beyond the region where most of the nodes are located. After a TME, the specimen is typically shiny and bilobed in contrast to the irregular and rough surface after a blunt dissection, where much of the mesorectal fat is left behind. TME attempts not only to clear involved LNs but also to adequately manage the radial margins of the rectal tumor. These radial margins have been shown to be more important with respect to the risk of local regional recurrence than the distal mucosal margin.[66,74] Distal mucosal margins of ≥1 cm are adequate for local control; however, the margin on the mesorectum should extend beyond the distal mucosal margin in order to ensure a successful surgical outcome.[64,66] Numerous studies have demonstrated the benefit of TME, and it is now considered the standard of care for the surgical management of middle and lower third rectal cancers.[5,75–77] Although some studies have suggested that an adequate TME might in and of itself be sufficient management for T2 and T3 rectal cancers, the majority of the literature still supports the use of adjuvant chemoradiation for stages II and III disease even when combined with TME.

Large studies of proctectomy with TME have demonstrated a reduction in the overall incidence of local recurrence to <10%.[4] The consequences of TME can be impairment in erectile and bladder function because of disruption of parasympathetic nerves that are located in proximity to the mesorectum. Several authors have stressed the importance of the experience of the surgeon performing the procedure, and some have suggested specific techniques for monitoring modalities that can be used during this procedure to minimize morbidity.[5,6] A careful understanding of the anatomy and adequate visualization during sharp dissection will help in minimizing injury to the parasympathetic nerves and the consequent morbidity.[3,4]

Adequate visualization in the deep pelvis can often be a challenge. This may be a situation where the visual magnification and ability to enter tight spaces that are unique to the laparoscopic approach may be an advantage. Several groups have demonstrated the feasibility of laparoscopic TME for low rectal cancer as part of a sphincter-preserving operation.[78–80] Some of the larger series, while demonstrating that TME using laparoscopic techniques can be performed safely, do not have adequate follow-up to demonstrate whether there were any oncologic disadvantages to such an approach. Unfortunately, the prospective random assignment trial conducted in the United States to evaluate the role of laparoscopic surgery for colon cancer excluded patients with low rectal lesions. In addition, subgroup analysis from the UK CLASICC trial reported a 34% conversion rate and double the frequency of positive margins compared to open cases (12% versus 6%), prompting the authors to advise against routine practice of laparoscopic proctectomy outside of the research setting.[81] While these results have raised serious concerns regarding oncologic outcomes, follow-up reports are more encouraging. Multiple single-institution experiences have now been published demonstrating not only similar surgical parameters (margin status, LN harvest numbers) but also comparable recurrence and 5-year survival data.[82–86] Furthermore, in a study based on National Surgical Quality Improvement Program data from 5,420 patients, Greenblatt et al.[87] reported significant short-term advantages to laparoscopy, including decreased length of stay (5 days versus 7 days; $p <0.0001$) and 30-day morbidity (20.5% versus 28.8%; $p <0.0001$). Smaller randomized trials as well as two recent large meta-analyses of randomized controlled trials also support the oncologic equivalence of the two approaches, although short-term benefits are mixed.[88–90] In 10-year follow-up data from a pooled analysis of three randomized controlled trials (including 136 laparoscopic and 142 open cases), continued long-term oncologic safety of the laparoscopic approach was demonstrated with no significant differences compared to open in terms of locoregional recurrence (5.5% versus 9.3%), cancer-specific survival (82.5% versus 77.6%), or OS (63% versus 61.1%). Additionally, there was a trend toward lower recurrence among stage III patients in the laparoscopic group (17.7% versus 25.3%), though this did not reach statistical significance.[91] Lujan et al.[92] also reported similar rates of local recurrence and OS in a prospective cohort of 4,405 patients but found decreased complication rates (38.3% versus 45.6%) and improved oncologic parameters with laparoscopy, including decreased margin involvement and more complete TME. Finally, in a smaller study by Westerholm et al.,[93] laparoscopic surgery was found to be an independent predictor of DFS on multivariate analysis with 5-year DFS rates of 50.3% compared to 71.0% after open resection. Definitive recommendations await the results of three ongoing multicenter phase 3 randomized trials: the European COLOR II, the Japanese JCOG 0404, and the ACOSOG Z6051 from the United States.[94]

While laparoscopic TME may be technically feasible, it requires a high level of expertise and can be particularly challenging to perform within the confines of a deep and narrow pelvis. More recently, robotic technology has been applied to rectal dissection, overcoming many of the limitations associated with conventional laparoscopy including limited dexterity, inadequate visualization, and tremor. Robotic surgery offers the advantages of a stable, three-dimensional image, enhanced ergonomics and articulating instruments with seven degrees of freedom, in addition to operator-controlled camera and retraction.[95] Embraced by urologists and gynecologists over the past decade, this technology is ideally suited to pelvic procedures and has the potential to yield enhanced oncologic and functional outcomes in rectal cancer surgery as well. Limited studies so far have demonstrated feasibility and acceptable short-term outcomes.[95–99] In a case-control analysis of 118 patients undergoing laparoscopic versus robotic resection, Kwak et al.[100] reported no differences in surgical oncologic

parameters, postoperative complications, or recurrence rates at a median of 15 months follow-up. When compared to open TME in another case-matched study, the robotic approach was superior in terms of LN harvest, distal margin length, blood loss, and length of stay.[101] Other potential benefits include decreased conversion rates in three large meta-analyses as well as a trend toward reduced anastomotic leaks and CRM positivity with complete autonomic preservation in a recent systematic review of 1,549 patients.[102–105] Whether this data will translate into meaningful long-term advantages that justify the significantly higher cost of this approach remains to be seen.

The Robotic versus Laparoscopic Resection for Rectal Cancer (ROLARR) trial is a prospective, randomized, controlled, multicenter superiority trial that began enrollment in 2010, with a target recruitment of 400 patients. It will evaluate differences in conversion rates; CRM positivity, 3-year local recurrence, DFS and OS, as well as operative morbidity and mortality, quality of life, and cost-effectiveness. Investigators also wish to explore the purported clinical benefits of robotics including preservation of normal bladder and sexual function. Results from this ambitious trial are anxiously awaited.[106]

Resection of Contiguous Organs and Total Pelvic Exenteration

Although aggressive surgical approaches to rectal cancer have resulted in improvement in locoregional recurrence rates, these rates can still be as high as 33%. Not infrequently, large rectal lesions will invade through the wall of the rectum into contiguous structures such as the bladder, prostate, vagina, and uterus. Carefully selected patients with recurrent or locally advanced rectal cancers may benefit from an aggressive approach such as a total pelvic exenteration. Local recurrences remain localized to the pelvis in a significant number of patients, with autopsy studies demonstrating the incidence of pelvic recurrence to be as high as 50%.[107]

Recurrences in the pelvis can result in significant morbidity such as tenesmus, pain, bowel obstruction, and fistula. Although some of these can be ameliorated with radiation, these problems are best managed by preventing their occurrence. Although the impact of total pelvic exenteration on survival has been debated, the potential benefits on controlling locoregional disease and preventing morbidity keeps this technique as one of the tools in the surgeon's armamentarium when approaching large rectal lesions.

Existing literature on multivisceral resection of both primary and recurrent tumors has been recently evaluated in a systematic review of 22 studies comprising 1,575 patients. The authors reported a 4.2% perioperative mortality rate with morbidity of 42.5%. The overall 5-year survival rate was 50.3% with, not surprisingly, worse outcomes in patients with recurrent compared to primary disease (19.5% versus 52.8%). R0 resection was achieved in 79.5% of cases and, also not surprisingly, was the strongest factor associated with long-term survival.[108] Another review focusing only on locally recurrent tumors, reported R0 resection rates from 30% to 45% and 5-year global survival ranging from 30% to 40%, with authors stressing the importance of careful patient selection.[109] To this end, a panel of 36 colorectal surgeons were recently recruited to establish a scoring system for determining patient suitability for pelvic exenteration. A comprehensive list of clinicopathologic and radiographic criteria were considered and ranked by importance and utility in predicting negative resection margin. The authors hope to apply this quantitatively toward improving outcomes for this highly invasive and morbid intervention.[110]

For symptomatic tumors that are not resectable, other palliative options to consider include debulking and ablation. Ripley et al.[111] reported some benefit associated with sequential open radiofrequency ablation and surgical debulking in 16 patients, achieving a median survival of 12 months, with OS 24% at 36 months, and 3 patients remaining with no evidence of disease at 9,

48, and 84 months. There were four cases of significant postoperative morbidity, however, and variable levels of symptom relief.[111] Pusceddu et al.[112] reported far better palliation with CT-guided radiofrequency ablation in 12 patients with painful pelvic recurrence. At the end of follow-up (23±23 months), 92% of patients were symptom free, with a 16% treatment-related morbidity (one rectovesical fistula and one rectal abscess).[112] Finally, transrectal high-intensity focused ultrasonography has now been described in the palliative treatment of rectal cancer. As the only completely noninvasive thermal therapy, it can be delivered by either an intracavitary or extracorporeal device, causing focal ablation via coagulative necrosis. In the first case report, it was well-tolerated and led to immediate symptom relief.[113]

Combined Modality Therapy (Stage II and III)

The use of adjuvant radiation therapy is based on the substantial incidence of locoregional failure with surgical therapy alone. Older studies demonstrate local failure rates of up to 50% in patients with T3-4 or node-positive disease (Table 60.1).[114–120] The locoregional recurrence rates in these studies are in the range of 25% to 50% for patients with T3-4 and/or node-positive disease and is a dominant pattern of failure, although distant recurrence is also of great importance. Local failure is related not just to the stage of the disease, but also the location of the tumor in the rectum (tumors located low in the rectum have a higher incidence of local failure) and the experience and ability of the surgeon. However, the relevance of these older local recurrence data has been brought into question with the advent of the use of TME, as previously described. It is important to realize that the data on local recurrence after primary surgical resection come from selected series with operations performed by experienced surgeons who have been specially trained in TME and may not be relevant to the operations performed by general surgeons who perform the operation only occasionally and who are not specially trained.

Although initial studies reported locoregional failure rates of <5% after TME without the use of any adjuvant therapy,[75,77,121–123] there was concern that these excellent results could not be replicated in larger population-based studies. A number of European countries or regions have shown that the overall locoregional

recurrence risks could be decreased by limiting the surgeons who were authorized to perform rectal surgery to those who were trained and certified in the procedure, and by having educational sessions for those who were performing the surgery.[5] This raised the question of what is the true rate of local failure after TME to help define which patients really require adjuvant therapy.

The most important analysis on local recurrence rates with TME are the data from the Dutch TME study in which patients were randomized to receive either TME alone or a short course of preoperative radiation therapy followed by TME.[77] All patients with rectal cancer were eligible, including those with early-stage disease. Special attempts were made to have good surgical and pathology quality control. The early results (2 years) relating to local tumor recurrence have been reported and are summarized in Table 60.2. The study demonstrates that there are subsets of

TABLE 60.1

Results of Dutch Total Mesorectal Excision Trial

Technique	Preoperative Radiotherapy (5 Gy × 5) + Total Mesorectal Excision	Total Mesorectal Excision Alone
Percentage of Patients		
Stage 0 or I		30
Local failure (2 y)	2.4	8.2
Local failure (4 y)	3	10
Local Failure (Distance from Anal Verge)		
0–5 cm	5.8	10
5–10 cm	1	10.1
10–15 cm	1.3	3.8
Stage III (4-y estimate)		20

From Kapiteijn E, Marijnen CA, Nagtegall ID, et al, Preoperative radiotherapy combined with total mesorectal excision for resectable rectal cancer. *N Eng J Med* 2001;345:638–646, with permission.

TABLE 60.2

Local Failure of Rectal Cancer Surgery Alone (Local Failure Rate Percentage/Number of Patients in Cohort)

Analysis	Gunderson and Sosin[117] Reoperation (Crude)	Rich et al.[119] Clinical Exam + Surgery (Crude)	Minsky et al.[211] First Failure—Clinical Exam + Surgery (5-y Actuarial)	Martling et al.[120] Total Local Recurrence	Mendenhall, Million, and Pfaff[114] Total Local Recurrence—5-y Follow-up Clinical	Pilipshen et al.[116] First Failure—Clinical	Bonadeo et al.[228] Total Local Recurrence—Clinical[a]
T1N0		8%/39	11%/11	9%/78	0/6	0%/5	3%/103
T2N0			3%/36		38%/16	14%/128	
T3N0	67%/6	24%/42	23%/60	34%/80	40%/30	30%/111	4%/181
T4N0		53%/15	11%/9				
T1-2N+	24%/17	50%/4	14%/11	37%/93	71%/17	22%/49	24%/133
T3N+	83%/40	47%/34	25%/31		65%/17	49%/89	
T4N+		67%/6	22%/10				
Total	64%/75	30%/142	15%/168	27%/251	46%/90		

[a] Local recurrence highly dependent on site in rectum—18% overall for tumors ≤7 cm from anal verge.

TABLE 60.3

Local Control and Survival with and without Radiotherapy—Preoperatively, Postoperatively, and with or without Chemotherapy

Study/Institution[a] (Ref.)	No. of Patients	Local Failure (%)	Disease-Free Survival (%)	Survival (5 y) (%)
NSABP RO-1[129] Surg/Surg + RT (postoperative RT)	184/187	25/16	No difference	No difference
NSABP RO-2[130] Surg + chemo/Surg + chemo + RT (postoperative RT)	348/346	13/8		
GITSG[127] Surg/Surg + RT/Surg + chemo + RT (postoperative RT)	58/50/46	25/20/10	44/50/65	26/33/45
Swedish[215] Surg/Surg + RT (preoperative RT)		27/11		48/58
Stockholm II[120] Surg/Surg + RT (preoperative RT)		34/16 Stage II 37/21 Stage II		
MRC[132] Surg/Surg + RT (postoperative RT)	235/234	34/21		38/41

NSABP, National Surgical Adjuvant Breast and Bowel Project; Surg, surgery; RT, radiotherapy; chemo, chemotherapy; GITSG, Gastrointestinal Study Group; MRC, Medical Research Council.
[a] Randomized studies in either all patients or patients with stage II and III disease.

patients in whom TME alone is likely sufficient for obtaining good pelvic control, including patients with high rectal tumors (some of these may have been sigmoid cancers, rather than rectal) and low-stage tumors (T1-2, N0). On the other hand, low-lying rectal tumors that are moderately advanced (T3-4 and/or node-positive) had a higher incidence of locoregional failure. Local failure after TME alone was 15% in node-positive patients at 2 years, not corrected for site of the primary, and longer-term follow-up will undoubtedly demonstrate higher local failure rates. In addition, as these results were obtained in a controlled setting, one would likely not obtain similarly good results when surgery is done with less careful quality control. There was a consistent decrease in local failure rate by the addition of preoperative radiation therapy, but the absolute magnitude of the effect varied by the tumor characteristics previously discussed. Long-term results from the Dutch TME study have now been published demonstrating a stable, persistent >50% reduction in recurrence risk for the radiotherapy group after a median follow-up of 12 years. For patients with a negative circumferential margin, the benefit was even greater, with the 10-year cumulative incidence of local recurrence 3% after radiotherapy versus 9% after surgery alone (p <0.0001) and the incidence of distant recurrence 19% versus 24% (p = 0.06). In addition, the incidence of cancer-specific death at 10 years was 17% for the irradiated group versus 22% for surgery alone (p = 0.04). OS rates, however, were equivalent.[124]

A trial similar to the Dutch TME study was recently reported. This phase 3 trial randomized 1,350 patients with operable adenocarcinoma of the rectum to short-course preoperative radiotherapy (25 Gy in five fractions; n = 674) or to initial surgery with selective postoperative chemoradiotherapy (CRT; 45 Gy in 25 fractions with concurrent 5-fluorouracil [5-FU]) restricted to patients CRM involvement (n = 676). The primary outcome measure was local recurrence. At the time of analysis, 330 patients had died (157 preoperative radiotherapy group versus 173 selective postoperative CRT), and median follow-up of surviving patients was 4 years. A total of 99 patients developed local recurrence (27 preoperative radiotherapy versus 72 selective postoperative CRT). A reduction was noted of 61% in the relative risk of local recurrence for patients receiving preoperative radiotherapy (hazard ratio [HR] = 0.39; 95% confidence

interval [CI] = 0.27 to 0.58; p <0.0001) and an absolute difference at 3 years of 6.2% (4.4% preoperative radiotherapy versus 10.6% selective postoperative CRT; 95% CI = 5.3–7.1). A relative improvement in DFS of 24% for patients receiving preoperative radiotherapy (HR = 0.76; 95% CI = 0.62 to 0.94; p = 0.013), and an absolute difference at 3 years of 6.0% (77.5% versus 71.5%; 95% CI = 5.3 to 6.8) was observed. OS did not differ between the groups (HR = 0.91; 95% CI = 0.73 to 1.13; p = 0.40). These findings provide further evidence that short-course preoperative radiotherapy is an effective treatment for patients with operable rectal cancer.[125]

The data are excellent that radiation therapy, especially when combined with chemotherapy, can decrease the local failure rate. This is shown by a Swedish study of preoperative radiation therapy compared with surgery,[126] the Dutch TME trial in the preoperative setting,[76] and by multiple studies in the postoperative setting.[127–132] There are also excellent data to show that locoregional failure is decreased by the use of radiation therapy and is further decreased by the use of concurrent 5-FU–based chemotherapy (Table 60.3).[127,128,133] Most studies have demonstrated that local failure decreases by about 50% with the use of adjuvant radiation therapy, with a greater effect when concurrent 5-FU is used with irradiation. This appears to provide a strong justification for the use of adjuvant radiation therapy. What is less clear is whether trimodality therapy with radiation therapy improves survival, if radiochemotherapy should be given preoperatively or postoperatively, and precisely which patients should be irradiated. To that effect, Schrag et al.[134] investigated the use of a neoadjuvant chemotherapy utilizing a 5-FU–leucovorin-oxaliplatin (FOLFOX)-based regimen, with selective use of chemoradiation therapy only in those patients who had failed to demonstrate tumor improvement on neoadjuvant chemotherapy. Of the 30 patients treated without radiation therapy in this small pilot trial, none experienced local recurrence with a minimum follow-up of 4 years.[134] Three patients experienced distant failure, all in the lungs. This interesting pilot trial has led to the current phase 3 cooperative group trial comparing this approach of neoadjuvant chemotherapy plus selective use of radiation versus standard neoadjuvant chemoradiation therapy. Pending any new information from this randomized trial, neoadjuvant chemoradiation therapy remains appropriate standard practice.

TABLE 60.4

Results of Meta-Analysis, Preoperative Radiotherapy Versus Surgery Alone

Result	Preoperative Radiotherapy vs. Surgery
Overall 5-y mortality	OR = 0.84 (p = 0.03)
5-y cancer mortality	OR = 0.71 (p <0.001)
5-y local recurrence	OR = 0.49 (p <0.001)
5-y distant metastases	OR = 0.93 (p = 0.54)

OR, overall recovery.
From Camma C, Giunta M, Fiorica F, et al. Preoperative radiotherapy for resectable rectal cancer: A meta-analysis. *JAMA* 2000;284:1008–1015, with permission.

DOES ADJUVANT RADIATION THERAPY IMPACT SURVIVAL?

Although there have been multiple randomized trials addressing the use of adjuvant radiation therapy or chemoradiation therapy, and although they consistently show an improvement in local control with adjuvant radiation therapy, the survival outcome data have been mixed. In the past, there have been two meta-analyses performed.[135,136] Table 60.4 shows the results of a meta-analysis by Camma et al.[136] showing a decreased local recurrence rate, cancer mortality rate, and overall mortality rate with the use of preoperative radiation therapy, although without a decrease in distant metastasis rate. The Colorectal Cancer Collaborative Group study (Table 60.5) demonstrates no improvement in the likelihood of curative surgery with preoperative therapy or of OS with all types of radiation therapy combined.[135] Preoperative radiation therapy, however, was shown to improve local control, DFS, and OS compared with surgery alone, although deaths within the first year after surgery were higher after radiation therapy. Local recurrence with preoperative radiation therapy was 46% lower than surgery alone, and cancer deaths were decreased from 50% to 45%. Postoperative radiation therapy was shown to improve local control (although less than preoperative therapy), but did not impact long-term survival. Lending substantial strength to the conclusion that there was a true advantage to radiation therapy is the fact that there was a dose response demonstrated for the radiation effect on local control (i.e., better control was obtained with higher radiation dose). This observation strengthens the conclusion, as it demonstrates a direct correlation between the amount of therapy and outcome. The data from this analysis are heavily influenced by the results of a single Swedish study that showed a long-term survival advantage to the use of preoperative radiation therapy compared with surgery alone.[126] Thus, these data show that improving local control

TABLE 60.5

Colorectal Cancer Collaborative Group 2001 Adjuvant Radiation Therapy in Rectal Cancer

	Preoperative RT vs. Surgery	Postoperative RT vs. Surgery
Yearly risk of local recurrence	46% decrease with RT	37% decrease with RT
Death rate	5% less than with surgery	No difference from surgery

RT, radiotherapy.
From Colorectal Cancer Collaborative Group. Adjuvant radiotherapy for rectal cancer: a systematic overview of 8507 patients from 22 randomised trials. *Lancet* 2001;358:1291–1304, with permission.

with the use of radiation therapy (and presumably with concurrent chemoradiation therapy) is beneficial, and that trimodality therapy, especially when chemoradiation therapy is used preoperatively, can improve survival.

PREOPERATIVE RADIATION THERAPY

The second issue of importance is whether adjuvant therapy should be given preoperatively or postoperatively and the exact timing of the chemotherapy. Current data clearly favor the preoperative approach.

Perhaps the most important study addressing the issue of pre- versus postoperative adjuvant therapy is a German trial of preoperative versus postoperative chemoradiation with radiation therapy given at 1.8 Gy per fraction and using continuous-infusion 5-FU chemotherapy as a 120-hour infusion, for which results have been reported by Sauer et al.[137] This study demonstrates an advantage in sphincter preservation with the use of preoperative therapy. Of the patients thought to need an APR at initial assessment, only 19% had a sphincter-preserving surgery when operation was done immediately versus 39% after preoperative radiation therapy, although there was no difference in the overall sphincter preservation rate. There was a statistically significant decrease in local failure with preoperative radiation therapy compared to postoperative treatment (6% versus 13%; p = 0.006). The relative risk of local failure in the pre- versus postoperative treatment group was 0.46. The 5-year DFS showed a small advantage to preoperative therapy (68% versus 65%; p = 0.32), which was not statistically significant. There was a decrease in late anastomotic strictures with preoperative therapy, and acute toxicity was also decreased by the use of preoperative radiation and chemotherapy, both statistically significant. This provides strong evidence of the superiority of preoperative adjuvant treatment in patients in whom it is determined that adjuvant therapy is needed. Eleven-year follow-up data for this study have just been published, demonstrating a persistently significant improvement in local control for pre- versus postoperative chemoradiation (local relapse rates 7.1% versus 10.1%; p = 0.48). However, there was still no effect on OS or distant metastases, highlighting the need for more effective systemic therapy than just 5-FU–based regimens.[138]

As multimodality treatment regimens are intensified to achieve even better outcomes, it is important to identify subgroups of patients at higher risk for severe toxicity and treatment interruption, both through investigation of predictive markers as well as attention to basic clinical parameters. In an unplanned analysis of the German trial data, Wolff et al.[139] found female gender to be significantly associated with CRT-induced acute toxicity but also associated with improved 10-year OS (62.7% versus 58.4%; p = 0.066). Men with no acute organ toxicities had much poorer OS compared to the rest, leading the authors to conclude that acute toxicity was a significant prognostic parameter and possibly a surrogate for treatment response. Future efforts will need to focus on mitigating this toxicity in susceptible patients without compromising treatment intensity.[139]

Similar to the goals of the German trial, the National Surgical Adjuvant Breast and Bowel Project (NSABP) R-03 trial compared neoadjuvant versus adjuvant CRT in the treatment of locally advanced rectal carcinoma. Patients with clinical T3 or T4 or node-positive rectal cancer were randomly assigned to preoperative or postoperative CRT. Chemotherapy consisted of 5-FU and leucovorin with 45 Gy in 25 fractions with a 5.40-Gy boost within the original margins of treatment. In the preoperative group, surgery was performed within 8 weeks after completion of radiotherapy. In the postoperative group, chemotherapy began after recovery from surgery but no later than 4 weeks after surgery. The primary end points were DFS and OS. A total of 267 patients were randomly assigned to NSABP R-03. The intended sample size was 900 patients. Excluding 11 ineligible and 2 eligible patients without follow-up data, the analysis used data on 123 patients randomly assigned to preoperative and 131 to postoperative CRT. Surviving patients were observed for a median of 8.4 years. The 5-year DFS for preoperative patients was 64.7% versus 53.4% for postoperative patients ($p = 0.011$). The 5-year OS for preoperative patients was 74.5% versus 65.6% for postoperative patients ($p = 0.065$). A pCR was achieved in 15% of preoperative patients. No preoperative patient with a pCR has had a recurrence. The investigators concluded that preoperative CRT, compared with postoperative CRT, significantly improved DFS and showed a trend toward improved OS.[140]

In addition to improving survival, another reason for using preoperative chemoradiation therapy is to increase the chance for sphincter preservation for patients with low-lying tumors of the rectum, where an abdominoperineal resection would be conventionally used. The NSABP R-03 trial was able to obtain worthwhile information regarding this issue. When a patient was first seen, the surgeon was asked (for both preoperative and postoperative patients) what operation was needed. In the patients randomized to postoperative radiation therapy (i.e., immediate surgery), the determination in the office corresponded extremely well to the operation actually performed. However, in the patients who received preoperative radiation therapy, sphincter-preserving surgery was done in 50% of patients compared with 33% of those who had initial surgery.[141] However, the data have been inconsistent overall in demonstrating an advantage to preoperative therapy in terms of sphincter preservation. The analyses are complicated because the decision as to whether sphincter-preserving surgery should be done is heavily dependent on the biases of the surgeon. If the surgeon believes that the same operation should be done regardless of tumor regression, then clearly the same surgery will be done. There are some surgeons who will do sphincter-preserving operations after preoperative irradiation, when they would not have done so if the surgery had been done first.

If one is using preoperative radiotherapy to try to improve the likelihood of sphincter preservation, the radiation must be given in such a way as to maximize the likelihood of this occurring. Specifically, a "standard" long course of irradiation to a dose of approximately 50 Gy at 18 to 20 Gy per fraction over 5 to 5.5 weeks (as given in the German trial mentioned previously) has been thought by most US investigators to be optimal. The short-course therapy with immediate surgery (typically 50 Gy for five fractions given over 1 week), as often used in Europe, followed by immediate surgery is not likely to produce enough tumor shrinkage to allow for sphincter preservation in patients with very low-lying tumors. Bujko et al.[142] have published data that suggest that the short course is as effective in producing local control as the longer course of therapy. A total of 312 patients were randomized to either 25 Gy in 5 fractions followed by surgery within 1 week, or 50.4 Gy in 28 fractions with concurrent bolus 5-FU and leucovorin and surgery 4 to 6 weeks later. DFS was respectively (short- versus long-course therapy) 58.4% versus 55.6%; local recurrence, 9% versus 14.2%; severe late toxicity, 10.1% versus 7.1%; and acute toxicity, 3.2% versus 18.2%. There was no improvement in sphincter preservation with long-course treatment. Although this was a relatively small study, it provides important evidence to support the value of short-course preoperative therapy. A second randomized trial from the Australian Intergroup randomized 326 patients with T3 rectal cancer within 12 cm of the anal verge to short-course radiotherapy (25 Gy in five fractions) or CRT (50.4 Gy with continuous infusion 5-FU). Both arms received adjuvant chemotherapy. The primary end point, locoregional recurrence at 3 years, was not significantly different at 7.5% for short-course radiotherapy and 4.4% for CRT with no difference in distant recurrence rates or OS. At median follow-up of 6 years, there were no differences in late toxicity rates.[143]

Both the Polish and Australian Intergroup trials were relatively small and not powered to show equivalence of long-course CRT and short-course radiotherapy. Both trials have relatively short follow-up and, as indicated by other randomized trials, locoregional

recurrence continues to increase with time. In addition, late toxicities may manifest many years following treatment.

Another question is whether the time interval between radiation and surgery is more important than the duration of the preoperative treatment itself. Pettersson et al.[144] evaluated 112 patients who underwent short-course radiotherapy (25 Gy over 5 to 7 days) with delayed surgery >4 weeks and found a significant downstaging effect not previously seen with immediate resection.[144] Another study in which 154 patients receiving short-course radiation were prospectively randomized to immediate surgery (7-day to 10-day interval) versus delayed (4 weeks to 5 weeks) also demonstrated a higher downstaging rate in the latter group (13% versus 44.2%; $p = 0.0001$). In addition, there was reduced systemic recurrence (2.8% versus 12.3%; $p = 0.035$) and a trend toward improved 5-year survival (73% versus 63%). Interestingly, however, delayed surgery was not associated with superior locoregional control or increased rates of sphincter-saving procedures and curative resections.[145] Further trials are necessary to determine the ideal schedule of radiotherapy and surgery that optimizes both downstaging and overall oncologic outcomes. Some clinicians are advocating even more extended intervals between radiation and surgery. In a review of 1,593 patients, the median interval from the start of radiotherapy was 14 weeks (range, 6 weeks to 85 weeks; interquartile range, 12 weeks to 16 weeks) with the highest pCR rate found in patients undergoing resection at 15 weeks to 16 weeks (18%; $p = 0.013$).[146]

There are theoretical reasons to believe that radiation therapy delivered preoperatively would decrease the toxicity of therapy. With postoperative radiation therapy, the soft tissues of the perineum are at risk for involvement after an APR because of surgical manipulation and, therefore, need to be irradiated with its attendant acute skin toxicity. This is not needed with preoperative therapy. With postoperative radiation therapy, normal bowel is moved into the pelvis for the anastomosis after a low anterior resection and therefore is irradiated and at risk for late toxicity. In the preoperative setting, much of the irradiated bowel is removed with the surgical specimen and therefore is not at risk for producing late bowel injury. There is also likely to be a higher risk of having small bowel fixed in the pelvis after surgery secondary to adhesions, which could also lead to late toxicity. On the other hand, many studies have demonstrated that acute surgical morbidity and mortality are not substantially increased with the use of preoperative irradiation, although many surgeons routinely perform a temporary diverting colostomy in order to avoid the problems associated with an anastomotic leak. Except for the German trial previously mentioned, which shows decreased acute and late toxicity, data on late toxicity are not available to directly compare the two techniques when used with concurrent chemotherapy and the commonly used dose/fractionation schedules.

To better evaluate the impact of preoperative chemoradiation on long-term functional outcome, Loos et al.[147] performed a systematic review and meta-analysis of 25 studies and 6,548 patients, including six randomized controlled trials and previously published data from the Dutch TME trial. Although there was substantial heterogeneity of the included trials and low methodologic quality, the authors suggest that preoperative treatment has a largely negative impact on long-term anorectal function but does not significantly affect sexual or urinary performance compared to surgery alone. Without better designed trials, however, that include standardized pre- and postoperative assessment of these parameters as well as direct comparison to postoperative treatment, no definitive conclusions can be drawn.[147]

As the retrospective meta-analyses have generally shown better tumor control locally and better evidence of a survival advantage secondary to preoperative irradiation, many gastrointestinal oncologists prefer preoperative CRT for the patient who clearly requires adjuvant radiation therapy. A reasonable strategy at present is to use preoperative CRT for patients in whom there is little doubt about the advisability of adjuvant therapy (T3 node-positive or T4 disease) or patients with low-lying tumors in whom an APR may still be avoided, but to use initial surgery for other patient cohorts, with postoperative CRT used based on the operative and pathologic findings.

Another issue of importance is the timing of chemotherapy. It has been assumed by many investigators that concurrent preoperative chemotherapy and postoperative adjuvant chemotherapy is the proper way of delivering treatment. A study by the European Organization for Research and Treatment of Cancer, however, questions these assumptions.[148] Patients were randomized to receive either preoperative radiation therapy alone, preoperative CRT, preoperative radiation therapy and postoperative chemotherapy, or preoperative CRT and postoperative chemotherapy. Chemotherapy was bolus 5-FU (350 mg/m² per day for 5 days) and leucovorin (20 mg/m² for 5 days) with two cycles given with radiation therapy and four cycles postoperatively for the appropriate groups. Local recurrence rates were roughly similar for all patients receiving chemotherapy regardless of timing (7% to 9%) and significantly improved compared with those patients not receiving any chemotherapy (17%). There was no difference in survival outcomes based on the timing of chemotherapy. The 5-year DFS rates were 52.2% and 58.2% in the no adjuvant treatment groups and the adjuvant treatment groups, respectively ($p = 0.13$).

Two recent Cochrane reviews have addressed the role of adding chemotherapy to preoperative radiation regimens. The first included six randomized controlled trials, with a total of 247 patients, comparing preoperative CRT to radiation alone in the treatment of stage III cancers. Thirty-day mortality, sphincter preservation rates, and late toxicity events were similar between groups. A significant increase in acute grade 3/4 toxicity was seen in patients who received CRT versus radiation alone. While there was no difference in OS, CRT was associated with significantly less local recurrence (OR = 0.56; $p < 0.0001$).[149] A second meta-analysis, including five randomized controlled trials, addressed similar questions in stage II-III disease and reported similar findings. The addition of chemotherapy increased grade 3/4 toxicity with no impact on postoperative mortality, anastomotic leak rate, or sphincter preservation. There was also a significant reduction in 5-year local recurrence rate (OR = 0.39 to 0.72; $p < 0.001$) as well as an increase in pCR (OR = 2.12 to 5.84; $p < 0.00001$) in the CRT group, but again no differences in survival. Additional studies with longer follow-up are needed to determine the full benefit of preoperative chemotherapy as well its impact on functional outcome and quality of life.[150]

WHICH PATIENTS SHOULD RECEIVE ADJUVANT THERAPY?

For either pre- or postoperative therapy, the physician needs to address the issue of precisely which patients need to receive adjuvant radiation therapy and chemotherapy. At the present time, these two modalities have been completely linked in US clinical trials, so it is not possible to determine if there are subsets of patients who might benefit from one modality and not the other. In addition, recent US trials have all used chemotherapy concurrent with the radiation therapy in addition to postradiation chemotherapy, so it is not possible to determine the relative importance of each modality.

Based on the historical patterns of failure data, which demonstrated high local failure rates with surgery alone for patients with T3 and/or node-positive disease, virtually all US studies have evaluated this entire patient population. However, many of these studies predate the routine use of now-standard TME surgery, and more detailed analyses have allowed us to define characteristics that help define relatively low-risk and relatively high-risk patient subsets. As mentioned earlier, among the patients conventionally treated with adjuvant CRT, a number of relatively lower risk categories have been identified. Those include patients with T3N0 or

T1-2N1 disease,[17,18,151] those with primary tumors located high in the rectum, those with wide circumferential margins on the final pathology specimen,[29,30] those with node-negative disease after multiple (12 to 14 or more) nodes have been evaluated,[19–21,152] and those in whom TME surgery had been performed by an experienced colorectal oncologic surgeon.[153,154] In the preoperative setting, only some of this information will be available at the time a therapeutic decision must be made, but some information will be available (including knowledge of the surgeon). In addition, one must consider the known inaccuracy of transrectal ultrasound in staging and the experience of the ultrasonographer.[33,60] However, if most of these conditions are met, it is possible that routine adjuvant radiation therapy, and perhaps chemotherapy, is not required for the lower-stage tumors.

Another question is which patients are unlikely to respond to chemoradiation at all and would only be disadvantaged by the toxicities and delay in surgical treatment. Numerous biomarkers and tumor-related features are under investigation as potential predictive factors of response, and this will have important implications for preoperative patient selection as well.[155–165] Among these biomarkers, KRAS has received quite a lot of attention, but results are conflicting. Previous reports suggest that mutated tumors are less likely to develop a pCR compared to wild-type. Duldulao et al.[166] has recently published follow-up data that support this (13% versus 33% pCR in KRAS mutant versus wild-type; $p = 0.006$).[166] However, a larger meta-analysis of eight series and 696 patients showed no association between KRAS status and pCR, tumor downstaging, or cancer-related mortality. Although limited by the heterogeneity of its included studies, this report highlights the need for caution when considering biomarkers in the context of clinical decision making.[167] Another newly described method for predicting response to neoadjuvant therapy involves measuring histologic changes in the tumor soon after the initiation of treatment. Suzuki et al.[168] evaluated biopsies obtained 7 days into the CRT course, comparing expression levels of various apoptotic markers and cellular changes to pretreatment findings as well as to the final surgical specimen. Markers and cellular features of apoptosis at 7 days were strongly correlated with pCR and tumor regression. This study offers another potential strategy for identifying patients who might benefit from early alternative interventions.[168] At the present time, most patients treated outside clinical trials that have T3-4 and/or node-positive disease should probably receive neoadjuvant CRT if there are no extenuating circumstances. However, for patients who meet the previously mentioned favorable criteria, especially those with high rectal T3 N0 tumors, avoiding neoadjuvant radiation therapy and perhaps chemotherapy can be considered. Clinical trials will need to be performed to help resolve which subsets of patients do not require routine adjuvant radiation therapy. New data suggests that for the subset of patients who are confirmed to be node-negative after neoadjuvant chemoradiation and curative surgery, little benefit may be derived from additional postoperative treatment. In two studies, long-term survival and recurrence outcomes were compared between patients with ypN0 rectal cancer who did and did not receive adjuvant chemotherapy. Overall, there was minimal difference between the two groups with prognosis primarily determined by pathologic stage.[169,170] However, these nonrandomized data should be regarded as preliminary and hypothesis-generating; postoperative chemotherapy should be the default position in these patients, and deviations from this plan should only be made on an individual basis after a detailed review of the patient's comorbidities, relative risks, and benefits, and a detailed discussion of this with the patient.

Another important area of investigation is whether patients who have a complete clinical response to neoadjuvant therapy can be safely managed with a nonoperative, "watch and wait" approach. In other words, can the organ-preserving multidisciplinary algorithm, which is now the standard of care for anal cancer, be adopted for rectal malignancy as well? This "wait and see" approach was first seriously addressed in a seminal study by Habr-Gama et al.,[171] which compared the outcomes of 71 clinically complete responders who were observed without surgery to a well-matched group of patients with pCR who were resected. After a mean follow-up of 57 months, there were no cancer-related deaths in the observation group and recurrence rates were extremely low regardless of treatment strategy.[171] Another more recently published study from a different group reported similar results. In this report, 21 patients who achieved a clinical complete response were followed without surgery for a mean of 25 ± 19 months and compared to 20 patients who underwent resection with pCR.[172] There was one local recurrence in the observed group, treated with local excision, and two deaths in the control group. In addition (not surprisingly) functional outcome was significantly better in the patients who did not undergo surgery. Despite the small sample size and short follow-up, these results lend further credibility to the "wait and see" approach in carefully selected patients with rectal cancer. A similar report from yet a third group noted that in 32 patients carefully selected over a 5-year period, with a median follow-up of 28 months, 6 patients experienced local recurrence (3 of whom also had distant recurrence), and all 6 patients were able to undergo resection of the recurrent primary to achieve local control. When compared in an exploratory analysis to a control group of patient treated in the same institution who had undergone resection and had been found to have a pCR, 2-year distant DFS and OS appeared to be similar. Of course, these numbers are small and nonrandomized, and follow-up is short; however, the experience further supports the investigation of selective nonoperative management in patients who achieve a clinical complete response.[173]

Given continued improvements in adjuvant therapies as well as the increasingly sophisticated imaging modalities available for follow-up, a new organ-sparing algorithm for treatment warrants further consideration. At present such an approach outside a clinical trial represents a clear departure from standard practice, and should only be considered in a fully informed patient who is willing and able to comprehend and accept the inherent risks. Logically, this approach seems most appropriate for consideration in those patients with distal tumors, in whom either an APR or a low anastomosis with poor functional outcome would be required. As noted previously, PET scans have insufficient sensitivity and specificity to be relied on in terms of determining the presence or absence of a complete clinical response, and should not be used for this purpose.

One aspect of combined modality therapy, which is undergoing reconsideration at some centers, is the order of administration of modalities of therapy. As noted in detail previously, preoperative chemoradiation followed by surgery followed by postoperative chemotherapy is the most commonly used approach. The role of administering all therapy, both chemotherapy and CRT prior to surgery has become of increasing interest, however. Chau et al.[174] were the first to publish an experience using induction capecitabine plus oxaliplatin (Cape/Ox) for 3 months prior to radiation plus capecitabine in 77 patients with poor-risk rectal cancer.[174] The response rate to Cape/Ox chemotherapy alone was 88%, with 86% of patients achieving symptomatic relieve within a median of 32 days of starting therapy. Fernandez-Martos et al.[175] published a small randomized phase 2 trial in which a total of 108 patients with rectal cancer were randomly assigned to either standard order chemoradiation followed by surgery followed by Cape/Ox chemotherapy, or to Cape/Ox chemotherapy first, followed by surgery. As might be anticipated from the small size of this trial, there were no differences between the arms in terms of efficacy, with pCR rates and R0 resection rates being essentially the same; however, greater dose intensity of both oxaliplatin and capecitabine was achieved in the group receiving preoperative chemotherapy, and higher grades 3 and 4 adverse events were seen during postoperative versus preoperative chemotherapy. The toxicities and dose intensities during the combined CRT were essentially the same in the two arms. Subsequently, several other single-institution experiences with this total neoadjuvant approach

have been reported. Cercek et al.[176] reported a retrospective series of 61 patients who received some or all of their planned chemotherapy as initial treatment for rectal cancer. Of these 61, 19 (31%) had either a pCR (14 patients) or had a complete clinical response and elected to pursue nonoperative management (5 patients). Perez et al.[177] reported preliminary results of a prospective trial of this approach in 36 patients and concluded that a larger proportion of patients were able to complete all planned FOLFOX chemotherapy than would have been expected from postoperative administration. Given the expense of a large-scale trial of initial versus postoperative chemotherapy, it is clear that an adequately powered trial comparing these two approaches will never be done. The potential benefits of initial chemotherapy are several. Firstly, it allows for administration of full-dose chemotherapy earlier in the course of treatment and appears to permit greater dose intensity, which may improve treatment of distant micrometastases and so improve long-term outcome. It also allows for patients requiring temporary ostomies after resection to have those ostomies closed after only 2 months and to not have to tolerate chemotherapy during the time they have an ostomy. In addition, the approach of delivering all planned chemotherapy and radiation therapy preoperatively allows for a favorable platform from which to consider nonoperative management in carefully selected patients.

A critical component of the "wait and see" approach is the ability to accurately identify pathologic complete responders in the preoperative setting. While many strategies have been utilized toward this end, including endoscopic evaluation, imaging, and tissue biopsy, there is no consensus on the optimal method and each has significant limitations. Endoscopic evaluation and close surveillance have long been considered important tools for detecting residual or recurrent malignancy. A recent expert consensus article described the cardinal signs of incomplete tumor response: deep ulceration with or without necrosis, superficial ulceration or mucosal irregularity, a palpable nodule despite mucosal integrity, or significant stenosis.[178] Using these criteria, Smith et al.[179] reported that an endoscopic, or "clinically complete," response was 90% predictive of pCR. Sensitivity of this assessment was low, however, with 61% of the pathologic complete responders demonstrating ultimately false signs of incomplete clinical response.[179]

A variety of imaging modalities have been applied to evaluate tumor burden after neoadjuvant therapy as well. Most are limited by the inability to differentiate postradiation fibrosis from residual cancer cells. Guillem et al.[180] found PET and CT equally inadequate in distinguishing complete from partial pathologic responders in a prospective analysis of 121 patients. Among the 26 patients with a complete response, only 54% and 19% were correctly classified by PET and CT scans, respectively. And of the 95 patients with an incomplete response, 66% and 95% were appropriately recognized by these techniques.[180] Perez et al.[181] also found PET/CT lacking in its ability to definitively identify pCR. In a series of 99 patients, imaging yielded 5 false-negative and 10 false-positive results, giving PET/CT a 93% sensitivity, 53% specificity, 73% negative predictive value, and 87% positive predictive value for the detection of residual cancer. Accuracy of PET/CT was 85%, which was inferior to that of clinical assessment alone at 91%.[181] Much attention has focused on the role of MRI in evaluating tumor burden at all stages of rectal cancer management. Diffusion-weighted MRI has been particularly useful for predicting tumor response in multiple sites and has the advantage of providing a quantitative measurement (apparent diffusion coefficient), which can be tracked longitudinally and compared to pretreatment values. However, this modality is also limited in its ability to distinguish residual solitary tumor cells from a complete response.[182]

Endoscopic biopsies seem to be the most unreliable measure of tumor response, with one study reporting a negative predictive value of 11% (only 3 of the 28 negative biopsies were associated an actual tumor-free specimen after definitive resection).[183] These disappointing results might be explained by the fact that residual tumor cells do not necessarily reside in the most superficial layers of the bowel wall. In fact, Duldulao et al.[184] reports that, in analysis of 94 patients with yPT2-4 tumors, only 13% had cancer cells remaining in the mucosa and only 56% in the submucosa. The majority of tumor burden after neoadjuvant therapy appears to be located at the invasive front, or deepest layer of the bowel wall, suggesting that only a full-thickness or excisional biopsy could accurately detect residual malignancy.[184] The question then becomes where to perform this biopsy. In a recent study, Hayden et al.[185] found that a significant amount of "tumor scatter" occurs after neoadjuvant therapy, with 49.1% of cancer cells located outside the visible ulcer or deep to normal-appearing mucosa. Moreover, the mean distance of distal scatter was 1.0 cm from the visible edge to a maximum of 3 cm, indicating that neither gross ulceration nor the traditional 2 cm margin can be used to adequately guide biopsy or excision of the potential residual tumor.[185] Additionally, even if complete full-thickness excision of the tumor site and all remaining potential cancer cells within the bowel wall were accomplished, a sterile specimen does not guarantee complete nodal response. While the rate of LN involvement in patients with a ypT0 lesion is small, it is not zero (7.7% and 9.1% in recent reports), and therefore there is ultimately no conclusive method for determining a pCR short of total mesenteric excision.[186,187]

CONCURRENT CHEMOTHERAPY

The use of adjuvant chemotherapy has centered on the use of 5-FU chemotherapy, although this drug has been in use for over 50 years and is not very effective for colon or rectal cancer. The initial trials of trimodality therapy in rectal cancer used bolus 5-FU at a dose of 500 mg/m^2 per day for 3 days during weeks 1 and 5 of the radiation therapy. This was the approach routinely used until the results of the North Central Cancer Treatment Group study testing the use of long-term continuous infusion 5-FU with postoperative radiation therapy (bolus 5-FU was used both before and after the radiation therapy) were reported.[133] This study demonstrated an advantage to continuous infusion 5-FU (only during radiation therapy) compared with bolus 5-FU in terms of local control, DFS, and OS. Because of this result and the encouraging results found with more aggressive therapy in colon cancer, it was logical to think that further intensification of chemotherapy would be of value both for local and systemic control.

Unfortunately, this expectation has not been borne out. Two large US Gastrointestinal Intergroup trials have been run testing intensification with either more aggressive 5-FU and leucovorin, additional continuous infusion 5-FU, and other combinations, with data demonstrating no advantage.[188,189] Thus, we are left with evidence that continuous infusion 5-FU during radiation therapy is of value in improving local control, distant metastases, and survival, but no evidence that anything other than simple 5-FU or 5-FU plus leucovorin should be used during the chemotherapy portion of the therapy. As will be discussed in the following, at present we do not have compelling evidence that addition of other agents, such as oxaliplatin, irinotecan, bevacizumab, cetuximab, or panitumumab, should be included with fluoropyrimidines concurrently with radiation therapy.

In practice, most gastrointestinal oncologists now use capecitabine or continuous infusion 5-FU during radiation therapy. The 1,608-patient phase 3 randomized NSABP R-04 trial has definitively established that capecitabine is noninferior to infusional 5-FU when used concurrently with preoperative radiation therapy in patents with rectal cancer.[190] There were no statistically significant differences in pCR rates, rate of sphincter-sparing surgery, surgical downstaging, or treatment-related toxicities. This study also was a 2 × 2 randomization to include concurrent oxaliplatin with radiation therapy or not. This large

trial showed no benefit for the inclusion of oxaliplatin, with substantially increased toxicity in the oxaliplatin-containing arm. A large trial of capecitabine versus bolus 5-FU confirmed that capecitabine is noninferior to 5-FU in this setting. Final results from this trial are now published, demonstrating superior 5-year OS (76% versus 67%; $p = 0.05$) and 3-year DFS (75% versus 67%; $p = 0.07$) for patients who received capecitabine in both adjuvant and neoadjuvant cohorts. There were similar rates of local recurrence in each group (6% versus 7%), but fewer patients receiving capecitabine developed distant metastases (19% versus 28%; $p = 0.04$).[191] These findings suggest greater systemic efficacy of capecitabine compared to bolus 5-FU and mirror the conclusions drawn from the most recent X-ACT trial data for stage III colon cancer. Long-term follow-up from this study over a median of 6.9 years demonstrated that capecitabine significantly improved both DFS and OS with a better overall safety profile than 5-FU/folinic acid in the adjuvant setting.[192]

There has been greater interest in the use of oxaliplatin added to 5-FU and radiation therapy, although thus far the results have been disappointing. A phase 1/2 study performed by the Cancer and Leukemia Group B demonstrated the feasibility of concurrent oxaliplatin, 5-FU, and radiation therapy,[193] as did a German multicenter phase 2 trial,[194] and the previously mentioned Radiation Therapy Oncology Group randomized phase 2 trial.[195] The NSABP, as part of their R-04 trial, is doing a second randomization to the use of weekly oxaliplatin (50 mg/m^2 per day) with an evaluation of pCR and local control as end points. However, phase 3 results have begun to emerge, and they are not as encouraging as had been hoped.[196] The French ACCORD cooperative group reported a trial in which 598 patients with locally advanced rectal cancer were randomly assigned to preoperative treatment with 5 weeks of radiation therapy (45 Gy in 25 fractions) with concurrent capecitabine 800 mg/m^2 twice daily 5 days per week or the same regimen plus oxaliplatin 50 mg/m^2 once weekly.[197] There was not a statistically significant difference in the primary end point of the trial, the pCR rate, which was 13.9% without and 19.2% with oxaliplatin ($p = 0.09$). More preoperative grade 3–4 toxicity occurred in the oxaliplatin group (25% versus 1%; $p < 0.001$). There were no statistically significant differences between groups in the rate of sphincter-preserving operations (75%), and no differences in terms of rates of serious medical or surgical complications or postoperative deaths at 60 days (0.3%). The authors concluded that the trial did not support the addition of oxaliplatin to this regimen, and that oxaliplatin should not be used with concurrent irradiation in standard practice. They did not detect an improvement in the frequency of clear circumferential radial margins, and they speculated that further investigations are warranted in selected populations. Secondary end point data from this trial have just been published demonstrating no advantage in clinical outcomes with the addition of oxaliplatin either. At 3 years follow-up, there were no significant differences in local recurrence, OS, or DFS.[198]

A large Italian cooperative group phase 3 trial reached a similar result.[199] A total of 747 patients were randomly assigned to either 5-FU infusion (225 mg/m^2 per day) concomitant with external beam pelvic radiation (50.4 Gy in 28 daily fractions) or the same regimen plus weekly oxaliplatin (60 mg/m^2 × 6). The primary end point was OS. Data are not yet mature for this end point; however, a secondary end point of primary tumor response to preoperative treatment, as well as toxicity data, have been reported. Overall grade 3–4 toxicity rates on treated patients (mainly diarrhea) were 8% without oxaliplatin and 24% in the oxaliplatin-containing arm ($p < 0.001$). Eighty-two percent of patients receiving oxaliplatin got five or more doses of this drug. pCR rates were 15% and 16% in the 5-FU only and 5-FU–oxaliplatin arms, respectively. The authors concluded that the addition of weekly oxaliplatin to standard 5-FU–based preoperative CRT significantly increases toxicity without affecting local tumor response. Survival data requires further maturation.

As a follow-up to the seminal publication by Sauer et al.,[137] another German trial has been initiated to better evaluate the integration of oxaliplatin into neoadjuvant and adjuvant regimens for rectal cancer. This randomized phase 3 study, entitled CAO/ARO/AIO-04, hopes to achieve an impact on DFS not seen in previous reports. Only preliminary data has been published thus far supporting the feasibility of an oxaliplatin-based regimen, with good compliance and acceptable toxicity and surgical morbidity. Interestingly, in an unplanned analysis, the pCR rate was found to be significantly higher in the oxaliplatin group compared to 5-FU alone (17% versus 13%; $p = 0.038$). Longer follow-up is needed to address the primary end point of DFS, and the finding must be considered in the context of the multiple negative trials regarding concurrent use of oxaliplatin and radiation therapy previously noted.[200]

Postresection use of adjuvant chemotherapy based on the results in colon cancer has become a widespread practice, with oncologists using primarily FOLFOX (biweekly oxaliplatin, 5-FU, and leucovorin; see Chapter 57) as the postradiation chemotherapy. This is based on the reasonable, albeit unproven, extrapolation from data showing that the addition of oxaliplatin to 5-FU/leucovorin improves DFS and OS in the postoperative management of patients with colon cancer (see Chapter 57). In addition to studies that have substituted fluoropyrimidines, there is also substantial interest in the use of other agents added to fluoropyrimidines with concurrent radiation therapy. There have been studies with the addition of irinotecan,[201] but because of the overlapping toxicity of diarrhea with radiation therapy and 5-FU, plus the demonstrated lack of efficacy of irinotecan in the adjuvant treatment of colon cancer, use of irinotecan in the combined mode has not been, and most likely ought not be, heavily pursued. A small randomized phase 3 study showed no benefit to the addition of irinotecan to 5-FU/leucovorin in the nonradiation portion of the treatment.[202] The Radiation Therapy Oncology Group completed a small randomized phase 2 trial of concurrent capecitabine, irinotecan, and radiation therapy versus concurrent oxaliplatin, capecitabine, and radiation therapy.[195] Both on the basis of a lack of data supporting adjuvant irinotecan and a superior pCR rate in the oxaliplatin-containing arm, no further development of the irinotecan-containing schedule is planned.

As biologic agents have a substantial appeal when used in combination with conventional cytotoxics, they also have a large appeal in combination with radiation therapy. There is evidence for a beneficial effect of both cetuximab and bevacizumab when combined with cytotoxics in patients with metastatic colon and rectal cancer (see Chapter 57). There are good laboratory data demonstrating radiation sensitization when these (and similar) agents are used in vitro, and a substantial improvement has been shown in survival in patients with head and neck cancer when cetuximab is added to radiation therapy.[203] Only preliminary studies have been done,[204] but given the lack of encouraging complete responses and the negative results with cetuximab in adjuvant colon cancer (see Chapter 57), it is unlikely that there will be substantial further investigations in this area, and neither cetuximab nor panitumumab should be used in standard practice with radiation therapy for rectal cancer. Similarly, bevacizumab has failed to demonstrate a benefit in adjuvant colon cancer, and should not be used in the routine management of locally advanced rectal cancer.

The literature on this topic continues to grow with a number of new phase 2 trials reporting on the feasibility, safety, and even potential superiority of neoadjuvant regimens that incorporate these agents. Kim et al.[205] found that adding cetuximab to preoperative radiotherapy with irinotecan and capecitabine was well tolerated in 39 patients and achieved a much higher pCR rate of 23.1%, compared to 10% to 15% with conventional 5-FU regimens. Pinto et al.[206] reported a similarly improved pCR rate of 21.1% in the StarPan/STAR-02 Study, which evaluated panitumumab, oxaliplatin, and 5-FU with concurrent radiotherapy. While this did

not reach their anticipated goal, it was a substantial improvement over both 5-FU–only regimens and 5-FU/oxaliplatin combinations from previous reports. The high incidence of grade 3-4 diarrhea with one toxic death, however, mandates modification of this regimen in future trials.[206]

Most recently, in a study evaluating pre- and postoperative Cape/Ox regimens with and without weekly cetuximab, the addition of cetuximab significantly improved radiologic response as well as OS (HR = 0.27; $p = 0.34$).[207] These results are tempered by the negative phase 2 trial of cetuximab in the adjuvant treatment of KRAS wild-type stage III colon cancer. Outside of a clinical trial, neither cetuximab nor panitumumab should be used in the adjuvant or neoadjuvant treatment of locally advanced rectal cancer.

The role of bevacizumab in neoadjuvant therapy is also promising, although dosing schedules, appropriate use of synergistic medications, and patient selection have yet to be defined. When combined with 5-FU ± oxaliplatin in the most recent studies, toxicity levels were manageable and pCR rates ranged from 13% to 36%. In addition, Spigel et al.[208] reported an 85% 1-year DFS.[209,210] However, the negative outcomes of bevacizumab trials in colon cancer adjuvant therapy have greatly dampened enthusiasm for pursuing this approach. Outside of a clinical trial, the use of bevacizumab in the adjuvant treatment of rectal cancer is not recommended.

SYNCHRONOUS RECTAL PRIMARY AND METASTASES

The use of pelvic radiotherapy in patients with synchronous presentation of primary and metastatic disease is controversial. Primary combination chemotherapy can provide substantial palliation and can be considered as initial therapy in many patients with rectal cancer and metastatic disease.[211] Endoscopically placed expandable metal stents can be considered for palliation or protection from impending obstruction. Control of disease in the pelvis can have important implications for patient quality of life; therefore, combined modality therapy, including radiation, chemotherapy, and in some cases palliative surgery, can be appropriate, especially when extrapelvic metastatic disease is small volume and the patient's prognosis is favorable enough that pelvic complications could be anticipated as a long-term problem. No firm guidelines can be made in the management of these complex patients, and treatment decisions must be made on an individual basis.

MANAGEMENT OF UNRESECTABLE PRIMARY AND LOCALLY ADVANCED DISEASE (T4)

Although the majority of patients who present with stage II and III disease have primary tumors that are technically easily resectable, there are a group of patients who have T4 tumors with deep local invasion into adjacent structures, which makes primary resection for cure difficult, if not impossible. Some T4 tumors invade into the vagina, which is easily resectable, but others invade into pelvic sidewall or sacrum, where a complete surgical resection may be impossible (the coccyx and distal sacrum can be resected, if appropriate), and others invade into bladder or prostate, where a more extensive surgical resection can be done, but often at the expense of major morbidity or functional loss. Although there are few randomized trials to define optimal therapy in this group of patients, there are data suggesting that it is appropriate to treat these patients with preoperative radiation therapy combined with chemotherapy, in a manner similar to that described for T3 disease, generally with concurrent 5-FU–based chemotherapy. This will often result in a good clinical response that will allow for a potentially curative resection to be performed. It is preferable to treat a patient preoperatively to try to avoid leaving residual disease rather than attempting to salvage a patient after a clearly inadequate operation.

The use of adjuvant radiation therapy in this clinical situation also allows for treatment of the lymphatics draining the locally invaded organ, such as the internal or external iliacs, that are not typically resected in a low anterior resection or APR, but which may be at substantial risk of secondary involvement from an invaded organ, such as the bladder. Although the definition of "unresectable" is very subjective, a number of studies have shown that preoperative radiation therapy can convert a substantial number of these patients to having resectable disease with substantial cure rates.[212-215]

In a randomized phase 3 trial of 207 patients with locally nonresectable T4 primary rectal carcinoma or local recurrence from rectal cancer, patients received chemotherapy (5-FU/leucovorin) administered concurrently with radiotherapy (50 Gy) and adjuvant for 16 weeks after surgery (98 patients) or radiation therapy (50 Gy) alone (109 patients). The two groups were well balanced according to pretreatment characteristics. An R0 resection was performed in 82 patients (84%) in the CRT group and in 74 patients (68%) in the radiation therapy group ($p = 0.009$). Local control (82% versus 67% at 5 years; log-rank $p = 0.03$), time to treatment failure (63% versus 44%; $p = 0.003$), cancer-specific survival (72% versus 55%; $p = 0.02$), and OS (66% versus 53%; $p = 0.09$) all favored the CRT group. There was no difference in late toxicity.[216] Although the use of preoperative radiation therapy with concurrent 5-FU–based chemotherapy, as described earlier, appears of value in patients with locally advanced disease, there is still a substantial incidence of local failure. Therefore, a number of investigators have explored ways to increase the radiation dose to the highest risk region to try to improve local tumor control. Three main techniques have been used: supplemental postoperative external beam radiation boost, intraoperative electron beam radiation therapy boost, and intraoperative brachytherapy boost.

There are relatively few data on the use of postoperative external beam as a boost, largely because of concerns of normal tissue tolerance after the use of the relatively large fields delivered preoperatively, extensive surgical resection, and the prolonged delay between initial external beam therapy and the final boost after recovery from surgery. The two intraoperative techniques are philosophically the same, although the technique of radiation delivery is different. After a high dose (50 Gy) of preoperative CRT and then a 4- to 6-week break, surgical resection is performed, the extent of which depends on the location and extent of tumor. Areas considered at high risk for residual tumor are determined both by the surgical findings and frozen section pathologic evaluation. For electron beam intraoperative radiotherapy, a treatment cylinder is placed over the high-risk region, often on a pelvic sidewall or the sacrum, and the cylinder is then aligned to the radiation machine, which is either in the operating room or in the radiation therapy department. The cylinder acts both to hold normal tissues outside the radiation beam and to confine the electron beam. The use of electrons allows the radiation oncologist to adjust the depth of penetration of the beam to conform to the local tumor extent. When using brachytherapy, carriers for the radioactive sources are placed over the high-risk region, and the radiation is then given either during the surgery (high-dose rate) or the radioactive sources are inserted approximately 5 days after surgery and left in place for 1 or 2 days (low-dose rate). In all situations, the radiation dose is in the range of 10 to 20 (most commonly 15) Gy when used as a boost to conventional therapy. In both approaches, care must be taken to ensure that normal tissues such as small bowel are out of the irradiated volume.

Techniques similar to this have been used for a number of years and have shown encouraging results, although formal randomized trials have not been performed. Data suggest fairly good levels of local control and long-term survival if a gross total resection can be accomplished, with poorer results if there is gross residual (Table 60.6).[217-220] Use of intraoperative radiotherapy boosts often requires specialized radiation facilities and expertise as well as an experienced team of radiation oncologists, surgical oncologists, urologists, and plastic surgeons. Similar types of surgical and radiation therapy approaches can produce surprisingly good results. For patients who still cannot have a surgical resection performed, either because of the tumor extent or because of coexisting medical problems, attempts should be made to maximize palliation and perhaps local control. Boost doses of radiation are appropriately delivered to the residual tumor to doses of >60 Gy if sensitive normal tissues (primarily small bowel) can be removed from the radiation fields. Only a small percentage (5%) of patients with these advanced tumors will be locally controlled and cured by such an approach, but a substantial percentage will obtain good palliation.[221-223]

RADIATION THERAPY TECHNIQUE

There have been primarily two dosing schemes for radiation therapy that have been used in the treatment of rectal cancer. In the preoperative setting, many European centers have favored a rapid short-course treatment of doses of approximately 25 Gy in five fractions followed by immediate surgery, whereas US centers have generally favored doses of 50.4 Gy given at 1.8 Gy per fraction

---

TABLE 60.6

Intraoperative Radiation Therapy for Locally Advanced Rectal Cancer[a]

Resection	Mayo Clinic			Massachusetts General Hospital		
	No. of Patients	Local Failure (%)	Overall Survival (5 y) (%)	No. of Patients	Local Failure (%)	Disease-Specific Survival (%)
Complete resection	18[b]	7	69	40	9	63
Partial resection	35	~20	~40	24	37	35
No resection	1	—	0	—	—	—
Total	56	16	46	64	—	—
Recurrent locally advanced tumor	42	40	19	—	—	—

[a] External beam radiotherapy + resection + intraoperative radiotherapy, no prior radiation therapy.
[b] Two additional patients with no tumor in specimen—both without any tumor recurrence. These are included in the totals.

with a delay of 4 to 8 weeks until surgery. As previously mentioned, an advantage of the long-course therapy is that it provides time to have tumor regression, which appears to facilitate sphincter preservation, although it is more expensive and time-consuming for the patient. In addition, there was substantial late toxicity from the short-course treatment in earlier series, although this was most evident when the radiation therapy techniques were less sophisticated and simple anteroposterior/posteroanterior fields alone were used, which were at times quite large[224]; those techniques are not used at present.

Although major late toxicity is relatively uncommon, functional gastrointestinal disturbances are relatively common. These relate to both surgical effects on bowel with lack of a good reservoir function and possible nerve dysfunction, as well as long-term radiation effects on bowel compliance and neural functioning.[225,226] Many patients continue to have some rectal urgency and food intolerance (especially to roughage), but symptoms tend to improve over time and most patients can live a relatively normal life regarding their gastrointestinal tract. Detailed discussions with the patient about the type of foods likely to cause worsening bowel symptoms, attention to the superimposed problems that can occur from other difficulties such as lactose intolerance, and use of agents such as loperamide all can help the patient deal with bowel problems.

Small bowel–related complications are directly proportional to the volume of small bowel in the radiation field and the radiation dose. In patients receiving combined modality therapy, the volume of irradiated small bowel limits the ability to escalate the dose of 5-FU. A number of simple radiotherapeutic techniques are available to decrease radiation-related small bowel toxicity. First, small bowel contrast or CT scanning during treatment planning allows identification of the location of the small bowel so that fields can be designed to minimize its treatment. Multiple-field techniques (preferably a three- or four-field technique) are now standard to minimize normal tissue irradiation. The use of lateral fields for the boost as well as positioning the patient in the prone position can further decrease the volume of small bowel in the lateral radiation fields.

The treatment should be designed with the use of computerized radiation dosimetry and be delivered by high-energy linear accelerators that deliver a higher dose to the target volume while relatively sparing surrounding normal structures. The advantage of combining a multiple-field technique, high-energy photons, and computerized dosimetry produces a homogenous dose distribution throughout the target volume and minimizes the dose to the small bowel. Although not well studied to date, newer developments in intensity-modulated radiation therapy may allow more conformal radiation dose distributions and a decrease in the irradiation of small bowel. To date, intensity-modulated radiation therapy has not been shown to be of additional value in the adjuvant treatment of rectal cancer.

After pelvic surgery, the small bowel commonly fills the pelvis. Adhesions can form, resulting in fixed loops of small bowel in the radiation fields. In this situation, despite treatment of the patient in the prone position, the use of multiple-field techniques may be of limited value. In contrast, when radiation therapy is delivered preoperatively to a patient who has not undergone prior pelvic surgery, the small bowel is usually mobile. When no small bowel fixation is present, treatment in the prone position can exclude much of the small bowel from the posteroanterior field and completely from the lateral fields.

Various physical maneuvers to exclude small bowel from the pelvis have been examined. Gallagher et al.[227] determined the volume, distribution, and mobility of small bowel in the pelvis after a variety of maneuvers. Regardless of the prior surgical history, a significant decrease was seen in the average small bowel volume when the patients were treated in the prone position with abdominal wall compression and bladder distention compared with the supine position. Treatment in the prone position without abdominal wall compression was not consistently effective in displacing small bowel and, in some patients (most commonly, obese), the volume of small bowel increased.

Radiation Fields

The precise radiation fields that are used should depend on the individual clinical situation, although the principles of the radiation treatment remain the same. The locoregional failures in rectal cancer occur both because of residual disease in the soft tissues of the pelvis as well as from residual pelvic nodal disease. The nodal disease can be in the internal iliac chain for very low-lying lesions, but only involves the external iliac nodes if the anal canal or sphincter is involved or if an organ is involved that drains into the external iliac system. The internal iliac nodes are not usually dissected by the surgeon, so it is important to treat these for low rectal cancers, but the external iliacs should not be routinely irradiated. The proximal extent of nodal radiation is arbitrary, but the primary drainage of all rectal cancers is along the mesenteric system, and those nodes should primarily be treated surgically. Extending radiation fields to cover para-aortic nodes is not indicated unless there is evidence of disease in those chains.

Because many of the local recurrences occur in the soft tissues of the pelvis, the radiation oncologist must be sure to treat the regions that are least well treated by the surgeon. These include extension to the pelvic sidewall and presacral space, and to the prostate in men and vagina in women. The proximal extent of the radiation field should generally extend to the sacral promontory, as that is the level at which there is an attachment of the posterior peritoneum and where the retroperitoneal rectum becomes the intraperitoneal colon. Above this level, there is little risk of pelvic soft tissue invasion for standard rectal cancer.

The lower extent of the radiation field is more complex. Often, the surgeon will rely on the radiation oncologist to sterilize the most distal extent of the primary tumor in order to perform a sphincter-preserving operation, so the distal margins should be at least a couple of centimeters below the primary tumor mass. Although rectal tumors tend to have only a minimal amount of longitudinal spread along the mucosal margin, they can spread further distally in the perirectal fat and in the LNs in the mesorectum. In fact, this is part of the rationale for a TME. Attempts should thus be made for treatment to at least the level of the dentate line for most low-lying rectal cancers, although this is likely not necessary for rectal cancers in the proximal third. However, it is also likely true that a substantial part of the late toxicity from pelvic radiation therapy is related to dysfunction of the anal sphincter. Thus, it is important to try to minimize the amount of sphincter that is irradiated. Although many textbooks define the lower edge of the radiation field relative to the bones of the pelvis, this is not the proper way to think about irradiating such tumors. The locations of bony anatomic landmarks such as the ischial tuberosity have no consistent relationship to the anal sphincter, anal verge, dentate line, or the rectal cancer. The radiation oncologist must identify the location of these structures as best as possible using radiopaque markers and rectal contrast, and then determine the balance between adequate distal coverage of the tumor as well as minimizing irradiation of the anal sphincter and the perineum (acute toxicity). For anteroposterior or posteroanterior fields, the lateral borders should extend to treat the pelvic sidewall, a possible region for soft tissue extension. The lateral fields should have a similar superior and inferior margin. The posterior border should include all of the presacral soft tissue so the posterior extent of the field should cover the anterior border of the sacrum with at least a 1.5-cm margin for patient motion and dosimetric variation. The anterior border of the lateral fields should cover at least the posterior border of the vagina or the prostate, the anterior extent of the primary rectal tumor, and the anterior edge of the sacral promontory. Examples of typical radiation fields as depicted by a CT simulation are shown in Figure 60.4.

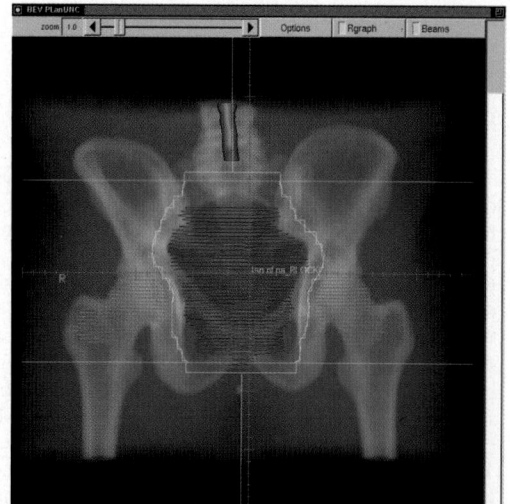

A

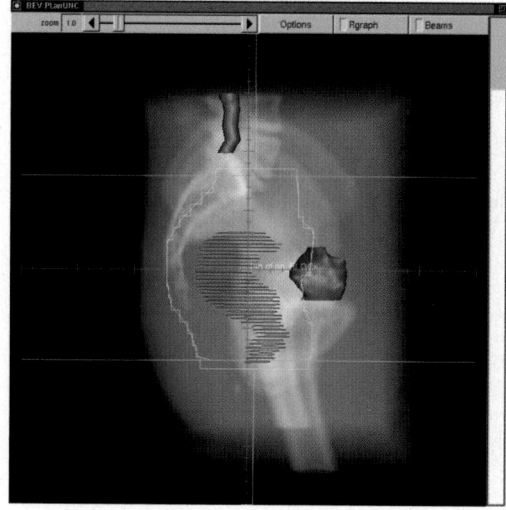

B

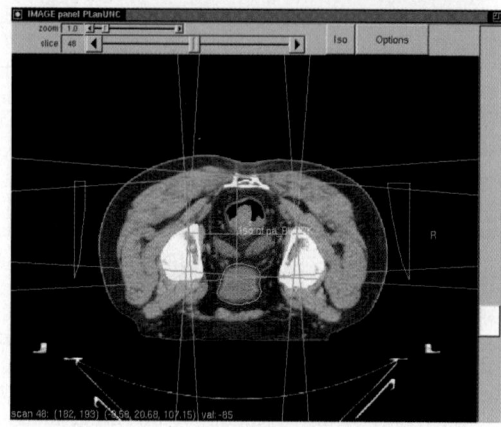

C

Figure 60.4 Posteroanterior **(A)** and lateral digitally **(B)** reconstructed radiograph of the radiation fields for preoperative radiation therapy of a T3N1 rectal adenocarcinoma. The clinical target volume and rectum are *outlined*. There is a marker at the anal verge to help avoid irradiating the entire anal canal. The field treats the mesorectum and the lymph nodes to the level of the sacral promontory. **(C)** Transverse cut at the middle of the radiation field.

SELECTED REFERENCES

The full reference list can be accessed at lwwhealthlibrary.com/oncology.

5. Wibe A, Eriksen MT, Syse A, et al. Total mesorectal excision for rectal cancer—what can be achieved by a national audit? *Colorectal Dis* 2003;5: 471–477.

7. Watanabe T, Wu TT, Catalamo PJ, et al. Molecular predictors of survival after adjuvant chemotherapy for colon cancer. *N Engl J Med* 2001;344: 1196–1206.

8. Compton CC. Surgical pathology of colorectal cancer. In Saltz LB, ed. *Colorectal Cancer: Multimodality Management.* Totowa, NJ: Humana Press; 2002:247–265.

16. Ayez N, Alberda WJ, Burger JW, et al. Is restaging with chest and abdominal CT scan after neoadjuvant chemoradiotherapy for locally advanced rectal cancer necessary? *Ann Surg Oncol* 2013;20:155–160.

17. Gunderson LL, Sargent DJ, Tepper JE, et al. Impact of T and N substage on survival and disease relapse in adjuvant rectal cancer: a pooled analysis. *Int J Radiat Oncol Biol Phys* 2002;54:386–396.

19. Tepper JE, O'Connell MJ, Niedzwiecki D, et al. Impact of number of nodes retrieved on outcome in patients with rectal cancer. *J Clin Oncol* 2001;19:157–163.

25. de Campos-Lobato LF, Stocchi L, de Sousa JB, et al. Less than 12 nodes in the surgical specimen after total mesorectal excision following neoadjuvant chemoradiation: it means more than you think! *Ann Surg Oncol* 2013;20:3398–3406.

29. Quirke P, Durdey P, Dixon MF, et al. Local recurrence of rectal adenocarcinoma due to inadequate surgical resection: histopathological study of lateral tumour spread and surgical excision. *Lancet* 1986;2:996–999.

34. MERCURY Study Group. Diagnostic accuracy of preoperative magnetic resonance imaging in predicting curative resection of rectal cancer: prospective observational study. *BMJ* 2006;333:779.

38. Patel UB, Taylor F, Blomqvist L, et al. Magnetic resonance imaging-detected tumor response for locally advanced rectal cancer predicts survival outcomes: MERCURY experience. *J Clin Oncol* 2011;29:3753–3760.

39. Taylor FG, Quirke P, Heald RJ, et al. Preoperative high-resolution magnetic resonance imaging can identify good prognosis stage I, II, and III rectal cancer best managed by surgery alone: a prospective, multicenter, European study. *Ann Surg* 2011;253:711–719.

47. Cipe G, Ergul N, Hasbahceci M, et al. Routine use of positron-emission tomography/computed tomography for staging of primary colorectal cancer: does it affect clinical management? *World J Surg Oncol* 2013;11:49.

49. Saraste D, Gunnarsson U, Janson M. Predicting lymph node metastases in early rectal cancer. *Eur J Cancer* 2013;49:1104–1108.

51. Greenberg JA, Shibata D, Herndon JE 2nd, et al. Local excision of distal rectal cancer: an update of cancer and leukemia group B 8984. *Dis Colon Rectum* 2008;51:1185–1191, discussion 1191–1194.

53. Garcia-Aguilar J, Shi Q, Thomas CR Jr, et al. A phase II trial of neoadjuvant chemoradiation and local excision for T2N0 rectal cancer: preliminary results of the ACOSOG Z6041 trial. *Ann Surg Oncol* 2012;19:384–391.

54. Lezoche E, Baldarelli M, Lezoche G, et al. Randomized clinical trial of endoluminal locoregional resection versus laparoscopic total mesorectal excision for T2 rectal cancer after neoadjuvant therapy. *Br J Surg* 2012;99: 1211–1218.

55. Sgourakis G, Lanitis S, Gockel I, et al. Transanal endoscopic microsurgery for T1 and T2 rectal cancers: a meta-analysis and meta-regression analysis of outcomes. *Am Surg* 2011;77:761–772.

56. Wu Y, Wu YY, Li S, et al. TEM and conventional rectal surgery for T1 rectal cancer: a meta-analysis. *Hepatogastroenterology* 2011;58:364–368.

58. Ramirez JM, Aquilella V, Valencia J, et al. Transanal endoscopic microsurgery for rectal cancer. Long-term oncologic results. *Int J Colorectal Dis* 2011;26:437–443.

62. Libutti SK, Forde KA. Surgical considerations III: bowel anastomosis. In Cohen A, Weaver S, eds. *Cancer of the Colon, Rectum and Anus.* New York, NY: McGraw Hill; 1995:445–456.

67. Pahlman L, Bujko K, Rutkowski A, et al. Altering the therapeutic paradigm towards a distal bowel margin of < 1 cm in patients with low-lying rectal cancer: a systematic review and commentary. *Colorectal Dis* 2013;15:e166–e174.

71. Barisic G, Markovic V, Popovic M, et al. Function after intersphincteric resection for low rectal cancer and its influence on quality of life. *Colorectal Dis* 2011;13:638–643.

76. Kapiteijn E, Marijnen CA, Nagtegaal ID, et al. Preoperative radiotherapy combined with total mesorectal excision for resectable rectal cancer. *N Eng J Med* 2001;345:638–646.

87. Greenblatt DY, Rajamanickam V, Pugely AJ, et al. Short-term outcomes after laparoscopic-assisted proctectomy for rectal cancer: results from the ACS NSQIP. *J Am Coll Surg* 2012;212:844–854.

89. Huang MJ, Liang JL, Wang H, et al. Laparoscopic-assisted versus open surgery for rectal cancer: a meta-analysis of randomized controlled trials on oncologic adequacy of resection and long-term oncologic outcomes. *Int J Colorectal Dis* 2011;26:415–421.

91. Ng SS, Lee JF, Yiu RY, et al. Long-term oncologic outcomes of laparoscopic versus open surgery for rectal cancer: a pooled analysis of 3 randomized controlled trials. *Ann Surg* 2014;259:139–147.

92. Lujan J, Valero G, Biondo S, et al. Laparoscopic versus open surgery for rectal cancer: results of a prospective multicentre analysis of 4,970 patients. *Surg Endosc* 2013;27:295–302.

94. Soop M, Nelson H. Laparoscopic-assisted proctectomy for rectal cancer: on trial. *Ann Surg Oncol* 2008;15:2357–2359.

103. Trastulli S, Farinella E, Cirocchi R, et al. Robotic resection compared with laparoscopic rectal resection for cancer: systematic review and meta-analysis of short-term outcome. *Colorectal Dis* 2012;14:e134–e156.

106. Collinson FJ, Jayne DG, Pigazzi A, et al. An international, multicentre, prospective, randomised, controlled, unblinded, parallel-group trial of robotic-assisted versus standard laparoscopic surgery for the curative treatment of rectal cancer. *Int J Colorectal Dis* 2012;27:233–241.

108. Mohan HM, Evans MD, Larkin JO, et al. Multivisceral resection in colorectal cancer: a systematic review. *Ann Surg Oncol* 2013;20:2929–2936.

110. Chew MH, Brown WE, Masya L, et al. Clinical, MRI, and PET-CT criteria used by surgeons to determine suitability for pelvic exenteration surgery for recurrent rectal cancers: a Delphi study. *Dis Colon Rectum* 2013;56:717–725.

111. Ripley RT, Gajdos C, Reppert AE, et al. Sequential radiofrequency ablation and surgical debulking for unresectable colorectal carcinoma: thermo-surgical ablation. *J Surg Oncol* 2013;107:144–147.

112. Pusceddu C, Sotgia B, Melis L, et al. Painful pelvic recurrence of rectal cancer: percutaneous radiofrequency ablation treatment. *Abdom Imaging* 2013;38:1225–1233.

117. Gunderson LL, Sosin H. Areas of failure found at reoperation (second or symptomatic look) following "curative surgery" for adenocarcinoma of the rectum. *Cancer* 1974;34:1278–1292.

121. Heald RJ. The "Holy Plane" of rectal surgery. *J Royal Soc Med* 1988;81:503–508.

125. Sebag-Montefiore D, Stephens RJ, Steele R, et al. Preoperative radiotherapy versus selective postoperative chemoradiotherapy in patients with rectal cancer (MRC CR07 and NCIC-CTG C016): a multicentre, randomised trial. *Lancet* 2009;373:811–820.

126. Swedish Rectal Cancer Trial. Improved survival with preoperative radiotherapy in resectable rectal cancer. *N Engl J Med* 1997;336:980–987.

127. Prolongation of the disease-free interval in surgically treated rectal carcinoma. Gastrointestinal Tumor Study Group. *N Engl J Med* 1985;312:1465–1472.

128. Krook JE, Moertel CG, Gunderson LL, et al. Effective surgical adjuvant therapy for high-risk rectal carcinoma. *N Engl J Med* 1991;324:709–715.

133. O'Connell MJ, Martenson JA, Wieand HS, et al. Improving adjuvant therapy for rectal cancer by combining protracted-infusion fluorouracil with radiation therapy after curative surgery. *N Engl J Med* 1994;331:502–507.

134. Schrag D, Weiser M, Goodman K, et al. Neoadjuvant chemotherapy without routine use of radiation therapy for patients with locally advanced rectal cancer: a pilot trial. *J Clin Oncol* 2014;32:513–518.

138. Sauer R, Liersch T, Merkel S, et al. Preoperative versus postoperative chemoradiotherapy for locally advanced rectal cancer: results of the German CAO/ARO/AIO-94 randomized phase III trial after a median follow-up of 11 years. *J Clin Oncol* 2012;30:1926–1933.

139. Wolff HA, Conradi LC, Beissbarth T, et al. Gender affects acute organ toxicity during radiochemotherapy for rectal cancer: long-term results of the German CAO/ARO/AIO-94 phase III trial. *Radiother Oncol* 2013;108:48–54.

140. Roh MS, Colangelo LH, O'Connell MJ, et al. Preoperative multimodality therapy improves disease-free survival in patients with carcinoma of the rectum: NSABP R-03. *J Clin Oncol* 2009;27:5124–5130.

143. Ngan SY, Burmeister B, Fisher RJ, et al. Randomized trial of short-course radiotherapy versus long-course chemoradiation comparing rates of local recurrence in patients with T3 rectal cancer: Trans-Tasman Radiation Oncology Group trial 01.04. *J Clin Oncol* 2012;30:3827–3833.

147. Loos M, Quentmeier P, Schuster T, et al. Effect of preoperative radio(chemo)therapy on long-term functional outcome in rectal cancer patients: a systematic review and meta-analysis. *Ann Surg Oncol* 2013;20:1816–1828.

148. Bosset JF, Collette L, Calais G, et al. Chemotherapy with preoperative radiotherapy in rectal cancer. *N Engl J Med* 2006;355:1114–1123.

153. Stocchi L, Nelson H, Sargent DJ, et al. Impact of surgical and pathologic variables in rectal cancer: a United States community and cooperative group report. *J Clin Oncol* 2001;19:3895–3902.

154. Martling AL, Holm T, Rutqvist LE, et al. Effect of a surgical training programme on outcome of rectal cancer in the Country of Stockholm. *Lancet* 2000;356:93–96.

157. Nishioka M, Shimada M, Kurita N, et al. Gene expression profile can predict pathological response to preoperative chemoradiotherapy in rectal cancer. *Cancer Genomics Proteomics* 2011;8:87–92.

159. Grimminger PP, Danenberg P, Dellas K, et al. Biomarkers for cetuximab-based neoadjuvant radiochemotherapy in locally advanced rectal cancer. *Clin Cancer Res* 2011;17:3469–3477.

162. Edden Y, Wexner SD, Berho M. The use of molecular markers as a method to predict the response to neoadjuvant therapy for advanced stage rectal adenocarcinoma. *Colorectal Dis* 2012;14:555–561.

163. Casado E, Garcia VM, Sanchez JJ, et al. A combined strategy of SAGE and quantitative PCR Provides a 13-gene signature that predicts preoperative chemoradiotherapy response and outcome in rectal cancer. *Clin Cancer Res* 2011;17:4145–4154.

171. Habr-Gama A, Perez RO, Nadalin W, et al. Operative versus nonoperative treatment for stage 0 distal rectal cancer following chemoradiation therapy: long-term results. *Ann Surg* 2004;240:711–717, discussion 717–718.

172. Maas M, Beets-Tan RG, Lambregts DM, et al. Wait-and-see policy for clinical complete responders after chemoradiation for rectal cancer. *J Clin Oncol* 2011;29:4633–4640.

173. Smith JD, Ruby JA, Goodman KA, et al. Nonoperative management of rectal cancer with complete clinical response after neoadjuvant therapy. *Ann Surg* 2012;256:965–972.

174. Chau I, Brown G, Cunningham D, et al. Neoadjuvant capecitabine and oxaliplatin followed by synchronous chemoradiation and total mesorectal excision in magnetic resonance imaging–defined poor-risk rectal cancer. *J Clin Oncol* 2006;24:668–674.

176. Cercek A, Goodman KA, Hajj C, et al. Chemotherapy first, followed by chemoradiation and then surgery, in the management of locally advanced rectal cancer. *J Natl Compr Canc Netw* 2014;12:513–519.

180. Guillem JG, Ruby JA, Leibold T, et al. Neither FDG-PET Nor CT can distinguish between a pathological complete response and an incomplete response after neoadjuvant chemoradiation in locally advanced rectal cancer: a prospective study. *Ann Surg* 2013;258:289–295.

184. Duldulao MP, Lee W, Streja L, et al. Distribution of residual cancer cells in the bowel wall after neoadjuvant chemoradiation in patients with rectal cancer. *Dis Colon Rectum* 2013;56:142–149.

190. Roh MS, Yothers GA, O'Connell MJ, et al. The impact of capecitabine and oxaliplatin in the preoperative multimodality treatment in patients with carcinoma of the rectum: NSABP R-04. *J Clin Oncol* 2011;29:Abstr 3503.

191. Hofheinz RD, Wenz F, Post S, et al. Chemoradiotherapy with capecitabine versus fluorouracil for locally advanced rectal cancer: a randomised, multicentre, non-inferiority, phase 3 trial. *Lancet Oncol* 2012;13:579–588.

192. Twelves C, Scheithauer W, McKendrick J, et al. Capecitabine versus 5-fluorouracil/folinic acid as adjuvant therapy for stage III colon cancer: final results from the X-ACT trial with analysis by age and preliminary evidence of a pharmacodynamic marker of efficacy. *Ann Oncol* 2012;23:1190–1197.

198. Gerard JP, Azria D, Gourgou-Bourgade S, et al. Clinical outcome of the ACCORD 12/0405 PRODIGE 2 randomized trial in rectal cancer. *J Clin Oncol* 2012;30:4558–4565.

199. Aschele C, Pinto C, Cordio S, et al. Preoperative fluorouracil (FU)-based chemoradiation with and without oxaliplatin in locally advanced rectal cancer: pathologic response analysis of the Studio Terapia Adiuvante Retto (STAR)-01 randomized phase III trial. *J Clin Oncol* 2009;27:Abstr CRA4008.

204. Willett CG, Boucher Y, di Tomaso E, et al. Direct evidence that the VEGF-specific antibody bevacizumab has antivascular effects in human rectal cancer. *Nat Med* 2004;10:145–147.

207. Dewdney A, Cunningham D, Tabernero J, et al. Multicenter randomized phase II clinical trial comparing neoadjuvant oxaliplatin, capecitabine, and preoperative radiotherapy with or without cetuximab followed by total mesorectal excision in patients with high-risk rectal cancer (EXPERT-C). *J Clin Oncol* 2012;30:1620–1627.

209. Nogue M, Salud A, Vicente P, et al. Addition of bevacizumab to XELOX induction therapy plus concomitant capecitabine-based chemoradiotherapy in magnetic resonance imaging-defined poor-prognosis locally advanced rectal cancer: the AVACROSS study. *Oncologist* 2011;16:614–620.

211. Saltz L, Raben D, Minsky BD, et al. Rectal cancer: presentation with metastatic and locally advanced disease. American College of Radiology. ACR Appropriateness Criteria. *Radiology* 2000;215:1491–1499.

216. Braendengen M, Tveit KM, Berglund A, et al. Randomized phase III study comparing preoperative radiotherapy with chemoradiotherapy in nonresectable rectal cancer. *J Clin Oncol* 2008;26:3687–3694.

217. Gunderson LL, Nelson H, Martenson JA, et al. Locally advanced primary colorectal cancer: intraoperative electron and external beam irradiation +/− 5-FU. *Int J Radiat Oncol Biol Phys* 1997;37:601–614.

220. Harrison LB, Minsky BD, Enker WE, et al. High dose rate intraoperative radiation therapy (HDR-IORT) as part of the management strategy for locally advanced primary and recurrent rectal cancer. *Int J Radiat Oncol Biol Phys* 1998;42:325–330.

223. Brierley JD, Cummings BJ, Wong CS, et al. Adenocarcinoma of the rectum treated by radical external radiation therapy. *Int J Radiat Oncol Biol Phys* 1995;31:255–259.

225. Frykholm GJ, Glimelius B, Pahlman L. Preoperative or postoperative irradiation in adenocarcinoma of the rectum: final treatment results of a randomized trial and an evaluation of late secondary effects. *Dis Colon Rectum* 1993;36:564–572.

61 Cancer of the Anal Region

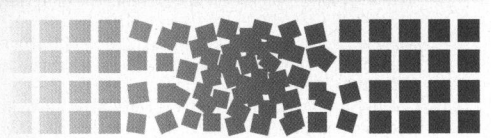

Brian G. Czito, Shahab Ahmed, Matthew Kalady, and Cathy Eng

INTRODUCTION

Carcinoma of the anal canal is a rare malignancy, although its incidence is steadily increasing. The development of anal cancer is a multifocal process largely associated with the human papillomavirus (HPV). The treatment approach to this disease has evolved significantly over recent decades and serves as a model for organ-preserving therapy, transitioning from radical surgery by abdominal perineal resection (APR, entailing permanent colostomy placement with associated high pelvic recurrence rates) to a nonsurgical approach of definitive chemoradiotherapy with 5-fluorouracil (5-FU) and mitomycin C (MMC), leading to successful preservation of anorectal function in the majority of patients. Anal cancer is relatively unique amongst gastrointestinal malignancies in that it has a low propensity for metastatic spread, making local–regional control a paramount endpoint in the approach to this disease. Over the past 2 decades, published randomized trials have demonstrated the superiority of chemoradiotherapy with 5-FU and MMC over radiation therapy alone, radiation with concurrent 5-FU, as well as induction cisplatin/5-FU alone followed by concurrent radiotherapy using the same regimen. Additionally, randomized trials have failed to demonstrate a definitive benefit for radiation dose escalation nor superiority when substituting cisplatin for MMC. Treatment with chemoradiotherapy is associated with significant acute and chronic toxicity rates, and improvement in radiation therapy techniques has been shown to decrease such. Current investigations include the use of novel cytotoxic and inhibitor targeted agents, including epidermal growth factor receptor, in efforts to improve outcomes in patients with more advanced disease, as well as further understanding the molecular etiology and resistance of this disease. This chapter provides an overview of the background, epidemiology, diagnosis, multidisciplinary treatment, and outcomes of tumors arising in the anal canal and perianal skin, as well as anal canal adenocarcinoma and melanoma.

EPIDEMIOLOGY AND ETIOLOGY

Anal cancer is the least prevalent among all gastrointestinal (GI) cancers. It has been reported that anal cancers account for 1% to 2% of all large bowel malignancies. According to the 2014 American Cancer Society statistics, about 7,210 men and women (37% men and 63% women, a ratio of almost 1:2 for men to women) will be diagnosed with anal cancer, and it is estimated that 950 (or 13%) of those diagnosed with anal cancers will die from their disease.[1]

The median age at diagnosis for anal, anal canal, and anorectal cancers was 60 years during 2006 to 2010. This data showed that among all races, Caucasian females experienced the highest incidence rate (2.1 out of 100,000), whereas Asian males had the lowest incidence rate (0.5 out of 100,000) during that time frame (Fig. 61.1). The median age at death was 64 years during this period. It was estimated that African American males

and Caucasian females had the highest mortality rate (0.3 out of 100,000 each) among all races, whereas at the same time, both male and female Asians had the lowest mortality rate (0.1 out of 100,000 each) (see Fig. 61.1).

The incidence of anal cancer has been increasing over the last 30 years in the United States as well as globally.[2,3] This is likely related to the increase in infections by the sexually transmitted HPV and HIV, which may have a significant impact on anal cancer incidence. In one large case-control series, an increasing number of sexual partners was associated with the development of anal cancer in both men and women (odds ratio of 4.5 for women and 2.5 for men with ≥10 sexual partners). This study also demonstrated that a history of anal warts was associated with a higher risk of developing anal cancer, as was receptive anal intercourse in women.[3]

Human Papillomavirus Infection

High-risk HPV type-16 has been detected in almost 90% of cases of squamous cell carcinoma of the anus.[4] A recent meta-analysis suggests that HPV-16 is found more frequently (75%) and HPV-18 less frequently (10%) in anal carcinomas than in cervical carcinomas. Moreover, approximately 80% of anal cancers demonstrated more than one HPV genotype.[5] Anal cancer, now considered to be a predominantly HPV-related cancer, has an incidence 15 times higher in homosexual men than in heterosexual men.[6] In most cases, anal infection with HPV is sexually transmitted, and the risk for cancer is increased in patients with a history of receptive anal intercourse in women and homosexual activity in men.[7] It is also been shown that women with high-grade cervical or vulvar dysplasia are more susceptible to develop anal cancer, as cervical or vulvar HPV infection escalates anal HPV infection risk.[8]

HIV Infection

The incidence of anal cancer in patients who are infected with HIV is estimated to be twice that of HIV-negative patients. Highly active antiretroviral therapy (HAART) has resulted in patients with HIV living longer and the development of related malignancies. In contrast to other HIV-associated malignancies, the incidence of anal cancer has actually risen following implementation of HAART.[9–11] According to the National Cancer Institute (NCI), the rise in anal cancer incidence rates during 1980 to 2005 was predominantly seen in male patients with HIV, relative to their female counterparts.[12] Although HIV has been considered to be a major factor in anal cancer incidence, it is also suggested that HIV may have an impact on the survival of patients with anal cancer, with one report demonstrating that HIV-positive patients with anal cancer tended to develop earlier recurrences than HIV-negative patients by 20 months, although the median survival for HIV-positive patients (34 months) and HIV-negative patients (39 months) were similar (non-significant) (discussed as follows).[13]

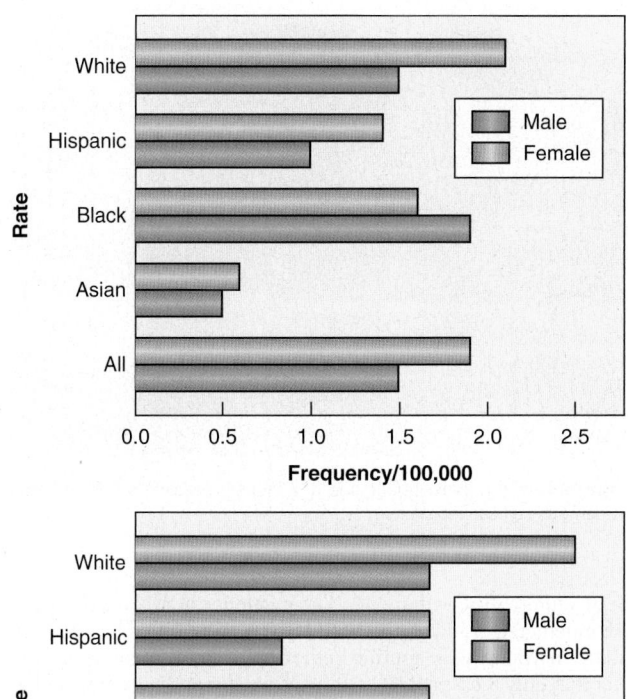

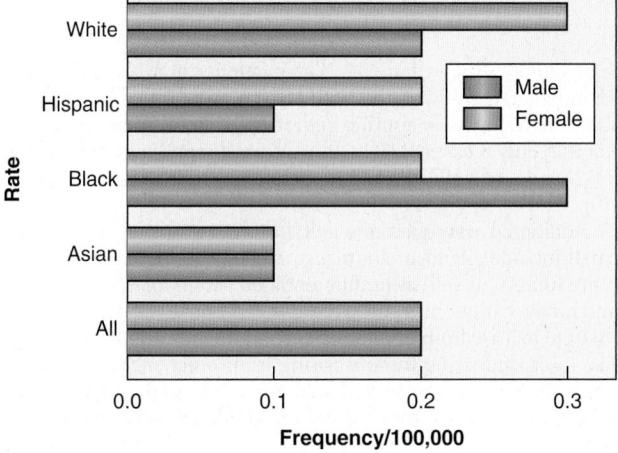

Figure 61.1 Anal cancer distribution among different races. *(Top)* Incidence rate. *(Bottom)* Death rate.

Other Risk Factors

According to the American Society of Colon and Rectal Surgeons (ASCRS), risk factors other than HIV and HPV infections include:

- Age: 67% >55 years.
- Smoking: There are reports demonstrating that that smoking is a risk factor for anal cancer development. According to one study, the relationship between smoking and anal cancer persists for both gender types (adjusted odds ratio for women = 3.8, 95% confidence interval [CI], 2.3 to 6.2; adjusted odds ratio for men = 3.9, 95% CI, 1.9 to 8.0). Similarly, the risk of anal cancer appears to be related to the pack-year history of smoking, with more extensive histories associated with a higher risk.[14]
- Immunosuppression: Solid organ transplant recipients with chronic immunosuppressive therapy have a six times higher risk to develop anal cancer relative to the general population.[15]

Benign anal lesions are no longer thought to contribute to the development of this disease, although anal cancers are frequently misdiagnosed as these conditions.

SCREENING AND PREVENTION

Anal squamous intraepithelial lesions (SIL) or anal intraepithelial neoplasia (AIN) have been recognized as precursors that can progress to anal squamous cell carcinoma (SCC).[16] Although there are no published guidelines that recommend screening of

the general population for anal cancer, there are high-risk groups that may benefit from such, most prominently patients infected with HIV. Although the natural history of SIL is still being unraveled, studies show increased rates of progression in HIV-positive patients with a relative risk of 2.4 and increasing to 3.1 for those with CD4 counts below 200.[17,18] The rationale for screening for SIL is based on the following: there is a high incidence of the anal cancer within the proposed screening population (i.e., HIV-positive patients), available screening tests are effective and cost-efficient, and early detection can change the outcome of the disease. The initial recommended screening test is an "anal Pap smear" that evaluates cells in the anal canal for abnormal cytology through swabbing. Patients with abnormal cytology should then be evaluated by high-resolution anoscopy, which facilitates the visualization of abnormal lesions, allowing biopsy and/or removal.[19,20] Algorithms for the management of low-grade and high-grade SILs remain controversial as more data are needed to determine the effectiveness of intervention on decreasing long-term rates of anal SCC.

Treatment options of high-grade AIN include ablation with electrocautery, topical trichloroacetic acid, topical 5-FU, or imiquimod,[21–23] with estimated lesion control rates ranging from 60% to 80%. A 2012 Cochrane Review highlights the dearth of evidence addressing the efficacy of available interventions for SIL. This review resulted in one randomized trial being identified. This trial evaluated the medication imiquimod versus placebo. Although underpowered, results showed no statistically significant benefit for treatment. The authors concluded that, given the rising incidence of AIN and anal cancer, well-designed randomized controlled trials are urgently needed to address this topic, with emphasis on AIN resolution, downstaging, recurrence, and progression to invasive disease in both HIV-positive and -negative populations.[24]

A promising strategy for the prevention of anal dysplasia and malignancy is HPV vaccination. Two vaccines (Cervarix and Gardasil) are now approved by the U.S. Food and Drug Administration and have been shown to protect against cervical cancer in women.[25,26] The quadrivalent HPV vaccine Gardasil has demonstrated efficacy for prevention of HPV 6-, 11-, 16-, and 18-related genital warts and has been shown to protect against cancers of the anus, vagina, and vulva.[27] In a large, double blind study, 602 healthy men who have sex with men were randomized to receive the quadrivalent HPV vaccine versus placebo. With a 36-month median follow-up for the development of AIN and/or high-risk HPV infection, significantly reduced rates of high-grade anal dysplasia and high-risk HPV infection were demonstrated in the vaccinated group.[28] No cases of anal cancer or vaccine-related serious events were noted. In the context of limited availability and suboptimal outcomes of AIN screening programs, vaccination may reflect the best long-term approach for reducing anal cancer risk and is recommended for girls and boys at age 11 or 12 years and girls 13 to 26 years of age who have not been previously vaccinated.

PATHOLOGY

A variety of malignancies can arise in the anal canal and perianal skin. The typical gross appearance of SCC of the anal canal consists of a lesion with rolled edges, often with central ulceration, with a minority consisting of polypoid lesions (Fig. 61.2). On a practical level, these can be divided into squamous and nonsquamous histologies. The vast majority of anal canal tumors are classified as SCC, which encompasses tumors previously described as basaloid, cloacogenic, transitional, mucoepidermoid, and verrucous mucoepidermoid varieties (Fig. 61.3). These subtypes generally referred to tumors arising in the anal transitional zone, where the anal squamous histology transitions into the glandular epithelium seen in the colorectum. From a treatment standpoint, these are all approached as SCC. The current World Health Organization (WHO)[29] classification does not include these subtypes. The majority of these are

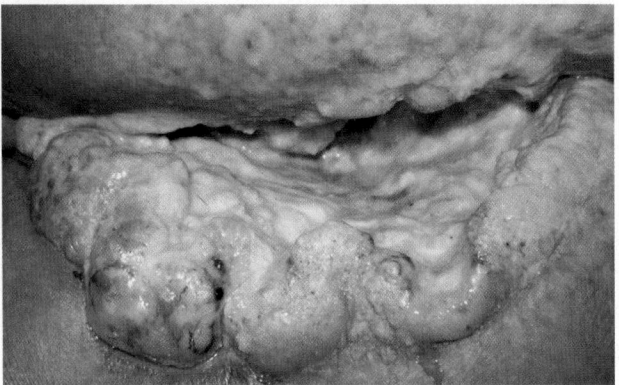

Figure 61.2 A 60-year-old male with advanced squamous cell carcinoma of the anal verge, exhibiting rolled edges with central ulceration.

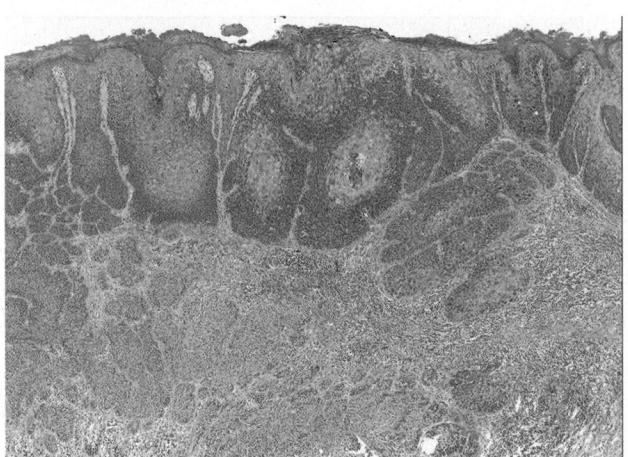

Figure 61.3 A microscopic image of a biopsy revealing nonkeratinizing squamous cell carcinoma.

nonkeratinizing, although tumors arising below the dentate line often display keratinizing properties. Most squamous lesions are moderately to poorly differentiated and display koilocytic changes consistent with HPV infection.

It is believed that most anal cancers arise from precancerous changes (i.e., AIN) of the anal canal and perianal skin epithelium. AIN is a multifocal process associated with HPV, analogous to cervical dysplasia. There is a progression from normal epithelium to condyloma and grade I AIN (associated with mild dysplasia), later progressing to grade II AIN (with moderate dysplasia), and ultimately grade III AIN with severe dysplasia, as well as in situ disease. Once disease has reached grade III AIN, it rarely regresses. It has been estimated that approximately 5% of AIN III patients progress to invasive malignancy, often occurring over a multiyear period. This incidence of progression of AIN III is substantially increased in patients who are immunocompromised.[17,30] The prevalence of AIN among HIV-negative homosexual men is high (>36%), and almost universal among HIV-positive men who have

sexual intercourse with men.[31] The incidence of AIN is believed to be much greater in patients with HIV as exemplified by a French study analyzing 8,153 routine hemorrhoidectomy specimens, finding that only 3 cases of AIN (0.04%) were seen,[32] as compared to 20 cases out of a 103 (19.4%) in specimens from HIV-positive men (Fig. 61.4).[33]

Additional nonsquamous cell histologies arising in the anal canal include adenocarcinoma, small cell carcinoma/neuroendocrine tumors, as well as undifferentiated carcinomas, melanomas, and rarely, lymphomas and sarcomas. Neuroendocrine tumors are thought to arise from endocrine cells in the transitional zone and, like neuroendocrine tumors arising from other sites, tend to disseminate widely. A suspected anal adenocarcinoma may actually reflect an extension from a distal rectal adenocarcinoma in some situations. Mucinous adenocarcinoma is generally thought to arise

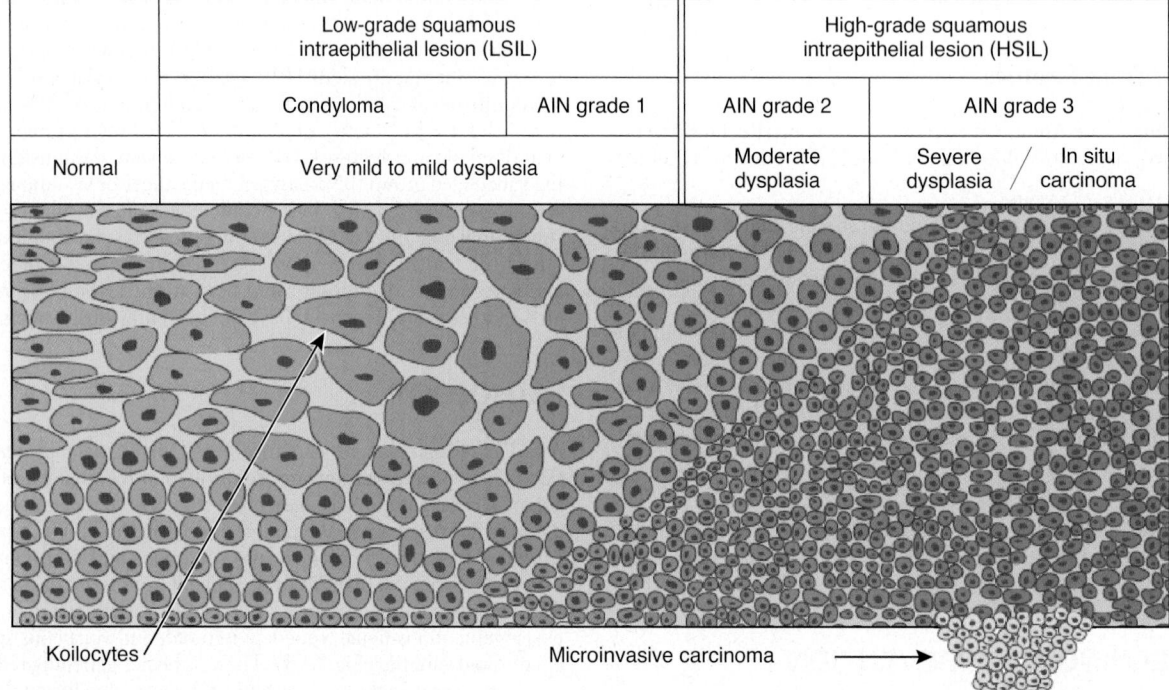

	Low-grade squamous intraepithelial lesion (LSIL)		High-grade squamous intraepithelial lesion (HSIL)	
	Condyloma	AIN grade 1	AIN grade 2	AIN grade 3
Normal	Very mild to mild dysplasia		Moderate dysplasia	Severe dysplasia / In situ carcinoma

Koilocytes   Microinvasive carcinoma →

Figure 61.4 A schematic representation of an anal intraepithelial neoplasia progression. Note that the increasing severity as a proportion of epithelium is replaced by progressive increase in immature-appearing cells, ultimately leading to invasive disease with violation of the basement membrane. (Goldstone SE. Diagnosis and treatment of HPV related squamous intraepithelial neoplasia in men who have sex with men. *PRN Notebook* 2005;10:11–16.)

in the anal glands and ducts and is uncommon. It should be noted that histology is generally more important than location within the anal canal and usually dictates overall patient management.

Tumors of the perianal skin are similar to that seen in the anal canal, primarily comprised of SCC. These tumors are generally well differentiated and keratinizing. Verrucous carcinoma—also sometimes known as a giant condyloma or Buschke-Lowenstein tumor—was initially described in 1925. These tumors are sometimes mistakenly considered to be benign and misdiagnosed as condylomata acuminata, with a subsequent histologic analysis revealing invasion. These are often locally destructive and HPV related. They are often slow growing and can be present for many years before coming to medical attention. Local recurrence rates following excision are high and malignant transformation can be seen in up to 50%.[34] Additional precursor lesions seen in the perianal skin include Bowen disease, which consist of a slow growing intraepidermal SCC that may mimic perianal dermatitis, as well as Paget disease, which is similar to the entity seen associated with breast cancer, with an eczematous appearance. Approximately half of Paget disease patients will harbor an underlying adenocarcinoma, notably in the colorectum.

CLINICAL PRESENTATION AND STAGING

Symptoms of anal cancer can be diverse and include bleeding, pain, sensation of a mass, itching, anal discharge, tenesmus, and a sense of fullness or a lump in the anal canal. The most common presentation is bleeding from the anus. More extensive lesions may present with more ominous symptoms such as incontinence, passage of gas or stool from the vagina, or significant change in bowel habits. Less frequently, an enlarged inguinal lymph node is reported, and 20% of patients are initially asymptomatic. Symptoms may often be dismissed as hemorrhoids or other benign causes, and it is crucial to further evaluate by a physical examination and anoscopy. Any mass should be biopsied for a diagnosis.

Clinical staging is performed by a combination of clinical, endoscopic, and radiographic examinations (Table 61.1). History should include an assessment of anal sphincter function as well as HIV risk factors. Digital rectal examination can identify fixation to the sphincter complex or adjacent organs such as the vagina and prostate. Proctoscopy provides information about the extent of mucosal spread, including the relationship to the dentate line, and facilitates biopsy. It may be necessary to examine patients under anesthesia secondary to pain and sphincter muscle spasms. Female patients should undergo a gynecologic examination to determine vaginal involvement and to exclude other HPV-associated cancers, including evaluation of the cervix. Imaging is used to better delineate the local extent of disease and regional adenopathy, and to determine the presence of distant metastases. An endoanal

---

TABLE 61.1

Recommended Diagnostic Evaluation in Newly Diagnosed Anal Cancer

- Digital rectal examination with tumor characterization (location, fixation, extent)
- Examination of inguinal lymph nodes; consideration of biopsy if deemed suspicious
- Endoscopy/proctoscopy
- Gynecologic examination in females to rule out vaginal invasion as well as exclude gynecologic primary
- Positron-emission tomography/computed tomography (PET-CT) scan
- Complete blood count with serum chemistries as well as HIV testing/CD4 levels in the presence of risk factors

---

ultrasound or pelvic magnetic resonance imaging (MRI) can be considered to assess tumor size and involvement with local structures such as the anal sphincters and vagina or prostate. Computed tomography (CT) scans of the chest, abdomen, and pelvis are commonly employed to evaluate distant disease and adenopathy, particularly in the inguinal regions. Of all patients presenting with palpable inguinal lymph nodes, only 50% are malignant; therefore, fine-needle aspiration is often recommended in suspected cases, and a positive result may guide radiation field design and dose. Some oncologists have suggested a routine sentinel lymph node (SLN) evaluation as a staging technique. A systematic review of 16 published series evaluating the outcome of SLN biopsy of inguinal nodes included 323 patients, and the success in identifying the SLN was 86%. However, the exact role of SNL in the pretreatment evaluation remains undetermined.[35]

A number of recent studies have investigated the role of positron-emission tomography (PET)-CT scans for staging anal cancer. One review described outcomes of patients undergoing conventional staging with ultrasound as well as PET-CT scans. Of 95 patients, the authors found that PET-CT scans were particularly valuable in detecting more extensive nodal and metastatic disease as well as the detection of synchronous malignancies. Upstaging was noted in 14% of patients, and 23% had a change in treatment plan relative to ultrasound staging.[36] Another study comparing the use of conventional imaging with CT scans and MRI found that the addition of PET-CT scans upstaged patients in 20%, downstaged 25%, and altered management in 37%. These authors concluded that PET-CT scans should be a routine part of initial staging of all anal cancers. A lesser impact was seen in patients evaluated in follow-up where PET-CT scans upstaged 11% and downstaged in 6% of cases; however, these changes also led to an altered management in 17%, indicating a potential role for selected PET-CT scan use when there is a question of recurrence or salvage surgery is planned.[37] A study by Vercellino and colleagues[38] similarly found that PET-CT scans were useful in the avoidance of unnecessary biopsies and surgery, with a negative predictive value of 94%, ultimately impacting on treatment plans in 22% of follow-up cases. Finally, PET-CT scans may have prognostic value as well, with one study demonstrating a significant correlation between metabolic response posttreatment and progression-free as well as overall survival.[39] National Comprehensive Cancer Network (NCCN) treatment guidelines include the use of FDG-PET scans with CT scans as part of the staging evaluation, notably for patients with T2-4N0 disease or those with involved lymph nodes.[40] After the previously mentioned evaluation, staging is assigned according to the American Joint Committee on Cancer 2010 (AJCC) (Table 61.2).

PROGNOSTIC FACTORS

Clinical

T and N stages are the most important prognostic factors for anal cancer. According to the AJCC, the 5-year observed overall survival (OS) rates of anal cancer for stage I, II, IIIA, IIIB, and IV are 69.5%, 68.1%, 45.6%, 39.6%, and 15.3%, respectively. It has also been demonstrated that the 5-year OS rates for T1, T2, T3, T4, N0, and node-positive anal cancer are 86%, 86%, 60%, 45%, 76%, and 54%.[41]

There are relatively few studies available that analyze prognostic factors for anal cancer. According to the Radiation Therapy Oncology Group (RTOG) 98-11 study, tumor size (>5 cm), involved lymph nodes (N+), and male sex were associated with worse 5-year disease-free survival (DFS) and OS.[42] Results from European Organisation for Research and Treatment of Cancer (EORTC) 22861 study indicated that skin ulceration, lymph node involvement, and male sex were independent variables associated with local–regional failure (LRF) and OS in multivariate analysis.[43] A secondary analysis of the UK Coordinating Committee on

TABLE 61.2

TNM Anus Staging According to the American Joint Committee on Cancer

Primary Tumor (T)

TX	Primary tumor cannot be assessed
T0	No evidence of primary tumor
Tis	Carcinoma in situ (Bowen disease, high-grade squamous intraepithelial lesion [HISL], anal intraepithelial neoplasia [AIN] II–III)
T1	Tumor 2 cm or less in greatest dimension
T2	Tumor more than 2 cm but not more than 5 cm in greatest dimension
T3	Tumor more than 5 cm in greatest dimension
T4	Tumor of any size invades adjacent organ(s) (e.g., vagina, urethra, bladder) (direct invasion of rectal wall, perirectal skin, subcutaneous tissue or sphincter muscle is not classified as T4)

Regional Lymph Nodes (N)

NX	Regional lymph nodes cannot be assessed
N0	No regional lymph node metastasis
N1	Metastasis in perirectal lymph nodes(s)
N2	Metastasis in unilateral internal iliac and/or unilateral inguinal lymph node(s)
N3	Metastasis in perirectal and inguinal lymph nodes and/or bilateral internal iliac and/or inguinal lymph nodes

Distant Metastases (M)

M0	No distant metastasis
M1	Distant metastasis

Anatomic Stage/Prognostic Group

Stage 0	Tis	N0	M0
Stage I	T1	N0	M0
Stage II	T2	N0	M0
	T3	N0	M0
Stage IIIA	T1, T2, T3	N1	M0
	T4	N0	M0
Stage IIIB	T4	N1	M0
	Any T	N2, N3	M0
Stage IV	Any T	Any N	M1

From Edge SB, Byrd DB, Compton CC, et al., eds. *AJCC Cancer Staging Manual*, 7th ed. New York: Springer-Verlag; 2010: 171.

Cancer Research (CCCR) Anal Cancer Trial (ACT) 1 trial indicated that palpable lymph nodes as well as male sex portended a poor prognosis, similar to previous studies. In addition, after adjusting for these factors, these investigators also reported that lower hemoglobin and higher white blood cell counts were also prognostic in terms of anal cancer death and worsened overall survival, respectively. Tumor site, T classification, and platelet levels had no influence on outcomes.[44] However, not all studies have confirmed gender as an independent prognostic factor in terms of local control, metastasis, or overall survival.[45,46]

Although well-differentiated histologies have been shown to portend more favorable outcomes in other cancers, the histologic subtypes of anal cancer have not yet been demonstrated as substantial prognostic factors.[47] According to a study by Schlienger and

colleagues,[48] there was no significant difference found in survival analysis among cloacogenic, well-differentiated, and moderately or poorly differentiated anal carcinomas.

Molecular

Prognostic biomarkers provide information on patient outcomes regardless of therapy, whereas predictive biomarkers provide information about the effect of specific therapeutic intervention.[49] The ultimate goal of determining prognostic factors is to improve patient survival. Disease processes and progression result from molecular and pathologic pathways, and by targeting altered pathways, potential avenues for therapeutic interventions that could facilitate improvements in survival may emerge. Similarly, molecular analyses of anal cancer to predict treatment response and survival outcomes are essential. Lampejo and colleagues[50] performed a systematic review on anal cancer prognostic biomarkers after reviewing 29 studies for final analysis. The authors found that 13 biomarkers were associated with anal cancer outcomes in only one study, whereas the tumor suppressor genes p53 and p21 as prognostic markers were established by more than one study.

The p53 gene is located in the short arm of chromosome 17 (17p13.1), which encodes a protein (393-amino acid nuclear phosphoprotein) that regulates the cell cycle and is responsible for cell apoptosis.[51,52] Accumulation of nuclear proteins was seen by immunohistochemistry in the cases of muted p53 genes in some studies.[53–55] These studies found that in anal carcinoma, p53 was overexpressed with a range of 34% to 100%. Wong et al.[52] described that increased p53 expression was associated with worse local–regional control ($p = 0.02$) and DFS ($p = 0.01$). Another study of 64 patients suggested that mutant p53 was responsible for inferior LRF rates relative to wild type, although nonsignificant (48 versus 27%, $p = 0.14$).[56] Allal and colleagues[57] reported that anal cancer patients with p53-positive lesions had a lower local–regional control rate (relative risk [RR], 0.38; $p = 0.03$) and shorter DFS (RR, 0.29; $p = 0.003$).

The p21 gene protein, a cyclin-dependent kinase (CDK) inhibitor, is considered to be a mediator of the p53 gene function.[58] Some studies have indicated that the lack of p21 expression is associated with poor prognosis in patients with squamous cell carcinoma of the anal canal (SCCA). Holm et al.[59] reported that a lack of p21 expression was associated with reduced OS ($p = 0.013$), whereas Nilsson and colleagues[60] reported that absence of the same p21 expression was also responsible for an increased LRF rate ($p < 0.05$).

Ajani and colleagues[55] reported epidermal growth factor receptor (EGFR) expression was observed in 86% of patients with anal cancer, but the study was unable to determine the significant correlation between degree of staining and DFS. The same study's multivariate models suggested that Ki67 (negatively, coefficient: −0.04), nuclear factor kappa B (NF-κB) (positively, coefficient: 0.07), Sonic Hedgehog (SHH) (positively, coefficient: 0.05), and Gli-1 (positively, coefficient: 0.03) were associated with DFS ($p = 0.005, 0.002, 0.02,$ and 0.02, respectively). Further investigation into the molecular prognostic factors of anal carcinoma is needed.[50]

TREATMENT OF LOCALIZED SQUAMOUS CELL CARCINOMA

Surgery

As with any disease, treatment decisions in anal cancer are made following a consideration of the risks and benefits. Wide local excision may be considered in a highly select subset of patients of anal cancer patients. This approach should generally be reserved for small, well-differentiated, superficial lesions confined to the anal margin, not involving the internal sphincter, and without nodal involvement.[61] For lesions that have residual microscopic disease or have close surgical margins less than 1 mm, further local excision, if technically possible, may be pursued, or adjuvant chemoradiation should be considered.[40]

Prior to the mid 1970s, the standard surgical approach to anal cancer was abdominal perineal resection (APR), which required a permanent colostomy following the removal of the rectum, ischiorectal fat, levator sling, perirectal and superior hemorrhoidal nodes, as well as a wide area of perianal skin, with associated long-term sequelae of sexual and urinary dysfunction. Collectively, long-term DFS results with a surgery alone approach were approximately 50%. A review at the Mayo Clinic of 118 anal cancers treated with APR reported an OS rate of 70% and overall recurrence rate of 40%. Of these, greater than 80% established recurrence sites had either local recurrence alone or some component of such.[62] Similarly, other surgical series using surgery alone results suggested high rates of regional recurrence (up to 60%) following local excision or APR alone across a variety of stages.[63]

Definitive Chemoradiotherapy

Given the relatively poor outcomes obtained with APR alone, Nigro et al., from Wayne State University pioneered incorporating concurrent pelvic radiation therapy and chemotherapy (5-FU and MMC) prior to surgical resection, resulting in high rates of pathologic complete response and survival, later verified by other investigators.[64–69] This led to significant interest in a *definitive* chemoradiotherapy approach.

Initially, the UK CCCR conducted the ACT I study. In this study, 585 patients with SCC of the anal canal or perianal skin were randomized to receive radiation therapy alone (45 Gy in 20 or 25 fractions), followed by additional radiation dose in patients achieving at least a 50% response (delivering an additional 15 to 25 Gy using either external beam radiation therapy or brachytherapy following a 6-week break) versus a similar radiation approach delivered concurrently with infusional 5-FU (750 mg/m^2 or 1,000 mg/m^2 for 5 days given during the first and last weeks of radiation therapy) along with MMC (12 mg/m^2 delivered on day 1 of treatment). Note that ACT I local failure rates captured several events, including persistence of primary disease following combined modality therapy, the requirement for surgery or colostomy because of treatment failure, as well as ongoing requirement for colostomy at 6 months following the completion of treatment. On the initial report, following a median follow-up of 42 months, the 3-year local failure rate was significantly lower in patients receiving chemoradiotherapy (39% versus 61%; p <0.0001), although at the expense of increased treatment-related morbidity. In particular, hematologic, skin, GI, and genitourinary toxicities were higher with the addition of chemotherapy, with six (2%) treatment-related deaths in the chemoradiation arm versus two (0.7%) for the radiation-alone arm. Although no statistically significant advantage was seen in terms of OS (3-year OS 72% versus 65%; p = 0.17), with the addition of chemotherapy, anal cancer-related mortality was significantly improved (28% versus 39%; p = 0.02), leading the authors to conclude that patients with SCC of the anal canal could be treated with definitive chemoradiotherapy with surgery reserved for salvage. In a report of long-term follow-up of this trial, no significant differences were seen in terms of long-term morbidity, although an excess in non–anal cancer deaths was seen in the combined modality group in the first 10 years following treatment (cardiovascular, treatment related, pulmonary disease, and second malignancy), but not beyond. LRF rates remained significantly higher in patients treated with radiation therapy alone (25% absolute difference at 12 years), with a corresponding improvement in relapse-free survival (12% absolute at 12 years) through the addition of chemotherapy, with no significant difference reported between the

two groups in terms of late morbidity.[70,71] Although not statistically significant, an absolute improvement in 12-year survival of 5.6% was seen.

A similar but smaller trial conducted by the EORTC randomized 103 patients with T3-4N0-3 or T1-2N1-3 anal cancer to radiation therapy (45 Gy, with a boost dose of 15 to 20 Gy following a 6-week break, based on disease response), with or without concurrent chemotherapy using infusional 5-FU (750 mg/m^2 per day, days 1 through 5 and days 29 through 33) with MMC (given on day 1 at 15 mg/m^2). Surgery was reserved for patients with less than a partial response. Outcomes from this study revealed that patients treated with concurrent chemotherapy had a higher complete response rate (80% versus 54%) with significant improvement in local–regional control (68 versus 50%), colostomy-free (72% versus 40%) and event-free survival with the addition of chemotherapy at 5 years. Similarly, OS was improved in patients receiving chemotherapy (3 year: 72% versus 65%), although this did not reach statistical significance. Rates of high-grade toxicity were deemed similar between the two groups, although rates of late anal ulceration were higher with the use of concurrent chemotherapy.[43]

The results from these two trials demonstrated that the addition of chemotherapy to definitive radiation therapy significantly improves LRF rates as well as relapse-free and colostomy-free survival rates, although at the expense of increased toxicity.

The Role of Mitomycin in the Combined Modality Therapy Approach of Anal Cancer

Although MMC was delivered concurrently with 5-FU in the aforementioned trials, it's necessity was questioned given the association with significant toxicities, including significant myelosuppression, dermatitis, as well as less common side effects of pulmonary fibrosis, hemolytic-uremic syndrome and therapy-related myelodysplastic syndrome. Given this, a randomized trial conducted by the RTOG and ECOG attempted to deintensify therapy by omitting MMC in efforts to preserve oncologic efficacy while eliminating MMC-related toxicity. In this study, patients with anal cancer of any T or N stage were randomized to radiation therapy (45 to 50.4 Gy, with an additional 9 Gy to patients with biopsy-proven persistence of disease 4 to 6 weeks following the completion of initial therapy) with infusional 5-FU (1,000 mg/m^2 per day on days 1 to 4 and days 29 to 32), with patients randomized to MMC (10 mg/m^2 days 1 and 29) versus not. Note that in patients with a positive biopsy following the first 4- to 6-week treatment, an additional cycle of cisplatin and 5-FU with radiotherapy was delivered. A second biopsy was later obtained and, if positive for residual tumor, patients proceeded to APR. This study enrolled 310 patients, of which 291 were analyzable. Colostomy-free and disease-free survival rates were significantly higher in patients receiving MMC (71% versus 59% and 73% versus 51%, respectively) with significantly lower colostomy (9% versus 22%) and local failure rates (16% versus 34%). OS was not improved, although as in the previously described randomized studies, was numerically superior (76% versus 67%). Also of note is that all grade 4 and 5 toxicities were considerably higher in patients receiving MMC.[47] Table 61.3 summarizes the results of randomized phase III clinical trials evaluating combined modality therapy with radiation, 5-FU, and mitomycin versus radiation therapy alone or radiation therapy with 5-FU.

The Role of Cisplatin Concurrent with Radiation Therapy in Anal Cancer

Given the aforementioned toxicities associated with MMC, there has been interest in substituting with a platinum-based chemotherapy when delivered concurrently with radiation therapy. Initial results using this approach from a Cancer and Leukemia Group B (CALGB) pilot study demonstrated that the use of induction 5-FU with cisplatin for advanced anal cancers (T3 to 4, or

TABLE 61.3

Summary of Randomized Phase III Clinical Trials Evaluating Combined Modality Treatment with Mitomycin-C/5-FU Versus Radiation Therapy Alone Or Radiation Therapy/5-FU for Anal Cancer

Study (Reference)	Treatment Arms[a]	Local–Regional Failure	Relapse-Free Survival	Colostomy-Free Survival	Overall Survival	Acute Toxicity
UKCCR/ ACT I[70,71]	(1) Radiation	(1) 59.1%	(1) 17.7%	(1) 20.1%	(1) 27.5%	(1) "Severe" skin toxicity = 39%; "severe" GI toxicity = 5%
	(2) Radiation + 5-FU + MMC	(2) 33.8% (at 12 years)	(2) 29.7% (at 12 years)	(2) 29.6% (at 12 years)	(2) 33.1% (at 12 years) p = NS	(2) "Severe" skin toxicity = 50%; "severe" GI toxicity = 14%
EORTC[43]	(1) Radiation	18% improvement in arm 2	N/A	32% improvement in arm 2	7% improvement in arm 2 p = NS	(1) Grade 3–4 diarrhea = 8%; grade 3–4 Dermatologic = 50%
	(2) Radiation + 5-FU + MMC					(2) Grade 3–4 diarrhea = 20%; grade 3–4 dermatologic = 57%
RTOG/ ECOG[47]	(1) Radiation + 5-FU	(1) 34%	(1) 51%	(1) 59%	(1) 67%	(1) Grade 4–5 heme = 3%; grade 4–5 nonheme = 4%
	(2) Radiation + 5-FU + MMC	(2) 16%	(2) 73% (disease-free survival at 4 years)	(2) 73% (at 4 years)	(2) 76% (at 4 years) p = NS	(2) Grade 4–5 heme = 18%; grade 4–5 nonheme = 7%

NS, not stated.

Note: [+] P values significant for comparisons unless otherwise noted.

[a] Details of treatment arms noted in text.

node positive) followed by definitive chemoradiotherapy (45 Gy, with or without a 9 Gy boost) with 5-FU and MMC resulted in an 80% complete response rates with 56% and colostomy-free survival.[72] These and other data led to increasing interest in substituting cisplatin for MMC. The RTOG subsequently conducted a phase III trial (RTOG 98-11), which randomized 644 patients to (1) a standard arm of concurrent chemoradiotherapy (45 to 59 Gy) with continuous infusional 5-FU (1,000 mg/m^2 per day) and bolus MMC (10 mg/m^2) weeks 1 and 5 versus (2) an experimental arm of two cycles of induction continuous 5-FU (1,000 mg/m^2 per day) and bolus cisplatin (75 mg/m^2) alone on weeks 1 and 5, followed by concurrent chemoradiotherapy with two cycles of continuous 5-FU (1,000 mg/m^2 per day) and bolus cisplatin (75 mg/m^2) on weeks 9 and 13. The trial primary endpoint was DFS and secondary endpoint included toxicity analysis. On the initial report, no significant difference was seen in 5-year DFS (60% versus 54%; p = 0.17), OS (75% versus 70%; p = 0.10), or local–regional relapse (25% versus 33%; p = 0.07). However, the 5-year colostomy rate was 10% in the mitomycin group versus 19% in the cisplatin-containing arm (p = 0.02).[73] An update of this trial demonstrated a significant improvement in 5-year DFS (68% versus 58%; p = 0.005), OS (78% versus 71%; p = 0.02), and borderline colostomy-free survival (72% versus 65%; p = 0.05) in the MMC-containing arm, albeit at the expense of increased grade 3 and higher hematologic toxicities (61% versus 42%; p < 0.001). However, nonhematologic toxicity rates were equivalent in both arms, with similar rates of late toxicity.[74] Critics of this study have pointed out that the prolonged the overall treatment duration associated with the use of induction chemotherapy with cisplatin may have allowed for accelerated tumoral repopulation prior to radiation therapy initiation.

A follow-up study from the UK CCCR (the ACT II trial) performed a more direct comparison of the use of cisplatin in conjunction with radiation therapy compared to MMC. In this largest of anal cancer randomized trials, 950 patients with anal or perianal skin cancer were randomized using a 2 × 2 factorial design, with patients randomized to receive infusional 5-FU (1,000 mg/m^2 per day, on days 1 to 4 and days 29 to 32) with

pelvic radiation therapy (50.4 Gy) plus MMC (12 mg/m^2 on day 1) versus cisplatin (60 mg/m^2 on day 1 and 29) with the same 5-FU–radiation regimen. A second randomization was performed following completion of the combined treatment course to no further therapy versus two additional cycles of cisplatin and 5-FU. Grade 3 to 4 acute nonhematologic toxicity rates were similar between the regimens (60% versus 65%; p = 0.17). Not unexpectantly, grade 3 and higher hematologic toxicity rates were greater in the mitomycin group (25% versus 13%; p < 0.001), although no toxic deaths were reported in the trial. In terms of the trial primary endpoint of complete clinical response at 6 months, there was no significant difference between the two groups, and at a median follow-up of 5.1 years, clinical complete response at 26 weeks was 91% in the MMC group compared to 90% in the cisplatin group. Additionally, the 3-year colostomy rate was similar between the two groups (14% mitomycin versus 11% cisplatin). The use of maintenance therapy in this trial showed no obvious benefit, with 3-year recurrence-free survival of 75% in both arms, similar OS rates between the maintenance versus no maintenance groups (85% versus 84%), with 3-year PFS rates of 74% in the maintenance group versus 73% in the nonmaintenance group. The authors concluded that MMC given concurrently with 5-FU and radiation therapy should remain the standard in the treatment of anal cancer, given the following: (1) the high grade hematologic toxicity seen with MMC did not significantly increase sepsis rates; (2) the MMC course was delivered over approximately 10 minutes compared to two courses of either all day or overnight intravenous (IV) hydration with cisplatin, with similar efficacy and overall toxicities between the regimens; (3) fewer chemotherapy cycles were required; (4) there was requirement for fewer nonchemotherapy drugs; (5) there was lesser expense; and (6) there was no risk of neuropathy.[75]

Another phase III trial conducted by the French Federation Nationale des Centres de Lutte Contre La Cancer ACCORD (the ACCORD-03 trial) randomized patients with stage II to III anal cancer to one of four treatment arms: (1) neoadjuvant 5-FU + cisplatin alone followed by 5-FU cisplatin radiation therapy (45 Gy) with a radiation therapy boost (15 Gy) using either external beam or brachytherapy techniques; (2) same as the first arm, except utilizing a higher dose radiation boost (20 to 25 Gy); (3) same as the first arm, but no neoadjuvant chemotherapy; and (4) same as the second arm, but no neoadjuvant chemotherapy. Of note is that a 3-week break was mandated following the completion of the initial 45 Gy, prior to boost treatments. Following a median 50-month follow-up, there was no significant difference in 5-year colostomy-free survival rates (70% to 82%). Similarly, no significant differences were seen between the arms in terms of LRF, cause-specific survival, and OS. The most intensified treatment arm of induction chemotherapy with high-dose radiation boost demonstrated a numerically improved local control (88% versus 72% to 83% on the additional arms). The trial authors indicated that induction chemotherapy does not improve outcomes, with the role of radiation dose escalation in this disease remaining uncertain, but felt that that the combination of induction chemotherapy and radiation dose escalation should be explored further.[76] The results of randomized trials evaluating cisplatin are shown in Table 61.4.

Novel Biologic Radiosensitizing Agents

To date, no biologic agent has been granted U.S. Food and Drug Administration (FDA) approval as an effective radiosensitizer in anal cancer. Early reports have described outcomes of combined treatment modality with EGFR inhibitors, with varying degrees of response and toxicity.[79,80] These and other studies are warranted to assess the role of treatment intensification, particularly in more advanced disease where outcomes are less favorable.

Traditional Radiation and Intensity Modulated Radiation Therapy

The use of combined modality therapy in the definitive treatment of anal cancer results in significant acute as well as late toxicities. All the previously mentioned randomized trials used radiation therapy planned and delivered using either conventional 2-dimensional or 3-dimensional radiation planning techniques. This approach frequently entails treating large volumes of nontarget tissues (bowel, bladder, bone, genitalia), leading to the aforementioned morbidities. Although 3-dimensional planning results in potentially improved normal tissue sparing through the use of axial CT images to define the target volume as well as normal tissue structures, results remain suboptimal. Intensity-modulated radiation therapy is an advanced form of 3-dimensional conformal radiation therapy that implements multiple beams using a nonuniform dose delivery. This can be accomplished in a variety of ways, all of which entail the use of collimating leafs that sweep across the beam path during treatment delivery. Through inverse computer planning techniques, the radiation dose can be more tightly conformed to target tissues with dose reductions to adjacent, nontarget organs. With this technique, there is a significant potential to reduce both acute and long-term morbidity associated with anal cancer treatments. Multiple institutional studies have indicated that, compared to patients treated with non–intensity-modulated radiation therapy (IMRT) techniques, a significant reduction of treatment-related toxicity can be accomplished.[81,82] Additionally, with corresponding reductions in acute toxicity, there may be a reduction in the need for treatment breaks, with the potential to further influence disease-related outcomes.[83] A prospective trial evaluating IMRT for anal cancer was conducted through the RTOG (0529 study). In this phase II trial, patients received concurrent 5-FU with MMC. Radiation therapy was delivered through a *dose-painting* technique, whereby differing target volumes received differing doses of radiation therapy during any one treatment as defined by the study. The primary endpoint of this study included an assessment of grade 2 or higher GI and genitourinary toxicities as compared to the previously described RTOG 98-11 trial (MMC-containing arm). In 52 analyzable patients (out of 63 accrued), rates of grade 3 or higher dermatologic toxicity

were improved in the IMRT study (20% versus 47%; p < 0.001) as were rates of grade 3 or higher GI and genitourinary toxicity (22% versus 36%; p = 0.014). Additionally, median radiation duration was 42.5 days in the IMRT study compared to 49 days in 98-11, with similar 2-year disease-related outcomes when compared to RTOG 98-11.[84,85] An important caveat to this trial was that a central reviewer performed pretreatment quality assurance on all patients. Of initially submitted plans, 81% required planning revisions, with 46% of plans requiring two or more revisions. Although this trial did not formally meet its primary endpoints in reduction and acute toxicities, it does suggest that the use of IMRT can significantly reduce high-grade GI, genitourinary, and skin toxicities without compromising treatment-related outcomes, and that there is also a significant learning curve for the use of IMRT in the treatment of anal cancer. Figure 61.5 demonstrates an example of an anal cancer plan implementing IMRT.

Follow-Up Management

Given that SCC of the anus can regress slowly following treatment completion (up to 12 months), it is generally recommended that patients who have regressive disease do not undergo repeat biopsies given this may lead to nonhealing ulceration and chronic wound infection in previously irradiated tissues.[45,86] Exemplifying this phenomena, in a preliminary report from the ACT II trial, 72% of patients who had not achieved a clinical complete response at 11 weeks ultimately achieved such at 26 weeks from treatment initiation,[87] indicating that premature biopsy following definitive chemoradiotherapy may result in the aforementioned complications as well as premature *salvage* surgery in some cases. Of the 265 patients in the ACT II trial not in complete response at week 11, only 83 ultimately had progression/persistent disease.

Approximately 20% to 25% of patients with SCC treated by chemoradiation will either fail to completely respond or relapse within the first 3 years after treatment. Posttreatment evaluation is critical to assess the effectiveness of therapy and to detect a persistent or recurrent tumor.[86] The first evaluation typically is between 8 to 12 weeks after the completion of chemoradiation. The physical examination should include a visual inspection, a digital rectal exam, an anoscopy, and palpation of the inguinal nodal regions. Ongoing clinical evaluation typically occurs every 3 to 6 months for the first 2 years, then every 6 to 12 months until 5 years following completion of chemoradiation. It may be appropriate to conduct less intense follow-ups following 3 years, given that only 7% of relapses occur beyond this time point.[88] Lesions persisting beyond 3 months following treatment are more concerning for residual disease; however, as stated previously, it is important to assess changes over time. If a tumor continues to shrink, then close clinical surveillance is advised. Chronically persistent or recurrent tumors should be biopsied for confirmation of SCC.[61] Discretion regarding the size and depth of biopsies is needed because extensive biopsies may result in nonhealing ulcers and chronic wound infection.[45] As an adjunct to physical examination, imaging studies for posttreatment surveillance should be considered.[61] Current NCCN guidelines recommend a CT scan of the chest, abdomen, and pelvis annually for 3 years for patients who had T3 or T4 disease or positive inguinal nodes.

Treatment for HIV Population

Unfortunately, the majority of pivotal phase III trials did not allow the inclusion of HIV-positive patients. There are studies suggesting that anal cancer patients with HIV comorbidities have comparable rates of response to HIV-negative patients while being treated with chemoradiation.[89–91] Earlier studies suggested that there was a potential for HIV-positive patients to experience higher toxicities and inferior treatment compliance, which could ultimately alter their outcomes.[92,93] Most studies addressing the application

TABLE 61.4

Phase III Randomized Trials Evaluating the Role of Cisplatin in Anal Cancer

Study (Reference)	Primary site	N	Stage	Treatments	Colostomy-Free Survival (%)[a]	Overall Survival (%)[a]	Grade 3 or 4 Hematological Toxic Effects (%; n/N)[b]	Grade 3 or 4 Nonhematological Toxic Effects (%; n/N)[b]	Late Toxic Effects (%; n/N)[b]
RTOG 98-11[77,78]	Anal canal	682	T2 to T4, N0 to N3	Group 1: EBRT (45–59 Gy) + fluorouracil and mitomycin Group 2: fluorouracil and cisplatin→ EBRT (45–59 Gy) + fluorouracil and cisplatin	Group 1: 71.9% Group 2: 65.0%	Group 1: 78.3% Group 2: 70.7%	Group 1: 61% (199/324) Group 2: 42% (134/320)	Group 1: 74% (240/324) Group 2: 74% (239/320)	Grade 4 small or large bowel: 1% (6/625)
ACCORD[76]	Anal canal	307	≥4cm, <4cm plus N1 to N3	Group 1: fluorouracil and cisplatin →EBRT (45 Gy) + fluorouracil and cisplatin→rest→15 Gy Group 2: fluorouracil and cisplatin →EBRT (45 Gy) + fluorouracil and cisplatin→rest→20–25Gy Group 3: EBRT (45 Gy) + fluorouracil and cisplatin →rest→15 Gy Group 4: EBRT (45 Gy) + fluorouracil and cisplatin →rest→20–25 Gy	Group 1: 69.6% Group 2: 82.4% Group 3: 77.1% Group 4: 72.7%	Group 1 + Group 2: 75% Group 3 + Group 4: 71% Group 1 + Group 3: 71% Group 2 + Group 4: 74%	Group 1 + Group 2: 19% (29/150) Group 3 + Group 4: 12% (19/157)	Group 1 + Group 2 diarrhea: 9% (14/150) Group 3 + Group 4 diarrhea: 12% (18/157)	Grade 4 colostomy: 3% (9/307)
ACTII[75]	Anal canal or anal margin	940	T1 to T4, N– or N+	Group1: EBRT (50.4 Gy) + fluorouracil and cisplatin Group 2: EBRT (50.4 Gy) + fluorouracil and mitomycin Group 3: EBRT (50.4 Gy) + fluorouracil and cisplatin→fluorouracil and cisplatin Group 4: EBRT (50.4 Gy) + fluorouracil and mitomycin→fluorouracil and cisplatin	Group 1: 72% Group 2: 75% Group 3: 75% Group 4: 73%	Group 1: 84% Group 2: 86% Group 3: 83% Group 4: 82%	Mitomycin: 26% (124/472) Cisplatin: 16% (73/468)	Mitomycin: 62% (294/472) Cisplatin: 68% (316/468)	Colostomy: 2% (14/844)

[a] At 5 years in RTOG 98-11 and ACCORD3; at 3 years in ACT II.
[b] (n/N) = affected population/total population.

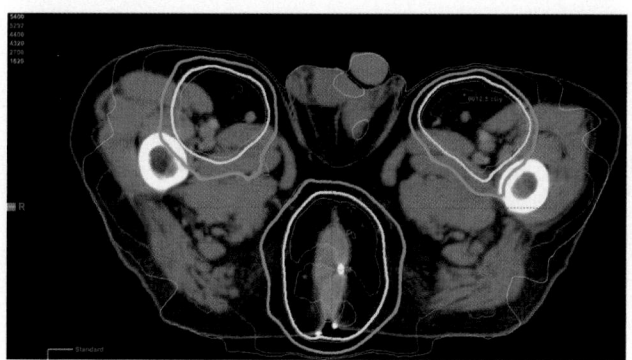

Figure 61.5 An axial CT slice of an intensity-modulated radiation therapy plan of a 56-year-old male with clinical T3N3 squamous cell carcinoma of the anal canal treated with definitive chemoradiotherapy. Note relative organ sparing and *bending* of isodose curves around normal structures including anteriorly based (genitalia) and femora bilaterally while still encompassing the primary target volume of his gross tumor *(red)* as well as local–regional lymph nodes basins (perirectal and inguinal). Note that *colored lines* (isodose curves) represent varying radiation doses.

and outcomes of standard combined regimens for the treatment of anal cancer with HIV-positive patients describe small sample sizes. There are several studies where investigators endeavored to describe the outcomes of treatment modalities for anal carcinomas based on CD4 cell count.[94,95] According to Hoffman et al.,[94] patients with CD4 count ≥200/mm³ tolerated combined therapy (5-FU/MMC/radiation) better (decreased likelihood of toxicity) compared with patients who had CD4 counts <200/mm³. In the Cook County Hospital AIDS Malignancy Project (CHAMP) study, median survival in the HIV-positive versus HIV-negative patients was 34 versus 39 months (p > 0.5). In the HIV-negative population, 22% survived 120 months, whereas no HIV patient survived over 90 months, and time to local recurrence was 20 months shorter in the HIV-positive arm (p < 0.5), with the authors speculating this may imply more aggressive disease. OS based on CD4 count did not differ.[13]

Preliminary safety and efficacy results were presented on the administration of two doses of cetuximab, cisplatin, 5-FU and with radiation therapy (45 to 54 Gy) in immunocompetent (ECOG 3205, n = 28) and HIV-positive (AMC045, n = 45) patients with non-metastatic (stage I to III) squamous cell carcinoma of anal canal.[96] These results showed that the PFS and OS rates in the subsequent 2 years were 80% and 89% for HIV-positive patients with anal cancer, compared to 92% and 93%, respectively for HIV-negative patients. The authors concluded that combined cetuximab, cisplatin, 5FU and radiation combination therapy in HIV positive patients with anal cancer yielded favorable outcomes based on feasibility, safety and efficacy. Further data on these two companion studies are indicated and evaluation within a randomized clinical trial would be required to determine whether patients with anal cancer benefit from an EGFR-targeted therapeutic agent.

HAART is important for bolstering CD4 cell counts in patients with HIV. To analyze the impact of HAART on patients with anal cancer receiving combined modality therapy (CMT), Place and colleagues[95] completed a small study in which patients were divided into two groups: one group received CMT before HAART implementation, and the other group received CMT following HAART therapy. The authors concluded that the patients who received CMT after the advent of HAART had better outcomes, although it was speculated interpretation could be hampered by the fact HAART alone might have altered the immune status of the patients.[95] In a French study, clinical outcomes of anal cancer patients with HIV treated with HAART and chemoradiation were similar to immunocompetent (HIV

negative) controls.[97] More recently, however, a single institution French study[98] reported significantly poorer outcomes for their HIV-positive compared to HIV-negative patients. Local control was achieved in 50% versus 77%, with corresponding 5-year OS rates of 30% versus 84% and DFS rates of 37% versus 75%, respectively. In addition, HIV-infected patients were more likely to be younger and male, although no significant differences were seen in terms of stage or other tumor characteristics. These investigators postulated that the worsened outcomes may have resulted from a higher frequency of advanced disease in their population relative to other studies and a reflection of lack of routine and local screening programs. However, a follow-up study at Case Western University showed that both HIV-positive and HIV-negative patients treated with HAART had comparable treatment efficacy and toxicity rates.[99] Finally, a pooled analysis of 121 patients with anal cancer treated in the HAART era revealed similar complete response and OS rates among HIV-positive and HIV-negative patients, although HIV-positive patients were much more likely to experience local failure (5-year 62% versus 13%; p = 0.008) along with increased acute dermatologic and hematologic toxicities with treatment.[100]

There is a general concern that cancer patients receiving chemotherapy are predisposed to develop immunosuppression, particularly in the setting of an immunodeficiency disease such as HIV, thus complicating the treatment choice and follow-up plan. There is also a potentially greater chance of experiencing adverse treatment reactions that can hinder treatment compliance. Although it is usually not necessary to alter standard management recommendations, HIV-infected patients, especially those with a CD4 count less than 200/μL, should be monitored for an increased risk of toxicity when treated with chemoradiation. Given the previously described ACT I and EORTC trial results, chemotherapy omission is generally not recommended. Thus, factors including pretreatment CD4 cell count, HAART compliance, posttreatment CD4 cell count, and performance status, must come into account in order to formulate a favorable combined treatment modality for anal cancer patients on a personalized, case-by-case basis.

Salvage Therapy for Local Recurrence

APR is recommended for patients who have chronically persistent disease or who develop recurrence. Restaging is performed to evaluate the extent of the disease and determine the presence of extrapelvic metastases. Curative surgery must attain negative margins for oncologic success, and tumor invasion into adjacent organs warrants en bloc resection. Invasion of local structures, including the vagina or prostate, should be approached with an intent of resecting with negative margins. This may involve a multivisceral resection. In instances where there may be close or involved margins at resection, the use of intraoperative radiotherapy or brachytherapy may enhance local control rates. In highly selected cases, there may be a role for low-dose reirradiation with concurrent chemotherapy followed by resection and intraoperative radiotherapy. The majority of published series describing outcomes with salvage surgery have small patient numbers given the relative rarity of such. Five-year survival following resection generally ranges between 30% to 70%, with DFS rates ranging from 30% to 40% (Table 61.5). The most important prognostic factor of survival after resection is margin status, and patients with negative margins (R0) have up to a 75% 5-year OS.[101] Further predictors of a poor OS outcome following surgery include inguinal lymph node involvement, tumor size greater than 5 cm, adjacent organ involvement, male gender, and comorbidities.[102,103] In one of the largest series describing salvage surgery in anal cancer, Correa et al.[104] proposed a scoring system predicting postoperative survival. The three factors included were lymph

---

TABLE 61.5

Results of Salvage Surgery for Residual or Recurrent Anal Cancer

Study	Patient Number	Negative Margin After Surgery (R0)	5-Year Survival Based on Margin Status	Overall 5-Year Survival
Akbari et al., 2004[102]	62	85%	R0 = 38% R½ = 0%	33%
Nilsson et al., 2002[105]	35	91%	NS	52%
Ghouti et al., 2005[106]	36	NS	NS	69.4% (DFS, 31.1%)
Renehan et al., 2005[107]	73	75%	R0 = 61.4% R½ = 0%	40%
Schiller et al., 2007[103]	40	83%	NS	39% (DFS, 30%)
Ferenschild et al., 2005[109]	18	78%	NS	30%
Sunesen et al., 2009[101]	45	78%	R0 = 75% R1 = 40% R2 = 0%	61%
Eeson et al., 2011[110]	51	63%	R0 = 42% R½ = 0%	29%
Lefevre et al., 2012[111]	105	82%	R0 = 69% R1 = 0%	61%

R0, clear margin; R1, microscopic positive margin; R2, grossly positive margin; NS, not stated.

node involvement, involved surgical margins, and perineural and/or lymphovascular invasion.[104] Patients who had none of these factors (i.e., a score of 0), had an estimated 5-year survival of 55%; however, those with scores of 1 to 3 did much worse, with 5-year survival of 0.03% in patients with all of the factors. The utility of such a system is to define a subgroup that would potentially benefit from additional postoperative treatments. The majority of reported series describing salvage surgery indicate that persistence of disease (as opposed to recurrence) following combined modality therapy was the primary reason for such an approach. In patients undergoing salvage surgery, even with R0 resection, patients with disease persistence tend to have worse outcomes, with 5-year overall survival rates ranging from 31% to 33% as compared to 51% to 82% for truly recurrent patients.[102,105] It is been hypothesized that persistent tumors may harbor a more aggressive tumor biology resistant to chemoradiotherapy, leading to worse outcomes. Overall, length of time to recurrence following resection varies from 1 to 50 months.[101,103,106,107]

Salvage resection is associated with significant morbidity in up to 72% of patients, including side effects of delayed perineal wound healing, pelvic abscesses, perineal wound hernia, urinary retention, as well as the development of impotence. Perineal wound healing difficulties are a result of both the large soft tissue defect created in fully excising these tumors as well as potentially impacted by prior radiation therapy. Closure of the wound by primary intention produces suboptimal results if not combined with flap placement. In one series of 22 patients undergoing salvage APR with primary closure, 59% experience perineal wound break down, with 1 requiring reconstructive operation.[107] Commonly used tissue flaps include an omental pedicle flap, a gracilis muscle flap, and the vertical rectus abdominis myocutaneous flap (VRAM). In one series of 95 patients undergoing salvage APR, patients undergoing an omental pedicle flap, as compared to a VRAM flap, had more perineal wound complications and slower healing.[108] In another smaller series, the perineal wound breakdown rate with the use of omental flap reconstruction was 36% versus 0% with a VRAM flap following APR.[110] Finally, a series

of 48 patients who underwent salvage APR reported no delays in wound healing or infectious complications when a VRAM flap was used.[101]

Management of Metastatic Disease

Randomized studies have demonstrated that patients treated with chemoradiation can develop metastatic disease in 10% to 17% of cases.[43,70] Currently, systemic chemotherapy is the treatment of choice for metastatic anal cancer. However, there is little published data in the setting of metastatic disease. Much of the treatment has been extrapolated from more common squamous cell cancers such as head and neck cancer, cervical cancer, etc. A 5-FU/cisplatin combination is recommended by the NCCN[40] guidelines as the first-line regimen to treat metastatic anal SCC.

There are a few small studies that report the benefit of administration of the previous mentioned regimen in patients with metastatic SCCA.[86,112–115] Most notably, according to Faivre et al.,[112] survival at 1 and 5 years were 62.2% and 32.2%, respectively, whereas the median survival was 34.5 months.

MMC and 5-FU may also be considered for first-line therapy[116] for metastatic SCCA. One study showed that patients treated with this regimen ultimately achieved better response that included tumor size shrinkage, pain management, and performance improvement. There are additional combination chemotherapy trials and single agent case reports available that are described briefly in Table 61.6.[117]

Cetuximab has shown favorable outcomes for the treatment of SCC of the head and neck while delivered concurrently with radiation therapy.[125] However, the data supporting the administration of cetuximab in metastatic SCCA is scant. According to a few small studies and case reports, the maximum clinical response achieved was a partial response, with varying ranges of PFS with cetuximab/irinotecan combination therapy.[126–128] Due to the very small sample sizes of these studies, a further evaluation is warranted.

TABLE 61.6

Studies Demonstrating Survival and Response Data on Metastatic Anal Cancer.

Study Type (Reference)	Patient Number	Agent(s)	Response Rate or Clinical Response	Progression-Free Survival in Months
Combination[118]	15	Vincristine/bleomycin/methotrexate	25%	2
Combination[119]	7 (anal only)	Paclitaxel/carboplatin/5-FU	65%	26
Combination[120]	20	Mitomycin-C/Adriamycin/cisplatin/bleomycin	60%	8
Combination[121]	77	5-FU/cisplatin versus Carboplatin/paclitaxel		8 versus 4
Single-agent case report[122]		Carboplatin	Partial	9
Single-agent case report[123]		Semustine	Partial	15
Single-agent case report[124]		Irinotecan	Partial	Not reported

Like other GI cancers, the liver is the primary site of metastasis from anal cancer. Data on the resection of an isolated hepatic lesion are sparse, and currently, a definitive surgical treatment protocol remains largely undefined in the metastatic setting. That said, surgical resection of metastatic disease can be considered when appropriate, based on the extent of disease and performance status. According to Eng et al.,[121] the median PFS and OS of 33 out of 77 patients with metastatic anal SCCA who received curative surgical treatment for their metastatic disease were 16 (95% CI, 9.2 to 22.8) and 53 months (95% CI, 28.3 to 77.6), respectively. Previously, a multicenter study[129] comprising of 52 patients also suggested that a subset of patients might benefit from surgical resection. According to the study, among 27 metastatic squamous cell anal carcinoma patients pretreated with systemic therapy, the median PFS and OS were 9.6 and 22.3 months, respectively, although definitive selection criteria for surgical resection were lacking.

Outcome, benefit, and toxicity analysis on chemoradiation for metastatic anal cancer is limited. A small study[130] (n = 6) from the M.D. Anderson Cancer Center of patients with para-aortic nodal involvement was reported. In this study, all the patients were treated with IMRT with concurrent infusional 5-FU and cisplatin. The results showed that 3-year actuarial local–regional control, distant control, and survival rates were 100%, 56%, and 63%, respectively. In another study, a short course of chemoradiation comprised of 30 Gy with concurrent 5-FU demonstrated good local–regional control (73% at the median follow-up of 16 months) in elderly patients (median age 81 years).[131] Combined chemoradiation may also be used to palliate symptoms related to metastatic disease.

The International Rare Cancer Initiative (IRCI) in collaboration with the NCI has expressed interest specifically focusing on establishing guidelines for metastatic anal cancer squamous carcinoma patients, including diagnostic imaging, staging, surveillance, and survivorship. The first initiative is an international collaboration with the United Kingdom, EORTC, and ECOG/ACRIN on a randomized phase II trial of 5-FU/cisplatin versus carboplatin/paclitaxel in treatment-naïve patients (InterAACT).

TREATMENT OF OTHER SITES AND PATHOLOGIES

Squamous Cell Carcinoma of the Anal Margin

The definition of anal margin tumors has varied over time, ranging from perianal skin to the distal aspect of the anal canal.

A generally accepted, contemporary definition includes the area extending from the anal verge radially 5 cm outward on the perianal skin. The onset of this disease is frequently seen in the 7th and 8th decades of life, with a slight female predominance.[116,132,133] The majority of these tumors are well differentiated, indicating a slow growing nature with the development of distant metastases rare.[116,134,135] The primary drainage is to the inguinal region and regional nodal metastases directly related to tumoral size. Once series[136] describes that tumors less than 2 cm rarely exhibit lymph node metastases, 2 to 5 cm tumors associated with an approximately 23% node positive rate, and in tumors larger than 5 cm, rates as high as 67%. Therefore, it is important that these tumors be approached on an individual basis based on size, location, and histologic characteristics. Tumors whose epicenter is distal to the anal verge may be managed as skin tumors. Potential treatment options for these patients include local excision with or without adjuvant radiation therapy, or radiation with or without chemotherapy. Treatment considerations in these patients must take into account expected morbidity with such approaches. For smaller tumors, wide local excision with a 1-cm margin is often sufficient. However, surgery for larger tumors may require more aggressive removal, which may entail APR; combined modality therapy may be an appropriate alternative in such cases, particularly where the risk of lymph node involvement is high. Therefore, surgery is often reserved for tumors <2 cm in greatest dimension without adverse histologic features and no involvement of the anal sphincter. APR should generally be reserved for patients with recurrent disease following radiation/chemoradiation or recurrence not amenable to local excision. Chapet and colleagues[137] reviewed an experience of 26 patients with tumors of the perianal skin, 5 with involvement of the anal canal. Most were ≤5 cm in diameter. Fourteen received definitive radiation therapy, with or without chemotherapy, and 12 received radiation therapy following initial local excision. Actuarial local control rate was 61%, and with salvage surgical treatment, this increased to 81%, with a 5-year cause-specific survival of 88%. Khanfir et al.[138] reported similar results in a series of 45 patients. Twenty-nine patients underwent local excision prior to radiation therapy. Five-year local–regional control was 78% with 5-year DFS of 86%. Balmucki et al.[139] updated at University of Florida experience with definitive radiotherapy and chemoradiotherapy in 26 patients with SCC of the perianal skin. Two patients developed local recurrence and two developed regional nodal recurrence, resulting in a 10-year cause-specific survival of 92%. Of note, two patients who had clinically node-negative disease who did not receive prophylactic inguinal nodal radiation developed inguinal recurrences.

Anal Canal Adenocarcinoma

Primary adenocarcinoma of the anal canal is an uncommon tumor. In many situations, this will represent growth of a distal rectal adenocarcinoma into the anal canal and is managed as such. In some instances, this disease is believed to arise from glandular epithelium in the anal canal, accounting for less than 5% of all anal malignancies.[140] Occasionally, adenocarcinoma may occur in patients with ulcerative colitis or Crohn's disease who have ileal pouch–anal anastomosis.[141–143] A study from the Rare Cancer Network registry of 82 patients diagnosed with anal adenocarcinoma was analyzed based on the treatment approach. The actuarial local–regional relapse rate at 5 years was 37%, 36%, and 20%, respectively, in the radiation/surgery, combined chemoradiation therapy alone, and APR alone groups. The 5-year OS rate was 29%, 58%, and 21% and 5-year DFS rate 25%, 54%, and 22%, respectively. A multivariate analysis revealed four independent prognostic factors for survival: T stage, N stage, histologic grade, and treatment modality (chemoradiotherapy). The authors concluded that they observed better survival rates after combined chemoradiotherapy and recommended using APR only for salvage treatment.[144] In contrast, a Surveillance, Epidemiology, and End Results (SEER) study evaluated 165 patients with nonmetastatic adenocarcinoma of the anal canal. Of these, 30 patients were treated with an APR only, 42 patients with an APR and radiation, and 93 patients with radiation alone. The 5-year survival for APR only, APR and radiation, and radiation alone was 58%, 50%, and 30%, respectively (p = 0.04). A multivariate analysis confirmed factors accounting for the survival differences included age, nodal stage, and treatment groups. The authors concluded definitive surgical treatment in the form of an APR with or without radiation is associated with improved survival in these patients.[145] An institutional report from the M. D. Anderson Cancer Center analyzed 16 patients with anal adenocarcinoma and compared outcomes with definitive chemoradiotherapy to similarly treated patients with squamous cell tumors.[146] At 5-years, local failure rate was 54% in the adenocarcinoma group compared to 18% for patients with SCC, with corresponding 5-year DFS of 19% versus 77%, respectively, and OS rates of 64% versus 85%. Given this, patients with primary anal adenocarcinoma are generally treated as if they had rectal adenocarcinomas of similar stage, with surgery remaining as a cornerstone therapy and neoadjuvant radiation therapy or combined modality therapy generally implemented in patients with high-risk features (T3 or T4 and/or nodal involvement).

Anal Paget disease is an intraepithelial adenocarcinoma arising from the dermal apocrine sweat glands, most commonly found in females and in older patients.[34] Although progression from perianal Paget disease to invasive disease is seen in approximately 5% of cases, invasive cancers have been reported up to 40% of patients with untreated Paget disease. Association with tubo-ovarian adenocarcinoma was seen in 7% to 24% and GI cancers in 12% to 14%

of cases.[34] Therefore, appropriate imaging and fiber-optic endoscopy studies are recommended to rule out synchronous underlying malignancies.

Melanoma of the Anorectal Region

Anorectal melanoma is a rare disease that accounts for approximately 1% of all malignant melanomas and 0.5% of tumors of anorectal area.[147–149] Symptoms are rather nondescript, with bleeding manifesting as the most common complaint.[150] The gross appearance varies from a small, pigmented lesion to an ulcerated mass. Anal canal melanomas are usually pigmented lesions, but can be amelanotic in as many as 29% of cases.[151] A SEER database review reported a 5-year OS of 2.5%,[152] although some series report up to a 20% survival.[149,150,153] Surgery is the cornerstone of treatment with debate regarding the optimal approach. Traditionally, surgeons adopted a more radical approach utilizing APR with a radical lymph node dissection. However, this approach was associated with significant morbidity without improving OS. Kiran et al.[154] reviewed 109 patients with anorectal melanoma from the SEER database between 1982 and 2002 and reported no significant difference between patients treated by APR or local resection. A retrospective review of 251 patients from the Swedish National Cancer Registry between 1960 and 1999 demonstrated similar findings.[155] A recent systematic review comparing APR to wide local excision in anal melanoma patients reported similar median survivals regardless of treatment approach (21 months for APR, N = 369; 20 months for local excision, N = 324). Similarly, the treatment approach did not significantly impact 5-year survival (14% for APRs, 15% for local excision).[156]

There are some centers that advocate more aggressive treatment for localized disease, arguing for better oncologic outcomes in select subsets. In an older Memorial Sloan Kettering experience, factors associated with long-term survival following APR included female gender, negative lymph nodes, and tumor size less than 2.5 cm, concluding APR may be considered in the subset of patients with these features.[150] A Japanese study that included 79 patients with anorectal melanoma reported 3- and 5-year survival rates of 34.8% and 28.8%, respectively (median survival 22 months), for patients treated by APR.[157] Therefore, the authors of that study recommended local excision for patients with stage 0 melanoma, whereas those with stage 1 cancers or T1 tumors should undergo an APR with lymph node dissection. Ballo et al.[158] reported on 23 patients treated at the M. D. Anderson Cancer Center with sphincter sparing excision and adjuvant radiation therapy using a hypofractionated regimen of 30 Gy delivered in five fractions. Nine patients received systemic therapy. Five-year actuarial overall, disease-free, distant metastases-free, local, and regional nodal control rates were 31%, 37%, 35%, 74%, and 84%, respectively, comparing favorably to varying reports using local excision alone.

SELECTED REFERENCES

The full reference list can be accessed at lwwhealthlibrary.com/oncology.

1. Siegel R, Ma J, Zou Z, et al. Cancer statistics, 2014. *CA Cancer J Clin* 2014;64:9–29.
2. Johnson LG, Madeleine MM, Newcomer LM, et al. Anal cancer incidence and survival: the surveillance, epidemiology, and end results experience, 1973-2000. *Cancer* 2004;101:281–288.
3. Frisch M, Melbye M, Moller H. Trends in incidence of anal cancer in Denmark. *BMJ* 1993;306:419–422.
4. Grulich AE, Poynten IM, Machalek DA, et al. The epidemiology of anal cancer. *Sex Health* 2012;9:504–508.
5. Machalek DA, Poynten M, Jin F, et al. Anal human papillomavirus infection and associated neoplastic lesions in men who have sex with men: a systematic review and meta-analysis. *Lancet Oncol* 2012;13:487–500.
7. Frisch M, Glimelius B, van den Brule AJ, et al. Sexually transmitted infection as a cause of anal cancer. *N Engl J Med* 1997;337:1350–1358.
8. Goodman MT, Shvetsov YB, McDuffie K, et al. Sequential acquisition of human papillomavirus (HPV) infection of the anus and cervix: the Hawaii HPV Cohort Study. *J Infect Dis* 2010;201:1331–1339.
10. Crum-Cianflone NF, Hullsiek KH, Marconi VC, et al. Anal cancers among HIV-infected persons: HAART is not slowing rising incidence. *AIDS* 2010;24:535–543.
11. Shiels MS, Pfeiffer RM, Gail MH, et al. Cancer burden in the HIV-infected population in the United States. *J Natl Cancer Inst* 2011;103:753–762.
12. Shiels MS, Pfeiffer RM, Chaturvedi AK, et al. Impact of the HIV epidemic on the incidence rates of anal cancer in the United States. *J Natl Cancer Inst* 2012;104:1591–1598.

14. Daling JR, Madeleine MM, Johnson LG, et al. Human papillomavirus, smoking, and sexual practices in the etiology of anal cancer. *Cancer* 2004; 101:270–280.

15. Grulich AE, van Leeuwen MT, Falster MO, et al. Incidence of cancers in people with HIV/AIDS compared with immunosuppressed transplant recipients: a meta-analysis. *Lancet* 2007;370:59–67.

21. Fox PA, Nathan M, Francis N, et al. A double-blind, randomized controlled trial of the use of imiquimod cream for the treatment of anal canal high-grade anal intraepithelial neoplasia in HIV-positive MSM on HAART, with long-term follow-up data including the use of open-label imiquimod. *AIDS* 2010;24:2331–2335.

22. Richel O, Wieland U, de Vries HJ, et al. Topical 5-fluorouracil treatment of anal intraepithelial neoplasia in human immunodeficiency virus-positive men. *Br J Dermatol* 2010;163:1301–1307.

23. Singh JC, Kuohung V, Palefsky JM. Efficacy of trichloroacetic acid in the treatment of anal intraepithelial neoplasia in HIV-positive and HIV-negative men who have sex with men. *J Acquir Immune Defic Syndr* 2009;52:474–479.

24. Macaya A, Munoz-Santos C, Balaguer A, et al. Interventions for anal canal intraepithelial neoplasia. *Cochrane Database Syst Rev* 2012;12:CD009244.

25. FUTURE II Study Group. Quadrivalent vaccine against human papillomavirus to prevent high-grade cervical lesions. *N Engl J Med* 2007;356: 1915–1927.

26. Paavonen J, Jenkins D, Bosch FX, et al. Efficacy of a prophylactic adjuvanted bivalent L1 virus-like-particle vaccine against infection with human papillomavirus types 16 and 18 in young women: an interim analysis of a phase III double-blind, randomised controlled trial. *Lancet* 2007;369:2161–2170.

27. Villa LL, Costa RL, Petta CA, et al. High sustained efficacy of a prophylactic quadrivalent human papillomavirus types 6/11/16/18 L1 virus-like particle vaccine through 5 years of follow-up. *Br J Cancer* 2006;95:1459–1466.

28. Palefsky JM, Giuliano AR, Goldstone S, et al. HPV vaccine against anal HPV infection and anal intraepithelial neoplasia. *N Engl J Med* 2011;365: 1576–1585.

30. Scholefield JH, Castle MT, Watson NF. Malignant transformation of high-grade anal intraepithelial neoplasia. *Br J Surg* 2005;92:1133–1136.

31. Glynne-Jones R, Renehan A. Current treatment of anal squamous cell carcinoma. *Hematol Oncol Clin North Am* 2012;26:1315–1350.

34. Wietfeldt ED, Thiele J. Malignancies of the anal margin and perianal skin. *Clin Colon Rectal Surg* 2009;22:127–135.

35. Tehranian S, Treglia G, Krag DN, et al. Sentinel node mapping in anal canal cancer: systematic review and meta-analysis. *J Gastrointestin Liver Dis* 2013;22:321–328.

36. Sveistrup J, Loft A, Berthelsen AK, et al. Positron emission tomography/computed tomography in the staging and treatment of anal cancer. *Int J Radiat Oncol Biol Phys* 2012;83:134–141.

37. Wells IT, Fox BM. PET/CT in anal cancer—is it worth doing? *Clin Radiol* 2012;67:535–540.

40. National Comprehensive Cancer Network (NCCN). NCCN Clinical Practice Guidelines in Oncology - Anal Carcinoma (Version 2.2014). http://www.nccn.org/professionals/physician_gls/pdf/anal.pdf. Accessed June 20, 2014.

41. Touboul E, Schlienger M, Buffat L, et al. Epidermoid carcinoma of the anal canal. Results of curative-intent radiation therapy in a series of 270 patients. *Cancer* 1994;73:1569–1579.

42. Ajani JA, Winter KA, Gunderson LL, et al. Prognostic factors derived from a prospective database dictate clinical biology of anal cancer: the intergroup trial (RTOG 98-11). *Cancer* 2010;116:4007–4013.

43. Bartelink H, Roelofsen F, Eschwege F, et al. Concomitant radiotherapy and chemotherapy is superior to radiotherapy alone in the treatment of locally advanced anal cancer: results of a phase III randomized trial of the European Organization for Research and Treatment of Cancer Radiotherapy and Gastrointestinal Cooperative Groups. *J Clin Oncol* 1997;15:2040–2049.

44. Glynne-Jones R, Sebag-Montefiore D, Adams R, et al. Prognostic factors for recurrence and survival in anal cancer: generating hypotheses from the mature outcomes of the first United Kingdom Coordinating Committee on Cancer Research Anal Cancer Trial (ACT I). *Cancer* 2013;119:748–755.

45. Cummings BJ, Keane TJ, O'Sullivan B, et al. Epidermoid anal cancer: treatment by radiation alone or by radiation and 5-fluorouracil with and without mitomycin C. *Int J Radiat Oncol Biol Phys* 1991;21:1115–1125.

46. Das P, Bhatia S, Eng C, et al. Predictors and patterns of recurrence after definitive chemoradiation for anal cancer. *Int J Radiat Oncol Biol Phys* 2007; 68:794–800.

47. Flam M, John M, Pajak TF, et al. Role of mitomycin in combination with fluorouracil and radiotherapy, and of salvage chemoradiation in the definitive nonsurgical treatment of epidermoid carcinoma of the anal canal: results of a phase III randomized intergroup study. *J Clin Oncol* 1996;14:2527–2539.

50. Lampejo T, Kavanagh D, Clark J, et al. Prognostic biomarkers in squamous cell carcinoma of the anus: a systematic review. *Br J Cancer* 2010;103: 1858–1869.

55. Ajani JA, Wang X, Izzo JG, et al. Molecular biomarkers correlate with disease-free survival in patients with anal canal carcinoma treated with chemoradiation. *Dig Dis Sci* 2010;55:1098–1105.

56. Bonin SR, Pajak TF, Russell AH, et al. Overexpression of p53 protein and outcome of patients treated with chemoradiation for carcinoma of the anal canal: a report of randomized trial RTOG 87-04. Radiation Therapy Oncology Group. *Cancer* 1999;85:1226–1233.

61. Steele SR, Varma MG, Melton GB, et al. Practice parameters for anal squamous neoplasms. *Dis Colon Rectum* 2012;55:735–749.

62. Boman BM, Moertel CG, O'Connell MJ, et al. Carcinoma of the anal canal. A clinical and pathologic study of 188 cases. *Cancer* 1984;54:114–125.

63. Singh R, Nime F, Mittelman A. Malignant epithelial tumors of the anal canal. *Cancer* 1981;48:411–415.

64. Nigro ND, Vaitkevicius VK, Considine B Jr. Combined therapy for cancer of the anal canal: a preliminary report. *Dis Colon Rectum* 1974;17:354–356.

65. Nigro ND, Vaitkevicius VK, Buroker T, et al. Combined therapy for cancer of the anal canal. *Dis Colon Rectum* 1981;24:73–75.

66. Nigro ND, Seydel HG, Considine B, et al. Combined preoperative radiation and chemotherapy for squamous cell carcinoma of the anal canal. *Cancer* 1983;51:1826–1829.

67. Leichman L, Nigro N, Vaitkevicius VK, et al. Cancer of the anal canal. Model for preoperative adjuvant combined modality therapy. *Am J Med* 1985;78:211–215.

70. Epidermoid anal cancer: results from the UKCCCR randomised trial of radiotherapy alone versus radiotherapy, 5-fluorouracil, and mitomycin. UKCCCR Anal Cancer Trial Working Party. UK Co-ordinating Committee on Cancer Research. *Lancet* 1996;348:1049–1054.

71. Northover J, Glynne-Jones R, Sebag-Montefiore D, et al. Chemoradiation for the treatment of epidermoid anal cancer: 13-year follow-up of the first randomised UKCCCR Anal Cancer Trial (ACT I). *Br J Cancer* 2010;102:1123–1128.

72. Meropol NJ, Niedzwiecki D, Shank B, et al. Induction therapy for poor-prognosis anal canal carcinoma: a phase II study of the cancer and Leukemia Group B (CALGB 9281). *J Clin Oncol* 2008;26:3229–3234.

73. Ajani JA, Winter KA, Gunderson LL, et al. Fluorouracil, mitomycin, and radiotherapy vs fluorouracil, cisplatin, and radiotherapy for carcinoma of the anal canal: a randomized controlled trial. *JAMA* 2008;299:1914–1921.

74. Gunderson LL, Winter KA, Ajani JA, et al. Long-term update of US GI intergroup RTOG 98-11 phase III trial for anal carcinoma: survival, relapse, and colostomy failure with concurrent chemoradiation involving fluorouracil/mitomycin versus fluorouracil/cisplatin. *J Clin Oncol* 2012;30:4344–4351.

75. James RD, Glynne-Jones R, Meadows HM, et al. Mitomycin or cisplatin chemoradiation with or without maintenance chemotherapy for treatment of squamous-cell carcinoma of the anus (ACT II): a randomised, phase 3, open-label, 2 × 2 factorial trial. *Lancet Oncol* 2013;14:516–524.

76. Peiffert D, Tournier-Rangeard L, Gerard JP, et al. Induction chemotherapy and dose intensification of the radiation boost in locally advanced anal canal carcinoma: final analysis of the randomized UNICANCER ACCORD 03 trial. *J Clin Oncol* 2012;30:1941–1948.

77. Ajani JA, Winter KA, Gunderson LL, et al. Intergroup RTOG 98-11: a phase III randomized study of 5-fluorouracil (5-FU), mitomycin, and radiotherapy versus 5-fluorouracil, cisplatin and radiotherapy in carcinoma of the anal canal. *J Clin Oncol* 2006;24:180s.

78. Gunderson LL, Winter KA, Ajani JA, et al. Intergroup RTOG 9811 phase III comparison of chemoradiation with 5-FU and mitomycin vs 5-FU and cisplatin for anal canal carcinoma: impact of disease-free, overall and colostomy-free survival (abstract). *Int J Radiat Oncol Biol Phys* 2006;66:S24.

81. Salama JK, Mell LK, Schomas DA, et al. Concurrent chemotherapy and intensity-modulated radiation therapy for anal cancer patients: a multicenter experience. *J Clin Oncol* 2007;25:4581–4586.

82. Pepek JM, Willett CG, Wu QJ, et al. Intensity-modulated radiation therapy for anal malignancies: a preliminary toxicity and disease outcomes analysis. *Int J Radiat Oncol Biol Phys* 2010;78:1413–1419.

83. Ben-Josef E, Moughan J, Ajani JA, et al. Impact of overall treatment time on survival and local control in patients with anal cancer: a pooled data analysis of Radiation Therapy Oncology Group trials 87-04 and 98-11. *J Clin Oncol* 2010;28:5061–5066.

84. Kachnic LA, Tsai HK, Coen JJ, et al. Dose-painted intensity-modulated radiation therapy for anal cancer: a multi-institutional report of acute toxicity and response to therapy. *Int J Radiat Oncol Biol Phys* 2012;82:153–158.

85. Kachnic LA, Winter K, Myerson RJ, et al. RTOG 0529: a phase 2 evaluation of dose-painted intensity modulated radiation therapy in combination with 5-fluorouracil and mitomycin-C for the reduction of acute morbidity in carcinoma of the anal canal. *Int J Radiat Oncol Biol Phys* 2013;86:27–33.

86. Tanum G. Treatment of relapsing anal carcinoma. *Acta Oncol* 1993;32: 33–35.

87. Glynne-Jones R, James R, Meadows H, et al, eds. Optimum time to assess complete clinical response (CR) following chemoradiation (CRT) using mitomycin (MMC) or cisplatin (CisP), with or without maintenance CisP/5FU in squamous cell carcinoma of the anus: Results of ACT II. Paper presented at: 2012 ASCO Annual Meeting; 2012; Chicago, IL.

88. Sebag-Montefiore D, James R, Meadows H, et al. The pattern and timing of disease recurrence in cancer of the anus: mature results from the NCRI ACT II trial. *J Clin Oncol.* 2012;30. 2012 ASCO Annual Meeting.

92. Oehler-Janne C, Seifert B, Lutolf UM, et al. Local tumor control and toxicity in HIV-associated anal carcinoma treated with radiotherapy in the era of antiretroviral therapy. *Radiat Oncol* 2006;1:29.

93. Kauh J, Koshy M, Gunthel C, et al. Management of anal cancer in the HIV-positive population. *Oncology (Williston Park)* 2005;19:1634–1638.

94. Hoffman R, Welton ML, Klencke B, et al. The significance of pretreatment CD4 count on the outcome and treatment tolerance of HIV-positive patients with anal cancer. *Int J Radiat Oncol Biol Phys* 1999;44:127–131.

98. Munoz-Bongrand N, Poghosyan T, Zohar S, et al. Anal carcinoma in HIV-infected patients in the era of antiretroviral therapy: a comparative study. *Dis Colon Rectum* 2011;54:729–735.

99. Seo Y, Kinsella MT, Reynolds HL, et al. Outcomes of chemoradiotherapy with 5-Fluorouracil and mitomycin C for anal cancer in immunocompetent versus immunodeficient patients. *Int J Radiat Oncol Biol Phys* 2009;75:143–149.

100. Oehler-Janne C, Huguet F, Provencher S, et al. HIV-specific differences in outcome of squamous cell carcinoma of the anal canal: a multicentric cohort study of HIV-positive patients receiving highly active antiretroviral therapy. *J Clin Oncol* 2008;26:2550–2557.

102. Akbari RP, Paty PB, Guillem JG, et al. Oncologic outcomes of salvage surgery for epidermoid carcinoma of the anus initially managed with combined modality therapy. *Dis Colon Rectum* 2004;47:1136–1144.

103. Schiller DE, Cummings BJ, Rai S, et al. Outcomes of salvage surgery for squamous cell carcinoma of the anal canal. *Ann Surg Oncol* 2007;14:2780–2789.

104. Correa JH, Castro LS, Kesley R, et al. Salvage abdominoperineal resection for anal cancer following chemoradiation: a proposed scoring system for predicting postoperative survival. *J Surg Oncol* 2013;107:486–492.

108. Lefevre JH, Parc Y, Kerneis S, et al. Abdomino-perineal resection for anal cancer: impact of a vertical rectus abdominis myocutaneous flap on survival, recurrence, morbidity, and wound healing. *Ann Surg* 2009;250:707–711.

110. Eeson G, Foo M, Harrow S, et al. Outcomes of salvage surgery for epidermoid carcinoma of the anus following failed combined modality treatment. *Am J Surg* 2011;201:628–633.

111. Lefevre JH, Corte H, Tiret E, et al. Abdominoperineal resection for squamous cell anal carcinoma: survival and risk factors for recurrence. *Ann Surg Oncol* 2012;19:4186–4192.

112. Faivre C, Rougier P, Ducreux M, et al. [5-fluorouracile and cisplatinum combination chemotherapy for metastatic squamous-cell anal cancer]. *Bull Cancer* 1999;86:861–865.

117. Dewdney A, Rao S. Metastatic squamous cell carcinoma of the anus: time for a shift in the treatment paradigm? *ISRN Oncol* 2012;2012:756591.

119. Hainsworth JD, Burris HA 3rd, Meluch AA, et al. Paclitaxel, carboplatin, and long-term continuous infusion of 5-fluorouracil in the treatment of advanced squamous and other selected carcinomas: results of a Phase II trial. *Cancer* 2001;92:642–649.

121. Eng C, Rogers J, Chang GJ, et al. Choice of chemotherapy in the treatment of metastatic squamous cell carcinoma of the anal canal. *J Clin Oncol* 2012;30:abstr 4060.

125. Bonner JA, Harari PM, Giralt J, et al. Radiotherapy plus cetuximab for squamous-cell carcinoma of the head and neck. *N Engl J Med* 2006;354:567–578.

129. Pawlik TM, Gleisner AL, Bauer TW, et al. Liver-directed surgery for metastatic squamous cell carcinoma to the liver: results of a multi-center analysis. *Ann Surg Oncol* 2007;14:2807–2816.

130. Hodges JC, Das P, Eng C, et al. Intensity-modulated radiation therapy for the treatment of squamous cell anal cancer with para-aortic nodal involvement. *Int J Radiat Oncol Biol Phys* 2009;75:791–794.

131. Charnley N, Choudhury A, Chesser P, et al. Effective treatment of anal cancer in the elderly with low-dose chemoradiotherapy. *Br J Cancer* 2005;92:1221–1225.

132. Cutuli B, Fenton J, Labib A, et al. Anal margin carcinoma: 21 cases treated at the Institut Curie by exclusive conservative radiotherapy. *Radiother Oncol* 1988;11:1–6.

133. Peiffert D, Bey P, Pernot M, et al. Conservative treatment by irradiation of epidermoid carcinomas of the anal margin. *Int J Radiat Oncol Biol Phys* 1997;39:57–66.

134. Chawla AK, Willett CG. Squamous cell carcinoma of the anal canal and anal margin. *Hematol Oncol Clin North Am* 2001;15:321–344.

136. Papillon J, Chassard JL. Respective roles of radiotherapy and surgery in the management of epidermoid carcinoma of the anal margin. Series of 57 patients. *Dis Colon Rectum* 1992;35:422–429.

137. Chapet O, Gerard JP, Mornex F, et al. Prognostic factors of squamous cell carcinoma of the anal margin treated by radiotherapy: the Lyon experience. *Int J Colorectal Dis* 2007;22:191–199.

138. Khanfir K, Ozsahin M, Bieri S, et al. Patterns of failure and outcome in patients with carcinoma of the anal margin. *Ann Surg Oncol* 2008;15:1092–1098.

139. Balamucki CJ, Zlotecki RA, Rout WR, et al. Squamous cell carcinoma of the anal margin: the university of Florida experience. *Am J Clin Oncol* 2011;34:406–410.

144. Belkacemi Y, Berger C, Poortmans P, et al. Management of primary anal canal adenocarcinoma: a large retrospective study from the Rare Cancer Network. *Int J Radiat Oncol Biol Phys* 2003;56:1274–1283.

145. Kounalakis N, Artinyan A, Smith D, et al. Abdominal perineal resection improves survival for nonmetastatic adenocarcinoma of the anal canal. *Ann Surg Oncol* 2009;16:1310–1315.

150. Brady MS, Kavolius JP, Quan SH. Anorectal melanoma. A 64-year experience at Memorial Sloan-Kettering Cancer Center. *Dis Colon Rectum* 1995;38:146–151.

151. Quan SH, White JE, Deddish MR. Malignant melanoma of the anorectum. *Dis Colon Rectum* 1959;2:275–283.

152. Metildi C, McLemore EC, Tran T, et al. Incidence and survival patterns of rare anal canal neoplasms using the surveillance epidemiology and end results registry. *Am Surg* 2013;79:1068–1074.

153. Slingluff CL Jr, Seigler HF. Anorectal melanoma: clinical characteristics and the role of abdominoperineal resection. *Ann Plast Surg* 1992;28:85–88.

154. Kiran R, Rottoli M, Pokala N, et al. Long-term outcomes after local excision and radical surgery for anal melanoma: data from a population database. *Dis Colon Rectum* 2010;53:402.

155. Nilsson PJ, Ragnarsson-Olding BK. Importance of clear resection margins in anorectal malignant melanoma. *Br J Surg* 2010;97:98–103.

156. Kanaan Z, Mulhall A, Mahid S, et al. A systematic review of prognosis and therapy of anal malignant melanoma: a plea for more precise reporting of location and thickness. *Am Surg* 2012;78:28–35.

158. Ballo MT, Gershenwald JE, Zagars GK, et al. Sphincter-sparing local excision and adjuvant radiation for anal-rectal melanoma. *J Clin Oncol* 2002;20:4555–4558.

62 Molecular Biology of Kidney Cancer

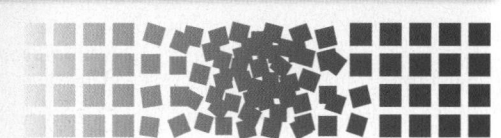

W. Marston Linehan and Laura S. Schmidt

INTRODUCTION

Kidney cancer or renal cell carcinoma (RCC) affects more than 271,000 people annually worldwide, resulting in 116,000 deaths each year.[1] A variety of risk factors, including obesity, hypertension, tobacco smoking, and certain occupational exposures, have been shown to increase one's risk for developing RCC. Our current understanding of the molecular genetics of kidney cancer has come from studies of families with an inherited predisposition to develop renal tumors. Individuals with a family history of RCC have a 2.5-fold greater chance for developing renal cancer during their lifetimes[2] and comprise about 4% of all RCCs.

Kidney cancer is not a single disease, but rather is classified into tumor subtypes based on histology.[3] Over the past 2 decades, studies of families with inherited renal carcinoma enabled the identification of five inherited renal cancer syndromes and their predisposing genes (Table 62.1), which implicate diverse biologic pathways in renal cancer tumorigenesis.[4] The von Hippel-Lindau (VHL) tumor suppressor gene was discovered in 1993.[5] Subsequently, activating mutations were identified in the MET protooncogene in patients with hereditary papillary renal carcinoma (HPRC).[6] More recently, germ-line mutations in the gene for Krebs cycle enzyme fumarate hydratase (FH), responsible for hereditary leiomyomatosis and renal cell carcinoma (HLRCC),[7] and in FLCN, the gene for Birt–Hogg–Dubé (BHD) syndrome, were identified.[8] Germ-line mutations in the genes encoding subunits B, C, and D of another Krebs cycle enzyme, succinate dehydrogenase (SDHB/SDHC/SDHD), have been found in patients with familial renal cancer.[9–11] Discovery of the genes for the inherited forms of renal cancer has enabled the development of diagnostic genetic tests for presymptomatic diagnosis and improved prognosis for at-risk individuals.

VON HIPPEL-LINDAU DISEASE

Von Hippel-Lindau (VHL) disease is an autosomal-dominant inherited multisystem neoplastic disorder that is characterized by clear cell renal tumors, retinal angiomas, central nervous system hemangioblastomas, tumors of the adrenal gland (pheochromocytoma), endolymphatic sac and pancreatic islet cell, and cysts in the pancreas and kidney. VHL occurs in about 1 in 36,000 and develops during the 2nd to 4th decades of life with nearly 70% penetrance by age 60. Bilateral, multifocal renal tumors with clear cell histology develop in 25% to 45% of VHL patients[12] that can have metastatic potential when they reach 3 cm.

Genetics of VHL

Loss of heterozygosity (LOH) on chromosome 3p in clear cell renal tumors suggested the location of a predisposing gene for RCC.[13] Positional cloning in VHL kindreds defined the disease locus to chromosome 3p25-26, leading to the cloning of the VHL gene in 1993.[5] VHL is a tumor suppressor gene in which both copies of VHL must be inactivated for tumor initiation. Germ-line VHL mutations that predispose individuals to VHL encompass the entire mutation spectrum, including large deletions, protein-truncating mutations, and missense mutations that exchange the amino acid in the VHL protein. Over 700 different VHL mutations have been identified in more than 945 VHL families worldwide. Mutations are located throughout the entire gene with the exception of the first 35 residues in the acidic domain.[12] With the development of new methods for detection of deletions, VHL mutation detection rates are approaching 100%.[14,15] VHL subclasses based on the predisposition to develop pheochromocytomas and a high or low risk of RCC have been established with clear genotype–phenotype associations emerging.[16]

Gene Mutated in Renal Cancer Families with Chromosome 3p Translocations

In 1979, Cohen et al.[17] described a family with a constitutional t(3;8)(p14;q24) balanced translocation that cosegregated with bilateral multifocal clear cell renal tumors. Loss of the derivative chromosome carrying the 3p segment and different somatic mutations in the remaining copy of VHL were identified in the tumors from this translocation family. Based on these data, Schmidt et al.[18] proposed a three-step tumorigenesis model in 3p translocation families: (1) inheritance of the constitutional translocation, (2) loss of the derivative chromosome bearing 3p25, and (3) mutation of the remaining copy of VHL, resulting in inactivation of both copies of VHL and predisposing individuals to clear cell RCC. A number of chromosome 3 translocation families have been described.[19,20] Loss of the derivative chromosome concomitant with the somatic mutation of the remaining copy of VHL in these families provides strong evidence for the three-step tumorigenesis model and implicates VHL loss in clear cell RCC that develops in chromosome 3 translocation kindreds.

Gene for Sporadic Clear Cell Kidney Cancer

Somatic mutation of the VHL gene with associated loss of the wild-type allele is found in a high percentage of tumors from patients with clear cell kidney cancer.[21] Nickerson et al.[22] recently identified mutation or methylation of the VHL gene in 92% of clear cell kidney cancers. The VHL gene mutation is not found in papillary, chromophobe, collecting duct, medullary, or other types of kidney cancer.

Function of the VHL Protein

The most well-understood function of the VHL protein pVHL is the substrate recognition site for the hypoxia-inducible factor

TABLE 62.1

Hereditary Renal Cancer Syndromes

Syndrome	Chromosome Location	Predisposing Gene	Histology	Frequency of Gene Mutations	
				Germ Line	Sporadic RCC
Von Hippel-Lindau (VHL) disease	3p25	VHL	Clear cell	100%[14]	92%[22]
Hereditary papillary renal carcinoma type 1 (HPRC)	7q31	MET	Type 1 papillary	100%[6,41,42]	13%[45]
Birt-Hogg-Dubé syndrome (BHD)	17p11.2	FLCN	Chromophobe, hybrid	90%[65]	11%[76]
Hereditary leiomyomatosis and renal cell carcinoma (HLRCC)	1q42–43	FH	Type 2 papillary	93%[105]	TBD
Succinate dehydrogenase (SDH)–associated familial renal cancer	1p35–36 1q23.3 11q23	SDHB SDHC SDHD	Clear cell, chromophobe, oncocytic neoplasm	TBD	TBD
Tuberous sclerosis complex (TSC)	9q34 16p13.3	TSC1 TSC2	Angiomyolipoma, all histologies	80%–90%	TBD

TBD, to be determined.

(HIF)-α family of transcription factors targeting them for ubiquitin-mediated proteasomal degradation (Fig. 62.1).[16] pVHL binds through its α domain to elongin C and forms an E3 ubiquitin ligase complex with elongin B, cullin-2, and Rbx-1. Under normal oxygen conditions, HIF-α becomes hydroxylated on critical prolines by a family of HIF prolyl hydroxylases (PHD) that require α-ketoglutarate, molecular oxygen, ascorbic acid, and iron as cofactors. pVHL then binds to hydroxylated HIF-α through its β domain, targeting HIF-α for ubiquitylation by the E3 ligase complex. Under hypoxic conditions when PHDs are unable to function or when pVHL is mutated—thereby altering its binding to HIF-α or elongin C—HIF-α cannot be recognized by pVHL. HIF-α accumulates and transcriptionally upregulates a number of genes important in blood vessel development (*EPO*, *VEGF*), cell proliferation (*PDGFβ*, *TGFα*), and glucose metabolism

(*GLUT-1*).[16] HIF-α–dependent upregulation of target genes involved in neovascularization provides an explanation for the increased vascularity of central nervous system (CNS) hemangioblastomas and clear cell renal tumors in VHL. Germ-line *VHL* mutations frequently occur in the pVHL binding domains for HIF-α and elongin C.[23] HIF-2α (rather than HIF-1α) stabilization appears to be critical for renal tumor development.[24,25] Additional HIF-independent functions for pVHL have been reported,[12,16,26] including an increase of p53 activity through the suppression of MDM2-mediated ubiquitination and nuclear export,[27] modulation of nuclear factor κ B (NF-κB) through casein kinase 2 binding and inhibitory phosphorylation of NF-κB agonist CARD9,[28] microtubule stabilization,[29] maintenance of primary cilium,[30] and extracellular matrix formation affecting cell–cell adhesion.[31,32]

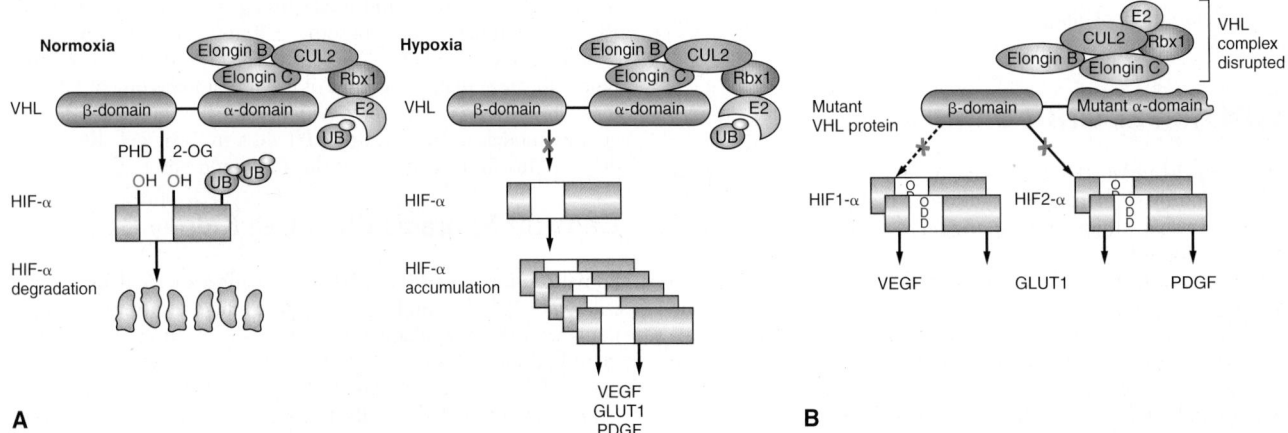

Figure 62.1 The von Hippel-Lindau (VHL) E3 ubiquitin ligase complex targets hypoxia-inducible factor (HIF)-α for ubiquitin-mediated degradation. **(A)** Under normal oxygen conditions, HIF-α is hydroxylated on critical prolines by HIF prolyl hydroxylase (PHD), requiring molecular oxygen, α-ketoglutarate (2-OG), and iron as cosubstrates. The VHL protein (pVHL) can then recognize and bind hydroxylated HIF-α, enabling ubiquitylation by the VHL E3 ligase complex and degradation by the proteasome. Under hypoxic conditions, PHD is unable to function properly, pVHL cannot recognize HIF-α, and HIF-α accumulates, leading to the upregulation of HIF-target genes (*VEGF, GLUT1, PDGF*) that support tumor growth and neovascularization. **(B)** When *VHL* is mutated and pVHL is unable to bind HIF-α, HIF-α stabilization leads to transcriptional upregulation of HIF target genes. (From Linehan WM, Srinivasan R, Schmidt LS. The genetic basis of kidney cancer: a metabolic disease. *Nat Rev Urol* 2010;7:277–285.)

Additional Genes for Clear Cell Kidney Cancer

Studies using next-generation sequencing approaches to identify the genetic basis of clear cell kidney cancer have revealed a considerable number of genetic alterations in chromatin remodeling genes important for the maintenance of chromatin states. Significantly mutated genes identified in sporadic clear cell kidney cancer in addition to *VHL* include *PBRM1*, a subunit of the PBAF SWI/SNF chromatin remodeling complex (41%),[33] histone methyl transferase *SETD2* (4%)[34] histone demethylases *JARID1C* (*KDM5C*; 3%)[35] and *UTX* (*KMD6A*; 3%),[35] and the novel tumor suppressor gene, *BAP1* (15%),[36] a histone deubiquitinase. *BAP1* is also mutated, albeit rarely, in the germ line of inherited clear cell kidney cancer families[37,38] and is associated with poor survival outcome.[39]

HEREDITARY PAPILLARY RENAL CARCINOMA TYPE 1

HPRC is an autosomal-dominant hereditary cancer syndrome in which affected individuals are at risk for the development of multifocal, bilateral papillary type 1 kidney cancer.[40] HPRC develops in the 5th and 6th decades, with age-dependent penetrance estimated at 67% by 60 years of age[41]; however, early-onset HPRC has been described.[42] This rare disorder has been reported in less than 40 kindreds worldwide.[40]

Genetics of Hereditary Papillary Renal Carcinoma: *MET* Proto-oncogene

In 1995, Zbar et al.[43] described 10 families in which multifocal, bilateral papillary renal tumors were inherited in an autosomal-dominant fashion and suggested that these families might represent a hereditary counterpart to sporadic papillary tumors. Schmidt et al.[6] localized the HPRC disease locus to chromosome 7q31.1-34 by genetic linkage analysis. Because the trisomy of chromosome 7 was described as a hallmark feature of papillary renal tumors,[44] a gain-of-function oncogene seemed a likely candidate disease gene; in fact, germ-line missense mutations were identified in the tyrosine-kinase domain of the *MET* protooncogene located at 7q31 in affected HPRC family members.[6] Mutations of the *MET* gene have been detected in 13% of sporadic papillary renal tumors.[6,45] Further studies to determine the role of *MET* and related genes in papillary type 1 kidney cancer are currently under way.

Hereditary Papillary Renal Carcinoma: Functional Consequences of *MET* Mutations

The *MET* protooncogene encodes the hepatocyte growth factor/scatter factor (HGF/SF) receptor tyrosine kinase. Binding of ligand HGF to MET triggers autophosphorylation of critical tyrosines in the intracellular tyrosine kinase domain, subsequent phosphorylation of tyrosines in the multifunctional docking site, and recruitment of a variety of transducers of downstream signaling cascades that regulate cellular programs leading to cell growth, branching morphogenesis, differentiation, and "invasive growth."[46] Although MET overexpression has been demonstrated in a number of epithelial cancers,[47] HPRC was the first cancer syndrome for which germ-line *MET* mutations were identified. The missense *MET* mutations in HPRC are constitutively activating without ligand stimulation, display oncogenic potential in vitro,[48,49] and are predicted by molecular modeling to stabilize active MET kinase.[50] Nonrandom duplication of the chromosome 7 bearing the mutant *MET* allele was demonstrated in papillary renal tumors from HPRC patients[51] and may represent the second step in HPRC tumor pathogenesis. The presence of two copies of mutant *MET* may give kidney cells a proliferative growth advantage and lead to tumor progression.

XP11.2 TRANSLOCATION RENAL CELL CANCER

Xp11.2 translocation renal cell carcinomas, typically presenting with papillary architecture and clear or eosinophilic cytoplasm, are rare tumors in adults (1.6%), but are the cause of 20% to 45% of renal cancers in children and young adults. Translocations involving Xp11.2 and 1q21.2 associated with sporadic papillary renal carcinoma, and first described in a 2-year-old child,[52] generate a fusion between a novel gene, *PRCC*, and the basic helix-loop-helix-leucine zipper transcription factor gene, *TFE3*, a member of the microphthalmia (MiT) family of transcription factors.[53] The encoded fusion protein, PRCC-TFE3, acts as a stronger transcriptional activator than native TFE3, and a loss of the majority of native TFE3 transcripts is observed in these tumors. This deregulation of normal TFE3 transcriptional control caused by the chromosomal translocation may be important to the development of sporadic papillary renal cell carcinoma.[54,55] Xp11.2 translocation renal cell carcinomas involving at least five different TFE3 gene fusions and resulting in deregulation of TFE3 transcription activity have been described, including *NonO-TFE3*, *PSF-TFE3*, *CLTC-TFE3*, and *ASPL-TFE3*.[56] Tsuda et al.[57] have shown that these TFE3 fusion proteins are strong transcriptional activators of the *MET* gene, resulting in inappropriate MET-directed cell proliferation and invasive growth. Given the physiologic consequences of TFE3 fusion protein expression, therapeutic targeting of MET may be an effective treatment for Xp11.2 translocation renal tumors.

The fusion of another member of the MiT family, *TFEB*, with the *Alpha* gene has been described in renal tumors harboring t(6;11)(p21;q13) chromosomal translocation.[58] The first case of renal cancer involving a third MiT family member, MITF, was recently reported, in which an activating *MITF* mutation was identified in the germ-line of family members affected with renal tumors.[59]

BIRT-HOGG-DUBÉ SYNDROME

BHD syndrome is a rare autosomal-dominant inherited cancer syndrome characterized by benign tumors of the hair follicle (fibrofolliculoma), pulmonary cysts and spontaneous pneumothorax, and a sevenfold increased risk for renal cancers.[60–63] Fibrofolliculomas and lung cysts are the most common manifestations (>85%) of BHD patients.[64–66] Renal tumors with variable histologies develop in about 30% of BHD-affected individuals (median age, 48 to 50 years), most frequently chromophobe renal carcinoma and hybrid oncocytic tumors.[64,67] Metastases may develop from BHD renal tumors, but they are uncommon.

Genetics of Birt-Hogg-Dubé Syndrome: Folliculin Gene

A genetic linkage analysis performed in BHD kindreds led to the localization of the disease locus on the short arm of chromosome 17[68,69] and the identification of the BHD gene, *FLCN*.[8] Almost all BHD-associated *FLCN* mutations are predicted to truncate the BHD protein, folliculin, including insertion or deletion, nonsense, and splice-site mutations,[8,64,65,70] but recently, several missense mutations located in conserved amino acid residues and partial gene deletions have been described.[65,71–73] The mutation detection rate in several large BHD cohorts approached 90%, and germ-line mutations were distributed throughout the entire length of the *FLCN* gene with no clear genotype–phenotype correlations.[64,65,74] Vocke et al.[75] identified second "hit" somatic mutations or LOH in 70% of renal tumors from BHD patients, supporting a role for *FLCN* as a tumor suppressor gene that predisposes individuals to renal tumors when both copies are inactivated. *FLCN* mutations have

PRACTICE OF ONCOLOGY

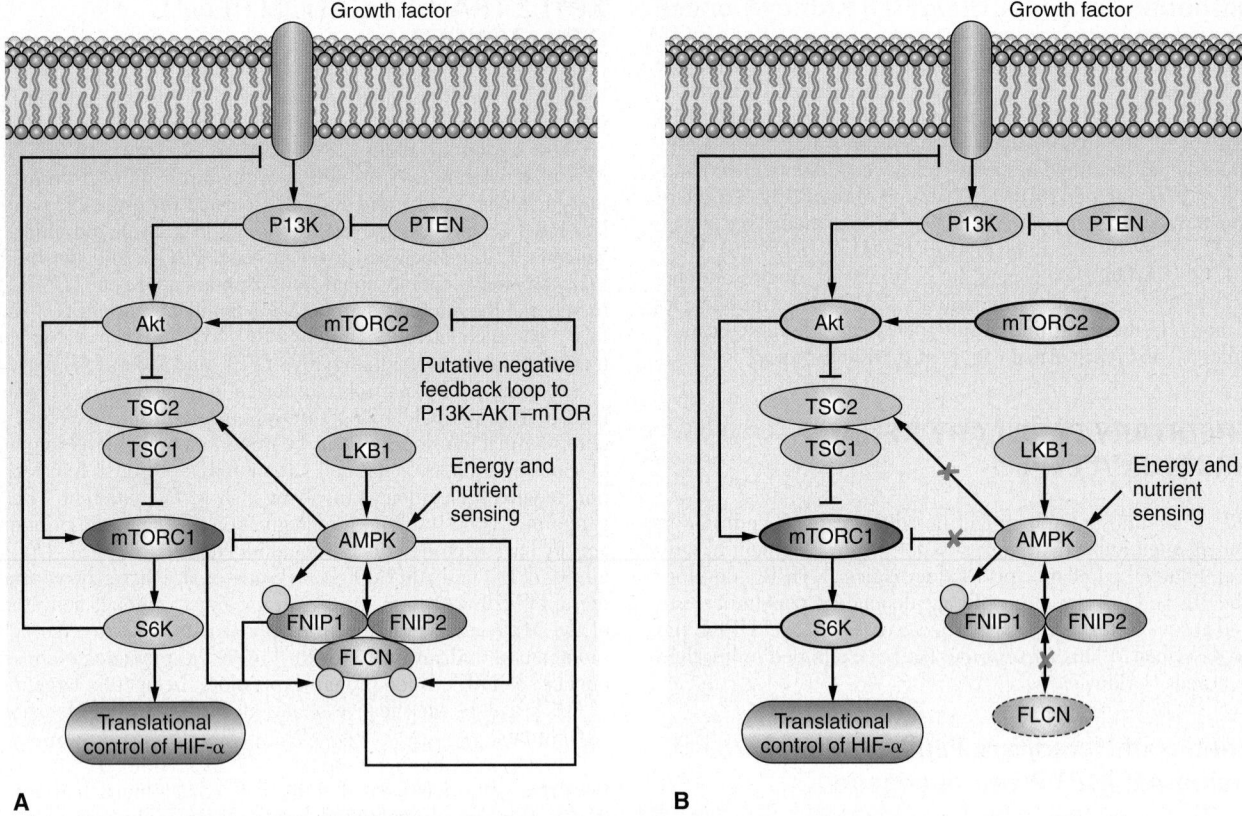

A

B

Figure 62.2 The putative Birt-Hogg-Dubé gene (*FLCN*) pathway. **(A)** *FLCN* binds through FNIP1/2 to AMP–activated protein kinase (AMPK) and may become phosphorylated by AMPK or by a rapamycin-sensitive kinase (i.e., mTOR). **(B)** When *FLCN* is inactivated and, presumably, FLCN protein is absent, mTOR is dysregulated, potentially driving kidney tumor formation in BHD patients. (From Linehan WM, Srinivasan R, Schmidt LS. The genetic basis of kidney cancer: a metabolic disease. *Nat Rev Urol* 2010;7:277–285.)

been found infrequently in chromophobe renal cell carcinomas (11%),[76] and only rarely in other histologic variants of RCC.[77–79]

Function of the Birt-Hogg-Dubé Protein: Folliculin

The *FLCN* gene encodes a novel protein, folliculin (FLCN), with no characteristic functional domains. Baba et al.[80] identified a novel FLCN-interacting protein, FNIP1, and showed that FNIP1 interacts with the γ subunit of 5' adenosine monophosphate (AMP)–activated protein kinase (AMPK), an energy sensor in cells that negatively regulates mammalian target of rapamycin (mTOR), the master switch for protein translation and cell proliferation, through TSC1/2.[81,82] A second folliculin interacting protein, FNIP2, was subsequently identified that displayed similar biochemical properties to FNIP1.[83,84] FLCN, through FNIP1/2, may play a role in the regulation of the AMPK-TSC1/2–mTOR signaling pathway (Fig. 62.2). Published data from in vivo models and BHD renal tumors, supporting mTOR activation[85,86] as well as mTOR inhibition[87–89] as a consequence of *FLCN* inactivation, has led to the hypothesis that the mechanism by which FLCN interacts with and modulates mTOR is context dependent.[89]

Additional functional roles for FLCN in transforming growth factor β (TGF-β) signaling,[90,91] modulation of HIF-α and its target genes,[92] ciliogenesis,[93] peroxisome proliferator-activated receptor γ coactivator 1α (PGC-1α) regulation and mitochondrial biogenesis,[94,95] cell–cell adhesion,[96,97] exit from embryonic stem cell pluripotency,[98] and regulation of lysosome function through cytoplasmic sequestration of the transcription factors TFE3[99] and TFEB[100] have been reported. The resolution of C-terminal FLCN crystal structure has demonstrated structural homology to the

DENN domain, which has guanine exchange factor (GEF) activity toward RabGTPases.[101] Two recent reports have shown FLCN/FNIP1/FNIP2 interaction with RagGTPases and proposed a role of this complex in amino acid sensing for mTOR activation.[100,102] In addition to a role for FNIP1 in facilitating FLCN interaction with AMPK, *Fnip1* knockout mice displayed a defect in pro- to preB cell differentiation demonstrating a unique requirement for the FLCN-FNIP1 complex in B-cell development.[103]

HEREDITARY LEIOMYOMATOSIS AND RENAL CELL CARCINOMA

HLRCC is an autosomal-dominant inherited disorder that predisposes individuals to the development of skin and uterine leiomyomas and an aggressive form of type 2 papillary renal carcinoma. Fewer than 150 HLRCC families have been reported worldwide.[104,105] Renal tumors, which are often unilateral and solitary,[104,106] may develop with early age of onset in 15% to 25% of affected individuals[104,105] and can be aggressive, metastasize, and cause death within 5 years of diagnosis.

Genetics of Hereditary Leiomyomatosis and Renal Cell Carcinoma: Fumarate Hydratase Gene

A genetic linkage analysis localized the HLRCC disease locus to chromosome 1q42-43,[107] but an association with renal cancer was not appreciated until Launonen et al.[108] demonstrated a linkage to chromosome 1q in two Finnish multiple cutaneous and uterine leiomyomata (MCUL) kindreds with solitary, highly aggressive papillary type 2 renal tumors. The disorder was renamed *hereditary leiomyomatosis and renal cell carcinoma* and the locus was subsequently mapped to a 1.6-Mb region of 1q42. Germ-line mutations were identified in the fumarate hydratase (*FH*) gene, a Krebs cycle enzyme that converts fumarate to malate in HLRCC-affected family members.[7] *FH* mutations in HLRCC include missense, frameshift, nonsense, and splice-site mutations, as well as partial and complete gene deletions.[104,106,109,110] Missense mutations are the most common (57%) and occur mainly at evolutionarily conserved residues.[106,109,110] Mutations are found throughout the entire length of the *FH* gene excluding exon 1, which encodes a mitochondrial signal peptide, and no clear genotype–phenotype associations have been reported.[104] *FH* acts as a classic tumor suppressor gene with a loss or somatic mutation of the wild-type *FH* allele at high frequency in renal tumors and skin and uterine leiomyomata.[7] *FH* mutations are rarely detected in sporadic uterine and skin leiomyomata or sporadic RCCs.[111]

Functional Consequences of Fumarate Hydratase Mutations

FH mutations reduce FH activity by 20% to 80%[7,109,112] in lymphoblastoid cell lines from HLRCC patients. HLRCC-associated missense mutations significantly lowered FH activity compared to truncating mutations,[109] suggesting that mutant FH monomers might act in a dominant negative manner to alter proper conformation of FH tetramers. Loss of FH activity in HLRCC leads to accumulation of fumarate and, to a lesser extent, succinate, due to a block in the Krebs cycle.[113,114] Pollard et al.[113] have confirmed that the accumulation of fumarate and succinate resulted in the elevation of HIF-1α and HIF-target genes (*VEGF*, *BNIP*), and increased microvessel density[115] in HLRCC-associated uterine fibroids. Isaacs et al.[114] showed that stabilization of HIF-1α resulted from the competitive inhibition of the HIF PHD cosubstrate, α-ketoglutarate, by fumarate accumulation, leading to the abrogation of PHD function and release of HIF-1α from proteasomal degradation. This pseudohypoxic drive, resulting from loss of FH activity, HIF-1α stabilization, and upregulation of HIF-inducible genes, contributes to the aggressive nature of HLRCC-associated renal tumors (Fig. 62.3). Xiao et al.[116] have demonstrated that accumulated fumarate and succinate can act as competitive inhibitors of multiple α-ketoglutarate–dependent dioxygenases, including histone demethylases and the ten-eleven translocation (TET) family of 5-methylcytosine hydroxylases leading to more global alterations in histone and DNA methylation. Additionally, Sudarshan et al.[117] showed that *FH* mutations in an HLRCC-derived cell line led to glucose-mediated generation of

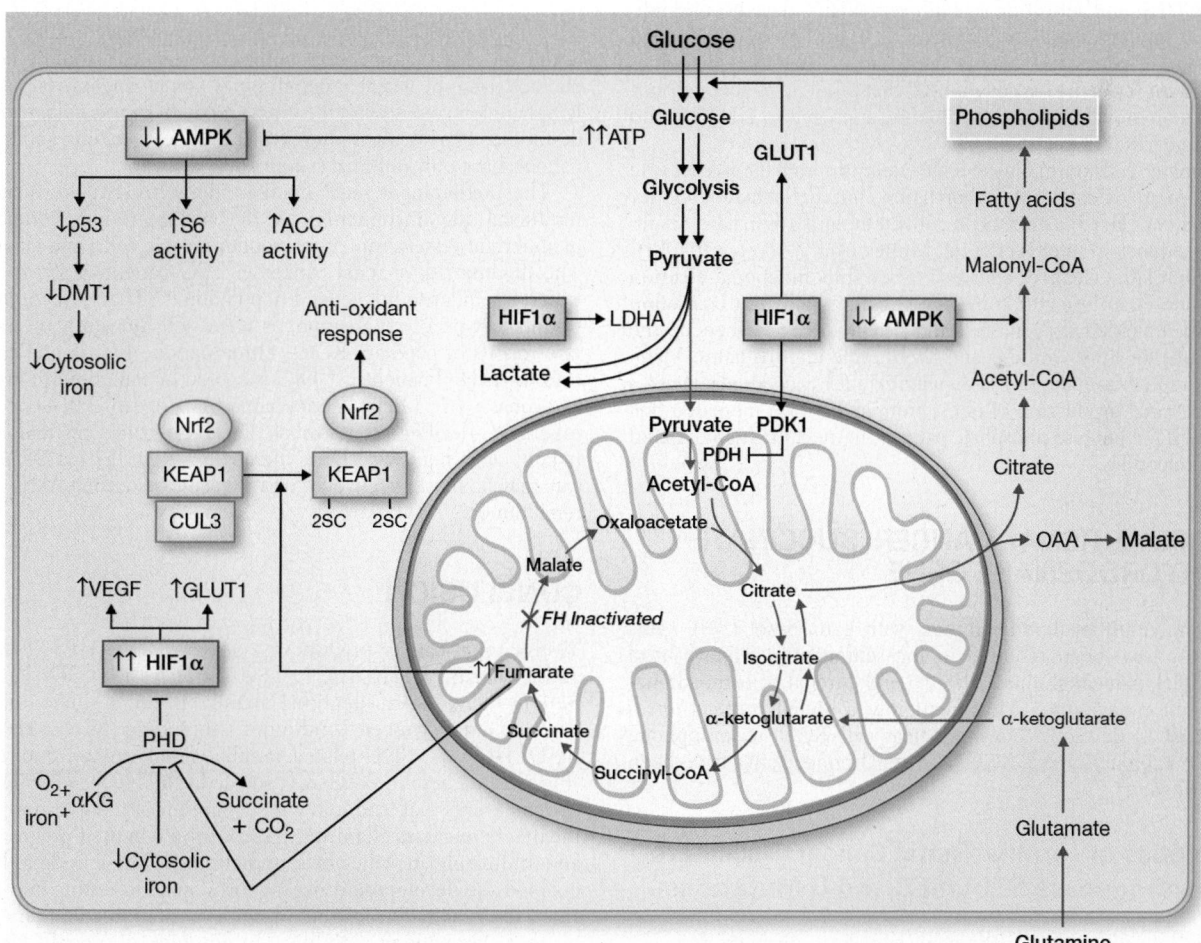

Figure 62.3 Fumarate hydratase (FH)–deficient kidney cancer, an aggressive form of type 2 papillary kidney cancer, is found in patients affected with the hereditary cancer syndrome, HLRCC. FH-deficient kidney cancer is characterized by a metabolic shift to aerobic glycolysis. Mitochondrial function is impaired by a decrease in FH function, and the cell depends on aerobic glycolysis for adenosine triphosphate (ATP) production needed for rapid growth. The increased ATP leads to decreased activation of AMPK, which results in increased mTOR/phosphoS6 activity and increased Acetyl CoA carboxylase (ACC)/fatty acid production. Increased fumarate, a result of decreased fumarate hydratase activity, inhibits HIF PHD, resulting in increased HIF1α levels. The increased fumarate also inhibits KEAP1 activity, resulting in increased Nrf2 transcriptional activity that is critical for the survival of these cells, which are characterized by high oxidative stress. (From Linehan WM, Rouault TA. Molecular pathways: fumarate hydratase-deficient kidney cancer: targeting the Warburg effect in cancer. *Clin Cancer Res* 2013;19:3345–3352.)

reactive oxygen species (ROS) and ROS-dependent HIF-1α stabilization, supporting an alternate mechanism by which pseudohypoxic drive could support renal tumorigenesis in HLRCC. Further, Sullivan et al.[118] determined that the increase in ROS was due to the succination of antioxidant glutathione by accumulated fumarate (see the following) to produce the oncometabolite succinated glutathione, an alternate substrate to glutathione reductase, resulting in a decrease in NADPH levels, enhanced ROS and HIF1-α activation.

Recent in vivo and in vitro evidence supports a role for fumarate accumulation in activation of the nuclear factor (erythroid-derived 2)–like 2 (Nrf2)-mediated antioxidant signaling pathway.[119] Kelch-like erythroid-derived Cap-n-Collar homology (ECH)–associated protein 1 (KEAP1), an electrophile sensor and substrate recognition site for cullin-3 (CUL3)–based E3 ubiquitin ligase, binds to Nrf transcription factors under low electrophile conditions facilitating interactions with CUL3 for ubiquitin-mediated degradation. However, intracellular accumulated fumarate in FH-deficient kidney cancer (HLRCC) reacts with exposed cysteines on the KEAP1 protein (*succination*), resulting in a conformational change that inhibits KEAP1–Nrf2 binding (see Fig. 62.3). Consequently Nrf2 becomes available for transcriptional activation of its target genes that are regulated through antioxidant response elements (ARE) in their promoters.[120,121] In support of this model, somatic inactivating mutations in *KEAP1* and *CUL3*, and activating mutations in *NRF2*, have been identified in sporadic papillary RCC type 2.[122] Inhibiting upregulated Nrf2-target genes (i.e., heme oxygenase1 [HMOX1], which is important for heme oxygenation)[123] that promote cancer cell survival may provide a novel therapeutic approach to HLRCC and sporadic PRCC2 treatment.

Finally, cells normally generate energy through the Krebs cycle coupled to oxidative phosphorylation, but FH-deficient kidney cancer cells lack the enzyme to convert fumarate to malate, resulting in a block in the Krebs cycle. Mullen et al.[124] showed that FH-deficient kidney cancer cells that lack a fully functional electron transport chain use glutamine-dependent reductive carboxylation via isocitrate dehydrogenases 1 and 2 to produce acetyl coenzyme A (CoA) for lipid synthesis and Krebs cycle intermediates. Metabolic reprogramming of FH-deficient kidney cancer cells enables the elevated production of ribose from glucose via increased flux through the pentose phosphate pathway to meet the high demand for nucleotides.[125]

FAMILIAL RENAL CANCER: SUCCINATE DEHYDROGENASE GENE

Bilateral multifocal renal tumors with early onset (<40 years of age) have been reported in the setting of hereditary head and neck paragangliomas (HPGL) and adrenal or extra-adrenal pheochromocytomas.[9] Most frequently, a unique form of oncocytic RCC develops; however, clear cell RCC, chromophobe RCC, papillary type 2 RCC, and renal oncocytoma have been described.[126–128]

Genetics of Familial Renal Cancer: Succinate Dehydrogenase Subunit B and D Mutations

Germ-line mutations in the gene encoding succinate dehydrogenase subunit D (SDHD) were initially associated with HPGL

and later with familial and sporadic pheochromocytomas.[129,130] Subsequently, inactivating mutations in *SDHB* were found in kindreds with familial pheochromocytoma only and with HPGL, and in one case of sporadic pheochromocytoma.[131] Later, early onset clear cell RCC was diagnosed in two individuals with HPGL and germ-line *SDHB* mutations.[9] Renal carcinomas with various histologies have been reported in patients with germline missense, frameshift, and nonsense mutations in *SDHB, C,* and *D*.[10,11,126–128,132]

Functional Consequences of Succinate Dehydrogenase Subunit B and D Mutations

Mutational inactivation of the *SDH* gene results in reduced SDH enzyme activity and the accumulation of succinate in renal tumors. In a mechanism similar to *FH* mutations in HLRCC (see Fig. 62.3), the accumulation of succinate serves to competitively inhibit α-ketoglutarate and block PHD activity.[113,114] In the absence of PHD, HIF-α accumulates and drives transcriptional activation of HIF-α target genes that support tumor neovascularization, growth, and invasion.

TUBEROUS SCLEROSIS COMPLEX

The tuberous sclerosis complex (TSC) is a multisystem, autosomal-dominant disorder affecting both children and adults and is characterized by facial angiofibromas, renal angiomyolipomas, lymphangiomyomatosis of the lung, and disabling neurologic manifestations. The disease is phenotypically heterogeneous, and many patients have only minimal symptoms of disease.[133]

The predominant renal manifestations in TSC are bilateral multifocal angiomyolipomas (AML), benign tumors composed of abnormal vessels, immature smooth muscle cells, and fat cells. The lifetime risk of renal cancer in TSC patients is 2% to 3%, which is similar to the general population.[133] The most common histologic type of renal tumor is clear cell; however, there are rare reports of papillary RCCs, chromophobe RCCs, and oncocytoma in TSC patients.[133] TSC is caused by mutations in one of two genes—*TSC1* that encodes hamartin[134] or *TSC2* that encodes tuberin[135]—leading to a loss of TSC1/2-negative regulation of mTOR signaling.[81,82,136] Drug therapy targeting the mTOR pathway may be most effective for treating TSC-associated AMLs and renal tumors.[137]

CONCLUSION

Twelve renal cancer predisposing genes—*VHL, MET, FLCN, TFE3, TFEB, MITF, TSC1, TSC2, PTEN, FH, SDHB,* and *SDHD*—have been identified mainly through studies of inherited renal cancer syndromes, including VHL, HPRC, BHD, HLRCC, SDH-related familial renal cancer, and TSC (Fig. 62.4). These studies have provided valuable insight into the genetic events that lead to the development of renal tumors and the biochemical mechanisms that contribute to their progression and, ultimately, in some cases, to metastasis. These findings have enabled the development of diagnostic genetic testing and provided the foundation for the development of targeted therapeutic agents for patients with the common form of sporadic kidney cancer.

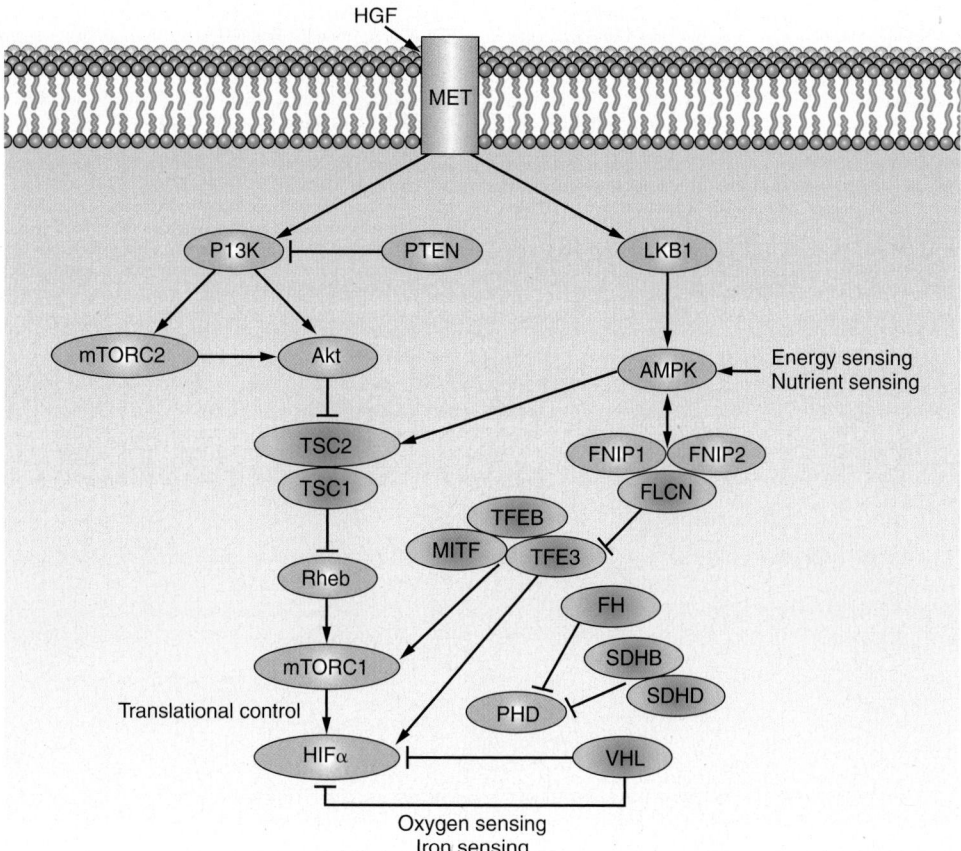

Figure 62.4 The genetic basis of kidney cancer. Twelve renal cancer predisposing genes—*VHL, MET, FLCN, TFE3, TFEB, MITF, TSC1, TSC2, PTEN, FH, SDHB,* and *SDHD*— have been identified mainly through studies of inherited kidney cancer syndromes. These genes interact through common oxygen, iron, nutrient, and energy sensing pathways and demonstrate that kidney cancer is fundamentally a metabolic disease. Our understanding of the molecular mechanisms by which these genes interact in these pathways has enabled the development of targeted therapeutic agents to benefit kidney cancer patients. (From Linehan WM, Ricketts CJ. The metabolic basis of kidney cancer. *Semin Cancer Biol* 2013;23:46–55.)

SELECTED REFERENCES

The full reference list can be accessed at lwwhealthlibrary.com/oncology.

4. Linehan WM, Srinivasan R, Schmidt LS. The genetic basis of kidney cancer: a metabolic disease. *Nat Rev Urol* 2010;7:277–285.
5. Latif F, Tory K, Gnarra JR, et al. Identification of the von Hippel-Lindau disease tumor suppressor gene. *Science* 1993;260:1317–1320.
6. Schmidt LS, Duh FM, Chen F, et al. Germline and somatic mutations in the tyrosine kinase domain of the MET proto-oncogene in papillary renal carcinomas. *Nat Genet* 1997;16:68–73.
7. Tomlinson IP, Alam NA, Rowan AJ, et al. Germline mutations in FH predispose to dominantly inherited uterine fibroids, skin leiomyomata and papillary renal cell cancer. *Nat Genet* 2002;30:406–410.
8. Nickerson ML, Warren MB, Toro JR, et al. Mutations in a novel gene lead to kidney tumors, lung wall defects, and benign tumors of the hair follicle in patients with the Birt-Hogg-Dubé syndrome. *Cancer Cell* 2002;2:157–164.
9. Vanharanta S, Buchta M, McWhinney SR, et al. Early-onset renal cell carcinoma as a novel extraparaganglial component of SDHB-associated heritable paraganglioma. *Am J Hum Genet* 2004;74:153–159.
10. Ricketts CJ, Shuch B, Vocke CD, et al. Succinate dehydrogenase kidney cancer: an aggressive example of the Warburg effect in cancer. *J Urol* 2012;188:2063–2071.
11. Malinoc A, Sullivan M, Wiech T, et al. Biallelic inactivation of the SDHC gene in renal carcinoma associated with paraganglioma syndrome type 3. *Endocr Relat Cancer* 2012;19:283–290.
16. Kaelin WG Jr. The von Hippel-Lindau tumour suppressor protein: O2 sensing and cancer. *Nat Rev Cancer* 2008;8:865–873.
17. Cohen AJ, Li FP, Berg S, et al. Hereditary renal-cell carcinoma associated with a chromosomal translocation. *N Engl J Med* 1979;301:592–595.

23. Stebbins CE, Kaelin WG, Pavletich NP. Structure of the VHL-ElonginC-ElonginB complex: implications for VHL tumor suppressor function. *Science* 1999;284:455–461.
26. Li M, Kim WY. Two sides to every story: the HIF-dependent and HIF-independent functions of pVHL. *J Cell Mol Med* 2011;15:187–195.
33. Varela I, Tarpey P, Raine K, et al. Exome sequencing identifies frequent mutation of the SWI/SNF complex gene PBRM1 in renal carcinoma. *Nature* 2011;469:539–542.
35. Dalgliesh GL, Furge K, Greenman C, et al. Systematic sequencing of renal carcinoma reveals inactivation of histone modifying genes. *Nature* 2010;463:360–363.
37. Farley MN, Schmidt LS, Mester JL, et al. A novel germline mutation in BAP1 predisposes to familial clear-cell renal cell carcinoma. *Mol Cancer Res* 2013;11:1061–1071.
48. Jeffers M, Schmidt LS, Nakaigawa N, et al. Activating mutations for the met tyrosine kinase receptor in human cancer. *Proc Natl Acad Sci U S A* 1997;94:11445–11450.
53. Sidhar SK, Clark J, Gill S, et al. The t(X;1)(p11.2;q21.2) translocation in papillary renal cell carcinoma fuses a novel gene PRCC to the TFE3 transcription factor gene. *Hum Mol Genet* 1996;5:1333–1338.
56. Armah HB, Parwani AV. Xp11.2 translocation renal cell carcinoma. *Arch Pathol Lab Med* 2010;134:124–129.
57. Tsuda M, Davis IJ, Argani P, et al. TFE3 fusions activate MET signaling by transcriptional up-regulation, defining another class of tumors as candidates for therapeutic MET inhibition. *Cancer Res* 2007;67:919–929.
59. Bertolotto C, Lesueur F, Giuliano S, et al. A SUMOylation-defective MITF germline mutation predisposes to melanoma and renal carcinoma. *Nature* 2011;480:94–98.
62. Zbar B, Alvord WG, Glenn GM, et al. Risk of renal and colonic neoplasms and spontaneous pneumothorax in the Birt-Hogg-Dubé syndrome. *Cancer Epidemiol Biomarkers Prev* 2002;11:393–400.

PRACTICE OF ONCOLOGY

63. Menko FH, van Steensel MA, Giraud S, et al. Birt-Hogg-Dubé syndrome: diagnosis and management. *Lancet Oncol* 2009;10:1199–1206.

80. Baba M, Hong SB, Sharma N, et al. Folliculin encoded by the BHD gene interacts with a binding protein, FNIP1, and AMPK, and is involved in AMPK and mTOR signaling. *Proc Natl Acad Sci U S A* 2006;103: 15552–15557.

109. Alam NA, Rowan AJ, Wortham NC, et al. Genetic and functional analyses of FH mutations in multiple cutaneous and uterine leiomyomatosis, hereditary leiomyomatosis and renal cancer, and fumarate hydratase deficiency. *Hum Mol Genet* 2003;12:1241–1252.

114. Isaacs JS, Jung YJ, Mole DR, et al. HIF overexpression correlates with biallelic loss of fumarate hydratase in renal cancer: novel role of fumarate in regulation of HIF stability. *Cancer Cell* 2005;8:143–153.

120. Ooi A, Wong JC, Petillo D, et al. An antioxidant response phenotype shared between hereditary and sporadic type 2 papillary renal cell carcinoma. *Cancer Cell* 2011;20:511–523.

122. Ooi A, Dykema K, Ansari A, et al. CUL3 and NRF2 mutations confer an NRF2 activation phenotype in a sporadic form of papillary renal cell carcinoma. *Cancer Res* 2013;73:2044–2051.

133. Crino PB, Nathanson KL, Henske EP. The tuberous sclerosis complex. *N Engl J Med* 2006;355:1345–1356.

134. van Slegtenhorst M, de Hoogt R, Hermans C, et al. Identification of the tuberous sclerosis gene TSC1 on chromosome 9q34. *Science* 1997;277:805–808.

135. The European Chromosome 16 Tuberous Sclerosis Consortium. Identification and characterization of the tuberous sclerosis gene on chromosome 16. *Cell* 1993;75:1305–1315.

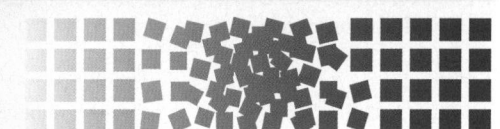

63 Cancer of the Kidney

Brian R. Lane, Daniel J. Canter, Brian I. Rini, and Robert G. Uzzo

INTRODUCTION

Cancer of the kidney is neither common enough to cause a large percentage of cancer-related deaths nor uncommon enough to be considered an "orphan" malignancy. In that context, the progress made in uncovering the genetic basis of renal cell carcinoma (RCC), its molecular pathways, and the approval of novel therapies to perturb those pathways over the last decade is indeed remarkable. Over a relatively short time, the management options for localized kidney cancer have evolved from near universal acceptance of open radical nephrectomy (RN) to the routine use of minimally invasive partial nephrectomy (PN), thermal ablation (TA), and active surveillance (AS). Concurrently, metastatic RCC has progressed from marginally treatable, with a low incidence of spontaneous and/or immune-induced durable regression, to overall response rates (complete response + partial response + stable disease) of >50% and a near doubling of cancer-specific survival. Looking forward, it is anticipated that kidney cancer will soon become a chronic disorder as we better understand the biologic heterogeneity and systemic therapies for RCC. Herein, we review the current and rapid evolution in our understanding and management of cancer of the kidney.

EPIDEMIOLOGY, DEMOGRAPHICS, AND RISK FACTORS

Kidney cancer accounts for approximately 2% of malignancies worldwide with about 300,000 cases diagnosed per year and 100,000 deaths.[1] Data suggest the incidence of RCC is more common in industrialized countries, which may be related to increased incidental detection. In the United States, tumors of the kidney account for 3% to 4% of all cancer diagnoses with an estimated 65,000 cases and 14,000 deaths.[2] There is a male-to-female predominance with the lifetime risk of a RCC diagnosis of 1:69 in men and 1:116 in women.[3] While kidney cancer remains predominantly a tumor of the elderly (median age at diagnosis of 65 years), the number of new kidney cancer cases appears to be rising in younger individuals.[2] This may be explained by either the increasing use of noninvasive imaging in younger patients[4–6] or perhaps true biologic differences in the disease.[7] Similarly, racial differences have also been described with increased rates and decreased survival noted in African Americans and improved survival in Asian populations.[8] Whether this represents differences in health-care access or disease biology is unclear.

The most commonly cited risk factors for the development of RCC include smoking, obesity, and hypertension.[9] The data regarding smoking as a risk factor for RCC appear strong. In a meta-analysis evaluating 19 case control studies and 5 cohort studies, Hunt et al.[10] found a 38% increased risk in current and former smokers, noting not only a dose-risk relationship, but also an abatement of risk with smoking cessation >10 years. The relationship between obesity and RCC is less well studied, although the epidemiology seems to point to a causal association. In a quantitative review of the literature between 1966 and 1998, Renehan et al.[11]

calculated a relative risk of 1.07 per increase in unit body mass index and concluded that nearly a third of RCC cases may be attributable to obesity. Data suggesting a stronger association of obesity and RCC in women lead to hypotheses that the relationship may be due to dysregulation of sex hormones, insulin metabolism, or the immune system.[3] The relationship between hypertension and RCC is based largely upon retrospective and/or population-based epidemiologic data. In an analysis of 13 case controlled studies, Grossman et al.[12] noted hypertensive patients exhibited a pooled odds ratio of 1.75 of having RCC. While there may be a relationship between severity and duration of hypertension, given the limits of the data, if such an association exists it is difficult to ascertain.[3] Finally, exposure to chronic diuretics,[13] nonsteroidal analgesics,[14] and tricholorethylene, a cleaning agent, have all been associated with an increased risk of RCC.[3]

While screening for kidney and other potentially lethal diseases is enticing, a risk benefit analysis argues against it given the low overall prevalence of RCC in the general population. One large study, in which over 200,000 adults were screened for abdominal malignancy with ultrasound, found only 192 cases of RCC (0.09%).[15] Screening has, therefore, been proposed in target populations, including individuals with familial RCC syndromes such as von Hippel-Lindau disease (VHL) and those on hemodialysis, who are known to be more likely to be diagnosed with RCC. In patients on dialysis, while there appears to be an increased incidence of RCC in the native kidneys or even in a transplanted allograft, this may be due to their medical follow-up. Indeed, most patients with end-stage renal disease will have been "screened" during the evaluation and management of their renal failure/allograph, making the reasons for this association difficult to dissect. This is distinctively different than an emerging population of patients with increased genetic risk for cancer, but whose kidneys have not yet been imaged. In families who carry known mutations in the genes responsible for VHL, hereditary papillary RCC, hereditary leiomyoma RCC, Birt-Hogg-Dubé syndrome (BHD), potentially tuberous sclerosis, and/or autosomal dominant polycystic kidney disease, a renal ultrasound may be an inexpensive, low-risk, and judicious means of targeted screening. The initial timing, frequency, and effectiveness of screening in these at-risk populations are not yet established.

PATHOLOGY OF RENAL CELL CARCINOMA

Pathologic classifications assist in diagnosis and prognosis, and inform therapy. Most pathologic classifications emphasize a tumor's morphology and histology—although, increasingly they are incorporating genetic characteristics.[16] There are 10 tumor subtypes in the current World Health Organization classification system for RCC (Table 63.1). The major histologic variants include clear cell, papillary, chromophobe, and collecting duct tumors, which account for 90% to 95% of renal carcinomas,[17] although less common subtypes and an "unclassified" category also exist. Uncommon subtypes of RCC, not included in the World Health Organization classification, include tubulocystic carcinoma, clear

TABLE 63.1

2004 World Health Organization Classification of Sporadic Renal Cell Carcinoma with Genetic and Clinical Correlates

Type	Genetics	Clinical
ccRCC (70% to 80%)	Deletion, mutation or methylation of 3p25-26 (VHL)	Most common variant Prognosis predicted by stage and grade
Multilocular cystic ccRCC (uncommon)	Deletion, mutation, or methylation of 3p25-26 (VHL)	Variant of ccRCC Distant metastases uncommon
Papillary RCC (10% to 15%)	Gain of 7 or 17 (trisomy or tetrasomy), loss of Y, deletion of 9p. Mutations of 7q31 when associated with hereditary papillary RCC	10% to 15% of RCC 95%+ 5-year cancer-specific survival in type I papillary RCC Response to tyrosine-kinase inhibitors less robust
Chromophobe RCC (3% to 5%)	Extensive chromosomal loss of Y, 1, 2, 6, 10, 13, 17, 21 Mutations of 17p11.2 when associated with BHD	5% of RCC Affects men and women equally with overall excellent prognosis
Collecting duct carcinoma (Bellini tumor) (<1%)	Highly variable Losses of 1q, 6p, 8p, 9p, 13q, 19q, 21q	Male preponderance (2:1) Mean age 55 Microscopically high grade, may resemble urothelial spectrum of cancers, Overall poor prognosis
Renal medullary carcinoma (rare)	Not defined	Associated with sickle cell trait Aggressive and lethal within 12 mo Mean age 19 y Male>female
Xp11 translocation carcinoma (rare)	Translocation of TFE3 gene on XP11.2	Children and young adults May present at advanced state and act more aggressively in adults
Renal carcinoma associated with neuroblastoma (rare)	Not defined	Morphologically and microscopically similar to ccRCC
Mucinous tubular and spindle cell carcinoma (rare)	Not defined	Female preponderance (4:1) Rarely metastasize
Unclassified RCC (1% to 3%)	Varied	Generally poor prognosis

ccRCC, clear cell renal cell carcinoma; RCC, renal cell carcinoma.
Adapted from Deng FM, Melamed J, Zhou M. Pathology of renal cell carcinoma. In: Libertino JA, ed. In *Renal Cancer: Contemporary Management*. New York: Springer; 2013:51–69.

cell tubulopapillary RCC, thyroid-like follicular carcinoma, and acquired cystic disease–associated RCC. The relatively rapid movement in RCC toward molecular classification follows advances in our molecular understanding of these variants and may soon supplant simple morphologic classification.

Other pathologically relevant variables in RCC include nuclear grade, sarcomatoid and rhabdoid differentiation, tumor necrosis, and vascular invasion. Nuclear grade usually follows the Fuhrman grading system[18] and is most often and best used for clear cell RCC (ccRCC) as the prognostic value in non-ccRCC remains largely unproven. Sarcomatoid differentiation exists in 5% of RCC and can be seen in any subtype. As such it is not considered a distinct entity, but rather a high-grade or poorly differentiated component. The presence and extent of micro- or macronecrosis has been correlated with prognosis in ccRCC.[19] Micro- or macrovascular invasion is thought to be a requisite step toward systemic disease; however, correlation between the extent of invasion and prognosis remains imprecise.

DIFFERENTIAL DIAGNOSIS AND STAGING

Most patients with RCC present with an incidental, radiographically detected renal mass (Fig. 63.1). While symptoms including microscopic or gross hematuria, flank pain, gastrointestinal disturbances and/or pain, bleeding or systemic disturbances related to metastases may lead to the diagnosis, the use of routine cross-sectional imaging has led to the more common scenario of

an incidentally detected renal mass. While the suspicion for RCC may be high in cases such as these, RCC is a pathologic/tissue diagnosis, not a clinical one (Fig. 63.2). Proper radiographic evaluation of a renal mass requires a pre- and postcontrast computed tomography or magnetic resonance imaging (MRI) to assess enhancement.[20] Duplex ultrasound, renal mass biopsy, and noncontrast diffusion-weighted MRI with antibody drug conjugates mapping may be useful adjunctive tests in various clinical settings. deoxy-2[^{18}F]fluoro-d-glucose positron emission tomography exhibits a low sensitivity for the diagnosis of RCC and is therefore not recommended for the evaluation of RCC. ImmunoPET with G-250 using an iodine-labeled antibody against carbonic anhydrase IX (CA-IX), which is known to be overexpressed in ccRCC, exhibits near 90% sensitivity and specificity for this RCC subtype.[21]

The differential diagnosis of the renal mass is broad and includes a long list of benign, malignant, and inflammatory conditions. Clinical and radiographic features can assist the astute clinician in narrowing down the diagnosis of the renal mass, particularly for benign and inflammatory lesions. Cystic lesions, for example, are frequently benign,[22] and fat-containing solid lesions are most commonly found to be angiomyolipomas (also benign). About 20% of enhancing renal masses and 15% of surgically removed masses are nonmalignant, with the most common diagnoses being oncocytoma and fat-poor angiomyolipoma.[23–25] Young to middle-aged women, in particular, are more likely to have benign pathology, as high as 40% in some series, while the likelihood of malignancy gradually decreases with age in men.[24,26] Tumor size is the most

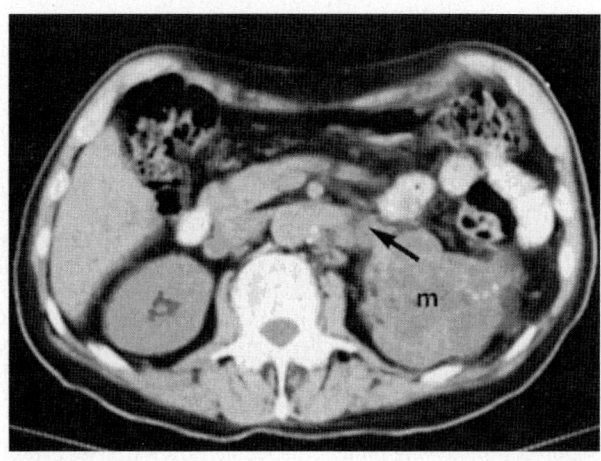
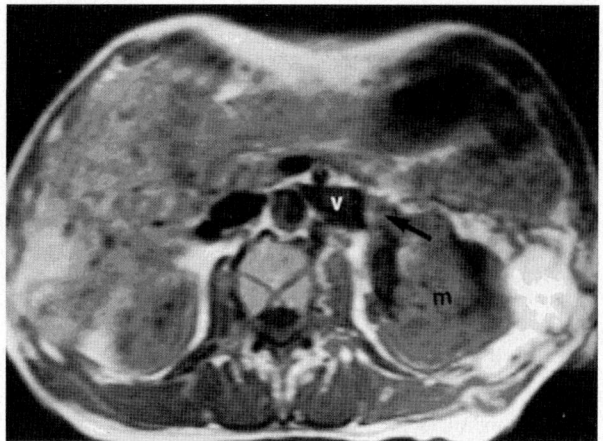

Figure 63.1 Cross-sectional imaging of kidney cancer using computed tomography and magnetic resonance imaging. **(A)** Contrast-enhanced computed tomography imaging (parenchymal phase) reveals a left renal mass with tumor thrombus within the left renal vein. **(B)** Magnetic resonance imaging in the same patient shows that the renal vein thrombus extends within the renal vein, but not to the confluence with the inferior vena cava (level 0 thrombus). m, mass; v, vein.

important determinant of pathology and biologic aggressiveness with larger tumors more likely to be high grade, locally invasive, and/or of adverse histologic subtype.[23,24,27] Incorporation of readily available features can allow the physician to provide an individualized risk of cancer (ranging between ~50% and ~99%), but a certain diagnosis requires pathologic confirmation.[24,28] The most accurate nomogram currently available gives estimates of preoperative prediction of tumor histology with an area under the curve of 0.76 and high-grade malignancy with an area under the curve of 0.73.[28]

Percutaneous renal mass sampling is now being performed with increased regularity at many centers.[29] There is a strong rationale for biopsy when the findings will change management, such as when there is reason to suspect lymphoma/leukemia or abscess or to guide systemic therapy for metastatic disease. Even for clinically localized renal tumors, conventional renal mass biopsy can provide a definitive diagnosis in 80% to 90% of cases, and the ability to subtype and grade RCC can increase with the use of immunohistochemical and other molecular analyses.[30,31] Therefore, renal mass sampling should be considered in patients with enhancing renal masses who are candidates for a wide range of management strategies.[30–34] However, younger, healthier patients who are unwilling to accept the uncertainty associated with renal mass biopsy as well as elderly, frail patients who will be managed conservatively (independent of biopsy results) should still be managed without a biopsy.

Clinical and pathologic staging systems provide a basis of standardized communication, comparison, and prognostication. They are used to communicate risk for treatment decision making and clinical trials planning. There have been several staging systems for RCC proposed. The most widely used is version 7 of the TNM (tumor, node, metastasis) staging system of the American Joint Committee on Cancer and the Union for International Cancer Control, updated in 2010 (Table 63.2). It distinguishes T1a from T1b and T2a from T2b based on tumor size.[35] Additionally, adrenal involvement was changed from pathologic stage T3a to T4 and venous invasion was separated into renal vein/segmental branches (T3a) and inferior vena cava (IVC) below (T3b) or above the diaphragm (T3c). Nodal and metastatic disease are only classified as negative (N0/M0) or positive (N1/M1). Other potential prognostic features of the primary tumor not included in the TNM classification include necrosis, urothelial involvement, microvascular invasion and molecular features. Review of these and other prognostic features of RCC are available.[36]

HEREDITARY KIDNEY CANCER SYNDROMES, GENETICS, AND MOLECULAR BIOLOGY

While most renal cancers are believed to occur sporadically, familial clusters have led to the discovery of at least seven RCC susceptible syndromes (Table 63.3). It is estimated that approximately 4% of RCC have a hereditary basis.[37] In these cases, in addition to a provocative family history, tumors tend to be bilateral,

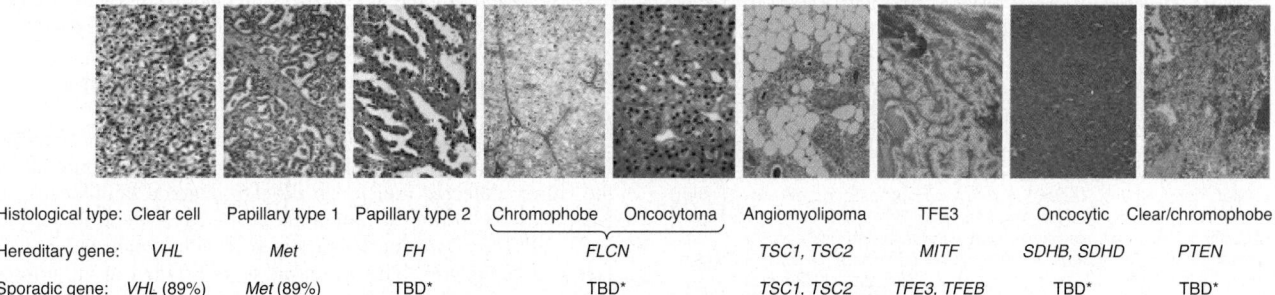

Histological type:	Clear cell	Papillary type 1	Papillary type 2	Chromophobe	Oncocytoma	Angiomyolipoma	TFE3	Oncocytic	Clear/chromophobe
Hereditary gene:	*VHL*	*Met*	*FH*	*FLCN*		*TSC1, TSC2*	*MITF*	*SDHB, SDHD*	*PTEN*
Sporadic gene:	*VHL* (89%)	*Met* (89%)	TBD*	TBD*		*TSC1, TSC2*	*TFE3, TFEB*	TBD*	TBD*

Figure 63.2 Human renal epithelial neoplasms. Renal cortical tumors do not conform to a single pathology. There are a number of different tumor subtypes that display the full range of oncologic activity, ranging from benign to indolent to aggressive. Each histologic type is characterized by distinct gross and microscopic appearance, gene associated with their familial forms, and genetic changes commonly detected in sporadic cases. (Used with permission from Linehan WM, Ricketts CJ. The metabolic basis of kidney cancer. *Semin Cancer Biol* 2013;23:46–55.)

TABLE 63.2

International Tumor, Node, Metastasis Staging System for Renal Cell Carcinoma and Survival Rates

T: Primary Tumor		Five-Year Survival (%)
TX	Primary tumor cannot be assessed	
T0	No evidence of primary tumor	
T1a	Tumor ≤4 cm and confined to the kidney	90–100
T1b	Tumor >4 cm and ≤7 cm and confined to the kidney	80–90
T2a	Tumor >7 cm and ≤10 cm and confined to the kidney	65–80
T2b	Tumor >10 cm and confined to the kidney	50–70
T3a	Tumor grossly extends into the renal vein or its segmental (muscle containing) branches, or tumor invades perirenal and/or renal sinus fat but not beyond Gerota fascia	40–65
T3b	Tumor grossly extends into the vena cava below the diaphragm	30–50
T3c	Tumor grossly extends into the vena cava above the diaphragm or invades the wall of the vena cava	20–40
T4	Tumor invades beyond Gerota fascia (including contiguous extension into the ipsilateral adrenal gland)	0–20
N: Regional Lymph Nodes		
NX	Regional lymph nodes cannot be assessed	
N0	No regional lymph nodes metastasis	
N1	Metastasis in regional lymph node(s)	0–20
M: Distant Metastases		
MX	Distant metastasis cannot be assessed	
M0	No distant metastasis	
M1	Distant metastasis present	0–10

Stage Grouping

Stage I	T1	N0	M0
Stage II	T2	N0	M0
Stage III	T3	Any N	M0
	T1 or T2	N1	M0
Stage IV	T4	Any N	M0
	Any T	Any N	M1

Modified from American Joint Committee on Cancer. Edge S, Byrd DR, Compton CC, et al, eds. *AJCC Cancer Staging Manual.* 7th ed. New York: Springer-Verlag; 2010. Data from Hafez KS, Fergany AF, Novick AC. Nephron sparing surgery for localized renal cell carcinoma: impact of tumor size on patient survival, tumor recurrence, and TNM staging. *J Urol* 1999;162(6): 1930-1933; Leibovich BC, Cheville JC, Lohse CM, et al. Cancer specific survival for patients with pT3 renal cell carcinoma—can the 2002 primary tumor classification be improved? *J Urol* 2005;173(3):716–719; Thompson RH, Cheville JC, Lohse CM, et al. Reclassification of patients with pT3 and pT4 renal cell carcinoma improves prognostic accuracy. *Cancer* 2005;104:53–60; Lane BR, Kattan MW. Prognostic models and algorithms in renal cell carcinoma. *Urol Clin North Am* 2008;35:613–625; Campbell L, Nuttall R, Griffiths D, et al. Activated extracellular signal-regulated kinase is an independent prognostic factor in clinically confined renal cell carcinoma. *Cancer* 2009; 115:3457–3467; Martinez-Salamanca JI, Huang WC, Millán I, et al; International Renal Cell Carcinoma-Venous Thrombus Consortium. Prognostic impact of the 2009 UICC/AJCC TNM staging system for renal cell carcinoma with venous extension. *Eur Urol* 2011;59:120–127; Haddad H, Rini BL. Current treatment considerations in metastatic renal cell carcinoma. *Curr Treat Options Oncol* 2012;13:212–229.

multifocal, and arise at an early age of onset. Importantly, the study of hereditary kidney cancer has dramatically changed our understanding of the genetic and molecular basis of RCC and has led to the development of effective, approved therapeutic agents as similar cytogenetic and molecular alterations appear to be shared between sporadic and hereditary RCC (see Fig. 63.2).[38]

The molecular alterations in RCC appear to converge on similar pathways involved in dysregulated oxygen sensing/angiogenesis, iron metabolism, and energy/nutrient sensing.[39,40] The predominant genetic and molecular defects in RCC known to date include VHL loss of function (ccRCC), neurofibromatosis type 2 loss of function (ccRCC), MET gain of function (papillary type I RCC), NRF2 gain of function and alterations in fumarate hydratase (papillary type II RCC), CCND1 gain of function and folliculin loss of function (oncocytoma/chromophobe RCC), and MiTF-TFE3 gain of function (translocation RCC). Additionally, inactivation of chromatin modifying proteins including *PBRM1*, *BAP1*, and histone methylases/demethylases, as well as inactivation of electron transporters, may represent early or common events in multiple subtypes.[41] While important, the associations of these aberrant pathways with various subtypes of RCC likely represent an overly simplified model of renal tumor development.[42] A variety of small nucleotide mutations, structural mutations, and large chromosomal abnormalities characterizes RCC, with as many as 5 to 70 small somatic mutations found in individual renal tumor cells.[42] Moreover, variable gene expressions may reflect differences in cell types from which RCC originates, suggesting that genetic aberrations require a specific cellular context for dysregulated growth. The development of rapid sequencers continues to redefine the molecular characterization of RCC from which a genetic profile/classification is emerging with important implications for the development of the next generation of targeted therapeutic molecules.[43,44]

Von Hippel-Lindau Disease

VHL is a syndrome characterized by the development of highly vascular tumors of the retina, central nervous system, pancreas, adrenal, and kidney (ccRCC). It is inherited in an autosomal dominant fashion with an incidence of 1:35,000.[39] Loss of VHL function (3p25.1) by genetic or epigenetic means in a classic tumor suppressor fashion is the known cause. In an established genotype-phenotype relationship, type 1 VHL (absence of pheochromocytoma) is due to germline deletions, insertions, and nonsense mutations, whereas type II VHL (with pheochromocytoma) is associated with missense mutations.[45] Between 25% to 60% of patients with VHL develop bilateral multifocal cystic and solid RCC, which represents a common cause of death (Fig. 63.3). Management of renal tumors in patients with VHL now includes surveillance of smaller tumors (<3 cm) and resection of larger ones (>3 cm) by PN with the goal of preventing metastases and optimizing renal function by "resetting the biologic clock" through appropriately timed surgeries.[46] The goal of complete tumor removal with wide negative surgical margins is less appropriate for these patients where management of localized lesions supplants cure.[39,46] Patients should be evaluated and followed by a team of clinicians familiar with the complexities of multisystem genetic disorders.

Hereditary Papillary Renal Cell Carcinoma

Hereditary papillary RCC is perhaps the least common familial RCC syndrome, with manifestations that appear to only affect the kidney. Affected individuals develop bilateral multifocal type I papillary RCC due to mutations in the *MET* gene located at 7q31. MET is a tyrosine kinase receptor with hepatocyte growth factor as its ligand.[47] The syndrome is transmitted in an autosomal dominant fashion and tumors usually appear after the age of 30.[39] As with VHL, management of renal tumors recognizes the need to remove larger lesions and observe smaller ones. While no size cutoff for intervention has been established, the biology of type I papillary RCC appears to be more indolent that ccRCC,

TABLE 63.3

Familial Renal Cell Carcinoma Syndromes

Syndrome	Gene (Chromosome)	Major Clinical Manifestations
von Hippel-Lindau	*VHL* gene (3p25-26)	Clear cell RCC Retinal angiomas Central nervous system hemangioblastomas Pheochromocytoma Other tumors
Hereditary papillary RCC	*c-met* proto-oncogene (7q31)	Multiple, bilateral type 1 papillary RCCs
Familial leiomyomatosis and RCC	*Fumarate hydratase* (1q42-43)	Type 2 papillary RCC Collecting duct RCC Leiomyomas of skin or uterus Uterine leiomyosarcomas
Birt-Hogg-Dubé	*Folliculin* (17p11)	Multiple chromophobe RCC, hybrid oncocytic tumor, oncocytomas Occasional clear cell (occasionally) Papillary RCC (occasionally) Facial fibrofolliculomas Lung cysts Spontaneous pneumothorax
Succinate dehydrogenase RCC	Succinate dehydrogenase complex subunits: *SDHB* (1p36.1-35) or *SDHD* (11q23)	Chromophobe, clear cell, type 2 papillary RCC, oncocytoma Paragangliomas (benign and malignant) Papillary thyroid carcinoma
Tuberous sclerosis	*TSC1* (9q34) or *TSC2* (16p13)	Multiple renal angiomyolipomas Clear cell RCC (occasionally) Renal cysts/polycystic kidney disease Cutaneous angiofibromas Pulmonary lymphangiomyomatosis
PTEN hamartoma tumor syndrome (Cowden syndrome)	*PTEN* (10q23)	Breast tumors (malignant and benign) Epithelial thyroid carcinoma Papillary RCC or other histology

PTEN, phosphatase and tensin homolog; RCC, renal cell carcinoma.
Adapted from Linehan WM, Walther MM, Zbar B. The genetic basis of cancer of the kidney. *J Urol* 2003; 170(6 Pt 1):2163-2172. and Linehan WM, Ricketts CJ. The metabolic basis of kidney cancer. *Semin Cancer Biol* 2013;23:46–55.

suggesting the risk of death from kidney cancer in these patients is low. Again, PN with renal preservation is emphasized despite the diffuse micro- and macromultifocality of these lesions.

Birt-Hogg-Dubé Syndrome

BHD is characterized by cutaneous fibrofolliculomas, a 50-fold increased risk of pneumothorax, and bilateral multifocal solid renal tumors. It is an autosomal dominant disorder with an incidence of around 1:200,000. Linkage analysis has mapped the gene for BHD (*folliculin*), a tumor suppressor, to 17p11.2. Folliculin is thought to be a downstream effector of activated protein kinase and mammalian target of rapamycin (mTOR).[39] Renal tumors associated with BHD are more indolent in nature, occurring in approximately 20% of individuals, with <5% developing metastases. While the histology of renal tumors associated with BHD is most often chromophobe RCC, oncocytoma, or hybrids of both, clear cell or papillary tumors may rarely occur as well.

Hereditary Leiomyomatosis Renal Cell Carcinoma

Hereditary leiomyomatosis RCC is also characterized by dermatologic manifestations. Patients with HLRCC exhibit cutaneous leiomyomas, early onset of uterine fibroids, macronodular adrenal hyperplasia, and kidney cancer. Linkage analysis has localized the HLRCC gene (*fumarate hydratase*), a key Kreb cycle enzyme, to 1p42.3 (FN).[48]

Renal tumors in HLRCC tend to be aggressive and lethal. The most common histology observed is type II (eosinophilic) papillary RCC.[39] Unlike other hereditary forms of RCC, given the aggressive nature of these tumors, AS with delayed intervention is not recommended.

TREATMENT OF LOCALIZED RENAL CELL CARCINOMA

Greater use of cross-sectional imaging has contributed to earlier detection of RCC in many cases.[2,49,50] Between 50% to 70% of RCC are detected incidentally,[51] and the majority are "small renal masses (SRM)," or clinically localized renal cortical tumors up to 4 cm in size. Our perspectives about treatment of clinical T1 renal masses have changed substantially in the past 20 years. While all had been presumed to be malignant and managed aggressively, we now recognize the tremendous biologic heterogeneity of these lesions, and multiple management strategies are now available, including RN, PN, TA, and AS.[52–57] Once controversial, elective PN is now accepted as a standard of care, based in part on the appreciation of the deleterious renal functional consequences of RN (Fig. 63.4).[53,55,58] Ongoing analysis of the relative merits of PN, RN, and other management strategies has produced vibrant literature over the past few years.[46,59–62] Both the American Urologic Association (AUA) and the European Association of Urology have released guidelines for the management of localized renal masses in recent years providing a robust analysis of the available studies.[9,63–67] Each approach has associated risks and benefits, and no one approach is best in all circumstances

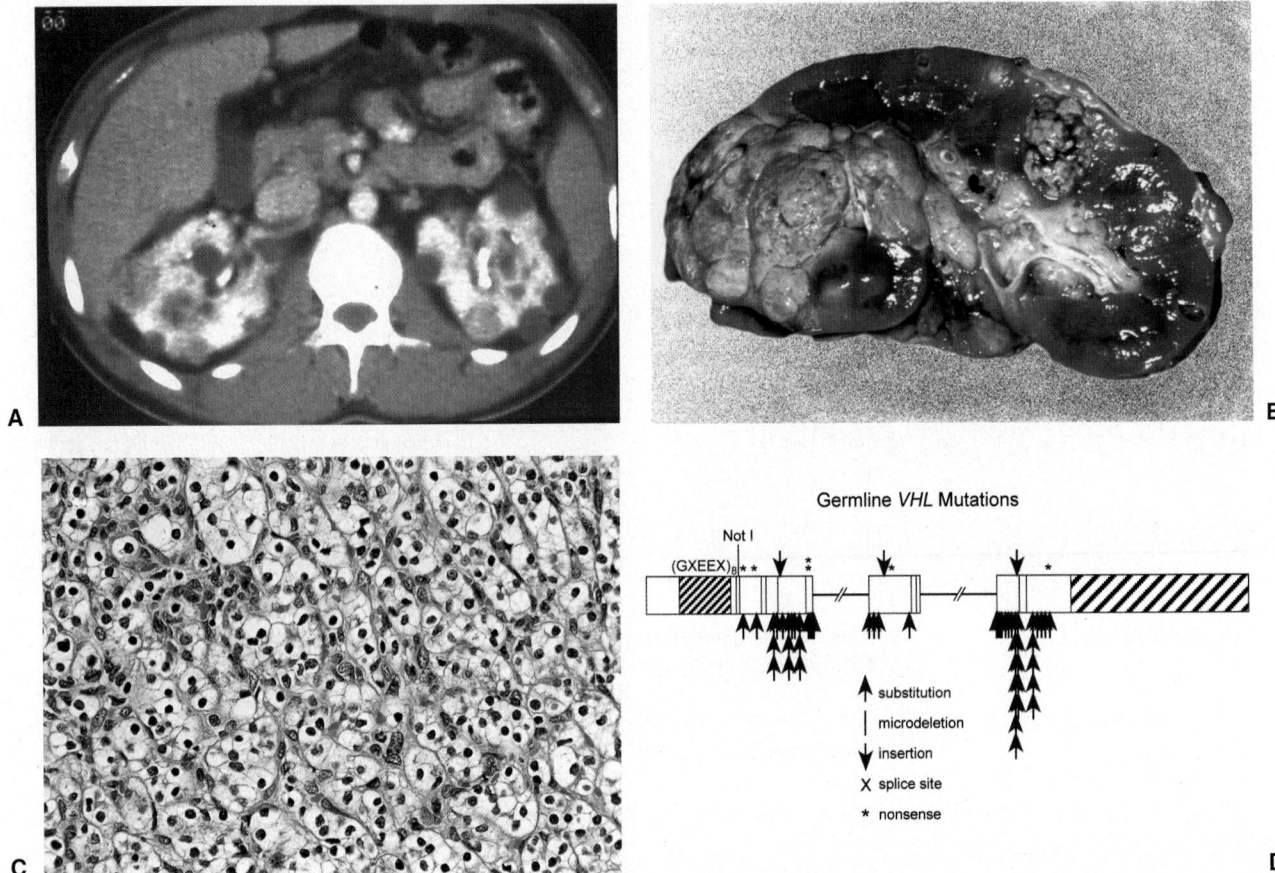

Figure 63.3 The von Hippel-Lindau (*VHL*) gene is responsible for the inherited form of clear cell renal cell carcinoma (ccRCC): VHL syndrome. **(A)** Axial computed tomography image showing multifocal and bilateral renal tumors and cysts. **(B)** Gross image of nephrectomy specimen showing typical yellow-gold appearance of ccRCC present in multiple portions of this kidney from a patient with VHL. **(C)** Histologic appearance of ccRCC, showing the clearing of the cytoplasm around the darker nuclei typical of these "clear cells." **(D)** Structure of the VHL gene with sites of point mutations and truncations indicated. (Used with permission from Linehan and colleagues' prior work. DeVita VT, Lawrence TS, Rosenberg SA, et al, eds. *DeVita, Hellman, and Rosenberg's Cancer: Principles and Practice of Oncology.* 9th ed. Philadelphia, PA: Lippincott Williams & Wilkins; 2011.)

(Table 63.4). The involvement of an urologist with expertise in the management of RCC is essential for selection of the optimal strategy based on the individual features of each patient and tumor.

Radical Nephrectomy for Renal Cell Carcinoma

The objective of surgical therapy for RCC is to excise all of the cancer with an adequate surgical margin. Simple nephrectomy was practiced for many decades, but was replaced by RN when Robson and colleagues (1969) established this procedure as the "gold standard" approach for localized RCC.[68] "RN" as currently practiced may be better termed "total nephrectomy," as it often omits several of the components of the original, "radical" nephrectomy, which always included extrafascial nephrectomy, adrenalectomy, and extended lymphadenectomy from the crus of the diaphragm to the aortic bifurcation. Perifascial dissection is still routinely practiced for larger tumors, as ≥25% of these tumors extend into the perinephric fat.[69,70] Removal of the ipsilateral adrenal gland is no longer recommended, unless there is suspicion of direct invasion of the gland by tumor or a radiographically or clinically suspicious adrenal tumor, because of the similar propensity of RCC to metastasize to the ipsilateral or contralateral adrenal gland.[71–73] Finally, extended lymphadenectomy has been shown to be of no benefit for patients with clinically localized RCC and remains controversial for those with higher-risk disease.[74–77]

RN is still a preferred option for many patients with localized RCC, such as those with very large tumors (most clinical T2

tumors) or the relatively limited subgroup of patients with clinical T1 tumors that are not amenable to nephron-sparing approaches.[78] The surgical approach for RN depends on the size and location of the tumor, as well as the patient's habitus and medical/surgical history. For locally advanced disease and/or bulky lymphadenopathy, an open surgical approach using either an extended subcostal, midline, or thoracoabdominal incision is generally used.[79]

Current minimally invasive approaches allow all of the essential steps of RN to be performed, with the associated benefits of shorter convalescence and reduced morbidity.[80–83] Laparoscopic RN is now established as a preferred approach for moderate to large volume tumors (≤10 cm to 12 cm), without invasion of adjacent organs, with limited (or no) venous involvement, and having manageable (or no) lymphadenopathy. Therefore, a minimally invasive approach is suitable for most patients with renal tumors, even including some patients with features previously thought to mandate open RN.

On the other hand, RN has fallen out of favor for smaller renal tumors due to concerns about chronic kidney disease (CKD), and it should only be performed when necessary in this population.[53,58,78,84] Several studies have shown an increased risk of CKD on longitudinal follow-up after RN.[58,85,86] Huang et al. first reported that 26% of patient populations with a small renal mass, normal opposite kidney, and "normal" serum creatinine had pre-existing grade 3 CKD (estimated glomerular filtration rate [eGFR] <60 ml/min per 1.73 m^2). After surgery, stage 3b or higher CKD (eGFR <45 ml/min per 1.73 m^2) was more common after RN than PN (36% versus 5%, p <0.001). CKD has been proven to lead to increased rates of cardiovascular events and death, with

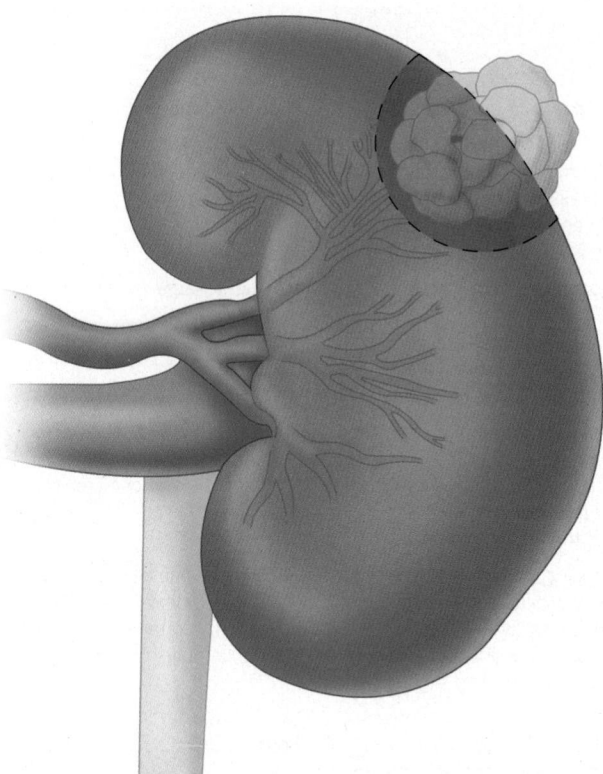

Figure 63.4 Partial nephrectomy. The intention of kidney-sparing surgery, or "nephron-sparing surgery," is to achieve complete local resection of the tumor while leaving as much functioning parenchyma in the involved kidney as possible. An assessment of volume preservation can be made by accounting for both the amount of parenchyma replaced by tumor and the adjacent uninvolved parenchyma removed or devascularized during the procedure.[61] The amount of volume preservation and the quality of the functioning renal remnant are the most important determinants of renal function after renal surgery. Partial nephrectomy and other kidney-sparing alternatives provide definite renal functional benefits that must be weighed against the potential for increased risk of cancer recurrence, when compared with radical nephrectomy.[287] (Artwork courtesy of Kristen Tobert.)

proportionally greater impact with higher CKD stage (and lower GFR). For example, in a population-based study of >1 million subjects, the relative death rates were 1.2, 1.8, 3.2, and 5.9 for eGFR (ml/min per 1.73 m²) of 45 to 60, 30 to 45, 15 to 30, and <15, respectively, even after controlling for hypertension, diabetes, and other potential confounding factors.[87] Coupled with the biologic heterogeneity of small renal masses, many of which will never lead to compromised survival, the potential negative consequences of RN on renal function have highlighted the importance of nephron-sparing approaches.[53,58,72,88–90]

Partial Nephrectomy for Renal Cell Carcinoma

Kidney-sparing surgery for renal tumors was first described by Czerny in 1890; however, significant morbidity limited its use for the next half century.[91] Vermooten (1950) revisited the concept of local excision with a margin of normal parenchyma for encapsulated and peripherally located renal tumors.[92] The use of PN for RCC has subsequently been stimulated by experience with renal vascular surgery for other conditions, advances in renal imaging, growing numbers of incidentally discovered small renal masses, greater appreciation of the deleterious effects of CKD, introduction of minimally invasive techniques, and encouraging long-term survival in patients undergoing this form of treatment during the

last 50 years.[93–95] Kidney-sparing surgery entails complete local resection of the tumor while leaving the largest possible amount of normal functioning parenchyma in the involved kidney (see Fig. 63.4).

Initially described for patients with an "absolute" indication for kidney-sparing surgery or for the "elective" indication of a small renal tumor in the setting of a normal contralateral kidney, PN is now strongly considered whenever preservation of renal function is potentially important. Common indications include conditions that pose a threat to future renal function, such as hypertension, diabetes mellitus, peripheral or coronary artery disease, or nephrolithiasis, and patients with baseline CKD, an abnormal contralateral kidney, or those with multifocal or familial RCC.[96,97] PN is generally considered feasible for the vast majority of localized renal masses <5 cm in size and often for tumors ≥7 cm by those with expertise with kidney-sparing surgery.[98–101] Particularly for those with a strong rationale for nephron-sparing surgery, PN can even be performed for tumors that deeply invest the renal vascular structures or with limited venous thrombus, but such procedures clearly carry higher perioperative morbidity.[95,102] Local recurrence rates after PN for imperative indications have averaged 3% to 5% or higher in historical series.[103] The decision to perform a PN in such circumstances should be individualized, weighing the potential increased technical and oncologic risks of such an operation with the renal functional consequences of RN (see Fig. 63.4).

PN clearly leads to improved functional outcomes, when compared with RN, even for complicated situations.[104,105] Temporary or permanent renal replacement therapy has been reported to be necessary in <5% of patients undergoing PN in a solitary kidney and is rarely needed for patients with a functioning contralateral kidney.[106,107] In fact, the vast majority of patients will avoid permanent dialysis, even following multiple surgeries for multiple tumors in both kidneys, so long as at least 30% of a well-functioning remnant kidney is preserved.[95] For situations in which PN is deemed impossible, RN with ensuing hemodialysis is sometimes necessary, but presurgical therapy with a tyrosine-kinase inhibitor is an alternative approach that has proven successful in some patients.[108–111]

For patients with clinical T1 renal masses, local recurrence rates are 1% to 2% after PN and most commonly located distant from the initial resection. Cancer-free survival is achieved in well above 90% of patients.[104] The contralateral kidney is also at risk for metachronous disease, which also occurs in 1% to 2% of patients, even with contemporary imaging modalities. This provides further rationale to avoid unnecessary RN for tumors amenable to nephron-sparing surgery. The goal of PN is resection of all grossly appreciated tumor with negative microscopic surgical margins; this is generally performed with a thin rim of normal parenchyma based on prior literature indicating that margin width is immaterial.[67,112–117] Some centers now routinely perform enucleation of renal tumors with excellent oncologic outcomes, although enthusiasm for more widespread use of this approach has been tempered by the somewhat higher recurrence rate among patients with RCC with positive margins and the propensity of some RCC subtypes to invade the pseudocapsule that is generally present.

Within the last decade, substantial progress has been made with minimally invasive PN, which is now the most commonly performed procedure for small renal masses. Laparoscopic PN, with or without robotic assistance, is performed according to the same principles as open PN. Margin status and oncologic outcomes with laparoscopic and open PN appear equivalent in series of patients in which patients were selected appropriately for each of these approaches.[101,118] Although early to intermediate experience with laparoscopic PN suggested increased urologic complications compared with open RN,[119] subsequent experience with pure laparoscopic PN and more prevalent use of robotic PN have substantially reduced perioperative morbidity.[104,120–125] Tumor complexity remains a major predictor for intraoperative and postoperative complications, regardless of surgical approach, and open PN should be considered for particularly challenging situations.[126]

TABLE 63.4

Treatments for Localized Renal Cell Carcinoma

	Advantages	Disadvantages	Main Indications
ORN	Traditional surgical approach for renal cancer, effective in removing tumor with surrounding structures and lymph nodes when indicated	Morbidity of surgical incision (flank, subcostal, midline, thoracoabdominal) Renal functional implications of removing entire kidney (average 35% decrease in GFR)	Large tumor (>12 cm) Locally advanced tumor Bulky adenopathy
MIRN	Reproducible and effective surgery for most localized renal tumors Minimally invasive surgery, with decreased pain, morbidity and convalescence compared to ORN	Many tumors up to 7 cm can be treated with PN Renal functional implications of removing entire kidney (average 35% decrease in GFR)	Medium to large tumor (up to 10 to 12 cm) High tumor complexity
OPN	Oncologic outcomes appear similar to RN, although selection biases limit this conclusion Maximizes renal functional preservation when performed with precise tumor excision and judicious use of regional hypothermia	Morbidity of flank incision (bulge, longer recovery) Potential for local recurrence due to incomplete excision or de novo tumors in the renal remnant	Small to medium tumors (up to 7 cm and occasionally larger) Moderate to high-complexity tumors
MIPN	Kidney-sparing surgery, with preservation of renal function when warm ischemia kept to limited duration (<20 to 25 min) Minimally invasive surgery, with decreased pain, morbidity, and convalescence compared to OPN	Higher complication rate for high complexity tumors and in less-experienced hands Positive surgical margins and local recurrence rates may be higher in such situations	Small renal masses (up to 5 cm and occasionally larger) Low to moderate (and selected high) complexity tumors
TA	Kidney-sparing approach, with renal functional benefits versus RN Can be performed outside of OR (percutaneous) or with minimally invasive approach (laparoscopic) For small (<3 cm) tumors, provides comparable control of metastasis to PN and RN	Relatively high rate of local failure Imprecision of histopathologic diagnosis Increased and challenging radiographic follow-up	Prior ipsilateral surgery for renal tumor Poorer surgical candidates unwilling to undergo surveillance
AS	Least invasive and kidney-sparing of all strategies Most SRMs have limited oncologic potential and can be safely managed with initial short interval follow-up imaging Intensity of surveillance can be tailored to patient and tumor characteristics	Tumor remains in place and untreated Oncologic nature of tumor unknown (without biopsy)	Poor surgical candidates Limited life expectancy

ORN, open radical nephrectomy; GFR; glomerular filtration rate; MIRN, minimally invasive radical nephrectomy; OPN, open partial nephrectomy; RN, radical nephrectomy; MIPN, minimally invasive partial nephrectomy; TA, thermal ablation; OR, operating room; PN, partial nephrectomy; AS, active surveillance; SRM, small renal mass.

Thermal Ablation of Renal Cell Carcinoma

TA, including renal cryosurgery and radiofrequency ablation (RFA) have emerged as alternative kidney-sparing treatments for patients with small (<3 cm) renal tumors.[127,128] Both can be administered percutaneously or with laparoscopic exposure and thus offer the potential for reduced morbidity and more rapid recovery compared with extirpative approaches.[128,129] In general, the long-term efficacy of TA has not been well established when compared to surgical excision, and current data suggest that the local recurrence rates are somewhat higher than that reported with extirpative approaches.[55,63] Another concern has been the lack of accurate histologic and pathologic information obtained with these modalities because the treated lesion is left in situ.

The ideal candidates for TA are patients with advanced age and/or significant comorbidities who prefer a proactive approach (over surveillance), but are not optimal candidates for conventional surgery, patients with local recurrence after previous kidney-sparing surgery, and patients with hereditary renal cancer who present with multifocal lesions for which multiple PNs might be cumbersome.[55] Patient preference must also be considered as some patients not fitting these criteria may select TA after balanced counseling about the current status of these modalities.[130,131] Tumor size is an important factor in patient selection because the current technology does not allow for reliable treatment of lesions >4 cm and success rates appear to be highest for tumors <2.5 cm to 3 cm.[132–135]

Clinical experience and follow-up of patients after renal cryosurgery suggests successful local control in about 90% of patients, although many studies provide limited and often incomplete, follow-up.[136–140] Diagnosis of local recurrence after TA can be challenging because evolving fibrosis within the tumor bed can be difficult to differentiate from residual cancer. In general, central or nodular enhancement within the tumor bed on extended follow-up has been considered diagnostic of local recurrence and the clinical experience with cryoablation has thus far supported this.[141,142] Other findings that suggest local recurrence include failure of the treated lesion to regress over time, a progressive increase in size of an ablated neoplasm, new nodularity in or around the treated zone, or satellite or port site lesions.[143] If these features are found, biopsy and possible retreatment should be considered. The AUA guidelines for surveillance after TA include cross-sectional scanning (computed tomography or MRI) with and without intravenous contrast at 3 and 6 months following ablative therapy and annually with chest X-ray for 5 years thereafter.[143]

More mature data from a limited number of studies now provide encouraging outcomes for smaller tumors, particularly those <3 cm, yet the cumulative experience continues to suggest that local control after cryoablative therapy remains suboptimal when compared to surgical excision.[55,138] The 5-year local recurrence rates in two series were 8% to 9%,[52,144] which is significantly higher than the 1% to 2% consistently reported with surgical excision of analogous small renal masses.[53] Other concerns with TA relate to surgical salvage and potential morbidity. Most local recurrences can be salvaged with repeat ablation, but some patients with progressive disease eventually require surgical extirpation. Nguyen and colleagues (2008b) have shown that PN and minimally invasive approaches are occasionally precluded in this setting due to the extensive fibrotic reaction induced by TA.[78] As expected, the incidence of treatment failure or complications after TA correlates with tumor size and complexity.[145]

The experience with RFA has been even more variable, likely related to surgeon experience, the availability of different platforms for the procedure, and inability to monitor treatment progress.[128] Local control after RFA is estimated to be 80% to 90%, although the definitions of local recurrence within the literature have been inconsistent.[53,55] Although loss of enhancement on cross-sectional imaging within the lesion has generally been accepted as an indicator of success, viable cancer cells have been detected at biopsy of the tumor bed even in the absence of enhancement on the MRI 6 months after treatment.[142] The issue of potential false-negative and false-positive imaging findings after TA remains a concern, and more strict definitions of local control after TA were recently advocated by an AUA guidelines panel.[143,146] The technology for RFA continues to improve with most contemporary series reporting relatively low rates of local recurrence. Some patients require repeat treatments to achieve local control, which is an infrequent event with cryoablation and rarely required with conventional surgical treatments for localized RCC.[128] One recent series documented local control in 91% of 179 patients with biopsy proven RCC at median follow-up of 27 months.[135] Some RFA series report even more encouraging results, particularly for tumors <3 cm diameter,[132] but others have reported 5-year local recurrence rates as high as 39%.[147]

Complications from ablation are uncommon, but have included acute renal failure, stricture of the ureteropelvic junction, necrotizing pancreatitis, and lumbar radiculopathy; therefore, careful and judicious selection of patients is essential.[128] Direct comparisons between cryoablation and RFA are inevitable, but perhaps unfair because RFA is earlier in its development and recent reports suggest great promise.[128,132] Other new technologies, such as high-intensity focused ultrasound and frameless, image-guided radiosurgical treatments (CyberKnife), are also under development and may allow extracorporeal treatment of small renal tumors in the future.[148–150] However, at present cell kill with these modalities is not sufficiently reliable and they should still be considered developmental.[151]

Active Surveillance of Clinically Localized Renal Cell Carcinoma

The concept of overdiagnosis and overtreatment of kidney cancers is a relatively new concept. The risks and consequences associated with unnecessary treatment of low-risk RCC are an unintentional, yet underappreciated harm associated with incidental detection of these tumors. While early detection leads to "cure," lead time biases in reported surgical series and the growing recognition that some localized renal tumors exhibit an indolent natural history have challenged the "find it, excise it" practice pattern. As the data emerge, AS remains a rational therapeutic option, particularly in the elderly or infirm where competing health, surgical, or renal functional risks may exceed that of the tumor's biology.[152,153]

Objectifying and comparing the risks of treatment (excision/ablation) versus AS remains difficult as the data upon which competing risks models are based remain largely retrospective and incomplete.[28] Nonetheless, data have emerged to suggest

that radiographically localized small renal masses, most of which are RCC,[154,152] exhibit slow linear/volumetric growth (0.3 cm/year on average) with a low metastatic potential (1.1% to 1.4%) over the first 24 to 36 months following diagnosis.[154,152] Moreover, in patients with localized small renal tumors at diagnosis, the risk of metastases appears to be related to both the size of the primary tumor and perhaps more importantly the growth kinetics of the lesion.[155] Interestingly, as many as 20% to 30% of small renal tumors exhibit zero radiographic growth over the initial 24 months following diagnosis.[55] Given these data, the practice of AS with delayed intervention informed by an objective assessment of risk in the elderly, infirm, and/or well-informed is emerging.[156] This practice is a calculated risk accepted by the patient and managed by the physician. Percutaneous biopsy and emerging biologic and genetic markers will continue to improve the decision-making process. In the meantime, AS remains a viable option for highly motivated patients and highly engaged physicians.

Follow-Up for Localized Renal Cell Carcinoma

Follow-up for cancer survivors focuses broadly on early detection of cancer recurrence. With earlier diagnosis of many cancers and a longer length of life after diagnosis and treatment, an increasing number of survivors remain under the care of cancer specialists and primary care physicians. Wide variations in recommended practice have led to the development of guidelines by various organizations. The AUA released guidelines for follow-up of clinically localized RCC in 2013 that reflect a consistent approach that also takes into account the heterogeneity of the population of cancer survivors (Table 63.5).[143] Clinicians should be aware that in managing adult cancer survivors they are not only looking for RCC recurrence, but also monitoring for secondary malignancy and the effects of cancer treatment, implementing therapies to prevent recurrences or new tumors, understanding the consequences of cancer and its treatment effects, and coordinating the overall care between cancer specialists and the primary care physician to meet each individual's needs.

TREATMENT OF LOCALLY ADVANCED RENAL CELL CARCINOMA

Surgery for Tumor Thrombus in the Inferior Vena Cava

Renal tumors are unique in their ability to form tumor thrombi that can propagate from the ipsilateral renal vein into the IVC and extend as far as the patient's right atrium. Approximately 4% to 10% of patients who present with renal masses will have a concomitant tumor thrombus. The level of tumor thrombus is classified as level 0 (thrombus limited to the renal vein), level I (thrombus extending into the inferior vena cava ≤2 cm above the renal vein), level II (thrombus extending into the inferior vena cava >2 cm above the renal vein, but below the hepatic veins), level III (thrombus extending into the inferior vena cava to or above the level of the hepatic veins, but still remaining below the diaphragm), and level IV (thrombus extending into the inferior vena cava and above the level of the diaphragm) (Fig. 63.5). A tumor thrombus should be suspected in a patient with a renal tumor who also have new onset lower extremity edema, an isolated right-sided varicocele or one that does not collapse with recumbency, dilated superficial abdominal veins, proteinuria, pulmonary embolism, right atrial mass, or nonfunction of the involved kidney.

Five-year cancer-specific survival for patients with RCC and venous extension ranges from 45% to 70%, and surgical therapy in the form of RN and IVC thrombectomy can be curative. Interestingly, many patients with vena cava extension will present

TABLE 63.5

Guidelines for Follow-Up of Clinically Localized Renal Cell Carcinoma

Follow-up Measure	Recommendation
Physical exam and history	History and physical examination directed at detecting signs and symptoms of metastatic spread or local progression
Laboratory testing	Basic laboratory testing including blood urea nitrogen/creatinine, urinalysis and estimated glomerular filtration rate for all patients Progressive renal insufficiency should prompt nephrology referral Complete blood count, lactate dehydrogenase, liver function tests, alkaline phosphatase, and serum calcium per discretion of the physician
Abdominal imaging	Obtain a baseline abdominal scan (CT or magnetic resonance imaging) within 3 to 6 mo following surgery, and periodically thereafter based on individual risk factors (e.g., every 6 mo for 3 y for moderate to high-risk RCC) Perform site-specific imaging as symptoms warrant Imaging beyond 5 y may be performed at the discretion of the clinician
Chest imaging	Low-risk RCC: Chest X-ray annually for 3 y and only as clinically indicated beyond that time period Moderate to high-risk RCC: baseline chest CT 3 to 6 mo after surgery with continued imaging (chest X-ray or CT) every 6 mo for at least 3 y Imaging beyond 5 y is optional and should be based on individual patient characteristic and tumor risk factors
Bone scan	Elevated alkaline phosphatase, clinical symptoms such as bone pain, and/or radiographic findings suggestive of a bony neoplasm should prompt a bone scan Bone scan should not be performed in the absence of these signs and symptoms
Central nervous system imaging	Acute neurologic signs should lead to prompt neurologic cross-sectional imaging of the head or spine based on localized symptoms

CT, computed tomography; RCC, renal cell carcinoma.
Adapted from Donat SM, Diaz M, Bishoff JT, et al. Follow-up for clinically localized renal neoplasms: AUA guideline. *J Urol* 2013;190:407–416.

without metastatic disease.[157,158] The prognostic significance of IVC thrombus level has been controversial. Most studies suggest that the incidence of locoregional or systemic progression is higher in patients with level III-IV IVC thrombus, which may account for the reduced survival reported in this subgroup in some series.[159–162] Other series have shown that any IVC involvement is worse than renal vein involvement without distinction with regard to IVC level; in these series, other factors, such as nodal or metastatic involvement and tumor grade, have more impact on overall survival (OS).[163,164] Despite this debate, patients with any tumor thrombus

level can be cured with surgical resection, even level IV, in the absence of metastases and other adverse features.[165–168]

More recent series have re-evaluated the clinical variables predictive of survival after surgery for patients with tumor thrombi. In a single institutional series of 99 patients, median survival for patients with level I/II tumor thrombus was 6.6 years compared to 1.4 years for patients with level III/IV tumor thrombi. Higher level of tumor thrombus ([III/IV versus I/II], hazard ratio [HR] = 1.84 95% confidence interval [CI] = 1.03 to 3.30, p = 0.041) and the presence of metastatic disease at the time of surgery (HR = 2.97, 95% CI = 1.65 to 5.36, p <0.001) both portended a worse OS on multivariate analysis.[169] Other investigators have examined the impact of tumor histology on clinical and pathologic outcomes in patients with venous tumor extension. Authors at the Mayo Clinic found that patients with non–clear cell histology presented with a significantly larger tumor size, greater rate of lymph node disease, higher nuclear grade, and more frequent sarcomatoid differentiation.[170] As a result of these clinical and pathologic variables, these patients had a considerably worse 5-year cancer-specific survival as compared with patients with clear cell histology (p = 0.03).[170] Similarly, a recent international multi-institutional retrospective study analyzed the role of tumor histology on survival in patients undergoing RN and caval thrombectomy. In this series of 1,774 patients, the overall 5-year cancer-specific survival was 53.4%.[171] In this series' multivariable analysis, papillary histology (HR = 1.62, 95% CI = 1.01 to 2.61, p <0.05), fat invasion (HR = 1.49, 95% CI = 1.10 to 2.03, p <0.01), and thrombus level (p <0.01) were all independent predictors of a poor cancer-specific survival.[171] In contrast to the Mayo series, when the authors restricted their analysis to only N0M0 patients, thrombus level and papillary histology were still significantly associated with a decreased cancer-specific survival.[170,171]

Surgery remains an integral part in the treatment paradigm for patients with tumor venous extension because of the sequelae of such vascular involvement. The surgical approach and technique to treat these challenging tumors are tailored to the level of IVC thrombus, but uniformly begin with careful mobilization of the kidney and early ligation of the arterial blood supply.[164,172,173] With an increasing tumor thrombus level, more advanced surgical techniques are required for vasculature control and complete tumor extirpation, including veno-venous bypass and cardiopulmonary bypass potentially with hypothermic circulatory arrest for some cases. Specifically for level III and level IV thrombi, a multidisciplinary surgical team is often required for advanced surgical maneuvers, including a liver surgeon to aid in mobilization of the liver and exposure of the intrahepatic IVC and a vascular and/or cardiac surgeon if bypass is required.

Despite the surgical ability to resect these tumor thrombi, perioperative mortality rates associated with RN and IVC thrombectomy have been reported to be as high as 5% to 10% in some series, depending on patient comorbidities and tumor characteristics.[164,166] Although there may be a palliative role for surgery in some patients with metastasis who experience severe disability from intractable edema, ascites, cardiac dysfunction, or associated local symptoms such as abdominal pain and hematuria, most such patients will not benefit due to risk of perioperative morbidity and limited life expectancy.[174,175]

Lymphadenectomy

The need for extensive lymphadenectomy in patients undergoing RN remains a subject of debate. Despite the fact that multiple prior studies have shown a survival benefit with a lymph node dissection performed at the time of nephrectomy,[75,176,177] a recent randomized trial failed to show a distinct advantage.[74] Although this trial represents level I evidence, its generalizability is limited since the trial included many patients at low risk for nodal metastasis (81% of patients had grade 1 or 2 tumors and 72% had organ-confined

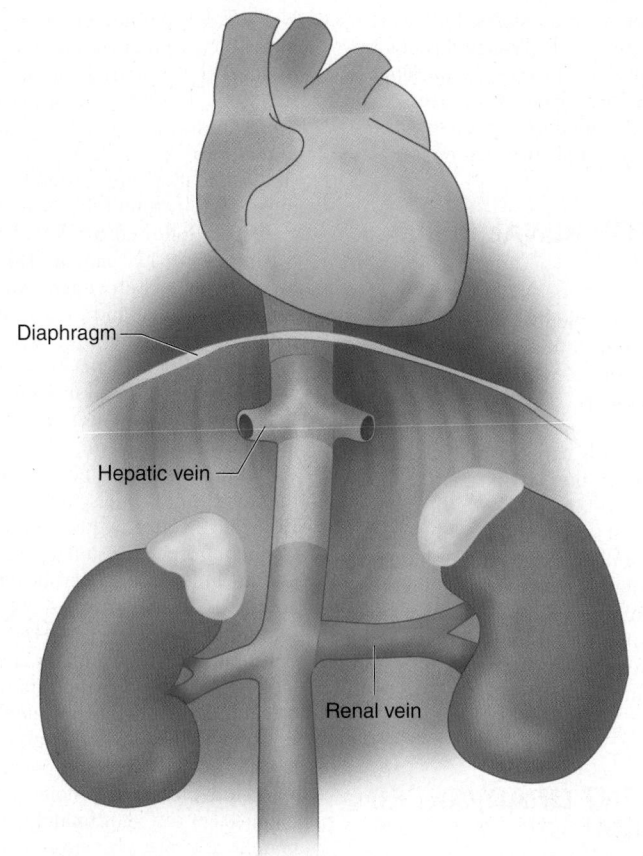

Prognostic and surgical staging systems of IVC tumor thrombus

Anatomic landmark	Staging systems				
	TNM	Neves	Novick	Hinman	Robson
RV	T3b	0	I	I	IIIa
IVC <2 cm above RV		I	II		
IVC >2 cm above RV and below hepatic veins		II			
IVC above hepatic veins and below diaphragm		III	III	II	
IVC above diaphragm	T3c	IV	IV	III	

Figure 63.5 Classification of renal cell carcinoma venous tumor thrombi. Level 0 (*green*): Thrombus within main renal vein (RV) or its branches and not reaching into the inferior vena cava (IVC). Level I (*yellow*): IVC thrombus is present within the IVC, <2 cm above renal vein. Level II (*orange*): IVC thrombus extends along the IVC, but not to the level of the main hepatic veins. Level III (*purple*): IVC thrombus extends within the IVC above the level of the main hepatic veins, but below the diaphragm. Level IV (*red*): IVC thrombus extends above the diaphragm, near to or into the right atrium and occasionally beyond. TNM, tumor, node, metastasis. (Reproduced with permission from Pouliot F, Shuch B, Larochelle JC, et al. Contemporary management of renal tumors with venous tumor thrombus. *J Urol* 2010;184:833–841.)

disease).[74] Furthermore, in the entire cohort, lymph node metastases were present in only 4% of patients undergoing complete lymph node dissection.[74] Based on this trial, a compelling argument for lymph node dissection in patients with clinically localized RCC cannot be supported.

Of greater impact is the study from Blute and colleagues[164] who elucidated pathologic features associated with increased risk for nodal metastases: tumor grade (grade 3 or 4), presence of a sarcomatoid component, tumor size ≥10 cm, tumor stage pT3 or pT4, and histologic tumor necrosis. Based on this study and a subsequent prospective evaluation of this approach, patients with two or more of these risk factors should be considered for extensive lymph node dissection incorporating the ipsilateral renal hilar region, the ipsilateral great vessel, and the interaortocaval region. This dissection should extend from the crus of the diaphragm to the common iliac artery. In a retrospective study, 45% of patients had positive lymph nodes outside of the renal hilar region, mandating a broader template.[177] Finally, a recently published retrospective study of 1,983 patients treated for RCC assessed the factors predictive of lymph node invasion and/or progression. In this study, the overall prevalence of lymph node invasion was 6.1% and the clinical factors that were independently predictive of lymph node involvement were tumor stage (T3-T4), clinical nodal status, the presence of metastatic disease, and tumor size as a continuous variable.[178] Using these variables, the authors created a nomogram that calculates a patient's probability of having lymph

PRACTICE OF ONCOLOGY

node disease at the time of nephrectomy or in disease follow-up.[178] It appears fair to conclude that a lymph node dissection is not routinely needed for organ-confined disease; however, the presence of multiple adverse pathologic features (e.g., large tumor size, locally advanced disease, etc.) seems to favor performing a lymph node dissection that is more extensive than simply the hilar region.

ADJUVANT THERAPY FOR RENAL CELL CARCINOMA

Although a significant proportion of patients can be considered to be cured or in remission after surgical treatment for nonmetastatic RCC, distant metastases are detected in 20% to 35% and local recurrence in 2% to 5% of patients.[54,94] Patients with locally advanced RCC and other high-risk features are at greater risk of recurrence and various predictive tools can be used to provide an individualized estimate.[54] Despite the significant likelihood of recurrence in patients with poor-risk features, no therapy has ever been shown to be of benefit in the adjuvant setting. Prior trials have evaluated hormone therapy, radiotherapy, immunotherapy, and tumor vaccines, all with essentially negative results. Based on the significant antitumor activity of targeted molecular therapies in advanced RCC, a number of randomized trials evaluating the ability of these agents to prevent metastasis have completed enrollment and results of these trials can be expected as early as 2015 (Table 63.6).

SURGICAL MANAGEMENT OF ADVANCED RENAL CELL CARCINOMA

Cytoreductive Nephrectomy

Approximately 30% to 40% of patients will present with metastatic or advanced RCC.[179] For these patients, multimodal therapy, which includes surgery, has produced improved progression-free survival (PFS) and OS. The National Comprehensive Cancer Network Guidelines for kidney cancer list cytoreductive nephrectomy (CN) with or without metastasectomy prior to systemic treatment as the primary treatment option for patients with stage IV RCC.[180] The data supporting this recommendation come from three randomized trials demonstrating a survival benefit for patients who received systemic immunotherapy with interferon (IFN)-alfa after surgical removal of the primary tumor.[181–183] Flanigan et al.[181] found the median survival of 120 patients assigned to surgery followed by IFN-alfa to be 11.1 months compared to 8.1 months in 121 patients assigned to IFN-alfa alone ($p = 0.05$). Similarly, Mickisch et al.[183] found time to progression (5 months versus 3 months) and median duration of survival to be better in patients randomized to surgery plus IFN-alfa compared to those randomized to IFN-alfa alone. Combining the survival data from all these trials resulted in a median survival of 13.6 months versus 7.8 months for patients undergoing surgery in addition to IFN-alfa as compared to IFN-alfa alone.[181,183–185]

More recent data accounting for the current use of targeted therapies as first-line systemic therapy for patients with metastatic RCC have confirmed the survival advantage associated with CN. In one retrospective study, patients ($n = 201$) who underwent CN had an independent statistically significant survival advantage as compared to patients ($n = 113$) who did not (HR = 0.68; 95% CI = 0.46 to 0.99, $p = 0.04$).[186] This survival advantage was present even when adjusting for contemporary adverse prognostic risk factors (e.g., performance status, time from diagnosis to therapy initiation, anemia, hypercalcemia, neutrophilia, and thrombocytosis).[187] Despite these promising results, other studies have shown that CN may not confer a survival advantage in patients with non–clear cell histology, especially those with sarcomatoid features.[172,188,189] Fortunately, a prospective study evaluating the benefit of surgery in combination with sunitinib versus sunitinib alone is currently ongoing in patients with metastatic RCC.

Although the use of laparoscopic/minimally invasive techniques in patients with advanced disease can potentially provide a less invasive and less morbid method for cytoreduction as preparation for administration of systemic therapies, CN is still not without risk, and surgical risk assessment needs to be considered preoperatively. According to prior reports, patients that are most

---

TABLE 63.6

Clinical Trials of Adjuvant Treatment for Nonmetastatic Renal Call Carcinoma

Trial	Study Groups	Treatment Duration	Inclusion Criteria
ASSURE: Adjuvant Sorafenib or Sunitinib for Unfavorable Renal Cell Carcinoma	Sunitinib vs. sorafenib vs. placebo	1 y	Clear cell and non–clear cell RCC eligible pT1b and G3-4; pT2/pT3/pT4; N1 if complete dissection performed
SORCE: Sorafenib for Patients with Resected Primary Renal Cell Carcinoma	Sorafenib (for 1 or 3 y) vs. placebo	3 y	Clear cell and non–clear cell RCC eligible Mayo Clinic progression score 3–11
S-TRAC: Sunitinib vs. Placebo for the Treatment of Patients at high risk for Recurrent Renal Cell Cancer	Sunitinib vs. placebo	1 y	Clear cell predominant histology eligible High-risk RCC according to UISS
EVEREST: Everolimus for Renal Cancer Ensuing Surgical Therapy	Everolimus vs. placebo	1 y	Clear cell and non–clear cell RCC eligible pT1b and G3-4; pT2/pT3/pT4; N1 if complete dissection performed
ATLAS: Adjuvant Axitinib Treatment of Renal Cancer	Axitinib vs. placebo	3 y	Clear cell predominant (>50%) eligible pT2 and G3-4; pT3a and >4 cm; pT3b/pT3c/pT4; N1
PROTECT: Pazopanib as an Adjuvant Treatment for Locally Advanced Renal Cell Carcinoma	Pazopanib vs. placebo	1 y	Clear cell predominant (>50%) eligible pT2 and G3-4; pT3/pT4; N1

RCC, renal cell carcinoma; pT: pathologic T stage; G: Fuhrman nuclear grade; . UISS: University of California, Los Angeles, integrated staging system.
Source: Zisman A, Pantuck AJ, Chao DH, et al. Renal cell carcinoma with tumor thrombus: is cytoreductive nephrectomy for advanced disease associated with an increased complication rate? *J Urol* 2002;168:962–967.

likely to benefit from CN are those patients with lung-only metastatic disease, good prognostic features as defined by Motzer (or other) criteria, and a good performance status.[175,190] Conversely, predictors of short survival for patients with advanced RCC include an elevated serum lactate dehydrogenase (LDH; >1.5 times upper limit of normal), a hemoglobin level <lower limit of normal, a corrected serum calcium level >10 mg/dl, an interval of <1 year from original diagnosis to the start of systemic therapy, a Karnofsky performance score ≤70, and two or more sites of organ metastasis.[191] However, the challenge associated with these risk criteria is that they mostly account for the risk associated with the disease and do not consider the perioperative risk to the patient, which is not insignificant.

For example, Abdollah et al.[192] identified 17,688 patients within the Florida Inpatient Database that underwent nephrectomy between the years 1999 to 2008. They identified 1,063 (6%) patients who underwent a CN and found that these patients were more likely to have a longer length of stay (8.4 versus 5.7 days, *p* <0.001), a secondary surgical procedure (28.3% versus 10%, *p* <0.001), an in-hospital mortality (2.4% versus 0.9%, *p* <0.001), and a postoperative complication (26.5% versus 18.9%, *p* <0.001). In this report, increasing age was predictive of increasing in-hospital mortality and complications for patients undergoing CN. A similar analysis was conducted by Trinh et al[193] using the Nationwide Inpatient Sample registry. Thirty one percent of the study population (n = 16,285) experienced a perioperative complication, and patients ≥75 years old who had a comorbidity score ≥3 were more likely to experience a complication after CN (both *p* <0.001).[193] Of the patients (n = 4,974) that experienced an adverse event, 5% (n = 245 patients) died during their hospitalization.[193] Finally, it is worth noting that despite the survival advantage garnered from a CN followed by targeted therapy, it is not universally received. In a single institutional study from the Fox Chase Cancer Center, only 69.5% of patients actually received systemic therapy after surgery.[194] The most common reason in this study for patients not to receive systemic therapy was rapid disease progression, which occurred in 30% of patients. Also, there were eight perioperative deaths, accounting for 19% of patients who did not receive systemic treatment.[194]

In summary, CN offers patients with metastatic RCC a survival advantage and the National Comprehensive Cancer Network Guidelines recommend a CN for patients with an Eastern Cooperative Oncology Group performance status <2 who have no evidence of brain metastasis.[180] Despite these recommendations, recent data has shown that surgical risk associated with CN is not insignificant, especially in the elderly and comorbid, and should be weighed against the patient's disease biology (presence of poor-risk disease) before reflexively proceeding with surgery.

Surgical Management of Recurrent and Metastatic Disease

Approximately one-third of patients initially diagnosed with RCC will present with metastatic disease.[179] An additional 40% of patients that present with localized disease will ultimately develop metastatic disease.[179,195] As these statistics illustrate, the biology of RCC is unique and variable and as such the treatment of patients with metastatic RCC is as well. In patients with diffuse metastatic disease, metastatectomy is not routinely used for therapeutic purposes. However, for the subset of patients who either present with or develop low-volume, radiographically solitary, or limited metastases, whether it be synchronous or metachronous, resection is often an integral part of the treatment paradigm and can confer a survival advantage.[180,196,197] Complete metastasectomy has been associated with a two-fold reduction in the risk of death from RCC.[162]

Of the approximately 30% of patients with RCC who present with metastases, only 1.5% to 3.5% have a solitary metastasis.[198]

Patients with a solitary synchronous metastatic lesion have decreased survival when compared with patients who develop metastasis after the primary tumor is removed.[199] Nevertheless, surgical resection of metastatic disease either alone or in combination with immunotherapy/targeted therapy has been shown to be curative or to confer a survival advantage compared to patients who did not undergo consolidative metastasectomy. However, these data must be interpreted in the context that only a small subset of patients will be optimal candidates for surgical extirpation of metastatic lesions. In a large series from the Mayo Clinic, 887 patients were identified with multiple metastatic sites of disease from RCC who underwent surgical resection. Of this large cohort, only 125 (14%) patients underwent a complete resection of their metastatic disease, whereas 698 (78.7%) patients had died of RCC at a median of 1.2 years after the first occurrence of their metastatic disease.[200] In this analysis, the authors demonstrated that complete surgical resection of metastatic disease, across all subgroups, was predictive of improved survival. For example, the median RCC specific and OS for patients who underwent complete metastatectomy were 4.8 and 4.0 years, respectively.[200] Comparative RCC-specific and OS rates for patients where complete surgical resection was not achieved were 1.3 and 1.3 years, respectively. Also, patients experienced an improved survival if they underwent complete surgical resection regardless of metastatic sites (lung versus nonlung, *p* <0.001), number of metastatic sites (*p* <0.001), and timing of metastatic disease—synchronous (*p* <0.001) and asynchronous (*p* = 0.002).[200] Finally, on multivariate analysis, patients in whom surgery did not achieve a complete metastasectomy were almost three times more likely to die of RCC (HR = 2.91; 95% CI = 2.17 to 3.90, *p* <0.001).[200] In this series, approximately half of the patients (45.6%) received some form of systemic therapy during their treatment course and the receipt of systemic therapy was associated with a significant improvement in survival only in patients who did not undergo complete metastasectomy, highlighting the importance of surgery in the treatment of metastatic/recurrent RCC.[200]

In patients treated with immunotherapy, there are multiple retrospective series demonstrating that patients who underwent metastasectomy had better outcomes than those who did not undergo resection of metastatic sites. In these series, 24% to 100% of patients were disease free 1 to 4 years postsurgery.[201–206] More recent data in patients who have received targeted therapies has shown similar results, albeit in small patient cohorts. In a retrospective, multi-institutional study, only 22 patients with metastatic RCC who underwent metastasectomy after targeted therapy were identified. At a median follow-up of 42 weeks after surgery, 50% of patients had experienced a tumor recurrence; however, only one patient died of RCC 105 weeks after surgery.[207]

Surgical management of recurrent and metastatic RCC plays an important role in the treatment paradigm of this group of patients and appears to confer a survival advantage in retrospective series. However, not all patients will ultimately be optimal surgical candidates and the ability to achieve a complete surgical resection is paramount in helping to guide preoperative surgical decision making.

SYSTEMIC THERAPY FOR ADVANCED RENAL CELL CARCINOMA

Prognostic Factors

Clinical characteristics have been extensively studied as potential prognostic factors in metastatic RCC. Performance status is a measure of overall well-being and is the most consistently reported factor associated with survival in advanced RCC, while other demographic features, such as age, gender, and race, are of limited value.[208–211] Some studies have found the presence of visceral (i.e., lung, liver, and adrenal), bone, and brain metastases to be associated with poor survival,[208,211,212] whereas others have found no relationship between these sites and prognosis.[210,213] A more reliable finding is the number of metastatic sites present, which provides a rough estimate of tumor burden. Most studies have found that patients with higher number of metastatic sites (more than two) are independently associated with at least two-fold greater probability of death. Similarly, patients with a short interval from initial RCC diagnosis to metastases have been found to have a worse outcome, likely as a reflection of faster-growing disease.[209,211,214,215] Those with synchronous metastases have outcomes intermediate between those with metastases developing within 1 year of diagnosis and those with asynchronous metastases that develop later.[216] Investigators have evaluated the effects of several laboratory parameters in patients with advanced RCC. Erythrocyte sedimentation rate, C-reactive protein, hemoglobin, white blood cell, and platelet parameters have been evaluated. Elevated erythrocyte sedimentation rate and C-reactive protein were consistently found to be independent poor prognostic factors.[64,214,217,218] Patients with thrombocytosis (defined as platelet counts >400,000/μL), another potential marker of inflammation, have been reported to have a negative impact on survival mostly in patients with localized RCC. Studies overall have been inconsistent in the metastatic setting, especially when other markers of inflammation were considered. Anemia has also consistently been found to be an independent prognostic factor for an adverse outcome. Patients with pretreatment hemoglobin below the lower limit of laboratory normal values were found to have twice the risk of death compared with patients with normal hemoglobin in several large studies.[210,211] The mechanism of effect of such blood parameters is unknown—whether these markers reflect an underlying inflammatory disease and/or somehow contribute to the disease process itself is unclear. Other biochemical factors that have been implicated in RCC prognosis include pretreatment serum LDH and calcium (corrected for albumin), while serum alkaline phosphatase, creatinine, gamma glutamyltransfrease, and triglycerides have not been found to have prognostic value. Corrected serum calcium >10 mg/dL and LDH >1.5 times the upper limit of normal have been associated with a two- to three-fold higher risk of death, respectively.[210,211,214]

Prognostic Schema

Using the previously identified variables, investigators have combined these variables to stratify patients into "risk groups" to predict outcome. Such schema serve to aid in individual patient counseling, stratify patients for randomized clinical trial entry, and aid in interpretation of nonrandomized clinical trials (Table 63.7). The most commonly employed schema from Memorial Sloan-Kettering Cancer Center was developed from patients treated with IFN-based regimens.[219] This schema uses Eastern Cooperative Oncology Group performance status, anemia, LDH, corrected serum calcium, and time from diagnosis to metastatic disease to segregate patients into three risk groups. This schema is still widely used today despite the limited IFN use currently and has been shown to also segregate patients treated with newer agents. More recent efforts have developed prognostic variables and risk groups based on patients treated with targeted agents. This schema uses hemoglobin, corrected calcium, performance status, and time from diagnosis to treatment, but additionally neutrophil and platelet count.[187] Both Memorial Sloan-Kettering Cancer Center and Heng criteria are used to describe patient populations treated in the targeted therapy era.

Predictive Markers

With the shift in systemic therapy for RCC to molecularly targeted agents, looking at the molecular characteristics of tumors

TABLE 63.7

Prognostic System in Metastatic Renal Cell Carcinoma

Schema	Factors	Comments
MSKCC[215]	▪ Low Karnofsky performance status ▪ High lactate dehydrogenase ▪ Low serum hemoglobin ▪ High corrected serum calcium ▪ Time from initial RCC diagnosis to start of therapy <1 y	Developed from patients with metastatic RCC patients treated with IFN-based therapy on clinical trials at MSKCC
Heng et al.[187]	▪ Low Karnofsky performance status ▪ Low serum hemoglobin ▪ High corrected serum calcium ▪ Time from initial RCC diagnosis to start of therapy <1 y ▪ Elevated neutrophils ▪ Elevated platelets	Developed from retrospective data for a global multicenter consortium of patients receiving targeted therapy for metastatic RCC

MSKCC, Memorial Sloan-Kettering Cancer Center; RCC, renal cell carcinoma; IFN, interferon.

has occurred to identify additional prognostic factors. VHL gene status has been investigated for an association with clinical outcome. Over multiple retrospective series and prospective trials, VHL status (and other VHL pathway elements, such as hypoxia-inducible factor expression) has not been consistently associated with response to vascular endothelial growth factor (VEGF)-targeted agents.[220–222] CA-IX, a member of the carbonic anhydrase family, regulates pH during hypoxia and is a product of the hypoxia inducible transcription factor (HIF) complex overexpression. The vast majority of ccRCC tumor samples stain positive for CA-IX and high CA-IX staining (>85% staining by immunohistochemical analysis) was found to be an independent favorable prognostic indicator of survival in patients with metastatic ccRCC.[223] Retrospective data initially suggested CA-IX to be potentially associated with response to high-dose interleukin (IL)-2.[224] However, the prospective SELECT trial failed to confirm this finding and thus there remain no predictive biomarkers to identify the small percentage of patients who will have a complete response to high-dose IL-2.[225] Single nucleotide polymorphisms, which are natural variations in tumor and/or germline DNA sequences, have also been investigated in relation to targeted therapy efficacy and toxicity in RCC.[226–228] While several retrospective series have found associations between single nucleotide polymorphisms associated with the VEGF pathway and/or drug metabolism with outcome, none have been consistent or robust enough to currently affect clinical practice. Finally, clinical markers, such as treatment-induced hypertension, have been explored. Several retrospective data sets have identified a strong association of treatment-induced hypertension and clinical outcome in response to VEGF-targeting agents.[229,230] This has been identified across mechanism of agent and including non-RCC diseases.[231] The precise biologic mechanism underlying this observation remains to be elucidated. In addition, this observation requires treatment of all patients initially and as a result does not spare ineffective therapy for patients who will not benefit.

Systemic Therapy

Although several active agents now exist for metastatic RCC (as discussed subsequently), they are considered noncurative for the majority of patients and thus require chronic therapy. Thus, benefits must be weighed against the toxicity, time commitment, and cost. There exists a subset of patients with metastatic RCC with low-volume slow-growing disease in which withholding systemic therapy until radiographic progression has occurred may be a reasonable approach. Further investigation into this strategy is ongoing.

Historically, progestational agents such as medroxyprogesterone acetate were investigated in metastatic RCC.[232,233] These reports documented some tumor regression and symptom reduction, largely applied to a very advanced, symptomatic population of RCC patients. Multicenter randomized trials demonstrate uniformly low response rates.[234] In the current era, progestational agents may be useful for symptom palliation, but do not appear to have any significant antitumor effects.

Due to success in other solid tumors, chemotherapy for advanced RCC has been extensively studied during the last four decades. A summary of clinical trials from 1983 to 1993 noted a 6% overall response rate in 4,093 patients with advanced RCC.[235] Another report of 51 published phase 2 clinical trials ($n = 1,347$) involving 33 chemotherapeutic agents noted an overall response rate of 5.5%.[236] Combinations of 5-fluorouracil and analogues with gemcitabine have produced modestly higher response rates, on the order of 10% to 15%.[237,238] Similarly, the addition of chemotherapy to cytokine regimens has not resulted in significant benefit over cytokines alone when investigated in phase 3 trials.[239,240] A report of 18 metastatic RCC patients with sarcomatoid histologic features and/or rapidly progressing disease treated with doxorubicin and gemcitabine noted a 28% objective response rate (ORR), potentially identifying a subset of patients with RCC where chemotherapy may have some utility.[241] Overall, chemotherapy currently has little to no role in the treatment of metastatic RCC pending further study of novel chemotherapeutic agents or combinations, or perhaps through additional patient selection efforts.

Immunotherapy

IL-2 and IFN had been the standard of care for patients with metastatic RCC until the development of targeted therapy. These agents are nonspecific cytokines that presumably have an antitumor effect through stimulation of an antitumor immune response that is not adequate in the patient prior to therapy. Specific insights into mechanism(s) of action are still lacking after decades of use and further clinical and/or molecular markers to predict benefit are lacking.

Bolus high-dose intravenous IL-2 treatment, as initially described many years ago, leads to sustained responses in a small subset of patients.[242] However, later randomized trials failed to demonstrate a benefit over lower-dose cytokine regimens for the entire cohort, likely reflecting the small number of patients benefitting.[243,244] The durable complete remissions that occur in 5% to 7% of patients, however, served as the basis for US Food and Drug Administration (FDA) approval of high-dose IL-2 in the United States in 1992.[245–247] Thus, given the noncurative nature of targeted therapy and considering only a small fraction of patients are eligible for this toxic treatment, IL-2 remains a viable treatment option for patients with ccRCC and a good performance status.

IFN (given only in low doses in RCC) has also been employed. While never approved by the FDA specifically for this indication, two large randomized trials demonstrated that IFN improved OS compared with medroxyprogesterone[234] or vinblastine.[248] IFN thus was a community standard for metastatic RCC prior to targeted therapy and served as the comparator arm in many trials. Single-agent IFN is generally no longer used. As noted in the following, IFN combined with bevacizumab is a currently approved regimen for metastatic RCC, although in practice many oncologists use bevacizumab monotherapy as the IFN likely adds some benefit, but significantly more toxicity. Multiple attempts over many decades to improve on the modest effects of IL-2 and IFN, including combinations of cytokines, combinations with chemotherapy, and cytokine sequencing, have failed.[249–252]

Investigational Immunotherapy

RCC has long been considered responsive to immune manipulation due to the modest response to cytokines noted previously. Additional efforts are ongoing to expand the application of immunotherapy. Specifically, IMA901, a vaccine composed of multiple tumor-associated peptides, has been found to be safe and to induce antitumor immunity in patients with metastatic RCC.[253] Based in part on data that sunitinib may favorably modulate the immune repertoire,[254] a phase 3 trial that randomized patients with metastatic RCC to sunitinib alone or sunitinib in combination with IMA901 has completed accrual. In addition, an autologous dendritic cell vaccine derived from primary patient tumor-specific antigens demonstrated favorable results in phase 2 studies and is currently in phase 3 testing.[255]

In addition, checkpoint inhibitors, agents that stimulate antitumor immunity by releasing the natural "brake" of the immune system, have entered clinical testing in metastatic RCC with promising initial results.[256,257] Nivolumab, which binds to programmed death receptor 1 is one such checkpoint inhibitor. A phase I expansion RCC cohort reported a 30% ORR associated with durable responses even after therapy was stopped. Additional phase II trials and a phase III registration trial are ongoing. In addition, several anti–programmed death receptor 1 agents and antibodies against its ligand, PD-L1, are being investigated in metastatic RCC.

Vascular Endothelial Growth Factor–Targeted Therapy

RCC presents a unique clinical setting for the application of antiangiogenic approaches. Through mutations in the *VHL* gene and/or other genetic events that result in the deregulated expression of the hypoxia inducible transcription factors, HIF-1α and/or HIF-2α, a large cohort of hypoxia-responsive genes is induced, including VEGF as one of the classic transcriptional targets.[258] There is a direct link between *VHL* mutation and upregulation of angiogenesis-promoting proteins, including VEGF and platelet-derived growth factor (PDGF). Thus, increased expression of these proteins and the consequences of that increased expression are central events in the development of most RCC tumors. VEGF is the major factor responsible for tumor angiogenesis. Several treatment strategies have thus been investigated in metastatic RCC to block components of the angiogenic signaling pathway components, such as VEGF.

Sunitinib

Sunitinib (Sutent, Pfizer Inc., New York, NY) is an oral drug with in vitro and cellular inhibitory activity against several related protein tyrosine kinase receptors, including PDGF-receptor-beta, stem cell factor receptor (KIT), and Fms-like tyrosine kinase-3 (FLT-3), as well as VEGF receptors 1, 2, and 3.[259,260] Sunitinib was initially studied in metastatic RCC in two sequential phase 2 trials in cytokine-refractory patients that demonstrated an ORR of approximately 40% with a combined median PFS of 8.2 months (Table 63.8).[261,262] The most common adverse events with sunitinib are fatigue, diarrhea, mucositis, hand-foot syndrome, and hypertension. A phase 3 randomized trial of first-line sunitinib versus IFN-alfa in 750 patients with metastatic ccRCC showed statistically significant improvements in ORR and PFS with sunitinib compared with IFN. Median PFS as assessed by an

TABLE 63.8

TABLE 63.8

Summary of Target Agents in Metastatic Renal Cell Carcinoma

Treatment	Response Rate	Progression-Free Survival	Overall Survival
VEGF Receptor Inhibitors			
Sunitinib	30% to 47%	9.5 to 11 mo in treatment-naïve patients 8.4 mo in cytokine refractory patients	29.3 mo in untreated patients
Pazopanib	30%	8.4 to 9.2 mo (11.1 mo in treatment-naïve patients)	28.4 mo in untreated patients
Sorafenib	2% to 10%	5.7 to 9 mo in treatment-naïve patients 5.5 mo in treatment-refractory patients	17.8 to 19.2 mo in treatment-refractory patients
Axitinib	19%	6.7 mo (second-line)	20.1 mo in treatment-refractory patients
VEGF Ligand-Binding Agents			
Bevacizumab	10% to 13% as monotherapy 26% to 31% in combination with IFNA	8.5 mo in treatment-naïve patients as monotherapy 8.5 to 10.2 mo in treatment-naïve patients in combination with IFNA 4.8 mo in cytokine-refractory patients	18.3 to 23.3 mo
mTOR-Inhibiting Agents			
Temsirolimus	7% to 9%	3.7 mo (vs. 1.9 mo for IFNA monotherapy; $p = 0.0001$) in treatment-naïve patients 5.8 mo in treatment-refractory patients	10.9 mo (vs. 7.3 mo for IFNA; $p = 0.008$)
Everolimus	1%	4.9 mo (vs. 1.9 mo for placebo-treated patients) in refractory patients	14.8 mo (vs. 14.4 mo for placebo-treated patients; $p = 0.177$)

VEGF, vascular endothelial growth factor; IFNA, interferon-alfa; mTOR, mammalian target of rapamycin.

independent review was 11 months in the sunitinib arm versus 5 months in the IFN arm, and ORR was 31% versus 6%, respectively ($p < 0.000001$; see Table 63.8).[263] Median OS was 26.4 months for sunitinib versus 21.8 months for IFN ($p = 0.051$).[264] The OS data are a reflection of not only sunitinib activity, but several other active drugs that patients received upon progression, resulting in notably prolonged median survival times compared to historical controls. Sunitinib was approved by the FDA as monotherapy for advanced RCC in January 2006 and remains an initial standard of care in metastatic RCC.

Pazopanib

Pazopanib is an oral multitargeted tyrosine kinase inhibitor that targets VEGF receptors 1 to 3, PDGF receptor, and c-kit. A phase 2 study initially designed as a randomized discontinuation study was revised to an open-label study based on the response rate of a planned interim analysis. This study evaluated 255 patients with metastatic RCC who received pazopanib 800 mg once daily; 69% had no prior treatment and 31% had received one prior treatment. The overall response rate was 35%, the median PFS was 52 weeks, and the median duration of response was 68 weeks. The main adverse effects were diarrhea and fatigue, and the most common grade 3-4 side effect was hypertension. Alanine transaminase and aspartate transaminase elevation occurred in 54% of patients. In October 2009, the FDA approved pazopanib for the treatment of metastatic RCC, based on the results of a phase 3 trial. This study evaluated 435 patients with advanced ccRCC with either no previous treatment or with one prior cytokine treatment. Patients were randomized (2:1) to receive pazopanib 800 mg daily or placebo. The response rate for patients treated with pazopanib was 30% and the median duration of response was 58.7 weeks. Median PFS was 9.2 months in the pazopanib group and 4.2 months in the placebo group (HR = 0.46; $p <0.0001$; see Table 63.8). PFS was prolonged in both treatment naïve patients (11.1 months versus 2.8 months;

$p <0.0001$) and in cytokine-pretreated patients (7.4 months versus 4.2 months; $p <0.001$).

Pazopanib has been further studied in a noninferiority study compared to sunitinib in the front-line treatment of metastatic RCC (COMPARZ study).[265] Over 1,100 patients with previously untreated ccRCC were randomized to either pazopanib or sunitinib (1:1) in a noninferiority design. Median PFS was 9.5 months with sunitinib and 8.4 months with pazopanib, with a hazard ratio of 1.047 (95% CI = 0.898 to 1.220). The upper bound of the confidence interval was <1.25, satisfying the predefined boundary for noninferiority. OS was approximately 29 months in both arms. Certain toxicities were more common with sunitinib including fatigue and hand-foot syndrome, while pazopanib produced greater hepatic abnormalities. This trial demonstrated that both sunitinib and pazopanib are appropriate front-line treatment options in metastatic RCC and that a differing toxicity profile may allow the physician to tailor therapy to each individual patient.

Sorafenib

Sorafenib (Nexavar, Bayer Pharmaceuticals and Onyx, Leverkusen, Germany) is an oral multikinase inhibitor that inhibits VEGF receptors 1 to 3, PDGF-receptor-beta, and the serine threonine kinase Raf-1, which acts through the RAF/MEK/ERK signaling pathway and plays a role in cellular proliferation and tumorigenesis.[266,267] In an initial sorafenib trial, metastatic RCC patients ($n = 202$) were treated with 12 weeks of continuous oral sorafenib 400 mg bid and patients with tumor burden increase or decrease within 25% of baseline were randomized to placebo or to continuation of sorafenib. A PFS advantage of 24 versus 6 weeks ($p = 0.0087$) was demonstrated in the randomized cohort of 65 patients at 12 weeks postrandomization.[268] A subsequent 905 patient, placebo-controlled, randomized trial of sorafenib 400 mg bid in treatment-refractory, metastatic RCC reported a PFS advantage in the sorafenib arm of 5.5 months versus 2.8 months for placebo (p <0.000001; see Table 63.8). A 2% RECIST-defined ORR was seen in the sorafenib arm, but 74% of patients overall had some degree of tumor burden shrinkage thus accounting for the PFS benefit. The median OS was 19.3 months for patients in the sorafenib group and 15.9 months for patients in the placebo group (HR = 0.77; 95% CI = 0.63 to 0.95; p = 0.02), which did not reach prespecified statistical boundaries for significance.[269] Common toxicity in the sorafenib trials has included dermatologic (hand-foot syndrome), fatigue, diarrhea, and hypertension. Sorafenib was approved by the FDA as monotherapy for advanced RCC in December 2005. A randomized phase 2 trial of sorafenib versus IFN in untreated metastatic RCC failed to demonstrate a difference in median PFS between the two treatment arms.[270] Sorafenib has thus assumed a small, salvage role in the treatment of metastatic RCC.

Bevacizumab

Bevacizumab (Avastin, Genentech, South San Francisco, CA) is a monoclonal antibody that binds and neutralizes circulating VEGF protein.[271] The activity of this agent in RCC was initially identified by small randomized trials.[272,273] Two phase 3 trials were subsequently reported and led to FDA approval of bevacizumab plus IFN for advanced RCC. One phase 3 trial randomized 649 untreated patients with metastatic RCC to treatment with IFN (Roferon, Roche, Basel, Switzerland) plus placebo infusion or to IFN plus bevacizumab infusion 10 mg/kg every 2 weeks.[274] A significant advantage for bevacizumab plus IFN was observed for ORR (31% versus 13%, p <0.0001) and PFS (10.2 months versus 5.4 months, p <0.0001; see Table 63.8). A second multicenter phase 3 trial, conducted in the United States and Canada through the Cancer and Leukemia Group B, was nearly identical in design with the exception of lacking a placebo infusion and not requiring prior nephrectomy.[275] In this trial, the median PFS was 8.5 months in patients receiving bevacizumab plus IFN (95% CI = 7.5 to 9.7) versus 5.2 months (95% CI = 3.1 to 5.6) for IFN monotherapy (p <0.0001; see Table 63.8). Also, among patients with measurable disease, the ORR was higher in patients treated with bevacizumab plus IFN (25.5%) than for IFN monotherapy (13.1%; p <0.0001). OS data are similar to the other agents with a numerical advantage in median survival not meeting statistical significance, reflecting the large proportion of patents who receive subsequent active therapy. The contribution of IFN to the antitumor effect of this regimen is unclear at present, although preliminary results indicate a longer PFS and higher response rate than expected with bevacizumab monotherapy.[272] Combination IFN and bevacizumab therapy is more toxic than either as monotherapy, notable for fatigue, anorexia, hypertension, and proteinuria. Thus, the use of IFN with bevacizumab requires evaluation of the risk/benefit ratio for each patient.

Axitinib

Axitinib is a potent VEGF receptor family inhibitor studied in several setting in metastatic RCC. Initial studies in cytokine- and sorafenib-refractory patients demonstrated objective responses and disease control, which prompted further development.[276,277] The phase 3 AXIS trial randomized 723 patients with metastatic RCC (refractory to either sunitinib, cytokines, bevacizumab, or temsirolimus) to axitinib or sorafenib.[278] The median PFS was 6.7 months for axitinib versus 4.7 months for sorafenib (HR for disease progression or death of 0.665 [95% CI = 0.544 to 0.812]; p <0.0001). ORR was 19.4% versus 9.4% with axitinib and sorafenib, respectively. This trial resulted in FDA approval of axitinib for previously treated metastatic RCC. A separate trial examined axitinib versus sorafenib in the front-line setting.[279] Despite a numerical advantage for PFS for axitinib, this trial did not meet its stringent predefined efficacy endpoint, and thus axitinib is largely used in the second-line setting in RCC.

Mammalian Target of Rapamycin–Targeted Therapy

Temsirolimus

Temsirolimus is an inhibitor of mTOR, a molecule implicated in multiple tumor-promoting intracellular signaling pathways, including regulation of transcription factors involved in VEGF expression, such as HIF.[280] A phase 2 trial in patients with treatment-refractory, metastatic RCC randomized 111 patients to temsirolimus at one of multiple dose levels (25 mg, 75 mg, or 250 mg intravenously weekly).[281] The ORR was 7% with additional patients demonstrating minor responses (see Table 63.8). Retrospective assignment of risk criteria to patients in this study identified a poor-prognosis group with a median OS of 8.2 months compared to 4.9 months for historical IFN-treated patients.[215] Loss of phosphatase and tensin homolog and/or activation of Akt (upstream regulators of the mTOR expression) may be more common in poor-risk patients and thereby potentially increase the relevance of mTOR-targeted therapy in this subgroup.

A subsequent randomized phase 3 trial was conducted in patients with metastatic RCC (n = 626) and three or more adverse risk features as defined by existing prognostic schema (see Table 63.7).[211,215] Patients were randomized equally to receive IFN (18 million units subcutaneously) three times a week, temsirolimus 25 mg intravenously weekly, or temsirolimus 15 mg intravenously weekly and IFN (6 million units subcutaneously) three times a week. The primary study endpoint was OS and the study was powered to compare each of the temsirolimus arms to the IFN arm. Both temsirolimus-containing arms demonstrated a PFS advantage versus IFN (3.7 months for each arm versus 1.9 months; p = 0.0001 for temsirolimus monotherapy and p = 0.0019 for temsirolimus plus IFN). Patients treated with temsirolimus monotherapy had a statistically longer survival than those treated with IFN alone (10.9 months versus 7.3 months, p = 0.0069). OS of patients treated with IFN and temsirolimus + IFN were not statistically different (7.3 months versus 8.4 months, p = 0.6912). Even though temsirolimus has demonstrated activity in poor-risk RCC, it is not clear that this agent has more activity than the VEGF-targeted agents in this subset, as VEGF-targeted agents have shown activity, albeit in limited subsets, in poor-risk patients.

Everolimus

Everolimus is an oral rapamycin analogue that inhibits mTOR. A phase 3 study evaluated 410 patients previously treated with sorafenib, sunitinib, or both who were randomized (2:1) to receive everolimus 10 mg once daily or placebo.[282] PFS was significantly longer in the everolimus group (HR = 0.30, 95% CI = 0.22 to 0.40; p <0.0001). Median PFS in the everolimus group was 4.9 months versus 1.9 months in the placebo group. Partial response in the everolimus group occurred in 1% of the patients, and 63% (versus 32% in the placebo group) had disease stabilization for at least 56 days. Most common adverse effects of everolimus were stomatitis, rash, fatigue, asthenia, and diarrhea. Stomatitis, fatigue, infection, and pneumonitis were the most common grade 3/4 toxicities. On the basis of these results, everolimus was approved for the treatment of metastatic RCC refractory to sunitinib and/or sorafenib.

A recent trial (RECORD-3) randomized 471 patients with previously untreated metastatic RCC to either sunitinib or everolimus, with crossover at progression.[283] This trial, reported to date only in abstract form, demonstrated an advantage to sunitinib in response rate (27% versus 8%), PFS (10.7 months versus 7.9 months), and OS (32 months versus 22 months). In addition, all subsets examined (non–clear cell, clear cell, and prognostic groups) favored sunitinib. These data support the use of everolimus only in a refractory setting and confirm a hypothesis that VEGF targeting is a superior initial strategy for RCC therapy.

PRACTICE OF ONCOLOGY

Second-Line Therapy

As noted previously, axitinib has been studied and FDA-approved as second-line therapy in metastatic RCC with a PFS advantage over sorafenib. Still debated is the role of everolimus versus a VEGF agent in this setting. The INTORSECT trial randomized patients with metastatic RCC refractory to prior sunitinib to receive either temsirolimus or sorafenib.[254] Although there was no significant difference in PFS (approximately 4 months in both arms), an OS advantage to sorafenib was observed. These data lend support to the hypothesis that continued VEGF targeting is of benefit in metastatic RCC, although no PFS advantage was demonstrated and the mTOR inhibitor used in this trial had not been specifically shown to have benefits in this setting.

Current Status of Systemic Therapy in Metastatic Renal Cell Carcinoma

Of note, several trials have been conducted attempting to combine the targeted therapies discussed previously. None have demonstrated an advantage over monotherapy, in large part due to excessive toxicity in the combination arms.[285,286] Sunitinib and pazopanib are the most commonly used front-line agents based in large part on the COMPARZ efficacy data as well as their tolerability and oral formulation. There is no proven sequence of agents or ability to predict response to any given agent, and thus the current standard of care is an empiric sequence of targeted therapy monotherapy, notwithstanding the select patient who initially receives high-dose IL-2.

CONCLUSION AND FUTURE DIRECTIONS

The last 20 years have seen a tremendous increase in our understanding of the tumor biology of the heterogeneous tumors within the family of renal cancers. Insights beginning with the clinical observation of the hypervascularity of these tumors, continuing with rigorous scientific investigation of familial cases of RCC, and culminating in the development of treatments based on the VEGF pathway, have made the last decade a rich period of expansion in treatment options for RCC. With increasing availability of next generation sequencing, the potential for subsequent discoveries to advance our understanding of and therapies for this often lethal malignancy remains considerable. Through multidisciplinary explorations of these fascinating neoplasms, renal cancer can continue to pace oncologic discoveries for the next 20 years as well.

ACKNOWLEDGMENTS

The authors would like to thank Sabrina Noyes for administrative support and technical editing.

SELECTED REFERENCES

The full reference list can be accessed at lwwhealthlibrary.com/oncology.

2. Siegel R, Naishadham D, Jemal A. Cancer statistics, 2013. *CA Cancer J Clin* 2013;63:11–30.
3. Lipsky MJ, Deibert CM, McKiernan JM. Epidemiology, screening, and clinical staging. In: Libertino JA, ed. *Renal Cancer: Contemporary Management.* New York: Springer Science + Business Media; 2013:1–18.
9. Ljungberg B, Campbell SC, Cho HY, et al. The epidemiology of renal cell carcinoma. *Eur Urol* 2011;60:615–621.
16. Algaba F, Akaza H, Lopez-Beltran A, et al. Current pathology keys of renal cell carcinoma. *Eur Urol* 2011;60:634–643.
17. Deng F-M, Melamed J, Zhou M. Pathology of renal cell carcinoma. In: Libertino JA, ed. *Renal Cancer: Contemporary Management.* New York: Springer Science + Business Media; 2013:51–69.
20. Kang SK, Chandarana H. Contemporary imaging of the renal mass. *Urol Clin North Am* 2012;39:161–170.
21. Divgi CR, Uzzo RG, Gatsonis C, et al. Positron emission tomography/computed tomography identification of clear cell renal cell carcinoma: results from the REDECT trial. *J Clin Oncol* 2013;31:187–194.
22. Bosniak MA. The Bosniak renal cyst classification: 25 years later. *Radiology* 2012;262:781–785.
23. Corcoran AT, Russo P, Lowrance WT, et al. A review of contemporary data on surgically resected renal masses—benign or malignant? *Urology* 2013;81:707–713.
24. Lane BR, Babineau D, Kattan MW, et al. A preoperative prognostic nomogram for solid enhancing renal tumors 7 cm or less amenable to partial nephrectomy. *J Urol* 2007;178:429–434.
27. Frank I, Blute ML, Cheville JC, et al. Solid renal tumors: an analysis of pathological features related to tumor size. *J Urol* 2003;170:2217–2220.
28. Kutikov A, Smaldone MC, Egleston BL, et al. Anatomic features of enhancing renal masses predict malignant and high-grade pathology: a preoperative nomogram using the RENAL Nephrometry score. *Eur Urol* 2011;60:241–248.
31. Samplaski MK, Zhou M, Lane BR, et al. Renal mass sampling: an enlightened perspective. *Int J Urol* 2011;18:5–19.
34. Volpe A, Finelli A, Gill IS, et al. Rationale for percutaneous biopsy and histologic characterisation of renal tumours. *Eur Urol* 2012;62:491–504.
35. Edge SB, Byrd DR, Compton CC. *AJCC Cancer Staging Manual.* Vol 7. New York, NY: Springer; 2010.
36. Meskawi M, Sun M, Trinh QD, et al. A review of integrated staging systems for renal cell carcinoma. *Eur Urol* 2012;62:303–314.
38. Linehan WM, Ricketts CJ. The metabolic basis of kidney cancer. *Semin Cancer Biol* 2013;23:46–55.
40. Keefe SM, Nathanson KL, Rathmell WK. The molecular biology of renal cell carcinoma. *Semin Oncol* 2013;40:421–428.
41. Jonasch E, Futreal PA, Davis IJ, et al. State of the science: an update on renal cell carcinoma. *Mol Cancer Res* 2012;10:859–880.

42. Klomp J, Dykema K, Teh BT, et al. Molecular biology and genetics. In: Libertino JA, ed. *Renal Cancer: Contemporary Management.* New York: Springer Science + Business Media; 2013:19–37.
44. Cancer Genome Atlas Research Network. Comprehensive molecular characterization of clear cell renal cell carcinoma. *Nature* 2013;499:43–49.
46. Shuch B, Singer EA, Bratslavsky G. The surgical approach to multifocal renal cancers: hereditary syndromes, ipsilateral multifocality, and bilateral tumors. *Urol Clin North Am* 2012;39:133–148, v.
53. Campbell SC, Thomas AA, Rini BI, et al. Response of the primary tumor to neoadjuvant sunitinib in patients with advanced renal cell carcinoma. *J Urol* 2009;181:518–523.
55. Kunkle DA, Chen DYT, Greenberg RE, et al. Metastatic progression of enhancing renal masses under active surveillance is associated with rapid interval growth of the primary tumor. *J Urol* 2008;179(4 Suppl):375.
58. Russo P, Huang W. The medical and oncological rationale for partial nephrectomy for the treatment of T1 renal cortical tumors. *Urol Clin North Am* 2008;35:635–643; vii.
59. Van Poppel H, Da Pozzo L, Albrecht W, et al. A prospective, randomised EORTC intergroup phase 3 study comparing the oncologic outcome of elective nephron-sparing surgery and radical nephrectomy for low-stage renal cell carcinoma. *Eur Urol* 2011;59:543–552.
60. Tan HJ, Norton EC, Ye Z, et al. Long-term survival following partial vs radical nephrectomy among older patients with early-stage kidney cancer. *JAMA* 2012;307:1629–1635.
61. Tobert CM, Riedinger CB, Lane BR. Do we know (or just believe) that partial nephrectomy leads to better survival than radical nephrectomy for renal cancer? *World J Urol* 2014 (Epub ahead of print).
62. Kim SP, Thompson RH, Boorjian SA, et al. Comparative effectiveness for survival and renal function of partial and radical nephrectomy for localized renal tumors: a systematic review and meta-analysis. *J Urol* 2012;188:51–57.
65. Ljungberg B, Cowan NC, Hanbury DC, et al. EAU guidelines on renal cell carcinoma: the 2010 update. *Eur Urol* 2010;58:398–406.
67. Campbell SC, Novick AC, Belldegrun A, et al. Guideline for management of the clinical T1 renal mass. *J Urol* 2009;182:1271–1279.
70. Thompson RH, Blute ML, Krambeck AE, et al. Patients with pT1 renal cell carcinoma who die from disease after nephrectomy may have unrecognized renal sinus fat invasion. *Am J Surg Pathol* 2007;31:1089–1093.
71. Bratslavsky G, Linehan WM. Surgery: Routine adrenalectomy in renal cancer—an antiquated practice. *Nat Rev Urol* 2011;8:534–536.
72. Lane BR, Tiong HY, Campbell SC, et al. Management of the adrenal gland during partial nephrectomy. *J Urol* 2009;181:2430–2437.
74. Blom JH, van Poppel H, Marechal JM, et al. Radical nephrectomy with and without lymph-node dissection: final results of European Organization for Research and Treatment of Cancer (EORTC) randomized phase 3 trial 30881. *Eur Urol* 2009;55:28–34.

75. Leibovich BC, Blute ML. Lymph node dissection in the management of renal cell carcinoma. *Urol Clin North Am* 2008;35:673–678; viii.

77. Phillips CK, Taneja SS. The role of lymphadenectomy in the surgical management of renal cell carcinoma. *Urol Oncol* 2004;22:214–224.

78. Nguyen CT, Campbell SC. Salvage of local recurrence after primary thermal ablation for small renal masses. *Expert Rev Anticancer Ther* 2008;8:1899–1905.

85. Huang WC, Levey AS, Serio AM, et al. Chronic kidney disease after nephrectomy in patients with renal cortical tumours: a retrospective cohort study. *Lancet Oncol* 2006;7:735–740.

86. Lane BR, Russo P, Uzzo RG, et al. Comparison of cold and warm ischemia during partial nephrectomy in 660 solitary kidneys reveals predominant role of nonmodifiable factors in determining ultimate renal function. *J Urol* 2011;185:421–427.

87. Go AS, Chertow GM, Fan D, et al. Chronic kidney disease and the risks of death, cardiovascular events, and hospitalization. *N Engl J Med* 2004;351: 1296–1305.

95. Uzzo RG, Novick AC. Nephron sparing surgery for renal tumors: indications, techniques and outcomes. *J Urol* 2001;166:6–18.

101. Lane BR, Golan S, Eggener S, et al. Differential use of partial nephrectomy for intermediate and high complexity tumors may explain variability in reported utilization rates. *J Urol* 2013;189:2047–2053.

103. Fergany AF, Hafez KS, Novick AC. Long-term results of nephron sparing surgery for localized renal cell carcinoma: 10-year followup. *J Urol* 2000;163:442.

104. Lane BR, Campbell SC, Gill IS. Ten-year oncologic outcomes after laparoscopic and open partial nephrectomy. *J Urol* 2013;190:44–49.

105. Lane BR, Fergany AF, Weight CJ, et al. Renal functional outcomes after partial nephrectomy with extended ischemic intervals are better than after radical nephrectomy. *J Urol* 2010;184:1286–1290.

106. Fergany AF, Saad IR, Woo L, et al. Open partial nephrectomy for tumor in a solitary kidney: experience with 400 cases. *J Urol* 2006;175:1630–1633.

111. Lane BR, Derweesh IH, Kim HL, et al. Presurgical sunitinib reduces tumor size and may facilitate partial nephrectomy in patients with renal cell carcinoma. *Urology* (In press).

115. Marszalek M, Carini M, Chlosta P, et al. Positive surgical margins after nephron-sparing surgery. *Eur Urol* 2012;61:757–763.

119. Gill IS, Kavoussi LR, Lane BR, et al. Comparison of 1,800 laparoscopic and open partial nephrectomies for single renal tumors. *J Urol* 2007;178:41–46.

120. Dulabon LM, Kaouk JH, Haber GP, et al. Multi-institutional analysis of robotic partial nephrectomy for hilar versus nonhilar lesions in 446 consecutive cases. *Eur Urol* 2011;59:325–330.

123. Kaouk JH, Khalifeh A, Hillyer S, et al. Robot-assisted laparoscopic partial nephrectomy: step-by-step contemporary technique and surgical outcomes at a single high-volume institution. *Eur Urol* 2012;62:553–561.

124. Mullins JK, Feng T, Pierorazio PM, et al. Comparative analysis of minimally invasive partial nephrectomy techniques in the treatment of localized renal tumors. *Urology* 2012;80:316–321.

130. Faddegon S, Cadeddu JA. Does renal mass ablation provide adequate long-term oncologic control? *Urol Clin North Am* 2012;39:181–190.

132. Atwell TD, Schmit GD, Boorjian SA, et al. Percutaneous ablation of renal masses measuring 3.0 cm and smaller: comparative local control and complications after radiofrequency ablation and cryoablation. *AJR Am J Roentgenol* 2013;200:461–466.

133. Tracy CR, Raman JD, Donnally C, et al. Durable oncologic outcomes after radiofrequency ablation: experience from treating 243 small renal masses over 7.5 years. *Cancer* 2010;116:3135–3142.

142. Weight CJ, Kaouk JH, Hegarty NJ, et al. Correlation of radiographic imaging and histopathology following cryoablation and radio frequency ablation for renal tumors. *J Urol* 2008;179:1277–1281.

143. Donat SM, Diaz M, Bishoff JT, et al. Follow-up for clinically localized renal neoplasms: AUA guideline. *J Urol* 2013;190:407–416.

154. Corcoran AT, Russo P, Lowrance WT, et al. A review of contemporary data on surgically resected renal masses—benign or malignant? *Urology* 2013; 81:707–713.

155. Smaldone MC, Kutikov A, Egleston BL, et al. Small renal masses progressing to metastases under active surveillance: a systematic review and pooled analysis. *Cancer* 2012;118:997–1006.

164. Blute ML, Leibovich BC, Cheville JC, et al. A protocol for performing extended lymph node dissection using primary tumor pathological features for patients treated with radical nephrectomy for clear cell renal cell carcinoma. *J Urol* 2004;172:465–469.

165. Libertino JA, Zinman L, Watkins E Jr. Long-term results of resection of renal cell cancer with extension into inferior vena cava. *J Urol* 1987;137:21–24.

170. Kutikov A, Uzzo RG. The R.E.N.A.L. nephrometry score: a comprehensive standardized system for quantitating renal tumor size, location and depth. *J Urol* 2009;182:844–853.

173. Ciancio G, Gonzalez J, Shirodkar SP, et al. Liver transplantation techniques for the surgical management of renal cell carcinoma with tumor thrombus in the inferior vena cava: step-by-step description. *Eur Urol* 2011;59:401–406.

175. Culp SH, Tannir NM, Abel EJ, et al. Can we better select patients with metastatic renal cell carcinoma for cytoreductive nephrectomy? *Cancer* 2010;116:3378–3388.

176. Margulis V, Master VA, Cost NG, et al. International consultation on urologic diseases and the European Association of Urology international consultation on locally advanced renal cell carcinoma. *Eur Urol* 2011;60:673–683.

177. Crispen PL, Breau RH, Allmer C, et al. Lymph node dissection at the time of radical nephrectomy for high-risk clear cell renal cell carcinoma: indications and recommendations for surgical templates. *Eur Urol* 2011;59:18–23.

180. Motzer RJ, Agarwal N, Beard C, et al. Kidney cancer. *J Natl Compr Canc Netw* 2011;9:960–977.

181. Flanigan RC, Salmon SE, Blumenstein BA, et al. Nephrectomy followed by interferon alfa-2b compared with interferon alfa-2b alone for metastatic renal-cell cancer. *N Engl J Med* 2001;345:1655–1659.

183. Mickisch GH, Garin A, van Poppel H, et al. Radical nephrectomy plus interferon-alfa-based immunotherapy compared with interferon alfa alone in metastatic renal-cell carcinoma: a randomised trial. *Lancet* 2001;358:966–970.

186. Choueiri TK, Xie W, Kollmannsberger C, et al. The impact of cytoreductive nephrectomy on survival of patients with metastatic renal cell carcinoma receiving vascular endothelial growth factor targeted therapy. *J Urol* 2011;185:60–66.

187. Heng DY, Xie W, Regan MM, et al. Prognostic factors for overall survival in patients with metastatic renal cell carcinoma treated with vascular endothelial growth factor-targeted agents: Results From a large, multicenter study. *J Clin Oncol* 2009;27:5794–5799.

191. Hudes G, Carducci M, Tomczak P, et al. Temsirolimus, interferon alfa, or both for advanced renal-cell carcinoma. *N Engl J Med* 2007;356:2271–2281.

193. Trinh QD, Bianchi M, Hansen J, et al. In-hospital mortality and failure to rescue after cytoreductive nephrectomy. *Eur Urol* 2013;63:1107–1114.

196. Eggener SE, Yossepowitch O, Kundu S, et al. Risk score and metastasectomy independently impact prognosis of patients with recurrent renal cell carcinoma. *J Urol* 2008;180:873–878; discussion 878.

200. Alt AL, Boorjian SA, Lohse CM, et al. Survival after complete surgical resection of multiple metastases from renal cell carcinoma. *Cancer* 2011;117: 2873–2882.

207. Karam JA, Rini BI, Varella L, et al. Metastasectomy after targeted therapy in patients with advanced renal cell carcinoma. *J Urol* 2011;185:439–444.

210. Motzer RJ, Mazumdar M, Bacik J, et al. Survival and prognostic stratification of 670 patients with advanced renal cell carcinoma. *J Clin Oncol* 1999;17:2530–2540.

211. Mekhail TM, Abou-Jawde RM, Boumerhi G, et al. Validation and extension of the Memorial Sloan-Kettering prognostic factors model for survival in patients with previously untreated metastatic renal cell carcinoma. *J Clin Oncol* 2005;23:832–841.

216. Leibovich BC, Blute ML, Cheville JC, et al. Prediction of progression after radical nephrectomy for patients with clear cell renal cell carcinoma: a stratification tool for prospective clinical trials. *Cancer* 2003;97:1663–1671.

230. Rini BI, Cohen DP, Lu DR, et al. Hypertension as a biomarker of efficacy in patients with metastatic renal cell carcinoma treated with sunitinib. *J Natl Cancer Inst* 2011;103:763–773.

234. Interferon-alpha and survival in metastatic renal carcinoma: early results of a randomised controlled trial. Medical Research Council Renal Cancer Collaborators. *Lancet* 1999;353:14–17.

242. Rosenberg SA, Lotze MT, Muul LM, et al. Observations on the systemic administration of autologous lymphokine-activated killer cells and recombinant interleukin-2 to patients with metastatic cancer. *N Engl J Med* 1985;313: 1485–1492.

243. McDermott DF, Regan MM, Clark JI, et al. Randomized phase III trial of high-dose interleukin-2 versus subcutaneous interleukin-2 and interferon in patients with metastatic renal cell carcinoma. *J Clin Oncol* 2005;23: 133–141.

249. Negrier S, Escudier B, Lasset C, et al. Recombinant human interleukin-2, recombinant human interferon alfa-2a, or both in metastatic renal-cell carcinoma. Groupe Francais d'Immunotherapie. *N Engl J Med* 1998;338: 1272–1278.

253. Walter S, Weinschenk T, Stenzl A, et al. Multipeptide immune response to cancer vaccine IMA901 after single-dose cyclophosphamide associates with longer patient survival. *Nat Med* 2012;18:1254–1261.

254. Finke JH, Rini B, Ireland J, et al. Sunitinib reverses type-1 immune suppression and decreases T-regulatory cells in renal cell carcinoma patients. *Clin Cancer Res* 2008;14:6674–6682.

256. McDermott DF, Drake CG, Sznol M, et al. Clinical activity and safety of anti-PD-1 (BMS-936558, MDX-1106) in patients with previously treated metastatic renal cell carcinoma (mRCC). *J Clin Oncol* 2012;30(15 Suppl):4505.

258. Shweiki D, Itin A, Soffer D, et al. Vascular endothelial growth factor induced by hypoxia may mediate hypoxia-initiated angiogenesis. *Nature* 1992;359: 843–845.

260. Mendel DB, Laird AD, Xin X, et al. In vivo antitumor activity of SU11248, a novel tyrosine kinase inhibitor targeting vascular endothelial growth factor and platelet-derived growth factor receptors: determination of a pharmacokinetic/pharmacodynamic relationship. *Clin Cancer Res* 2003;9:327–337.

263. Motzer RJ, Hutson TE, Tomczak P, et al. Sunitinib versus interferon alfa in metastatic renal-cell carcinoma. *N Engl J Med* 2007;356:115–124.

265. Motzer RJ, Hutson TE, Cella D, et al. Pazopanib versus sunitinib in metastatic renal-cell carcinoma. *N Engl J Med* 2013;369:722–731.

270. Escudier B, Eisen T, Stadler WM, et al. Sorafenib in advanced clear-cell renal-cell carcinoma. *N Engl J Med* 2007;356:125–134.

272. Bukowski RM, Kabbinavar FF, Figlin RA, et al. Randomized phase II study of erlotinib combined with bevacizumab compared with bevacizumab alone in metastatic renal cell cancer. *J Clin Oncol* 2007;25:4536–4541.

PRACTICE OF ONCOLOGY

273. Yang JC, Haworth L, Sherry RM, et al. A randomized trial of bevacizumab, an anti-vascular endothelial growth factor antibody, for metastatic renal cancer. *N Engl J Med* 2003;349:427–434.

274. Escudier B, Pluzanska A, Koralewski P, et al. Bevacizumab plus interferon alfa-2a for treatment of metastatic renal cell carcinoma: a randomised, double-blind phase III trial. *Lancet* 2007;370:2103–2111.

277. Rixe O, Bukowski RM, Michaelson MD, et al. Axitinib treatment in patients with cytokine-refractory metastatic renal-cell cancer: a phase II study. *Lancet Oncol* 2007;8:975–984.

278. Rini BI, Escudier B, Tomczak P, et al. Comparative effectiveness of axitinib versus sorafenib in advanced renal cell carcinoma (AXIS): a randomised phase 3 trial. *Lancet* 2011;378:1931–1939.

279. Hutson TE, Lesovoy V, Al-Shukri S, et al. Axitinib versus sorafenib as first-line therapy in patients with metastatic renal-cell carcinoma: a randomised open-label phase 3 trial. *Lancet Oncol* 2013;14:1287–1294.

280. Barthelemy P, Hoch B, Chevreau C, et al. mTOR inhibitors in advanced renal cell carcinomas: From biology to clinical practice. *Crit Rev Oncol Hematol* 2013;88:42–56.

282. Motzer RJ, Bukowski RM, Figlin RA, et al. Prognostic nomogram for sunitinib in patients with metastatic renal cell carcinoma. *Cancer* 2008;113: 1552–1558.

283. Motzer RJ, Barrios CH, Kim TM, et al. Record-3: Phase II randomized trial comparing sequential first-line everolimus (EVE) and second-line sunitinib (SUN) versus first-line SUN and second-line EVE in patients with metastatic renal cell carcinoma (mRCC). *J Clin Oncol* 2013;31: abstr 4504.

284. Hutson TE, Escudier B, Esteban E, et al. Randomized phase III trial of temsirolimus versus sorafenib as second-line therapy after sunitinib in patients with metastatic renal cell carcinoma. *J Clin Oncol* 2014;32:760–767.

286. Ravaud A, Barrios CH, Anak Ö, et al. Randomized phase II study of first-line everolimus (EVE) + bevacizumab (BEV) versus interferon alfa-2A (IFN) + BEV in patients (PTS) with metastatic renal cell carcinoma (MRCC): record-2. Abstract #7830. *Ann Oncol* 2012;23:ixe1–ixe30.

287. Weight CJ, Miller DC, Campbell SC, et al. The management of a clinical T1b renal tumor in the presence of a normal contralateral kidney: the case for nephron sparing surgery. *J Urol* 2013;189:1198–1202.

64 Molecular Biology of Bladder Cancer

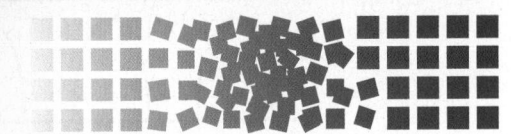

Margaret A. Knowles and Carolyn D. Hurst

INTRODUCTION

There has been rapid progress in elucidating the molecular changes that underlie bladder cancer development. A wealth of data is now available that identifies several critical drivers of the malignant urothelial phenotype, some of which have clear potential for therapeutic targeting. Most studies have focused on urothelial carcinomas (UC), which comprise the majority (>90%) of tumors diagnosed in the Western world. This chapter will provide an overview of somatic molecular features of UC identified by genomic, epigenomic, and expression profiling. There is also much information about germline variants that confer increased risk of UC development and the reader is referred to recent reviews on this topic.[1,2]

At diagnosis, approximately 60% of UCs are noninvasive (stage Ta) papillary lesions. These commonly recur, but progression to muscle invasion is infrequent (10% to 15%) and prognosis is good. In contrast, tumors that are muscle invasive at diagnosis (≥T2) have poor prognosis (<50% survival at 5 years). Stage T1 tumors, which have penetrated the epithelial basement membrane but not invaded muscle, represent a clinically challenging and molecularly heterogeneous group with features related to each of the two major groups. The distinction of the two major groups is supported by a wealth of molecular information, and a "two-pathway" model for UC pathogenesis has long dominated thinking about this cancer type and its clinical management. Many genomic alterations and expression of specific genes relate directly to these groups and will be discussed in this context here. Global expression and epigenetic alterations show less direct relationships and will be discussed together. Importantly, recent molecular information provides strong evidence for multiple molecular subgroups that are independent of tumor grade and stage. This new molecular classification, which shows great promise of clinical relevance, is described in a separate section.

KEY MOLECULAR ALTERATIONS IN STAGE Ta UROTHELIAL CARCINOMA

Low-grade stage Ta papillary UC ("superficial" UC) are genomically stable, often with near-diploid karyotype. Common features are activation of FGFR1, FGFR3, PIK3CA, and CCND1 genes by mutation or upregulated expression and mutational inactivation of CDKN2A, STAG2, and TSC1. The most common event recorded to date is mutation of the promoter region of telomerase reverse transcriptase (TERT).

FGF Receptors

Activating point mutations in FGF receptor 3 (FGFR3) are present in ≥ 70% of cases.[3] These are in hot-spot codons in exons 7, 10, and 15 (Fig. 64.1A) and are all predicted to constitutively activate the receptor.[4] Mutations are also found in urothelial papilloma, a likely precursor of superficial UC.[5] Increased expression of mutant FGFR3 is common in these tumors.[6] MicroRNAs (miRNAs) miR-99a/100, which are commonly downregulated in non–muscle-invasive (NMI)

tumors, are negative regulators of FGFR3 expression.[7] Transcriptional regulation by the p53 family member p63 has also been demonstrated.[8] In cultured normal human urothelial cells (NHUC), expression of mutant FGFR3 leads to activation of the RAS-MAPK pathway and PLCγ, leading to overgrowth of cells at confluence,[9] and suggesting a possible contribution of FGFR3 activation to urothelial hyperplasia in vivo. An alternative mechanism of FGFR3 activation in a subset of cases (2% to 5%) is chromosomal translocation to generate a fusion protein. All FGFR3 fusions identified to date show loss of the final exon of FGFR3 and fusion in-frame to TACC3 (transforming acid coiled-coil containing protein 3), or in one case to BAIAP2L1 (BAI1-associated protein 2-like 1) also known as IRTKS (insulin receptor tyrosine-kinase substrate).[10] It is not yet clear whether this activation mechanism is related to tumor grade or stage. These fusion proteins are highly activated and transforming oncogenes. FGF1 and FGF2 are expressed in UC tissues and cell lines,[11,12] FGF2 is detected in the urine of patients with bladder cancer,[13] and expression has been detected in the urothelial stroma.[14] Thus, it is also likely that both autocrine and paracrine FGF production contributes to FGFR3 activation in UC, particularly in those tumors with expression of wild-type protein (Fig. 64.1B).

Activation of the RAS-MAPK pathway in Ta tumors may also be achieved by mutation of one of the RAS genes (most commonly HRAS or KRAS2), and this is mutually exclusive with FGFR3 mutation.[15] More than 80% of noninvasive bladder tumors are predicted to have RAS-MAPK pathway activation via these mechanisms (Fig. 64.2A). Compatible with this, urothelial expression of an activated Ras transgene in mice leads to hyperplasia and papillary tumors,[16] suggesting an important role for activation of the RAS-MAPK pathway in the generation of urothelial hyperplasia.

In NMI UC, FGFR3 mutation is associated with favorable outcome.[17–19] High FGFR3 expression, normal staining pattern for CK20, and low proliferative index in papillary urothelial neoplasms of low malignant potential[20] is reported to identify tumors that do not recur.[21]

FGFR3 is considered a good therapeutic target in superficial UC, though early clinical application is most likely in muscle invasive rather than superficial UC (see the following). Several studies indicate that inhibition of mutant FGFR3 by knockdown or inhibition using small molecules or antibodies has a profound effect on UC cell phenotype, including inhibition of xenograft growth in vivo.[22]

Upregulated expression of the related receptor FGFR1 is also found in Ta tumors.[23] No mutations have been detected, and there is infrequent gene amplification.[24] Ectopic expression of FGFR1 in NHUC in the presence of FGF2 ligand, activates the RAS-MAPK pathway and PLCγ, and promotes cell survival.[23] Currently, there is no information on the prognostic significance of these alterations.

PIK3CA

The phosphatidylinositol-3 kinase (PI3K) pathway plays a pivotal role in signaling from receptor tyrosine kinases (Fig. 64.2A). Activating mutations of the p110α catalytic subunit (PIK3CA) are found in UC, most commonly in low-grade, stage Ta tumors (~25%).[25–28]

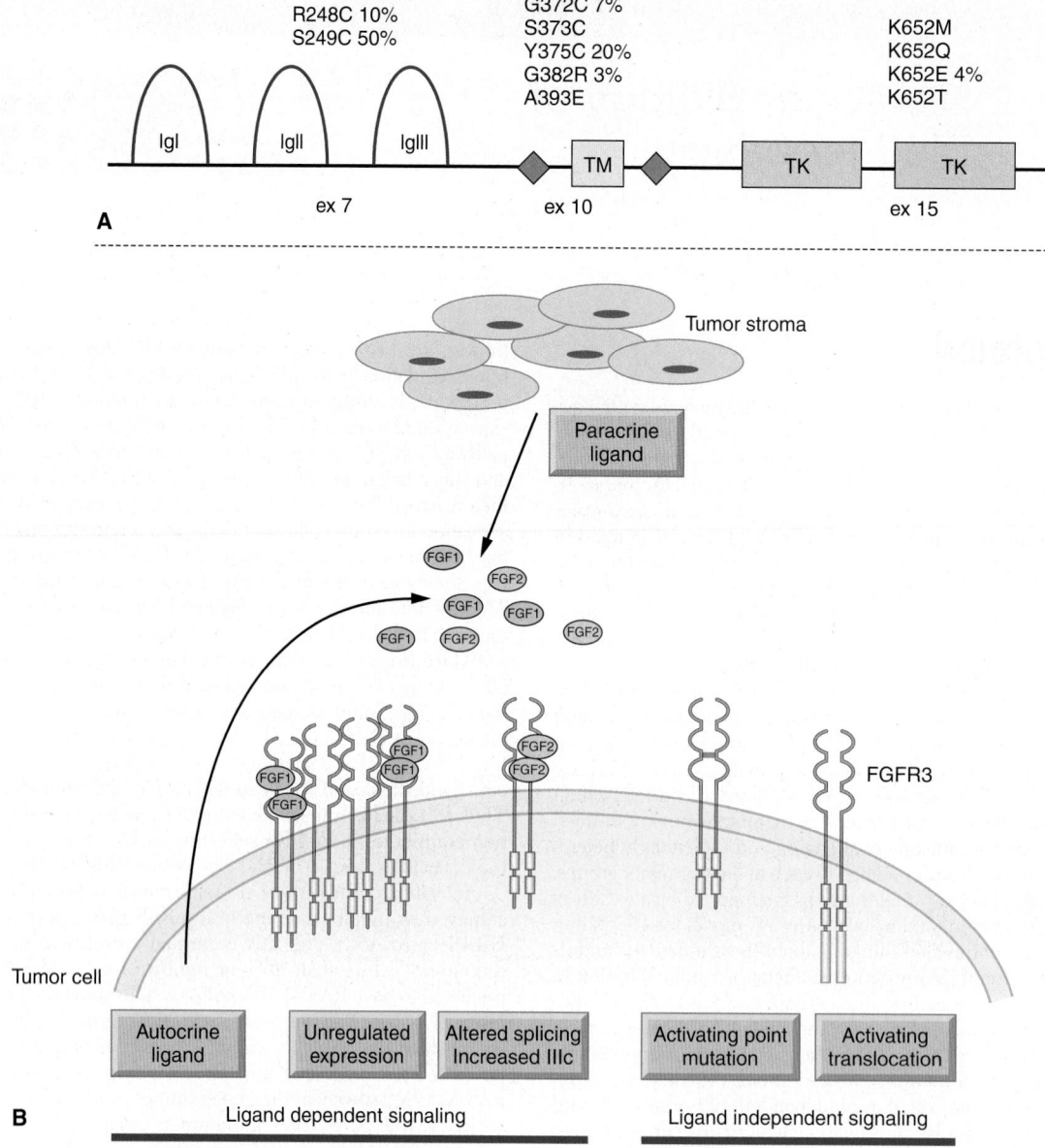

Figure 64.1 (A) *FGFR3* mutations identified in bladder cancer. Positions of hot-spot mutations in exons 7, 10, and 15 that are found in bladder cancer are shown in relation to protein structure. The relative frequency of the more common mutations is given as a percentage. IgI, IgII, IgIII, immunoglobulinlike domains; TM, transmembrane domain; TK, tyrosine-kinase domain. **(B)** Mechanisms of FGFR3 activation in bladder cancer. FGFR3 can be activated by ligand-dependent and -independent mechanisms. Ligand-dependent activation may be via increased expression of wild-type FGFR3, increased production of FGFs by tumor or stromal cells, with or without upregulated FGFR3 expression, or through expression of splice variants with the ability to bind a wider range of FGF ligands. Ligand independent activation can be achieved by point mutation that facilitates receptor dimerization or by the generation of fusion proteins that constitutively dimerise.

The mutation spectrum (Fig. 64.2B) differs significantly from that found in other cancers. Mutations E542K and E545K in the helical domain are most common (22% and 60%, respectively) and the kinase domain mutation H1047R, which is the most common mutation in other cancers, is less frequent. The selective pressure for helical domain mutation in UC is not fully understood. E542K and E545K forms require interaction with RAS-GTP but not binding to p85, the regulatory subunit of PI3K, whereas H1047R depends on p85 binding and is active in the absence of RAS binding.[29] This suggests potential cooperation between helical domain PIK3CA mutant proteins and events in UC that activate RAS. Compatible with this, *PIK3CA* and *FGFR3* mutations are commonly found together.[25–28] Mutant PIK3CA confers a proliferative advantage at confluence and stimulates intraepithelial movement in NHUC,

with higher activity of helical domain than kinase domain mutants in this cell context.[30] Several other mechanisms of PI3K pathway activation have been identified in UC, though none of these are common in noninvasive tumors (Table 64.1).

STAG2

Inactivating mutations in the cohesin complex component *STAG2* (Xq25) have been identified in UC.[31–34] Mutations are most common in stage Ta tumors (20% to 36%) and are predominantly inactivating, suggesting a tumor suppressor function. The cohesin complex, which in human cells contains SMC1A, SMC3, RAD21, and either STAG2 or STAG1, mediates

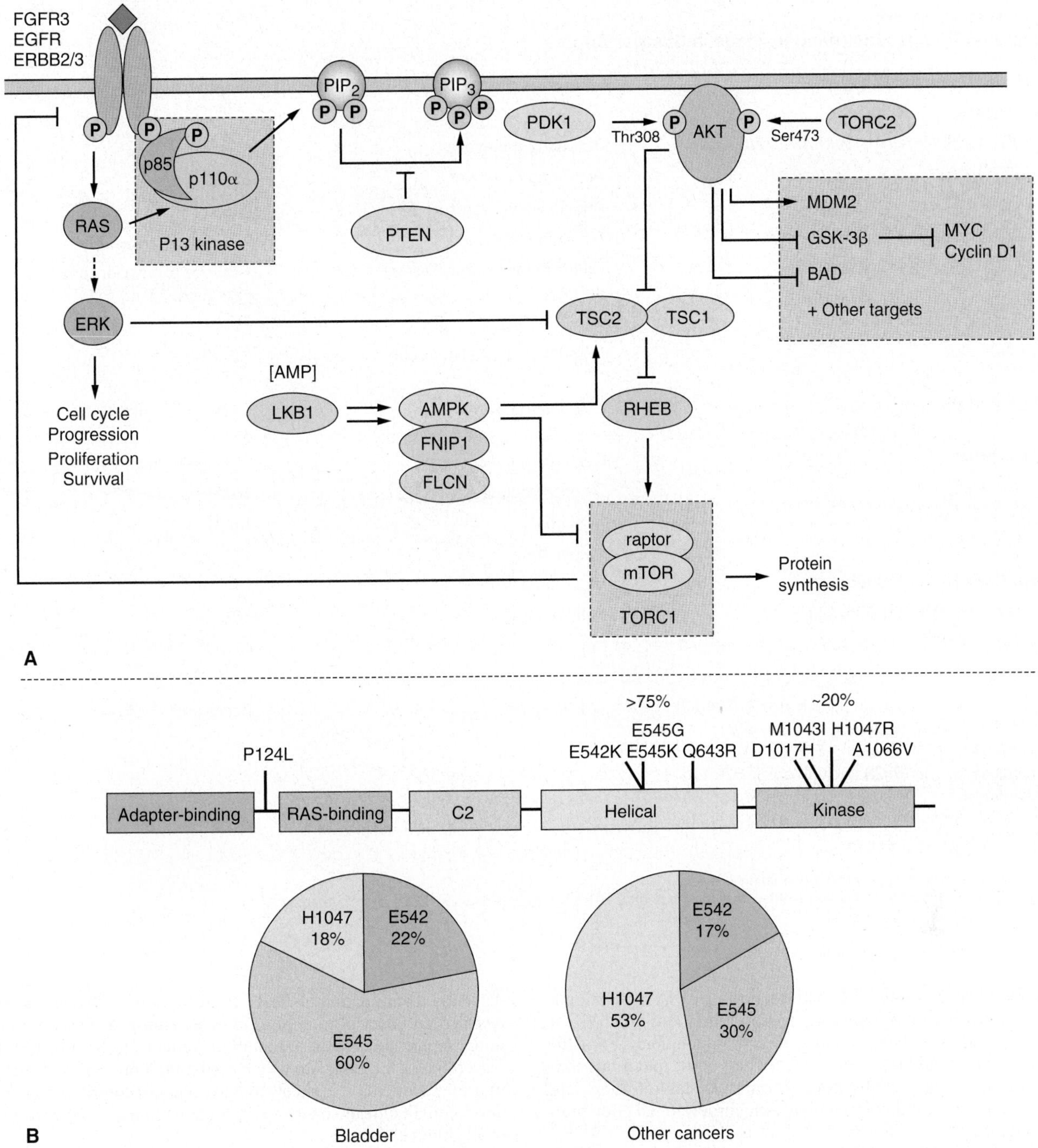

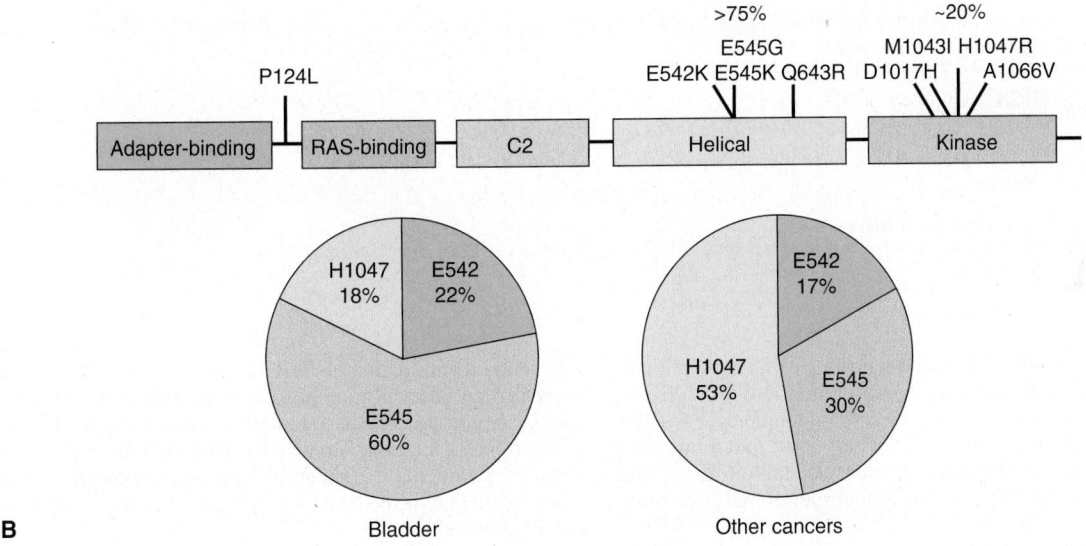

Figure 64.2 (A) Oncogenic signaling via the RAS-MAPK and PI3K pathways. Growth factor–mediated signaling or mutational activation of RAS oncogenes can activate both of these pathways. Signaling via the RAS/RAF/MEK/ERK cascade leads to phosphorylation of many substrates that can have multiple cellular effects depending on the intensity and duration of signaling. In many situations, proliferation is induced. Activated receptor tyrosine kinases bind p85, the regulatory subunit of PI3K, and recruit the enzyme to the membrane where it phosphorylates phosphatidyinositol-4, 5-bisphosphate (PIP2) to generate PIP3, which in turn recruits PDK1 and AKT to the membrane, where AKT is activated by phosphorylation to regulate a wide range of target proteins (not all shown). Among these are cyclin D1 and MDM2, which are upregulated either directly or indirectly, resulting in a positive stimulus via the RB or p53 pathways, respectively. AKT also phosphorylates and inactivates tuberin the *TSC2* gene product, leading to activation of mTOR complex 1 (TORC1), which controls protein synthesis. The *TSC1* product hamartin forms an active complex with tuberin, and loss of function of either protein leads to dysregulated mTOR signaling. MYC expression is induced as a consequence of both by ERK and AKT signaling. Many genes in these pathways show mutation [*FGFR3, PIK3R1* (p85α), *PIK3CA* (p110α), *HRAS, KRAS2, PTEN, AKT1, TSC1, TSC2*] or upregulated expression (EGFR, ERRB2, ERRB3, FGFR1) in bladder cancer. **(B)** *PIK3CA* mutations identified in bladder cancer in relation to protein structure. Pie charts show proportions of common helical domain (E542, E545) and kinase domain (H1047) mutations in bladder and other cancers. Data from COSMIC (http://cancer.sanger.ac.uk/cancergenome/projects/cosmic/; accessed November 15, 2013).

TABLE 64.1

TABLE 64.1

Genetic Changes Identified in Stage Ta Bladder Tumors

Gene (Cytogenetic Location)	Alteration	Frequency (%)
Oncogenes		
HRAS (11p15)/*NRAS* (1p13)/*KRAS2* (12p12)	Activating mutations	15[15,27,28,221]
FGFR3 (4p16)	Activating mutations	60–80[3,222]
CCND1 (11q13)	Amplification/overexpression	10–20[58,223–225]
PIK3CA (3q26)	Activating mutations	27 PUNLMP; 16–30 Ta[25,26]
MDM2 (12q13)	Overexpression/amplification	~30 overexpression; amplification infrequent[58,85,226]
Tumor Suppressor Genes		
CDKN2A (9p21)	Homozygous deletion/mutation/methylation	HD 20–30[40,41,227,228] LOH ~60[229]
PTCH (9q22)	Deletion/mutation	LOH ~ 60; mutation frequency low[43,44]
TSC1 (9q34)	Deletion/mutation	LOH ~ 60; mutation ~12[26,27,48,230]
STAG2 (Xq25)	Deletion/mutation	34–36[33,34]
KDM6A (Xp11)	Mutation	10–30[31,32,140]
ARID1A	Mutation	10[31,32]
DNA Copy Number Changes[a]		
8p, 10q, 11p, 11q, 13q, 17p, 18q	Deletion	>15[57,135,231,232]
9p, 9q	Deletion	46–53[57,135,231,232]
1q, 20q	Gain	>15[57,135,231,232]
1q13, 1q21-q24, 3p25 (including *RAF1*, *PPARG*), 3q25, 3q26, 4p16 (including *FGFR3*), 4q21, 5p13.3-p12, 6p22 (including *E2F3*, *SOX4*), 8p12, 8q24 (including *MYC*), 10q26 (including *FGFR2*), 11q13 (including *CCND1*), 11q24, 12q15 (including *MDM2*), 17q12-q21 (including *ERBB2*), 20q11-q13 (including *YWHAB*, *MYBL2*)	Amplification	Occasional[57,58,232]

[a]Array-based comparative genomic hybridization analyses.
PUNLMP, papillary urothelial neoplasms of low malignant potential; HD, homozygous deletion; LOH, loss of heterozygosity.

cohesion between sister chromatids following DNA replication to ensure correct chromosomal segregation. Mutations in STAG2 in glioblastoma have been reported to cause aneuploidy[35] but this relationship is not apparent in UC, where most mutations have been found in low grade/stage, genomically stable tumors, and there is no association of mutation with chromosomal copy number changes.[31,34]

In addition to its well-documented functions during cell division, cohesin regulates gene expression through mechanisms involving DNA looping and interactions with transcriptional regulators such as CTCF, though evidence to date suggests that these roles are mainly related to STAG1-cohesin.[36] Functional studies are now required to elucidate the consequences of STAG2 loss of function in UC.

Telomerase Reverse Transcriptase Gene Promoter

The most common genomic alterations identified in UC of all grades and stages are mutations in the promoter of the telomerase reverse transcriptase gene (*TERT*) in more than 80% of cases.[37,38] Mutations are predominantly in two hotspot positions [-124 bp (G>A) and -146 bp (G>A) relative to the ATG translational start site], and this has facilitated the design of robust methods of detection. Examination of TERT expression in UC tissues has not revealed an effect of mutation on expression,[37] so that the functional significance of these mutations remains to be determined. Nevertheless, the ease with which these mutations can be detected in urine sediments[37,38] is likely to make a major contribution to the development of urine-based assays for detection of bladder tumors of all grades and stages.

Other Genomic Alterations in Noninvasive Urothelial Carcinoma

These tumors are often near diploid. The most common genomic alteration is loss of heterozygosity (LOH) or copy number loss of chromosome 9, often an entire homolog. More than 50% of UC of all of grades and stages show chromosome 9 LOH. A critical region on 9p21 and at least three regions on 9q (9q22, 9q32–q33, and 9q34) have been identified. Candidate genes within these regions are *CDKN2A* (p16/p14ARF) and *CDKN2B* (p15) at 9p21,[39–42] *PTCH* (Gorlin syndrome gene) at 9q22,[43,44] *DBC1* at 9q32–q33,[45–47] and *TSC1* (tuberous sclerosis syndrome gene 1) at 9q34[26,48,49] (Table 64.1).

CDKN2A (9p21) encodes the two cell-cycle regulators, p16 and p14ARF. p16 is a negative regulator of the RB pathway and p14ARF, a negative regulator of the p53 pathway (Fig. 64.3).

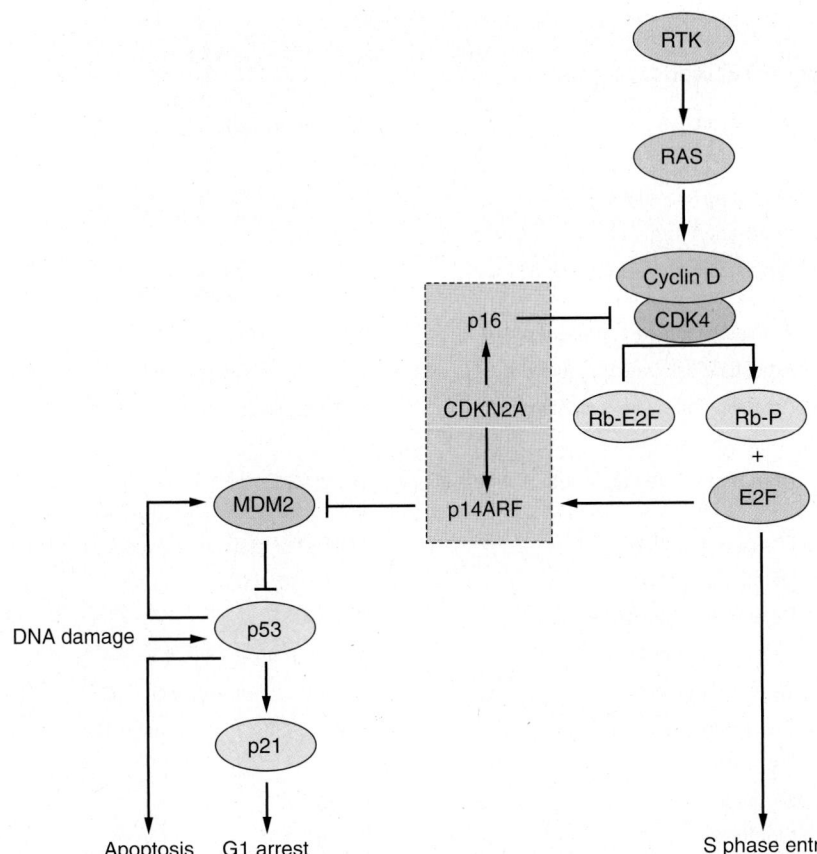

Figure 64.3 Key interactions in the RB and p53 pathways. The *CDKN2A* locus encodes p16 and p14ARF that act as negative regulators of the RB and p53 pathways, respectively. This interrelated signaling network is central to tumor suppression via the mechanisms of cell-cycle arrest and apoptosis. Stimulation by mitogens induces cyclin D1 expression. Phosphorylation of RB1 by CDK4-cyclin D1 complexes releases E2F family members to induce expression of genes required for progression into S phase. The cyclin D-CDK4 complexes also sequester p27 and p21 (not shown). This allows formation of cyclin E-CDK2, which reinforces the inactivation of RB1. p16 negatively regulates this process by interacting with CDK4. The p53 pathway responds to stress signals (e.g., DNA damage). p21 expression is induced and this leads to cell-cycle arrest. MDM2 is a ubiquitin ligase responsible for inactivation of p53. In turn, p53 regulates MDM2 expression providing a negative feedback loop. The p53 and RB pathways are connected by p14ARF, which sequesters (inactivates) MDM2 in the nucleus and is upregulated by E2Fs and in response to mitogenic signaling. Overexpression of E2Fs and oncogenes such as *MYC* can both result in p53-triggered cell-cycle arrest via p14ARF. RTK; receptor tyrosine kinase.

Inactivation of this locus in UC is commonly by homozygous deletion (HD). LOH of 9p, HD of *CDKN2A*, and loss of expression of p16 in NMI UC is predictive of reduced recurrence-free interval.[50–52] Mouse knockout and in vitro experiments indicate that p16 and/or p14ARF may be haploinsufficient.[53,54] In human UC, this may affect the biology of approximately 45% of cases that have LOH or reduced copy number of 9p21.

On 9q, three genes are implicated. *PTCH*, the Gorlin syndrome gene (9q22), shows infrequent mutation,[44] but many tumors have reduced mRNA expression.[43] *DBC1* (9q33) shows HD in a few tumors[55] and no mutations, but is commonly silenced by hypermethylation.[45,56] *TSC1* is the best-validated 9q tumor suppressor gene. TSC1 in complex with TSC2 negatively regulates the mTOR branch of the PI3K pathway (Fig. 64.2A).

Biallelic inactivation of *TSC1* is found in 12% to 16% of UC with no relationship to grade or stage.[26,27]

Cyclin D1

CCND1 (11q13) is amplified in some superficial and invasive UC,[57,58] and the protein is overexpressed in an even larger number.[59,60] Overexpression in many cases may be the consequence of other alterations, such as activation of the MAPK or PI3K pathways (Fig. 64.2A). In Ta tumors, upregulated expression is associated with higher risk of progression to muscle invasion.[60]

KEY MOLECULAR ALTERATIONS IN INVASIVE UROTHELIAL CARCINOMA

Many genomic alterations are found in muscle-invasive (MI) UC, including alterations to known genes and genomic alterations for which the target genes are currently unknown (Table 64.2).

Oncogenes

Overexpression of EGFR, ERBB2, and/or ERBB3 is associated with higher tumor grade and stage and with clinical outcome.[61–63] *ERBB2* (17q23) is amplified in 10% to 20% and overexpressed in 10% to 50% of MI UC.[64–66] Amplification is more common in metastatic lesions than in the related primary tumor.[67] As this receptor cannot bind ligand and relies on heterodimerization with ERBB3, it is likely that ERBB3 status and/or ligand expression may have significant influence.[65,68,69] Up to 70% of MI tumors overexpress EGFR, and this is associated with poor prognosis.[61,70,71] Both ERBB2 and EGFR represent potential therapeutic targets in advanced UC.[72] These changes may activate the RAS-MAPK and/or PI3K pathways (Fig. 64.2A).

RAS gene mutation is not associated with either invasive or noninvasive disease (mutations in ~13% overall).[15] Although mice expressing mutant H-ras in the urothelium develop superficial papillary tumors rather than MI tumors,[73] in vitro experiments in human tumor cells indicate that HRAS can induce an invasive phenotype.[74] Thus, RAS mutation may contribute to development of both major forms of UC.

PIK3CA and *FGFR3* are mutated less frequently than in NMI UC. Approximately 15% of T2 tumors show *FGFR3* mutation.[3,6,75] However, protein expression is upregulated in 40% to 50% of nonmutant MI UC.[6] Thus FGFR3 is considered a good therapeutic target in invasive and metastatic disease and preclinical studies have shown that gene knockdown[76] or treatment with FGFR-selective small molecules and antibodies inhibits cell proliferation and tumorigenicity of UC cell lines with mutant or upregulated FGFR3.[77–79] Potential predictive biomarkers include mutation, overexpression, or detection of an FGFR3 fusion protein. The presence of FGFR3 fusion proteins in UC cell lines[10] is associated with good response to FGFR inhibitors.[77] Epithelial phenotype may provide an additional biomarker as in vitro assays indicate that

Genetic Changes Identified in Invasive (Stage ≥T2) Bladder Tumors

Gene (Cytogenetic Location)	Alteration	Frequency (%)
Oncogenes		
HRAS (11p15)/*NRAS* (1p13)/*KRAS2* (12p12)	Activating mutations	4–15[15,27,28,32,221]
FGFR3 (4p16)	Activating mutations	0–20[3,6,28,222,233]
ERBB2 (17q)	Amplification/overexpression	10–14 amplification 10–50 overexpression[64–66]
CCND1 (11q13)	Amplification/overexpression	10–20 amplification[223,224,234]
MDM2 (12q13)	Amplification/overexpression	4–11 amplification[85,235,236]
E2F3 (6p22)	Amplification/overexpression	9–11 amplification in ≥T1[89,91]
Tumor Suppressor Genes		
CDKN2A (9p21)	Homozygous deletion/mutation/methylation	HD 20–30[40–42,228] LOH ~60[229]
PTCH (9q22)	Deletion/mutation	LOH ~60; mutation frequency low[43,44]
TSC1 (9q34)	Deletion/mutation	LOH ~60; mutation ~12[26,27,48,230]
STAG2 (Xq25)	Deletion/mutation/methylation	9–13[31–34]
TP53 (17p13)	Deletion/mutation	Mutation 50–70[237–239]
RB1 (13q14)	Deletion/mutation	LOH or loss of expression 37[96,99]
PTEN (10q23)	Deletion/mutation	LOH 30–35[106–109]; mutation 17[111]
ARID1A	Mutation	~10[32,240]
KDM6A	Mutation	11–15[31,32]
CREBBP	Mutation	10–15[31,32]
EP300	Mutation	6–8[31,32]
DNA Copy Number Changes[a]		
2q, 3p, 3q, 4p, 4q, 5q, 6p, 6q, 8p, 9p, 9q, 10p, 10q, 11p, 11q, 12q, 13q, 14q, 15q, 16p, 16q, 17p, 18q, 19p, 19q, 22q	Deletion	>15[57,135,231,232]
1p, 1q, 2p, 2q, 3p, 3q, 4p, 4q, 5p, 5q, 6p, 7p, 7q, 8p, 8q, 9p, 10p, 10q, 11q, 12p, 12q, 13q, 14q, 15q, 16p, 16q, 17p, 17q, 18p, 19p, 19q, 20p, 20q, 21q, 22q	Gain	>15[57,135,231,232]
1q23, 3p25 (including *RAF1*, *PPARG*), 6p22 (including *E2F3*, *SOX4*), 8p12-p11.2 (including *FGFR1*, *TACC1*, *POLB*), 8q24 (including *MYC*), 8q22 (including *YWHAZ*), 11q13 (including *CCND1*), 12q15 (including *MDM2*), 17q12-q21 (including *ERBB2*), 20q12-q13.2 (including *YWHAB*, *MYBL2*), 20q13.32-q13.33	Amplification	3–12 [57,232]

[a] Array-based comparative genomic hybridization analyses.
HD, homozygous deletion; LOH, loss of heterozygosity.

UC cells with epithelial phenotype have enhanced sensitivity to FGFR inhibition compared to those with mesenchymal phenotype.[80] A recent RNAi screen in UC cell lines indicated that up-regulated EGFR signaling provides a mechanism of escape from FGFR inhibition and can mediate de novo resistance. A reciprocal relationship was found when EGFR was inhibited and both in vitro and in a preclinical in vivo model, combined inhibition showed improved anti-tumor activity.[81] Thus, assessment of both FGFR3 and EGFR status may be required to predict response and combined EGFR and FGFR3 inhibition may be essential. Several clinical trials of FGFR inhibitors are now planned or in progress in advanced UC.

FGFR1 is also overexpressed in many of these cancers.[23] An increased ratio of the FGFR1-β : FGFR1-α splice variants is found in MI tumors. The β isoform, lacking the first immunoglobulin-like domain, has increased sensitivity to FGF1.[82] FGF2 stimulation of ectopically expressed FGFR1-β in some UC-derived cell lines induces an epithelial-mesenchymal transition (EMT), a major feature of which is PLCγ-mediated upregulation of COX-2.[83] This is in contrast to the effect of FGFR1 signaling in NHUC, where increased proliferation and reduced apoptosis but no EMT is induced,[23] suggesting that FGFR1 plays different roles in NMI and MI UC. Compatible with this, UC cell lines with highest FGFR1 expression show a mesenchymal (EMT) phenotype (low E-cadherin expression) and upregulated FGF2 expression, and those with epithelial phenotype show higher FGFR3 and E-cadherin and lower FGFR1.[84] In an animal model of UC metastasis using an FGFR1-dependent cell line, an FGFR inhibitor reduced the development of circulating tumor cells and metastasis but not primary tumor growth.[84] Currently, there is no information on the prognostic significance of FGFR1 upregulation, and FGFR1 has not yet been examined independently of FGFR3 as a potential therapeutic target.

Several other oncogenes are implicated in MI UC. Four to six percent have amplification of *MDM2* (12q14).[57,85,86] MDM2 regulates p53 levels, and overexpression provides an alternative mechanism to inactivate p53 function (Fig. 64.3). There is no consensus on the relationship of upregulated MDM2 to tumor grade, stage, or prognosis. MYC is upregulated in many bladder tumors, although the mechanism for this is unclear.[87] Although amplifications of 8q are found in invasive UC, MYC is not the major target. However, additional copies of the whole of 8q are common and may lead to overexpression.[24,57] MYC is also upregulated in response to other molecular events (e.g., MAPK pathway stimulation). An amplicon on 6p in 14% of MI UC and cell lines contains *E2F3*, and functional studies indicate that *E2F3* can drive urothelial cell proliferation.[88–92] E2F transcription factors interact with and are regulated by RB1 (Fig. 64.3) and in accord with this, tumors with *E2F3* amplification have RB1 or p16 inactivated.[89]

Tumor Suppressor Genes

As in other aggressive cancers, the tumor suppressor genes *TP53*, *RB1*, *CDKN2A*, and *PTEN* are implicated in MI UC. The pathways controlled by TP53 and RB1 regulate cell-cycle progression and responses to stress (Fig. 64.3). *TP53* mutation is common in invasive UC and detection of mutation or TP53 protein accumulation is associated with poor prognosis. Although immunohistochemical detection of TP53 protein with increased half-life identifies many mutant TP53 proteins and is commonly used as a surrogate marker for mutation, some *TP53* mutations (~20%) yield unstable or truncated proteins that cannot be detected in this way. Thus, TP53 protein accumulation is not a useful prognostic marker. Two meta-analyses indicate only a small association between TP53 positivity and poor prognosis.[93,94] However, examination of both protein expression and mutation of *TP53* provides useful prognostic information.[95]

The RB pathway regulates cell-cycle progression from G1 to S phase (Fig. 64.3). HD, LOH of 13q14, and loss of RB1 protein expression are common in MI UC.[96–99] Loss of p16 expression is inversely related to positive RB1 expression,[100] and high-level p16 expression results from negative feedback in tumors with loss of RB1.[101] Thus, both loss of expression and high-level expression of p16 are associated with RB pathway deregulation, and these are adverse prognostic biomarkers found in >50% of MI tumors.[102] Interestingly, in MI UC with *FGFR3* mutation, a high frequency of *CDKN2A* HD has been reported, which may identify a progression pathway for NMI *FGFR3*-mutant tumors to muscle invasion via loss of *CDKN2A*.[103] As indicated previously, amplification and overexpression of E2F3, which is normally repressed by RB1, is associated with RB1 or p16 loss in MI tumors.[89] p16 and p14[ARF] proteins link the RB and p53 pathways (Fig. 64.3), and due to multiple regulatory feedback mechanisms, inactivation of both pathways together is predicted to have greater impact than inactivation of either pathway alone. This is borne out by the achievement of greater predictive power in studies using concurrent analyses of multiple changes that deregulate the G1 checkpoint.[102,104,105]

Altered PTEN expression is the most frequent mechanism for deregulation of the PI3K pathway in MI UC. PTEN (phosphatase and tensin homolog deleted on chromosome 10) (10q23) is a lipid and protein phosphatase whose major lipid substrate is phosphatidylinositol (3,4,5)-triphosphate (PIP3) generated by PI3K (Fig. 64.2A). *PTEN* LOH is found in 24% to 58% of invasive UC,[106–108] and copy number analysis has identified a relationship of PTEN loss to metastatic disease.[57] Mutation of the retained copy is infrequent but HD has been detected in tumor cell lines.[26,109–111] Overall, 46% of UC lines (largely derived from MI tumors) had PTEN alterations.[26] Reduced expression is common

in tumors[26,112] and is associated with TP53 alteration. Many tumors (41%) with altered TP53 show downregulation of *PTEN*, and this combined alteration is associated with poor outcome.[113] As *PTEN* is haploinsufficient in mouse models,[114] loss of one allele in UC may lead to altered phenotype. In mice, conditional deletion of *Pten* in the urothelium led to early urothelial hyperplasia[112,115] and late development of tumors resembling human papillary superficial tumors. A study that induced stochastic deletion of *p53* and/or *Pten* showed that deletion of either gene alone did not lead to tumor formation, but dual deletion led to early development of aggressive UC, with frequent metastases.[113] PTEN loss may affect proliferation, apoptosis, and migration. Reexpression in PTEN-null UC cells has revealed effects on cell chemotaxis, anchorage-independent growth, and tumor growth in vivo.[116–118] UC cell invasion can be inhibited by the protein phosphatase activity of PTEN alone.[116] Thus, loss of lipid and protein phosphatase activities of PTEN may contribute in different ways to urothelial tumorigenesis.

The *TSC1* product hamartin acts in the PI3K pathway downstream of PTEN (Fig. 64.2A), providing an alternative mechanism of pathway activation in 13% of invasive UCs that have mutational inactivation.[26,27] Whereas good response to mTOR inhibitors has been reported in some patients and UC cell lines with mutant *TSC1*, mutation alone is not a sufficient predictive biomarker.[119,120]

The Rho GDP dissociation inhibitor RhoGDI2 has been implicated as a tumor suppressor in UC. Expression is reduced in an isogenic cell line model of metastasis and low expression is associated with reduced survival in patients with UC.[121] Potential downstream effectors of RhoGDI2 are endothelin and versican, which are upregulated upon loss of RhoGDI2 expression. In an experimental model of metastasis, endothelin 1 was required for lung colonization by UC cells and pharmacologic inhibition of the endothelin axis reduced colonization.[122] RhoGDI2-regulated versican levels are implicated in enhancing macrophage recruitment and chemokine CCL1 levels.[123] As both of these proteins enhance the inflammatory response, the major role of RhoGDI2 may be to inhibit this. RhoGDI2 is phosphorylated by SRC, and this enhances its membrane localization and metastasis-suppression activity.[124] Compatible with this, and unlike the situation in many tumors, SRC levels in UC are highest in NMI tumors where RhoGDI2 function is intact.[125,126] SRC contributes to suppression of metastasis via regulation of p190Rho GAP, which in turn downregulates the activity of RHOA, RHOC, and ROCK.[127]

The WNT signaling pathway is also implicated in UC. Mutations in *APC* have been reported,[27,128] mainly in MI tumors. The frequency of mutations in *CTNNB1* is low, but altered beta-catenin expression (reduced expression or increased nuclear localization) is frequent in MI UC,[128–131] though this is not associated with *APC* mutation.[128] Other alterations in the WNT pathway include epigenetic silencing of the antagonists of WNT signaling, secreted frizzled receptor proteins,[132] and the Wnt inhibitory factor 1 (WIF1).[133]

Other Genomic Alterations in Invasive Urothelial Carcinoma

Invasive UC is often genomically unstable, with significant genetic divergence of related tumors in the same patient over time. Array-based comparative genomic hybridization and single nucleotide polymorphism array analyses have identified many copy number alterations[57,134–137] (Table 64.2). These include numerous losses and gains in DNA copy number and many regions of high-level amplification that may contain novel oncogenes. To date, the target genes within many of these regions have not been identified. Many regions of copy number alteration show significant association with high tumor grade, stage, and/or outcome. These include amplicons at 1q21–24, 3p25, 6p22, 8p11, 8q22, 11q12, 12q15, and 17q12. Plausible candidate oncogenes within these are *PPARG* (3p25), *E2F3* and *SOX4* (6p22), *FGFR1*, *TACC1* and *POLB* (8p11), *YWHAZ* (8q22),

PRACTICE OF ONCOLOGY

CCND1 (11q12), *MDM2* (12q15), and *ERBB2* (17q12).[57,135,138,139] On 1q21–24, at least three regions have been defined, two of which contain plausible candidates (*BCL9* and *CHD1L* in one, and *MCL1*, *SETDB1*, and *HIF1B* in a second).[139] Regions of HD include 1p34, 2q36, 9p21, 11p11, 18p11, and 19q13.[57] On 9p22, *CDKN2A* is one target and two further regions of HD have been identified.[57] Candidates within the other regions are less obvious.

It is notable that some stage T1 tumors show similar profiles to MI tumors (T2 or greater), suggesting that these tumors with the ability to break through the basement membrane may be aggressive lesions. However, other T1 tumors show remarkable similarity in their copy number profiles to Ta tumors, suggesting that distinct biologic subgroups exist.[57]

INFORMATION FROM EXOME SEQUENCING

At the time of writing, three studies have reported sequencing of whole UC exomes.[31,32,140] In total, these have sequenced 12 Ta, 41 T1, and 72 T2 tumors. In two studies, selected genes were assessed in larger sample sets to examine prevalence.[31,140] Whereas the overall numbers of tumors studied remains relatively small, several important conclusions can be drawn. The first is that UC contains a relatively high frequency of somatic single nucleotide mutations, with estimates ranging from 50 to 170 per sample on average but with wide variability between samples. Many of the mutations ($\geq$ 30%) were nonsynonymous, a large proportion of which are predicted to be damaging (~60% estimated in one study[31]). To date, significant differences in mutation rates between non-aggressive and aggressive tumors are not apparent, though it is notable that very few stage Ta tumors have been studied so far. The most common base change reported is C:G>T:A transition followed by C:G>G:A transversion.

The most significant finding is that in addition to genes already implicated in UC (*TP53*, *FGFR3*, *HRAS*, *KRAS*, *PIK3CA*, *RB1*, *TSC1*), a large number of genes involved in chromatin modification show mutation. In the largest study, 58% of tumors had mutation in chromatin remodeling genes,[32] indicating that altered regulation of chromatin is a major oncogenic driver in UC. Mutated genes include histone demethylases (*KDM6A*, *KDM5A*, *KDM5B*, *UTY*), chromatin remodeling genes (*ARID1A*, *ARID4A*), histone lysine methyltransferases (*MLL*, *MLL2*, *MLL3*, *MLL5*), histone acetyltransferases (*CREBBP*, *EP300*, *EP400*), and SWI/SNF complex-related genes (*SMARCA4*, *SMARCA1*). Many of the mutations are predicted to impair function, suggesting tumor suppressor roles. Mutations were also found in DNA repair genes including *ATM*, *FANCA*, and *ERCC2*. Overall, in MI tumors the most frequently mutated genes were *KDM6A* (30%), *TP53* (24%), *ARID1A* (15%), *CREBBP* (15%), *EP300* (13%), *HRAS* (13%), *RB1* (13%), *PIK3CA* (12%), *STAG2* (11%), and *FGFR3* (11%).[32] In all three studies, relatively large numbers of genes were mutated at low frequency, suggesting that there is considerable biologic heterogeneity.

EPIGENETIC ALTERATIONS

Epigenetic alterations, mainly those involving DNA methylation, have been widely reported. Most studies have analyzed single genes or small series of genes.[141–144] Genome-wide analyses have identified novel candidates, some with clinicopathologic associations.[145–149] In general, hypermethylation in CpG islands is more common in MI tumors and hypomethylation in regions distinct from CpG islands in NMI tumors.[147,148] Integrated analysis of methylation and gene expression indicates that CpG island hypermethylation is associated with loss of expression and CpG methylation within genes or at transcription factor binding sites with increased expression.[149] Hypermethylation-associated disease progression biomarkers in NMI tumors include *TBX2*, *TBX3*, *TBX4*, *GATA2*, and *ZIC2*.[145,147] These genes, which encode transcription factors

involved in lineage decisions during development, are implicated in EMT, stem cell phenotype, and differentiation. In the high-risk group of T1 grade 3 tumors treated with BCG, combined methylation of *MSH6* and *THBS1* is associated with disease progression.[150] Hypermethylation of several miRNAs is associated with tumor grade and stage. Some of these have prognostic value (e.g., the miR-200 family and miR-205) and are frequently silenced in MI tumors, and this is correlated with disease progression in T1 tumors.[151]

There are many reports of improved detection of UC by analysis of methylation biomarkers in urine. Examples include a panel of five biomarkers (*MYO3A*, *CA10*, *NKX6-2*, *DBC1*, and *SOX11* or *PENK*),[152] two panels each of four biomarkers (*ZNF154*, *POU4F2*, *HOXA9*, and *EOMES*),[147] (*APC*, 2 *TERT* CpGs, and *EDNRB*),[153] one of two markers (*TWIST1* and *NID2*),[154] and one of three markers (*OTX1*, *ONECUT*, and *OSR1*), used in combination with *FGFR3* mutation.[155]

To date, chromatin modification has not been extensively studied. In UC cell lines, the active histone mark H3K9Ac and the repressive mark H3K27me3 are associated with miR-200/miR-205 expression or methylation, respectively.[151] Genomewide analysis has identified UC-specific differences in the distribution of histone marks and indicated the importance of both DNA and H3K27 methylation in gene silencing in cell lines.[156] In tumor tissues, seven genomic regions where transcriptional deregulation is independent of DNA copy number[157] were shown to be silenced by a mechanism associated with histone H3K9 and H3K27 trimethylation and histone H3K9 hypoacetylation, a pattern of silencing also found in a subgroup of UC with a carcinoma in situ (CIS)–associated expression signature.[158] With the recent identification of many mutations in chromatin remodeling genes in UC,[31,32,140] more extensive analysis of chromatin modifications and assessment of potential therapeutic opportunities are now needed.

INFORMATION FROM EXPRESSION PROFILING

mRNA expression signatures associated with UC grade, stage, progression, nodal involvement, response to chemotherapy, and survival have been derived,[134,159–171] and some signatures have performed well in independent validation studies.[172,173] Overlap between signatures from different studies is generally low, but there is significant overlap in the cellular processes implicated.[174] Clinical application of these signatures requires the development of robust polymerase chain reaction–based assays or identification of antibodies suitable for immunohistochemistry. Already polymerase chain reaction–based gene signatures have been derived to predict progression in NMI tumors.[169,175] Recently, a novel system of classification for UC based on global analysis of expression data has been developed, and this is discussed in detail in a following section.

There are several reports of altered miRNA expression in UC.[176,177] Changes in apparently "normal" urothelium from patients with UC indicate that such alterations may occur early in disease development.[7] Global analyses using array-based methods or deep sequencing have revealed common upregulation of miRNAs in MI tumors and downregulation in NMI tumors.[7,178] Clustering analysis of miRNA data generated three clusters containing mainly Ta, T1, and T2-T4 tumors.[179] miRNAs downregulated in Ta tumors include miRs 7, 99a/100, 125b, 143, 146, 188, and 29c.[176,179,180] Many miRNA alterations are found in MI UC.[151,176,178–183] Examples include upregulation of miR-21,[7,182] which negatively regulates *TP53*,[7] and the miR-200 family, which are implicated in regulation of EMT.[184] Several miRNAs that are downregulated in MI UC (e.g., miR-145, miR-143, miR-203, miR-1, miR-133a, miR-195, and miR-125b) can induce apoptosis, reduce cell proliferation or migration in cultured UC cells, and show reciprocal expression with their targets in tumor tissues.[185–191] Upregulated miRNAs include miR-222 and miR-452, which are associated with adverse outcome.[192] Downregulation of miR-138 was shown to increase cisplatin sensitivity in UC cell lines.[193] Together, these data indicate that miRNA expression profiles may be valuable prognostic biomarkers.

UROTHELIAL TUMOR–INITIATING CELLS

There is evidence for the existence of highly tumorigenic subpopulations of cells with stem cell–like characteristics within UC populations. As cancer stem cells in other tumor types show resistance to chemotherapy agents and are predicted to be the cause of posttreatment disease relapse, there is great interest in characterizing these cells and identifying markers that may allow specific targeting. Isolation of bladder cancer "stem" or "tumor-initiating" cells has been attempted from fresh tumor tissues and UC cell lines, using a range of assays. The putative stem cells express a range of markers including 67kD laminin receptor (67LR), CD44, CD90, ALDH1A1, and keratins 5, 14, and 17.[194,195] The majority of these are markers expressed by normal urothelial basal cells and in low-grade tumors, cells expressing these markers reside at the tumor-stromal interface.[196] Cell surface markers have been used to great effect to sort putative stem cells from mass cell populations. Cells from tumor samples that expressed CD44+, CK5+, CK20− had enhanced tumor-initiating ability compared to CD44−, CK5−, CK20+ cells and could generate tumors that contained both CD44+ and CD44− cells.[197] In UC cell lines, a subpopulation of CD44+, ALDH1A1+ cells is reported to have higher tumorigenicity than CD44−, ALDH1A1− cells, and in UC tissues higher ALDH1A1 expression was an independent prognostic factor for overall survival.[198] However, the finding that 58% of UC do not express CD44[197] has suggested that not all UC stem cells are derived from the basal compartment. Combinations of markers related to different urothelial differentiation states were found to stratify UC into clinically relevant subgroups; in each group, it was found that the least differentiated cell type showed stem cell–like characteristics.[199] This implies that UC stem cells can be derived from urothelial cells of different differentiation states. This diversity in stem cell phenotype may influence subsequent disease development and may have prognostic value.

MOLECULAR PATHOGENESIS AND TUMOR CLONALITY

Multifocality and/or development of multiple recurrent tumors in the same patient is a common feature of UC. Although some patients develop more than one molecularly distinct tumor (oligoclonal disease),[200] most commonly tumors from the same patient are molecularly related,[201–203] with evidence for subclonal genomic evolution in different lesions.[204] Chromosome 9 LOH has been proposed as an early event in UC development as it is found in "normal" urothelium and hyperplasia in tumor-bearing patients.[205,206] Compatible with this, loss of the same allele is commonly shared by all related tumors.[207] Construction of phylogenetic trees from multiple related NMI tumors confirms the early loss of chromosome 9 with later events including 11p−, 20q+, 17p−, and 11q−.[203] Interestingly, tumors with highest genomic complexity are not necessarily the last to appear in the patient.[208,209] Urothelial dysplasia and CIS, predicted precursors of MI UC, show frequent chromosome 9 LOH and TP53 mutation,[210–212] and multiple other chromosomal alterations.[213] Detailed genomic mapping of cystectomy specimens has indicated that prior to detectable morphologic abnormality, large areas of urothelium show LOH of specific chromosomal regions. Areas of dysplasia showed more complex patterns of LOH, suggesting sequential evolutionary changes associated with acquisition of growth advantage. Thus, it is suggested that development of MI UC involves displacement of the normal urothelium by a molecularly altered clone, within which subclones with additional alterations arise. Six critical regions of LOH (3q22, 5q22–23, 9q21, 10q26, and 17p13) were identified.[214,215] Biallelic inactivation of ITM2B and P2RY5, genes close to RB1, implicate these in driving early clonal expansion.[214]

Polyclonal hypermethylation detected throughout the "normal" urothelium in tumor-bearing bladders also suggests widespread pre-malignant epigenetic "field change."[148] The genes affected, which may represent early "drivers" of UC, include ZO2, MYOD1, CDH13, and many polycomb repressive complex 2 (PRC2) targets, all of which have plausible functional significance and showed hypermethylation in the related invasive tumors.

MULTIPLE TUMOR SUBGROUPS DEFINED BY MOLECULAR PROFILING

Bladder tumors of similar grade and stage commonly show divergent clinical behavior. In particular, stage T1 tumors show considerable molecular and clinical diversity. Until recently, molecular features have failed to explain or predict this heterogeneity. The two tumor groupings that have for so long dominated the bladder cancer literature are insufficient for this. Recent studies have begun to unravel this complexity, revealing multiple subgroups that are independent of conventional grade and stage groupings (Fig. 64.4).

Initial assessment of mRNA expression profiles of UC of all grades and stages identified the two major molecular subtypes, separated mainly though not entirely, according to grade and stage with stage T1 tumors distributed relatively equally between the two.[134,135] More recent analysis has defined additional subtypes. Five major subtypes were termed urobasal A (UroA), UroB, GU, squamous cell carcinoma–like (SCCL), and "infiltrated"[216] (Fig. 64.4A). Tumors in the latter group are highly infiltrated with nontumor cells, whereas the definition of the other groups reflects tumor cell–specific criteria. Clear differences in expression of cell cycle regulators, keratins, receptor tyrosine kinases, and cell adhesion molecules are evident. UroA and UroB subtypes express high levels of FGFR3, CCND1, and TP63; GU tumors show low levels of these proteins but high levels of ERBB2 and E-cadherin; and SCCL tumors express P-cadherin and high levels of KRT5, KRT14, and proteins involved in keratinization. These subtypes showed distinct clinical outcome. UroA had good prognosis, GU had intermediate prognosis, and SCCL and UroB, the worst prognosis. UroB tumors share epithelial characteristics with UroA tumors including FGFR3 mutation, but they also show TP53 mutation and are often invasive. T1 tumors appear evenly distributed between molecular subtypes.[216]

Robust assays, ideally based on immunohistochemical detection of proteins in formalin-fixed, paraffin-embedded tissues are required to apply these findings in the clinic. Immunohistochemistry of a panel of markers selected from the defined mRNA subgroup signatures has recently been assessed in combination with morphologic criteria.[217] Histopathologic and immunohistochemical profiles were examined in all subtypes except "infiltrated," with excellent correlation between mRNA and protein expression for the majority of markers. Importantly, the distribution of protein expression within the tissues also provided valuable information. For example, UroA tumors show restriction of KRT5, P-cadherin, EGFR, and CCNB1 expression to the basal cell layer, reminiscent of normal urothelium, implying retention of dependence on stromal interactions, whereas many UroB tumor show expression of these proteins in suprabasal layers. The keratin expression profile (KRT14+, KRT5+, KRT20−) of SCCL tumors is characteristic of the least differentiated class of tumor initiating cells described by Chan et al.[197] and termed "basal" in the study of Volkmer et al.[199] Their phenotype is also similar to basal-like breast carcinoma,[218] and it has been suggested that these UC could in future be defined as "basal-like."[217]

A simple classifier based on grade and urothelial differentiation pattern and expression of KRT5 and CCNB1 was able to reproduce the original genomewide expression classification with an accuracy of 0.88.[217] The three major subgroups, urobasal (UroA + UroB), GU, and SCCL, showed highly significant association with disease-specific survival. However, a simple method to distinguish UroA from the small, related UroB subset, many of which are MI, proved difficult.[217] The common features of UroA and UroB may indicate that MI UroB tumors have their origins as non-invasive

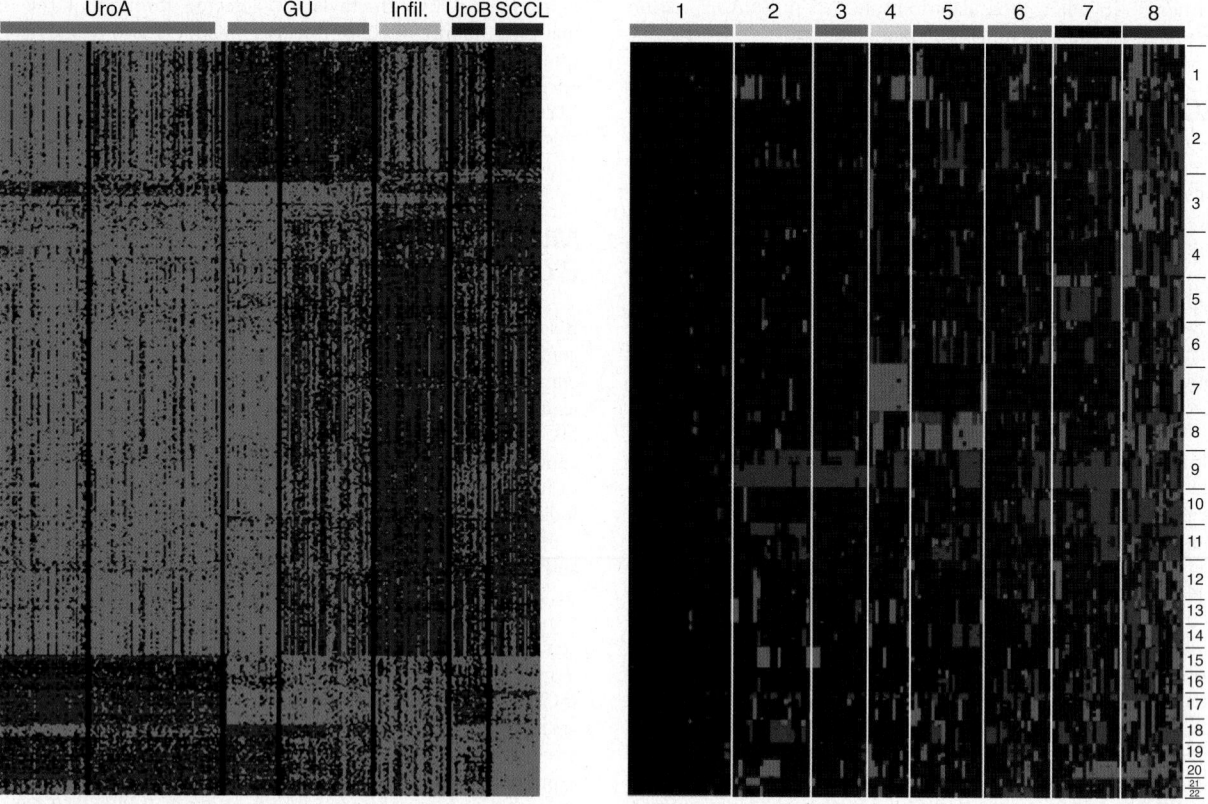

Figure 64.4 Tumor subgroups defined by molecular profiling. **(A)** Major bladder cancer subtypes identified by mRNA expression profiling (adapted with permission from Sjodahl et al.[216]). Hierarchical cluster analysis of 308 samples generated five major tumor clusters. Each column of the heatmap represents one sample, and each row represents one gene. *Green* represents low gene expression, and *red* represents high gene expression. The five major subtypes are indicated by the *color bars* at the top of figure. GU, genomically unstable; SCCL, squamous cell carcinoma–like; UroA, urobasal A; UroB, urobasal B; Infil, "Infiltrated". **(B)** Major bladder cancer subtypes identified by array-based comparative genomic hybridization.[57] Hierarchical cluster analysis was performed using copy number data from 160 tumors. *Red* represents copy number loss, and *green* represents copy number gain. Chromosome number is shown down the right-hand side of the figure. Eight main clusters of tumors were identified, and these are indicated by the *color bars* at the top of the figure.

UroA tumors. Interestingly, UroB showed common loss of p16 expression, which as discussed previously, may represent a means by which NMI *FGFR3*-mutant tumors can progress.[103] In common with NMI tumors, UroB retains TP63 expression and may represent the aggressive subset of TP63-expressing advanced UC reported by Choi et al.[219] Further studies of this subtype are essential to allow development of a clinically applicable classification assay.

Similarly, DNA copy number and mutation status has identified multiple subgroups of tumors within the conventional grade and stage groupings[57] (Fig 64.4B), though these have not been as extensively studied as expression-based subtypes and classification signatures are not yet defined. DNA methylation profiles also identify several subtypes.[148,149,220] Four "epitypes" showed broad alignment with expression subtypes.[149] One epitype showed methylation pattern similar to immune cells and represented the heavily infiltrated group of tumors. Two others corresponded to the two major expression subtypes,[134,135] one of which contained many aggressive

tumors with upregulation of EZH2 and corresponding DNA methylation of polycomb target genes and several HOX genes, whose hypermethylation is implicated in aggressive growth of other cancer types. As for expression subtypes, these epitypes do not align absolutely with tumor grade and stage. Integration of information from all genome-wide platforms, including miRNA expression data, is now needed to provide optimum prognostic and predictive biomarkers. As DNA and miRNA are more robust molecules than RNA in formalin-fixed, paraffin-embedded specimens, a combination of these and protein biomarkers may ultimately be most useful.

ACKNOWLEDGEMENTS

We acknowledge the valuable advice of Professor M Höglund and Dr KS Chan on the sections on tumor subgroups and urothelial tumor-initiating cells.

SELECTED REFERENCES

The full reference list can be accessed at lwwhealthlibrary.com/oncology.

2. Chang DW, Gu J, Wu X. Germline prognostic markers for urinary bladder cancer: obstacles and opportunities. *Urol Oncol* 2012;30:524–532.
3. Billerey C, Chopin D, Aubriot-Lorton MH, et al. Frequent FGFR3 mutations in papillary non-invasive bladder (pTa) tumors. *Am J Pathol* 2001;158:1955–1959.
6. Tomlinson DC, Baldo O, Harnden P, et al. FGFR3 protein expression and its relationship to mutation status and prognostic variables in bladder cancer. *J Pathol* 2007;213:91–98.

7. Catto JW, Miah S, Owen HC, et al. Distinct microRNA alterations characterize high- and low-grade bladder cancer. *Cancer Res* 2009;69:8472–8481.
9. di Martino E, L'Hôte CG, Kennedy W, et al. Mutant fibroblast growth factor receptor 3 induces intracellular signaling and cellular transformation in a cell type- and mutation-specific manner. *Oncogene* 2009;28:4306–4316.
10. Williams SV, Hurst CD, Knowles MA. Oncogenic FGFR3 gene fusions in bladder cancer. *Hum Mol Genet* 2012.
15. Jebar AH, Hurst CD, Tomlinson DC, et al. FGFR3 and Ras gene mutations are mutually exclusive genetic events in urothelial cell carcinoma. *Oncogene* 2005;24:5218–5225.

18. Hernandez S, Lopez-Knowles E, Lloreta J, et al. Prospective study of FGFR3 mutations as a prognostic factor in nonmuscle invasive urothelial bladder carcinomas. *J Clin Oncol* 2006;24:3664–3671.

22. di Martino E, Tomlinson DC, Knowles MA. A decade of FGF receptor research in bladder cancer: Past, present, and future challenges. *Adv Urol* 2012;2012:429213.

23. Tomlinson DC, Lamont FR, Shnyder SD, et al. Fibroblast growth factor receptor 1 promotes proliferation and survival via activation of the mitogen-activated protein kinase pathway in bladder cancer. *Cancer Res* 2009;69:4613–4620.

26. Platt FM, Hurst CD, Taylor CF, et al. Spectrum of phosphatidylinositol 3-kinase pathway gene alterations in bladder cancer. *Clin Cancer Res* 2009;15:6008–6017.

27. Sjodahl G, Lauss M, Gudjonsson S, et al. A systematic study of gene mutations in urothelial carcinoma; inactivating mutations in TSC2 and PIK3R1. *PloS One* 2011;6:e18583.

31. Balbas-Martinez C, Sagrera A, Carrillo-de-Santa-Pau E, et al. Recurrent inactivation of STAG2 in bladder cancer is not associated with aneuploidy. *Nat Genet* 2013;45:1464–1469.

32. Guo G, Sun X, Chen C, et al. Whole-genome and whole-exome sequencing of bladder cancer identifies frequent alterations in genes involved in sister chromatid cohesion and segregation. *Nat Genet* 2013;45:1459–1463.

34. Taylor C, Platt F, Hurst C, et al. Frequent inactivating mutations of STAG2 in bladder cancer are associated with low tumor grade and stage and inversely related to chromosomal copy number changes. *Hum Mol Genet* 2014;23:1964–1974.

37. Allory Y, Beukers W, Sagrera A, et al. Telomerase reverse transcriptase promoter mutations in bladder cancer: High frequency across stages, detection in urine, and lack of association with outcome. *Eur Urol* 2014;65:360–366.

38. Hurst CD, Platt FM, Knowles MA. Comprehensive mutation analysis of the TERT promoter in bladder cancer and detection of mutations in voided urine. *Eur Urol* 2014;65:367–369.

51. Kruger S, Mahnken A, Kausch I, et al. P16 immunoreactivity is an independent predictor of tumor progression in minimally invasive urothelial bladder carcinoma. *Eur Urol* 2005;47:463–467.

57. Hurst CD, Platt FM, Taylor CF, et al. Novel tumor subgroups of urothelial carcinoma of the bladder defined by integrated genomic analysis. *Clin Cancer Res* 2012;18:5865–5877.

60. Fristrup N, Birkenkamp-Demtroder K, Reinert T, et al. Multicenter validation of cyclin D1, MCM7, TRIM29, and UBE2C as prognostic protein markers in non-muscle-invasive bladder cancer. *Am J Pathol* 2013;182:339–349.

64. Chow NH, Chan SH, Tzai TS, et al. Expression profiles of ErbB family receptors and prognosis in primary transitional cell carcinoma of the urinary bladder. *Clin Cancer Res* 2001;7:1957–1962.

67. Fleischmann A, Rotzer D, Seiler R, et al. Her2 amplification is significantly more frequent in lymph node metastases from urothelial bladder cancer than in the primary tumours. *Eur Urol* 2011;60:350–357.

76. Tomlinson DC, Hurst CD, Knowles MA. Knockdown by shRNA identifies S249C mutant FGFR3 as a potential therapeutic target in bladder cancer. *Oncogene* 2007;26:5889–5899.

77. Lamont FR, Tomlinson DC, Cooper PA, et al. Small molecule FGF receptor inhibitors block FGFR-dependent urothelial carcinoma growth in vitro and in vivo. *Br J Cancer* 2011;104:75–82.

78. Qing J, Du X, Chen Y, et al. Antibody-based targeting of FGFR3 in bladder carcinoma and t(4;14)-positive multiple myeloma in mice. *J Clin Invest* 2009;119:1216–1229.

81. Herrera-Abreu MT, Pearson A, Campbell J, et al. Parallel RNA interference screens identify EGFR activation as an escape mechanism in FGFR3 mutant cancer. *Cancer Discovery* 2013;3:1058–1071.

83. Tomlinson DC, Baxter EW, Loadman PM, et al. FGFR1-induced epithelial to mesenchymal transition through MAPK/PLCgamma/COX-2-mediated mechanisms. *PloS One* 2012;7:e38972.

88. Feber A, Clark J, Goodwin G, et al. Amplification and overexpression of E2F3 in human bladder cancer. *Oncogene* 2004;23:1627–1630.

89. Hurst CD, Tomlinson DC, Williams SV, et al. Inactivation of the Rb pathway and overexpression of both isoforms of E2F3 are obligate events in bladder tumours with 6p22 amplification. *Oncogene* 2008;27:2716–2727.

93. Malats N, Bustos A, Nascimento CM, et al. P53 as a prognostic marker for bladder cancer: A meta-analysis and review. *Lancet Oncol* 2005;6:678–686.

95. George B, Datar RH, Wu L, et al. p53 gene and protein status: the role of p53 alterations in predicting outcome in patients with bladder cancer. *J Clin Oncol* 2007;25:5352–5358.

97. Cordon-Cardo C, Wartinger D, Petrylak D, et al. Altered expression of the retinoblastoma gene product: Prognostic indicator in bladder cancer. *J Natl Cancer Inst* 1992;84:1251–1256.

98. Logothetis CJ, Xu H-J, Ro JY, et al. Altered expression of retinoblastoma protein and known prognostic variables in locally advanced bladder cancer. *J Natl Cancer Inst* 1992;84:1256–1261.

103. Rebouissou S, Herault A, Letouze E, et al. CDKN2A homozygous deletion is associated with muscle invasion in FGFR3-mutated urothelial bladder carcinoma. *J Pathol* 2012;227:315–324.

105. Chatterjee SJ, Datar R, Youssefzadeh D, et al. Combined effects of p53, p21, and pRb expression in the progression of bladder transitional cell carcinoma. *J Clin Oncol* 2004;22:1007–1013.

109. Cairns P, Evron E, Okami K, et al. Point mutation and homozygous deletion of PTEN/MMAC1 in primary bladder cancers. *Oncogene* 1998;16:3215–3218.

113. Puzio-Kuter AM, Castillo-Martin M, Kinkade CW, et al. Inactivation of p53 and Pten promotes invasive bladder cancer. *Genes Dev* 2009;23:675–680.

119. Iyer G, Hanrahan AJ, Milowsky MI, et al. Genome sequencing identifies a basis for everolimus sensitivity. *Science* 2012;338:221.

120. Guo Y, Chekaluk Y, Zhang J, et al. TSC1 involvement in bladder cancer: diverse effects and therapeutic implications. *J Pathol* 2013;230:17–27.

121. Griner EM, Theodorescu D. The faces and friends of RhoGDI2. *Cancer Metastasis Rev* 2012;31:519–528.

128. Kastritis E, Murray S, Kyriakou F, et al. Somatic mutations of adenomatous polyposis coli gene and nuclear β-catenin accumulation have prognostic significance in invasive urothelial carcinoma: evidence for Wnt pathway implication. *Int J Cancer* 2009;124:103–108.

135. Lindgren D, Sjodahl G, Lauss M, et al. Integrated genomic and gene expression profiling identifies two major genomic circuits in urothelial carcinoma. *PloS One* 2012;7:e38863.

140. Gui Y, Guo G, Huang Y, et al. Frequent mutations of chromatin remodeling genes in transitional cell carcinoma of the bladder. *Nat Genet* 2011;43:875–878.

143. Sanchez-Carbayo M. Hypermethylation in bladder cancer: Biological pathways and translational applications. *Tumour Biol* 2012;33:347–361.

147. Reinert T, Modin C, Castano FM, et al. Comprehensive genome methylation analysis in bladder cancer: Identification and validation of novel methylated genes and application of these as urinary tumor markers. *Clin Cancer Res* 2011;17:5582–5592.

148. Wolff EM, Chihara Y, Pan F, et al. Unique DNA methylation patterns distinguish noninvasive and invasive urothelial cancers and establish an epigenetic field defect in premalignant tissue. *Cancer Res* 2010;70:8169–8178.

149. Lauss M, Aine M, Sjodahl G, et al. DNA methylation analyses of urothelial carcinoma reveal distinct epigenetic subtypes and an association between gene copy number and methylation status. *Epigenetics* 2012;7:858–867.

150. Agundez M, Grau L, Palou J, et al. Evaluation of the methylation status of tumour suppressor genes for predicting bacillus Calmette-Guerin response in patients with T1G3 high-risk bladder tumours. *Eur Urol* 2011;60:131–140.

151. Wiklund ED, Bramsen JB, Hulf T, et al. Coordinated epigenetic repression of the miR-200 family and miR-205 in invasive bladder cancer. *Int J Cancer* 2011;128:1327–1334.

155. Kandimalla R, Masius R, Beukers W, et al. A 3-Plex methylation assay combined with the FGFR3 mutation assay sensitively detects recurrent bladder cancer in voided urine. *Clin Cancer Res* 2013;19:4760–4769.

158. Vallot C, Stransky N, Bernard-Pierrot I, et al. A novel epigenetic phenotype associated with the most aggressive pathway of bladder tumor progression. *J Natl Cancer Inst* 2011;103:47–60.

172. Dyrskjot L, Zieger K, Real FX, et al. Gene expression signatures predict outcome in non-muscle-invasive bladder carcinoma: a multicenter validation study. *Clin Cancer Res* 2007;13:3545–3551.

173. Takata R, Katagiri T, Kanehira M, et al. Validation study of the prediction system for clinical response of M-VAC neoadjuvant chemotherapy. *Cancer Science* 2007;98:113–117.

176. Catto JW, Alcaraz A, Bjartell AS, et al. MicroRNA in prostate, bladder, and kidney cancer: A systematic review. *Eur Urol* 2011;59:671–681.

194. Ho PL, Kurtova A, Chan KS. Normal and neoplastic urothelial stem cells: getting to the root of the problem. *Nat Rev Urol* 2012;9:583–594.

196. He X, Marchionni L, Hansel DE, et al. Differentiation of a highly tumorigenic basal cell compartment in urothelial carcinoma. *Stem Cells* 2009;27:1487–1495.

197. Chan KS, Espinosa I, Chao M, et al. Identification, molecular characterization, clinical prognosis, and therapeutic targeting of human bladder tumor-initiating cells. *Proc Natl Acad Sci* 2009;106:14016–14021.

199. Volkmer JP, Sahoo D, Chin RK, et al. Three differentiation states risk-stratify bladder cancer into distinct subtypes. *Proc Natl Acad Sci* 2012;109:2078–2083.

203. Kawanishi H, Takahashi T, Ito M, et al. Genetic analysis of multifocal superficial urothelial cancers by array-based comparative genomic hybridisation. *Br J Cancer* 2007;97:260–266.

208. van Tilborg AA, de Vries A, de Bont M, et al. Molecular evolution of multiple recurrent cancers of the bladder. *Hum Mol Genet* 2000;9:2973–2980.

215. Majewski T, Lee S, Jeong J, et al. Understanding the development of human bladder cancer by using a whole-organ genomic mapping strategy. *Lab Invest* 2008;88:694–721.

216. Sjodahl G, Lauss M, Lovgren K, et al. A molecular taxonomy for urothelial carcinoma. *Clin Cancer Res* 2012;18:3377–3386.

217. Sjodahl G, Lovgren K, Lauss M, et al. Toward a molecular pathologic classification of urothelial carcinoma. *Am J Pathol* 2013;183:681–691.

219. Choi W, Shah JB, Tran M, et al. p63 expression defines a lethal subset of muscle-invasive bladder cancers. *PloS One* 2012;7:e30206.

220. Wilhelm-Benartzi CS, Koestler DC, Houseman EA, et al. DNA methylation profiles delineate etiologic heterogeneity and clinically important subgroups of bladder cancer. *Carcinogenesis* 2010;31:1972–1976.

PRACTICE OF ONCOLOGY

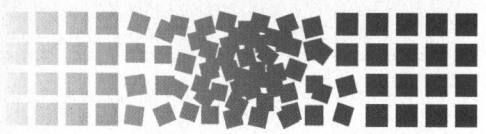

Adam S. Feldman, Jason A. Efstathiou, Richard J. Lee, Douglas M. Dahl, M. Dror Michaelson, and Anthony L. Zietman

INTRODUCTION

This chapter details the incidence, epidemiology, pathology, and treatment of cancers of the bladder, ureter, and renal pelvis. Transitional cell carcinomas (TCC) constitute 90% to 95% of all the urothelial tumors diagnosed in North America and Europe. TCCs occur throughout the lining of the urinary tract from the renal calyceal system to the proximal two-thirds of the urethra, at which point squamous epithelium predominates. In this 10th edition, cancers of the renal pelvis and ureter are grouped with bladder cancer rather than with cancers of the kidney. This is a natural fit, because approximately 90% of the urothelial cancers of the renal pelvis, ureter, and bladder are transitional cell cancers, all of which share similarities in epidemiology, pathology, biology, patterns of spread, molecular tumor markers, and treatment. The chapter presents the common characteristics of urothelial cancers in an initial section and then deals in subsequent sections with the separate characteristics of these organs. The multidisciplinary treatment of this chapter reflects the current approach to patients with these diseases.

UROTHELIAL CANCERS

Epidemiology

Bladder cancer is almost three times more common in males than in females and more common in whites than in blacks. In 2013, there were approximately 72,570 new cases in the United States, over a 20% increase from 20 years ago. The incidence increases with age and peaks in the 6th, 7th, and 8th decades of life.[1]

Simultaneous or subsequent development of TCC of the urethra in patients with TCC of the bladder occurs with an incidence of 6% to 16% more commonly in women than men and in those with recurrent multifocal bladder cancers, and bladder neck or trigonal involvement with either invasive cancer or carcinoma in situ (CIS).[2,3]

The incidence of ureteral TCC is 0.7 per 100,000, whereas renal pelvic TCCs have an incidence of 1 per 100,000.[4] Renal pelvic tumors constitute 5% of all renal tumors, and 90% of them are TCCs. Squamous cell carcinoma and adenocarcinoma constitute the majority of the remainder. Renal pelvic transitional cell cancers constitute 5% of all TCCs of the urinary tract. Patients who have primary TCCs of the renal pelvis or ureter have a 20% to 40% incidence of either synchronous or metachronous bladder cancer. Conversely, patients with bladder cancer have a 1% to 4% incidence of synchronous or metachronous upper tract urothelial tumors.[5,6] However, if the bladder cancer is grade 3, there is associated CIS, or the patient has failed intravesical chemotherapy, some reports suggest a doubling of the incidence of upper tract tumors.[7] Patients with Balkan nephropathy have an increased incidence of upper tract tumors; these tumors are usually low grade and multiple.[8]

Recently, aristolochic acid, a component of all *Aristolochia* plants, was identified as the etiologic agent causing Balkan nephropathy and the associated urothelial carcinoma.[9–11] In the Balkan region, the exposure seems to occur via consumption of bread made from flour contaminated with *Aristolochia clematitis* seeds.[12] There are also specific areas of Taiwan where TCC of the renal pelvis accounts for 40% of all renal tumors, whereas in other nonendemic areas, the upper tract tumors account for only 1% or 2% of renal tumors.[13] Aristolochic acid has also recently been identified as the etiology in this population due to widespread use of *Aristolochia* herbal remedies.[14,15]

Risk factors for urothelial cancer may be classified into one of three categories: (1) gene abnormalities that result in perturbations in cell cycle regulatory processes, (2) chemical exposure, or (3) chronic irritation. Those risk factors that involve genetic abnormalities include chromosome deletions or duplications, proto-oncogene expression, tumor suppressor gene mutation, and abnormalities of specific cell cycle regulatory proteins. In non–muscularis propria–invasive transitional cell cancers, deletions of part or all of chromosome 9 and alterations in the gene encoding for fibroblast growth factor receptor 3 (FGFR3) are often encountered. Inactivation of the cohesion subunit stromal antigen 2 (Stage 2), which regulates sister chromatid cohesion and segregation, is frequently found in low-grade and low-stage bladder cancer.[16–18] Other proto-oncogenes that have been implicated in bladder cancer include the RAS and p21 proteins.[19] Genetic abnormalities associated with CIS include alterations in the retinoblastoma gene (Rb), p53, and phosphatase and tensin homolog (PTEN). In muscularis propria–invasive disease, the tumor suppressor genes that have been associated with an altered biology and more aggressive behavior include the *p53* and the *Rb* gene.[20] Abnormalities in specific cell-cycle regulatory proteins such as epidermal growth factor (EGF), Ki-67, cyclin D1, metalloproteinase (MMP), and tissue inhibition of metalloproteinase (TIMP) have also been implicated.[20–25] At this time, there is no single molecular marker that is capable of predicting the tumor with a high degree of accuracy, which may result in muscularis propria invasion or distant metastases.

Chemical exposure has perhaps the most epidemiologic evidence to support it as an inciting agent. Aromatic amines, aniline dyes, and nitrites and nitrates have all been implicated. There are genetic polymorphisms that appear to increase the susceptibility of affected patients exposed to carcinogens. N-acetyltransferase, which detoxifies nitrosamines and glutathione-S transferase, which conjugates reactive chemicals, have been implicated in increasing the risk for the development of bladder cancer in patients so afflicted. Tobacco use carries with it, for those who continue to smoke, a threefold increased risk of developing bladder cancer, and even ex-smokers have a twofold increased risk.[26] Numerous reports have shown strong associations between the development of both bladder and upper tract TCCs with industrial contact to chemicals, plastics, coal, tar, and asphalt, and aristolochic acid, as discussed previously. Cyclophosphamide administration over the long term, particularly in patients who have upper tract or bladder outlet obstructions, results in an increased risk of bladder cancer. These cancers, when discovered, tend to be particularly aggressive. Coffee, tea, analgesics, alcohol, and artificial sweeteners have not been shown to act as independent risk factors.

Chronic irritants include catheters, recurrent urinary track infections, *Schistosoma haematobium*, and irradiation. Chronic irritation due to indwelling catheters associated with chronic infection increases the risk for the development of squamous cell carcinoma; a *S. haematobium* infestation results in an increased risk of squamous cell and TCCs; pelvic irradiation also carries with it an increased risk of developing a urothelial cancer.

There are many studies that suggest high water consumption, vitamin intake, and various diets as beneficial in preventing bladder cancer. However, none of these have shown any clear benefit with respect to prevention.

Screening and Early Detection

Screening has not been particularly useful in the detection of bladder cancer and the most recent statement from the U.S. Preventive Services Task Force concludes that the current data are insufficient to make a definitive recommendation on screening for bladder cancer in asymptomatic adults.[27] The only test of proven usefulness is a urinalysis to detect microhematuria. If significant microhematuria is detected, then specific diagnostic studies are performed. When individuals are screened, 4% to 20% are found to have microhematuria. Of those with microhematuria, 0.5% to 8.1% have bladder tumors.[28–30] In these particular studies, high-grade disease was identified in 2.4% to 3.5% of those presenting with dipstick microhematuria, and invasive disease was identified in 0.4% to 1%. Although one of these studies suggests that routine screening results in a reduced mortality from bladder cancer, the data are unconvincing due to a lack of randomization and likely significant selection bias.[30] Others have suggested that screening in high-risk populations increases the early detection rate of high-grade cancers. Early treatment of these would be expected to be associated with an increased survival, although this hypothesis in this group of patients has not been substantiated. Screening does not generally improve the detection rate of low-grade tumors because the methods used for screening have a large number of false-negative findings for low-grade tumors. When urothelial cancer is suspected, noninvasive screening may be performed using cytology, nuclear matrix protein, telomerase, or fluorescence in situ hybridization analysis, but the definitive diagnosis is made only by cystoscopy and biopsy.

Cytology has been regarded as the gold standard for noninvasive screening of urine for bladder cancer. It has a sensitivity of 40% to 60% and specificity in excess of 90%. Nuclear matrix protein[31] fibrin or fibrinogen degradation products,[32] urinary bladder cancer antigen,[33] and basic fetoprotein[34] have all been compared with cytology in bladder cancer screening studies. Other methods used include fluorescence in situ hybridization,[35] microsatellite analysis of free DNA,[36] and telomerase reverse transcriptase determination.[37] Unfortunately, all of these tests have a sensitivity that ranges from only 40% to 75% with a specificity of 50% to 90%, thus making it impossible to eliminate the need for cystoscopy by the use of these tests.[38] These urinary biomarkers have not been studied yet for sensitivity and specificity in detecting upper tract TCCs.

Cytology remains the preferred bladder tumor marker for specificity[39]; however, many of the other bladder tumor markers have a better sensitivity.[40]

Pathology

More than 90% of the TCCs throughout the lining of the urinary tract occur in the urinary bladder and of the remaining 10%, most are in the renal pelvis and fewer than 2% are in the ureter and urethra. Squamous cell carcinomas, defined by the presence of keratinization, account for 5% of bladder tumors. Other, even less common bladder tumor types include adenocarcinoma and undifferentiated carcinoma variants such as small-cell carcinoma, giant-cell carcinoma, and lymphoepitheliomas.[41–43] A TCC histology can also demonstrate areas of a variant subtype within a tumor, including micropapillary, squamous, glandular, or sarcomatoid differentiation. These are considered variants of TCC, and stage for stage, they do not portend a worse prognosis,[44,45] likely with the exception of sarcomatoid carcinoma, which presents with a higher stage and more distant metastases than conventional TCC.[46] Pure adenocarcinoma of the bladder may also arise in the embryonal remnant of the urachus on or above the bladder dome. Other adenocarcinomas may closely resemble intestinal adenocarcinoma and must be distinguished from direct spread to the bladder from an intestinal primary by careful clinical evaluation. Rarely, these demonstrate a signet ring cell or clear cell histology.

Primary Tumors of the Bladder

The differential diagnosis of TCC usually does not pose a diagnostic difficulty for experienced pathologists, but tumors that are grade 1 and invasive are occasionally difficult to distinguish from von Brunn nests.[47] Also, rarely, an invasive TCC may be overdiagnosed when the glandular component of a nephrogenic adenoma is mistaken for TCC with glandular differentiation or for a pure adenocarcinoma. When invasion of the lamina propria has occurred, the pathologist must report whether muscularis propria is present in the submitted tissue and whether there is invasion of the muscularis propria. If muscularis propria is not present in the submitted tissue, this should be noted by the pathologist. Identification of invasion of the muscularis propria by the tumor may occasionally be difficult, because it may be confused with involvement of the muscularis mucosa, which is in the lamina propria.[48] More than two-thirds of newly diagnosed cases of bladder tumors are exophytic papillary TCCs that are confined to the epithelium (stage Ta) or invade only into the lamina propria (stage T1). These tumors are generally managed endoscopically and, in some cases, with the addition of intravesical therapy (discussed in the following paragraphs). Approximately one-half to two-thirds of patients with such tumors have a recurrence or a new TCC in the bladder within 5 years.

Bladder tumors are also classified by their cytologic characteristics as low grade (G1) or high grade (G2, G3).[43] Low-grade tumors may also be referred to as papillary tumors of low malignant potential (PNLMP). Tumor grade is clinically more significant for noninvasive tumors because nearly all of the invasive neoplasms are high grade at diagnosis. Papillary carcinomas of low grade are considered to be relatively benign tumors that histologically resemble the normal urothelium. They show only very slight pleomorphism or loss of polarity and rarely progress to a higher stage. On the contrary, CIS is cytologically synonymous with high-grade disease and carries a high risk of progression to invasive disease. Primary CIS (stage Tis) that presents without a concurrent exophytic tumor constitutes only 1% to 2% of newly detected cases of bladder cancer, but CIS is found accompanying more than half of bladders presenting with multiple papillary tumors. CIS, in this instance, is either adjacent to or involves mucosal sites remote from papillary lesions.[49] CIS is believed to be an important precursor of invasive cancer and, if untreated, will develop into muscularis propria–invasive disease within 5 years from the initial diagnosis in more than 50% of patients.

Upper Tract Tumors

Like bladder tumors, 90% of upper tract tumors are TCCs with similar morphology.[50] Squamous cell carcinomas account for most of the remaining carcinomas, with adenocarcinoma representing, at most, 1% of upper tract malignancies. The cytologic characteristics for the classification of TCC by grade are the same for upper tract TCCs as they are for those in the bladder.

PRACTICE OF ONCOLOGY

Molecular Tumor Markers

Because the natural history of superficial urothelial tumors is that of recurrence, an area of controversy is if tumors that occur at separate sites or at separate times in the urothelial tract are derived from the same clone or are polyclonal in origin. A report by Sidransky et al.[51] demonstrated the clonality of multiple bladder tumors from different sites. Miyao et al.[52] showed concordant genetic alterations in asynchronous tumors from individual patients. These studies suggest that urothelial TCCs appearing at different times and sites can be derived from the same neoplastic clone. Moreover, many studies have reported an increasing frequency of specific genetic abnormalities in bladder tumors of more advanced stages.[53–56] Many tumor suppressor gene modifications, including those of *p53*, *pRB*, *p16*, *p21*, thrombospondin-1, glutathione, and factors controlling the expression and function of the epidermal growth factor receptor (EGFR), have been shown in retrospective analyses to be adverse prognostic factors in patients with TCC after various treatments.[58–62] However, even in the most intensively studied tumor suppressor gene in advanced TCC, the *p53* gene, retrospective analyses give. There is conflicting retrospective data on the association of *p53* mutation status and responsiveness to chemotherapy or radiation[59,60] led to a phase III trial that randomized 114 postcystectomy patients with p53 alteration to three cycles of adjuvant methotrexate, vinblastine, doxorubicin, and cisplatin (MVAC) or observation. Neither p53 status nor MVAC adjuvant chemotherapy impacted the risk of recurrence.[57]

The enthusiasm engendered by the development of novel biologic agents targeted against tumor-specific growth factor pathways or against angiogenesis has been fortified by positive studies in a variety of solid tumors. Two classes of agents that have received great attention are inhibitors of EGFR, including EGFR1 and EGFR2 (or HER2/neu), and inhibitors of vascular endothelial growth factor (VEGF) or its receptors. Ample preclinical evidence has shown that (1) many, if not most, bladder tumors express products of the EGFR family, (2) overexpression correlates with an unfavorable outcome, and (3) inhibition of these pathways may have an antitumor effect.[64–69]

Evidence suggests that *p53*, *p16*, and *pRB* altered expression are of no prognostic significance in patients treated with chemoradiation, but that overexpression of *HER2* correlated with a significantly inferior complete response rate. The recently closed Radiation Therapy Oncology Group (RTOG) 0524 protocol evaluated the addition of trastuzumab to chemoradiation for Her2 overexpressing tumors. EGFR overexpression, which occurred in only 19% of the patients, was associated with improved disease-specific survival.[70]

Another potential therapeutic avenue is the inhibition of angiogenesis. Several studies have correlated elevated VEGF levels or cyclooxygenase-2 (COX-2) expression with disease recurrence or progression, often as an independent prognostic factor by multivariate analysis.[69,71]

Preclinical data support the concept that COX-2 inhibitors may inhibit the development of non–muscle-invasive bladder cancer. A randomized, double-blind, placebo-controlled trial sought to determine whether celecoxib, a COX-2 inhibitor, could reduce the time-to-recurrence of superficial tumors. No benefit was observed in patients receiving daily celecoxib.[72]

The major challenge for clinical and translational investigators is to design appropriate trials that will identify which molecular tumor markers will be prognostic of outcome *and* also be predictive of whether a patient will do better treated by surgery, radiation, chemotherapy, molecular targeted therapy, or a combination of these. An example of recent encouraging results include the identification of MRE11, a protein involved in DNA damage double-strand break repair, as a predictive marker of disease specific survival following radiation or chemoradiation for muscle invasive bladder cancer.[73,74] Only when such molecular biomarkers are validated and incorporated into clinical decision making will

physicians be able to make better treatment choices on behalf of their patients.

CANCER OF THE BLADDER

Cancers of the bladder can be grouped into three general categories by their stages at presentation: (1) those that do not invade the muscularis propria, (2) muscularis propria–invasive cancers, and (3) metastatic cancers. Each differs in clinical behavior, primary management, and outcome. When treating non–muscularis-invasive tumors, the aim is to prevent recurrences and progression to a stage that is life threatening. With muscularis propria–invasive disease, the main issue is to determine which tumors require cystectomy, which can be successfully managed by bladder preservation using combined modality therapy, and which tumors, by virtue of a high metastatic potential, require an integrated systemic chemotherapeutic approach from the outset. Combination chemotherapy is the standard for treating metastatic disease. Despite reports of complete responses (CR) in more than 40% of cases, the duration of response and overall cure rates remain low.

Clinical Presentations and Staging

Bladder cancer is rarely incidentally discovered at autopsy. Indeed, almost all cases show symptoms in the premortem period. The most common presentation is gross painless hematuria. Unexplained urinary frequency and irritative voiding symptoms should alert one to the possibility of CIS of the bladder or, less commonly, muscularis propria–invasive cancer.

Workup

The workup of suspected bladder cancer should include urine cytology, a cystoscopy, and an upper tract study. The preference for the upper tract study is a renal computed tomography (CT) urogram because both ureters and renal pelves as well as the relevant lymph nodes and the kidney parenchyma can be particularly well visualized.

Careful staging is important, because treatment depends on the initial stage of the disease. The clinical stage of the primary tumor is determined by transurethral resection of the bladder tumor (TURBT). This resection should include a sample of the muscularis propria for appropriate diagnosis, particularly if the tumor appears sessile or high grade. Once the specimen has been resected, the base of the resected area should be separately biopsied. Any suspicious areas in the remainder of the bladder should be biopsied, and many advocate additional selected biopsies of the bladder mucosa and a prostatic urethral biopsy as well. Urethral biopsies are clearly indicated in patients with risk factors for urethral involvement, as previously discussed, and in those who have persistent positive cytologies in the absence of a demonstrated bladder lesion. Patients who have T1, G3 tumors on biopsy without muscularis propria in the specimen require a second biopsy in order to obtain muscularis propria to reduce the risk of understaging. Indeed, the authors rebiopsy all patients with T1, G3 disease, because it has been shown that even if muscularis propria is in the initial specimen, a significant number of patients will be upstaged (T2) on the second biopsy.

5-Alpha amino levulinic acid installation into the bladder, resulting in porphyrin-induced fluorescence of vascular lesions when viewed with blue light, and narrow band imaging, which increases the contrast between vascular lesions and normal mucosa, have been recommended by some to increase the yield of positive biopsies. Several studies have shown a slight advantage to these techniques in reducing disease recurrence, but it remains difficult to differentiate inflammatory lesions from urothelial carcinomas with either technique, and not all well-designed clinical trials have shown a benefit.[75–78]

Staging

The primary bladder cancer is staged according to the depth of invasion into the bladder wall or beyond (Table 65.1).[70,79] The urothelial basement membrane separates non–muscularis propria bladder cancers into Ta (noninvasive) and T1 (invasive) tumors. Stage T2 and higher T-stage tumors invade the muscularis propria, the true muscle of the bladder wall. If the tumor extends through the muscle to involve the full thickness of the bladder and into the serosa, it is classified as T3. If the tumor involves contiguous structures such as the prostate, the vagina, the uterus, or the pelvic sidewall, the tumor is classified as stage T4 (nonstromal invasive urothelial tumors of the prostate are not classified as T4, because the prognosis in this group is quite good). In a fragmented TURBT specimen, in contrast to a cystectomy specimen, it is relatively infrequent for the pathologist to be able to make an accurate assessment as to the depth of invasion of the tumor into the muscularis propria. Thus, the primary pathologic substages of the TNM (tumor, nodes, metastasis) staging system shown in Table 65.1, such as pT2a and pT2b, cannot be determined from TURBT specimens. Of note, significant rates of clinical–pathologic stage discrepancy and clinical (TURBT) understaging have been described.[138] CT scans or magnetic resonance images (MRI), even those done prior to the TURBT, are not reliable for staging of

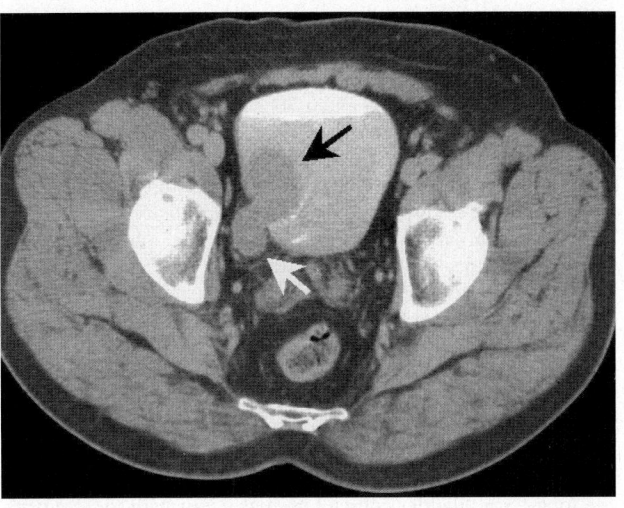

Figure 65.1 A computed tomography scan of a patient with a muscularis propria–invasive bladder cancer performed before a transurethral tumor resection, unequivocally showing an extravesical extension of tumor (stage T3). The tumor projecting into the bladder lumen (*black arrow*); portion of the tumor extending into the ureter outside the bladder (*white arrow*).

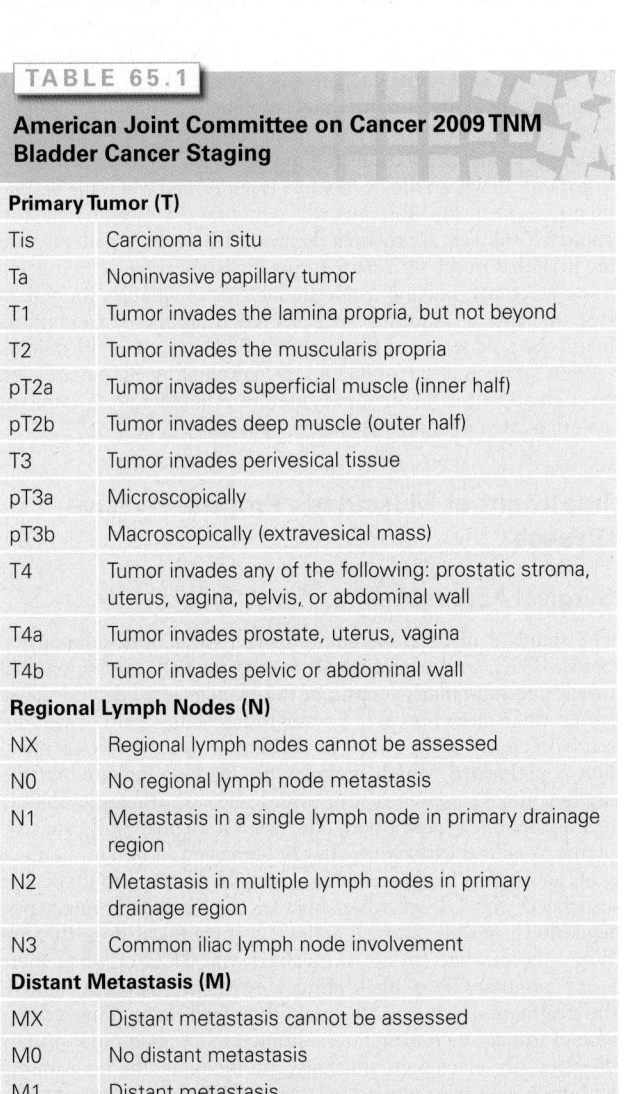

TABLE 65.1	

American Joint Committee on Cancer 2009 TNM Bladder Cancer Staging

Primary Tumor (T)	
Tis	Carcinoma in situ
Ta	Noninvasive papillary tumor
T1	Tumor invades the lamina propria, but not beyond
T2	Tumor invades the muscularis propria
pT2a	Tumor invades superficial muscle (inner half)
pT2b	Tumor invades deep muscle (outer half)
T3	Tumor invades perivesical tissue
pT3a	Microscopically
pT3b	Macroscopically (extravesical mass)
T4	Tumor invades any of the following: prostatic stroma, uterus, vagina, pelvis, or abdominal wall
T4a	Tumor invades prostate, uterus, vagina
T4b	Tumor invades pelvic or abdominal wall
Regional Lymph Nodes (N)	
NX	Regional lymph nodes cannot be assessed
N0	No regional lymph node metastasis
N1	Metastasis in a single lymph node in primary drainage region
N2	Metastasis in multiple lymph nodes in primary drainage region
N3	Common iliac lymph node involvement
Distant Metastasis (M)	
MX	Distant metastasis cannot be assessed
M0	No distant metastasis
M1	Distant metastasis

Used with the permission of the American Joint Committee on Cancer (AJCC), Chicago, Illinois. The original source for this material is the *AJCC Cancer Staging Manual*, Seventh Edition (2010) published by Springer Science and Business Media LLC, www.springer.com, page 500.

the primary tumor. Neither scan can differentiate a Ta/T1 tumor from a T2/T3 tumor because neither can visualize the depth of invasion of the primary tumor into the bladder wall. These scans are helpful, however, when they show unequivocal tumor extension outside the bladder (stage T3) (Fig. 65.1). CT scans or MRIs following a TURBT also are not reliable for staging of the primary tumor because either surgically induced edema in the resected portion of the bladder wall or postsurgical extravesical inflammatory stranding may be confused with extravesical tumor extension. For this reason, it is preferable and recommended to perform a staging CT or MRI prior to TURBT.

Patients who have documented muscularis propria–invasive bladder cancer require an additional set of studies: a chest x-ray or CT scan, liver function studies, creatinine and electrolytes level studies, and a CT evaluation of the pelvic and retroperitoneal lymph nodes. A bimanual examination is also performed at the time the tumor is transurethrally resected to evaluate for possible extravesical extension of the tumor and to determine mobility of the pelvic contents. An MRI lymphangiography, using a lymphotropic iron nanoparticle administered intravenously, shows potential.[80] Nodes that appear to be enlarged on a CT may be differentiated by this technique as to whether they are inflammatory or malignant. The sensitivity and specificity of the test are quite high.

If there is a history of functional bowel abnormality, a barium study of the segment of bowel to be used for the diversion should be performed. It is the authors' practice when using colon in the reconstruction of the urinary tract to obtain a barium enema or colonoscopy so that there are no surprises at the time of surgery. Finally, patients with muscularis propria–invasive bladder cancer must have a prostatic urethra and bulbous urethra biopsy to determine whether an orthotopic bladder may be placed or whether the procedure should encompass the urethra—that is, a cystoprostatourethrectomy in males or a cystourethrectomy and anterior exenteration in females.

Treatment of Non–Muscularis Propria–Invasive Bladder Cancer (Ta, Tis, T1)

Of patients with bladder cancer, 70% have disease that does not involve the muscularis propria at presentation. Approximately 15% to 20% of these patients will progress to stage T2 disease or greater over time. Of those presenting with Ta or T1 disease, 50% to 70% will have a recurrence following initial therapy. Low-grade tumors

(G1 or G2) and low-stage (Ta) disease tend to have a lower recurrence rate at about 50% and a 5% progression rate, whereas high-risk disease (G3, T1 associated with CIS, and multifocal disease) has a 70% recurrence rate and a 30% to 50% progression rate to stage T2 disease or greater. Less than 5% of patients with non–muscularis propria–invasive bladder cancer will develop metastatic disease without developing evidence of muscularis propria invasion (stage T2 disease or greater) of the primary lesion.

Patients who are at significant risk for developing progressive or recurrent disease following TURBT are generally considered candidates for adjuvant intravesical drug therapy. This includes those with multifocal CIS, CIS associated with Ta or T1 tumors, any G3 tumor, multifocal tumors, and those whose tumors rapidly recur following TURBT of the initial bladder tumor. A number of drugs have been used intravesically, including bacillus Calmette-Guérin (BCG), interferon (IFN) and BCG, thioTEPA, mitomycin C, doxorubicin, and gemcitabine. Complications generally include frequency, dysuria, and irritative voiding symptoms. Over the long term, bladder contracture may occur with these agents. Other complications, which are specific for each drug, are as follows: BCG administration may result in fever, joint pain, granulomatous prostatitis, sinus formation, disseminated tuberculosis, and death; thioTEPA may cause myelosuppression; mitomycin C may cause skin desquamation and rash; and doxorubicin may cause gastrointestinal upset and allergic reactions. The proposed benefit of intravesical chemotherapy is to lessen the rate of recurrences and reduce the incidence of progression. Unfortunately, it cannot be clearly stated that any of these drugs accomplish these goals over the long term.

The use of electromotive installation as an adjunct to intravesical therapy remains controversial. A randomized trial sought to clarify the benefit of electromotive installation of mitomycin. Patients were randomized to TURBT alone (n = 124), immediate post-TURBT mitomycin (n = 126), or pre-TURBT electromotive mitomycin (n = 124). Trial results demonstrated that intravesical electromotive installation of mitomycin before TURBT reduced recurrence and improved the disease-free interval compared with intravesical mitomycin after TURBT and TURBT alone.[81]

Intravesical BCG therapy is typically initiated with an induction course of 6 weekly instillations, followed by a cystoscopic evaluation 1 month after induction. In cases in which CIS is present or suspected, only a biopsy can differentiate this from inflammatory change secondary to treatment. For those who respond to induction, maintenance BCG therapy for up to 3 years is a standard of care, although patients frequently discontinue therapy early due to bladder toxicity.[82]

A European Organisation for Research and Treatment of Cancer (EORTC) phase III trial in over 1,300 patients sought to evaluate whether a third of a dose versus a full dose and a 1-year treatment versus a 3-year treatment could suffice.[83] The trial thus had four different doses and schedules of BCG maintenance therapy. No meaningful differences in toxicity, progression, or survival were observed across dose and schedules. However, the recurrence rate was lowest in high-risk patients treated with the full dose therapy for 3 years, supporting current treatment recommendations.

A number of studies have compared one intravesical chemotherapeutic agent with another. For the most part, BCG in these comparisons has a slight advantage in reducing recurrences.[84] However, when the follow-up is more than 5 years, it appears that there is minimal overall effect at reducing the recurrence rate when compared with no treatment. BCG and epirubicin are the most commonly used agents in this setting and both are considered effective for the treatment of superficial bladder cancer. However, superiority of one over the other is unknown. A meta-analysis of over 1,100 patients treated with either drug reported that intravesical BCG was more efficacious, although also more toxic.[85]

BCG failure is a clinical concern and a treatment dilemma with limited truly effective nonsurgical options. The precise definitions of BCG failure are well outlined by the 2005 International Consensus Panel on T1 bladder cancer and include four subtypes of BCG failure.[86] BCG refractory T1 disease should be of paramount concern and raises the concern for understaged diseases. Options for further intravesical treatment after BCG failure include BCG plus IFNα-2B, gemcitabine, valrubicin, docetaxel, and other novel agents.[85–92] Unfortunately, however, no single agent has yet proven to be more reliably or durably effective than another, and a true consensus on continued intravesical treatment in this setting remains to be determined.

Approximately 70% of patients with high-grade disease will experience recurrence whether or not they are treated with intravesical therapy. Moreover, there is no well-documented evidence that the use of these agents prevents disease progression, for example, from stage Ta/T1 disease to stage T2 or greater disease. One-third of patients who are at high risk for disease progression (those with G3, T1 disease) will progress to stage T2 or greater disease whether or not they are treated with BCG.[93] One-third of patients at 5 years who have disease progression and undergo a cystectomy die of metastatic disease. Thus, approximately 15% of patients with superficial disease at high risk for disease progression (CIS with associated Ta or T1 disease, rapidly recurrent disease, or G3 disease), irrespective of treatment modality, will die of their disease.[94] If definitive therapy (cystectomy) is performed when the disease is found to progress into the muscularis propria (T2 or greater), there is no difference in cure rate when these patients are compared with those who present primarily with T2 or greater disease. These statistics have encouraged some to perform a preemptive cystectomy in those patients at high risk for progression before muscularis propria invasion is documented. Ten-year cancer-specific survivals of 80% are given as justification for this approach, as compared with 50% in patients in whom the cystectomy is performed when the disease progresses to involve the muscularis propria.[95] Unfortunately, this approach subjects approximately two-thirds of these patients who are included in the 80% cancer-specific survival figure to a needless cystectomy, making it questionable as to whether there is in fact any survival advantage whatsoever. Although cystectomy remains the gold standard for recurrent BCG refractory T1 disease, there is an open protocol RTOG 0926 evaluating chemoradiation for such patients who opt for an attempt at bladder preservation or are otherwise not good cystectomy candidates.[96]

Treatment of Muscularis Propria–Invasive Disease

Surgical Approaches

The standard of care for squamous cell carcinoma, adenocarcinoma, TCC, and sarcomatoid or spindle cell carcinoma that invade the muscularis propria of the bladder is a bilateral pelvic lymph node dissection and a cystoprostatectomy, with or without a urethrectomy in the male. In the female, an anterior exenteration is performed, which includes the bladder and urethra (the urethra may be spared if uninvolved and an orthotopic bladder reconstruction is performed), the ventral vaginal wall, and the uterus. A radical cystectomy may be indicated in non–muscularis propria–invasive bladder cancers when G3 disease is multifocal or associated with CIS or when bladder tumors rapidly recur, particularly in multifocal areas following intravesical drug therapy. When the prostate stroma is involved with TCC or when there is concomitant CIS of the urethra, a cystoprostatourethrectomy is the treatment of choice.[97] If the urethra needs to be removed, the type of urinary reconstruction is limited to an abdominal urinary diversion. In selected circumstances in the male, the neurovascular bundles coursing along the lateral side of the prostate caudally and adjacent to the rectum more cephalad may be preserved, sometimes preserving potency. Partial cystectomies may rarely be performed in selected patients, thus preserving bladder function and affording in the properly selected patient the same cure rate as a radical cystectomy.[98] Patients who are candidates for such procedures must have focal disease located far enough away from the ureteral orifices and bladder neck to achieve at least a 2-cm margin around the tumor and a margin sufficient around the ureteral orifices and bladder neck to reconstruct the bladder. Practically, this limits partial cystectomies to those patients who have small tumors located in the dome of the bladder and in whom random bladder biopsies show no evidence of CIS or other bladder tumors.

Survival

The probability of survival from bladder cancer following a cystectomy is determined by the pathologic stage of the disease. Survival is markedly influenced by the presence or absence of positive lymph nodes. Some have argued that the number of positive nodes impacts survival in that, when resected, there is a potential for cure provided there are less than four to eight positive nodes.[99,100] Positive perivesical nodes have a less ominous prognosis when compared with involvement of iliac or para-aortic nodes. Pathologic type may also impact outcome, but in most series, survival is more dependent on pathologic stage than on the cell type of the cancer. Most large series of survival statistics following treatment include all patients regardless of cell type. These series are generally constituted as to histologic type as follows: TCC, 85% to 90%; combination of TCC and either squamous cell or adenocarcinoma, 6%; pure squamous cell carcinoma, 3%; pure adenocarcinoma, 3%; small-cell and sarcomatoid or spindle cell carcinoma, 2% (Table 65.2).

Types of Urinary Diversion

Urinary diversions may be divided into continent and incontinent. Incontinent urinary diversions or conduits involve the use of a segment of ileum or colon and, less commonly, a segment of jejunum. The distal end is brought to the skin, and the ureters are implanted into the proximal end. The patient wears a urinary collection appliance. The advantages of a conduit (ileal or colonic) are its simplicity and the reduced number of immediate and long-term

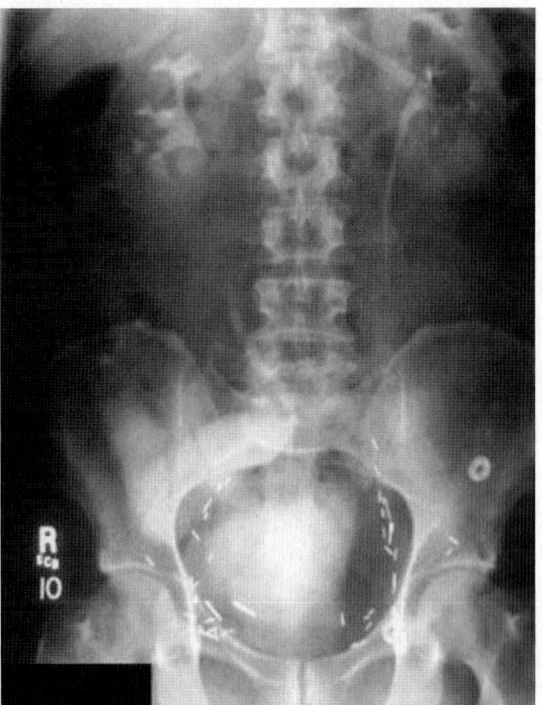

Figure 65.2 An intravenous urogram of a patient with an orthotopic bladder after a radical cystoprostatectomy. The orthotopic bladder was constructed of the right colon and distal ileum.

postoperative complications. In most series, 13% of patients who undergo a cystectomy and urinary diversion of this type will have a significant complication that impacts on hospital stay or recovery. Generally, the distal ileum is used for the urinary conduit or reservoir; however, if it has been irradiated or is otherwise involved, one may select the right colon or a short segment of jejunum. The latter is the least desirable choice because electrolyte problems may be significant. On occasion, during exenterative surgery when an end colostomy is created, a segment of distal bowel is used, thus obviating the need for an intestinal anastomosis.

Continent diversions may be divided into two types: abdominal and orthotopic. Abdominal diversions require a continence valve, whereas an orthotopic neobladder depends on the urethral sphincter for continence. The reservoir is made of bowel that is fashioned into a globular configuration. In the abdominal type of continent diversion, the stoma is brought through the abdominal wall to the skin. The patient catheterizes the pouch every 4 hours. Orthotopic urinary diversions entail the use of bowel brought to the urethra, thus allowing the patient to void by Valsalva (Fig. 65.2). Patients must have the facility to catheterize themselves, because it is mandatory in the abdominal continent diversion and occasionally necessary in the orthotopic reconstruction. The advantage of continent diversions is the avoidance of a collection device. The advantage of an orthotopic bladder over all other types of continent diversions is that it rehabilitates the patient to normal voiding through the urethra, often without the need for intermittent catheterization or the need to wear a collection device. Postoperative and long-term complications of continent diversion are increased over the conduit types of diversions. Indeed, in some series, postoperative complications range from 13% to 30%. Long-term metabolic complications are also increased.

Complications of Cystectomy and Urinary Diversion

The complications of all types of urinary diversion may be divided into three groups: metabolic, neuromechanical, and surgical.

TABLE 65.2

Survival After Radical Cystectomy According to Pathologic Stage at 10 Years

Pathologic Stage	Disease-Specific Survival (%)	Overall Survival (%)
pTa, Tis, T1 with high risk of progression	82	—
Organ confined, negative nodes (pT2, pN0)	73	49
Non–organ confined (pT3–4a or pN1–2)	33	23
Lymph node positive (any T, pN1–2)	28, 34	21

From Gschwend JE, Dahm P, Fair WR. Disease specific survival as endpoint of outcome for bladder cancer patients following radical cystectomy. *Eur Urol* 2002;41:440–448; Stein JP, Cai J, Groshen S, et al. Risk factors for patients with pelvic lymph node metastases following radical cystectomy with en bloc pelvic lymphadenectomy: concept of lymph node density. *J Urol* 2003;170:35–41; Stein JP, Lieskovsky G, Cote R, et al. Radical cystectomy in the treatment of invasive bladder cancer: long-term results in 1,054 patients. *J Clin Oncol* 2001;19:666–675; Dalbagni G, Genega E, Hashibe M, et al. Cystectomy for bladder cancer: a contemporary series. *J Urol* 2001;165:1111–1116; Grossman HB, Natale RB, Tangen CM, et al. Neoadjuvant chemotherapy plus cystectomy compared with cystectomy alone for locally advanced bladder cancer. *N Engl J Med* 2003;349:859–866; and Zehnder P, Studer UE, Skinner EC, et al. Super extended versus extended pelvic lymph node dissection in patients undergoing radical cystectomy for bladder cancer: a comparative study. *J Urol* 2011;186:1261–1268.

PRACTICE OF ONCOLOGY

Metabolic Complications of Urinary Intestinal Diversion.
When the intestine is interposed in the urinary tract, there is the potential for a number of metabolic complications.[104] These may involve electrolyte abnormalities and altered drug metabolism, which may result in altered sensorium, infection, osteomalacia, growth retardation, calculi both within the reservoir as well as in the kidney, short bowel syndrome, cancer, and altered bile metabolism.

Depending on the segment used, different specific electrolyte abnormalities may occur. When the ileum and colon are used, hyperchloremic metabolic acidosis may result; when jejunum is used, hypochloremic or hyperkalemic metabolic acidosis may follow.

Hypokalemia is more common when the colon is used, whereas hypocalcemia is more common when the ileum and colon are used, and hypomagnesemia is more common when the ileum and the colon are used.

The most pervasive detrimental effect created by all urinary intestinal diversions is due to acidosis. Acidosis may result in electrolyte abnormalities, osteomalacia, growth retardation, altered sensorium, altered hepatic metabolism, renal calculi, and abnormal drug metabolism. In general, patients with normal renal function as well as normal hepatic function are less prone to acidosis and its complications.

Treatment for the metabolic acidosis is straightforward and can be accomplished with bicarbonate or with Bicitra solution, which is sodium citrate and citric acid. Polycitra, which is a combination of potassium citrate, sodium citrate, and citric acid, may also be employed. It has the advantage of supplying potassium, which, on occasion, is deficient. Chlorpromazine and nicotinic acid have been used to block the chloride bicarbonate exchanger, and thus lessen the potential for the acidosis.

Decreased renal function is seen in a majority of patients in the decade following a radical cystectomy, and choice of diversion does not predict the decline. Postoperative hydronephrosis, pyelonephritis, and uretero-enteric strictures represent factors that, if addressed, may mitigate the loss of function.[105]

Patients with conduits may have a 3% to 4% incidence of renal calculi over the long term. Those with reservoirs have up to a 20% incidence of calculi within the reservoir. The pathogenesis may be a metabolic alteration or infection, whereas reservoir stones are most commonly due to a surgical foreign body or mucus serving as a nidus.

There is a high incidence of bacteriuria in patients with either conduits or pouches, and the incidence of sepsis is 13%. There appears to be diminished antibacterial activity of the intestinal mucosa, with the immunoglobulins, which are normally secreted by the mucosa, being altered. In addition to this, when the bowel is distended, there can be a translocation of bacteria from the lumen into the bloodstream.

Because the intestine is interposed in the urinary tract, drugs that are eliminated unchanged from the body through the kidney and have the potential to be reabsorbed by the gut can in fact result in significant alterations in metabolism of that drug. Patients with a urinary diversion, when given systemic chemotherapy, have a higher incidence of complications and are more likely to have their chemotherapy limited when compared with patients without diversion who receive the same drugs and dose.[106]

The loss of the distal ileum may result in vitamin B_{12} malabsorption, which then manifests itself as anemia and neurologic abnormalities. Bile salt malabsorption may occur and result in diarrhea. Loss of the ileocecal valve may result in diarrhea with bacterial overgrowth of the ileum and malabsorption of vitamin B_{12} and fat-soluble vitamins A, D, E, and K. Loss of the colon may result in diarrhea and bicarbonate loss.

Neuromechanical Complications. Neuromechanical complications may be of two types: atonic, resulting in an atonic segment with urinary retention, and hyperperistaltic contractions. The latter is relevant in continent diversions, as this may result in incontinence and a low-capacity reservoir.

Surgical Complications. There are a number of complications that occur following any major surgical procedure, which include thrombophlebitis, pulmonary embolus, wound dehiscence, pneumonia, atelectasis, myocardial infarction, and death. Complications specific to cystectomy and urinary diversion are divided into short term and late. The short-term complications include acute acidosis (16%), urine leak (3% to 16%), bowel obstruction or fecal leak (10%), and pyelonephritis (5% to 15%). The longer term complications include ureteral or intestinal obstruction (15%), renal deterioration (15%), renal failure (5%), stoma problems (15%), and intestinal stricture (10% to 15%).[107,108]

The morbidity of salvage cystectomy for a recurrence following bladder sparing chemoradiation has also been described and appears acceptable when compared to primary cystectomy series.[109]

Selective Bladder-Preserving Approaches

The treatment options for muscularis propria–invasive bladder tumors can broadly be divided into those that remove the bladder and those that spare it. In the United States, a radical cystectomy with pelvic lymph node dissection remains the standard method used to treat patients with this tumor. Several reports from North America and Europe have described long-term results using multimodality treatment of muscularis propria–invading bladder cancer, with appropriate safeguards for early cystectomy should this treatment fail. For bladder-conserving therapy to be more widely accepted, this treatment approach must have a high likelihood of eradicating the primary tumor, must preserve good organ function, and must not result in compromised patient survival. It does appear that, for selected patients, bladder sparing therapy with salvage cystectomy reserved for tumor recurrence represents a safe and effective alternative to immediate radical cystectomy.[110]

Successful bladder-preserving approaches have evolved during the past 3 decades. They began with the use of radiation therapy but expanded when the National Bladder Cancer Group first demonstrated the safety and efficacy of cisplatin as a radiation sensitizer in patients with muscle-invasive bladder cancer that was unsuitable for cystectomy.[111] The long-term survival with stage T2 tumors (64%) and stage T3 to T4 tumors (22%) was encouraging. This was validated by the National Cancer Institute–Canada randomized trial of radiation (either definitive or precystectomy) with or without concurrent cisplatin for patients with T3 bladder cancer, which showed a significant improvement in long-term survival with pelvic tumor control (67% versus 47%) in the patients who were assigned cisplatin.[112] Additional single-institution studies showed that the combination of a visibly complete TURBT followed by radiation therapy or radiation therapy concurrent with chemotherapy safely improved local control.[113,114] These findings led the RTOG to develop protocols for bladder preservation beginning with a TURBT of as much of the tumor as is safely possible, followed by the combination of radiation with concurrent radiosensitizing chemotherapy. One key to the success of such a program is the selection of patients for bladder preservation on the basis of the initial response of each individual patient's tumor to therapy. Thus, bladder conservation is reserved for those patients who have a clinical CR to concurrent chemotherapy and radiation. A prompt cystectomy is recommended for those patients whose tumors respond only incompletely or who subsequently develop an invasive tumor (Fig. 65.3). Up to 30% of the patients entering a potential bladder-preserving protocol with trimodality therapy (initial TURBT followed by concurrent chemoradiation) will ultimately require a salvage radical cystectomy.

For over 2 decades, the Massachusetts General Hospital (MGH), the RTOG, and several centers in Europe have evaluated in phase II and III protocols concurrent chemoradiation plus neoadjuvant or adjuvant chemotherapy (Table 65.3). Radiosensitizing drugs studied in these series, either singly or in various combinations, include cisplatin, carboplatin, paclitaxel, 5-fluorouracil (5-FU), mitomycin C,

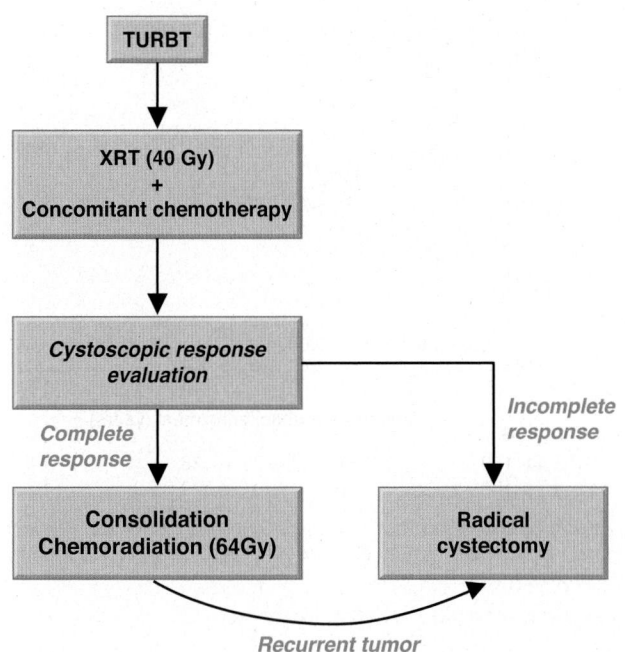

Figure 65.3 Schema for trimodality treatment of muscularis propria–invasive bladder cancer with selective bladder preservation. XRT, radiation therapy.

and gemcitabine.[113] The first RTOG study of patients treated with once-daily radiation treatment and concurrent cisplatin yielded a 5-year survival of 52% (42% with intact bladder).[115] RTOG studies 8802 and 8903 used methotrexate, cisplatin, and vinblastine (MCV) chemotherapy as neoadjuvant treatment.[116] In the latter study, the neoadjuvant therapy was tested in a randomized fashion.[117] No improvement was seen in survival or in local tumor eradication as a result of neoadjuvant therapy, although the trial was closed early and underpowered to give a definitive answer. The toxicity of the MCV arm was considerable, with only 67% of patients able to complete the planned treatment. The use of contemporary neoadjuvant

chemotherapy (dose-dense methotrexate, vinblastine, adriamycin, cisplatin [ddMVAC] or gemcitabine and cisplatin [GC]) regimens with appropriate supportive therapy in well-selected bladder-sparing patients may warrant further investigation.

Other studies from Paris and Germany have reported their large experience with bladder sparing.[118,119] The CR rate in the German study was 72%, and local control of the bladder tumor after the CR without a muscle-invasive relapse was maintained in 64% of the patients at 10 years. The 10-year disease-specific survival was 42%, and more than 80% of these survivors preserved their bladder. This series reported the sequential use of radiation with no chemotherapy (126 patients), followed by concurrent cisplatin (145 patients), then concurrent carboplatin (95 patients), and finally concurrent cisplatin with 5-FU (49 patients). The CR rates in these four protocols were 51%, 81%, 64%, and 87%, respectively.[120,121] The 5-year actuarial survival with an intact bladder in these studies was 38%, 47%, 41%, and 54%, respectively. These results strongly suggest that radiochemotherapy, when given concurrently, is superior to radiation therapy alone; that carboplatin is less radiosensitizing than cisplatin; and that cisplatin plus 5-FU may be superior to cisplatin alone.

The RTOG protocols have subsequently explored both twice-daily radiation therapy and novel radiosensitization using cisplatin with or without 5-FU or paclitaxel.[62,122,123,124] Complete response and bladder preservation rates are consistently high, with no one regimen clearly superior.[62]

Gemcitabine has been also tested in bladder-treatment protocols. In a phase I trial from the University of Michigan, 23 patients, mostly T2, were treated with gemcitabine and concurrent daily radiation. At a median follow-up of 5.6 years, an impressive 91% CR rate was observed, and the 5-year actuarial estimates of survival include a bladder-intact survival of 62%, an overall survival of 76%, and a disease-specific survival of 82%.[125] A phase II study from the United Kingdom of 50 patients treated with concurrent weekly gemcitabine and hypofractionated radiation reported an 88% complete endoscopic response rate, a 3-year overall survival of 75%, and cancer-specific survival of 82%.[126] Twice weekly low-dose gemcitabine was recently evaluated as a radiosensitizer with daily radiation in protocol RTOG 0712.

Cisplatin is not always an ideal drug for bladder cancer patients, because it may cause impaired renal function in many. A British group observed high response rates using the combination of 5-FU

TABLE 65.3

Results of Multimodality Treatment for Muscle-Invading Bladder Cancer

Series (Ref.)	Multimodality Therapy Used	Number of Patients	5-Year Overall Survival (%)	5-Year Survival with Intact Bladder (%)
RTOG 8512, 1993[115]	External-beam radiation with cisplatin	42	52	42
RTOG 8802, 1996[116]	TURBT, MCV, external-beam radiation with cisplatin	91	51	44 (4 y)
RTOG 8903, 1998[117]	TURBT with or without MCV, external-beam radiation with cisplatin	123	49	38
University of Paris, 1998[118]	TURBT, 5-FU, external-beam radiation with cisplatin	120	63	N/A
Erlangen, 2002[119]	TURBT, external-beam radiation, cisplatin, carboplatin, or cisplatin and 5-FU	415 (cisplatin, 82; carboplatin, 61; 5-FU/cisplatin, 87)	51	42
RTOG 9906, 2009[122]	TURBT, TAX plus CP plus XRT; adjuvant CP plus GEM	80	56	47
MGH, 2012[130]	TURBT, external-beam radiation and cisplatin *with or without* 5-FU or TAX; neoadjuvant or adjuvant chemotherapy	348	52	42

MCV, methotrexate, cisplatin, vinblastine; 5-FU, 5-fluorouracil; N/A, not available; TAX, paclitaxel; CP, cisplatin; GEM, gemcitabine.

and mitomycin C with pelvic radiotherapy.[127] These results led to the phase III Bladder Cancer 2001 (BC2001) trial, in which 360 patients with muscle-invasive bladder cancer were randomized to either radiotherapy alone or to radiotherapy with concomitant 5-FU and mitomycin C chemotherapy. Local–regional disease-free survival was superior for those patients receiving chemotherapy (67% versus 54% at 2 years; hazard ratio [HR] 0.68, $p = 0.03$ with median follow-up of 70 months). Survival at 5 years was higher with chemoradiotherapy (48% versus 35%), but did not reach statistical significance (HR 0.82; $p = 0.16$).[128]

Predictors of Outcome

A common feature of all the RTOG protocols was early bladder tumor response evaluation and the selection of patients for bladder conservation on the basis of their initial response to TURBT combined with chemotherapy and radiation.[130] Bladder conservation was reserved for those who had a complete clinical response at the midpoint in therapy (after a radiation dosage of 40 Gy). Complete responders to induction therapy then received consolidation with additional chemotherapy and radiation to a total tumor dose of 64 to 65 Gy. Incomplete responders were advised to undergo a radical cystectomy, as were patients whose invasive tumors persisted or recurred after treatment. The current schema for trimodality treatment of muscle-invading bladder cancer is provided in Figure 65.3. Other tumor presentations associated with successful bladder-sparing therapy include: solitary T2 or early T3 tumors (typically <6 cm in size), no tumor-associated hydronephrosis, tumors allowing a visibly complete TURBT, invasive tumors not associated with extensive carcinoma in situ, and urothelial carcinoma histology (because alternative histologies have not been rigorously evaluated in bladder sparing protocols).

In the MGH series,[130] the median follow-up for all surviving patients was 7.7 years. Of patients, 72% (78% with stage T2) had CR to induction therapy. The 10-year actuarial overall survival was 35% (T2, 43%; T3–T4a, 27%) and the 10-year disease-specific survival was 59% (T2, 67%; stage T3–T4a, 49%) (Figs. 65.4 and 65.5). The clinical stage and achieving a CR were significantly associated with both overall survival and disease-specific survival. A nomogram predicting response has been developed from this data.[129] The use of neoadjuvant chemotherapy with MCV, however, was not associated with survival or incidence of metastases, although this may warrant further investigation in the modern era.

The 10-year disease-specific survival rate for the 102 patients (29%) undergoing a cystectomy was 44%, illustrating the very

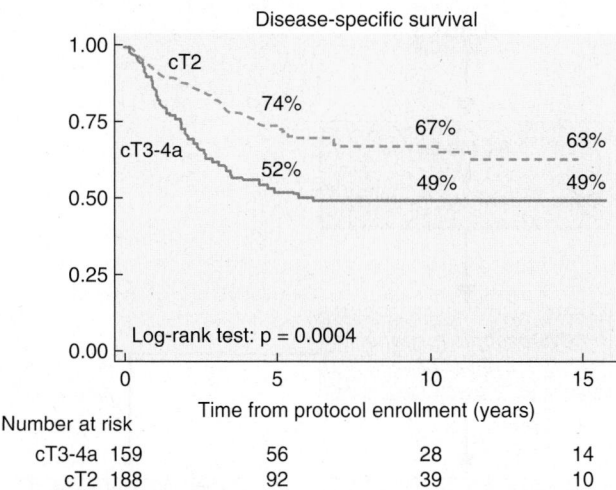

Figure 65.5 Massachusetts General Hospital Selective Bladder Preservation Series 1986 to 2002 disease-specific survival reported by intention to treat.

important contribution of prompt salvage cystectomy. The 10-year disease-specific survival with an intact bladder was 45% (T2, 52%; T3–T4a, 36%). No patient required a cystectomy due to bladder morbidity. The overall survival and disease-specific survival for all 348 patients and for some clinically important subgroups are shown in Table 65.4. The value of complete TURBT in bladder-sparing therapy is demonstrated in this report. Of the 348 patients followed, 227 underwent a complete TURBT and 116 had an incomplete TURBT. Patients who underwent a complete TURBT had improved CR, overall survival, disease-specific survival, and lower rates of cystectomy (22% versus 42%) compared to those with an incomplete TURBT. In a review of the patients who were complete responders after induction therapy, 55% developed no further bladder tumors, 29% subsequently developed a superficial occurrence, and 16% developed an invasive tumor.[132] Most patients with superficial recurrence were treated successfully by TURBT and intravesical chemotherapy. For these individuals, the overall survival was comparable to those who had no failure. However, one-quarter of these patients ultimately required a salvage cystectomy.

Notably, age is not a contraindication to successful bladder sparing therapy, and indeed, results are favorable in patients aged 75 years or older.[130] This is an important consideration given that the elderly generally appear to be undertreated for invasive bladder cancer in the United States.[131] Bladder-sparing chemoradiation remains a good option for those patients who are not cystectomy candidates and, often, such patients would be treated with daily radiation and appropriate concurrent chemotherapy without a break.

Radiation Treatment

The most common approach with external-beam irradiation reported from North America and Europe involves the treatment of the pelvis to include the bladder, the prostate (in men), and often, the low external and internal iliac lymph nodes for a total dose of 40 to 45 Gy in 1.8- to 2.0-Gy fractions during 4 to 5 weeks. Subsequently, the target volume is reduced to deliver a final boost dose of 20 to 25 Gy in 15 fractions to the primary bladder tumor. Some protocols call for partial bladder radiation as the boost volume if the location of the tumor in the bladder can be satisfactorily identified by the use of cystoscopic mapping, selected mucosal biopsies, and imaging information from CT or MRI. Figure 65.6 is an isodose color wash of a partial bladder boost in a three-dimensional–conformal plan. Plans using conventional fractionation that result in a whole bladder dose of 50 to 55 Gy and a bladder tumor volume dose of 65 Gy in combination with concurrent

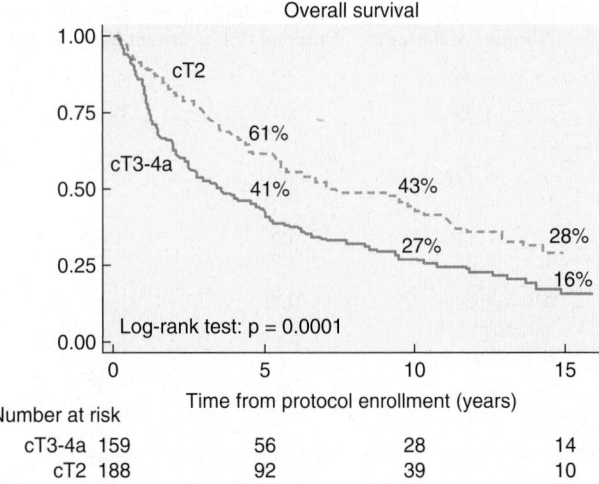

Figure 65.4 Massachusetts General Hospital Selective Bladder Preservation Series 1986 to 2002 overall survival reported by intention to treat.

TABLE 65.4

Survival Outcomes by Patient and Tumor Characteristics: Massachusetts General Hospital

Patient Group	n	Overall Survival (%)				Disease-Specific Survival (%)			
		5 Year	10 Year	15 Year	P value	5 Year	10 Year	15 Year	P value
All patients	348	52 ± 5.3[a]	35 ± 5.6[a]	22 ± 5.6[a]		64 ± 5.8[a]	59 ± 6.2[a]	57 ± 6.6[a]	
Age at Entry (y)									
<75	262	54	39	27	0.004	65	59	58	0.59
>75	86	45	23	2.9		63	60	52	
Sex									
Female	91	55	37	17	0.72	64	55	55	0.59
Male	257	51	35	24		64	60	58	
Clinical Stage									
T2	188	61	43	28	0.0001	74	67	63	0.0004
T3–T4a	159	41	27	16		52	49	49	
Hydronephrosis									
No	289	55	39	24	0.0004	68	63	61	0.0005
Yes	58	34	17	10		44	38	38	

[a] 95% confidence interval.
Source: Efstathiou JA, Spiegel DY, Shipley WU, et al. Long-term outcomes of selective bladder preservation by combined-modality therapy for invasive bladder cancer: the MGH experience. *Eur Urol* 2012;61:705–711.

cisplatin-containing chemotherapy have been widely used. The available information suggests that higher doses per fraction may lead to a higher rate of significant late complications. Data looking at toxicity from urodynamic and quality-of-life studies indicate that lower dose per fraction irradiation given once or twice a day concurrent with chemotherapy results in excellent long-term bladder function and low rates of late pelvic toxicity.[133,134]

Because the bladder is not a fixed organ, its location and volume can vary considerably from day to day. This results in a number of

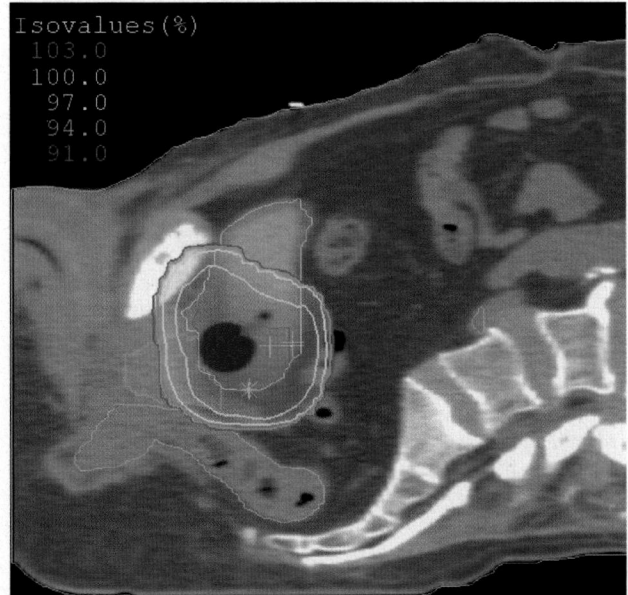

Figure 65.6 Display of a sagittal section through the three-dimensional (3-D) data set, with dose displayed in color wash, for a patient with bladder cancer treated with a partial bladder tumor boost with 3-D conformal radiotherapy. Note sparing of the anterior, non–tumor bearing portion of bladder.

logistic problems to ensure adequate coverage of the bladder. Studies have identified substantial movement of the bladder during the course of external-beam radiation therapy, and as a result of these findings, many have recommended that the bladder be emptied when simulated and prior to each treatment to maximize reproducibility and avoid a geographic miss. Forms of image-guided delivery (including daily cone-beam CT and fiducials) have also been employed for accurate localization. Another acceptable approach often employed in the United Kingdom, is for radiation to be delivered to 55 Gy in 20 fractions or 64 Gy in 32 fractions to the whole bladder without a tumor boost and without fields to specifically cover the pelvic lymph nodes.[135]

Brachytherapy is another technique to deliver a higher dose of radiation to a limited area of the bladder within a short period. This approach has been reported from institutions in the Netherlands, Belgium, and France. It is reserved for patients with solitary bladder tumors and as part of combined modality therapy with transurethral resection and external-beam radiation therapy as well as interstitial radiation therapy. External-beam doses of 30 Gy are used in combination with an implant tumor dose of 40 Gy. These groups report that for patients with solitary clinical stage T2 to T3a tumors less than 5 cm in diameter, local control rates at 5 to 10 years range from 72% to 84% with disease-specific survivals of approximately 75%.[136]

Comparison of Treatment Outcomes of Contemporary Cystectomy Series with Contemporary Selective Bladder-Preserving Series

Comparing the results of selective bladder-preserving approaches with those of radical cystectomy series is confounded by selection bias and the discordance between clinical (TURBT) staging and pathologic (cystectomy) staging. Clinical staging will understage the extent of disease 40% of the time with regard to penetration into the muscularis propria or beyond when compared to pathologic staging.[137,138] The University of Southern California and Memorial Sloan-Kettering Cancer Center have reported their large cystectomy experience,[102,136,139] and the national phase III protocol by Southwest Oncology Group (SWOG), Eastern Cooperative Oncology Group, and Cancer and Leukemia Group B (CALGB)

TABLE 65.5

Muscle-Invasive Bladder Cancer: Survival Outcomes in Contemporary Series

Series (Ref.)	Stages	Number of Patients	Overall Survival (%) 5 Year	10 Year
Cystectomy				
University of Southern California, 2001[101]	pT2–pT4a	633	48	32
Memorial Sloan-Kettering, 2001[102]	pT2–pT4a	181	36	27
SWOG/ECOG/CALGB,[a,b] 2003[103]	cT2–cT4a	303	49	34
Selective Bladder Preservation (Chemoradiation)				
University of Erlangen,[a] 2002[119]	cT2–cT4a	326	45	29
MGH,[a] 2012[130]	cT2–cT4a	348	52	35
RTOG,[a] 1998[117]	cT2–cT4a	123	49	—
BC2001,[a] 2012[128]	cT2–4a	182	48	

[a] These series include all patients by their intention to treat.
[b] Fifty percent of patients were randomly assigned to receive three cycles of neoadjuvant MVAC (methotrexate, vinblastine, doxorubicin, cisplatin).
ECOG, Eastern Cooperative Oncology Group; CALGB, Cancer and Leukemia Group B; RTOG, Radiation Therapy Oncology Group, Bladder Cancer 2001 (BC2001) trial.

has also reported valuable prospective data.[103] The overall survival rates from these contemporary cystectomy series are comparable to those reported from single-institution and cooperative group results using contemporary selective bladder-preserving approaches with trimodality therapy and prompt salvage cystectomy for the minority of patients who recur (Table 65.5). An attempt to compare cystectomy to bladder-sparing therapy in a randomized fashion in the United Kingdom failed to accrue.

Bladder-Preservation Treatments with Less than Trimodality Therapy

It has been argued that trimodality therapy might represent excessive treatment for many patients with invasive bladder cancer and that comparable results could be obtained by TURBT, either alone or with chemotherapy. Herr[140] reported the outcome of 432 patients initially evaluated by repeat TURBT for muscle-invasive bladder tumors. In that series, 99 patients (23% of the original 432 patients) initially treated conservatively without immediate cystectomy had a 34% rate of progression to a recurrent muscle-invading tumor at 20 years. In series combining TURBT and MVAC chemotherapy, only 50% of those found to have a clinical CR proved to be tumor-free at cystectomy.[141] By comparison, one of the clearest examples of the improved success of trimodality treatment was reported in the study from the University of Paris.[142] TURBT followed by concurrent cisplatin, 5-FU, and accelerated radiation was used by this group initially as a precystectomy regimen. In the first 18 patients, all of whom demonstrated no residual tumor on cystoscopic evaluation and rebiopsy (a CR) but who all underwent a cystectomy, none had any tumor in the cystectomy specimen (100% had a pathologic CR). Comparing approaches by TURBT plus MVAC chemotherapy alone with trimodality therapy, the 5-year survival rates are comparable (50%), but the preserved bladder rate for all patients studied ranged from 20% to 33% when radiation therapy was not used and from 41% to 45% when radiation therapy was used.[142] Thus, trimodality therapy increases the probability of surviving with an intact bladder by 30% to 40% compared with the results reported with TURBT and chemotherapy alone.

Herr[143] reported on 63 patients who had achieved a complete clinical response to neoadjuvant chemotherapy with a cisplatin-based regimen, who then refused to undergo a planned cystectomy. He reported that the most significant predictor of improved survival was complete resection of the tumor before starting chemotherapy. Over 90% of surviving patients had small low-stage invasive tumors that were completely resected. Thus, he concluded, selected patients with T2 bladder cancers may do well after a transurethral resection and chemotherapy.

Systemic Chemotherapy with Radical Therapy

Neoadjuvant Chemotherapy

The advantage of neoadjuvant chemotherapy is its potential to downsize and downstage tumors and to attack occult metastatic disease early, especially given the frequent postoperative complications and prolonged recovery that can delay or derail plans for adjuvant chemotherapy. Moreover, although trials described as follows suggest a survival advantage for neoadjuvant chemotherapy, there have been no contemporary studies supporting a benefit with adjuvant chemotherapy. The disadvantages of neoadjuvant therapy include the inherent difficulties in assessing response, the fact that clinical rather than pathologic criteria must be relied on, the debilitating effects of chemotherapy in some patients, increasing the risks of surgery and possibly complicating or delaying full recovery from surgery, and the possibility of the deleterious effects of the delay in cystectomy or radiation associated with neoadjuvant chemotherapy.[144]

Although downstaging of the primary tumor has been demonstrated, randomized studies using single-agent neoadjuvant chemotherapy have failed to demonstrate a survival benefit. Studies in patients with measurable metastatic disease clearly showed the superiority of MVAC over single-agent cisplatin on survival, inspiring further studies of multiagent neoadjuvant therapy.[145]

The study by Grossman et al.[143] randomly assigned patients with muscularis propria–invasive bladder cancer (stage T2 to T4a) to radical cystectomy alone or three cycles of MVAC followed by radical cystectomy. During an 11-year period, 317 patients were enrolled. The authors reported that MVAC can be given before radical cystectomy, but the side effects are appreciable. One-third of patients had severe hematologic or gastrointestinal reactions, but, on the positive side, there were no drug-related deaths and the chemotherapy did not adversely affect the performance of surgery. The authors concluded:

1. The survival benefit associated with MVAC appeared to be strongly related to downstaging of the tumor to pT0. Of the chemotherapy-treated patients, 38% had no evidence of cancer at cystectomy, as compared with 15% of patients in the cystectomy-only group. In both groups, improved survival was associated with the absence of residual cancer in the cystectomy specimen.

2. The median survival was 77 months for the chemotherapy-treated patients compared with 46 months for the cystectomy-only group.
3. The 5-year actuarial survival was 43% in the cystectomy group, which was not significantly different from 57% in the chemotherapy-treated group.

Stratification by tumor stage indicated greater improvement in median survival with chemotherapy in subjects with T3–T4a disease (65 versus 24 months, chemotherapy versus observation) than in subjects with T2 disease (105 versus 75 months). The authors point out that their study is different from seven previous negative studies that used either single-agent cisplatin (demonstrated to be inferior to MVAC in measurable metastatic disease) or a two-drug combination. They also acknowledged problems of interpretation created by slow accrual and a lack of pathologic review.

The Medical Research Council and the EORTC performed a prospective randomized trial of neoadjuvant cisplatin, methotrexate, and vinblastine in patients undergoing cystectomy or full-dose external-beam radiotherapy for muscularis propria–invasive bladder cancer.[146,147] In the initial report with a median follow-up of 7.4 years, the difference in 5-year survival between those who received chemotherapy (49%) and those who did not (43%) just reached clinical significance with a probability value of 0.048.[147] However, the survival benefit did not reach the prespecified study goal. Long-term follow-up of the study with median follow-up of 8 years and more death events demonstrated that systemic chemotherapy plus local treatment improved overall 10-year survival by 6% and reduced the risk of bladder cancer death by 17% compared to local treatment alone. For patients whose local treatment included a cystectomy, the use of cisplatin, methotrexate, and vinblastine (CMV) resulted in a 26% reduction in the risk of death compared to surgery alone.[148] Based on their interpretation of the data as presented, Sharma and Bajorin[149] now recommend neoadjuvant chemotherapy, although others are concerned that the "number needed to treat" is very high.

A third randomized trial was the Nordic Cystectomy Trial 1.[150] Patients were treated with two cycles of neoadjuvant doxorubicin and cisplatin. All patients received 5 days of radiation followed by cystectomy. A subgroup analysis was performed and showed a 20% difference in disease-specific survival at 5 years in patients with T3 and T4 disease, but there was no difference in stages T1 and T2, nor a difference when all entered patients were compared.

The Nordic Cystectomy Trial 2 included only stage T3 or T4a patients in an attempt to confirm the positive results in Nordic 1 in this subgroup of patients.[151] This trial eliminated radiation therapy and substituted methotrexate for doxorubicin in order to lower toxicity. In 317 patients studied, no survival benefit was noted in the chemotherapy arm. The authors concluded that despite substantial downstaging, no survival benefit was seen with neoadjuvant chemotherapy after 5 years of follow-up, although the choice of chemotherapy was unconventional by contemporary standards.

Raghavan et al.[152] published a meta-analysis of all completed randomized trials of neoadjuvant chemotherapy for invasive bladder cancer (2,688 patients). They concluded that single-agent neoadjuvant chemotherapy is ineffective and should not be used; current combination chemotherapy regimens improve the 5-year survival by 5%, which reduces the risk of death by 13% compared with the use of definitive local treatment alone (from 43% to 38%).

Additional meta-analyses have been published[144,153–155] that showed a 4% to 6% absolute increase in 5-year survival. Many phase II studies are now investigating alternative neoadjuvant combinations including cisplatin/gemcitabine and dose-dense or accelerated MVAC, and time will tell whether any have superiority.[156–162]

In the 2014 National Comprehensive Cancer Network *Clinical Practice Guidelines in Oncology: Bladder Cancer*, neoadjuvant chemotherapy is a category 1 recommendation for localized stage T2–T4a disease. According to the National Cancer Data Base in the United States, only 11.6% of patients underwent any perioperative chemotherapy, with most in the adjuvant setting.[162] In the future, gene profiling may identify those most likely to respond to chemotherapy.[163]

Adjuvant Chemotherapy

The advantage of adjuvant, as opposed to neoadjuvant, chemotherapy is that pathologic staging allows for a more accurate selection of patients. This approach facilitates the separation of patients in stage pT2 from those in stages pT3 or pT4 or node-positive disease, all at a high risk for metastatic progression.

Adjuvant chemotherapy has been studied in two major clinical settings: (1) following bladder-sparing chemoirradiation and (2) following a radical cystectomy. In the former case, there is no guidance from pathologic staging, but experience has shown that up to 50% of those with invasive cancers have, in truth, a systemic disease.[164] Respecting this, the RTOG studies have added adjuvant chemotherapy at first with MCV, later using cisplatin plus gemcitabine, and more recently adding paclitaxel.[165] The results thus far do not indicate whether adjuvant chemotherapy is affecting survival.

The place of adjuvant chemotherapy after cystectomy has been studied more thoroughly, but again, the results are not clear. Investigators generally agree that in the face of positive nodes, and even with negative nodes and high pathologic stage of the primary tumor, adjuvant chemotherapy is likely to be important in improving survival. In reviewing existing reports of adjuvant trials in bladder cancer, there are five randomized trials using adjuvant chemotherapy.[166–170] Three studies found no difference between adjuvant chemotherapy and cystectomy alone, but all three were seriously flawed in design or accrual.[149] Two of the five studies[169,170] showed a survival benefit for cystectomy and adjuvant chemotherapy over cystectomy alone, but both are subject to criticism for both method considerations and small accrual.

Nonetheless, in a follow-up report by Stockle et al.[171] an analysis of 166 patients, including the 49 initially randomized patients, a difference was noted in the 80 patients who received adjuvant chemotherapy as compared with 86 patients who underwent cystectomy alone. The extent of nodal involvement proved important, and when patients were stratified by the number of nodes involved, adjuvant chemotherapy was most effective in patients with N1 disease.

In an important review of the current status of adjuvant chemotherapy in muscle-invasive bladder cancer, the Advanced Bladder Cancer Meta-Analysis Collaboration examined 491 patients from six trials, representing 90% of all patients randomized in cisplatin-based combination chemotherapy trials. They concluded that there is insufficient evidence on which to base reliable treatment decisions, and they recommended further research.[172]

More recent studies have used different adjuvant chemotherapy regimens or molecular stratification. A randomized trial performed in Italy randomized patients after cystectomy either to four courses of gemcitabine plus cisplatin (n = 102) or to the same treatment at time of relapse (n = 92). There was no difference in the 5-year overall survival across treatment arms. However, due to poor accrual, the study was insufficiently powered to detect a survival difference.[173]

As described earlier, p53 alteration status was hypothesized to be both prognostic for recurrence after cystectomy and predictive for a survival benefit conferred by adjuvant chemotherapy. A phase III trial separated patients based on p53 status, with all p53-negative patients followed with observation alone. Patients with p53 alteration (n = 114) were randomized postcystectomy to three cycles of adjuvant MVAC or observation. Neither p53 status nor MVAC adjuvant chemotherapy impacted risk of recurrence.[57]

Gallagher et al.[174] studied adjuvant, sequential chemotherapy in a nonrandomized design, using as a basis the improvement in survival in breast cancer when sequential adjuvant chemotherapy was used. In this study and others similarly designed,[175,176] adjuvant, sequential chemotherapy for patients with high-risk urothelial cancer did not appear to improve disease-specific survival over that observed with surgery alone.

Dreicer,[161] in reviewing the published literature, made the case for adjuvant chemotherapy as the standard of care given the lethality of radical cystectomy alone in muscle-invasive bladder cancer, but he acknowledges that "suboptimal trial design, insufficient numbers of patients, and lack of standardization of the chemotherapy regimens used have plagued adjuvant studies."

Combined Modality Treatment of Local–Regionally Advanced Disease

The place of combined modality therapy for advanced disease has not been settled. Several series have suggested an improvement in long-term survival in selected patients undergoing resection of persistent cancer deposits after MVAC or CMV.[164,177]

In our experience, carefully selected patients with locally advanced unresectable bladder cancer, including some patients with pelvic nodal masses, may experience long-term survival with the combination of chemotherapy and radiation. To be selected for this combined modality treatment, patients must have (1) an excellent performance status, (2) locally advanced measurable disease, (3) normal kidney function tests, and (4) no evidence of distant metastases beyond the common iliac lymph nodes. The initial treatment consists of four to six cycles of combination chemotherapy. If a significant regression of tumor is achieved, radiation treatment is administered in combination with radiosensitizing chemotherapy. These patients were carefully selected, but in the majority of patients so treated, excellent tumor shrinkage and long-term survival were achieved in patients who would otherwise have been expected to succumb rapidly if treatment had consisted of chemotherapy alone.

Quality of Life After Cystectomy or Bladder Preservation

Evaluating the quality of life in long-term survivors of bladder cancer has been difficult, and only recently have attempts been made to assess this in an objective and quantitative fashion.[134,178–191] A number of problems arise in the interpretation of the published studies. Tools to assess quality-of-life variables were developed early for common prostate and gynecologic cancers, but until very recently no such instruments existed for bladder cancer. The instruments in use for bladder cancer have thus been adaptations of uncertain validity. The published studies are all cross-sectional and patients have follow-ups of varying lengths. This matters in a surgical series in which functional outcome improves with time and in a radiation series in which it may deteriorate. Despite these limitations, some conclusions can now be drawn.

A radical cystectomy causes changes in many areas of quality of life, including urinary, sexual, and social function, daily living activities, and satisfaction with body image.[166–171,192] During the past decade, researchers have concentrated on the relative merits of continent and incontinent diversions. Available data have been mixed with some groups, surprisingly, reporting few differences between the quality of life of those with an ileal conduit and those with continent diversions. Hart et al.[182] have compared outcome in cystectomy patients who have either ileal conduits, cutaneous Koch pouches, or urethral Koch pouches. Regardless of the type of urinary diversion, the majority of patients reported good overall quality of life, little emotional distress, and few problems with social, physical, or functional activities. Problems with their diversions and with sexual function were most commonly reported. After controlling for age, no significant differences were seen among urinary diversion subgroups in any quality-of-life area. It might be anticipated that those receiving the urethral Koch

diversions would be the most satisfied, and the explanation why this is not so is unclear. It may be that the subgroups were too small to detect differences, but perhaps it is more likely that each group adapts in time to the specific difficulties presented by that type of diversion. Somani et al.[184] reviewed 40 published studies that evaluated overall quality of life, reporting on 3,645 patients. Only two studies reported a better quality of life for those who had neobladder and only two reported a better body image.[184] Another prospective study reported by Mansson et al.[185] suggested that there may be a large cultural component to the response with big differences seen between Egyptian and Swedish men followed prospectively through trials of chemotherapy and cystectomy.

Porter and Penson[183] attempted a systematic review of the literature, testing the premise that continent diversions result in improved health-related quality-of-life outcomes. They concluded that, whatever our assumptions, there is no literature to support the use of one urinary diversion over another. Reviews by Gerharz et al.[187] and Somani et al.[184] came to the same conclusion. It appears that women have more problems with continent diversions, particularly the need to catheterize, than do men.[186]

Zietman et al.[188] have performed a study on patients treated with chemoradiation for muscle-invasive bladder cancer. Patients underwent a urodynamic study and completed a quality-of-life questionnaire with a median time from therapy of 6.3 years. This long follow-up is sufficient to capture the majority of late radiation effects. Seventy-five percent of patients had normally functioning bladders by urodynamic studies. Reduced bladder compliance, a recognized complication of radiation, was seen in 22%, but in only one-third of these was it reflected in distressing symptoms. The questionnaire showed that bladder symptoms were uncommon, especially among men, with the exception of control problems. These were reported by 19%, with 11% using incontinence products (all women). Distress from urinary symptoms was half as common as their prevalence. Bowel symptoms occurred in 22% with only 14% recording any level of distress. The majority of men retained sexual function. Global health-related quality of life was high. A study reported by Herman et al.[189] showed that when low doses of gemcitabine are used as an alternative radiation-sensitizer to cisplatin, then treatment is also very tolerable. Thus, the great majority of patients treated by trimodality therapy retain good bladder function.

Two cross-sectional questionnaire studies, one from Sweden and one from Italy, have compared the outcome following radiation with the outcome following cystectomy.[190,191] The questionnaire results for urinary function following radiation were very similar to those recorded in the MGH study. More than 74% of patients reported good urinary function. Both studies compared bowel function in irradiated patients with that seen in patients undergoing cystectomy. In both, the bowel symptoms were greater for those receiving radiation than for those receiving cystectomy (10% versus 3% and 32% versus 24%, respectively), but in neither was this statistically significant.

Data on the assessment of sexual function are limited to men. The majority in the MGH series report adequate erectile function (full or sufficient for intercourse). These findings are in line with those obtained in the Swedish and Italian series in which three times as many men retained useful erections as compared with cystectomized controls.

A Bladder Cancer Index has now been developed and validated.[193] It has been shown to have high internal and retest consistency and can be used regardless of local treatment type and across the genders. This is the first such tool developed and it holds great promise for comparative treatment studies in the future.

Metastatic Bladder Cancer

An estimated 12,500 deaths per year in the United States are due to metastatic bladder cancer.[194] Through lymphatic and hematogenous means, bladder cancer metastasizes to distant organs, most commonly the lungs, bone, liver, and brain. The prognosis of metastatic bladder cancer, as with other metastatic solid tumors, is poor, with a median survival on the order of only 12 months. Nevertheless, since the discovery that platinum-containing agents have significant antitumor effect in bladder cancer, there has been great interest in the use of chemotherapy for advanced disease.

Compared with other solid-tumor malignancies, transitional cell cancer is chemosensitive. In phase II clinical trials, radiographic response rates may be as high as 70% to 80%, and in phase III clinical trials, response rates are often on the order of 50%. Moreover, a small but substantial minority of responding patients manifest a CR, and among these patients some long-term, durable responses are observed. Overall, however, the duration of response in TCC is short, with a median of 4 to 6 months, and therefore, the impact of chemotherapy on survival has been disappointing. As newer targeted agents come into clinical practice, the hope is that their incorporation into treatment regimens will lengthen the duration of response and, ultimately, will translate into a real change in survival.

Cisplatin

In 1976, a series of 24 patients with bladder cancer treated with single-agent cisplatin was reported.[195] The investigators observed eight partial responses in addition to four minor responses. Subsequent studies confirmed the activity of cisplatin in TCC, although the response rate to single-agent cisplatin has been lower than that of cisplatin-containing combination therapy.[196,197] Thus, most subsequent studies have explored combination regimens.

Cisplatin-Based Combination Chemotherapy

The standard chemotherapy regimen for advanced bladder cancer for more than a decade was MVAC.[198,199] MVAC is administered in 28-day cycles, with starting doses of methotrexate 30 mg/m^2 (days 1, 15, and 22), vinblastine 3 mg/m^2 (days 2, 15, and 22), doxorubicin 30 mg/m^2 (day 2), and cisplatin 70 mg/m^2 (day 2). Another commonly used regimen has been CMV, which omits the doxorubicin and has somewhat less toxicity.[200] The MVAC regimen has superior activity to cisplatin alone[196,197] and to other cisplatin-containing regimens.[201] The response rate to MVAC is 40% to 65%,[197,198,202] and there is improved progression-free and overall survival compared with either single-agent cisplatin or cisplatin, cyclophosphamide, and doxorubicin. Complete response is seen in 15% to 25% of patients, with an expected median survival of 12 months (Table 65.6).[196–201]

On the negative side, MVAC is associated with substantial toxicity, and most patients require dose adjustment at some point in their treatment. Toxic effects of MVAC in notable numbers of patients include neutropenia, anemia, thrombocytopenia, stomatitis, nausea, and fatigue.[136,149,202] The rate of chemotherapy-induced fatality among patients with metastatic disease may be as high as 3%, most often due to neutropenic sepsis.[202]

The doublet of gemcitabine and cisplatin showed encouraging results in phase II studies, with response rates of 42% to 66% and CR rates of 18% to 28%.[203,204] Primary toxicity was hematologic and was generally easily managed, with rare hospitalizations for febrile neutropenia and no toxic deaths. Based on these encouraging results, GC was compared with MVAC in a multicenter phase III study.[202,205] MVAC was administered as previously described, and GC was administered in 28-day cycles with gemcitabine 1,000 mg/m^2 (days 1, 8, and 15) and cisplatin 70 mg/m^2 (day 2). In the study, 405 patients were randomized to one of the two treatment arms, and the two groups exhibited similar characteristics. Median survival was 14 months with GC and 15.2 months with MVAC, which were statistically comparable.[205] Patients treated with GC, however, had significantly less toxicity and improved tolerability. Patients receiving GC gained more weight, reported less fatigue, and had better performance status than patients who received MVAC. As a result of this study, GC is generally considered the current standard of care for metastatic bladder cancer.

Taxane- and Platinum-Containing Regimens

The addition of taxanes to cisplatin-based regimens has been the subject of numerous phase II trials in bladder cancer (Table 65.7). The doublets of cisplatin and paclitaxel and cisplatin and docetaxel appear to have response rates comparable to that of GC.[211–214] Trials with carboplatin suggest that this agent has good activity, although likely not the same level of activity as cisplatin.[207,221]

Many patients with bladder cancer cannot receive cisplatin due to medical comorbidities. The EORTC reported a randomized phase III study comparing an historic standard of care in Europe, the three-drug regimen of methotrexate, carboplatin, and vinblastine (M-CAVI), to the doublet gemcitabine and carboplatin in patients who were felt to be unfit for cisplatin-based therapy. All had previously untreated locally advanced or metastatic urothelial cancer. Severe toxicity was greater in patients receiving the three-drug regimen. Responses were greater in the two-drug regimen, but this did not translate into a difference in survival between the two arms. The authors recommended gemcitabine plus carboplatin as the

TABLE 65.6

Standard Cisplatin-Containing Regimens for Transitional Cell Carcinoma

Agents (Ref.)	Regimen	Schedule	Composite Number of Assessable Patients	Complete Response (%)	Response Rate (%)	Median Survival (Mo)
MVAC[197,198,200]	Methotrexate	30 mg/m^2 d 1, 15, 22	374	12–35	39–65	12.5–14.8
	Vinblastine	3 mg/m^2 d 2, 15, 22				
	Doxorubicin	30 mg/m^2 d 2				
	Cisplatin	70 mg/m^2 d 2				
CMV[213]	Cisplatin	70 mg/m^2 d 2	104	10	36	7
	Methotrexate	30 mg/m^2 d 1, 8				
	Vinblastine	4 mg/m^2 d 1, 8				
GC[214]	Gemcitabine	1000 mg/m^2 d 1, 8, 15	203	12	49	13.8
	Cisplatin	70 mg/m^2 d 2				

CMV, cisplatin, methotrexate, vinblastine.

Phase II Trials of Taxane-Containing Chemotherapy Regimens

Regimen	Composite Number of Patients	Response Rate (%)	Median Survival (Mo)	Reference
Carboplatin/paclitaxel	104	21–65	8.5–9.5	206, 207, 209
Cisplatin/paclitaxel	52	50	10.6	211
Cisplatin/docetaxel	129	52–60	8.0–13.6	212–214
Cisplatin/gemcitabine/paclitaxel	61	78	15.8	168, 215
Carboplatin/gemcitabine/paclitaxel	49	68	14.7	216
Cisplatin/gemcitabine/docetaxel	35	66	15.5	217
Gemcitabine/paclitaxel	94	54–60	14.4	218–220

new standard of care based on a better safety profile in this patient population.[208]

A phase III trial compared MVAC with carboplatin and paclitaxel.[209] The study failed to reach its accrual goal, with only 85 patients randomized, although no significant differences in efficacy were seen. It is of note that the MVAC group exhibited a trend toward higher response rate (36% versus 28%), progression-free survival (8.7 versus 5.2 months), and overall survival (15.4 versus 13.8 months).

To date, there has been no consensus regarding those patients who should not receive cisplatin-based chemotherapy. A review of trial eligibility shows marked variation across studies. To address this concern, criteria for trials for "cisplatin-ineligible" patients were reviewed, and a set of criteria for all future studies was proposed by an international group of investigators.[210]

The complete omission of platinum has been studied as well. The doublet of gemcitabine and paclitaxel appears to have good activity, with phase II studies suggesting that this regimen has response rates and survival comparable to GC, with minimal toxicity.[218–220,222] Gemcitabine with paclitaxel may be a reasonable regimen to consider in patients unfit for platinum therapy. Gemcitabine and docetaxel demonstrated a response rate of 33% and median survival of 12 months in a trial of 27 patients with advanced TCC.[223]

Triplet Chemotherapy

Because of the activity of each of these agents in TCC, investigators then asked whether triplet combinations of platinum, taxanes, and gemcitabine might have increased activity over the doublets. In phase II trials, three such combinations, including cisplatin/gemcitabine/paclitaxel,[168] carboplatin/gemcitabine/paclitaxel,[224] and cisplatin/gemcitabine/docetaxel,[217] demonstrated high CR rates of 28% to 32%, and overall response rates of 66% to 78%, although the number of patients with visceral metastases was relatively low. A second study of carboplatin/gemcitabine/paclitaxel showed a more modest response rate of 43% and overall survival of 11 months in a more typical population of metastatic TCC.[216] A triplet of paclitaxel, cisplatin, and infusional high-dose 5-FU with leucovorin has also been studied. The response rate was 75%, with 28% CRs, and a median overall survival of 17 months. Significant toxicity included frequent myelosuppression, gastrointestinal disturbances, infections, and two treatment-related deaths.[225]

A randomized phase III trial compared the standard GC regimen with GC plus paclitaxel (PCG).[215] Preliminary results and updated data are available. Despite a response rate that was superior in the three drug arm (55.5% versus 43.6%, $p = 0.0031$) and a median overall survival that was slightly longer in patients receiving the third drug (15.8 months versus 12.7 months), the HR for survival did not achieve statistical significance (HR, 0.85; $p = 0.075$). Thus, the standard of care remains the doublet of gemcitabine plus cisplatin.[226]

Biologic Agents

The enthusiasm engendered by the development of novel biologic agents targeted against tumor-specific growth factor pathways or angiogenesis has been fortified in recent years by positive studies in a variety of solid tumors. Two classes of agents that may be of interest in TCC are inhibitors of EGFR, including EGFR1 and EGFR2 (HER2/neu), and inhibitors of VEGF or its receptors. There is ample preclinical evidence that many bladder tumors express members of the EGFR family, that overexpression may correlate inversely with prognosis, and that inhibition of these pathways may have an antitumor effect.[63–69] A number of groups are conducting studies with inhibitors of EGFR1 and HER2/neu in the treatment of advanced bladder cancer. Similarly, the utility of angiogenesis inhibitors in TCC is currently being explored in a cooperative group trial in metastatic TCC studying GC with or without the addition of bevacizumab.

Second-Line Therapy and Beyond

There is no U.S. Food and Drug Administration (FDA)-approved therapy or regimen for second-line chemotherapy for progressive bladder cancer. One phase III trial randomized 370 patients with advanced TCC who had received prior platinum-based chemotherapy 2:1 to single-agent vinflunine or best supportive care. Median survival favored the vinflunine population (6.9 versus 4.6 months), but the difference was not statistically significant ($p = 0.287$).[226] These findings were confirmed at longer follow-up.[228] The lack of benefit combined with adverse effects have not led to broad approval of vinflunine worldwide or approval by the FDA in the United States. In practice, treatment beyond first-line chemotherapy typically employs doublet regimens described previously, single-agent chemotherapy, or clinical trials, where available.

CANCERS OF THE RENAL PELVIS AND URETER

The majority of tumors of the upper urinary collecting system are TCCs. However, these are uncommon, with fewer than 3,000 cases diagnosed annually in the United States. The incidence has remained constant, but there has recently been a slight stage migration toward a higher proportion of earlier stage tumors.[229] Because of the challenge in gaining access to them, initial diagnosis and staging are less accurate than for cancer of the bladder. Histologically, 90% of upper tract tumors are TCC. Squamous cell carcinoma accounts for nearly all of the remainder. There is a predilection for these tumors to arise in the renal pelvis; primary tumors of the ureter occur only half as frequently as do tumors of the renal pelvis.[230] Men develop upper tract TCC two to three times more often than women, with the peak age of development of these tumors in the 7th and 8th decades of life.[211] Women, however, are more likely than men to have a more advanced and higher grade tumor at nephroureterectomy.[231] As discussed in the first section of this chapter, the majority of these tumors arise as a result of, or at least in association with, environmental exposures and stresses.[7–13,25]

Clinical Presentation, Diagnosis, and Staging

Gross hematuria is the presenting symptom in 75% to 95% of all patients who present with tumors of the renal pelvis and ureter. Hematuria may be accompanied by colicky flank pain if the tumor or blood clots cause obstruction of the upper urinary tract. Patients often describe the passage of vermiform clots, which are unusual in bleeding from a lower tract source. Hydronephrosis may also be a presenting sign. Urinary cytology is an important part of the workup for an upper tract tumor. Voided urine cytology, however, has only 10% to 40% sensitivity in the detection of low-grade TCC lesions. Cytology is far more useful for high-grade tumors, for which the sensitivity may be as high as 70%.[232,233]

Improvements in endoscopic technology allow the urologist to view directly and to obtain tissue in many of the TCCs of the upper tract. A pathologic confirmation may be obtained prior to treatment. Also, the grade may be a useful predictor of advanced stage disease.[234,235]

Historically, intravenous urography was the mainstay of a radiographic evaluation of upper tract tumors, but now, in most major centers, a CT urogram is preferred (Fig. 65.7).[236] An MRI urography may also be useful in patients when sensitivity to iodinated contrast prevents the use of that agent.[237,238] When a patient is found or judged to have a TCC more aggressive than a G1 stage I tumor, additional staging of the patient is indicated, including CT scans of the chest, abdomen, and pelvis. Because standard therapy is radical excision of the kidney and the ipsilateral ureter, an evaluation of the total remaining renal function prior to a proposed nephrectomy is indicated. Isotope renal scanning can accurately estimate the function of the uninvolved kidney.

The current American Joint Committee on Cancer TNM staging for tumors of the upper urinary tract is shown in Figure 65.8 and in Table 65.8. The staging is determined by the extent of invasion by the primary tumor and by microscopic evaluation of the regional lymph nodes.

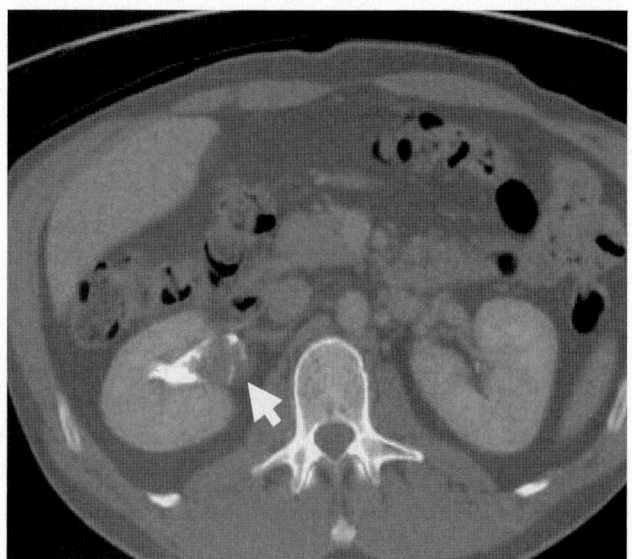

Figure 65.7 Abdominal computed tomographic scan of a stage T3 transitional cell carcinoma of the right renal pelvis, with intravenous contrast showing a large filling defect in the right renal pelvis (*arrow*).

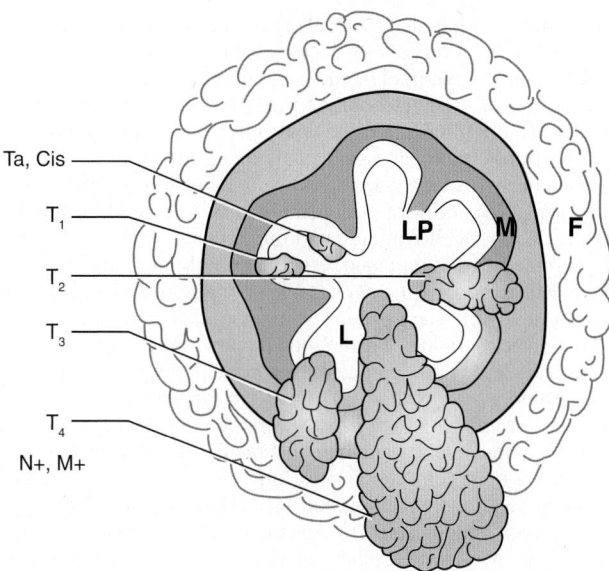

Figure 65.8 Schematic diagram of the American Joint Committee on Cancer TNM (tumor, necrosis, metastasis) staging of cancers of the renal pelvis; LP, lamina propria; M, muscularis propria; F, peripelvic fat; L, lumen.

Surgical Treatment

The standard surgical treatment for patients with transitional cell cancer of the upper urinary tract of all grades and stages is radical nephroureterectomy. This involves a complete removal of the kidney with its surrounding perirenal fat contained within Gerota fascia and en bloc removal of the ureter down to, and including, the portion of ureter within the urinary bladder (the ureteral orifice and the intramural ureter).[239] A retroperitoneal lymph node dissection along the ipsilateral great vessel (the vena cava for right-sided tumors; the aorta for left-sided tumors) is performed for more complete surgical staging, especially for higher grade and invasive cancers (Fig. 65.9). A lymphadenectomy and complete bladder cuff excision may not be necessary in cases of upper tract TCC, particularly at a low stage and grade.[240] When TCC of the renal pelvis invades the renal vein or the vena cava, an extensive surgical procedure, including thrombus extraction or partial vena cava dissection, may be required. A nephroureterectomy may be performed via open or laparoscopic surgical techniques. Common open approaches employ either a single extended midline abdominal incision or nephrectomy via a thoracoabdominal incision and a separate incision in the lower abdomen to accomplish the distal ureterectomy with a cuff of the contiguous urinary bladder.

Open surgical approach had long been the standard of treatment for the majority of patients with tumors of the renal pelvis and ureter, although morbidity may be reduced by using a laparoscopic technique.[241,242] The operative time and blood loss with the laparoscopic technique may be substantially less and the hospital stay shorter than those of an open surgical technique. With proper technique in resecting the distal ureter, laparoscopic or robotic-assisted nephroureterectomy is equally oncologically effective.[243,244] Invasive TCC may seed the abdomen if spilled, allowing tumor implantation, and this has led to concern among surgical oncologists about the laparoscopic approach. One group has reported three cases of laparoscopic port-site recurrence; however, in all three of these cases, the tumor was spilled from the operative specimen, allowing growth of the tumor tissue at the trocar sites.[245]

In patients in whom radical excision of the tumor would result in severe renal insufficiency that required dialysis (such as patients with a solitary kidney or in a patient with substantially diminished renal function), other surgical therapies may be considered. Endoscopic resection techniques have been developed and shown to be effective when done selectively and in experienced hands.[246] Endoscopic ablation via laser or electrocautery may be used to treat small tumors of the ureter and renal collecting system. However, the success of focal resection can be thwarted by the multicentricity of these tumors and the common concurrent existence of CIS.[247] Furthermore, although small, low-grade tumors can often be effectively treated endoscopically, high-grade tumors are often understaged by endoscopic assessment only, and therefore, may be treated inadequately without nephroureterectomy.[248]

Percutaneous endoscopic surgery of renal pelvic and calyceal TCC with access via the flank has been developed as a treatment option in highly select patients who have poor renal function or who medically could not withstand an open surgical procedure.[249] Using standard endoscopic tools, it is possible to resect tumors in the fashion similar to that which is used for bladder tumors. All limited resection endoscopic procedures require vigilant follow-up with an endoscopic reevaluation on a regular schedule because recurrence is quite common. In one study, 33% of patients ultimately required nephroureterectomy and 11% of patients died of TCC.[250]

Although endoscopic management of high-grade tumors can result in undertreatment and poorer oncologic outcomes, a

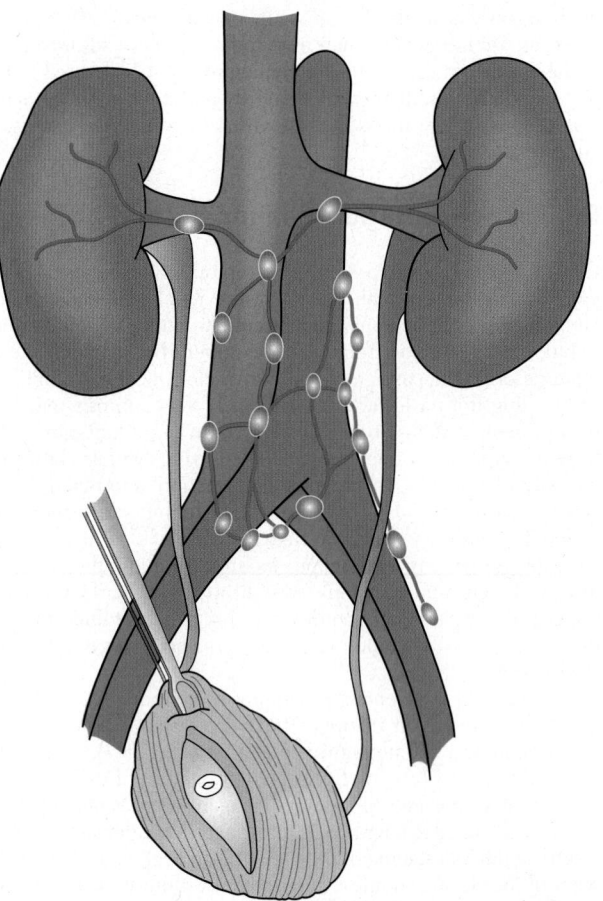

Figure 65.9 Diagram of the kidneys, ureters, bladder, and retroperitoneal lymph nodes to demonstrate that a nephroureterectomy for upper tract transitional cell carcinoma requires a complete excision of the distal ureter, including the portion within the wall of the bladder. The bladder here is open to reveal the distal ureter, which tunnels within the wall of the bladder.

kidney-sparing approach to appropriately selected isolated ureteral tumors using surgical resection is becoming a more accepted alternative to nephroureterectomy with similar oncologic outcomes.[251,252] This involves segmental resection of the ureter incorporating the tumor and the entire ureter distally, including the ureteral orifice/bladder cuff, and appropriate lymphadenectomy. Because recurrences and urothelial atypia are usually distal in the ureter to the index lesion, it is reasonable to spare the kidney without undue risk of recurrent disease. Surgically, it is possible to remove approximately half of the distal ureter and reimplant it in the bladder. For upper ureteral tumors, replacement of the ureter with a segment of the ileum may be considered. Although segmental resection is becoming more accepted for mid and distal ureteral tumors, radical nephroureterectomy does remain the gold standard, especially for tumors in the proximal ureter and tumors with extensive ureteral involvement.

Results of Surgical Therapy

The success rate of surgical procedures is primarily influenced by the pathologic stage of the disease at the resection (Table 65.9). Tumors lower in the urinary tract have a better prognosis when matched by stage with tumors higher in the ureter and pelvis.[254] Within the upper tract, the location of the tumor in the ureter versus the renal pelvis does not seem to affect the prognosis.[255,256] In a report with a long follow-up from the University of Texas Southwestern Medical Center, of 252 patients treated surgically for upper tract TCC, disease-specific and overall survival were strongly influenced by the pathologic stage of the primary tumor.[253] The

TABLE 65.8

American Joint Committee on Cancer 2009 TNM Staging of Renal Pelvis and Ureter Cancers: Definition of TNM

Primary Tumor (T)

TX	Primary tumor cannot be assessed
T0	No evidence of primary tumor
Ta	Papillary noninvasive carcinoma
Tis	Carcinoma in situ
T1	Tumor invades subepithelial connective tissue
T2	Tumor invades the muscularis
T3	(For renal pelvis only) Tumor invades beyond muscularis into peripelvic fat or the renal parenchyma
T3	(For ureter only) Tumor invades beyond muscularis into periureteric fat
T4	Tumor invades adjacent organs or through the kidney into the perinephric fat

Regional Lymph Nodes (N)[a]

NX	Regional lymph nodes cannot be assessed
N0	No regional lymph node metastasis
N1	Metastasis in a single lymph node 2 cm or less in greatest dimension
N2	Metastasis in a single lymph node more than 2 cm but not more than 5 cm in greatest dimension or multiple lymph nodes; none more than 5 cm in greatest dimension
N3	Metastasis in a lymph node, more than 5 cm in greatest dimension

Distant Metastasis (M)

MX	Distant metastasis cannot be assessed
M0	No distant metastasis
M1	Distant metastasis

[a] Laterality does not affect the N classification.
Used with the permission of the American Joint Committee on Cancer (AJCC), Chicago, Illinois. The original source for this material is the *AJCC Cancer Staging Manual*, Seventh Edition (2010) published by Springer Science and Business Media LLC, www.springer.com, page 493.

TABLE 65.9

Five-Year Disease-Specific Survival by Primary Tumor Pathologic Stage After Surgical Resection of Transitional Cell Carcinoma of the Upper Urinary Tract

Tumor Stage	Number of Patients	Percentage (%)
pTa/pTis	38	100
pT1	99	92
pT2	34	73
pT3	53	41
pT4	19	0

From Hall MC, Womack S, Sagalowsky AI, et al. Prognostic factors, recurrence, and survival in transitional cell carcinoma of the upper urinary tract: a 30-year experience in 252 patients. *Urology* 1998;52:594–601, with permission

5-year actuarial disease-specific survival rates by primary tumor pathologic stage were 100% for noninvasive tumors (Ta and Tis), 92% for pathologic stage T1, 73% for pathologic stage T2, and 41% for pathologic stage T3. There were no long-term survivors for those with stage T4 tumors (Table 65.9). The type of open surgical procedure used (nephroureterectomy in 77% of the patients compared with a kidney-sparing approach used in 17%) was evaluated by a univariate and multivariate analysis. Patients undergoing nephroureterectomy were found to have a significantly improved recurrence-free and disease-specific survival on multivariate analysis but not on the univariate analysis. However, as discussed previously, in other more recent series, patients with ureteral cancers who were appropriately selected for kidney-sparing resections did not have a poorer outcome.

Adjuvant Topical Therapy Following Local Excision Only

In cases in which endoscopic resection is performed, topical immunotherapy or topical chemotherapy may be important in preventing or delaying local tumor recurrence. BCG appears to be useful in treating carcinomas of the upper tract that are stage Tis.[247] Adriamycin given prophylactically following conservative resection of upper tract TCCs, using an antegrade infusion, also has been judged to be of some benefit in reducing recurrence.[257] The risk of systemic absorption of BCG or the chemotherapeutic agents is substantially higher than in treatment of the bladder and should be considered in therapeutic decision making.

Adjuvant Combined-Modality Therapy: Advanced Primary Tumors

The most appropriate treatment for invasive transitional cell cancers of the upper urinary tract is nephroureterectomy. Despite aggressive surgery, cure rates are low when the disease has spread beyond the muscularis, with 5-year survival rates varying between zero and 34%.[257–262] Whether these low survival rates can be improved by adjuvant therapy depends on the pattern of failure and the efficacy of the available treatment. Metastatic relapse appears to predominate over local relapse when systemic cisplatin-based chemotherapy has been used, extrapolating from the experience with locally advanced bladder cancer. The true rate of local–regional failure is, however, unknown because many of the published series are old and employed pre-CT methods of intra-abdominal evaluation. The available data suggest an overall local–regional failure of 2% to 27%, although these figures may be underestimated.[263–265] Cozad et al.[266] report local failure rates of 50% in stage T3 disease,

rising to 60% if the tumors were high grade. Brookland and Richter[267] have reported local–regional recurrence in 45% and 62%, respectively. Most series report a close association between local failure and distant metastasis, although whether the association is causal or simply synchronous cannot be determined from the small numbers in the series.

Radiation has been employed as an adjuvant therapy with mixed results reported in the literature (Table 65.10). Several small phase II studies have suggested a local control and perhaps survival advantage for adjuvant radiation.[267–273] One study reported no benefit, although their treated population was diluted with 30% early stage patients. Another study showed no advantage to radiation, but the radiation doses given were inadequate. In others, chemotherapy was given in addition. Therefore, it is difficult to determine the true benefit of adjuvant radiation, if any. However, in a recent retrospective report by Chen et al.,[273] a survival advantage was seen in patients with T3/T4 disease of the renal pelvis or ureter receiving postoperative radiation with a median dose of 50 Gy to the tumor bed.

At the MGH, a more aggressive approach has been taken during the past 20 years in which patients with high-risk disease were treated first with adjuvant radiation alone and then more recently with concomitant radiation-sensitizing chemotherapy and, if tolerable, further combination chemotherapy.[271] Although the authors' series of 31 patients is nonrandomized and small, local failure was lower if chemotherapy was combined with radiation and the survival rate at 5 years was higher (see Table 65.10). Kwak et al.[272] also suggested that cisplatin-based adjuvant chemotherapy may reduce the rate of relapse and death from disease at 5 years. The small size of these two series and the biases inherent in this kind of retrospective review make it difficult to draw conclusions.

Very little published data exist to guide physicians managing patients with a local relapse following a nephroureterectomy. If the relapse is bulky and metastases are present elsewhere, then palliation with chemotherapy would be the most appropriate course. When the relapse appears isolated and the patient relatively vigorous, consideration can be given to an aggressive approach that holds out the chance for cure. The first step would be to downsize and perhaps improve the respectability of the recurrence using external radiation to a modest preoperative dose of 30 to 45 Gy along with sensitizing chemotherapy. An attempt could then be made at resection or debulking and, if the facility were available, intraoperative radiation could then be given directly onto the tumor bed or onto an unresectable mass, with the bowel and other critical organs displaced out of the field. Such an approach allows for the delivery of high doses of radiation to the target without the risk of bowel injury that is present when managing such disease using external radiation treatment alone (Fig. 65.10).

Advanced Transitional Cell Carcinoma of the Upper Tract

Most patients with upper tract TCC have superficial disease, with a favorable prognosis.[274,275] However, patients with disease that invades beyond the muscularis propria have a significantly worse prognosis. The most consistent prognostic variables for the outcome of patients with upper tract TCC, including renal pelvic and ureteral carcinomas, are tumor stage and grade.[276–279] Molecular markers are being studied, and a poor outcome may be predicted by overexpression of $p53$ and a higher Ki-67 labeling index.[280–282]

In a series of 252 patients with mostly localized disease, relapse occurred in 67 patients (27%) after a median of 12 months.[265] Survival was highly stage specific, with 5-year disease-specific survival of 92% for T1, 73% for T2, 41% for T3, and zero for T4. In a series of 126 patients with nonmetastatic but more advanced renal pelvic or ureteral tumors, relapsed disease was noted in 81 patients (64%) after a median of 9 months.[268] Overall, 5- and 10-year survival rates

TABLE 65.10

Larger Published Series Using Surgery with or without Adjuvant Radiation for Carcinoma of the Upper Urinary Tract

Method/Study (Ref.)	Number of Patients	Median Dose (Gy)	Local–Regional Failure % (Absolute)	Overall 5-Year Survival (%)
Surgery with Radiotherapy				
Ozsahin et al.[268]	45	50	38 (17/45)	21
Maulard-Durdux et al.[269]	26[a]	45	19 (5/26)	49 (T2, 60%; T3, 19%)
Catton et al.[270]	86[b]	35	34 (29/86)	43 (T3N0, 45%; N+, 15%)
Brookland and Richter[267]	11	50	9 (1/11)	27
Cozad et al.[266]	9	50	11 (1/9)	44
Czito et al.[271]	31	47	23 (7/31)	39 (67% in combined-modality group)
Chen[273]	67	50	22 (15/67)	50
Surgery Only				
Ozsahin et al.[268]	81		65 (53/81)	33
Cozad et al.[266]	17[c]		53 (9/17)	24
Brookland and Richter[267]	11		45 (5/11)	17
Chen[273]	66		35 (23/66)	45

[a] Thirty percent stage T2.
[b] Twenty-seven percent stage T1 to T2.
[c] All stages ≥T3.

were 29% and 19%, respectively. The most common sites of distant metastases were liver, bone, or lung. Utilization of postoperative radiation therapy did not impact on local or distant relapse. Factors that influenced survival outcomes in a multivariate analysis were initial tumor stage, residual postsurgery tumor, and the location of the initial tumor, with renal pelvic cancer being more favorable than ureteral cancer. The role of adjuvant chemotherapy in reducing relapse has not been explored in randomized fashion in this uncommon disease.

The biology of upper tract TCC is considered to be identical to that of bladder TCC. Consequently, the chemotherapy regimens recommended for advanced or metastatic upper tract TCC are the same as that for bladder cancer, as previously described. Standard treatment is cisplatin-based combination therapy, such as gemcitabine and cisplatin or methotrexate, vinblastine, doxorubicin, and cisplatin. As with bladder cancer, upper tract TCC is highly responsive to chemotherapy but has a short median duration of response.

Coronal pretreatment

Coronal posttreatment

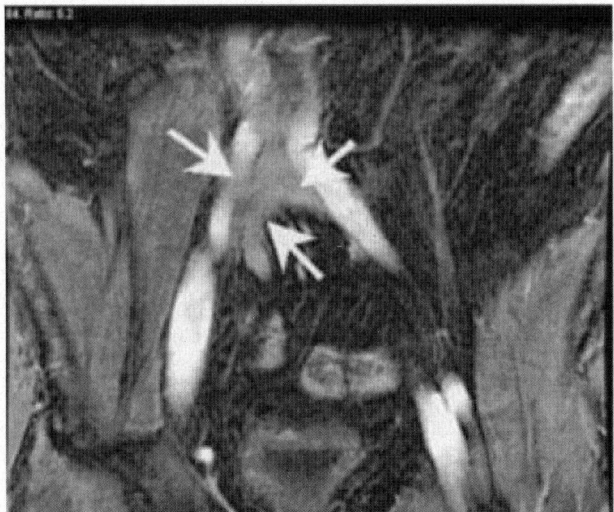 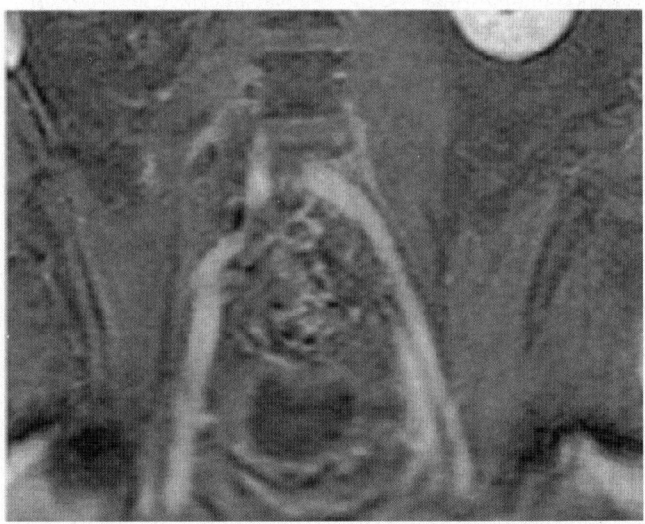

Figure 65.10 Sequential coronal MRI of a patient with an unresectable ureteral tumor mass. The mass shown on the MRI on the **left** (*arrows*) was at the bifurcation of the aorta; it was initially judged unresectable because of involvement of the vessels. A partial resection, however, became possible as part of a combined-modality treatment approach that included preoperative conformal external-beam radiation. Intraoperative electron-beam radiation was given to the entire tumor bed after resection. On the **right** is the repeat MRI 1 year after treatment without any visible tumor.

SELECTED REFERENCES

The full reference list can be accessed at lwwhealthlibrary.com/oncology.

1. Siegal R, Naishadham D, Jemal A. Cancer statistics 2013. *CA Cancer J Clin* 2013;63:11–30.

2. Maralani S, Wood DP Jr, Grignon D, et al. Incidence of urethral involvement in female bladder cancer: an anatomic pathologic study. *Urology* 1997;50:537–541.

6. Rabbani F, Perrotti M, Russo P, et al. Upper-tract tumors after an initial diagnosis of bladder cancer: argument for long-term surveillance. *J Clin Oncol* 2001;19:94–100.

7. Hurle R, Losa A, Manzetti A, et al. Upper urinary tract tumors developing after treatment of superficial bladder cancer: 7-year follow-up of 591 consecutive patients. *Urology* 1999;53:1144–1148.

9. Nortier JL, Martinez MC, Schmeiser HH, et al. Urothelial carcinoma associated with the use of a Chinese herb (*Aristolochia fangchi*). *N Engl J Med* 2000;342:1686–1692.

10. Grollman AP, Shibutani S, Moriya M, et al. Aristolochic acid and the etiology of endemic (Balkan) nephropathy. *Proc Natl Acad Sci U S A* 2007; 104:12129–12134.

26. Zeegers MP, Goldbohm RA, van den Brandt PA. A prospective study on active and environmental tobacco smoking and bladder cancer risk (The Netherlands). *Cancer Causes Control* 2002;13:83–90.

27. Moyer VA. Screening for bladder cancer: US Preventive Services Task Force recommendation statement. *Ann Intern Med* 2011;133:246–251.

29. Mishriki SF, Nabi G, Cohen NP, et al. Diagnosis of urologic malignancies in patients with asymptomatic dipstick hematuria: prospective study with 13 years' follow-up. *Urology* 2008;71:13–16.

30. Messing EM, Madeb R, Young T, et al. Long-term outcome of hematuria home screening for bladder cancer in men. *Cancer* 2006;107:2173–2179.

39. Lokeshwar VB, Habuchi T, Grossman HB, et al. Bladder tumor markers beyond cytology: international consensus panel on bladder tumor markers. *Urology* 2005;66:35–63.

51. Sidransky D, Frost P, Von Eschenbach A, et al. The clonal origin of bladder cancer. *N Engl J Med* 1992;326:737–740.

56. Cordon-Cardo C. Molecular alterations associated with bladder cancer initiation and progression. *Scand J Urol Nephrol Suppl* 2008;218:154–165.

57. Stadler WM, Lerner SP, Groshen S, et al. S Phase II study of molecularly targeted adjuvant therapy in locally advanced urothelial cancer of the bladder based on p53 status. *J Clin Oncol* 2011;29:3443–3449.

69. Jimenez RE, Hussain M, Bianco FJ Jr, et al. Her-2/neu over-expression in muscle-invasive urothelial carcinoma of the bladder: prognostic significance and comparative analysis in primary and metastatic tumors. *Clin Cancer Res* 2001;7:2440–2447.

71. Lautenschlaeger T, George A, Klimowicz AC, et al. Bladder preservation therapy for muscle-invading bladder cancers on Radiation Therapy Oncology Group trials 8802, 8903, 9506, and 9706: vascular endothelial growth factor B overexpression predicts for increased distant metastasis and shorter survival. *Oncologist* 2013;18:685–686.

72. Sabichi AL, Lee JJ, Grossman HB, et al. A randomized controlled trial of celecoxib to prevent recurrence of nonmuscle-invasive bladder cancer. *Cancer Prev Res (Phila)* 2011;4:1580–1589.

73. Choudhury A, Nelson LD, Teo MT, et al. MRE11 expression is predictive of cause-specific survival following radical radiotherapy for muscle-invasive bladder cancer. *Cancer Res* 2010;70:7017–7026.

75. Daniltchenko DI, Riedl CR, Sachs MD, et al. Long-term benefit of 5-aminolevulinic acid fluorescence assisted transurethral resection of superficial bladder cancer: 5-year results of a prospective randomized study. *J Urol* 2005;174:2129–2133.

76. Denzinger S, Burger M, Walter B, et al. Clinically relevant reduction in risk of recurrence of superficial bladder cancer using 5-aminolevulinic acid-induced fluorescence diagnosis: 8-year results of prospective randomized study. *Urology* 2007;69:675–679.

77. Naselli A, Introini C, Timossi L, et al. A randomized prospective trial to assess the impact of transurethral resection in narrow band imaging modality on non-muscle-invasive bladder cancer recurrence. *Eur Urol* 2012;61:908–913.

78. Stenzl A, Penkoff H, Dajc-Sommerer E, et al. Detection and clinical outcome of urinary bladder cancer with 5-aminolevulinic acid-induced fluorescence cystoscopy: A multicenter randomized, double-blind, placebo-controlled trial. *Cancer* 2011;117:938–947.

79. American Joint Committee on Cancer. *Cancer Staging Manual*, 7th ed. New York: Springer-Verlag; 2008.

80. Harisinghani MG, Barentsz J, Hahn PF, et al. Noninvasive detection of clinically occult lymph-node metastases in prostate cancer. *N Engl J Med* 2003;348:2491–2499.

81. Di Stasi SM, Valenti M, Verri C, et al. Electromotive instillation of mitomycin immediately before transurethral resection for patients with primary urothelial non-muscle invasive bladder cancer: a randomised controlled trial. *Lancet Oncol* 2011;12:891–899.

82. Lamm DL, Blumenstein BA, Crissman JD, et al. Maintenance bacillus Calmette-Guerin immunotherapy for recurrent TA, T1 and carcinoma in situ transitional cell carcinoma of the bladder: a randomized Southwest Oncology Group Study. *J Urol* 2000;163:1124–1129.

84. Bohle A, Jocham D, Bock PR. Intravesical bacillus Calmette-Guerin versus mitomycin C for superficial bladder cancer: a formal meta-analysis of comparative studies on recurrence and toxicity. *J Urol* 2003;169:900.

85. Shang PF, Kwong J, Wang ZP, et al. Intravesical BCG vs epirubicin for Ta and T1 bladder cancer. *Cochrane Database Syst Rev* 2011;(5):CD006885.

90. Addeo R, Caraglia M, Bellini S, et al. Randomized phase III trial on gemcitabine versus mytomicin in recurrent superficial bladder cancer: evaluation of efficacy and tolerance. *J Clin Oncol* 2010;28:543–548.

91. Skinner EC, Goldman B, Sakr WA, et al. 1666 SWOG S0353 phase II trial of intravesical gemcitabine in patients with non-muscle invasive bladder cancer who recurred following at least two prior courses of BCG. *J Urol* 2012;187:e673.

98. Knoedler JJ, Boorjian SA, Kim SP, et al. Does partial cystectomy compromise oncologic outcomes for patients with bladder cancer compared to radical cystectomy? A matched case-control analysis. *J Urol* 2012;188:1115–1119.

100. Stein JP, Cai J, Groshen S, et al. Risk factors for patients with pelvic lymph node metastases following radical cystectomy with en bloc pelvic lymphadenectomy: concept of lymph node density. *J Urol* 2003;170:35–41.

101. Stein JP, Lieskovsky G, Cote R, et al. Radical cystectomy in the treatment of invasive bladder cancer: long-term results in 1,054 patients. *J Clin Oncol* 2001;19:666–675.

102. Dalbagni G, Genega E, Hashibe M, et al. Cystectomy for bladder cancer: a contemporary series. *J Urol* 2001;165:1111–1116.

103. Grossman HB, Natale RB, Tangen CM, et al. Neoadjuvant chemotherapy plus cystectomy compared with cystectomy alone for locally advanced bladder cancer. *N Engl J Med* 2003;349:859–866.

105. Eisenberg M, Thompson R, Frank I, et al. Long-term renal function outcomes after radical cystectomy. *J Urol* 2014;191:1–7

107. Chahal R, Sundaram SK, Iddenden R, et al. A study of the morbidity, mortality and long-term survival following radical cystectomy and radical radiotherapy in the treatment of invasive bladder cancer in Yorkshire. *Eur Urol* 2003;43:246–257.

108. Shabsigh A, Korets R, Vora KC, et al. Defining early morbidity of radical cystectomy for patients with bladder cancer using a standardized reporting methodology. *Eur Urol* 2009;55:164–174.

110. Gakis G, Efstathiou J, Lerner SP, et al. ICUD-EAU International Consultation on Bladder Cancer 2012: Radical cystectomy and bladder preservation for muscle-invasive urothelial carcinoma of the bladder. *Eur Urol* 2013; 63:45–57.

116. Tester W, Caplan R, Heaney J, et al. Neoadjuvant combined modality program with selective organ preservation for invasive bladder cancer: results of Radiation Therapy Oncology Group phase II trial 8802. *J Clin Oncol* 1996; 14:119–126.

117. Shipley WU, Winter KA, Kaufman DS, et al. Phase III trial of neoadjuvant chemotherapy in patients with invasive bladder cancer treated with selective bladder preservation by combined radiation therapy and chemotherapy: initial results of Radiation Therapy Oncology Group 89-03. *J Clin Oncol* 1998;16:3576–3583.

119. Rodel C, Grabenbauer GG, Kuhn R, et al. Combined-modality treatment and selective organ preservation in invasive bladder cancer: long-term results. *J Clin Oncol* 2002;20:3061–3071.

124. Mitin T, Hunt D, Shipley WU, et al. Transurethral surgery and twice-daily radiation plus paclitaxel-cisplatin or fluorouracil-cisplatin with selective bladder preservation and adjuvant chemotherapy for patients with muscle invasive bladder cancer (RTOG 0233): a randomised multicentre phase 2 trial. *Lancet Oncol* 2013;14:863–872

125. Oh KS, Soto DE, Smith DC, et al. Combined-modality therapy with gemcitabine and radiation therapy as a bladder preservation strategy: long-term results of a phase I trial. *Int J Radiat Oncol Biol Phys* 2009;74:511–517.

128. James ND, Hussain SA, Hall E, et al. Radiotherapy with or without chemotherapy in muscle-invasive bladder cancer. *N Engl J Med* 2012;366:1477–1488.

130. Efstathiou JA, Spiegel DY, Shipley WU, et al. Long-term outcomes of selective bladder preservation by combined-modality therapy for invasive bladder cancer: the MGH experience. *Eur Urol* 2012;61:705–711.

132. Zietman AL, Grocela J, Zehr E, et al. Selective bladder conservation using transurethral resection, chemotherapy, and radiation: management and consequences of Ta, T1, and Tis recurrence within the retained bladder. *Urology* 2001;58:380–385.

133. Horwich A, Dearnaley D, Huddart R, et al. A randomised trial of accelerated radiotherapy for localised invasive bladder cancer. *Radiother Oncol* 2005;75:34–43.

138. Gray PJ, Lin CC, Jemal A, et al. Clinical-pathologic stage discrepancy in bladder cancer patients treated with radical cystectomy: results from the National Cancer Data Base. *Int J Radiat Biol Phys* 2014;88:1048–1056.

139. Zehnder P, Studer UE, Skinner EC, et al. Super extended versus extended pelvic lymph node dissection in patients undergoing radical cystectomy for bladder cancer: a comparative study. *J Urol* 2011;186:1261–1268.

140. Herr HW. Transurethral resection of muscle-invasive bladder cancer: 10-year outcome. *J Clin Oncol* 2001;19:89–93.

143. Herr HW. Outcome of patients who refuse cystectomy after receiving neoadjuvant chemotherapy for muscle-invasive bladder cancer. *Eur Assoc Urol* 2008;54:126–132.

PRACTICE OF ONCOLOGY

147. Hall RR. Updated results of a randomized controlled trial of neoadjuvant cisplatin, methotrexate and vinblastine chemotherapy for muscle invasive bladder cancer. *Proc Am Soc Clin Oncol* 2002;21:178.

148. International Collaboration of Trialists. International phase III trial assessing neoadjuvant cisplatin, methotrexate, and vinblastine chemotherapy in muscle-invasive bladder cancer. Long-term results of the BA06 30894 trial. *J Clin Oncol* 2011;29:2171–2177.

150. Malmstrom PU, Rintala E, Wahlqvist R, et al. Five-year follow-up of a prospective trial of radical cystectomy and neoadjuvant chemotherapy: Nordic Cystectomy Trial I. The Nordic Cooperative Bladder Cancer Study Group. *J Urol* 1996;155:1903.

151. Sherif A, Rintala E, Mestad O, et al. Neoadjuvant cisplatin-methotrexate chemotherapy for invasive bladder cancer. Nordic Trial 2. *Scand J Urol Nephrol* 2002;36:419–425.

153. Advanced Bladder Cancer Overview Collaboration. Neoadjuvant chemotherapy for invasive bladder cancer. *Cochrane Database Syst Rev* 2005;2:CD005246.

160. Weight CJ, Garcia JA, Hansel DE, et al. Lack of pathologic down-staging with neoadjuvant chemotherapy for muscle-invasive urothelial carcinoma of the bladder: a contemporary series. *Expert Rev Anticancer Ther* 2009;9: 792–799.

161. Dreicer R. Chemotherapy for muscle-invasive bladder cancer in the perioperative setting: current standards. *Urol Oncol* 2007;25:72–75.

162. Donat SM. Integrating perioperative chemotherapy into the treatment of muscle-invasive bladder cancer: strategy versus reality. *J Natl Compr Canc Netw* 2009;7:40–47.

166. Studer UE, Bacchi M, Biedermann C, et al. Adjuvant cisplatin chemotherapy following cystectomy for bladder cancer: results of a prospective randomized trial. *J Urol* 1994;152:81–84.

167. Bono AV, Benvenuti C, Reali L, et al. Adjuvant chemotherapy in advanced bladder cancer. Italian Uro-Oncologic Cooperative Group. *Prog Clin Biol Res* 1989;303:533–540.

168. Freiha F, Reese J, Torti FM. A randomized trial of radical cystectomy versus radical cystectomy plus cisplatin, vinblastine and methotrexate chemotherapy for muscle invasive bladder cancer. *J Urol* 1996;155:495–499.

169. Skinner DG, Daniels JR, Russell CA, et al. The role of adjuvant chemotherapy following cystectomy for invasive bladder cancer: a prospective comparative trial. *J Urol* 1991;145:459–464.

171. Stockle M, Meyenburg W, Wellek S, et al. Adjuvant polychemotherapy of nonorgan-confined bladder cancer after radical cystectomy revisited: long-term results of a controlled prospective study and further clinical experience. *J Urol* 1995;153:47–52.

172. Advanced Bladder Cancer (ABC) Meta-analysis Collaboration. Adjuvant chemotherapy in invasive bladder cancer: a systematic review and meta-analysis of individual patient data Advanced Bladder Cancer (ABC) Meta-analysis Collaboration. *Eur Urol* 2005;48(2):189–199.

173. Cognetti F, Ruggeri EM, Felici A, et al. Adjuvant chemotherapy with cisplatin and gemcitabine versus chemotherapy at relapse in patients with muscle-invasive bladder cancer submitted to radical cystectomy: an Italian multicenter phase III trial. *Ann Oncol* 2012;23:695–700.

175. Calabro F, Sternberg CN. Neoadjuvant and adjuvant chemotherapy in muscle-invasive bladder cancer. *Eur Urol* 2009;55:303–358.

181. Bjerre BD, Johansen C, Steven K. Health related quality of life after cystectomy: bladder substitution compared with ileal conduit diversion. A questionnaire survey. *Br J Urol* 1995;75:200–205.

182. Hart S, Skinner EC, Meyerowitz BE, et al. Quality of life after radical cystectomy for bladder cancer in patients with an ileal conduit, or cutaneous or urethral Kock pouch. *J Urol* 1999;162:77–81.

183. Porter MP, Penson DF. Health related quality of life after radical cystectomy and urinary diversion for bladder cancer: a systematic review and critical analysis of the literature. *J Urol* 2005;173:1318–1322.

184. Somani BK, Gimlin D, Fayers P, et al. Quality of life and body image for bladder cancer patients undergoing radical cystectomy and urinary diversion—a prospective cohort study with systematic review of the literature. *Urology* 2009;74:1138–1143.

186. Bartsch G, Daneshmand S, Skinner E, et al. Urinary functional outcomes in female neobladder patients. *World J Urol* 2014;32:221–228.

188. Zietman AL, Sacco D, Skowronski U, et al. Organ-conservation in invasive bladder cancer treated by trans-urethral resection, chemotherapy, and radiation: results of a urodynamic and quality of life study on long-term survivors. *J Urol* 2003;170:1772–1776.

189. Herman JM, Smith DC, Montie J, et al. Prospective quality of life assessment in patients receiving concurrent gemcitabine and radiotherapy as a bladder preservation strategy. *Urology* 2004;64:69–73.

193. Gilbert SM, Dunn RL, Hollenbeck BK, et al. Development and validation of the Bladder Cancer Index: a comprehensive, disease specific measure of health related quality of life in patients with localized bladder cancer. *J Urol* 2010;183:1764–1769.

196. Saxman SB, Propert KJ, Einhorn LH, et al. Long-term follow-up of a phase III intergroup study of cisplatin alone or in combination with methotrexate, vinblastine, and doxorubicin in patients with metastatic urothelial carcinoma: a cooperative group study. *J Clin Oncol* 1997;15:2564–2569.

205. Roberts JT, von der Maase H, Sengelov L, et al. Long-term survival results of a randomized trial comparing gemcitabine/cisplatin and methotrexate/vinblastine/doxorubicin/cisplatin in patients with locally advanced and metastatic bladder cancer. *Ann Oncol* 2006;17:v118.

206. Johannsen M, Sachs M, Roigas J, et al. Phase II trial of weekly paclitaxel and carboplatin chemotherapy in patients with advanced transitional cell cancer. *Eur Urol* 2005;48:246–251.

208. De Santis M, Bellmunt J, Mead G, et al. Randomized phase II/III trial assessing gemcitabine/carboplatin and methotrexate/carboplatin/vinblastine in patients with advanced urothelial cancer "unfit" for cisplatin-based chemotherapy: phase II—results of EORTC study 30986. *J Clin Oncol* 2009: 5634–5639.

209. Dreicer R, Manola J, Roth BJ, et al. Phase III trial of methotrexate, vinblastine, doxorubicin, and cisplatin versus carboplatin and paclitaxel in patients with advanced carcinoma of the urothelium. *Cancer* 2004;100:1639–1645.

221. Dogliotti L, Carteni G, Siena S, et al. Gemcitabine plus cisplatin versus gemcitabine plus carboplatin as first-line chemotherapy in advanced transitional cell carcinoma of the urothelium: results of a randomized phase 2 trial. *Eur Urol* 2007;52:134–141.

226. Bellmunt J, von der Maase H, Mead GM, et al. Randomized phase III study comparing paclitaxel/cisplatin/gemcitabine and gemcitabine/cisplatin in patients with locally advanced or metastatic urothelial cancer without prior systemic therapy: EORTC Intergroup Study 30987. *Clin Oncol* 2012;30: 1107–2213.

228. Bellmunt J, Fougeray R, Rosenberg J, et al. Long-term survival results of a randomized phase III trial of vinflunine plus best supportive care versus best supportive care alone in advanced urothelial carcinoma patients after failure of platinum-based chemotherapy. *Ann Oncol* 2013;24:1466–1472.

232. Walsh IK, Keane PF, Ishak LM, et al. The BTA stat test: a tumor marker for the detection of upper tract transitional cell carcinoma. *Urology* 2001; 58:532–535.

233. Skacel M, Fahmy M, Brainard JA, et al. Multitarget fluorescence in situ hybridization assay detects transitional cell carcinoma in the majority of patients with bladder cancer and atypical or negative urine cytology. *J Urol* 2003;169:2101–2105.

237. Jung P, Brauers A, Nolte-Ersting CA, et al. Magnetic resonance urography enhanced by gadolinium and diuretics: a comparison with conventional urography in diagnosing the cause of ureteric obstruction. *BJU Int* 2000;86:960–965.

244. Ambani SN1, Weizer AZ2, Wolf JS Jr, et al. Matched comparison of robotic vs laparoscopic nephroureterectomy: an initial experience. *Urology* 2014;83:345–349.

248. Cutress ML, Stewart GD, Tudor EC, et al. Endoscopic versus laparoscopic management of noninvasive upper tract urothelial carcinoma: 20-year single center experience. *J Urol.* 2013;189:2054–2060.

250. Thompson RH, Krambeck AE, Lohse CM, et al. Endoscopic management of upper tract transitional cell carcinoma in patients with normal contralateral kidneys. *Urology* 2008;71:713–717.

252. Colin P, Ouzzane A, Pignot G, et al. Comparison of oncological outcomes after segmental ureterectomy or radical nephroureterectomy in urothelial carcinomas of the upper urinary tract: results from a large French multicentre study. *BJU Int* 2012;110:1134–1141.

254. Van der Poel HG, Antonini N, Van Tinteren H, et al. Upper urinary tract cancer: location is correlated with prognosis. *Eur Urol* 2005;48:438–444.

266. Cozad SC, Smalley SR, Austenfeld M, et al. Transitional cell carcinoma of the renal pelvis or ureter: patterns of failure. *Urology* 1995;46:796–800.

268. Ozsahin M, Zouhair A, Villa S, et al. Prognostic factors in urothelial renal pelvis and ureter tumours: a multicentre Rare Cancer Network study. *Eur J Cancer* 1999;35:738–743.

271. Czito B, Zietman AL, Kaufman DS, et al. Adjuvant combined modality therapy in locally advanced upper urinary tract malignancies. *J Urol* 2004; 172:1271.

272. Kwak C, Lee SE, Jeong IG, et al. Adjuvant systemic chemotherapy in the treatment of patients with invasive transitional cell carcinoma of the upper urinary tract. *Urology* 2006;68:53–57.

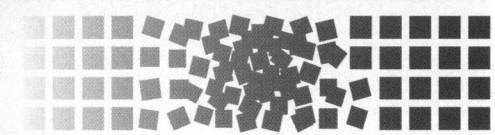

66 Genetic Testing in Urinary Tract Cancers

Gayun Chan-Smutko

PRACTICE OF ONCOLOGY

INTRODUCTION

Cancers of the urinary tract include renal cell carcinoma (RCC) and transitional cell carcinoma, or urothelial carcinoma (UC). About 64,770 cases of invasive cancer of the kidney and renal pelvis, 74,510 cases of urinary bladder cancer, and 2,860 cases of cancer of the ureter and other urinary organs are expected to be diagnosed in men and women in the United States in 2012.[1] The lifetime risk of cancer of the kidney and renal pelvis is 1.6%, with an average age at diagnosis (based on statistics from 2005 to 2009) of 64 years.[2] A family history of RCC is associated with a 2.2- to 2.8-fold increased risk for developing RCC.[3] Most cases of RCC are sporadic, and approximately 4% are due to a hereditary susceptibility.

RCC is a heterogeneous disease, which has been divided into the following subtypes based on the World Health Organization 2004 classification system: Clear cell (80%), papillary types 1 and 2 (10%), chromophobe (5%), collecting duct (1%), and RCC unclassified (4% to 6%). Additional rarer types that collectively account for <2% of RCCs have been described as well.[4] The molecular pathways driving tumorigenesis in hereditary syndromes such as von Hippel-Lindau (VHL) disease, Birt-Hogg-Dubé (BHD) syndrome, hereditary leiomyomatosis and RCC, and hereditary papillary renal cell carcinoma (HPRCC) have provided greater insight into the molecular mechanisms behind the four major subtypes of RCC. This understanding has led to targeted therapies aimed at specific molecular pathways such as the hypoxia-inducible factor (HIF) pathway. This review is devoted primarily to the discussion of renal neoplasms in the adult population and their associated hereditary syndromes (Table 66.1). Genetic testing for susceptibility to urothelial cancers of the upper urinary tract is also presented.

GENETIC SUSCEPTIBILITY TO RENAL CELL CARCINOMA

von Hippel-Lindau Disease

VHL disease is an autosomal dominant condition that affects approximately 1 in 36,000 live births worldwide. The *VHL* gene is located on the short arm of chromosome 3 (3p25) and is the only known susceptibility locus associated with the condition. It is a well-studied tumor suppressor gene that demonstrates loss of heterozygosity in RCCs of patients with VHL disease and sporadic clear cell RCC as well.

VHL disease is a multisystem condition, and an affected individual is at risk to develop any of the following lesions: (1) hemangioblastoma of the cerebellum, spine, or retina; (2) papillary cystadenoma of the epididymis, the adnexal organs, or the endolymphatic sac; (3) adrenal pheochromocytoma and occasionally extra-adrenal paraganglioma; (4) pancreatic cysts, serous cystadenomas, and neuroendocrine tumors (NET); and (5) multiple and/or bilateral RCC and cysts.

Although the penetrance of VHL disease is 100%, where individuals will develop at least one associated lesion by their sixth decade of life, the expressivity is highly variable even among individuals

sharing the same gene mutation. The disease is phenotypically categorized into type 1 and type 2 based on risk for developing pheochromocytoma, with the latter further divided into three subtypes (2A, 2B, and 2C) based on risk for developing RCC. The genotype/phenotype correlations within each type are described in Table 66.2.

Renal Lesions

RCCs of patients with VHL disease are of exclusively clear cell histology. The lifetime risk for developing RCC is 25% to 45%, and when renal cysts are included, the risk rises to 60%.[5] Renal cysts and RCCs develop at an earlier age in patients with VHL in comparison to sporadic counterparts, with an average age of 39 years (range, 16 to 67 years).[5] Cystic lesions are typically asymptomatic; however, complex cysts must be monitored closely with computed tomography (CT) or magnetic resonance imaging as they will harbor a visibly solid RCC component. RCC will often arise from noncystic parenchyma as well.

Nonrenal Clinical Features

With the exception of RCC and pancreatic NETs, the malignancy risk with VHL-associated tumors is very low. Renal lesions and hemangioblastoma of the cerebellum, spine, or retina are common presenting lesions in VHL. The risk for developing a single hemangioblastoma of the spine, cerebellum, and brainstem is 60% to 80%, and the average age is 33 years (range, 9 to 73 years),[5] although most patients can develop multiple lesions at any point in their lifetime. Patients may remain completely asymptomatic, especially during periods of no growth or slow growth. Surgical resection is delayed until onset of symptoms.

Retinal hemangioblastomas (retinal angiomas) are usually multifocal and bilateral. These hypervascular tumors can lead to retinal detachment and vision loss. Retinal hemangioblastomas have been observed in 25% to 60% of patients with an average age of 25 years (range, 1 to 67 years). Approximately 5% of lesions are seen younger than 10 years, making genetic testing of at-risk children essential as affected children should undergo annual retinal examinations beginning at birth. Pheochromocytoma has also been observed in young children and can present as a hypertensive crisis. The average age at presentation is 30 years (range, 5 to 58 years), and the risk is 10% to 20%.[5]

Pancreatic manifestations include multiple simple cysts and serous cystadenomas (47% and 11%, respectively), which follow a benign course and are almost always asymptomatic in patients. Pancreatic NETs are less common (15%); however, approximately 2% undergo malignant transformation.[6] A NET tends to be indolent and is seldom the initial presenting lesion; however, close monitoring is indicated for timing of surgical resection. A less common manifestation of VHL is a papillary cystadenoma of the endolymphatic sac, or inner ear, which is extremely rare in the general population but more prevalent in VHL disease (~11%). Papillary cystadenomas may also arise in the epididymis in men and less commonly in the adnexal organs in women.

917

TABLE 66.1

Genetic Susceptibility to Renal Cell Carcinoma

Syndrome	Acronym	Gene(s)	Phenotype	RCC Type	Genetic Testing Sensitivity
von Hippel-Lindau syndrome	VHL	*VHL*	Hemangioblastoma (cerebellum, spine, retina), pheochromocytoma, papillary cystadenoma (pancreas, epididymis, adnexal organs, endolymphatic sac pancreatic NET, and cysts)	Clear cell	Nearly 100%[a]
Birt-Hogg-Dubé syndrome	BHD	Folliculin, *FLCN*	Fibrofolliculoma, trichodiscoma, acrochordon, lung cysts, spontaneous pneumothorax	50% chromophobe/oncocytic hybrid, 34% chromophobe, 9% clear cell, 5% oncocytoma, 2% papillary	~88%[20]
Hereditary leiomyomatosis and RCC	HLRCC	*FH*	Cutaneous leiomyoma, uterine leiomyoma	Papillary type 2	~93%[25]
Hereditary papillary RCC	HPRCC	*MET*	No additional features	Papillary type 1	Not well established as families are rare
Hereditary paraganglioma/pheochromocytoma	HPGL	*SDHB*, possibly *SDHD* and *SDHC*	Pheochromocytoma and paraganglioma	Not well defined, but clear cell and papillary types reported	Unknown in families with RCC and no paraganglioma or pheochromocytoma

RCC, renal cell carcinoma; NET, neuroendocrine tumor.
[a] Stolle C, Glenn G, Zbar B, et al. Improved detection of germline mutations in the von Hippel–Lindau disease tumor suppressor gene. *Hum Mutat* 1998;12:417–423.

von Hippel-Lindau Molecular Genetics

The *VHL* gene was cloned by Latif et al.[7] in 1993 and is the most well studied of the familial RCC syndromes. Loss of *VHL* function has been demonstrated to cause RCC formation in VHL disease as well as in the majority of sporadic clear cell RCCs.[8,9] The *VHL* gene encodes the pVHL protein, which in normoxic conditions forms a complex with elongin B, elongin C, Cullin 2, and Rbx1. The VHL complex targets HIF-1α and HIF-2α for ubiquitin-mediated degradation. The HIF-1α and HIF-2α genes, along with HIF-3α, encode the α subunit of the HIF heterodimer. In hypoxic conditions, the VHL complex does not interact with HIF-1α and HIF-2α, leading to an accumulation of these subunits and downstream transcription of HIF-dependent genes. Loss of VHL protein

function in renal tumors simulates low tissue oxygen levels, or "pseudohypoxia," where HIF-1α and HIF-2α accumulate, causing upregulation of many genes involved in tumorigenesis such as vascular endothelial growth factor (proangiogenesis), epidermal growth factor receptor (cell proliferation and survival), and glucose transporter 1 (regulation of glucose uptake).

von Hippel-Lindau Genetic Testing

Genetic testing of the VHL gene is available on a clinical basis and involves full-gene sequencing and large gene rearrangement analysis. When both methods are used, the mutation detection rate is nearly 100% in patients with a clinical diagnosis of VHL.[10] Approximately 80% of patients have a parent with VHL, and ~20% represent de

---

TABLE 66.2

von Hippel-Lindau Genotype Phenotype Correlations

VHL Phenotype	Pheo	RCC	HB	Predominant Mutation Type
Type 1	Rare or absent	High	High	Large deletions, nonsense, frameshift
Type 2A	High	Rare	High	Missense
Type 2B	High	High	High	Missense
Type 2C (uncommon)	High	Absent	Absent	Missense

Note: The majority of type 1 mutations are partial or complete deletions and protein truncating (nonsense and frameshift), whereas 96% of type 2 mutations are missense. Missense mutations that disrupt amino acid residues on the surface of the VHL protein confer a higher Pheo risk than missense mutations that disrupt protein structure.
VHL, von Hippel-Lindau; Pheo, pheochromocytoma; RCC, renal cell carcinoma; HB, hemangioblastoma.
From Maher ER, Webster AR, Richards FM, et al. Phenotypic expression in von Hippel–Lindau disease: Correlations with germline VHL gene mutations. *J Med Genet* 1996;33:328–332; and Ong KR, Woodward ER, Killick P, et al. Genotype–phenotype correlations in von Hippel–Lindau disease. *Hum Mutat* 2007;28:143–149.

novo cases where neither parent carries the mutation. Genetic testing is recommended for a proband with a personal and family history of VHL, as the identification of causative mutations aids in determining disease subtype (see Table 66.2). Disease subtype information along with a careful, detailed family history aids in guiding screening and surveillance of patients with VHL. In simplex cases, where a patient has two or more VHL-associated lesions and a negative family history, genetic testing is recommended to establish a diagnosis. When a mutation is identified in a proband, at-risk family members should be offered predictive testing. Since young children with VHL are known to be at risk for retinal lesions and pheochromocytoma, genetic testing should be offered any time after birth.

Birt-Hogg-Dubé Syndrome

In 1977, Drs. Birt, Hogg, and Dubé first described a multigenerational kindred showing autosomal dominant transmission of fibrofolliculomas with trichodiscomas and acrochordons.[11] The phenotype was later expanded beyond dermatologic manifestations to include lung cysts and pneumothorax and renal tumors.[12] The number of families with BHD syndrome described in the literature to date is small, and therefore, the exact incidence is unknown. Inherited mutations in the folliculin (FLCN) gene are associated with BHD syndrome.

Renal Lesions

An individual with BHD syndrome is at increased risk of developing multiple and bilateral renal tumors, frequently of more than one histologic type even within the same renal unit, and at younger ages compared with the general population. The lifetime risk is in the range of 27% to 45%,[13,14] and the wide range may be a reflection of ascertainment bias introduced when families are recruited predominantly through dermatology clinics versus urology. The most common tumor pathology found in patients is a hybrid oncocytic RCC, which contains a mixture of oncocytic and chromophobe cells. Furthermore, radical nephrectomy specimens of patients have demonstrated oncocytosis where tiny nodules of cells similar to the larger hybrid tumors are diffusely scattered throughout the renal parenchyma. A retrospective study by Pavlovich et al.[15] examined 130 tumor specimens from 30 patients (25 males, 5 females) in 19 different BHD families. The authors found that hybrid oncocytic (50%) and chromophobe (34%) were the more common histologic findings, followed by clear cell (9%), benign oncocytoma (5%), and papillary (2%). The average age at first tumor was 50.7 years, and patients averaged 5.3 tumors each (range, 1 to 28). Other studies reporting histologic subtypes of BHD syndrome–related renal tumors have similar findings.

Nonrenal Manifestations

Skin findings associated with BHD syndrome are benign and consist of fibrofolliculoma, trichodiscoma (which are histologically and clinically indistinguishable from angiofibroma), perifollicular fibroma, and acrochordons. Fibrofolliculoma is highly specific for BHD syndrome, whereas trichodiscomas and acrochordons are not. Onset for skin lesions is typically at older than 25 years, and a dermatologic diagnosis of BHD syndrome can be made on the basis of the presence of five or more facial or truncal papules with at least one histologically confirmed fibrofolliculoma.

Approximately 83% to 89% of patients with BHD syndrome will have multiple pulmonary cysts[14,16,17] identified upon chest CT. The lifetime risk of spontaneous pneumothorax is 24% to 32%,[14,18] and the majority of patients have their first event by age 50 years. The presence of lung cysts is strongly associated with risk of pneumothorax,[17] but the mechanism behind this is not known. A possible association between BHD syndrome and parotid oncocytoma has also been reported in a small number of cases.[14]

FLCN Molecular Genetics

The FLCN gene is located on chromosome 17p11.2 and was cloned by Nickerson et al.[12] in 2002. The gene has 14 exons and encodes the protein folliculin. The role of FLCN and tumorigenesis has not been fully established, but animal studies and loss of heterozygosity studies in renal tumors provide some evidence that it is a tumor suppressor gene. Folliculin binds with folliculin-interacting proteins (FNIP1 and FNIP2) and then binds AMP-activated protein kinase, which is part of the cellular energy and nutrient sensing system. AMP-activated protein kinase also helps regulates mTOR activity (mTORC1 and mTORC2). Studies of renal tumors from heterozygous BHD knockout mice and renal tumors from patients with BHD syndrome show mTOR activation. Therapeutic agents inhibiting mTOR activity in sporadic chromophobe tumors are currently under investigation and may have implications for patients with BHD syndrome–related renal tumors.[19]

The mutation detection rate for FLCN clinical testing is approximately 89%, and nearly all of the mutations described to date have been truncating point mutations (frameshift and nonsense). Splice-site mutations have also been reported in a small number of BHD families, and one missense mutation in a patient with bilateral renal tumors has been reported as well.[20] A mutational hotspot in a polycytosine tract in exon 11 has been suggested.[14]

Hereditary Papillary Renal Cell Carcinoma

HPRCC is inherited in an autosomal dominant manner with reduced penetrance where patients with HPRCC are at risk of developing multiple and/or bilateral papillary RCCs at a young age. The phenotype is limited to the risk of papillary RCC alone, particularly papillary type 1, although the distinction between type 1 and type 2 is not always made on initial pathology review.

Germ-line mutations in the c-met or MET proto-oncogene on chromosome 7q31.2 have been associated with HPRCC.[21] This is a comparatively uncommon condition, and few families with a MET mutation have been reported to date. Missense mutations found in HPRCC families occur in exons 16, 17, 18, and 19 of the MET proto-oncogene, which encodes the tyrosine-kinase domain of the protein product. These mutations have been shown to be activating or gain-of-function mutations, unlike most hereditary cancer susceptibility syndromes, which are associated with loss-of-function mutations in tumor suppressor genes. Papillary tumors obtained from patients with HPRCC typically show duplication of chromosome 7, as do their sporadic counterparts.[22] Furthermore, HPRCC-associated tumors show nonrandom duplication of the chromosome 7 copy harboring the mutation MET allele,[22,23] suggesting that overexpression of MET may lead to cellular proliferation, although the exact mechanism has not yet been elucidated.

Analysis by Lindor et al.[24] of 59 apparently sporadic patients with papillary type 1 tumors, including 13 cases with multifocal or bilateral disease, found no germ-line mutations in MET. This suggests differing etiology in sporadic versus papillary type 1 cancers. The rarity of the disease and low likelihood of identifying mutation carriers in isolated cases poses a challenge for genetic counseling of these patients. In the setting of a positive family history, MET genetic testing should be offered to patients with papillary type 1 RCC. A negative genetic test result, however, does not exclude the possibility of a hereditary susceptibility.

Hereditary Leiomyomatosis and Renal Cell Carcinoma

Susceptibility to papillary type 2 RCC has been associated with hereditary leiomyomatosis and RCC (HLRCC) syndrome demonstrating autosomal dominant transmission. Most individuals with HLRCC-associated renal lesions present with unilateral, solitary tumors; however, bilateral and multifocal disease has also been observed.[25] The tumors tend to be highly aggressive with poor prognosis, which has implications for screening and early detection in at-risk patients. Although papillary type 2 is the predominant histology, collecting duct RCC and mixed cystic, papillary, and tubulopapillary RCC have also been reported. The incidence of RCC in individuals with HLRCC is approximately 25% to 40%.[25,26]

Cutaneous leiomyomatosis and uterine leiomyomatosis are additional features of the disease. Leiomyomas of the skin appear as firm skin-colored to light brown papules and can be distributed anywhere along the trunk, extremities, head, or neck. Uterine leiomyomas (fibroids) are common in the general population; however, HLRCC-associated burden tends to be greater in women with HLRCC. Compared with the general population, the average age at onset is younger where many women become symptomatic before the age of 30 years, significantly impacting their childbearing years. The fibroids tend to be multiple (ranging from 1 to 15 in one series of 22 women from 16 families studied) and large (1 to 8 cm), often requiring myomectomy or hysterectomy for treatment.[25] Not all individuals with HLRCC will have cutaneous manifestations, although it is worthwhile to note that the presence of cutaneous leiomyomas has a strong concordance with uterine leiomyoma. A very small number of cases have been reported of cutaneous and uterine leiomyosarcoma in HLRCC families. The fumarate hydratase gene, or *FH*, is the only gene associated with the disease to date. Fumarate hydratase functions in the Krebs cycle to convert fumarate to malate. Alteration of the *FH* gene results in accumulation of fumarate, which inhibits HIF-a prolyl hydroxylase enzymes (HPH). HIF-a is hydroxylated by HPH in normoxic conditions, but when HPH is inhibited, HIF-a levels rise, leading to increased transcription of downstream genes involved in tumorigenesis.[19]

Hereditary Paraganglioma and Pheochromocytoma Associated with SDHB

Several genes have been implicated in hereditary paraganglioma with and without pheochromocytoma, such as the succinate dehydrogenase complex genes (*SDHB*, *SDHD*, and *SDHC*), as well as *TMEM127*, *SDHAF2*, *VHL*, *MEN2*, and others. The reader is referred to Chapter 88 "Genetic Testing in the Endocrine System" in this book for a detailed discussion of these genes.

Earlier reports of families with mutations in *SDHB* also noted renal tumors in a minority of these families with a paraganglioma/pheochromocytoma phenotype.[27] Different renal tumor histologic findings have been reported including clear cell, chromophobe, carcinoma not classifiable, papillary type 2, or oncocytoma.[27-31] Gill et al.[32] examined five renal tumors from four families with an *SDHB* mutation and suggest that *SDHB*-associated renal tumors share common morphologic features such as bubbly eosinophilic cytoplasm with intracytoplasmic inclusions and indistinct cell borders.

Genetic testing of *SDHB* should be considered in patients presenting with early-onset and/or multifocal/bilateral RCC and a family history of paraganglioma or pheochromocytoma. Testing can also be considered in familial RCC especially in multigeneration and early-onset families, although there are not enough data at this time to suggest whether many *SDHB* carriers will be identified in the absence of known paraganglioma or pheochromocytoma. Ricketts et al.[29] studied a cohort of 68 patients with RCC and no evidence of syndromic RCC susceptibility and identified three *SDHB* mutation carriers (4.4%). One had a personal history of RCC at 24 years and a positive family history; two had a history of bilateral disease, one at the age of 30 years and the other at the age of 38 years; none of the three cases had a personal or family history of paraganglioma or pheochromocytoma.[29]

GENETIC SUSCEPTIBILITY TO UROTHELIAL CANCERS

Hereditary Nonpolyposis Colorectal Cancer, or Lynch Syndrome

Hereditary nonpolyposis colorectal cancer, or Lynch syndrome, is an inherited syndrome characterized by an increased risk for carcinoma of the colon, uterus, stomach, ovary, pancreas, and upper urinary tract. Inherited mutations in the DNA mismatch repair genes (*MLH1*, *MSH2*, *MSH6*, and *PMS2*) are associated with the syndrome. A detailed discussion of Lynch syndrome and genetic testing can be found in Chapter 59 "Genetic Testing in Colon Cancer (Nonpolyposis Syndromes)" of this book.

Upper urinary tract cancers are the third most common cancer in Lynch syndrome, with a 5% to 6% lifetime risk. The associated cancers are mainly UCs of the ureter and renal pelvis with a relative risk of 22 times higher than that of the general population and a median age at onset of 56 years, or 10 to 15 years earlier.[33] Upper urinary UC may be the initial presenting feature in some patients from Lynch families. Most of the reported cases are in families with *MSH2* mutations, but have been observed in smaller number of *MLH1* and *MSH6* families as well. Bladder UC has been reported in patients with Lynch syndrome, with some studies reporting a relative risk similar or slightly higher to that of the general population.[34] In a cohort of Dutch families with Lynch syndrome, the relative risk of bladder cancer compared with the Dutch population was higher: 4.2 for men and 2.5 for women. *MSH2* mutation carriers in this cohort showed an even higher risk of 7 for men and 5.8 for women.[35]

Upper urinary tract cancers may be an underrecognized entity in Lynch syndrome, particularly in the urology specialty setting. Patients with UC of the ureter and renal pelvis may warrant a referral to genetics for risk assessment when presenting at young ages and/or synchronous or metachronous disease. Family history positivity for upper urinary tract cancers and other Lynch-associated tumors should be an indication for referral as well.

INDICATIONS FOR GENETIC TESTING

One or more of the indicators listed in the following should prompt a referral for evaluating a patient for genetic susceptibility to RCC. Possible entry points for the patient include a diagnosis of RCC, pheochromocytoma or paraganglioma, spontaneous pneumothorax, bilateral cystic kidneys, cystic pancreas, or suspicious cutaneous lesions. A proposed guide to making a differential diagnosis is depicted in Figure 66.1.

■ Syndromic features: A thorough medical history and physical examination may provide supporting evidence of syndromic features. Review of available radiology examinations is warranted. Patients with suspicious cutaneous lesions should be referred to dermatology for biopsy and histologic confirmation.
■ Personal diagnosis of RCC: Even in the absence of known family history, early-onset (<40 years) and/or presence of multifocal or bilateral lesions warrants referral.
■ Family history: Obtaining and reviewing pathology reports on renal tumors from family members is essential. Patients should be queried for a positive family history of related tumors such as pheochromocytoma, skin findings, and colon cancer.

GENETIC TESTING AND COUNSELING

Genetic testing for *VHL*, *FLCN*, *MET*, *FH*, and *SDHB* is clinically available for approximately $1,000 to $1,200 per gene, although the per-gene cost is anticipated to decrease as the cost of sequencing technologies decreases and more multigene panels are offered.

Approach to diagnosis of familial RCC

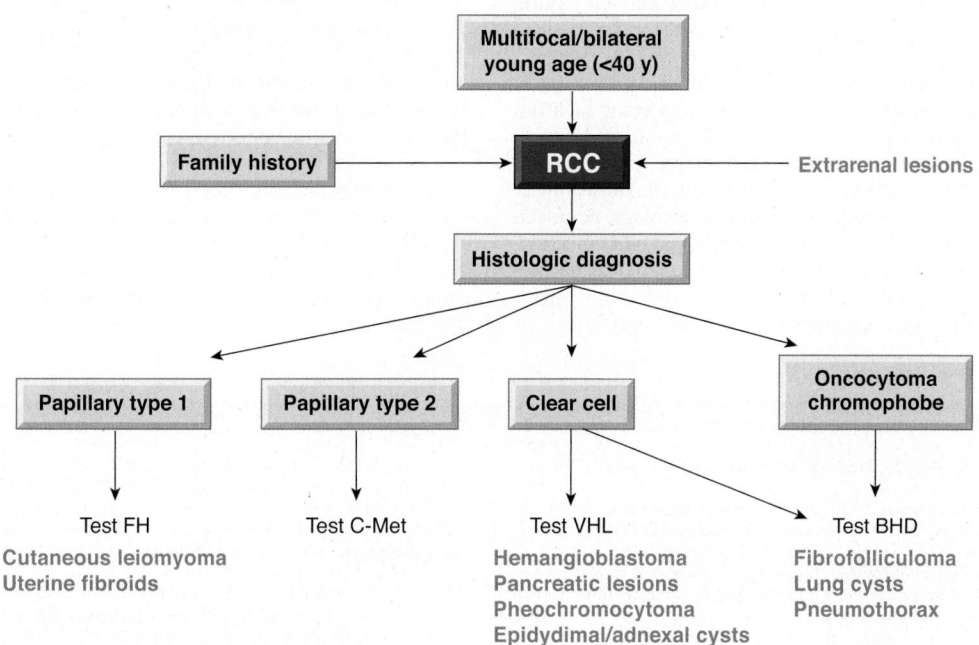

Figure 66.1 Proposed approach for evaluation and testing for inherited susceptibility to RCC. Family history, age at onset, extrarenal lesions, and renal histology guide testing. RCC, renal cell carcinoma; FH, fumarate hydratase; VHL, von Hippel-Lindau; BHD, Birt-Hogg-Dubé.

Lynch syndrome testing is also available; however, it is a genetically heterogeneous disease, and tumor screening with microsatellite instability analysis and immunohistochemistry of the DNA mismatch repair genes can help guide germline testing (see "Colon Nonpolyposis" section of this book). A summary of the mutation detection rates for each gene can be found in Table 66.1. Testing sensitivity is predictably highest in syndromic cases with uncommon tumors that are highly specific for the syndrome such as hemangioblastoma (VHL) and fibrofolliculoma (BHD). Genetic testing is still warranted in less suspicious cases as a positive test result in a patient (i.e., germline mutation) prompts close monitoring in a rational, targeted manner. This includes screening for new renal tumors and nonrenal manifestations such as pheochromocytoma and paraganglioma. High-risk, aggressive papillary type 2 tumors are associated with HLRCC and warrant prompt intervention. Early detection and monitoring of nonpapillary type 2 renal lesions provide the patient and physician with information on disease burden, tumor size, and doubling time. Because patients with hereditary conditions such as VHL are at high risk of developing multiple RCC over their lifetime, close surveillance provides necessary clinical information for timing surgical intervention and increases the likelihood that nephron-sparing approaches can be used.

When a deleterious mutation is identified, at-risk family members should be offered predictive genetic testing. Genetic counseling regarding the natural history of the condition, the risk of carrying the mutation, age-appropriate screening, and the limitations of genetic testing is essential. In the case of BHD, HPRCC, and HLRCC, there is no consensus for a minimum age at which genetic testing should be considered. Timing of testing of asymptomatic relatives may be guided by ages at onset within the family. Each first-degree relative of a mutation carrier has an empiric risk of 50%. A negative test effectively rules out the disease and spares the individual from unnecessary imaging and screening. A positive test prompts close monitoring, such as regular imaging of the kidneys with CT or magnetic resonance imaging. With respect to limitations, it is important for patients to understand that a positive test result does not predict which tumors they will develop over their lifetime, age at onset of tumors, or severity of their disease.

VHL disease represents an exception where genetic testing should be offered anytime after a child is born. When a child tests negative for the familial VHL mutation, he/she is spared unnecessary screening; a child who carries the mutation must begin annual retinal examinations within the first year of life, with additional imaging examinations of the abdomen and brain around the onset of puberty. Multiple cases of retinal hemangioblastomas (angioma) in young children have been reported, and the morbidity of undiagnosed retinal tumors is high. Similarly, childhood-onset pheochromocytoma is also known to be associated with VHL and hereditary paraganglioma/pheochromocytoma syndromes.

Predictive testing of minors in their teenage years should be treated with a greater sensitivity to the minor's intellectual and emotional capacity. Some parents include their child on the decision to test, depending on the age and emotional maturity of their child. This helps maintain trust between the child and the parent, and lays a foundation for greater comprehension of the test result and the implications, whether the results are positive or negative. In the setting of genetic predisposition counseling, the concept of risk and the struggle to cope with risk information is a tenuous position for any adult patient. This is no less stressful for a teenager and his/her parents demanding elevated sensitivity and awareness from the provider and genetic counselor caring for the family.

Not including an older child in the testing decision is also the parents' prerogative; however, the health-care provider or genetic counselor working with the family should help parents consider the potential ramifications of initiating testing without the child's knowledge. Questions to consider include when and how they would disclose the results to their child in an age-appropriate way. When we consider a teenaged minor who is intellectually capable of giving assent for genetic testing, the process of obtaining the minor's assent involves the health-care professional who, together with the parents, provides age-appropriate information about the genetic disease, what is involved in carrying out the test, and how results will be disclosed. Parents may wish to test their teenage minor without his/her knowledge primarily because they are hoping for a "good news" scenario of a negative test result where both the teen and the parents can be worry-free. When parents request testing for their teenager without his/her knowledge, the provider should help parents anticipate that they may be putting their child's trust in them (and their child's trust in the medical community) at risk, particularly if it results in a positive diagnosis.

The role of the genetic counselor and health-care provider is to support the patient and family with a focus on improving their understanding of their disease and on helping the family find a common language with which to communicate their fears, concerns, and needs. Families often benefit from participating in multidisciplinary practices staffed by a combination of medical oncology, advanced practice nursing, genetic counseling, urosurgery, and other practitioners.[36] These disease specialty clinics are geared toward meeting the medical and informational needs of the patient and family, which are expected to evolve with age and with major life transitions.

SUMMARY

The genetic basis of heritable susceptibility to cancers of the urinary tract is a complex problem composed of many different genes and molecular pathways. Careful inspection of family medical history, tumor histology, and physical findings such as cutaneous lesions provide the opportunity for a stepwise approach to genetic risk assessment of the patient with cancer. Genetic testing of cancer susceptibility genes has downstream implications for surveillance and treatment of disease, and identification of causative mutations provides valuable information for patients and their at-risk family members. Genetic counseling of patients and their family members allows for enhanced understanding of the disease and treatment.

REFERENCES

1. Siegel R, Naishadham D, Jemal A. Cancer statistics. *CA Cancer J Clin* 2012; 62:10–29.
2. National Cancer Institute. SEER Stat Fact Sheets: Kidney and Renal Pelvis Cancer. SEER Web site. http://seer.cancer.gov/statfacts/html/kidrp.html#risk. Accessed May 2, 2012.
3. Clague J, Lin J, Cassidy A, et al. Family history and risk of renal cell carcinoma: Results from a case-control study and systematic meta-analysis. *Cancer Epidemiol Biomarkers Prev* 2009;18:801–807.
4. Deng FM, Melamed J. Histologic variants of renal cell carcinoma: Does tumor type influence outcome? *Urol Clin North Am* 2012;39:119–132.
5. Lonser RR, Glenn GM, Walther M, et al. von Hippel–Lindau disease. *Lancet* 2003;361:2059–2067.
6. Charlesworth M, Verbeke CS, Falk GA, et al. Pancreatic lesions in von Hippel–Lindau disease? A systematic review and meta-synthesis of the literature. *J Gastrointest Surg* 2012;16:1422–1428.
7. Latif F, Tory K, Gnarra J, et al. Identification of the von Hippel–Lindau disease tumor suppressor gene. *Science* 1993;260:1317–1320.
8. Gnarra JR, Tory K, Weng Y, et al. Mutations of the VHL tumour suppressor gene in renal carcinoma. *Nat Genet* 1994;7:85–90.
9. Shuin T, Kondo K, Torigoe S, et al. Frequent somatic mutations and loss of heterozygosity of the von Hippel–Lindau tumor suppressor gene in primary human renal cell carcinomas. *Cancer Res* 1994;54:2852–2855.
10. Schimke RN, Collins DL, Stolle CA. Von-Hippel Lindau Syndrome. GeneReviews at GeneTests: Medical Genetics Information Resource (website) http://www.genetests.org. Updated December 22, 2009. Accessed April 11, 2012.
11. Birt AR, Hogg GR, Dube WJ. Hereditary multiple fibrofolliculomas with trichodiscomas and acrochordons. *Arch Dermatol* 1977;113:1674–1677.
12. Nickerson ML, Warren MB, Toro JR, et al. Mutations in a novel gene lead to kidney tumors, lung wall defects, and benign tumors of the hair follicle in patients with the Birt–Hogg–Dube syndrome. *Cancer Cell* 2002;2:157–164.
13. Pavlovich CP, Grubb RL 3rd, Hurley K, et al. Evaluation and management of renal tumors in the Birt–Hogg–Dube syndrome. *J Urol* 2005;173: 1482–1486.
14. Schmidt LS, Nickerson ML, Warren MB, et al. Germline BHD-mutation spectrum and phenotype analysis of a large cohort of families with Birt–Hogg–Dube syndrome. *Am J Hum Genet* 2005;76:1023–1033.
15. Pavlovich CP, Walther MM, Eyler RA, et al. Renal tumors in the Birt–Hogg–Dube syndrome. *Am J Surg Pathol* 2002;26:1542–1552.
16. Zbar B, Alvord WG, Glenn G, et al. Risk of renal and colonic neoplasms and spontaneous pneumothorax in the Birt–Hogg–Dube syndrome. *Cancer Epidemiol Biomarkers Prev* 2002;11:393–400.
17. Toro JR, Pautler SE, Stewart L, et al. Lung cysts, spontaneous pneumothorax, and genetic associations in 89 families with Birt–Hogg–Dube syndrome. *Am J Respir Crit Care Med* 2007;175:1044–1053.
18. Houweling AC, Gijezen LM, Jonker MA, et al. Renal cancer and pneumothorax risk in Birt–Hogg–Dube syndrome; an analysis of 115 FLCN mutation carriers from 35 BHD families. *Br J Cancer* 2011;105:1912–1919.
19. Singer EA, Bratslavsky G, Middelton L, et al. Impact of genetics on the diagnosis and treatment of renal cancer. *Curr Urol Rep* 2011;12:47–55.

20. Toro JR, Wei MH, Glenn GM, et al. BHD mutations, clinical and molecular genetic investigations of Birt–Hogg–Dube syndrome: A new series of 50 families and a review of published reports. *J Med Genet* 2008;45:321–331.
21. Schmidt L, Duh FM, Chen F, et al. Germline and somatic mutations in the tyrosine kinase domain of the MET proto-oncogene in papillary renal carcinomas. *Nat Genet* 1997;16:68–73.
22. Fischer J, Palmedo G, von Knobloch R, et al. Duplication and overexpression of the mutant allele of the MET proto-oncogene in multiple hereditary papillary renal cell tumours. *Oncogene* 1998;17:733–739.
23. Zhuang Z, Park WS, Pack S, et al. Trisomy 7–harbouring non-random duplication of the mutant MET allele in hereditary papillary renal carcinomas. *Nat Genet* 1998;20:66–69.
24. Lindor NM, Dechet CB, Greene MH, et al. Papillary renal cell carcinoma: Analysis of germline mutations in the MET proto-oncogene in a clinic-based population. *Genet Test* 2001;5:101–106.
25. Wei MH, Toure O, Glenn GM, et al. Novel mutations in FH and expansion of the spectrum of phenotypes expressed in families with hereditary leiomyomatosis and renal cell cancer. *J Med Genet* 2006;43:18–27.
26. Gardie B, Remenieras A, Kattygnarath D, et al. Novel FH mutations in families with hereditary leiomyomatosis and renal cell cancer (HLRCC) and patients with isolated type 2 papillary renal cell carcinoma. *J Med Genet* 2011;48:226–234.
27. Vanharanta S, Buchta M, McWhinney SR, et al. Early-onset renal cell carcinoma as a novel extraparaganglial component of SDHB-associated heritable paraganglioma. *Am J Hum Genet* 2004;74:153–159.
28. Henderson A, Douglas F, Perros P, et al. SDHB-associated renal oncocytoma suggests a broadening of the renal phenotype in hereditary paragangliomatosis. *Fam Cancer* 2009;8:257–260.
29. Ricketts C, Woodward ER, Killick P, et al. Germline SDHB mutations and familial renal cell carcinoma. *J Natl Cancer Inst* 2008;100:1260–1262.
30. Ricketts CJ, Forman JR, Rattenberry E, et al. Tumor risks and genotype–phenotype–proteotype analysis in 358 patients with germline mutations in SDHB and SDHD. *Hum Mutat* 2010;31:41–51.
31. Srirangalingam U, Walker L, Khoo B, et al. Clinical manifestations of familial paraganglioma and pheochromocytomas in succinate dehydrogenase B (SDH-B) gene mutation carriers. *Clin Endocrinol (Oxf)* 2008;69:587–596.
32. Gill AJ, Pachter NS, Chou A, et al. Renal tumors associated with germline SDHB mutation show distinctive morphology. *Am J Surg Pathol* 2011;35:1578–1585.
33. Rouprêt M, Yates DR, Comperat E, et al. Upper urinary tract urothelial cell carcinomas and other urological malignancies involved in the hereditary nonpolyposis colorectal cancer (Lynch syndrome) tumor spectrum. *Eur Urol* 2008;54:1226–1236.
34. Crockett DG, Wagner DG, Holmäng S, et al. Upper urinary tract carcinoma in Lynch syndrome cases. *J Urol* 2011;185:1627–1630.
35. van der Post RS, Kiemeney LA, Ligtenberg MJ, et al. Risk of urothelial bladder cancer in Lynch syndrome is increased, in particular among MSH2 mutation carriers. *J Med Genet* 2010;47:464–470.
36. VHL Alliance. A list of VHL specialty clinics in the United States and other countries. www.vhl.org. Accessed September 3, 2014.

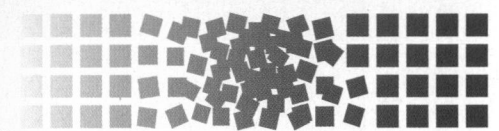

67 Molecular Biology of Prostate Cancer

Felix Y. Feng, Arul M. Chinnaiyan, and Edwin M. Posadas

INTRODUCTION

Prostate cancer is the most common malignancy and the second leading cause of cancer death in men in the United States.[1] It also poses a global problem, with recent significant increases in incidence outside the Western world.[2] This malignancy is marked by extremely clinical and biological heterogeneity, which creates the opportunity for resistant clones to emerge, leading to eventual relapse and disease progression, and thus presenting problems for both patients and their physicians.

A major limitation in the management of this disease has been in the nomenclature used to describe the nature of each patient's underlying disease. The currently employed staging system and the histopathologic scores established by Gleason reflect neither our current understanding of prostate cancer biology, nor the implications of this biology for outcomes and management. There has remained a need to further refine the pathologic classification of prostate cancers to account for the various families of molecular aberrations that exist within this disease. It is hoped that this refinement of classification may allow for more precise or "personalized" management of prostatic adenocarcinomas.

Systemic therapy for this disease begins with the reduction of circulating testosterone levels by medical or surgical castration. In most cases, this results in clinical benefit. However, progression to castration-resistant prostate cancer (CRPC) eventually occurs. A number of effective CRPC therapies have recently emerged. Regretfully, none are curative and all have a limited benefit, as shown in clinical trials. Refining our understanding of the molecular nature of this disease will hopefully lead to better characterization and, ultimately, more effective assignment of treatments to improve outcomes for patients.

OVERVIEW OF THE GENOMIC LANDSCAPE OF PROSTATE CANCER

The advent of next-generation sequencing technology has significantly broadened our understanding of the genomic landscape of prostate cancer. Recent studies have characterized the complete prostate cancer genome from 75 patients and have reported on the exomes of hundreds of additional cases.[3-7] In combination with gene expression and copy number data previously interrogated from thousands of tumors, these studies provide a relatively comprehensive profile of the prostate cancer genome and transcriptome. Like other epithelial tumors, prostate cancers harbor genomic lesions, such as amplifications and deletions; point mutations; and translocations, as well as transcriptional changes leading to overexpression of oncogenes and underexpression of tumor suppressor genes.

Subsets of tumors have been shown to harbor recurrent amplifications and deletions ranging from focal alternations (one to a few genes) to others that span entire chromosomal arms (Fig. 67.1). These alterations tend to increase in prevalence with higher grade and stage. The most common deletions occur on chromosomes 8p,

10q, and 13q, and include genes such as *NKX3-1*, *PTEN*, and *RB1*. Metastatic tumors harbor amplifications of chromosome X and 8q, which include the androgen receptor (AR) and *MYC* oncogenes (see Fig. 67.1). Although the prostate cancer genome exhibits an overall low mutation rate (~1 per MB), the landscape of prostate cancer can also be defined by copy number and mutational alterations along several key oncogenic and tumor suppressor pathways, which are commonly involved when the individual genes in each pathway are considered collectively. Three of these pathways—the AR pathway, the phosphatidylinositol 3-phosphate kinase (PI3K)/AKT pathway, and the retinoblastoma (RB) pathway—are altered in more than one-third of primary cancers and in the vast majority of metastatic lesions.[3-7] Frequent alterations in these pathways suggest that, in prostate cancer, different individual genes in the pathway may be targeted to activate or suppress a common pathway lesion (Fig. 67.2).

In addition to pathway-based analyses, prostate cancer can be defined by recurrent lesions of single genes. Approximately 50% of prostate-specific antigen (PSA)-screened prostate cancers harbor gene fusions involving E26 transformation specific (ETS) transcription factors, which represent oncogenic drivers.[8,9] Strikingly, ETS fusions and certain other lesions, such as mutation of the E3 ubiquitin ligase *SPOP* and fusions involving *RAF*, appear to be mutually exclusive, suggesting a framework for molecular subtyping of prostate cancer.[5,10,11] The sections that follow further describe the altered pathways and recurrent genetic lesions most validated in prostate cancer.

ANDROGEN RECEPTOR BIOLOGY AND THERAPY

Introduction to the Androgen Receptor

AR has remained one of the most important and most studied proteins in prostate cancer. The dependence of most prostate cancers on AR activation has served as a basis for important therapeutic approaches, such as luteinizing hormone releasing hormone (LHRH) analogs, antiandrogens, and androgen biosynthesis inhibitors.

AR is a 110-kb steroid receptor transcription factor, located on Xq12.[12] Upon binding to an androgen, AR mediates the transcription of a number of genes involved in survival and differentiation of prostate epithelial cells, starting at development of the normal gland. Expression of AR is high in the luminal epithelial cells but lower in the basal epithelial cells that define glandular structure.[13]

In conjunction with *NKX3.1* and *FOXA1*, AR plays a critical role in normal prostate organogenesis and disease progression.[14] *NKX3.1* is an AR-regulated prostatic tumor suppressor gene that is located on chromosome 8p and present through development.[15] It is the earliest marker of organogenesis and is involved with ductal morphogenesis and secretory function.[16] Mutations are infrequent in human cancers, but loss of heterozygosity in 8p becomes more frequent during cancer progression, with 86% loss in prostate cancers (see Fig. 67.1).[17] Loss of *NKX3.1* has been associated with

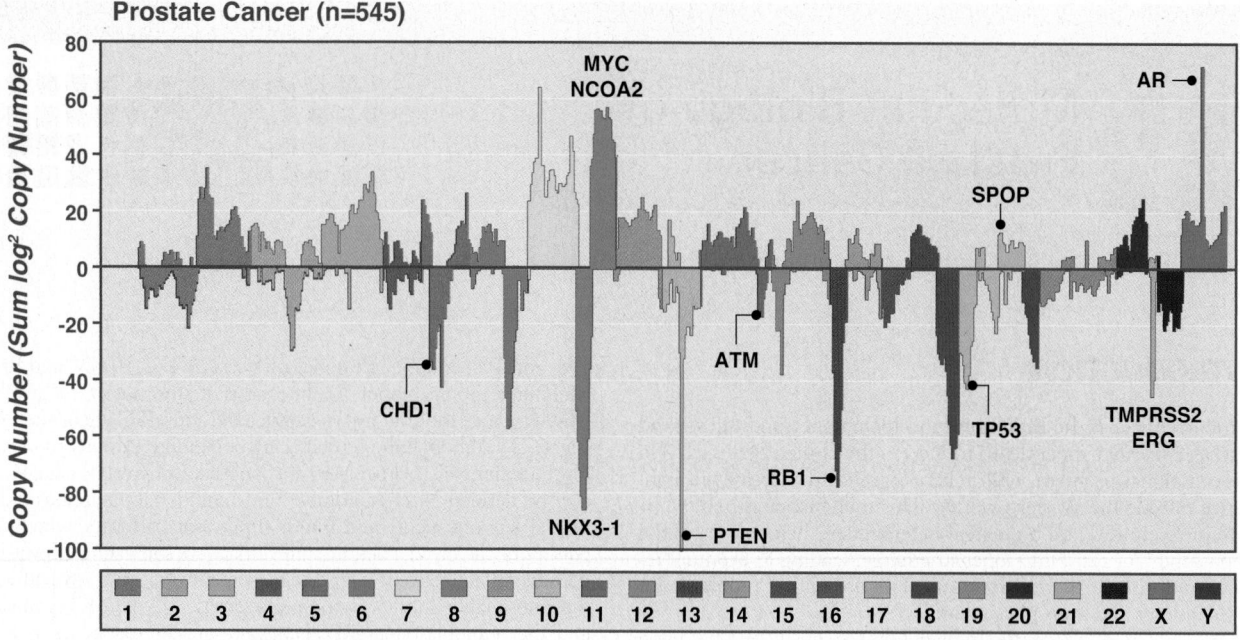

Figure 67.1 Copy number alterations found in prostate cancer. Genomewide copy number profiles were plotted from four publicly available datasets including 545 prostate cancers, using the Oncomine Powertools DNA Copy Number Browser (Life Technology). Each chromosome is color coded (see legend), and the locations of key genes harboring recurrent copy number gains/losses or mutations are labeled. The y axis indicates the sum of the log2 copy number for each segmented sample, as plotted in genomic order.

activation of the TMPRSS2-ERG gene fusion, which promotes tumorigenesis.[18] *FOXA1* is a member of the forkhead transcription factor family that opens compacted chromatin to facilitate AR recruitment.[19] It is known to play a pivotal role in AR and steroid receptor function.[20] It is now recognized that mutation and overexpression of FOXA1 can promote progression to CRPC (see Fig. 67.2).[3,5]

Polymorphisms of *AR* as well as *CYP17* and *SRD5A2* are low penetrant risk factors for prostate cancer development in some but not all studies.[21] AR-pathway alterations exist in 60% of primary tumors and nearly 100% of metastatic tumors. *NCOA2* (also called *SRC2*) is the most commonly altered member of this pathway (see Fig. 67.2) and is an AR coactivator that potentiates transcriptional output. Several other AR coactivators, including *NCOA1, TNK2,* and *EP300,* are upregulated in metastatic disease, whereas AR corepressors, including *NRIP1, NCOR1,* and *NCOR2,* are downregulated (see Fig. 67.2).

Targeting Androgen Receptor Activity: GnRH-Targeting Therapies and Androgen Biosynthesis Inhibitors

The inhibition of androgen synthesis has been used a means of suppressing AR activity. Gonadotropin-releasing hormone-luteinizing hormone (GnRH) agonists or antagonists represent the first-line approach for inhibiting androgen synthesis (Fig. 67.3). These therapies work by suppressing the hypothalamic–pituitary–gonadal axis by eventually causing luteinizing hormone (LH) levels to fall, thereby minimizing testicular production of testosterone and its subsequent conversion to dihydrotestosterone (DHT) by 5-alpha reduction. DHT is the most potent activator of AR and binds to the AR, resulting in translocation to the nucleus and activation of transcription (see Fig. 67.3).

These strategies, although initially highly effective, are often overcome during tumor progression. Alternative sources of DHT and alternative means of AR activity have been identified as mechanisms of resistance. GnRH-targeting agents have no impact on

nongonadal androgen synthesis (i.e., suppression of adrenocorticotropic hormone [ACTH] and, hence, adrenal androgen synthesis) (see Fig. 67.3). The adrenal glands can synthesize adequate levels of androgens to promote cancer growth. CYP17 is a key P450 enzyme in the androgen biosynthesis pathway that generates dehydroepiandrosterone (DHEA) and androstenedione in the adrenal glands. These weak androgens can be further converted into testosterone or alternative steroid substrates that are reduced to DHT.[22,12] This step is recognized as a particular bottleneck in androgen production. The specific inhibition of CYP17 decreases androgen synthesis, with less effect on the production of other essential steroids. Abiraterone acetate is a pregnenolone derivative that is a high-affinity, irreversible inhibitor of CYP17, and results in decreased adrenal androgen synthesis. At higher doses, this agent inhibits other DHT synthetic pathways such as 3β-hydroxysteroid dehydrogenase.[23]

Intratumoral androgens may be increased in CRPC.[24] Measurements of intratumoral androgens showed that CRPC tumors have more testosterone than primary tumors in untreated men.[25] Expression profiling studies comparing CRPC with primary tumors have shown that androgen synthesis enzymes are upregulated in CRPC.[26,27] Patient samples at all stages of disease contain an abundance of AKR1C3 and SRD5A1, which are necessary for the conversion of androstenedione to DHT. However, the samples lacked high expression of enzymes necessary for de novo steroidogenesis.[28] These data suggest that autocrine androgen synthesis may allow tumors to grow despite low serum androgen levels, but that this process may, in part, be dependent on adrenal precursors.

Targeting Androgen Receptor Activity: Antiandrogens

Antiandrogens compete with endogenous androgens for the ligand binding pocket of AR (see Fig. 67.3). Older agents promote translocation of AR from the cytoplasm into the nucleus and DNA binding, but induce conformational changes that prevent optimal transcriptional activity. In the United States, there have been

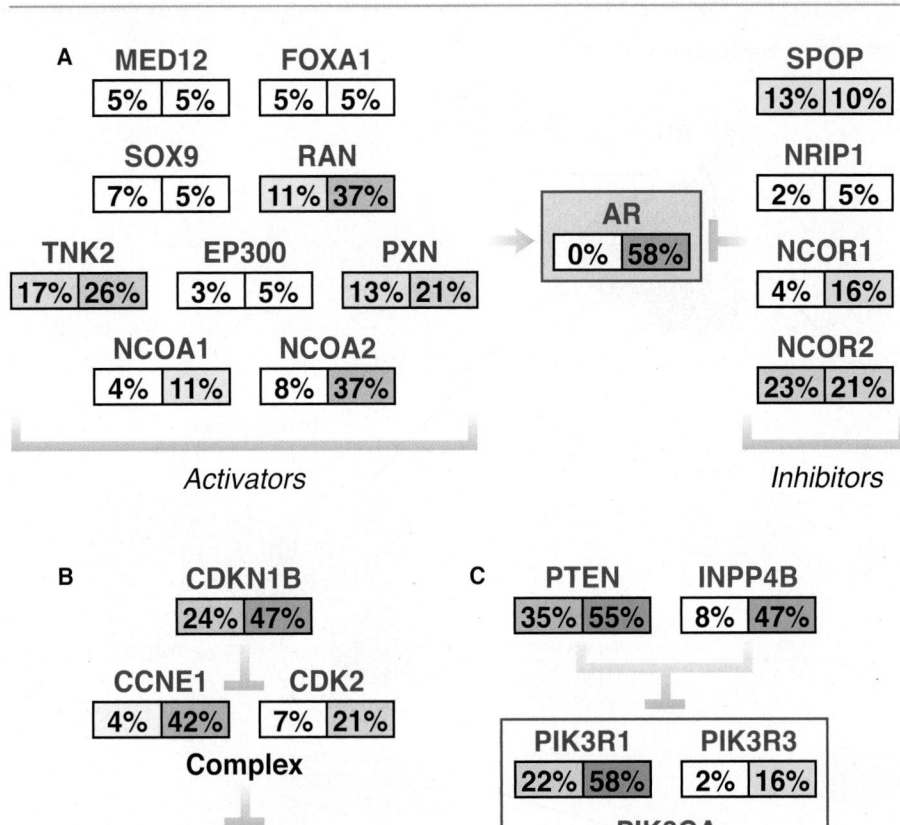

Figure 67.2 Alterations in common pathways dysregulated in prostate cancer. The androgen receptor *(AR)* **(A)**, retinoblastoma **(B)**, and phosphatidylinositol 3-kinase *(PI3K)* **(C)** pathways are altered in more than one-third of primary cancers and in the vast majority of metastatic lesions. This schematic depicts alteration frequencies for individual genes and for the entire pathway in primary and metastatic tumors. Alterations are defined as those having significant up- or downregulation compared with normal prostate samples, or by somatic mutations, and are interpreted as activation *(red)* or inactivation *(blue)* of protein function. (Figure adapted from the 9th edition of Devita, Hellman, and Rosenberg's *Cancer: Principles and Practice of Oncology*.)

three historic nonsteroidal antiandrogens (NSAA): flutamide, bicalutamide, and nilutamide. Each has been associated with an antiandrogen withdrawal effect, whereby treated patients experiencing disease progression on treatment derive clinical benefit when the antiandrogen is stopped.[29] Although this was initially believed to be related to AR mutation, later studies have shown this is due to AR activation by these NSAAs.[30,31]

Newer NSAAs have now been developed that lack agonist effects on the AR. Enzalutamide (MDV3100) was approved by the U.S. Food and Drug Administration (FDA) in 2012.[32] Other next-generation NSAAs are in development, including ARN-509.

Finally, new approaches are being taken to inhibit AR at the amino terminus.[33] As opposed to interrupting ligand binding, agents such as EPI-001 interfere with transcriptional activity of AR. These agents are still in early development, but appear very promising because they display activity even when the ligand-binding domain of AR has been altered.

Alterations in the Androgen Receptor During Prostate Cancer Progression

Prostate cancers eventually progress to a more lethal state: castration resistance. The time to development of resistance and the molecular pathways to CRPC differ from patient to patient. Progression of CRPC usually accompanied by the restoration of PSA secretion, indicating a reactivation of AR activity in these cases.[12]

Gene amplification and increased protein expression represent the most common mechanisms of means of reactivating AR signaling in the face of castration therapy. These changes allow cancer cells to respond to subphysiologic concentrations of androgen.[34] AR mutations are detected in up to 10% of CRPC cases and allow for activation by alternative ligands.[35] Overexpression of AR is seen in approximately 30% of cases of CRPC.[36] Alternative splicing of *AR* mRNA can lead to a truncated protein missing the ligand-binding domain. These increase in number in the face of many second-line NSAAs.[37,38] Some of these variants have constitutive transcriptional activity in the absence of androgens. Overexpression of these variants can confer castration resistance in preclinical models.[39] More recent studies show that these variants impact sensitivity to taxanes[40] and even next-generation antiandrogens such as enzalutamide.[41]

ADDITIONAL PATHWAYS FREQUENTLY ALTERED DURING DISEASE PROGRESSION

The Phosphatidylinositol 3-Phosphate Kinase (*PI3K*) Pathway

Progression to CRPC is characterized by gain of function in *AR* and activation of the phosphatidylinositol 3-phosphate kinase

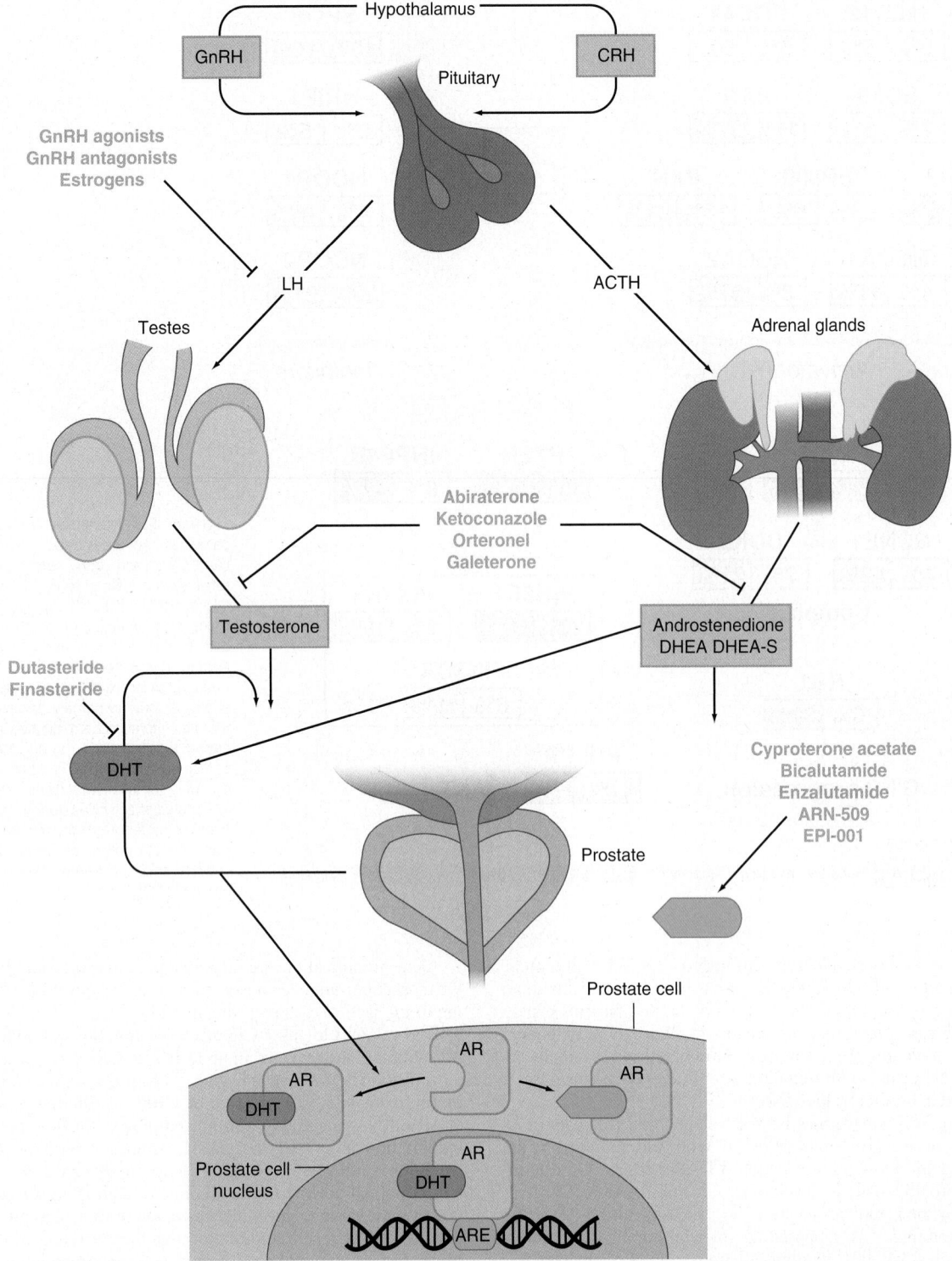

Figure 67.3 The androgen-signaling axis and its inhibitors. Testicular androgen synthesis is regulated by the gonadotropin-releasing hormone-luteinizing hormone (GnRH–LH) axis. Pharmacologic inhibitors are labeled in *red* at respective steps. GnRH-driven activity can be inhibited by both GnRH agonists and antagonists, as well as estrogens. Adrenal androgen synthesis is regulated by the corticotrophin-releasing hormone (CRH)–adrenocorticotropic hormone (ACTH) axis. CYP17 is a critical enzyme in androgen synthesis inhibited by abiraterone, orteronel, and galeterone. CYP17 inhibitors decrease synthesis of androgen from the adrenal glands, testes, and (in advanced disease) the tumors themselves. 5-Alpha reductase inhibitors prevent reduction of testosterone and other androgen intermediates to DHT. Antiandrogens such as enzalutamide and ARN-509 block activation of AR by inhibiting the binding of androgens to androgen receptors. DHEA-S, dehydroepiandrosterone sulfate; ARE, androgen-response element.

(PI3K) pathway. Cross-talk between these pathways has been proposed[42,43] because a loss of *PTEN* and subsequent PI3K activation is associated with repression of androgen responsive genes. Conversely, AR inhibition results in the upregulation of PI3K activity.[42,43] As such, combination therapy with PI3K and AR inhibition are currently being evaluated in clinical trials.

The PI3K signaling cascade is one of the most commonly altered pathways in human malignancy. *PTEN* is a tumor suppressor that deactivates PI3K signaling. *PTEN* deletions are present in nearly 30% of primary prostate cancers, and inactivating mutations of *PTEN* occur in another 5% to 10%; both are more common in advanced disease (see Fig 67.2).[3,5,7,44,45] Functional studies across multiple preclinical model systems of prostate cancer consistently reinforce the role of *PTEN* in suppressing tumorigenesis and prostate cancer progression.[46,47] Dysregulation of *PTEN* represents a poor prognostic factor. There is significant evidence that *PTEN* deletion is associated with higher stage, higher Gleason grade, and higher rates of progression, recurrence after therapy, and disease-specific mortality.[48,49]

Amplification and point mutations in *PIK3CA*, encoding a catalytic subunit of PI3K, also result in overactivation of the pathway and are enriched in metastatic versus localized prostate cancer (see Fig 67.2).[3,50] Activating *PIK3CA* lesions and inactivation of *PTEN* are usually mutually exclusive, supporting a similar endpoint in driving downstream signaling.

Recent studies have also identified the presence of rarer events that affect PI3K signaling. These lesions include the rearrangement of *MAGI2*, the deletion of *PHLPP1*, mutations in *GSK3B*, and point mutations and genomic deletions of *CDKN1B*.[3,4,44,47,51] Recurrent alterations in multiple nodes along the PI3K pathway emphasize its critical importance in the pathogenesis of prostate cancer and support the rationale for therapies targeting this pathway.

The Retinoblastoma Pathway

Another tumor suppressor pathway that is frequently inactivated in epithelial malignancies is the RB pathway (see Fig. 67.2). The p130 RB protein regulates cell cycle progression by binding to E2F family members and repressing E2F-mediated gene transcription. RB is inactivated via phosphorylation by cyclin-dependent kinases (CDK), resulting in E2F-mediated cell cycle progression.[52] The absence of RB signaling results in aberrant cell cycle progression and tumor proliferation.

Similar to *PTEN* deletion, the loss of *RB* is enriched in prostate cancer metastases compared to primary disease (see Fig. 67.2).[53] Within preclinical prostate cancer models, the inactivation of RB confers castration-resistant tumor growth via E2F1-mediated activation of AR gene transcription.[53] RB status is currently being explored as a stratification variable for treatment strategies on ongoing clinical trials.

E26 TRANSFORMATION SPECIFIC (ETS) GENE FUSIONS AND THE MOLECULAR SUBTYPES OF PROSTATE CANCER

E26 Transformation Specific (ETS) Gene Fusions

In addition to pathway-based analyses, prostate cancer can be defined by recurrent lesions of single genes. The most common molecular abnormality in prostate cancer is a gene fusion involving an ETS transcription factor.[8,9] These genetic rearrangements, found in approximately 50% of prostate cancers, occur when genes encoding an ETS transcription factor are translocated downstream of the regulatory, usually androgen-responsive, element of a second gene.[8,9,54] These fusions result in AR-driven overexpression of an ETS transcription factor, causing transcriptional dysregulation of downstream oncogenic pathways, increased invasion, and carcinogenesis in preclinical models of prostate cancer.[8,9,54,55] The most prevalent ETS gene rearrangement involves either chromosomal deletion or insertion of chromosome 21, resulting in fusion of the 5′ untranslated region of the androgen-regulated gene *TMPRSS2* with the ETS family member *ERG*. Over 90% of ETS rearrangements involve *ERG*, whereas the remaining ETS fusions include *ETV1* (chromosome 7), *ETV5* (chromosome 3), or *ETV4* (chromosome 17) as common 3′ partners (Fig. 67.4). Although *TMPRSS2* is the most common 5′ partner for *ERG*, over 10 androgen-regulated genes, including *SLC45A3* and *NDRG1*, have been identified as 5′ fusion partners in ETS rearrangements (see Fig. 67.4).

Several studies have investigated the prognostic value of ETS fusion status, with conflicting results likely stemming from the heterogeneity of study cohorts, screening practices, and management

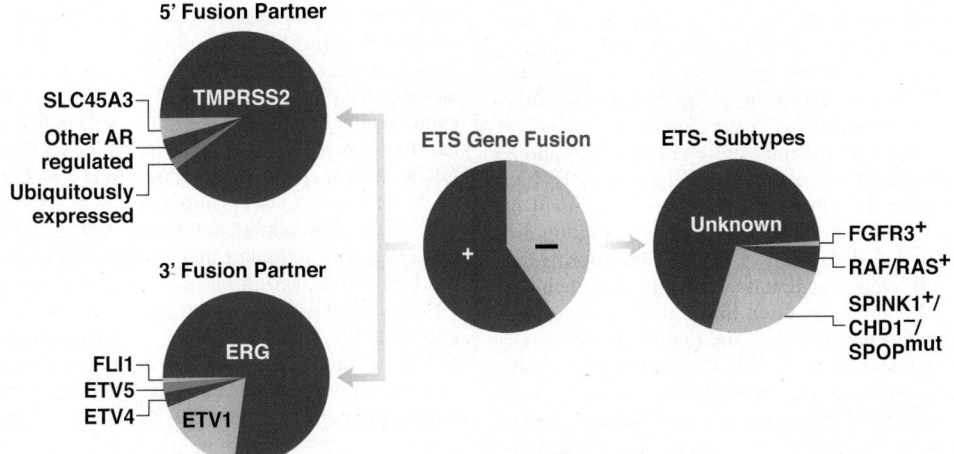

Figure 67.4 The molecular subtypes of prostate cancer subtypes. The approximate distribution of prostate cancer subtypes, as defined by driving molecular lesions, is presented for PSA-screened Caucasian populations. Approximately 50% to 60% of all prostate cancers harbor ETS gene fusions *(central pie chart)*. ETS gene fusions are nearly mutually exclusive with other alterations, such as *FGFR3* fusions, *RAF* fusions, *SPOP* mutations, *CHD1* deletions, and SPINK1 overexpression *(right pie chart)*. The predominant 5′ fusion partner in ETS fusions is the androgen-regulated promoter of the TMPRSS2 gene *(top left pie chart)*. The primary 3′ fusion partner is ERG, though other genes encoding ETS transcription factors, such as ETV1, ETV4, ETV5, and FLI1, are involved at lower frequencies *(bottom left pie chart)*.

strategies, as well as the variability in tumor sampling, disease multifocality, and measured clinical outcomes. In the context of non–PSA-screened populations managed conservatively, population-based studies have demonstrated a significant association between ETS fusion status and adverse clinicopathologic predictors, metastases, or disease-specific mortality.[56,57,58] However, in the context of patients treated with radical prostatectomy, the prognostic impact of ETS fusions is uncertain, with some studies demonstrating an association between ETS fusion status and features of aggressive prostate cancer, and other studies finding no such associations. The largest report, a prospective cohort study involving over 1,100 patients treated with radical prostatectomy, found that ETS related gene (ERG) rearrangement or overexpression was associated with tumor stage, but not recurrence or mortality.[59] Overall, ETS fusions are associated with poorer prognosis in population-based studies of watchful waiting cohorts, but are of uncertain prognostic value in radical prostatectomy patients.

The Molecular Subtypes of Prostate Cancer

Although the prognostic value of ETS fusions remains unclear, the molecular characterization of prostate cancer often begins with the determination of ETS fusion status, by either fluorescence in situ hybridization or immunohistochemical approaches. Transcriptomic, genomic, and epigenetic profiling studies have demonstrated that ETS fusion-positive prostate cancers are biologically distinct from ETS fusion-negative disease.[4,60] For example, certain lesions, such as deletions or mutations of the *PTEN* or *TP53* tumor suppressors, are significantly enriched in ETS-positive cancers.[4,44,61] Strikingly, other alterations, such as *RAF* fusions, *SPOP* mutations, *CHD1* deletions, and SPINK1 overexpression, occur exclusively in ETS-negative cancers,[3,5,62] (Fig. 67.4) providing evidence that these alterations define distinct biologic subsets of prostate cancer and may provide a framework for defining molecular subtypes of prostate cancer.[3,10,11] The potential subtypes are described in the following paragraphs.

Gene fusions and known activating mutations in *RAF* and *RAS* family members have also been identified in approximately 1% to 2% of all prostate cancers (see Fig. 67.4).[3,5,11] *RAF* encodes for a serine/threonine-specific protein kinase, and *RAS* encodes for a GTPase. *RAF-RAS*[+] tumors are exclusively negative for ETS fusions, *SPOP* mutations, *CHD1* deletions, and SPINK1 overexpression. Both RAF and RAS serve as signaling intermediates in the mitogen activated protein kinase (MAPK) pathway, and activation of RAF and RAS may enhance the transcriptional activity of the androgen receptor.[63] Of note, activating events in the *RAF/RAS/MAPK* pathway may be targetable by existing kinase inhibitors.

SPOP mutations represent the most prevalent point mutations in localized prostate cancer, occurring at a frequency of 10% to 15%.[3,4] *SPOP* codes for the substrate-recognition component of a Cullin3-based E3-ubiquitin ligase. Recurrent mutations are located exclusively within the region of *SPOP*, which forms the substrate-binding cleft, suggesting that they prevent substrate binding.[3,64] Previous studies have suggested that SPOP substrates include AR and its coactivator SRC-3,[65,66] and that *SPOP* mutations result in increased androgen signaling. *SPOP*-mutant prostate cancers have a distinct genomic profile; in addition to occurring only in ETS-negative cases, *SPOP* mutations are also mutually exclusive with *TP53* mutations/deletions, and generally lack PI3K pathway alterations. Additionally, *SPOP* mutations are significantly associated with deletions of the *CHD1* gene, which is a DNA binding protein that functions in remodeling chromatin states. Of note, cases with *CHD1* deletions are significantly enriched in the number of genomic rearrangements that they harbor, compared to other prostate cancers.[67,68] Thus, *SPOP* mutations and *CHD1* deletions appear to define a distinct ETS fusion–negative subtype of prostate cancer.

SPINK1 is a secreted protease that is overexpressed in approximately 10% of prostate cancers.[62] Although SPINK1 overexpression is present in only ETS fusion–negative cases, SPINK1 overexpression can co-occur with *SPOP* mutations and *CHD1* deletions, suggesting that multiple aberrations can define this subset of ETS-negative prostate cancer (see Fig. 67.4). SPINK1 interacts with epidermal growth factor receptor (EGFR) to mediate its neoplastic effects, suggesting that SPINK1-positive prostate cancers may be targeted via EGFR inhibition.[69]

Lastly, a recent study has identified a potential new subset of ETS-negative prostate cancers, defined by the presence of a fibroblast growth factor receptor (FGFR) fusion, in which the FGFR2 gene is translocated downstream of an androgen-regulated promoter, resulting in androgen-driven overexpression of FGFR2.[70] Although these FGFR fusions are rare, they have, to date, not been found to co-occur with the other subtypes described previously. In total, results described previously suggest the presence of molecular subtypes of prostate cancer, several of which are mutually exclusive and represent biologically distinct diseases. As the biology underlying these subtypes is elucidated and as therapeutic approaches are further investigated for each subtype, the hope is that physicians will eventually be able to utilize a simple molecular barcode (i.e., ETS/SPINK1/SPOP/CHD1/RAS-RAF/FGFR status) to better personalize therapy.

EMERGING AREAS IN PROSTATE CANCER BIOLOGY AND THERAPY

Our growing understanding of prostate cancer biology has opened a variety of potential therapeutic venues (Fig. 67.5) These opportunities range from kinase inhibition to immunotherapy, which impact both the tumor and microenvironment.

Kinase Targeting in Castration-Resistant Prostate Cancer

Multiple kinase signaling pathways beyond those listed previously have been implicated in CRPC. Examples of these pathways and targets include mesenchymal epithelial transition factor (MET) and the Src-family kinases (SFKs). MET is a transmembrane receptor tyrosine kinase activated by hepatocyte growth factor that plays a crucial role in the development of the normal prostate as well as in the progression of cancer. Activation of MET has been associated with increased proliferation, survival, motility, invasiveness, and angiogenesis in several tumor models, as well as clinical aggressiveness.[71,72] AR blockade also appears to promote the expression of MET.[73] These findings have led to a series of clinical studies exploring the utility of MET as a therapeutic target for CRPC with agents such as cabozantinib (see Fig. 67.5).

SFKs have also been implicated in the progression to CRPC. SRC, FYN, and Lck-Yes novel tyrosine kinase (LYN) have all been associated with prostate cancer progression.[74,75] In particular, SRC has been implicated as playing a role in tumorigenesis,[76] whereas FYN and LYN have been implicated in the progression of metastatic and castration-resistant disease.[74,77] Initial therapeutic trials with SFK inhibitors such as dasatinib have been difficult to interpret because the appropriate means of manipulating SFK biology in CRPC remain under investigation (see Fig. 67.5).

Targeting Chromatin Regulatory Pathways in Castration-Resistant Prostate Cancer

Recent studies have demonstrated that chromatin regulation and remodeling leads to disease progression across a wide range of human cancers. Overexpression of the Enhancer of Zest Homolog 2 (EZH2) gene, which encodes a histone methyltransferase,

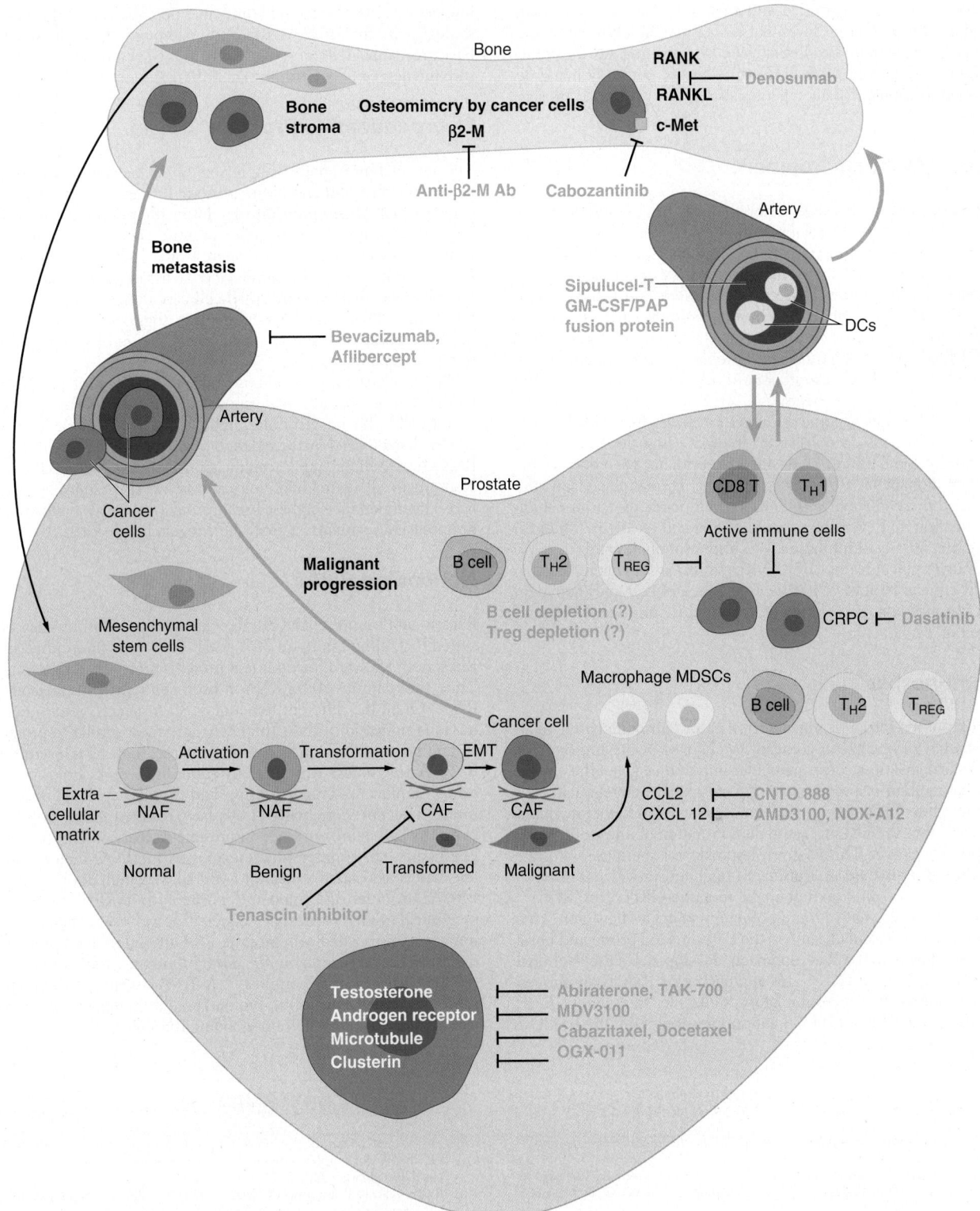

Figure 67.5 The tumor microenvironment (TME) and agents targeting the tumor–TME interaction. The TME is a complex biome of interactions between the prostate cancer tumor cell and various environmental components, including cancer-associated fibroblasts (CAF) and mesenchymal stem cells (MSC) in the local prostatic stroma, as well as bone stromal cells and MSCs in the metastatic TME in areas such as bone. The TME also includes neovasculature and the immune microenvironment. Inhibitors are shown in *red* at respective sites of action. Events in the TME that promote metastasis include osteomimicry by cancer cells, transformation of normal fibroblasts to protumorigenic/prometastatic CAFs, and alternations of endothelial cell function allowing for vascular invasion and hematogenous dissemination of tumor cells. β2-M, beta-2 microglobulin; DC, dendritic cells; EMT, epithelial-to-mesenchymal transition; NAF, normal fibroblast; RANKL, receptor-activated nuclear factor κB (Ligand); Treg, T-regulatory cells.

PRACTICE OF ONCOLOGY

is associated with aggressive and metastatic disease in prostate cancer.[78] Studies have shown that EZH2 may function via silencing gene expression, or alternatively, by activating AR and other transcription factors.[79,80] EZH2 inhibitors are currently being developed as a potential therapeutic strategy for advanced prostate cancer.

Tumor Microenvironment

It has become increasingly clear that the tumor microenvironment (TME) plays a crucial role in disease initiation and progression.[81–83] Reactive stroma, including fibroblasts, endothelial cells, osteoblasts, osteoclasts, and mesenchymal stem cells, have been associated with prostate cancer development and tumorigenesis (see Fig. 67.5).[84,85] Studies of human prostate cancers have revealed a loss of transforming growth factor beta type receptor 2 (TGFβRII) in cancer-associated fibroblasts. In a murine model, stromal TGFβRII knockout alone results in the development of spontaneous prostate cancers.[86]

The TME has become an target for newer therapies because host stromal cells do not exhibit the same high level of genetic instability as the tumor.[87] Considerable work has been done in the area of angiogenesis. A greater emphasis is now placed on stromal and mesenchymal cells and their influence on epithelial differentiation and even the prostate cancer cell of origin.[88,89] As an example, osteoclast inhibition with bisphosphonates and receptor-activated nuclear factor κB (RANKL) inhibitors has been shown to yield clinical benefit. With the emergence of therapies active on the immune microenvironment, this field is continues to expand (see Fig. 67.5).

Immunotherapy

Unlike other forms of anticancer therapy, immune-based treatments have the capacity to adapt to changes in the tumor. This biological advantage bears particular importance given the emerging recognition of progressive temporal-spatial heterogeneity and chromoplexy in cancer.[6,90] The dendritic cell–based therapy, sipuleucel-T, was the first successful demonstration of immunotherapy in prostate cancer. This relatively nontoxic treatment used prostate alkaline phosphatase as a primary target and provided a survival benefit for men with asymptomatic metastic CRPC (mCRPC).[91] A number of alternative immunotherapy strategies have gone into advanced development, such as the PSA-directed prime and boost vaccinia/fowlpox ProstVac approach developed by the National Cancer Institute (NCI).[92] This approach uses PSA as an antigen and employs three costimulatory molecule transgenes: *B7.1*, *ICAM-1*, and *LFA-3*. CTLA-4 and suppression of the PD-L1/PD-1

interaction have also been identified as potentially useful immune strategies in metastatic CRPC.[93,94] Although these approaches have great appeal, there remains an absence of biomarkers to measure the degree of benefit that such therapies may provide.

Neuroendocrine Prostate Cancer

The use of more potent suppressors of AR activation has raised concerns over neuroendocrine prostate cancer. There is growing concern that AR suppression may foster the development of this particularly aggressive subtype of prostate cancer. The approach to these cancers has been hampered by a lack of consensus on nomenclature. The term *neuroendocrine* has been used to describe those cancers that are pure small-cell carcinomas to those clearly differentiated with biochemical features suggesting some level of neuroendocrine differentiation (e.g., expression of synaptophysin or chromogranin A).

Small-cell carcinoma composes only 0.5% to 2% of all primary tumors.[95] This is a pathologic diagnosis histologically marked by small round cells with no glandular architecture. Molecularly, this disease is characterized by the deletion of *RB1*,[96] increased MET and RANKL activation,[97] and amplification of *AURKA* and *MYCN*.[98] Non–small-cell neuroendocrine cancers are also clinically identified. The importance of these findings and their impact on therapeutic approaches remains an area where research is needed.

Noncoding RNAs

Recent data from the ENCODE sequencing consortium has suggested that, although up to 70% of the genome is transcribed into RNA, only 1.5% of the genome represents protein-coding genes.[99] Thus, the majority of the RNA in each cell represents *noncoding* RNAs. Of all the different noncoding RNA species, genes encoding long noncoding RNAs (lncRNAs) are most similar to protein-coding genes, based on common features, such as transcription by RNA polymerase II, polyadenylation, the presence of multiple exons, similar splicing patterns, and similar epigenetic signatures.[100] Recent sequencing efforts have resulted in the discovery of lncRNAs that are enriched in prostate cancer compared to normal tissue. These differentially expressed lncRNAs include prostate cancer associated transcript 1 (PCAT-1), which downregulates BRCA2 to confer *BRCAness* and sensitivity to PARP1 inhibitors in preclinical models of prostate cancer,[101] as well as second chromosome locus associated with prostate 1 (SChLAP1), which promotes metastases by antagonizing the Switch/Sucrose NonFermentable (SWI-SNF) epigenetic complex.[102] As RNA targeting strategies improve, it is likely that future biomarker and therapeutic strategies will begin to focus on these noncoding RNA elements.

SELECTED REFERENCES

The full reference list can be accessed at lwwhealthlibrary.com/oncology.

3. Barbieri CE, Baca SC, Lawrence MS, et al. Exome sequencing identifies recurrent SPOP, FOXA1 and MED12 mutations in prostate cancer. *Nat Genet* 2012;44:685–689.

4. Berger MF, Lawrence MS, Demichelis F, et al. The genomic complexity of primary human prostate cancer. *Nature* 2011;470:214–220.

5. Grasso CS, Wu YM, Robinson DR, et al. The mutational landscape of lethal castration-resistant prostate cancer. *Nature* 2012;487:239–243.

6. Baca SC, Prandi D, Lawrence MS, et al. Punctuated evolution of prostate cancer genomes. *Cell* 2013;153:666–677.

8. Tomlins SA, Rhodes DR, Perner S, et al. Recurrent fusion of TMPRSS2 and ETS transcription factor genes in prostate cancer. *Science* 2005;310:644–648.

11. Palanisamy N, Ateeq B, Kalyana-Sundaram S, et al. Rearrangements of the RAF kinase pathway in prostate cancer, gastric cancer and melanoma. *Nat Med* 2010;16:793–798.

12. Feldman BJ, Feldman D. The development of androgen-independent prostate cancer. *Nat Rev Cancer* 2001;1:34–45.

14. Abate-Shen C, Shen MM, Gelmann E. Integrating differentiation and cancer: the Nkx3.1 homeobox gene in prostate organogenesis and carcinogenesis. *Differentiation* 2008;76:717–727.

16. Bhatia-Gaur R, Donjacour AA, Sciavolino PJ, et al. Roles for Nkx3.1 in prostate development and cancer. *Genes Dev* 1999;13:966–977.

17. Bova GS, Carter BS, Bussemakers MJ, et al. Homozygous deletion and frequent allelic loss of chromosome 8p22 loci in human prostate cancer. *Cancer Res* 1993;53:3869–3873.

20. Augello MA, Hickey TE, Knudsen KE. FOXA1: master of steroid receptor function in cancer. *Embo J* 2011;30:3885–3894.

21. Nelson WG, De Marzo AM, Isaacs WB. Prostate cancer. *N Engl J Med* 2003;349:366–381.

22. Chang KH, Li R, Papari-Zareei M, et al. Dihydrotestosterone synthesis bypasses testosterone to drive castration-resistant prostate cancer. *Proc Natl Acad Sci U S A* 2011;108:13728–13733.

23. Li R, Evaul K, Sharma KK, et al. Abiraterone inhibits 3beta-hydroxysteroid dehydrogenase: a rationale for increasing drug exposure in castration-resistant prostate cancer. *Clin Cancer Res* 2012;18:3571–3579.

24. Mostaghel EA, Page ST, Lin DW, et al. Intraprostatic androgens and androgen-regulated gene expression persist after testosterone suppression: therapeutic implications for castration-resistant prostate cancer. *Cancer Res* 2007;67:5033–5041.

25. Montgomery RB, Mostaghel EA, Vessella R, et al. Maintenance of intratumoral androgens in metastatic prostate cancer: a mechanism for castration-resistant tumor growth. *Cancer Res* 2008;68:4447–4454.

27. Stanbrough M, Bubley GJ, Ross K, et al. Increased expression of genes converting adrenal androgens to testosterone in androgen-independent prostate cancer. *Cancer Res* 2006;66:2815–2825.

30. Tran C, Ouk S, Clegg NJ, et al. Development of a second-generation antiandrogen for treatment of advanced prostate cancer. *Science* 2009;324:787–790.

31. Chen CD, Welsbie DS, Tran C, et al. Molecular determinants of resistance to antiandrogen therapy. *Nat Med* 2004;10:33–39.

32. Scher HI, Fizazi K, Saad F, et al. Increased survival with enzalutamide in prostate cancer after chemotherapy. *N Engl J Med* 2012;367:1187–1197.

36. Linja MJ, Savinainen KJ, Saramaki OR, et al. Amplification and overexpression of androgen receptor gene in hormone-refractory prostate cancer. *Cancer Res* 2001;61:3550–3555.

38. Yuan X, Cai C, Chen S, et al. Androgen receptor functions in castration-resistant prostate cancer and mechanisms of resistance to new agents targeting the androgen axis. *Oncogene* 2014;33:2815–2825.

39. Dehm SM, Schmidt LJ, Heemers HV, et al. Splicing of a novel androgen receptor exon generates a constitutively active androgen receptor that mediates prostate cancer therapy resistance. *Cancer Res* 2008;68:5469–5477.

42. Carver BS, Chapinski C, Wongvipat J, et al. Reciprocal feedback regulation of PI3K and androgen receptor signaling in PTEN-deficient prostate cancer. *Cancer Cell* 2011;19:575–586.

43. Mulholland DJ, Tran LM, Li Y, et al. Cell autonomous role of PTEN in regulating castration-resistant prostate cancer growth. *Cancer Cell* 2011;19: 792–804.

44. Taylor BS, Schultz N, Hieronymus H, et al. Integrative genomic profiling of human prostate cancer. *Cancer Cell* 2010;18:11–22.

46. Carver BS, Tran J, Gopalan A, et al. Aberrant ERG expression cooperates with loss of PTEN to promote cancer progression in the prostate. *Nat Genet* 2009;41:619–624.

48. McMenamin ME, Soung P, Perera S, et al. Loss of PTEN expression in paraffin-embedded primary prostate cancer correlates with high Gleason score and advanced stage. *Cancer Res* 1999;59:4291–4296.

53. Sharma A, Yeow WS, Ertel A, et al. The retinoblastoma tumor suppressor controls androgen signaling and human prostate cancer progression. *J Clin Invest* 2010;120:4478–4492.

54. Tomlins SA, Laxman B, Dhanasekaran SM, et al. Distinct classes of chromosomal rearrangements create oncogenic ETS gene fusions in prostate cancer. *Nature* 2007;448:595–599.

57. Demichelis F, Fall K, Perner S, et al. TMPRSS2:ERG gene fusion associated with lethal prostate cancer in a watchful waiting cohort. *Oncogene* 2007;26: 4596–4599.

59. Pettersson A, Graff RE, Bauer SR, et al. The TMPRSS2:ERG rearrangement, ERG expression, and prostate cancer outcomes: a cohort study and meta-analysis. *Cancer Epidemiol Biomarkers Prev* 2012;21:1497–1509.

61. Demichelis F, Setlur SR, Beroukhim R, et al. Distinct genomic aberrations associated with ERG rearranged prostate cancer. *Genes Chromosomes Cancer* 2009;48:366–380.

62. Tomlins SA, Rhodes DR, Yu J, et al. The role of SPINK1 in ETS rearrangement-negative prostate cancers. *Cancer Cell* 2008;13:519–528.

66. An J, Wang C, Deng Y, et al. Destruction of full-length androgen receptor by wild-type SPOP, but not prostate-cancer-associated mutants. *Cell Rep* 2014;6:657–669.

68. Liu W, Lindberg J, Sui G, et al. Identification of novel CHD1-associated collaborative alterations of genomic structure and functional assessment of CHD1 in prostate cancer. *Oncogene* 2012;31:3939–3948.

70. Wu YM, Su F, Kalyana-Sundaram S, et al. Identification of targetable FGFR gene fusions in diverse cancers. *Cancer Discov* 2013;3:636–647.

71. Knudsen BS, Gmyrek GA, Inra J, et al. High expression of the Met receptor in prostate cancer metastasis to bone. *Urology* 2002;60:1113–1117.

74. Jensen AR, David SY, Liao C, et al. Fyn is downstream of the HGF/MET signaling axis and affects cellular shape and tropism in PC3 cells. *Clin Cancer Res* 2011;17:3112–3122.

75. Varkaris A, Katsiampoura AD, Araujo JC, et al. Src signaling pathways in prostate cancer. *Cancer Metastasis Rev* 2014;33(2–3):595–606.

76. Cai H, Smith DA, Memarzadeh S, et al. Differential transformation capacity of Src family kinases during the initiation of prostate cancer. *Proc Natl Acad Sci U S A* 2011;108:6579–6584.

78. Varambally S, Dhanasekaran SM, Zhou M, et al. The polycomb group protein EZH2 is involved in progression of prostate cancer. *Nature* 2002; 419:624–629.

79. Xu K, Wu ZJ, Groner AC, et al. EZH2 oncogenic activity in castration-resistant prostate cancer cells is Polycomb-independent. *Science* 2012;338: 1465–1469.

82. Kiskowski MA, Jackson RS 2nd, Banerjee J, et al. Role for stromal heterogeneity in prostate tumorigenesis. *Cancer Res* 2011;71:3459–3470.

86. Bhowmick NA, Chytil A, Plieth D, et al. TGF-beta signaling in fibroblasts modulates the oncogenic potential of adjacent epithelia. *Science* 2004; 303:848–851.

90. Gerlinger M, Rowan AJ, Horswell S, et al. Intratumor heterogeneity and branched evolution revealed by multiregion sequencing. *N Engl J Med* 2012; 366:883–892.

91. Kantoff PW, Higano CS, Shore ND, et al. Sipuleucel-T immunotherapy for castration-resistant prostate cancer. *N Engl J Med* 2010;363:411–422.

92. Kantoff PW, Schuetz TJ, Blumenstein BA, et al. Overall survival analysis of a phase II randomized controlled trial of a Poxviral-based PSA-targeted immunotherapy in metastatic castration-resistant prostate cancer. *J Clin Oncol* 2010;28:1099–1105.

94. Kwek SS, Cha E, Fong L. Unmasking the immune recognition of prostate cancer with CTLA4 blockade. *Nat Rev Cancer* 2012;12:289–297.

98. Beltran H, Rickman DS, Park K, et al. Molecular characterization of neuroendocrine prostate cancer and identification of new drug targets. *Cancer Discov* 2011;1:487–495.

102. Prensner JR, Iyer MK, Sahu A, et al. The long noncoding RNA SChLAP1 promotes aggressive prostate cancer and antagonizes the SWI/SNF complex. *Nat Genet* 2013;45:1392–1398.

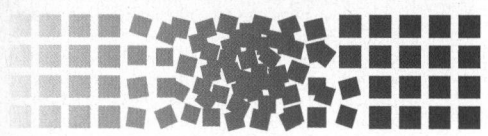

68 Cancer of the Prostate

Howard I. Scher, Peter T. Scardino, and Michael J. Zelefsky

INTRODUCTION

The approach to prostate cancer diagnosis and treatment has changed dramatically across the spectrum of the illness. Recognizing the need to reduce overdiagnosis and overtreatment of clinically insignificant cancers, new diagnostic algorithms have become available to identify which men have a higher likelihood of having a clinically significant cancer and benefit from early detection and early treatment. New clinical and biologic biomarkers are being validated to determine, once localized prostate cancer is diagnosed, which tumors can be optimally treated using an active surveillance (AS) approach that closely monitors the cancer—based on the likelihood that the tumor will or has metastasized, putting the patient at risk for an impaired quality of life (QOL) and a shortened life expectancy. The techniques of surgery have evolved and more patients are being treated with robot-assisted approaches with the aims of reducing morbidity and shortening hospital stays without compromising cancer control. The ability to deliver higher doses of radiation safely has improved disease control rates without compromising long-term QOL. The past 4 years have also seen unparalleled progress in the treatment of castration-resistant metastatic tumors, as five agents with different mechanisms of action were proven to prolong life. At the same time that more patients and physicians recognize there are effective treatments for metastatic disease, these agents are also being tested earlier in minimal disease settings where they have the potential to provide even greater benefit.

In contrast to other tumor types, the paradigm of early detection leading to increased cure rates must be cautiously applied to prostate cancer. The widespread use of prostate-specific antigen (PSA)-based detection strategies has resulted, unfortunately, in increased treatment of clinically insignificant cancers, to the point where the morbidity and mortality associated with making a diagnosis and the therapy utilized to treat it can exceed that of the cancer itself. The high prevalence of prostate cancer in the general population, coupled with a natural history that can range from a few years to decades, mandates a different framework than that provided by the more traditional tumor, node, and metastasis (TNM) staging. There are also many prostate cancers from which a relapse after primary treatment does not require any intervention because the probability is low that the cancer will become metastatic, symptomatic, or lethal.

Many of these issues are addressed by describing the spectrum of the disease as a series of clinical states, ranging from prediagnosis to the lethal metastatic castration-resistant phenotype (Fig. 68.1).[1] Each state represents a milestone in the disease that is easily recognizable by patients and physicians, enabling them to define therapeutic objectives based on the manifestations present at a particular point in time or the likelihood that specific disease manifestations might occur in the future. The utility of specific diagnostic tests needed to maximally inform a treatment decision for a specific context of use at a particular point in time is considered analogously; in short, how the performance and the result of the test guide management. This chapter will refer throughout to this clinical states model.

INCIDENCE AND ETIOLOGY

Incidence and Mortality

In 2014, some 233,000 men in the United States are expected to be diagnosed with prostate cancer and 29,480 to die of the disease,[2] accounting for 14% of all new cancers in men and women[3] and 11% of male cancer deaths.[4] Over the past decade, men in the United States had a 15.4% chance of being diagnosed with prostate cancer and a 2.7% chance of dying of it.[2] Worldwide, there were an estimated 899,100 new cases and 258,100 deaths from prostate cancer in 2008.[5] Histologic cancers, found in the prostate at autopsy in men who die of other causes, are even more common, and their age-adjusted frequency varies relatively little from country to country, about 2.4-fold.[6] In contrast, the mortality rate from prostate cancer varies by 10.8-fold among different countries, suggesting different mechanisms of carcinogenesis and progression, and supporting the concept of distinct "indolent" and "aggressive" forms of the disease.[6–8] There are significant age, ethnic, racial, geographic, and familial differences in incidence and mortality rates.[9]

Risk Factors

Age

Clinically detected prostate cancer is rare before age 40, but then the incidence increases with age faster than that of any other cancer, and continues to rise through the ninth decade of life. Histologic evidence of invasive cancer can be found in the prostates of men as early as the third decade of life, and its prevalence increases dramatically with age to reach 50% to 60% by age 90. As life expectancy increases throughout the world, morbidity and mortality from prostate cancer will impose increasing burdens in developing countries.[5]

Family History and Genetic Susceptibility

A family history of prostate cancer increases the risk that a man will develop the disease. The level of risk when a family member is affected is similar in breast and prostate cancers. Men with a first-degree relative with prostate cancer have a 2- to 3-fold increased risk, and those with two or more first-degree relatives affected have a 5- to 11-fold increased risk compared with the general population.[10] Nevertheless, familial factors have been thought to play a role in only 11% of prostate cancers, although studies of twins suggest that inherited factors may be involved in as many as 42% of all cases.[11] While over 70 risk alleles (single nucleotide polymorphisms [SNP]) have been associated with prostate cancer in genome-wide association studies, few are associated with the risk of aggressive or lethal cancer. Many such SNPs are in genes that code for PSA or related kallikreins, blood levels of which are widely used for diagnosis.[12] For these SNPs, the increased risk is for a diagnosis of prostate cancer, not metastases or death from the disease. Several high-penetrance mutated genes have been identified, such

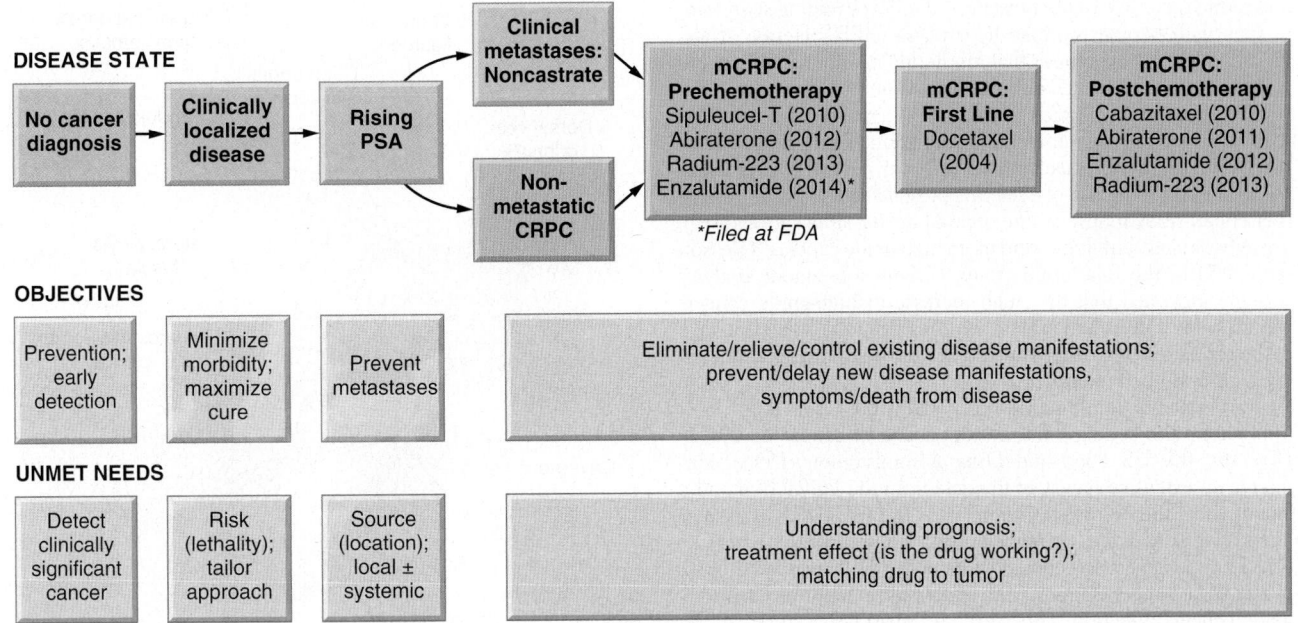

Figure 68.1 Clinical states model of prostate cancer progression. *Green boxes* indicate castration-resistant prostate cancer (CRPC) and *blue* indicate noncastrate disease. PSA, prostate-specific antigen; mCA RPC, metastatic castration-resistant prostate cancer. (Modified from Scher HI, Heller G. Clinical states in prostate cancer: towards a dynamic model of disease progression. *Urology* 2000;55:323–327.)

as HOX13B, which are more common in patients with early-onset and familial disease, but this variant is rare (occurring in 0.1% of the population) and it is not associated with the lethal form of the disease.[13] In contrast, men who carry BRCA2 mutations are more likely to develop early-onset prostate cancer, which is more likely to be aggressive and lethal.[14]

Race and Ethnicity

The incidence and frequency of diagnosed clinical cancers are similar in most Western countries, with the highest age-adjusted mortality rates in Scandinavia and significantly lower rates in non-Western countries. Both genetic susceptibility and exposure to causative environmental factors contribute to these variations.

Men of African ancestry in the United States and Caribbean have the highest incidence of prostate cancer in the world, with striking differences in incidence (1.8-fold) and mortality (2.4-fold) relative to American men of European descent. African American men are diagnosed at a younger age and have higher tumor burdens within each stage category,[15] a two-fold higher frequency of metastatic disease at presentation,[16] and lower survival rates.[17] Incidence and mortality rates are significantly lower for Americans of Asian descent and somewhat lower for those of Hispanic descent.

Environmental factors also affect mortality risk.[7] Asians who immigrate to the United States have a higher incidence of and mortality from the disease than in their countries of origin, which increases with each succeeding generation, but remains below the rates in men of African or European descent.[18]

Other Risk Factors

Diet, Supplements, and Lifestyle Factors. The increased incidence and mortality from prostate cancer evident in immigrants moving from low- to high-risk countries supports an important role for environmental in addition to genetic risk factors. Many epidemiologic studies support an association between high fat intake and breast, colon, and prostate cancer incidence and mortality.[19,20] Adult obesity has been associated with aggressive prostate cancer, adverse outcomes after therapy, and increased mortality.[11,21,22] The risk of death from prostate cancer has been reported to increase

15% to 20% for each 5 kg/m² increase in body mass index (BMI).[23] Among men diagnosed with prostate cancer, the risk of death from the disease is significantly associated with increased BMI (1.5-fold for overweight men and 2.7-fold for obese men).[24] Physical activity may reduce the risk of mortality from prostate cancer; the data are inconsistent for development of the disease, but convincing once the diagnosis has been established.[25] Smoking has not been shown to alter incidence rates, but it may be associated with the risk of prostate cancer death, especially when assessed in men after diagnosis.[25]

Despite many indications that certain micronutrients, minerals, and vitamins have a protective effect on the development of prostate cancer or mortality from the disease, firm evidence is sparse. In the large Selenium and Vitamin E Cancer Prevention Trial (SELECT), vitamin E and selenium, alone or in combination, failed to reduce the incidence of prostate cancer. In fact, men who took vitamin E alone may have had a greater risk of the disease,[26] although there is some suggestion that aggressive, potentially lethal cancer may be reduced among smokers taking vitamin E supplements.[27] There is no evidence that ingestion of calcium or administration of vitamin D affects incidence or mortality from prostate cancer. Diets rich in tomato-based products, which contain high amounts of carotenoids and lycopene, may reduce the risk of advanced prostate cancer.[28,29]

Alcohol use, blood group, body hair distribution, sexual activity, urban versus rural residence, and vasectomy do not affect risk.[30] There are no data supporting a viral origin of prostate cancer.[31]

Prevention

While the evidence is incomplete and there are no large intervention trials addressing the role of diet and exercise in preventing prostate cancer, it is reasonable to recommend a low-fat diet, regular exercise, and maintenance of a normal BMI as likely having a modest effect in reducing the risk of developing prostate cancer. More evidence suggests there may be some benefit for such lifestyle changes after the diagnosis of prostate cancer is established.[11,21,22]

Finasteride, a competitive inhibitor of type II 5α-reductase (5αRI) that blocks the conversion of testosterone to dihydrotestosterone (DHT) within prostatic cells, is a safe and effective drug that reduces the size of the prostate and relieves voiding symptoms in men with benign prostatic hyperplasia (BPH). Hence, it was logical to test the hypothesis that finasteride, or other 5αRIs, could prevent prostate cancer. The Prostate Cancer Prevention Trial (PCPT) randomly assigned 18,882 men, age 55 years or older, who had a normal digital rectal examination (DRE) and PSA, to receive finasteride or placebo over a 7-year period.[32] Finasteride reduced by 25% the risk of detecting prostate cancer on biopsy (either end-of-study biopsy or one ordered during study "for cause"). Toxicity was low, but there were more high-grade cancers (Gleason score ≥7) in the finasteride group.[33] Many subsequent analyses strongly suggested that the small increase in high-grade cancers was probably a detection artifact resulting from the 20% shrinkage of the prostate by the drug,[34] and there were no differences in long-term survival in either arm.[35]

In a separate randomized trial (REDUCE), the dual 5αRI dutasteride also reduced the detection rate of cancer by 23%.[36] However, the US Food and Drug Administration (FDA) conducted an extensive review of the data from the PCPT trial and a reanalysis of the biopsy specimens from the REDUCE trial after Gleason grades were reassigned using contemporary criteria.[37] The FDA reviewers agreed that while both 5αRIs reduced the risk of a prostate cancer diagnosis, the effect was seen only among low-grade cancers (Gleason score ≤6), and there was a small (0.5%) but significant absolute increase in the risk of the highest-grade cancers (Gleason score 8 to 10). The FDA concluded that the tradeoff for using a 5αRI in healthy, asymptomatic men would be the occurrence of one additional high-grade cancer for every three or four low-grade cancers (of uncertain clinical potential) prevented, and recommended against the approval of these drugs for chemoprevention of prostate cancer.[34]

Other agents, such as statins, metformin, and resveratrol, may have protective effects,[38] but to demonstrate their benefit will require studies focusing on populations at high risk of developing clinically significant cancers.[38] PSA levels at midlife hold great promise for identifying men most likely to benefit from aggressive prevention strategies (see "Prostate-Specific Antigen: A Powerful Tool For Risk Stratification").

ANATOMY AND PATHOLOGY

The prostate is an exocrine organ weighing 20 g to 25 g, which consists of lobular tubuloalveolar glands that secrete fluid through ducts that empty into the prostatic urethra. The fluid comprises

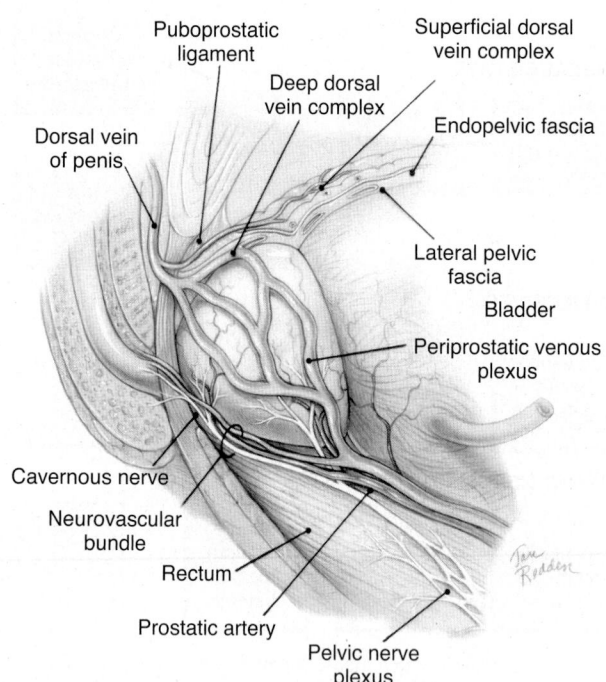

Figure 68.2 Lateral view of normal anatomy of the pelvis. (Redrawn from Ohori M, Scardino PT. Localized prostate cancer. *Curr Probl Surg* 2002;39: 833–957.)

the bulk of seminal emissions and is rich in PSA. The prostate is located deep in the pelvis between the bladder and the external urinary sphincter, anterior to the rectum and below the pubis (Fig. 68.2).[39] The cavernous nerves, which control blood flow to the penis and hence erectile function, run from the pelvic plexus lateral to the rectum along the posterolateral prostate and external urinary sphincter to enter the corpora cavernosa. Because the prostate is located at this critical anatomic juncture, cancers of the prostate and the treatment of these cancers place urinary, sexual, and bowel function at risk.

The prostate has three anatomic zones and an anterior fibromuscular stroma (Fig. 68.3). The central zone surrounds the ejaculatory

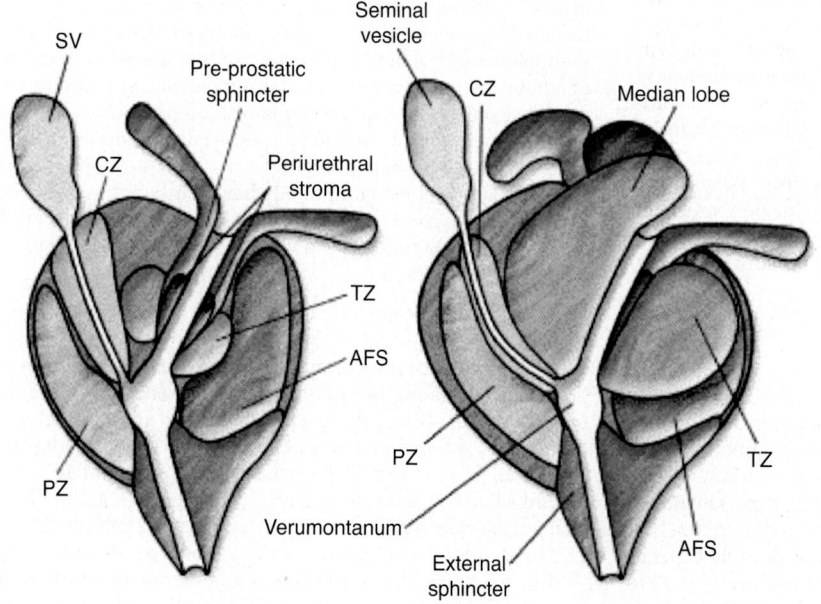

Figure 68.3 Zonal anatomy of the prostate. **(A)** Young male with minimal transition zone hypertrophy. Note that preprostatic sphincter and periejaculatory duct zone (central zone of McLean) are clearly defined. **(B)** Older male with transition zone hypertrophy, which effaces the preprostatic sphincter and compresses the periejaculatory duct zone. SV, seminal vesicle; CZ, central zone; PZ, peripheral zone; TZ, transition zone; AFS, anterior fibromuscular stroma. (From McLaughlin PW, Troyer S, Berri S, et al. Functional anatomy of the prostate: implications for treatment planning. *Int J Radiat Oncol Biol Phys* 2005;63:479, with permission.)

ducts, the transition zone surrounds the urethra, and the peripheral zone makes up the bulk of the normal gland. The posterior peripheral zone lies against the rectum and is the area that is palpable by DRE. These zonal boundaries are indistinct in the prostate of a normal postpubescent male, but as men age the transition zone enlarges from nonmalignant growth (BPH). The frequency of malignancy in the different zones is disproportionate to the glandular tissue present. Very few cancers originate in the central zone, and only 15% originate in the transition zone; most originate in the peripheral zone.

Patterns of Spread

Localized prostate cancer is typically multifocal, in 85% of patients. Most cancers arise near the capsule in the peripheral zone; the surrounding capsule is invaded early and frequently, in up to 80% of cancers detected clinically. Local extension occurs through the capsule (termed "focal" or "established" extracapsular extension [ECE], depending on extent, when observed in a radical prostatectomy [RP] specimen), but may also extend through defects in the capsule where the neurovascular structures and ejaculatory ducts enter the gland, or in the region of the bladder neck. Local invasion can progress to involve the seminal vesicles or the bladder, or to invade the levator muscles. Rarely does tumor invade through Denonvilliers' fascia to reach the rectal wall. Lymphatic dissemination can involve the hypogastric, obturator, external iliac, presacral, common iliac, or retroperitoneal nodes, with no consistent sentinel landing zone. Hematogenous spread most commonly involves the bones of the axial skeleton and, less commonly, the lung, liver, and other soft tissue organs. The predilection for bone seems to result from a unique bidirectional interaction between tumor cells and the marrow stroma.

Histopathology

Two main growth-related diseases develop in the prostate: BPH, which affects both the epithelial and mesenchymal components, and cancer.[40] There is no direct etiologic relationship between BPH and cancer; they are related only by their close anatomic site of origin and high incidence in men over 40 years of age. More than 95% of malignant tumors of the prostate are adenocarcinomas that arise in acinar and proximal ductal epithelium. Grossly, carcinoma appears as pale yellow or gray flecks of tissue coalesced into a firm, poorly defined mass that is difficult to distinguish from surrounding normal tissue. Adenocarcinomas are often multifocal, heterogeneous, and follow a papillary, cribriform, comedo, or acinar pattern. Immunohistochemistry may assist the diagnosis when atypical areas, suspicious for carcinoma, are present in a biopsy sample, particularly in the differentiation of high-grade prostatic intraepithelial neoplasia (PIN) and atypical adenomatous hyperplasias from low-grade carcinoma. A hallmark of prostate cancer is the loss of basal cells, highlighted by negative staining for basal cell markers (high molecular weight/basal-specific cytokeratin) and p63, and positive staining for alpha-methyl-CoA racemase, which is upregulated in cancer.[41]

Pathogenesis

Prostate cancers develop from the accumulation of genetic alterations that result in an increase in cell proliferation relative to cell death, arrest differentiation, and confer the ability to invade, metastasize, and proliferate in a distant site. Histologic changes can be found in the prostates of men in their 20s, yet the diagnosis is typically made three to four decades later, which suggests that the development of the disease is a multistep process resulting from a variety of genetic and epigenetic alterations.[42] The accumulation of changes acting synergistically seems to be more critical than the order in which the alterations occur. Identifying and understanding the events has implications for control of the disease at the earliest stages of transformation, for progression to an invasive tumor, for prognostication, and for points of therapeutic attack. Men who are castrated or who become hypopituitary before the age of 40 rarely develop prostate cancer.[43] The evolution of the tumor is heavily influenced by hormonal factors; it is also influenced by environmental, infectious/inflammatory factors, and given the long history once the diagnosis is established, the response to specific treatments.

Premalignant Lesions

The phenotypic alterations that occur during prostate carcinogenesis and progression are shown in Figure 68.4. The earliest precursor lesion is the subject of debate, as is the cell type that

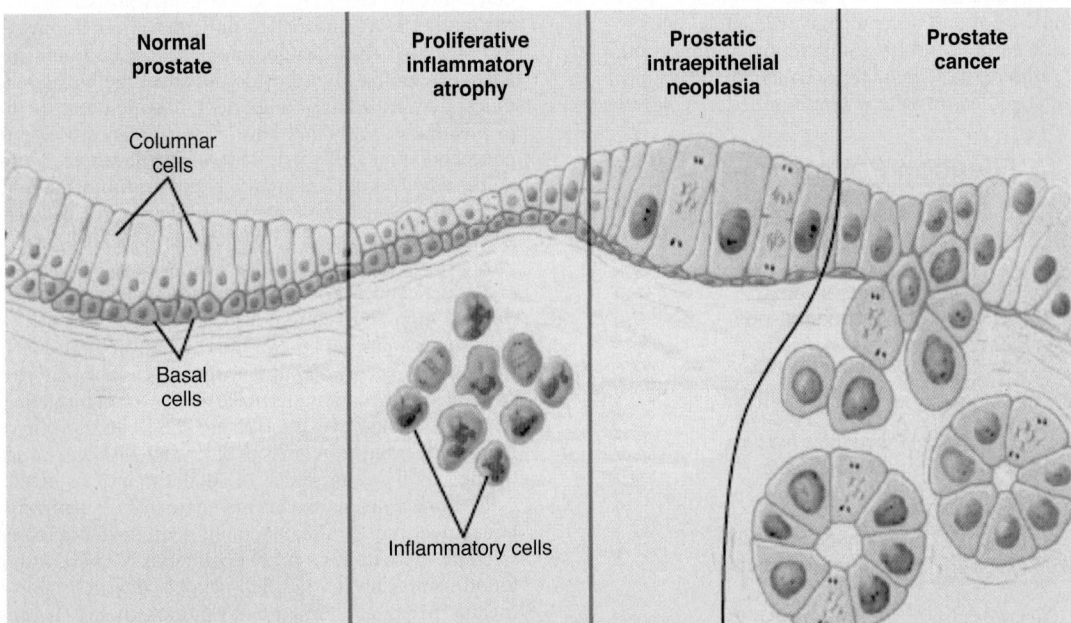

Figure 68.4 Proliferative inflammatory atrophy is hypothesized to be a precursor to prostatic intraepithelial neoplasia, which in turn is the precursor of prostate cancer. (From Nelson WG, De Marzo AM, Isaacs WB. Prostate cancer. *N Engl J Med* 2003;349:366, with permission.)

is actually transformed. Recognizable changes begin with proliferation of cells within glands, termed PIN, often found adjacent to areas of proliferative inflammatory atrophy.[44] PIN is defined by the presence of cytologically atypical or dysplastic epithelial cells within architecturally benign-appearing acini, and is subdivided into low- and high-grade. Only high-grade PIN is considered a precursor for some invasive carcinomas.[45,46] Because high-grade PIN develops preferentially in the peripheral zone where most cancers originate, it precedes the development of cancer by 10 years or more,[47] and prostates with extensive high-grade PIN tend to have multifocal tumors. With subsequent loss of the basal cell layer surrounding prostatic glands and the development of anaplastic cellular morphology with nuclear pleomorphism and prominent nuclei, the tumor invades the basement membrane, spreads locally, and begins to metastasize. Not all lesions progress to invasive prostatic cancer during the lifetime of the host. Foci of small atypical acini that display some but not all features diagnostic of adenocarcinoma are referred to as atypical small acinar proliferation, a significant predictor of invasive cancer on subsequent prostate biopsy.[48,49] Atypical adenomatous hyperplasia, on the other hand, is not considered a malignant precursor lesion.

Gleason Grade

For adenocarcinomas, the degree of differentiation has prognostic significance and pathologists judge biopsy specimens using the Gleason grading system, which assesses the architectural details of malignant glands under low to medium magnification.[50–52] Cytologic features under high magnification are not considered.[53,54] Five distinct patterns of growth from well- to poorly differentiated were originally described by Gleason using a scale from 1 to 5 (Fig. 68.5). Pattern 1 tumors were considered the most differentiated with discrete glandular formation, while pattern 5 lesions were the most undifferentiated with strands of disorganized, free-floating cells and complete loss of the glandular architecture. Prostate cancers tend to be heterogeneous, with two or three patterns occurring within a typical prostate. So the final Gleason *score* is the sum of the grades of the primary (largest) and secondary patterns, ranging from 2 (1 + 1) to 10 (5 + 5).

The prognostic importance of Gleason's scoring system has been difficult to improve on, but the system has been modified several times, most recently by a consensus of expert pathologists, to reflect current data and best practices.[55,56] In biopsy specimens, patterns 1 and 2 are almost never recognized, so Gleason 3 + 3 = 6 cancers are the earliest, most well-differentiated tumors currently reported by pathologists. Careful reassessment of the histologic criteria for assigning Gleason pattern 3 has resulted in reclassification

of many grade 3 cancers as grade 4, and some grade 4 variants are now considered grade 3. As a result, there has been "grade inflation" over the last decade, and the prognosis for both Gleason 3 + 3/well-differentiated cancers and for 3 + 4/moderately differentiated cancers is better than in historical series.

If three Gleason patterns are seen within a single biopsy, the accepted approach is to designate the largest area as the primary grade and the highest grade as the secondary grade to arrive at a score. So a biopsy with a large area of pattern 3, a smaller area of pattern 4, and an even smaller area of pattern 5 would be designated 3 + 5 = 8. Multiple cores are typically taken during each biopsy session, and the Gleason score assigned to the patient is the score of the highest single core. In contemporary biopsy series, 25% to 50% of tumors are low-grade (Gleason 3 + 3 = 6 or less), 40% to 70% are intermediate grade (Gleason 3 + 4 or 4 + 3 = 7), and 5% to 10% are high grade (Gleason 8 to 10).[55]

The Gleason grading system is also used to assign grade in RP specimens, with some modifications. When the pathologist inspects all areas of cancer within the prostate, it is not unusual to identify more than two Gleason patterns.[57] The original system ignored patterns that represented <5% of the cancer, but the presence of a small amount of high-grade tumor has subsequently been shown to worsen prognosis. The current recommendation is to report a tertiary grade (i.e., 3 + 4 = 7 with tertiary 5).[40] Transition zone cancers tend to have lower Gleason grades than peripheral zone cancers of comparable size, and they are less likely to extend to the seminal vesicles or lymph nodes (LN).[58] Despite its apparent complexity, the Gleason grading system has proven reliable and reproducible, it is strongly associated with prognosis, and it is accepted worldwide.

Other Histologic Types

Although other tumors and histologic variants of adenocarcinoma rarely develop within the prostate, the most notable include ductal carcinomas (now considered a variant of poorly differentiated adenocarcinoma), small cell or neuroendocrine tumors, and transitional cell carcinomas. Pure ductal carcinomas comprise <1% of prostate cancers, but ductal elements are present in ~5%. These tumors are biologically similar to high-grade prostate adenocarcinomas, are clinically aggressive, and are associated with lower PSA levels than comparable adenocarcinomas.[59] Small cell or neuroendocrine tumors of the prostate typically comprise small, round, undifferentiated cells.[60] Distinguishing these tumors from lymphomas or round cell sarcomas can be difficult without immunohistochemical analysis.[40] Neuroendocrine cells can be found in almost all adenocarcinomas, but they do not affect the biology of the tumor unless they are a large component, in which case the tumors tend to metastasize early and have a poor prognosis. The presence of neuroendocrine cells may raise serum levels of neuroendocrine markers such as chromogranin-A, and the tumors should be treated with immediate chemotherapy as well as androgen ablation (androgen deprivation therapy [ADT]). Transitional cell carcinoma of the prostate is most frequently associated with and may be an extension of bladder cancer. When found in isolation, as a primary tumor on prostate biopsy without an associated bladder cancer, transitional cell carcinoma may be confined to periurethral ducts, but often invades stroma. Treatment may require cystoprostatectomy. Malignant mesenchymal tumors make up <0.3% of prostatic neoplasms, of which rhabdomyosarcomas are most common in younger patients and leiomyosarcomas in older patients. Carcinosarcomas are defined by the coexistence of adenocarcinomas of the epithelial cells, along with malignant mesenchymal elements that have differentiated into identifiable chondrosarcoma, osteosarcoma, myosarcoma, liposarcoma, or angiosarcoma.[61] These tumors may be found in previously irradiated patients and are highly resistant to therapy. Metastatic tumors to the prostate include lymphomas, leukemias, adenocarcinomas of the lung, melanoma, seminoma, and malignant rhabdoid tumors, whereas tumors of the bladder and colon may sometimes involve the gland by direct extension.

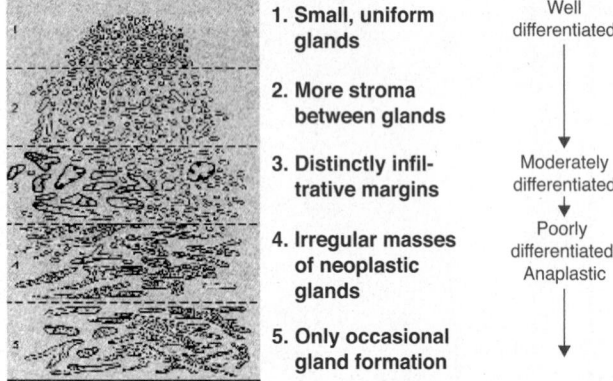

Gleason Pattern

1. Small, uniform glands — Well differentiated
2. More stroma between glands
3. Distinctly infiltrative margins — Moderately differentiated
4. Irregular masses of neoplastic glands — Poorly differentiated/Anaplastic
5. Only occasional gland formation

Figure 68.5 Gleason histologic grading of prostate cancer demonstrating progressive loss of glandular formation with increasing score. (Adapted from Gleason DF. Histologic grade, clinical stage, and patient age in prostate cancer. *NCI Monogr* 1988:15.)

SCREENING

Screening and Early Detection

The clinical states model (see Fig. 68.1) can also be applied to men without a cancer diagnosis by considering an individual's need for screening or other diagnostic tests designed to detect cancer on the likelihood that he already has or will develop a clinically significant prostate cancer. Operationally, a "clinically significant" cancer can be defined as one that, left untreated, would lead to symptoms, metastases, or a premature death from cancer—but for each individual, these risks must be balanced against his competing risks of noncancer-related morbidity and mortality, and the risk of suffering harm from overtreatment or unnecessary treatment.

PSA level and DRE are commonly used for screening and early detection, although both are limited by low specificity: only one-quarter of men with an abnormal DRE or a PSA level >3 ng/ml are found to have cancer on biopsy.[62,63]

Prostate-Specific Antigen: A Powerful Tool for Risk Stratification

PSA is a 28 kDa protein of the kallikrein family, a group of serine proteases whose genes are found on chromosome 19q13. PSA is abundant in seminal fluid, at concentrations up to 3 mg/ml, a million times higher than in serum.[64] The enzymatic activity of PSA induces liquefaction of seminal fluid and the release of mobile spermatozoa. PSA is synthesized in the ductal and acinar epithelium and is secreted into the lumina of the prostate gland. PSA is organ-specific but not cancer-specific; normal prostatic tissue (and BPH) produces more PSA per gram than cancer, and well-differentiated cancer produces more PSA than poorly differentiated cancer.[65] Under pathologic conditions, PSA is thought to reach the circulation through the disrupted epithelial basement membranes. Circulating levels of PSA are inherently variable, fluctuating spontaneously by 15% from year to year.[66] When cancer is present, each gram of tumor raises the serum PSA level above background by approximately 3 ng/ml, whereas each gram of BPH contributes an average of only 0.3 ng/ml. Thus, there is considerable overlap in values between patients with cancer and those with benign conditions such as BPH and prostatitis. Acute urinary retention, urethral catheterization, urinary tract infection, and prostatic manipulation by needle biopsy, or transurethral resection of the prostate (TURP) may raise serum PSA levels dramatically. Performance of DRE does not.

A commonly used threshold for a normal PSA level in adult men is 4.0 ng/ml. But there is no "normal" level; the risk of cancer rises directly with PSA levels as a continuum.[67] PSA levels in healthy men vary with age. The population median PSA at age 45 to 50 is 0.6 ng/ml (interquartile range, 0.4 to 1.0), at age 60 the median is 1.1 (interquartile range, 0.6 to 2.0), and at age 70, 1.6 (interquartile range, 0.9 to 2.6).[68–70]

PSA levels at midlife predict with remarkable accuracy the risk that a man will develop advanced prostate cancer or die of the disease.[68,70,71] For example, in the Malmö Preventive Medicine cohort of 60-year-old men followed to age 85, stored blood samples from 1981 were retrieved and analyzed for PSA. Ninety percent of deaths from prostate cancer were in men in the top quartile of PSA levels (>2 ng/ml). In contrast, the risk of death from prostate cancer was only 0.2% by age 85 for those with a PSA below median (<1.1 ng/ml) at age 60.[70] PSA levels in men as young as 44 to 50 years were also prognostic, with 81% of advanced cancers diagnosed within 30 years occurring in men with PSA levels above the median (0.65 ng/ml).[68]

In fact, PSA levels at midlife are more informative than family history or ethnicity (Table 68.1), and can be used to stratify the intensity of screening over the next two to three decades of life, an approach that could substantially reduce false-positive test results without delaying detection of potentially lethal cancers.[17,72]

TABLE 68.1

Proportion of Prostate Cancer Deaths in Men Defined as at High Risk by Family History, Race, or Prostate-Specific Antigen in Middle Age

Risk Factor (scenario)	% High Risk/ % Death	Risk Group Size/ No. Risk Group Deaths
Prostate-specific antigen	10/44	4.4
Family history	10/14	1.4
African American	12.6/28	2.2

Adapted from Vertosick EA, Poon BY, Vickers AJ. Relative value of race, family history and prostate-specific antigen as indications for early initiation of prostate cancer screening. *J Urol* 2014 [Epub ahead of print], with permission.

Prostate-Specific Antigen for Screening

Although PSA has proved to be a valuable test for early detection, prognosis, and monitoring the response to therapy, its use for population-based screening for prostate cancer remains controversial. The widespread adoption of PSA testing in the United States shifted the stage at diagnosis away from metastases in 20% of patients in the 1980s to 5% in the 1990s, with a corresponding increase in frequency of early-state cancers that are potentially curable with surgery or radiation. Over the last two decades, the age-adjusted mortality rate for prostate cancer in the United States has declined by 42% from its peak in 1992, a more rapid decline than in any other country.[2] In the largest randomized trials, PSA screening reduced the risk of dying from prostate cancer by 21% to 44% (29% to 56% among men actually screened).[71,73] With long-term follow-up, the number needed to screen to prevent one prostate cancer death declined from 1,410 at 9 years to 293 at 14 years, and is estimated in models to be 98 over the lifetimes of men screened at ages 55 to 69.[63,71,74] The number of men who need to be diagnosed or treated (40% were managed expectantly on AS) was estimated to be 48 at 9 years, but falls to 12 at 14 years and 5 over the lifetime of men screened.[63,71,74] These numbers compare favorably with other screening programs. With mammography screening from age 50 to 70, 111 to 235 women need to be screened and 10 to 14 diagnosed to avert one death from breast cancer.[75–77] For colorectal cancer screening, 850 need to be screened with flexible sigmoidoscopy to prevent one colorectal cancer death.[78]

Nevertheless, PSA has low specificity: three of four men who have a biopsy for a PSA >3 ng/ml are not found to have cancer,[63] and 10% to 56% of those in whom cancer is found would probably have lived out their lives with no symptoms from the disease, and are therefore considered "overdetected."[79] An additional consideration is that the prostate biopsy itself carries a risk of bleeding and infection in 3% to 4% of those undergoing the procedure, which increases with the number of cores obtained. In cases where "saturation" biopsies are performed, in which upwards of 24 to 30 cores are sampled in the same session, the risk is higher and mortalities have resulted. Most cancers detected have been treated immediately with radical surgery or radiation,[80] with substantial risk of adverse effects on bowel, urinary, and sexual function.

In screening large populations, the lack of specificity of PSA leads to overdiagnosis, the discovery of incidental, clinically insignificant cancers that pose little or no immediate threat to life or health,[81] which often leads to overtreatment with accompanying morbidities that may be permanent and compromise QOL. With rare exceptions, low-risk cancers managed expectantly, as well as intermediate-risk cancers in older men, have a good prognosis when carefully observed on an "AS" protocol, rather than proceeding to immediate treatment.[82–86] AS is treatment that is designed to detect changes in the cancer that indicate it has become more aggressive and therefore requires more definitive intervention(s).

But most men with low-risk prostate cancer are treated, especially in the United States,[80] with all the attendant risks of bothersome side effects and altered QOL. These findings led the US Preventive Services Task Force (USPSTF) to conclude that "there is moderate or high certainty that this service has no net benefit or that the harms outweigh the benefits" (grade D recommendation).[87] Rather than screening all men or no men, a risk-adapted approach is clearly preferable (see "Clinical States Model").

Screening Trials

Two large, prospective randomized trials of screening for prostate cancer have been published, with conflicting results.[79,88] Both studies were recently updated.[89,90] The European Randomized Study of Screening for Prostate Cancer (ERSPC) compared screening with PSA every 2 to 4 years to no screening in a core group of 162,243 men age 55 to 69 years in seven European countries. At a median of 9 years, prostate cancer was diagnosed more often in the screened (8.2%) than in the control (4.8%) group (relative risk [RR] = 1.63), while the risk of dying of prostate cancer was reduced by 20% (RR = 0.80; p = 0.04). The number of men needed to be screened to prevent one death from prostate cancer was 1,410 (1,068 among those actually screened), comparable to the data for breast cancer and colorectal cancer screening.[75–78] However, the number needed to diagnose to prevent one death

was high, 48, probably because the full impact of prostate cancer on mortality was not manifest within 9 years, and because some of the cancers detected were indolent. With further follow-up, the reduction in prostate cancer mortality at a median of 11 years was 21% in the screening arm (p <0.0001), and 29% among those actually screened. The number needed to be screened fell to 1,055 and the number needed to diagnose to 37.

The Göteborg randomized population-based prostate cancer screening trial was planned and initiated independently of the ERSPC in 1995, although the investigators subsequently agreed to include a subset of participants in the ERSPC. In Göteborg, 20,000 men ages 50 to 64 were randomly assigned to be screened with PSA every 2 years up to age 69, or to a control group with no screening. After a median of 14 years, cancer was detected in 12.7% of the screened group and 8.2% of the controls (RR = 1.64), and the risk of death from prostate cancer was reduced by 44% (RR = 0.56; p <0.002) in the screening group (56% among the 76% who were actually screened at least once, RR = 0.44) (Fig. 68.6). At 14 years, the number needed to be screened fell to 293, while the number needed to diagnose to prevent one death from prostate cancer was only 12. (Forty percent of the men diagnosed with cancer were monitored expectantly and not treated.)[74]

In contrast, screening with PSA and DRE in a US cohort did not reduce mortality from prostate cancer.[88,89] The Prostate, Lung, Colorectal and Ovarian Cancer (PLCO) Screening Trial enrolled 76,685 men ages 55 to 74 in a prospective randomized trial from 1993–2001, comparing annual PSA for 6 years and DRE for 4 years

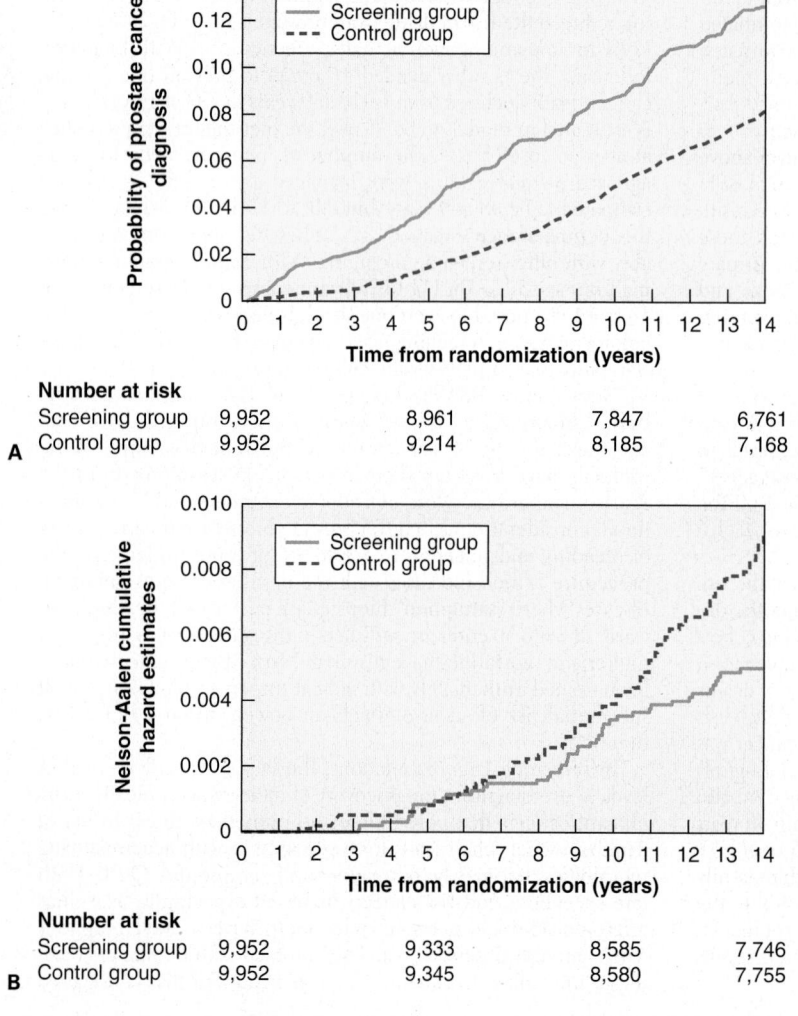

Figure 68.6 (A) Cumulative incidence of prostate cancer in the screening group and in the control group. **(B)** Cumulative risk of death from prostate cancer using Nelson-Aalen cumulative hazard estimates. (From Hugosson J, Carlsson S, Aus G, et al. Mortality results from the Goteborg randomised population-based prostate-cancer screening trial. *Lancet Oncol* 2010;11:725–732, with permission.)

with opportunistic screening. At the most recent (13-year) follow-up, the cancer detection rate was slightly higher (RR = 1.12) in the screened arm, but there was no difference in the risk of dying of prostate cancer.

The difference in outcomes of the US and European trials largely stems from the very different contexts in which the trials were conducted. The American trial was initiated in the 1990s, when PSA screening had already become widespread in the United States. In fact, 44% of the PLCO study subjects had had at least one PSA test before randomization, which would have excluded many men with potentially lethal cancers. The mortality rate from prostate cancer in both arms of the PLCO trial (1.7 and 2 per 10,000 person-years in the control and screened arms) was much lower than in the ERSPC (3.9 and 3.2, respectively), suggesting a heavily prescreened population. Many men (45% to 85%) in the PLCO control arm had at least one PSA test after randomization, compared with <20% in the ERSPC control arm, further diluting the potential for a difference between the arms.

Screening Recommendations

The USPSTF's recent recommendation against screening[87,91] has been understandably criticized as based on a one-time analysis of a rapidly changing field.[92] The USPSTF justifiably raised concerns about the high level of overdetection and overtreatment inherent in PSA screening, which can lead to the immediate risks of harm from invasive prostate biopsies and subsequent radical therapy when cancer is found. But the potential harms from PSA screening can be greatly reduced by risk-adjusting screening so that it focuses on men at high risk of otherwise dying of prostate cancer; incorporating into screening newer, more specific biomarkers; and avoiding radical treatment of low-risk cancers.[93] In a recently published computer simulation model of PSA screening, prostate cancer mortality was reduced by 28% over the lifetime of men screened annually from ages 55 to 69. Over the lifetime of this population of 1,000 men, only 98 men would need to be screened and five cancers detected (three treated and two managed expectantly) to prevent one death from prostate cancer.[94]

In response to the changes in the USPSTF recommendations, a number of professional organizations have revised their guidelines for prostate cancer screening. The American Society of Clinical Oncology recommends that men with a life expectancy >10 years have a discussion with their physician about whether screening for prostate cancer is appropriate, including a clear statement that screening may save lives but is associated with harms, including complications from unnecessary biopsies, surgery, or radiation treatments. Men with a shorter life expectancy should not be screened.[95] The American Urological Association recommends that men ages 55 to 69 years engage in shared decision making with their physicians and proceed based on each man's values and preferences. For men younger than 55 years at higher risk (e.g., African American men, or those with a positive family history), the decision about screening should be individualized.[96]

The American Cancer Society recommends that men have an opportunity to make an informed decision with their health-care providers about whether to be screened. This decision should be made after the patients have received information about the uncertainties, risks, and potential benefits of screening; men should not be screened unless they have received this information. The American Cancer Society further recommends that discussion about screening should take place at age 50 for men who are at average risk of prostate cancer and are expected to live at least 10 more years, and at age 45 for men at high risk of developing prostate cancer (e.g., African American men and those with a first-degree relative diagnosed with prostate cancer at an early age [<65 years]). This discussion should occur at age 40 for men at even higher risk, that is, those with more than one first-degree relative who had prostate cancer at an early age.[97]

DIAGNOSIS, RISK ASSESSMENT, AND STATE ASSIGNMENT

Signs and Symptoms

The most common symptoms arising from the prostate in men over 40 years are bladder outlet obstruction, including hesitancy; nocturia; incomplete emptying; and a diminished urinary stream. The occurrence of these symptoms, although more commonly related to BPH, should prompt a careful DRE and a PSA determination. The acute development of pelvic or perineal pain, erectile dysfunction, or hematuria should prompt further evaluation of the prostate. Today, men rarely present with symptoms of metastatic disease such as bone pain, pathologic fracture, anemia, or pancytopenia from bone marrow replacement, or disseminated intravascular coagulation.

Digital Rectal Examination

The physical examination should focus on a thorough DRE of the prostate, although palpable nodes can sometimes be detected in the inguinal or supraclavicular areas. Special attention should be paid to detect areas of induration within the prostate, extension through the capsule, or involvement of the seminal vesicles. If there is bladder outlet obstruction, the bladder may be palpable. Although not uniformly accurate or reproducible, DRE results are associated with pathologic stage and prognosis, and are the principal basis for assigning the clinical T stage of the cancer.[98]

Prostate-Specific Antigen and Related Biomarkers

PSA levels are best considered as a continuum: the higher the level, the greater the likelihood that any cancer, or high-grade cancer, will be found on biopsy. The most commonly used threshold for recommending a biopsy is 3 ng/ml.[72] A level this high is found in only 5% to 10% of men age 45 to 69 years. As PSA levels vary,[66] a rise in PSA to a newly "elevated" level should be verified 2 to 3 months later, after the patient has been evaluated by a medical history, DRE, and appropriate laboratory tests to exclude causes other than cancer for the "rise." The likelihood of finding cancer is about 15% to 20% in men with a normal DRE and a PSA level between 2.5 to 4 ng/ml. Among men with a PSA level of 4 to 10 ng/ml, 20% to 30% will have cancer. If the PSA level is >10 ng/ml, 60% of men will have cancer on biopsy. Many of these cancers will be low risk and can be managed conservatively without radical therapy.

Higher circulating PSA levels prior to treatment are associated with larger, more extensive cancers, although there may be a wide range of levels within any clinical T, N, or M category.[99,100] Although poorly differentiated cancers produce less PSA per gram than well-differentiated cancers, higher PSA levels indicate a more extensive cancer and a poorer prognosis across all Gleason scores. Rare, highly aggressive, poorly differentiated cancers are found in men with low PSA levels (<2 ng/ml), but patients with these cancers usually present with rapidly progressive voiding symptoms and palpably abnormal DRE.

PSA levels rise with age because of age-related increases in prostate volume due to BPH. Adjusting the upper limit of normal for age, PSA should be <2.5 ng/ml for men age 40 to 49 years, <3.5 for men aged 50 to 59, <4.5 for men aged 60 to 69, and <6.5 for men aged 70 to 79.[101] The utility of *age-specific PSA levels* has been challenged in screening trials because sensitivity is lost for a small increase in specificity in older men.[102]

PSA levels can also be adjusted for the volume of the prostate gland. *PSA density* (PSAD) is the ratio of PSA to gland volume, measured in ng/ml per cm³.[103] As more PSA is released into the serum by cancer (3 ng/g) than by BPH (0.3 ng/g),[104] PSAD can help to discriminate cancer from BPH. Because DRE correlates poorly with gland volume, an imaging study (transrectal ultrasound [TRUS] or magnetic resonance imaging [MRI]) is required to measure PSAD accurately, so PSAD is generally useful only in men who have had an ultrasound during a biopsy. PSAD has proved to be more valuable in prognosis than in detection, where it has been largely replaced by the *free/total PSA ratio*. The percent-free PSA in serum is higher in men with BPH than in men with cancer and can be used to discriminate cancer from BPH. Percent-free PSA values <10% are more indicative of cancer in men with values in the 4 to 10 ng/ml range.[62,105]

PSA levels rise more rapidly over time in men with cancer than in those without cancer, even within the normal range.[106] The rate of change, termed *PSA velocity*, may indicate the presence of cancer, but normal biologic variations in PSA levels over time create many more false positives and lessen the accuracy of the calculated results.[107] Once a man's PSA level is known, PSA velocity contributes no additional information to predict the presence of a cancer,[107] except in the rare case of an unusually aggressive, high-grade cancer that produces little PSA.

Panels of Kallikrein Markers

The major limitation of PSA for screening and early detection of prostate cancer is the high proportion of false-positive tests: 70% to 80% of men with a PSA >3 ng/ml and a normal DRE do not have cancer on biopsy. The specificity of PSA testing can be increased substantially at any given level of sensitivity by incorporating additional kallikreins into a panel of markers. There are two commercially available panels: the 4Kscore test (OPKO Lab, Nashville, TN) and the *phi* (Prostate Health Index; Beckman Coulter, Brea, CA). To baseline measurements of PSA and free-PSA levels the 4Kscore adds "intact" PSA and hK2, and the *phi* adds -2(pro) PSA.[108–111] All three of these kallikreins are elevated in cancer, relative to BPH. Both the 4Kscore and *phi* panels increase specificity, reducing the indication for biopsy among men with an elevated PSA level. In published studies, the number of biopsies was reduced by 40% to 50% while missing few high-grade cancers. The 4Kscore preserves sensitivity for high-grade (Gleason ≥7) cancer while reducing the number of negative biopsies and biopsies finding only low-grade (Gleason ≤6), small-volume cancer.[110,111]

Urinary Molecular Biomarkers

Prostatic fluid may contain shed cells from prostate cancer that can be recognized by measuring the level of RNA for prostate cancer antigen-3 (PCA-3) relative to that for PSA in urinary sediment using reverse transcription–polymerase chain reaction technology. Urinary PCA-3 has been approved by the FDA to determine the likelihood of cancer in men with an elevated PSA level and a previously negative biopsy,[112] but is also useful in comparable men with no previous biopsy to avoid unnecessary biopsies. The test requires collection of urine after a prostatic massage by DRE, and the levels of PCA-3 do not reflect the volume, grade, and extent of cancer,[113] limiting its clinical utility, especially when the goal is to avoid biopsy in men with only low-risk cancers. Other urinary assays for molecular markers are being explored, including one for the TMPRSS fusion gene, which may be more prognostic than PCA-3.[113]

Biopsy

Because prostate cancer is rarely curable when it causes symptoms, and rises in incidence with age, detection has focused on evaluating asymptomatic men between the ages of 50 and 70. The principal indications for biopsy are either an abnormal DRE or, more commonly, an elevated PSA level. Any palpable induration

TABLE 68.2

Probability of a Positive Prostate Biopsy Based on the Results of the Digital Rectal Examination and Serum Prostate-Specific Antigen Level

DRE Status (%)	PSA (ng/ml)			
	0–2	2–4	4–10	>10
DRE−	1	15	25	>50
DRE+	5	20	45	>75

PSA, prostate-specific antigen; DRE, digital rectal examination; DRE−, normal findings on the digital rectal examination; DRE+, findings on digital rectal examination suspicious for prostate cancer.
Modified from Thompson IM, Pauler DK, Goodman PJ, et al. Prevalence of prostate cancer among men with a prostate-specific antigen level < or = 4.0 ng per milliliter. *N Engl J Med* 2004;350:2239–2246; Catalona W, Richie J, deKernion JB, et al. Comparison of prostate specific antigen concentration versus prostate specific antigen density in the early detection of prostate cancer. *J Urol* 1994;152:2031–2036.

should be evaluated further, but only about a third of men with an abnormal DRE prove to have prostate cancer. Similarly, a normal DRE does not exclude the presence of cancer. The likelihood that cancer will be found on biopsy depends on the results of the DRE and PSA test (Table 68.2).[67,114]

The diagnosis of prostate cancer is typically established by TRUS-guided transrectal needle biopsy. TRUS is most useful for identifying the regions within the prostate for needle biopsy and for determining prostate volume; it is not used routinely for screening. When cancers are seen on TRUS, they are typically hypoechoic relative to normal prostate tissue, but the sensitivity of detection is low and MRI has proven to be more accurate and is the preferred imaging modality for identifying suspicious lesions for TRUS-guided biopsies within the prostate.

A needle biopsy of the prostate is usually performed transrectally with an 18-gauge needle mounted on a spring-loaded gun directed by ultrasound. Any palpable abnormality on DRE should be targeted for biopsy using finger guidance. In addition, abnormal areas visible on TRUS or MRI should be sampled, along with a total of at least 10 systematic biopsies of the prostate taken from the left and right apex, middle, and base of the peripheral zone. Each core or group of cores from a single region should be identified separately as to location and orientation so that the pathologist can report the extent and grade of cancer in each region and the presence of any perineural invasion or extraprostatic extension. Higher Gleason scores are strongly associated with larger tumor volume, extension outside the prostate, probability of metastases, and duration of response to therapy.[115,116] Biopsy results are used not only to assign a Gleason score to the cancer, but also to assess the volume and extent of the cancer by determining the number and percent of cores involved by cancer,[117,118] the amount of cancer in each core, and the total length of cancer in all cores. Each of these features adds important additional staging and prognostic information.[119–122]

Because patient selection for AS is critically dependent on the results of the prostate biopsy, some investigators have suggested more extensive biopsy strategies to better assess the true extent of cancer within the prostate. Transperineal "mapping" biopsies use a brachytherapy template, with needle cores taken at 5 mm to 10 mm intervals throughout the gland.[123] These template biopsies more accurately reflect the grade and extent of cancer. One study collected a median of 46 individual cores and found bilateral cancer in 55% of patients and an increased Gleason score in 23%. However, the risk of acute urinary retention, hematuria, and erectile dysfunction are increased with mapping biopsy, compared with standard transrectal needle biopsy. Further experience is needed before extensive mapping biopsies can be recommended as routine. Today, more attention is being focused on targeted biopsies of suspicious lesions seen on MRI.[124]

Imaging for Diagnosis and Staging

The overwhelming majority of men diagnosed with prostate cancer today do not have metastases at the time of diagnosis, so imaging studies to detect metastases are usually not indicated. Neither bone scans nor computed tomography (CT) are helpful for patients with clinically localized cancer unless they have a poorly differentiated tumor (Gleason score 8 to 10) or a PSA >20 ng/ml.[125] Consequently, most patients diagnosed with a clinically localized prostate cancer need no further studies to rule out metastases. Patients with very aggressive tumors (PSA >20 ng/ml and biopsy Gleason score >7), advanced local lesions (T3-4), or symptoms suggestive of metastatic disease should have imaging studies, including a bone scan and a CT of the chest, abdomen, and pelvis.

Magnetic Resonance Imaging

With current magnet strengths of 3 Tesla (3T), a multiparametric MRI, which provides T1- and T2-weighted images as well as diffusion-weighted and contrast images, permits excellent visualization of the prostate and surrounding tissues and the pelvic LN (in which case CT imaging of the pelvis is unnecessary).[126] The endorectal coil is helpful for enhanced visualization of the internal anatomy of the prostate when the magnetic strength is ≤1.5T, but magnetic resonance spectroscopy is rarely used today despite early promising results. On T1-weighted images, the prostate should appear homogenous and low intensity; cancers are not visible, but high-intensity areas resulting from recent biopsy should be noted to avoid misinterpreting corresponding low-intensity areas on T2 images as malignant lesions. On T2-weighted images, cancers can be recognized by their low signal intensity relative to the normal peripheral zone.

Diffusion-weighted imaging is a promising MRI technique that takes advantage of the known variability of random movements of water molecules observed between normal tissues and tumors. The rate of diffusion of water molecules is more restricted within tumors than in normal tissues and allows for an important metric known as the apparent diffusion coefficient. In one study comparing MRI with combined MRI and diffusion-weighted MRI, the sensitivity and specificity were 86% and 84%, respectively.[127] Dynamic contrast-enhancement MRI may also identify malignant lesions within the prostate.[128] In one study, the combination of T2-weighted imaging and dynamic contrast-enhancement MRI findings had sensitivity and specificity rates of 77% and 91% for detecting tumor foci that measured 0.2 cm^3, but these values improved to 90% and 88%, respectively, when detecting tumors >0.5 cm^3.[129–131]

Opinions vary regarding the value of MRI in routine staging and imaging of the prostate, and a wide range in specificity and sensitivity has been reported for the detection of extraprostatic extension and seminal vesicle invasion (SVI). In general, multiparametric MRI permits excellent visualization of the prostate and is more sensitive than DRE, TRUS, and CT for identifying extraprostatic extension and SVI (Fig. 68.7). MRI also allows accurate estimates of the size and shape of the prostate, the proximity of cancer to the neurovascular bundles and the urethral sphincter, the presence of a large anterior tumor that may be invading the anterior fibromuscular stroma or bladder neck, and the length of the membranous urethral sphincter, making MRI a valuable adjunct to the preoperative evaluation of patients with apparently localized prostate cancer.[132]

Computed Tomography

CT scans of the abdomen and pelvis are ordered far too frequently in the initial evaluation of men with prostate cancer, as they have limited capability to detect cancer within the prostate or the presence of extraprostatic extension or SVI. CT scans can detect LN metastases within the pelvis, but these can be detected equally well with pelvic/prostatic MRI, which provides more information about the primary tumor.

Bone Scan

A radionuclide bone scan is the standard imaging study used to identify the presence of osseous metastases,[130] but is not generally indicated in patients with clinically localized cancer because true positive results are much less common than false positives. In patients with a baseline PSA level <10 ng/ml, a bone scan identifies metastases in <1% of men who have no symptoms of bone pain.

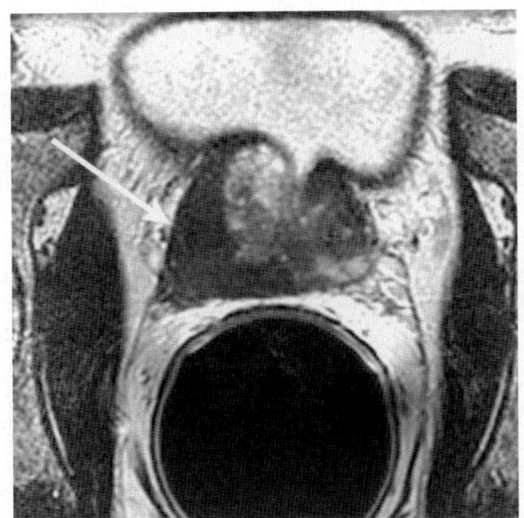 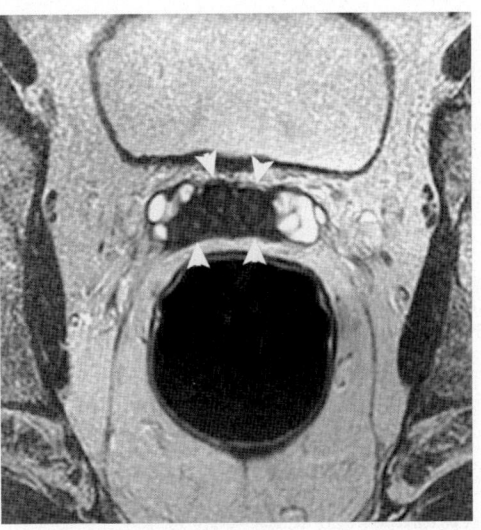

Figure 68.7 Clinical stage T2a prostate cancer. On the transverse image **(A)**, the patient was noted to have a dominant tumor at the right base with loss of normal contour and irregular bulging consistent with extracapsular extension (*arrow*). Image **(B)** indicates the evidence of seminal vesicle involvement (*arrowheads*) demonstrating mild enlargement of the seminal vesicles and low signal intensity tissue replacing normal thin walls and obliterating the lumen. (From Hricak H, Choyke PL, Eberhardt SC, et al. Imaging prostate cancer: a multidisciplinary perspective. *Radiology* 2007;243:28, with permission of the Radiological Society of America.)

For patients with PSA levels between 10 ng/ml and 50 ng/ml or >50 ng/ml, the probability of a positive bone scan is 10% and 50%, respectively.[131] Bone scans are frequently used to assess the response to hormonal therapy and chemotherapy in men with metastatic disease.

Risk Assessment

Characterization of the Local Tumor

A thorough evaluation of the extent of the local tumor should include a diagram of the area of induration and a recording of the clinical T stage, which reflects the size, location, and extent of the cancer (determined by DRE and imaging), histologic grade (Gleason score) in the biopsy specimen, baseline serum PSA level, and systematic biopsy results. These factors are used to predict pathologic stage, assist in treatment planning, and determine prognosis.

Tumor, Node, and Metastasis Classification

At the time of initial diagnosis, prostate cancers are staged using the TNM classification developed by the American Joint Committee on Cancer and the Union for International Cancer Control.[50–52,133,134] We recommend the use of the seventh edition published in 2010[51] (Table 68.3). With the TNM system, designations for the primary tumor, regional nodes, and distant metastases are noted separately. A distinct category, T1c, is used to describe cancers that are neither palpable nor visible, but were detected by a biopsy performed after an abnormal PSA test or for other reasons. Cancers that are not palpable but visible on imaging such as TRUS or MRI are classified appropriately along with palpable cancers in the T2-4 categories. However, the TNM system does not fully reflect prognosis because it does not include PSA levels, Gleason grade, or the extent of cancer in the biopsy specimen.

Staging Tables and Risk Groups

While individual prognostic factors can be informative, combining multiple factors together produces more accurate estimates of pathologic stage and prognosis. Partin et al.[135] developed a nomogram reported as a series of staging tables (Partin tables) that combine clinical tumor stage, biopsy Gleason grade, and PSA to predict pathologic stage. The accuracy of these tables has been widely validated.[136]

As pathologic stage is only a proxy for prognosis, a classification scheme has been developed to predict the risk of recurrence after treatment of the primary tumor using the same key prognostic factors (clinical stage, Gleason grade, and PSA).[137] The D'Amico classification, now adopted by the American Urological Association, assigns patients to one of three logical (rather than empirical) risk groups according to their clinical T stage, Gleason grade, and PSA.[137] Although it is intuitive to group patients into such risk-group categories, each "group" actually contains a heterogeneous population.[138] For example, patients with a clinical stage T1c, Gleason grade 3 + 3, and PSA 9.9 ng/ml would be classified as low risk, but if the PSA were 10.1 ng/ml, the same patient would be considered intermediate risk. Using categorical values

TABLE 68.3

Comparison of the 1992, 1997, 2002, and 2010 American Joint Committee on Cancer/International Union Against Cancer Tumor, Node, Metastasis Staging System

Stage	1992[50]	1997[52]	2002[133]	2010[51]
TX	Primary tumor cannot be assessed			
T0	No evidence of primary tumor			
T1	Clinically inapparent, not palpable or visible by imaging			
T1a	Incidental histologic finding, ≤5% of resected tissue			
T1b	Incidental histologic finding, >5% of resected tissue			
T1c	Tumor identified by needle biopsy, for any reason (e.g., elevated PSA)			
T2	Palpable or visible tumor, confined within the prostate[a]			
T2a	≤ Half one lobe	One lobe	≤ Half one lobe	≤ Half one lobe
T2b	One lobe	Both lobes	One lobe	> Half one lobe, not both
T2c	Both lobes	No T2c classification	Both lobes	Both lobes
T3	Tumor extends through prostate capsule[b]			
T3a	Unilateral ECE	ECE, unilateral or bilateral		ECE, unilateral or bilateral
T3b	Bilateral ECE	Seminal vesicle involvement		Seminal vesicle involvement
T3c	Seminal vesicle involvement	No T3c classification		No T3c classification
T4	Tumor is fixed or invades adjacent structures			Tumor is fixed or invades adjacent structures other than seminal vesicles, such as external sphincter, rectum, bladder, levator muscles, and/or pelvic wall
T4a	Invades bladder neck, external sphincter, or rectum			No T4a classification
T4b	Invades levator muscles or fixed to pelvic sidewalls			No T4b classification

PSA, prostate-specific antigen; ECE, extracapsular extension.
[a] Tumor found in one or both lobes by needle biopsy, but not palpable or reliably visible by imaging, is classified as T1c.
[b] Invasion into the prostatic apex or into (but not beyond) the prostatic capsule is classified not as T3 but as T2.
Modified from Beahrs OH, Henson DE, Hutter RVP, et al. *American Joint Committee on Cancer. AJCC Cancer Staging Manual.* 4th ed. Philadelphia, PA: Lippincott-Raven; 1992; Edge S, Byrd DR, Compton CC, et al. *American Joint Committee on Cancer. AJCC Cancer Staging Manual.* 7th ed. New York: Springer; 2010; Fleming ID, Cooper JS, Henson DE, et al. *American Joint Committee on Cancer. AJCC Cancer Staging Manual.* 5th ed. Philadelphia: JB Lippincott; 1997; Greene FL, Page DL, Fleming ID, et al. *American Joint Committee on Cancer. AJCC Cancer Staging Manual.* 6th ed. New York: Springer; 2002; and Ohori M, Wheeler TM, Scardino PT. The New American Joint Committee on Cancer and International Union against Cancer TNM classification of prostate cancer. *Cancer* 1994;74:104–114.

(e.g., PSA 10 to 20 ng/ml) rather than continuous values, and assigning a patient to an increased risk group if any single variable is high (e.g., tumor stage cT2c, Gleason 8 to 10, or PSA >20 ng/ml), is inherently inaccurate. Predictions are much more accurate when nomograms are used to combine individual prognostic factors into a single prognostic score assigned to an individual patient. Consequent comparisons of the results of different treatments are also more accurate when patients are more precisely matched.

Nomograms

Nomograms now widely available to predict prognosis in men with prostate cancer combine clinical and pathologic prognostic factors as continuous rather than categorical variables.[139] The prognosis or probability of recurrence after definitive therapy of an apparently localized prostate cancer depends on the clinical stage and grade of the cancer, the number or percent of positive biopsy cores, as well as the PSA level before treatment. Nomograms have proved highly useful in clinical practice and have been developed for external beam radiation therapy (EBRT)[140] and brachytherapy as well as surgery.[141] These nomograms may provide clues about the relative efficacy of different treatment modalities in patients with comparable tumors. All these nomograms are available at http://www.mskcc.org/cancer-care/prediction-tools (accessed June 13, 2014).

Molecular Profiles

Genomic testing has recently been introduced to characterize the level of aggressiveness of prostate cancer, and, as in breast cancer,[142–144] can help to guide treatment decisions.[145] There are currently two commercially available genomic tests for risk-stratification of prostate cancer, the Cell Cycle Progression assay (Prolaris, Myriad Genetic Laboratories Inc., Salt Lake City, UT) and the Genomic Prostate Score assay (Oncotype DX, Genomic Health, Redwood City, CA).[146–149] Both these tests use reverse transcription–polymerase chain reaction techniques to assay the expression level of a panel of genes that reflect the biologic activity of the cancer relative to the level of housekeeper genes. The Cell Cycle Progression-Prolaris assay was developed on a cohort of men with a wide spectrum of prostate cancer managed conservatively; the molecular profile added significantly to the ability of standard clinicopathologic features (stage, grade, PSA, and extent of cancer in biopsy specimens) to predict time to death from prostate cancer.[147] When needle biopsy specimens from men who were candidates for AS were assayed with Genomic Prostate Score-Oncotype DX, the assay independently predicted the risk of adverse pathology (extraprostatic extension or Gleason grade 4 + 3 or greater) in RP specimens. Both tests can successfully assay expression profiles from as little as 1 mm of cancer in an 18-g needle core obtained as long as 10 to 15 years previous to the assay, and both show a wide range of expression levels, and therefore prognoses, within any clinicopathologic risk group.

The clinical utility of these molecular profiles is under active investigation; today, the assays are largely used to recommend AS in men with low- or intermediate-risk, low-volume cancer and favorable expression profiles. Assay results tend to be concordant with the clinicopathologic risk classification in approximately 45% of patients, whereas it is higher or lower in the remaining 55%. In a recent study, 14% of patients considered low risk and suitable for AS were reclassified as higher risk patients for whom active intervention was warranted, and 7% of those with clinically aggressive tumors were reclassified as low-risk and suitable for AS by the Cell Cycle Progression-Prolaris assay.[150]

Pathologic Stage

Several other indices have been developed that improve the biologic characterization of a given tumor. Pathologic stage, determined by examining the RP specimen, predicts recurrence much more accurately than clinical stage.[151] Independent prognostic factors include the level of invasion through the capsule of the prostate, SVI, LN metastases, and positive surgical margins, as well as the Gleason score in the RP specimen and the preoperative serum PSA level. Some investigators have considered tumor volume an important prognostic factor, but others have found that it has no independent prognostic significance. Stephenson et al.[152] combined these independent prognostic factors into postoperative nomograms to predict biochemical recurrence (BCR)[153] 10 years after RP and 15-year cancer-specific survival.[139,154] These nomograms are more accurate than the preoperative nomogram, because they incorporate the final Gleason grade and pathologic stage as well as preoperative PSA.[154]

Stage Assignment

Clinical States Model

Given the range of prognoses among men within each of the TNM-defined stages at diagnosis, a risk-adapted approach to diagnosis and treatment is mandated. To facilitate this approach, a model was developed that divides the disease continuum from prediagnosis to advanced metastatic disease into a series of clinical states. Each state represents a distinct clinical milestone defined by the status of the tumor in the primary site, the presence or absence of metastatic disease on imaging, whether the testosterone levels in the blood are in noncastrate or castrate (<50 ng/dl) range, and prior therapy. This model differs from staging algorithms in that it applies to both the newly diagnosed, untreated patient and to the patient who has received treatment as his disease evolves. Unmet needs in diagnosis, defining treatment objectives, and assessing outcomes vary by clinical state (see Fig. 68.1). Applied clinically to men without a cancer diagnosis, this approach accommodates the need to assess an individual's cancer based on the risk of harboring or developing clinically significant disease.

In the clinical states model, an individual is assigned to only one state and he remains in that state until his disease has progressed. He can only move forward, never back, even if his disease has been eradicated completely. Each assessment is considered a new evaluation in which the patient's symptoms and overall tumor status are reviewed, and the decision to offer treatment, and the specific form of treatment, are based on the current state of the disease or the future risk posed by the cancer relative to comorbid conditions.

For example, the rising PSA states include patients who have a rising PSA following treatment of the primary tumor with either surgery or radiation, an indication that the disease has recurred. Issues for these patients include whether the recurrence is systemic or limited to the prostate bed (following surgery) or the prostate itself (following radiation). A more important consideration is whether any treatment is needed, based on the likelihood in the long term that the cancer will cause symptoms, local or distant, or shorten a patient's life. Patients with rising PSA who are considered to have disease in the prostate bed (or the prostate itself) are discussed in the sections of this chapter that review the primary treatment modalities for prostate cancer. Treatment objectives and the means to assess outcomes vary by clinical state and will be considered separately. The more rapidly the disease is progressing or the more advanced the disease state, the greater the need for treatment.

Principles of Treatment and Assessing Outcomes

Treatment is offered with therapeutic intent that considers (1) why the treatment should be administered, (2) the potential benefits it can provide relative to potential morbidity, and (3) financial cost. Changing established practice paradigms requires demonstrating that a new therapy or approach provides incremental clinical benefit relative to a previous standard (if one exists) or to a suitable control in prospective randomized trials. Clinical benefit in regulatory terms represents an improvement in the way a patient functions or feels, or in how long he survives.[155] Examples of clinical benefits include prolonging life, relieving pain or other symptoms, and/or reducing toxicity relative to an established standard. It is also important to demonstrate that a new approach, whether it is a therapeutic procedure or a drug, is safe and well tolerated in an elderly population.

Assessing Treatment Effects

It has long been recognized that the most common manifestations of prostate cancer, which include disease in the primary site, a rising PSA, and metastasis to bone, are not evaluable by the traditional measures of tumor regression used to monitor disease status in other solid malignancies (Response Evaluation Criteria In Solid Tumors [RECIST] 1.1).[156] Changes in nodal and visceral sites that can be assessed reliably using RECIST occur less often. To address this unmet need, the Prostate Cancer Working Group (PCWG2) was formed to develop guidelines for clinical trial design in castration-resistant prostate cancer (CRPC) that also apply to earlier disease states.[157]

In the clinical states framework, treatment objectives are divided into early outcomes representing the control, relief, or elimination of disease manifestations present when a treatment is being considered or initiated, and later outcomes representing the delay or prevention of future manifestations. Existing manifestations may include disease limited to the prostate (localized disease), a biochemical recurrence following local treatment (rising PSA), or cancer in the extrapelvic LN, bone, or viscera with or without a rising PSA (clinical metastases). Potential manifestations that might be delayed or prevented from occurring include growth in the primary site, BCR, growth in an existing site, new sites of spread, pain, or other complications of progressive osseous disease described as skeletal-related events (SRE),[158] and death from disease. SREs, first used in the regulatory filing of zoledronate, include fractures, pain requiring a change in therapy, epidural disease, and/or surgery to bone.[159]

"Control/relieve/eliminate" outcomes representing "response" are reported individually by the change in each disease manifestation present—PSA level, soft tissue disease, bone disease, and/or symptoms when treatment was started—rather than by grouped categorizations, such as complete and partial remission, that include all sites of disease. For example, a key PSA-based outcome for patients treated with RP is the proportion of patients who achieve an undetectable PSA level postoperatively, whereas for patients with CRPC treated with a systemic approach, a waterfall plot showing the percent change from baseline for each patient treated, or the proportion of patients achieving a defined degree of decline (e.g., ≥50%), is more informative. "Delay/prevent" outcomes focusing on time-to-event progression are also measured individually. For a patient with localized disease, outcomes from surgery or radiation include a response measure that demonstrates whether the disease was eliminated completely (e.g., a negative biopsy of the prostate at a certain time after radiotherapy) or time-to-event outcomes that include time to PSA recurrence, metastases, symptoms, or death from disease. This approach to evaluating outcomes enables the physician to focus on the specific therapeutic objective for a single patient or group of patients in a given disease state, rather than on changes in other, less-relevant measures, and at the same time enables clinical trial investigators to explore the relation between changes in individual disease manifestations and other measures of clinical benefit such as overall survival.

MANAGEMENT BY CLINICAL STATES

Clinically Localized Disease

The clinical course of newly diagnosed prostate cancer is difficult to predict. Men with similar clinical stage, serum PSA levels, and biopsy features can have markedly different outcomes. Although prostate cancer is unequivocally lethal in some patients, most men die with, rather than of, their cancer. The challenge to physicians is to identify those men with aggressive, localized prostate cancer with a natural history that can be altered by definitive local therapy, while sparing the remainder the morbidity of unnecessary treatment. Not all men with clinically localized prostate cancer require or benefit from therapy. Depending on the characteristics of their cancer, their age, and comorbidities, some men would benefit greatly by aggressive treatment, whereas others would suffer harm.

Well-established prognostic factors for clinically localized prostate cancer include age, PSA level, clinical stage based on DRE and imaging, Gleason grade, and extent of the cancer on biopsy. Prognosis can be estimated more accurately by combining these risk factors into nomograms[99] that calculate the probability of a clinically important endpoint, such as freedom from BCR 10 years after surgery[153] or cancer-specific survival 15 years after surgery.[139]

Active Surveillance

AS is a planned treatment of monitoring a patient with a potentially curable prostate cancer based on the likelihood that the cancer will progress, delaying active treatment until signs of progression to a more aggressive, potentially lethal cancer are detected. AS attempts to avoid the adverse effects of treatment in the majority of men, intervening with curative therapy for selected men only for specific indications. AS is now widely recommended for most men with low-risk cancer, based on the lack of survival benefit of immediate surgery versus observation at 12 years in the PIVOT trial[160] and the low risk of prostate cancer death at 10 years in large phase 2 studies of AS.[84] In this and other AS trials, the risk of progression or treatment for men with low-risk cancer is about 20% to 40% within 5 years and 35% to 60% within 10 years, depending on the initial eligibility criteria and the indications for delayed intervention.

A recommendation for AS assumes that the risk posed by the cancer at diagnosis can be assessed accurately, that progression can be identified by regular monitoring, and that deferring treatment until it is necessary will offer cancer control and survival rates similar to immediate treatment. Achieving all of these goals has not yet been realized. Standard assessment at diagnosis includes PSA, clinical stage, Gleason grade, and extent of cancer in biopsy results. This limited evaluation underestimates the grade and extent of the cancer in 15% to 25% of patients.[161] A multiparametric MRI of the prostate can detect large, more aggressive cancers in some patients, and these findings can be confirmed by biopsies targeting the suspicious lesions.[162] Alternatively, one can depend on annual repeat biopsies[163] or PSA velocity[84] to detect progression in time for effective intervention. In either case, patients under AS must accept frequent, regular, detailed evaluations of the status of their cancer for as long as they are healthy and young enough to be candidates for definitive therapy. Patients under AS are generally monitored every 6 months with DRE and measurement of free and total PSA, with repeat imaging and biopsy every 2 to 3 years after the baseline evaluation. The goal is to detect progression of the cancer while cure is still possible.

Outcomes of Active Surveillance with Selective Delayed Intervention

There are few reports of long-term outcomes of AS for localized prostate cancer. Klotz et al.[84] conducted a prospective phase 2 study of AS in men with low-risk cancer (or those over 70 with Gleason 7 [3 + 4] and PSA <15 ng/ml). The indications for intervention were a short PSA doubling time (PSADT) or grade progression on repeat biopsy. At 8 years, overall survival was 85% and disease-specific and metastasis-free survival 99%. Some 25%

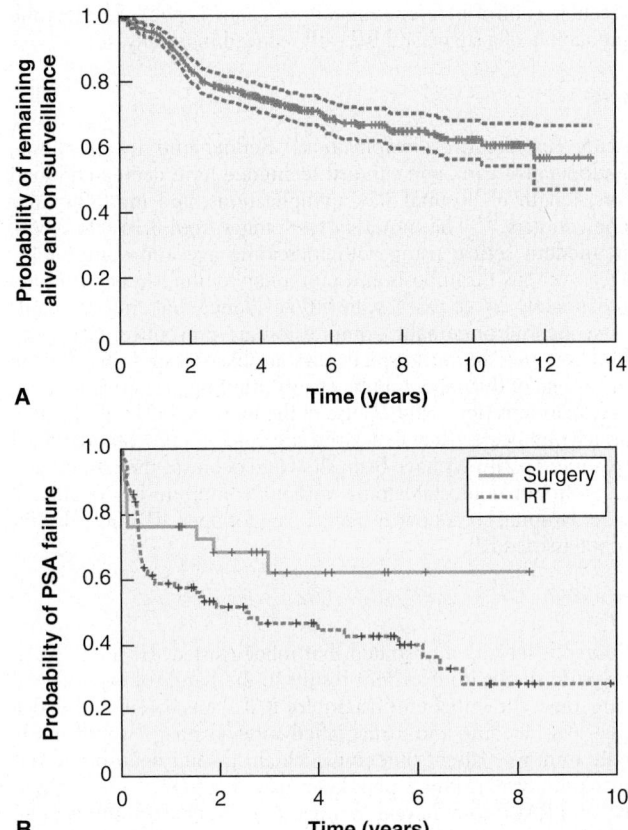

Figure 68.8 Long-term follow-up of active surveillance cohort with localized prostate cancer. **(A)** Likelihood of remaining alive and on surveillance in 450 patients. *Green lines* indicate 95% confidence intervals. **(B)** Prostate-specific antigen (PSA) failure in 117 patients treated with surgery or radiation after a period of surveillance. RT, radiotherapy. (From Klotz L, Zhang L, Lam A, et al. Clinical results of long-term follow-up of a large, active surveillance cohort with localized prostate cancer. *J Clin Oncol* 2010;28:126–131, with permission.)

is necessary to determine the long-term risk of progression. The National Comprehensive Cancer Network recommends AS as the appropriate initial management strategy for patients with low-risk cancer and a life expectancy <10 years, as well as for patients with very low-risk cancer and a life expectancy <20 years.[125]

Radical Prostatectomy

The modern anatomic technique for RP was developed nearly 35 years ago and has proven safe and effective in many large cohort studies and randomized clinical trials. The retropubic technique originally described by Walsh[165] for open surgery is equally suitable for laparoscopic and robot-assisted RP. Initially focused on patients with early-stage, organ-confined cancers, RP with pelvic LN dissection (PLND) is now recommended primarily for patients with aggressive cancers (intermediate- and high-risk), whereas low-risk tumors are generally managed with AS (see previous discussion). Because of the risk inherent in major surgery, RP should be reserved for patients without serious systemic comorbidity. Although the risk of recurrence after RP rises with higher clinical stage, Gleason grade, and serum PSA level, no absolute cutoff values exclude a patient as a candidate.

Surgical Technique. The goals of modern RP are to remove the entire cancer with negative surgical margins, minimal blood loss, no serious perioperative complications, and complete recovery of continence and potency. Achieving these goals requires careful surgical planning. Because no single test provides a reliable estimate of the size, location, and extent of the cancer, we rely on the results of DRE, serum PSA levels, and a detailed analysis of the amount and grade of cancer in each individually labeled biopsy core, along with multiparametric MRI. The results are used to plan the steps necessary to remove the cancer completely and to assess the likelihood that one or both of the neurovascular bundles will have to be resected partially or fully to minimize the risk of a positive surgical margin. The retropubic procedure is performed either through a suprapubic incision (open RP) or using a minimal access (laparoscopic or robot-assisted laparoscopic) approach. The operation should be exactly the same internally, regardless of the method of access.

Selecting Patients for Pelvic Lymph Node Dissection

Cancer that has spread to the pelvic LN carries a worse prognosis than when the nodes are negative, enhancing accurate staging. However, the therapeutic benefit of PLND is uncertain. Overall rates of pelvic LN metastases found at RP vary from 2% to 35% depending on the extent of the node dissection, whether the cancer was discovered after screening, and the stage and grade of the cancer.[166] Men with low-risk screen-detected cancer are rarely found to have nodal metastases (0.5% to 2%),[166–168] so PLND is generally unnecessary, but it may be indicated if imaging studies or intraoperative findings suggest a more advanced cancer. The limited PLND commonly performed today, especially with robot-assisted RP, has underestimated the rate of nodal metastases.[169] In men with intermediate-risk prostate cancer, LN metastases are found in 5% (screen-detected) to 20%, whereas in men with high-risk cancer, the rates are 20% to 50%, respectively, when a full or extended PLND is performed.[166,170–173] The incidence of LN metastases increases with increasing PSA, clinical stage, and Gleason score.[168] Our current practice is to restrict PLND at the time of RP to men with a ≥2% risk of positive nodes according to a contemporary nomogram.[174] Even so, controversy persists concerning the role of PLND in patients with prostate cancer.

Limited Versus Extended Pelvic Lymph Node Dissection

No prospective studies have demonstrated the optimal anatomic limits of a PLND for prostate cancer. However, lymphatic drainage of the prostate is known to be highly variable and involves

of patients were treated within 5 years, and 40% by 10 years (Fig. 68.8). Delayed intervention was associated with a relatively low rate of cancer control, raising concerns that treatment for men with a short PSADT (<2 years) was too late.

Carter et al.[96] observed a cohort of 769 men with very-low-risk prostate cancer and low PSA density (<0.15) from 1 to 15 years after diagnosis with DRE, measurements of total and free PSA every 6 months, and an annual surveillance biopsy. Treatment was recommended based on biopsy changes (any Gleason pattern 4 or 5, more than two cores that were positive for cancer, or >50% of any one core that was involved with cancer) or if a patient requested a change in management, but not for changes in PSA alone. A total of 41% of patients had been treated at 5 years, and 59% at 10 years, and the median time to treatment was 6.5 years. Cancer control after delayed therapy was excellent. The large number of men who required delayed intervention suggested that many tumors were underestimated at baseline, and the high cure rates at delayed intervention call into question the clinical significance of the criteria for delayed intervention. Many physicians now recommend more comprehensive initial evaluation of candidates for AS with multiparametric MRI and/or early confirmatory biopsies.[164]

These and other studies confirm that in appropriately selected men, AS is associated with an extremely low rate of progression to metastatic disease and/or death, and that the majority of patients do not require intervention over the first decade. Further follow-up regions not sampled during an external iliac–only PLND.[166] Some surgeons resect only the external iliac LN unless imaging suggests abnormal LN in other regions, whereas other surgeons routinely perform a more extensive dissection that includes the obturator, external iliac, and hypogastric areas.[175] No sentinel LN has been identified in prostate cancer. The more extensive the PLND, the greater the number of LN removed, and the greater the number of positive nodes.[166,168,171–173] Nevertheless, the total number of positive LN is one in 50% of patients, two in 30%, and three or more in only 20% of patients who have an extended LN dissection.[166] A PLND that includes the external iliac, hypogastric, and obturator node packets is feasible in both open and minimally invasive RP, and carries no greater risk than a PLND limited to the external iliac nodes alone.

Therapeutic Benefit of Pelvic Lymph Node Dissection

Evidence from several surgical series of patients undergoing RP demonstrates a potential therapeutic benefit of extended PLND, particularly in men with only one or two positive nodes and Gleason score ≤7 in cancer identified in the RP specimen (Fig. 68.9).[170–172,176–178] In a series of patients with positive LN treated at Johns Hopkins Hospital, men who had an extended PLND were less likely to develop BCR at 5 years, compared with men who underwent a limited PLND when 15% or fewer of the removed LN were involved.[170] In the Memorial Sloan Kettering Cancer Center (MSKCC) series, 25% to 30% of patients with positive nodes remained free of BCR 10 years after surgery with no additional therapy.[179]

Radical Prostatectomy: Surgical Approach

RP is one of the most complex operations performed by urologists. The outcomes—cancer control, urinary continence, and erectile function—are exquisitely sensitive to fine details in surgical technique. No surgeon achieves perfect results, and outcomes vary dramatically among individual surgeons.[180,181] Technical refinements have resulted in lower rates of urinary incontinence and higher rates of recovery of erectile function, less blood loss and fewer transfusions, shorter hospital stays, and lower rates of positive surgical margins. Laparoscopic and robot-assisted RP promised better cancer control and functional recovery, but numerous studies have confirmed that the only consistent advantages of "minimally invasive" surgery are shorter hospital stays and fewer blood transfusions.[182] A thorough understanding of periprostatic anatomy and

vascular control by contemporary surgeons further increases the probability of a successful RP with reduced morbidity.

Open Radical Prostatectomy

Acute Postoperative Complications. Refinements in anesthesia, perioperative care, and surgical technique have decreased blood loss, length of hospital stay, complications, and mortality after open surgery.[183] The mortality rate ranges from 0.16% to 0.66% in modern series, rising with increasing age and comorbidity. Deep venous thrombosis and pulmonary embolism occur in approximately 2% of cases, with little evidence that anticoagulants or sequential pneumatic compression are preventive. Early ambulation and shorter hospital stays are likely responsible for the lower rate of thromboembolic events. Routine perioperative anticoagulation is not used because of the increased risks of bleeding and lymphocele. Rectal injuries are uncommon. Standardized treatment pathways have been shown to decrease the cost of radical retropubic prostatectomy without compromising quality of care. Hospital stays now average 2 days for open RP and 1 day for robot-assisted RP.

Robot-Assisted Radical Prostatectomy

Surgeons have demonstrated that robot-assisted RP (RALP) can be performed with excellent results in the hands of experienced surgeons. The initial enthusiasm for RALP was based on the idea that less bleeding and a magnified surgical image would markedly improve patient outcomes, which has not been borne out in carefully performed population-based studies.[182,184,185] Open RP and RALP each have a number of theoretical advantages and disadvantages (Table 68.4).[186] No prospective randomized trials have yet compared the two techniques, and it is now clear that variations in outcomes among individual surgeons are much greater than variations between technologic approaches.[181] Hu et al.[184] have suggested that the rapid increase in utilization of minimally invasive RP despite insufficient data demonstrating superiority over the well-established open operation may be a reflection of a society and a health-care system enamored of a new technology that has increased health-care costs but has yet to uniformly realize marketed or potential benefits during early adoption. As with open surgical techniques, laparoscopic RP and RALP outcomes, including surgical margin status, continence, and potency, reflect surgical technique (the actions and expertise of the surgeon) more than surgical approach. Current data suggest that the best way to improve outcomes after RP is to have the procedure performed by a skilled surgeon, regardless of the approach he or she uses.[181,187]

Cancer Control with Radical Prostatectomy

Benefits of Surgery Relative to Active Surveillance. The most compelling evidence that selected patients with prostate cancer benefit from active treatment compared with watchful waiting comes from the Scandinavian randomized trial (SPCG-4) of 695 unscreened men with clinically localized prostate cancer.[188,189] Over 23 years of follow-up, RP (compared with watchful waiting) reduced the risk of death from any cause by 29% and risk of death from prostate cancer by 44% (an absolute difference of 11%). The need for subsequent ADT was reduced by 51%, and clinical local recurrence was reduced by 66%. At 18 years of follow-up, the number needed to treat to prevent one death from prostate cancer was eight overall and four in men under age 65. This elegant study firmly documents the overall benefit of RP in patients with clinically localized prostate cancer diagnosed in the absence of systematic screening.[188,189]

In a population of men subjected to widespread PSA screening, the benefit of surgery for prostate cancer was tested in the Prostate Cancer Intervention Versus Observation Trial (PIVOT).[160] This

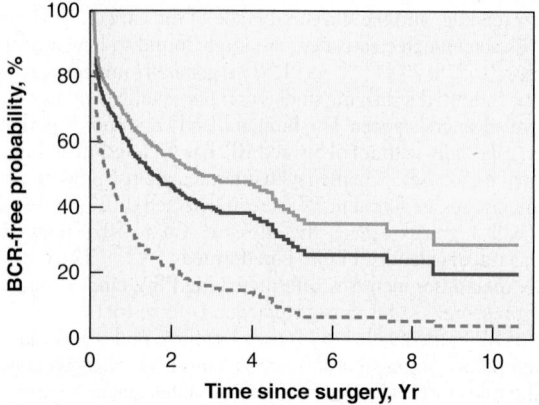

Figure 68.9 Probability of freedom from biochemical recurrence (BCR) by number of positive nodes. *Orange line,* one positive node; *blue line,* two positive nodes; *red line,* three or more positive nodes. (From Touijer KA, Mazzola CR, Sjoberg DD, et al. Long-term outcomes of patients with lymph node metastasis treated with radical prostatectomy without adjuvant androgen-deprivation therapy. *Eur Urol* 2014;65:20–25, with permission.)

TABLE 68.4

Advantages and Disadvantages of Various Surgical Approaches to Radical Prostatectomy

Claims by Minimally Invasive Surgeons: Advantages	Rebuttal by Open Surgeons
Magnification improves visualization	Magnification achieved with surgical loupes
Less blood loss	Transfusion rates are similar
Improved visualization permits more precise dissection of the prostatic apex and neurovascular bundles	Outcomes fail to demonstrate any advantage in terms of continence and potency
Less pain and quicker recovery	Postoperative pain and recovery are comparable
Watertight anastomosis allows earlier catheter removal	No difference noted in most large series
Claims by Open Surgeons: Disadvantages	**Rebuttal by Minimally Invasive Surgeons**
Lack of proprioception compromises cancer control	Positive margin rates are equivalent
Complication rates are lower with open surgery	Complication rates with laparoscopic surgery decrease with experience
Mobilization of the neurovascular bundles with electrocautery compromises potency	Potency rates are similar
Significant learning curve	Proctoring reduces learning curve
Longer operative time	No rebuttal
Increased cost	No rebuttal

trial was conducted in the United States and randomly assigned 731 men with clinically localized prostate cancer to RP or observation. The mean age was 67, the median PSA level was 7.8 ng/ml, and approximately three-quarters of the men had a biopsy as a consequence of an elevated PSA; half had no palpable tumor (cT1c) and 70% had low-grade (Gleason ≤6) cancer on biopsy. With a median of 10 years of follow-up, 48% of the patients had died, but only 7% had died from prostate cancer. There were no differences in overall or cancer-specific mortality between the two arms of the trial. But there were clear indications that RP reduced the risk of dying of cancer in the subset of men who had aggressive cancers, including those whose PSA was >10.0 ng/ml and those with high-risk cancers.

Taken together, these two trials indicate that most men with cancers detected without screening and those with screen-detected intermediate- and high-risk cancers have less risk of metastases and of death from prostate cancer when treated with early RP than with observation alone. In contrast, men with screen-detected low-risk cancer can be managed safely with AS and do not need immediate surgery or radiotherapy. Life expectancy should be considered in

the choice of immediate therapy or AS, as the risks of RP increase and benefits decline progressively with age and comorbidity.[190] A UK-based trial (ProtecT) is currently assessing treatment versus no treatment in a PSA-screened population in >1,500 patients.[191]

Progression rates after RP depend on the clinical stage, biopsy Gleason score, and serum PSA level before surgery, as well as pathologic findings in the surgical specimen. After RP, the PSA level should become undetectable. Cancer control, as measured by freedom from BCR, is excellent after RP and is reproducible among many large series (Table 68.5).[179, 192–196] Of 12,086 patients treated with RP between 1966 and 2003, 69% to 84% were free of progression at 5 years, and 47% to 78% at 10 years.[179, 192–196]

Fifteen-year outcomes have been reported after RP based on preoperative and pathologic factors (Table 68.6). Bianco, Scardino, and Eastham[179] calculated the risk of recurrence in 1,743 consecutive patients with clinical stage T1-T3, N0 or X, M0 cancer treated with RP and followed with serum PSA levels for a mean of 72 months (range, 1 month to 240 months). Failure after RP was defined as a rising serum PSA >0.2 ng/ml, clinical evidence of local or distant recurrence, or the initiation of adjuvant radiotherapy or

TABLE 68.5

Freedom from Prostate-Specific Antigen Progression After Radical Retropubic Prostatectomy

Group (Ref.)	No. of Patients	Clinical Stage	Years of RP	PSA Nonprogression (%) Five-Y	Ten-Y	Fifteen-Y
Han et al.[193]	2,091[a]	T1c-2NX	1982–1999	84	72	61
Trapasso et al.[195]	601[b]	T1-3NX	1987–1992	69	47	—
Zincke et al.[196]	3,170[c]	T1-2NX	1966–1991	70	52	40
Roehl et al.[192]	3,478[c]	T1-3NX	1983–2003	80	68	—
Hull et al.[194]	1,000[d]	T1-2NX	1983–1998	78	75	—
Bianco, Scardino, and Eastham[179]	1,746[e]	T1-3NX	1983–2003	82	77	75

PSA, prostate-specific antigen; RP, radical prostatectomy.
[a] Progression defined as a serum PSA ≥0.2 ng/ml.
[b] Progression defined as a serum PSA >0.4 ng/ml.
[c] Progression defined as a serum PSA >0.3 ng/ml.
[d] Progression defined as a serum PSA ≥0.4 ng/ml.
[e] Progression defined as a serum PSA ≥0.4 ng/ml before 1996 and ≥0.2 ng/ml afterward.

TABLE 68.6

Actuarial 5-, 10-, and 15-Year (Prostate-Specific Antigen–Based) Nonprogression Rates (%) After Radical Retropubic Prostatectomy for Clinically Localized Prostate Cancer According to Preoperative and Pathologic Factors

	Johns Hopkins University[a]			MSKCC SPORE in Prostate Cancer Database[b]		
	Five-Y	**Ten-Y**	**Fifteen-Y**	**Five-Y**	**Ten-Y**	**Fifteen-Y**
No. of patients	2,404	2,404	2,404	4,037	4,037	4,037
BCR	412	412	412	630	630	630
BCR-free (%)	84	74	66	82	75	73
Actuarial Nonprogression Rate (95% CI) by Preoperative Serum PSA (ng/ml)						
≤4	94 (92–96)	91 (87–93)	67 (34–86)	92 (89–95)	89 (85–93)	86 (80–92)
>4 and ≤10	89 (86–91)	79 (74–83)	75 (69–80)	87 (85–89)	80 (77–83)	78 (74–81)
>10 and ≤20	73 (68–78)	57 (48–64)	54[c] (44–63)	75 (72–78)	68 (64–71)	66 (62–70)
>20	60 (49–69)	48 (36–59)	48 (36–59)	58 (54–62)	52 (47–57)	50 (43–56)
Actuarial Nonprogression Rate (95% CI) by Clinical Stage						
cT1ab	90 (83–95)	85 (76–91)	75 (58–86)	90 (85–95)	85 (79–92)	83 (76–90)
cT1c	91 (88–93)	76 (48–90)	76[c] (48–90)	88 (86–90)	79 (73–85)	NA
cT2a	86 (83–88)	75 (71–79)	66 (59–72)	85 (82–88)	77 (71–83)	75 (70–80)
cT2b	75 (70–79)	62 (56–68)	50 (41–58)	74 (70–79)	69 (64–75)	69 (64–75)
cT2c	71 (61–79)	57 (45–68)	57 (45–68)	71 (68–75)	64 (59–68)	62 (57–67)
cT3	60 (45–72)	49 (34–63)	NA	54 (44–64)	51 (40–62)	NA
Actuarial Nonprogression Rate (95% CI) by Specimen Gleason Sum						
2–4	100	100	100	100	100	100
5	98 (96–99)	94 (90–96)	86 (78–92)	92 (90–94)	89 (86–92)	88 (84–92)
6	95 (93–97)	88 (83–92)	73 (59–82)	91 (89–93)	83 (80–86)	81 (78–85)
7 (All)	73 (69–76)	54 (48–59)	48 (41–56)	77 (75–79)	70 (66–74)	67 (63–72)
3 + 4	81 (77–84)	60 (53–67)	59 (51–65)	82 (79–84)	74 (69–79)	72 (62–82)
4 + 3	53 (44–61)	33 (22–43)	33 (22–43)	60 (50–70)	53 (44–64)	53 (44–64)
8–10	44 (36–52)	29 (22–37)	15 (5–28)	41 (35–47)	33 (24–42)	NA
Actuarial Nonprogression Rate (95% CI) by Pathologic Stage						
Organ confined	97 (95–98)	93 (90–95)	84 (77–90)	93 (92–94)	89 (87–91)	87 (85–89)
EPE+, GS <7, SM−	97 (94–98)	93 (89–96)	84 (70–92)	92 (89–94)	89 (84–94)	86 (79–92)
EPE+, GS <7, SM+	89 (80–94)	73 (61–82)	58 (41–71)	74 (64–84)	65 (54–76)	65 (54–76)
EPE+, GS ≥7, SM−	80 (75–85)	61 (52–68)	59 (50–67)	76 (66–86)	68 (61–75)	65 (56–74)
EPE+, GS ≥7, SM+	58 (49–66)	42 (32–52)	33 (23–44)	60 (53–67)	55 (44–66)	55 (44–66)
SV+, LN−	48 (38–58)	30 (19–41)	17 (5–35)	44 (38–50)	31 (24–38)	28 (19–37)
LN+	26 (19–35)	10 (5–18)	0	25 (18–32)	15 (5–25)	0
Negative margins	NA	NA	NA	87 (86–88)	81 (79–83)	79 (76–82)
Positive margins	NA	NA	NA	66 (63–69)	56 (52–60)	54 (49–59)

MSKCC SPORE, Memorial Sloan Kettering Cancer Center Specialized Programs of Research Excellence; BCR, biochemical recurrence; CI, confidence interval; PSA, prostate-specific antigen; NA, not applicable; EPE, extraprostatic extension; GS, Gleason sum; SM, surgical margin; SV, seminal vesicles; LN, lymph node.
[a] Single surgeon series. From Han M, Partin AW, Pound CR, et al. Long-term biochemical disease-free and cancer-specific survival following anatomic radical retropubic prostatectomy. The 15-year Johns Hopkins experience. *Urol Clin North Am* 2001;28:555–565.
[b] Includes 1,092 radical prostatectomies performed by a single surgeon.
[c] Fourteen-year data.

hormonal treatment. At 5 years 84% of patients, at 10 years 78%, and at 15 years 73% were free of progression (see Table 68.5).

Of particular interest are patients with high-grade cancers (Gleason sum 7 to 10). Of patients with Gleason 3 + 4 = 7 cancers in the RP specimen, 68% were free of progression at 15 years. When the tumor was Gleason 4 + 3 = 7, 51% were free of progression at 15 years.[179] Even patients with Gleason sum 8 to 10 cancers fared well, with 27%

free of progression at 10 years. These progression rates are substantially lower than the 15-year cancer mortality rates reported for patients with Gleason sum 7 to 10 cancers managed with watchful waiting.[197]

Once the prostate is removed, the most powerful prognostic factor is the pathologic stage (see Table 68.6). When the cancer is confined to the prostate (defined as cancer not extending into the periprostatic soft tissue), 92% to 98% of patients remain free of progression at 5 years and 88% to 96% remain free 10 years after RP.[194] Focal penetration through the capsule into the periprostatic soft tissue alone, in the absence of SVI, results in a 73% 10-year nonprogression rate. Established (extensive) penetration through the prostatic capsule into the periprostatic soft tissue, in the absence of SVI, results in a 42% 10-year nonprogression rate. Even some patients with SVI (pT3cN0) can be cured with surgery, with 30% being free of disease recurrence at 10 years (see Table 68.6).

The slow clinical progression of prostate cancer after RP has led to the widespread use of PSA recurrence as the primary end point for evaluating treatment outcome. However, doing so ignores the fact that the prognosis of men in the rising PSA state is highly variable, and that the rising PSA by itself does not necessarily mean that a patient will develop metastatic disease, develop symptoms, or die of his cancer. For many, the threat posed to a man's duration and quality of survival is limited at best.

Reports of long-term, prostate cancer–specific survival rates after RP have clearly shown that many patients with PSA recurrence live out their lives free of cancer.[179,193,194,196,198] The long-term risk of prostate cancer–specific mortality (PCSM) after RP for patients treated in the era of widespread PSA screening has

recently been estimated based on a multi-institutional cohort of 12,677 patients treated with RP between 1987 and 2005.[139] Fifteen-year PCSM and all-cause mortality were 12% and 38%, respectively. The estimated PCSM ranged from 5% to 38% for patients in the lowest and highest quartiles of nomogram-predicted risk of PSA-defined recurrence (Table 68.7). Only 4% of contemporary patients had a predicted 15-year PCSM of >5%.

Clearly, few patients will die from prostate cancer within 15 years of RP, despite the presence of adverse clinical features. It is not known whether this favorable prognosis is related to the effectiveness of RP (with or without secondary therapy) or to the low lethality of cancers detected by early screening. Although year of surgery, biopsy Gleason grade, and PSA level are associated with PCSM risk, an individual patient's risk cannot be predicted on the basis of clinical features alone. Further research is needed to identify novel markers specifically associated with the biology of lethal prostate cancer.

High-Risk Prostate Cancer

Monotherapy is often believed to be inadequate for high-risk cancers, and some clinicians are reluctant to consider RP in high-risk

TABLE 68.7

Risk of Prostate Cancer–Specific Mortality at 10 and 15 Years After Radical Prostatectomy[a]

Variable	Patients[b] No.	%	Events[b] No.	%	Ten-Y PCSM %	95% CI	Fifteen-Y PCSM %	95% CI
Nomogram-Predicted 5-y PFP (%)								
76–99	8,555	73	51	26	1.8	1.2–2.4	5	3–7
51–75	2,228	19	75	38	6	4–7	15	10–21
26–50	656	6	40	21	9	6–12	16	9–22
1–25	209	2	29	15	15	9–22	38	19–56
Risk Group								
PSA <10, Gleason score 6, T1c or T2a	5,200	46	14	7	0.9	0.3–1.5	2	0.3–4
PSA 10–20, Gleason score 7, T2b	4,184	37	64	32	4	2–5	10	6–14
PSA >20, Gleason score 8–10, T2c-T3	1,962	17	121	61	8	7–10	19	14–24
Pretreatment PSA (ng/ml)								
<4	2,285	18	18	9	2	1–4	4	1–7
4–10	7,574	61	75	37	3	2–4	9	5–12
10.1–20	1,874	15	50	24	4	3–6	11	6–15
20.1–50	726	6	62	30	10	7–12	22	15–30
1992 TNM Clinical Stage								
T1ab	174	2	4	2	2	0–4	6	0–12
T1c	6,413	56	28	14	2	1–3	6	5–7
T2a	2,520	22	42	21	3	2–4	7	4–10
T2b	1,461	13	57	29	5	3–7	14	9–19
T2c	714	6	38	19	7	4–9	12	8–17
T3	254	2	28	14	15	9–21	38	22–54
Biopsy Gleason Score								
2–6	7,454	65	78	40	2	1–3	6	4–8
7	3,292	29	55	28	5	3–7	17	8–26
8–10	702	6	61	32	16	11–20	34	23–46

PCSM, prostate cancer–specific mortality; CI, confidence interval; PFP, progression-free probability; PSA, prostate-specific antigen; TNM, tumor, node, metastasis.
[a] Values were based on a previously validated nomogram, risk groups, clinical stage, pretreatment PSA, and biopsy Gleason score.
[b] Percentages refer to proportion of total in each category.
From Stephenson AJ, Kattan MW, Eastham JA, et al. Prostate cancer-specific mortality after radical prostatectomy for patients treated in the prostate-specific antigen era. *J Clin Oncol* 2009;27:4300–4305, with permission.

TABLE 68.8

Estimates of 5- and 10-Year Progression-Free Probability in Men Undergoing Radical Prostatectomy for High-Risk Prostate Cancer

High-Risk Definition	BCR/No. of Patients	Five-Y PFP (95% CI)	Ten-Y PFP (95% CI)
Biopsy Gleason 8–10	109/274	53 (46,60)	42 (38,56)
Preoperative PSA ≥20	121/275	56 (50,62)	47 (40,54)
1992 TNM stage T3	62/144	49 (39,58)	41 (29,53)
PSA ≥20 or ≥T2c or GS ≥8	299/957	68 (65,71)	59 (55,63)
Nomogram 5-y PFP ≤50%	180/391	53 (47,57)	43 (36,49)
PSA ≥20 or ≥T3 or GS ≥8	234/605	57 (53,62)	50 (44,55)
PSA ≥15 or ≥T2b or GS ≥8	466/1,752	73 (71,75)	65 (62,68)
PSA velocity >2 ng/ml/y	161/952	80 (77,83)	74 (70,78)

BCR, biochemical relapse; PFP, progression-free probability; CI, confidence interval; PSA, prostate-specific antigen; TNM, tumor, node, metastasis; GS, Gleason score.
From Yossepowitch O, Eggener SE, Bianco FJ Jr, et al. Radical prostatectomy for clinically localized, high risk prostate cancer: critical analysis of risk assessment methods. *J Urol* 2007;178:493–499, with permission.

TABLE 68.9

Estimated 10-Year Disease-Specific Mortality After Radical Prostatectomy for Patients with High-Risk Cancer by Various Definitions

High-Risk Definition	Ten-Y DSM (95% CI)
Biopsy Gleason 8–10	12 (7–19)
Preoperative PSA ≥20	9 (6–13)
1992 TNM stage T3	11 (7–19)
PSA ≥20 or ≥T2c or GS ≥8	7 (5–9)
Nomogram 5-y PFP ≤50%	8 (6–12)
PSA ≥20 or ≥T3 or GS ≥8	8 (6–11)
PSA ≥15 or ≥T2b or GS ≥8	5 (4–7)
PSA velocity >2 ng/ml/y	3 (2–6)

DSM, disease-specific mortality; CI, confidence interval; PSA, prostate-specific antigen; TNM, tumor, node, metastasis; GS, Gleason score; PFP, progression-free probability.
From Yossepowitch O, Eggener SE, Serio AM, et al. Secondary therapy, metastatic progression, and cancer-specific mortality in men with clinically high-risk prostate cancer treated with radical prostatectomy. *Eur Urol* 2008;53:950–959, with permission.

patients. However, there are no standardized criteria to define high-risk before definitive treatment. Among 4,708 patients undergoing RP, high-risk patients were identified based on eight established definitions, and their pathologic characteristics and PSA outcomes were examined (Table 68.8). Depending on the definition used, high-risk patients composed 3% to 38% of the study population. Among patients defined as high-risk, 22% to 63% of tumors proved to be confined to the prostate on pathologic examination. Although high-risk patients had a 1.8- to 4.8-fold increased hazard of PSA relapse, their 10-year relapse-free probability after RP alone was 41% to 74% (see Table 68.8).[199] Disease-specific survival at 12 years was between 78% to 94% (Table 68.9).[200] Of the high-risk patients who relapsed, 25% (across all definitions) relapsed more than 2 years after surgery, and in 26% to 39% the PSADT at recurrence was ≥10 months. These results show that the commonly used definitions of high risk have the potential to deny patients potentially curative treatment. New criteria are needed to identify those patients who need the integration of systemic therapy to improve outcomes beyond what can be achieved with monotherapies directed to the prostate itself.[201]

Impact of the Surgeon on Outcomes After Radical Prostatectomy

Recent research has focused on the ways in which surgical volume and the individual surgeon influence results after RP. Begg et al.[202] used the Surveillance, Epidemiology, and End Results–Medicare-linked database to evaluate health-related outcomes after RP. The rates of postoperative complications, late urinary complications (strictures or fistulas 31 days to 365 days after the procedure), and long-term incontinence (>1 year after the procedure) were inferred from the Medicare claims records of 11,522 patients who underwent RP between 1992 and 1996. These rates were analyzed in relation to hospital volume and surgeon volume (the number of procedures performed at individual hospitals and by

individual surgeons, respectively). Neither hospital volume nor surgeon volume was significantly associated with surgery-related death. Significant trends in the relation between volume and outcome were observed with respect to postoperative complications and late urinary complications. Postoperative morbidity was lower in very-high-volume hospitals than in low-volume hospitals (27% versus 32%; $p = 0.03$) and was also lower when the prostatectomy was performed by very-high-volume surgeons than when it was performed by low-volume surgeons (26% versus 32%; $p < 0.001$). The rates of late urinary complications followed a similar pattern. Results for long-term preservation of continence were less clear-cut. In a detailed analysis of the 159 surgeons who performed a high or very high volume of procedures, wide surgeon-to-surgeon variations in clinical outcomes were observed, and these variations were much greater than would have been predicted on the basis of chance or observed variations in the case mix. These findings suggest that, in general, high-volume surgeons have superior results compared with low-volume surgeons, in terms of early postoperative morbidity and urinary complications after RP. However, the much better than anticipated outcomes among the highest-volume surgeons suggest that individual surgical technique also influences clinical outcomes.

Individual patient data from four institutions was used to study the association between a surgeon's prior experience and BCR after RP (the principal reason that patients visit an oncologic surgeon).[181] This relationship has often been termed the *learning curve* and probably reflects differences in surgical skill. A retrospective cohort study of consecutive patients treated from 1987 to 2003 was conducted at four academic, tertiary referral centers in the United States. In this study, 7,850 patients with localized prostate cancer received no neoadjuvant therapy and underwent open radical retropubic prostatectomy by 1 of 73 different surgeons.[179] For each patient, surgeon experience was coded as the total number of RPs conducted by the surgeon prior to the incident case, and cancer control was defined as a corroborated rising PSA level >0.4 ng/ml. The study demonstrated that cancer control improved with increasing surgeon experience (Fig. 68.10), and this relationship[181] remained highly significant ($p < 0.001$) after adjustment for tumor characteristics and year of surgery. The learning curve for cancer control after radical retropubic prostatectomy was steep but did not begin to plateau until a surgeon had completed approximately 250 prior operations. Five-year probability of BCR was 17.8% for patients treated by surgeons in the early phase of their career (10 prior operations),

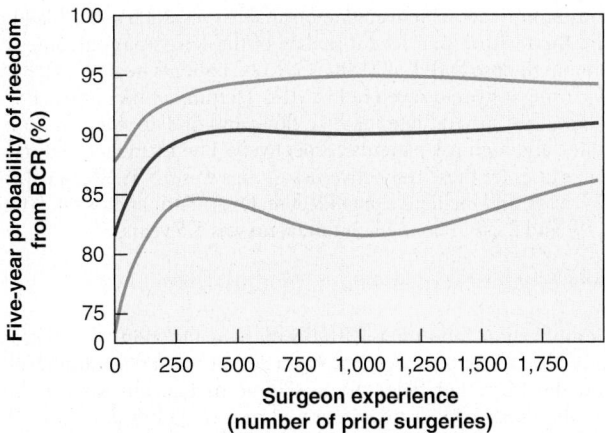

Figure 68.10 The surgical learning curve for cancer control after radical prostatectomy. Predicted probability (*purple curve*) and 95% confidence intervals (*orange curves*) for freedom from biochemical recurrence (BCR) at 5 years after radical prostatectomy are plotted against increasing surgeon experience. Probabilities are for a patient with typical cancer severity (mean prostate-specific antigen level, pathologic stage, and grade) treated in 1997 (approximately equal numbers of patients were treated before and after 1997). (From Vickers AJ, Bianco FJ, Serio AM, et al. The surgical learning curve for prostate cancer control after radical prostatectomy. *J Natl Cancer Inst* 2007;99:1171–1177, with permission.)

compared with 10.9% when surgeons had performed 250 operations (absolute risk difference, 6.9%; 95% confidence interval [CI] = 4.3% to 9.5%) (see Fig. 68.10). We saw no evidence that patient risk attenuates the learning curve: there was a statistically significant association between BCR and surgeon experience in all analyses. The relative risk for a patient receiving treatment from a surgeon with 10 rather than 250 prior RP was 2.5, 1.8, and 1.3 for low-, medium-, and high-risk patients, respectively.

Radiotherapy for Localized Prostate Cancer

Radiotherapy given by external beam or brachytherapy techniques is a second treatment option for men with clinically localized prostate cancers. With the availability of sophisticated treatment planning systems and image-guided approaches, there have been significant advances in radiotherapy enabling higher doses to be delivered more safely, and concomitant improvements in disease-free survival outcomes. Intensity-modulated external beam radiotherapy (IMRT) has become a standard mode of treatment delivery and has facilitated the application of higher radiation dose levels of ≥ 80 Gy, with lower risks of late rectal and urinary toxicities. Such treatments coupled with image guidance have enabled the routine use of tighter margins, incorporating less normal tissue within the high-dose region and leading to further decrements in late toxicities. Brachytherapy using permanent or temporary radioactive implants within the prostate alone or combined with IMRT is another commonly used radiotherapeutic approach. This approach has also improved with more accurate image guidance and intraoperative real-time planning for brachytherapy, resulting in more highly conformal dose distributions, which in turn has resulted in better outcomes and lower toxicity rates, relative to what has been previously reported. In some cases, ADT is used in several contexts: to improve local eradication of locally advanced tumors by reducing tumor size, to eliminate tumor clonogens inherently resistant to radiotherapy by impairing DNA repair pathways, and/or reducing prostate volumes by 30% to 40%, which improves the ability to deliver maximal radiation dose levels without exceeding the tolerance for the surrounding normal tissue. Hormone therapy also has a favorable effect on micrometastatic disease that may be present at the time of diagnosis in men with high-risk tumors.

Although there are no randomized trials comparing modern, sophisticated high-dose EBRT to brachytherapy for the treatment of localized prostate cancer, there are several criteria used to help select the most appropriate form of therapy for the patient. For patients with low-risk disease in whom AS may not be considered—owing to PSA velocity, the presence of a dominant lesion on imaging studies, or a larger volume of disease determined by biopsy—high-dose IMRT alone (in the range of 80 Gy) or brachytherapy alone are excellent treatment options.

Larger prostate volumes, the presence of urinary obstructive symptoms, and medical comorbidities may influence the selection away from a brachytherapy-based treatment. In contrast, brachytherapy may be the preferred choice for patients without these factors because of its excellent ablative capabilities (leading to long-term PSA relapse-free survival outcomes) and its convenience (as a treatment accomplished in a single outpatient setting). For patients with intermediate- and higher-risk disease, combined modality treatments including brachytherapy and supplemental IMRT are preferred to allow for the delivery of a high and concentrated dose of radiation to the prostate. Ultrahypofractionated EBRT regimens have generated increasing interest as another therapeutic option for patients with localized disease; however, the long-term results of this approach are not available, and the results of ongoing trials are awaiting more mature follow-up.

External Beam Radiotherapy

Intensity-Modulated Radiotherapy and Image-Guided Techniques

IMRT, a type of conformal radiotherapy (CRT), has become a standard mode of treatment planning for patients with localized prostate cancer and takes advantage of inverse-planning methods to optimize dose distribution. Inverse planning is part of a mathematical optimization algorithm that creates a treatment plan based on predefined, desired dose-distribution parameters for the target and dose constraints imposed on the normal tissues. The highly conformal radiation beam is produced with the ability to vary the intensities of the X-rays from each treatment field over the entire cross-section of the beam.

More recently, image-guided approaches have enhanced IMRT delivery. Acquisition of CT images or kilovoltage images on the treatment machine immediately before the radiation treatment allows for visualization of the target and correction of its position, which can fluctuate on a daily basis, related to bladder or rectal filling. Linac-based kilovoltage image guidance systems have become commercially available; they possess capabilities for kilovoltage two-dimensional projection imaging (radiographs), fluoroscopy, and three-dimensional cone beam CT, and are thus ideally suited for monitoring inter- and intrafractional motion. The use of image-guided radiotherapy and enhanced target localization could lead to a further reduction of safety margins and a decrease in morbidity related to ultrahypofractionated regimens. A recent retrospective report demonstrated reduced urinary-related treatment toxicities and improved tumor control outcomes among patients with clinically localized prostate cancer treated with image-guided approaches, compared with patients not treated with image-guided therapy.[203] Among a cohort of patients treated to dose levels of 86.4 Gy, the incidence of late grade 2 urinary toxicities was 20% for those treated with daily image guidance, compared with 10% for patients treated with daily image guidance and target positional corrections ($p = 0.02$)

Definition of Target Volume

The multifocal nature of prostate cancer and the well-documented risk of microscopic ECE, even for patients with early clinical stages of disease, are important considerations that influence the design of the target volume for radiation treatment planning. The clinical target volume (CTV) includes the entire prostate gland and immediate periprostatic tissues, as well as the seminal vesicles, as visualized on CT. For patients with low-risk disease with unremarkable imaging studies, the CTV may exclude the seminal vesicles, owing to the low likelihood of disease involvement. The planning target volume places an additional margin around the CTV to take into account patient setup uncertainties and organ motion. With the use of image-guided approaches, the margin can be safely reduced to 5 mm to 6 mm around the CTV, except at the prostate-rectal interface, where an even tighter margin (3 mm to 5 mm) is used.

Role of Dose Escalation in Patients with Clinically Localized Disease

Findings from several randomized phase 3 trials (Table 68.10)[204–208] and the long-term results of single-institution studies[209–212] demonstrate a significant improvement in treatment outcomes with higher radiation doses in patients with clinically localized disease. As shown in Table 68.10, these studies have generally demonstrated a 10% to 20% improvement in 5- to 10-year PSA survival outcomes when higher doses of 78 Gy to 80 Gy are applied, compared with dose levels of 70 Gy, and such benefits have been observed for low-, intermediate-, and high-risk cohorts. Although overall survival benefits have not been demonstrated with dose escalation, improvements in distant metastases–free survival are emerging with longer follow-up, suggesting that survival benefits will be seen as these studies mature. In one report, a reduction in death due to prostate cancer was noted at 10 years for intermediate- and high-risk patients treated with doses of 78 Gy, compared with those treated at 70 Gy.[213]

For patients with intermediate- and especially high-risk disease, doses beyond 80 Gy may be required to achieve optimal tumor control outcomes. To do so requires ultra-high-dose IMRT, which constrains the dose delivered to normal tissues, such as the bladder and the rectum. In a recent update of the long-term outcomes of ultra-high-dose IMRT at MSKCC, 1,002 patients treated with 86.4 Gy, using a five- to seven-field IMRT technique, had 7-year PSA-relapse-free survival rates of 99%, 86%, and 68% for low-, intermediate-, and high-risk patients, respectively. The incidence of distant metastases for these respective risk groups was 0.5%, 6%, and 18% at 7 years, and incidence of grade 3 rectal and urinary toxicities was 0.7% and 2.2%. The median follow-up was 5.5 years.[214]

Sequelae of External Beam Radiotherapy

Complication rates after EBRT vary as a function of the dose, the volume of normal tissues irradiated at particular dose levels, and the treatment field. Acute symptoms typically appear during the third week of treatment and resolve within days to weeks after its completion. Acute intestinal symptoms, especially those associated with whole pelvic irradiation, are most commonly relieved with dietary manipulations. Otherwise, medications such as loperamide hydrochloride (Imodium; McNEIL-PPC, Inc., Fort Washington, PA) or diphenoxylate hydrochloride and atropine sulphate (Lomotil; Pfizer, New York, NY) are appropriate to relieve symptoms. Internal and external hemorrhoids, which may become inflamed during the course of therapy, are often best treated with sitz baths and hydrocortisone suppositories. Patients may also experience changes in the consistency of their bowel movements or an increase in mucous discharge. Acute urinary symptoms are treated with phenazopyridine hydrochloride (Pyridium; Warner Chilcott, Rockaway, NJ), nonsteroidal anti-inflammatory agents, or alpha-blockers, such as tamsulosin hydrochloride (Flomax; Boehringer Ingelheim Pharmaceuticals, Inc., Ridgefield, CT). Alpha-blockers have been reported to be significantly more effective than nonsteroidal anti-inflammatory agents, resulting in significant resolution of urinary symptoms in 66% of patients and moderate improvement in 22%.[215]

TABLE 68.10

Phase 3 External Beam Radiotherapy Dose Escalation Studies

Study (Ref.)	No. of Patients	Median Follow-Up	Treatment Arms	PSA Relapse-Free Survival Outcome	P Value
Beckendorf et al.[204]/ GETUG 06	306	5 y	80 Gy vs. 70 Gy	At 5 y: Overall results High dose, 72% Low dose, 61%	0.039
Al-Mamgani et al.[205]	669	70 mo	78 vs. 68 Gy (neoadjuvant short-term and long-term ADT used in two participating institutions for high-risk patients)	At 7 y: Intermediate- and high-risk patients High dose, 54% Low dose, 47%	<0.04
Kuban et al.[206]	301	8.7 y	78 vs. 70 Gy (no ADT given)	At 8 y: Overall results High dose, 78% Low dose, 59% At 8 y: PSA >10 ng/ml High dose, 78% Low dose, 39%	0.004 <0.001
Zietman et al.[207]	393	8.9 y	79.2 Gy equivalent vs. 70.2 Gy equivalent (dose delivered with combination of protons/photons)	At 10 y: Overall results High dose, 83% Low dose, 68% At 10 y: Low-risk patients High dose, 93% Low dose, 72%	<0.001 <0.001
Dearnaley et al.[208]/ MRC-RT01	843	10 y	74 vs. 64 Gy 30-CRT (3–6 mo neoadjuvant + concurrent ADT administered)	At 10 y: Low-risk patients High dose, 55% Low dose, 43%	0.0003

PSA, prostate-specific antigen; GETUG, Genitourinary Tumor Group; ADT, androgen deprivation therapy; MRC, Medical Research Council; CRT, conformal radiotherapy.

Late rectal toxicities attributed to radiotherapy typically manifest 12 months to 18 months after completion of treatment and may persist for several years thereafter; the development of rectal complications after 5 years is rare. Late rectal toxicities may include rectal bleeding, mucous discharge, and mild incontinence of stool. The more-severe toxicities, including ulcer development and fistula formation, are observed in ≤1% of patients. Grade 2 rectal bleeding can be effectively treated with steroid suppositories, sitz baths, and an increase in dietary fiber. Because of the increased risk of further trauma to the rectal mucosa and the risk of fistula formation, deep rectal biopsies and cauterization procedures should be avoided unless absolutely necessary. For radiation-induced proctitis not responsive to conservative measures, argon-beam plasma laser coagulation can decrease the frequency of rectal bleeding episodes.[216] Hyperbaric oxygen treatments, at a pressure of 2.4 atmospheres for a median of 36 sessions (90 minutes per session), may be helpful; in one study, they were associated with a complete resolution of rectal bleeding in 48% of patients and a reduction in bleeding episodes in 28% of patients.[217] It is assumed that hyperbaric oxygen improves the delivery of oxygen to ischemic rectal mucosa, promoting angiogenesis and advancing mucosal healing and fibroblast proliferation.

Late urinary toxicities include chronic urethritis, which occurs in approximately 10% to 15% of patients, and urethral strictures, which occur in 2% to 3%. Hemorrhagic cystitis is uncommon with conformal radiation techniques, which reduce the dose to the bladder. Current treatment approaches for hemorrhagic cystitis include intravesical formalin therapy and selective embolization of the hypogastric arteries. For patients refractory to such measures, hyperbaric oxygen therapy can be considered for radiation-induced hemorrhagic cystitis. In one report, 49 of 57 patients (86%) experienced complete resolution or marked improvement of hematuria following hyperbaric oxygen treatment.[218]

Whereas any form of radiotherapy can increase the risk of developing a secondary cancer, the incidence after prostate radiotherapy appears to be lower than expected. One report comparing the risks of secondary cancers among patients treated with RP, EBRT, and brachytherapy did not find the therapeutic intervention to be a significant predictor of secondary cancer at 10-year follow-up.[219] Longer follow-up will be required to determine whether any significant differences eventually develop between the treatment arms. Nonetheless, given the risk of secondary cancer with any form of radiotherapy, close monitoring is important. Colonoscopy every 5 years and careful evaluation of patients who present with hematuria after radiotherapy are recommended to rule out the possibility of a secondary bladder cancer.

IMRT is also associated with a reduced risk of rectal-related toxicities after high-dose radiotherapy. In the initial cohort of patients treated with 81 Gy, late rectal and urinary complications were significantly reduced with IMRT relative to conventional three-dimensional CRT (Fig. 68.11). In 561 patients treated with IMRT (81 Gy) at MSKCC,[220] the 8-year actuarial likelihood of developing grade 2 rectal bleeding was 1.6% with no grade 4 events and late grade 2 and 3 (urethral strictures) urinary toxicities were 9% and 3%, respectively. Among patients who were potent before IMRT, 49% developed erectile dysfunction.[220]

Factors predictive of late urinary toxicities after high-dose IMRT included a lower baseline urinary symptom score (International Prostate Symptoms Score) ($p = 0.006$) and an increased maximal dose beyond the prescribed dose to the bladder trigone region ($p = 0.003$).[221] When high-dose radiotherapy is used, efforts should be made to restrict the high-dose region from receiving >15% to 20% of the prescription doses for the urethra and, in particular, for the bladder neck and the region of the bladder trigone. These and other data indicate that patients with significant urinary symptoms before treatment may be better served by surgery, rather than radiotherapy.

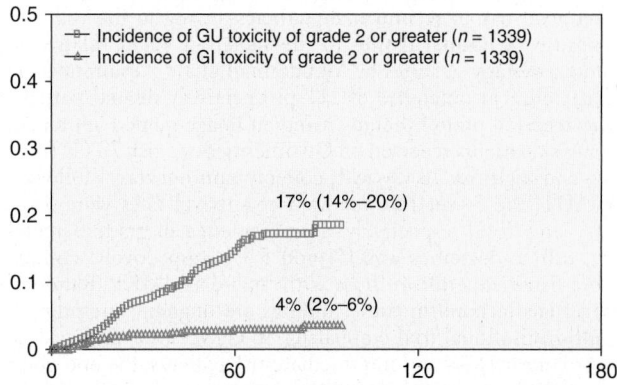

Figure 68.11 Incidence of grade 2 or greater genitourinary (GU) and gastrointestinal (GI) toxicities for patients receiving intensity-modulated radiation therapy only for patients treated at Memorial Sloan Kettering Cancer Center. *X-axis* represents months from completion of treatment. *Y-axis* represents the percentage incidence of toxicity.

Potency Preservation with External Beam Radiotherapy

The reported rates of impotence at 3 years or longer after EBRT ranges widely from 36% to 68%,[222] a reflection of the differences in methodologies used to assess this end point and the heterogeneity of the EBRT patient population. Factors such as advanced age and the presence of medical comorbidities (coronary artery disease, diabetes, and use of antihypertensive medications) can have a profound effect on erectile function. Besides erectile dysfunction, aspects of sexual dysfunction that occur after radiotherapy include decreased volume of ejaculate, absence of ejaculate, decreased intensity of orgasm, and decreased libido.

Hypofractionated External Beam Radiotherapy

The administration of larger doses for each treatment fraction has potential radiobiologic advantages (hypofractionated radiotherapy) that can result in a greater degree of cell kill.[223,224] One approach is stereotactic body radiosurgery, which has been used increasingly during the last several years. Unfortunately, most reports to date are uncontrolled single-center series of selected patients which, despite recognized limitations, are showing promising results using PSA-based outcomes.[225–227] These treatments are delivered with a linear accelerator mounted with an image-guided device to achieve greater precision of the dose delivery. With tight margins used, high doses per fraction allow completion of the course of therapy in 1 week. A pooled analysis of 1,100 patients treated from 2003 to 2011 at eight institutions was recently reported.[228] The median dose delivered for these patients was 36.25 Gy in five fractions. The median follow-up was 3 years; the 5-year PSA-relapse-free survival rates were 95%, 84%, and 81% for low-, intermediate-, and high-risk patients, repsectively. Stereotactic radiosurgery appears promising, but this form of treatment cannot be considered an established form of radiotherapy delivery, and ongoing studies will define its role better in the years ahead.

The Role of Proton Therapy for Localized Prostate Cancer

Recently, there has been increasing interest in the use of proton therapy for clinically localized disease because of the known physical advantages of this charged particle—namely, the Bragg peak—by which the majority of the energy of the beam is deposited at the end of its track, creating a rapid falloff of dose beyond the target. The result is that exit dose beyond the target volume is eliminated, providing the potential to achieve greater sparing of normal tissues with dose escalation. Theoretically, physical advantages of the proton beam may also translate into a reduced risk of second malignancies, owing to the reduced exposure of normal tissues to the radiation beam relative to photon therapy. A series by Mendenhall et al.[229] examined the 5-year clinical outcomes of 211 prospectively treated patients who received proton therapy using an image-guided approach. Low-risk patients received 78 Gy, intermediate-risk 78 Gy to 82 Gy, and high-risk 78 Gy with concomitant docetaxel followed by ADT; the 5-year PSA-relapse-free survival rates were 99%, 99%, and 76%, respectively. The incidence of grade 3 rectal and urinary toxicities was 1% and 5.4%, respectively, comparable if not superior to those with high-dose IMRT. Randomized trials to confirm these findings are ongoing, including a multi-institutional trial comparing 80 Gy versus a similar dose of protons for low- and intermediate-risk patients; the end point is 2-year QOL and late toxicities.

Reports addressing the question of whether protons are associated with reduced long-term toxicities relative to high-dose photon therapy are conflicting. One recent study of 1,242 patients treated with either proton therapy at doses of 76 Gy to 82 Gy or IMRT at doses of 75.6 Gy to 79.4 Gy showed similar QOL scores for the bowel, urinary incontinence, urinary irritative symptoms, and sexual domains at the last follow-up evaluation. Further exploration of specific function outcomes showed that patients treated with proton therapy had less frequent bowel movements and rectal urgency, compared with patients treated with IMRT.[230] However, an analysis of the relative toxicities of IMRT and proton therapy in patients with localized prostate cancer based on the Surveillance, Epidemiology, and End Results–Medicare-linked database showed that IMRT was associated with fewer gastrointestinal (GI)-related toxicities and hip fractures, whereas proton therapy was associated with a lower risk of erectile dysfunction.[231] It is anticipated that future improvements in intensity-modulated proton therapy will also improve the conformality of the proton beam, resulting in fewer complications with proton dose escalation. To date, however, there is no established evidence that proton therapy provides superior tumor control outcomes, compared with well-delivered high-dose IMRT or image-guided radiotherapy, for the treatment of prostate cancer.

Prostate Brachytherapy

Excellent long-term tumor control can be achieved with brachytherapy, and the approach is considered a standard treatment intervention associated with outcomes comparable to those with prostatectomy and EBRT for patients with clinically localized disease.[232–237] By category, low-risk disease is managed with seed implantation alone (i.e., monotherapy), whereas intermediate- and selected high-risk disease is managed with a combination of brachytherapy (low-dose-rate [LDR] permanent interstitial implantation or high-dose-rate [HDR] brachytherapy via after-loading catheters) and EBRT. Whether the addition of EBRT is necessary in all patients with intermediate-risk prostate cancer is being studied in a phase 3 randomized trial (Radiation Therapy Oncology Group [RTOG] 0232).

Technical Aspects of Prostate Brachytherapy

Transperineal ultrasound-guided approaches have facilitated image-guided placement of the seeds and are credited with improved long-term outcomes and reduced treatment-related complications. These approaches have further improved the accuracy and consistency of the dose delivery to the target, with a concomitant reduction of dose to the urethra and rectum. The use of adjunctive intraoperative CT scanning to verify the actual deposited seed coordinates may eliminate the need for postimplantation assessments and may allow for opportunities, if necessary, to correct suboptimal implanted regions within the gland before the reversal of anesthesia. Close collaboration between the radiation oncologist and the medical physicist in

the design of the pre- or intraoperative treatment plan is critical for a successful outcome.

The two most commonly used radioisotopes for permanent seed brachytherapy are iodine-125 (^{125}I) and palladium-103 (^{103}Pd). The half-life of ^{125}I is 60 days, with a mean photon energy of 27 KeV and an initial dose rate of 0.07 Gy/h. In contrast, the half-life of ^{103}Pd is 17 days, with a mean photon energy of 21 KeV and an initial dose rate of 0.19 cGy/h. The active periods for ^{125}I and ^{103}Pd are 10 months and 3 months, respectively. When ^{125}I is used, the typical prescription dose is 144 Gy; 125 Gy is routinely used for ^{103}Pd.

The quality of the implant and dose distributions are routinely evaluated using CT scans obtained on the day of the implant or 30 days later. Postimplantation CT scans are used to generate dose-volume histograms, which allow detailed analysis of the radiation dose distribution relative to the prostate and surrounding normal tissues. Dosimetric parameters include V100 for the target (volume of the prostate receiving 100% of the prescription dose), D90 of the target (dose delivered to 90% of the prostate), and the average and maximum rectal and urethral doses.[238]

Table 68.11 summarizes the published biochemical control outcomes after LDR interstitial seed implantation, according to prognostic risk groups.[235,237,239–243] The size of the prostate gland should preferably be <60 cm^3 and optimally <50 cm^3. In larger gland sizes, the pubic arch may interfere with needle placement reaching the anterolateral portions of the gland, resulting in inadequate dose coverage of the target volume. Larger glands require more seeds and activity to achieve coverage of the gland with the prescription dose, which may result in an increase in the central urethral doses and potentially increase the risk of urinary morbidity.[244] The size of the prostate can be effectively addressed with combined androgen-blockade therapy. An approximately 30% reduction in volume is commonly observed after 3 months of ADT. For patients who have imaging findings consistent with gross ECE or SVI not detected on rectal examination, monotherapy is not sufficient, and supplemental EBRT should be considered.

Patients with a significant degree of urinary obstructive symptoms are more prone to develop prolonged morbidity after brachytherapy and would be better suited to other treatment interventions. A previous TURP may increase the risk of urinary morbidity after seed implantation[245]; brachytherapy should be performed with caution in such patients. Careful attention to dose-volume considerations to the periurethral region and the area of the TURP defect should reduce the likelihood of long-term morbidities.

Seed implantation may be a more suitable intervention for patients with bilateral hip replacements, in whom CT-based treatment planning is technically difficult because of the substantial artifact created by the prosthesis, precluding adequate visualization of the target volume. Ultrasound-based seed implantation would be an appropriate alternative for such patients, as artifacts would not pose a difficulty with this imaging modality. In most cases, patients with hip prostheses are able to tolerate the extended dorsal lithotomy position for adequate perineal exposure during seed implantation. Patients with small bowel in close proximity to the prostate volume are also better suited to brachytherapy, owing to the lower doses to the bowel expected with brachytherapy. Brachytherapy may be safe for patients with a history of inflammatory bowel disease, a condition that represents a relative contraindication for EBRT. Of 24 patients with a history of inflammatory bowel disease who were treated with brachytherapy, none experienced grade 3 or higher rectal toxicities (median follow-up, 4 years), but late grade 2 rectal bleeding (19%) was significantly higher than among patients without a history of inflammatory bowel disease.[246]

Transient urinary morbidity related to radiation-induced urethritis or prostatitis represents the most common side effect following seed implantation. Symptoms include urinary frequency, urgency,

TABLE 68.11

Prostate-Specific Antigen Relapse-Free Survival Outcomes for Low-Dose–Rate Brachytherapy

Study (Ref.)	No. of Patients	Median Follow-Up (y)	Treatment	Five-Y Biochemical Outcome According to Risk Group	Comments
Stock et al.[239]	1,377	4.2	MT/CMT	Low, 94% Intermediate, 89.5% High, 78%	Interactive real-time planning
Zelefsky et al.[237]	2,693	5.2	MT	Low, 82% Intermediate, 70% High, 48%	D90 ≥130 Gy 8-y PSA control, 93% D90 <130 Gy 8-y PSA control, 76%
Guedea et al.[240]	1,050	2.5	MT	Low, 93% Intermediate, 88% High, 80%	—
Khaksar et al.[241]	300	4	MT	Low, 96% Intermediate, 89% High, 93%	—
Zelefsky et al.[242]	367	5.3	MT	Low, 96% Intermediate, 89%	Real-time intraoperative planned implants
Sylvester et al.[243]	232	9.4	CMT	Low, 86% Intermediate, 80% Unfavorable, 68%	—
Potters et al.[235]	1,449	7	MT/CMT	Low, 89% Intermediate, 78% Unfavorable, 63%	—

MT, monotherapy; CMT, combined-modality therapy (implant + external beam); D90, the dose received by 90% of the prostate; PSA, prostate-specific antigen.

and dysuria, which usually peak 1 to 3 months after the implant procedure and gradually resolve during the subsequent months. The incidence of urinary symptoms persisting after 1 year is 15% to 25%; the risk of urethral strictures ranges from 1% to 12%. The incidence of grade 3 and 4 rectal or urinary toxicities, including urinary or rectal incontinence, is ≤1% (Table 68.12).[239,242,247–255]

The incidence of grade 2 rectal toxicity after prostate brachytherapy ranges from 2% to 5%[247,256,257]; grade 3 or 4 rectal toxicity is unusual (<2%). These results are similar to late toxicities observed after high-dose EBRT. Meticulous attention to needle and seed placement, as well as to the intraoperative dose-volume histogram data on normal tissue, should reduce rectal doses and lower risks of toxicity to minimal levels.

Erectile Function After Brachytherapy

Impotence rates after prostate brachytherapy and EBRT are likely underestimated in the literature. With longer follow-up, observations and responses from patient surveys indicate that approximately 40% to 50% of patients maintain erectile function after prostate brachytherapy.[258,259] Preimplant erectile-function score and the dose to 50% of the proximal crura of the penis have been shown to be significant predictors of erectile dysfunction.[258]

Excellent responses have been observed with sildenafil citrate in the treatment of impotence after brachytherapy and EBRT. In one report,[259] 80% of patients responded to the medication. With long-term follow-up, 37% of patients discontinued use of the medication. Similar responses have been reported for patients who developed erectile dysfunction after EBRT and were treated with sildenafil citrate. There has been increasing interest in the use of sildenafil before the development of erectile dysfunction to reduce the risk of erectile dysfunction after treatment. The RTOG randomized patients to receive sildenafil following radiotherapy but before the development of erectile dysfunction and found no

demonstrable benefit.[260] However, a recent randomized trial from MSKCC showed improvements in sexual function parameters 12 months and 24 months after therapy among patients treated with prophylactic sildenafil, compared with those who received placebo.[261]

Combined Brachytherapy and External Beam Radiotherapy

Combined brachytherapy and EBRT is considered to be a more suitable treatment option than implantation alone for patients with unfavorable intermediate- or high-risk disease. The combined approach effectively delivers an increased dose of radiation that has been estimated to have a biologic equivalent that well exceeds a 100-Gy dose of EBRT. Conventional or conformal-based techniques are used to deliver 45 Gy to 50 Gy of EBRT to the prostate and periprostatic tissues. If an LDR boost is used, the brachytherapy prescription dose is 90 Gy to 100 Gy for ^{103}Pd implants and 110 Gy for ^{125}I implants. In the absence of clinical trials comparing HDR brachytherapy boosts with LDR boosts or establishing the optimal sequence of therapy (brachytherapy boost preceding EBRT or vice versa) or the preferred isotope to be used for combined-modality therapy, there is no definitive evidence demonstrating the superiority of a particular treatment strategy over another.

The phase 3 trial RTOG 0232 is comparing permanent-source brachytherapy as monotherapy with EBRT followed by brachytherapy for patients with intermediate-risk prostate cancer. The study is ongoing but no longer recruiting patients. The primary end point of this study is survival; secondary end points include PSA-relapse-free survival, distant metastases–free survival, and QOL. Eligibility criteria for this study include clinical stage T1c–T2b and either Gleason score <7 with a PSA level of 10 ng/ml to 20 ng/ml, or Gleason score of 7 with a PSA level <10 ng/ml. The American Urological Association voiding symptom score should be ≤15, and prostate volume should be <60 g.

Late Toxicity Outcomes After Prostate Brachytherapy

Study (Ref.)	No. of Patients	Median Follow-Up (y)	Genitourinary	Gastrointestinal
Stock et al.[239]	325 Incontinence, 1%	7	Grade 3, 2% (urethral stricture)	Grade ≤2, 24% Grade 3–4, 0%
Waterman and Dicker[248]	98	3		Grade 2, 10%
Merrick et al.[247]	1,186	4.3	Grade 3, 3.6% Urethral stricture	
Gelblum et al.[249,250]	825	4	Grade 3, 4.7% 17% post TURP developed incontinence	Grade 1, 9% Grade 2, 6.6% Grade 3, 0.5%
Bottomley et al.[251]	667	2.5	Acute retention, 14.5% Late retention, 1% Urethritis at 6 months, 13.5% Urethritis at 24 months, 2.5%	Grade 4, <1%
Lee et al.[252] (RTOG 0019)	138	4	Late ≥ grade 3 gastrointestinal/ genitourinary, 15% (combined-modality therapy)	
Shah et al.[253]	135	3.5		Diarrhea, 7.3% Urgency, 6.5% Bleeding, 7.3%
Keyes et al.[254]	805	3.3	AUR: IPSS 0–5, 8% IPSS 10–15, 15% IPSS >16, 21%	
Albert et al.[255]	201	2.8	Radiation-cystitis Monotherapy, 0% Combined-modality therapy, 5%	Grade 3 Monotherapy, 8% Combined-modality therapy, 30%
Zelefsky et al.[242]	367	5.2	Grade 2, 19% Grade 3, 4%	Grade 2, 7% Grade 3, 1%

TURP, transurethral resection of the prostate; RTOG, Radiation Therapy Oncology Group; AUR, acute urinary retention; IPSS, International Prostate Symptom Score.

High-Dose-Rate Brachytherapy

HDR brachytherapy has been used in combination with EBRT for the treatment of prostate cancer.[262–266] Patients undergo ultrasound-guided transperineal placement of afterloading catheters in the prostate. After CT-based treatment planning, several high-dose fractions, ranging from 4 Gy to 6 Gy each, are administered during an interval of 24 hours to 36 hours using ^{192}Ir, followed by supplemental EBRT directed to the prostate and periprostatic tissues at a dose of 45 Gy to 50.4 Gy using conventional fractionation. The results of a randomized trial[267] comparing hypofractionated EBRT at 55 Gy in 20 fractions with EBRT at 35.75 Gy in 13 fractions followed by an HDR brachytherapy boost of 17 Gy in two fractions delivered over 24 hours showed a 7-year likelihood of biochemical control of 66% in the combined-modality group versus 48% in the EBRT group (*p* = 0.04).

HDR brachytherapy offers several potential advantages over other techniques. Taking advantage of an afterloading approach, the radiation oncologist and physicist can more easily optimize the delivery of radiotherapy to the prostate, reducing the potential for underdosage ("cold spots"). This technique also reduces radiation exposure to the radiation oncologist and others involved in the procedure, compared with that from permanent interstitial implantation. Finally, HDR brachytherapy boosts may be radiobiologically more efficacious in terms of tumor cell kill for patients with increased tumor bulk or adverse prognostic features, compared with LDR boosts using ^{125}I or [103]Pd.

Selecting the Optimal Radiotherapeutic Approach for Localized Disease Adapted for Risk Group

For patients with low-risk disease who have significant volume of disease (≥50% cores involved by cancer on the diagnostic biopsy), increasing PSA velocity, or a dominant lesion noted on MRI, a treatment intervention would be often indicated. For such patients, brachytherapy as monotherapy or IMRT at dose levels of 80 Gy would be appropriate and associated with biochemical outcomes of approximately 90% at 10 years. In these cases, brachytherapy is preferred over IMRT, given the convenience of a single treatment accomplished in an outpatient setting. Patients with significant urinary obstructive symptoms or other medical comorbidities may be better suited to IMRT. Patients with enlarged prostate glands of 60 ml to 90 ml are best treated with ADT to reduce the size of the gland before brachytherapy which in most cases, will result in a 30% volume reduction in 3 to 4 months.

For patients with intermediate- or high-risk disease, doses higher than 80 Gy may be necessary to achieve further improvement in local tumor control. In the absence of randomized trials comparing the efficacy of various forms of radiotherapy to deliver high dose levels for patients with intermediate- and high-risk disease, it has been our preference to recommend for these patients brachytherapy in combination with image-guided EBRT. In a recent study from MSKCC comparing intermediate-risk patients treated with brachytherapy combined with supplemental

IMRT versus IMRT alone to levels of 86.4 Gy, the 7-year actuarial prostate PSA-relapse-free survival rates were 81.4% versus 92.0% (p <0.001) and distant metastases–free survival rates were 93.0% versus 97.2% (p = 0.04) for IMRT alone versus brachytherapy combined with IMRT, respectively. Multivariate analysis demonstrated that brachytherapy combined with IMRT boost was associated with better PSA-relapse-free survival (hazard ratio [HR] = 0.40; 95% CI = 0.24 to 0.66; p <0.001) and better distant metastases–free survival (HR = 0.41 [0.18 to 0.92]; p = 0.03). The tradeoff was a higher rate of acute urinary grade 2 symptoms in the combined treatment arm, which in most cases gradually resolved with time. Late toxicity outcomes were 4.6% versus 4.1% for grade 2 GI toxicity (p = 0.89), 0.4% versus 1.4% for grade 3 GI toxicity (p = 0.36), 19.4% versus 21.2% for grade 2 genitourinary toxicity (p = 0.14), and 3.1% versus 1.4% for grade 3 genitourinary toxicity (p = 0.74) for the IMRT versus the combination RT groups, respectively.

Androgen Deprivation Therapy and Radiotherapy

ADT has been used as part of a combined modality approach with radiation, and randomized trials have demonstrated improved outcomes, including an overall survival benefit for this combination, compared with radiotherapy alone. The uses include neoadjuvant and concurrent; neoadjuvant, concurrent, and adjuvant; and concurrent and adjuvant. It is routinely recommended for patients with high-risk disease and selected patients with intermediate-risk disease when used in combination with EBRT. Reported trials, however, vary in the total dose of radiation used to the primary site, whether pelvic radiation was utilized, as well as the duration and timing of ADT. The end points also vary from PSA recurrence alone, whether a biopsy of the gland was performed to assess for local disease control, to the documentation of metastatic disease or death. For many, follow-up is simply too short to draw definitive conclusions. Recognizing these caveats, outcomes and indications for use in practice are summarized.

Randomized Trials for High-Risk Disease

Table 68.13[268–270] summarizes the outcomes of randomized trials comparing radiotherapy alone to radiotherapy combined with ADT for patients with locally advanced high-risk prostate cancer. These trials have consistently demonstrated improved outcomes when ADT is combined with EBRT and the administered dose is ≥70 Gy (see Table 68.10).

Several trials have used adjuvant hormonal therapy for various durations after EBRT and demonstrated long-term disease-free survival benefits. In another important randomized trial, the European Organization for Research and Treatment of Cancer (EORTC) 22863, node-negative patients with clinical stage T3 disease or T1–T2 patients with high-grade disease received adjuvant ADT on the first day of radiotherapy (prescribed dose of 70 Gy) and continued for 3 years. Improved outcomes were observed for all parameters, including absolute survival (median follow-up, 9 years).[271] The 10-year overall survival was 58% versus 40% for patients treated with ADT plus EBRT and EBRT alone, respectively (p = 0.0004). In addition, the 10-year PCSM rates for these respective cohorts of patients were 10% and 30% (p <0.0001).

The duration of ADT was addressed in RTOG 92-02, the first ADT trial performed with baseline PSA information available, which randomized patients with clinical T2–T4 disease with PSA baseline levels <150 ng/ml to receive either neoadjuvant and concurrent ADT for a total of 4 months or the same therapy plus an additional 24 months of adjuvant ADT for a total of 28 months. The prescribed radiation dose levels used in this study ranged from 65 Gy to 70 Gy. At a median follow-up of 5.8 years, the results showed that all outcomes were improved for patients who received 28 months with the exception of overall survival. A subset analysis,

however, showed a 10% overall survival advantage for patients with Gleason scores of 8 to 10 who were treated with the longer course of ADT.[272]

RTOG 94-13 evaluated two sequencing regimens of adjuvant ADT as well as the role of pelvic radiotherapy in the setting of treatment with ADT in patients with T2c–T4 disease or those with an estimated LN risk ≥15%. The radiation dose administered was 70.2 Gy in 39 fractions. Patients were randomized to receive either 4 months of ADT before and during radiotherapy or 4 months of ADT as adjuvant therapy following the completion of EBRT. Patients were also randomized to receive either whole-pelvic radiotherapy or treatment directed to the prostate only. Neoadjuvant and concurrent ADT in conjunction with whole-pelvic radiotherapy was associated with a trend for an improved progression-free survival (PFS) compared to the other study arms (48% PFS for neoadjuvant ADT and whole-pelvic radiotherapy versus 40% for prostate only radiotherapy and adjuvant ADT; p = 0.065).[273]

Randomized Trials for Intermediate-Risk Disease

Recent studies have explored the role of ADT for patients with earlier stages of disease. D'Amico et al.[274] reported the results of a randomized trial comparing 70 Gy of three-dimensional CRT alone or a similar dose of radiotherapy combined with 6 months of ADT (initiated 2 months before radiotherapy). Of note, most of the patients included in this study had intermediate-risk disease—namely, pretreatment PSA levels 10 ng/ml to 40 ng/ml or Gleason score >7 with T1–T2 disease. Overall 5-year (median follow-up, 4.5 years) survival advantage was demonstrated for the combination-therapy regimen, compared with radiotherapy alone (88% versus 78%; p = 0.04). RTOG 9408[269] compared radiation alone with radiation plus 4 months of ADT (starting 2 months before radiation) in 1,979 patients with stage T1b, T1c, T2a, or T2b prostate cancer and a PSA level ≤20 ng/ml. The total EBRT dose was 66.6 Gy, 46.8 Gy delivered to the pelvis (prostate and regional LN), followed by 19.8 Gy to the prostate (see Table 68.13). Low-risk disease was defined as a Gleason score ≤6, PSA level ≤10 ng/ml, and clinical stage T2a or lower; intermediate-risk disease was defined as a Gleason score of 7, Gleason score ≤6 and PSA level from 10 ng/ml to 20 ng/ml, or clinical stage T2b; and high-risk disease was defined as a Gleason score of 8 to 10. The 10-year overall survival (median follow-up, 9.1 years) was 62% for EBRT + ADT, compared with 57% for EBRT alone (p = 0.03). The addition of ADT decreased 10-year PCSM from 8% to 4% (p = 0.001). The reduction in risk was primarily observed in intermediate-risk patients; no significant reductions in mortality were noted among low-risk patients. Conclusions from this trial are limited by the dose of radiation administered, which was far lower than contemporary standards. Nevertheless, this study provides further level I evidence that short-course ADT is associated with a survival benefit when combined with subtherapeutic doses of EBRT. A subsequent trial in a similar patient population showed that 8 months of ADT was not superior to 3 months of therapy. This multi-institutional phase 3 study from Canada[275] randomized 378 patients to receive either 3 months or 8 months of total androgen blockade. Conventional radiotherapy at 66 Gy was initiated within 2 weeks of completion of the ADT regimen. In this trial, 31% of the patients were considered to have high-risk disease; the remaining patients had low- or intermediate-risk disease. No differences in any of the end points, including BCR-free survival, were observed.

The various trials have used different sequences to deliver ADT, and the eligibility criteria have not been consistent. Nevertheless, some broad conclusions can be drawn regarding the optimal integration of ADT with radiotherapy. For patients with high-risk cancers, and in particular high-grade cancers, ADT is indicated and adjuvant courses of hormonal therapy that extend ≥2 years

TABLE 68.13

Randomized Trials Involving Hormone Therapy and Radiation Therapy for Locally Advanced Prostate Cancer

Trial	Eligibility	Arms	LF (%)	DM (%)	bNED (%)	DFS (%)	OS (%)
RTOG 85-31	T3 (15%) or T1-2, N+ or path T3 and (+) margin or (+) SV	RT (HT at failure) vs. RT + AHT indefinite	10-y: 38 vs. 23 (p <0.0001)	10-y: 39 vs. 24 (p <0.0001)	10-y: 9 vs. 31 (p <0.0001)	10-y: 23 vs. 37 (p <0.0001)	10-y: 39 vs. 49 (p = 0.002)
EORTC 22863	T3-4 (89%) or T1-2 WHO 3	RT vs. RT + CAHT 3 y	5-y: 16.4 vs. 1.7 (p <0.0001)	5-y: 29.2 vs. 9.8 (p <0.0001)	5-y: 45 vs. 76 (p <0.0001)	5-y: 40 vs. 74 (p <0.0001)	5-y: 62 vs.78 (p = 0.0002)
RTOG 86-10	Bulky T2b, T3-4, N+ allowed	RT vs. RT + NHT (TAB) 3.7 mo	8-y: 42 vs. 30 (p = 0.016)	8-y: 45 vs. 34 (p = 0.04)	8-y: 3 vs. 16 (p <0.0001)	8-y: 69 vs. 77 (p = 0.05)	8-y: 44 vs. 53 (p = 0.10)
RTOG 92-02	T2c-4 w/PSA <150, N+ allowed	RT + NHT (TAB) 4 mo vs. RT + NHT + AHT × 28 mo	5-y: 12.3 vs. 6.4 (p = 0.0001)	5-y: 17 vs. 11.5 (p = 0.0035)	5-y: 45.5 vs. 72 (p <0.0001)	5-y: 28.1 vs. 46.4 (p <0.0001)	5-y: 78.5 vs. 80 (p = 0.73)
RTOG 94-13	T2c-4 w/Gleason ≥6, or >15% risk of N+	WP + NHT, WP + AHT, PO + NHT, PO + AHT	4-y: 9.1 WP vs. 8.0 PO (p = 0.78)	4-y: 8.2 WP vs. 6.6 PO (p = 0.54)	4-y: 69.7, 63.3, 57.2, 63.5 (p = 0.048)	4-y: 59.6, 48.9, 44.3, 49.8 (p = 0.008)	4-y: 84.7 vs. 84.3 (p = 0.94)
Brigham and Women's Hospital[274]	PSA ≥10, Gleason ≥7, T1-T2b	RT 70 Gy 30-CRT vs. RT + 6 mo ADT	NS	NS		5-y: 82 vs. 57 (p = 0.002)	5-y: 88 vs.78 (p = 0.04)
RTOG 94-08[269]	PSA ≥20, Gleason any, T1b-T2b	RT 66.6 Gy vs. RT + 4 mo ADT	NS	10-y: 8 vs. 6 (p = 0.04)	10-y (biochemical failure): 41 vs. 26 (p <0.001)	10-y (disease-specific mortality): 8 vs. 4 (p = 0.001)	10-y: 57 vs 62 (p = 0.03)

LF, local failure; DM, distant metastasis; bNED, biochemical failure-free survival; DFS, disease-free survival; OS, overall survival; RTOG, Radiation Therapy Oncology Group; SV, seminal vesicle; RT, radiation therapy; HT, hormone therapy; AHT, adjuvant HT; EORTC, European Organisation for Research and Treatment of Cancer; WHO, World Health Organization; CAHT, concurrent adjuvant HT; NHT, neoadjuvant HT; TAB, total androgen blockade; PSA, prostate-specific antigen; WP, whole pelvis; PO, prostate only; CRT, conformal RT; ADT, androgen deprivation therapy; NS, not significant.
Adapted from D'Amico AV. Radiation and hormonal therapy for locally advanced and clinically localized prostate cancer. *Urology* 2002;60:32–37; D'Amico AV, Manola J, Loffredo M, et al. 6-month androgen suppression plus radiation therapy vs radiation therapy alone for patients with clinically localized prostate cancer: a randomized controlled trial. *JAMA* 2004;292:821–827. Jones CU, Hunt D, McGowan DG, et al. Radiotherapy and short-term androgen deprivation for localized prostate cancer. *N Engl J Med* 2011;365:107–118; Lee AK. Radiation therapy combined with hormone therapy for prostate cancer. *Semin Radiat Oncol* 2006;16:20–28.

appear to be associated with disease-free survival improvements compared to shorter courses. The preliminary results of the EORTC phase 3 trial 22961,[276] comprising 970 patients with locally advanced prostate cancer who were randomized to receive either 6 months or 3 years of ADT in conjunction with 70 Gy of EBRT, show that biochemical control and PFS were shorter for patients treated with the 6-month ADT regimen than for those treated with the longer course. No differences in survival have been noted so far between the two treatment arms. These data suggest that, for high-risk patients, longer courses of ADT may be critical in the setting of subtherapeutic doses of EBRT (i.e., 70 Gy). One cannot extrapolate from the published randomized trials whether 2-year or longer courses for high-risk disease are necessary when using modern dose escalated radiotherapy in the range of 78 Gy to 80 Gy. Nevertheless, longer courses of ADT are routinely used in clinical practice for high-risk patients in combination with dose-escalated radiotherapy. For patients with lower Gleason scores but with larger-volume disease, or for select patients with intermediate-risk disease, a shorter course of 6 months may be sufficient to provide a significant clinical benefit. In a meta-analysis of studies using various durations of ADT in conjunction with radiotherapy, a two-fold reduction in prostate cancer mortality was observed among patients treated with longer courses of ADT.[277]

As all of the previously mentioned trials used doses of radiotherapy ≤70 Gy, the role of ADT in the setting of an escalated dose of radiotherapy (≥75.6 Gy) remains uncertain. Higher doses of radiotherapy have been shown to improve local tumor control and may obviate the need for ADT. Nevertheless, in the absence of a randomized trial in this setting, it remains uncertain whether ADT should be avoided in the treatment of high-risk patients. Retrospective data from MSKCC showed that, among intermediate-risk patients treated with high-dose IMRT, short-course ADT (6 months) was associated with improved PSA-relapse-free survival, distant metastases–free survival, and PCSM, compared with high-dose radiotherapy alone.[278] The 10-year incidence of distant metastases and PCSM rates were 6.5% and 2.4%, respectively, for patients treated with high-dose IMRT and ADT compared to 12.3% and 5%, respectively, for patients treated with IMRT alone (p <0.001).

Definitive trials addressing the role of ADT in combination with brachytherapy are lacking, but its use is supported by basis extrapolating the results of randomized trials of patients treated with EBRT. Several reports[262,279,280] have suggested that, in the setting of brachytherapy (LDR or HDR brachytherapy boosts), ADT may be less beneficial than EBRT, whereas others[239] have suggested a benefit for higher-risk patients. It is possible that the primary role of ADT is to act as a radiosensitizer of EBRT when lower radiation doses, such as 70 Gy, are used. When higher radiation doses were used, or with the incorporation of brachytherapy boosts, several retrospective reports found no benefit of hormone therapy, except in high-grade, high-risk patients. In the absence of randomized trials in this setting, it is reasonable to recommend the use of ADT in high-risk patients, even when higher radiation doses are used. Many reports have not confirmed the role of ADT in conjunction with brachytherapy for intermediate-risk disease. The phase 3 RTOG 0815 trial will address the role of short-course ADT for intermediate-risk patients who receive dose-escalated radiotherapy and brachytherapy as well; 1,520 patients will be randomized to receive either 6 months of ADT with high-dose radiotherapy or radiotherapy alone. High-dose radiotherapy will be administered either at 79.2 Gy in conventional fractionation or as combined brachytherapy with EBRT.

Morbidities for Androgen Deprivation Therapy and Radiotherapy

Finally, there is a growing awareness that the use of ADT in conjunction with radiation therapy is not without cost, as outcomes suggest an increased risk of subsequent congestive heart failure

or myocardial infarction. Although most of the previously cited randomized trials did not report an increase in cardiac-related events, a meta-analysis of patients with unfavorable-risk prostate cancer with moderate to severe medical or cardiac-related comorbidities showed no survival difference between the two groups due to a relative increase in noncancer-related deaths in the ADT-treated group.[281] In a report of 12,792 men treated with brachytherapy, the use of a 4-month course of ADT was associated with an increased risk of all-cause mortality among those with a history of coronary artery disease–induced heart failure or myocardial infarction.[282] The effect of longer courses of ADT in patients with moderate or severe comorbidities is unclear. These data suggest that the use of ADT among favorable-risk patients, in whom its oncologic benefit is unproven, should be carefully considered (particularly in those with severe cardiac comorbidities), owing to its potential morbidity.[283] Future, well-designed prospective studies will be needed to elucidate these issues.

Adjuvant Radiation Therapy for High-Risk Patients After Radical Prostatectomy

Adjuvant Radiotherapy

Randomized Studies

The long-term (median follow-up, 14 years) results of Southwest Oncology Group (SWOG) trial 8794, which included 425 patients with high-risk localized disease who were randomized to receive either 60 Gy to 64 Gy to the prostatic fossa or only observation, have demonstrated a survival benefit of adjuvant radiotherapy in high-risk patients after RP.[284] The 10-year distant metastases–free survival and overall survival rates were 71% and 74% for the adjuvant radiotherapy arm, compared with 61% and 66% for the observation arm, respectively (p = 0.01; HR = 0.71 and 0.72, respectively). The differences between the treatment groups were detected only after 10 years, highlighting the importance of long-term follow-up in these patients (Fig. 68.12).

EORTC 22911 included 1,005 patients with positive surgical margins or pT3 (ECE and SVI) disease; these patients were randomized to receive either adjuvant EBRT (50 Gy to the prostatic

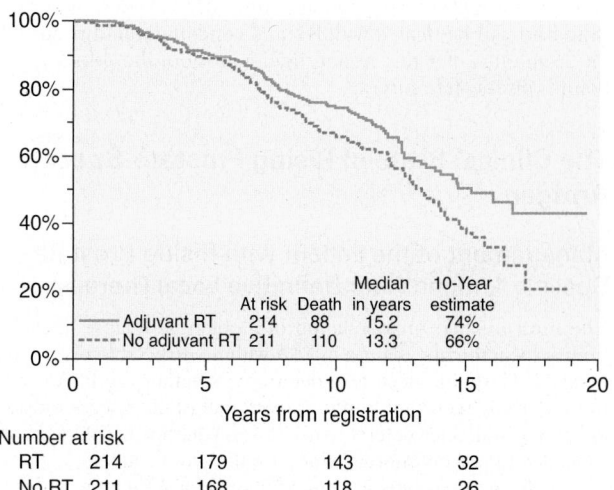

	At risk	Death	Median in years	10-Year estimate
Adjuvant RT	214	88	15.2	74%
No adjuvant RT	211	110	13.3	66%

Number at risk

RT	214	179	143	32
No RT	211	168	118	26

Figure 68.12 Overall survival advantage demonstrated for high-risk postoperative patients receiving adjuvant radiation therapy (RT) versus observation in the Southwest Oncology Group 8794 trial. (From Thompson IM, Tangen CM, Paradelo J, et al. Adjuvant radiotherapy for pathological T3N0M0 prostate cancer significantly reduces risk of metastases and improves survival; long-term followup of a randomized clinical trial. *J Urol* 2009;181:956–962, with permission.)

fossa and periprostatic tissue plus a 10-Gy to 14-Gy boost to the prostatic fossa only) or no immediate treatment.[285] A published update of this study (median follow-up, 10.6 years) showed that adjuvant radiotherapy improved the biochemical PFS rate from 40.1% to 60.6% (p <0.0001); the 10-year rate of locoregional relapse was 7.3% for the adjuvant radiotherapy group and 16.6% for the control group. There was no difference in prostate cancer mortality (HR = 0.78; p = 0.34): 10-year prostate cancer mortality was 3.9% for the adjuvant irradiation group versus 5.4% for the observation group.[286]

The results of adjuvant radiation therapy trials show improvements in shorter term end points, including PSA PFS and locoregional relapse free survival, as anticipated. A meaningful improvement in PCSM has not been shown. Noteworthy as well is that PCSM rate in the nonadjuvant radiation therapy group was only 5.4%,[286] reinforcing that preventing a BCR alone does not necessarily translate into a significant survival benefit and that deferring treatment until the disease has declared itself as being more aggressive is an option.

Similar results were observed in a phase 3 trial from Germany (ARO 96-02) which randomized 388 patients with pathologic T3 prostate cancer with undetectable postoperative PSA levels to receive either adjuvant radiotherapy or observation. The 10-year PFS was 56% for the adjuvant radiotherapy group and 35% for the observation group (p <0.0001) with no survival benefit.[287]

These trials provide evidence that adjuvant postprostatectomy radiotherapy reduces the risk of BCR and in one trial, an improvement in distant metastases–free survival. Yet it remains unproven that deferring radiotherapy until manifestation of an early biochemical relapse would compromise the outcome of patients, compared with subjecting all high-risk patients to salvage radiotherapy. To address this issue, the RADICALS (NCT00541047) trial is randomizing patients to receive either immediate radiotherapy or salvage radiotherapy on detection of PSA during follow-up observations. In this trial, patients with positive margins after RP or pathologic stage T3 disease with a postoperative PSA ≤0.2 ng/ml would be randomized to receive early adjuvant radiotherapy or deferred radiotherapy on manifestation of a PSA relapse (defined as a detectable and rising PSA >0.1 ng/ml or three consecutive rising PSA values). The primary end point of this study is distant metastases–free survival. A second randomization will evaluate the role of ADT with salvage radiotherapy and will randomize patients to be treated with RT alone versus RT with concomitant/adjuvant ADT for 6 months; a third arm will be treated with RT and concomitant/adjuvant RT for 24 months. For this second randomization, the primary end point is disease-free survival.

The Clinical State of Rising Prostate-Specific Antigen

Management of the Patient with Rising Prostate-Specific Antigen After Definitive Local Therapy

The most frequent manifestation of a potential relapse after definitive local therapy is a rise in PSA with no detectable disease on imaging. Here, the need is to determine whether the PSA rise is from a locally recurrent tumor or micrometastatic disease outside the pelvis, and, once determined, to assess whether an intervention is needed to prevent morbidity or mortality from cancer.

The former may benefit from additional local therapy, whereas the latter would require a systemic approach. Patients who develop a rising PSA following RP may be candidates for potentially curative salvage radiation, particularly those who have an undetectable PSA after surgery and develop the rising PSA later (see "Salvage Radiotherapy for the Patient with Rising Prostate-Specific Antigen After Prostatectomy"). Patients who develop a rising PSA after radiation therapy may be candidates for salvage RP, salvage cryotherapy, or

brachytherapy, assuming the sole source of the PSA is the gland itself. Here we consider salvage local therapy. Systemic options are considered later.

Salvage Therapies

Salvage Radiotherapy for the Patient with Rising Prostate-Specific Antigen After Prostatectomy

Numerous nonrandomized studies have shown improved biochemical control outcomes with salvage EBRT, yet the overall PSA-relapse-free survival outcome at ≥5 years is approximately 50%.[288–292] Prognostic factors associated with relapse include surgical Gleason score, the presence of SVI, absolute preradiotherapy PSA level, and preradiotherapy PSADT. Improved outcomes are achieved with salvage radiotherapy when preradiotherapy PSA values are ≤0.5 ng/ml.[290]

At MSKCC, 285 patients with increasing PSA levels after prostatectomy[291] were treated with either salvage three-dimensional CRT or IMRT. The median dose delivered to the prostate fossa was 70.2 Gy. Neoadjuvant and concurrent ADT were used in 31% of treated patients. The 7-year (median follow-up, 5 years) PSA-relapse-free survival and distant metastases–free survival rates were 37% and 77%, respectively. Multivariate analysis demonstrated that predictors of postradiotherapy failure included the presence of vascular invasion, negative surgical margins, presalvage PSA level >0.4 ng/ml, and radiotherapy alone (i.e., without ADT). Patients treated without any adverse prognostic features had a 5-year PSA-relapse-free survival of 70%, compared with 30% for those with any adverse feature. In a multi-institutional cohort of 472 patients treated with salvage radiotherapy for a BCR after prostatectomy,[292] the overall PSA-relapse-free survival at 5 years (median follow-up, 4 years) was 73%. Variables significant as predictors of biochemical tumor control included Gleason score, surgical margin status, and preradiotherapy PSA level. Although it is difficult to compare retrospective series, it would appear that this latter multi-institutional cohort comprised a more favorable group with fewer adverse pathologic features.

The efficacy of salvage EBRT alone for clinically palpable local disease or imaging evidence of disease within the prostatic bed is suboptimal in part due to the inability to deliver full therapeutic doses of radiation safely.[293,294] Here, ADT can be used to improve local tumor eradication by reducing the size of a mass, by the concurrent elimination of tumor clonogens inherently resistant to radiotherapy, or both. The 30% to 40% size reduction also increases the ability to deliver maximal radiation dose levels without exceeding the tolerance for the surrounding normal tissue. As such, it is our policy that neoadjuvant and concurrent ADT should be considered in patients with palpable local recurrence, imaging evidence of recurrent disease, especially if biopsy proven, or an immediate detectable PSA after surgery, extrapolating from randomized trials showing the benefit of ADT in patients treated with the prostate intact. Further studies are needed in this setting.

There is limited information on the role of ADT in combination with salvage radiotherapy in the postprostatectomy setting. RTOG 0534 is accruing patients with an increasing PSA level after prostatectomy to receive either radiotherapy alone to the prostate bed, radiotherapy to the prostate bed plus 4 to 6 months of ADT, or radiotherapy to the pelvis and prostate bed plus 6 months of ADT. The previously mentioned RADICALS study incorporates a second randomization of all patients that will explore the role of ADT in the setting of salvage or adjuvant therapy.

The American Society for Radiation Oncology and American Urological Association guidelines recommend that, among patients with adverse pathologic features after prostatectomy (such as positive surgical margins and SVI), adjuvant radiotherapy should be used to reduce the risk of biochemical failures and clinical progression, although its impact on overall survival is unclear. The level of evidence grade was C. The guidelines also recommend that salvage radiotherapy should be offered to patients with an increasing PSA level or with evidence of local recurrence in the absence of metastatic disease. The recommended definition of biochemical failure after surgery is a detectable or rising PSA level >0.2 ng/ml, with a second confirmatory increase >0.2 ng/ml. Once documented, earlier administration of salvage radiotherapy is appropriate, as disease control is improved when salvage radiotherapy is administered at lower PSA levels.[295]

Salvage Therapy for Locally Recurrent Disease After Radiation

Patients with persistent disease in the prostate after radiation therapy can be considered for salvage local therapies including a salvage RP, brachytherapy, or cryosurgery. Patient selection requires a performance status of 80 or more, histologic confirmation of disease in the gland, and no evidence of metastatic disease by imaging.

Salvage RP is technically challenging. Reported short-term and long-term complication rates exceed those of standard RP, but with appropriate patient selection and surgical expertise, the procedure has become less hazardous. Despite these advances, complications including bladder-neck contractures and anastomotic strictures have continued to be problematic.[296] Urinary incontinence rates remain high and in an MSKCC series,[152] only 74% (95% CI = 54% to 94%) recover urinary control and 20% require a sling procedure or artificial urinary sphincters. The 15-year nonprogression rate was 29% and the 15-year cancer-specific survival rate was 64% after salvage RP. The 5-year actuarial nonprogression rate was 86% for patients with organ-confined cancer (pT2N0), 61% for those with ECE, and 48% for those with SVI.

Salvage Brachytherapy

Initial efforts to use brachytherapy in the salvage setting were restricted because of concerns about treatment-related complications. Improvements in imaging, dosimetry, and approaches (including HDR brachytherapy) have significantly lowered the risks of treatment-related complications to an acceptable level. After recurrent disease in the prostate is documented histologically, preferred candidates include those with no clinical or radiologic evidence of distant disease, adequate urinary function, age and overall health indicative of a >5- to 10-year life expectancy, prolonged disease-free interval (>2 years) from primary radiotherapy, and a long PSADT (>6 to 9 months) at the time of recurrence. Salvage brachytherapy should be avoided in patients with evidence of SVI recurrence and extracapsular disease, as these patients are poorly treated in the conventional setting.

Therapeutic approaches include permanent interstitial seed implantation,[297–299] with reported 5- to 10-year PSA-relapse-free survival rates ranging from 10% to 53%. In a second series of 37 patients with a median follow-up of 86 months, 10-year PSA-relapse-free survival and cause-specific survival rates were 54% and 96%, respectively. Improved biochemical tumor control was associated with a presalvage PSA level of ≤0.6 ng/ml in multivariate analysis.[297] In another report, 69 patients were treated with salvage permanent seed implantation using [103]Pd with a planned D90 dose of 100 Gy as monotherapy of whom 90% received concurrent ADT. With a median follow-up of 5 years, 5-year PSA-relapse-free survival rates were 86%, 75%, and 66% for patients with low-, intermediate-, and high-risk disease, respectively. Grade 3 urinary toxicity was observed in 9% of patients.[298]

In 52 patients treated with salvage HDR brachytherapy after radiotherapy failure delivering 36 Gy in six fractions using two TRUS-guided HDR prostate implants, separated by 1 week, the 5-year PSA-relapse-free survival was 51% (median follow-up, 60 months). The incidence of grade 3 urinary toxicity was 2%,

and that of grade 2 rectal toxicity was 4%.[300] A prospective phase 2 protocol at MSKCC assessed the safety and efficacy of salvage HDR brachytherapy after EBRT failure in 42 patients; the median dose was 81 Gy. The 5-year PSA-relapse-free survival and distant metastasis–free survival rates were 69% and 82%, respectively. Late grade rectal toxicity was 8%; grade 2 urethral toxicity was 7%. One patient developed urinary incontinence.[301]

Caution and meticulous treatment planning are necessary when considering repeat irradiation, especially in the setting of previous high-dose EBRT. Given the radiation dose previously delivered to the prostate and nearby normal tissue structures, side effects can manifest, including chronic urinary retention, hematuria, rectal ulcers, rectal bleeding, and permanent sexual dysfunction. Yet in the absence of randomized trials, the nonrandomized published studies suggest salvage brachytherapy as potentially less toxic relative to salvage RP.

Salvage Cryotherapy

With the development of second- and third-generation probes, real-time TRUS for intraoperative monitoring, thermocouplers, and urethral warmers, cryotherapy is potentially less toxic and a feasible alternative for salvage local therapy after radiation failure. Case selection criteria include a prostate volume between 20 g to 30 g. The procedure is not advised for patients in whom the gland is ≥60 g. Patients with a prior TURP have an increased risk of urethral sloughing and urinary retention. Reported biochemical disease-free survival rates range from 34% to 98%.[302–307] Reported long-term complications include erectile dysfunction (77% to 100%), rectal pain (10% to 40%), urinary incontinence (4% to 20%), urinary retention (0% to 7%), and urethral sloughing (0% to 5%).[302–307] Rectourethral fistulas, the most serious complication following cryotherapy, are relatively uncommon (0% to 4%).

A second series of 187 patients with local follow-up[306] showed that patients with precryotherapy PSA levels <4 ng/ml had 5- and 8-year (mean follow-up, 49 months) BCR-free survival rates of 56% and 37%, respectively, whereas those with precryotherapy levels ≥10 ng/ml had 5- and 8-year BCR-free survival rates of only 1% and 7%, respectively. A total of 17% of patients overall had a positive four-quadrant prostate biopsy after salvage cryotherapy.

Advanced Prostate Cancer: Rising Prostate-Specific Antigen and Clinical Metastases—Noncastrate and Castrate

The core principle of treatment of advanced prostate cancer is to deplete androgens or inhibit signaling through the androgen receptor (AR). The approach was first described in the 1940s by Huggins and Hodges,[308] who showed that surgical removal of the testes or the administration of exogenous estrogen could induce tumor regressions, reduce the level of acid phosphatase in the blood, and palliate symptoms of the disease.[308,309] Both remained the standard of care until the luteinizing hormone–releasing hormone (LHRH) agonists were introduced in the 1980s.[310,311] The palliative role of surgical adrenalectomy for disease that was progressing following orchiectomy was first described in 1945,[312] later replaced by the first-generation enzymatic inhibitors of adrenal steroid biosynthesis (aminoglutethimide and ketoconazole).[313,314] Nonsteroidal antiandrogens were introduced in the 1980s.[315,316] All these agents lower androgen levels, with the exception of the nonsteroidal antiandrogens that block the binding of androgens to the AR.

The "combined androgen blockade" era followed, during which various hormone combinations were explored in an attempt to increase the degree of AR signaling inhibition and thereby response. The first combined a LHRH agonist with flutamide,[317] others with adrenal androgen synthesis inhibitors; none of these meaningfully improved survival.[318,319]

Other approaches to treating advanced prostate cancer include cytotoxic agents, biologic agents, and immunotherapy. In 1996, the first cytotoxic drug, mitoxantrone, was approved for the palliation of pain secondary to progressive osseous disease based upon a trial that was not specifically designed to show a survival benefit.[320] But it was not until 2004 that the first systemic therapy, docetaxel, was shown to prolong the lives of men with progressive CRPC,[321,322] setting a new benchmark for drug approvals that has not been exceeded by any docetaxel-based combination, several of which have proved inferior to docetaxel alone (Table 68.14).[322–337]

Efforts were also focused on better understanding of the biology of the disease. This effort has led to the approval of six new treatments with diverse mechanisms of action since 2010. Five were shown to prolong life (see Table 68.14), including a biologic agent (sipuleucel-T),[323] a cytotoxic (cabazitaxel),[325] a bone-seeking alpha-emitting radionuclide (radium-223),[326] and two hormonal agents, the CYP17 inhibitor abiraterone acetate that inhibits androgen biosynthesis in combination with prednisone and a next-generation antiandrogen, enzalutamide, which is mechanistically unique from the first-generation compounds.[327,328] The sixth agent, denosumab, a monoclonal antibody that binds the cytokine RANKL (receptor activator of nuclear factor-κB ligand), was shown to reduce the morbidity associated with skeletal metastases relative to a previously established standard (zoledronate).[338]

Taken together, the results of these new treatments showed that survival could be prolonged by targeting different aspects of the malignant process in addition to direct targeting of the tumor, and demonstrated the complexity of measuring success for these new agents. Separately, the success of hormonal agents that inhibit the AR and AR signaling confirmed that prostate cancers progressing despite castrate levels of testosterone are not uniformly hormone-refractory; instead, they are more accurately described as castration-resistant.

Efficacy End Points

Prostate cancer treatment outcomes are reported based on the changes in individual disease manifestations that are present when therapy is initiated and the prevention of development of subsequent manifestations. The appropriateness of one metric over another depends on the class and mechanism of the drug or therapy being used, the disease state of the patients being treated, and the clinical benefit or outcome the therapy is expected to achieve. Measurements of PSA levels alone are not sufficient to gauge efficacy for several classes of agents. For example, AR and AR signaling inhibitors may, in some patients, produce declines in PSA without affecting tumor growth. Conversely, bone-seeking radiopharmaceuticals may relieve pain without decreasing PSA levels. A drug that inhibits cell proliferation without inducing an apoptotic effect may lead to a prolonged period of disease stability or "nonprogression," preventing disease manifestations such as the development of new metastatic lesions or pain that were expected to occur. Such a drug might be beneficial independent of its effect on PSA. In contrast, a hormonal agent or cytotoxic drug that

---

TABLE 68.14

(A) Phase 3 Trials of Single Agents Leading to Regulatory Approval in Castration-Resistant Prostate Cancer. (B) Completed or Ongoing Phase 3 Studies Examining Docetaxel-Based Combinations in the First-Line Treatment of Metastatic Castration-Resistant Prostate Cancer

Trial: Therapy (Approved Date)	N	Disease State	Comparator	HR	OS	*P* Value
(A) Phase 3 Trials of Single Agents Leading to Regulatory Approval						
IMPACT: Provenge vaccine (2010)[323]	512	Prechemotherapy Asymptomatic	Placebo	0.775	25.8 vs. 21.7	0.032
COU-AA-302: Abiraterone acetate (2013)[324]	1,088	Prechemotherapy	Placebo Prednisone	0.75	NYR vs. 27.2	0.01
TAX327: Docetaxel (2004)[322]	1006	First-line	Mitoxantrone Prednisone	0.76	18.9 vs. 16.5	0.009
TROPIC: Cabazitaxel (2010)[325]	755	Postchemotherapy Symptoms	Mitoxantrone Prednisone	0.70	15.1 vs. 12.7	<0.0001
COU-AA-301: Abiraterone acetate (2011)[327]	1195	Postdocetaxel	Placebo Prednisone	0.646	14.8 vs. 10.9	<0.0001
AFFIRM: Enzalutamide (2012)[328]	1199	Postdocetaxel	Placebo	0.631	18.4 vs. 13.6	<0.0001
ALYMPTA: Alpharadin (2013)[326]	922	Pre- and postsymptomatic	Placebo	0.695	14.0 vs. 11.2	0.00085
(B) Phase 3 Trials with Docetaxel-Based Combinations						
CALGB 90401: Docetaxel ± bevacizumab[329]	1,050	First-line	Placebo	0.091	22.6 vs. 21.5	0.181
VENICE: Docetaxel ± aflibercept[330]	1,224	First-line	Placebo	0.94	22.1 vs. 21.2	0.38
SWOG S0421: Docetaxel ± atrasentan[331]	994	First-line	Placebo	1.04	17.8 vs. 17.6	0.64
ENTHUSE: Docetaxel ± zibotentan[332]	1,052	First-line	Placebo	1.00	20.0 vs. 19.2	0.963
READY: Docetaxel ± dasatinib[333]	1,380	First-line	Placebo	0.99	21.5 vs. 21.2	0.90
VITAL-2: Docetaxel ± GVAX[334]	408	First-line Symptomatic	Placebo	1.70	12.2 vs. 14.1	0.0076
MAINSAIL: Docetaxel ± lenalidomide[335]	1,059	First-line	Placebo	1.53	17.7 vs. NYR	0.0017
ASCENT: Docetaxel ± calcitriol[336]	953	First-line	Placebo	1.42	17.8 vs. 20.2	0.002
SYNERGY: Docetaxel ± custirsen[337]	1,022	First-line	Placebo	0.93	23.4 vs. 22.2	0.207

HR, hazard ratio; OS, overall survival (mo); NYR, not yet reached.

does not produce a decline in PSA is likely to be inactive. Examples of agents that provide clinical benefit without PSA declines include the delay and prevention benefit of zoledronate[159] and denosumab[338] on SREs, and separately, the survival benefit shown for sipuleucel-T[323] and radium-223.[326]

It is for these reasons that the PCWG2 recommended focusing less on whether a treatment was "working" and more on when it was "not working," and to carefully consider the potential significance of an apparent adverse change in PSA before stopping therapy.[157] Rather than discontinue treatment based on a PSA change alone, it is preferable to wait until there is evidence of radiographic or clinical progression. Figure 68.13 shows examples where (1) a significant initial rise in PSA or (2) a slow rise following an initial decline did not associate with radiographic or clinical progression for a considerable period of time (2 years and 3.5 years, respectively, in Fig. 68.13).[339] In each case, reliance on the PSA change alone to guide management would have resulted in the premature discontinuation of therapy and denied the patient durable disease control.

Noncastrate Prostate Cancer (Rising Prostate-Specific Antigen and Noncastrate Metastases)

Hypothalamic-Pituitary-Gonadal Axis

The regulation of androgen production begins with LHRH being secreted from the hypothalamus, which acts on the pituitary gland to release follicle-stimulating hormone, which acts on Sertoli cells, and luteinizing hormone (LH), which acts on Leydig cells to control androgen synthesis and spermatogenesis in the testes (Fig. 68.14).[340]

Bilateral orchiectomy is an inexpensive standard treatment that reliably reduces testosterone levels to the "castrate" range (<50 ng/dl). Estrogens inhibit the production of LHRH, which decreases the release of follicle-stimulating hormone and LH, and reduces androgen levels in a dose-dependent manner. A dose of diethylstilbesterol (DES), 3 mg/d, generally achieves castrate testosterone levels.

PRACTICE OF ONCOLOGY

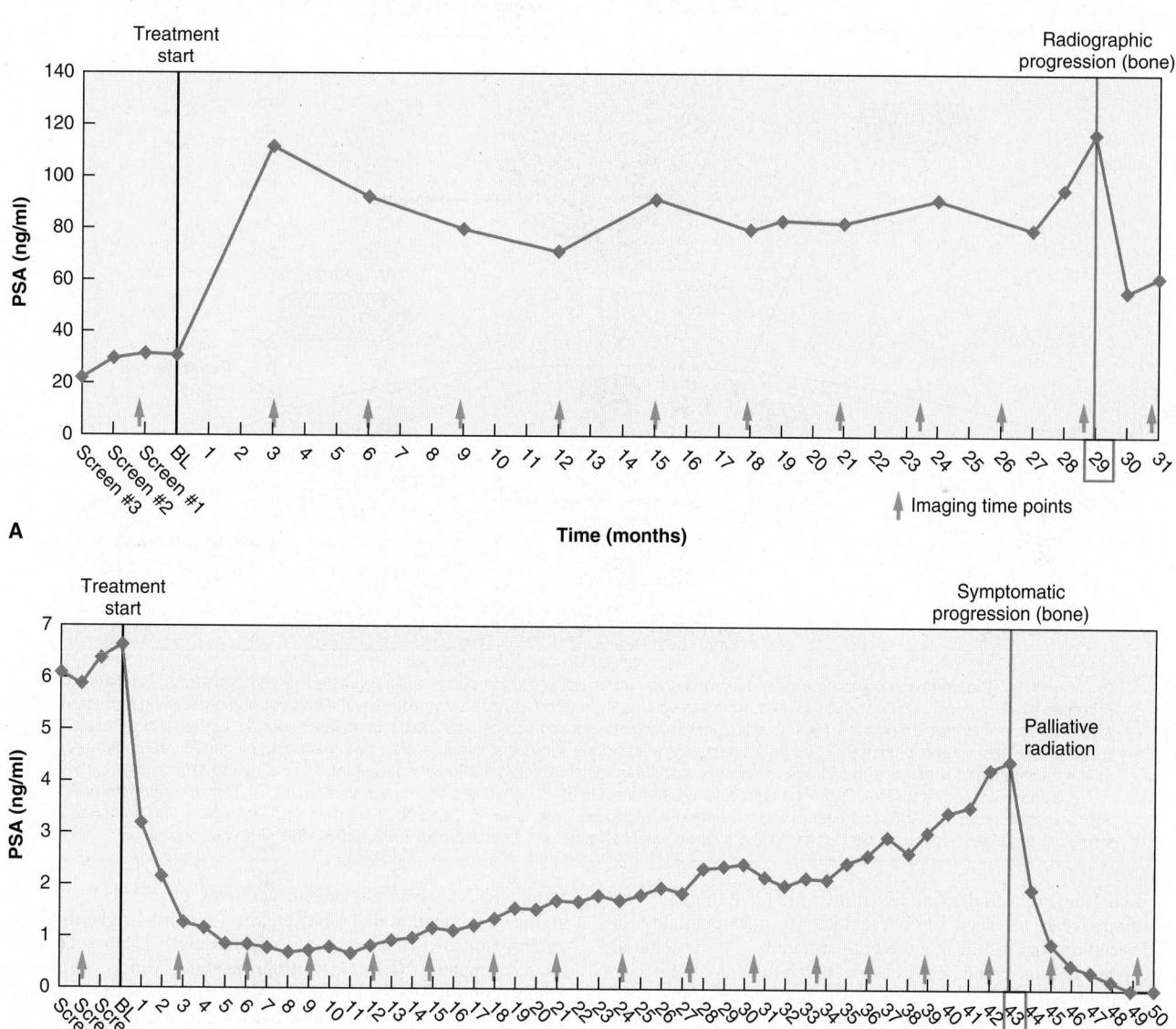

Figure 68.13 Prostate-specific antigen (PSA) rise alone is not sufficient reason to discontinue treatment; there must also be radiographic or clinical evidence of progression. **(A)** An initial rapid rise in PSA, with subsequent decline above baseline on a second value, in a patient who remained biochemically, radiographically, and clinically stable for 22 months on abiraterone acetate. **(B)** A slow rise in PSA after an initial rapid decline, with no evidence of radiographic or clinical progression for 28 months while receiving enzalutamide. (From Scher HI, Morris MJ, Basch E, et al. End points and outcomes in castration-resistant prostate cancer: from clinical trials to clinical practice. *J Clin Oncol* 2011;29:3695–3704, with permission.)

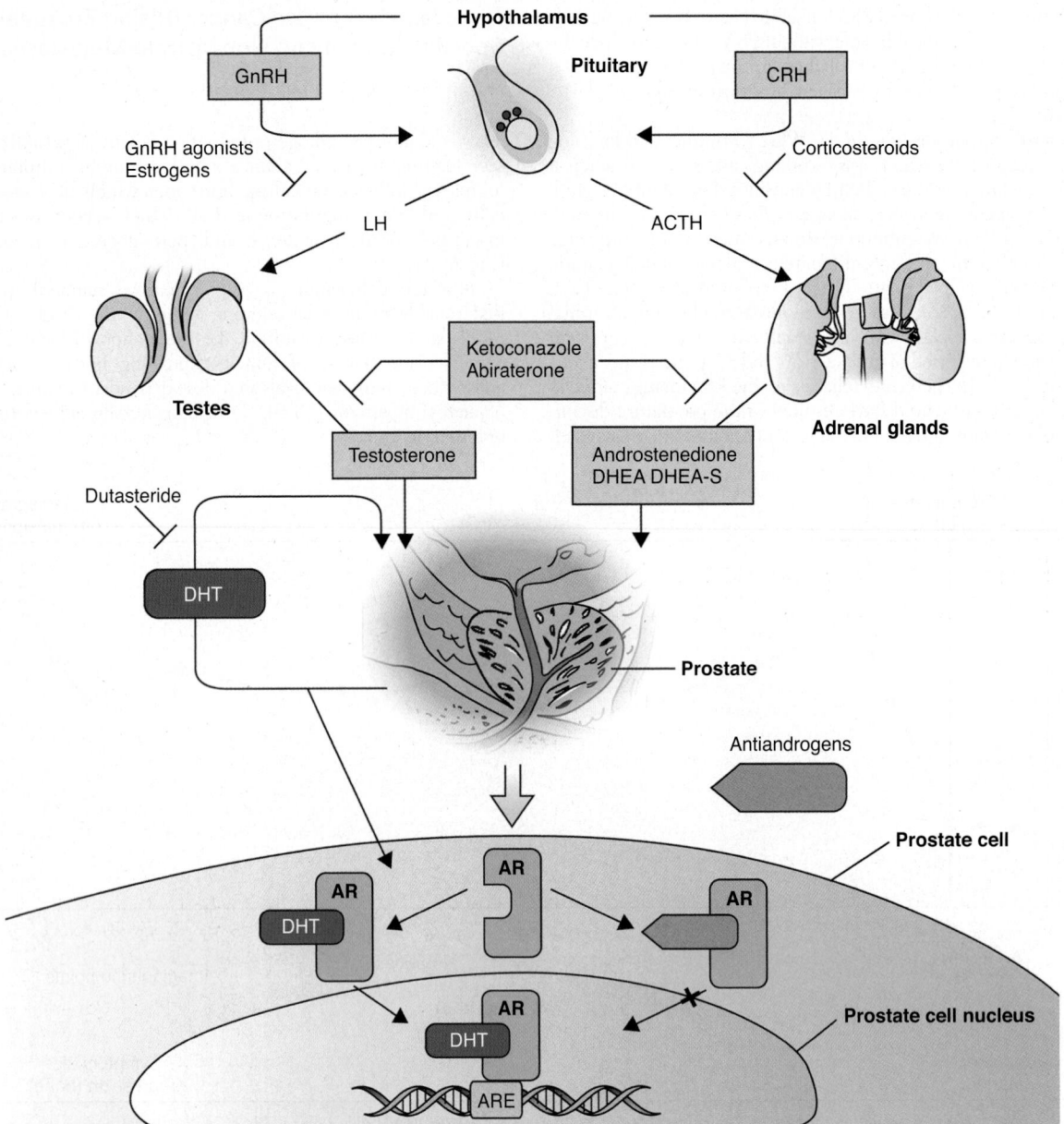

Figure 68.14 The androgen-signaling axis and its inhibitors. Testicular androgen synthesis is regulated by the gonadotropin-releasing hormone (GnRH)–luteinizing hormone (LH) axis, whereas adrenal androgen synthesis is regulated by the corticotrophin-releasing hormone (CRH)-adrenocorticotropic hormone (ACTH) axis. GnRH agonists and corticosteroids inhibit stimulation of the testes and adrenals, respectively. Abiraterone inhibits CYP17, a critical enzyme in androgen synthesis. Bicalutamide, flutamide, and nilutamide competitively inhibit the binding of androgens to androgen receptors; enzalutamide also blocks the translocation of the ligand bound AR complex to the nucleus and from binding to DNA. DHEA, dehydroepiandrosterone; DHEA-S, dehydroepiandrosterone sulphate; DHT, dihydrotestosterone; AR, androgen receptor; ARE, androgen-response element. (Adapted from Chen Y, Clegg NJ, Scher HI. Anti-androgens and androgen-depleting therapies in prostate cancer: new agents for an established target. *Lancet Oncol* 2009;10:981–991, with permission.)

LHRH agonists produce an initial rise in LH that increases testosterone levels, followed 1 to 2 weeks later by downregulation of LH receptors that results in a medical castration.[310,311] The initial rise in testosterone can flare the disease, precipitating or exacerbating symptoms such as pain, obstructive uropathies, and spinal cord compromise. These agents were first approved on the basis of trials showing an improved safety profile compared with oral estrogens, most notably the reduction in cardiovascular-related events such as edema, thrombosis and thromboembolism, myocardial infarction, and stroke.[341–343] Several are approved for use in the United States, including leuprolide acetate (Lupron, given intramuscularly [AbbVie, North Chicago, IL]; Eligard, given subcutaneously [TOLMAR Pharmaceuticals, Inc., Fort Collins, CO]; Viadur, implanted subcutaneously [Bayer HealthCare Pharmaceuticals Inc.,

Montville, NJ]), goserelin acetate (Zoladex, given subcutaneously in the abdominal wall [AstraZeneca, London, England]), triptorelin pamoate (Trelstar, given intramuscularly [Actavis Pharma, Inc., Parsippany, NJ]), and histrelin acetate (Vantas, implanted subcutaneously [Endo Pharmaceuticals Inc., Dublin, Ireland]). These drugs are available as daily or monthly injections, and 3-, 4-, 6-, or 12-month depot injections.

In contrast, LHRH antagonists produce castrate levels of testosterone in 48 hours without the initial rise (Fig. 68.15), making them a compelling choice for the initial treatment of patients with symptoms. At present, degarelix, available as monthly subcutaneous injections, is the only LHRH antagonist that is approved in the United States. Reported outcomes suggest a comparable to slightly improved efficacy relative to the agonists/antagonists discussed

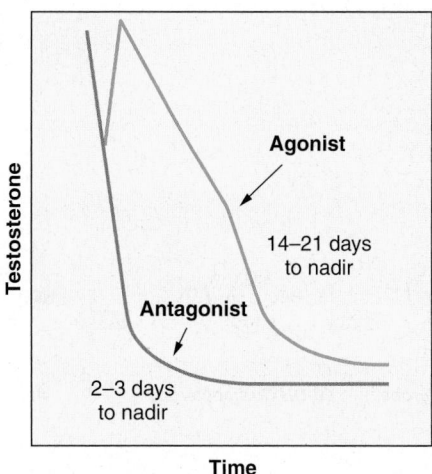

Figure 68.15 Testosterone levels following treatment with a luteinizing hormone–releasing hormone agonist and antagonist. Nadir is achieving castrate range.

previously.[344] The tradeoff is the need for monthly injections and a higher frequency of injection-site reactions.

Antiandrogens

Antiandrogens block the binding of testosterone to the AR (see Fig. 68.14). There are two types: the steroidal type I agents such as cyproterone acetate have progestational properties that suppress LH levels and lower serum testosterone; these are not widely used. The nonsteroidal type II agents bind to the AR and act as competitive antagonists for ligands that might otherwise bind and activate the ligand-dependent transcriptional activity of the receptor. The three first-generation type II agents approved are flutamide, which has a short half-life requiring multiple daily doses, and bicalutamide and nilutamide, which have weekly half-lives and are administered once daily. All three were approved initially in combination with a LHRH analog: flutamide to prevent the flare that can result from the initial rise in testosterone that occurs with LHRH analogs,[345,346] bicalutamide (50 mg daily) on the basis of an improved safety profile relative to flutamide,[347] and nilutamide in combination with surgical orchiectomy based on greater efficacy relative to orchiectomy alone.[348] Type II agents given as monotherapy do not inhibit LH synthesis in the hypothalamus or pituitary, and circulating testosterone levels rise. None of these antiandrogens are approved as monotherapy in the United States, although bicalutamide 150 mg is approved in the European Union.[349]

Enzymatic Inhibitors of Androgen Synthesis

All steroidal hormones are derived from pregnenolone and subsequently metabolized via several CYP450 class enzymes. Within the adrenal gland, CYP17 mediates the synthesis of weak androgens dehydroepiandrosterone (DHEA) and androstenedione (Fig. 68.16), whereas in the testes, the presence of 17-keto reductase generates testosterone that can be further converted to DHT in peripheral tissues by 5α-reductase. Ketoconazole is a nonspecific P450 inhibitor that, at a dose of 1,200 mg/d, produces castrate levels of testosterone in 24 hours through inhibition of adrenal and testicular steroidogenesis. The effect is not durable, limiting the drug's use as first-line treatment. It was useful for patients who presented with acute spinal cord compression or disseminated intravascular coagulation, when LHRH analogs are contraindicated and the risk of hemorrhage from surgery is significant.[314]

Toxicities of Androgen Deprivation Therapy

The adverse effects associated with ADT include those associated with the hypogonadal state and others that are unique to the specific drugs utilized. Symptoms associated with castration, whether medical or surgical, can be grouped under the "androgen deprivation syndrome," and include hot flashes, a decrease in libido, erectile dysfunction, impotence, fatigue, anemia, weight gain and alterations in fat metabolism, loss of muscle mass and weakness, bone loss, a decrease in mental acuity, mood swings, personality changes, memory loss, depression, and insomnia. Consequently, to relieve patients' anxiety and minimize stress, it is essential to inform them of the goals of treatment and the potential adverse events that may occur. Many of the adverse effects of ADT can be relieved by exercise.[350–352] Table 68.15 shows the frequency and methods of amelioration. Hot flashes occur in more than 80% of patients at any time, even during sleep, and may last for several seconds or an hour or more. They are bothersome in about 25% of cases, and if significant, can be reduced in frequency and intensity with estrogens at doses as low as 0.3 mg/d by patch[353] or progestins (e.g., megestrol acetate or medroxyprogesterone acetate).[354]

Erectile dysfunction and loss of libido are almost universal. Penile and testicular size may diminish and facial and body hair decrease, but male-pattern baldness may improve. Fatigue, in part related to anemia, is also frequent, as 90% of men on ADT show a decrease in hemoglobin of 10%, and 25% show a decrease of 18% or more.[355] Weight gain is also frequent (most of which is fat, as lean body mass decreases) and exceeded 6 kg on average at 12 months in one study.[356] Other factors contributing to weight gain include an increase in appetite and sedentary lifestyle.

Metabolic changes include an increase in cholesterol in 10% of patients, increase in triglycerides in 26%, and incident diabetes,[357] a consequence of insulin resistance. It is uncertain whether glucose intolerance results from an increase in weight or adiposity, a decrease in exercise tolerance, or a combination of these or other factors.

Osteopenia and osteoporosis are well documented, and in one prospective trial bone mass decreased by 2% to 5% after 1 year of ADT, leading to an increased rate of fracture,[358] although few fractures occur in patients treated for <1 year (Fig. 68.17).[359] Changes in bone can be monitored by bone densitometry and bone turnover markers such as urinary N-telopeptide (a breakdown product of collagen), bone-specific alkaline phosphatase, and osteocalcin.[360] Bone loss and fracture rates can be reduced by bisphosphonates such as zoledronate[361] or denosumab, blocking osteoclast maturation, function, and survival,[362,363] and toremifene,[364] a selective estrogen receptor modulator.[364] Supplemental calcium (1,000 mg/d to 1,500 mg/d) and vitamin D (400 international units) daily are also advised to prevent bone loss, but data to support their use are limited. Integral parts of the maintenance of bone integrity are exercise, reduction in caffeine, and smoking cessation.

Other adverse effects of ADT include depression, mood swings, emotional lability, decreased mental acuity, and memory loss.[365] Psychological tests for cognitive dysfunction suggest that certain aspects of spatial reasoning and spatial ability,[366] along with memory and attention, can be impaired by ADT.[367]

Cardiovascular issues are also a concern, given the multiplicity of risk factors that are worsened by ADT, including weight gain, increased adipose tissue, decreased exercise tolerance, hyperlipidemia, decreased insulin sensitivity, and glucose intolerance. The literature on the effects of ADT on cardiovascular mortality shows that this remains an area of controversy. A recent advisory panel from the American Heart Association concluded that links between ADT and cardiovascular mortality remain controversial, and that there is no reason at present to initiate cardiac testing in patients with cardiovascular disease before initiation of ADT.[368,369]

Antiandrogen Toxicity

Antiandrogens do not lower serum androgens, and as a result, there is less loss of libido, fewer hot flashes, and potency may be spared, while muscle and bone mass are retained. Unique toxicities relative to testosterone-lowering approaches include GI events such as

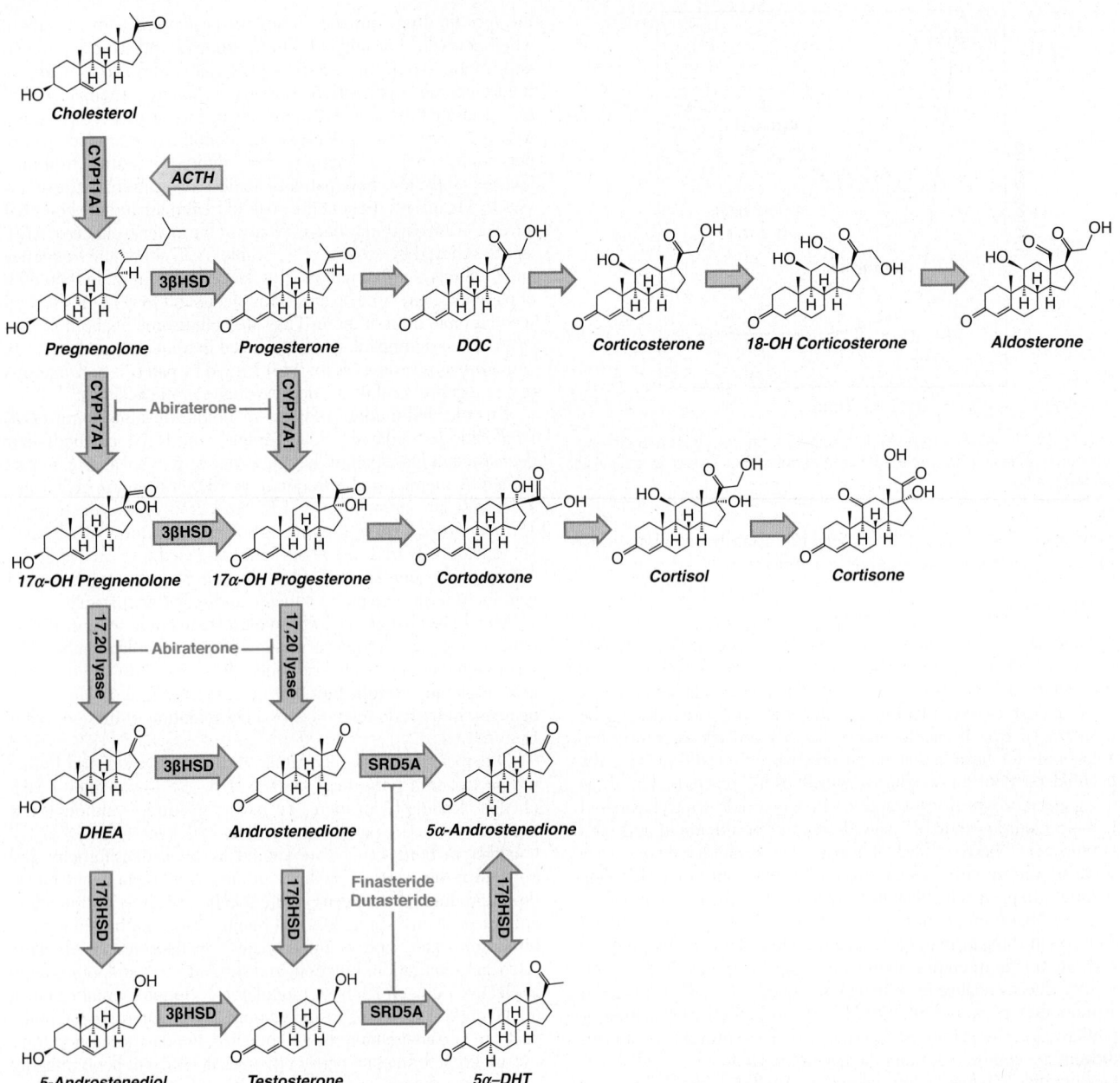

Figure 68.16 The effects of abiraterone acetate on steroid biosynthesis. ACTH, adrenocorticotropic hormone; DOC, 11-deoxycorticosterone; DHEA, dehydroepiandrosterone; DHT, dihydrotestosterone.

elevations in hepatic enzymes, stomach upset and diarrhea,[347] and pulmonary complications such as fibrosis; these toxicities are a rare class effect of the first-generation antiandrogens,[370] which occur most frequently with nilutamide. Gynecomastia and/or breast tenderness may also develop, which, if severe, might require a reduction mammoplasty. Prophylactic breast irradiation can reduce the frequency and severity of these effects.[350,351]

Contemporary Management

For the patient with metastatic disease and/or symptoms, or the patient in the rising PSA state for whom treatment is advised based on the absolute level of PSA or PSA kinetics, standard practice is to initiate therapy and monitor the disease with serial PSA measurements and imaging as appropriate until there are signs that the disease has started to progress, at which point it is considered "castration-resistant." In most patients, this is manifested first by a rise in PSA despite castrate (<50 ng/dl) levels of testosterone.

Androgen deprivation and/or blockade produces declines in PSA, regression of measurable tumor masses if present, and a period of clinical quiescence or stability in which PSA levels and tumor size does not change, followed in a variable period of time by a rise in PSA, tumor proliferation, and clinically detectable changes on imaging. Applying the control/relieve–delay/prevent metric, approximately 60% to 70% of patients with an abnormal PSA will show a normalization to a value of ≤4 ng/ml, 30% to 50% of measurable tumor masses will regress by ≥50%, 30% to 40% of bone scans will improve while the majority remain stable, and >60% of patients with symptoms will show palliation, be the symptoms urinary or osseous in origin.

The complete elimination of disease in any site with ADT is rare, be it in bone or the prostate itself, although in many cases, LN disease that was present when hormone therapy is initiated does not recur. When ADTs are used as neoadjuvant therapy prior to surgery for upwards of 8 months, <5% of prostates removed subsequently are pathologically free of tumor,[371] which suggests that hormone therapy

TABLE 68.15

Adverse Effects of Androgen Deprivation, Approximate Frequency, and Potential Therapeutic Options for Amelioration[a]

Effect	Approximate Frequency	Potential Corrective Actions
Libido loss	Universal	None known
Erectile dysfunction	Universal	None known
Hot flashes	50%–80%	Venlafaxine, estrogens, progestins
Muscle loss	Common, duration-dependent	Exercise
Weight gain	Common	Exercise/diet
Facial/body hair loss	Very common	None known
Fatigue	Not defined	Exercise
Emotional lability	Not defined	None known
Depression	0%–30%	Various antidepressants
Cognitive dysfunction	Not defined	None known
Gynecomastia	Up to 20%	Preemptive radiation
Breast tenderness	Not defined	Aromatase inhibitors
Osteoporosis	Common, duration-dependent	Exercise/bisphosphonates
Anemia	5%–13%	Erythropoietin not recommended
Hyperlipidemia	10%	Diet, statins
Diabetes	0.8%/year increase	Exercise, oral agents
Myocardial infarction	0.25%/year increase	Treatment of risk factors
Coronary heart disease	1%/year increase	Treatment of risk factors

[a] A number of events are poorly defined in frequency as a consequence of a lack of controlled studies, quantitative assessments, and/or agreed on definitions.

PRACTICE OF ONCOLOGY

alone does not cure the disease. Prognosis varies by the disease state, grade of the tumor, rapidity of growth, and extent of disease when hormone therapy was started. Adverse features from multiple series include a high Gleason score (8 to 10), low performance status, bone pain, low hemoglobin, high alkaline phosphatase, low testosterone level, and extensive as opposed to minimal disease.[372,373] The number of metastases[344] or percentage of the skeleton involved by tumor[345] is also prognostic. In one series, 2-year survival times were 94%, 71%,

61%, and 40% for men with 0 to 5, 6 to 10, 19, and ≥20 lesions, respectively.[374,375] Using a different classification, patients with minimal disease (involvement confined to the axial skeleton [pelvis and/or spine] and/or LN) and extensive disease (disease in long bones, skull or ribs, and/or viscera) had median PFS of 46 months and 16 months, respectively, and overall survival times of 51 months and 27.5 months, respectively.[376]

Prognosis can be estimated in part by the degree and rapidity of response determined by the posttreatment PSA nadir and the timing of the nadir. In a trial enrolling 1,345 patients, failure to achieve a PSA nadir of ≤4 ng/ml within 7 months was associated with a median survival of 13 months, whereas those with a nadir between 0.2 to 4.0 ng/ml had a median survival of 44 months, and patients with a nadir ≤0.2 ng/ml had a median survival of 75 months.[377] With respect to the timing of the nadir, those who achieved a nadir in <6 months had a median survival of 4.5 years versus 7.8 years for those with a nadir after 6 months from the start of treatment.[378]

Unfortunately, more contemporary natural history studies for patients with metastatic disease are lacking, in part because fewer men are presenting with metastatic disease, and because this approach has been the standard of care for over seven decades, fewer randomized trials are being conducted. As a result, comparing different treatments outside of dedicated trials is difficult due to the different methods used to determine and define disease extent, the posttreatment monitoring schema, and how outcomes were reported, leaving several basic questions in management incompletely resolved.

Is one form of monotherapy that suppresses testosterone levels superior to another? No. All single-therapy hormonal interventions that lower serum testosterone levels to castrate levels had similar overall survival times after 2 years of treatment.[379] An EORTC study, powered for a 13% difference around the medians, showed similar outcomes between DES 1 mg and orchiectomy.[380] In a meta-analysis of 10 randomized controlled trials that included

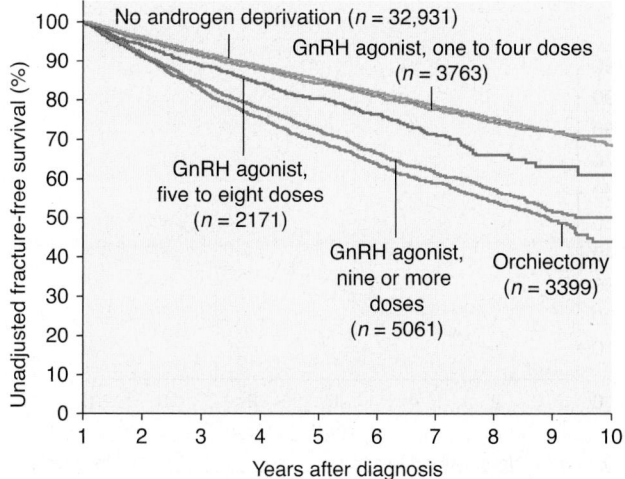

Figure 68.17 Fracture rate as a function of time after androgen deprivation therapy in men older than age 68 in the United States. Number of doses is the number administered within 12 months after diagnosis. GnRH, gonadotropin-releasing hormone. (From Shahinian VB, Kuo YF, Freeman JL, et al. Risk of fracture after androgen deprivation for prostate cancer. *N Engl J Med* 2005;352:154, with permission.)

LHRH agonists/antagonists, orchiectomy, DES, or choice of DES or orchiectomy, outcomes were similar.

Is more complete androgen suppression superior? Geller et al.[381] were the first to document elevated DHT levels in patients treated by orchiectomy, a finding validated later when more sensitive and specific mass spectroscopy–based assays became available,[382] and the demonstration of persistent PSA and TMPRSS2:ERG expression in posthormone treated RP specimens indicating continued AR signaling.[383,384] This led to trials testing the hypothesis that more complete androgen suppression using a combination of an antiandrogen (flutamide, bicalutamide, or nilutamide) to inhibit adrenal androgens with a LHRH agonist/antagonist or orchiectomy would provide greater benefit.[317] Adrenal androgens can contribute 5% to 45% of the residual androgens present in tumors after surgical castration alone. Early results were promising,[385] but subsequent meta-analyses have been conducted showing that the first-generation antiandrogens did not add significantly to the antitumor effects of surgical castration.[319,341,386,387] One, summarizing 27 randomized trials with 8,275 patients, showed a 2% difference in mortality at 5 years: 72.4% for monotherapy versus 70.4% for the combined approach[386]; a second meta-analysis limited to trials of a nonsteroidal antiandrogen showed a 2.9% difference: 75.3% versus 72.4% at 5 years.[341] Other combinations explored to effect more complete androgen suppression included low-dose DES and megestrol acetate; an LHRH analog and ketoconazole plus hydrocortisone; an LHRH analog, antiandrogen and ketoconazole, plus hydrocortisone or aminoglutethimide and hydrocortisone.[387] None proved meaningfully superior.

When should hormone therapy be initiated? Early versus late? This question is difficult to answer because of methodologic differences in the trials designed to address it. The differences include the clinical state of the patient group studied, whether the primary tumor has been treated and how (no treatment, surgery, or radiation including dose and treatment field), the specific hormones used, the duration they were administered, and the patient follow-up including the frequency of visits and the specific clinical, laboratory, and imaging assessments performed. Critical to the discussion as well is the "trigger" used to start treating patients randomized to the "no immediate treatment" arm of the study, which range from a predefined degree or level of PSA rise alone, the documentation of metastases, or the development of symptoms. Further confounding the issue is that in some studies, a significant proportion of patients in the "no immediate treatment" group were never treated.

A complete review of all of the trials designed to assess this question is beyond the scope of this chapter. In general, randomized trials

that address this question show "early" hormone therapy delays the time to metastases and symptoms, but the effect on overall survival is less clear. A key consideration in formulating a recommendation for patients at a particular point in the illness is to balance the likelihood that a patient would require treatment based on the development of metastatic disease or symptoms and when, with the likelihood that no treatment would ever be required based on these same metrics.

Trials in patients who did not receive treatment of the primary tumor were reported by the Veterans Administration Research Service Cooperative Urological Research Group, the Medical Research Council (MRC), and the Early Prostate Cancer Trials Group. The Veterans Administration Research Service Cooperative Urological Research Group trials enrolled 1,900 patients staged primarily by DRE and showed that DES or orchiectomy could delay the development of metastatic disease in patients with locally advanced stage C tumors,[388,389] although overall survival was worse due to cardiovascular complications. There was also no overall survival benefit for patients with metastatic disease.

The MRC PR03 trial randomized 998 patients with locally advanced or asymptomatic metastatic prostate cancer to "immediate" treatment (orchiectomy or LHRH analog) or to the same treatment deferred until there was an "indication." The trigger to initiate treatment was "clinically significant progression," which was as frequent locally as metastatic. The trial showed that patients treated with early therapy were less likely to require a TURP or develop ureteral obstruction, progress from M0 to M1 disease ($P < 0.001$, two-tailed), to develop pain ($P < 0.001$), or to die of prostate cancer relative to those in whom therapy was "deferred." Even so, survival times were similar between the two groups. An important caveat limiting the extrapolation of the results to the question of "early" versus "late" was that half of the men who died in the deferred arm never received therapy.[390]

The Early Prostate Cancer Trials Group trial ($n = 985$) randomized men with T0-4N0-2M0 prostate cancer who were not candidates for local therapy to immediate or to deferred treatment until symptomatic progression was documented. The results showed an increased risk of death in the deferred arm (HR = 1.25; 95% CI = 1.05 to 1.48), which remained after adjusting for baseline factors. Notable was that only 49.7% of men in the deferred arm began anticancer therapy during the median 7.8-year follow-up period, suggesting that a significant proportion of men on the immediate arm were overtreated. The median time to treatment for those who required it, however, was 3.2 years. Deaths were equally balanced between prostate cancer ($n = 193$, 18.8% of the population) and cardiovascular disease ($n = 185$) (Fig. 68.18).[391]

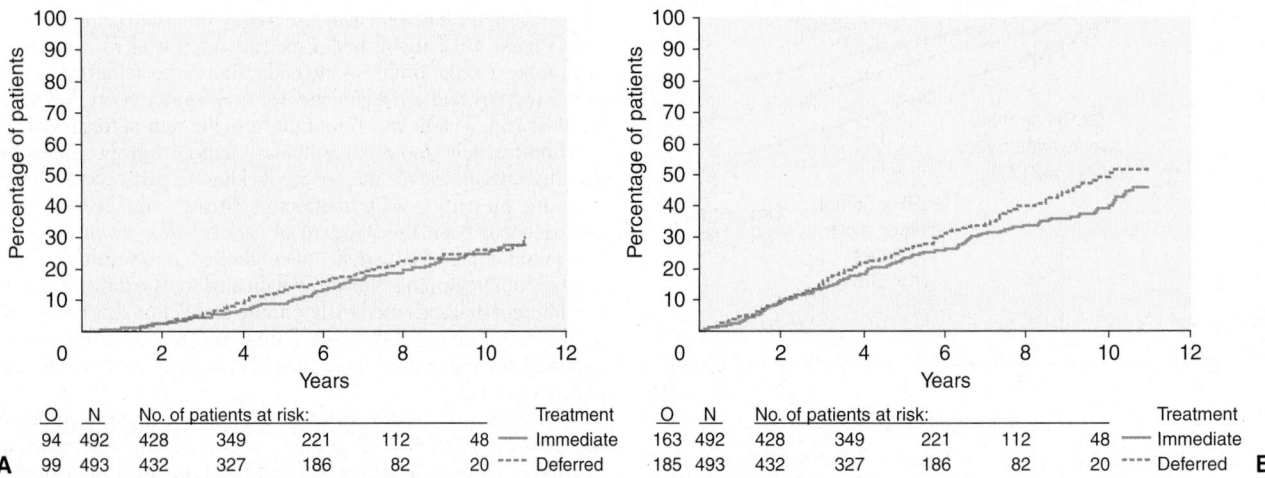

Figure 68.18 Immediate versus deferred hormonal therapy in patients with M0 prostate cancer who either refused local therapy or were deemed unsuitable for local therapy. **(A)** Prostate cancer–specific mortality. **(B)** Non-prostate cancer mortality. (From Studer UE, Whelan P, Albrecht W, et al. Immediate or deferred androgen deprivation for patients with prostate cancer not suitable for local treatment with curative intent: European Organisation for Research and Treatment of Cancer [EORTC] Trial 30891. *J Clin Oncol* 2006;24:1868, with permission.)

Rising Prostate-Specific Antigen (Extrapelvic Disease)

For the patient presumed to have microscopic nodal or more distant disease that would not respond or which cannot be addressed by additional treatment to the primary site, the optimal timing of ADT initiation is controversial. The first issue is to determine the risk of developing metastatic disease and in what time frame. One series that addressed this question included 1997 RP-treated patients, of whom 315 (15%) developed a rising PSA and were followed with annual imaging and PSA assessment until metastatic disease was documented. Of these patients, metastatic disease was subsequently documented in 103 at a median actuarial time of 8 years, of whom 44 (44%, or 2% of the 1997) died of disease.[392] Factors associated with the development of metastasis included the grade of the primary tumor, the time interval between the start of the treatment to the date of first recurrence, the absolute PSA value, and the rate that it was rising, typically expressed in terms of the PSADT.[393] In a separate study, virtually all cancer-related deaths occurred in men who had PSADT ≤6 months, independent of whether the patient received radiation or surgery as primary treatment.[394] In practice, many physicians consider treating patients when the PSADT is ≤12 months, although there remains no absolute PSA level mandating that treatment be started.

Strategies to Reduce the Toxicities Associated with Androgen Deprivation Therapy. Now, with the widespread use of PSA-based detection and monitoring, fewer men are diagnosed with or develop symptoms of advanced prostate cancer. For these individuals, the tolerance of castration is less than for men who receive treatment to relieve the symptoms of urinary obstruction or bone pain from osseous spread. This, coupled with the adverse events that can occur with longer use, has led to the evaluation of noncastrating approaches in an effort to improve patient tolerance without compromising efficacy.

Antiandrogen Monotherapy. Several randomized trials have compared antiandrogens alone to conventional testosterone-lowering forms of castration. Bicalutamide 50 mg daily, the dose approved for use in combination with an LHRH analog, was inferior to surgical orchiectomy.[395] Bicalutamide 150 mg, which produces a higher frequency of PSA normalization than does the 50 mg dose (97% versus 73% of cases), showed mixed results: inferiority to castration for patients with metastatic disease but equivalence for patients with M0 disease (rising PSA values with no detectable metastases on imaging studies).[396] Another approach is to begin with the antiandrogen alone and add a testosterone-lowering therapy when PSA levels rise. Unfortunately, only 30% of patients treated in this fashion respond to the addition of the LHRH analog.[397] Nevertheless, some patients may be willing to accept this risk

rather than experience the impotence and other adverse effects of testosterone-lowering treatment, as long as symptoms of disease are controlled.

Intermittent Androgen Depletion/Blockade. A second approach that is now used widely is intermittent androgen deprivation (IAD). It evolved somewhat empirically in the era of estrogen therapy, pre-PSA, when it was recognized that patients in whom therapy was stopped for noncancer-related reasons would often respond when the treatment was resumed to control the disease.[398] The central hypothesis, based on studies in murine tumors, is that by minimizing the exposure time to a castrate environment, the sensitivity to subsequent androgen depletion would be retained.[399,400] An additional advantage is the potential for an improved QOL during the "off" intervals.

Applied today, the approach is considered for patients who respond well to ADT, typically defined as a PSA nadir ≤4 ng/ml for those with metastatic disease, and is restarted when PSA levels return to a predetermined level (typically 10 ng/ml to 20 ng/ml). Multiple phase 3 trials have been reported that differ in the patient population treated (BCR only, metastatic disease only, or both), the type and duration of treatment (3 months to 8 months), the criteria for discontinuation and for restarting it, and the primary end point. Most report a time to progression measure but do not use the same criteria. Few are powered for survival. Several large randomized trials have been reported recently: none showed the intermittent approach to be superior to continuous therapy in terms of cancer control, but most show a better QOL during the off intervals, which patients prefer.

In one trial enrolling 1,386 patients, median survival in the intermittent versus continuous arms was 8.8 years and 9.1 years, respectively, with more prostate cancer deaths in the intermittent arm and more deaths from other causes, including cardiovascular events, in the continuous arm. In this trial, a slight increase in cancer-related deaths in the intermittent arm was counterbalanced by an increase in nonprostate cancer deaths in the continuous arm.[401]

In the largest trial reported to date, 3,040 men with noncastrate metastatic disease were enrolled, of whom 1,535 met the criteria for discontinuation. The trial was designed as a noninferiority study to show that the intermittent approach was no more than 20% inferior to continuous therapy. No significant different in survival was observed overall, but for the subset of men with disease limited to the axial skeleton and no visceral disease at presentation, the median survival was 7.1 years for continuous therapy and 5.1 years for the intermittent group (HR = 1.23; 95% CI = 1.02 to 1.48); the study did not exclude IAD to be inferior.[402] Three meta-analyses were recently reported based on 8 trials enrolling a total of 4,664 patients,[403] nine trials of 5,508 patients,[404] and 13 trials

Study or Subgroup	log[Hazard Ratio]	SE	Weight	Hazard Ratio IV, Fixed, 95% CI
Calais da Silva 2009/2011	0.04082199	0.09302291	13.4%	1.04 [0.87, 1.25]
Crook 2012	0.01980263	0.08705543	15.3%	1.02 [0.86, 1.21]
Hussain 2013	0.09531018	0.06416923	28.2%	1.10 [0.97, 1.25]
Irani 2008	0.51082562	0.26909671	1.6%	1.67 [0.98, 2.82]
Miller 2007	0.03922071	0.0969628	12.4%	1.04 [0.86, 1.26]
Mottet 2012	0.13102826	0.22048025	2.4%	1.14 [0.74, 1.76]
Salonen 2012/2013	−0.13976194	0.10287809	11.0%	0.87 [0.71, 1.06]
Silva 2013	−0.10536052	0.08626502	15.6%	0.90 [0.76, 1.07]
Total (95% CI)			**100.0%**	**1.02 [0.95, 1.09]**

Heterogeneity: $Chi^2 = 9.57$, df = 7 (P = 0.21); $I^2 = 27\%$
Test for overall effect: Z = 0.58 (P = 0.56)

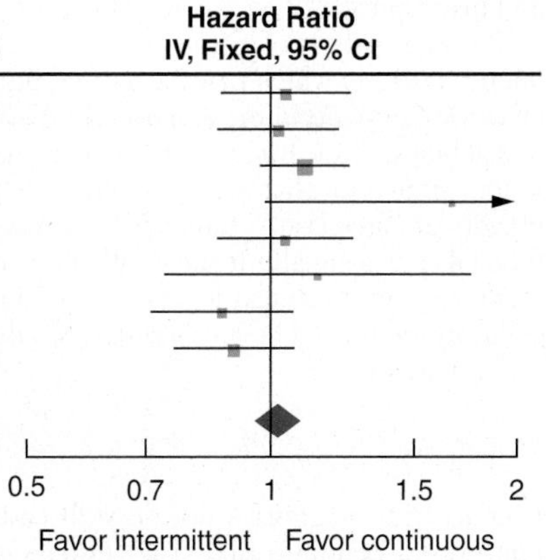

Favor intermittent   Favor continuous

Figure 68.19 Overall survival with intermittent versus continuous androgen deprivation in prostate cancer. This figure is licensed under a Creative Commons Attribution 4.0 license. (From Botrel TE, Clark O, dos Reis RB, et al. Intermittent versus continuous androgen deprivation for locally advanced, recurrent or metastatic prostate cancer: a systematic review and meta-analysis. *BMC Urol* 2014;14:9.)

of 6,419 men[405] (Fig. 68.19). All showed no difference in overall survival, two showed no significant differences in disease-specific survival,[403,405] and one showed more deaths with IAD offset by more prostate cancer deaths with continuous therapy.[404] IAD was superior with respect to overall QOL and sexual function with significantly reduced costs.

While some controversy remains whether a patient will accept the tradeoff of a potentially higher risk of a prostate cancer death in return for time off therapy, it is important to recognize that the approach should only be considered for patients who respond well to ADT. In the recently reported SWOG study, only 1,535 of the 3,040 enrolled patients (51%) reached the defined PSA nadir of ≤4 ng/ml.[402]

Castration-Resistant Disease: Metastatic and Nonmetastatic

A rising PSA despite castrate levels of testosterone represents the transition to a castration-resistant (CRPC) state, which is lethal for most men. Clinically, there are several phenotypes: nonmetastatic that includes a rising PSA or disease limited to the prostate or prostate bed, and metastatic which includes the patterns of osseous disease and no soft tissue disease, nodal spread and no bone or visceral spread, and visceral spread with or without osseous disease. In some cases, the pattern of spread is observed with no increase in PSA. Symptoms may or may not be present. Disease in other sites, including the adrenal glands, omentum, kidney, pancreas, or brain, is rare. Which pattern develops in a patient is influenced in part by the extent of disease at the time ADT was first initiated. The patient who initially received hormones for a rising PSA alone is likely to relapse with a rising PSA and negative imaging studies—the nonmetastatic-CRPC state. A therapeutic objective for these patients is to prevent the development of bone metastases, the likelihood of which is highly variable between patients. In the placebo arm of one metastasis prevention study evaluating denosumab, the median time to metastasis was 25.2 months,[406] whereas in a second evaluating zoledronate, only one-third of patients had evidence of radiologic spread after 2 years of follow-up.[407] In Smith et al.,[408] men with a PSADT of ≤6 months had a median time to first bone metastases of 18.5 months.

In both trials, overall risk of developing visible metastases by imaging was most informed by the PSA level at baseline and the PSADT: men with higher PSA levels and faster PSADT had a shorter time to first bone metastasis. In contrast, the patient who first receives hormones for symptomatic osseous disease is more likely to develop recurrent symptoms and is at higher risk of death from prostate cancer. Considered by site of spread based on trials enrolling patients with progressing metastatic CRPC, 85% to 90% have osseous disease, 20% to 40% have measurable pelvic or retroperitoneal nodal disease, and 5% to 10% have visceral (lung and liver) spread.[409–411]

A unique pattern of spread being recognized with increasing frequency is one in which new metastases, predominantly in the lung or viscera, develop in the absence of a PSA rise. Histologically on repeat biopsy, these tumors may be pure small cell/neuroendocrine lesions similar to what is seen in other sites, or are classified more broadly as "anaplastic" tumors.[409,410] These entities, when documented, are generally treated with platinum-containing chemotherapy regimens similar to what is used in small cell tumors that occur in the lung. The responses are similar: rapid improvements of short duration.[412]

Patient Management

Patients with progressive disease with castrate levels of testosterone should continue LHRH agonist/antagonist therapies recognizing that no randomized trials have prospectively addressed this issue. Although not direct evidence, the survival benefits seen with the recently approved agents that inhibit AR signaling would

suggest that allowing testosterone levels to rise may adversely affect outcome. A retrospective analysis of 341 patients treated on four trials of secondary therapies suggested an improved survival for continuous androgen suppression when corrected for other factors,[413] but another did not.

The first consideration is to document castrate levels of testosterone. In rare cases, approximately 1% in prospective trials, LHRH analogs do not effect complete testosterone suppression.[414] The second is whether the patient has been on long-term antiandrogen therapy in combination with an LHRH analog or surgical orchiectomy, and if so, whether to discontinue the antiandrogen (continuing LHRH analog therapy) and to monitor the patient for a withdrawal response. The withdrawal response, consistent with the conversion of an antagonist to an agonist, was first reported in 1993 with flutamide discontinuation and later shown to occur with bicalutamide, nilutamide, cyproterone acetate, estrogens, glucocorticoids, and progestational agents.[415,416] The onset of the withdrawal response, when it occurs, is directly related to the half-life of the drug: early for flutamide with its short half-life and 6 weeks to 8 weeks for agents such as bicalutamide, which has a 7-day half-life. The disease flare that can occur with megestrol acetate prescribed to increase appetite is consistent with an agonist effect.[397,417–419]

Previously, if no withdrawal response was observed, patients were often treated with a different antiandrogen to which they had not been exposed, with limited benefit. The approaches included estrogens such as oral DES at a dose of 1 mg/d to 3 mg/d,[420] Premarin (1.25 mg three times daily; Wyeth Pharmaceuticals Inc., Philadelphia, PA),[421] estramustine, the first agent with a formal indication in this setting, [422] and various parenteral formulations.[423] All provided PSA decline rates in the 24% to 42% range, although durable responses were rare.[422,424] Attempts to reduce the thromboembolic risk of estrogens by using transdermal estrogen delivery systems have been made; however, efficacy in these trials has generally been less than anticipated.[425,426]

Ketoconazole, 600 to 1,200 mg/d in combination with hydrocortisone to minimize adrenal insufficiency, produces PSA declines by ≥50% in up to 71% of patients,[427] the response correlating with higher serum androgen levels at baseline.[428] Absorption requires an acidic environment and so it is typically taken with juice. Proton-pump inhibitors and H_2 antagonists potentially interfere with absorption. Caution is urged with ketoconazole use as it is a potent inhibitor of CYP3A4. Cancer progression is associated with rises in androstenedione and DHEA sulfate,[429] implying that steroidogenic compensatory mechanisms contribute to escape from ketoconazole.

Prednisone 10 mg daily was shown to palliate symptoms of the disease in one-third of patients by Tannock et al.[430] in the pre-PSA era. Based on this, prednisone became an integral part of the "control" arms of many phase 3 trials in this disease. Similar results have been reported with hydrocortisone 30 mg/d to 40 mg/d and low-dose dexamethasone 0.5 mg to 2 mg daily in the PSA era, with reported decline rates ranging from 16% to 59% of patients.[431] These agents also lower serum androgen levels and, in a recent phase 3 trial in which patients were treated with prednisone 10 mg daily plus placebo, median survival times increased with each quartile increase in baseline serum androgen levels. PSA levels at baseline strongly associated with survival ($p < 0.0001$) in bivariate and multivariable analyses.[432]

Cytotoxic Therapy

Mitoxantrone. Building on the palliative benefits observed with prednisone alone, its combination with mitoxantrone 12 mg/m^2 every 3 weeks suggested superiority to prednisone monotherapy. The definitive phase 3 trial enrolling 160 patients, small by today's standard, used a primary end point of pain palliation assessed with a patient-reported outcome scale and measuring daily analgesic consumption.[320] The trial was not designed nor was it powered to show a survival benefit. The results showed that a higher proportion of patients treated with the combination had a decrease in pain (29% versus 12%) and overall palliative response (38% versus 21%). Consistent with the findings was a decrease in analgesic consumption, improved bowel function, and increased patient mobility. Disease control shown by the duration of pain relief among mitoxantrone responders was 43 weeks versus 18 weeks for the control group. Similar results were obtained in a second trial,[433] leading to the approval of mitoxantrone and prednisone for the treatment of CRPC in 1996 and establishing the regimen as the first cytotoxic-containing standard and the standard to which other treatments would be compared. Common toxicities with mitoxantrone at doses of 12 mg/m^2 every 3 weeks included nausea (61%), fatigue (39%), alopecia (29%), and anorexia (25%). Grade 3/4 neutropenia is reported in approximately 20% of patients, but febrile neutropenia is relatively unusual (2% of patients). Cardiac function is a concern; decreased cardiac function was reported in 5% to 7% of patients.

Docetaxel. Two pivotal trials were reported in 2004 showing that docetaxel plus prednisone could palliate symptoms, delay progression, and definitively prolong life relative to mitoxantrone and prednisone. TAX327 compared docetaxel 75 mg/m^2 every 3 weeks for up to 10 cycles (group 1), docetaxel 30 mg/m^2 weekly for 5 cycles (group 2), or mitoxantrone 12 mg/m^2 every 3 weeks for 10 cycles (group 3). Prednisone (10 mg daily) was added to all regimens. The primary end point was overall survival; secondary end points included changes in pain, PSA, and overall QOL. Median survival for the respective arms was 18.9 months, 17.4 months, and 16.5 months, respectively, which led to the approval of docetaxel plus prednisone for "androgen-independent (hormone-refractory)" disease. The 2.4-month difference in median survival (18.9 months versus 16.5 months) for the every-three-week docetaxel versus the mitoxantrone schedule established the every-three-week regimen as the de facto standard.[322]

SWOG 99-16 randomized 770 patients to estramustine (280 mg orally three times daily on days 1 to 5), docetaxel (60 mg/m^2 every 3 weeks), and dexamethasone (60 mg every 3 weeks) versus mitoxantrone and prednisone (5 mg twice a day) to a maximum of 12 cycles with no crossover at progression. The primary end point was overall survival. PSA declines, soft tissue response, and PFS were secondary end points. Here again, a 2-month difference in median survival was observed for docetaxel/estramustine (17.5 months versus 15.6 months), representing a 20% reduction in mortality (HR = 0.8). A higher incidence of neutropenia and fever, nausea, vomiting, and vascular events with docetaxel/estramustine was noted despite the lower dose of docetaxel. The results further supported docetaxel 70 mg/m^2 every 3 weeks as the standard regimen.[321]

With docetaxel established as the first-line cytotoxic standard, drug development efforts focused on three discrete clinical contexts: the prechemotherapy space, the first-line cytotoxic chemotherapy space to build on the results of docetaxel, and the postchemotherapy space for which there was no standard of care at the time. Notable is that none of the docetaxel-based combination trials showed an improvement over single-agent therapy, whereas, in several trials, outcomes were inferior with the combination arm (see Table 68.14).[329–337]

Cabazitaxel is a next-generation taxane with an improved therapeutic index relative to docetaxel that is noncross-resistant with the parent compound in selected contexts.[434] Following successful early phase trials showing antitumor activity in docetaxel-refractory metastatic CRPC, a randomized phase 3 trial comparing cabazitaxel plus prednisone (*n* = 377) to mitoxantrone plus prednisone (*n* = 378) was developed in this setting. At the final analysis, median survival and median PFS for the cabazitaxel and mitoxantrone cohorts was 15.1 months and 12.7 months (HR =0.70; 95% CI = 0.59 to 0.83; *p* <0.0001) and 2.8 months and 1.4 months (HR = 0.74; 95% CI = 0.64 to 0.86; *p* <0.0001), respectively.[325] In 2010, the FDA approved cabazitaxel plus prednisone for the treatment of metastatic CRPC previously treated with a docetaxel-containing regimen.

Further progress was not achieved until there was a more complete understanding of the biology of the disease. Through profiling studies of prostate cancers representing different clinical states, a series of oncogenic changes in the AR signaling pathway were identified that showed CRPC remained hormone driven, while serving as points for therapeutic attack. These changes included amplification of a wild-type AR gene, overexpression of the enzymes involved in androgen synthesis, and alterations in the ligand-binding domain and co-activator/co-repressor protein interactions leading to promiscuous activation by other steroid hormones and antiandrogens.[435] Consistent with the upregulation of the androgen biosynthetic machinery, and with the development of mass spectroscopy based assays for serum and tissue androgens,[436] came the demonstration that intratumoral androgen levels in metastatic CRPC tumor samples could exceed those present in the prostates of men in a eugonadal state.[437] This finding, coupled with overexpression of the receptor itself, enabled an intracrine signaling mechanism to sustain growth.

Abiraterone acetate plus prednisone: The cytochrome P450 (17) inhibitor abiraterone was developed to inhibit testicular and adrenal androgen production,[438] and shown in a series of three dose-escalating studies to achieve androgen suppression in both noncastrate and castrate men.[439] A subsequent phase 1 trial in men with CRPC who had not received chemotherapy showed a sustained decrease in testosterone to the 1 ng/dl to 2 ng/dl range as well as a reduction in estradiol, DHEA, and androstenedione, confirming the dependence of CRPC on ligand-activated AR signaling. Antitumor effects included significant declines in PSA, tumor regressions, and favorable changes in circulating tumor cell number. Adverse clinical and laboratory events consistent with mineralocorticoid excess including hypertension, fluid retention, and hyperkalemia were identified, which could be reduced by eplerenone or prednisone.[440] A second phase 1 trial showed similar results in the same patient group and established a dose of 1,000 mg daily for phase 2 investigations.[441]

Phase 2 trials of abiraterone acetate alone[442] or abiraterone acetate plus prednisone[443] in postchemotherapy-treated CRPC followed based on the hypothesis that the decision to treat a patient with chemotherapy would not change the underlying biology of the disease significantly, and that if efficacy were shown, the track to approval would be shorter because the prognosis of these patients was inferior to that of patients who had not received prior chemotherapy. The unmet need for effective therapy was also greater in this population because there was no standard of care that had been shown to prolong life. Two phase 2 trials followed, one that excluded prior ketoconazole exposure[442] and one which did not[443]; both trials showed significant activity leading to the definitive phase 3 trial, Cougar AA-301, comparing the combination of abiraterone acetate (1,000 mg daily) plus prednisone (5 mg twice a day) to placebo plus prednisone (5 mg twice a day). The primary end point was overall survival, and secondary end points were radiographic PFS (rPFS), PSA response, time to PSA progression, and changes in QOL. Superiority of the combination relative to the placebo combination with respect to overall survival was shown in both interim (median 14.8 months versus 10.9 months; HR = 0.65; 95% CI = 0.54 to 0.77; *p* <0.001) and final (15.8 months versus 11.2 months; HR = 0.74; 95% CI = 0.64 to 0.86) analyses. The drug was approved in 2011 for postchemotherapy-treated CRPC.[327,444]

Subsequently, there was an abiraterone phase 3 trial in chemotherapy-naïve patients that used a coprimary end point of rPFS and overall survival. Notably, the rPFS end point included the PCWG2 definition of bone scan progression, which enabled 72% (166 of 229) of patients with apparent progression on a first follow-up to continue treatment because no additional new lesions were documented on the confirmatory scan. In the final analysis with a median follow-up period of 27.1 months, rPFS was

8.3 months in the placebo arm and not yet reached in the abiraterone arm (HR = 0.43; 95% CI = 0.35 to 0.52; p <0.0001). Improvement in overall survival (35.3 months versus 30.1 months; HR = 0.78; 95% CI = 0.66 to 0.95; p = 0.0151) did not reach the prespecified statistical efficacy boundary but was supported by significant improvements in time-to-opiate-use and time-to-cytotoxic-chemotherapy end points.[324,445] Abiraterone plus prednisone gained expanded approval for chemotherapy-naïve metastatic CRPC in 2012.[324]

Next-Generation Antiandrogens

Enzalutamide (previously MDV3100) was rationally designed with the aim of developing an antiandrogen active in prostate cancers with overexpressed AR, a setting in which the tumor is both resistant and growth is stimulated by bicalutamide, consistent with an antagonist-agonist conversion.

In the phase 1/2 enzalutamide clinical trial that enrolled patients with pre- and postchemotherapy CRPC treated with a variety of dose levels, there were PSA declines of ≥50% in 71% and 37% of patients who were prechemotherapy or postchemotherapy treated, respectively, along with soft tissue regressions, and a posttherapy conversion of circulating tumor cell counts from unfavorable to favorable in 49% (25 of 51) of patients.[446] The results led to the phase 3 AFFIRM trial in which 1,199 men with progressive postchemotherapy-treated CRPC were randomized in a 2:1 ratio to enzalutamide 160 mg daily (n = 800) or placebo (n = 399). The primary end point was overall survival and at the first interim analysis, a statistically significant reduction in mortality was seen (HR = 0.63; 95% CI = 0.53 to 0.74; p <0.001), with a median overall survival of 18.4 months (95% CI = 17.3 to not yet reached) for enzalutamide versus 13.6 months (95% CI = 11.3 to 15.8) in the placebo group. All secondary end points favored enzalutamide including rPFS (8.3 months versus 2.9 months; HR = 0.40; p <0.001), the time to the first SRE (16.7 months versus 13.3 months; HR = 0.69; p <0.001), and QOL response rate (43% versus 18%; p <0.001). The results led to FDA approval in 2012.[328]

More recently, the results of the prechemotherapy enzalutamide trial PREVAIL were reported; PREVAIL randomized 1,717 patients with prechemotherapy CRPC to enzalutamide 160 mg daily or placebo using the coprimary end points of rPFS and overall survival. This study was stopped by the data and safety monitoring board after 540 deaths based on the superiority of enzalutamide in delaying radiographic progression or death (HR = 0.19; 95% CI = 0.15 to 0.23; p <0.001) and risk of death (HR = 0.71; 95% CI = 0.60 to 0.84; p <0.001) relative to placebo. The benefit of enzalutamide was consistent for all secondary end points including rate of ≥50% PSA decline (78% versus 3%;), overall soft tissue response (59% versus 5%), time to PSA progression (HR = 0.17), time to initiation of cytotoxic chemotherapy (HR = 0.35), and time to first SRE (HR = 0.72) (p <0.001 for all comparisons).[447] These results have been submitted to the FDA, and an expanded indication is pending.

New antiandrogens in development include ARN-509 and galeterone. ARN-509 was more potent than enzalutamide in preclinical models,[448] has shown significant activity in a phase 1 trial,[449] and is now in phase 3 testing in nonmetastatic CRPC (NCT01946204). Galeterone (previously TOK-001) has multiple effects, including blocking and degrading AR,[450] and will be entering phase 3 testing shortly.

Targeting the Tumor Microenvironment

Immunotherapy

Sipuleucel-T (Provenge; Dendreon Corporation, Seattle, WA) is an autologous active cellular immunotherapy that includes an acid phosphatase specific, replication-competent adenovirus that is cotransfected with granulocyte macrophage–colony-stimulating factor. Mononuclear cells are harvested by leukopheresis, transfected with the viral construct, and maintained in culture under an adequate number of the defined mononuclear cell fraction has developed to enable re-infusion to the patient. A phase 1 dose-ranging study showed that injection of the primed cells into the prostates of patients with recurrent disease after radiation therapy was safe, and declines in PSA were observed that correlated with the administered dose of the virus.[451]

A randomized phase 3 trial in which patients received either primed and unprimed mononuclear cells was then performed; the trial failed to meet the primary end point of PFS,[452] but with longer follow-up, an overall survival benefit was observed.[453] A pivotal trial was then designed in which 512 patients with asymptomatic or minimally symptomatic metastatic CRPC were randomized to three doses of the biologic product or autologous cells that had been treated similarly but not exposed to the granulocyte macrophage–colony-stimulating factor/prostatic acid phosphatase fusion protein. The results showed a significant improvement in survival for the immunized patients (HR = 0.77; 95% CI = 0.61 to 0.97; p = 0.02), median 25.8 months in the sipuleucel-T arm and 21.7 months in the control arm. Adverse reactions were primarily related to the infusion of the activated cells and included chills (53%), fatigue (41%), fever (31%), back pain (30%), nausea (21%), joint aches (20%), and headaches (18%). Most of these reactions had resolved within 2 days of infusion. Grade 3–4 events were <3% for each of these conditions. No improvement in PFS or response rate was seen in the large randomized trial, suggesting either that these parameters were not accurately measured or that slower kinetics of the disease were manifest after progression was initially measured. FDA approval was granted in 2010.[324]

PROSTVAC (Bavarian Nordic, Kvistgaard, Denmark) is a vaccinia and fowlpox immunization approach that includes the gene sequence for PSA and three costimulatory molecules (B7-1, ICAM-1, and LFA-3) collectively designated as TRICOM. In the phase 1 trial, patients received the recombinant vaccinia virus vaccine first, which was followed by a booster injection with recombinant fowlpox virus; all patients generated an immune response to vaccinia.[454] A randomized phase 2 trial was then performed with a primary end point of PFS, which showed no difference between the groups, but 3 years post study, 30% (25 of 82) of the vaccine-treated versus 17% (7 of 40) of the placebo-treated patients were alive (median survival 25.1 months versus 16.6 months; HR = 0.56; 95% CI = 0.37 to 0.85).[453] A phase 3 trial is ongoing.

Ipilimumab: Cytotoxic T-lymphocyte antigen-4 is a T-cell coinhibitory and immune checkpoint molecule expressed by activated and regulatory T cells that plays a critical role in maintaining immune homeostasis and peripheral tolerance to self-antigens. In preclinical studies, cytotoxic T-lymphocyte antigen-4 blockade augmented T cell–mediated immune responses against tumors. This led to the development of ipilimumab, a fully humanized immunoglobulin G_1 monoclonal antibody to cytotoxic T-lymphocyte antigen-4 in malignant melanoma, renal cell carcinoma, prostate cancer, and other tumors. Two phase 3 trials demonstrated an overall survival benefit in malignant melanoma leading to FDA approval, and of particular note is the durable, complete remission of over 4 years in approximately 20% to 25% of patients.[455,456] Antitumor activity was shown in a phase 1/2 trial of ipilimumab alone or in combination with EBRT in prostate cancer,[457] which led to a phase 3 trial in patients with CRPC who had received prior treatment with docetaxel of radiation therapy alone versus radiation therapy plus ipilimumab.[458] This study failed to meet the primary overall survival end point but did show evidence of activity at later time points. A second trial in prechemotherapy treated CRPC has fully accrued.

There are two randomized, double-blind, phase 3 registration trials in metastatic CRPC, which have fully accrued. One trial, comparing the efficacy of ipilimumab versus placebo in asymptomatic or minimally symptomatic patients with chemotherapy-naïve metastatic CRPC (NCT01057810), fell short of the primary end point. Results from preclinical studies and early clinical trials suggest synergistic effect of ipilimumab and next-generation drugs targeting the AR signaling axis, cytotoxics and other immune modulators (poxvirus).

Cabozantinib (previously XL-184) is an orally bioavailable tyrosine kinase inhibitor with potent activity against MET and vascular endothelial growth factor receptor 2 shown in preclinical bone metastatic CRPC models to inhibit osteoblasts and osteoclasts function. In the clinic, the drug produced dramatic improvements in radionuclide bone scans which were associated with relief of pain. In a subsequent phase 2 randomized discontinuation study (nonrandomized extension),[459] 122 patients with postdocetaxel CRPC with measurable disease received cabozantinib 100 mg daily for 12 weeks and were then randomized based on response: subjects with response by modified RECIST criteria continued open-label cabozantinib, subjects with progressive disease discontinued therapy, and subjects with stable disease were randomized to either placebo or continued cabozantinib (primary end point: PFS). The results showed improvements on bone scan in 68% of patients, including complete resolution in 12%, declines in total alkaline phosphatase and plasma cross-linked C-terminal telopeptide of type I collagen of ≥50% in 57% of patients, and 67% showed reductions in pain. Notable was that improvements in pain and changes in PSA were in 40% of patients.

A subsequent nonrandomized extension was conducted in 85 patients evaluable for bone scan response, and 51 (60%) had a partial resolution, 24 (28%) stable disease, 5 (6%) progressive disease, and 5 (6%) discontinued prior to follow-up scan. Measurable disease was reduced in 21/30 patients (70%). Of the 33 patients with a Brief Pain Inventory score ≥4, 16 (49%) had pain reduction durable for ≥6 weeks; 46% had decreased narcotic use, including 27% who discontinued use completely.

The results led to the design of two, currently ongoing, phase 3 trials of cabozantinib in patients with metastatic CRPC who have progressed on docetaxel-containing chemotherapy and abiraterone or enzalutamide. In COMET-1 (NCT01605227), the effect of cabozantinib on overall survival is being compared to prednisone. COMET-2 (NCT01522443) explores the effect of cabozantinib versus mitoxantrone plus prednisone on pain response and bone scan response.

Tasquinimod (formerly ABR-215050) is a quinoline carboxamide that binds to the immunomodulatory protein S100A9 with antiangiogenic activity in xenograft models through a vascular endothelial growth factor–independent mechanism.[460–462] A randomized placebo-controlled phase 2 trial of 201 men with chemotherapy-naïve CRPC showed improvement in median PFS (7.6 months versus 3.3 months; HR = 0.57; 95% CI = 0.39 to 0.85; $p = 0.0042$)[463] and a trend toward improvement in median overall survival (33.4 months versus 30.4 months; $p = 0.49$).[464] The results led to a phase 3 trial (10TASQ10) in men with asymptomatic to mildly symptomatic metastatic CRPC. Other ongoing studies include the phase 1 CATCH trial combining tasquinimod and cabazitaxel in postchemotherapy metastatic CRPC (NCT01513733) and a phase 2 trial evaluating the drug as a maintenance therapy for men with metastatic CRPC who are not progressing after first-line docetaxel-based therapy (NCT01732549).

PALLIATION

Bone-Directed Therapy

The high propensity for prostate cancers to metastasize to the skeleton puts patients at a high risk for significant morbidity from SREs. This can be complicated further by the bone loss associated with ADT itself, and the frequent use of corticosteroids for antitumor effects, to reduce the toxicities of anticancer agents such as the taxanes and CYP17 inhibitors, and for palliation of pain or

symptoms related to neurologic compromise. Targeting the bone microenvironment can provide palliation of symptoms, delay SREs, and prolong life.

Targeting Growth Factors and Cytokines

Bisphosphonates localize to the bone tumor interface and inhibit osteoclast activity to reduce bone turnover. The bisphosphonate zoledronate is the only FDA-approved agent for CRPC with bone metastases. In randomized trials, zoledronate (4 mg intravenously every 3 to 4 weeks) reduced the frequency of SREs (defined as pathologic fractures, radiation to bone, spinal cord compression, and/or surgery to bone) by 25% (33% with zoledronate versus 44%; $p = 0.021$). Time to first SRE was prolonged, whereas skeletal morbidity rate and the proportion of patients with an individual SRE were lowered. There was no effect on overall survival.[159] Bisphosphonates are also used in patients with prostate cancer to reduce the risk of osteoporosis, exacerbated by ADT, that increases the susceptibility to fracture or collapse of a vertebra in nontumor-bearing areas.[159] Nephrotoxicity can occur with these agents, and doses must be adjusted on the basis of renal function.

Denosumab is a monoclonal antibody that binds RANKL, inhibiting osteoclast function. Initial trials showed a decrease in bone loss and reduction in fracture rate for patients on ADT.[465] A subsequent phase 3 trial enrolled 1,904 patients and compared denosumab (120 mg subcutaneous monthly) to zoledronate (4 mg every 3 weeks). The primary end point, delay in time to first SRE, showed a benefit in favor of denosumab (20.7 months versus 17.1 months; HR = 0.82; $p <0.001$ for noninferiority and $p = 0.008$ for superiority). The denosumab arm had a slightly higher frequency of serious adverse events (63% versus 60%), Common Terminology Criteria for Adverse Events grade 3-4 adverse events (72% versus 66%; $p = 0.01$), and grade ≥3 hypocalcemia (5% versus 1%). There was no significant difference in the rate of serious adverse events, disease progression, or overall survival. The frequency of osteonecrosis of the jaw was similar (2% versus 1%). This relatively rare but serious side effect seems associated with bisphosphonate or denosumab use in combination with dental disease, dental surgery (e.g., tooth extraction), oral trauma, periodontitis, poor dental hygiene, glucocorticoid use, or chemotherapy use.[338]

Denosumab 120 mg every 4 weeks was also shown to delay the development of bone metastases relative to placebo in patients with nonmetastatic CRPC at a high risk of bone metastases (baseline PSA ≥8 ng/ml or PSADT ≤10 months). In this trial, bone metastasis–free survival was increased by a median of 4.2 months (median 29.5 months, 95% CI = 25.4 to 33.3 for denosumab versus 25.2 months, 95% CI = 22.2 to 29.5 for placebo). Denosumab also prolonged the time to first bone metastasis. Osteonecrosis was observed in 5% of patients receiving denosumab. Although statistically significant, denosumab's effect upon bone metastases was deemed insufficient for FDA approval.[406]

Pain

Optimal palliation of pain requires careful attention to the pain frequency, pattern, and precipitating factors. It also requires early performance of appropriate diagnostic studies to establish an etiology.

Critical for pain management is a low threshold for recommending an MRI if there should be any of the following: back pain suggestive of neurologic compromise of the spinal cord or cauda equina; diplopia, dysarthria, difficulty swallowing, or facial weakness suggestive of involvement of the base of the skull; or numbness in the jaw or chin suggestive of mental nerve compromise that may interfere with eating.[466] If neurologic encroachment is documented in any of these areas, radiotherapy should be administered on an urgent basis to preserve function and to maximize the chance of recovery. Corticosteroids are also administered to provide more immediate palliation, and to reduce the risk of further compromise secondary to swelling that can occur after radiotherapy is initiated.[467] An MRI can also be recommended for patients with extensive bony disease in the absence of symptoms, as one series showed occult cord compromise in 11% of patients, which involved multiple locations in several patients.[468] Metastases to the base of the skull leading to cranial nerve palsies can also severely compromise function unless diagnosed and treated expeditiously.

For one or more painful lesions that can be encompassed by a single or regional radiation port, EBRT offers excellent palliation. A variety of fractionation schemes and administered daily doses have been studied: 30 Gy administered as 300 cGy in 10 fractions is considered standard, although randomized trials have shown a single administered dose of 8 Gy in 1 fraction to be equivalent but not as durable. Patients treated with 30 Gy are less likely to require repeat treatment (18% versus 9%). High-dose hypofractionation regimens have also been studied, including 20 Gy or 24 Gy as a single dose, or 500 cGy to 800 cGy in three separate doses. A limitation of EBRT is that the disease is often diffuse and that lacking some form of systemic control, patients often experience recurrence in a relatively short interval after a first lesion is treated. In such cases of patients with recurrence of painful lesions outside of radiated areas, a systemic approach is preferred. Retreatment of a site previously irradiated is also necessary in approximately 25% of cases.[469–471]

Radiopharmaceuticals

Therapies to control more diffuse pain include those directed at the tumor/bone interface with little effect on tumor, those directed at specific cytokines and growth factors produced by tumor cells and the host that contribute to the progression and survival of prostate cancer cells in the skeleton, and those directed at the tumor itself.

Bone-seeking radiopharmaceuticals are taken up rapidly at the tumor/bone interface with maximal deposition at the site of maximal bone turnover. The distribution of the isotope through the tumor is uncertain, making dosimetry difficult to calculate, but estimates are that the administered dose to the tumor itself is typically below that achieved with EBRT. Three such agents are currently approved in the United States on the basis of phase 3 trials.[326,472–474]

Strontium-89 is a low-energy beta-emitter with a long (50-day) half-life. It was approved on the basis of a trial enrolling patients with symptomatic skeletal metastasis randomized to EBRT alone or EBRT plus the radiopharmaceutical, showing patients treated with strontium were less likely to have pain in new metastatic sites.[474]

Samarium (^{153}Sm) lexidronam,[475,476] with a 2.9-day half-life, relies on the diphosphonate moiety for targeting, while the radionuclide simultaneously emits gamma energies that can be imaged and short-range beta energies that can be therapeutic. Technetium (99mTc) methyl diphosphonate bone imaging can identify tumors with high uptake.

^{153}Sm-EDTMP exhibits pharmacokinetic, toxicity, and pain response using an escalating dose schedule in treatment of metastatic bone cancer. This agent was approved on the basis of a trial that randomized patients to radioactive (^{153}Sm) versus nonradioactive (^{152}Sm) drug, showing a reduction in both opioid analgesic consumption and improvement in patient-reported visual analog scales and pain descriptor scales. The most common side effects were pain flare in approximately 10% of cases that could last for several days and myelosuppression which varies with the extent of disease and with the amount of bone marrow that has received radiation in the past.[472,477] ^{153}Sm lexidronam has also been safely administered on a repetitive basis in combination with docetaxel.[478]

As beta-emitters, both strontium-89 and ^{153}Sm lexidronam have a penetration energy up to 2.4 mm in bone that disrupts normal hematopoiesis leading to myelosuppression and anemia. Tumor cell kill results from the inability to repair single-strand DNA breaks induced by the agent.

Radium-223 dichloride (radium-223) is a high linear energy transfer radiation that has a very short (<0.1 mm) range and induces double-strand DNA breaks, rendering cellular repair mechanisms ineffective. Exposure of the surrounding tissues is minimized. After activity was shown in a phase 1 trial,[479] a phase 3, randomized, double-blind, placebo-controlled study was completed that enrolled, in a 2:1 ratio, 922 patients with symptomatic bone metastases and no visceral disease who had either received, were not eligible to receive, or declined docetaxel. Patients were randomized to receive six injections of radium-223 (at a dose of 50 kBq per kg of body weight intravenously) or matching placebo; one injection was administered every 4 weeks. The primary end point was overall survival. Secondary end points included time to the first symptomatic SRE; time to bone-specific alkaline phosphatase progression, response, and normalization; PSA progression; and changes in several biochemical measures. Relative to placebo, radium-223 significantly improved overall survival (median, 14 months versus 11.2 months; HR = 0.66; 95% CI = 0.58 to 0.83; two-sided p = 0.00007). Assessments of all main secondary efficacy end points also showed a benefit for radium-233 compared with placebo, including the time to first SRE, which was prolonged from a median 9.8 months for placebo to 15.6 months (HR = 0.66; 95% CI = 0.52 to 0.83). Notable was that the drug was associated with low myelosuppression rates and fewer adverse events.[326]

FUTURE DIRECTIONS

The key to prostate cancer diagnosis and management is the assessment of risk based on the continuous reassessment of the disease at the current point in time and projecting the likelihood of disease-specific events in the future. Now, advances in our understanding of prostate cancer biology have changed diagnostic and treatment paradigms and improved the outcomes for patients across the clinical spectrum of the disease. The diagnostic algorithms used to detect disease are increasingly incorporating biologic determinants to better enable the detection of clinically significant cancers rather than all cancers. Many of the prognostic models used to define the metastatic and lethal potential of a tumor are also including molecular measures in addition to the standard clinicopathologic measures such as T stage (plagued by interobserver variability), PSA (lacks sensitivity and specificity), and Gleason score based on morphology. All prognostic models aim to ensure that only those tumors with the potential to cause symptoms, metastasize, or shorten patient survival are treated, while recognizing that for the tumors that are not treated, close monitoring using an AS approach is the "treatment."

Technologic advances in surgery and radiation therapy have resulted in better cancer control rates, particularly for "high-risk" patients, with fewer and lesser short- and long-term morbidities. In these cases, the focus of treatment centers on two objectives: control of the primary tumor and of metastatic disease. A range of biomarkers are in development to better inform prognosis (who needs treatment), prediction (what type of treatment), treatment efficacy (if it is working), and regulatory approval (providing clinical benefit). Missing in many biomarker studies is clinical utility—showing the incremental information provided by the "test" relative to what is currently available, a key factor in whether a test will be used in practice.

The same needs apply to patients who have experienced recurrence after primary therapy: to determine the likelihood that a tumor can be cured if still localized, independent of whether the primary treatment was surgery or radiation, and if not still localized, to guide the need for a systemic intervention based on the likelihood that metastatic disease might develop and when. Equally important is that we have learned that prostate cancer in an individual is more than one disease that can have different drivers of growth in different tumors as well as within one individual site of disease. The heterogeneity increases even further with the increasing number of drugs to which the cancer has been exposed. To address this will require the continued characterization of disease biology. However, the necessary repeated tissue- or blood-based diagnostics to do so are presently not part of routine clinical practice.

Unfortunately, the field is still plagued by the use of end points of convenience that occur early as opposed to end points that take longer to observe but which more accurately reflect clinical benefit. Few reports include a clearly defined statistical design, and those that do rarely define a level of improvement to justify the development of a large-scale definitive trial to generate the evidence required to change practice standards.

The recent approval of several life-prolonging therapies as well as agents that reduce morbidity is particularly encouraging. However, it also presents an additional challenge because the use of effective treatments *after* a patient has been treated on a clinical trial reduces the trial's ability to show a survival benefit for an experimental drug. The failure to show a survival benefit in the phase 3 trials in CRPC with the Cyp 17 inhibitor orteronel[480] and custirsen,[481] an antisense molecule that reduces the levels of the antiapoptotic protein clusterin, are recent examples. The latter represents another docetaxel-based combination that failed to show a survival benefit relative to docetaxel alone. Yet, both agents showed promising effects in phase 2 studies[482–484] and show that it is essential to carefully consider the regulatory path to approval for any prostate cancer drug. Critical here is the discovery, validation, and qualification of predictive biomarkers of sensitivity. Such biomarkers will enable the enrollment of patients most likely to respond to the treatment being evaluated and will supply trial end points short of survival that could potentially lead to regulatory approvals.

A challenge now is to design trials that show how to maximize patient benefit with the available agents, used alone in sequence or in combination, and to understand cross-resistance and synergies. Strategies to improve outcomes with AR and AR signaling inhibitors include the development of new antiandrogens such as ARN-509 and galeterone (previously TOK-001). An analysis of the posttherapy PSA patterns of patients treated with AR and AR signaling inhibitors shows that a proportion of tumors are intrinsically resistant, a proportion show a pattern consistent with acquired resistance, and others show durable response followed later by progression.[485] Studies in preclinical models have associated intrinsic resistance with reciprocal feedback between the AR and phosphatidylinositol kinase signaling pathways,[486] and AR splice variants,[487] in particular the AR-V7 variant,[488] whereas acquired resistance has been associated with an acquired mutation in the ligand-binding domain of the AR at position 876L.[489] Cooptation of the AR by the glucocorticoid receptor[490] and a number of new agents and combinations are being evaluated in the clinic based on activity demonstrated in these models.

The efficacy seen with newer agents in late-stage disease also suggests that the time is now to shift our paradigm from palliation to cure by evaluating available life-prolonging therapies in noncastrate settings with low disease burdens. Several trials exploring combinations of ADT and radiation therapy have been completed and have shown significant survival improvements. Such has not been the case with trials of ADT and RP as, to date, only one trial that enrolled patients with node-positive disease following RP showed a survival improvement.[491] More recently, another trial, CHAARTED, showed that early use of docetaxel in combination with standard ADT conferred a 13.6-month improvement in median survival for patients with high-grade, high-volume, noncastrate disease.[492] Two ongoing randomized trials are awaited that will evaluate a similar combination in the high-risk neoadjuvant setting (NCT00430183) and in patients with a rising PSA with rapid PSADT (NCT01813370). An important consideration in the design of such studies is to demonstrate that the "experimental" treatment proposed has sufficient activity to justify large-scale testing. Here, neoadjuvant studies are particularly important because they ensure that adequate amounts of tumor material are available for analysis.[493] One promising approach reported recently was a randomized trial in which abiraterone acetate and prednisone in combination with leuprolide acetate was shown to provide a higher pathologic complete response rate relative to leuprolide acetate alone.[494] To test this further, the trial in patients with a rising PSA and rapid PSADT is comparing degarelix in combination with abiraterone acetate and prednisone to degarelix alone, with the end point of an undetectable PSA (NCT01813370). Trials of this type can be useful to support larger-scale studies to address whether even greater benefit can be provided to patients with potentially lethal disease if treated early, an approach that has been shown to be effective in many cancer types.

SELECTED REFERENCES

The full reference list can be accessed at lwwhealthlibrary.com/oncology.

1. Scher HI, Heller G. Clinical states in prostate cancer: towards a dynamic model of disease progression. *Urology* 2000;55:323–327.

5. Center MM, Jemal A, Lortet-Tieulent J, et al. International variation in prostate cancer incidence and mortality rates. *Eur Urol* 2012;61:1079–1092.

7. Haenszel W, Kurihara M. Studies of Japanese migrants. I. Mortality from cancer and other diseases among Japanese in the United States. *J Natl Cancer Inst* 1968;40:43–68.

10. Smith JR, Freije D, Carpten JD, et al. Major susceptibility locus for prostate cancer on chromosome 1 suggested by a genome wide search. *Science* 1996;274:1371–1374.

11. Wilson KM, Giovannucci EL, Mucci LA. Lifestyle and dietary factors in the prevention of lethal prostate cancer. *Asian J Androl* 2012;14:365–374.

12. Scardino PT. Prostate cancer: improving PSA testing by adjusting for genetic background. *Nat Rev Urol* 2013;10:190–192.

13. Ewing CM, Ray AM, Lange EM, et al. Germline mutations in HOXB13 and prostate-cancer risk. *N Engl J Med* 2012;366:141–149.

14. Gallagher DJ, Gaudet MM, Pal P, et al. Germline BRCA mutations denote a clinicopathologic subset of prostate cancer. *Clin Cancer Res* 2010;16:2115–2121.

17. Vertosick EA, Poon BY, Vickers AJ. Relative value of race, family history and prostate-specific antigen as indications for early initiation of prostate cancer screening. *J Urol* 2014 [Epub ahead of print]. doi: 10.1016/j.juro.2014.03.032

21. Allott EH, Masko EM, Freedland SJ. Obesity and prostate cancer: weighing the evidence. *Eur Urol* 2013;63:800–809.

22. Muller RL, Gerber L, Moreira DM, et al. Obesity is associated with increased prostate growth and attenuated prostate volume reduction by dutasteride. *Eur Urol* 2013;63:1115–1121.

24. Ma J, Li H, Giovannucci E, et al. Prediagnostic body-mass index, plasma C-peptide concentration, and prostate cancer-specific mortality in men with prostate cancer: a long-term survival analysis. *Lancet Oncol* 2008;9:1039–1047.

26. Klein EA, Thompson IM Jr, Tangen CM, et al. Vitamin E and the risk of prostate cancer: the Selenium and Vitamin E Cancer Prevention Trial (SELECT). *JAMA* 2011;306:1549–1556.

31. Paprotka T, Delviks-Frankenberry KA, Cingoz O, et al. Recombinant origin of the retrovirus XMRV. *Science* 2011;333:97–101.

32. Thompson IM, Goodman PJ, Tangen CM, et al. The influence of finasteride on the development of prostate cancer. *N Engl J Med* 2003;349:215–224.

34. Theoret MR, Ning YM, Zhang JJ, et al. The risks and benefits of 5alpha-reductase inhibitors for prostate-cancer prevention. *N Engl J Med* 2011;365:97–99.

35. Thompson IM Jr, Goodman PJ, Tangen CM, et al. Long-term survival of participants in the prostate cancer prevention trial. *N Engl J Med* 2013;369:603–610.

36. Andriole GL, Bostwick DG, Brawley OW, et al. Effect of dutasteride on the risk of prostate cancer. *N Engl J Med* 2010;362:1192–1202.

37. US Food and Drug Administration. FDA Drug Safety Communication: 5-alpha reductase inhibitors (5-ARIs) may increase the risk of a more serious form of prostate cancer. June 9, 2011. Accessed May 21, 2014. http://www.fda.gov/Drugs/DrugSafety/ucm258314.htm.

38. Schmitz-Drager BJ, Schoffski O, Marberger M, et al. Risk adapted chemoprevention for prostate cancer: an option? *Recent Results Cancer Res* 2014;202:79–91.

39. Ohori M, Scardino PT. Localized prostate cancer. *Curr Probl Surg* 2002;39:833–957.

45. Bostwick DG. Prospective origins of prostate carcinoma. Prostatic intraepithelial neoplasia and atypical adenomatous hyperplasia. *Cancer* 1996;78:330–336.

48. De Marzo AM, Platz EA, Epstein JI, et al. A working group classification of focal prostate atrophy lesions. *Am J Surg Pathol* 2006;30:1281–1291.

50. Beahrs OH, Henson DE, Hutter RVP, et al. *American Joint Committee on Cancer. AJCC Cancer Staging Manual.* 4th ed. Philadelphia, PA: Lippincott-Raven, 1992.

51. Edge S, Byrd DR, Compton CC, et al. *American Joint Committee on Cancer. AJCC Cancer Staging Manual.* 7th ed. New York: Springer, 2010.

52. Fleming ID, Cooper JS, Henson DE, et al. *American Joint Committee on Cancer. AJCC Cancer Staging Manual.* 5th ed. Philadelphia: JB Lippincott, 1997.

53. Gleason DF. Classification of prostatic carcinomas. *Cancer Chemother Rep* 1966;50:125–128.

54. Gleason DF, Mellinger GT. Prediction of prognosis for prostatic adenocarcinoma by combined histological grading and clinical staging. *J Urol* 1974;111:58–64.

55. Epstein JI. Prognostic significance of tumor volume in radical prostatectomy and needle biopsy specimens. *J Urol* 2011;186:790–797.

59. Morgan TM, Welty CJ, Vakar-Lopez F, et al. Ductal adenocarcinoma of the prostate: increased mortality risk and decreased serum prostate specific antigen. *J Urol* 2010;184:2303–2307.

60. Nadal R, Schweizer M, Kryvenko ON, et al. Small cell carcinoma of the prostate. *Nat Rev Urol* 2014;11:213–219.

62. Catalona WJ, Richie JP, Ahmann FR, et al. Comparison of digital rectal examination and serum prostate specific antigen in the early detection of prostate cancer: results of a multicenter clinical trial of 6,630 men. *J Urol* 1994;151:1283–1290.

64. Lilja H, Piironen TP, Rittenhouse HG, et al. Value of molecular forms of prostate-specific antigen and related kallikreins, hk2, in diagnosis and staging of prostate cancer. In Vogelzang NA, Scardino PT, Shipley WU, et al. *Comprehensive Textbook of Genitourinary Oncology.* 2nd ed. Philadelphia: Lippincott Williams & Wilkins; 2000:638–650.

66. Eastham JA, Riedel E, Scardino PT, et al. Variation of serum prostate-specific antigen levels: an evaluation of year-to-year fluctuations. *JAMA* 2003;289:2695–2700.

67. Thompson IM, Pauler DK, Goodman PJ, et al. Prevalence of prostate cancer among men with a prostate-specific antigen level < or =4.0 ng per milliliter. *N Engl J Med* 2004;350:2239–2246.

68. Lilja H, Cronin AM, Dahlin A, et al. Prediction of significant prostate cancer diagnosed 20 to 30 years later with a single measure of prostate-specific antigen at or before age 50. *Cancer* 2011;117:1210–1219.

69. Orsted DD, Bojesen SE, Kamstrup PR, et al. Long-term prostate-specific antigen velocity in improved classification of prostate cancer risk and mortality. *Eur Urol* 2013;64:384–393.

70. Vickers AJ, Cronin AM, Bjork T, et al. Prostate specific antigen concentration at age 60 and death or metastasis from prostate cancer: case-control study. *BMJ* 2010;341:c4521.

71. Orsted DD, Nordestgaard BG, Jensen GB, et al. Prostate-specific antigen and long-term prediction of prostate cancer incidence and mortality in the general population. *Eur Urol* 2012;61:865–874.

72. MSKCC Prostate Cancer: Screening Guidelines. Accessed May 6, 2014. http://www.mskcc.org/cancer-care/adult/prostate/screening-guidelines-prostate.

74. Hugosson J, Carlsson S, Aus G, et al. Mortality results from the Goteborg randomised population-based prostate-cancer screening trial. *Lancet Oncol* 2010;11:725–732.

79. Schroder FH, Hugosson J, Roobol MJ, et al. Screening and prostate-cancer mortality in a randomized European study. *N Engl J Med* 2009;360:1320–1328.

80. Cooperberg MR, Cowan JE, Hilton JF, et al. Outcomes of active surveillance for men with intermediate-risk prostate cancer. *J Clin Oncol* 2011;29:228–234.

82. Bellardita L, Rancati T, Alvisi MF, et al. Predictors of health-related quality of life and adjustment to prostate cancer during active surveillance. *Eur Urol* 2013;64:30–36.

83. Cooperberg MR, Broering JM, Carroll PR. Time trends and local variation in primary treatment of localized prostate cancer. *J Clin Oncol* 2010;28:1117–1123.

84. Klotz L, Zhang L, Lam A, et al. Clinical results of long-term follow-up of a large, active surveillance cohort with localized prostate cancer. *J Clin Oncol* 2010;28:126–131.

85. Taneja SS. Re: active surveillance for low-risk prostate cancer worldwide: the PRIAS study. *J Urol* 2013;189:1322.

86. Tosoian JJ, Trock BJ, Landis P, et al. Active surveillance program for prostate cancer: an update of the Johns Hopkins experience. *J Clin Oncol* 2011;29:2185–2190.

87. Moyer VA, U.S. Preventive Services Task Force. Screening for prostate cancer: U.S. Preventive Services Task Force recommendation statement. *Ann Intern Med* 2012;157:120–134.

88. Andriole GL, Crawford ED, Grubb RL 3rd, et al. Mortality results from a randomized prostate-cancer screening trial. *N Engl J Med* 2009;360:1310–1319.

89. Andriole GL, Crawford ED, Grubb RL 3rd, et al. Prostate cancer screening in the randomized Prostate, Lung, Colorectal, and Ovarian Cancer Screening Trial: mortality results after 13 years of follow-up. *J Natl Cancer Inst* 2012;104:125–132.

90. Schroder FH, Hugosson J, Roobol MJ, et al. Prostate-cancer mortality at 11 years of follow-up. *N Engl J Med* 2012;366:981–990.

91. Chou R, Croswell JM, Dana T, et al. Screening for prostate cancer: a review of the evidence for the U.S. Preventive Services Task Force. *Ann Intern Med* 2011;155:762–771.

92. Carlsson S, Vickers AJ, Roobol M, et al. Prostate cancer screening: facts, statistics, and interpretation in response to the US Preventive Services Task Force Review. *J Clin Oncol* 2012;30:2581–2584.

93. Vickers AJ, Roobol MJ, Lilja H. Screening for prostate cancer: early detection or overdetection? *Annu Rev Med* 2012;63:161–170.

94. Heijnsdijk EA, Wever EM, Auvinen A, et al. Quality-of-life effects of prostate-specific antigen screening. *N Engl J Med* 2012;367:595–605.

95. Basch E, Oliver TK, Vickers A, et al. Screening for prostate cancer with prostate-specific antigen testing: American Society of Clinical Oncology Provisional Clinical Opinion. *J Clin Oncol* 2012;30:3020–3025.

96. Carter HB, Albertsen PC, Barry MJ, et al. Early detection of prostate cancer: AUA Guideline. *J Urol* 2013;190:419–426.

97. American Cancer Society. Can prostate cancer be found early? Updated March 12, 2014. Accessed June 6, 2014. http://www.cancer.org/cancer/prostate cancer/detailedguide/prostate-cancer-detection.

100. Pound CR, Partin AW, Epstein JI, et al. Prostate-specific antigen after anatomic radical retropubic prostatectomy. Patterns of recurrence and cancer control. *Cancer* 1997;79:528–537.

101. Oesterling JE, Jacobsen SJ, Chute CG, et al. Serum prostate-specific antigen in a community-based population of healthy men: establishment of age-specific reference ranges. *JAMA* 1993;270:860–864.

102. Petteway J, Brawer MK. Age specific versus 4.0 ng/ml as a PSA cutoff in the screening population: impact on cancer detection (abstract). *J Urol* 1995;153:465A.

107. O'Brien MF, Cronin AM, Fearn PA, et al. Pretreatment prostate-specific antigen (PSA) velocity and doubling time are associated with outcome but neither improves prediction of outcome beyond pretreatment PSA alone in patients treated with radical prostatectomy. *J Clin Oncol* 2009;27:3591–3597.

108. Loeb S, Sokoll LJ, Broyles DL, et al. Prospective multicenter evaluation of the Beckman Coulter Prostate Health Index using WHO calibration. *J Urol* 2013;189:1702–1706.

109. Catalona WJ, Partin AW, Sanda MG, et al. A multicenter study of [-2]proprostate specific antigen combined with prostate specific antigen and free prostate specific antigen for prostate cancer detection in the 2.0 to 10.0 ng/ml prostate specific antigen range. *J Urol* 2011;185:1650–1655.

111. Vickers AJ, Gupta A, Savage CJ, et al. A panel of kallikrein marker predicts prostate cancer in a large, population-based cohort followed for 15 years without screening. *Cancer Epidemiol Biomarkers Prev* 2011;20:255–261.

112. Heidenreich A, Abrahamsson PA, Artibani W, et al. Early detection of prostate cancer: European Association of Urology recommendation. *Eur Urol* 2013;64:347–354.

114. Catalona W, Richie J, deKernion JB, et al. Comparison of prostate specific antigen concentration versus prostate specific antigen density in the early detection of prostate cancer. *J Urol* 1994;152:2031–2036.

117. Porten SP, Whitson JM, Cowan JE, et al. Changes in prostate cancer grade on serial biopsy in men undergoing active surveillance. *J Clin Oncol* 2011;29:2795–2800.

118. Whitson JM, Porten SP, Hilton JF, et al. The relationship between prostate specific antigen change and biopsy progression in patients on active surveillance for prostate cancer. *J Urol* 2011;185:1656–1660.

123. Barqawi AB, Rove KO, Gholizadeh S, et al. The role of 3-dimensional mapping biopsy in decision making for treatment of apparent early stage prostate cancer. *J Urol* 2011;186:80–85.

125. Mohler JL, Kantoff PW, Armstrong AJ, et al. NCCN Guidelines: Prostate cancer, version 2.2014. *J Natl Compr Canc Netw* 2014;12:686–718.

126. Vargas HA, Akin O, Shukla-Dave A, et al. Performance characteristics of MR imaging in the evaluation of clinically low-risk prostate cancer: a prospective study. *Radiology* 2012;265:478–487.

131. Lin K, Szabo Z, Chin BB, et al. The value of a baseline bone scan in patients with newly diagnosed prostate cancer. *Clin Nucl Med* 1999;24:579–582.

132. Sciarra A, Barentsz J, Bjartell A, et al. Advances in magnetic resonance imaging: how they are changing the management of prostate cancer. *Eur Urol* 2011;59:962–977.

133. Greene FL, Page DL, Fleming ID, et al. *American Joint Committee on Cancer. AJCC Cancer Staging Manual.* 6th ed. New York: Springer, 2002.

134. Ohori M, Wheeler TM, Scardino PT. The New American Joint Committee on Cancer and International Union against Cancer TNM classification of prostate cancer. *Cancer* 1994;74:104–114.

136. Eifler JB, Feng Z, Lin BM, et al. An updated prostate cancer staging nomogram (Partin tables) based on cases from 2006 to 2011. *BJU Int* 2013;111:22–29.

137. D'Amico AV, Whittington R, Malkowicz SB, et al. Biochemical outcome after radical prostatectomy, external beam radiation therapy, or interstitial radiation therapy for clinically localized prostate cancer. *JAMA* 1998;280:969–974.

139. Stephenson AJ, Kattan MW, Eastham JA, et al. Prostate cancer-specific mortality after radical prostatectomy for patients treated in the prostate-specific antigen era. *J Clin Oncol* 2009;27:4300–4305.

146. Cuzick J, Berney DM, Fisher G, et al. Prognostic value of a cell cycle progression signature for prostate cancer death in a conservatively managed needle biopsy cohort. *Br J Cancer* 2012;106:1095–1099.

148. Bishoff JT, Freedland SJ, Gerber L, et al. Prognostic utility of the cell cycle progression score generated from biopsy in men treated with prostatectomy. *J Urol* 2014;192:409–414.

149. Klein EA, Cooperberg MR, Magi-Galluzzi C, et al. A 17-gene assay to predict prostate cancer aggressiveness in the context of Gleason grade heterogeneity, tumor multifocality, and biopsy undersampling. *Eur Urol* 2014 [Epub ahead of print]. doi: 10.1016/j.eururo.2014.05.004.

151. Stephenson AJ, Scardino PT, Eastham JA, et al. Postoperative nomogram predicting the 10-year probability of prostate cancer recurrence after radical prostatectomy. *J Clin Oncol* 2005;23:7005–7012.

152. Stephenson AJ, Scardino PT, Bianco FJ Jr, et al. Morbidity and functional outcomes of salvage radical prostatectomy for locally recurrent prostate cancer after radiation therapy. *J Urol* 2004;172:2239–2243.

153. Stephenson AJ, Scardino PT, Eastham JA, et al. Preoperative nomogram predicting the 10-year probability of prostate cancer recurrence after radical prostatectomy. *J Natl Cancer Inst* 2006;98:715–717.

154. Eggener SE, Scardino PT, Walsh PC, et al. Predicting 15-year prostate cancer specific mortality after radical prostatectomy. *J Urol* 2011;185:869–875.

155. Food and Drug Administration. *Guidance for Industry: Clinical Trial Endpoints for the Approval of Cancer Drugs and Biologics.* May 2007. Accessed May 21, 2014. http://www.fda.gov/downloads/Drugs/.../Guidances /ucm071590.pdf.

156. Eisenhauer EA, Therasse P, Bogaerts J, et al. New response evaluation criteria in solid tumours: revised RECIST guideline (version 1.1). *Eur J Cancer* 2009;45:228–247.

157. Scher HI, Halabi S, Tannock I, et al. Design and end points of clinical trials for patients with progressive prostate cancer and castrate levels of testosterone: recommendations of the Prostate Cancer Clinical Trials Working Group. *J Clin Oncol* 2008;26:1148–1159.

158. Smith MR. Bisphosphonates to prevent skeletal complications in men with metastatic prostate cancer. *J Urol* 2003;170:S55–S57.

160. Wilt TJ, Brawer MK, Jones KM, et al. Radical prostatectomy versus observation for localized prostate cancer. *N Engl J Med* 2012;367:203–213.

161. Berglund A, Garmo H, Tishelman C, et al. Comorbidity, treatment and mortality: a population based cohort study of prostate cancer in PCBaSe Sweden. *J Urol* 2011;185:833–839.

162. Vargas HA, Akin O, Afaq A, et al. Magnetic resonance imaging for predicting prostate biopsy findings in patients considered for active surveillance of clinically low risk prostate cancer. *J Urol* 2012;188:1732–1738.

163. Liu D, Lehmann HP, Frick KD, et al. Active surveillance versus surgery for low risk prostate cancer: a clinical decision analysis. *J Urol* 2012;187: 1241–1246.

164. Mullins JK, Bonekamp D, Landis P, et al. Multiparametric magnetic resonance imaging findings in men with low-risk prostate cancer followed using active surveillance. *BJU Int* 2013;111:1037–1045.

166. Godoy G, von Bodman C, Chade DC, et al. Pelvic lymph node dissection for prostate cancer: frequency and distribution of nodal metastases in a contemporary radical prostatectomy series. *J Urol* 2012;187:2082–2086.

169. Feifer AH, Elkin EB, Lowrance WT, et al. Temporal trends and predictors of pelvic lymph node dissection in open or minimally invasive radical prostatectomy. *Cancer* 2011;117:3933–3942.

172. Heidenreich A, Varga Z, Von Knobloch R. Extended pelvic lymphadenectomy in patients undergoing radical prostatectomy: high incidence of lymph node metastasis. *J Urol* 2002;167:1681–1686.

175. Touijer KA, Ahallal Y, Guillonneau BD. Indications for and anatomical extent of pelvic lymph node dissection for prostate cancer: practice patterns of uro-oncologists in North America. *Urol Oncol* 2013;31:1517–1521.

176. Touijer KA, Mazzola CR, Sjoberg DD, et al. Long-term outcomes of patients with lymph node metastasis treated with radical prostatectomy without adjuvant androgen-deprivation therapy. *Eur Urol* 2014;65:20–25.

177. Carlsson SV, Tafe LJ, Chade DC, et al. Pathological features of lymph node metastasis for predicting biochemical recurrence after radical prostatectomy for prostate cancer. *J Urol* 2013;189:1314–1318.

179. Bianco FJ Jr, Scardino PT, Eastham JA. Radical prostatectomy: long-term cancer control and recovery of sexual and urinary function ("trifecta"). *Urology* 2005;66:83–94.

180. Vickers A, Savage C, Bianco F, et al. Cancer control and functional outcomes after radical prostatectomy as markers of surgical quality: analysis of heterogeneity between surgeons at a single cancer center. *Eur Urol* 2011;59:317–322.

181. Vickers AJ, Bianco FJ, Serio AM, et al. The surgical learning curve for prostate cancer control after radical prostatectomy. *J Natl Cancer Inst* 2007;99:1171–1177.

182. Gandaglia G, Sammon JD, Chang SL, et al. Comparative effectiveness of robot-assisted and open radical prostatectomy in the postdissemination era. *J Clin Oncol* 2014;32:1419–1426.

184. Hu JC, Gu X, Lipsitz SR, et al. Comparative effectiveness of minimally invasive vs open radical prostatectomy. *JAMA* 2009;302:1557–1564.

186. Lepor H. Open versus laparoscopic radical prostatectomy. *Rev Urol* 2005; 7:115–127.

187. Murphy DG, Bjartell A, Ficarra V, et al. Downsides of robot-assisted laparoscopic radical prostatectomy: limitations and complications. *Eur Urol* 2010; 57:735–746.

188. Bill-Axelson A, Holmberg L, Garmo H, et al. Radical prostatectomy or watchful waiting in early prostate cancer. *N Engl J Med* 2014;370:932–942.

189. Bill-Axelson A, Holmberg L, Ruutu M, et al. Radical prostatectomy versus watchful waiting in early prostate cancer. *N Engl J Med* 2005;352: 1977–1984.

190. Vickers A, Bennette C, Steineck G, et al. Individualized estimation of the benefit of radical prostatectomy from the Scandinavian Prostate Cancer Group randomized trial. *Eur Urol* 2012;62:204–209.

191. Lane JA, Hamdy FC, Martin RM, et al. Latest results from the UK trials evaluating prostate cancer screening and treatment: the CAP and ProtecT studies. *Eur J Cancer* 2010;46:3095–3101.

193. Han M, Partin AW, Zahurak M, et al. Biochemical (prostate specific antigen) recurrence probability following radical prostatectomy for clinically localized prostate cancer. *J Urol* 2003;169:517–523.

196. Zincke H, Oesterling JE, Blute ML, et al. Long-term (15 years) results after radical prostatectomy for clinically localized (stage T2c or lower) prostate cancer. *J Urol* 1994;152:1850–1857.

197. Lu-Yao GL, Albertsen PC, Moore DF, et al. Outcomes of localized prostate cancer following conservative management. *JAMA* 2009;302:1202–1209.

198. Han M, Partin AW, Pound CR, et al. Long-term biochemical disease-free and cancer-specific survival following anatomic radical retropubic prostatectomy. The 15-year Johns Hopkins experience. *Urol Clin North Am* 2001;28: 555–565.

199. Yossepowitch O, Eggener SE, Bianco FJ Jr, et al. Radical prostatectomy for clinically localized, high risk prostate cancer: critical analysis of risk assessment methods. *J Urol* 2007;178:493–499.

200. Yossepowitch O, Eggener SE, Serio AM, et al. Secondary therapy, metastatic progression, and cancer-specific mortality in men with clinically high-risk prostate cancer treated with radical prostatectomy. *Eur Urol* 2008;53: 950–959.

201. Chang AJ, Autio KA, Roach M 3rd, et al. High-risk prostate cancer-classification and therapy. *Nat Rev Clin Oncol* 2014;11:308–323.

203. Zelefsky MJ, Kollmeier M, Cox B, et al. Improved clinical outcomes with high-dose image guided radiotherapy compared with non-IGRT for the treatment of clinically localized prostate cancer. *Int J Radiat Oncol Biol Phys* 2012;84:125–129.

204. Beckendorf V, Guerif S, Le Prise E, et al. 70 Gy versus 80 Gy in localized prostate cancer: 5-year results of GETUG 06 randomized trial. *Int J Radiat Oncol Biol Phys* 2011;80:1056–1063.

205. Al-Mamgani A, van Putten WL, Heemsbergen WD, et al. Update of Dutch multicenter dose-escalation trial of radiotherapy for localized prostate cancer. *Int J Radiat Oncol Biol Phys* 2008;72:980–988.

206. Kuban DA, Tucker SL, Dong L, et al. Long-term results of the M. D. Anderson randomized dose-escalation trial for prostate cancer. *Int J Radiat Oncol Biol Phys* 2008;70:67–74.

207. Zietman AL, Bae K, Slater JD, et al. Randomized trial comparing conventional-dose with high-dose conformal radiation therapy in early-stage adenocarcinoma of the prostate: long-term results from Proton Radiation Oncology Group/American College of Radiology 95-09. *J Clin Oncol* 2010;28: 1106–1111.

208. Dearnaley DP, Jovic G, Syndikus I, et al. Escalated-dose versus control-dose conformal radiotherapy for prostate cancer: long-term results from the MRC RT01 randomised controlled trial. *Lancet Oncol* 2014;15:464–473.

213. Kuban DA, Levy LB, Cheung MR, et al. Long-term failure patterns and survival in a randomized dose-escalation trial for prostate cancer. Who dies of disease? *Int J Radiat Oncol Biol Phys* 2011;79:1310–1317.

214. Spratt DE, Pei X, Yamada J, et al. Long-term survival and toxicity in patients treated with high-dose intensity modulated radiation therapy for localized prostate cancer. *Int J Radiat Oncol Biol Phys* 2013;85:686–692.

219. Zelefsky MJ, Pei X, Teslova T, et al. Secondary cancers after intensity-modulated radiotherapy, brachytherapy and radical prostatectomy for the treatment of prostate cancer: incidence and cause-specific survival outcomes according to the initial treatment intervention. *BJU Int* 2012;110: 1696–1701.

221. Ghadjar P, Zelefsky MJ, Spratt DE, et al. Impact of dose to the bladder trigone on long-term urinary function after high-dose intensity modulated radiation therapy for localized prostate cancer. *Int J Radiat Oncol Biol Phys* 2014;88:339–344.

225. Anwar M, Weinberg V, Chang AJ, et al. Hypofractionated SBRT versus conventionally fractionated EBRT for prostate cancer: comparison of PSA slope and nadir. *Radiat Oncol* 2014;9:42.

227. King CR, Brooks JD, Gill H, et al. Long-term outcomes from a prospective trial of stereotactic body radiotherapy for low-risk prostate cancer. *Int J Radiat Oncol Biol Phys* 2012;82:877–882.

228. King CR, Freeman D, Kaplan I, et al. Stereotactic body radiotherapy for localized prostate cancer: pooled analysis from a multi-institutional consortium of prospective phase II trials. *Radiother Oncol* 2013;109:217–221.

229. Mendenhall NP, Hoppe BS, Nichols RC, et al. Five-year outcomes from 3 prospective trials of image-guided proton therapy for prostate cancer. *Int J Radiat Oncol Biol Phys* 2014;88:596–602.

230. Hoppe BS, Michalski JM, Mendenhall NP, et al. Comparative effectiveness study of patient-reported outcomes after proton therapy or intensity-modulated radiotherapy for prostate cancer. *Cancer* 2014;120:1076–1082.

231. Sheets NC, Goldin GH, Meyer AM, et al. Intensity-modulated radiation therapy, proton therapy, or conformal radiation therapy and morbidity and disease control in localized prostate cancer. *JAMA* 2012;307:1611–1620.

234. Morris WJ, Keyes M, Spadinger I, et al. Population-based 10-year oncologic outcomes after low-dose-rate brachytherapy for low-risk and intermediate-risk prostate cancer. *Cancer* 2013;119:1537–1546.

235. Potters L, Morgenstern C, Calugaru E, et al. 12-year outcomes following permanent prostate brachytherapy in patients with clinically localized prostate cancer. *J Urol* 2005;173:1562–1566.

236. Zelefsky MJ, Chou JF, Pei X, et al. Predicting biochemical tumor control after brachytherapy for clinically localized prostate cancer: The Memorial Sloan-Kettering Cancer Center experience. *Brachytherapy* 2012;11:245–249.

237. Zelefsky MJ, Kuban DA, Levy LB, et al. Multi-institutional analysis of long-term outcome for stages T1-T2 prostate cancer treated with permanent seed implantation. *Int J Radiat Oncol Biol Phys* 2007;67:327–333.

238. Nag S, Bice W, DeWyngaert K, et al. The American Brachytherapy Society recommendations for permanent prostate brachytherapy postimplant dosimetric analysis. *Int J Radiat Oncol Biol Phys* 2000;46:221–230.

239. Stock RG, Stone NN, Cesaretti JA, et al. Biologically effective dose values for prostate brachytherapy: effects on PSA failure and posttreatment biopsy results. *Int J Radiat Oncol Biol Phys* 2006;64:527–533.

240. Guedea F, Aguilo F, Polo A, et al. Early biochemical outcomes following permanent interstitial brachytherapy as monotherapy in 1050 patients with clinical T1-T2 prostate cancer. *Radiother Oncol* 2006;80:57–61.

241. Khaksar SJ, Laing RW, Henderson A, et al. Biochemical (prostate-specific antigen) relapse-free survival and toxicity after 125I low-dose-rate prostate brachytherapy. *BJU Int* 2006;98:1210–1215.

242. Zelefsky MJ, Yamada Y, Cohen GN, et al. Five-year outcome of intraoperative conformal permanent I-125 interstitial implantation for patients with clinically localized prostate cancer. *Int J Radiat Oncol Biol Phys* 2007;67:65–70.

243. Sylvester JE, Grimm PD, Blasko JC, et al. 15-Year biochemical relapse free survival in clinical Stage T1-T3 prostate cancer following combined external beam radiotherapy and brachytherapy; Seattle experience. *Int J Radiat Oncol Biol Phys* 2007;67:57–64.

247. Merrick GS, Butler WM, Wallner KE, et al. Risk factors for the development of prostate brachytherapy related urethral strictures. *J Urol* 2006;175:1376–1380.

248. Waterman FM, Dicker AP. Probability of late rectal morbidity in 125I prostate brachytherapy. *Int J Radiat Oncol Biol Phys* 2003;55:342–353.

249. Gelblum DY, Potters L. Rectal complications associated with transperineal interstitial brachytherapy for prostate cancer. *Int J Radiat Oncol Biol Phys* 2000;48:119–124.

250. Gelblum DY, Potters L, Ashley R, et al. Urinary morbidity following ultrasound-guided transperineal prostate seed implantation. *Int J Radiat Oncol Biol Phys* 1999;45:59–67.

251. Bottomley D, Ash D, Al-Qaisieh B, et al. Side effects of permanent I125 prostate seed implants in 667 patients treated in Leeds. *Radiother Oncol* 2007;82:46–49.

252. Lee WR, Bae K, Lawton C, et al. Late toxicity and biochemical recurrence after external-beam radiotherapy combined with permanent-source prostate brachytherapy: analysis of Radiation Therapy Oncology Group study 0019. *Cancer* 2007;109:1506–1512.

253. Shah JN, Wuu CS, Katz AE, et al. Improved biochemical control and clinical disease-free survival with intraoperative versus preoperative preplanning for transperineal interstitial permanent prostate brachytherapy. *Cancer J* 2006;12:289–297.

254. Keyes M, Schellenberg D, Moravan V, et al. Decline in urinary retention incidence in 805 patients after prostate brachytherapy: the effect of learning curve? *Int J Radiat Oncol Biol Phys* 2006;64:825–834.

255. Albert M, Tempany CM, Schultz D, et al. Late genitourinary and gastrointestinal toxicity after magnetic resonance image-guided prostate brachytherapy with or without neoadjuvant external beam radiation therapy. *Cancer* 2003;98:949–954.

260. Pisansky TM, Pugh SL, Greenberg RE, et al. Tadalafil for prevention of erectile dysfunction after radiotherapy for prostate cancer: the Radiation Therapy Oncology Group [0831] randomized clinical trial. *JAMA* 2014;311:1300–1307.

261. Zelefsky MJ, Shasha D, Branco RD, et al. Prophylactic sildenafil citrate improves selected aspects of sexual function in men treated by radiotherapy for prostate cancer. *J Urol* 2014;192:868–874.

267. Hoskin PJ, Rojas AM, Bownes PJ, et al. Randomised trial of external beam radiotherapy alone or combined with high-dose-rate brachytherapy boost for localised prostate cancer. *Radiother Oncol* 2012;103:217–222.

268. D'Amico AV. Radiation and hormonal therapy for locally advanced and clinically localized prostate cancer. *Urology* 2002;60:32–37.

269. Jones CU, Hunt D, McGowan DG, et al. Radiotherapy and short-term androgen deprivation for localized prostate cancer. *N Engl J Med* 2011;365:107–118.

270. Lee AK. Radiation therapy combined with hormone therapy for prostate cancer. *Semin Radiat Oncol* 2006;16:20–28.

271. Bolla M, Van Tienhoven G, Warde P, et al. External irradiation with or without long-term androgen suppression for prostate cancer with high metastatic risk: 10-year results of an EORTC randomized study. *Lancet Oncol* 2010;11:1066–1073.

272. Hanks GE, Pajak TF, Porter A, et al. Phase III trial of long-term adjuvant androgen deprivation after neoadjuvant hormonal cytoreduction and radiotherapy in locally advanced carcinoma of the prostate: the Radiation Therapy Oncology Group Protocol 92-02. *J Clin Oncol* 2003;21:3972–3978.

274. D'Amico AV, Manola J, Loffredo M, et al. 6-month androgen suppression plus radiation therapy vs radiation therapy alone for patients with clinically localized prostate cancer: a randomized controlled trial. *JAMA* 2004;292:821–827.

277. Sasse AD, Sasse E, Carvalho AM, et al. Androgenic suppression combined with radiotherapy for the treatment of prostate adenocarcinoma: a systematic review. *BMC Cancer* 2012;12:54.

278. Zumsteg ZS, Spratt DE, Pei I, et al. A new risk classification system for therapeutic decision making with intermediate-risk prostate cancer patients undergoing dose-escalated external-beam radiation therapy. *Eur Urol* 2013;64:895–902.

280. Zumsteg ZS, Zelefsky MJ. Short-term androgen deprivation therapy for patients with intermediate-risk prostate cancer undergoing dose-escalated radiotherapy: the standard of care? *Lancet Oncol* 2012;13:e259–e269.

281. Nguyen PL, Je Y, Schutz FA, et al. Association of androgen deprivation therapy with cardiovascular death in patients with prostate cancer: a meta-analysis of randomized trials. *JAMA* 2011;306:2359–2366.

286. Bolla M, van Poppel H, Tombal B, et al. Postoperative radiotherapy after radical prostatectomy for high-risk prostate cancer: long-term results of a randomised controlled trial (EORTC trial 22911). *Lancet* 2012;380:2018–2027.

287. Wiegel T, Bartkowiak D, Bottke D, et al. Adjuvant radiotherapy versus wait-and-see after radical prostatectomy: 10-year follow-up of the ARO 96-02/AUO AP 09/95 trial. *Eur Urol* 2014 [Epub ahead of print]. doi: 10.1016/j.eururo.2014.03.011.

288. Stephenson AJ, Scardino PT, Kattan MW, et al. Predicting the outcome of salvage radiation therapy for recurrent prostate cancer after radical prostatectomy. *J Clin Oncol* 2007;25:2035–2041.

290. Pfister D, Bolla M, Briganti A, et al. Early salvage radiotherapy following radical prostatectomy. *Eur Urol* 2014;65:1034–1043.

291. Goenka A, Magsanoc JM, Pei X, et al. Long-term outcomes after high-dose postprostatectomy salvage radiation treatment. *Int J Radiat Oncol Biol Phys* 2012;84:112–118.

292. Briganti A, Karnes RJ, Joniau S, et al. Prediction of outcome following early salvage radiotherapy among patients with biochemical recurrence after radical prostatectomy. *Eur Urol* 2013 [Epub ahead of print]. doi: 10.1016/j.eururo.2013.11.045.

295. Valicenti RK, Thompson I Jr, Albertsen P, et al. Adjuvant and salvage radiation therapy after prostatectomy: American Society for Radiation Oncology/American Urological Association guidelines. *Int J Radiat Oncol Biol Phys* 2013;86:822–828.

296. Eastham JA, Kattan MW, Rogers E, et al. Risk factors for urinary incontinence after radical prostatectomy. *J Urol* 1996;156:1707–1713.

297. Burri RJ, Stone NN, Unger P, et al. Long-term outcome and toxicity of salvage brachytherapy for local failure after initial radiotherapy for prostate cancer. *Int J Radiat Oncol Biol Phys* 2010;77:1338–1344.

298. Vargas C, Swartz D, Vashi A, et al. Salvage brachytherapy for recurrent prostate cancer. *Brachytherapy* 2014;13:53–58.

299. Lahmer G, Lotter M, Kreppner S, et al. Protocol-based image-guided salvage brachytherapy. Early results in patients with local failure of prostate cancer after radiation therapy. *Strahlenther Onkol* 2013;189:668–674.

300. Chen CP, Weinberg V, Shinohara K, et al. Salvage HDR brachytherapy for recurrent prostate cancer after previous definitive radiation therapy: 5-year outcomes. *Int J Radiat Oncol Biol Phys* 2013;86:324–329.

301. Yamada Y, Kollmeier MA, Pei X, et al. A Phase II study of salvage high-dose-rate brachytherapy for the treatment of locally recurrent prostate cancer after definitive external beam radiotherapy. *Brachytherapy* 2014;13:111–116.

305. Finley DS, Pouliot F, Miller DC, et al. Primary and salvage cryotherapy for prostate cancer. *Urol Clin North Am* 2010;37:67–82.

308. Huggins C, Hodges CV. Studies on prostatic cancer. I. The effect of castration, of estrogen and of androgen injection on serum phosphatases in metastatic carcinoma of the prostate. *Cancer Res* 1941;1:293–297.

309. Huggins C, Stevens RE Jr, Hodges CV. Studies on prostatic cancer. II. The effect of castration on advanced carcinoma of the prostate gland. *Arch Surg* 1941;43:209–223.

310. Schally AV, Redding TW, Comaru-Schally AM. Inhibition of prostate tumors by agonistic and antagonistic analogs of LH-RH. *Prostate* 1983;4:545–552.

318. Maximum androgen blockade in advanced prostate cancer: an overview of 22 randomised trials with 3283 deaths in 5710 patients. Prostate Cancer Trialists' Collaborative Group. *Lancet* 1995;346:265–269.

320. Tannock IF, Osoba D, Stockler MR, et al. Chemotherapy with mitoxantrone plus prednisone or prednisone alone for symptomatic hormone-resistant prostate cancer: a Canadian randomized trial with palliative end points. *J Clin Oncol* 1996;14:1756–1764.

321. Petrylak DP, Tangen CM, Hussain MH, et al. Docetaxel and estramustine compared with mitoxantrone and prednisone for advanced refractory prostate cancer. *N Engl J Med* 2004;351:1513–1520.

322. Tannock IF, de Wit R, Berry WR, et al. Docetaxel plus prednisone or mitoxantrone plus prednisone for advanced prostate cancer. *N Engl J Med* 2004;351:1502–1512.

323. Kantoff PW, Higano CS, Shore ND, et al. Sipuleucel-T immunotherapy for castration-resistant prostate cancer. *N Engl J Med* 2010;363:411–422.

324. Ryan CJ, Smith MR, de Bono JS, et al. Abiraterone in metastatic prostate cancer without previous chemotherapy. *N Engl J Med* 2013;368:138–148.

325. de Bono JS, Oudard S, Ozguroglu M, et al. Prednisone plus cabazitaxel or mitoxantrone for metastatic castration-resistant prostate cancer progressing after docetaxel treatment: a randomised open-label trial. *Lancet* 2010;376:1147–1154.

326. Parker C, Nilsson S, Heinrich D, et al. Alpha emitter radium-223 and survival in metastatic prostate cancer. *N Engl J Med* 2013;369:213–223.

327. de Bono JS, Logothetis CJ, Molina A, et al. Abiraterone and increased survival in metastatic prostate cancer. *N Engl J Med* 2011;364:1995–2005.

328. Scher HI, Fizazi K, Saad F, et al. Increased survival with enzalutamide in prostate cancer after chemotherapy. *N Engl J Med* 2012;367:1187–1197.

338. Fizazi K, Carducci M, Smith M, et al. Denosumab versus zoledronic acid for treatment of bone metastases in men with castration-resistant prostate cancer: a randomised, double-blind study. *Lancet* 2011;377:813–822.

339. Scher HI, Morris MJ, Basch E, et al. End points and outcomes in castration-resistant prostate cancer: from clinical trials to clinical practice. *J Clin Oncol* 2011;29:3695–3704.

340. Chen Y, Clegg NJ, Scher HI. Anti-androgens and androgen-depleting therapies in prostate cancer: new agents for an established target. *Lancet Oncol* 2009;10:981–991.

350. Ahmadi H, Daneshmand S. Androgen deprivation therapy: evidence-based management of side effects. *BJU Int* 2013;111:543–548.

359. Shahinian VB, Kuo YF, Freeman JL, et al. Risk of fracture after androgen deprivation for prostate cancer. *N Engl J Med* 2005;352:154–164.

361. Saad F, Higano CS, Sartor O, et al. The role of bisphosphonates in the treatment of prostate cancer: recommendations from an expert panel. *Clin Genitourin Cancer* 2006;4:257–262.

362. Hanley DA, Adachi JD, Bell A, et al. Denosumab: mechanism of action and clinical outcomes. *Int J Clin Pract* 2012;66:1139–1146.

363. Smith MR, Egerdie B, Hernandez Toriz N, et al. Denosumab in men receiving androgen-deprivation therapy for prostate cancer. *N Engl J Med* 2009; 361:745–755.

364. Smith MR, Morton RA, Barnette KG, et al. Toremifene to reduce fracture risk in men receiving androgen deprivation therapy for prostate cancer. *J Urol* 2013;189:S45–S50.

368. Conteduca V, Di Lorenzo G, Tartarone A, et al. The cardiovascular risk of gonadotropin releasing hormone agonists in men with prostate cancer: an unresolved controversy. *Crit Rev Oncol Hematol* 2013;86:42–51.

369. Levine GN, D'Amico AV, Berger P, et al. Androgen-deprivation therapy in prostate cancer and cardiovascular risk: a science advisory from the American Heart Association, American Cancer Society, and American Urological Association: endorsed by the American Society for Radiation Oncology. *CA Cancer J Clin* 2010;60:194–201.

373. Sylvester RJ, Denis L, de Voogt H. The importance of prognostic factors in the interpretation of two EORTC metastatic prostate cancer trials. European Organization for Research and Treatment of Cancer (EORTC) Genito-Urinary Tract Cancer Cooperative Group. *Eur Urol* 1998;33:134–143.

376. Eisenberger MA, Blumenstein BA, Crawford ED, et al. Bilateral orchiectomy with or without flutamide for metastatic prostate cancer. *N Engl J Med* 1998;339:1036–1042.

377. Hussain M, Tangen CM, Higano C, et al. Absolute prostate-specific antigen value after androgen deprivation is a strong independent predictor of survival in new metastatic prostate cancer: data from Southwest Oncology Group Trial 9346 (INT-0162). *J Clin Oncol* 2006;24:3984–3990.

378. Choueiri TK, Xie W, D'Amico AV, et al. Time to prostate-specific antigen nadir independently predicts overall survival in patients who have metastatic hormone-sensitive prostate cancer treated with androgen-deprivation therapy. *Cancer* 2009;115:981–987.

383. Mostaghel EA, Page ST, Lin DW, et al. Intraprostatic androgens and androgen-regulated gene expression persist after testosterone suppression: therapeutic implications for castration-resistant prostate cancer. *Cancer Res* 2007;67:5033–5041.

384. Ryan CJ, Smith A, Lal P, et al. Persistent prostate-specific antigen expression after neoadjuvant androgen depletion: an early predictor of relapse or incomplete androgen suppression. *Urology* 2006;68:834–839.

392. Pound CR, Partin AW, Eisenberger MA, et al. Natural history of progression after PSA elevation following radical prostatectomy. *JAMA* 1999;281:1591–1597.

393. Antonarakis ES, Feng Z, Trock BJ, et al. The natural history of metastatic progression in men with prostate-specific antigen recurrence after radical prostatectomy: long-term follow-up. *BJU Int* 2012;109:32–39.

394. Zhou P, Chen MH, McLeod D, et al. Predictors of prostate cancer-specific mortality after radical prostatectomy or radiation therapy. *J Clin Oncol* 2005;23: 6992–6998.

401. Crook JM, O'Callaghan CJ, Duncan G, et al. Intermittent androgen suppression for rising PSA level after radiotherapy. *N Engl J Med* 2012;367:895–903.

402. Hussain M, Tangen CM, Berry DL, et al. Intermittent versus continuous androgen deprivation in prostate cancer. *N Engl J Med* 2013;368:1314–1325.

403. Tsai HT, Penson DF, Makambi KH, et al. Efficacy of intermittent androgen deprivation therapy vs conventional continuous androgen deprivation therapy for advanced prostate cancer: a meta-analysis. *Urology* 2013;82:327–333.

404. Niraula S, Le LW, Tannock IF. Treatment of prostate cancer with intermittent versus continuous androgen deprivation: a systematic review of randomized trials. *J Clin Oncol* 2013;31:2029–2036.

405. Botrel TE, Clark O, dos Reis RB, et al. Intermittent versus continuous androgen deprivation for locally advanced, recurrent or metastatic prostate cancer: a systematic review and meta-analysis. *BMC Urol* 2014;14:9.

406. Smith MR, Saad F, Coleman R, et al. Denosumab and bone-metastasis-free survival in men with castration-resistant prostate cancer: results of a phase 3, randomised, placebo-controlled trial. *Lancet* 2012;379:39–46.

407. Smith MR, Eastham J, Gleason DM, et al. Randomized controlled trial of zoledronic acid to prevent bone loss in men receiving androgen deprivation therapy for nonmetastatic prostate cancer. *J Urol* 2003;169:2008–2012.

408. Smith MR, Saad F, Oudard S, et al. Denosumab and bone metastasis-free survival in men with nonmetastatic castration-resistant prostate cancer: exploratory analyses by baseline prostate-specific antigen doubling time. *J Clin Oncol* 2013;31:3800–3806.

409. Beltran H, Tomlins S, Aparicio A, et al. Aggressive variants of castration-resistant prostate cancer. *Clin Cancer Res* 2014;20:2846–2850.

410. Epstein JI, Amin MB, Beltran H, et al. Proposed morphologic classification of prostate cancer with neuroendocrine differentiation. *Am J Surg Pathol* 2014;38:756–767.

411. Pond GR, Sonpavde G, de Wit R, et al. The prognostic importance of metastatic site in men with metastatic castration-resistant prostate cancer. *Eur Urol* 2014;65:3–6.

412. Aparicio AM, Harzstark AL, Corn PG, et al. Platinum-based chemotherapy for variant castrate-resistant prostate cancer. *Clin Cancer Res* 2013;19:3621–3630.

419. Courtney KD, Taplin ME. The evolving paradigm of second-line hormonal therapy options for castration-resistant prostate cancer. *Curr Opin Oncol* 2012;24:272–277.

428. Ryan CJ, Halabi S, Ou SS, et al. Adrenal androgen levels as predictors of outcome in prostate cancer patients treated with ketoconazole plus antiandrogen withdrawal: results from a cancer and leukemia group B study. *Clin Cancer Res* 2007;13:2030–2037.

429. Small EJ, Halabi S, Dawson NA, et al. Antiandrogen withdrawal alone or in combination with ketoconazole in androgen-independent prostate cancer patients: a phase III trial (CALGB 9583). *J Clin Oncol* 2004;22:1025–1033.

431. Montgomery B, Cheng HH, Drechsler J, et al. Glucocorticoids and prostate cancer treatment: friend or foe? *Asian J Androl* 2014;16:354–358.

432. Ryan CJ, Molina A, Li J, et al. Serum androgens as prognostic biomarkers in castration-resistant prostate cancer: results from an analysis of a randomized phase III trial. *J Clin Oncol* 2013;31:2791–2798.

436. Tamae D, Byrns M, Marck B, et al. Development, validation and application of a stable isotope dilution liquid chromatography electrospray ionization /selected reaction monitoring/mass spectrometry (SID-LC/ESI/SRM/MS) method for quantification of keto-androgens in human serum. *J Steroid Biochem Mol Biol* 2013;138:281–289.

444. Fizazi K, Scher HI, Molina A, et al. Abiraterone acetate for treatment of metastatic castration-resistant prostate cancer: final overall survival analysis of the COU-AA-301 randomised, double-blind, placebo-controlled phase 3 study. *Lancet Oncol* 2012;13:983–992.

445. Rathkopf DE, Smith MR, de Bono JS, et al. Updated interim efficacy analysis and long-term safety of abiraterone acetate in metastatic castration-resistant prostate cancer patients without prior chemotherapy (COU-AA-302). *Eur Urol* 2014 [Epub ahead of print]. doi: 10.1016/j.eururo.2014.02.056.

446. Scher HI, Beer TM, Higano CS, et al. Antitumour activity of MDV3100 in castration-resistant prostate cancer: a phase 1-2 study. *Lancet* 2010;375: 1437–1446.

447. Beer TM, Armstrong AJ, Rathkopf DE, et al. Enzalutamide in metastatic prostate cancer before chemotherapy. *N Engl J Med* 2014;371:424–433.

448. Clegg NJ, Wongvipat J, Joseph JD, et al. ARN-509: a novel antiandrogen for prostate cancer treatment. *Cancer Res* 2012;72:1494–1503.

449. Rathkopf DE, Morris MJ, Fox JJ, et al. Phase I study of ARN-509, a novel antiandrogen, in the treatment of castration-resistant prostate cancer. *J Clin Oncol* 2013;31:3525–3530.

450. Stein MN, Patel N, Bershadskiy A, et al. Androgen synthesis inhibitors in the treatment of castration-resistant prostate cancer. *Asian J Androl* 2014;16:387–400.

452. Small EJ, Schellhammer PF, Higano CS, et al. Placebo-controlled phase III trial of immunologic therapy with sipuleucel-T (APC8015) in patients with metastatic, asymptomatic hormone refractory prostate cancer. *J Clin Oncol* 2006;24:3089–3094.

453. Kantoff PW, Schuetz TJ, Blumenstein BA, et al. Overall survival analysis of a phase II randomized controlled trial of a Poxviral-based PSA-targeted immunotherapy in metastatic castration-resistant prostate cancer. *J Clin Oncol* 2010;28:1099–1105.

454. DiPaola RS, Plante M, Kaufman H, et al. A phase I trial of pox PSA vaccines (PROSTVAC-VF) with B7-1, ICAM-1, and LFA-3 co-stimulatory molecules (TRICOM) in patients with prostate cancer. *J Transl Med* 2006;4:1.

458. Kwon ED, Drake CG, Scher HI, et al. Ipilimumab versus placebo after radiotherapy in patients with metastatic castration-resistant prostate cancer that had progressed after docetaxel chemotherapy (CA184-043): a multicentre, randomised, double-blind, phase 3 trial. *Lancet Oncol* 2014;15:700–712.

461. Gupta N, Ustwani OA, Shen L, et al. Mechanism of action and clinical activity of tasquinimod in castrate-resistant prostate cancer. *Onco Targets Ther* 2014;7:223–234.

463. Pili R, Haggman M, Stadler WM, et al. Phase II randomized, double-blind, placebo-controlled study of tasquinimod in men with minimally symptomatic metastatic castrate-resistant prostate cancer. *J Clin Oncol* 2011;29:4022–4028.

464. Armstrong AJ, Haggman M, Stadler WM, et al. Long-term survival and biomarker correlates of tasquinimod efficacy in a multicenter randomized study of men with minimally symptomatic metastatic castration-resistant prostate cancer. *Clin Cancer Res* 2013;19:6891–6901.

465. Smith MR, Saad F, Egerdie B, et al. Effects of denosumab on bone mineral density in men receiving androgen deprivation therapy for prostate cancer. *J Urol* 2009;182:2670–2675.

PRACTICE OF ONCOLOGY

473. Gartrell BA, Saad F. Managing bone metastases and reducing skeletal related events in prostate cancer. *Nat Rev Clin Oncol* 2014;11:335–345.

474. Porter AT, McEwan AJ, Powe JE, et al. Results of a randomized phase-III trial to evaluate the efficacy of strontium-89 adjuvant to local field external beam irradiation in the management of endocrine resistant metastatic prostate cancer. *Int J Radiat Oncol Biol Phys* 1993;25:805–813.

478. Autio KA, Pandit-Taskar N, Carrasquillo JA, et al. Repetitively dosed docetaxel and (1)(5)(3)samarium-EDTMP as an antitumor strategy for metastatic castration-resistant prostate cancer. *Cancer* 2013;119:3186–3194.

480. Dreicer R, Jones R, Oudard S, et al. Results from a phase 3, randomized, double-blind, multicenter, placebo-controlled trial of orteronel (TAK-700) plus prednisone in patients with metastatic castration-resistant prostate cancer (mCRPC) that has progressed during or following docetaxel-based therapy (ELM-PC 5 trial). *J Clin Oncol* 2014;32;Abstr 7.

481. OncoGenex Pharmaceuticals, Inc. OncoGenex Announces Top-Line Survival Results of Phase 3 SYNERGY Trial Evaluating Custirsen for Metastatic Castrate-Resistant Prostate Cancer [press release]. April 28, 2014. Accessed June 20, 2014. http://ir.oncogenex.com/releasedetail.cfm?ReleaseID=842949.

482. Dreicer R, MacLean D, Suri A, et al. Phase I/II trial of orteronel (TAK-700)—an investigational 17,20-lyase inhibitor—in patients with metastatic castration-resistant prostate cancer. *Clin Cancer Res* 2014;20:1335–1344.

484. Saad F, Hotte S, North S, et al. Randomized phase II trial of Custirsen (OGX-011) in combination with docetaxel or mitoxantrone as second-line therapy in patients with metastatic castrate-resistant prostate cancer progressing after first-line docetaxel: CUOG trial P-06c. *Clin Cancer Res* 2011;17:5765–5773.

485. Rathkopf D, Scher HI. Androgen receptor antagonists in castration-resistant prostate cancer. *Cancer J* 2013;19:43–49.

486. Carver BS, Chapinski C, Wongvipat J, et al. Reciprocal feedback regulation of PI3K and androgen receptor signaling in PTEN-deficient prostate cancer. *Cancer Cell* 2011;19:575–586.

487. Sprenger CC, Plymate SR. The link between androgen receptor splice variants and castration-resistant prostate cancer. *Horm Cancer* 2014;5:207–217.

488. Antonarakis ES, Lu C, Luber B, et al. AR-V7 and resistance to enzalutamide and abiraterone in prostate cancer. *N Engl J Med* 2014 [Epub ahead of print].

489. Balbas MD, Evans MJ, Hosfield DJ, et al. Overcoming mutation-based resistance to antiandrogens with rational drug design. *Elife* 2013;2:e00499.

490. Arora VK, Schenkein E, Murali R, et al. Glucocorticoid receptor confers resistance to antiandrogens by bypassing androgen receptor blockade. *Cell* 2013;155:1309–1322.

491. Messing EM, Manola J, Sarosdy M, et al. Immediate hormonal therapy compared with observation after radical prostatectomy and pelvic lymphadenectomy in men with node-positive prostate cancer. *N Engl J Med* 1999;341:1781–1788.

493. McKay RR, Choueiri TK, Taplin ME. Rationale for and review of neoadjuvant therapy prior to radical prostatectomy for patients with high-risk prostate cancer. *Drugs* 2013;73:1417–1430.

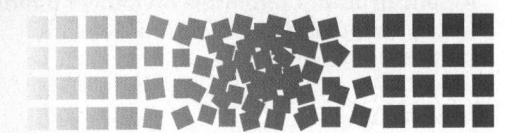

69 Cancer of the Urethra and Penis

Edouard J. Trabulsi and Leonard G. Gomella

INTRODUCTION

Penile and urethral carcinomas are uncommon malignancies, with a peak incidence in the 6th decade of life. Often overshadowed by more common genitourinary cancers, penile and urethral cancers represent difficult challenges for the treating physician. Squamous cell carcinoma is the most frequent type of cancer in the penis and the urethra. Carcinoma of the penis is a slow-growing tumor with a usually well-defined pattern of dissemination. This orderly spread allows definitive local–regional management of the primary tumor in most cases. In contradistinction, urethral carcinoma in men and women tends to invade locally and metastasize to regional nodes early. Depending on the site of the urethra involved and disease extent, a multimodal treatment approach may be required to treat this aggressive tumor.[1]

CANCER OF THE MALE URETHRA

Carcinoma of the male urethra is uncommon. Chronic irritation and infection are the strongest risk factors. The incidence of urethral stricture in men with development of urethral cancer ranges from 24% to 76%, and most of these strictures involve the bulbomembranous urethra, also the most frequent site of cancer.[2] Human papillomavirus-16 (HPV-16) likely has a causative role in the development of squamous cell carcinoma of the urethra.[3] No racial predisposition has been noted.

The onset of malignancy in a patient with a longstanding urethral stricture disease is often insidious, and a high index of suspicion is needed to diagnose these tumors early. The new onset of urethrorrhagia or urethral stricture in a man without a history of trauma or venereal disease should raise the possibility of urethral carcinoma. A palpable urethral mass associated with obstructive voiding symptoms is the most common presenting symptom.[4] Pain associated with a periurethral abscess or urethral fistula may be the harbinger of a male urethral cancer.

Pathology

Overall, 80% of male urethral cancers are squamous cell, 15% are urothelial (transitional cell), and approximately 5% are adenocarcinomas or undifferentiated tumors.[5] The anatomic location of urethral cancer largely determines the histologic type. Carcinomas of the prostatic urethra are urothelial in 90% and squamous in 10%; conversely, carcinomas of the penile urethra are squamous in 90% and urothelial in 10%. Adenocarcinomas of the urethra arise from metaplasia of mucosa or from periurethral glands, but direct invasion of rectal adenocarcinoma must be ruled out. Adenocarcinoma has the same prognosis, stage for stage, as the other histologies.[4]

The bulbomembranous urethra is most commonly involved (60%), followed by the penile urethra (30%) and the prostatic urethra (10%).[4] The incidence of urethral involvement associated with carcinoma of the bladder has been estimated to be approximately 6%,[6] and urethral recurrences after radical cystectomy occur in 4% to 17%.[7]

Male urethral cancer may spread locally to involve the corpus spongiosum or may metastasize to regional nodes. The lymphatics of the anterior urethra drain into the superficial and deep inguinal lymph nodes and occasionally to the external iliac nodes. The lymphatics from the posterior urethra drain into the external iliac, obturator, and hypogastric nodes. Palpable inguinal nodes are found in approximately 20% and almost always suggest metastatic disease, in contrast to penile cancer, where 50% of palpable nodes are inflammatory. Bulbomembranous urethral cancer in particular spreads to the urogenital diaphragm, prostate, perineum, and scrotum. Hematogenous spread is rare except in advanced disease and in primary transitional cell carcinoma of the prostatic urethra.

Evaluation and Staging

The 2010 American Joint Committee on Cancer (AJCC) tumor, node, metastasis (TNM) staging system[8] is based on the depth of invasion of the primary tumor and the presence or absence of regional lymph node involvement and distant metastasis (Table 69.1). The 2010 AJCC system subdivides T1 lesions into T1a (no lymphovascular invasion or poorly differentiated tumors) and T1b (the presence of lymphovascular invasion or poorly differentiated histology); prostatic invasion is now reclassified as T4 disease (previously T3). Examination under anesthesia is useful to evaluate the local extent of disease. Cystoscopy and transurethral or needle biopsy of the lesion, and of the prostate if indicated, are also performed at the time of examination under anesthesia. A complete blood count and serum chemistry analysis coupled with urine culture and cytology are routinely obtained. Cytology is particularly helpful in patients with transitional cell carcinoma. A computed tomography (CT) scan with contrast is useful in local staging with magnetic resonance imaging (MRI) scan with gadolinium the ideal staging modality for evaluating local soft tissue, lymph node, and bone involvement.[9]

Treatment

Surgery is the mainstay of treatment of carcinoma of the male urethra. In general, anterior urethral cancers are more amenable to surgical extirpation, and the prognosis is better than that of posterior urethral tumors, which are more often associated with extensive local invasion and distant metastasis.[10] Radiation therapy is reserved for patients with early-stage lesions of the anterior urethra who refuse surgery. Although it preserves the penis, radiation may cause urethral stricture or chronic penile edema and may not prevent new tumor occurrence. Multimodal treatment combining chemotherapy and radiation therapy with surgical excision for locally advanced urethral carcinomas has yielded promising results (disease-free survival 60% in one series).[11] The median survival without treatment or with palliation is approximately 3 months.

Site-Specific Treatment

Carcinoma of the Distal Urethra. Superficial tumors (Ta, Tis, and T1) are usually treated with transurethral resection and fulguration with close follow-up. Tumors invading the corpus

TABLE 69.1

American Joint Committee on Cancer Tumor, Node, Metastasis Classification System for Urethral Cancer

Stage Grouping

0a	Ta	N0	M0
0is	Tis	N0	M0
	Tis (prostatic urethra)	N0	M0
	Tis (prostatic ducts)	N0	M0
I	T1	N0	M0
II	T2	N0	M0
III	T1	N1	M0
	T2	N1	M0
	T3	N0	M0
	T4	N1	M0
IV	T4	N0	M0
	T4	N1	M0
	Any T	N2	M0
	Any T	Any N	M1

From American Joint Committee on Cancer. *AJCC Cancer Staging Manual.* 7th ed. New York: Springer-Verlag; 2010, with permission.

spongiosum (T2) and localized to the distal half of the penis are best treated with a partial penile amputation with a 2-cm margin proximal to the visible or palpable tumor. If infiltrating tumor is confined to the proximal penile urethra or involves the entire urethra, total penectomy is indicated. Isolated reports of penile-sparing surgery (urethrectomy with corpora cavernosa sparing) have a high incidence of failure.[12] Ilioinguinal node dissection is indicated only in the presence of palpable adenopathy. Prophylactic groin dissection has no proven role in this site.

Carcinoma of the Bulbomembranous Urethra. Early superficial tumors (Ta, Tis, and T1) can be treated with transurethral fulguration or segmental resection with end-to-end anastomosis; however, such cases are rare. Invasive tumors (T2, T3) are best treated with radical cystoprostatectomy with en bloc penectomy and pelvic lymphadenectomy. Despite this aggressive approach, the prognosis remains dismal, with a 5-year disease-free survival of 26% in patients with invasive bulbomembranous carcinomas.[13] Isolated reports of penile preservation surgery for invasive bulbomembranous cancers have used adjuvant radiation therapy (45 Gy) and concurrent chemotherapy with 5-fluorouracil (5-FU) and mitomycin C with acceptable results.[14]

Carcinoma of the Prostatic Urethra. Primary carcinoma arising from the prostatic urethra is rare. Adenocarcinomas and urothelial carcinomas are found. Although superficial lesions (Tis-pu, Tis-pd, T1) can be managed by transurethral resection, such tumors are rare. Invasive urothelial carcinoma of the prostatic stroma (T2) carries a poor prognosis despite aggressive surgical therapy. Extravesical extension of disease has a worse prognosis than intraurethral disease, with a higher chance of nodal involvement and a 5-year survival rate of only 32%.[15]

Advanced carcinoma (T3-4N1 to N3) of the prostatic urethra is best treated with a combination of neoadjuvant chemotherapy (methotrexate sodium, vinblastine sulfate, doxorubicin hydrochloride [Adriamycin, Pharmacia S.p.A, Milan, Italy], and cisplatin [MVAC]) with consolidative surgery or irradiation. One series of five patients (with T2-4N0M0 lesions) treated with neoadjuvant

MVAC chemotherapy had a complete response rate of 60%.[16] MVAC chemotherapy preoperatively was ineffective against nonurothelial carcinoma.

Radiation and Multimodal Therapy

Radiation therapy alone has poor results in male urethral carcinoma. Patients who receive radiation therapy followed by salvage surgery seem to fare worse than with surgery in an integrated fashion. The most common approach has been external-beam radiotherapy of 50 to 60 Gy with best results for *distal* urethral lesions. Multimodal therapy with chemoradiation has shown the efficacy of 5-FU, mitomycin C, and cisplatin with radiation for squamous cell carcinoma of the urethra.[17,18]

CARCINOMA OF THE FEMALE URETHRA

Carcinoma of the urethra is the only genitourinary neoplasm that is more common in women than in men (four-to-one ratio). The peak incidence is in the sixth decade, more commonly in white women. Chronic irritation, recurrent urinary tract infections, and a host of proliferative lesions (caruncles, papillomas, polyps) are predisposing factors, and HPV may play a role. Leukoplakia of the urethra is considered a premalignant condition. In females, the urethra is approximately 4 cm long, mostly buried in the anterior vaginal wall, and divided into the distal one-third (anterior urethra) and the proximal two-thirds (posterior urethra). The most common presenting symptom (greater than 50%) is urethrorrhagia. Urinary frequency, obstructive voiding, a foul-smelling discharge, and a palpable urethral mass are other modes of presentation. Initially, it may be difficult to distinguish fungating tumors of the urethra from those of the vagina or vulva.

Spread of urethral carcinoma follows the anatomic subdivision: lymphatics of the anterior urethra drain into the superficial and deep inguinal nodes and the posterior urethra into the external iliac, hypogastric, and obturator nodes. At presentation, one-third of patients have inguinal lymph node metastases and 20% have pelvic node involvement. Palpable inguinal nodes in patients with urethral cancer invariably contain metastatic carcinoma. The most common sites of distant spread are the lungs, liver, and bone.[19]

An epidemiologic survey of female urethral cancer identified over 700 women in the Surveillance, Epidemiology, and End Results database.[20] No other study approaches this one in number of patients analyzed. The median overall survival in this large cohort was 42 months, with 5- and 10-year overall survival rates of 43% and 32%, respectively. The median cancer-specific survival was 78 months, and the 5- and 10-year cancer-specific survival was 53% and 46%, respectively. On multivariate analysis of nonmetastatic patients, variables predicting for worse cancer-specific survival were African-American race, stage T3 through T4 tumors, node-positive disease, nonsquamous cell histology, and advanced age.

Pathology

Stratified squamous epithelium lines the distal two-thirds of the female urethra, and transitional epithelium (urothelium) lines the proximal one-third. The majority (60%) of neoplasms of the female urethra are squamous cell carcinomas. Less common types are urothelial carcinoma (20%), adenocarcinoma (10%), undifferentiated tumors (8%), and melanoma (2%). Clear cell carcinoma is a distinctive clinical entity that has generated considerable interest with respect to its prognosis and relationship to urethral diverticulae.[21] Histology does not affect the prognosis, and all are treated similarly. In general, anterior urethral carcinomas are low grade and stage; carcinomas involving the proximal or entire urethra are of a higher grade and stage.

Evaluation and Staging

The workup for women with suspected urethral carcinoma includes a pelvic examination under anesthesia, cystourethroscopy, and biopsy. Radiographic evaluation includes a chest x-ray and CT of the pelvis and abdomen. MRI is particularly useful for staging of female urethral carcinoma. Although the 2010 AJCC TNM staging includes female urethral cancer,[8] the practical usefulness is limited. Clinically, it is more useful to stage, treat, and prognosticate female urethral cancers by stratifying patients based on anatomic location (anterior versus posterior urethra versus entire urethra) and clinical stage (low stage versus high stage).[22]

Treatment

The anatomic location and stage of the tumor are the most significant prognostic factors predicting local control and survival. Treatment is based on the stage at the time of initial presentation, with low-stage distal urethral tumors having a better prognosis than high-stage proximal urethral tumors. In one series, the 5-year disease-specific survival was 46%, with 89% survival for low-stage tumors and 33% for high-stage disease.[23]

Local surgical excision is often sufficient in selected patients with low-stage distal urethra carcinoma. With proximal urethra and for bulky locally advanced tumors, more aggressive treatment with an anterior pelvic exenteration is often needed (en bloc total urethrectomy, cystectomy, pelvic lymphadenectomy, hysterectomy with salpingectomy, removal of the anterior vaginal wall). Bulky proximal urethral tumors that invade the pubic symphysis may require resection of the pubic symphysis and inferior rami. Anterior exenteration alone has been reported to produce a 5-year survival rate of <20% in patients with invasive carcinoma of the female urethra.[24] Radiation therapy (brachytherapy alone or with external-beam radiation) is an alternative to surgery in low-stage urethral carcinoma with cure rates up to 75%. The reported doses have ranged from 50 to 60 Gy for brachytherapy alone and 40 to 45 Gy external-beam radiation to the whole pelvis followed by a brachytherapy boost of 20 to 25 Gy over 2 to 3 days. Proximal urethral tumors with bladder neck invasion and bulky tumors require combined external-beam and brachytherapy. Large primary tumor bulk and treatment with external radiation alone (no brachytherapy) were independent adverse prognostic factors. Brachytherapy reduced the risk of local recurrence, possibly as a result of the higher radiation dose.[25] Complications from radiation therapy occur in about 20% and include urethral strictures and stenosis, urethrovaginal fistulas, incontinence, and bowel obstruction.

Combined modality treatment with neoadjuvant chemotherapy and preoperative radiation therapy, followed by surgery, is recommended for advanced female urethral carcinoma. A 55% survival rate has been reported with advanced urethral carcinoma treated with radiotherapy plus surgery, as compared with a rate of 34% with radiation alone.[26] Although long-term results from multimodal therapy are not yet available, combination chemotherapy, radiation, and surgery is believed essential for local control and cure with larger or locally advanced urethral cancer.[23] The prognosis for women with carcinoma of the urethra is poor, regardless of the treatment modality used, and the median time to local recurrence for invasive carcinoma is 13 months.

Distal Urethral Carcinoma

Small superficial (Ta, Tis, and T1) tumors of the distal female urethra can be removed surgically with little risk of urinary incontinence. Spatulation of the urethra and approximation to the adjacent vagina preserve urinary continence and prevent meatal stenosis. For small invasive tumors of the distal urethra (T2), brachytherapy alone is an excellent therapeutic option.

Proximal Urethral Carcinoma

Proximal female urethral carcinomas tend to be more aggressive and bulky. For advanced (T3 and T4) lesions, a multimodal approach is preferred. Surgery consists of a radical cystourethrectomy or an anterior exenteration, depending on the extent of the disease. Radiation therapy with a combination of brachytherapy and external-beam irradiation is usually required. Neoadjuvant chemotherapy with 5-FU and mitomycin C has been noted to enhance the therapeutic ratio of radiation therapy.

CANCER OF THE PENIS

Carcinoma of the penis is an uncommon malignancy in Western countries, representing 0.4% of male malignancies and 3.0% of all genitourinary cancers. Penile cancer constitutes a major health problem in many countries in Asia, Africa, and South America, where it may comprise up to 10% of all malignancies. The incidence of penile cancer has been declining in many countries, partly because of increased attention to personal hygiene.[27] It most commonly presents in the sixth decade but may occur in men younger than 40 years. Analysis of the Surveillance, Epidemiology, and End Results database data shows no racial difference in the incidence of penile cancer among African American men and white men, but significant disparities exist in the mortality of invasive penile carcinoma in the United States.[28] Significantly lower rates of invasive penile cancer are seen in Asian American men and significantly higher rates are seen in Hispanic American men. Regional and socioeconomic differences are also noted, with higher rates in the southern area of the United States and in lower socioeconomic populations.

Etiology

Penile cancer is associated with phimosis and poor local hygiene, with phimosis found in more than half the patients. The irritative effect of smegma, a byproduct of bacterial action on desquamated epithelial cells in the preputial sac, is well known, although definitive evidence of its role in carcinogenesis is lacking. Neonatal circumcision as practiced by religious groups virtually eliminates the occurrence of penile carcinoma. While circumcision can reduce the risk of various sexually transmitted diseases such as HIV, and possibly HPV and herpes virus, delaying circumcision until puberty or adult circumcision does not have the same benefit with respect to penile cancer.[29]

HPV infection, particularly HPV-16, has been implicated in the development of invasive penile cancer, as has the number of sexual partners.[29] HPV infection accounts for about half of penile cancers, with HPV-16 and -18 the predominant subtypes.[30,31] Evidence now indicates that penile cancer has two primary etiologies: approximately half are related to HPV infection, with the other half related to inflammatory conditions such as phimosis, chronic balanitis, and lichen sclerosis.[32] The use of tobacco products is an independent risk factor.[33] Thus, avoidance of tobacco products and HPV infection, penile hygiene, and neonatal circumcision represent important preventive strategies against penile cancer. Vaccination of younger men against HPV is controversial but may change the incidence and burden of this disease.[34,35]

Symptoms

Local symptoms and signs often draw attention to penile cancer. The clinical spectrum of penile cancer is varied: subtle areas of erythema or induration to a frankly ulcerated, fungating, foul-smelling mass. Penile cancer is commonly associated with concomitant infection, with infection playing an important role in the pathogenesis and ultimately in the presentation of the disease. Pain usually is not a prominent feature and is not proportional to the extent of local destruction. The lesion primarily involves the prepuce and glans, often under a tight phimotic ring. In late stages, involvement and destruction of the shaft of the penis or urethra are seen. Urethral obstruction is rare. Instead, erosion of the urethra with multiple fistulas ("watering-can perineum") may be seen. Rarely, inguinal ulceration may be the presenting symptom, with the primary tumor concealed within a phimotic preputial sac.

Patients with penile cancer, more than with other types of cancer, delay seeking medical attention. Historically, up to 50% of patients delayed more than 1 year in seeking medical help; contemporary series, especially from the United States, fail to show such a trend.

Pathology

More than 95% of penile carcinomas are squamous cell. Nonsquamous cell carcinomas consist of melanomas, basal cell carcinomas, lymphomas, and sarcomas. Nearly 18% of patients with acquired immunodeficiency syndrome–related Kaposi sarcoma have penile involvement.[36]

Squamous cell carcinomas are graded using Broder classification. Low-grade tumors (grades I and II), typically confined to the prepuce and glans penis, constitute nearly 80% of penile cancers. Most lesions that involve the shaft of the penis are high grade (grade III), with grade and stage often correlated. The incidence of lymph node metastases from squamous cell carcinoma of the penis is related to histologic grade. Verrucous carcinoma, a particularly exuberant variant of squamous cell carcinoma, has low potential for lymph node spread and a good prognosis. Another important predictor of lymph node metastases and, hence, prognosis is the presence of vascular invasion.[37]

Premalignant Lesions

The description of early and premalignant lesions has been complicated by the rarity of the disease and a proliferation of eponyms.

Leukoplakia

Leukoplakia is characterized by the presence of solitary or multiple whitish plaques involving the glans or prepuce in the setting of chronic or recurrent balanoposthitis. Surgical excision in the form of circumcision or local wedge resection is usually curative.

Balanitis Xerotica Obliterans

Balanitis xerotica obliterans (BXO) is an inflammatory condition of the glans and prepuce of unknown cause; it is a form of lichen sclerosis isolated to the penis. BXO is a scaly, indurated, whitish plaque that produces significant phimosis and meatal stenosis. Although selected reports suggest an association with penile cancer, treatment remains controversial and consists of topical steroids and surgical excision. Meatoplasty may be required, with early circumcision the most effective treatment for BXO.[38]

Buschke-Löwenstein Tumor

The Buschke-Löwenstein tumor is a large exophytic mass involving the glans penis and prepuce; it is a giant condyloma acuminatum that has a good prognosis and does not metastasize. Except for unrestrained local growth, this lesion has malignant features. A viral etiology has been proposed, with identification of HPV-6 and -11 in some tumors. Treatment consists of local conservative resection. Recurrence is common. Systemic interferon-α therapy combined with neodymium: yttrium aluminum garnet (Nd:YAG) laser therapy is successful in some cases. Radiation therapy is contraindicated because rapid malignant degeneration has been described.

Diagnosis and Staging

The workup for penile cancer begins with physical examination of the genitalia and inguinal nodes to ascertain local extent of the

TABLE 69.2

American Joint Committee on Cancer Tumor, Node, Metastasis Classification System for Penile Cancer

Stage Grouping

0	Tis	N0	M0
	Ta	N0	M0
I	T1a	N0	M0
II	T1b	N0	M0
	T2	N0	M0
	T3	N0	M0
IIIa	T1-3	N1	M0
IIIb	T1-3	N2	M0
IV	T4	Any N	M0
	Any T	N3	M0
	Any T	Any N	M1

From American Joint Committee on Cancer. *AJCC Cancer Staging Manual.* 7th ed. New York: Springer-Verlag; 2010, with permission.

lesion and the presence of inguinal adenopathy. Nodal status is the most significant prognostic variable predicting survival. Approximately 50% of patients with penile cancer present with palpable inguinal nodes. Only half of these patients will have metastatic disease, with the remainder having inflammatory adenopathy secondary to infection of the primary lesion. Conversely, 20% of patients with clinically negative groin examination are found to have metastases on prophylactic node dissection. The most common distant metastatic sites are the lung, bone, and liver. The AJCC system (seventh edition) for staging penile cancer uses the TNM classification to determine the stage of the primary tumor and the extent of nodal metastases (Table 69.2).[8] After biopsy confirmation of the lesion, no further radiologic workup is generally needed in patients with early-stage disease and the absence of inguinal adenopathy on examination or other worrisome symptoms. Ultrasound and gadolinium-enhanced MRI are recommended for high-grade and high-stage lesions suspected of involving the corporal bodies, especially if partial penectomy is contemplated. Abdominal and pelvic CT scanning is recommended in obese patients to evaluate the inguinal nodes. In patients with known inguinal metastases, CT-guided biopsy of enlarged pelvic nodes, if positive, may be an indication for neoadjuvant chemotherapy. The role of positron emission tomography scan in the staging of penile cancer is unclear, with conflicting data.[39-41]

Treatment

Treatment of penile carcinoma depends on the local extent of the primary neoplasm and the regional lymph node status. For the primary lesion, a 2-cm proximal margin of resection is recommended. If an adequate margin can be obtained, a partial penectomy offers excellent local control. Leaving the patient with adequate penile length for hygienic upright micturition and sexual intercourse is the goal. Thus, depending on the extent of the primary tumor, resection may include a partial or total penectomy, with local recurrence rare.[42]

In advanced cases (T4), more aggressive resections (emasculation, hemipelvectomy, hemicorpectomy) have been reported with mixed results. Although surgery is the mainstay for treatment of the primary lesion, radiation therapy can be considered for a select group of patients. Radiation therapy allows preservation of the penis, obviating the psychosocial and physical morbidity caused by partial or total penectomy. External-beam and brachytherapy techniques have been used for treatment of the primary cancer. Circumcision is generally recommended before radiation therapy is initiated. This allows for further evaluation of the tumor extent and reduces morbidity associated with radiation (swelling, maceration, secondary infection), all of which may eventually result in secondary phimosis. Local control and penile preservation rates approaching 70% at 10 years have been reported for carefully selected early (T1 to T2) lesions.[43] Treatment of more advanced penile cancers has a much higher risk of local recurrence and progression to nodal and systemic disease.[44] Thus, radiation therapy, although cosmetically attractive, has disadvantages, and the number of patients for whom this treatment is appropriate is small.

Of paramount importance in treatment is consideration of the lymphatic drainage of the penis. The inguinal lymph nodes constitute the first echelon of drainage. Superficial and deep inguinal nodes are involved in a stepwise manner. Bilateral drainage occurs as a result of free anastomoses and crossover at the base of the penis. Therefore, the pattern of nodal metastasis is not limited to one side. The superficial inguinal nodes are located in the deep portion of Camper fascia above the deep fascia of the thigh (fascia lata). The superficial lymphatics drain into the deep inguinal lymphatics, which surround the femoral vessels deep to the fascia lata. Secondary drainage is to the iliac nodes, although direct drainage to these nodes (skip metastases) can occur rarely.

Five-year disease-free survival rates for palpably negative adenopathy (cN0) or low volume palpable groin disease (cN1) are similar and favorable at 93% and 84%, respectively, with a markedly worse survival for palpably bulky disease (cN2 or cN3) of 32% and 0%, respectively.[45] When stratified by pathologic stage, low volume nodal involvement (pN1) had favorable and similar 5-year disease-free survival rates when compared to pathologically negative nodes (pN0) at 93% and 90%, respectively. Pathologically confirmed bulky adenopathy (pN2 and pN3) had very poor long-term outcomes with 5-year disease-free survival rates of 31% and 0%, respectively.

Based on the rarity of advanced penile carcinoma in the Western world, there is growing awareness that these men may receive better outcomes if they are directed to tertiary care centers with expertise in penile carcinoma and inguinal lymphadenectomy. In the United Kingdom, the National Institute for Clinical Excellence published guidelines in 2002 that included the treatment of penile carcinoma and advocated the creation of regional multidisciplinary teams.[46] These guidelines have increased the rate of penis-preserving procedures and inguinal lymphadenectomy, with decreased mortality.[47]

Treatment of Primary Lesion

Surgery for penile carcinoma ranges from circumcision, conservative local resection, laser ablation, and Mohs micrographic surgery to partial and total penectomy. Radiation therapy can be used in selected patients with early superficial lesions.

Carcinoma In Situ (Tis). Penile squamous cell carcinoma in situ, also known as erythroplasia of Queyrat, is a red, velvety, well-marginated lesion of the glans penis or the prepuce of uncircumcised men. After confirmatory biopsy, a conservative approach that spares penile anatomy and function is preferred. Preputial lesions are adequately treated with circumcision. Topical 5-FU cream and imiquimod have been used with excellent cosmetic results for glandular and meatal lesions (imiquimod 5% cream for 5 days per week for 4 to 6 weeks or 5-FU 5% cream every other day for 4 to 6 weeks). A prospective study of carbon dioxide and Nd:YAG lasers has shown good local tumor control and satisfactory cosmetic results.[48] Mohs micrographic surgery has been described as a less-deforming alternative, with local control rates up to 86% in selected patients with early penile cancer.[49] Radiation therapy can often eradicate these lesions with minimal morbidity.

Verrucous Carcinoma (Ta). Penile verrucous carcinoma is characterized by aggressive local growth and a low metastatic potential. Partial or total penectomy is usually overtreatment, and conservative therapeutic approaches are favored. Laser ablation or Mohs micrographic surgical technique has yielded acceptable results. Intra-aortic infusion with methotrexate has been reported with reasonable results.[50] Radiation therapy is contraindicated as it has been shown to cause subsequent rapid malignant degeneration and metastases.

Invasive Penile Cancer (T1, T2, T3, and N1). Distal penile lesions, in which a serviceable penis for upright micturition and sexual function can be achieved, are best treated with a partial penectomy. Extensive lesions that approach the base of the penis usually require total penectomy with corporal body excision and perineal urethrostomy. Local recurrence after a partial penectomy in properly selected cases is rare. Most relapses occur within the first 12 to 18 months after penectomy, and salvage surgery is beneficial.

The effectiveness of radiation therapy in the treatment of penile cancer is hindered by a lack of uniformity of radiation treatment in terms of type of delivery and doses. Radiation therapy is effective for local control of small, 2- to 4-cm, T1 and T2 lesions but also for more advanced T-stage tumors. Local recurrence is higher in those with T3 and T4 tumors, but a significant percentage can be salvaged by adjuvant surgical resection.[51] Before treatment, patients should have a circumcision to allow direct inspection and staging of the tumor and to facilitate management of the acute side effects of radiation. External-beam and brachytherapy techniques have been used. External-beam radiotherapy can be delivered by a direct field method that uses a low-energy photon beam or an electron beam applied directly to the tumor, with a safety margin of 2 cm beyond the visible and palpable extent of the tumor. This approach is suitable only for very superficial tumors (Tis and T1). For T2 and T3 lesions, a parallel opposed field method is used. Using this approach, the entire thickness of the penis can be irradiated by encasing the lesion in a wax mold to ensure uniform dosage and to negate the skin-sparing effects of supervoltage beams with a total dose of 60 Gy recommended. A 65% to 80% local success rate has been reported with radiation therapy for small T1 and T2 tumors.[43] Brachytherapy involves placement of radioactive material (usually iridium-192 wire) within the tumor (interstitial brachytherapy) or molded around the tumor (plesio-brachytherapy) and is limited to T1 and T2 tumors. This form of therapy is not suitable for patients with bulky tumors, deeply infiltrating tumors, and obese patients with a short penis. Radiation therapy as primary treatment for invasive penile carcinoma has significant disadvantages: acute effects of skin edema, maceration, and dysuria may persist for 6 to 8 weeks. Telangiectasia and fibrosis are found in more than 90% of cases. The most serious late effects are urethral fistula, meatal stenosis, and penile necrosis. Postradiation fibrosis, scar, and necrosis may be difficult to distinguish from recurrent cancer. Infection is very often associated with penile cancer and reduces the therapeutic efficacy of radiation while increasing the risk of penile necrosis. Thus, in summary, radiation therapy for primary penile cancer should be considered only in a select group of patients: young patients with small (2 to 4 cm) superficial lesions of the distal penis who wish to maintain penile integrity, patients who refuse surgery, and patients with inoperable cancer or those unsuitable for major surgery.

Advanced Penile Cancer (T4, N2-3, and M1). Large proximal shaft tumors require a total penectomy with a perineal urethrostomy. For extensive, proximal tumors with invasion of adjacent structures, total emasculation (total penectomy, scrotectomy, and orchiectomy) is recommended. In extreme cases, a hemipelvectomy or even a hemicorporectomy has been described. Multimodal therapy with chemoradiation and salvage surgery has also been used in this setting.

Management of Regional Lymph Nodes

The presence and extent of inguinal lymph node metastases are the most important prognostic factors in penile cancer. Although 50% of patients with a penile lesion have clinically palpable inguinal nodes at presentation, in more than half of these the adenopathy is inflammatory. A 4- to 6-week course of antibiotics (e.g., first- or second-generation cephalosporin) after treatment of the primary lesion is recommended. Persistent palpable adenopathy after antibiotic therapy should be biopsied. Unlike many other genitourinary malignancies that require systemic chemotherapy, once lymph node metastases are discovered, inguinal metastases from penile cancer are potentially curable by lymphadenectomy alone. Inguinal lymphadenectomy therefore should be performed at the earliest suspicion of metastases.

Clinical Node Negative (N0). Although there is no controversy in the literature regarding management of the patient with clinically positive inguinal lymph nodes after a course of antibiotics, considerable controversy surrounds the management of the clinically N0 patient. Approximately 20% of these clinically negative groins harbor occult lymphatic metastases on prophylactic lymph node dissection. Stated another way, approximately 80% of patients with clinically negative groins would be subjected to the morbidity of inguinal lymph node dissection without benefit. To resolve this dilemma, a risk-based approach to management of the clinically negative groin has been recommended in most contemporary series. Analysis of histopathologic data from the primary penile cancer allows stratification of patients into high- and low-risk groups for lymph node metastases.[52]

Low-Risk Group. Patients with carcinoma in situ (Tis), verrucous carcinoma (Ta), and T1 tumors who have grade 1 or 2 tumor histology have a <10% chance of developing lymph node metastases and are best served by surveillance and a low incidence of lymphovascular invasion, a risk for nodal metastasis.[37]

High-Risk Group. Patients with invasive penile cancer (T2 and T3) with grade 3 tumors and the presence of vascular invasion have a >50% incidence of inguinal lymph node metastases in various series. Vascular invasion is strongly correlated with lymph node metastases. In pT2 patients, the incidence of lymph node metastases was found to be 75% in the presence of vascular invasion and only 25% when vascular invasion was absent.[52] In this cohort of patients, a prophylactic lymphadenectomy is reasonable.

The timing of surgery in the clinically negative groin has been debated in the past. Most contemporary series favor *early adjunctive* lymphadenectomy, especially in the high-risk group, over surveillance and *delayed therapeutic* lymphadenectomy. Sentinel lymph node biopsy, originally described by Cabanas,[53] is no longer recommended in view of the high false-negative rate. Intraoperative lymphatic mapping using dynamic scintigraphy with technetium-labeled sulfur colloid have decreased the false-negative rate considerably.[54] Other approaches that use sentinel lymph node biopsy have also been advocated, including measurement of the size of the micrometastatic sentinel lymph node to determine whether to perform lymphadenectomy.[55] Sentinel node biopsy remains controversial, with recent studies demonstrating a much lower false negative rate,[56,57] but further data are required.[58] Lymphotropic nanoparticle-enhanced MRI has been investigated to detect micrometastasis but awaits validation.[59]

Inguinal lymph node dissection superficial to the fascia lata has been found to be adequate for the N0 patient. Superficial inguinal lymph node dissection should include a frozen section, and if positive, a modified complete dissection should be carried out. Creation of thicker skin flaps, control of infection, and preservation of the areolar fat superficial to the Scarpa fascia have greatly decreased the complications of flap necrosis, scrotal and extremity edema, lymphocele, and lymphorrhea.

Prediction Models. Ficarra et al.[60] and Kattan et al.[61] have developed predictive nomograms to help determine an individual patient's risk of nodal involvement and cancer-specific survival. One nomogram to predict the probability of lymph node involvement uses eight clinical and pathologic variables (tumor thickness, growth pattern, grade, lymphovascular invasion, corpora cavernosal involvement, spongiosal involvement, urethral involvement, palpable lymph nodes).[60] Not surprisingly, clinically suspicious inguinal lymph nodes are a powerful predictor of pathologic nodal involvement. For cancer-specific survival of patients who undergo surgery for squamous cell carcinoma of the penis, two separate nomograms were created, depending on whether clinical or pathologic staging of inguinal lymph nodes was used.[61] These nomograms may guide patients and clinicians alike on the appropriate treatment and can potentially avoid the risks of lymph node dissection in low-risk patients.

Clinical Node Positive (N1, N2, or N3). The modified inguinal lymph node dissection as described by Catalona[62] has replaced the standard complete inguinal lymphadenectomy as the procedure of choice with clinically persistent nodes after antibiotics. It involves a smaller incision, limited field of inguinal dissection, and preservation of the saphenous vein in an effort to reduce the morbidity of the standard procedure while adhering to standard oncologic principles. Unlike superficial dissection, the deep nodes within the fossa ovalis are also removed. In the face of synchronous unilateral N+ disease, it is standard practice to proceed with a bilateral lymph node dissection in view of the high incidence of bilateral drainage. The exception to this rule is the patient with a clinically negative groin in whom metachronous unilateral inguinal lymphadenopathy develops sometime after treatment of the primary tumor. In these patients, a unilateral dissection of the clinically positive groin usually suffices. The value of pelvic lymphadenectomy in the presence of positive inguinal lymph nodes is for the purposes of staging and identifying patients who would be candidates for adjuvant chemotherapy and had little therapeutic efficacy (5-year survival with pelvic lymph node metastases is <5%).

Patients with advanced nodal disease or bulky fixed inguinal nodes (N3) may require neoadjuvant radiation or chemotherapy before any surgery. Groin lymph nodes adherent to or fungating through the skin require wide excision with myocutaneous flaps to cover the skin defect. The published literature unequivocally favors surgical resection as superior to radiation therapy for the treatment of inguinal lymph nodes. Clinical evaluation of the groin is difficult because of postradiation tissue changes, and the inguinal area tolerates radiation rather poorly. Radiation therapy can be used as a palliative measure in patients with fixed inoperable inguinal nodes or in those with advanced unresectable penile cancer in which the primary and the ilioinguinal region can be treated with radiation therapy.

Role of Chemotherapy and Multimodality Therapy

The role of chemotherapy in the management of penile carcinoma is evolving, and the exact role of chemotherapy has not been established. Data suggest that penile cancer is sensitive to chemotherapy.[63] Besides the use of 5-FU in the treatment of superficial penile cancer, single-agent chemotherapy with cisplatin, methotrexate, and bleomycin has modest activity in advanced penile cancer. The combination of methotrexate, bleomycin, and cisplatin is more active than cisplatin alone but is associated with marked toxicity. Anti–epidermal growth factor receptor therapy may also hold some promise in this disease.[64]

The Southwest Oncology Group reported on the largest prospective clinical trial in patients with penile cancer.[65] In 40 evaluable patients treated with a combination of methotrexate, bleomycin, and cisplatin, an overall response of 32.5% and a complete response of 12.5% were observed. The median response duration was 16 weeks, and the median survival was 28 weeks. Toxicity was formidable, with 11% treatment-related mortality, and 17% of the remaining patients experiencing life-threatening toxicity. Another prospective trial from a UK consortium reported on 29 patients treated with three 21-day cycles of TPF (docetaxel 75 mg/m^2 and cisplatin 60 mg/m^2 on day 1 and 5-FU 750 mg/m^2 per day days 1 to 5) in patients with locally advanced or metastatic penile cancer. The objective response rate was 28.5% and 1-year overall survival rate was 55%, demonstrating activity of this regimen in advanced penile cancer. There was significant toxicity, however, with neutropenic fever in 25% and dose delays or reductions in nearly half

of patients.[66] Multimodality therapy, using a combination of chemotherapy and surgery or chemotherapy and radiation, has been used in isolated reports of advanced penile cancer. Small series in men with fixed, unresectable inguinal nodes had neoadjuvant vincristine, bleomycin, and methotrexate before surgery with some long-term responses.[67] Another small series of patients who underwent surgical resection after neoadjuvant chemotherapy for unresectable penile squamous cell were treated with several different chemotherapy combinations, including bleomycin, methotrexate, cisplatin; ifosfamide, paclitaxel, cisplatin; or paclitaxel/carboplatin with some responses.[68] Clearly, more tolerable and active regimens are needed for unresectable or metastatic penile cancer.

SELECTED REFERENCES

The full reference list can be accessed at lwwhealthlibrary.com/oncology.

1. Tefilli MV, Gheiler EL, Shekarriz B, et al. Primary adenocarcinoma of the urethra with metastasis to the glans penis: successful treatment with chemotherapy and radiation therapy. *Urology* 1998;52:517–519.
3. Wiener JS, Liu ET, Walther PJ. Oncogenic human papillomavirus type 16 is associated with squamous cell cancer of the male urethra. *Cancer Res* 1992;52:5018–5023.
5. Grabstald H. Proceedings: Tumors of the urethra in men and women. *Cancer* 1973;32:1236–1255.
6. Erckert M, Stenzl A, Falk M, et al. Incidence of urethral tumor involvement in 910 men with bladder cancer. *World J Urol* 1996;14:3–8.
8. American Joint Committee on Cancer. *AJCC Cancer Staging Manual.* 7th ed. New York: Springer-Verlag; 2010.
10. Zeidman EJ, Desmond P, Thompson IM. Surgical treatment of carcinoma of the male urethra. *Urol Clin North Am* 1992;19:359–372.
11. Gheiler EL, Tefilli MV, Tiguert R, et al. Management of primary urethral cancer. *Urology* 1998;52:487–493.
12. Davis JW, Schellhammer PF, Schlossberg SM. Conservative surgical therapy for penile and urethral carcinoma. *Urology* 1999;53:386–392.
13. Dalbagni G, Zhang ZF, Lacombe L, et al. Male urethral carcinoma: analysis of treatment outcome. *Urology* 1999;53:1126–1132.
14. Christopher N, Arya M, Brown RS, et al. Penile preservation in squamous cell carcinoma of the bulbomembranous urethra. *BJU Int* 2002;89:464–465.
15. Shen SS, Lerner SP, Muezzinoglu B, et al. Prostatic involvement by transitional cell carcinoma in patients with bladder cancer and its prognostic significance. *Hum Pathol* 2006;37:726–734.
16. Scher HI, Yagoda A, Herr HW, et al. Neoadjuvant M-VAC (methotrexate, vinblastine, doxorubicin and cisplatin) for extravesical urinary tract tumors. *J Urol* 1988;139:475–477.
17. Oberfield RA, Zinman LN, Leibenhaut M, et al. Management of invasive squamous cell carcinoma of the bulbomembranous male urethra with co-ordinated chemo-radiotherapy and genital preservation. *Br J Urol* 1996;78:573–578.
18. Licht MR, Klein EA, Bukowski R, et al. Combination radiation and chemotherapy for the treatment of squamous cell carcinoma of the male and female urethra. *J Urol* 1995;153:1918–1920.
19. Srinivas V, Khan SA. Female urethral cancer—an overview. *Int Urol Nephrol* 1987;19:423–427.
20. Champ CE, Hegarty SE, Shen X, et al. Prognostic factors and outcomes after definitive treatment of female urethral cancer: a population-based analysis. *Urology* 2012;80:374–381.
22. Sailer SL, Shipley WU, Wang CC. Carcinoma of the female urethra: a review of results with radiation therapy. *J Urol* 1988;140:1–5.
23. Dalbagni G, Zhang ZF, Lacombe L, et al. Female urethral carcinoma: an analysis of treatment outcome and a plea for a standardized management strategy. *Br J Urol* 1998;82:835–841.
24. Grabstald H, Hilaris B, Henschke U, et al. Cancer of the female urethra. *JAMA* 1966;197:835–842.
25. Milosevic MF, Warde PR, Banerjee D, et al. Urethral carcinoma in women: results of treatment with primary radiotherapy. *Radiother Oncol* 2000;56:29–35.
28. Hernandez BY, Barnholtz-Sloan J, German RR, et al. Burden of invasive squamous cell carcinoma of the penis in the United States, 1998–2003. *Cancer* 2008;113:2883–2891.

29. Maden C, Sherman KJ, Beckmann AM, et al. History of circumcision, medical conditions, and sexual activity and risk of penile cancer. *J Natl Cancer Inst* 1993;85:19–24.
30. Miralles-Guri C, Bruni L, Cubilla AL, et al. Human papillomavirus prevalence and type distribution in penile carcinoma. *J Clin Pathol* 2009;62:870–878.
32. Chaux A, Cubilla AL. The role of human papillomavirus infection in the pathogenesis of penile squamous cell carcinomas. *Sem Diagn Pathol* 2012;29:67–71.
33. Harish K, Ravi R. The role of tobacco in penile carcinoma. *Br J Urol* 1995;75:375–377.
37. Lopes A, Hidalgo GS, Kowalski LP, et al. Prognostic factors in carcinoma of the penis: multivariate analysis of 145 patients treated with amputation and lymphadenectomy. *J Urol* 1996;156:1637–1642.
41. Leijte JA, Graafland NM, Valdes Olmos RA, et al. Prospective evaluation of hybrid 18F-fluorodeoxyglucose positron emission tomography/computed tomography in staging clinically node-negative patients with penile carcinoma. *BJU Int* 2009;104:640–644.
42. Korets R, Koppie TM, Snyder ME, et al. Partial penectomy for patients with squamous cell carcinoma of the penis: the Memorial Sloan-Kettering experience. *Ann Surg Oncol* 2007;14:3614–3619.
43. Crook JM, Haie-Meder C, Demanes DJ, et al. American Brachytherapy Society-Groupe Europeen de Curietherapie-European Society of Therapeutic Radiation Oncology (ABS-GEC-ESTRO) consensus statement for penile brachytherapy. *Brachytherapy* 2013;12:191–198.
48. Windahl T, Andersson SO. Combined laser treatment for penile carcinoma: results after long-term followup. *J Urol* 2003;169(6):2118–2121.
52. Slaton JW, Morgenstern N, Levy DA, et al. Tumor stage, vascular invasion and the percentage of poorly differentiated cancer: independent prognosticators for inguinal lymph node metastasis in penile squamous cancer. *J Urol* 2001;165:1138–1142.
56. Leijte JA, Hughes B, Graafland NM, et al. Two-center evaluation of dynamic sentinel node biopsy for squamous cell carcinoma of the penis. *J Clin Oncol* 2009;27:3325–3329.
57. Jensen JB, Jensen KM, Ulhoi BP, et al. Sentinel lymph-node biopsy in patients with squamous cell carcinoma of the penis. *BJU Int* 2009;103:1199–1203.
60. Ficarra V, Zattoni F, Artibani W, et al. Nomogram predictive of pathological inguinal lymph node involvement in patients with squamous cell carcinoma of the penis. *J Urol* 2006;175:1700–1704; discussion 1704–1705.
61. Kattan MW, Ficarra V, Artibani W, et al. Nomogram predictive of cancer specific survival in patients undergoing partial or total amputation for squamous cell carcinoma of the penis. *J Urol* 2006;175:2103–2108; discussion 2108.
62. Catalona WJ. Modified inguinal lymphadenectomy for carcinoma of the penis with preservation of saphenous veins: technique and preliminary results. *J Urol* 1988;140:306–310.
63. Trabulsi EJ, Hoffman-Censits J. Chemotherapy for penile and urethral carcinoma. *Urol Clin North Am* 2010;37:467–474.
65. Haas GP, Blumenstein BA, Gagliano RG, et al. Cisplatin, methotrexate and bleomycin for the treatment of carcinoma of the penis: a Southwest Oncology Group study. *J Urol* 1999;161:1823–1825.
67. Pizzocaro G, Piva L. Adjuvant and neoadjuvant vincristine, bleomycin, and methotrexate for inguinal metastases from squamous cell carcinoma of the penis. *Acta Oncol* 1988;27:823–824.
68. Bermejo C, Busby JE, Spiess PE, et al. Neoadjuvant chemotherapy followed by aggressive surgical consolidation for metastatic penile squamous cell carcinoma. *J Urol* 2007;177:1335–1338.

PRACTICE OF ONCOLOGY

70 Cancer of the Testis

Lance C. Pagliaro and Christopher J. Logothetis

INTRODUCTION

Testicular cancers are the most common malignant neoplasm affecting men ages 15 to 35 years. Approximately 90% of testicular cancers are germ cell tumors, which can be broadly classified as seminoma or nonseminomatous germ cell tumors (NSGCT). Male extragonadal germ cell tumors are also discussed in this chapter. Analogous germ cell and sex cord stromal tumors in women are not included here, but in many cases the male and female counterparts share a common biology and therapeutic approach.

INCIDENCE AND EPIDEMIOLOGY

In the United States, 8,820 new cases of testicular cancer per year is estimated for 2014.[1] This figure greatly underestimates the prevalence of testicular cancer survivors. This is because the cancer-specific survival rate for testicular cancer with standard treatment is >95%.[2] The incidence varies among geographic areas, being highest in Scandinavia, Switzerland, and Germany, and lowest in Africa and Asia.[3] Although testicular germ cell tumors are most common among adolescent and young adult men, they can potentially occur in males of any age or genetic background. For reasons that have yet to be discovered, the incidence of testicular germ cell tumors has increased over the preceding 30 years in the United States and United Kingdom.[4]

Risk Factors

Men whose family history includes a first-degree relative with testicular germ cell tumor or who have a personal history of cryptorchidism are at increased risk of developing germ cell tumor.[5,6] Testicular cancer survivors are also at increased risk of a second primary cancer in the contralateral testicle.[7] These risk factors suggest a genetic or developmental etiology for testicular germ cell tumors. No postnatal environmental risk factors have yet been identified.[8]

In the United States, testicular cancer is rare among African Americans and most common among Caucasian men.[9] This racial disparity in testicular cancer diagnosis and its geographic distribution suggest a genetic linkage with the Caucasian phenotype, but no high penetrance allele has yet been identified.[4] Testicular germ cell tumors are commonly accompanied by intratubular germ cell neoplasia (ITGCN). It is thought that all adult germ cell tumors, with the exception of spermatocytic seminoma, arise from ITGCN.[10] The widely accepted theory is that ITGCN begins in utero.[11] The multifocality of ITGCN suggests a field effect within the testicle and provides a mechanistic explanation for cases of bilateral testicular cancer.

Men without a history of testicular cancer are occasionally found to have ITGCN on testicular biopsy or orchiectomy that was performed for other reasons. The incidental finding of testicular microlithiasis on ultrasound may also provide evidence of ITGCN in an otherwise healthy man.[12,13] The risk of testicular cancer for such individuals has not been determined, but they should be counseled regarding a potential increased risk and to report any new testicular symptoms.[14]

INITIAL PRESENTATION AND MANAGEMENT

Symptoms and Signs

Testicular swelling is the most common presenting complaint and in most cases is detected by the patient himself. Patients may also report a pressure-like sensation, heaviness, or mild-to-moderate testicular pain. This will sometimes be confused with orchitis or epididymitis and treated initially with antibiotics. Acute or severe pain is rarely caused by testicular cancer and suggests a different etiology such as testicular torsion. Testicular ultrasound should be obtained as soon as a neoplasm is suspected, and it will appear as one or more hypoechoic lesions within the testicle. Ultrasound distinguishes a solid from cystic mass, and intratesticular from intrascrotal/extratesticular location. A solid intratesticular mass on ultrasound is presumed to be a neoplasm and is an indication for radical inguinal orchiectomy.[15]

Approximately half of patients present with a testicular mass and no clinical evidence of metastasis (clinical stage I). Others present with metastatic disease that may also be symptomatic. Primary tumors can be small and asymptomatic, even in the presence of metastatic disease, and occasionally they "burn out" leaving only a fibrotic scar (burned-out primary). Metastases can be the source of clinical symptoms on presentation in such cases, and include back pain, shortness of breath, cough, gynecomastia, hemoptysis, and weight loss.[16] Ultrasound of the testicles is helpful in establishing the diagnosis even if there is no palpable testicular mass.[15] The detection of elevated serum tumor markers can also be helpful when an occult testicular primary or extragonadal germ cell tumor is suspected.[17]

Diagnosis

Radical inguinal orchiectomy is the standard diagnostic and therapeutic procedure for a solid intratesticular mass.[18] Transscrotal orchiectomy or biopsy is specifically contraindicated because of the risk of tumor cell seeding of the inguinal and pelvic lymphatic drainage. Biopsy is also of limited value because testicular germ cell tumors are heterogeneous. Removal of the entire organ is necessary to properly identify the histologic type(s) present and to select the appropriate therapy. It is reasonable to perform needle biopsy of a metastatic site in cases of occult testicular primary, burned-out primary, or extragonadal germ cell tumor; although, the results of needle biopsy must always be interpreted with caution due to sampling error. The pattern of serum tumor marker elevation is also informative about the likely cell types present (seminoma or nonseminoma), as discussed in the next section.[17]

HISTOLOGY

Male germ cell tumors are broadly classified as seminoma and NSGCT (Table 70.1).[19,20] Patients with pure seminoma are

TABLE 70.1

World Health Organization Histologic Classification of Testicular Germ Cell Tumors

Germ Cell Tumors
Intratubular germ cell neoplasia, unclassified
Other types

Tumors of One Histologic Type (Pure Forms)
Seminoma
Seminoma with syncytiotrophoblastic cells
Spermatocytic seminoma
Spermatocytic seminoma with sarcoma
Embryonal carcinoma
Yolk sac tumor
Trophoblastic tumors
Choriocarcinoma
Trophoblastic neoplasms other than choriocarcinoma
Teratoma
Dermoid cyst
Monodermal teratoma
Teratoma with somatic type malignancies

Tumors of More Than One Histologic Type (Mixed Forms)
Mixed embryonal carcinoma and teratoma
Mixed teratoma and seminoma
Choriocarcinoma and teratoma/embryonal carcinoma
Others

Source: Eble JN, Sauter G, Epstein JI, et al., eds. *Pathology and Genetics of Tumours of the Urinary System and Male Genital Organs.* Lyon, France: IARC Press; 2004.

managed differently than patients with NSGCT or mixed histology tumors, although mixed tumors may have a component of seminoma. In that sense, when we refer to seminoma as a clinical diagnosis it is meant as pure seminoma, whereas seminoma as a histologic pattern may also be present in mixed NSGCT.

Seminoma

The microscopic appearance of seminoma is characterized by sheets of neoplastic cells with abundant cytoplasm, round, hyperchromatic nuclei and prominent nucleoli (Fig. 70.1). A prominent lymphocytic infiltrate is common, such that it is sometimes confused with lymphoma until the surface immunophenotype has been determined. Most seminomas do not produce serum tumor

markers, but the presence of syncytiotrophoblastic giant cells in a minority of cases accounts for modest elevations of serum human chorionic gonadotropin (hCG).[21] Seminomas never produce alpha-fetoprotein (AFP), and patients whose tumors have the histologic appearance of seminoma and whose serum AFP is elevated should be considered to have a mixed NSGCT, even if a nonseminomatous histologic pattern cannot be identified.[22] Exceptions are cases in which there is another explanation for the elevated AFP, such as liver disease or a chronic nonspecific elevation.

Immunohistochemistry is usually positive for placental alkaline phosphatase (PLAP), negative for CD30, AFP, and epithelial membrane antigen, and either negative or weak/focally positive for cytokeratin.[23]

Histologic variations of seminoma such as "anaplastic" or "atypical" seminoma are of no known clinical relevance. Spermatocytic seminoma, however, is the one variant of seminoma that has a different natural history and is even of uncertain relation to other germ cell tumors. Spermatocytic seminoma usually occurs in older individuals and has low metastatic potential.[24] Orchiectomy is the only treatment required. Unlike all other germ cell tumors, spermatocytic seminoma is not associated with ITGCN.

Nonseminomatous Histologies

Germ cell tumors may be composed of a single histology or multiple histologic patterns.[19] Through poorly understood processes of mutation and differentiation, a single clone beginning as ITGCN can develop into an undifferentiated neoplasm (seminoma), or to a primitive zygotic neoplasm (embryonal carcinoma).[25] Further differentiation from embryonal carcinoma results in somatically differentiated tumors (teratoma) or extraembryonal-differentiated tumors (yolk sac and choriocarcinoma).[26] Nonseminomatous histologies are found in 55% of germ cell tumors. Male germ cell tumors that contain any histologic cell type other than seminoma or syncytiotrophoblasts are collectively referred to as NSGCT.

Embryonal Carcinoma

Embryonal carcinoma is the most undifferentiated type of germ cell tumor and is thought to be pluripotent. Cells are characterized by indistinct borders and scant cytoplasm, which can be arranged in solid sheets or in glandular or tubular structures (Fig. 70.2). On immunohistochemical staining, embryonal carcinoma can be positive for cytokeratin, CD30, PLAP, AFP, and hCG. Modest elevations of serum AFP and/or hCG can be seen, and frequently it is marker-negative. Lactate dehydrogenase (LDH) concentration in the serum is an important prognostic factor in metastatic embryonal carcinoma that is marker negative.

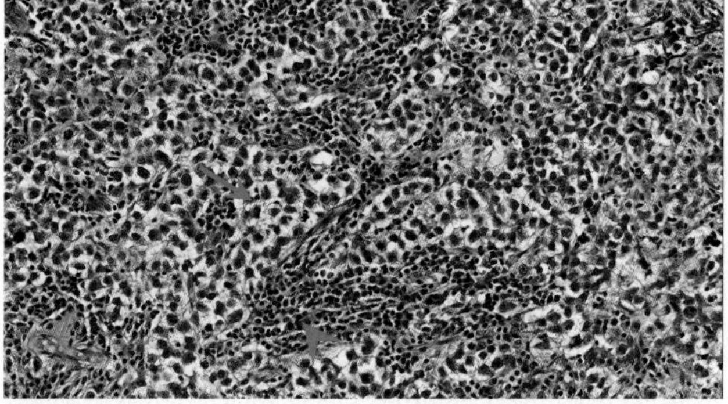

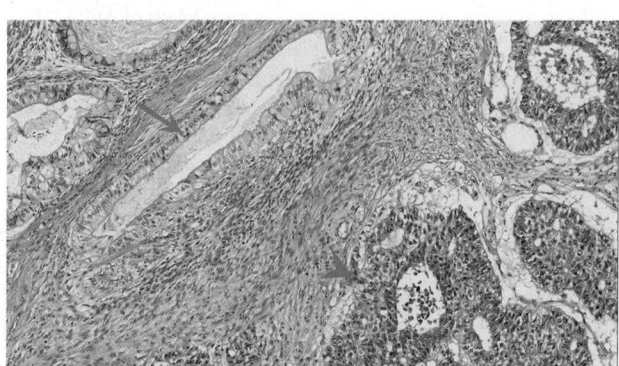

Figure 70.1 Seminoma, classic type, with neoplastic cells (*arrow*) and the typical accompanying lymphocytic infiltrate (*arrowhead*). (Source: Rao B, Pagliaro LC. Testicular germ cell tumors. In. Silverman PM, ed. *Oncologic Imaging: A Multidisciplinary Approach.* Philadelphia: Elsevier; 2012:335–357.)

Figure 70.2 Mixed nonseminomatous germ cell tumor comprised of teratoma (*arrow*) and embryonal carcinoma (*arrowhead*). (Source: Rao B, Pagliaro LC. Testicular germ cell tumors. In. Silverman PM, ed. *Oncologic Imaging: A Multidisciplinary Approach.* Philadelphia: Elsevier; 2012:335–357.)

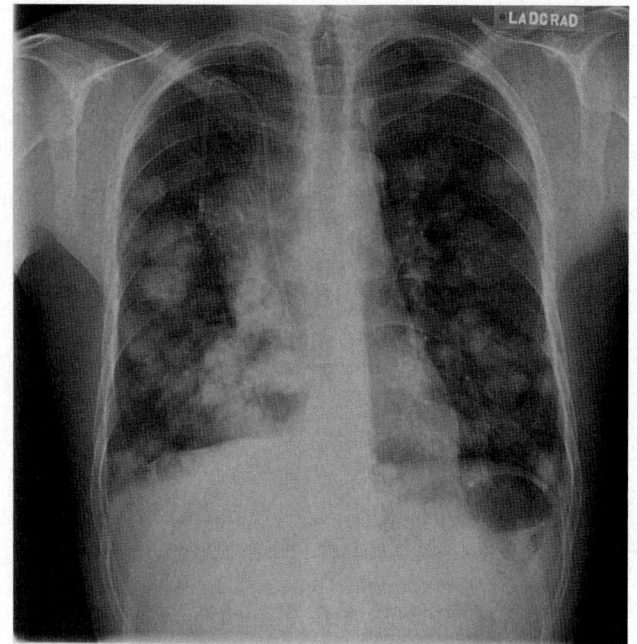
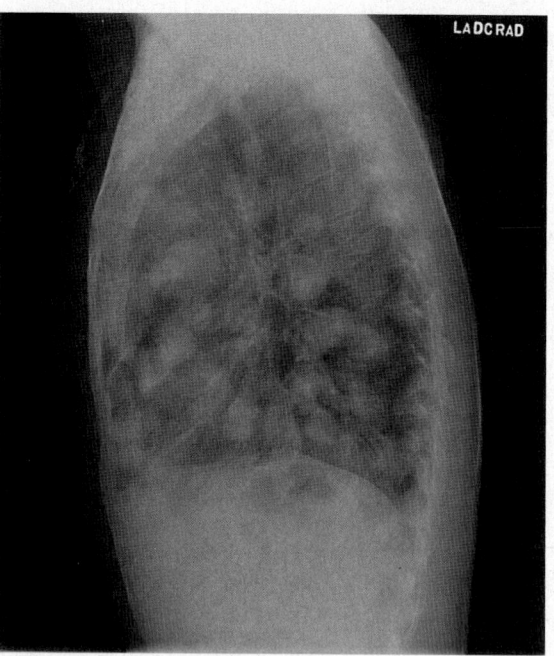

Figure 70.3 Chest radiograph of a man with primary mediastinal choriocarcinoma and pulmonary metastases.

Choriocarcinoma

Choriocarcinoma is composed of both cytotrophoblasts and syncytiotrophoblasts.[27] The cells strongly express hCG. The clinical presentation of a choriocarcinoma-predominant or pure choriocarcinoma tumor often includes very high serum hCG levels, widespread hematogenous metastases, and tumor hemorrhage (Fig. 70.3). Syncytiotrophoblasts and syncytiotrophoblastic giant cells can be associated with other germ cell histologies, so the presence of cytotophoblasts is required for the diagnosis.

Yolk Sac Tumor

Yolk sac tumor (endodermal sinus tumor) is commonly seen as a component of mixed NSGCT. Pure yolk sac tumors represent a significant proportion of mediastinal germ cell tumors, but are rarely seen in adult testicular cancer. Histologic patterns include papillary, solid, glandular, hepatoid, macrocystic, and microcystic types. Perivascular arrangements of epithelial cells can be seen in yolk sac tumor and are known as glomeruloid or Schiller-Duval bodies. Immunostains are diffusely positive for AFP and may also be positive for cytokeratin, SALL4, glipican-3, PLAP, and CD117. Yolk sac tumor is associated with high serum levels of AFP.

Teratoma

Teratoma arises from a pluripotent malignant precursor (embryonal carcionoma or yolk sac tumor) and contains somatic cells from at least two germ cell layers (ectoderm, endoderm, or mesoderm). Teratoma is commonly seen as a component of adult mixed NSGCT (see Fig. 70.2). A small percentage (2% to 3%) of postpubertal male germ cell tumors appear to have teratoma as the only histologic type, but these are always assumed to harbor a minor component of pluripotent NSGCT and are treated the same as a mixed NSGCT.

Immature teratoma shows partial somatic differentiation, whereas mature teratoma has terminally differentiated tissues such as cartilage, skeletal muscle, or nerve tissue, and frequently forms cystic structures. Although these cells can resemble normal tissues, teratoma is a low-grade malignancy and if untreated will grow until it is unresectable. Moreover, teratomas can give rise to secondary somatic malignancy, such as rhabdomyosarcoma, poorly

differentiated carcinoma, or primitive neuroectodermal tumor.[28] These typically display the biology of their de novo counterparts and are treated accordingly.[29,30]

Teratoma does not produce elevated serum AFP or hCG. Patients with elevated serum AFP and/or hCG should be assumed to have a nonteratoma germ cell tumor component, unless the elevation can be otherwise explained.

BIOLOGY

Mechanism of Germ Cell Transformation

ITGCN is thought to derive from malignant transformation of primordial germ cells or gonocytes during fetal development.[31] Primordial germ cells migrate from the proximal epiblast (yolk sac) through the hindgut and mesentery to the genital ridge, and become gonocytes. The precise molecular events underlying transformation to ITGCN are not well understood. The most consistent genetic finding in germ cell tumors is a gain of material from chromosome 12p. The majority of NSGCT and seminomas contain i(12p), an isochromosome comprised of two fused short arms of chromosome 12. The remaining i(12p)-negative germ cell tumors also have a gain of 12p sequences in the form of tandem duplications that may be transposed elsewhere in the genome.

Gain of 12p sequences has been found in ITGCN, indicating that it is an early event in testicular cancer pathogenesis. The acquisition of i(12p) is not thought to be the initiating event, however, because it is preceded by polyploidization.[32] Overexpressed genes on 12p are likely to be important, and there are candidate genes on 12p including several that confer growth advantage (KRAS2, CCND2 [cyclin D2]), and others that establish or maintain the stem cell phenotype (NANOG, DPPA3, GDF3). The exact genes that are critical to this step have not yet been identified.

Seminomas are usually hypertriploid, whereas NSGCT is more commonly hypotriploid.[33] Other chromosome regions were found to have nonrandom gains or losses in germ cell tumors with less frequency than 12p. Single gene mutations are uncommon in germ cell tumors. The most commonly mutated genes are BRAF, KIT, KRAS, NRAS, and TP53.[11] The KIT/kit ligand (KITLG) pathway

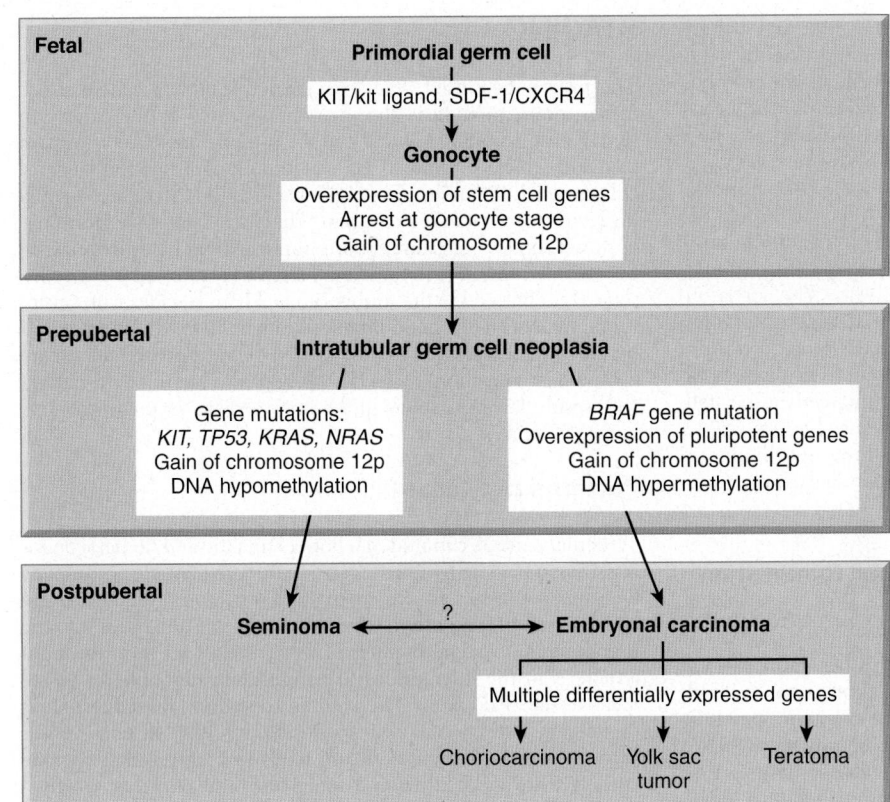

Figure 70.4 Pathogenesis of testicular germ cell tumors. (Adapted from Sheikine Y, Genega E, Melamed J, et al. Molecular genetics of testicular germ cell tumors. *Am J Cancer Res* 2012;2:153–167.)

has special relevance for gonadal development. The biologic function of this pathway is broad and includes development of hematopoietic cells, melanocytes, and germ cells.[34] *KITLG* is essential for primordial germ cell survival and motility, as are the chemokine *SDF-1* (CXCL12) and its receptor CXCR4.[11] Immunohistochemical markers found on primordial germ cells and gonocytes (PLAP, CD117 [*KIT*], OCT3/4 [*POU5F1*]) are also found on ITGCN, suggesting a transformation from these cells during fetal development (Fig. 70.4). The biallelic expression of imprinted genes in germ cell tumors has been reported, showing that they likely arose from primordial germ cells where the genomic imprinting is temporarily erased.[31]

Somatic mutations in *KIT* as well as increased copy number have been described in 9% of testicular germ cell tumors and 20% of seminomas.[4] The somatic alterations in *KIT* found in germ cell tumors are predicted to upregulate pathway activity. *KITLG* plays a role in determining skin pigmentation and has undergone strong selection in European and Asian populations. Difference in the frequency of risk alleles for *KITLG* between European and African populations may provide an explanation for the difference in germ cell tumor incidence between Caucasian and African Americans.

There is evidence that epigenetic regulation of gene expression plays a role in the pathogenesis of germ cell tumors. The DNA methylation patterns are different among histologic types. Global hypomethylation is more common in seminomas than in NSGCT.[31] In a study of 16 germ cell tumors, the methylation of CpG islands in NSGCT was similar to that observed in other tumor types, whereas it was virtually absent in seminomas.[35] Aberrant promoter methylation is generally associated with absent or downregulated expression of the methylated genes. This can result, for example, in the silencing of tumor suppressor genes.[31] Methylation has also been correlated with germ cell tumor differentiation. The more differentiated tumors (yolk sac tumor, choriocarcinoma, teratoma) were consistently hypermethylated, whereas seminoma and ITGCN were hypomethylated.[36] Some of the observed methylation patterns may reflect normal development rather than germ cell tumor pathogenesis.

Pluripotency of Embryonal-Like Differentiation in Germ Cell Tumors

Embryonal carcinoma has a six-gene signature (*DNMT3B, DPPA4, GAL, GPC4, POU5F1, TERF1*), which was detected in three of five independent studies.[11] All six of these genes are involved in establishing and maintaining pluripotency. *SOX2* encodes a transcription factor essential for maintaining self-renewal of embryonic stem cells and is upregulated in embryonal carcinoma. Two additional genes that encode transcription factors associated with stem cell pluripotency, *NANOG* and *POU5F1*, are upregulated in both seminoma and embryonal carcinoma.[26] Lineage differentiation takes place in NSGCT, mimicking the development of a normal zygote. Thus, embryonal carcinoma can be thought of as the transformed counterpart of embryonic stem cells, displaying self-renewal, pluripotency, and lineage differentiation.

Familial Predisposition to Germ Cell Tumors

Approximately 1.4% of patients with newly diagnosed germ cell tumor report a family history of germ cell tumor.[34] First-degree male relatives of patients with testicular cancer have a 6- to 10-fold increased risk of developing testicular cancer. These observations point to the likely existence of a hereditary germ cell tumor subset. The inheritable effect is mild, and the most common number of affected relatives in a family is two. The age at diagnosis among familial cases is 2 to 3 years younger than sporadic cases, and there is a higher incidence of bilateral tumors.

The gr/gr deletion on chromosome Y, common among infertility patients and associated with a two- to threefold increased risk of testicular cancer, was studied as a candidate region for hereditary risk.[4] The frequency of gr/gr variant is low, however, such that it could only account for a small component of hereditary risk. Genome-wide association studies (GWAS) for testicular cancer have been hampered by relatively small sample sizes. Nevertheless, five loci of interest were identified in a GWAS study from the

United Kingdom, on chromosomes 1, 4, 5q31.3, 6, and 12p22, including confirmatory data for the chromosome 6 locus. The single nucleotide polymorphism (SNP) associations on chromosomes 1 and 4 were not convincingly replicated in an independent US study, whereas the associations on chromosomes 5 and 12 were confirmed. The strongest associated SNPs were at 12q22 within the *KITLG* gene, for which there is a >2.5 risk of disease per major allele. For the chromosome 5 and 6 loci, a 1.5-fold increased risk was identified per major allele. The loci on chromosome 5 implicate the gene *SPRY4*, which encodes an inhibitor of the mitogen-activated protein kinase pathway. The locus on chromosome 6 falls within the intron of *BAK1*, which promotes apoptosis. The location of a disease-associated SNP near or within a gene does not definitively implicate that gene, yet all three of the genes identified in GWASs are directly or indirectly associated with the KIT/KITLG pathway.[11] These genes may be responsible for an estimated 15% of genetic predisposition to germ cell tumors, whereas the genetic basis of the other 85% of familial aggregations remains unexplained.

Cisplatin Sensitivity and Acquired Resistance in Adult Germ Cell Tumors

Exquisite sensitivity to chemotherapy distinguishes germ cell tumors from most other cancers. Levels of p53 protein are elevated in all germ cell tumors except teratoma.[31] To maintain genomic integrity, embryonic stem cells have a high sensitivity to DNA damage, suggesting that the high levels of wild-type p53 seen in germ cell tumors may be intrinsic to their germ cell nature. *TP53* gene mutations are uncommon in germ cell tumors, however, and the role of acquired *TP53* mutations in the emergence of chemotherapy resistance has not been established.[11] Moreover, levels of p53 protein assessed by immunohistochemistry were not associated with outcome. While mutations in *TP53* have been observed in about 7% of seminomas, its significance in germ cell tumors remains unclear.

Mutations of *BRAF* including V600E mutations have been detected in a small percentage of NSGCT. *BRAF* mutations were most prevalent in mediastinal primary tumors, late relapse, and cisplatin-resistant NSGCT, suggesting a role in chemoresistance. Further study is needed to define the prognostic significance of *BRAF* mutation and whether the V600E mutation can be therapeutically targeted. A high ratio of proapoptotic Bax to antiapoptotic Bcl-2 was found in invasive germ cell tumors and may explain the rapid apoptotic response to DNA-damaging drugs; however, the Bax:Bcl-2 ratio was not associated with treatment outcome.[31] Finally, the emergence of cisplatin resistance may be intimately associated with the expression of genes and pathways responsible for lineage differentiation in NSGCT, in other words, intrinsic to the germ cell biology rather than the result of specific mutations.

IMMUNOHISTOCHEMICAL MARKERS

SALL4 is expressed in almost all germ cell tumors and has been reported to be positive in ITGCN, classic seminoma, spermatocytic seminoma, embryonal carcinoma, yolk sac tumor, choriocarcinoma, and teratoma.[37,38] OCT3/4 is variably expressed in ITGCN, classic seminoma, embryonal carcinoma, and yolk sac tumor. Spermatocytic seminoma, choriocarcinoma, and teratoma are usually negative for OCT3/4. CD117 (KIT) helps highlight ITGCN and classic seminoma. CD30, SOX2, and keratin are helpful in the diagnosis of embryonal carcinoma, whereas SALL4 and Glypican-3 are often positive in yolk sac tumor.[39] In tumors of unknown primary or those presenting as a retroperitoneal or mediastinal mass, SALL4, OCT3/4, CD117, SOX2, CD30, and low-molecular-weight keratins all may be useful in distinguishing germ cell tumors from non–germ cell tumors.

STAGING

The most widely used system for staging testicular cancer is the tumor, node, metastasis classification endorsed by the American Joint Commission on Cancer and the International Union Against Cancer (Tables 70.2 and 70.3).[40] An important distinction for germ cell tumors is the inclusion of "S" classification (S0 to S3), signifying serum tumor marker elevation. There are three stage groupings of tumor, node, metastasis/serum tumor marker elevation classifications whereby, in general, stage I disease is confined to the testis, stage II is confined to the retroperitoneal lymph nodes with serum tumor markers in the good-prognosis range (S0 to S1), and stage III includes metastases that extend beyond the retroperitoneum or are extranodal in location. Stage III NSGCT also includes any patient with serum tumor markers in the intermediate- or poor-prognosis range (S2 to S3).

Patterns of Metastasis

Testicular cancers can undergo both lymphatic and hematogenous dissemination. The lymphatics arising from the testicle accompany the gonadal vessels in the spermatic cord. Some follow the gonadal vessels to their origin while others diverge and drain into the retroperitoneum. The landing zone for metastasis from the right testicle is in the interaortocaval lymph nodes just inferior to the renal vessels (Fig. 70.5). The landing zone from the left testicle is in the para-aortic lymph nodes just inferior to the left renal vessels (Fig. 70.6). Large volume disease tends to progress in retrograde fashion to the aortic bifurcation and below, along the iliac vessels.[41]

Seminoma

Seminoma can spread extensively through the lymphatic system to include retroperitoneal, retrocrural, mediastinal, supraclavicular, and cervical lymph nodes, often in the absence of hematogenous metastasis.[42] Metastasis to lungs (stage IIIA) is common; metastasis to nonpulmonary organs (stage IIIB) is less common.[43] Serum tumor markers do not affect the stage (except in stage IS) or prognosis in seminoma. Hematogenous metastasis to extrapulmonary organs (e.g., bone) in seminoma carries an intermediate prognosis. There is no stage IIIC or poor-prognosis designation in seminoma.[44]

Nonseminomatous Germ Cell Tumors

Similar to seminoma, lymphatic spread is the most common and usually the earliest type of dissemination in NSGCT. Stage groupings depend on both the anatomic extent of disease and serum tumor markers.[40] Stage IIIB is distinguished from stage II or IIIA on the basis of tumor markers being in the intermediate-prognosis range (S2). Stage IIIC NSGCT carries a poor prognosis, and more often than seminoma it involves multiple organs such as liver and brain.[44]

Embryonal carcinoma, in some cases, exhibits hematogenous metastasis to lungs or nonpulmonary viscera without clinical involvement of retroperitoneal lymph nodes.[45] Computed tomography (CT) of the chest is necessary for complete staging workup of tumors that have a high percentage of embryonal carcinoma.

Serum Tumor Markers

Serum tumor markers are an important part of the staging system for germ cell tumors. Three markers, namely AFP, hCG, and total LDH, are considered for establishing the correct prognostic classification (good, intermediate, or poor prognosis).[44] Markers should be assessed after orchiectomy and before the start of chemotherapy. Markers that are elevated prior to orchiectomy and then normalize appropriately have no prognostic significance. Markers that do not normalize in a patient without any other clinical evidence of metastatic disease are considered stage IS.[40] In the absence of residual disease, the expected half-life of postoperative serum tumor marker decline is 2 to 3 days for hCG and 5 to 7 days for AFP.

TABLE 70.2

Definition of TNM

TNM Category	Description
Primary Tumor (T)	
pTX	Primary tumor cannot be assessed.
pT0	No evidence of primary tumor (e.g., histologic scar in testis).
pTis	Intratubular germ cell neoplasia (carcinoma in situ)
pT1	Tumor limited to the testis and epididymis without vascular/lymphatic invasion. Tumor may invade into the tunica albuginea but not the tunica vaginalis.
pT2	Tumor limited to the testis and epididymis with vascular/lymphatic invasion or tumor extending through the tunica albuginea with involvement of the tunica vaginalis.
pT3	Tumor invades the spermatic cord with or without vascular/lymphatic invasion.
pT4	Tumor invades the scrotum with or without vascular/lymphatic invasion.
Note: Except for pTis and pT4, extent of primary tumor is classified by radical orchiectomy. TX may be used for other categories in the absence of radical orchiectomy.	
Regional Lymph Nodes (N)	
Clinical	
NX	Regional lymph nodes cannot be assessed.
N0	No regional lymph node metastasis
N1	Metastasis with a lymph node mass 2 cm or less in greatest dimension or multiple lymph nodes; none >2 cm in greatest dimension.
N2	Metastasis with a lymph node mass >2 cm but not >5 cm in greatest dimension, or multiple lymph nodes, any one mass >2 cm but not >5 cm cm in greatest dimension.
N3	Metastasis with a lymph node mass >5 cm in greatest dimension.
Pathologic (pN)	
pNX	Regional lymph nodes cannot be assessed.
pN0	No regional lymph node metastasis
pN1	Metastasis with a lymph node mass 2 cm or less in greatest dimension and ≤5 nodes positive; none >2 cm in greatest dimension.
pN2	Metastasis with a lymph node mass >2 cm but not >5 cm in greatest dimension, or >5 nodes positive, none >5 cm, or evidence of extranodal extension of tumor.
pN3	Metastasis with a lymph node mass >5 cm in greatest dimension.
Distant Metastases (M)	
M0	No distant metastasis.
M1	Distant metastasis
M1a	Nonregional nodal or pulmonary metastases
M1b	Distant metastasis other than to nonregional lymph nodes and lungs
Serum Tumor Markers (S)	
SX	Marker studies not available or not performed
S0	Marker study levels within normal limits
S1	LDH <1.5 × N[a] **AND** hCG (mIU/mL) <5,000 **AND** AFP (ng/mL) <1,000
S2	LDH 1.5–10 × N **OR** hCG (mIU/mL) 5,000–50,000 **OR** AFP (ng/mL) 1,000–10,000
S3	LDH >10 × N **OR** hCG (mIU/mL) >50,000 **OR** AFP (ng/mL) >10,000

TNM, tumor, node, metastasis; LDH, lactate dehydrogenase; hCG, human chorionic gonadotropin; AFP, α-fetoprotein; S, serum tumor markers.
[a] N indicates upper limit of normal for the LDH assay.
Used with the permission of the American Joint Committee on Cancer (AJCC), Chicago, Illinois. The original source for this material is the Edge SB, Byrd DR, Compton CC, et al., eds. *AJCC Cancer Staging Manual*, 7th ed. New York: Springer Science and Business Media LLC; 2010: 471–472.

PRACTICE OF ONCOLOGY

TABLE 70.3

Stage Grouping

Group	T	N	M	S[a]
Stage 0	pTis	N0	M0	S0
Stage I	pT1–4	N0	M0	SX
IA	pT1	N0	M0	S0
IB	pT2	N0	M0	S0
	pT3	N0	M0	S0
	pT4	N0	M0	S0
IS	Any pT/Tx	N0	M0	S1–3
Stage II	Any pT/Tx	N1-3	M0	SX
IIA	Any pT/Tx	N1	M0	S0
	Any pT/Tx	N1	M0	S1
IIB	Any pT/Tx	N2	M0	S0
	Any pT/Tx	N2	M0	S1
IIC	Any pT/Tx	N3	M0	S0
	Any pT/Tx	N3	M0	S1
Stage III	Any pT/Tx	Any N	M1	SX
IIIA	Any pT/Tx	Any N	M1a	S0
	Any pT/Tx	Any N	M1a	S1
IIIB	Any pT/Tx	N1–3	M0	S2
	Any pT/Tx	Any N	M1a	S2
IIIC	Any pT/Tx	N1–3	M0	S3
	Any pT/Tx	Any N	M1a	S3
	Any pT/Tx	Any N	M1b	Any S

[a] Measured after orchiectomy.
Used with the permission of the American Joint Committee on Cancer
(AJCC), Chicago, Illinois. The original source for this material is the Edge SB,
Byrd DR, Compton CC, et al., eds. *AJCC Cancer Staging Manual*, 7th ed.
New York: Springer Science and Business Media LLC; 2010: 471–472.

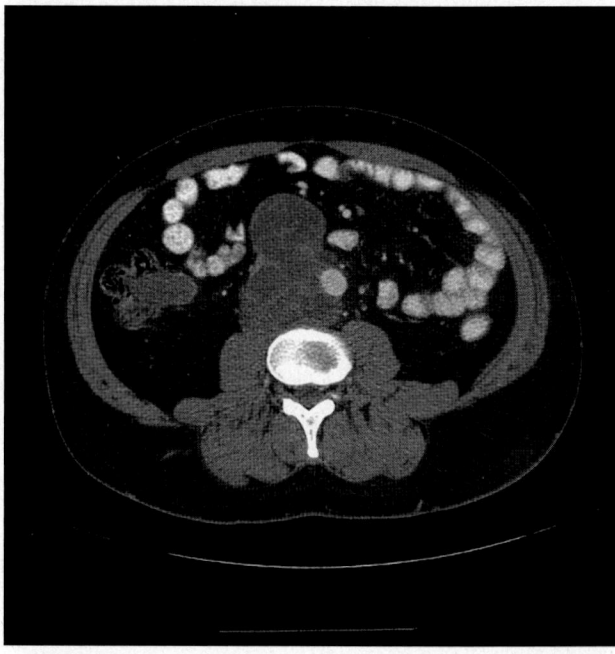

Figure 70.5 Lymph node metastasis from nonseminomatous germ cell tumor of the right testicle. Postchemotherapy resection showed metastatic teratoma.

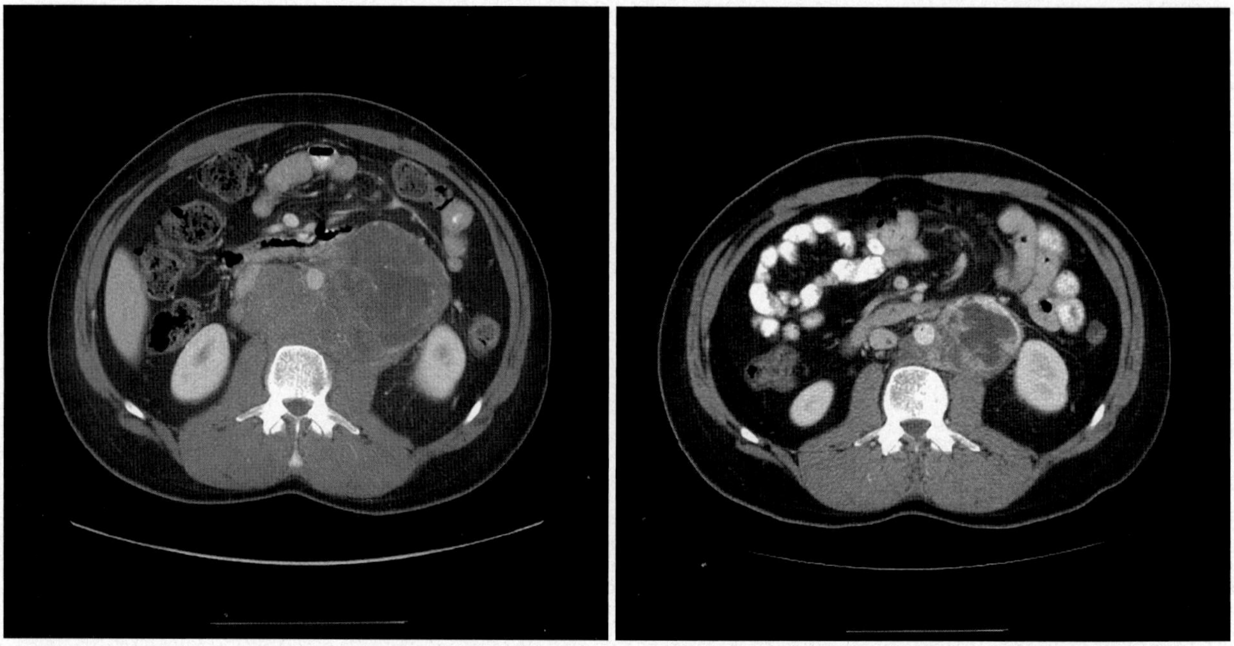

Figure 70.6 Lymph node metastasis from nonseminomatous germ cell tumor of the left testicle **(A)** at diagnosis, and **(B)** upon completion of chemotherapy. Postchemotherapy resection showed metastatic teratoma with somatic transformation to primitive neuroectodermal tumor.

TABLE 70.4		
Germ CellTumor Risk Classification		
Risk Group	**Seminoma**	**Nonseminoma**
Good	Any hCG Any LDH Nonpulmonary visceral metastases absent Any primary site	AFP <1,000 ng/mL hCG <5,000 mIU/mL LDH <1.5 × ULN Nonpulmonary visceral metastases absent Gonadal or retroperitoneal primary site
Intermediate	Nonpulmonary visceral metastases present Any hCG Any LDH Any primary site	AFP 1,000–10,000 ng/mL hCG 5,000–50,000 mIU/mL LDH 1.5–10.0 × ULN Nonpulmonary visceral metastases absent Gonadal or retroperitoneal primary site
Poor	Does not exist	Mediastinal primary site Nonpulmonary visceral metastases present (e.g., bone, liver, brain) AFP >10,000 ng/mL hCG >50,000 mIU/mL LDH >10 × ULN

hCG, human chorionic gonadotropin; LDH, lactate dehydrogenase; AFP, α-fetoprotein; ULN, upper limit of normal range.
Source: International Germ Cell Consensus Classification: a prognostic factor-based staging system for metastatic germ cell cancers. International Germ Cell Cancer Collaborative Group. *J Clin Oncol* 1997;15:594–603.

Elevated AFP has special significance in seminoma because it is only produced by NSGCT. Germ cell tumors that histologically appear to be pure seminoma with elevated serum AFP are given the clinical diagnosis of NSGCT, and are treated as such.[22] HCG can be elevated in either seminoma or NSGCT, but has prognostic significance only for NSCGT.

Total LDH concentration prior to chemotherapy functions as a prognostic factor in NSGCT and helps to determine stage. In seminoma with bulky metastases, LDH can be markedly elevated but has no prognostic significance.

There are several potential causes of spurious elevation of tumor markers. AFP is not cancer specific; it may be elevated in the presence of liver disease or as a nonspecific chronic elevation. Stability of AFP over time suggests a benign etiology. HCG is cancer specific in men, but it is not specific to germ cell tumors. It can be associated with other neoplasms and with exposure to cannabis products. Patients should be questioned about the use of marijuana. A positive hCG test can also occur as a laboratory artifact in patients with low serum testosterone, owing to the increased secretion of luteinizing hormone and its sequence similarity to hCG.[46,47]

Clinical Staging

The most commonly used methods for detecting metastatic disease are serum tumor markers and CT scan.[15] Positron emission tomography (PET) scan can be helpful in the staging evaluation of a seminoma patient by distinguishing hypermetabolic lymph node metastases from reactive lymph nodes. PET is not as useful in NSGCT, where CT scan with oral and intravenous contrast is the preferred technique for detecting retroperitoneal adenopathy.

Pathologic Staging

The T classification is determined by pathology of the orchiectomy specimen.[40] The presence of lymphovascular invasion (LVI) or invasion through the tunica albuginea with involvement of the tunica vaginalis are pT2, invasion of the spermatic cord is pT3, and involvement of the scrotum constitutes pT4 (see Table 70.2).

Prophylactic retroperitoneal lymph node dissection (RPLND) is performed for surgical staging in some patients with clinical stage I NSGCT. In such cases, if no metastatic germ cell tumor is found, the stage is pathologic stage I; when disease is found, it is designated pathologic stage II.

Factors Affecting Outcome

In clinical stage I NSGCT, the presence of LVI (pT2) is associated with an approximately 50% risk of recurrence with surveillance alone. A high percentage of embryonal carcinoma has also been associated with high risk in some series, but embryonal carcinoma is often seen together with LVI and has not been validated as an independent risk factor.[48]

In clinical stage I seminoma, tumor size ≥4 cm is associated with approximately 30% risk of recurrence with surveillance alone. Involvement of rete testis has not been validated as a risk factor, although it is often mentioned.[49]

The classification of patients with metastatic germ cell tumors as good, intermediate, or poor prognosis, based on serum tumor markers and extent of disease, was proposed in 1997 by The International Germ Cell Cancer Collaborative Group (Table 70.4).[44] In this system, the presence or absence of nonpulmonary, extranodal metastasis was validated as an independent prognostic factor for progression-free survival. For NSGCT, the degree of marker elevation and mediastinal primary (versus testis or retroperitoneal primary) were also validated as prognostic factors. The threshold values for tumor markers (hCG, AFP, and LDH) have been incorporated into the American Joint Commission on Cancer/International Union Against Cancer staging system as the "S" classification. These prognostic groupings are used to make treatment decisions and are discussed in the following sections.

MANAGEMENT OF CLINICAL STAGE I DISEASE

Virtually all patients with clinical stage I germ cell tumors survive (cancer specific survival 98% to 99%).[49] In general, patients managed with observation have the same life expectancy as those who receive adjuvant intervention. Treatment decisions must therefore be based on considerations of cost, burden of therapy, and patient preference.[48]

Seminoma

Clinical stage I seminoma is grouped into high-risk and average-risk based on tumor size, but similar options exist for all patients with stage I seminoma, regardless of risk.[48,49] Stage I is a common presentation, accounting for approximately 70% of patients diagnosed with pure seminoma.

Surveillance

The average risk of recurrence with surveillance for stage I seminoma is 15% to 20%. Recurrences are temporally distributed over a 10-year period.[50] High-risk tumors have a recurrence probability of 30% to 35%, whereas tumors <4 cm without rete testis involvement may have a risk as low as 12%.[51] Observation is heavily dependent on CT scanning because the region at highest risk is in the retroperitoneum, and most seminomas do not secrete tumor markers.

Adjuvant Chemotherapy

Carboplatin is a simple and apparently safe form of adjuvant chemotherapy that is very similar in efficacy to prophylactic radiotherapy. In a randomized trial of carboplatin given as a single infusion (area under curve equals 7) versus radiotherapy to the para-aortic lymph nodes, there was no significant difference in progression-free survival (94.7% and 96%, respectively).[52,53] There was only one death from seminoma (N = 1,447) reported at a median follow-up of 6.5 years. Recurrences after adjuvant carboplatin were frequently retroperitoneal in location, meaning that follow-up CT scans are mandatory. There has been no reported evidence of second malignant neoplasms (SMN), and there have been fewer contralateral germ cell tumors reported in the patients treated with chemotherapy versus radiotherapy at medium-term follow-up. Two courses of carboplatin have also been shown to be effective in the adjuvant setting, and in its 2014 guidelines the National Comprehensive Cancer Network (NCCN) endorsed one or two courses as a standard of care for clinical stage I seminoma, regardless of the estimated risk of recurrence.[54] Observation is also standard and is the preferred option.

Prophylactic Radiotherapy

Treatment of para-aortic lymph nodes to a dose of 20 Gy was associated with excellent local control approaching 100%. A randomized trial of 20 Gy versus 30 Gy showed no difference in rate of recurrence.[55] Omission of ipsilateral iliac lymph nodes from the treatment field resulted in less toxicity (infertility, gastrointestinal effects) and minimal loss of efficacy. The recurrence rate after prophylactic radiotherapy for clinical stage I seminoma is about 4%, and most of those patients survive with additional treatment (combination chemotherapy). Recurrences tend to occur below the radiation field (pelvic lymph nodes) or above it (lungs). Radiotherapy is contraindicated for patients with horseshoe kidney or inflammatory bowel disease.

Radiotherapy was once popularized because it reduced the number of CT scans that were necessary for follow-up, with a net reduction in the cost of treatment.[56] There is, however, a different type of cost with radiotherapy, and that is the risk of SMN.[57] Studies of testicular cancer survivors 20 or more years after treatment have revealed an increase in midline cancers such as gastrointestinal and genitourinary malignancies.[58] This has brought about a reassessment of prophylactic radiotherapy, specifically, whether it is warranted when 80% of seminoma patients will be treated unnecessarily, there is a risk of SMN, and there is no survival benefit. While it continues to be offered, the use of prophylactic radiotherapy for seminoma is declining.[59]

Nonseminomatous Germ Cell Tumor

Clinical stage I NSGCT is broadly categorized as high risk and average risk. Although there are many differences in presentation,

including tumor size, histology, and tumor marker pattern, only LVI has been validated as a risk factor. NSGCT with LVI has a recurrence rate of approximately 50% with observation.[60] Most recurrences are seen within 2 to 3 years of the orchiectomy.[50] The average risk is 30%, and most patients with LVI-negative ("good risk") stage I NSGCT probably have a risk of recurrence <30%. The risk of recurrence for LVI-negative stage I NSGCT with predominantly embryonal carcinoma histology, however, may be higher (30% to 50%).[61]

Surveillance

Approximately two-thirds of relapses among patients on surveillance are in retroperitoneal lymph nodes and one-third occur in lungs or by marker elevation alone. Recurrences in nonpulmonary viscera are rare. Most relapses occur within 2 to 3 years of orchiectomy, and patients need to remain on follow-up for at least 5 years. The ability to cure systemic disease with cisplatin-based chemotherapy in those who relapse makes observation an attractive option. It avoids unnecessary therapy for about two-thirds of patients.

Criteria for selecting patients for observation have been suggested in the literature and in the NCCN guidelines.[54] Selection based on whether the patient is "reliable" (i.e., likely to be compliant with follow-up) was once the prevalent view, but this has been largely replaced by a more objective risk-adapted approach. Observation is the standard of care for patients with stage IA NSGCT. The alternative is nerve-sparing RPLND, which is an unnecessary procedure for the majority of these patients. There is no subgroup of stage IA for whom RPLND is preferred, but patients who choose observation should agree to be compliant with follow-up and to receive chemotherapy in the event of recurrence. Patients with stage IA embryonal carcinoma–predominant tumors are probably the least likely to benefit from RPLND because of the tendency for hematogenous spread and associated risk of recurrence in lungs.[61,62]

Most patients with LVI-negative, clinical stage I NSGCT are candidates for observation. There is less of a consensus on management of patients with pT2-pT4 tumors (including LVI-positive). A minority of patients with pT2 tumors may choose observation, but they must understand that the risk of recurrence is 50% and they should agree (as in stage IA) to comply with follow-up. The preferred treatment for LVI-positive or advanced T classification NSGCT is adjuvant chemotherapy.

Adjuvant Chemotherapy

Primary chemotherapy for NSGCT consists of bleomycin, etoposide, and cisplatin (BEP) (Table 70.5).[63,64] There are several published studies using either one or two courses of adjuvant BEP or similar regimens in patients with clinical stage I NSGCT.[65–68] A phase II study by the Medical Research Council found 98% relapse-free survival after two courses of bleomycin, vincristine, and cisplatin, although chemotherapy-induced neurotoxicity (CIN) remained a problem.[68] Two courses of BEP are similarly effective in preventing recurrence with less CIN; however, etoposide causes transient myelosuppression and is associated with a low but real risk of treatment-induced leukemia. The toxicity of two courses of BEP makes it unacceptable for stage IA NSGCT, but reasonable for stage IB where the relapse rate on observation is 50%.[48] One limitation of adjuvant chemotherapy is the continuing risk of growing teratoma syndrome. Only RPLND can remove foci of teratoma from the retroperitoneum, where they may persist and grow following chemotherapy.[69]

One strategy for lowering the toxicity of adjuvant chemotherapy is by shortening treatment to one course of BEP. Two European studies provide data collected prospectively; in one study, patients were randomized to a single course of BEP or RPLND (none were observed), and in a second study, the patients with LVI-negative tumors were offered surveillance or one course of BEP, while

TABLE 70.5		
Chemotherapy Regimens for Stage II/III Germ Cell Tumor		
Previously Untreated—Good Risk[a]		
Etoposide	100 mg/m^2 IV daily × 5 days	
Cisplatin	20 mg/m^2 IV daily × 5 days; *Four cycles administered at 21-day intervals*	
Etoposide	100 mg/m^2 IV daily × 5 days	
Cisplatin	20 mg/m^2 IV daily × 5 days	
Bleomycin	30 units IV weekly (e.g., days 1, 8, 15); *Three cycles administered at 21-day intervals*	
Previously Untreated—Intermediate and Poor Risk		
Etoposide	100 mg/m^2 IV daily × 5 days	
Cisplatin	20 mg/m^2 IV daily × 5 days	
Bleomycin	30 units IV weekly (e.g., days 1, 8, 15); *four cycles administered at 21-day intervals*	
Previously Treated—1st-Line Salvage Therapy		
Ifosfamide	1.2 g/m^2 IV daily × 5 days	
Mesna	400 mg/m^2 IV every 8 h × 5 days	
Cisplatin	20 mg/m^2 IV daily × 5 days	
Vinblastine	0.11 mg/kg IV days 1 and 2; *Four cycles administered at 21-day intervals*	
Paclitaxel	250 mg/m^2 IV by continuous infusion over 24 h on day 1	
Ifosfamide	1.5 g/m^2 IV daily on days 2–5	
Cisplatin	25 mg/m^2 IV daily on days 2–5	
Mesna	500 mg/m^2 IV every 8 h on days 2–5; *Four cycles administered at 21-day intervals*	

IV, intravenous.

[a] Good risk regimens (BEP or EP) can also be used for stage I adjuvant or stage IS.

patients with LVI-positive tumors were offered one or two courses of adjuvant BEP.[66,67] Both of these studies showed a <5% recurrence rate after one course of BEP and an acceptably low rate of growing teratoma. The 2014 NCCN guideline endorses either one or two courses of adjuvant BEP for stage IB NSGCT.[54]

Retroperitoneal Lymph Node Dissection

RPLND performed in clinical stage I NSGCT is done to accurately stage the patient (as pathologic stage I or stage II) and remove all viable disease. RPLND is curative for teratoma, which has been reported in 21% to 30% of cases with viable disease.[70] Mortality from RPLND is <1%; minor complications include prolonged ileus, wound infection, and lymphocele. Major complications (hemorrhage, ureteral injury, chylous ascites, pulmonary embolus, wound dehiscence, bowel obstruction) are rare. A notable long-term morbidity is sympathetic nerve damage leading to failure of ejaculaton.[71]

For optimal outcomes, RPLND should be performed at a referral center with an experienced surgeon. A bilateral infrahilar RPLND includes the precaval, retrocaval, paracaval, interaortocaval, retroaortic, preaortic, paraortic, and common iliac lymph nodes.

There are two types of nerve-sparing RPLND: the modified template RPLND and nerve-dissection bilateral RPLND.[70,72,73] The template dissection helps the surgeon avoid regions where the risk of metastasis may be less. The nerve-dissection technique identifies and preserves both sympathetic chains, postganglionic sympathetic fibers, and the hypogastric plexus, which are necessary for anterograde ejaculation. The reported incidence of retrograde ejaculation with this technique is <5%. Another innovation is the robot-assisted RPLND, in which robotic instruments are inserted through a series of trocar entry sites and controlled remotely by the surgeon.[74–76] Patients have less pain, shorter hospitalization time, rapid recovery, and smaller surgical scars.

The relapse rate following RPLND is variable. It may be as low as 4% with a low-risk patient and an experienced surgeon. Most series include patients who also received adjuvant chemotherapy, typically with two courses of BEP, for pathologic stage II disease. Thus, the success of RPLND comes at the expense of double therapy for some patients. The LVI-positive and other high-risk patients have higher reported failure rates (10% to 14%) with prophylactic RPLND alone.[62] The greatest advantage of RPLND is the early control of teratoma when it exists. The randomized trial of RPLND versus one course of BEP found a recurrence rate of 8.3% in the RPLND arm and 1.1% in the BEP arm.[66] With median follow-up of 4.7 years, only one patient had growing teratoma after BEP. Limitations of the study were that unilateral dissections were performed (nonstandard) and that the experience level of surgeons varied, as it was a community-based study. The low incidence (1% to 2%) of growing teratoma seen among patients on observation or adjuvant chemotherapy is lower than one would expect based on results of surgical staging, and this suggests that not all teratoma has the same potential for growth or malignant transformation.

MANAGEMENT OF CLINICAL STAGE II (LOW TUMOR BURDEN)

The anatomic definition of stage II germ cell tumor is metastasis confined to retroperitoneal lymph nodes. For NSGCT, there is the further requirement that tumor markers be in the good-prognosis range (S0 to S1).[40] For both seminoma and NSGCT, the majority of these patients are cured with standard treatment.

Seminoma

Seminoma is exquisitely sensitive to both chemotherapy and radiation. Radiotherapy to the retroperitoneum with a boost to the involved nodes is standard for disease with a transverse measurement of 3 cm or less.[77–79] The fields include the landing zone and proximal ipsilateral iliac lymph nodes (dog-leg field). Radiotherapy is curative in 80% to 90% of patients, with recurrence owing largely to occult disease outside the radiation field.[80] Nevertheless, prophylactic radiotherapy to the mediastinum or supraclavicular nodes is not recommended because of toxicity concerns.[81] There is an excellent rate of success with combination chemotherapy in the patients who do relapse after radiotherapy.[82]

For patients with bulky (>3 cm transverse dimension) retroperitoneal disease, primary treatment with cisplatin-based chemotherapy is standard.[54,82] As in the adjuvant setting, patients with horseshoe kidney or inflammatory bowel disease should not receive radiotherapy; chemotherapy is the primary treatment for such patients regardless of nodal size.

Nonseminomatous Germ Cell Tumor (Low Tumor Burden)

Stage IS

Serum tumor markers that do not normalize after radical orchiectomy are evidence of micrometastases. Treatment is with three courses BEP followed by surveillance.

Pathologic Stage II after Retroperitoneal Lymph Node Dissection

In the case of low-volume metastatic NSGCT, a prophylactic RPLND may be curative without additional therapy.[69,83] Patients with fewer than six lymph nodes involved, no focus >2 cm, and without extranodal extension (pN1) have an estimated 10% to 20% risk of recurrence and can be managed with surveillance. Adjuvant chemotherapy with BEP or EP (two courses) is an option for selected patients based on their access to follow-up, psychological factors, and tumor histology. Although there is no strong evidence to support adjuvant decision making based on the histology, metastases with predominantly teratoma or yolk sac tumor may have lower post-RPLND risk of recurrence than those that have predominantly embryonal carcinoma or choriocarcinoma. Nevertheless, surveillance and treatment with three or four courses of chemotherapy at recurrence is likely to yield a similar overall survival as adjuvant treatment. Adjuvant chemotherapy should be recommended for patients with pN2-N3 disease.

Clinical Stage IIA

Primary chemotherapy with three courses of BEP is the standard treatment for patients with enlarged retroperitoneal lymph nodes and elevated serum tumor markers (S1).[63] Patients with enlarged lymph nodes and normal serum tumor markers (N1, S0) may be appropriate for nerve-sparing bilateral RPLND or chemotherapy. A primary RPLND can be considered if the primary tumor contains teratoma and is not embryonal carcinoma–predominant, tumor markers are not elevated, and there is no back pain. Elevated tumor markers, back pain, or nodal size >2 cm suggest multifocal or unresectable disease, and chemotherapy is preferred.[84]

Embryonal carcinoma can be marker negative and also requires chemotherapy. If metastatic embryonal carcinoma is suspected on clinical grounds (enlarged retroperitoneal lymph nodes), chemotherapy is the treatment of choice, whether or not the markers are elevated.

MANAGEMENT OF STAGE II WITH HIGH TUMOR BURDEN AND STAGE III DISEASE

Patients with metastatic germ cell tumor and high tumor burden are curable, but they can be critically ill at presentation. The chance of survival improves with early recognition of the diagnosis by medical providers, often on clinical grounds, and the prompt administration of chemotherapy. Whenever possible, patients with

stage IIIC NSGCT should be treated by an experienced team at a tertiary care center.[85,86]

Good Prognosis

The International Germ Cell Cancer Collaborative Group risk classification identifies a "good prognosis" subset with overall survival of 90% to 95% with standard therapy.[44] These patients include most of those with metastatic seminoma, including mediastinal seminoma, excluding only seminoma with nonpulmonary visceral metastasis; and NSGCT stages II and IIIA (metastasis confined to lymph nodes and lungs and tumor markers below the intermediate- [S2] or high-risk [S3] levels).[87] For good prognosis NSGCT, three courses of BEP results in normalization of tumor markers for the majority of patients.[63] Postchemotherapy surgery is necessary for some patients with NSGCT who have a residual mass, as this can harbor teratoma or other viable disease (see Fig. 70.6).[88]

An alternative to three courses of BEP, for the good prognosis patients only, is etoposide and cisplatin (EP) given for four courses.[89–91] For selected patients, the added risk of CIN and other complications from a fourth course of EP may be balanced by avoidance of the pulmonary toxicity risk of bleomycin. In practice, patients with seminoma are less tolerant of bleomycin because of older age, and four courses of EP is a reasonable standard for the majority of these patients.

Intermediate and Poor Prognosis

The intermediate prognosis subset (stage IIIB) accounts for 25% of patients with metastatic germ cell tumors and has an overall survival of approximately 75% with standard therapy.[44] The poor prognosis group (stage IIIC) is exclusively NSGCT, accounts for 15% of metastatic germ cell tumors, and has 5-year progression-free survival of 45%. These include any patient with mediastinal primary NSGCT, nonpulmonary visceral metastasis, or tumor markers in the S3 range. Four courses of BEP is the standard primary treatment for stage IIIB and IIIC germ cell tumors.[92–94] Patients with seminoma with intermediate prognosis are unlikely to tolerate bleomycin, and addition of ifosfamide to etoposide and cisplatin (VIP) is a reasonable standard for these patients.[82] In NSGCT, VIP can also be used instead of BEP if there is an increased risk of bleomycin lung toxicity because of respiratory distress, age 50 years or older, smoking or other chronic respiratory disease, or anticipated major thoracic surgery.

Personalized Strategy Based on Tumor Marker Decline

Serum tumor markers (AFP, hCG) virtually always decline during the initial two to three cycles of chemotherapy. Failure of either marker to normalize is a well-recognized feature of chemotherapy resistance.[95] The rate of tumor marker decline has also been studied as a predictor of poor outcome. For patients presenting with stage IIIC NSGCT, it is possible to identify a subgroup of about 25% who will do comparatively well, and a larger group of about 75% whose outcome with standard therapy is poor.[96] This observation led to a phase III clinical trial in which patients with stage IIIC NSGCT received BEP in the first cycle; based on the tumor marker decline in the first cycle, those with favorable decline remained on BEP (four courses total) and the rest were randomized (1:1) to BEP or an intensified regimen. Preliminary results of this study confirmed the superior progression-free and overall survival of the group with favorable decline compared to unfavorable decline (treated with BEP), and demonstrated a statistically significant improvement in progression-free survival for patients randomized to intensified treatment based on unfavorable marker decline.[97]

Central Nervous System Metastases

Patients with brain metastasis are curable.[98] Imaging of the brain, preferably with magnetic resonance imaging, is appropriate at baseline for stage II or III disease. The initial management for most patients with asymptomatic brain metastases is with systemic chemotherapy. Responses tend to occur swiftly (Fig. 70.7), but there is a risk of intracranial hemorrhage. The risk of bleeding can be minimized by modifying the first cycle of chemotherapy (e.g., EP given for 3 days). Tumors with active bleeding may require craniotomy. Radiotherapy is useful for postchemotherapy consolidation of residual lesions in the brain. Gamma knife is preferable to whole brain radiotherapy in these patients with potentially long survival and risk of cognitive impairment.

The brain is a potential sanctuary site. This can manifest as a solitary recurrence in the brain shortly after the completion of chemotherapy, for which surgical resection may be curative.

Choriocarcinoma Syndrome

Metastatic choriocarcinoma is characterized by rapid hematogenous spread.[27] It usually starts as a component of a mixed testicular NSGCT, but can then proliferate and dominate the clinical picture.[27] Choriocarcinoma syndrome is recognizable by very high serum hCG levels in the range of 10^5 to 10^6 mIU/mL, and occasionally over 1 million, a testicular mass (or mediastinal mass), diffuse lung metastases, involvement of nonpulmonary viscera (brain, liver), tumor hemorrhage (hemoptysis, hemoperitoneum, intracranial bleed), and hyperthyroidism. The hyperthyroidism occurs at very high levels of hCG because hCG has sequence similarity to thyroid stimulating hormone.[99,100]

Patients with choriocarcinoma syndrome have a high rate of mortality caused by complications such as hemorrhage or as a result of recurrent/refractory disease. At the time of diagnosis, however, the clinical condition rapidly stabilizes with the administration of chemotherapy. It is not recommended to use bleomycin for the first course in most cases because of high volume pulmonary metastases and the risk of pulmonary hemorrhage. To avoid destabilizing the patient, EP chemotherapy can be shortened to 3 days for the first course only. For subsequent courses, EP is not sufficient for stage IIIC NSGCT and either BEP or an ifosfamide-containing regimen should be given. Administration of a beta blocker during the first course alleviates symptoms of hyperthyroidism (hypertension, tachycardia).

A male patient with testicular mass or anterior mediastinal mass, serum hCG over 50,000 mIU/mL, and clinical picture of choriocarcinoma syndrome does not require orchiectomy or biopsy prior to the start of treatment. The clinical diagnosis of choriocarcinoma should be recognized and treated as a medical emergency. Immediate chemotherapy offers the best chance for survival. Resection of the involved testis should be performed between cycles when the patient has stabilized, or at the time of RPLND.

Mediastinal Nonseminomatous Germ Cell Tumor

Extragonadal germ cell tumors are the result of arrested migration of germ cells along the urogenital ridge during embryogenesis. This aberrant germinal tissue is usually located along the craniocaudal axis in adult life, and malignant transformation can occur in both women and men. The most common presentation is in the anterior mediastinum of an adult man.[101] Patients with Klinefelter syndrome are at increased risk for mediastinal germ cell tumors.[102,103]

Mediastinal NSGCT is curable but at a lower rate than most testicular germ cell tumors.[104] The 3-year progression-free survival described in recent series was 48% to 54%.[105-108] The first-line chemotherapy is the same as other stage IIIC germ cell tumors, consisting of four courses of BEP for patients with good pulmonary function, and four courses of VIP for those who are unlikely to tolerate bleomycin. Some authors have advocated that VIP is the preferred regimen because most patients will undergo postchemotherapy thoracic surgery.[109] In a prospective multicenter study, however, 66 patients with mediastinal NSGCT were treated with bleomycin-containing regimens and excessive pulmonary complications were not seen.[97] Mediastinal primary tumors have a high incidence of viable germ cell malignancy, teratoma, and transformation to somatic malignancy in postchemotherapy resections, so surgical consolidation is essential.[105,110]

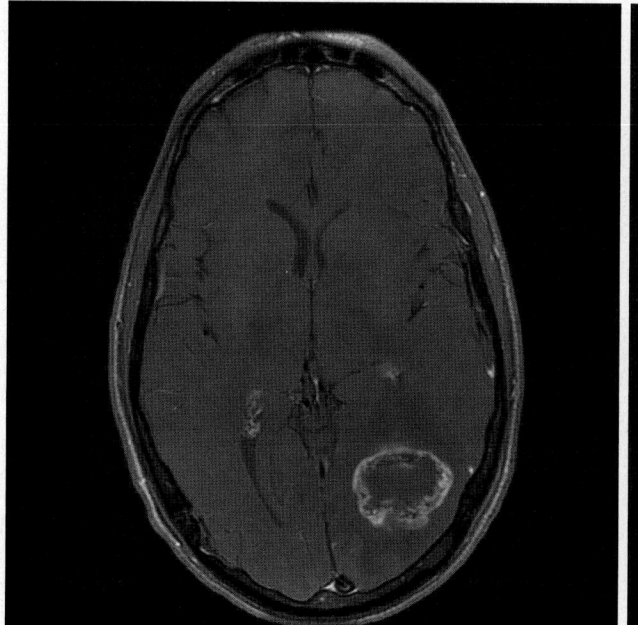 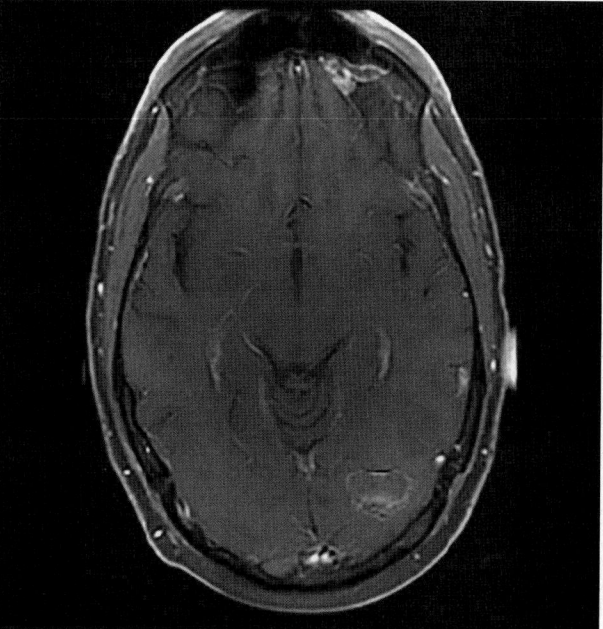

Figure 70.7 Brain metastasis in a patient with testicular nonseminomatous germ cell tumor and clinical features of choriocarcinoma syndrome. Magnetic resonance images were acquired **(A)** at diagnosis and **(B)** after three cycles of cisplatin-based chemotherapy (9 weeks), using modified regimens to avoid thrombocytopenia.

Management of Residual Mass

Patients with high tumor burden frequently have one or more sites of residual disease after chemotherapy and normalization of tumor markers. The management of a residual mass is critical to the curative management of germ cell tumors. There are different treatment considerations based on the setting of seminoma or NSGCT and the size of the lesion.

Residual Nodal Size <1 cm

For either seminoma or NSGCT, a radiographic complete response does not require consolidative treatment. The size criterion for absence of residual mass in a site of lymph node metastasis is a transverse dimension <1 cm (on CT imaging). There is a potential benefit to some patients with NSGCT from the surgical consolidation of residual masses >0.5 cm and <1.0 cm, based on the possibility of teratoma.[69] By some estimates, as many as 20% of nodes <0.5 cm and 29% of nodes <1.0 cm harbor teratoma. As noted previously, however, the incidence of growing teratoma syndrome among patients observed without RPLND is lower (1% to 2%) and these can be detected on follow-up with CT imaging. Most are treated successfully, and RPLND for a residual mass <1 cm is the exception rather than the rule.

Residual Mass >1 cm

A persistent mass in a nodal site after chemotherapy is of concern for residual germ cell malignancy in both seminoma and NSGCT, and for teratoma in NSGCT. The same applies for residual masses in extranodal organs.

For NSGCT, the standard management of a residual mass >1 cm in the retroperitoneum is a bilateral RPLND.[88] Modified template RPLND is not appropriate in this setting, as it may leave behind disease in 7% to 32% of cases. Robot-assisted RPLND is an option for some patients resulting in less short-term morbidity of the procedure compared to an open RPLND.[75] The principal long-term morbidity is retrograde ejaculation.[111] After the standard three or four courses of BEP, viable germ cell malignancy is found in only 15% of specimens. A total of 40% contain teratoma, and 45% contain only necrosis and fibrosis. There is no reliable method for determining preoperatively whether teratoma is present. Twenty-five to forty-five percent of patients with no teratoma in the primary tumor can still have teratoma in a residual mass. Biopsy is useless for ruling out the presence of teratoma because of sampling error. Complete excision is the standard of care. For the minority of patients with viable germ cell malignancy (other than teratoma) in a residual mass, the standard treatment is postoperative administration of two additional courses of chemotherapy. Residual teratoma requires no further therapy.

Seminoma

Unlike NSGCT, seminoma does not produce teratoma. A residual mass is common, however, owing to the fibrotic reaction that occurs in the treated lymph nodes. Surgery is technically difficult and in most cases unnecessary. Patients with very high volume seminoma or residual mass >3 cm can suffer relapse from residual seminoma. The optimal consolidation for these patients is an unsettled question. Patients with residual mass <3 cm can remain on observation. For those with a mass >3 cm, radiotherapy is one means to reduce the risk of relapse. An overall survival benefit from postchemotherapy radiation has not been demonstrated. This may be in part due to the overall high survival rate for seminoma and the relatively small proportion of patients at risk for relapse after chemotherapy. The 2014 NCCN guidelines recommend surgery (RPLND), if technically feasible, for residual mass >3 cm with PET positivity.

MANAGEMENT OF RECURRENT DISEASE

Patients in first relapse after BEP chemotherapy can be successfully salvaged in about 50% of cases. The relapse-free survival with high-dose chemotherapy and autologous stem cell transplant (HDC-ASCT) in one retrospective study was 60% (90 of 149 patients with recurrent/refractory NSGCT). Whether this was an improvement in outcome over conventional chemotherapy or a reflection of patient selection is unknown. A randomized trial for patients in first relapse with four courses of paclitaxel, ifosfamide, and cisplatin versus HDC-ASCT will hopefully answer this question.

Conventional Dose Chemotherapy

Standard-dose regimens have resulted in a complete response rate of 35% to 70% in the second line without the use of HDC-ASCT. The most effective regimens for first recurrence after BEP have been combinations with ifosfamide and cisplatin.[112,113] Examples are vinblastine, ifosfamide, and cisplatin (VeIP), and paclitaxel, ifosfamide, and cisplatin, typically four courses with consolidation surgery (see Table 70.5).[114,115]

High-Dose Chemotherapy and Stem Cell Transplant

In a retrospective study of patients treated at Indiana University from 1996 to 2004, 135 patients in first recurrence received one to two cycles of standard VeIP followed by two cycles of high-dose carboplatin plus etoposide ("tandem transplant").[116] At a median follow-up of 4 years, 94 of 135 (70%) remained continuously disease-free. This study included 61 patients who relapsed from a complete response (favorable), but excluded mediastinal NSGCT, late relapses, and other nongonadal primary sites (unfavorable). In a prospective trial from Memorial Sloan-Kettering Cancer Center, 81 patients received one to two cycles of paclitaxel plus ifosfamide followed by three cycles of high-dose carboplatin plus etoposide as first salvage.[117] At a median of 5 years, 56% remained free of disease. This study excluded patients with a testicular primary tumor who either had a prior complete response to first-line chemotherapy or a partial response with negative markers, but included patients with mediastinal NSGCT, late relapse, and other nongonadal primary sites.

Second and Subsequent Relapse

Patients with recurrence after conventional second-line chemotherapy such as VeIP or TIP can be considered for HDC-ASCT.[116] Compared to the patients in first relapse, however, these patients have more chemotherapy sequelae such as CIN, renal insufficiency, and decreased performance status, leading to a high complication rate and mortality from HDC-ASCT. Conventional chemotherapy after second-line or HDC-ASCT is usually palliative. Regimens endorsed by NCCN guidelines include gemcitabine and oxaliplatin, gemcitabine and paclitaxel, gemcitabine/oxaliplatin/paclitaxel, and oral etoposide.[118-121]

Molecular targeted therapies do not yet have an established role in the treatment of germ cell tumors. There are two published studies of sunitinib in relapsed/refractory germ cell tumors.[122,123] A study from the Canadian Urologic Oncology Group and the German Testicular cancer study group found three confirmed and one unconfirmed partial responses (13%) among 32 patients with refractory germ cell tumors treated with sunitinib. Another study from Memorial Sloan-Kettering Cancer Center found no responses among 10 men with highly refractory germ cell tumors treated with sunitinib, although 4 patients had some decline in serum tumor markers. An inhibitor of cyclin-dependent kinase 4/6 showed activity in patients with unresectable teratoma, leading to clinical trials.[124] Patients with chemotherapy-refractory germ cell tumors should be encouraged to participate in clinical trials.

Surgery after Salvage Chemotherapy

Residual lesions that persist after chemotherapy should be resected whenever feasible. There is often viable tumor in the setting of recurrent/refractory disease, even when tumor markers have normalized on chemotherapy.[125] When tumor markers decline to a plateau but do not normalize, surgery to remove all viable disease is a consideration. Surgical salvage is successful in about 20% of patients.[126,127] Patients with elevated AFP and normal hCG have better prognosis with surgery than patients with elevated or rising hCG. Adjuvant chemotherapy is not known to improve the outcome when surgery reveals viable germ cell malignancy after salvage chemotherapy.

Late Recurrence Nonseminomatous Germ Cell Tumor

Most NSGCT recurrences after chemotherapy are seen within 2 to 3 years. Only about 2% of patients experience a relapse after 2 years. These late recurrences appear to be less sensitive to subsequent chemotherapy than the earlier recurrences.[128,129] Surgery can be curative in cases that are slowly growing and anatomically resectable. Treatment must be individualized. Although late recurrences are less chemosensitive as a group, complete responses have been described. Surgery should always be considered and integrated as a component of the overall treatment plan.

TREATMENT SEQUELAE

Both chemotherapy and radiotherapy have long-term adverse effects on survivors of testicular cancer.[2,57,58,81] With posttreatment life expectancy of 40 years or more, the morbidity attributable to chronic and late effects of treatment can exceed that of the cancer itself.

Cardiovascular Effects

One of the most significant delayed effects of chemotherapy is an increased risk of cardiovascular disease.[81] The risk of suffering a cardiac event is two- to seven-fold higher in survivors of testicular cancer who received cisplatin-based chemotherapy than the general population.[130,131] Other risk factors such as hyperlipidemia, obesity, and hypertension (metabolic syndrome) are also more common among survivors of testicular cancer. The health and longevity of survivors of testicular cancer can be maximized through early treatment of hypertension and hyperlipidemia, and by interventions such as diet, exercise, and tobacco cessation.

Chemotherapy-Induced Neurotoxicity

Peripheral neurotoxicity is a common adverse effect of cisplatin. Approximately 20% to 40% of patients treated with neurotoxic chemotherapy drugs develop CIN, which can cause painful and permanent sensory disturbance. Drug therapy for CIN is only partially effective in relieving symptoms.[132] The mechanisms of CIN are not well understood, and they appear to include damage to neuronal cell bodies in dorsal root ganglia.[133] Circulating platinum levels remain elevated for many years after chemotherapy, and it is not known whether this also contributes to long-term morbidity.[134] The severity of CIN is influenced by the cumulative dose of cisplatin, exposure to other neurotoxic drugs (e.g., paclitaxel), and other medical conditions such as diabetes.

Hypogonadism and Infertility

Chemotherapy can damage the germinal epithelium and increase the risk of abnormal sperm morphology, motility, and number. Oligospermia has been associated with prior radiotherapy for seminoma, presumably due to scatter radiation to the contralateral testis. It is also recognized that at the time of diagnosis, the percentage of men with germ cell tumor who are subfertile or infertile is greater than the general male population. Thus, sperm banking should be offered to all patients undergoing chemotherapy or radiotherapy, and to patients undergoing RPLND because they are at risk for retrograde ejaculation.

The risk of infertility from treatment is proportional to the type and duration of treatment. In a study of paternity following treatment, 71% of unselected survivors of testicular cancer were successful at 15 years. For treatment subgroups, successful paternity was 81% with surveillance, 77% after RPLND, 65% after radiotherapy, 62% after chemotherapy, and 38% after high-dose salvage chemotherapy. The risk to patients receiving fewer than four cycles of chemotherapy has not been studied, particularly in the adjuvant setting (one or two cycles), or with carboplatin in the setting of seminoma. While the risk of infertility may be lower in the adjuvant setting, these patients should receive fertility counseling and an opportunity for cryopreservation of semen.

Hypogonadism, or low testosterone, is also a common finding. Testicular dysfunction is more common among survivors of testicular cancer than the general male population. Persistent low testosterone in a patient who has completed therapy is an indication of a functional deficit in the contralateral testis. Testosterone replacement therapy can prevent complications such as weight gain, gynecomastia, erectile dysfunction, loss of libido, fatigue, depression, and osteoporosis.

Ototoxicity

Cisplatin can result in permanent, bilateral sensorineural hearing loss in 19% to 77% of patients, and tinnitus in 19% to 42%.[135] The incidence and severity of ototoxicity is related to the cumulative dose and dose intensity of cisplatin.[136] The mechanism is thought to be through overproduction of reactive oxygen species in the cochlea, causing irreversible free radical–related apoptosis of outer hair cells, spiral ganglion cells, and the stria vascularis.[135] There may be genetic underpinnings to the susceptibility to ototoxicity from chemotherapy. There is no effective method for treating or preventing cisplatin-induced ototoxicity.[137]

Psychosocial Functioning

There are potential short-term and long-term psychological consequences in the posttreatment period.[138] Anxiety and depression are common in the first 6 months, whereas most patients are well adjusted by 1 year. Certain patients (10% to 30%) continue to suffer moderate to severe nervousness, anxiety, or depression. Patients who have sexual difficulties, are unemployed, or have financial difficulties appear to be at greatest risk. Strain in relationships can be due to a perception of sexual dysfunction; however, some studies suggest that in married couples the patient is more concerned than the spouse, and divorce rates are no higher than the general population.[139]

Second Malignant Neoplasms

Both radiotherapy and chemotherapy increase the risk of SMN later in life. Second malignancies can occur 20 years after treatment or later. An exception is acute leukemia, which occurs 2 to 4 years after chemotherapy. The risk of treatment-related leukemia is proportional to the cumulative dose of etoposide, and is estimated to be <0.5% for two courses (1,000 mg/m^2), less than 1% for three or four courses (1,500 to 2,000 mg/m^2), and as high as

6% for cumulative etoposide doses >3,000 mg/m². Chromosomal translocations involving 11q are characteristic of etoposide-related acute leukemia.[140]

Acute leukemia is also seen in a small percentage of patients with mediastinal NSGCT. While chemotherapy may be a contributing factor, the leukemia associated with mediastinal primary tumors has a separate etiology. Megakaryocytic leukemia has been described and may be more common in this setting.[141] Studies have identified the clonal marker i(12p) in leukemic cells, indicating that they are clonally descended from the primary germ cell tumor.[142,143] One hypothesis is that yolk sac tumor (a common histology among mediastinal germ cell tumors) retains the pluripotency of the normal yolk sac, which functions as a hematopoietic organ during embryogenesis.[144] This association has not been described in yolk sac tumor of testicular origin.

Second primary germ cell tumor of the contralateral testicle occurs in approximately 2% of survivors, and occasionally as a synchronous (bilateral) presentation. The risk of second germ cell tumor is present over the lifetime of the individual, making it especially important that the patient is counseled to report any testicular symptoms, and that long-term follow-up includes surveillance of the contralateral testicle. Prophylactic radiation of the contralateral testicle has been promoted in Europe as a means to reduce the risk, and surveillance alone is standard in the United States. Although adjuvant carboplatin for stage I seminoma appeared to reduce the incidence of second primary tumors, longer follow-up is needed to determine whether it is merely a delay in clinical presentation.[53]

LONG-TERM FOLLOW-UP

The mandatory duration of follow-up for detection and management of recurrence of germ cell tumors is 5 years for NSGCT and 10 years for seminoma. There is wide consensus, however, that survivors of testicular cancer should have lifelong follow-up, whether it is at the primary treatment center or with a general internist who is knowledgeable about survivorship issues. Long-term follow-up is necessary for detection of late recurrences, second testicular primaries, and SMN. Survivors require management of cardiovascular effects and symptoms of neurotoxicity. Special care may be required for maintenance of sexual health, fertility issues, and psychosocial functioning.

MIDLINE TUMORS OF UNCERTAIN HISTOGENESIS

Tumors of unknown primary site in young patients occasionally respond well to cisplatin-based chemotherapy. This can be the presentation of an extragonadal germ cell tumor. The diagnosis should be considered in relatively young patients in whom the tumor has predominantly midline distribution and histologic appearance of poorly differentiated carcinoma. Serum tumor markers may or may not be elevated. Molecular cytogenetic analysis for 12p genetic content can help to confirm the diagnosis, but is often inconclusive. Immunohistochemical markers SALL4, OCT3/4, CD117, SOX2, CD30, and low-molecular-weight keratins can also facilitate the diagnosis.

OTHER TESTICULAR TUMORS

Sex Cord/Gonadal Stromal Tumors

Leydig and Sertoli Cell Tumors

The most common sex cord stromal tumors in men are Leydig cell and Sertoli cell tumors (Table 70.6). These tumors are occasionally

TABLE 70.6
World Health Organization Histologic Classification of Testicular Sex Cord/Gonadal Stromal Tumors
Leydig cell tumor
Malignant Leydig cell tumor

Sertoli cell tumor
  Sertoli cell tumor lipid rich variant
  Sclerosing Sertoli cell tumor
  Large cell calcifying Sertoli cell tumor

Malignant Sertoli cell tumor

Granulosa cell tumor
  Adult type granulosa cell tumor
  Juvenile type granulosa cell tumor

Tumors of the thecoma/fibroma group
  Thecoma
  Fibroma

Sex cord/gonadal stromal tumor: Incompletely differentiated
Sex cord/gonadal stromal tumors, mixed forms
Malignant sex cord/gonadal stromal tumors

Tumors containing both germ cell and sex cord/gonadal stromal elements
  Gonadoblastoma
  Germ cell-sex cord/gonadal stromal tumor, unclassified

Source: Eble JN, Sauter G, Epstein JI, et al., eds. *Pathology and Genetics of Tumours of the Urinary System and Male Genital Organs.* Lyon, France: IARC Press; 2004.

metastatic, but the majority are benign. Treatment is radical orchiectomy. The risk of metastasis has been associated with vascular invasion, cellular atypia, tumor necrosis, infiltrative margins, increased mitotic rate, tumor size >5 cm, older age at presentation, increased proliferation index, and aneuploidy. The pattern of metastasis is initially to the retroperitoneal lymph nodes.[20,145,146]

Leydig and Sertoli cell tumors are associated with steroid hormone hypersecretion. Sertoli cell tumors may be accompanied by precocious puberty in boys. Patients with Leydig cell tumors may have decreased libido and gynecomastia, or virilization in prepubertal boys.

Chemotherapy and radiotherapy are not known to be effective for metastatic sex cord stromal tumors. There are several reports of treatment with mitotane, which was used because it is known to be effective in adrenocortical carcinoma, another steroid-producing tumor. Reported results with mitotane treatment of metastatic sex cord stromal tumors have been mixed, but it can be considered, especially for functional tumors with symptom of steroid hormone excess.

Granulosa Cell Tumors

Granulosa cell tumors of the testicle are rare.[147] They resemble granulosa cell tumors of the ovary. Tumors secrete estrogen, and patients may present with gynecomastia. Treatment is radical orchiectomy, which is usually curative. Granulosa cell tumor (juvenile type) is the most common testicular neoplasm in neonates.

Gonadoblastoma

Gonadoblastoma contains both germ cell and sex cord stromal elements.[20] It is associated with testicular dysgenesis and karyotypic anomalies. It has potential for metastasis of the germ cell component of the primary tumor.

Mesothelioma

Mesothelioma of the tunica vaginalis can invade the testis and spermatic cord.[148] Treatment is radical orchiectomy with complete excision of the spermatic cord and hemiscrotum. RPLND should be considered in patients with LVI or invasion of the testicular parenchyma.

Adenocarcinoma of the Rete Testis

Adenocarcinoma of the rete testis has a poor prognosis.[149] It is not responsive to radiotherapy or chemotherapy. Treatment is radical orchiectomy, and 30% to 50% of patients die within 1 year of metastatic disease. RPLND should be considered for selected patients and may be curative for low-volume metastatic disease.

Epidermoid Cyst

Epidermoid cyst is often asymptomatic.[150] On palpation, it is firm and sharply demarcated, and it appears cystic on ultrasound. It is of uncertain relation to germ cell tumors and is not associated with ITGCN. Histologically, the cyst is lined with squamous epithelium and the adjacent testicular parenchyma is benign. The clinical course is benign. Treatment with enucleation of the tumor or radical orchiectomy is curative.

Lymphoma

Lymphoma presents as painless enlargement of the testicle and may be bilateral.[20] It is the most common secondary malignancy of the testis in men older than 50 years. It typically occurs in the setting of advanced systemic disease, often accompanied by central nervous system or bone marrow involvement.

Metastatic Carcinoma

Metastatic carcinoma is rarely confused with primary testicular cancer. It occurs most commonly in the setting of advanced disseminated disease. Treatment is determined by the type of primary tumor.

SELECTED REFERENCES

The full reference list can be accessed at lwwhealthlibrary.com/oncology.

2. Travis LB, Beard C, Allan JM, et al. Testicular cancer survivorship: research strategies and recommendations. *J Natl Cancer Inst* 2010;102:1114–1130.
4. Rapley EA, Nathanson KL. Predisposition alleles for testicular germ cell tumour. *Curr Opin Genet Dev* 2010;20:225–230.
8. Looijenga LH, Van Agthoven T, Biermann K. Development of malignant germ cells—the genvironmental hypothesis. *Int J Dev Biol* 2013;57:241–253.
11. Sheikine Y, Genega E, Melamed J, et al. Molecular genetics of testicular germ cell tumors. *Am J Cancer Res* 2012;2:153–167.
12. Tan MH, Eng C. Testicular microlithiasis: recent advances in understanding and management. *Nat Rev Urol* 2011;8:153–163.
20. Eble JN, Sauter G, Epstein JI, et al., eds. *Pathology and Genetics of Tumours of the Urinary System and Male Genital Organs.* Lyon, France: IARC Press; 2004.
27. Alvarado-Cabrero I, Hernandez-Toriz N, Paner GP. Clinicopathologic analysis of choriocarcinoma as a pure or predominant component of germ cell tumor of the testis. *Am J Surg Pathol* 2014;38:111–118.
28. Ehrlich Y, Beck SD, Ulbright TM, et al. Outcome analysis of patients with transformed teratoma to primitive neuroectodermal tumor. *Ann Oncol* 2010;21:1846–1850.
29. Rabbani F, Farivar-Mohseni H, Leon A, et al. Clinical outcome after retroperitoneal lymphadenectomy of patients with pure testicular teratoma. *Urology* 2003;62:1092–1096.
30. Donadio AC, Motzer RJ, Bajorin DF, et al. Chemotherapy for teratoma with malignant transformation. *J Clin Oncol* 2003;21:4285–4291.
31. Ma YT, Cullen MH, Hussain SA. Biology of germ cell tumors. *Hematol Oncol Clin North Am* 2011;25:457–471, vii.
34. Greene MH, Kratz CP, Mai PL, et al. Familial testicular germ cell tumors in adults: 2010 summary of genetic risk factors and clinical phenotype. *Endocr Relat Cancer* 2010;17:R109–R121.
44. International Germ Cell Consensus Classification: a prognostic factor-based staging system for metastatic germ cell cancers. International Germ Cell Cancer Collaborative Group. *J Clin Oncol* 1997;15:594–603.
46. Germa JR, Arcusa A, Casamitjana R. False elevations of human chorionic gonadotropin associated to iatrogenic hypogonadism in gonadal germ cell tumors. *Cancer* 1987;60:2489–2493.
47. Morris MJ, Bosl GJ. Recognizing abnormal marker results that do not reflect disease in patients with germ cell tumors. *J Urol* 2000;163:796–801.
48. Pagliaro LC. Testicular cancer: when less is more. *Curr Oncol Rep* 2010;12:271–277.
49. Beard CJ, Travis LB, Chen MH, et al. Outcomes in stage I testicular seminoma: a population-based study of 9193 patients. *Cancer* 2013;119:2771–2777.
50. Chung P, Parker C, Panzarella T, et al. Surveillance in stage I testicular seminoma—risk of late relapse. *Can J Urol* 2002;9:1637–1640.
52. Oliver RT, Mason MD, Mead GM, et al. Radiotherapy versus single-dose carboplatin in adjuvant treatment of stage I seminoma: a randomised trial. *Lancet* 2005;366:293–300.
53. Oliver RT, Mead GM, Rustin GJ, et al. Randomized trial of carboplatin versus radiotherapy for stage I seminoma: mature results on relapse and contralateral testis cancer rates in MRC TE19/EORTC 30982 study (ISRCTN27163214). *J Clin Oncol* 2011;29:957–962.
57. Travis LB, Curtis RE, Storm H, et al. Risk of second malignant neoplasms among long-term survivors of testicular cancer. *J Natl Cancer Inst* 1997;89:1429–1439.
58. Travis LB, Fossa SD, Schonfeld SJ, et al. Second cancers among 40,576 testicular cancer patients: focus on long-term survivors. *J Natl Cancer Inst* 2005;97:1354–1365.
62. Stephenson AJ, Bosl GJ, Bajorin DF, et al. Retroperitoneal lymph node dissection in patients with low stage testicular cancer with embryonal carcinoma predominance and/or lymphovascular invasion. *J Urol* 2005;174:557–560; discussion 560.
63. Williams SD, Birch R, Einhorn LH, et al. Treatment of disseminated germ-cell tumors with cisplatin, bleomycin, and either vinblastine or etoposide. *N Engl J Med* 1987;316:1435–1440.
64. Behnia M, Foster R, Einhorn LH, et al. Adjuvant bleomycin, etoposide and cisplatin in pathological stage II non-seminomatous testicular cancer. the Indiana University experience. *Eur J Cancer* 2000;36:472–475.
65. Swanson DA. Two courses of chemotherapy after orchidectomy for high-risk clinical stage I nonseminomatous testicular tumours. *BJU Int* 2005;95:477–478.
66. Albers P, Siener R, Krege S, et al. Randomized phase III trial comparing retroperitoneal lymph node dissection with one course of bleomycin and etoposide plus cisplatin chemotherapy in the adjuvant treatment of clinical stage I nonseminomatous testicular germ cell tumors: AUO trial AH 01/94 by the German Testicular Cancer Study Group. *J Clin Oncol* 2008;26:2966–2972.
67. Tandstad T, Dahl O, Cohn-Cedermark G, et al. Risk-adapted treatment in clinical stage I nonseminomatous germ cell testicular cancer: the SWENOTECA management program. *J Clin Oncol* 2009;27:2122–2128.
69. Stephenson AJ, Bosl GJ, Motzer RJ, et al. Retroperitoneal lymph node dissection for nonseminomatous germ cell testicular cancer: impact of patient selection factors on outcome. *J Clin Oncol* 2005;23:2781–2788.
77. Classen J, Schmidberger H, Meisner C, et al. Radiotherapy for stages IIA/B testicular seminoma: final report of a prospective multicenter clinical trial. *J Clin Oncol* 2003;21:1101–1106.
81. van den Belt-Dusebout AW, de Wit R, Gietema JA, et al. Treatment-specific risks of second malignancies and cardiovascular disease in 5-year survivors of testicular cancer. *J Clin Oncol* 2007;25:4370–4378.
82. Fizazi K, Delva R, Caty A, et al. A risk-adapted study of cisplatin and etoposide, with or without ifosfamide, in patients with metastatic seminoma: results of the GETUG S99 multicenter prospective study. *Eur Urol* 2014;65:381–386.
83. Rabbani F, Sheinfeld J, Farivar-Mohseni H, et al. Low-volume nodal metastases detected at retroperitoneal lymphadenectomy for testicular cancer: pattern and prognostic factors for relapse. *J Clin Oncol* 2001;19:2020–2025.
87. Moran CA, Suster S, Przygodzki RM, et al. Primary germ cell tumors of the mediastinum: II. Mediastinal seminomas—a clinicopathologic and immunohistochemical study of 120 cases. *Cancer* 1997;80:691–698.
89. Kondagunta GV, Bacik J, Bajorin D, et al. Etoposide and cisplatin chemotherapy for metastatic good-risk germ cell tumors. *J Clin Oncol* 2005;23:9290–9294.
90. Culine S, Kerbrat P, Kramar A, et al. Refining the optimal chemotherapy regimen for good-risk metastatic nonseminomatous germ-cell tumors: a randomized trial of the Genito-Urinary Group of the French Federation of Cancer Centers (GETUG T93BP). *Ann Oncol* 2007;18:917–924.

PRACTICE OF ONCOLOGY

91. Bajorin DF, Sarosdy MF, Pfister DG, et al. Randomized trial of etoposide and cisplatin versus etoposide and carboplatin in patients with good-risk germ cell tumors: a multiinstitutional study. *J Clin Oncol* 1993;11:598–606.

94. Motzer RJ, Nichols CJ, Margolin KA, et al. Phase III randomized trial of conventional-dose chemotherapy with or without high-dose chemotherapy and autologous hematopoietic stem-cell rescue as first-line treatment for patients with poor-prognosis metastatic germ cell tumors. *J Clin Oncol* 2007;25: 247–256.

95. Beck SD, Patel MI, Sheinfeld J. Tumor marker levels in post-chemotherapy cystic masses: clinical implications for patients with germ cell tumors. *J Urol* 2004;171:168–171.

96. Fizazi K, Culine S, Kramar A, et al. Early predicted time to normalization of tumor markers predicts outcome in poor-prognosis nonseminomatous germ cell tumors. *J Clin Oncol* 2004;22:3868–3876.

99. Goodarzi MO, Van Herle AJ. Thyrotoxicosis in a male patient associated with excess human chorionic gonadotropin production by germ cell tumor. *Thyroid* 2000;10:611–619.

100. Giralt SA, Dexeus F, Amato R, et al. Hyperthyroidism in men with germ cell tumors and high levels of beta-human chorionic gonadotropin. *Cancer* 1992;69:1286–1290.

101. Moran CA, Suster A. Primary germ cell tumors of the mediastinum: I. Analysis of 322 cases with special emphasis on teratomatous lesions and a proposal for histopathologic classification and clinical staging. *Cancer* 1997;80: 681–690.

102. McNeil MM, Leong AS, Sage RE. Primary mediastinal embryonal carcinoma in association with Klinefelter's syndrome. *Cancer* 1981;47:343–345.

103. Nichols CR, Heerema NA, Palmer C, et al. Klinefelter's syndrome associated with mediastinal germ cell neoplasms. *J Clin Oncol* 1987;5:1290–1294.

105. Rodney AJ, Tannir NM, Siefer-Radtke AO, et al. Survival outcomes for men with mediastinal germ-cell tumors: the University of Texas M. D. Anderson Cancer Center experience. *Urol Oncol* 2012;30:879–885.

106. Nichols CR, Saxman S, Williams SD, et al. Primary mediastinal nonseminomatous germ cell tumors. A modern single institution experience. *Cancer* 1990;65:1641–1646.

107. Fizazi K, Culine S, Droz JP, et al. Primary mediastinal nonseminomatous germ cell tumors: results of modern therapy including cisplatin-based chemotherapy. *J Clin Oncol* 1998;16:725–732.

108. Bokemeyer C, Nichols CR, Droz JP, et al. Extragonadal germ cell tumors of the mediastinum and retroperitoneum: results from an international analysis. *J Clin Oncol* 2002;20:1864–1873.

109. Radaideh SM, Cook VC, Kesler KA, et al. Outcome following resection for patients with primary mediastinal nonseminomatous germ-cell tumors and rising serum tumor markers post-chemotherapy. *Ann Oncol* 2010;21: 804–807.

110. Moran CA, Suster S, Koss MN. Primary germ cell tumors of the mediastinum: III. Yolk sac tumor, embryonal carcinoma, choriocarcinoma, and combined nonteratomatous germ cell tumors of the mediastinum—a clinicopathologic and immunohistochemical study of 64 cases. *Cancer* 1997;80:699–707.

112. Loehrer PJ Sr, Einhorn LH, Williams SD. VP-16 plus ifosfamide plus cisplatin as salvage therapy in refractory germ cell cancer. *J Clin Oncol* 1986;4: 528–536.

114. Loehrer PJ Sr, Gonin R, Nichols CR, et al. Vinblastine plus ifosfamide plus cisplatin as initial salvage therapy in recurrent germ cell tumor. *J Clin Oncol* 1998;16:2500–2504.

115. Kondagunta GV, Bacik J, Donadio A, et al. Combination of paclitaxel, ifosfamide, and cisplatin is an effective second-line therapy for patients with relapsed testicular germ cell tumors. *J Clin Oncol* 2005;23:6549–6555.

116. Einhorn LH, Williams SD, Chamness A, et al. High-dose chemotherapy and stem-cell rescue for metastatic germ-cell tumors. *N Engl J Med* 2007; 357:340–348.

117. Feldman DR, Sheinfeld J, Bajorin DF, et al. TI-CE high-dose chemotherapy for patients with previously treated germ cell tumors: results and prognostic factor analysis. *J Clin Oncol* 2010;28:1706–1713.

118. Kollmannsberger C, Beyer J, Liersch R, et al. Combination chemotherapy with gemcitabine plus oxaliplatin in patients with intensively pretreated or refractory germ cell cancer: a study of the German Testicular Cancer Study Group. *J Clin Oncol* 2004;22:108–114.

119. Einhorn LH, Brames MJ, Juliar B, et al. Phase II study of paclitaxel plus gemcitabine salvage chemotherapy for germ cell tumors after progression following high-dose chemotherapy with tandem transplant. *J Clin Oncol* 2007;25:513–516.

121. Cooper MA, Einhorn LH. Maintenance chemotherapy with daily oral etoposide following salvage therapy in patients with germ cell tumors. *J Clin Oncol* 1995;13:1167–1169.

124. Vaughn DJ, Flaherty K, Lal P, et al. Treatment of growing teratoma syndrome. *N Engl J Med* 2009;360:423–424.

127. Eastham JA, Wilson TG, Russell C, et al. Surgical resection in patients with nonseminomatous germ cell tumor who fail to normalize serum tumor markers after chemotherapy. *Urology* 1994;43:74–80.

128. Carver BS, Motzer RJ, Kondagunta GV, et al. Late relapse of testicular germ cell tumors. *Urol Oncol* 2005;23:441–445.

129. Ronnen EA, Kondagunta GV, Bacik J, et al. Incidence of late-relapse germ cell tumor and outcome to salvage chemotherapy. *J Clin Oncol* 2005;23:6999–7004.

131. Huddart RA, Norman A, Shahidi M, et al. Cardiovascular disease as a long-term complication of treatment for testicular cancer. *J Clin Oncol* 2003;21:1513–1523.

133. Argyriou AA, Bruna J, Marmiroli P, et al. Chemotherapy-induced peripheral neurotoxicity (CIPN): an update. *Crit Rev Oncol Hematol* 2012;82:51–77.

134. Gietema JA, Meinardi MT, Messerschmidt J, et al. Circulating plasma platinum more than 10 years after cisplatin treatment for testicular cancer. *Lancet* 2000;355:1075–1076.

135. Travis LB, Fossa SD, Sesso HD, et al. Chemotherapy-induced peripheral neurotoxicity and ototoxicity: new paradigms for translational genomics. *J Natl Cancer Inst* 2014;106.

136. Rademaker-Lakhai JM, Crul M, Zuur L, et al. Relationship between cisplatin administration and the development of ototoxicity. *J Clin Oncol* 2006;24:918–924.

140. Kollmannsberger C, Beyer J, Droz JP, et al. Secondary leukemia following high cumulative doses of etoposide in patients treated for advanced germ cell tumors. *J Clin Oncol* 1998;16:3386–3391.

143. Ladanyi M, Samaniego D, Reuter VE, et al. Cytogenetic and immunohistochemical evidence for the germ cell origin of a subset of acute leukemias associated with mediastinal germ cell tumors. *J Natl Cancer Inst* 1990;82:221–227.

144. Orazi A, Neiman RS, Ulbright TM, et al. Hematopoietic precursor cells within the yolk sac tumor component are the source of secondary hematopoietic malignancies in patients with mediastinal germ cell tumors. *Cancer* 1993;71:3873–3881.

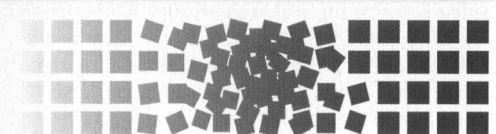

71 Molecular Biology of Gynecologic Cancers

Tanja Pejovic, Michael J. Birrer, Matthew L. Anderson, and Kunle Odunsi

INTRODUCTION

Gynecologic cancer research has mirrored all cancer research programs in that it has focused largely on molecular defects in oncogenes, tumor-suppressor genes, and DNA repair mechanisms. Several research groups have also channeled their resources into various carcinogenic phenomena, such as apoptotic pathway defects, growth signaling, angiogenesis, tissue invasion, or metastasis. These efforts have led to a broad understanding of the chromosomal and molecular abnormalities that underlie malignancies of the female genital tract (vulva, vagina, cervix, uterus, ovaries, and fallopian tubes). It is clear that an improvement in outcome of these malignancies can only be achieved if: (1) early diagnosis is achieved, (2) there is accurate prediction of progression and response, and (3) new treatment options reflecting the molecular pathogenesis and progression are developed. This requires detailed disease-specific understanding of the diverse molecular changes in gynecologic malignancies that ultimately lead cells to develop the following hallmarks of cancer: abnormalities in self-sufficiency of growth signals, evasion of apoptosis, insensitivity to antigrowth signals, limitless replicative potential, sustained angiogenesis, and tissue invasion and metastases. Moreover, there is growing evidence for the concept of cancer immunosurveillance and immunoediting based on (1) protection against development of spontaneous and chemically induced tumors in animal systems and (2) the identification of targets for immune recognition of human cancer.[1] This concept is supported by several studies in gynecologic cancers and has opened new avenues for the development of novel biomarkers and therapeutic targets. It is the purpose of this chapter to highlight and summarize some of the recent basic findings in gynecologic malignancies, with an emphasis on clinically applicable developments.

OVARIAN CANCER

Origins of Epithelial Ovarian Cancer

Until recently, epithelial ovarian cancer (EOC) was thought to arise primarily from the ovarian surface epithelium (OSE), with a subset likely originating in the adjacent fimbria.[2,3] The OSE forms a monolayer surrounding the ovary, but is composed of relatively few cuboidal cells (107 cells per ovary, or 0.05% of the entire organ). Developmentally, it derives from the coelomic epithelium, which also gives rise to the peritoneal mesothelium and oviductal epithelium.[4] The OSE appears generally stable, uniform, and quiescent, although it can undergo proliferation in vivo.[5] Despite the small number of cells within the OSE and their apparent inactivity, the risk for EOC is nearly 2%, suggesting a high malignant potential. The basis for such a high potential is poorly understood. No physiologic role for the primate OSE has been established,[6] and the lack of any obvious function could contribute to the asymptomatic nature of early-stage EOC.

In other organs, such as the colon, distinct premalignant lesions have been identified and found to accumulate genetic defects that ultimately result in malignancy. However, the search to identify similar epithelial precursors in the human ovary has proven only partially fruitful, in large part because normal ovaries are only rarely biopsied or examined. Histologic findings consistent with a preinvasive lesion for ovarian cancer have been described by a number of studies where ovaries were removed from women who eventually developed peritoneal carcinomas, ovaries from high-risk women who were undergoing prophylactic oophorectomy, and in areas of ovarian epithelium adjacent to early-stage ovarian cancers that demonstrate a transition from normal to malignant cells.[7] Surprisingly, occult noninvasive and invasive carcinomas in the fallopian tubes, typically in the fimbria, have been discovered in women undergoing prophylactic salpingo-oophorectomies because of a family history or germ-line mutations of *BRCA1* and *BRCA2*.[8] This led to the hypothesis that these occult tubal carcinomas might shed malignant cells, which then implant and grow on the ovary, simulating primary ovarian cancer. Moreover, gene expression studies have demonstrated that the expression profiles of ovarian high-grade serous cancers (HGSCs) more closely resembled fallopian tube epithelium (FTE) than the OSE.[9] Because the tubal carcinomas were associated with serous and not endometrioid, clear cell, or mucinous carcinomas, the noninvasive tubal carcinomas have been designated *serous tubal intraepithelial carcinoma* (STIC).

The new paradigm for the pathogenesis of ovarian serous cancer based on a dualistic model and the recognition that the majority of these tumors originate outside the ovary facilitates the development of novel approaches to prevention, screening, and treatment. The low-grade serous tumors (type I) are generally indolent, present in stage I (tumor confined to the ovary) and develop from well-established precursors, and are characterized by specific mutations, including *KRAS*, *BRAF* and *ERBB2*, but rarely *TP53*. They are relatively genetically stable. In contrast, the HGSCs (type II) are aggressive, present in advanced stage, and develop from STICs. They have a very high frequency of *TP53* mutations, but rarely harbor the mutations detected in the low-grade serous tumors. Although low-grade serous and HGSCs develop along different molecular pathways, both types may develop from FTE and secondarily involve the ovary.[10]

Molecular Pathways to Ovarian Cancer

Inherited Syndromes of Ovarian Cancers

A family history of the disease is the most significant known risk factor for EOC. There is a threefold increased risk of developing the disease for an individual with a first-degree relative affected with ovarian cancer.[11] Inherited EOC most often occurs as part of families with both ovarian and breast cancer cases or in families with only multiple ovarian cancer cases. Inherited ovarian cancer is also part of Lynch syndrome or hereditary nonpolyposis colorectal cancer (HNPCC), found in families with multiple cases of colon cancer. It is estimated that 5% to 10% of EOC cases are due to these familial syndromes.[12]

A linkage analysis of familial breast and ovarian cancers provided some of the first insights into the molecular basis of ovarian cancer, ultimately leading to the identification of two genes, *BRCA1* and *BRCA2*, each associated with a significant increased incidence of ovarian cancer. The frequency of *BRCA1* and *BRCA2* mutations in the general population is estimated to be 1 in 800 and 1 in 500, respectively,[11] whereas population-based ovarian cancer studies revealed that the frequency of *BRCA1* mutations was 3% to 10% and for *BRCA2*, 0.6% to 6%.[12]

The *BRCA1* gene was cloned in 1994[13] and was found to have 24 exons spanning 80 kb of genomic DNA, and had a 7.8 kb transcript coding for an 1,863 amino acid protein. The *BRCA2* gene mapped to chromosome 13q12-13, had 27 exons (26 coding), spanning 70 kb of genomic DNA, and had an 11.4-kb transcript and coded a 3,418 amino acid protein.[14] Hundreds of mutations in *BRCA1* have now been identified, most commonly, loss of function nonsense or frameshift mutations. Two specific mutations, 185delAG and 5382insC, are found in 1% and 0.1%, respectively, of Ashkenazi Jewish women. Some missense changes have been found to be pathogenic, but the majority are polymorphisms or unclassified variants (UV), also known as variants of uncertain significance (VUS). A high frequency of large genomic rearrangements (LGR) have been identified in both *BRCA1* and the *BRCA2* gene.[15]

The position of mutations within large *BRCA1* and *BRCA2* genes determines the risk of ovarian cancer. The *BRCA1* gene mutation within nucleotides 2402 and 4190 carries the high risk of ovarian cancer (and a lower risk of breast cancer). Both genes show an autosomal-dominant transmission of highly penetrant germ-line mutations and behave as tumor suppressor genes. Both proteins function in the double-strand DNA break repair pathway but may have additional functions; *BRCA1* functions in both checkpoint activation and DNA repair, and *BRCA2* is a mediator of homologous recombination.

Functionally, *BRCA1* regulates *p53*, an oncogene frequently implicated in ovarian cancer. Thus, the loss of *BRCA1* allows DNA damage to accumulate via a loss of its activation of *p53*. However, mutations in *BRCA1* also likely contribute to ovarian cancer by mechanisms other than its interactions with *p53*. Any understanding of the role of *BRCA1* in ovarian cancer is further complicated by reports of women with high-risk mutations in *BRCA1* who fail to develop ovarian cancer. These observations speak clearly to the role of genetic modifiers in determining whether *BRCA1* or *BRCA2* mutations ultimately lead to malignancy. For example, the CAG repeat polymorphism in the androgen receptor has been shown to modify the subsequent risk of ovarian cancer in women with known mutations in *BRCA1*.

High penetrance *BRCA1* and *BRCA2* gene mutation accounts for about 40% of ovarian cancer risk.[16] The remaining risk is due to very rare high risk genes, very few moderate risk genes, and/or multiple low risk genes. The Ovarian Cancer Association Consortium (OCAC) was established in 2005 to investigate the risk of SNP in ovarian cancer. So far, an additional six loci associated with a risk of ovarian cancer have been reported: 2q31, 3q25, 8q24, 9p22.2, 17q21, and 19p13.1.[11]

Genomic Instability, Fanconi Anemia/BRCA DNA Repair Pathway, and Rare Mutations

BRCA1 indirectly and *BRCA2* directly are associated with maintaining the genome stability (i.e., a cell's ability to tolerate DNA damage). *BRCA2* is a member of BRCA/Fanconi anemia (FA) DNA repair pathway. Studies on the pathogenesis of FA, a rare inherited DNA repair disorder, have helped define the molecular basis of defective DNA damage responses linked to cancer risk. FA is a genetic disorder characterized by skeletal anomalies,

progressive bone marrow failure, cancer susceptibility, and cellular hypersensitivity to DNA cross-linking agents. To date, 15 FA genes have been cloned: *FANCA, -B, -C, -D1, -D2, -E, -F, -G, -J, -L, -M, -N,* and *-I, -O,* and *-P.* Of these, *FANCA, FANCB, FANCC, FANCE, FANCF, FANCG, FANCL,* and *FANCM* form a nuclear core complex. Although the functional scope of this complex has not been fully defined, it is clear that it must be completely intact to facilitate monoubiquitination of the downstream FANCD2 and FANCI proteins, a change that allows FANCD2 and FANCI to colocalize with *BRCA1, BRCA2* (and presumably FANCJ and FANCN), and *RAD51* in damage-induced nuclear foci.[17]

Four lines of evidence link the FA pathway with ovarian carcinogenesis. First, *BRCA2* has been identified as the FA gene, *FANCD1.* As a result, heterozygotes for *BRCA2* mutations have a high risk of tissue-specific epithelial cancers, whereas homozygotes develop FA. Second, an increased prevalence of ovarian malignancies has been observed in FANCD2 nullizygous mice. Functionally silencing *FANCF* in ovarian cancer through promoter hypermethylation has also been described. Lastly, low levels of the FANCD2 protein are found in ovarian surface epithelia from women at risk for ovarian cancer. Taken together, these data suggest that the FA pathway is important in defining a predisposition to ovarian (and breast) cancer, and that aberrations of FA genes may account for some familial ovarian cancer cases not accounted for by *BRCA1* and *BRCA2* mutations.

In sporadic ovarian cancers, the epigenetic silencing of the FA pathway through methylation of the FA gene promoter region is one of the frequent mechanisms of inactivation. One study found that 4 of 19 primary ovarian carcinomas had *FANCF* methylation, although a larger study of 106 ovarian tumors did not identify the loss of FANCF expression. Loss of the *BRCA2* mRNA and protein has been reported in 13% of ovarian carcinomas and, in contrast to other FA genes, methylation is not a cause of the protein loss. Epigenetic silencing of *BRCA1* through methylation was found in 23% of advanced ovarian carcinomas.

Interestingly, tumors with inactivated *BRCA2* are responsive to cisplatin. However, due to their low accuracy of DNA repair, these cells accumulate secondary genetic modifications that can lead to a reversal of the *BRCA2* mutation, allowing these cells to acquire resistance to cross-linking agents.[18]

Recently, mutations have been identified in four genes: *RAD51C, RAD51D, BRIP1* and *PALB2* in the FA-BRCA pathway. Mutations in the *RAD51C* and *RAD51D* genes were found in approximately 1% of breast/ovarian cancer families. The relative risk (RR) of ovarian cancer in *RAD51D* carriers was 6.3 (95% confidence interval [CI], 2.9 to 13.9). Mutations in *PALB2 (FANCN)* were found in 3.4% of breast cancer families, and 55% of these families had family members with ovarian cancer. An Icelandic mutation in *BRIP1 (FANCJ)* with a frequency of 0.41% increased the risk ovarian cancer, OR 8.1 (95% CI, 4.7 to 14.0). A Spanish *BRIP1* mutation had a frequency of 1.3% in ovarian cancer cases and the risk of ovarian cancer was OR 25 (95% CI, 1.8 to 340).[11]

In 2010, Walsh et al.[19] screened 21 tumor suppressor genes in mutations in 360 unselected ovarian, fallopian tube, or peritoneal cancer cases and found mutations in six additional genes (*BARD1, CHEK2, MRE11A, NBN, RAD50,* and *TP53*).[19] These findings suggest that a careful and comprehensive mutational screen of all women may identify that the inherited risk of ovarian cancer is higher than originally thought and that an early identification of the risk may ultimately lead to prevention in 24% of ovarian cancer cases.

Role of Poly (ADP-Ribose)-Polymerase (PARP) and PARP Inhibitors in Gynecologic Cancers

Abnormalities in DNA repair have been identified in many human epithelial cancers. Gynecologic cancers are not an exception, with ovarian cancer being the most extensively studied. Serous ovarian cancer has been characterized as having a major defect in homologous recombination resulting from mutations within Fanconi pathway, as noted previously. DNA repair is a complex process designed to repair specific abnormalities within the DNA. Single-stranded DNA breaks are repaired by a protein complex containing poly (ADP-ribose)-polymerase (PARP). In contrast, double-stranded breaks that are lethal for the cell require a different complex, which contains the BRCA proteins.

Because PARP proteins are intimately involved in the repair of single-stranded DNA breaks, the inhibition of PARP function impedes single-stranded DNA break repair, leading to the formation of double-stranded breaks. Research performed in multiple laboratories suggested that the inhibition of PARP would be a lethal event in cells that have inactivation of *BRCA1* or *BRCA2*. This concept, called *synthetic lethality* (first proposed for cancer therapeutics in 1997), was tested early in the development of PARP inhibitors.[20] Preclinical data strongly supported this concept, with *BRCA*-mutated cell lines showing a 100- to 1,000-fold sensitivity to PARP inhibitors compared with wild-type control cell lines. This laboratory proof of principle led to a rapid transition into the clinic.

The clinical development of PARP inhibitors began in earnest in the mid-2000s where they were tested in early phase trials. The first phase I trial focused on women with germ-line *BRCA* mutation of and yielded encouraging results. The expansion cohort of this study treated woman with ovarian cancer and recorded a 46% response rate in platinum-sensitive patients and a 33% response rate in platinum-resistant patients. Of note, the drug was well tolerated and its oral delivery made it quite convenient. This landmark trial led to a follow-up study that examined doses of 100 mg to 400 mg and involved ovarian cancer mutation carriers. The response rate was dose dependent (13% to 33%) and again demonstrated significant activity in the platinum-resistant disease. PARP inhibitors have also been tested in the maintenance setting after the effective treatment of platinum-sensitive recurrent disease. A dramatic improvement in progression-free survival was demonstrated with a hazard ratio (HR) of 0.15 for mutation carriers.[21]

Despite these results, the development of PARP inhibitors has been slow. Difficulties in formulation, precise dose determination, and the identification of pharmacodynamic endpoints have impeded determining the effective role of these agents. Further, a randomized phase II trial directly comparing a PARP inhibitor to doxorubicin in germ-line mutation patients with recurrent ovarian cancer showed no difference between the arms. Despite these setbacks, continued enthusiasm for these agents has led three companies to recently design phase III trials to establish their role in the treatment of ovarian cancer.

It is important to note that most of these trials have tested the effectiveness of PARP inhibitors in mutation carriers. Recent work form large genomic studies support that a much larger percentage of serous ovarian cancers have homologous recombination deficiencies. Estimates have been as high as 50% of all sporadic ovarian cancers. The precise genomic or protein biomarkers, which predict for responsiveness, is the focus of intense research.

There are important unanswered questions and challenges involving the effective use of PARP inhibitors. The precise optimal dose, duration, and sequence are yet to be determined. Should PARP inhibitors be used up-front with chemotherapy or later in maintenance or relapse disease? At present, there are little long-term safety data on PARP inhibition and, given their mechanisms of action, there is concern about secondary malignancies such as leukemia. This may be dependent on the mode of administration with chronic use versus intermittent being more problematic. Further, the mechanism(s) of PARP inhibitor resistance remains essentially unknown. Recent work has demonstrated an in-frame mutation in the *BRCA* gene that restored the protein function in a small number of resistant tumors. Other mechanisms are surely present and need to be determined. Finally, other potential clinical settings for PARP inhibitors, such as radiation sensitizers in combination with chemotherapy, for cervical or endometrial cancers will need to be evaluated.

Ovarian Cancer Microenvironment, Metastases, and Angiogenesis

The ovarian cancer microenvironment consists of any biologic component that interacts with tumor cells, and it includes stromal components, extracellular matrix (ECM) molecules, and cytokines.[22] Together, these components create a microenvironment that interacts with the tumor and influences tumor behavior. Two hallmarks of cancer, angiogenesis and metastatic potential, are dependent on the tumor microenvironment. Targeting the interactions between the tumor and its environment has the potential to revolutionize the treatment for ovarian cancer patients.

Inflammatory Cytokines

Cytokine-mediator molecules have a profound effect on tumors. Tumor necrosis factor alpha (TNF-α) is a cytokine that is expressed on ovarian cancer cells and macrophages and is implicated in inflammation. It works through affecting other cytokines and angiogenesis.[23] Animal studies showed that suppressing TNF-α resulted in lower plasma levels of interleukin (IL)-6, reduced IL-17 levels in the ascites, and reduced tumor burden.[24] In a phase I clinical trial with the TNF-α antibody, infliximab, patients with ovarian cancer showed decreased IL-17 ascitic levels.[24] In addition to TNF-α, high levels of IL-6, IL-8, and macrophage inflammatory protein are also found in ascites. In a multivariate analysis, IL-6 has shown to be a predictor of poor prognosis. A monoclonal antibody siltuximab, which abrogates the IL-6 signaling pathway, had been tested in a phase II clinical trial in platinum-resistant ovarian cancer with one third of the patients showing a clinically meaningful response.[25]

Particular attention has recently focused on the role of lysophosphatidic acid (LPA) in promoting the metastasis of ovarian cancers. LPA is constitutively produced by mesothelial cells lining the peritoneal cavity; its levels are increased in the ascites of women with both early- and late-stage ovarian cancers.[26] When applied to ovarian cancer cell lines in vitro, LPA promotes both the migration of these cells in a manner dependent on Ras MEK kinase-1 as well as their invasion across artificial barriers analogous to a basement membrane. At a molecular level, exogenous LPA enhances ovarian cancer invasiveness both by activating matrix metalloproteinase-2 via membrane type 1-matrix metalloproteinase (MT1-MMP) and downregulating the expression of specific tissue inhibitors of metalloproteinases (TIMP-2 and -3).[27] Its application to cultured ovarian cancer cells has also been shown to promote disassembly of intracellular stress fibers and focal adhesions,[28] observations that are consistent with the idea that LPA promotes the dissemination of ovarian cancer by a loss of cell adhesion. However, LPA has also been shown to promote the invasiveness of ovarian cancers by additional mechanisms dependent on IL-8. The G12/13-RhoA and cyclooxygenase pathways have also been implicated in the LPA-induced migration of ovarian cancers. These mechanisms appear to be independent of the ability of LPA to induce changes in *MMP2* expression. Lastly, it should be noted that LPA appears to promote ovarian cancer metastasis by stimulating *fas*-ligand expression and the shedding of *fas*-ligand–containing microvesicles, potentially leading to an evasion of tumor immunity.

Stromal Cells

A subset of host cells are typically recruited to tumor site. These include tumor-infiltrating lymphocytes, macrophages, fibroblasts, mesenchymal stem cells (MSC), and adipocytes as a body response to a solid tumor. For example, a distinct population of T cells recruited to the tumor site exhibit a cytotoxic effect, although some tumor cells escape detection by the immune system, possibly through immunosuppression of T cells by stromal cells in the ascites.[29] In addition, macrophages are recruited to tumor sites and establish bidirectional interaction with tumor cells via chemokines and MMPs. Chemokines activate tumor-associated macrophages (TAM) M2 immunosuppressive cells, which is found in ovarian cancer. The M2 phenotype is also induced by colony stimulation factor-1 (CSF-1). CSF-1 is highly expressed in ovarian cancer and associated with poor prognosis.[30] In 2004, Turk et al.[31] have described a method that targets both cancer cells and TAMs and involves the folate receptor that are typically expressed on both TAM and cancer cells. Folate-conjugated liposomes showed greater affinity toward TAMs then to cancer cells, highlighting this method of drug delivery to tumor microenvironment. More recently, trabectedin, a compound that prevents differentiation of monocytes to macrophages, was developed against TAM. In a phase II randomized clinical trial that compared the efficacy of doxorubicin versus trabectedin + doxorubicin combination in patients with platinum-sensitive ovarian cancer. The trabectedin + doxorubicin combination showed improved progression-free survival and response rates.[32] Preclinical studies are now assessing if clear cell ovarian carcinoma, a subtype characterized by rich TAM infiltrates, may have a more favorable response to trabectidin.[33]

Cancer-Associated Fibroblasts

Fibroblasts are a major component of tissue stroma; cancer-associated fibroblasts (CAF or myofibroblasts) remain activated, forming reactive tumor stroma. They are characterized by an altered phenotype and expression of alpha-smooth muscle actin (alpha-SMA) and fibroblast activation protein (FAP). The interaction between cancer cells and FAPs results in a release of cytokines and signals that promote cancer cells invasiveness via paracrine signaling. Targeting FAP and its paracrine signaling may also be a promising new venue for ovarian therapeutics.

Mesenchymal Stem Cells

MSCs are components of the tumor microenvironment with the ability to differentiate into many different cell types, including CAFs. They have been investigated for their potential use as vehicles for cancer drug delivery by exploiting their ability to migrate to the site of tumor proliferation. For example, such an approach used MSCs transduced with recombinant virus encoding endostatin, an inhibitor of angiogenesis.[34]

Metastases

Changes in ECM components are associated with cell adhesion and tumor invasion. Malignant cells constantly alter their cells' adhesion molecules in response signals, which favors their ability to disseminate and invade locally. Cell membrane integrins have been shown to be important in the progression of ovarian cancer. Beta 1 integrins and alpha 5B1-integrin mediate the attachment of tumor aggregates to the mesothelium. Targeting alpha 5B1-integrin interactions had been attempted in platinum-resistant ovarian cancer without clinically meaningful results. Khanna et al.[35] using a high-throughput, small-molecule inhibitor screen, identified several components that are able to inhibit cell adhesion, thus paving the way to further test these molecules as strategies to minimize cancer invasion/spread.[35]

Angiogenesis

The growth of both primary ovarian cancers and their metastases requires the formation of new blood vessels to support adequate perfusion. This process, known as *angiogenesis*, mechanistically involves both the branching of new capillaries as well as the remodeling of larger vessels. Other processes, such as vasculogenic mimicry, have also been implicated in tumor angiogenesis.

Angiogenesis is tightly regulated by a balance of pro- and antiangiogenic factors. These include growth factors, such as transforming growth factor (TGF)-β, vascular endothelial growth factor (VEGF), and platelet-derived growth factor; prostaglandins, such as prostaglandin E2; cytokines, such as IL-8; and other factors, such as the angiopoietins (Ang-1, Ang-2) and hypoxia-inducible factor-1α (HIF-1α). Many of these angiogenic factors have been implicated in ovarian cancer. For example, VEGF is a family of secreted polypeptides with critical roles in both normal development and human disease. Many cancers, including ovarian carcinomas, release VEGF in response to the hypoxic or acidic conditions typical in solid tumors. Near universal, albeit variable, levels of VEGF expression have been reported in ovarian cancers, in which higher levels correlate with advanced disease and poor clinical prognosis.[36] Circulating levels of VEGF have also been reported to be higher in the serum of women with ovarian cancers when compared with those with benign tumors. Expression of HIF-1 correlates well with microvessel density in ovarian cancers and has been proposed to upregulate VEGF expression.[37] Culturing ovarian cancer cell lines under hypoxic conditions stimulates the expression of both HIF-1α and VEGF expression, and the addition of prostaglandin E2 potentiates the ability of hypoxia to induce the expression of both proangiogenic factors.[38]

Ironically, many of the molecules implicated in regulating angiogenesis in cancer, such as c-met, also regulate other processes critical for cancer metastasis, such as cell migration and invasiveness. The inhibition of PI3K decreases the transcription of VEGF in ovarian cancer cells, an effect that is reversed by the forced expression of AKT. Such observations are consistent with reports that hypoxia not only induces angiogenesis, but also increases the invasiveness of ovarian cancer cells.[39] Likewise, an acidic environment induces increased IL-8 expression in ovarian cancer in a manner dependent on transcription factors AP-1 and nuclear factor-κB (NF-κB)–like factor, suggesting that the feedback between these pathways may also determine how tumors interact with their external environment. Undoubtedly, better insight into these interactions will help to define the suitability of these molecules as therapeutic targets.

So far, antiangiogenic-targeting treatments have been used in combination with conventional chemotherapy in ovarian cancer. Phase III clinical trials have investigated the potential of the VEGF inhibitor bevacizumab as an addition to carboplatin + paclitaxel for improving progression-free survival in ovarian cancer patients at high risk for progression by approximately 4 months.[40]

Epigenetics

It has become increasingly apparent that epigenetic events can lead to cancer as frequently as a loss of gene function due to mutations or loss of heterozygosity. The overall level of genomic methylation is reduced in cancer (global hypomethylation), but hypermethylation of promoter regions of specific genes is a common event that is often associated with the transcriptional inactivation of specific genes.[41] This is critical because the silenced genes are often tumor suppressor genes, and their loss of function can be evident in early stages of cancer and can also drive neoplastic progression and metastasis. Epigenetic gene silencing is a complex series of events that includes DNA hypermethylation of CpG islands within gene-promoter regions, histone deacetylation, methylation or phosphorylation, or histone demethylation. Global hypermethylation of CpG islands appears to be prevalent but highly variable in ovarian cancer tissue.[42] Multiple genes are abnormally methylated in ovarian cancer compared with normal ovarian tissue, including p16, retinoic acid receptor beta (RAR-β), H-cadherin, GSTP1, MGMT, RASSF1A, leukotriene B4 receptor, MTHFR, progesterone receptor, CDH1, IGSF4, BRCA1, TMS1, estrogen receptor-α, the putative tumor suppressor km23 (TGF-β component), and others.[42,43] The degree of DNA methylation, the demethylation activity of chemotherapeutic drugs, the degree of histone acetylation, and the specificity of demethylation of select genes are all critical to ensuring the success of treatment and the prevention of ovarian cancer recurrence.[43]

Role of Specific Immune Responses

The novel observation by William Coley in the 1890s that severe bacterial infections could induce an antitumor response in patients with partially resected tumors has evolved into an understanding that the immune system can recognize tumor-associated antigens and direct a targeted response. The concept of *cancer immunoediting* suggests that the immune system not only protects the host against the development of primary cancers, but also dynamically sculpts tumor immunogenicity.[44] In epithelial ovarian cancer, support for the role of immune surveillance of tumors comes from observations that the presence of tumor-infiltrating lymphocytes (TIL) in tumors is associated with improved survival of patients with the disease.[44,45] A recent meta-analysis of 10 studies with 1,815 ovarian cancer patients confirmed the observation that a lack of intraepithelial lymphocytes (TILs) is significantly associated with a worse survival among ovarian cancer patients (pooled HR, 2.24, 95% CI, 1.71 to 2.91).[9] This effect was evident regardless of tumor grade, stage, or histologic subtype. In addition, encouraging results from large-scale clinical trials of immune system–provoking therapies[10–13] have rekindled the promise of harnessing the immune system to attack cancers.

Finally, advanced-stage ovarian cancer patients can have detectable tumor-specific cytotoxic T-cell and antibody immunity. This was illustrated in a study that indicated that immunity to p53 predicted improved overall survival in patients with advanced-stage disease.[46] All of these observations support clinical trials of immunotherapy for epithelial ovarian cancer in an effort to elicit effective antitumor responses. Major obstacles include the identification of tumor-restricted immunogenic targets, the generation of a sufficient immune response to cause tumor rejection, and approaches to overcome tumor evasion of an immune attack.

Ovarian Cancer-Specific Antigens

Human tumor antigens defined to date can be classified into one or more of the following categories: (1) differentiation antigens, such as tyrosinase, Melan-A/MART-1, and gp100; (2) mutational antigens, such as CDK4, β-catenin, caspase-8, and P53; (3) amplification antigens, such as Her2/neu and p53; (4) splice variant antigens, such as NY-CO-37/PDZ-45 and ING1; (5) viral antigens, such as human papillomavirus (HPV) and Epstein-Barr virus; and (6) cancer-testis antigens, such as MAGE, NY-ESO-1, and LAGE-1. Thus, it is clear that some antigens may play a crucial role in the progression of tumor cells (e.g., Her2/neu) and could be useful as biomarkers of disease progression and targets of therapy. On the other hand, in considering an antigenic target for ovarian cancer immunotherapy, an ideal candidate antigen should not only demonstrate high-frequency expression in the tumor tissues and restricted expression in normal tissues, but should also provide evidence for inherent immunogenicity. In this regard, the cancer-testis antigens are a distinct and unique class of differentiation antigens with high levels of expression in adult male germ cells, but generally not in other normal adult tissues, and aberrant expression in a variable proportion of a wide range of different cancer types. Among cancer-testis antigens, NY-ESO-1, initially defined by a serologic analysis of recombinant cDNA expression (SEREX) libraries in esophageal cancer, is particularly immunogenic, eliciting both cellular and humoral immune responses in a high proportion of patients with advanced NY-ESO-1–expressing ovarian cancer.[47]

The reasons for the aberrant expression of cancer-testis antigens in cancer are currently unknown. Nevertheless, the fact that the expression of these antigens is restricted to cancers, gametes, and trophoblasts suggests a link between cancer and gametogenesis. Although possible mechanisms include global demethylation and histone deacetylation, the induction of a *gametogenic* program in cancer has also been proposed.[48] Although several lines of evidence have shown that spontaneous or vaccine-induced tumor

antigen–specific T cells can recognize ovarian cancer targets, prolonged survival in patients treated with immunization has only rarely been observed. This is probably a reflection of several in vivo immunosuppressive mechanisms in tumor-bearing hosts. A recently described mechanism in ovarian cancer is the expression of inhibitory molecules such as programmed death-1 (PD-1) and lymphocyte activation gene-3 (LAG-3).[49] Together, these molecules render ovarian tumor infiltrating CD8+ T cells hyporesponsive, wherein effector function is most impaired in antigen-specific LAG-3+PD-1+CD8+ TILs.

Immunotherapy Clinical Trials in Ovarian Cancer

Several groups have launched clinical trials testing various vaccination strategies of generating antitumor immune responses, either against specific tumor antigens[50,51] or against autologous tumor lysate.[52,53] Studies on vaccination combined with immune checkpoint blockade and studies of adoptive T-cell therapy utilizing engineered T cells are ongoing at several institutions.

ENDOMETRIAL CANCER

The current concept of endometrial cancer integrates histopathology with molecular genetic mechanisms of cancer development. Two major pathogenetic variants of endometrial carcinoma, type I (endometrioid) and type II (serous), evolve via divergent pathways and different precursor lesions, different genetic abnormalities, and ultimately, different clinical outcomes parallel their distinct histology.

Type I Cancers

More than 90% of uterine cancers arise in the self-renewing glandular epithelium that lines the uterine cavity. The endometrium epithelium responds to steroid hormones with well-characterized patterns of growth and maturation critical for its role in normal reproduction. Estrogen is a well-recognized growth factor for the endometrium, promoting glandular proliferation. Subsequent exposure to the progestin-rich environment that follows ovulation results in an arrest of endometrial proliferation accompanied by glandular luteinization. Several decades of epidemiologic evidence has convincingly demonstrated that continued, unopposed exposure to estrogen is associated with an increased risk of developing endometrial cancer. These risks are particularly notable among postmenopausal women treated with estrogen-only hormone replacement. Following the introduction of hormone replacement therapy, the incidence of endometrial cancer among women in the United States rose steadily. An association between the growth-promoting effects of estrogen and endometrial carcinomas is thought to underlie the epidemiologic associations found for endometrial cancers, medical conditions such as anovulation, obesity, and other epidemiologically defined risk factors, including early age at menarche and nulliparity.

The estrogen-related endometrioid adenocarcinomas account for 80% of endometrial cancer, demonstrate a large number of genetic changes, and appear to arise via a progression pathway. Common genetic changes in this type of endometrial carcinoma include microsatellite instability (MSI), or specific mutations of *PTEN, K-ras,* and βB-catenin genes.

Microsatellite Instability

Microsatellites are short segments of repetitive DNA found predominately in noncoding DNA and scattered through the genome. The MSI phenotype is expressed in the cells with changes in the number of repeat elements as compared with normal tissue because of DNA repair error during replication. Approximately 20% of type I endometrial cancers demonstrate MSI phenotype, whereas MSI in type II cancers is very rare and is only present in less than 5% of the cases.[54] MSI is due to the inactivation of any of the mismatch repair genes and proteins: *MLH1*, *MSH2*, *MSH3*, and *MSH6*. The most common mechanism of MSI in the endometrium is inactivation of *MLH1* by epigenetic silencing of its promoter through hypermethylation of CpG islands, followed by *MSH6* mutation and *MSH3* frameshift mutations. In contrast, the MSI present in colon cancer is predominantly due to mutations in *MSH2*, followed by *MLH1* and *MSH6* mutations. MSI is an early event in type I cancers and it has been described in precancerous lesions. Once established, MSI may specifically target or inactivate genes with susceptible repeat elements, such as TGF-β1 receptors and IGFIIR, resulting in new subclones with an altered capacity to invade and metastasize.

PTEN

Inactivation of the phosphatase and tensin homolog (*PTEN*) tumor suppressor gene, located at 10q23, is the most common genetic defect in type I endometrial cancers, and it is present in more than 80% of tumors that are preceded by the histologically distinct premalignant phase.[55] The predominant *PTEN* activity is a lipid phosphatase that converts inositol triphosphates into inositol biphosphate, thus inhibiting survival and proliferative pathways that are activated by inositol triphosphatase. PTEN protein functions in maintaining G1 arrest and enabling apoptosis via an AKT-dependent mechanism. *PTEN* inactivation is caused by various mechanisms. The most common *PTEN* defect in endometrial cancer is its complete loss of function through the inactivation of both alleles. Mutations or deletions that result in loss of heterozygosity at the *PTEN* locus are also observed with high frequency. The *PTEN* mutations pattern is different in microsatellite-stable and MSI cancers. MSI tumors have a higher frequency of deletions, involving three or more base pairs, as compared with the microsatellite-stable tumors. In addition, the mutations in MSI tumors only rarely involve the polyadenine repeat of exon 8, which is the expected target.

KRAS mutations have been found in up to 30% of type I endometrial cancers. The frequency of *KRAS* mutations is particularly high in MSI-positive tumors.[56]

β-Catenin

β-Catenin (3p21) is a component of the E-cadherin–catenin complex essential for cell differentiation and maintenance of normal tissue architecture, and it also plays a role in signal transduction. The APC protein downregulates β-catenin levels, inducing the phosphorylation of serine-threonine residues coded in exon 3 of the β-catenin and its degradation via the ubiquitin–proteasome pathway. Gain of function mutations in β-catenin exon 3 are seen in 25% to 38% of type I cancers.[57] These mutations result in protein stabilization, accumulation, and transcriptional activation. β-Catenin mutations have also been found in premalignant endometrial lesions. β-Catenin changes may characterize pathways of endometrial cancer separate from *PTEN* mutations and are characterized by squamous differentiation. Several genes may be targets of the dysregulated β-catenin pathway. Although in colon cancer, elevated β-catenin levels trigger cyclin D1 expression and uncontrolled progression of tumor cells into the cell cycle, in type I endometrial cancers, β-catenin may regulate the expression of MMP-7, which has a role in the establishment of microenvironment necessary for the maintenance of tumor growth.

Type II Endometrial Cancer

The more aggressive, non-estrogen–related, nonendometrioid cancers (predominantly serous and clear cell carcinomas) are characterized by p53 mutations and Her2/neu amplification and Bcl-2 changes. These high-grade tumors are known to be associated in some cases with an identifiable intraepithelial neoplasia component. The same pattern of genetic changes is seen in the preneoplastic atrophic endometrium, suggesting that these are early events in type II tumors carcinogenesis.[58]

CERVIX, VAGINAL, AND VULVAR CANCERS

Role of Human Papillomavirus

Persistent infections with specific high-risk HPV genotypes (e.g., HPV-16, HPV-18, HPV-31, HPV-33, and HPV-45) have been identified as an essential, although not sufficient, factor in the pathogenesis of a majority of cancers of the cervix, vagina, and vulva.[59] The existence of papilloma viruses was first demonstrated by Shope[60] in the 1930s using an ultrafiltrate of warts from rabbits. Since then, papilloma viruses with an epithelial tropism have been demonstrated in nearly every mammalian species, including humans. The HPVs are encapsulated DNA viruses containing a double-stranded DNA genome of approximately 7,800 base pairs. After infecting a suitable epithelium, viral DNA replication takes place in the basal cells of the epidermis, where the HPV genome is stably retained in multiple copies, guaranteeing its persistence in the epithelium's proliferative cells. This occurs early in preneoplastic lesions, when the viral genome still persists in an episomal state. In most invasive cancers and also in a few high-grade dysplastic lesions, however, integration of high-risk HPV genomes into the host genome is observed. Integration seems to be a direct consequence of chromosomal instability and an important molecular event in the progression of preneoplastic lesions. In a review of more than 190 reported integration loci, HPV integration sites are found to be randomly distributed over the whole genome with a clear predilection for genomic fragile sites. No evidence for targeted disruption or functional alteration of critical cellular genes by the integrated viral sequences could be found.[61]

The ability of high-risk HPVs to transform human epithelia relates to the transcription of specific viral gene products. Transcription from the HPV genome occurs in two waves: an early phase with seven to eight gene products, and a late phase with two gene products (L1, L2). Early-phase gene products play a critical role in viral DNA replication (E1, E8) and in the regulation of transcription (E2, E8). In contrast, the L1 and L2 genes code for the capsid's primary and secondary proteins, respectively. The ability of different high-risk HPVs to transform human epithelia has been primarily associated with the expression of two specific viral gene products, E6 and E7. The transformation of human genital tract epithelium likely requires the expression of both E6 and E7; the transfection of human keratinocytes in vitro with either is insufficient to accomplish this phenomenon.

At a molecular level, E6 and E7 interfere with important control mechanisms of the cell cycle, apoptosis, and the maintenance of chromosomal stability by directly interacting with p53 and pRB, respectively. Moreover, recent studies demonstrated that the two viral oncoproteins cooperatively disturb the mechanisms of chromosome duplication and segregation during mitosis and thereby induce severe chromosomal instability associated with centrosome aberrations, anaphase bridges, chromosome lagging, and breaking.[62] They have also been shown to interact with a number of other cellular proteins, whose role in epithelial transformation remains unclear, including transcriptional coactivators, such as p300, and components of junctional complexes, such as hDlg1. The altered expression of hDlg1 has been observed in high-grade cervical dysplasias, which is consistent with the hypothesis that these gene products play an early role in the HPV-induced progression to cervical cancer. Specific sequence differences have been associated with different levels of risk for ultimately developing cervical cancers. For example, recent evidence demonstrates that the sequence of E6 found in Ashkenazi populations confers a protective advantage against developing cervical cancer, which was previously attributed to the practice of circumcision. Although much less understood, other early genes, such as E2, have also been implicated in the transformation.

In addition to HPV, somatic mutations in PIK3CA, PTEN, TP53, STK11, and KRAS as well as several copy-number alterations have also been implicated in the pathogenesis of cervical carcinomas. A recent study included a whole-exome sequencing analysis of 115 cervical carcinoma–normal paired samples, transcriptome sequencing of 79 cases, and whole-genome sequencing of 14 tumor-normal pairs.[63] Previously unknown somatic mutations in 79 primary squamous cell carcinomas include recurrent E322K substitutions in the MAPK1 gene (8%), inactivating mutations in the HLA-B gene (9%), and mutations in EP300 (16%), FBXW7 (15%), NFE2L2 (4%), TP53 (5%), and ERBB2 (6%) were noted. Moreover, there were somatic ELF3 (13%) and CBFB (8%) mutations in 24 adenocarcinomas.[63] Overall, squamous cell carcinomas have higher frequencies of somatic nucleotide substitutions occurring at cytosines preceded by thymines (Tp*C sites) than adenocarcinomas. HPV integration sites were found within or in close proximity to several fragile sites as well as previously reported genes, including MYC, ERBB2, TP63, FANCC, RAD51B, and CEACAM5.[63] HPV integration also occurred closer to amplified regions than expected by chance, with 21 of 51 (41%) integration sites overlapping with amplified regions, supporting the hypothesis that viral integration may trigger genome amplification. Interestingly, recurrent HPV integration into the RAD51B locus was noted in some tumors, involving HPV16, HPV18, and HPV52.[63]

Immune Evasion by Human Papillomavirus

HPV infection has a transitory pattern, whereby most individuals (70% to 90%) eliminate the virus 12 to 24 months after the initial diagnosis.[64] HPV has evolved several strategies to evade immune attack. Most obviously, papillomaviruses do not infect and replicate in antigen-presenting cells that are located in the epithelium, nor do they lyse keratinocytes, so there is no opportunity for antigen-presenting cells to engulf virions and present virion-derived antigens to the immune system. Furthermore, there is no blood- borne phase of infection, so the immune system outside of the epithelium has little opportunity to detect the virus. Additionally, HPVs have exploited the redundancy of the genetic code to keep the levels of "late" proteins low.[65] Papillomavirus capsid protein production in mammalian cells is markedly upregulated if the "viral" codons are replaced by the ones that are used by mammals, thereby limiting opportunities for the host to mount an effective immune attack. Following viral integration and subsequent malignant change, the local tumor environment at the cervical lesion is immunosuppressive. Thus, antigen-loaded dendritic cells (DCs) fail to mature, and immature DCs transmit a tolerogenic, rather than an immunogenic, signal to T cells, bearing antigen-directed T-cell receptors in draining lymph nodes.

Human Papillomavirus Vaccines

The aim of the prophylactic vaccination is to generate neutralizing antibodies against the HPV L1 and L2 capsid proteins. Prophylactic vaccine development against HPV has focused on the ability of the L1 and L2 virion structural proteins to assemble into viruslike particles (VLP). VLPs mimic the natural structure of the virion and generate a potent immune response. Because the VLPs are devoid of DNA, they are not infectious or harmful. HPV VLPs can be generated by expressing the HPV capsid protein L1 in Baculoviruses or yeast. They consist of five L1 subunits that multimerize into immunogenic pentamers. Seventy-one L1 pentamers, in turn, multimerize into an HPV VLP. Initial studies have shown that VLPs are capable of inducing high titers of neutralizing antibodies to L1 and L2 epitopes.[66] Furthermore, VLPs have proven effective at generating HPV type–specific protection from viral challenge in animal papillomavirus models.

With the approval of preventive HPV vaccines that encompass HPV-16, -18, -6, and -11, large prevention clinical trials targeting the most prevalent HPV types in different regions of the world are warranted. Questions such as the necessity of repeat vaccinations and the longevity of protection from an HPV infection remain to be determined. It is estimated that if women were vaccinated against all high-risk types of HPV before they become sexually active, there should be a reduction of at least 85% in the risk of cervical cancer and a decline of 44% to 70% in the frequency of abnormal Papanicolaou (Pap) smears attributable to HPV.[67] Unfortunately, even after vaccination is implemented, a reduction in the incidence of cervical cancer could not be expected to become apparent for at least a decade.[68] Therefore, therapeutic vaccines are still very much needed to reduce the morbidity and mortality associated with cervical cancer.

The therapeutic approach to patients with preinvasive and invasive cervical cancers is to develop vaccine strategies that induce specific CD8+ cytotoxic T-lymphocyte responses aimed at eliminating virus-infected or transformed cells. The majority of cervical cancers express the HPV-16–derived E6 and E7 oncoproteins, which are thus attractive targets for T-cell–mediated immunotherapy. Several HPV vaccine strategies have successfully elicited immune responses against HPV E6 and E7 epitopes and have prevented tumor growth on challenge with HPV-16–positive tumor cells in mice. Early-phase human trials using therapeutic vaccines have shown that they are safe; no serious adverse effects have been reported. Other approaches currently undergoing preclinical development include the use of recombinant alpha viruses such as Venezuelan equine encephalitis virus, Semliki Forest virus, and naked DNA vaccination.

SELECTED REFERENCES

The full reference list can be accessed at lwwhealthlibrary.com/oncology.

1. Dunn GP, Old LJ, Schreiber RD. The immunobiology of cancer immunosurveillance and immunoediting. *Immunity* 2004;21:137–148.
3. Levanon K, Crum C, Drapkin R. New insights into the pathogenesis of serous ovarian cancer and its clinical impact. *J Clin Oncol* 2008;26:5284–5293.
7. Schlosshauer PW, Cohen CJ, Penault-Llorca F, et al. Prophylactic oophorectomy: a morphologic and immunohistochemical study. *Cancer* 2003;98:2599–2606.
8. Callahan MJ, Crum CP, Medeiros F, et al. Primary fallopian tube malignancies in BRCA-positive women undergoing surgery for ovarian cancer risk reduction. *J Clin Oncol* 2007;25:3985–3990.
9. Tone AA, Begley H, Sharma M, et al. Gene expression profiles of luteal phase fallopian tube epithelium from BRCA mutation carriers resemble high-grade serous carcinoma. *Clin Cancer Res* 2008;14:4067–4078.
11. Ramus SJ. Current status of inherited predisposition to ovarian cancer: lessons from familial ovarian cancer registries in the UK and USA. In: Odunsi K, Pejovic T, eds. *Gynecologic Cancer: A Multidisciplinary Approach to Diagnosis and Management.* New York: Demos Medical; 2013.
13. Miki Y, Swensen J, Shattuck-Eidens D, et al. A strong candidate for the breast and ovarian cancer susceptibility gene BRCA1. *Science* 1994;266:66–71.
14. Wooster R, Bignell G, Lancaster J, et al. Identification of the breast cancer susceptibility gene BRCA2. *Nature* 1995;378:789–792.
18. Sakai W, Swisher EM, Karlan BY, et al. Secondary mutations as a mechanism of cisplatin resistance in BRCA2-mutated cancers. *Nature* 2008;451:1116–1120.
19. Walsh T, Lee MK, Casadei S, et al. Detection of inherited mutations for breast and ovarian cancer using genomic capture and massively parallel sequencing. *Proc Natl Acad Sci U S A* 2010;107:12629–12633.
21. Bradford L, Ambrosio A, Birrer MJ. PARP Inhibitors in gyecologic malignancies. In: Odunsi K, Pejovic T, eds. *Gynecologic Cancers: A Multidisciplinary Approach to Diagnosis and Management.* New York: Demos Medical; 2013.
22. Musrap N, Diamandis EP. Revisiting the complexity of the ovarian cancer microenvironment—clinical implications for treatment strategies. *Mol Cancer Res* 2012;10:1254–1264.
24. Charles KA, Kulbe H, Soper R, et al. The tumor-promoting actions of TNF-alpha involve TNFR1 and IL-17 in ovarian cancer in mice and humans. *J Clin Invest* 2009;119:3011–3023.

25. Coward J, Kulbe H, Chakravarty P, et al. Interleukin-6 as a therapeutic target in human ovarian cancer. *Clin Cancer Res* 2011;17:6083–6096.
28. Do TV, Symowicz JC, Berman DM, et al. Lysophosphatidic acid down-regulates stress fibers and up-regulates pro-matrix metalloproteinase-2 activation in ovarian cancer cells. *Mol Cancer Res* 2007;5:121–131.
32. Monk BJ, Herzog TJ, Kaye SB, et al. Trabectedin plus pegylated liposomal Doxorubicin in recurrent ovarian cancer. *J Clin Oncol* 2010;28:3107–3114.
35. Khanna M, Chelladurai B, Gavini A, et al. Targeting ovarian tumor cell adhesion mediated by tissue transglutaminase. *Mol Cancer Ther* 2011;10: 626–636.
40. Burger RA, Brady MF, Bookman MA, et al. Incorporation of bevacizumab in the primary treatment of ovarian cancer. *N Engl J Med* 2011;365:2473–2483.
42. Wei SH, Chen CM, Strathdee G, et al. Methylation microarray analysis of late-stage ovarian carcinomas distinguishes progression-free survival in patients and identifies candidate epigenetic markers. *Clin Cancer Res* 2002;8:2246–2252.
44. Zhang L, Conejo-Garcia JR, Katsaros D, et al. Intratumoral T cells, recurrence, and survival in epithelial ovarian cancer. *N Engl J Med* 2003;348: 203–213.
45. Smyth MJ, Dunn GP, Schreiber RD. Cancer immunosurveillance and immunoediting: the roles of immunity in suppressing tumor development and shaping tumor immunogenicity. *Adv Immunol* 2006;90:1–50.
47. Odunsi K, Jungbluth AA, Stockert E, et al. NY-ESO-1 and LAGE-1 cancer-testis antigens are potential targets for immunotherapy in epithelial ovarian cancer. *Cancer Res* 2003;63:6076–6083.
48. Old LJ. Cancer/testis (CT) antigens - a new link between gametogenesis and cancer. *Cancer Immun* 2001;1:1.
49. Matsuzaki J, Gnjatic S, Mhawech-Fauceglia P, et al. Tumor-infiltrating NY-ESO-1-specific CD8+ T cells are negatively regulated by LAG-3 and PD-1 in human ovarian cancer. *Proc Natl Acad Sci U S A* 2010;107:7875–7880.
50. Odunsi K, Qian F, Matsuzaki J, et al. Vaccination with an NY-ESO-1 peptide of HLA class I/II specificities induces integrated humoral and T cell responses in ovarian cancer. *Proc Natl Acad Sci U S A* 2007;104:12837–12842.
51. Odunsi K, Matsuzaki J, Karbach J, et al. Efficacy of vaccination with recombinant vaccinia and fowlpox vectors expressing NY-ESO-1 antigen in ovarian cancer and melanoma patients. *Proc Natl Acad Sci U S A* 2012;109:5797–5802.
52. Chiang CL, Kandalaft LE, Tanyi J, et al. A dendritic cell vaccine pulsed with autologous hypochlorous acid-oxidized ovarian cancer lysate primes effective broad antitumor immunity: from bench to bedside. *Clin Cancer Res* 2013;19:4801–4815.
53. Kandalaft LE, Chiang CL, Tanyi J, et al. A Phase I vaccine trial using dendritic cells pulsed with autologous oxidized lysate for recurrent ovarian cancer. *J Transl Med* 2013;11:149.
54. Mutter GL, Boynton KA, Faquin WC, et al. Allelotype mapping of unstable microsatellites establishes direct lineage continuity between endometrial precancers and cancer. *Cancer Res* 1996;56:4483–4486.
57. Mirabelli-Primdahl L, Gryfe R, Kim H, et al. Beta-catenin mutations are specific for colorectal carcinomas with microsatellite instability but occur in endometrial carcinomas irrespective of mutator pathway. *Cancer Res* 1999;59:3346–3351.
59. zur Hausen H. Papillomaviruses causing cancer: evasion from host-cell control in early events in carcinogenesis. *J Natl Cancer Inst* 2000;92:690–698.
63. Ojesina AI, Lichtenstein L, Freeman SS, et al. Landscape of genomic alterations in cervical carcinomas. *Nature* 2014;506:371–375.
64. Ho GY, Bierman R, Beardsley L, et al. Natural history of cervicovaginal papillomavirus infection in young women. *N Engl J Med* 1998;338:423–428.
67. Walboomers JM, Jacobs MV, Manos MM, et al. Human papillomavirus is a necessary cause of invasive cervical cancer worldwide. *J Pathol* 1999;189: 12–19.

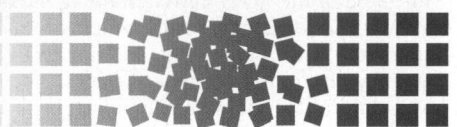

72 Cancer of the Cervix, Vagina, and Vulva

Ann H. Klopp, Patricia J. Eifel, Jonathan S. Berek, and Panagiotis A. Konstantinopoulos

CARCINOMA OF THE VAGINA

Carcinomas of the vagina are rare, accounting for only about 2% of gynecologic malignancies. The American Cancer Society estimated that in the United States in 2014, 3,170 new cases of invasive vaginal cancer will be diagnosed and there will be 880 deaths due to vaginal cancer.[1] According to the International Federation of Gynecology and Obstetrics (FIGO), cases should be classified as vaginal carcinomas only when "the primary site of the growth is in the vagina."[2] Any tumor that has extended to the cervical portio and has reached the area of the external os should be classified as a cervical carcinoma, and a tumor that has extended from the vulva to involve the vagina should be classified as a primary vulvar cancer.[2] In patients with an intact uterus, it is probable that many tumors that originate in the apical vagina are classified as cervical cancers because they have reached the area of the external os by the time of diagnosis. This may explain why a large percentage (30% to 50%) of patients diagnosed with vaginal carcinoma have previously undergone hysterectomy, which prevents classification of tumors as primary cervical cancers.[3,4]

More commonly, the vagina is a site of metastasis, direct extension, or recurrence of tumors originating in other genital sites, such as the cervix or endometrium, or from extragenital sites, including the rectum and bladder.

Epidemiology

Vaginal intraepithelial neoplasia (VAIN) often accompanies cervical intraepithelial neoplasia (CIN) and is thought to have a similar etiology.[5] Kalogirou et al.[6] found 41 cases of VAIN in 993 patients followed with cytologic examination and colposcopy after hysterectomy for CIN. Most VAIN lesions were in the upper vagina, particularly in the vault angles of the suture line.

Investigators have reported a human papillomavirus (HPV) infection rate of 60% to 65% in women with vaginal carcinoma.[7] Population-based studies indicate that the prevalence of HPV infection is similar in the vaginas of women who have undergone hysterectomy and the cervixes of women who still have their uterus.[8] The much lower rate of carcinoma in the vagina is thought to reflect the fact that the vagina does not have a transformation zone of immature epithelial cells susceptible to transformation; HPV-induced vaginal lesions are thought to arise in areas of squamous metaplasia that develop during healing of mucosal abrasions caused by coitus, tampon use, chronic pessary use, or other trauma.[5] Most vaginal cancers arising in patients who used pessaries are located in the posterior wall.[9] Pelvic irradiation might be a predisposing factor in some cases of vaginal cancer.[10] However, viral and other nontreatment-related factors probably play a role in the etiology of vaginal cancers that arise after treatment of another malignancy.

Primary invasive carcinoma of the vagina is predominantly a disease of elderly women; 70% to 80% of cases are diagnosed in women older than 60 years.[11] Except for clear cell carcinomas, which are associated with maternal diethylstilbestrol (DES) exposure, invasive vaginal carcinomas are extremely rare in women younger than 40 years.[2,11] African American women have been reported to have significantly poorer survival compared with whites when controlling for age, histology, stage, grade, and treatment modality.

In 1971, Herbst et al.[12] first reported a highly significant association between clear cell carcinoma of the vagina and maternal ingestion of DES during pregnancy. The peak number of DES-associated cases occurred in 1975, when 33 cases were reported to a US registry.[12] The peak risk period for exposed women in the United States was between the ages of 15 and 22 years; few cases were diagnosed after the age of 40 years. Obesity, oral contraceptive use, and pregnancy were suggested as possible risk factors for development of clear cell carcinoma in DES-exposed women, but larger case-matched studies generally failed to confirm these associations.[13] Infection with HPV may be a cofactor in some cases. Among 14 cases of clear cell carcinoma studied by Waggoner et al.,[14] 3 contained HPV-31 DNA; 10 of the remaining HPV-negative tumors had p53 protein detected by immunohistochemistry, suggesting a TP53 gene mutation.

DES-related clear cell carcinomas appear to have a better prognosis with less likelihood of distant metastasis than other vaginal adenocarcinomas. Because many DES-exposed women with clear cell carcinoma were young at the time of diagnosis, treatment of early lesions has emphasized preservation of vaginal and ovarian function. Senekjian et al.[15] reported successful treatment of early lesions with excision or local radiotherapy only. However, retroperitoneal lymphadenectomy may be indicated when local treatment is considered for stage I lesions, which are reported to have an overall rate of pelvic lymph node metastases of 15% to 20%.[16]

There is as yet no evidence that DES-exposed women are at risk for genital tract malignancies other than clear cell carcinoma,[17] although recent studies suggest that they may have an increased risk of developing breast cancer after the age of 40 years.[18,19]

Natural History and Pattern of Spread

Approximately 50% of vaginal cancers arise in the upper third of the vagina, and there is a fairly even distribution of lesions arising on the anterior, posterior, and lateral walls. Tumors may exhibit an exophytic or ulcerative, infiltrating pattern of growth.

Tumors may invade directly to involve adjacent structures such as the urethra, bladder, and rectum, although <10% of vaginal cancers are found to be stage IVA (spread to adjacent organs and/or direct extension beyond the true pelvis) at presentation.[4,20,21]

Vaginal cancers may also spread laterally to the paravaginal space and pelvic wall. Although tumors arising in the vagina undoubtedly can spread superiorly to involve the cervix and uterus, such tumors are usually classified as cervical cancers according to FIGO criteria.

The vagina is supplied with a fine anastomosing network of lymphatics in the mucosa and submucosa. Despite the continuity of lymphatic vessels within the vagina, Plentl and Friedman[22]

found a regular pattern of regional drainage from specific regions of the vagina. The lymphatics of the vaginal vault communicate with those of the lower cervix, draining laterally to the obturator and hypogastric nodes. The lymphatics of the posterior wall anastomose with those of the anterior rectal wall, draining to the superior and inferior gluteal nodes. The lymphatics of the lower third of the vagina communicate with those of the vulva and drain either to the pelvic nodes or to the inguinofemoral lymph nodes.

Few data are available concerning the incidence of spread of vaginal cancer to the pelvic lymph nodes. However, studies suggest that the incidence of positive pelvic nodes in patients with stage II disease is at least 25% to 30%, emphasizing the importance of regional treatment for these patients.[23]

The most frequent site of hematogenous metastasis is the lung. Less frequently, vaginal cancers may metastasize to liver, bone, or other sites.[2,4]

Pathology

Eighty to ninety percent of primary vaginal malignancies are squamous cell carcinomas.[24] Grossly, these tumors may be nodular, ulcerative, exophytic, or form plaques. Histologically, they are similar to squamous tumors at other sites. Approximately one-third of vaginal squamous cell carcinomas are keratinizing, and more than half are nonkeratinizing, moderately differentiated lesions.

Approximately 5% to 10% of primary vaginal neoplasms are adenocarcinomas.[24,25] The differential diagnosis of adenocarcinoma occurring in the vagina is often difficult, as it must be distinguished from metastatic tumors originating at other sites. Histologic patterns include clear cell, mucinous, adenosquamous, papillary, and undifferentiated. During the 1970s and 1980s, clear cell carcinomas of the vagina were sometimes seen in young women in association with maternal DES exposure. Today, these are extremely rare, and most adenocarcinomas occur in postmenopausal women. The prognosis of patients with adenocarcinoma appears to be poorer than that of patients with squamous carcinoma of the vagina.[26]

Primary small cell carcinomas of the vagina are very rare, with <30 cases reported in the literature.[26] They are histologically indistinguishable from neuroendocrine small cell carcinomas of the lung or cervix and, like these tumors, may coexist with squamous or adenocarcinoma elements.

Primary vaginal melanomas represent about 3% of primary vaginal cancers and <20% of genital melanomas.[24] Primary vaginal melanomas are thought to arise from melanocytes in areas of melanosis or atypical melanocytic hyperplasia. They usually originate in the distal third of the vagina and occur at a mean age of 55 years. Vaginal melanomas tend to be associated with a poorer prognosis than vulvar melanomas; 5-year survival rates are 15% to 20% after treatment with surgery, radiation, or both.[27]

About 3% of vaginal cancers are sarcomas; about two-thirds of these are leiomyosarcomas, but endometrial stromal sarcomas, malignant mixed Müllerian tumors, and other types have been reported.[28] Embryonal rhabdomyosarcoma (sarcoma botryoides) is a highly malignant sarcoma that occurs in girls, usually before 6 years of age. This tumor usually forms soft nodules that fill and protrude from the vagina. The prognosis for children with this tumor has improved with the use of appropriate multimodality therapy.[29]

Diagnosis, Clinical Evaluation, and Staging

Most patients with VAIN and about 10% to 20% of patients with invasive vaginal carcinoma are asymptomatic at presentation; in these cases, carcinoma is usually diagnosed during investigation of an abnormal Papanicolaou (Pap) smear finding. Colposcopic evaluation in the case of abnormal cytologic findings should always include a detailed examination of the entire vagina and cervix, even when there is an obvious cervical lesion, because patients can present with multiple areas of abnormality. Women who have persistent positive Pap smear findings after treatment of CIN should be examined carefully for VAIN.

About 50% to 60% of patients with invasive vaginal cancer present with abnormal vaginal bleeding. Patients may also present with complaints of vaginal discharge, a palpable mass, dyspareunia, or pain in the perineum or pelvis.[4,20,30]

The initial workup of patients with vaginal cancer should include a pelvic examination including thorough visualization of the entire vagina. Examination under anesthesia can be useful to ensure adequate visualization of the full extent of disease and to place marker seeds to delineate the extent of involvement for brachytherapy planning. All patients should have chest radiography, a complete blood cell count, and a biochemical profile. Computed tomography (CT) is useful to evaluate for possible regional spread and to evaluate the kidneys but usually does not provide accurate information about the extent of primary disease. Magnetic resonance imaging (MRI) provides much more detailed information about the extent of paravaginal infiltration but frequently underestimates the extent of superficial vaginal involvement, which is often better appreciated on pelvic examination. 18-Fluorodeoxyglucose (FDG)–positron emission tomography (PET)/CT is useful to evaluate for evidence of nodal involvement. If involvement of adjacent structures is suspected on physical examination or imaging, further evaluation with cystoscopy, ureteroscopy, and/or proctoscopy is recommended.

The FIGO stage categories for vaginal cancers are listed in Table 72.1.[2] Because this is a clinical staging system, the classification of lesions as stage I or II tends to be somewhat subjective. In general, thin (<0.5 cm), relatively exophytic tumors tend to be classified as stage I, and thicker, infiltrating tumors and those with obvious paravaginal nodularity tend to be classified as stage II.

FIGO recommendations for staging of disease associated with positive lymph nodes are somewhat ambiguous.[2,31] Although clinical staging is recommended, with rules similar to those used for cervical cancer (e.g., disallowing use of imaging or surgical information about lymph node involvement in assignment of stage), the most recent FIGO manual quoted stage groupings based on nodal involvement. A more specific method of nodal evaluation is elaborated in the American Joint Committee on Cancer staging manual,[31] which suggests options for pathologic or clinical TNM

TABLE 72.1

International Federation of Gynecology and Obstetrics Clinical Staging of Carcinoma of the Vagina

Stage	Description
0	Carcinoma in situ, intraepithelial carcinoma.
I	The carcinoma is limited to the vaginal wall.
II	The carcinoma has involved the subvaginal tissues but has not extended onto the pelvic wall.
III	The carcinoma has extended onto the pelvic wall.
IV	The carcinoma has extended beyond the true pelvis or has clinically involved the mucosa of the bladder or rectum. Bullous edema as such does not permit a case to be allotted to stage IV.
IVA	Spread of the growth to adjacent organs and/or direct extension beyond the true pelvis.
IVB	Spread to distant organs.

(tumor, node, metastases) staging. According to the American Joint Committee on Cancer, results of biopsy or fine needle aspiration of lymph nodes may be included in the clinical staging[31]; FIGO states that such results can be used for treatment planning only.[2] Although the FIGO system could be interpreted to assign patients who have clinically evident inguinal involvement to stage IV, patients with inguinal metastases are sometimes cured with locoregional treatment; Kucera and Vavra[30] reported uncorrected 5-year survival rates of 29% for patients with clinically suspicious inguinal nodes and 44% for patients with clinically negative groins.

Prognostic Factors

The rates of local control, distant metastasis, and survival in vaginal carcinoma are all correlated strongly with FIGO stage (Table 72.2).[4,20,21,30] Tumor size also is an important predictor of outcome.[4,20,21,32]

Most investigators have been unable to find a correlation between tumor site and outcome.[20,21,33] However, tumors that involve the entire vagina tend to be associated with a poorer prognosis, probably reflecting the larger size of these lesions. Exophytic tumors may be associated with a better prognosis than infiltrating or necrotic lesions.[21]

Frank et al.[25] reported significantly poorer survival and pelvic disease control rates for patients with non–DES-related adenocarcinomas than for patients with squamous cell carcinomas; at 5 years, the overall survival and pelvic disease control rates were 34% and 39%, respectively, for patients with adenocarcinomas versus 58% and 81%, respectively, for patients with squamous carcinomas of the vagina. Although other investigators[20,34] found no difference in outcome between patients with squamous carcinoma and those with adenocarcinoma, this may reflect inclusion of DES-related clear cell carcinomas, which appear to be associated with a better prognosis than other adenocarcinomas.[15]

Treatment

Technical aspects of the treatment of vaginal cancer are highly specialized and vary widely according to the site, size, and distribution of tumor within the vagina and adjacent structures. To achieve the best results for patients with these rare cancers, treatment should be delivered at a center that has a strong multidisciplinary team, including a radiation oncologist well versed in the specialized brachytherapy and external beam techniques used to treat these cancers.

Vaginal Intraepithelial Neoplasia

Patients with only HPV infection, or VAIN 1, do not require treatment. These lesions often regress spontaneously, are frequently multifocal, and recur quickly after attempts at ablative therapy. VAIN 2 may be treated with observation or topical estrogen. The malignant potential of VAIN 1–2 is uncertain. However, VAIN 3 may progress to an invasive lesion. Thus, when VAIN 3 is found, a careful evaluation should be done to rule out the presence of occult invasive disease.

VAIN 3 lesions that have been adequately sampled to rule out invasion can be treated with laser ablation. Cryosurgery should not be used in the vagina because the depth of injury cannot be controlled and inadvertent injury to the bladder or rectum may occur. Superficial fulguration with electrosurgical ball cautery may be used under careful colposcopic control. Local excision is an excellent method of treatment for small upper vaginal lesions. Intravaginal 5-fluorouracil (5-FU) has been used to treat patients who have persistent disease after resection.

Most authors report that about 5% to 10% of patients who undergo excision of VAIN develop subsequent invasive cancers,[35,36] and Hoffman et al.[5] reported finding occult invasive disease in upper vaginectomy specimens from 9 of 32 patients (28%) who had surgery for VAIN 3. These risks are sufficient to warrant close follow-up of patients treated for VAIN.

VAIN can also be treated effectively with intracavitary brachytherapy,[20,21,34] but this treatment is usually reserved for patients with multifocal, multiply recurrent disease or high operative risk. Although most experiences have been with low-dose-rate (LDR) brachytherapy, MacLeod et al.[37] reported a high control rate without major complications using high-dose-rate (HDR) intracavitary brachytherapy; the vaginal surface was treated with a total dose of 34 to 45 Gy in 4 to 10 fractions. In contrast, Ogino et al.[38] reported adhesive vaginitis and rectal bleeding in two patients treated to the entire vagina with a less conservative HDR fractionation schedule.

TABLE 72.2

Carcinoma of the Vagina: Survival Rates According to Clinical Stage

	Stage I		Stage II		Stage III		Stage IV		
Study (Ref.)	No. of Patients	Survival (%)	No. of Patients	Survival (%)	No. of Patients	Survival (%)	No. of Patients	Survival (%)	Calculation Method
Perez et al.[21]	59	80	64 (IIa)[a] 34 (IIb)	55 35	20	38	15	0	10-y, actuarial, disease free
Davis et al.[23]	44	82	45	53					5-y, actuarial, uncorrected
Eddy et al.[3]	25	73	39	39	15	38	12	25	5-y, actuarial, corrected
Kucera and Vavra[30]	73	77	110	45	174	31	77	14	5-y, crude, uncorrected
Kirkbride et al.[20]	40	77	38	78	42	60	19	41	5-y, actuarial, cause-specific
Chyle et al.[34]	59	55 76	104	51 69	55	37 47	16	40 27	10-y, actuarial, uncorrected 10-y freedom from relapse
Stock et al.[32]	23	67	58	53	9	0	10	15	5-y, actuarial, disease-free
Frank et al.[4]	50	85	97	78	46[b]	58[b]			5-y, actuarial, disease-specific

[a] IIa, paravaginal submucosal extension only; IIb, parametrial involvement.
[b] Stages III and IVA combined.

Stage I Disease

Radiotherapy is often the treatment of choice for stage I disease because if surgery is used, total vaginectomy or even exenteration may be needed to obtain satisfactory resection margins. However, surgery has a definite role in selected cases.[23,32] Early tumors that involve the upper posterior vagina can be removed with a radical hysterectomy and partial (proximal) vaginectomy if the uterus is intact or with a radical upper (proximal) vaginectomy if the patient has previously undergone hysterectomy; in both situations, bilateral pelvic lymphadenectomy is also performed. For patients with a prior history of pelvic irradiation, radical surgery (usually pelvic exenteration) is indicated and is often curative.

Disease-specific survival rates for patients with stage I disease treated with definitive irradiation range from 75% to 95%.[4,21,30,39] Although some authors have suggested that selected patients with small, very superficial tumors may be treated with brachytherapy alone,[21] others have noted unacceptable rates of paravaginal recurrence after treatment with brachytherapy alone and suggest that external beam irradiation should be used to treat at least the distal pelvis.[4] Thicker stage I tumors always should be treated with a combination of external beam irradiation and brachytherapy with an aim to deliver 40 to 50 Gy to the pelvic nodes and 70 to 75 Gy to the tumor.

Stage II Disease

Because investigators rarely define their criteria for distinguishing stage I from stage II vaginal carcinoma or for selecting patients for various treatments, different institutional experiences cannot easily be compared. Disease-specific survival rates for patients with stage II disease range from 50% to 80%. To control possible regional disease, patients with stage II disease should receive 40 to 50 Gy to the whole pelvis delivered using conventional fields or intensity-modulated radiotherapy (IMRT). This should be followed by additional irradiation of sites of initial gross disease.[4] In most cases, brachytherapy is used to supplement the dose to the primary vaginal tumor site. Perez et al.[21] achieved pelvic tumor control in only 4 of 11 patients (36%) with stage II tumors treated with brachytherapy alone, compared with 54 of 81 patients (67%) treated with a combination of external beam irradiation and brachytherapy.[21]

Brachytherapy should be tailored to the volume and distribution of the tumor and its response to external beam irradiation. For apical tumors that flatten to <5 mm in thickness, the dose to the vagina may be boosted using intracavitary sources in a vaginal cylinder, although interstitial brachytherapy or conformal external beam techniques may still be useful in selected cases. Examination under anesthesia, transvaginal sonography, or MRI may be helpful in evaluation of disease extent for treatment planning. Larger tumors usually require a boost with interstitial brachytherapy or with additional external beam irradiation (taking into account the influence of internal organ motion on external beam radiation doses). Most authors emphasize the importance of brachytherapy in the treatment of vaginal cancer.[21,39] However, brachytherapy must be designed to treat the entire vaginal tumor. Frank et al.[4] argue that tumors that cannot be covered adequately with brachytherapy can often be cured with external beam irradiation alone using carefully designed conformal fields.

Selected patients with stage II disease may be cured with radical surgery.[32] However, total radical vaginectomy or pelvic exenteration is often required to remove the tumor, and results with radical surgery do not appear to be better than those with radiotherapy alone. Primary radical surgery is usually indicated for patients who have previously had pelvic radiotherapy.

Stage III and IVA Disease

Reported 5-year disease-specific survival rates range from 30% to 60% for patients with stage III disease and from 15% to 40% for patients with stage IVA disease.[4,20,21,30] Stage III and IVA tumors are usually bulky, highly infiltrative lesions involving most or all of the vagina as well as the pelvic wall, bladder, or rectum. The extent of these tumors and the proximity of critical normal tissue structures make their management a formidable technical challenge. Pelvic recurrence rates are high in many series; the risk of distant metastasis is also relatively high, although distant relapse is often accompanied by locoregional recurrence.

All patients require treatment with external beam irradiation. Most authors advocate the use of brachytherapy whenever possible. However, Frank et al.[4] reported a high disease-specific survival rate (58% at 5 years) in a series of patients with stage III and IVA disease in which the majority of patients (31 of 46) were treated with external beam irradiation alone. Brachytherapy is undoubtedly an important part of disease management in some patients. However, in certain cases, interstitial brachytherapy does not provide adequate coverage of tumors that are very large and intimately associated with critical structures. In these cases, it may be appropriate to place greater emphasis on external beam treatment. Conformal radiotherapy techniques such as IMRT may help to increase the dose to tumor while limiting the dose to critical structures.

For selected patients with relatively small, mobile stage IVA cancers who are in otherwise good medical condition, pelvic exenteration with vaginal reconstruction using a gracilis myocutaneous flap or rectus abdominis myocutaneous flap may be the treatment of choice, particularly if a rectovaginal or vesicovaginal fistula is present.[40] Radical radiotherapy is also curative in some cases; Frank et al.[4] reported an 86% pelvic control rate in seven patients treated with radiotherapy for stage IVA disease.

Radiotherapy Technique

Pelvic external beam fields must be individualized according to the primary tumor site and potential sites of regional spread. Radiopaque markers placed at the distal edge of the tumor help to define the lower border and facilitate studies of internal organ motion. Treating the patient in an open ("frog-leg") position can often reduce the severity of vulvar cutaneous reactions when coverage of distal lesions necessitates inclusion of the introitus in the radiation field.

When tumors involve the distal third of the vagina, pelvic fields should be designed to include at least the medial inguinal-femoral lymph nodes. When four fields are used to treat the pelvis, care must be taken to cover all the draining lymph nodes. Lateral fields should adequately cover posterior perirectal nodes, particularly when the primary lesion involves the posterior vaginal wall.

Intracavitary brachytherapy is of limited value in the treatment of locally advanced vaginal cancer because the dose falls off very rapidly from the surface of a vaginal cylinder. In general, the dose at a 5-mm depth is only 60% to 70% of the dose at the vaginal surface. Interstitial brachytherapy can provide better coverage of thick vaginal tumors. Vaginal implants can be inserted freehand. Successful use of this technique requires experience, but direct palpation during needle insertion permits excellent control of the position of sources with respect to the vaginal surface and rectal mucosa (Fig. 72.1). Vaginal implants may also be positioned using a perineal template. This technique provides a more homogeneous dose distribution because it facilitates parallel positioning of sources, but the template interferes somewhat with the ability of the brachytherapist to monitor the placement of needles with respect to the rectal and vaginal mucosa. When tumors involve the vaginal apex in patients who have had a hysterectomy, laparoscopic or laparotomy guidance may be needed to ensure accurate needle placement.

Interstitial needles can be placed transperineally while monitoring the position of the needles by direct palpation with fingers in the vagina and rectum. A plastic cylinder in the vagina can be

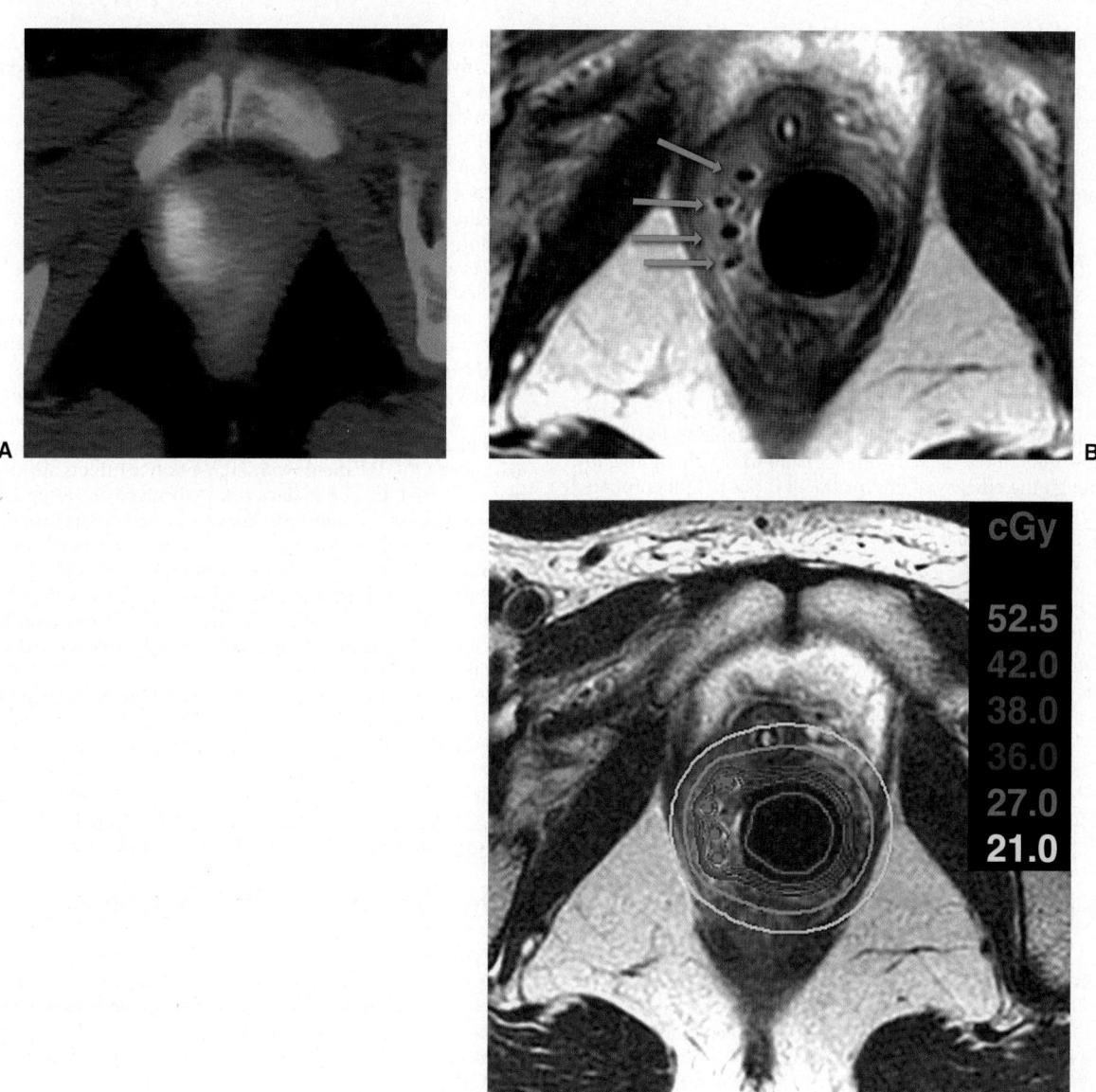

Figure 72.1 Interstitial implant of a squamous carcinoma involving the right lateral walls of the vagina. Positron emission tomography **(A)** demonstrated uptake in right lateral wall of vagina. After 50 Gy of external beam radiation with weekly cisplatin, four interstitial needles were placed in the right lateral vaginal wall which could be visualized on magnetic resonance imaging (*blue arrows* shown in **B**). **(C)** Brachytherapy treatment plan was optimized to deliver 26 Gy over 72 hours to the residual disease. Isodose contours represent the dose rates (in centigray per hour) delivered to tissues in the axial plane at the approximate center of the implant.

used to displace uninvolved tissues away from the needles, which are loaded with iridium-192 (^{192}Ir) sources. MRI after placement of MRI-compatible applicators allows visualization of residual tumor and can be used to shape the dose distribution.

Efforts to correlate radiation dose with tumor control have yielded inconsistent results and may be misleading because the total dose of radiation prescribed for a vaginal tumor is often influenced by the tumor's size, extent, and initial response to irradiation, all of which determine the feasibility of delivering high-dose brachytherapy.[4,21,39] When good brachytherapy coverage of the tumor can be accomplished, an effort should be made to treat the tumor to a dose of 75 to 85 Gy. When brachytherapy is not possible, some patients may be cured with external beam irradiation alone using shrinking pelvic fields or IMRT to deliver a tumor dose of 60 to 70 Gy. Treatment can usually be completed in <6 to 7 weeks and should not be protracted unnecessarily. Lee et al.[41] reported a significantly lower pelvic

recurrence rate in patients whose entire treatment course was completed in ≤9 weeks.

Complications of Radiotherapy

The close proximity of the bladder and rectum to the vagina makes them vulnerable to damage when invasive vaginal cancers are treated with radiotherapy. In their review of 193 patients treated with definitive irradiation, Frank et al.[4] reported a 10% actuarial incidence of serious complications at 5 years. The most frequent complications were proctitis, hemorrhagic cystitis, and fistulae. Complication rates were significantly correlated with FIGO stage and with a history of smoking; major complications rates were 4%, 9%, and 21% for patients with stage I, II, or III–IVA disease, respectively. Other authors have reported similar major complication rates.[20,21,30] There have been no comprehensive studies of vaginal function in women with vaginal cancer treated with radiotherapy, although some degree of vaginal stenosis or shortening is common.[20] The severity of vaginal morbidity is probably related to the damage to vaginal mucosa and submucosa from tumor infiltration, ulceration, and infection; the age and menopausal status of the patient; and the radiation dose and the amount of vaginal tissue treated to high doses.

Role of Chemotherapy

Because primary vaginal carcinomas are rare, few reports have specifically addressed the role of chemotherapy in the treatment of this disease. Chemotherapeutic management is usually based on extrapolations from experience with the treatment of carcinomas of the cervix. For this reason, patients who have metastatic or recurrent vaginal carcinoma that is no longer amenable to local treatment are sometimes treated with cisplatin-based chemotherapy, even though the efficacy of this treatment is not well documented in the literature. Thigpen et al.[42] noted several responses among 16 patients with vaginal cancers treated with cisplatin (50 mg/m² every 3 weeks).

Because vaginal carcinoma resembles cervical carcinoma in its location, pattern of spread, histologic appearance, relationship to HPV infection, and response to radiotherapy, it may be reasonable to extrapolate from randomized trials demonstrating a benefit from concurrent chemoradiation in patients with locally advanced cervical cancer to justify a similar approach in selected patients with high-risk invasive vaginal cancer.[43,44] A retrospective analysis of 71 patients treated with or without chemotherapy for vaginal cancer found that chemotherapy delivery concurrent with radiation was independently predictor of survival.[45]

CARCINOMA OF THE VULVA

Epidemiology

Invasive vulvar carcinoma is a rare disease that accounts for about 4% of gynecologic cancers.[46,47] The American Cancer Society estimated that in the United States in 2014, 4,850 new cases of invasive vulvar cancer will be diagnosed and there will be 1,030 deaths due to vulvar cancer.[1] The median age at diagnosis of patients with invasive vulvar cancer is about 65 to 70 years. In contrast, vulvar intraepithelial neoplasia (VIN) tends to occur in younger women; the median age at diagnosis of women with VIN is 45 to 50 years. The incidence of VIN has more than doubled since the early 1970s.[46,47] This increase has been particularly marked in

women younger than 55 years. In the past, the incidence of invasive vulvar cancer was thought to be stable; however, recent data suggest that the median age of women presenting with invasive vulvar cancer may be decreasing, probably reflecting an increase in HPV-related vulvar cancers in young women.[48] This change has also been associated with an increase in the proportion of vulvar cancers involving the periurethral and clitoral region rather than the labia.[48]

Only 30% to 50% of invasive vulvar carcinomas are associated with evidence of HPV infection.[49,50] However, 80% to 90% of VIN lesions contain HPV-16 or other HPV types. On the basis of these statistics, it has been estimated that HPV vaccination could prevent about half of the vulvar carcinomas in young women and about two-thirds of the VIN lesions.

HPV-positive vulvar cancers are usually basaloid or warty carcinomas with little keratin formation, are often associated with VIN, are frequently multifocal, and tend to occur in younger women (35 to 55 years).[48,49,51] Patients with HPV-positive tumors are also more likely to have CIN and to have risk factors typically associated with cervical cancer.[51] In contrast, HPV-negative tumors usually occur in older women (55 to 85 years), are often associated with vulvar inflammation or lichen sclerosis (but rarely with VIN), are generally unifocal, and are usually well differentiated with exuberant keratin formation.[52,53] Although a number of investigators have reported this distinct grouping of patients with vulvar cancer, others have found greater overlap.[54]

Several investigators have reported a high incidence of TP53 mutations in HPV-negative tumors.[55,56] Lee et al.[55] found missense mutations of TP53 in 4 of 9 (44%) HPV-negative tumors but in only 1 of 12 (8%) HPV-positive tumors. They postulated that alteration in *p53* activity, either through point mutations or through E6-mediated loss of *p53* function in HPV-infected cells, could be important in the development of vulvar neoplasms.

Natural History and Pattern of Spread

The vulva includes the mons pubis, labia majora, labia minora, clitoris, vestibular bulb, vestibular glands (including Bartholin glands), and vestibule of the vagina. The region between the posterior commissure of the labia and the anus is termed the *gynecologic perineum*. About 70% of vulvar squamous carcinomas involve the labia majora or minora, most frequently the labia majora. Vulvar tumors may extend locally to invade adjacent structures, including the vagina, urethra, and anus; advanced vulvar tumors may invade adjacent pelvic bones.

A rich network of anastomosing lymphatics that frequently cross the midline drains the vulva. Even minimally invasive vulvar tumors may spread to regional lymph nodes (Table 72.3).[57–61] For most lesions, initial regional metastasis is to the inguinal lymph

---

TABLE 72.3

Relationship Between Depth of Stromal Invasion and Inguinal Lymph Node Metastases in Patients with Squamous Cell Carcinoma of the Vulva

Study (Ref.)	≤1.0	1.1–2.0	2.1–3.0	3.1–5.0	≤5
No. of Patients with Positive Lymph Nodes/Total No. of Patients by Depth of Invasion (mm)					
Binder et al.[58]	0/7	0/23	3/14	6/25	15/31
Ross and Ehrmann[61]	0/17	1/9	1/13	4/15	0/1
Hoffman et al.[60]	0/24	0/19	2/17	8/15	7/13
Hacker et al.[59]	0/34	2/19	2/17	1/7	3/7
Andreasson and Nyboe[57]	0/8	1/13	3/12	5/32	19/57
Total	0/90	4/83 (5%)	11/73 (15%)	24/94 (26%)	44/109 (40%)

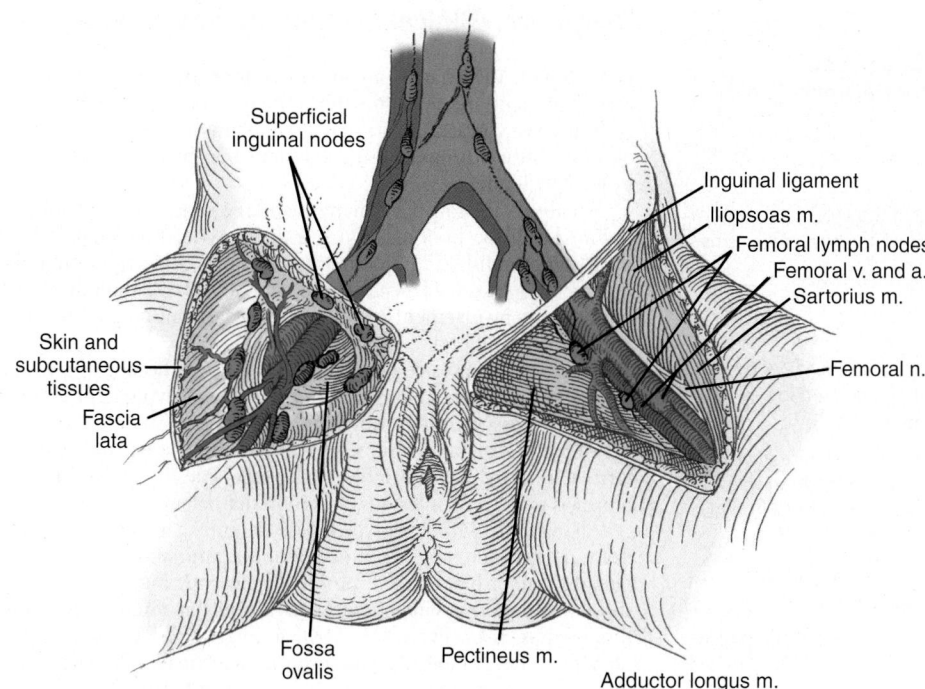

Figure 72.2 Inguinal-femoral lymph nodes.

nodes that are superficial to Camper's fascia; tumors may then metastasize secondarily to deeper femoral lymph nodes and to the pelvic lymph nodes (Fig. 72.2). However, some lesions, particularly those involving the clitoris and other medial structures, metastasize directly to medial femoral lymph nodes that lie in the region of the fossa ovalis, a gap in the cribriform fascia.[62] Theoretically, tumors involving the clitoris can spread directly to the obturator nodes through lymphatics that follow the dorsal vein of the clitoris, although evidence of this route is rarely seen in practice. Despite the extensive anastomosis of lymphatics in the region, metastasis of vulvar carcinoma to contralateral lymph nodes is uncommon in patients with well-lateralized T1 lesions. The lungs are the most common sites of hematogenous metastasis.

Pathology

As classified by the International Society for the Study of Vulvar Disease, nonneoplastic epithelial disorders of the vulva (previously termed *vulvar dystrophies*) include lichen sclerosis, squamous hyperplasia, and other dermatoses.[63] About 10% of these lesions have cellular atypia and are termed *vulvar intraepithelial neoplasia*. Histologically, VIN is characterized by disruption of the normal epithelial architecture, varying degrees of cytoplasmic and nuclear maturation, and giant cells with abnormal nuclei.[49] VIN lesions are assigned a grade from 1 to 3 according to their degree of maturation. The most common VINs contain nuclear atypia throughout the epithelial layers and are frequently associated with HPV.[49] A second subset of VINs have atypia that is largely confined to the basal layers of the epithelium. These lesions tend to occur in older women and are not usually associated with HPV but are commonly adjacent to areas of lichen sclerosis or hyperplasia. Buscema and Woodruff[64] estimated that approximately 4% of patients treated for VIN develop a subsequent invasive cancer.

Paget disease of the vulva, a rare intraepithelial lesion located in the epidermis and skin adnexa, accounts for 1% to 5% of vulvar neoplasms. Histologically, vulvar Paget disease is characterized by large, pale, mucopolysaccharide-rich cells that are positive for periodic acid-Schiff. The lesions are usually negative for HPV.[65] Electron microscopic studies have suggested that Paget cells derive from apocrine cells in the stratum germinativum of the epidermis.[66] Paget disease usually occurs in postmenopausal women, who

often present with symptoms of vulvar pruritus and discomfort.[67] Grossly, Paget lesions appear eczematoid or, when extensive, may be raised and velvety with persistent weeping. About 5% to 10% of newly diagnosed Paget lesions are associated with underlying adenocarcinoma arising locally in a vulvar vestibular gland or skin appendage or from a distant site such as the breast or rectum.[67]

The term *microinvasive carcinoma of the vulva* should be used with caution. Stromal invasion by vulvar carcinomas is not measured in a uniform manner, and strict criteria for the diagnosis of microinvasive vulvar cancer have not been defined. VIN is not routinely seen adjacent to invasive vulvar cancer, and the transition from normal tissue to invasive cancer can be abrupt. Elongated rete pegs may extend 6 mm or more from the basement membrane and are sometimes misconstrued as invasive cancer. The International Society of Gynecologic Pathologists recommends that the depth of stromal invasion be measured vertically from the most superficial basement membrane to the deepest extent of tumor. Tumor thickness is defined as the distance between the granular layer of the epidermis and the deepest extent of tumor. Lymph node metastases from tumors <1 mm in depth or thickness are extremely rare (see Table 72.3). For this reason, FIGO now includes in its vulvar carcinoma staging system a stage IA subcategory for tumors that invade no more than 1 mm (Table 72.4).[68] However, the risk of inguinal lymph node metastasis rises steeply as the depth of invasion exceeds 1 mm.

More than 90% of invasive vulvar cancers are squamous cell carcinomas. Atypical keratinization is the hallmark of invasive vulvar cancer. Most squamous cell carcinomas are well differentiated, but mitoses may be noted. About 5% of vulvar cancers are anaplastic carcinomas, which may consist of large immature cells, spindle sarcomatoid cells, or small cells. Vulvar carcinomas consisting of small cells may resemble small cell anaplastic carcinomas of the lung or Merkel cell tumors, and have demonstrated an aggressive biologic behavior in the few reported cases.[69]

The diagnosis of Bartholin gland carcinoma is based on clinical findings of a tumor arising in the anatomic location of Bartholin glands and on the histologic appearance. Biopsy of a tumor arising from a Bartholin gland usually reveals squamous cell carcinoma, but adenocarcinoma, transitional cell carcinomas (arising from the duct and histologically indistinguishable from transitional cell carcinoma of the bladder), and adenoid cystic carcinomas have also been reported.

International Federation of Gynecology and Onstetrics Staging of Carcinoma of the Vulva (2009)

Stage	Description
I	Tumor confined to the vulva.
IA	Lesions ≤2 cm in size, confined to the vulva or perineum and with stromal invasion ≤1 mm,[a] no nodal metastasis.
IB	Lesions >2 cm in size or with stromal invasion >1 mm,[a] confined to the vulva or perineum, with negative nodes.
II	Tumor of any size with extension to adjacent perineal structures (one-third lower urethra, one-third lower vagina, anus) with negative nodes.
III	Tumor of any size with or without extension to adjacent perineal structures (one-third lower urethra, one-third lower vagina, anus) with positive inguinofemoral lymph nodes.
IIIA	(i) With one lymph node metastasis (≥5 mm), or (ii) One or two lymph node metastasis(es) (<5 mm).
IIIB	(i) With two or more lymph node metastases (≥5 mm), or (ii) Three or more lymph node metastases (<5 mm).
IIIC	With positive nodes with extracapsular spread.
IV	Tumor invades other regional (two-thirds upper urethra, two-thirds upper vagina) or other distant structures.
IVA	Tumor invades any of the following (i) Upper urethral and/or vaginal mucosa, bladder mucosa, rectal mucosa, or fixed to pelvic bone, or (ii) Fixed or ulcerated inguinofemoral nodes.
IVB	Any distant metastasis including pelvic lymph nodes.

[a] The depth of invasion is defined as the measurement of the tumor from the epithelial-stromal junction of the adjacent most superficial dermal papilla to the deepest point of invasion.

Rare cases of primary mammary adenocarcinoma of the vulva have been reported, presumably arising in aberrant mammary tissue occurring along the embryonic milk line.[70] Other rare carcinomas that may occur in the vulva include basal cell carcinomas,[71] verrucous carcinomas,[72] and sebaceous carcinomas.[73]

Malignant melanomas of the vulva account for approximately 2% to 4% of primary vulvar malignancies and 1% to 3% of melanomas arising in women.[74] Vulvar melanoma occurs most frequently in women older than 60 years of age, but 10% to 20% of vulvar melanomas occur in women younger than 40 years. In a large Swedish series,[75] 57% of vulvar melanomas were of the mucosal lentiginous type, 22% were nodular, and 16% were superficial spreading or lentiginous. Most investigators have reported a correlation between higher depth of invasion or Breslow thickness and poorer outcome.[75,76] However, because the vulvar epithelium sometimes lacks a well-developed papillary dermis, which makes it difficult to assign Clark's levels of invasion, a modification of the Clark system is often used to categorize patients with vulvar melanoma.[77] Other factors that have been associated with a poorer prognosis are ulceration, clinical amelanosis, and older age.[75]

Vulvar sarcomas constitute 1% to 2% of vulvar malignancies and include leiomyosarcomas, rhabdomyosarcomas, angiosarcomas, neurofibrosarcomas, and epithelioid sarcomas. The prognosis appears to depend on three main determinants: lesion size, tumor contour, and mitotic activity. Lesions >5 cm in diameter with infiltrating margins, extensive necrosis, and more than five mitotic figures per 10 high-power fields are the most likely to recur after surgical resection.[78,79]

Diagnosis, Clinical Evaluation, and Staging

Patients with VIN may complain of vulvar pruritus, irritation, or a mass, but many are asymptomatic at the time of diagnosis. Patients with invasive vulvar cancer usually complain of a vulvar mass and chronic vulvar pruritus. Advanced lesions may bleed and are often exquisitely tender.

Because VIN can have many manifestations, any new vulvar lesion should be biopsied. Once a diagnosis of high-grade VIN has been established, the entire vulva, cervix, and vagina should be carefully examined because patients often have multifocal or multicentric involvement.[80] Colposcopic examination may help to define the extent of disease.

Diagnosis of invasive vulvar lesions requires a wedge biopsy of the lesion with surrounding skin and with underlying dermis and connective tissue so that the pathologist can adequately evaluate the depth of stromal invasion. This procedure can usually be performed in the physician's office under local anesthesia. Excisional biopsy is preferred for lesions <1 cm in diameter.

All patients with invasive disease require a careful physical examination including a detailed pelvic examination, chest radiography, and a biochemical profile. Cystoscopy and proctoscopy should be performed in patients with tumors that are near the urethra or anus, respectively. CT, MRI, and FDG-PET/CT scans can be obtained to evaluate deep inguinal and pelvic lymph nodes and possible local extension of disease to adjacent structures. FDG-PET/CT has relatively poor sensitivity but high specificity in the prediction of lymph node metastases.[81]

The correlation between clinical assessment of the inguinal lymph nodes and pathologic findings is poor.[82] Homesley et al.[82] reported that 24% of patients with clinically negative nodes had inguinal lymph node metastases and 24% of patients with suspicious but mobile nodes had negative findings at lymphadenectomy. For this reason, in 1988, the FIGO staging system was changed from a clinical staging system to one that incorporates the more accurate information gained from surgical assessment of regional lymph nodes; a subsequent amendment provided a definition of minimally invasive vulvar cancer.[83]

Studies also suggest that, when corrected for the number of involved lymph nodes, lymph node bilaterality and local factors such as tumor size and early involvement of adjacent structures have little impact on survival.[84,85] However, extracapsular nodal extension was found to be a powerful prognostic indicator.[86,87] In 2009, to incorporate these findings and to improve the prognostic accuracy of the FIGO staging system, another major revision was implemented.[84] In this revision, the role of tumor diameter was diminished; distal urethral, vaginal, and anal involvement were removed as indications for upstaging; and stage III was subdivided to include more detailed information about the number of positive lymph nodes and the presence of extracapsular nodal extension (see Table 72.4).[68]

Prognostic Factors

Our understanding of the importance of various prognostic indicators in vulvar carcinoma has shifted with the increased use of adjuvant radiotherapy and the accumulation of outcome data. In a 1991 retrospective review of 586 patients entered in Gynecologic Oncology Group (GOG) trials between 1977 and 1984, the presence and number of lymph nodes and tumor diameter were the only independent predictors of survival.[85] Five-year survival rates were 91% for patients with negative inguinal lymph nodes and 75%, 36%, and 24%, respectively, for patients with one or two, three or four, or five or six positive nodes. Using these data, the authors suggested a classification system that categorized patients according to tumor size and number of involved lymph nodes (Table 72.5). Although treatment details were not given, postoperative radiotherapy was not standard in the years of this study, and

TABLE 72.5

Relationship Between International Federation of Gynecology and Obstetrics Risk Groups and Outcome in Patients with Invasive Vulvar Cancer

Risk Group	Surgical Findings	Five-Y Survival Rate (No. of Patients)	
		GOG 36[85]	Landrum et al.[88]
Minimal	Tumor ≤2 cm in diameter and negative lymph nodes	97.9%, $n = 154$	100%, $n = 89$
Low	Tumor 2.1–8 cm in diameter and negative lymph nodes or	87.4%, $n = 232$	97.1%, $n = 69$
	Tumor ≤2 cm in diameter and one positive lymph node		
Intermediate	Tumor >8 cm in diameter and negative lymph nodes or	74.8%, $n = 104$	81.8%, $n = 11$
	Tumor >2 cm in diameter and one positive lymph node or		
	Tumor ≤8 cm in diameter and two unilaterally positive lymph nodes		
High	Tumor >8 cm in diameter and two unilaterally positive lymph nodes	29%, $n = 87$	100%, $n = 6$

GOG, International Federation of Gynecology and Obstetrics.

it is likely that most patients did not receive radiotherapy; more recent reviews suggest that modern adjuvant radiotherapy may reduce the influence of tumor size and number of positive nodes on outcome (see Table 72.5).[68] Nevertheless, the GOG risk classification was a major influence on recent modifications of the FIGO staging system. In addition to the number of lymph nodes, the presence of extracapsular extension has been found to be an important predictor of outcome.[88,89] However, in a review of patients treated with radiation after lymphadenectomy, Katz et al.[90] found no correlation between extracapsular extension and inguinal node recurrence if the dose of radiation was ≥56 Gy.

The presence of pelvic lymph node metastases is generally considered to be a predictor of very poor prognosis.[91] However, this impression comes largely from decades-old studies of outcome in patients who had pelvic lymph node dissection without adjuvant radiotherapy. The generalizability of these data to current practice, in which most patients who have nodal involvement receive radiotherapy, is uncertain.

Other factors that have consistently been correlated with lymph node metastasis and outcome include depth of invasion, tumor thickness, and the presence or absence of lymph-vascular space invasion (LVSI).[82,85,92] More than 75% of patients with LVSI have positive inguinal nodes.[82] Studies of the relationship between tumor grade and outcome have supported various conclusions, possibly reflecting the inconsistent criteria used to grade vulvar tumors.[82,89,93] Other factors that have been associated with poorer prognosis include high mitotic rate, aneuploidy, an infiltrative growth pattern, and a basaloid histologic pattern.[93-95] Several authors have reported that tumors containing HPV DNA have a poorer prognosis than HPV-negative tumors.[53,96] Some investigators have reported a worse prognosis for patients age 70 years or older, whereas others have found no correlation between prognosis and age.[82,93]

Studying the relationship between surgical margins and tumor recurrence, Heaps et al.[92] reported no local failures in 91 patients whose narrowest tumor margin (deep or at the skin surface) was ≥8 mm in the fixed specimen. A total of 10 of 23 patients (43%) with margins of ≤4.8 mm experienced a local recurrence, as did 8 of 13 patients (62%) with margins between 4.8 and 8 mm. The risk of recurrence in patients with narrow margins may be diminished when postoperative radiotherapy is given.[97]

Treatment

During the last 30 years, the treatment of vulvar cancer has evolved away from radical en bloc surgical resection, which was standard before the 1980s, toward a multidisciplinary approach that emphasizes tissue-sparing operations and selective use of radiotherapy or chemoradiation to optimize local control, survival, and organ function.

High-Grade Vulvar Intraepithelial Neoplasia

After invasive carcinoma has been excluded by a sufficient number of excisional biopsies, the treatment of high-grade VIN (VIN 3) should be as conservative as possible. Focal lesions can be simply excised. Multiple lesions can be excised separately or, if confluent, with a larger single excision. This approach is generally well tolerated and provides material for histologic assessment. When there is more extensive high-grade VIN, the lesions can be vaporized with a CO_2 laser. This method may provide an alternative to more extensive operations but does not yield a specimen for histologic inspection.

Extensive, diffuse VIN 3 may necessitate a wider excision, particularly if the lesion involves the perianal skin. These lesions are sometimes treated with a partial vulvectomy of the superficial skin ("skinning vulvectomy"). Whenever possible, the vulvar skin should be sutured primarily, but a split-thickness skin graft is sometimes needed to close the defect.

VIN 3 often recurs at or near the margins of resection, even when the histopathology analysis demonstrates that the initial lesions were completely resected. Presumably, this phenomenon reflects the multifocal nature of the condition.[80] VIN 3 can also recur within the donor skin from split-thickness grafts.[98]

Women with HPV-16–positive high-grade VIN showed that vaccination with a mix of long peptides from the HPV-16 viral oncoproteins E6 and E7 induced clinical responses (including sustained complete responses in 47% of patients at 24 months of follow-up) and relief of symptoms.[99] Complete responses were associated with induction of HPV-16–specific immunity.

Invasive Disease

The optimal treatment of invasive disease requires careful consideration of the potential benefits of various local and regional treatment options to find an overall treatment strategy that will maximize locoregional disease control with as little acute and long-term morbidity as possible.

Treatment of the Vulva. Most small lesions (approximately <4 cm) that do not involve the urethra, anus, or other adjacent structures can be controlled locally with a radical local excision. A wide and deep excision of the lesion is performed, with the incision extended down to the inferior fascia of the urogenital diaphragm. An effort should be made to remove the lesion with a 1-cm margin of normal tissue in all directions unless this would compromise of the anus or urethra. Small lesions that invade ≤1 mm can be managed with local resection alone because the risk of regional spread is very small. Patients with more invasive tumors must also have surgical or radiation treatment of the inguinal nodes, as discussed in the next section.

Primary tumors that involve the anus, rectum, rectovaginal septum, or urethra pose a difficult problem because adequate surgical clearance can often be obtained only by sacrificing organ function. Some patients who have tumors that minimally involve the external urethra or anus can undergo initial vulvectomy without sacrifice of major organ function if close margins are accepted near critical structures. Postoperative radiotherapy can then be delivered to prevent local recurrence.[100] Although local recurrences are frequently successfully controlled with additional surgery, Faul et al.[101] reported an overall 5-year survival rate of only 40% after the first local recurrence and emphasized the importance of achieving local control. These authors reported a significant reduction in the local failure rate (from 58% to 16%) when tumors that were within 8 mm of the operative margins were treated with radiotherapy after surgery.[101] Although some patients with more extensive organ involvement may be cured with ultraradical operations, in some cases with pelvic exenteration, the risks of acute and long-term complications of these procedures are substantial.[102,103] For this reason, a number of investigators have explored the use of radiotherapy with or without surgery and chemotherapy to spare critical structures in patients with locally advanced disease.

In the 1980s, several investigators[104–106] reported results of preoperative radiotherapy in small series of patients with locally advanced disease. These reports indicated that modest doses of radiation (45 to 55 Gy) produced dramatic tumor responses in some patients with locally advanced disease, permitting organ-sparing surgery without sacrifice of tumor control. Hacker et al.[106] reported that four of eight patients with T3 or T4 tumors treated preoperatively with 44 to 54 Gy had no residual tumor in the vulvectomy specimen, and that seven of these eight had local control of their disease. More recently, investigators have emphasized the use of concurrent chemoradiation, as discussed later in this section.

Treatment of Regional Disease. Effective treatment of regional disease is the single most important element in the curative management of early vulvar cancer. Although patients with vulvar recurrences may have their disease successfully controlled with additional local treatment, patients who suffer inguinal recurrences are rarely curable.

All patients with primary tumors that invade >1 mm must have their inguinal lymph nodes treated. In the past, this treatment usually included a bilateral radical inguinal-femoral lymphadenectomy, which initially was combined with vulvectomy using a single incision and, more recently, was performed through separate groin incisions. At one time, pelvic lymphadenectomy was also performed in most patients with invasive vulvar cancer. When subsequent studies demonstrated that pelvic node metastases were found only in patients with positive inguinal nodes, use of the procedure was limited to patients found intraoperatively to have inguinal node metastases.

Then, in 1986, Homesley et al.[91] published results of a prospective randomized study that compared pelvic lymphadenectomy with inguinal and pelvic irradiation in patients with inguinal node metastases from carcinoma of the vulva. All patients were initially treated with radical vulvectomy and inguinal-femoral lymphadenectomy. Patient randomization was done intraoperatively after frozen-section evaluation of the inguinal-femoral lymph nodes. This trial was closed prematurely, after 114 eligible patients had been entered, when interim analysis revealed a survival advantage for the radiotherapy arm ($p = 0.03$; Fig. 72.3). The difference was most marked for patients with clinically positive or multiple histologically positive groin nodes. The initial preliminary report was finally updated in 2009,[107] confirming marked reductions in the risks of recurrence and cancer-related death in patients who had radiotherapy. There were 3 inguinal recurrences in the radiation arm versus 13 in the control arm. Although no differences were seen in the number of pelvic recurrences, competing risks and the lack of high-quality tomographic imaging in this early study may have led to underestimates of the risks of pelvic recurrence. In the updated report, the relative risk of disease progression with radiation was 39% (95% confidence interval = 0.17 to 0.88; $p = 0.02$); the relative risk of death was less impressive, with a hazard ratio of 0.61 (95% confidence interval = 0.3 to 1.3; $p = 0.18$), apparently because of a marked difference in the rate of deaths from other causes: 14 in the radiation arm versus 2 in the control arm. With the 1986 publication of this study, most practitioners abandoned routine pelvic lymphadenectomy, and postoperative radiotherapy became standard for most patients with inguinal lymph node metastases.

Although radical inguinal-femoral lymphadenectomy was historically considered the treatment of choice for regional management of invasive vulvar carcinoma, a number of groups have investigated the possibility that regional radiotherapy may be an effective and less morbid way of preventing recurrence in patients with clinically negative groins.[90,108–110]

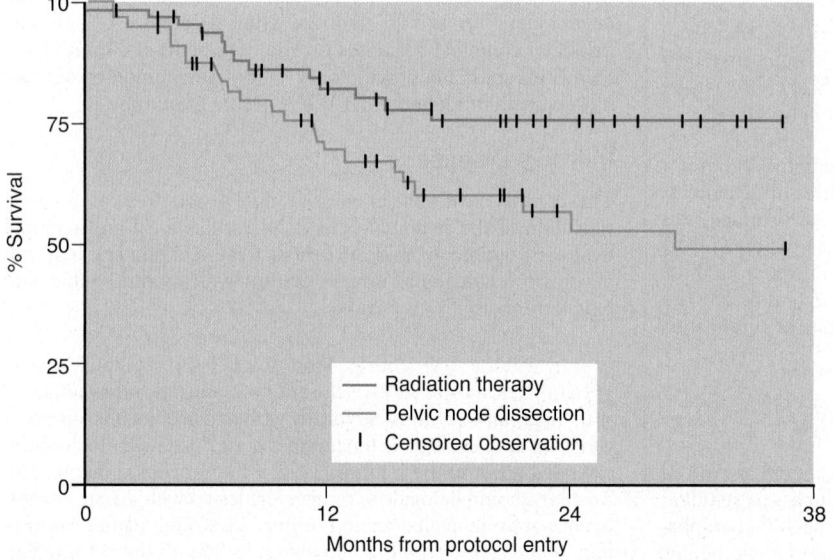

Figure 72.3 Survival rates of 114 patients with invasive squamous cell carcinoma of the vulva who were entered on a Gynecologic Oncology Group protocol in which patients with positive groin nodes after radical vulvectomy and bilateral inguinal lymphadenectomies were randomly assigned to undergo pelvic lymph node dissection or postoperative irradiation of the pelvis and inguinal nodes ($p = 0.004$). (From Homesley HD, Bundy BN, Sedlis A, et al. Radiation therapy versus pelvic node resection for carcinoma of the vulva with positive groin nodes. *Obstet Gynecol* 1986;68:733, with permission.)

In 1992, the GOG reported the results of a trial that randomly assigned patients with clinically negative inguinal nodes to receive inguinal lymph node irradiation or inguinal-femoral lymphadenectomy (followed by inguinopelvic irradiation in patients with positive lymph nodes) after resection of the primary tumor.[110] The study was closed after entry of only 58 patients, when an interim analysis demonstrated a significantly higher rate of inguinal recurrence and death in the radiotherapy group. The authors concluded that lymphadenectomy was the superior treatment, although the morbidity rate of lymphadenectomy was greater than that of groin irradiation. However, the radiotherapy techniques used in this study have since been criticized. Preirradiation CT scans were not consistently obtained to verify the position and size of inguinal nodes. Patients were treated with anterior appositional fields, the dose was prescribed at a depth of 3 cm, and the use of electrons (usually 12 MeV) was emphasized. This method of treatment can lead to significant underdosage of the inguinal-femoral nodes, which frequently extend to a depth of >5 to 8 cm.[111]

In contrast, retrospective studies have indicated that patients who have negative inguinal nodes (by tomographic imaging) and careful radiotherapy treatment planning rarely experience a regional recurrence after inguinal-pelvic irradiation to 40 to 50 Gy.[90,108,109] Katz et al.[90] emphasized the importance of careful technique. They reported three recurrences in 29 patients treated with radiotherapy alone for clinically negative inguinal nodes; two of these recurrences occurred adjacent to radiation fields that had not fully encompassed the lateral inguinal nodes. It appears that, with careful radiotherapy technique, microscopic disease in the inguinal lymph nodes can be readily controlled with radiation alone. Radiation alone appears to be a reasonable treatment to prevent inguinal recurrence, particularly for patients who have clinically and radiographically negative groins but require radiation for locally advanced disease.

Some surgeons have tried to reduce the incidence and severity of surgical complications by reducing the extent of lymph node dissections. In the 1990s, several groups reported the use of a more limited "superficial" inguinal lymphadenectomy for patients with early disease; patients who had positive lymph nodes were referred for radiotherapy. Although many of the complications usually associated with radical lymphadenectomy were avoided, inguinal recurrence rates were higher than expected, ranging from 7% to 16% in patients who had negative dissections.[90,112] It has been suggested that the procedure used in these studies did not remove medial inguinal-femoral nodes, which may be the primary site of drainage of some vulvar cancers[113,114]; for this reason, many gynecologic oncologists now recommend removal of at least the superficial and medial inguinofemoral nodes.

During the last decade, a number of investigators have explored the use of intraoperative lymphatic mapping to identify a "sentinel" node that would predict the presence or absence of regional metastases. A number of studies have evaluated the results from sentinel lymph node biopsy followed by regional lymphadenectomy. From the pooled results for 383 patients entered in 10 trials, the authors concluded that the negative predictive value of sentinel node biopsy was 99.3% and the false-negative rate was 2.4%.[115] The GROningen INternational Study on Sentinel nodes in Vulvar cancer (GROINSS)-V[116] study assessed the efficacy of sentinel lymph node evaluation alone in patients with invasive vulvar cancers <4 cm in diameter. Of 402 patients registered in this trial, 231 patients with negative sentinel nodes did not undergo lymphadenectomy; at the time of the analysis, groin recurrences had been observed in 9 (3.9%) of these 231 patients, and 7 patients (3.0%) had died. Patients with sentinel lymph node metastasis >2 mm had significantly lower disease-specific survival (69.5% versus 94.4%; $p = 0.001$).[117] Robison et al[118] reported long-term follow-up after sentinel lymph node evaluation. With a median follow-up of 58 months, only 3 of 57 patients who were observed after a negative sentinel lymph node developed an inguinal recurrence. A large GOG trial designed to estimate the sensitivity of sentinel lymph node biopsy

in a community-based setting enrolled 452 women who underwent intraoperative lymphatic mapping, sentinel lymph node biopsy, and inguinal femoral lymphadenectomy. Ninety-two percent of patients had at least one sentinel node identified. The sensitivity was 91.7% and the false-negative predictive value (1-negative predictive value) was 3.7%, which was even lower in women whose tumors were <4 cm. These data suggest that sentinel lymph node biopsy is a reasonable alternative to inguinal femoral lymphadenectomy in selected women with squamous cell carcinoma of the vulva.[119] On the subsequent observational (GROINSS)-VI study, patients with a positive sentinel nodes received postoperative radiation therapy without undergoing a full lymphadenectomy. The currently enrolling (GROINSS)-VII study uses the same approach for patients with <2 mm of disease in the sentinel node, but patients with >2 mm focus of disease undergo a lymphadenectomy followed by postoperative radiation.

Participants in a 2008 expert panel at an International Sentinel Node Society Meeting concluded that sentinel lymph node biopsy "is a reasonable alternative to complete inguinal lymphadenectomy when [it] is performed by a skilled multidisciplinary team in well-selected patients."[115] They concluded that patients who have tumors that invade >1 mm, no obvious metastatic disease, and a tumor diameter of <4 cm are good candidates for the procedure.

Radiotherapy Technique. Comprehensive regional radiotherapy for vulvar cancer requires adequate coverage of at least the inguinofemoral and distal pelvic lymph nodes. Patients who have extensive inguinal or pelvic disease may require larger fields that encompass the common iliac nodes. If the vulvar cancer has been excised with widely negative margins, some clinicians choose to not treat the primary site. Several techniques have been used to reduce the dose given to the femoral head and neck during treatment of the groin. One approach is to use a combination of photons and electrons; this technique requires careful image-based planning to assure that the treatment is delivering an adequate dose to the superficial and deep inguinal lymph nodes. Alternatively, IMRT can be used to spare soft tissue, bladder, bowel, and other critical structures, but this method is technically challenging and requires a sound understanding of the local and regional anatomy.[120]

Patients who have local risk factors for recurrence but pathologically negative lymph nodes may be treated with local radiation alone using conformal photon fields or, in selected cases, appositional electron beam techniques. Whenever photons are used to treat the vulvar surface, tissue-equivalent materials may need to be applied to ensure that the surface dose is adequate. Thermoluminescent dosimeters can be used to verify that the surface of the vulva is receiving the prescribed dose of radiation.

Chemoradiation in Locoregionally Advanced Disease. To reduce the need for morbid ultraradical surgery and to improve locoregional control rates, a number of investigators have explored combinations of chemotherapy with radiation and surgery in patients with locally advanced vulvar carcinoma.[121–128] Most studies have used combinations of cisplatin, 5-FU, and mitomycin-C (Table 72.6), extrapolating from the high response rates observed with such combinations for locally advanced carcinomas of the cervix and head and neck and from studies that have demonstrated the efficacy of these drugs as radiosensitizers in the treatment of carcinomas of the anus. Although studies have usually included small numbers of patients with very advanced local or regional disease, most investigators have observed impressive responses that often appear to be better than would be expected with radiation alone. Randomized trials have not been done and may be difficult to perform because of the small number of patients with locally advanced vulvar cancer. However, results of trials in other types of cancer are encouraging: trials that demonstrated improved local control and survival when concurrent cisplatin-containing chemotherapy was added to radiation treatment of cervical cancers[129,130] and improved colostomy-free survival when mitomycin-C and

TABLE 72.6

Concurrent Chemoradiotherapy in the Management of Locally Advanced or Recurrent Carcinoma of the Vulva (Series Including 20 or More Patients)

Study (Ref.)	No. of Patients	Chemotherapy	Radiotherapy Dose (Gy)	No. (%) with Recurrent or Persistent Local Disease after Radiotherapy ± Surgery	Follow-Up (mo)
Moore et al.[125]	71	5-FU + CDDP	47.6	11 (16)	22–72
Landoni et al.[122]	58	5-FU + Mito	54	13 (22)	4–48
Lupi et al.[124]	31	5-FU + Mito	54	7 (23)	22–73
Koh et al.[121]	20	5-FU ± CDDP or Mito	30–54	9 (45)	1–75
Russell et al.[126]	25	5-FU ± CDDP	47–72	6 (24)	4–52
Scheistroen and Trope[127]	42	Bleomycin	45	39 (93)	7–60
Thomas et al.[128]	24	5-FU ± Mito	44–60	10 (42)	5–43
Landrum et al.[123]	33	CDDP ± 5-FU	37–63	4 (12)	NS

5-FU, 5-fluorouracil; CDDP, cisplatin; Mito, mitomycin-C; NS, not stated.

5-FU were added to radiation treatment of anal cancer[131] suggest that this approach may be also be useful in the treatment of women with vulvar cancer. In a single-arm phase 2 study, the GOG investigated the use of cisplatin with daily radiation therapy to a total dose of 57.6 Gy in locally advanced vulvar cancer.[132] Overall, 50% of patients achieved a complete pathologic response with this regimen. The current GOG trial will utilize IMRT and deliver gemcitabine in addition to cisplatin.

Several investigators have explored the use of neoadjuvant chemotherapy for locally advanced vulvar cancer.[133,134] Although partial responses to multiagent chemotherapy have been observed, response rates appear to be lower than for cervical cancers, and survival rates have been discouraging.[134]

Caution is warranted in designing aggressive treatment protocols for patients with vulvar cancers, as these patients typically are elderly and often have concurrent medical problems. Serious pulmonary damage has been observed in a number of patients treated in studies that included bleomycin.[127] In the largest published series of patients treated with mitomycin-C and 5-FU, hematologic tolerance was acceptable, but the administered dose of mitomycin-C was somewhat lower than that generally used in the treatment of anal cancers.[128] Although chemotherapy may improve control rates, radiation alone can produce impressive responses and should be considered in patients who are poor surgical candidates and who cannot tolerate chemotherapy.

Complications of Treatment

Most of the serious acute and subacute complications of radical vulvectomy are related to the lymphadenectomy, although these risks have decreased somewhat with the use of separate groin incisions. Acute complications include wound seroma, disruption, or infection in up to 50% to 75% of cases, chronic lymphedema in 20% to 50%, and perioperative death in 2% to 5%.[109,112,135,136] Other acute complications include urinary tract infection, wound cellulitis, temporary anterior thigh anesthesia from femoral nerve injury, thrombophlebitis, and, rarely, pulmonary embolus.[91,137] The risk of chronic leg edema decreased from approximately 30% to 15% with the use of separate groin incisions and is rare after sentinel lymph node dissection only.[116,138] Other chronic complications include genital prolapse, urinary stress incontinence, temporary weakness of the quadriceps muscle, and introital stenosis. These risks are less when radical local excision of the primary lesion is done instead of radical vulvectomy.[139,140] Patients who undergo vulvectomy without inguinal lymphadenectomy have significantly shorter hospital stays and fewer complications.[109,112]

The most prominent acute complication of radical radiotherapy for vulvar carcinoma is radiation dermatitis. Moist desquamation is commonly seen in the final weeks of treatment but resolves within 2 to 3 weeks after completion; sitz baths and appropriate use of pain medications are helpful during the acute phase. Skin reactions that occur in the first 2 to 4 weeks of treatment are frequently due to superinfection with *Candida albicans* and should be treated presumptively with antifungal agents. Other acute side effects of radiation include diarrhea, dysuria, and painful defecation. Late complications result from a combination of radiation, surgery, and tissue destruction from locally advanced tumors. Introital or vaginal stenosis, tissue atrophy, and other effects of combined therapy may cause sexual dysfunction. Vulvar edema, tissue atrophy, hyperpigmentation, fibrosis, and telangiectasia may occur and are related to the dose of radiation and the volume of tissue irradiated. Combined effects of treatment may also cause bladder or rectal incontinence, urethral or anal stenosis, ulceration, or fistula.

Treatment of Metastatic Disease

Unfortunately, reports of chemotherapy activity in the treatment of metastatic or recurrent squamous cell carcinoma of the vulva are largely anecdotal. In the absence of reliable data specific to this cancer, clinicians often use single agents and combination regimens that have had some activity in the treatment of cervical cancer. However, there are, as yet, few data to indicate that chemotherapy can provide effective palliation for patients with metastatic or recurrent vulvar carcinomas that are not amendable to locoregional treatments. In terms of molecular-targeted agents, erlotinib has shown promising activity and may represent one of the most active agents for the management of squamous cell carcinoma of the vulva. Specifically, in a phase 2 study, erlotinib exhibited a 67.5% overall clinical benefit rate (i.e., 27.5% partial response and 40.0% stable disease by response evaluation criteria in solid tumors).[141]

CARCINOMA OF THE CERVIX

Epidemiology

The American Cancer Society estimated that in the United States in 2014, 12,360 new cases of invasive cervical cancer would be diagnosed and there would be 4,020 deaths due to cervical cancer, representing approximately 1.5% of all cancer deaths in women.[1] In the United States and other developed countries, age-adjusted death rates from cervical cancer have declined steadily since the

1930s. However, global cervical cancer incidence increased from 378,000 cases per year in 1980 to 528,000 new cases in 2012; during that period, the annual death rate increased by 7.5% with 266,000 deaths per year in 2012.[142] The decrease in incidence in developed countries is primarily the result of the adoption of routine screening programs; however, the death rates from cervical cancer had begun to decrease before the implementation of Pap screening, suggesting that other, unknown factors may have played some role.[143]

International incidences of cervical cancer tend to reflect differences in cultural attitudes toward sexual practices and differences in the penetration of mass screening programs. The highest incidences tend to occur in populations that have low screening rates combined with a high background prevalence of HPV infection.[144] Rates of invasive cervical cancer are particularly high in Latin America, southern and eastern Africa, India, and Polynesia. In many of these developing countries, cervical cancer is the leading cause of cancer deaths among women. Differences in age-specific incidences between developed and medically underserved countries illustrate the probable impact of mass screening on the development of invasive disease. For example, a comparison between data from Brazil and the United Kingdom showed similar rates of cervical cancer in young women, suggesting similar levels of exposure to HPV, but rapidly diverging rates in older women, probably reflecting differences in the availability of mass screening in the two countries (Fig. 72.4).

Although the overall incidence of cervical cancer is low in the United States, the incidence in black Americans is about 30% higher than the incidence in white Americans, and the incidence in Hispanic women is about twice the incidence in white Americans.[145] Barriers to cervical cancer screening, including lack of insurance, low income, and cultural factors, probably contribute to higher incidences and mortality rates in black and Hispanic women.[146]

Molecular and human epidemiologic studies have demonstrated a strong relationship between HPV, CIN, and invasive carcinoma of the cervix. HPV can be identified in >99% of cervical cancers, and infection with HPV is now accepted as a necessary cause of most cervical cancers.[144] It appears that most of the covariables historically associated with an increased risk of cervical cancer are surrogates for sexually transmitted HPV infection. Women who have coitus at a young age, who have multiple sexual partners, have partners with multiple partners, or who bear children at a young age are at increased risk. A pooled analysis of 26 epidemiologic studies showed a strong inverse association between use of intrauterine devices and cervical cancer, perhaps due to a cellular immune response triggered by the device.[147] Castellsague et al.[148] have reported that circumcised males have a lower incidence of HPV infection than uncircumcised males and a correspondingly lower incidence of cervical cancer in their female partners.

A number of studies suggest that the incidence of cervical adenocarcinoma has been increasing, particularly among women in their 20s and 30s.[149] In a study based on Surveillance, Epidemiology, and End Results program data, Smith et al.[149] found that the age-adjusted incidence of cervical adenocarcinoma in the United States increased by 29.1% during a period (1973–1996) when the overall incidence of cervical cancer decreased by 41.9%. Several investigators have reported a correlation between cervical adenocarcinoma and prolonged oral contraceptive use.[150] However, this relationship may not be causative, given the many potential confounding risk factors and possible changes in diagnostic criteria over time.[149,151] Another possible explanation for the increase in incidence of cervical adenocarcinoma is that cytologic screening methods may be less effective in detecting preinvasive adenocarcinomas than they are in detecting preinvasive squamous lesions, resulting in a less dramatic reduction in the incidence of invasive adenocarcinomas.

In 1993, the Centers for Disease Control and Prevention added cervical cancer to the list of AIDS-defining neoplasms.[152] However, the relationship between immunosuppression (particularly HIV-related immunosuppression) and the risk of HPV-related disease is complex and incompletely understood.[153,154] Current data strongly suggest that women infected with HIV have an increased incidence and are more likely to have persistence of cervical HPV infection, even when studies are corrected for confounding risk factors; women infected with HIV also tend to have a faster rate

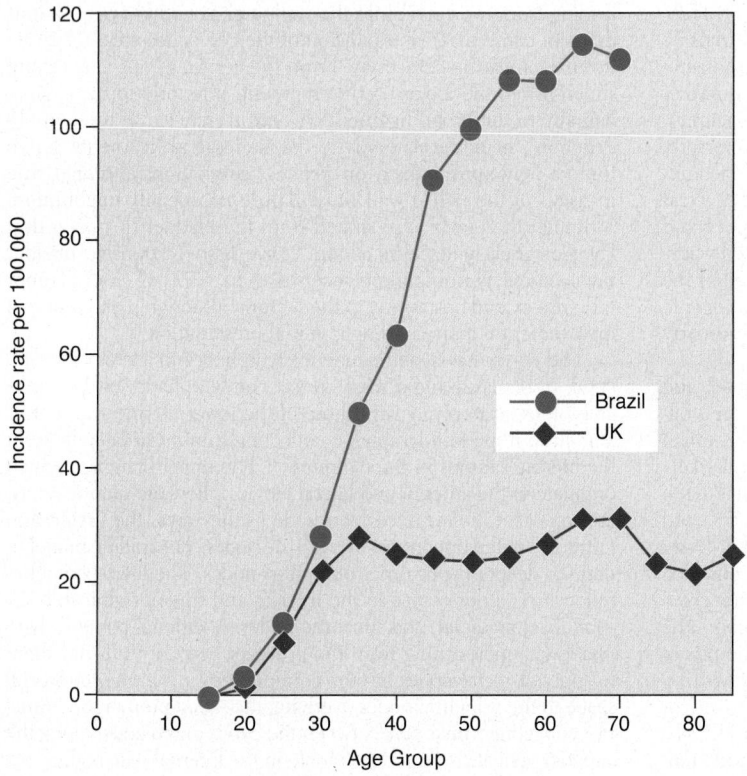

Figure 72.4 Age-specific incidences of invasive cervical cancer in Brazil and in the United Kingdom (*UK*). (From Bosch FX, de Sanjose S. Human papillomavirus and cervical cancer—burden and assessment of causality. *J Natl Cancer Inst Monogr* 2003;31:3, with permission.)

of progression to high-grade CIN.[153,154] Iatrogenic immunosuppression in organ transplant recipients is also associated with an increased prevalence of CIN.[155] Although less definitive, evidence linking HIV infection with invasive cervical cancer has also been increasing.[154] Some investigators[156] have suggested that cervical cancer is a more aggressive disease in immunosuppressed patients, but other studies have failed to reveal an independent linkage.[153,154] In most cases, antiretroviral therapy does not appear to affect HPV levels, nor does it appear to decrease the risks of high-grade squamous intraepithelial lesions (HSILs) or invasive cancer.[154] Because of the increased risk of HPV infection in women infected with HIV, vigilant surveillance with Pap smears, pelvic examinations, and colposcopy (when indicated) should be part of the routine care of these women.

Human Papillomavirus

HPV is associated with nearly all cases of cervical cancer. Examination of tumor DNA from cervical cancers reveals integration of one the high-risk HPV subtypes, including 16, 18, 31, 33, and 45. The most common subtypes in human cancers are HPV-16 and -18, which are found in 70% of cases. Although cervical cancer is relatively rare in the United States, HPV is highly prevalent in the US population. Vaginal swab testing demonstrated that 26% of US women and 44% of women between 20 and 24 testing positive for HPV.[157] However, in only a small percentage of women does HPV infection lead to the development of premalignant or malignant lesions. This suggests that viral infection is essential, but not sufficient, for the development of high-grade dysplasia or invasive cancers.

In the initial infection, viral DNA remains episomal in the basal cell of the epidermis. Viral DNA integration occurs preferentially into areas of genomic instability, such as fragile sites, and oncogenesis does not appear to require disruption of any critical tumor suppressor genes. Rather, expression of viral genes, E6 and E7, disrupts the function of critical tumor suppressor genes, p53 and pRB, respectively, leading to enhanced cell cycle proliferation, impaired apoptosis, and loss of genome maintenance leading to increased genomic instability.

The strong correlation between high-risk HPV types and cervical carcinoma has led to the development of prophylactic HPV vaccines that have proven highly effective in randomized trials.[158] In response to these studies, the US Food and Drug Administration approved a prophylactic HPV vaccine for women between the ages of 9 and 26 years in 2006. Currently, two vaccines, Guardasil (Merck & Co, White House Station, NJ) and Cervarix (GlaxoSmithKline, Brentford, UK), are available. Both vaccines target HPV subtypes 16 and 18, which account for 70% of cervical cancers. Guardasil also includes antigen from HPV subtypes 6 and 11, which are associated with 90% of cases of benign genital warts. Both of these vaccines deliver viral-like particles composed of the L1 capsid protein that has assembled into the highly immunogenic viral-like particle form. The vaccines are DNA-free and thus carry no risk of infection.

Both vaccines are highly effective at generating a robust and durable immune response, including the production of neutralizing antibodies to the HPV viral capsid protein.[159] The effect appears to be highly durable, lasting at least 5 years and likely significantly longer.[159] The efficacy of these vaccines has been tested in large prospective randomized trials: FUTURE I[160] and FUTURE II[161,162] for Guardasil, and PATRICIA and the Costa Rica HPV vaccine trial[160,163] for Cervarix. FUTURE II enrolled 12,167 women between the ages of 15 and 26 years who received three doses of either HPV-6/-11/-16/-18 vaccine or placebo. The study was designed to determine if the vaccine reduced the rate of malignant or premalignancy cervical lesions. In women with no previous infection, the vaccine eliminated 98% of CIN grade 2 or 3, adenocarcinoma in situ, or cervical cancer related to HPV-16 or -18. Among all women, including those with previous infection

with HPV-16 and -18, the vaccine efficacy was significantly lower, just 44%. Other studies have confirmed that the HPV vaccine does not appear to speed clearance of the HPV virus for women who have previous exposure to HPV.[164] As a result, the vaccine is recommended for girls aged 11 to 12 years, with the goal of vaccinating prior to exposure to HPV. Analysis of the Costa Rica HPV vaccine trial has demonstrated that HPV vaccination also prevents oral and anal infection with HPV-16 and -18. Future analysis will determine if this translates to a reduction of HPV-associated oral and anal cancers.

The impact of widespread vaccination programs on HPV infection and HPV-associated disease is now being reported. In Scotland, HPV testing performed prior to and after introduction of the HPV vaccine revealed a reduction in the rate of HPV-16 and -18 positivity on cervical swabs from 29.8% (95% confidence interval = 28.3 to 31.3) to 13.6% (95% confidence interval = 11.7 to 15.8). A reduction in other HPV subtypes, including -31, -33, and -45 was also seen, suggesting cross-protection.

Natural History and Pattern of Spread

Most cervical carcinomas arise at the junction between the primarily columnar epithelium of the endocervix and the squamous epithelium of the ectocervix. This junction is a site of continuous metaplastic change, which is greatest in utero, at puberty, and during first pregnancy, and declines after menopause. Long before the relationship between HPV and cervical cancer was known, Richart and Barron[165] demonstrated that invasive squamous cell cancer of the cervix was the end result of progressive intraepithelial dysplastic changes within metaplastic epithelium of the transformation zone. The greatest risk of neoplastic transformation of virally induced atypical squamous metaplasia coincides with periods of greatest metaplastic activity. The approximately 15-year difference in the mean ages of women with CIN and women with invasive cervical cancer indicates a generally slow progression of CIN to invasive carcinoma.[166]

Once tumor has broken through the basement membrane, it may penetrate the cervical stroma directly or through vascular channels. Invasive tumors may develop as exophytic growths protruding from the cervix into the vagina or as endocervical lesions that can cause massive expansion of the cervix despite a relatively normal-appearing ectocervix. From the cervix, tumor may extend superiorly to the lower uterine segment, inferiorly to the vagina, laterally to the broad ligaments (where it may cause ureteral obstruction), or posterolaterally to the uterosacral ligaments. Large tumors may appear fixed on pelvic examination, although true invasion of the pelvic wall musculature is probably uncommon. Although the cervix is separated from the bladder by only a thin layer of fascia and cellular connective tissue, extensive bladder involvement is uncommon, occurring in <5% of cases. Tumor may also extend posteriorly to the rectum, although rectal mucosal involvement is a rare finding at initial presentation.

The cervix has a rich supply of lymphatics that drain the mucosal, muscularis, and serosal layers. The lymphatics of the cervix anastomose extensively with those of the lower uterine segment.[167] The most important lymphatic collecting trunks exit laterally from the uterine isthmus in three groups.[167] The upper branches, which originate in the anterior and lateral cervix, follow the uterine artery, are sometimes interrupted by a node as they cross the ureter, and terminate in the uppermost hypogastric nodes. The middle branches drain to deeper hypogastric (obturator) nodes. The lowest branches follow a posterior course to the inferior and superior gluteal, common iliac, presacral, and subaortic nodes. Additional posterior lymphatic channels arising from the posterior cervical wall may drain to superior rectal nodes or may continue upward in the retrorectal space to the subaortic nodes overlying the sacral promontory. Anterior collecting trunks pass between the cervix and bladder along the superior vesical artery and terminate in the internal iliac nodes.

The incidence of pelvic and para-aortic node involvement is correlated with tumor stage, size, histologic subtype, depth of invasion, and presence of LVSI. Reported rates of regional metastasis, which come primarily from series of patients who underwent lymphadenectomy as part of radical surgical treatment or before radiotherapy, vary widely. For patients with stage I disease treated with radical hysterectomy, most investigators report an incidence of positive pelvic nodes of 15% to 20% and an incidence of positive para-aortic nodes of 1% to 5%. For patients with stage I disease treated with radiation, reported rates of positive para-aortic nodes tend to be higher—usually 10% to 25%—reflecting the fact that stage I tumors selected for treatment with radiation are usually more advanced. Variations in the completeness of lymphadenectomies and histologic processing may lead to underestimates of the true incidence of regional spread from carcinomas of the cervix.[168]

Cervical cancer usually follows a relatively orderly pattern of metastatic progression, initially to primary echelon nodes in the pelvis and then to para-aortic nodes and distant sites. Initial presentation with hematogenous metastases is uncommon. FDG-PET scanning is probably the most accurate noninvasive method for the diagnosis of nodal metastasis, with a sensitivity of 82% and specificity of 95% as reported in a 2010 meta-analysis.[169] PET-positive pelvic nodes are frequently identified along the lymphatics that extend from the obturator vessels to the bifurcation of the common iliac vessels. Nodes that lie along the common iliac vessels lie most frequently between the psoas muscle and the common iliac artery and vein.[170] In the para-aortics, the nodes are closely associated with the aorta and are rarely identified to the left of the vena cava. The anatomic distribution of FDG-avid nodal metastasis in the pelvis and para-aortic nodes in a series of patients with cervical cancer demonstrates the areas where lymphatic metastasis are most commonly identified (Fig. 72.5).

The most frequent sites of distant recurrence are lung, left supraclavicular and mediastinal nodes, liver, and bone.

Pathology

Cervical Intraepithelial Neoplasia

Several systems have been developed for classifying premalignant cytologic and histologic cervical findings (Table 72.7). Following

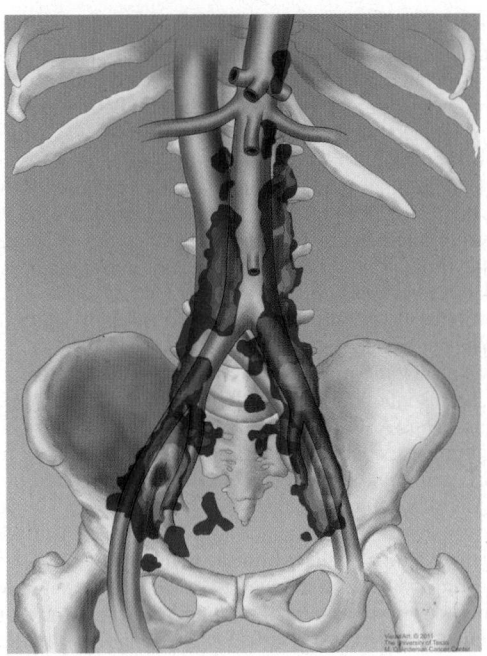

Figure 72.5 Anatomic distribution of positron emission tomography–positive lymph nodes based on a volume probability map. A color gradient corresponding to the visible-light spectrum is used to indicate the frequency of lymph node involvement. *Red*, high frequency; *green*, moderate frequency; *blue*, low frequency. (© 2011 The University of Texas M.D. Anderson Cancer Center.)

a 1988 National Cancer Institute Consensus Conference, the Bethesda system of classification was developed in an effort to further standardize reporting. The Bethesda system divides cytologic specimens into two groups: low-grade squamous intraepithelial lesions (LSIL) and HSILs. LSILs have low-grade dysplasia or changes associated with HPV. They are typically associated with low-risk HPV types and have a low likelihood of progressing to invasive cancers. These are to be distinguished from HSILs, which

TABLE 72.7

Comparison of Cytology Classification Systems for Cervical Neoplasms

Bethesda System	Dysplasia/CIN System		Papanicolaou System
Within normal limits	Normal		Class I
Infection (specify organism)	Inflammatory atypia (organism)		Class II
Reactive and reparative changes	—		—
Squamous cell abnormalities	—		—
Atypical squamous cells of undetermined significance	Squamous atypia		Class IIR
	HPV atypia		
Low-grade squamous intraepithelial lesion			
	Mild dysplasia	CIN 1	
			Class III
—	Moderate dysplasia	CIN 2	
High-grade squamous intraepithelial lesion	Severe dysplasia		
		CIN 3	
	Carcinoma in situ		Class IV
Invasive squamous carcinoma	Invasive squamous carcinoma		Class V

CIN, cervical intraepithelial neoplasia; HPV, human papillomavirus.

have findings of moderate of high-grade dysplasia such as abnormal mitoses, coarse chromatin, and loss of polarity. HSILs are usually associated with high-risk HPV types and have a higher likelihood of progressing to invasive cancer. The Bethesda system was meant to replace the Papanicolaou system and is now widely used in the United States. However, its use is still controversial. Some groups[171] argue that the new nomenclature has failed to improve diagnostic accuracy and believe that with dichotomization of the spectrum of atypical lesions, lesions that were formerly classified as CIN 2 (now HSIL) may be overtreated despite their relatively low risk of progression.

The Bethesda system also introduced the term *atypical squamous cells of undetermined significance* (ASC-US). This uncertain diagnosis is now the most common abnormal Pap smear result in United States laboratories,[172] with 1.6% to 9% of Pap smears reported as having ASC-US. Although most cases of ASC-US reflect a benign process, about 5% to 10% are associated with an underlying HSIL and one-third or more of HSILs are heralded by a finding of ASC-US on a Pap smear.[173] There has been considerable controversy about the evaluation and management of ASC-US, leading the National Cancer Institute to initiate the ASC-US-LSIL Triage Study.[174] This multicenter, randomized trial compared three methods of management—immediate colposcopy, cytological follow-up, and triage by HPV DNA testing—in 5,060 patients who were recruited to the study following a community-based Pap smear report of ASC-US or LSIL. Preliminary analyses of this study[174] demonstrated that in patients with LSIL, the prevalence of high-risk HPV was too high to permit useful triage based on HPV DNA testing, but that in the 3,488 patients with ASC-US, HPV DNA testing had a sensitivity in the detection of HSIL similar to that of immediate colposcopy and reduced the number of referrals for colposcopy by 50%. After exclusion of patients who had a diagnosis of CIN 2 or 3 at initial colposcopy, the cumulative risk of subsequent progression to CIN 2 or 3 was equivalent for women with LSIL (27.6%) or high-risk HPV-positive ASC-US (26.7%).[175]

Biopsy specimens that allow evaluation of tissue architecture can be scored as CIN I-III based on the Bethesda system.[176] Although criteria for the diagnosis of CIN and degree of neoplasia vary somewhat between pathologists, the important features of CIN are cellular immaturity, cellular disorganization, nuclear abnormalities, and increased mitotic activity. If mitoses and immature cells are present only in the lower third of the epithelium, the lesion is usually designated *CIN 1*. Lesions involving only the lower and middle thirds are designated *CIN 2*, and those involving the upper third are designated *CIN 3*. The term *cervical intraepithelial neoplasia*, as proposed by Richart,[177] refers only to a lesion that may progress to invasive carcinoma. Although CIN 1 and CIN 2 are sometimes referred to as *mild-to-moderate dysplasia*, the term *CIN* is now preferred over *dysplasia*.

Adenocarcinoma in Situ

Adenocarcinoma in situ is diagnosed when normal endocervical gland cells are replaced by tall, irregular columnar cells with stratified, hyperchromatic nuclei and increased mitotic activity but the normal branching pattern of the endocervical glands is maintained and there is no obvious stromal invasion. About 20% to 50% of women with cervical adenocarcinoma in situ also have squamous CIN.[178] Because adenocarcinoma in situ is frequently multifocal, cone biopsy margins are unreliable.[179] Although some investigators have described a possible precursor lesion termed *endocervical glandular dysplasia*, the reproducibility and clinical value of this designation are uncertain.[180]

Microinvasive Carcinoma

Microinvasive carcinoma is defined by FIGO as "invasive carcinoma which can be diagnosed only by microscopy, with deepest invasion ≤5 mm and largest extension ≥7 mm" (stage IA in Table 72.8). Thus, this diagnosis can be made only after examination of

TABLE 72.8

International Federation of Gynecology and Obstetrics Staging of Carcinoma of the Cervix (2009)

Stage	Description
I	The carcinoma is strictly confined to the cervix (*extension to the corpus should be disregarded*).
IA	Invasive carcinoma THAT can be diagnosed only by microscopy, with deepest invasion ≤5 mm and largest extension ≥7 mm.
IA1	Measured stromal invasion of ≤3 mm in depth and extension of ≤7 mm.
IA2	Measured stromal invasion >3 mm and not >5 mm in depth with an extension of not >7 mm.
IB	Clinically visible lesions limited to the cervix uteri or preclinical cancers greater than stage IA.[a]
IB1	Clinically visible lesion ≤4 cm in greatest dimension.
IB2	Clinically visible lesion >4 cm in greatest dimension.
II	Cervical carcinoma invades beyond the uterus, but not to the pelvic wall or to the lower third of the vagina.
IIA	Without parametrial invasion.
IIA1	Clinically visible lesion ≤4 cm in greatest dimension.
IIA2	Clinically visible lesion >4 cm in greatest dimension.
IIB	With obvious parametrial invasion.
III	The tumor extends to the pelvic wall and/or involves the lower third of the vagina and/or causes hydronephrosis or nonfunctioning kidney.[b]
IIIA	Tumor involves lower third of the vagina, with no extension to the pelvic wall.
IIIB	Extension to the pelvic wall and/or hydronephrosis or nonfunctioning kidney.
IV	The carcinoma has extended beyond the true pelvis or has involved (biopsy-proven) the mucosa of the bladder or rectum. A bullous edema, as such, does not permit a case to be allotted to stage IV.
IVA	Spread of the growth to adjacent organs.
IVB	Spread to distant organs.

[a] All macroscopically visible lesions—even with superficial invasion—are allotted to stage IB carcinomas. Invasion is limited to a measured stromal invasion with a maximal depth of 5 mm and a horizontal extension of not >7 mm. Depth of invasion should not be >5 mm taken from the base of the epithelium of the original tissue—superficial or glandular. The depth of invasion should always be reported in millimeters, even in those cases with "early (minimal) stromal invasion" (~1 mm). The involvement of vascular/lymphatic spaces should not change the stage allotment.
[b] On rectal examination, there is no cancer-free space between the tumor and the pelvic wall. All cases with hydronephrosis or nonfunctioning kidney are included, unless they are known to be the result of another cause.
Data from Pecorelli S, Zigliani L, Odicino F. Revised FIGO staging for carcinoma of the cervix. *Int J Gynaecol Obstet* 2009;105:107.

a specimen that includes the entire neoplastic lesion and cervical transformation zone. This requires a cervical cone biopsy. Following the advent of cytologic screening, the proportion of invasive carcinomas that invade <5 mm increased more than 10-fold to about 20% in the United States.[181]

The earliest invasion appears as a blurring of the stromoepithelial junction with a protrusion of cells into the stroma. These cells are less well differentiated than the adjacent noninvasive cells and have abundant pink-staining cytoplasm, hyperchromatic nuclei, and prominent nucleoli. They also exhibit a loss of polarity at the stromoepithelial junction.[181] Early microinvasion is usually characterized by a desmoplastic response in adjacent stroma with scalloping or duplication of the neoplastic epithelium or formation of pseudoglands (nests of invasive carcinoma that can mimic crypt involvement). In a study of cone specimens, Reich et al.[182] reported that 12% of microinvasive carcinomas were multifocal. The depth of invasion should be measured with a micrometer from the base of the epithelium to the deepest point of invasion. Lesions that have invaded <3 mm (FIGO stage IA1) are rarely associated with metastases; 5% to 10% of tumors that have invaded 3 to 5 mm (FIGO stage IA2) are associated with positive pelvic lymph nodes.[183] Until FIGO refined its definition of microinvasive carcinoma (see Table 72.8), most clinicians in the United States used a different definition of microinvasive carcinoma formulated by the Society of Gynecologic Oncologists: cancers that invaded <3 mm with no evidence of LVSI. The importance of LVSI remains somewhat controversial; the risk of metastatic regional disease appears to be exceedingly low for any tumor that invades <3 mm, even in the presence of LVSI.[181] Although most clinicians have adopted the FIGO definitions, many think that the risk of regional spread from tumors that have invaded 3 to 5 mm is sufficiently high to warrant evaluation or treatment of the parametria and regional nodes.

For adenocarcinoma, in particular, measuring the depth of invasion can be difficult. Because invasive adenocarcinomas may originate anywhere along the profile of architecturally complex glands that course through the cervical stroma, no reproducible method has been found for measuring the depth of invasion of these tumors. Some authors have measured the extent of invasion from the basement membrane or from the nearest abnormal glandular epithelium; others have defined early adenocarcinomas according to the volume of tumor (in cubic millimeters).[180] Despite these differences in measurement method, it is apparent that a subset of patients with very small adenocarcinomas have a low likelihood of lymph node metastasis or recurrence.[180]

Invasive Squamous Cell Carcinoma

Between 80% and 90% of cervical carcinomas are squamous cell carcinomas. Although squamous neoplasms are often subclassified as large cell keratinizing, large cell nonkeratinizing, or small cell carcinomas, these designations do not correlate well with prognosis.[184] Small cell squamous carcinomas have small- to medium-sized nuclei, open chromatin, small or large nucleoli, and abundant cytoplasm, and are believed by most authorities to have a somewhat poorer prognosis than large cell neoplasms with or without keratin. However, small cell squamous carcinomas should not be confused with the much more aggressive anaplastic small cell neuroendocrine carcinomas discussed later. Papillary variants of squamous carcinoma may be well differentiated (occasionally confused with immature condylomata) or very poorly differentiated (resembling high-grade transitional carcinoma).[181] Verrucous carcinoma is a very rare warty-appearing variant of squamous carcinoma that may be difficult to differentiate from benign condyloma without multiple biopsies or hysterectomy.[185] Sarcomatoid squamous carcinoma is another very rare variant, demonstrating areas of spindle-cell carcinomatous tumor confluent with poorly differentiated squamous cell carcinoma; immunohistochemistry demonstrates expression of cytokeratin as well as vimentin. The natural history of this uncommon tumor is not well understood.[186]

Adenocarcinoma

Invasive adenocarcinoma may be pure or mixed with squamous cell carcinoma (adenosquamous carcinoma). About 80% of cervical adenocarcinomas are endocervical-type adenocarcinomas, which are composed predominantly of cells with eosinophilic cytoplasm, brisk mitotic activity, and frequent apoptotic bodies, although many other patterns and cell types have also been observed. Endocervical-type adenocarcinomas are frequently referred to as *mucinous*; however, although some have abundant intracytoplasmic mucin, most have little or none.[187]

Minimal-deviation adenocarcinoma (adenoma malignum) is a rare, extremely well-differentiated adenocarcinoma that is sometimes associated with Peutz-Jeghers syndrome.[188] Because the branching glandular pattern strongly resembles normal endocervical glands and the mucin-rich cells can be deceptively benign-appearing, minimal-deviation adenocarcinoma may not be recognized as malignant in small biopsy specimens.[187] Earlier studies reported a poor outcome for women with this tumor, but more recently, patients have been reported to have a favorable prognosis if the disease is detected early.[188]

Glassy cell carcinoma[187] is a variant of poorly differentiated adenosquamous carcinoma characterized by cells with abundant eosinophilic, granular, ground-glass cytoplasm with large round to oval nuclei and prominent nucleoli. Adenoid basal carcinoma is a well-differentiated tumor that histologically resembles basal cell carcinoma of the skin and tends to have a favorable prognosis.[189] Adenoid cystic carcinoma consists of basaloid cells in a cribriform or cylindromatous pattern; metastases are frequent, although the natural history of these tumors may be long.[189] Rarely, primary carcinomas of the cervix are composed of endometrioid, serous, or clear cells; mixtures of these cell types may be seen, and histologically, some of these tumors are indistinguishable from those arising elsewhere in the endometrium or ovary. In a study of 17 cases, Zhou et al.[190] found that serous carcinomas of the cervix have an aggressive course, similar to that of high-grade serous tumors originating in the other Müllerian sites.

Anaplastic Small Cell/Neuroendocrine Carcinoma

Anaplastic small cell carcinomas resemble oat cell carcinomas of the lung and are made up of small tumor cells that have scanty cytoplasm, small round to oval nuclei, and high mitotic activity; they frequently display neuroendocrine features.[191] Anaplastic small cell carcinomas behave more aggressively than poorly differentiated small cell squamous carcinomas; most investigators report survival rates of <50% even for patients with early stage I disease, although recent studies of aggressive multimodality treatments have been somewhat more encouraging.[192–195] Widespread hematogenous metastases are frequent, but brain metastases are rare unless preceded by pulmonary involvement.[195]

Other Rare Neoplasms

A variety of neoplasms may infiltrate the cervix from adjacent sites, and this makes differential diagnosis difficult. In particular, it may be difficult or impossible to determine the origin of adenocarcinomas involving the endocervix and uterine isthmus. Although endometrioid histology suggests endometrial origin and mucinous tumors in young patients are most often of endocervical origin, both histologic types can arise in either site.[196] Metastatic tumors from the colon, breast, or other sites may involve the cervix secondarily. Malignant mixed Müllerian tumors, adenosarcomas, and leiomyosarcomas occasionally arise in the cervix but more often involve it secondarily. Primary lymphomas and melanomas of the cervix are extremely rare. Despite the different prognostic implications of the histologic subtypes of cervical cancer, the treatment approach generally remains the same.

Clinical Manifestations

Preinvasive disease is usually detected during routine cervical cytologic screening. Early invasive disease may not be associated with any symptoms and is also usually detected during screening examinations. The earliest symptom of invasive cervical cancer is usually abnormal vaginal bleeding, often following coitus or vaginal douching. This may be associated with a clear or foul-smelling vaginal discharge. Pelvic pain may result from locoregionally invasive disease or from coexistent pelvic inflammatory disease. Flank pain may be a symptom of hydronephrosis, which may be complicated by pyelonephritis. Patients with very advanced tumors may have hematuria or incontinence from a vesicovaginal fistula caused by direct extension of tumor to the bladder. External compression of the rectum by a massive primary tumor may cause constipation, but the rectal mucosa is rarely involved at initial diagnosis.

Diagnosis, Clinical Evaluation, and Staging

Diagnosis

The long preinvasive stage of cervical cancer, the relatively high prevalence of the disease in unscreened populations, and the sensitivity of cytologic screening make cervical carcinoma an ideal target for cancer screening. In the United States, screening with cervical cytologic examination and pelvic examination has led to a decrease of >50% in the incidence of cervical cancer since 1975.[197] Only nations with well-developed screening programs have experienced substantial decreases in cervical cancer incidence.

The American Cancer Society, in conjunction with multidisciplinary working groups, recently updated the guidelines for cervical cancer screening.[198,199] The guidelines are as follows: screening is recommended to begin at age 21 years; screening should be avoided before this age because screening at younger ages may lead to unnecessary and harmful evaluation and treatment in women at very low risk of cancer. Between ages 21 and 29, Pap tests are recommended every 3 years. Between ages 30 and 65, both Pap test and HPV testing is recommended every 5 years. A single negative test for HPV is sufficient to reassure against cervical cancer over 5 years, so women aged 30 years and older who are negative for HPV testing have normal cytology can now safely extend the screening interval.[200,201] Women with a normal Pap test result who test positive for oncogenic HPV should be rescreened annually. The 5-year screening interval may be also recommended for women infected with HIV who are cytologically normal and are oncogenic HPV-negative based on a recent study showing that the 5-year cumulative incidence of HSIL and CIN-2 is similar in women infected with HIV and women not infected with HIV who are cytologically normal and oncogenic HPV-negative.[202] Women who have had a total hysterectomy for benign conditions and who have no history of high-grade CIN may discontinue routine screening. It is also reasonable to discontinue screening for women older than 65 to 70 years who have three or more consecutive negative studies and have had no abnormal test results in the past 10 years. Women previously treated for high-grade CIN or for cancer should continue to have annual screening for at least 20 years and periodic screening indefinitely. Annual gynecologic examination might still be appropriate even if cytologic screening is not performed.[197]

Accurate calculation of false-negative rates for the Pap test is difficult; estimates range from <5% to ≥20%. The sensitivity of individual tests may be improved by ensuring adequate sampling of the squamocolumnar junction and the endocervical canal; smears without endocervical or metaplastic cells are inadequate, and in such cases the test must be repeated. The sensitivity of a screening program is increased by repeated testing; studies of the test frequency required to optimize the sensitivity of screening formed the basis of the American College of Obstetrics and Gynecology recommendations.

Most US gynecologists currently prefer newer liquid-based screening methods to conventional Pap tests. A meta-analysis of available data concluded that "liquid-based cervical cytology is neither more sensitive nor more specific for detection of high-grade CIN compared with the conventional Pap,"[203] but liquid based tests are more widely used based on the ability to perform HPV typing on fluid remaining after cytologic examination. HPV testing of ASC-US smears followed by colposcopy in patients with HPV-positive lesions has been shown to be a highly accurate and cost-effective means of detecting HSIL in cases of equivocal smears and may also be used to triage postmenopausal women with LSIL.[203,204]

Patients with abnormal findings on cytologic examination who do not have a gross cervical lesion must be evaluated with colposcopy and directed biopsies. Following application of a 3% acetic-acid solution, the cervix is examined under 10- to 15-fold magnification with a bright, filtered light that enhances the acetowhitening and vascular patterns characteristic of dysplasia or carcinoma. The skilled colposcopist can accurately distinguish between low- and high-grade dysplasia,[205] but microinvasive disease cannot consistently be distinguished from intraepithelial lesions on colposcopy.[206]

In patients with a high-grade Pap smear finding, if no abnormalities are found on colposcopic examination or if the entire squamocolumnar junction cannot be visualized, an additional endocervical sample should be collected. Although some authorities advocate the routine addition of endocervical curettage to colposcopic examination, it is probably reasonable to omit this step in previously untreated women if the entire squamocolumnar junction is visible with a complete ring of unaltered columnar epithelium in the lower canal.[207] The rate of detection of endocervical lesions may be higher when specimens are collected using a cytobrush rather than by curettage.[208]

Cervical cone biopsy is used to diagnose occult endocervical lesions and is an essential step in the diagnosis and management of microinvasive carcinoma of the cervix. Cervical cone biopsy yields an accurate diagnosis and decreases the incidence of inappropriate therapy when (1) the squamocolumnar junction is poorly visualized on colposcopy and a high-grade lesion is suspected, (2) high-grade dysplastic epithelium extends into the endocervical canal, (3) the cytologic findings suggest high-grade dysplasia or carcinoma in situ, (4) a microinvasive carcinoma is found on directed biopsy, (5) the endocervical curettage specimens show high-grade CIN, or (6) the cytologic findings are suggestive of adenocarcinoma in situ.[209]

Clinical Evaluation of Patients with Invasive Carcinoma

All patients with invasive cervical cancer should be evaluated with a detailed history and physical examination, with particular attention paid to inspection and palpation of the pelvic organs with bimanual and rectovaginal examinations. Standard laboratory studies should include a complete blood cell count and renal function and liver function tests. All patients should have chest radiography to rule out lung metastases. Additional imaging of the abdomen and pelvis should be performed for all patients who have stage IB2 or greater disease and is generally recommended for patients with stage IB1 disease. MRI can be used to evaluate the size and extent of the cervical mass as well as suggest invasion into the parametria, bladder, or rectum. Cystoscopy and proctoscopy should be considered in patients with bulky tumors and patients with imaging findings suggestive of organ involvement.

Many clinicians obtain CT or MRI scans to evaluate regional lymph nodes, but these studies have suboptimal accuracy because they fail to detect small metastases and because patients with bulky necrotic tumors often have enlarged reactive lymph nodes that may be free of metastasis.[210,211] In a large GOG study that compared the results of radiographic studies with subsequent histologic findings, Heller et al.[211] found that the sensitivity of CT in the detection of positive para-aortic nodes was only 34%. PET appears to be a more sensitive, specific, and noninvasive method of evaluating the regional nodes of patients with cervical cancer.[169,212]

Clinical Staging

The FIGO staging system is the most widely accepted staging system for carcinomas of the cervix.[213,214] The latest (2009) update of this system is summarized in Table 72.8.[213] (Since the earliest versions of the cervical cancer staging system, there have been numerous changes: the designation of preinvasive disease as a separate category [1950], designation and changes in the definition of microinvasive disease [1962, 1985, and 1994], and subdivisions of the stage I and II categories according to tumor or cervical diameter [1994 and 2009]). Although these changes have gradually improved the discriminatory value of the staging system, the many fluctuations in the definitions of stages IA and IB have complicated efforts to compare the outcomes of patients whose tumors were staged and treated during different periods.[215]

FIGO stage is based primarily on careful clinical examination. The use of diagnostic imaging techniques to assess tumor size and local extent is encouraged but not mandatory in the 2009 staging system. However, FIGO still does not incorporate evidence of lymph node metastasis gained by surgical staging or advanced imaging studies in the 2009 staging system. Some form of imaging must be performed to evaluate the presence or absence of hydronephrosis, but intravenous pyelography is no longer required. Cystoscopy, sigmoidoscopy, and examination under anesthesia are also optional. However, suspected bladder or rectal involvement must be confirmed by biopsy. Stage should be assigned before any definitive therapy is administered. The clinical stage should never be changed on the basis of subsequent findings. When the stage to which a particular case should be allotted is in doubt, the case should be assigned to the earlier stage.

Although surgically treated patients are sometimes classified according to a TNM pathologic staging system, this practice has not been widely accepted because it cannot be applied to patients who are treated with primary radiotherapy.[216]

Surgical Evaluation of Regional Spread

Lymphadenectomy is performed as part of the surgical treatment of most patients with early carcinomas of the cervix. Early studies of diagnostic preradiotherapy lymph node staging were discouraging because of the high complication rates observed when transperitoneal lymph node dissections were combined with large radiation fields. In 1989, Weiser et al.[217] reported that the proportion of patients with postradiotherapy bowel complications was reduced to <5% if lymphadenectomy was performed using a retroperitoneal approach. Today, laparoscopic methods are often used to reduce the perioperative morbidity and hospitalization times associated with surgical staging.[218–220] The rate of late complications from radiotherapy following laparoscopic lymphadenectomy is probably less than with transperitoneal surgery but has not yet been fully evaluated. The use of sentinel lymph node evaluation is expanding in cervical cancer, with high rates of detection of positive nodes in most studies reported.[221,222] In the prospective SENTICOL study, the sensitivity and negative predictive values of sentinel node biopsy in early cervical cancer were 92% and 98.2%, respectively.[223] In patients where sentinel lymph nodes were identified bilaterally, sensitivity and negative predictive value were 100%.

Pelvic lymphadenectomy is indicated for patients undergoing radical hysterectomy but is controversial in other settings. The detection of microscopic para-aortic or common iliac node involvement may identify patients who will benefit from extended-field irradiation, but lymphadenectomy can also add to the morbidity of treatment. Because patients with radiographically positive pelvic nodes are at greatest risk for occult metastasis to para-aortic nodes, these patients may have the greatest chance of benefiting from surgical staging. An ongoing randomized study, LiLACs, will compare retroperitoneal node dissection with PET staging of para-aortic nodes in patients with IB2-IVA cervical cancer undergoing definitive chemoradiation.[224] Some investigators advocate for resection of large pelvic nodes before radiotherapy to improve the rate of pelvic disease control.[225,226]

Prognostic Factors

Prognosis is strongly influenced by a number of tumor characteristics that are not included in the staging system. Although FIGO now subdivides the stage IB and IIA categories according to size greater or less than 4 cm (see Table 72.8), specific information about clinical tumor diameter remains an important prognostic indicator even within these stage categories (Fig. 72.6).[227] Although FIGO stage is correlated with outcome, assessment by clinical examination tends to be inaccurate, and operative findings often do not agree with clinical estimates of parametrial or pelvic wall involvement. Furthermore, some authors have found that the predictive power of stage diminishes or is lost when comparisons are corrected for differences in clinical tumor diameter.[227]

Lymph node metastasis is one of the most important predictors of prognosis. Survival rates for patients treated with radical hysterectomy with or without postoperative radiotherapy for stage IB disease were usually reported as 85% to 95% for patients with negative nodes and 45% to 55% for those with lymph node metastases.[228,229] Survival has also been correlated with the size of the largest lymph node and with the number of involved pelvic lymph nodes.[229–231] Survival rates for patients with positive para-aortic nodes treated with extended-field radiotherapy range from 10% to 50% depending on the extent of pelvic disease and para-aortic lymph node involvement.

For patients treated with radical hysterectomy, other histologic parameters that have been associated with a poor prognosis are LVSI, deep stromal invasion (≥10 mm or >70% invasion), and parametrial extension.[231–236] Roman et al.[234] reported a correlation between the percentage of histopathologic sections containing LVSI and the incidence of lymph node metastases. Uterine-body involvement has been associated with an increased rate of distant metastases.[237] A strong inflammatory response in the cervical stroma tends to predict a good outcome.[238]

Although some investigators have reported no difference in outcome between patients with squamous carcinomas and those with adenocarcinomas of the cervix, most investigators have concluded that adenocarcinomas confer a poorer prognosis.[239–249] The evidence for a poorer prognosis is particularly strong for patients whose tumors are stage IB2 or greater. In a multivariate analysis of 1,767 patients treated with radiation for stage IB disease, Eifel et al.[242] found that the relative risk of death from cancer for 106 patients with adenocarcinomas ≥4 cm in diameter was 1.9 times that for patients with squamous tumors of the same size (p <0.01). Pelvic disease control rates were not correlated with histology, but the incidence of distant metastases was significantly higher in patients with adenocarcinomas. For patients with adenocarcinoma of the cervix, outcome appears to be correlated with the degree of tumor differentiation.[240,241,244] In a population-based analysis of 24,562 patients from the Surveillance, Epidemiology, and End Results database, women with adenocarcinomas were younger, more often white, more frequently married, and more likely to present with early stage disease than patients with squamous cell tumors. Furthermore, adenocarcinomas were associated with worse survival than squamous cell carcinomas in both early (IB1-IIA) and advanced-stage (IIB-IVA) disease (39% and 21% higher risk of death for early and advanced-stage carcinomas, respectively).[250]

In patients with squamous carcinomas, the serum concentration of squamous cell carcinoma antigen appears to correlate with stage and tumor size, the presence of lymph node metastases, and the presence of recurrent disease; however, the value of this antigen as an independent predictor of prognosis and the cost-effectiveness of measurement of this antigen as a screening modality have been disputed.[251,252]

Many studies have demonstrated a relationship between hemoglobin level and prognosis in patients with locally advanced cervical cancer, although the independent influence of hemoglobin on outcome can be difficult to estimate because of numerous confounding prognostic factors.[253] The strongest evidence that anemia plays a causative role in pelvic recurrence comes from a small 1978 randomized study conducted at the Princess Margaret Hospital; in that study, anemic patients who were transfused to a hemoglobin

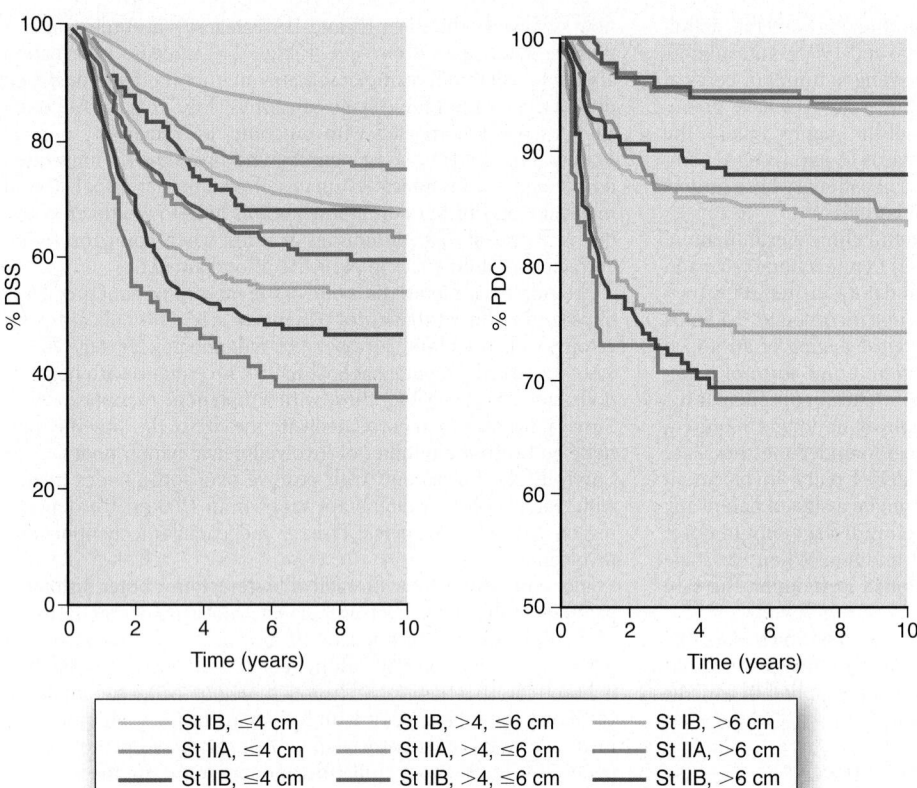

Figure 72.6 Disease-specific survival (*DSS*) and pelvic disease control (*PDC*) rates for 4,490 patients with stage I or II carcinomas of the cervix divided according to clinical tumor diameter and International Federation of Gynecology and Obstetrics (1988) stage. (From Eifel PJ, Jhingran A, Levenback CF, et al. Predictive value of a proposed subclassification of stages I and II cervical cancer based on clinical tumor diameter. *Int J Gynecol Cancer* 2009;19:2, with permission.)

level of at least 12.5 g/dl had a lower rate of locoregional recurrence than those who were maintained at a hemoglobin level of at least 10 g/dl.[254] Studies aimed at overcoming the theoretical radiobiologic consequences of intratumoral hypoxia with hypoxic cell sensitizers,[255,256] hyperbaric oxygen breathing,[257] or neutron therapy[258] have not been successful. Several investigators have correlated low intratumoral oxygen tension levels with a high rate of regional and distant metastasis and poor survival.[259,260] A recent GOG study designed to test the value of erythropoietin-induced hemoglobin elevation was closed early because of erythropoietin-related thrombotic events; however, overall survival rates of 74% and 60%, respectively, for patients receiving chemoradiation alone or with erythropoietin were not encouraging.[261]

Other clinical and biologic features have been reported to correlate with outcome but none of these have been incorporated into routine clinical practice.[262] Clinical and pathologic factors investigated include patient age,[229,263] peritoneal cytology,[264] and platelet count.[265] Molecular markers such as tumor vascularity, cyclooxygenase-2 expression,[266] galectin expression[267] (and other growth factor receptors) have been reported to correlate with outcome.[268,269] Several investigators have found the presence of HPV DNA in histologically cancer-free lymph nodes to be correlated with poor outcome.[270,271] Tumor PIK3CA mutation status has also been identified as a prognostic factor in cervical cancer.[272] Specifically, 23% of cervical cancers harbor exon 9 or exon 20 PIK3CA mutations; of these 84% are squamous cell carcinomas. PIK3CA mutation status is strongly associated with poor overall survival in patients with stage IB/II cervical cancer, but not stage III/IVa patients.

Functional imaging approaches, such as FDG-PET, may also be used to refine prognosis. Kidd et al.[273] developed a pretreatment FDG-PET–based prognostic nomogram that identified extent of lymph node metastases, tumor volume, and primary tumor maximum standardized uptake value as three significant independent prognostic variables.[274]

Treatment

A number of factors may influence the choice of local treatment for cervical cancer, including tumor size, stage, histologic features, evidence of lymph node metastasis, risk factors for complications of surgery or radiotherapy, and patient preference. However, as a rule, HSILs are managed with a loop electroexcision procedure (LEEP); microinvasive cancers invading <3 mm (stage IA1) are managed with conservative surgery (excisional conization or extrafascial hysterectomy); early invasive cancers (stage IA2 and IB1 and some small stage IIA tumors) are managed with radical or modified radical hysterectomy, radical trachelectomy (if fertility preservation is desired), or radiotherapy; and locally advanced cancers (stages IB2 through IVA) are managed with combined chemotherapy and radiotherapy. Selected patients with centrally recurrent disease after maximum radiotherapy may be treated with radical exenterative surgery; isolated pelvic recurrence after hysterectomy is treated with irradiation.

Preinvasive Disease

LEEP is the preferred treatment for HSIL.[274] With this technique, a charged electrode is used to excise the entire transformation zone and distal canal. Although control rates are similar to those achieved with cryotherapy or laser ablation, LEEP is more easily learned, is less expensive than laser ablation, and preserves the excised lesion and transformation zone for histologic evaluation.[274,275] LEEP is an outpatient procedure that preserves fertility. LEEP conization or excisional conization with a scalpel should be performed when microinvasive or invasive cancer is suspected and in patients with adenocarcinoma in situ. Although recurrence rates are low (1% to 5%) and progression to invasion rare (<1% in most series), patients treated with LEEP require careful post-LEEP surveillance.

Treatment with total hysterectomy currently is reserved for women who have other gynecologic conditions that justify the procedure; invasive cancer still must be excluded before surgery to rule out the need for a more extensive operative procedure.

Microinvasive Carcinoma (Stage IA)

The standard treatment for patients with stage IA1 disease is cervical conization or total (type I) hysterectomy. Because the risk of pelvic lymph node metastases from these minimally invasive tumors is <1%,[232,276] pelvic lymphadenectomy is not usually recommended.

Patients who have FIGO stage IA1 disease without LVSI and who wish to maintain fertility may be adequately treated with a therapeutic cervical conization if the margins of the cone are negative. Although reports suggest that recurrences are infrequent,[277,278] patients who have this conservative treatment must be followed very closely with periodic cytologic evaluation, colposcopy, and endocervical curettage.

The likelihood of residual invasive disease after cone biopsy is correlated with the status of the internal cone margin and the results of an endocervical curettage performed after cone biopsy.[279,280] Roman et al.[281] reported the surgical findings in 87 patients who underwent a conization that showed microinvasive squamous carcinoma, followed by either a repeat conization or hysterectomy. Residual invasive disease was present in only 4% of patients whose cone margins were free of CIN and who had no disease detected on endocervical curettage. However, residual invasive disease was present in 13% of women who had either CIN in cone margins or positive endocervical curettage findings, and 33% of women who had both of these features (*p* <0.015), suggesting the need for a second procedure in any patient who has one of these findings. The authors did not find any correlation between the depth of invasion or the number of invasive foci and residual invasive disease.

Therapeutic conization for microinvasive disease is usually performed with a scalpel while the patient is under general or spinal anesthesia. Because an accurate assessment of the maximum depth of invasion is critical, the entire specimen must be sectioned and carefully handled to maintain its original orientation for microscopic assessment. Complications occur in 2% to 12% of patients, are related to the depth of the cone, and include hemorrhage, sepsis, infertility, stenosis, and cervical incompetence.[281] The width and depth of the cone should be tailored to produce the least amount of injury while providing clear surgical margins.

For patients whose tumors invade 3 to 5 mm into the stroma (FIGO stage IA2), the risk of nodal metastases is approximately 5%.[183,233,276] Therefore, in such patients, bilateral pelvic lymphadenectomy should be performed in conjunction with modified radical (type II) hysterectomy. Modified radical hysterectomy is a less extensive procedure than classic radical (type III) hysterectomy (Fig. 72.7). The uterus, cervix, upper vagina, and paracervical tissues are removed after careful dissection of the ureters to the point of their entry to the bladder. The medial halves of the cardinal ligament and the uterosacral ligaments are also removed. With this treatment, significant urinary tract complications are rare, and cure rates exceed 95%.[139]

The potential for fertility-conserving surgery is being investigated for patients with low-risk features and stage IA2-IB1 tumors.[282] A radical trachelectomy removes the cervix and parametrial tissues while retaining the uterine corpus. Outcomes appear to be similar for patients treated with radical hysterectomy or radical trachelectomy,[283] and successful pregnancies are reported in a significant percentage of patients after radical trachylectomy. However, it is not clear that removal of the parametria tissue is needed for all patients with low-risk stage IA2-IBI tumors, as few patients with low-risk early stage cervical cancers have extension to the parametria and many have no residual tumor in the trachelectomy specimen. This has led to the question of whether more conservative surgery, such as simple trachelectomy or cone with or without a nodal assessment, could be performed. An ongoing international study, ConCerv, is currently testing the safety and feasibility of conservative surgery in patients with low-risk features.[282] Eligible patients have stage IA2 or IB1 disease, tumor size of ≤2 cm, and squamous cell carcinoma (any grade) or adenocarcinoma (grades

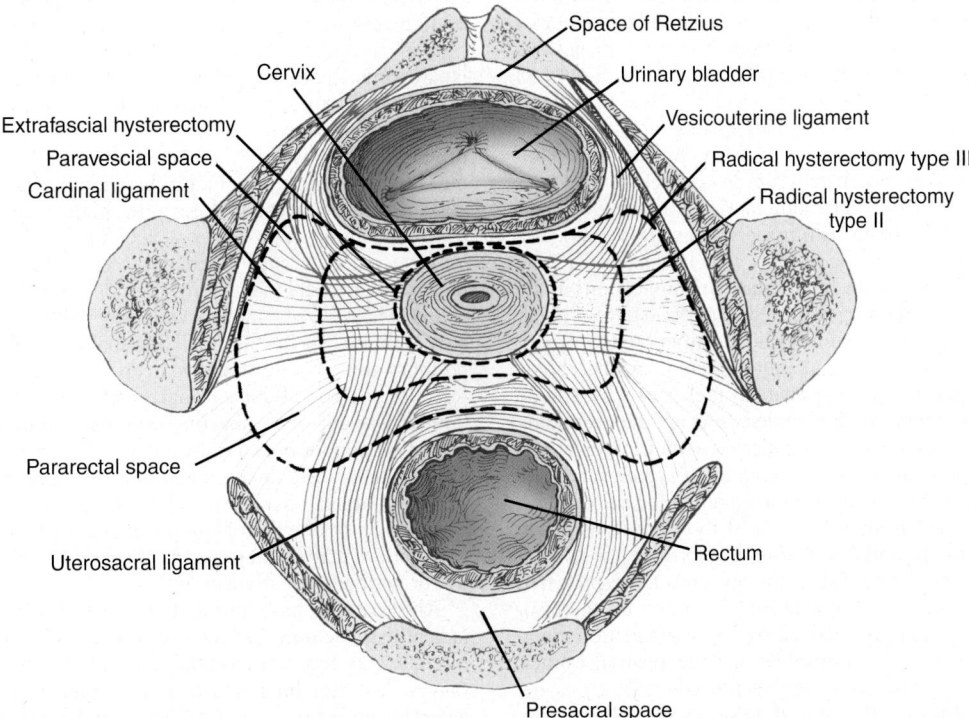

Figure 72.7 The pelvic ligaments and spaces. *Dotted lines* indicate the tissues removed with a modified radical (type II) or radical (type III) hysterectomy. (From Berek JS, Hacker NF. *Practical Gynecologic Oncology.* Philadelphia, PA: Lippincott Williams & Wilkins; 2005, with permission.)

1 or 2) and no evidence of LVSI. Patients who wish to conserve fertility receive cervical cone with lymph node dissection and lymphatic mapping while patients who do not wish to conserve fertility undergo a simple hysterectomy with nodal assessment.

Although surgical treatment is standard for in situ and microinvasive cancer, patients with severe medical problems or other contraindications to surgical treatment can be successfully treated with radiotherapy. Depending on the depth of invasion, these early lesions are treated with brachytherapy alone or brachytherapy combined with external beam irradiation, and cure rates exceed 95%.[284,285]

Stage IB and IIA Disease

Early stage IB cervical carcinomas can be treated effectively with combined external beam irradiation and brachytherapy or with radical hysterectomy and bilateral pelvic lymphadenectomy. The goal of both treatments is to destroy malignant cells in the cervix, paracervical tissues, and regional lymph nodes. Patients who are treated with radical hysterectomy whose tumors are found to have high-risk disease features may benefit from postoperative radiotherapy or chemoradiation.[286,287]

Disease-specific survival rates for patients with stage IB cervical cancer treated with surgery or radiation usually range between 80% and 90%, suggesting that the two treatments are equally effective.[288–291] However, biases introduced by patient selection, variations in the definition of stage IA disease, and variable indications for postoperative radiotherapy, concurrent chemotherapy, or adjuvant hysterectomy confound comparisons of efficacy between radiotherapy and surgery. Because young women with small, clinically node-negative tumors tend to be favored candidates for surgery and because tumor diameter and nodal status are inconsistently described in published series, it is difficult to compare the results reported for patients treated with surgery and those treated with radiotherapy.

In 1997, Landoni et al.[292] reported results from the only prospective trial comparing radical surgery with radiotherapy alone for cervical cancer. In their study, 343 patients with stage IB or IIA disease were randomly assigned to treatment with radical (type III) hysterectomy or a combination of external beam and LDR intracavitary brachytherapy. In the surgery arm, findings of parametrial involvement, positive margins, deep stromal invasion, or positive nodes led to the use of postoperative pelvic irradiation in 54% of patients with tumors ≤4 cm in diameter and in 84% of patients with larger tumors. Patients in the radiotherapy arm received a relatively low median dose to point A of 76 Gy. With a median follow-up of 87 months, the 5-year actuarial disease-free survival rates for patients in the surgery and radiotherapy groups were 80% and 82%, respectively, for patients with tumors that were ≤4 cm, and 63% and 57%, respectively, for patients with larger tumors. The authors reported a significantly higher rate of complications in the patients treated with initial surgery, and they attributed this finding to the frequent use of combined-modality treatment in this group.

For patients with stage IB1 squamous carcinomas, the choice of treatment is based primarily on patient preference, anesthetic and surgical risks, physician preference, and an understanding of the nature and incidence of complications with hysterectomy and radiotherapy. For patients with similar tumors, the overall rate of major complications is similar with surgery and radiotherapy, although urinary tract complications tend to be more common after surgical treatment and bowel complications are more common after radiotherapy. Surgical treatment tends to be preferred for young women with small tumors because it permits preservation of ovarian function and may cause less vaginal shortening. Radiotherapy is often selected for older, postmenopausal women to avoid the morbidity of a major surgical procedure.

For patients with stage IB2 tumors, some surgeons have advocated the use of radical hysterectomy as initial treatment.[293–295] Patients who have tumors measuring >4 cm in diameter are at high risk for lymph node involvement and parametrial extension.

Because patients with these risk factors have an increased rate of pelvic disease recurrence, surgical treatment is usually followed by postoperative irradiation or chemoradiation, increasing the overall length of treatment and side effects of treatment. Consequently, many gynecologic and radiation oncologists believe that patients with stage IB2 carcinomas are better treated with primary chemoradiation.

Two prospective randomized trials[43,296] demonstrated that patients who are treated with radiation for bulky stage I cancers benefit from concurrent administration of cisplatin-containing chemotherapy. A third study suggested that patients who require postoperative radiotherapy because of findings of lymph node metastasis or involved surgical margins also benefit from concurrent chemoradiation.[286] Patients who have stage IB1 cancers without evidence of regional involvement have excellent pelvic control rates with radiotherapy alone (about 97% at 5 years) and probably do not require chemotherapy when they are treated with primary radiotherapy.[290,291]

Radical and Modified Radical Hysterectomy

The standard surgical treatment for stage IB and IIA cervical carcinomas is radical (type III) hysterectomy and bilateral pelvic lymphadenectomy. This procedure involves en bloc removal of the uterus, cervix, and paracervical, parametrial, and paravaginal tissues to the pelvic sidewalls bilaterally, with removal of as much of the uterosacral ligaments as possible (see Fig. 72.7). The uterine vessels are ligated at their origin, and the proximal third of the vagina and the paracolpium are resected. Modified radical (type II) hysterectomy may be used for IA2 and selected small (<2 cm in diameter) stage IB lesions; with this procedure, the parametrial and paracervical tissue is removed medial to the ureter, the uterosacral ligaments are partially resected, and only the proximal 1 to 2 cm of the vagina are removed. The decision of whether to remove the ovaries should be individualized and based on the patient's age, menopausal status, and other factors. Ovarian metastases are rare in the absence of metastases to lymph nodes or other sites. If intraoperative findings suggest a need for postoperative pelvic irradiation, the ovaries may be transposed out of the pelvis.

Radical hysterectomy is increasingly being performed using a laparoscopic approach with or without robotic assistance.[297–299] In experienced hands, these methods may result in reduced blood loss and quicker postoperative recovery times, although operative times may be somewhat longer. Preliminary results suggest that outcomes of laparoscopic radical hysterectomy are similar to those achieved with radical hysterectomy performed using the traditional abdominal approach.

Intraoperative and immediate postoperative complications of radical abdominal hysterectomy include blood loss, ureterovaginal fistula (1% to 2% of patients), vesicovaginal fistula (<1%), pulmonary embolus (1% to 2%), small bowel obstruction (1% to 2%), and postoperative fever secondary to deep vein thrombosis, pulmonary infection, pelvic cellulitis, urinary tract infection, or wound infection (25% to 50%).[300] Subacute complications include lymphocyst formation and lower extremity edema, the risk of which is related to the extent of the node dissection.[301] Lymphocysts may obstruct a ureter, but hydronephrosis usually improves with drainage of the lymphocyst.[302] The risk of complications, particularly small bowel obstruction, may be increased in patients who undergo preoperative or postoperative irradiation.[294]

Most patients have transient decreased bladder sensation after radical hysterectomy. Severe long-term bladder complications are infrequent and are related to the extent of the parametrial and paravaginal dissection but not to the type of surgical approach (abdominal or laparoscopic).[303,304] Even with careful postoperative bladder drainage, chronic bladder hypotonia or atony occurs in approximately 3% to 5% of patients.[303,305,306] Radical hysterectomy may be complicated by stress incontinence, but reported incidences vary widely and may be influenced by the addition of postoperative radiotherapy.[305,306] Patients may also experience constipation and, rarely, chronic obstipation after radical hysterectomy.

Radical Trachelectomy

In 1994, Dargent et al.[307] pioneered the use of radical trachelectomy and laparoscopic pelvic lymphadenectomy as a means of sparing fertility in young women with early cervical cancer. Since then, it has been demonstrated that when these procedures are performed by experienced surgeons, the cure rates are high and many women are able to carry subsequent pregnancies to viability.[308] Successful pregnancies have also been reported after radical abdominal trachelectomy.[309] In order to keep the residual uterine segment intact, a nonabsorbable cervical cerclage is placed around the uterine isthmus at the time of the trachelectomy. Alexander-Sefre et al.[310] reported that radical trachelectomy was associated with shorter operative times and hospital stays, less blood loss, and a lower incidence of bladder hypotony than radical hysterectomy. However, patients who had radical trachelectomy had more problems with dysmenorrhea, irregular menstruation, and vaginal discharge; in addition, 14% had cervical suture problems, 10% had isthmic stenosis, and 7% had prolonged amenorrhea.

The use of radical vaginal or abdominal trachelectomy and laparoscopic lymphadenectomy may be indicated in carefully selected women with small IB1 (≤2 cm) lesions who are eager to preserve fertility. Patients with extensive endocervical extension are poor candidates for fertility-sparing surgery. Preoperative MRI is a relatively sensitive and specific method to evaluate the possibility of tumor extension beyond the internal os.[311] A recent review of 504 women who underwent radical trachelectomy summarized the outcome of 200 pregnancies.[312] Although 84 of 200 pregnancies (42%) produced full-term viable infants, 37% of third-trimester deliveries were preterm, indicating that these women are at high risk for complicated pregnancies.

Radiotherapy After Radical Hysterectomy

Retrospective and prospective studies clearly demonstrate that irradiation decreases the risk of pelvic recurrence after radical hysterectomy in patients with high-risk disease features (lymph node metastasis, deep stromal invasion, positive or close surgical margins, or parametrial involvement).[287,313] However, because the patients who received postoperative radiotherapy in most studies were selected because they had high-risk features, it has been difficult to determine the impact of adjuvant irradiation on survival.

GOG-92, a randomized trial first reported in 1999 and updated in 2006,[287,313] tested the benefit of adjuvant pelvic irradiation in patients with an intermediate risk of recurrence after radical hysterectomy for stage IB carcinoma. Patients were eligible for this study if they had at least two of the following risk factors: greater than one-third stromal invasion, LVSI, or clinical tumor diameter of at least 4 cm. Patients with involvement of the pelvic lymph nodes, parametria, or surgical margins were excluded. Patients who received adjuvant radiotherapy experienced a 46% reduction in the risk of recurrence ($p = 0.007$). Although there was a 30% reduction in the risk of death for patients who received radiotherapy, this difference was not statistically significant ($p = 0.07$). A subset analysis suggested that the benefit of postoperative radiotherapy was particularly striking for patients who had adenocarcinomas or adenosquamous carcinomas.[287,313]

Although pelvic irradiation reduces the risk of recurrence for patients with pelvic lymph node metastases or parametrial involvement, the risk of pelvic and distant recurrence remains high for these women after radiotherapy. In an attempt to improve the results of combined-modality treatment, the Southwest Oncology Group conducted a prospective trial comparing postoperative pelvic radiotherapy alone versus administration of cisplatin and 5-FU during and after postoperative pelvic radiotherapy for patients with

lymph node metastases, parametrial involvement, or involved surgical margins. Initial results of this trial, published in 2000, demonstrated significantly improved rates of pelvic disease control and survival for patients who received chemotherapy (Table 72.9).[286]

The use of adjuvant radiotherapy undoubtedly increases the rate of posttreatment small bowel and genitourinary complications in patients who have had radical hysterectomy[292,313]; however, inconsistencies in the methods of analysis, selection biases, and the relatively small number of patients in most series make studies of this subject difficult to interpret.[314]

Definitive Radiotherapy

Radiotherapy alone also achieves excellent survival and pelvic disease control rates in patients with stage IB cervical cancer.[227,290,315] Eifel et al.[290] reported 5-year disease-specific survival and pelvic control rates of 90% and 98%, respectively, for 701 patients treated with radiation alone for stage IB1 disease. Although outcomes are poorer for patients with larger tumors, even these are frequently curable with a combination of external beam irradiation and brachytherapy. However, patients with stage IB2 and bulky stage IIA cancers are usually treated with concurrent cisplatin-based chemoradiation, which has been demonstrated in randomized trials to yield better outcomes than radiotherapy alone.[129,296]

As with radical surgery, the goal of radical radiotherapy is to sterilize disease in the cervix, paracervical tissues, and regional lymph nodes in the pelvis. Patients are usually treated with a combination of external beam irradiation to the pelvis and brachytherapy. Even relatively small tumors that involve multiple quadrants of the cervix are usually treated with total doses of 80 to 85 Gy to point A. The dose may be reduced by 5% to 10% for very small superficial tumors. Although patients with small tumors may be treated with somewhat smaller fields than patients with more advanced locoregional disease, care must still be taken to adequately cover the obturator, external iliac, low common iliac, and presacral nodes. Radiation technique, which is similar for patients who have bulky stage I or more advanced cancers, is discussed further in "Stage IIB, III, and IVA Disease."

Irradiation Followed by Hysterectomy

Although early studies from the MD Anderson Cancer Center suggested that local recurrence rates for patients with bulky stage IB cancers were decreased when radiotherapy was followed by adjuvant hysterectomy, subsequent retrospective studies were less convincing and suggested that selection bias may have been responsible for the observed differences.[316,317] In a study of 1,526 patients with stage IB squamous carcinomas, Eifel et al.[290] reported central tumor recurrence rates of <10% for tumors as large as 7 to 7.9 cm treated with radiation alone, suggesting that the margin for possible improvement with adjuvant hysterectomy is small.

In 2003, the GOG reported results of a prospective randomized trial of irradiation with or without adjuvant extrafascial hysterectomy in patients with stage IB tumors ≥4 cm in diameter[318]; the study demonstrated no significant improvement in the survival rate among patients who had adjuvant hysterectomy (relative risk of death = 0.89; 95% confidence interval = 0.65 to 1.21).

These results, combined with those of more recent studies demonstrating low pelvic recurrence rates after concurrent treatment with chemotherapy and radiation,[129] suggest that there is little role for routine treatment with adjuvant hysterectomy. However, adjuvant hysterectomy may still play a role in selected cases in which uterine fibroids or other anatomic variations limit the dose of radiation deliverable with brachytherapy and in patients who have involvement of the uterine fundus with cancer. In these cases, extrafascial (type I) hysterectomy is usually performed, in which the uterus, cervix, adjacent tissues, and a small cuff of the upper vagina in a plane outside the pubocervical fascia are removed. Radical

TABLE 72.9

Prospective Randomized Trials that Investigated the Role of Concurrent Radiotherapy and Chemotherapy for Patients with Locoregionally Advanced Cervical Cancer

Study (Ref.)	Protocol Designation	No. of Patients	Eligibility	Chemotherapy in Investigational Arm	Chemotherapy in Control Arm	Relative Risk of Recurrence (95% CI)	P Value
Rose et al.[130]	GOG-120	526	FIGO IIB–IVA, PA nodes negative (dissection)	Cisplatin 40 mg/m² (wk 1–6)	Hydroxyurea 3 g/m² (twice weekly, wk 1–6)	0.57 (0.42–0.78)	<0.001
				Cisplatin 50 mg/m² (days 1 and 29) 5-FU 4 g/m² (96-hr infusion days 1, 29) Hydroxyurea 2 g/m² (twice weekly, wk 1–6)	Hydroxyurea 3 g/m² (twice weekly, wk 1–6)	0.55 (0.40–0.75)	<0.001
Eifel[369]	RTOG 90-01	403	FIGO IB–IIA (≥5 cm), IIB–IVA, or pelvic lymph node positive PA nodes negative (dissection or lymphangiogram)	Cisplatin 75 mg/m² (days 1 and 22 and with second brachytherapy) 5-FU 4 g/m² (96-hr infusion days 1 and 22 and with second brachytherapy)	None[a]	0.51 (0.36–0.66)	<0.001
Keys et al.[296]	GOG-123	369	FIGO IB (≥4 cm) PA nodes negative (CT or lymphangiogram)	Cisplatin 40 mg/m² (wk 1–6)[b]	None[b]	0.51 (0.34–0.75)	0.001
Whitney et al.[268]	GOG-85	368	FIGO IIB–IVA, PA nodes negative (dissection)	Cisplatin 50 mg/m² days 1 and 29) 5-FU 4 g/m² (96-hr infusion days 1 and 29)	Hydroxyurea 80 mg/kg (twice weekly during external radiotherapy)	0.79 (0.62–0.99)	0.03
Peters et al.[286]	SWOG 87–97	268	FIGO I–IIA after radical hysterectomy with findings of pelvic lymph node metastases and/or positive margins and/or parametrial involvement PA nodes negative	Cisplatin 70 mg/m² 5-FU 4 g/m² (96-hr infusion) Every 21 days for 4 cycles beginning on day 1 of radiation therapy	None	0.50 (0.29–0.84)	0.01
Pearcey et al.[371]	NCI Canada	259	FIGO IB–IIA (≥5 cm), IIB–IVA, or pelvic lymph nodes positive	Cisplatin 40 mg/m² (wk 1–6)	None	0.91 (0.62–1.35)	0.33
Wong et al.[374]		220	FIGO IB–IIA (>4 cm), IIB–III	Epirubicin 60 mg/m² then 90 mg/m² every 4 wk for five more cycles[c]	None	Not stated	0.02
Thomas et al.[372]		234	FIGO IB–IIA (≥5 cm), IIB–IVA	5-FU 4 g/m²/96 hr × 2	None[d]	Not stated	Not significant
Lorvidhaya et al.[373]		926	FIGO IIB–IVA	Mitomycin 10 mg/m² and oral 5-FU 300 mg/m²/d × 14 days (two cycles); ± adjuvant 5-FU	None or adjuvant 5-FU only	Not stated	0.0001
Lanciano et al.[373]	GOG-165	316	FIGO IIB–IVA	5-FU 225 mg/m²/d for 5 days per week (protracted venous infusion)	Cisplatin 40 mg/m² (wk 1–6)	1.29 (0.93–1.8)	Not stated
Dueñas-González et al.[376]	International Multicenter	515	FIGO IIB–IVA	Cisplatin 40 mg/m² + Gemcitabine 125mg/m² (wk 1–6) followed by adjuvant cisplatin 50 mg/m² on day 1 plus gemcitabine 1,000 mg/m² on days 1 and 8, every 3 weeks for two cycles	Cisplatin 40 mg/m² (wk 1–6)	0.68 (0.49–0.95)	0.0227

CI, confidence interval; GOG, Gynecologic Oncology Group; FIGO, FIGO, International Federation of Gynecology and Obstetrics; PA, para-aortic; 5-FU, 5-fluorouracil; RTOG, Radiation Therapy Oncology Group; CT, computed tomography; SWOG, Southwest Oncology Group; NCI, National Cancer Institute.
[a] Patients in the control arm had prophylactic para-aortic irradiation.
[b] All patients had extrafascial hysterectomy after radiotherapy.
[c] Chemotherapy was begun on day 1 and continued every 4 weeks during and after radiotherapy.
[d] Patients were also randomly assigned to receive standard or hyperfractionated radiotherapy in a four-arm trial.

hysterectomy is avoided after high-dose irradiation because of an increased risk of fistula and other complications.

Chemotherapy Followed by Radical Surgery

A number of researchers have investigated the use of neoadjuvant chemotherapy followed by radical hysterectomy to treat patients with bulky stage IB or stage II cervical carcinoma. Neoadjuvant regimens have usually included cisplatin and bleomycin plus one or two other drugs.

In an early trial of this approach, Sardi et al.[319] reported better projected 4-year disease-free survival rates when neoadjuvant chemotherapy was added to radical hysterectomy plus postoperative radiotherapy in patients whose tumors were >4 cm. However, in a subsequent randomized trial,[320] the GOG reported no significant difference in recurrence rates (relative risk = 0.998) or death rates (relative risk = 1.008) for patients who did or did not receive neoadjuvant chemotherapy before radical hysterectomy. In their trial, patients who underwent hysterectomy were treated with postoperative irradiation if they had high-risk disease features; the proportion requiring postoperative irradiation was similar in the two arms (45% for those who did and 52% for those who did not receive neoadjuvant chemotherapy). Several trials have compared radiotherapy alone versus neoadjuvant chemotherapy followed by hysterectomy plus or minus postoperative radiotherapy with conflicting results.[321,322] However, these trials, conceived before 1999, did not include concurrent chemotherapy in the radiotherapy arms.

Ultimately, the cost and morbidity of triple-modality treatment can only be justified if it proves to be more effective than treatment with the current standard of concurrent chemotherapy and radiotherapy.

Stage IIB, III, and IVA Disease

Radiotherapy is the primary local treatment for most patients with locoregionally advanced cervical carcinoma. The success of radiotherapy depends on a careful balance between external beam radiotherapy and brachytherapy, optimizing the dose to tumor and normal tissues and the overall duration of treatment. For patients treated with radiotherapy alone for stage IIB, IIIB, and IV disease, 5-year survival rates of 65% to 75%, 35% to 50%, and 15% to 20%, respectively, have been reported.[227,323–325] Results of major clinical trials reported at the end of the 1990s indicate that, barring medical contraindications, patients with locally advanced tumors should also receive concurrent chemotherapy along with radiotherapy. With appropriate chemoradiotherapy, even patients with massive locoregional disease have a significant chance for cure.

External beam irradiation is used to deliver a homogeneous dose to the primary cervical tumor and to potential sites of regional spread and may also improve the efficacy of subsequent intracavitary brachytherapy by shrinking bulky tumor and bringing it within the range of the high-dose portion of the brachytherapy dose distribution. To facilitate brachytherapy, patients with locally advanced disease usually begin with a course of external beam treatment with concurrent chemotherapy. Subsequent brachytherapy exploits the inverse square law to deliver a high dose to the cervix and paracervical tissues while minimizing the dose to adjacent normal tissues.

Breaks during or between external beam and intracavitary treatments should be discouraged, and every effort should be made to complete the entire radiation treatment in <7 to 8 weeks. Several studies have suggested that treatment courses >8 weeks are associated with decreased pelvic disease control and survival rates.[326–328] A recently analysis of patterns of care for patients with cervical cancer treated across the United States in radiation oncology facilities revealed that a concerningly high percentage of patients were not completing treatment within this time frame. Approximately 40% of patients treated in nonacademic facilities failed to complete treatment within 10 weeks.[329] Although treatment protraction also

tended to be a problem in academic centers, the percentage of patients completing treatment in <10 weeks (83%) was significantly greater. These findings highlight the logistical and therapeutic challenges associated with delivery of multimodality cervical cancer treatment and suggest that facilities with experience in treating cervical cancer are more successful at managing these issues to prevent treatment delays.

External Beam Radiotherapy Technique. High-energy photons (15 to 18 MV) are usually preferred for standard three-dimensional conformal pelvic treatment because they spare superficial tissues that are unlikely to be involved with tumor. At these energies, the pelvis can be treated either with four fields (anterior, posterior, and lateral fields) or with anterior and posterior fields alone (Fig. 72.8). When high-energy beams are not available, four fields are usually used because less-penetrating 4- to 6-mV photons often deliver an unacceptably high dose to superficial tissues when only two fields are used.

When lateral fields are used to treat intact cervical cancers, particular care must be taken to adequately encompass the primary tumor and potential sites of regional spread in the radiation fields. Representative axial and sagittal dose distributions obtained with this technique are shown in Figures 72.8C and 72.8D, respectively.

CT simulation is recommended to confirm adequate coverage of the uterus and draining lymphatics. Information gained from radiologic studies such as MRI, CT, and PET can improve estimates of disease extent and assist in localization of regional nodes and paracervical tissues that may contain microscopic disease. The caudad extent of disease can be determined by inserting radiopaque markers in the cervix or at the lowest extent of vaginal disease. It is usually wise to cover the entire presacrococcygeal region when locally advanced cancers are treated to account for internal organ motion.

Tumor response should be evaluated with periodic pelvic examinations. Some practitioners prefer to maximize the brachytherapy component of treatment and begin it as soon as the tumor has responded enough to permit a good placement of the brachytherapy applicators, delivering subsequent pelvic irradiation with a central shield. This technique may reduce the volume of normal tissue treated to a high dose but can also result in overdoses to medial structures such as the ureters or underdosage of posterior uterosacral disease. For these reasons, most clinicians prefer to give an initial dose of 40 to 45 Gy to the whole pelvis, believing that the ability to deliver a homogeneous distribution to the entire region at risk for microscopic disease outweighs other considerations. External beam doses of >40 to 45 Gy to the central pelvis tend to compromise the dose deliverable to paracentral tissues and increase the risk of late complications.

A total dose (external beam and intracavitary) of 45 to 55 Gy appears to be sufficient to sterilize microscopic disease in the pelvic nodes in most patients. It is customary to treat lymph nodes known to contain gross disease and heavily involved parametria to a total dose of 60 to 66 Gy (including the contribution from brachytherapy treatments).

Intensity-Modulated Radiotherapy. The use of IMRT and other forms of highly conformal radiotherapy in patients with gynecologic tumors is increasing.[330–332] Unlike standard two-field and four-field techniques, IMRT makes it possible to deliver a lower daily dose to the intrapelvic contents than to surrounding pelvic lymph nodes (Fig. 72.9). With standard techniques, the close proximity of bowel has made it difficult to sterilize disease in nodes >2 cm; IMRT allows delivery of doses exceeding 60 Gy to regional nodes with relative sparing of adjacent critical structures.

When the para-aortic region requires treatment, IMRT can reduce the dose of radiation to the small bowel, including the duodenum. IMRT is particularly adventagous when there are grossly involved para-aortic nodes, which can be treated with an integrated

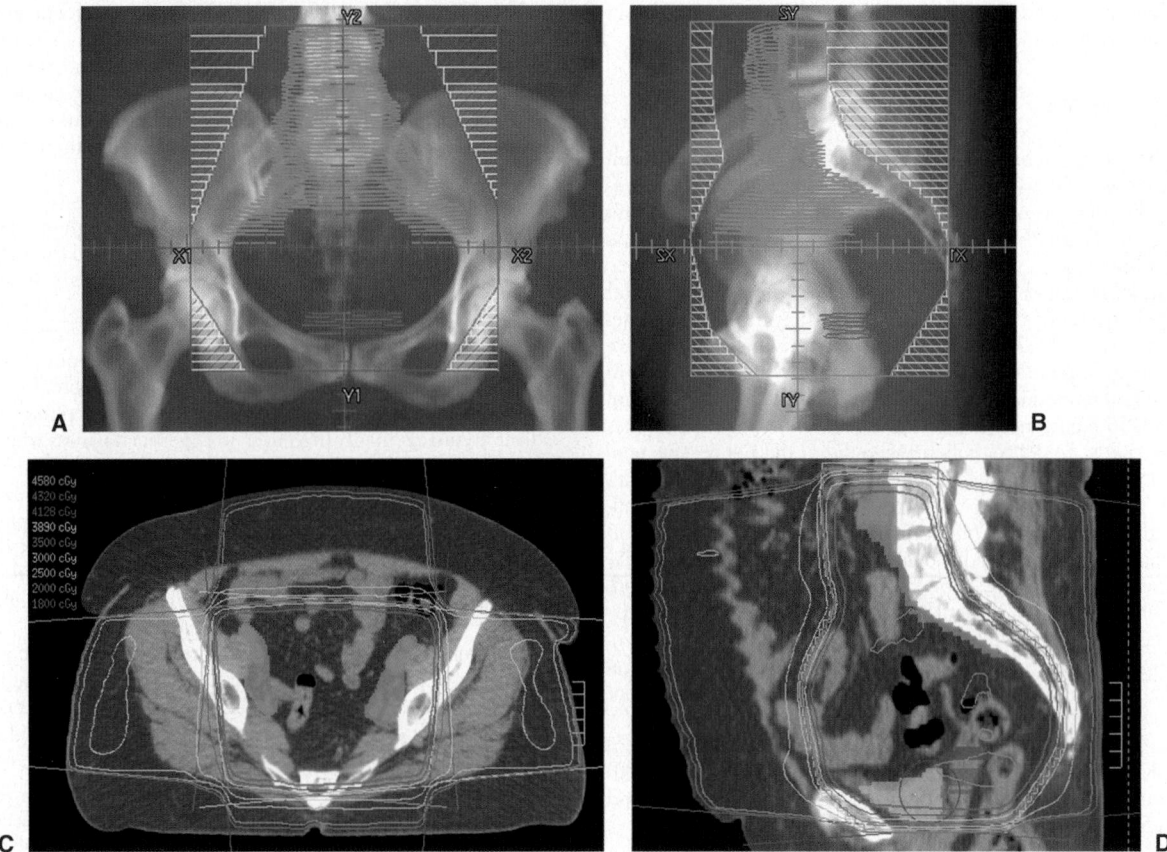

Figure 72.8 Typical anterior **(A)** and lateral **(B)** fields used to treat the pelvis with a four-field technique. When lateral fields are used to treat intact cervical cancers, particular care must be taken to adequately encompass the primary tumor and potential sites of regional spread in the radiation fields. Representative axial and sagittal dose distributions obtained with this technique are shown in panels **C** and **D**, respectively.

boost. The duodenum should be contoured and avoided in such situations; reducing the volume receiving 55 Gy has been reported to reduce toxicity.[333] IMRT to the para-aortics can be matched to a four-field or anteroposterior/posteroanterior pelvic field. Alternatively, IMRT can be used to treat the pelvis, but great care should be used to define the volume at risk and to account for the potential for significant uterine motion.

Although IMRT is an extremely useful tool in the treatment of gynecologic cancers, the highly conformal dose distributions achievable with IMRT also increase the potential for error and require considerable experience and attention to detail on the part of the radiation oncologist. In particular, great attention must be paid to the influence of internal organ motion and intratreatment tumor response on the doses to tumor and critical structures. The uterus and vagina can move 3 to 4 cm with bladder and rectal filling, and even greater excursion is possible with anterversion or retroversion of the uterus, which can occur spontaneously.[334] Daily image guidance with CT or kV imaging should be used with IMRT to

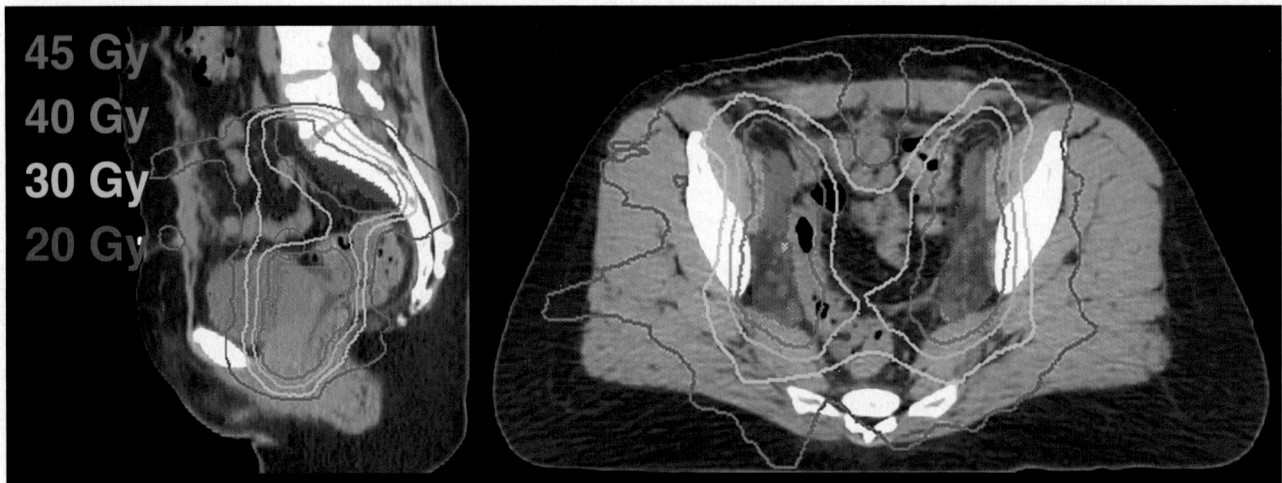

Figure 72.9 Axial and midline sagittal views of an intensity-modulated radiation therapy plan for postoperative pelvic radiotherapy in a patient with adenocarcinoma of the cervix. The target volume was extended to the top of S1 rather than L5 due to an extensive negative node dissection.

ensure that the uterus remains within the target volume. Although some investigators have begun to explore the use of IMRT to treat patients with intact cervical cancers, large inter- and intratreatment variations in the position and size of the target volume raise serious concerns about the risk of missing tumor with these highly conforming treatments; if very ample margins are used to account for variability in the target, the gain relative to simpler treatments may not justify such complex treatment. There is no evidence that IMRT can safely be used as an alternative to brachytherapy for routine treatment of intact cervical cancer. Although IMRT achieves very conformal dose distributions, it cannot accurately reproduce the high-dose gradients produced with intracavitary brachytherapy. More importantly, the large, unpredictable variations that occur in the positions of the bladder, rectum, and target mandate the use of large treatment margins that inevitably encompass adjacent critical structures and reduce the dose deliverable to tumor.

Role of Para-Aortic Irradiation.

Two prospective randomized trials conducted during the 1980s addressed the role of prophylactic para-aortic irradiation in patients without known para-aortic node involvement.[335,336] In a Radiation Therapy Oncology Group study of 367 patients, Rotman et al.[337] demonstrated a significantly better survival rate for patients treated with extended fields than for those treated with standard pelvic radiotherapy (67% versus 55% at 5 years; $p = 0.02$). A second trial, from the European Organization for Research and Treatment of Cancer,[335] involved a similar randomization but included patients with somewhat more advanced disease; in that study, 4-year disease-free survival rates for patients treated with pelvic radiotherapy and those treated with extended fields were not significantly different, although the rate of para-aortic node recurrence was significantly higher in the pelvic-field group. Both studies revealed an increased rate of enteric complications in patients treated with extended fields.

Numerous small series of patients with documented para-aortic node involvement suggest that 25% to 50% have long-term survival after extended-field irradiation. Survival is correlated with the bulk of central disease and the extent and size of involved lymph nodes. Cunningham et al.[338] reported a 48% 5-year survival rate in patients who had para-aortic node involvement discovered at exploration for radical hysterectomy that was then aborted. This experience with patients who had relatively small primary disease demonstrates that extensive regional spread can occur without distant metastases and that patients with para-aortic node metastases can often be cured. The side effects of extended-field radiotherapy, particularly when combined with concurrent chemotherapy,[339,340] can be substantial, and the management of such patients requires close multidisciplinary collaboration.

Brachytherapy.

Brachytherapy was first used to treat cervical cancers in the early 20th century and continues to play a central role in their curative management. The goal of brachytherapy is to deliver a high dose to disease in the cervix and paracervical tissues while preserving function of adjacent critical structures.

The uterine cavity provides an ideal receptacle for radioactive sources, which are positioned using specially designed applicator systems that capitalize on the distinctive anatomy of the distal female genital tract and the physical advantages of the inverse square law. Most applicator systems consist of an angled or curved intrauterine tandem with some form of intravaginal applicator; vaginal applicators used in various clinical settings include several versions of the Fletcher-Suit afterloading colpostats, vaginal rings, French molds, vaginal cylinders, and others.[341,342] Vaginal packing is used to hold the applicator in place and to maximize the distance between the sources and the bladder and rectum. Radiographs should be obtained at the time of insertion to verify accurate placement, and the system should be repositioned if radiographs indicate that positioning can be improved.

Treatments may be delivered over several days at a continuous LDR or with frequent pulses (pulsed dose rate [PDR]); alternatively,

treatment may be administered in several fractions of radiation delivered at a HDR. For LDR treatments, cesium-137 sources are usually loaded manually after applicator placement has been optimized. In contrast, the remote afterloading units commonly used for HDR or PDR treatments employ a single "stepping" source of ^{192}Ir that travels through the applicator tubes, pausing for varying times in a series of "dwell" positions to deliver the desired dose to adjacent tissues. The activity of sources used for HDR is approximately 10 Ci; the activity of sources used for PDR is approximately 0.5 to 1 Ci. However, because a computer controls insertion of the source, exposure to personnel is negligible with these methods. Although the nominal dose of radiation needs to be adjusted for treatment delivered at different dose rates, the applicator systems and rules of optimal brachytherapy placement are similar for LDR, HDR, and PDR treatment. The importance of radiation dose rate and fraction size is discussed in more detail later in this section.

Brachytherapy Dose. The paracentral dose from intracavitary brachytherapy is most frequently expressed at a single reference point, usually designated *point A*. Although point A has been specified in a number of different ways, the most widely accepted definition is a point 2 cm lateral to the cervical collar and 2 cm above the top of the colpostats, measured at their intersection with the tandem midpoint on the lateral radiograph (Fig. 72.10).[343] Point A usually lies approximately at the crossing of the ureter and the uterine artery, but it bears no consistent relationship to the tumor or target volume. Originally developed as part of the Manchester treatment system, point A was meant to be used in the context of a detailed set of rules governing the placement and loading of the intracavitary system and was intended to be used primarily as a means of reporting treatment intensity, not as the sole parameter for treatment prescription. Today, this context is often lost. Other measures have been used to describe the intensity of intracavitary treatment. "Mg-hr" or "mgRaEq-hr" are proportional to the dose of radiation at relatively distant points from the system and therefore give a sense of the dose to the whole pelvis. Total reference air kerma—expressed in micrograys at 1 m—is an alternative measure that allows for the use of various radionuclides.[344] Reference points have also been used to estimate the doses to the bladder and rectum. Although normal tissue reference points provide useful information about the dose to a portion of normal tissue, volumetric studies have demonstrated that they consistently underestimate the maximum dose to normal tissue.[345] Volumetric MRI-guided dose specification for tumor and normal tissue doses is increasingly being used and is discussed in more detail below.[346] The use of volumetric measurements yields much more accurate information about the relationships between dose, treatment volume, and outcome than has been possible with traditional methods.

Whatever system of dose specification is used, emphasis should always be placed on optimizing the relationship between the intracavitary applicators and the cervical tumor and other pelvic tissues. Source strengths and positions should be carefully chosen to provide optimal tumor coverage without exceeding normal tissue tolerance limits. However, optimized source placement can rarely correct for a poorly positioned applicator.

Factors that influence source strength and position are beyond the scope of this chapter and can be found elsewhere.[344,347] An effort should be made to deliver a dose to point A of at least 85 Gy (with LDR brachytherapy) or its biologic equivalent (with HDR brachytherapy) for patients with bulky central disease. If the intracavitary placement has been optimized, this can usually be accomplished without exceeding a dose of 75 Gy to the bladder reference point or 70 Gy to the rectal reference point, doses that are usually associated with an acceptably low risk of major complications. Suboptimal placements occasionally force compromises in the dose to tumor or normal tissues. To choose a treatment that optimizes the therapeutic ratio in these circumstances requires experience and a detailed understanding of factors that influence tumor control and normal tissue complications.

PRACTICE OF ONCOLOGY

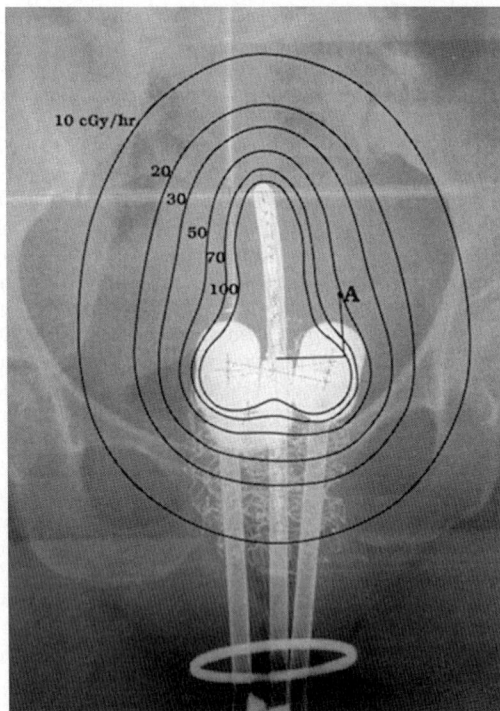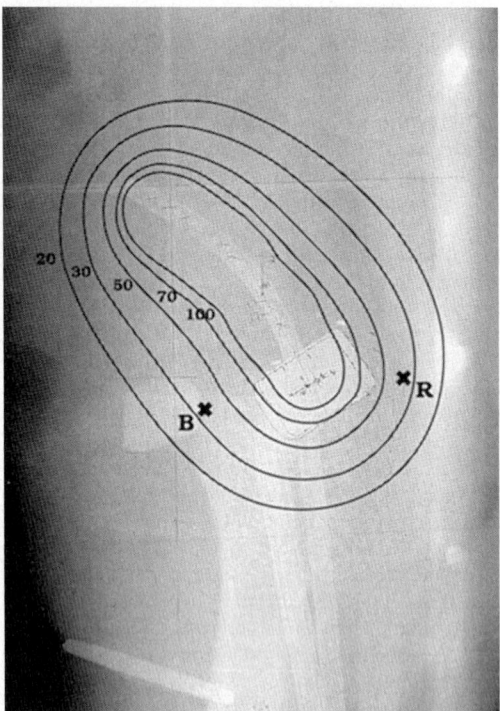

Figure 72.10 Posteroanterior and lateral views of a Fletcher-Suit-Delclos applicator system in a patient with invasive carcinoma of the cervix. Units on the isodose contours are centigray per hour. *A*, point A; *B*, bladder reference point; *R*, rectal reference point.

Image-Based Brachytherapy Treatment Planning. The use of CT and MRI for brachytherapy treatment planning has expanded significantly in the past 10 years. Both modalities can be used to verify appropriate placement of the applicator and evaluate the dose to normal tissues. CT has the advantage of being more widely available than MRI and does not require the use of special MRI-compatible applicators. However, MRI provides much better visualization of soft tissues and more accurate appreciation of the extent of tumor within the cervix and paracervical tissues. Despite this significant advantage, the more limited availability of MRI limited the adoption of MRI-based treatment planning. A survey of radiation oncologists performing brachytherapy in 2007 for cervical cancer reported that 70% of respondents obtained a CT postapplicator placement while only 2% of respondents reviewed images from an MRI with the brachytherapy applicator in place.[348] Although most physicians surveyed obtained a CT at the time of brachytherapy planning, most respondents specified a treatment dose to point A rather than contouring and specifying dose to an image-based target volume.

The Groupe Européen de Curiethérapie-European Society of Therapeutic Radiation Oncology (GEC-ESTRO) consortium has developed a series of guidelines on the optimal approach for imaging, delineating target and avoidance volumes and treatment planning using MRI.[349–352] According to their guidelines, T2 multiplanar images should be obtained after applicator placement to allow delineation of the gross tumor volume that is typically hyperintense on T2 images. The high-risk clinical target volume (CTV) encompasses the entire cervix and and gross residual macroscopic disease at the time of brachytherapy. An intermediate-risk CTV includes the initial extent of disease plus 1-cm margin on the high-risk CTV. Using these methods, Georg et al.[353] reported a strong correlation between the dose to the high-risk CTV and local control with a 96% control rate when the equivalent dose at 2 Gy per fractions (EQD2) to 90% of the target volume (D90) was >87 Gy. The GEC-ESTRO recommendation suggests delivering a total dose equivalent of 60 Gy to the intermediate-risk CTV D90. In

addition, organs at risk including the bladder, rectum, and sigmoid should be delineated. Current recommendations suggest limiting the D2cc (minimum dose to the maximally irradiated 2 ml) of the bladder to <90 Gy and the rectum and sigmoid to <70,[353] although these dose relationships have only been convincingly demonstrated for the rectum. An example of a MRI-based plan, optimized to cover the high-risk CTV while minimizing dose to normal tissues, is shown in Fig. 72.11.

The advantage of image-guided brachytherapy was evaluated in the prospective multicenter nonrandomized STIC study that

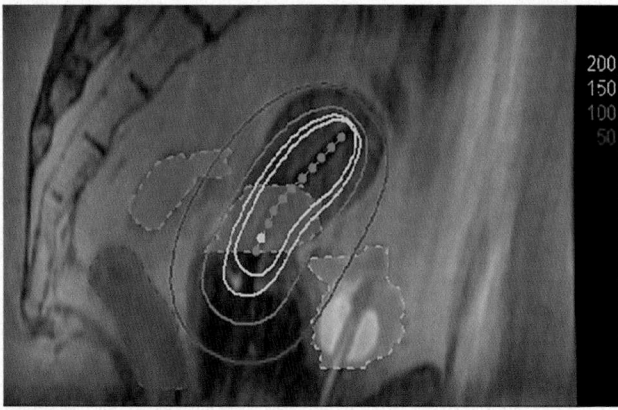

Figure 72.11 Sagittal and axial images of a T2-weighted magnetic resonance imaging obtained in a patient with invasive squamous cell carcinoma of cervix receiving pulsed dose rate brachytherapy with tandem and ovoid implant. Dwell times within the tandem and ovoids were optimized to deliver 22 Gy over 44 hours to the high-risk clinical target volume (*peach*). *Isodose lines* represent percentages of the prescribed dose. The dose the D2cc rectum (*green*), bladder (*yellow*), and sigmoid (*blue*) was 6 Gy, 11 Gy, and 12 Gy, respectively.

compared treatment with standard two-dimensional approach to image-guided brachytherapy in 705 patients.[354] Patients were assigned to one of three groups: patients receiving brachytherapy alone followed by surgery; patients receiving external beam, brachytherapy, and surgery; or patients with more advanced cervical cancers treated with external beam and brachytherapy. Treatment in the three-dimensional group was performed according to GEC-ESTRO guidelines that were adapted for CT. In all three groups, the local-relapse free survival was higher in the three-dimensional group and the rates of grade 3 or 4 complications were lower. Of note, this benefit was observed despite the low total dose to point A, 70 Gy, in patients receiving definitive radiation.

Brachytherapy Dose Rate and Treatment Schedule. Cervical cancer brachytherapy can be delivered with LDR, PDR, or HDR approach. LDR is typically delivered with a cesium source in two implants over 48 hours, separated by 2 weeks after completion of primary external beam fields. PDR treatment follows a similar treatment schedule as LDR but utilizes a stepping iridium source, which delivers treatment over in hourly pulses. HDR brachytherapy uses a higher activity iridium source to deliver four to seven treatments that are delivered over several minutes and spaced over 2 to 5 weeks. HDR brachytherapy is typically delivered after the completion of primary external beam fields or can be started during external beam for smaller or rapidly responding tumors.

Traditional LDR brachytherapy has been performed with sources that yield a dose rate at point A of approximately 0.45 Gy/h. These low dose rates permit repair of sublethal cellular injury with preferential sparing of normal tissues. In a randomized trial, Haie-Meder et al.[355] reported a significant increase in complications when the dose rate was doubled from 0.4 to 0.8 Gy/h, indicating that the total dose must be reduced and the therapeutic ratio of treatment may be compromised with higher dose rates. Differences in the magnitude of the dose-rate effect between tumor and normal tissues may partly reflect differences in the half-times for repair of sublethal radiation damage.[356]

HDR brachytherapy can be delivered in an outpatient setting, which can make treatment more convenient for patients and physicians. In the past decade, the use of HDR brachytherapy has expanded significantly. The most recent patterns of care study that surveyed practice patterns between 2005 and 2007 found that 68.5% of patients were treated using HDR intracavitary brachytherapy as compared with 15.4% in the 1992 to 1994 survey. HDR brachytherapy may lose the radiobiologic advantage of LDR treatment, potentially narrowing the therapeutic window for complication-free cure, particularly for patients with unfavorable anatomy. Published experiences suggest that survival rates are roughly similar to those achieved with traditional LDR treatment, although these experiences are difficult to compare because of the same potential problems of selection bias that confound other nonrandomized comparisons. Prospective trials suggest that LDR and HDR treatment produce similar results, but these trials have been criticized for methodologic flaws. However, logistical advantages, including increasingly scarce availability of cesium for LDR brachytherapy, have contributed to a steady increase in the proportion of patients treated using HDR techniques. HDR is probably similar to LDR brachytherapy in terms of therapeutic efficacy and side effects when the patient's anatomy permits displacement of the bladder, rectosigmoid, and other critical structures away from intrauterine and intravaginal radiation sources, making it possible to prevent exposure of these tissues to high fractional doses.

As with LDR treatment, successful HDR brachytherapy depends on optimized applicator position, balanced use of external beam therapy and brachytherapy, compact overall treatment duration, and delivery of an adequate dose to tumor with respect for normal tissue tolerance limits. The advent of image-guided treatment planning may contribute to further improvements in the safety of high-dose-per-fraction intracavitary brachytherapy by providing a more realistic understanding of the doses delivered by brachytherapy to critical structures.

Some clinicians advocate the use of interstitial brachytherapy for patients whose anatomy or tumor distribution make it difficult to obtain an ideal intracavitary placement. Template-based interstitial implants are usually placed transperineally, guided by an acrylic glass template that encourages parallel placement of hollow needles that penetrate the cervix and paracervical spaces; needles are usually loaded with [193]Ir. Advocates of the procedure describe the relatively homogeneous dose distribution achieved with this method, the ease of inserting implants in patients in whom the uterus is difficult to probe, and the ability to place sources directly into the parametrium.[357,358] In a 1995 review of the combined experiences of Stanford University and the Joint Center for Radiation Therapy,[359] the 3-year disease-free survival rates for patients with stage IIB and IIIB disease were only 36% and 18%, respectively; local control rates were 22% and 44%, respectively; and the rate of complications requiring surgical intervention was high. A 1997 report from the University of California, Irvine, described 5-year survival rates of only 21% and 29%, respectively, for patients with stage IIB and IIIB disease, again with a high rate of major complications.

Some treating physicians have explored the use of laparoscopic or image-guided techniques to improve local control and complication rates with interstitial brachytherapy.[360,361] However, outside of an investigational setting, template-based interstitial treatment of primary cervical cancers should probably be limited to patients who cannot accommodate intrauterine brachytherapy and patients with distal vaginal disease that requires a boost with interstitial brachytherapy. Newer applicators allow the placement of interstitial needles through an ovoid or ring for treatment of bulky cervical tumors. CT or MRI is needed with these applicators to ensure that needles are safely placed.

Complications of Radiotherapy. During pelvic radiotherapy, most patients have mild fatigue and mild-to-moderate diarrhea that usually is controllable with antidiarrheal medications; some patients have mild bladder irritation. When extended fields are treated, patients may have nausea, gastric irritation, and depression of peripheral blood cell counts. Hematologic and gastrointestinal complications are significantly increased in patients receiving concurrent chemotherapy. Unless the ovaries have been transposed, all premenopausal patients who receive pelvic radiotherapy experience ovarian failure by the completion of treatment.

Perioperative complications of intracavitary brachytherapy include uterine perforation, fever, and the usual risks of anesthesia. Thromboembolisms are rare. In a review of 4,043 patients who had 7,662 intracavitary applications for cervical cancer, Jhingran and Eifel[362] reported 11 patients (0.3%) with thromboembolisms, 4 of whom—all with pulmonary embolisms—died. All four fatal pulmonary embolisms were in patients with advanced pelvic wall disease.

Estimates of the risk of late complications of radical radiotherapy vary according to the grading system, duration of follow-up, method of calculation, treatment method, and prevalence of risk factors in the study population. However, most reports quote an overall risk of major complications (requiring transfusion, hospitalization, or surgical intervention) of 5% to 15%.[129,130,355,363,364] In a study of 1,784 patients with stage IB disease, Eifel et al.[363] reported an overall actuarial risk of major complications of 7.7% at 5 years. Although the actuarial risk was greatest during the first 3 years of follow-up, there was a continuing risk to surviving patients of approximately 0.3% per year, resulting in an overall actuarial risk of 14% at 20 years.

During the first 3 years after treatment, rectal complications are most common and include bleeding, stricture, ulceration, and fistula. In the study by Eifel et al.,[363] the risk of major rectosigmoid complications was 2.3% at 5 years. Major gastrointestinal complications were rare 3 years or more after treatment, but a constant low risk of urinary tract complications persisted for many years (Fig. 72.12). The actuarial risk of developing a fistula of any

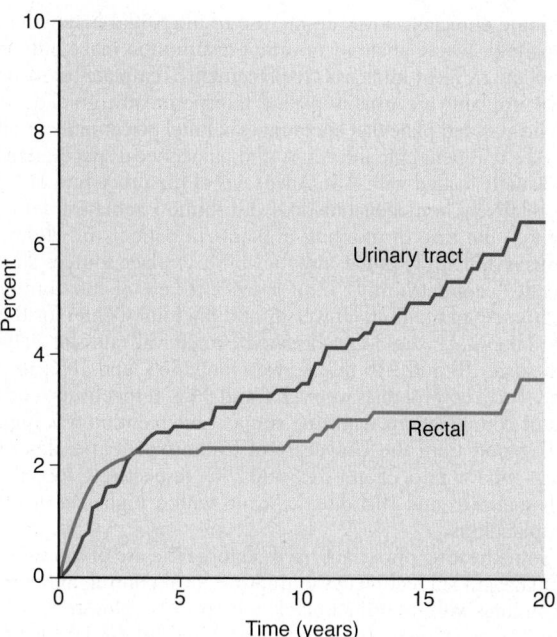

Figure 72.12 Rates of major rectal and urinary tract complications in 1,784 patients with stage IB carcinomas of the cervix treated with radiotherapy. Complication rates were calculated actuarially, and patients who died without experiencing a major complication were censored at the time of death. (From Eifel PJ, Levenback C, Wharton JT, et al. Time course and incidence of late complications in patients treated with radiation therapy for FIGO stage IB carcinoma of the uterine cervix. *Int J Radiat Oncol Biol Phys* 1995;32:1289, with permission.)

type was 1.7% at 5 years. Complication rates were calculated actuarially, and patients who died without experiencing a major complication were censored at the time of death.

Small bowel obstruction is an infrequent complication of standard radiotherapy for patients without special risk factors. The risk of small bowel obstruction is increased dramatically in patients who have undergone transperitoneal lymph node dissection.[217,365] However, there appears to be little increase in risk if the operation is performed with a retroperitoneal approach.[217] Other factors that can increase the risk of small bowel complications in patients treated for cervical cancer include pelvic inflammatory disease, thin body habitus, heavy smoking, and the use of high doses or large volumes for external beam irradiation, particularly with low-energy treatment beams and large daily fraction sizes.[365] Most patients treated with high-dose radiotherapy have some agglutination and telangiectasia of the apical vagina. More significant vaginal shortening can occur, particularly in elderly, postmenopausal women and those with extensive tumors treated with a high dose of radiation.[363,366] Vaginal function can be optimized with appropriate estrogen support and vaginal dilatation.

Concurrent Chemoradiation. At the end of the 1990s, publication of a series of prospective randomized trials provided compelling evidence that the addition of concurrent cisplatin-containing chemotherapy to standard radiotherapy reduces the risk of disease recurrence by as much as 50% (see Table 72.9).[129,130,227,296,367-369]

Some of the earliest trials of chemoradiation studied the concurrent use of hydroxyurea with radiation; although the validity of these small trials has since been questioned, encouraging results led to the use of hydroxyurea-containing regimens as controls in two subsequent GOG trials.[130,368,370] In these trials,[364,368] the GOG randomly assigned patients with stage IIB–IVA disease to receive either hydroxyurea or cisplatin-containing chemotherapy during external beam irradiation. All three of the cisplatin-containing regimens produced local control and survival rates superior to

those for the control arms (hydroxyurea and radiation). In a third study,[297] patients with stage IB tumors measuring at least 4 cm in diameter were randomly assigned to receive radiation alone or radiation plus weekly cisplatin before extrafascial hysterectomy. Patients who received cisplatin were more likely to have a complete histologic response and were more likely to be disease-free at the time of preliminary analysis. A fourth study, cosponsored by the Southwest Oncology Group and the GOG,[286] included patients who were treated with radical hysterectomy and were found to have pelvic lymph node metastases, positive margins, or parametrial involvement. In this study, patients who were randomly assigned to receive postoperative pelvic irradiation combined with concurrent and postradiation cisplatin and 5-FU had a better disease-free survival rate than those treated with postoperative radiotherapy alone.

During this time, the Radiation Therapy Oncology Group also conducted a trial in which radiotherapy alone (including prophylactic para-aortic irradiation) was compared with pelvic irradiation plus concurrent cisplatin and 5-FU.[129,369] The results of this trial also demonstrated highly significant differences in the rates of local control, distant metastasis, overall survival, and disease-free survival, favoring the treatment arm that included chemotherapy. Although acute toxic effects of treatment were greater with chemotherapy, the dose of radiation and duration of radiotherapy were similar in the two arms, and there was no significant difference in the incidence of late treatment-related complications. Although the magnitude of benefit appeared greatest for patients with earlier-stage disease, those with stage III and IVA cancers also had improved disease-free survival when treated with concurrent chemotherapy.[129,365]

Only one large randomized trial, published by Pearcey et al.[371] in 2002, has failed to demonstrate a significant advantage from concurrent cisplatin-based chemotherapy in patients with cervical cancer. Although the authors suggested that differences in technique could explain the difference between their results and the results of the earlier trials, the survival rate in their control arm indicated that the margin for improvement was similar to that in the earlier trials. This trial also was the smallest of the six, resulting in relatively large confidence intervals, which may have contributed to the lack of significant difference between the treatment arms.

These studies raise interesting questions that will undoubtedly be the subjects of future studies. Of four different cisplatin-containing regimens, only two were compared directly. It is unclear from the results which regimen achieves the most favorable therapeutic ratio and whether the inclusion of 5-FU in several of the studies contributed importantly to the results. Although an early trial suggested that 5-FU delivered by protracted venous infusion with radiation might be of benefit,[372] a subsequent GOG trial showed no benefit of 5-FU over a control treatment of weekly cisplatin plus radiation.[373] Although North American studies have emphasized cisplatin-containing regimens, investigators in Southeast Asia have reported improved outcome when radiation was combined with epirubicin[374] or mitomycin and 5-FU.[375] A recently reported study indicates that the addition of gemcitabine to concurrent and adjuvant cisplatin may have greater benefit in terms of both progression-free survival and overall survival than chemoradiation with weekly cisplatin alone (hazard ratio of 0.68 for both progression-free survival and overall survival).[376] However, this regimen had significant acute toxicity even with the limited radiation fields used. In addition, the benefit in the experimental arm may be due to the use of adjuvant chemotherapy in general and may not require use of gemcitabine, which is associated with higher rates of hematologic and gastrointestinal toxicity than the more commonly used carboplatin and taxol regimen. The impact of adjuvant chemotherapy following chemoradiation is being tested in the currently enrolling Australia New Zealand Gynaecological Oncology Group outback trial. Other drugs that are being studied for their radiosensitizing effects in patients with advanced disease are paclitaxel,[377] carboplatin,[378] and several biologic response modifiers.

Several groups have attempted to develop models that predict distant recurrence in locally advanced cervical cancer after platinum-based chemoradiation. In a Korean gynecology oncology group study, a four-parameter model consisting of pelvic and para-aortic nodal positivity on FDG-PET, nonsquamous cell histology, and pretreatment serum squamous cell carcinoma antigen levels was able to predict 5-year probability of distant recurrence.[379]

Taken together, the randomized trials provide strong evidence that the addition of concurrent chemotherapy to pelvic radiotherapy benefits selected patients with locoregionally advanced cervical cancer. A meta-analysis of randomized trials confirmed the benefit of concurrent chemoradiation, showing an advantage for both cisplatin- and non–cisplatin-containing regimens.[380] However, most trials have explicitly excluded patients with evidence of para-aortic lymph node metastases, poor performance status, or impaired renal function. In the future, clinicians will be challenged to determine whether favorable results can be generalized to patients with cervical cancer who differ from those included in the prospective trials because of serious medical or social problems. A large Canadian population-based study that demonstrated a significant improvement in survival of women with cervical cancer after the 1999 adoption of chemoradiation as a standard did indicate that the benefits of chemoradiation can be generalized beyond the trial setting.[381]

Neoadjuvant Chemotherapy with Radiotherapy.

Although investigators were initially encouraged by high response rates of untreated cervical cancer to multiple-agent, cisplatin-containing chemotherapy regimens, these results have not translated to a clear advantage when neoadjuvant chemotherapy is given before radiotherapy. Of seven phase 3 trials of this approach, five[382–386] demonstrated no benefit from neoadjuvant therapy and two[387] demonstrated a significantly better survival rate with radiotherapy alone. Combinations of neoadjuvant followed by concurrent chemoradiotherapy have not yet been tested in large randomized trials. Such combinations should probably be avoided outside an investigational setting because neoadjuvant chemotherapy could compromise patients' tolerance of subsequent chemoradiation.

Stage IVB Disease

Patients who present with disease in distant organs are almost always incurable. The care of these patients must emphasize palliation of symptoms with use of appropriate pain medications and localized radiotherapy. Tumors may respond to chemotherapy, but responses are usually brief.

Single-Agent Chemotherapy.

Cisplatin has been studied in a variety of doses and schedules in the management of recurrent or metastatic cervical cancer and is considered the most active agent against this malignancy.[388,389] Although a number of other agents (e.g., ifosfamide, carboplatin, irinotecan, and paclitaxel) have exhibited a modest level of biologic activity in cervical cancer (producing response rates of 10% to 15%),[390] the clinical utility of these drugs in patients who have not responded to cisplatin or who have experienced recurrence or progression after chemoradiation is uncertain. Further, it is well recognized that the objective rate of response to chemotherapy is lower in previously irradiated areas (e.g., pelvis) than in nonirradiated sites (e.g., lung).[391]

Combination Chemotherapy.

Most reports of combination chemotherapy for carcinoma of the cervix have described small, uncontrolled phase 2 trials of drug combinations. The results of two phase 3 randomized trials, published in 2004 and 2005, have provided the first solid evidence that combination chemotherapy can improve both progression-free survival (cisplatin plus paclitaxel versus single-agent cisplatin,[392] cisplatin plus topotecan versus single-agent cisplatin[393]) and overall survival (cisplatin plus topotecan versus single-agent cisplatin[393]) when it is administered

for recurrent or metastatic carcinoma of the cervix. However, a recently reported phase 3 trial comparing combinations of cisplatin with either topotecan, paclitaxel, gemcitabine, or vinorelbine revealed no significant differences in outcome between patients treated with the four cisplatin-based regimens.[394]

Carboplatin is less toxic than cisplatin in terms of nephrotoxicity, neurotoxicity, and emetogenicity, so the combination of carboplatin and paclitaxel has been evaluated in this setting. A multicenter phase 2 study showed that the carboplatin and paclitaxel regimen was feasible and with similar efficacy as other cisplatin-based doublets for the treatment of metastatic or recurrent cervical cancer.[395] Furthermore, preliminary data from a randomized phase 3 trial of paclitaxel plus carboplatin versus paclitaxel plus cisplatin in stage IVb, persistent, or recurrent cervical cancer performed by the Japan Clinical Oncology Group (JCOG0505 study) showed that the carboplatin doublet was noninferior to the cisplatin doublet in terms of overall survival.

Molecular Targeted Agents.

Several recently reported studies have addressed the role of molecular targeted agents in recurrent or metastatic cervical cancer. Bevacizumab was recently shown to improve overall survival in women with recurrent, persistant, or metastatic cervical cancer.[396] Median survival was 3.7 months longer in women who received bevacizumab in addition to chemotherapy with cisplatin and paclitaxel or topotecan with paclitaxel. No difference in outcome was seen between the two chemotherapy regimens. Pazopanib, another antiangiogenic agent that targets vascular endothelial growth factor receptor and platelet-derived growth factor receptor, was shown to be well-tolerated and demonstrated activity in recurrent or metastatic cervical cancer.[397] However, agents that target the epidermal growth factor receptor and/or the human epidermal growth factor receptor 2 such as cetuximab or lapatinib have demonstrated limited activity in recurrent or metastatic cervical cancer.[397,398]

Palliative Radiotherapy.

Localized radiotherapy can provide effective relief of pain caused by metastases in bone, brain, lymph nodes, or other sites. A rapid course of pelvic radiotherapy can also provide excellent relief of pain and bleeding for patients who present with incurable disseminated disease.

Special Treatment Problems

Treatment of Locally Recurrent Carcinoma of the Cervix.

Patients should be evaluated for possible recurrent disease if a new mass develops; if, in irradiated patients, the cervix remains bulky or nodular or cervical cytologic findings are abnormal ≥3 months after irradiation; or if symptoms of leg edema, pain, or bleeding develop after initial treatment. The diagnosis must be confirmed with a tissue biopsy, and the extent of disease should be evaluated with appropriate radiographic studies, cystoscopy, proctoscopy, and serum chemistry studies before treatment is administered.

After Radical Surgery. The treatment of choice for patients who have an isolated pelvic recurrence after initial treatment with radical hysterectomy alone is aggressive radiotherapy. Treatment using external beam radiotherapy with or without brachytherapy is similar to that for patients with a primary carcinoma of the vagina. Pelvic wall recurrences are often treated with external beam irradiation alone, although surgery and intraoperative radiotherapy may contribute to local control in selected patients.[399] Patients with vaginal recurrence usually have a better prognosis than those with pelvic wall recurrence. Ijaz et al.[400] reported a survival rate of 69% 5 years after radical radiotherapy for 16 patients who had isolated vaginal recurrences that did not involve the pelvic wall. Only 18% of patients who had recurrences that were fixed to the pelvic wall or that involved pelvic lymph nodes survived 5 years. Several authors have reported significantly lower rates of successful salvage therapy for patients with locally recurrent adenocarcinoma.[401,402] Thomas et al.[403] reported encouraging results in a group of patients with recurrent cervical carcinoma treated with radiation and concurrent chemotherapy, but further studies will be needed to determine whether this approach is superior to radiotherapy alone.

After Definitive Irradiation. Some patients who have an isolated central recurrence after radiotherapy can be cured with surgical treatment. Because the extent of disease may be difficult to evaluate and the risk of serious urinary tract complications of pelvic surgery is high after high-dose radiotherapy, surgical salvage treatment usually requires a pelvic exenteration, most often an anterior exenteration. Less extensive operations, such as radical hysterectomy, are reserved for selected patients with small tumors confined to the cervix or lesions that do not encroach on the rectum.[403,404]

In all cases, preparation for total pelvic exenteration must involve a detailed medical and imaging evaluation as well as careful counseling of the patient and family regarding the extent of surgery and postoperative expectations. Tumor involvement of the pelvic sidewall is a contraindication for exenteration but may be difficult to assess if there is extensive radiation fibrosis. Although advanced age may be a contraindication to pelvic exenteration, studies have suggested that, with careful selection, good outcomes can be achieved with pelvic exenteration even in women aged 65 years or older.[405]

The operation begins with a thorough inspection of the abdomen for evidence of intraperitoneal spread, lymph node metastases, or pelvic sidewall infiltration. Despite careful preoperative evaluation, about 30% of operations are aborted intraoperatively.[406] Frozen section biopsies are done of suspicious areas. If the biopsy findings are negative, the surgeon proceeds to remove the bladder, rectum, vagina, uterus, ovaries, fallopian tubes, and all other supporting tissues in the true pelvis. A urinary conduit, a transverse or sigmoid colostomy, and a neovagina are created.

Postoperative recuperation may take as long as 3 months. The surgical mortality rate is <10%, with most postoperative complications and deaths related to sepsis, pulmonary thromboembolism, and intestinal complications such as small bowel obstruction and fistula formation.[407,408] The rate of gastrointestinal complications may be reduced by using unirradiated segments of bowel and by closing pelvic floor defects with omentum, rectosigmoid colon, or myocutaneous flaps.[407] Advances in low colorectal anastomosis and techniques for creating continent urinary reservoirs have improved the quality of life for selected patients.[406,409]

Several investigators have studied the quality of patients' lives after surgical salvage treatment for recurrent cervical cancer.[406,410,411] In the first years after exenteration, patients' quality of life is heavily influenced by worries about the progression of tumor.[410] Most investigators report that the most common problems for survivors relate to their adjustment to urostomy or colostomy. Women with vaginal reconstruction tend to report fewer sexual problems and better quality of life than those without reconstruction.[407,410] However, vaginal dryness and discharge still may interfere with intercourse.[411] In a retrospective study of 75 exenterations, Berek et al.[406] found that the approach that produced the best outcome included the creation of a neovagina using a pedicled transverse rectus abdominis myocutaneous flap, the creation of a continent urinary conduit using a colonic (Miami) pouch, and the performance of a primary colon reanastomosis or the creation of a rectal J-pouch. All of these findings indicate the importance of adequate counseling following the exenterative surgery. The 5-year survival rate for patients who undergo anterior pelvic exenteration is 33% to 60%; the 5-year survival rate for those who undergo total pelvic exenteration is 20% to 46%.[406,410,411] For patients who have unresectable recurrent disease after definitive irradiation, treatment options are limited. Several groups are exploring the role of intraoperative irradiation in the treatment of selected patients with recurrent disease that involves the pelvic wall.[412] However, most patients who have unresectable pelvic recurrences after radiotherapy are treated with chemotherapy alone; response rates and prognosis are generally poor.

Treatment After Simple Hysterectomy that Reveals Unsuspected Invasive Cancer. Every patient who undergoes a planned hysterectomy should be carefully screened before the procedure to rule out invasive cervical cancer. When unexpected invasive cancer is detected in a hysterectomy specimen, the patient should be referred for consideration of additional treatment.[413] Patients with invasion of <3 mm without LVSI usually require no treatment after simple hysterectomy. However, patients with more extensive disease should undergo treatment of the paracolpal tissues and nodes.

Patients who have negative margins usually are treated with pelvic radiotherapy to 45 or 50 Gy. Most clinicians follow this with vaginal intracavitary brachytherapy, delivering an additional vaginal surface dose of 30 to 50 Gy. Patients with positive margins may benefit from a somewhat higher dose of external beam irradiation through reduced fields designed to include the region at highest risk (e.g., parametria and posterior bladder wall).[413,414] In a report of the results of radiotherapy in 123 patients in whom hysterectomy revealed unsuspected invasive cancer, Roman et al.[413] reported 5-year survival rates of 79% for patients with negative margins and 59% for those with microscopically positive margins. In contrast, the 5-year survival rate for 30 patients with gross residual disease was only 41% (*p* = 0.0001). Results of studies of treatment for high-risk cervical cancer after radical hysterectomy suggest that concurrent treatment with chemotherapy and radiation should probably be considered for patients who have positive margins or gross residual disease.

Carcinoma of the Cervical Stump. Supracervical hysterectomy was once a popular treatment for benign uterine conditions. Although enthusiasm for the procedure declined after the 1950s, its use has increased somewhat in recent years. The natural history, staging, and workup for cervical stump carcinomas are the same as those for carcinomas of the intact uterus.

Patients with stage IA1 disease may be treated with simple trachelectomy, and selected patients with stage IA2 or small stage IB tumors may be treated with radical trachelectomy and pelvic lymph node dissection. However, most patients are treated with irradiation alone using a combination of external beam therapy and brachytherapy. The altered geometry and short uterine canal in these patients complicate treatment planning. MRI may be an important aid to treatment planning in these patients. However, in most cases, the endocervical canal is 2 cm or longer, and after a course of external beam irradiation, patients can be adequately treated with intracavitary therapy. If the endocervical canal cannot accommodate any sources, a boost dose may be delivered to the tumor with interstitial therapy or transvaginal irradiation. Vaginal ovoids alone rarely deliver an adequate dose to the cervix. If brachytherapy is impossible, some patients can be cured using external beam irradiation with reduced fields. However, brachytherapy should be used whenever possible. Barillot et al.[415] reported a survival rate of 81.5% for patients treated with combined brachytherapy and external beam irradiation versus 38.5% for those treated with external beam irradiation alone. When brachytherapy is used, most investigators have reported survival rates similar to those for patients with carcinomas of the intact cervix.[415,416]

Carcinoma of the Cervix During Pregnancy. Estimates of the incidence of invasive cervical cancer during pregnancy range from 0.02% to 0.9%.[417,418] Estimates of the incidence of pregnancy in patients with invasive cervical cancer usually range between 0.5% and 5%. Hacker et al.[417] reported an incidence of cervical carcinoma in situ of 0.013% in pregnant women.

Any suspicious cervical lesion observed during pregnancy should be biopsied. If the Pap smear is positive for malignant cells and the diagnosis of invasive cancer cannot be made with colposcopy and biopsy, a diagnostic conization may be necessary. Because conization subjects the mother and fetus to complications, it should be performed only in the second trimester and only in patients with inadequate colposcopy findings and strong cytologic evidence of invasive cancer. Conization in the first trimester of pregnancy is associated with an abortion rate of up to 33%.[416] Conservative conization under colposcopic guidance may reduce this risk.[419]

It appears to be safe to delay definitive treatment of patients with carcinoma in situ or stage IA disease until the fetus has matured.[417-419] Patients whose disease invades <5 mm may be followed to term. The infant may be delivered by a cesarean section, which is followed immediately by modified radical hysterectomy or radical trachelectomy and pelvic lymph node dissection.

Treatment of patients with more advanced cancers depends on the stage of gestation and the wishes of the patient. Modern neonatal care affords a very high survival rates for infants delivered at >28 weeks of gestational age. Fetal pulmonary maturity can be determined by amniocentesis, and, when pulmonary maturity is documented, the infant can be delivered and prompt treatment of the mother can be instituted. It is probably wise to avoid delays in therapy of >4 weeks whenever possible, although this guideline is controversial.[418,420] For most women with stage IB1 tumors, the recommended approach is classic cesarean section followed by radical hysterectomy with pelvic lymph node dissection. There

should be a thorough discussion of the risks and options with both parents before any treatment is undertaken.

Patients with stage II–IV tumors and some patients with bulky stage IB cervical cancers will require radiotherapy to treat their cancer. If the fetus is viable at the time of diagnosis, it is delivered by classic cesarean section and radiotherapy is begun postoperatively. In the second trimester, a delay of therapy may be entertained to improve the chances of fetal survival. If the patient wishes to delay therapy, it is important to ensure fetal pulmonary maturity before delivery is undertaken.

Compared with other patients with cervical cancer, those with cervical cancer during pregnancy have slightly better overall survival because an increased proportion have stage I disease. Although studies differ in their conclusions about whether pregnancy has an independent influence on the prognosis of patients with cervical cancer, case-matched studies have suggested similar survival rates for pregnant and nonpregnant patients.[421]

Patients who are diagnosed with invasive cervical cancer shortly after a vaginal delivery and who had an episiotomy appear to be at risk for recurrence at the site of their episiotomy. At least 13 cases demonstrating this unusual pattern of failure have been reported.[422]

SELECTED REFERENCES

The full reference list can be accessed at lwwhealthlibrary.com/oncology.

1. American Cancer Society. *Cancer Facts and Figures 2014.* Atlanta, GA: American Cancer Society; 2014.
2. Shepherd J, Sideri M, Benedet J, et al. Carcinoma of the vagina. *J Epidemiol Biostat* 1998;3:103–109.
4. Frank SJ, Jhingran A, Levenback C, et al. Definitive radiation therapy for squamous cell carcinoma of the vagina. *Int J Radiat Oncol Biol Phys* 2005;62:138–147.
7. International Agency for Research on Cancer (IARC). *Monographs on the Evaluation of Carcinogenic Risks to Humans. Human Papillomaviruses.* Vol 64. Lyon, France: IARC; 1995.
13. Palmer JR, Anderson D, Helmrich SP, et al. Risk factors for diethylstilbestrol-associated clear cell adenocarcinoma. *Obstet Gynecol* 2000;95:814–820.
19. Hoover RN, Hyer M, Pfeiffer RM, et al. Adverse health outcomes in women exposed in utero to diethylstilbestrol. *N Engl J Med* 2011;365:1304–1314.
20. Kirkbride P, Fyles A, Rawlings GA, et al. Carcinoma of the vagina—experience at the Princess Margaret Hospital (1974–1989). *Gynecol Oncol* 1995;56:435–443.
24. Creasman WT, Phillips JL, Menck HR. The National Cancer Data Base report on cancer of the vagina. *Cancer* 1998;83:1033–1040.
25. Frank SJ, Deavers MT, Jhingran A, et al. Primary adenocarcinoma of the vagina not associated with diethylstilbestrol (DES) exposure. *Gynecol Oncol* 2007;105:470–474.
33. Kucera H, Mock U, Knocke TH, et al. Radiotherapy alone for invasive vaginal cancer: outcome with intracavitary high dose rate brachytherapy versus conventional low dose rate brachytherapy. *Acta Obstet Gynecol Scand* 2001;80:355–360.
45. Miyamoto DT, Viswanathan AN. Concurrent chemoradiation for vaginal cancer. *PLoS One* 2013;8:e65048.
46. Beller U, Quinn M, Benedet J, et al. Carcinoma of the vulva. *Int J Gynaecol Obstet* 2006;95:S7–S26.
48. Hampl M, Deckers-Figiel S, Hampl JA, et al. New aspects of vulvar cancer: changes in localization and age of onset. *Gynecol Oncol* 2008;109:340–345.
50. Hampl M, Sarajuuri H, Wentzensen N, et al. Effect of human papillomavirus vaccines on vulvar, vaginal, and anal intraepithelial lesions and vulvar cancer. *Obstet Gynecol* 2006;108:1361–1368.
55. Lee YY, Wilczanski SP, Chumakov A, et al. Carcinoma of the vulva: HPV and p53 mutations. *Oncogene* 1994;9:1655–1659.
82. Homesley HD, Bundy BN, Sedlis A, et al. Prognostic factors for groin node metastasis in squamous cell carcinoma of the vulva (a Gynecologic Oncology Group study). *Gynecol Oncol* 1993;49:279–283.
83. International Federation of Gynecology and Obstetrics. Staging announcement. FIGO staging of gynecologic cancers; cervical and vulva. *Int J Gynaecol Cancer* 1995;5:319.
84. Hacker NF. Revised FIGO staging for carcinoma of the vulva. *Int J Gynaecol Obstet* 2009;105:105–106.
85. Homesley HD, Bundy BN, Sedlis A, et al. Assessment of current International Federation of Gynecology and Obstetrics staging of vulvar carcinoma relative to prognostic factors for survival (a Gynecologic Oncology Group study). *Am J Obstet Gynecol* 1991;164:997–1003, discussion 1003–1004.
88. Landrum LM, Lanneau GS, Skaggs VJ, et al. Gynecologic Oncology Group risk groups for vulvar carcinoma: improvement in survival in the modern era. *Gynecol Oncol* 2007;106:521–525.

90. Katz A, Eifel PJ, Jhingran A, et al. The role of radiation therapy in preventing regional recurrences of invasive squamous cell carcinoma of the vulva. *Int J Radiat Oncol Biol Phys* 2003;57:409–418.
91. Homesley HD, Bundy BN, Sedlis A, et al. Radiation therapy versus pelvic node resection for carcinoma of the vulva with positive groin nodes. *Obstet Gynecol* 1986;68:733–740.
92. Heaps JM, Fu YS, Montz FJ, et al. Surgical-pathologic variables predictive of local recurrence in squamous cell carcinoma of the vulva. *Gynecol Oncol* 1990;38:309–314.
97. Faul C, Mirmow D, Gerszten K, et al. Isolated local recurrence in carcinoma of the vulva: prognosis and implications for treatment. *Int J Gynecol Cancer* 1998;8:409–414.
98. Berek JS, Hacker NF. *Practical Gynecologic Oncology.* Philadelphia, PA: Lippincott Williams & Wilkins; 2005.
99. Kenter GG, Welters MJ, Valentijn AR, et al. Vaccination against HPV-16 oncoproteins for vulvar intraepithelial neoplasia. *N Engl J Med* 2009;361: 1838–1847.
101. Faul CM, Mirmow D, Huang Q, et al. Adjuvant radiation for vulvar carcinoma: improved local control. *Int J Radiat Oncol Biol Phys* 1997;38:381–389.
107. Kunos C, Simpkins F, Gibbons H, et al. Radiation therapy compared with pelvic node resection for node-positive vulvar cancer: a randomized controlled trial. *Obstet Gynecol* 2009;114:537–546.
113. Levenback C, Morris M, Burke TW, et al. Groin dissection practices among gynecologic oncologists treating early vulvar cancer. *Gynecol Oncol* 1996;62:73–77.
115. Levenback CF, van der Zee AG, Rob L, et al. Sentinel lymph node biopsy in patients with gynecologic cancers Expert panel statement from the International Sentinel Node Society Meeting, February 21, 2008. *Gynecol Oncol* 2009;114:151–156.
116. Van der Zee AG, Oonk MH, De Hullu JA, et al. Sentinel node dissection is safe in the treatment of early-stage vulvar cancer. *J Clin Oncol* 2008;26:884–889.
117. Oonk MH, van Hemel BM, Hollema H, et al. Size of sentinel-node metastasis and chances of non-sentinel-node involvement and survival in early stage vulvar cancer: results from GROINSS-V, a multicentre observational study. *Lancet Oncol* 2010;11:646–652.
119. Levenback CF, Ali S, Coleman RL et al. Lymphatic mapping and sentinel lymph node biopsy in women with squamous cell carcinoma of the vulva: a gynecologic oncology group study. *J Clin Oncol* 2012;30:3786–3791.
125. Moore DH, Thomas GM, Montana GS, et al. Preoperative chemoradiation for advanced vulvar cancer: a phase II study of the Gynecologic Oncology Group. *Int J Radiat Oncol Biol Phys* 1998;42:79–85.
129. Eifel PJ, Winter K, Morris M, et al. Pelvic irradiation with concurrent chemotherapy versus pelvic and para-aortic irradiation for high-risk cervical cancer: an update of Radiation Therapy Oncology Group trial (RTOG) 90-01. *J Clin Oncol* 2004;22:872–880.
130. Rose PG, Bundy BN, Watkins J, et al. Concurrent cisplatin-based chemotherapy and radiotherapy for locally advanced cervical cancer. *N Engl J Med* 1999;340:1144–1153.
132. Moore DH, Ali S, Koh WJ, et al. A phase II trial of radiation therapy and weekly cisplatin chemotherapy for the treatment of locally-advanced squamous cell carcinoma of the vulva: a gynecologic oncologic group study. *Gynecol Oncol* 2012;124:529–533.

PRACTICE OF ONCOLOGY

134. Domingues AP, Mota F, Durao M, et al. Neoadjuvant chemotherapy in advanced vulvar cancer. *Int J Gynecol Cancer* 2010;20:294–298.

139. Magrina JF, Goodrich MA, Weaver AL, et al. Modified radical hysterectomy: morbidity and mortality. *Gynecol Oncol* 1995;59:277–282.

141. Horowitz NS, Olawaiye AB, Borger DR, et al. Phase II trial of erlotinib in women with squamous cell carcinoma of the vulva. *Gynecol Oncol* 2012; 127:141–146.

147. Castellsagué X, Díaz M, Vaccarella S, et al. Intrauterine device use, cervical infection with human papillomavirus, and risk of cervical cancer: a pooled analysis of 26 epidemiological studies. *Lancet Oncol* 2011;12:1023–1031.

152. Buehler JW, Ward JW. A new definition for AIDS surveillance. *Ann Intern Med* 1993;118:390–392.

153. Chirenje ZM. HIV and cancer of the cervix. *Best Pract Res Clin Obstet Gynaecol* 2005;19:269–276.

157. Dunne EF, Unger ER, Sternberg M, et al. Prevalence of HPV infection among females in the United States. *JAMA* 2007;297:813–819.

158. Roden R, Wu TC. How will HPV vaccines affect cervical cancer? *Nat Rev Cancer* 2006;6:753–763.

159. Harper DM, Franco EL, Wheeler CM, et al. Sustained efficacy up to 4.5 years of a bivalent L1 virus-like particle vaccine against human papillomavirus types 16 and 18: follow-up from a randomised control trial. *Lancet* 2006;367:1247–1255.

160. Garland SM, Hernandez-Avila M, Wheeler CM, et al. Quadrivalent vaccine against human papillomavirus to prevent anogenital diseases. *N Engl J Med* 2007;356:1928–1943.

161. The Future II Study Group. Quadrivalent Vaccine against Human Papillomavirus to Prevent High-Grade Cervical Lesions. *N Engl J Med* 2007;356: 1915–1927.

162. Paavonen J, Naud P, Salmeron J, et al. Efficacy of human papillomavirus (HPV)-16/18 AS04-adjuvanted vaccine against cervical infection and precancer caused by oncogenic HPV types (PATRICIA): final analysis of a double-blind, randomised study in young women. *Lancet* 2009;374:301–314.

163. Herrero R, Hildesheim A, Rodriguez AC, et al. Rationale and design of a community-based double-blind randomized clinical trial of an HPV 16 and 18 vaccine in Guanacaste, Costa Rica. *Vaccine* 2008;26:4795–4808.

164. Hildesheim A, Herrero R, Wacholder S, et al. Effect of human papillomavirus 16/18 L1 viruslike particle vaccine among young women with preexisting infection: a randomized trial. *JAMA* 2007;298:743–753.

169. Choi HJ, Ju W, Myung SK, et al. Diagnostic performance of computer tomography, magnetic resonance imaging, and positron emission tomography or positron emission tomography/computer tomography for detection of metastatic lymph nodes in patients with cervical cancer: meta-analysis. *Cancer Sci* 2010;101:1471–1479.

170. Fontanilla HP, Klopp AH, Lindberg ME, et al. Anatomic distribution of [(18) F] fluorodeoxyglucose-avid lymph nodes in patients with cervical cancer. *Pract Radiat Oncol* 2013;3:45–53.

174. Schiffman M, Solomon D. Findings to date from the ASCUS-LSIL Triage Study (ALTS). *Arch Pathol Lab Med* 2003;127:946–949.

175. Cox JT, Schiffman M, Solomon D. Prospective follow-up suggests similar risk of subsequent cervical intraepithelial neoplasia grade 2 or 3 among women with cervical intraepithelial neoplasia grade 1 or negative colposcopy and directed biopsy. *Am J Obstet Gynecol* 2003;188:1406–1412.

176. Solomon D, Davey D, Kurman R, et al. The 2001 Bethesda System: terminology for reporting results of cervical cytology. *JAMA* 2002;287:2114–2119.

179. Wolf JK, Levenback C, Malpica A, et al. Adenocarcinoma in situ of the cervix: significance of cone biopsy margins. *Obstet Gynecol* 1996;88:82–86.

183. Creasman WT, Zaino RJ, Major FJ, et al. Early invasive carcinoma of the cervix (3 to 5 mm invasion): risk factors and prognosis. A Gynecologic Oncology Group study. *Am J Obstet Gynecol* 1998;178:62–65.

191. Albores-Saavedra J, Gersell D, Gilks CB, et al. Terminology of endocrine tumors of the uterine cervix: results of a workshop sponsored by the College of American Pathologists and the National Cancer Institute. *Arch Pathol Lab Med* 1997;121:34–39.

192. Wang Y, Mei K, Xiang MF, et al. Clinicopathological characteristics and outcome of patients with small cell neuroendocrine carcinoma of the uterine cervix: case series and literature review. *Eur J Gynaecol Oncol* 2013;34:307–310.

195. Viswanathan AN, Deavers MT, Jhingran A, et al. Small cell neuroendocrine carcinoma of the cervix: outcome and patterns of recurrence. *Gynecol Oncol* 2004;93:27–33.

197. ACOG Committee on Practice Bulletins—Gynecology. ACOG Practice Bulletin no. 109: Cervical cytology screening. *Obstet Gynecol* 2009;114: 1409–1420.

198. Saslow D, Solomon D, Lawson HW, et al. American Cancer Society, American Society for Colposcopy and Cervical Pathology, and American Society for Clinical Pathology screening guidelines for the prevention and early detection of cervical cancer. *Am J Clin Pathol* 2012;137:516–542.

199. Moyer VA, U.S. Preventive Services Task Force. Screening for cervical cancer: U.S. Preventive Services Task Force recommendation statement. *Ann Intern Med* 2012;156:880–891.

200. Katki HA, Kinney WK, Fetterman B, et al. Cervical cancer risk for women undergoing concurrent testing for human papillomavirus and cervical cytology: a population-based study in routine clinical practice. *Lancet Oncol* 2011;12:663–672.

201. Rijkaart DC, Berkhof J, Rozendaal L, et al. Human papillomavirus testing for the detection of high-grade cervical intraepithelial neoplasia and cancer:

final results of the POBASCAM randomised controlled trial. *Lancet Oncol* 2012;13:78–88.

202. Keller MJ, Burk RD, Xie X, et al. Risk of cervical precancer and cancer among HIV-infected women with normal cervical cytology and no evidence of oncogenic HPV infection. *JAMA* 2012;308:362–369.

203. Arbyn M, Bergeron C, Klinkhamer P, et al. Liquid compared with conventional cervical cytology: a systematic review and meta-analysis. *Obstet Gynecol* 2008;111:167–177.

209. Nanda K, McCrory DC, Myers ER, et al. Accuracy of the Papanicolaou test in screening for and follow-up of cervical cytologic abnormalities: a systematic review. *Ann Intern Med* 2000;132:810–819.

212. Grigsby PW. PET/CT imaging to guide cervical cancer therapy. *Future Oncol* 2009;5:953–958.

213. Pecorelli S. Revised FIGO staging for carcinoma of the vulva, cervix, and endometrium. *Int J Gynaecol Obstet* 2009;105:103–104.

214. Pecorelli S, Zigliani L, Odicino F. Revised FIGO staging for carcinoma of the cervix. *Int J Gynaecol Obstet* 2009;105:103–104.

217. Weiser EB, Bundy BN, Hoskins WJ, et al. Extraperitoneal versus transperitoneal selective paraaortic lymphadenectomy in the pretreatment surgical staging of advanced cervical carcinoma (a Gynecologic Oncology Group study). *Gynecol Oncol* 1989;33:283–289.

218. Schlaerth J, Spiritos N, Carson LF, et al. Laparoscopic retroperitoneal lymphadenectomy followed by immediate laparotomy in women with cervical cancer: a Gynecologic Oncology Group study. *Gynecol Oncol* 2002;85:81–88.

222. Gortzak-Uzan L, Jimenez W, Nofech-Mozes S, et al. Sentinel lymph node biopsy vs. pelvic lymphadenectomy in early stage cervical cancer: is it time to change the gold standard? *Gynecol Oncol* 2010;116:28–32.

223. Lécuru F, Mathevet P, Querleu D, et al. Bilateral negative sentinel nodes accurately predict absence of lymph node metastasis in early cervical cancer: results of the SENTICOL study. *J Clin Oncol* 2011;29:1686–1691.

224. Frumovitz M, Querleu D, Gil-Moreno A, et al. Lymphadenectomy in locally advanced cervical cancer study (LiLACS): Phase III clinical trial comparing surgical with radiologic staging in patients with stages IB2-IVA cervical cancer. *J Minim Invasive Gynecol* 2014;21:3–8.

227. Eifel PJ, Jhingran A, Levenback CF, et al. Predictive value of a proposed subclassification of stages I and II cervical cancer based on clinical tumor diameter. *Int J Gynecol Cancer* 2009;19:2–7.

229. Delgado G, Bundy B, Zaino R, et al. Prospective surgical-pathological study of disease-free interval in patients with stage IB squamous cell carcinoma of the cervix: a Gynecologic Oncology Group study. *Gynecol Oncol* 1990;38:352–357.

234. Roman LD, Felix JC, Muderspach LI, et al. Influence of quantity of lymph-vascular space invasion on the risk of nodal metastases in women with early-stage squamous cancer of the cervix [see comments]. *Gynecol Oncol* 1998;68:220–225.

239. Noh JM, Park W, Kim YS, et al. Comparison of clinical outcomes of adenocarcinoma and adenosquamous carcinoma in uterine cervical cancer patients receiving surgical resection followed by radiotherapy: a multicenter retrospective study (KROG 13-10). *Gynecol Oncol* 2014;132:618–623.

242. Eifel PJ, Burke TW, Morris M, et al. Adenocarcinoma as an independent risk factor for disease recurrence in patients with stage IB cervical carcinoma. *Gynecol Oncol* 1995;59:38–44.

250. Galic V, Herzog TJ, Lewin SN, et al. Prognostic significance of adenocarcinoma histology in women with cervical cancer. *Gynecol Oncol* 2012;125:287–291.

251. Chan YM, Ng TY, Ngan HY, et al. Monitoring of serum squamous cell carcinoma antigen levels in invasive cervical cancer: is it cost-effective? *Gynecol Oncol* 2002;84:7–11.

252. Zanagnolo V, Minig LA, Gadducci A, et al. Surveillance procedures for patients for cervical carcinoma: a review of the literature. *Int J Gynecol Cancer* 2009;19:306–313.

261. Thomas G, Ali S, Hoebers FJ, et al. Phase III trial to evaluate the efficacy of maintaining hemoglobin levels above 12.0 g/dL with erythropoietin vs above 10.0 g/dL without erythropoietin in anemic patients receiving concurrent radiation and cisplatin for cervical cancer. *Gynecol Oncol* 2008;108:317–325.

262. Klopp AH, Eifel PJ. Biological predictors of cervical cancer response to radiation therapy. *Semin Radiat Oncol* 2012;22:143–150.

267. Tsai CJ, Sulman EP, Eifel PJ, et al. Galectin-7 levels predict radiation response in squamous cell carcinoma of the cervix. *Gynecol Oncol* 2013; 131:645–649.

270. Pilch H, Gunzel S, Schaffer U, et al. Human papillomavirus (HPV) DNA in primary cervical cancer and in cancer free pelvic lymph nodes—correlation with clinico-pathological parameters and prognostic significance. *Zentralbl Gynakol* 2001;123:91–101.

272. McIntyre JB, Wu JS, Craighead PS, et al. (2013) PIK3CA mutational status and overall survival in patients with cervical cancer treated with radical chemoradiotherapy. *Gynecol Oncol* 2012;128:409–414.

273. Kidd EA, El Naqa I, Siegel BA, et al. FDG-PET-based prognostic nomograms for locally advanced cervical cancer. *Gynecol Oncol* 2012;127:136–140.

274. Alvarez RD, Helm CW, Edwards R, et al. Prospective randomized trial of LLETZ versus laser ablation in patients with cervical intraepithelial neoplasia. *Gynecol Oncol* 1994;52:175–179.

275. Mitchell MF, Tortolero-Luna G, Cook E, et al. A randomized clinical trial of cryotherapy, laser vaporization, and loop electrosurgical excision for treatment of squamous intraepithelial lesions of the cervix. *Obstet Gynecol* 1998;92:737–744.

276. Kolstad P. Follow-up study of 232 patients with stage Ia1 and 411 patients with stage Ia2 squamous cell carcinoma of the cervix (microinvasive carcinoma). *Gynecol Oncol* 1989;33:265–272.

282. Ramirez PT, Pareja R, Rendon GJ, et al. Management of low-risk early-stage cervical cancer: should conization, simple trachelectomy, or simple hysterectomy replace radical surgery as the new standard of care? *Gynecol Oncol* 2014;132:254–259.

283. Xu L, Sun FQ, Wang ZH. Radical trachelectomy versus radical hysterectomy for the treatment of early cervical cancer: a systematic review. *Acta Obstet Gynecol Scand* 2011;90:1200–1209.

286. Peters WA 3rd, Liu PY, Barrett RJ II, et al. Concurrent chemotherapy and pelvic radiation therapy compared with pelvic radiation therapy alone as adjuvant therapy after radical surgery in high-risk early-stage cancer of the cervix. *J Clin Oncol* 2000;18:1606–1613.

287. Rotman M, Sedlis A, Piedmonte MR, et al. A phase III randomized trial of postoperative pelvic irradiation in Stage IB cervical carcinoma with poor prognostic features: follow-up of a gynecologic oncology group study. *Int J Radiat Oncol Biol Phys* 2006;65:169–176.

292. Landoni F, Maneo A, Colombo A, et al. Randomised study of radical surgery versus radiotherapy for stage Ib–IIa cervical cancer. *Lancet* 1997;350:535–540.

296. Keys HM, Bundy BN, Stehman FB, et al. Cisplatin, radiation, and adjuvant hysterectomy for bulky stage IB cervical carcinoma. *N Engl J Med* 1999;340:1154–1161.

297. Pellegrino A, Vizza E, Fruscio R, et al. Total laparoscopic radical hysterectomy and pelvic lymphadenectomy in patients with Ib1 stage cervical cancer: analysis of surgical and oncological outcome. *Eur J Surg Oncol* 2009;35:98–103.

298. Ramirez PT, Soliman PT, Schmeler KM, et al. Laparoscopic and robotic techniques for radical hysterectomy in patients with early-stage cervical cancer. *Gynecol Oncol* 2008;110:S21–S24.

301. Bergmark K, Avall-Lundqvist E, Dickman PW, et al. Lymphedema and bladder-emptying difficulties after radical hysterectomy for early cervical cancer and among population controls. *Int J Gynecol Cancer* 2006;16:1130–1139.

303. Landoni F, Maneo A, Cormio G, et al. Class II versus class III radical hysterectomy in stage IB-IIA cervical cancer: a prospective randomized study. *Gynecol Oncol* 2001;80:3–12.

304. Uccella S, Laterza R, Ciravolo G, et al. A comparison of urinary complications following total laparoscopic radical hysterectomy and laparoscopic pelvic lymphadenectomy to open abdominal surgery. *Gynecol Oncol* 2007;107:S147–S149.

307. Dargent D, Brun JL, Roy M, et al. Pregnancies following radical trachelectomy for invasive cervical cancer. *Gynecol Oncol* 1994;52:105 (abstract).

308. Covens A, Shaw P, Murphy J, et al. Is radical trachelectomy a safe alternative to radical hysterectomy for patients with stage IA-B carcinoma of the cervix? *Cancer* 1999;86:2273–2279.

318. Keys HM, Bundy BN, Stehman FB, et al. Radiation therapy with and without extrafascial hysterectomy for bulky stage IB cervical carcinoma: a randomized trial of the Gynecologic Oncology Group. *Gynecol Oncol* 2003;89:343–353.

325. Logsdon MD, Eifel PJ. FIGO IIIB squamous cell carcinoma of the cervix: an analysis of prognostic factors emphasizing the balance between external beam and intracavitary radiation therapy. *Int J Radiat Oncol Biol Phys* 1999;43:763–775.

326. Fyles A, Keane TJ, Barton M, et al. The effect of treatment duration in the local control of cervix cancer. *Radiother Oncol* 1992;25:273–279.

329. Eifel PJ, Ho A, Khalid N, et al. Patterns of radiation therapy practice for patients treated for intact cervical cancer in 2005 to 2007: a quality research in radiation oncology study. *Int J Radiat Oncol Biol Phys* 2014;89:249–256.

332. Small W Jr, Mell LK, Anderson P, et al. Consensus guidelines for delineation of clinical target volume for intensity-modulated pelvic radiotherapy in postoperative treatment of endometrial and cervical cancer. *Int J Radiat Oncol Biol Phys* 2008;71:428–434.

333. Verma J, Sulman EP, Jhingran A, et al. Dosimetric predictors of duodenal toxicity after intensity modulated radiation therapy for treatment of the para-aortic nodes in gynecologic cancer. *Int J Radiat Oncol Biol Phys* 2014;88:357–362.

334. Beadle BM, Jhingran A, Salehpour M, et al. Cervix regression and motion during the course of external beam chemoradiation for cervical cancer. *Int J Radiat Oncol Biol Phys* 2009;73:235–241.

335. Haie C, Pejovic MH, Gerbaulet A, et al. Is prophylactic para-aortic irradiation worthwhile in the treatment of advanced cervical carcinoma? Results of a controlled clinical trial of the EORTC radiotherapy group. *Radiother Oncol* 1988;11:101–112.

342. Eifel PJ, Moughan J, Erickson B, et al. Patterns of radiotherapy practice for patients with carcinoma of the uterine cervix: a patterns of care study. *Int J Radiat Oncol Biol Phys* 2004;60:1144–1153.

346. Potter R, Haie-Meder C, Van Limbergen E, et al. Recommendations from gynaecological (GYN) GEC ESTRO working group (II): concepts and terms in 3D image-based treatment planning in cervix cancer brachytherapy-3D dose volume parameters and aspects of 3D image-based anatomy, radiation physics, radiobiology. *Radiother Oncol* 2006;78:67–77.

348. Viswanathan AN, Erickson BA. Three-dimensional imaging in gynecologic brachytherapy: a survey of the American Brachytherapy Society. *Int J Radiat Oncol Biol Phys* 2010;76:104–109.

349. Dimopoulos JC, Petrow P, Tanderup K, et al. Recommendations from Gynaecological (GYN) GEC-ESTRO Working Group (IV): Basic principles and parameters for MR imaging within the frame of image based adaptive cervix cancer brachytherapy. *Radiother Oncol* 2012;103:113–122.

350. Hellebust TP, Kirisits C, Berger D, et al. Recommendations from Gynaecological (GYN) GEC-ESTRO Working Group: considerations and pitfalls in commissioning and applicator reconstruction in 3D image-based treatment planning of cervix cancer brachytherapy. *Radiother Oncol* 2010;96:153–160.

351. Pötter R, Haie-Meder C, Van Limbergen E, et al. Recommendations from gynaecological (GYN) GEC ESTRO working group (II): concepts and terms in 3D image-based treatment planning in cervix cancer brachytherapy-3D dose volume parameters and aspects of 3D image-based anatomy, radiation physics, radiobiology. *Radiother Oncol* 2006;78:67–77.

352. Haie-Meder C, Pötter R, Van Limbergen E, et al. Recommendations from Gynaecological (GYN) GEC-ESTRO Working Group (I): concepts and terms in 3D image based 3D treatment planning in cervix cancer brachytherapy with emphasis on MRI assessment of GTV and CTV. *Radiother Oncol* 2005;74:235–245.

353. Georg P, Lang S, Dimopoulos JC, et al. Dose-volume histogram parameters and late side effects in magnetic resonance image-guided adaptive cervical cancer brachytherapy. *Int J Radiat Oncol Biol Phys* 2011;79:356–362.

354. Charra-Brunaud C, Harter V, Delannes M, et al. Impact of 3D image-based PDR brachytherapy on outcome of patients treated for cervix carcinoma in France: results of the French STIC prospective study. *Radiother Oncol* 2012;103:305–313.

355. Haie-Meder C, Kramar A, Lambin P, et al. Analysis of complications in a prospective randomized trial comparing two brachytherapy low dose rates in cervical carcinoma. *Int J Radiat Oncol Biol Phys* 1994;29:953–960.

359. Hughes-Davies L, Silver B, Kapp D. Parametrial interstitial brachytherapy for advanced or recurrent pelvic malignancy: the Harvard/Stanford experience. *Gynecol Oncol* 1995;58:24–27.

361. Erickson B, Gillin MT. Interstitial implantation of gynecologic malignancies. *J Surg Oncol* 1997;66:285–295.

363. Eifel PJ, Levenback C, Wharton JT, et al. Time course and incidence of late complications in patients treated with radiation therapy for FIGO stage IB carcinoma of the uterine cervix. *Int J Radiat Oncol Biol Phys* 1995;32:1289–1300.

365. Eifel PJ, Jhingran A, Bodurka DC, et al. Correlation of smoking history and other patient characteristics with major complications of pelvic radiation therapy for cervical cancer. *J Clin Oncol* 2002;20:3651–3657.

367. Morris M, Eifel PJ, Lu J, et al. Pelvic radiation with concurrent chemotherapy compared with pelvic and para-aortic radiation for high-risk cervical cancer. *N Engl J Med* 1999;340:1137–1143.

368. Whitney CW, Sause W, Bundy BN, et al. A randomized comparison of fluorouracil plus cisplatin versus hydroxyurea as an adjunct to radiation therapy in stages IIB–IVA carcinoma of the cervix with negative para-aortic lymph nodes: a Gynecologic Oncology Group and Southwest Oncology Group study. *J Clin Oncol* 1999;17:1339–1348.

371. Pearcey R, Brundage M, Drouin P, et al. Phase III trial comparing radical radiotherapy with and without cisplatin chemotherapy in patients with advanced squamous cell cancer of the cervix. *J Clin Oncol* 2002;20:966–972.

372. Thomas G, Dembo A, Ackerman I, et al. A randomized trial of standard versus partially hyperfractionated radiation with or without concurrent 5-fluorouracil in locally advanced cervical cancer. *Gynecol Oncol* 1998;69:137–145.

373. Lanciano R, Calkins A, Bundy BN, et al. Randomized comparison of weekly cisplatin or protracted venous infusion of fluorouracil in combination with pelvic radiation in advanced cervix cancer: a gynecologic oncology group study. *J Clin Oncol* 2005;23:8289–8295.

375. Lorvidhaya V, Chitapanarux I, Sangruchi S, et al. Concurrent mitomycin C, 5-fluorouracil, and radiotherapy in the treatment of locally advanced carcinoma of the cervix: a randomized trial. *Int J Radiat Oncol Biol Phys* 2003;55:1226–1232.

376. Dueñas-González A, Zarbá JJ, Patel F, et al. Phase III, open-label, randomized study comparing concurrent gemcitabine plus cisplatin and radiation followed by adjuvant gemcitabine and cisplatin versus concurrent cisplatin and radiation in patients with stage IIB to IVA carcinoma of the cervix. *J Clin Oncol* 2011;29:1678–1685.

380. Chemoradiotherapy for Cervical Cancer Meta-Analysis Collaboration. Reducing uncertainties about the effects of chemoradiotherapy for cervical cancer: a systematic review and meta-analysis of individual patient data from 18 randomized trials. *J Clin Oncol* 2008;26:5802–5812.

381. Pearcey R, Miao Q, Kong W, et al. Impact of adoption of chemoradiotherapy on the outcome of cervical cancer in Ontario: results of a population-based cohort study. *J Clin Oncol* 2007;25:2383–2388.

395. Kitagawa R, Katsumata N, Ando M, et al. A multi-institutional phase II trial of paclitaxel and carboplatin in the treatment of advanced or recurrent cervical cancer. *Gynecol Oncol* 2012;125:307–311.

396. Tewari KS, Sill MW, Long HJ, et al. Improved survival with bevacizumab in advanced cervical cancer. *N Engl J Med* 2014;370:734–743.

397. Monk BJ, Mas Lopez L, Zarba JJ, et al. Phase II, open-label study of pazopanib or lapatinib monotherapy compared with pazopanib plus lapatinib combination therapy in patients with advanced and recurrent cervical cancer. *J Clin Oncol* 2010;28:3562–3569.

398. Santin AD, Sill MW, McMeekin DS, et al. Phase II trial of cetuximab in the treatment of persistent or recurrent squamous or non-squamous cell carcinoma of the cervix: a Gynecologic Oncology Group study. *Gynecol Oncol* 2011;122:495–500.

406. Berek JS, Howe C, Lagasse LD, et al. Pelvic exenteration for recurrent gynecologic malignancy: survival and morbidity analysis of the 45-year experience at UCLA. *Gynecol Oncol* 2005;99:153–159.

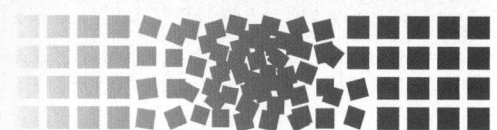

73 Cancer of the Uterine Body

Kaled M. Alektiar, Nadeem R. Abu-Rustum, and Gini F. Fleming

ENODOMETRIAL CARCINOMA

Epidemiology

Endometrial cancer is the most common gynecologic malignancy and the fourth most frequently diagnosed cancer in women in the United States. The American Cancer Society[1] estimates there will be 52,630 new cases and 8,590 deaths in 2014. The median age of diagnosis for endometrial cancer is 61 years, with 20% diagnosed before menopause, including 5% who develop the disease before age 40.

The exact etiology of endometrial cancer remains unknown, but chronic unopposed estrogenic stimulation is considered the main risk factor. The normal endometrium is a hormonally responsive tissue; estrogenic stimulation produces cellular growth and glandular proliferation, which is cyclically balanced by the maturational effects of progesterone.[2] Because menarche and menopause are commonly associated with absent or irregular ovulation, women who experience *early menarche* or *late menopause* are more likely to have additional estrogenic exposure, thus higher risk of developing endometrial cancer.[3] *Nuliparity* is also associated with increased risk of endometrial cancer,[4] due in part to anovulatory menstrual cycles. Morbidly obese women are at greatest risk of endometrial cancer, presumably because their adipocytes are able to convert androstenedione of adrenal origin to estrone, a weak circulating estrogen. Obesity may also influence endometrial cancer risk via chronic hyperinsulinemia, which appears to be a key factor for the development of ovarian hyperandrogenism, associated with anovulation and progesterone deficiency, especially for premenopausal women.[5] *Non–insulin-dependent diabetes mellitus* and *hypertension* also increase the risk of endometrial cancer, in large part secondary to obesity, but there are data showing that these risk factors could operate independently.[6–8] The use of *estrogen-only hormone-replacement therapy* and *sequential oral contraceptives* significantly increase endometrial cancer risk (relative risk, 10 to 20), while combined preparations (i.e., that contain progestagen) have a protective effect (relative risk, 0.3 to 0.5).[9–11]

The use of *tamoxifen* in patients with breast cancer has been associated with increased risk of endometrial cancer.[12–14] In premenopausal women, tamoxifen has an antiestrogenic effect, but in postmenopausal women it has a weak estrogenic effect because of the upregulation of estrogen receptors. In a meta-analysis about adjuvant tamoxifen and endometrial cancer, for patients who were <55 years, there was little absolute risk. In contrast, for patients in the 55 to 69 years age group, the 15-year incidence was 3.8% in the tamoxifen group versus 1.1% in the control group (absolute increase, 2.6%), highlighting the influence of age on the risk of endometrial cancer from tamoxifen use.[15] Initial data seem to indicate that the majority of endometrial cancers associated with tamoxifen use were early stage with favorable features.[16] Other data, however, point to a change in the profile of these endometrial cancers with a rise in the rate of serous carcinoma, clear cell carcinoma, carcinosarcoma, and sarcoma.[17,18] The risk of endometrial cancer from tamoxifen, including the duration of its use,

has to be weighed against its benefit in reducing mortality from breast cancer.[19]

About 5% of endometrial cancers are associated with *Lynch syndrome* or hereditary nonpolyposis colorectal cancer. Lynch syndrome is an autosomal dominant inherited cancer susceptibility syndrome caused by a germline mutation in one of the DNA mismatch repair genes (*MSH2, MLH1, MSH6, PMS2*). Women with this syndrome have a 40% to 60% risk of endometrial cancer, which equals or exceeds their risk of colorectal cancer. In a study of 537 families with Lynch syndrome,[20] the estimated cumulative risks for endometrial cancer by age 70 years were 54% for MLH1 mutation carriers, 21% for MSH2, and 16% for MSH6. The mean age at endometrial cancer diagnosis in women with Lynch syndrome has been reported to be 46 to 54 years, compared with a mean age of 60 years in the general population.[21,22] There seems to be a high rate of lower uterine segment involvement in patients with Lynch syndrome associated endometrial cancer.[23] In terms of histology, endometrioid is the most common, but other histology, such as uterine serous carcinoma, clear cell carcinoma, and carcinosarcoma, have been reported in patients with Lynch syndrome.[21]

Natural History and Routes of Spread

The most common presentation for endometrial cancer is postmenopausal vaginal bleeding, which is reported by 80% to 90% of patients. The incidence of endometrial cancer in women presenting with postmenopausal bleeding, however, is only 10% to 15%. This incidence could vary from 1% up to 25% depending on patient's age, the number of vaginal bleeding episodes, and presence of other risk factors such as diabetes and high body mass index.[24] Other patterns of presentations include vaginal discharge, abnormal Papanicolaou smear, or thickened endometrium on routine transvaginal ultrasound. Presenting with urinary or rectal bleeding, pain, lower extremity lymphedema, ascites, and cough and/or hemoptysis is rare and often indicative of advanced disease.

The uterus has a rich and complex lymphatic network. The main body of the uterus drains via lymphatic trunks that condense in the parametria and end up in pelvic nodes. Channels draining the superior portion of the fundus and fundal uterine serosa parallel the ovarian vessels and empty into the para-aortic lymph nodes in the upper abdomen. A few small lymphatic vessels course through the round ligaments to the superficial inguinal nodes. Invasion into adjacent organs such as bladder and rectum may occur, although not frequent. Tumor cells may gain access to the peritoneal cavity and at times leading to peritoneal implants, similar to ovarian cancers. Sites of distant spread include lungs, liver, and bone.

Diagnosis and Pretherapy Evaluation

Office endometrial biopsy is the preferred approach to establish the diagnosis of endometrial cancer. Its sensitivity in detecting endometrial cancer in postmenopausal women is 99.6%, compared to 91% in premenopausal women, and its specificity is >98% for both groups.[25] However, if symptoms persist, the biopsy sampling is inadequate, or patient is being considered for conservative fertility-sparing approaches, a dilatation and curettage should be performed instead. In order to confirm a diagnosis of endometrial cancer, a tissue diagnosis is required and it must not be substituted by imaging studies. *Transvaginal ultrasonography* may be a useful imaging modality, particularly in patients who are medically compromised in whom obtaining a tissue sample is not feasible. Normal endometrium looks thin and homogenously hyperechoic, but it becomes thickened and heterogenous with hyperplasia, polyps, and cancer.[26] The consensus statement from the Society of Radiologists in Ultrasound has defined an endometrial thickness of ≥5 mm as being abnormal.[27] If the thickness of the endometrium is <5 mm, the risk of endometrial cancer is minimal; the false negative rate is about 4% in general.[28] Recent meta-analysis seems to indicate that perhaps a cut-off of 3 mm thickness provides even better diagnostic accuracy.[29]

The utility of *computed tomography (CT) imaging* in changing the management of patients with endometrial cancer has been evaluated prospectively. When patients have a preoperative diagnosis of endometrial hyperplasia or endometrioid low-grade carcinoma, CT scan imaging changed the planned treatment only 4% of the time. By contrast, in patients with higher grade histology and high-risk histologic subtypes such as papillary serous or clear cell carcinoma, CT scan imaging changed treatment in 11% of the time.[30]

Magnetic resonance imaging (MRI), especially dynamic contrast-enhanced MRI, is very useful in detecting myometrial invasion,[31] with an accuracy of 85% to 93%. In patients with suspected cervical involvement, preoperative MRI may also facilitate determining if the uterine tumor involves the lower uterine segment or if there is true extension into the cervix. Documenting gross cervical involvement from endometrial cancer, albeit a rare finding, is important since radical hysterectomy as opposed to simple hysterectomy might be the preferred surgical approach. *Position emission tomography (PET)/CT* is of little benefit in assessing the primary tumor extension. With regard to regional lymph nodes metastasis, the reported sensitivity is 50% to 100%, specificity 87 to 100, and accuracy 78% to 100%. The main limitation of PET/CT is its inability to detect metastasis in lymph nodes ≥5 mm in size.[32] *Serum CA 125* levels may be a predictor of extrauterine disease.[33] In a study of 214 endometrial cancer patients, serum CA 125 was found to be an independent risk factor for pelvic and para-aortic lymph node metastasis.[34] Elevated levels of CA 125 may also assist in predicting treatment response or in posttreatment surveillance.[35]

Pathology

Endometrial *hyperplasia* is the precursor lesion of the most common endometrial cancer, endometrioid adenocarcinoma. The World Health Organization classifies endometrial hyperplasia into four subtypes: simple hyperplasia, complex hyperplasia, simple atypical hyperplasia, and complex atypical hyperplasia.[36] The risk of progressing to endometrial cancer is only 1% for simple hyperplasia, but increases up to 29% for complex hyperplasia associated with atypia.[37] The Gynecologic Oncology Group (GOG) conducted a prospective trial in which all patients with atypical hyperplasia of the uterus underwent an immediate hysterectomy. The rate of underlying concurrent carcinoma in the uterus was 42.6% in these patients.[38] The standard recommended treatment for atypical hyperplasia of the uterus is hysterectomy. In patients who desire future fertility or have an absolute contraindication to surgery, progestational therapies may be used with caution.[39]

The most common histologic subtype of endometrial cancer is *endometrioid*. The grading is primarily driven by the architectural grading, which is determined by the amount of solid masses of tumor cells compared to well-defined glands. Grade 1 is an endometrioid cancer in which <5% of the tumor growth is in

TABLE 73.1

Pathologic Classificaton of Endometrial Cancers

Endometrioid adenocarcinoma
  Not otherwise specified
  Adenocarcinoma with squamous differentiation
  Secretory adenocarcinoma
  Ciliated carcinoma
  Villoglandular
Serous
Clear cell carcinoma
Undifferentiated carcinoma
Mucinous carcinoma
Squamous cell carcinoma
Transitional cell carcinoma
Mixed cell type

solid sheets. Grade 2 is an adenocarcinoma in which 6% to 50% of the tumor is composed of solid sheets of cells. Grade 3 occurs when >50% of the tumor is made up of solid sheets. There are several subtypes of endometrioid adenocarcinoma, as shown in Table 73.1. *Serous carcinoma*, also known as uterine papillary serous cancer, is seen in about 10% of endometrial cancers. The presence of marked cellular atypia in addition to papilla is what distinguishes serous carcinoma from others. This is an aggressive subtype with a high propensity for early lymphatic and intraperitoneal dissemination, often despite little myometrial penetration.[40] Other histologies include clear cell carcinoma and undifferentiated carcinomas. The latter can also be associated with an endometrioid carcinoma component, and such tumors have been referred to as "dedifferentiated carcinomas," which may belong to the spectrum of gynecologic neoplasms seen in the setting of microsatellite instability and possibly Lynch syndrome.[41]

Prognostic Factors

Several clinicopathologic factors have been identified in patients with endometrial carcinoma to help predict the prognosis and individualize the treatment plan.[42,43] At Memorial Sloan Kettering Cancer Center (MSKCC), a nomogram was developed for predicting overall survival of women with endometrial cancer (n = 1,735) following primary therapy.[44] Five prognostic factors (age, grade, histologic type, number of lymph nodes removed, and International Federation of Gynecology and Obstetrics [FIGO] 1988 surgical stage) were used to predict overall survival (OS) with high concordance probability (Fig. 73.1).

The adverse prognostic factors in endometrial cancer that are part of the staging system include depth of myometrial invasion, cervical stromal involvement, adnexal involvement, pelvic/para-aortic node involvement, extension into bladder or rectum, and distant spread.[42,43] Other prognostic factors include age, grade, histologic type, and lymphovascular invasion (LVI). The adverse impact of *older age* is often explained away by pointing out that older patients tend to present with aggressive histologies and more advanced disease and are generally treated less aggressively. Age of ≥60 years, however, has been shown to be predictive of local-regional recurrence (hazard ratio [HR] 3.9; p = 0.0017) and death (HR: 2.66; p = 0.01) in a randomized trial limited to stage I and where patients with deep myometrial invasion and grade 3 were excluded.[45] Further, the adverse impact of advanced age persists even when older patients are treated as aggressively as younger patients.[46] It is unclear if the prognosis differs significantly between grade 1 and 2 patients. What is clear is the adverse impact of *grade 3* on outcome. In the FIGO annual report,[47] *grade 3* was an independent predictor of poor survival on multivariate analysis within each stage: stage I (HR: 2.45), II (HR: 2.14), III (HR: 2.44), and

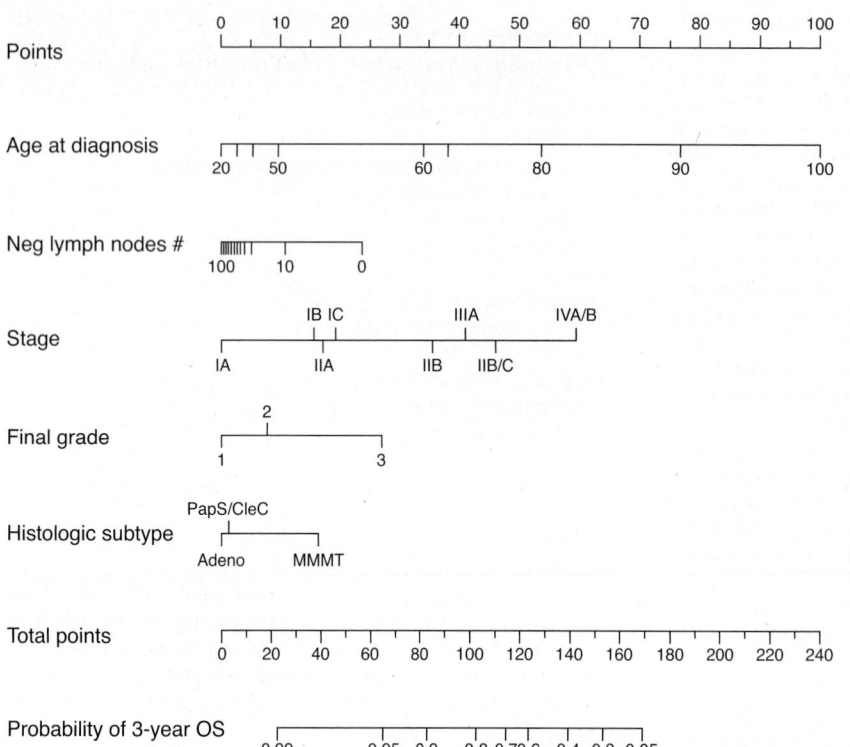

Points

0 10 20 30 40 50 60 70 80 90 100

Age at diagnosis

20 50 60 80 90 100

Neg lymph nodes #

100 10 0

Stage

IB IC   IIIA   IVA/B

IA   IIA   IIB   IIB/C

Final grade

2

1   3

Histologic subtype

PapS/CleC

Adeno   MMMT

Total points

0 20 40 60 80 100 120 140 160 180 200 220 240

Probability of 3-year OS

0.99   0.95 0.9   0.8 0.70.6   0.4 0.2 0.05

Figure 73.1 Overall survival (OS) nomogram.

stage IV (HR: 2.55). In that report, the 5-year survival rates based on *histology* were 83.2% for endometrioid adenocarcinoma, compared to 52.6% for serous and 62.5% for clear cell in 8,033 surgically staged patients.[47] LVI is seen in about 15% of patients with clinically stage I (confined to uterus) endometrial cancer.[42] Its presence causes a four- to six-fold increase in the rate of pelvic and para-aortic nodal metastases.[42] This translates into more frequent relapses, including vaginal recurrences[48,49] and a poorer outcome.[50]

On the basis of a prospective study of 366 patients with endometrial carcinoma, Bokhman[51] postulated that there are two different pathogenetic types of endometrial carcinoma. Type I disease arises in women with obesity and signs of hyperestrogenism: anovulatory uterine bleeding, infertility, late onset of the menopause, and hyperplasia of the endometrium. The tumors tend to be well to moderately differentiated, with minimal invasion, and tend to carry good prognosis. Type II arises in women who lack signs of hyperestrogenism and tend to be older. The tumors are often poorly differentiated, with deep myometrial invasion and frequent occurrence of extrauterine spread.[51] What is remarkable is that this clinical observation can now be confirmed at the molecular level. In a review by Dedes et al.,[52] the most frequently altered molecular pathway in type I endometrial carcinomas is the phosphatidylinositol-3 kinase (PI3K)/phosphatase and tensin homolog (PTEN)/protein kinase B (AKT) pathway, whereas alterations in type II endometrial cancers involve the tumor suppressors p53 and/or p16. More recent genomics data seem to show that there are in fact four distinct types of endometrial cancer with different prognosis based on number of mutations (ultramutated versus hypermutated) and copy numbers (low versus high) observed.[53]

Staging

In 2009, the FIGO Committee on Gynecologic Oncology (Table 73.2) revised the 1988 staging for endometrial cancer.[54] There were several modifications in the new staging system. Patients who used to be staged as IB (i.e., <50% myometrial invasion) are now considered IA. Those with ≥50% myometrial

TABLE 73.2	
Revised International Federation of Gynecology and Obstetrics Staging for Endometrial Cancer	
Stage I[a]	Tumor confined to the corpus uteri
IA[a]	No or less than half myometrial invasion
IB[a]	Invasion equal to or more than half of the myometrium
Stage II[a]	Tumor invades cervical stroma but does not extend beyond the uterus[b]
Stage III[a,c]	Local and/or regional spread of the tumor
IIIA[a]	Tumor invades the serosa of the corpus uteri and/or adnexae[a]
IIIB[a]	Vaginal and/or parametrial involvement[a]
IIIC[a]	Metastases to pelvic and/or para-aortic lymph nodes[a]
IIIC1	Positive pelvic nodes
IIIC2	Positive para-aortic lymph nodes with or without positive pelvic nodes
Stage IV[a]	Tumor invades bladder and/or bowel mucosa, and/or distant metastases
IVA[a]	Tumor invasion of bladder and/or bowel mucosa
IVB[a]	Distant metastases, including intra-abdominal metastases and/or inguinal lymph nodes

[a] Either G1, G2, or G3.
[b] Endocervical glandular involvement only should be considered as stage I and no longer as stage II.
[c] Positive cytology has to be reported separately without changing the stage.
From Pecorelli S. International Federation of Gynecology and Obstetrics: Revised FIGO staging for carcinoma of the vulva, cervix, and endometrium. *Int J Gynecol Obstet* 2009;105:103–104.

invasion are designated as stage IB. The discriminating power of the new FIGO staging system is being debated. Page et al.[55] evaluated a total of 10,839 cases from 1998 to 2006 using the Surveillance, Epidemiology, and End Results program. The analysis demonstrated the usefulness of two divisions rather than three for stage I in the new FIGO staging system.[55] In contrast, a study from MSKCC of 1,307 patients with FIGO 1988 stage I disease showed that the revised system for stage I did not improve its predictive ability over the 1988 system.[56] Endocervical glandular involvement does not affect staging anymore; only patients with cervical stromal invasion are considered stage II. Having positive peritoneal cytology does not affect staging either. But it is important to continue to obtain peritoneal cytology because of its prognostic impact, especially in patients with other extrauterine features. Milgrom et al.[57] reported on 196 patients with stage III (2009 FIGO staging system) endometrial cancer, where positive peritoneal cytology was associated with an increased hazard for relapse (HR 2.3; $p = 0.002$) and death (HR 2.9; $p < 0.001$). Parametrial extension is now considered IIIB. Patients with stage IIIC are now subdivided into IIIC1 if pelvic nodes are involved and IIIC2 if para-aortic nodes are involved.

Treatment of Early-Stage (I-II) Disease

Surgery

The main treatment is simple hysterectomy/bilateral salpingo-oophorectomy (BSO), peritoneal cytology, and some form of regional lymph node assessment. Salpingo-oophorectomy is recommended since 5% of patients with clinically stage I (confined to uterus) endometrial cancer may have adnexal involvement.[42] There is also the concern about synchronous ovarian cancer[58]; among all women with endometrial cancer, 3.1% have a synchronous ovarian cancer, but among women <50 years of age, the rate is as high as 9.4%. Differentiating between metastasis to ovary as opposed to synchronous ovarian cancer is not always easy. The use of genetic profiling may represent a powerful tool for use in clinical practice for distinguishing between metastatic and dual primaries in patients with simultaneous ovarian/endometrial cancer and predicting disease outcome.[59] The revised staging system requires that cytology be obtained and be reported separately without changing the stage. Positive peritoneal cytology is seen in about 12% of patients with clinically stage I (confined to uterus) endometrial cancer.[42] The simple hysterectomy could be done with an open approach (i.e., *total abdominal hysterectomy* [TAH/BSO]) or with a minimally invasive approach (i.e., *laproscopic-assisted hysterotomy/BSO or robotic assisted hysterectomy/BSO*). The GOG completed a trial where patients with clinical stage I to occult IIA uterine cancer were randomly assigned to laparoscopy ($n = 1,696$) or open laparotomy ($n = 920$), including hysterectomy, salpingo-oophorectomy, pelvic cytology, and pelvic and para-aortic lymphadenectomy. Laparoscopy had fewer moderate to severe postoperative adverse events than laparotomy (14% versus 21%, respectively; $p < 0.0001$). Hospitalization of >2 days was significantly lower in laparoscopy versus laparotomy patients (52% versus 94%, respectively; $p < 0.0001$). The conversion rate to laparotomy was 25.8%. The estimated 5-year OS was 89.8% for laparoscopy and 89.8% for laparotomy.[60,61] In 2005, the US Food and Drug Administration (FDA) approved the da Vinci robotic system for gynecologic procedures. In a recent systematic review of robotic surgery in gynecology, investigators found that the proficiency plateau seems to be lower for robotic surgery than for conventional laparoscopy. The conclusion from this analysis was that the specific method of minimally invasive surgery, whether conventional laparoscopy or robotic surgery, should be tailored to patient selection, surgeon ability, and equipment availability.[62]

With regards to regional lymph node assessment, the options range from removing only grossly suspicious nodes to routine lymphadenectomy for all comers. Based on GOG 33 surgical-pathologic assessment,[42] the rate of positive pelvic lymph node in patients who are otherwise clinically stage I (confined to uterus) is 9% and the rate of positive para-aortic node is 6%. Two randomized trials addressed the role of *lymphadenectomy* in early-stage endometrial cancer. In both trials, patients with clinically stage I disease were randomized to pelvic lymphadenectomy versus none. Para-aortic node sampling was optional. In the first trial, 514 patients were randomized and with a median follow-up of 49 months, the 5-year disease-free and OS rates, in an intention-to-treat analysis, were similar between arms (81.0% and 85.9% in the lymphadenectomy arm and 81.7% and 90.0% in the no-lymphadenectomy arm, respectively).[63,64]

These two trials have been criticized extensively due to multiple flaws in design and to numerous study deviations. Nonetheless, most gynecologic oncologists agree that staging of apparent uterine-confined endometrial cancer is to help guide adjuvant therapy and potentially limit toxic additional therapy but by itself is not therapeutic. A middle ground approach between removing only grossly suspicious node to routine lymphadenectomy is emerging. It is sentinel lymph node (SLN) mapping (Fig. 73.2). In a prospective trial from France, regarding the role of SLN in early-stage endometrial cancer, at least one SLN was detected in 111 of the 125 eligible patients. Of the 111 patients, 19 (17%) had pelvic-lymph-node metastases. Three patients had false-negative results (two had metastatic nodes in the contralateral pelvic area and one in the para-aortic area), giving a negative predictive value of 97% (95% confidence interval = 91 to 99) and sensitivity of 84% (62% to 95%). SLN biopsy upstaged 10% of patients with low-risk and 15% of those with intermediate-risk endometrial cancer.[65] Currently at MSKCC *sentinel node mapping algorithm* is utilized to further refine the utility of such technique.[66] SLN mapping is for *normal-appearing nodes*. Any grossly enlarged or suspicious nodes must be evaluated irrespective of mapping. In fact such nodes, while being the sentinel nodes, often do not absorb the injected dye or radiocolloid (i.e. don't map). Similarly, a failed mapping on a hemipelvis cannot be considered a "negative, healthy pelvic sidewall." A failed mapping should be accompanied by a side-specific lymphadenectomy to include the iliac and obturator nodes (Fig. 73.3). In a recent study from MSKCC, 498 patients received a blue dye cervical injection for SLN mapping. At least one lymph node was removed in 95% of cases (474/498); at least one SLN was identified in 81% (401/498). SLN correctly diagnosed 40/47 patients with nodal metastases who had at least one SLN mapped, resulting in a 15% false-negative rate. However, after applying the algorithm mentioned previously, the false-negative rate dropped to 2%. Only one patient, whose lymph node spread would not have been caught by the algorithm, had an isolated positive right para-aortic lymph node with a negative ipsilateral SLN and pelvic lymph node dissection.[67] In general, isolated para-aortic nodal metastasis in the absence of pelvic nodal metastasis is rare and only seen in 1% to 3% of cases.[68] Further, there is no definitive, well-documented association between para-aortic nodal assessment and improved OS in endometrial cancer.[69]

In summary, minimally invasive simple hysterectomy/BSO (laproscopic or robotic), peritoneal cytology, and SLN mapping seems to provide the highest prognostic/therapeutic yield while maintaining a low morbidity profile.

Radiation

Indications and types of radiation for early-stage endometrioid adenocarcinoma are shown in Table 73.3. For patients with *stage IA grade 1 and 2* endometrioid adenocarcinoma (no or <50% myometrial invasion), adjuvant radiotherapy (RT) is not routinely recommended. In a trial reported by Sorbe et al.,[70] 645 such patients were randomized after surgery to observation ($n = 326$) or intravaginal RT ($n = 319$). Surgery consisted of TAH/BSO (laproscopic was allowed), pelvic washing, and removal of enlarged nodes. The

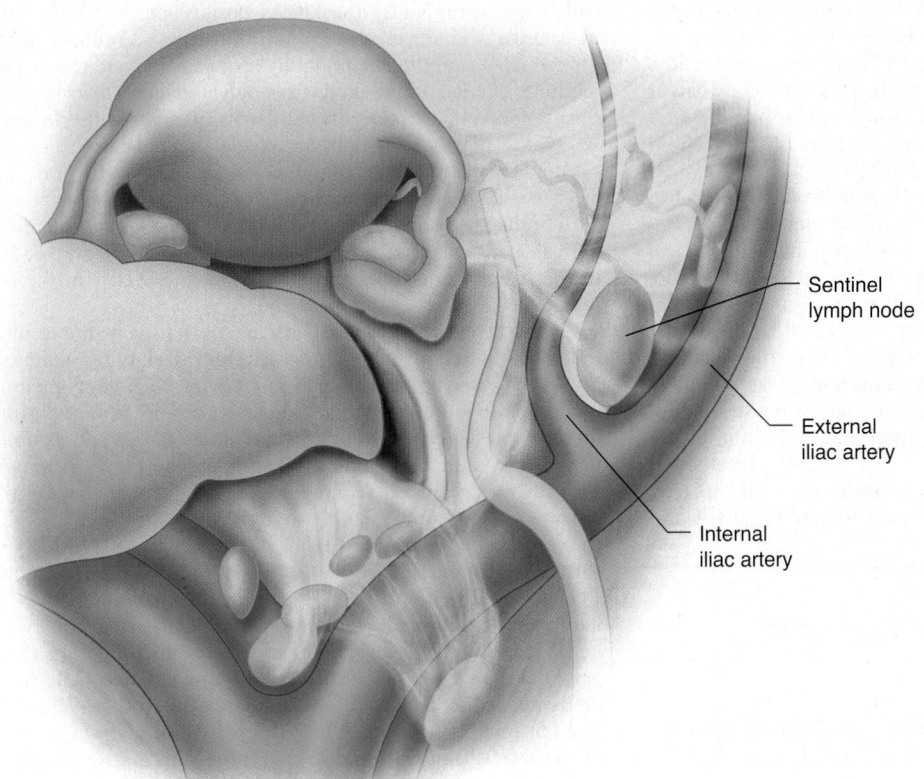

Figure 73.2 Diagrammatic illustration of the location of the sentinel lymph nodes (*blue* in relationship to vessels between internal and external iliac arteries).

rate of vaginal recurrence was 3.1% in the observation arm compared to 1.2% for the intravaginal RT arm ($p = 0.114$). The rate of pelvic recurrence was 0.9% in the observation arm and 0.3% in the treatment arm ($p = 0.326$). There was no significance difference between the two arms in terms of OS.[70] Since the data from this trial did not report outcome based on myometrial invasion, it is difficult to determine the true impact of intravaginal RT on patients with <50% invasion as opposed to those without any invasion. Therefore, while observation is still a valid option for patient with grade 1-2 and myometrial invasion that is <50%, age of patient and the presence of LVI should be taken into account. In the randomized trial by Sorbe et al.[70] mentioned previously, patients with vaginal recurrences were significantly ($p = 0.018$) older (mean age: 68.6 years) compared to patients without vaginal recurrences (mean: 62.6 years). Mariani et al.[48] reported on 508 patients (152

without any invasion) with stage I endometrial cancer treated with surgery alone. LVI significantly increased the vaginal relapse rate from 3% to 7% ($p = 0.02$). At MSKCC, patients who are ≥60 years old or have LVI are recommended to have intravaginal RT.

For patients with *stage IA grade* 3 endometrioid adenocarcinoma, those without myometrial invasion could be observed or treated with postoperative intravaginal RT, while patients with <50% invasion are often treated with adjuvant radiation. In PORTEC-1 trial, 715 patients with stage I (excluded were patients with <50% myometrial invasion grade 1 and patients with >50% grade 3) endometrial cancer were randomized after TAH/BSO to observation or pelvic RT.[71] In the subset of patients with <50% myometrial invasion grade 3 endometrioid tumors ($n = 37$), the 5-year vaginal recurrence rate was 14% with surgery alone compared to 0% for those treated with pelvic RT. In contrast, none

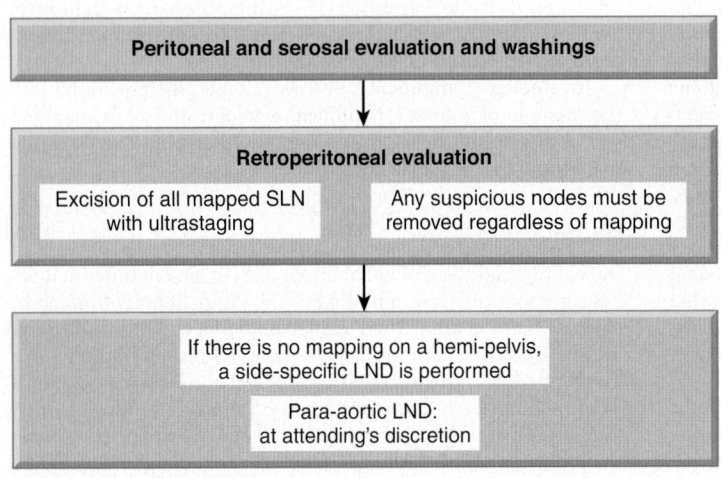

Figure 73.3 Sentinel lymph node mapping algorithm. SLN, sentinel lymph node; LND, lymphadenectomy.

TABLE 73.3

Treatment Recommendations for Early-Stage (FIGO 2009) Endometrioid Adenocarcinoma of the Uterus

	Grade 1/2	Grade 3
IA	Observation[a]	Observation versus IVRT
IB	IVRT	IMRT versus IVRT plus CT
II[b] (<50% cervical stromal invasion)	IVRT	IMRT versus IVRT plus CT
II (>50% cervical stromal invasion)	IMRT	IMRT versus IVRT plus CT

[a] Consider IVRT for patients with <50% myometrial invasion who are also ≥60 years or have lymphovascular invasion.
[b] Patients with endocervical gland involvement, although no longer considered stage II, should be treated in a similar fashion to this subgroup of stage II.
IVRT, intravaginal radiation; IMRT, intensity modulated radiation therapy; CT, chemotherapy, generally paclitaxel/carboplatin.

of 37 patients in this subset relapsed in the pelvis irrespective of the treatment.[72] Horowitz et al.[73] (n = 31) and Fanning et al.[74] (n = 21) reported no vaginal or pelvic recurrence in their series of patients with <50% myometrial invasion grade 3 treated with post-operative intravaginal RT. Such data indicates that intravaginal RT is the preferred approach in these patients.

For patients with *stage IB grade 1 and 2* endometrioid adeno-carcinoma in PORTEC-1 trial, the 5-year vaginal recurrence for patients treated with surgery alone was 10% for those with grade 1 and 13% for grade 2. In contrast, the corresponding 5-year vaginal recurrence rates for patients treated with pelvic RT were 1% and 2%, respectively. The risk of pelvic recurrence at 5 years after surgery alone for these patients (>50% invasion) was 2% for grade 1 and 6% for grade 2 tumors.[72] One of the important questions in patients with IB grade 1 and 2 is whether pelvic RT could be safely omitted. There are two randomized trials comparing pelvic RT to intravaginal RT. Neither trial required pelvic lymphadenectomy. In PORTEC 2 trial, 427 patients were randomized to pelvic RT (n = 214) or intravaginal RT (n = 213) after TAH/BSO. Inclusion criteria in this trial differed from that in PORTEC-1. For patients with stage I, they needed to be ≥60 years old and have either grade 3 tumors with <50% myometrial invasion or >50% invasion grade 1 and 2 tumors. Patients with endocervical mucosal involvement were also added. The 5-year vaginal recurrence rates were 1.8% in the intravaginal RT arm and 1.6% in the pelvic RT arm (p = 0.74). The pelvic recurrence was 3.8% in the intravaginal RT arm compared to only 0.5% in the pelvic RT arm (p = 0.02). There was no significant difference in disease-free or OS between the two arms.[75] The other trial reported by Sorbe et al.,[76] patients with stage I endometrioid adenocarcinoma with at least one of the following risk factors (grade 3, ≥50% myometrial invasion, or DNA aneuploidy) were randomized to adjuvant intravaginal RT (n = 263) or pelvic plus intravaginal RT (n = 264). The vaginal recurrence rate was 2.7% (7/263) in the intravaginal RT alone arm compared to 1.9% (5/264) in the pelvic RT arm (p = 0.555). Pelvic recurrence rate, however, was different: 5.3% in the intravaginal RT alone arm compared to 0.4% in the pelvic RT arm (p = 0.0006). There was no significant difference in OS between the two arms (90% versus 89%, respectively).[76] The data from these trials indicate that the omission of pelvic RT in favor of intravaginal RT did not significantly increase the risk of vaginal recurrence. The reported risk of pelvic recurrence after lymphadenectomy or pelvic RT in patients with >50% invasion grade 1 and 2 tumors is about 1.5% on average.[73,77–79] But that is not a sufficient reason to recommend routine lymphadenectomy or pelvic RT for two reasons. First, neither pel-

vic RT nor lymphadenectomy have been shown to improve survival in patients with early-stage endometrial cancer. Second, in the PORTEC-2 trial,[75] most patients with pelvic recurrences had simultaneous distant metastasis. The 5-year rate of isolated pelvic recurrence was only 1.5% in the intravaginal RT arm compared to 0.5% for pelvic RT (p = 0.3). At MSKCC, most of these patients (IB, grade 1 and 2) undergo SLN mapping, and if the nodes are pathologically negative, they receive intravaginal RT alone.

Patients with *stage IB grade 3* endometrioid adenocarcinoma were not enrolled in PORTEC 1 or 2 trials, because it was felt that omitting pelvic RT when lymphadenectomy was not performed could not be justified. In the registry study reported by Creutzberg et al.,[72] 99 patients with ≥50% myometrial invasion grade 3 were treated with postoperative pelvic RT. The 5-year rate of vaginal recurrence was 5%, pelvic recurrence 8%, and distant relapse 31%. Very few investigators would recommend surgery alone for these patients. In fact, an argument could be made that pelvic RT might be needed even after a negative lymphadenectomy especially for older patients and those with LVI. In a GOG 99 trial, 190 patients with stage I-II (patients without myometrial invasion were excluded) underwent TAH/BSO, pelvic washing, and pelvic/para-aortic lymph nodes sampling and then were randomized to observation versus pelvic RT.[80] At 2 years, there was a statistically significant difference in the rates of relapse in favor of the adjuvant pelvic RT arm (3% versus 12%, p = 0.007). There was, however, no significant difference in 4-year OS (92% RT versus 86% with surgery alone, p = 0.557). The benefit of pelvic RT was predominantly seen in a subset of patients designated "high-intermediate risk (HIR)" based on advancing age, grade 2 or 3 tumors, outer third myometrial invasion, and LVI. Those on the pelvic RT arm demonstrated a somewhat lower overall death rate when compared to those on the observation arm (hazard ratio = 0.73, 90% confidence interval = 0.43 to 1.26) in the HIR subgroup.[80] AT MSKCC, patients with >50% myometrial invasion grade 3 who are HIR per GOG 99 would be offered postoperative pelvic RT even in the setting of negative lymphadenectomy. If they are not HIR, then intravaginal RT could be considered but only with adequate pelvic lymphadenectomy and/or SLN mapping.

Patients with *endocervical mucosal invasion* are no longer considered stage II per the FIGO 2009 staging system. However, there are no data to indicate that observation is safe; in fact such patients were randomized to either pelvic RT or intravaginal RT in PORTEC 2 trial.[75] At MSKCC, these patients are treated with postoperative intravaginal RT. Having cervical involvement, especially stromal invasion, increases the risk of lymph node involvement. In the GOG 33 surgical-pathologic assessment study, the rate positive pelvic lymph node was 8% when the cervix-isthmus was not involved versus16% when it was involved.[42] For patients with *stage II* (cervical stromal invasion) omitting pelvic RT could be justified, in the setting of negative lymphadenectomy, based on an average rate of vaginal recurrence of 1.47% and a similar pelvic recurrence rate of 1.47% reported in the literature for patients who underwent lymphadenectomy and intravaginal RT.[49,73,81,82] However, patients in these series were highly selected. At MSKCC, intravaginal RT alone as opposed to pelvic RT is considered only for stage II patients who meet the following criteria: grade 1 and 2 endometriod histology, depth of cervical stromal invasion of <50%, and adequate lymphadenectomy/SLN mapping. Patients with stage II grade 3 or those with cervical stromal invasion >50% are treated with pelvic RT.

It is clear from the data mentioned thus far that if postoperative radiation is needed in early-stage endometrioid adenocarcinoma, the preferred approach is intravaginal RT rather than pelvic RT in most cases. Intravaginal RT targets the most likely site of recurrence in patients with early-stage disease (about 80% of recurrences are vaginal) and its morbidity profile is better than pelvic RT (Fig. 73.4). In the PORTEC 2 trial randomizing patients to pelvic RT versus intravaginal RT, the rate of grade 1 and 2 acute gastrointestinal toxicity was 53% versus 12% (p <0.001) in favor of intravaginal RT.[75] Furthermore, the increased risk of secondary

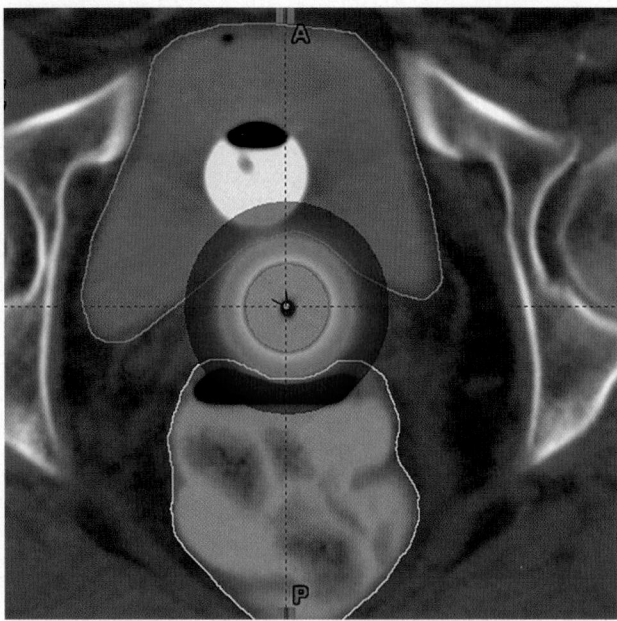

Figure 73.4 Intravaginal radiation therapy conformal dose distribution.

malignancies after pelvic RT for patients who are <60 years old has to be taken into consideration.[83]

In summary, intravaginal RT provides the best therapeutic ration for most patients with early-stage endometrial cancer. At MSKCC, intravaginal RT is given as an outpatient treatment using a high dose rate Ir-192. The dose is 18-21 Gy given in three fractions with 1 to 2 weeks between fractions.

Chemotherapy

Adjuvant *chemotherapy* is not routinely recommended for patients with stage I-II endometrioid adenocarcinoma. In the PORTEC-2 trial,[75] where only the high-risk patients from PORTEC-1 were included, the 5-year rate of distant relapse was 8.3% in the intravaginal RT arm and 5.7% in the pelvic RT arm ($p = 0.46$). In contrast, for patients with deep myometrial invasion grade 3 tumors in the PORTEC registry (all received pelvic RT), the 5-year rate of distant relapse was 31%, indicating the need for effective systemic therapy in this group of patients.[72] The results of recently completed trial for early-stage high-risk patients with endometrial cancer (GOG249), where patients were randomized to pelvic RT versus intravaginal RT plus three cycles of paclitaxel/carboplatin, are eagerly awaited. At MSKCC, intravaginal RT and chemotherapy are offered as an option for patients with endometrioid adenocarcinoma stage IB grade 3 and stage II grade 3. There are more data in the literature on adjuvant chemotherapy in patients with serous endometrial cancer and to a lesser extent clear cell carcinoma. In a study from MSKCC, 41 patients with stage I-II serous cancer (those with no residual disease in hysterectomy were excluded) were treated with postoperative intravaginal RT and six cycles of paclitaxel/carboplatin. Of the 41 patients, 85% completed treatment as prescribed. With a median follow-up time of 58 months, the 5-year disease-free and OS rates were 85% and 90%, respectively. The 5-year actuarial recurrence rates were 9% in the pelvis, 5% in the para-aortic nodes, and 10% at distant sites. None of the patients developed vaginal recurrence.[84]

Treatment of Stage III Disease

There are three randomized trials comparing adjuvant chemotherapy to adjuvant radiation alone. The Japanese Gynecology Oncology Group trial randomized 385 patients with stage I (deep invasion)-III endometrial cancer patients to pelvic RT (193 patients) or to chemotherapy (192 patients). Chemotherapy consisted of cyclophosphamide (333 mg/m²), cisplatin (50 mg/m²), and doxorubicin (40 mg/m²) every 4 weeks for three cycles or more. There was no significant difference in progression-free survival (PFS; $p = 0.726$) or OS ($p = 0.462$) between the two groups.[85] The trial from Italy had similar design and inclusion criteria, where 340 patients were randomized to RT or to chemotherapy. With a median follow-up of 95.5 months, the 5-year disease-free survival was 63% in both arms ($p = 0.44$) and the 5-year overall survival rates were 69% in the radiation arm compared to 66% in the chemotherapy arm ($p = 0.77$). Again, there was no significant difference in outcome despite using five cycles of cyclophosphamide, cisplatin, and doxorubicin.[86] In GOG 122, 396 patients with stage III-IV disease were randomized to whole abdomen radiation ($n = 202$) versus doxorubicin/cisplatin ($n = 194$) for eight cycles. Progression-free survival was the primary end point of this study. With a median follow-up of 74 months, there was significant improvement in both PFS (50% versus 38%; $p = 0.007$) as well as OS (55% versus 42%; $p = 0.004$), respectively, in favor of chemotherapy.[87]

There are two trials comparing adjuvant RT to chemotherapy plus RT. One trial from Finland,[88] randomized 156 patients with stage I-IIIA (FIGO 1988) to RT only or RT combined with three cycles of cisplatin (50 mg/m²), epirubicin (60 mg/m²), and cyclophosphamide (500 mg/m²) chemotherapy ($n = 84$). The disease-specific overall 5-year survival was 84.7% in the RT arm versus 82.1% in the chemoradiation arm ($p = 0.148$). The second trial by Hogberg et al.[89] is a report on two trials. In the MaNGO trial portion, there were 157 patients; 76 were randomized to pelvic RT (45 Gy) and 80 to chemoradiation. The chemotherapy consisted of three cycles of doxorubicin (60 mg/m²) and cisplatin (50 mg/m²). The 5-year PFS was 61% in the RT group compared to 74% for chemoradiation but that difference was not significant ($p = 0.1$). The 5-year OS was also not significant (73% versus 78%, respectively, $p = 0.41$). In the Nordic Society of Gynaecological Oncology/European Organization for Research and Treatment of Cancer (EORTC) trial portion, 383 patients were randomized to RT ($n = 191$) versus chemoradiation ($n = 187$). The type of chemotherapy varied and only a handful of patients were stage III. The 5-year PFS was better for the chemoradiation arm (79% versus 72% for RT, $p = 0.04$) but OS was not significantly better (83% versus 76%, respectively, $p = 0.1$).

Unlike in cervical cancer where the addition of chemotherapy to radiation has been clearly demonstrated in several large-scale randomized trials, the superiority of chemotherapy over radiation alone in endometrial cancer is not conclusive. In fact, even the results from GOG 120 trial are not that definitive. The chemotherapy arm has more patients with stage IIIC disease, therefore PFS and OS were adjusted accordingly. Without that adjustment, there would be no difference between the two arms.[87] The crude rate of relapse in the radiation arm was 54% compared to 50% in the chemotherapy arm, indicating the need for improvements in both arms of the study. Therefore, the question is no longer chemotherapy versus radiation, but rather what is the optimal way of combining the two modalities? Greven et al.[90] reported the results of RTOG 9708 phase 2 study on 44 patients with stage I-III endometrial cancer who were treated with pelvic radiation and intravaginal RT given concurrently with cisplatin (50 mg/m²) on day 1 and 28 of radiation followed by four cycles of cisplatin (50 mg/m²) and paclitaxel (175 mg/m²). The 4-year disease-free and OS was 85% and 81%, respectively. In the subset of patients with stage III disease (66% of patients), the corresponding rates were 72% and 77%, respectively.[90] Currently, the GOG is comparing chemoradiation (similar to RTOG 9708) to six cycles of carboplatin/paclitaxel in patients with stage III disease. The PORTEC 3 randomized trial is comparing chemoradiation to RT alone. Until the results of these trials are available, the decision on whether to give chemoradiation or chemotherapy alone should be based on risk factors. Patients with stage III endometrial cancer represent a heterogenous group of patients. In a report from MSKCC on 192 patients with stage III (FIGO 2009) endometrial cancer, three factors emerged as independent predictors of relapse and death from endometrial cancer.[91] These factors were >50% myometrial invasion, positive peritoneal cytology, and aggressive histology defined as grade 3 endometrioid, serous, clear cell, or undifferentiated. The 5-year relapse rate for patients with no risk factors was 13%, one risk factor 27%, and two or more risk factors 62% (p <0.001). The corresponding 5-year rates of death from endometrial cancer were 11%, 20%, and 56% (p <0.001). Therefore, for patients with stage III with two or more risk factors, especially positive peritoneal cytology in the setting of serous endometrial cancer, full systemic chemotherapy (six cycles of paclitaxel/carboplatin) is preferred over chemoradiation. For those with no more than one risk factor (lymph node involvement only, for example), using an approach similar to RTOG 9708 seems feasible. In a report from MSKCC, 40 patients with stage III disease were treated as such. Of the 40 patients, 78% completed chemoradiation followed by four cycles of paclitaxel/carboplatin. With a median follow-up of 49 months, the 5-year rate of freedom from relapse and OS were 79% and 85%, respectively.[92] When using radiation in stage III endometrial cancer, the preferred approach is intensity modulated (IM)RT because of its favorable morbidity profile. In a report from MSKCC, 46 patients with stage I-III (78% stage III) endometrial cancer were treated with postoperative radiation using IMRT. With a median follow-up of 52 months, the 5-year disease-free survival was 88% and OS was 97%. Chemotherapy was given to 30/46 patients; 5 had grade 3 leukopenia, 8 grade 2 anemia, and 2 grade 2 thrombocytopenia.[93]

In summary, patients with stage III endometrial cancer are very heterogenous; the treatment recommendations thus need to be individualized. Concurrent chemoradiation followed by four cycles of paclitaxel/carboplatin seems to provide excellent outcome for most patients. The preferred form of radiation at MSKCC is pelvic/extended-field IMRT to 50.4 Gy in 28 fractions. Patients who are at high risk for peritoneal relapse should be treated with full systemic therapy.

Treatment of Distant Recurrence

Patients with distant recurrence are not generally curable, and treatment choices should take both efficacy and toxicity into account, particularly as many patients with recurrent endometrial cancer are elderly.

Endocrine Therapy

Progestins have been used in the management of recurrent endometrial cancer since the 1961 report by Kelley and Baker[94] describing a response rate of 29% with various progestational agents, generally parenterally administered hydroxyprogesterone caproate. Subsequent trials generally have used medroxyprogesterone acetate or megestrol acetate (MA), which are available in pill form (Table 73.4).[95–99] Results in unselected patient groups show limited activity with short median PFS, and a recent Cochrane analysis found no evidence that hormonal therapy as a single agent or in combination prolonged overall or 5-year disease-free survival.[100] Nonetheless, some patients will have their disease controlled for several years on hormonal therapy with minimal toxicity. In early reports, patients with well-differentiated tumors, a long disease-free interval, and lung metastases were noted to have the best results. Subsequent work suggested that tumors expressing estrogen receptors (ER) and/or progesterone receptors (PR) had the highest chance of response to progestin therapy, and some more recent trials of endocrine therapy have been limited to tumors expressing ERs or PRs.[95,101]

Sequentially alternating tamoxifen and medroxyprogesterone acetate or MA was tested based on the hypothesis that the antiestrogen therapy could upregulate the progesterone receptor.[102,103] Response

rates were promising, in the range of 30% in a chemotherapy-naïve population; however, median PFS, as with single agent progestin therapy, was short (approximately 3 months). A small randomized trial of MA alone or with concomitant tamoxifen showed no difference between the two regimens.[104] Phase 2 trials with other agents, including aromatase inhibitors,[105,160] tamoxifen,[107] and luteinizing hormone-releasing hormone (LHRH) agonists,[108–110] have mostly yielded lower response rates than seen with progestins, although results may not be truly comparable, as some of these more recent trials were conducted in patients who had prior chemotherapy or hormonal therapy. It seems likely that results would be inferior in a pretreated population. A recent randomized phase 2 trial comparing the mTOR inhibitor ridaforolimus to control treatment (control treatment consisting of progestin therapy with either medroxyprogesterone [200 mg/day] or megestrol [60 mg/day] in 53 patients and chemotherapy in 13 patients) in women with one or two prior chemotherapy regimens reported a response rate of only 4.3% for control therapy.[111]

Preclinical data have suggested that inhibiting the PI3K/Akt pathway reverses progestin resistance in endometrial cancer,[112] and attempts have been made to improve results of endocrine therapy by combining it with an mTOR inhibitor (analogous to the FDA-approved use of everolimus with exemestane in patients with breast cancer). GOG conducted a randomized phase 2 trial testing the mTOR inhibitor temsirolimus with or without a regimen of MA alternating with tamoxifen in patients with no more than one prior chemotherapy regimen. Unfortunately, the combination of temsirolimus with MA/tamoxifen resulted in an unacceptable rate of venous thrombosis (seven events in 22 patients), and the combination arm was closed to accrual after the first stage. Three of twenty-one patients had a response (14%), which is in the range of reported with temsirolimus alone (see the following).[113] A phase 2 open-label single arm study of the combination of everolimus and letrozole enrolled 28 patients who had received one or two prior chemotherapy regimens[114] and showed a somewhat more promising objective response rate of 21%.

In summary, hormonal therapy should be considered for women with low grade ER-positive tumors, particularly if they have a long interval from diagnosis to recurrence. Commonly used regimens in the United States are MA 80 mg twice a day and MA 80 mg twice a day for 3 weeks alternating with tamoxifen 20 mg twice a day for 3 weeks.

Cytotoxic Chemotherapy

First-Line Chemotherapy. Most women with recurrent or stage IV endometrial carcinoma should be assessed for treatment with cytotoxic chemotherapy. Current combination chemotherapy regimens can yield response rates of 50% to 60% with median OS about 12 to 15 months.

Historically, doxorubicin showed reproducible activity in multiple phase 2 and phase 3 studies of patients with chemotherapy-naïve disease (Table 73.5),[115–118] with response rates in the range of 20% to 30%. Single-agent cisplatin[119] and carboplatin[120,121] therapy subsequently produced similar results. As the combination of doxorubicin plus cisplatin (AP) appeared more active than single agent doxorubicin,[115,122] it became the standard for use in both adjuvant and metastatic disease settings. Taxanes were next found to have meaningful activity and, indeed, remain the class of agents that have produced the highest response rates in the setting of pretreated disease (see Table 73.5).[123] In a phase 3 trial of women with recurrent or stage IV endometrial cancer, the triplet of paclitaxel, cisplatin, and doxorubicin (TAP) produced a superior response rate (57% versus 34%), PFS (median, 8.3 versus 5.3 months), and OS (median, 15.3 versus 12.3 months; p = 0.037) when compared to AP.[124] TAP is the only treatment proven to produce a survival benefit in women with recurrent or stage IV endometrial disease. However, a subsequent phase 3 trial comparing TAP to AP as adjuvant therapy after surgery and radiation for stage III and resected stage IV disease

TABLE 73.4

Selected Trials of Hormone Therapy in Advanced Endometrial Cancer

Author	Regimen	Prior Chemotherapy	HR status	N	RR (%)	Median OS (mo)
	Progestins					
Lentz 1996[96]	MGA 800 mg/day	No	Unselected	54	24	7.6
Thigpen 1999[95]	MPA 200 mg/day MPA 1,000 mg/day	No	Unselected	145 154	25 15	11.1 7.0
Whitney 2004[103]	MPA 200 mg/day qo wk and TAM 40 mg daily	No	Unselected	61	33	13
Fiorica 2004[102]	MGA 160 mg/day × 3 wk followed by TAM 40 mg/day × 3 wk	No	Unselected	61	27	14
Pandya 2001[104]	MGA 160 mg/day versus MGA 160 mg/day + TAM 20 mg/day	Yes (6%)	Unselected	20 42	20 19	12.6 8.6
Oza 2012[111]	MPA 200 mg/day or Megestrol 60 mg/day (13 patients had chemotherapy)	One or two regimens	Unselected	66	4.3	8.9
	SERMs					
Thigpen 2001[107]	TAM 40 mg/day	No	Unselected	68	10	8.8
McMeekin 2003[97]	Arzoxifene 20 mg/day	Adjuvant only (9%)[a]	HR positive or Grade 1/2	9	31	n/a Median duration of response 13.9 mo
	GnRH Agonists					
Covens 1997[108]	Leuprolide 7.5 mg IM q 28 d	Yes (two patients)[a]	Unselected	25	0	6
Lhomme 1999[109]	Triptorelin 3.75 mg IM q 28 d	Yes (three patients)[a]	Unselected	25	8.7	7.2
Asbury 2002[110]	Goserelin 3.6 mg SQ q 28 d	Yes (one patient)[a]	Unselected	40	11	7.3
	Aromatase Inhibitors					
Rose 2000[105]	Anastrozole 1 mg/day	No[a]	Unselected	23	9	6
Ma 2004[106]	Letrozole 2.5 mg/day	Adjuvant only[a]	Unselected	28	9.4	n/a
	ER Antagonist					
Covens 2011[98]	Fulvestrant 250 mg IM q 4 wk	Adjuvant (32%)[a]	ER negative ER positive	22 31	0 16	3 26
Emons 2013[99]	Fulvestrant 250 mg IM q 4 wk	Yes (40%)	HR positive 80% HR unknown 20%	35	11.4	13.2

[a] Prior hormonal therapy allowed.
HR, hormone receptors; OS, overall survival; RR, relative risk; MGA, megestrol acetate; MPA, medroxyprogesterone acetate; TAM, tamoxifen; IM, intramuscular; SQ, subcutaneous; SERM, selective estrogen receptor modulator; GnRH, gonadotropin-releasing hormone; n/a, not available; ER, estrogen receptor.

showed no difference between the two regimens, although the subset of women with gross residual disease had a 50% reduction in the risk of recurrence or death with the addition of paclitaxel.[125]

The TAP regimen required growth factor support and produced grade 2 or higher neurotoxicity in 25% to 40% of patients. As phase 2 studies had shown good tolerability and activity with paclitaxel/carboplatin (TC), a 1,300-woman phase 3 noninferiority trial for those with stage III, IV, or recurrent disease was conducted comparing TC to TAP. Preliminary results showed no significant difference in median PFS (14 months in each arm) or median OS (32 months for TC, 38 months for TAP; not statistically significant). Regarding toxicity, study treatment was discontinued due to toxicity in 18% of subjects on TAP and 12% on TC.[126]

One interesting alternative option for front-line therapy might be the combination of liposomal doxorubicin/carboplatin. Considering the well-reproduced activity of free doxorubicin, single-agent liposomal doxorubicin produced a disappointingly low response rate of 11.5% in patients with chemotherapy-naïve endometrial

cancer.[127] Oddly, almost the same level of activity was reported[128] in women with pretreated disease (9.5%), raising the question of whether some unknown adverse selection factors were operating in the front-line trial (e.g., since upfront combination chemotherapy was already established at the time, perhaps less fit patients elected to participate in the trial of single-agent liposomal doxorubicin). The Multicentre Italian Trials in Ovarian Cancer and Gynecologic Malignancies Group conducted a single arm phase 2 trial of pegylated liposomal doxorubicin plus carboplatin in the front-line therapy of advanced endometrial cancer and reported a response rate of 59.5% and a median survival of 80.1 weeks.[129] While the combination of carboplatin/liposomal doxorubicin has performed well compared to TC in a randomized trial for women with ovarian cancer,[130] it has not been compared to other options in women with endometrial cancer. Nonetheless, the carboplatin/liposomal doxorubicin regimen, which produces minimal alopecia and neuropathy, might be a reasonable choice, particularly for patients with contraindications to taxane therapy.

TABLE 73.5

Selected Randomized Trials of Combination Chemotherapy in Chemotherapy Naïve Endometrial Cancer

Author	Regimen	N	RR (%)	Median PFS (mo)	Median OS (mo)
Thigpen 1994[115]	Dox 60 mg/m² q 3 wk versus Dox 60 mg/m² + CTX 500 mg/m² q 3 wk	132 144	22 30	3.2 3.9	6.7 7.3
Pawinski 1999[116]	CTX 1,200 mg/m² q 3 wk IFX 5 mg/m² q 3 wk	14 16	14 25	n/a n/a	n/a n/a
Aapro 2003[117]	Dox 60 mg/m² q 4 wk Dox 60 mg/m² + CDDP 50 mg/m² q 4 wk	87 90	17 43	7 8	7 9
Thigpen 2004[122]	Dox 60 mg/m² q 3 wk Dox 60 mg/m² + CDDP 50 mg/m² q 3 wk	150 131	25 42	3.8 5.7	9.2 9.0
Fleming 2004[118]	Dox 60 mg/m² + CDDP 50 mg/m² q 3 wk Dox 50 mg/m² + PTX 150 mg/m²/24 h + G-CSF	157 160	40 43	7.2 6	12.6 13.6
Fleming 2004[124]	Dox 60 mg/m² + CDDP 50 mg/m² q 3 wk Dox 45 mg/m² + CDDP 50 mg/m² + PTX 160 mg/m² + G-CSF	129 134	34 57	5.3 8.3	12.3 15.3
Miller 2012[a,126]	PTX 175 mg/m² + CPL AUC 6 q 3 wk Dox 45 mg/m² + CDDP 50 mg/m² + PTX 160 mg/m² + G-CSF	663 532	51 51	14 14	36.5 40.3

[a] Including patients with stage III disease.
RR, relative risk; PFS, progression-free survival; OS, overall survival; Dox, doxorubicin; CTX, cyclophosphamide; IFZ, ifosphamide; n/a, not available; CDDP, cisplatin; PTX, paclitaxel; G-CSF, granulocytic colony-stimulating factor; CPL, carboplatin; AUC, area under the curve.

In summary, TC therapy every 3 weeks is the usual first-line chemotherapy treatment in the United States for women with stage IV endometrial cancer. Issues of duration of therapy, optimal treatment after adjuvant TC (which is increasingly used, particularly for women with serous carcinomas), and of paclitaxel scheduling (weekly versus every three weeks) remain to be addressed.

Second (and Later)-Line Chemotherapy. The efficacy of second-line cytotoxic chemotherapy remains very limited. Women who have a prolonged disease-free interval after prior carboplatin/taxane therapy can be retreated with a similar regimen. Nagao et al.[131] reviewed 262 patients, 49% of whom had a platinum-free interval of ≥12 months, and 51% of whom had a platinum-free interval of ≥12 months. Over half received their initial chemotherapy regimen in the adjuvant setting. They found response rates to retreatment with a platinum-based regimen for platinum-free intervals of <6 months, 6 to 11 months, 12 to 23 months, and ≥24 months to be 25%, 38%, 61%, and 65%, respectively, suggesting that the general concept of "platinum sensitivity" in selection of second-line therapy can be applied to endometrial cancer as well as ovarian cancer. However, trials of second-line treatments for endometrial cancer have not traditionally been prospectively stratified along these lines (which may contribute to some of the variability seen in response rates of small phase 2 studies in endometrial cancer to agents such as pegylated liposomal doxorubicin).

Results of selected trials with standard available cytotoxic agents in patients who have received prior chemotherapy are shown in Table 73.6.[132–149] Taxanes showed good activity in the days before taxane-containing therapy was the standard first-line approach.[123] Neither doxorubicin nor platinum agents have generally produced high response rates when used second-line. Other agents such as topotecan and gemcitabine have likewise shown minimal efficacy in previously treated populations.[150]

In summary, women with a prolonged disease-free interval from their front-line platinum therapy can be retreated with a platinum-containing combination. However, in general, response rates to second-line cytotoxic therapy (and noncytotoxic agents) are low.

Predictors of Response to Cytotoxic Therapy. As discussed previously, endometrial carcinoma is composed of several biologically different subsets, including endometrioid (high and low grade), serous, and clear cell. The proportions of the subtypes with advanced recurrent/disease different than in early-stage disease, where low-grade tumors are most common. These histologic subtypes have been shown to have very different genetic makeup, but to date, differences in response to standard front-line cytotoxic therapy have not been observed. McMeekin et al.[151] published results showing that histologic subtype was not an independent predictor of response to doxorubicin/cisplatin/doxorubicin–based regimens. The overall response rate to treatment was 42% (endometrioid 44%, serous 44%, clear cell 32%). The effect of grade was not considered in this analysis.[151] A primary endpoint of the 1,300 patient GOG 209 trial comparing TC to TAP is to determine whether ER status of the tumor has any effect on chemotherapy outcomes, and these data should be available soon.

An integrated genomic analysis of serous and endometrioid endometrial carcinomas by the The Cancer Genome Atlas has revealed that 19.6% of histologically classified high-grade endometrioid endometrial carcinomas had genomic profiles that resemble those of serous carcinomas. Four molecular subgroups were described: a POLE ultramutated subgroup, a hypermutated/microsatellite-unstable subgroup, a copy number-low microsatellite-stable group, and a copy number-high subgroup.[53] Hopefully, improved classifications will eventually help select those tumors most likely to respond to conventional agents as well as identifying targets for novel therapies.

Therapeutic Agents in Development

Antiangiogenic Agents. Antiangiogenic therapies have shown some activity in the treatment of endometrial cancer (see Table 73.6). Bevacizumab, an antivascular endothelial growth factor monoclonal antibody, produced a response rate of 13.5% in patients with one or two prior cytotoxic regimens, and 40% of subjects were progression-free at 6 months.[152] A front-line randomized phase 2 GOG trial randomly assigning patients to TC with either bevacizumab or temsirolimus or to carboplatin plus ixabepilone with bevacizumab has completed accrual and results should be available soon.

TABLE 73.6

Representative Single Agent Trials in Chemotherapy-Pretreated Endometrial Cancer

Cytotoxic Agents	Dose	RR
Cisplatin[132]	50 mg/m² q 3 wk	4%
Etoposide oral[133]	50 mg/m²/d × 21 q 28 d[a]	0
Ifosfamide[134]	1.2 mg/m²/d × 5 q 28 d	15%
Ifosfamide[116]	5 g/m²/24 h q 3 wk	0
Ixabepilone[135]	40 mg/m² q 21 d	12%
Oxaliplatin[136]	130 mg/m² q 21 d	13.5%
Gemcitabine[137]	800 mg/m² d1,8 q 21 d	4%
Paclitaxel[123]	200 mg/m² q 3 wk	27%
Pegylated liposomal doxorubicin[128]	50 mg/m² q 4 wk	9.5%
Pegylated liposomal doxorubicin[138]	40 mg/m² q 28 d	21%
Nonpegylated liposomal doxorubicin[139]	60 mg/m² q 4 wk	0
Topotecan[140]	0.5–1.5 mg/m²/d × 5 q 21 d	9%
Docetaxel[141]	70 mg/m² q 3 wk	23%
Pemetrexed[142]	900 mg/m² q 21 d	3.8%
Antiangiogenic Agents		
Bevacizumab[152]	15 mg/kg IV q 3 wk	13.5%
Aflibercept[143]	4 mg/kg IV q 14 d	7%
Sorafenib[144]	400 mg po bid	5%
Sunitinib[153]	50 mg/d po 4 wk on 2 wk off	15%
mTOR Inhibitors		
Temsirolimus[145]	25 mg IV q wk	4%
Temsirolimus (no prior chemotherapy)[145]	25 mg IV q wk	14%
Everolimus[146]	10 mg po qd	0
Everolimus[147]	10 mg po qd	5%
Ridaforolimus[148]	12.5 mg IV qd × 5 q 14d	11%
Ridaforolimus[149]	40 mg po qd × 5 q 4 wk	8%
Anti-EGFR1/2 Agents		
Trastuzumab[164]	2 mg/kg IV q wk	0
Lapatinib[162]	1,500 mg po qd	3%
Gefitinib[159]	500 mg po qd	3%
Erlotinib[160]	150 mg po qd	12.5%

[a] 30 mg/m²/d in patients with prior radiotherapy.
RR, relative risk.

Other antiangiogenic agents tested have generally not appeared quite as active, although a preliminary report suggested that sunitinib produced a 15% response rate.[153] Trials of multiple other multitargeted antiangiogenic agents, including cediranib, brivanib, cabozantanib, nintedanib, lenvatinib, and AMG 386 (trebananib), are ongoing or completed but not yet reported.

Phosphatidylinositol-3 Kinase/mTOR Pathway. Endometrial cancers harbor the highest rates of PI3K pathway alterations reported to date. Germline mutations in PTEN, which deactivates

the PI3K-AKT signaling pathway, are the etiology of Cowden syndrome, for which endometrial cancer is a diagnostic criterion. PTEN mutations are extremely common in sporadic type I endometrial cancer. There has therefore been widespread interest in testing PI3K pathway inhibitors in endometrial cancer.

Numerous trials involving the rapamycin analogs have been published, and in general modest activity is seen in patients with chemotherapy-naïve disease, but response rates in patients with prior therapy are low (see Table 73.6). The randomized phase 2 trial comparing ridaforolimus progestins as second-line therapy reported improved PFS with ridaforolimus (3.6 versus 1.9 months), but no objective responses in the ridaforolimus arm.[111] Nonetheless, sporadic patients treated with mTOR inhibitors have prolonged responses, and these responses are seen across histologic subtypes, including endometrioid, serous, and clear cell cancers. Several studies have explored the association between molecular biomarkers and response. No association between clinical benefit and any marker, including PTEN mutation, PIK3CA mutation, PTEN protein expression or mutation, or stathmin protein expression, has been observed. One analysis noted that K-Ras mutation was associated with decreased PFS and OS.[154]

Trials of newer PI3K pathway agents, including pan-PI3K, dual PI3K/mTOR, AKT, and catalytic mTOR inhibitors, are underway or have been completed, and results are expected soon. A preliminary report of a phase 2 trial of the allosteric AKT inhibitor, MK-2206, noted a 5.5% response rate with no clear association between PIC3CA mutation and response.[155]

Combinations of mTOR inhibitors with other agents are also being explored. Combinations of mTOR inhibitors with hormonal therapy and chemotherapy are described previously (see "Endocrine Therapy" and "Antiangiogenic Agents"). Two trials have combined temsirolimus with bevacizumab. In previously treated patients, the combination produced a 24.5% response rate, but there was significant toxicity, with two gastrointestinal-vaginal fistulas, one grade 3 epistaxis, two intestinal perforations, and one grade 4 thrombosis/embolism. Three patient deaths were possibly treatment related.[156] When the same combination was tested in patients with no prior chemotherapy for metastatic disease, a 20% response rate was reported with only two grade 4 events that were possibly related, a duodenal perforation, and an anorectal infection.[157]

Anti-HER1/2 Agents. Endometrial cancer can overexpress epidermal growth factor receptor (EGFR) (HER1), and EGFR overexpression has been correlated with poor survival.[158] However, phase 2 trials of single agent anti-EGFR agents have not shown meaningful activity in unselected populations with reported response rates of 3% for the anti-EGFR tyrosine kinase inhibitor (TKI) gefitinib,[159] 12.5% for the anti-EGFR TKI erlotinib,[160] 3% for the anti-EGFR monoclonal antibody cetuximab,[161] and 3% for the dual HER1/2 inhibitor lapatinib.[162] Association of biomarkers with response has been explored in several of these trials. In the lapatinib trial, exons 18 to 21 of EGFR from tumor specimens were sequenced. Three mutations in EGFR were identified. Two of these were not associated with response or PFS, but a newly identified mutation in exon 18, E690K, was found in the tumor of the patient with a partial response. Only 8% of tumors expressed HER2 in the primary specimen, and the HER2 expression was weak. In the erlotinib trial, there was no association between EGFR gene amplification by fluorescence in situ hybridization, and none of the responders had an EGFR mutation. Responses were seen in subsets both with and without EGFR expression by IHC. There was also no correlation between severity of rash and response. In the gefitinib trial, the single responding tumor did not have an EGFR mutation.

HER2 overexpression and amplification is found in 20% to 30% of serous carcinomas, and a percentage of high-grade endometrioid tumors; it is rare in lower grade endometrioid tumors. This has been confirmed in multiple reports, including The Cancer Genome Atlas analysis.[53] While there is at least one case report suggesting activity of trastuzumab,[163] a phase 2 trial of single-agent trastuzumab in women with HER2-overexpressing or amplified disease reported no responses.[164] This trial allowed unlimited prior chemotherapy, and this may have simply been too resistant a population to demonstrate benefit. A randomized trial of TC with or without trastuzumab in women with HER2-positive, platinum-sensitive endometrial cancer is ongoing. It is also possible that there are biologic differences between endometrial cancer and breast cancer that would inhibit the effectiveness of single-agent trastuzumab. One major determinant of resistance to trastuzumab in breast cancer is believed to be activation of downstream signaling via the PI3K/AKT pathway.[165] As discussed previously, a large fraction of endometrial carcinomas have upregulated PI3K signaling; if this were the cause of resistance to trastuzumab it might be overcome by combinations of PI3K pathway blockade and anti-HER2 therapy, or by conjugation of a cytotoxic agent to an anti-HER2 antibody. A trial with the cytotoxic-HER2 conjugate ado-trastuzumab emtansine has been approved by the GOG.

Luteinizing Hormone-Releasing Hormone Conjugates.
Over 80% of endometrial cancers are reported to have functional binding sites for LHRH.[166] Unmodified LHRH agonists (see Table 73.4) have produced low response rates in the treatment of advanced endometrial carcinoma. AEZS-108 is a LHRH agonist chemically linked to doxorubicin designed for specific uptake by tumors expressing LHRH receptors. Phase 1 and 2 studies showed some activity against ovarian and endometrial cancers,[167] and there is an ongoing phase 3 trial comparing AEZA-108 to free doxorubicin as second-line therapy for recurrent/metastatic endometrial carcinoma.

Other Targets

Fibroblast growth factor receptor 2 inhibitors. The fibroblast growth factor receptor 2 (FGFR2) tyrosine kinase is somatically mutated in approximately 10% of endometrioid carcinomas, and in preclinical studies endometrial cancer cell lines expressing activating FGFR2 mutations were sensitive to FGFR inhibitors.[168,169] Dovitinib, a multikinase inhibitor targeting FGFRs as well as vascular endothelial growth factor receptors, is currently being evaluated in a phase 2 study.

MEK inhibitors. Activation of the mitogen-activated protein kinase pathway is a frequent event in endometrial cancer. However, results from a phase 2 trial of the selective MEK-1/2 inhibitor AZD6244 showed only a 6% response rate.[170]

Poly (adenosine diphosphate ribose) polymerase inhibitors. Poly (adenosine diphosphate ribose) polymerase (PARP) inhibitors may be a therapeutic option for some endometrial carcinomas. In addition to regulating the PI3K pathway, it has been suggested that PTEN has a role in the repair of DNA damage via homologous recombination; PTEN-deficient endometrial cancer cell lines have been reported to show increased sensitivity to PARP inhibition.[171] There is a case report of tumor shrinkage with single-agent olaparib in a patient whose cancer was negative for somatic BRCA1 or 2 mutations but had loss of PTEN.[172]

Metformin. Retrospective studies have suggested that patients with diabetes and endometrial cancer who use metformin have superior OS and relapse-free survival compared to patients with endometrial cancer with or without diabetes who do not use metformin.[173,174] In preclinical models, metformin inhibited cell proliferation, induced apoptosis, and decreased tumor growth, with one study showing the greatest response in cells harboring activating mutations in K-Ras.[175] In the everolimus/letrozole trial described previously, higher response rates were observed in patients who used metformin. These data have led to a phase 2 trial of combined everolimus, letrozole, and metformin. In addition, the GOG has proposed a randomized trial of carboplatin/paclitaxel/metformin versus carboplatin/paclitaxel/placebo in the front-line setting.

In summary, single-agent bevacizumab has modest activity in pretreated endometrial cancer, and its role in front-line therapy is being explored. Multiple other newer agents are under investigation, but none have yet produced high response rates as single agents in unselected (or selected) populations.

Treatment of Locally Recurrent Disease

Treatment for locally recurrent endometrial cancer should be individualized. Factors to consider include location of recurrence (vaginal versus pelvic), and whether the patient had prior radiation. Creutzberg et al.[176] reported on survival after relapse in patients with endometrial cancer who were randomized to observation versus postoperative pelvic RT (PORTEC-1 trial). The 3-year survival rate was 73% for patients with vaginal recurrence compared to 8% for pelvic recurrence (p <0.001). The 3-year survival rate for patients who relapsed after surgery alone was 51% compared to 19% who relapsed after postoperative pelvic RT ($p = 0.004$).

Surgery

Surgery should be reserved for patients with recurrent disease in an irradiated area (i.e., received external beam radiation). Achieving complete gross resection is important.[177] Awtrey et al.[178] evaluated patients with recurrent endometrial cancer who underwent non-exenterative surgery and found that patients with residual disease ≤2 cm had a median disease-specific survival of 43 months compared with 10 months for those with >2-cm residual.[178]

Pelvic exenteration may be considered in women with isolated central pelvic recurrences who had prior pelvic radiation. Five-year survival rates for such patients range between 17% and 62%. Poor prognostic factors include age >69 years, recurrence within 3 years of prior treatment, and positive resection margins.[179,180] A study by Barakat et al.[181] showed that the complication rate in 44 patients undergoing pelvic exenteration for recurrent endometrial cancer is 80% and the 5-year survival rate was only 20%.

Radiation

Radiotherapy is commonly used in patients with locally recurrent disease.[183–188] Survival rates range from 24.1% to 96%, with patients with isolated vaginal recurrences representing a particularly favorable group. Pai et al.[183] evaluated the outcome of 20 patients with isolated vaginal involvement treated with salvage radiotherapy. The 10-year actuarial local control and cause-specific survival were 74% and 71%, respectively. Favorable prognostic factors include long disease-free intervals, low-grade disease, adenocarcinoma histology, and no prior RT. Particularly poor outcomes have been reported in women with high-grade disease even when the recurrence is limited to the vagina.[187]

Local control is achieved in 65% to 100% of patients treated with salvage RT, with the majority of series reporting rates between 40% and 70%. A major determinant of local control is tumor size. Wylie et al.[185] reported 5-year local control rates of 80% for tumors <2 cm as opposed to 54% in tumors >2 cm ($p = 0.02$).

Select small volume *vaginal recurrence* can be treated with intravaginal RT alone following excision. But for most vaginal recurrence, the optimal RT approach is a combination of pelvic RT and brachytherapy. The type of brachytherapy to be used in combination with pelvic RT depends on the size of vaginal recurrence. For those with disease >2 cm, interstitial brachytherapy is the preferred approach, while intravaginal RT could be used instead in those with smaller volume disease and especially in those who responded well to pelvic RT. The dose of radiation is typically 45 Gy with pelvic RT plus additional 20 to 30 Gy with brachytherapy. With such high doses being required, severe complications may occur, primarily related to the gastrointestinal tract and vaginal mucosa. In a study by Jhingran et al.[186] on 91 patients with isolated vaginal recurrence who were treated with definitive radiation (median dose 75 Gy), the rate of grade 4 complications (requiring surgery) was 9%. Therefore, when considering observation after surgery for early-stage endometrial cancer, the potential for such complications should be considered. Currently, PORTEC is performing a randomized trial comparing postoperative intravaginal RT to observation with radiation reserved for salvage.

Data regarding radiation for *nodal (pelvic/para-aortic) recurrence* are more limited and less encouraging than that for vaginal recurrence. Typically, external beam radiation is used, with very limited role for brachytherapy. In the PORTEC-1 trial,[176] the 3-year survival rate for pelvic recurrence was only 8%. In an attempt to improve outcome, a combined modality approach is warranted. Viswanathan et al.[189] reported on a phase 2 trial on 15 patients with endometrial cancer who were treated with concurrent radiation and bevacizumab. The 3-year PFS and OS rates were 67% and 80%, respectively. Of 15 patients, 7 had some component of pelvic and/or para-aortic disease at time of enrollment. With a median follow-up of 45.4 months, five of seven patients were alive without evidence of disease.[189]

UTERINE SARCOMAS

Uterine sarcomas are uncommon representing about 3% to 7% of all uterine cancers.[190] The World Health Organization classification includes endometrial stromal tumors, smooth muscle tumors, and miscellaneous mesenchymal tumors. In the mixed epithelial and mesenchymal tumors category, the World Health Organization classification includes adenosarcoma and malignant mixed müllerian tumors or carcinosarcoma.[36]

Carcinosarcoma

Uterine carcinosarcoma (also referred to as mixed mullerian tumor) accounts for approximately 15% of uterine cancer–associated deaths in the United States.[191] It is more common in African Americans.[192] Tamoxifen is a risk factor[193]; among women treated with tamoxifen for breast cancer, the relative risk for carcinosarcomas was found to be 4.62. Approximately 5% to 30% of carcinosarcomas arise in women with previous pelvic RT. Carcinosarcomas are rare in women under the age of 40, and the incidence rises sharply after age 50.[194]

Uterine carcinosarcomas are currently regarded as metaplastic carcinomas, with the sarcomatous element being derived as a result of dedifferentiation.[195] Most series suggest that the carcinomatous component tends to predominate in metastases.[196] Review of pathology slides may be important for accurate diagnosis; one GOG trial reported that 23% (5 of 22) subjects entered on a trial for advanced or recurrent uterine carcinosarcoma were excluded after central pathology review.[197]

Complete surgical staging is recommended as 10% to 15% of patients with apparent early-stage disease with have involvement of pelvic lymph nodes,[198] and the number of positive lymph nodes correlates with risk for recurrence and death.[199] The FIGO 2009 staging for endometrial cancer is used for carcinosarcomas.

Uterine carcinosarcomas are aggressive tumors with a generally poor prognosis; 5-year OS has been reported to be about 30%, and for those with stage I disease it is about 50%.[200] Carcinosarcomas have a generally worse prognosis than even high-grade endometrial carcinomas. One review matched cases with carcinosarcoma and controls with grade 3 endometrioid, serous, or clear cell carcinomas. Median survival was 26 months for women with stage I or II carcinosarcoma and 95 months for control patients with stage I or II disease; there was no difference in median survival for patients with stage III/IV disease.[201]

Adjuvant radiotherapy is frequently used for early-stage disease. The EORTC preformed a prospective randomized trial addressing the role of postoperative pelvic RT in stage I-II uterine sarcomas. There were a total of 224 patients in the trial who underwent TAH/BSO and peritoneal washings (*n* = 166 patients). Lymphadenectomy was optional. There were 103 leiomyosarcomas,

91 carcinosarcomas, and 28 endometrial stromal sarcomas. The 5-year cumulative incidence of locoregional recurrence was 18.8% in the pelvic RT arm compared to 35.9% in the surgery alone arm (*p* = 0.0013). The 5-year cumulative incidence of distant relapse was 45.3% for the pelvic RT and 33.6% for surgery alone, but the difference was not statistically significant (*p* = 0.2569). There was no significant difference in PFS (*p* = 0.3254) or OS (*p* = 0.923) between the two arms. For patients with carcinosarcoma, the rate of pelvic recurrence only was 4% in the pelvic RT arm compared to 24% for the surgery alone arm.[202]

There are few randomized trials of *adjuvant chemotherapy* in early-stage carcinosarcoma, and results of small single institution series are difficult to interpret, although platinum-based therapy generally appears to be of benefit.[203] A very small early trial including stage I or II carcinosarcomas and leiomyosarcomas found no difference for the administration of single-agent doxorubicin (60 mg/m^2 every 3 weeks for eight courses) versus observation in either tumor type.[204] GOG-150 is a phase 3 randomized study of whole abdominal irradiation (WAI) versus three cycles of cisplatin, ifosfamide, and mesna (CIM). Eligible patients (*n* = 206) included stage I-IV uterine carcinosarcoma, no more than 1 cm postsurgical residuum, and/or no extra-abdominal spread. The estimated crude probability of recurring within 5 years was 58% (WAI) and 52% (CIM). Adjusting for stage and age, the recurrence rate was 21% lower for CIM patients than for WAI patients (relative hazard = 0.789, *p* = 0.245). The estimated death rate was 29% lower among the CIM group (relative hazard = 0.712, *p* = 0.085). The conclusion was that there was not a statistically significant advantage in recurrence rate or survival for adjuvant chemotherapy over WAI. However, the observed differences favor the use of combination chemotherapy in future trials.[205] The rate of vaginal recurrence was 3.8% in the WAI compared to 9.9% in the chemotherapy arm. Based on the higher rate of vaginal recurrence in the chemotherapy arm, combining intravaginal RT with chemotherapy seems warranted. In a recent study from MSKCC, 31 patients with stage I-II carcinosarcoma were treated with intravaginal RT and chemotherapy (84% TC). With a median follow-up of 48 months, the 5-year disease-free survival and OS rates were 66% and 79%, respectively.[206] National Comprehensive Cancer Network guidelines recommend that adjuvant therapy for carcinosarcomas be similar to that of poorly differentiated adenocarcinomas.[207]

Systemic therapy for relapsed disease is noncurative. Ifosfamide, cisplatin, and paclitaxel are the only drugs studied with clear cut activity in the therapy of carcinosarcoma. Ifosfamide produces significant toxicity, including granulocytopenia and central nervous system toxicity in the regimens tested. Trials of doxorubicin have produced inconsistent results. Combination therapy generally produces higher response rates, but median survival is not always improved and is generally <1 year (Tables 73.7 and 73.8).[182–188,208–215] There is no evidence for effectiveness of antiangiogenic agents. The GOG has an ongoing trial, GOG #261, comparing the regimens of TC and ifosfamide/paclitaxel, and accrual is nearing completion.

Uterine Leiomyosarcoma

Leiomyosarcomas are the most common of the uterine sarcomas. They are malignant smooth muscle tumors that are believed to arise de novo; for most cases, evidence does not show transition from benign leiomyoma (uterine fibroids) to leiomyosarcoma.[216] They usually present as stage I disease with abnormal bleeding or a pelvic mass, and are more common in African Americans than in Caucasians. The median age at diagnosis is in the early 50s. About 0.5% of patients undergoing hysterectomy for presumed benign leiomyoma will be found to have leiomyosarcoma.[217] Leiomyosarcomas must be distinguished from atypical leiomyomas and smooth-muscle tumors of uncertain malignant potential. Smooth-muscle tumors of uncertain malignant potential rarely metastasize and have an intermediate histology between benign leiomyoma and leiomyosarcoma. Mitotic rate alone does

TABLE 73.7

Salvage Radiotherapy, Locally Recurrent Endometrial Cancer

Study (Ref.)	Year	No. of Patients (n)	Local Control (%)	Five-Year Survival (%)
Nag et al.[182]	1997	15	66.6	42.3
Pai et al.[183]	1997	20	74	71 (10 y)
Hart et al.[184]	1998	26	65	53
Wylie et al.[185]	2000	58	65	53
Jhingran, Burke, and Eifel[186]	2003	91	75	43
Lin et al.[187]	2005	50	80	55
Petignat et al.[188]	2006	22	100	96

not distinguish leiomyosarcomas from tumors of low or uncertain malignant potential; cytologic atypia and coagulative necrosis are important criteria for making the diagnosis.[198]

Surgery including simple hysterectomy/BSO is the standard primary treatment for stage I disease. Lymph node involvement is rare, and lymph node dissection is not required.[218] Chest imaging at time of diagnosis is warranted, as 10% of patients will have lung metastases at time of diagnosis. Five-year survival for stage I disease is 50% to 60%; for stage II, it is about 25%.[219] A nomogram to predict survival has been developed and validated; factors included were age (older age is associated with worse prognosis), tumor size, tumor grade, cervical involvement, locoregional and distant metastases, and mitotic index.[220] The current FIGO (2009) recognizes the importance of tumor size in leimyosarcoma.

In the EORTC phase 3 randomized trial comparing observation to *adjuvant pelvic RT*, 103 patients with leiomyosarcoma were included.

RT produced no improvement in survival or local control (20% local recurrence in RT arm compared to 24% for surgery alone).[202]

Only very limited data exist on the effect of *adjuvant chemotherapy* on survival. The GOG performed a small prospective trial of eight cycles of adjuvant doxorubicin versus observation after tumor resection. Stage I or II leiomyosarcomas and carcinosarcomas were included, and radiation was at the discretion of the treating physician. Of the 25 patients with leiomyosarcoma in the doxorubicin group 11 (44%) recurred, compared with 14 out of 23 (61%) in the observation group.[204] The French Sarcoma Group conducted a randomized clinical trial of adjuvant chemotherapy with doxorubicin, ifosfamide, and cisplatin followed by RT versus RT alone in patients with localized uterine sarcomas. Eighty-one patients were included of whom, fifty-three had leiomyosarcoma. The 3-year disease-free survival was 55% in patients receiving chemoradiation versus 41% for RT alone ($p = 0.048$). The corresponding 3-year overall survival rates were 81% versus 69%, respectively ($p = 0.41$).[221]

The recent 3-year follow-up update of SaRC 005, a nonrandomized trial prescribing four cycles of gemcitabine/docetaxel followed by four cycles of doxorubicin to 47 patients with high-risk uterine leiomyosarcoma, showed a PFS rate of 57% at 3 years, which compares favorably with historic controls without adjuvant chemotherapy.[222] There is an ongoing randomized trial adjuvant gemcitabine/docetaxel followed by doxorubicin versus no further treatment after surgery for early-stage uterine leiomyosarcoma, which will hopefully provide a definitive answer regarding the benefits of chemotherapy.

For patients with multifocal metastatic disease, treatment is usually *systemic chemotherapy*. Active agents include gemcitabine, ifosfamide, doxorubicin, dacarbazine, and temozolomide (Tables 73.9 and 73.10).[223–238] A frequent front-line regimen is the combination of gemcitabine with docetaxel, which is reasonably well tolerated although it requires the administration of granulocyte colony-stimulating factor and is associated with occasional severe pulmonary toxicity.[239] Trials of antiangiogenic agents have produced limited response rates to date, but there a percentage of patients experience prolonged stable disease. Pazopanib, an orally available mul-

TABLE 73.8

Selected Phase 2 and 3 Trials of Systemic Therapy in Uterine Carcinosarcoma with No Prior Systemic Therapy

Trial	Regimen[a]	No. of Patients (n)	RR	Median OS/Comments
Omura et al.[208]	Doxorubicin	41	10%	One arm of a randomized trial
Muss et al.[209]	Doxorubicin 60 mg/m^2 versus Doxorubicin 60 m/m^2 + cyclophosphamide 500 mg/m^2 q 3 wk	51	25%	OS n/a RR 25% for arms combined, no difference between arms
Thigpen et al.[210]	Cisplatin 50 mg/m^2 q 3 wk	63	19%	7 mo
Sutton et al.[211]	Ifosfamide 1.5 g/m^2/d × 5 q 4 wk	29	32%	n/a
Van Rijswijk et al.[212]	Cisplatin + doxorubicin + ifosfamide	32	56%	26 mo
Sutton et al.[213]	Ifosfamide 1.5 g/m^2/d × 5 q 3wk versus Ifosfamide + cisplatin 20 mg/m^2/d × 5 q 3 wk	102 / 92	36% / 54%	7.6 mo / 9.4 mo
Homesley et al.[214]	Ifosfamide 2.0 g/m^2/d × 3 q 3 wk versus Ifosfamide 1.6 g/m^2/d × 3 + paclitaxel 135 mg/m^2/d q 3 wk	91 / 88	29% / 45%	8.4 mo / 13.5 mo; $p = 0.03$
Powell et al.[215]	Carboplatin (AUC 6) + paclitaxel 175 mg/m^2 q 3 wk	46	52%	14.7 mo
Aghajanian et al.[197]	Carboplatin (AUC 6) + paclitaxel 175 mg/m^2 q 3 wk + iniparib 4 mg/kg twice weekly	17	23.5%	11.3 mo

[a] Many trials used initial dose reductions in patients with prior pelvic radiotherapy.
RR, relative risk; OS, overall survival; n/a, not available; AUC, area under the curve.

Selected Phase 2 and 3 Trials of Systemic Therapy in Uterine Carcinosarcome with Prior Systemic Therapy

Trial	Regimen[a]	No. of Patients (n)	RR	Median OS
Slayton et al[223]	Etoposide IV d 1,3,5 q 3 wk	31	6%	n/a
Thigpen[224]	Cisplatin 50 mg/m² q 3 wk	28	18%	n/a
Gershenson[225]	Cisplatin 75–100 mg/m² q 4 wk	18	42%	9 mo[b]
Sutton et al.[226]	Ifosfamide 1.2 g/m²/d × 5	32	17.9%	n/a
Curtin et al.[227]	Paclitaxel 170 mg/m²	44	18.2%	n/a
Miller et al.[228]	Gemcitabine 600 mg/m² d 1,8,15 + docetaxel 35 mg/m² d 1,8,15 q 28 d	24	8.3%	4.9 mo
Miller et al.[229]	Topotecan 1.5 mg/m²/day × 5	48	10%	n/a
Mackay et al.[230]	Aflibercept 4 mg/kg q 2 wk	19	0	3.2 mo
Nimeiri et al.[231]	Sorafenib 400 mg bid	16	0	5 mo

[a] Many trials used initial dose reductions in patients with prior pelvic radiotherapy.
[b] Nine months for patients with prior chemotherapy. Eleven months for chemotherapy naïve cohort.
RR, relative risk; OS, overall survival; IV, intravenous; n/a, not available.

tikinase angiogenesis inhibitor, has recently been approved by the FDA for the treatment of soft tissue sarcomas including uterine leiomyosarcoma. A phase 2 trial of pazopanib 800 mg by mouth daily showed a PFS at 12 weeks of 44% in patients with leiomyosarcoma treated with two or fewer prior cytotoxic regimens (all primary sites), although there was only one PR in a leiomyosarcoma patient (of 41 treated).[240] A subsequent randomized phase 3 trial (PALETTE) in pretreated patients showed a PFS of 4.6 months (all sarcoma subtypes) versus 1.6 months for placebo.[241] A randomized trial of gemcitabine/docetaxel with or without bevacizumab in the treatment of advanced or recurrent uterine leiomyosarcoma has been completed by the GOG, and results should be available soon.

Leiomyosarcomas express ER or PR in a significant number of cases, and hormone receptor expression has been reported to be prognostic. One study reported that only 1/10 early-stage PR(+) cases recurred and died while 9/10 PR(−) cases recurred, and 5 died.[242] It has been suggested that hormonal therapy may be of benefit in patients with advanced-stage leiomyosarcoma that expresses ER or PR, but this remains hypothetical.[243] One prospective phase 2 trial treated 27 patients with leiomyosarcoma whose tumors expressed ER and/or PR with the aromatase inhibitor letrozole at a dose of 2.5 mg daily. The patients had received a median of two prior treatment regimens. There were no objective responses, but the 12-week PFS rate was 50% (90% confidence interval = 30% to 67%), and three

Selected Prospective Phase 2 and 3 Trials of Systemic Therapy in Advanced/Recurrent Uterine Leiomyosarcoma with No Prior Systemic Therapy

Trial	Regimen[a]	No. of Patients (n)	RR	Median OS
Omura et al.[208]	Doxorubicin 60 mg/m² q 3 wk versus	28	25%	12.1 mo for both arms combined
	Doxorubicin + dacarbacin 250 mg/m²/d × 5	30	30%	
Muss et al.[209]	Doxorubicin 60 mg/m² versus	21	13%	n/a
	Doxorubicin 60 m/m² + Cyclophosphamide 500 mg/m² q 3 wk	17		response rate is for both arms combined, no difference seen
Sutton et al.[232]	Liposomal doxorubicin 50 mg/m² q 4 wk	35	16.1%	n/a
Miller et al.[233]	Topotecan 1.5 mg/m²/d × 5 q 21 d	36	11%	n/a
Thigpen et al.[210]	Cisplatin 50 mg/m² q 3 wk	33	3%	7.8 mo
Thigpen et al.[234]	Etoposide IV 100 mg/m²/d × 3 q 21 d	28	0	n/a
Monk et al.[235]	Trabectedin 1.5 mg/m² IV over 24 hr q 3 wk	20	10%	n/a
Sutton et al.[236]	Ifosfamide 1.5 g/m²/d × 5 q 3 wk	35	17.2%	6 mo
Sutton, Blessing, and Malfetano[237]	Ifosfamide 5 g/m²/24 hr + doxorubicin 50 mg/m² q 21 d	35	30.3%	9.6 mo
Hensley et al.[238]	Gemcitabine 900 mg/m² over 90 min d 1,8 plus Docetaxel 100 mg/m² d 8 with G-CSF q 21 d	42	35.8%	16+ mo

[a] Regimens often dose reduced in patients with prior pelvic radiotherapy.
RR, relative risk; OS, overall survival; n/a, not available; IV, intravenous; G-CSF, granulocytic colony-stimulating factor.

TABLE 73.11

Selected Prospective Phase 2 and 3 Trials of Systemic Therapy in Advanced/Recurrent Uterine Leimyosarcoma with Prior Systemic Therapy

Trial	Regimen[a]	No. of Patients (n)	RR	Median OS
Rose et al.[245]	Oral etoposide 50 mg/m^2/d × 21 d then 7 d off	36	6.9%	7.6+ mo One case AML
Garcia Del Muro et al.[246]	Temozolomide 75–100 mg/m^2/d	11	45%	n/a
Gallup et al.[247]	Paclitaxel 175 mg/m^2/3 hr q 21 d	53	8.4%	12.1 mo
Look et al.[248]	Gemcitabine 1,000 mg/m^2/30 min d 1,8,15 q 21 d	44	20.5%	n/a
Hensley et al.[238]	Gemcitabine 900 mg/m^2 over 90 min d 1,8 + docetaxel 100 mg/m^2 d 8 with G-CSF q 21 d	48	27%	14.7 mo
Hensley et al.[249]	Sunitinib 50 mg po qd × 4 wk then 2 wk off	23	8.7%	15.1 mo
Mackay et al.[230]	Aflibercept 4 mg/kd IV q 2 wk	41	0	18.1 mo 17% 6 mo PFS

[a] Regimens often dose reduced in patients with prior pelvic radiotherapy.
RR, relative risk; OS, overall survival; AML, acute myeloid leukemia; n/a, not available; G-CSF, granulocytic colony-stimulating factor; IV, intravenous; PFS, progression-free survival.

patients, all of whom had tumors expressing ER and PR in >90% of tumor cells, continued to receive letrozole for >24 weeks.[244] However, this may merely reflect the indolent natural biology of certain strongly receptors positive uterine leiomyosarcomas.

See Table 73.11 for more information about trials in the system therapy of uterine leiomyosarcoma.[245–249]

Endometrial Stromal Sarcoma

Endometrial stromal sarcomas (also known as low-grade endometrial stromal sarcomas) are uncommon low-grade malignancies comprising approximately 0.2% of all uterine malignancies and 6% to 20% of uterine sarcomas.[250] They usually occur in women 40 to 55 years of age. The tumor cells are usually positive for CD 10 and ERs or PRs.[251]

Translocation of t(7; 17)(p15; q21), resulting in the juxtaposition of two zinc finger genes JAZF1-SUZ12, been described in endometrial stromal sarcomas. The exact role this fusion gene plays in the pathogenesis of endometrial stromal sarcomas is not well understood.[251]

In most patients, the disease is diagnosed at an early stage; 65% to 86% of endometrial stromal sarcomas are confined to the uterus at diagnosis. Estimates of the rate of lymph node metastasis range from 10% to 45%, and positive lymph nodes are associated with shorter survival.[250] As in leiomyosarcoma, the FIGO (2009) recognizes the importance of tumor size. Approximately one-third of stage I patients eventually develop recurrent disease.[252] Recurrences can occur 10 to 20 years after diagnosis. In one study, 5- and 10-year crude survival rates for women with stage I disease were 84% and 77%, respectively; for women with stage II disease, it was 62% and 40%, respectively.[253] Survival after recurrence may be relatively long; in one series, the estimated median survival after recurrence was 133 months.[252]

The primary treatment for early-stage endometrial stromal sarcoma is hysterectomy. Lymph node dissection may offer prognostic information, but it has not been shown to improve survival. In general, removal of the ovaries is recommended, as estrogen has been noted to be a proliferative stimulus. However, some,[250] though not all,[252] more recent series have suggested that preservation of ovaries may not be associated with worse survival.

Regarding the role of *adjuvant radiation*, in the EORTC randomized phase 3 trial, only 28 cases of endometrial stromal sarcoma were included: relapse rate was 12.5% among patients treated with radiotherapy versus 21.4% for the observation group.[202] Sampath et al.[254] performed a retrospective review of patients with uterine sarcoma using the National Oncology Database. The impact of adjuvant radiation was assessed in patients who presented with nonmetastatic disease and underwent definitive surgery (n = 2,206). For endometrial stromal sarcoma, the rate was 97% with RT (109) versus 93% for surgery alone (n = 252, p <0.05). There are no prospective data for the use of *adjuvant hormonal therapy*, but given its efficacy in advanced or recurrent disease, it is often recommended for women with stage III or higher disease.

Surgical resection of limited metastases (e.g., lung) should be considered. In recurrent disease, progestins and aromastase inhibitors can both produce prolonged responses. The role of chemotherapy is unclear, and studies using chemotherapy have not clearly separated out endometrial stromal sarcomas and undifferentiated endometrial sarcomas (which were previously referred to as high-grade endometrial stromal sarcomas).[251]

Undifferentiated endometrial sarcomas are less common than endometrial stromal sarcoma tumors and usually occur in postmenopausal women.[251] They lack a signature chromosomal translocation and are aggressive tumors with a poor overall prognosis. Half of patients present with stage IV disease. Progression after resection of early-stage disease may occur within months.[125] Surgery is the primary therapy for early-stage disease; as with endometrial stromal sarcoma, the role of lymph node dissection is uncertain. Gemcitabine/docetaxel-, doxorubicin-, and ifosfamide-based regimens have been reported to achieve short-lived responses.[255]

SELECTED REFERENCES

The full reference list can be accessed at lwwhealthlibrary.com/oncology.

8. Friedenreich CM, Biel RK, Lau DC, et al. Case–control study of the metabolic syndrome and metabolic risk factors for endometrial cancer. *Cancer Epidemiol Biomarkers Prev* 2011;20:2384–2395.

17. DeMichele A, Troxel AB, Berlin JA, et al. Impact of raloxifene or tamoxifen use on endometrial cancer risk: a population-based case-control study. *J Clin Oncol* 2008;26:4151–4159.

20. Bonadona V, Bonaïti B, Olschwang S, et al. Cancer risks associated with germline mutations in MLH1, MSH2, and MSH6 genes in Lynch syndrome. *JAMA* 2011;305:2304–2310.

21. Broaddus RR, Lynch HT, Chen LM, et al. Pathologic features of endometrial carcinoma associated with HNPCC: a comparison with sporadic endometrial carcinoma. *Cancer* 2006;106:87–94.

26. Bell DJ, Pannu HK. Radiological assessment of gynecologic malignancies. *Obstet Gynecol Clin North Am* 2011;38:45–68.

38. Trimble CL, Kauderer J, Zaino R, et al. Concurrent endometrial carcinoma in women with a biopsy diagnosis of atypical endometrial hyperplasia: a Gynecologic Oncology Group study. *Cancer* 2006;106:812–819.

42. Creasman WT, Morrow CP, Bundy BN, et al. Surgical pathologic spread patterns of endometrial cancer. A Gynecologic Oncology Group study. *Cancer* 1987;60:2035–2041.

43. Morrow CP, Bundy BN, Kurman RJ, et al. Relationship between surgical-pathological risk factors and outcome in clinical stage I and II carcinoma of the endometrium: a Gynecologic Oncology Group study. *Gynecol Oncol* 1991;40:55–65.

44. Abu-Rustum NR, Zhou Q, Gomez JD, et al. A nomogram for predicting overall survival of women with endometrial cancer following primary therapy: toward improving individualized cancer care. *Gynecol Oncol* 2010; 116:399–403.

52. Dedes KJ, Wetterskog D, Ashworth A, et al. Emerging therapeutic targets in endometrial cancer. *Nat Rev Clin Oncol* 2011;8:261–271.

53. Cancer Genome Atlas Research Network, Kandoth C, Schultz N, Cherniack AD, et al. Integrated genomic characterization of endometrial carcinoma. *Nature* 2013;497:67–73.

57. Milgrom SA, Kollmeier MA, Abu-Rustum NR, et al. Positive peritoneal cytology is highly predictive of prognosis and relapse patterns in stage III (FIGO 2009) endometrial cancer. *Gynecol Oncol* 2013;130:49–53.

60. Walker JL, Piedmonte MR, Spirtos NM, et al. Laparoscopy compared with laparotomy for comprehensive surgical staging of uterine cancer: Gynecologic Oncology Group study LAP2. *J Clin Oncol* 2009;27:5331–5336.

61. Walker JL, Piedmonte MR, Spirtos NM, et al. Recurrence and survival after random assignment to laparoscopy versus laparotomy for comprehensive surgical staging uterine cancer: Gynecology Oncolgy Group LAP2 study. *J Clin Oncol* 2012;30:695–700.

63. Benedetti Panici P, Basile S, Maneschi F, et al. Systematic pelvic lymphadenectomy vs. no lymphadenectomy in early-stage endometrial cancer: randomized clinical trial. *J Natl Cancer Inst* 2008;100:1707–1716.

64. ASTEC study group, Kitchener H, Swart AM, Qian Q, et al. Efficacy of systematic pelvic lymphadenectomy in endometrial cancer (MRC ASTEC trial): a randomised study. *Lancet* 2009;373:125–136.

67. Barlin JN, Khoury-Collado F, Kim CH, et al. The importance of applying a sentinel lymph node mapping algorithm in endometrial cancer staging: beyond removal of blue nodes. *Gynecol Oncol* 2012;125:531–535.

70. Sorbe B, Nordström B, Mäenpää J, et al. Intravaginal brachytherapy in FIGO stage I low-risk endometrial cancer: a controlled randomized study. *Int J Gynecol Cancer* 2009;19:873–878.

71. Creutzberg CL, van Putten WL, Koper PC, et al. Surgery and postoperative radiotherapy versus surgery alone for patients with stage-1 endometrial carcinoma: multicentre randomised trial. PORTEC Study Group. Post Operative Radiation Therapy in Endometrial Carcinoma. *Lancet* 2000;355:1404–1411.

72. Creutzberg CL, van Putten WL, Warlam-Rodenhuis CC, et al. Outcome of high-risk stage IC, grade 3, compared with stage I endometrial carcinoma patients: the Postoperative Radiation Therapy in Endometrial Carcinoma Trial. *J Clin Oncol* 2004;22:1234–1241.

75. Nout RA, Smit VT, Putter H, et al. PORTEC Study Group. Vaginal brachytherapy versus pelvic external beam radiotherapy for patients with endometrial cancer of high-intermediate risk (PORTEC-2): an open-label, non-inferiority, randomised trial. *Lancet* 2010;375:816–823.

76. Sorbe B, Horvath G, Andersson H, et al. External pelvic and vaginal irradiation versus vaginal irradiation alone as postoperative therapy in medium-risk endometrial carcinoma-a prospective randomized study. *Int J Radiat Oncol Biol Phys* 2012;82:1249–1255.

80. Keys HM, Roberts JA, Brunetto VL, et al. A phase III trial of surgery with or without adjunctive external pelvic radiation therapy in intermediate risk endometrial adenocarcinoma: a Gynecologic Oncology Group study. *Gynecol Oncol* 2004;92:744–751.

84. Kiess AP, Damast S, Makker V, et al. Five-year outcomes of adjuvant carboplatin/paclitaxel chemotherapy and intravaginal radiation for stage I-II papillary serous endometrial cancer. *Gynecol Oncol* 2012;127:321–325.

85. Susumu N, Sagae S, Udagawa Y, et al. Randomized phase III trial of pelvic radiotherapy versus cisplatin-based combined chemotherapy in patients with intermediate- and high-risk endometrial cancer: a Japanese Gynecologic Oncology Group study. *Gynecol Oncol* 2008;108:226–233.

86. Maggi R, Lissoni A, Spina F, et al. Adjuvant chemotherapy vs radiotherapy in high-risk endometrial carcinoma: results of a randomised trial. *Br J Cancer* 2006;95:266–271.

87. Randall ME, Filiaci VL, Muss H, et al. Randomized phase III trial of whole-abdominal irradiation versus doxorubicin and cisplatin chemotherapy in advanced endometrial carcinoma: a Gynecologic Oncology Group study. *J Clin Oncol* 2006;24:36–44.

90. Greven K, Winter K, Underhill K, et al. Final analysis of RTOG 9708: adjuvant postoperative irradiation combined with cisplatin/paclitaxel chemotherapy following surgery for patients with high-risk endometrial cancer. *Gynecol Oncol* 2006;103:155–159.

92. Milgrom SA, Kollmeier MA, Abu-Rustum NR, et al. Postoperative external beam radiation therapy and concurrent cisplatin followed by carboplatin/paclitaxel for stage III (FIGO 2009) endometrial cancer. *Gynecol Oncol* 2013;130:436–440.

93. Shih KK, Milgrom SA, Abu-Rustum NR, et al. Postoperative pelvic intensity-modulated radiotherapy in high risk endometrial cancer. *Gynecol Oncol* 2013;128:535–539.

118. Fleming GF, Filiaci VL, Bentley RC, et al. Phase III randomized trial of doxorubicin + cisplatin versus doxorubicin + 24-h paclitaxel + filgrastim in endometrial carcinoma: a Gynecologic Oncology Group study. *Ann Oncol* 2004;15:1173–1178.

124. Fleming GF, Brunetto VL, Cella D, et al. Phase III trial of doxorubicin plus cisplatin with or without paclitaxel plus filgrastim in advanced endometrial carcinoma: a Gynecologic Oncology Group Study. *J Clin Oncol* 2004;22:2159–2166.

125. Homesley HD, Filiaci V, Gibbons SK, et al. A randomized phase III trial in advanced endometrial carcinoma of surgery and volume directed radiation followed by cisplatin and doxorubicin with or without paclitaxel: a Gynecologic Oncology Group study. *Gynecol Oncol* 2009;112:543–552.

126. Miller D, Filiaci V, Fleming G, et al. Randomized phase III noninferiority trial of first line chemotherapy for metastatic or recurrent endometrial carcinoma: a Gynecologic Oncology Group study. *Gynecol Oncol* 2012;125:771.

164. Fleming GF, Sill MW, Darcy KM, et al. Phase II trial of trastuzumab in women with advanced or recurrent, HER2-positive endometrial carcinoma: a Gynecologic Oncology Group study. *Gynecol Oncol* 2010;116:15–20.

189. Viswanathan AN, Lee H, Berkowitz R, et al. A prospective feasibility study of radiation and concurrent bevacizumab for recurrent endometrial cancer. *Gynecol Oncol* 2014;132:55–60.

190. D'Angelo E, Prat J. Uterine sarcomas, a review. *Gynecol Oncol* 2010;1162: 131–139.

198. Sutton G. Uterine sarcomas 2013. *Gynecol Oncol* 2013;130:3–5.

202. Reed NS, Mangioni C, Malmstrom H, et al. Phase III randomised study to evaluate the role of adjuvant pelvic radiotherapy in the treatment of uterine sarcomas stages I and II: an European Organisation for Research and Treatment of Cancer Gynaecological Cancer Group Study (protocol 55874). *Eur J Cancer* 2008;44:808–818.

205. Wolfson AH, Brady MF, Rocereto T, et al. A gynecologic oncology group randomized phase III trial of whole abdominal irradiation (WAI) vs. cisplatin-ifosfamide and mesna (CIM) as post-surgical therapy in stage I-IV carcinosarcoma (CS) of the uterus. *Gynecol Oncol* 2007;107:177–185.

214. Homesley HD, Filiaci V, Markman M, et al. Phase III trial of ifosfamide with or without paclitaxel in advanced uterine carcinosarcoma: a Gynecologic Oncology Group Study. *J Clin Oncol* 2007;25:526–531.

221. Pautier P, Floquet A, Gladieff L, et al. A randomized clinical trial of adjuvant chemotherapy with doxorubicin, ifosfamide, and cisplatin followed by radiotherapy versus radiotherapy alone in patients with localized uterine sarcomas (SARCGYN study). A study of the French Sarcoma Group. *Ann Oncol* 2013;24:1099–1104.

222. Hensley ML, Wathen JK, Maki RG, et al. Adjuvant therapy for high-grade, uterus-limited leiomyosarcoma: results of a phase 2 trial (SARC 005). *Cancer* 2013;119:1555–1561.

238. Hensley ML, Blessing JA, Mannel R, et al. Fixed-dose rate gemcitabine plus docetaxel as first-line therapy for metastatic uterine leiomyosarcoma: a Gynecologic Oncology Group phase II trial. *Gynecol Oncol* 2008;109:329–334.

254. Sampath S, Schultheiss TE, Ryu JK, et al. The role of adjuvant radiation in uterine sarcomas. *Int J Radiat Oncol Biol Phys* 2010;76:728–734.

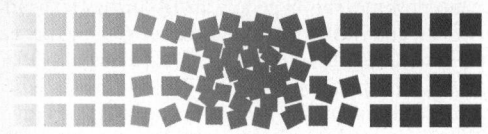

74 Genetic Testing in Uterine Cancer

Molly S. Daniels

INTRODUCTION

Uterine cancer is the most common invasive gynecologic cancer in the United States.[1] The median age at diagnosis of uterine cancer in the general population is 60 years.[1] The average woman's lifetime risk of developing uterine cancer is approximately 2.6%.[2] The vast majority of uterine cancers are endometrial in origin. Five percent or less of uterine cancers are nonendometrial; examples include endometrial stromal sarcoma and uterine leiomyosarcoma.[3]

Endometrial cancers can be further subdivided into type I and type II. Type I endometrial cancers are endometrioid in histology and account for more than 75% of endometrial cancers. Type II endometrial cancers include all nonendometrioid histologies, such as uterine papillary serous carcinoma (UPSC), clear cell carcinoma, and carcinosarcoma (also called malignant mixed Müllerian tumor).[4] Type II endometrial cancers are generally diagnosed at later stages and have a poorer prognosis than type I endometrial cancers.[5]

Type I endometrial cancers, in particular, are associated with personal medical history risk factors, likely due to their impact on the amount of estrogen to which the endometrium is exposed. Other than long-term use of unopposed estrogen (which is no longer prescribed for women with an intact uterus because of the associated endometrial cancer risk) and hereditary cancer predisposition (which will be discussed subsequently), the biggest risk factor for endometrial cancer is obesity. Obese women have up to a six-fold risk of endometrial cancer when compared with women at ideal body weight.[6] Other risk factors include nulliparity, early age at menarche, late age at menopause, and tamoxifen use.[6] Use of combination oral contraceptives decreases risk of endometrial cancer in the general population, with a relative risk of 0.6.[1]

This review also discusses uterine leiomyomas, commonly referred to as uterine fibroids. Uterine leiomyomas are benign smooth muscle tumors that are common in the general population. A US study found that more than 80% of black women and almost 70% of white women develop uterine leiomyomas, although not all were symptomatic.[7] Symptoms of uterine leiomyomas can include pelvic pain, infertility, pregnancy complications, and menometrorrhagia.[7]

LYNCH SYNDROME (ALSO KNOWN AS HEREDITARY NONPOLYPOSIS COLORECTAL CANCER SYNDROME)

Since Lynch syndrome has been extensively described elsewhere in this book, this section focuses on Lynch syndrome–associated endometrial cancer. Lynch syndrome is an autosomal dominant hereditary cancer predisposition syndrome characterized by significantly increased risks of colorectal, endometrial, and other cancers. Mutations in the DNA mismatch repair genes *MLH1*, *MSH2*, *MSH6*, *PMS2*, and *EPCAM* (via disruption of *MSH2* expression) have been associated with Lynch syndrome.

Two to three percent of women with endometrial cancer have Lynch syndrome.[8,9] Average age at diagnosis of endometrial cancer for women with Lynch syndrome is in the 40s to 50s in many[8–10]

but not all[11] studies, younger than the general population. The likelihood of Lynch syndrome is increased in women with endometrial cancer, diagnosed at younger than 50 years,[12,13] who have also had colorectal cancer,[14] with lower body mass index,[12] with lower uterine segment tumors,[15] or with family history of colorectal and/or endometrial cancers.[16,17] Models to assess risk of Lynch syndrome based on personal and family history are available.[16,17] The identification of Lynch syndrome in the patient with endometrial cancer allows her to take steps to reduce her colorectal cancer risk and also allows family members to benefit from predictive genetic testing and subsequent targeted cancer risk reduction strategies.

The optimal way to screen patients with endometrial cancer for Lynch syndrome is an area of active discussion. Historically, patients with endometrial cancer with personal and/or family histories suggestive of Lynch syndrome have been referred for cancer genetic risk assessment. More recently, some institutions have undertaken universal screening of all patients with endometrial cancer by immunohistochemistry (IHC) and/or microsatellite instability (MSI) analysis of the endometrial tumor.[18] The advantage to this approach is that it has the potential to detect all Lynch syndrome–associated endometrial cancers, some of which occur in the absence of a known family history and would be missed by any strategy that screens patients by family history.[8,9] Limitations to the universal screening approach include high cost per mutation identified[19] and lower than expected uptake of genetic counseling and genetic testing among patients with endometrial cancer identified via universal screening.[18]

By whatever method patients with endometrial cancer are selected for Lynch syndrome evaluation, the recommended first step in genetic testing is tumor studies: IHC for the mismatch repair proteins and/or MSI analysis.[20,21] Nearly all Lynch syndrome–associated endometrial cancers will demonstrate high MSI (MSI-H) and/or IHC loss of one or more mismatch repair proteins, and the IHC results often allow genetic testing to be targeted to one Lynch syndrome gene.[20] *MLH1* promoter hypermethylation analysis is recommended as a follow-up study when an endometrial tumor is MSI-H, and IHC shows loss of *MLH1* and *PMS2*, because 15% to 20% of sporadic endometrial cancers exhibit *MLH1* promoter hypermethylation.[22] Whereas sporadic MSI-H colorectal cancers often have somatic *BRAF* mutations, sporadic MSI-H endometrial cancers usually do not,[23] and therefore, *BRAF* mutation analysis is not recommended for distinguishing sporadic MSI-H endometrial cancers from Lynch syndrome–associated endometrial cancers. Lynch syndrome is confirmed by the finding of a germline mutation in a mismatch repair gene through molecular genetic testing, and family members can subsequently undergo predictive genetic testing. Currently, molecular genetic testing is not always able to identify a pathogenic Lynch syndrome mutation when tumor studies are suggestive of Lynch syndrome; possible explanations in these cases include limited genetic test sensitivity for the known mismatch repair genes, other as yet unidentified Lynch syndrome genes, and as yet unidentified other epigenetic causes for the tumor phenotype. Given that Lynch syndrome has not been ruled out in a patient with suggestive tumor studies and negative genetic test results, consideration should be given to following Lynch syndrome management guidelines in these cases.[20,21]

The lifetime risk of endometrial cancer for women with Lynch syndrome has been recently reported as 33% to 40%.[10,24] Endometrial cancer risk may vary by gene, with risks highest for women with *MLH1*, *MSH2*, and *MSH6* mutations. Lower endometrial cancer risks have been reported for women with *PMS2* mutations (15% lifetime risk[25]) or *EPCAM* mutations (up to 12% lifetime risk[26,27]). Lynch syndrome–associated endometrial cancers can be both type I (endometrioid) and type II (nonendometrioid); nonendometrioid histologies observed in women with Lynch syndrome include clear cell carcinoma, UPSC, and malignant mixed Müllerian tumor (carcinosarcoma).[28]

Given the high risk of endometrial cancer for women with Lynch syndrome, both cancer screening and risk reduction options should be considered. Patient education regarding endometrial cancer symptoms (such as abnormal vaginal bleeding) and the importance of reporting them promptly are also important.[21] In terms of risk reduction, hysterectomy (plus bilateral salpingo-oophorectomy [BSO], because ovarian cancer risk is also elevated) is clearly effective in preventing endometrial cancer[29] and can be considered if childbearing is completed and/or after menopause.[21,30,31] If a woman with Lynch syndrome is undergoing surgery for colon cancer, concomitant hysterectomy/BSO can be considered.[30,31] Risk-reducing hysterectomy/BSO has not been demonstrated to reduce mortality in women with Lynch syndrome. Oral contraceptives reduce risk of endometrial and ovarian cancer in the general population[1]; their efficacy in women with Lynch syndrome has not been determined. There is no proven benefit to endometrial cancer screening in women with Lynch syndrome; screening guidelines are based on expert opinion. Transvaginal ultrasound alone does not appear to be an effective screening test in this population[32,33]; endometrial biopsy plus transvaginal ultrasound may be more effective.[34] The National Comprehensive Cancer Network currently recommends considering annual endometrial biopsy as an option.[21]

PHOSPHATASE AND TENSIN HOMOLOG HAMARTOMA TUMOR SYNDROME (ALSO KNOWN AS COWDEN SYNDROME, BANNAYAN-RUVALCABA-RILEY SYNDROME)

Since phosphatase and tensin homolog (PTEN) hamartoma tumor syndrome (PHTS) has also been extensively described elsewhere in this book, this section focuses on uterine manifestations of PHTS. PHTS is a rare autosomal dominant syndrome defined by the presence of a pathogenic *PTEN* mutation. PHTS can manifest in many organ systems, with phenotypic effects ranging from autism[35,36] to increased cancer risk[37,38] to characteristic mucocutaneous lesions.[39]

Uterine leiomyomas have been described as a common finding in women with PHTS,[40] and uterine leiomyomas are included as a minor diagnostic criterion of PHTS.[39] However, given the high prevalence of uterine leiomyomas in the general population,[7] it is not clear whether the prevalence is actually elevated in PHTS.[38,41] Uterine leiomyomas are a nonspecific finding and should not by themselves be considered particularly suggestive of PHTS.[38,41]

Endometrial cancer has been reported to occur at increased frequency in women with PHTS.[37,41] Reported ages at endometrial cancer diagnosis have been mostly in the 30s to 50s.[39,42] Endometrial cancer has been reported in adolescence in PHTS.[43] Endometrial cancer has been observed in 12 (17%) of 69[41] and 25 (16%) of 158[39] of adult women who were referred for *PTEN* genetic testing and tested positive. Data regarding lifetime risk of endometrial cancer in PHTS are sparse; studies to date have focused on probands and are thus subject to significant ascertainment bias. Therefore, a recent estimate of lifetime endometrial cancer risk in PHTS of 28%[37] is likely a significant overestimation. PHTS appears to account for a very small proportion of unselected endometrial cancers; a study by Black et al.[44] found no germline *PTEN* mutations in a series of 240 patients with endometrial cancer.

In light of the limited data regarding lifetime risk of endometrial cancer for women with PHTS, the National Comprehensive Cancer Network does not currently recommend a specific endometrial cancer screening strategy beyond educating women to respond promptly to symptoms and considering enrollment in a clinical trial to determine effectiveness and necessity of screening.[45] Others have suggested that women with PHTS undergo annual endometrial biopsy and/or transvaginal ultrasound.[37,40] To date, there is no proven benefit to these screening strategies in the context of PHTS. Based on the lack of efficacy of transvaginal ultrasound as an endometrial cancer screening test for women with Lynch syndrome discussed previously, if screening is undertaken, ultrasound may not be the ideal modality. The National Comprehensive Cancer Network also notes that risk-reducing hysterectomy can be discussed as an option on a case-by-case basis.[45]

HEREDITARY LEIOMYOMATOSIS AND RENAL CELL CARCINOMA

Hereditary leiomyomatosis and renal cell carcinoma (HLRCC) (OMIM 150800) is characterized by increased risk of type 2 papillary renal cell carcinoma, cutaneous leiomyomas, and uterine leiomyomas. The fumarate hydratase (*FH*) gene is the only gene that has been associated with HLRCC. HLRCC exhibits autosomal dominant inheritance. Both point mutations and large rearrangements of the *FH* gene have been reported in individuals with HLRCC.[46] If germline mutations in both copies of the *FH* gene are present, this causes the severe autosomal recessive condition fumarase deficiency (OMIM 606812), which is characterized by encephalopathy and psychomotor retardation, and is frequently lethal in infancy or childhood.

The uterine leiomyomas seen in the context of HLRCC tend to occur at younger ages than in the general population, with a mean age at diagnosis around 30 years.[47,48] Women with HLRCC frequently report complications from uterine leiomyomas, including symptoms of menorrhagia, pelvic pain, and reduced fertility,[49] and are more likely than women with uterine leiomyomas who do not have HLRCC to have had treatment, including hysterectomy.[48] In a study of North Americans with HLRCC, 98% of women had uterine leiomyomas, and 89% had undergone hysterectomy, often before the age of 30 years.[47]

Uterine leiomyosarcoma has been reported in Finnish women with HLRCC, but a recent review notes that only one clinically malignant uterine leiomyosarcoma has been confirmed in a patient with an *FH* germline mutation.[50] Therefore, to what extent the risk of uterine leiomyosarcoma may be elevated over that in the general population is not yet clear. It also appears that germline *FH* mutations are not common in women with isolated uterine leiomyosarcoma; a series of 67 uterine leiomyosarcomas diagnosed in Finland were tested for *FH* mutations, and only one patient was found to have a *FH* missense sequence variant, which was present in both tumor and normal tissue but is of uncertain significance.[51]

The presence of multiple cutaneous leiomyomas should prompt consideration of HLRCC; studies of patients with multiple cutaneous leiomyomas have found *FH* mutations in 80% to 89%.[47,49,52] Cutaneous leiomyomas vary in appearance; biopsy is required for diagnosis.[49] Pain and paresthesias associated with cutaneous leiomyomas are frequently reported.[47] Ages at onset were reported to be from 10 to 47 years, with mean age at onset of 25 years.[47] The absence of cutaneous leiomyomas does not exclude the possibility of HLRCC; some patients with HLRCC showed no evidence of cutaneous leiomyoma after detailed skin examination.[47,53] Rarely, cutaneous leiomyosarcoma has been reported with HLRCC.[47,53]

The type 2 papillary renal cell carcinomas associated with HLRCC are usually unilateral and unifocal but nonetheless appear to be aggressive in that they can already be metastatic when the primary tumor is still small (<1 cm).[50] Penetrance of renal cell carcinoma in HLRCC has been reported as approximately 20%.[52] Age at diagnosis of renal cell carcinoma has been reported as early as 11 years[54] and 16 years,[49] with average age at diagnosis in the 40s.[47,52] Other types of kidney cancer have also been reported in patients with HLRCC, including collecting duct carcinoma, oncocytoma, clear cell renal cell carcinoma, and Wilms tumor.[50]

Given the relative rarity of HLRCC (estimated approximately 180 families identified worldwide[50]), guidelines for screening and management are still evolving and are based on expert opinion only. Pediatric kidney cancers have been reported in HLRCC but appear to be rare; thus, there is some debate regarding at what age predictive genetic should be offered as well as at what age screening should begin. Proposed kidney cancer screening recommendations have included magnetic resonance imaging, computed tomography, or positron emission tomography–computed tomography; annual or biannual; and beginning at age 18 to 20 or as early as the age of 5 years (perhaps particularly if pediatric kidney cancer has occurred in a family member).[50] Ultrasound may not be effective at detecting HLRCC-associated kidney cancers and is not recommended.[47] The aggressive nature of the type 2 papillary renal cell carcinomas also makes designing an effective screening program challenging, and there is not yet evidence that instituting screening favorably impacts morbidity or mortality for patients with HLRCC.

UTERINE CANCER AND OTHER HEREDITARY CANCER SYNDROMES

UPSC is histologically similar to ovarian serous carcinoma[5] and has been observed in Ashkenazi Jewish women with *BRCA1/BRCA2* mutations who also had personal and/or family histories of breast and/or ovarian cancer.[55] However, other studies of consecutive series of Jewish patients with endometrial cancer found a *BRCA*-positive rate that is similar to that of the general Jewish population.[56,57] It therefore seems unlikely that a personal history of endometrial cancer, UPSC or otherwise, increases the likelihood for a woman to have a germline *BRCA1/BRCA2* mutation.

Patients with hereditary retinoblastoma are at increased risk to develop a variety of second malignancies. A recent study found that women with hereditary retinoblastoma are at significantly increased risk for uterine leiomyosarcoma in particular.[58]

CONCLUSION

Approximately 2% to 3% of endometrial cancers are attributable to Lynch syndrome. Early age at diagnosis, low body mass index, and personal and/or family history of Lynch syndrome–associated cancers increase the likelihood for a patient with endometrial cancer to have Lynch syndrome, but not all Lynch syndrome–associated endometrial cancers occur in the presence of these risk factors. MSI and IHC analyses are the recommended first step in Lynch syndrome evaluation. The identification of Lynch syndrome in the patient with endometrial cancer allows her to take steps to reduce her colorectal cancer risk and also allows family members to benefit from predictive genetic testing and subsequent targeted cancer risk reduction strategies. Unaffected women with Lynch syndrome are at significantly increased risk to develop endometrial cancer and should be educated regarding signs and symptoms of endometrial cancer and should be offered screening and prevention options.

The proportion of endometrial cancer attributable to PHTS (Cowden syndrome) is not precisely known but appears to be <1%. The risk for endometrial cancer is likely elevated in women with PHTS, but the magnitude of this risk is not well defined at this time. Women with PHTS should be educated regarding signs and symptoms of endometrial cancer. Endometrial cancer screening and surgical risk reduction can be considered for women with PHTS.

Symptomatic uterine leiomyomas are more common in those with HLRCC than in the general population, with a tendency toward earlier age at diagnosis. Multiple cutaneous leiomyomas are a characteristic finding in HLRCC. Uterine leiomyosarcoma has occurred in the context of HLRCC, but whether and to what extent this risk exceeds that in the general population remains to be determined. Individuals with HLRCC are at increased risk to develop an aggressive subtype of kidney cancer, and therefore, should consider periodic kidney cancer screening.

PRACTICE OF ONCOLOGY

REFERENCES

1. National Cancer Institute. Endometrial cancer prevention (PDQ). http://www.cancer.gov/cancertopics/pdq/prevention/endometrial/. Accessed September 3, 2014.
2. National Cancer Institute. SEER stat fact sheets: Corpus and uterus, NOS. http://seer.cancer.gov/statfacts/html/corp.html#risk. Accessed April 16, 2012.
3. National Cancer Institute. Uterine sarcoma. http://www.cancer.gov/cancertopics/types/uterinesarcoma. Accessed April 16, 2012.
4. Broaddus R. Pathology of Lynch syndrome–associated gynecological cancers. In: Lu KH, ed. *Hereditary Gynecologic Cancer: Risk, Prevention, and Management.* New York: Informa Healthcare; 2008:149–162.
5. Mendivil A, Schuler KM, Gehrig PA. Non-endometrioid adenocarcinoma of the uterine corpus: A review of selected histological subtypes. *Cancer Control* 2009;16:46–52.
6. Buchanan EM, Weinstein LC, Hillson C. Endometrial cancer. *Am Fam Physician* 2009;80:1075–1080.
7. Day Baird D, Dunson DB, Hill MC, et al. High cumulative incidence of uterine leiomyoma in black and white women: Ultrasound evidence. *Am J Obstet Gynecol* 2003;188:100–107.
8. Hampel H, Frankel W, Panescu J, et al. Screening for Lynch syndrome (hereditary nonpolyposis colorectal cancer) among endometrial cancer patients. *Cancer Res* 2006;66:7810–7817.
9. Hampel H, Panescu J, Lockman J, et al. Comment on: Screening for Lynch syndrome (hereditary nonpolyposis colorectal cancer) among endometrial cancer patients. *Cancer Res* 2007;67:9603.
10. Stoffel E, Mukherjee B, Raymond VM, et al. Calculation of risk of colorectal and endometrial cancer among patients with Lynch syndrome. *Gastroenterology* 2009;137:1621–1627.
11. Hampel H, Stephens JA, Pukkala E, et al. Cancer risk in hereditary nonpolyposis colorectal cancer syndrome: Later age of onset. *Gastroenterology* 2005;129:415–421.
12. Lu KH, Schorge JO, Rodabaugh KJ, et al. Prospective determination of prevalence of Lynch syndrome in young women with endometrial cancer. *J Clin Oncol* 2007;25:5158–5164.

13. Berends MJ, Wu Y, Sijmons RH, et al. Toward new strategies to select young endometrial cancer patients for mismatch repair gene mutation analysis. *J Clin Oncol* 2003;21:4364–4370.
14. Millar AL, Pal T, Madlensky L, et al. Mismatch repair gene defects contribute to the genetic basis of double primary cancers of the colorectum and endometrium. *Hum Mol Genet* 1999;8:823–829.
15. Westin SN, Lacour RA, Urbauer DL, et al. Carcinoma of the lower uterine segment: A newly described association with Lynch syndrome. *J Clin Oncol* 2008;26:5965–5971.
16. Balmana J, Stockwell DH, Steyerberg EW, et al. Prediction of MLH1 and MSH2 mutations in Lynch syndrome. *JAMA* 2006;296:1469–1478.
17. Chen S, Wang W, Lee S, et al. Prediction of germline mutations and cancer risk in the Lynch syndrome. *JAMA* 2006;296:1479–1487.
18. Backes FJ, Leon ME, Ivanov I, et al. Prospective evaluation of DNA mismatch repair protein expression in primary endometrial cancer. *Gynecol Oncol* 2009;114:486–490.
19. Kwon JS, Scott JL, Gilks CB, et al. Testing women with endometrial cancer to detect Lynch syndrome. *J Clin Oncol* 2011;29:2247–2252.
20. Weissman SM, Bellcross C, Bittner CC, et al. Genetic counseling considerations in the evaluation of families for Lynch syndrome—a review. *J Genet Couns* 2011;20:5–19.
21. National Comprehensive Cancer Network. Colorectal cancer screening, V1. 2012. http://www.nccn.org/professionals/physician_gls/pdf/colorectal_screening.pdf. Accessed April 16, 2012.
22. Esteller M, Levine R, Baylin SB, et al. MLH1 promoter hypermethylation is associated with the microsatellite instability phenotype in sporadic endometrial carcinomas. *Oncogene* 1998;17:2413–2417.
23. Kawaguchi M, Yanokura M, Banno K, et al. Analysis of a correlation between the BRAF V600E mutation and abnormal DNA mismatch repair in patients with sporadic endometrial cancer. *Int J Oncol* 2009;34:1541–1547.
24. Bonadona V, Bonaiti B, Olschwang S, et al. Cancer risks associated with germline mutations in MLH1, MSH2, and MSH6 genes in Lynch syndrome. *JAMA* 2011;305:2304–2310.

25. Senter L, Clendenning M, Sotamaa K, et al. The clinical phenotype of Lynch syndrome due to germ-line PMS2 mutations. *Gastroenterology* 2008;135:419–428.

26. Kempers MJ, Kuiper RP, Ockeloen CW, et al. Risk of colorectal and endometrial cancers in EPCAM deletion-positive Lynch syndrome: A cohort study. *Lancet Oncol* 2011;12:49–55.

27. Lynch HT, Riegert-Johnson DL, Snyder C, et al. Lynch syndrome–associated extracolonic tumors are rare in two extended families with the same EPCAM deletion. *Am J Gastroenterol* 2011;106:1829–1836.

28. Broaddus RR, Lynch HT, Chen LM, et al. Pathologic features of endometrial carcinoma associated with HNPCC: A comparison with sporadic endometrial carcinoma. *Cancer* 2006;106:87–94.

29. Schmeler KM, Lynch HT, Chen LM, et al. Prophylactic surgery to reduce the risk of gynecologic cancers in the Lynch syndrome. *N Engl J Med* 2006; 354:261–269.

30. Lindor NM, Petersen GM, Hadley DW, et al. Recommendations for the care of individuals with an inherited predisposition to Lynch syndrome: A systematic review. *JAMA* 2006;296:1507–1517.

31. Vasen HF, Moslein G, Alonso A, et al. Guidelines for the clinical management of Lynch syndrome (hereditary non-polyposis cancer). *J Med Genet* 2007;44:353–362.

32. Rijcken FE, Mourits MJ, Kleibeuker JH, et al. Gynecologic screening in hereditary nonpolyposis colorectal cancer. *Gynecol Oncol* 2003;91:74–80.

33. Dove-Edwin I, Boks D, Goff S, et al. The outcome of endometrial carcinoma surveillance by ultrasound scan in women at risk of hereditary nonpolyposis colorectal carcinoma and familial colorectal carcinoma. *Cancer* 2002;94:1708–1712.

34. Renkonen-Sinisalo L, Butzow R, Leminen A, et al. Surveillance for endometrial cancer in hereditary nonpolyposis colorectal cancer syndrome. *J Int Cancer* 2007;120:821–824.

35. Butler MG, Dasouki MJ, Zhou XP, et al. Subset of individuals with autism spectrum disorders and extreme macrocephaly associated with germline PTEN tumour suppressor gene mutations. *J Med Genet* 2005;42:318–321.

36. Varga EA, Pastore M, Prior T, et al. The prevalence of PTEN mutations in a clinical pediatric cohort with autism spectrum disorders, developmental delay, and macrocephaly. *Genet Med* 2009;11:111–117.

37. Tan MH, Mester JL, Ngeow J, et al. Lifetime cancer risks in individuals with germline PTEN mutations. *Clin Cancer Res* 2012;18:400–407.

38. Pilarski R. Cowden syndrome: A critical review of the clinical literature. *J Genet Couns* 2009;18:13–27.

39. Tan MH, Mester J, Peterson C, et al. A clinical scoring system for selection of patients for PTEN mutation testing is proposed on the basis of a prospective study of 3042 probands. *Am J Hum Genet* 2011;88:42–56.

40. Eng C. PTEN hamartoma tumor syndrome (PHTS). In: Pagon RA, Bird TD, Dolan CR, et al., eds. *Gene Reviews*. Seattle, WA: University of Washington, Seattle; 1993.

41. Pilarski R, Stephens JA, Noss R, et al. Predicting PTEN mutations: An evaluation of Cowden syndrome and Bannayan–Riley–Ruvalcaba syndrome clinical features. *J Med Genet* 2011;48:505–512.

42. Starink TM, van der Veen JP, Arwert F, et al. The Cowden syndrome: A clinical and genetic study in 21 patients. *Clin Genet* 1986;29:222–233.

43. Schmeler KM, Daniels MS, Brandt AC, et al. Endometrial cancer in an adolescent: A possible manifestation of Cowden syndrome. *Obstet Gynecol* 2009;114:477–479.

44. Black D, Bogomolniy F, Robson ME, et al. Evaluation of germline PTEN mutations in endometrial cancer patients. *Gynecol Oncol* 2005;96:21–24.

45. National Comprehensive Cancer Network. Genetic/familial high-risk assessment: breast and ovarian. V1.2011. www.nccn.org. Accessed April 7, 2011.

46. Bayley JP, Launonen V, Tomlinson IP. The FH mutation database: An online database of fumarate hydratase mutations involved in the MCUL (HLRCC) tumor syndrome and congenital fumarase deficiency. *BMC Med Genet* 2008;9:20.

47. Toro JR, Nickerson ML, Wei MH, et al. Mutations in the fumarate hydratase gene cause hereditary leiomyomatosis and renal cell cancer in families in North America. *Am J Hum Genet* 2003;73:95–106.

48. Stewart L, Glenn GM, Stratton P, et al. Association of germline mutations in the fumarate hydratase gene and uterine fibroids in women with hereditary leiomyomatosis and renal cell cancer. *Arch Dermatol* 2008;144:1584–1592.

49. Alam NA, Barclay E, Rowan AJ, et al. Clinical features of multiple cutaneous and uterine leiomyomatosis: An underdiagnosed tumor syndrome. *Arch Dermatol* 2005;141:199–206.

50. Lehtonen HJ. Hereditary leiomyomatosis and renal cell cancer: Update on clinical and molecular characteristics. *Fam Cancer* 2011;10:397–411.

51. Ylisaukko-oja SK, Kiuru M, Lehtonen HJ, et al. Analysis of fumarate hydratase mutations in a population-based series of early onset uterine leiomyosarcoma patients. *Int J Cancer* 2006;119:283–287.

52. Gardie B, Remenieras A, Kattygnarath D, et al. Novel FH mutations in families with hereditary leiomyomatosis and renal cell cancer (HLRCC) and patients with isolated type 2 papillary renal cell carcinoma. *J Med Genet* 2011;48:226–234.

53. Wei MH, Toure O, Glenn GM, et al. Novel mutations in FH and expansion of the spectrum of phenotypes expressed in families with hereditary leiomyomatosis and renal cell cancer. *J Med Genet* 2006;43:18–27.

54. Alrashdi I, Levine S, Paterson J, et al. Hereditary leiomyomatosis and renal cell carcinoma: Very early diagnosis of renal cancer in a paediatric patient. *Fam Cancer* 2010;9:239–243.

55. Lavie O, Hornreich G, Ben-Arie A, et al. BRCA germline mutations in Jewish women with uterine serous papillary carcinoma. *Gynecol Oncol* 2004;92: 521–524.

56. Barak F, Milgram R, Laitman Y, et al. The rate of the predominant Jewish mutations in the BRCA1, BRCA2, MSH2 and MSH6 genes in unselected Jewish endometrial cancer patients. *Gynecol Oncol* 2010;119:511–515.

57. Levine DA, Lin O, Barakat RR, et al. Risk of endometrial carcinoma associated with BRCA mutation. *Gynecol Oncol* 2001;80:395–398.

58. Francis JH, Kleinerman RA, Seddon JM, et al. Increased risk of secondary uterine leiomyosarcoma in hereditary retinoblastoma. *Gynecol Oncol* 2012;124:254–259.

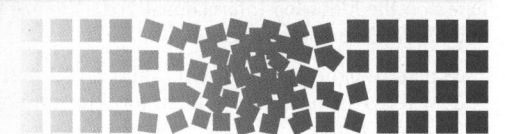

75 Gestational Trophoblastic Diseases

Donald P. Goldstein, Ross S. Berkowitz, and Neil S. Horowitz

INTRODUCTION

Gestational trophoblastic neoplasia (GTN) comprise a group of interrelated conditions that arise from trophoblastic tissue and consist of six distinct clinicopathologic entities: complete hydatidiform mole (CHM), partial hydatidiform mole (PHM), invasive mole (IM), choriocarcinoma (CCA), placental site trophoblastic tumors (PSTT), and epithelioid trophoblastic tumors (ETT). All trophoblastic tumors produce human chorionic gonadotropin (hCG), which can be used as a tumor marker for diagnosis, monitoring the effects of therapy and follow-up to detect relapse.[1] Although these tumors represent <1% of gynecologic malignancies, it is important that medical oncologists understand their natural history and management because of their life-threatening potential in reproductive-age females and their high curability with preservation of reproductive potential if treated early and according to well-established guidelines.

INCIDENCE

GTN arises most commonly after a molar pregnancy, but can also occur after normal or ectopic pregnancies and spontaneous or induced abortions. Molar pregnancy occurs in approximately 1:1000 gestations.[1] GTN after spontaneous miscarriage is estimated to occur in 1:15,000 pregnancies, while the incidence after a term pregnancy is 1:150,000 pregnancies. The overall incidence of GTN following all types of pregnancies is estimated at 1:40,000.[2]

PATHOLOGY AND NATURAL HISTORY

CHM is characterized by clusters of hydropic villi with trophoblastic hyperplasia and atypia. CHMs are diploid and have a chromosomal pattern of either 46XX or 46XY. All chromosomes are androgenetic, that is, of paternal origin, and arise from fertilization of an empty ovum by a haploid sperm that then undergoes duplication. Occasionally, CHMs arise from fertilization of an empty ovum by two sperm. Maternally transcribed nuclear genome is lost, although one can identify maternal mitochondrial DNA.[3]

PHM shows a variable amount of abnormal villous swelling and focal trophoblastic hyperplasia in association with identifiable fetal or embryonic tissue. PHM contains both maternal and paternal chromosomes and are triploid, typically 69XXY, which occurs by fertilization of a normal ovum by two sperm.[4]

IM occurs when molar tissue invades the myometrial wall. Deep myometrial invasion can lead to uterine rupture and severe intraperitoneal hemorrhage. IM develops in approximately 15% of patients with CHM and about 1% to 5% of patients with PHM.[5] Most IM remain localized to the uterus, but metastases to distant sites have been reported.

CCA consists of invasive, highly vascular, and anaplastic trophoblastic tissue made up of cytotrophoblasts and syncytiotrophoblasts without villi. CCA metastasizes hematogenously and can follow any type of pregnancy, but most commonly develops after CHM.

Approximately 50% of cases follow a molar pregnancy, 25% follow an abortion or ectopic pregnancy, and 25% follow a term delivery. The most common metastatic site is the lungs, which are involved in >80% of patients with metastases. Vaginal metastases are noted in 30% of patients with metastases. Distant sites such as the liver, brain, kidney, gastrointestinal tract, and spleen occur in about 10% of patients with metastatic disease, and these women are at the highest risk of death from disease. Metastatic disease is most commonly encountered in postpartum patients in whom diagnosis is frequently delayed.[6]

PSTT is a rare and unique form of GTN accounting for only 0.25% of all cases and is derived from neoplastic transformation of intermediate trophoblastic cells that normally play a critical role in implantation. PSTT can occur after any gestational event, but unlike CCA occurs more commonly after a nonmolar or term pregnancy. Microscopically, these tumors show no chorionic villi and are characterized by a proliferation of cells with oval nuclei and abundant eosinophilic cytoplasm. They are slow-growing and tend to locally infiltrate the myometrium, at which point they can metastasize both via the hematogenous and lymphatic systems. PSTT display a wide clinical spectrum and when metastatic, can be difficult to control even with surgery and chemotherapy. Unlike other forms of GTN, these tumors tend to remain localized in the uterus for long periods before metastasizing to regional lymph nodes or other metastatic sites.[7] PSTT is characterized by low beta-hCG levels because it is a neoplastic proliferation of intermediate trophoblastic cells.[8] Therefore, a large tumor burden may be present before the disease is diagnosed. Expression, however, of human placental lactogen is increased on immunochemical histologic sections as well as in the serum. PSTT are also characterized by high levels of free beta-hCG.[8]

ETT is a very rare but distinctive form of GTN also derived from intermediate trophoblastic cells that typically presents as a discrete, hemorrhagic, solid, and cystic lesion that is located either in the fundus, lower uterine segment, or endocervix. Microscopically, the tumor is composed of a relatively uniform population of mononucleate intermediate trophoblastic cells forming nests and solid masses. The cells resemble the trophoblastic cells in the chorion laeve, and are therefore designated as "chorionic-type intermediate trophoblast." Typically, islands of trophoblastic cells are surrounded by extensive necrosis and associated with a hyaline-like matrix creating a "geographic" pattern that is quite characteristic of this lesion.[9] Patients with ETT are in the reproductive age group and present with abnormal vaginal bleeding. It is not uncommon for ETT to be diagnosed long after an antecedent pregnancy. Patients may also present with extrauterine ETT without evidence of prior gestational trophoblastic disease in the uterus. Serum beta-hCG levels are generally in a low range, but may be absent.

INDICATIONS FOR TREATMENT

Following a Molar Pregnancy

The early diagnosis of molar pregnancy with ultrasound has led to changes in the histologic characteristics and clinical presentation

PRACTICE OF ONCOLOGY

1069

of CHM without changing the potential for developing persistent disease.[10] Following molar evacuation, the diagnosis of GTN is based on the following International Federation of Gynecologists and Obstetricians (FIGO) guidelines[11]:

1. A plateau in beta-hCG of four values ±10% over 3 weeks
2. A ≥10% rise in beta-hCG levels for three or more values over at least 2 weeks
3. Persistence of beta-hCG levels for >6 months after molar evacuation
4. Histologic evidence of choriocarcinoma
5. Presence of metastatic disease

Following a Nonmolar Pregnancy

Patients who develop rising hCG titers following a nonmolar pregnancy have GTN (CCA, PSTT, or ETT) until proven otherwise. Serum hCG levels are not routinely obtained after nonmolar pregnancies (except in following ectopic pregnancies), unless the woman has had a previous molar pregnancy when it becomes the standard of care because of the increased risk of developing GTN. *However, any woman in the reproductive age group who presents with abnormal vaginal bleeding or evidence of metastatic disease should undergo hCG screening to rule out GTN.* At this point, a thorough clinical and radiologic evaluation of the patient should be carried out to determine the extent of disease. Rapid growth, widespread dissemination, and a high propensity for hemorrhage make CCA a medical emergency. Metastases are found in the lungs (80%), vagina (30%), pelvis (20%), brain (10%), and liver (10%), as well as other sites (<5%).[12]

MEASUREMENT OF HUMAN CHORIONIC GONADOTROPIN

The serial quantitative measurement of hCG is essential for the diagnosis, monitoring the efficacy of treatment, and follow-up of patients with molar pregnancy and GTN. hCG is a glycoprotein that consists of an alpha subunit common to other glycoproteins, and a beta subunit that is hormone-specific. Therefore, the measurement of hCG in patients with GTN should be performed by assays that measure the beta subunit only.[13] hCG is synthesized by syncytiotrophoblastic cells of the developing placenta and hydatidiform moles. In contrast, the hyperglycosylated form of hCG (H-hCG) is produced by the cytotrophoblastic cells of the developing placenta during early gestation and by malignant GTN (i.e., invasive moles and CCA).[14] After evacuation of a molar pregnancy, beta-hCG levels usually disappear in 8 to 12 weeks. After normal delivery or nonmolar miscarriage, hCG levels become undetectable within 3 to 6 weeks.[15] Persistence of hCG levels indicates local or metastatic disease, which allows for early detection and timely intervention. During treatment, beta-hCG response is used as a guide to determine whether to continue treatment with an agent or switch to another agent. Beta-hCG monitoring after treatment allows for identification of patients who relapse and require additional treatment.

Hyperglycosylated Human Chorionic Gonadotropin

H-hCG is now believed to be a marker for malignant GTN, and its presence is associated with response to chemotherapy.[14] Some patients treated for molar pregnancy or GTN will have persistent (weeks or months) low levels (<200 mIU/ml) of real hCG, but low or absent concentrations of H-hCG. Characteristically, these women have no radiographic or clinical evidence of active disease, and do not appear to respond to chemotherapy. This condition of persistent low-level non–H-hCG is called *quiescent GTN.*[16] Careful follow-up is necessary because 6% to 10% of these patients will

ultimately relapse with evidence of active disease and rising hCG levels with a high concentration (>30%) of H-hCG, at which point chemotherapy becomes effective.

Phantom Human Chorionic Gonadotropin

False-positive findings on hCG tests can occur with the presence of heterophile antibodies that interfere with the immunoassay. Although a rare occurrence, false-positive hCG tests can be confusing to clinicians when attempting to diagnose disorders of pregnancy such as ectopic and GTN. Misinterpretations of false-positive tests have led to inappropriate treatment, including surgery and chemotherapy, when based only on the persistently elevated serum beta-hCG levels. A false-positive hCG result should be suspected if the clinical picture and the laboratory results are discordant, if there is no identifiable antecedent pregnancy, or if patients under treatment with persistent low levels do not respond appropriately. When a false-positive hCG test is suspected, a urinary assay should be performed because heterophile antibodies do not cross the renal tubules. In rare instances, particularly in women approaching menopause or in women treated with multiagent chemotherapy that may suppress ovarian function, the source of the hCG is the pituitary gland.[17]

PRETREATMENT EVALUATION

Once the diagnosis of GTN has been made, the following pretreatment evaluation is recommended to determine the extent and location of disease:

1. A complete history and physical examination including a speculum examination to detect vaginal metastases occurring in approximately 30% of patients with metastatic disease.
2. Biopsy of the vaginal lesion is not recommended given the highly vascular nature of the tumor and the risk of uncontrollable hemorrhage.
3. Baseline measurement of the serum hCG value.
4. Hepatic, thyroid, and renal function tests.
5. Baseline peripheral white blood cell and platelet counts.
6. Stool guaiac to screen for the rare gastrointestinal metastasis.
7. Chest X-ray, essential since the lungs are involved in 80% of patients who develop metastatic disease.
8. Pelvic ultrasound to confirm absence of a new pregnancy and to detect pelvic disease, myometrial invasion and retained issue.[18]

If there is evidence of metastatic disease on initial evaluation, the workup should be expanded to include the following studies:

1. Chest computed tomography (CT), if chest X-ray is positive. Although pulmonary metastases can be detected by chest CT in up to 40% of patients with a negative chest X-ray, it is not required initially when a plain film is negative since the presence of micrometastases does not affect outcome and are not considered a risk factor.[19]
2. Ultrasound or CT scan of the abdomen and pelvis, with special attention to the liver, kidneys, and spleen.
3. Magnetic resonance imaging or CT scan of the head.[20]
4. Measurement of cerebrospinal fluid hCG level is recommended to confirm central nervous system metastases if the patient exhibits neurologic signs and the head magnetic resonance imaging or CT scan is negative.[21,22]
5. Selective angiography of abdominal and pelvic organs, if indicated.
6. Whole-body deoxy-2[^{18}F]fluoro-d-glucose positron emission tomography (PET) scan to identify active disease site for occult disease, if indicated.[23,24]
7. Review of all available pathology. Histologic confirmation of the diagnosis of GTN is not required for treatment. However, biopsy of a metastatic site may be indicated if the diagnosis is in doubt.

TABLE 75.1

International Federation of Gynecologists and Obstetricians Staging of Gestational Trophoblastic Neoplasia and World Health Organization Scoring System Based on Prognostic Factors

Stage I	Disease confined to the uterus
Stage II	GTN extends outside of the uterus, but is limited to the genital structures
Stage III	GTN extends to the lungs, with or without genital tract involvement
Stage IV	All other metastatic sites

A risk factor score (see below) should be assigned to each patient.

The stage should be followed by the sum of the risk factor score (e.g., II:4).

	Score			
Prognostic factors	0	1	2	4
Age in years	<40	≥40	—	—
Antecedent pregnancy	Mole	Abortion	Term	—
Interval (months)[a]	<4	≥4 but <7	≥7 but <13	≥13
Pretreatment serum hCG (mIU/mL)	<1,000	1,000 to <10,000	10,000 to <100,000	≥100,000
Largest tumor, including uterine	—	3 to <5 cm	≥5 cm	—
Site of Metastases	**Lung**	**Spleen, Kidney**	**GI Tract**	**Brain, Liver**
Number of metastases	—	1–4	5–8	>8
Prior failed chemotherapy	—	—	Single drug	Two or more drugs

GTN, gestational trophoblastic neoplasm; hCG, human chorionic gonadotropin; GI, gastrointestinal.
[a] Interval (in months) between end of antecedent pregnancy and start of chemotherapy.

STAGING AND PROGNOSTIC SCORE

Table 75.1 summarizes the staging of GTN adopted by FIGO in 2002.[25] In addition to anatomic staging, a prognostic scoring system has also been adopted by FIGO to help determine the appropriate chemotherapy regimen that affords the patient optimal management by reducing the risk of developing resistance to chemotherapy.[26] Patients with a score <7 are considered at low risk of developing resistance and generally achieve remission with single-agent therapy. Patients with scores of ≥7 are at high risk of developing resistance to single-agent therapy and should be treated primarily with multiple-agent regimens. All patients with stage IV disease are considered high risk. However, recent data from Charing Cross Hospital indicate that only 30% of patients with low-risk GTN with a risk score of 5 to 6 are cured with monotherapy. Patients who prove resistant to sequential single-agent therapy are more likely to be older, have hCG levels >100,000 mIU/ml, develop GTN following a nonmolar antecedent pregnancy with an histologic diagnosis of choriocarcinoma, have metastatic disease, and are found to have ultrasound evidence of large uterine tumor burden.[27] A similar "intermediate-risk group" (scores 5–6, etc.) was seen in the Gynecologic Oncology Group trial evaluating two single-agent regimens. For those women with risk scores of 5 to 6, the response rates to single-agent chemotherapy was about 10% to 40%.[28]

TREATMENT

Chemotherapy is highly effective in most patients with GTN. Cure rates of 100% in low-risk disease and 80% to 90% in high-risk cases are reported from a number of treatment centers.[29] Despite the success of chemotherapy, the role of other modalities such as surgery and radiation therapy should not be overlooked. The best results are achieved when patients are treated under the auspices of a multidisciplinary team.

Low-Risk Disease

Most patients with low-risk GTN (risk score <7) including all cases of nonmetastatic disease and most cases of postmolar metastatic disease have survival rates that approach 100% when treated with monotherapy with either methotrexate (MTX) or actinomycin D (actD).[29] A number of different regimens are currently in use (Table 75.2). A recently reported study compared biweekly intrave-

TABLE 75.2

Single-Agent Regiments for Low-Risk Gestational Trophoblastic Neoplasms

MTX
- MTX 0.4–0.5 mg/kg IV or IM daily for 5 days (not to exceed 25 mg/d)
- Pulse MTX 50 mg/m² IM weekly

MTX/FA
- MTX 1 mg/kg IM or IV on days 1, 3, 5, 7
- FA 0.1 mg/kg PO on days 2, 4, 6, 8

High-dose MTX/FA
- MTX 100 mg/m² IV bolus
- MTX 200 mg/m² 12-h infusion
- FA 15 mg q 12 h in four doses IM or PO beginning 24 h after starting MTX

Actinomycin regimens
- actD 10–12 mcg/kg IV push daily for 5 days (not to exceed 1,000 mcg/d)
- actD 1.25 mg/m² IV push q 2 weeks

MTX, methotrexate; IV, intravenous; IM, intramuscular; FA, folinic acid (calcium leucovorin); PO, by mouth; actD, actinomycin-D (Cosmegan, Whitehouse Station, NJ).

nous actD and weekly intramuscular MTX regimens, and showed that the biweekly actD regimen was associated with a statistically significantly higher complete response rate.[28] Overall, the weekly intramuscular or intermittent continuous intravenous infusion MTX regimens are thought to be less effective than the daily (for 5 days) MTX or the 8-day alternating MTX/leucovorin regimens.[30] Lurain et al.[31] analyzed their experience using secondary actD in patients with MTX resistance and found a 75% complete response rate. The patients who were resistant to both MTX and actD ultimately achieved complete response with multiagent salvage therapy.[31] Maesta et al.,[32] using multivariate analysis, studied prognostic factors that affect time to remission in low-risk GTN and concluded that complete molar histology, metastases, the use of multiagent therapy, and higher FIGO score were the main factors associated with longer time to remission. Chapman-Davis et al.[33] stressed the importance of dose-intensive treatment in patients with low-risk GTN treated initially with 5-day MTX. Shah et al.[34] performed a cost analysis of single-agent chemotherapy in low-risk GTN and concluded that 8-day MTX-folinic acid was consistently less expensive than actD.

MTX with folinic acid is the initial choice at the New England Trophoblastic Disease Center for low-risk GTN because it has the least toxicity and a high rate of response.[35] Courses are administered at 2-week intervals until the serum beta-hCG level becomes undetectable. The results of a recent study from the Netherlands and United Kingdom suggest that three rather than two additional courses of consolidation therapy should be administered after patients achieve remission to reduce the likelihood of relapse.[36] ActD is used when the patient develops resistance to MTX or if there is evidence of MTX-induced abnormal liver function tests. Patients with low-risk GTN who develop resistance to sequential monotherapy should be switched to a multidrug regimen such as MTX, actD, and cyclophosphamide in lower-

volume disease (Table 75.3); or etoposide, MTX, actD, cyclophosphamide, and vincristine (EMA/CO) for large-volume disease (Table 75.4).[37] Remission is defined as an undetectable hCG level for 3 consecutive weeks. Hysterectomy with ovarian preservation should also be considered as primary therapy for patients with stage I disease who have completed their family. It is advisable to administer adjunctive chemotherapy at the time of surgery because of the risk of occult disease.[38]

After attaining undetectable hCG levels, patients should be followed with monthly hCG levels for 12 months. During this time, effective contraception is mandatory and also serves the useful purpose of suppressing pituitary hCG which can falsely suggest residual disease.[39] Pregnancy may be undertaken after 1 year of normal hCG titers.

TABLE 75.3

Protocols for Modified Triple Therapy for Methotrexate, Actinomycin D, and Cyclophosphamide

Days 1–5	Actinomycin D (Cosmegan, Whitehouse Station, NJ), 12 mcg/kg, IV push[a] Cyclophosphamide, 3 mg/kg, IV bolus over 45–60 min
Days 1, 3, 5, 7	Methotrexate, 1 mg/kg IM or IV
Days 2, 4, 6, 8	Leucovorin calcium, 0.1 mg/kg PO
Repeat cycles every 2 to 3 wk, toxicity permitting.	

IV, intravenous; IM, intramuscular; PO, by mouth.
[a] Vesicant: Administer through free-flowing IV.

TABLE 75.4

Protocols for Etoposide, Methotrexate, Actinomycin D, Cyclophosphamide, and Vincristine, and Etoposide, Methotrexate, Actinomycin D, and Cisplatin Regimens

Day	Drug	Dose
		Protocol for EMA/CO Regimen
1	Etoposide actD MTX	100 mg/m² by infusion in 200 ml saline over 30 min 0.5 mg IV push 100 mg/m² IV push 200 mg/m² by infusion over 12 h
2	Etoposide actD Folinic acid	100 mg/m² by infusion in 200 ml saline over 30 min 0.5 mg IV push 15 mg q 12 h × four doses IM or PO beginning 24 h after starting MTX
8	Cyclophosphamide Vincristine	600 mg/m² by infusion in saline over 30 min 1.0 mg/m² IV push
		Protocol for EMA/EP Regimen
1	Etoposide actD MTX	100 mg/m² by infusion in 200 ml saline over 30 min 0.5 mg IV push 100 mg/m² IV push 200 mg/m² by infusion over 12 h
2	Etoposide actD Folinic acid	100 mg/m² by infusion in 200 ml saline over 30 min 0.5 mg IV push 15 mg q 12 h × four doses IM or PO beginning 24 h after starting MTX
8	Cisplatin Etoposide	60 mg/m² with prehydration 100 mg/m² by infusion in 200 ml saline over 30 min

EMA/CO, etoposide, methotrexate, and dactinomycin alternating with cyclophosphamide and vincristine; actD, actinomycin-D (Cosmegan, Whitehouse Station, NJ); IV, intravenous; MTX, methotrexate; IM, intramuscular; PO, by mouth; EMA/EP, etoposide, methotrexate, actinomycin D, and cisplatin.

High-Risk Disease

Dose-intensive multiple-agent chemotherapy should be used initially in all patients with stage II and III disease whose prognostic scores are >6 and all patients with stage IV disease.[40] Table 75.4 summarizes the most widely used regimens including EMA/CO and etoposide, MTX, actD, and cisplatin (EMA/EP), which are associated with cure rates ranging from 70% to 90%. Cagayan[41] reported a remission rate of 72% with the primary use of EMA/CO and an overall survival rate of 86%. Despite the success of EMA/CO, roughly 30% to 40% of women with high-risk disease will have an incomplete response to first-line multiagent therapy or will relapse from remission and will need additional multiagent chemotherapy with potentially other multimodality treatment. An alternative regimen containing cisplatin (EMA/EP) should be used as salvage therapy for patients who develop resistance to EMA/CO.[42] A recent Cochrane Database review of chemotherapy for resistant or recurrent GTN recognizes the efficacy of a number of platinum/etoposide combinations.[43] 5-Fluorouracil has also been shown to be an active agent in the management of this disease in both low-risk and high-risk patients.[44] The Charing Cross group has reported that the use of induction low-dose etoposide 100 mg/m[2], and cisplatin 20 mg/m[2] (days 1 and 2 every 7 days) in selected patients with high tumor burden may almost completely eliminate early mortality that may result from respiratory compromise and hemorrhage.[45] They also report a 94% remission rate with EMA/CO by carefully excluding nongestational tumors in patients with atypical presentation using genetic analysis. Treatment should be dose-intensive every 2 to 3 weeks, toxicity permitting. The use of granulocyte colony-stimulating factor and, when absolutely necessary, platelet transfusions are important to maintain adequate dose-intensity and to prevent unnecessary dose reduction. Treatment should be continued until the hCG level becomes undetectable and remains undetectable for 3 consecutive weeks. The administration of four courses of the remission regimen after the patient achieves remission is recommended to reduce relapse.[46]

Role of Radiation Therapy

Radiation therapy has little application in patients with GTN except in selected patients with cerebral metastases. The use of whole brain or localized radiation therapy in conjunction with chemotherapy can prevent a life-threatening or debilitating hemorrhage and should be initiated promptly.[47] An alternative to the use of radiation for cerebral metastases is the use of intrathecal MTX in combination with multiagent chemotherapy, particularly in the presence of meningeal involvement.[48]

Role of Surgery

Surgery also plays an important role in the management of high-risk patients.[49] Hysterectomy in patients with heavy bleeding, large bulky intrauterine disease, or in the presence of significant pelvic sepsis should be performed regardless of the patient's parity.[38] Removal of tumor masses in the bowel should also be performed because of the risk of hemorrhage. Unresponsive masses in the liver, kidneys, and spleen should be removed, although embolization has been used with some success in controlling liver metastases.

Although pulmonary disease is usually chemosensitive, resection of persistent lung nodules can be curative and should be considered when the metastasis is solitary, limited to one lung, and the beta-hCG <1,000.[50] Normalization of beta-hCG within 1 to 2 weeks after resection of a pulmonary lesion is a good indication of a positive outcome. Alifrangis et al.[51] confirmed the criteria for thoracotomy but also reported that multiple resections over time or resection of more than one lesion can result in salvage after failure of standard or high-dose chemotherapy. When evaluating patients for thoracotomy, it is important to remember that lung nodules can persist for several months or years after completion of chemotherapy and normalization of beta-hCG. These nodules may represent areas of scar tissue or viable tumor which the use of PET or PET/CT may help to determine.[23]

Surgery can also play a role in the management of cerebral metastases. Multimodality therapy including chemotherapy with surgical resection and irradiation (whole brain and/or stereotactic radiation) has improved overall survival from 46% to 64% in the last 14 years, even when metastases developed during chemotherapy.[52] Craniotomy is indicated for the resection of peripheral, solitary, drug-resistant lesions and can be life-saving in the management of intracranial hemorrhage or increased intracranial pressure.

Patients with high-risk disease who achieve remission should be followed for 24 months before pregnancy is attempted. There is no contraindication to the use of oral contraceptives in these patients.

PLACENTAL SITE OR EPITHELIOID TROPHOBLASTIC TUMORS

Patients with PSTT and ETT confined to the uterus can be cured with hysterectomy.[53] If deep myometrial involvement is noted, we believe it is advisable to also perform a pelvic lymphadenectomy. Metastatic PSTT/ETT are recognized as having a high fatality rate[54]; FIGO stage and interval from antecedent pregnancy appear to be two important prognostic factors. Although universally accepted guidelines on how to manage PSTT/ETT are not available, given its aggressive clinical behavior, multimodality therapy with surgery and chemotherapy, preferably with EMA/EP, has been shown to improve survival.[55]

SUBSEQUENT PREGNANCY AFTER TREATMENT FOR GESTATIONAL TROPHOBLASTIC NEOPLASIA

Patients with GTN treated successfully with chemotherapy can expect normal reproductive function.[56] The New England Trophoblastic Disease Center database has follow-up on 668 subsequent pregnancies in patients treated between July 1, 1965 and May 1, 2013 that resulted in 446 term live births (66.8%), 44 premature deliveries (6.6%), 7 ectopic pregnancies (1.0%), 10 stillbirths (1.5%), and 10 repeat molar pregnancies (1.5%). First- and second-trimester spontaneous abortions occurred in 123 pregnancies (18.4%). There were 28 therapeutic abortions (4.2%). Major and minor congenital anomalies were detected in only 12 of 500 births (2.4%). These values are comparable to the general gestational population. The low incidence of congenital malformations is reassuring in spite of the fact that chemotherapeutic agents are known to have teratogenic and mutagenic potential.

Although we advise patients to practice strict contraception during follow-up, patients occasionally become pregnant, either accidentally or intentionally, before their follow-up has been completed. When this occurs and the pregnancy is desired, we monitor the developing fetus and placenta with sonograms at 6 and 10 weeks of gestation. If the 10-week sonogram appears normal, there is little likelihood of recurrence. We strongly advise these patients to undergo hCG testing at the 6 week postpartum or postabortal check-up to ensure complete remission.

PSYCHOSOCIAL ISSUES

Women who develop GTN can experience significant mood disturbance, marital and sexual problems, and concerns over future fertility.[57] Because GTN is a consequence of pregnancy, patients and their partners must confront the loss of a pregnancy at the same time they face concerns regarding malignancy. Patients can experience clinically significant levels of anxiety, fatigue, anger, confusion, sexual problems, and concern for future pregnancy that last for protracted periods of time. Patients with metastatic disease, in particular, are at risk of psychological disturbances; these patients need assessments and interventions both during treatment and after remission is attained.

SELECTED REFERENCES

The full reference list can be accessed at lwwhealthlibrary.com/oncology.

9. Shih IM, Kurman RJ. Epitheliod trophoblastic tumor: A neoplasm distinct from choriocarcinoma and placental site trophoblastic tumor. *Am J Surg Pathol* 1998;223:1393–1403.
10. Berkowitz RS, Goldstein DP. Clinical practice. Molar pregnancy. *N Engl J Med* 2009;360:1639–1645.
11. Kohorn EI. The new FIGO 2000 staging system and risk factor scoring system for gestational trophoblastic disease: description and critical assessment. *Int J Gynaecol Cancer* 2001;11:73–77.
12. Berkowitz RS, Goldstein DP. Current management of gestational trophoblastic disease. *Gynecol Oncol* 2009;112:654–662.
19. Garner EI, Garrett A, Goldstein DP, et al. Significance of chest computed tomography findings in the evaluation and treatment of persistent gestational trophoblastic neoplasms. *J Reprod Med* 2004;49:411–414.
27. McGrath S, Short D, Harvey R, et al. The management and outcome of women with post-hydatidiform mole 'low-risk' gestational trophoblastic neoplasia, but hCG levels in excess of 100,000 IU/L. *Brit J Cancer* 2010;102:810–814.
30. Agahjanian C. Treatment of low-risk gestational trophoblastic neoplasia. *J Clin Oncol* 2011;29:786–788.
31. Lurain JR, Chapman-Davis E, Hoekstra AV, et al. Actinomycin D for methotrexate-failed low-risk gestational trophoblastic neoplasia. *J Reprod Med* 2012;57:283–287.
32. Maesta I, Growdon WB, Goldstein DP, et al. Prognostic factors associated with time to hCG remission in patients with low-risk post-molar gestational trophoblastic neoplasia. *Gynecol Oncol* 2013;130:312–316.
33. Chapman-Davis E, Hoekstra AV, Rademaker AW, et al. Treatment of non-metastatic and metastatic low-risk gestational trophoblastic neoplasia: factors associated with resistance to single agent methotrexate chemotherapy. *Gynecol Oncol* 2012;125:572–575.
35. Berkowitz RS, Goldstein DP. Chorionic tumors. *N Engl J Med* 1996;335:1740–1748.
36. Lybol C, Sweep FC, Harvey R, et al. Relapse rates after two versus three consolidation courses of methotrexate in the treatment of low-risk gestational trophoblastic neoplasia. *Gynecol Oncol* 2012;125:576–579.
38. Clark RM, Nevadunsky N, Ghosh S, et al. The evolving role of hysterectomy in gestational trophoblastic neoplasia at the New England Trophoblastic Disease Center. *J Reprod Med* 2010;55:194–198.
40. Lurain JR, Schink JC. Importance of salvage therapy in the management of high-risk gestational trophoblastic neoplasia. *J Reprod Med* 2012;57:219–224.
41. Cagayan MS. High-risk metastatic gestational trophoblastic neoplasia. Primary management with EMAC-CO (etoposide, methotrexate, actinomycin D, cyclophosphamide and vincristine) chemotherapy. *J Reprod Med* 2012;57:231–236.
42. Xiang Y, Sun Z, Wan X, et al. EMA/EP chemotherapy for chemorefractory gestational trophoblastic tumors. *J Reprod Med* 2004;49:443–446.
43. Alazzam M, Tidy J, Osborne J, et al. Chemotherapy for resistant or recurrent gestational trophoblastic neoplasia. *Cochrane Database Syst Rev* 2012;12:CD008891.
46. Lurain JR. Gestational trophoblastic disease. II. Classification and management of gestational trophoblastic neoplasia. *Am J Obstet Gynecol* 2011;204:11–18.
48. Newlands ES, Holden L, Seckl MJ, et al. Management of brain metastases in patients with high risk gestational trophoblastic tumors. *J Reprod Med* 2002;47:465–471.
49. Lurain JR, Singh DK, Schink JC. Role of surgery in the management of high-risk gestational trophoblastic neoplasia. *J Reprod Med* 2006;51:773–776.
51. Alfrangis C, Wilkinson MJ, Stefanou DC, et al. Role of thoracotomy and metastatectomy in gestational trophoblastic neoplasia. A single center experience. *J Repro Med* 2012;57:350–358.
52. Neubauer NL, Latif N, Kalakota K, et al. Brain metastasis in gestational trophoblastic neoplasia. An update. *J Reprod Med* 2012;57:288–292.
54. Kingdon SJ, Coleman RE, Ellis L, et al. Deaths from gestational trophoblastic neoplasia. Any Lessons to be learned? *J Reprod Med* 2012;57:293–296.
55. Hyman DM, Bakios L, Gualtiere G, et al. Placental site trophoblastic tumor: analysis of presentation, treatment, and outcome. *Gynecol Oncol* 2013;129:58–62.
56. Garrett LA, Garner EIO, Feltmate CM, et al. Subsequent pregnancy outcomes in patients with molar pregnancy and persistent gestational trophoblastic neoplasia. *J Reprod Med* 2008;53:481–486.
57. Wenzel LB, Berkowitz RS, Habbal R, et al. Predictors of quality of life among long-term survivors of gestational trophoblastic disease. *J Reprod Med* 2004;49:589–594.

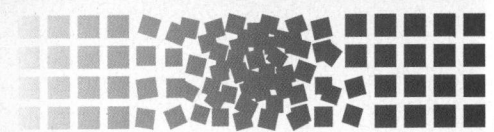

76 Ovarian Cancer, Fallopian Tube Carcinoma, and Peritoneal Carcinoma

Stephen A. Cannistra, David M. Gershenson, and Abram Recht

Stephen A. Cannistra, David M. Gershenson, and Abram Recht

PRACTICE OF ONCOLOGY

INTRODUCTION

Ovarian cancer is not a single entity but instead represents tumors of epithelial, germ cell, or sex cord–stromal origin. Epithelial ovarian cancer typically occurs in postmenopausal women, most germ cell tumors present in younger women, and sex cord–stromal tumors may occur at any age. Approximately 90% of ovarian cancer is epithelial in origin and poses significant therapeutic challenges due to the advanced stage of most patients with this disease. In contrast, other types of ovarian cancer such as germ cell and sex cord–stromal tumors are often localized in distribution, more amenable to surgical resection, and have a more favorable prognosis. Although primary peritoneal serous carcinoma and fallopian tube carcinoma do not originate in the ovary, they are discussed in this chapter because their clinical and management considerations are similar to those of epithelial ovarian cancer.

EPITHELIAL OVARIAN CANCER

Epidemiology

Epithelial ovarian cancer is expected to occur in 22,240 women and cause 14,030 deaths in the United States in 2013, which makes this tumor the leading cause of gynecologic cancer mortality.[1] The lifetime risk of developing sporadic epithelial ovarian cancer is approximately 1.7%, although patients with a familial predisposition have a much higher lifetime risk, in the range of 10% to 40%.[2] The median age at diagnosis for sporadic disease is 60 years, although patients with a genetic predisposition may develop this tumor earlier, often in their fifth decade. The age-specific incidence of sporadic disease increases with age, from 15 to 16 per 100,000 in the 40- to 44-year-old age group to a peak rate of 57 per 100,000 in the 70- to 74-year-old age group.[1] There has been a statistically significant improvement in 5-year survival over the past decades, with a rate of 36% in 1977, 39% in 1986, and 45% in 2002.[1] This improvement in survival is likely the result of more effective chemotherapy options and surgical techniques for tumor debulking. African American women in the United States have a lower incidence of ovarian cancer (10.3 per 100,000 women) compared to white women, but both have a similar stage distribution and overall survival rate.[1] A higher risk for developing epithelial ovarian cancer is observed for nulliparous women and a lower risk for those who have had children, who have breastfed, who have undergone tubal ligation, or who have taken oral contraceptives.[3]

Pathogenesis and Patterns of Metastases

Some epithelial ovarian neoplasms are thought to arise from the surface epithelium covering the ovary, which is contiguous with peritoneal mesothelium. In some cases, malignant transformation appears to occur within epithelium that becomes trapped within ovarian inclusion cysts during ovulation, where it can develop into a variety of Müllerian-type histologies.[4] However, emerging evidence suggests that a subset of epithelial ovarian cancers may instead originate in the fallopian tube fimbria, subsequently spreading to the ovary or peritoneal cavity.[5] Germ cell tumors most likely originate in cells derived from the primitive streak that ultimately migrated to the gonads. The ovarian stroma consists of granulosa cells, theca cells, and fibroblasts, which give rise to the sex cord–stromal tumors.

Several molecular abnormalities have been identified in patients with epithelial ovarian cancer, although their contribution to early malignant transformation is poorly understood. Cytogenetic analysis may reveal complex abnormalities, including deletions of 3p, 6q, 8p, and 10q, and loss of heterozygosity is commonly observed on 11p, 13q, 16q, 17p, and 17q.6 Mutation in the $p53$ protooncogene occurs in over 50% of cases, predominantly involving tumors in patients with advanced-stage and high-grade serous histology.[6] In contrast, mutations in B-raf, K-ras, $PTEN$, or β-catenin may be seen in endometrioid, mucinous, or low-grade histologies.[5] Mutations in the $ARID1A$ gene occur in 50% of patients with clear cell ovarian cancer.[7] Amplification of the $HER2/neu$ gene is observed in only approximately 8% of patients and confers a poorer prognosis.[8] Overexpression of proapoptotic genes such as BAX is associated with chemoresponsiveness and a more favorable prognosis, although the r-zole of BAX in the pathogenesis of this tumor has not been well studied.[9] Surface adhesion proteins such as CD44H and β-1 integrins have been shown to mediate transperitoneal spread of this tumor by promoting the attachment of cancer cells to the peritoneal mesothelial lining.[10] Expression of angiogenic cytokines such as the vascular endothelial growth factor (VEGF) is frequently observed in epithelial ovarian cancer, with high serum levels conferring a worse prognosis.[11]

The ability of tumor cells to exfoliate from the ovarian surface and to spread in an asymptomatic fashion impedes the development of successful screening approaches that would allow for early diagnosis. The tumor typically spreads to the omentum and to peritoneal surfaces such as the underside of the diaphragm, paracolic gutters, and bowel serosa (Fig. 76.1). The lymphatic drainage of the ovary follows its blood supply through the infundibulopelvic ligament to nodes in the para-aortic region. Lymphatic drainage through the broad ligament and parametrial channels can also result in involvement of pelvic sidewall lymphatics, including the external iliac, obturator, and hypogastric chains. Spread may rarely occur along the course of the round ligament, resulting in involvement of inguinal lymph nodes. Approximately 10% to 15% of patients with ovarian cancer that appears to be localized to the ovaries have metastases to para-aortic lymph nodes, and retroperitoneal lymph node involvement is found in >50% of patients with advanced disease.[2]

Although epithelial ovarian cancer typically spreads in a locoregional fashion to involve the peritoneal cavity and retroperitoneal nodes, it can be found outside the abdomen as well. The most common site of extra-abdominal spread is the pleural space (thought to occur via transdiaphragmatic lymphatics), where it causes a malignant pleural effusion in some patients. Hematogenous metastases

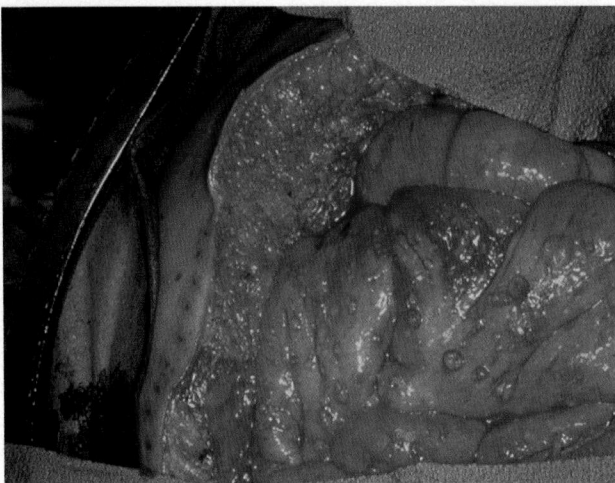

Figure 76.1 Intraoperative appearance of advanced epithelial ovarian cancer, with multiple tumor implants involving the peritoneal surface of the upper abdomen. (Courtesy of Dr. Jonathan Niloff, Beth Israel Deaconess Medical Center, Boston, MA.)

to the liver, spleen, or lung can also occur during the course of the disease, but are relatively uncommon at presentation. Bone or central nervous system metastases may rarely be observed in patients who have lived for many years after initial diagnosis, during which unusual patterns of disease spread may occur.

Histologic Classification of Epithelial Tumors

Table 76.1 outlines the classification of common epithelial tumors that has been accepted by the World Health Organization (WHO) and the International Federation of Gynecology and Obstetrics (FIGO).[4] The nomenclature for these tumors reflects the cell type, location of the tumor, and degree of malignancy, ranging from benign lesions to tumors of low malignant potential (LMP) to invasive carcinomas.

Tumors of LMP (borderline tumors) have an excellent prognosis compared with invasive carcinomas.[12,13] They are characterized by epithelial papillae with atypical cell clusters, cellular stratification, nuclear atypia, and increased mitotic activity. In contrast to epithelial ovarian carcinoma, borderline tumors lack stromal invasion.[13]

Epithelial carcinomas are characterized by histologic cell type and degree of differentiation (tumor grade). The histologic cell type has limited prognostic significance independent of clinical stage, although patients with clear cell and mucinous types of epithelial ovarian cancer fare less well due to the relative chemoresistance of these histologies.[14] Conversely, low-grade serous carcinoma is associated with a better prognosis despite relative chemoresistance.[15,16] High tumor grade appears to be an important prognostic factor, especially in patients with early stage epithelial tumors.

Certain pathologic and clinical features are characteristic of distinct histologic subtypes of epithelial carcinoma (Table 76.2). For instance, concentric rings of calcification called psammoma bodies (Fig. 76.2) are often observed in the papillary serous variety of epithelial ovarian cancer, although they are not pathognomonic for this disease and may also be seen, for example, in breast, lung, and papillary thyroid cancers. The endometrioid variant of ovarian cancer is associated with endometriosis in about 20% to 30% of cases, with a separate endometrioid uterine cancer (often stage I and low grade) simultaneously present in 15% of cases.[17] Likewise, clear cell histology may also be associated with endometriosis, as well as humorally mediated hypercalcemia (which can also be observed with the rare small cell variant of ovarian cancer). Clear cell cancers are relatively resistant to chemotherapy compared to

From Young RH. A brief history of the pathology of the gonads. *Mod Pathol* 2005;18:S3.

TABLE 76.1

World Health Organization Classification of Malignant Ovarian Tumors

Common Epithelial Tumors

Malignant serous tumor
- Adenocarcinoma, papillary adenocarcinoma, papillary cystadenocarcinoma
- Surface papillary carcinoma
- Malignant adenofibroma, cystadenofibroma

Malignant mucinous tumor
- Adenocarcinoma, cystadenocarcinoma
- Malignant adenofibroma, cystadenofibroma

Malignant endometrioid tumor
- Carcinoma
- Adenocarcinoma
- Adenoacanthoma
- Malignant adenofibroma, cystadenofibroma
- Endometrioid stromal sarcoma
- Mesodermal (mullerian) mixed tumor: homologous and heterologous

Other
- Clear cell (mesonephroid) tumor, malignant
- Carcinoma and adenocarcinoma
- Brenner tumor, malignant
- Mixed epithelial tumor, malignant
- Undifferentiated carcinoma
- Unclassified

Sex Cord–Stromal Tumors

Granulosa–stromal cell tumor
- Granulosa cell tumor
- Tumor in the thecoma-fibroma group
- Fibroma
- Unclassified

Androblastoma: Sertoli-Leydig cell tumor
- Well differentiated
- Tubular androblastoma, Sertoli cell tumor (tubular adenoma of Pick)
- Tubular androblastoma with lipid storage, Sertoli cell tumor with lipid storage
- Sertoli-Leydig cell tumor (tubular adenoma with Leydig cells)
- Leydig cell tumor, hilus cell tumor
- Of intermediate differentiation
- Poorly differentiated (sarcomatoid)
- With heterologous elements
- Gynandroblastoma
- Lipid (lipoid) cell tumors
- Unclassified

Germ Cell Tumor
- Dysgerminoma
- Endodermal sinus tumor
- Embryonal carcinoma
- Polyembryoma
- Choriocarcinoma
- Immature teratoma
- Mature dermoid cyst with malignant transformation
- Monodermal and highly specialized
- Struma ovarii
- Carcinoid
- Struma ovarii and carcinoid
- Others
- Mixed forms

Gonadoblastoma
- Pure
- Mixed with dysgerminoma or other form of germ cell tumor

TABLE 76.2

Common Histologic Types of Epithelial Ovarian Cancer

Histology	Features
Papillary serous	The most common type of epithelial ovarian cancer. May contain psammoma bodies (see Fig. 76.3) and is often associated with CA 125 elevation. Identical histology is observed for primary peritoneal serous cancer.
Endometrioid	Sometimes associated with endometriosis or an independent uterine cancer of similar histology. May occur with early-stage disease in younger patients, although advanced disease is also possible.
Mucinous	May rarely be associated with pseudomyxoma peritoneii. CA 125 levels may not be markedly elevated. Relatively chemoresistant. Differential diagnosis of a mucinous ovarian tumor includes metastatic disease from an appendiceal primary.
Clear cell	The most chemoresistant type of ovarian cancer. Often contains "hobnail" cells with cleared out cytoplasm due to glycogen. Sometimes associated with endometriosis or humorally mediated hypercalcemia.

CA, cancer antigen.

their more common papillary serous counterparts. Finally, primary mucinous ovarian cancers are also relatively chemoresistant, are sometimes associated with pseudomyxoma peritonei, and may not be associated with dramatic elevations of the cancer antigen (CA) 125 serum tumor marker.

Gastric, breast (especially infiltrating lobular carcinoma), mesothelioma, and colorectal cancers may occasionally present with diffuse peritoneal implants, ascites, and ovarian metastases that mimic primary ovarian cancer. It is usually possible to distinguish between these possibilities on routine light microscopic histologic evaluation, although immunohistochemistry can be most helpful when the histologic diagnosis is ambiguous. Staining for cytokeratin CK7 is positive and CK20 is negative in most cases of primary serous ovarian cancer, whereas the reverse staining pattern is typically observed for colorectal cancer. Staining for gross cystic disease fluid protein (GCDFP) may be positive in up to 50% of patients with breast cancer, whereas this marker should be negative in patients with gastric, colorectal, or ovarian cancer. Finally, calretinin is usually expressed in mesothelioma but is typically negative in epithelial ovarian cancer.

Diagnosis

Most patients with epithelial ovarian cancer experience no signs or symptoms of the disease until it spreads to the upper abdomen.

Approximately 70% of patients with this tumor present with advanced disease (stage III or IV, Table 76.3), whereas the majority of patients with borderline, germ cell, and sex cord–stromal tumors present with early stage disease limited to the pelvis.[2] Occasionally, patients with epithelial ovarian cancer will be diagnosed with early stage disease due to discovery of a mass on routine pelvic examination or because of pelvic pain caused by ovarian torsion. Unlike epithelial cancers, which are generally asymptomatic at an early stage, ovarian germ cell malignancies tend to stretch and twist the infundibulopelvic ligament, causing severe pain while the disease is still confined to the ovary.

Abdominal discomfort, bloating, and early satiety are the most common symptoms experienced by women with epithelial ovarian cancer. Patients presenting with such nonspecific complaints may be found to have ascites and a pelvic mass on physical examination. Occasionally an umbilical lymph node metastasis will be present (Sister Mary Joseph node) or a pleural effusion will be found. The mass on pelvic examination is frequently firm and fixed, with multiple nodularities palpable in the cul-de-sac.

The CA 125 serum level is elevated in >80% of serous epithelial ovarian cancers.[18] However, it is not a reliable diagnostic test, as it can also be elevated in a variety of benign gynecologic conditions (such as endometriosis, pelvic inflammatory disease, or pregnancy) and nongynecologic malignancies (such as breast, lung, and gastrointestinal cancers). Furthermore, the CA 125 level is elevated in only approximately 50% of patients with early stage epithelial ovarian cancer, which also limits its value as a screening test.[18] Other tumor markers, such as CA 19-9, which is elevated in some mucinous ovarian carcinomas, and carcinoembryonic antigen (CEA) are less frequently useful. It is typical for a patient with epithelial ovarian cancer to have a normal CEA level in the setting of a significantly elevated CA 125 level. Postoperatively, the CA 125 level provides a sensitive way to monitor treatment response and development of disease recurrence. Because relapsed epithelial ovarian cancer is usually incurable, however, there is currently no evidence that early detection of recurrence through CA 125 surveillance confers either a quality of life or a survival advantage in this disease.[19]

Transvaginal ultrasonography (TVU) is an important diagnostic tool in the evaluation of patients with a pelvic mass. TVU is more sensitive at detecting ovarian tumors compared to other tests such as computed tomography (CT), and it can provide qualitative information about the mass that might suggest malignancy. The classic sonographic finding of malignancy is a "complex" cyst, defined as containing both solid and cystic components, sometimes with septations and internal echogenicity (Fig. 76.3). Finding a complex cyst on sonography, especially in the presence of signs and symptoms consistent with ovarian cancer, often requires surgery for further evaluation. It is best to avoid percutaneous biopsy during the initial evaluation, which can result in cyst rupture and spillage of malignant cells into the peritoneal cavity. Bilateral

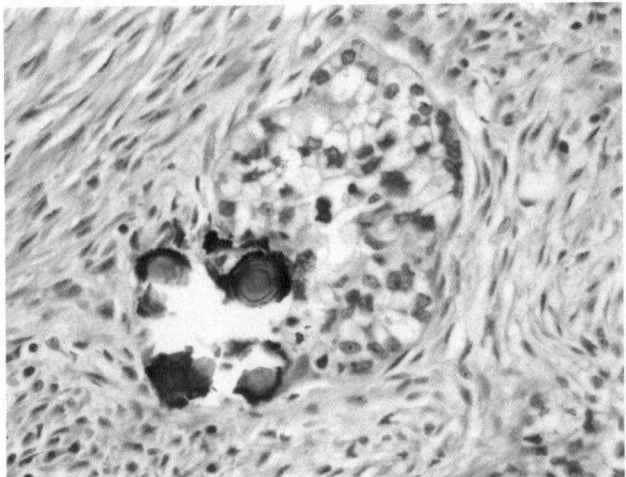

Figure 76.2 Photomicrograph of a hematoxylin and eosin-stained section of papillary serous ovarian cancer, showing psammoma bodies. (Courtesy of Dr. Jonathan Hecht, Beth Israel Deaconess Medical Center, Boston, MA.)

TABLE 76.3

International Federation of Gynecology and Obstetrics Staging System for Epithelial Ovarian Cancer

Stage I	*Tumor limited to ovary or ovaries[a]*
IA	One ovary, without malignant ascites, positive peritoneal washings, surface involvement, or rupture
IB	Both ovaries, without malignant ascites, positive peritoneal washings, surface involvement, or rupture
IC	Malignant ascites, positive peritoneal washings, surface involvement, or rupture present IC1: Surgical spill IC2: Capsule rupture before surgery or tumor on ovarian or fallopian tube surface IC3: Malignant cells in ascites or peritoneal washings
Stage II	*Ovarian tumor with pelvic extension[a]*
IIA	Involvement of the uterus or fallopian tubes
IIB	Involvement of other pelvic organs (e.g., bladder, rectum, or pelvic sidewall)
Stage III	*Tumor involving the upper abdomen or lymph nodes*
IIIA	Positive retroperitoneal nodes only or microscopic peritoneal disease outside of the pelvis. IIIA1: Positive retroperitoneal nodes as the only site of extrapelvic spread 　　IIIA1(i): Metastases up to 10 mm in greatest dimension 　　IIIA1(ii): Metastases >10 mm in greatest dimension IIIA2: Microscopic extrapelvic peritoneal involvement (with or without nodal involvement)
IIIB	Macroscopic peritoneal metastases ≤2 cm in diameter (with or without nodal involvement)[b]
IIIC	Macroscopic peritoneal metastases >2 cm in diameter (with or without nodal involvement)[b]
Stage IV	*Distant organ involvement, including pleural space[c] or hepatic/splenic parenchyma*
	IVA: Pleural effusion with positive cytology IVB: Parenchymal metastases (e.g., hematogenous spread to liver) or metastases to extra-abdominal sites such as inguinal lymph nodes

[a] Patients with disease that appears to be confined to the ovaries or pelvis require nodal biopsy for complete staging, in order to exclude the possibility of occult nodal involvement.
[b] Disease measurements for staging purposes are made before debulking has been attempted.
[c] Pleural effusion must be cytologically proven to be malignant if used to define stage IV disease.

ovarian involvement and ascites are sometimes detected by sonography as well. Color Doppler imaging evaluates blood flow to an ovarian mass and can potentially identify a malignant process based on the presence of abnormal neovascularization.[20]

In contrast to complex cysts, "simple" cysts are defined as being thin-walled, fluid-filled, without a mass component, septations, or internal echogenicity on TVU examination. Simple cysts are most often benign in nature and may be found in 5% to 10% of asymptomatic postmenopausal women during TVU examination, especially in the first decade after menopause. Simple cysts do not always require surgical evaluation if they are associated with normal CA 125 levels, although management must be individualized.[21] Postmenopausal women with simple cysts in association with elevated serum CA 125 levels, simple cysts that are >5 to 10 cm in diameter, or simple cysts in association with abnormal color Doppler flow studies are often referred for surgery.

In premenopausal women, simple cysts detected on TVU examination may be functional (i.e., a corpus luteum cyst) or represent a benign process such as a serous cystadenoma. Such cysts may generally be followed through several menstrual cycles, during which they often resolve. Functional cysts may also disappear when oral contraceptives are used. However, premenopausal women with simple cysts that are persistent or enlarging, especially in the setting of a rising CA 125 level, are reasonable candidates for surgical evaluation to exclude malignancy.[21] As previously mentioned, several benign conditions in premenopausal women may also be associated with elevated CA 125 levels, such as pregnancy or endometriosis, and there is no absolute CA 125 cutoff to distinguish benign from malignant pathologies.[22]

CT or magnetic resonance imaging may sometimes be helpful in defining the extent of peritoneal disease in patients with suspected ovarian cancer. However, for the patient with a complex

ovarian cyst and clinical signs and symptoms to suggest ovarian cancer, these studies generally do not obviate the need for surgical exploration. Occasionally, CT may sometimes be helpful in distinguishing a gynecologic malignancy from a metastatic pancreatic neoplasm, for instance, for which an exploratory laparotomy may not be warranted. In selected patients, CT may also assist in surgical planning by locating the site of suspected bowel

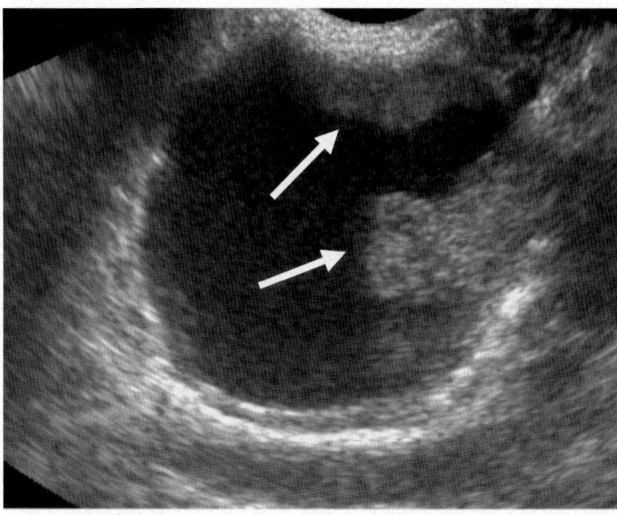

Figure 76.3 Transvaginal ultrasound of a complex cyst, containing both solid (*arrows*) and fluid components. (Courtesy of Dr. Ann McNamara, Beth Israel Deaconess Medical Center, Boston, MA.)

obstruction. Magnetic resonance imaging has not been shown to have a clear advantage over CT in patients with an ovarian mass, except for pregnant patients when ultrasonography is inconclusive and there is a desire to avoid radiation exposure. Positron emission tomography (PET) is a form of functional imaging that most frequently uses the positron-emitting glucose analogue fluorodeoxyglucose. Tumor masses are imaged based on their relatively increased glucose metabolism compared to normal tissues. However, there is currently no proven role for PET in the diagnosis or subsequent follow-up of patients with ovarian cancer.[23] Chest radiographs may sometimes be performed to evaluate the presence of pleural effusions, which occur in 10% of patients with epithelial ovarian cancer at diagnosis.

Screening and Early Detection

A successful screening test for ovarian cancer should be capable of identifying the majority of patients with precancerous lesions or early disease. Because a positive screening test for ovarian cancer would result in major surgery with associated morbidity, costs, and even mortality, the false-positive rate of such a screening test must be low, and its positive predictive value (PPV) relatively high (at least 10%). At present, there are no screening tests for epithelial ovarian cancer that convincingly meet these criteria.

Ovarian palpation has not been established as a useful screening procedure, and most screening studies have used serum tumor marker levels, ultrasonography, or both. The CA 125 serum level is not a useful screening test when used alone, as elevations are not specific for ovarian cancer and may be observed in cirrhosis, peritonitis, pleuritis, pancreatitis, endometriosis, uterine leiomyomata, benign ovarian cysts, and pelvic inflammatory disease. In addition, CA 125 serum levels may be elevated in other malignancies such as breast, lung, colorectal, pancreatic, and gastric cancers. Finally, although the CA 125 level is elevated in the majority of patients with advanced epithelial ovarian cancer, it is abnormal in only half of patients with early stage disease.[18] Therefore, by itself this test would fail to detect a sizable fraction of patients with curable disease. More recently, a number of candidate markers have been discovered that show promise for enhancing the accuracy of CA 125 levels, such as human epididymis 4, osteopontin, mesothelin, and osteoblast-stimulating factor-2. Algorithms that define the behavior of these markers have also been developed, incorporating biologic characteristics of tumor growth and marker behavior.[24] Levels of OVX-1 and macrophage colony-stimulating factor have been found to be elevated in patients with clinically evident ovarian cancer but normal CA 125 levels, which suggests that these markers may be complementary to CA 125.[25] Lysophosphatidic acid level has also been reported to discriminate patients with ovarian cancer from controls, including cases with early stage disease.[26] None of these tests has been proven to have sufficient sensitivity and specificity for routine screening at the current time.

Measurement of the CA 125 level has been combined with performance of TVU in an attempt to improve screening.[20,27,28] Early studies of TVU suggested a sensitivity of close to 100% but a specificity of 98%, which is insufficient to achieve a PPV of 10%. More recent reports suggest that use of color Doppler imaging improves the specificity of TVU, but it is uncertain whether this will achieve the desired PPV. Investigators at the University of Kentucky improved the specificity of TVU by using a morphologic index. They screened 6,470 women, including high-risk premenopausal women and average-risk postmenopausal women.[28] Of 90 women who underwent surgery, 6 were found to have an ovarian malignancy, for a PPV of 6.7%. One interval cancer was found at prophylactic oophorectomy 11 months after screening, for a sensitivity of 86%. All but one of these cancers were stage I, and no deaths due to ovarian cancer were noted in this group.

Two randomized controlled trials are currently under way to evaluate a multimodal screening approach using both CA 125 and

TVU. In the United States, the Prostate, Lung, Colorectal, Ovarian Cancer Screening Trial uses measurement of CA 125 level (single threshold elevation of >35 U/mL) and TVU together, performed annually, as a first-line screen.[29] If either test is positive, the woman is referred for surgical consultation. In this two-arm, randomized controlled trial involving 10 centers, 78,216 of general US women aged 55 to 74 years were randomly assigned to the screening arm or to a standard-care control arm. After a median follow-up of 12.4 years, no mortality reduction was observed for patients randomized to the screening arm.[30]

The second randomized screening trial is currently being conducted in the United Kingdom and uses CA 125 levels (or rate of rise of CA 125) as a trigger for performing TVU. This trial is based on an earlier study by Jacobs et al.[31] in which 21,935 average-risk postmenopausal women were assigned to undergo three annual screenings or no screening. The screening protocol used CA 125 level as a first-line screen and referred the patient for TVU if the CA 125 level was >30 U/mL. If the TVU revealed an ovarian mass, the patient was referred for surgical consultation. Findings from this trial support the notion that this stepwise approach can yield high specificity and an acceptable PPV.[31] Specifically, when the decision rule for surgical referral requires that results of both tests be positive, the PPV is 20%. Furthermore, there were one-half as many deaths in the screened group as there were among controls, and there was a statistically significant improvement in survival. Individuals with index cancers survived an average of 72.9 months in the screening group and 41.8 months in the control group. However, the multimodal screening strategy originally described by Jacobs et al.[31] is limited by the sensitivity of the CA 125 level, which serves as a trigger for performing ultrasound. Accordingly, these investigators are exploring ways to improve on these results by detecting changes in CA 125 levels over time. Skates et al.[32] suggested fitting an exponential model that uses data from several prior CA 125 screens, with an exponential rise triggering a callback for additional ultrasound testing. This screening strategy forms the basis of the three-arm randomized trial currently being conducted in the United Kingdom.

Hereditary Ovarian Carcinoma

Approximately 5% to 10% of patients with epithelial ovarian carcinoma carry a germline mutation that places them at substantially increased risk of developing this disease. The breast–ovarian cancer syndrome accounts for approximately 90% of hereditary ovarian cancer and is often suspected whenever the pedigree reveals multiple affected family members with ovarian cancer, bilateral or early onset breast cancer, both breast and ovarian cancer in the same individual, or a male relative with breast cancer.[33,34] Fallopian tube cancer and primary peritoneal serous cancer (PPSC) are also recognized to be part of this syndrome.[35] The high incidence of breast and ovarian cancers in these families is due to inherited germline mutations in the BRCA1 or BRCA2 genes, which may be transferred by either parent, meaning that both maternal and paternal family histories must be obtained to determine risk.[36] The BRCA1 gene, located on chromosome band 17q12-21, and the BRCA2 gene, located on chromosome band 13q12-13, were identified and linked to hereditary breast and ovarian cancers in the 1990s. Emerging evidence suggests that these genes act as tumor suppressors and play a critical role in the repair of double-stranded DNA breaks.[36]

Many mutations have been described throughout the BRCA1 and BRCA2 genes, with nonsense and frameshift mutations being predominant.[36] Nonsense mutations occur when a nucleotide substitution results in a stop codon, and frameshift mutations occur when one or more nucleotides are deleted to produce a downstream stop codon. Certain ethnic groups have higher frequencies of distinctive BRCA mutations, thought to be due to a founder effect in which certain mutations are preserved within a genetically isolated population. Three such founder mutations (185delAG *BRCA1*, 5382insC *BRCA1*, and 6174delT *BRCA2*) are carried by 2% to 2.4% of the Ashkenazic Jewish population.[37] Furthermore, up to 40% of patients of Jewish descent with epithelial ovarian cancer may carry one of these mutations (regardless of their family histories).[37] This is compared to a carrier frequency of approximately 5% among non-Jewish women with ovarian cancer.

The lifetime risk of ovarian cancer is approximately 20% to 40% for patients with *BRCA1* mutations, and 10% to 20% for *BRCA2* mutation carriers.[38] Ovarian cancer associated with germline mutations of *BRCA1* appears to present with distinct clinical and pathologic features compared with sporadic ovarian cancer.[39] The majority of *BRCA1*-associated cancers are serous adenocarcinomas, with an average age at diagnosis of 48 years, whereas the mean age for *BRCA2*-associated ovarian cancers is 60 years.[40] Other histologies may also occur, including endometrioid and clear cell tumors, although mucinous ovarian cancer appears to be underrepresented in these genetic syndromes. Furthermore, *BRCA*-associated cancers may have a more favorable course than sporadic ovarian cancer. In a study by Rubin et al.,[39] the median survival of 43 patients with advanced *BRCA1*-associated disease was 77 months, compared with 29 months for matched controls. Cass et al.[41] noted a similar survival advantage for carriers in their matched cohort study and suggested that this was a result of having an improved response to platinum-based chemotherapy compared to women with sporadic disease. This increased chemosensitivity may be partly due to the inability of tumor cells to repair platinum-induced DNA damage in the setting of a *BRCA1* or *BRCA2* mutation.[36] The more favorable survival of patients with *BRCA1* or *BRCA2* mutations when compared to their sporadic counterparts is not necessarily related to a higher rate of cure, but may also be related to a longer duration of responsiveness to chemotherapy agents used in the relapsed setting. The Gynecologic Oncology Group (GOG) is conducting a prospective study to better compare the clinical course of sporadic ovarian cancer with that associated with *BRCA1* and *BRCA2* mutations.

The hereditary nonpolyposis colorectal cancer (HNPCC) syndrome accounts for approximately 5% to 10% of all hereditary ovarian cancer cases.[17] It is an autosomal dominant genetic syndrome characterized by nonpolyposis colon cancer, often involving the right colon, as well as an increased risk of developing endometrial, ovarian, hepatobiliary, upper gastrointestinal, and genitourinary cancers.[42] Colorectal and uterine cancers comprise the majority of tumors developing in affected families. The risk of endometrial cancer among women in HNPCC syndrome families is estimated to be 40% to 60% by age 70, compared to 1.5% in the general population. Limited studies have reported a 3.5-fold increase in the risk of ovarian cancer in members of these families.[42] A germline mutation in one of five genes involved in DNA mismatch repair is responsible for the HNPCC phenotype: *hMSH2* (chromosome arm 2p), *hMLH1* (chromosome arm 3p), *hPMS1* (chromosome arm 2q), *hPMS2* (chromosome arm 7p), and *hMSH6* (chromosome arm 2p).[36] The majority of affected patients are found to have defects in either *hMSH2* or *hMLH1*. Patients with HNPCC due to germline mutation of *hMSH6* may be particularly predisposed to uterine cancer. In addition, HNPCC may account for approximately 7% of cases with synchronous uterine and ovarian cancers, which are often (but not always) low grade and of endometrioid histology.[17] The estimated cumulative risks for ovarian cancer by age 70 years can be as high as 24% for those with germline mutations in *MLH1* and *MSH2*.[43]

Patients at high risk of having a hereditary cancer typically undergo genetic counseling, so that the ramifications of genetic testing can be discussed. Multidisciplinary services available in such a setting often include pretest and posttest counseling, screening, treatment, and psychosocial counseling.[44] The most direct approach to determine whether a cancer-associated mutation is present is to test the patient affected with the disease (the proband), because he or she is the most likely to carry a deleterious mutation.

The first family member to be tested will often require comprehensive gene sequencing. Other individuals can then be tested for the identified mutation, which may be unique to this particular family. In the Ashkenazic Jewish population, genetic testing for the three founder mutations is required because the carrier frequency in this population is high, and individuals may occasionally harbor germline mutations in both *BRCA1* and *BRCA2*.

Test results may reveal an identifiable mutation, no identifiable mutation, or a polymorphism of indeterminate clinical significance. If the proband has tested positive for a recognized mutation, then a relative with a negative result has likely not inherited the deleterious mutation, and her cancer risk approximates that of the general population. However, if no identifiable mutation is found in the proband, it is still possible that a cancer-associated mutation exists that is not detectable with current testing methods. This is especially the case for probands with a highly suggestive family history of breast, ovarian, or both cancers. In this regard, it has been shown that approximately 12% of probands who test negative for a germline mutation using standard gene sequencing techniques are found to have a clinically significant mutation in *BRCA1* or *BRCA2* when tested by the technique of multiplex ligation dependent probe amplification.[45] Finally, a minority of test results represent genetic variants or polymorphisms in *BRCA1* or *BRCA2* that are of indeterminate clinical significance. Further study of these genetic variants and associated cancer risks in large populations will help reduce the number of reports of indeterminate findings.

The management of patients with an inherited genetic predisposition to ovarian cancer is complex due to the variable penetrance of genetic alterations and the lack of effective early detection methods for ovarian cancer. Although annual pelvic examinations, serum CA 125 determinations, and TVU are sometimes considered in affected individuals, there is currently no conclusive evidence that ovarian cancer mortality is reduced as a result of these interventions.[27] In contrast, the efficacy of prophylactic, risk reduction bilateral salpingo-oophorectomy (RRSO) for patients with the hereditary breast–ovarian cancer syndrome has been more convincingly demonstrated.[46,47] One study of 259 patients who underwent RRSO found a 96% decrease in ovarian cancers and an approximately 50% reduction in subsequent breast cancer compared to age-matched controls.[46] More recent studies also confirm the benefit of RRSO in this patient population.[48] Even after RRSO, *BRCA* mutation carriers are still at small risk for developing PPSC, which is histologically and clinically similar to epithelial ovarian cancer. Such cancers represent malignant transformation of the peritoneal mesothelium, which is contiguous with ovarian surface epithelium.

RRSO is generally considered for patients at high risk for developing ovarian cancer and who have completed childbearing, especially if they are at least 35 years of age.[27,49] A laparoscopic approach is frequently possible, but the surgical options must be individualized, as must the decision for concomitant hysterectomy (which is an especially relevant consideration for patients with HNPCC undergoing this procedure). It is important to remove the fallopian tubes as part of prophylactic surgery, as the tubal epithelium may harbor dysplasia or may develop in situ cancers in this setting.[50] The surgical pathologist must perform a careful examination of the surgical specimens, as occult ovarian and tubal carcinoma have been found in 2% to 10% of RRSO specimens.[51] Some patients with occult disease discovered after careful pathologic evaluation may require a second operation to complete surgical staging in order to determine the need for postoperative treatment, as described later in the chapter. Significant issues regarding RRSO remain unresolved, such as the physiologic adjustments to premature surgical menopause and the safety of hormone replacement therapy in this group, especially in those at high risk for breast cancer.[52]

It has been suggested that chemoprophylaxis with oral contraceptives for 5 years might decrease ovarian cancer risk by 50% in both the general population and in high-risk women. For example, a case-controlled study of 207 known *BRCA* mutation carriers and their sister controls found a 60% reduction of ovarian cancer risk with oral contraceptive use.[53] Other risk-reducing strategies such as tubal ligation and hysterectomy have also been associated with a reduced incidence of ovarian cancer among high-risk women.[3] Nonetheless, RRSO is currently the most effective preventative strategy to reduce ovarian cancer risk in patients with *BRCA* mutations.

Staging

Exploratory laparotomy serves three main purposes in the management of patients with suspected ovarian cancer. First, laparotomy permits histologic confirmation of disease, as a complex cyst may not only represent primary ovarian cancer, but may also be caused by metastatic gastric cancer to the ovary (Krukenberg tumor), metastatic disease to the ovary from a gastrointestinal or breast primary (especially infiltrating lobular breast cancer), or benign conditions such as endometriosis.[54] Surgery is also necessary to determine the extent of disease (staging), which is critical in determining whether postoperative treatment will be necessary, as well as to assess prognosis. Finally, exploratory laparotomy is necessary to permit debulking of as much tumor as possible, as patients who are optimally cytoreduced (defined as having ≤1-cm diameter residual tumor) have a better prognosis compared to those with greater amounts of residual disease.[55]

The staging system for ovarian cancer was updated in 2014 by FIGO and is based on the findings at exploratory laparotomy (see Table 76.3).[56,56a] Proper surgical staging via exploratory laparotomy requires a midline incision large enough to permit inspection of the peritoneal cavity, including the upper abdomen, as well as evaluation of the retroperitoneal spaces and lymph nodes.[57] When the peritoneal cavity is entered, ascitic fluid is aspirated and the peritoneal surfaces are irrigated, with the samples sent for cytologic evaluation. The pelvis and paracolic spaces should be irrigated and the fluid sent for cytologic examination. If intraperitoneal (IP) carcinomatosis is absent, it may be most appropriate to first resect the ovarian tumor and then to proceed with surgical staging to avoid rupturing the mass. The grossly normal, opposite ovary may undergo biopsy, or any visible benign-appearing cysts may be excised. Pelvic and para-aortic retroperitoneal lymph nodes are generally evaluated in patients whose tumors do not grossly extend outside the ovary, as approximately 10% to 15% of patients with otherwise stage I disease will have occult nodal involvement that places them in the stage III category.[57] Any enlarged pelvic retroperitoneal lymph nodes should be removed if technically feasible in order to achieve optimal cytoreduction.

It is frequently necessary to extend the vertical incision above the umbilicus in order to fully inspect the upper abdomen. If gross disease is not present in the omentum, an infracolic omentectomy is usually sufficient for diagnostic purposes. When the omentum demonstrates diffuse infiltration by tumor (an omental cake), it should be excised from the greater curvature of the stomach as completely as possible. The upper abdominal evaluation continues with a careful inspection of the right hemidiaphragm, liver serosa, and liver parenchyma. The spleen is then carefully inspected, as is the left diaphragm. A splenectomy could be considered if this procedure would lead to an optimal surgical cytoreduction. The paracolic spaces and large bowel are then carefully inspected. The small intestine and mesentery are evaluated, and any tumor implants are removed as much as possible. If luminal narrowing is present, especially in the area of the terminal ileum, a small bowel resection and reanastomosis are performed. Similarly, if tumor appears to invade the large bowel, a resection may be performed if the mass is large enough to pose a threat for bowel obstruction. Lymphadenectomy is considered if this procedure is technically feasible and would lead to a maximally cytoreductive result. In

postmenopausal women or in women in whom fertility is no longer desired, a bilateral salpingo-oophorectomy and total abdominal hysterectomy are typically performed.

For women who wish to preserve fertility, which is sometimes possible when the tumor is limited to one ovary, staging may be performed without removal of the contralateral ovary and tube and without hysterectomy.[58] In that regard, patients with endometrioid ovarian cancer may have a synchronous endometrioid uterine cancer in up to 15% of cases, which may not always be appreciated preoperatively.[17] In such cases, the tumor is often minimally invasive and low grade, and the prognosis is often favorable. Therefore, for patients with early stage, endometrioid ovarian cancer in whom a fertility sparing operation is considered, it is reasonable to perform an endometrial biopsy to exclude the presence of a separate uterine cancer that would alter the surgical approach.

On occasion, the initial surgical staging is incomplete due to lack of lymph node or upper abdominal evaluation in a patient with presumptive stage I disease. In this situation, it is reasonable to consider completing the surgical staging if the findings would alter postoperative management. For instance, if a patient has stage IA, grade 1 or 2 disease (see Table 76.3) after complete surgical staging, no further postoperative treatment would generally be indicated.[59] However, if a patient is already known to have at least stage IC or stage II disease, or if the tumor is grade 3, then postoperative chemotherapy is generally required, and the impact of additional staging procedures might be less important (except perhaps for the patient who is discovered to have stage III disease on re-exploration, in which case IP chemotherapy might play a role if she is optimally cytoreduced (as noted subsequently)). Laparoscopic or robotic surgical techniques may allow para-aortic lymph node dissections and omentectomies to be performed with less morbidity, which is an important consideration in a patient who might have undergone recent, albeit incomplete, surgical evaluation. If this is not possible or practical, an alternative is to obtain a CT scan in an attempt to identify the presence of any subclinical bulky disease that might be amenable to surgical resection. However, CT is not capable of detecting small volume or microscopic disease that could affect decisions regarding the need for postoperative chemotherapy.

Prognostic Factors for Epithelial Ovarian Cancer

Clinicopathologic findings of prognostic value include FIGO stage, volume of residual disease after cytoreductive surgery, histologic subtype, histologic grade, age, and malignant ascites.[14] Tumor stage remains the most important prognostic factor, although only 30% of patients have early stage disease (defined as having stage I or stage II tumors). Stage IA disease is completely encapsulated, without involvement of the ovarian surface, without rupture, malignant ascites, or positive washings (see Table 76.3). The 5-year survival of patients with stage IA disease and grade 1 or 2 histology is >90% after surgery alone, and several investigators include patients with stage IB, grade 1 or 2 disease, in this good prognostic group.[59] However, the relapse rate without postoperative adjuvant treatment is 30% to 40% for patients with stage IC disease (defined by the presence of rupture, surface involvement, malignant ascites, or positive washings), those with stage I, grade 3 disease, or those with stage II tumors. These patients comprise a high-risk group of early stage tumors and experience a 5-year survival rate of approximately 80% after receiving postoperative adjuvant therapy.[59] It should be noted that the prognostic significance of rupture as the sole criterion for stage IC disease is somewhat controversial, as some investigators report that rupture alone does not appear to confer a worse prognosis if it occurred intraoperatively, as opposed to preoperatively.[60]

The majority of patients with epithelial ovarian cancer present with advanced disease (stage III or IV). After postoperative treatment, the 5-year survival rate of patients with stage III optimally debulked, gross residual disease (≤1-cm diameter residual tumor) is approximately 20% to 30%, and this decreases to <10% for patients with suboptimally debulked stage III disease or those with stage IV tumors.[61,62] Patients who have stage IIIA disease on the basis of microscopic upper abdominal involvement (usually detected on omental biopsy) have survivals in the range of 50% after postoperative adjuvant therapy.[63] Patients with advanced-stage disease who have mucinous or clear cell histologic also have a worse prognosis, which appears to be related to the relative chemoresistance of these histologies. In a GOG study, no patient with advanced clear cell or mucinous histology achieved a pathologic complete response after chemotherapy, as defined by performance of second-look laparotomy.[14]

Preoperative serum CA 125 levels frequently reflect the volume of disease and do not appear to have an independent effect on survival, after correcting for stage and debulking status. However, postoperative CA 125 levels, both during and after completion of first-line chemotherapy, have prognostic value.[64,65] Some investigators have demonstrated that normalization of the serum CA 125 levels after three cycles of chemotherapy is associated with more favorable outcome, as well as achievement of a CA 125 nadir of ≤10 U/mL upon completion of treatment.[64,65] Although this information has prognostic significance, it has limited therapeutic value in the absence of effective salvage regimens with curative potential.

Germline mutation in *BRCA1* or *BRCA2* genes is associated with an improved prognosis. A pooled analysis of 26 observational studies on the survival of women with ovarian cancer showed that having a germline mutation in *BRCA1* or *BRCA2* was associated with improved 5-year overall survival (for *BRCA1*: hazard ratio [HR] = 0.73; for *BRCA2*: HR = 0.49).[66] In addition, several other molecular prognostic factors have been investigated in ovarian cancer. These include markers of proliferation or drug resistance, levels of serum cytokines or growth factor receptors, and expression of genes associated with metastases.[67] More recently, it has been possible to use microarray analysis, which provides a global snapshot of gene expression, to assess prognosis and response to therapy in this disease. At least two profiles have been defined, referred to as the Ovarian Cancer Prognostic Profile and the Chemo Response Profile, that provide information of independent prognostic and predictive value for patients with advanced disease.[68,69] However, it remains to be determined how best to incorporate such new techniques into the management of patients with this tumor. In the future, it is hoped that gene expression profiling will be capable of identifying patients who might benefit from novel forms of treatment (such as antiangiogenic therapy) or those with poor prognosis who might be appropriate for clinical trial participation.

Management of Early Stage Disease

Postoperative Chemotherapy

The results of two randomized European trials (International Collaborative Ovarian Neoplasm Trial [ICON] 1 and Adjuvant ChemoTherapy in Ovarian Neoplasm Trial) suggest that adjuvant chemotherapy can improve both progression-free survival (PFS) and overall survival in patients with high-risk, early stage ovarian cancer.[70] Such patients include those with stage I, grade 3, stage IC, or any stage II disease. These two studies collectively enrolled 925 patients, although they differed in eligibility criteria, requirements for surgical staging, and the specific adjuvant chemotherapy program used. Overall survival was superior for platinum-based adjuvant therapy in the entire patient cohort, although subset analysis revealed that the benefit appeared to be restricted to those patients who did not undergo adequate surgical staging. This observation suggested that the observed survival benefit might be due to unintentional enrollment of a subset of patients who actually had occult stage III disease. Nonetheless, caution must be used

when interpreting the results of an unplanned subset analysis, and most physicians feel that these data support the use of adjuvant chemotherapy for patients with high-risk, early stage disease.[71]

A study performed by the GOG compared three cycles of carboplatin and paclitaxel to six cycles of this regimen in patients with high-risk, early stage ovarian cancer in order to determine whether a shorter duration of treatment is equally effective and less toxic.[72] The relapse rate and PFS were not statistically different between these two treatment arms, which led some investigators to conclude that administering three cycles of adjuvant chemotherapy was as effective as six cycles in this setting. However, a recent subset analysis of this trial involving patients with serous histology showed that the 5-year recurrence-free survival for patients who received six cycles was 83%, compared with 60% for those who received three cycles (p = 0.007).[73] In addition, this study was not sufficiently powered to determine whether three cycles was equivalent to six cycles in terms of an overall survival benefit. In view of these issues, administration of six cycles of adjuvant carboplatin plus paclitaxel chemotherapy can still be considered a reasonable approach for high-risk, early stage patients, unless more definitive data supporting lesser amounts of chemotherapy become available.[74] The rationale for choosing carboplatin and paclitaxel is based on the experience gained from management of advanced disease, which will be described in detail later in the chapter.

Postoperative Radiation Therapy

The role of radiation therapy in the treatment of patients with primary ovarian cancer has changed markedly over time. For several decades, it was used as the sole modality of treatment. As experience with chemotherapy grew, randomized trials were conducted to compare different chemotherapy regimens to whole abdominal radiotherapy (WAR) or to IP administration of radioactive phosphorus (^{32}P). Most are now of only historical interest, as the chemotherapy regimens used did not contain platinum compounds, and they will not be reviewed here. In general, these studies showed that WAR and ^{32}P had similar efficacy compared to prolonged courses of melphalan or chlorambucil, given with or without pelvic irradiation.

The first trial to compare radiation therapy to a platinum-based regimen was conducted from 1981 to 1987 in Birmingham, England. This trial randomized 40 patients with stages IC to III ovarian cancer with no macroscopic residual disease following surgery to either WAR using a moving-strip technique or to cisplatin (100 mg/m², given every 3 weeks for five cycles). With a median follow-up of 84 months, the 5-year survival rates in the two groups were 58% and 62%, respectively.[75]

A trial conducted in Genoa, Italy, from 1985 to 1989 included 70 patients with high-risk stage I or II ovarian carcinoma.[76] They received either WAR using an open-field technique (24 fractions delivering 43.2 Gy to the pelvis and 30.2 Gy to the upper abdomen) or cisplatin (50 mg/m²) plus cyclophosphamide (600 mg/m²), given every 4 weeks for six cycles. Eight patients randomized to WAR received chemotherapy because of their own or their physicians' preference. Because protocol compliance was poor and accrual low, the study was prematurely closed. At a median follow-up of 60 months, the 5-year overall survival rates in the radiation and chemotherapy arms were 53% and 71%, respectively (p = 0.16); relapse-free survival rates were 50% and 74%, respectively (p = 0.07). Of note, late bowel obstruction requiring surgery occurred in only one patient.

From 1982 to 1988, 340 eligible patients with stages I through III ovarian carcinoma without residual disease after surgery seen at the Norwegian Radium Hospital in Oslo were randomized to receive either IP radioactive chromic phosphate (7 to 10 mCi, or 260 to 370 MBq) or six cycles of intravenous (IV) cisplatin (50 mg/m²) given every 3 weeks.[77] Twenty-eight patients with peritoneal adhesions who were randomized to IP ^{32}P were treated instead with WAR. The 5-year overall survival rates in the two arms were 83% and 81%, respectively; disease-free survival rates were 81% and

75%, respectively. Patients with stage II or III tumors had superior survival when treated with cisplatin, although the difference was not statistically significant. The long-term risk of bowel obstruction without recurrence in radiation and chemotherapy arms was 11% and 2%, respectively.

Finally, a trial conducted between 1986 and 1994 by the GOG randomly allocated 229 eligible patients with stage IA-B grade 3 or stage II tumors without macroscopic residual disease after surgery to either IP ^{32}P (15 mCi) or three cycles every 3 weeks of cyclophosphamide (1,000 mg/m^2) and cisplatin (100 mg/m^2).[78] With a median follow-up of nearly 10 years in survivors, the 10-year relapse rates in the radiation and chemotherapy arms were 35% and 28%, respectively, which was not statistically significant. There was a relative reduction of 17% in the overall death rate in the chemotherapy arm, which was not statistically significant. The incidence of nonhematologic grade 3 or 4 toxicities was similar in both arms.

One question not addressed in these trials is whether patients with certain subtypes of ovarian cancer might have better outcome if treated with WAR instead of chemotherapy. A retrospective study of patients with predominantly early-stage clear cell carcinomas treated in Okinawa from 1996 to 2004 found superior 5-year overall survival (82%) and disease-free survival (82%) compared to patients treated with platinum-based chemotherapy (rates of 33% and 25%, respectively), although interpretation is difficult to small patient numbers and the possibility of selection bias.[79]

In summary, these randomized trials generally found WAR or IP ^{32}P was less effective or more toxic than platinum-containing regimens. Hence, adjuvant radiation therapy has fallen out of use as the primary treatment for patients with high-risk, early stage ovarian cancer.

Management of Advanced-Stage Disease

Debulking Surgery

The theoretical benefits of debulking surgery include removal of large, necrotic tumors with poor blood supply that might lead to impaired chemotherapy delivery. It has also been postulated that tumor debulking may permit residual tumor to proliferate more rapidly and thereby enhance sensitivity to postoperative chemotherapy. Although neither of these mechanisms has been proven, the association between successful surgical cytoreduction and more favorable outcome has been demonstrated in many surgical series.[14,55,63]

The definition of *optimal cytoreduction* achieved through debulking surgery has varied through the years, but residual disease of ≤1 cm in maximum individual tumor diameter is most widely accepted. Recently, however, there has been a trend toward redefining *optimal cytoreduction* to refer more specifically to those patients who have no gross residual disease, reflecting complete cytoreduction to microscopic residual status.[80]

Primary debulking surgery refers to performance of surgery prior to administration of first-line chemotherapy and is the standard approach for managing most patients with suspected epithelial ovarian cancer. Despite the importance of primary debulking surgery, some patients with advanced disease are not ideal surgical candidates due to a poor performance status, or extensive amounts of bulky intra-abdominal disease as assessed by radiographic studies, and therefore may not be appropriate candidates for this procedure. In these cases, initiating neoadjuvant chemotherapy is a reasonable approach, followed by an interval attempt at surgical cytoreduction in responding patients after three cycles of chemotherapy have been administered. In this instance, surgery is referred to as *interval debulking surgery*.[81,82] Theoretical advantages of neoadjuvant chemotherapy in this setting are a more rapid improvement in quality of life, and, if interval debulking surgery is ultimately performed, a technically more feasible operation with shorter hospitalization and less morbidity. Prospective randomized trials incorporating neoadjuvant chemotherapy in the management of advanced-

stage ovarian cancer are under way to better define the value of this strategy. The first of these to be reported was conducted by the European Organisation for Research and Treatment of Cancer (EORTC)-National Cancer Institute of Canada (NCIC), involving 632 patients who were randomized to receive either primary debulking surgery followed by six cycles of platinum-based chemotherapy, or neoadjuvant chemotherapy for three cycles, followed by interval debulking surgery in responding or stable patients, followed by an additional three cycles of chemotherapy.[83] Eligibility for this study included stage IIIC and IV disease, performance status ≤2, and no disease in the upper abdomen measuring <2 cm in greatest diameter as assessed by CT or laparoscopy. Patients with retroperitoneal lymph node involvement as their only site of stage III disease were not included.[84] In addition, confirmation of the clinical impression of ovarian cancer was required prior to instituting neoadjuvant therapy, using either core biopsy or fine needle aspiration, with supportive serology including a CA 125:CEA ratio of ≥25. For patients whose CA 125:CEA ratio was <25, appropriate studies were performed to exclude the possibility of a breast or gastrointestinal primary. The results of this trial show that the overall survival was equivalent between the two treatment approaches, despite the fact that the rate of optimal cytoreduction was higher in patients undergoing neoadjuvant chemotherapy. There was a trend toward less postoperative morbidity in those who received neoadjuvant therapy, although this did not reach statistical significance. However, for the subset of patients whose disease was <5 cm in greatest diameter at study entry, their overall survival was improved with primary cytoreduction compared to neoadjuvant therapy.[84] Based upon the results of this study, the approach of neoadjuvant therapy and interval debulking surgery is a reasonable option for patients with bulky upper abdominal peritoneal disease >5 cm in diameter, or those with medical comorbidities that preclude safe performance of primary surgical cytoreduction. Preliminary results from a second randomized trial of neoadjuvant chemotherapy and interval debulking surgery being performed in the United Kingdom are supportive of this approach, and we await the results of a third confirmatory trial being performed by the Japanese Clinical Oncology Group.[85] Despite the value of neoadjuvant chemotherapy and interval debulking surgery in appropriately selected patients, primary cytoreduction should still be the preferred initial option for patients with stage IIIC and IV disease with good performance status who have <5 cm upper abdominal disease, who have retroperitoneal only disease preoperatively, or who might otherwise be considered ideal candidates for IP therapy if optimally cytoreduced (see the following).

Postoperative Chemotherapy for Epithelial Ovarian Cancer

Advanced-stage epithelial ovarian cancer is a chemoresponsive disease in the majority of cases, although relapse often occurs and resistance eventually develops to most forms of treatment. The platinum compounds remain the single most active drugs in the treatment of this disease. Cisplatin was the most frequently used platinum compound in the late 1970s and early 1980s, although it was soon recognized that the use of carboplatin instead of cisplatin conferred an equivalent survival advantage, but with less neuropathy, nephropathy, and emesis.[86]

Although numerous combination chemotherapy regimens have been studied over the past three decades, the combination of an IV platinum compound and a taxane such as paclitaxel is now accepted as an appropriate first-line, postoperative option for many patients. The response rate of this combination is as high as 70% for patients with suboptimally debulked disease, and over 80% for patients who are optimally cytoreduced.[61,62] Platinum agents exert their effects by forming intrastrand DNA adducts with guanosine bases, whereas taxanes mediate cytotoxicity by binding to and stabilizing the tubulin polymer, thereby preventing physiologic dissociation of the mitotic spindle at the completion of M phase. Given these nonoverlapping mechanisms of action, it was not surprising to find that taxanes were active agents in the treatment of some patients with relapsed, platinum-resistant ovarian cancer.[87] These observations formed the basis for investigating the platinum and taxane combination in the first-line setting.

Two phase 3 randomized trials begun in the early 1990s compared a cisplatin and paclitaxel combination to a cisplatin and cyclophosphamide regimen (Table 76.4). In the GOG study, patients with suboptimally resected stage III or IV ovarian cancer were randomized to receive six cycles of either cisplatin and cyclophosphamide or the experimental arm of cisplatin and paclitaxel.[62] Women treated with the paclitaxel-containing program experienced a statistically significant improvement in response rate (73% versus 60%; p <0.01), median PFS (18 months versus 13 months; p <0.001), and median overall survival (38 months versus 24 months; p <0.001).

These results were confirmed in a trial conducted in Europe and Canada that used a similar but not identical study design.[88] In this trial, paclitaxel was delivered as a 3-hour infusion of 175 mg/m², whereas in the GOG study a dose of 135 mg/m² was administered over 24 hours. In addition, a much larger percentage of patients in the control arm of the European-Canadian study received paclitaxel as second-line therapy after relapse, compared to the control arm of the GOG trial. Despite these differences, this study also revealed a statistically significant improvement in both PFS and overall survival associated with the paclitaxel-containing regimen (see Table 76.4).

Neither the GOG nor the European-Canadian trials was able to address whether the survival benefit observed with the platinum-taxane doublet was related to the use of combination chemotherapy or whether it could also be achieved through the use of sequential monotherapy. In an attempt to address this issue, the GOG conducted a randomized trial in which patients with suboptimally debulked advanced disease received either single-agent cisplatin (100 mg/m²), single-agent paclitaxel (200 mg/m² administered over 24 hours), or the combination of cisplatin (75 mg/m²) and paclitaxel (135 mg/m² administered over 24 hours).[89] Survival was similar between the three study arms, despite a superior objective response rate to both platinum-containing regimens (67%), compared to single-agent paclitaxel (42%). This result is likely explained by the fact that approximately 50% of patients in the single-agent arms were switched to the alternative agent before

TABLE 76.4

Randomized Trials of Paclitaxel Versus Nonpaclitaxel First-Line Therapy in Advanced Epithelial Ovarian Cancer

Trial and Randomization	Patient Number	Stage	CCR (%)	Median PFS (mo)	Median OS (mo)
GOG-111[62]	386	III, IV			
Paclitaxel (135 mg/m²)			51	18	38
Cisplatin (75 mg/m²)					
				$p < 0.001$	$p < 0.001$
Cyclosphosphamide (750 mg/m²)			31	13	24
Cisplatin (75 mg/m²)					
OV10[86]	668	IIB–IV			
Paclitaxel (175 mg/m²)			40.7	15.5	35.6
Cisplatin (75 mg/m²)					
				$p = 0.0005$	$p = 0.0016$
Cyclophosphamide (750 mg/m²)			27.3	12	25.8
Cisplatin (75 mg/m²)					
ICON-3[90]	2074	I–IV			
Paclitaxel (175 mg/m²)			NA	17.3	36.1
Carboplatin (AUC 5 to 6)					
				$p = 0.16$	$p = 0.74$
Carboplatin (AUC 5 to 6)			NA	16.1	35.4[a]
Cisplatin (50 mg/m²)					
Doxorubicin (50 mg/m²)					
Cyclophosphamide (500 mg/m²)					
GOG-132[89]	614	III–IV			
Paclitaxel (135 mg/m²)			NA	16	35[b]
Cisplatin (75 mg/m²)					
Cisplatin (100 mg/m²)			NA	16.4	30.2
Paclitaxel (200 mg/m²)			NA	10.8	25.9

CCR, clinical complete remission; PFS, progression-free survival; OS, overall survival; GOG, Gynecologic Oncology Group; ICON-3, International Collaborative Ovarian Neoplasm trial 3; NA, not available; AUC, area under the curve.
[a] For ICON-3, patients in the control arms could receive either carboplatin alone, or cisplatin, doxorubicin, and cyclophosphamide.
[b] There was no significant difference in OS between any of the three treatment arms of GOG-132 ($p = 0.31$).

documented disease progression. These results support the concept that sequential treatment with a platinum agent, followed by paclitaxel, may be therapeutically equivalent to combination therapy with both agents in advanced ovarian cancer. However, as crossover to the alternative agent was not a formal part of this study's design, this interpretation should be viewed with caution, and combination first-line chemotherapy with a taxane and platinum compound remains the standard of care.

A third European randomized trial (ICON-3) compared a nonpaclitaxel, platinum-based control regimen (either single-agent carboplatin or the combination of cisplatin, doxorubicin, and cyclophosphamide) to an experimental arm of carboplatin and paclitaxel.[90] Surprisingly, this study failed to reveal a difference in survival between either control arm and the paclitaxel-containing experimental arm. Perhaps the most likely explanation for this observation is that one-third of the patients in the control arms of ICON-3 ultimately received paclitaxel at some point in their disease course.[91] Thus, as in the previously mentioned three-arm GOG study,[89] this outcome provides circumstantial evidence to suggest that the sequential administration of these two active agents may be therapeutically equivalent to combination drug delivery in this setting.

Three randomized trials have directly compared a carboplatin and paclitaxel combination to cisplatin and paclitaxel (Table 76.5).[61,92,93] These studies found equivalent PFS and overall survivals for either carboplatin- or cisplatin-containing regimens, but with a more favorable toxicity profile associated with carboplatin-based treatment. Thus, the carboplatin-based combination (carboplatin, area under the curve [AUC] = 5 to 6, and paclitaxel, 175 mg/m^2, administered over 3 hours) is preferred when systemic

chemotherapy is indicated, due to reduced toxicity and the ability to give paclitaxel over a shorter infusion time. For individuals who may have difficulty tolerating a combination regimen (e.g., those with marginal performance status or significant comorbid medical conditions), it is reasonable to initiate treatment with IV single-agent carboplatin and later add IV paclitaxel to the regimen or deliver the drugs as sequential single agents. For appropriate patients with stage III disease who are optimally cytoreduced, *IP* chemotherapy is an important new option, which will be described in detail subsequently.

The optimal choice of taxane has also been investigated in the first-line setting. A randomized trial comparing IV carboplatin (AUC = 5) plus paclitaxel (175 mg/m^2) to IV carboplatin (AUC = 5) and docetaxel (75 mg/m^2) has shown equivalent response rates and PFS and overall survival for the two programs, although their toxicity profiles differed.[94] More grade 4 neutropenia occurred with the docetaxel-containing regimen, and a greater incidence of grade 2 or 3 neuropathy was observed with the paclitaxel-containing program. These data indicate that a carboplatin and docetaxel combination is an acceptable first-line regimen for patients with advanced ovarian cancer, especially in the setting of preexisting neuropathy (where paclitaxel may be difficult to tolerate).

There appears to be no value in extending platinum-based first-line therapy beyond six cycles.[95,96] Furthermore, there is no convincing evidence to suggest a benefit to the addition of cytotoxic drugs such as liposomal doxorubicin, epirubicin, topotecan, or gemcitabine to the platinum and taxane doublet.[97] A recent randomized trial performed by the Japanese GOG demonstrated a PFS and overall survival advantage for the use of weekly paclitaxel (in conjunction with day 1 carboplatin) in newly diagnosed

TABLE 76.5

Randomized Trials of Carboplatin and Paclitaxel Versus Cisplatin and Paclitaxel in Advance Epithelial Ovarian Cancer

Trial and Randomization[a]	Patient Number	Stage	Median PFS (mo)	Median OS (mo)
GOG-158[61]	792	III[b]		
Paclitaxel (175 mg/m^2)				
Carboplatin (AUC 7.5)			20.7	57.4
			0.88 (0.75–1.03)[c]	0.84 (0.70–1.02)
Paclitaxel (135 mg/m^2)			19.4	48.7
Cisplatin (75 mg/m^2)				
AGO[92]	798	IIB–IV		
Paclitaxel (185 mg/m^2)			17.2	43.3
Carboplatin (AUC 6)				
			1.05 (0.89–1.23)	1.05 (0.87–1.26)
Paclitaxel (185 mg/m^2)			19.1	44.1
Cisplatin (75 mg/m^2)				
Netherlands-Denmark[93]	208	IIB–IV		
Paclitaxel (175 mg/m^2)				
Carboplatin (AUC 5)				
			16	31[d]
Paclitaxel (175 mg/m^2)				
Cisplatin (75 mg/m^2)				

PFS, progression-free survival; OS, overall survival; GOG, Gynecologic Oncology Group; AUC, area under the curve; AGO, Arbeitsgemeinschaft Gynaekologische Onkologie.
[a] Six cycles of chemotherapy were administered in each trial unless otherwise stated.
[b] Patients enrolled in GOG-158 were required to have an optimal cytoreduction, as defined as residual disease ≤1 cm in greatest diameter.
[c] Hazard ratio followed by 95% confidence interval in parentheses.
[d] The Netherlands-Denmark trial was not sufficiently powered to assess noninferiority. Therefore, the survival data shown reflect the entire patient cohort, as opposed to the individual treatment groups.

patients with ovarian cancer, and confirmatory trials are under way.[98] Given the activity of bevacizumab in relapsed disease, there is interest in investigating the value of this agent in the first line and maintenance setting (see the following).

Intraperitoneal Chemotherapy

Epithelial ovarian cancer is largely confined to the peritoneal space during most of its natural history.[2] Given this relatively localized distribution, efforts to instill chemotherapy directly into the peritoneal cavity have received a great deal of attention over the past two decades. The rationale for this approach is based on the observation that many active drugs such as cisplatin and paclitaxel have favorable peritoneal-to-plasma concentrations, on the order of 20 to 1 and 1,000 to 1, respectively.[99] The ability to deliver high local concentrations of active drugs, with generally acceptable systemic side effects, suggested that it may be possible to achieve more effective cytoreduction of disease that is present at the peritoneal surface. Given the rather limited penetration of such drugs into peritoneal tumor, to a depth of only a few millimeters, patients with optimally cytoreduced disease are theoretically most likely to benefit from this approach.

Three randomized trials have addressed the role of IP chemotherapy in the first-line management of patients with optimally debulked stage III disease (Table 76.6). Two of these trials showed a statistically significant improvement in both PFS and overall survival rates for patients treated with IP chemotherapy, and the other demonstrated improvement in PFS only (although a nonsignificant trend for improved overall survival in the IP arm was noted). The first of these was an intergroup trial performed in 546 optimally debulked stage III patients with ≤2-cm residual disease (GOG 104).[100] Note that this definition of "optimally debulked" was widely accepted at the time, although subsequently a 1-cm cutoff has been adopted. Patients were randomized to receive either IP cisplatin or IV cisplatin, in combination with IV cyclophosphamide, every 3 weeks for six cycles (note that paclitaxel was not an approved drug at the time of this study's design). The median survival of all eligible patients was 49 months for the IP cisplatin arm compared to 41 months for the IV cisplatin group ($p = 0.02$; HR = 0.76). There was also a trend toward a higher likelihood of pathologic complete remission in the IP arm compared to IV treatment (47% versus 36%, respectively). However, the positive results of this study were overshadowed by the emerging value of the IV paclitaxel and platinum combination in the first-line setting,[62] and the added benefit of the IP route remained uncertain. Specifically, it was argued that perhaps the use of IV paclitaxel might negate the benefit of IP therapy, and this issue led to a second randomized IP trial that included paclitaxel.

The second study performed by the GOG (GOG 114) involved optimally debulked patients with stage III disease (≤1-cm diameter residual) who were randomized to receive either IV paclitaxel (135 mg/m² over 24 hours) and IV cisplatin (75 mg/m²) for six cycles, or IV carboplatin (AUC = 9) for two cycles followed by IV paclitaxel (135 mg/m² administered over 24 hours) and IP cisplatin (100 mg/m²) for six cycles.[101] The median PFSs for the IP and IV arms were 28 months and 22 months, respectively ($p = 0.01$; one-sided t test). However, there was only a borderline significant trend in overall survival in favor of the IP treatment arm (63.2 months versus 52.5 months, respectively; $p = 0.05$, one-sided t test), but with substantial toxicity partly due to the use of high-dose, single-agent carboplatin in the experimental arm. The significant toxicity of this regimen, coupled with only a borderline significant survival difference, did not provide convincing enough evidence to adopt this regimen for widespread use.

TABLE 76.6

Selected Randomized Trials of Intraperitoneal First-Line Therapy in Optimally Debulked Stage III Ovarian Cancer

Trial and Randomization[a]	Patient Number	Median PFS (mo)	Median OS (mo)	Hazard Ratio (95% CI, *p* value)
GOG-104/SWOG-8501[100,b]	546			
Cisplatin IP (100 mg/m²)		NA	49	
Cyclophosphamide IV (600 mg/m²)				0.76 (0.61–0.96; p = 0.02)
Cisplatin IV (100 mg/m²)		NA	41	
Cyclophosphamide IV (600 mg/m²)				
GOG-114[101]	462			
Carboplatin (AUC 9 for two cycles)		28	63	
Paclitaxel IV (135 mg/m²)				
Cisplatin IP (100 mg/m²)				0.81 (0.65–1.0; p = 0.056)[c]
Paclitaxel IV (135 mg/m²)		22	52	
Cisplatin IV (75 mg/m²)				
GOG-172[102]	429			
Paclitaxel IV day 1 (135 mg/m²)		23.8	65.6	
Cisplatin IP day 2 (100 mg/m²)				
Paclitaxel IP day 8 (60 mg/m²)				0.75 (0.58–0.97; p = 0.03)
Paclitaxel IV (135 mg/m²)		18.3	49.7	
Cisplatin IV (75 mg/m²)				

PFS, progression-free survival; OS, overall survival; CI, confidence interval; GOG, Gynecologic Oncology Group; SWOG, Southwest Oncology Group; IP, intraperitoneal; NA, not available; IV, intravenous; AUC, area under the curve.
[a] Six cycles of chemotherapy were administered in each trial unless otherwise stated.
[b] Optimal cytoreduction in GOG-104/SWOG-8501 was defined as ≤2-cm diameter residual disease, whereas a 1-cm cutoff was used for GOG-114 and GOG-172.
[c] P value determined using a one-sided t test.

carboplatin, epirubicin, and prednimustine to observation or WAR (30 Gy in 1.5-Gy fractions, using 12 to 18 MeV photons), followed by pelvic and para-aortic and partial diaphragm boosts (total doses to these regions, 51.6 Gy and 42.6 Gy, respectively).[114] The 5-year relapse-free survival and overall survival rates in the observation arm were 26% and 33%, respectively, compared to rates of 49% and 59%, respectively, in the WAR arm. One patient in the WAR arm developed a small bowel obstruction.

A trial conducted by the GOG and North Central Cancer Treatment Group from 1987 to 1996 enrolled 202 patients with initial stage III disease in complete clinical remission following chemotherapy (almost all had received a platinum-containing agent, and 39% also received paclitaxel) who then had a second-look laparotomy that found no gross residual disease.[115] They were either observed or treated with IP chromic phosphate (15 mCi). Of note, 15% of patients assigned to the ^{32}P arm did not receive it for various reasons. With a median follow-up time of 63 months, the 5-year relapse-free survival rates in the two arms were 36% and 42%, respectively, and the 5-year overall survival rates were 63% and 67%, respectively. These differences were not statistically significant. Results were not analyzed according to whether the patient had microscopic or no pathologic evidence of disease at second-look surgery. A total of 2 of 98 patients in the control arm and 3 of 104 in the ^{32}P arm developed long-term grade 3 or 4 gastrointestinal complications.

A trial conducted in Sweden and Norway from 1988 to 1993 enrolled patients with initial stage III ovarian carcinoma who had no evidence of disease after initial surgery or who responded to induction chemotherapy (four courses of cisplatin 50 mg/m^2 with either doxorubicin or epirubicin) who then underwent second-look laparotomy.[116] Ninety-eight patients with no gross or microscopic residual disease were randomly allocated to observation, six further cycles of the same chemotherapy, or WAR (20 Gy in 1-Gy fractions using an open field technique) followed by an extended pelvic boost (from the L3-4 interspace to the pelvic floor, 20.4 Gy in 1.7-Gy fractions using opposed anterior-posterior fields). Seventy-four patients with microscopic residual disease were randomized to the same chemotherapy or WAR. The length of follow-up was not stated, but data were collected up to early 2002. The 5-year PFS rates in the patients with no residual microscopic disease were 36%, 36%, and 56% in the observation, chemotherapy, and WAR arms, respectively; the difference was statistically significant. However, the 5-year overall survival rates were 65%, 57%, and 69%, respectively, and these differences were not statistically significant. In patients with microscopic residual disease, the 5-year PFS rates in the chemotherapy and WAR arms were 25% and 16%, respectively, and the 10-year rates were 22% and 5%, respectively. The 5-year overall survival rates were 41% for the chemotherapy arm and 32% for the WAR arm; 10-year rates were 23% and 10%, respectively. None of these differences was statistically significant. A total of 4 of 69 patients receiving WAR (6%) required bowel diversion due to bowel obstruction or adhesions, compared to no such complications occurring in the chemotherapy or observation group.

Finally, an international trial conducted from 1998 to 2003 enrolled 447 patients with a negative second-look laparotomy following initial treatment with surgery and platinum-based chemotherapy. Patients were randomly assigned to receive or not to receive a single IP injection of a radiolabeled monoclonal antibody directed against the MUC1 antigen using yttrium-90 (18 mCi, or 666 MBq/m^2).[117] Two-thirds of patients had stage III disease; 90% had no microscopic residual disease at second-look. With a median follow-up of 3.5 years, there was no difference in relapse or survival rates between the arms.

Despite these negative results, it is possible that patients with certain subtypes of ovarian cancer might derive benefit from consolidation radiation therapy. For instance, retrospective studies from the British Columbia Cancer Agency in Canada suggested that patients with stage I-II clear cell, mucinous, or endometriod cancers had reduced failure rates and better overall survival

when patients received WAR in addition to three or six cycles of platinum-containing chemotherapy, compared to chemotherapy alone.[118] It is also possible that clear cell histology may predict for benefit of radiotherapy, although data from prospective randomized trials are lacking.[119]

In conclusion, the value of radiation therapy as consolidation therapy following chemotherapy for patients with ovarian cancer is uncertain. The available randomized studies have conflicting results, especially in the subgroup of patients with no detectable residual disease after platinum-based chemotherapy. However, these studies were relatively small, with heterogeneous patient characteristics and treatments, and hence their statistical power to show clinically meaningful differences was limited. Further, no trials have been conducted for patients treated initially with both platinum compounds and paclitaxel. It seems likely that any benefits of consolidation radiation therapy are quite small in this setting. These must be weighed against their potential toxicity, although modern radiation techniques may reduce the toxicity of WAR compared to past approaches.[120] Hence, routine use of consolidation radiotherapy after chemotherapy is not generally recommended.

Maintenance Therapy

Several investigators have explored the value of maintenance or consolidation approaches after achievement of a clinical complete remission in patients with advanced epithelial ovarian cancer. In a randomized trial conducted by the Southwest Oncology Group and the GOG, women with advanced disease who experienced a clinically defined complete response were randomly assigned to receive either 3 cycles or 12 cycles of single-agent paclitaxel (175 mg/m^2 over 3 hours) administered every 28 days.[121] The study was stopped early when an interim analysis revealed a 50% reduction in the risk of recurrence associated with the 12-month maintenance strategy (median PFS for the 12-month and 3-month paclitaxel arms was 28 months and 21 months, respectively; $p = 0.0023$). However, there was no difference in overall survival between the two regimens, which was also true in a subsequent analysis with longer follow-up. Interpretation of long-term data from this study will be confounded by crossover, whereby patients randomized to the three-cycle arm received additional maintenance paclitaxel after study closure. Likewise, a more recent randomized trial conducted in Europe showed no survival benefit to the use of six cycles of maintenance single-agent paclitaxel in this setting.[122] Based on these data, maintenance single-agent paclitaxel cannot be recommended as a standard approach in patients who achieve a complete clinical remission after a platinum-based first-line chemotherapy.

The GOG has conducted a three-arm, placebo-controlled randomized trial investigating the role of maintenance bevacizumab (anti–VEGF-A neutralizing antibody) for 1 year in newly diagnosed patients with stage III or IV disease (GOG 218). This study showed that median PFS was significantly increased by 3.8 months ($p < 0.0001$) in patients receiving bevacizumab during first-line chemotherapy, followed by single-agent maintenance bevacizumab for approximately 1 year thereafter, compared with chemotherapy alone.[123] No improvement in quality of life or overall survival was noted at the time of publication. A similar question was addressed in a two-arm European trial (ICON-7) for newly diagnosed patients with either optimally or suboptimally debulked disease. Analysis of mature PFS data from that study showed a 2.4-month median PFS benefit ($p = 0.04$) associated with bevacizumab, without improvement in quality of life or overall survival at the time of publication.[124] More recently, a randomized trial investigating maintenance pazopanib (a VEGF-receptor tyrosine kinase inhibitor) showed similar results, with extension of PFS but without an overall survival advantage thus far.[125] Neither bevacizumab nor pazopanib are currently approved by the US Food and Drug Administration for maintenance use in ovarian cancer due to the lack of either an overall survival advantage or quality-of-life improvement, although additional follow-up of these studies is ongoing.

Surveillance After First-Line Chemotherapy

Over 50% of newly diagnosed patients with advanced-stage epithelial ovarian cancer will achieve a clinical complete remission after platinum and taxane induction chemotherapy.[2] Clinical complete remission is defined as no evidence of disease on physical examination, a normal CA 125 level, and normal radiographic studies such as CT. Patients with advanced-stage disease who achieve a clinical complete remission have a high chance of relapse and are typically followed with serial physician visits, including pelvic examinations and CA 125 determinations. The value of routine CA 125 surveillance after completion of first-line chemotherapy has recently been challenged by the OV05 randomized trial.[19] Patients who underwent CA 125 surveillance, with early institution of cytotoxic chemotherapy for serologic relapse, did not experience improved quality of life or survival compared with those followed solely on the basis of physical examination and symptoms. Despite these negative results, it is possible that CA 125 surveillance may prove to be valuable once more effective salvage therapies become available or for those settings in which clinical trials might be available for patients with early relapse. In addition, CA 125 surveillance may still play an important role in well-informed patients who may feel empowered by knowing their CA 125 levels. Thus, the use of this test for surveillance purposes should be individualized. Routine performance of CT in the absence of symptoms, findings on physical examination, or an elevated CA 125 level has no proven value in the management of patients with this disease. This is partly due to the lack of sensitivity of CT compared to serologic testing with CA 125, which is currently the most sensitive method for detection of early relapse. Thus, CT is typically reserved for further evaluation of signs, symptoms, or serologic evidence of relapse. Likewise, there is currently no proven benefit for routine surveillance with other radiographic tests such as PET scans in the posttreatment setting.[23] Although performance of a second-look laparotomy after completion of first-line therapy will reveal residual disease in over half of all patients with advanced ovarian cancer who have achieved a complete clinical remission, this procedure does not appear to confer a survival advantage.[61] This is due to the current lack of curative treatment options for patients with disease that persists after platinum-based, first-line therapy. In addition, a negative second-look laparotomy does not guarantee against the development of disease relapse, which occurs in 50% of patients with advanced-stage disease who have a negative second-look procedure.[2] For these reasons, second-look laparotomy is no longer considered a standard procedure in the assessment of patients after completion of first-line therapy, although it is sometimes used as an investigation tool in the context of clinical trials.

Management of Recurrent Disease

Hormonal Therapy

Most patients with advanced ovarian cancer will recur after first-line chemotherapy.[2] Recurrence is often manifested by a rising CA 125 in the absence of symptoms or objective evidence of disease as assessed by examination or CT (marker-only relapse). Unfortunately, the majority of patients with recurrent ovarian cancer are destined to die of their tumors, regardless of the second-line treatment modality used. Patients who demonstrate marker-only evidence of relapse, without symptoms or findings on examination or CT, are often initially managed with a drug like tamoxifen or an aromatase inhibitor. These drugs are potentially active in ovarian cancer[126,127] and are generally well tolerated. The response to hormonal agents is typically slow and may require approximately 2 to 3 months before a reduction in the CA 125 level is evident.

Chemotherapy

Chemotherapy for recurrent disease is usually indicated for the development of tumor-related symptoms, objective evidence of

significant disease on examination or CT, or failure of hormonal therapy. Platinum is the most active agent in the management of patients with epithelial ovarian cancer, and retreatment with this drug may produce valuable responses that translate into improvement in quality of life. However, the likelihood of benefit depends on the interval between the last dose of platinum and the time of relapse (i.e., the platinum-free interval, PFI). Patients with a PFI of <6 months are less likely to respond to second-line platinum and are often managed with an alternative agent, as described subsequently.[128] Such patients are referred to as platinum resistant, although a small percentage may still derive benefit from platinum rechallenge. Patients with a PFI of between 6 and 24 months have an approximately 30% chance of benefit from second-line platinum used at the time of relapse. In patients with a very prolonged PFI (e.g., >2 years), the response rate with second-line platinum may be as high as 60% to 70%.[128] Patients with a PFI of >6 months are referred to as potentially platinum sensitive and are often treated with either single-agent platinum or a combination of platinum with another agent such as paclitaxel, gemcitabine, or liposomal doxorubicin.

Three randomized trials have investigated the value of combination chemotherapy in the setting of potentially platinum-sensitive relapse (PFI >6 months). The ICON-4 trial compared combination chemotherapy with paclitaxel and platinum to single-agent platinum in patients with potentially platinum-sensitive disease, with most patients having a PFI of $\geq$12 months.[129] This study demonstrated a statistically significant improvement in overall survival for the combination regimen, with an absolute difference at 2 years of 7% ($p = 0.023$). However, 58% of patients in the single-agent platinum arm never received a taxane as part of first-line therapy, and 69% of patients in the single-agent platinum arm never received a taxane as part of relapse management (i.e., after progression on single-agent platinum). Thus, 40% of patients in the single-agent platinum arm never received a taxane at any point during the course of their disease. Given the proven survival benefit of taxanes in this disease, the imbalance in the use of taxanes between these two treatment arms makes the results of ICON-4 difficult to interpret.

The second trial performed by the Arbeitsgemeinschaft Gynaekologische Onkologie from Germany randomized patients with potentially platinum-sensitive relapse to either gemcitabine and carboplatin or carboplatin alone.[130] PFS was 8.6 months for the combination versus 5.8 months for single-agent carboplatin ($p = 0.0038$), although overall survival was not improved in the combination chemotherapy arm. Quality of life appeared to be equivalent between the two arms, despite a higher incidence of thrombocytopenia, neutropenia, and anemia with combination chemotherapy.

The third trial compared paclitaxel and carboplatin with liposomal doxorubicin and carboplatin in patients with platinum-sensitive relapse.[131] There was a statistically significant improvement in median PFS (11.3 months versus 9.4 months; $p = 0.005$), with a lower incidence of severe hypersensitivity reactions (5% versus 18%), in favor of the liposomal doxorubicin-containing arm. No difference in overall survival was noted at the time of this report. More frequent grade 2 or greater alopecia (83.6% versus 7%) and sensory neuropathy (26.9% versus 4.9%) were observed in the paclitaxel-containing arm, while more hand-foot syndrome (grade 2 to 3, 12.0% versus 2.2%), nausea (35.2% versus 24.2%), and mucositis (grade 2-3, 13.9% versus 7%) in the liposomal doxorubicin-containing arm.

Because the primary goal of relapse management is palliation of symptoms, the decision to use combinations in this setting should be based on a number of factors, including patient age, amount of disease, kinetics of relapse, and patient preference after a discussion of the issues.[132] For older patients who require chemotherapy for asymptomatic, minimal volume, potentially platinum-sensitive relapse, it is still reasonable to use single-agent carboplatin as a first step. As described subsequently, liposomal doxorubicin is a generally well-tolerated alternative if there is a contraindication to the use of carboplatin, if carboplatin fails to induce a response, or if an allergic reaction develops to carboplatin that precludes further administration. With either single-agent carboplatin or liposomal doxorubicin, patients have minimal problems with alopecia or myelosuppression, and their quality of life is generally well preserved. For younger patients who wish to adopt an aggressive approach to the management of potentially platinum-sensitive relapse, combination chemotherapy with either paclitaxel and carboplatin, gemcitabine and carboplatin, or liposomal doxorubicin and carboplatin is reasonable. This is especially the case for the symptomatic patient with kinetically brisk relapse or the patient who has undergone a successful secondary cytoreduction after a very long PFI.[132] There are currently no data supporting a role for combination chemotherapy regimens in the management of patients with platinum-resistant relapse.

Patients who are platinum resistant, as defined by a short PFI of <6 months or progression during platinum-based chemotherapy, or those who tolerate second-line platinum poorly, are typically treated with a variety of single agents. Potentially non–cross-resistant drugs with activity in the platinum-resistant setting include liposomal doxorubicin, paclitaxel, docetaxel, topotecan, gemcitabine, pemetrexed, ixabepilone, or oral etoposide.[133] Liposomal doxorubicin is often well tolerated in doses of 40 mg/m^2 given every 4 weeks, although the development of palmer-planar erythrodysesthesia (hand-foot syndrome) or mucositis may require dose reductions and treatment delays.[134] Topotecan may cause significant myelosuppression and fatigue, although this agent is generally well tolerated through the use of weekly dosing schedules.[135] Unfortunately, the likelihood of obtaining a response to any of these agents in the platinum-resistant setting is <20%, responses are generally short lived (median PFS in the range of 4 to 6 months), and they tend to become progressively shorter with each subsequent regimen.[132]

Several investigational agents are being studied in the relapsed setting. Bevacizumab is a humanized antibody that recognizes and neutralizes VEGF, an angiogenic factor that is often secreted by ovarian cancer cells. Randomized data in metastatic colorectal, breast, and lung cancers have shown a survival advantage for the use of this drug in combination with chemotherapy.[136–138] As a single agent, bevacizumab has been shown by the GOG to induce responses in 18% of patients with relapsed ovarian cancer (either platinum sensitive or platinum resistant, treated with less than or equal to two prior regimens), with 39% of patients progression-free at 6 months.[139] A recent multi-institutional nationwide study restricted to platinum-resistant patients reported a response rate of 16%, with 27% of patients progression free at 6 months.[140] However, there was an 11% incidence of potentially life-threatening bowel perforation, prompting early closure of this study. Compared to the GOG study, all patients in this trial were platinum resistant and heavily pretreated, with 50% having received three prior regimens. It has been suggested that the risk of bowel perforation with bevacizumab in the recurrent ovarian cancer setting might be related to a higher number of prior treatment regimens, radiographic evidence of bowel wall involvement by tumor, or the presence of bowel obstruction.[140] These and other possible risk factors for this complication will require further evaluation.

In addition to its use as a single agent, bevacizumab has also been combined with cytotoxic chemotherapy in the relapsed setting. In patients with platinum-sensitive relapse, the OCEANS study randomized patients to receive either the combination of carboplatin, gemcitabine, and placebo, or the combination of carboplatin, gemcitabine, and bevacizumab, for up to 10 cycles, followed by with single-agent placebo or bevacizumab until progression.[141] A 4-month improvement in median PFS in favor of the bevacizumab combination ($p < 0.0001$) was observed, but without an overall survival advantage. The overall response rate was also improved in the bevacizumab-containing arm compared to placebo (78.5% and 57.4%, respectively, $p < 0.0001$), associated with

prolongation of median response duration by 3 months. In patients with platinum-resistant relapse, the combination of bevacizumab with either liposomal doxorubicin, topotecan, or weekly paclitaxel has been studied in the AURELIA trial.[142] As for the OCEANS study, the combination of bevacizumab with either of these single agents was associated with statistically significant prolongation of median PFS, a higher response rate, but no improvement in overall survival. Although not yet approved by the US Food and Drug Administration for these indications, these studies suggest that there may be a role for combining bevacizumab with these specific chemotherapy regimens in the relapsed setting.

Other investigational agents with reported activity in platinum-sensitive (and, to a lesser degree, platinum-resistant) disease include ET743 (trabectedin), halichondrin B, pertuzumab, epothilones, and AMG386.[143,144] Receptor tyrosine kinase inhibitors that target the VEGF receptor such as AZD2171 (cediranib) appear to have activity and are being studied in combination with platinum-based chemotherapy.[145] In contrast, epidermal growth factor–receptor inhibitors such as gefitinib appear to have low activity in the recurrent disease setting. An exciting new class of agents that inhibit poly-adenosine diphosphate-ribose polymerase is demonstrating important activity in patients with recurrent disease, especially those who harbor a germline mutation in BRCA1 or BRCA2.[146,147] Poly-adenosine diphosphate-ribose polymerase inhibitors such as olaparib have also been studied as a maintenance strategy in unselected patients with platinum-sensitive relapse, with an improvement in median PFS but without an overall survival benefit.[148] Whether selection of patients on the basis of germline BRCA mutation status will enrich for those most likely to derive benefit with maintenance olaparib, in either the first line or recurrent disease setting, is under investigation. At present, none of these agents is currently approved by the US Food and Drug Administration for treating patients with relapsed ovarian cancer, and their ultimate value needs to be better defined.

The agents mentioned previously have largely been studied in patients who have relapsed with high-grade serous disease. Within the past few years, based on a greater understanding of the heterogeneity of epithelial ovarian cancer, particularly the molecular biology of uncommon subtypes, the GOG has initiated clinical trials for women with recurrent low-grade serous carcinoma and clear cell carcinoma. Low-grade serous cancer is a distinct entity characterized by advanced stage, molecular features such as K-ras (30%) or BRAF (5%) mutation, as opposed to p53 mutation more typical of high-grade disease, and it is relatively chemoresistant. In the relapsed setting, the response rate to conventional cytotoxic chemotherapy options is in the range of only 5%, whereas the response to hormonal agents like tamoxifen or aromatase inhibitors is generally higher, in the range of 10% to 15%.[149,150] A recent retrospective review suggests that there may be value in combining bevacizumab with conventional cytotoxic agents in patients who relapse with low-grade serous ovarian cancer, although this requires additional prospective validation.[151] Finally, given the presence of K-ras mutation, and to a lesser extent BRAF mutation, in low-grade serous cancer, it is reasonable to expect that downstream mediators of the MAP-kinase pathway such as MEK might serve as therapeutic targets. In that regard, the MEK 1/2 inhibitor selumetinib was recently shown to yield a 15% response rate in patients with relapsed low-grade serous ovarian or primary peritoneal cancer, although no predictive biomarkers could be identified.[152] In 2014, the GOG has launched a randomized phase 2/3 study of a similar MEK inhibitor, trametinib, in patients with relapsed low-grade serous cancer, comparing the activity of this agent with that of cytotoxic chemotherapy.

Recurrent clear cell carcinoma of the ovary appears also to be relatively chemoresistant.[153,154] Potential targets for clear cell carcinoma of the ovary include VEGF, the PI3K/AKT/mTOR pathway, c-MET, and the IL-6/STAT3/HIF pathway. Thus, the GOG has initiated a clinical trial with sunitinib for women with recurrent clear cell carcinoma, with two other trials in development.

Surgery

Secondary cytoreductive surgery refers to an attempt at surgical debulking of disease at the time of relapse and is performed in selected patients prior to the administration of second-line chemotherapy. The ability to perform a successful secondary cytoreduction, as generally defined by having no gross residual disease >1 cm in diameter, is associated with a median survival advantage in retrospective studies.[155] However, it is possible that the *ability* to perform a successful secondary cytoreduction may simply identify those patients with biologically less aggressive disease or those with a lower tumor burden at the time of relapse. The only way to determine whether secondary cytoreduction has intrinsic therapeutic value is to conduct a randomized trial of this procedure, which has not yet been performed.

Patients who relapse within 6 to 12 months after completion of first-line therapy, especially if they have ascites, are generally not candidates for this procedure.[155] Occasional patients with late relapses (i.e., >2 to 3 years after finishing chemotherapy) or those with apparently isolated relapses may experience a prolonged disease-free interval after successful secondary cytoreduction followed by additional chemotherapy. The value of secondary cytoreduction is currently being investigated in two prospective, randomized trials: GOG 213 and the Arbeitsgemeinschaft Gynaekologische Onkologie Desktop III study.

Palliative surgery may be of benefit for patients with recurrent ovarian cancer. Common operations performed in this setting include colostomy for relief of a large bowel obstruction, lysis of adhesions, and management of small bowel obstruction. The decision to perform surgery to relieve small bowel obstruction should take into account the time elapsed from the original diagnosis to the development of obstruction, as well as the likelihood for continued responsiveness to chemotherapy postoperatively. Women who develop small bowel obstruction during first-line chemotherapy have biologically aggressive tumors that are usually not amenable to surgical intervention. A palliative gastrostomy tube may be most appropriate in this situation, and frequently this can be inserted endoscopically or under CT guidance. In contrast, women who have had prolonged periods of freedom from disease, usually lasting >1 year from the original diagnosis, may benefit from small bowel surgery to relieve obstruction. Surgery generally plays no role in management of patients with a pseudo-obstructive pattern due to intra-abdominal carcinomatosis, with infiltration of the myoenteric plexus of the small bowel. Metoclopramide, which improves motility of the upper gastrointestinal tract without stimulating gastric, biliary, or pancreatic secretions, may at times be helpful for this condition. Large bowel obstruction (particularly sigmoid colon obstruction) is often relieved by performing a colostomy, which can provide significant prolongation of survival and improved quality of life in appropriate patients.

Radiation Therapy

A minority of patients with localized recurrences may experience prolonged survival after WAR or limited-field irradiation.[156–158] For example, a study from the MD Anderson Cancer Center included 102 patients treated with doses of ≥45 Gy to localized nodal or extranodal recurrences.[158] With a median follow-up of 37 months, the 5-year PFS and overall survival rates were 24% and 40%, respectively. Results were better for the eight patients with clear cell carcinoma (5-year PFS and overall survival rates of 75% and 88%, respectively) than for patients with other histologies (20% and 33%, respectively). The 5-year in-field disease control rate was higher for the 16 patients who had complete gross tumor resection (88%) than for the 73 patients with gross residual disease (68%) or the 13 patients with a complete response to chemotherapy who did not undergo surgery (68%). However, the small number of highly selected patients in these series, their heterogeneous presentations, and the highly variable treatments they received before and after

radiation make it difficult to adequately assess whether radiation therapy truly improves long-term outcome in this setting.

Although rarely curative, radiation therapy can play a role in the palliation of some patients with recurrent ovarian cancer. Symptoms from a growing pelvic mass can cause pain, bleeding, and rectal narrowing. Palliative pelvic radiotherapy can provide rapid relief and, in some cases, may prevent or delay the need for diverting colostomy. Doses of 8 to 10 Gy in a single fraction, 20 Gy in 5 fractions, 30 Gy in 10 fractions, or higher total doses given in smaller fractions have produced acceptable short-term results, with serious complications in 5% or fewer patients. Finally, patients with epithelial ovarian cancer may rarely develop isolated cerebral or bone metastases that can often be successfully palliated with radiotherapy.

BORDERLINE TUMORS

Definition and Clinical Features

Ovarian borderline tumors are epithelial neoplasms that are histologically distinguished from ovarian carcinomas by the absence of stromal invasion. These neoplasms are also referred to as tumors of LMP, which reflects their indolent natural history.[159] Although borderline tumors generally do not exhibit stromal invasion within the ovary, cells from the primary tumor mass can be shed into the peritoneal cavity and eventually form serosal implants that involve the bowel, omentum, and upper abdomen. Nonetheless, the majority of patients with borderline tumors present with early stage disease.[12]

The median age of women developing borderline tumors is 40 years, approximately 20 years younger than the median age for women with epithelial ovarian cancer. Women may be diagnosed with an asymptomatic mass on routine pelvic examination or may come to medical attention due to pelvic pain. Nonspecific gastrointestinal symptoms such as abdominal bloating or early satiety may rarely occur.

As with epithelial cancers of the ovary, borderline tumors may exhibit serous or mucinous features. Serous borderline tumors are more common and may be bilateral in 10% to 20% of cases.[159] Mucinous borderline tumors tend to be larger than their serous counterparts, are infrequently bilateral, and are occasionally associated with pseudomyxoma peritonei. Pseudomyxoma peritonei is characterized by a hypocellular, gelatinous material secreted by an intra-abdominal tumor, eventually filling the peritoneal cavity and encasing abdominal contents such as bowel. This condition may be associated with mucinous borderline ovarian tumor, mucinous ovarian carcinoma, or gastrointestinal tumors such as appendiceal mucinous cystadenocarcinoma. The latter diagnosis may occur synchronously with a primary ovarian mucinous neoplasm or may mimic a primary ovarian tumor by metastasizing to the ovary (often right sided, reflecting the proximity of the appendix to the right ovary). The mainstay of treatment for pseudomyxoma peritonei is intermittent surgery to remove the gelatinous material, although this is not curative in the majority of cases, and repeated debulking attempts are associated with increased potential for adhesions and complications such as bowel obstruction.

The distinctive pathologic and biologic behaviors of these tumors were recognized by the WHO in 1973 (see Table 76.1).[4] Borderline malignant potential tumors are distinguished from benign cystadenomas by the presence of epithelial budding, multilayering of the epithelium, increased mitotic activity, and nuclear atypia. They are distinguished from epithelial carcinomas by the absence of stromal invasion. In the spectrum of aggressiveness between epithelial ovarian carcinoma and benign ovarian tumors such as cystadenoma, borderline tumors are closer to benign ovarian tumors in their clinical behavior. However, they are accorded their own classification based on distinctive histologic features, their potential to occasionally spread beyond the ovary, and their ability to recur and lead to death in a minority of patients.

Because the absence of stromal invasion is a criterion for making this diagnosis, careful examination of the tissue blocks is necessary to exclude a component of invasive carcinoma. In this regard, approximately 20% of ovarian tumors diagnosed as borderline on frozen-section analysis prove to be carcinomas on review of the permanent section. The presence of microinvasion (as opposed to deep stromal invasion) is sometimes observed in a borderline tumor, in association with more typical histologic features. In such cases, the microinvasive component is typically no greater than 3 mm in depth, in which case it most likely does not impact on prognosis.[160] Mucinous borderline tumors are characterized by multiloculated cystic masses, with smooth outer surfaces and areas of papulations and solid thickening on the inner surface. Microscopically, the epithelial lining of cysts within a mucinous borderline tumor consists of tall, columnar, mucin-secreting cells, resembling the epithelium of the endocervix or intestine. Although mucinous borderline tumors lack stromal invasion, they are sometimes difficult to distinguish from their invasive mucinous carcinoma counterparts. Most mucinous borderline tumors have fewer than four layers of stratified mucinous cells and lack invasion, whereas mucinous carcinomas often demonstrate an infiltrative or expansile pattern of stromal involvement.[161]

Greater than 90% of patients with early stage borderline tumors are alive at 10 years, and >50% of patients with advanced disease experience long-term survival.[12] The fact that survival does not appear to be improved by postoperative adjuvant treatment with either chemotherapy or radiation attests to the slow growth rate of this tumor, which confers indolent behavior but at the same time results in resistance to modalities that target actively dividing cells. Nevertheless, a small fraction of patients with borderline tumors exhibits a more aggressive course, and attempts have been made to identify histologic correlates that might predict for worse outcome. Some investigators have proposed that borderline serous tumors may behave more aggressively if they are associated with micropapillary features or invasive implants elsewhere in the peritoneal cavity.[13,162,163] Micropapillary serous carcinoma is characterized by thin, elongated micropapillae with minimal or no fibrovascular support. Patients with invasive implants in the setting of a primary borderline tumor typically have a desmoplastic reaction within the implant, associated with an irregular, infiltrative border that invades underlying structures and replaces the fatty tissue of the underlying omentum.[163] An implant that simply shows desmoplasia, without these other features, should be referred to as a desmoplastic *noninvasive* implant and does not appear to predict a worse outcome, in contrast to its invasive counterpart. Patients with serous borderline tumors without invasive implants have expected 10-year survival rates of >95%, whereas those with serous borderline tumors and invasive implants have survival rates of approximately 60% to 70% at 10 years.[164] Of interest, the majority of patients with invasive implants, or those with recurrences that progressed to invasive carcinoma, have been found to have micropapillary features within the primary ovarian tumor on careful sectioning. Thus, it is possible that micropapillary features portend a poorer prognosis because of their association with invasive implants, although this is still an area of controversy.

Surgical Management

Surgery for patients with borderline tumors who have completed childbearing is identical to that recommended for epithelial ovarian cancer, including a total abdominal hysterectomy, bilateral salpingo-oophorectomy, tumor debulking, and full staging. Although unusual, patients with borderline tumors may sometimes have retroperitoneal nodal involvement that can benefit from debulking. In such cases, the tumor typically involves the sinusoidal nodal spaces, as opposed to nodal parenchyma. An appendectomy is considered in patients with suspected mucinous borderline tumors because of its occasional association with a primary appendiceal carcinoma.

In younger patients with early stage borderline tumor who wish to preserve fertility, conservative surgery with preservation of the uterus, the contralateral ovary and fallopian tube, and in some cases the ipsilateral ovary (i.e., cystectomy) may be appropriate treatment. Several studies have reported excellent outcomes with conservative management of such patients. One of the largest studies found a 12% recurrence rate for patients treated conservatively with either unilateral salpingo-oophorectomy ($n = 110$) or ovarian cystectomy ($n = 74$), compared to 2.5% for patients treated with hysterectomy and bilateral salpingo-oophorectomy.[165] Recurrences or progression to carcinoma (1.5%) were more common among patients with invasive implants or advanced-stage disease.

Borderline ovarian tumors have also been diagnosed during pregnancy. Conservative surgery is usually performed, and pregnancy does not appear to affect the prognosis. Most patients go on to deliver at full term without any complications.

Postoperative Management

There is currently no convincing evidence that postoperative adjuvant chemotherapy or radiation confers a survival advantage for patients with borderline tumors of any stage.[12] In the absence of effective postoperative adjuvant therapy, in a disease where long-term survival is generally excellent, simple observation with serial examinations is reasonable, with radiographic studies as needed to investigate new symptoms or findings on examination. Late relapses may occur and reveal persistent borderline histology, although transformation to low-grade invasive serous cancer is a more common occurrence in this setting.[166] Surgery is the mainstay of treating recurrent disease and can lead to long-term survival. Some patients who recur with borderline histology may respond to a hormonal option such as tamoxifen.[167] However, for patients with borderline tumors who recur with low-grade invasive serous cancer, surgical debulking followed by platinum-based chemotherapy is often recommended.

GERM CELL TUMORS OF THE OVARY

Definition and Clinical Features

Germ cell tumors of the ovary are much less common than epithelial ovarian neoplasms, accounting for 2% to 3% of all ovarian cancers in Western countries and usually occurring in younger women, with a peak incidence in women in their early 20s. An increased incidence of germ cell tumors is found in Asian and black populations, where these tumors may represent as many as 15% of all ovarian cancers. It is often possible to cure these malignancies while preserving fertility, which is an especially important consideration given the young age of most patients.

The WHO classification for germ cell tumors of the ovary is shown in Table 76.1.[4] These tumors are often divided into dysgerminoma, which is the female counterpart of male seminoma, and nondysgerminoma. Abdominal pain, distention, pelvic fullness, and urinary symptoms are common in patients with germ cell tumors of the ovary. In a minority of patients, abdominal pain can be severe, usually the result of hemorrhage, rupture, or ovarian torsion.

The rapid growth of most ovarian germ cell tumors causes pain due to stretching of the ovarian capsule, often prompting the patient to seek medical attention while the tumor is still confined to the ovary. Patients frequently have a palpable adnexal mass that is typically evaluated by TVU, which may show a complex cyst comprised of solid and cystic regions. Serum levels of α-fetoprotein (AFP) and β–human chorionic gonadotropin (HCG) are often helpful in recognizing the presence of an endodermal sinus tumor (AFP elevation only), embryonal carcinoma (both AFP and HCG elevation), or choriocarcinoma (HCG elevation only). Patients with pure immature teratoma of the ovary typically have normal levels of AFP and HCG, although the AFP may be elevated in 30% of cases. Patients with mature cystic teratoma (dermoid cyst), which is a benign germ cell tumor, usually have normal levels of AFP and HCG. Measurement of AFP and HCG levels is also useful to gauge the effectiveness of postoperative therapy and in monitoring for disease recurrence.

Occasionally, patients with choriocarcinoma have extreme elevation of the β-HCG that results in hyperthyroidism due to homology between β-HCG and thyroid-stimulating hormone. Patients with mature cystic teratoma may also present with hyperthyroidism related to tumor-derived secretion of thyroxine, produced by mature thyroid tissue present within the tumor itself (struma ovarii). Rare patients with mature cystic teratoma will experience a Coomb's positive hemolytic anemia that resolves after surgical resection of the mass.

In contrast to epithelial tumors, 60% to 70% of germ cell tumors are stage I at diagnosis. Stages II and IV tumors are relatively uncommon, and stage III disease accounts for about 25% to 30% of tumors. Bilateral ovarian involvement in most germ cell histologies is uncommon, although dysgerminoma and mature cystic teratoma may be bilateral in 10% to 15% of cases. More advanced disease may involve retroperitoneal lymph nodes and multiple peritoneal surfaces, although ascites is infrequent. Hematogenous spread to the liver, lung, and brain can be observed, especially with choriocarcinoma.

Surgical Management

The principles for surgical management of germ cell tumors are similar to those described for epithelial tumors, with the important caveat that in most patients with germ cell cancer, fertility can be preserved by sparing the contralateral ovary and fallopian tube and the uterus. Even in dysgerminoma, in which bilaterality is more common, bilateral oophorectomy is not routinely necessary because postoperative chemotherapy is often capable of eradicating disease that could not be entirely removed at the time of initial surgery. In cases in which the contralateral ovary is grossly abnormal, cystectomy or biopsy can be performed, and bilateral salpingo-oophorectomy can be undertaken in the case of a dysgenetic gonad.

Once the peritoneal cavity is opened, peritoneal washings are obtained, and all fluids are sent for histologic examination. If disease is grossly confined to the pelvis, random biopsies are often performed as in the surgical staging of early stage epithelial ovarian carcinomas. Particular attention is paid to para-aortic and pelvic lymph node enlargement, because these sites are frequently involved in patients with advanced ovarian germ cell tumors. Although lymph node sampling is often performed for staging, no evidence suggests that lymphadenectomy is beneficial. Although the conventional approach among gynecologic oncologists consists of comprehensive surgical staging (with the possible exception of lymphadenectomy) for patients with apparent early-stage malignant ovarian germ cell tumors, the standard surgical management for children who undergo primary surgery by pediatric surgeons has been less extensive. Billmire et al.,[168] reporting the outcomes of 131 patients with malignant ovarian germ cell tumors who were enrolled in two intergroup studies, found that less comprehensive surgical staging did not compromise survival. Clearly, further study of the extent of surgical staging is warranted.

Cytoreductive surgery is recommended as for epithelial tumors of the ovary. However, whether such an aggressive approach is necessary in selected patients with extensive disease that is generally much more chemosensitive that epithelial ovarian cancer remains unresolved.

There is no role for routine second-look operations in patients with germ cell tumors who are clinically free of disease after chemotherapy. In particular, if the primary tumor is completely resected and does not contain teratomatous elements, second-look procedures after chemotherapy are of no established benefit. In some patients whose tumor contains teratomatous elements, however, a second-look procedure may be beneficial. Such patients may have residual mature teratoma, which is chemotherapy insensitive, making it reasonable to consider a second-look procedure in selected cases for resection of such residual disease if technically possible. The rationale for this is derived from the experience with testicular germ cell cancer, in which residual teratoma has been known to enlarge and cause local complications or rarely transform to an undifferentiated sarcoma or carcinoma. However, the extent to which residual teratoma may transform to a more aggressive histology in patients with ovarian germ cell tumors has not been well studied.

Postoperative Management of Dysgerminoma

Dysgerminoma is the most common malignant germ cell tumor of the ovary. In contrast to nondysgerminomatous tumors (which contain embryonal, yolk sac, or choriocarcinoma elements), dysgerminomas are more frequently stage I, may involve both ovaries, more often spread to retroperitoneal lymph nodes, and are markedly sensitive to radiotherapy. Because these tumors are also exquisitely sensitive to cisplatin-based chemotherapy, the role of curative radiation therapy has significantly decreased, especially in view of its propensity to cause sterility.

The majority of patients with dysgerminomas are diagnosed with early stage disease. Because preservation of fertility is an important issue for most patients, those with stage IA disease can be observed without further postoperative treatment. Approximately 15% to 25% of such patients will experience recurrence, although salvage chemotherapy is almost always successful.[169] Dysgerminoma in patients with higher than stage IA disease is typically treated with platinum-based chemotherapy. In the early 1980s, ovarian germ cell tumors were treated with the cisplatin, vinblastine, and bleomycin (PVB) regimen, similar to the regimens used in the treatment of testicular cancer. The MD Anderson Cancer Center group began to use the bleomycin, etoposide, and cisplatin (BEP) combination for patients with metastatic dysgerminoma in 1984 and subsequently reported their findings, with all 14 BEP-treated patients disease free at a median follow-up of 22.4 months.[170] The GOG also reported their experience of 20 patients with incompletely resected dysgerminoma who received either PVB or BEP followed by the combination of vincristine, dactinomycin, and cyclophosphamide.[169] With a median follow-up of 26 months, 19 of the 20 patients were disease free.

In an update of the MD Anderson series, Brewer et al.[171] reported 26 patients with ovarian dysgerminoma who received BEP chemotherapy, with all patients being disease free at the time of the report. Of the 14 evaluable patients who underwent fertility-sparing surgery, 93% had normal menstrual function, with five pregnancies reported. In an attempt to identify a less-toxic regimen, the GOG conducted a clinical trial in which 39 eligible patients with completely resected, stages IB through III ovarian dysgerminoma received the combination of etoposide and carboplatin; all 39 patients were in sustained remission (median follow-up 7.8 years), with myelosuppression being the most severe toxicity.[172] Although BEP is still considered the preferred regimen for use in this setting, with the etoposide and carboplatin combination being reserved for those patients with completely resected, stages IC through III dysgerminoma who have a contraindication to BEP (such as significant neuropathy or renal dysfunction), there appears to be renewed interest in development of a regimen less toxic than BEP.

Postoperative Management of Nondysgerminoma

Nondysgerminomas include tumors that contain embryonal, yolk sac, choriocarcinoma, and immature teratoma elements. The vast majority of these histologic subtypes require treatment with surgery followed by combination chemotherapy, as even patients with early stage nondysgerminomas have a significant risk of relapse that can be reduced by postoperative adjuvant therapy. The current regimen of choice is BEP. The GOG reported that 89 of 93 patients with stages I, II, and III disease whose tumors were completely resected remained disease free after three courses of this regimen.[173] Toxicities of BEP include the risk of bleomycin-induced pulmonary damage, etoposide-induced leukemia, and platinum-induced neuropathy and nephropathy. Many patients who receive the BEP regimen will regain fertility after completion of treatment. Several series have reported that at least 80% of patients with germ cell tumors of the ovary who were treated with fertility-sparing surgery and postoperative chemotherapy regained normal menstrual function, and there are several documented normal pregnancies.[174] However, patients are known to be at increased risk for development of premature menopause following chemotherapy.[175]

Although most patients with nondysgerminomatous germ cell cancer will require postoperative chemotherapy, a subset of patients with pure immature teratoma of the ovary has an excellent prognosis after surgery alone. Specifically, patients with stage IA, grade 1 immature teratoma experience 5-year survivals >90%, and there is no evidence to suggest that chemotherapy improves outcome. Patients with stage IA, grades 2 and 3 immature teratoma have a higher relapse rate, which generally warrants consideration of postoperative chemotherapy.

Several investigators have examined the feasibility of surgery followed by close surveillance in a much broader group of patients. Dark et al.[176] reported 24 patients with stage IA germ cell tumors of the ovary who underwent postoperative surveillance. Fifteen of these had nondysgerminomas, with nine immature teratomas and six yolk sac tumors. Three of these fifteen (20%) patients relapsed. The two patients with yolk sac tumor each relapsed at 4 months, and both were salvaged with combination chemotherapy. The third patient became pregnant; she presented with ascites and hepatic metastases during the third trimester, 13 months after diagnosis, and died of a pulmonary embolus 4 weeks after starting chemotherapy.

Cushing et al.[177] reported 44 patients with completely resected ovarian immature teratoma, grades 1 through 3 (31 pure and 13 with yolk sac tumor elements). Ten of twelve patients had elevated levels of serum AFP. The 4-year event-free and overall survival rates for the two groups were 97.7% and 100%, respectively. One patient with a mixed tumor relapsed 18 weeks after primary surgery with a rising AFP level; she was treated with four cycles of BEP and was disease free 57 months after completing chemotherapy. Two other studies reported a total of 39 patients with stage I disease who were treated with surgery alone.[178,179] The overall survival for the combined studies was 97.4%; 13 patients relapsed, and 12 were salvaged with chemotherapy.

The Children's Oncology Group is currently studying the approach of surgery followed by surveillance in patients with stage I germ cell tumors of the ovary. Although this strategy appears to be potentially promising, further study, particularly in adult patients, is warranted to ensure its safety and efficacy.

SEX CORD–STROMAL TUMORS

Definition and Clinical Features

Ovarian sex cord–stromal tumors represent approximately 5% of all ovarian cancers.[56] Patients often present with stage I disease, which has an excellent prognosis. However, the potential for late relapse, sometimes occurring more than 10 years after diagnosis, mandates long-term follow-up. Granulosa cell tumors are the most common type of sex cord–stromal malignancy. Such tumors typically present as a solid mass with occasional cystic features, which

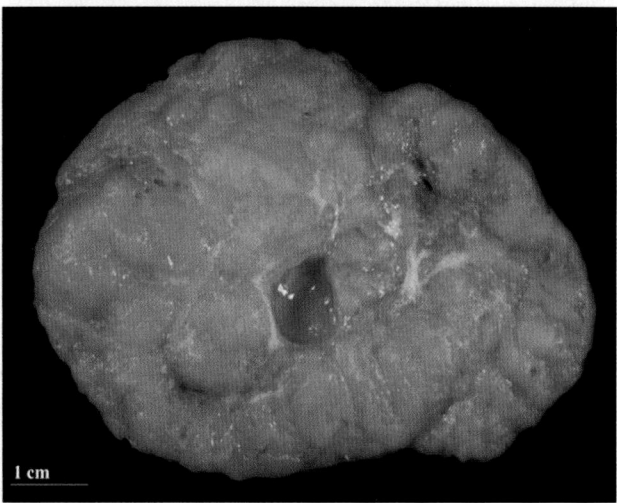

Figure 76.5 Cross-section of a granulosa cell tumor, showing the tan-yellow appearance characteristic of steroid production. (Courtesy of Dr. Marisa Nucci, Brigham and Women's Hospital, Boston, MA.)

is often yellow on cross-section due to the presence of cholesterol (Fig. 76.5). In addition, the cells of granulosa cell tumors are characterized by a longitudinal cleft that resembles a coffee bean (Fig. 76.6), and they may be organized into fluid-filled spherical structures known as Call-Exner bodies. These tumors may produce estrogenic or, less commonly, androgenic steroids. The estradiol in such cases is due to production of androstenedione by normal theca cells within the ovarian stroma, which is then converted to estradiol under the influence of aromatase present in the granulosa cell tumor.[56] In addition to estradiol, sex cord–stromal tumors such as granulosa cell tumors may secrete other factors such as inhibin and Müllerian inhibitory substance, which can sometimes be useful as tumor markers during the surveillance phase of management.[56,180]

The hormonal manifestations of sex cord–stromal neoplasms such as granulosa cell tumors vary depending on the age of the patient. Thus, granulosa cell tumors occurring in premenarchal girls may present with precocious puberty, whereas women in the reproductive years may present with amenorrhea or abnormal

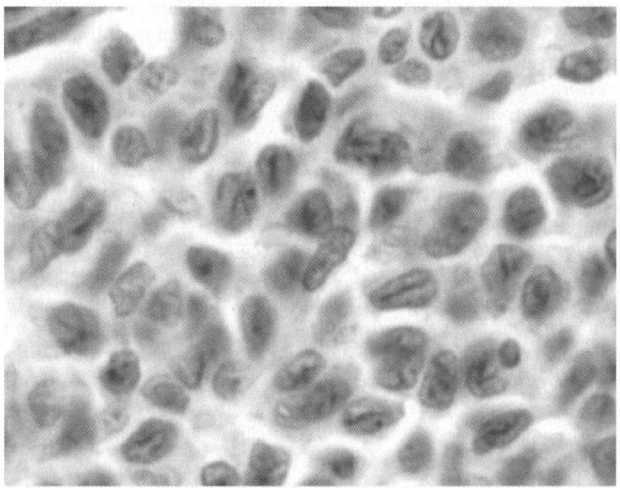

Figure 76.6 Photomicrograph of a hematoxylin and eosin-stained section of granulosa cell tumor, showing characteristic nuclear grooves (coffee bean nuclei). (Courtesy of Dr. Jonathan Hecht, Beth Israel Deaconess Medical Center, Boston, MA.)

menses or may occasionally develop intra-abdominal hemorrhage that mimics an ectopic pregnancy. Postmenopausal women with granulosa cell tumor may present with postmenopausal bleeding due to endometrial hyperplasia (or a separate uterine carcinoma), resulting from tumor-derived estrogen. Sertoli-Leydig cell tumors may present with symptoms of virilization, but none of these hormonal effects is a reliable diagnostic criterion, and many patients with sex cord–stromal tumors have no hormonal manifestations of their disease. The tumor may present as a mass discovered on routine pelvic examination or during the evaluation of pelvic pain due to ovarian torsion.

Surgical Management

Surgical staging of sex cord–stromal tumors is the same as that for epithelial ovarian cancer, with the exception of management of the retroperitoneum. In two reported series, no lymph node metastases were observed in patients who underwent pelvic and/or paraaortic lymphadenectomy.[181,182] Furthermore, recurrence involving lymph nodes is uncommon. Surgical management of sex cord–stromal tumors is based on the stage of the tumor as well as the age of the patient. As the tumor is rarely bilateral, premenarchal women or patients presenting in the reproductive years with stage I disease are often managed with unilateral salpingo-oophorectomy in an attempt to preserve fertility. In women who have completed childbearing, initial surgery for sex cord–stromal tumors typically consists of bilateral salpingo-oophorectomy and total abdominal hysterectomy, along with standard surgical staging.

Postoperative Management

Stage is the most important prognostic factor, with 10-year survivals of over 85% for stage I tumors, decreasing to 50% to 65% for stage II disease, and to 17% to 33% for stages III and IV.[56] Based on these considerations, patients with stages II to IV sex cord–stromal tumors are reasonable candidates for additional therapy after initial surgery, although the survival benefit of such therapy has not been proven due to the rarity of this tumor and resultant lack of randomized trials. Approximately 30% to 50% of patients will respond to platinum-based chemotherapy, and some patients may be rendered into a clinical and pathologic complete response at the time of second-look laparotomy (usually performed in the context of a clinical trial).[56,183] The most commonly studied platinum combinations are cyclophosphamide, doxorubicin, and cisplatin; PVB; and BEP. The single-agent activity of drugs such as bleomycin or etoposide has not been well established in this disease, and combinations such as PVB or BEP have been used by analogy with germ cell cancer (which derives from a completely different cell lineage). Although randomized comparisons are lacking, the highest response rates and the best tolerance among these three regimens has been observed with BEP, which is often used for sex cord–stromal tumors that require chemotherapy.[183] However, the BEP regimen is still associated with the potential for serious toxicity, including bleomycin-induced lung damage, etoposide-induced leukemia, renal dysfunction, hypertension, and Raynaud phenomenon. Furthermore, the added benefit of BEP when compared to etoposide and cisplatin (without bleomycin) or even single-agent platinum has not been formally demonstrated. Thus, there may be circumstances in which the clinician may choose other platinum-based regimens in this disease, as opposed to BEP, especially in the older patient who cannot tolerate bleomycin due to underlying pulmonary disease, or in the young patient who is not willing to accept the small chance of etoposide-induced leukemia. In this regard, it has been shown that combined paclitaxel and carboplatin has significant activity in patients with sex cord–stromal tumors, with generally improved tolerance compared to BEP.[184] Whether paclitaxel and carboplatin will eventually become the preferred regimen for this disease will require additional study, although it is

a consideration in patients who wish to avoid the toxicity of BEP or those who cannot tolerate BEP due to side effects. A randomized trial comparing paclitaxel and carboplatin with BEP in patients with newly diagnosed, advanced-stage sex cord–stromal tumors of the ovary is currently under way (GOG 264).

Selected patients with stage I disease may be at higher risk of relapse due to the presence of features such as large tumor size (>10 to 15 cm in diameter) and high mitotic count (>4 to 10 mitoses per 10 high-power fields).[56] Based on the retrospective nature and small size of most series, it is difficult to know whether the prognostic value of tumor size and mitotic rate is independent of stage. The prognostic value of rupture, surface involvement, or age is even less certain. Nonetheless, it is reasonable to consider some form of adjuvant, platinum-based therapy for selected patients with stage I disease who have high-risk features, although the data to support a survival benefit to this approach are lacking at the present time. In such cases, the uncertain benefits of treatment must be weighed against the potential for side effects.

Sex cord–stromal tumors may recur several years after the original diagnosis. Relapses may be associated with abdominal or pelvic discomfort, a mass on pelvic examination, or an asymptomatic rise in serum tumor markers such as estradiol or inhibin. Such recurrences are often limited to the abdomen or pelvis, although may occasionally present with hematogenous spread to the liver, lung, or bone. Locoregional recurrences are treated with surgical resection followed by postoperative therapy such as platinum-based treatment or radiotherapy. In cases in which the recurrence is isolated and can be encompassed in a radiation field, older literature suggests that radiation therapy may be of value for granulosa cell histology. Eventually, patients become resistant to platinum-based chemotherapy, in which case single-agent paclitaxel, or the use of progestational agents or leuprolide, may be considered.[56]

PRIMARY PERITONEAL SEROUS CARCINOMA

PPSC is histologically identical to serous carcinoma of ovarian origin, but typically presents with diffuse peritoneal implants in the absence of a dominant ovarian mass. This entity is thought to represent malignant transformation of peritoneal surface epithelium, which, like ovarian surface epithelium, is derived from coelomic mesoderm.[2] Another possibility is that PPSC represents secondary seeding of the peritoneal cavity from an occult primary lesion residing in the fallopian tube fimbria.[5] Initial reports of PPSC involved patients who underwent a prophylactic oophorectomy for a family history of ovarian cancer, but who later developed diffuse intra-abdominal carcinomatosis that resembled ovarian cancer.[185] In other patients with intact ovaries, diffuse carcinomatosis developed that histologically resembled papillary serous ovarian cancer, but without a dominant ovarian mass. In such cases, it is not unusual to observe small tumor implants involving the ovarian surface, although these are the result of generalized peritoneal seeding from a primary tumor mass in the omentum or deep within the pelvis. These two types of clinical presentations eventually led to the recognition that PPSC is a distinct clinical entity that resembles ovarian cancer histologically, clinically, and in its response to treatment.

Some investigators using molecular markers of clonality have proposed that PPSC is more likely to develop in a multifocal fashion, as opposed to most cases of ovarian cancer, which are clonal in origin.[186] Cases of PPSC that are multifocal may reflect a field defect within the peritoneal mesothelial lining. PPSC occurs at a higher incidence in patients with germline mutations in BRCA1 and BRCA2.[35]

The differential diagnosis for PPSC is similar to that of epithelial ovarian carcinoma. On occasion, poorly differentiated PPSC may be difficult to distinguish from other entities such as metastatic breast cancer to the abdominal cavity. In such cases, expression of

GCDFP may be helpful, as this marker is highly specific for breast and salivary gland tumors and is usually negative for Müllerian origin tumors such as PPSC or ovarian primaries. The utility of GCDFP as a marker for breast cancer is limited by rather low sensitivity, being positive in only about 50% of cases. Other entities that may rarely be confused with PPSC include peritoneal mesothelioma, gastric or pancreatic cancers, and hepatobiliary tumors.

Patients with PPSC present in a similar fashion to those with epithelial ovarian cancer, although they may not have an adnexal mass on ultrasound or pelvic examination. The abdominal examination may reveal ascites and an omental mass. The stool does not contain blood, and the hematocrit usually does not suggest an iron deficiency anemia (features that would be more suggestive of a gastrointestinal primary site).

In appropriate surgical candidates, an exploratory laparotomy is usually necessary to establish the histologic diagnosis and to perform tumor cytoreduction. Given the more diffuse nature of this entity, almost all patients with PPSC present with stage III or IV disease. The principles of treatment are the same as those for epithelial ovarian cancer. Primary surgical cytoreduction should be performed, followed by combination chemotherapy with paclitaxel and carboplatin. The prognosis of patients with PPSC is likely to be the same, when corrected for stage and debulking status, as for epithelial ovarian cancer.

As PPSC may sometimes be associated with germline mutations in *BRCA1* and *BRCA2*, a careful family history is important in patients with this entity. In addition, individuals with germline *BRCA1* or *BRCA2* mutations who have undergone prophylactic bilateral salpingo-oophorectomy should be informed that there is a risk for developing PPSC, sometimes many years after the prophylactic procedure has been performed. In a series reported by Piver et al.,[187] 6 of 324 women developed PPSC from 1 to 27 years after prophylactic surgery. There is currently no effective screening procedure that enables early detection of PPSC in this clinical setting.

FALLOPIAN TUBE CANCER

Fallopian tube cancer is a rare disease, with only a few hundred new cases diagnosed annually in the United States.[1] Most tubal carcinomas represent papillary serous adenocarcinoma arising within the lumen of the tube, although other Müllerian histologies such as endometrioid tumors may occur. A minority of fallopian tube carcinomas are bilateral at the time of diagnosis. In contrast to patients with ovarian cancer, the majority of patients with tubal carcinoma are diagnosed with disease confined to the tubes and pelvic structures. However, fallopian tube cancer appears to have

a higher propensity for retroperitoneal lymph node spread compared to epithelial ovarian cancer. Advanced-stage disease may occur with a pattern of IP dissemination similar to that observed for epithelial ovarian cancer.

Postmenopausal vaginal bleeding may bring patients with fallopian tube cancer to medical attention. Hydrops tubae profluens, characterized by colicky lower abdominal pain relieved by profuse serous yellow intermittent vaginal discharge, occurs in a minority of cases, but intermittent abdominal pain and leucorrhea are common presentations. Tubal distention produces more intense pain than is usually reported by patients with ovarian cancer. Occasionally, a Papanicolaou smear revealing abnormal glandular cells with negative cervical or endometrial findings may lead to the diagnosis of fallopian tube carcinoma. As for ovarian cancer and PPSC, fallopian tube cancer occurs at higher frequency in patients with germline mutations of *BRCA1* and *BRCA2*, thus requiring a careful family history in affected individuals.[50]

Differentiation of a primary fallopian tube cancer from metastatic ovarian carcinoma can sometimes be difficult. Apart from a dominant mass arising within the fallopian tube lumen, the main criterion used to establish the diagnosis of a primary fallopian tube carcinoma is histologic evidence of a transition between in situ carcinoma and invasive malignancy within the fallopian tube epithelium. In cases where it is impossible to determine whether the tumor began in the fallopian tube and spread to the ovary, or began in the ovary and spread to the lumen of the fallopian tube, the tumors are referred to as *tubo-ovarian carcinoma*.

Survival is partly dependent on the depth of invasion of the primary lesion.[177] For intramucosal lesions, the 5-year survival is 91%, compared with 53% for tumors that invade the muscular wall, and <25% for tumors that have penetrated the tubal serosa. Histologic differentiation and lymphatic capillary space involvement may also have prognostic significance.[188]

The surgical management and staging system of fallopian tube carcinoma is identical to that of patients with epithelial ovarian cancer. Patients rendered into a minimal residual disease state after cytoreductive surgery appear to have an improved prognosis. Postoperatively, it is reasonable to use combination chemotherapy with paclitaxel and carboplatin in patients with fallopian tube carcinoma that has spread beyond the tube. In addition, patients with disease limited to the tubal lumen may also be reasonable candidates for postoperative adjuvant treatment, based on features such as muscle wall invasion, serosal extension, or high-grade histology. However, the survival benefit of platinum-based adjuvant therapy for early stage fallopian tube cancer has not been formally demonstrated in randomized trials due to the rarity of this disease.

SELECTED REFERENCES

The full reference list can be accessed at lwwhealthlibrary.com/oncology.

1. Siegel R, Naishadham D, Jemal A. Cancer Statistics, 2013. *CA Cancer J Clin* 2013;63:11–30.
2. Cannistra SA. Cancer of the ovary. *N Engl J Med* 2004;351:2519–2529.
6. The Cancer Genome Atlas. Integrated genomic analyses of ovarian carcinoma. *Nature* 2011;474:609–615.
7. Wiegand KC, Shah SP, Al-Agha OM, et al. ARID1A mutations in endometriosis-associated ovarian carcinomas. *N Engl J Med* 2010;363:1532–1543.
12. Leake JF, Currie JL, Rosenshein NB, et al. Long-term follow-up of serous ovarian tumors of low malignant potential. *Gynecol Oncol* 1992;47:150–158.
14. Omura GA, Brady MF, Homesley HD, et al. Long-term follow-up and prognostic factor analysis in advanced ovarian carcinoma: the Gynecologic Oncology Group experience. *J Clin Oncol* 1991;9:1138–1150.
15. Gershenson DM, Sun CC, Lu KH, et al. Clinical behavior of stage II-IV low-grade serous carcinoma of the ovary. *Obstet Gynecol* 2006;108:361–368.
16. Gershenson DM, Sun CC, Bodurka D, et al. Recurrent low-grade serous ovarian carcinoma is relatively chemoresistant. *Gynecol Oncol* 2009;114:48–52.
18. Bast RC Jr, Knapp RC. Use of the CA 125 antigen in diagnosis and monitoring of ovarian carcinoma. *Euro J Obstet Gynecol Reprod Biol* 1985;19:354–356.

24. Jacobs I. Genetic, biochemical, and multimodal approaches to screening for ovarian cancer. *Gynecol Oncol* 1994;55:S22–S27.
31. Jacobs IJ, Skates SJ, MacDonald N, et al. Screening for ovarian cancer: a pilot randomised controlled trial. *Lancet* 1999;353:1207–1210.
33. Ford D, Easton DF, Bishop DT, et al. Risks of cancer in BRCA1-mutation carriers. Breast Cancer Linkage Consortium. *Lancet* 1994;343:692–695.
34. Tavtigian SV, Simard J, Rommens J, et al. The complete BRCA2 gene and mutations in chromosome 13q-linked kindreds. *Nat Genet* 1996;12:333–337.
35. Levine DA, Argenta PA, Yee CJ, et al. Fallopian tube and primary peritoneal carcinomas associated with BRCA mutations. *J Clin Oncol* 2003;21:4222–4227.
38. Struewing JP, Hartge P, Wacholder S, et al. The risk of cancer associated with specific mutations of BRCA1 and BRCA2 among Ashkenazi Jews. *N Engl J Med* 1997;336:1401–1408.
39. Rubin SC, Benjamin I, Behbakht K, et al. Clinical and pathological features of ovarian cancer in women with germ-line mutations of BRCA1 [see comment]. *N Engl J Med* 1996;335:1413–1416.
40. Frank TS, Deffenbaugh AM, Reid JE, et al. Clinical characteristics of individuals with germline mutations in BRCA1 and BRCA2: analysis of 10,000 individuals. *J Clin Oncol* 2002;20:1480–1490.

PRACTICE OF ONCOLOGY

42. Watson P, Butzow R, Lynch HT, et al. The clinical features of ovarian cancer in hereditary nonpolyposis colorectal cancer. *Gynecol Oncol* 2001;82: 223–228.

43. Bonadona V, Bonaiti B, Olschwang S, et al. Cancer risks associated with germline mutations in mlh1, msh2, and msh6 genes in lynch syndrome. *JAMA* 2011;305:2304–2310.

44. American Society of Clinical Oncology. American Society of Clinical Oncology policy statement update: genetic testing for cancer susceptibility. *J Clin Oncol* 2003;21:2397–2406.

45. Walsh T, Casadei S, Coats KH, et al. Spectrum of mutations in BRCA1, BRCA2, CHEK2, and TP53 in families at high risk of breast cancer. *JAMA* 2006;295:1379–1388.

46. Rebbeck TR, Lynch HT, Neuhausen SL, et al. Prophylactic oophorectomy in carriers of BRCA1 or BRCA2 mutations. *N Engl J Med* 2002;346:1616–1622.

47. Kauff ND, Satagopan JM, Robson ME, et al. Risk-reducing salpingo-oophorectomy in women with a BRCA1 or BRCA2 mutation. *N Engl J Med* 2002;346:1609–1615.

48. Domchek SM, Friebel TM, Singer CF, et al. Association of risk-reducing surgery in brca1 or brca2 mutation carriers with cancer risk and mortality. *JAMA* 2010;304:967–975.

51. Lu KH, Garber JE, Cramer DW, et al. Occult ovarian tumors in women with BRCA1 or BRCA2 mutations undergoing prophylactic oophorectomy. *J Clin Oncol* 2000;18:2728–2732.

53. Narod SA, Dube MP, Klijn J, et al. Oral contraceptives and the risk of breast cancer in BRCA1 and BRCA2 mutation carriers. *J Natl Cancer Inst* 2002;94:1773–1779.

54. Holtz F, Hart WR. Krukenberg tumors of the ovary: a clinicopathologic analysis of 27 cases. *Cancer* 1982;50:2438–2447.

55. Bristow RE, Tomacruz RS, Armstrong DK, et al. Survival effect of maximal cytoreductive surgery for advanced ovarian carcinoma during the platinum era: a meta-analysis. *J Clin Oncol* 2002;20:1248–1259.

56a. Prat J; FIGO Committee on Gynecologic Oncology. Staging classification for cancer of the ovary, fallopian tube, and peritoneum. *Int J Gynaecol Obstet* 2014;124:1–5.

56. Schumer ST, Cannistra SA. Granulosa cell tumor of the ovary. *J Clin Oncol* 2003;21:1180–1189.

57. Young RC, Decker DG, Wharton JT, et al. Staging laparotomy in early ovarian cancer. *JAMA* 1983;250:3072–3076.

58. Gershenson DM. Fertility-sparing surgery for malignancies in women. *J Natl Cancer Inst Monogr* 2005;34:43–47.

59. Young RC, Walton LA, Ellenberg SS, et al. Adjuvant therapy in stage I and stage II epithelial ovarian cancer. Results of two prospective randomized trials. *N Engl J Med* 1990;322:1021–1027.

60. Ahmed F, Wiltshaw E, A'Hern R, et al. Natural history and prognosis of untreated stage I epithelial ovarian carcinoma. *J Clin Oncol* 1996;14:2968–2975.

61. Ozols RF, Bundy BN, Greer BE, et al. Phase III trial of carboplatin and paclitaxel compared with cisplatin and paclitaxel in patients with optimally resected stage III ovarian cancer: a Gynecologic Oncology Group study. *J Clin Oncol* 2003;21:3194–3200.

62. McGuire WP, Hoskins WJ, Brady MF, et al. Cyclophosphamide and cisplatin compared with paclitaxel and cisplatin in patients with stage III and stage IV ovarian cancer. *N Engl J Med* 1996;334:1–6.

63. Hoskins WJ, Bundy BN, Thigpen JT, et al. The influence of cytoreductive surgery on recurrence-free interval and survival in small-volume stage III epithelial ovarian cancer: a Gynecologic Oncology Group study. *Gynecol Oncol* 1992;47:159–166.

64. Lavin PT, Knapp RC, Malkasian G, et al. CA 125 for the monitoring of ovarian carcinoma during primary therapy. *Obstet Gynecol* 1987;69:223–227.

65. Crawford SM, Paul J, Reed NS, et al. The prognostic significance of the CA 125 nadir in patients that achieve a CA 125 response. *Proc Am Soc Clin Oncol* 2004;23:448 (Abstr 5001).

66. Bolton KL, Chenevix-Trench G, Goh C, et al. Association between brca1 and brca2 mutations and survival in women with invasive epithelial ovarian cancer. *JAMA* 2012;307:382–390.

70. Trimbos JB, Parmar M, Vergote I, et al. International Collaborative Ovarian Neoplasm trial 1 and Adjuvant ChemoTherapy in Ovarian Neoplasm trial: two parallel randomized phase III trials of adjuvant chemotherapy in patients with early-stage ovarian carcinoma [comment]. *J Natl Cancer Inst* 2003;95:105–112.

72. Bell J, Brady M, Lage JM, et al. A randomized phase III trial of three versus six cycles of carboplatin and paclitaxel as adjuvant treatment in early stage ovarian epithelial carcinoma: a Gynecologic Oncology Group study. *Gynecol Oncol* 2003;88:156.

73. Chan JK, Tian C, Fleming GF, et al. The potential benefit of 6 vs. 3 cycles of chemotherapy in subsets of women with early-stage high-risk epithelial ovarian cancer: an exploratory analysis of a Gynecologic Oncology Group study. *Gynecol Oncol* 2010;116:301–306.

80. Chang SJ, Bristow RE. Evolution of surgical treatment paradigms for advanced-stage ovarian cancer: redefining "optimal" residual disease. *Gynecol Oncol* 2012;125:483–492.

81. Van Der Burg ME, van Lent M, Buyse M, et al. The effect of debulking surgery after induction chemotherapy on the prognosis in advanced epithelial ovarian cancer. Gynecological Cancer Cooperative Group of the European Organization for Research and Treatment of Cancer. *N Engl J Med* 1995;332:629–634.

83. Vergote I, Trope CG, Amant F, et al. Neoadjuvant chemotherapy or primary surgery in stage IIIC or IV ovarian cancer. *N Engl J Med* 2010;363: 943–953.

84. Vergote I, du Bois A. Neoadjuvant chemotherapy in advanced ovarian cancer: on what do we agree and disagree? *Gynecol Oncol* 2013;128:6–11.

88. Piccart MJ, Bertelsen K, James K, et al. Randomized intergroup trial of cisplatin-paclitaxel versus cisplatin-cyclophosphamide in women with advanced epithelial ovarian cancer: three-year results. *J Natl Cancer Inst* 2000;92:699–708.

89. Muggia FM, Braly PS, Brady MF, et al. Phase III randomized study of cisplatin versus paclitaxel versus cisplatin and paclitaxel in patients with suboptimal stage III or IV ovarian cancer: a gynecologic oncology group study [see comment]. *J Clin Oncol* 2000;18:106–115.

90. International Collaborative Ovarian Neoplasm Group. Paclitaxel plus carboplatin versus standard chemotherapy with either single-agent carboplatin or cyclophosphamide, doxorubicin, and cisplatin in women with ovarian cancer: the ICON3 randomised trial. *Lancet* 2002;360:505–515.

100. Alberts DS, Liu PY, Hannigan EV, et al. Intraperitoneal cisplatin plus intravenous cyclophosphamide versus intravenous cisplatin plus intravenous cyclophosphamide for stage III ovarian cancer. *N Engl J Med* 1996;335:1950–1955.

101. Markman M, Bundy BN, Alberts DS, et al. Phase III trial of standard-dose intravenous cisplatin plus paclitaxel versus moderately high-dose carboplatin followed by intravenous paclitaxel and intraperitoneal cisplatin in small-volume stage III ovarian carcinoma: an intergroup study of the Gynecologic Oncology Group, Southwestern Oncology Group, and Eastern Cooperative Oncology Group. *J Clin Oncol* 2001;19:1001–1007.

102. Armstrong DK, Bundy B, Wenzel L, et al. Intraperitoneal cisplatin and paclitaxel in ovarian cancer. *N Engl J Med* 2006;354:34–43.

121. Markman M, Liu PY, Wilczynski S, et al. Phase III randomized trial of 12 versus 3 months of maintenance paclitaxel in patients with advanced ovarian cancer after complete response to platinum and paclitaxel-based chemotherapy: a Southwest Oncology Group and Gynecologic Oncology Group trial. *J Clin Oncol* 2003;21:2460–2465.

123. Burger RA, Brady MF, Bookman MA, et al. Incorporation of bevacizumab in the primary treatment of ovarian cancer. *N Engl J Med* 2011;365:2473–2483.

124. Perren TJ, Swart AM, Pfisterer J, et al. A phase 3 trial of bevacizumab in ovarian cancer. *N Engl J Med* 2011;365:2484–2496.

126. Ahlgren JD, Ellison NM, Gottlieb RJ, et al. Hormonal palliation of chemoresistant ovarian cancer: three consecutive phase II trials of the Mid-Atlantic Oncology Program. *J Clin Oncol* 1993;11:1957–1968.

129. Parmar MK, Ledermann JA, Colombo N, et al. Paclitaxel plus platinum-based chemotherapy versus conventional platinum-based chemotherapy in women with relapsed ovarian cancer: the ICON4/AGO-OVAR-2.2 trial. *Lancet* 2003;361:2099–2106.

130. Pfisterer J, Plante M, Vergote I, et al. Gemcitabine plus carboplatin compared with carboplatin in patients with platinum-sensitive recurrent ovarian cancer: an intergroup trial of the AGO-OVAR, the NCIC CTG, and the EORTC GCG. *J Clin Oncol* 2006;24:4699–4707.

131. Pujade-Lauraine E, Wagner U, Aavall-Lundqvist E, et al. Pegylated liposomal doxorubicin and carboplatin compared with paclitaxel and carboplatin for patients with platinum-sensitive ovarian cancer in late relapse. *J Clin Oncol* 2010;28:3323–3329.

132. Cannistra SA. Is there a "best" choice of second-line agent in the treatment of recurrent, potentially platinum-sensitive ovarian cancer? *J Clin Oncol* 2002;20:1158–1160.

139. Burger RA, Sill MW, Monk BJ, et al. Phase II trial of bevacizumab in persistent or recurrent epithelial ovarian cancer or primary peritoneal cancer: a Gynecologic Oncology Group Study. *J Clin Oncol* 2007;25: 5165–5171.

140. Cannistra SA, Matulonis UA, Penson RT, et al. Phase II study of bevacizumab in patients with platinum-resistant ovarian cancer or peritoneal serous cancer. *J Clin Oncol* 2007;25:5180–5186.

141. Aghajanian C, Blank SV, Goff BA, et al. OCEANS: a randomized, double-blind, placebo-controlled phase III trial of chemotherapy with or without bevacizumab in patients with platinum-sensitive recurrent epithelial ovarian, primary peritoneal, or fallopian tube cancer. *J Clin Oncol* 2012;30: 2039–2045.

142. Pujade-Lauraine E, Hilpert F, Weber B, et al. AURELIA: A randomized phase III trial evaluating bevacizumab (BEV) plus chemotherapy (CT) for platinum (PT)-resistant recurrent ovarian cancer (OC). *J Clin Oncol* 2012; 30:Abstr LBA5002.

146. Fong PC, Boss DS, Yap TA, et al. Inhibition of poly(ADP-ribose) polymerase in tumors from BRCA mutation carriers. *N Engl J Med* 2009;361:123–134.

147. Gelmon KA, Tischkowitz M, Mackay H, et al. Olaparib in patients with recurrent high-grade serous or poorly differentiated ovarian carcinoma or triple-negative breast cancer: a phase 2, multicentre, open-label, non-randomised study. *Lancet Oncol* 2011;12:852–861.

148. Ledermann J, Harter P, Gourley C, et al. Olaparib maintenance therapy in platinum-sensitive relapsed ovarian cancer. *N Engl J Med* 2012;366: 1382–1392.

149. Gershenson DM, Sun CC, Bodurka D, et al. Recurrent low-grade serous ovarian cancer is relatively chemoresistant. *Gynecol Oncol* 2009;114:48–52.

152. Farley J, Brady WE, Vathipadiekal V, et al. Selumetinib in women with recurrent low-grade serous carcinoma of the ovary or peritoneum: an open-label, single-arm, phase 2 study. *Lancet Oncol* 2013;14:134–140.

155. Berek JS, Hacker NF, Lagasse LD, et al. Survival of patients following secondary cytoreductive surgery in ovarian cancer. *Obstet Gynecol* 1983;61:189–193.

156. Firat S, Erickson B. Selective irradiation for the treatment of recurrent ovarian carcinoma involving the vagina or rectum. *Gynecol Oncol* 2001;80:213–220.

157. Albuquerque KV, Singla R, Potkul RK, et al. Impact of tumor volume-directed involved field radiation therapy integrated in the management of recurrent ovarian cancer. *Gynecol Oncol* 2005;96:701–704.

159. Trimble CL, Kosary C, Trimble EL. Long-term survival and patterns of care in women with ovarian tumors of low malignant potential. *Gynecol Oncol* 2002;86:34–37.

160. Bell DA, Scully RE. Ovarian serous borderline tumors with stromal microinvasion: a report of 21 cases. *Hum Pathol* 1990;21:397–403.

163. Bell DA, Weinstock MA, Scully RE. Peritoneal implants of ovarian serous borderline tumors. Histologic features and prognosis. *Cancer* 1988;62:2212–2222.

166. Silva EG, Gershenson DM, Malpica A, et al. The recurrence and the overall survival rates of ovarian serous borderline neoplasms with noninvasive implants is time dependent. *Am J Surg Pathol* 2006;30:1367–1371.

170. Gershenson DM, Morris M, Cangir A, et al. Treatment of malignant germ cell tumors of the ovary with bleomycin, etoposide, and cisplatin. *J Clin Oncol* 1990;8:715–720.

171. Brewer M, Gershenson DM, Herzog CE, et al. Outcome and reproductive function after chemotherapy for ovarian dysgerminoma. *J Clin Oncol* 1999;17:2670–2675.

173. Williams S, Blessing JA, Liao SY, et al. Adjuvant therapy of ovarian germ cell tumors with cisplatin, etoposide, and bleomycin: a trial of the Gynecologic Oncology Group. *J Clin Oncol* 1994;12:701–706.

174. Gershenson DM, Miller AM, Champion VL, et al. Reproductive and sexual function after platinum-based chemotherapy in long-term ovarian germ cell tumor survivors: a Gynecologic Oncology Group study. *J Clin Oncol* 2007;25:2792–2797.

182. Brown J, Sood AK, Deavers MT, et al. Patterns of metastasis in sex cord-stromal tumors of the ovary: can routine staging lympadenectomy be omitted? *Gynecol Oncol* 2009;113:86–90.

183. Homesley HD, Bundy BN, Hurteau JA, et al. Bleomycin, etoposide, and cisplatin combination therapy of ovarian granulosa cell tumors and other stromal malignancies: a Gynecologic Oncology Group study. *Gynecol Oncol* 1999;72:131–137.

185. Tobacman JK, Greene MH, Tucker MA, et al. Intra-abdominal carcinomatosis after prophylactic oophorectomy in ovarian-cancer-prone families. *Lancet* 1982;2:795–797.

187. Piver MS, Jishi MF, Tsukada Y, et al. Primary peritoneal carcinoma after prophylactic oophorectomy in women with a family history of ovarian cancer. A report of the Gilda Radner Familial Ovarian Cancer Registry. *Cancer* 1993;71:2751–2755.

PRACTICE OF ONCOLOGY

77 Genetic Testing in Ovarian Cancer

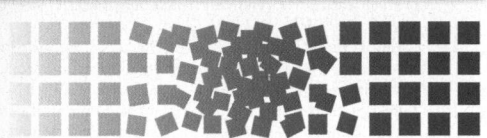

Scott M. Weissman, Shelly M. Weiss, and Anna C. Newlin

INTRODUCTION

Ovarian cancer is responsible for ~3% of all cancers among women, and in 2014, there will be ~21,980 new cases and 14,270 deaths from this cancer.[1] Given this fact, it is of critical importance to identify women who face an elevated risk for ovarian cancer to allow for early detection or prevention. A number of risk factors (e.g., nulliparity, early menarche, late menopause) for ovarian cancer have been identified and reviewed by others.[2–4] By far, the most important risk factor is family history. Having one first-degree relative with ovarian cancer increases the lifetime risk from 1.4% (average risk) to 5% and at least 7% with two or more first-degree relatives.[5] However, in families with two or more cases of ovarian cancer, there may be a hereditary cause for the cancer, which in turn would result into higher lifetime ovarian cancer risks. Historically, it was believed that ~10% of ovarian cancers were due to an underlying hereditary syndrome, but more recent data indicate that just two syndromes (hereditary breast and ovarian cancer syndrome and Lynch syndrome) account for at least 20% of ovarian cancers, and overall, at least 25% of newly diagnosed cases are due to a hereditary mutation in a single gene[6–8]; this suggests that a much larger proportion of ovarian cancer cases is hereditary in nature than originally thought (Fig. 77.1). This chapter reviews ovarian cancer within the context of known hereditary cancer syndromes. In addition, we address some of the newer genes ovarian cancer has been linked to as clinical genetic testing for some of these genes are quickly becoming available to health-care professionals.

HEREDITARY BREAST AND OVARIAN CANCER SYNDROM (THE *BRCA1* AND *BRCA2* GENES)

Hereditary breast and ovarian cancer syndrome due to mutations in the *BRCA1* and *BRCA2* (*BRCA1/2*) genes is the most common cause of hereditary ovarian cancer, including fallopian tube and primary peritoneal cancer. Anywhere from 0.125% to 0.20% of the general population carry mutations in *BRCA1/2* compared with 15% of women with a diagnosis of invasive ovarian cancer.[6,8–10] The contribution of the *BRCA1/2* genes to ovarian cancer is even greater in certain ethnicities that have higher *BRCA1/2* mutation prevalence rates (e.g., Polish, Ashkenazi Jewish [AJ], French Canadian). For example, the prevalence of *BRCA1/2* mutations in individuals of AJ ancestry and women of AJ ancestry with ovarian cancer is ~2.3% and ~30% to 40%, respectively.[11–13] Because of the strong connection between ovarian cancer and *BRCA1/2*, multiple professional societies and organizations recommend genetic counseling and testing for any woman with ovarian cancer regardless of age at onset or family history (Table 77.1). The current sensitivity of *BRCA1/2* genetic testing at the commercial laboratory is ~90% for identifying mutations in either gene.

The lifetime risk of developing ovarian cancer differs between the two genes. A number of studies over the years have quantified the lifetime risk[20–26]; however, two large meta-analyses suggest an ~40% and 20% lifetime risk for *BRCA1* and *BRCA2* mutation carriers, respectively.[27,28] In 1997, Gayther et al.,[29] in an effort to determine whether there were any genotype–phenotype correlations associated with *BRCA2* mutations, identified a region in exon 11 of *BRCA2* between nucleotides 3,035 and 6,629 that appeared to confer a further increased risk of ovarian cancer; they coined this region the "ovarian cancer cluster region" (OCCR). A follow-up study of the OCCR in families from the Breast Cancer Linkage Consortium (which included the families from the study by Gayther et al.[29]) further refined the OCCR to nucleotides 3,059 to 4,075 and 6,503 to 6,629, but found that the phenotype of increased ovarian cancer may actually be due to a reduced breast cancer risk.[30] Regardless, the potential difference in ovarian cancer risk was not significant enough to affect management recommendations. In addition to genotype–phenotype associations, researchers have studied other genetic modifiers (e.g., single-nucleotide polymorphisms) that can influence ovarian cancer risk in *BRCA1/2* mutation carriers, but these data need maturation before testing for genetic modifiers can be used clinically.[31–34]

The average age at onset of ovarian cancer is between 49 and 53 years for *BRCA1* and 55 and 58 years for *BRCA2* compared with 63 years in the general population.[6,8,35–37] Unlike breast cancer, women with a diagnosis of very early-onset ovarian cancer (>40 years) are significantly less likely to harbor *BRCA1/2* mutations.[8,26,35,38,39] This is in part due to the fact that early-onset ovarian cancers are more likely to be associated with borderline tumors, earlier stages, and more favorable histologic characteristics, none of which are typical of *BRCA1/2*-related ovarian cancer.[40]

BRCA1/2-associated ovarian cancers are almost uniformly epithelial in origin and, for the most part, are invasive and nonmucinous; there are case reports of germ cell and stromal tumors in *BRCA1/2* mutation carriers. Mucinous and borderline tumors individually account for ~2% of ovarian tumors identified in *BRCA1/2* mutation carriers; this percentage is the same for both prospective and retrospective analyses, which are nicely summarized by Evans et al.[41] Compared with sporadic ovarian cancers, *BRCA1/2* ovarian cancers are more often of serous histology, higher grade, and solid type, and have intact p53 staining on immunohistochemistry (IHC).[39,41–44] It is important to note that other histologic findings are seen in mutation carriers (e.g., endometrioid, clear cell, papillary), and one study found more giant cell–type cancers in *BRCA1* mutation carriers compared with controls.[42] Several smaller studies have found that *BRCA1/2*-related ovarian cancers have a better prognosis compared with ovarian cancers in nonmutation carriers.[39,45–48] This finding seems to have been confirmed as a recent large pooled analysis of 26 observational studies comparing 3,879 *BRCA1/2* ovarian cancers and 2,666 noncarriers found the 5-year survival for *BRCA2* carriers was 52%, 44% for *BRCA1* carriers, and 36% for noncarriers.[44] The survival difference remained after adjusting for age at diagnosis, stage, histology, and grade.

One potential reason for the differences in survival may be that *BRCA1/2*-related ovarian cancers respond better to platinum-based agents.[45,48] *BRCA1/2* repair DNA damage through homologous recombination and platinum agents are particularly active

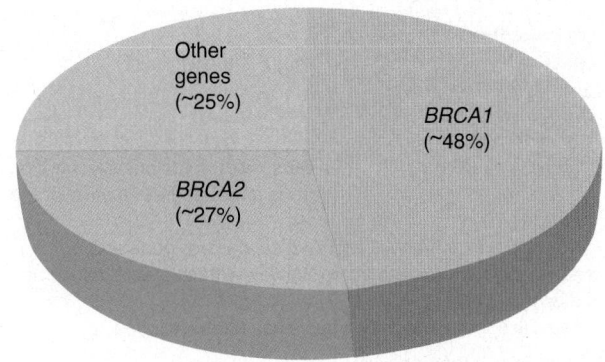

Figure 77.1 Genes responsible for hereditary ovarian cancer (including fallopian tube and primary peritoneal cancer). Other genes include *BARD1, BRIP1, CHEK2, MRE11, MSH6, NBN, PALB2, RAD50, RAD51C,* and *TP53*. (Data derived from Walsh T, Casadei S, Lee MK, et al. Mutations in 12 genes for inherited ovarian cancer, fallopian tube, and peritoneal carcinoma identified by massively parallel sequencing. *Proc Natl Acad Sci U S A* 2011;108:18032–18037.)

in cells deficient in homologous recombination.[48,49] It is through this pathway that another class of drugs called poly(ADP-ribose) polymerase (PARP) inhibitors has been developed to help treat *BRCA1/2*-related cancers. Unlike platinum agents targeting homologous recombination, PARP inhibitors block repair of single-strand DNA breaks through base excision repair, which in turn can lead to double-strand breaks that cannot be repaired by *BRCA1/2*-deficient tumor cells at the same time sparing normal cells.[50–52] A number of phase 1 and phase 2 trials have been reported, and clinical trials continue to study PARP inhibitors in both ovarian and breast cancers.[53–56]

Identifying women who have a *BRCA1/2* mutation would ideally lead to women either being diagnosed with ovarian cancer at earlier stages or preventing ovarian cancer altogether. When counseling women who have tested positive for a *BRCA1/2* mutation, it is these central tenets, ovarian cancer screening versus prevention, that guide discussions. Current National Comprehensive Cancer Network® Guidelines for managing ovarian cancer risk include the recommendation for risk-reducing bilateral salpingo-oophorectomy (RRSO) between the ages of 35 and 40 years when

TABLE 77.1

Societies or Organizations with Position Statements Recommending *BRCA1/2* Genetic Counseling and/or Testing Related to Ovarian Cancer

Society Organization	Year	Recommendation
American College of Medical Genetics[14]	2005	One or more cases of OC and at least one relative on the same side of the family with BC (at any age)
American College of Obstetrics and Gynecology[15]	2009	Genetic risk assessment is recommended for patients with ≥20%–25% chance of having a predisposition to OC (FT and PPC included), which include women with a personal history of OC; women with OC and an FDR or SDR with OC, premenopausal BC or both; women with BC ≤50 y and an FDR or SDR with OC Genetic risk assessment is helpful for patients with a 5%–10% chance of having a predisposition to OC, which include women at any age with OC, PPC, or FT of high grade, serous histology
American Society of Breast Surgeons[16]	2006	A personal or family history of OC (particularly nonmucinous types) should have access to *BRCA* testing
National Comprehensive Cancer Network[17]	2012	Genetic risk assessment should be offered to any woman with BC who has an FDR, SDR, or TDR with epithelial OC, FT, or PPC at any age; any woman with OC, FT, or PPC; any unaffected individual with a family history of more than one OC from the same side of the family *BRCA1/2* genetic testing should be offered to any woman with BC <50 y with more than one FDR, SDR, or TDR with epithelial OC, FT, or PPC at any age; any woman with BC regardless of age when there are more than two FDR, SDR, or TDR with epithelial OC, FT, or PPC at any age; any woman with epithelial OC, FT, or PPC; any individual with PC at any age with more than two FDR, SDR, or TDR with BC and/or OC and/or PC at any age; an unaffected individual who has an FDR or SDR who meet any of the above criteria or a TDR with BC and/or OC/FT/PPC with more than two FDR, SDR, or TDR with BC (one <50 y) and/or OC
Society of Gynecologic Oncologists[18]	2007	Genetic risk assessment is recommended for patients with ≥20%–25% chance of having a predisposition to OC (FT and PPC included), which include women with a personal history of OC and BC; women with OC and an FDR, SDR, or TDR with OC or BC ≤50 y; women with OC at any age who are AJ; women with BC ≤50 y and an FDR, SDR, or TDR with OC Genetic risk assessment is helpful for patients with a 5%–10% chance of having a predisposition to OC, which include women with OC or BC at any age and two or more FDR, SDR, or TDR with BC at any age (particularly if at least one BC is ≤50 y); unaffected women with an FDR or SDR who meet the above criteria
US Preventative Services Task Force[19]	2005	Unaffected women whose family history is suggestive of a *BRCA1/2* mutation should be referred for genetic counseling and evaluation for *BRCA1/2* testing; this includes: Non-AJ women—a combination of both BC and OC among FDR and SDR; a combination of two or more FDR or SDR with OC regardless of age at onset; an FDR or SDR with both BC and OC at any age AJ women—any FDR (or two SDRs on the same side of the family) with OC

OC, ovarian cancer; BC, breast cancer; FT, fallopian tube cancer; PPC, primary peritoneal cancer; PC, pancreatic cancer; FDR, first-degree relative (parent, child, sibling); SDR, second-degree relative (aunt/uncle, grandparent, grandchild, niece/nephew, half-sibling); TDR, third-degree relative (first cousin, great aunt/uncle, great grandparent, great grandchild); AJ, Ashkenazi Jewish.

childbearing is complete; for women not choosing RRSO, transvaginal ultrasound and CA-125 are recommended every 6 months starting at age 30 years or 5 to 10 years before the earliest age at onset of ovarian cancer in the family.[17] Surgical prevention is recommended over screening for two main reasons. First, many women can receive a dual risk reduction with one surgery. RRSO has been shown to reduce ovarian cancer risk by 80% to 95%,[57–60] and breast cancer risk by 50% (for premenopausal women) in *BRCA1/2* mutation carriers.[59–62] Anywhere from 2.5% to 17%[63–65] of women who undergo RRSO are found to have an occult ovarian, fallopian tube, or primary peritoneal cancer upon pathology review, emphasizing the need for a "high-risk" pathologic examination of the tissues.[66] However, after surgery, women may still face an ~4% risk of developing primary peritoneal cancer over the course of 20 years.[57] The second major reason surgery is recommended over screening is that ovarian cancer screening is ineffective at detecting ovarian cancer at early stages[67]; the pros and cons of ovarian cancer screening with transvaginal ultrasound and CA-125 have been reviewed elsewhere.[4] A second option for reducing ovarian cancer risk is through oral contraceptive (OCP) use. OCPs use can reduce ovarian cancer risk by ~50% with 5 years of use; the benefit has been shown for both *BRCA1* and *BRCA2* carriers.[68,69] However, it is worth noting that data are conflicting about whether OCP use can increase breast cancer risk, so it is important to take into account a woman's age, family history, and genetic test results before making recommendations to use OCPs.[70–73] Recently, researchers at Stanford created an online decision tool to aid female *BRCA1/2* mutation carriers in conjunction with a health-care provider making decisions with respect to cancer screening and surgical prevention[74]; the tool is available at http://brcatool.stanford.edu.

LYNCH SYNDROME

Approximately 2% to 4% of ovarian cancer is believed to be associated with Lynch syndrome, also referred to as hereditary nonpolyposis colorectal cancer syndrome.[7,75] Lynch syndrome is an autosomal dominant cancer predisposition syndrome characterized by a significantly increased lifetime risk of colorectal cancer (~30% to 70%) and extracolonic malignancies of the endometrium (28% to 60%), stomach (6% to 9%), small bowel (3% to 4%), urinary tract (3% to 8%), central nervous system (4%), hepatobiliary tract (1%), and sebaceous skin lesions (1% to 9%).[76]

Lynch syndrome is caused by germline mismatch repair (MMR) gene mutations in *MLH1, MSH2, MSH6,* and *PMS2.* Alterations in these four genes account for approximately 36%, 38%, 14%, and 15% of Lynch syndrome, respectively.[77] In addition, germline deletions in *EPCAM* inactivate *MSH2* through epigenetic silencing in a small proportion of individuals with Lynch syndrome.[78] Variations in cancer risk have been noted among the four *MMR* genes. An increased risk for endometrial cancer and slightly decreased risk for colorectal cancer are observed in families with germline *MSH6* mutations compared with families with *MLH1* and *MSH2* mutations.[79] Germline mutations in *PMS2* are associated with the lowest overall risk for Lynch syndrome–associated malignancies.[80]

Lynch syndrome is diagnosed clinically within families meeting either the Amsterdam I or Amsterdam II criteria[81,82] (Table 77.2). Although fulfillment of the Amsterdam criteria is a significant predictor of identifying a germline MMR gene mutation in a family, it is well known that at least 25% of families affected with Lynch syndrome do not meet the Amsterdam criteria.[83]

The lifetime risk of ovarian cancer in Lynch syndrome is estimated to be anywhere between 4% and 11%,[78,84,85] with a mean age of diagnosis at 42.7 years.[75] In this series, approximately one-third of the individuals were younger than 40 years at the time of diagnosis (*n* = 80). Approximately 94% of ovarian tumors in Lynch syndrome are invasive epithelial in origin, with borderline

Amsterdam Criteria for Clinical Diagnosis of Lynch Syndrome

Amsterdam I Criteria[81]
- Three affected family members with histologically verified colorectal cancer, one of whom is a first-degree relative of the other two
- Colorectal cancer in at least two successive generations
- At least one of the affected relatives with colorectal cancer is diagnosed at <50 y
- Familial adenomatous polyposis has been excluded

Amsterdam II Criteria[82]
- Three affected family members with a Lynch syndrome–associated cancer (colon, endometrial, small bowel, ureter, or renal pelvis), one of whom is a first-degree relative of the other two
- Cancer diagnoses in at least two successive generations
- At least one of the affected relatives with a Lynch syndrome–associated cancer is diagnosed at <50 y
- Familial adenomatous polyposis has been excluded

and granulosa cell tumors representing ~4% of cases. Lynch-related ovarian tumors are most frequently moderately or well differentiated. Of note, synchronous endometrial cancer was identified in 21.5% of cases. In a meta-analysis of 159 cases of MMR-related ovarian cancers, histologic subtypes included serous (32%), endometrioid (29%), mixed (24%), mucinous (19%), and clear cell (18%).[87] In a study of individuals with Lynch-related ovarian cancer compared with individuals with sporadic ovarian cancer, no significant difference was observed in survival rate, although the total number of Lynch-related ovarian cancers was small (*n* = 277).[87]

Lynch syndrome is one of a few hereditary cancer syndromes that have more than one method available to make a genetic diagnosis by identifying MMR deficiency including (1) tumor studies, specifically microsatellite instability (MSI) and IHC, and (2) germline genetic testing (typically includes DNA sequencing and a technology to look for large structural rearrangements). In initiating a genetic evaluation for Lynch syndrome, tumor studies are generally the recommended first-line tests.[78] However, because the majority of available data on performing MSI and IHC pertain to colorectal and endometrial tumors,[76–78] it is not certain whether tumor studies on ovarian cancers as a first-line approach are valid. Approximately 12% of unselected ovarian cancers will have an MSI-high phenotype.[75] In an analysis of 52 ovarian carcinomas in a population who received a diagnosis at younger than 50 years, defects in MMR expression were identified in 10% of cases using MSI and IHC.[88] Domanska et al.[89] evaluated ovarian carcinomas in a population who received a diagnosis at younger than 40 years and found MMR deficiency with IHC in ~6% of cases. If tumor studies are indicative of Lynch syndrome (results show the tumor to be MSI-high and/or loss of ≥1 MMR proteins), germline genetic testing should be offered and will identify a deleterious mutation anywhere from 20% to 70% of the time.[78] Molecular analysis is widely available for the four MMR genes and *EPCAM.* However, if tumor studies are performed on an ovarian cancer, and the results are not indicative of Lynch syndrome, given the paucity of data, Lynch syndrome cannot conclusively be ruled out, and germline genetic testing may still be warranted, depending on the patient's age at onset and family history.

If a tumor specimen is not available, germline genetic testing may be initiated at the outset. A recent abstract showed that up to 4% of unselected ovarian cancers may be found to have a germline mutation in *MLH1, MSH2,* or *MSH6.*[7] If a patient with ovarian cancer needs a genetic evaluation for Lynch syndrome, the ideal approach would be for the health-care provider to have a detailed discussion about the pros and cons of each testing methodology with the patient, so that the patient and provider can jointly come to a decision about the best approach given the rest of the family history of cancer.

Current ovarian cancer management guidelines for women with Lynch syndrome include prophylactic hysterectomy and bilateral salpingo-oophorectomy after completion of childbearing; there is not enough data to support routine ovarian cancer screening with transvaginal ultrasound and CA-125 blood tests for women, although it may be considered at the clinician's discretion.[90]

PEUTZ–JEGHERS SYNDROME

Peutz–Jeghers syndrome (PJS) is a rare autosomal dominant inherited disorder characterized by gastrointestinal hamartomatous polyposis, mucocutaneous melanin pigmentation, and benign and malignant tumors of the gastrointestinal tract, breast, ovary, cervix, and testis. The incidence of PJS is unknown but has been estimated between 1:8,300 and 1:200,000 births.[91,92]

In contrast to the other hamartomatous syndromes in which polyps occur most commonly in the colon, PJS-related polyps occur most commonly in the small intestine (90%), although they can also occur elsewhere in the gastrointestinal tract including the stomach (25%) and large bowel (33%), and may also develop outside the digestive tract in the uterus, bladder, lungs, and nasal passages.[93] Gastrointestinal polyps can result in chronic bleeding and anemia, and cause recurrent obstruction and intussusception requiring repeated laparotomy and bowel resection. Polyposis usually becomes symptomatic in early adolescence, although intestinal obstruction has been reported in infancy.[94] Polyps may be of mixed histologic types (hyperplastic, adenomatous) but are mostly hamartomatous and may number from one to dozens.

The characteristic mucocutaneous hyperpigmentation presents in childhood as dark blue to dark brown macules around the mouth, eyes, and nostrils; in the perianal area; and on the buccal mucosa. Hyperpigmented macules on the fingers are common and can also occur on the feet and in the axillae. The macules may fade in puberty and adulthood; however, pigmented areas inside the mouth or on the gums tend to persist into adulthood.[95]

In a single individual, a clinical diagnosis of PJS may be made when any one of the following is present[96]:

- Two or more histologically confirmed PJS polyps
- Any number of PJS polyps detected in one individual who has a family history of PJS in close relative(s)
- Characteristic mucocutaneous pigmentation in an individual who has a family history of PJS in close relative(s)
- Any number of PJS polyps in an individual who also has characteristic mucocutaneous pigmentation

Individuals with PJS are at increased risk for a wide variety of epithelial malignancies (colorectal, gastric, pancreatic, breast, and ovarian cancers). The estimated incidence of cancer among patients with PJS was identified as 18-fold higher than that in the general population by Giardello et al.,[97] although a recent meta-analysis by van Lier et al.[98] placed the lower end of the range at close to 10-fold.

Females with PJS are at risk for sex cord tumors with annular tubules (SCTAT), a distinctive benign ovarian neoplasm, the predominant component of which has morphologic features intermediate between those of the granulosa cell tumor and those of the Sertoli cell tumor; focal differentiation into either tumor may occur. Up to 36% of women who have SCTATs are found to have PJS.[99] SCTATs may cause sexual precocity and infertility, and they are generally considered benign, but may become malignant. Of the 74 cases that formed the basis of the investigation of Young et al.,[99] 27 were associated with PJS; these tumors were all benign and were typically multifocal, bilateral, very small or even microscopic in size, and calcified. Although SCTATs predominate

as the ovarian tumors identified in PJS, other histologic findings have been identified including granulosa cell tumors, cystadenomas, nonneoplastic cysts, Brenner tumors, dysgerminomas, and Sertoli cell tumors.[100] Patients have ranged in age from 4.5 to 60 years at the time their ovarian tumors were diagnosed; more than half were 22 years or younger.

In 1998, investigators discovered that mutations in the serine threonine kinase 11 gene (*STK11*, also known as *LKB1* gene) cause PJS.[101,102] Genetic testing for clinical practice is now widely available; mutations in the *STK11* gene are detected in 50% to 90% of individuals with PJS.[103–106] The variability in detection rates is likely due to differences in selection criteria and testing methodologies. The majority of mutations are truncating or missense mutations, which eliminate the kinase function of the protein. However, up to 30% of mutations may be large deletions, which would not be detected by sequencing alone.[107] Therefore, the optimal approach for genetic testing would include both full sequencing and analysis for large deletions and duplications. Although the addition of large deletion analysis to *STK11* testing has greatly increased the mutation detection rate, there is still a very small portion of individuals and families meeting the clinical diagnostic criteria in which a deleterious mutation cannot be identified.[108,109] There are reports of families with a clinical diagnosis of PJS who do not link to 19p13.3, suggesting that there might be another genetic locus causing PJS in rare families.[110]

Current management guidelines for individuals with PJS are reflected in the current National Comprehensive Cancer Network Guidelines® (NCCN Guidelines®) (Table 77.3)[90] and with respect to ovarian cancer screening include consideration of an annual transvaginal ultrasound starting between the ages of 18 and 20 years. These recommendations reflect expert opinion as no controlled trials have been published on the effectiveness of surveillance in PJS.[96] With respect to uncontrolled data, German investigators recently reported a surveillance strategy that led to the early detection of 50% of all cancers (5/10) diagnosed in 31 patients with PJS.[104] Malignancies that occur in PJS, including SCTATs, should be treated in a standard manner, and conservative management of gonadal tumors in females is deemed appropriate.

NEWER GENES

RAD51C

RAD51C, a RAD51 paralog, is an integral part of the DNA double-strand break repair through homologous recombination. Biallelic *RAD51C* mutations have recently been identified in patients with Fanconi anemia, and subsequently, monoallelic mutations have been identified in up to 2.9% of highly penetrant breast and ovarian cancer families who previously screened negative for *BRCA1/2* mutations.[111–114] *RAD51C* families show major similarities in ovarian cancer occurrence with families carrying *BRCA1/2* mutations. Moreover, as these families show apparently complete segregation of the mutation with the cancer phenotype, the penetrance of *RAD51C* mutations is predicted to be at least comparable to that of *BRCA1/2* mutations.

In comparison to the younger age at onset of *BRCA1/2*-associated ovarian cancers, the reported mean age at onset for ovarian cancer in women with *RAD51C* mutations ranges from 57.7 to 770 years (range, 50 to 81 years).[112,115,116] *RAD51C*-associated ovarian tumors are almost uniformly epithelial in origin and, for the most part, are invasive and nonmucinous.[112,115,116] Other reported histologic findings include invasive endometrioid adenocarcinoma, malignant cystadenoma, and fallopian tube carcinoma.[116]

Two recurrent founder mutations in the *RAD51C* gene have been identified in Finnish breast and/or ovarian cancer families, suggesting that founder mutations in this gene may exist in other ethnic groups.[116]

TABLE 77.3

Adapted National Comprehensive Cancer Network Guidelines for Peutz-Jeghers Cancer Screening

Site	Screening Procedure and Interval	Initiation Age
Breast	Mammogram and breast magnetic resonance imaging (MRI) annually Clinical breast examination every 6 mo	~25 y
Colon	Colonoscopy every 2–3 y	~Late teens
Stomach	Upper endoscopy every 2–3 y	~Late teens
Pancreas	Magnetic resonance cholangiopancreatography or endoscopic ultrasound every 1–2 y CA-19-9 at similar intervals	~30–35 y
Small intestine	Small-bowel visualization (computed tomography or MRI enterography) baseline at 8–10 y with follow-up interval based on findings but at least by age 18 y, then every 2–3 y, although this may be individualized, or with symptoms	~8–10 y
Ovary	Pelvic examination and Papanicolaou smear annually	~18–20 y
Cervix Uterus	Consider transvaginal ultrasound	
Testes	Annual testicular examination and observation for feminizing changes	~10 y
Lung	Provide education about symptoms and smoking cessation No other specific recommendations have been made	

RAD51D

Identification of *RAD51C* mutations in families with breast and ovarian cancer prompted investigations into the role of another RAD51 paralog, *RAD51D*, in cancer susceptibility. Monoallelic mutations have been identified in up to 0.9% of highly penetrant breast and ovarian cancer families who previously screened negative for *BRCA1/2* mutations; it is estimated that ~0.6% of unselected individuals with ovarian cancer will harbor *RAD51D* mutations.[117] Loveday et al.[117] found that mutations were more prevalent in families with more than one ovarian cancer: Four mutations were identified in 235 families (1.7%) with two or more ovarian cancer cases. Remarkably, three mutations were found in 59 families (5.1%) with three or more ovarian cancer cases.

RAD51D-associated ovarian tumors are almost uniformly epithelial in origin, with one report of a clear-cell ovarian carcinoma.[118] The relative risk of ovarian cancer for *RAD51D* mutation carriers is estimated to be 6.3, which equates to ~10% cumulative risk by age 80 years.[117]

The current studies, although few in number, clearly show that *RAD51D* is an ovarian cancer predisposition gene, but further studies in familial and sporadic ovarian cancer series would be of value to further clarify the risks of ovarian cancer. Cells deficient in *RAD51D* are sensitive to treatment with a PARP inhibitor, suggesting a possible therapeutic approach for cancers arising in *RAD51D* mutation carriers.[117]

Given the recent identification of their contribution to ovarian cancer susceptibility, *RAD51C*, as well as *RAD51D*, has to be validated in larger mutation positive cohorts to generate reliable estimations of the clinical implications of carrying germline mutations as well as determine appropriate screening and cancer prevention strategies.

CONCLUSION

The puzzle of identifying genes causative of hereditary ovarian cancer continues to be deciphered. Historically, *BRCA1* and *BRCA2* have been the only genes considered when evaluating families suggestive of a hereditary ovarian cancer syndrome, but new studies have linked ovarian cancer to other known hereditary syndromes such as Lynch syndrome as well as new genes such as *RAD51C/D*. As genetic testing advances and newer technologies such as next-generation sequencing and whole-exome sequencing are used, additional genes will continue to be discovered. With these discoveries, new insights into ovarian cancer pathogenesis will be understood and hopefully lead to better and more effective treatments such as PARP inhibitors, but more importantly, more women can be identified as being at risk before developing ovarian cancer, leading to increased ovarian cancer prevention.

REFERENCES

1. American Cancer Society. Cancer facts & figures 2014. http://www.cancer.org/acs/groups/content/@research/documents/webcontent/acspc-042151.pdf. Accessed September 5, 2014.
2. Nelson HD, Westhoff C, Piepert J, et al. Screening for ovarian cancer: Brief evidence update. http://www.uspreventiveservicestaskforce.org/uspstf/uspsovar.htm. Accessed April 7, 2012.
3. Roett MA, Evans P. Ovarian cancer: An overview. *Am Fam Physician* 2009;80:609–616.
4. Schorge JO, Modesitt SC, Coleman RL, et al. SGO white paper on ovarian cancer: Etiology, screening and surveillance. *Gynecol Oncol* 2010;119:7–17.
5. Kerlikowske K, Brown JS, Grady DG. Should women with familial ovarian cancer undergo prophylactic oophorectomy? *Obstet Gynecol* 1992;80:700–707.
6. Pal T, Permuth-Wey J, Betts JA, et al. BRCA1 and BRCA2 mutations account for a large proportion of ovarian carcinoma cases. *Cancer* 2005;104:2804–2816.
7. Pal T, Mohammad R, Sun P, et al. The frequency of MLH1, MSH2 and MSH6 mutations in a population-based sample of ovarian cancers [abstract]. In: *Proceedings of the 102nd Annual Meeting for the American Association for Cancer Research*; April 2–6, 2011; Orlando, FL. Philadelphia, PA: AACR; 2011. Abstract 5617.
8. Walsh T, Casadei S, Lee MK, et al. Mutations in 12 genes for inherited ovarian, fallopian tube, and peritoneal carcinoma identified by massively parallel sequencing. *Proc Natl Acad Sci U S A* 2011;108:18032–18037.
9. Wooster R, Bignel G, Lancaster J, et al. Identification of the breast cancer susceptibility gene BRCA2. *Nature* 1995;378:789–792.

10. Ford D, Easton DF, Peto J. Estimates of the gene frequency of BRCA1 and its contribution to breast and ovarian cancer incidence. *Am J Hum Genet* 1995;57:1457–1462.
11. Struewing JP, Hartge P, Wacholder S, et al. The risk of cancer associated with specific mutations of BRCA1 and BRCA2 among Ashkenazi Jews. *N Engl J Med* 1997;336:1401–1408.
12. Moslehi B, Chu W, Karlan B, et al. BRCA1 and BRCA2 mutation analysis of 208 Ashkenazi Jewish women with ovarian cancer. *Am J Hum Genet* 2000;66:1259–1272.
13. Modan B, Hartge P, Hirsh-Yechezkel G, et al. Parity, oral contraceptives and the risk of ovarian cancer among carriers and non-carriers of a BRCA1 or BRCA2 mutation. *N Engl J Med* 2001;345:235–240.
14. American College of Medical Genetics Foundation. ACMG genetic susceptibility to breast and ovarian cancer: Assessment, counseling and testing guidelines. http://www.health.ny.gov/diseases/cancer/obcancer/pp27-35.htm. Accessed April 21, 2012.
15. American College of Obstetricians and Gynecologists, ACOG Committee on Practice Bulletins—Gynecology, ACOG Committee on Genetics, et al. ACOG Practice Bulletin No. 103: Hereditary breast and ovarian cancer syndrome. *Obstet Gynecol* 2009;113:957–966.
16. American Society of Breast Surgeons. BRCA genetic testing for patients with and without breast cancer. http://www.breastsurgeons.org/statements/PDF_Statements/BRCA_Testing.pdf. Accessed April 21, 2012.
17. Daly MB, Pilarski R, Axilbund JE, et al. NCCN Clinical Practice Guidelines in Oncology (NCCN Guidelines®). Genetic/Familial High-Risk Assessment: Breast and Ovarian V2.2014. © 2014 National Comprehensive Cancer Network, Inc. www.nccn.org. Accessed September 25, 2014.
18. Lancaster JM, Powell CB, Kauff ND, et al. Society of Gynecologic Oncologists Education Committee statement on risk assessment for inherited gynecologic cancer predispositions. *Gynecol Oncol* 2007;107:159–162.
19. U.S. Preventative Services Task Force. Genetic risk assessment and BRCA mutation testing for breast and ovarian cancer susceptibility: Recommendation statement. *Ann Intern Med* 2005;143:355–361.
20. Easton DF, Bishop DT, Ford D, et al. Genetic linkage analysis in familial breast and ovarian cancer: Results from 214 families. *Am J Hum Genet* 1993;52:678–701.
21. Ford D, Easton DF, Bishop DT, et al. Risks of cancer in BRCA1-mutation carriers. Breast Cancer Linkage Consortium. *Lancet* 1994;343:692–695.
22. Easton DF, Ford D, Bishop DT, et al. Breast and ovarian cancer incidence in BRCA1-mutation carriers. *Am J Hum Genet* 1995;56:265–271.
23. Narod SA, Ford D, Devilee P, et al. An evaluation of genetic heterogeneity in 145 breast-ovarian cancer families: Breast Cancer Linkage Consortium. *Am J Hum Genet* 1995;56:254–264.
24. Ford D, Easton DF, Stratton M, et al. Genetic heterogeneity and penetrance analysis of the BRCA1 and BRCA2 genes in breast cancer families. *Am J Hum Genet* 1998;62:676–689.
25. The Breast Cancer Linkage Consortium. Cancer risks in BRCA2 mutation carriers. *J Natl Cancer Inst* 1999;91:1310–1316.
26. Antoniou A, Pharoah PD, Narod S, et al. Average risks of breast and ovarian cancer associated with BRCA1 or BRCA2 mutations detected in a case series unselected for family history: A combined analysis of 22 studies. *Am J Hum Genet* 2003;72:1117–1130.
27. Chen S, Iversen ES, Friebel T, et al. Characterization of BRCA1 and BRCA2 mutations in a large United States sample. *J Clin Oncol* 2006;24:863–871.
28. Chen S, Parmigiani G. Meta-analysis of BRCA1 and BRCA2 penetrance. *J Clin Oncol* 2007;25:1329–1333.
29. Gayther SA, Mangion J, Russell P, et al. Variation of risks of breast and ovarian cancer associated with different germline mutations of the BRCA2 gene. *Nat Genet* 1997;15:103–105.
30. Thompson D, Easton D. Variation in cancer risks, by mutation position, in BRCA2 mutation carriers. *Am J Hum Genet* 2001;68:410–419.
31. Chenevix-Trench G, Milne RL, Antoniou AC, et al. An international initiative to identify genetic modifiers of cancer risk in BRCA1 and BRCA2 mutation carriers: The Consortium of Investigators of Modifiers of BRCA1 and BRCA2 (CIMBA). *Breast Cancer Res* 2007;9:104.
32. Rebbeck TR, Mitra N, Domchek SM, et al. Modification of ovarian cancer risk by BRCA1/2-interacting genes in a multicenter cohort of BRCA1/2 mutation carriers. *Cancer Res* 2009;69:5801–5810.
33. Jakubowska A, Rozkrut D, Antoniou A, et al. The Leu33Pro polymorphism in the ITGB3 gene does not modify BRCA1/2-associated breast or ovarian cancer risks: Results from a multicenter study among 15542 BRCA1 and BRCA2 mutation carriers. *Breast Cancer Res Treat* 2009;121:639–649.
34. Ramus SJ, Kartsonaki C, Gayther SA, et al. Genetic variation at 9p22.2 and ovarian cancer risk for BRCA1 and BRCA2 mutation carriers. *J Natl Cancer Inst* 2011;103:105–116.
35. Risch HA, McLaughlin JR, Cole DE, et al. Prevalence and penetrance of germline BRCA1 and BRCA2 mutations in a population series of 649 women with ovarian cancer. *Am J Hum Genet* 2001;68:700–710.
36. Frank TS, Deffenbaugh AM, Reid JE, et al. Clinical characteristics of individuals with germline mutations in BRCA1 and BRCA2: Analysis of 10000 individuals. *J Clin Oncol* 2002;20:1480–1490.
37. National Cancer Institute. SEER stat fact sheets: Ovary. http://seer.cancer.gov/statfacts/html/ovary.html. Accessed April 8, 2012.
38. Stratton JF, Thompson D, Bobrow L, et al. The genetic epidemiology of early-onset epithelial ovarian cancer: A population-based study. *Am J Hum Genet* 1999;65:1725–1732.
39. Boyd J, Sonoda Y, Federici MG, et al. Clinicopathologic features of BRCA-linked and sporadic ovarian cancer. *JAMA* 2000;283:2260–2265.
40. Friedlander ML, Dembo AJ. Prognostic factors in ovarian cancer. *Semin Oncol* 1991;18:205–212.
41. Evans DGR, Young K, Bulman M, et al. Probability of BRCA1/2 mutation varies with ovarian histology: Results from screening 442 ovarian cancer families. *Clin Genet* 2008;73:338–345.
42. Lakhani SR, Manek S, Penault-Llorca F, et al. Pathology of ovarian cancers in BRCA1 and BRCA2 carriers. *Clin Cancer Res* 2004;10:2473–2481.
43. Mavaddat N, Barrowdale D, Andrulis IL, et al. Pathology of breast and ovarian cancers among BRCA1 and BRCA2 mutation carriers: Results from the Consortium Investigators of Modifiers of BRCA1/2 (CIMBA). *Cancer Epidemiol Biomarkers Prev* 2012;21:134–147.
44. Bolton KL, Chenevix-Trench G, Goh C, et al. Association between BRCA1 and BRCA2 mutations and survival in women with invasive epithelial ovarian cancer. *JAMA* 2012;307:382–390.
45. Ben David Y, Chetrit A, Hirsh-Yechezkel G, et al. Effect of BRCA mutations on the length of survival in epithelial ovarian cancers. *J Clin Oncol* 2002;20:463–466.
46. Cass I, Baldwin RL, Varkey T, et al. Improved survival in women with BRCA-associated ovarian carcinoma. *Cancer* 2003;97:2187–2195.
47. Chetrit A, Hirsh-Yechezkel G, Ben-David Y, et al. Effect of BRCA1/2 mutations on long term survival of patients with invasive ovarian cancer: The national Israeli study of ovarian cancer. *J Clin Oncol* 2008;26:20–25.
48. Tan DS, Rothermundt C, Thomas K, et al. "BRCAness" syndrome in ovarian cancer: A case-control study describing clinical features and outcome of patents with epithelial ovarian cancer associated with BRCA1 and BRCA2 mutations. *J Clin Oncol* 2008;26:5530–5536.
49. Roy R, Chun J, Powell SN. BRCA1 and BRCA2: Different roles in a common pathway of genome protection. *Nat Rev Cancer* 2012;12:68–78.
50. Bryant HE, Schultz N, Thomas HD, et al. Specific killing of BRCA2-deficient tumors with inhibitors of poly(ADP-ribose) polymerase. *Nature* 2005;434:913–917.
51. Fong PC, Boss DS, Yap TA, et al. Inhibition of poly(ADP-ribose) polymerase in tumors from BRCA mutation carriers. *N Engl J Med* 2009;361:123–134.
52. Rouleau M, Patel A, Hendzel MJ, et al. PARP inhibition: PARP1 and beyond. *Nat Rev Cancer* 2010;10:293–301.
53. Fong PC, Yap TA, Boss DS, et al. Poly(ADP-ribose) polymerase inhibition: Frequent durable responses in BRCA carrier ovarian cancer correlating with platinum-free interval. *J Clin Oncol* 2010;28:2512–2519.
54. Audeh MW, Carmichael J, Penson RT, et al. Oral poly(ADP-ribose) polymerase inhibitor olaparib in patients with BRCA1 or BRCA2 mutations and recurrent ovarian cancer: A proof-of-concept trial. *Lancet* 2010;376:245–251.
55. Gelmon KA, Tischkowitz M, Mackay H, et al. Olaparib in patients with recurrent high-grade serous or poorly differentiated ovarian carcinoma or triple-negative breast cancer: A phase 2, multicentre, open-label, non-randomized study. *Lancet Oncol* 2011;12:852–861.
56. Ledermann J, Harter P, Gourley C, et al. Olaparib maintenance therapy in platinum-sensitive relapsed ovarian cancer. *N Engl J Med* 2012;366:1382–1392.
57. Finch A, Beiner M, Lubinski J, et al. Salpingo-oophorectomy and the risk of ovarian, fallopian tube and peritoneal cancers in women with a BRCA1 or BRCA2 mutation. *JAMA* 2006;296:185–192.
58. Kauff ND, Domchek SM, Friebel TM, et al. Risk-reducing salpingo-oophorectomy for the prevention of BRCA1- and BRCA2-associated breast and gynecologic cancer: A multicenter, prospective study. *J Clin Oncol* 2008;26:1331–1337.
59. Rebbeck TR, Kauff ND, Domchek SM. Meta-analysis of risk reduction estimates associated with risk-reducing salpingo-oophorectomy in BRCA1 and BRCA2 mutation carriers. *J Natl Cancer Inst* 2009;101:80–87.
60. Domchek SM, Friebel TM, Singer CF, et al. Association of risk-reducing surgery in BRCA1 or BRCA2 mutation carriers with cancer risk and mortality. *JAMA* 2010;304:967–975.
61. Rebbeck TR, Levin AM, Eisen A, et al. Breast cancer risk after bilateral prophylactic oophorectomy in BRCA1 mutation carriers. *J Natl Cancer Inst* 1999;91:1475–1479.
62. Eisen A, Lubinski J, Klijn J, et al. Breast cancer risk following bilateral oophorectomy in BRCA1 and BRCA2 mutation carriers: An international case-control study. *J Clin Oncol* 2005;23:7491–7496.
63. Powell CB, Kenley E, Chen L, et al. Risk-reducing salpingo-oophorectomy in BRCA mutation carriers: Role of serial sectioning in the detection of occult malignancy. *J Clin Oncol* 2005;23:127–132.
64. Finch A, Shaw P, Rosen B, et al. Clinical and pathologic findings of prophylactic salpingo-oophorectomy in 159 BRCA1 and BRCA2 carriers. *Gynecol Oncol* 2006;100:58–64.
65. Domchek SM, Friebel TM, Garber JE, et al. Occult ovarian cancers identified at risk-reducing salpingo-oophorectomy in a prospective cohort of BRCA1/2 mutation carriers. *Breast Cancer Res Treat* 2010;124:195–203.

66. Movahedi-Lankarani S, Baker PM, Giks B, et al. Protocol for the examination of specimens from patients with carcinoma of the ovary. http://www.cap.org/apps/docs/committees/cancer/cancer_protocols/2009/Ovary_09protocol.pdf. Accessed April 14, 2012.
67. Stirling D, Evans DGR, Pichert G, et al. Screening for familial ovarian cancer: Failure of current protocols to detect ovarian cancer at an early stage according to the International Federation of Gynecology and Obstetrics System. *J Clin Oncol* 2005;23:5588–5596.
68. Narod SA, Risch H, Moslehi R, et al. Oral contraceptives and the risk of hereditary ovarian cancer. Hereditary Ovarian Cancer Clinical Study Group. *N Engl J Med* 1998;39:424–428.
69. Iodice S, Barile M, Rotmensz N, et al. Oral contraceptive use and breast or ovarian cancer risk in BRCA1/2 carriers: A meta-analysis. *Eur J Cancer* 2010;46:2275–2284.
70. Narod SA, Dube MP, Klijn J, et al. Oral contraceptives and the risk of breast cancer in BRCA1 and BRCA2 mutation carriers. *J Natl Cancer Inst* 2002;94:1773–1779.
71. Milne RL, Knight JA, John EM, et al. Oral contraceptive use and risk of early-onset breast cancer in carriers and noncarriers of BRCA1 and BRCA2 mutations. *Cancer Epidemiol Biomarkers Prev* 2005;14:350–356.
72. Haile RW, Thomas DC, McGuire V, et al. BRCA1 and BRCA2 mutation carriers, oral contraceptive use, and breast cancer before age 50. *Cancer Epidemiol Biomarkers Prev* 2006;15:1863–1870.
73. Lee E, Ma H, McKean-Cowdin R, et al. Effect of reproductive factors and oral contraceptives on breast cancer risk in BRCA1/2 mutation carriers and noncarriers: Results from a population based study. *Cancer Epidemiol Biomarkers Prev* 2008;17:3170–3178.
74. Kurian AW, Munoz DF, Rust P, et al. Online tool to guide decisions for BRCA1/2 mutation carriers. *J Clin Oncol* 2012;30:497–506.
75. Watson P, Bützow R, Lynch HT, et al. The clinical features of ovarian cancer in hereditary nonpolyposis colorectal cancer. *Gynecol Oncol* 2001;82:223–228.
76. Weissman SM, Bellcross C, Bittner CC, et al. Genetic counseling considerations in the evaluation of families for Lynch syndrome—a review. *J Genet Counsel* 2011;20:5–19.
77. Palomaki GE, McClain MR, Melillo S, et al. EGAPP supplementary evidence review: DNA testing strategies aimed at reducing morbidity and mortality from Lynch syndrome. *Genet Med* 2009;11:42–65.
78. Weissman SM, Burt R, Church J, et al. Identification of individuals at risk for Lynch syndrome using targeted evaluations and genetic testing: National Society of Genetic Counselors and the Collaborative Group of the Americans on Inherited Colorectal Cancer Joint Practice Guideline. *J Genet Counsel* 2012;21:484–493.
79. Hendriks YM, Wagner A, Morreau H, et al. Cancer risk in hereditary nonpolyposis colorectal cancer due to MSH6 mutations: Impact on counseling and surveillance. *Gastroenterology* 2004;127:17–25.
80. Senter L, Clendenning M, Sotamaa K, et al. The clinical phenotype of Lynch syndrome due to germ-line PMS2 mutations. *Gastroenterology* 2008;135:419–428.
81. Vasen HF, Mecklin JP, Khan PM, et al. The International Collaborative Group on hereditary non-polyposis colorectal cancer (ICG-HNPCC). *Dis Colon Rectum* 1991;34:424–425.
82. Vasen HF, Watson P, Mecklin JP, et al. New clinical criteria for hereditary nonpolyposis colorectal cancer (HNPCC, Lynch syndrome) proposed by the International Collaborative group on HNPCC. *Gastroenterology* 1999;116:1453–1456.
83. Hampel H, Frankel WL, Martin E, et al. Feasibility of screening for Lynch syndrome among patients with colorectal cancer. *J Clin Oncol* 2008;26:5783–5788.
84. Barrow E, Alduaij W, Robinson L, et al. Colorectal cancer in HNPCC: Cumulative lifetime incidence, survival and tumour distribution. A report of 121 families with proven mutations. *Clin Genet* 2008;74:233–242.
85. Watson P, Vasen HF, Mecklin JP, et al. The risk of extra-colonic, extra-endometrial cancer in the Lynch syndrome. *Int J Cancer* 2008;123:444–449.
86. Pal T, Permuth-Wey J, Kumar A, et al. Systematic review and meta-analysis of ovarian cancers: Estimation of microsatellite-high frequency and characterization of mismatch repair deficient tumor histology. *Clin Cancer Res* 2008;14:6847–6854.
87. Crijnen TE, Janssen-Heijnen ML, Gelderblom H, et al. Survival of patients with ovarian cancer due to a mismatch repair defect. *Fam Cancer* 2005;4:301–305.
88. Jensen KC, Mariappan MR, Putcha GV, et al. Microsatellite instability and mismatch repair protein defects in ovarian epithelial neoplasms in patients 50 years of age and younger. *Am J Surg Pathol* 2008;32:1029–1037.
89. Domanska K, Malander S, Måsbäck A, et al. Ovarian cancer at young age: The contribution of mismatch-repair defects in a population-based series of epithelial ovarian cancer before age 40. *Intl J Gynecol Cancer* 2007;17:789–793.
90. NCCN Clinical Practice Guidelines in Oncology (NCCN Guidelines®). Genetic/Familial High Risk Assessment: Colorectal. V2.2014. © 2014 National Comprehensive Cancer Network, Inc. www.nccn.org. Accessed September 25, 2014.
91. Allen BA, Terdiman JP. Hereditary polyposis syndromes and hereditary non-polyposis colorectal cancer. *Best Pract Res Clin Gastroenterol* 2003;17:237–258.
92. Lindor NM, McMaster ML, Lindor CJ, et al. Concise handbook of familial cancer susceptibility syndromes—second edition. *J Natl Cancer Inst Monogr* 2008;(38):1–93.
93. Schreibman IR, Baker M, Amos C, et al. The hamartomatous polyposis syndromes: A clinical and molecular review. *Am J Gastroenterol* 2005;100:476–490.
94. Boardman LA. Heritable colorectal cancer syndromes: Recognition and preventive management. *Gastroenterol Clin North Am* 2002;31:1107–1131.
95. McGarrity TJ, Kulin HE, Zaino RJ. Peutz–Jeghers syndrome. *Am J Gastroenterol* 2000;95:596–604.
96. Beggs AD, Latchford AR, Vasen HF, et al. Peutz–Jeghers syndrome: A systematic review and recommendations for management. *Gut* 2010;59:975–986.
97. Giardello FM, Brensinger JD, Tersmette AC. Very high risk of cancer in familial Peutz–Jeghers syndrome. *Gastroenterology* 2000;119:1447–1453.
98. van Lier MGF, Mathus-Vliegen FMH, Wagner A, et al. High cancer risk in Peutz–Jeghers syndrome: A systematic review and surveillance recommendations. *Am J Gastroenterol* 2010;105:1258–1264.
99. Young RH, Welch WR, Dickersin GR, et al. Ovarian sex cord tumor with annular tubules: Review of 74 cases including 27 with Peutz–Jeghers syndrome and four with adenoma malignum of the cervix. *Cancer* 1982;50:1384–1402.
100. Dozois RR, Kempers RD, Dahlin DC, et al. Ovarian tumors associated with the Peutz–Jeghers syndrome. *Ann Surg* 1970;172:233–238.
101. Hemminki A, Markie D, Tomlinson I, et al. A serine/threonine kinase gene defective in Peutz–Jeghers syndrome. *Nature* 1998;391:184–187.
102. Jenne DE, Reimann H, Nezu J, et al. Peutz–Jeghers syndrome is caused by mutations in a novel serine threonine kinase. *Nat Genet* 1998;18:38–43.
103. Volikos E, Robinson J, Aittomäki K, et al. LKB1 exonic and whole gene deletions are a common cause of Peutz–Jeghers syndrome. *J Med Genet* 2006;43:e18.
104. Salloch H, Reinacher-Schick A, Schulmann K, et al. Truncating mutations in Peutz–Jeghers syndrome are associated with more polyps, surgical interventions and cancers. *Int J Colorectal Dis* 2010;25:97–107.
105. Amos CI, Keitheri-Cheteri MB, Sabripour M, et al. Genotype–phenotype correlations in Peutz–Jeghers. *J Med Genet* 2004;41:327–333.
106. Mehenni H, Resta N, Guanti G, et al. Molecular and clinical characteristics in 46 families affected with Peutz–Jeghers syndrome. *Dig Dis Sci* 2007;52:1924–1933.
107. Aretz S, Steinen D, Uhlhaas S, et al. High proportion of large genomic STK11 deletions in Peutz–Jeghers syndrome. *Human Mutat* 2005;26:513–519.
108. Hearle N, Lucassen A, Wang R, et al. Mapping of a translocation breakpoint in a Peutz–Jeghers hamartoma to the putative PJS locus at 19q13.4 and mutation analysis of candidate genes in polyp and STK11-negative PJS cases. *Genes Chromosomes Cancer* 2004;41:163–169.
109. Mehenni H, Gehrig C, Nezu J, et al. Loss of LKB1 kinase activity in Peutz–Jeghers syndrome, and evidence for allelic and locus heterogeneity. *Am J Hum Genet* 1998;63:1641–1650.
110. Boardman LA, Couch FJ, Burgart LJ, et al. Genetic heterogeneity in Peutz–Jeghers syndrome. *Human Mutat* 2000;16:23–30.
111. Vaz F, Hanenberg H, Schuster B, et al. Mutation of the RAD51C gene in a Fanconi anemia-like disorder. *Nat Genet* 2010;42:406–409.
112. Meindl A, Hellebrand H, Wiek C, et al. Germline mutations in breast and ovarian cancer pedigrees establish RAD51C as a human cancer susceptibility gene. *Nat Genet* 2010;42:410–414.
113. Vuorela P, Pylkäs K, Hartikainen JM, et al. Further evidence for the contribution of the RAD51C gene in hereditary breast and ovarian cancer susceptibility. *Breast Cancer Res Treat* 2011;130:1003–1010.
114. Thompson ER, Boyle SE, Johnson J, et al. Analysis of RAD51C germline mutations in high-risk breast and ovarian cancer families and ovarian cancer patients. *Hum Mutat* 2012;33:95–99.
115. Osorio A, Endt D, Fernández F. Predominance of pathogenic missense variants in the RAD51C gene occurring in breast and ovarian cancer families. *Hum Mol Genet* 2012;21(13)2889–2898.
116. Pelttari LM, Heikkinen T, Thompson D, et al. RAD51C is a susceptibility gene for ovarian cancer. *Hum Mol Genet* 2011;20:3278–3288.
117. Loveday C, Turnbull C, Ramsay E, et al. Germline mutations in RAD51D confer susceptibility to ovarian cancer. *Nat Genet* 2011;43:879–882.
118. Osher DJ, De Leeneer K, Michils G, et al. Mutation analysis of RAD51D in non-BRCA1/2 ovarian and breast cancer families. *Br J Cancer* 2012;106:1460–1463.

78

Molecular Biology of Breast Cancer

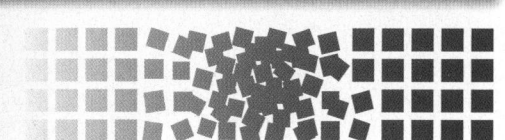

Shaveta Vinayak, Hannah L. Gilmore, and Lyndsay N. Harris

INTRODUCTION

It has been said that cancer is a genetic disease and can be best understood by studying the DNA alterations that lead to the development of cancer. However, a deeper understanding of carcinogenesis requires insight into how these genetic changes alter cellular programs that lead to growth, invasion, and metastasis. This chapter is presented following the logical progression of DNA to RNA to protein, and it describes, at each step, the lesions that contribute to breast cancer carcinogenesis. The chapter also introduces concepts in epigenetics, microRNAs, and gene expression analyses that illustrate how new biologic discoveries and novel technologies have profoundly affected our understanding of breast cancer pathogenesis and influenced the treatment of patients.

GENETICS OF BREAST CANCER

Breast cancer is a heterogeneous disease fundamentally caused by the progressive accumulation of genetic aberrations, including point mutations, chromosomal amplifications, deletions, rearrangements, translocations, and duplications.[1,2] Germ-line mutations account for only about 10% of all breast cancers, whereas the vast majority of breast cancers appear to occur sporadically and are attributed to somatic genetic alterations (Fig. 78.1).[3]

HEREDITARY BREAST CANCER

One of the most important risk factors for breast cancer is family history. Although familial forms comprise nearly 20% of all breast cancers, most of the genes responsible for familial breast cancer have yet to be identified. Breast cancer susceptibility genes can be categorized into three classes according to their frequency and level of risk they confer: rare high-penetrance genes, rare intermediate-penetrance genes, and common low-penetrance genes and loci (Table 78.1).[4]

High-Penetrance, Low-Frequency Breast Cancer Predisposition Genes

BRCA1 and BRCA2

BRCA1 and *BRCA2* mutations account for approximately half of all dominantly inherited hereditary breast cancers. These mutations confer a relative risk of breast cancer 10 to 30 times that of women in the general population, resulting in a nearly 85% lifetime risk of breast cancer development.[5] *BRCA1* and *BRCA2* mutation carriers are quite rare among the general population; however, the prevalence is substantially higher in certain founder

populations, most notably in the Ashkenazi Jewish population, where the carrier frequency is 1 in 40.

More than a thousand germ-line mutations have been identified in *BRCA1* and *BRCA2*. Pathogenic mutations most often result in truncated protein products, although mutations that interfere with protein function also exist.[4,5] Interestingly, the penetrance of pathogenic *BRCA1* and *BRCA2* mutations and age of cancer onset appear to vary both within and among family members. Specific *BRCA* mutations as well as gene–gene and gene–environment interactions as potential modifiers of *BRCA*-related cancer risk are areas of active investigation.[6,7] Variation in risk may be explained by genetic modifiers that are different for both *BRCA1* and *BRCA2* mutation carriers. These alleles have been primarily identified from studies of the Consortium of Investigators of Modifiers of *BRCA1/2* (CIMBA).[8] The commonly identified single-nucleotide polymorphisms (SNP) that modify *BRCA1/2* are listed in Table 78.2 with their gene location, associated risks, and frequency. Evidence from published studies shows that these modifying SNPs combine multiplicatively, and therefore, may significantly alter a mutation carrier's risk depending on the number of risk alleles present.[9,10] In addition to retrospective studies, more recently, common breast cancer susceptibility alleles were evaluated prospectively to assess cancer risk conferred among unaffected *BRCA1/2* mutation carriers.[11] A risk score was constructed and divided into tertiles for seven *BRCA2*-associated variants and four *BRCA1*-associated variants. Among *BRCA2* mutation carriers, breast cancer risks were significantly different when stratified by tertiles; women in the highest tertile had a breast cancer risk of 72% by age 70 compared to 20% for those in the lowest tertile. There was no significant difference by risk score for *BRCA1* mutation carriers.

BRCA1-related breast cancers are characterized by features that distinguish them from both *BRCA2*-related and sporadic breast cancers.[4] *BRCA1*-related tumors typically occur in younger women and have more aggressive features, with high histologic grade, high proliferative rate, aneuploidy, and absence of estrogen and progesterone receptors and human epidermal growth factor receptor 2 (HER2). This *triple-negative* phenotype of *BRCA1*-related breast cancers is further characterized by a *basallike* gene expression profile of cytokeratins 5/6, 14, and 17, epidermal growth factor, and P-cadherin.[12] Although *BRCA1* and *BRCA2* genes encode large proteins with multiple functions, they primarily act as classic tumor suppressor genes that function to maintain genomic stability by facilitating double-strand DNA repair through homologous recombination.[12,13] When loss of heterozygosity (LOH) occurs via loss, mutation, or silencing of the wild-type *BRCA1* or *BRCA2* allele, the resultant defective DNA repair leads to rapid acquisition of additional mutations, particularly during DNA replication, and ultimately sets the stage for cancer development.

The integral role of *BRCA1* and *BRCA2* in double-strand DNA repair holds potential as a therapeutic target for *BRCA*-related breast cancers. For example, platinum agents cause interstrand cross-links, thereby blocking DNA replication and leading

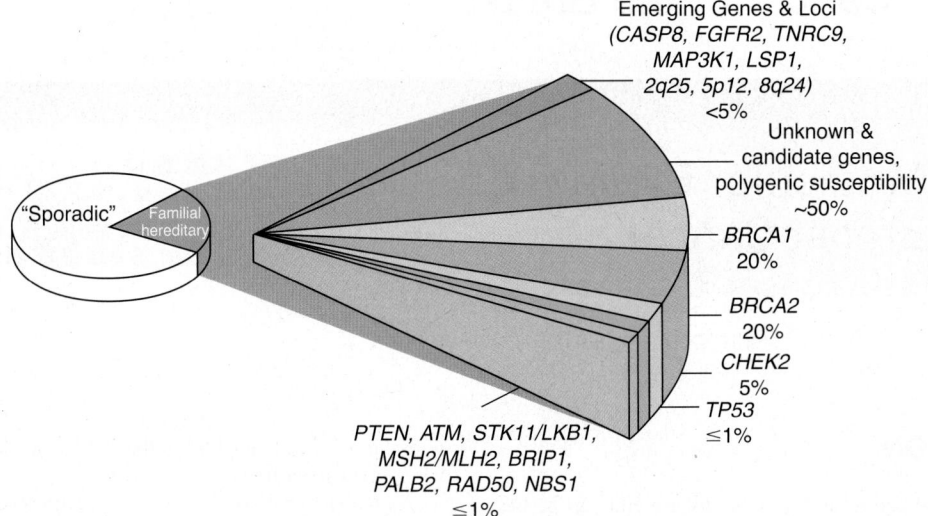

Figure 78.1 Genetic susceptibility to breast cancer. Familial breast cancer comprises approximately 20% to 30% of all breast cancers. *BRCA1* and *BRCA2* are the two major high-penetrance genes associated with hereditary breast and ovarian cancer syndrome, which together account for nearly half of inherited breast cancers. Other rare breast cancer susceptibility genes have been identified, such as *CHEK2*, *TP53*, *PTEN*, and *STK11*. Several emerging low-penetrance genes and loci recently discovered by genomewide association studies account for a small proportion of familial breast cancers (<5%). To date, about half of familial breast cancers remain unexplained but are likely attributable to as yet unknown genes and/ or polygenic susceptibility. (From Olopade O, Grushko TA, Nanda R, Huo D. Advances in breast cancer: pathways to personalized medicine. *Clin Cancer Res* 2008;14:7988–7999, Fig 1.)

to stalled replication forks. Poly (adenosine diphosphate [ADP]-ribose) polymerase-1 (PARP1) inhibitors additionally show promise as specific therapy for *BRCA*-related tumors. PARP1 is a cellular enzyme that functions in single-strand DNA repair through base excision and represents a major alternative DNA repair pathway in the cell.[14,15] When PARP inhibition is applied to a background deficient in double-strand DNA repair, as is the case in *BRCA*-related tumor cells, the cells are left without adequate DNA repair mechanisms and ultimately undergo cell cycle arrest, chromosome instability, and cell death.[4] Given their phenotypic similarities to *BRCA1*-related breast cancers, sporadic basallike breast tumors may display sensitivity to PARP inhibition as well.[15] Phase II studies are currently under way to explore the use of PARP inhibitors in both *BRCA*- and basallike, non–*BRCA*-related breast tumors. There is much that remains to be understood about the optimal use of PARP inhibitors. Current challenges include, but are not limited to, identifying robust predictive biomarkers of response that can guide patient selection and understanding variations among PARP inhibitors in clinical development. Differences in potency and the mechanism of action have been well elucidated in recent preclinical studies,[16–20] and the results of ongoing clinical trials will need to be interpreted in this context. Additionally, recent studies have also identified mechanisms of resistance to PARP inhibitors. One of these important mechanisms includes secondary mutations in the *BRCA1/2* gene that can restore the open reading frame, and therefore, DNA repair functional activity,[21–23] which renders tumors resistant to PARP inhibitors. Secondly, loss of tumor protein p53 binding protein 1 (TP53BP1) in *BRCA1*-deficient cells can restore DNA repair activity,[24,25] and this may confer resistance.

Other High-Penetrance Genes

A small number of other high-risk, low-frequency breast cancer susceptibility genes exist, and they include *TP53*, *PTEN*, *STK11/LKB1*, and *CDH1*.[4–6] These high-penetrance genes confer an eight- to tenfold increase in the risk of breast cancer as compared to noncarriers, but they collectively account for less than 1% of breast cancer cases. Like *BRCA1* and *BRCA2*, these genes are in-

herited in an autosomal-dominant fashion and function as tumor suppressors.[26] The hereditary cancer syndromes associated with each gene are usually characterized by multiple cancers in addition to breast cancer, as summarized in Table 78.1.

Moderate-Penetrance, Low-Frequency Breast Cancer Predisposition Genes

Four genes have been identified that confer an elevated but moderate risk of developing breast cancer, namely *CHEK2*, *ATM*, *BRIP1*, and *PALB2* (see Table 78.1). Each of these genes confers approximately a two- to threefold relative risk of breast cancer in mutation carriers, although this risk may be higher in select clinical settings.[5] Mutation frequencies in the general population are rare, on the order of 0.1% to 1%, although some founder mutations have been identified. Together, these genes account for approximately 2.3% of inherited breast cancer. The moderate relative risk of breast cancer of these genes in conjunction with the low population frequency renders this class of genes very difficult to detect with typical association studies. However, these genes were specifically selected for study as candidate breast cancer genes based on their known roles in signal transduction and DNA repair in close association with *BRCA1* and *BRCA2*.[6]

Low-Penetrance, High-Frequency Breast Cancer Predisposition Genes and Loci

Both candidate gene and genome-wide association studies (GWAS) have identified a low-risk panel of approximately 10 different alleles and loci in 15% to 40% of women with breast cancer (see Table 78.1).[5] Despite their frequency, the relative risk of breast cancer conferred by any one of these genetic variants alone is minimal, on the order of less than 1.5.[4] Nevertheless, these alleles and loci may become clinically relevant in their suggestion of interactions with other high-, moderate-, and low-risk genes; these additive or multiplicative relationships could account for a measurable

TABLE 78.1

Breast Cancer Susceptibility Genes and Loci

Gene/Locus	Associated Syndrome and Clinical Features	Breast Cancer Risk	Mutation/Minor Allele Frequency
High-Penetrance Genes			
BRCA1 (17q21)	**Hereditary breast/ovarian cancer:** Bilateral/multifocal breast tumor, prostate, colon, liver, bone cancers	60%–85% (lifetime); 15%–40% risk of ovarian cancer	1/400
BRCA2 (13q12.3)	**Hereditary breast/ovarian cancer:** Male breast cancer, pancreas, gall bladder, pharynx, stomach, melanoma, prostate cancer; also causes D1 Fanconi anemia (biallelic mutations)	60%–85% (lifetime); 15%–40% risk of ovarian cancer	1/400
TP53 (17p13.1)	**Li-Fraumeni syndrome:** Breast cancer, soft tissue sarcoma, central nervous system tumors, adrenocortical cancer, leukemia, prostate cancer	50%–89% (by age 50); 90% in Li-Fraumeni survivors	<1/10,000
PTEN (10q23.3)	**Cowden syndrome:** Breast cancer, hamartoma, thyroid, oral mucosa, endometrial, brain tumor	25%–50% (lifetime)	<1/10,000
CDH1 (16q22.1)	**Familial diffuse gastric cancer:** Lobular breast cancer, gastric cancer	RR 6.6	<1/10,000
STK11/LKB1 (19p13.3)	**Peutz-Jeghers syndrome:** Breast, ovary, testis, pancreas, cervix, uterine, colon cancers; melanocytic macules of lips/digits; gastrointestinal hamartomatous polyps	30%–50% (by age 70)	<1/10,000
Moderate-Penetrance Genes			
CHEK2 (22q12.1)	**Li-Fraumeni 2 syndrome:** Breast, prostate, colorectal, and brain tumors, sarcomas	OR 2.6 (for 1100delC mutation)	1/100–200 (in certain populations)
BRIP1 (17q22)	**Breast cancer:** Also causes FA-J Fanconi anemia (biallelic mutations)	RR 2.0	<1/1000
ATM (11q22.3)	**Ataxia telangiectasia:** Breast, ovarian, leukemia, lymphoma, possible stomach/pancreas/bladder cancers; immunodeficiency	RR 2.37	1/33–333
PALB2 (16p12)	**Breast, pancreatic, prostate cancers:** Also causes FA-N Fanconi anemia (biallelic mutations)	RR 2.3	<1/1000
Low-Penetrance Genes and Loci			
FGFR2 (10q26)	Breast cancer	OR 1.26	0.38
TOX3 (16q12.1)	Breast cancer	OR 1.14	0.46
LSP1 (11p15.5)	Breast cancer	OR 1.06	0.3
TGFB1 (19q13.1)	Breast cancer	OR 1.07	0.68
MAP3K1 (5q11.2)	Breast cancer	OR 1.13	0.28
CASP8 (2q33–34)	Breast cancer (protective)	OR 0.89	0.13
6q22.33	Breast cancer	OR 1.41	0.21 (in Ashkenazi Jewish)
2q35	Breast cancer	OR 1.11	0.11–0.52
8q24	Breast cancer	OR 1.06	0.4
5p12	Breast cancer	OR 1.19	0.2–0.31

OR, overall risk; RR, relative risk.

fraction of population risk. For example, association studies of fibroblast growth factor receptor 2 (FGFR2) and mitogen-activated protein kinase kinase kinase 1 (MAP3K1) within BRCA families showed that these SNPs conferred an increased risk in the presence of BRCA2 mutations.

Microsatellite Instability in Breast Cancer

There is emerging data that Lynch syndrome, an autosomal-dominant inherited disorder of cancer susceptibility caused by germ-line mutations in the DNA mismatch repair (MMR) genes

including, MLH1, MSH2, MSH5, and PMS2, may increase the risk of breast cancer.[27] Mutation carriers are at increased risk of colorectal and other cancers, but its association with breast cancer risk has been controversial. A prospective cohort study using the Colon Cancer Family Registry evaluated cancer risks among unaffected carriers and noncarriers with a pathogenic MMR gene mutation; notably, breast cancer risk was estimated to be fourfold among mutation carriers compared to the general population.[27] A systematic review of breast cancer risk studies for Lynch syndrome mutation carriers showed mixed results; 13 studies did not observe an increased risk, whereas 8 studies observed an increased risk of breast cancer ranging from 2- to 18-fold compared to the

TABLE 78.2

High Penetrance: Modifiers of *BRCA1/2*

	Gene or Region	SNP	Frequency	Hazard Ratio
BRCA1	CASP8	D302H	12%	0.85
	TOX3/TNRC9	rs3803662	28%	1.09
	TERT (5p15)	rs10069690	27%	1.16
	TERT (5p15)	rs2736108	26%	0.92
	1q32	rs2290854	33%	1.14
	2q35	rs1337042	52%	1.11
	6q25.1	rs2046210	35%	1.17
	6q25.1	rs9397435	7%	1.28
	19p13	rs8170	17%	1.26
	19p13	rs2363956	52%	0.84
BRCA2	FGFR2	rs2981582	39%	1.3
	LSP1	rs3817198	33%	1.14
	MAP3K1	rs889312	29%	1.10
	RAD51	rs1801320	6%	3.18
	SLC4A7/NEK10	rs4973768	49%	1.10
	TOX3/TNRC9	rs3803662	28%	1.17
	ZNF365	rs16917302	11%	0.75
	1p11.2	rs11249433	40%	1.09
	2q35	rs1337042	52%	1.15
	5p12	rs10941679	23%	1.09
	6p24	rs9348512	35%	0.85
	6q25.1	rs9397435	8%	1.14

SNP, single nucleotide polymorphism.

general population.[28] Further studies are needed to determine more precise estimates of breast cancer risk in Lynch syndrome carriers with longer follow-ups. These studies may also guide future breast cancer screening guidelines for this population.

MicroRNA and Cancer Susceptibility

Recent studies suggest that microRNA (miRNA) SNPs may also contribute to breast cancer susceptibility, and miRNAs appear to regulate many tumor suppressor genes and oncogenes via degradation of target miRNAs or repression of their translation. Thus, genetic variations in miRNA genes or miRNA binding sites could affect the expression of tumor suppressor genes or oncogenes and, thereby, affect cancer risk. For example, specific SNPs located within *pre-mir-27a* and *mir-196a-2* genes have been associated with reduced breast cancer risk, which has been confirmed in a recent meta-analysis.[29,30]

SOMATIC CHANGES IN BREAST CANCER

The vast majority of breast cancers are sporadic in origin, ultimately caused by an accumulation of numerous somatic genetic alterations.[1] Recent data suggest that a typical individual breast cancer harbors anywhere from 50 to 80 different somatic mutations.[2] Many of these mutations occur as a result of erroneous DNA replication; others may occur through exposure to exogenous and endogenous mutagens. To date, hundreds of candidate somatic breast cancer genes have been identified through GWAS.[31,32]

Determining the role of each identified mutation in the development of breast cancer remains a substantial challenge. Data suggest that the vast majority of identified somatic DNA mutations in a given tumor are *passenger* mutations, representing harmless, biologically neutral changes that do not contribute to oncogenesis.[1,2] Conversely, *driver* mutations confer a growth advantage on the cell in which they occur and appear to be implicated in cancer development. By definition, driver mutations are found in candidate cancer genes (CAN).[32] A comprehensive catalog of somatic mutations and CAN genes has been accumulated through multiple studies. When specific driver mutations are cataloged among several different breast tumors, a bimodal cancer *genomic landscape* appears, comprising a small number of commonly mutated gene *mountains* among hundreds of infrequently mutated gene *hills*.[1,2] Gene mountains correspond to the most frequently mutated genes found within breast tumors, such as *TP53*, *CDH1*, phosphatidylinositol 3-kinase (*PI3K*), cyclin D, *PTEN*, and *AKT*.[6] Each individual gene hill, on the other hand, is typically found in less than 5% of breast tumors.[1,33] This substantial heterogeneity of DNA mutations among breast tumors may explain the wide variations in phenotypes, both in terms of tumor behavior as well as responsiveness to therapy.

Historically, the focus of genetic research has been on the gene mountains, in part because they were the only mutations that available technology could identify. However, emerging data suggest that it is actually the gene hills that play a much more pivotal role in breast cancer, which is consistent with the idea that having a large number of mutations, each associated with a small survival advantage, drives tumor progression. Recent studies have shown that a substantial number of these infrequent somatic mutations sort out among a much smaller number of biologic groups and cell signaling pathways that are known to be pathogenic in breast cancer, thereby vastly reducing the complexity of the genomic landscape. Examples of such pathways include interferon signaling, cell cycle checkpoint, *BRCA1/2*-related DNA repair, p53, AKT, transforming growth factor β (TGF-β) signaling, Notch, epidermal growth factor receptor (EGFR), FGF, ERBB2, RAS, and PI3K. In short, it appears that common pathways, rather than individual gene mutations, govern the course of breast cancer development.[33]

Although recurrent point mutations are less common in breast cancer than other solid tumors, emerging data show that particular regions of the genome are commonly amplified, and these regions contain genes that drive cancer progression. The best example of an important amplified region is the 17q12 amplicon that harbors the *HER2* oncogene. This amplicon leads to a more aggressive tumor phenotype, now the target of a highly successful antibody therapy, trastuzumab (Herceptin). It has been observed that RNA-mediated interference (RNAi) knockdown of coamplified genes within the 17q12 amplicon results in decreased cell proliferation and increased apoptosis.[34] Thus, the 17q12 amplicon appears to encode a concerted genetic program that contributes to the oncogenesis.

There are several other amplicons, in addition to 17q12 (*HER2*), that seem to drive the cancer phenotype and have prognostic significance in breast cancers, for example, 11q13 (*CCND1*) and 8q24 (*MYC*), 20q13.[35] These regions contain gene sets that are important in DNA metabolism and in the maintenance of chromosomal integrity, suggesting that a response to DNA damaging agents used as anticancer therapy might be modulated by the presence of particular amplicons. Indeed, these coamplicons are frequent in *HER2*-amplified tumors and may modify tumor behavior and patient outcome.[36,37] The contribution of these genomic alterations to functional consequences may lie not in the overexpression of individual genes, but of gene cassettes on the amplicon.

Direct clinical translation of the growing catalog of somatic alterations in breast cancer has yet to evolve. However, with advancing technology and further identification and categorization of genetic mutations, new opportunities for individualized diagnosis and treatment options are likely to emerge.

TRANSCRIPTIONAL PROFILING OF BREAST CANCER

The cellular programs that are encoded by DNA are enacted by transcription into messenger RNA (mRNA) and translated into protein. Not surprisingly, the DNA alterations described previously lead to either under- or overexpression of their associated mRNAs; consequently, abnormal gene expression patterns are a common finding in breast tumors. Gene expression profiling has been introduced into the clinical literature during the past decade because research suggests that assessing the expression of multiple genes in a tumor sample may reflect programs turned on by DNA alternations and predict tumor behavior. So-called molecular signatures hold promise for improving the diagnosis, the prediction of recurrence, and the selection of therapies for individual patients.

Several technologies have been developed to generate molecular signatures, including cDNA and oligonucleotide arrays and multiplex polymerase chain reaction (PCR) technologies. These technologies and newly developed statistical methodologies now allow for evaluations of hundreds and even thousands of mRNAs simultaneously with groupings of samples based on coexpressedgenes.

Molecular Classification of Breast Cancer

The seminal work by Perou et al.[38] and Sorlie et al.[39] suggests a classification of breast cancer subtypes based on gene expression patterns they termed *molecular portraits* of breast cancer. Among the categories they defined were the luminal A and B tumor types (typically estrogen-receptor [ER] or progesterone-receptor [PR] positive), HER2 gene-amplified tumors, and a class termed *basal-like* due to the expression of basal keratins. Recent large scale efforts by The Cancer Genome Atlas Network (TCGA)[40] and the Molecular Taxonomy of Breast Cancer International Consortium (METABRIC)[41] groups have confirmed these earlier findings in addition to providing more detailed molecular portraits.

Luminal Subtypes

The luminal subtypes comprise the majority of breast cancers and are characterized by the expression of genes that are normally expressed in the luminal epithelial of the breast such as cytokeratins 8 and 18 and the luminal expression signature (*ESR1, GATA3, FOXA1, XPB1,* and *MYB*). Luminal subtypes comprise the majority of clinical ER-positive breast cancers and can be divided into two subgroups: luminal A and luminal B. Luminal A tumors are more common and are characterized by high expression levels of ER-related genes and low expression of the HER2 cluster and proliferation-associated genes. In contrast, luminal B tumors are characterized by lower expression levels of ER-related genes, variable expression of the HER2 cluster, and higher levels of proliferation-associated genes. Luminal A tumors have an overall better prognosis than luminal B tumors.

HER2-Enriched Subtype

The HER2-enriched subtype comprises approximately 10% to 15% of all breast cancers and overexpresses both HER2 and proliferation-associated genes and has lower expression of ER-related genes. Interestingly, more recent work by the TCGA demonstrates that not all cancers that are clinically HER2-positive as defined by an immunohistochemical (IHC) analysis and/or fluorescent in situ hybridization (FISH) fall into the HER2-enriched molecular subtype and vice versa. The majority of clinically HER2-positive breast cancers that are not considered part of the HER2-enriched subgroup by gene expression profiling fall into the luminal intrinsic subtype with overexpression of HER2.

Estrogen Receptor–Negative Subtypes

The ER-negative subtypes comprise a heterogeneous group of tumors that clinically are termed triple negative breast cancer (TNBC) because they typically lack ER, PR, and *HER2*, and are often referred to as *triple negative*, although not all basallike tumors are triple negative and visa versa. The basallike category of the ER-negative subsets were first identified with first-generation microarray technology and show a high expression of proliferation genes and basal cytokeratins[5,31,34] and a loss of genes associated with cell cycle control, which confer an overall poor prognosis. Though basallike tumors are the most common of the ER-negative subtypes (50% to 75% of all ER-negative tumors) and comprise 15% to 20% of all types of breast cancer, other ER-negative subtypes also exist, which include the recently described claudin-low group, as well as interferon-rich, androgen receptor, normallike groups. Though the claudin-low subgroup has some similarities to basallike breast cancer, it is distinct because these tumors have low expression of the claudin genes that are involved in epithelial cell tight-tight junctions. The claudin-low tumors have been of particular interest because they posses stem cell–like features of epithelial–mesenchymal transition (EMT).[42] To further characterize the heterogeneity of TNBC, a recent study did a clustering analysis of gene expression profiling of primary tumors and identified six distinct subtypes.[43] Major clusters included two basallike, an immunomodulatory, a mesenchymal, a mesenchymal stem–like, and a luminal androgen receptor subtype. Of further significance, this group provided preclinical evidence that these molecular subtypes were sensitive to different therapies.[43] This has direct translational relevance and should be validated further.

Although the exact definition of molecular subtypes is an area of active debate, it is clear that these subtypes are reproducible in multiple, unrelated data sets, and their prognostic impact has been validated in these settings.[38,40,44,45] As a result, clinical trials are now being designed to subdivide patients by ER/PR and *HER2* status to validate claims that therapeutic approaches should address these groups rather than the population of breast cancer patients as a whole. In 2011, the St. Gallen International Breast Cancer Conference recognized that breast cancer should not be treated as a single disease and recommended defining disease by molecular subtype using genetic array testing or approximated by ER/PR/HER2 status in conjunction with markers of proliferation, such as Ki-67. The panel reaffirmed this position again in 2013.[46]

Genetic Changes in Breast Cancer by Molecular Subtype

Mutational profiling of all types of breast cancer has demonstrated the marked heterogeneity that exists across the entire spectrum of tumors. Data from the TCGA highlights the fact that somatic mutations in just three genes (*TP53, PIK3A,* and *GATA3*) occurred at an incidence of greater than 10%.[40] However, when the mutation profile of breast cancers is analyzed by intrinsic subgroup, certain patterns continue to emerge. Although the rate of significantly mutated genes is the lowest in the luminal subgroup, it is also the most heterogeneous group in terms of mutational spectrum. The most frequent mutation in luminal A tumors was in *PIK3CA* (45%) followed by *MAP3K1, GATA3, TP53, CDH1,* and *MAP2K4*. Like luminal A cancers, luminal B cancers also showed a wide range, with the most frequently mutation genes being *TP53* and *PIK3CA* (both 29%). However, the TP53 pathway appears to be differentially inactivated with lower *TP53* mutations in luminal A (12%) and higher mutations in luminal B (29%). Although the HER2-enriched subgroup also shows a high frequency of mutations in *TP53* (72%) and *PIK3CA* (39%), unlike the luminal subtypes, HER2-enriched tumors appear to have a much lower frequency of other significantly mutated genes. Basallike tumors commonly harbor mutations in *TP53* (80%), and there seems to be little overlap with the mutations seen in the luminal subtypes. In addition, the TP53 mutations present in the basallike group were mostly nonsense and frameshift–type mutations as opposed to more missense mutations seen in the luminal group. In fact, the mutations seen in the basallike group showed significant similarities to serous cancers of the ovary.[42]

Prognostic and Predictive Genomic Signatures

Prognostic Signatures

Gene expression molecular signatures are currently in clinical use for both defining prognosis and for determining the benefit of systemic therapies, including chemotherapy and endocrine treatment, for breast cancer. Van't Veer et al.[45] and van de Vijver et al.[47] were the first to apply gene expression analysis to define a subgroup of breast cancer patients with an increased likelihood of metastasis. The estimated hazard ratio for distant metastases in the group with a poor prognosis signature, as compared to the group with the good prognosis signature, was 5.1 (95% confidence interval [CI], 2.9 to 9.0; p <0.001). The European Organisation for Research and Treatment of Cancer (EORTC) and the Breast International Group (BIG) are currently conducting a prospective clinical trial to validate the utility of this assay for sparing patients from systemic chemotherapy (the MINDACT study).[48] In a preliminary analysis, the 70-gene profile signature was strongly prognostic, outperforming classic prognostic criteria such as those used by the St. Gallen consensus panel[49]; however, the magnitude of effect was much less than previously reported, with hazard ratios for time to distant metastases of 1.85 (1.14 to 3.0) and for overall survival of 2.5 (1.4 to 4.5). The 70-gene signature is now commercialized as the MammaPrint and has received clearance by the U.S. Food and Drug Administration (FDA) as a class 2, 510(k) product.

Other groups have developed prognostic gene expression signatures, including the 76-gene Rotterdam signature, which identifies a high-risk group of node-negative patients, and the Genomic Grade Index (GGI), which distinguishes poor and good prognosis groups in breast tumors of intermediate histologic grade.[50] The potential value of these signatures has yet to be clearly defined, but it emphasizes the role of gene expression profiling at distinguishing prognostic groups not otherwise recognizable by standard histologic or clinical parameters.

Predictive Signatures

Endocrine Therapy. Several groups have applied a gene expression profiling analysis to better define the likelihood of benefit from therapy. Such predictive signatures may have particular value as they help oncologists counsel patients about appropriate choices for treatment. Genomics Health Inc. (Redwood City, California) developed the Oncotype DX assay as a predictor of benefit from antiestrogen therapy using multiple real-time reverse transcriptase polymerase chain reaction (RT-PCR) assays in formalin-fixed paraffin-embedded tissue. The assay was developed from 250 candidate genes selected from published literature, genomic databases, and in-house experiments performed on frozen tissue. From these data, a panel of 16 cancer-related genes and 5 reference genes were used to develop an algorithm to compute a recurrence score, ranging from 0 to 100, that can be used to estimate the odds of recurrence over 10 years from the diagnosis.[51] Paik et al.[51] reported an analysis of two randomized controlled trials: the National Surgical Adjuvant Breast and Bowel Project NSABP-B14, in which node-negative patients with ER-positive tumors were randomly assigned to tamoxifen or nil; and NSABP-B20, in which node-negative patients with ER-positive tumors were randomly assigned to tamoxifen alone or with cyclophosphamide, methotrexate, and fluorouracil (CMF) chemotherapy. Using the tissue samples from NSABP-B20, patients were categorized into three recurrence score groups: low risk (recurrence score less than 18), intermediate risk (recurrence score 18 to 30), and high risk (recurrence score 31 to 100). Samples from NSABP-B14 were then analyzed and found to be 6.8% (4.0% to 9.6%), 14.3% (8.3% to 20.3%), and 30.5% (23.6% to 37.4%). Paik et al.[51] further analyzed the performance of the Oncotype DX assay to include patients in the other arms of NSABP-B14 and NSABP-B20 and found that the

Oncotype DX assay was a strong predictor of benefit from CMF in NSABP-B20, with little or no benefit from chemotherapy for patients with low or intermediate recurrence scores but substantial benefit for those with high recurrence scores. Conversely, in NSABP-B14, the benefit from tamoxifen versus observation was confined to the low and intermediate risk categories (p value for interaction of 0.001). These data suggest that in patients who have an apparent favorable prognosis based on clinical features (negative nodes, positive ER), the Oncotype DX assay helps determine those most likely to benefit from tamoxifen only (low recurrence scores) versus those most likely not to benefit from tamoxifen but likely to benefit from chemotherapy (high recurrence scores). The benefits of chemotherapy in the 25% of patients who have intermediate recurrence scores remains uncertain and are the basis of an ongoing prospective randomized trial (Tailor Rx) where those with high recurrence scores will receive endocrine therapy and chemotherapy, those with low recurrence scores will receive endocrine therapy alone, and those with intermediate recurrence scores are randomly assigned to endocrine therapy versus endocrine and chemotherapy. A study by Albain et al.[52] suggested that a low recurrence score predicts a lack of benefit of fluorouracil (5-FU), adriamycin (doxorubicin), and cyclophosphamide (FAC) chemotherapy in node-positive breast cancer patients treated on Southwest Oncology Group SWOG-8814. Although these provocative data suggest a similar utility for Oncotype DX in node-positive patients, they require additional validation with modern-day regimens. The value of the Oncotype DX assay in predicting a benefit from hormonal therapy in patients treated with aromatase inhibitor therapy has recently been published, demonstrating that the assay performs equally with both tamoxifen and anastrozole but does not distinguish a benefit of one over the other.[53] Given the independent prognostic utility of both the Oncotype DX recurrence score and the clinicopathologic factors, such as tumor size and grade, a recent study formally integrated each of these measures to determine whether prognostic and predictive value is improved over using a single measure.[54] The use of an integrated score, recurrence score-pathology-clinical (RSPC), among ER-positive, node-negative patients provided a more significant prognostic value for distant recurrence when compared to the recurrence score alone. This score also resulted in better risk stratification and reduced the number of patients classified as intermediate risk. However, the addition of clinicopathologic factors to the recurrence score did not improve its predictive value for chemotherapy benefit.[54]

Several other additional predictors for ER-positive breast cancer include the Breast Cancer Index (AvariaDx Inc., Carlsbad, California), a quantitative RT-PCR–based assay that measures the ratio of the *HOXB6* and *IL17BR* genes, and includes a proliferation score. It was shown to be a marker of recurrence risk in untreated ER-positive/node-negative patients[55,56] in two studies of lymph node–negative, ER-positive, tamoxifen-treated patients with breast cancer and was more recently found to predict late recurrence after adjuvant endocrine therapy.[57] The breast cancer index (BCI) was compared with Onctoype DX recurrence score, and IHC4, a score based on four protein markers detected by immunohistochemistry. In ER-positive, node-positive breast cancer patients given either tamoxifen or anastrozole in the Arimidex, Tamoxifen, or Alone or in Combination (ATAC) trial, the BCI index was the only prognostic index that identified populations at risk of both early and late recurrences.[57] This may be of clinical value in postmenopausal patients, who have undergone 5 years of endocrine therapy because the test was defined in this population.

Chemotherapy. Defining predictors of response to chemotherapy and targeted therapies has been more challenging. Ayers et al.[58] from the M.D. Anderson Cancer Center were the first to report that a multigene analysis of fine needle aspiration specimens predicts a response to neoadjuvant Taxol, 5-fluouracil, Adriamycin, and cyclophosphamide (TFAC) chemotherapy.[59] Validation of gene signatures is of utmost importance in the future to determine the value of these expression profiles at predicting treatment response and clinical outcome in breast cancer patients. National organizations such as the American Society of Clinical Oncology, the National Comprehensive Cancer Network, and the College of American Pathologists have ongoing efforts to interpret the data from the burgeoning field of multigene biomarker tests to help the practicing clinician interpret their clinical utility.[60]

EPIGENETICS OF BREAST CANCER

Cells maintain their stable identity and phenotype over many generations without external stimuli or signaling events. This cellular memory is encoded in the epigenome, a collection of heritable information that exists alongside the genomic sequence. DNA methylation and chromatin modification are major epigenetic mechanisms in higher eukaryotes and are tightly coupled to basic genetic processes, such as DNA replication, transcription, and repair. It is well documented that cancers, including breast cancer, have altered patterns of DNA methylation and histone acetylation, leading to alterations in transcription that appear to be oncogenic.[61,62] Recent work from TCGA demonstrates different patterns of methylation by breast cancer subtypes as defined by gene expression profiling. Among these subtypes, luminal B subtype had a hypermethylated phenotype, whereas basallike subtype had a hypomethylated phenotype.[40] Ongoing initiatives, including the Epigenome Project, and further analyses of the TCGA data will likely enhance our understanding of epigenetics in breast cancer.

Major epigenetic cancer drugs include DNA methyltransferase (DNMT) and histone deacetylase (HDAC) inhibitors. Preclinical studies show promise that HDAC inhibitors may have activity in breast cancer cells, and many clinical phase I and II studies are in progress.[63–65]

MicroRNAs

miRNAs are small noncoding RNAs that belong to a novel class of regulatory molecules that control the expression of hundreds of target mRNA transcripts[66] in two ways. First, miRNAs that bind to protein-coding mRNA sequences that are exactly complementary to the miRNA induce the RNAi pathway. Messenger RNA targets are then cleaved by ribonucleases in the RNA-induced silencing complex (RISC). Second, miRNAs bind to imperfect complementary sites within the 3′ untranslated regions (3′UTR) of their target protein-coding mRNAs and repress the expression of these genes at the level of translation.[67]

miRNAs are known to be associated with breast cancer in both cell lines and clinical samples. For example, *miR-21*, *miR-155*, *miR-7*, and *miR-210* are overexpressed in aggressive human breast cancers,[68,69] whereas *let-7* and *miR-125a* have been shown to be downregulated in breast cancers.[70] It has also been shown that *miR-125a* may function as a tumor suppressor by inhibiting ERBB2 and ERBB3. More recently, the TCGA identified seven subtypes by microRNA expression profiling. Among all of these microRNA clusters, only two of them had a positive correlation with TP53 mutation and overlap with the basallike subtype. No additional correlation with mutation status or mRNA-defined breast cancer subtypes was identified.[40]

MicroRNAs and Response to Cancer Treatment

miRNA misexpression patterns were found to be associated with cancer outcome and response to treatment, including radiation and chemotherapy. Certain miRNAs associated with hypoxia, such as *miR-210*, have been shown to be biomarkers of poor outcome in breast cancer.[68] Furthermore, in vitro data show that certain miRNAs are associated with resistance to doxorubicin[71] or tamoxifen.[72] In patient samples, an association of miRNA's tumor subtypes have specific miRNA patterns and this is associated with a poor outcome. Defining the role of miRNAs as biomarkers for prognosis and prediction, as well as their potential as targeted therapies, is an active area of research in breast cancer.

PROTEIN/PATHWAY ALTERATIONS

The molecular mechanisms that lead to cancer have been characterized as the hallmarks of cancer, as proposed by Hanahan and Weinberg and revised in 2011.[73] They include sustained proliferative signaling, evading growth suppressors, resisting cell death, replicative immortality through telomerase inhibition, angiogenesis, invasion and metastasis, genomic instability, deregulated metabolism, and avoiding immune destruction. The effectors of genetic and epigenetic abnormalities are, in most cases, reflected in the abnormal levels, functions, and interactions of proteins and signaling pathways. Recent studies of the genome have generated new insights into the proteome associated with specific breast cancer subtypes and suggest important targets for therapy, in addition to those canonical drivers ER and HER2.[40] Undoubtedly, numerous alterations coordinate to result in the malignant phenotype; however, a number of key proteins and their pathways have emerged as critical drivers of breast cancer development and growth as well as potential therapeutic targets.

ESTROGEN RECEPTOR PATHWAY

Therapeutic Targets in Breast Cancer

Estrogen Signaling

Most breast cancers are intimately linked with exposure to estrogen and alterations in the estrogen receptor signaling pathway. Estrogen is a steroid hormone that exerts its actions by binding to the nuclear ER. Upon activation by its ligand, ER binds in a coordinated fashion with a number of coregulatory proteins to estrogen response elements in the promoter region of estrogen-responsive genes. This in turn directs the transcription of numerous growth-promoting genes, including PR. The level of ER expression is not only of biologic interest, but it is also a highly effective predictor for response to antiestrogens, which is a recommended treatment for all ER-expressing tumors.

Although ER is overexpressed in as many as 70% of invasive breast cancers, the precise mechanism by which this occurs is unclear. Amplification of the gene appears to be one mechanism (approximately 50% of cases with ER overexpression in one study), suggesting that transcriptional deregulation and posttranscriptional modifications (such as alteration of mRNA levels by miRNAs) may also play a role. In addition, recent studies suggest ER mutations can lead to constitutive activation of the pathway and may be a mechanism of resistance to antiestrogen treatment.[74]

Estrogen exerts its actions through both genomic (described previously) and nongenomic mechanisms. In contrast to the genomic actions of ER, nongenomic actions of ER are extremely rapid (within seconds to minutes of estrogen exposure) and are believed to result from the hormone-dependent activation of membrane-bound or cytosolic ERs. These nonnuclear ER actions result in rapid phosphorylation and activation of important growth regulatory kinases, including EGFRs, insulinlike growth factor 1R (IGF-1R), c-Src, Shc, and the p85α regulatory subunit of PI3K.[5] This *cross-talk* between ER and growth factor receptors is bidirectional; for example, constitutive HER2 can increase ER signaling to the point where it is unresponsive to antiestrogen treatments. These findings suggest a role for HER2/IGF-1R/EGFR activation in both acquired and de novo resistance to treatment with antiestrogens.[75]

The ER pathway has proven to be an invaluable target for therapeutic treatments in breast cancer. A number of agents have been developed over the prior decades that can inhibit this pathway by either binding to the receptor itself (e.g., selective ER modulators such as tamoxifen, raloxifene, fulvestrant) or by decreasing the production of endogenous estrogen (e.g., aromatase inhibitors, ovarian ablation).

Recent data suggest that a longer duration of tamoxifen (10 years) is superior to 5 years, and 5 years of Aromatase Inhibitor (AI) are standard of care after any duration of tamoxifen in postmenopausal women.[76] Although these agents are highly effective and have made a significant impact on breast cancer morbidity and mortality, *de novo* and acquired resistance are also quite common. Recent studies suggest that the inhibition of growth factor pathways in conjunction with antiestrogen therapy can overcome resistance to these agents; for example, the mammalian target of rapamycin (mTOR) inhibitor temsirolimus with a steroidal inhibitor (exemestane) is a new standard of care after progression on a nonsteroidal aromatase inhibitor in the metastatic setting.[77] The challenge for the oncology community is to define optimal biomarkers to predict patients most likely to benefit from longer tamoxifen or AI + mTOR therapy. As described previously, the Oncotype DX assay, IHC4, and Breast Cancer Index provide insight into the behavior of ER-positive tumors and help in treatment decision making.[55–57]

Growth Factor Receptor Pathways

Growth factor receptor pathways—in particular, tyrosine-kinase receptors—play an essential role in initiating both proliferative and cell survival pathways in tissues and are tightly regulated. In breast cancer biology, the ErbB family has been studied most extensively, but an expanding number of other growth factors, such as insulin-like growth factor receptors, have also been the subject of intense scrutiny in hopes of identifying effective therapeutic targets.[78] These growth factor receptor pathways can be constitutively activated by a number of mechanisms, including excessive ligand levels, gain-of-function mutations, overexpression with or without gene amplification, and

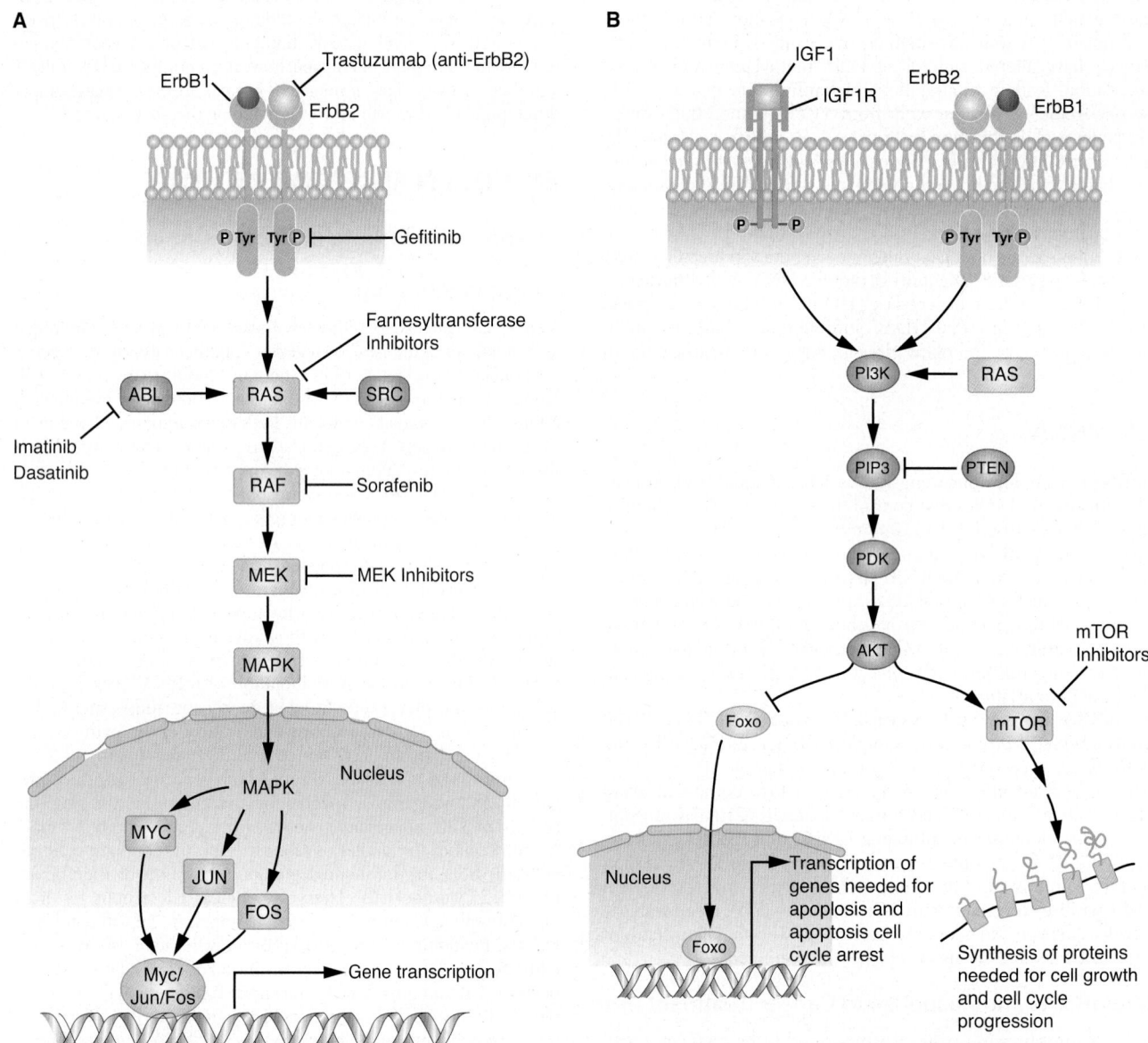

Figure 78.2 (A) The ras/raf/MEK/MAPK pathway is activated by multiple growth factor receptors (here exemplified by ErbB1 and ErbB2) as well as several intracellular tyrosine kinases such as SRC and ABL. Activated RAS stimulates a sequence of phosphorylation events mediated by RAF, MEK, and ERK (MAP) kinases. Activated MAP kinase (MAPK) translocates to the nucleus and activates proteins such as MYC, JUN, and FOS, which promote the transcription of numerous genes involved in tumor growth. **(B)** The phosphatidylinositol 3-kinase (PI3K) pathway is activated by RAS and by a number of growth factor receptors (here exemplified by IGF1R and the ErbB1/ErbB2 heterodimer). Activated PI3K generates phosphatidylinositol-3,4,5-triphosphate (PIP3), which activates phosphoinositide-dependent kinase-1 (PDK). In turn, PDK phosphorylates AKT. PTEN is an endogenous inhibitor of AKT activation. Phosphorylated AKT transduces multiple downstream signals, including the mTOR and the inhibition of the FOXO family of transcription factors. mTOR activation promotes the synthesis of proteins required for cell growth and cell cycle progression. (Redrawn from Golan DE, Tashjian AH, Armstrong EJ. *Principles of Pharmacology: The Pathophysiologic Basis of Drug Therapy.* 2nd ed. Baltimore: Lippincott Williams & Wilkins; 2008.)

gene rearrangements and resultant fusion proteins with oncogenic potential. This can ultimately lead to inappropriate kinase activity and growth promoting second messenger activation (Fig. 78.2).

Human Epidermal Growth Factor Receptor 2

HER2 (EGFR2 or ErbB2) is a member of a family of receptor tyrosine kinases that also includes EGFR (HER1, ErbB1), ErbB3, and ErbB4. Ligand binding to the extracellular domains of the ErbB1, ErbB3, or ErbB4 receptors induces homo- and heterodimerization and kinase activation. The HER2 protein exists in a closed conformation and has no ligand, but it is the preferred partner for dimerization with HER1, -3, and -4. At a molecular level, HER2 amplification is associated with deregulation of G1/S phase cell cycle control via the upregulation of cyclins D1, E, and cdk6, as well as p27 degradation. HER2 also interacts with important second messengers, including SH2-domain–containing proteins (e.g., Src kinases).

Importantly, HER2 amplification or protein overexpression (found in 20% of invasive breast cancers) is clearly associated with accelerated cell growth and proliferation, poor clinical outcome, and response to the monoclonal anti-HER2 antibody, trastuzumab. Numerous randomized trials have shown that the addition of trastuzumab to chemotherapy improves survival in both metastatic and early stage disease, leading to its inclusion in the standard of care for all patients with HER2-positive breast cancer.[79] In addition, several other HER2-targeted agents have been approved for metastatic HER2-positive breast cancer and are being evaluated in the early stage setting. One of these, the monoclonal antibody pertuzumab, which targets the HER2-3 heterodimerization site, has recently been approved for use in the preoperative setting for stage II and III HER2-positive breast cancer.[80] These rapid advances in the setting of targeted therapy for HER2-positive disease illustrate the profound effect that targeting an important molecular *driver* can have on clinical practice.

The precise mechanism of action of the FDA-approved HER2-targeted therapies trastuzumab, pertuzumab, lapatinib, and trastuzumab emtansine (TDM-1) are not well understood.[79,81] In preclinical studies, the first three appear to inhibit signal transduction through the canonical signaling pathways for the HER2 receptor, but may vary in their degree of ras-MAPK versus PI3K-AKT pathway inhibition. This may largely be due to different degrees of inhibition of the coreceptors HER1, 3, and 4 that have a different predilection for each pathway. For instance, lapatinib inhibits both HER2 and EGFR (HER1) with a greater effect on the ras-MAPK pathway. Pertuzumab interferes with the HER3 heterodimer and hence has more effect on the AKT pathway. The new targeted therapy TDM-1 is an antibody–drug conjugate, and its effects are more cytotoxic than signal transduction. All three antibody therapies are thought to activate natural killer cells involved in antibody-dependent cellular cytotoxicity (ADCC); however, there is little evidence from clinical studies to support this or any mechanism of action. As a result, mechanisms of resistance are poorly understood; current hypotheses include activation of alternate receptors (e.g., IGF-1R, c-met) or the AKT pathway via a loss of phosphatase and tensin homolog (PTEN) or PI3K mutation (see Fig. 78.2).[78,79,81,82]

Ras And Phosphatidylinositol 3-Kinase Pathways

Redundancies and cross-talk of numerous different signaling pathways are a common theme. Several downstream messengers, however, bear special consideration due to their functional importance and therapeutic implications. Recent data from TCGA Breast Cancer publication suggest that the PI3K/AKT and ras-MAP kinase pathways are particularly relevant in breast cancer based on frequent mutation, amplification, and/or activation of these pathways as measured by genomic technologies.[40]

PI3K-AKT is a central signaling pathway downstream of many receptor tyrosine kinases and regulates cell growth and proliferation (see Fig. 78.2B). Activating mutations in the gene encoding the p110α catalytic subunit of PI3K (*PI3CKA*) may be an important contributing factor to mammary tumor progression, and the site of mutation differs depending on the breast cancer molecular subtype as noted previously. Activating mutations of the *AKT* gene family are seen in 2% to 4% of breast cancers, excluding the basal-like subtype, where they are rare.[42]

PTEN dephosphorylates—and therefore inactivates—the p110 catalytic domain of PI3K and is either mutated or underexpressed (e.g., via methylation) in many breast cancers. Activation of the PI3K pathway, in turn, results in the 3-phosphoinositide–dependent kinase-mediated activation of several known kinases, including AKT1, AKT2, and AKT3. Interestingly, activated AKT1 appears to be antiapoptotic but also plays an anti-invasive role in tumor formation. In addition to the AKTs, downstream proliferative effectors of the PI3K pathway also include the mTOR complex 1 (TORC1), which consists of mTOR, raptor, and mLst8. It is currently believed that TORC1 mediates its progrowth effects through the activation of S6-kinase 1 and suppression of 4E-BP1, an inhibitor of cap-dependent translation. These observations all point to mTOR-raptor as a critical target in cancer therapy, and indeed, several mTOR inhibitors known as rapamycin analogs (e.g., CCI-779, RAD-001, AP-23576) are in clinical trials, and temsirolimus (Affinitor) has been approved for use with aromatase inhibitor therapy.

The ras/raf/MEK/MAPK pathway is also a critical signaling pathway for numerous growth factor receptors (see Fig. 78.2A). Thus far in breast cancer, agents that target the MEK pathway (e.g., raf inhibitor sorafenib) have had modest success as single agents, but studies in combination with other treatments hold more promise.

Angiogenesis

Angiogenesis is normally a tightly regulated process of vessel formation during physiologic events, such as wound healing and pregnancy. It has also been shown to be an important part of tumor growth and spread. In contrast to physiologic angiogenesis, tumor-associated angiogenesis is highly dysregulated with disorganized and distorted vasculature and increased vascular permeability. Thus, in recent years, angiogenesis has become a frequent target for the treatment of many cancers.

Central to this process is the proangiogenic factor, vascular endothelial growth factor (VEGF), which together with its receptors, regulate endothelial cell growth and new vessel formation.[81] VEGF receptors (VEGFR), like EGFRs, are also tyrosine-kinase receptors. VEGF-A binds to both VEGFR1 (Flt-1) and VEGFR2 (KDR/Flk1). VEGFR2 appears to mediate most of the known cellular responses to VEGFs, whereas the function of VEGFR1 is less well defined. Bevacizumab, a humanized monoclonal antibody directed against VEGF-A, has been the most extensively studied thus far. To date, three large randomized trials have shown a statistically significant benefit in progression-free survival when bevacizumab was added to a variety of different chemotherapies in the first-line metastatic setting. However, the lack of survival advantage in any study has led to the withdrawal of bevacizumab's approval, and studies in early stage breast cancer are required to be positive in order to reconsider its use in breast cancer. Multitargeted VEGFR tyrosine-kinase inhibitors such as sunitinib (VEGFR, platelet-derived growth factor receptor (PDGFR), and c-kit blockade) and sorafenib (VEGFR and RAF kinase blockade) have also been studied extensively in breast and other cancers. Despite the success of some of these agents, the identification of predictive factors for an antiangiogenic response have thus far proven to be elusive.

SUMMARY

Breast cancer is a heterogeneous malignancy, with multiple molecular subtypes and clinical presentations ranging from aggressive to indolent, and varying in distribution by age, menopausal status, and racial group. Recent molecular analyses have shed light on this heterogeneity by mapping patterns that correspond to clinical phenotypes. These studies include, but are not limited to, the study of germ-line variations in breast cancer susceptibility genes, gene expression, copy number and somatic mutations, epigenetic modifications, and alterations in protein pathways associated with the malignant phenotype. This review attempts to summarize the current state of the science with an emphasis on the insights provided by these studies on prognosis and prediction for therapy and potential new therapeutic targets. It is only through ongoing research that this disease will one day be cured.

SELECTED REFERENCES

The full reference list can be accessed at lwwhealthlibrary.com/oncology.

2. Wood LD, Parsons DW, Jones S, et al. The genomic landscapes of human breast and colorectal cancers. *Science* 2007;318:1108–1113.
4. Turnbull C, Rahman N. Genetic predisposition to breast cancer: past, present, and future. *Annu Rev Genomics Hum Genet* 2008;9:321–245.
8. Chenevix-Trench G, Milne RL, Antoniou AC, et al. An international initiative to identify genetic modifiers of cancer risk in BRCA1 and BRCA2 mutation carriers: the Consortium of Investigators of Modifiers of BRCA1 and BRCA2 (CIMBA). *Breast Cancer Res* 2007;9:104.
11. Mavaddat N, Peock S, Frost D, et al. Cancer risks for BRCA1 and BRCA2 mutation carriers: results from prospective analysis of EMBRACE. *J Natl Cancer Inst* 2013;105:812–822.
12. Turner NC, Reis-Filho JS. Basal-like breast cancer and the BRCA1 phenotype. *Oncogene* 2006;25:5846–5853.
14. Fong PC, Boss DS, Yap TA, et al. Inhibition of poly(ADP-ribose) polymerase in tumors from BRCA mutation carriers. *N Engl J Med* 2009;361:123–134.
15. Iglehart JD, Silver DP. Synthetic lethality—a new direction in cancer-drug development. *N Engl J Med* 2009;2:189–191.
19. Patel AG, De Lorenzo SB, Flatten KS, et al. Failure of iniparib to inhibit poly(ADP-Ribose) polymerase in vitro. *Clin Cancer Res* 2012;18:1655–1662.
20. Shen Y, Rehman FL, Feng Y, et al. BMN 673, a novel and highly potent PARP1/2 inhibitor for the treatment of human cancers with DNA repair deficiency. *Clin Cancer Res* 2013;19:5003–5015.
21. Edwards SL, Brough R, Lord CJ, et al. Resistance to therapy caused by intragenic deletion in BRCA2. *Nature* 2008;451:1111–1115.
22. Norquist B, Wurz KA, Pennil CC, et al. Secondary somatic mutations restoring BRCA1/2 predict chemotherapy resistance in hereditary ovarian carcinomas. *J Clin Oncol* 2011;29:3008–3015.
23. Sakai W, Swisher EM, Karlan BY, et al. Secondary mutations as a mechanism of cisplatin resistance in BRCA2-mutated cancers. *Nature* 2008;451:1116–1120.
24. Bouwman P, Aly A, Escandell JM, et al. 53BP1 loss rescues BRCA1 deficiency and is associated with triple-negative and BRCA-mutated breast cancers. *Nat Struct Mol Biol* 2010;17:688–695.
26. Stratton MR, Rahman N. The emerging landscape of breast cancer susceptibility. *Nat Genet* 2008;40:17–22.
27. Win AK, Young JP, Lindor NM, et al. Colorectal and other cancer risks for carriers and noncarriers from families with a DNA mismatch repair gene mutation: a prospective cohort study. *J Clin Oncol* 2012;30:958–964.
28. Win AK, Lindor NM, Jenkins MA. Risk of breast cancer in Lynch syndrome: a systematic review. *Breast Cancer Res* 2013;15:R27.
31. Forbes SA, Bhamra G, Bamford S, et al. The Catalogue of Somatic Mutations in Cancer (COSMIC). *Curr Protoc Hum Genet* 2008;Chapter 10:Unit 10.11.
32. Stratton MR, Campbell PJ, Futreal PA. The cancer genome. *Nature* 2009; 458:719–724.
38. Perou CM, Sorlie T, Eisen MB, et al. Molecular portraits of human breast tumours. *Nature* 2000;406:747–752.
39. Sorlie T, Perou CM, Tibshirani R, et al. Gene expression patterns of breast carcinomas distinguish tumor subclasses with clinical implications. *Proc Natl Acad Sci U S A* 2001;98:10869–10874.
40. Cancer Genome Atlas Network. Comprehensive molecular portraits of human breast tumours. *Nature* 2012;490:61–70.
41. Curtis C, Shah SP, Chin SF, et al. The genomic and transcriptomic architecture of 2,000 breast tumours reveals novel subgroups. *Nature* 2012;486: 346–352.
42. Perou CM. Molecular stratification of triple-negative breast cancers. *Oncologist* 2010;15:39–48.
43. Lehmann BD, Bauer JA, Chen X, et al. Identification of human triple-negative breast cancer subtypes and preclinical models for selection of targeted therapies. *J Clin Invest* 2011;121:2750–2767.
45. van't Veer LJ, Dai H, van de Vijver MJ, et al. Gene expression profiling predicts clinical outcome of breast cancer. *Nature* 2002;415:530–536.

46. Goldhirsch A, Winer EP, Coates AS, et al. Personalizing the treatment of women with early breast cancer: highlights of the St Gallen International Expert Consensus on the Primary Therapy of Early Breast Cancer 2013. *Ann Oncol* 2013;24:2206–2223.
47. van de Vijver MJ, He YD, van't Veer LJ, et al. A gene-expression signature as a predictor of survival in breast cancer. *N Engl J Med* 2002;25:1999–2009.
48. Piccart M, Loi S, Van't Veer L, et al. Multi-center external validation study of the Amsterdam 70-gene prognostic signature in node negative untreated breast cancer: Are the results still outperforming the clinical-pathological criteria? Presented at: 2004 27th San Antonio Breast Cancer Symposium; December 2004; San Antonio, TX.
50. Sotiriou C, Wirapati P, Loi S, et al. Gene expression profiling in breast cancer: understanding the molecular basis of histologic grade to improve prognosis. *J Natl Cancer Inst* 2006;98:262–272.
51. Paik S, Shak S, Tang G, et al. A multigene assay to predict recurrence of tamoxifen-treated, node-negative breast cancer. *N Engl J Med* 2004;351: 2817–2826.
52. Albain KS, Barlow WE, Shak S, et al. Prognostic and predictive value of the 21-gene recurrence score assay in postmenopausal women with node-positive, oestrogen-receptor-positive breast cancer on chemotherapy: a retrospective analysis of a randomised trial. *Lancet Oncol* 2010;11:55–65.
53. Mamounas EP, Tang G, Fisher B, et al. Association between the 21-gene recurrence score assay and risk of locoregional recurrence in node-negative, estrogen receptor-positive breast cancer: results from NSABP B-14 and NSABP B-20. *J Clin Oncol* 2010;10:1677–1683.
54. Tang G, Cuzick J, Costantino JP, et al. Risk of recurrence and chemotherapy benefit for patients with node-negative, estrogen receptor-positive breast cancer: recurrence score alone and integrated with pathologic and clinical factors. *J Clin Oncol* 2011;29:4365–4372.
55. Ma XJ, Hilsenbeck SG, Wang W, et al. The HOXB13:IL17BR expression index is a prognostic factor in early-stage breast cancer. *J Clin Oncol* 2003; 28:4611–4619.
56. Ma XJ, Wang Z, Ryan PD, et al. A two-gene expression ratio predicts clinical outcome in breast cancer patients treated with tamoxifen. *Cancer Cell* 2004;5:607–616.
57. Sgroi DC, Sestak I, Cuzick J, et al. Prediction of late distant recurrence in patients with oestrogen-receptor-positive breast cancer: a prospective comparison of the breast-cancer index (BCI) assay, 21-gene recurrence score, and IHC4 in the TransATAC study population. *Lancet Oncol* 2013;14: 1067–1076.
60. Harris L, Fritsche H, Mennel R, et al. American Society of Clinical Oncology 2007 update of recommendations for the use of tumor markers in breast cancer. *J Clin Oncol* 2007;33:5287–5312.
61. Barski A, Cuddapah S, Cui K, et al. High-resolution profiling of histone methylations in the human genome. *Cell* 2007;129:823–837.
62. Veeck J, Esteller M. Breast cancer epigenetics: from DNA methylation to microRNAs. *J Mammary Gland Biol Neoplasia* 2010;15:5–17.
70. Iorio MV, Casalini P, Tagliabue E, et al. MicroRNA profiling as a tool to understand prognosis, therapy response and resistance in breast cancer. *Eur J Cancer* 2008;18:2753–2759.
75. Massarweh S, Schiff R. Unraveling the mechanisms of endocrine resistance in breast cancer: new therapeutic opportunities. *Clin Cancer Res* 2007;13:1950–1954.
76. Davies C, Pan H, Godwin J, et al. Long-term effects of continuing adjuvant tamoxifen to 10 years versus stopping at 5 years after diagnosis of oestrogen receptor-positive breast cancer: ATLAS, a randomised trial. *Lancet* 2013;9869:805–816.
77. Baselga J, Campone M, Piccart M, et al. Everolimus in postmenopausal hormone-receptor-positive advanced breast cancer. *N Engl J Med* 2012;366: 520–529.
79. Hudis CA. Trastuzumab—mechanism of action and use in clinical practice. *N Engl J Med* 2007;1:39–51.

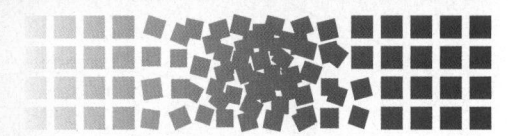

79 Malignant Tumors of the Breast

Monica Morrow, Harold J. Burstein, and Jay R. Harris

INTRODUCTION

Breast cancer is a major public health problem for women throughout the world. In the United States, breast cancer remains the most frequent cancer in women and the second most frequent cause of cancer death. In 2012, it was estimated there were 226,870 new cases of breast cancer, with 39,510 deaths.[1] Worldwide, breast cancer is the most frequently diagnosed cancer and the leading cause of cancer death among females, accounting for 23% of the total cancer cases and 14% of the cancer deaths, although there is a five-fold variation in incidence between high-incidence areas such as the United States and Western Europe, and low incidence areas such as Africa and Asia.[2] Since 1990, the death rate from breast cancer has decreased in the United States by 24%, and similar reductions have been observed in other countries.[3,4] The adoption of screening mammography, and the use of adjuvant therapy, have contributed approximately equally to this improvement.[5] Although breast cancer has traditionally been less common in nonindustrialized nations, its incidence in these areas is increasing.[6] This chapter examines the salient features of breast cancer, stressing practical information of importance to clinicians and the results of prospective randomized trials that guide therapeutic decisions.

ANATOMY OF THE BREAST

The adult female breast lies between the second and sixth ribs, and between the sternal edge and the midaxillary line. The breast is composed of skin, subcutaneous tissue, and breast tissue, with the breast tissue including both epithelial and stromal elements. Epithelial elements make up 10% to 15% of the breast mass, with the remainder being stroma. Each breast consists of 15 to 20 lobes of glandular tissue supported by fibrous connective tissue. The space between lobes is filled with adipose tissue, and differences in the amount of adipose tissue are responsible for variations in breast size. The blood supply of the breast is derived from the internal mammary and lateral thoracic arteries. The breast lymphatic drainage occurs through a superficial and deep lymphatic plexus, and >95% of the lymphatic drainage of the breast is through the axillary lymph nodes, with the remainder via the internal mammary nodes. The axillary nodes are variable in number and have traditionally been divided into three levels based on their relationship to the pectoralis minor muscle, as illustrated in Figure 79.1. The sentinel axillary node is almost always found in the level 1 axillary nodes. The internal mammary nodes are located in the first six intercostal spaces within 3 cm of the sternal edge, with the highest concentration of internal mammary nodes in the first three intercostal spaces.

RISK FACTORS FOR BREAST CANCER

Multiple factors are associated with an increased risk of developing breast cancer, but the majority of these factors convey a small to moderate increase in risk for any individual woman. It has been estimated that approximately 50% of women who develop breast cancer have no identifiable risk factor beyond increasing age and female gender. The importance of age as a breast cancer risk factor is sometimes overlooked. In 2009, it was estimated that 18,640 invasive breast cancers and 2,820 breast cancer deaths occurred in US women under age 45 compared with 173,730 cancers and 37,350 deaths in women aged 45 years and older.[7]

Familial Factors

A family history of breast cancer has long been recognized as a risk factor for the disease, but only 5% to 10% of women who develop breast cancer have a true hereditary predisposition. Many women with a family history overestimate their risk of developing breast cancer or harboring a predisposing genetic mutation. Overall, the risk of developing breast cancer is increased 1.5-fold to 3-fold if a woman has a mother or sister with breast cancer. Family history, however, is a heterogeneous risk factor with different implications depending on the number of relatives with breast cancer, the exact relationship, the age at diagnosis, and the number of unaffected relatives. Even in the absence of a known inherited predisposition, women with a family history of breast cancer face some level of increased risk, likely from some combination of shared environmental exposures, unexplained genetic factors, or both.

Inherited Predisposition to Breast Cancer

Mutations in the breast cancer susceptibility genes BRCA1 and BRCA2 are associated with a significant increase in the risk of breast and ovarian carcinoma, and account for 5% to 10% of all breast cancers. These mutations are inherited in an autosomal dominant fashion and have varying penetrance. As a result, the estimated lifetime risk of breast cancer development in mutation carriers ranges from 26% to 85%, and the risk of ovarian cancer from 16% to 63% and 10% to 27%, respectively, in carriers of BRCA1 and BRCA2.[8] In a meta-analysis of 10 international studies, the cumulative risks to age 70 for breast cancer were 57% for BRCA1 and 40% for BRCA2 carriers.[9] More than 700 different mutations of BRCA1 and 300 different mutations of BRCA2 have been described, and the position of the mutation within the gene has been shown to influence the risk of both breast and ovarian cancers.

Other cancers associated with BRCA1 or BRCA2 mutations include male breast cancer, fallopian tube cancer, and prostate cancer. Carriers of BRCA2 may also have an elevated risk of melanoma and gastric cancer. Management strategies available for risk reduction in BRCA1/2 mutation carriers include intensive surveillance, chemoprevention with selective estrogen receptor modulators (SERM), and prophylactic (breast and salpingo-ovarian) surgery, and these are discussed in a later section. There is a great interest in the role of environmental and lifestyle factors in the modification of cancer risk among BRCA1 or BRCA2 carriers; at present, however, the available data are inconsistent. It is worth

PRACTICE OF ONCOLOGY

1117

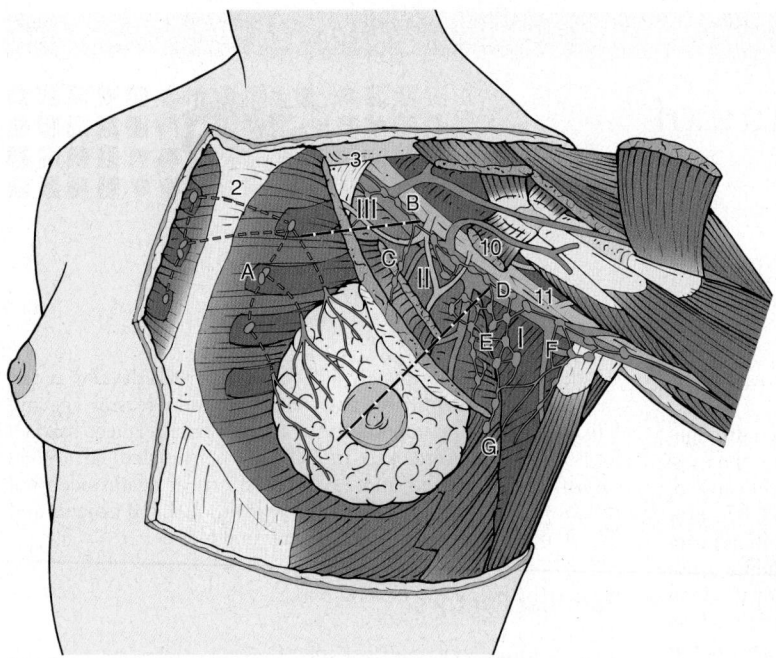

Figure 79.1 Lymphatic drainage of the breast showing lymph node groups and levels. *1*, Internal mammary artery and vein; *2*, substernal cross-drainage to contralateral internal mammary lymphatic chain; *3*, subclavius muscle and Halsted ligament; *4*, lateral pectoral nerve (from the lateral cord); *5*, pectoral branch from thoracoacromial vein; *6*, pectoralis minor muscle; *7*, pectoralis major muscle; *8*, lateral thoracic vein; *9*, medial pectoral nerve (from the medial cord); *10*, pectoralis minor muscle; *11*, median nerve; *12*, subscapular vein; *13*, thoracodorsal vein. Internal mammary lymph nodes *(A)*, apical lymph nodes *(B)*, interpectoral (Rotter) lymph nodes *(C)*, axillary vein lymph nodes *(D)*, central lymph nodes *(E)*, scapular lymph nodes *(F)*, external mammary lymph nodes *(G)*. Level I lymph nodes: lateral to lateral border of pectoralis minor muscle; level II lymph nodes: behind pectoralis minor muscle; level III lymph nodes: medial to medial border of pectoralis minor muscle.

noting that women with a significant family history of breast cancer (i.e., two or more breast cancers under the age of 50 years, or three or more breast cancers at any age), but who test negative for *BRCA* mutations have approximately a four-fold risk of breast cancer.[10] In contrast, women in families where a *BRCA* mutation is present who test negative for the mutation are not at increased risk for breast cancer development in the absence of other risk factors, and do not require special surveillance.[11]

Women with *BRCA1* mutations have a higher incidence of triple-negative/basal-like breast cancers (see the following), and cancers are more likely to be grade 3 tumors and to lack expression of the estrogen receptor (ER), progesterone receptor (PR), and *HER2* overexpression than sporadic cancers.[12] The phenotype of *BRCA2* cancers does not differ from that seen in sporadic cancers. The presence of a *BRCA1* or *BRCA2* mutation may be suggested by the family history on either the maternal or paternal side of the family. The features considered by the 2005 US Preventive Services Task Force[13] are listed in Table 79.1. Less-rigorous criteria for referral for genetic counseling are used for individuals of Ashkenazi Jewish ancestry, because the carrier frequency of specific *BRCA1* (187delAG, 5385 ins C) and *BRCA2* (6174delT) mutations in this group is 1:40, compared with 1:500 in the general population. These guidelines are particularly useful for individuals not affected with breast cancer. In the patient with newly diagnosed breast cancer, young age at diagnosis (≤40 years), bilateral breast cancer, Ashkenazi ancestry, or a malignancy consistent with the *BRCA1* phenotype all constitute reasons for referral to a genetic counselor, particularly in the woman with a small number of female relatives. Models are available to estimate the likelihood of a *BRCA1* or *BRCA2* mutation based on family history. The implications of genetic testing for both individuals and their family members are considerable, and these issues should be discussed prior to undertaking genetic testing.

Other genetic mutations have been associated with breast cancer risk, although with a lower prevalence or penetrance than *BRCA1* and *BRCA2*. *TP53* and *PTEN* each account for <1% of cases, while mutations in CDH1 are associated with an autosomal dominant predisposition to diffuse gastric cancer and lobular breast cancer.[14] Young women with TP53 mutations (Li-Fraumeni syndrome) seem to have a greater propensity for *HER2*+ breast cancers.[15] Mutations in low-penetrance genes are thought to account for a significant number of non-*BRCA1* or -*BRCA2* breast

cancers. A specific mutation of the checkpoint kinase 2 (*CHEK2*) gene was found in 11.4% of families with three or more cases of breast cancer diagnosed before age 60,[16] but in a large study of 10,860 unselected breast cancer patients from five countries, the *CHEK2* mutation was identified in only 1.9% of cases[17] and 0.7% of controls (odds ratio, 2.34), and testing for *CHEK2* is not routine. The increasing availability of next-generation sequencing has already resulted in commercially available panels of high and moderate penetrance genes, and is likely to change the approach to genetic screening in future years.

Hormonal Factors

The development of breast cancer in many women appears to be related to female reproductive hormones, particularly endogenous estrogens. Early age at menarche, nulliparity or late age at first full-term pregnancy, and late age at menopause increase the risk of developing breast cancer. In postmenopausal women, obesity and postmenopausal hormone replacement therapy (HRT), both of which are positively correlated with plasma estrogen levels and

TABLE 79.1
Factors Suggestive of *BRCA1* or *BRCA2* Mutation

- Non-Ashkenazic Jewish women
  - Two first-degree relatives[a] with breast cancer, one diagnosed ≤50 y
  - Three or more first- or second-degree relatives with breast cancer, any age
  - Breast and ovarian cancer among first- and second-degree relatives
  - First-degree relative with bilateral breast cancer
  - Breast cancer in a male relative
  - Two or more first- or second-degree relatives with ovarian cancer
- Ashkenazic Jewish women
  - First-degree relative with breast or ovarian cancer
  - Two second-degree relatives with breast or ovarian cancer

[a] Relatives on the same side of the family.

plasma estradiol levels, are associated with increased breast cancer risk. Most hormonal risk factors have a relative risk (RR) of ≤2 for breast cancer development.

The age-specific incidence of breast cancer increases steeply with age until menopause, and then plateaus. There is substantial evidence that estrogen deprivation via iatrogenic premature menopause can reduce breast cancer risk. Premenopausal women who undergo oophorectomy without hormone replacement have a markedly reduced risk of breast cancer later in life, with an increasing magnitude of risk reduction as the age at oophorectomy decreases.[18] Data from women with *BRCA1* and *BRCA2* mutations suggest that early oophorectomy has a substantial protective effect on breast cancer risk in this population also.[19]

Age at menarche and the establishment of regular ovulatory cycles are strongly linked to breast cancer risk; the total duration of exposure to endogenous estrogens seems important. There appears to be a 20% decrease in breast cancer risk for each year that menarche is delayed. Of note, hormone levels through the reproductive years in women who experience early menarche may be higher than in women who undergo a later menarche.[20] Additionally, late onset of menarche results in a delay in the establishment of regular ovulatory cycles, which may contribute to protective effects.

The relationship between pregnancy and breast cancer risk appears more complicated. Women whose first full-term pregnancy occurs after age 30 have a two- to five-fold increase in breast cancer risk in comparison with women who have a first full-term pregnancy before approximately age 18.[20,21] Nulliparous women are at greater risk for the development of breast cancer than parous women, with a RR of about 1.4. Breast cancer risk increases transiently for the 10 years after a pregnancy, but then declines.[21] Abortion, whether spontaneous or induced, does not increase breast cancer risk.[22] Breastfeeding, particularly for longer duration, lowers the risk of breast cancer diagnosis. The combined effects of reproductive history and breastfeeding may account for substantial fractions of the difference in breast cancer risk between developed and developing nations.

The use of combined estrogen and progestin HRT also increases breast cancer risk. In the Women's Health Initiative, use of combined estrogen and progestin HRT was associated with a hazard ratio (HR) of 1.24 (*p* <0.001) for breast cancer development as compared to placebo.[23] The effects of HRT were noted after a relatively short duration of use. An excess of abnormal mammograms was observed after 1 year of HRT use and persisted throughout the study, and an increase in breast cancer incidence was noted after 2 years. The cancers occurring in HRT users were larger and more likely to have nodal or distant metastases than those occurring in the placebo group (25.4% versus 16%; *p* = 0.04), although they were of similar histology and grade.[23] The observational UK Million Women Study found that current use of HRT was associated with a RR of breast cancer development of 1.66 (*p* <0.001) and a RR of breast cancer death of 1.22 (*p* = 0.05).[24]

Dietary and Lifestyle Factors

Observational studies suggested that high-fat diets were associated with higher rates of breast cancer than low-fat diets. However, a meta-analysis of eight prospective epidemiologic studies failed to identify an association between fat intake and breast cancer risk in adult women in developed countries.[25] Consistent with these findings, a randomized dietary modification in 48,835 women in the Women's Health Initiative study did not result in a statistically significant reduction in breast cancer incidence after 8 years of follow-up.[26] Breast cancer risk increases linearly with the amount of alcohol consumed.[27] Decreased intake of nutrients such as vitamin C, folate, and β-carotene may enhance the risk related to alcohol consumption.

Obesity is associated with both an increased risk of breast cancer development in postmenopausal women and increased breast cancer mortality. Women with a body mass index of ≥31.1 have a 2.5-fold greater risk of developing breast cancer than those with a body mass index of ≤22.6.[23] Weight and weight gain appear to play an important but complex role in breast cancer risk. During childhood, rapid growth rates decrease the age of menarche, an established risk factor, and result in greater attained stature, which has been consistently associated with increased risk. During early adult life, obesity is associated with a lower incidence of breast cancer before menopause, but no reduction in breast mortality. Weight gain after age 18 is associated with a graded and substantial increase in postmenopausal breast cancer, particularly in the absence of HRT.[28]

Benign Breast Disease

Benign breast lesions are classified as proliferative or nonproliferative. Nonproliferative disease is not associated with an increased risk of breast cancer, whereas proliferative disease without atypia results in a small increase in risk (RR = 1.5 to 2.0). Proliferative disease with atypical hyperplasia is associated with a greater risk of cancer development (RR = 4.0 to 5.0).[29] Dupont and Page[30] found a marked interaction between atypia and a family history of a first-degree relative with breast cancer. This subgroup of patients had a risk 11-fold that of women with nonproliferative breast disease, and an absolute risk of breast cancer development of 20% at 15 years, compared with 8% in women with atypical hyperplasia and a negative family history of breast carcinoma. Proliferative breast disease appears to be more common in women with a significant family history of breast cancer than in controls, further supporting its significance as a risk factor. Of note, however, the majority of breast biopsies done for clinical indications demonstrate nonproliferative disease. In the study of 10,000 breast biopsies by Dupont and Page,[30] 69% had nonproliferative changes and only 3.6% demonstrated atypical hyperplasia.

Breast Density

Mammographic breast density has emerged as an important predictor of breast cancer risk, and makes detection of cancer more difficult. A significant component of breast density is genetically determined, although density has also been shown to vary with the initiation and discontinuation of postmenopausal HRT. Women with >75% breast density have 4.7-fold increase in the odds of breast cancer development compared with those with >10% breast density.[31] The risk was apparent even after adjustment for other risk factors.

Environmental Factors

Exposure to ionizing radiation increases breast cancer risk, and the increase is particularly marked for exposure at a young age. This pattern has been observed in survivors of the atomic bombings, those undergoing multiple diagnostic X-ray examinations, and in women receiving therapeutic irradiation. A markedly increased risk of breast cancer development has been reported in women who received mantle irradiation for the treatment of Hodgkin lymphoma before age 15 years.[32] Additionally, in women with Hodgkin lymphoma who develop unilateral breast cancer, the risk of a contralateral cancer approximates the level of risk seen in *BRCA* mutation carriers.[32] Well-conducted studies do not suggest that exposure to electromagnetic fields and organochlorine pesticides increase breast cancer risk. A summary of the magnitude of risk associated with known breast cancer risk factors is provided in Table 79.2.

PRACTICE OF ONCOLOGY

TABLE 79.2

Magnitude of Risk of Known Breast Cancer Risk Factors

Relative Risk <2	Relative Risk 2–4	Relative Risk >4
Early menarche Late menopause	One first-degree relative with breast cancer	Mutation *BRCA1* or *BRCA2* LCIS
Nulliparity	*CHEK2* mutation	Atypical hyperplasia
Estrogen plus progesterone	Age >35 y for first birth	Radiation exposure before 30
HRT	Proliferative breast disease	
Alcohol use	Mammographic breast density	
Postmenopausal obesity		

LCIS, lobular carcinoma in situ; HRT, hormone replacement therapy.

MANAGEMENT OF THE HIGH-RISK PATIENT

There is no formal definition of what constitutes *high risk*. Without question, women who carry mutations in either *BRCA1* or *BRCA2*, or who have a family history consistent with genetically transmitted breast cancer, are considered to be at higher risk than those in the general population. Other high-risk groups include women who have received mantle irradiation, usually for treatment of Hodgkin lymphoma, and those with lobular carcinoma in situ (LCIS) or atypical hyperplasia. Although a variety of hormonal factors (e.g., early menarche, late age at first full-term pregnancy) affect breast cancer risk on a population basis, these conditions have a relatively small effect on risk for any individual woman.

Many women overestimate their risk of developing breast cancer, so providing an accurate assessment of breast cancer risk will often allay anxiety and facilitate management decisions. It can be helpful to provide women who are concerned about their breast cancer risk with a numeric risk estimate. The Gail et al. model,[33] which calculates a woman's risk of developing breast cancer based on age at menarche, age at first live birth, number of previous breast biopsies, the presence or absence of atypical hyperplasia, and the number of first-degree female relatives with breast cancer, has been used in the National Surgical Adjuvant Breast and Bowel Project (NSABP) breast cancer prevention trials. Efforts to validate the Gail et al. model in different settings have produced variable results. It was highly accurate in the NSABP P1 prevention trial,[34] with a ratio of observed to predicted cancers in study participants of 1.03. In general, the Gail et al.[33] model is thought to underestimate risk in women with strong family histories, at least in part because it only incorporates a family history in first-degree relatives and does not include ovarian carcinoma. The Claus et al.[35] model takes into account both first- and second-degree relatives, although it does not include other risk factors, and may be more useful for women at risk on the basis of family history.

Management strategies available for high-risk women include intensive surveillance, chemoprevention with endocrine agents, and prophylactic surgery. Surveillance, consisting of monthly breast self-examination, annual screening mammography, and clinical breast examinations once or twice yearly, did not clearly result in early detection in high-risk women in the placebo arm of the NSABP P1 prevention trial where 29% of the women who developed breast cancer had axillary node metastases at diagnosis.[34] Women at risk as a result of known or suspected *BRCA1* or *BRCA2* mutations warrant screening with magnetic resonance imaging (MRI), which results in earlier detection of breast cancer than conventional surveillance strategies, and has a higher specificity and sensitivity among high-risk women.[36] Because the cancers detected by MRI are smaller and less likely to be associated with nodal positivity, it is likely that a survival benefit is present. However, there is no benefit for MRI screening in women

with atypical hyperplasia or LCIS.[37] An expert panel convened by the American Cancer Society in 2007 to develop guidelines for MRI screening recommended the use of MRI in addition to mammography for a small group of women at very high risk of breast cancer development, either due to genetic factors or a history of prior thoracic irradiation (Table 79.3). It has been estimated that only 1% of the population would be eligible for MRI screening using these criteria.[38] For women with a <15% risk of breast cancer development, the American Cancer Society recommended against the use of MRI screening.[39] In the remainder, they thought that the evidence was insufficient to recommend for or against MRI screening. Chemoprevention is an option in addition to surveillance strategies. Two SERMs, tamoxifen and raloxifene, have been shown to reduce the incidence of ER⁺ breast cancer. Four prospective, randomized trials have examined the effect of tamoxifen on breast cancer incidence (Tables 79.4 and 79.5).[34,40–42] There is considerable heterogeneity in outcome among the trials, much of which can be attributed to differences in the populations studied. In an overview of the four studies, tamoxifen produced a 38% reduction in breast cancer incidence (95% confidence interval [CI], 8 to 46; p <0.001), and a 48% reduction in the incidence of ER⁺ breast cancers.[43] No effect on the incidence of ER⁻ cancers was seen in any of the trials, and the cancers occurring in women taking tamoxifen were not

TABLE 79.3

American Cancer Society Guidelines for Magnetic Resonance Imaging Screening

- Annual MRI recommended based on evidence
  - *BRCA* mutation
  - Untested first-degree relative of *BRCA* carrier
  - Lifetime risk of breast cancer 20% to 25%
- Annual MRI recommended based on expert opinion
  - Radiation to chest between age 10 and 30 y
  - Li-Fraumeni syndrome and first-degree relatives
  - Cowden and Bannayan-Riley-Ruvalcaba syndromes and first-degree relatives
- Insufficient evidence to recommend for or against MRI
  - Lifetime breast cancer risk 15% to 20%
  - Lobular carcinoma in situ
  - Atypical hyperplasia (lobular or ductal)
  - Extremely or heterogeneously dense breasts on mammogram
  - Personal history of breast cancer, including ductal carcinoma in situ

MRI, magnetic resonance imaging.

TABLE 79.4

A Comparison of Tamoxifen Chemoprevention Studies

Study[(Ref.)]	Age Range (y)	Family History (%)	HRT Use (%)	Lost to Follow-Up (%)
Royal Marsden[41] (n = 2,471)	30–70, median 47	100	26	11
NSABP P-1[34] (n = 13,388)	>35, median NS	76	0	1.6
Italian[42] (n = 5,408)	35–70, median 51	21	24.7	0.8
IBIS[40] (n = 7,152)	35–70, median 50.8	97	39.7	NS

HRT, hormone replacement therapy; NSABP, National Surgical Adjuvant Breast and Bowel Project; NS, not stated; IBIS, International Breast Cancer Intervention Study.

found to have had more positive nodes or to be larger in size than those in the placebo arm, providing reassurance that tamoxifen chemoprevention does not result in the occurrence of biologically more-aggressive cancers.

In the largest of these studies, the NSABP P1 trial, a 49% risk reduction was seen with tamoxifen, with 43.4 cancers per 1,000 women occurring in the placebo arm compared with 22.0 per 1,000 in the tamoxifen arm.[34] The benefits of tamoxifen were observed for both invasive and noninvasive carcinoma, and were seen in women of all ages. A particular benefit was seen in those at risk because of atypical hyperplasia, with an 84% reduction in cancer incidence in this group. The risk reductions were similar in those at risk on the basis of a family history of breast cancer and those at risk from other factors. Controversy exists over the benefit of tamoxifen in BRCA mutation carriers,[44,45] but it appears that it is the likelihood of expressing the ER that determines the efficacy of tamoxifen as a chemopreventive agent rather than the presence of a BRCA mutation.

The side effects of tamoxifen were well known from its use as a cancer treatment and were again observed in the prevention trials. In the combined analysis of the four studies, the RR of thromboembolic events in tamoxifen users was 1.9 (95% CI = 1.4 to 2.6; p <0.0001) and the RR of endometrial cancer was 2.4 (95% CI = 1.5 to 4.0; p = 0.0005).[43] Significant elevation in endometrial cancer and thromboembolic events was limited to postmenopausal women. Thus, women most likely to have a favorable risk-benefit ratio for tamoxifen prevention include premenopausal women, younger postmenopausal women without a uterus, and those at risk on the basis of atypical hyperplasia or LCIS. Despite the proven efficacy, use of tamoxifen as chemoprevention has been limited because of concerns about side effects and the small absolute differences in outcomes.

Raloxifene is a SERM used for the treatment and prevention of osteoporosis that was noted to reduce the incidence of ER$^+$ breast cancer in this population. The NSABP P2 trial, the Study of Tamoxifen and Raloxifene (STAR) trial, directly compared the chemopreventive actions and side effects of tamoxifen and raloxifene in 19,747 postmenopausal women at increased risk of breast cancer development.[36] No difference in the incidence of invasive cancer was seen between women taking tamoxifen and those taking raloxifene (RR = 1.02; 95% CI = 0.82 to 1.28). More cases of noninvasive cancer were noted in the raloxifene group, with a cumulative incidence of 11.7 per 1,000 compared with 8.1 per 1,000 in the tamoxifen group at 6 years (RR = 1.4; p = 0.052). A more favorable side-effect profile was seen for raloxifene, with a reduction in the number of hysterectomies and endometrial cancers in the raloxifene group (RR = 0.62; 95% CI = 0.35 to 1.08), although the difference did not reach statistical significance. Significantly fewer thromboembolic events and cataracts occurred with raloxifene. Raloxifene is thus a viable alternative to tamoxifen for the chemoprevention of breast cancer in postmenopausal women at increased risk for the disease. In addition, the use of raloxifene in women with osteoporosis has the potential to lower breast cancer incidence in a group of women not considered at high risk.

Trials of aromatase inhibitors (AI) for breast cancer prevention suggest qualitatively similar results as seen with SERMs. The MAP.3 trial examined the use of the AI exemestane in postmenopausal women with a Gail risk score of 1.66, atypical hyperplasia, LCIS, or unilateral ductal carcinoma in situ (DCIS) treated with mastectomy. After a median follow-up of 3 years, a 65% reduction in invasive breast cancer was seen with exemestane (p = 0.002).[46] The reduction in cancer incidence was also limited to ER$^+$ cancers. At present, there are no chemopreventive agents that have been proven to be effective in reducing the incidence of ER$^-$ breast cancer.

The 2013 American Society of Clinical Oncology (ASCO) guideline on pharmacologic agents for breast cancer risk reduction[47] recommends discussion of tamoxifen for breast cancer risk reduction with premenopausal women age 35 and older at increased risk for breast cancer development, and discussion of tamoxifen, raloxifene, and exemestane with high-risk

TABLE 79.5

Outcome of Tamoxifen Chemoprevention Studies

Study[(Ref.)]	Median Follow-Up (mo)	Total Cancers	Breast Cancer Rate (per 1,000 women-y)		RR (95% CI)
			Placebo	Tamoxifen	
Royal Marsden[41]	70	70	5.0	4.7	0.94 (0.59–1.43)
NSABP P-1[34]	54.6	368	6.8	3.4	0.51 (0.39–0.66)
Italian[42]	81.2	79	2.3	2.1	0.87 (0.62–2.14)
IBIS[40]	96	337	6.8	5.0	0.73 (0.58–0.91)

RR, relative risk tamoxifen to placebo; CI, confidence interval; NSABP, National Surgical Adjuvant Breast and Bowel Project; IBIS, International Breast Cancer Intervention Study

TABLE 79.6

Outcome of Bilateral Prophylatic Mastectomy in High-Risk Women

Author[Ref.]	Population	No. of Women	Follow-Up (y)	Risk Reduction (%)
Hartmann et al.[48]	Women with a family history of breast cancer	639	14 (median)	90–94
Meijers-Heijboer et al.[49]	*BRCA1/2* mutation carriers	139	3 (mean)	100
Rebbeck et al.[50]	*BRCA1/2* mutation carriers	105	6.4 (mean)	90–95

postmenopausal women. Histories of deep vein thrombosis, stroke, pulmonary embolism, or transient ischemic attacks are considered contraindications to the use of both tamoxifen and raloxifene.

Prophylactic surgery, in the form of bilateral mastectomy or bilateral salpingo-oophorectomy, is another option for breast cancer risk reduction. The efficacy of prophylactic mastectomy has never been studied in a prospective, randomized trial. In a retrospective study of 639 women who had bilateral prophylactic mastectomy due to a family history of breast cancer,[48] a 90% to 94% reduction in breast cancer incidence (95% CI = 71% to 99%) and an 81% to 100% reduction in breast cancer mortality with prophylactic mastectomy compared to unaffected sisters or Gail model predictions was observed. Prospective studies in *BRCA* mutation carriers (Table 79.6) demonstrate similar levels of risk reduction.[48–50]

Prophylactic bilateral salpingo-oophorectomy is an alternative risk-reduction strategy in women at risk on the basis of *BRCA* mutations, which has the added benefit of reducing the risk of ovarian carcinoma, a disease for which effective screening is not available. In a prospective study of the benefits of prophylactic salpingo-oophorectomy in 170 *BRCA* mutation carriers, Kauff et al.[19] observed that the HR for breast cancer was reduced to 0.32 (95% CI = 0.08 to 1.20) and to 0.25 for gynecologic cancer (95% CI = 0.08 to 0.74) at a mean follow-up of 24 months. In a meta-analysis[51] of risk-reduction estimates associated with risk-reducing salpingo-oophorectomy in *BRCA1* or *BRCA2* mutation carriers, statistically significant reductions in breast cancer (HR = 0.49; 95% CI = 0.37 to 0.65 with similar risk reductions in *BRCA1* and *BRCA2* mutation carriers) and in the risk of *BRCA1/2*-associated ovarian or fallopian tube cancer (HR = 0.21; 95% CI = 0.12 to 0.39) were observed. More recently, recognition that *BRCA*-associated cancers arise in the fallopian tube rather than the ovary has led some to propose bilateral salpingectomy, with ovarian preservation, as a risk-reducing strategy, but the efficacy of this approach is uncertain.

DIAGNOSIS AND BIOPSY

The presence or absence of carcinoma in a suspicious clinically or mammographically detected abnormality can only be reliably determined by tissue biopsy. An abnormal MRI does not reliably indicate the presence of cancer, and a nonworrisome MRI does not reliably exclude carcinoma.[52] Available biopsy techniques include fine needle aspiration (FNA), core needle biopsy, and excisional biopsy. Needle biopsy techniques (FNA or core biopsy) are preferred because they are more cost-effective than surgical excision, and because most breast lesions are benign, they avoid a surgical scar and potential cosmetic deformity.

FNA is easily performed, but requires a trained cytopathologist for accurate specimen interpretation and does not reliably distinguish invasive cancer from DCIS, a particular drawback for nonpalpable abnormalities, which are often DCIS. Core-cutting needle biopsy has many of the advantages of FNA, but provides a histologic specimen suitable for interpretation by any pathologist, and facilitates ER, PR, and *HER2* testing. False-negative results from sampling error may occur with both core-cutting needle biopsy and FNA. When concordance between the core biopsy or

FNA diagnosis, and the clinical and imaging findings is not present, additional tissue should be obtained, usually by excisional biopsy. Concerns about the false-negative rate of image-guided core biopsy have been resolved with the availability of large, vacuum-assisted biopsy devices that increase the extent of lesion sampling, coupled with the development of clearly defined indications for follow-up surgical biopsy. False-negative rates of core biopsy are now reliably <1%. Indications for surgical biopsy following core biopsy are listed in Table 79.7. Although the finding of atypical ductal hyperplasia on a core biopsy is uniformly accepted as an indication for open surgical biopsy, the need for surgical excision of all lesions showing atypical lobular hyperplasia (ALH) or LCIS remains controversial (discussed in the section "Lobular Carcinoma in Situ"). Papillary carcinoma in situ cannot always be readily distinguished from benign papillary lesions on a core biopsy, and radial scar may be difficult to distinguish from tubular carcinoma without complete removal of the lesion.

The use of core biopsy for the diagnosis of mammographic abnormalities is cost-effective and increases the likelihood that the patient will be able to undergo a single surgical procedure for definitive cancer treatment.[53] Excisional biopsy as a diagnostic technique should be reserved for patients with imaging abnormalities that cannot be targeted for core biopsy. A core biopsy diagnosis permits a complete discussion of treatment options prior to the placement of an incision on the breast and allows the breast procedure and the axillary surgery to take place at a single operation.

When excisional biopsy is performed for diagnosis, a small margin of grossly normal breast should be excised around the tumor, orienting sutures should be placed, and the specimen should be inked to allow margin evaluation.

LOBULAR CARCINOMA IN SITU

In 1941, Foote and Stewart[54] published their landmark study of LCIS, describing a relatively uncommon entity characterized by an "alteration of lobular cytology." They hypothesized that LCIS was a precursor lesion of invasive cancer, and, based on this, treatment with mastectomy was recommended. More recently, the term ALH has been introduced to describe morphologically

TABLE 79.7

Indications for Surgical Biopsy After Core Needle Biopsy

- Failure to sample calcifications
- Diagnosis of atypical ductal hyperplasia
- Diagnosis of atypical lobular hyperplasia or lobular carcinoma in situ[a]
- Lack of concordance between imaging findings and histologic diagnosis
- Radial scar
- Papillary lesions

[a] See text for details.

similar, but less well-developed, lesions. Some centers use the term *lobular neoplasia* (LN) to cover both ALH and LCIS. Morphologically, LN is defined as "a proliferation of generally small and often loosely cohesive cells originating in the terminal duct-lobular unit, with or without pagetoid involvement of terminal ducts."[55]

In the past, LCIS was most frequently diagnosed in women aged 40 to 50, a decade earlier than DCIS, but recent literature indicates that the incidence in postmenopausal women is increasing.[56] Determining the true incidence of LCIS is difficult, as there are no specific clinical or mammographic abnormalities associated with the lesion and the diagnosis of LCIS is often made as an incidental, microscopic finding in a breast biopsy performed for other indications. The prevalence of LN in an otherwise benign breast biopsy has been reported as between 0.5% and 4.3%.[57] LCIS is both multifocal and bilateral in a large percentage of cases.

In an analysis of nine studies including 172 patients with LCIS who were treated by biopsy alone, 15% developed invasive carcinoma in the ipsilateral breast and 9.3% carcinoma in the contralateral breast after 10 years of follow-up.[58] This corresponds to a risk of development of invasive carcinoma of about 1% to 2% per year, with a lifetime risk of 30% to 40%. In this study (conducted prior to effective breast imaging), 5.7% of the patients developed metastatic breast cancer. In a more recent study of 776 women with LCIS followed in a high-risk screening program at Memorial Sloan-Kettering Cancer Center, King et al.[37] reported that 13% had developed cancer at a median follow-up of 58 months, a rate similar to that seen in older studies. Cancers were detected at a median size of 0.8 cm (0.1 cm to 3.5 cm), and 78% were node negative. MRI screening had no significant impact on cancer stage at diagnosis in this cohort. Subsequent cancers are more often invasive ductal carcinoma than invasive lobular carcinoma (ILC), but the incidence of subsequent ILC is substantially increased compared with women without LCIS. Although the risk for development of breast cancer is bilateral, subsequent ipsilateral carcinoma is more likely than contralateral breast cancer, supporting the view that ALH and LCIS act both as precursor lesions and as risk indicators. The RR for development of subsequent breast cancer is lower in women diagnosed with ALH compared with LCIS. Therefore, although LN is a helpful term for collectively describing this group of lesions, specific classification into ALH and LCIS is preferable in terms of risk assessment and management.

LCIS is typically positive for ER and PR staining and negative for *HER2/neu* staining. LN (and ILC) characteristically lacks expression of E-cadherin, an epithelial cell membrane molecule involved in cell-cell adhesion. E-cadherin negativity serves as a fairly reliable means of distinguishing ductal from lobular disease, both in situ and invasive. Pleomorphic LCIS is a relatively uncommon variant of LCIS characterized by medium-to-large pleomorphic cells containing eccentric nuclei, prominent nucleoli, and eosinophilic cytoplasm. As with classic LCIS, it is usually ER$^+$ and negative for E-cadherin; it also tests positive by immunohistochemistry (IHC) for gross cystic disease fluid protein-15. Pleomorphic LCIS can be associated with central necrosis, may be associated with mammographic microcalcifications, and may be difficult to distinguish from DCIS. Although pleomorphic LCIS has a more aggressive histologic appearance than classic LCIS, the relative rarity of this lesion and the lack of uniform diagnostic criteria make it difficult to know if pleomorphic LCIS has a different natural history than classic LCIS.

Genetic changes in LN have been evaluated in a number of studies using comparative genomic hybridization. In both ALH and LCIS, there was loss at 16q21-q23.1, an altered region previously identified in invasive carcinoma.[59] This genomic signature, common to LN and ILC, further suggests that LN is a precursor lesion in some women.

Management of LN must address the bilateral risk, and options therefore include surveillance, chemoprevention, and prophylactic bilateral mastectomy. Surveillance is the strategy selected by most patients. Mammographic screening is the standard breast

imaging technique for patients selecting surveillance. Breast MRI has been used, but, as noted previously, existing evidence does not support its routine use for patients with LCIS. Prophylactic mastectomy reduces breast cancer risk among high-risk women by approximately 90%. Chemoprevention with tamoxifen in patients with LCIS has been evaluated as part of the NSABP P1 study.[34] Overall, tamoxifen reduced the incidence of breast cancer by 49% ($p < 0.00001$), and a similar level of risk reduction was seen in the 826 participants with a history of LCIS. In the NSABP P2 (STAR) trial,[36] 893 participants gave a history of LCIS, and their rates of subsequent breast cancer were similar with tamoxifen and raloxifene. Benefit for exemestane in women with LCIS was also seen in the MAP.3 study.[46]

In the past, the finding of LN on a core needle biopsy usually led to a recommendation for surgical biopsy to rule out coexisting DCIS or invasive cancer. Recent studies have demonstrated that when the diagnosis of LN is concordant with the imaging findings, upgrade rates with surgical excision are ≤3%.[60] Discordance between the pathology and imaging, and the presence of pleomorphic LCIS in a core biopsy remain indications for surgical excision. The recent recognition that, in some cases, LCIS may be a precursor lesion has led to confusion as to whether it should be treated like DCIS (i.e., excised to negative margins and irradiated). At this time, there are no data indicating that the incidence of subsequent cancer is reduced with this approach. When LCIS is seen on an excised tissue, it is not necessary to obtain negative margins of resection, and there is no established role for radiation therapy in patients with LN.

DUCTAL CARCINOMA IN SITU

DCIS is defined as the proliferation of malignant-appearing mammary ductal epithelial cells without evidence of invasion beyond the basement membrane. Prior to the widespread use of screening mammography, <5% of mammary cancers were DCIS. At present, 15% to 30% of the cancers detected in mammography screening programs are DCIS, and the greatest increase in the incidence of DCIS has been seen in women aged 49 to 69 years. DCIS can present as a palpable or nonpalpable mass, Paget disease of the nipple, an incidental finding at biopsy, or, most commonly, as mammographically detected calcifications.

A central problem in the management of DCIS is the lack of understanding of its natural history and the inability to determine which DCIS will progress to invasive carcinoma during a woman's lifetime. The concordance between risk factors for DCIS and invasive carcinoma suggests that they are part of the same disease process.[61] Attempts to better characterize the natural history of DCIS on the basis of pathologic features have not been particularly successful. The traditional morphologic classification into comedo, papillary, micropapillary, solid, and cribriform types is confounded by the observation that as many as 30% to 60% of DCIS lesions display more than one histologic pattern. To overcome this difficulty, a number of classifications based on nuclear grade and the presence or absence of necrosis have been developed. No single classification scheme has been widely adopted and, most importantly, none of the classification systems have been prospectively demonstrated to predict the risk of development of invasive carcinoma. Molecular profiling studies in DCIS have been limited by the need for histologic examination of the entire lesion to reliably exclude the presence of invasive carcinoma. The Oncotype DX (Genomic Health, Redwood City, CA) assay using paraffin-embedded tissue was modified for DCIS, and an initial study suggested usefulness in predicting the risk of invasive in-breast recurrence. This finding has not been validated in other populations, nor has this test been shown to predict the benefit of radiotherapy (RT).[62] The available data indicate that DCIS lesions share many of the genetic alterations of invasive carcinoma, but predictors of progression to invasion remain to be identified.

Treatment of the Breast

Cancer-specific survival for the woman diagnosed with DCIS exceeds 95%, regardless of the type of local therapy employed.[63,64] Mastectomy, excision and RT, and excision alone have all been proposed as management strategies for DCIS. The appropriate therapy for the woman with DCIS depends on the extent of the DCIS lesion, the risk of local recurrence (LR) with each form of treatment, and the patient's attitude toward the risks and benefits of a particular therapy.

Total or simple mastectomy is curative in approximately 98% of patients regardless of age, DCIS presentation, size, or grade.[65] The primary medical indication for mastectomy in DCIS is a lesion too large to be excised to negative margins with a cosmetically acceptable outcome.[66] The extent of DCIS is most accurately estimated preoperatively with the use of magnification mammography.[67] Studies indicate that MRI both overestimates and underestimates the size of DCIS lesions, does not improve surgical planning when compared with diagnostic mammography, and does not decrease the rate of ipsilateral breast tumor recurrence (IBTR).[68]

For women with localized DCIS, management by excision alone and excision plus RT have both been employed. Four published prospective, randomized trials have directly compared these two approaches in >4,500 patients.[63,64,69,70] In all four trials, the majority of participants had mammographically detected DCIS, and in all but the Swedish trial,[70] negative margins (no ink on tumor) were required. A dose of 50 Gy of radiation was delivered to the whole breast in 25 fractions, and a boost dose to the tumor bed was not required. The results of these trials are summarized in Table 79.8. No differences in overall survival (OS) were seen between treatment arms. In all four studies, the use of RT resulted in a highly significant reduction in the risk of an IBTR, with proportional risk reductions ranging from 47% to 63%.[40,63] Consistent with observations from many retrospective studies, approximately 50% of the recurrences in both groups were invasive carcinoma, and a benefit for RT was seen in the reduction of both invasive and noninvasive recurrences.

A meta-analysis by the Early Breast Cancer Trialists' Collaborative Group (EBCTCG) provides a concise overview of RT effect following lumpectomy for DCIS.[71] With a median follow-up of 8.9 years, RT approximately halved the rate of ipsilateral breast events (rate ratio = 0.46; standard error [SE] = 0.05; 2p <0.00001). RT was effective in all subgroups. There were 291 "low-risk" cases of DCIS that were low-grade, >20 mm in size, and with negative surgical margins identified. Among them, the 10-year risk of an ipsilateral event in those allocated to lumpectomy alone was substantial at 30.1%, and even with this relatively small number of women, the effect of RT was highly significant (rate ratio = 0.48; SE = 0.17; 2p =0.002), with a 10-year absolute gain of 18.0% (SE = 5.5%).

The Radiation Therapy Oncology Group (RTOG) study 9804 sought to determine RT benefit after lumpectomy for patients with low-risk DCIS.[72] In comparison to the other randomized trials, RTOG 9804 enrolled patients with smaller lesions, all low- or intermediate-grade DCIS, and had a much higher rate of adjuvant tamoxifen use (62%). Recurrence rates were 6.7% in the observation arm, compared to 0.9% in the RT arm, after a median follow-up of 7.2 years (HR = 0.11; 95% CI = 0.03 to 0.47; p = 0.0003).[72] This suggests that even in low-risk DCIS, RT can lower the risk of in-breast recurrence. LR rates after excision and RT have decreased over time due to improvements in imaging and pathologic analysis. In a retrospective review of 246 consecutive patients treated at Dana-Farber Cancer Institute and Brigham and Women's Hospital from 2001 to 2007, there were no LRs with a median follow-up time of 58 months.[73]

Despite the clear benefit of RT seen in these five trials, there was considerable interest in identifying patients who could be spared RT for DCIS. The Dana-Farber/Harvard Cancer Center conducted a single-arm, prospective trial of wide excision alone from 1995 to 2002 among 158 patients.[74] Entry criteria included DCIS of predominant grade 1 or 2 with a mammographic extent of no greater than 2.5 cm and final margin width of at least 1 cm. Tamoxifen was not permitted. The study was closed to further accrual because the number of LRs (n = 13) met the predefined stopping rules. The median patient age was 51 years, and 94% had mammographically detected DCIS. The median follow-up was 11 years, and 143 patients were followed for >8 years. Nineteen patients developed an LR. Fourteen recurrences were in the same quadrant as the initial DCIS, and five were elsewhere in the ipsilateral breast. A total of 32% recurred with invasive disease. No patient developed distant metastasis. The 10-year cumulative incidence of LR was 15.6%.

Similar results were seen in the Eastern Cooperative Oncology Group single-arm trial of excision alone for DCIS. Eligibility criteria for this study included DCIS at least 3 mm in size, excised with a margin width of ≥3 mm as determined by sequential sectioning, and complete embedding. The study enrolled patients with low- or intermediate-grade DCIS ≤2.5 cm in size and high-grade DCIS (defined as nuclear grade 3 with necrosis) up to 1 cm in size. A postexcision mammogram was required for

---

TABLE 79.8

Randomized Trials of Excision with or without Radiotherapy in Ductal Carcinoma In Situ

Trial[(Ref.)]	No. of Patients	Ipsilateral Local Recurrence				Breast Cancer–Specific Survival		
		Without RT	With RT	Risk Reduction	P Value	Without RT	With RT	P Value
NSABP B-17[64] 12-y results	813	35	19.8	44	<0.00005	96.9	95.3	NS
EORTC 10853[63] 10.5-y results	1,010	26	15	47	<0.0001	96	96	NS
UK/ANZ[69] Median FU = 12.7-y crude incidence	1,030	19.4	7.1	63	<0.0001	97.5	98.5	NS
Swedish[70] 8 y = mean FU; 10-y cumulative incidence	1,046	27.1	12.1	55	<0.0001	99.4	99.8	NS

RT, radiotherapy; NSABP, National Surgical Adjuvant Breast and Bowel Project; NS, not stated; EORTC, European Organisation for Research and Treatment of Cancer; UK/ANZ, United Kingdom/Australia New Zealand; FU, follow-up.

all patients. At a median follow-up of 8.8 years, the 10-year LR rate was 19.0% for patients with high-grade DCIS, and 14.6% for those with low- or intermediate-grade DCIS.[62] Taken together, these prospective studies indicate that even patients with small low- to immediate-grade DCIS treated with excision to widely negative margins of resection have about a 15% 10-year risk of a LR in the absence of RT. No reduction in recurrence was observed for patients excised to margins of ≥1 cm compared to those with margins of 3 to 9 mm.

The 2014 National Comprehensive Cancer Network (NCCN) Guidelines® endorse lumpectomy and whole breast radiation therapy or total mastectomy as category 1 recommendations, and lumpectomy without RT as a category 2B recommendation.[66] Clearly, patients should be included in the treatment decision making to learn what magnitude of risk reduction is meaningful to them. A detailed discussion of the pros and cons of the various treatment options is needed to allow each woman with DCIS to make an informed treatment choice.

Treatment of the Axilla

In situ carcinoma by definition does not metastasize, so theoretically, axillary staging should be unnecessary for DCIS. Studies of axillary dissection (ALND) in DCIS have demonstrated axillary nodal metastases in only 1% to 2% of patients, presumably due to unrecognized microinvasion. Data from the NSABP B-17 and B-24 studies confirm that the risk of isolated axillary recurrence with no axillary surgery is <0.1%, regardless of whether RT and tamoxifen are administered.[75] These low rates of axillary recurrence argue against routine use of sentinel lymph node biopsy in DCIS. Selective use of sentinel node biopsy in patients with DCIS who are at significant risk of having coexistent invasive carcinoma is appropriate. Approximately 15% of patients diagnosed as having DCIS with large vacuum-assisted biopsy devices are found to have invasive cancer after complete excision of the lesion. The diagnosis of DCIS in a palpable breast mass and pathologic interpretation of a core biopsy specimen as suspicious, but not diagnostic, of microinvasion are circumstances in which invasive cancer is frequently found when the lesion is completely examined and so sentinel node biopsy should be considered.

Because patients undergoing mastectomy forfeit the opportunity for sentinel node biopsy if not performed concurrently, patients receiving mastectomy for DCIS should undergo sentinel node biopsy.

Endocrine Therapy

The ER is present in about 80% of DCIS lesions and is more frequent in noncomedo than comedo DCIS.[76] Endocrine therapy might reduce LR after breast-conserving therapy (BCT) and prevent development of new primary breast cancers in the contralateral breast. Two trials have examined the use of tamoxifen in women with DCIS. In the NSABP B-24 trial,[64] patients with DCIS were treated with excision and RT and randomized to tamoxifen 20 mg daily or a placebo for 5 years. Patients in the tamoxifen arm had a 32% reduction in the risk of an invasive LR ($p = 0.025$), a 16% reduction in the risk of a DCIS LR ($p = 0.33$), and a 32% reduction in contralateral breast cancer ($p = 0.023$) compared to the patients in the placebo arm. In the subset of women with ER$^+$ DCIS, tamoxifen reduced the risk of any breast cancer event by 51% (RR = 0.41; 95% CI = 0.25 to 0.65; $p = 0.0002$); there was no benefit seen if the DCIS lesion was ER$^-$.[76] The United Kingdom/Australia New Zealand trial[69] that randomized women to tamoxifen or to no tamoxifen and with a median follow-up of 12.7 years found that tamoxifen reduced ipsilateral events (HR = 0.78; 95% CI = 0.62 to 0.99), but more significantly, reduced contralateral events (HR = 0.44; 95% CI = 0.25 to 0.77) (In a subset analysis, the benefit of tamoxifen appeared restricted to

patients who did not receive RT.) Taken together, these trials suggest that tamoxifen modestly reduces ipsilateral events with or without RT, and substantially reduce contralateral events. The addition of tamoxifen to RT is particularly attractive in young patients with ER$^+$ DCIS, in whom the risk of LR is higher and the toxicity of tamoxifen is less than in older patients.

Evidence that the AIs reduce the incidence of contralateral breast cancer to a greater extent than tamoxifen has led to interest in their use in DCIS. Ongoing trials (NSABP B53 and IBIS II) are comparing tamoxifen with an AI; however, at present, there are no data for use of AIs in management.

In summary, patients with localized DCIS have treatment options ranging from simple excision to mastectomy, all of which have high survival rates but different risks of LR. Patient preference plays a major role in treatment selection, but available evidence indicates that patients have limited understanding of the nature of DCIS. In one study, women with DCIS estimated their risk of breast cancer death to be 39%.[77] Perhaps related to this, Katz et al.[78] found that although patients reported that their surgeon infrequently recommended mastectomy for DCIS, greater involvement of patients in the decision-making process was associated with higher rates of mastectomy.

STAGING

The staging system for breast cancer was last updated in 2010.[79] The American Joint Committee on Cancer (AJCC) system is both a clinical and pathologic staging system, and is based on the TNM system in which "T" refers to tumor, "N" to nodes, and "M" to metastasis. The current version is the seventh edition of the system and is provided in the following.[79]

The major changes in this edition were the inclusion of a new classification system for patients after neoadjuvant therapy and the creation of a new M0(i+) category for patients found to have circulating tumor cells, tumor in the bone marrow, or incidentally detected tumor deposits in other tissues not exceeding 0.2 mm in size. Patients in this category are staged according to T and N, and are not classified as stage IV.

The AJCC staging system provides a strategy for grouping patients with respect to prognosis. However, TNM staging, while still important, has been superseded by rapidly evolving molecular characterizations of breast cancers, which more precisely define subgroups with different outcomes, both in terms of prognosis and response to specific treatments. Increasingly, multigene diagnostic tests, such as Oncotype DX and MammaPrint (Agendia Inc. USA, Irvine, CA), are employed as part of treatment decision making for invasive breast cancer.

Tumor, Node, and Metastases Definitions

Definitions for classifying the primary tumor (T) are the same for clinical and for pathologic classification. If the measurement is made by physical examination, the examiner will use the major headings (T1, T2, or T3). If other measurements are used, such as mammographic or pathologic measurements, the subsets of T1 can be used. Tumors should be measured to the nearest 0.1 cm increment. The AJCC TNM staging system is illustrated in Table 79.9. Stage IIIC breast cancer includes patients with any T stage who have pN3 disease. Patients with pN3a and pN3b disease are considered operable and are managed as described in the section on stage I, II, IIIA, and operable IIIC breast cancer. Patients with pN3c disease, in which the ipsilateral supraclavicular nodes are affected by cancer, are considered inoperable and are managed as described in the section on inoperable stage IIIB or IIIC or inflammatory breast cancer (IBC).[79] Pathologic stage after neoadjuvant therapy is designated with the prefix "yp." Complete response is defined as the absence of invasive carcinoma in the breast and axillary nodes.

TABLE 79.9

TABLE 79.9

American Joint Committee on Cancer Staging

Primary Tumor (T)

- TX: Primary tumor cannot be assessed
- T0: No evidence of primary tumor
- Tis: Carcinoma in situ
  - Tis: DCIS
  - Tis: LCIS
  - Tis (Paget): Paget disease of the nipple NOT associated with invasive carcinoma and/or carcinoma in situ (DCIS and/or LCIS) in the underlying breast parenchyma. Carcinomas in the breast parenchyma associated with Paget disease are categorized based on the size and characteristics of the parenchymal disease, although the presence of Paget disease should still be noted.
- T1: Tumor ≤20 mm in greatest dimension
  - T1mi: Tumor ≤1 mm in greatest dimension
  - T1a: Tumor >1 mm but ≤5 mm in greatest dimension
  - T1b: Tumor >5 mm but ≤10 mm in greatest dimension
  - T1c: Tumor >10 mm but ≤20 mm in greatest dimension
- T2: Tumor >20 mm but ≤50 mm in greatest dimension
- T3: Tumor >50 mm in greatest dimension
- T4: Tumor of any size with direct extension to the chest wall and/or to skin (ulceration or skin nodules). (Note: Invasion of the dermis alone does not qualify as T4.)
  - T4a: Extension to chest wall, not including only pectoralis muscle adherence/invasion
  - T4b: Ulceration and/or ipsilateral satellite nodules and/or edema (including peau d'orange) of the skin, which do not meet the criteria for inflammatory carcinoma
  - T4c: Both T4a and T4b
  - T4d: Inflammatory carcinoma

Regional Lymph Nodes (N)

- NX: Regional lymph nodes cannot be assessed (e.g., previously removed)
- N0: No regional lymph node metastases
- N1: Metastases to movable ipsilateral level I, II axillary lymph node(s)
- N2: Metastases in ipsilateral level I, II axillary lymph nodes that are clinically fixed or matted; or in clinically detected[a] ipsilateral internal mammary nodes in the *absence* of clinically evident lymph node metastases
- N2a: Metastases in ipsilateral level I, II axillary lymph nodes fixed to one another (matted) or to other structures.
- N2b: Metastases only in clinically detected[a] ipsilateral internal mammary nodes and in the *absence* of clinically evident level I, II axillary lymph node metastases
- N3: Metastases in ipsilateral infraclavicular (level III axillary) lymph node(s) with or without level I, II axillary lymph node involvement; or in clinically detected[a] ipsilateral internal mammary lymph node(s) with clinically evident level I, II axillary lymph node metastases; or metastases in ipsilateral supraclavicular lymph node(s) with or without axillary or internal mammary lymph node involvement
- N3a: Metastases in ipsilateral infraclavicular lymph node(s)
- N3b: Metastases in ipsilateral internal mammary lymph node(s) and axillary lymph node(s)
- N3c: Metastases in ipsilateral supraclavicular lymph node(s)

Pathologic (pN)[b]

- pNX: Regional lymph nodes cannot be assessed (e.g., previously removed, or not removed for pathologic study)
- pN0: No regional lymph node metastasis identified histologically
- [Note: ITC clusters are defined as small clusters of cells not >0.2 mm, or single tumor cells, or a cluster of <200 cells in a single histologic cross-section. ITCs may be detected by routine histology or by IHC methods. Nodes containing only ITCs are excluded from the total positive node count for purposes of N classification but should be included in the total number of nodes evaluated.]
- pN0(i−): No regional lymph node metastases histologically, negative IHC
- pN0(i+): Malignant cells in regional lymph node(s) no >0.2 mm (detected by H&E or IHC including ITC)
- pN0(mol−): No regional lymph node metastases histologically, negative molecular findings (RT-PCR)
- pN0(mol+): Positive molecular findings (RT-PCR), but no regional lymph node metastases detected by histology or IHC
- pN1: Micrometastases; or metastases in one to three axillary lymph nodes; and/or in internal mammary nodes with metastases detected by SLNB but not clinically detected[c]
  - pN1mi: Micrometastases (>0.2 mm and/or >200 cells, but none >2.0 mm)
  - pN1a: Metastases in one to three axillary lymph nodes, at least one metastasis >2.0 mm
  - pN1b: Metastases in internal mammary nodes with micrometastases or macrometastases detected by SLNB but not clinically detected[c]
  - pN1c: Metastases in one to three axillary lymph nodes and in internal mammary lymph nodes with micrometastases or macrometastases detected by SLNB but not clinically detected
  - pN2: Metastases in four to nine axillary lymph nodes; or in clinically detected[d] internal mammary lymph nodes in the *absence* of axillary lymph node metastases
  - pN2a: Metastases in four to nine axillary lymph nodes (at least one tumor deposit >2.0 mm)
  - pN2b: Metastases in clinically detected[d] internal mammary lymph nodes in the *absence* of axillary lymph node metastases
  - pN3: Metastases in 10 or more axillary lymph nodes; or in infraclavicular (level III axillary) lymph nodes; or in clinically detected[d] ipsilateral internal mammary lymph nodes in the *presence* of one or more positive level I, II axillary lymph node(s); or in more than three axillary lymph nodes and in internal mammary lymph nodes with micrometastases or macrometastases detected by SLNB but not clinically detected[c]; or in ipsilateral supraclavicular lymph nodes

(continued)

TABLE 79.9

American Joint Committee on Cancer Staging *(continued)*

■ pN3a: Metastases in 10 or more axillary lymph nodes (at least one tumor deposit >2.0 mm); or metastases to the infraclavicular (level III axillary) lymph nodes
■ pN3b: Metastases in clinically detected[d] ipsilateral internal mammary lymph nodes in the *presence* of one or more positive axillary lymph nodes; or in more than three axillary lymph nodes and in internal mammary lymph nodes with micrometastases or macrometastases detected by SLNB but not clinically detected[c]
■ pN3c: Metastases in ipsilateral supraclavicular lymph nodes

Distant Metastases (M)
■ M0: No clinical or radiographic evidence of distant metastases
■ cM0(i+): No clinical or radiographic evidence of distant metastases, but deposits of molecularly or microscopically detected tumor cells in circulating blood, bone marrow, or other nonregional nodal tissue that are no greater than 0.2 mm in a patient without symptoms or signs of metastases
■ M1: Distant detectable metastases as determined by classic clinical and radiographic means and/or histologically proven >0.2 mm

Anatomic Stage/Prognostic Groups

Stage 0
Tis, N0, M0

Stage IA
T1,[e] N0, M0

Stage IB
T0, N1mi, M0
T1,[e] N1mi, M0

Stage IIA
T0, N1,[f] M0
T1,[e] N1,[f] M0
T2, N0, M0

Stage IIB
T2, N1, M0
T3, N0, M0

Stage IIIA
T0, N2, M0
T1,[e] N2, M0
T2, N2, M0
T3, N1, M0
T3, N2, M0

Stage IIIB
T4, N0, M0
T4, N1, M0
T4, N2, M0

Stage IIIC
Any T, N3, M0

Stage IV
Any T, Any N, M1

DCIS, ductal carcinoma in situ; LCIS, lobular carcinoma in situ; ITC, isolated tumor cells; IHC, immunohistochemical; H&E, hematoxylin and eosin stain; RT-PCR, reverse transcriptase-polymerase chain reaction; SLNB, sentinel lymph node biopsy.
[a] Clinically detected is defined as detected by imaging studies (excluding lymphoscintigraphy) or by clinical examination and having characteristics highly suspicious for malignancy or a presumed pathologic macrometastasis based on fine needle aspiration biopsy with cytologic examination. Confirmation of clinically detected metastatic disease by fine needle aspiration without excision biopsy is designated with an (f) suffix, for example, cN3a(f). Excisional biopsy of a lymph node or biopsy of a sentinel node, in the absence of assignment of a pT, is classified as a clinical N, for example, cN1. Information regarding the confirmation of the nodal status will be designated in site-specific factors as clinical, fine needle aspiration, core biopsy, or SLNB. Pathologic classification (pN) is used for excision or SLNB only in connection with a pathologic T assignment.
[b] Classification is based on axillary lymph node dissection with or without SLNB. Classification based solely on SLNB without subsequent axillary lymph node dissection is designated (sn) for "sentinel node" [for example, pN0(sn)].
[c] "Not clinically detected" is defined as not detected by imaging studies (excluding lymphoscintigraphy) or by clinical examination.
[d] "Clinically detected" is defined as detected by imaging studies (excluding lymphoscintigraphy) or by clinical examination and having characteristics highly suspicious for malignancy or a presumed pathologic macrometastasis based on fine needle aspiration biopsy with cytologic examination.
[e] T1 includes T1mi.
[f] T0 and T1 tumors with nodal micrometastases only are excluded from stage IIA and are classified as stage IB.
From Edge SB, Byrd DR, Compton CC, eds. *AJCC Cancer Staging Manual*, 7th ed. New York: Springer, 2010; used with the permission of the American Joint Committee on Cancer, Chicago, Illinois.

PRACTICE OF ONCOLOGY

PATHOLOGY OF BREAST CANCER

Historically, classification of invasive breast cancers has been based on the morphologic appearance of the cancer as seen by light microscopy.[80] The most widely used such classification is that of the World Health Organization (second edition),[55] based on the growth pattern and cytologic features of the invasive tumor cells. Although the classification system recognizes invasive "ductal" and "lobular" carcinomas, this is not meant to indicate that the former originates in the ducts and the latter in the lobules of the breast. Most invasive breast cancers arise in the terminal duct lobular unit, regardless of histologic type.

The most common histologic type of breast cancer is invasive (infiltrating) ductal carcinoma, comprising 70% to 80% of cases. The diagnosis of invasive ductal carcinoma is a diagnosis by exclusion (i.e., this tumor type is defined as a type of cancer not classified into any of the other special categories of invasive mammary carcinoma, such as invasive lobular, tubular, mucinous, medullary, and other special types). To emphasize this point, most classification systems use the term *infiltrating ductal carcinoma, not otherwise specified* (NOS) or *infiltrating carcinoma of no special type*. In practice, the terms invasive ductal carcinoma, infiltrating ductal carcinoma, and infiltrating or invasive carcinoma of no special type are used interchangeably.

Special types of cancers comprise approximately 20% to 30% of invasive carcinomas. At least 90% of a tumor should demonstrate the defining histologic characteristics of a special type of cancer to be designated as that histologic type. Breast cancer histologic classifications recommended by the *AJCC Staging Manual* include NOS; ductal; inflammatory; medullary, NOS; medullary with lymphoid stroma; mucinous; papillary (predominantly micropapillary pattern); tubular; lobular; Paget disease and infiltrating; undifferentiated; squamous cell; adenoid cystic; secretory; and cribriform. Tumor subtypes that occur in the breast, but that are not considered to be typical breast cancers, include cystosarcoma phyllodes, angiosarcoma, and primary lymphoma.

Invasive breast cancers can be further subclassified based on microscopic features. The most common subclassification has been grading, based either solely on nuclear features (nuclear grading) or on a combination of architectural and nuclear characteristics (histologic grading). In nuclear grading, the appearance of the tumor cell nuclei is compared with those of normal breast epithelial cells, and the tumor nuclei are classified as well differentiated, intermediately differentiated, or poorly differentiated. In current practice, histologic grading is the most commonly used method of grading. In histologic grading, breast carcinomas are categorized based on the evaluation of (1) tubule formation, (2) nuclear pleomorphism, and (3) mitotic activity. The grading system by Elston and Ellis,[81] a modification of the grading system proposed by Bloom and Richardson in 1957, is recommended as part of AJCC staging. Tubule formation (>75%, 10% to 75%, and <10%), nuclear pleomorphism (small and uniform, moderate variation in size and shape, and marked nuclear pleomorphism), and mitotic activity (per field area) are each scored on a scale of 1 to 3. The sum of the scores for these three parameters is the overall histologic grade. Tumors with a sum of the scores of 3 to 5 are designated grade 1 (well differentiated), those with sums of 6 and 7 are designated grade 2 (moderately differentiated), and those with sums of 8 and 9 are designated grade 3 (poorly differentiated). Histologic grading, particularly the distinction between grades 1 and 3, has prognostic significance as discussed in the section "Prognostic and Predictive Factors in Breast Cancer." In addition, breast cancers with pure tubular, mucinous, papillary, or cribriform features are recognized to have a more favorable outcome than the more common types of breast cancer.[80] Micropapillary tumors are a recently recognized entity with a high incidence of lymphatic and vascular invasion, and systemic recurrence.[82]

LOCAL MANAGEMENT OF INVASIVE CANCER

The evaluation of the patient newly diagnosed with breast cancer begins with a determination of operability. The presence of distant metastases at diagnosis has traditionally been considered a contraindication to surgery. Some retrospective studies have suggested a survival benefit for surgery of the primary tumor in the patient presenting with metastatic disease,[83,84] but systemic therapy remains the initial therapeutic approach. Extensive evaluations to look for metastatic disease are not warranted in asymptomatic patients with stage I and II cancer because of the low likelihood of identifying metastatic disease.[85] In patients with stage III disease, occult metastases are more frequent, often estimated at 20% of cases, and staging studies are recommended.[85]

Patients with T4 tumors and those with N2 or N3 nodal disease are also not candidates for surgery as the first therapeutic approach and should be treated with systemic therapy initially (discussed in the section "Locally Advanced Breast Cancer and Inflammatory Breast Cancer" on page 1147). In the patient with clinical stage I, II, and T3N1 disease, the initial management is usually surgical. In these patients, the evaluation consists of a determination of their suitability for BCT and a discussion of the options of mastectomy with and without reconstruction. Initial systemic therapy may be used to shrink the primary tumor to allow BCT in a woman who would otherwise require mastectomy, but is not mandatory, as it is for women with locally advanced and inflammatory carcinoma. The current status of management approaches for primary operable breast cancer is discussed in detail in the following sections.

Breast-Conserving Therapy

The goal of BCT using conservative surgery (CS) and RT is to provide survival equivalent to mastectomy with preservation of the cosmetic appearance and a low rate of recurrence in the treated breast. Because of the wide acceptance of the Halstedian dogma, a relatively large number of randomized clinical trials were conducted comparing mastectomy and BCT, and they demonstrated equivalent survival. The long-term stability of this equivalence was confirmed by the 20-year follow-up reports of the two largest studies, the NSABP B-06 and Milan I trials.[86,87] An overview of all the trials has also demonstrated comparable survival,[88] indicating that survival for most patients with breast cancer does not depend on the choice of mastectomy versus BCT.

Medical contraindications to BCT are infrequent. In a population-based study of 1984 patients with DCIS, stage I and II breast cancer, only 13.4% were advised by their surgeon that mastectomy was medically necessary.[89] In the 1,459 women in whom BCT was attempted, conversion to mastectomy occurred in 12%, and re-excision was not attempted in the majority. Thus, the available data indicate that a minority of patients have contraindications to BCT, and these are readily identified with standard clinical tools. Patient participation in the surgical decision-making process is an important factor in mastectomy use. In a population-based study of patients diagnosed with breast cancer in 2002 in two large metropolitan areas (Los Angeles and Detroit), more patient involvement in decision making was associated with a *greater* likelihood of undergoing mastectomy.[90,91] The incidence of LR after BCT has declined over time, from 10-year rates of 8% to 19% seen in retrospective studies and the initial randomized trials of BCT, to 2% to 7% in patients excised to negative margins in more recent studies. Table 79.10 shows the 10-year rates of LR in node-negative NSABP trials.[92] This decrease in LR rates is the result of a combination of improved mammographic and pathologic evaluation, and the more frequent use of adjuvant systemic therapy (discussed in detail in the section "Risk Factors for Local Recurrence Following Conservative Surgery and Radiation Therapy" on page 1129). In contrast, rates of LR after mastectomy have remained stable over the same time period.

Recurrences in the breast are typically classified by their location in relation to the original tumor. Recurrences at or near the primary site (presumably representing a recurrence of the original tumor) are classified as either a *true recurrence* (within the boosted region), a *marginal miss* (adjacent to the boosted region), or *elsewhere* in the breast (occurring at a distance from the original tumor and presumably representing a new primary). The time course to LR in the patient undergoing BCT is prolonged. In one study, the annual incidence rate for a true recurrence/marginal miss recurrence was between 1.3% and 1.8% for years 2 through 7 after treatment and then decreased to 0.4% by 10 years after

TABLE 79.10

Ten-Year Local Recurrence Rates in Recent National Surgical Adjuvant Breast and Bowel Project Trials

Trial	Systemic Therapy	ER Status	10-Year LR (%)
B-13	No chemo	−	13.3
	Chemo	−	3.5
B-14	No tamoxifen	+	11.0
	Tamoxifen	+	3.6
B-19	Chemo	−	6.5
B-20	Tamoxifen	+	4.7
B-23	Chemo	−	4.3

ER, estrogen receptor; LR, local recurrence; chemo, chemotherapy.
From Anderson SJ, Wapnir I, Dignam JJ, et al. Prognosis after ipsilateral breast tumor recurrence and locoregional recurrences in patients treated by breast-conserving therapy in five National Surgical Adjuvant Breast and Bowel Project protocols of node-negative breast cancer. *J Clin Oncol* 2009;27:2466–2473.

treatment. The annual incidence rate for recurrence elsewhere in the breast increased slowly to a rate of approximately 0.7% per year at 8 years and remained stable. It also appears that just as the time to development of distant metastases is more rapid in patients with ER^- or $HER2^+$ cancers than in those with ER^+ and PR^+ cancers, the time to LR also varies with receptor status. (These results have been contrasted to those seen after mastectomy, in which most LRs occur in the first 3 to 5 years after surgery.) In the Milan I trial, after 20 years of follow-up, the risk of any type of recurrence in the treated breast was 0.63 per 100 woman-years compared with a risk of 0.66 per 100 woman-years for contralateral cancer.[87] This suggests that although whole-breast irradiation (WBI) is effective at eradicating subclinical multicentric foci of breast carcinoma present at the time of diagnosis, it does not prevent the subsequent development of new cancers. Thus, patients who elect BCT require lifelong follow-up to screen for the development of new cancers in both the treated and the contralateral breast.

Risk Factors for Local Recurrence Following Conservative Surgery and Radiation Therapy

Risk factors for recurrence after CS and RT can be subdivided into patient, tumor, and treatment factors.

Patient Risk Factors

The most important patient risk factors for LR recurrence are age and inherited susceptibility. *Age* (<35 or 40) is associated with an increased risk of LR after BCT. Young patient age is associated with an increased frequency of various adverse pathologic features, such as lymphatic vessel invasion, grade 3 histology, absence of ER/presence of *HER2*, and the presence of an extensive intraductal component (EIC). However, even when correction is done for the differing incidence of the pathologic features of the primary tumor between the age groups, young age is still associated with an increased likelihood of recurrence in the breast.[93] However, young age is also a risk factor for LR after mastectomy and should not be considered a contraindication to BCT.

An *inherited susceptibility* to breast and ovarian cancer, and other cancers has been mainly linked to germline mutations in *BRCA1* and *BRCA2*. Patients with breast cancer with a mutation have a substantial risk of contralateral and late ipsilateral breast cancers. In a retrospective study, outcome following CS and RT was compared for 302 stage I-III patients with breast cancer with germline *BRCA1* or *BRCA2* mutations and 353 stage I-III patients treated with mastectomy.[94] With a follow-up time of 8.2 and 8.9 years for BCT and mastectomy patients, respectively, LR was significantly more likely in those treated with BCT compared to mastectomy, with a cumulative estimated risk of 23.5% versus 5.5%, respectively, at 15 years (p <0.0001); the 15-year estimate in carriers treated with BCT and chemotherapy was 11.9% (p = 0.08 when compared to mastectomy). Most LR events appeared to be second primary cancers. The risk of contralateral breast cancer was high in all groups, exceeding 40%. It is important to consider genetic testing in a patient with newly diagnosed breast cancer with a personal and family history suggestive of a *BRCA1* or *BRCA2* germline mutation. In patients with a mutation, the option of bilateral mastectomy should be strongly considered to avoid the long-term risk of a second breast cancer in either breast. Patients with breast cancer most likely to benefit from bilateral mastectomy are those who are young and have early-stage disease. Given the high risk of a contralateral breast cancer, unilateral mastectomy is generally not performed in a patient who is a candidate for BCT.

Tumor-Based Risk Factors

An important *tumor risk factor* is the *margin of resection*. A negative margin is defined by absence of cancer cells at inked surfaces, but

there is no standard definition of a close margin. Margins need to be interpreted in conjunction with the operative findings. A close deep margin is not significant if the breast resection was carried down to the pectoral fascia; the same is true for a close anterior margin if the resection extended to the deep dermal surface. Patients with negative margins of excision have low rates of LR after treatment with CS and RT. The impact of close margins of resection on LR has been more controversial, resulting in the frequent use of re-excision to obtain margins more widely clear than no ink on tumor. A 2013 multidisciplinary consensus panel considered a meta-analysis of margin width and IBTR from a systematic review of 33 studies including 28,162 patients. The results of randomized trials, reproducibility of margin assessment, and current patterns of multi-modality care were also considered. The panel concluded that positive margins (ink on invasive carcinoma or DCIS) were associated with a two-fold increase in the risk of IBTR compared to negative margins. This increased risk was not mitigated by favorable biology, endocrine therapy, or a radiation boost. The panel also concluded that more widely clear margins beyond "no ink on tumor" do not significantly decrease the rate of IBTR. There is no evidence that more widely clear margins reduce IBTR for young patients, unfavorable biology, lobular cancers, or cancers with an EIC. (When an EIC is present, young age and multiple close margins are associated with an increased risk of IBTR and can be used to select patients who might benefit from re-excision). Therefore, the use of no ink on tumor as the standard for an adequate margin in invasive cancer in the era of multidisciplinary therapy is associated with low rates of IBTR and has the potential to decrease re-excision rates, improve cosmetic outcomes, and decrease health-care costs.[95]

The underlying molecular subtype of the tumor is the most significant determinant of the likelihood of LR after BCT (and mastectomy), particularly among those treated in the modern era with surgery to achieve negative margins.[96-98] Higher risks of LR are observed in patients with triple-negative breast cancer than in those with other subtypes, regardless of whether they are treated with BCT or mastectomy.[99]

There is interest in identifying molecular predictors of the risk of LR. The 21-gene recurrence score (Oncotype DX) predicts local-regional recurrence (LRR) in node-negative, ER^+ breast cancer, regardless of type of surgery.[100] The 10-year LR rate was 4.3% for patients with a low recurrence score (<18), 7.2% with an intermediate recurrence score (18 to 30), and 15.8% with a high recurrence score (>30).

Treatment-Based Risk Factors

Other important *treatment risk factors* are the use of a boost and the use of adjuvant systemic therapy. A *boost* or supplementary irradiation to the area of the primary site is generally used. It is standard in RT after lumpectomy for patients to receive 45 to 50 Gy of WBI followed by a 10 to 16 Gy boost to the region of the tumor bed (Fig. 79.2). The use of a boost is supported by the large European Organisation for Research and Treatment of Cancer (EORTC) trial in which 5,318 patients with negative margins were randomized to a boost of 16 Gy or no boost following 50 Gy to the whole breast.[101] With a median follow-up of 10.8 years, the cumulative incidence of ipsilateral breast recurrence was 10.2% without a boost and 6.2% with a boost (p <0.0001). This 41% proportional reduction in LR was similar in all age groups; however, the absolute benefit of the boost was greatest in young patients aged 40 years or less (24% decreased to 14%) and was smallest in patients over age 60 (7% decreased to 4%). Severe fibrosis was increased from 2% to 4% with the boost. Survival at 10 years was the same in both arms. A clinicopathologic study was performed on 1,616 patients in the EORTC trial. In multivariate analysis, high-grade invasive ductal carcinoma was associated with an increased risk of LR (HR = 1.67; p = 0.026), and the boost was effective in reducing LR in this subgroup.[102]

The use of *adjuvant systemic therapy* is a very important factor associated with recurrence in the treated breast in conjunction

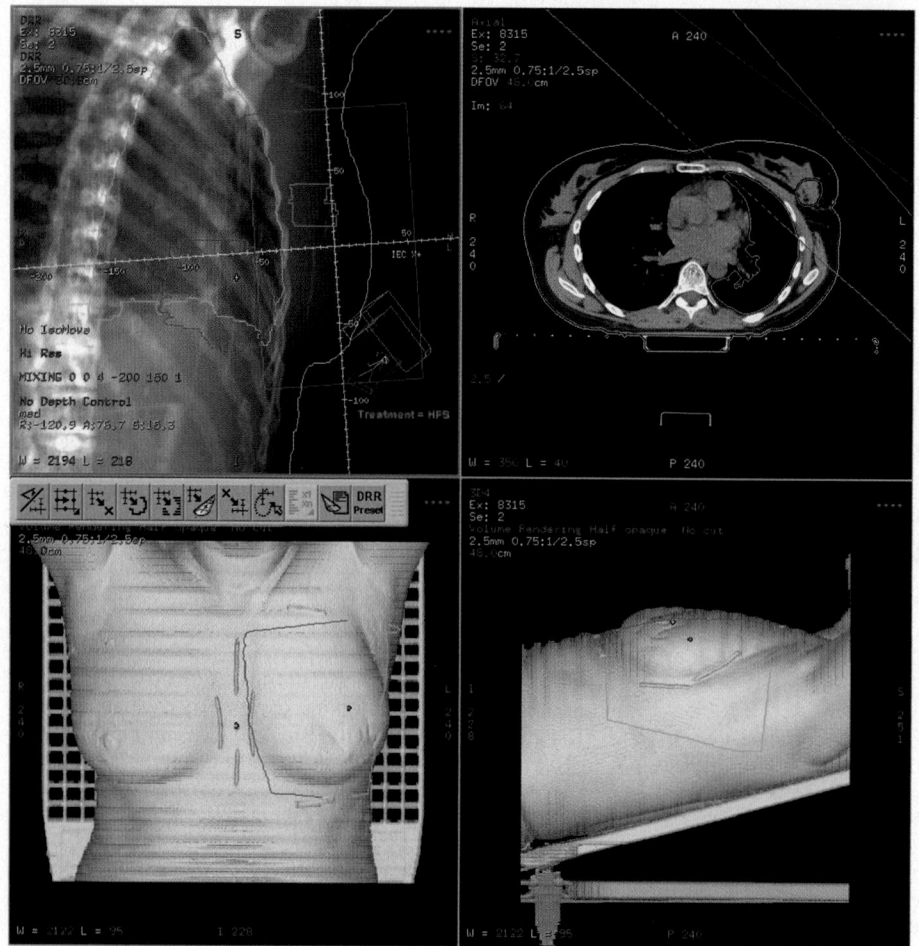

Figure 79.2 Computed tomography simulation for a left-sided breast cancer with medial and lateral tangential fields. Left upper is the beam's eye view with the large rectangle being the treatment field. The area of the primary in the upper outer quadrant is contoured in *magenta* and the heart is contoured in *red*. Note that for the actual treatment a block was used to block irradiation of her heart, which also blocked out some breast tissue well away from the primary cancer. Right upper is an axial view of the treatment fields in the center of the treatment fields. Left lower shows (in *red*) the medial tangent borders on the patient's skin. Right lower shows (in *green*) the lateral tangent borders on the patient's skin.

with CS and RT. This effect is clearly demonstrated in three randomized clinical trials. In the NSABP B-14 trial, node-negative, ER$^+$ patients were randomized to receive tamoxifen or to a placebo. The 10-year rate of recurrence in the ipsilateral breast was 14.7% without tamoxifen and only 4.3% with tamoxifen.[103] A similar result was seen in the Stockholm Breast Cancer Study Group among node-negative patients randomized to receive tamoxifen or a placebo.[104] In the NSABP B-21 trial, patients with node-negative breast cancer measuring ≤1 cm treated with lumpectomy were randomized to tamoxifen alone, RT, or RT and tamoxifen. With a mean follow-up of 87 months, the 8-year rate of ipsilateral LR was 9.3% in the patients treated with RT and 2.8% in the patients treated with RT and tamoxifen.[105] Similar results are seen with adjuvant chemotherapy. In the NSABP B-13 trial, node-negative, ER$^-$ patients were randomized to chemotherapy or to a no-treatment control group. Among the 235 patients treated with CS and RT, the 8-year rate of recurrence in the ipsilateral breast was 13.4% without chemotherapy and only 2.6% with chemotherapy given concurrently with the RT.[106] The net result of the benefit of systemic therapy on local control is that between 1990 and 2011, LRR decreased from 30% to 15% of all recurrences seen in a population of 86,598 women enrolled in 53 randomized phase 3 trials.[107]

The standard approach is to use sequential chemotherapy and RT. Given the primary importance of preventing systemic relapse, it has been the standard to use initial chemotherapy followed by RT. Although concerns have been expressed about an increased rate of LR with this approach, the results of clinical trials in patients with negative margins have not shown this to be a problem even following 6 months of chemotherapy as with four cycles of doxorubicin and cyclophosphamide followed by four cycles of taxol, both given every 3 weeks.[108]

Preservation of a Cosmetically Acceptable Breast

A major goal of BCT is the preservation of a cosmetically acceptable breast. When modern treatment techniques are used, an acceptable cosmetic outcome can be achieved in almost all patients (without compromise of local tumor control) (Fig. 79.3). Treatment-related changes in the breast stabilize at around

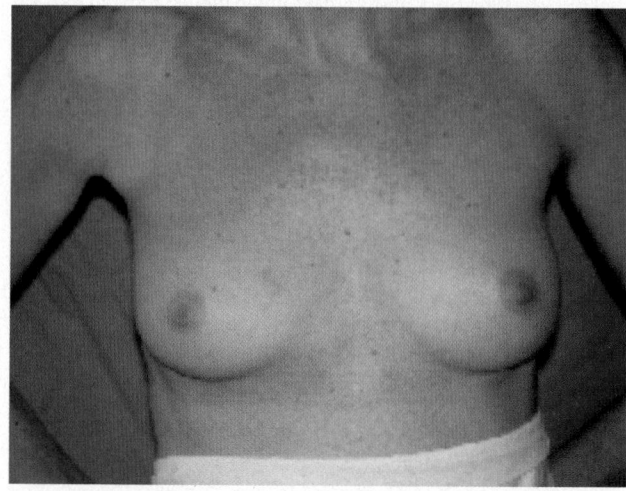

Figure 79.3 Cosmetic outcome of breast-conserving therapy. Other than the surgical scar, there is minimal difference between the treated and the untreated breast.

3 years. Evolution of the untreated breast, such as change in size because of weight gain and the normal ptosis seen with aging, continue to affect the symmetry. The major factor determining the cosmetic result is the extent of surgical resection.[109] A variety of factors must be considered together (the size of the patient's breast, the size of the tumor, the depth of the tumor within the breast, and the quadrant of the breast in which the tumor is located) to judge the feasibility of a cosmetically acceptable resection. For example, although the removal of a large tumor in the lower portion of the breast often results in distortion of the breast contour, this is only apparent with the arms raised and is acceptable to most women. A similar distortion in the upper inner quadrant of the breast, which is visible in most types of clothing, might not be as acceptable.

Guidelines for Patient Selection

Because of the potential options for treatment of early-stage breast cancer, careful patient selection and a multidisciplinary approach are necessary. Critical elements in patient selection for BCT are (1) history and physical examination, (2) mammographic evaluation, (3) histologic assessment of the resected breast specimen, and (4) assessment of the patient's needs and expectations.

Recent (i.e., usually within 3 months) preoperative mammographic evaluation is necessary to determine a patient's eligibility for BCT by defining the extent of a patient's disease, the presence or absence of multicentricity, and other factors that might influence the treatment decision. If the mass is associated with microcalcifications, an assessment of the extent of the calcifications within and outside the mass should be made using magnification views. Mammography of the contralateral breast is also standard at the time of diagnosis to exclude synchronous lesions.

There is controversy regarding the role of additional imaging studies, particularly MRI of the breast, in selecting patients for BCT. A meta-analysis of 3,112 patients in nine studies with comparison cohorts treated with and without MRI found no difference in the need for re-excision or unexpected conversion to mastectomy, after age adjustment, in patients managed with and without MRI.[110] The age-adjusted rate of initial mastectomy was increased three-fold in patients having MRI. Several other studies have shown an association between MRI use and greater, but unwarranted, use of mastectomy.[111,112] MRI frequently identifies additional areas of involvement in the breast, but long-term clinical experience has demonstrated that the majority of this disease is controlled with RT. In addition, MRI has a substantial false-positive rate. Ideally, prospective trials demonstrating a clinical benefit in patients selected for BCT with MRI are needed before these examinations are routinely used for patient selection.

The patient and her physician must discuss the benefits and risks of mastectomy compared with those of BCT in her individual case. The following factors should be discussed:

1. The absence of a long-term survival difference between treatments
2. The possibility and consequences of LR with both approaches
3. Psychological adjustment (including the fear of cancer recurrence), cosmetic outcome, sexual adaptation, and functional competence

Psychological research comparing patient adaptation after mastectomy with that after BCT shows no significant differences in global measures of emotional distress. However, women whose breasts are preserved have more positive attitudes about their body image and experience fewer changes in their frequency of breast stimulation and feelings of sexual desirability. In addition, patients treated with BCT have better physical functioning compared with patients treated with mastectomy at the end of primary treatment.[113]

Absolute and Relative Contraindications to Breast-Conserving Therapy (National Comprehensive Cancer Network 2014)

Contraindications for BCT requiring radiation therapy include the following:
Absolute:

- Radiation therapy during pregnancy
- Diffuse suspicious or malignant-appearing microcalcifications
- Widespread disease that cannot be incorporated by local excision through a single incision that achieves negative margins with a satisfactory cosmetic result
- Positive pathologic margin

Relative:

- Active connective tissue disease involving the skin (especially scleroderma and lupus)
- Tumors >5 cm
- Focally positive margin
- Women with a known or suspected genetic predisposition to breast cancer:
    - May have an increased risk of ipsilateral breast recurrence or contralateral breast cancer with BCT
    - Prophylactic bilateral mastectomy for risk reduction may be considered

Preoperative Systemic Therapy for Operable Cancer

Women who desire BCT but are not candidates for the procedure because of a large tumor relative to the size of the breast should be considered for preoperative or neoadjuvant therapy. This approach does not allow BCT for patients with multicentric carcinoma or those with an EIC that precludes a cosmetic resection. Patients most likely to be converted to BCT with neoadjuvant chemotherapy are those with unicentric, higher-grade, HER2+ or triple-negative cancers, as such cancers often respond dramatically to chemotherapy.

Pathologic complete response (pCR)—defined as the absence of residual invasive cancer in the breast and axilla following preoperative therapy—is a common endpoint for clinical trials of preoperative treatment. Multiple studies have shown that patients who experience pCR with neoadjuvant treatment have, on average, better long-term outcomes, with lower risk of cancer recurrence, than women with residual cancer following neoadjuvant chemotherapy. The US Food and Drug Administration has recently indicated that pCR may be a surrogate for accelerated drug approval in neoadjuvant treatment of operable breast cancer.[114]

Prospective, randomized trials of patients with operable breast cancer have demonstrated that clinical response rates to neoadjuvant chemotherapy are high, ranging from 50% to 85% in many studies. pCRs in the breast range from 15% to 40%. Despite these high response rates, only 25% to 30% of patients who were not candidates for BCT at presentation were able to undergo the procedure after preoperative therapy.[115,116] This is a reflection of both the difficulty of assessing the extent of residual viable tumor after preoperative chemotherapy and the often patchy nature of cancer cell death in response to chemotherapy. This type of response significantly decreases the total number of viable tumor cells, but viable tumor remains scattered throughout the same volume of breast tissue, precluding BCT. MRI is better than mammography or ultrasonography in evaluating the extent of viable tumor and its distribution, but may both underestimate and overestimate the extent of residual disease.

In patients who overexpress HER2, the preoperative administration of anti-HER2 therapy in combination with chemotherapy has been associated with high rates of pCR. Clinical trials have confirmed that adding trastuzumab to chemotherapy improves the pCR rate among women with *HER2*[+] breast cancer receiving neoadjuvant therapy and improves long-term survival,[117] consistent with the survival benefit observed for trastuzumab when given with chemotherapy in the adjuvant setting.

In 2013, the US Food and Drug Administration approved concurrent use of a second anti-*HER2* antibody, pertuzumab, for use in combination with trastuzumab and chemotherapy in women receiving neoadjuvant therapy for *HER2*[+] breast cancer, after it was shown that pertuzumab enhanced the rates of pCR.[118]

A meta-analysis of nine randomized trials of preoperative chemotherapy demonstrated no increase, or decrease, in survival with preoperative compared with postoperative treatment,[119] but an elevated risk of LRR (RR = 1.22; 95% CI = 1.04 to 1.45) was noted. Some of the increase in LR was due to the inclusion of studies in the meta-analysis in which patients who had a clinical complete response did not have surgery. Even in patients undergoing surgery, an elevated risk of LR has been observed. In the NSABP B-18 study,[115] LR rates were 15% in patients who required chemotherapy to undergo BCT compared with only 7% in those who were initially candidates for BCT. The increased rates of LR after neoadjuvant therapy likely reflect that in this setting, a negative margin may still be associated with a clinically significant residual tumor burden that is unlikely to be controlled by RT. Thus, an evaluation of both surgical margins and the extent of viable tumor elsewhere in the specimen is essential and may dictate resection of additional breast tissue even when margins are apparently tumor-free. Among women who have mastectomy after neoadjuvant chemotherapy, a pCR is a favorable prognostic finding, associated with a far lower risk of LRR than seen in women with residual cancer.[120] Percutaneous placement of marker clips within the primary tumor prior to the initiation of chemotherapy will provide a landmark for localization and excision should a clinical and radiographic complete response occur. The lack of a survival benefit for neoadjuvant therapy and the increased complexity in determining the appropriate extent of resection suggest that for women who are candidates for breast conservation at presentation, neoadjuvant therapy outside the context of a clinical trial offers little benefit.

Neoadjuvant endocrine therapy has also been used to increase rates of BCT. In trials of postmenopausal women with ER[+] cancers who were not considered candidates for BCT at presentation, roughly 30% to 40% of those who received 4 months of endocrine therapy were able to undergo BCT.[121,122] These studies indicate that in postmenopausal women with hormone receptor-positive tumors, the preoperative use of an AI or tamoxifen significantly increases the likelihood of breast conservation. However, despite the proven survival benefit seen with adjuvant endocrine therapy, pCR is rare with the short duration of treatment used in the neoadjuvant setting. Patients who experience substantial tumor shrinkage with endocrine therapy, even short of pCR, may also have a more favorable prognosis.[123] For women with ER[+] breast cancer, a small randomized trial has suggested that either endocrine or chemotherapy can be equally effective.[124] In clinical practice, neoadjuvant endocrine therapy is typically reserved for women not considered to be candidates for neoadjuvant chemotherapy.

Conservative Surgery Without Radiation Therapy

An unresolved question is whether RT is necessary in all patients with invasive breast cancer after CS. It is well known that RT after CS reduces LR by about 70%, but there has been uncertainty about whether this improvement in LR is important to survival and whether there is a subgroup of patients with a low risk of LR following CS alone. The impact of improving local control on overall long-term survival was greatly clarified with the findings of the EBCTCG meta-analysis[125] first published in 2005, and updated in 2011.[125] In this updated analysis, 17 trials including

10,801 women, 3,143 deaths, and 9.5 median woman-years at risk were included. Importantly, the EBCTCG moved from assessing the effect of RT on LR to its effect on first failure (or first recurrence, either LR or distant metastasis). (Although commonly employed in studies on the local treatment of breast cancer, actuarial calculation of time to LR is, strictly, not statistically valid.) RT proportionally reduced the annual rate of any failure (LR or distant metastases) over the first 10 years by about half (RR = 0.52) and proportionally reduced the annual rate of breast cancer death by about one-sixth. The absolute benefit of RT was greater in patients with the greater risk of recurrence. In node-negative patients, the absolute benefit was strongly correlated with age (inversely), tumor grade and size, and ER status, with very small absolute benefit seen in some subgroups. The updated EBCTCG analysis still demonstrates that RT after CS is not only important for local control, but also for maximizing long-term survival.

Attempts to identify a subgroup of patients (based on various clinical and histologic features) within the available clinical trials who have a low risk of LR after CS alone have been unsuccessful. LR rates are generally lower in trials that use more extensive surgery than in those using lumpectomy, and in older patients than in younger patients. The Joint Center for Radiation Therapy in Boston conducted a prospective single-arm trial of wide excision alone for patients with a tumor size of ≤2 cm, histologically negative axillary nodes, absence of either lymphatic vessel invasion or an EIC in the cancer, and no cancer cells within 1 cm of inked margins.[126] The median age of patients in this trial was 66 years, 75% of cancers were detected by mammography alone, and the median pathologic size of the cancers was 9 mm. None of the patients received adjuvant endocrine therapy or chemotherapy. This trial was stopped shortly before it reached its accrual goal of 90 patients because of stopping rules ensuring against an excessively high LR rate. With a median follow-up time of 86 months among the 81 eligible patients, the crude rate of LR was 23%. The average LR rate was 2.8% per year. Of note, of the six patients with a tubular cancer, three had an LR. Examination of subsets of patients by age and tumor size did not find any statistically significant differences. Similar results were seen in a small randomized clinical trial from Finland. Based on the results of these prospective studies, it was concluded that even highly selected patients with breast cancer (based on patient and tumor characteristics) have a substantial risk of early LR after treatment with wide excision alone. Newer markers are needed to more reliably identify patients who can be safely treated with wide excision alone.

More recently, there have been five trials that have compared tamoxifen with and without RT after breast-conserving surgery (BCS; largely in ER[+] patients), and their details are shown in Table 79.11.[105,127-130] The LRR rates for these trials are shown in Table 79.12. The 5-year results seem reasonable, but the rate of LR appears increased after 5 years. In the Canadian trial,[128] LR was 7.7% at 5 years, but 17.6% at 8 years. This raises the question of whether tamoxifen is merely delaying LR. As previously discussed,

TABLE 79.11

Trials of Tamoxifen with or without Radiotherapy After Breast-Conserving Therapy

Study[(Ref.)]	No. of Patients: Selection	FU (median mo)
NSABP B-21[105]	1,009: ≤1 cm; pN0	87
Canadian[128]	769: >50, T1,2; pN0	67
Scottish[127]	427: <70, T1,2; pN0	67
CALGB[129]	636: >70, T1; pN0	151
Austrian[130]	869: ≤3 cm, grade 1, 2, pN0	54

FU, follow-up; NSABP, National Surgical Adjuvant Breast and Bowel Project; CALGB, Cancer and Leukemia Group B

TABLE 79.12

Five-Year Rates of Local Recurrence in Tamoxifen with or without Radiotherapy Trials

Study[(Ref.)]	Tamoxifen (%)	Tamoxifen + RT (%)	End Point
NSABP B-21[105]	8.4	1.1	5-yr LR
Canadian[128]	7.7	0.6	5-yr LR
Canadian[128]	13.2	1.1	5-yr L-RR
Scottish[127]	25.0	3.1	5-yr L-RR
CALGB[129]	4	1	10-yr L-RR
Austrian[130]	5.1	0.4	5-yr LR

RT, radiotherapy; NSABP, National Surgical Adjuvant Breast and Bowel Project; LR, local recurrence; L-RR, local-regional recurrence; CALGB, Cancer and Leukemia Group B.

the combination of tamoxifen and RT provides a very low rate of LR. Tamoxifen alone has its greatest appeal in older patients (older than 70 years)[129] where competing risks of other illnesses are substantial. In a prospective randomized trial of 636 patients age 70 and above with stage 1, ER$^+$ breast cancers treated by lumpectomy and randomized to tamoxifen or tamoxifen plus WBI, no differences in OS or rates of breast preservation were observed at 10 years. WBI reduced the incidence of LRR from 10% to 2% in this population.[129] In elderly patients, it is critical for the clinician to assess the patient's particular cancer characteristics (especially tumor grade) as well as her comorbid illnesses and individual value system in determining the advisability of adding RT. (The website ePrognosis.com is useful is estimating life expectancy in older patients.)

Hypofractionated Whole-Breast and Accelerated Partial-Breast Irradiation

There have been a growing number of studies attempting to decrease the overall treatment time for RT after lumpectomy through the administration of fewer, but larger daily doses (hypofractionation) of RT delivered to the whole breast or only to the portion of the breast containing the primary tumor, typically given twice a day (accelerated).

Hypofractionated WBI was studied[131] among women with invasive breast cancer who had undergone BCS and in whom resection margins were clear and axillary lymph nodes were negative. Women were randomly assigned to receive WBI either at a standard dose of 50 Gy in 25 fractions over a period of 35 days (the control group) or at a dose of 42.5 Gy in 16 fractions over a period of 22 days (the hypofractionated-radiation group). The risk of LR at 10 years was 6.7% with standard irradiation as compared to 6.2% in the hypofractionated regimen (95% CI = −2.5 to 3.5). At 10 years, 71.3% of women in the control group compared with 69.8% of the women in the hypofractionated-radiation group had a good or excellent cosmetic outcome. In a subset analysis, conventional fractionation had better results in patients with high-grade cancers. This trial was initiated before the value of a boost was established, and it is not clear how best to give a boost in patients treated with hypofractionated WBI. As noted previously, the value of a boost is very small in patients aged 60 years and greater, so at a minimum, it seems reasonable to treat patients aged 60 and greater with grade 1 or 2 node-negative breast cancer with accelerated WBI without a boost. A task force of the American Society for Radiation Oncology (ASTRO) developed guidelines for the use of hypofractionated WBI in 2011.[132] The task force favored a dose schedule of 42.5 Gy in 16 fractions ("Canadian") and its use in patients aged 50 years or older with pT1-2N0 cancer treated with BCS, and not treated with

adjuvant chemotherapy where the dose homogeneity is within ±7% and the heart can be excluded from direct irradiation. There was no agreement on the use of a boost.

Ten-year results are now available from the similar START-B trial fully corroborating the results of the Canadian trial.[133] In START-B, a regimen of 50 Gy in 25 fractions over 5 weeks was compared with 40 Gy in 15 fractions over 3 weeks. START-B enrolled 2,215 women. A boost dose was allowed in this trial. Median follow-up was 9.9 years, after which 95 LRRs had occurred. The proportion of patients with LRR at 10 years did not differ significantly between the 40 Gy group (4.3%; 95% CI = 3.2 to 5.9) and the 50 Gy group (5.5%; 95% CI = 4.2 to 7.2; HR = 0.77; 95% CI = 0.51 to 1.16; p = 0.21). In START-B, breast shrinkage, telangiectasia, and breast edema were significantly less-common normal tissue effects in the 40 Gy group than in the 50 Gy group. It is anticipated that the use of hypofractionated WBI will increase.

There are several potential benefits for accelerated partial-breast irradiation (APBI), including the following: (1) the quality of life of patients could be improved by relieving patients of the necessity of daily treatments for 5 to 6 weeks, (2) the underutilization of BCT could be reduced by making it more feasible for patients to receive RT, (3) the integration of local and systemic therapies could be simplified, and (4) long-term complications of RT could be decreased by limiting the volume of critical structures irradiated to high dose. The rationale for APBI is based on studies of the patterns of recurrence after standard whole-breast RT and after excision alone that demonstrate that the large majority of recurrences are in the immediate vicinity of the tumor bed.[134] In addition, pathologic studies on the distribution of tumor cells in relation to the primary tumor demonstrate in most cases that the vast majority of tumor cells in the breast are found near the primary tumor.

These are a number of different APBI techniques, including interstitial brachytherapy, (three-dimensional conformal) external-beam irradiation, intracavitary brachytherapy, and intraoperative limited RT. At present, there are few long-term data, especially from randomized clinical trials, for APBI, and appropriate patient selection remains controversial. Successful application of this approach requires technical expertise. Two cooperative group studies—the recently completed NSABP/RTOG phase 3 trial comparing conventional RT versus APBI (allowing implant or external-beam techniques) and the National Cancer Institute of Canada RAPID study, which permitted external beam technique—will answer important questions about APBI. To provide some direction during this time of uncertainty, an ASTRO expert panel has defined a "suitable" group, for whom APBI outside a clinical trial was acceptable, as being patients[135] meeting all of the following criteria: age 60 years or greater, BRCA1/2 mutation not present, unicentric invasive ductal carcinoma measuring ≤2 cm, margins negative by at least 2 mm, without lymphatic vessel invasion or an EIC, ERs present, and node-negative on pathologic examination. The panel also identified "cautionary" and "unsuitable" groups.

The most widely used form of APBI is with external beam irradiation. There is controversy whether cosmetic results are compromised relative to conventional whole breast external beam treatment. An interim cosmetic and toxicity analysis from the RAPID trial was published in 2013.[136] Between 2006 and 2011, 2,135 women had been randomly assigned to APBI or WBI. Median follow-up was 36 months. Adverse cosmesis at 3 years was increased among those treated with APBI compared with WBI as assessed by trained nurses (29% versus 17%; p <0.001), by patients (26% versus 18%; p = 0.0022), and by physicians reviewing digital photographs (35% versus 17%; p <0.001). Grade 3 toxicities were rare in both treatment arms (1.4% versus 0%), but grade 1 and 2 toxicities were increased among those who received APBI compared with WBI (p <0.001). The authors concluded that external beam APBI increased rates of adverse cosmesis and late radiation toxicity compared with standard WBI.

The first results of a trial from the European Institute of Oncology in Milan testing APBI using intraoperative radiation with electron beam versus conventional whole-breast radiation were published in 2013. A total of 1,305 patients were randomized, and after a median follow-up of 5.8 years, the 5-year rate of LR (IBTR) was 4.4% in the APBI arm and only 0.4% in the conventional whole breast arm (HR = 9.3; 95% CI = 3.3 to 26.3). OS did not differ.[137]

Toxicities of Breast Radiotherapy

Breast RT is generally very well tolerated with very few long-term toxicities. Evidence has long been accumulating that RT involving the heart can result in premature ischemic heart disease, but interest peaked in 2013 when a case-control study found an increased risk for cardiac-related deaths in patients with breast cancer who received RT.[138] This was a population-based case-control study involving 2,168 Scandinavian women treated between 1958 and 2001. It found that rates of major coronary events increased linearly with the mean dose to the heart by 7.4% per Gy (p <0.001), with no apparent threshold. The increase started within the first 5 years after RT and continued into the third decade after RT. The proportional increase in the rate of major coronary events per Gy was similar in women with and without cardiac risk factors at the time of RT, but the absolute increase was greater in patients with cardiac risk factors. The overall average of the mean doses to the whole heart in this study was 4.9 Gy.

It is important to note the major limitations of the study; mainly, it is a case-control study and as such, it does not provide the highest level of evidence. Also, there were limitations in design. The investigators developed virtual simulations of RT dose based on CT scans of patients with "typical anatomy," which they used to construct idealized radiation fields and with which they estimated the doses to the heart.

It is also important to emphasize that despite the proportional relationship between RT dose to the heart and heart disease, the *absolute* increase was very small. For 50-year-old women without cardiac risk factors, the lifetime increased risk was 0.5% after 0.5 Gy, 0.2% after 1 Gy, and just 0.5% after 3 Gy delivered as a mean heart dose. Today, for most node-negative women having BCT, the mean heart dose is only about 1 Gy, although higher doses (still only about 2 Gy) are more common for women with left-sided postmastectomy RT.

It should also be noted that any cardiac mortality risk in current practice is small compared to the survival benefit from RT both in the setting of BCT and PMRT. The survival benefit seen for RT in these older trials includes the deleterious effects on the heart seen with doses as high as 10 Gy. This means that using current techniques that spare the heart, RT will provide even greater survival benefit. The issue of cardiac irradiation, however, has more importance in patients with DCIS, where the survival impact of RT is small at best.

Notwithstanding these study limitations and improvements in technique, radiation oncologists should operate on the principle that there is no totally safe radiation dose to the heart, and that the heart dose should be kept as low as possible. A number of maneuvers, such as using cardiac blocks, prone techniques, and deep inspiration breath holds, make radiation delivery much safer in current practice.

Mastectomy

Mastectomy, with or without immediate breast reconstruction, is the surgical approach for the patient with breast cancer who has contraindications to BCT or who prefers treatment with mastectomy. The mastectomy used today is a total or complete mastectomy, with removal of the breast tissue from the clavicle to the rectus abdominous and between the sternal edge and the latissimus dorsi muscles. A total mastectomy also removes the nipple-areolar complex (NAC), the excess skin of the breast, and the fascia of the pectoralis major muscle. When accompanied by an ALND, the procedure is termed a *modified radical mastectomy*. Mastectomy is an extremely safe operation. The 30-day mortality is approximately 0.25%, and the 30-day incidence of major complications is about 5%, the majority of which are related to wound healing. In contemporary American practice, roughly 30% of women underwent mastectomy for breast cancer owing to either contraindications to BCT or patient choice.[90]

Advances in plastic surgical technique have made immediate reconstruction an option for most patients who undergo mastectomy. There have been no prospective trials comparing mastectomy alone with mastectomy with immediate reconstruction, but the available retrospective data do not support concerns about the incidence or detection of LR in the reconstructed patient. The majority of postmastectomy recurrences occur in the skin or subcutaneous fat of the chest wall and present as palpable masses in the skin flap, so detection is not affected by the presence of the reconstruction.[139] Skin-sparing mastectomy in which skin excision is limited to the NAC and the excisional biopsy scar (if present) is now routinely used to preserve the skin envelope of the breast and facilitate reconstruction. The reported rates of LR after skin-sparing mastectomy are comparable to those of patients treated with conventional mastectomy. This finding is consistent with prior observations that the extent of skin removal in patients treated with mastectomy alone is not a major determinant of the risk of chest wall recurrence. Traditionally, skin-sparing mastectomy has included resection of the NAC due to the need to leave breast tissue on the NAC to provide a blood supply and the risk of leaving behind malignancy within the ducts of the nipple. Nipple sparing mastectomy (NSM) preserves the NAC and is being used with increasing frequency due to the excellent cosmetic results that can be obtained with this technique. Intraoperative frozen section of the tissue beneath the nipple is often used to minimize the risk of residual cancer. To date, most studies of this procedure have consisted of highly selected patients who had relatively short follow-up periods, making the long-term safety of NSM, particularly in high-risk women such as those with *BRCA* mutations, difficult to ascertain. The reported incidence of occult involvement of the NAC in patients with known breast cancer ranges from 0% to 58%.[140] Despite this, a review of 10 studies including 1,148 NSMs reported a 2.8% rate of LRR after a median follow-up of only 2 years.[141] In a large series from the European Institute of Oncology, including 772 patients with invasive cancer, and 162 with DCIS treated with NSM and intraoperative RT to the NAC, at a median follow-up of 50 months, the 5-year rate of LR was 4.4% in the invasive cancer group and 7.8% in patients with DCIS.[142] The majority of recurrences were at a distance from the NAC, suggesting that the more difficult exposure with this operation may result in retained breast tissue on the skin flaps. These studies indicate that NSM may be a viable option in highly selected women, specifically, patients with small, peripherally located, node-negative tumors with favorable histologic features. Most women in this category, however, are candidates for conventional BCT. The eligible population for NSM is further limited by the requirement that the nipple be in the appropriate position on the reconstructed breast. This is rarely the case for women with large, ptotic breasts, further limiting the application of this procedure.

In summary, immediate reconstruction with preservation of the skin envelope of the breast has not been shown to alter the outcome of mastectomy or to delay the administration of systemic therapy. Immediate reconstruction has the advantages of avoiding the need for a second major operative procedure and the psychological morbidity of the loss of the breast. The two major reconstructive techniques involve the use of implants and/or tissue expanders or the use of myocutaneous tissue flaps to create a new breast mound. The advantages and disadvantages

TABLE 79.13

Common Reproductive Options After Mastectomy

Type	Advantages	Disadvantages
Implant	One-stage procedure, minimal prolongation, hospitalization, or recovery Low cost	Poor symmetry if skin removed or in large ptotic breasts Capsular contracture, leakage, rupture possible
Tissue expander	Short operative time Hospitalization, recovery not prolonged Low cost	Multiple physician visits postoperatively Poor symmetry large or ptotic breasts Capsular contracture, leakage rupture possible
Latissimus dorsi flap	Very low risk of flap loss Natural contour with autogenous tissue	Donor site scar Usually requires an implant Moderate prolongation hospitalization and recovery
TRAM flap	Natural contour Good match for large or ptotic breasts Abdominoplasty	Donor site scar Fat necrosis, flap loss possible Abdominal wall weakness plus hernia Significant prolongation hospitalization plus recovery
DIEP flap	Natural contour Muscle-sparing Abdominoplasty	Donor site scar Need for microsurgeon Flap loss possible Moderate prolongation hospitalization plus recovery
Superior gluteal artery perforator flap	Natural contour Alternative donor site	Donor site scar Need for microsurgeon Flap loss possible Moderate prolongation hospitalization plus recovery

TRAM, transverse rectus abdominous myocutaneous; DIEP, deep inferior epigastric perforator.

of the techniques are summarized in Table 79.13. Implant reconstructions are best suited for women with small- to moderate-sized breasts with minimal ptosis, while flap reconstructions allow more flexibility in the size and shape of the reconstructed breast (Fig. 79.4). In the past, most breast implants were filled with silicone gel. However, after reports from uncontrolled studies suggested an increased incidence of connective tissue disease in women with silicone implants, the US Food and Drug Administration declared a moratorium on their use. Since that time, several epidemiologic studies have failed to demonstrate an increased incidence of connective tissue disorders in women with implants compared with matched control populations. Silicone implants are again available for use in patients with breast cancer, but many patients opt for saline implants or flap reconstructions as a result of the adverse publicity surrounding silicone implants.

Reconstructive choices may be influenced by the possible need for postmastectomy RT. As indications for postmastectomy RT have expanded, the impact of RT on reconstruction has also become an issue. Immediate reconstruction can negatively impact the technical delivery of RT, possibly resulting in greater irradiation of the heart (in left-sided cancers) and lung, and undercoverage of the chest wall.[143] There are a variety of strategies that have been proposed for selecting the type of reconstruction for a patient with a significant likelihood of requiring postmastectomy RT. There is considerable variability in outcome reported in the medical literature for the same approaches, and there are no prospective studies reported to date. The use of RT in patients who have been reconstructed with implants is associated with a higher risk of encapsulation and implant loss than in nonirradiated patients. In one study, however, Cordeiro et al.[144] reported that after a mean follow-up of 34 months in 68 patients reconstructed with tissue expanders or implants who received RT, 80% had good to excellent aesthetic results and 72% would have chosen the same form of reconstruction again. The figures for nonirradiated patients were 88% ($p =$ not significant) and 85%, respectively. Implant loss occurred in 11% of patients with irradiated implants and 6% of nonirradiated pa-

tients. The finding that the majority of patients who require RT after implant reconstruction have good cosmesis and are satisfied with their reconstruction choice has led some to advocate insertion of an expander at the time of mastectomy, which is inflated during chemotherapy and exchanged for a permanent implant prior to RT. In patients who are satisfied with the cosmetic outcome

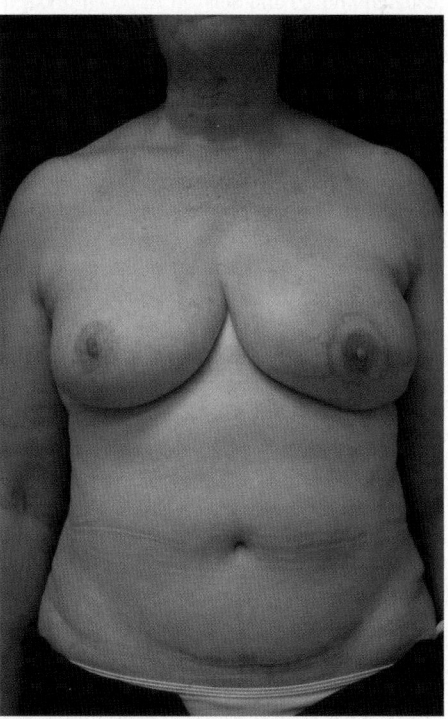

Figure 79.4 Cosmetic outcome of transverse rectus abdominis muscle flap reconstruction after skin-sparing mastectomy.

after RT, no further surgery is required. In patients with significant cosmetic deformity, a secondary flap reconstruction is performed. This approach has the advantage of allowing preservation of the breast skin and providing the patient with a breast mound during what may be a prolonged course of postoperative cancer therapy. However, additional favorable experience with irradiation of expanders or implants at other institutions is needed.

A primary flap reconstruction is another alternative for the patient who may require postmastectomy RT. Variable outcomes have been reported for patients who receive RT after transverse rectus myocutaneous flap or latissimus dorsi flap reconstruction. Complete flap loss is rare, but fat necrosis, fibrosis, and volume loss can occur. As in the native breast, the full cosmetic impact may not be evident until 3 years posttreatment. In one study, the 5-year incidence of major complications after transverse rectus myocutaneous reconstruction was 0% ($n = 35$) and 5% after tissue expander/implant ($n = 50$) reconstruction followed by RT.[145] In contrast, 4 of 47 (9%) patients reconstructed with flaps and 6 of 15 (40%) implant patients underwent major corrective surgery a median of 8 months after RT in another series.[146] An alternative approach is to perform sentinel node biopsy prior to mastectomy to identify patients with nodal involvement at highest risk for requiring postmastectomy RT and delay reconstruction in this subset of women until after the completion of oncologic therapy. This is an area that continues to evolve, and multidisciplinary consultation between the oncologic surgeon, reconstructive surgeon, and radiation oncologist will help to ensure optimal patient outcomes.

MANAGEMENT OF THE AXILLA

For many years, standard management of the axilla for patients with invasive breast carcinoma consisted of a complete ALND. Initially, this was thought to be a critical component of the surgical cure of breast cancer. This changed when studies such as the NSABP B-04 trial, in which clinically node-negative patients were randomized to radical mastectomy, total mastectomy with RT to the regional lymphatics, or total mastectomy with observation of the axillary nodes and delayed ALND if nodal metastases developed, showed no survival benefit for the axillary surgery.[147] ALND came to be regarded as a staging procedure that provided prognostic information and maintained local control in the axilla. However, the observation that 25% to 30% of long-term survivors treated with radical mastectomy alone had positive nodes,[148] coupled with the decreased survival observed after inadequate axillary treatment in the Guys Hospital trial,[149] suggested that ALND was therapeutic for some patients with axillary nodal metastases.

Lymphatic mapping and sentinel node biopsy has replaced ALND as the staging procedure of choice in clinically node-negative women. A sentinel node can be identified in 97% of women.[150,151] In the American College of Surgeons Oncology Group (ACOSOG) Z10 trial, participating surgeons chose the method of lymphatic mapping, and no significant differences were seen in the rate of sentinel node identification with the use of blue dye alone, radiocolloid alone, or the combination of the two.[150] Increasing body mass index, increasing age, and <50 patients accrued to the trial were all associated with a significant decrease in sentinel node identification rate, but a sentinel node was successfully identified in >95% of patients in all groups. Complications of sentinel node biopsy are infrequent, with anaphylaxis to lymphazurin blue dye observed in 0.1% of patients in the ACOSOG Z10 trial[152] and axillary paresthesias 6 months postoperatively in 8.6%. Lymphedema can occur after sentinel node biopsy, but at a much lower rate than after ALND. In the randomized Axillary Lymphatic Mapping Against Nodal Axillary Clearance trial, the absolute incidence of lymphedema in the sentinel node biopsy group was 5% at 12 months, with an RR of 0.37 (95% CI = 0.23 to

0.60) compared with the axillary clearance group in an intention-to-treat analysis.[153]

The majority of patients with stage I and II cancer are candidates for sentinel node biopsy. Contraindications to the procedure include pregnancy, lactation, and locally advanced breast cancer (LABC). Care should be taken to excise any palpably abnormal nodes intraoperatively because lymph nodes that contain a heavy tumor burden may not take up the mapping agent. In the patient with clinically positive nodes, confirmation of metastases preoperatively with needle biopsy allows an immediate ALND. Caution should be used in proceeding directly to dissection without pathologic confirmation because the false-positive rate of physical examination is approximately 20%. Multicentric cancers and T3 primary tumors were initially thought to be contraindications to lymphatic mapping, but studies have shown that sentinel node biopsy is accurate in these circumstances.[154] Early in the experience with sentinel node biopsy, the false-negative rates of approximately 10%, determined by completing an ALND after the sentinel node(s) were removed, were a source of concern. However, three randomized studies directly comparing the identification of axillary metastases with ALND and sentinel node biopsy found no difference in the likelihood of identifying nodal disease.[151,153,155] Follow-up studies of patients treated by sentinel node biopsy alone demonstrate that the rate of LR in the axilla is extremely low if the sentinel node does not contain metastases, despite the 10% false-negative rate. In one study with a median follow-up of 31 months, isolated axillary first failure was seen in only 3 of 4,008 patients (0.07%) who had a sentinel node biopsy.[156]

In clinically node-negative patients receiving neoadjuvant chemotherapy, sentinel node biopsy after chemotherapy offers the patient the potential benefit of axillary downstaging and avoidance of ALND. A meta-analysis of 27 studies involving 2,148 patients undergoing sentinel node biopsy after chemotherapy reported a sentinel node identification rate of 90.5% (95% CI = 88% to 92%) and a false-negative rate of 10.5% (8% to 14%), comparable to what is seen in the primary surgical setting,[157] and in the NSABP B18 trial,[158] the rate of nodal positivity was reduced from 57 to 41% with neoadjuvant chemotherapy ($p < 0.001$). The accuracy of sentinel node biopsy in patients with clinically evident axillary nodal metastases at presentation who receive neoadjuvant therapy with resolution of clinically apparent adenopathy has been addressed in two multi-institutional prospective studies, as summarized in Table 79.14.[159,160] These studies demonstrate false-negative rates <10% only when three or more sentinel nodes are identified, a circumstance present in only 28% of patients in the German multi-institutional Sentinel Neoadjuvant trial.[160] These findings suggest that ALND should remain the standard approach for patients presenting with clinically evident nodal involvement unless three or more sentinel nodes are identified. Ongoing trials are examining whether nodal irradiation could replace ALND in this setting.

TABLE 79.14

Accuracy of Sentinel Node Biopsy After Neoadjuvant Chemotherapy in Patients with Lymph Node Involvement at Presentation

# of Sentinel Nodes Removed	% False-Negative Rate	
	ACOSOG Z1071	SENTINA
1	32	24
2	21	19
≥3	9	7

ACOSOG, American College of Surgeons Oncology Group; SENTINA, German multi-institutional Sentinel Neoadjuvant.

The ability to perform a more detailed examination of the sentinel node has significantly increased the identification of small tumor deposits in the axillary nodes. The presence of isolated tumor cells (<0.2 mm deposits) and micrometastases (>0.2 mm, <2.0 mm) was initially thought to identify patients at increased risk for distant metastases. However, prospective trials in the modern era, including systemic therapy, have failed to identify an OS difference associated with micrometastases.[161,162] A prospective randomized trial addressing the need for completion ALND in patients with sentinel node micrometastases[163] found no significant difference in local, regional, or distant recurrence rates among patients with sentinel node micrometastases treated with sentinel node biopsy alone versus completion ALND, despite the finding of additional nodal metastases in 13% of the ALND group. Based on these findings, the routine use of serial sections and IHC to detect micrometastases is not warranted.

ALND has been the standard approach to patients with axillary nodal metastases. Studies comparing sentinel node biopsy with ALND have provided important information on the morbidity of the procedure. In the Axillary Lymphatic Mapping Against Nodal Axillary Clearance trial, moderate to severe lymphedema was reported by 13% of patients 12 months after ALND as well as sensory loss in 31%.[155] Decreases in shoulder flexion and abduction were present 1 month after surgery but resolved rapidly after that time. ALND provides excellent long-term local control, with only 1.4% of patients treated by radical mastectomy in the NSABP B-04 trial[147] having an isolated axillary recurrence at 10-year follow-up. The use of axillary irradiation as an alternative to ALND was studied in the presentinel node era in a randomized trial in clinically node-negative patients performed at the Institute Curie. After 15 years of follow-up, the axillary failure rate was 3% in the radiated group and 1% in the surgical group ($p = 0.03$),[164] indicating that this is an acceptable alternative in patients with contraindications to axillary surgery or those who refuse the procedure. The recognition that patients in the modern era who are eligible for BCT often have smaller cancers with lower nodal disease burdens, coupled with the recognition that systemic therapy significantly reduces LR,[165] led to the ACOSOG Z0011 trial, a prospective randomized study to address the need for ALND in clinically node-negative women found to have macrometastases in less than three sentinel nodes. The study was designed to identify a 5% difference in survival between patients undergoing a completion ALND and those treated with sentinel node biopsy alone. It closed prematurely because of a low event rate, but 891 patients were randomized. After a median follow-up of 6.2 years, the 5-year nodal recurrence rate was 0.5% in the dissection arm and 0.9% in the sentinel node biopsy alone arm ($p = 0.11$). No difference in 5-year DFS or OS was seen between groups, and no evidence of a trend toward a survival benefit for dissection, which might have been evident with a larger sample size, was observed. Morbidity, including wound infection, paresthesia, and patient-reported lymphedema, was significantly lower in the sentinel node group. All patients in this study were treated with BCT, 97% received some type of systemic therapy, and irradiation of an axillary field was not permitted, but it is likely that the low rate of axillary failure in the sentinel node biopsy alone group is at least in part related to irradiation of the low axilla with the breast tangents.[166] These findings do not apply to women with clinically positive nodes or extensive nodal involvement, or those undergoing partial breast irradiation or treatment with mastectomy. Investigators from Memorial Sloan-Kettering Cancer Center applied the ACOSOG Z0011 eligibility criteria to a consecutive series of 287 women, and ALND was avoided in 84%.[167] Patient age, hormone receptor status, and *HER2* status did not differ between patients requiring ALND and those who did not.

The After Mapping of the Axilla: Radiotherapy or Surgery trial examined alternative management approaches for the patient with a positive sentinel node, in this case, irradiation of the axillary and supraclavicular fields instead of dissection.[168] At

	ACOSOG Z0011	AMAROS	MA.20
No. of patients	891	1425	1832
Surgery	BCS	BCS, Mastectomy	BCS
Control arm	ALND	ALND	ALND
Experimental arm	SN Only	SN, RT Axilla and SC nodes	ALND, RT SC, IM nodes, axillary apex
Significant survival differences			
DFS	No	No	Yes
OS	No	No	No

TABLE 79.15

Recent Trials of Axillary Management

ACOSOG, American College of Surgeons Oncology Group; AMAROS, After Mapping of the Axilla: Radiotherapy or Surgery; MA, National Cancer Institute of Canada MA; BCS, breast-conserving surgery; ALND, axillary lymph node dissection; SN, sentinel node; RT, radiotherapy; SC, supraclavicular; IM, internal mammary; DFS, disease-free survival; OS, overall survival.

5 years, axillary recurrence was seen in 0.54% of patients undergoing ALND and 1.03% of those having RT, without significant differences in 5-year DFS. There was a lower risk of lymphedema among women treated with axillary RT instead of surgery (14% versus 28%, $p < 0.0001$). This study indicates that RT is an alternative to dissection, but does not prove that all patients with metastases to one or two sentinel nodes require nodal irradiation as similar rates of local control were observed in ACOSOG Z0011 after sentinel node biopsy alone. In marked contrast to these two studies are the results of the MA.20 trial, a study randomizing patients with T1 and T2 tumors undergoing WBI to ALND or ALND plus nodal RT. The majority of patients included in the study (85%) had involvement of one to three axillary nodes. The 5-year LR-free survival was improved from 94.5% to 96.8% ($p = 0.02$) with the addition of nodal RT, the distant DFS was improved from 87% to 92.4% ($p = 0.002$), and OS from 90.7% to 92.3% ($p = 0.07$).[169] These trials are summarized in Table 79.15. At present, the optimal approach to the patient with positive sentinel nodes treated with BCS and whole-breast RT is a matter of debate, but ALND should no longer be considered the standard approach for all patients. Future research to clarify which subsets of patients are best managed with sentinel node biopsy alone versus sentinel node biopsy and axillary RT, and which high-risk groups require dissection and nodal RT, is needed.

POSTMASTECTOMY RADIATION THERAPY

The use of postmastectomy radiation therapy (PMRT) is in evolution based on emerging data from clinical trials. The 2005 publication from the EBCTCG suggested a 4:1 ratio between reduction in LRR at 5 years and improved mortality at 15 years with RT both after BCS and after mastectomy, and confirmed that LRR was reduced by 70% with RT after either BCS or mastectomy.[88] This established LRR as a convenient intermediate endpoint for the survival benefit of PMRT.

ASTRO[170] and ASCO[171] have endorsed the routine use of PMRT in women with four or more involved nodes and node-positive women with tumors >5 cm, who have a high (>20% to 25%) risk of LRR without RT. There is uncertain benefit of PMRT in patients with T1/T2 primaries and one to three positive nodes (stage II) in whom the risk of LRR is intermediate (around 10% to 20%). Current NCCN guidelines give a category 1

PRACTICE OF ONCOLOGY

TABLE 79.16

Five-Year Local-Regional Recurrence Rates and Fifteen-Year Breast Cancer Mortality Rates in the Three Groups for Patients Randomly Assigned to Postmastectomy Radiation Therapy or Not

Prognostic Group	Five-Year LRR No RT	Five-Year LRR RT	Fifteen-Year Breast Cancer Mortality – No RT	Fifteen-Year Breast Cancer Mortality – RT
Good	11%	0%	33%	22%
Intermediate	26%	5%	61%	50%
Poor	50%	14%	81%	81%

LRR, local-regional recurrence; RT, radiotherapy.

recommendation for PMRT for patients with four or more positive nodes and a category 2A recommendation for PMRT for patients with one to three positive nodes.

However, in more recent analyses, the EBCTCG has focused on first recurrence of any type (LRR or distant) rather than LRR as a first event.[125] This difference was partly because it is now clear that RT after BCT or mastectomy reduces breast cancer death, so it must also reduce distant recurrence. In addition, it is because women with a higher risk of LRR also have a higher risk of distant recurrence (i.e., the probabilities of LRR and of distant recurrence are not statistically independent), so valid estimates of the separate effects of RT on LRR and distant recurrence cannot be obtained.[172] As a practical matter, this means that LRR is not an intermediate endpoint for the survival benefit of RT and that the survival benefit can only be learned in long-term follow-up of clinical trials testing RT.

This interplay between LRR and distant recurrence and its effect on survival was illustrated in a post hoc analysis of the Danish PMRT trials.[173] Patients were assigned to one of three prognostic groups based on number of positive axillary nodes, tumor size, histologic grade, and receptor status. The 5-year LRR rates and the 15-year breast cancer mortality rates were analyzed in the three groups for patients randomly assigned to PMRT or not (Table 79.16). It is noteworthy that the "poor" group had the biggest absolute reduction in LRR with RT (36%), but had no improvement in 15-year breast cancer mortality. In contrast, the "good" group had the smallest absolute reduction in LRR with RT (11%), but the biggest absolute reduction in 15-year breast cancer mortality (11%). The EBCTCG data on trials of PMRT was updated in 2007.[174] Although the data are still preliminary, they demonstrate that the benefit of PMRT was greater in the patients with one to three positive nodes than in patients with four or more positive nodes. In the subgroup of patients with one to three positive lymph nodes, the 15-year gain in breast cancer mortality was 10.2% (51.3 versus 41.1%, $2p$ <0.0001), and the 15-year gain in all-cause mortality was 7.3% (57.2% versus 49.9%, $2p$ = 0.004) with PMRT. The reduction in the rate of any first recurrence in the one to three positive node group at 10 years was 13.5% ($2p$ <0.0001). In contrast, the reduction in the rate of any first recurrence in the four or more positive node group at 10 years was 11.5% ($2p$ <0.0001). Thus, these and other data demonstrated that reduction in LRR is not a valid intermediate endpoint for the benefit in long-term survival and that the biggest benefit for PMRT might be in intermediate-risk, not high-risk, patients.

A critically important but unresolved issue is whether the use of effective adjuvant systemic therapy makes PMRT more or less useful. It is clear that effective adjuvant systemic therapy reduces the risk of LRR, but if this is no longer an important endpoint, then this does not provide a justification for less PMRT. We and others have argued that it is in context of effective systemic therapy that eradicates micrometastatic disease that improved local therapy might be most beneficial.[175]

A number of preliminary findings support the use of regional RT in intermediate-risk patients. The MA.20 trial[169] randomized high-risk node-negative or node-positive patients to WBI alone or WBI plus regional RT including internal mammary node and medial supraclavicular (IM-MS) fields after BCS. Most patients had one to three positive nodes. With a median follow-up of 62 months, the addition of IM-MS RT improved LR DFS (LR DFS, 96.8% versus 94.8%), distant DFS (distant DFS, 92.4% versus 87%; p = 0.002), and overall DFS (DFS, 89.7% versus 84.0%), and had a borderline effect on OS (91.9% versus 89.5%). The HR reduction with RT for DFS was 0.67 (p = 0.003) and the HR reduction with RT for survival was 0.76 (p = 0.07).

The EORTC randomized patients to WBI plus IM-MS RT versus WBI alone.[176] The patients in this trial were more heterogeneous than in the Canadian trial: 76% had BCT and 24% had mastectomy, and 44% were pN0, 43% were pN1, and 10% were pN2. With a median follow-up of 10.9 years, IM-MS RT improved DFS and distant DFS, and had a borderline effect on OS, the primary endpoint; but the magnitude of benefit in this larger study with longer follow-up was less than that seen in the MA.20 trial. The HR reduction with RT for DFS was 0.89 (p = 0.04) and the HR reduction with RT for survival was 0.87 (p = 0.056).

It will be important to examine the data in published manuscripts, but the evolving evidence suggests that a serious discussion of PMRT is warranted in the majority of women with intermediate-risk breast cancer treated with mastectomy, including those with one to three positive lymph nodes. There are a number of points about PMRT worth stressing. One is that, similar to the previous discussion on BCT, minimizing cardiac irradiation is critical but can be more difficult in PMRT, because unlike in BCT, the target volume includes the whole chest wall. The use of the deep inspiration breath hold technique is encouraged for left-sided patients. The other point relates to the multidisciplinary collaboration needed when reconstruction, particularly immediate reconstruction, is planned.

PROGNOSTIC AND PREDICTIVE FACTORS IN BREAST CANCER

The AJCC staging system reviewed elsewhere in this chapter[79] is based on established clinical and pathologic prognostic factors, and stage—particularly the *extent of axillary lymph node involvement* by breast cancer—is the most established and reliable prognostic factor for subsequent metastatic disease and survival. Tumor size and histologic grading also have established prognostic significance. *Tumor size* is typically given as the microscopic size of the invasive cancer. *Histologic grade* is best determined by an established methodology, such as the Nottingham combined histologic grading system. However, persistent challenges in interpretation of grade either under the microscope or in genomic assays, especially intermediate grade, tend to diminish some of its prognostic impact.[177]

Estrogen and progesterone receptor expression are important and useful predictive factors. Patients with invasive breast cancer whose tumors are totally lacking in ER and PR do not derive benefit from hormonal treatment. Assays for ER and PR are performed using IHC techniques. Laboratories need to adhere to well-described techniques to ensure accurate determination of ER and PR as a centerpiece for quality care in breast cancer.[178] Using tumor size and grade, ER status, and the number of involved axillary nodes, online services such as Adjuvant Online (www.adjuvantonline.com) can give accurate estimates of recurrence risk and treatment benefit.[179]

Patient age has also consistently been shown to be a prognostic factor. Very young breast cancer patients (≤35 years) have a poorer prognosis than older patients. The cancers in these patients tend to be higher grade, less often ER/PR+, and more likely to have lymphovascular invasion than cancers in older patients—differences that likely explain much of the worse outcomes in very young patients.[180,181] A retrospective review of patients in clinical trials examining prognosis based on age, ER, PR, and HER2 status found that patients <35 years of age with ER/PR+, HER2− tumors had no different risk of local or distant relapse than their older counterparts, but differences in LRR and survival persisted among other subgroups.[182]

Approximately 20% of patients with breast cancer have *HER2/neu gene amplification*, which results in glycoprotein overexpression. Approximately 5% of patients have overexpression without gene amplification, but otherwise, gene amplification and expression are highly correlated. HER2 amplification or overexpression has been associated with higher tumor grade, lower expression or lack of hormone receptors, higher levels of tumor proliferation, heavier nodal tumor burden, and poorer prognosis. HER2 status is the major predictive factor for benefit from anti-HER2 targeted therapies, which is discussed later in this chapter. There is some evidence that suggests that HER2 status is predictive for benefit from anthracycline-based chemotherapy, although this relationship is not certain, particularly with the availability of trastuzumab.[183] Measurements of HER2 can be performed by either IHC or fluorescent in situ hybridization. Similar to ER, laboratories need to adhere to well-described techniques to ensure accurate determination of HER2. In clinical practice, tumors that are considered HER2 3+ by IHC, or show evidence of HER2 gene amplification with ratios ≥2, warrant treatment with anti-HER2 therapies.[184]

Involvement of lymphovascular spaces is associated with a greater likelihood of lymph node metastases and is an independent adverse prognostic factor in both node-negative and node-positive patients. Rigid pathologic criteria are required for this factor to be reliable.

Other Factors

Numerous other prognostic and predictive factors have been evaluated, but have not been widely adopted in routine clinical use in the United States and include (1) markers of *proliferation*, such as S-phase fraction, the percentage of cells labeling with thymidine or bromodeoxyuridine or cellular expression of Ki-67 or MIB-1 (which measure the percentage of cells in the G_1 phase of the cell cycle), and mitotic index; (2) measures of the *plasminogen activator system*, such as the concentrations of urokinase plasminogen activator and its inhibitor, plasminogen activator inhibitor-1; and (3) the detection of *occult micrometastases* in the bone marrow using IHC techniques.[185] Sources are available for a more detailed discussion of these and other factors.[186]

Molecular and Genomic Factors

Breast cancer is a heterogeneous disease, and it has long been appreciated that tumors with different biologic features have different clinical outcomes and responses to therapy. At present,

prognosis and treatment selection in breast cancer are based on characterization of tumor growth factor receptor status—ER, PR, and HER2. These markers can be used to define four functional groups of tumors: hormone receptor-positive, HER2−, hormone receptor-negative, HER2− ("triple-negative" tumors), and HER2-overexpressing tumors with or without hormone receptor expression.

Recent advances in molecular biology have resulted in further refinement of these breast cancer subsets. Sorlie et al.[187] and Perou et al.[188] were able to classify breast cancers into tumor subtypes that had different prognoses using complementary DNA microarrays. These studies used hierarchical clustering analysis to identify tumor subtypes with distinct gene expression patterns. The differences in gene expression patterns among these subtypes reflect basic differences in the cell biology of the tumors and are manifest in differences in clinical outcome; clinicians are increasingly viewing these molecular subtypes as separable diseases. The subtypes are luminal A, luminal B, HER2/neu, and basal-like (or basaloid, or triple-negative). The subtypes are commonly approximated using routine tumor markers, such as luminal A: ER and/or PR+/HER2−; luminal B: ER and/or PR+/HER2+; HER2+: ER−/PR−/HER2+; and basal-like ER−/PR−/HER2− and/or CK5/6+ and/or epidermal growth factor-positive. Differences in gene expression pattern affecting hundreds of genes are found between the various subgroups; these differences appear to persist through the natural life history of the breast cancer,[189] and neoadjuvant treatment of breast tumors appears to have little bearing on the gene expression patterns that contribute to the intrinsic tumor subtype.[188,190] Subgroup affects both the likelihood and timing of cancer recurrence.[191] Triple-negative/basal-like, HER2-associated, and luminal B breast cancers are at greater risk for early recurrence relative to luminal A cancers, which have a longer latency period of possible recurrence.

Complete genetic sequencing of human breast cancers has reinforced the idea that discrete subtypes of breast cancer exist.[192] There is strong correlation between histologic subtypes of breast cancers, genomic profiles, and mutations identified by genomic sequencing. This information is beginning to influence clinical practice in breast cancer management.

In addition to defining biologic tumor subsets, gene expression profiling has been used to stratify tumors as having good-risk or poor-risk prognostic signatures.[193,194] Several of these assays are now commercially available. MammaPrint is a 70-gene signature developed in the Netherlands.[193] Prosigna (NanoString Technologies, Seattle, WA) is a 50-gene intrinsic subtype classifier that categories cancers into luminal A, luminal B, HER2, or basal-like subtypes.[195] Retrospective analyses suggest that these gene signatures contribute independent prognostic information above and beyond that achieved with use of traditional pathologic markers, such as stage, grade, lymphovascular invasion, and ER/PR/HER2 status.

One molecular test that is of use clinically is the Oncotype DX recurrence score. The recurrence score is based on a quantitative assessment of 21 genes thought to be relevant to breast cancer biology, including hormone receptors, Ki67, and HER2, among others. In contrast to gene expression profiles that classify tumors into specific subsets or dichotomize tumors into good/poor prognostic groups, the recurrence score calculates a continuous, numeric result that correlates with distant metastatic recurrence in tamoxifen-treated patients with node-negative breast cancer,[196] and has been shown to be a prognostic marker in postmenopausal women with node-negative or node-positive tumors receiving either tamoxifen or an AI.[197] Although the recurrence score tends to correlate with features like tumor grade, size, nodal status, and quantitative levels of hormone receptor expression, multivariate analyses demonstrate that the score provides significant independent prognostic information. Oncotype DX has been applied to a common clinical question: whether a patient with ER+ breast cancer should receive chemotherapy in addition to hormonal therapy. Retrospective analyses from NSABP B-20—a trial of tamoxifen alone versus tamoxifen plus chemotherapy for ER+, node-negative

Association of Clinicopathologic Features of Breast Cancer with Intrinsic Subtype

Intrinsic Subtype	Luminal A	Luminal B	*HER2* Enriched	Basal-like
Estrogen/progesterone receptor expression	Positive – strong	Positive – variable	Positive or negative	Negative
HER2 amplification	Rare	Rare though small percentage positive	Common	Negative
Grade	Low-intermediate	Intermediate-high	Intermediate-high	High
P53 mutation	Rare	Uncommon	Common	Common
Ki67%	Low	Intermediate-high	High	High
DNA copy number	Diploid	Aneuploid	Aneuploid; high genomic instability	Aneuploid; high genomic instability
mRNA expression signature	High ER cluster; low proliferation	Lower ER cluster, high proliferation	High *HER2* amplicon, high proliferation	Basal signature, high proliferation

Adapted from Cancer Genome Atlas Network. Comprehensive molecular portraits of human breast tumours. *Nature* 2012;490:61–70.

patients—demonstrated that the recurrence score was a predictive factor for benefit from chemotherapy. Patients with tumors that had a low recurrence score had a very favorable overall prognosis that was not meaningfully improved by chemotherapy, while patients with high recurrence scores derived a substantial benefit from chemotherapy.[198] Qualitatively similar findings were seen in the Southwest Oncology Group (SWOG) 8814 study, a randomized trial of tamoxifen alone or tamoxifen plus cyclophosphamide/doxorubicin/5-fluorouracil chemotherapy for postmenopausal women with ER+, node-positive breast cancer, although the overall prognosis in this node-positive cohort was less favorable than in node-negative cases.[199]

There is substantial overlap between the various molecular diagnostic assays used to gauge prognosis and treatment for early-stage breast cancer.[200] In particular, many assays appear capable of distinguishing node-negative, lower-grade tumors that are strongly ER+ and *HER2*−, and are unlikely to benefit from adjuvant chemotherapy[201] (Table 79.17). Collectively, these molecular tools have led to the evolution of specific treatment algorithms based on subtype classification, and clinical trials are increasingly designed for specific tumor types.

ADJUVANT SYSTEMIC THERAPY

The goal of adjuvant systemic therapy is to prevent the recurrence of breast cancer by eradicating occult, micrometastatic deposits of tumor present at the time of diagnosis. The rationale for adjuvant treatment stems from the systemic hypothesis of breast tumorigenesis, which argues that in the early stages of breast cancer development, tumor cells are disseminated throughout the body. To a large extent, this hypothesis has been validated through decades of clinical investigation, and approximately half of the

recent decline in breast cancer mortality in the United States and Western Europe has been attributed to the widespread use of adjuvant therapy.[5]

In current practice, three systemic treatment modalities are widely used as adjuvant therapy for early-stage breast cancer. These modalities are (1) endocrine treatments such as tamoxifen, AIs, or ovarian suppression; (2) anti-*HER2* therapy with the humanized monoclonal antibody, trastuzumab; and (3) chemotherapy. Selection of adjuvant treatment is determined by the biologic features of the breast cancer (Table 79.18). Patients with tumors that are hormone receptor positive (either for ER, PR, or both) are candidates for adjuvant endocrine therapy; patients with tumors that are *HER2* overexpressing are candidates for trastuzumab. Chemotherapy is used for tumors that are hormone receptor negative, alongside trastuzumab in *HER2*+ tumors, and in addition to endocrine therapy in ER+ patients, based largely on features such as tumor size, nodal status, and the patient's other health considerations.

Adjuvant Endocrine Therapy

Tamoxifen is the historic standard for adjuvant endocrine therapy for breast cancer. The EBCTCG has performed an overview of the randomized trials of adjuvant tamoxifen therapy.[202] These results reflect data with 15 years of follow-up, from over 60 adjuvant trials including >80,000 women. Tamoxifen administered for 5 years results in a 41% reduction in the annual rate of breast cancer recurrence (HR = 0.59) and a 34% reduction in the annual death rate (HR = 0.66) for women with ER+ breast cancer. The gains associated with tamoxifen are achieved independent of patient age or menopausal status, with and without the use of adjuvant chemotherapy, and are durable, contributing to improved survival through at least 15 years of follow-up. Shorter durations of tamoxifen therapy are also beneficial, but appear to have less impact than

Overview of Adjuvant Treatment Approaches in Breast Cancer

Tumor HER Status	Tumor Hormone Receptor Status	
	Positive	Negative
HER2 negative/normal	Endocrine therapy ± chemotherapy	Chemotherapy
HER2 positive/overexpressed	Endocrine therapy + chemotherapy + trastuzumab	Chemotherapy + trastuzumab

5-year treatment duration. Until recently, data had suggested that the optimal duration of tamoxifen therapy was 5 years; extending tamoxifen therapy beyond 5 years in patients with no evidence of tumor recurrence had not led to further improvements in DFS or OS.[203] However, the Adjuvant Tamoxifen: Longer Against Shorter trial compared 10 years versus 5 years of adjuvant tamoxifen, and found an improvement in overall and DFS with the longer duration of tamoxifen treatment.[204] This finding is of particular relevance for premenopausal women who lack the option of receiving extended adjuvant endocrine therapy with an AI (see the following). Based on the Adjuvant Tamoxifen: Longer Against Shorter trial, premenopausal women should consider longer duration of tamoxifen up to 10 years as adjuvant endocrine treatment. Tamoxifen is not effective in preventing recurrence of hormone receptor–negative breast cancer.[205,206]

Multiple clinical trials have examined the role of AIs as adjuvant endocrine therapy for early breast cancer. Although tamoxifen works by binding to the ER, AIs function through inhibition of the aromatase enzyme that converts androgens into estrogens,[207] resulting in profound estrogen depletion. In postmenopausal patients, where only nonovarian, baseline levels of aromatase activity are present, AIs lower estrogen production by 90% to nearly undetectable levels.[208] AIs are not appropriate for premenopausal patients, as residual ovarian function can lead to enhanced production of aromatase and thus overcome the effects of AIs.

Major trials have studied whether the incorporation of an AI improves the results seen with 5 years of tamoxifen in postmenopausal women with hormone receptor–positive breast cancer (Table 79.19). AI treatment has been explored as primary or upfront therapy *instead* of tamoxifen,[209–211] as *sequential* therapy after 2 or 3 years of tamoxifen,[212,213] and as *extended* therapy after 5 years of tamoxifen.[214–216] In each setting, the use of an AI achieved modest improvements in DFS as a result of a lower risk of both distant metastasis as well as of in-breast recurrences and contralateral tumors. Two trials, BIG 1-98[217] and the Tamoxifen and Exemestane in Early Breast Cancer study,[218] have compared up-front use of an AI against a sequential treatment with tamoxifen followed by an AI. These studies demonstrate equal rates of tumor recurrence with either 5 years of an AI or 2 to 3 years of tamoxifen followed by 2 to 3 years of an AI for a total of 5 years of therapy. Randomized trials have shown no important clinical differences between nonsteroidal or steroidal AIs as adjuvant therapy, demonstrating that different commercially available AIs can be used interchangeably.[219]

For women who begin taking an AI at the time of diagnosis, the appropriate duration of endocrine treatment is unknown, although at present, a maximum of 5 years is the only duration for which safety and efficacy data exist. Studies are ongoing to address this question. The option of starting with either an AI or tamoxifen appears reasonable for any patient. The up-front trials[210,211]

limited treatment to a total of 5 years' duration, and the sequential trials[212,213] used AI therapy for only 2 or 3 years as part of a total of 5 years of adjuvant endocrine treatment. The studies of extended endocrine therapy beyond 5 years[204,214,216] underscore the long natural history of hormone receptor–positive breast cancer and demonstrate that antiestrogen treatments have ongoing benefits well beyond 5 years after diagnosis.

The recently updated ASCO guidelines on adjuvant endocrine therapy recommend that postmenopausal women consider an AI at some point in their treatment program as either initial therapy or as sequential therapy after several years of tamoxifen.[220] Differences in side effect profiles between tamoxifen and AI therapy may inform treatment selection. Tamoxifen is associated with rare risks of thromboembolism and uterine cancer.[203,210,211] AI treatment is associated with accelerated osteoporosis and an arthralgia syndrome[221]; patients receiving AI therapy require serial monitoring of bone mineral density.[222] Both treatments are associated with menopausal symptoms, such as hot flashes, night sweats, and genitourinary symptoms, including sexual dysfunction. Postmenopausal women who are intolerant of either tamoxifen or AI therapy should be offered the alternative type of treatment. Because AI therapy is only effective in postmenopausal women, tamoxifen remains the treatment of choice in women who are pre- or perimenopausal, or in whom there is question of residual ovarian function. In particular, women with chemotherapy-induced amenorrhea may have recovery of ovarian function and are not suitable candidates for AI treatment.[223]

Despite longstanding interest in ovarian suppression as adjuvant therapy, its role in addition to tamoxifen or chemotherapy remains unclear because of confounding clinical factors. Early studies of ovarian suppression were not limited to patients with hormone receptor–positive tumors, did not necessarily include tamoxifen, and frequently included chemotherapy, which led to a high incidence of chemotherapy-induced menopause.[224] Thus, despite the fact that multiple randomized trials have demonstrated that ovarian suppression can be effective adjuvant therapy for premenopausal women[202] and have demonstrated that ovarian suppression is frequently at least as effective as adjuvant chemotherapy in preventing breast cancer recurrence,[225] there remains little consensus on whether ovarian suppression adds meaningfully to results seen with tamoxifen with or without adjuvant chemotherapy.

Very young women—typically those <35 years of age—who do not routinely experience amenorrhea with adjuvant chemotherapy, appear to have a substantially worse prognosis than patients who do enter menopause with chemotherapy.[226] A randomized trial has compared chemotherapy alone, chemotherapy plus ovarian suppression and tamoxifen, and ovarian suppression plus tamoxifen as adjuvant treatment. The addition of tamoxifen clearly

PRACTICE OF ONCOLOGY

TABLE 79.19

Major Studies Comparing Adjuvant Therapy Incorporating Aromatase Inhibitors with Five Years of Tamoxifen

Timing/Setting	Trial(Ref.)	AI	No. of Patients	Hazard Ratio for Disease-Free Survival	Absolute Difference in Disease-Free Survival (%)
Upfront; y 0	ATAC[209]	ANA	9,366	0.87[a]	2.8 at 5 y
	BIG 1-98[217]	LET	8,010	0.81	2.6 at 5 y
Sequential; after 2–3 y of TAM	IES[212]	EXE	4,742	0.68	4.7 at 3 y
	ARNO/ABCSG[213]	ANA	3,224	0.60	3.1 at 3 y
Extended; after 5 y of TAM	MA.17[214]	LET	5,187	0.58	4.6 at 4 y
	NSABP B-33[216]	EXE	1,598	0.68	2.0 at 4 y

AI, aromatase inhibitor; ATAC, arimidex, tamoxifen, alone or in combination; ANA, anastrozole; BIG, Breast International Group; LET, letrozole; TAM, tamoxifen; IES, Intergroup Exemestane Study; EXE, exemestane; ARNO/ABCSG, Arimidex-Nolvadex/Austrian Breast and Colorectal Cancer Study Group; MA, National Cancer Institute of Canada MA; NSABP, National Surgical Adjuvant Breast and Bowel Project.
[a] Comparison for ANA versus TAM. The third arm of the trial, combined therapy with ANA plus TAM, yielded outcomes similar to those of TAM alone.

improved results compared to chemotherapy with or without ovarian suppression. In subset analyses, younger women (<40 years of age) who were less likely to experience chemotherapy-induced amenorrhea did appear to benefit from ovarian suppression in addition to chemotherapy.[227] The Adjuvant Breast Cancer Ovarian Ablation or Suppression Trial compared tamoxifen alone versus tamoxifen with ovarian suppression in premenopausal women and did not show a substantial improvement in DFS with the addition of ovarian suppression.[228] However, in this study, only 40% of patients were known to have ER⁺ breast cancer, and 80% of patients additionally received adjuvant chemotherapy, profoundly limiting study interpretation. Ongoing trials are specifically testing the role of ovarian suppression in addition to tamoxifen for premenopausal patients.

Tamoxifen is metabolized by the cytochrome P-450 system into biologically active metabolites. Pharmacogenomic variation in P-450 alleles or the concurrent use of tamoxifen and P-450 inhibitors might affect tamoxifen metabolism, with clinically significant effects.[229–233] Larger retrospective studies have not found consistent relationships between CYP2D6 metabolism and long-term outcomes with tamoxifen treatment.[234,235] At present, neither the full significance of pharmacogenomic allelic variation nor the adequacy of testing for such variation is well characterized.

Multiple studies have documented high rates of noncompliance and early termination of adjuvant endocrine treatments.[236] Factors associated with limited compliance or adherence to tamoxifen and AIs include age, treatment-related symptoms, costs of therapy, and patient-specific perceptions of therapeutic benefit. While the precise impact of noncompliance or nonpersistence with adjuvant endocrine treatment is unclear, clinicians should inquire about treatment utilization given the importance of these agents at improving survival.

Adjuvant Chemotherapy

Adjuvant chemotherapy consisting of multiple cycles of polychemotherapy is well established as an important strategy for lowering the risk of breast cancer recurrence and improving survival. Initial studies of adjuvant chemotherapy were conducted in women with higher-risk, lymph node–positive breast cancer. Subsequent trials have extended the benefits of adjuvant chemotherapy into lower risk, node-negative patient populations.[237] Long-term follow-up from the EBCTCG overview demonstrated benefit from chemotherapy for women irrespective of age, tumor ER status, or whether patients also receive adjuvant endocrine therapy. In addition, the overview suggests that there are advantages for multiple cycles (four to eight) of chemotherapy compared with single-cycle regimens, and demonstrates the superiority of taxane-based and anthracycline-based chemotherapy over cyclophosphamide, methotrexate, 5-fluorouracil (CMF)-based, nonanthracycline regimens.

Multiple cycles of adjuvant chemotherapy, typically including taxanes and anthracyclines as part of the regimen, are recommended for the majority of patients with node-positive and higher-risk node-negative tumors.[238] The current challenges in adjuvant chemotherapy treatment are to select subsets of patients that might preferentially benefit from chemotherapy or conversely be spared adjuvant chemotherapy and to optimize the dosing and scheduling of chemotherapy to achieve the best clinical results and improve the side effect profile of treatment.

The introduction of taxanes into early-stage breast cancer treatment constitutes an important advance over the historic experience with alkylator and anthracycline-based chemotherapy. The first report on adjuvant taxane therapy, Cancer and Leukemia Group B 9344, demonstrated that the addition of sequential paclitaxel therapy improved both DFS and OS among women with node-positive breast cancer compared to women receiving four cycles of cyclophosphamide-doxorubicin (AC) chemotherapy.[239] Since that time, nearly one dozen studies have reported on breast cancer outcomes with the incorporation of taxanes—either paclitaxel or docetaxel—either as substitutes or sequential additions to anthracycline-based regimens. Studies to define the optimal taxane-based regimen have yielded the following important results. The Cancer and Leukemia Group B 9741 trial compared AC followed by paclitaxel given either every 3 weeks or every 2 weeks at the same doses and schedules.[240] Accelerated, every 2-week treatment (so-called dose-dense) led to lower risk of recurrence and improved survival. A randomized comparison of AC followed by either docetaxel or paclitaxel, with taxanes given either every 3 weeks or on a weekly schedule, did not show significant differences between the taxanes with respect to breast cancer recurrence, though weekly paclitaxel was the best tolerated option.[241] Sequential therapy with anthracyclines/alkylators followed by taxanes proved superior to concurrent taxane-anthracycline-alkylator treatments.[242] Sequential dose-dense AC followed by paclitaxel was at least as effective, and better tolerated, than concurrent docetaxel/doxorubicin/cyclophosphamide chemotherapy.[243]

Meanwhile, neither additional chemotherapy doses nor agents have improved outcomes. Multiple studies have failed to demonstrate that dose escalation of cyclophosphamide[244] or doxorubicin[239] results in a lower risk of recurrence. The addition of capecitabine or gemcitabine to anthracycline- and taxane-based chemotherapy regimens did not improve efficacy.[243,245]

For women who warrant chemotherapy, sequential anthracycline- and taxane-based treatment remains the "gold standard." While multiple possible variations on this regimen exist, the experience to date has not demonstrated that any regimen is better tolerated or more effective than AC for four cycles followed by paclitaxel chemotherapy, with paclitaxel given as either four cycles every 2 weeks, or as 12 weeks of weekly therapy.

There is growing interest in adjuvant chemotherapy regimens that might spare patients exposure to anthracycline-based chemotherapy. Historical options include CMF chemotherapy, which was shown to be equivalent to doxorubicin/cyclophosphamide.[240] The two-drug combination regimen of docetaxel plus cyclophosphamide was superior to doxorubicin/cyclophosphamide (each regimen given for a total of four cycles)[246] in a trial of 1,016 women with node-negative or one to three positive lymph nodes, establishing docetaxel plus cyclophosphamide as an option for these intermediate-risk patients. Six cycles of chemotherapy with AC or taxanes is not better than four cycles of the same regimen.[247] Among higher-risk patients, it is unclear that anthracyclines can be safely omitted.

Clinical studies have shown that chemotherapy can be of benefit to women with node-positive and node-negative breast cancers, with tumors that are either hormone receptor–positive or –negative, regardless of age or menopausal status. Retrospective analyses have even shown that chemotherapy can be beneficial to women with tumors as small as ≤1 cm, including both ER⁺ and ER⁻ tumors.[248] However, not all patients warrant chemotherapy. While chemotherapy often leads to statistically significant risk reduction, the differences in the absolute risk of recurrence for patients, especially patients with small cancers[249] or ER⁺ cancers who also receive adjuvant endocrine therapy, tend to be very small (single percentage points). Third, most benchmark trial results did not take into account the existence of molecularly defined breast cancer subsets and may overestimate the benefits of chemotherapy in certain subtypes of breast cancer, while underestimating the benefits in others. Finally, for patients in whom the absolute advantages of chemotherapy are modest, efforts to weigh patient preferences and directly quantify chemotherapy benefits for specific patients, as opposed to large cohorts in clinical trials, have led to further individualization of chemotherapy choices.

Hormone receptor status may be an important predictor of benefit from chemotherapy. Tumors that are low or nonexpressors of ER derive substantial benefit from the addition of chemotherapy to tamoxifen; by contrast, tumors with high quantitative levels of ER do not appear to gain substantially from adding chemotherapy to endocrine therapy.[205] A retrospective review of trials for node-positive breast cancer found the gains associated with chemotherapy innovations in anthracycline- and taxane-based treatments were most noticeable among patients with ER⁻ tumors, while patients with ER⁺ tumors derived more limited benefit.[250] However, not all retrospective studies have shown a clear relationship between ER status and the benefit of chemotherapy,[251] and precise thresholds of ER expression and chemotherapy benefit are not well established.

HER2 is also a marker that has been widely studied as a predictor of benefit from adjuvant chemotherapy. HER2 overexpression is associated with a relative benefit from anthracycline-based chemotherapy,[252] and HER2⁻ tumors do not selectively benefit from anthracyclines, as opposed to CMF-type chemotherapy treatments. Other retrospective work based on characterizing both HER2 status and ER status of tumors suggests that chemotherapy with taxanes may be especially critical in tumors that either lack ER expression or express HER2.[253] However, these chemotherapy trials all predate the widespread use of adjuvant trastuzumab, which may render moot the details of chemotherapy selection for HER2⁺ tumors.

Molecular assays that integrate larger numbers of biomarkers can clarify the role of chemotherapeutic agents in adjuvant treatment. The 21-gene recurrence score (Oncotype DX, discussed in the section "Prognostic and Predictive Factors in Breast Cancer" on page 1138) predicts outcome for ER⁺, node-negative breast cancers treated with tamoxifen[196] or tamoxifen plus chemotherapy in node-negative[197] and node-positive[199] patients. Patients with tumors with higher recurrence scores derive substantial benefit from the addition of chemotherapy to endocrine treatment, while patients with low recurrence scores have both a more favorable overall prognosis and do not appear to benefit meaningfully from the addition of chemotherapy. Pathologic features such as low or no expression of hormone receptors, expression of HER2, and high tumor grade all tend to be predictors of likely sensitivity of tumors to chemotherapy.[177,200] Tumors at the other end of the molecular spectrum—low grade, high levels of hormone receptors, lack of HER2 expression—tend to be more sensitive to endocrine therapies and less sensitive to adjuvant chemotherapy. Various chemotherapy regimens have distinctive side effect profiles that can inform regimen selection for an individual patient. For example, anthracyclines are associated with a low risk of cardiomyopathy and may not be appropriate for patients with previous anthracycline exposure or preexisting cardiac disease. Taxane-based treatments are associated with neuropathy that may be worse in patients with preexisting peripheral neuropathy.

Patients and doctors should gauge the absolute gains associated with chemotherapy by considering rigorously the tumor stage, comorbid conditions, age of the patient, and the biologic features of the tumor. Adjuvant!, an online tool that quantifies the benefits of adjuvant treatment, integrates tumor size and biomarker information, patient age and health status, and the relative benefits of chemotherapy as measured in clinical trials, and reports in bar graph format the absolute benefits that the given patient is likely to achieve with adjuvant chemotherapy.[179,254] There are limitations to Adjuvant!, which neither factors into account intrinsic subtypes, nor the efficacy of adjuvant trastuzumab for HER2⁺ tumors. Nonetheless, Adjuvant! can be valuable for framing the realistic benefits of chemotherapy for a variety of clinical situations. Patient surveys, inevitably performed after patients have endured adjuvant chemotherapy, suggest that many women would prefer adjuvant chemotherapy for extraordinarily small gains (1% improvement in outcome), and most women would accept chemotherapy for modest differences on the order of a 3% to 5% improvement in chance of recurrence.[255]

Adjuvant Trastuzumab Therapy for HER2-Overexpressing Breast Cancer

HER2 expression was historically an adverse prognostic factor associated with a higher risk of recurrence, lack of or lower levels of ER expression, and relative resistance to endocrine therapy and CMF-based chemotherapy.[256,257] In 2005, reports became available from five randomized clinical trials that examined the addition of trastuzumab, the humanized monoclonal antibody against the HER2 protein, to chemotherapy as adjuvant treatment for HER2-overexpressing breast cancer (Table 79.20).[258–261] Although these trials used a variety of different adjuvant chemotherapy regimens and employed trastuzumab in different schedules and sequences, they all showed significant improvements in DFS (reduction in risk of 50% on average) and OS. Subset analyses demonstrated comparable RR reduction regardless of tumor size, nodal status, or hormone receptor status, resulting in the rapid incorporation of trastuzumab into standard treatment recommendations for women with HER2+ breast cancer.

Cardiomyopathy is a novel side effect of trastuzumab therapy.[260] Cardiac dysfunction is more frequent in patients receiving anthracycline-based than nonanthracycline adjuvant chemotherapy (2% versus 1%) in addition to trastuzumab. Other risk factors for cardiac dysfunction with adjuvant trastuzumab include preexisting cardiac disease, such as borderline normal left ventricular ejection fraction or hypertension, and age >65 years. All patients being considered for adjuvant trastuzumab require baseline determination of left ventricular ejection fraction and serial monitoring of cardiac function.

Adjuvant trastuzumab is only known to be effective in tumors with aberrant expression of HER2.[262] The optimal duration of

TABLE 79.20

Adjuvant Trials of Trastuzumab

Trial[(Ref.)]	No. of Patients	Chemotherapy Regimen	Trastuzumab Regimen	Hazard Ratio—DFS	Hazard Ratio—OS
NSABP B-31[260]/ NCCTG N9831	3,351	AC → P	1 y beginning concurrently with P	0.48	0.67
HERA[259]	3,401	Various	1 y beginning sequentially after chemotherapy	0.64	0.63
FinHER[258]	232	V or D → FEC	9 wk beginning concurrently with V or D	0.42	0.41
BCIRG 006[261]	3,222	AC → D	1 y beginning concurrently with D	0.61	0.59
		CbD[a]	1 y beginning concurrently with CbD	0.67	0.66

DFS, disease-free survival; OS, overall survival; NSABP, National Surgical Adjuvant Breast and Bowel Project; NCCTG, North Central Cancer Treatment Group; A, doxorubicin; C, cyclophosphamide; P, paclitaxel; HERA, Herceptin Adjuvant; FinHER, Finland Herceptin; V, vinorelbine; D, docetaxel; FEC, a regimen of fluorouracil, epirubicin, and cyclophosphamide; BCIRG, Breast Cancer International Research Group; Cb, carboplatin.
[a] In comparison to AC → D chemotherapy.

trastuzumab therapy is 1 year. While short exposure (9 weeks) of concurrent chemotherapy-trastuzumab treatment is better than no trastuzumab,[258] a comparison of 6 months versus 12 months of trastuzumab therapy showed superiority for the 12 month duration.[263] The HERA (Herceptin Adjuvant) trial compared 1 year versus 2 years of therapy and found no benefit for a second year of treatment.[259,264]

Trastuzumab is active when delivered sequentially after chemotherapy (as done in the HERA trial[259]) or concurrently with chemotherapy (as done in the NSABP B-31/North Central Cancer Treatment Group N9831,[260] and Breast Cancer International Research Group trials[261]). However, concurrent trastuzumab-chemotherapy administration yielded superior results compared to sequential therapy.[265] All of the adjuvant trastuzumab trials gave chemotherapy; there are no data on whether trastuzumab would be effective without adjuvant chemotherapy.

The optimal chemotherapy backbone for trastuzumab-based adjuvant treatment is uncertain.[266] Most patients treated on the extant clinical trials received sequential anthracyclines and taxane-based treatment, with concurrent use of trastuzumab during taxane treatment. The results from Breast Cancer International Research Group 006 suggest that the nonanthracycline trastuzumab/docetaxel/carboplatin regimen is superior to chemotherapy given without trastuzumab.[261] However, the study was not powered to adequately compare trastuzumab/docetaxel/carboplatin against the doxorubicin and cyclophosphamide followed by docetaxel and trastuzumab treatment arms, and numerically, the anthracycline-based regimen followed by trastuzumab was associated with a lower risk of cancer recurrence.[261] Trastuzumab/docetaxel/carboplatin is an important treatment option, particularly in patients with contraindications to anthracycline-based treatment. Concomitant RT and maintenance trastuzumab can be safely delivered after chemotherapy.

Most of the patients in the major trastuzumab trials had node-positive or high-risk, node-negative breast cancers. The role of trastuzumab treatment for women with smaller, node-negative tumors, particularly tumors <1 cm, remains unproven in randomized trials. Historical studies have suggested that these smaller, $HER2^+$ breast cancers still carried a substantial risk of tumor recurrence (on the order of 15% to 20% through 5 to 10 years of therapy).[267] Recent retrospective analyses of small $HER2^+$ tumors suggest a benefit may exist for this subgroup with the addition of trastuzumab.[268] A prospective trial of 12 weeks of paclitaxel plus trastuzumab, followed by conclusion of 1 year of adjuvant trastuzumab, yielded a remarkably low risk of recurrence when studied in stage 1, $HER2^+$ breast cancers.[269] Patients with $HER2^+$ tumors ≥5 mm are likely to benefit substantially from adjuvant chemotherapy and trastuzumab.

INTEGRATION OF MULTIMODALITY PRIMARY THERAPY

Current consensus recommendations for adjuvant therapy are summarized in Table 79.21. The majority of women with breast cancer receive some form of adjuvant therapy, which requires integration of systemic treatments with local therapy including surgery and RT. Low rates of LR are seen regardless of the sequence of RT and chemotherapy.[270] A nonsignificant trend toward a greater risk of distant recurrence in patients receiving RT first was seen in one study,[270] and because of the primary importance of preventing distant relapse, the convention has been to administer chemotherapy first. Tamoxifen therapy should not be given concurrently with chemotherapy because in one randomized study, concurrent tamoxifen and chemotherapy was associated with greater risk of recurrence than sequential treatment of chemotherapy followed by tamoxifen.[271] There are no compelling data that the concurrent administration of endocrine therapy and RT has deleterious consequences, nor that it has particular advantages.[272] The timing of surgery either before (neo) or after adjuvant chemotherapy does not alter long-term survival for women with breast cancer.[119] Thus, patients may comfortably proceed in a linear fashion of treatment, receiving one therapeutic modality (surgery, RT, chemotherapy, biologic therapy) after another, as they receive definitive treatment for early-stage breast cancer.

FOLLOW-UP FOR BREAST CANCER SURVIVORS

Following initial treatment for breast cancer, patients require surveillance for local-regional tumor recurrence, contralateral breast cancer, and the development of distant metastatic disease. In addition, medical follow-up allows clinicians to monitor for late effects of chemotherapy, RT, or surgery, to gauge ongoing side effects from cancer treatments, such as antiestrogen therapies, and to facilitate opportunities to update patients on new developments that

---

TABLE 79.21

International Recommendations for Adjuvant Chemotherapy

	St. Gallen Consensus Conference 2013	National Comprehensive Cancer Network 2013
HER2 positive tumors	Adjuvant chemotherapy (no specific size threshold) and trastuzumab	Adjuvant chemotherapy and trastuzumab for tumors >0.5 cm and/or node-positive
HER2 negative tumors	ER negative: ■ Adjuvant chemotherapy (no specific size threshold)	ER negative: ■ Adjuvant chemotherapy for tumors ≥1.0 cm and/or node-positive; ■ Consider for tumors 0.5 to 1.0 cm if adverse prognostic factors (lymphovascular invasion, high-grade features) are present
HER2 negative tumors	ER positive: ■ Adjuvant chemotherapy if four or more lymph nodes are positive ■ Consider if tumor >2 cm, or grade 2–3, or age <35, or lymphovascular invasion is present ■ Risk stratify by ER/PR/Ki67/intrinsic subtype/Oncotype DX	ER positive: ■ Adjuvant chemotherapy if node-positive ■ Risk stratify by Oncotype DX (Genomic Health, Redwood City, CA) for node-negative ■ Consider if tumor >1 cm, or if tumor 0.6 to 1.0 cm and lymphovascular invasion or grade 2–3 features are present

ER, estrogen receptor.

may affect their treatment plan.[273] Although the greatest risk of recurrence is in the first 5 years after breast cancer diagnosis, women remain at risk for many years after their treatment, especially those with hormone receptor–positive breast cancer. (These experiences justify ongoing follow-up with breast cancer specialists, although particularly in later years, follow-up is often shared with primary care physicians.)

LR and new contralateral cancers are potentially cureable, so women should undergo regular breast examinations and annual mammography, with supplemental breast imaging as clinically indicated. LR is often associated with concurrent metastatic disease, and evaluation for distant metastases is indicated prior to local therapy in this setting. By contrast, it is not clear that early detection of distant metastatic disease contributes to substantial improvement in clinically important end points. Most distant recurrences are detected following patient-reported symptoms, such as bone discomfort, lymphadenopathy, chest wall/breast changes, or respiratory symptoms; asymptomatic detection through screening laboratory tests or radiology studies occurs in only a modest fraction of patients, even with intensive surveillance.[273] Randomized trials have compared vigorous surveillance with radiologic imaging (chest radiography, bone scanning, and liver ultrasound) and laboratory testing (blood counts, liver function tests, and serum tumor markers) against standard care consisting of regular physical examination and mammography, with additional testing performed only if indicated by symptoms or physical examination.[274,275] More intensive surveillance achieved modest gains in early detection of metastatic breast cancer, with a small increase in the fraction of patients diagnosed while asymptomatic, but no improvement in OS was noted.

Based on these data, ASCO has issued surveillance guidelines for women with early-stage breast cancer[276] (Table 79.22). These guidelines emphasize the importance of a careful history and examination to elicit symptoms or signs of recurrent breast cancer, but minimize the role of routine imaging studies including plain films and CT scans, and do not recommend routine laboratory testing in the absence of symptoms. Patients should be encouraged to perform breast self-examination and to contact their physicians if they develop symptoms possibly suggestive of breast cancer recurrence. Understandably, patients often request additional testing to provide reassurance and to "catch" early recurrences. Clinical experience suggests, however, that patients respond well to discussions regarding optimal testing strategies, the role of surveillance for breast cancer recurrence, the challenges of false-positive and false-negative test results, and the limited need for testing in the absence of symptoms or physical examination findings.[277]

SPECIAL THERAPEUTIC PROBLEMS

Paget Disease

Paget disease represents in situ carcinoma in the nipple epidermis. The classic pathologic finding is the presence of Paget cells (large cells with clear cytoplasm and atypical nuclei) within the epidermis of the nipple. The clinical manifestations of Paget disease include eczematoid changes, crusting, redness, irritation, erosion, discharge, retraction, and inversion. Rarely, Paget disease is bilateral or occurs in a male patient.

Paget disease may occur in the nipple (1) in conjunction with an underlying invasive cancer (staged by the invasive cancer), (2) with underlying DCIS (staged Tis), or (3) alone without any underlying invasive breast carcinoma or DCIS (also staged Tis). The associated underlying cancer may be located centrally in the breast adjacent to the nipple or it may be located peripherally. It is uncertain whether the origin of Paget disease is primarily an in situ intraepidermal malignancy with secondary extension to adjacent structures (intraepidermal theory) or migration of tumor cells into the nipple epidermis from an underlying carcinoma of the breast (epidermotropic theory).

The age-adjusted incidence rates of female Paget disease peaked in 1985 and have decreased yearly thereafter through 2002,[278] perhaps because of earlier detection of breast lesions by mammography prior to the development of pagetoid changes. More recently, Paget disease has been observed as a form of recurrence after nipple-sparing mastectomy.

The workup for the patient with Paget disease includes mammography and physical examination of the breast to rule out an underlying invasive cancer or DCIS. In patients with negative findings on physical examination and mammogram, breast MRI should be considered for patients who are candidates for BCT.

Historically, Paget disease was treated with mastectomy. Prognosis is determined by the stage of the underlying malignancy, if present. Small studies examining the use of excision and WBI for Paget disease have reported LR rates of 5% to 8%[279,280] and no survival differences between BCT and mastectomy, suggesting that BCT with WBI is a reasonable alternative to mastectomy. Local excision alone, without RT, has been used to treat a small number

TABLE 79.22

Breast Cancer Follow-Up

Recommended for Routine Surveillance	
History/physical examination	Every 3 to 6 mo for the first 3 y, every 6 to 12 mo y 4 and 5, annually thereafter
Mammography	Annually, beginning no earlier than 6 mo after radiation therapy
Breast self-examination	All women should be counseled to perform monthly
Pelvic examination	Annually
Coordination of care	Continuity of care with breast cancer specialist and appropriate other health care providers
Not Recommended for Routine Surveillance	
Routine blood tests	Complete blood cell count and liver function tests are not recommended
Imaging studies	Chest radiograph, bone scans, liver ultrasound, computed tomography scans, fluorodeoxyglucose-positron emission tomography scans, and breast magnetic resonance imaging are not recommended for routine breast cancer surveillance
Tumor markers	Cancer antigen 15-3, 27.29, and carcinoembryonic antigen are not recommended

Adapted from Khatcheressian JL, Wolff AC, Smith TJ, et al. American Society of Clinical Oncology 2006 update of the breast cancer follow-up and management guidelines in the adjuvant setting. *J Clin Oncol* 2006;24:5091–5097.

of patients. In one series of 33 patients prospectively treated with local excision alone, the LR rate was 33%[281] and 10 of 11 recurrences were invasive carcinoma. Because of the small numbers of patients treated without RT and the high rate of local failure, such treatment must be considered as nonstandard at the present time.

For patients treated with BCT, surgery should include excision of the full NAC with a cone of underlying retroareolar tissue and complete excision of any tissue with abnormal radiologic findings. For patients with positive margins after central lumpectomy, additional surgery is indicated. Patients with negative surgical margins should undergo irradiation based on criteria generally used to select patients with DCIS and invasive cancer for RT and discussed previously. The decision for axillary node surgery should be based on the presence of an invasive breast cancer; sentinel node biopsy has been used successfully in this setting. Recommendations for adjuvant systemic therapy are based on the final pathology.

Occult Primary with Axillary Metastases

Axillary metastases in the absence of a clinically or mammographically detectable breast tumor are an uncommon presentation of breast carcinoma, seen in <1% of cases. The initial evaluation should include a detailed history and physical examination, bilateral mammogram, breast MRI (if the mammogram is unrevealing), and a chest radiograph. The presence of ER, PR, or *HER2* overexpression is strongly suggestive of metastatic breast carcinoma, although their absence does not exclude a primary breast tumor. MRI identifies the primary tumor in the breast in a significant number of patients with a normal mammogram and breast examination. In a meta-analysis of 220 patients with occult primary tumors, MRI identified a suspicious lesion in 72% with a sensitivity of 90% and a specificity of 31%. The size of tumors identified on pathologic exam ranged from 5 mm to 16 mm.[282] The identification of the primary tumor within the breast simplifies local management, allowing these patients to be treated with BCT or mastectomy according to standard guidelines.

In cases in which a primary tumor cannot be identified, treatment has traditionally been with mastectomy. This strategy was based on the observation that approximately 50% of patients who do not receive therapy to the breast will develop clinically evident disease in the breast. In addition, prior to the era of modern mammography and the availability of MRI, the occult cancers found in the breast at mastectomy were sometimes quite large.[283] More recently, WBI has been used in these patients. Fourquet et al.[283] treated 54 patients with WBI without removal of the primary tumor. The 5- and 10-year rates of IBTR were 7.5% and 20%, respectively. Other small studies antedating the use of MRI confirm that although rates of LR after BCT are higher than in patients treated with excision of a known primary tumor and a boost dose of RT to the tumor bed, WBI with a dose of about 50 Gy is an acceptable alternative to mastectomy in this patient population.

Regardless of the management approach chosen for the breast, ALND should be carried out because of the limited ability of radiation to control gross axillary disease. OS for women with occult primary tumors is similar to that of patients with comparable axillary involvement and a known primary tumor, and some investigators have suggested that survival is actually superior for those with occult primary tumors.[284] Because of the small size of most studies of occult primary cancer, the heterogeneous treatments employed, and the variable durations of follow-up, this claim is difficult to substantiate. Systemic treatment for patients with occult primary breast cancer and axillary involvement should follow the current guidelines for patients with node-positive breast cancer.

Breast Cancer and Pregnancy

Breast carcinoma is one of the most commonly diagnosed malignancies during pregnancy. Older studies estimated that breast cancer developed in 2.2 in 10,000 pregnancies[285]; however, the trend toward later age at first childbirth has increased the number of breast cancer cases coexistent with pregnancy, and breast cancer is now estimated to occur in 1 in 1,000 pregnancies.[286] Delay in diagnosis remains a problem due to the nodularity of the pregnant breast and the assumption that new breast masses are normal physiologic changes. Dominant breast masses developing during pregnancy require biopsy before assuming that they are benign. This can be readily accomplished with a core-cutting needle biopsy in the majority of women. If excisional biopsy is necessary, it should be undertaken; concerns about the development of a milk fistula appear to be overstated.[287] Mammography is not as useful in pregnant patients as in those who are not pregnant because of the increased density in the breast parenchyma associated with pregnancy. Ultrasound may be helpful in confirming the presence of a dominant mass, but, as in the nonpregnant patient, normal imaging studies should not lead to a decision to forgo biopsy in the patient with a dominant breast mass.

After a diagnosis is made, the initial evaluation should include an assessment of the extent of the disease. Computed tomography and bone scans are not recommended during pregnancy because of concerns about radiation exposure to the fetus. In patients with symptoms suggestive of metastases, MRI without contrast can be used to evaluate bony sites and the intra-abdominal viscera.[287]

Breast cancers occurring during pregnancy are usually high-grade infiltrating ductal carcinomas. In a prospective study of 38 pregnant women who developed breast cancer, only 28% had ER+ tumors and 24% had PR+ tumors.[288] In general, the characteristics of cancers occurring during pregnancy are similar to those of nonpregnant women of the same age. Data from retrospective case-control series suggest that after adjusting for age and disease stage, the prognosis of women with breast cancer occurring during pregnancy differs little from that of nonpregnant patients.[287]

For women diagnosed in the first or second trimester, the question of pregnancy termination is inevitably raised. Although some treatment approaches are feasible during pregnancy, others are contraindicated. Depending on the patient's specific situation, continuing the pregnancy may or may not compromise the breast cancer treatment. Even when deviations from standard treatment are required, it is unclear to what extent such changes or delays affect a woman's odds of remaining free from recurrent breast cancer. The concerns about compromising care must be balanced by the woman, her family, and her physicians, with the desire to continue the pregnancy. The woman facing these issues must also consider the possibility that if she receives chemotherapy, her ability to conceive another child could be compromised.[224] There is no clear evidence that pregnancy termination changes OS.[289]

Breast surgery can be safely performed during any trimester of pregnancy. Mastectomy is the treatment that has traditionally been undertaken because of the inability to safely deliver RT to the breast without excessive fetal exposure during any trimester. The effect of delaying RT on LR, in the absence of systemic therapy, is unknown and is of concern. Guidelines for BCS[66] consider this an appropriate approach for cancers diagnosed in the third trimester and one that must be considered on a case-by-case basis for cancers diagnosed earlier in pregnancy. In the woman who will receive systemic chemotherapy, the delay in the delivery of RT is often no greater than in the nonpregnant patient. The success rate of lymphatic mapping and sentinel node biopsy in the pregnant woman is unknown. Isosulfan blue dye is not approved by the US Food and Drug Administration for use during pregnancy. The radiation exposure to the fetus from the use of technetium has been estimated to be low, and it has been suggested that mapping with technetium alone could be discussed with patients as an appropriate management strategy.[290] In the absence of definitive data on the safety and accuracy of sentinel node biopsy in the pregnant woman, ALND remains the standard management strategy.

The risk of congenital malformation from cytotoxic chemotherapy varies with the fetal age at exposure and the agent used.

Exposure in the first trimester is associated with risks of 10% to 20% and should be avoided. Risks decline to <2% with exposure in the second and third trimesters, enabling chemotherapy administration in those trimesters.[291] Chemotherapy during pregnancy may also contribute to intrauterine growth retardation, and the long-term consequences of exposure remain uncertain. In a prospective study of 24 pregnant women treated with fluorouracil, doxorubicin, and cyclophosphamide during the second and third trimesters of pregnancy, no complications were observed for the fetus or infant.[292] Experience with the taxanes in pregnancy is limited, but appears feasible after the first trimester.[293]

The use of trastuzumab in pregnancy is associated with oligohydramnios,[294] and more information on the safety of this agent in pregnancy is needed. Methotrexate should be avoided during pregnancy because of the risk of abortion and severe fetal malformation. Similarly, tamoxifen should be withheld until after delivery because its safety is uncertain. When chemotherapy or tamoxifen is given postpartum, breastfeeding should be avoided, as these agents may be excreted in the breast milk.

The management of breast cancer during pregnancy is difficult, as there is often a conflict between optimal therapy for the mother and the fetus. Multidisciplinary management by a team including medical, surgical, and radiation oncologists, an obstetrician, a maternal-fetal medicine specialist, and a psychologist will facilitate the development of a strategy that optimizes the outcome for both mother and child.

Male Breast Cancer

The incidence of male breast cancer varies on a worldwide basis, with the highest rates in some sub-Saharan countries. In the United States, it is estimated that in 2012, 2,190 men were diagnosed with breast cancer, and 410 died of the disease. Worldwide, the female to male incidence ratio is 122:1.[295] In recent years, as the incidence of female breast cancer has declined by 42%, a 28% decline in male breast cancer has been observed.[296] The risk of male breast cancer is related to an increased lifelong exposure to estrogen (as with female breast cancer) or to reduced androgen. The strongest association is in men with Klinefelter syndrome (XXY); they have a 14- to 50-fold increased risk of developing male breast cancer and account for about 3% of all male breast cancer cases. Also, men who carry a *BRCA1* or, particularly, a *BRCA2* mutation, have an increased risk of developing breast cancer. The following conditions have been reported to be associated with an increased risk of breast cancer in men: chronic liver disorders, such as cirrhosis, chronic alcoholism, and schistosomiasis; a history of mumps orchitis, undescended testes, or testicular injury; and feminization, genetically or by environmental exposure. In contrast, gynecomastia alone does not appear to be a risk factor.[297]

The clinical presentation of male breast cancer is similar to that of female breast cancer, but the median age of onset is later than in women (60 years versus 53 years). Because the diagnosis of breast cancer is often not considered as promptly in men and screening mammography is not used, men often present with more advanced stage than do women. All known histopathologic types of breast cancer have been described in men, with infiltrating ductal carcinoma accounting for at least 70% of cases. However, ILC in men is rare. A majority of male breast cancers are ER/PR+, and the percentage positive is greater than for female breast cancer. As for women, stage is the predominant prognostic indicator, and most studies report that stage for stage, men with breast cancer have the same outcome following treatment as women with breast cancer. A recent study, however, from the Veterans Affairs reports a worse prognosis for men than women in early-stage breast cancer.[298] There appears to be a substantial negative disparity in outcome for blacks with male breast cancer compared with whites.[299]

Primary local treatment is typically total mastectomy. In some patients with early disease, BCT can be considered. However, the subareolar location of most male breast cancers and the small amount of breast tissue present in most men limits eligibility for BCT. The same considerations regarding nodal surgery pertain for men as for women, with sentinel node biopsy the preferred treatment in clinically node-negative patients. The use of postmastectomy RT follows the same guidelines as for female breast cancer. Similarly, the use of systemic therapy follows the same guidelines as for women with postmenopausal breast cancer. Adjuvant systemic chemotherapy is used in men, although no controlled trials have confirmed its value.[300] Tamoxifen is the mainstay for adjuvant systemic therapy in ER+ male breast cancer; a study of 257 male breast cancer patients demonstrated a 1.5-fold increase in mortality in those treated with an AI versus tamoxifen.[301] Metastatic breast cancer in men is treated identically to metastatic disease in women.

Phyllodes Tumor

The term *phyllodes tumor* includes a group of lesions of varying malignant potential, ranging from completely benign tumors to fully malignant sarcomas. Clinically, phyllodes tumors are smooth, rounded, usually painless multinodular lesions that may be indistinguishable from fibroadenomas. The average age at diagnosis is in the fourth decade. Skin ulceration may be seen with large tumors, but this is usually due to pressure necrosis rather than invasion of the skin by malignant cells. Histologically, phyllodes tumor, like fibroadenoma, is composed of epithelial elements and a connective tissue stroma.

Phyllodes tumors are classified as benign, borderline, or malignant on the basis of the nature of the tumor margins (pushing or infiltrative) and presence of cellular atypia, mitotic activity, and overgrowth in the stroma. There is disagreement about which of these criteria is most important, although most experts favor stromal overgrowth. The percentage of phyllodes tumors classified as malignant ranges from 23% to 50%. Local excision to negative margins is an appropriate management strategy for both benign and malignant phyllodes tumors if this can be accomplished with a satisfactory cosmetic outcome. The optimal margin width is not known, but wider excisions appear to reduce the risk of LR. Approximately 20% of phyllodes tumors recur locally if excised with no margin or a margin of a few millimeters of normal breast tissue, regardless of whether they are benign or malignant.[302] In a review of 821 patients with nonmetastatic malignant phyllodes tumors reported to the Surveillance, Epidemiology, and End Results registry between 1983 and 2002, 52% were treated with mastectomy and the remainder with local excision. The 10-year cause-specific survival was 89%, and no survival benefit for mastectomy was observed.[302]

The role of RT and systemic therapy in phyllodes tumor is unclear. RT is not used for benign or borderline lesions, but has been combined with wide excision in the management of malignant phyllodes tumors. When phyllodes tumors metastasize, they tend to behave like sarcomas, with the lung as the most common site. Axillary metastases are seen in <5% of cases, and axillary surgery is not indicated unless worrisome nodes are clinically evident. When systemic therapy is used for malignant phyllodes tumors, treatment is based on the guidelines for treating sarcomas.

Locally Advanced Breast Cancer and Inflammatory Breast Cancer

LABC and IBC refer to a heterogeneous group of breast cancers without evidence of distant metastases (M0) and represent only 2% to 5% of all breast cancers in the United States. The term LABC encompasses patients with (1) operable disease at presentation (clinical stage T3N1), (2) inoperable disease at presentation (clinical stage T4 and/or N2-3), and (3) IBC (clinical stage

T4dN0-3, also inoperable). (All stages refer to the *AJCC Cancer Staging Manual*, seventh edition, 2010).[79] Subdividing patients into these three broad groups facilitates clinical management.

Comparison of studies of LABC and IBC is problematic due to a high degree of heterogeneity within T and N classification, small numbers of patients in stage subgroups, and variation in the definition of LABC according to AJCC staging criteria over time.[79] For example, supraclavicular lymphadenopathy, now classified as N3 disease, was previously classified as M1.[303] IBC accounts for 1% to 5% of all cases of breast cancer in the United States and is an aggressive variant of LABC. IBC is a clinicopathologic entity characterized by diffuse erythema and edema (peau d'orange) of the skin of the breast, often without a discreet, underlying palpable mass, although the breast is usually diffusely thickened. IBC typically has a rapid onset and is often initially mistaken as infection and treated with antibiotics before the diagnosis is established. The clinical presentation results from tumor emboli in the dermal lymphatics. According to the AJCC staging rules,[79] IBC is primarily a clinical diagnosis. Involvement of dermal lymphatics in the absence of clinical findings does not indicate IBC. A skin biopsy may be performed to confirm the clinical impression of IBC, but the absence of dermal lymphatic involvement does not affect staging. IBCs are more likely to be high-grade, *HER2*-overexpressing, and lacking in hormone receptor expression compared with other presentations of breast cancer. Because both LABC and IBC are associated with substantial risk of metastatic disease, patients with these cancers should undergo full workup for distant metastases prior to initiation of therapy.

Patients with LABC or IBC should be evaluated by a multidisciplinary team (ideally, around the time of diagnosis). Treatment typically includes neoadjuvant chemotherapy, surgery, and RT. Prior to the use of neoadjuvant chemotherapy, long-term survival was uncommon. Long-term survival has been greatly improved with aggressive trimodality treatment. As with early-stage breast cancer, biologic tumor markers should affect treatment selection: patients with *HER2*+ cancers should receive trastuzumab-based therapy, and patients with hormone receptor–positive cancers should receive adjuvant endocrine therapy. Anthracycline- and taxane-based chemotherapy regimens are appropriate as induction chemotherapy for women with LABC or IBC. The vast majority of patients will have clinical response to therapy, and roughly 15% to 25% will experience a pCR. The addition of paclitaxel to anthracycline-based therapy appears to improve long-term disease outcomes for women with LABC and IBC.[304] There are no studies of trastuzumab specifically for LABC/IBC; however, by extrapolation of results using trastuzumab for early-stage breast cancer, it should be incorporated into the treatment of women with *HER2*+ LABC or IBC. As with other experiences using neoadjuvant chemotherapy, complete pathologic eradication of the tumor is associated with superior outcomes among women with LABC or IBC.[305] However, even among patients with pCR to neoadjuvant chemotherapy, those with LABC or IBC at baseline have a higher risk of recurrence than patients with earlier-stage breast cancer at baseline.[306] Patients with LABC or IBC should be routinely treated with postmastectomy RT, regardless of the pathologic response.[307]

Some women with LABC may be candidates for BCT following neoadjuvant chemotherapy. In one series, local-regional control following this approach appeared to be excellent except in patients with one or more of the following features: (1) clinical N2-3 disease, (2) lymphovascular invasion, (3) residual primary pathologic size >2 cm and (4) multifocal residual disease.[308] However, there is still limited experience with this approach. In contrast, BCT is contraindicated in patients with IBC, even after a complete clinical response to neoadjuvant therapy. In a small study of 13 patients with IBC treated with preoperative chemotherapy and BCT, 7 of 13 experienced LR.[309] This, coupled with the diffuse nature of IBC, indicates that BCT is contraindicated in women with this diagnosis.

Although most women have a clinical response to neoadjuvant chemotherapy, some patients will experience tumor progression or remain inoperable. Such patients may be candidates for non–cross-resistant chemotherapy or novel treatments. Surgery is contraindicated in IBC unless there is complete resolution of the inflammatory skin changes. In modern studies, 85% to 90% of patients become operable after initial chemotherapy.[310] RT may facilitate conversion of inoperable to operable disease. Despite modern multimodality therapy, approximately 20% of patients with IBC treated with chemotherapy, surgery, and RT will experience LRR.[310] Patients with chest wall recurrence after chemotherapy, surgery, and RT are at high risk for both extensive local-regional tumor spread and for developing metastatic disease to visceral organ sites, and are treated according to guidelines for metastatic breast cancer.

MANAGEMENT OF LOCAL-REGIONAL RECURRENCE

LRR after primary therapy for breast cancer includes in-breast recurrence after BCS, chest wall recurrence after mastectomy, and regional nodal recurrences, and accounts for about 15% of all breast cancer recurrences.[107] Predictors of LR include higher initial tumor stage, young patient age involved, surgical margins, and intrinsic subtype (greater risk with basal-like, luminal B, or *HER2*+ cancers). More than 60% of patients with LRR after either BCT or mastectomy will eventually develop metastatic disease.[311,312] Short disease-free intervals, lymph node recurrence, skin lesions, and tumor lack of ER expression all portend greater risk of disseminated cancer. Patients with LRR warrant comprehensive restaging to exclude concurrent metastatic disease.

Despite the high-risk nature of LRR, patients are treated with curative intent in multidisciplinary fashion, with treatment plans individualized based on the nature of the LRR, prior local therapy, and prior adjuvant systemic therapy. The initial management step is usually surgical resection. Women previously treated with BCS are offered salvage mastectomy. Patients with localized chest wall recurrences should undergo surgical excision, while ALND is indicated for axillary nodal recurrences occurring after sentinel lymph node biopsy. RT to sites of regional recurrence and additional regional lymph nodes is standard. Patients with prior RT after either BCS or mastectomy need careful planning to minimize overlap with prior RT fields.

Current treatment standards for LRR recommend introduction of systemic therapy following local management. Recurrences that are ER+ warrant introduction or switching of endocrine therapy. Patients with recurrence on tamoxifen should consider treatment with AIs. Patients who have recurrences on AI therapy may consider tamoxifen or fulvestrant. Patients with *HER2*+ tumors should consider initiation or re-institution of anti-*HER2* therapy in an adjuvant fashion. The role of chemotherapy in the management of LRR has been controversial, especially among those previously treated with adjuvant chemotherapy. The Chemotherapy as Adjuvant for Locally Recurrent Breast Cancer study was a randomized trial of "adjuvant" chemotherapy following optimal resection of LRR.[313] Chemotherapy reduced the risk of subsequent cancer recurrence and improved OS, especially in ER− tumors, though modest benefits were seen among patients with ER+ tumors. Patients without prior chemotherapy exposure would be suitable for any standard adjuvant chemotherapy regimen. Those patients with prior chemotherapy treatment may consider nonoverlapping regimens.

METASTATIC DISEASE

Metastatic (stage IV) breast cancer is defined by tumor spread beyond the breast, chest wall, and ipsilateral regional lymph nodes. The most common sites for breast cancer metastasis include the bone, lung, liver, lymph nodes, chest wall, and brain. However, case reports have documented breast cancer dissemination to almost every organ in the body. Hormone receptor–positive tumors are more likely to spread to bone as the initial site of metastasis; hormone receptor–negative and/or $HER2^+$ tumors are more likely to recur initially in viscera.[314] Lobular (as opposed to ductal) cancers are more often associated with serosal metastases to the pleura and abdomen. Most women with metastatic disease will have been initially diagnosed with early-stage breast cancer, treated with curative intent, and then experience metastatic recurrence. Only about 10% of patients with newly diagnosed breast cancer in the United States have metastatic disease at presentation; this proportion is far higher in areas where screening programs are not available.

Symptoms of metastatic breast cancer are related to the location and extent of the tumor. Common symptoms or physical examination findings include bone discomfort, lymphadenopathy, skin changes, cough or shortness of breath, and fatigue. These clinical findings are all nonspecific, and appropriate evaluation is warranted in patients with breast cancer with new or evolving symptoms. In some cases, physical examination or radiologic findings will demonstrate unequivocal evidence of metastatic breast cancer. In instances when radiologic or clinical findings are equivocal, tissue biopsy is imperative. If a biopsy is performed, ER, PR, and $HER2$ should be redetermined.

The treatment goals in women with advanced breast cancer include prolongation of life, control of tumor burden, reduction in cancer-related symptoms or complications, and maintenance of quality of life and function. Therapy is not generally considered curative. A small fraction of patients, often those with limited sites of metastatic disease or bearing tumors with exquisite sensitivity to treatment, may experience very long periods of remission and tumor control. Treatment of metastatic breast cancer, like treatment of early-stage breast cancer, is based on consideration of tumor biology and clinical history. Thus, characterization of tumor ER, PR, and $HER2$ status is critical for all patients, and a detailed assessment of past treatment, including timing of therapies as well as patient symptoms and functional assessment, is essential. Patients with endocrine-sensitive tumors, particularly those with minimal symptoms and limited visceral involvement, are candidates for initial treatment with endocrine therapy alone; initial treatment using combined chemoendocrine therapy has not been shown to improve survival compared with sequential treatment programs. Patients with hormone receptor–negative tumors or those with hormone receptor–positive tumors progressing despite the use of endocrine therapy are candidates for chemotherapy. If the tumor is $HER2+$, then anti-$HER2$ treatment is employed in combination with chemotherapy.

Well-established clinical factors can inform the likelihood of response to therapy and long-term outcomes in women with metastatic breast cancer. Patients who have received less therapy, a longer disease-free interval since initial diagnosis, soft tissue or bone metastases, fewer symptoms and better performance status, and tumors that are hormone receptor–positive or $HER2^+$ are likely to experience longer survival with metastatic disease than more heavily treated patients with shorter intervals since treatment, visceral metastases, and greater symptoms.

In clinical trials, the measured end points for defining efficacy of therapy for metastatic breast cancer are response rate, time to tumor progression, and OS. These landmarks are important for guiding clinical practice as well, although formal measures of response/progression are often difficult to apply owing to inconsistencies in imaging studies, the prevalence of nonmeasurable disease such as bone lesions, subcentimeter tumor deposits, and pleural effusions or ascites. The art of treating patients with metastatic breast cancer involves careful, thoughtful repetition of a process of treatment initiation, evaluation including assessment of patient functional status and symptom profile, and serial measurement of tumor burden and response to therapy, through multiple lines of therapy. Clinical guidelines for the management of

metastatic carcinoma[66] are often quite open-ended, acknowledging the multiple treatment pathways that might be legitimately pursued, arguing for judicious use of clinical decision making and treatment selection based on tumor biology, and focusing clinicians on the continuous considerations of patient preference and illness experience.

Endocrine Therapy for Metastatic Breast Cancer

Endocrine treatment is a key intervention for women with hormone receptor–positive, metastatic breast cancer. Table 79.23 lists available endocrine drugs for treating advanced breast cancer. Single-agent therapy is the standard approach; combining endocrine agents has not in general been shown to improve outcomes. Many women will be candidates for multiple lines of endocrine therapy to control metastatic breast cancer. On average, first-line treatment is associated with 8 to 12 months of tumor control, and second-line treatment with 4 to 6 months. Individual patients may experience substantially longer time to progression. Sequential single-agent second- and third-line endocrine treatments are often effective, although typically for shorter durations than initial therapy. Patients with either overt tumor shrinkage or stabilization of disease in response to endocrine treatment can have equivalent long-term tumor control. Endocrine therapy can cause regression of soft tissue and bone and visceral metastases.

Recently, several studies have examined the combined use of an AI with fulvestrant for de novo or progressive, ER^+, metastatic breast cancer.[315–317] In treatment-naïve patients, the SWOG 0226 trial suggested that combining anastrozole with fulvestrant improved progression-free survival and OS. By contrast, in patients who had received prior tamoxifen in the SWOG and Fulvestrant and Anastrozole Combination Therapy trials, or prior AI therapy in the Study of Faslodex vs Exemestane with/without Arimidex trial, the combination of fulvestrant plus an AI was not superior to monotherapy approaches. Thus, the combined use of an AI with fulvestrant is appropriate primarily among women with endocrine-naïve cancers.

Eventually, most women with hormone receptor–positive metastatic breast cancer will progress despite first-line endocrine therapy, and be candidates for second-, third-, and even subsequent lines of endocrine therapy. Resistance to treatment does not seem to be associated with loss of hormone receptor expression by the tumor cells. The results of the Breast Cancer Trials of Oral Everolimus-2 trial have recently led to the approval of the mammalian target of rapamycin inhibitor everolimus in the advanced setting.[318] In this randomized clinical trial, patients with advanced disease resistant to letrozole or anastrozole were assigned to exemestane plus everolimus or placebo. The combination of exemestane and everolimus extended progression-free survival, but

---

TABLE 79.23

Endocrine Therapies for Metastatic Breast Cancer

- Ovarian suppression/ablation (premenopausal women)
- Selective estrogen receptor modulators (tamoxifen, toremifene)
- Aromatase inhibitors (anastrozole, letrozole, exemestane; postmenopausal women)
- Antiestrogens (fulvestrant; postmenopausal women)
- Progestins (megestrol and medroxyprogesterone)
- Other steroid hormones (high-dose estrogens, androgens; principally of historical interest)

was associated with significant side effects, including stomatitis, hyperglycemia, and pneumonitis.

Indications for chemotherapy include symptomatic tumor progression, pending visceral crisis, or resistance to multiple endocrine therapies. Patients presenting with extensive visceral metastases or profound symptoms from breast cancer may benefit from induction chemotherapy, which should then be followed with endocrine therapy.

Tamoxifen was the historic standard as treatment for ER$^+$ metastatic breast cancer, associated with a 50% response rate and median duration of response of 12 to 18 months among treatment-naïve patients. A "tamoxifen flare" reaction, typically characterized by intensification of bone pain, transient tumor progression, and hypercalcemia, can arise in 5% to 10% of patients within the first days or weeks of tamoxifen treatment. Flare reactions are often harbingers of exquisite tumor sensitivity to endocrine manipulation, but must be distinguished from overt tumor progression. Flare reactions are not frequently seen with other endocrine therapies.

In premenopausal women with metastatic breast cancer, combined endocrine therapy with ovarian suppression and tamoxifen can improve survival compared with treatment with either tamoxifen or ovarian suppression alone.[319] Thus, the first intervention for premenopausal women with breast cancer recurrence is ovarian suppression or ablation, with initiation of tamoxifen treatment. Premenopausal women with metastatic tumor despite tamoxifen use are candidates for ovarian suppression/ablation and AI therapy. Postmenopausal women are candidates for either tamoxifen, AIs, fulvestrant, or progestational agents as palliation for metastatic breast cancer. AIs appear to be the preferred initial agents for women who received prior tamoxifen treatment in the adjuvant setting,[319,320] and may have modest clinical advantages over tamoxifen as initial treatment for metastatic disease.[321,322] Fulvestrant appears to have comparable activity to AIs in women previously treated with tamoxifen.[323,324]

The optimal sequencing of endocrine therapy for postmenopausal women treated with adjuvant AIs is not clear, as few trials have rigorously explored different treatments among such patients. Tamoxifen, fulvestrant, progestins, and possibly different AIs are all reasonable options among such patients.

Chemotherapy for Metastatic Breast Cancer

Cytotoxic chemotherapy remains a mainstay of treatment for women with metastatic breast cancer, irrespective of hormone receptor status, and is the backbone of many novel treatments incorporating biologic therapy.[325] Chemotherapy has substantial side effects, including fatigue, nausea, vomiting, myelosuppression, neuropathy, diarrhea, and alopecia, making for tradeoffs between cancer palliation and toxicities of therapy. Chemotherapy is used in patients with hormone-refractory or hormone-insensitive tumors.

Tumor response to chemotherapy is a surrogate for longer cancer control and survival.[326,327] First-line chemotherapy is associated with higher response rates and longer tumor control than second-line, and so forth. There are relatively few studies of fourth or higher lines of chemotherapy, although patients often receive many lines of treatment. Trials have demonstrated palliative benefits of chemotherapy in patients with refractory tumors receiving third-line or subsequent chemotherapy treatment, but the magnitude of such gains must be realistically weighed against the side effects of treatment. Chemotherapy treatment can be interrupted in patients who have had significant response or palliation following initiation of therapy and reintroduced when there is tumor progression or symptom recurrence.

Since the advent of chemotherapy administration for metastatic breast cancer, it has been debated whether single-agent sequential treatment or combination treatment with multiple agents is the best strategy. Combination chemotherapy may be associated with higher response rates and improved time to progression compared with single-agent therapy. However, studies that have specifically planned for crossover treatment with second-line sequential therapy have not shown improved survival compared with a sequential treatment program.[328] Patients with extensive visceral disease or pending visceral crisis may preferentially require initiation of combination chemotherapy, but this has not been demonstrated in prospective studies. Because single-agent chemotherapy facilitates better understanding of which drugs are contributing to benefit or side effects and is generally associated with less toxicity, it remains the preferred approach.

A large number of chemotherapy agents and combinations are effective in treatment of metastatic breast cancer (Table 79.24).[66]

TABLE 79.24

Common Chemotherapy Agents and Combinations for Advanced Breast Cancer

Single Agents	Combination Regimens
Anthracyclines (doxorubicin, epirubicin, pegylated liposomal doxorubicin)	Cyclophosphamide/anthracycline ± 5-fluorouracil regimens (such as AC, EC, CEF, CAF, FEC, FAC)
Taxanes (paclitaxel, docetaxel, albumin nano-particle bound paclitaxel)	CMF
5-fluorouracil[a] (continuous-infusion 5-fluorouracil, capecitabine)	Anthracyclines/taxanes (such as doxorubicin/paclitaxel or doxorubicin/docetaxel)
Vinca alkaloids (vinorelbine, vinblastine[a])	Docetaxel/capecitabine
Gemcitabine	Gemcitabine/paclitaxel
Platinum salts (cisplatin, carboplatin)	Taxane/platinum regimens[b] (such as paclitaxel/carboplatin or docetaxel/carboplatin)
Ixabepilone	Ixabepilone/capecitabine[b]
Cyclophosphamide	
Eribulin	

A, doxorubicin; C, cyclophosphamide; E, epirubicin; F, 5-fluorouracil; M, methotrexate; NCCN, National Comprehensive Cancer Network.
[a] Not listed in NCCN Guidelines as a single agent.
[b] Combination not listed in NCCN Guidelines.

A variety of specific drugs and combinations are considered preferred based on a large historical experience, results from randomized trials, and consideration of toxicity profiles. A single "best" approach for all patients with metastatic cancer is not supported by the literature. Although anthracycline- and taxane-based treatments are generally considered to be among the most active in treatment of metastatic breast cancer, their utility has led to their incorporation into adjuvant chemotherapy regimens. Thus, many women with metastatic breast cancer will already have been treated with anthracyclines and/or taxanes, diminishing the utility of these agents in the palliation of metastatic disease.

Capecitabine is an orally available fluoropyrimidine, metabolized in tissues into 5-fluorouracil. Capecitabine has clinical activity in anthracycline- and taxane-resistant breast cancer,[329] and improves response and survival as first-line treatment when added to single-agent docetaxel.[329] The antimetabolite gemcitabine similarly yields higher response rates and survival when paired with paclitaxel compared with paclitaxel therapy alone.[330] Ixabepilone, an epothilone chemotherapy agent, has substantial activity as a single agent or in combination with capecitabine in patients previously treated with anthracyclines and taxanes.[331,332] Eribulin, a synthetic analog of halochondrin B, is a nontaxane microtubule dynamics inhibitor that was evaluated against physician's choice of chemotherapy in a randomized phase 3 study, the 30-Day Cardiac Event Monitor Belt for Recording Atrial Fibrillation After a Cerebral Ischemic Event trial,[333] and led to improved OS in patients with locally recurrent or metastatic breast cancer with at least two prior regimens.

Dose escalation of taxane therapy with paclitaxel has not been shown to result in clinically important improvements. However, weekly administration of paclitaxel therapy does appear to improve response rate and time to progression compared with less frequent, every-3-week administration.[334,335]

As a strategy to overcome chemotherapy resistance, many investigators in the 1990s explored high-dose chemotherapy with autologous bone marrow or stem cell support as treatment for breast cancer. Preliminary studies suggested favorable clinical outcomes, prompting both widespread use of high-dose chemotherapy in clinical practice and randomized trials for patients with either metastatic or high-risk, node-positive breast cancer. Despite initial hopes, clinical trials found no difference in outcome between standard chemotherapy followed by treatment with either high-dose chemotherapy and autologous stem cell rescue or maintenance chemotherapy at conventional doses.[336] There is no current role for bone marrow or stem cell transplant in management of either early- or late-stage breast cancer.

Anti-*HER2* Therapy for Metastatic Breast Cancer

First-Line Treatment

Just as hormonal therapy radically alters that natural history of ER$^+$ metastatic breast cancer, so has anti-*HER2* treatment revolutionized outcomes for patients with *HER2*$^+$ breast cancer. Trastuzumab, the humanized anti-*HER2* monoclonal antibody, was the first anti-*HER2* agent to enter clinical practice. When added to first-line chemotherapy for *HER2*$^+$ metastatic breast cancer, trastuzumab improved response rates, time to progression, and OS.[337,338] Cardiomyopathy is a known side effect of trastuzumab therapy, and concurrent administration of trastuzumab and anthracyclines should be avoided. Serial determinations of left ventricular ejection fraction should be performed to screen for changes related to trastuzumab.[339]

Pertuzumab is a different anti-*HER2* antibody than trastuzumab, which binds to both *HER2* and *HER3* proteins, and is believed to prevent dimerization of those receptors. Clinically, the activity of pertuzumab seems dependent on coadministration of

trastuzumab.[340] The Placebo + Trastuzumab + Docetaxel in Previously Untreated HER2-positive Metastatic Breast Cancer study compared docetaxel/trastuzumab versus docetaxel/trastuzumab/pertuzumab as first-line treatment for *HER2*$^+$ breast cancer, and showed improvement in both progression-free survival and OS with the addition of pertuzumab.[341]

As the first anti-*HER2* agent, trastuzumab has served as the model for treatment principles for anti-*HER2*–based therapy. While responses can be seen with either single-agent trastuzumab or trastuzumab plus pertuzumab anti-*HER2* therapy,[340,342] the major benefits of these therapies have only been proven in combination with chemotherapy. The addition of anti-*HER2* treatments to endocrine therapy yields modest improvements in progression-free survival.[343,344] After an induction phase of therapy, the chemotherapy can be withheld, and endocrine therapy initiated (if appropriate), while continuing maintenance treatments with the antibodies. Currently, data for use of pertuzumab and trastuzumab are limited to concurrent administration with taxane-based chemotherapy. A variety of chemotherapy agents have shown clinical activity and safety when paired with trastuzumab, including taxanes, vinorelbine, and platinum analogs.

Refractory, *HER2*$^+$ Breast Cancer

A variety of clinical approaches are used to treat trastuzumab-refractory, *HER2*$^+$ metastatic breast cancer. Continuation of trastuzumab treatment beyond progression is associated with improvements in time to progression,[344,345] and justifies the practice of continued anti-*HER2* blockade in association with multiple lines of treatment for *HER2*$^+$ metastatic breast cancer. Lapatinib is a dual-kinase inhibitor that targets both the *HER2* and *EGFR* tyrosine kinase signaling pathways. Lapatinib has been studied as second-line anti-*HER2* therapy for patients progressing after chemotherapy and trastuzumab.[346] In comparison with the administration of capecitabine chemotherapy alone, the combination of lapatinib plus capecitabine was associated with a longer period of tumor control and improvement in response rate, but not survival.

Trastuzumab emtansine (TDM1) is a novel antibody-drug conjugate in which the trastuzumab antibody has been linked chemically to a potent chemotherapy moiety. The resulting conjugated antibody has been shown to have substantial activity in trastuzumab-refractory breast cancer, without the traditional side effects of chemotherapy, such as neutropenia or alopecia.[347] In a randomized trial of trastuzumab-resistant breast cancer, TDM1 was found to be superior to the combination of lapatinib/capecitabine with respect to progression-free survival, OS, and tolerability.[348] A study of first-line therapy for *HER2*$^+$ breast cancer found that TDM1 was more effective than docetaxel/trastuzumab, and led to dramatic improvements in quality of life.[349] Ongoing studies are examining the combination of TDM1 with pertuzumab, and assessing whether treatment beyond progression will prove clinically valuable.

Patients with *HER2*$^+$ metastatic breast cancer continue to receive clinical benefit from multiple lines of anti-*HER2* therapy,[350] and can have tumor responses even following progression on TDM1.[351]

Emerging Options for *BRCA1*- or *BRCA2*-Associated Breast Cancer

A novel class of therapeutics, drugs that inhibit the poly(adenosine diphosphate-ribose) polymerase (PARP) enzyme, are emerging as potentially valuable drugs in treatment of advanced breast cancer, particularly in hereditary breast cancer. In a proof of principle open-label phase 2 study, the PARP inhibitor olaparib was studied in patients with *BRCA1*- or *BRCA2*-associated cancers. This select group of patients was chosen because of preclinical data that suggested that tumors with *BRCA* deficiency might be particularly dependent on the DNA repair function of the PARP enzyme complex, and thus suitable targets for PARP inhibition. Initial observations have suggested robust responses among *BRCA*-associated breast cancers when patients are given single-agent therapy with olaparib.[352,353] In addition to PARP inhibitors, platinum-based chemotherapy may have a clinical role in hereditary breast cancers. Limited experience using platinum-based chemotherapy as neoadjuvant treatment for early-stage breast cancer has shown dramatic rates of pCR.[354] It remains unclear how important these findings are for either the long-term natural history of *BRCA*-associated breast cancer or treatment of metastatic disease.

Treatment of Special Metastatic Sites in Patients with Breast Cancer

Specialized treatment options are available for patients with breast cancer with metastases to selective anatomic sites. Patients with lytic bone metastases should receive bone targeted therapy either with intravenous bisphosphonate therapy, such as pamidronate or zoledronic acid, or the RANK-ligand inhibitor, denosumab.[355] These agents lessen the pain associated with bone lesions and prevent complications of skeletal metastases, including fracture and hypercalcemia.[356] Extended therapy can be associated with osteonecrosis of the jaw, so patients should be monitored for atypical oral lesions. Patients with focal pain at sites of skeletal metastases, pending fracture, or pathologic fracture may also benefit from external-beam RT at selected tumor sites and, when necessary, surgical stabilization or repair of the bone or joint.

Improvements in survival in metastatic breast cancer achieved through chemotherapy and trastuzumab-based treatment have led to an increase in the incidence of central nervous system metastases, especially those with *HER2*-overexpressing or hormone receptor–negative tumors.[357] Therapy for brain metastases remains inadequate, but generally includes WBI. Patients with isolated lesions, dominant masses, or recurrence after WBI may additionally be candidates for surgical resection or stereotactic RT to specific lesions. Patients with leptomeningeal disease may achieve symptomatic improvement with WBI or, in some cases, intrathecal chemotherapy with methotrexate or cytarabine. Very limited clinical experience suggests that some

systemic therapies, including endocrine treatments, chemotherapy agents including anthracyclines, alkylators, and capecitabine, and lapatinib, may have antitumor activity in the brain.[358] However, none of these are a substitute for local therapy to the brain.

Some patients with breast cancer will have limited sites of metastatic disease, such as isolated pulmonary nodules, isolated contralateral lymph node recurrence, or bone lesions. Single-institutional experience from the MD Anderson Cancer Center suggests that a fraction of such patients may be treated "aggressively" with curative intent, with favorable long-term results.[359] In a cohort of patients without previous adjuvant therapy and with oligometastatic disease that could be definitively treated with local therapy, "stage IV–NED" (no evidence of disease) the use of adjuvant chemotherapy, and, where appropriate, endocrine therapy resulted in 25% to 30% of patients remaining free of further recurrence through 10 years of follow-up.[359]

The treatment of the primary tumor in the breast in women who present with metastatic disease is another area of controversy. Historically, surgery or RT to the breast was limited to patients with local tumor complications, such as pain or skin erosion, and systemic drug therapy was the primary form of treatment. An analysis of 16,023 patients presenting with stage IV disease and an intact primary tumor compared outcomes between patients having surgery of the primary tumor to negative margins or no surgery. In a multivariate analysis adjusting for known prognostic factors, surgery reduced the HR for death to 0.61 (95% CI = 0.58 to 0.65).[83] Multiple other retrospective studies from single institutions, registries, and population-based cohorts have confirmed this initial observation, but it is uncertain whether these studies reflect a real benefit for surgery or consistent selection bias. Three prospective randomized trials are examining the role of surgery in patients presenting with stage IV disease and an intact primary tumor. While awaiting the results of these trials, it is not known precisely how or when to integrate such surgical management into standard medical therapy for metastatic breast cancer or which patients in particular are most likely to benefit from such treatment. Local therapy should not be used as an initial approach to the patient with metastatic disease, but may be considered in a highly selected group of patients with a good response to systemic therapy and a limited number of metastatic sites.

SELECTED REFERENCES

The full reference list can be accessed at lwwhealthlibrary.com/oncology.

5. Berry DA, Cronin KA, Plevritis SK, et al. Effect of screening and adjuvant therapy on mortality from breast cancer. *N Engl J Med* 2005;353:1784–1792.

9. Chen S, Parmigiani G. Meta-analysis of BRCA1 and BRCA2 penetrance. *J Clin Oncol* 2007;25:1329–1333.

10. Metcalfe KA, Finch A, Poll A, et al. Breast cancer risks in women with a family history of breast or ovarian cancer who have tested negative for a BRCA1 or BRCA2 mutation. *Br J Cancer* 2009;100:421–425.

11. Kurian AW, Gong GD, John EM, et al. Breast cancer risk for noncarriers of family-specific BRCA1 and BRCA2 mutations: findings from the Breast Cancer Family Registry. *J Clin Oncol* 2011;29:4505–4509.

13. U.S. Preventive Services Task Force. Genetic risk assessment and BRCA mutation testing for breast and ovarian cancer susceptibility: recommendation statement. *Ann Intern Med* 2005;143:355–361.

19. Kauff ND, Satagopan JM, Robson ME, et al. Risk-reducing salpingo-oophorectomy in women with a BRCA1 or BRCA2 mutation. *N Engl J Med* 2002;346:1609–1615.

23. Chlebowski RT, Hendrix SL, Langer RD, et al. Influence of estrogen plus progestin on breast cancer and mammography in healthy postmenopausal women: the Women's Health Initiative Randomized Trial. *JAMA* 2003;289: 3243–3253.

25. Alexander DD, Morimoto LM, Mink PJ, et al. Summary and meta-analysis of prospective studies of animal fat intake and breast cancer. *Nutr Res Rev* 2010;23:169–179.

26. Prentice RL, Caan B, Chlebowski RT, et al. Low-fat dietary pattern and risk of invasive breast cancer: the Women's Health Initiative Randomized Controlled Dietary Modification Trial. *JAMA* 2006;295:629–642.

28. Willett WC, Tamini RM, Hankinson SE, et al. Non-genetic factors in the causation of breast cancer. In: Harris JR, Lippman ME, Morrow M, et al., eds. *Diseases of the Breast*, 4th ed. Philadelphia: Wolters Kluwer/Lippincott Williams and Wilkins; 2010:248.

30. Dupont WD, Page DL. Risk factors for breast cancer in women with proliferative breast disease. *N Engl J Med* 1985;312:146–151.

31. Boyd NF, Guo H, Martin LJ, et al. Mammographic density and the risk and detection of breast cancer. *N Engl J Med* 2007;356:227–236.

32. Elkin EB, Klem ML, Gonzales AM, et al. Characteristics and outcomes of breast cancer in women with and without a history of radiation for Hodgkin's lymphoma: a multi-institutional, matched cohort study. *J Clin Oncol* 2011; 29:2466–2473.

33. Gail MH, Brinton LA, Byar DP, et al. Projecting individualized probabilities of developing breast cancer for white females who are being examined annually. *J Natl Cancer Inst* 1989;81:1879–1886.

34. Fisher B, Costantino JP, Wickerham DL, et al. Tamoxifen for prevention of breast cancer: report of the National Surgical Adjuvant Breast and Bowel Project P-1 Study. *J Natl Cancer Inst* 1998;90:1371–1388.

37. King TA, Muhsen S, Patil S, et al. Is there a role for routine screening MRI in women with LCIS? *Breast Cancer Res Treat* 2013;142:445–453.

39. Saslow D, Boetes C, Burke W, et al. American Cancer Society guidelines for breast screening with MRI as an adjunct to mammography. *CA Cancer J Clin* 2007;57:75–89.

40. Cuzick J, Forbes J, Edwards R, et al. First results from the International Breast Cancer Intervention Study (IBIS-I): a randomised prevention trial. *Lancet* 2002;360:817–824.

43. Cuzick J, Powles T, Veronesi U, et al. Overview of the main outcomes in breast-cancer prevention trials. *Lancet* 2003;361:296–300.

46. Goss PE, Ingle JN, Ales-Martinez JE, et al. Exemestane for breast-cancer prevention in postmenopausal women. *N Engl J Med* 2011;364:2381–2391.

47. Visvanathan K, Hurley P, Bantug E, et al. Use of pharmacologic interventions for breast cancer risk reduction: American Society of Clinical Oncology clinical practice guideline. *J Clin Oncol* 2013;31:2942–2962.

50. Rebbeck TR, Friebel T, Lynch HT, et al. Bilateral prophylactic mastectomy reduces breast cancer risk in BRCA1 and BRCA2 mutation carriers: the PROSE Study Group. *J Clin Oncol* 2004;22:1055–1062.

51. Rebbeck TR, Kauff ND, Domchek SM. Meta-analysis of risk reduction estimates associated with risk-reducing salpingo-oophorectomy in BRCA1 or BRCA2 mutation carriers. *J Natl Cancer Inst* 2009;101:80–87.

60. Murray MP, Luedtke C, Liberman L, et al. Classic lobular carcinoma in situ and atypical lobular hyperplasia at percutaneous breast core biopsy: outcomes of prospective excision. *Cancer* 2013;119:1073–1079.

62. Solin LJ, Gray R, Baehner FL, et al. A multigene expression assay to predict local recurrence risk for ductal carcinoma in situ of the breast. *J Natl Cancer Inst* 2013;105:701–710.

63. EORTC Breast Cancer Cooperative Group, EORTC Radiotherapy Group, Bijker N, et al. Breast-conserving treatment with or without radiotherapy in ductal carcinoma-in-situ: ten-year results of European Organisation for Research and Treatment of Cancer randomized phase III trial 10853—a study by the EORTC Breast Cancer Cooperative Group and EORTC Radiotherapy Group. *J Clin Oncol* 2006;24:3381–3387.

64. Wapnir IL, Dignam JJ, Fisher B, et al. Long-term outcomes of invasive ipsilateral breast tumor recurrences after lumpectomy in NSABP B-17 and B-24 randomized clinical trials for DCIS. *J Natl Cancer Inst* 2011;103:478–488.

68. Pilewskie M, Kennedy C, Shappell C, et al. Effect of MRI on the management of ductal carcinoma in situ of the breast. *Ann Surg Oncol* 2013;20:1522–1529.

69. Cuzick J, Sestak I, Pinder SE, et al. Effect of tamoxifen and radiotherapy in women with locally excised ductal carcinoma in situ: long-term results from the UK/ANZ DCIS trial. *Lancet Oncol* 2011;12:21–29.

70. Holmberg L, Garmo H, Granstrand B, et al. Absolute risk reductions for local recurrence after postoperative radiotherapy after sector resection for ductal carcinoma in situ of the breast. *J Clin Oncol* 2008;26:1247–1252.

71. Early Breast Cancer Trialists' Collaborative Group, Correa C, McGale P, et al. Overview of the randomized trials of radiotherapy in ductal carcinoma in situ of the breast. *J Natl Cancer Inst Monogr* 2010;2010:162–177.

72. McCormick B, Stock K, Moughan VJ, et al. Low-risk breast ductal carcinoma in situ (DCIS): results from the Radiation Therapy Oncology Group 9804 phase 3 trial. *Int J Radiat Oncol* 2012;84:S5.

74. Wong JS, Chen YH, Gadd MA, et al. Eight-year update of a prospective study of wide excision alone for ductal carcinoma in situ (DCIS). *Breast Cancer Res Treat* 2014;143:343–350.

76. Allred DC, Anderson SJ, Paik S, et al. Adjuvant tamoxifen reduces subsequent breast cancer in women with estrogen receptor-positive ductal carcinoma in situ: a study based on NSABP protocol B-24. *J Clin Oncol* 2012;30:1268–1273.

83. Khan SA, Stewart AK, Morrow M. Does aggressive local therapy improve survival in metastatic breast cancer? *Surgery* 2002;132:620–626, discussion 626–627.

86. Fisher B, Anderson S, Bryant J, et al. Twenty-year follow-up of a randomized trial comparing total mastectomy, lumpectomy, and lumpectomy plus irradiation for the treatment of invasive breast cancer. *N Engl J Med* 2002;347:1233–1241.

87. Veronesi U, Cascinelli N, Mariani L, et al. Twenty-year follow-up of a randomized study comparing breast-conserving surgery with radical mastectomy for early breast cancer. *N Engl J Med* 2002;347:1227–1232.

88. Clarke M, Collins R, Darby S, et al. Effects of radiotherapy and of differences in the extent of surgery for early breast cancer on local recurrence and 15-year survival: an overview of the randomised trials. *Lancet* 2005;366:2087–2106.

89. Morrow M, Jagsi R, Alderman AK, et al. Surgeon recommendations and receipt of mastectomy for treatment of breast cancer. *JAMA* 2009;302:1551–1556.

90. Katz SJ, Lantz PM, Janz NK, et al. Patient involvement in surgery treatment decisions for breast cancer. *J Clin Oncol* 2005;23:5526–5533.

92. Anderson SJ, Wapnir I, Dignam JJ, et al. Prognosis after ipsilateral breast tumor recurrence and locoregional recurrences in patients treated by breast-conserving therapy in five National Surgical Adjuvant Breast and Bowel Project protocols of node-negative breast cancer. *J Clin Oncol* 2009;27:2466–2473.

95. Moran MS, Schnitt SJ, Giuliano AE, et al. SSO-ASTRO consensus guideline on margins for breast-conserving surgery with whole breast irradiation in stage I and II invasive breast cancer. *J Clin Oncol* 2014;21(5):1512–1514.

96. Arvold ND, Taghian AG, Niemierko A, et al. Age, breast cancer subtype approximation, and local recurrence after breast-conserving therapy. *J Clin Oncol* 2011;29:3885–3891.

100. Mamounas EP, Tang G, Fisher B, et al. Association between the 21-gene recurrence score assay and risk of locoregional recurrence in node-negative, estrogen receptor-positive breast cancer: results from NSABP B-14 and NSABP B-20. *J Clin Oncol* 2010;28:1677–1683.

101. Bartelink H, Horiot JC, Poortmans PM, et al. Impact of a higher radiation dose on local control and survival in breast-conserving therapy of early breast cancer: 10-year results of the randomized boost versus no boost EORTC 22881-10882 trial. *J Clin Oncol* 2007;25:3259–3265.

104. Dalberg K, Johansson H, Johansson U, et al. A randomized trial of long term adjuvant tamoxifen plus postoperative radiation therapy versus radiation therapy alone for patients with early stage breast carcinoma treated with breast-conserving surgery. Stockholm Breast Cancer Study Group. *Cancer* 1998;82:2204–2211.

105. Fisher B, Bryant J, Dignam JJ, et al. Tamoxifen, radiation therapy, or both for prevention of ipsilateral breast tumor recurrence after lumpectomy in women with invasive breast cancers of one centimeter or less. *J Clin Oncol* 2002;20:4141–4149.

109. de la Rochefordiere A, Abner AL, Silver B, et al. Are cosmetic results following conservative surgery and radiation therapy for early breast cancer dependent on technique? *Int J Radiat Oncol Biol Phys* 1992;23:925–931.

110. Houssami N, Turner R, Morrow M. Preoperative magnetic resonance imaging in breast cancer: meta-analysis of surgical outcomes. *Ann Surg* 2013;257:249–255.

114. Prowell TM, Pazdur R. Pathological complete response and accelerated drug approval in early breast cancer. *N Engl J Med* 2012;366:2438–2441.

116. van der Hage JA, van de Velde CJ, Julien JP, et al. Preoperative chemotherapy in primary operable breast cancer: results from the European Organization for Research and Treatment of Cancer trial 10902. *J Clin Oncol* 2001;19:4224–4237.

117. Gianni L, Eiermann W, Semiglazov V, et al. Neoadjuvant chemotherapy with trastuzumab followed by adjuvant trastuzumab versus neoadjuvant chemotherapy alone, in patients with HER2-positive locally advanced breast cancer (the NOAH trial): a randomised controlled superiority trial with a parallel HER2-negative cohort. *Lancet* 2010;375:377–384.

118. Gianni L, Pienkowski T, Im YH, et al. Efficacy and safety of neoadjuvant pertuzumab and trastuzumab in women with locally advanced, inflammatory, or early HER2-positive breast cancer (NeoSphere): a randomised multicentre, open-label, phase 2 trial. *Lancet Oncol* 2012;13:25–32.

120. Mamounas EP, Anderson SJ, Dignam JJ, et al. Predictors of locoregional recurrence after neoadjuvant chemotherapy: results from combined analysis of National Surgical Adjuvant Breast and Bowel Project B-18 and B-27. *J Clin Oncol* 2012;30:3960–3966.

122. Smith IE, Dowsett M, Ebbs SR, et al. Neoadjuvant treatment of postmenopausal breast cancer with anastrozole, tamoxifen, or both in combination: the Immediate Preoperative Anastrozole, Tamoxifen, or Combined with Tamoxifen (IMPACT) multicenter double-blind randomized trial. *J Clin Oncol* 2005;23:5108–5116.

125. Early Breast Cancer Trialists' Collaborative Group, Darby S, McGale P, et al. Effect of radiotherapy after breast-conserving surgery on 10-year recurrence and 15-year breast cancer death: meta-analysis of individual patient data for 10,801 women in 17 randomised trials. *Lancet* 2011;378:1707–1716.

128. Fyles AW, McCready DR, Manchul LA, et al. Tamoxifen with or without breast irradiation in women 50 years of age or older with early breast cancer. *N Engl J Med* 2004;351:963–970.

129. Hughes KS, Schnaper LA, Bellon JR, et al. Lumpectomy plus tamoxifen with or without irradiation in women age 70 years or older with early breast cancer: long-term follow-up of CALGB 9343. *J Clin Oncol* 2013;31:2382–2387.

131. Whelan TJ, Pignol JP, Levine MN, et al. Long-term results of hypofractionated radiation therapy for breast cancer. *N Engl J Med* 2010;362:513–520.

132. Smith BD, Bentzen SM, Correa CR, et al. Fractionation for whole breast irradiation: an American Society for Radiation Oncology (ASTRO) evidence-based guideline. *Int J Radiat Oncol Biol Phys* 2011;81:59–68.

133. Haviland JS, Owen JR, Dewar JA, et al. The UK Standardisation of Breast Radiotherapy (START) trials of radiotherapy hypofractionation for treatment of early breast cancer: 10-year follow-up results of two randomised controlled trials. *Lancet Oncol* 2013;14:1086–1094.

134. Russo AL, Arvold ND, Niemierko A, et al. Margin status and the risk of local recurrence in patients with early-stage breast cancer treated with breast-conserving therapy. *Breast Cancer Res Treat* 2013;140:353–361.

135. Smith BD, Arthur DW, Buchholz TA, et al. Accelerated partial breast irradiation consensus statement from the American Society for Radiation Oncology (ASTRO). *Int J Radiat Oncol Biol Phys* 2009;74:987–1001.

136. Olivotto IA, Whelan TJ, Parpia S, et al. Interim cosmetic and toxicity results from RAPID: a randomized trial of accelerated partial breast irradiation using three-dimensional conformal external beam radiation therapy. *J Clin Oncol* 2013;31:4038–4045.

137. Veronesi U, Orecchia R, Maisonneuve P, et al. Intraoperative radiotherapy versus external radiotherapy for early breast cancer (ELIOT): a randomised controlled equivalence trial. *Lancet Oncol* 2013;14:1269–1277.

138. Darby SC, Ewertz M, McGale P, et al. Risk of ischemic heart disease in women after radiotherapy for breast cancer. *N Engl J Med* 2013;368:987–998.

142. Petit JY, Veronesi U, Orecchia R, et al. Risk factors associated with recurrence after nipple-sparing mastectomy for invasive and intraepithelial neoplasia. *Ann Oncol* 2012;23:2053–2058.

143. Motwani SB, Strom EA, Schechter NR, et al. The impact of immediate breast reconstruction on the technical delivery of postmastectomy radiotherapy. *Int J Radiat Oncol Biol Phys* 2006;66:76–82.

147. Fisher B, Jeong JH, Anderson S, et al. Twenty-five-year follow-up of a randomized trial comparing radical mastectomy, total mastectomy, and total mastectomy followed by irradiation. *N Engl J Med* 2002;347:567–575.

150. Posther KE, McCall LM, Blumencranz PW, et al. Sentinel node skills verification and surgeon performance: data from a multicenter clinical trial for early-stage breast cancer. *Ann Surg* 2005;242:593–599, discussion 599–602.

151. Krag DN, Anderson SJ, Julian TB, et al. Sentinel-lymph-node resection compared with conventional axillary-lymph-node dissection in clinically node-negative patients with breast cancer: overall survival findings from the NSABP B-32 randomised phase 3 trial. *Lancet Oncol* 2010;11:927–933.

153. Mansel RE, Fallowfield L, Kissin M, et al. Randomized multicenter trial of sentinel node biopsy versus standard axillary treatment in operable breast cancer: the ALMANAC Trial. *J Natl Cancer Inst* 2006;98:599–609.

155. Veronesi U, Paganelli G, Viale G, et al. Sentinel-lymph-node biopsy as a staging procedure in breast cancer: update of a randomised controlled study. *Lancet Oncol* 2006;7:983–990.

157. van Deurzen CH, Vriens BE, Tjan-Heijnen VC, et al. Accuracy of sentinel node biopsy after neoadjuvant chemotherapy in breast cancer patients: a systematic review. *Eur J Cancer* 2009;45:3124–3130.

159. Boughey JC, Suman VJ, Mittendorf EA, et al. Sentinel lymph node surgery after neoadjuvant chemotherapy in patients with node-positive breast cancer: the ACOSOG Z1071 (Alliance) clinical trial. *JAMA* 2013;310:1455–1461.

160. Kuehn T, Bauerfeind I, Fehm T, et al. Sentinel-lymph-node biopsy in patients with breast cancer before and after neoadjuvant chemotherapy (SENTINA): a prospective, multicentre cohort study. *Lancet Oncol* 2013;14:609–618.

161. Giuliano AE, Hawes D, Ballman KV, et al. Association of occult metastases in sentinel lymph nodes and bone marrow with survival among women with early-stage invasive breast cancer. *JAMA* 2011;306:385–393.

163. Galimberti V, Cole BF, Zurrida S, et al. Axillary dissection versus no axillary dissection in patients with sentinel-node micrometastases (IBCSG 23-01): a phase 3 randomised controlled trial. *Lancet Oncol* 2013;14:297–305.

165. Morrow M, Harris JR, Schnitt SJ. Surgical margins in lumpectomy for breast cancer—bigger is not better. *N Engl J Med* 2012;367:79–82.

166. Giuliano AE, Hunt KK, Ballman KV, et al. Axillary dissection vs no axillary dissection in women with invasive breast cancer and sentinel node metastasis: a randomized clinical trial. *JAMA* 2011;305:569–575.

167. Dengel LT, Van Zee KJ, King TA, et al. Axillary dissection can be avoided in the majority of clinically node-negative patients undergoing breast-conserving therapy. *Ann Surg Oncol* 2014;21:22–27.

168. Rutgers EJ, Donker M, Straver ME, et al. Radiotherapy or surgery of the axilla after a positive sentinel node in breast cancer patients: Final analysis of the EORTC AMAROS trial (10981/22023). *J Clin Oncol* 2013;31:Abstr LBA1001.

169. Whelan TJ, Olivotto I, Ackerman I, et al. NCIC CTG MA.20: An intergroup trial of regional nodal irradiation in early breast cancer. *J Clin Oncol* 2011;29:Abstr LBA1003.

173. Kyndi M, Overgaard M, Nielsen HM, et al. High local recurrence risk is not associated with large survival reduction after postmastectomy radiotherapy in high-risk breast cancer: a subgroup analysis of DBCG 82 b&c. *Radiother Oncol* 2009;90:74–79.

175. Punglia RS, Morrow M, Winer EP, et al. Local therapy and survival in breast cancer. *N Engl J Med* 2007;356:2399–2405.

176. Poortmans P, Struikmans H, Kirkove C, et al. Irradiation of the internal mammary and medial supraclavicular lymph nodes in stage I to III breast cancer: 10 years results of the EORTC Radiation Oncology and Breast Cancer Groups phase III trial 22922/10925. Proceedings of the 2013 ECCO Conference. Abstract No. 2.

178. Hammond ME, Hayes DF, Dowsett M, et al. American Society of Clinical Oncology/College Of American Pathologists guideline recommendations for immunohistochemical testing of estrogen and progesterone receptors in breast cancer. *J Clin Oncol* 2010;28:2784–2795.

182. Cancello G, Maisonneuve P, Rotmensz N, et al. Prognosis and adjuvant treatment effects in selected breast cancer subtypes of very young women (<35 years) with operable breast cancer. *Ann Oncol* 2010;21:1974–1981.

183. Piccart-Gebhart MJ. Anthracyclines and the tailoring of treatment for early breast cancer. *N Engl J Med* 2006;354:2177–2179.

184. Perez EA, Dueck AC, McCullough AE, et al. Predictability of adjuvant trastuzumab benefit in N9831 breast cancer using the ASCO/CAP HER2-positivity criteria. *J Natl Cancer Inst* 2012;104:159–162.

187. Sorlie T, Tibshirani R, Parker J, et al. Repeated observation of breast tumor subtypes in independent gene expression data sets. *Proc Natl Acad Sci U S A* 2003;100:8418–8423.

188. Perou CM, Sorlie T, Eisen MB, et al. Molecular portraits of human breast tumours. *Nature* 2000;406:747–752.

192. Cancer Genome Atlas Network. Comprehensive molecular portraits of human breast tumours. *Nature* 2012;490:61–70.

193. van de Vijver MJ, He YD, van't Veer LJ, et al. A gene-expression signature as a predictor of survival in breast cancer. *N Engl J Med* 2002;347:1999–2009.

196. Paik S, Shak S, Tang G, et al. A multigene assay to predict recurrence of tamoxifen-treated, node-negative breast cancer. *N Engl J Med* 2004;351:2817–2826.

197. Dowsett M, Cuzick J, Wale C, et al. Prediction of risk of distant recurrence using the 21-gene recurrence score in node-negative and node-positive postmenopausal patients with breast cancer treated with anastrozole or tamoxifen: a TransATAC study. *J Clin Oncol* 2010;28:1829–1834.

198. Paik S, Tang G, Shak S, et al. Gene expression and benefit of chemotherapy in women with node-negative, estrogen receptor-positive breast cancer. *J Clin Oncol* 2006;24:3726–3734.

199. Albain KS, Barlow WE, Shak S, et al. Prognostic and predictive value of the 21-gene recurrence score assay in postmenopausal women with node-positive, oestrogen-receptor-positive breast cancer on chemotherapy: a retrospective analysis of a randomised trial. *Lancet Oncol* 2010;11:55–65.

200. Fan C, Oh DS, Wessels L, et al. Concordance among gene-expression-based predictors for breast cancer. *N Engl J Med* 2006;355:560–569.

202. Early Breast Cancer Trialists' Collaborative Group. Effects of chemotherapy and hormonal therapy for early breast cancer on recurrence and 15-year survival: an overview of the randomised trials. *Lancet* 2005;365:1687–1717.

204. Davies C, Pan H, Godwin J, et al. Long-term effects of continuing adjuvant tamoxifen to 10 years versus stopping at 5 years after diagnosis of oestrogen-receptor-positive breast cancer: ATLAS, a randomised trial. *Lancet* 2013;381:805–816.

209. Baum M, Budzar AU, Cuzick J, et al. Anastrozole alone or in combination with tamoxifen versus tamoxifen alone for adjuvant treatment of postmenopausal women with early breast cancer: first results of the ATAC randomised trial. *Lancet* 2002;359:2131–2139.

211. Thurlimann B, Keshaviah A, Coates AS, et al. A comparison of letrozole and tamoxifen in postmenopausal women with early breast cancer. *N Engl J Med* 2005;353:2747–2757.

212. Coombes RC, Hall E, Gibson LJ, et al. A randomized trial of exemestane after two to three years of tamoxifen therapy in postmenopausal women with primary breast cancer. *N Engl J Med* 2004;350:1081–1092.

213. Jakesz R, Jonat W, Gnant M, et al. Switching of postmenopausal women with endocrine-responsive early breast cancer to anastrozole after 2 years' adjuvant tamoxifen: combined results of ABCSG trial 8 and ARNO 95 trial. *Lancet* 2005;366:455–462.

214. Goss PE, Ingle JN, Martino S, et al. Randomized trial of letrozole following tamoxifen as extended adjuvant therapy in receptor-positive breast cancer: updated findings from NCIC CTG MA.17. *J Natl Cancer Inst* 2005;97:1262–1271.

216. Mamounas EP, Jeong JH, Wickerham DL, et al. Benefit from exemestane as extended adjuvant therapy after 5 years of adjuvant tamoxifen: intention-to-treat analysis of the National Surgical Adjuvant Breast And Bowel Project B-33 trial. *J Clin Oncol* 2008;26:1965–1971.

217. Mouridsen H, Giobbie-Hurder A, Goldhirsch A, et al. Letrozole therapy alone or in sequence with tamoxifen in women with breast cancer. *N Engl J Med* 2009;361:766–776.

218. Rea D, Hasenburg A, Seynaeve C, et al. Five years of exemestane as initial therapy compared to 5 years of tamoxifen followed by exemestane: the TEAM Trial, a prospective, randomized, phase III trial in postmenopausal women with hormone-sensitive early breast cancer. *Cancer Res* 2009;69:11.

219. Goss PE, Ingle JN, Pritchard KI, et al. Exemestane versus anastrozole in postmenopausal women with early breast cancer: NCIC CTG MA.27—a randomized controlled phase III trial. *J Clin Oncol* 2013;31:1398–1404.

220. Burstein HJ, Prestrud AA, Seidenfeld J, et al. American Society of Clinical Oncology clinical practice guideline: update on adjuvant endocrine therapy for women with hormone receptor-positive breast cancer. *J Clin Oncol* 2010;28:3784–3796.

226. Aebi S, Gelber S, Castiglione-Gertsch M, et al. Is chemotherapy alone adequate for young women with oestrogen-receptor-positive breast cancer? *Lancet* 2000;355:1869–1874.

227. Davidson NE, O'Neill AM, Vukov AM, et al. Chemoendocrine therapy for premenopausal women with axillary lymph node-positive, steroid hormone receptor-positive breast cancer: results from INT 0101 (E5188). *J Clin Oncol* 2005;23:5973–5982.

228. Adjuvant Breast Cancer Trialists' Group. Ovarian ablation or suppression in premenopausal early breast cancer: results from the international adjuvant breast cancer ovarian ablation or suppression randomized trial. *J Natl Cancer Inst* 2007;99:516–525.

236. Murphy CC, Bartholomew LK, Carpentier MY, et al. Adherence to adjuvant hormonal therapy among breast cancer survivors in clinical practice: a systematic review. *Breast Cancer Res Treat* 2012;134:459–478.

237. Peto R, Davies C, Godwin J, et al. Comparisons between different polychemotherapy regimens for early breast cancer: meta-analyses of long-term outcome among 100,000 women in 123 randomised trials. *Lancet* 2012;379:432–444.

238. Goldhirsch A, Winer EP, Coates AS, et al. Personalizing the treatment of women with early breast cancer: highlights of the St Gallen International Expert Consensus on the Primary Therapy of Early Breast Cancer 2013. *Ann Oncol* 2013;24:2206–2223.

239. Henderson IC, Berry DA, Demetri GD, et al. Improved outcomes from adding sequential Paclitaxel but not from escalating Doxorubicin dose in an adjuvant chemotherapy regimen for patients with node-positive primary breast cancer. *J Clin Oncol* 2003;21:976–983.

240. Fisher B, Jeong JH, Anderson S, et al. Treatment of axillary lymph node-negative, estrogen receptor-negative breast cancer: updated findings from National Surgical Adjuvant Breast and Bowel Project clinical trials. *J Natl Cancer Inst* 2004;96:1823–1831.

241. Sparano JA, Wang M, Martino S, et al. Weekly paclitaxel in the adjuvant treatment of breast cancer. *N Engl J Med* 2008;358:1663–1671.

243. Swain SM, Tang G, Geyer CE Jr, et al. Definitive results of a phase III adjuvant trial comparing three chemotherapy regimens in women with operable, node-positive breast cancer: the NSABP B-38 trial. *J Clin Oncol* 2013;31:3197–3204.

245. Joensuu H, Kellokumpu-Lehtinen PL, Huovinen R, et al. Adjuvant capecitabine, docetaxel, cyclophosphamide, and epirubicin for early breast cancer: final analysis of the randomized FinXX trial. *J Clin Oncol* 2012;30:11–18.

246. Jones S, Holmes FA, O'Shaughnessy J, et al. Docetaxel with cyclophosphamide is associated with an overall survival benefit compared with doxorubicin and cyclophosphamide: 7-year follow-up of US Oncology Research Trial 9735. *J Clin Oncol* 2009;27:1177–1183.

247. Shulman LN, Cirrincione CT, Berry DA, et al. Six cycles of doxorubicin and cyclophosphamide or Paclitaxel are not superior to four cycles as adjuvant chemotherapy for breast cancer in women with zero to three positive axillary nodes: Cancer and Leukemia Group B 40101. *J Clin Oncol* 2012;30:4071–4076.

248. Fisher B, Dignam J, Tan-Chiu E, et al. Prognosis and treatment of patients with breast tumors of one centimeter or less and negative axillary lymph nodes. *J Natl Cancer Inst* 2001;93:112–120.

250. Berry DA, Cirrincione C, Henderson IC, et al. Estrogen-receptor status and outcomes of modern chemotherapy for patients with node-positive breast cancer. *JAMA* 2006;295:1658–1667.

258. Joensuu H, Kellokumpu-Lehtinen PL, Bono P, et al. Adjuvant docetaxel or vinorelbine with or without trastuzumab for breast cancer. *N Engl J Med* 2006;354:809–820.

259. Piccart-Gebhart MJ, Procter M, Leyland-Jones B, et al. Trastuzumab after adjuvant chemotherapy in HER2-positive breast cancer. *N Engl J Med* 2005;353:1659–1672.

260. Tan-Chiu E, Yothers G, Romond E, et al. Assessment of cardiac dysfunction in a randomized trial comparing doxorubicin and cyclophosphamide followed by paclitaxel, with or without trastuzumab as adjuvant therapy in node-positive, human epidermal growth factor receptor 2-overexpressing breast cancer: NSABP B-31. *J Clin Oncol* 2005;23:7811–7819.

261. Slamon D, Eiermann W, Robert N, et al. Adjuvant trastuzumab in HER2-positive breast cancer. *N Engl J Med* 2011;365:1273–1283.

263. Pivot X, Romieu G, Debled M, et al. 6 months versus 12 months of adjuvant trastuzumab for patients with HER2-positive early breast cancer (PHARE): a randomised phase 3 trial. *Lancet Oncol* 2013;14:741–748.

264. Goldhirsch A, Gelber RD, Piccart-Gebhart MJ, et al. 2 years versus 1 year of adjuvant trastuzumab for HER2-positive breast cancer (HERA): an open-label, randomised controlled trial. *Lancet* 2013;382:1021–1028.

265. Perez EA, Suman VJ, Davidson NE, et al. Sequential versus concurrent trastuzumab in adjuvant chemotherapy for breast cancer. *J Clin Oncol* 2011;29:4491–4497.

268. McArthur HL, Mahoney KM, Morris PG, et al. Adjuvant trastuzumab with chemotherapy is effective in women with small, node-negative, HER2-positive breast cancer. *Cancer* 2011;117:5461–5468.

273. Burstein HJ, Winer EP. Primary care for survivors of breast cancer. *N Engl J Med* 2000;343:1086–1094.

274. GIVIO Investigators. Impact of follow-up testing on survival and health-related quality of life in breast cancer patients. A multicenter randomized controlled trial. The GIVIO Investigators. *JAMA* 1994;271:1587–1592.

275. Rosselli Del Turco M, Palli D, Cariddi A, et al. Intensive diagnostic follow-up after treatment of primary breast cancer. A randomized trial. National Research Council Project on Breast Cancer follow-up. *JAMA* 1994;271:1593–1597.

276. Khatcheressian JL, Wolff AC, Smith TJ, et al. American Society of Clinical Oncology 2006 update of the breast cancer follow-up and management guidelines in the adjuvant setting. *J Clin Oncol* 2006;24:5091–5097.

279. Bijker N, Rutgers EJ, Duchateau L, et al. Breast-conserving therapy for Paget disease of the nipple: a prospective European Organization for Research and Treatment of Cancer study of 61 patients. *Cancer* 2001;91:472–477.

282. de Bresser J, de Vos B, van der Ent F, et al. Breast MRI in clinically and mammographically occult breast cancer presenting with an axillary metastasis: a systematic review. *Eur J Surg Oncol* 2010;36:114–119.

284. Merson M, Andreola S, Galimberti V, et al. Breast carcinoma presenting as axillary metastases without evidence of a primary tumor. *Cancer* 1992;70:504–508.

287. Loibl S, von Minckwitz G, Gwyn K, et al. Breast carcinoma during pregnancy. International recommendations from an expert meeting. *Cancer* 2006;106:237–246.

289. Litton JK, Theriault RL. Breast cancer during pregnancy and subsequent pregnancy in breast cancer survivors. In: Harris JR, Lippman ME, Morrow M, et al., eds. *Diseases of the Breast*, 5th ed. Philadelphia: Lippincott Williams and Wilkins (In Press).

292. Berry DL, Theriault RL, Holmes FA, et al. Management of breast cancer during pregnancy using a standardized protocol. *J Clin Oncol* 1999;17:855–861.

294. Zagouri F, Sergentanis TN, Chrysikos D, et al. Trastuzumab administration during pregnancy: a systematic review and meta-analysis. *Breast Cancer Res Treat* 2013;137:349–357.

296. Anderson WF, Jatoi I, Tse J, et al. Male breast cancer: a population-based comparison with female breast cancer. *J Clin Oncol* 2010;28:232–239.

300. Walshe JM, Berman AW, Vatas U, et al. A prospective study of adjuvant CMF in males with node positive breast cancer: 20-year follow-up. *Breast Cancer Res Treat* 2007;103:177–183.

301. Eggemann H, Ignatov A, Smith BJ, et al. Adjuvant therapy with tamoxifen compared to aromatase inhibitors for 257 male breast cancer patients. *Breast Cancer Res Treat* 2013;137:465–470.

302. Asoglu O, Ugurlu MM, Blanchard K, et al. Risk factors for recurrence and death after primary surgical treatment of malignant phyllodes tumors. *Ann Surg Oncol* 2004;11:1011–1017.

304. Cristofanilli M, Gonzalez-Angulo AM, Buzdar AU, et al. Paclitaxel improves the prognosis in estrogen receptor negative inflammatory breast cancer: the M. D. Anderson Cancer Center experience. *Clin Breast Cancer* 2004;4:415–419.

305. Hennessy BT, Gonzalez-Angulo AM, Hortobagyi GN, et al. Disease-free and overall survival after pathologic complete disease remission of cytologically proven inflammatory breast carcinoma axillary lymph node metastases after primary systemic chemotherapy. *Cancer* 2006;106:1000–1006.

308. Huang EH, Strom EA, Perkins GH, et al. Comparison of risk of local-regional recurrence after mastectomy or breast conservation therapy for patients treated with neoadjuvant chemotherapy and radiation stratified according to a prognostic index score. *Int J Radiat Oncol Biol Phys* 2006;66:352–357.

313. Aebi S, Gelber S, Lang I, et al. Chemotherapy prolongs survival for isolated local or regional recurrence of breast cancer: The CALOR trial (Chemotherapy as Adjuvant for Locally Recurrent breast cancer; IBCSG 27-02, NSABP B-37, BIG 1-02). *Cancer Res* 2012;72:3227–3231.

315. Bergh J, Jonsson PE, Lidbrink EK, et al. FACT: an open-label randomized phase III study of fulvestrant and anastrozole in combination compared with anastrozole alone as first-line therapy for patients with receptor-positive postmenopausal breast cancer. *J Clin Oncol* 2012;30:1919–1925.

316. Johnston SR, Kilburn LS, Ellis P, et al. Fulvestrant plus anastrozole or placebo versus exemestane alone after progression on non-steroidal aromatase inhibitors in postmenopausal patients with hormone-receptor-positive locally advanced or metastatic breast cancer (SoFEA): a composite, multicentre, phase 3 randomised trial. *Lancet Oncol* 2013;14:989–998.

317. Mehta RS, Barlow WE, Albain KS, et al. Combination anastrozole and fulvestrant in metastatic breast cancer. *N Engl J Med* 2012;367:435–444.

318. Baselga J, Campone M, Piccart M, et al. Everolimus in postmenopausal hormone-receptor-positive advanced breast cancer. *N Engl J Med* 2012;366:520–529.

319. Buzdar AU, Jonat W, Howell A, et al. Anastrozole versus megestrol acetate in the treatment of postmenopausal women with advanced breast carcinoma: results of a survival update based on a combined analysis of data from two mature phase III trials. Arimidex Study Group. *Cancer* 1998;83:1142–1152.

320. Buzdar A, Douma J, Davidson N, et al. Phase III, multicenter, double-blind, randomized study of letrozole, an aromatase inhibitor, for advanced breast cancer versus megestrol acetate. *J Clin Oncol* 2001;19:3357–3366.

321. Bonneterre J, Thurlimann B, Robertson JF, et al. Anastrozole versus tamoxifen as first-line therapy for advanced breast cancer in 668 postmenopausal women: results of the Tamoxifen or Arimidex Randomized Group Efficacy and Tolerability study. *J Clin Oncol* 2000;18:3748–3757.

322. Mouridsen H, Gershanovich M, Sun Y, et al. Superior efficacy of letrozole versus tamoxifen as first-line therapy for postmenopausal women with advanced breast cancer: results of a phase III study of the International Letrozole Breast Cancer Group. *J Clin Oncol* 2001;19:2596–2606.

323. Robertson JF, Llombart-Cussac A, Rolski J, et al. Activity of fulvestrant 500 mg versus anastrozole 1 mg as first-line treatment for advanced breast cancer: results from the FIRST study. *J Clin Oncol* 2009;27:4530–4535.

325. Mayer EL, Burstein HJ. Chemotherapy for metastatic breast cancer. *Hematol Oncol Clin North Am* 2007;21:257–272.

328. Sledge GW, Neuberg D, Bernardo P, et al. Phase III trial of doxorubicin, paclitaxel, and the combination of doxorubicin and paclitaxel as front-line chemotherapy for metastatic breast cancer: an intergroup trial (E1193). *J Clin Oncol* 2003;21:588–592.

329. O'Shaughnessy J, Miles D, Vukelja S, et al. Superior survival with capecitabine plus docetaxel combination therapy in anthracycline-pretreated patients with advanced breast cancer: phase III trial results. *J Clin Oncol* 2002;20:2812–2823.

331. Thomas E, Tabernero J, Fornier M, et al. Phase II clinical trial of ixabepilone (BMS-247550), an epothilone B analog, in patients with taxane-resistant metastatic breast cancer. *J Clin Oncol* 2007;25:3399–3406.

332. Thomas ES, Gomez HL, Li RK, et al. Ixabepilone plus capecitabine for metastatic breast cancer progressing after anthracycline and taxane treatment. *J Clin Oncol* 2007;25:5210–5217.

333. Cortes J, O'Shaughnessy J, Loesch D, et al. Eribulin monotherapy versus treatment of physician's choice in patients with metastatic breast cancer (EMBRACE): a phase 3 open-label randomised study. *Lancet* 2011;377:914–923.

334. Gradishar WJ, Krasnojon D, Cheporov S, et al. Phase II trial of nab-paclitaxel compared with docetaxel as first-line chemotherapy in patients with metastatic breast cancer: final analysis of overall survival. *Clin Breast Cancer* 2012;12:313–321.

PRACTICE OF ONCOLOGY

335. Seidman AD, Berry D, Cirrincione C, et al. Randomized phase III trial of weekly compared with every-3-weeks paclitaxel for metastatic breast cancer, with trastuzumab for all HER-2 overexpressors and random assignment to trastuzumab or not in HER-2 nonoverexpressors: final results of Cancer and Leukemia Group B protocol 9840. *J Clin Oncol* 2008;26:1642–1649.

336. Stadtmauer EA, O'Neill A, Goldstein LJ, et al. Conventional-dose chemotherapy compared with high-dose chemotherapy plus autologous hematopoietic stem-cell transplantation for metastatic breast cancer. Philadelphia Bone Marrow Transplant Group. *N Engl J Med* 2000;342:1069–1076.

338. Slamon DJ, Leyland-Jones B, Shak S, et al. Use of chemotherapy plus a monoclonal antibody against HER2 for metastatic breast cancer that overexpresses HER2. *N Engl J Med* 2001;344:783–792.

339. Seidman A, Hudis C, Pierri MK, et al. Cardiac dysfunction in the trastuzumab clinical trials experience. *J Clin Oncol* 2002;20:1215–1221.

340. Cortes J, Fumoleau P, Bianchi GV, et al. Pertuzumab monotherapy after trastuzumab-based treatment and subsequent reintroduction of trastuzumab: activity and tolerability in patients with advanced human epidermal growth factor receptor 2-positive breast cancer. *J Clin Oncol* 2012;30:1594–1600.

341. Baselga J, Cortes J, Kim SB, et al. Pertuzumab plus trastuzumab plus docetaxel for metastatic breast cancer. *N Engl J Med* 2012;366:109–119.

342. Vogel CL, Cobleigh MA, Tripathy D, et al. Efficacy and safety of trastuzumab as a single agent in first-line treatment of HER2-overexpressing metastatic breast cancer. *J Clin Oncol* 2002;20:719–726.

343. Johnston S, Pippen J Jr, Pivot X, et al. Lapatinib combined with letrozole versus letrozole and placebo as first-line therapy for postmenopausal hormone receptor-positive metastatic breast cancer. *J Clin Oncol* 2009;27: 5538–5546.

344. von Minckwitz G, du Bois A, Schmidt M, et al. Trastuzumab beyond progression in human epidermal growth factor receptor 2-positive advanced breast cancer: a german breast group 26/breast international group 03-05 study. *J Clin Oncol* 2009;27:1999–2006.

346. Geyer CE, Forster J, Lindquist D, et al. Lapatinib plus capecitabine for HER2-positive advanced breast cancer. *N Engl J Med* 2006;355:2733–2743.

348. Verma S, Miles D, Gianni L, et al. Trastuzumab emtansine for HER2-positive advanced breast cancer. *N Engl J Med* 2012;367:1783–1791.

351. Olson EM, Lin NU, DiPiro PJ, et al. Responses to subsequent anti-HER2 therapy after treatment with trastuzumab-DM1 in women with HER2-positive metastatic breast cancer. *Ann Oncol* 2012;23:93–97.

352. Fong PC, Boss DS, Yap TA, et al. Inhibition of poly(ADP-ribose) polymerase in tumors from BRCA mutation carriers. *N Engl J Med* 2009;361:123–134.

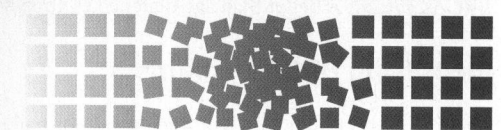

80 Genetic Testing in Breast Cancer

Kristen M. Shannon and Anu Chittenden

INTRODUCTION

Women in the United States have a 12% lifetime risk of developing breast cancer.[1] Although only about 5% to 10% of all cases of breast cancer are attributable to a highly penetrant cancer predisposition gene, individuals who carry a mutation in one of these genes have a significantly higher risk of developing breast cancer, as well as other cancers, over their lifetime compared with the general population. The ability to distinguish those individuals at high risk allows health-care providers to intervene with appropriate counseling and education, surveillance, and prevention with the overall goal of improved survival for these individuals. This chapter focuses on the identification of patients at high risk for breast cancer and provides an overview of the clinical features, cancer risks, causative genes, and medical management for the most clearly described hereditary breast cancer syndromes.

IDENTIFICATION OF HIGH-RISK INDIVIDUALS

An accurate and comprehensive family history of cancer is essential for identifying individuals who may be at risk for inherited breast cancer. As with any family history, it is important to gather a three-generation family history with information on both maternal and paternal lineages.[2,3] Particular focus should be on individuals with malignancies (affected), but those family members without a personal history of cancer (unaffected) should also be included. It is also important to include the presence of nonmalignant findings in the proband and family members, as some inherited cancer syndromes have other physical characteristics associated with them (e.g., trichilemmomas with Cowden syndrome [CS]).

When taking the family history, the accuracy of the information obtained from an individual patient should be considered. Many factors can influence an individual's knowledge of his/her family history, and errors in the reporting of family history have been documented.[4,5] A recent study indicates that individuals are often confident that a family member has had cancer but are typically unsure of the details surrounding that diagnosis.[6,7] Reports of breast cancer tend to be accurate, whereas reports of ovarian cancer are less trustworthy.[8,9] It is important to note that family histories can change over time, with clinically relevant diagnoses arising in family members, especially between the ages of 30 and 50 years.[10] Finally, the physical examination of the proband and family members can be incredibly helpful in the identification of some inherited breast cancer syndromes, such as CS.

GENETIC TESTING

Although some published guidelines for genetic testing exist, much of the time the decision to offer genetic testing is based on clinical judgment. The National Comprehensive Cancer Network® (NCCN®) provides guidelines for individuals who should be offered genetic testing for some of the genes mentioned in this text (NCCN 2011). In the end, however, it is up to the individual provider's judgment as to whether genetic testing is indicated.

Genetic testing for breast cancer susceptibility is rapidly changing. The classic method includes pursuing genetic testing for individual cancer predisposition gene(s) that the clinical suspects may be the cause of breast cancer in the family. In this scenario, finding the appropriate laboratory to perform the testing is very important because laboratory techniques (as well as sensitivity of the technique) vary. Most genetic testing includes sequencing of the gene in question. However, there are emerging data that suggest deletion/duplication studies are imperative for genetic testing as the mutational spectra include various rare, yet important genomic rearrangements.[11]

Recent changes in genetic testing, and specifically the advent of next-generation sequencing tests, have led various genetic testing companies to establish "panel" testing for multiple breast cancer susceptibility genes. In this scenario, up to 14 different breast cancer susceptibility genes are analyzed from one blood specimen. These genes vary in clinical significance from the very highly penetrant breast cancer susceptibility gene *TP53* to the low penetrant breast cancer gene *CHEK2*. How this testing will evolve and the role it will play in clinical care remains to be seen.

BRCA1 AND BRCA2

Description

Mutations in the *BRCA1* and *BRCA2* genes give rise to the "classic" inherited breast cancer syndrome "hereditary breast and ovarian cancer (HBOC) syndrome." The vast majority of cases of HBOC are due to mutations in the *BRCA1* and *BRCA2* genes,[12,13] which were cloned in 1994 and 1995, respectively.[14,15] *BRCA1* and *BRCA2* mutations are rare in most populations, occurring in approximately 1 of 400 individuals, but much more common in the Ashkenazi Jewish population in which 1 of 40 individuals carries one of three main disease-causing mutations: two in *BRCA1* (185delAG and 5382insC) and the 6174delT mutation in *BRCA2*.[16,17] Other founder mutations have been identified, but the utility of these in the US population is minimal.[18,19]

There has been a great deal of research into the tumor biology associated with *BRCA1/2* mutation carriers. *BRCA2*-associated breast cancers are similar in phenotype and clinical behavior in comparison to sporadic cancers.[20,21] *BRCA1*-related breast cancers are often of higher histologic grade, show an excess of medullary histopathology, and are more likely than sporadic tumors to be "triple negative" (i.e., estrogen receptor–negative, progesterone receptor–negative, and are less likely to demonstrate HER2/neu overexpression).[22] Serous papillary ovarian carcinoma is a key feature of hereditary cancers in *BRCA1* mutation carriers; it is less common in *BRCA2* carriers. Endometrioid and clear-cell subtypes of ovarian cancer have been observed,[23] but borderline ovarian tumors do not seem to be a part of the phenotype.[24] Both primary tumors of the fallopian tubes and peritoneum occur with increased frequency in mutation carriers.[25] The prognosis of ovarian cancer in BRCA1 and BRCA2 carriers is better than age-matched controls.[23,26,27]

Identifying BRCA1/2 Carriers

Identifying those individuals at highest risk for harboring a mutation in BRCA1 or BRCA2 is of utmost importance so that they can benefit from surveillance and prevention options. There exist various models designed to estimate the likelihood of identifying a mutation in the BRCA1 or BRCA2 gene[13,28–31]; these models have strengths and limitations that health-care providers need to be familiar with to use and interpret them appropriately.[32–34] The BRCAPRO model, likely the most often used in clinical cancer genetics, estimates the probability that an individual is a carrier of a BRCA mutation using family history and Bayes theorem.[28] It is important when using these risk models to understand the limitations of these risk calculations and to place risk estimates into the appropriate context. It is important to note that risk estimates calculated by different models may vary, a factor that complicates the use of quantitative thresholds for making screening recommendations.[35] The health-care provider should use clinical judgment in conjunction with estimates from models to provide the most precise risk assessment for an individual patient.

Cancer Risks

The penetrance associated with mutations in BRCA1 and BRCA2 remains an active area of research. The risks of developing specific cancers can be found in Table 80.1. The range of breast cancer risk is influenced by the population under study: Higher risk estimates have come from studies with affected families and somewhat lower risk estimates from studies in populations. Also, the risk of ovarian cancer is not the same for all BRCA2 mutations, with mutations in the central ovarian cancer cluster region conferring a higher lifetime risk.[42] Other factors, such as birth cohort, oral contraceptive use, age at first pregnancy, and exercise, have all been shown to influence penetrance risk in populations.[36] There has been a report of increased risk of gallbladder and bile duct cancer, stomach cancer, and melanoma with BRCA2 mutation, none of which seem to be clinically actionable.[37,43]

TABLE 80.1		
BRCA1/2 Cancer Risks		
Cancer Site	**BRCA1 Mutation (%)**	**BRCA2 Mutation (%)**
Female breast	50–80	40–70
Ovarian	<40	<20
Prostate	<30	<39
Pancreatic	1.3–3.2	2.3–7

From Ford D, Easton DF, Stratton M, et al. Genetic heterogeneity and penetrance analysis of the BRCA1 and BRCA2 genes in breast cancer families. The Breast Cancer Linkage Consortium. *Am J Hum Genet* 1998;62:676–689; King MC, Marks JH, Mandell JB. Breast and ovarian cancer risks due to inherited mutations in BRCA1 and BRCA2. *Science* 2003;302:643–646; Ozcelik H, Schmocker B, Di Nicola N, et al. Germline BRCA2 6174delT mutations in Ashkenazi Jewish pancreatic cancer patients. *Nat Genet* 1997;16:17–18; Antoniou A, Pharoah PD, Narod S, et al. Average risks of breast and ovarian cancer associated with BRCA1 or BRCA2 mutations detected in case series unselected for family history: a combined analysis of 22 studies. *Am J Hum Genet* 2003;72:1117–1130; Risch HA, McLaughlin JR, Cole DE, et al. Prevalence and penetrance of germline BRCA1 and BRCA2 mutations in a population series of 649 women with ovarian cancer. *Am J Hum Genet* 2001;68:700–710; The Breast Cancer Linkage Consortium. Cancer risks in BRCA2 mutation carriers. *J Natl Cancer Inst* 1999;91:1310–1316; Thompson D, Easton DF. Cancer incidence in BRCA1 mutation carriers. *J Natl Cancer Inst* 2002;94:1358–1365.

Management

The current recommendations for the screening of women at risk for HBOC is based on the best available evidence and is expected to change as more specific features of BRCA1- and BRCA2-related disease become available. The current screening recommendations for women are listed in Table 80.2.

Risk-reduction mastectomies are an appropriate consideration for women at the highest hereditary risk for breast cancer. Studies have shown a 90% to 95% reduction in breast cancer risk following prophylactic mastectomy.[44–47] The evidence for the use of tamoxifen or raloxifene as a chemopreventive agent in BRCA carriers is limited; however, tamoxifen has been shown to reduce the risk of contralateral breast cancers in BRCA carriers.[48,49] Two recent studies support the role of risk-reducing salpingo-oophorectomy: The hazard ratio for ovarian cancer for women who underwent prophylactic surgery and that for those who chose close surveillance were 0.15 and 0.04, respectively.[50,51] Women should be informed about the potential for the subsequent development of peritoneal carcinomatosis, which has been reported up to 15 years after risk-reducing bilateral salpingo-oophorectomy.[25,52] Combination oral contraceptives containing estrogen and progestin result in a protective effect against ovarian cancer in some studies, but not in others.[53–55]

Male BRCA mutation carriers are advised to undergo training in breast self-examination with regular monthly practice and semiannual clinical breast examinations, and workup of any suspected breast lesions is recommended. The NCCN Clinical Practice Guidelines In Oncology (NCCN Guidelines®) also recommend that a baseline mammogram be considered, with an annual mammogram if gynecomastia or parenchymal/glandular breast density is identified on baseline study.[56] The NCCN Guidelines® recommend that male BRCA mutation carriers should adhere to the current prostate cancer screening guidelines.[56,57]

Psychosocial Considerations

The psychosocial needs of BRCA-positive women have been studied fairly widely. Studies have shown that although there is slight worsening of distress symptoms following cancer genetic counseling in BRCA1/BRCA2 mutation carriers, these symptoms were minimal, did not affect everyday life activities, and had almost disappeared at 1-year follow-up.[58–62] Approximately 20% of BRCA1/2 mutation carrier women experience high distress after learning their test result.[63,64] Factors that are related to high posttest distress include a high level of pretest anxiety, higher pretest perceived risk, and whether they are opting for prophylactic surgery to reduce their risk.[5] It is important to note, however, that even in women who experienced distress after receipt of genetic test information, women do not "regret" their decision to be tested.[66] It has been suggested that health-care providers consider including a brief pretest psychological assessment before initiating genetic testing for BRCA1 and BRCA2[67] so that these women can be targeted for more comprehensive support once test results are available.[68]

The anxiety-associated symptoms reported by BRCA1/2 carriers include sleeplessness and "bad mood."[60,69,70] One other psychosocial issue reported by single women with BRCA1/2 mutations is that they experience increased urgency at finding a life partner capable of handling the emotional strain of the cancer world and open to pursuing multiple paths toward parenthood.[71]

Various studies have suggested that existing social support networks are inadequate for BRCA1/2 mutation carriers and that formal services are unavailable or underutilized.[66,70,72] To address this lack of formal support services, a retreat for BRCA1/2 carriers that includes educational updates about medical management, genetic privacy, and discrimination and addresses psychological and family issues may provide a valuable opportunity for BRCA carriers and their families to receive updated medical information, share personal experiences, provide and receive support, and change health behaviors.[73]

TABLE 80.2

National Comprehensive Cancer Network Guidelines for Management of BRCA1/2 Carriers

Women

- Breast awareness starting at age 18 y
- Clinical breast examination, every 6–12 mo, starting at age 25 y
- Breast screening
  - Age 25–29 y, annual breast magnetic resonance imaging (MRI) screening (preferred) or mammogram if MRI is unavailable or individualized based on earliest age of onset in family.
  - Age ≥30–75 y, annual mammogram and breast MRI screening.
  - Age >75 y, management should be considered on an individual basis.
- Discuss option of risk-reducing mastectomy and counsel regarding degree of protection, reconstruction options, and risks
- Recommend risk-reducing salpingo-oophorectomy, ideally between 35 and 40 y and upon completion of childbearing, or individualized based on earliest age at onset of ovarian cancer in the family; counseling includes a discussion of reproductive desires, extent of cancer risk, degree of protection for breast and ovarian cancer, management of menopausal symptoms, possible short-term hormone replacement therapy to a recommended maximum age at natural menopause, and related medical issues
- Address psychosocial, social, and quality-of-life aspects of undergoing risk-reducing mastectomy and/or salpingo-oophorectomy.
- For those patients who have not elected risk-reducing salpingo-oophorectomy, consider concurrent transvaginal ultrasound (preferably days 1–10 of menstrual cycle in premenopausal women) and CA-125 (preferably after day 5 of menstrual cycle in premenopausal women), every 6 mo starting at age 30 y or 5–10 y before the earliest age at first diagnosis of ovarian cancer in the family
- Consider chemoprevention options for breast and ovarian cancer, including discussing risks and benefits
- Consider investigational imaging and screening studies, when available (e.g., novel imaging technologies and more frequent screening interval[s] in the context of a clinical trial)

Men

- Breast self-examination training and education starting at the age of 35 y
- Clinical breast examination, every 6–12 mo, starting at the age of 35 y
- Consider baseline mammogram at the age of 40 y; annual mammogram if gynecomastia or parenchymal/glandular breast density on baseline study
- Starting at age 40:
  - Recommend prostate cancer screening for *BRCA2* carriers
  - Consider prostate cancer screening for *BRCA1* carriers

TABLE 80.3

Tumors Reported to Be Associated with Li-Fraumeni Syndrome

Wilms Tumor	Bladder Cancer	Prostate Cancer
Malignant phyllodes tumor	Hepatoblastoma	Pancreatic cancer
Lung cancer	Lymphomas	Neuroblastoma
Choroid plexus tumor	Nasopharyngeal cancer	Testicular cancer
Colorectal cancer	Ureteral tumors	Ovarian cancer
Stomach cancer	Laryngeal cancer	Melanoma
Gonadal germ cell tumors	Teratomas	

From Gonzalez KD, Noltner KA, Buzin CH, et al. Beyond Li-Fraumeni syndrome: Clinical characteristics of families with p53 germline mutations. *J Clin Oncol* 2009;27:1250–1256; Nichols KE, Malkin D, Garber JE, et al. Germ-line p53 mutations predispose to a wide spectrum of early-onset cancers. *Cancer Epidemiol Biomarkers Prev* 2001;10:83–87; Hwang SJ, Lozano G, Amos CI, et al. Germline p53 mutations in a cohort with childhood sarcoma: sex differences in cancer risk. *Am J Hum Genet* 2003;72:975–983; Kleihues P, Schäuble B, zur Hausen A, et al. Tumors associated with p53 germline mutations: a synopsis of 91 families. *Am J Pathol* 1997;150:1–13; Olivier M, Goldgar DE, Sogda N, et al. Li-Fraumeni and related syndromes: correlation between tumor type, family structure, and TP53 genotype. *Cancer Res* 2003;63:6643–6650; Birch JM, Alston RD, McNally RJ, et al. Relative frequency and morphology of cancers in carriers of germline TP53 mutations. *Oncogene* 2001;20:4621–4628; Strong LC, Williams WR, Tainsky MA. The Li-Fraumeni syndrome: From clinical epidemiology to molecular genetics. *Am J Epidemiol* 1992;135:190–199.

Distress in male *BRCA* carriers has not be studied quite as widely, but one study noted that high distress after disclosure of the result was reported by one of four male mutation carriers.[74]

TP53

Description

Germline mutations in the *TP53* gene give rise to a disease called Li-Fraumeni syndrome (LFS), which is a rare cancer predisposition syndrome thought to be responsible for ~1% of breast cancers.[75] LFS is often thought of as a hereditary predisposition to cancer in general, involving many tumor types and occurring at any point in an individual's lifetime, including childhood. The majority of cases of LFS are due to mutations in the *p53* gene.[76–79] The component tumors of LFS include bone sarcomas (primarily osteosarcomas and chondrosarcomas), soft tissue sarcomas, breast cancer, brain tumors, leukemia, and adrenocortical carcinomas.[80] The classic component tumors are thought to account for 63% to 77% of cancer diagnoses in individuals with LFS.[80–83] Breast cancer is the most common tumor in *p53* mutation carriers (24% to 31.2%), followed by soft tissue sarcomas (11.6% to 17.8%), brain tumors (3.5% to 14%), osteosarcomas (12.6% to 13.4%), and adrenocortical tumors (6.5% to 9.9%).[84,85] Other tumors that have been argued to be component tumors of LFS are listed in Table 80.3.

There are some data regarding common histology of LFS component tumors. Breast cancers are most commonly invasive ductal carcinomas.[80] Rhabdomyosarcomas account for 55% of soft tissue sarcomas, followed by fibrosarcomas (13%) and then malignant fibrous histiocytomas.[84] For LFS-associated brain tumors, 69% are astrocytic (astrocytoma or glioblastoma), followed by medulloblastoma/primitive neuroectodermal tumors (17%).[84]

Identifying Li-Fraumeni Syndrome

Li et al.[80] first defined LFS in 1988 at which point clinical criteria were established, now known as classic LFS criteria (Table 80.4). In 1994, Birch et al.[77] went on to define less stringent criteria (see Table 80.4) in an attempt to capture families with *p53* mutations

TABLE 80.4

TABLE 80.4

Clinical Criteria for Classic Li-Fraumeni Syndrome

LFL Syndrome and Chompret Criteria

Classic LFS criteria
- Proband diagnosed with a sarcoma before 45 y of age and
- A first-degree relative[a] with cancer diagnosed before 45 y of age and
- A first- or second-degree relative[b] on the same side of the family with cancer diagnosed before 45 y of age or a sarcoma at any age

LFL syndrome criteria
- Proband with any childhood cancer or sarcoma, brain tumor, or adrenocortical carcinoma diagnosed before 45 y of age and
- First- or second-degree relative with a component LFS cancer (sarcoma, breast cancer, brain tumor, leukemia, or adrenocortical carcinoma) diagnosed at any age and
- One first- or second-degree relative on the same side of the family with any cancer diagnosed before age 60 y

Chompret criteria
- Proband diagnosed with a narrow spectrum cancer (sarcoma, brain tumor, breast cancer, or adrenocortical carcinoma) before the age of 36 y, and at least one first- or second-degree relative affected by a narrow-spectrum tumor (other than breast cancer if the proband was affected by breast cancer) before 46 y or a relative with multiple primary tumors at any age
- A proband with multiple primary tumors, two of which belong to the narrow spectrum and the first of which occurred before 36 y, regardless of family history
- A proband with adrenocortical carcinoma, regardless of age at diagnosis or family history

LFL, LFS-like; LFS, Li-Fraumeni syndrome.
[a] First-degree relative is defined as parent, sibling, or child.
[b] Second-degree relative is defined as grandparent, aunt, uncle, niece, nephew, or grandchild.

who did not necessarily conform to the classic criteria. Families who met the broader criteria of Birch et al.[77] were referred to as "LFS-like (LFL)" families. Both classic and LFL criteria are based on family history and fail to recognize potential $p53$ mutation carriers who have de novo germline $p53$ mutations. Although the de novo rate is not well defined for $p53$, one study showed as high as a 24% rate.[88]

More recently in 2001, Chompret et al.[89] developed criteria for identifying patients likely to carry $p53$ mutations (see Table 80.4) and included criteria that address families who display a collection of component tumors but also address individuals whose personal histories are suggestive of $p53$ mutation even in the absence of a suggestive family history. The Chompret criteria were designed to include individuals who may potentially carry de novo $p53$ mutations.

Fifty to seventy percent of individuals who meet the classic definition of LFS will have a mutation in $p53$.[77,89–92] Individuals who meet the LFL criteria are less likely to be $p53$ mutation carriers, estimated at 21% to 40%.[79,90] Twenty percent of individuals meeting the Chompret criteria will be identified as $p53$ mutation carriers.[89]

Cancer Risks

Typically, LFS-associated tumors occur at significantly younger ages than when they occur sporadically. However, depending on tumor type, the mean age at diagnosis varies from childhood well into adulthood.[84] Understanding cancer risk for LFS is somewhat complicated as the ranges of risk vary greatly between studies and depend largely on study population. When pooling studies that examine overall cancer risk in $p53$ mutation carriers (both female and male), the risk of developing cancer by ages 15 to 20 years is 12% to 42%, by ages 40 to 45 years is 52% to 66%, by age 50 years is 80%, and by age 85 years is 85%.[82,83,88,93] When separating out

the sexes, it is apparent that female $p53$ mutation carriers have generally a higher lifetime cancer risk in comparison to males.[83,88,94]

Individuals with a diagnosis of LFS are also at markedly increased risk of developing multiple primary tumors. Hisada et al.[95] found that, following a first cancer diagnosis, there is a 57% risk for a second primary tumor within 30 years of the first diagnosis, followed by a 38% risk for a third primary tumor within 10 years of the second cancer diagnosis. In addition, it has been widely observed that second, third, and so on primary cancers commonly occur in the radiation field of previously treated cancers.[76,80,88,95]

Psychosocial Issues

The psychosocial effects of being a member of an LFS family and/or being affected with LFS have not been widely studied.[96,97] The nature of the disease itself leads to unique psychosocial implications with individual members of LFS families often experiencing many cancer diagnoses (and deaths) in their immediate and extended family. These cancer diagnoses will be throughout the life span, with many parents having to deal with a child's diagnosis and many children needing to deal with a parent's diagnosis. It is likely that these repeated experiences of grief and stress pose a significant psychological burden for the members of LFS families.[98] Although no data exist, this psychosocial burden may also impact individuals' relationships with their family members including, but not limited to, children and spouses.

Because of the rarity of the syndrome, many individuals with LFS may feel isolated. Other inherited syndromes, in general, and inherited cancer syndromes, in particular, have "support groups" that can help with the coping process when an individual is diagnosed with the disease. Unfortunately, no such group exists in the United States today. An online discussion group/support group for individuals with LFS is available (http://listserv.acor.org/SCRIPTS/WA-ACOR.EXE?OK=53111E8B&L=LI-FRAUMENI). Members of the listserv include patients with LFS, health-care providers, and spouses and friends of individuals with LFS. The listserv serves as a place not only to share information about the disease but also to discuss fears, anxiety, grief, and other psychological manifestations of the disease.

COWDEN SYNDROME (PHOSPHATE AND TENSIN HOMOLOG)

Description

CS is a rare hereditary cancer syndrome that is characterized by overgrowth in different organ systems. The incidence of CS is thought to be about 1 in 200,000, but it may be underdiagnosed.[99] CS belongs to the set of syndromes known as the phosphatase and tensin homolog (PTEN) hamartoma tumor syndromes.[100] PTEN mutations are found in the vast majority of patients with CS, although mutations in other genes such as BMPR1A and the succinate dehydrogenase genes have been reported in a small number of patients who have features of CS but do not meet diagnostic criteria (CS-like).[101,102]

Diagnostic Criteria Testing Criteria

Traditionally, one of the hallmark features of CS is the development of multiple hamartomas of the skin and mucosa. A thorough physical examination, including head circumference measurement and examination for skin manifestations, is an important component of assessing for CS. However, a lack of hamartomas does not exclude CS; diagnostic criteria are complicated.[103] The NCCN®'s most recent guidelines (v.1.2014) for testing for CS are in Table 80.5.

Identifying Cowden Syndrome

In 2011, the Cleveland Clinic made available an online calculator for risk of a PTEN mutation in adults, as well as a set of pediatric criteria (http://www.lerner.ccf.org/gmi/ccscore/). Risk estimates

TABLE 80.5

National Comprehensive Cancer Network Guidelines (V.1.2014): Testing Criteria for Cowden Syndrome

Individual from a family with a known *PTEN* mutation or

Individual meeting clinical diagnostic criteria for CS/PHTS or
- At risk individual with a relative with a clinical diagnosis of CS/PHTS or BRRS for whom testing has not been performed
  - The at-risk individual must have the following:
    - Any one major criterion or
    - Two minor criteria

or

Individual with a personal history of
- Bannayan–Riley–Ruvalcaba syndrome or
- Adult Lhermitte-Duclos disease (dysplastic gangliocytoma of the cerebellum) or
- Autism spectrum disorder and macrocephaly or
- Two or more biopsy-proven trichilemmomas or
- Two or more major criteria (one must be macrocephaly) or
- Three or more major criteria, without macrocephaly or
- One major and three or more minor criteria or
- Four or more minor criteria or
- Fewer criteria are needed when an individual has a relative with a clinical diagnosis of Cowden syndrome or Bannayan–Riley–Ruvalcaba syndrome (any one major criterion or two minor criteria)

Major criteria
- Breast cancer
- Mucocutaneous lesions
  - Biopsy-proven trichilemmoma
  - Multiple palmoplantar ÿeratosis
  - Multifocal or extensive oral mucosal papillomatosis
  - Multiple cutaneous facial papules (often verrucous)
- Macular pigmentation of glans penis
- Macrocephaly (≥97th percentile, 58 cm in adult women, 60 cm in adult male)
- Endometrial cancer
- Follicular thyroid cancer
- Multiple gastrointestinal hamartomas or ganglioneuromas

Minor criteria
- Thyroid structural lesions (e.g., adenoma, multinodular goiter)
- Papillary or follicular variant of papillary thyroid cancer
- Mental retardation (intelligence quotient ≤75)
- Autism spectrum disorder
- Single gastrointestinal hamartoma or ganglioneuroma
- >3 esophageal glycogenic acanthoses
- Lipomas
- Testicular lipomatosis
- Renal cell carcinoma
- Colon cancer
- Vascular anomalies (including multiple intracranial developmental venous anomalies)

TABLE 80.6

Cancer Risks Associated with Cowden Syndrome

	Pilarski et al.[105] (2009) (%)	Tan et al.[104] (2012) (%)
Breast cancer risk	25–50	85
Thyroid cancer	3–10	35
Endometrial cancer	5–10	28
Renal cell cancer	Unknown	34
Melanoma	Unknown	6
Colorectal cancer	Unknown	9

Cancer Risks

The highest risk of cancer associated with CS is for female breast cancer. Other cancers that are thought to be a part of the spectrum of cancers seen in CS include thyroid cancer and uterine cancer; more recently, renal cell cancer, melanoma, and colorectal cancer have also been reported. The magnitude of risk for the cancers associated with CS varies widely.[104,105] A recent article from Cleveland Clinic estimated the lifetime risks of cancer to be much higher than previously reported; however, it is likely that there is significant ascertainment bias present in this cohort.[104] A comparison of two publications reviewing the cancer risks associated with CS is presented in Table 80.6.

Management

CS is a complex diagnosis to make and to receive. Because of the degree of variability in CS, it is difficult for clinicians to make a firm diagnosis except in the most obvious of cases. In situations where there is a high suspicion, a negative genetic test result may be uninformative for the patient and her family. Conversely, a positive result or variant of uncertain significance in an individual without classic features of Cowden can lead to uncertainty regarding how aggressive to be about screening and prevention measures. The NCCN guidelines for management are in Table 80.7.

Psychosocial Issues

There is a dearth of literature addressing the psychological issues for individuals and families with a clinical and/or genetic diagnosis of CS, possibly due to its rarity. However, there are several factors associated with CS that could add to the psychological burden of having a hereditary syndrome. These include variability in clinical presentation, difficulty screening (especially for breast cancer), disfigurement due to mucocutaneous lesions and surgical procedures, the possibility of intellectual disabilities and/or autism in children, lack of knowledge about how often *PTEN* mutations are found de novo versus inherited in a family, a large number of uncertain variants found through genetic testing, and overall lack of knowledge about the syndrome.

Because of the association of CS with autism and macrocephaly, many children are now undergoing genetic testing for alterations in the *PTEN* gene; a small number of them will be found to have CS or a related disorder.[106] When the child is the index case in the family, testing him/her may provide information for adult family members about cancer risks. In addition, parents may find value in knowing that there is an underlying genetic cause to their child's issues and in finding a community with a shared diagnosis. There is also the hope that the development of targeted therapies may help ameliorate the disease in children and, going forward, in adults.

The benefit of testing an asymptomatic child whose parent has a known mutation in *PTEN* is still unknown. Although childhood cancers have been reported in CS, these cancers appear to be rare. Some experts argue that thyroid and other screening is warranted in

were based on data from the largest prospective cohort of patients collected with a potential diagnosis of CS. Information on physical findings, specific cancer diagnoses, intestinal polyps, and other benign conditions is collected. If a patient has a risk of mutation greater than 3%, testing for *PTEN* is recommended.[104]

National Comprehensive Cancer Network Guidelines (V.1.2014) for Cowden Syndrome Management

Women

- Breast awareness starting at the age of 18 y
- Clinical breast examination, every 6–12 mo, starting at the age of 25 y or 5–10 y before the earliest known breast cancer in the family
- Annual mammography and breast magnetic resonance imaging screening starting at the age of 30–35 y or individualized based on earliest age of onset in family. For endometrial cancer screening, encourage patient education and prompt response to symptoms. Consider annual random endometrial biopsies and/or ultrasound beginning at age 30–35 y
- Discuss option of risk-reducing mastectomy and hysterectomy on a case-by-case basis and counsel regarding degree of protection, extent of cancer risk, and reconstruction options

Men and Women

- Annual comprehensive physical examination starting at the age of 18 y or 5 y before the youngest age at diagnosis of a component cancer in the family (whichever comes first), with particular attention to breast and thyroid examinations
- Annual thyroid ultrasound at the age of 18 y, or 5–10 y before the earliest known thyroid cancer in the family, whichever is earlier
- Colonoscopy starting at the age of 35 y, then every 5 y or more frequently if patient is symptomatic or polyps found
- Consider renal ultrasound starting at age 40 y, then every 1–2 y. Dermatologic management may be indicated for some patients
- Consider psychomotor assessment in children at diagnosis and brain MRI if there are symptoms.
- Education regarding the signs and symptoms of cancer

Risk to Relatives

- Advise about possible inherited cancer risk to relatives and options for risk assessment and management
- Recommend genetic counseling and consideration of genetic testing for at-risk relatives

Adapted with permission from the National Comprehensive Cancer Network's (NCCN) *NCCN Clinical Practice Guidelines in Oncology (NCCN Guidelines) for Genetic/Familial High-Risk Assessment: Breast and Ovarian* V.1.2014. © 2014 National Comprehensive Cancer Network, Inc. All rights reserved. The NCCN Guidelines and illustrations herein may not be reproduced in any form for any purpose without the expressed written permission of the NCCN. To view the most recent and complete version of the NCCN Guidelines, go online to www.NCCN.org. National Comprehensive Cancer Network, NCCN, NCCN Guidelines, and all other NCCN content are trademarks owned by the National Comprehensive Cancer Network, Inc.

children for the early detection and prevention of related cancers[107]; however, others would say that the psychological burden of screening outweighs any small medical benefit that may be derived from discovering benign lesions that are unlikely to become cancerous at a young age. Testing unaffected children for CS remains controversial.

OTHER GENETIC MUTATIONS AND BREAST CANCER

STK11

Peutz–Jeghers syndrome (PJS) is a rare autosomal dominant gastrointestinal hamartomatous polyposis syndrome. It is estimated that the incidence is approximately 1 in 150,000 in North America and Western Europe.[108,109] PJS is characterized by the development of Peutz–Jeghers polyps in the intestine in conjunction with pigmentation

Clinical Criteria for Peutz-Jeghers Syndrome and Hereditary Diffuse Gastric Cancer Syndrome

PJS Clinical Diagnostic Criteria

Any one of the following is present

- Two or more histologically confirmed Peutz–Jeghers polyps
- Any number of Peutz–Jeghers polyps detected in one individual who has a family history of PJS in close relative(s)
- Characteristic mucocutaneous pigmentation in an individual who has a family history of PJS in close relative(s)
- Any number of Peutz–Jeghers polyps in an individual who also has characteristic mucocutaneous pigmentation

Beggs et al.[110] (2010)

Hereditary Diffuse Gastric Cancer Clinical Criteria

Any of the following:

- Two gastric cancer cases in a family, one individual aged <50 y with confirmed DGC
- Three confirmed DGC cases in first- or second-degree relatives independent of age
- Simplex case (i.e., a single occurrence in a family) of DGC occurring before the age of 40 y
- Personal or family history of DGC and lobular breast cancer, one diagnosed before the age of 50 y

PJS, Peutz–Jeghers syndrome; DGC, diffuse gastric cancer.
Fitzgerald RC, Hardwick R, Hunstman D, et al. Hereditary diffuse gastric cancer: Updated consensus guidelines for clinical management and directions for future research. *J Med Genet* 2010;47:436–444.

(brown or bluish spots) around and inside the mouth, nose and lips, and perianal area, as well as other parts of the body. These lesions are often most prominent in childhood and fade with age.

Most families with PJS have mutations in the *STK11* gene, although this gene does not explain all inherited cases of PJS as well as many simplex cases.[110] The lifetime risk of breast cancer in females is reported in a wide range, with the most consistent risks being in the 30% to 50% range.[111,112] Other cancers that can be seen in PJS include cancers of the colon, pancreas, stomach, ovary, small intestine, lung, cervix, testes, uterus, and esophagus.[110] Consensus diagnostic criteria were published in 2010 and are listed in Table 80.8.[110]

CDH1

Hereditary diffuse gastric cancer is a rare autosomal dominant hereditary syndrome characterized by diffuse (or signet ring cell pathology) stomach cancer. The incidence of this syndrome is not well known but likely to be rare. The lifetime risk of stomach cancer is thought to be approximately 80% compared with <1% in the general population.[114,115] The second most common cancer in families with this syndrome is lobular breast cancer, with a lifetime risk of about 40% in women.[116–120] Cleft lip and palate have also been reported in some families.[121] The International Gastric Cancer Linkage Consortium published clinical criteria in 2010, shown in Table 80.8.[113] The incidence of *CDH1* mutations in lobular breast cancer cases is thought to be low in the absence of a family history of gastric cancer.[122] Please see Chapter 59 ("Genetic Testing in Colon Cancer [Nonpolyposis Syndrome]") for more detailed information.

MODERATE- AND LOW-PENETRANCE BREAST CANCER GENES

There are several genes that have already been described in families with breast cancer including *CHEK2* and *ATM*. The risk of breast cancer associated with alterations in these genes is thought to be lower than with traditional hereditary breast cancer syndromes; other factors are likely to interact with the effects of changes in these genes and result in a more moderate increase in risk for breast cancer.

Recently, a US group published a study on 12 genes linked to hereditary ovarian cancer, which are also being analyzed in families with hereditary breast cancer.[123–125] More laboratories are beginning to offer genetic testing for panels of genes that are important in DNA repair pathways.[126] There are several categories of these genes.

1. Category 1—genes functionally related to *BRCA1* and *BRCA2* (*ATM, BARD1, CHEK2, MRE11A, NBN, RAD50, RAD51D*)

   - *ATM* (ataxia telangiectasia mutated)
   - *BARD1* (*BRCA1*-associated RING domain 1)
   - *CHEK2* (cell cycle checkpoint kinase 2)
   - *MRE11A* (meiotic recombination 11 homolog A)
   - *NBN* (nibrin; aka *NBS1*)
   - *RAD50*
   - *RAD51D*

2. Category 2—(other) genes in the Fanconi anemia pathway that increase breast cancer risk (*BRIP1, PALB2, RAD51C*)

   - *BRIP1* (*BRCA*-interacting protein C-terminal helicase 1; *FANCJ*)
   - *PALB2* (partner and localizer of *BRCA2*; *FANCN*)
   - *RAD51C* (*FANCO*)

3. Category 3—genes involved in hereditary colorectal cancer (*MLH1, MSH2, MSH6, PMS2, EPCAM, MYH*)

For many of the genes in categories 1 and 2, risks of breast cancer are not well defined, and it is unclear if women who test negative for a mutation that was found in an affected relative ("true negatives") are really at general population risk.

Lynch Syndrome and MYH-Associated Polyposis

Lynch syndrome (LS) is the most common hereditary form of colorectal cancer, accounting for about 2% to 3% of colorectal cancer cases. It is caused by mutations in genes involved in DNA mismatch repair, including *MLH1, MSH2, MSH6, PMS2*, and, indirectly, *EPCAM*. LS is typically characterized by the development of relatively early-onset colorectal and uterine cancer; risks for other cancers including stomach cancer, cancer of the small intestine, pancreatic cancer, sebaceous carcinomas, ovarian cancer, and cancers of the urinary collecting tract. Rarely, brain tumors are thought to be increased.[127] Most studies have not shown a significant increase in breast cancer risk for *MMR* mutation carriers versus noncarriers,[128] although a more recent article studying a cohort of LS families prospectively did show a fourfold increase in breast cancer risk.[129] It is clear that defective mismatch repair can be seen in some breast cancers in women from LS families.[130–131] Whether there is a true increase in risk (and the magnitude of this risk) remains to be seen. Please see "Genetic Testing in Colon Cancer (Nonpolyposis Syndrome)" for more detailed information.

MYH-associated polyposis (MAP) is the lesser known of the adenomatous polyposis syndromes (versus familial adenomatous polyposis). *MYH* is involved in base excision repair; without *MYH*, oxidative DNA damage leads to the formation of 8-oxo-G, which mispairs with adenine. This leads to an increase in G:C>T:A transversions in *APC* and other genes.[132] MAP is associated with an attenuated phenotype; fewer adenomas (generally in the range of 10 to 100) and a mixture of polyp types (serrated adenomas, hyperplastic polyps) and duodenal polyps are often seen.[133,134] Extraintestinal manifestations, including breast cancer, have been reported in MAP.[135,136] However, *MYH* does not appear to be a common cause of breast cancer.[137] Please see "Genetic Testing in Colon Cancer (Nonpolyposis Syndrome)" for more detailed information.

CONCLUSION

This chapter has provided a synopsis of the genes linked to the most well-defined syndromes associated with breast cancer and an introduction to breast cancer gene panels. It is important for clinicians to be able to identify the classic breast cancer syndromes, know the relevant genes, and understand the medical management and psychosocial issues associated with the syndromes. The advent of whole genome sequencing and the ability to analyze the estimated 22,000 genes in the human genome with cheap and efficient technology bring the hope that all of the genes involved in hereditary and familial breast cancer will be found. However, making this information clinically relevant will require much more research. Elucidating the interaction of mutations in these genes with modifying factors could help clarify risks in families and lead to targeted screening and prevention measures. It is clear that genetic testing will become more complicated over time and that the interpretation of test results will require continuing education and expertise in the field.

REFERENCES

1. Howlander N, Noone AM, Krapcho M, et al, eds. *SEER Cancer Statistics Review, 1975–2008*. Bethesda, MD: National Cancer Institute; 2011.
2. Bennett RL, French KS, Resta RG, et al. Standardized human pedigree nomenclature: Update and assessment of the recommendations of the National Society of Genetic Counselors. *J Genet Couns* 2008;17:424–433.
3. Bennett RL, Steinhaus KA, Uhrich SB, et al. Recommendations for standardized human pedigree nomenclature. Pedigree Standardization Task Force of the National Society of Genetic Counselors. *Am J Hum Genet* 1995;56:745–752.
4. Love RR, Evans AM, Josten DM. The accuracy of patient reports of a family history of cancer. *J Chronic Dis* 1985;38:289–293.
5. Theis B, Boyd N, Lockwood G, et al. Accuracy of family cancer history in breast cancer patients. *Eur J Cancer Prev* 1994;3:321–327.
6. Reid GT, Walter FM, Brisbane JM, et al. Family history questionnaires designed for clinical use: a systematic review. *Public Health Genomics* 2009;12:73–83.
7. Jefferies S, Goldgar D, Eeles R. The accuracy of cancer diagnoses as reported in families with head and neck cancer: A case-control study. *Clin Oncol (R Coll Radiol)* 2008;20:309–314.
8. Murff HJ, Spigel DR, Syngal S. Does this patient have a family history of cancer? An evidence-based analysis of the accuracy of family cancer history. *JAMA* 2004;292:1480–1489.
9. Chang ET, Smedby KE, Hjalgrim H, et al. Reliability of self-reported family history of cancer in a large case-control study of lymphoma. *J Natl Cancer Inst* 2006;98:61–68.
10. Ziogas A, Horick NK, Kinney AY, et al. Clinically relevant changes in family history of cancer over time. *JAMA* 2011;306:172–178.
11. Walsh T, Casadei S, Coats KH, et al. Spectrum of mutations in BRCA1, BRCA2, CHEK2, and TP53 in families at high risk of breast cancer. *JAMA* 2006;295:1379–1388.
12. Ford D, Easton DF, Stratton M, et al. Genetic heterogeneity and penetrance analysis of the BRCA1 and BRCA2 genes in breast cancer families. The Breast Cancer Linkage Consortium. *Am J Hum Genet* 1998;62:676–689.
13. Frank TS, Manley SA, Olopade OI, et al. Sequence analysis of BRCA1 and BRCA2: Correlation of mutations with family history and ovarian cancer risk. *J Clin Oncol* 1998;16:2417–2425.
14. Miki Y, Swensen J, Shattuck-Eidens D, et al. A strong candidate for the breast and ovarian cancer susceptibility gene BRCA1. *Science* 1994;266:66–71.
15. Wooster R, Bignell G, Lancaster J, et al. Identification of the breast cancer susceptibility gene BRCA2. *Nature* 1995;378:789–792.
16. Struewing JP, Hartge P, Wacholder S, et al. The risk of cancer associated with specific mutations of BRCA1 and BRCA2 among Ashkenazi Jews. *N Engl J Med* 1997;336:1401–1408.
17. Kauff ND, Perez-Segura P, Robson ME, et al. Incidence of non-founder BRCA1 and BRCA2 mutations in high risk Ashkenazi breast and ovarian cancer families. *J Med Genet* 2002;39:611–614.
18. Thorlacius S, Olafsdottir G, Tryggvadottir L, et al. A single BRCA2 mutation in male and female breast cancer families from Iceland with varied cancer phenotypes. *Nat Genet* 1996;13:117–119.

19. Unger MA, Nathanson KL, Calzone K, et al. Screening for genomic rearrangements in families with breast and ovarian cancer identifies BRCA1 mutations previously missed by conformation-sensitive gel electrophoresis or sequencing. *Am J Hum Genet* 2000;67:841–850.

20. Chappuis PO, Nethercot V, Foulkes WD. Clinico-pathological characteristics of BRCA1- and BRCA2-related breast cancer. *Semin Surg Oncol* 2000;18:287–295.

21. Phillips KA, Andrulis IL, Goodwin PJ. Breast carcinomas arising in carriers of mutations in BRCA1 or BRCA2: Are they prognostically different? *J Clin Oncol* 1999;17:3653–3663.

22. Rakha EA, Reis-Filho JS, Ellis IO. Basal-like breast cancer: A critical review. *J Clin Oncol* 2008;26:2568–2581.

23. Boyd J, Sonoda Y, Federici MG, et al. Clinicopathologic features of BRCA-linked and sporadic ovarian cancer. *JAMA* 2000;283:2260–2265.

24. Lakhani SR, Manek S, Penault-Llorca F, et al. Pathology of ovarian cancers in BRCA1 and BRCA2 carriers. *Clin Cancer Res* 2004;10:2473–2481.

25. Levine DA, Argenta PA, Yee CJ, et al. Fallopian tube and primary peritoneal carcinomas associated with BRCA mutations. *J Clin Oncol* 2003;21: 4222–4227.

26. Cass I, Baldwin RL, Varkey T, et al. Improved survival in women with BRCA-associated ovarian carcinoma. *Cancer* 2003;97:2187–2195.

27. Arun B, Bayraktar S, Liu DD, et al. Response to neoadjuvant systemic therapy for breast cancer in BRCA mutation carriers and noncarriers: A single-institution experience. *J Clin Oncol* 2011;29:3739–3746.

28. Berry DA, Iversen ES Jr, Gudbjartsson DF, et al. BRCAPRO validation, sensitivity of genetic testing of BRCA1/BRCA2, and prevalence of other breast cancer susceptibility genes. *J Clin Oncol* 2002;20:2701–2712.

29. Tyrer J, Duffy SW, Cuzick J. A breast cancer prediction model incorporating familial and personal risk factors. *Stat Med* 2004;23:1111–1130.

30. Couch FJ, DeShano ML, Blackwood MA, et al. BRCA1 mutations in women attending clinics that evaluate the risk of breast cancer. *N Engl J Med* 1997;336:1409–1415.

31. Shattuck-Eidens D, Oliphant A, McClure M, et al. BRCA1 sequence analysis in women at high risk for susceptibility mutations. Risk factor analysis and implications for genetic testing. *JAMA* 1997;278:1242–1250.

32. Kang HH, Williams R, Leary J, et al. Evaluation of models to predict BRCA germline mutations. *Br J Cancer* 2006;95:914–920.

33. Barcenas CH, Hosain GM, Arun B, et al. Assessing BRCA carrier probabilities in extended families. *J Clin Oncol* 2006;24:354–360.

34. James PA, Doherty R, Harris M, et al. Optimal selection of individuals for BRCA mutation testing: A comparison of available methods. *J Clin Oncol* 2006;24:707–715.

35. Saslow D, Castle PE, Cox JT, et al. American Cancer Society Guideline for human papillomavirus (HPV) vaccine use to prevent cervical cancer and its precursors. *CA Cancer J Clin* 2007;57:7–28.

36. King MC, Marks JH, Mandell JB. Breast and ovarian cancer risks due to inherited mutations in BRCA1 and BRCA2. *Science* 2003;302:643–646.

37. Özçelik H, Schmocker B, Di Nicola N, et al. Germline BRCA2 6174delT mutations in Ashkenazi Jewish pancreatic cancer patients. *Nat Genet* 1997; 16:17–18.

38. Antoniou A, Pharoah PD, Narod S, et al. Average risks of breast and ovarian cancer associated with BRCA1 or BRCA2 mutations detected in case series unselected for family history: a combined analysis of 22 studies. *Am J Hum Genet* 2003;72:1117–1130.

39. Risch HA, McLaughlin JR, Cole DE, et al. Prevalence and penetrance of germline BRCA1 and BRCA2 mutations in a population series of 649 women with ovarian cancer. *Am J Hum Genet* 2001;68:700–710.

40. The Breast Cancer Linkage Consortium. Cancer risks in BRCA2 mutation carriers. *J Natl Cancer Inst* 1999;91:1310–1316.

41. Thompson D, Easton DF. Cancer incidence in BRCA1 mutation carriers. *J Natl Cancer Inst* 2002;94:1358–1365.

42. Thompson D, Easton D. Variation in cancer risks, by mutation position, in BRCA2 mutation carriers. *Am J Hum Genet* 2001;68:410–419.

43. van Asperen CJ, Brohet RM, Meijers-Heijboer EJ, et al. Cancer risks in BRCA2 families: Estimates for sites other than breast and ovary. *J Med Genet* 2005;42:711–719.

44. Hartmann LC, Sellers TA, Schaid DJ, et al. Efficacy of bilateral prophylactic mastectomy in BRCA1 and BRCA2 gene mutation carriers. *J Natl Cancer Inst* 2001;93:1633–1637.

45. Rebbeck TR, Friebel T, Lynch HT, et al. Bilateral prophylactic mastectomy reduces breast cancer risk in BRCA1 and BRCA2 mutation carriers: The PROSE Study Group. *J Clin Oncol* 2004;22:1055–1062.

46. Meijers-Heijboer H, van Geel B, van Putten WL, et al. Breast cancer after prophylactic bilateral mastectomy in women with a BRCA1 or BRCA2 mutation. *N Engl J Med* 2001;345:159–164.

47. Robson M, Svahn T, McCormick B, et al. Appropriateness of breast-conserving treatment of breast carcinoma in women with germline mutations in BRCA1 or BRCA2: A clinic-based series. *Cancer* 2005;103:44–51.

48. Narod SA, Brunet JS, Ghadirian P, et al. Tamoxifen and risk of contralateral breast cancer in BRCA1 and BRCA2 mutation carriers: a case-control study. Hereditary Breast Cancer Clinical Study Group. *Lancet* 2000;356:1876–1881.

49. Gronwald J, Tung N, Foulkes WD, et al. Tamoxifen and contralateral breast cancer in BRCA1 and BRCA2 carriers: an update. *Int J Cancer* 2006;118: 2281–2284.

50. Kauff ND, Satagopan JM, Robson ME, et al. Risk-reducing salpingo-oophorectomy in women with a BRCA1 or BRCA2 mutation. *N Engl J Med* 2002;346:1609–1615.

51. Rebbeck TR, Lunch HT, Neuhausen SL, et al. Prophylactic oophorectomy in carriers of BRCA1 or BRCA2 mutations. *N Engl J Med* 2002;346:1616–1622.

52. Piver MS, Jishi MF, Tsukada Y, et al. Primary peritoneal carcinoma after prophylactic oophorectomy in women with a family history of ovarian cancer. A report of the Gilda Radner Familial Ovarian Cancer Registry. *Cancer* 1993;71:2751–2755.

53. Modan B, Hartge P, Hirsh-Yechezkel G, et al. Parity, oral contraceptives, and the risk of ovarian cancer among carriers and noncarriers of a BRCA1 or BRCA2 mutation. *N Engl J Med* 2001;345:235–240.

54. Narod SA, Risch H, Moslehi R, et al. Oral contraceptives and the risk of hereditary ovarian cancer. Hereditary Ovarian Cancer Clinical Study Group. *N Engl J Med* 1998;339:424–428.

55. Narod SA, Dubé MP, Klihn J, et al. Oral contraceptives and the risk of breast cancer in BRCA1 and BRCA2 mutation carriers. *J Natl Cancer Inst* 2002;94:1773–1779.

56. Daly MB, Pilarski R, Axilbund JE, et al. NCCN *Clinical Practice Guidelines in Oncology (NCCN Guidelines®). Genetic/Familial High-Risk Assessment: Breast and Ovarian* V1.2014. © 2014 National Comprehensive Cancer Network, Inc. www.nccn.org. Accessed September 18, 2014.

57. Liede A, Karlan BY, Narod SA. Cancer risks for male carriers of germline mutations in BRCA1 or BRCA2: A review of the literature. *J Clin Oncol* 2004;22:735–742.

58. DiCastro M, Frydman M, Friedman I, et al. Genetic counseling in hereditary breast/ovarian cancer in Israel: Psychosocial impact and retention of genetic information. *Am J Med Genet* 2002;111:147–151.

59. Lodder LN, Frets PG, Trisburg RW, et al. One year follow-up of women opting for presymptomatic testing for BRCA1 and BRCA2: Emotional impact of the test outcome and decisions on risk management (surveillance or prophylactic surgery). *Breast Cancer Res Treat* 2002;73:97–112.

60. Crotser CB, Boehmke M. Survivorship considerations in adults with hereditary breast and ovarian cancer syndrome: State of the science. *J Cancer Surviv* 2009;3:21–42.

61. Hamilton JG, Lobel M, Moyer A. Emotional distress following genetic testing for hereditary breast and ovarian cancer: A meta-analytic review. *Health Psychol* 2009;28:510–518.

62. Reichelt JG, Møller P, Heimdal K, et al. Psychological and cancer-specific distress at 18 months post-testing in women with demonstrated BRCA1 mutations for hereditary breast/ovarian cancer. *Fam Cancer* 2008;7:245–254.

63. Lodder L, Frets PG, Trijsburg RW, et al. Psychological impact of receiving a BRCA1/BRCA2 test result. *Am J Med Genet* 2001;98:15–24.

64. Power TE, Robinson JW, Bridge P, et al. Distress and psychosocial needs of a heterogeneous high risk familial cancer population. *J Genet Couns* 2011; 20:249–269.

65. O'Neill SC, Rini C, Goldsmith RE, et al. Distress among women receiving uninformative BRCA1/2 results: 12-month outcomes. *Psychooncology* 2009;18:1088–1096.

66. Di Prospero LS, Seminsky M, Honeyford J, et al. Psychosocial issues following a positive result of genetic testing for BRCA1 and BRCA2 mutations: Findings from a focus group and a needs-assessment survey. *CMAJ* 2001;164:1005–1009.

67. Ertmanski S, Metcalfe K, Trempała J, et al. Identification of patients at high risk of psychological distress after BRCA1 genetic testing. *Genet Test Mol Biomarkers* 2009;13:325–330.

68. Roussi P, Sherman KA, Miller S, et al. Enhanced counselling for women undergoing BRCA1/2 testing: Impact on knowledge and psychological distress-results from a randomised clinical trial. *Psychol Health* 2010;25:401–415.

69. Shochat T, Dagan E. Sleep disturbances in asymptomatic BRCA1/2 mutation carriers: Women at high risk for breast-ovarian cancer. *J Sleep Res* 2010;19: 333–340.

70. Werner-Lin A. Formal and informal support needs of young women with BRCA mutations. *J Psychosoc Oncol* 2008;26:111–133.

71. Werner-Lin A. Beating the biological clock: The compressed family life cycle of young women with BRCA gene alterations. *Soc Work Health Care* 2008;47:416–437.

72. Metcalfe KA, Liede A, Hoodfar E, et al. An evaluation of needs of female BRCA1 and BRCA2 carriers undergoing genetic counselling. *J Med Genet* 2000;37:866–874.

73. McKinnon W, Naud S, Ashikaga T, et al. Results of an intervention for individuals and families with BRCA mutations: a model for providing medical updates and psychosocial support following genetic testing. *J Genet Couns* 2007;16:433–456.

74. Lodder L, Frets PG, Trijsburg RW, et al. Men at risk of being a mutation carrier for hereditary breast/ovarian cancer: An exploration of attitudes and psychological functioning during genetic testing. *Eur J Hum Genet* 2001;9:492–500.

75. Sidransky D, Tokino T, Helzlsouer K, et al. Inherited p53 gene mutations in breast cancer. *Cancer Res* 1992;52:2984–2986.

76. Malkin D, Li FP, Strong LC, et al. Germ line p53 mutations in a familial syndrome of breast cancer, sarcomas, and other neoplasms. *Science* 1990;250:1233–1238.

77. Birch JM, Hartley AL, Tricker KJ, et al. Prevalence and diversity of constitutional mutations in the p53 gene among 21 Li-Fraumeni families. *Cancer Res* 1994;54:1298–1304.

78. Srivastava S, Zou ZQ, Pirollo K, et al. Germ-line transmission of a mutated p53 gene in a cancer-prone family with Li-Fraumeni syndrome. *Nature* 1990;348:747–749.

79. Varley JM, McGown G, Thorncraft M, et al. Germ-line mutations of TP53 in Li-Fraumeni families: An extended study of 39 families. *Cancer Res* 1997;57:3245–3252.

80. Li FP, Fraumeni JF Jr, Mulvihill JJ, et al. A cancer family syndrome in twenty-four kindreds. *Cancer Res* 1988;48:5358–5362.

81. Gonzalez KD, Noltner KA, Buzin CH, et al. Beyond Li Fraumeni syndrome: Clinical characteristics of families with p53 germline mutations. *J Clin Oncol* 2009;27:1250–1256.

82. Nichols KE, Malkin D, Garber JE, et al. Germ-line p53 mutations predispose to a wide spectrum of early-onset cancers. *Cancer Epidemiol Biomarkers Prev* 2001;10:83–87.

83. Hwang SJ, Lozano G, Amos CI, et al. Germline p53 mutations in a cohort with childhood sarcoma: sex differences in cancer risk. *Am J Hum Genet* 2003;72:975–983.

84. Kleihues P, Schäuble B, zur Hausen A, et al. Tumors associated with p53 germline mutations: a synopsis of 91 families. *Am J Pathol* 1997;150:1–13.

85. Olivier M, Goldgar DE, Sodha N, et al. Li-Fraumeni and related syndromes: Correlation between tumor type, family structure, and TP53 genotype. *Cancer Res* 2003;63:6643–6650.

86. Birch JM, Alston RD, McNally RJ, et al. Relative frequency and morphology of cancers in carriers of germline TP53 mutations. *Oncogene* 2001;20:4621–4628.

87. Strong LC, Williams WR, Tainsky MA. The Li-Fraumeni syndrome: From clinical epidemiology to molecular genetics. *Am J Epidemiol* 1992;135:190–199.

88. Chompret A, Brugières L, Ronsin M, et al. P53 germline mutations in childhood cancers and cancer risk for carrier individuals. *Br J Cancer* 2000;82:1932–1937.

89. Chompret A, Abel A, Stoppa-Lyonnet D, et al. Sensitivity and predictive value of criteria for p53 germline mutation screening. *J Med Genet* 2001;38:43–47.

90. Varley JM, Evans DG, Birch JM. Li-Fraumeni syndrome—a molecular and clinical review. *Br J Cancer* 1997;76:1–14.

91. Frebourg T, Barbier N, Yan YX, et al. Germ-line p53 mutations in 15 families with Li-Fraumeni syndrome. *Am J Hum Genet* 1995;56:608–615.

92. Brugières L, Gardes M, Moutou C, et al. Screening for germ line p53 mutations in children with malignant tumors and a family history of cancer. *Cancer Res* 1993;53:452–455.

93. Le Bihan C, Moutou C, Brugières L, et al. ARCAD: A method for estimating age-dependent disease risk associated with mutation carrier status from family data. *Genet Epidemiol* 1995;12:13–25.

94. Wu CC, Shete S, Amos CI, et al. Joint effects of germ-line p53 mutation and sex on cancer risk in Li-Fraumeni syndrome. *Cancer Res* 2006;66:8287–8292.

95. Hisada M, Garber JE, Fung CY, et al. Multiple primary cancers in families with Li-Fraumeni syndrome. *J Natl Cancer Inst* 1998;90:606–611.

96. Dorval M, Patenaude AF, Schneider KA, et al. Anticipated versus actual emotional reactions to disclosure of results of genetic tests for cancer susceptibility: findings from p53 and BRCA1 testing programs. *J Clin Oncol* 2000;18:2135–2142.

97. Peterson SK, Pentz ED, Marani SK, et al. Psychological functioning in persons considering genetic counseling and testing for Li-Fraumeni syndrome. *Psychooncology* 2008;17:783–789.

98. Oppenheim D, Brigieres L, Chompret A, et al. The psychological burden inflicted by multiple cancers in Li-Fraumeni families: Five case studies. *J Genet Couns* 2001;10:169–183.

99. Nelen MR, Kremer H, Konings IB, et al. Novel PTEN mutations in patients with Cowden disease: Absence of clear genotype-phenotype correlations. *Eur J Hum Genet* 1999;7:267–273.

100. PTEN hamartoma tumor syndrome (PHTS). 2011. http://www.ncbi.nlm.nih.gov/books/NBK1488/. Accessed April 23, 2012.

101. Zhou XP, Woodford-Richens K, Lehtonen R, et al. Germline mutations in BMPR1A/ALK3 cause a subset of cases of juvenile polyposis syndrome and of Cowden and Bannayan-Riley-Ruvalcaba syndromes. *Am J Hum Genet* 2001;69:704–711.

102. Ni Y, Zbuk KM, Sadler T, et al. Germline mutations and variants in the succinate dehydrogenase genes in Cowden and Cowden-like syndromes. *Am J Hum Genet* 2008;83:261–268.

103. Eng C. Will the real Cowden syndrome please stand up: Revised diagnostic criteria. *J Med Genet* 2000;37:828–830.

104. Tan MH, Mester JL, Ngeow J, et al. Lifetime cancer risks in individuals with germline PTEN mutations. *Clin Cancer Res* 2012;18:400–407.

105. Pilarski R. Cowden syndrome: A critical review of the clinical literature. *J Genet Couns* 2009;18:13–27.

106. Conti S, Condò M, Posar A, et al. Phosphatase and tensin homolog (PTEN) gene mutations and autism: Literature review and a case report of a patient with Cowden syndrome, autistic disorder, and epilepsy. *J Child Neurol* 2012;27:392–397.

107. Smith JR, Margusee E, Webb S, et al. Thyroid nodules and cancer in children with PTEN hamartoma tumor syndrome. *J Clin Endocrinol Metab* 2011;96:34–37.

108. Zbuk KM, Eng C. Hamartomatous polyposis syndromes. *Nat Clin Pract Gastroenterol Hepatol* 2007;4:492–502.

109. Kutscher AH, Zegarelli EV, Rankow RM, et al. Incidence of Peutz-Jeghers syndrome. *Am J Dig Dis* 1960;5:576–577.

110. Beggs AD, Latchford AR, Vasen HF, et al. Peutz-Jeghers syndrome: A systematic review and recommendations for management. *Gut* 2010;59:975–986.

111. Lim W, Olschwang S, Keller JJ, et al. Relative frequency and morphology of cancers in STK11 mutation carriers. *Gastroenterology* 2004;126:1788–1794.

112. Hearle N, Schumacher V, Menko FH, et al. Frequency and spectrum of cancers in the Peutz-Jeghers syndrome. *Clin Cancer Res* 2006;12:3209–3215.

113. Fitzgerald RC, Hardwick R, Hunstman D, et al. Hereditary diffuse gastric cancer: Updated consensus guidelines for clinical management and directions for future research. *J Med Genet* 2010;47:436–444.

114. Kluijt I, Sijmons RH, Hoogerbrugge N, et al. Familial gastric cancer: Guidelines for diagnosis, treatment and periodic surveillance. *Fam Cancer* 2012;11:363–369.

115. Howlader N, Noone AM, Krapcho M, et al. (eds). SEER Cancer Statistics Review, 1975-2008, National Cancer Institute. Bethesda, MD. http://seer.cancer.gov/csr/1975_2008/, based on November 2010 SEER data submission, posted to the SEER web site, 2011. Accessed September 3, 2014.

116. Kaurah P, MacMillan A, Boyd N, et al. Founder and recurrent CDH1 mutations in families with hereditary diffuse gastric cancer. *JAMA* 2007;297:2360–2372.

117. Brooks-Wilson AR, Kaurah P, Suriano G, et al. Germline E-cadherin mutations in hereditary diffuse gastric cancer: Assessment of 42 new families and review of genetic screening criteria. *J Med Genet* 2004;41:508–517.

118. Pharoah PD, Guilford P, Caldas C, et al. Incidence of gastric cancer and breast cancer in CDH1 (E-cadherin) mutation carriers from hereditary diffuse gastric cancer families. *Gastroenterology* 2001;121:1348–1353.

119. Keller G, Vogelsang H, Becker I, et al. Diffuse type gastric and lobular breast carcinoma in a familial gastric cancer patient with an E-cadherin germline mutation. *Am J Pathol* 1999;155:337–342.

120. Oliveira C, Bordin MC, Grehan N, et al. Screening E-cadherin in gastric cancer families reveals germline mutations only in hereditary diffuse gastric cancer kindred. *Hum Mutat* 2002;19:510–517.

121. Frebourg T, Oliveira C, Hochain P, et al. Cleft lip/palate and CDH1/E-cadherin mutations in families with hereditary diffuse gastric cancer. *J Med Genet* 2006;43:138–142.

122. Schrader KA, Masciari S, Boyd N, et al. Germline mutations in CDH1 are infrequent in women with early-onset or familial lobular breast cancers. *J Med Genet* 2011;48:64–68.

123. Walsh T, Casadei S, Lee MK, et al. Mutations in 12 genes for inherited ovarian, fallopian tube, and peritoneal carcinoma identified by massively parallel sequencing. *Proc Natl Acad Sci U S A* 2011;108:18032–18037.

124. Ripperger T, Gadzicki D, Meindl A, et al. Breast cancer susceptibility: Current knowledge and implications for genetic counselling. *Eur J Hum Genet* 2009;17:722–731.

125. Lalloo F, Evans DG. Familial breast cancer. *Clin Genet* 2012;82:105–114.

126. Shuen AY, Foulkes WD. Inherited mutations in breast cancer genes—risk and response. *J Mammary Gland Biol Neoplasia* 2011;16:3–15.

127. Weissman SM, Bellcross C, Bittner CC, et al. Genetic counseling considerations in the evaluation of families for Lynch syndrome—a review. *J Genet Couns* 2011;20:5–19.

128. Watson P, Vasen HF, Mecklin JP, et al. The risk of extra-colonic, extra-endometrial cancer in the Lynch syndrome. *Int J Cancer* 2008;123:444–449.

129. Win AK, Young JP, Lindor NM, et al. Colorectal and other cancer risks for carriers and noncarriers from families with a DNA mismatch repair gene mutation: a prospective cohort study. *J Clin Oncol* 2012;30:958–964.

130. Walsh MD, Buchanan DD, Cummings MC, et al. Lynch syndrome-associated breast cancers: Clinicopathologic characteristics of a case series from the colon cancer family registry. *Clin Cancer Res* 2010;16:2214–2224.

131. Buerki N, Gautier L, Kovac M, et al. Evidence for breast cancer as an integral part of Lynch syndrome. *Genes Chromosomes Cancer* 2012;51:83–91.

132. Lefevre JH, Colas C, Coulet F, et al. MYH biallelic mutation can inactivate the two genetic pathways of colorectal cancer by APC or MLH1 transversions. *Fam Cancer* 2010;9:589–594.

133. Sieber OM, Lipton L, Crabtree M, et al. Multiple colorectal adenomas, classic adenomatous polyposis, and germ-line mutations in MYH. *N Engl J Med* 2003;348:791–799.

134. Boparai KS, Dekker E, Van Eeden S, et al. Hyperplastic polyps and sessile serrated adenomas as a phenotypic expression of MYH-associated polyposis. *Gastroenterology* 2008;135:2014–2018.

135. Vogt S, Jones N, Christian D, et al. Expanded extracolonic tumor spectrum in MUTYH-associated polyposis. *Gastroenterology* 2009;137:1976–1985.e1–e10.

136. Nielsen M, Franken PF, Reinards TH, et al. Multiplicity in polyp count and extracolonic manifestations in 40 Dutch patients with MYH associated polyposis coli (MAP). *J Med Genet* 2005;42:e54.

137. Beiner ME, Zhang WW, Zhang S, et al. Mutations of the MYH gene do not substantially contribute to the risk of breast cancer. *Breast Cancer Res Treat* 2009;114:575–578.

PRACTICE OF ONCOLOGY

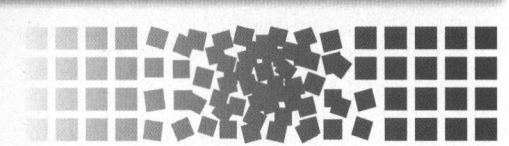

81 Molecular Biology of Endocrine Tumors

Samuel A. Wells, Jr.

INTRODUCTION

Over the last two decades, advances in molecular biology have provided a deeper understanding of the etiology and pathogenesis of endocrine diseases. Studies of hereditary endocrinopathies have been particularly instructive in this regard and have led to significant improvements in the diagnosis and treatment of patients with both hereditary and sporadic endocrine cancers. The introduction of a new class of drugs, molecular targeted therapeutics (MTT), has been a particularly notable achievement in the treatment of patients with advanced endocrine cancers, a disease stage for which there had been no effective therapy.

THE MULTIPLE ENDOCRINE NEOPLASIA SYNDROMES

Most endocrine tumors involve a single gland, are usually benign, and occur sporadically. Rarely, however, two or more endocrine tumors occur together in a familial pattern designated as the multiple endocrine neoplasias (MEN) syndromes. The genetic mutations causing the two most common of these disorders, MEN1 and MEN2, have been identified, which led to improved management of patients with these syndromes as well as patients with the related sporadic endocrine tumors.

Multiple Endocrine Neoplasia Type 1

Clinical Features

In 1954, Wermer described a family with hyperparathyroidism and tumors of the pancreatic islet cells and the pituitary gland.[1] This hereditary syndrome has since been named MEN1 (Online Mendelian Inheritance in Man [OMIM] #131100), and it may include over 20 separate endocrine and nonendocrine tumors. The prevalence of MEN1 is 1 per 30,000 to 100,000 persons. Males and females are equally affected, although women are more prone to develop pituitary tumors and men are more prone to develop gastrinomas and thymus tumors.[2-6] MEN1 is characterized by high penetrance but variable expressivity. While parathyroid hyperplasia occurs in virtually all patients by age 40 years, other endocrine tumors develop less frequently. Pancreatic islet cell tumors (usually gastrinomas, less often insulinomas, and rarely glucagonomas, or vasoactive intestinal polypeptide secreting tumors, occur in 50% to 70% of patients) Pituitary tumors (usually prolactinomas, adrenal cortical tumors, and thymus tumors, occur in 20% to 40%, 20% to 40%, and 10% of patients, respectively. The diagnosis of MEN1 is established when a patient with hyperparathyroidism develops a pituitary tumor or a pancreatic islet cell tumor, when a previously unaffected member of a family with MEN1 develops a single characteristic endocrine tumor, or when a germline MEN1 mutation is detected in an individual who may or may not have an endocrine tumor associated with MEN1. The severity of the disease is unpredictable; although recently, an interaction between menin and JunD was shown to be significantly associated with a higher death rate, primarily due to thymus and pancreatic tumors.[7]

Molecular Genetics of MEN1

Chandrasekharappa et al. discovered MEN1, the genetic mutation for MEN1.[8] The MEN1 gene spans a 9.8 kb segment of chromosome 11q13 and consists of 10 exons with a 1,830 base pair region that encodes transcripts of 2.7 and 3.1 kb. MEN1 is a putative tumor suppressor gene, residing in the nucleus of nondividing cells and in the cytoplasm of diving cells.[9,10] Homozygous mice null for MEN1 die during embryogenesis, while heterologous mice, $MEN1^{+/-}$, develop a pattern of endocrine tumors very similar to that occurring in patients with MEN1.[11] The transcripts, expressed in almost all tissues, encode a novel, highly conserved, ubiquitously expressed, 610 amino acid, 67kDa protein, named menin. The biochemical mechanism underlying the tumor-suppressing function of menin is unknown, however, it appears to play a critical role in the regulation of gene transcription, apoptosis, and genome stability.[12] Menin's crystal structure indicates that it is a scaffold protein that interacts with distinct partner proteins, approximately 40 of which have been identified, the most common including JunD, MLL1, LEDGF, and H3K4m3.[13] Epigenetic regulation of gene expression is a central aspect of menin's function, thus alteration of epigenetic targets holds promise for the treatment of MEN1-related tumors.[14]

More than 1,000 distinct and presumed pathologic mutations have been identified over the coding region of the MEN1 gene; approximately 70% are germline mutations and 30% are somatic mutations (Fig. 81.1).[12] The mutations are diverse in type (including frame-shift, deletions or insertions, nonsense, missense, splice-site alterations, in-frame deletions or insertions, and large deletions), and occur throughout the 1,830 base pair coding region with no evidence of clustering or "hot spots," as is seen in MEN2.[15] Although large deletions have been reported in the MEN1 gene, no mutations have been reported in the promoter region.[16] Screening of the coding region of the MEN1 gene has identified a heterozygous germline mutation in 70% of sporadic or familial index cases of MEN1.[15] There is no association between genotype and phenotype, and even families with the same base pair deletion can display a wide range of MEN1-associated tumors.[17] The first "hit" leading to tumorogenesis involves small mutations in one or several bases, broadly distributed across the MEN1 open reading frame. Approximately 75% of first-hit mutations lead to premature truncation of the menin protein. Most often, a large chromosomal rearrangement causes a deletion of the normal MEN1 gene resulting in loss of heterozygosity, compromising the second hit in the Knudson two-hit hypothesis.[18]

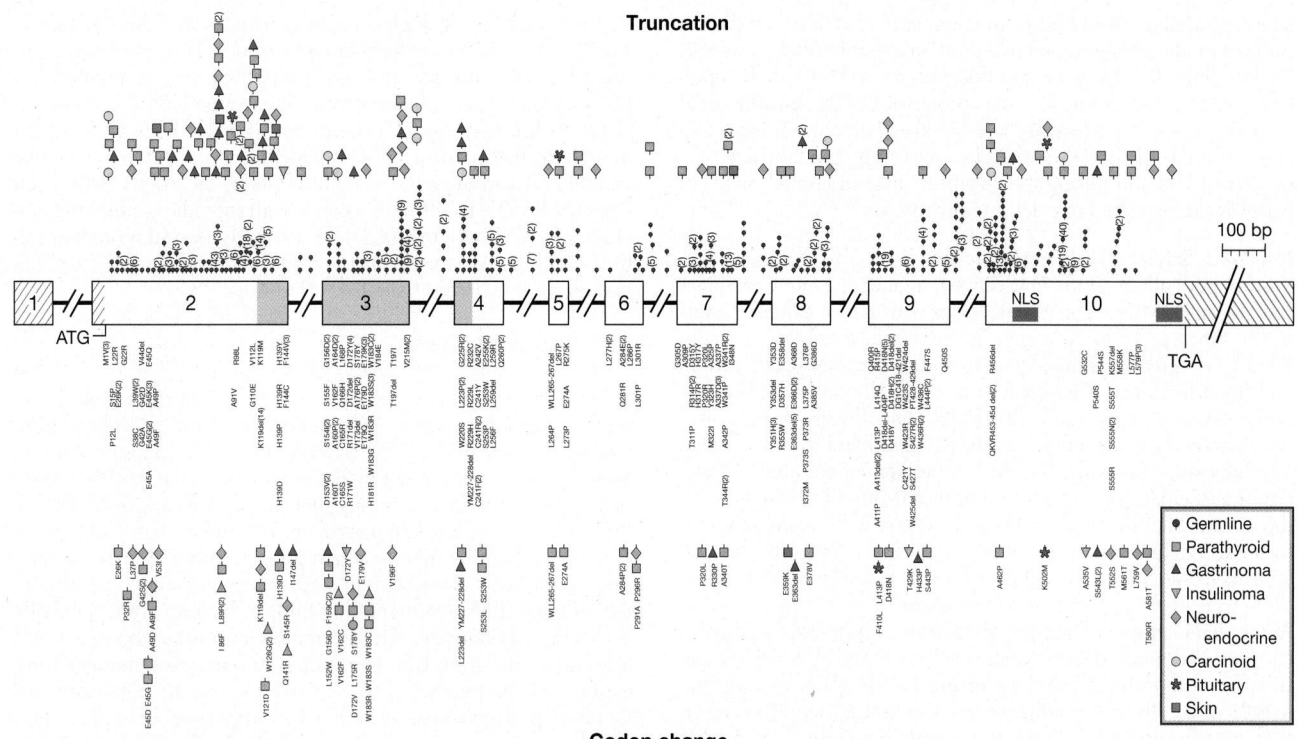

Figure 81.1 Germline and somatic mutations of the *MEN1* gene. Unique germline *MEN1* mutations in families, sporadic cases, and nonhereditary tumors. The figure shows 670 unique mutations identified by 2006. Repeating mutations within the germline or somatic category (common ancestry versus hot spots for mutation) are shown only once, with a small number in parentheses to indicate total occurrences. Germline mutations are shown as *black lollipops* or as code about the messenger RNA (mRNA). Somatic *MEN1* mutations in diverse tumors are shown separately as *flags* along the upper and lower border and as code. *MEN1* mRNA is diagrammed with exons numbered; untranslated regions are *crosshatched*. Truncating mutations (frameshift mutations, splice errors, and nonsense [stop codon] mutations) are shown above the mRNA; they account for 75% of all mutations. Codon change mutations (missense mutations or small in-frame deletions) are shown below the mRNA with their three-letter amino acid code. *Stippling* about exon 3 represents the main zone of menin interaction with JunD. Several large deletions, probably of the entire *MEN1* gene, are not shown. NLS, nuclear localization sequence; ATG, a transcription factor; TGA, a stop codon; bp, base pair. (Reprinted from Melmed S, Polonsky KS, Larsen PR, et al., eds. The multiple endocrine neoplasia syndromes. In: *Williams Textbook of Endocrinology*. 12th ed. Amsterdam: Elsevier; 2011:1728–1756, Figure 41-7. With permission from Elsevier.)

Mutational analysis is important in confirming the diagnosis in patients with clinically evident MEN1 and in identifying first-degree relatives who have inherited, or have not inherited, the MEN1 mutation so that respectively they can either be followed for the development of endocrine tumors or cease to be followed. Half of newly diagnosed index cases are found to have novel mutations, and more than 10% of *MEN1* mutations arise de novo and will be passed to subsequent generations.[17,19,20] It is important to note that the absence of an *MEN1* mutation in a patient with tumors characteristic of MEN1 does not exclude that the patient has MEN1.

The endocrine tumors associated with MEN1 occur more commonly in a sporadic setting, and it is of interest that 25% of gastrinomas, 10% to 20% of insulinomas, 50% of VIPomas, 25% to 35% of bronchial carcinoids, and 20% of parathyroid adenomas express somatic *MEN1* mutations. Conversely, somatic *MEN1* mutations rarely if ever occur in sporadic adrenocortical tumors, pituitary tumors, or thymus tumors.[21]

Hereditary Endocrinopathies, Other than MEN1, Involving the Parathyroid and Pituitary Glands

The Parathyroid Gland

Primary hyperparathyroidism occurs in 1 of every 1,000 persons, and 5% to 10% of cases occur in a familial pattern, most often as MEN1, MEN2A, familial hypocalciuric hypercalcemia (FHH),

the hyperparathyroidism jaw-tumor syndrome (HPT-JT), and familial isolated hyperparathyroidism (FIHP).

Familial Hypocalciuric Hypercalcemia, Neonatal Severe Hyperparathyroidism, Autosomal Dominant Hypoparathyroidism, and Familial Isolated Hyperparathyroidism

Familial Hypocalciuric Hypercalcemia. The calcium-sensing receptor *CASR* gene is a seven-transmembrane-spanning G protein–coupled receptor that is expressed in cells of the parathyroid gland and the kidney tubule. *CASR* plays a critical role in regulating extracellular calcium homeostasis. The discovery of *CASR* was a surprise, since previously no small cation had been shown capable of acting as a ligand for a G-protein coupled receptor.[22] The human *CASR*, located on chromosome 3q113.3-q21, is sensitive to changes in the ambient calcium concentration and when activated inhibits parathyroid hormone (PTH) secretion and the renal reabsorption of calcium. With heterogeneous inactivating mutations of the *CASR* gene, the parathyroid cell fails to sense properly an increased serum calcium concentration; the resulting increase in PTH secretion causes FHH (OMIM #145980), an autosomal dominant disease characterized by hypocalciuria, hypercalcemia, mild hypermagnesemia, and parathyroid hyperfunction.[23] Bone density levels are not decreased, and patients are generally asymptomatic. It is important for clinicians to recognize this relatively mild form of familial hyperparathyroidism, as it is not cured by parathyroidectomy.[24] More than 250 different mutations have been reported to affect *CASR* function, and mutational analysis is utilized to identify family members who have inherited a mutated *CASR* allele. It is important to note, however, that *CASR* mutations are detected in only 65% of patients with FHH and additional mapping studies have revealed additional loci on chromosome 19p and chromosome 19q13.3, thereby suggesting genetic heterogeneity for FHH and raising the possibility that additional or signal pathways are involved in calcium homeostasis.[25–27]

Neonatal Severe Hyperparathyroidism. With inactivating mutations in both alleles of the *CASR* gene, neonatal severe hyperparathyroidism (OMIM #239200) develops with serum calcium levels in the range of 15 to 20 mg/dl, up to 10-fold increases in serum PTH levels, greatly enlarged parathyroid glands, demineralization, and bone fractures. The disease was originally described in consanguineous parents, each with FHH. This disease represents a life-threatening emergency, and urgent parathyroidectomy is usually indicated. Recently, however, there are reports that the calcimimetic cinacalcet produces robust and durable reductions in the serum calcium concentrations of patients with neonatal severe hyperparathyroidism. However, the response is not uniform and appears to depend on the patient's specific *CASR* mutation.[24,28]

Autosomal Dominant Hypoparathyroidism. The related syndrome, autosomal dominant hypoparathyroidism (OMIM #146200) results from activating mutations of the *CASR* gene, causing the parathyroid cells to sense that serum calcium is "elevated" when it is actually normal.[29] There is a resulting suppression of PTH secretion (even though it remains within the reference range), enhanced urinary Ca^{++} secretion, hypomagnesemia, and increased fractional excretion of magnesium. More than 70 activating mutations have been reported in autosomal dominant hypoparathyroidism, and both familial cases and sporadic cases with de novo mutations have been described.[30]

Familial Isolated Hyperparathyroidism. FIHP (OMIM #146200) is a heterogeneous condition, and some kindreds thought to have this disease have been shown to have germline mutations of *MEN1*, *CASR*, *CDC73*, and *CDKN1B* suggesting that the disease represents incompletely expressed forms of MEN1, FHH, or the HPT-JT.[31] Over 100 families with FIHP have been reported, and in most cases the causative genetic mutation is unknown although there are convincing data that it resides on chromosome 2p13.3-14.[32]

Hyperparathyroidism-Jaw Tumor Syndrome. HPT-JT (OMIM #145001) is characterized by the autosomal dominant occurrence of hyperparathyroidism, ossifying fibromas of the mandible or maxilla, renal cysts or solid tumors, and uterine fibromas.[33] Approximately 50 families with HPT-JT have been reported, and 80 percent of patients have hyperparathyroidism. In 15% of patients with HPT-JT, the parathyroid tumors are malignant. It is noteworthy that the age-related penetrance of HPT-JT is approximately 40% by age 40 years in contrast to MEN1 where the age-related penetrance is 98% by age 40.[34] Members of kindreds with this disease need lifelong surveillance by physical examination and biochemical evaluation. It has even been suggested that serial ultrasound examination of the neck should be performed beginning at a young age as parathyroid carcinoma has been reported in normocalcemic family members.[35]

Inactivating mutations of the HRPT2 tumor suppressor gene, also known as *CDC73*, causes HPT-JT. The gene is located on chromosome 1q25-q31 and codes for the 531 amino acid tumor suppressor protein, parafibromin (named for parathyroid tumors and jaw fibromas).[36] The function of parafibromin is unknown but it is thought to regulate posttranscriptional events and histone modification. There is recent evidence that parafibromin has proapoptotic activity, important as a tumor suppressor function.[37]

The *CDC73* gene consists of 17 exons, and the mutations are scattered throughout the coding region, with the majority resulting in functional loss through premature truncation.[38] Approximately 100 germline and somatic mutations of *CDC73* have been identified but there are no "hot spot" mutations and no relationship between genotype and phenotype.[39] Germline *CDC73* mutations occur in the majority of patients with the HPT-JT, and surprisingly they also occur in 20% of patients with apparently sporadic parathyroid carcinomas. Somatic *CDC73* mutations have been detected in 50% to 100% of patients with sporadic parathyroid carcinoma.[40,41] Mutations in *CDC73* are rarely seen in sporadic parathyroid adenomas, an important diagnostic finding distinguishing benign from malignant parathyroid tumors.[37,42]

The Pituitary Gland

Familial Isolated Pituitary Adenomas. Approximately 5% of pituitary tumors occur in a familial pattern. Familial isolated pituitary adenomas (FIPA [OMIM #102200]) is an autosomal dominant disease characterized by the occurrence of at least two cases of pituitary tumors in a family that has no features of MEN1 or the Carney complex.[43] In a study of 64 families with FIPA, 55 of 138 affected family members had prolactinomas, 47 had somatotropinomas, 28 had nonsecreting adenomas, and eight had adrenocorticotropic hormone–secreting tumors.[44] There are two equally occurring phenotypes, where families are either homogenous, expressing the same type of pituitary tumors, or heterogeneous, expressing different types of pituitary tumors. In heterogeneous families, prolactinomas exhibit more aggressive behavior, compared to their sporadic counterparts, with higher rates of subsella expansion and cavernous sinus invasion. Conversely, somatotropinomas are more aggressive in the homogenous setting.

Germline mutations in the *aryl hydrocarbon receptor interacting protein (AIP)* gene occur in 20% (range 15% to 40%) of patients with FIPA; however, in the remainder, the causative gene is unknown.[45] The *AIP* gene consists of six exons encoding a 330 amino acid (37 kDa) cytoplasmic co-chaperone phosphoprotein (XAP2).[46] The gene is located at 11q13, which is 2.7 Mb downstream from the *MEN1* gene. *AIP* forms a complex with the aryl hydrocarbon receptor and two 90-kD heat-shock proteins (HSP90). The aryl hydrocarbon receptor is a ligand-activated transcription factor and also participates in cellular signaling pathways.[47] The mean age at diagnosis is 13 years earlier in *AIP*-positive FIPA families compared to *AIP*-negative families, and the majority of patients in *AIP*-positive families are male, where there is equal gender balance in *AIP*-negative families. The pituitary tumors in *AIP*-positive patients are large, frequently invade surrounding structures, and respond poorly to somatostatin analogues.[48,49]

Multiple Endocrine Neoplasia Type 2

Multiple Endocrine Neoplasia Type 2A and Multiple Endocrine Neoplasia 2B

Clinical Features. In 1968, Steiner and associates described a large family with medullary thyroid carcinoma (MTC), pheochromocytomas (PHEO), hyperparathyroidism (HPTH), and Cushing syndrome.[50] The disease was named MEN type 2, and we now it as MEN2A. Until recently, there were three related syndromes of hereditary MTC: MEN2A (OMIM #171400), MEN2B (OMIM #162300), and familial MTC (FMTC) (OMIM #155240).[51,52] Most endocrinologists now feel that FMTC represents a variant of MEN2A and should not stand alone as a disease entity. It has recently been suggested that there be two MEN2 syndromes: MEN2A and MEN2B. In addition, within MEN2A, it has been suggested that there be four variants: classical MEN2A, MEN2A with Hirschsprung disease, MEN2A with cutaneous lichen amyloidosis, and FMTC.[53]

Of patients with hereditary MTC, 95% have MEN2A and 5% have MEN2B. Virtually all patients with these syndromes develop MTC, and up to half of the patients with MEN2A and MEN2B develop PHEOs. The PHEOs are almost always benign and confined to the adrenal gland. Patients with a unilateral PHEO usually develop a contralateral PHEO within 10 years.[54] Prior to the development of biochemical and genetic test to establish the early diagnosis of hereditary MTC, PHEO, not MTC, was the most common cause of death in patients with MEN2A.[55] Approximately 30% of patients with MEN2A develop HPTH, which is usually mild and asymptomatic.

Patients with MEN2B have a typical physical appearance with a Marfanoid habitus and atypical facies. They also have a generalized ganglioneuromatosis and ocular and skeletal abnormalities.

MTC originates from the neural crest–derived C-cells. The MTC cells secrete the polypeptide hormone calcitonin (CTN) and the glycoprotein carcinoembryonic antigen. Serum levels of CTN and carcinoembryonic antigen are excellent tumor markers, most useful in detecting persistent or recurrent disease following thyroidectomy for MTC. The most effective therapy for MTC is thyroidectomy, preferentially performed before MTC develops or while it is still confined to the thyroid gland.

Molecular Genetics of MEN2A and MEN2B. In 1985, Takahashi and associates discovered the *RET* (REarranged during Transfection) protooncogene.[56] The gene is located in the pericentromeric region of chromosome 10q11.2 and includes 21 exons. *RET* encodes a receptor tyrosine kinase, which is expressed in neuroendocrine cells (including thyroid C cells and adrenal medullary cells), neural cells (including parasympathetic and sympathetic ganglion cells), urogenital tract cells, and branchial arch cells. *RET* is essential for the development, survival, and regeneration of neuronal cells in the gut, the kidney, and the nervous system.

The *RET* gene has an extracellular portion containing four cadherin-like repeats, a calcium binding site and a cysteine–rich region, a transmembrane portion, and an intracellular portion containing two tyrosine kinase domains.[53] Alternate splicing of *RET* produces three isoforms with either 9, 43, or 51 amino acids at the C terminus, referred to as *RET9*, *RET43*, and *RET51*.[57,58] Mice lacking *RET51* are normal; however, mice lacking *RET9* have renal malformation and defects in innervation of the gut.[59] *RET51* and *RET9* have transforming activity but *RET51* is the stronger of the two.

A tripartite complex is necessary for *RET* signaling. One of four glial-derived neurotrophic factors (GDNF) family ligands; GDNF, neurturin, persephin, or artemin binds *RET* in conjunction with one of four glycosylphosphatidylinositol-anchored co-receptors, designated GDNF family receptors (GFR): GFR-α1, GFR-α2, GFR-α3, or GFR-α4.[60–62] The GDNF family ligand–GFR complex causes dimerization of *RET* with activation of autophosphorylation and intracellular signaling. The molecular pathways associated with activation of the *RET* protooncogene are shown in Fig. 81.2.[53]

MEN2A and MEN2B are caused by mutations in the *RET* protooncogene; the most common are shown in Fig. 81.3.[63,64] In

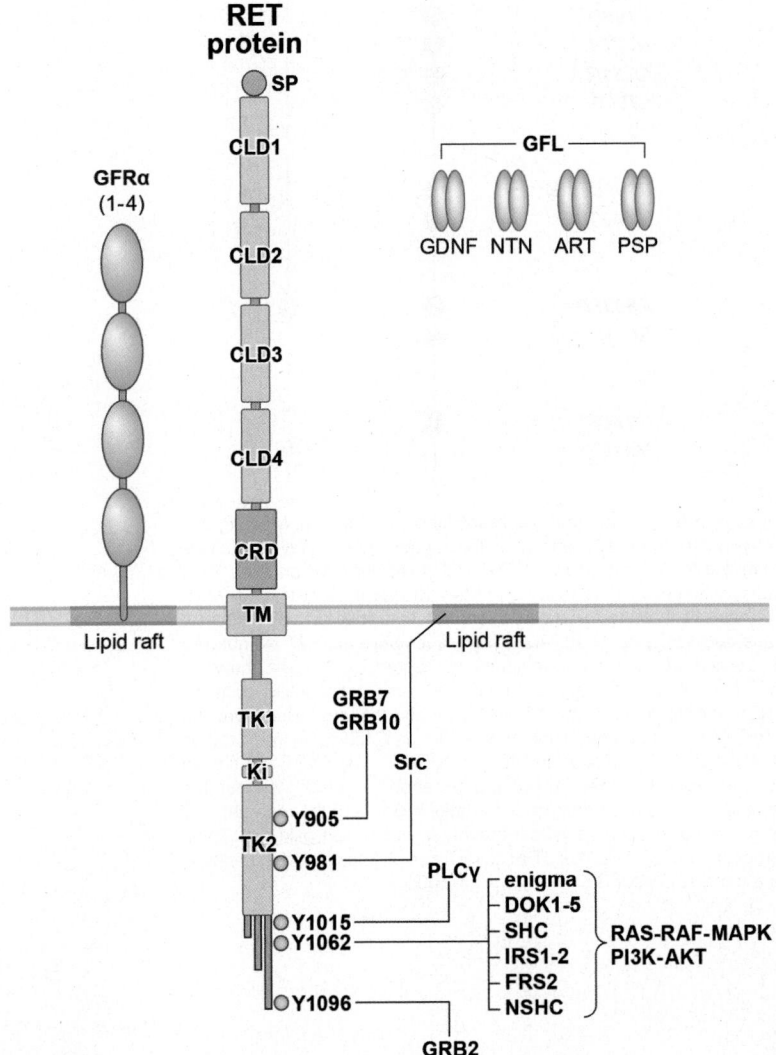

Figure 81.2 The RET protein. The position of major RET phosphorylation sites (Y905, Y1015, and Y1062) are marked, as are other phosphorylation sites and signaling pathways. SP, signal peptide; CLD, cadherin-like domains; CRD, cysteine-rich domain; TM, transmembrane domain; TK, tyrosine kinase domain; Ki, kinase insert region; GFRα (1–4), GDNF family alpha receptors; GFL, glial derived neurotrophic factor family ligands; GDNF, glial derived neurotrophic factor; NTN, neuturin; ART, artemin; PSP, persephin. (Reproduced from Wells SA Jr, Pacini F, Robinson BG, et al. Multiple endocrine neoplasia type 2 and familial medullary thyroid carcinoma: an update. *J Clin Endocrinol Metab* 2013;98:3149–3164, Figure 1, Copyright 2013; With permission from the Endocrine Society, *http://jcem.endojournals.org/site/author/itoa.xhtml.*)

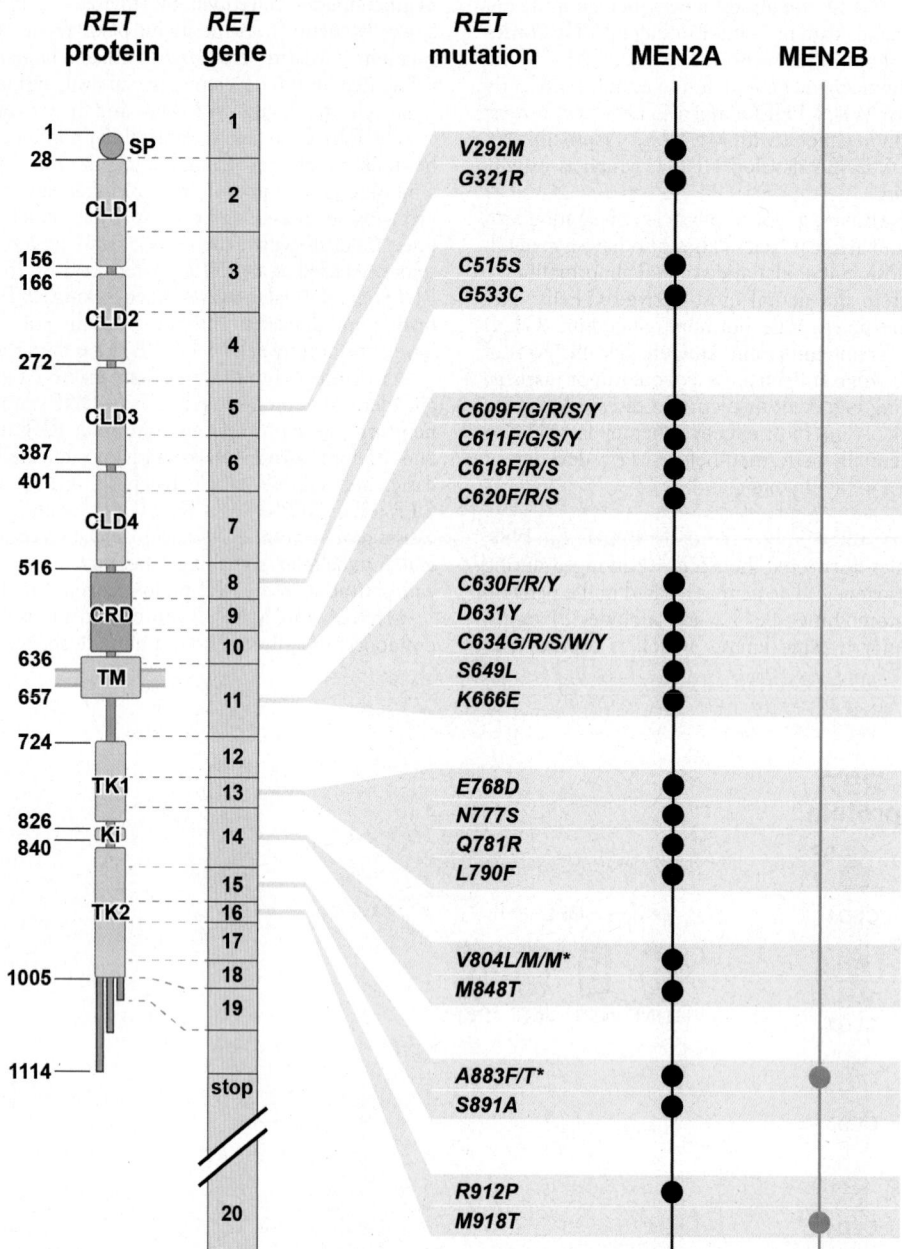

Figure 81.3 The *RET* gene, the RET protein, and *RET* point mutations associated with MEN2A, MEN2B, and FMTC. RET gene structure with coding exons numbered 1–20 is shown as the central figure in *gray*. Alternative splicing in exon 19 generates two alternative mRNAs, coding for RET-51 (1,114 residues) when exon 19 is spliced to exon 20, or RET-9 (1,072 residues), when exon 19 remains unspliced. Moreover, alternative splicing to a further exon (exon 21) causes the synthesis of the C-terminal part of another less abundant RET isoform, RET-43. In this figure, only RET-51 is represented, while RET-9, RET-43 and the alternative exon 21 are not. The RET protein is represented on the left in *blue* and *red*. Amino acid residues, numbered 1–1,114, are shown to the left of the figure. The extracellular RET domain (with the signal peptide [SP], four cadherin-like domains [CLD1–4], and a cysteine-rich domain [CRD]), the transmembrane domain (TM), and the intracellular tyrosine kinase domain (TK) are represented. The RET TK is split into two subdomains (TK1 and TK2) by an insert region (Ki). The positions of reported *RET* point mutations associated with MEN2A, MEN2B, and FMTC are shown to the right of the *RET* gene. The mutations causing MEN2A and MEN2B are shown in *black*, whereas the mutations for FMTC are shown in *red*. An *asterisk* denotes homozygous mutations. Some of the reported RET mutations have no function studies demonstrating that the specific mutation is a bona fide gain-of-function mutation. (Modified from Figure 5 in de Groot JW, Links TP, Plukker JT, et al. RET as a diagnostic and therapeutic target in sporadic and hereditary endocrine tumors. *Endocr Rev* 2006; 27:535–560.)

approximately 50% of patients with MEN2B and 10% of patients with MEN2A, the *RET* mutation arises de novo and virtually always from the paternal allele. Furthermore, in MEN2B there is a gender preference such that the first offspring of transmitting males is almost always an affected female.[65]

In patients with MEN2A, there is a correlation between genotype and phenotype. In 98% of patients with MEN2A, mutations occur in *RET* codons 609, 611, 618, 620, and 634. *RET* codon 634 accounts for 80% of mutations in MEN2A. The frequency of PHEO depends on the *RET* codon mutation: (634 [50%], 609 [4% to 26%], 611 [10% to 25%], 618 [12% to 23%], and 620 [13% to 24%]).[66,67] A *RET* codon 634 mutation is associated with a 30% incidence of HPTH; however, the frequency ranges between 2% and 10% in patients with mutations in *RET* codons 609, 611, 618, and 620.[68] Patients with MEN2A may also develop cutaneous lichen amyloidosis, which is almost always associated with a *RET* codon 634 mutation.[69] Less commonly, patients with MEN2A develop Hirschsprung disease, which is associated with *RET* codon mutations in exon 10: 609 (15%), 611 (5%), 618 (30%), and 620 (50%).[70]

Approximately 95% of patients with MEN2B have mutations in *RET* codon M918T, and most of the remainder have mutations in *RET* codon A833F.[71,72] Rarely, patients with MEN2B have double mutations appearing in tandem on the same allele involving *RET* codon V804M and either codon Y806C, S904C, E805K, or Q781R. The MEN2B syndrome in patients with these double mutations is atypical, and MTC presents at a later age than in patients with typical MEN2B.[73–76] Approximately half of the patients with sporadic MTC have a somatic *RET* M918T mutation, which it appears is associated with a more aggressive clinical phenotype.[77] Recently, it was discovered that the majority of patients with sporadic MTC who have no somatic *RET* mutations have somatic mutations of *HRAS*, *KRAS*, or rarely *NRAS*.[78] There is no indication that the presence of somatic *RAS* mutations is associated with a pattern of clinical behavior of the MTC.

Of patients with presumed sporadic MTC, 7% will be found on direct DNA analysis to have germline *RET* mutations, characteristic of MEN2A, meaning that they and their first-degree relatives should be evaluated for the presence of all components of this syndrome.[79]

APPLICATION OF MOLECULAR GENETICS TO CLINICAL MEDICINE

The discovery that mutations in the *RET* protooncogene cause MEN2A, MEN2B, and FMTC changed the management of patients with both sporadic and hereditary MTC and represents a paradigm for personalized genomic medicine.

Prophylactic Thyroidectomy

In patients with MEN2A and MEN2B who are shown to have inherited a mutated *RET* allele, it is important to remove the thyroid before MTC develops or while it is still confined to the gland.[80] The question in family members with hereditary MTC who have inherited a mutated *RET* allele is not whether the thyroid gland should be removed but at what age? At the MEN Consortium Meeting in 2000, a consensus panel evaluated the relationship between the *RET* codon mutation and the biologic aggressiveness of hereditary MTC.[81] Based on combined clinical data, the panel defined three levels of thyroid cancer severity on which to base the timing of thyroidectomy. Subsequently, three professional organizations published guidelines defining the management of patients with MEN2A and MEN2B, including the timing of recommended thyroidectomy in patients who had inherited a mutated *RET* allele.[82–84] Generally, the

recommendations among the groups were similar and the timing of thyroidectomy was based on the clinical aggressiveness of patients with a specific *RET* mutation. This was not a problem for patients with some mutations. For example, patients with *RET* M918T mutations, which occur in the large majority of patients with MEN2B, should have thyroidectomy as soon as the diagnosis is established, even in the first months of life. Also, patients with MEN2A who have mutations in codon 634 have an aggressive MTC and the thyroid should be removed at or before 5 years of age. Decisions regarding thyroidectomy in patients with other *RET* mutations are based on knowledge of behavior of MTC in the patient's family, or in other families with the same *RET* mutation, or more importantly on measurements of basal or stimulated serum CTN levels.

Molecular Targeted Therapeutics

There has been no effective therapy for patients with locally advanced or metastatic MTC, as single-agent or combined chemotherapy has been characterized by low response rates of short duration.[85] With the discovery that the MTT imatinib induced striking and prolonged remissions in patients with chronic myelogenous leukemia, it was hoped that similar therapeutics would be developed for solid tumors, including thyroid cancer, where the specific mutated gene was known and druggable.[86] In phase 2 clinical trials the MTT vandetanib, known to inhibit RET and vascular endothelial growth factor receptors, showed significant clinical activity in patients with advanced MTC.[87,88] In a subsequent phase 3 prospective, randomized, clinical trial of patients with locally advanced or metastatic MTC, vandetanib induced significant progression-free survival compared to placebo.[89] Based on the trial the US Food and Drug Administration (FDA) approved vandetanib for the treatment of patients with advanced MTC. Subsequently, also based on results of a phase 3 clinical trial, the FDA approved the MTT cabozantinib for the treatment of patients with advanced MTC.[90] Despite the fact that these drugs have shown efficacy in the treatment of advanced MTC, most patients in time become resistant to the drug, and their disease progresses. Hopefully, an understanding at the molecular level of mechanisms of resistance to various MTTs will provide the basis for the development of promising regimens of combinatorial therapy.

THYROID CARCINOMAS

Papillary Thyroid Carcinoma

Malignant tumors of the thyroid gland have a great range of biologic behavior, ranging from the relatively slow-growing papillary thyroid carcinoma (PTC) and follicular thyroid carcinoma (FTC) to the highly aggressive anaplastic thyroid carcinoma (ATC). Over the last three decades, it has become clear that mutations or chromosomal rearrangements in the mitogen-activated-protein kinase (MAPK) and the phosphatidylinositol 3-kinase (PI3K)/protein kinase B pathways cause the most common forms of thyroid cancer (Fig. 81.4). For example, mutually exclusive activating mutations of *HRAS*, *KRAS*, *NRAS*, or *BRAF*, or chromosomal rearrangements of genes encoding *RET* (*RET/PTCs*) or *NTRK1* (*TRK-Ts*) occur in 70% of patients with PTC.[91] The most common mutation, *BRAF*^{V600E}, occurs in approximately 50% of patients with PTC and is most common in patients with classic PTC (60%) and the tall cell variant of PTC (90%). The mutation also occurs in poorly differentiated thyroid carcinomas and ATCs, derived from PTC. Mutations in *HRAS*, *KRAS*, or more commonly *NRAS* occur in 25% of FTCs, 15% of PTCs (almost always the follicular variant of PTC), and 5% of follicular adenomas.[92] Mutations in

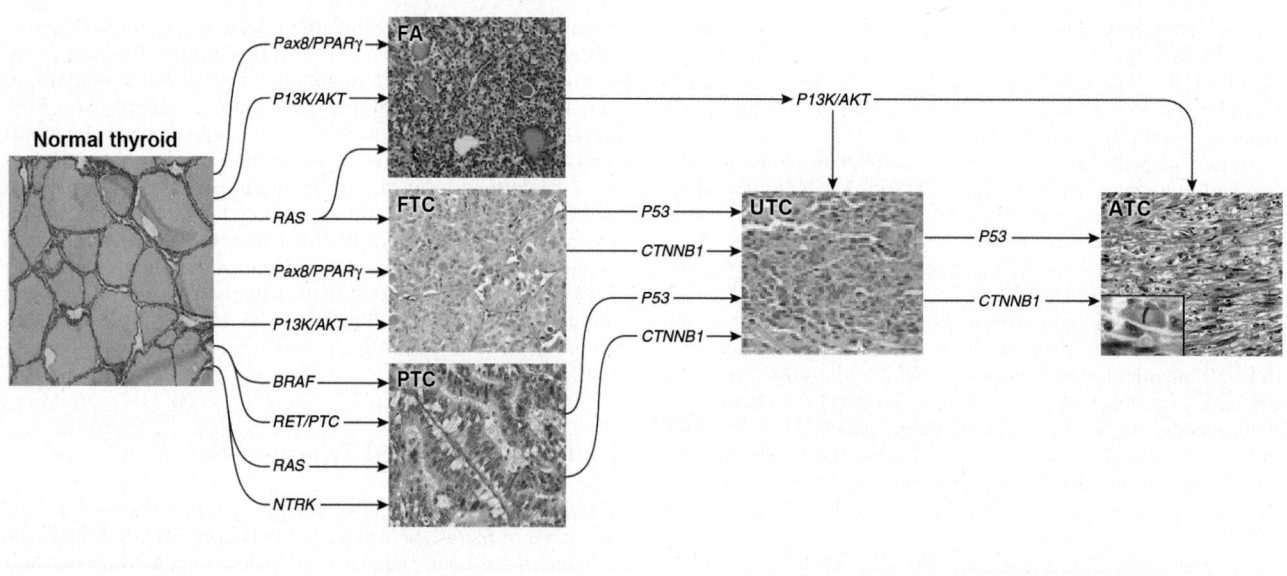

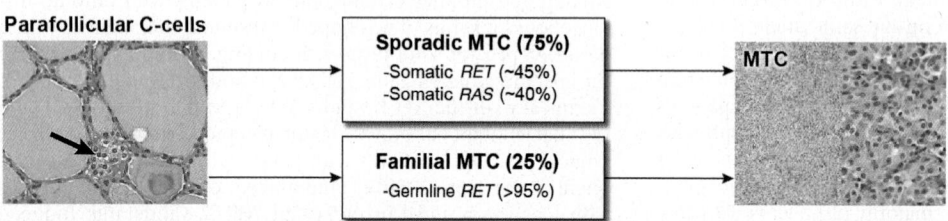

Figure 81.4 Subtypes of thyroid neoplasms, either arising from follicular (*top*) or parafollicular (*bottom*) cells are depicted together with genes bearing the most prevalent oncogenic driving lesions (see text for details). FA, follicular adenoma; FTC, follicular thyroid carcinoma; PTC, papillary thyroid carcinoma; UTC, undifferentiated thyroid carcinoma; ATC, anaplastic thyroid carcinoma; MTC, medullary thyroid carcinoma. *Arrow*: area of parafollicular thyroid C cells. (Reproduced from Wells SA Jr, Sanoto M. Update: the status of clinical trials of kinase inhibitors in thyroid cancer. *J Clin Endocrinol Metab* 2014;99:1543–1555, Figure 1, Copyright 2013; With permission from the Endocrine Society, http://jcem.endojournals.org/site/author/itoa.xhtml.)

p53 and *CTNNB1* (B-catenin) occur commonly in patients with poorly differentiated thyroid carcinoma and ATC.[93]

The first chromosomal rearrangement associated with thyroid cancer was described in 1985 with the discovery of the *RET* protooncogene.[56] In 1987, Fusco and associates demonstrated that approximately 30% of PTCs have a chromosomal translocation, resulting in the fusion of the C-terminal *RET* tyrosine kinase–encoding domain to the promoter and N-terminal portion of unrelated genes.[94] The creation of these heterologous partners results in the illegitimate expression of a constitutively active chimeric oncogene termed *RET/PTC*. Subsequently, more than 15 molecular fusion oncogenes in PTCs have been identified, all of which differ according to the 5′-terminal region of the heterologous gene (Fig. 81.5).[95] The most common of these chimeric oncogenes are *H4 (CCDC6)-RET*, also known as *RET/PTC1* (60% to 70%), and *ELE1-RET*, also known as *RET/PTC3* (20% to 30%). The prevalence of *RET/PTC* in the thyroid cancers of children is >50%; in youngsters in Kiev and Belarus who developed PTC following exposure to radiation from the Chernobyl accident, the prevalence of such rearrangements is 67% to 87%.[96,97]

There have been several clinical trials of MTTs in patients with differentiated thyroid carcinoma. Most of the drugs have targeted *BRAF*[V6003] and have induced partial remissions (modified RECIST) ranging from 0% to 60%.[98,99] A phase 3 prospective, randomized, clinical trial of sorafenib, compared to placebo, was conducted in patients with progressive, locally advanced or metastatic,

and ^{131}I refractory differentiated thyroid carcinoma. Based on significantly improved progression-free survival in patients receiving sorafenib compared to placebo, the FDA approved the drug for the treatment of patients with advanced PTC.[100]

Follicular Thyroid Carcinoma

The peroxisome proliferators-activated receptor-γ (PPAR-γ), a member of the steroid-nuclear hormone receptor superfamily, is encoded by *PPARG* located on 3p25. Rearrangements involving the thyroid-specific transcription factor paired-box gene 8 (*PAX8*) with the peroxisome proliferators-activated receptor-γ (*PPAR-γ*) were first identified in FTC as a cytogenetically detectable translocation t (2,3)(q13; p25).[101] The *PAX8–PPARγ* appears to be confined to atypical follicular adenomas and FTC, and has not been detected in PTC or either poorly differentiated or undifferentiated (anaplastic) thyroid carcinomas. In an evaluation of 88 conventional follicular and Hürthle cell tumors analyzed for *RAS* mutations and *PAX8-PPARγ* re-arrangements, 49 percent of FTC had *RAS* mutations, 36 percent had *PAX8-PPARγ* rearrangements, and one had both. *RAS* mutations occurred in almost half of the follicular adenomas, and *PAX8-PPARγ* translocations were present in only 4%. Overt tumor invasiveness was associated with *PAX8-PPARγ* translocations and not *RAS* mutations.[102]

Even though there have been significant advances with MTTs in the treatment of patients with differentiated thyroid

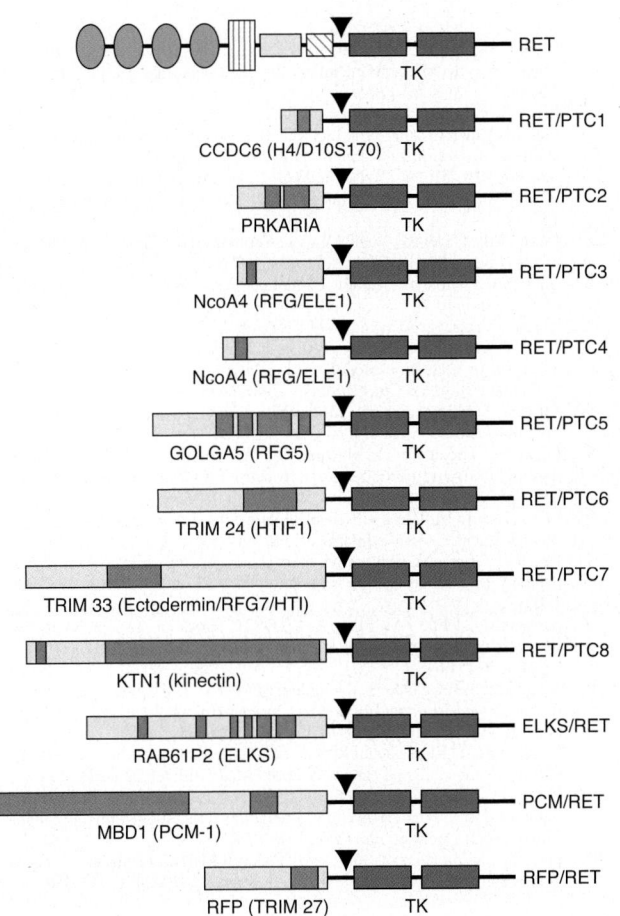

Figure 81.5 RET/PTC translocations associated with papillary thyroid carcinoma. TK, tyrosine kinase domain. (Reprinted with permission from Santoro M, Melillo RM, Fusco A. RET/PTC activation in papillary thyroid carcinoma: European Journal of Endocrinology Prize Lecture. *Eur J Endocrinol* 2006;155:645–653.)

carcinomas and MTCs, virtually all patients become resistant to the therapy, develop progressive disease, and die. It is hoped that new single-agent therapeutics will improve survival beyond what has been achieved with the current drugs, but clinical investigators need to focus attention on the development of combinatorial therapies based on molecular studies of tumor cells in vitro and in vivo. There have already been examples of successful combined therapies, such as the demonstrated effectiveness of combined imatinib and nilotinib in the treatment of patients with imatinib-refractory blast phase chronic myelogenous leukemia who were initially unresponsive to, or intolerant of, either agent alone.[103,104]

FUTURE DIRECTIONS

Advances in molecular genetics have elucidated the oncogenic event(s) of many solid tumors; this is nowhere more evident than in endocrine tumors. The discovery of the mutations causing MEN1 and MEN2 has been most important as it has led to an understanding of the pathogenesis, not only of the component hereditary tumors but their sporadic counterparts as well. These discoveries have already been of great benefit in the diagnosis and treatment of patients with endocrine tumors, as evidenced most clearly in families with hereditary MTC.

Another therapeutic benefit of the molecular research has been the identification of molecular targets for MTTs. Recently, prospectively randomized placebo controlled trials have been completed in patients with differentiated thyroid carcinoma and MTC. With the demonstration of progression-free survival in treated patients, compared to controls, in each of these trials, the FDA approved the drugs for the treatment of patients with advanced thyroid cancer, a stage of disease for which there had been no effective therapy. The use of MTTs for the treatment of patients with endocrine tumors will expand with the introduction of new more potent compounds and with the design of effective combinatorial regimens.

PRACTICE OF ONCOLOGY

SELECTED REFERENCES

The full reference list can be accessed at lwwhealthlibrary.com/oncology.

1. Wermer P. Genetic aspects of adenomatosis of endocrine glands. *Am J Med* 1954;16:363–371.
8. Chandrasekharappa SC, Guru SC, Manickam P, et al. Positional cloning of the gene for multiple endocrine neoplasia-type 1. *Science* 1997;276:404–407.
12. Lemos MC, Thakker RV. Multiple endocrine neoplasia type 1 (MEN1): analysis of 1336 mutations reported in the first decade following identification of the gene. *Hum Mutat* 2008;29:22–32.
15. Agarwal SK. Multiple endocrine neoplasia type 1. *Front Horm Res* 2013;41:1–15.
16. Thakker RV. Multiple endocrine neoplasia type 1 (MEN1). *Best Pract Res Clin Endocrinol Metab* 2010;24:355–370.
18. Knudson AG Jr, Strong LC, Anderson DE. Heredity and cancer in man. *Prog Med Genet* 1973;9:113–158.
22. Brown EM, Gamba G, Riccardi D, et al. Cloning and characterization of an extracellular Ca(2+)-sensing receptor from bovine parathyroid. *Nature* 1993;366:575–580.
23. Foley TP Jr, Harrison HC, Arnaud CD, et al. Familial benign hypercalcemia. *J Pediatr* 1972;81:1060–1067.
24. Pollak MR, Brown EM, Chou YH, et al. Mutations in the human Ca(2+)-sensing receptor gene cause familial hypocalciuric hypercalcemia and neonatal severe hyperparathyroidism. *Cell* 1993;75:1297–1303.
29. Pollak MR, Brown EM, Estep HL, et al. Autosomal dominant hypocalcaemia caused by a Ca(2+)-sensing receptor gene mutation. *Nat Genet* 1994;8:303–307.
33. Jackson CE, Norum RA, Boyd SB, et al. Hereditary hyperparathyroidism and multiple ossifying jaw fibromas: a clinically and genetically distinct syndrome. *Surgery* 1990;108:1006–1012; discussion 1012–1013.

34. Cavaco BM, Guerra L, Bradley KJ, et al. Hyperparathyroidism-jaw tumor syndrome in Roma families from Portugal is due to a founder mutation of the HRPT2 gene. *J Clin Endocrinol Metab* 2004;89:1747–1752.
35. Guarnieri V, Scillitani A, Muscarella LA, et al. Diagnosis of parathyroid tumors in familial isolated hyperparathyroidism with HRPT2 mutation: implications for cancer surveillance. *J Clin Endocrinol Metab* 2006;91:2827–2832.
36. Carpten JD, Robbins CM, Villablanca A, et al. HRPT2, encoding parafibromin, is mutated in hyperparathyroidism-jaw tumor syndrome. *Nat Genet* 2002;32:676–680.
40. Howell VM, Haven CJ, Kahnoski K, et al. HRPT2 mutations are associated with malignancy in sporadic parathyroid tumours. *J Med Genet* 2003;40:657–663.
43. Carney JA, Gordon H, Carpenter PC, et al. The complex of myxomas, spotty pigmentation, and endocrine overactivity. *Medicine (Baltimore)* 1985;64:270–283.
44. Daly AF, Jaffrain-Rea ML, Ciccarelli A, et al. Clinical characterization of familial isolated pituitary adenomas. *J Clin Endocrinol Metab* 2006;91:3316–3323.
45. Igreja S, Chahal HS, King P, et al. Characterization of aryl hydrocarbon receptor interacting protein (AIP) mutations in familial isolated pituitary adenoma families. *Hum Mutat* 2010;31:950–960.
48. Daly AF, Tichomirowa MA, Petrossians P, et al. Clinical characteristics and therapeutic responses in patients with germ-line AIP mutations and pituitary adenomas: an international collaborative study. *J Clin Endocrinol Metab* 2010;95:E373–E383.
50. Steiner AL, Goodman AD, Powers SR. Study of a kindred with pheochromocytoma, medullary thyroid carcinoma, hyperparathyroidism and Cushing's disease: multiple endocrine neoplasia, type 2. *Medicine (Baltimore)* 1968;47:371–409.

52. Farndon JR, Leight GS, Dilley WG, et al. Familial medullary thyroid carcinoma without associated endocrinopathies: a distinct clinical entity. *Br J Surg* 1986;73:278–281.

53. Wells SA Jr, Santoro M. Targeting the RET pathway in thyroid cancer. *Clin Cancer Res* 2009;15:7119–7123.

54. Lairmore TC, Ball DW, Baylin SB, et al. Management of pheochromocytomas in patients with multiple endocrine neoplasia type 2 syndromes. *Ann Surg* 1993;217:595–601; discussion 601–603.

55. Lips CJ, Landsvater RM, Hoppener JW, et al. Clinical screening as compared with DNA analysis in families with multiple endocrine neoplasia type 2A. *N Engl J Med* 1994;331:828–835.

56. Takahashi M, Ritz J, Cooper GM. Activation of a novel human transforming gene, ret, by DNA rearrangement. *Cell* 1985;42:581–588.

63. Donis-Keller H, Dou S, Chi D, et al. Mutations in the RET proto-oncogene are associated with MEN 2A and FMTC. *Hum Mol Genet* 1993;2:851–856.

64. Mulligan LM, Kwok JB, Healey CS, et al. Germ-line mutations of the RET proto-oncogene in multiple endocrine neoplasia type 2A. *Nature* 1993;363:458–460.

65. Carlson KM, Bracamontes J, Jackson CE, et al. Parent-of-origin effects in multiple endocrine neoplasia type 2B. *Am J Hum Genet* 1994;55:1076–1082.

67. Frank-Raue K, Rybicki LA, Erlic Z, et al. Risk profiles and penetrance estimations in multiple endocrine neoplasia type 2A caused by germline RET mutations located in exon 10. *Hum Mutat* 2011;32:51–58.

68. Herfarth KK, Bartsch D, Doherty GM, et al. Surgical management of hyperparathyroidism in patients with multiple endocrine neoplasia type 2A. *Surgery* 1996;120:966–973; discussion 973–974.

69. Gagel RF, Levy ML, Donovan DT, et al. Multiple endocrine neoplasia type 2a associated with cutaneous lichen amyloidosis. *Ann Intern Med* 1989;111:802–806.

70. Borst MJ, VanCamp JM, Peacock ML, et al. Mutational analysis of multiple endocrine neoplasia type 2A associated with Hirschsprung's disease. *Surgery* 1995;117:386–391.

71. Eng C, Smith DP, Mulligan LM, et al. Point mutation within the tyrosine kinase domain of the RET proto-oncogene in multiple endocrine neoplasia type 2B and related sporadic tumours. *Hum Mol Genet* 1994;3:237–241.

72. Smith DP, Houghton C, Ponder BA. Germline mutation of RET codon 883 in two cases of de novo MEN 2B. *Oncogene* 1997;15:1213–1217.

77. Elisei R, Cosci B, Romei C, et al. Prognostic significance of somatic RET oncogene mutations in sporadic medullary thyroid cancer: a 10-year follow-up study. *J Clin Endocrinol Metab* 2008;93:682–687.

78. Moura MM, Cavaco BM, Pinto AE, et al. High prevalence of RAS mutations in RET-negative sporadic medullary thyroid carcinomas. *J Clin Endocrinol Metab* 2011;96:E863–E868.

79. Elisei R, Romei C, Cosci B, et al. RET genetic screening in patients with medullary thyroid cancer and their relatives: experience with 807 individuals at one center. *J Clin Endocrinol Metab* 2007;92:4725–4729.

80. Skinner MA, Moley JA, Dilley WG, et al. Prophylactic thyroidectomy in multiple endocrine neoplasia type 2A. *N Engl J Med* 2005;353:1105–1113.

81. Brandi ML, Gagel RF, Angeli A, et al. Guidelines for diagnosis and therapy of MEN type 1 and type 2. *J Clin Endocrinol Metab* 2001;86:5658–5671.

82. American Thyroid Association Guidelines Task Force, Kloos RT, Eng C, et al. Medullary thyroid cancer: management guidelines of the American Thyroid Association. *Thyroid* 2009;19:565–612.

89. Wells SA Jr, Robinson BG, Gagel RF, et al. Vandetanib in patients with locally advanced or metastatic medullary thyroid cancer: a randomized, double-blind phase III trial. *J Clin Oncol* 2012;30:134–141.

90. Elisei R, Schlumberger MJ, Muller SP, et al. Cabozantinib in progressive medullary thyroid cancer. *J Clin Oncol* 2013;31:3639–3646.

91. Fagin JA. The Jeremiah Metzger Lecture: intelligent design of cancer therapy: trials and tribulations. *Trans Am Clin Climatol Assoc* 2007;118:253–261.

93. Lee J, Hwang JA, Lee EK. Recent progress of genome study for anaplastic thyroid cancer. *Genomics Inform* 2013;11:68–75.

94. Fusco A, Grieco M, Santoro M, et al. A new oncogene in human thyroid papillary carcinomas and their lymph-nodal metastases. *Nature* 1987;328:170–172.

95. Santoro M, Melillo RM, Fusco A. RET/PTC activation in papillary thyroid carcinoma: European Journal of Endocrinology Prize Lecture. *Eur J Endocrinol* 2006;155:645–653.

96. Klugbauer S, Lengfelder E, Demidchik EP, et al. High prevalence of RET rearrangement in thyroid tumors of children from Belarus after the Chernobyl reactor accident. *Oncogene* 1995;11:2459–2467.

98. Ho AL, Grewal RK, Leboeuf R, et al. Selumetinib-enhanced radioiodine uptake in advanced thyroid cancer. *N Engl J Med* 2013;368:623–632.

100. Brose MS, Nutting C, Jarzarb B, et al. Sorafenib in locally advanced or metastatic patients with radioactive iocine-refractory differentiated thyroid cancer: The phase III Decision trial. *J Clin Oncol* 2013;31:4.

101. Kroll TG, Sarraf P, Pecciarini L, et al. PAX8-PPARgamma1 fusion oncogene in human thyroid carcinoma [corrected]. *Science* 2000;289:1357–1360.

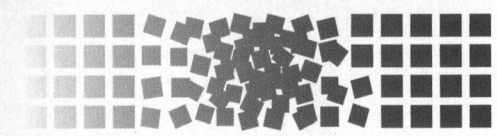

82 Thyroid Tumors

Caroline J. Davidge-Pitts and Geoffrey B. Thompson

ANATOMY AND PHYSIOLOGY

The name "thyroid" is derived from the Greek term "shield-shaped," which was first introduced by Thomas Wharton in 1656 due to the shape of the nearby thyroid cartilage. The thyroid is one of the largest endocrine organs weighing between 10 and 25 g. This bilobed gland is derived from foregut endoderm that finds its final position in the anterior neck after fusion with the ventral aspect of the fourth ventral pouch. The thyroglossal duct is formed during the thyroid's caudal descent into the neck, a canal between the gland and the pharyngeal floor. The duct subsequently undergoes degeneration, leaving behind the foramen cecum at the base of the tongue. The distal duct differentiates into thyroid tissue that becomes the pyramidal lobe. Parafollicular or C cells are derived from neural crest cells in the ultimobranchial body that fuse with the thyroid diverticulum during the descent into the neck. By gestational age 18 to 20 weeks, thyroid hormone is produced.

The thyroid is made up of two lobes, connected by the isthmus. Each lobe is approximately 2 cm thick and 4 cm in length, although the right lobe may be larger than the left. The gland is made up of follicular cells arranged in a spherical manner (follicles) that are filled with a proteinaceous substance called colloid. The principle function of the thyroid gland is to produce thyroid hormone (thyroxine [T4] and 3,5,3'-triiodothyronine [T3]), which is synthesized by the follicular cells. Production of thyroid hormone by the thyroid gland is controlled by thyrotropin-stimulating hormone (TSH) secreted from the anterior pituitary in response to thyrotropin-releasing hormone secreted by the hypothalamus. C cells are found in the thyroid interstitium surrounding the follicles, and secrete calcitonin. Additional cells within the thyroid include lymphocytes, fibroblasts, and adipocytes.

The thyroid is a very vascular gland (Fig. 82.1), with the right lobe exhibiting more vascularity than the left. Arterial supply is from the superior and inferior thyroid arteries. The thyroid drains into the superior, middle, and inferior thyroid veins through a venous plexus on the surface of the gland. These veins then drain into the internal jugular and innominate veins. The thyroid is innervated by the middle and inferior cervical ganglia of the sympathetic nervous system.

THYROID NODULES

A thyroid nodule is defined as a discrete lesion in the thyroid gland that is radiologically distinct from the surrounding parenchyma.[1] Thyroid nodules are very common in the general population, ranging from 20% to 76%. Nodules discovered at autopsy typically reflect this prevalence.[2] Nodules are more common with increasing age, particularly in women.[1] Up to 90% of women older than 70 years and 60% of men older than 80 years have thyroid nodules. Other risk factors include radiation exposure, particularly during childhood, family history of thyroid nodules, and iodine deficiency. Nodules may also occur in the setting of Hashimoto disease, where chronic inflammation leads to destruction of the thyroid gland with a rise in TSH in response to reduction in thyroid hormone. This rise in TSH stimulates growth of thyroid cells, forming nodules.

Thyroid nodules may be discovered by palpation during a physical exam in 3% to 7% of patients.[3,4] Nodules may also be found incidentally on imaging studies such as neck ultrasounds, computed tomography (CT) scans, and deoxy-2[^{18}F]fluoro-d-glucose positron emission tomography (^{18}FDG-PET) scans performed for unrelated reasons. Risk of malignancy is the same in nodules discovered by palpation and those discovered incidentally.[5]

The proportion of thyroid nodules that prove to be malignant is 10% to 15%.[6] Part of determination of malignancy is evaluation of individual risk assessment, which includes a detailed history and examination. Patients with the following histories may be at increased risk for malignancy:

1. Age. Patients age >70 years and <14 years have increased risk of malignancy.[7] Nodules discovered during childhood have a three- to four-fold higher risk of malignancy than adults.[8]
2. Head and neck radiation, particularly during childhood. Nodules carry a 33% to 37% chance of malignancy.[9]
3. ^{18}FDG-PET–positive lesion. See "Incidental ^{18}FDG-PET Positive Lesions."
4. Family history of thyroid cancer, particularly first-degree relatives.
5. Personal history of genetic syndromes commonly associated with thyroid cancer (multiple endocrine neoplasia 2, familial papillary thyroid cancer, familial polyposis coli, Gardner syndrome, and Cowden disease; Table 82.1).
6. Physical examination findings of a fixed, hard, solid nodule, cervical lymphadenopathy, and vocal cord paralysis.

In addition to history and physical examination, a TSH level should be performed on discovery of a thyroid nodule. If the TSH is suppressed, then a radionuclear thyroid scan should be performed to ascertain whether the nodule is hyperfunctioning. Hyperfunctioning nodules are rarely malignant; therefore, further cytologic evaluation is not needed if the patient's risk profile is otherwise low.[7] It is generally accepted that if a cold nodule is present on radionuclear thyroid scan, cytologic assessment is performed. If the TSH is in the upper range of normal, there may be an increased risk of malignancy,[10] although this association is poorly understood.

Routine measurement of calcitonin is controversial but is supported by the European Thyroid Association.[11] The American Thyroid Association (ATA) cannot recommend for or against routine testing of calcitonin.[1] It seems reasonable to perform, however, if there is a history of familial medullary thyroid cancer (MTC) as measurement may provide earlier diagnosis and more focused operative management.

A real-time two-dimensional, high-resolution ultrasound of the neck should be performed if thyroid nodules are discovered or suspected. Certain features may help distinguish benign from malignant lesions, although these signs are not independently predictive. These features include presence of microcalcifications, nodular hypoechogenicity, irregular borders, nodular vascularity, and a nodule that is taller than wide on transverse view.[1] Purely

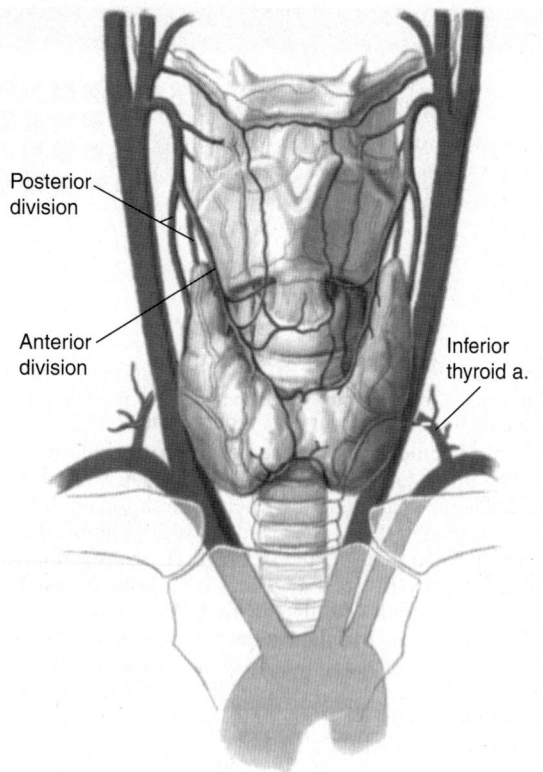

Figure 82.1 The thyroid gland and its arterial supply. (Drs. L.J. Rizzolo and W.B. Stewart, Section of Anatomy, Department of Surgery, Yale University School of Medicine, are acknowledged for providing the figure. With permission from Springer, Berlin-Heidelberg-New York.)

cystic nodules are likely to be benign.[12] Solitary nodules may not have a higher malignant risk than a nodule embedded in a multinodular goiter[13,14]; however, this still remains controversial.

Fine needle aspiration (FNA) is a very sensitive, low-risk procedure to help distinguish benign from malignant nodules.

According to the Mayo Clinic experience from 1979 to 1990, FNA reduced the proportion of operations for benign nodules by 50% and increased detection of malignancy.[15] The nondiagnostic rate is lower when performed in conjunction with neck ultrasound. Accuracy of the FNA will rely on an experienced team, and the cytopathologist should have an interest in thyroid disease. The ATA and American Association of Clinical Endocrinologists have provided guidelines to help clinicians decide which nodules require biopsy. Generally, routine FNA is recommended if the nodule is >1 cm with solid, hypoechoic features. Smaller nodules should also be considered for FNA if the nodule has suspicious features as described previously or if the patient has risk for thyroid cancer based on history or physical examination. The cytopathology may be reported as benign (60% to 80%), malignant (3.5% to 10%), suspicious for papillary thyroid cancer (2.5% to 10%), suspicious for follicular lesion/neoplasm or indeterminate (10% to 20%), and nondiagnostic (10% to 15%).[7] Follicular or Hürthle cell adenomas and carcinomas appear identical on cytologic examination. Malignancy is found in approximately 20% of these neoplasms. Capsular or vascular invasion seen in the surgical specimen needs to be present for diagnosis of follicular or Hürthle cell carcinoma (HCC).

The use of genetic markers could help improve diagnostic accuracy of indeterminate lesions.[16,17] Many centers now use these markers routinely to help guide management of indeterminate lesions, particularly in patients who do not want to undergo surgery. If the molecular profile suggests a low rate of malignancy (<5%), then observation may be recommended over surgical intervention.[18] Long-term follow up studies are still needed before this technology is widely adopted.

Figure 82.2 shows the evaluation of thyroid nodule in a euthyroid patient based on FNA results. Benign nodules can be followed conservatively by physical examination or ultrasound, unless there are compressive symptoms such as dysphagia or respiratory compromise, at which time surgical management should be considered. Lesions suspicious for follicular or Hürthle cell neoplasm typically are treated at Mayo Clinic with thyroid lobectomy and intraoperative frozen section. If the lesion is benign, no further thyroid resection is needed. If the lesion is malignant, completion thyroidectomy is performed. Molecular profiling can also be used to guide management decisions as described previously.

TABLE 82.1

Clinical and Genetic Characteristics of Familial Thyroid Follicular Cell Carcinoma Susceptibility Syndromes

Syndrome	Chromosome Linkage/Gene	Characteristics
Papillary thyroid carcinoma with papillary renal neoplasia	1q21/?	Associated with papillary renal neoplasia Autosomal dominant with partial penetrance
Familial nonmedullary thyroid carcinoma	2q21/? and 19p13/?	Two genetic loci identified Autosomal dominant with partial penetrance
Familial thyroid tumors with cell oxyphilia	19p13.2/?	Characteristic oxyphilic cells Autosomal dominant with partial penetrance
Familial adenomatous polyposis	5q21–22/APC	Papillary thyroid carcinoma with ~10× increased prevalence Colorectal carcinoma, ampullary carcinoma, hepatoblastoma, medulloblastoma Autosomal dominant
Cowden disease (multiple hamartoma syndrome)	10q23.3/PTEN	Follicular and papillary thyroid carcinoma Multiple hamartomas, breast and endometrial cancer Autosomal dominant
Carney complex 1	17q/PRKAR1A	Follicular and papillary thyroid carcinoma Skin pigmentation, and cardiac, endocrine, cutaneous, and neural myxomatous tumors Autosomal dominant

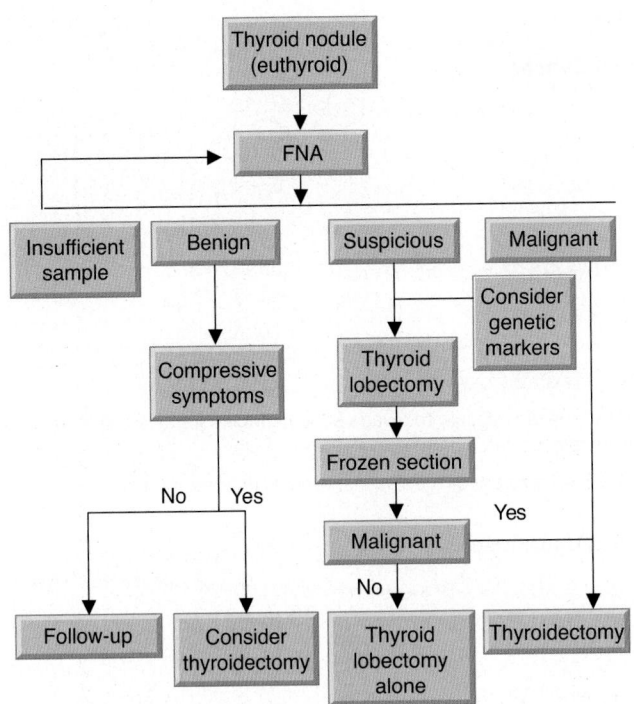

Figure 82.2 Flow diagram for the evaluation of thyroid nodule based on the results of fine needle aspiration (FNA) biopsy.

Nondiagnostic specimens require repeat FNA, particularly if there are suspicious features on ultrasound. Repeated nondiagnostic FNAs may lead to surgical excision in order to obtain a diagnosis. Malignant lesions will be discussed in the chapter to follow.

Incidental ¹⁸FDG-PET Positive Lesions

Fluorodeoxyglucose whole-body positron emission tomography is frequently used in oncology to evaluate and follow-up malignancies. High concentrations of ¹⁸FDG occur in most malignant tumors; however, high glucose uptake may also be nonspecific. Normal thyroid tissue has diffuse, low accumulation of ¹⁸FDG. Incidental focal increased uptake in the thyroid may occur and has been reported in 1.1% of ¹⁸FDG-PET imaging in a recent series.[19] Both primary and secondary thyroid malignancies have increased metabolic activity including lymphoma; therefore, an ¹⁸FDG-PET–positive solitary thyroid lesion has increased risk of malignancy of approximately 30% to 50%[19–22] compared to the 5% risk of malignancy of an incidental thyroid nodule found by other imaging. Therefore, solitary ¹⁸FDG-PET–positive thyroid lesions should be referred for ultrasound-guided FNA to exclude a primary or metastatic lesion in the thyroid. Hot nodules have also been reported to have increased ¹⁸FDG uptake; therefore, if the TSH is suppressed, further imaging with a thyroid uptake and scan may be indicated. Some studies have advocated the use of maximum standardized uptake value to differentiate benign from malignant lesions[20,21,23,24]; however, this approach has not been supported by all studies.[19,25] Diffuse thyroid uptake that does not correlate to a lesion on CT or ultrasound may be seen in autoimmune thyroid disease such as Hashimoto[26] or Graves thyroiditis,[27] and often do not require further evaluation unless other risk factors for malignancy are present.

Malignancies of the Thyroid

Risk Factors for Thyroid Malignancy

Although many risk factors have been evaluated in thyroid cancer, few clear associations have been found. Exposure to radiation, particularly in childhood, is associated with an increased risk of well-differentiated thyroid cancer.[9] Relative risk is related to exposure dose, starting as low as 0.1 Gy.[9] The latency period after childhood exposure is at least 3 to 5 years, and the risk remains apparent even 40 years after the radiation exposure.[9] The majority of cases occur between 20 and 40 years after exposure. However, even after 40 years, the relative risk as compared to a nonirradiated population is still increased. In addition to those who are exposed to radiation for medical reasons, patients who have been exposed to nuclear disasters or who are atomic bomb survivors are also at increased risk for thyroid cancer. On the other hand, ¹³¹I for treatment of positive thyroid scans or hyperthyroidism has not been associated with this risk.

Family history is also an important risk factor, particularly if well-differentiated cancer is present in first-degree relatives[28] or there is a family history of thyroid cancer syndromes as mentioned previously (see Table 82.1). MTC is also associated with distinct familial syndromes, which will be discussed in more detail later in the chapter.

The only known risk factor for thyroid lymphoma is Hashimoto's thyroiditis,[29] particularly the non-Hodgkin lymphoma derived from mucosa-associated lymphoid tissue.

THYROID TUMOR CLASSIFICATION AND STAGING SYSTEMS

The follicular cells give rise to well-differentiated cancers and anaplastic thyroid cancer (ATC). The C or parafollicular cell gives rise to medullary thyroid carcinoma. Immune cells and stromal cells of the thyroid are responsible for lymphoma and sarcoma, respectively. A total of 90% are well-differentiated cancers, 5% to 9% are medullary, 1% to 2% are anaplastic, 1% to 3% are lymphoma, and <1% are sarcomas or other rare tumors.[30]

Thyroid carcinoma can be categorized as tumors derived from follicular epithelium including differentiated thyroid carcinoma (DTC; papillary thyroid carcinoma, follicular carcinoma, including more aggressive forms such as HCC, some rare variants of papillary carcinoma, including the tall cell variant, columnar cell variant, and diffuse sclerosing variant), poorly differentiated thyroid carcinoma, and anaplastic carcinoma. Medullary thyroid carcinoma is derived from the C cells.

Many systems have been proposed for staging thyroid cancer. In the absence of a universally accepted system, it is recommended that the TNM (tumor-node-metastasis) staging system, introduced by the International Union Against Cancer and promoted by the American Joint Committee on Cancer, the American Cancer Society, the National Cooperative Cancer Network, and the American College of Surgeons, be adopted as the international staging system (Table 82.2). The system stages the malignant lesions based on tumor size, invasiveness, nodal spread, and distant metastases. Based on this system, all patients younger than 45 years of age with papillary or follicular carcinoma are stage I unless distant metastases are present. Patients older than 45 years of age with papillary or follicular microcarcinoma without nodal disease are stage I, whereas any tumor >2 cm is considered stage II. Stage III is classified in older patients with nodal disease or extrathyroidal invasion. Staging of MTC is similar, although there are no age distinctions and extrathyroidal invasion is classified as stage II. In papillary, follicular, and MTC, distant metastases are considered stage IV disease.

DIFFERENTIATED THYROID CANCER

Incidence and Prognosis

In the United States, the diagnosis of thyroid cancer has tripled in the past three decades, likely secondary to increased detection rates. Papillary thyroid cancer (PTC) is by far the most

TABLE 82.2

American Joint Committee on Cancer Classification of Thyroid Cancer, Seventh Edition (2010)

Primary Tumor (T)[a]

TX	Primary tumor cannot be assessed
T0	No evidence of primary tumor
T1	Tumor ≤2 cm confined to the thyroid 　T1a　Tumor ≤1 cm confined to the thyroid 　T1b　Tumor 1–2 cm confined to the thyroid
T2	Tumor >2 cm and <4 cm confined to the thyroid
T3	Tumor >4 cm confined to the thyroid or tumor of any size with minimal extrathyroid extension
T4a	Moderately advanced disease; tumor of any size extending beyond the thyroid capsule to invade subcutaneous soft tissues, larynx, trachea, esophagus, or recurrent laryngeal nerve or intrathyroidal anaplastic carcinoma[b]
T4b	Very advanced disease; tumor invades prevertebral fascia or encases carotid artery or mediastinal vessels or extrathyroidal anaplastic carcinoma[b]

Regional Lymph Nodes (N) (Central Compartment, Lateral Cervical, and Upper Mediastinal)

NX	Regional lymph nodes cannot be assessed
N0	No regional lymph node metastasis
N1	Regional lymph node metastasis
	N1a　Metastasis to level VI (pretracheal, paratracheal, and prelaryngeal/Delphian lymph nodes) N1b　Metastasis to unilateral, bilateral, or contralateral cervical (levels I, II, III, IV, or V) or retropharyngeal or superior mediastinal lymph nodes (level VII)

Distant Metastasis (M)

MX	Distant metastasis cannot be assessed
M0	No distant metastasis
M1	Distant metastasis

Stage Groupings

PAPILLARY AND FOLLICULAR

Under 45 y of age				Medullary carcinoma			
Stage I	Any T	Any N	M0	Stage I	T1	N0	M0
Stage II	Any T	Any N	M1	Stage II	T2	N0	M0
45 y of age and over					T3	N0	M0
Stage I	T1	N0	M0	Stage III	T1	N1a	M0
Stage II	T2	N0	M0		T2	N1a	M0
Stage III	T3	N0	M0		T3	N1a	M0
	T1	N1a	M0	Stage IVA	T4a	N0	M0
	T2	N1a	M0		T4a	N1a	M0
	T3	N1a	M0		T1	N1b	M0
Stage IVA	T4a	N0	M0		T2	N1b	M0
	T4a	N1a	M0		T3	N1b	M0
	T1	N1b	M0		T4a	N1b	M0
	T2	N1b	M0	Stage IVB	T4b	Any N	M0
	T3	N1b	M0	Stage IVC	Any T	Any N	M1
	T4a	N1b	M0	Anaplastic carcinoma			
	T4a	N1b	M0	Stage IVA	T4a	Any N	M0
Stage IVB	T4b	Any N	M0	Stage IVB	T4b	Any N	M0
Stage IVC	Any T	Any N	M1	Stage IVC	Any T	Any N	M1

[a] All categories may be subdivided: (a) solitary tumor, (b) multifocal tumor (the largest determines the classification).
[b] All anaplastic carcinomas are considered T4 tumors.
Used with the permission of the American Joint Committee on Cancer (AJCC), Chicago, Illinois. The original source for this material is the *AJCC Cancer Staging Manual*, Seventh Edition (2010) published by Springer Science and Business Media LLC, www.springer.com, page 89.

common (80% to 85%) compared to 10% to 15% follicular and 3% to 5% HCC.[31]

Several databases define prognostic risk factors for well-differentiated thyroid cancer.[32] Most prognostic indicators are derived from uncontrolled retrospective trials. The most widely used systems include AGES (age, tumor grade, tumor extent, tumor size), AMES (age, metastatic disease, extrathyroidal extension, size), and MACIS (metastasis, patient age, completeness of resection, local invasion, and tumor size) (Table 82.3). Evaluation of 859 patients treated at Mayo clinic between 1946 and 1970 revealed that age of the patient, histologic grade of the tumor, and extent and size of the tumor were associated with worse prognosis.[33] These variables were combined into a prognostic score (AGES) with high-risk patients having a score ≥4 and low risk patients <4. Cause-specific mortality in low-risk patients was 1.1% at 20 years compared to 39% in the high-risk group. The AMES system was developed after a subsequent analysis of 821 patients with DTC treated at Lahey Clinic between 1941 and 1980.[34] This system was based on age, distant metastases, and extent and size of

primary tumor. Twenty-year mortality rates were 1.2% and 39.5% for low- and high-risk patients, respectively. Worse prognostic indicators included male sex, older age, major capsular invasion for follicular carcinoma, tumors >5 cm in size, extrathyroidal extension of the tumor, and distant metastases at presentation. Mayo Clinic developed the MACIS system after analyzing 1,779 patients with PTC.[35] A low-risk score is considered <6 with a 20-year mortality of 1%. This scoring system is the current predominant system to determine risk of death and postoperative outcome at Mayo Clinic, and is the only system to take gross residual disease after primary resection into account. These three staging systems allow the clinician to determine risk following the initial cancer operation.

Lymph node status has not been associated with cause-specific mortality; however, positive nodal involvement at presentation increases the risk of locoregional recurrence.[36]

A single point mutation (V600E) of the BRAF protooncogene is recognized as the initiating oncogenic trigger in up to 40% to 50% of PTC.[37–39] Less commonly, RET rearrangements and RAS mutations may be present.[40,41] When compared to papillary cancers that do not have BRAF mutations, PTCs with this mutation are more advanced at the time of diagnosis, more likely to be invasive beyond the thyroid capsule, more likely to metastasize to regional lymph nodes, more likely to exhibit distant metastatic spread, and therefore less likely to be surgically curable.[37,42–46] It remains unclear whether BRAF V600E status provides incremental prognostic information beyond that available based on surgical and pathologic information obtained at the time of initial surgery. Nevertheless, some investigators suggest that assessment of V600E BRAF status could be a standard part of the workup for patients with PTC.[47] For further discussion on the clinical and molecular genetics of endocrine tumorigenesis, see Chapter 81.

The majority (35% to 70%) of patients with follicular cell carcinoma and HCC present with stage II disease. In patients older than 45 years of age, stage III disease accounts for 4% to 7% of follicular thyroid carcinoma (FTC) and 8% to 10% of HCC. Stage IV disease with distant metastases is seen in 7% to 15% of FTC and 4% to 6% of HCC. Predictors of cause-specific mortality include age >50 years, marked vascular invasion, and metastatic disease at presentation.[32] A retrospective review from Memorial Sloan-Kettering from 1930 to 1985[48] showed that age >45 years, Hürthle cell subtype, extrathyroidal extension, tumor >4 cm, and distant metastases were associated with worse prognosis. Patients were divided into low-, intermediate-, and high-risk groups. The 10-year survival for low-, intermediate-, and high-risk groups were 98%, 88%, and 76%, respectively. HCC is considered a more aggressive subtype, and studies evaluating flow cytometry show that tumors with DNA aneuploidy are associated with increased tumor-related mortality.[49] Although originally designed for PTC, prognostic scoring systems AMES and AGES have been used in FTC, although it is important to point out that these scoring systems do not include important prognostic factors just described, namely vascular invasion or flow cytometry.

Pathology

PTC constitutes approximately 80% to 85% of malignant epithelial thyroid tumors. Grossly, papillary carcinomas have a variable appearance, from subcapsular white scars to large tumors >5 to 6 cm that invade nearby structures outside the thyroid gland. Cystic change, calcification, and even ossification may be identified. Microscopically, papillary carcinomas are characterized by the presence of papillae, but some variants contain no papillary areas, are totally follicular in pattern, and are identified as a follicular variant. Biologically, all these tumors, independent of their degree of follicular pattern, show similar clinical characteristics. The major cytologic feature shared by all members of this papillary group is the characteristic nucleus containing

---

TABLE 82.3

Prognostic Scoring Systems for AGES, AMES, and MACIS

AGES (age, tumor grade, tumor extent, tumor size)

Prognostic score = 0.05 × age (if age ≥40 y)
+ 1 (if grade 2)
+ 3 (if grade 3 or 4)
+ 1 (if extrathyroid)
+ 3 (if distant spread)
+ 0.2 × tumor size (cm maximum diameter)

Survival by AGES score (20-y):
≤3.99 = 99%
4–4.99 = 80%
5–5.99 = 67%
   ≥6 = 13%

AMES (age, metastatic disease, extrathyroidal extension, size)

Low risk: Younger patients (men ≤40 y, women ≤50 y) with no metastases
Older patients (intrathyroid papillary, minor capsular invasion for follicular lesions)
Primary cancers <5 cm
No distant metastases

High risk: All patients with distant metastases
Extrathyroid papillary, major capsular invasion follicular
Primary cancers ≥5 cm in older patients (men >40 y, women >50 y)

Survival by AMES risk groups (20-y):
Low risk = 99%
High risk = 61%

MACIS (metastasis, patient age, completeness of resection, local invasion, and tumor size)

Score = 3.1 (if age <40 y) or 0.08 × age (if age ≥40 y)
+ 0.3 × tumor size (cm maximum diameter)
+ 1 (if incompletely resected)
+ 1 (if locally invasive)
+ 3 (if distant spread)

Survival by MACIS score (20-y):
<6 = 99%
6–6.99 = 89%
7–7.99 = 56%
≥8 = 24%

Adapted from Dean DS, Hay ID. Prognostic indicators in differentiated thyroid carcinoma. *Cancer Control* 2000;7(3):229–239. Reprinted with permission by *Cancer Control: Journal of the Moffitt Cancer Center.*

PRACTICE OF ONCOLOGY

Orphan-Annie nuclei, nuclear grooves, and intranuclear pseudoinclusions. Because the nuclei are enlarged, they frequently overlap one another. Papillary carcinoma has a propensity to invade lymphatic spaces and, therefore, leads to microscopic multimodal lesions in the gland as well as a high incidence of regional lymph node metastases.

In contrast to the overall indolent behavior of the classical DTC, subtypes of these tumors have been identified as being more aggressive. These tumors comprise approximately 10% to 15% of all thyroid cancers.[50] These include HCCs (oncocytic, oxyphilic) as well as variants of PTC such as the tall cell variant, columnar cell variant, and diffuse sclerosing variant. These variants exhibit unique histopathologic features. However, they do share some commonalities, such as a high rate of extrathyroidal extension and nodal metastasis at diagnosis, as well as locoregional recurrence and development of synchronous and metachronous metastasis.[50]

True FTC is a tumor comprising approximately 5% to 10% of thyroid malignancies in nonendemic goiter areas of the world.[51] Most of the follicular pattern of thyroid malignancies represent the follicular variant of papillary carcinoma and share the biologic features, natural history, and prognosis of PTC.[52] FTC is unifocal, thickly encapsulated, and shows invasion of the capsule and/or vessels.

The Hürthle cell neoplasm is considered by most to be a variant of follicular neoplasms. Historically, all such lesions, despite the histologic features, were considered to be malignant; hence, it was recommended that they all be treated aggressively. However, many studies have evaluated the clinical pathologic features of thyroid Hürthle cell tumors and have shown that, on average, only 20% to 33% show histologic evidence of malignancy or invasive growth and may metastasize.[52] However, the size of the lesion is related to the risk of malignancy, and 65% of tumors >4 cm are found to be malignant.[52] Hürthle cell tumors that do not demonstrate invasion microscopically behave as adenomas and may be treated conservatively.

TREATMENT OF DIFFERENTIATED THYROID CANCER

Surgery

Mayo Clinic has been observing the treatment of PTC since 1940.[53] Over the decades, our management of PTC has become more aggressive. Seventy percent of patients treated for PTC in the 1940s underwent unilateral lobectomy. By the 1950s, the frequency dropped to 22% and by the 1960s, only 5% of patients with PTC underwent unilateral lobectomy. In contrast, by the 1980s, total or near-total thyroidectomy was performed in 92% of patients with PTC.[53] In current day practice, a patient diagnosed with PTC will undergo either total or near-total thyroidectomy as the preferred initial treatment.

Preoperative ultrasonography of the neck allows for evaluation of suspicious neck node metastases (NNM) that should be resected with a modified neck dissection at time of initial thyroidectomy (Fig. 82.3). Of 1,916 patients undergoing primary surgery for PTC at Mayo Clinic during 1940 through 1991, 23% of patients had suspicious nodes by palpation. More than 50% of those with PTC had neck nodes removed at surgery; 38% of the patients with PTC had nodes that were positive for metastatic disease. Only 4% of patients with FTC and 6% of those with HCC had NNM at initial surgical diagnosis.[54] Patients with DTC may be found to have recurrent NNM on long-term follow-up after initial surgery. The proportion of patients who present with these recurrences varies among histologic types of DTC. In 2,172 patients with DTC who underwent complete surgical resection at Mayo during 1940 to 1991, neck node recurrence occurred in 8% of PTC (1,801), 2% of FTC (124), and 18% of HCC (87) by 20 years. Definition of recurrence was 180 days after initial surgery.[54] In 2,370 patients with PTC treated with curative intent during 1940 to 2000 at Mayo Clinic, the cumulative occurrence rates for postoperative NNM at both 25 and 40 years were 10%.[55]

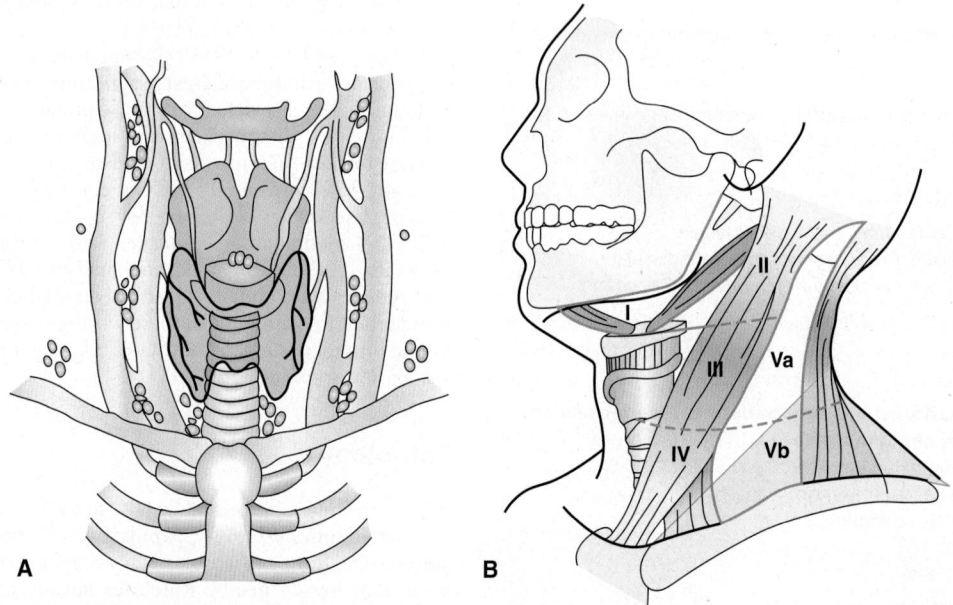

Figure 82.3 The thyroid gland and lymphatic node basins. **(A)** Schematic representation of the lymphatic node basins of the neck. The lateral neck lymph node compartments (levels II to V) and the central neck compartment (level IV). **(B)** Schematic illustration of the anatomic borders of the central neck compartment (level VI). The superior margin is at the level of the hyoid bone, the inferior margin is at the level of the brachiocephalic vessels, and the lateral margins are at the medial aspect of the common carotid arteries **(A)**. The central neck (level VI) contains the precricoid (Delphian), pretracheal, paratracheal, and perithyroidal nodes, including those along the recurrent laryngeal nerves, and the external branch of the superior laryngeal nerve. The parathyroid glands are also normally located in the central neck **(B)**.

According to the European Thyroid Association,[11] ATA,[1] and National Comprehensive Cancer Network,[18] therapeutic neck dissection is performed with initial thyroidectomy for patients with PTC with NNM. Prophylactic lateral neck dissection is not recommended; however, prophylactic central neck dissection remains controversial. At Mayo Clinic, we routinely dissect the central neck compartment at time of initial thyroidectomy considering the high risk of NNM in DTC. Contrast-enhanced CT scanning is indicated in patients with locally advanced disease or vocal cord paralysis to rule out invasion of the aerodigestive tree which will alter surgical management.

Adjuvant Therapy

Adjuvant therapy includes postoperative TSH suppression with thyroxine therapy, usually to a level around 0.1 mIU/L. If the patient is considered low risk, TSH levels are acceptable into the low range of normal. High-risk patients are often maintained at ≤0.1 mIU/L. This has been standard practice in PTC and FTC for many years; however, risks of thyroid hormone suppression should be weighed against individual patients' cardiovascular risk.

The trends in surgical management of DTC have been described previously. Similar changes have been seen in the management of DTC with radioactive iodine (RAI), particularly with respect to postoperative radioiodine remnant ablation (RRA) in low-risk patients. At Mayo Clinic, approximately 60% of patients underwent RRA within 6 months of initial surgery in the 1980s. This is in comparison to only 6% in the 1970s.[53] The ATA guidelines recommend RRA for patients with stage II disease older than 45 years of age and patients with stage III and IV disease. Only selected patients with stage I disease should be considered for RRA (aggressive histologies, multifocal disease, nodal metastases, extrathyroidal or vascular invasion).[1] Analysis of 1,163 patients at Mayo Clinic with low-risk PTC (defined as MACIS <6) between 1970 and 2000 showed no statistical difference was seen in 20-year tumor recurrence and cause-specific mortality between those that received surgical treatment alone versus those who received surgical treatment with RRA.[53] In addition, the National Thyroid Cancer Treatment Cooperative Study group[56] and a multivariate analysis performed in Toronto, Canada,[57] did not show improvement in recurrence and cause-specific mortality in patients with low-risk disease. It has therefore become clearer that RRA in low-risk disease does not change long-term outcomes and should be reserved for higher risk patients. At Mayo Clinic, we reserve postoperative RRA for patients with high-risk PTC (MACIS >6) or patients with a diagnosis of follicular or HCC. In those elected to receive RAI, quantitation of uptake is assessed by whole-body ^{131}I scan and customization of dose is decided based on this quantitation and distribution of disease.

Postoperative RRA is typically performed approximately 6 weeks after near-total or total thyroidectomy. Most centers perform a pretherapy whole-body iodine scan. If performed, a pretherapy scan should use a low dose of [131]I (1 to 3 mCi) or [123]I. To optimize uptake by both normal residual thyroid and thyroid cancer, patients are rendered hypothyroid with a goal of increasing serum TSH. To accomplish this, thyroid replacement after thyroidectomy is often performed with the administration of triiodothyronine (T_3), as it has a much shorter half-life than thyroxine (T_4), and it is discontinued 2 weeks before treatment. In response to this hypothyroid state, TSH must be >30 mU/L to obtain optimal uptake of radioiodine. It is also recommended that a serum thyroglobulin level is obtained during this period of hypothyroid state (see "Long-Term Surveillance"). A low-iodine diet is recommended 1 to 2 weeks before scanning or ablative ^{131}I therapy to enhance the uptake and retention of radioiodine. Alternatively, imaging and treatment employing TSH stimulation with recombinant human TSH (rhTSH; Thyrogen, Genzyme, Cambridge, MA) is presently performed with increased frequency. This way is preferred if rendering the

patient frankly hypothyroid is potentially hazardous, for example, metastatic PTC in the central nervous system. Posttherapy whole-body iodine scanning is typically performed 1 week after ^{131}I treatment to identify metastases.

The most common side effects from radioiodine therapy include sialadenitis, nausea, and temporary bone marrow suppression. Women undergoing ^{131}I treatment should be advised to avoid pregnancy during and 6 to 12 months after treatment due to risk of miscarriage and fetal malformation. There is a weak, but dose-dependent relationship between ^{131}I therapy and the development of second malignancies, such as bone and soft tissue tumors, colorectal cancer, salivary tumors, and leukemia.[58]

Papillary Thyroid Microcarcinoma

Papillary thyroid microcarcinomas (PMC) are defined as PTC with a maximum diameter of ≤10 mm.[59] In contrast with ATC with a poor prognosis, PTC generally has an excellent prognosis, with majority of patients with small primary tumors alive at 20 years. Prior to the advent of high-resolution ultrasound, most PTCs were discovered by palpation. With improved ultrasound imaging techniques and the ability to perform guided biopsies in the office setting, subclinical papillary cancers are now being discovered. In addition, these micropapillary carcinomas are often incidentally found on imaging performed for other reasons. Autopsy studies reveal an incidence of 6% to 36%.[60] The treatment of these microcarcinomas remains very controversial in the thyroid field. Mayo Clinic reported treatment outcomes of 900 patients with PMC over 60 years.[61] Prognosis was excellent with cause-specific mortality of only 0.3%. A total of 30% of patients had cervical lymph node involvement, with only 0.3% having distant spread at the time of diagnosis. Bilateral lobar resections were performed in 86% with unilateral lobectomy performed in 14%. By 20 years, 5.7% of patients recurred within the neck or at distant sites. Eighty percent of recurrences occurred within cervical lymph nodes, whereas the remainder occurred in the nonresected contralateral lobe or soft tissues of the thyroid bed. However, cervical recurrences were not associated with increased mortality. Of the recurrences, 4% were to distant sites. Higher recurrences were seen in patients with multifocal tumors and positive NNM at primary resection. Recurrence rates did not differ whether primary resection included bilateral or unilateral lobar resection. RRA did not improve mortality or recurrence rate. In summary of this large series, as long as complete resection is possible, more extensive surgery and RRA do not seem to influence recurrence risk or mortality. The most common site of recurrent disease is the cervical lymph nodes, and central compartment exploration can be performed at the time of initial surgery to remove involved nodes. Future recurrence is higher in those with positive nodes at initial resection, and those with multifocal disease.

In a Japanese observational study of 1,395 patients with PMC, patients were given the choice of surgery versus observation if no unfavorable features were present.[62] Less than a quarter chose observation, and these patients were followed with frequent ultrasounds over an average of 74 months. Tumor enlargement was considered growth of ≥3. At 5- and 10-year follow-up, the proportion of patients with tumor growth was 6.4% and 15.9%, respectively. Eighteen of the thirty-one patients with tumor enlargement underwent surgery after observation, two of which were found to have lymph node metastases. Of the 13 patients who continued with observation, 7 tumors decreased in size. Tumor enlargement was not related to the original size of the tumor, multicentricity, or TSH suppression. Tumors of patients under the age of 45 tended to enlarge, but this did not reach statistical significance. The proportion of patients with new node metastases at 5- and 10-year follow-up was 1.4% and 3.4%, respectively. This author therefore summarized that observation of papillary microcarcinoma without unfavorable characteristics is a potential therapeutic option, with progression to surgical resection if tumor enlargement or lymph node metastases occur.

Treatment of PMC is largely based on observational and epidemiologic studies. Further large trials are needed to rest this controversy. Recently, authors have advocated for a change in the name of PMC to try and prevent overtreatment of these small tumors.[63] However, it is important to note that not all PMCs may be "created equal," with more aggressive variants of PTC possibly behaving differently.[64] It is currently unknown whether these aggressive variants change survival risk.

Long-Term Surveillance

The goal of long-term surveillance is to identify recurrence in patients thought to be free of disease. Thyroglobulin (Tg), an important serum tumor marker in the surveillance of patients with thyroid cancer, is the protein that provides a matrix for thyroid hormone synthesis within thyroid follicles and is critical in the storage of thyroid hormone within the thyroid gland. After successful thyroidectomy and ablation of residual normal or malignant thyroid tissue by radioiodine, the Tg should be in the athyreotic range. Both normal thyroid tissue as well as follicular cell–derived thyroid cancer will produce Tg. Levels above the athyreotic range are indicative of persistent, functioning thyroid tissue or carcinoma.

Follow-up protocols have also been a controversial issue in the management of PTC. At Mayo Clinic, we typically order a TSH with Tg testing (including Tg tumor marker and antibody) yearly for at least 5 years as this is the period of time where most recurrences occur. The presence of autoantibodies to Tg, which occurs in 25% of patients with thyroid cancer and 10% of the general population, will falsely lower serum Tg levels. Thus, such antibodies should quantitatively be determined at every measurement of serum Tg levels. We do not routinely order a TSH-stimulated Tg level. In patients with low-risk disease, a TSH-suppressed Tg level <0.5 ng/mL likely represents absence of clinically relevant disease.

In addition to Tg and TSH monitoring, follow-up imaging after initial surgery and adjuvant therapy is required. High-sensitivity ultrasonography has become the mainstay of imaging surveillance in patients with low-risk disease, with the ability to pick up small NNM that are millimeters in size. Neck ultrasound should be performed 6 and 12 months after surgery, and then annually for 3 to 5 years, depending on the patient's risk for recurrence and Tg status.[1] At Mayo Clinic, routine posttherapeutic radioiodine whole-body scanning (WBS) in the absence of recurrence by ultrasound or positive Tg is not performed. A report from Mayo Clinic Jacksonville looked at 194 patients with follicular cell–derived thyroid cancer with a TSH suppressed Tg of 0.1 ng/mL who subsequently underwent TSH stimulation and radioiodine scanning.[65] The Tg rarely stimulated above 2 ng/mL and none of the 194 patients had radioiodine scanning that was positive for locoregional recurrence or distant metastases. Therefore, radioiodine scanning is reserved for patients with recurrence or metastatic disease that may be amenable to therapeutic doses of RAI.

Management of Local Recurrence and Distant Metastasis

Patients with significant nodal locoregional recurrence in the neck should undergo modified radical neck dissection or central compartment (level VI) neck dissection, depending on the location of the recurrence. More aggressive surgery may be warranted in selected patients with invasion of the aerodigestive tract.[66] Tracheal stents and tracheotomy can be used as palliative measures in the case of unresectable disease or poor performance status. For smaller regional lymph node metastasis or patients who are not amenable to surgical therapy or have distant metastasis, locoregional disease control can also be achieved using ultrasound-guided percutaneous ethanol ablation, which will be discussed in more detail in the following.

Metastatic disease that is detected with whole-body iodine scan, and is considered radioiodine avid, is treated with ^{131}I therapy. Similar to the discussion of initial treatment, no consensus exists regarding dosing of ^{131}I, although most authors use a high dose ranging between 150 to 300 mCi. Pulmonary metastases are frequently detected exclusively on radioiodine scanning and tend to respond to ^{131}I treatment. Treatment can be performed every 6 to 12 months as long as the disease continues to respond. It should be noted, however, that pulmonary fibrosis may limit further ^{131}I treatment.[67] For select patients with incurable pulmonary disease, palliative treatments using metastasectomy, laser ablation, and external beam radiation therapy (EBRT) may be considered. Complete surgical resection of isolated symptomatic bone metastases and[131]I treatment for radioiodine avid, widespread disease have both been associated with an increased survival and are recommended especially in younger patients.[67] A combination of treatments may be considered for symptomatic bone lesions when surgery or ^{131}I treatment is not possible nor effective. Similarly, complete surgical resection of central nervous system metastasis seem to be the most efficacious treatment, whereas EBRT and gamma knife therapy may be considered in those not candidates for surgery.

There has been a great deal of debate regarding the optimal management of patients who are Tg positive with negative imaging including negative whole-body iodine scans and ultrasonography. It is important to rule out technical factors that could lead to a false negative scan including iodine contamination and suboptimal TSH elevation. If the scan is truly negative in the setting of positive Tg, management is controversial. Previous reports have indicated benefit from empiric RAI of 100 to 200 mCi ^{131}I in these patients.[68,69] If the posttherapy scan is positive, then repeated RAI is given until the scan is negative. The idea is that metastases may be too small to visualize on pretherapy scan or the tumor has reduced ability to concentrate iodine. A study from Mayo Clinic looking at 24 high-risk patients with detectable Tg and negative WBSs and known macrometastases, treated with RAI between 1997 and 2000, showed that only 2 patients had evidence of uptake on the posttherapy scan.[70] The study showed that high-risk patients with known metastases who have been treated with RAI for remnant ablation, with subsequent negative WBS and positive Tg, are unlikely to benefit from empiric high-dose RAI due to reduced ^{131}I accumulation in the persistent disease. In addition, the adverse effects of high-dose RAI should be considered. This study did not look at patients without evidence of metastases on conventional imaging. [18]FDG-PET has been used in restaging of residual or recurrent advanced disease in patients with negative WBS but with increased Tg. FDG-avid lesions are associated with increased cancer-associated mortality, with negative [18]FDG-PETs indicating a better prognosis.[71,72] A recent retrospective study by van Dijk et al.[73] showed that PET scanning performed early after negative WBS lead to additional tumor localization in 17% (9 of 52 patients). Ninety percent of patients with positive PET scan had a Tg of >2 ng/ml. Due to the retrospective nature of this study, both stimulated and unstimulated Tg were included.[73] [18]FDG-PET is best performed with a high Tg.[74]

Ultrasound-Guided Percutaneous Ethanol Ablation

Many well-differentiated thyroid carcinomas present with NNM at diagnosis, approaching or exceeding 40% in both medullary and PTC. In addition, NNM may develop many years after the primary surgery, despite complete surgical resection. In the past, these lymph node recurrences have been treated with repeat surgical excision, which may include neck dissection or the less favored "berry picking" approach. High-resolution ultrasound has also allowed us to discover subcentimeter NNM that are too small for surgical intervention. These small lesions present a dilemma to the treating clinician. Percutaneous ethanol ablation was used to treat benign disease in the 1980s, including parathyroid adenomas and benign thyroid nodules.[75] In the early 1990s, Mayo Clinic successfully started treating neck node recurrences with ultrasound-guided percutaneous ethanol ablation in both medullary and PTC.[76,77] This procedure has subsequently been adopted by institutions around the United States and the world.[78–80] In a series of 14 patients at the Mayo Clinic, 29 NNM were treated with ultrasound-guided percutaneous ethanol ablation between 1993 and 2000. Over a follow-up period of 18 months, all treated nodes reduced in volume, and blood flow within the metastases disappeared.[76] Long-term studies have revealed similar successes.[80,81] The procedure can be repeated if needed, either on the same treated node or in new nodes. Figure 82.4 shows an example of a treated NNM in a patient with locoregional recurrence of PTC. We recommend this procedure for patients who are poor surgical candidates, patients who prefer to not undergo repeated neck surgery, or disease that is resistance to radioactive iodine ablation. If performed by an experienced center, the procedure has few complications, with pain at injection being the most common. Hoarseness has also been reported, but this is usually transient.[76]

Systemic Agents

Approximately 25% to 50% of patients with advanced DTC are refractory to radioactive iodine therapy (RAI-R). Five- and ten-year survival may decrease to <50% and <10%, respectively. In these circumstances, systemic therapies should be considered, particularly in patients with rapidly progressive disease. Treatment options for these patients include doxorubicin, palliative EBRT, targeted molecular therapies such as tyrosine kinase inhibitors, and enrollment in clinical trials.

The role of EBRT and chemotherapy in thyroid cancer is limited. EBRT should be considered in patients with unresectable gross residual cervical disease, painful bone metastases, and for metastases in critical locations that are not amenable to surgery and that would likely result in fracture, neurologic, or compressive symptoms (such as metastases in the central nervous system, vertebral bodies, selected mediastinal lymph nodes, and pelvis). Doxorubicin is approved by the US Food and Drug Administration for the treatment of RAI-R DTC; however, significant partial and complete responses are lacking. In addition, doxorubicin has many toxicities, limiting its durability. It is clear that more established evidence is needed in order to provide therapeutic agents that reduce disease progression and increase survival without the burden of cost and morbidity associated with these agents. Anderson et al.[82]

performed an extensive literature review of current clinical trials involving treatment of advanced thyroid cancer. The majority of evidence came from nonrandomized single arm phase 2 clinical trials, begging for more rigorous trial designs. In the last decade, vascular endothelial growth factor receptor tyrosine kinase inhibitors (TKI) appear to be the most promising agents in the treatment of advanced thyroid cancer, with disease regression seen in many patients. Impact of these agents on quality of life and overall survival is still unknown. Sorafenib was recently approved by the US Food and Drug Administration in November 2013. This was based on a double-blind, placebo-controlled phase 3 trial of 417 patients with locally recurrent or progressive, metastatic DTC that is refractory to radioactive iodine, presented at the American Society of Clinical Oncology annual meeting in June 2013. The majority of the patients had papillary carcinoma (57%); however, patients with follicular (25%) and poorly differentiated carcinomas (10%) were also included. Ninety-six percent of patients had metastases (pulmonary, 86%; lymph nodes, 51%; and bone, 27%). The median progression-free survival was 10.8 and 5.8 months for the sorafenib and placebo arms, respectively, with no complete responses. The overall survival was not significantly different. Another TKI, vandetanib, has shown progression-free survival advantage of 5.2 months in patients with RAI-R DTC,[83] and a phase 2 study with pazopanib showed a 49% partial Response Evaluation Criteria in Solid Tumors (RECIST) response rate in patients with RAI-R DTC.[84] Many questions still remain in the treatment of RAI-R DTC, including adaptation of therapy based on genetic profiling or tumor histology. Also, questions about economic factors, quality of life, overall survival, and disease progression despite treatment with these agents still need to be answered.

Another interesting area of research is the use of MEK inhibitors to "reverse" the loss of RAI avidity seen in many advanced tumors, particularly those with RAS mutations. A recent study published in the *New England Journal of Medicine* showed that the MEK1/MEK2 inhibitor selumetanib induced iodine incorporation into previously RAI-R tumors allowing a therapeutic RAI dose to be delivered to the metastatic lesion. Of 20 patients evaluated, 12 patients had increased uptake of iodine and 8 patients received a therapeutic dose of RAI.[85]

ANAPLASTIC THYROID CARCINOMA

ATC is an undifferentiated thyroid malignancy of the follicular epithelium. ATC is fortunately rare, but is aggressive and has a very poor prognosis with median overall survival of <6 months.[86] Median age at diagnosis is older than other thyroid cancers, and female

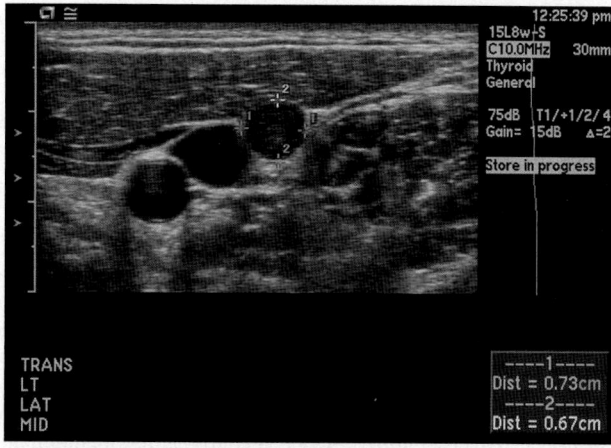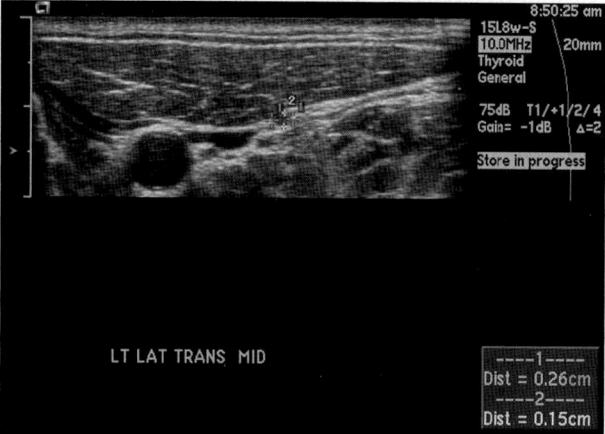

Figure 82.4 Transverse sonogram of a left lateral neck papillary thyroid carcinoma neck node metastasis (*indicated markers*). **(A)** Before ultrasound-guided percutaneous ethanol ablation and **(B)** 1 year after. The lesion has become indistinct and avascular.

patients predominate. All ATCs are classified as stage IV, with stage IVA limited to the thyroid, stage IVB with local invasion, and stage IVC with distant metastases.[87] Death is mainly caused by distant metastases (51.5%), local complications (24.7%), or both (26.2%).[86] Only 10% of patients will have intrathyroidal tumors at diagnosis, with 40% having extrathyroidal extension and lymph node involvement and 50% with distant metastases.[88] Lungs and bones are the most common sites of distant spread.

ATC may occur in synchrony with other thyroid malignancies including papillary, follicular, and HCC,[89] leading to the question about development of ATC through dedifferentiation of these well-differentiated cancers, possibly through activating mutations of BRAF and RAS. ATC typically presents with a rapidly enlarging thyroid mass, which frequently involves cervical lymph nodes and surrounding neck structures leading to compressive symptoms. Ultrasonography may be helpful to determine lymph node status and invasion; however, there are no specific ultrasound features to ATC. FNA is usually adequate to make the diagnosis, as long as the sample is taken from nonnecrotic areas. If the FNA is nondiagnostic, then core biopsy or incisional biopsy should be performed. Cytopathology shows significant necrosis in addition to morphologic patterns such as pleomorphic giant cell, spindle cell, and squamoid. Once the diagnosis has been established, imaging should be performed to assess local invasion as well as distant metastases. Per the ATA guidelines,[88] initial imaging includes a neck ultrasound, cross-sectional imaging of the neck and chest, imaging of the brain, and [18]FDG-PET. [18]FDG-PET has been shown to be very useful in the management of ATC, with intense uptake seen in both primary tumors and metastases.[90]

Treatment involves a multidisciplinary approach involving endocrinologists, surgeons, medical oncologists, and radiation oncologists. Considering the aggressive nature of the disease, palliative care teams should be involved early. The first step in management is to assess if the resectability with the imaging modalities described previously. For patients with locoregional disease and in which a grossly negative margin is achievable, initial appropriate management includes surgical resection. In circumstances when the disease is considered unresectable or high risk, neoadjuvant radiation and/or chemotherapy can be considered permitting delayed primary resection if needed. Resection after neoadjuvant therapy may reduce local relapse.

Adjuvant therapy with radiation, with or without chemotherapy, should be considered in patients with both resectable and unresectable disease and has been shown to improve outcomes in ATC. Due to rapid growth of anaplastic carcinoma, adjuvant therapy should be started as soon as possible after surgery. Palliative radiotherapy can be offered to patients with poor performance status. Traditionally, doxorubicin-based chemotherapy has been used, with or without platins. Encouraging results have also been seen with taxanes (both paclitaxel and docetaxel).[91–93] The TKI pazopanib has less activity against ATC than DTC as a single agent; however, ongoing trials are evaluating pazopanib in combination therapy with paclitaxel.[94]

An important decision to make in patients with metastatic disease is aggressiveness of therapy. Although there is no clear evidence that survival is prolonged with the addition of systemic therapy, some therapies may have disease-modifying effects including taxanes, doxorubicin, and possibly the platins. These agents, in single or combination therapies, can be considered first line in patients with advanced ATC who require a more aggressive approach. If a palliative approach is preferred, therapy should be aimed at local disease control to prevent demise from invasion of vital structures such as the trachea, including surgery and/or palliative radiation.

Better understanding of the biology of the ATC has led to investigation into newer targeted agents. Patients should be enrolled in clinical trials if possible. Newer agents include imatinib, an inhibitor of C-kit, platelet-derived growth factor receptor, and Bcr-Abl tyrosine kinases. Imatinib has produced partial remissions in two patients with stable disease in four patients.[95] Fosbretabulin,

a microtubule disrupting agent, has shown to produce stable disease in 26 patients.[96] Erlotinib, an epidermal growth factor receptor antagonist, has shown tumor reduction in several patients,[97,98] and gefitinib led to stable disease in one of five patients for 12 months.[99] Due to the lack of randomized controlled trials, many management questions unfortunately remain unanswered.

MEDULLARY THYROID CANCER

MTC was first described as a "malignant goiter with amyloid" by Jaquet in the German literature.[100] MTC is derived from the parafollicular or C cells, and is therefore classified as a neuroendocrine tumor. Embryologically, C cells are derived from neural crest and are located in the upper and middle portions of the thyroid. Therefore, most tumors are found in this location. Histologically, MTC resembles other neuroendocrine tumors, such as islet cell tumors.

MTC comprises approximately 4% of thyroid malignancies[101] and can be challenging to manage. Radiation is not associated with increased risk of MTC, but rather is associated with distinct familial syndromes. Both sporadic and familial MTC may have mutations in the RET (REarranged during Transfection) gene.

Sporadic Medullary Thyroid Cancer

Sporadic MTC comprises the majority of MTC: approximately 80%.[102] In 6% to 7% of cases, a RET germline mutation may be present. Up to 60% of MTC tumor cells may have a RET somatic mutation that is only limited to the C cells.[103–105] Tumors with these somatic mutations may have a poorer prognosis.[106]

Patients typically present with an asymptomatic thyroid mass but if the disease is locally advanced, patients may develop systemic symptoms such as diarrhea and flushing secondary to calcitonin secretion. Rarely, tumors may be a source of ectopic corticotropin production, leading to clinical evidence of Cushing syndrome.

Unfortunately, many presentations have evidence of local metastases at the time of diagnosis. Local invasion can present with cervical lymph node involvement (50% of patients) or invasion of local structures such as the nerves, trachea, and esophagus. Approximately 5% of patients will have distant metastatic disease; the sites favored include liver, bone, and lungs.[107]

Familial Medullary Thyroid Cancer

Autosomal dominant inherited MTC comprises 20% to 25% of MTC.[102] These syndromes consist of multiple endocrine neoplasia (MEN)2A, MEN2B, and familial MTC (FMTC) (Table 82.4). All three genetic syndromes are associated with gain of function mutations in the RET proto-oncogene, which leads to overexpression of Ret protein in the affected tissues, subsequent C cell hyperplasia, and progression to MTC over time.[100] MTC associated with familial syndromes is usually bilateral and multicentric. MEN2A is the most common of the MEN2 subtypes and usually presents in the third or fourth decade of life. Ninety five percent will have an identifiable RET mutation.[108] MEN2A is comprised of MTC, primary hyperparathyroidism (PHPT), and pheochromocytoma (PHEO), with MTC occurring in 90% of gene carriers.[108] It may be difficult to differentiate MEN2A from FMTC. FMTC has MTC in at least two generations, in the absence of PHPT and PHEO.[109] This is an important distinction to make as PHEOs can be missed if misclassification occurs. Presentation of disease in FMTC is later than MEN2A and has lower penetrance.[110,111] MEN2B is the more aggressive subtype of MEN2 syndromes, with many patients presenting with more advanced disease. MEN2B comprises of MTC and PHEO, but lacks the PHPT seen in MEN2A. In addition, patients with MEN2B have musculoskeletal abnormalities including marfanoid habitus, ganglioneuromatosis of the gut and oral mucosa, and medullated corneal nerve fibers (see Table 82.3).[100]

PRACTICE OF ONCOLOGY

TABLE 82.4

Clinical and Genetic Characteristics of Familial Medullary Thyroid Cancer Syndromes

Syndrome	Characteristic Features
FMTC	MTC
MEN2A	MTC Adrenal medulla (pheochromocytoma) Parathyroid hyperplasia
MEN2A with cutaneous lichen amyloidosis	MEN2A and a pruritic cutaneous lesion located over the upper back
MEN2A or FMTC with Hirschsprung disease	MEN2A or FMTC with Hirschsprung disease

MEN2B	MTC
	Adrenal medulla
	  (pheochromocytoma)
	Intestinal and mucosal
	  ganglioneuromatosis
	Characteristic Marfanoid habitus

FMTC, familial MTC; MTC, medullary thyroid cancer; MEN, multiple endocrine neoplasia.

Diagnosis and Staging

Ultrasound is a common modality utilized in the diagnosis of thyroid cancer. MTC may appear solid and hypoechoic on ultrasound, with some having microcalcifications as seen in PTC (varying frequency depending on study).[112–115] In sporadic MTC, diagnosis is made by FNA of the thyroid mass. Considering the sensitivity of FNA in MTC is 50% to 80%, calcitonin washout of the FNA needle may improve sensitivity.[116,117]

Once the diagnosis is made, an ultrasound of the neck should be performed to evaluate for nodal disease. In addition, the tumor markers calcitonin and carcinoembryonic antigen (CEA) should be measured, which can be used for comparison in the postoperative period. Additional imaging for metastatic disease should be performed if neck nodal disease is present or if the calcitonin is >400 pg/ml. The additional imaging should concentrate on the lungs, liver, and bones, as these are the most common sites of metastases. Imaging modalities include CT scans of the neck, chest, and abdomen. Bone magnetic resonance imaging can be performed if there is clinical suspicion of bony metastases. MTC does not concentrate iodine; therefore, ^{131}I thyroid scans are of no utility. Similarly, thallium as well as technetium scans have been used with minimal efficacy.[118] ^{18}FDG-PET and octreotide scans have low sensitivity, especially if the calcitonin is not very high; therefore, they are not used in routine metastatic evaluation.

Testing for germline mutations in *RET* proto-oncogene should be considered in all patients diagnosed with C cell hyperplasia or MTC, as mutations may occur in both sporadic and familial MTC. If a germline mutation is present, family members should also be screened for the mutation. In addition, patients with a germline mutation should be screened for other diseases associated with the familial syndromes including PHPT and PHEO, particularly prior to any surgical intervention. This screening will include serum calcium for PHPT and plasma-fractionated metanephrines for PHEO. Plasma-fractionated metanephrines are very sensitive but have a high false positive rate. If abnormal, we recommend confirmation with 24-hour urine-free metanephrines and catecholamines. Screening for PHEO and PHPT is usually not necessary if there is no evidence of *RET* mutation and no family history of MTC.

Prognosis

Recent studies show a 5-year survival between 80% and 90% and 10-year survival between 70% and 80% for combined series of familial and sporadic MTC.[119] The natural history and prognosis for the various subtypes of MTC correlate with described genetic changes. Poor prognostic factors include advanced age, large primary tumors, nodal disease, and distant metastases.

Treatment of Medullary Thyroid Cancer

Initial surgical management of MTC includes total thyroidectomy with central compartment node dissection. Total extracapsular thyroidectomy is always indicated in familial MTC due to incidence of bilateral tumors with metastatic disease. As mentioned previously, the anatomic position of primary MTC is in the upper thyroid lobes. This anatomic position of the primary tumor can make complete resection with a difficult due to close proximity of the recurrent laryngeal nerve. The ATA published guidelines on the management of sporadic and familial MTC.[100] The ATA recommends routine level VI compartment dissection with normal ultrasound of the lateral neck. On the other hand, if the lateral compartment has evidence of disease, without distant metastases, or limited distant metastases, level IIA, III, IV, and V neck dissection in addition to the central neck compartment dissection is recommended. At Mayo Clinic, 32% of 182 patients with MTC had palpable nodes and 40% of the patients with MTC had nodes involved with metastatic disease by pathologic examination.[54]

Postoperatively, patients should begin replacement levothyroxine therapy to maintain euthyroidism. Because C cells are not responsive to TSH, suppressive doses of levothyroxine are not indicated. Postoperative radioactive iodine is also not indicated as MTC tissue does not take up iodine. Serum calcitonin and CEA should be measured 3 to 6 months after surgery. It may take a long time for tumor markers to fall after surgery; however, if they remain elevated 6 months after surgery, prognosis is generally poorer. On the other hand, if the postoperative calcitonin and CEA are undetectable, the 5-year recurrence rate is only 5%.[119] Calcium stimulation testing has diminished over the years, and pentagastrin is no longer available in the United States. In those patients with evidence of biochemical cure, imaging is repeated 6 to 12 months after surgery to establish a baseline. Calcitonin and CEA should be measured every 6 months for the first 2 years and yearly thereafter.

A challenge in the surgical management of patients with MTC is the approach to patients who have persistently elevated basal or stimulated calcitonin after resection of all gross disease.[100,118] In many of these cases, imaging studies fail to demonstrate areas of disease. Excision attempts generally do not produce normalization of calcitonin levels. Tisell et al.[120] advocated meticulous 12-hour neck dissections, often removing 40 to 60 additional cervical lymph nodes in patients with occult MTC. In a series of 11 patients, 4 demonstrated normalization of calcitonin levels, with another 4 who had dramatic improvement in their calcitonin levels. However, even these improvements in the calcitonin levels do not necessarily translate into improved survival. In another report, only 9 of 32 patients developed biochemical cure after microdissection of the central and bilateral compartments.[121–123] Prognosis of postoperative hypercalcitonemia is dependent on extent of disease at initial surgery as well as the patient's age, with younger age and lack of nodal metastases having a better prognosis. In a large series of 899 patients, the 10-year survival rate of patients with postoperative hypercalcitonemia was 70% compared to 98% in those patients who had evidence of biochemical cure.[119] Therefore, considering biochemical cure is only achieved in approximately 25% of patients with repeat neck dissections, observation should be considered with periodic imaging and tumor marker evaluation in patients with limited locoregional disease. Surgery can be reconsidered if the locoregional disease progresses.

If calcitonin remains detectable but <150 pg/ml, imaging of the neck should be performed to evaluate for persistent disease.

If disease is evident on imaging, repeat neck dissection may be indicated to provide locoregional disease control as long as metastatic disease is not suspected. If imaging of the neck is negative for locoregional recurrence, then calcitonin should be monitored for stability. If the calcitonin remains stable, imaging can be performed yearly. If the calcitonin or CEA begins to rise, further imaging may be required to look for metastatic disease.

If the calcitonin is >150 pg/ml postoperatively, evaluation for distant metastases can be considered, particularly if the calcitonin is >300 pg/ml. Imaging should include CT evaluation of the neck, chest, and abdomen. Bone magnetic resonance imaging can be performed if there are any skeletal complaints. PET scanning is not very sensitive in detecting recurrent disease, with one study reporting a sensitivity of 78% in MTC with calcitonin >1,000 pg/ml.[124]

Assessment of tumor progression rate can be evaluated using RECIST or tumor marker surrogates such as calcitonin and CEA doubling time (DT). Barbet et al.[125] studied 41 patients with MTC with postoperative abnormal calcitonin levels. When the calcitonin DT was <6 months, the 5- and 10-year survivals were 25% and 8%, respectively; when 6 to 24 months, the 5- and 10-year survivals were 92% and 37%, respectively, and all patients with a calcitonin DT of >2 years were alive at the end of the study. Calcitonin DT using the first four measurements is an independent predictor of survival.[126] Reliable estimates include at least four data points over a minimum of 2 years. However, DT <6 months can be reliably estimated in the first 12 months. A calcitonin DT calculator is available on the ATA website (www.thyroid.org).

If disease is evident on imaging, the goal of treatment is to prevent complications of progressive local or metastatic disease. The first approach to neck nodal metastases may include neck dissection attempting to obtain surgical cure in the setting of limited disease. The second approach includes palliative debulking in the setting of metastatic disease to prevent locoregional complications including compression and pain. Ultrasound-guided percutaneous ethanol ablation of metastatic lymph nodes has been used successfully in patients who are poor surgical candidates (see "Ultrasound-guided Percutaneous Ethanol Ablation").

Systemic Therapy in Medullary Thyroid Cancer

The role of EBRT is limited. EBRT to the neck may be considered in patients who have extensive locoregional disease without complete resection of gross disease as this approach may provide increased time to recurrence or progression.[127] EBRT may also be used to treat skeletal metastases that are symptomatic or are located in sites prone to fracture.

Systemic therapy may be associated with significant toxicity and should be reserved for patients who have unresectable, locally advanced, or progressive disease (growing diameter >20% per year). TKIs have been of great interest in the treatment of advanced MTC and have changed the standard approach to therapy. Two TKIs have been recently approved for the treatment of MTC: vandetanib (2011) and cabozantinib (2012). Vandetanib is currently approved in the United States for treatment of unresectable locally advanced or progressive sporadic and familial MTC, and is available to prescribers who are part of the Risk Evaluation Mitigation Strategy (REMS) program. Vandetanib targets vascular endothelial growth factor receptor, RET, and the epidermal growth factor receptor, all of which are responsible for a tumor's ability to proliferate, invade, and metastasize. Approval was based on the phase 3 ZETA trial of 331 patients, with 300 mg of vandetanib daily versus placebo.[128] Median follow-up was 24 months. Patients treated with vandetanib had increased progression-free survival of 30.5 months compared to 19.3 months. In addition, reduction in calcitonin and CEA was seen. No overall survival benefit has been reported as of yet. Common side effects were present in approximately 20% of patients, including diarrhea, rash, nausea, and fatigue. Severe side effects were present in approximately 5% and included sudden cardiac death and

torsades des pointes. In the phase 3 EXAM trial, 330 patients were randomized to cabozantinib versus placebo.[129] Median progression-free survival was 11.2 months in the cabozantinib arm compared to 4 months in the placebo arm. Many other TKIs are under investigation in advanced MTC, including sorafenib and sunitinib.

Traditional cytotoxic agents have been used in MTC but the results are disappointing. Chemotherapeutic agents used in the treatment of MTC include doxorubicin, dacarbazine, cyclophosphamide, vincristine, streptozocin, and 5-fluorouracil. Combination regimens are preferred. These agents are considered second-line therapy and should be reserved for patients who fail or cannot tolerate TKIs. Other investigational approaches have included immunotherapy.

THYROID LYMPHOMA

Primary lymphoma of the thyroid is rare, only accounting for 1% to 5% of thyroid malignancies[130] and 2% of all extranodal lymphomas. There is a strong female predominance, with median age of diagnosis in the seventh decade. Approximately 50% of patients of primary thyroid lymphoma have underlying Hashimoto's thyroiditis, the only known risk factor.[29] Patients frequently present with a rapidly enlarging goiter[131]; however, smaller tumors may present as a solitary or dominant nodule. Between 10% and 30% of patients report a symptom or combination of symptoms relating to local invasion, including hoarseness, dyspnea with stridor, or dysphagia. Examination may reveal a firm, possibly tender thyroid that may be fixed. Thyroid function may be compromised, with many patients having hypothyroidism, either due to underlying Hashimoto's thyroiditis or due to infiltration of the thyroid with lymphoma. Hyperthyroidism is rare but has been described. Systemic symptoms associated with lymphoma or "B" symptoms including fever, weight loss, and night sweats may be present in 10% of patients with primary thyroid lymphoma.

Diagnosis may be difficult, particularly if the clinical suspicion is not high. Primary thyroid lymphomas may be indistinguishable from Hashimoto's thyroiditis and have low echogenicity on ultrasound. Lesions are commonly described as pseudocystic. Borders may be ill or well defined depending on the underlying lymphoma subtype.[132] There is no role for other radiographic imaging in differentiating thyroid lymphoma from other thyroid pathologies. However, imaging can be useful in staging once the diagnosis of lymphoma has been made.

FNA has led to great advancement in the diagnosis of thyroid cancer; however, in thyroid lymphoma the FNA is frequently nondiagnostic. If clinical suspicion for lymphoma is high, then core or incisional biopsies should be performed to allow for flow cytometry and immunohistochemical staining to be performed. The most common histologic subtype is diffuse large B cell lymphoma, whereas the remaining are mucosa-associated lymphoid tissue or follicular subtype.[131,133] The majority of patients with thyroid lymphoma have disease on one side of the diaphragm with approximately 50% confined to the thyroid (stage IE). Approximately 45% have thyroid disease plus cervical or mediastinal lymph nodes (stage IIE). Only 5% have disease both sides of the diaphragm (stage IIIE) or diffuse organ involvement (stage IV).[29,134,135]

According to the Surveillance, Epidemiology and End Results (SEER) database on thyroid lymphoma, decreased disease-specific survival is associated with advanced age >80 years, advanced stage of disease, lack of chemotherapy and radiotherapy, and diffuse large B cell lymphoma or follicular subtype.[136] Five-year survival ranges from 52% to 90%.

Surgery is predominantly used as a diagnostic tool in the treatment of primary thyroid lymphoma. In stage IE disease, surgery may help differentiate intrathyroidal tumors from extrathyroidal extension, which is an important distinction to make with respect to treatment decisions. If the tumor remains intrathyroidal, treatment with surgery and radiation alone may be appropriate. If the tumor extends outside the thyroid, combination chemotherapy is required.[137] Thyroidectomy in patients with stage IIE or IIIE is less commonly performed as cause-specific survival is not improved in patients who received thyroidectomy with radiation versus those who receive radiation alone.[138] Diffuse large B-cell lymphoma is treated with three courses of combination chemotherapy, followed by radiation, or six to eight cycles of combination chemotherapy without radiation. In localized, low-grade, or indolent lymphomas, radiation therapy can be used alone unless systemic disease is present, at which time chemotherapy can be used alone.

CHILDREN WITH THYROID CARCINOMA

Differentiated Thyroid Carcinoma

PTC accounts for 1.5% of childhood malignancy but >90% of childhood thyroid cancers.[139] Due to low incidence, current treatment strategies for pediatric patients with well-differentiated thyroid carcinoma are derived from single institution clinical cohorts, reports of extensive personal experience, and extrapolation of several common therapeutic practices in adults. PTC has a higher incidence of metastases to the lymph nodes and lungs at presentation than in adults.[140,141] However, PTC in childhood tends to be indolent with low death rates. Children with well-differentiated thyroid carcinoma more often than their adult counterparts have a history of external irradiation to the head and neck, although the majority present without such a history.[142] In the past, >50% of patients had exposure to ionizing radiation. Outside of the Chernobyl accident region, this exposure has dropped to <3% of cases.

Most authors agree that aggressive initial management with total thyroidectomy and cervical lymph node dissection should be performed in most children with well-differentiated thyroid carcinoma. Routine radioactive remnant ablation has become more controversial over time. A study of 215 patients <21 years of age with PTC at Mayo Clinic showed that the initial surgery had the greatest impact on recurrence that was not further influenced by RRA.[143] In addition, there is concern about nonthyroid secondary malignancies, which occurred in patients 30 to 50 years after initial treatment, most commonly in patients that were exposed to various forms of radiation. At Mayo Clinic, we therefore restrict adjuvant RAI to patients who are considered high risk with distant metastases or incomplete resection with gross residual disease. Due to the limited experience in the management of thyroid cancer in the pediatric population, consideration should be made for referral to centers with experience in managing these challenging cases.

Medullary Thyroid Carcinoma

With the introduction of genetic screening for *RET* gene mutations, an increasing number of patients are diagnosed with inherited forms of MTC during childhood or even infancy. Depending on genotype, the current recommendations advise that individuals with *RET* gene mutations associated with MEN2A and FMTC undergo prophylactic thyroidectomy between ages 5 to 6 years, whereas affected individuals in kindreds with MEN2B should undergo thyroidectomy during infancy due to the aggressiveness and earlier age at onset of MTC in these patients.[100] At the MD Anderson Cancer Center, 86 patients with inherited MTC were stratified into three *RET* gene mutation risk groups: level 1, low risk for MTC (mutations in codons 609, 768, 790, 791, 804, and 891); level 2, intermediate risk (mutations in codons 611, 618, 620, and 634); and level 3, highest risk (mutations in codons 883 and 918).[100] All patients in the level 3 group (all with MEN2B) had MTC present at initial thyroidectomy performed at a median age of 13.5 years. With increased knowledge of genotype–phenotype correlations, more individualized management can be used in the treatment of familial variants of MTC.

SELECTED REFERENCES

The full reference list can be accessed at lwwhealthlibrary.com/oncology.

2. Mortensen JD, Woolner LB, Bennett WA. Gross and microscopic findings in clinically normal thyroid glands. *J Clin Endocrinol Metab* 1955;15:1270–1280.
5. Hagag P, Strauss S, Weiss M. Role of ultrasound-guided fine-needle aspiration biopsy in evaluation of nonpalpable thyroid nodules. *Thyroid* 1998;8:989–995.
7. Gharib H, Papini E, Valcavi R, et al. American Association of Clinical Endocrinologists and Associazione Medici Endocrinologi medical guidelines for clinical practice for the diagnosis and management of thyroid nodules. *Endocr Pract* 2006;12:63–102.
9. Schneider AB, Sarne DH. Long-term risks for thyroid cancer and other neoplasms after exposure to radiation. *Nat Clin Pract Endocrinol Metab* 2005;1:82–91.
11. Pacini F, Schlumberger M, Dralle H, et al. European consensus for the management of patients with differentiated thyroid carcinoma of the follicular epithelium. *Eur J Endocrinol* 2006;154:787–803.
14. Tan GH, Gharib H, Reading CC. Solitary thyroid nodule. Comparison between palpation and ultrasonography. *Arch Intern Med* 1995;155:2418–2423.
15. Bisi H, de Camargo RY, Longatto Filho A. Role of fine-needle aspiration cytology in the management of thyroid nodules: review of experience with 1,925 cases. *Diagn Cytopathol* 1992;8:504–510.
16. Nikiforov YE, Ohori NP, Hodak SP, et al. Impact of mutational testing on the diagnosis and management of patients with cytologically indeterminate thyroid nodules: a prospective analysis of 1056 FNA samples. *J Clin Endocrinol Metab* 2011;96:3390–3397.
18. Tuttle RM, Ball DW, Byrd D, et al. Thyroid carcinoma. *J Natl Compr Canc Netw* 2010;8:1228–1274.
19. Bogsrud TV, Karantanis D, Nathan MA, et al. The value of quantifying 18F-FDG uptake in thyroid nodules found incidentally on whole-body PET-CT. *Nucl Med Commun* 2007;28:373–381.
20. Cohen MS, Arslan N, Dehdashti F, et al. Risk of malignancy in thyroid incidentalomas identified by fluorodeoxyglucose-positron emission tomography. *Surgery* 2001;130:941–946.
21. Kang KW, Kim SK, Kang HS, et al. Prevalence and risk of cancer of focal thyroid incidentaloma identified by 18F-fluorodeoxyglucose positron emission tomography for metastasis evaluation and cancer screening in healthy subjects. *J Clin Endocrinol Metab* 2003;88:4100–4104.
28. Pal T, Vogl FD, Chappuis PO, et al. Increased risk for nonmedullary thyroid cancer in the first degree relatives of prevalent cases of nonmedullary thyroid cancer: a hospital-based study. *J Clin Endocrinol Metab* 2001;86:5307–5312.
30. Jemal A, Siegel R, Ward E, et al. Cancer statistics, 2009. *CA Cancer J Clin* 2009;59:225–249.
31. Jossart GH, Clark OH. Well-differentiated thyroid cancer. *Curr Probl Surg* 1994;31:933–1012.
32. Dean DS, Hay ID. Prognostic indicators in differentiated thyroid carcinoma. *Cancer Control* 2000;7:229–239.
33. Hay ID, Grant CS, Taylor WF, et al. Ipsilateral lobectomy versus bilateral lobar resection in papillary thyroid carcinoma: a retrospective analysis of surgical outcome using a novel prognostic scoring system. *Surgery* 1987;102:1088–1095.
34. Cady B, Rossi R. An expanded view of risk-group definition in differentiated thyroid carcinoma. *Surgery* 1988;104:947–953.
35. Hay ID, Bergstralh EJ, Goellner JR, et al. Predicting outcome in papillary thyroid carcinoma: development of a reliable prognostic scoring system in a cohort of 1779 patients surgically treated at one institution during 1940 through 1989. *Surgery* 1993;114:1050–1057; discussion 1057–1058.
36. Hay ID. Papillary thyroid carcinoma. *Endocrinol Metab Clin North Am* 1990;19:545–576.
37. Nikiforova MN, Kimura ET, Gandhi M, et al. BRAF mutations in thyroid tumors are restricted to papillary carcinomas and anaplastic or poorly differentiated carcinomas arising from papillary carcinomas. *J Clin Endocrinol Metab* 2003;88:5399–5404.
42. Xing M, Clark D, Guan H, et al. BRAF mutation testing of thyroid fine-needle aspiration biopsy specimens for preoperative risk stratification in papillary thyroid cancer. *J Clin Oncol* 2009;27:2977–2982.
49. Hay ID, Ryan JJ, Grant CS, et al. Prognostic significance of nondiploid DNA determined by flow cytometry in sporadic and familial medullary thyroid carcinoma. *Surgery* 1990;108:972–979; discussion 979–980.
50. Carling T, Ocal IT, Udelsman R. Special variants of differentiated thyroid cancer: does it alter the extent of surgery versus well-differentiated thyroid cancer? *World J Surg* 2007;31:916–923.
51. LiVolsi VA, Asa SL. The demise of follicular carcinoma of the thyroid gland. *Thyroid* 1994;4:233–236.
52. Carling T, Udelsman R. Follicular neoplasms of the thyroid: what to recommend. *Thyroid* 2005;15:583–587.

53. Hay ID, Thompson GB, Grant CS, et al. Papillary thyroid carcinoma managed at the Mayo Clinic during six decades (1940–1999): temporal trends in initial therapy and long-term outcome in 2444 consecutively treated patients. *World J Surg* 2002;26:879–885.

54. Grebe SK, Hay ID. Thyroid cancer nodal metastases: biologic significance and therapeutic considerations. *Surg Oncol Clin N Am* 1996;5:43–63.

55. Hay ID, McConahey WM, Goellner JR. Managing patients with papillary thyroid carcinoma: insights gained from the Mayo Clinic's experience of treating 2,512 consecutive patients during 1940 through 2000. *Trans Am Clin Climatol Assoc* 2002;113:241–260.

56. Jonklaas J, Sarlis NJ, Litofsky D, et al. Outcomes of patients with differentiated thyroid carcinoma following initial therapy. *Thyroid* 2006;16:1229–1242.

57. Brierley J, Tsang R, Panzarella T, et al. Prognostic factors and the effect of treatment with radioactive iodine and external beam radiation on patients with differentiated thyroid cancer seen at a single institution over 40 years. *Clin Endocrinol (Oxf)* 2005;63:418–427.

60. Baudin E, Travagli JP, Ropers J, et al. Microcarcinoma of the thyroid gland: the Gustave-Roussy Institute experience. *Cancer* 1998;83:553–559.

61. Hay ID, Hutchinson ME, Gonzalez-Losada T, et al. Papillary thyroid microcarcinoma: a study of 900 cases observed in a 60-year period. *Surgery* 2008;144:980–987; discussion 987–988.

62. Ito Y, Uruno T, Nakano K, et al. An observation trial without surgical treatment in patients with papillary microcarcinoma of the thyroid. *Thyroid* 2003;13:381–387.

65. Smallridge RC, Meek SE, Morgan MA, et al. Monitoring thyroglobulin in a sensitive immunoassay has comparable sensitivity to recombinant human tsh-stimulated thyroglobulin in follow-up of thyroid cancer patients. *J Clin Endocrinol Metab* 2007;92:82–87.

67. Durante C, Haddy N, Baudin E, et al. Long-term outcome of 444 patients with distant metastases from papillary and follicular thyroid carcinoma: benefits and limits of radioiodine therapy. *J Clin Endocrinol Metab* 2006;91:2892–2899.

68. Clark OH, Hoelting T. Management of patients with differentiated thyroid cancer who have positive serum thyroglobulin levels and negative radioiodine scans. *Thyroid* 1994;4:501–505.

69. Schlumberger MJ. Papillary and follicular thyroid carcinoma. *New Engl J Med* 1998;338:297–306.

70. Fatourechi V, Hay ID, Javedan H, et al. Lack of impact of radioiodine therapy in tg-positive, diagnostic whole-body scan-negative patients with follicular cell-derived thyroid cancer. *J Clin Endocrinol Metab* 2002;87:1521–1526.

73. van Dijk D, Plukker JT, Phan HT, et al. 18-fluorodeoxyglucose positron emission tomography in the early diagnostic workup of differentiated thyroid cancer patients with a negative post-therapeutic iodine scan and detectable thyroglobulin. *Thyroid* 2013;23:1003–1009.

74. Leboulleux S, Schroeder PR, Schlumberger M, et al. The role of PET in follow-up of patients treated for differentiated epithelial thyroid cancers. *Nat Clin Pract Endocrinol Metab* 2007;3:112–121.

75. Livraghi T, Paracchi A, Ferrari C, et al. Treatment of autonomous thyroid nodules with percutaneous ethanol injection: preliminary results. Work in progress. *Radiology* 1990;175:827–829.

76. Lewis BD, Hay ID, Charboneau JW, et al. Percutaneous ethanol injection for treatment of cervical lymph node metastases in patients with papillary thyroid carcinoma. *AJR Am J Roentgenol* 2002;178:699–704.

77. Hay ID, Charboneau JW. The coming of age of ultrasound-guided percutaneous ethanol ablation of selected neck nodal metastases in well-differentiated thyroid carcinoma. *J Clin Endocrinol Metab* 2011;96:2717–2720.

80. Heilo A, Sigstad E, Fagerlid KH, et al. Efficacy of ultrasound-guided percutaneous ethanol injection treatment in patients with a limited number of metastatic cervical lymph nodes from papillary thyroid carcinoma. *J Clin Endocrinol Metab* 2011;96:2750–2755.

81. Hay ID, Lee RA, Davidge-Pitts C, et al. Long-term outcome of ultrasound-guided percutaneous ethanol ablation of selected "recurrent" neck nodal metastases in 25 patients with TNM stages III or IVA papillary thyroid carcinoma previously treated by surgery and I therapy. *Surgery* 2014;154:1448–1454.

82. Anderson RT, Linnehan JE, Tongbram V, et al. Clinical, safety, and economic evidence in radioactive iodine-refractory differentiated thyroid cancer: a systematic literature review. *Thyroid* 2013;23:392–407.

83. Leboulleux S, Bastholt L, Krause T, et al. Vandetanib in locally advanced or metastatic differentiated thyroid cancer: a randomised, double-blind, phase 2 trial. *Lancet Oncol* 2012;13:897–905.

84. Bible KC, Suman VJ, Molina JR, et al. Efficacy of pazopanib in progressive, radioiodine-refractory, metastatic differentiated thyroid cancers: results of a phase 2 consortium study. *Lancet Oncol* 2010;11:962–972.

85. Ho AL, Grewal RK, Leboeuf R, et al. Selumetinib-enhanced radioiodine uptake in advanced thyroid cancer. *New Engl J Med* 2013;368:623–632.

86. Granata R, Locati L, Licitra L. Therapeutic strategies in the management of patients with metastatic anaplastic thyroid cancer: review of the current literature. *Curr Opin Oncol* 2013;25:224–228.

87. Smallridge RC. Approach to the patient with anaplastic thyroid carcinoma. *J Clin Endocrinol Metab* 2012;97:2566–2572.

88. Smallridge RC, Ain KB, Asa SL, et al. American Thyroid Association guidelines for management of patients with anaplastic thyroid cancer. *Thyroid* 2012;22:1104–1139.

90. Bogsrud TV, Karantanis D, Nathan MA, et al. 18F-FDG PET in the management of patients with anaplastic thyroid carcinoma. *Thyroid* 2008;18:713–719.

91. Ain KB, Egorin MJ, DeSimone PA. Treatment of anaplastic thyroid carcinoma with paclitaxel: phase 2 trial using ninety-six-hour infusion. Collaborative Anaplastic Thyroid Cancer Health Intervention Trials (CATCHIT) Group. *Thyroid* 2000;10:587–594.

92. Higashiyama T, Ito Y, Hirokawa M, et al. Induction chemotherapy with weekly paclitaxel administration for anaplastic thyroid carcinoma. *Thyroid* 2010;20:7–14.

93. Bhatia A, Rao A, Ang KK, et al. Anaplastic thyroid cancer: Clinical outcomes with conformal radiotherapy. *Head Neck* 2010;32:829–836.

94. Isham CR, Bossou AR, Negron V, et al. Pazopanib enhances paclitaxel-induced mitotic catastrophe in anaplastic thyroid cancer. *Sci Transl Med* 2013;5:166ra3.

95. Ha HT, Lee JS, Urba S, et al. A phase II study of imatinib in patients with advanced anaplastic thyroid cancer. *Thyroid* 2010;20:975–980.

96. Mooney CJ, Nagaiah G, Fu P, et al. A phase II trial of fosbretabulin in advanced anaplastic thyroid carcinoma and correlation of baseline serum-soluble intracellular adhesion molecule-1 with outcome. *Thyroid* 2009;19:233–240.

97. Hogan T, Jing Jie Yu, Williams HJ, et al. Oncocytic, focally anaplastic, thyroid cancer responding to erlotinib. *J Oncol Pharm Pract* 2009;15:111–117.

98. Masago K, Miura M, Toiyama Y, et al. Good clinical response to erlotinib in a patient with anaplastic thyroid carcinoma harboring an epidermal growth factor somatic mutation, L858R, in exon 21. *J Clin Oncol* 2011;29:e465–e467.

99. Pennell NA, Daniels GH, Haddad RI, et al. A phase II study of gefitinib in patients with advanced thyroid cancer. *Thyroid* 2008;18:317–323.

102. Pelizzo MR, Boschin IM, Bernante P, et al. Natural history, diagnosis, treatment and outcome of medullary thyroid cancer: 37 years experience on 157 patients. *Eur J Surg Oncol* 2007;33:493–497.

103. Wohllk N, Cote GJ, Bugalho MM, et al. Relevance of RET proto-oncogene mutations in sporadic medullary thyroid carcinoma. *J Clin Endocrinol Metab* 1996;81:3740–3745.

107. Pacini F, Castagna MG, Cipri C, et al. Medullary thyroid carcinoma. *Clin Oncol (R Coll Radiol)* 2010;22:475–485.

108. Brandi ML, Gagel RF, Angeli A, et al. Guidelines for diagnosis and therapy of MEN type 1 and type 2. *J Clin Endocrinol Metab* 2001;86:5658–5671.

118. Moley JF. Medullary thyroid carcinoma. *Curr Treat Options Oncol* 2003;4:339–347.

119. Modigliani E, Cohen R, Campos JM, et al. Prognostic factors for survival and for biochemical cure in medullary thyroid carcinoma: results in 899 patients. The GETC Study Group. Groupe d'etude des tumeurs a calcitonine. *Clin Endocrinol (Oxf)* 1998;48:265–273.

121. Moley JF, Wells SA, Dilley WG, et al. Reoperation for recurrent or persistent medullary thyroid cancer. *Surgery* 1993;114:1090–1095; discussion 1095–1096.

122. Fialkowski E, DeBenedetti M, Moley J. Long-term outcome of reoperations for medullary thyroid carcinoma. *World J Surg* 2008;32:754–765.

123. van Veelen W, de Groot JW, Acton DS, et al. Medullary thyroid carcinoma and biomarkers: past, present and future. *J Intern Med* 2009;266:126–140.

124. Ong SC, Schöder H, Patel SG, et al. Diagnostic accuracy of 18F-FDG PET in restaging patients with medullary thyroid carcinoma and elevated calcitonin levels. *J Nucl Med* 2007;48:501–507.

125. Barbet J, Campion L, Kraeber-Bodéré F, et al. Prognostic impact of serum calcitonin and carcinoembryonic antigen doubling-times in patients with medullary thyroid carcinoma. *J Clin Endocrinol Metab* 2005;90:6077–6084.

126. Laure Giraudet A, Al Ghulzan A, Aupérin A, et al. Progression of medullary thyroid carcinoma: assessment with calcitonin and carcinoembryonic antigen doubling times. *Eur J Endocrinol* 2008;158:239–246.

127. Brierley J, Tsang R, Simpson WJ, et al. Medullary thyroid cancer: analyses of survival and prognostic factors and the role of radiation therapy in local control. *Thyroid* 1996;6:305–310.

128. Wells SA Jr, Robinson BG, Gagel RF, et al. Vandetanib in patients with locally advanced or metastatic medullary thyroid cancer: a randomized, double-blind phase III trial. *J Clin Oncol* 2012;30:134–141.

129. Elisei R, Schlumberger MJ, Müller SP, et al. Cabozantinib in progressive medullary thyroid cancer. *J Clin Oncol* 2013;31:3639–3646.

130. Graff-Baker A, Sosa JA, Roman SA. Primary thyroid lymphoma: a review of recent developments in diagnosis and histology-driven treatment. *Curr Opin Oncol* 2010;22:17–22.

133. Junor EJ, Paul J, Reed NS. Primary non-Hodgkin's lymphoma of the thyroid. *Eur J Surg Oncol* 1992;18:313–321.

136. Graff-Baker A, Roman SA, Thomas DC, et al. Prognosis of primary thyroid lymphoma: demographic, clinical, and pathologic predictors of survival in 1,408 cases. *Surgery* 2009;146:1105–1115.

137. Friedberg MH, Coburn MC, Monchik JM. Role of surgery in stage IE non-Hodgkin's lymphoma of the thyroid. *Surgery* 1994;116:1061–1066; discussion 1066–1067.

138. Pyke CM, Grant CS, Habermann TM, et al. Non-Hodgkin's lymphoma of the thyroid: is more than biopsy necessary? *World J Surg* 1992;16:604–609; discussion 609–610.

143. Hay ID, Gonzalez-Losada R, Reinalda MS, et al. Long-term outcome in 215 children and adolescents with papillary thyroid cancer treated during 1940 through 2008. *World J Surg* 2010;34:1192–1202.

83 Parathyroid Tumors

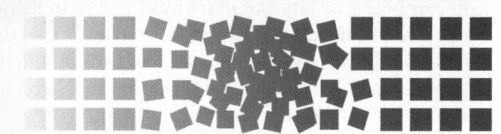

Marcio L. Griebeler and Geoffrey B. Thompson

INCIDENCE AND ETIOLOGY

Parathyroid tumors are one of the most common endocrine neoplasms. Hyperparathyroidism may be primary, secondary, or rarely, tertiary. Primary hyperparathyroidism (PHP) is one of the most common endocrine disorders along with diabetes mellitus, osteoporosis, thyroid nodules, and the most common cause of hypercalcemia in the outpatient setting.[1,2]

PHP occurs as a result of inappropriate parathyroid hormone (PTH) secretion from an enlarged gland. A total of 85% of the cases are caused by a parathyroid adenoma, parathyroid hyperplasia involving the four glands (10%), double parathyroid adenoma (2% to 5%), and parathyroid cancer in <1% of the cases.[3] Secondary hyperparathyroidism occurs when the parathyroid glands appropriately respond to a reduced level of extracellular calcium and elevated levels of serum phosphorus. It is characterized by an elevation of PTH with normal or low calcium concentration, which usually is associated with renal failure and vitamin D deficiency. Finally, in tertiary hyperparathyroidism there is a continued autonomous hypersecretion of PTH from one or more enlarged parathyroid gland. PHP may also be associated with some familial syndromes, like multiple endocrine neoplasia (MEN) type 1 and type 2A, familial isolated hyperparathyroidism, and the hyperparathyroidism-jaw tumor syndrome (HPT-JT).[4,5]

PHP was diagnosed less often when the diagnosis was dependent on overt symptoms related to long-standing disease. The epidemiology of this disease has shown significant changes over the last several decades, with the majority of the patients remaining relatively asymptomatic with only mild hypercalcemia, being diagnosed by routine calcium measurements instead of symptoms.[6] Recent studies from Europe and the United States have demonstrated that the incidence of PHP is higher than previously reported, suggesting that the incidence has increased from 2000 to 2010.[7–9] There are approximately 100,000 new cases diagnosed each year in the United States. It is more common in women (1 in 500) than in men (1 in 1,000) and occurs in approximately 0.3% of the general population. PHP occurs most often in perimenopausal or postmenopausal women and is rare in children.

Parathyroid cancer is a rare cause of PHP and one of the rarest of malignancies.[10] The estimated prevalence is 0.005% of all solid malignancies.[11,12] The majority of cases often coexist with PHP, but there are reports of cancers occurring in secondary hyperparathyroidism and with nonfunctioning tumors. The incidence of parathyroid cancer ranges from 0.5% to 5% of cases of PHP. The majority of studies show a prevalence of <1% of all cases of PHP.[11,13–15] Variable rates in parathyroid cancer are likely the result of the fact that most studies take place at tertiary referral centers where rare diagnoses are more likely to be encountered. Hundahl et al.,[16] in their review of the National Cancer Data Base, reported 286 cases of parathyroid cancer between the years 1985 and 1995. Lee et al.,[12] who used the Surveillance, Epidemiology and End Results (SEER) cancer registry database for years 1988 through 2003, reported 224 cases of parathyroid cancer.[12] Talat and Schulte[17] recently compiled information on 330 patients collected from case reviews and 706 patients from other studies providing clustered data between 1961 and February 2009. Based on some of these studies, which capture approximately 60% to 80% of all cancer diagnoses in the United States, between 30 and 50 cases of parathyroid carcinoma occur annually.

The majority of patients with parathyroid cancer present with symptoms, severe hypercalcemia, and metabolic complications of PHP, like bone and renal disease. The levels of PTH are usually very high. The clinical behavior of parathyroid cancer is quite variable but usually the tumor is very aggressive, and most patients develop locoregional recurrence; distant metastasis to lung, bone, and liver occur late. Most patients with parathyroid cancer succumb to uncontrollable hypercalcemia, not to direct tumor burden.

Different than the benign parathyroid tumors (female-to-male ratio of 3 to 4:1), parathyroid cancer occurs with equal frequency in men and women. The male sex is associated with worse overall survival. Parathyroid carcinoma typically will develop between ages 45 to 59 years. More than 75% of patients will present after the age of 45 where the median age of presentation is 55 years old.[12,16] Patients with benign parathyroid tumors are on average a decade older than patients with parathyroid carcinoma. There is no ethnic or racial disparity in the incidence of parathyroid cancer.[12,16]

There are few risk factors associated with parathyroid cancer. Genetic syndromes associated with parathyroid cancer include MEN1 and MEN2A, but benign parathyroid tumors remain much more common in these syndromes as well.[18,19] Another very important genetic syndrome is the HPT-JT syndrome, where up to 15% of affected individuals develop parathyroid cancer. The gene that predisposes to tumor is an inactivating germ line mutation of the HRPT2 gene (CDC73).[20] There are a few case reports of carcinoma occurring in patients with a history of neck irradiation and end-stage renal disease; however, there is very little clinical evidence to support this association.[18,21–23] A retrospective cohort study from Swedish Family Cancer Database reported an association of parathyroid cancer in patients with history of thyroid cancer and parathyroid adenoma, but despite these associations the evidence of parathyroid carcinoma arising from malignant transformation has not been found.[24,25]

ANATOMY AND PATHOLOGY

It can be difficult to distinguish parathyroid cancer from parathyroid adenoma. At the time of neck exploration, malignant tumors are often large (usually >3 cm), weighing between 2 and 10 g (the combined weight of all four normal parathyroid glands is approximately 150 mg). They are often hard, firm, and whitish-gray, and with invasion or adherence to the adjacent tissues such as the strap muscles, thyroid gland, recurrent laryngeal nerve, trachea, or esophagus.[11] For an unequivocal diagnosis of parathyroid cancer, the presence of gross local invasion, lymph node or distant (lung, liver, or bone) metastasis, or local recurrence after complete resection (not as a result of tumor spillage at the initial resection) is needed.

Even by histopathology the diagnosis of parathyroid carcinoma is challenging. In 1973 after 70 cases of parathyroid cancer were examined, Schantz and Castleman[25] reported histologic criteria that are still commonly used. This includes the presence of fibrous bands intersecting the tumors forming trabecular architecture, along with capsular invasion, vascular invasion, and increased mitotic activity. These features are not unique to parathyroid carcinoma and can also be found in benign parathyroid tumors (adenoma, atypical adenoma, parathyromatosis, and hyperplasia). Overall, there is not one histopathologic sign that can distinguish between parathyroid cancer and benign disease; definitive diagnosis can be made only with the presence of loco regional invasion or distant metastases.[4]

Several other markers of malignancy have been studied besides routine hematoxylin and eosin histology to help distinguish parathyroid cancer from parathyroid adenoma. Electron microscopy does not add proof of malignancy when compared to light microscopy.[26] Flow-cytometric analysis of parathyroid tumors are more likely to be aneuploid than adenomas (60% versus 9%, respectively). Determination of DNA ploidy may add valuable information to routine histology, even though some studies have shown that variables rates of DNA ploidy can also be seen in parathyroid adenoma.[27] Analysis of human telomerase expression in parathyroid tumors may be a helpful adjunct to histology as 100% of parathyroid cancers are positive on immunohistochemistry examination as compared with 6% of parathyroid adenomas (6%).[28]

Increased Ki-67 and galectin 3 expression in association with absent parafibromin expression may help distinguish parathyroid cancer from benign parathyroid tumors.[29] A combination of these three markers showed that 15 of 16 parathyroid cancers were correctly identified with only a 3% false positive rate.[4] Recently, Starker et al.[30] demonstrated that a comprehensive analysis of epigenetic alteration in parathyroid tumors shows distinct DNA methylation profiles between benign and malignant lesions.

Molecular classification of parathyroid cancer by gene expression profiling comes from inherited disorders of PHP, especially HPT-JT syndrome. Identification of the molecular markers associated with parathyroid carcinoma will prove to be an important tool for the improvement of the often difficult diagnostic dilemma. HPT-JT is an autosomal-dominant disease, and the majority of patients are heterozygous for germline CDC 73 mutations, located on chromosome 1q31.2.[31] The gene encodes parafibromin, a tumor suppressor protein. Parafibromin inhibits mitogenic functions of cyclin D1 and c-myc pathway.[32] The most common mutations are frame-shift and nonsense mutations. Patients with HPT-JT syndrome have ossifying fibromas of the maxilla and mandible, less frequently hamartomas and renal cysts, and develop parathyroid tumors that are mostly malignant.[33]

Cyclin D1 is an oncogene located on chromosome 11q13 and is involved in cell cycle regulation. Overexpression of the oncogene CCND1 (or BCL1 or PRad1) that encodes cyclin-D1 was found in many benign tumors and the vast majority of parathyroid cancers.[20,34] Although cyclin D1 overexpression has been seen in parathyroid cancer, it appears that the increase in expression may be related to increased proliferation and not to the pathogenesis of parathyroid cancer.[5] Furthermore, it appears that parafibromin regulates cyclin D1 and thus may be a downstream effector of parafibromin. P27kip1 (cell-cycle progression regulator) is also downregulated in parathyroid cancer cells.[35]

The importance of underlying germline mutations in susceptibility genes was recently underscored by the presence of *MEN1*, *CASR*, and *HRPT2/CDC73* gene mutations in about 10% of young patients (<45 years of age) with no family history suggestive of familial hyperparathyroidism.[36] Finding mutations in these genes implies that the parathyroid lesion in this specific subset of patient should be treated with a high index of suspicion.

CLINICAL MANIFESTATIONS AND SCREENING

The majority of patients with parathyroid cancer will be hormonally functional, presenting with symptoms of hypercalcemia, while

TABLE 83.1

Sites of Parathyroid Cancer at Presentation and at Recurrence

Initial Presentation	
Local invasion	40%
Lymph node metastases	15%–30%
Distant metastases	1.8%
Recurrence	
Local	33%–82%
Lymph node	17%–32%
Distant	10%–40%

the benign forms of PHP may be relatively asymptomatic.[15,37] Some of the patients with parathyroid cancer may present already with complications, such as renal (polyuria, renal colic, nephrocalcinosis, nephrolithiasis) and skeletal involvement (bone pain, osteopenia, pathologic fractures). Concomitant renal and bone involvement can be seen in half of the patients and can lead to chronic renal insufficiency. Manifestations of bone disease include osteitis fibrosa cystica, subperiosteal bone resorption, and "salt and pepper" skull.[38,39] Other symptoms seen in patients with hypercalcemia, like nausea, abdominal pain, peptic ulcer, pancreatitis, psychiatric complaints, fatigue and depression, may also be present. The overall symptoms can be exactly the same for benign parathyroid disease, and the challenge for the physician remains to differentiate between hyperparathyroidism due to benign disease versus parathyroid cancer. Less than 10% of parathyroid carcinomas will be hormonally nonfunctional.[40] Calcium is markedly elevated, usually >14 mg/dL, and PTH levels may be >5 to 10 times greater than normal levels.[38,41] Hypercalcemic crisis is not uncommon in parathyroid carcinoma.[29] PHP due to benign parathyroid disease usually will have milder elevation of calcium and PTH levels. It should be noted that very high calcium and PTH levels are seen more often in benign disease due to their relative frequency.

On the physical examination, a neck mass is palpable in >40% of patients, while in benign parathyroid disease this is much less frequent[15] (Table 83.1). Lymph node disease occurs in 15% to 30% of the patients at initial presentation.[42] Most commonly, parathyroid cancer invades the adjacent thyroid lobe, but invasion into the esophagus, trachea, carotid sheath, strap muscles, and mediastinum is not uncommon.[11,43] Parathyroid cancer may also cause local symptoms such as dysphagia, dyspnea, dysphonia, odynophagia, and/or ear pain from local invasion.[39] Recurrent laryngeal nerve paralysis can also be seen, and a preoperative laryngoscopy should be performed in patients with voice change, as a vocal cord paralysis may be present from tumor invasion of the recurrent laryngeal nerve and should be recognized before operative intervention. Common sites of distant metastasis are lung, bone, and liver.

DIAGNOSIS

It is often difficult to diagnose parathyroid cancer prior to surgery as the clinical features are very similar with benign disease. On the other hand, PHP can easily be established with an abnormal level of total calcium and an inappropriate or high level of PTH. As part of the differential diagnosis of PHP, it is important to exclude benign familial hypercalcemic hypocalciuria. This disease will present with hypercalcemia, usually normal PTH levels, and hypocalciuria with calcium to creatinine clearance ration <0.01. Genetic testing is also available for evaluation of CASR mutations.

Making a preoperative diagnosis of parathyroid cancer as the cause of PHP is often difficult. As said before, there is no single laboratory finding that is pathognomonic of parathyroid cancer. Findings of severe hypercalcemia (calcium levels usually >14 mg/dL), extreme elevated levels of PTH (5 to 10 times the upper limit of the normal range), and a palpable neck mass may suggest the diagnosis. About 60% to 65% of patients present with a calcium level >14 mg/dL.[14,39,44] Patients with parathyroid cancer often have elevated alkaline phosphatase and low serum phosphorus levels. Some tests like human chorionic gonadotropin and N-terminal parathyroid hormone can be ordered, but they can also be elevated in benign parathyroid disease.[45–47]

Patients that present with severe hypercalcemia, metabolic complications (like bone and renal), and a neck mass have a higher likelihood of parathyroid cancer. Preoperative imaging may help with tumor localization but cannot reliable distinguish benign and malignant disease. A heterogeneous mass with irregular borders may increase the suspicious of malignancy, but these characteristics are not always present in parathyroid cancers.[48] Fine needle aspiration should be avoided in patients with suspected parathyroid cancer because of the possibility of cutaneous seeding along the needle track.[49]

Parathyroid cancer remains a diagnostic dilemma. There are no definitive histologic diagnostic criteria, and the diagnosis can only be made in a patient who has either locoregional or distant metastasis at the time of initial neck exploration. A patient presenting with severe symptoms, a palpable mass, and metabolic complications has a higher likelihood of having parathyroid cancer, but this is not pathognomonic.[11]

STAGING

At the present time, there is a lack of a TNM (tumor, node, metastases) staging system available for parathyroid cancer. Shaha and Shah[50] have proposed a staging system in the past taking in consideration the size of the tumor, invasion to adjacent tissues, lymph node involvement, and distant metastases (Table 83.2). Talat and Schulte[17] in 2010 suggested an anatomy-based TNM system that showed that patient prognosis could be predicted with their model. They used the same principles established for other endocrine tumors.[17]

TABLE 83.2	
Proposed Staging System	
Proposed Staging System	
T1	Primary tumor <3 cm
T2	Primary tumor >3 cm
T3	Primary tumor of any size with invasion of the surrounding soft tissues (thyroid gland, strap muscles, etc.)
T4	Massive central compartment disease invading trachea and esophagus or recurrence parathyroid cancer
N0	No regional lymph node metastases
N1	Regional lymph node metastases
M0	No evidence of distant metastases
M1	Evidence of distant metastases
Stage	
I	T1N0M0
II	T2N0M0
IIIa	T3N0M0
IIIb	T3N0M0
IIIc	Any T, N1M0
IV	Any T, Any N, M1

MANAGEMENT OF PARATHYROID CANCER

Surgery is the treatment of choice for parathyroid cancer. It is helpful to have a high index of suspicion prior to the surgical procedure to better enable the surgeon to perform the appropriate operation, including a complete resection with microscopically negative margins as this offers the best chance of cure. An en bloc resection of the tumor and the involved structure(s) has been associated with decreased risk of recurrent disease. At the very least, the surgical resection should include en bloc removal of the tumor without compromising the tumor capsule. Systemic chemotherapy, embolization, and radiofrequency ablation have been attempted but in general are not effective in patients with parathyroid cancer.

Hypercalcemia can be very challenging to manage and correction of electrolyte imbalance is paramount to avoid irreversible cardiac and renal complications. Several therapies may be instituted including rehydration, repletion of electrolytes, and loop diuretics after adequate hydration to improve urinary excretion of calcium.[11] Other treatment options include calcitonin and bisphosphonates in an attempt to lower calcium levels. Less common treatment includes amifostine (agent that inhibits PTH release) but use has been limited due to side effect profile.[51] A new drug called cinacalcet (a calcimimetic) is more effective in lowering serum calcium levels and with fewer side effects. This medication is preferred when compared to the older drugs.

Surgical Treatment

As patients are often not assessed for the risk of parathyroid cancer, the initial surgery may not completely address the need for wide resection. If during the resection the adenoma shows suspicious features like a large mass, whitish capsule, and adherence to adjacent structures, an en bloc resection of the tumor and adjacent structures involving the neck, including the ipsilateral thyroid lobe with gross clear margins should be attempted.[18,50,52]

En bloc resection is the modality of choice and is associated with improved outcome.[11] It includes removal of the parathyroid lesion with avoidance of capsular disruption (rupture can cause tumor spread leading to parathyromatosis)[53] and resection of all involved tissues, including the ipsilateral thyroid lobe, trachea, and esophageal wall. Suspicious ipsilateral regional lymph nodes should also be removed. Patients with untreated hypercalcemic crisis should have their surgery delayed until the electrolyte imbalance is corrected. Those with diffuse metastatic disease are less likely to benefit from surgical resection.

Common surgical complications include recurrent laryngeal nerve (RLN) injury, esophageal and tracheal injury, neck hematoma, and infection. If the patient presents with a hoarse voice, invasion of the RLN should be suspected. Preoperative laryngoscopy can confirm vocal cord paralysis. It is appropriate to resect the nerve in symptomatic patients or the ones at high risk of RLN invasion, as the risk of recurrence outweighs the benefit of preserving the nerve.[54]

Patients with poor outcome usually are the ones with incomplete resection, tumor seeding, and a history of recurrence. The finding of positive surgical margins predicts recurrence.[55] Studies have shown that patients with local excision rather than en bloc resection have poor outcomes.[56] For localized recurrent tumors, a cervical and/or mediastinal exploration with wide resection is recommended.[42] Radical surgical procedures will reduce the risk of local recurrence but will not prevent distant metastasis secondary to vascular invasion.

Lymph node metastasis occurs in up to 8% of patients with parathyroid cancer but can be as high as 17% to 32% (see Table 83.1).[38,44,57] If cervical nodes are involved, a modified neck dissection should be performed. Prophylactic neck dissection does not seem to improve survival and has increased morbidity.[58] En bloc resection has an 8% local recurrence rate and long-term overall survival rate of 89%.[18] Usually, parathyroid carcinoma will recur 2 to 5 years after surgery with a local recurrence rate of 33%

to 82% at 5 years.[11] Metastases may occur via lymphatic spread or hematogenously; the most common sites include lung and liver (40% and 10% incidence, respectively).[37,52,59]

Radiotherapy

Usually, parathyroid cancer is radioresistant and radiation treatment as primary therapy has not been shown to have any significant effect either locally or at distant sites. External-beam adjuvant radiotherapy therapy may be considered in high-risk patients or those with positive surgical margins.[60] One study showed that the local recurrence rate is lower with radiation independent of the surgical procedure or stage, in addition to improved disease-free survival. These findings, however, were not statistically significant.[43] Another study showed that patients with aggressive tumors who received radiation postsurgery achieved better locoregional disease control, but all patients had negative margins.[60] Patients with parathyroid cancer have been treated with doses as high as 70 Gy.[42] The efficacy of radiotherapy is difficult to evaluate as the current evidence in the literature is scarce and most of the studies have a small number of patients. In addition, parathyroid cancer is a rare diagnosis. Resection in bloc with negative margins is still the best chance of cure in parathyroid carcinoma, and the use of adjuvant radiotherapy should be decided on an individual basis. Adjuvant radiation therapy does not affect the survival of patients with parathyroid cancer.

Chemotherapy

There is no standard chemotherapy regimen for parathyroid carcinoma, and such treatment usually is ineffective. Most of the experience comes from a limited number of case reports without randomized clinical trials.[13,15,37,39] Regimens used include dacarbazine as monotherapy; a combination of fluorouracil, cyclosphosphamide, and dacarbazine; or a combination of methotrexate, doxorubicin, cyclophosphamide, and lomustine. There is no survival benefit associated with chemotherapy in patients with parathyroid cancer.

Other Treatment Modalities of Parathyroid Cancer

Patients with parathyroid cancer will usually succumb to the complications of severe hypercalcemia. The primary goal in patients with metastatic disease is controlling the PTH-driven hypercalcemia. Some of the drugs that may be used include bisphosphonates, calcitonin, glucocorticoids, mitramycin, plicamycin, and gallium nitrate as well as hemodialysis in addition to generous hydration. These medications help decrease the calcium levels in the short term, but long-term remission rarely is seen.[61] Studies with intravenous pamidronate and zoledronate have shown good calcium response in the short term, but gradually the effect diminishes with subsequent infusions.[61–63] Oral bisphosphonates are not effective.

A new drug called cinacalcet (a calcimimetic) is more effective in lowering serum calcium levels and with less side effects. This drug is preferred when compared to the other drugs. Cinacalcet modulates calcium receptors on the surface of parathyroid cells directly decreasing PTH synthesis and secretion, consequently lowering serum calcium levels. It usually is started at a dose of 30 mg twice daily.[64–67] A study showed that cinacalcet decreased serum calcium by 1 mg/dL in 62% of patients with parathyroid cancer.[66] Patients tolerated total daily doses up to 360 mg. In responders, the magnitude of decrease in calcium levels was greatest in those with the highest baseline calcium levels. Interestingly, decreases in serum calcium have been achieved despite no significant decrease in serum PTH levels.[66]

Other modalities that have been attempted include radiofrequency ablation and transcatheter arterial embolization for diffuse metastatic disease.[68,69] These reports showed improved control in both serum calcium and PTH levels after treatment. Use of ultrasound-guided percutaneous alcohol injection for unresectable disease has also been reported.[70] Another approach is the induction of anti-PTH antibodies by immunization with PTH fragments, with an attempt to shrink tumors and halt the progression of metastases. No clinical trials are available at this time.[71–74] The adjuvant therapies mentioned previously are described in small case series or cases reports, so insufficient information is available to determine the effects of these therapies on long-term survival. These therapeutic options should be decided on a case-by-case basis.

FOLLOW-UP AND NATURAL HISTORY

Patients with parathyroid cancer will require lifelong follow-up. At least half of patients with parathyroid cancer will develop recurrent disease, the neck being the most common site of recurrence (80%).[60] The average time to recurrence is slightly over 33 months.[37] The rate of recurrence is higher when the diagnosis is not initially known and en bloc parathyroidectomy is not performed. Disruption of the parathyroid capsule also leads to higher rates of recurrence.

PTH and calcium monitoring is the best way to follow these patients. If there is biochemical evidence of persistent disease, high-resolution ultrasound of the neck is the best next approach. Whole-body sestamibi scan and other images like computed tomography or magnetic resonance imaging of the chest, neck, and abdomen can be performed for evaluation of metastatic disease. The most common sites of metastasis include lungs, bone, and mediastinum. A study showed that the ultrasound of the neck has a sensitivity of 69% while the sestamibi, computed tomography, and magnetic resonance imaging have 93%, 79%, and 67%, respectively.[54]

Once biochemical recurrence has been confirmed, the next step is to distinguish between local and distant recurrence. Noninvasive localizing studies are used to rule out lung and bone metastasis. If noninvasive studies are nondiagnostic, selective venous sampling for PTH can be performed in an attempt to localize the site of recurrence. If isolated distant metastases are confirmed, resection might be helpful in controlling disease both clinically and biochemically. Local recurrence is usually treated with reoperation and resection of cervical and/or mediastinal disease. This often helps to improve symptoms and calcium levels in up to 75% of the patients.[54] Patients with disseminated disease are less likely to benefit. These patients are usually treated with medical management that includes bisphosphonates and, more recently, cinacalcet.

PROGNOSIS

In a mean follow-up of 6.1 years, Talat and Schulte[17] showed that 35% patients died of disease and 64% experienced recurrence. The relative risk of recurrence is 1.7 in males and 4.3 when there is presence of vascular invasion. In addition, failure to perform an oncologic operation (en bloc resection) carries with it a relative risk of 2.0 for reoperative surgery. Studies have shown that recurrence is detected on average 2 to 4 years after the initial operation, and these patients have a median survival of 5 to 6 years after the initial diagnosis.[37,39,43,44,57] Patients will usually succumb to uncontrolled hypercalcemia and its sequelae. The 10-year survival is quite variable and institution-dependent (Table 83.3). The best survival seems to occur most often in patients presenting with a high index of suspicious for parathyroid carcinoma prior to surgery thus recognizing the need for en bloc resection. Once a patient has recurrent parathyroid cancer, the 5-year survival is <15%. Patients with parathyroid cancer may have long survival but this will typically involve multiple reoperations and a high rate of complications.[42]

TABLE 83.3

Demographics and Clinical Characteristics of Primary Hyperparathyroidism due to Parathyroid Cancer

Article	Gender (M:F)	Age (y) (mean, range)	Size (cm) (mean, range)	Weight (g) (mean, range)	PTH (mean, range)	Calcium (mM) (mean, range)	Lymph Node	Follow-up (mo) (mean, range)	Death
Talat and Schulte[17]	152:169	49 (13–83)	2.9 (0.2–12)	14.1 (0.4–152)	8 (1–71.6)	3.6 (2.2–6.0)	Positive: 27 Negative: 15 Unknown: 287	73 (3–320)	117
Hundahl et al.[16]	146:140	—	—	—	—	—	Positive: 16 Negative: 89 Unknown: 181	—	140
Kebebew et al.[54]	13:5	46 (23–63)	—	—	— (1.6–20)	— (2.4–4.6)	Positive: 2 Negative: — Unknown: 16	97.2 (12–240)	0
Wynne et al.[39]	21:22	54 (29–74)	—	— (0.6–110)	— (1.5–36)	3.6 (2.8–>5.0)	—	— (3–312)	17
Iihara et al.[29]	17:21	— (13–74)	—	— (0.8–67)	— (1.8–33)	— (2.8–5.0)	Positive: 3 Negative: 19 Unknown: 16	119 (18–96)	9
Cordeiro et al.[75]	3:6	51 (21–74)	—	—	— (1–16.5)	— (2.7–4.2)	Positive: 1 Negative: 1 Unknown: 7	3.8 (18–96)	5
Ippolito et al.[76]	4:7	— (25–69)	—	—	—	—	Positive: 0 Negative: 7 Unknown: 40	—	4
Fernandez et al.[14]	19:9	15.3 (23–70)	— (1.7–3.1)	—	—	? (2.7–6.0)	Positive: 3 Negative: 0 Unknown: 25	58	18
Wang and Gaz[77]	14:14	45 (28–72)	3 (1.5–6)	6.7 (1.5–27)	—	3.2 (2.5–5.1)	Positive: 1 Negative: — Unknown: 27	36–264	9
Agarwal et al.[78]	1:3	37 (22–56)	—	—	—	—	—	46.7 (16–108)	2
Lee et al.[12]	112:112	? (23–90)	—	—	—	—	Positive: 9 Negative: — Unknown: 215	— (12–192)	72
Mucci-Hennekinne et al.[79]	7:10	61 (41–74)	—	8.13	— (2.4–44.6)	—	—	84 (3–180)	4

SELECTED REFERENCES

The full reference list can be accessed at lwwhealthlibrary.com/oncology.

2. Fraser WD. Hyperparathyroidism. *Lancet* 2009;374:145–158.
3. Kebebew E, Clark OH. Parathyroid adenoma, hyperplasia, and carcinoma: localization, technical details of primary neck exploration, and treatment of hypercalcemic crisis. *Surg Oncol Clin N Am* 1998;7:721–748.
6. Wermers RA, Khosla S, Atkinson EJ, et al. Incidence of primary hyperparathyroidism in Rochester, Minnesota, 1993–2001: an update on the changing epidemiology of the disease. *J Bone Miner Res* 2006;21:171–177.
10. Wei CH, Harari A. Parathyroid carcinoma: update and guidelines for management. *Curr Treat Options Oncol* 2012;13:11–23.
11. Kebebew E. Parathyroid carcinoma. *Curr Treat Options Oncol* 2001;2:347–354.
12. Lee PK, Jarosek SL, Virnig BA, et al. Trends in the incidence and treatment of parathyroid cancer in the United States. *Cancer* 2007;109:1736–1741.
13. Dudney WC, Bodenner D, Stack BC Jr. Parathyroid carcinoma. *Otolaryngol Clin North Am* 2010;43:441–453, xi.
14. Fernandez-Ranvier GG, Khanafshar E, Jensen K, et al. Parathyroid carcinoma, atypical parathyroid adenoma, or parathyromatosis? *Cancer* 2007;110:255–264.
15. Givi B, Shah JP. Parathyroid carcinoma. *Clin Oncol (R Coll Radiol)* 2010;22:498–507.
16. Hundahl SA, Fleming ID, Fremgen AM, et al. Two hundred eighty-six cases of parathyroid carcinoma treated in the U.S. between 1985–1995: a National Cancer Data Base Report. The American College of Surgeons Commission on Cancer and the American Cancer Society. *Cancer* 1999;86:538–544.
17. Talat N, Schulte KM. Clinical presentation, staging and long-term evolution of parathyroid cancer. *Ann Surg Oncol* 2010;17:2156–2174.
19. Kebebew E. Parathyroid carcinoma, a rare but important disorder for endocrinologists, primary care physicians, and endocrine surgeons. *Thyroid* 2008;18:385–386.
24. Fallah M, Kharazmi E, Sundquist J, et al. Nonendocrine cancers associated with benign and malignant parathyroid tumors. *J Clin Endocrinol Metab* 2011;96:E1108–E1114.
25. Schantz A, Castleman B. Parathyroid carcinoma. A study of 70 cases. *Cancer* 1973;31:600–605.
29. Iihara M, Okamoto T, Suzuki R, et al. Functional parathyroid carcinoma: Long-term treatment outcome and risk factor analysis. *Surgery* 2007;142:936–943; discussion 943.e1.

38. Holmes EC, Morton DL, Ketcham AS. Parathyroid carcinoma: a collective review. *Ann Surg* 1969;169:631–640.
39. Wynne AG, van Heerden J, Carney JA, et al. Parathyroid carcinoma: clinical and pathologic features in 43 patients. *Medicine (Baltimore)* 1992;71:197–205.
40. Wilkins BJ, Lewis JS Jr. Non-functional parathyroid carcinoma: a review of the literature and report of a case requiring extensive surgery. *Head Neck Pathol* 2009;3:140–149.
41. Schaapveld M, Jorna FH, Aben KK, et al. Incidence and prognosis of parathyroid gland carcinoma: a population-based study in The Netherlands estimating the preoperative diagnosis. *Am J Surg* 2011;202:590–597.
42. Harari A, Waring A, Fernandez-Ranvier G, et al. Parathyroid carcinoma: a 43-year outcome and survival analysis. *J Clin Endocrinol Metab* 2011;96:3679–3686.
43. Busaidy NL, Jimenez C, Habra MA, et al. Parathyroid carcinoma: a 22-year experience. *Head Neck* 2004;26:716–726.
44. Obara T, Fujimoto Y. Diagnosis and treatment of patients with parathyroid carcinoma: an update and review. *World J Surg* 1991;15:738–744.
50. Shaha AR, Shah JP. Parathyroid carcinoma: a diagnostic and therapeutic challenge. *Cancer* 1999;86:378–380.
52. Owen RP, Silver CE, Pellitteri PK, et al. Parathyroid carcinoma: a review. *Head Neck* 2011;33:429–436.
54. Kebebew E, Arici C, Duh QY, et al. Localization and reoperation results for persistent and recurrent parathyroid carcinoma. *Arch Surg* 2001;136:878–885.
56. Wiseman SM, Rigual NR, Hicks WL Jr, et al. Parathyroid carcinoma: a multicenter review of clinicopathologic features and treatment outcomes. *Ear Nose Throat J* 2004;83:491–494.
57. Sandelin K, Auer G, Bondeson L, et al. Prognostic factors in parathyroid cancer: a review of 95 cases. *World J Surg* 1992;16:724–731.
58. Vetto JT, Brennan MF, Woodruf J, et al. Parathyroid carcinoma: diagnosis and clinical history. *Surgery* 1993;114:882–892.
59. Witteveen JE, Haak HR, Kievit J, et al. Challenges and pitfalls in the management of parathyroid carcinoma: 17-year follow-up of a case and review of the literature. *Horm Cancer* 2010;1:205–214.
60. Munson ND, Foote RL, Northcutt RC, et al. Parathyroid carcinoma: is there a role for adjuvant radiation therapy? *Cancer* 2003;98:2378–2384.
77. Wang CA, Gaz RD. Natural history of parathyroid carcinoma. Diagnosis, treatment, and results. *Am J Surg* 1985;149:522–527.

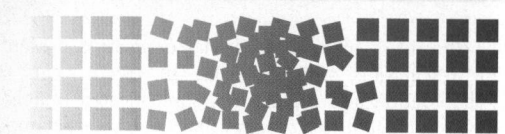

84 Adrenal Tumors

Roy Lirov, Tobias Else, Antonio M. Lerario, and Gary D. Hammer*

INTRODUCTION

The focus of this chapter is the evaluation and management of primary malignant adrenal neoplasia. Other etiologies of adrenal tumors include primary benign neoplasms, which will be discussed briefly, metastatic nonadrenal tumors, and nonneoplastic masses, such as adrenal cysts, tuberculosis, and histoplasmosis.[1-5] Additionally, many disease processes in close proximity may mimic adrenal tumors.[3] Primary benign or malignant neoplasms of the adrenal may derive from the adrenal cortex or medulla. Evaluation and management of adrenal neoplasms depends on clinical suspicion of malignancy and biochemical evidence of autonomous hormone production.[6,7] Although malignancy is extremely rare, a missed opportunity for appropriate management of early-stage cancer can be devastating. Much more common are functional (hormone-producing) benign lesions, which may be symptomatic or indolent, but can still cause morbidity and mortality unless properly addressed. Therefore, the most important primary adrenal neoplasms to consider are functional adrenocortical adenoma (ACA), adrenocortical carcinoma (ACC), and benign or malignant pheochromocytoma. Surgery is the cornerstone of management in most cases, although therapy is often multimodal and highly individualized. Review by a multidisciplinary team of experts is essential because management algorithms are complex and rapidly evolving. Early referral to specialized centers at tertiary care facilities is recommended.

OVERVIEW AND PATHOPHYSIOLOGY OF THE ADRENAL GLAND

The adrenal cortex and medulla are developmentally and physiologically distinct organs. The adrenogonadal primordium begins to form in the third week of intrauterine life, eventually giving rise to the three-layered adrenal cortex and structures of the gonad. As its outer capsule forms during the eighth week, the gland is infiltrated by cells of the neural crest, which migrate to the center of the gland and differentiate into the chromaffin cells of the adrenal medulla. The gland continues to develop during early life and does not reach its mature form until ages 10 to 20 with formation of the zona reticularis.[8] The adrenal medulla is closely related to the paraganglia associated with the autonomic nervous system and found in the head, neck, mediastinum, and retroperitoneum. The paraganglia associated with the sympathetic system are often para-aortic[9]; the largest of these is the organ of Zuckerkandl, located anterior and superior to the aortic bifurcation.[10]

The adrenals are paired glands of the retroperitoneum with a rich blood supply. Their venous drainage is asymmetric: the right gland drains directly into the inferior vena cava while the left drains into the left renal vein.[11,12] Steroidogenic cells of the adrenal cortex produce hormones by incremental modifications to cholesterol catalyzed by a complement of enzymes that are specific to each concentric cortical layer. The outer zona glomerulosa synthesizes the mineralocorticoid aldosterone, the middle zona fasciculata synthesizes the glucocorticoid cortisol, and the inner zona reticularis synthesizes the androgen precursor dehydroepiandrosterone sulfate. The synthetic pathway involves multiple intermediate hormones that can sometimes mimic the activity of mature hormones if produced in sufficient quantity by tumors of the adrenal cortex.[12] Norepinephrine is synthesized in the adrenal medulla and peripheral sympathetic nerves from tyrosine or phenylalanine by way of dopa and dopamine intermediates. The adrenal medulla additionally converts norepinephrine into epinephrine.[13]

ACAs are benign neoplasms of the adrenal cortex. The majority are functionally silent, but these tumors can produce steroid hormones, which in excess may cause typical clinical syndromes.[14] Cortisol-producing ACAs are the usual cause of adrenocorticotropic hormone (ACTH)-independent hypercortisolism.[15] Primary hyperaldosteronism was recently shown to have a prevalence of >10% in unselected patients with newly diagnosed hypertension, and an aldosterone-producing ACA, previously thought to be rare, was identified in almost half of those patients.[16] ACAs rarely produce significant amounts of androgens or estrogens. Hence, the presence of virilization or feminization should alert the clinician to the possibility of ACC.[6,14]

ACC is a malignant neoplasm of the adrenal cortex. Although classically these are thought to be distinct from ACA, recent evidence suggests that a transition from ACA to ACC can occur, albeit such an event is extremely rare.[17-19] ACC may behave aggressively with high rates of invasion, metastasis, and recurrence.[20] Histologically, these tumors can be heterogeneous with atypia, deranged architecture, and chromosomal instability.[9] They may produce an excess of one or several steroid hormones, including intermediates that may produce a mixed clinical picture.[21,22]

Pheochromocytoma (PC) is a tumor of the chromaffin cells of the adrenal medulla. These tumors typically produce a combination of epinephrine, norepinephrine, and rarely dopamine.[23-25] Paraganglioma (PGL) is an extra-adrenal tumor of the autonomic nervous system. Those of sympathetic origin are typically mediastinal or abdominal and can produce norepinephrine, whereas those of parasympathetic origin are found in the head and neck and are functionally silent.[23,26] Occasionally PC or PGL can produce dopamine, a feature that might be associated with malignancy. Although these catecholamines can be released intermittently and degraded rapidly, their metabolites normetanephrine and metanephrine are typically released from PC in a less variable fashion and hence are more reliable in the assessment of medullary neoplasms.[26,27] PGLs are often considered together with PCs (PCPGL) because of their shared neural crest origin, similar histology, pathogenesis, biological behavior, and therapy.[28,29]

*Disclosure Summary:

Gary D. Hammer consults for ISIS, Orphagen, Embara, Atterocor; holds stock in Orphagen, Embara, Atterocor; and is part owner of Atterocor. All other authors do not have disclosures relevant to this publication.

PRACTICE OF ONCOLOGY

MOLECULAR GENETICS OF ADRENAL NEOPLASMS

The rarity of malignant adrenal neoplasms presents challenges for researchers and clinicians. In recent years, international collaboration and increasingly sophisticated biologic techniques have elucidated many genes that appear to be important in the pathogenesis of these diseases.[30–42]

The association of several important genes with adrenocortical neoplasia, both benign and malignant, derives from the study of heritable syndromes. Studies of families with Carney complex, which can include primary pigmented nodular adrenocortical hyperplasia, identified a mutation in *PRKAR1A*, the gene encoding a regulatory subunit of protein kinase A. Although somatic mutations in *PRKAR1A* in cortisol-producing ACAs are rare, other disruptions of the protein kinase A pathway in these tumors are frequent.[43] High-throughput techniques used in the study of aldosterone-producing ACAs led to the discovery of an inactivating mutation in the potassium-channel gene *KCNJ5* (found in up to 40% of samples), as well as mutations in *ATP1A1*, *ATP2B3*, and *CACNA1D*.[44–47] Study of families with syndromes associated with ACC such as Li-Fraumeni syndrome, Beckwith-Wiedemann syndrome, and familial adenomatous polyposis led to recognition of the importance of *TP53*, *IGF2*, and *APC* genes in ACC. Somatic mutations in these genes or their regulatory elements and others are present in many cases of sporadic ACC.[40] Particularly, the very high expression of *IGF2* as well as methylation changes of its locus on 11p15 have emerged as a molecular hallmark separating benign from malignant tumors.[48]

PCs are classically associated with von Hippel-Lindau disease (*VHL*, often bilateral and norepinephrine producing), neurofibromatosis type 1 (*NF1*), and multiple endocrine neoplasia type 2 (*RET*, almost always epinephrine producing).[9,30–38,49] PCs and in particular PGLs clinically define the different hereditary PGL syndromes (PGL1 to 5), in which several germline mutations of the genes encoding the succinate dehydrogenase complex (*SDHA*, *SDHB*, *SDHC*, *SDHD*, *SDHAF2*) have recently been discovered (Table 84.1).[33,34,36,37,39,41] Mutations in the *SDHx* genes lead to slightly different phenotypes in terms of localization, biochemistry, and biologic behavior, with *SDHB* conferring a higher risk of malignancy.[37,50] More recently, exome sequencing has identified new germline mutations in *MAX* and *TMEM127* predisposing to PC (see Table 84.1).[35,38]

INCIDENCE AND EPIDEMIOLOGY

While the overall prevalence of adrenal tumors is estimated to be 3% in those >50 years of age and 6% in those >60 years of age, primary malignancies of the adrenal glands are extremely rare.[14,51,52] When discovered during imaging for reasons other than an evaluation for suspected adrenal diseases or staging for a different primary tumor, adrenal tumors are referred to as adrenal incidentalomas. The vast majority of adrenal incidentalomas are benign, but up to 15% can be functional, autonomously secreting adrenal hormones leading to clinical or subclinical hormone excess, making clinical exam and biochemical evaluation for hormone excess mandatory.[3,6,7,14]

The estimated incidence of ACC is 0.5 to 2 per million per year. It has a slight predilection for women (female:male, 1.5:1) with a relative bimodal age distribution peaking in early childhood and in the fifth decade of life.[3,53,54–56] Although there are no established risk factors for sporadic ACC, smoking and early contraceptive use have been suggested.[57,58] Up to 10% to 15% of all ACCs arise in patients with familial cancer syndromes, such as Li-Fraumeni syndrome, Lynch syndrome, multiple endocrine neoplasia type 1, and less commonly familial adenomatous polyposis, Beckwith-Wiedemann syndrome, or Carney complex.[59,60]

The overall rate of PCPGL in the general population has been estimated at between 0.05% to 0.1%.[61,62] The estimated incidence of malignant PCPGL is 1 to 5 per million per year.[26] Between 3% to 36% of PCPGL are malignant, with higher rates of malignancy in children, those with *SDHB* mutations, and those with extra-adrenal tumors.[26,29,62,63] The average age at presentation is 44 in sporadic cases, compared with 25 for hereditary disease.[62,64,65] Although historically only 10% of PCs were assumed to be associated with a familial syndrome, this is now estimated at 25% to 30%, particularly when also including PGLs.[26,63] The relatively high contribution of hereditary conditions predisposing to all adrenal neoplasms warrants evaluation of every patient by a cancer geneticist and genetic counselor.

TABLE 84.1

Pheochromocytoma/Paraganglioma-Associated Syndromes[41,196–209]

Gene	Syndrome	% Malignant	Clinical Features	Adrenal	Abdominal	Thoracic	Head/Neck
					Localization		
VHL	Von Hippel-Lindau	<5	Clear cell renal carcinoma, CNS/retinal hemangioblastomas, neuroendocrine pancreatic tumors	+++	+	+	+
RET	MEN2	<5	Medullary thyroid carcinoma, primary hyperparathyroidism	++++			
NF1	Neurofibromatosis type 1	<10	Neurofibromas, schwanomas, gliomas, Lisch nodules	++++	+		
SDHB	PGL4	35–70	Renal cell carcinoma, GIST, neuroblastoma	++	+++	++	++
SDHD	PGL1	<5	GIST	+	++++	++	++++
SDHC	PGL3	<5	GIST				++++
SDHA	—	—	GIST	+	++	+	++
SDHAF2	PGL2	—					++++
TMEM127	—	<5		++++	+		+
MAX	—	~10		++++	++		+

CNS, central nervous system; GIST, gastrointestinal stromal tumor.

SCREENING IN SPECIAL POPULATIONS

There are no current screening recommendations for adrenal tumors in the general population. As such, screening should only be considered for patients with a known or suspected familial syndrome that predisposes to adrenal neoplasia. Of all familial syndromes associated with ACC, Li-Fraumeni syndrome has the highest lifetime risk at up to 6.5% to 9.9%.[66,67] Adrenal lesions identified in imaging obtained in patients with any of the other predisposing syndromes should be evaluated carefully for signs of malignancy. All patients diagnosed with PCPGL should undergo evaluation for predisposing familial syndromes caused by mutations in *SDHx*, *VHL*, *NF1*, *TMEM127*, *MAX*, and *RET*. Demonstration of a genetic mutation allows for identification of other affected family members and disease-specific screening and surveillance for adrenal neoplasms and other associated tumors in all gene carriers.[49,68,69]

DIAGNOSIS OF ADRENAL NEOPLASIA

Patients with adrenal neoplasia may seek medical attention because of symptoms related to the size of their mass, hormone excess, or be referred for an incidentally discovered tumor (Fig. 84.1).[64,70] Evaluation should begin with a thorough history and physical exam, including specific questions regarding symptoms of hormone excess, systemic illness, and a careful family history. The classic symptom triad of PC is headache, palpitations,

and diaphoresis, but presentation is highly variable and the complete triad is not observed in all cases.[26,64] Patients with functional cortical neoplasms may present with overt hypercortisolism, hyperaldosteronism, virilization, or rarely feminization. Cortisol is the most commonly produced hormone in both benign and malignant functional cortical neoplasms.[14,15,70] Mild hypercortisolism may be challenging to recognize given the absence of obvious signs.[6,7] Hypertension may be caused by aldosterone-producing ACA, although aldosterone secretion by ACC is rare. Hypertension in ACC is more often related to mineralocortioid effects of cortisol or secreted steroid intermediates.[14,70] Virilization or feminization should increase suspicion for malignancy, as adrenal androgens are the next most common steroid hormone secreted by ACC, and up to half of hormone-producing ACCs produce both cortisol and androgen.[70] Likewise, hypercortisolism of rapid onset should increase concern for ACC.

Basic laboratory evaluation of a patient presenting with an adrenal mass or syndrome of hormone excess includes a complete blood count and comprehensive metabolic panel with liver enzymes. Those presenting with an incidental adrenal mass require comprehensive hormonal evaluation including tests for hypercortisolism, androgen excess, hyperaldosteronism in hypertensive patients, and catecholamine production in all patients.[71,72] The most sensitive test for hypercortisolism is a 1 mg dexamethasone suppression test. Overt hypercortisolism is most often associated with morning (8 a.m.) cortisol levels >5 μg/dL following dexamethasone testing, while a value of <1.8 μg/dL excludes endogenous hypercortisolism.[7] Conversely, spontaneous morning (8 a.m.)

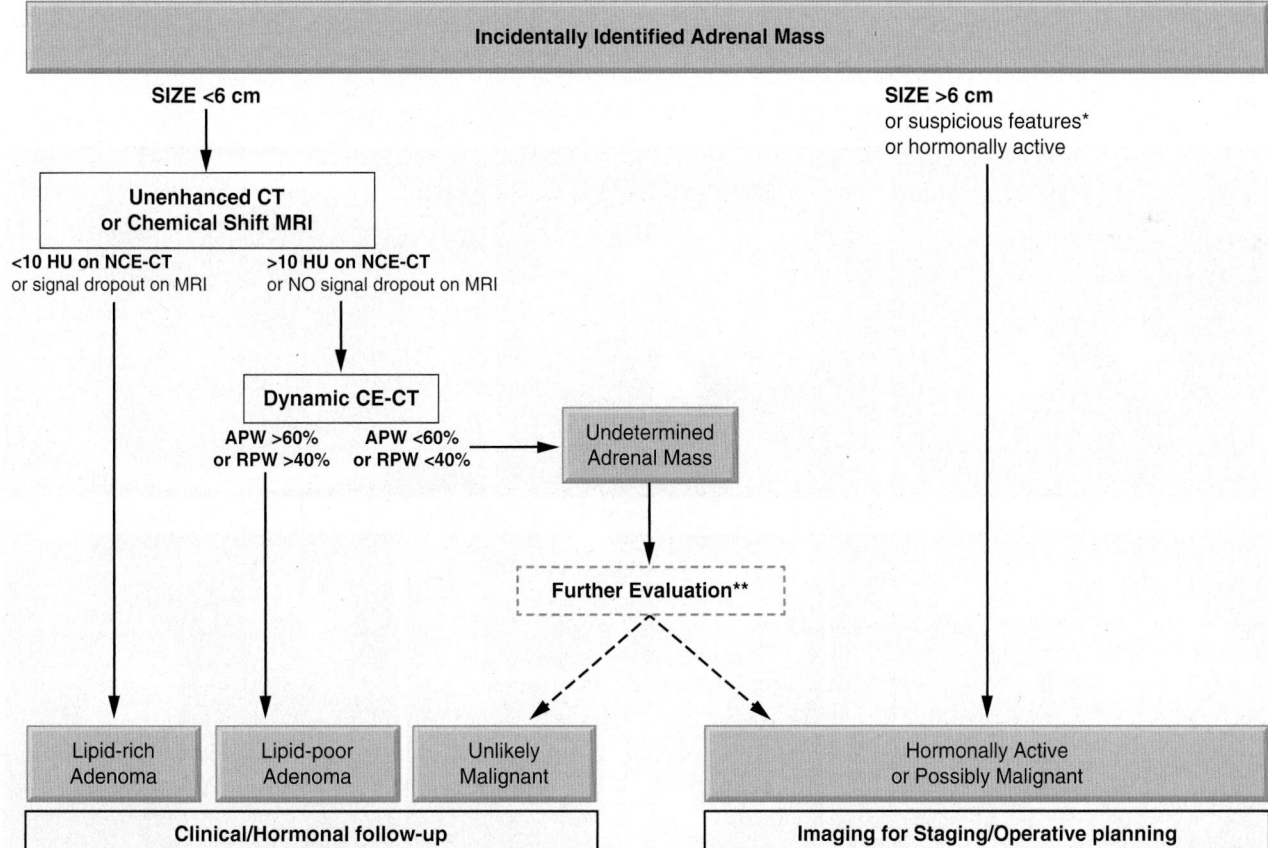

Figure 84.1 Imaging evaluation of an incidentally identified adrenal mass.[6,7,26,62,71,78–88] CT, computed tomography; MRI, magnetic resonance imaging; NCE, non–contrast-enhanced; CE, contrast-enhanced; APW, absolute percentage washout; RPW relative percentage washout.
*Suspicious features include heterogeneity, irregular margins, and calcifications.
**Functional imaging with positron emission tomography/computed tomography or follow-up with magnetic resonance imaging or computed tomography has been described; however, emerging evidence of substantially increased lifetime risk of cancer death related to radiation exposure should be considered when developing a follow-up or surveillance plan.[194,195]

PRACTICE OF ONCOLOGY

ACTH levels of <10 pg/ml will be demonstrated for most cortisol-secreting tumors due to suppression of the hypothalamic-pituitary axis (HPA).[6] Bioavailable or total testosterone and dehydroepiandrosterone sulfate are obtained to evaluate potential androgen excess, the latter produced only in the adrenal gland and therefore helpful in differentiating adrenal from gonadal neoplasia. Hypertensive or hypokalemic patients should have serum aldosterone concentration and plasma renin activity (PRA) measured. Hyperaldosteronism is typically diagnosed with a ratio of serum aldosterone concentration/PRA >20 to 40, provided the absolute level of aldosterone is also elevated, since mineralocorticoid effects of intermediates or volume repletion may also suppress renin.[7] Plasma free metanephrine and normetanephrine are the most sensitive tests for PCPGL.[73] Positive screening hormonal evaluation dictates additional confirmatory hormonal studies, which may include 24-hour urine free cortisol to measure the extent of hypercortisolism,[6] serum aldosterone levels following saline-infusion or 24-hour urine aldosterone under salt loading conditions, or measurement of additional steroid hormones such as progesterone, androstenedione, estradiol, 17-hydroxyprogesterone, or 17-hydroxypregnenolone for further characterization.[6,7,72] The initial steroid profile can be useful for surveillance in ACC.[21,72] For PCPGL, chromogranin A should be obtained, as it can be followed in surveillance.[26,74–76] (Fig. 84.2) with computed tomography (CT) or magnetic resonance imaging (MRI) is important for establishing the extent of disease and identifying features concerning for malignant cortical lesions. Benign cortical lesions tend to be small, fat-containing, and homogeneous, with smooth borders. Conversely, large, heterogeneous lesions with irregular margins and calcifications are strongly suggestive of ACC. The risk of ACC increases with size, and is estimated at <2% for lesions <4 cm, 2%

to 6% for lesions 4 to 6 cm, and 25% for lesions >6 cm. Lesions with enhancement of <10 Hounsfield units (HU) are indicative of lipid-rich ACA, although up to 30% of ACAs may be lipid-poor with intermediate enhancement between 10 and 30 HU.[6,7,62,77] Lipid-containing lesions may also be identified on MRI by signal dropout on opposed-phase sequences. PCPGL are often bright as cerebrospinal fluid on T2-weighted MRI, but can be variable in appearance. They tend to be homogeneous when smaller and heterogeneous when larger with features overlapping lipid-poor ACAs, but no imaging features predict malignancy.[7,26,62]

Suspicious tumors or those with indeterminate characteristics require additional imaging to further characterize the lesion in question and to evaluate for metastatic disease.[78] If the initial CT was non–contrast enhanced or optimized for another purpose, a dedicated adrenal-protocol CT with thin slices, oral contrast, and careful timing of intravenous contrast should be obtained for lesions that are homogeneous on the initial scan.[62] Absolute percentage enhancement washout above a threshold of 60% (or relative washout above 40%) at 15 minutes has high sensitivity and specificity for lipid-poor ACA (Fig. 84.3).[79–82] Compared with CT, contrast-enhanced MRI is more sensitive for vascular invasion and is occasionally obtained as a complementary study in patients with larger tumors.[71] Contrast-enhanced CT of the chest, abdomen, and pelvis is appropriate to evaluate for metastases and hence complete staging.[71] Imaging of the head should only be obtained if neurologic symptoms are present, and bone scintigraphy can be obtained for those presenting with skeletal pain. Neither test is required in the initial evaluation of the asymptomatic patient.

Functional imaging can be useful in evaluating both cortical and medullary tumors of the adrenal gland. Deoxy-2[18F]fluoro-d-glucose positron emission tomography (18FDG-PET) (Fig. 84.2F) is a useful, complementary modality that can sometimes alter

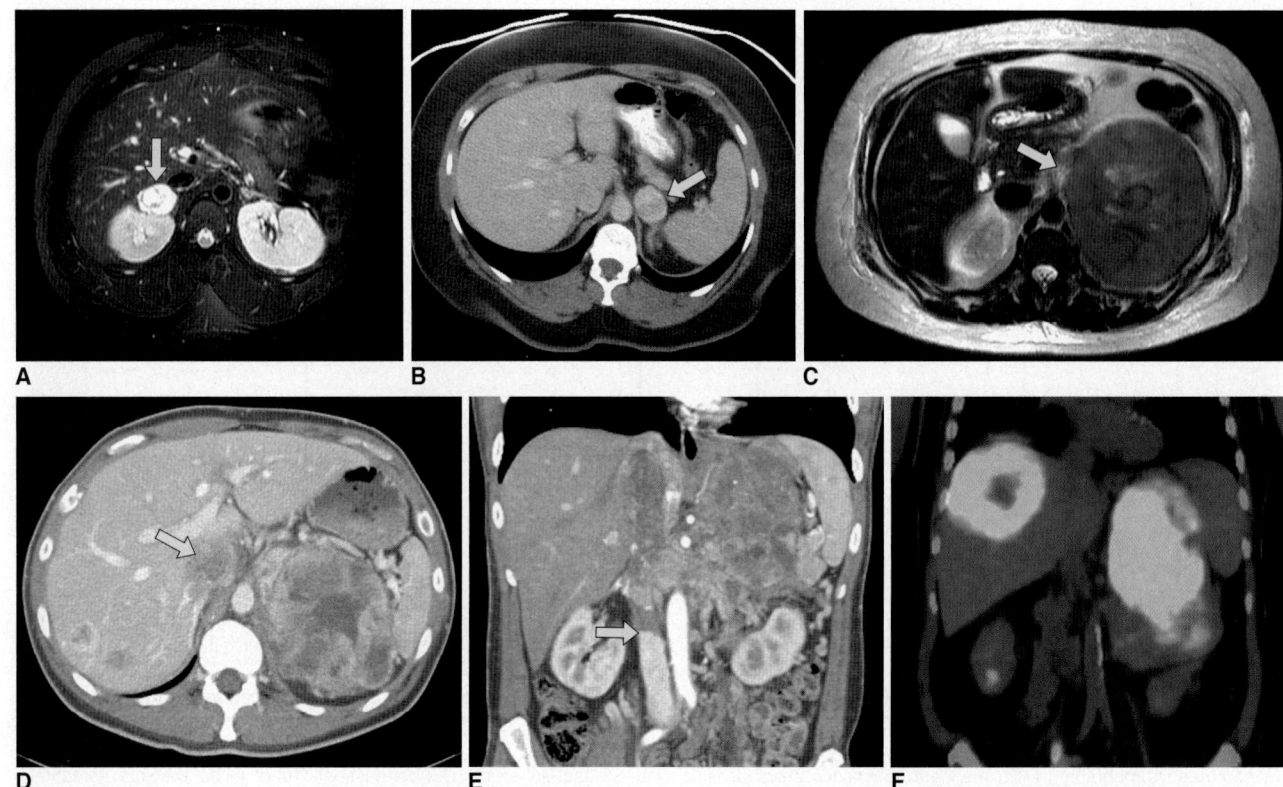

Figure 84.2 **(A)** T2-weighted magnetic resonance imaging demonstrating pheochromocytoma (*arrow*). **(B)** Computed tomography of heterogeneous-appearing small left adrenocortical carcinoma (ACC) (*arrow*). **(C)** Large left ACC on T1-weighted magnetic resonance imaging (*arrow*). **(D, E)** Computed tomography demonstrating large, heterogeneous left ACC with contrast demarcation of caval thrombus (*arrows*). **(F)** Coronal section of positron emission tomography/computed tomography demonstrating high uptake in a patient with ACC locoregional recurrence in left adrenal fossa and dome of liver.

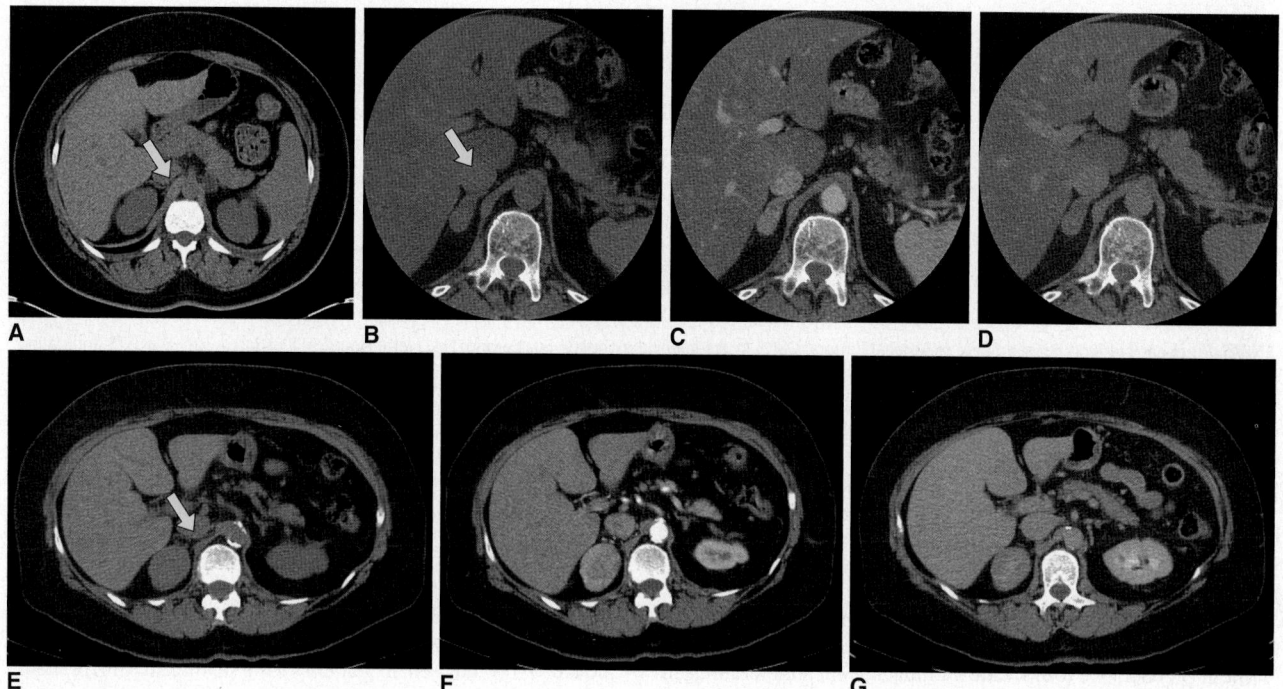

Figure 84.3 **(A)** Non–contrast-enhanced computed tomography of lipid-rich adrenocortical adenoma (2 HU, *arrow*). **(B–D)** Dynamic contrast-enhanced computed tomography of lipid-poor adrenocortical adenoma demonstrating density of 27 HU without contrast **(B**, *arrow*), 79 Hu at 1 minute **(C)**, and 40 HU at 15 minutes **(D)**. After infusion of intravenous contrast (absolute percentage washout = 75%, relative percentage washout = 49%).[82] **(E–G)** Contrast-enhanced computed tomography of suspicious lesion showing heterogeneity and density of 45 HU without contrast **(E)**, followed by 70 to 100 HU at 1 minute **(F)** and 60 to 90 HU at 15 minutes **(G)**. Absolute percentage washout ≈ 18%.

management of an indeterminate lesion (i.e., one that is unable to be characterized with a high degree of certainty as benign or malignant). However, no validated quantitative criteria exist for reliably predicting whether a lesion that is indeterminate by anatomic imaging in a patient without a known primary cancer will be benign or malignant.[78,83–88] Furthermore, metastatic disease from nonadrenal primary, PC (benign or malignant), and up to 10% of ACA can be positive on [18]FDG-PET scan.[79,89–93] ^{123}I-metaiodobenzylguanidine (^{123}I-MIBG) scans have high positive-predictive value for PCPGL and can be used for the identification of additional foci of disease, including multicentric tumors or metastasis, especially in patients with inherited syndromes.[26,94] However, the use of ^{123}I-MIBG for diagnostic purposes is of rather limited utility as the diagnosis of PCPGL is often made through simple biochemistry and cross-sectional imaging. Moreover, for PGL of the head and neck ^{111}In-pentetreotide scintigraphy has better sensitivity.[95] It is worth mentioning that functional imaging will rarely discover any tumor that is not evident on cross-sectional imaging. In such cases where biochemical testing suggests PCPGL but imaging is negative, there are often other causes for clinical symptoms and/or elevated metanephrines (e.g., use of tricyclic antidepressants, congestive heart failure).

Percutaneous biopsy of adrenal tumors is almost never indicated because cytology is unhelpful in characterizing adrenal neoplasia, and biopsy has significant risk of complications including hemorrhage and pneumothorax.[6,7,96–98] Careful consideration should be given to how the test will influence management and whether alternative approaches, such as PET/CT, can suffice, as most single adrenal masses can be diagnosed by imaging and endocrine evaluation.[71,89] Only in the setting of a patient with a nonadrenal primary cancer should an adrenal biopsy be considered if it remains unclear whether the adrenal mass is a primary adrenal tumor versus a metastasis of the nonadrenal primary tumor. PCPGL should always be excluded prior to an attempted biopsy due to the high morbidity and mortality of biopsy-associated catecholamine surges.[97,98]

GRADING AND STAGING OF MALIGNANCY

Establishing malignancy of adrenal neoplasms can be challenging. Histopathologic criteria established by Weiss predict malignancy in adrenocortical neoplasms when three or more of nine criteria are present.[71,99] Mitotic rate is a particularly important criterion and indicates malignancy when greater than five mitoses are observed in 50 high-powered fields. Mitotic activity >20/50 high-powered fields defines a high-grade ACC.[71,100,101] Several staging systems have been proposed for ACC, but the European Network for the Study of Adrenal Tumors staging system (Table 84.2) has become widely adopted as it best reflects outcome.[102–105]

Differentiation between benign and malignant PCPGL is a challenging clinical problem as well. Indeed, because even extensive invasion does not accurately predict malignancy, the only criterion adopted by the World Health Organization for defining malignant PCPGL is metastasis.[73] No single histologic criterion predicts malignant PCPGL. The Pheochromocytoma of the Adrenal Gland Scaled Score system has been proposed for assessing malignant potential by using 12 histopathologic criteria,[106] but validation studies have produced conflicting results.[107–109] At present, there is no staging system for PCPGL. Tumors are categorized as local, regional, or metastatic.[62]

IMPORTANT CONSIDERATIONS IN PERIOPERATIVE MANAGEMENT OF ADRENAL TUMORS

Patients with adrenal neoplasms present unique perioperative challenges. In addition to hemodynamic and metabolic instability due to intraoperative catecholamine fluctuation, patients with PCPGL may have established cardiovascular sequelae related to chronic catecholamine excess.[110] Those with cortisol-secreting tumors are at higher risk for infectious, metabolic, and wound-healing complications,

TABLE 84.2

Staging for Adrenocortical Carcinoma and Five-Year Cause-Specific Mortality

Stage	ENSAT 2008[74]	Five-Year CSM (Eu)[103]	Five-Year CSM (NA)[104]
Stage I	T1N0M0	82%	74%
Stage II	T2N0M0	61%	64%
Stage III	T1-2,N1,M0	50%	44%
	T3-4,N0-1,M0		
Stage IV	T1-4,N0-1,M1	13%	6.9%

ENSAT, European Network for the Study of Adrenal Tumors; CSM, cause-specific mortality; Eu, Europe; NA, North America; T1 ≤5 cm; T2 >5 cm; T3, infiltrating surrounding tissue; T4, invading organs, tumor thrombus in renal vein or vena cava; N0, no positive lymph nodes; N1, positive lymph node(s); M1, distant metastasis.[103]

and will require careful glucocorticoid replacement following complete surgical resection due to suppression of the HPA.[70]

Historically, perioperative mortality related to resection of PCPGL was as high as 45%. The introduction of α-blockade and volume repletion has reduced mortality to 0% to 3% in contemporary series.[69,111] It is important to recognize that even patients with asymptomatic PCPGL are at risk for cardiovascular complications without preoperative α-blockade and that significant elevations in blood pressure may still occur intraoperatively despite adequate α-blockade.[29,112] Either selective or nonselective α antagonists can be used to establish α-blockade. Selective α_1-blockade has been used to avoid some undesirable α_2-mediated side effects including reflex tachycardia, hypoglycemia, and somnolence, but these agents are less well studied compared with nonselective agents. Traditionally, phenoxybenzamine is the preferred nonselective α-blocker for PCPGL. Dosage can be titrated on an outpatient basis for adequate blockade, which often takes 2 weeks or longer. During this time, salt- and fluid-loading are recommended for volume optimization to minimize postoperative hypotension.[69] Other α-blocking agents can serve as an alternative to phenoxybenzamine and are preferred by some institutions.[113] Initiation of a β-blocker for reflex tachycardia may be considered, but not before α-blockade is established. Data regarding the use of calcium channel blockers and angiotensin-converting enzyme inhibitors preoperatively in patients with PC are limited.[114–116] It is important to recognize that α-adrenergic vasopressors may not be helpful in treating hypotension resulting from α-blockade and that volume expansion should be the treatment of choice.[69]

Resection of cortisol-producing tumors may present unique perioperative challenges as well. Aggressive preoperative control of hypercortisolism is advocated but should not delay surgery.[70] Postoperative adrenal insufficiency should be anticipated in all patients with preoperative hypercortisolism and replacement should be initiated preemptively postoperatively, with surveillance of the HPA and treatment adjustment as necessary. Recovery of the HPA might take up to 6 to 24 months, and additional steroid replacement during times of stress to prevent Addisonian crisis is necessary.[71,117,118]

MANAGEMENT OF BENIGN-APPEARING ADRENOCORTICAL TUMORS AND PHEOCHROMOCYTOMA

Before pursuing surgical management, an assessment of the likelihood of malignancy based on size, imaging, and clinical presentation must be made.[119] The surgeon should strictly adhere to oncologic principles when resecting tumors not meeting criteria for being benign.[70]

Although its role in potentially malignant lesions is controversial, minimally invasive adrenalectomy has lower morbidity, decreased pain, and shorter hospital stay, and is the procedure of choice for benign-appearing adrenocortical tumors or PCPGL if technically feasible.[120–122] Minimally invasive approaches for adrenalectomy may be performed laparoscopically by an anterior abdominal approach or by a posterior retroperitoneal approach.[120,123] The posterior retroperitoneal approach is advantageous in patients with prior abdominal operations because the potential need for adhesiolysis is obviated; however, the posterior retroperitoneal approach is not advised in patients with significant subcutaneous or perinephric fat, unfavorable anatomy, or tumors >8 cm.[124,125] Partial (i.e., cortical-sparing) adrenalectomy is the preferred approach for patients with familial bilateral benign diseases, such as bilateral PCPGL in patients with von Hippel-Lindau disease or multiple endocrine neoplasia type 2.[29,126,127]

SURVEILLANCE AFTER RESECTION OF PHEOCHROMOCYTOMA

There are no standard recommendations for surveillance for malignant PCPGL after resection of apparently benign disease. However, most endocrine neoplasia groups suggest that all patients receive some form of long-term follow-up.[29,69] Surveillance strategies must be individualized and may depend on overall impression of risk for malignancy (e.g., *SDHB*), operative findings, and genetic predisposition to additional primary tumors.[128] Initially, all patients should undergo surveillance reevaluation with history, physical exam, laboratories, and imaging. Postoperative biochemical testing at 2 to 6 weeks and 6 months is appropriate, and chromogranin A may be useful if elevated preoperatively.[29,69,94] The preferred imaging modality for surveillance is CT or MRI of the site of the initial tumor, as local recurrence is the most common form of relapse. Particularly in patients with hereditary syndromes, MRI should be preferred as the number of scans might otherwise lead to excessive radiation doses.[94]

MANAGEMENT OF RECURRENT OR METASTATIC MALIGNANT PHEOCHROMOCYTOMA

Diagnosis of malignant PCPGL is made based on recurrence or identification of metastasis on initial presentation.[129] In a retrospective review of 176 patients with PCPGL initially presenting without evidence of malignancy, up to 17% of patients developed recurrence at either the primary site or another location. Recurrences were malignant in half of all cases and more commonly occurred in patients with familial syndromes or larger tumors.[130] The most common sites of metastasis of PCPGL are to bones, lungs, liver, and lymph nodes.[69,94] Five-year survival is 34% to 60%, although this is dependent on location of metastasis, as those with lung and liver lesions have shorter survival compared with those who have osseous metastasis only.[29]

Treatment options for malignant PCPGL are limited and the goal of therapy is palliative, with a focus on controlling catecholamine secretion, pain, and tumor burden.[72,131,132] Options include supportive medications, modalities for locoregional control, external-beam radiation, radiopharmaceuticals, and chemotherapy. Quality of life must be considered because in some cases observation and supportive medication alone is the best option.[72,131] Debulking and metastasectomy can be considered in patients who have significant resectable tumor burden in the context of slowly progressive disease.[26,72,131,132] Radiofrequency ablation (RFA) and transarterial chemoemoblization (TACE) have been described for unresectable metastases. Similar to any surgery, these procedures require sufficient preparative α-blockade.[26] External-beam radiation has been particularly useful in treating osseous metastases but can provoke hypertensive crises.[26] In patients with disease not amenable to surgery but with acceptable overall clinical status, ^{131}I-MIBG can be used for locoregional control, provided ^{123}I-MIBG imaging demonstrates good avidity.[26,131,132]

In patients with symptomatic unresectable disease for which other modalities have failed or are not indicated, cytotoxic chemotherapy can be considered.[26,132] Cyclophosphamide-dacarabzine–based regimens are the most thoroughly evaluated.[72] Three nonrandomized studies have shown radiographic and symptomatic responses in 40% to 50% of patients treated with these regimens, and 22-year follow-up of one nonrandomized prospective study published similar results with cyclophosphamide, vincristine, and dacarbazine.[131] After therapy is discontinued, however, refractory disease tends to recur.[26] Cytotoxic chemotherapy has also been used in borderline resectable cases, with sufficient response allowing patients to proceed with surgery.[72] During treatment surveillance, imaging with CT, MRI, and bone scan as indicated every 3 months to evaluate response is recommended.[131]

MANAGEMENT OF LOCAL AND LOCOREGIONALLY ADVANCED ADRENOCORTICAL CARCINOMA

Surgery is the cornerstone of management for ACC in stages I to III and should always follow the principles of an oncologic resection, which requires careful preoperative planning with an appreciation for the rapid growth potential of aggressive ACCs.[70,71,133] Preoperative imaging can underestimate tumor size by as much as 40%, and relationships to surrounding structures are subject to change during the interval between imaging and operation.[70,133] The surgeon should be prepared for concomitant resection of liver, kidney, spleen, pancreas, stomach, colon, diaphragm, or vena cava, as suggested by imaging. Although there is no evidence that prophylactic nephrectomy of an uninvolved ipsilateral kidney improves survival, threshold for en bloc resection should be low, and nephrectomy is indicated for involvement of renal capsule or vein.[71,72] The celiac axis and root of the superior mesenteric artery may be partially encased by tumor, which may be a contraindication to surgery if resection and reconstruction is not feasible.[133]

Locally advanced tumors of questionable resectability or behavior can be considered for systemic preoperative therapy with close monitoring. Patients with rapidly progressive disease may not derive sufficient benefit to justify a large resection, whereas tumors that respond to therapy may subsequently be deemed resectable.[72,133]

Adrenalectomy is traditionally performed through a midline or subcostal incision, depending on preoperative assessment of need for multivisceral resection.[70] A thoracoabdominal incision may provide better exposure for diaphragmatic resection and repair or in those with prior abdominal surgery.[133,134] Access to the retrohepatic inferior vena cava is necessary if it is infiltrated by tumor directly or harbors tumor thrombus requiring venotomy or resection.[133] On rare occasions, median sternotomy and cardiopulmonary bypass are necessary for extracting tumor thrombus extending into the right atrium.[135]

The role of locoregional lymphadenectomy is not established, but one study suggests improvements in staging and possibly survival.[9,72,136] Lymph node metastasis is not uncommon in ACC, and en bloc lymphadenectomy, when feasible, to clear nodes of the celiac axis, superior mesenteric artery, and renal hilum has been advocated.[70,137]

Consideration of laparoscopy for resection of potentially malignant low-stage ACC <8 cm is advocated by some, provided an R0 resection can be achieved and the operation is conducted by an expert surgeon.[72] This issue is highly controversial, and failure to achieve an R0 resection can rarely be overcome by additional operations or adjuvant treatments.[70,72,133] Independent of approach, strict adherence to oncologic principles is necessary for optimal outcome, including a complete and systematic evaluation of the entire peritoneal cavity, full mobilization of overlying uninvolved organs, and en bloc resection including the entire retroperitoneal fat pad surrounding the tumor without directly manipulating the tumor to prevent rupture of the fragile capsule and consequential peritoneal seeding.[70,71,133,138] Surgical specimens should be submitted to pathology carefully marked and intact, and clips should be placed in the tumor bed for targeting of adjuvant radiotherapy if necessary.[70]

Patients undergoing adrenalectomy at high-volume centers have better oncologic outcome; therefore, referral to an experienced facility is advised.[20,70,102,139]

SURVEILLANCE AND ADJUVANT THERAPY FOR ADRENOCORTICAL CARCINOMA

Recommendations for surveillance and adjuvant therapy depend on behavior and appearance of the tumor, stage at presentation, and operative findings. Pathologic findings should be carefully reviewed as it has been reported that 25% of patients diagnosed with stage III disease by pathologic evaluation after resection were thought pre- and intraoperatively to have a lower-stage tumor.[133]

Data from the National Cancer Database show that 19% of patients undergoing surgery do not receive an R0 resection.[137] In patients who remain good operative candidates, repeat resection by an expert surgeon should be considered, especially after an R2 resection.[140] Those who are not candidates for reoperation can be considered for radiotherapy.[71]

In those who do undergo R0 resection, rates of local recurrence remain high at 19% to 34%, with the overwhelming majority of recurrences occurring in the first 5 years.[20,70,141] Close surveillance is mandatory, and a complete evaluation every 3 months for 2 to 3 years has been advocated. Subsequently, this can be reduced to biannually until 5 years and annually thereafter. Evaluation in this setting should include a history and physical exam, a complete blood count and metabolic profile, including liver enzymes, as well as steroid profile, and cross-sectional imaging of the chest, abdomen, and pelvis.[71,72] Steroid profiles should be carefully evaluated as recurrence of preoperative patterns of elevation raise concern for recurrence.[21] Additional laboratories are necessary for monitoring mitotane therapy in patients receiving this treatment.[142] [18]FDG-PET scan is not a standard modality for surveillance but is useful in characterizing newly discovered lesions on surveillance imaging as ACCs are almost invariably PET-positive.[71,72,88]

Evidence-based guidelines for adjuvant therapy after completely resected disease are lacking. Radiotherapy has historically been avoided because of a pervasive impression that ACC is radioresistant.[70] Although there is no convincing evidence corroborating this notion, <10% of patients with ACC receive radiotherapy.[20] Modern series have reported conflicting results on adjuvant radiotherapy, raising the possibility that radiotherapy may be a useful modality.[143–145] In general, radiotherapy has been shown to provide good local control and decrease the risk of local recurrence following primary resection, but its effect on survival parameters is not well researched. Current expert consensus opinion and practice guidelines recommend radiotherapy in the adjuvant setting, especially in those who have previously undergone R1 or R2 resection.[71,72,146]

Similarly, there are conflicting data regarding the benefits of mitotane as adjuvant therapy, with an ongoing prospective, randomized clinical trial designed to address this issue (ADIUVO trial). In patients undergoing R0 resection, immunohistochemistry for Ki67 can be used to inform decision making. A large retrospective study showed significant improvement in median tumor-free survival with adjuvant mitotane therapy in patients with Ki67 >10%, and therefore mitotane therapy should be offered to all of these patients.[72,147–150] Although there is no robust evidence for the use of combination radiotherapy and mitotane as adjuvant treatment, this should be considered in patients with stage III disease or those who have undergone repeated resection. Mitotane is routinely started within 3 months of resection and continued for at least 2 years in lower-risk patients, and if tolerated up to 5 years or longer, especially for higher-risk patients. Mitotane requires careful monitoring as the therapeutic window is tight and complications may be dose limiting.[70–72,142,150]

MANAGEMENT OF LOCOREGIONAL RECURRENCE OF ADRENOCORTICAL CARCINOMA

Failure of primary treatment may manifest as locoregional recurrence detected during surveillance. The extent and timing of recurrence, as well as the histologic appearance of the tumor from surgical specimens, are important predictors for survival.[70,71,101,105,151] Repeat resection is not a curative modality but may prolong survival and should be considered in patients with excellent performance status who have recurrence confined to a minimal number of sites and can undergo resection of all remaining tumor.[71,101,151,152] Other situations in which repeat resection can be considered include patients with long disease-free intervals and low-grade appearance, as patients with high-grade tumors or rapidly progressive disease may benefit less than those with more indolent disease. For questionably resectable lesions, systemic therapy including mitotane followed by repeated evaluation after 3 months can be considered. Although complete remission is rare, up to 30% of patients show stable disease or partial remission with mitotane therapy.[70,71,133,141] In situations where local recurrence is symptomatic and not amenable to surgical management, definitive radiotherapy can be considered. In patients with asymptomatic recurrence, this modality is controversial.[70–72]

MANAGEMENT OF ISOLATED METASTASES OF ADRENOCORTICAL CARCINOMA

All therapy for metastatic ACC is palliative, and appropriate counseling of patients regarding expectations of additional therapies is paramount.[70] When recurrence presents as an isolated metastasis, surgery can be considered in highly selected patients when complete resection is possible without undue morbidity.[71,72] Metastasectomy has shown promise particularly with limited pulmonary disease, and can be repeated in selected patients when technically feasible.[153–155] In other circumstances, additional palliative modalities are available, including RFA, TACE, and external-beam radiation.[70–72] Radiotherapy has been particularly useful in treating osseous metastasis and has also been utilized in treating metastases to the brain and other locations. Although there are no robust clinical trial data available to support the use of RFA or TACE, these options can be used in combination with surgery

for isolated metastases that are difficult to access or for situations when surgery is not indicated or desired. RFA has demonstrated success in liver metastasis and has also shown promise in other locations, with better outcomes in lesions <5 cm that are not near large blood vessels to avoid a heat-sink effect, which can inhibit efficacy.[71,156–158] TACE, which involves selective embolization and intratumoral infusion of high concentrations of cytotoxic chemotherapy, is used often to treat isolated metastases with few reported complications, although published experience is limited and treatment of primary tumors has been reported to cause hemorrhage.[159–161] More information regarding both modalities is needed before definitive recommendations can be made.

MANAGEMENT OF METASTATIC OR UNRESECTABLE ADRENOCORTICAL CARCINOMA

Goals of palliative care for metastatic ACC are control of pain, symptoms of hormone excess, side effects of treatments, and prevention of fractures.[70] Patients presenting with widespread metastasis in multiple organs or unresectable deposits in a single organ system do not typically undergo surgery and all therapy is palliative. Debulking for control of symptomatic hormone excess can be performed in patients with excellent functional status but is not expected to provide a durable response and may not be advisable in situations where only limited debulking is feasible (e.g., patients with rapidly growing tumors or expected debulked load of <80% to 90%).[70,71] Furthermore, steroidogenic inhibitors are replacing surgical debulking as a growing means of lowering steroid levels (see the following).[162–164]

The mainstay of therapy for widely metastatic disease is cytotoxic chemotherapy.[70] Initial studies of single agents led to most common contemporary regimens. In the past few decades, the two most promising cytotoxic chemotherapeutic regimens used in combination with mitotane have been etoposide, doxorubicin, and cisplatin, or streptozotocin.[165–171] Recently, these regimens (etoposide, doxorubicin, and cisplatin with mitotane, and streptocotozin with mitotane, respectively) were compared in a randomized controlled trial (FIRM-ACT) that demonstrated a modest but significant increase in progression-free survival of 5 months in the etoposide, doxorubicin, and cisplatin with mitotane compared with 2 months in the streptocotozin with mitotane group. Although significant comparative improvements were demonstrated, objective response and median duration of survival remained dismal.[172]

Although cytotoxic chemotherapy is often administered concurrently with mitotane, the latter causes CYP3A4 induction with attendant catabolism of many drugs. This has led some to question whether mitotane therapy has confounded earlier studies of chemotherapeutics (as well as recent trials of targeted therapy), but prospective studies of regimens with and without mitotane are heterogeneous and have not convincingly resolved this issue.[70]

Patients suffering from metastatic ACC experience debilitating hormonal symptoms, necessitating effective control. The adrenolytic and steroidogenic inhibitory effects of mitotane are often successful in mitigating these symptoms in patients who have achieved therapeutic levels. In others, however, steroidogenic inhibitors such as ketoconazole or metyrapone are commonly required.[142] Typically, 24-hour urine cortisol is used to guide therapy, but titration is challenging because cortisol levels are often unreliable in this setting. Furthermore, patients undergoing systemic therapy or treatment with inhibitors of steroidogenesis may require supplementary glucocorticoid treatment during times of stress. Alternatively, hypercortisolism can be controlled by using mifepristone, a direct glucocorticoid receptor antagonist. However, under mifepristone therapy, cortisol and ACTH levels rise and cannot be used to guide therapy; therefore, doses are usually titrated clinically. Patients with mineralocorticoid excess can be treated with spironolactone, which may also benefit females with virilizing symptoms due to its antiandrogenic effect. Males suffering from feminization may benefit from aromatase inhibitors or estrogen receptor antagonists.[70]

EMERGING DIAGNOSTIC TECHNIQUES AND TREATMENT STRATEGIES FOR ADRENAL TUMORS

Ongoing effort in basic science, translational, and clinical research is expected to yield improved diagnostic tools and therapies. Rigorous evaluation of currently available therapeutics is necessary to identify optimal treatment regimens. With regard to surgical management, this includes addressing the controversy surrounding operative approach (open versus laparoscopic) for presumed low-grade ACC, necessity for lymphadenectomy, and utility of debulking procedures. The role of radiotherapy both in the adjuvant setting and for unresectable disease needs further clarification.[173] Novel strategies for optimal delivery of radionuclide treatment including non–carrier-added techniques, new ligands, sensitizing agents, and combination delivery are undergoing evaluation.[70,131,138,139,174] Many questions regarding mitotane treatment remain, including its utility in the adjuvant setting for low-intermediate–risk disease (ADIUVO trial) and implications of its profound, lasting induction of CYP3A4 on concomitantly delivered therapeutics. Although early trials of targeted therapeutics in both PCPGL and ACC have not been promising, further study has resulted in increased appreciation for the complexity of the pathways involved and offered some explanations for past failures. Additional innovations are also necessary in diagnostic techniques to address the challenge of accurately predicting malignant potential of adrenal neoplasms. A variety of promising molecular imaging agents need to be rigorously evaluated.[175] Urine steroid profiling is an intriguing tool that may be useful in diagnosis and surveillance but requires validation.[21,78,107,173] Upcoming genome-wide expression studies and international collaboration may suggest additional biomarkers for diagnosis and surveillance or potential therapeutic targets.

SPECIAL CONSIDERATIONS IN PREGNANCY

Adrenal neoplasms considered in this chapter (PCPGL, ACA, ACC) have all been described in pregnancy, albeit rarely, and management is often complex.[176] Many typical physiologic changes or common complications of pregnancy can mask signs and symptoms of an underlying adrenal neoplasm, resulting in the potential for mortality as high as 29% without an antenatal diagnosis.[176] The preferred imaging study is MRI, because radioisotope studies, CT scans, and gadolinium are contraindicated in pregnancy.[176,177] Biochemical diagnosis of PCPGL is established as for nonpregnant patients, and α-blockade is essential to prevent hypertensive crises. Adrenalectomy for patients diagnosed with PCPGL within the first two trimesters is advocated.[177] When diagnosed in the third trimester, caesarean section is recommended, with adrenalectomy immediately after, or at a later date.[176,177]

Similarly, diagnosis of adrenocortical tumors may be more challenging due to significant physiologic elevations in adrenocortical steroid hormones with pregnancy.[178] Furthermore, in the case of hypercortisolism, symptoms such as weight gain, striae, and fatigue may similarly be misattributed to normal pregnancy. Although hypercortisolism in pregnancy is rare, 50% of cases are caused by cortisol-producing ACA and 10% by ACC.[178] Surgical management is preferred due to significant fetal morbidity of untreated hypercortisolism.[178] Conversely, most reported cases of aldosterone-producing ACA are managed medically until delivery.[179,180] Finally, poor outcomes are reported for pregnancies in

the setting of ACC or mitotane therapy; therefore, effective contraceptive in such patients is recommended.[181]

ADRENAL NEOPLASIA IN CHILDHOOD

Many diagnostic and management considerations for ACC and PCPGL in children parallel their adult counterparts, but several important distinctions deserve special attention. PCPGL is a rare diagnosis in children, estimated at 1 in 2 million overall.[182] Several small series suggest a slight male preponderance and presentation in early adolescence on average.[183–185] Genetic mutations (including *SDHB* and *VHL*, as described previously) are reported in up to 33%,[183,185] though this may be an underestimate. Presentation appears variable but symptoms such as diaphoresis may be more prevalent and severe compared with adults.[183,184] Reported complications of sustained hypertension in these patients include hypertensive retinopathy and hypertonic cardiomyopathy.[182] As in adults, the biochemical diagnosis is established with plasma metanephrines and normetanephrines; however, careful consideration should be given to choice of imaging modality to limit radiation exposure if possible. Definitive treatment is surgical, with mandatory preoperative α-blockade and volume expansion. Laparoscopic and cortex-sparing procedures are commonly utilized, especially for patients with bilateral disease or hereditary syndromes.[183,184,186] As a caution, PCPGL can be mistaken for the far more commonly encountered neuroblastoma preoperatively;[182,186,187] this can have adverse consequences because preoperative α-blockade is not usually initiated for resection of neuroblastoma.[185,188]

ACC is also a rare diagnosis in children, accounting for 0.2% of childhood cancers.[189] An early peak at ages 3 to 4 years is described, with another smaller increase in incidence in adolescence.[189] Although there is a slight overall female predilection, gender distribution appears age dependent.[189,190] In contrast to their adult counterparts, adrenocortical tumors in children are malignant in >60% of cases.[186] In general, a predisposing genetic mutation is identified in >50% of all childhood ACC, and most are mutations in *TP53*.[189] A cohort of patients in southern Brazil has been identified with 10 to 50 times higher rate of ACC, of whom 95% have a specific germline mutation in *TP53*.[189] Many other genomic changes have been described that appear distinct from the adult population.[189] Intriguingly, histopathologic features, molecular signature, clinical presentation, and prognosis of ACC appear distinct in tumors from young children compared with those from adolescents. Features characteristic of the fetal adrenal cortex have been demonstrated in specimens of early childhood ACC by microscopy and microarray analysis.[189,190] Moreover, the overwhelming majority of early childhood ACC present with virizilation, compared with those presenting in adolescence, when hypercortisolism is more common.[190] Either way, 90% of childhood ACC are functional and virilization alone or in combination with hypercortisolism has been described in 80%.[189] In some cases, subtle signs or laboratory evidence of hormone excess have been documented years before diagnosis.[191] Approximately one-third of patients with childhood ACC present with unresectable disease, and overall 5-year survival is reported at 54% to 74%,[189,190,192,193] although prognosis for younger children is better, especially in those with smaller tumors after complete resection.[190] As in adults, surgery is the primary treatment modality with multimodal therapy for more advanced disease including mitotane and cytotoxic chemotherapy.[189]

ACKNOWLEDGMENTS

The authors wish to acknowledge Barbra S. Miller, MD, and Anca M. Avram, MD, at the University of Michigan for carefully reviewing this manuscript and generously sharing their scientific and clinical insights.

SELECTED REFERENCES

The full reference list can be accessed at lwwhealthlibrary.com/oncology.

6. Young WF. Clinical practice. The incidentally discovered adrenal mass. *N Engl J Med* 2007;356:601–610.

16. Rossi GP, Bernini G, Caliumi C, et al. A prospective study of the prevalence of primary aldosteronism in 1,125 hypertensive patients. *J Am Coll Cardiol* 2006;48:2293–2300.

21. Arlt W, Biehl M, Taylor AE, et al. Urine steroid metabolomics as a biomarker tool for detecting malignancy in adrenal tumors. *J Clin Endocrinol Metab* 2011;96:3775–3784.

22. Icard P, Goudet P, Charpenay C, et al. Adrenocortical carcinomas: surgical trends and results of a 253-patient series from the French Association of Endocrine Surgeons study group. *World J Surg* 2001;25:891–897.

28. Goffredo P, Sosa JA, Roman SA. Malignant pheochromocytoma and paraganglioma: a population level analysis of long-term survival over two decades. *J Surg Oncol* 2013;107:659–664.

29. Pacak K, Eisenhofer G, Ahlman H, et al. Pheochromocytoma: recommendations for clinical practice from the First International Symposium. October 2005. *Nat Clin Pract Endocrinol Metab* 2007;3:92–102.

36. Astuti D, Laitf F, Dallol A, et al. Gene mutations in the succinate dehydrogenase subunit SDHB cause susceptibility to familial pheochromocytoma and to familial paraganglioma. *Am J Hum Genet* 2001;69:49–54.

42. Giordano TJ, Thomas DG, Kuick R, et al. Distinct transcriptional profiles of adrenocortical tumors uncovered by DNA microarray analysis. *Am J Pathol* 2003;162:521–531.

43. Lerario AM, Moraitis A, Hammer GD. Genetics and epigenetics of adrenocortical tumors. *Mol Cell Endocrinol* 2014;386:67–84.

46. Åkerström T, Crona J, Delgado Verdugo A, et al. Comprehensive resequencing of adrenal aldosterone producing lesions reveal three somatic mutations near the KCNJ5 potassium channel selectivity filter. *PLoS ONE* 2012;7(7):e41926.

48. Gicquel C, Raffin-Sanson ML, Gaston V, et al. Structural and functional abnormalities at 11p15 are associated with the malignant phenotype in sporadic adrenocortical tumors: study on a series of 82 tumors. *J Clin Endocrinol Metab* 1997;82:2559–2565.

59. Raymond VM, Else T, Everett JN, et al. Prevalence of germline TP53 mutations in a prospective series of unselected patients with adrenocortical carcinoma. *J Clin Endocrinol Metab* 2013;98:E119–E125.

65. Neumann HPH, Bausch B, McWhinney SR, et al. Germ-line mutations in nonsyndromic pheochromocytoma. *N Engl J Med* 2002;346:1459–1466.

69. Kinney MAO, Narr BJ, Warner MA. Perioperative management of pheochromocytoma. *J Cardiothorac Vasc Anesth* 2002;16:359–369.

71. Schteingart DE, Doherty GM, Gauger PG, et al. Management of patients with adrenal cancer: recommendations of an international consensus conference. *Endocr Relat Cancer* 2005;12:667–680.

72. Berruti A, Baudin E, Gelderblom H, et al. Adrenal cancer: ESMO Clinical Practice Guidelines for diagnosis, treatment and follow-up. *Ann Oncol* 2012; 23:vii131–vii138.

73. Lenders JWM, Pacak K, Walther MM, et al. Biochemical diagnosis of pheochromocytoma: which test is best? *JAMA* 2002;287:1427–1434.

81. Caoili EM, Korobkin M, Francis IR, et al. Adrenal masses: characterization with combined unenhanced and delayed enhanced CT. *Radiology* 2002; 222:629–633.

83. Groussin L, Bonardel G, Silvéra S, et al. 18F-fluorodeoxyglucose positron emission tomography for the diagnosis of adrenocortical tumors: a prospective study in 77 operated patients. *J Clin Endocrinol Metab* 2009;94:1713–1722.

95. Taieb D, Timmers HJ, Hindié E, et al. EANM 2012 guidelines for radionuclide imaging of phaeochromocytoma and paraganglioma. *Eur J Nucl Med Mol Imaging* 2012;39:1977–1995.

98. Vanderveen KA, Thompson SM, Callstrom MR, et al. Biopsy of pheochromocytomas and paragangliomas: potential for disaster. *Surgery* 2009;146: 1158–1166.

99. Weiss LM. Comparative histologic study of 43 metastasizing and nonmetastasizing adrenocortical tumors. *Am J Surg Pathol* 1984;8:163–169.

102. Lebastchi AH, Kunstman JW, Carling T. Adrenocortical carcinoma: current therapeutic state-of-the-art. *J Oncol* 2012;2012:234726.

103. Fassnacht M, Johanssen S, Quinkler M, et al. Limited prognostic value of the 2004 International Union Against Cancer staging classification for adrenocortical carcinoma: proposal for a Revised TNM Classification. *Cancer* 2009;115:243–250.

104. Lughezzani G, Sun M, Perrotte P, et al. The European Network for the Study of Adrenal Tumors staging system is prognostically superior to the international union against cancer-staging system: a North American validation. *Eur J Cancer* 2010;46:713–719.

109. Wu D, Tischler AS, Lloyd RV, et al. Observer variation in the application of the Pheochromocytoma of the Adrenal Gland Scaled Score. *Am J Surg Pathol* 2009;33:599–608.

122. Lee J, El-Tamer M, Schifftner T, et al. Open and laparoscopic adrenalectomy: analysis of the National Surgical Quality Improvement Program. *J Am Coll Surg* 2008;206:953–959, discussion 959–961.

123. Nigri G, Rosman AS, Petrucciani N, et al. Meta-analysis of trials comparing laparoscopic transperitoneal and retroperitoneal adrenalectomy. *Surgery* 2013;153:111–119.

124. Walz MK, Alesina PF, Wenger FA, et al. Posterior retroperitoneoscopic adrenalectomy—results of 560 procedures in 520 patients. *Surgery* 2006;140: 943–948, discussion 948–950.

132. Scholz T, Eisenhofer G, Pacak K, et al. Clinical review: Current treatment of malignant pheochromocytoma. *J Clin Endocrinol Metab* 2007;92: 1217–1225.

136. Reibetanz J, Jurowich C, Erdogan I, et al. Impact of lymphadenectomy on the oncologic outcome of patients with adrenocortical carcinoma. *Ann Surg* 2012;255:363–369.

137. Bilimoria KY, Shen WT, Elaraj D, et al. Adrenocortical carcinoma in the United States: treatment utilization and prognostic factors. *Cancer* 2008; 113:3130–3136.

139. Fassnacht M, Kroiss M, Allolio B. Update in adrenocortical carcinoma. *J Clin Endocrinol Metab* 2013;98:4551–4564.

142. Veytsman I, Nieman L, Fojo T. Management of endocrine manifestations and the use of mitotane as a chemotherapeutic agent for adrenocortical carcinoma. *J Clin Oncol* 2009;27:4619–4629.

144. Fassnacht M, Hahner S, Polat B, et al. Efficacy of adjuvant radiotherapy of the tumor bed on local recurrence of adrenocortical carcinoma. *J Clin Endocrinol Metab* 2006;91:4501–4504.

148. Morimoto R, Satoh F, Murakami O, et al. Immunohistochemistry of a proliferation marker Ki67/MIB1 in adrenocortical carcinomas: Ki67/MIB1 labeling index is a predictor for recurrence of adrenocortical carcinomas. *Endocr J* 2008;55:49–55.

149. Berruti A, Fassnacht M, Baudin E, et al. Adjuvant therapy in patients with adrenocortical carcinoma: a position of an international panel. *J Clin Oncol* 2010;28(23):e401–e402, author reply e403.

151. Erdogan I, Deutschbein T, Jurowich C, et al. The role of surgery in the management of recurrent adrenocortical carcinoma. *J Clin Endocrinol Metab* 2013;98:181–191.

152. Schulick RD, Brennan MF. Long-term survival after complete resection and repeat resection in patients with adrenocortical carcinoma. *Ann Surg Oncol* 1999;6:719–726.

154. Kemp CD, Ripley RT, Mathur A, et al. Pulmonary resection for metastatic adrenocortical carcinoma: the National Cancer Institute experience. *Ann Thorac Surg* 2011;92:1195–1200.

156. Wood BJ, Abraham J, Hvizda JL, et al. Radiofrequency ablation of adrenal tumors and adrenocortical carcinoma metastases. *Cancer* 2003;97:554–560.

160. Soga H, Takenaka A, Ooba T, et al. A twelve-year experience with adrenal cortical carcinoma in a single institution: long-term survival after surgical treatment and transcatheter arterial embolization. *Urol Int* 2009;82:222–226.

172. Fassnacht M, Terzolo M, Allolio B, et al. Combination chemotherapy in advanced adrenocortical carcinoma. *N Engl J Med* 2012;366:2189–2197.

175. Chen CC, Carrasquillo JA. Molecular imaging of adrenal neoplasms. *J Surg Oncol* 2012;106:532–542.

191. de Fraipont F, Atifi El M, Cherradi N, et al. Gene expression profiling of human adrenocortical tumors using complementary deoxyribonucleic Acid microarrays identifies several candidate genes as markers of malignancy. *J Clin Endocrinol Metab* 2005;90:1819–1829.

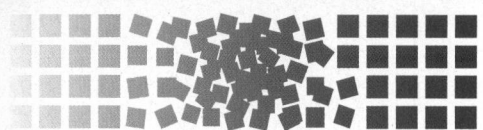

85 Pancreatic Neuroendocrine Tumors

James C. Yao and Douglas B. Evans

INTRODUCTION

Pancreatic neuroendocrine tumors (pNET), also known as pancreatic endocrine tumors, islet cell carcinoma, or pancreatic carcinoid, are low- to intermediate-grade neoplasms and have a more indolent course compared to pancreatic adenocarcinoma. pNETs can secrete hormones and be functional or nonfunctional. Functional status is generally influenced by several factors, including disease bulk, stage, secretory status, and whether the peptide secreted is intact and causes distinct clinical symptoms. pNETs are generally considered functional if they are associated with a hormonal syndrome. Regardless of tumor staining for hormones by immunohistochemistry (IHC) or serum levels of measured peptides in blood, those pNETs not causing a clinical hormonal syndrome are considered nonfunctional. It is also recognized that the functional status of these tumors may change over time or with treatment. Moreover, some of these tumors can produce multiple hormones simultaneously, although symptoms related to one of these hormones often will dominate.

Management of pNETs generally can be categorized into management of the problems caused by secreted hormone(s) and oncologic issues related to tumor growth and metastasis. The organization of this chapter parallels this paradigm. Following discussions of the epidemiology, pathology, and molecular genetics of these tumors, the oncologic issues common to the diagnosis and management of pNETs are discussed in the section on nonfunctional tumors. This is followed by discussions of issues unique to each functional "endocrinoma." Next is a section on additional clinical considerations, which includes hereditary cancer syndromes, pathology pitfalls, surgical pitfalls, and high-grade NETs. Our goal for this chapter is to provide a systematic, up-to-date, and practical approach to pNETs.

EPIDEMIOLOGY

pNETs are reputed to be relatively rare neoplasms, but their exact incidence and prevalence are somewhat elusive. This is in part because most registries, including the Surveillance, Epidemiology, and End Results (SEER) program, only include neoplasms that are deemed malignant. For pNETs, the definition of malignant behavior is complex. In the absence of malignant behavior such as direct invasion of adjacent organs or metastases to regional lymph nodes or distant sites, size is typically used to classify the malignant potential of pNETs. The age-adjusted incidence of pNETs has risen significantly over the last three decades (Fig. 85.1). The diagnosed incidence of pNETs in the United States was estimated to be 5.6 (95% confidence interval [CI], 5.1 to 6.2) per million in 2010.[1,2] The incidence of smaller pNETs in the general population, however, is likely to be much higher. In an analysis of 11,472 autopsies performed at a Hong Kong hospital, pNETs were found in 0.1% of all cases.[3] This suggests that the prevalence of small asymptomatic islet cell tumors, many of which are never diagnosed, may be 100-fold more common than the data suggested by SEER registries. It is yet unclear whether the observed increase in is purely due to better diagnosis and classification

or environmental factors including the use of certain medications, which may have led to a real increase in incidence.[4]

pNETs were slightly more common among men (53%) than women (47%), and the median age at diagnosis was 60 years.[1,5] At diagnosis, 14% had localized disease, 22% had regional disease, and 64% had distant disease. The survival of patients with pNETs has improved over time.[5,6] Among patients diagnosed from 1988 through 2004, the 5-year survival rates among patients with localized, regional, and distant pNETs were 79%, 62%, and 27%, respectively (Fig. 85.2).[1]

CLASSIFICATION, HISTOPATHOLOGY, MOLECULAR GENETICS

Criteria for Pathologic Diagnosis

A larger fraction of endocrine cells in the pancreas are insulin-producing (B) and glucagon-producing (A) cells. Relatively minor populations of cells produce somatostatin (D) and pancreatic polypeptide (PP). Rare cells also produce serotonin (EC) and ghrelin (P/D₁).[7] These endocrine cells are believed to be the source of pNETs. It is a matter of debate if tumors arise from islets or ducts. Transgenic mice expressing potent oncogenes in endocrine cells[8] and multiple endocrine neoplasia (MEN)1 knockout mice[9,10] point to an islet origin of tumors consistent with the auto-renewal properties of islet cells [11] and clinical observations in patients with MEN1.[12] Conversely, molecular evidence from islet microdissection in patients with MEN1 indicate a duct cell origin.[13] No matter where the truth lies, endocrine tumor cells largely display the same phenotype as their normal endocrine counterpart.

Aggressiveness of pNETs can be classified according to differentiation or proliferative rate. In the 2010 World Health Organization (WHO) classification, well-differentiated pancreatic neuroendocrine neoplasm is termed neuroendocrine tumor, whereas poorly differentiated neuroendocrine neoplasm is termed neuroendocrine carcinoma.[14] Histologically, well-differentiated tumors are characterized by bland features: trabecular, glandular, acinar, or mixed structures; the stroma is generally fine and rich in well-developed blood vessels, sometimes with hyalinised deposits of amyloid; tumor cells are monomorphic with abundant, variably eosinophilic cytoplasm, low cytological atypia and low mitotic index. Necrosis is usually absent or may be seen as spotty, limited areas in histologically more aggressive neoplasms. On the contrary, poorly differentiated neuroendocrine carcinomas are characterized by prevalent solid structure with abundant necrosis, often central, round tumor cell of small to medium size with severe cellular atypia and high mitotic index.

Fine Needle Aspiration Versus Core Needle Biopsy

The diagnosis of pNET is necessary (1) to meet the previously defined histologic and cytologic criteria, (2) to assess the status of endocrine differentiation, and (3) to evaluate prognostic markers (proliferative index). Fine needle aspiration (FNA) biopsy is

Age-adjusted Incidence per 1,000,000 Population

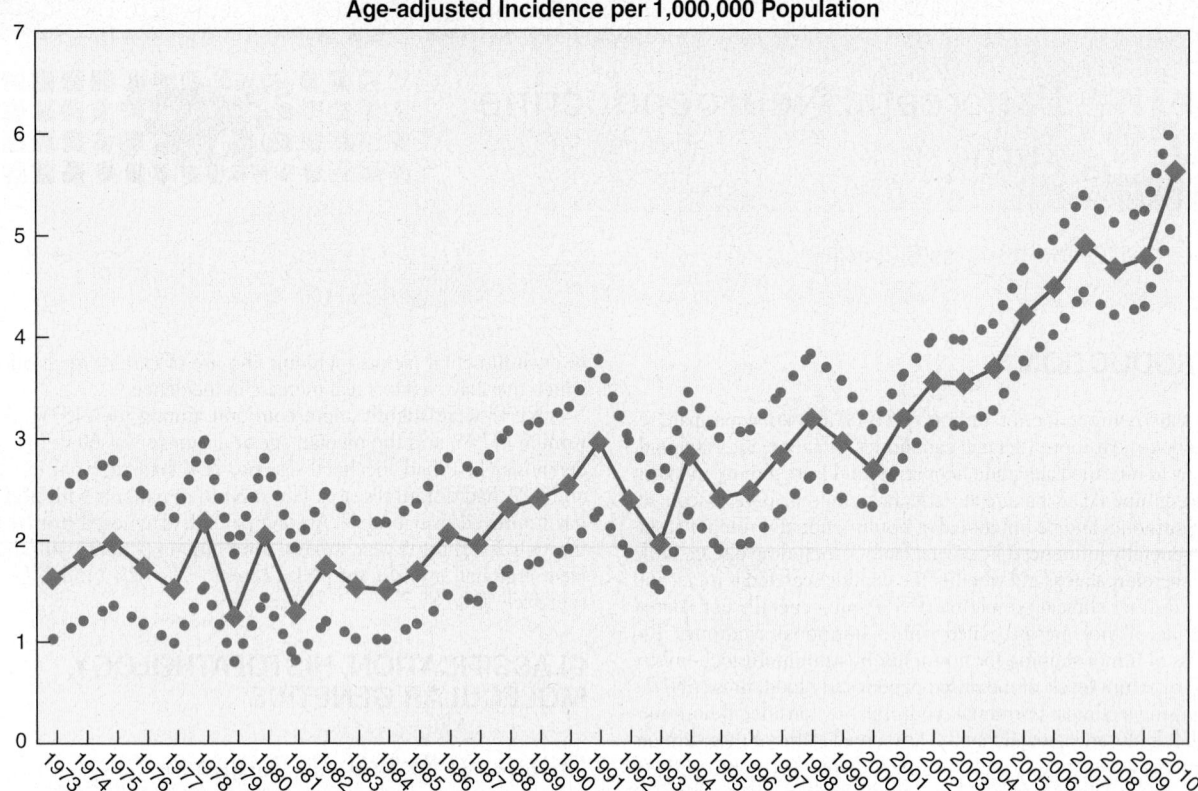

Figure 85.1 Age adjusted incidence rate per 1 million population.[2]

an effective technique in expert hands, allowing confirmation of the cytologic diagnosis on isolated or grouped cells with little information on tumor structure. The advantages of FNA are several, including its simplicity, low invasiveness, and cost. The disadvantages are mainly its operator-dependent efficacy and limited option for further study (small sample size) to include prognostic variables.

Conversely, the core needle biopsy (ideally 2 mm in diameter) produces a larger sized tumor sample, potentially allowing a cyto-/histologic diagnosis complete with all known prognostic parameters. Besides the easier diagnostic approach intrinsic to histology, its major advantage is certainly the potential for further studies to include all IHC studies and assessment of proliferative index.

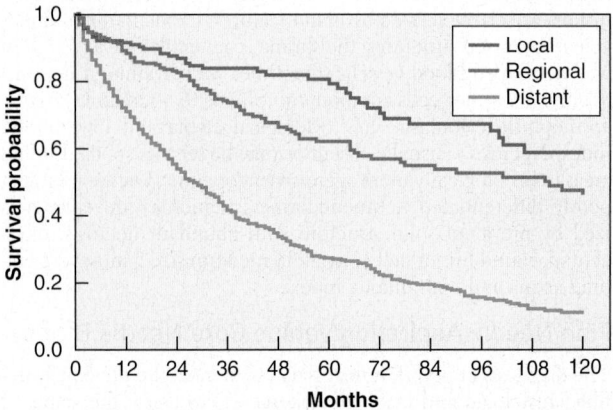

Figure 85.2 Survival by stage. Median survival for patients with localized, regional and distant metastatic disease were >10 years, 9.3 years, and 2.3 years, respectively.[1]

Disadvantages are the invasiveness of the procedure(s) and the relatively higher costs.

We typically recommend core needle when considering biopsy of liver metastases and FNA for biopsy of the pancreas.

Minimum Immunohistochemistry Markers

A large number of antigens, commonly defined as "neuroendocrine markers," are expressed in tumor cells.[7] They comprise markers dispersed in the cytosol including neuron-specific enolase (NSE) and protein gene product 9.5, and markers of the secretory compartment, either associated with electron-dense granules, large-dense-core vesicles such as chromogranins and related fragments (the most popular being chromogranin A [CgA]), or associated with small synaptic-like vesicles such as synaptophysin. These antigens are defined as "general markers," since they are widely expressed in cells of the diffuse endocrine system. Hormones and/or amines are produced by specific cell types and thus defined as "specific markers." The positive identification of the endocrine cell product(s) in tissue sections is obtained by IHC.

A minimal IHC histology panel is designed to (1) positively identify the degree of endocrine differentiation in tumor cells, and (2) determining the proliferation activity status. Determining the proliferation status is achieved by Ki67 IHC using the MIB1 antibody or it can be expressed as mitoses per 10 high power microscopic fields (or 2 mm^2).

Grade—World Health Organization 2010, American Joint Committee on Cancer, Union for International Cancer Control

Proliferative rate has been widely acknowledged as an important prognostic factor in pNETs. Though some controversies remain, the grading system based on mitotic rate and Ki 67 labeling

---

TABLE 85.1

Staging and Grading of Pancreatic Neuroendocrine Tumors[15]

AJCC, Seventh Edition	ENETS
Primary Tumor (T)	**Primary Tumor (T)**
TX Primary tumor cannot be assessed	TX Primary tumor cannot be assessed
T0 No evidence of primary tumor	T0 No evidence of primary tumor
T1 Tumor limited to the pancreas, ≤2 cm	T1 Tumor limited to the pancreas and size <2 cm
T2 Tumor limited to the pancreas, >2 cm	T2 Tumor limited to the pancreas and size 2–4cm
T3 Tumor extends beyond the pancreas but without involvement of the celiac axis or the superior mesenteric artery	T3 Tumor limited to the pancreas and size >4 cm or invading duodenum or bile duct
T4 Tumor involves the celiac axis or the superior mesenteric artery (unresectable primary tumor)	T4 Tumor invading adjacent organs (stomach, spleen, colon, adrenal gland) or the wall of large vessels (celiac axis or superior mesenteric artery)
Regional Lymph Nodes (N)	**Regional Lymph Nodes (N)**
NX Regional lymph nodes cannot be assessed	NX Regional lymph node cannot be assessed
N0 No regional lymph node metastasis	N0 No regional lymph node metastasis
N1 Regional lymph node metastasis	N1 Regional lymph node metastasis
Distant Metastases (M)	**Distant Metastases (M)**
—	MX Distant metastasis cannot be assessed
M0 No distant metastasis	M0 No distant metastases
M1 Distant metastasis	M1 Distant metastasis

AJCC				ENETs			
Stage	**T**	**N**	**M**	**Stage**	**T**	**N**	**M**
0	Tis	N0	M0	–	–	–	–
IA	T1	N0	M0	I	T1	N0	M0
IB	T2	N0	M0	IIA	T2	N0	M0
IIA	T3	N0	M0	IIB	T3	N0	M0
IIB	T1, T2, T3	N1	M0	IIIA	T4	N0	M0
III	T4	Any N	M0	IIIB	Any T	N1	M0
IV	Any T	Any N	M1	IV	Any T	Any N	M1

Grade	Mitotic Count[a]	Ki-67 Index (%)[b]
G1	<2	≤2
G2	2–20	3–20
G3	>20	>20

AJCC, American Joint Committee on Cancer; ENETS, European Neuroendocrine Tumor Society.
[a] 10 high-power field) = 2 mm^2, at least 40 fields (at 40× magnification) evaluated in areas of highest mitotic density.
[b] MIB1 antibody; % of 2,000 tumor cells in areas of highest nuclear labeling.

---

has been widely adopted by the American Joint Committee on Cancer (AJCC), International Union Against Cancer (UICC), and WHO (Table 85.1).[15,16] Low (G1) and intermediate (G2) grade neoplasms are termed pNETs, whereas aggressive high-grade (G3) neoplasm are termed pancreatic neuroendocrine carcinoma.

The general utility of such a grading scheme has been validated in a number of studies.[17–21] However, the optimal Ki-67 cut-off between G1 and G2 remains debated in the literature. Some authors have proposed 5% (instead of 2%) as a more discriminatory cut-point for important outcomes including overall survival (OS).[22] In one multivariate analysis that included lymph node ratio, a Ki-67 >5% was identified as the strongest predictor of recurrence after resection of malignant pNETs.[23] At the current time, G1 and G2 tumors are managed in a similar way. Therefore, the distinction between G1 and G2, while prognostic, does not have major therapeutic implications. A more important issue is the distinction between G2 and G3 as platinum-based chemotherapy is generally recommended for G3 tumors. In a recent review of a large Nordic series, response rate to platinum-based chemotherapy was low for the subgroup of G3 patients with Ki-67 between 20% and 55%. Tumors with a Ki-67 >55% appear more responsive to platinum-based chemotherapy.[24]

Tumor, Node, Metastases (TNM)

The recent European Neuroendocrine Tumor Society proposal of tumor node, metastases (TNM) for non functional pNETs is based on criteria previously identified by the WHO 2004 classification and implies a malignant potential for any tumor type.[15] The practical utility of this system was demonstrated in six independent studies.[17–21,25] In 2010, a TNM system was officially provided by AJCC and the UICC.[16] Their recommendation was to apply the same TNM system devised for exocrine pancreatic cancer to pNETs (see Table 85.1). The AJCC-UICC TNM scheme is based on a publication investigating a large tumor registry database.[26] As there is currently no adjuvant therapy available for pNETs, the distinction between the two staging system carries no practical therapeutic implications.

Molecular Genetics of Pancreatic Neuroendocrine Tumors

Advances in technology over the past 5 years have led to an explosion of new data emerging from high throughput molecular analyses. Recent exome sequencing studies have simultaneously

PRACTICE OF ONCOLOGY

confirmed the importance of genes associated with inherited cancer syndromes and discovered important novel genetic aberrations among patients with sporadic pNETs.[27]

The importance of the MEN1 gene in the carcinogenesis of pNETs has long been implicated by the genetic cancer syndrome bearing its name as well as studies showing frequent loss of 11q13 where the *MEN1* gene locus is found.[28–33] Studies using comparative genomic hybridization and high-resolution allelotyping have demonstrated frequent amplification and deletions across a large number of chromosomes compatible with karyotypic instability.[29–33] Exome sequencing studies identified three main groups (pathways) of mutations in sporadic pNETs. These include MEN1, DAXX or ATRX, and mammalian target of rapamycin (mTOR).[27] MEN1 is thought to be involved in epigenetic regulation and is implicated in the regulation of endocrine mass during pregnancy through a p27-dependent pathway.[34] DAXX and ATRX mutations are associated with alternative lengthening of telomeres and may offer escape from senescence.[35] mTOR pathway mutations suggest an attractive therapeutic target that has now been validated in a pivotal phase III study.[36]

DIAGNOSIS AND MANAGEMENT OF PANCREATIC NEUROENDOCRINE TUMORS

Nonfunctional Tumors

Symptoms and Diagnosis

Nonfunctioning pNETs and PP-secreting tumors do not cause a clinical syndrome. Rarely, case reports of PP-secreting tumors have been associated with watery diarrhea,[37–39] diabetes mellitus, ulcer diathesis,[40] or an erythematous pruritic skin rash different from that seen in patients with glucagonomas.[41] Until the tumor causes obstruction of the biliary tree or gastric outlet, the patients are usually asymptomatic unless the tumor bulk results in pain; this is in sharp contrast to pancreatic adenocarcinoma where very low tumor burden may be associated with profound symptoms and death. Jaundice may be the presenting symptom in patients with tumors to the right of the superior mesenteric artery (SMA) and superior mesenteric vein; these tumors originate in the pancreatic head or uncinate process, which may cause obstruction of the intrapancreatic portion of the common bile duct.[42,43] Tumors in this location may also cause gastric outlet obstruction and/or pain owing to invasion of the autonomic mesenteric plexus. Pain may also be secondary to tumor extension into the celiac ganglion (most commonly seen with tumors arising in the body of the pancreas) or to liver metastases that invade the liver capsule or extend to the parietal peritoneum. Occasional patients may experience gastrointestinal hemorrhage secondary to tumor erosion into the duodenum or secondary to splenic vein occlusion causing gastroesophageal varices (sinistral portal hypertension). Nonfunctioning pNETs can sometimes grow to an enormous size without producing jaundice or other symptoms. pNETs arising to the left of the SMA and superior mesenteric vein may cause vague, poorly localized upper abdominal pain or dyspepsia, but such tumors are usually asymptomatic until they reach a considerable size. In contrast to patients with adenocarcinoma of the pancreas, patients with pNETs may not experience significant weight loss, cachexia, or back pain, or show other signs of advanced disease.[42,43] In the absence of a large tumor or metastatic disease (of significant volume), pNETs are often detected incidentally on abdominal imaging studies.

On contrast-enhanced multidetector computed tomography (CT), pNETs characteristically appear hyperdense, as they are hypervascular. Therefore, imaging of the pancreas during the arterial phase is critically important to detect these lesions and their hypervascular liver metastases. However, similar to pancreatic adenocarcinomas, pNETs may occasionally appear hypodense compared with adjacent pancreatic parenchyma, and they may contain cystic components or microcalcifications. Importantly, intrapancreatic accessory splenic tissue can present as an asymptomatic, hypervascular mass involving the distal pancreatic tail, thus mimicking a pNET.

The current practice at our institutions is to obtain high-quality multidetector (multislice) CT images of the pancreatic tumor. We use objective CT criteria to determine a tumor's resectability based upon the relationship of the pancreatic tumor to the SMA and celiac axis.[44,45] Encasement (defined as >180-degree involvement of the vessel by tumor) of the SMA or occlusion of the superior mesenteric-portal venous confluence without the technical option of venous reconstruction are considered criteria for a tumor's unresectability. Similar to our philosophy on local-regional management of pancreatic adenocarcinomas,[46] we do not perform incomplete resection (debulking) of nonfunctioning pNETs. Some investigators have suggested that incomplete resection of the pancreatic tumor may provide relief of local tumor–related symptoms and improve survival, but most of these reports included patients with syndromes of hormone excess; no accurately reported data are available to support debulking in patients with unresectable nonfunctioning pNETs. However, in patients without distant metastases (or minimal liver metastases) extended resections to include complex vascular resection and reconstruction may be considered at these centers with experience in such complex operations.[47,48] Magnetic resonance imaging (MRI) is preferred over CT for patients with a history of allergy to iodine contrast material or for those with renal insufficiency. Moreover, MRI may be more sensitive than CT for the detection of small liver metastases. Endoscopic ultrasound (EUS) is currently considered the most sensitive modality for identifying small pNETs and is thus used for preoperative tumor localization in patients with MEN1, in which multifocal disease is common. In the absence of an inherited endocrine syndrome associated with multifocal disease, the role of EUS is limited to FNA biopsy of the tumor. In the current era of invasive gastroenterology, EUS is safe and is becoming more widely available.

Accurate preoperative diagnosis and staging of the primary tumor is necessary to ensure correct treatment. The oncologic (surgical *and* medical) approach to a pNET is different from that for pancreatic adenocarcinoma. Because of the poor prognosis associated with pancreatic adenocarcinoma, patients with pNETs who are incorrectly thought to have large, locally invasive or metastatic adenocarcinomas may not undergo surgery when it is indicated and also may receive incorrect chemotherapy. Unless a surgery first strategy is considered (in which preoperative biopsy may not be necessary) pretreatment FNA biopsy should always be performed to prevent an error in diagnosis; this is especially true when the clinical history, physical examination, and radiographic images are confusing and not consistent with the presumed clinical diagnosis.

Serum Tumor Markers

Several circulating tumor markers have been evaluated for the diagnosis and follow-up management of pNETs. While these can be very useful for follow-up, isolated elevation of marker levels is generally not sufficient for diagnosis. These markers usually can be divided into those associated with specific endocrine syndromes and those more general markers that may be present in functional as well as nonfunctional tumors. The most important of these markers, CgA, is a 49-kDa acidic polypeptide that is widely present in the secretory granules of neuroendocrine cells. CgA is elevated in the majority of patients with either functioning or nonfunctioning pNETs.[49–52] In a study where patients with advanced pNETs were treated with streptozotocin-based chemotherapy, 79% of patients had elevation of CgA at the time of diagnosis.[53] In addition, response to therapy was associated with a 30% decrease in serum CgA.[53] This concept was also tested in the RADIANT-1 study, which treated patients with progressive pNETs after cytotoxic chemotherapy with the mTOR inhibitor everolimus. In this study, a 30% decrease in

CgA, 4 weeks after initiation of therapy, was associated with significantly longer progression-free survival (PFS).[54] However, care should be taken in measuring CgA and interpreting the results. For example, as somatostatin analogues are known to affect blood levels of CgA, serial CgA levels should be measured at approximately the same interval from injection in patients receiving long-acting somatostatin analogues. Spuriously elevated levels of CgA have also been reported in patients using proton pump inhibitors, in patients with renal or liver failure, or in those with chronic gastritis.

Another general neuroendocrine marker, NSE, is a dimmer of the glycolytic enzyme enolase. NSE is present in the cytoplasmic compartment of the cell, and its serum level is thought to be unrelated to the secretory activity of the tumor.[52] While less specific as a diagnostic marker, it may be helpful in the follow-up of patients with unresectable disease. In the RADIANT-1 study, a 30% decrease in NSE at week 4 was associated with significantly longer PFS.[54]

PP levels also are frequently elevated in patients with pNETs. Elevation of PP is not associated with a distinct hormonal syndrome and is only considered significant when PP level is at least three times the age-matched normal basal level obtained in a fasting state.[55] A variety of other secreted amines can also be measured. These include other chromogranins such as chromogranin B and C, pancreastatin, substance P, neurotensin, neurokinin A, gastrin, glucagon, vasoactive intestinal peptide, insulin, proinsulin, and c-peptide. In general, blood markers should be drawn in the fasting state.

It is recognized that NETs sometimes can change what (if any) hormones and biomarkers are produced. The general principle of biomarker measurement is to evaluate a large panel of markers at key points in time (diagnosis or relapse) in order to identify the biomarkers that are elevated and then follow these over time. It is generally not necessary to check every biomarker at every visit.

Surgical Treatment

The majority of pNETs are malignant, with the exception of insulinomas, which are benign in 95% of patients. It is probably best to assume that if left untreated, all non–insulin-secreting pNETs have the biologic ability for uncontrolled local growth and metastasis to distant organs. pNETs frequently metastasize to regional lymph nodes, and the frequency of lymph node metastases depends on the extent of surgery and on the degree and accuracy of the pathologist's examination of the surgical specimen.[56]

Based on our experience and the reports from others, we have developed general guidelines for the surgical management of patients with nonfunctioning pNETs:

1. We establish the diagnosis with needle biopsy (EUS-guided FNA of the pancreas or image-guided core needle biopsy of the liver metastases is preferred) and decompress the biliary tree with an endobiliary stent if a distal bile duct obstruction is present. Once biliary obstruction is recognized and a stent is placed in the bile duct, an operation to remove the primary tumor or bypass the site of obstruction will likely be needed; in the absence of large volume distant metastases, the patient will most likely outlive the biliary stent and experience significant stent-related morbidity.
2. We resect localized, nonmetastatic disease confined to the pancreas if a gross complete resection can be performed. If radiographically occult liver metastases are found at the time of the operation, they are removed if possible. If the liver metastases are of small volume but diffuse, the primary tumor is usually removed due to the potential for major morbidity from the primary, which is a possibility because of the relatively long-anticipated survival of the patient.
3. There is an emerging body of literature to suggest that nonfunctioning pNETs < (approximately) 2 cm in diameter are of limited metastatic potential. This is especially important when dealing with patients of advanced age or clinically significant comorbidities (which increase operative risk even if the procedure

is performed laparoscopically). In this setting, if the pNET represents an incidental finding on CT/MRI obtained for an unrelated reason, observation may be the best approach.[57–59] Repeat imaging in 6 to 12 months will provide a window of opportunity to assess tumor biology. If observation is chosen and the diagnosis is confirmed on imaging, to include a functional study such as somatostatin receptor scintigraphy, biopsy may not be necessary.
4. In the setting of known metastatic disease or a large, borderline resectable primary tumor, we would first initiate systemic therapy as a bridge to eventual operation. Significant downstaging of the overall tumor burden can improve the safety of surgery in some patients.
5. The decision to operate on the primary pancreatic tumor is based upon the presence and/or extent of distant disease and the presence or absence of symptoms (bleeding, obstruction) from the primary tumor. For example, resection of an asymptomatic primary in the distal pancreas has a limited role, if any, in the presence of unresectable, moderate- to large-volume extrapancreatic metastatic disease. As treatments for metastatic disease become more effective, the rationale for aggressive management of the primary tumor despite the presence of extrapancreatic disease may become more compelling. However, treatment sequencing will likely emphasize a surgery-last strategy (after induction systemic therapy) to identify those patients most likely to benefit from large, multiorgan resections.
6. When dealing with a resectable primary tumor and resectable liver metastases, we usually remove the pancreatic tumor first; if that procedure goes well, we then consider resecting the liver under the same anesthesia induction.[60] However, we often use a two-stage procedure if all needed surgery cannot safely be performed at one operation.

The goals of surgery are to maximize local disease control and to increase the quality and length of patient survival. These goals must be tempered by the potential operative morbidity and the long-term complications of insulin dependence and gastrointestinal dysfunction. We previously reported survival data for 163 patients with nonfunctioning pNETs treated at our institution.[61] As expected, patients with localized or regional disease at diagnosis had a significantly superior median survival compared with those who had metastatic disease (7.1 years versus 2.2 years; $p < 0.0001$). Among patients with localized disease, those who underwent complete resection of the primary tumor demonstrated an additional survival advantage over those with locally advanced, unresectable tumors (median survivals of 7.1 years for patients with localized, resectable disease versus 5.2 years for patients with locally advanced, unresectable tumors).[61] However, only 48% of the 42 patients with localized, nonmetastatic disease who underwent resection of the primary tumor were alive and without evidence of recurrent disease at a median follow-up of 2.7 years (range, 1 to 8 years) from diagnosis. It is thus inappropriate to assume that complete resection of the primary tumor in the absence of metastatic disease corresponds to long-term cure.

Occasionally, an extended operation is required to achieve complete tumor resection of nonfunctioning pNETs. A high-risk operation (to include most that require complex vascular resection and reconstruction) should not be performed in a high-risk patient who because of age and medical comorbidities has a significant risk of perioperative mortality (=10%) or morbidity (=30%). In the absence of surgery, survival duration is often measured in years even in the presence of distant metastases and therefore surgery-related complications are to be avoided.[62] At present, we are highly selective in our use of extended pancreaticoduodenectomy or left-sided resections to include the celiac axis (Appleby procedure). Patients who undergo such high-risk operations must have limited to no medical comorbidities and have an excellent performance status. Decisions for or against surgical treatment are particularly difficult when dealing with large primary tumors, which require an extend resection, in the absence of distant metastases. The median survival duration for patients with unresectable, nonmetastatic, nonfunctioning pNETs is approximately 5 years. As survival time without operation increases and as potential operative morbidity and mortality increase, we are less accepting of the upfront risks of surgery. However, as mentioned previously, occasionally, locally advanced tumors of the pancreatic head or uncinate process are associated with significant patient morbidity due to complications such as biliary obstruction, gastric outlet obstruction, or gastrointestinal hemorrhage.[61] In contrast to the management of patients with pancreatic adenocarcinoma (where endoscopic stenting of the bile duct and occasionally the duodenum are fairly routine in the setting of locally advanced or metastatic disease), we would rarely use a duodenal stent in a patient with neuroendocrine carcinoma and would utilize endobiliary stents only for short-term (months, not years) biliary decompression. Because of the longer survival times of patients with pNETs (even advanced disease), we favor operative bypass of the bile duct and duodenum in most cases.

Oncologic Management of Advanced Pancreatic Neuroendocrine Tumors

Advanced, unresectable pNETs generally are not curable. The goals of oncologic management include palliation or prevention of symptoms and cytoreduction of bulky tumors in an effort to prolong survival. Although low- to intermediate-grade pNETs have a reputation of being indolent, most patients with advanced pNETs will not survive the disease.

Management of patients with advanced pNETs requires an understanding of the disease process and the importance of a multimodality approach. Treatment options include cytotoxic chemotherapy, everolimus, sunitinib, somatostatin analogues, peptide-receptor radiotherapy, as well as ablative approaches such as hepatic artery embolization and radiofrequency ablation (RFA). Occasionally, systemic therapy may also convert cases of unresectable tumors into cases wherein surgery may render the patients disease free. In such cases, we recommend that surgical options be considered in a multidisciplinary setting. Much of what is discussed here for non functional pNETs also holds true for managing the growth of functional tumors.

Systemic Therapy

Somatostatin Analogues

Somatostatin is a hormone that binds to specific high-affinity membrane receptors on target tissues. To date, five subtypes of somatostatin receptors (SSTR) have been identified. When activated, these receptors trigger differing biologic activity. The somatostatin analogues octreotide and lanreotide both bind with high affinity to SSTR 2 and with slightly lower affinity to SSTR 5. Pasireotide is a novel cyclohexapeptide in development that binds to SSRT 1, 2, 3, and 5.[63]

The somatostatin analogue octreotide is approved for the control of symptoms related to hormonal hypersecretion in NETs. More recently, randomized controlled studies have also demonstrated that somatostatin analogues can delay tumor growth. The PROMID study compared octreotide LAR 30 mg every 4 weeks to placebo among treatment-naïve patients with midgut NETs (carcinoid tumors). The study demonstrated significant benefit in time to progression (hazard ratio [HR] = 0.34; 95% CI, 0.20 to 0.59; $p < 0.0001$).[64] In a larger study that included a substantial number of pNETs, lanreotide 120 mg was compared to placebo in a population of patients with mostly stable disease (Table 85.2). Treatment with lanreotide was also associated with significant benefit in PFS (HR = 0.47; 95% CI, 0.30 to 0.73; $p = 0.0002$).[65] The long median PFS of 12 (95% CI, 9.4 to 18.3) months among patients with pNET receiving placebo suggests that many patients with known stable disease may not need immediate treatment.

Everolimus

mTOR is an intracellular protein that has a central role in cellular function. It acts as a nutrient sensor and mediates signaling downstream of receptor tyrosine kinases controlling cell growth, protein synthesis, autophagy, and angiogenesis. The association between aberrant mTOR pathway signaling and the pathogenesis of pNETs is suggested by the development of pNETs in patients with inherited genetic mutations in TSC2 and NF1. Loss of TSC2 and NF1 are both associated with mTOR activation. In an exome sequencing study, mTOR pathway mutations were also found in sporadic pNETs.[27] Finally on a protein level, low expression of PTEN and TSC2 were associated with poor prognosis.[66]

Phase 2 studies of the mTOR inhibitor everolimus have reported evidence of clinical activity.[54,67] In the initial report, the combination of octreotide LAR and everolimus was studied in 60 patients with NETs.[67] The response rate among 30 patients with pNET was 27%. In a subsequent multinational phase 2 study (RADIANT-1) in advanced pNETs with progression following chemotherapy, 160 patients were treated in two strata, with everolimus ($n = 115$) or everolimus plus octreotide ($n = 45$) based on whether patients were on octreotide at study entry.[54] By central radiology review, the response rate was lower at 9.6%. Durable disease stabilizations were, however, observed among patients with progression at study entry. The median PFS for patients receiving everolimus or

TABLE 85.2

Selected Phase 3 Studies In Pancreatic Neuroendocrine Tumors

Regimen	Number of Patients	Median PFS (Months)	Hazard Ratio (95% CI)	P
Study in patients with predominantly stable disease				
Lanreotide 120 mg q 4 weeks (overall)[65]	101	Not reached	0.47	0.0002
Placebo (overall)	103	18	(0.30–0.73)	
Lanreotide 120 mg q 4 weeks (pNET)	42	Not reached	0.58	0.06[a]
Placebo (pNET)	49	12.1	(0.32–1.04)	
Studies in patients with progressive disease				
Everolimus 10 mg daily[68]	204	11	0.35	<0.0001
Placebo	203	4.6	(0.27–0.45)	
Sunitinib 37.5 mg daily[70]	86	11.4	0.42	0.0001
Placebo	85	5.5	(0.26–0.66)	

PFS, progression-free survival; CI, confidence interval; pNET, pancreatic neuroendocrine tumor.
[a] Study not designed to test the treatment effect in pNET subgroup.

everolimus plus octreotide were 9.7 months and 16.7 months, respectively. In the largest phase 3 study to have been conducted in pNETs (RADIANT-3), 410 patients with progressive pNETs were randomly assigned to receive everolimus or placebo. The study demonstrated clinically and statistically significant benefit in PFS for patients receiving everolimus (see Table 85.2).[68] Everolimus prolonged median PFS from 4.6 months to 11 months leading to a 65% risk reduction for progression compared to placebo (HR = 0.35; 95% CI, 0.27 to 0.45; p <0.0001). Treatment also reduced the level of tumor-secreted hormones.

Sunitinib

pNETs are vascular tumors known to express vascular endothelial growth factor (VEGF). Recent studies have demonstrated the expression of VEGFR-FLK and VEGFR-FLT1 on tumor cells. Sunitinib is a novel tyrosine kinase inhibitor with activity against VEGF receptors, c-Kit, and platelet-derived growth factor receptor. In a multicenter phase 2 study, investigators treated patients with carcinoids and pNETs in separate strata and also observed evidence of clinical activity. Interestedly, in this study, the tumor response rate appeared to be higher among patients with pNETs than in patients with carcinoids (17% versus 2%).[69] A subsequent phase 3 study compared sunitinib to placebo in pNETs (see Table 85.2). Results of an early unplanned analysis showed improved PFS (5.5 months versus 11.4 months).[70] Although the study showed clinically meaningful benefit (HR = 0.42, 95% CI, 0.26 to 0.66), the type 1 error was uncontrolled. Due to the small number of events and unplanned nature of the analyses, the results failed to cross the O'Brian Fleming efficacy threshold for statistical significance.

Cytotoxic Chemotherapy

Systemic chemotherapy for advanced pNETs has been studied in many clinical trials over the last three decades. Despite the multitude of publications, the role of cytotoxic chemotherapy continues to be debated. Older studies often used criteria to measure outcome that are not accepted today. Older studies using cytotoxic agents have not documented improvements in PFS or OS versus best supportive care.[71,72]

Streptozocin-Based Chemotherapy. Streptozocin was originally isolated from streptomyces achromogenes in the 1950s. Its antitumor activity in pNETs was first reported in 1973; in a study that included 52 patients, a response rate of 50% was reported.[73] Streptozocin's single-agent activity in pNETs was subsequently confirmed in a study comparing that agent alone with streptozocin plus fluorouracil.[71] In this study, a higher response rate was reported for the combination of streptozocin and fluorouracil. The Eastern Cooperative Oncology Group subsequently compared this combination to streptozocin plus doxorubicin[72] and reported a significantly higher response rate (69% versus 45%), time to progression (median, 20 months versus 7 months), and OS (median, 2.2 years versus 1.4 years) for streptozocin plus doxorubicin than for streptozocin plus 5-FU. Based on these data, combination chemotherapy with streptozocin-based regimens is considered the standard treatment option by many.

However, two small retrospective series have recently cast doubt on the value of streptozocin-based chemotherapy. Each of these studies examined only 16 patients. Both reported a disappointing radiologic response rate of only 6%.[74,75] This 10-fold difference in response rates has aroused considerable controversy as to the role of chemotherapy in treating pNETs. Some of the disparity in response rate may be accounted for by differences in response criteria. For example, in a study reported by Eriksson et al.,[76] the response rates based on either decreased biochemical parameters or decreased tumor measurement were 36% for streptozocin plus doxorubicin and 58% for streptozocin plus 5-FU. When only radiologic response was counted, the respective response rates were 8% and 32%.[76]

A chemotherapeutic combination of 5-FU, streptozocin, and doxorubicin was studied in two small trials with 10 and 12 patients, and response rates were 40% and 55%, respectively.[53] In light of the continuing controversy regarding the role of chemotherapy in the management of pNETs, a larger retrospective study examined the outcome of 84 consecutive patients treated with the 5-FU-doxorubicin-streptozocin combination and observed a response rate of 39%.[53] The median PFS in that series was 18 months, and median OS was 37 months.

Dacarbazine- and Temozolomide-Based Chemotherapy. Dacarbazine was initially studied in a phase 2 study that included 42 patients with pNETs. A response rate of 33% was observed.[77] Temozolomide is an oral alkylating agent that metabolizes to the same active metabolite as dacarbazine, 5-(3-methyl-triazeno) imidazole-4-carboxamide. While a number of temozolomide-based doublets have been reported in clinical trials or retrospective series, the activity of single-agent temozolomide has not been prospectively evaluated.[18–20] In one large series, 18 (34%) of 53 patients with pNETs had objective response following temozolomide-based chemotherapy.[78] Although temozolomide-based therapy is generally well tolerated, absolute lymphopenia may occur and has been associated with opportunistic infections.[79] These studies suggest that temozolomide may have activity in pNETs. A randomized study comparing temozolomide versus temozolomide plus capecitabine is ongoing.

Cytotoxic chemotherapy continues to play an important role in the management of pNETs.

Peptide Receptor Radiotherapy

The presence of somatostatin receptors in high density on tumors cells has led to the development of peptide receptor radiotherapy for NETs. Early studies with ^{111}In-, ^{90}Y-, or ^{177}Lu-labeled somatostatin analogues have reported promising results in the control of hormone-associated symptoms.[80] The earliest studies were carried out with [^{111}In-DTPA^0] octreotide. Although symptomatic improvements were reported, objective tumor responses were rarely observed. Subsequently, ^{90}Yttrium was linked to octreotide to create [^{90}Y-DOTA^0,Tyr^3] octreotide. Several studies were carried out in patients with NETs and produced response rates of 10% to 30%.[80] In the largest prospective study of 90 patients with NETs, only a modest response rate of 4% was observed.[81]

Finally, a number of European centers are now using octreotate that substitutes the C-terminal threoninol with threonine. Octreotate is linked to ^{177}Lutetium to create 177Lu-DOTA0,Tyr3 octreotate. In the largest reported series, a response rate of 30% was found among a subset of 310 patients. However, if intent-to-treat analysis were performed, the objective response would be approximately 18%.[82] In general, expected toxicities with peptide receptor radiotherapy included nausea, vomiting, abdominal pain, cytopenia, and hair loss. More serious side effects, including renal failure, leukemia, and myelodysplastic syndrome, have also been reported. Large-scale random assignment trials are needed to define its role in the management of pNETs.

Liver-Directed Regional Therapy

Because the liver is the most common and sometimes the only site of metastasis, the development of liver-directed therapeutic approaches for pNETs is of obvious interest. These treatment approaches are generally palliative. In the absence of a hormonal syndrome, typical indications for liver-directed therapy include right upper quadrant pain, early satiety due to gastric compression by an enlarged left hepatic lobe, and the need to control slowly progressive but bulky disease.

Hepatic Artery Embolization and Chemoembolization. Hepatic artery embolization takes advantage of the liver's dual blood supply. The normal liver derives most of its blood supply from the portal circulation. pNET metastases, however, receive most of their blood supply from the hepatic artery. Thus, interruption of the blood supply from the hepatic artery preferentially causes ischemic necrosis of the metastases while sparing most of the normal liver. Currently, most procedures for occlusion of the hepatic artery involve the percutaneous intra-arterial infusion of small particles. The choice of embolic material varies by center and may include lipiodol or ethiodized oil, small plastic particles, or gelatin foam particles. Comparative studies of various embolic materials are lacking. In performing hepatic artery chemoembolization, cytotoxic agents are administered intra-arterially before the vessels are embolized, as this approach has the potential to enable delivery of a higher chemotherapy dose to liver metastases.

Most published studies of hepatic artery embolization or chemoembolization have included a mix of patients with carcinoids and pNETs. Studies have reported a wide range of response rates ranging from 8% to >60% using heterogeneous response criteria.[83,84] In a retrospective study from MD Anderson, where the outcome of patients with pNET were separately examined, the objective tumor response rate was 35%. When the bland embolization group was compared with the chemoembolization group, a trend was observed for improved response rate with the addition of chemotherapy (50% versus 25%; $p = 0.06$).[83] In a similar retrospective study of 67 patients with NETs (19 with pNETs) who underwent chemoembolization in France, investigators compared doxorubicin with streptozocin during embolization and reported a higher response rate with streptozocin-based chemoembolization after multivariate analyses.[85]

Based on these findings, we recommend hepatic artery chemoembolization in select patients with pNET with liver metastases. The procedure should be carried out in a hospital setting because treatment-related toxic effects are common and may be severe. A constellation of transient symptoms and laboratory abnormalities, sometimes referred to as "postembolization syndrome," occurs in most patients. These findings include abdominal pain, nausea, fever, fatigue, and elevated liver enzymes. Crises related to massive release of hormone(s) may occur in the presence of functional tumors; prophylactic administration of somatostatin analogues should always be considered. Major complications (even deaths) have been reported in clinical trials. To minimize the risk of hepatic insufficiency, embolization should be carried out in one liver lobe at a time. In patients with bulky disease or poor liver function, more limited embolization of liver segments should be considered; experience is clearly very important in the use of this treatment modality.

More recently, radioactive microsphere embolization is emerging as a well-tolerated outpatient procedure providing symptom relief and varying response rates.[86–88] However, prospective studies are lacking in patients with NETs and specifically those with pNETs.

Hepatic Metastasectomy and Transplantation. Because of the relatively indolent behavior of the disease, aggressive surgical resection has a role in the management of metastatic islet cell carcinoma. The largest published experience with pNETs involving liver resection was included in a series of 170 patients with NET at Mayo Clinic.[89] A total of 52 pNETs were included in this study. A separate analysis of pNETs was not performed, but the OS rate for all 170 patients was reported to be 61% and 35% at 5 and 10 years, respectively. It is, however, also clear from this study that liver resection is not curative in most patients; the disease recurrence rate was 85% at 5 years.[89]

We encourage resection for patients with a solitary metastasis. For patients with more extensive but still resectable disease, we advocate resection for those tumors with favorable biologic characteristics. Liver resection should be avoided in patients with a high-grade histologic subtype. A period of systemic chemotherapy may be used as part of a test-of-time approach to select patients whose disease is less likely to progress and who are therefore more likely to benefit from aggressive surgical intervention.

For those with clearly unresectable liver metastases, there has been some experience, although limited, with hepatic transplantation. However, following liver transplantation, survival of patients with pNETs was found to be inferior to that of patients who had carcinoid tumors (3-year survivals of 8% versus 80%).[90] Given the upfront operative risk and, as yet, the lack of data supporting a survival benefit, hepatic transplantation for the management of pNETs should be considered investigational. Further, the challenge of limited organ availability (at least in the United States) makes liver transplantation for pNET an unrealistic option in the absence of a living-related donor.

Radiofrequency Ablation. Given the natural history of nonfunctional pNETs, most patients are diagnosed with extensive disease. Those with unresectable disease often have diffuse liver involvement and/or have the primary tumor intact. The majority of these patients should receive systemic therapy or chemoembolization. Occasionally, patients may have liver metastases that are unresectable but still small and few enough to allow for an ablative approach. RFA can be carried out during laparoscopy, laparotomy, or via a percutaneous approach. Although RFA has not been systematically compared with other treatment modalities, an anecdotal description of the clinical benefit of RFA has been reported. In one series of 34 patients, including 9 with pNETs who underwent laparoscopic RFA, 79% of patients with symptoms at baseline reported either complete resolution or a significant reduction of tumor-related symptoms.[91]

Therapeutic Strategy for Advanced Unresectable Pancreatic Neuroendocrine Tumors

The past decade has seen rapid advances in the therapeutic options for pNETs. Agents approved by the US Food and Drug Administration include streptozocin, everolimus, and sunitinib. Recently, the somatostatin analogue lanreotide has also demonstrated significant antiproliferative activity in a phase 3 study. Surgical resection, regional therapy, and therapies not yet approved, including peptide receptor radiotherapy, selective internal radiotherapy, and temozolomide, offer additional options. Studies have also been completed in heterogeneous populations with the lanreotide study being conducted in an indolent (stable disease) population while the everolimus and sunitinib were studied among patients with progressive disease. None of these options have been compared in head-to-head clinical trials.

While the rarity of the pNETs precludes the large studies necessary to answer treatment sequencing questions, the relatively longer survival means patients will likely go through many of these options in varying sequence. A conceptual framework for choosing therapy at each stage should take into account the aggressiveness of the tumor, the burden (volume) of disease, and any symptoms due to tumor burden or hormonal secretion (Fig. 85.3). Depending on these variables, decisions can be made to prioritize the goals of therapy. For example, for a patient with low-volume, stable, and asymptomatic disease, quality of life can be prioritized by expectant observation or treatment with somatostatin analogues. Cytotoxic chemotherapy, on the other hand, may offer relief to a patient with bulky, progressive, and symptomatic disease. Everolimus or sunitinib can be suitable options for most patients in between the two extremes. The choice between everolimus and sunitinib can be considered based on the strength of published evidence, secretory status, and the matching of patient comorbidities to the adverse event profile of the drug. For example, everolimus has been more extensively studied among treatment-naïve patients and patients who have failed prior chemotherapy. It may also be preferred among patients with secretory (functional) tumors. Based on its safety profile, sunitinib would be a better choice for patients with uncontrolled diabetes or poor pulmonary function.

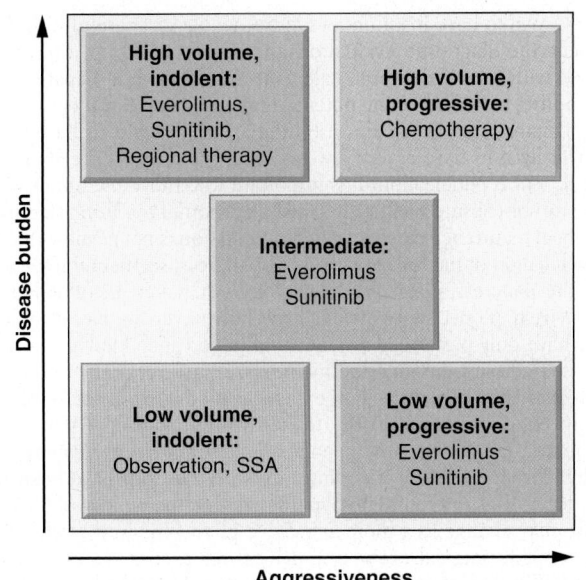

Figure 85.3 Management of patient with unresectable pancreatic neuroendocrine tumors. SSA, somatostatin analogue.

Conversely, everolimus may be safer in patients with hypertension or a history of heart disease.

Functional Tumors

Gastrinoma

Diagnosis and Management of Localized Disease. Gastrinoma, or Zollinger-Ellison syndrome (ZES), is a rare disease caused by a NET (gastrinoma) in the pancreas or duodenum. The hypersecretion of gastrin results in uncontrolled stimulation of parietal cells and production of gastric acid causing refractory peptic ulcer disease. Consequently, most patients have a long history of ulcers, abdominal pain, diarrhea, severe gastroesophageal reflux, and prolonged use of acid-suppressive medication and/or a history of gastric or duodenal surgery. However, the diagnosis of ZES is becoming more difficult owing to the frequent use of proton pump inhibitors (PPI), which usually control the symptoms of excess acid while the medication is taken.[92] Importantly, the vast majority of patients who are found to have an elevated level of serum gastrin do not have a gastrinoma. Hypergastrinemia is most commonly caused by acid-suppressive medications, especially PPIs. If the serum gastrin level is still elevated 1 week after the patient has stopped acid-suppressive therapy, it is then important to measure gastric pH. Basal gastric acid output analysis is not available in most centers, and gastric pH is rarely measured at the time of upper endoscopy (although at that time, the patient is usually tested for infection with *Helicobacter pylori*, which can also cause hypergastrinemia). Thus, the easiest way to measure gastric pH is to simply place a nasogastric tube and aspirate the gastric contents. These contents can be placed on litmus paper and the pH estimated; patients with ZES should have a gastric pH of <2. Elevated serum gastrin level and elevated gastric pH suggest a normal response of the gastric G cells (which produce gastrin) to parietal cell dysfunction associated with achlorhydria, atrophic gastritis, and pernicious anemia.

Patients with sporadic ZES usually have a fasting gastrin level of >600 pg/ml, and virtually all patients have a gastrin level of ≥100 pg/ml.[93] A serum gastrin ≥1,000 pg/ml or 10-fold above the normal range, and a gastric pH ≤2 secures the diagnosis of ZES. In patients with gastrin levels between 100 pg/ml and 1,000 pg/ml

and a gastric pH ≤2, a secretin or calcium stimulation test should be considered. A positive secretin test is associated with a postinjection serum gastrin level increase of >200 pg/ml, and a positive calcium stimulation test with a postinjection serum gastrin level increase of >395 pg/ml.[93]

Gastrinomas may reside in the duodenum (most often in the proximal duodenum) or pancreas, with duodenal location being the most common. Duodenal tumors are usually small (often <1 cm in diameter) and rarely associated with liver metastases. When located in the pancreas, gastrinomas are usually found in the pancreatic head or uncinate process; in the pancreas, that is to the right of the superior mesenteric vessels. Serum gastrin levels correlate with the extent of disease and are highest in those patients with locally advanced or metastatic disease.

Patients suspected to have ZES should be managed at a referral center experienced in the diagnosis and management of this disease. Once the diagnosis is established biochemically, tumor localization studies should be performed as part of the preoperative evaluation; these include upper endoscopy with EUS of the pancreatic head and duodenum, multidetector CT, and somatostatin receptor scintigraphy.[92,94] Because of the delay in diagnosing ZES in most patients combined with the improvements in imaging studies and EUS, gastrinomas seen today are usually successfully localized. When all localization studies are negative, the gastrinoma is most likely in the duodenum, which must be opened surgically (duodenotomy) to successfully locate and remove the tumor. For pancreatic gastrinomas, the operation is based on the anatomy of the tumor and may consist of enucleation or pancreaticoduodenectomy. Consistent with the operative management of most neuroendocrine carcinomas, regional lymphadenectomy is critically important. If the entire pancreatic head and duodenum are removed, regional lymphadenectomy is fairly easy to accomplish. If a less radical resection is performed, the lymph nodes located in the peripancreatic region, adjacent to the hepatic artery, and within the porta hepatis should be removed.

Management of Advanced Gastrinoma. As with other functional pNETs, the management of malignant gastrinoma has two goals: management of gastrin hypersecretion and its potential complications, and management of metastatic disease similar to the concern with advanced nonfunctional pNETs. Here, we will focus on issues unique to gastrinomas.

Prior to effective therapy for the control of gastric acid secretion, the principal therapy for ZES was gastrectomy to prevent gastric ulceration. Left unchecked, excessive acid secretion would frequently lead to massive gastrointestinal hemorrhage or gastric perforation. Early medical therapy for ZES included the use of histamine 2 receptor blockers such as cimetidine, ranitidine, and famotidine. The introduction of PPIs brought significant advances in the management of ZES, allowing for once or twice daily dosing. The dose of PPIs required to manage ZES is significantly higher than typically used in idiopathic peptic ulcer disease. In addition to careful monitoring for the absence of symptoms of acid hypersecretion, we have a low threshold for checking gastric pH prior to the next dose of PPI.

Another aspect that deserves special attention in patients with advanced gastrinoma is the development of type II gastric carcinoids in the setting of MEN1-associated ZES. These gastric carcinoids are often small, multifocal, and of low malignant potential. Occasionally, they can also become large, involve the stomach diffusely, and cause symptoms. When few in number, they can often be excised endoscopically. Regression of gastric carcinoids has been described in cases where somatostatin analogues or other treatment targeting the gastrinoma successfully reduced gastrin levels in a sustained manner.[95] Because gastric carcinoids are rarely seen in patients with sporadic ZES, the development of gastric carcinoids requires more than just hypergastrinemia (such as pernicious anemia or an additional genetic defect as is present in MEN1) and is likely unrelated to chronic administration of PPIs.

Insulinoma

Diagnosis and Management of Localized Disease. Insulinomas are seldom malignant and represent the most common functioning pNET. If metastatic disease is not found at the time of initial diagnosis, it is unlikely to develop in the future.[96] It is unknown whether this unique feature of insulinomas results from underlying tumor biology or simply because, owing to their profound symptom complex, these tumors are virtually always surgically excised early, when they are small. As with all functioning and nonfunctioning tumors of the pancreas, insulinoma may occur either as a unifocal sporadic event or as part of MEN1.[97] The uncontrolled secretion of insulin results in hyperglycemia, manifested by neuroglycopenic symptoms such as blurred vision, confusion, and abnormal behavior, which may progress to loss of consciousness and seizure. In response to hypoglycemia, the body releases catecholamines, which elicit perspiration, anxiety, palpitations, and hunger. Most patients with insulinoma associate the intake of food with the resolution of such symptoms very early in the disease process; this likely accounts for the weight gain experienced by most patients with insulinoma.

The diagnosis of insulinoma syndrome is established by supervised fasting of the patient, including laboratory evaluation and clinical observation. Serum levels of plasma glucose, C-peptide, proinsulin, insulin, and sulfonylurea are measured at intervals of 6 to 8 hours and when symptoms develop, patients with insulinoma have an insulin level >3 μIU/ml (usually >6 μIU/ml) when their blood glucose is <40 to 45 mg/dL. The insulin-to-glucose ratio is ≥0.3 reflecting the inappropriate secretion of insulin at the time of hypoglycemia. During the production of insulin, C-peptide is cleaved from proinsulin and thus, both are elevated in patients with insulinoma. In contrast, exogenous insulin does not contain C-peptide; therefore, an elevated insulin level combined with no detectable C-peptide would indicate exogenous administration of insulin. Detectable levels of sulfonylurea would indicate the administration of oral medications to induce hypoglycemia. When the patient is under observation as part of a supervised fast, symptomatic hypoglycemia and a serum glucose level <45 mg/dL should be treated with 1 mg of intravenous glucagon. If the hypoglycemia is insulin mediated, this will cause the release of glucose from the liver, resulting in an elevation of serum glucose (usually by 20 mg/dL) and the rapid resolution of symptoms.

In contrast to gastrinomas, which usually occur in the duodenum, pancreatic head, or uncinate process, insulinomas do not develop in the duodenum and may occur anywhere throughout the pancreas. In the absence of MEN1, insulinomas, similar to gastrinomas, are usually unifocal. Once the biochemical diagnosis is established, localization studies performed as part of the preoperative evaluation include contrast-enhanced, multidetector CT and usually upper endoscopy with EUS of the pancreas. In our practice, these studies will localize the overwhelming majority of sporadic insulinomas. For the very rare patient in whom tumor localization is not successful, we proceed with a regionalization study to determine whether the tumor is located to the right or left of the mesenteric vessels. Regionalization of an insulinoma is performed with selective arterial calcium stimulation and hepatic vein sampling.[98] Calcium is used as a secretagogue for insulin and is injected into the gastroduodenal artery, SMA, and splenic artery; a serum sample for insulin measurement is obtained from the right hepatic vein. An elevation of insulin in the hepatic vein following selective arterial injection regionalizes the insulinoma to that portion of the pancreas injected with calcium. It is therefore possible to determine whether the insulinoma is in the pancreatic head or uncinate process (elevation of hepatic vein insulin following calcium infusion of the gastroduodenal artery and/or SMA) or in the body or tail of the pancreas (elevation of insulin following calcium infusion into the splenic artery). Because tumor localization with a combination of multidetector CT and EUS is so successful, when these methods fail to localize the tumor in a patient

presumed to have insulinoma syndrome, we first carefully double check the diagnostic evaluation and if confirmed, we then proceed with selective arterial calcium stimulation and hepatic vein sampling to minimize the potential for an unsuccessful operation.

Because nonmetastatic insulinomas are thought to be benign (or at least to have a very low malignant potential), the standard treatment is enucleation. It is important to remove the tumor with the tumor capsule and not to leave a portion of the tumor behind, as local recurrence can occur.[99] If enucleation is not possible due to the location of the tumor within the pancreas, segmental resection of the pancreas, distal pancreatectomy, or pancreaticoduodenectomy may be necessary. In our experience over the past 20 years, we have only performed a handful of pancreaticoduodenectomies for sporadic insulinoma due to large size and proximity to the intrapancreatic bile duct. Large defects in the pancreas resulting from enucleation are usually treated with a Roux-en-Y pancreaticojejunostomy to prevent a pancreatic leak at the enucleation site. Metachronous distant metastases are very rare but have been reported.[100] It is interesting to hypothesize that the biology of the disease may change to a more aggressive phenotype in the setting of incomplete surgical excision and local recurrence. In contrast to the findings of a few reports in the literature,[100] we have not seen a patient with a surgically excised, nonmetastatic, isolated insulinoma develop metachronous tumor recurrence in a distant organ. The patients with metastatic insulinoma seen by these authors had liver metastases with or without bone metastases at the time of diagnosis.

Management of Advanced Insulinoma. In rare cases, insulinomas can be metastatic at diagnosis. These cases are challenging to manage often because of refractory hypoglycemia. There is no data to suggest that insulinomas respond differently to systemic or liver-directed therapy. Thus, the previously discussed strategies outlined for nonfunctional tumors can be applied. We will focus here on the aspects of malignant insulinoma that require special attention.

Glycemic control is a key aspect of managing malignant insulinomas. Mild symptoms sometimes can be controlled by diet. Patients may need to eat frequently; family members or caregivers may need to wake the patient at night for a snack to avoid early morning hypoglycemia. In selected cases, enteral feeding tubes may be required to provide continuous nocturnal caloric support. Medical therapy may include diazoxide, an antihypertensive agent known to increase blood sugar. It is typically administered in doses of 50 to 300 mg per day. Side effects include edema, weight gain, renal impairment, and hirsutism. Glucagon may also have a role in the management of insulinomas. A glucagon pen may be given to the patient's family and caregiver to be used in emergent cases. Not all insulinomas respond well to glucagon. We suggest that a test dose be given under supervision during a hypoglycemic episode before the drug is prescribed. While all of the aforementioned drugs may help control symptoms, eventual resistance may develop. These drugs are perhaps best used to maintain glycemic control while other therapeutic strategies are being applied.

Somatostatin analogues such as octreotide may be helpful for the control of insulin release, but they can also suppress counterregulatory hormones such as growth hormones, glucagon, and catecholamines. In this situation, somatostatin analogues can lead to worsening of hypoglycemia.[101] Therefore, we recommend that short-acting somatostatin analogues be initiated under direct medical supervision. Glucose and insulin levels should be checked before and after injection to assess the analogue's effect on hormonal production before committing the patient to long-term outpatient therapy.

Despite these measures, refractory hypoglycemia frequently occurs and can be difficult to manage. It has been recently observed that such patients often respond to the mTOR inhibitor everolimus. Data suggest that insulin triggers its own production and release via the insulin receptor.[102,103] The mTOR pathway mediates signal transduction downstream of the insulin receptor and mTOR inhibitors block insulin stimulated insulin synthesis, release, and proliferation.[102,103] In a series of four consecutive patients with malignant hypoglycemia treated with everolimus, all four patients experienced dramatic improvements in glycemic control.[104] Since this initial report, the efficacy of everolimus for the treatment of insulinoma has been confirmed in several case series.[105,106]

Finally, aggressive therapy targeting the tumor is needed. As malignant insulinomas can often be indolent in terms of tumor growth, surgical resection, hepatic artery chemoembolization, and RFA can all be considered. Streptozocin-based chemotherapy should also be considered based on tumor location and extent as data suggest that streptozocin is toxic to insulin-producing cells. In addition to its cytotoxic effect, streptozocin can decrease insulin production in beta cells. Indeed, our experience with some patients indicates that streptozocin may "turn off" the production of insulin for years, even in the absence of tumor response. Chemotherapy, however, may require intensive supportive care because the nausea, vomiting, and anorexia associated with treatment may transiently worsen hypoglycemia.

Rare Functional Endocrine Tumors

In addition to gastrinomas and insulinomas, several other less common functional tumors deserve special consideration. These include VIPomas, glucagonomas, somatostatinomas, adrenocorticotropic-secreting tumors, and parathyroid hormone–related peptide-secreting tumors. Similar to other functional pNETs, the bulk of these rare tumors are well differentiated (low Ki67 index). For the most part, the workup and management of these tumors are similar to those of nonfunctional pNETs. Thus, only the unique aspects of these tumors will be briefly discussed here.

VIPoma

VIPomas are the cause of the classic Verner-Morrison syndrome.[107] These endocrine tumors secrete vasoactive intestinal peptide, which can cause watery diarrhea, hypokalemia, and achlorhydria. Diarrhea in patients with VIPomas is often insidious at onset but extreme by the time the patient comes to diagnosis. Patients can have more than 20 bowel movements a day, with a daily stool volume exceeding 3 L. Thus, fluid and electrolyte replacement is often needed at the time of diagnosis. In adults, most VIPomas arise from the pancreas. In children, however, most vasoactive intestinal peptide–secreting tumors arise from an extrapancreatic location.

Control of diarrhea is an important part of management. These tumors are often quite sensitive, at least initially, to somatostatin analogues[108]; octreotide can promptly control diarrhea in 80% to 90% of patients. However, over time many patients will escape pharmacologic control. Dose escalation can be helpful in some cases. With short-acting octreotide, a dose of 50 to 400 mcg per day is typically used. With depot formulation, octreotide LAR doses exceeding 30 mg every 3 weeks have been advocated by some. Somatostatin analogues often cause exocrine pancreatic insufficiency, which can lead to malabsorptive diarrhea; pancrelipase and gastric acid suppression should be used in all patients who are receiving somatostatin analogues. Because of its toxicity, interferon is rarely used in the frontline setting, but it may have a role in cases refractory to somatostatin analogues. In general, measures aimed at cytoreduction should be initiated whenever possible.

Glucagonoma

Glucagon is a 29-amino acid peptide that causes glycogenolysis, gluconeogenesis, ketogenesis, lipolysis, and catecholamine secretion. Patients typically present with a syndrome that includes diabetes and a characteristic rash known as necrolytic migratory erythema. Weight loss, diarrhea, glossitis, and angular stomatitis

have also been reported.[43] These patients typically also have amino acid depletion due to the high level of glucagon. Somatostatin analogues may have a role in the management of the hormonal syndrome in patients with unresectable tumors.[109] Oral hypoglycemic agents and insulin can be used to control the diabetes. Necrolytic migratory erythema is thought to be related at least in part to amino acid depletion.[110] Thus, amino acid and zinc supplementation may also be helpful.[111]

Somatostatinoma

Somatotstatinomas are very rare functional endocrine tumors that can arise from the pancreas or the duodenum. Because of the insidious and nonspecific nature of the symptoms, most somatostatinomas are diagnosed at an advanced stage. Patients typically present with symptoms including diabetes, diarrhea, and jaundice due to biliary obstruction. Somatostatinomas may be associated with von Recklinghausen disease (neurofibromatosis); these tumors are usually duodenal or ampullary in origin, are less likely to be associated with a hormonal syndrome, and are usually small and localized (nonmetastatic) at the time of diagnosis.[112] The principles of management for somatostatinomas parallel those of nonfunctional pNETs.

Adrenocorticotropic-Secreting Tumors

Adrenocorticotropic hormone–secreting tumors are also among the rare functional tumors of the pancreas. Patients with adrenocorticotropic-secreting tumors often present with florid Cushing syndrome due to ectopic production of adrenocorticotropic hormone. Induction chemotherapy in these patients is fraught with difficulties owing to the patient's hypercortisolism causing immunosuppression and a debilitated state. Initial management should be aimed at controlling corticosteroid production. Metyrapone, ketoconazole, and mitotane tend to be more effective in this setting than for adrenal cortical carcinoma and can be used to suppress excess cortisol production. In rare cases, bilateral adrenalectomy may be needed.

ADDITIONAL CLINICAL CONSIDERATIONS

Hereditary Syndromes

It is known that pNETs can occur in the setting of several genetic syndromes. These include MEN1, tuberous sclerosis, neurofibromatosis, and von Hippel-Lindau disease (VHL). MEN1 is discussed in greater detail elsewhere in this book. Here, we will limit our discussion to special considerations involved in the surgical management of MEN1-related pNETs and selected aspects of tuberous sclerosis, neurofibromatosis, and VHL as they relate to pNETs. As in all genetic cancer syndromes, genetic counseling and cancer screening are necessary aspects of optimal patient management.

Multiple Endocrine Neoplasia Type 1

With regard to patients with MEN1 who have nonfunctioning pNETs, their surgical management remains controversial. Due to the characteristic multifocality of MEN1-associated pNETs and the desire to avoid total pancreatectomy, some investigators have discouraged early surgery in patients with MEN1.[113] It has been suggested that surgery for nonfunctioning pNETs should be limited to those tumors >2 to 3 cm in diameter.[98,113–118] In a single institution series, a trend was shown for larger tumors to be associated with the presence of synchronous distant metastases at the time of diagnosis.[119] None of the 19 pNETs that were 2.5 cm or less, in maximum dimension, had distant metastases at the time of diagnosis compared with 5 (23%) of the 22 pNETs >2.5 cm ($p = 0.05$).

However, tumor size may not be a completely reliable predictor of malignant behavior, as metastatic disease may be present in patients with MEN1 even when the primary tumors are small.[120]

Thompson[121,122] was the first to advocate a specific surgical procedure in patients with MEN1 with nonfunctioning pNETs >1 cm in diameter to include distal subtotal pancreatectomy, enucleation of any identified lesions in the pancreatic head or uncinate process, and regional lymphadenectomy.[121,122] Enthusiasm for this approach has waned largely due to an improved understanding of both the complex biology and often unpredictable natural history of MEN1-associated pNETs.

We currently operate on all patients with MEN1 who have evidence of a pNET(s) on CT imaging that are in the range of 1.5 to 2 cm in size or larger, or have demonstrated an increase in size on serial imaging. We agree that preservation of islet cell mass is important, especially in young patients, to hopefully prevent the complications of insulin-dependent diabetes associated with total pancreatectomy. The goal of the first operation is to delay the need for total pancreatectomy assuming that some patients may develop metachronous neoplasms in the remaining pancreas and require completion total pancreatectomy. In patients with large tumors within the head of the pancreas that are not amenable to enucleation, pancreaticoduodenectomy (with preservation of a portion of the pancreatic body and tail when possible) is an appropriate alternative. The extent to which removal of the duodenum and perhaps distal stomach reduce the level of trophic gastrointestinal hormones and prevent/retard tumor growth (in the remaining pancreas and in distant sites) is at present an unsupported theory based on anecdotal clinical observation. It is interesting to speculate if the historical emphasis on avoiding pancreaticoduodenectomy in MEN1-associated pNET may be misguided.

von Hippel-Lindau Syndrome

VHL is an autosomal dominant inherited familial cancer syndrome that was initially discovered in 1927.[123] It is associated with a variety of neoplasms, frequently including retinal, cerebellar, and spinal hemangioblastoma, as well as renal cell carcinoma, pheochromocytoma, and pNETs. The vHL gene is located on chromosome 3p26-p25. Tumors arising in the setting of VHL are often vascular likely due to the role of the vHL gene in regulating angiogenesis.

pNETs occur in approximately 15% of patients with VHL.[124] However, the vHL gene may be involved in sporadic cases of pNETs. Allelic deletion at chromosome 3p, the site of the vHL gene has also been described to occur frequently in sporadic pNETs.[30,125]

Tuberous Sclerosis and Neurofibromatosis

Tuberous sclerosis and neurofibromatosis are two other hereditary cancer syndromes associated with the development of pNETs. The genes responsible for tuberous sclerosis, TSC-1 and TSC-2, are located on chromosomes 9q34 and 16p13.3, respectively, and code for the proteins hamartin and tuberin. TSC1/2 complex is an inhibitor of mTOR, which is a key regulator of cellular proliferation and survival. TSC1/2 are normally expressed in neuroendocrine cells.[126] Although benign hamartomas are the most common manifestation of mutations in TSC1/2, patients with defects in the TSC2 gene have tuberous sclerosis and are known to develop islet cell carcinoma.[127]

Neurofibromatosis type 1 (NF1), also known as Von Recklinghausen disease, is an autosomal dominant disease associated with the development of cutaneous neurofibromas and skin lesions known as café au lait spots. The gene responsible for NF1 codes for the protein neurofibromin 1 and is located on chromosome 17. It has recently been discovered that NF1 regulates the activity of TSC2. The loss of NF1 in neurofibromatosis leads to constitutive mTOR activation and tumor formation.[128] NF1 is associated with the development of NETs in the region of the duodenum and ampulla of Vater.[127] Many of the endocrine tumors that arise from Von Recklinghausen disease (NF1) are somatostatinomas.

High-Grade Neuroendocrine Carcinoma

High-grade neuroendocrine carcinomas (also known as poorly differentiated neuroendocrine carcinomas)[129] rarely arise from the pancreas. These aggressive tumors are characterized by early systemic dissemination and rapid growth. Sometimes also described as small-cell carcinoma or large cell NET, high-grade neuroendocrine carcinomas share a similar pattern of clinical behavior with small-cell carcinomas of the lung. Although the diagnosis of poorly differentiated carcinoma is usually straightforward, when the diagnosis is made by FNA, the grade of the tumor may not be specified.

Owing to the rarity of these tumors, little prospective data is available to guide management. Much of the current practice has been based on experience with small-cell lung carcinoma. High-grade NETs of the pancreas are often diagnosed at advanced stages. We recommend induction chemotherapy even for localized potentially resectable cases due to the aggressive nature of this disease and the high rate of relapse.

These rare but aggressive tumors are initially chemosensitive. Treatment generally parallels the therapy developed for small-cell lung cancer. Platinum-based chemotherapy is recommended in the front-line setting; two-drug combinations such as etoposide plus cisplatin or irinotecan plus cisplatin have shown activity.[130,131]

SURGERY PITFALLS

For functioning tumors, it remains critically important to separate the diagnostic and the tumor localization phases of the evaluation. It is tempting to proceed with localization studies before the diagnosis of ZES or insulinoma is firmly established. In such cases, an incidental finding on cross-sectional imaging (now quite common due to the sensitivity of CT/MRI and their overuse) may prompt an ill-advised surgical procedure. If the diagnosis is biochemically confirmed but localization studies are negative, one should consider referring the patient to a specialty center and an experienced endocrine surgeon.

When dealing with a large, borderline resectable/locally advanced primary tumor (pNET) where there is a technical option for tumor removal, we frequently consider preoperative induction chemotherapy. In such patients, as well as those with both a pNET and liver metastases, determining the patient's candidacy for surgery has become very complex. For example, in the patient who has both local disease and liver metastases, we may follow induction chemotherapy with a two-staged surgical approach if imaging studies suggest that an adequate portion of the liver is uninvolved (or minimally involved) with disease. At the first operation, the primary tumor is removed, and the liver bisegment (or lobe) that is to remain in place is cleared of disease. This may then be followed by portal vein embolization of the hepatic lobe to be removed, with a second operation planned for liver resection.[132] Such multidisciplinary management requires a dedicated group of physicians and an infrastructure that can assist patients with treatment-related complications such as biliary stent occlusion, nutritional depletion, gastrointestinal and hematologic toxicity, and surgery-related morbidity.

Finally, all physicians must remember that pNETs usually grow slowly and, therefore, if patients have a good performance status, they will usually survive longer than we anticipate despite the presence of locally advanced or metastatic disease. Because of this, treatment-related mortality (especially surgery induced) should be avoided. An ill-advised operation with a bad outcome in an otherwise healthy patient (of any age and especially those of young age where the temptation/pressure to operate is often great) should be considered an act of poor judgment rather than heroism.

SELECTED REFERENCES

The full reference list can be accessed at lwwhealthlibrary.com/oncology.

1. Yao JC, Hassan M, Phan A, et al. One hundred years after "carcinoid": epidemiology of and prognostic factors for neuroendocrine tumors in 35,825 cases in the United States. *J Clin Oncol* 2008;26:3063–3072.

9. Crabtree JS, Scacheri PC, Ward JM, et al. A mouse model of multiple endocrine neoplasia, type 1, develops multiple endocrine tumors. *Proc Natl Acad Sci U S A* 2001;98:1118–1123.

10. Bertolino P, Tong WM, Galendo D, et al. Heterozygous Men1 mutant mice develop a range of endocrine tumors mimicking multiple endocrine neoplasia type 1. *Mol Endocrinol* 2003;17:1880–1892.

13. Vortmeyer AO, Huang S, Lubensky I, et al. Non-islet origin of pancreatic islet cell tumors. *J Clin Endocrinol Metab* 2004;89:1934–1938.

22. Khan MS, Luong TV, Watkins J, et al. A comparison of Ki-67 and mitotic count as prognostic markers for metastatic pancreatic and midgut neuroendocrine neoplasms. *Br J Cancer* 2013;108:1838–1845.

23. Boninsegna L, Panzuto F, Partelli S, et al. Malignant pancreatic neuroendocrine tumour: lymph node ratio and Ki67 are predictors of recurrence after curative resections. *Eur J Cancer* 2012;48:1608–1615.

24. Sorbye H, Welin S, Langer SW, et al. Predictive and prognostic factors for treatment and survival in 305 patients with advanced gastrointestinal neuroendocrine carcinoma (WHO G3): the NORDIC NEC study. *Ann Oncol* 2013;24:152–160.

27. Jiao Y, Shi C, Edil BH, et al. DAXX/ATRX, MEN1, and mTOR pathway genes are frequently altered in pancreatic neuroendocrine tumors. *Science* 2011;331:1199–1203.

30. Rigaud G, Missiaglia E, Moore PS, et al. High resolution allelotype of nonfunctional pancreatic endocrine tumors: identification of two molecular subgroups with clinical implications. *Cancer Res* 2001;61:285–292.

34. Karnik SK, Chen H, McLean GW, et al. Menin controls growth of pancreatic beta-cells in pregnant mice and promotes gestational diabetes mellitus. *Science* 2007;318:806–809.

35. Heaphy CM, de Wilde RF, Jiao Y, et al. Altered telomeres in tumors with ATRX and DAXX mutations. *Science* 2011;333:425.

36. Yao JC, Shah MH, Ito T, et al. Everolimus for advanced pancreatic neuroendocrine tumors. *N Engl J Med* 2011;364:514–523.

52. Bajetta E, Ferrari L, Martinetti A, et al. Chromogranin A, neuron specific enolase, carcinoembryonic antigen, and hydroxyindole acetic acid evaluation in patients with neuroendocrine tumors. *Cancer* 1999;86:858–865.

53. Kouvaraki MA, Ajani JA, Hoff P, et al. Fluorouracil, doxorubicin, and streptozocin in the treatment of patients with locally advanced and metastatic pancreatic endocrine carcinomas. *J Clin Oncol* 2004;22:4762–4771.

54. Yao JC, Lombard-Bohas C, Baudin E, et al. Daily oral everolimus activity in patients with metastatic pancreatic neuroendocrine tumors after failure of cytotoxic chemotherapy: a phase II trial. *J Clin Oncol* 2010;28:69–76.

56. Partelli S, Gaujoux S, Boninsegna L, et al. Pattern and clinical predictors of lymph node involvement in nonfunctioning pancreatic neuroendocrine tumors (NF-PanNETs). *JAMA Surg* 2013;148:932–939.

61. Solorzano CC, Lee JE, Pisters PW, et al. Nonfunctioning islet cell carcinoma of the pancreas: survival results in a contemporary series of 163 patients. *Surgery* 2001;130:1078–1085.

62. Mayo SC, Herman JM, Cosgrove D, et al. Emerging approaches in the management of patients with neuroendocrine liver metastasis: role of liver-directed and systemic therapies. *J Am Coll Surg* 2013;216:123–134.

64. Rinke A, Muller HH, Schade-Brittinger C, et al. Placebo-controlled, double-blind, prospective, randomized study on the effect of octreotide LAR in the control of tumor growth in patients with metastatic neuroendocrine midgut tumors: a report from the PROMID Study Group. *J Clin Oncol* 2009;27:4656–4663.

65. Caplin M, Ruszniewski P, Pavel ME, et al. A randomized double-blind placebo-controlled study of lanreotide antiproliferative response in patients with enteropancreatic neuroendocrine tumours (CLARINET), The European Cancer Congress. Amsterdam, EJC, 2013, pp abstract E17-7103.

67. Yao JC, Phan AT, Chang DZ, et al. Efficacy of RAD001 (everolimus) and octreotide LAR in advanced low- to intermediate-grade neuroendocrine tumors: Results of a phase II study. *J Clin Oncol* 2008;26:4311–4318.

68. Yao JC, Shah MH, Ito T, et al. Everolimus versus placebo in patients with advanced pancreatic neuroendocrine tumors (pNET) (RADIANT-3). *Ann Oncol* 2010;21.

69. Kulke MH, Lenz HJ, Meropol NJ, et al. Activity of sunitinib in patients with advanced neuroendocrine tumors. *J Clin Oncol* 2008;26:3403–3410.

70. Raymond E, Raoul J, Niccoli P, et al. Phase III, randomized, double-blind trial of sunitinib versus placebo in patients with progressibe well-differentiated pancreatic islet cell tumours. *Ann Oncol* 2009;20:vii1.

71. Moertel CG, Hanley JA, Johnson LA. Streptozocin alone compared with streptozocin plus fluorouracil in the treatment of advanced islet-cell carcinoma. *N Engl J Med* 1980;303:1189–1194.

72. Moertel CG, Lefkopoulo M, Lipsitz S, et al. Streptozocin-doxorubicin, streptozocin-fluorouracil or chlorozotocin in the treatment of advanced islet-cell carcinoma. *N Engl J Med* 1992;326:519–5230

78. Kulke M, Hornick J, Frauenhoffer C, et al. O6-methylguanine DNA methyltransferase deficiency and response to temozolomide-based therapy in patients with neuroendocrine tumors. *Clin Cancer Res* 2009;15:338–345.

81. Bushnell DL Jr, O'Dorisio TM, O'Dorisio MS, et al. 90Y-edotreotide for metastatic carcinoid refractory to octreotide. *J Clin Oncol* 2010;28:1652–1659.

82. Kwekkeboom DJ, de Herder WW, Kam BL, et al. Treatment with the radiolabeled somatostatin analog [177 Lu-DOTA 0,Tyr3]octreotate: toxicity, efficacy, and survival. *J Clin Oncol* 2008;26:2124–2130.

83. Gupta S, Johnson MM, Murthy R, et al. Hepatic arterial embolization and chemoembolization for the treatment of patients with metastatic neuroendocrine tumors. *Cancer* 2005;104:1590–1602.

86. Rhee TK, Lewandowski RJ, Liu DM, et al. 90Y Radioembolization for metastatic neuroendocrine liver tumors: preliminary results from a multi-institutional experience. *Ann Surg* 2008;247:1029–1035.

89. Sarmiento JM, Heywood G, Rubin J, et al. Surgical treatment of neuroendocrine metastases to the liver: a plea for resection to increase survival. *J Am Coll Surg* 2003;197:29–37.

95. Tomassetti P, Migliori M, Caletti GC, et al. Treatment of type II gastric carcinoid tumors with somatostatin analogues. *N Engl J Med* 2000;343:551–554.

98. Doppman JL, Chang R, Fraker DL, et al. Localization of insulinomas to regions of the pancreas by intra-arterial stimulation with calcium. *Ann Intern Med* 1995;123:269–273.

104. Kulke MH, Bergsland EK, Yao JC. Glycemic control in patients with insulinoma treated with everolimus. *N Engl J Med* 2009;360:195–197.

107. Verner JV, Morrison AB. Islet cell tumor and a syndrome of refractory watery diarrhea and hypokalemia. *Am J Med* 1958;25:374–380.

109. Altimari AF, Bhoopalam N, O'Dorsio T, et al. Use of a somatostatin analog (SMS 201-995) in the glucagonoma syndrome. *Surgery* 1986;100:989–996.

110. Norton JA, Kahn CR, Schiebinger R, et al. Amino acid deficiency and the skin rash associated with glucagonoma. *Ann Intern Med* 1979;91:213–215.

112. Mao C, Shah A, Hanson DJ, et al. Von Recklinghausen's disease associated with duodenal somatostatinoma: contrast of duodenal versus pancreatic somatostatinomas. *J Surg Oncol* 1995;59:67–73.

113. Norton JA, Fraker DL, Alexander HR, et al. Surgery to cure the Zollinger-Ellison syndrome. *N Engl J Med* 1999;341:635–644.

116. Doherty GM, Olson JA, Frisella MM, et al. Lethality of multiple endocrine neoplasia type I. *World J Surg* 1998;22:581–586; discussion 586–587.

118. Ruszniewski P, Rougier P, Roche A, et al. Hepatic arterial chemoembolization in patients with liver metastases of endocrine tumors. A prospective phase II study in 24 patients. *Cancer* 1993;71:2624–2630.

121. Thompson NW. Current concepts in the surgical management of multiple endocrine neoplasia type 1 pancreatic-duodenal disease. Results in the treatment of 40 patients with Zollinger-Ellison syndrome, hypoglycaemia or both. *J Intern Med* 1998;243:495–500.

130. Moertel CG, Kvols LK, O'Connell MJ, et al. Treatment of neuroendocrine carcinomas with combined etoposide and cisplatin. Evidence of major therapeutic activity in the anaplastic variants of these neoplasms. *Cancer* 1991;68:227–232.

PRACTICE OF ONCOLOGY

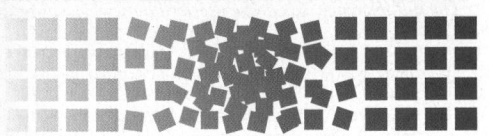

86 Carcinoid Tumors and the Carcinoid Syndrome

Jeffrey A. Norton and Pamela L. Kunz

INCIDENCE AND ETIOLOGY

Neuroendocrine tumors (NET) of the gastrointestinal tract (carcinoid tumors) are uncommon but are more common than other primary sites, followed by NETs of the lungs, thymus, and other less common sites like ovaries, testes, and hepatobiliary system.[1] The incidence of gastrointestinal (GI) NETs is 6.2 per 100,000 population and has been steadily increasing. The increasing incidence of NETs reported in many studies is likely multifactorial and includes increased awareness and improved endoscopic methods of detection.

Small bowel NETs (midgut carcinoids) are much more common than both foregut and hindgut.[2] The incidence is approximately 2 per 100,000 per year. In one study of 254 patients from Germany with GI NETs, the primary tumor was foregut, midgut, or hindgut in 44.1%, 43.7%, and 4.3%, respectively.[3] Midgut NETs can remain small (<1 cm) and still metastasize to regional lymph nodes and liver. Midgut carcinoids are the only primary site in which size does not directly correlate with metastatic disease, because these tumors may still spread despite a small size. Risk factors for the development of midgut carcinoid tumors include age, male sex, increased body mass index, and menopausal hormone therapy.[4]

As these tumors are indolent and patients survive a long time, the prevalence is quite high, making them the second most prevalent GI tract tumor, second only to colon cancer. Some are clinically silent and have been detected only at autopsy (incidence 8%). Further, patients with GI NETs have a higher risk of other noncarcinoid primary tumors.[5] The overall 5-year survival rate of all patients with GI NETs is 28.5%.

ANATOMY AND PATHOLOGY

In 1907, Oberndorfer first coined the term carcinoid, meaning "cancer-like," to describe a rare ileal tumor with less malignant behavior than the more commonly identified large bowel carcinomas. Now, it is clear that carcinoids are, indeed, malignant. They are derived from the diffuse neuroendocrine system that is composed of peptide- and amine-producing cells that may secrete different hormones depending on the site of origin.[6] The World Health Organization recently dropped the term carcinoid and now classifies these tumors as NETs, although carcinoid may likely remain in the vernacular.[7] NETs are composed of monotonous sheets of small round blue cells with uniform nuclei and cytoplasm.

The nomenclature, classification, and grading systems for NETs have historically been inconsistent, and there is currently no single system for NETs at all anatomic sites. Through critical evaluations of these systems, common principles have emerged.[8,9] Critical factors in NET pathology include key features that have been classified by various schema over the years. These are embryologic site of origin (foregut, midgut, hindgut), functional status (defined as hormone secretion associated with symptoms

of hormone excess), and grade. The recent 2010 World Health Organization pathology classification relies mainly on proliferation rates as measured by Ki67 antibody staining or mitotic index.[7] Low-grade tumors (grade 1) are the most common and have a mitotic index of fewer than two mitoses/10 high power field (hpf) and a Ki67 <3%. Intermediate-grade tumors (grade 2) have a mitotic index of 2 to 20 mitoses/10 hpf and a Ki67 3% to 20%. High-grade tumors (grade 3) have a mitotic index >20 mitoses/10 hpf and a Ki67 >20%. These numbers have clinical importance because extensive surgery including resection of locally advanced tumor and/or distant metastases is the treatment strategy of choice for low-grade tumors, whereas high-grade tumors are treated primarily with chemotherapy. Chromogranin A and synaptophysin immunostains identify proteins of neurosecretory granules and are specific immunologic markers for NETs. Other immunostains like gastrin and glucagon are sometimes performed but do not indicate whether a tumor is "functional" as defined by clinical symptoms of hormone excess. NET pathology guidelines have recently been updated and now recommend a set of minimum data elements to be included in all pathology reports for NETs[8,9] (Table 86.1).

Until recently, an understanding of the molecular basis of NETs has been elusive. Banck et al.[10] performed exome sequencing on 48 small intestine NETs. They reported an average of 0.1 somatic single nucleotide variants per 106 nucleotides (range, 0 to 0.59), mostly transitions (C>T and A>G). They discovered 197 protein-altering somatic single nucleotide variants affected mostly cancer genes, including FGFR2, MEN1, HOOK3, EZH2, MLF1, CARD11, VHL, NONO, and SMAD1. Alterations with potential therapeutic application were found in 35 patients, including SRC, SMAD family genes, AURKA, EGFR, HSP90, and PDGFR. Mutually exclusive amplification of AKT1 or AKT2 was the most common event in the 16 patients with alterations of phosphatidylinositol-3 kinase/protein kinase B/mammalian target of rapamycin (mTOR) signaling.[10]

Screening

The low NET incidence rates do not warrant population screening. For certain patients with an inherited predisposition for NETs (like in multiple endocrine neoplasia [MEN] syndromes), screening programs are often instituted. See Chapter 87 on MEN.

GENERAL PRINCIPLES OF NEUROENDOCRINE TUMOR DIAGNOSIS, STAGING, AND MANAGEMENT

General Diagnostic Principles

The diagnosis of GI and pulmonary NETs is often incidental, though patients with functional tumors can present with symptoms of hormone excess. The diagnostic approach for a patient with NETs is summarized by the North American

TABLE 86.1

Staging Criteria for Neuroendocrine Tumors

Grade	Low Grade	Intermediate Grade	High Grade
Old Terminology	Typical Carcinoid	Atypical Carcinoid	Small-Cell/ Large-Cell Carcinoma
Ki67	<3%	3% to 20%	>20%
Mitotic index	<2/10 hpf	2–20/10 hpf	>20/10 hpf
AJCC	T_1-T_2, N_0, M_0	T_3, N_1, M_0	$T_4 \pm M_1$
SEER	Localized	Regional	Distant

hpf, high power field; AJCC, American Joint Committee on Cancer; SEER, Surveillance, Epidemiology, and End Results.
AJCC definition: T_1 <2 cm, T_2 >2 cm, T_3 >4 cm, T_4 tumor extends outside structure. N_0 negative nodes, N_1 positive nodes, M_0 no distant metastases, M_1 distant metastases.

Neuroendocrine Tumor Society[11] and the National Comprehensive Cancer Network NET guidelines.[12]

Serum hormone markers are often elevated in NETs and can be a surrogate marker of symptoms of hormone excess or tumor growth, though none are sensitive enough to be used as a screening test. Chromogranin A levels are elevated in approximately 80% of patients with GI NETs; sensitivity is 75% and specificity is approximately 85%. Falsely positive elevated serum levels of chromogranin A may occur when patients take a commonly prescribed proton pump inhibitor (PPI) or H_2 receptor antagonist, so these medications should be discontinued for several days prior to testing and testing should be done fasting. Urine 5-hydroxyindoleacetic acid (5-HIAA), the primary metabolite of serotonin, is elevated in carcinoid syndrome. Test characteristics of this assay are sensitivity of 35% and specificity of 100%. Abnormal levels (>5 mg/24 hours) of 5-HIAA are diagnostic of carcinoid syndrome. Elevated levels of serum serotonin are also confirmatory and consistent with carcinoid syndrome, though more difficult to measure reproducibly. Patients need to be on a special diet in order to avoid false positive results. Bananas, pineapple, tomatoes, plums, eggplant, avocado, kiwi, fruits, and nuts must be avoided for 3 days. Medications such as PPIs, cough and antihistamine medications, thorazine and compazine, nasal drops and sprays, hypertension medications, acetaminophen, and muscle relaxants especially robaxin, valium, and flexeril can also lead to false positives and should be avoided.

Less common NETs may also be identified by the specific hormone and syndrome that is produced. For example, thymic carcinoid tumors may produce adrenocorticotropic hormone (ACTH) and corticotropin-releasing factor and result in ectopic Cushing syndrome.[5] Thirty percent of these tumors can also secrete catecholamines; therefore, 24-hour urinary catecholamine excretion should be measured as clinically indicated.

The diagnostic evaluation for GI and pulmonary NETs often begins with high-resolution cross-sectional imaging with either multiphasic computed tomography (CT) or magnetic resonance imaging (MRI). Small intestine NETs are often characterized by mesenteric masses that represent abnormal lymph nodes associated with cicatrization or desmoplastic changes and scarring (Fig. 86.1). Additionally, most NETs express somatostatin receptors that can bind and internalize the currently available octapeptide somatostatin analogues octreotide and lanreotide. This feature can be exploited both in terms of somatostatin receptor-based treatments and scintrigraphy (SRS). ^{111}In-pentetreotide scintigraphy (Octreoscan; Mallinckrodt, Dublin, Ireland) can image approximately 80% to 90% of patients and can unmask the primary tumor, regional lymph node metastases, and distant metastases. Positron emission tomography (PET) scanning with Ga-68 DOTATATE

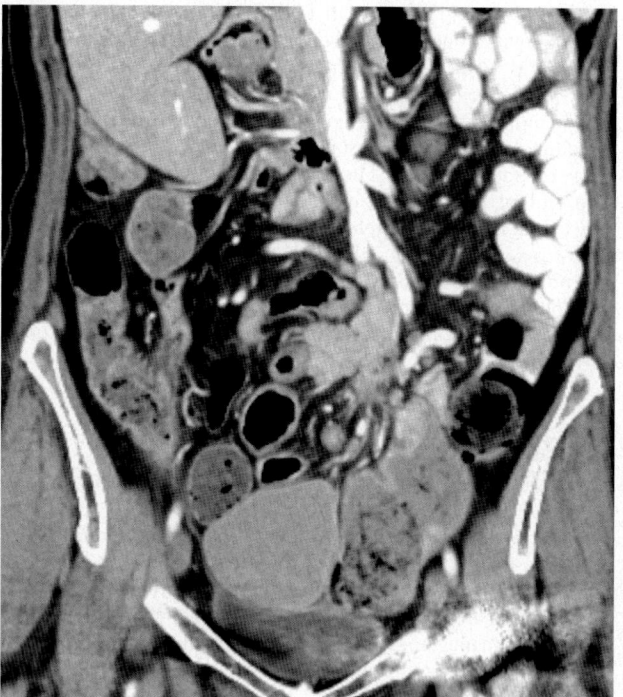

Figure 86.1 Coronal computed tomography of bulky mesenteric lymph node metastases from an ileal carcinoid (neuroendocrine) tumor. Nodes are centrally located near the superior mesenteric vein and are causing cicatrization and scarring. Patient needed an extended right hemicolectomy and distal ileal resection to completely remove the small primary (not shown) and bulky lymph node metastases.

is a newer somatostatin-based scintigraphy that is thought to be more sensitive than ^{111}In scans. At present, this imaging modality is available primary in Europe and select centers in the United States such that it is still considered experimental. Standard PET scanning with ^{18}F-deoxyglucose is disappointing in patients with well-differentiated GI and pulmonary NETs, although poorly differentiated NETs are often ^{18}F-deoxyglucose avid. [123]I- or ^{131}I-meta-iodobenzylguanidine is taken up and accumulated in some NET cells. Sensitivity of ^{131}I-meta-iodobenzylguanidine scan in patients with small intestine NETs is between 60% and 85%, and is especially useful in patients whose tumors secrete catecholamines. CT-enteroclysis is a newer imaging modality designed to image tumors of the small bowel. It has a sensitivity of 86% and a specificity of 100% for small bowel NETs.[13] Echocardiography is also included in the diagnostic workup to either confirm or exclude carcinoid heart disease.

General Staging Principles

The seventh edition of the American Joint Committee on Cancer (AJCC) *Staging Manual* is the first edition to include specific staging for GI NETs such as stomach, small bowel, appendix, colon, and rectum, and parallels staging for adenocarcinomas of those same sites.[14] Multiple papers have been published recently which both validate this AJCC staging and propose some additional modifications to enhance future AJCC versions[15,16] (see Table 86.1).

General Management Principles

Management of NETs falls under two main categories: therapies directed at tumor control and therapies directed at controlling symptoms of hormone excess. Additionally, therapies directed at tumor control are further divided based on biologic differences of well- versus poorly differentiated NETs. Unless noted, antitumor therapies will all be for well-differentiated tumors. Carcinoid syndrome and medical management of hormone-related symptoms will be addressed in detail later in this chapter.

Therapies directed at tumor control include surgery. Surgical resection remains the mainstay of treatment for resectable NETs of the GI tract and lungs. The primary goal of surgical intervention is to prolong survival. Yet, in addition to prolonged survival, surgery can also palliate symptoms of obstruction, diarrhea, flushing, and/or pain with eating.[17] In the setting of unresectable disease, antitumor therapy is only indicated in the setting of symptoms, tumor bulk, and/or disease progression. In newly diagnosed asymptomatic patients with unresectable or metastatic disease, it is often reasonable to monitor closely without any active treatment.

DIAGNOSIS, STAGING, AND MANAGEMENT BY PRIMARY TUMOR SITE

The previously mentioned general principles apply to most NETs of the GI tract and lungs. Following are some unique aspects of the diagnosis, staging, and management by primary tumor site. Management here focuses on surgical management of localized disease and management of hormone symptoms. Management of metastatic disease will be addressed separately.

Thymic Neuroendocrine Tumors

NETs of the thymus are rare. Thymic NETs make up between 2% and 7% of anterior mediastinal masses. CT or MRI is commonly used for imaging and the diagnosis. Patients may present with severe Cushing syndrome secondary to ectopic ACTH production.[18] Approximately 25% of patients with thymic carcinoids will have MEN-1. Patients typically present with either stage 1 well-differentiated neuroendocrine carcinoma previously termed typical carcinoid syndrome, or stage 2 moderately differentiated neuroendocrine carcinoma previously called atypical carcinoid tumor or stage 3 poorly differentiated or small cell neuroendocrine carcinoma. Surgery (radical thymectomy) is the primary treatment for stage 1 and 2 thymic NETs, whereas chemotherapy is best for stage 3. Five- and ten-year survival for resected thymic NETs is between 20% and 30%. Radiation may help with local control following incomplete resection.

Bronchial Neuroendocrine Tumors

Bronchial NETs appear histologically like intestinal NETs and are not related to cigarette smoking. These tumors are more common in patients with MEN-1. Poor prognostic factors include higher mitotic index, nuclear pleomorphism, vascular and lymphatic invasion, and poorly differentiated growth pattern. The bronchus is the site of a primary NET in approximately 2% of cases. These tumors occur close to the hilum on CT and MRI scan and may be confused with blood vessels. Bronchial NETs are divided into three categories: benign or low-grade malignant, which is the typical carcinoid form; low-grade malignant, which is the atypical carcinoid form; and poorly differentiated, either large cell or small cell. The grading system differs slightly when compared to GI NET grading. The three different categories of bronchial carcinoid tumors have different prognosis from excellent for typical well-differentiated carcinoids to poor for small cell neuroendocrine carcinomas. The well-differentiated tumors are surgically resected with a lobectomy while the small cell tumors are treated primarily with chemotherapy. SRS can be used to complement cross-sectional imaging with multiphasic CT or MRI. Atypical carcinoid tumors have more uptake of deoxyglucose on PET scan, while typical carcinoid tumors have more uptake of sandostatin (octreotide).[19] On bronchoscopy, NETs appear as a cherry red mass within the bronchus protruding into the lumen. It is recommended not to biopsy them as they can bleed excessively with biopsy. Bronchial carcinoids are the most common cause of ectopic ACTH syndrome, and Cushing syndrome is severe with usual clinical signs and symptoms plus severe weakness secondary to hypokalemia.[20]

Esophageal Neuroendocrine Tumors

Esophageal NETs are very uncommon (<1% of GI NETs). They occur predominantly in men at an age >60 years. Symptoms are nonspecific and vary from asymptomatic to indigestion and burning pain. Most tumors are seen in the distal esophagus just proximal to the esophageal-gastric junction. They are seen on endoscopy as a submucosal mass, and they usually dimple the mucosa. Endoscopic ultrasonography and SRS are indicated for staging because lymph node metastases occur in 50% of patients. Endoscopic mucosal resection (EMR) is done if there is no evidence of lymph node metastases and the tumor is amenable to complete excision. Open resection is done for patients with lymph node metastases. The operative procedure is most commonly an Ivor Lewis esophagogastrectomy that requires an upper midline incision and a right thoracotomy. Survival is dependent on stage of disease and adequacy of resection.

Gastric Neuroendocrine Tumors

Gastric NETs are rare tumors and constitute <1% of gastric tumors and 9% of GI NETs (Table 86.2). These tumors arise from the enterochromaffin-like (ECL) cells of the stomach that occur in the gastric fundus and body. Gastric NETs are immunoreactive to histamine, chromogranin A, and synaptophysin. Gastric NETs have three different forms: type 1, type 2, and type 3. Type 1 gastric carcinoids typically occur in a state of chronic atrophic gastritis that results in achlorhydria and hypergastrinemia.[21] They occur in 80% of gastric NETs. These tumors are typically multicentric consisting of multiple small gastric polyps and invariably develop from ECL cell hyperplasia and become small polypoid tumors.[22] Tumors vary in size from a few millimeters to 1.5 cm. These tumors are almost always benign with minimal risk of invasion or metastases. These are usually treated with repeat endoscopic examination, excision, and EMR of larger tumors. There is a very low risk of lymph node metastases (5%) or distant metastases (2%). Larger tumors (approximately >2 cm) require resection, either endoscopic or open surgery. If gastric surgery is performed, antrectomy is indicated as this will remove the source of the hypergastrinemia and the stimulus for ECL cell growth.

TABLE 86.2

Incidence and Prognosis of Different Stage Gastrointestinal Neuroendocrine Tumors

Site	Incidence (% GI NETs)	Five-Year Survival T_{1-2}, N_0	Five-Year Survival T_3, N_1	Five-Year Survival $T_4 \pm M_1$
Stomach	9	93	65	25
Duodenum	4	68	55	46
Ileum/jejunum	42	78	71	54
Appendix	8	98	78	25
Colon	4	85	46	14
Rectum	27	93	62–75	33

GI, gastrointestinal; NET, neuroendocrine tumor.

Type 2 gastric carcinoid tumors are rare and occur in only 6% to 8% of patients with gastric NETs. They are much less common than those seen in atrophic gastritis. Type 2 tumors occur in patients with MEN-1 with Zollinger-Ellison syndrome (ZES) who have been treated with PPIs for a long time period. They occur equally in both men and women with an age distribution of 45 to 50 years. The hypergastrinemia of ZES is exacerbated by the prolonged use of the PPI (approximately 10 years) to control symptoms related to excessive acid secretion. These NETs develop in a hyperplasia-dysplasia-neoplasia sequence. Moreover, there must be an effect of the menin gene defect, because non–MEN-1 patients with (sporadic) ZES have also been treated with prolonged use of PPI and have not developed similar tumors. Type 2 NETs of the stomach are often multiple and small (73% <1.5 cm), but are larger than the type 1 tumors. Lymph node metastases are present in 30% of patients with type 2 gastric carcinoid tumors, and distant metastases occur in 10% to 20%. Patients with MEN-1 may develop distant metastases from pancreatic NETs, so it is sometimes difficult to tell which primary NET led to the development of a liver NET. However, rare cases of highly malignant gastric NETs with a poor prognosis have been described in some patients with MEN-1/ZES. These patients have diffuse involvement of the entire stomach with NETs, and total gastrectomy with adjacent lymph node dissection is recommended.

Type 3 gastric NETs are those that occur sporadically with no association of hypergastrinemia. They represent 15% to 20% of gastric NETs and are markedly different from type 1 and 2 NETs. They occur sporadically, are solitary, and grow much more rapidly. Most have distant metastases at the time of diagnosis. These tumors have a male predominance and occur 3:1 in men. Mean age at presentation is 50 years. These tumors are large (mean size 3 cm). Most lesions invade the full thickness wall of the stomach. They are usually located in the body or fundus. Regional lymph node and liver metastases are present in 70% of patients. A total of 73% of patients with this disease are alive at 5 years, but those with liver metastasis have a 5-year survival of 10%. Sporadic type 3 gastric NETs usually have a Ki67 index of >2%. According to older classifications, these tumors may have typical or atypical histology. Atypical implies nuclear pleomorphism, more mitosis, and necrosis. Atypical tumors are larger (>5 cm) and have a more unfavorable prognosis. The atypical carcinoid syndrome occurs in these patients and is associated with tumor release of histamine. The atypical carcinoid syndrome has bright red cutaneous flushing, edema, itching, wheezing, and lacrimation. In patients with type 3 gastric NETs, tumor debulking of the primary and lymph node metastases may relieve symptoms. Hepatic metastases are treated with resection, hepatic artery embolization or chemoembolization, radiofrequency ablation, and sandostatin long-acting repeatable (LAR) that may ameliorate the symptoms of the atypical carcinoid syndrome. Chemotherapy is likely to be useful when the proliferation rate exceeds 5%. Response rates are between 20% to 40%.

Small Bowel Neuroendocrine Tumors

NETs of the duodenum are rare and comprise <4% of all GI NETs. Gastrinomas are the most common functional duodenal NET and represent 60% of duodenal NETs. These tumors are more common in the proximal duodenum and are less likely to arise in the distal duodenum. They are usually small <5 mm and multiple in MEN-1. They frequently (30% to 70%) spread to regional lymph nodes such that adjacent lymph node sampling is recommended but do not commonly spread to distant sites. Overall, the 10-year survival of duodenal NETs is 64%.[23] The 10-year survival rate for patients with duodenal gastrin-secreting NETs is 90%. Duodenotomy (opening the duodenum) at the time of surgery is the most effective method to identify these tumors. When found, complete excision of the duodenal wall around the tumor with lymph node

sampling is recommended. Some advocate Whipple procedure, but the prognosis is excellent with local tumor resection and the cure rate is 60%, so many think that Whipple resection is not indicated.

Periampullary duodenal NETs do not usually produce a hormonal syndrome.[23] Given their location, these tumors may cause obstructive jaundice or bleeding. The size of these tumors is small (between 1 to 2 cm in diameter). They are typically nodular, polypoid, and ulcerated. Periampullary NETs are associated with von Recklinghausen neurofibromatosis. A total of 50% of the patients have either lymph node or liver metastases. They require either local excision or Whipple pancreaticoduodenectomy, dependent on the size of the tumor, the age of the patient, and the relationship to the ampulla. Nonampullary duodenal NETs that are found during endoscopy have an excellent prognosis and can be removed by EMR if <1 cm. They are removed by surgical excision if the tumor is >2 cm. Lymph node metastases can occur in approximately 40% of patients, so lymph node sampling is recommended. For treatment of NETs >3 cm, Whipple pancreaticoduodenectomy is recommended. Small bowel NETs are most common GI NET, and they are most prevalent within the ileum. They account for 42% of all GI NETs. They usually occur within 20 cm of the ileal-cecal valve. They feel like a firm mobile nodule within the wall of the bowel. Patients typically have a long history of vague nonlocalizing abdominal pain before the tumor is detected. These symptoms may be borborygmi, episodic abdominal pain or cramping, and episodic diarrhea and constipation. Others may develop clinical signs of the typical carcinoid syndrome that include diarrhea, flushing, palpitations, intolerance of certain specific foods like cheese or red wine, intestinal venous congestion, and infarction, and these can occur as the tumor lymph node metastases enlarge and block the venous outflow. Intermittent severe episodes of abdominal pain or even intestinal obstruction can occur as the tumor progresses. Ileal NETs are commonly very small (2 to 4 mm) and multiple within the wall of the ileum, with adjacent large lymph node metastases that cause cicatrization and venous conjestion that can result in small bowel obstruction (see Fig. 86.1). Approximately 50% of patients will have liver metastases or peritoneal carcinomatosis at the time of diagnosis. The 10-year survival for jejunal and ileal NETs is 53% and 50%, respectively. Surgery includes wide resection of the small bowel with the primary tumors, its mesentery, and lymph node metastases. This usually requires an extended right hemicolectomy and may result in a relative short gut syndrome because the lymph node metastases can be very centrally located and require resection of proximal branches of the superior mesenteric artery and vein. Recent studies also suggest that surgery can be effectively done laparoscopically,[24] but commonly extensive nodal disease is present such that the superior mesenteric artery and vein must be skeletonized that usually requires open surgical techniques. Surgery for ileal NETs is the mainstay of treatment and surgical resection of the primary tumor even in the setting of numerous distant metastases has been recommended in order to avoid the cramping and bowel obstruction associated with primary NETs that are left to progress.[25] Patients with unknown primary metastatic NETs can often harbor occult primary ileal NETs. This is quite common, and careful exploration and palpation of the ileum allows detection of small submucosal primaries that feel like little peas within the bowel wall.[26] Cholecystectomy is also indicated because most of these patients with either lymph node or liver metastases will require the long-term use of somatostatin analogues that can cause gallstones when administered long-term.

Appendiceal Neuroendocrine Tumors

Appendiceal NETs represent between 5% to 8% of GI NETs. They occur in approximately 1 in 200 to 300 appendectomies.[27,28] Most are located in the tip of the appendix. They commonly present in younger patients who have a mean age of <50 years. They seldom metastasize; lymph node metastases occur in 3.8% and distant metastases in only 0.7%. The long-term survival is nearly 95% for all patients with appendiceal carcinoid tumors, 84% for those with lymph node metastases, and 28% for those with liver metastases. Appendectomy is adequate for tumors <2 cm and those that do not invade through the wall of the appendix or are present at the base. For patients with tumors >2 cm, invasion through the appendiceal wall, presence at the base, or lymph node metastases, a right hemicolectomy is indicated.

Colorectal Neuroendocrine Tumors

NETs of the colon are rare and account for only approximately 4% of GI NETs and 1% to 5% of colorectal tumors.[29] These tumors occur more commonly in older individuals >65 years. Tumors in the right colon are more common and can cause symptoms of carcinoid syndrome. The majority of colon NETs are well differentiated but some are large, less differentiated, and exophytic. These larger, less-differentiated tumors grow more rapidly and have a higher incidence of lymph node and liver metastases. The 5-year survival for colon NETs is 37%, which is only slightly better than all patients with colon cancer. In general, colon NETs should be treated with a hemicolectomy including adequate lymph node retrieval.

The incidence of rectal NETs is increasing.[30] They are among the most common NETs reported in recent series. They constitute 27% of GI NETs and 1% to 2% of all rectal tumors. These tumors are more common in Asian and Black populations. Most are small and discovered incidentally during endoscopy. The overall prognosis is favorable, and the 5-year survival for patients with stage 1 to 4 is 93%, 75%, 43%, and 33%, respectively.[30] Smaller tumors (<1 cm) can be treated by either EMR[31] or local excision. Larger tumors >1 cm may require a low anterior rectal resection or an abdominoperineal resection depending on the relationship to the distal rectum and anus.

DIAGNOSIS AND MANAGEMENT OF CARCINOID SYNDROME

Biogenic amines and vasoactive peptides in the systemic circulation cause symptoms of the carcinoid syndrome (Fig. 86.2). Serotonin, tachykinins, bradykinis, and histamine have each been measured in the systemic circulation of these patients. Enterochromaffin cells, precursors to NETs, have the ability to produce 5-hydroxytryptamine (serotonin). In the liver, serotonin is metabolized to 5-HIAA that eliminates the development of the signs and symptoms of the carcinoid syndrome. However, in patients with liver metastases or extrahepatic tumor in sites such as the ovary or the retroperitoneum, an excessive amount of serotonin enters the systemic circulation and causes carcinoid syndrome. Small bowel NETs are most often associated with carcinoid syndrome.

Symptoms of carcinoid syndrome include diarrhea, flushing, wheezing caused by bronchial obstruction, and carcinoid heart disease. Most patients complain of intermittent crampy abdominal pain. Flushing is the most common symptom, occurring in 94% of patients, and has been linked to secretion of tachykinins, serotonin, and histamine. Flushing has a uniform distribution and most commonly involves the upper chest, neck, and face. It may be provoked by certain foods like nuts, cheese, drugs, and alcohol, and during times of stress. Patients will develop skin thickening and redness in this distribution secondary to chronic flushing. Diarrhea occurs in 80% of patients with carcinoid syndrome. Serotonin is thought to be the most common cause of diarrhea, but other active amines like histamine, kallikrein, prostaglandin, substance P, and motilin may play a role. Further, a relative short gut

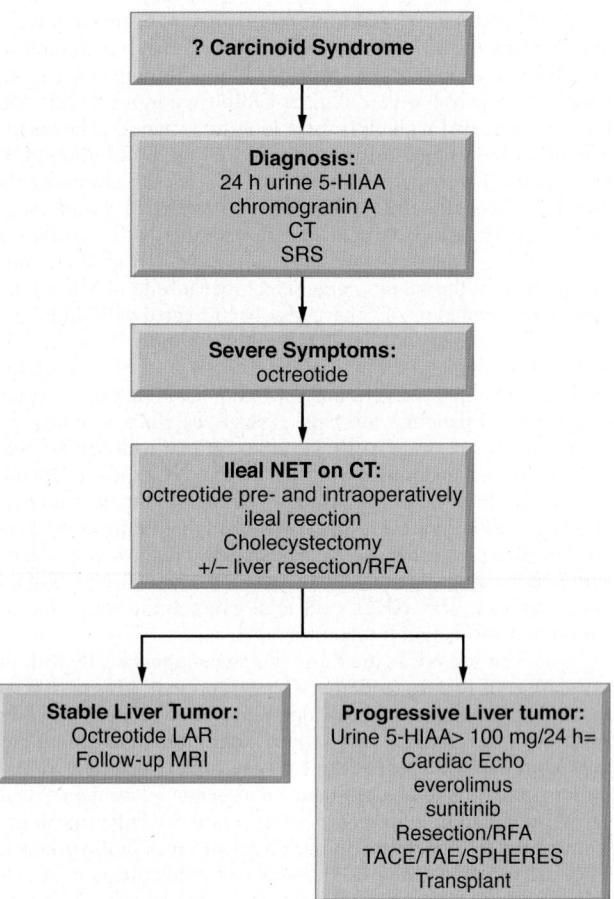

Figure 86.2 Flow diagram for the diagnosis and management of carcinoid syndrome. Diagram includes diagnosis and management of a primary ileal carcinoid tumor and liver metastases. HIAA, hydroxyindoleacetic acid; CT, computed tomography; SRS, somatostatin receptor-based treatments and scintrigraphy; NET, neuroendocrine tumor; RFA, radiofrequency ablation; MRI, magnetic resonance imaging; TACE, chemoembolization; TAE, transarterial embolization; SPHERES, Radioactive SPHERES.

syndrome may occur following removal of the primary tumor and malabsorption of bile salts and fat, as well as bacterial overgrowth, may also contribute to diarrhea.

Carcinoid heart disease develops in approximately 40% of patients with carcinoid syndrome. It is characterized by carcinoid plaques on the right side of the heart with involvement of the tricuspid and pulmonary valves and the endocardium.[32] The pathogenesis of these plaques and fibrosis is increased synthesis of collagen secondary to serotonin-induced transforming growth factor-beta secretion. The most common clinical manifestation is tricuspid and pulmonic valve insufficiency and stenosis. These valvular lesions can be significant and lead to right-sided heart failure. Several studies have shown that patients with carcinoid syndrome with valve disease have much greater levels of urinary 5-HIAA excretion. Cardiac surgery is indicated for valve replacement. Patients with urinary 5-HIAA excretion rates >100 mg/day should be screened by transthoracic echocardiography on a regular basis. Similarly, serotonin, histamine, and bradykinin also induce transforming growth factor-beta, collagen synthesis, and scarring in the mesentery of the bowel. This can lead to adhesions and bowel obstruction or venous obstruction that leads to inadequate venous outflow and bowel ischemia.

Intermittent bronchial obstruction and wheezing is present in 10% of patients with carcinoid syndrome. It usually occurs during episodes of flushing. It cannot be treated like asthma because

B₂-agonists that are used to treat asthma lead to additional release of biogenic amines and peptides.

Pellagra is also associated with carcinoid syndrome, though in a minority of patients (5%). The triad of dermatitis, diarrhea, and dementia characterizes pellagra. Pellagra is a direct result of niacin deficiency. Niacin is directly obtained from the diet or synthesized from tryptophan, a precursor of serotonin. Carcinoid tumors use a large proportion of the body tryptophan stores for overproduction of serotonin. Increased tryptophan consumption leads to impaired niacin synthesis and pellagra. Pellagra should be treated with niacin supplementation.

Finally, carcinoid crisis can occur in patients with carcinoid syndrome who undergo anesthesia or surgery and are not sufficiently blocked with somatostatin analogues. The clinical picture includes flushing, hypotension, bronchial obstruction, and cardiac arrhythmias. Of note, all patients with small bowel NET undergoing surgical intervention should be given perioperative octreotide to prevent carcinoid crisis. This may occur with anesthesia, surgery, and interventional radiology procedures like embolization, chemoembolization, dental procedures, and radiofrequency ablation. Basically, whenever an invasive procedure is planned on a patient with carcinoid syndrome, it is prudent to pretreat with a large dose of somatostatin analogue to avoid the development of carcinoid crisis. The recommended dose of octreotide is 25 to 500 mcg subcutaneously or intravenously 1 to 2 hours prior to the procedure.[33] For the same reason, adrenergic drugs should be avoided in patients with carcinoid syndrome. In a case of carcinoid crisis, the surgical or nonsurgical manipulation should be temporarily interrupted, intravenous volume administered under the guidance of hemodyamic monitoring, and additional doses of octreotide and steroids administered intravenously. Patients who develop intraoperative symptoms (hypotension or rash) should receive 500 to 1,000 mcg of octreotide intravenously until symptoms resolve and a continuous infusion of 50 to 200 mcg/hour.

Medical management of carcinoid syndrome centers around the use of somatostatin analogues.[6,34] Somatostatin analogs are the foundation of symptom management for patients with functional NETs and can both decrease the secretion of such hormones and inhibit their end-organ effects. Somatostatin is a naturally occurring polypeptide produced by paracrine cells that are scattered throughout the GI tract; it inhibits GI endocrine and exocrine function. Its effects are mediated through G-coupled protein somatostatin receptors (1 to 5). Short- and long-acting octreotide (with high affinity for somatostatin receptor 2) is available in the United States. Lanreotide, available in Europe, is a long-acting analog with similar binding affinity to octreotide. Pasireotide, a novel somatostatin analog with a different binding affinity profile compared to octreotide or lanreotide, is currently in development. Side effects are usually mild but include nausea, bloating, biliary sludge, and steatorrhea. Blockade of serotonin receptors via somatostatin analogues can greatly ameliorate the diarrhea of carcinoid syndrome in 40% to 80% of patients. Similarly, a reduction or normalization of biochemical markers can be seen in 40% to 70% of patients. Most patients can be managed with octreotide LAR, but 30% require either an increase in dose or frequency of administration to continue to control symptoms of hormone excess. Standard doses of octreotide LAR 20 to 30 mg every month intramuscularly[35] and depot-lanreotide 60 to 120 mg via deep subcutaneous injection.[36] Patients who experience recurrence of their symptoms toward the end of the treatment cycle may benefit from increased frequency of administration (every 3 weeks). Supplemental doses of standard subcutaneous octreotide can be given if patients develop breakthrough symptoms. Tachyphylaxis to somatostatin analogues often occurs between 8 and 12 months but can usually be overcome by increasing the dose.

Inhibitors of serotonin synthesis are emerging as a new class of agents to treat carcinoid syndrome. Telotristat etiprate is an oral inhibitor of tryptophan hydroxylase, a key enzyme in the synthesis of peripheral serotonin. A recent study randomized carcinoid patients with four or more bowel movements a day to receive telotristat etiprate or placebo as double-blind treatment. Treatment was associated with decreases in urine 5-HIAA and bowel movement frequency, and self-reported relief of bowel-related symptoms.[37] Phase 3 studies with telotristat etiprate for diarrhea and flushing are ongoing (NCT01677910).

Other methods for reducing diarrhea associated with carcinoid syndrome include drugs like cholestyramine that bind bile salts and increase bile absorption. Pancreatic enzymes are used to aid with fat absorption and reduce diarrhea. Antibacterial therapy can be used if there is evidence of bacterial overgrowth. Loperamide and tincture of opium are used to decrease transit time.

ANTITUMOR MANAGEMENT

Somatostatin Analogues

Clinical studies suggest that long-acting octreotide can also inhibit tumor growth. A total of 50% of patients with metastatic carcinoid who have had objective evidence of tumor progression had stabilization of tumor size when treated with long-acting octreotide. In vitro evidence suggests that octreotide interacts with somatostatin receptors that stimulate phosphotyrosine phosphatases that inhibit growth factors like insulin-like growth factor and vascular endothelial growth factor (VEGF) and thus inhibit tumor growth. The best clinical evidence came from the PROMID trial, which was a phase 3 study that randomized 85 patients with metastatic midgut carcinoids to octreotide LAR 30 mg versus placebo. The study demonstrated a significant improvement of median time to progression from 6 months in the placebo arm to 14.3 months in the treatment arm (hazard ratio = 0.34; p <0.01). On multivariate analysis, patients with low hepatic tumor burden (<10%) and resected primary tumor appeared to benefit most from octreotide treatment. Because the study had a crossover design and thus a small number of deaths, overall survival was not analyzed. The study has also been criticized for not requiring disease progression at the time of study entry. Despite these limitations, octreotide LAR is now considered an appropriate first-line therapy for patients with progressive metastatic midgut NETs regardless of the presence or absence of carcinoid syndrome.[38]

Interferon-Alpha

Interferons (IFN) exert antitumor effects through a variety of mechanisms including stimulation of T cells, inhibition of angiogenesis, and induction of cell cycle arrest in the G_1 and G_0 phases. IFN also induces somatostatin receptors. IFN was used in early trials prior to somatostatin analogues. Improvement of symptoms including palliation of diarrhea and flushing occurs in 50% of patients. However, objective antitumor responses occur in only 10% of patients. In vitro studies have suggested synergism between IFN and octreotide, prompting clinical trials to evaluate the combination. Three randomized trials have investigated octreotide alone versus the combination of octreotide with IFN. In one multicenter trial of 68 patients with metastatic midgut carcinoids, there was a strong suggestion of improvement with octreotide + IFN versus octreotide alone. The 5-year survival rate was 57% versus 37% but the difference was not significant (p = 0.13).[39] A three-arm trial compared subcutaneous lanreotide to IFN alone or the combination of both with a very small response rate (<7%) and no difference among the three groups.[40] A third randomized study of octreotide alone versus octreotide plus IFN demonstrated an increase in median survival with the combination (54 months versus 32 months), but the difference was not significant.[40] Response rates were low in both arms (<6%). The small number of patients accrued in these randomized trials preclude any meaningful conclusions on the role of IFN. Doses of IFN used were small and toxicity was minimal. A pivotal phase 3 study of octreotide and IFN versus octreotide and bevacizumab in advanced, high-risk NETs has recently been completed; results are anticipated in 2014 (NCT00569127). IFNs are commonly associated with flu-like symptoms, chronic fatigue, depression, thyroid dysfunction, mild hepatotoxicity, and cytopenias.

Mammalian Target of Rapamycin Inhibitors

The mTOR is a conserved serine/threonine kinase that regulates cell growth, metabolism, and proliferation. The mTOR enzyme lies downstream of the phosphatidylinositol-3 kinase/protein kinase B pathway and is activated in response to growth factors and cytokines. Pancreatic NETs have mutations in mTOR-associated genes (phosphatase and tensin homolog and phosphatidylinositol-3 kinase) in approximately 15% of cases, while it is not know if midgut NETs have similar mutations.[41]

Everolimus is an oral mTOR inhibitor that has been studied extensively in NETs.[42] Everolimus was approved by the US Food and Drug Administration for the treatment of metastatic pancreatic NETs based on improvement in progression-free survival from 4.6 months to 11 months in a randomized study of metastatic pancreatic NETs (RADIANT-3).[43] The phase 3 RADIANT-2 trial randomized 429 patients with metastatic NETs and evidence of carcinoid syndrome to treatment with everolimus plus octreotide LAR versus placebo plus octreotide LAR.[44] The majority of patients in each arm had primary small bowel NETs. Median progression-free survival was improved from 11.3 months in the placebo arm to 16.4 months in the everolimus arm (hazard ratio = 0.77; p = 0.026), though the result was not statistically significant because it failed to meet its prespecified p value. Overall survival was not improved in the treatment arm because of a crossover design. A major limitation of this study, contributing to its overall lack of statistical significance, was the issue of informative censoring and differences between central and investigator Response Evaluation Criteria In Solid Tumors reviews. Side effects of everolimus include oral aphthous ulcers, rash, hyperglycemia, cytopenias, and pneumonitis. Major guideline groups, like the National Comprehensive Cancer Network, do not currently recommend everolimus for management of small bowel NETs. Ongoing studies may expand the role of everolimus in other nonpancreatic NETs, particularly the RADIANT-4 study that is a non-crossover, randomized study of everolimus versus placebo in patients with NETs of lung or GI origin.

Angiogenesis Inhibitors

NETs are highly vascular tumors that frequently overexpress the VEGF receptor and its ligand. Consequently, inhibition of the VEGF pathway has been considered a promising target. In a randomized phase 2 trial, 44 patients with metastatic carcinoid tumors were randomly assigned to bevacizumab (a monoclonal antibody to circulating VEGF) versus pegylated IFN for 18 weeks, after which they received both agents in combination.[45] After 18 weeks of treatment, the progression-free survival was 95% in the bevacizumab arm versus 68% in the IFN arm. Moreover, the objective response rate was 18% in the bevacizumab arm, suggesting that the drug had significant clinical activity. This trial led to the development of a randomized phase 3 trial of octreotide and IFN versus octreotide and bevacizumab in advanced, high-risk NETs; it has recently completed accrual and results are anticipated in 2014 (NCT00569127).

Several other angiogenesis inhibitors have been evaluated in NETs, including tyrosine kinase inhibitors (TKI) of VEGF receptors. Sunitinib, an oral TKI, inhibits VEGF receptors 1, 2, and 3 as well as platelet-derived growth factor, cKIT, and Flt3. In a single-arm phase 2 study of patients with advanced NETs, only 1 of 41 (2%) patients with carcinoid had evidence of an objective radiographic response to sunitinib; however, the median time to progression was 10.2 months.[46] Sunitinib has since demonstrated improved progression-free survival compared to placebo in a randomized phase 3 study of advanced pancreatic NETs, which led to its approval by the US Food and Drug Administration for this indication in 2010.[47] A phase 3 study of pazopanib versus placebo in GI NETs is ongoing and is poised to definitely answer the question about effectiveness of oral TKIs in nonpancreatic NETs.

Cytotoxic Chemotherapy

Studies of cytotoxic chemotherapy in small bowel NETs have been disappointing. This is documented in modern clinical trials using radiographic response criteria. The combination of temozolomide and thalidomide has a response rate of 45% in pancreatic NETs but only 7% in carcinoid tumors.[48] Similarly, temozolomide plus bevacizumab have a response rate of 0/18 in carcinoid tumors but 33% in pancreatic NETs.[49] Cytotoxic agents are not recommended for the treatment of metastatic well-differentiated small bowel carcinoid tumors, except in the context of a clinical trial. Poorly differentiated NETs, regardless of primary site, are typically treated like small-cell lung cancer with a platinum/etoposide-based regimen.

Peptide Receptor Radionuclide Therapy

Nearly 80% of well-differentiated NETs express high levels of somatostatin receptors. This is the basis for the development of therapy using the somatostatin receptor as a radioligand, so called peptide receptor radionuclide therapy.[50] Selection criteria for peptide receptor radionuclide therapy include evidence of strong radiotracer uptake on SRS. Early trials used the same isotope that is used for SRS imaging, ^{111}In-pentetreotide. With this agent, clinical responses were rare. Next generation used ^{90}Y, a high-energy beta-particle emitter. A single-arm phase 2 trial of ^{90}Y-Edotreotide in 90 patients with metastatic carcinoid tumors reported an objective response rate of 4%, stable disease in 70%, and a high rate of symptom control. Adverse events include nausea and vomiting attributed to the amino acid infusions that were given to prevent nephrotoxicity.[51] The latest generation of radiolabelled somatostatin analogues utilizes ^{177}Lu-octreotate (^{177}Lu-DOTA-Tyr–[3]-octreotate), which is an alpha, beta, and gamma particle–emitting compound that has enhanced affinity for the somatostatin receptor 2. This compound provided an objective response rate of 23% in 188 patients with carcinoid tumors as reported in a large retrospective review.[50] Adverse effects were mild. Though this treatment is used routinely in Europe, it is not approved by the US Food and Drug Administration due to lack of prospective randomized data. The NETTER-1 study will hopefully provide a definitive answer to this question. In this randomized, multinational trial, patients with inoperable, progressive, somatostatin receptor–positive midgut carcinoid tumors are randomly assigned to receive high-dose octreotide (60 mg LAR monthly) versus ^{177}Lu-DOTA0-Tyr3-Octreotate (NCT01578239).

MANAGEMENT OF LIVER METASTASES

The liver is the predominant site of metastases in patients with GI NETs (Fig. 86.3). These patients typically have carcinoid syndrome, but they may also develop symptoms secondary to enlarging liver tumor burden including anorexia, weight loss, and pain. Liver-directed therapies include liver resection and/or ablation, transarterial embolization (TAE), chemoembolization (TACE), and liver transplantation. These therapies are reserved

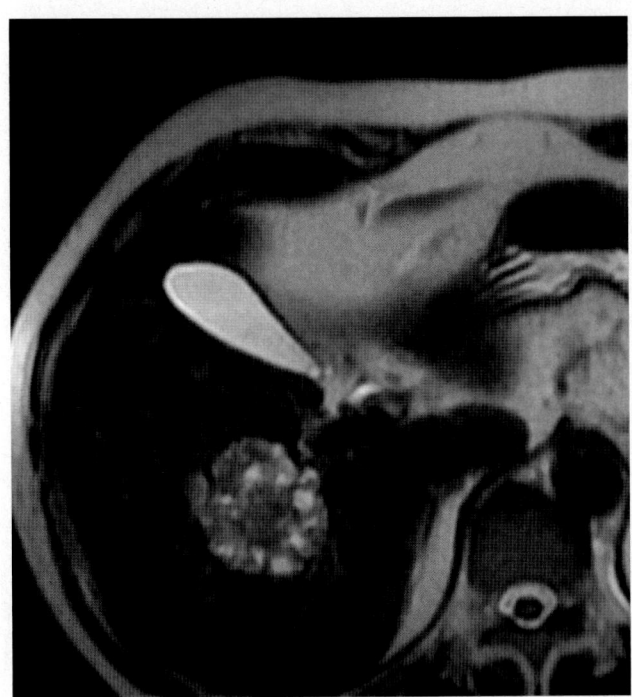

Figure 86.3 T2-weighted axial magnetic resonance image of a right lobe carcinoid tumor liver metastasis from an ileal carcinoid tumor. This patient had carcinoid syndrome. Surgical resection required preoperative and intraoperative treatment with octreotide. Patient underwent a cholecystectomy and right hepatic lobectomy. He has done well with long-term maintenance sandostatin-LAR intramuscularly on a monthly basis.

for patients whose sole or major tumor burden is confined to the liver.

Liver resection has been used in patients with limited liver disease if >90% of the tumor can be either resected or ablated[52–54] (see Fig. 86.2). Typically, resection is done with multiple wedge or segmental resections rather than anatomic resection so that reoperations remain feasible, if necessary. There are numerous single institution studies that suggest excellent palliation of carcinoid symptoms and prolonged survival of patients undergoing complete tumor resection; that is, surgery with curative or near-curative intent.[52,53,55] These studies clearly demonstrate that the surgery is feasible and can be done with minimal morbidity and mortality. However, none of these studies are randomized and none have a control group of similar patients who have not had surgery, thus the survival benefit conferred by surgical therapy remains speculative and controversial. The most common ablation technique is radiofrequency ablation that is used for centrally located tumors that are not near major blood vessels or ducts and are ≤3 cm.[56] Radiofrequency ablation involves conversion of radiofrequency waves to heat using an alternating current that generates ionic vibration.

TAE or TACE is usually performed in patients with diffuse or widely scattered diffuse bilateral liver metastases. The theoretical basis for this type of treatment is that the hepatic artery preferentially perfuses liver tumors, whereas normal hepatocytes are perfused primarily through the portal vein. In patients with bilobar liver metastases, staged lobar embolizations are typically performed at 4- to 6-week intervals. TACE is also done by combining cytotoxic drugs like cisplatin or doxorubicin with iodized oil and injecting it into the hepatic arterial branches until there is obliteration of blood flow. There is no clear advantage of TAE versus TACE. Response rates are similar. Major biomarker response is between 40% and 100%,

symptom response between 67% and 100%, and radiographic response between 33% and 67%. Median survival is 31 months. Side effects of TAE/TACE include abdominal pain, fever, and fatigue. Liver function studies typically demonstrate an increase in transaminase 2 to 3 days postembolization. One prospective study on small bowel NETs used TAE followed by sunitinib. Of 39 patients enrolled, 26 had primary intestinal NETs, 72% of patients had a partial radiographic response and the progression-free survival was 15 months.[57] Other trials combining liver-directed therapies and systemic therapies are in development. Carcinoid syndrome can also be palliated through TAE and TACE. Of 19 patients with carcinoid syndrome and elevated urinary 5-HIAA levels, 16 (84%) had a >50% decrease in levels and excellent palliation of carcinoid syndrome. Of note, liver-directed therapies following extensive liver resection should be approached with caution given increased risk of hepatic abscesses.

A novel approach to hepatic metastases involves radioembolization with [90]Yttrium embedded either as a resin microsphere (SIR-Sphere) or a glass microsphere (TheraSphere).[58,59] These techniques are also called selective intrahepatic radiotherapy. They provide delivery of radionuclide particles to hepatic metastases. Acute toxicities with this procedure appear to be less than the other procedures primarily because selective intrahepatic radiotherapy does not induce ischemic hepatitis. Therefore, it can be done on an outpatient basis. A rare, but significant, complication is radiation enteritis if the particles are accidentally infused into the enteric circulation. Chronic radiation hepatitis is another significant complication. Response rates are encouraging. This is becoming the procedure of choice for metastatic NETs to the liver. In several nonrandomized studies, the radiographic response rate with SIR-Spheres (Sirtex Medical Inc., North Ryde, Australia) and TheraSpheres (Nordion, Inc., Ottawa, Canada) is 51% and 63%, respectively, and the median survival is 70 months.

The role of liver transplantation in patients with metastatic NETs remains poorly defined and controversial. Data are retrospective. It is difficult to get live organs for these patients as they typically have a low priority on the transplantation list.[60] In the largest meta-analysis of 103 patients, the 5-year survival rate was 47% with only 24% free of disease recurrence.[61] Another study of 85 cases reported a 47% 5-year survival and a recurrence-free survival of 20% at 5 years. As recurrence-free survival results have not plateaued, it is unclear if liver transplantation can be curative. Negative prognostic factors for liver transplantation are high burden of hepatic tumor, pancreatic primary (not intestinal), and elevated Ki-67 index.

CONCLUSIONS

NETs of the lungs and GI tract (carcinoid tumors) are rare but given their indolent nature are quite prevalent. Some studies suggest that certain primary sites are increasing in incidence. Some of these tumors produce hormones that lead to symptoms, such as diarrhea and flushing of carcinoid syndrome. These tumors are, indeed, malignant and are often diagnosed in advanced stages. Somatostatin analogues have a profound impact on the management of small intestinal NETs. They are efficacious from both symptom management and tumor inhibition. Other systemic drugs with potential benefit include interferon-alpha and everolimus. Liver-directed therapies such as cytoreductive surgery and transarterial embolization are important options for liver-dominant disease. Other novel therapies, including VEGF tyrosine kinase inhibitors, are currently being investigated in clinical trials. The landscape of diagnostic and treatment options for NETs is rapidly changing which is cause for great optimism in this field.

REFERENCES

1. Yao JC, Hassan M, Phan A, et al. One hundred years after "carcinoid": epidemiology of and prognostic factors for neuroendocrine tumors in 35,825 cases in the United States. *J Clin Oncol* 2008;26:3063–3072.
2. de Herder WW, Kwekkeboom DJ, Feelders RA, et al. Somatostatin receptor imaging for neuroendocrine tumors. *Pituitary* 2006;9:243–248.
3. Fraenkel M, Kim MK, Faggiano A, et al. Epidemiology of gastroenteropancreatic neuroendocrine tumours. *Best Pract Res Clin Gastroenterol* 2012;26:691–703.
4. Cross AJ, Hollenback AR, Park Y. A large prospective study of risk factors for adenocarcinomas and malignant carcinoid tumors of the small intestine. *Cancer Causes Control* 2013;24:1737–1746.
5. Mocellin S, Nitti D. Gastrointestinal carcinoid: epidemiological and survival evidence from a large population-based study (n = 25 531). *Ann Oncol* 2013;24:3040–3044.
6. Strosberg J. Evolving treatment strategies for management of carcinoid tumors. *Curr Treat Options Oncol* 2013;14:374–388.
7. Bosman FT, Carneiro F, Hruban RH, et al., eds. *WHO Classification of Tumours of the Digestive System.* 4th ed. Lyon: International Agency for Research on Cancer; 2010.
8. Klimstra DS, Modlin IR, Adsay NV, et al. Pathology reporting of neuroendocrine tumors: application of the Delphic consensus process to the development of a minimum pathology data set. *Am J Surg Pathol* 2010;34:300–313.
9. Klimstra DS, Modlin IR, Coppola D, et al. The pathologic classification of neuroendocrine tumors: a review of nomenclature, grading, and staging systems. *Pancreas* 2010;39:707–712.
10. Banck MS, Kanwar R, Kulkarni AA, et al. The genomic landscape of small intestine neuroendocrine tumors. *J Clin Invest* 2013;123:2502–2508.
11. Kunz PL, Reidy-Lagunes D, Anthony LB, et al. Consensus guidelines for the management and treatment of neuroendocrine tumors. *Pancreas* 2013; 42:557–577.
12. Kulke MH, Benson AB 3rd, Bergsland E, et al. Neuroendocrine tumors. *J Natl Compr Canc Netw* 2012;10:724–764.
13. Soyer P, Dohan A, Eveno C, et al. Carcinoid tumors of the small-bowel: evaluation with 64-section CT-enteroclysis. *Eur J Radiol* 2013;82:943–950.
14. Edge SB, Byrd DR, Compton CC, et al., eds. *AJCC Cancer Staging Manual.* 7th ed. New York: Springer; 2010.
15. Strosberg JR, Weber JM, Feldman M, et al. Prognostic validity of the American Joint Committee on Cancer staging classification for midgut neuroendocrine tumors. *J Clin Oncol* 2013;31:420–425.
16. Chagpar R, Chiang YJ, Xing Y, et al. Neuroendocrine tumors of the colon and rectum: prognostic relevance and comparative performance of current staging systems. *Ann Surg Oncol* 2013;20:1170–1178.
17. Chambers AJ, Pasieka JL, Dixon E, et al. The palliative benefit of aggressive surgical intervention for both hepatic and mesenteric metastases from neuroendocrine tumors. *Surgery* 2008;144:645–651, discussion 651–653.
18. Dixon JL, Borgaonkar SP, Patel AK, et al. Thymic neuroendocrine carcinoma producing ectopic adrenocorticotropic hormone and Cushing's syndrome. *Ann Thorac Surg* 2013;96:e81–83.
19. Hunt BM, Horton MP, Vallieres E. Bronchogenic carcinoid tumours that are 18F-fluorodeoxyglucose avid on positron emission tomography. *Eur J Cardiothorac Surg* 2014;45:527–530.
20. Florez JC, Shepard JA, Kradin RL. Case records of the Massachusetts General Hospital. Case 17-2013. A 56-year-old woman with poorly controlled diabetes mellitus and fatigue. *N Engl J Med* 2013;368:2126–2136.
21. Nikou GC, Angelopoulos TP. Current concepts on gastric carcinoid tumors. *Gastroenterol Res Pract* 2012;2012:287825.
22. Thomas D, Tsolakis AV, Grozinsky-Glasberg S, et al. Long-term follow-up of a large series of patients with type 1 gastric carcinoid tumors: data from a multicenter study. *Eur J Endocrinol* 2013;168:185–193.
23. Nikou GC, Toubanakis C, Moulakakis KG, et al. Carcinoid tumors of the duodenum and the ampulla of Vater: current diagnostic and therapeutic approach in a series of 8 patients. Case series. *Int J Surg.* 2011;9:248–253.
24. Reissman P, Shmailov S, Grozinsky-Glasberg S, et al. Laparoscopic resection of primary midgut carcinoid tumors. *Surg Endosc* 2013;27:3678–3682.
25. Norlen O, Stalberg P, Oberg K, et al. Long-term results of surgery for small intestinal neuroendocrine tumors at a tertiary referral center. *World J Surg* 2012;36:1419–1431.
26. Bartlett EK, Roses RE, Gupta M, et al. Surgery for metastatic neuroendocrine tumors with occult primaries. *J Surg Res* 2013;184:221–227.
27. Landry CS, Woodall C, Scoggins CR, et al. Analysis of 900 appendiceal carcinoid tumors for a proposed predictive staging system. *Arch Surg* 2008;143:664–670, discussion 670.
28. Deschamps L, Couvelard A. Endocrine tumors of the appendix: a pathologic review. *Arch Pathol Lab Med* 2010;134:871–875.
29. Murray SE, Lloyd RV, Sippel RS, et al. Clinicopathologic characteristics of colonic carcinoid tumors. *J Surg Res* 2013;184:183–188.
30. Weinstock B, Ward SC, Harpaz N, et al. Clinical and prognostic features of rectal neuroendocrine tumors. *Neuroendocrinology* 2013;98:180–187.
31. Planting A, Phang PT, Raval MJ, et al. Transanal endoscopic microsurgery: impact on fecal incontinence and quality of life. *Can J Surg* 2013;56:243–248.
32. Bernheim AM, Connolly HM, Pellikka PA. Carcinoid heart disease in patients without hepatic metastases. *Am J Cardiol* 2007;99:292–294.
33. Seymour N, Sawh SC. Mega-dose intravenous octreotide for the treatment of carcinoid crisis: a systematic review. *Can J Anaesth* 2013;60:492–499.

34. Bergsland EK. The evolving landscape of neuroendocrine tumors. *Sem Oncol* 2013;40:4–22.
35. Strosberg J, Weber J, Feldman M, et al. Above-label doses of octreotide-LAR in patients with metastatic small intestinal carcinoid tumors. *Gastrointest Cancer Res* 2013;6:81–85.
36. Martin-Richard M, Massuti B, Pineda E, et al. Antiproliferative effects of lanreotide autogel in patients with progressive, well-differentiated neuroendocrine tumours: a Spanish, multicentre, open-label, single arm phase II study. *BMC Cancer* 2013;13:427.
37. O'Dorisio TM, Phan AT, Langdon RM, et al. Relief of bowel-related symptoms with telotristat etiprate in octreotide refractory carcinoid syndrome: Preliminary results of a double-blind, placebo-controlled multicenter study. *J Clin Oncol* 2012;30:Abstr 4085.
38. Rinke A, Muller HH, Schadwe-Brittinger C, et al. Placebo-controlled, double-blind, prospective, randomized study on the effects of octreotide LAR in the control of tumor growth in patients with metastatic neuroendocrine mid-gut tumors:a report from the PROMID study group. *J Clin Oncol* 2009;27:4656–4663.
39. Kolby L, Persson G, Franzen S, et al. Randomized clinical trial of the effect of interferon alpha on survival in patients with disseminated midgut carcinoid tumours. *Br J Surg* 2003;90:687–693.
40. Strosberg J. Neuroendocrine tumours of the small intestine. *Best Pract Res Clin Gastroenterol* 2012;26:755–773.
41. Oberg K, Casanovas O, Castano JP, et al. Molecular pathogenesis of neuroendocrine tumors: implications for current and future therapeutic approaches. *Clin Cancer Res* 2013;19:2842–2849.
42. Liu E, Marincola P, Oberg K. Everolimus in the treatment of patients with advanced pancreatic neuroendocrine tumors: latest findings and interpretations. *Ther Adv Gastroenterol* 2013;615:412–419.
43. Yao JC, Shah MH, Ito T, et al. Everolimus for advanced pancreatic neuroendocrine tumors. *N Engl J Med* 2011;364:514–523.
44. Pavel ME, Hainsworth JD, Baudin E, et al. Everolimus plus octreotide long-acting repeatable for the treatment of advanced neuroendocrine tumours associated with carcinoid syndrome (RADIANT-2): a randomised, placebo-controlled, phase 3 study. *Lancet* 2011;378:2005–2012.
45. Yao JC, Phan A, Hoff PM, et al. Targeting vascular endothelial growth factor in advanced carcinoid tumor: a random assignment phase II study of depot octreotide with bevacizumab and pegylated interferon alpha-2b. *J Clin Oncol* 2008;26:1316–1323.
46. Kulke MH, Lenz HJ, Meropol NJ, et al. Activity of sunitinib in patients with advanced neuroendocrine tumors. *J Clin Oncol* 2008;26:3403–3410.
47. Raymond E, Dahan L, Raoul JL, et al. Sunitinib malate for the treatment of pancreatic neuroendocrine tumors. *N Engl J Med* 2011;364:501–513.
48. Kulke MH, Stuart K, Enzinger PC, et al. Phase II study of temozolomide and thalidomide in patients with metastatic neuroendocrine tumors. *J Clin Oncol* 2006;24:401–406.
49. Chan JA, Stuart K, Earle CC, et al. Prospective study of bevacizumab plus temozolomide in patients with advanced neuroendocrine tumors. *J Clin Oncol* 2012;30:2963–2968.
50. Kwekkeboom DJ, de Herder WW, Kam BL, et al. Treatment with the radiolabeled somatostatin analog [177Lu-DOTA 0,Tyr3]octreotate: toxicity, efficacy, and survival. *J Clin Oncol* 2008;26:2124–2130.
51. Bushnell DL Jr, O'Dorisio TM, O'Dorisio MS, et al. 90Y-edotreotide for metastatic carcinoid refractory to octreotide. *J Clin Oncol* 2010;28:1652–1659.
52. Norton JA, Warren RS, Kelly MG, et al. Aggressive surgery for metastatic liver neuroendocrine tumors. *Surgery* 2003;134:1057–1063.
53. Frilling A. Systematic review of resection of primary midgut carcinoid tumour in patients with unresectable liver metastases (Br J Surg 2012; 99: 1480–1486). *Br J Surg* 2012;99:1486–1487.
54. Landry CS, Scoggins CR, McMasters KM, et al. Management of hepatic metastasis of gastrointestinal carcinoid tumors. *J Surg Oncol* 2008;97:253–258.
55. Norlen O, Stalberg P, Zedenius J, et al. Outcome after resection and radiofrequency ablation of liver metastases from small intestinal neuroendocrine tumours. *Br J Surg* 2013;100:1505–1514.
56. Henn AR, Levine EA, McNulty W, et al. Percutaneous radiofrequency ablation of hepatic metastases for symptomatic relief of neuroendocrine tumors. *AJR Am J Roentgenol* 2003;181:1005–1010.
57. Strosberg JR, Weber JM, Choi J, et al. A phase 2 clinical trial of sunitinib following hepatic transarterial embolization for metastatic neuroendocrine tumors. *Ann Oncol* 2012;23:2335–2341.
58. Kennedy A, Coldwell D, Sangro B, et al. Integrating radioembolization into the treatment paradigm for metastatic neuroendocrine tumors in the liver. *Am J Clin Oncol* 2012;35:393–398.
59. Kennedy AS, Dezarn WA, McNeillie P, et al. Radioembolization for unresectable neuroendocrine hepatic metastases using resin 90Y-microspheres: early results in 148 patients. *Am J Clin Oncol* 2008;31:271–279.
60. Frilling A, Malago M, Weber F, et al. Liver transplantation for patients with metastatic endocrine tumors: single-center experience with 15 patients. *Liver Transpl* 2006;12:1089–1096.
61. Lehnert T. Liver transplantation for metastatic neuroendocrine carcinoma: an analysis of 103 patients. *Transplantation* 1998;66:1307–1312.

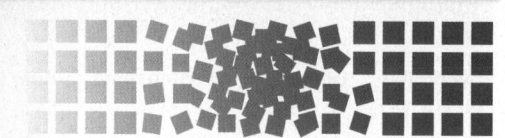

87 Multiple Endocrine Neoplasias

Jeffrey A. Norton and Pamela L. Kunz

INTRODUCTION

There are four multiple endocrine neoplasia (MEN) syndromes: MEN-1, MEN-2 (2a), MEN-3 (2b), familial medullary thyroid cancer (FMTC), and MEN-4 (Table 87.1). MEN-1 is inherited as an autosomal dominant syndrome caused by mutations of the menin gene. It is composed of multiple endocrine tumors classically affecting the parathyroid glands, anterior pituitary gland, and endocrine pancreas. It also may affect the adrenal cortex and thyroid gland. Neuroendocrine tumors (NET) of the bronchus, thymus, stomach, and small intestine (carcinoid tumors) are more common in patients with MEN-1. It also has some nonhormonal manifestations including facial angiofibromas, meningiomas, smooth muscle tumors, collagenomas, and lipomas.[1,2]

FMTC, MEN-2, and MEN-3 are caused by specific mutations of the RET proto-oncogene.[3,4] They are also inherited as an autosomal dominant condition. Patients with FMTC develop MTC usually late in adulthood with no other endocrine tumors. The MTC in this condition is indolent and nonmetastatic such that patients typically die from other causes. MEN-2 (also called MEN-2a) is characterized by medullary thyroid cancer (MTC), pheochromocytoma, and parathyroid hyperplasia. Cutaneous lichen amyloidosis has been described in several kindreds. MEN-3 (also called MEN-2b) is also associated with a RET mutation, but it is in the intracellular tyrosine kinase domain of the molecule. These patients develop a more aggressive form of MTC at a young age, and they have characteristic eye and bony changes. They also have bilateral pheochromocytomas usually in adulthood, but they do not have primary hyperparathyroidism (HPT). Finally, MEN-4 (also called MENX) is caused by a mutation in CDKN1B that encodes p27Kip1, a tumor suppressor gene that inhibits cell cycle progression.[5] These patients may be confused with MEN-1 because they develop pituitary and parathyroid adenomas.[6] This chapter will further characterize and describe these syndromes including specific molecular and genetic changes, epidemiology, screening, malignant potential, causes of death, and treatment.

MULTIPLE ENDOCRINE NEOPLASIA TYPE 1

Incidence and Etiology in Multiple Endocrine Neoplasia Type 1

Patients with MEN-1 develop parathyroid hyperplasia and primary HPT typically as the first manifestation of the syndrome (90% to 100%),[1,2] followed by pancreatic neuroendocrine tumors (pNET) either functional (20% to 70%) or nonfunctional (80% to 100%), pituitary adenomas (20% to 65%), adrenal tumors (10% to 73%), and thyroid adenomas (0% to 10%). Patients with MEN-1 also have a high occurrence of other endocrine and nonendocrine tumors including carcinoid tumors (thymic 0% to 8%, gastric 7% to 35%, bronchial 0% to 8%, and infrequently intestinal), skin and subcutaneous tumors (angiofibromas 88%, collagenomas 72%, lipomas

34%, and melanoma), central nervous system tumors (meningiomas, ependymomas, schwannomas 0% to 8%), and smooth muscle tumors (leiomyomas and leiomyosarcomas 1% to 7%). The main causes of death in these patients are the malignant potential of the pNET followed by the thymic carcinoid tumors[2] (Table 87.2).

Molecular and Genetic Basis in Multiple Endocrine Neoplasia Type 1

MEN-1 is inherited as an autosomal dominant disorder and has an incidence between 0.22% and 0.25% in autopsy studies. The gene causing MEN-1 is located on the long arm of chromosome 11 (11q13).[7] It encodes a 610 amino acid nuclear protein called menin that controls cell division, genomic stability, and transcriptional regulation. It is a tumor suppressor gene. Abnormalities of the gene can result in mutations, deletions, and truncations of menin protein. Menin acts as a scaffold protein and increases or decreases gene expression by epigenetic regulation via histone methylation. It complexes with trimethylate histone H3 at lysine, which subsequently facilitates activation of transcription in cyclin-dependent kinase inhibitors and silences transcriptional activity in other target genes. MEN-1–associated tumors harbor germline and somatic mutations.

Screening in Multiple Endocrine Neoplasia Type 1

Genetic screening for MEN-1 is recommended when an individual has two or more MEN-1–related tumors, multiple abnormal parathyroid glands before age 30 years, recurrent HPT at a young age, gastrinoma and HPT or multiple pNETs at any age, plus a family history of kidney stones or endocrine tumors that are part of the syndrome.[8] Genetic testing includes sequencing of the entire coding region of the MEN-1 gene (exons 2 to 10) and identifies mutations in about 80% of patients with familial MEN-1.

Primary Hyperparathyroidism in Multiple Endocrine Neoplasia Type 1

Primary HPT is the most common endocrine abnormality in MEN-1. It reaches nearly 100% penetrance by the age of 50 years. HPT is usually the first manifestation of MEN-1 with a typical age of onset of 20 to 25 years. Decreased bone density and kidney stones are common. HPT often occurs at the same time as Zollinger-Ellison syndrome (ZES) and surgery to correct the HPT greatly ameliorates the clinical findings of ZES.[9] As in sporadic cases, biochemical testing for HPT is critical to the diagnosis. Total or ionized serum level of calcium and intact serum parathyroid hormone levels are measured and both should be elevated. Twenty-four-hour urinary calcium should also be measured and will be elevated. Patients with MEN-1 and HPT typically have multiple abnormal glands. The tumors are asymmetric in size and should be considered as independent clonal adenomas.[8] Imaging studies are not useful for initial

TABLE 87.1

Multiple Endocrine Neoplasia Syndromes: Features and Genetics

Syndrome	Autosomal Dominant	Chromosome	Gene	Gene Function	Hormonal Syndrome	Nonendocrine Features
MEN-1	+	11q13	Menin	Tumor suppressor	■ Parathyroid adenomas (90%) ■ Enteropancreatic NET (70%) ■ Anterior pituitary (22%) ■ Carcinoid (4%)	■ Lipomas (30%) ■ Facial angiofibroma (85%) ■ Collagenomas (70%)
MEN-2 (2a)	+	10q11.2	RET	Oncogene	■ MTC (100%) ■ Pheochromocytomas (50%) ■ Parathyroid hyperplasia (20%)	■ Hisrchsprung ■ CLA
MEN-3 (2b)	+	10q11.2	RET	Oncogene	■ MTC (100%) ■ Pheochromocytomas (50%)	■ Marfanoid habitus ■ Skeletal changes ■ Mucosal neuromas ■ Corneal nerve hypertrophy
FMTC	+	10q11.2	RET	Oncogene	■ MTC (100%)	■ None
MEN-4 (MENX)	−	4	CDNK1B	Tumor suppressor	■ Parathyroid ■ Anterior pituitary ■ Adrenal	■ Kidney ■ Reproductive organs

MEN, multiple endocrine neoplasia; NET, neuroendocrine tumor; MTC, medullary thyroid cancer; CLA, cutaneous lichen amyloidosis; FMTC, familial medullary thyroid cancer.

operations because all four parathyroid glands must be identified. The current operation of choice is a subtotal parathyroidectomy (3.5 gland resection) with removal of the thymus. Intraoperative parathyroid hormone level monitoring is recommended to be certain that sufficient abnormal parathyroid tissue has been removed. A viable 50 mg amount of normal parathyroid tissue should be left in the neck and marked with a hemoclip. Because of the multiple abnormal parathyroid gland nature of this disease, there is a high probability of recurrent HPT years after surgery if <3.5 resections are performed. Calcium-sensing receptor agonists (calcimimetics) are a new class of drugs that can act directly on the parathyroid gland, decrease parathyroid hormone release, and may even decrease parathyroid tissue growth. These agents may play an important role in the management of these patients in the future.[8]

Enteropancreatic Neuroendocrine Tumors in Multiple Endocrine Neoplasia Type 1

The prevalence of enteropancreatic NETs in MEN-1 is between 30% to 75%.[1,2] The enteropancreatic pathology in MEN-1 is typically multicentric and multifocal with multiple endocrine tumors throughout the pancreas and the intestine. Tumors vary from microadenomas to carcinomas with lymph node and liver metastases. Duodenal gastrinomas in MEN-1 are usually small (<1 cm), submucosal, and multifocal. pNETs contain in decreasing frequency chromogranin, pancreatic polypeptide, glucagon, insulin, proinsulin, somatostatin, gastrin, vasoactive intestinal polypeptide, serotonin, calcitonin, growth hormone releasing factor, and neurotensin. Malignant enteropancreatic NETs are rare prior to the age of 30 years; however, 50% of middle-aged patients with MEN-1 have evidence for malignant pNETs. Recent studies identified the following factors as suggestive of poor prognosis: higher fasting serum levels of gastrin, presence of more than one functional hormonal syndrome, need for more than three parathyroid surgical procedures, presence of either liver metastases, aggressive primary tumor growth, large pNETs (>4 cm), pNETs with areas of poor vascular enhancement on computed tomography (CT), and serial imaging with evidence for progression.[2]

Gastrinomas (ZES) are the most common functional NET in MEN-1.[10] Approximately 40% of patients with MEN-1 will have ZES, and 25% of all ZES cases occur in patients with MEN-1. ZES is diagnosed by elevated fasting serum level of gastrin (>100 pg/ml,

off proton pump inhibitors) and concomitant increased gastric acid output (>10 meq/hr). Approximately one-third of patients with ZES will die from the malignant progression of the tumor. Correlates for a poor prognosis with MEN-1/ZES are pancreatic primary tumors, metastases, Cushing syndrome, and severe hypergastrinemia (defined as >3,000 pg/ml).[2] Surgery has been done to try to cure patients with MEN-1 of ZES. Local removal of tumors without duodenal/pancreatic resection are associated with persistent ZES; however, Whipple pancreaticoduodenectomy is more consistently associated with biochemical cure.[11] This approach is still controversial because those who favor less than Whipple argue that the symptoms of ZES are well controlled with proton pump inhibitors and the morbidity/mortality of Whipple procedure is too significant.

Insulinoma is the second most common functional pNET in MEN-1.[12] Approximately 10% of patients with MEN-1 will develop insulinoma, and 10% of insulinomas occur in the setting of

TABLE 87.2

Causes of Death in 194 Patients with Multiple Endocrine Neoplasia Type 1

Endocrine-related	**145 (75%)**
Malignant pancreatic NET	96 (49%)
Thymic carcinoid	31 (16%)
Pituitary adenoma	4 (2%)
Parathyroid hyperplasia	14 (7%)
Nonendocrine-related	**49 (25%)**
Heart attack	16 (8%)
Other cancers	21 (11%)
Stroke	9 (5%)
Hematologic	3 (2%)

NET, neuroendocrine tumor. Abstracted from Ito T, Igarashi H, Uehara H, et al. Causes of death and prognostic factors in multiple endocrine neoplasia type 1: a prospective study: comparison of 106 MEN1/Zollinger-Ellison syndrome patients with 1613 literature MEN1 patients with or without pancreatic endocrine tumors. *Medicine* 2013;92:135–181.

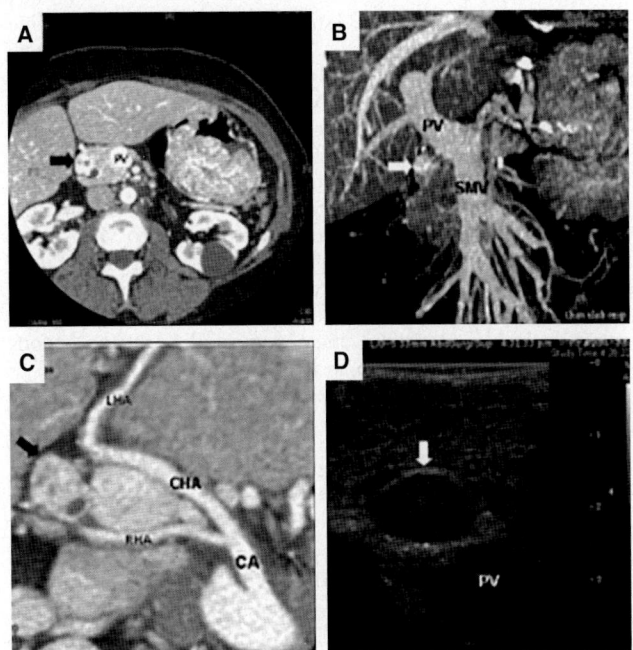

Figure 87.1 Insulinoma in a patient with multiple endocrine neoplasia type 1. **(A)** Computed tomography showing tumor (*arrow*) as hypervascular blush in head of pancreas. **(B)** The same tumor (*arrow*) on portal venogram. **(C)** The tumor (*arrow*) on angiogram. **(D)** The tumor (*arrow*) on intraoperative ultrasound. (Reprinted from Norton JA, Fang TD, Jensen RT. Surgery for gastrinoma and insulinoma in multiple endocrine neoplasia type 1. *J Natl Compr Canc Netw* 2006;4:148–153, with permission.)

MEN-1. Patients have hypoglycemia and neuroglycopenic symptoms (altered mental status and seizures). This occurs at a young age (<35 years). Fasting hypoglycemia (glucose <45 mg/dl) and concomitant hyperinsulinemia (levels >5 uU/ml) are diagnostic. Tumors are generally small (<2 cm) and distributed uniformly throughout the pancreas.[1,8] Since patients with MEN-1 have multiple pNETS, it may not be clear which tumor is secreting the excessive insulin. However, one study reported that the insulinoma is most commonly a dominant pNET that is easily identified by conventional imaging studies like CT or magnetic resonance imaging (MRI)[12] (Fig. 87.1).

For nonfunctional enteropancreatic NETS in asymptomatic patients with MEN-1, there is controversy over the role of surgery. Several groups advocate that surgery should be avoided unless the tumor is 2 cm or growing.[13] Other groups recommend surgery for tumors that are 1 cm.[14] The goal of surgery in MEN-1 appears to be control tumor to prevent cancerous progression. The standard operation is distal or subtotal (resection margin superior mesenteric vein) pancreatectomy with intraoperative ultrasound and enucleation of tumors from the pancreatic head and duodenum. Extensive pancreaticoduodenal procedures are associated with increased risk, thus the indication for the procedure, potential benefit, and surgeon experience must be considered.

Pituitary Tumors in Multiple Endocrine Neoplasia Type 1

Anterior pituitary adenomas are the initial clinical manifestation of MEN-1 in 25% of cases.[2,8] Its prevalence in MEN-1 is between 10% and 60%. Most anterior pituitary tumors are microadenomas (<1 cm in diameter). Every type of anterior pituitary tumor has been reported to occur in MEN-1 with the most common type being a prolactinoma. Screening for anterior pituitary tumors requires measuring serum levels of prolactin, insulin-like growth

factor 1, and MRI of the pituitary. Patients should be questioned for loss of peripheral vision and visual fields assessed formally if any suspicion. Treatment of pituitary tumors in MEN-1 is the same as sporadic pituitary tumors.

Less Common Tumors in Multiple Endocrine Neoplasia Type 1

Other primary sites of MEN-1 tumors include thymus, bronchus, and stomach. The most worrisome are thymic carcinoids because they are the second most common cause of death in patients with MEN-1.[2] Thymic carcinoids are seen more commonly in men with MEN-1 and are usually asymptomatic. Bronchial carcinoids also occur at a higher frequency and are more common in women with MEN-1. In patients with MEN-1 with ZES who have been taking proton pump inhibitors for a long time period, type II gastric enterochromaffin-like cell carcinoid tumors have been identified on upper gastrointestinal endoscopy. The tumors are usually multiple and may involve the entire stomach. These tumors may spread to lymph nodes and liver and may require total gastrectomy.[15] Each of these three foregut carcinoid tumors in MEN-1 has malignant potential, and physicians caring for these patients should be vigilant for early diagnosis in patients with known MEN-1.

Adrenal cortical tumors are common in MEN-1. The majority are bilateral, hyperplastic, and nonfunctional. Pathology may include cortical adenoma, diffuse hyperplasia, nodular hyperplasia, and carcinoma. Some patients may present with Cushing syndrome secondary to an adrenal tumor, but adrenocorticotropic hormone from a bronchial carcinoid or a pituitary adenoma may also cause hypercortisolism.[16] The adrenal cortical tumors are usually nonfunctional and benign so that surgical resection is not indicated; however, hormone production should be excluded. Multiple lipomas, both cutaneous and visceral, occur in one-third of patients with MEN-1. Lipomas in MEN-1 are small but can be large.[2,7,8] They are usually multicentric, cosmetically disturbing, and not malignant. If they are excised, they do not recur. Multiple facial angiofibromas occur in 40% to 80% of patients with MEN-1; collagenomas also are common.

Management of Metastatic Disease in Multiple Endocrine Neoplasia Type 1

Of the MEN-1–associated tumors, metastatic disease is common in pancreatic, small bowel, and bronchial NETs. For example, approximately 60% of patients with enteropancreatic NETs have metastatic disease at the time of diagnosis.[17] Patient selection is a critical first step in the treatment algorithm of these patients and is addressed extensively in other chapters. Management of metastatic disease in patients with MEN-1 is comparable to the management of patients without the syndrome. However, for patients with multiple primary endocrine tumors, vigilance must be taken when evaluating new findings on cross-sectional imaging to be certain which tumor is metastatic and/or progressing. The oncologic management of metastatic NETs has seen a recent renaissance, which is reflected in other chapters on pancreatic and small bowel NETs and MTC. Such advances include US Food and Drug Administration approval of two agents for the treatment of metastatic pNETs: everolimus[18] and sunitinib.[19] Additionally, multiple ongoing clinical trials are poised to address important questions in this field around the roles of chemotherapy and adjuvant treatment.

Follow-Up

CT and MRI are recommended for early diagnosis, but somatostatin receptor scintigraphy (octreoscan) is more sensitive. Recently Ga-68 DOTATOC positron emission tomography/CT scan may be even more sensitive for imaging ectopic or metastatic NETs.[20] It is a total body study, and these tumors have somatostatin receptors so there are few false positives. Further, once the diagnosis of MEN-1 is made, somatostatin receptor scintigraphy and DOTATOC positron emission tomography/CT may be useful to exclude unsuspected malignant tumors like bronchial and thymic carcinoids.

MULTIPLE ENDOCRINE NEOPLASIA TYPE 2, TYPE 3, AND FAMILIAL MEDULLARY THYROID CANCER

Incidence and Etiology in Multiple Endocrine Neoplasia Type 2, Type 3, and Familial Medullary Thyroid Cancer

MTC is a common feature of these three inherited syndromes. It is a rare type of thyroid cancer. It accounts for only 3% to 10% of all thyroid cancers. A total of 20% of all MTC is associated with one of these syndromes; 80% is sporadic. Familial forms of this disease present earlier in life. The mean age of sporadic MTC is 47 ± 17; for the familial forms, it is 25 ± 15 years. Patients who present with a thyroid nodule are seldom cured (Fig. 87.2). Thus in the familial form with 100% penetrance, screening for the inherited RET gene mutation is critical.

Molecular Genetic Basis of Multiple Endocrine Neoplasia Type 2, Type 3, and Familial Medullary Thyroid Cancer

RET is an oncogene composed of 21 exons located on the long-arm of chromosome 10 (10q11.2) encoding a transmembrane receptor tyrosine kinase. The RET protein is composed of three functional domains: an extracellular ligand-binding domain, a transmembrane domain, and a cytoplasmic tyrosine kinase domain. RET is involved in a number of cellular signaling pathways during development regulating the survival, proliferation, differentiation, and migration of the enteric nervous system progenitor cells, as well as the survival and regeneration of neural and kidney cells.

All MEN-2 cases have an identified mutation in the RET gene, and when tested no family with MEN-2 has failed to have a RET gene mutation.[3] MEN-2–associated mutations in RET have been identified on exons 10, 11, 13, 14, 15, and 16. The likelihood of a RET mutation in a patient with sporadic MTC is 1% to 7%. Recently, it has been shown that HRAS, KRAS, and NRAS mutations occur in approximately 10% to 45% of sporadic MTC cases. How-

ever, all cases of sporadic MTC should still be tested for a germline RET mutation. This should be performed through a laboratory that analyzes exons 10, 11, 14, 14, 15, and 16. If these exons are negative, the remaining 15 RET exons should be sequenced.[3]

Approximately 95% of patients with MEN-2 have RET mutations at 609, 611, 618, and 620 in exon10, or at codon 634 in exon11. The presence of mutations at codon 634 is associated with the development of primary HPT and pheochromocytoma. Most patients with MEN-3 have mutations in exon 16 M918T and less often exon 15 A883F. Patients with MEN-3 with mutations at A883F have a better prognosis, and rarely long-term cures have been reported following thyroidectomy in these patients. The most common FMTC mutations affect extracellular cysteine codons in RET exon 10 or intracellular RET codons other than A883 or M918[3] (Table 87.3).

Screening in Multiple Endocrine Neoplasia Type 2, Type 3, and Familial Medullary Thyroid Cancer

Screening for MTC in each of these syndromes is done by measuring the specific RET germline mutation. MTC arises from the calcitonin secreting cells or C-cells. C-cell hyperplasia is not itself malignant, but can transform to MTC; thyroidectomy during the hyperplasia stage can prevent development of MTC. Since C-cells make calcitonin, screening for MTC used to be done by measuring pentagastrin/calcium stimulated levels of calcitonin. However, since all of these patients have germline mutations in RET and all develop MTC, C-cell hyperplasia and MTC can be diagnosed in each affected individual by RET gene analysis. One cannot overemphasize the importance of direct DNA sequencing to detect RET mutations in kindred members at risk for MTC. Further, approximately 3% to 7% of patients with presumed sporadic MTC have familial MTC.[3]

A major issue is the age to perform screening and prophylactic thyroidectomy. In patients from a family with MEN-2 and a RET mutation, most clinicians recommend that the individual should be screened at age 5 and the thyroid gland be removed if affected. In this setting, central compartment lymph node dissection is unnecessary as it can increase the occurrence of postoperative hypoparathyroidism. In patients with MEN-3, the surgery should be done at any age as soon as the diagnosis is established. Since these patients commonly have a more aggressive tumor, central lymph node dissection should always be done. In patients with FMTC, screening should be done at age 21 and, if positive, thyroidectomy without central lymph node dissection. Postoperatively at 6 months, physical examination and serum levels of calcitonin and

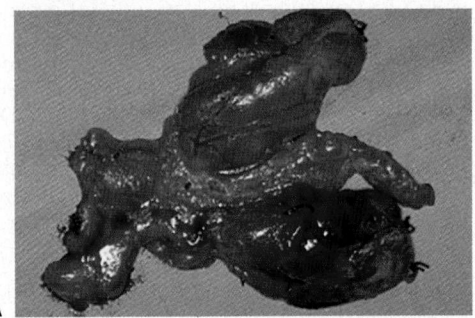

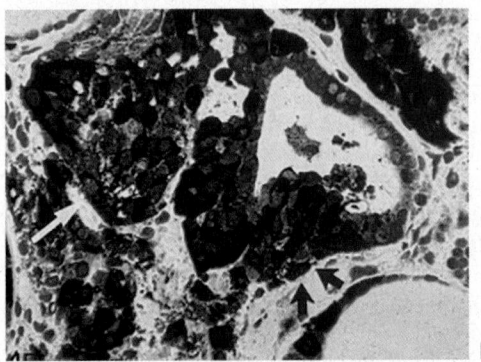

Figure 87.2 **(A)** Gross photography of thyroid with central lymph nodes in a patient with multiple endocrine neoplasia type 2a who presented with palpable thyroid nodules bilaterally. Note that the medullary thyroid cancer is bilateral and that the central lymph nodes are involved. **(B)** Immunohistochemistry for calcitonin of the same tumor showing malignancy of the parafollicular C-cells.

TABLE 87.3

RET Mutations in Multiple Endocrine Neoplasia: Genotype/Phenotype

Syndrome	Exon	Codon	Location	Phenotype
MEN-2 (2a)	10	609		MTC aggression ++
		611		
		618	Extra- and intracellular	
		620		
	11	634		Primary HPT/pheochromocytoma
MEN-3 (2b)	16	M918T	Intracellular	MTC aggression ++++
	15	A883F		Pheochromocytomas
FMTC	10	A883	Extra- and intracellular	MTC aggression +
		M918		

MEN, multiple endocrine neoplasia; MTC, medullary thyroid cancer; HPT, hyperparathyroidism. From Wells SA Jr, Pacini F, Robison BG, et al. Multiple endocrine neoplasia type 2 and familial medullary thyroid carcinoma: an update. *J Clin Endocrinol Metab* 2013;98:3149–3164.

PRACTICE OF ONCOLOGY

carcinoembryonic antigen (CEA) are measured. If calcitonin and CEA levels are undetectable or normal for 5 years, no additional studies are necessary.

Multiple Endocrine Neoplasia Type 2

MEN-2 (also termed MEN-2a) accounts for 80% of the FMTC syndromes. In MEN-2, beside MTC, 50% of patients develop pheochromocytomas, and 30% develop primary HPT depending on the RET codon mutation.[21] Patients with MEN-2 may also develop cutaneous lichen amyloidosis, Hirschsprung disease, and prominent corneal nerves. C-cells secrete calcitonin and CEA. Either calcitonin or CEA levels in the blood serve as an excellent marker for MTC. Pentagastrin or calcium stimulated serum calcitonin levels may serve as a more sensitive marker for MTC. Unlike sporadic MTC that is usually unilateral, familial forms of MTC are always bilateral (see Fig. 87.2). The tumor is multicentric and occupies the superior and central portion of each lobe. MTC initially remains confined to the thyroid gland but subsequently spreads to regional lymph nodes and then distant sites including the liver, lung, bone, and brain. The tumor is very firm and has a fibrous acellular stroma that has staining properties similar to amyloid, but it is immunohistochemically calcitonin.

Pheochromocytomas develop in 50% of patients with MEN-2 and -3.[22,23] The clinical findings and behavior is the same in both syndromes. The mean age at presentation is 36 years, and the diagnosis is made after MTC in 40% of cases and before MTC in 10%. In this setting, the pheochromocytomas are benign and confined to the adrenal gland. Sixty-five percent of the time, these tumors are bilateral; with 10-year follow-up, patients with a unilateral pheochromocytoma will develop a contralateral tumor. It is critical to exclude the diagnosis of pheochromocytoma in these patients before doing any invasive procedure because sudden death may occur if a pheochromocytoma is not detected and the patient is not appropriately prepared with alpha-adrenergic blocking agent. Deaths have been reported during surgical procedures and childbirth. Patients suspected of having a pheochromocytoma should have measurement of plasma-free metanephrine and normetanephrine levels or a 24-hour urine for vanillylmandelic acid, metanephrines, and total catecholamines. CT and MRI are used to image pheochromocytomas. The sensitivity and specificity are similar for the two procedures, 90% to 100% and 70% to 80%, respectively.

The pheochromocytoma should be resected before the thyroid surgery. Preoperative preparation with an alpha-adrenergic blocking drug like phenoxybenzamine is done. If necessary after the patient is well blocked and just before surgery, a beta-adrenergic drug is added. Despite the fact that the pheochromocytomas are usually bilateral, if on CT or MRI only one adrenal appears to contain tumor, unilateral adrenalectomy is recommended for the gland with the tumor.[22] This is recommended because there has been reported a significant risk of Addisonian crisis with bilateral adrenalectomy. Some other surgeons have recommended bilateral subtotal adrenalectomy for these patients to preserve cortical function. Although this approach may have merit, there have been limited follow-up and report of long-term function or recurrent pheochromocytomas with this procedure. Adrenalectomy can usually be accomplished laparoscopically, and this approach greatly reduces morbidity. In patients who undergo bilateral adrenalectomy, corticosteroid coverage is necessary both preoperatively and postoperatively.

Primary HPT develops in 20% to 30% of patients with MEN-2.[24] The mean age of onset is 36 years. It can occur prior to any manifestation of MTC in 5%. The hypercalcemia is minimal and most patients do not have symptoms. The parathyroid glands are asymmetrically enlarged and contain hyperplastic nodules. Pathologically, it is called pseudonodular hyperplasia. The operation of choice is subtotal parathyroidectomy or 3.5 gland parathyroidectomy.

Multiple Endocrine Neoplasia Type 3

MEN-3, also called MEN-2b, accounts for 5% of hereditary MTC.[25] These patients all have MTC, bilateral pheochromocytomas, and characteristic phenotype, but they do not develop primary HPT. Patients with MEN-3 have a characteristic phenotype that includes marfanoid habitus, prolonged facies, muscular skeletal abnormalities (pectus, saber shins, bowing of the extremities), ocular abnormalities (inability to cry tears and corneal nerve hypertrophy),[26] mucosal neuromas usually on the tip of the tongue (Fig. 87.3), and ganglioneuromatosis. Most have gastrointestinal symptoms characterized by pain, diarrhea, constipation, bloating, and megacolon. These symptoms may occur in children and young adults with this syndrome.

The MTC is uniformly aggressive and spreads to distant sites early in these patients. It occurs during infancy and early diagnosis is critical.[25] In approximately 50% of MEN-3 cases, de novo germline RET mutations give rise to the disease. In patients with de novo MEN-3, the mutated allele generally comes from the father. Babies are at a high risk in this setting because the parents are asymptomatic and the disease is not expected. This is unfortunate because there is only a narrow window during which thyroidectomy may be curative. Even in the most advantageous setting where thyroidectomy was performed during the neonatal period, most babies are not cured. These patients also get pheochromocytoma (usually bilateral), but they do not develop parathyroid disease.

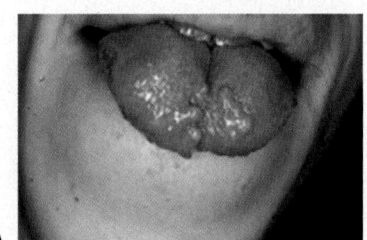
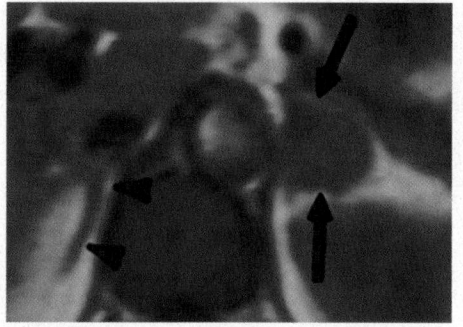

Figure 87.3 (A) Mucosal neuromas on the tip of the tongue in a patient with multiple endocrine neoplasia type 2a (MEN-3). **(B)** Patient had documented medullary thyroid cancer and needed a thyroidectomy, but the preoperative workup documented a pheochromocytoma that was localized to the left adrenal (*arrows*) by magnetic resonance imaging. A normal-appearing right adrenal (*arrows*) is also seen.

Familial Medullary Thyroid Carcinoma

FMTC accounts for 15% of hereditary MTC.[3] These patients only have MTC that occurs at a late age and is less aggressive than the other familial forms. They do not get pheochromocytomas or parathyroid disease. The diagnosis is made when an individual can identify 10 affected individuals occurring in kindred over the age of 50 years with an adequate history and biochemical data to exclude pheochromocytoma and primary HPT in affected individuals.

The strongest predictor of survival for patients with MTC is the stage of disease at the time of thyroidectomy. The 10-year disease-specific survival of MTC is 90% with localized disease, 78% with lymph node metastases, and 40% with distant metastases. Only 10% of patients with metastases to cervical lymph nodes are cured with extensive lymph node dissection. The prognosis is excellent for patients with FMTC who have a preoperative calcitonin level <150 pg/ml, an MTC <1 cm, and no lymph node metastases.[3] The 10-year survival approaches 100% if basal and stimulated calcitonin levels are undetectable after thyroidectomy. In patients with MTC confined to the thyroid gland, the standard operation is total thyroidectomy and resection of all lymph nodes in the central zone of the neck. The neck dissection is more extensive in patients with advanced nodal disease.

A reliable indicator of progression of MTC is the calcitonin or CEA doubling time. A calcitonin doubling time between 6 months and 2 years is associated with a 5-year survival of 92% and a 10-year survival of 37%, whereas a doubling rate of <6 months is associated with a 25% and 8% survival, respectively. In most patients, the calcitonin level is most predictive of prognosis, but in some patients the CEA level is more correlative so both should be measured. If the postoperative serum calcitonin level rises above 150 to 200 pg/ml, total body CT scan should be performed. In the absence of distant metastases and the presence of cervical lymph node disease, a neck dissection should be performed. Prior studies suggested that this strategy may cure approximately 30% of patients, but more recent long-term follow-up indicate that these patients will recur. Some studies suggest that external beam radiation should be administered after neck dissection; however, this treatment has not improved survival.

Management of Metastatic Disease in Multiple Endocrine Neoplasia Type 2, Type 3, and Familial Medullary Thyroid Cancer

Development of metastatic disease in patients not identified by screening is common in MTC. The survival of patients with distant metastases from MTC is 51% at 1 year, 26% at 5 years, and 10% at

10 years. When patients develop distant metastases from MTC and calcitonin levels increase, they may also develop secretory diarrhea that is difficult to control. Management of metastatic disease in patients with inherited forms of MTC is similar to management in sporadic MTC and is addressed extensively in the chapter on thyroid cancer (Chapter 82). Loperamide, codeine, or sandostatin may help control diarrhea in some cases. Tumor debulking or selective arterial embolization may provide symptomatic improvement in others. Two new compounds have recently been approved by the US Food and Drug Administration for the treatment of metastatic MTC and include vandetanib[27] and cabozantinib,[28] and were shown to prolong progression-free survival in phase 3 clinical trials.

MULTIPLE ENDOCRINE NEOPLASIA TYPE 4

MEN-4 (also known as MENX) has been recently identified.[5,29] It is characterized by the occurrence of parathyroid, anterior pituitary, and in possible association with tumors of the adrenal, kidneys, and reproductive organs (testicular cancer, neuroendocrine cervical carcinoma). It is caused by a heterozygous mutation of CDK1B that encodes the 196 amino acid CDK1 p27 Kip1 protein that is activated by H3K4 transmethylation.

There is a population of patients who are thought to have MEN-1, but they do not have mutations of menin and may have mutations of other genes. One of these other genes may be CDKN1B, which encodes a cyclin-dependent kinase inhibitor (CK1) p27^{kip1}. It was identified as causing a MEN-like syndrome in rats referred to as MENX. Rats with MENX have parathyroid adenomas, pancreatic islet cell hyperplasia, thyroid C-cell hyperplasia, bilateral pheochromocytomas, paragangliomas, and cataracts. The disorder is inherited as an autosomal recessive trait. Genetic mapping localized MENX to the distal part of rat chromosome 4, a region that contained the putative tumor suppressor CK1P27^{kip1}, which is also called p27. Mutation of this tumor suppressor gene resulted in a loss p27 protein in tumor cells. These findings prompted studies in patients with suspected MEN-1, who did not have MEN-1 mutations, for abnormalities of CDKN1B that in man is located on chromosome 12p13. These studies revealed that approximately 3% of patients with MEN-1 phenotype actually had CDKN1B mutations. These patients had parathyroid adenomas, pituitary adenomas, and pNETS, plus gonadal, adrenal, renal, and thyroid tumors. Currently, eight different heterozygous loss-of-function CDKN1B mutations have been identified in patients with MEN-1–like tumors. This indicates that MEN-4 in man is an autosomal dominant disorder, unlike MENX in rats. Further, germline mutations of CDKN1B have been identified in sporadic (nonfamilial) forms of primary HPT.

REFERENCES

1. Thakker RV, Newey PJ, Walls GV, et al. Clinical practice guidelines for multiple endocrine neopasia type 1 (MEN1). *J Clin Endocrinol Metab* 2012;97:2990–3001.
2. Ito T, Igarashi H, Uehara H, et al. Causes of death and prognostic factors in multiple endocrine neoplasia type 1: a prospective study: comparison of 106 MEN1/Zollinger-Ellison syndrome patients with 1613 literature MEN1 patients with or without pancreatic endocrine tumors. *Medicine* 2013;92:135–181.
3. Wells SA Jr, Pacini F, Robinson BG, et al. Multiple endocrine neoplasia Type 2 and familial medullary thyroid carcinoma: an update. *J Clin Endocrinol Metab* 2013;98:3149–3164.
4. Fox E, Widemann BC, Chuk MK, et al. Vandetanib in children and adolescents with multiple endocrine neoplasia type 2B associated medullary thyroid carcinoma. *Clin Cancer Res* 2013;19:4239–4248.
5. Lee M, Pellegata NS. Multiple endocrine neoplasia syndromes associated with mutation of p27. *J Endocrinol Invest* 2013;36:781–787.
6. Thakker RV. Multiple endocrine neoplasia type 1 (MEN1) and type 4 (MEN4). *Mol Cell Endocrinol* 2014;386:2–15.
7. Romei C, Pardi E, Cetani F, et al. Genetic and clinical features of multiple endocrine neoplasia type 1 and 2. *J Oncol* 2012;1–15.
8. Brandi M, Gagel RF, Angeli A, et al. Guidelines for diagnosis and therapy of MEN type 1 and type 2. *J Clin Endocrinol Metab* 2001;86:5658–6571.
9. Norton JA, Cornelius MJ, Doppman JL, et al. Effect of parathyroidectomy in patients with hyperparathyroidism and Zollinger-Ellison syndrome and multiple endocrine neoplasia type 1: a prospective study. *Surgery* 1987;102:958–966.
10. Singh MH, Fraker DL, Metz DC. Importance of surveillance for multiple endocrine neoplasia-1 and surgery in patients with sporadic Zollinger-Ellison syndrome. *Clin Gastroenterol Hepatol* 2012;10:1262–1269.
11. Lopez CL, Falconi M, Waldmann J, et al. Partial pancreaticoduodenectomy can provide cure for duodenal gastrinoma associated with multiple endocrine neoplasia type 1. *Ann Surg* 2013;257:308–314.
12. Norton JA, Fang TD, Jensen RT. Surgery for gastrinoma and insulinoma in multiple endocrine neoplasia type 1. *J Natl Compr Canc Netw* 2006;4:148–153.
13. Weber HC, Venzon DJ, Lin JT, et al. Determinants of metastatic rate and survival in patients with Zollinger-Ellison syndrome: a prospective long-term study. *Gastroenterology* 1995;108:1637–1649.
14. Skogseid B, Oberg K, Eriksson B, et al. Surgery for asymptomatic pancreatic lesions in multiple endocrine neoplasia type 1. *World J Surg* 1996;20:872–877.
15. Norton JA, Melcher ML, Gibril F, et al. Gastric carcinoid tumors in multiple endocrine neoplasia-1 patients with Zollinger-Ellison syndrome can be symptomatic, demonstrate aggressive growth, and require surgical treatment. *Surgery* 2004;136:1267–1274.
16. Simonds WF, Varghese S, Marx SJ, et al. Cushing's syndrome in multiple endocrine neoplasia type 1. *Clin Endocrinol* 2012;76:379–386.
17. Yao JC, Eisner MP, Leary C, et al. Population-based study of islet cell carcinoma. *Ann Surg Oncol* 2007;14:3492–3500.
18. Yao JC, Shah MH, Ito T, et al. Everolimus for advanced pancreatic neuroendocrine tumors. *N Engl J Med* 2011;363:514–523.
19. Raymond E, Dahan L, Raoul JL, et al. Sunitinib malate for the treatment of pancreatic neuroendocrine tumors. *N Engl J Med* 2011;364:501–513.
20. Froeling V, Elgeti F, Maurer MH, et al. Impact of Ga-68 DOTATOC PET/CT on the diagnosis and treatment of patients with multiple endocrine neoplasia. *Ann Nucl Med* 2012;26:738–743.
21. Schulte KM, Machens A, Fugazzola L, et al. The clinical spectrum of multiple endocrine neoplasia type 2a caused by the rare intracellular RET mutation S891A. *J Clin Endocrinol Metab* 2010;95:E92–E97.
22. Scholten A, Valk GD, Ulfman D, et al. Unilateral adrenalectomy for pheochromocytoma in multiple endocrine neoplasia type 2 patients. *Ann Surg* 2011;254:1022–1027.
23. Thosani S, Ayala-Ramirez M, Palmer L, et al. The characterization of pheochromocytoma and its impact on overall survival in multiple endocrine neoplasia type 2. *J Clin Endocrinol Metab* 2013;98:E1813–E1819.
24. Machens A, Lorenz K, Dralle H. Peak incidence of pheochromocytoma and primary hyperparathyroidism in multiple endocrine neoplasia 2: need for age-adjusted biochemical screening. *J Clin Endocrinol Metab* 2013;98:E336–E345.
25. Brauckhoff M, Machens A, Lorenz K, et al. Surgical curability of medullary thyroid cancer in multiple endocrine neoplasia 2B. *Ann Surg* 2014;259:800–806.
26. Lee R, Hyer J, Chowdhury H, et al. Ocular signs of multiple endocrine neoplasia type 2B (MEN2B). *J Clin Endocrinol Metab* 2012;97:725–726.
27. Wells SA Jr, Robinson BG, Gagel RF, et al. Vandetanib in patients with locally advanced or metastatic medullary thyroid cancer: a randomized, double-blind phase III trial. *J Clin Oncol* 2012;30:134–141.
28. Schoffski P, Elisei R, Muller S. An international, double-blind, randomized, placebo-controlled phase III trial (EXAM) of cabozantinib (XL184) in medullary thyroid carcinoma (MTC) patients with documented RECIST progression at baseline. *J Clin Oncol* 2012;30:Abstract 5508.
29. Lee M, Pellegata NS. Multiple endocrine neoplasia type 4. *Horm Res* 2013;41:63–78.

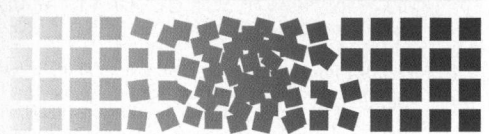

88 Genetic Testing in the Endocrine System

Robert Pilarski and Rebecca Nagy

INTRODUCTION

A number of hereditary syndromes, caused by mutations in an even larger number of tumor suppressor genes and oncogenes, can cause tumors in organs of the endocrine system. Table 88.1 summarizes the major syndromes, genes, and endocrine organs affected.

MULTIPLE ENDOCRINE NEOPLASIA TYPE 1

Syndrome Description

Multiple endocrine neoplasia (MEN) type 1 is an autosomal dominant syndrome with an estimated incidence in the general population on the order of 1/100,000 to 10/100,000.[1,2] The major endocrine features of MEN1 are parathyroid adenomas, entero-pancreatic endocrine tumors, and pituitary tumors. A diagnosis of MEN1 is made in a person with two of the three major endocrine tumors, or in an individual with at least one of these tumors if another relative has a diagnosis of MEN1.[3–5] The age-related penetrance of MEN1 is 45% at the age of 30 years, 82% at the age of 50 years, and 96% at the age of 70 years.[5–7]

The most common feature of MEN1 is parathyroid adenoma, which results in primary hyperparathyroidism (PHP). In approximately 50% to 85% of patients with MEN1, PHP will be the presenting manifestation. These tumors occur in 80% to 95% of patients by the age of 50 years,[5,8–10] and are typically multiglandular and often hyperplastic.[1] The average age at onset of PHP in MEN1 is 20 to 25 years, in contrast to that in the general population, which is in the 50s. Parathyroid carcinoma in MEN1 is rare but has been described.[11–13]

Pancreatic endocrine tumors are the second most common endocrine manifestation in MEN1, occurring in up to 30% to 80% of patients.[5,8] Gastrinomas and insulinomas are most common, followed by VIPomas (vasoactive intestinal peptide), glucagonomas, and somatostatinomas. These tumors are usually multicentric and can arise in the pancreas or more commonly as small (<0.5 cm) foci throughout the duodenum.[14] Gastrinomas represent 50% of the gastrointestinal neuroendocrine tumors in MEN1 and are the major cause of morbidity and mortality in patients with MEN1.[5,15] Most result in peptic ulcer disease (Zollinger–Ellison syndrome), and half are malignant at the time of diagnosis.[14–16] Nonfunctional tumors of the enteropancreas, some of which produce pancreatic polypeptide, are seen in 20% of patients.[17–19]

Approximately 15% to 50% of patients with MEN1 will develop a pituitary tumor.[5,8] Two-thirds are microadenomas (<1 cm in diameter), and the majority are prolactin secreting.[20] Other manifestations of MEN1 include carcinoids of the foregut (typically bronchial or thymic), skin lipomas, facial angiomas, and collagenomas and adrenal cortical lesions, including cortical adenomas, diffuse or nodular hyperplasia, or rarely carcinoma.[7,21] Thyroid adenomas, pheochromocytoma (PC) (usually unilateral), spinal ependymoma, and leiomyoma have also been reported.[22]

Genetic Testing

MEN1 is caused by mutations in the *MEN1* gene, which is located on chromosome 11q13. It is inherited in an autosomal dominant manner. Germline mutations are typically found in 80% to 95% of families with two or more affected members and in up to 65% of simplex cases (single case of MEN1 with no family history).[4,23] Menin, the protein encoded by the *MEN1* gene, functions as a tumor suppressor gene and is involved in multiple cellular functions including transcription regulation, genomic stability, cell division, and cell cycle control.[24]

More than 1,100 mutations have been identified in the *MEN1* gene to date, and these are scattered across the entire coding region.[24] The majority of these are nonsense or frameshift mutations, and the remainder are missense or in-frame deletions that lead to expression of an altered protein. Splice-site mutations have also been described. There is currently no evidence of genotype–phenotype correlations, and interfamilial and intrafamilial variability is the rule.[25,26]

Whereas the *MEN1* mutation detection rate is quite high in simplex and familial cases, the greater diagnostic challenge for the clinician is when to order genetic testing in an individual who does not meet diagnostic criteria, but has one of the three component tumors. The prevalence of MEN1 among patients with apparently sporadic component tumors varies widely by tumor type. Approximately one-third of patients with Zollinger–Ellison syndrome will carry an *MEN1* mutation.[27,28] In individuals with apparently isolated hyperparathyroidism (HPT) or pituitary adenomas, the mutation prevalence is lower, on the order of 2% to 5% for each,[20,29,30] but the prevalence is higher in individuals diagnosed with these tumors at younger ages (<30 years old). In a small series of patients with isolated foregut/midgut carcinoids, none of 68 were found to carry an *MEN1* mutation. Some authors suggest *MEN1* testing in those not meeting diagnostic criteria if one of the following is present: Gastrinoma at any age, multifocal pancreatic islet cell tumors at any age, parathyroid adenomas before the age of 30 years, multiglandular parathyroid adenomas, or recurrent HPT, or in individuals with one of the three main MEN1 tumors plus one of the less common tumors/findings.[31]

Management

Screening and surveillance for MEN1 should use a combination of biochemical screening and imaging as follows[3]:

- Annual serum prolactin and insulin-like growth factor 1 starting at the age of 5 years
- Annual fasting total serum calcium and/or ionized calcium and PTH starting at the age of 8 years
- Annual fasting serum gastrin starting at the age of 20 years; consider chromogranin A, glucagon, and proinsulin for other enteropancreatic tumors
- Annual fasting glucose starting at the age of 5 years

TABLE 88.1

Major Endocrine System Tumors and Associated Hereditary Syndromes

Tumor Site Type	*MEN1* (MEN 1)	*RET* (MEN 2)	Gene (Syndrome) *PTEN* (CS PHTS)	*SDHX* (HPCC/PGL)	*VHL* (VHL)
Adrenal (PC)		X		X	X
Carcinoid	X				X
Neuroendocrine	X			X	
Pancreas (islet cell)	X				X
Parathyroid	X	X			
Paraganglioma				X	X
Pituitary	X				
Thyroid		MTC	PTC, FTC		

MEN, multiple endocrine neoplasia; CS, Cowden syndrome; PHTS, *PTEN* hamartoma tumor syndrome; HPCC/PGL, hereditary pheochromocytoma/paraganglioma syndrome; VHL, von Hippel-Lindau disease; PC, pheochromocytoma; MTC, Medullary thyroid cancer; PTC, Papillary thyroid cancer; FTC, Follicular thyroid cancer.

■ Brain magnetic resonance imaging (MRI) at the age of 5 years, repeat every 3 to 5 years based on biochemical test results
■ Abdominal computed tomography or MRI starting at the age of 20 years, repeat every 3 to 5 years based on biochemical test results

Surgical management of MEN1 is complex and controversial given the multifocal and multiglandular nature of the disease and the high risk of tumor recurrence even after surgery. A full review of surgical options is outside the scope of this review, but this topic has been reviewed elsewhere.[32,33] Establishing the diagnosis of MEN1 before making surgical decisions and referring affected individuals to a surgeon with experience in treating MEN1 can be critical in preventing unnecessary surgeries or inappropriate surgical approaches.

MULTIPLE ENDOCRINE NEOPLASIA TYPE 2

Syndrome Description

MEN2, caused by germline mutations in the *RET* proto-oncogene, is an autosomal dominant syndrome characterized by medullary thyroid cancer (MTC), PC, and/or HPT. Historically, families were classified into one of the three clinical subtypes, MEN2A, MEN2B, and familial medullary thyroid carcinoma (FMTC) based on the presence or absence of certain endocrine tumors and other phenotypic features. However, there is debate about whether FMTC represents a separate entity or is a variation of MEN2A in which there is a lower lifetime risk and delay in the onset of the extrathyroidal manifestations.[34] Incorrect classification of families with MEN2A as having FMTC may result in delayed diagnosis of PC, a disease with significant morbidity and mortality. For this reason, current management recommendations include screening for all three tumors in individuals carrying a germline *RET* mutation, with the exception of parathyroid screening in MEN2B cases[35] (see section on management).

The endocrine tumors in MEN2 are often multifocal and bilateral/multiglandular and present at an early age. MTC is present in up to 95% of mutation carriers, and the age at presentation varies, somewhat depending on the specific mutation. Early diagnosis of MTC is critical, given the poor overall survival for individuals diagnosed with distant metastases.[36–38] PCs are present in up to 50% of carriers, and the lifetime risk is also dependent on genotype. Although the PCs in MEN2 rarely metastasize, they can be clinically significant because of intractable hypertension or anesthesia-induced hypertensive crises. Parathyroid abnormalities are the least common finding, occurring in up to 30% of patients. The parathyroid disease in MEN2 can include benign parathyroid adenomas or multiglandular hyperplasia, but is typically asymptomatic or associated with only mild elevations in calcium.[39,40]

MEN2A is diagnosed clinically by the occurrence of two or more of the specific endocrine tumors in a single individual or in close relatives. MEN2A may also be suspected when MTC occurs at an early age (<50 years) or is bilateral or multifocal even in the absence of family history. Several large series indicate a mutation frequency of 1% to 7% in isolated cases of MTC.[40,41] Based on these data, it is widely recommended that *RET* gene mutation testing be performed for all cases of MTC, regardless of age at diagnosis and family history.[3,35,42]

MEN2B, which makes up 5% of MEN2 cases, is characterized by the early development of an aggressive form of MTC in all patients.[43] Patients with MEN2B who do not undergo thyroidectomy at an early age (~1 year) are likely to develop metastatic MTC at an early age. PCs occur in about 50% of MEN2B cases, and clinically significant parathyroid disease is very uncommon.[44] Individuals with MEN2B can also have distinctive facies with enlarged lips, mucosal neuromas of the lips and tongue, medullated corneal nerve fibers, and an asthenic marfanoid body habitus.[44] About 40% of patients have diffuse ganglioneuromatosis of the gastrointestinal tract.[45]

Genetic Testing

MEN2 is the result of germline mutations in the *RET* gene, located on chromosome region 10q11.2.[46,47] The *RET* gene is a proto-oncogene encoding a receptor tyrosine kinase with extracellular, transmembrane, and intracellular domains. *RET* mutations causing MEN2 are activating mutations, resulting in a constitutively activated tyrosine kinase receptor.[48]

Genetic testing in MEN2 is considered an important part of the management of at-risk family members. As MTC and other tumors can develop in childhood, testing of children who have no symptoms is considered beneficial.[35] Timing of *RET* testing depends largely on the mutation present in the family. Several groups have developed mutation stratification systems to guide clinicians with regard to the appropriate timing of *RET* testing, prophylactic thyroidectomy, and biochemical screening.[3,35] These are based mainly on age at onset, aggressiveness of thyroid disease, and clinical phenotype, but have not been validated as clinical decision-making tools. The original stratification system was developed by the International RET Consortium.[3] A newer classification system by the American Thyroid Association[35] was published in 2009 (Table 88.2).

PRACTICE OF ONCOLOGY

Multiple Endocrine Neoplasia Type 2 Mutation Classification System and Management Guidelines of the American Thyroid Association

ATA Risk Level	Mutated Codon(s)	Age at RET Testing	Age at Prophylactic Thyroidectomy	Timing and Frequency of Other Surveillance
A	768, 790, 791, 804, 891	<age 3–5 y	May delay surgery after age 5 y if criteria are met[a]	Age 20 y, repeat periodically
B	609, 611, 618, 620, 630, compound heterozygote: V804M + V778I	<age 3–5 y	Consider surgery before age 5 y; may delay surgery after age 5 y if criteria are met[a]	Age 8 y for codon 630; age 20 y for all others; repeat periodically
C	634	<age 3–5 y	Before age 5 y	Age 8 y, annually
D	883 and 918 Compound heterozygotes V804M + S904C V804M + E805K V804M + Y806C	ASAP and within the first year of life	ASAP and within the first year of life	Age 8 y, annually for PC only

ATA, American Thyroid Association; ASAP, as soon as possible; PC, pheochromocytoma.
[a] Criteria include a normal annual basal and/or stimulated serum count, normal annual neck ultrasound, less aggressive medullary thyroid cancer family history, and family preference.
From Kloos RT, Eng C, Evans DB, et al. Medullary thyroid cancer: Management guidelines of the American Thyroid Association. *Thyroid* 2009;19:565–612.

Approximately 95% of patients with MEN2A or MEN2B will have an identifiable germline *RET* mutation.[43] As mentioned previously, 1% to 7% of apparently sporadic cases of MTC will carry a germline *RET* mutation, underscoring the importance of testing all cases of MTC.[3,35,42] A targeted exon approach is most commonly used in families with MEN2A. If the clinical suspicion is MEN2B, a targeted mutation analysis can be used. If targeted testing in a family with a high clinical suspicion for MEN2 is normal, sequencing of the remaining exons can then be performed. For families that do not have a detectable mutation, management recommendations can be based on the clinical features in the affected individual and in the family.

Management

Management of *RET* mutation carriers includes prophylactic thyroidectomy, as well as biochemical screening for PC and HPT.[3,35] The timing of these interventions has been largely based on genotype, but this remains controversial. Prophylactic thyroidectomy and parathyroidectomy with reimplantation of one or more parathyroid glands into the neck or forearm are a preventive option for all subtypes of MEN2. For those with mutations associated with early-onset aggressive MTC, genetic testing alone is used to determine timing of surgery.[3,35] For individuals carrying lower- or intermediate-risk mutations (see Table 88.2), some centers allow surgery to be delayed until biochemical screening becomes abnormal and/or the individual reaches a particular age.[35] This is still somewhat controversial, however, given the great intrafamilial variability and the fact that MTC can be present even in the absence of an elevated basal or stimulated calcitonin.

Biochemical screening for parathyroid disease and PC is recommended, and the timing and frequency depend on the genotype and, in some cases, presence/absence of these tumors in the family (see Table 88.2). Annual screening for HPT should include albumin-corrected calcium or ionized serum calcium with or without intact PTH measurement (American Thyroid Association, 2009). Screening for PC with plasma-free metanephrines and/or urinary fractionated metanephrines is recommended, given that these provide a higher diagnostic sensitivity than urinary catecholamines.[49,50] When biochemical screening suggests PC, MRI or computed tomography can be performed.[51,52] Confirmation of the diagnosis can be made using various anatomic and functional modalities.[52–54] Several reviews provide a succinct summary of the biochemical diagnosis, localization, and management of PC.[52,55] If surgical removal is required, laparoscopic adrenalectomy is the recommended approach for the treatment of unilateral PC.[56] For individuals with bilateral PC, cortical-sparing adrenalectomy is an option to minimize the risk of adrenal insufficiency.[56,57]

PHOSPHATASE AND TENSIN HOMOLOG ON CHROMOSOME 10

Clinical Features

Germline mutations in the *PTEN* (phosphatase and tensin homolog on chromosome 10) gene have been associated with a number of related clinical disorders, including Cowden syndrome (CS), Bannayan–Riley–Ruvalcaba syndrome, a Proteus-like syndrome, adult Lhermitte–Duclos disease, and autism-like disorders with macrocephaly. Although CS is the only one with a documented risk for endocrine (thyroid) cancer, it is possible that any person with a *PTEN* mutation is at increased risk.[58]

The prevalence of CS, an autosomal dominant disorder, has been estimated to be between 1/200,000 and 1/250,000.[59] Diagnostic criteria for CS were initially developed in 1996,[60] and subsequent modifications have been proposed.[61–63] A clinical diagnosis requires a requisite number of clinical features, which are divided into groups of "pathognomonic," "major," and "minor" criteria (Table 88.3).

Cancer rates in CS have historically been reported as 25% to 50% for breast cancer, 3% to 10% for thyroid cancer, and 5% to 10% for endometrial cancer, based on compilations of cases published in the early literature.[64–66] Thyroid cancer in CS is exclusively of follicular or papillary histology. More recently, an increased risk for colon cancer has been reported.[67] Although recent reports from two large cohorts found cancer rates similar to these,[67,68] a follow-up report on one of these cohorts projected lifetime cancer risks of 85% for breast cancer, 35% for thyroid cancer, 28% for endometrial cancer, 34% for kidney cancer, and 9% for colon cancer.[69] However, these high risks are subject to significant selection bias and should be considered with caution, given their discrepancy with clinical experience with patients with CS.

Benign lesions are also seen in CS and include mucocutaneous lesions (trichilemmomas, acral keratoses, and papillomatous papules, seen in most patients), thyroid abnormalities (goiter, adenoma in 50% to 67%), benign breast lesions (fibroadenomas,

TABLE 88.3

Cowden Syndrome Diagnostic Criteria

Pathognomonic criteria
- Lhermitte–Duclos disease—adult
- Mucocutaneous lesions
- Trichilemmomas, facial
- Acral keratoses
- Papillomatous lesions

Major criteria
- Breast cancer
- Thyroid cancer (papillary or follicular)
- Macrocephaly (≥97th percentile)
- Endometrial cancer

Minor criteria
- Other structural thyroid lesions (e.g., adenoma, multinodular goiter)
- Mental retardation (i.e., IQ ≤75)
- Gastrointestinal hamartomas
- Fibrocystic disease of the breast
- Lipomas
- Fibromas
- Genitourinary tumors (e.g., uterine fibroids, renal cell carcinoma) or
- Genitourinary structural malformations
- Uterine fibroids

Operational diagnosis in an individual (any of the following):
1. Mucocutaneous lesions alone, if
   a. There are six or more facial papules, of which three or more must be trichilemmoma, or
   b. Cutaneous facial papules and oral mucosal papillomatosis, or
   c. Oral mucosal papillomatosis and acral keratoses, or
   d. More than six palmoplantar keratosis
2. Two or more major criteria, but one must include macrocephaly or Lhermitte–Duclos disease; or
3. One major and three minor criteria; or
4. Four minor criteria

Operational diagnosis in a family where one individual is diagnostic for Cowden syndrome:
   a. One pathognomonic criterion; or
   b. Any one major criterion with or without minor criteria; or
   c. Two minor criteria; or
   d. History of Bannayan–Riley–Ruvalcaba syndrome[58]

---

fibrocystic disease in 40% to 75% of females), gastrointestinal polyps (≥80%), macrocephaly (≤80%), and uterine fibroids (25% to 44% of females).[68,69]

Genetic Testing

The *PTEN* tumor suppressor gene is a dual-specificity phosphatase with multiple and as yet incompletely understood roles in cellular regulation. It is known to signal down the PI3K/Akt pathway to cause G1 cell cycle arrest and apoptosis, and has also been shown to regulate cell-survival pathways, such as the mitogen-activated kinase pathway.[70] Although it is generally reported that germline *PTEN* mutations are found in 80% of patients with CS, based on initial reports in 1997,[71–73] more recent data suggest that it is much lower,[67–69] and there is reason to consider revising the diagnostic criteria.[68] A small number of studies suggest that gene deletions or rearrangements are rare in CS.[74,75] Approximately 2% of all patients with CS in one study had a variant in the *PTEN* promoter.[74] Although not definitive, protein expression studies suggested that these variants could be deleterious. The new mutation rate for *PTEN* is unknown.

Testing criteria for CS have been developed and are updated annually by the National Comprehensive Cancer Network.[76] Clinical *PTEN* testing is available in a number of national laboratories.

Germline genetic variants were found in the *SDHB* and *SDHD* genes in one report in a cohort of patients with CS- or a CS-like phenotype.[77] None of the patients with genetic variants met current CS diagnostic criteria, however, and the clinical significance of these variants has been questioned, given that most had previously been identified as benign polymorphisms.[78] More recently, germline methylation of the *KILLIN* gene has been suggested to be related to CS as well.[79]

Management

Management guidelines for individuals with CS have been adopted by the National Comprehensive Cancer Network[76] and include annual physical examinations, monthly breast self-examinations, and a baseline thyroid ultrasound (with consideration of repeating annually), starting at the age of 18 years; clinical breast examinations every 6 months, starting at the age of 25 years; annual mammography and breast MRI screening starting at the age of 30 to 35 years; consideration of colonoscopy every 5 to 10 years, starting at the age of 35 years; consideration of an annual dermatologic examination; and consideration of participation in clinical trials for endometrial cell cancer screening.

SDHX/TMEM127/MAX

Clinical Features

Mutations in four genes of the succinate dehydrogenase (SDH) complex, *SDHA*, *SDHB*, *SDHC*, and *SDHD* (collectively referred to as *SDHX*), and several interacting genes have been shown to cause the autosomal dominant hereditary paraganglioma (PGL)–pheochromocytoma (PCC) syndrome. The SDH complex is part of both the mitochondrial–respiratory chain (complex II) and the Krebs cycle.[80] The specific clinical phenotype varies, somewhat depending on the gene involved, as discussed in the following.

Individuals with *SDHB* mutations tend to present with sympathetic PGLs and less commonly PCC and parasympathetic PGL. There is a higher rate of malignancy and mortality with *SDHB* mutations compared with other SDH genes.[80] An analysis of 378 published cases with *SDHB* mutations found that 78% had PGL (71% sympathetic) and 25% had PCC (all unilateral), with a mean age at presentation of 33 years.[81] Up to 31% had malignant tumors. In one study of 32 patients with metastatic PCC/PGL whose tumor was diagnosed before age 20 years, 23 (72%) had *SDHB* mutations.[82] The penetrance of *SDHB* mutations has been estimated to be 77% by the age of 50 years.[83] The risks for renal cell carcinoma and oncocytoma also appear to be increased.[84,85]

SDHD mutations most commonly cause multifocal parasympathetic PGL. A review of the clinical features of 289 patients with *SDHD* mutations found that 92% had PGL (56% multiple), 24% had PCC (all unilateral), and only 4% had malignant disease.[81] The mean age at presentation is 35 years,[86] and the penetrance is estimated to be 86% by the age of 50 years.[83] *SDHD* mutations appear to be maternally imprinted such that tumors develop only when a mutation is inherited from the father.[87] However, several rare cases of maternal transmission have been reported.[88,89]

SDHC mutations are rare in patients with PCC/PGL. They mainly cause nonmalignant parasympathetic PGL (and rarely PCC) and were found in 4% of such patients in one study.[90] The average age at presentation is 43 years.[81]

More recently, mutations in the *SDHAF2* (also called *SDH5*), *SDHA*, *TMEM127*, and *MAX* genes have also been found in hereditary PGL/PCC. Given their rarity, and their recent discoveries, less is known about their clinical presentation. Mutations in *SDHAF2/SDH5* have been described in a number of families with head and neck PGL, but to date no cases with PCC have been reported.[91,92] It appears that there is genetic imprinting with paternal transmission required for tumor development.[91,92] Biallelic *SDHA* mutations have been known to cause inherited juvenile encephalopathy/Leigh syndrome,[93] but it was only recently that heterozygous mutations have been found in a few individuals with PCC or PGL.[94,95] Mutations in *TMEM127* were first identified in 2010[96] and were initially felt to be associated exclusively with PC.[97] However, several cases with extra-adrenal tumors have been reported.[98] *TMEM127* mutations are relatively rare causes of PCC and PGL—mutations were found in only 6 (1%) of 559 PCC cases and none of 72 PGL cases who did not carry mutations in *SDHB*, *SDHD*, *RET*, or *VHL*.[99] In addition, the age at diagnosis of PCC is not significantly earlier than average (41.5 years), and malignancy is infrequent.[96,97] Exome sequencing was used to identify *MAX* gene mutations in 12 individuals with hereditary PCC in one study.[100] Most cases (67%) were bilateral, and an association with malignancy was suggested, as was the possibility that paternal transmission was required for tumor development.

Genetic Testing

Although approximately 10% of patients with PCC have a clinically apparent hereditary syndrome, studies have shown that up to 25% of "sporadic" cases also have germline mutations in either *SDHB*, *SDHD*, *RET*, or *VHL*.[101] Similarly, analysis of 445 patients with PGL found mutations in *SDHB*, *SDHC*, or *SDHD* in 220 (50%).[102] Whereas some have called for genetic testing for all PCC/PGL, others have called for a targeted approach. A number of algorithms have been proposed whereby testing decisions are based on a variety of factors including presence of clinical features, early age at diagnosis, location and laterality of tumor(s), positive family history, and presence of malignancy.[81,103] Clinical testing is available in the United States for all of these genes except *MAX*.

Management

The management of PCC and PGL is primarily surgical, and it is critical that patients undergo preoperative catecholamine and metanephrine screening to detect functional disease, which could precipitate anesthesia-induced hypertensive crisis during surgery. For at-risk patients with known mutations, there are no consensus guidelines as to the appropriate screening protocols. Although it is generally felt that MRI and/or functional imaging and measurement of blood/urine metanephrines be performed on a regular basis, the specifics vary among centers.[104]

VON HIPPEL-LINDAU AND PHEOCHROMOCYTOMA

von Hippel-Lindau disease (VHL) is not often characterized as an endocrine-related disorder. However, the presence of PC and, rarely, pancreatic neuroendocrine tumors in VHL warrants a brief discussion in this section. Herein, we will also briefly review the genetic approach to the patient presenting with sporadic PC, as this is not an uncommon reason for referral for genetic counseling and risk assessment, and a significant proportion of these individuals will have an underlying hereditary condition. Additional information about other VHL and other VHL-related tumors (i.e., renal cell carcinoma) can be found in the section on urinary tract cancers.

VHL is an inherited multisystem disease predisposing to retinal and central nervous system hemangioblastomas, renal cell carcinoma, PC, pancreatic islet cell tumors, and endolymphatic sac tumors. It has an estimated birth incidence of 1 in 36,000 per year[105] and is inherited in an autosomal dominant manner with a high degree of interfamilial and intrafamilial variability.[106] The penetrance is age dependent, but reaches ~95% by the age of 65 years.[105,107] Four subtypes have been described on the basis of genotype–phenotype correlations.[107] PC is the main endocrine-related tumor associated with VHL. As in other hereditary syndromes, VHL-associated PCs are typically multifocal and/or bilateral and present at an earlier age than sporadic tumors and rarely metastatic.[107]

PC can be seen in several different hereditary conditions in addition to VHL, including neurofibromatosis type 1, MEN2, and the hereditary paraganglioma/PC syndromes.[108] One study of 271 patients with apparently sporadic PC analyzed the *NF1* (diagnosis made on the basis of clinical features, not genetic testing), *RET*, *VHL*, *SDHB*, and *SDHD* genes.[109] Upon further scrutiny, 166 (25.9%) of the 271 had a positive family history, and in these 166 families, germline mutations were detected in *RET* (n = 31), *VHL* (n = 56), *NF1* (n = 14), *SDHB* (n = 34), or *SDHD* (n = 31). Interestingly, 12.7% of those with no other syndromic features and/or family history (after rigorous clinical evaluation) also carried mutations.

These data indicate that a significant proportion of individuals presenting with apparently sporadic PC are carriers of germline genetic mutations. Referral to a genetic specialist may be warranted in all cases of apparently isolated PC, but is certainly appropriate in those diagnosed at or younger than 35 years and those with metastatic disease or multifocal and/or bilateral disease. Several clinical and genetic screening algorithms have been proposed to assist clinicians in deciding which genes to test and in which order,[52,109,110] as testing for mutations in five different genes in every patient may not be feasible or cost-effective.

REFERENCES

1. Chandrasekharappa S, Teh B. Clinical and molecular aspects of multiple endocrine neoplasia type 1. In: Dahia PLM, Eng C, eds. *Genetic Disorders of Endocrine Neoplasia*, Vol. 28. Front Horm Res. Basel: Switzerland: Karger; 2001:50–80.
2. Kouvaraki MA, Lee JE, Shapiro SE, et al. Genotype-phenotype analysis in multiple endocrine neoplasia type 1. *Arch Surg* 2002;137:641–647.
3. Brandi M, Gagel R, Angeli A, et al. Consensus guidelines for diagnosis and therapy of MEN type 1 and type 2. *J Clin Endocrinol Metab* 2001;86:5658–5671.
4. Chandrasekharappa SC, Guru SC, Manickam P, et al. Positional cloning of the gene for multiple endocrine neoplasia type 1 (MEN 1) gene. *Science* 1997;276:404–407.
5. Trump D, Farren B, Wooding C, et al. Clinical studies of multiple endocrine neoplasia type 1 (MEN1). *QJM* 1996;89:653–669.
6. Carty SE, Helm AK, Amico JA, et al. The variable penetrance and spectrum of manifestations of multiple endocrine neoplasia type 1. *Surgery* 1998;124:1106–1114.
7. Machens A, Schaaf L, Karges W, et al. Age-related penetrance of endocrine tumours in multiple endocrine neoplasia type 1 (MEN1): A multicentre study of 258 gene carriers. *Clin Endocrinol (Oxf)* 2007;67:613–622.
8. Thakker RV. Multiple endocrine neoplasia type 1 (MEN1). In: DeGroot LJ, Besser GK, Burger HG, et al, eds. *Endocrinology*. Philadelphia, PA: WB Saunders; 1995; 275–294.
9. Brandi ML, Marx SJ, Aurbach GD, et al. Familial multiple endocrine neoplasia type 1. A new look at pathophysiology. *Endocrinol Rev* 1987;8:391–405.
10. Benson L, Ljunghall S, Akerstrom G, et al. Hyperparathyroidism presenting as the first lesion in multiple endocrine neoplasia type 1. *Am J Med* 1987;82:731–737.
11. Agha A, Carpenter R, Bhattacharya S, et al. Parathyroid carcinoma in multiple endocrine neoplasia type 1 (MEN1) syndrome: Two case reports of an unrecognised entity. *J Endocrinol Invest* 2007;30:145–149.
12. Shih RY, Fackler S, Maturo S, et al. Parathyroid carcinoma in multiple endocrine neoplasia type 1 with a classic germline mutation. *Endocr Pract* 2009;15:567–572.
13. Sato M, Miyauchi A, Namihira H, et al. A newly recognized germline mutation of MEN1 gene identified in a patient with parathyroid adenoma and carcinoma. *Endocrine* 2000;12:223–226.
14. Pipeleers-Marichal M, Somers G, Willems G, et al. Gastrinomas in the duodenums of patients with multiple endocrine neoplasia type 1 and the Zollinger–Ellison syndrome. *N Engl J Med* 1990;322:723–727.

15. Norton JA, Fraker DL, Alexander HR, et al. Surgery to cure the Zollinger–Ellison syndrome. *N Engl J Med* 1999;341:635–644.
16. Weber H, Venzon D, Lin J, et al. Determinants of metastatic rate and survival in patients with Zollinger–Ellison syndrome: A prospective long-term study. *Gastroenterology* 1995;108:1637–1649.
17. Skosgeid B, Rastad J, Öberg K. Multiple endocrine neoplasia type 1. Clinical features and screening. *Endocrinol Metab Clin N Am* 1994;23:1–18.
18. Marx SJ. Multiple endocrine neoplasia type 1. In: Vogelstein B, Kinzler KW, eds. *The Genetic Basis of Human Cancer*. New York City: McGraw Hill; 2002:475–499.
19. Thomas-Marques L, Murat A, Delemer B, et al. Prospective endoscopic ultrasonographic evaluation of the frequency of nonfunctioning pancreaticoduodenal endocrine tumors in patients with multiple endocrine neoplasia type 1. *Am J Gastroenterol* 2006;101:266–273.
20. Corbetta S, Pizzocaro A, Peracchi M, et al. Multiple endocrine neoplasia type 1 in patients with recognized pituitary tumours of different types. *Clin Endocrinol (Oxf)* 1997;47:507–512.
21. Pieterman CR, Schreinemakers JM, Koppeschaar HP, et al. Multiple endocrine neoplasia type 1 (MEN1): Its manifestations and effect of genetic screening on clinical outcome. *Clin Endocrinol (Oxf)* 2009;70:575–581.
22. Gibril F, Schumann M, Pace A, et al. Multiple endocrine neoplasia type 1 and Zollinger–Ellison syndrome: A prospective study of 107 cases and comparison with 1009 cases from the literature. *Medicine (Baltimore)* 2004;83:43–83.
23. Larsson C, Skosgeid B, Öberg K, et al. Multiple endocrine neoplasia type 1 gene maps to chromosome 11 and is lost in insulinoma. *Nature* 1988;332:85–87.
24. Lemos MC, Thakker RV. Multiple endocrine neoplasia type 1 (MEN1): Analysis of 1336 mutations reported in the first decade following identification of the gene. *Hum Mutat* 2008;29:22–32.
25. Giraud S, Zhang CX, Serova-Sinilnikova OM, et al. Germ-line mutation analysis in patients with multiple endocrine neoplasia type 1 and related disorders. *Am J Hum Genet* 1998;63:455–467.
26. Wautot V, Vercherat C, Lespinasse J, et al. Germline mutation profile of MEN1 in multiple endocrine neoplasia type 1: Search for correlation between phenotype and the functional domains of the MEN1 protein. *Hum Mutat* 2002;20:35–47.
27. Roy PK, Venzon DJ, Shojamanesh H, et al. Zollinger-Ellison syndrome. Clinical presentation in 261 patients. *Medicine (Baltimore)* 2000;79:379–411.
28. Bardram L, Stage JG. Frequency of endocrine disorders in patients with the Zollinger-Ellison syndrome. *Scand J Gastroenterology* 1985;20:233–238.
29. Uchino S, Noguchi S, Sato M, et al. Screening of the MEN1 gene and discovery of germ-line and somatic mutations in apparently sporadic parathyroid tumors. *Cancer Res* 2000;60:5553–5557.
30. Scheithauer BW, Laws ERJ, Kovacs K, et al. Pituitary adenomas of the multiple endocrine neoplasia type 1 syndrome. *Semin Diagn Pathol* 1987;4:205–211.
31. Newey PJ, Thakker RV. Role of multiple endocrine neoplasia type 1 mutational analysis in clinical practice. *Endocr Pract* 2011;17:8–17.
32. Pieterman CR, van Hulsteijn LT, den Heijer M, et al. Primary hyperparathyroidism in MEN1 patients: A cohort study with longterm follow-up on preferred surgical procedure and the relation with genotype. *Ann Surg* 2012;255:1171–1178.
33. Pieterman CR, Vriens MR, Dreijerink KM, et al. Care for patients with multiple endocrine neoplasia type 1: The current evidence base. *Fam Cancer* 2010;10:157–171.
34. Pacini F, Castagna MG, Cipri C, et al. Medullary thyroid carcinoma. *Clin Oncol (R Coll Radiol)* 2010;22:475–485.
35. Kloos RT, Eng C, Evans DB, et al. Medullary thyroid cancer: Management guidelines of the American Thyroid Association. *Thyroid* 2009;19:565–612.
36. Fuchshuber PR, Loree TR, Hicks WL Jr, et al. Medullary carcinoma of the thyroid: Prognostic factors and treatment recommendations. *Ann Surg Oncol* 1998;5:81–86.
37. Dottorini ME, Assi A, Sironi M, et al. Multivariate analysis of patients with medullary thyroid carcinoma. Prognostic significance and impact on treatment of clinical and pathologic variables. *Cancer* 1996;77:1556–1565.
38. Kebebew E, Ituarte PH, Siperstein AE, et al. Medullary thyroid carcinoma: Clinical characteristics, treatment, prognostic factors, and a comparison of staging systems. *Cancer* 2000;88:1139–1148.
39. Kraimps JL, Denizot A, Carnaille B, et al. Primary hyperparathyroidism in multiple endocrine neoplasia type IIA: Retrospective French multicentric study. Groupe d'Etude des Tumeurs a Calcitonine (GETC, French Calcitonin Tumors Study Group), French Association of Endocrine Surgeons. *World J Surg* 1996;20:808–812; discussion 812–813.
40. Eng C, Mulligan LM, Smith DP, et al. Low frequency of germline mutations in the RET proto-oncogene in patients with apparently sporadic medullary thyroid carcinoma. *Clin Endocrinol (Oxf)* 1995;43:123–127.
41. Wohllk N, Cote GJ, Bugalho MM, et al. Relevance of RET proto-oncogene mutations in sporadic medullary thyroid carcinoma. *J Clin Endocrinol Metab* 1996;81:3740–3745.
42. National Comprehensive Cancer Network. *The NCCN Clinical Practice Guidelines in Oncology: Thyroid Cancer* (Version 2.2012). 2012. www.NCCN.org.
43. Eng C, Clayton D, Schuffenecker I, et al. The relationship between specific RET proto-oncogene mutations and disease phenotype in multiple endocrine neoplasia type 2. International RET mutation consortium analysis. *JAMA* 1996;2776:1575–1579.

44. Morrison PJ, Nevin NC. Multiple endocrine neoplasia type 2B (mucosal neuroma syndrome, Wagenmann-Froboese syndrome). *J Med Genet* 1996;33:779–782.
45. Brauckhoff M, Gimm O, Weiss CL, et al. Multiple endocrine neoplasia 2B syndrome due to codon 918 mutation: Clinical manifestation and course in early and late onset disease. *World J Surg* 2004;28:1305–1311.
46. Mole SE, Mulligan LM, Healey CS, et al. Localisation of the gene for multiple endocrine neoplasia type 2A to a 480 kb region in chromosome band 10q11.2. *Hum Mol Genet* 1993;2:247–252.
47. Gardner E, Papi L, Easton DF, et al. Genetic linkage studies map the multiple endocrine neoplasia type 2 loci to a small interval on chromosome 10q11.2. *Hum Mol Genet* 1993;2:241–246.
48. Takahashi M, Asai N, Iwashita T, et al. Molecular mechanisms of development of multiple endocrine neoplasia 2 by RET mutations. *J Intern Med* 1998;243:509–513.
49. Lenders JW, Pacak K, Walther MM, et al. Biochemical diagnosis of pheochromocytoma: Which test is best? *JAMA* 2002;287:1427–1434.
50. Boyle JG, Davidson DF, Perry CG, et al. Comparison of diagnostic accuracy of urinary free metanephrines, vanillyl mandelic acid, and catecholamines and plasma catecholamines for diagnosis of pheochromocytoma. *J Clin Endocrinol Metab* 2007;92:4602–4608.
51. Pacak K. Preoperative management of the pheochromocytoma patient. *J Clin Endocrinol Metab* 2007;92:4069–4079.
52. Pacak K, Eisenhofer G, Ahlman H, et al. Pheochromocytoma: recommendations for clinical practice from the First International Symposium. October 2005. *Nat Clin Pract Endocrinol Metab* 2007;3:92–102.
53. van der Harst E, de Herder WW, Bruining HA, et al. [(123)I]metaiodobenzylguanidine and [(111)In]octreotide uptake in benign and malignant pheochromocytomas. *J Clin Endocrinol Metab* 2001;86:685–693.
54. Timmers HJ, Taieb D, Pacak K. Current and future anatomical and functional imaging approaches to pheochromocytoma and paraganglioma. *Horm Metab Res* 2012;44:367–372.
55. Reisch N, Peczkowska M, Januszewicz A, et al. Pheochromocytoma: Presentation, diagnosis and treatment. *J Hypertens* 2006;24:2331–2339.
56. Yip L, Lee JE, Shapiro SE, et al. Surgical management of hereditary pheochromocytoma. *J Am Coll Surg* 2004;198:525–534; discussion 534–535.
57. Asari R, Scheuba C, Kaczirek K, et al. Estimated risk of pheochromocytoma recurrence after adrenal-sparing surgery in patients with multiple endocrine neoplasia type 2A. *Arch Surg* 2006;141:1199–1205; discussion 1205.
58. Pilarski R. Cowden syndrome: A critical review of the clinical literature. *J Genet Couns* 2009;18:13–27.
59. Nelen MR, Kremer H, Konings IB, et al. Novel PTEN mutations in patients with Cowden disease: Absence of clear genotype–phenotype correlations. *Eur J Hum Genet* 1999;7:267–273.
60. Nelen MR, Padberg GW, Peeters EAJ, et al. Localization of the gene for Cowden disease to 10q22-23. *Nat Genet* 1996;13:114–116.
61. Eng C. Will the real Cowden syndrome please stand up: Revised diagnostic criteria. *J Med Genet* 2000;37:828–830.
62. Pilarski R, Eng C. Will the real Cowden syndrome please stand up (again)? Expanding mutational and clinical spectra of the PTEN hamartoma tumour syndrome. *J Med Genet* 2004;41:323–326.
63. Zbuk KM, Stein, JL, Eng C. PTEN Hamartoma Tumor Syndrome (PHTS). GeneReviews at GeneTests: Medical Genetics Information Resource [database online]. http://www.genetests.org. Updated January 23, 2014. Accessed September 3, 2014.
64. Starink TM, van der Veen JPW, Arwert F, et al. The Cowden syndrome: A clinical and genetic study in 21 patients. *Clin Genet* 1986;29:222–233.
65. Starink TM. Cowden's disease: Analysis of fourteen new cases. *J Am Acad Dermatol* 1984;11:1127–1141.
66. Salem OS, Steck WD. Cowden's disease (multiple hamartoma and neoplasia syndrome). A case report and review of the English literature. *J Am Acad Dermatol* 1983;8:686–696.
67. Heald B, Mester J, Rybicki L, et al. Frequent gastrointestinal polyps and colorectal adenocarcinomas in a prospective series of PTEN mutation carriers. *Gastroenterology* 2010;139:1927–1933.
68. Pilarski R, Stephens JA, Noss R, et al. Predicting PTEN mutations: An evaluation of Cowden syndrome and Bannayan–Riley–Ruvalcaba syndrome clinical features. *J Med Genet* 2011;48:505–512.
69. Tan MH, Mester JL, Ngeow J, et al. Lifetime cancer risks in individuals with germline PTEN mutations. *Clin Cancer Res* 2012;18:400–407.
70. Tamguney T, Stokoe D. New insights into PTEN. *J Cell Sci* 2007;120:4071–4079.
71. Nelen MR, van Staveren CG, Peeters EAJ, et al. Germline mutations in the PTEN/MMAC1 gene in patients with Cowden disease. *Hum Mol Genet* 1997;6:1383–1387.
72. Liaw D, Marsh DJ, Li J, et al. Germline mutations of the PTEN gene in Cowden disease, an inherited breast and thyroid cancer syndrome. *Nat Genet* 1997;16:64–67.
73. Marsh DJ, Coulon V, Lunetta KL, et al. Mutation spectrum and genotype–phenotype analyses in Cowden disease and Bannayan–Zonana syndrome, two hamartoma syndromes with germline PTEN mutation. *Hum Mol Genet* 1998;7:507–515.
74. Zhou XP, Waite KA, Pilarski R, et al. Germline PTEN promoter mutations and deletions in Cowden/Bannayan–Riley–Ruvalcaba syndrome result in

PRACTICE OF ONCOLOGY

aberrant PTEN protein and dysregulation of the phosphoinositol-3-kinase/Akt pathway. *Am J Hum Genet* 2003;73:404–411.

75. Chibon F, Primois C, Bressieux JM, et al. Contribution of PTEN large rearrangements in Cowden disease: A MAPH screening approach. *J Med Genet* 2008;45:657–665.
76. National Comprehensive Cancer Network. The NCCN Genetic Familial High-Risk Assessment: Breast and Ovarian (Version 1.2012). Accessed September 3, 2014.
77. Ni Y, Zbuk KM, Sadler T, et al. Germline mutations and variants in the succinate dehydrogenase genes in Cowden and Cowden-like syndromes. *Am J Hum Genet* 2008;83:261–268.
78. Bayley JP. Succinate dehydrogenase gene variants and their role in Cowden syndrome. *Am J Hum Genet* 2011;88:674–675; author reply 676.
79. Bennett KL, Mester J, Eng C. Germline epigenetic regulation of KILLIN in Cowden and Cowden-like syndrome. *JAMA* 2011;304:2724–2731.
80. Gimenez-Roqueplo AP, Favier J, Rustin P, et al. Mutations in the SDHB gene are associated with extra-adrenal and/or malignant phaeochromocytomas. *Cancer Res* 2003;63:5615–5621.
81. Welander J, Soderkvist P, Gimm O. Genetics and clinical characteristics of hereditary pheochromocytomas and paragangliomas. *Endocr Relat Cancer* 2011;18:R253–R276.
82. King KS, Prodanov T, Kantorovich V, et al. Metastatic pheochromocytoma/paraganglioma related to primary tumor development in childhood or adolescence: Significant link to SDHB mutations. *J Clin Oncol* 2011;29:4137–4142.
83. Neumann HP, Pawlu C, Peczkowska M, et al. Distinct clinical features of paraganglioma syndromes associated with SDHB and SDHD gene mutations. *JAMA* 2004;292:943–951.
84. Ricketts C, Woodward ER, Killick P, et al. Germline SDHB mutations and familial renal cell carcinoma. *J Natl Cancer Inst* 2008;100:1260–1262.
85. Henderson A, Douglas F, Perros P, et al. SDHB-associated renal oncocytoma suggests a broadening of the renal phenotype in hereditary paragangliomatosis. *Fam Cancer* 2009;8:257–260.
86. Ricketts CJ, Forman JR, Rattenberry E, et al. Tumor risks and genotype–phenotype–proteotype analysis in 358 patients with germline mutations in SDHB and SDHD. *Hum Mutat* 2010;31:41–51.
87. van der Mey AG, Maaswinkel-Mooy PD, Cornelisse CJ, et al. Genomic imprinting in hereditary glomus tumours: Evidence for new genetic theory. *Lancet* 1989;2:1291–1294.
88. Pigny P, Vincent A, Cardot Bauters C, et al. Paraganglioma after maternal transmission of a succinate dehydrogenase gene mutation. *J Clin Endocrinol Metab* 2008;93:1609–1615.
89. Yeap PM, Tobias ES, Mavraki E, et al. Molecular analysis of pheochromocytoma after maternal transmission of SDHD mutation elucidates mechanism of parent-of-origin effect. *J Clin Endocrinol Metab* 2011;96:E2009–E2013.
90. Schiavi F, Boedeker CC, Bausch B, et al. Predictors and prevalence of paraganglioma syndrome associated with mutations of the SDHC gene. *JAMA* 2005;294:2057–2063.
91. Hao HX, Khalimonchuk O, Schraders M, et al. SDH5, a gene required for flavination of succinate dehydrogenase, is mutated in paraganglioma. *Science* 2009;325:1139–1142.
92. Bayley JP, Kunst HP, Cascon A, et al. SDHAF2 mutations in familial and sporadic paraganglioma and phaeochromocytoma. *Lancet Oncol* 2010;11:366–372.
93. Horvath R, Abicht A, Holinski-Feder E, et al. Leigh syndrome caused by mutations in the flavoprotein (Fp) subunit of succinate dehydrogenase (SDHA). *J Neurol Neurosurg Psychiatry* 2006;77:74–76.
94. Burnichon N, Briere JJ, Libe R, et al. SDHA is a tumor suppressor gene causing paraganglioma. *Hum Mol Genet* 2010;19:3011–3020.
95. Korpershoek E, Favier J, Gaal J, et al. SDHA immunohistochemistry detects germline SDHA gene mutations in apparently sporadic paragangliomas and pheochromocytomas. *J Clin Endocrinol Metab* 2011;96:E1472–E1476.
96. Qin Y, Yao L, King EE, et al. Germline mutations in TMEM127 confer susceptibility to pheochromocytoma. *Nat Genet* 2010;42:229–233.
97. Yao L, Schiavi F, Cascon A, et al. Spectrum and prevalence of FP/TMEM127 gene mutations in pheochromocytomas and paragangliomas. *JAMA* 2010;304:2611–2619.
98. Neumann HP, Sullivan M, Winter A, et al. Germline mutations of the TMEM127 gene in patients with paraganglioma of head and neck and extraadrenal abdominal sites. *J Clin Endocrinol Metab* 2011;96: E1279–E1282.
99. Abermil N, Guillaud-Bataille M, Burnichon N, et al. TMEM127 screening in a large cohort of patients with pheochromocytoma and/or paraganglioma. *J Clin Endocrinol Metab* 2012;97:E805–E809.
100. Comino-Mendez I, Gracia-Aznarez FJ, Schiavi F, et al. Exome sequencing identifies MAX mutations as a cause of hereditary pheochromocytoma. *Nat Genet* 2011;43:663–667.
101. Neumann HP, Bausch B, McWhinney SR, et al. Germ-line mutations in nonsyndromic pheochromocytoma. *N Engl J Med* 2002;346:1459–1466.
102. Burnichon N, Rohmer V, Amar L, et al. The succinate dehydrogenase genetic testing in a large prospective series of patients with paragangliomas. *J Clin Endocrinol Metab* 2009;94:2817–2827.
103. Jafri M, Maher ER. The genetics of phaeochromocytoma: using clinical features to guide genetic testing. *Eur J Endocrinol* 2012;166:151–158.
104. Rubinstein WS. Endocrine cancer predisposition syndromes: Hereditary paraganglioma, multiple endocrine neoplasia type 1, multiple endocrine neoplasia type 2, and hereditary thyroid cancer. *Hematol Oncol Clin North Am* 2010;24:907–937.
105. Maher ER, Iselius L, Yates JRW, et al. von Hippel-Lindau disease: a genetic study. *J Med Genet* 1991;28:443–447.
106. Neumann HPH, Wiestler OD. Clustering of features of von Hippel–Lindau syndrome: evidence for a complex genetic locus. *Lancet* 1991;337:1052–1054.
107. Maher ER, Neumann HP, Richard S. von Hippel–Lindau disease: a clinical and scientific review. *Eur J Hum Genet* 2011;19:617–623.
108. Maher ER, Eng C. The pressure rises: update on the genetics of phaeochromocytoma. *Hum Mol Genet* 2002;11:2347–2354.
109. Gimenez-Roqueplo AP, Lehnert H, Mannelli M, et al. Phaeochromocytoma, new genes and screening strategies. *Clin Endocrinol (Oxf)* 2006;65: 699–705.
110. Erlic Z, Rybicki L, Peczkowska M, et al. Clinical predictors and algorithm for the genetic diagnosis of pheochromocytoma patients. *Clin Cancer Res* 2009;15:6378–6385.

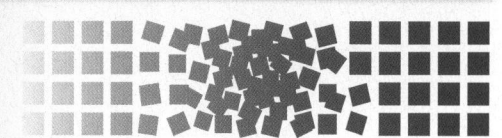

89 Molecular Biology of Sarcomas

Samuel Singer, Torsten O. Nielsen, and Cristina R. Antonescu

INTRODUCTION

Sarcomas are life-threatening mesenchymal neoplasms that account for approximately 1% of all human cancers. They pose a significant therapeutic challenge because about 50% of patients with newly diagnosed sarcoma eventually die of disease. Sarcomas also pose significant diagnostic challenges because there are more than 70 histologic subtypes with unique molecular, pathologic, clinical, prognostic, and therapeutic features.

SOFT TISSUE SARCOMAS

The molecular genetic and cytogenetic characterization of soft tissue sarcoma has improved classification and has divided sarcomas into two broad groups: those with simple karyotypes and those with highly complex karyotypes. Figure 89.1 shows the molecular alterations found in some of the subtypes in each group. The first group consists of sarcomas with near-diploid, simple karyotypes and simple genetic alterations (translocations, inversions, or specific activating mutations). Translocation-associated sarcomas typically occur in young adults, with the highest incidence at age 30 to 50 years. Oncogenesis mostly results from transcriptional deregulation induced by fusion genes. The second group consists of sarcomas with aberrant, highly complex genomes. The peak incidence for these complex sarcoma types is at age 50 to 70 years. These complex sarcoma subtypes commonly have alterations in cell-cycle genes *TP53*, *MDM2*, *RB1*, and *INK4a* and defects in specific growth-factor signaling pathways, but the critical subtype-specific molecular alterations that drive sarcomagenesis largely remain to be discovered. This information will be essential for the development of therapeutics that can selectively target the driver genetic alterations required for sarcoma survival. This idea is best illustrated by imatinib, a small molecule that inhibits ABL, KIT, and platelet-derived growth factor receptor alpha (PDGFRA) tyrosine kinases. The discovery that gastrointestinal stromal tumors (GIST) have activating mutations in *KIT* and *PDGFRA* led to rapid clinical development of imatinib for GIST, in which it proved to be an effective, low toxicity therapy (see Chapter 55 for a discussion of the molecular biology of GIST). This success illustrates how targeting a sarcoma-specific oncogenic mechanism can lead to dramatic responses.

Figure 89.2 shows the histologic appearance of the major soft tissue sarcoma subtypes, and Table 89.1 outlines diagnostic histologic characteristics and molecular and cytogenetic abnormalities.

TRANSLOCATION-ASSOCIATED SOFT TISSUE SARCOMAS

Myxoid/Round Cell Liposarcoma

Myxoid liposarcomas typically arise in the thigh or other deep soft tissues in adults (peak age, 30 to 50 years). Myxoid liposarcomas can usually be diagnosed with confidence by its characteristic morphology: a myxoid matrix, a plexiform vasculature, and lipoblasts. These features may, however, be partially lost in its high-grade form, *round cell liposarcoma*. Nearly all myxoid/round cell liposarcomas carry a balanced translocation, t(12;16)(q13;p11),[1] fusing *FUS* (also known as *TLS*) with *DDIT3* (aka *CHOP*, *GADD153*).[2] In rare cases, *EWSR1* substitutes for its homolog *FUS*. At least 12 *FUS-DDIT3* transcript variants have been reported,[3,4] and several are known to induce a sarcoma phenotype in model systems.[5,6] The translocations fuse 5' exons of *FUS* (encoding transcriptional regulatory domains that interact with the RNA polymerase II complex[7]) to the full coding sequence of *DDIT3*, a leucine-zipper transcription factor with roles in cell cycle control,[8] adipocytic differentiation,[9] and stress response.[10] The fusion oncoprotein binds cofactors including C/EBPβ to deregulate gene expression, although few direct targets have been validated to date.[11,12] One result is activation of critical pathways, including those related to angiogenesis (interleukin 8 [IL-8]), early adipose differentiation (PPARγ), growth factor signaling (insulinlike growth factor [IGF], RET), and cell-cycle control (cyclin D, CDK4).[12–15] Another result is repression of miR-486[16] and IL-24,[17] which might otherwise act as tumor suppressors.

Clinically, evidence for *FUS-DDIT3* translocations from reverse transcription polymerase chain reaction (RT-PCR)[3] or fluorescence in situ hybridization (FISH)[18] can help confirm the diagnosis and may be useful for small biopsies dominated by a round cell component. Fusion subtype, however, appears to have little prognostic value independent of stage and grade. In general, molecular markers in myxoid liposarcoma have been difficult to test for independent prognostic value, given the difficulty of assembling large series.[19] Nevertheless, high levels of p53, IGF1R/IGF2, AXL, and RET may be adverse factors.[13,20,21] In addition, mutations in *PIK3CA*, found in 18% of myxoid/round cell liposarcomas, were associated with a worse outcome.[22]

Myxoid liposarcomas have dense microvasculature and high expression of IL-8[12] and vascular endothelial growth factor (VEGF).[23] These characteristics suggest a value for antiangiogenic therapies and may underlie the observed sensitivity to radiotherapy[24] and trabectedin.[25] Trabectedin may also function by disrupting the binding of FUS-DDIT3 to target promoters.[11] Agents designed to target FUS-DDIT3 are not yet available.

Ewing Sarcoma

Ewing family tumors appear most commonly in adolescents and young adults; primary sites are most often in bone but can also be in soft tissues. A range of aggressive small blue round cell tumors have been subsumed under the general term *Ewing sarcoma family tumor* because of common pathognomonic chromosomal translocations.[26,27] *EWSR1*, the common 5' translocation partner, is fused to one of several ETS family transcription factor genes

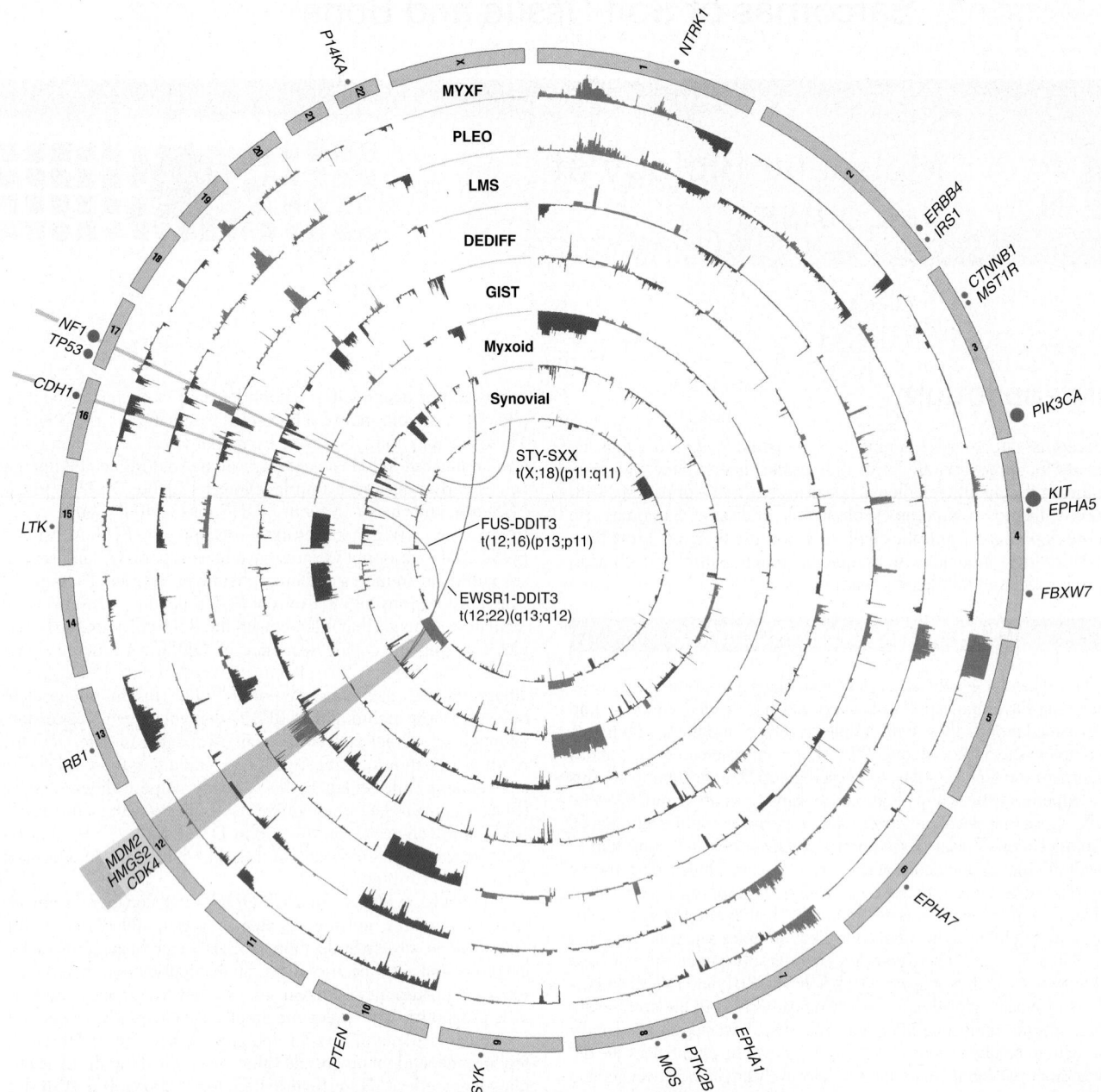

Figure 89.1 Nucleotide and copy number alterations in soft tissue sarcoma. The outer ring indicates the chromosomal position. The second through fifth rings represent four subtypes with complex karyotypes. The three inner rings represent subtypes with simple karyotypes. The plots show the statistical significance of genomic aberrations, with amplification in *red* and deletion in *blue*. *Green* curves indicate the chromosomal breakpoints of pathognomonic translocations in myxoid/round-cell liposarcoma and synovial sarcoma. Genes harboring somatic nucleotide alterations are indicated with *green circles* whose size is proportional to their frequency of occurrence. MYXF, myxofibrosarcoma; PLEO, pleomorphic liposarcoma; LMS, leiomyosarcoma; DEDIFF, dedifferentiated liposarcoma; Myxoid, myxoid/round cell liposarcoma. (Courtesy of Barry S. Taylor, Computational Biology Center, Memorial Sloan-Kettering Cancer. Adapted from Barretina J, Taylor BS, Banerji S, et al. Subtype-specific genomic alterations define new targets for soft tissue sarcoma therapy. *Nat Genet* 2010;42:715–721.)

(usually *FLI1*).[28] In the chimeric protein, EWSR1 provides, at minimum, its N-terminal transcriptional regulatory domain[29] and loses its RNA recognition domain. The ETS factor provides its C-terminal DNA-binding domain and loses its native transactivation domain. Several direct transcriptional targets for the fusion oncoprotein are supported by strong evidence. In Ewing sarcoma tissue, some of these targets are upregulated (*PTPL1*,[30] *PRKCB*,[31] *DAX1/NR0B1*[32]) and some repressed (*FOXO1*,[33] *TGFBR2*, *LOX*,[34] *IGFBP3*,[35] and the *Let*-7 microRNA precursor[36]), but gene repression, mediated by cofactors, appears to predominate.[37] The net result is the activation of pathways driving proliferation and

cell survival[38] and the repression of pathways promoting mesenchymal differentiation.[39,40]

Molecular confirmation of an *EWSR1* translocation can be critical for patient management because many of the clinical, morphologic, and immunophenotypic features of Ewing sarcoma are shared with entities such as mesenchymal chondrosarcoma and small cell osteosarcoma. Commercially available *EWSR1* split-apart FISH probes are valuable ancillary diagnostic tools (see Fig. 89.2)[41]; RT-PCR alternatives are complicated by the need to cover the many alternative fusion sites, but offer the advantage of identifying the specific fusion.[42]

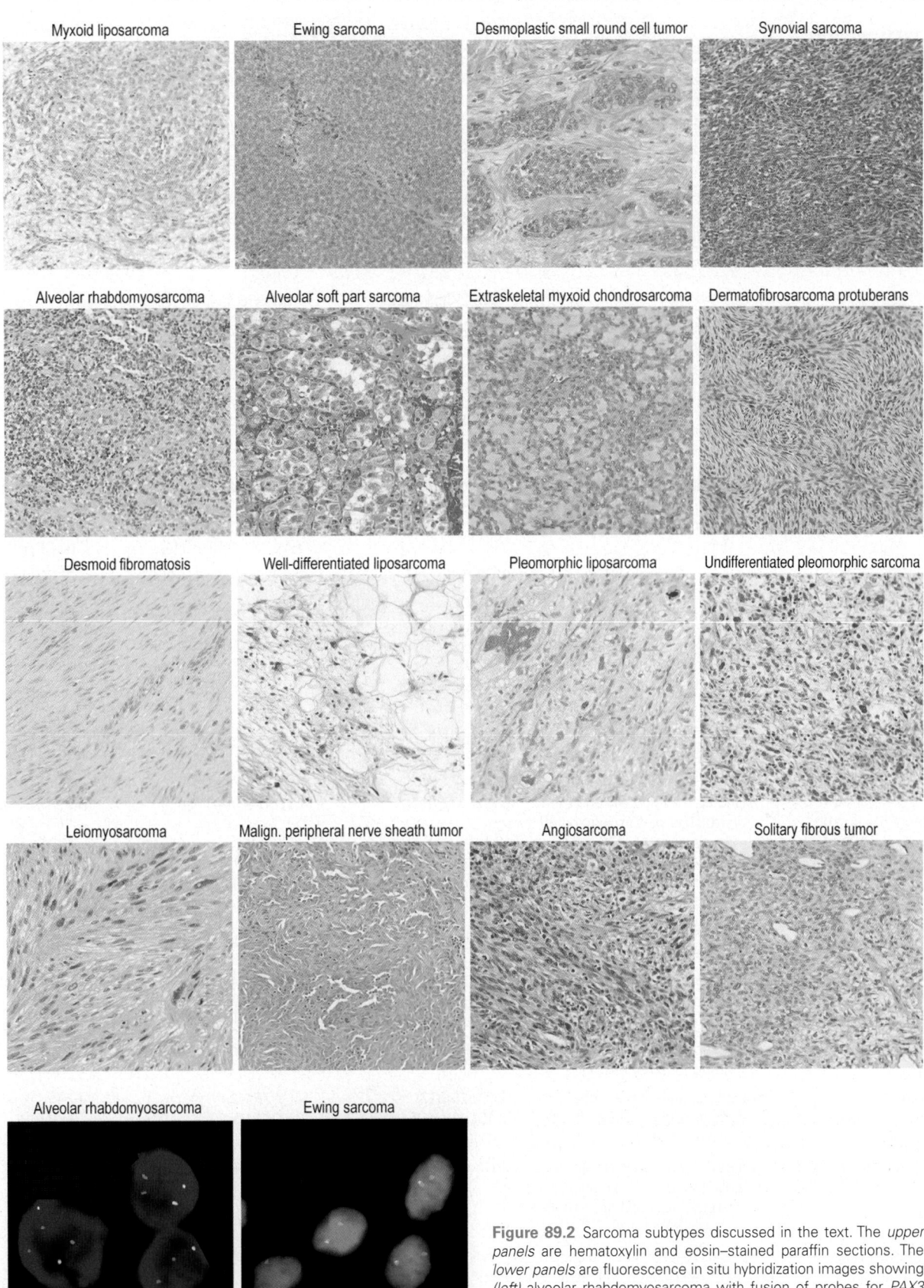

Figure 89.2 Sarcoma subtypes discussed in the text. The *upper panels* are hematoxylin and eosin–stained paraffin sections. The *lower panels* are fluorescence in situ hybridization images showing *(left)* alveolar rhabdomyosarcoma with fusion of probes for *PAX3 (red)* and *FOXO1 (green)*, and *(right)* Ewing sarcoma with break-apart of probes flanking the EWS breakpoint region, *EWSR1*. Malign., malignant.

TABLE 89.1

Cytogenetic and Molecular Abnormalities in Soft Tissue Sarcomas

Disease	Diagnostic Morphology or Immunohistochemistry	Cytogenetic Event	Molecular Abnormality	Molecular Diagnostic[a]
Myxoid/round cell liposarcoma	Lipoblasts, plexiform vasculature, myxoid matrix	t(12;16)(q13;p11) t(12;22)(q13;q12)	FUS-DDIT3 (>90%) EWSR1-DDIT3 (<5%)	DDIT3 breaks (FISH)[18,276]
Ewing sarcoma family tumor	Small, blue, round cells; CD99 and FLI1 expression; lack of lymphoid biomarker expression	t(11;22)(q24;q12) t(21;22)(q22;q12) Alternative events: fusions of 22q12 with 7p22, 17q22, 2q33; inv 22q12; t(16;21)(p11;q22)	EWSR1-FLI1 (>80%) EWSR1-ERG (10%–15%) Other ETS family partners: ETV1, ETV4, FEV, PATZ1 (~5%) FUS-ERG (<1%)	EWSR1 breaks (FISH)[41] or RT-PCR
Desmoplastic small round cell tumor	Small, blue, round cell islands in dense stroma; positive for keratin, desmin, vimentin, and WT1	t(11;22)(p13;q12)	EWSR1-WT1 (>75%)	EWSR1 breaks (FISH)[41]
Synovial sarcoma	Biphasic histology, positive for TLE1[61]	t(X;18)(p11;q11) (>90%)	SYT-SSX1 (66%), SYT-SSX2 (33%), SYT-SSX4 (<1%)	SYT breaks (FISH)[277]
Alveolar rhabdomyosarcoma	Small, blue cells expressing desmin, myogenin, myoD1	t(2;13)(q35;q14) t(1;13)(p36;q14)	PAX3-FOXO1 (~80%) PAX7-FOXO1 (~20%) PAX3-NCOA1 (<1%) PAX3-NCOA2 (<1%)	PAX3/7 type-specific FISH or RT-PCR[278]
Alveolar soft-part sarcoma	Nested polygonal cells in vascular network; positive for TFE3[279]	t(X;17)(p11;q25)	ASPSCR1-TFE3 (>90%)	ASPSCR1-TFE3 RT-PCR[280] or TFE3 FISH[93]
Dermatofibrosarcoma protuberans	Bland spindle cells, storiform and honeycomb growth in subcutis, positive for CD34	Rings derived from t(17;22) (>75%) t(17;22)(q22; q13.1)[103,104,281] (10%)	COL1A1-PDGFB	
Embryonal rhabdomyosarcoma	Spindle cells and rhabdomyoblasts, positive for desmin and myogenin	Trisomies 2q, 8 and 20 (>75%)	LOH at 11p15 (>75%)	
Extraskeletal myxoid chondrosarcoma	Bland epithelioid cells arranged in reticular pattern in myxoid stroma	t(9;22)(q22;q12) t(9;17)(q22;q11) t(9;15)(q22;q21) t(3;9)(q12;q22)	EWSR1-NR4A3 (75%) TAF15-NR4A3 (<10%) TCF12-NR4A3 (<10%) TFG–NR4A3 (<5%)	EWSR1 breaks (FISH); RT-PCR[112–114]
Endometrial stromal tumor	Bland spindle cells, positive for CD10 and ER	t(7;17)(p15;q21)	JAZF1-SUZ12 (30%)	
Clear cell sarcoma	Nested epithelioid cells with clear or amphophilic cytoplasm, positive for S100 and HMB-45	t(12;22)(q13;q12) t(2;22)(q34;q12)	EWSR1-ATF1 (>75%) EWSR1-CREB1 (<5%)	EWSR1 breaks (FISH)[41,282]
Infantile fibrosarcoma	Monomorphic spindle cells, herringbone pattern	t(12;15)(p13;q25)	ETV6-NTRK3 (>75%)	FISH, RT-PCR
Inflammatory myofibroblastic tumor	Myofibroblastic cells with lymphoplasmacytic infiltrate, positive for ALK	t(1;2)(q25;p23) t(2;19)(p23;p13) t(2;17)(p23;q23)	ALK-TPM34 ALK-TPM ALK-CLTC	ALK breaks (FISH)
Solitary fibrous tumor	Monomorphic spindle cells, collagenous stroma, and staghorn vasculature; STAT6 expression	12q13 inversion	NAB2-STAT6 (>95%)	RT-PCR
Gastrointestinal stromal tumor	Spindle (70%), epithelioid (20%) or mixed (10%) morphology, positive for CD117 (KIT), DOG1, and CD34	Monosomies 14 and 22 (>75%) Deletion of 1p (>25)		
			KIT or PDGFRA mutation (>90%)[283,284]	PCR mutation analysis

(continued)

TABLE 89.1

Cytogenetic and Molecular Abnormalities in Soft Tissue Sarcomas *(continued)*

Disease	Diagnostic Morphology or Immunohistochemistry	Cytogenetic Event	Molecular Abnormality	Molecular Diagnostic[a]
Desmoid fibromatosis	Bland myofibroblastic-type cells, fascicular growth, nuclear positivity for β-catenin	Trisomies 8 and 20 (30%)	*APC* inactivation by mutation/deletion (10%) *CTNNB1* (β-catenin) mutations (85%)	IHC for β-catenin expression
Well-differentiated/dedifferentiated liposarcoma	Atypical multinucleated stromal cells, lipoblasts, positive for MDM2, CDK4	12q13-15 rings and giant markers	*MDM2* and *CDK4* amplification (>85%)	*MDM2* amplification (FISH)
Pleomorphic liposarcoma	Pleomorphic spindle and giant cells, pleomorphic lipoblasts	Complex[b] (>90%)		None
Myxofibrosarcoma and undifferentiated pleomorphic sarcoma	Pleomorphic spindle and giant cells, storiform growth, variable myxoid stroma	Complex[b] >90%)	*SKP2* amplification	None
Leiomyosarcoma	Elongated fusiform cells with eosinophilic cytoplasm, in intersecting fascicles, positive for desmin and smooth muscle actin	Complex[b] (>50%) Deletions of 1p	*RB1* point mutations/deletions	None
Malignant peripheral nerve sheath tumor	Monomorphic spindle cells, high mitotic count, geographic necrosis	Complex[b] (90%)	*NF1* mutation, loss or deletion (>50%)	None

[a] Refers to molecular tests that can be run on formalin-fixed paraffin-embedded material for molecular confirmation of diagnosis: quantitative RT-PCR of transcripts,[278] or FISH to interphase genomic DNA.[285]
[b] Complex karyotypes containing multiple numerical and structural chromosomal aberrations.
FISH, fluorescence in situ hybridization; RT-PCR, reverse transcription polymerase chain reaction; LOH, loss of heterozygosity; IHC, immunohistochemistry.

Several agents (including inhibitors of IGF/mammalian target of rapamycin [mTOR], histone deacetylase, and cyclin-dependent kinase[43]) that target translocation-induced mechanisms and pathways are currently in clinical trials for Ewing sarcoma, and strategies to inhibit the oncoprotein itself are in active development.[43–45]

Desmoplastic Small Round Cell Tumor

In desmoplastic small round cell tumors, the same 5′ portions of *EWSR1* involved in Ewing sarcomas are fused to *WT1*,[46,47] a tumor suppressor deleted in Wilms tumor.[48] The chimeric protein includes the last three WT1 DNA-binding zinc finger domains. Despite some similarities to Ewing sarcoma family tumors, desmoplastic small round cell tumors are rarely cured with aggressive conventional chemotherapy combined with surgical debulking; prognosis is dismal, so new therapies are needed.[49,50] Several targets of EWSR1-WT1 have been identified. EWSR1-WT1 directly induces *PDGFA* expression,[51] which explains the desmoplastic background and, along with VEGFA and VEGFR2 overexpression, accounts for the observed partial responses to sunitinib.[52] *IL2RB* is also induced, and its downstream JAK/STAT and AKT/mTOR signaling pathways appear active,[46,53,54] representing potential targets for novel treatment approaches.

Synovial Sarcoma

Synovial sarcoma differs from most translocation-associated sarcomas in that the genes involved in its defining translocation, t(X;18)(p11;q11), encode epigenetic regulators, not transcription factors that bind DNA directly.[55] The translocation fuses the widely expressed

SS18 (aka *SYT*) gene with an *SSX* gene normally expressed only in testis.[56] In the fusion oncoprotein, SS18, which forms part of the BAF chromatin remodeling complex,[57] retains all but the last eight amino acids from its C-terminal transcriptional activation domain. The SSX partner (SSX1, 2, or 4) retains only its C-terminal 78-residue repressor domain, which confers nuclear localization in association with Polycomb proteins.[58] The forced expression of SS18-SSX in mesenchymal stem cells[59] or conditional expression in mice[55,60] recapitulates synovial sarcoma. Neither SS18 nor SSX carries a DNA-binding motif; however, the chimeric oncoprotein gains at least two abnormal functions affecting epigenetic gene regulation. The retained C-terminus of SSX binds TLE1, a highly expressed diagnostic marker of synovial sarcoma[61] that recruits Polycomb repressor complex proteins. SS18 binds the transcription factor ATF2, thereby directing the complex to promoters bearing cAMP response elements (CRE). The net result is Polycomb-mediated epigenetic repression of ATF2 target genes, including the tumor suppressors *EGR1* and *CDKN2A*.[62] Also, when SS18-SSX replaces native SS18 in BAF complexes, the SMARCB1 (SNF5) component is evicted.[63] This latter event increases Polycomb activity and induces hyperactivity of stem cell–associated programs,[64] a feature of synovial sarcoma.[65] Key genes and oncogenic pathways that become activated, directly or indirectly, in synovial sarcoma include histone deacetylases,[62] SOX2,[63] Wnt/β-catenin,[66] TWIST1,[67] FGFR2,[68] BCL2,[69] and the Akt/mTOR pathway[70] via IGF2.[59,71,72] Therefore, these represent candidates for targeted therapy approaches in the absence of known drugs that inhibit SS18-SSX directly.

Copy number alterations are more common in adult than in pediatric patients, and both copy number alterations and an expression signature of genes related to mitosis and chromosome function are associated with metastasis.[73]

Alveolar Rhabdomyosarcoma

In alveolar rhabdomyosarcoma, an aggressive cancer of older children and adolescents, the transcriptional activation domain of FOXO1 (i.e., FKHR) from 13q14 is fused to the DNA-binding domain of paired box transcription factor PAX3 (2q35) or PAX7 (1p36).[74,75] Until recently, about 20% of cases were thought to be translocation negative, but in fact, such tumors represent histologic variants of embryonal rhabdomyosarcoma.[76] Translocations involving PAX3 may be associated with a worse prognosis than those involving PAX7.[77] Thus, to optimize patient care, the diagnosis should be confirmed by FISH (see Fig. 89.2) and/or RT-PCR.[78] Either translocation results in a high-level nuclear expression of a chimeric transcription factor that abnormally activates PAX targets, many of which are involved in neurogenesis and are not expressed in normal skeletal muscle.[79,80] Recently, PAX3-FOXO1 fusion mRNA and chimeric protein were found to be expressed transiently during normal fetal muscle development (i.e., in cells without the DNA translocations).[81] Direct targets of PAX3-FOXO1 include P-cadherin (CDH3),[82] GREM1, DAPK1, and MYOD1,[83] as well as PDGFRA. Inhibitors of PDGFRA are effective in mouse models.[84] The list of targetable kinases expressed in alveolar rhabdomyosarcoma also includes IGF1R and ALK.[85–87] Another probable direct target of PAX3-FOXO1 is the cell-cycle regulator SKP2,[88] perhaps helping explain why alveolar rhabdomyosarcoma is responsive to conventional cytotoxic chemotherapy.

Alveolar Soft-Part Sarcoma

Alveolar soft-part sarcoma has a clinical presentation and pathognomonic molecular event with many similarities to other translocation-associated sarcomas.[89] In this disease, the 5' half of the widely expressed ASPSCR1 (i.e., ASPL) gene on 17q25 is fused to exon 3 or 4 of TFE3 on Xp11, the latter retaining its transcriptional activation, basic helix-loop-helix, and leucine zipper domains.[90] Interestingly, similar fusions are present in a subset of renal cell carcinomas, particularly those arising in younger patients,[91] and in a subset of perivascular epithelioid cell neoplasms.[92] Although alveolar soft-part sarcoma has distinctive histology, two useful diagnostic adjuncts are the detection of TFE3 rearrangements by FISH[93] and the detection of translocations by RT-PCR or by immunohistochemistry for TFE3.[94,95] Kobos et al.[96] combined expression profiling, chromatin immunoprecipitation, and functional validation to identify a CACGTG consensus motif in genes transcriptionally activated by the ASPSCR1-TFE3 oncoprotein. Their list of validated direct targets[97] includes MET and angiogenic mediators, which is consistent with previous studies.[97–99] Antiangiogenic therapy is effective in xenograft models.[100] A single-arm phase II study of the VEGFR inhibitor cediranib in metastatic alveolar soft-part sarcoma showed a high rate of disease control in association with downregulation of angiogenic genes (including ANGPT2), supporting advanced trials of antiangiogenic agents.[101]

Dermatofibrosarcoma Protuberans

A hallmark of dermatofibrosarcoma protuberans (DFSP) is supernumerary ring chromosomes that contain material from chromosomes 17 and 22,[102–104] or less commonly, an unbalanced der(22) t(17;22)(q21-23;q13). The molecular consequence of both types of aberration is the overexpression of the PDGF beta (PDGFB) gene on chromosome 22, through fusion with the collagen gene COL1A1 on chromosome 17.[105,106] The same fusion gene is also seen in two histologic variants: giant cell fibroblastoma and Bednar tumor (pigmented DFSP). FISH and comparative genomic hybridization (CGH) studies have indicated that increased COL1A1–PDGFB copy number is associated with fibrosarcomatous transformation of DFSP, although the copy number increase is not an invariable feature of these cases.[107,108]

The COL1A1-PDGFB fusion product signals through the PDGF receptor in an autocrine loop.[109] This signaling can be blocked using tyrosine-kinase inhibitors acting at PDGFR, such as imatinib. A number of clinical studies have shown a high response rate to imatinib therapy in both locally advanced and metastatic DFSP.[102,110,111] These results support the concept that DFSP cells depend on aberrant activation of PDGF signaling for proliferation and survival.

Extraskeletal Myxoid Chondrosarcoma

Most extraskeletal myxoid chondrosarcomas show reciprocal translocations that fuse NR4A3 in 9q22-q31.1 with one of four partners: EWSR1 in 22q12 (the most common), TAF15 in 17q11, TCF12 in 15q21, or TFG in 3q12.[112–114] Because these fusion genes have not been described in any other tumor type, they represent useful diagnostic markers. The four different fusion partners have unknown prognostic significance.

NR4A3 encodes a ubiquitously expressed orphan nuclear receptor also known as NOR-1, TEC, MINOR, or CHN.[115] The t(9;22) fuses the transactivation domain of EWSR1 to the full length of NR4A3. Analogous to EWSR1-ETS fusions, the EWSR1-NR4A3 fusion protein not only displays strong transcriptional activity, but also regulates RNA splicing.[116]

TAF15, like EWSR1 and FUS, belongs to the FET family, and contains a characteristic 87–amino acid RNA recognition motif implicated in protein-RNA binding.[117] The N-terminal regions of EWSR1, FUS, and TAF15 contain degenerate repeats of the SYGQ motif and mediate powerful transcriptional activation when fused to the heterologous DNA-binding domains of a variety of transcription factors.[118]

By gene profiling, extraskeletal myxoid chondrosarcomas constitute a distinct genomic entity, showing upregulation of several genes, including NMB, DKK1, DNER, and CLCN3.[119] In situ hybridization confirmed that NMB is highly expressed in extraskeletal myxoid chondrosarcoma but not in other sarcoma types, suggesting its potential value as a diagnostic marker.

Solitary Fibrous Tumor and Hemangiopericytoma

Solitary fibrous tumor (SFT) and hemangiopericytoma share similar histopathologic features and are now classified as a single biologic entity.[120] In a recent study using paired-end transcriptome sequencing, a recurrent NAB2-STAT6 fusion was identified in virtually all SFTs, regardless of anatomic location (pleura, meninges, or soft tissue).[121] In the normal genome, NAB2 and STAT6 are adjacent genes on chromosome 12q13 that are transcribed in opposite directions, but in SFT, the fusion is the result of a chromosomal inversion, fusing NAB2 and STAT6 in a common direction of transcription.

In contrast to the known activity of NAB2 as a repressor of early growth response protein 1 (EGR1) activity, the NAB2-STAT6 fusion induces expression of EGR1 target genes. In an RNA-sequencing analysis of seven SFTs and 282 other tumor samples, the SFTs showed a high-level expression of both EGR1 target genes, including NAB2, NAB1, IGF2, FGF2, and PDGFD, and receptor tyrosine kinases, such as FGFR1 and NTRK1.[121] Overexpression of other tyrosine-kinase receptor genes, such as DDR1 and ERBB2, has been seen in array-based profiling.[122]

IGF2 is uniformly overexpressed in SFT, regardless of anatomic location.[122] IGF2 is imprinted on the paternal allele in most adult tissues, and IGF2 overexpression in SFTs was related to a loss of imprinting. Although IGF2 acts by binding to IGF1R, SFTs do not show up-regulation of IGF1R, and it was suggested that IGF2 signaling occurs through the insulin receptor A pathway.[123] Overexpression of IGF2 and consequent activation of the insulin receptor may also explain why a subset of SFT patients presents with hypoglycemia. This syndrome, known as *Doege-Potter syndrome*, has been associated with large tumor size and aggressive clinical behavior and is resolved by surgical resection of the lesion.[124]

Although a *PDGFRB* mutation (D850V) was reported in a malignant pleural SFT,[125] none of the 39 SFTs tested subsequently showed mutation in this hot spot, nor did they show upregulation of PDGFRB mRNA.[122]

SOFT TISSUE SARCOMAS OF SIMPLE KARYOTYPE ASSOCIATED WITH MUTATIONS

Desmoid Fibromatosis

Desmoid-type fibromatoses are locally infiltrative, clonal fibroblastic proliferations that arise in the deep soft tissues and never metastasize. Although about 70% result from mutations in adenomatous polyposis coli (*APC*) or *CTNNB1*, tumorigenesis may be also be influenced by endocrine and physiologic factors such as pregnancy, trauma, and prior surgery. Desmoids are usually divided into two groups: sporadic desmoids and those in individuals with a heterozygous germ-line mutation in the *APC* gene (chromosome 5q). Although germ-line *APC* mutations also often result in familial adenomatous polyposis,[126] some desmoid patients harboring such a mutation have no polyposis. The desmoids in individuals with a germ-line *APC* mutation display inactivation of the second copy of *APC*, which usually occurs by point mutation or deletion.[126,127]

Among sporadic desmoids, only a minority display *APC* inactivation. A majority (52% to 85%) have an activating point mutation in the β-catenin gene, *CTNNB1*.[128,129] These *CTNNB1* mutations stabilize β-catenin, resulting in its overabundance. β-Catenin, a mediator of Wnt signaling, is negatively regulated by APC, so both *APC* inactivation and *CTNNB1* activating mutations result in the upregulation of the Wnt pathway. The specific *CTNNB1* mutation may have prognostic significance; patients with S45F-mutant desmoids were reported to have a 5-year recurrence-free survival of only 23%, compared with 57% for those with T41A-mutant tumors and 65% for those with wild-type *CTNNB1*.[128] These results raise the possibility that mutation status might aid in selecting patients for more aggressive therapy.

Based on the findings of *APC* inactivation or activating *CTNNB1* mutations in the majority of patients, the development of small-molecule β-catenin antagonists would be likely to provide significant benefit, particularly for patients with advanced disease in whom surgical resection is not feasible. Although such β-catenin–targeted agents are still in preclinical development, an inhibitor of matrix metalloproteinase, a downstream target of β-catenin, substantially reduced tumor volume and tumor invasion in a transgenic *Apc+/Apc*[1638N] mouse model of aggressive fibromatosis.[130] Hedgehog signaling is activated in human and murine desmoid tumors. Inhibiting Hedgehog signaling reduced cell proliferation and β-catenin protein levels in human desmoid cell cultures and reduced the tumor size and number in a murine model.[131] These results suggest Hedgehog antagonists as a promising therapy for desmoid patients.

Patients with desmoids were found to have elevated levels of PDGF-AA and PDGF-BB, leading to a trial of the tyrosine-kinase inhibitor imatinib in patients with advanced disease. Of 19 patients, 3 (16%) had a partial response to treatment and 4 additional patients had stable disease for more than 1 year; overall, the 1-year tumor control rate was 37%.[132] The response in these tumors was thought to be mediated by inhibition of PDGFRB kinase activity. Sorafenib, a multitargeted tyrosine-kinase inhibitor, results in tumor shrinkage in 25% of desmoid patients and stable disease in 70%, along with symptom relief in 70% of patients.[133]

COMPLEX SOFT TISSUE SARCOMA TYPES

Well-Differentiated and Dedifferentiated Liposarcoma

Well-differentiated and dedifferentiated liposarcomas represent the most common biologic group of liposarcoma. This group is characterized by amplification of 12q, which usually occurs in double minutes, ring chromosomes, and large marker chromosomes. In addition, the 12q13.2-q23.1 locus often harbors complex rearrangements (see Fig. 89.1).[22,134,135] The amplified region generally includes the oncogenes *MDM2*, *HMGA2*, and *CDK4*, but 12q may contain additional driver genes. On the basis of the rearrangements and correlated overexpression results, possibilities include *NAV3*, *WIF1*, *MDM1*, *DYRK2*, *ELK3*, *DUSP6*, *YEATS4*, *TBK1*, and *FRS2*, which are amplified in ~14% to 80% of tumors. Aside from 12q aberrations, dedifferentiated liposarcomas contain significant amplifications of 1p, 1q, 5p, 6q, and 20q.[22,134,135]

Amplification of *JUN* (on 1p32) has been suggested as the explanation for the block in adipocyte differentiation in undifferentiated sarcomas.[136] However, *JUN* is amplified or overexpressed in only a subset of dedifferentiated liposarcomas (DDLS).[22,137] Another gene that may be involved in the differentiation phenotype is C/EBPα, which is underexpressed in many DDLS tissues and cell lines. Exogenously expressing C/EBPα resulted in a 50% decrease in proliferation, a G2/M arrest, apoptosis, and restoration of the ability to induce early adipogenesis markers.[138] CCAAT-enhancer-binding protein alpha (C/EBPα) expression independently predicts distant recurrence–free survival for patients with primary liposarcoma,[139] and loss of the 19q region encompassing C/EBPα is associated with poor outcomes in primary retroperitoneal DDLS.[140] In addition, C/EBPα downregulation may result from epigenetic defects; 24% of DDLSs had C/EBPα promoter methylation and 8.3% had somatic mutations in the histone deacetylase HDAC1. Treating DDLS cells with a demethylating agent and the histone deacetylase inhibitor vorinostat increased C/EBPα expression 19-fold, decreased proliferation, induced apoptosis, and reduced xenograft tumor growth by 50% to 70%.[141] Taken together, these results suggest that C/EBPα acts as a tumor suppressor in DDLS and that its loss may explain the undifferentiated state of DDLS.

A microarray analysis of gene expression has demonstrated that well-differentiated liposarcomas and DDLS have activation of cell-cycle and checkpoint pathways, including the upregulation of CDK4, MDM2, CDK1, CDC7, TOP2A, PRC1, PLK1, and cyclins B1, B2, and E2.[142,143] Therefore, these pathways may be useful as therapeutic targets. In fact, nutlin-3a, a selective MDM2 antagonist, induces apoptosis and inhibits the proliferation of DDLS cell lines at concentrations that do not affect normal adipose-derived stem cells.[142] Furthermore, PD0332991, a selective CDK4/CDK6 inhibitor, inhibits proliferation by inducing G1 cell-cycle arrest and senescence in DDLS cell lines and xenografts.[22] In a recent phase II trial of PD0332991 in patients with advanced CDK4-amplified liposarcoma, 66% of patients were progression free at 12 weeks, and a subset had a radiographic response and prolonged stable disease.[144] These results provide a rationale for use of MDM2 antagonists and CDK4 inhibitors in patients with well-differentiated liposarcomas and DDLSs.

Pleomorphic Liposarcoma

Pleomorphic liposarcoma, accounting for 5% of all liposarcomas, is the least common subtype. It is characterized by high chromosome counts and complex rearrangements, with many unidentifiable marker chromosomes and nonclonal alterations. A high-resolution single nucleotide polymorphism (SNP) array analysis has revealed multiple regions of significant copy number amplification and deletion.[145] The most common alteration, found in approximately

60% of tumors, was a deletion of 13q14.2-q14.3, including the *RB1* tumor suppressor. The next most common alteration was a loss of 17p13.1, including *TP53*. Both *RB1* and *TP53* deletions were a mixture of hemizygous loss and, less frequently, homozygous deletion. In addition, *TP53* point mutations were found in 17% of tumors.[22] In *TP53*-mutant cells, antagonism of MDM2 by nutlin-3a enhances chemosensitivity,[146] suggesting the potential therapeutic utility of combining nutlin-3a with chemotherapy in *TP53*-mutant pleomorphic liposarcoma. Small molecules that reactivate mutant TP53, such as PRIMA-1 (APR-246),[147] are presently in phase I trials.

A third genetic alteration identified in an SNP analysis was the deletion of 17q11.2, including the tumor suppressor *NF1*. Among 24 pleomorphic liposarcomas, 9 (38%) had *NF1* loss, including 1 case of a homozygous deletion and 2 cases of a mutation of the nondeleted allele.[22] Because a loss of NF1 function appears to activate the RAS and mTOR pathways, the frequent *NF1* aberrations suggest that MEK or mTOR inhibitors may have clinical utility.

Myxofibrosarcoma and Undifferentiated Pleomorphic Sarcoma (Malignant Fibrous Histiocytoma)

Pathologists now regard myxofibrosarcoma as a distinct tumor type with clearly defined criteria for diagnosis.[120,148,149] Undifferentiated pleomorphic sarcoma, however, is less well defined, and it remains controversial whether it represents either (1) a pleomorphic sarcoma showing fibroblastic/myofibroblastic differentiation and thus sharing a common set of genomic alterations with myxofibrosarcoma, or (2) an end-stage undifferentiated morphologic pattern with genomic alterations distinct from those of myxofibrosarcoma.

Myxofibrosarcoma

Myxofibrosarcoma, also known as myxoid variant of malignant fibrous histiocytoma, is a malignant fibroblastic lesion with variably myxoid stroma (at least 10%) composed of hyaluronic acid and solid sheets of spindled and pleomorphic tumor cells. Karyotypes tend to be highly complex, often with multiple numerical and structural rearrangements and with chromosome numbers in the triploid or tetraploid range.[150–152] No consistent chromosomal aberration has emerged. In general, karyotype complexity is greater in high-grade lesions and in recurrences.[152]

In an SNP array analysis of 38 myxofibrosarcomas, approximately 55% harbored chromosome 5p amplification.[22] This region contains *RICTOR* (a binding partner of mTOR), *CDH9*, and *LIFR*. Other amplified regions included several discontinuous loci on 1p and 1q spanning *PI4KB*, *ETV3*, and *MCL1*, among others. *MCL1*, an antiapoptotic gene, was concomitantly overexpressed in these tumors. Myxofibrosarcomas also harbored deletions of tumor suppressors, including *CDKN2A/CDKN2B*, *RB1*, *TP53*, *NF1*, and *PTEN*. These events demonstrate an extensive loss of function in several known tumor suppressors.[22]

Undifferentiated Pleomorphic Sarcoma (Malignant Fibrous Histiocytoma)

Over 50% of soft tissue sarcomas occurring in older adults are histologically pleomorphic and high grade. Most have traditionally been classified as malignant fibrous histiocytoma (MFH).[153,154] MFH was originally defined as a malignant pleomorphic spindle cell neoplasm showing fibroblastic and histiocytic differentiation. More recently, pathologists have accepted that this morphology may be shared by a wide range of malignant neoplasms.[155] Many sarcomas that were previously classified as pleomorphic MFH, on careful immunohistochemical and histopathologic analyses, revealed a specific line of differentiation and could be reclassified as myxofibrosarcoma (30%), myogenic sarcoma (30%), liposarcoma (4%), malignant peripheral nerve sheath tumor (2%), or soft tissue osteosarcoma (3%), whereas about 30% had no specific line of differentiation or were myofibroblastic.[148] The term *undifferentiated pleomorphic sarcoma* (UPS) is now reserved for pleomorphic sarcomas that show no definable line of differentiation by current technology.

Because of this change in diagnostic criteria, the genetic basis of UPS is difficult to evaluate. Among the more than 60 cases in the Mitelman Database of Chromosome Alterations in Cancer described as storiform or pleomorphic MFH or MFH not otherwise specified, the karyotypes are highly complex. Most have chromosome numbers in the triploid or tetraploid range, but a few are near haploid.[156–160] Telomeric associations, ring chromosomes, and dicentric chromosomes are common. In a CGH study of 33 tumors, 25 of which were UPSs as currently defined, numerous copy number changes were found. The most frequent (found in 50% to 65% of tumors) were gains in chromosome 1p (1p33-p32, 1p31, and 1p21), 1q21, and 20q13 and losses in 1q41, 2q36-q37, 10q25-q26, 13q13-q14, 13q14-q21, and 16q12.[161] The copy number profiles of the majority of UPSs closely resembled those of leiomyosarcomas[161–164] or pleomorphic or dedifferentiated liposarcomas.[165–167] Mutations and/or deletions of *TP53*, *RB1*, and *INK4a* have been suggested to be drivers of oncogenesis.[162,168–171]

Recent work suggests that the stemlike tumor initiating cells (side population cells) isolated from UPS show activation of both the Hedgehog and Notch pathways. Inhibition of these pathways in UPS xenograft models decreased the proportion of side population cells and suppressed tumor self-renewal. This work shows that targeting signaling pathways activated in a small subpopulation of tumor-initiating cells has a dramatic effect on tumor self-renewal and may be a promising approach for these undifferentiated tumors.[172]

Leiomyosarcoma

Leiomyosarcoma is defined as a malignant tumor with evidence of smooth muscle differentiation. Karyotypes tend to be complex, with amplifications, gains, and losses involving multiple chromosomes.[173–175] Frequently observed aberrations include losses of 1p12-pter, 2p, 13q14-q21 (including *RB1*),[176] 10q (including *PTEN*),[177] and 16q and gains of 17p, 8q, and 1q21-31; these aberrations have been associated with aggressive clinical behavior. The myocardin (MYOCD) gene on 17p is significantly amplified and overexpressed in retroperitoneal tumors. Knockdown of MYOCD in leiomyosarcoma cell lines harboring this amplification decreases smooth muscle differentiation and inhibits cell migration.[178] In an analysis of copy number alterations in 27 leiomyosarcomas,[22] deletions, which were more common than amplifications, encompassed known tumor suppressors such as *TP53*, *BRCA2*, *RB1*, and *FANCA*. The most prominent changes were chromosome 10 deletions (50% to 70% of cases) (see Fig. 89.1). Indeed, genetic inactivation of *Pten* (human 10q23.21) in smooth muscle in mice recapitulates human leiomyosarcoma,[179] suggesting that 10q loss occurs early in leiomyosarcomagenesis. Moreover, partial inactivation of *Pten* and *Tp53* in the smooth muscle lineage in mice results in the development of high-grade pleomorphic sarcomas and leiomyosarcomas with complex karyotypes.[180] The sarcomas deficient in both *Pten* and *Tp53* showed upregulated notch signaling and a greater metastatic potential, which could be attenuated by a gamma-secretase inhibitor.[180] In addition to *PTEN* inactivation, we identified homozygous deletions in *MTOR*. Because PTEN is a repressor of Akt, both these events suggest a critical role for aberrant Akt-mTOR signaling in leiomyosarcoma. mTOR inhibitors such as everolimus (RAD001) and temsirolimus have shown some efficacy in patients with leiomyosarcoma in clinical trials.[181,182]

RB1 deletion is common in leiomyosarcomas, with 70% harboring heterozygous deletions and 8% harboring homozygous deletions. A role for *RB1* deletion in leiomyosarcoma fits with the high incidence of leiomyosarcoma in individuals with hereditary retinoblastoma.[183]

Malignant Peripheral Nerve Sheath Tumor

Malignant peripheral nerve sheath tumors (MPNST) are highly aggressive soft tissue sarcomas that rarely occur in the general population, but are much more common in patients with neurofibromatosis type 1 (NF1), a hereditary tumor predisposition syndrome caused by heterozygous mutations of the *NF1* gene. The MPNSTs in NF1 patients typically arise from neurofibromas. NF1 patients' lifetime risk of developing MPNST is 8% to 13%, contrasting with the 0.001% risk in the general population.[184,185]

The *NF1* gene is implicated in sporadic as well as NF1-associated MPNST. About 70% of sporadic and NF1-associated MPNSTs display monoallelic or biallelic loss at the *NF1* locus on 17q.[186–188] *NF1* encodes neurofibromin, a protein that accelerates Ras–GTP hydrolysis and thus negatively regulates Ras.[189] In individuals with NF1, neurofibromas develop when an unknown cell type in the Schwann cell lineage loses its remaining functional *NF1* gene (by mutation, deletion, or loss of heterozygosity), leading to neurofibromin loss and subsequent activation of Ras signaling.[190–192]

Both sporadic and NF1-associated MPNSTs display complex karyotypes and clonal chromosomal aberrations.[150,193,194] In CGH analyses of MPNSTs, the most frequent minimal regions of gain were 1q24.1-q24.2, 1q24.3-q25.1, 8p23.1-p12, 9q34.11-q34.13, and 17q23.2-q25.3.[195] The 17q gain was associated with poor survival and with the overexpression of genes previously implicated in cancer: *TOP2A*, *ETV4*, *ERBB2*, and *BIRC5*.[195–197] Other frequent alterations include rearrangement or loss of 9p21 and 13q14, resulting in inactivation of *CDKN2A* (encoding the p16INK4A and p14ARF cell cycle inhibitory proteins) and *RB1*, respectively. In fact, in a recent high-resolution CGH analysis of NF1-associated MPNST, the most frequently deleted locus (33% of cases) encompassed the *CDKN2A*, *CDKN2B*, and *MTAP* genes on 9p21.3.[191] Thus, these studies implicate the p16INK4A-RB1 pathway, as did another study.[198]

Other recent studies have implicated the p19ARF-MDM2-p53[199] and EGFR pathways in MPNST oncogenesis.[200,201] *TP53* (on 17p13) is frequently inactivated in MPNST through mutations or deletions, correlating with the frequent loss of 17p.[194] Building on these observations, MPNST driver genes were sought in a Sleeping Beauty (SB) transposon-based somatic mutagenesis screen in mice bearing transgenes that confer a somatic loss of p53 function and/ or overexpression of human EGFR.[202] EGFR overexpression and p53 mutation cooperated to significantly increase neurofibroma and MPNST formation, effects that were enhanced by SB mutagenesis. The mutations found in the highest percentage of MPNSTs in this genetic screen were in *Pten* and *Nf1*, suggesting that these mutations cooperate to drive MPNST development. In addition, the researchers found that *Foxr2* acts as a protooncogene by promoting anchorage-independent MPNST cell growth and tumorigenicity.[202]

NF1-deficient Schwann cells derived from human neurofibromas show an activation of mTOR, even in the absence of growth factors. Furthermore, both these cells and transformed mouse cells with knockdown of Nf1 are highly sensitive to the mTOR inhibitor rapamycin.[203] Finally, in a genetically engineered murine model, rapamycin potently suppresses the growth of aggressive NF1-associated malignancies by suppressing the mTOR target cyclin D1. These results demonstrate that mTOR inhibitors may be an effective targeted therapy for patients with neurofibromatosis and MPNST.

Recent work has shown that the chemokine receptor CXCR4 is highly expressed in NF1-associated MPNST and that CXCR4, along with its ligand CXCL12, promotes MPNST growth by stimulating cyclin D1 expression. The highly specific CXCR4 antagonist AMD3100 decreased growth of MPNST cell lines, MPNST allografts, and MPNST tumors in transgenic mouse models of spontaneous MPNST. These results suggest that targeting autocrine cell cycle progression regulated by CXCR4/CXCL12 may represent a promising therapy for MPNST.[204]

The inactivation of NF1 and the consequent activation of the Ras/Raf/MAPK pathway in the majority of MPNSTs supported targeting B-Raf with the B-Raf tyrosine-kinase inhibitor sorafenib.

MPNST cell lines are sensitive to sorafenib at nanomolar concentrations, and this was found to be mediated by the suppression of cyclin D1 and hypophosphorylation of RB1, resulting in G1 cell-cycle arrest.[205] A phase II trial of sorafenib in patients with metastatic MPNST was recently completed. Although none of the 12 patients with MPNST had Response Evaluation Criteria in Solid Tumors (RECIST) responses, 3 had stable disease and 2 had regression or cystification of metastatic disease.[206]

Angiosarcoma

Angiosarcomas are rare vascular malignancies of endothelial cell differentiation that arise either de novo or secondary to radiation therapy or chronic lymphedema. By expression profiling, angiosarcomas are characterized by upregulation of vascular-specific receptor tyrosine kinases, including *TIE1*, *KDR* (*VEGFR2*), *TEK* (*TIE2*), and *FLT1* (*VEGFR1*).[207] Full sequencing of these genes identified mutations in *KDR* in 10% of angiosarcoma patients, all of whom had tumors in the breast, with or without prior radiation. KDR was mutated in its extracellular immunoglobulinlike C2 domain, transmembrane domain, or kinase domain. *KDR* mutations were typically associated with strong KDR protein expression, although no gains in *KDR* copy number were detected. KDR mutants expressed in COS-7 cells showed ligand-independent activation of the kinase, which was inhibited with specific KDR inhibitors.[207] In contrast with other sarcoma types, angiosarcoma showed downregulation of VEGF ligand expression (VEGFA and VEGFB), in keeping with the constitutive activation of KDR independent of exogenous VEGF.[207] These results provide a basis for the activity of VEGFR-directed therapy in de novo and radiation-induced angiosarcoma.

In a recent array-CGH study, recurrent genetic abnormalities were identified in radiation- and lymphedema-associated angiosarcomas but not de novo angiosarcomas.[208] The most frequent recurrent changes were high-level amplifications on chromosome 8q24.21 (50%), followed by amplification on 10p12.33 (33%) and 5q35.3 (11%). A high-level amplification of *MYC* on 8q24.21 was confirmed by FISH in most angiosarcomas associated with radiation and chronic lymphedema, but only in a minority of de novo tumors.[209,210] *MYC* amplification was not found to predispose patients to a higher grade morphology or increased proliferation. These findings suggest that primary and secondary angiosarcoma, despite their similar morphology, are genetically distinct.

BONE AND CARTILAGINOUS TUMORS

CARTILAGINOUS TUMORS

Cartilaginous tumors represent the most common primary bone tumor. The cartilaginous tumors all produce chondroid matrix, at least focally.[120] The most common benign tumors are enchondromas and osteochondromas; they may serve as precursors to chondrosarcoma.

Enchondroma

Enchondromas may occur as solitary lesions in the metaphysis of bone or as multiple lesions, as is found in Ollier disease or Maffucci syndrome.[211] Enchondromas have constitutively active Hedgehog signaling, which blocks normal chondrocyte differentiation and drives proliferation.[212] Heterozygous somatic mutations in *PTHR1*, which encodes the receptor for parathyroid hormone–like hormone (PTHLH), have been found in approximately 15% of patients with Ollier disease.[213–215] *PTHR1* mutation disrupts the normal Indian Hedgehog–PTHLH feedback loop, leading to activated Hedgehog signaling[213] and, presumably, to pathogenesis of Ollier disease in some patients.[215] The genetic deficit in Maffucci syndrome is unknown.

Osteochondroma

Osteochondroma is a cartilage-capped bony outgrowth from the metaphysis of bone. Osteochondromas can be solitary or multiple, as seen in multiple osteochondromas syndrome (MO), which is caused by dominant germ-line mutations in the tumor-suppressor exostosin gene family, specifically *EXT1* (located on 8q) or *EXT2* (located on 11p).[216] Loss of the remaining wild-type allele is seen in about 38% of sporadic and in 25% of hereditary osteochondromas.[217,218] A mouse model having biallelic inactivation of *EXT1* recapitulates the morphology found in human MO.[219,220] *EXT1* and *EXT2* encode glycosyltransferases that catalyze chain elongation of heparan sulfate on proteoglycans[221]; defective heparan sulfate synthesis has been shown to affect the diffusion of Hedgehog ligands in the extracellular space, which in turn enables growth-plate chondrocyte growth in the wrong direction.[222] It also interferes with the ossification of the perichondrium so as to facilitate osteochondromagenesis.[223]

Chondrosarcoma

Chondrosarcoma is a malignant cartilaginous matrix–producing tumor with diverse morphologic features. It tends to occur in older patients with a peak incidence at ages 40 to 70. Low-grade chondrosarcomas rarely metastasize but may progress to high-grade chondrosarcoma, which metastasizes in about 70% of patients. Some chondrosarcomas arise from benign lesions (enchondromas or osteochondromas); these are termed secondary chondrosarcomas.[120]

A prominent genetic alteration detected in cartilaginous tumors is the somatic mutation of isocitrate dehydrogenase (IDH) genes. In the initial study, *IDH1* and *IDH2* were mutated in 81 of 145 cartilaginous tumors (56%).[224] A more recent study confirmed the presence of *IDH1* and *IDH2* mutations in 61% of chondrosarcomas.[225] Among cartilaginous tumors, *IDH* mutations appear to be confined to enchondromas, periosteal chondrosarcomas, and central (intramedullary) chondrosarcomas of conventional or dedifferentiated histology.[224,226] *IDH* mutations have not been found in secondary peripheral chondrosarcomas, which instead share some of the molecular characteristics of osteochondromas. *IDH1* and *IDH2* mutations also appear to be absent in osteochondromas or osteosarcomas, including chondroblastic osteosarcomas, and so mutation detection may be useful in diagnosis.

The common *IDH* mutations in chondrosarcoma affect IDH1 R132 (~90% of IDH mutant cases) and IDH2 at the homologous position, R172 (~10%). These mutations are also common in glioma and acute myeloid leukemia. The mutations block the ability of the enzymes to convert isocitrate to α-ketoglutarate, which in turn increases the levels of HIF1A, a subunit of a transcription factor that facilitates tumor growth in hypoxic environments.[227] HIF1A is highly expressed in high-grade central chondrosarcoma.[228,229]

IDH1 R132 and IDH2 R172 mutations confer on the enzymes a new ability to convert α-ketoglutarate to R($-$)-2-hydroxyglutarate (2HG), resulting in markedly elevated levels of 2HG.[230,231] 2HG itself appears to be oncogenic and has been shown to induce CpG island DNA hypermethylation in low-grade gliomas,[232] acute myeloid leukemia,[233] and chondrosarcoma[234] containing *IDH1* and *IDH2* mutations. Across all these cancer types, the increased production of 2HG is associated with the inhibition of ten-eleven translocation dioxygenase (TET)–mediated DNA demethylation, leading to a hypermethylation phenotype that affects genes of the retinoic acid receptor activation pathway[234] and, in chondrosarcoma, affects genes implicated in stem cell maintenance and differentiation.[235] The expression of an IDH2 mutant in mesenchymal progenitor cells is oncogenic in vitro and in vivo and leads to DNA hypermethylation and a differentiation block, which is reversible with DNA demethylating agents.[235] Thus, for patients with *IDH*-mutant chondrosarcomas, there may be a therapeutic potential for demethylating agents or for selective inhibitors of the mutant IDH proteins, such as an IDH1 R132 mutant inhibitor currently in development.[236]

A recent whole exome sequencing study[237] showed that 37% of chondrosarcomas have insertions, deletions, or rearrangements of *COL2A1*, which encodes the alpha chain of type II collagen fibers—the major collagen constituent of articular cartilage. The researchers postulated that such mutations may interfere with the production of mature collagen fibrils. They also identified mutations in *IDH1/2* (59%), *TP53* (20%), and genes of the RB1 pathway (33%) and the Hedgehog pathway (18%).

Other potentially targetable abnormalities in chondrosarcoma include the Hedgehog pathway, the IGF pathway, CDK4, MDM2, and SRC. Hedgehog signaling in primary central chondrosarcoma is constitutively activated, and activation is thought to occur early in tumorigenesis and serves to maintain chondrocytes in a proliferative state.[212,238] Hedgehog inhibitors such as cyclopamine and triparanol inhibit chondrosarcoma cell growth in vitro and in xenografts to varying degrees.[212] These results suggest that patients with conventional chondrosarcoma may benefit from some of the newer Hedgehog pathway inhibitors, such as the selective smoothened inhibitor vismodegib (GDC-0449, recently approved for basal cell carcinoma).[239–241] Unlike primary central chondrosarcoma, secondary peripheral chondrosarcoma actually has decreased Hedgehog signaling,[242] suggesting that Hedgehog blockade might not be effective for the peripheral subtype. Gli2 overexpression in a mouse model induces benign cartilage tumors, whereas Gli2 overexpression combined with p53 (*Trp53*) deficiency results in the development of tumors that resemble chondrosarcoma by negatively regulating apoptosis through activated IGF signaling.[243] Thus, the inhibition of IGF signaling may block chondrosarcoma progression and may also serve as an attractive therapeutic target. Kinome profiling has demonstrated SRC pathway activation in chondrosarcoma cell lines, and indeed, the SRC inhibitor dasatinib decreased chondrosarcoma cell viability.[244]

OSTEOSARCOMA

Osteosarcoma is a primary bone malignancy that arises most frequently in the long bones from osteoid-producing cells adjacent to growth plates, typically in children and adolescents.[245] Osteosarcomas are characterized by complex DNA copy number alterations with few recurrent alterations and a high level of genomic instability. Most osteosarcomas are sporadic. Risk factors include prior radiation therapy and chemotherapy.[246] Familial syndromes associated with osteosarcoma include Rothmund-Thomson syndrome,[247] Li-Fraumeni syndrome (associated with *TP53* mutation), and hereditary retinoblastoma. Children with hereditary retinoblastoma exhibit up to 1,000 times the incidence of osteosarcoma compared to the general population. In addition, alterations affecting *RB1* have been found in up to 80% of primary osteosarcoma samples.[248–250] About 20% of osteosarcomas have either a deletion of *CDKN2A* (encoding p16-INK4A) or an amplification of *CDK4*[251]; this finding, along with the reciprocal relationship between *RB1* and *CDKN2A* alterations,[252] suggests that G1/S deregulation by either *RB1* loss, *CDK4* amplification, or *CDKN2A* loss is nearly universal in osteosarcoma.

Another gene significantly associated with osteosarcoma is *TP53*. The frequency of somatic *TP53* mutations in osteosarcomas ranges from 19% to 38%,[253,254] and *TP53* mutations are associated with high levels of genomic instability.[254] An additional 5% to 10% of osteosarcomas harbor amplification of *MDM2*.[255] *TP53* mutations in osteosarcomas are frequently associated with hypermethylation of *HIC1* (hypermethylated in cancer 1). Specifically, *HIC1* was hypermethylated in 12 out of 29 human osteosarcomas with *TP53* mutations (41%) compared to 2 out of 24 tumors without *TP53* mutations (8%; p = 0.007).[256] Experiments in mice with heterozygous deletion of both *Hic1* and *Trp53* have demonstrated cooperation between these two genes in osteosarcomagenesis.[256] All these results suggest that the loss of HIC1 function may complement *TP53* mutations in the development of a subset of human osteosarcomas.

Array CGH of conventional osteosarcoma, which accounts for 75% of osteosarcomas, has shown that 1p36, 6p21, 8q24, 16p13, 17p11, and 19p13 are recurrently gained/amplified[257–260] and 2q, 6p, 8p, 10p, and 17p13 are recurrently lost/deleted.[258,261] High copy gains and/or amplifications of chromosome arms 6p, 8q, and 17p are frequently reported and are believed to confer a more aggressive disease course.[262] A high copy number gain of the *MYC* oncogene at 8q24 was found in 43% of osteosarcomas.[263] Other potential oncogenes on 8q24 include *RECQL4* and *EXT1*. Germ-line *RECQL4* helicase-inactivating mutations lead to Rothmund-Thomson syndrome[264] and *EXT1* mutations lead to multiple exostoses.[265] Both syndromes include a strong predisposition to osteosarcoma.

FUTURE DIRECTIONS: NEXT-GENERATION SEQUENCING AND FUNCTIONAL SCREENS

New targeted therapies are desperately needed for the ~5,800 patients who die each year from sarcoma in the United States.[266] A key challenge will be to identify the alterations that drive sarcomagenesis for each subtype of sarcoma. Once these driver alterations are identified, new small molecules to target them can be sought through a combination of functional screens, high-throughput compound screens, combinatorial chemistry, and structural biology information. Use of next-generation sequencing technologies can vastly expand our knowledge of the mutations, translocations, epigenetic alterations, and aberrant signaling pathways associated with specific sarcoma types and subtypes. Concurrent massively parallel sequencing experiments and integrative analysis now enable genomewide analysis of copy number alterations, structural rearrangements, expressed coding mutations, alternative splice forms, digital expression, chimeric/fusion transcripts, and DNA methylation status. This approach will provide a deeper view of the sarcoma genome than was previously possible. For example, on a single tumor sample, it is now possible to resequence all of the protein-coding regions of the human genome, generate detailed transcriptome profiles (RNA-seq),[267] and perform genomewide profiling of epigenetic marks and chromatin structures using other sequence-based methods (e.g., chromatin immunoprecipitation sequencing [ChIP-seq], methyl-seq, and DNase-seq).[268] In gene expression studies, microarrays are being replaced by sequence-based methods because RNA-seq provides far more precision on transcript levels, alternative splicing, and sequence variation in identified genes. RNA-seq has an additional advantage in that it can identify rare transcripts without prior knowledge of a particular gene.[267–270] These sequence-based methods, when integrated with data from high-throughput RNA interference screens in cell lines harboring the genetic alterations found in human sarcoma samples, will substantially enhance our ability to identify and target the signaling pathways and proteins driving sarcomagenesis.

Smart compounds, reflecting the three-dimensional structure of the targeted protein, may then be designed using high-throughput biochemical screens capable of identifying low-affinity compounds, together with sensitive biophysical techniques such as nuclear magnetic resonance, x-ray diffraction, and protein-ligand cocrystallography.[271–274] The resulting physicochemical data should facilitate the virtual screening of library structures for their three-dimensional fit with pharmacophores[275] and speed the discovery of new selective small-molecule inhibitors targeting the signaling pathways essential for sarcoma growth and survival.

SELECTED REFERENCES

The full reference list can be accessed at lwwhealthlibrary.com/oncology.

22. Barretina J, Taylor BS, Banerji S, et al. Subtype-specific genomic alterations define new targets for soft tissue sarcoma therapy. *Nat Genet* 2010;42: 715–721.
37. Owen LA, Kowalewski AA, Lessnick SL. EWS/FLI mediates transcriptional repression via NKX2.2 during oncogenic transformation in Ewing's sarcoma. *PloS One* 2008;3:e1965.
39. Bilke S, Schwentner R, Yang F, et al. Oncogenic ETS fusions deregulate E2F3 target genes in Ewing sarcoma and prostate cancer. *Genome Res* 2013;23:1797–1809.
46. Gerald WL, Haber DA. The EWS-WT1 gene fusion in desmoplastic small round cell tumor. *Semin Cancer Biol* 2005;15:197–205.
62. Su L, Sampaio AV, Jones KB, et al. Deconstruction of the SS18-SSX fusion oncoprotein complex: insights into disease etiology and therapeutics. *Cancer Cell* 2012;21:333–347.
63. Kadoch C, Crabtree GR. Reversible disruption of mSWI/SNF (BAF) complexes by the SS18-SSX oncogenic fusion in synovial sarcoma. *Cell* 2013;153:71–85.
78. Wexler LH, Ladanyi M. Diagnosing alveolar rhabdomyosarcoma: morphology must be coupled with fusion confirmation. *J Clin Oncol* 2010;28: 2126–2128.
88. Nishijo K, Chen QR, Zhang L, et al. Credentialing a preclinical mouse model of alveolar rhabdomyosarcoma. *Cancer Res* 2009;69:2902–2911.
96. Kobos R, Nagai M, Tsuda M, et al. Combining integrated genomics and functional genomics to dissect the biology of a cancer-associated, aberrant transcription factor, the ASPSCR1-TFE3 fusion oncoprotein. *J Pathol* 2013;229:743–754.
101. Kummar S, Allen D, Monks A, et al. Cediranib for metastatic alveolar soft part sarcoma. *J Clin Oncol* 2013;31:2296–2302.
102. McArthur GA, Demetri GD, van Oosterom A, et al. Molecular and clinical analysis of locally advanced dermatofibrosarcoma protuberans treated with imatinib: Imatinib Target Exploration Consortium Study B2225. *J Clin Oncol* 2005;23:866–873.
120. Fletcher CDM, Bridge JA, Hogendoorn P, et al eds. *WHO Classification of Tumours of Soft Tissue and Bone.* 4th ed. Lyon, France: IARC Press; 2013.
121. Robinson DR, Wu YM, Kalyana-Sundaram S, et al. Identification of recurrent NAB2-STAT6 gene fusions in solitary fibrous tumor by integrative sequencing. *Nat Genet* 2013;45:180–185.

132. Heinrich MC, McArthur GA, Demetri GD, et al. Clinical and molecular studies of the effect of imatinib on advanced aggressive fibromatosis (desmoid tumor). *J Clin Oncol* 2006;24:1195–1203.
133. Gounder MM, Lefkowitz RA, Keohan ML, et al. Activity of Sorafenib against desmoid tumor/deep fibromatosis. *Clin Cancer Res* 2011;17:4082–4090.
136. Mariani O, Brennetot C, Coindre JM, et al. JUN oncogene amplification and overexpression block adipocytic differentiation in highly aggressive sarcomas. *Cancer Cell* 2007;11:361–374.
142. Singer S, Socci ND, Ambrosini G, et al. Gene expression profiling of liposarcoma identifies distinct biological types/subtypes and potential therapeutic targets in well-differentiated and dedifferentiated liposarcoma. *Cancer Res* 2007;67:6626–6636.
144. Dickson MA, Tap WD, Keohan ML, et al. Phase II trial of the CDK4 inhibitor PD0332991 in patients with advanced CDK4-amplified well-differentiated or dedifferentiated liposarcoma. *J Clin Oncol* 2013;31:2024–2028.
179. Hernando E, Charytonowicz E, Dudas ME, et al. The AKT-mTOR pathway plays a critical role in the development of leiomyosarcomas. *Nat Med* 2007;13:748–753.
201. Ling BC, Wu J, Miller SJ, et al. Role for the epidermal growth factor receptor in neurofibromatosis-related peripheral nerve tumorigenesis. *Cancer Cell* 2005;7:65–75.
202. Rahrmann EP, Watson AL, Keng VW, et al. Forward genetic screen for malignant peripheral nerve sheath tumor formation identifies new genes and pathways driving tumorigenesis. *Nat Genet* 2013;45:756–766.
203. Johannessen CM, Reczek EE, James MF, et al. The NF1 tumor suppressor critically regulates TSC2 and mTOR. *Proc Natl Acad Sci U S A* 2005;102:8573–8578.
204. Mo W, Chen J, Patel A, et al. CXCR4/CXCL12 mediate autocrine cell-cycle progression in NF1-associated malignant peripheral nerve sheath tumors. *Cell* 2013;152:1077–1090.
205. Ambrosini G, Cheema HS, Seelman S, et al. Sorafenib inhibits growth and mitogen-activated protein kinase signaling in malignant peripheral nerve sheath cells. *Mol Cancer Ther* 2008;7:890–896.
206. Maki RG, D'Adamo DR, Keohan ML, et al. Phase II study of sorafenib in patients with metastatic or recurrent sarcomas. *J Clin Oncol* 2009;27: 3133–3140.
207. Antonescu CR, Yoshida A, Guo T, et al. KDR activating mutations in human angiosarcomas are sensitive to specific kinase inhibitors. *Cancer Res* 2009;69:7175–7179.

221. McCormick C, Leduc Y, Martindale D, et al. The putative tumour suppressor EXT1 alters the expression of cell-surface heparan sulfate. *Nat Genet* 1998;19:158–161.

224. Amary MF, Bacsi K, Maggiani F, et al. IDH1 and IDH2 mutations are frequent events in central chondrosarcoma and central and periosteal chondromas but not in other mesenchymal tumours. *J Pathol* 2011;224: 334–343.

227. Zhao S, Lin Y, Xu W, et al. Glioma-derived mutations in IDH1 dominantly inhibit IDH1 catalytic activity and induce HIF-1alpha. *Science* 2009;324:261–265.

232. Turcan S, Rohle D, Goenka A, et al. IDH1 mutation is sufficient to establish the glioma hypermethylator phenotype. *Nature* 2012;483:479–483.

234. Guilhamon P, Eskandarpour M, Halai D, et al. Meta-analysis of IDH-mutant cancers identifies EBF1 as an interaction partner for TET2. *Nat Commun* 2013;4:2166.

235. Lu C, Venneti S, Akalin A, et al. Induction of sarcomas by mutant IDH2. *Genes Dev* 2013;27:1986–1998.

237. Tarpey PS, Behjati S, Cooke SL, et al. Frequent mutation of the major cartilage collagen gene COL2A1 in chondrosarcoma. *Nat Genet* 2013;45:923–926.

256. Chen W, Cooper TK, Zahnow CA, et al. Epigenetic and genetic loss of Hic1 function accentuates the role of p53 in tumorigenesis. *Cancer Cell* 2004;6:387–398.

267. Wang Z, Gerstein M, Snyder M. RNA-Seq: a revolutionary tool for transcriptomics. *Nat Rev Genet* 2009;10:57–63.

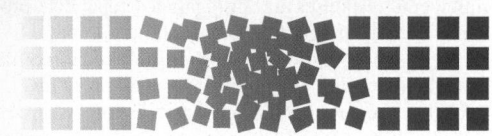

90 Soft Tissue Sarcoma

Samuel Singer, William D. Tap, Aimee M. Crago, and Brian O'Sullivan

INTRODUCTION

Tumors arising in the soft tissue form a diverse and complex group, as they may display varying degrees of mesenchymal differentiation. Most soft tissue tumors are benign and are usually cured with a simple surgical excision. Soft tissue sarcomas account for <1% of the overall human burden of malignant tumors but remain life-threatening, and approximately 40% of patients with newly diagnosed soft tissue sarcoma die of the disease, corresponding to approximately 4,000 deaths each year in the United States.[1] Soft tissue sarcoma, diagnosed at an early stage, is eminently curable. When diagnosed at the time of extensive local or metastatic disease, it is rarely curable. The relatively small number of cases and the great diversity in histopathologic features, anatomic sites, and biological behaviors have made comprehensive understanding of these disease entities difficult. A better understanding is urgently needed to accelerate the development of new treatments.

INCIDENCE AND ETIOLOGY

Epidemiology

Benign mesenchymal tumors are 100-fold more common than soft tissue sarcomas.[2] The annual international incidence of soft tissue sarcoma is estimated to be between 1.4 and 5.0 cases per 100,000; the true incidence remains difficult to determine because of variable reporting practices and inaccurate diagnosis.[3–8] Incidence patterns vary considerably by histologic type and subtype.[7,9] For most types of soft tissue sarcoma, incidence increases progressively with age from approximately 1 to 2 per 100,000 at age 15, to approximately 6 per 100,000 at age 49, and to as high as approximately 20 per 100,000 at age 80.[7,9]

Etiology and Risk Factors

Most soft tissue sarcomas are believed to be sporadic and have no clearly defined cause. In a small proportion of cases, researchers have identified predisposing or associated factors, including genetic factors, lymphedema, prior radiation therapy, and carcinogens.

Genetic Factors

A range of heritable genetic syndromes are associated with soft tissue neoplasms.[10] Desmoid tumors occur in patients with familial adenomatous polyposis, a disorder caused by germline mutations in the *APC* gene. Malignant peripheral nerve sheath tumors (MPNST) develop in neurofibromas in patients with neurofibromatosis 1 (NF1), caused by germline mutations in the *NF1* gene. Patients with NF1 have an estimated lifetime risk of MPNST of 8% to 13%.[11] Li-Fraumeni syndrome is a rare, highly penetrant familial cancer phenotype usually associated with germline mutations in *TP53*, the gene for tumor suppressor p53.[12] Eighty percent of patients with this syndrome develop cancer by age 45, and the index tumors in 36% of patients are soft tissue or bone sarcomas of diverse histology.[13] Heritable retinoblastoma gene (*RB1*) mutations are associated with an increased risk of bone and soft tissue sarcoma. For instance, patients with *RB1* mutations have a 36% cumulative incidence over 50 years of sarcoma in previously irradiated tissue.[14] Most of the excess cancer risk in *RB1* mutation carriers who survive retinoblastoma can probably be prevented by limiting exposure to DNA-damaging agents such as radiotherapy, tobacco, and ultraviolet light.[15] Similarly, radiotherapy should be avoided in patients with sarcoma with a known germline mutation in *RB1*.

Lymphedema

Lymphedema has long been established as a factor in the development of angiosarcoma. The best-recognized association is with the postmastectomy, postirradiated lymphedematous arm.[16] This is not a radiation-induced sarcoma because the tumors develop outside as well as inside the irradiated field. Similar advanced sarcomas have been seen after chronic lymphedema caused by filarial infection.[17] The oncogenic mechanism remains unknown, but one hypothesis, based on the frequent proliferation of lymphatic vessels in the edematous tissue, is that the block of the lymphatics stimulates growth factors and cytokines, leading to proliferation of vessels and lymphatics.[18] Others have postulated that the edematous tissue results in a regional immune deficiency that enables mutant cells to escape the host's immune surveillance.[19]

Radiation

It has been known since 1922 that radiation exposure can cause soft tissue and bone sarcoma. Soft tissue sarcomas are one of the more common types of radiation-associated tumors, both in the general population[20–23] and in individuals with cancer susceptibility syndromes.[14] Radiation-associated sarcomas are most often seen in diseases that are commonly treated with radiotherapy and in those in which patient survival is typically long. The prime candidate diseases are breast cancer, lymphoma, genitourinary cancer, and head and neck cancer.[24] Children are at risk due to the time latency involved. In a review of 130 patients with primary radiation-associated sarcoma, the median interval between radiotherapy and development of a radiation-associated sarcoma was 10 years (range, 1.3 to 74.0).[24] This interval varied significantly by histologic type, with the shortest latency observed in liposarcoma (median, 4.3 years) and longest in leiomyosarcoma (LMS) (median, 23.5 years). The most common histologic types of radiation-associated sarcomas were pleomorphic malignant histiocytoma (PMFH; also known as undifferentiated pleomorphic sarcomas [UPS]; 26%), angiosarcoma (21%), fibrosarcoma (12%), LMS (12%), and MPNST (9%).

The molecular mechanisms of radiation-associated sarcomas are poorly understood. Interestingly, they have a reputation for originating close to the penumbra of radiotherapy fields, perhaps because incomplete damage in normal tissues may result in mutagenic responses and disorganized reparative proliferation that can eventually trigger tumor induction.

Although uncommon, radiation-induced sarcomas usually have a poor prognosis.[24] A multivariate analysis of five common high-grade types of sarcoma showed that radiation-associated sarcoma had a worse disease-specific survival than sporadic soft tissue sarcoma ($p = 0.007$; hazard ratio = 1.7; 95% confidence interval [CI] = 1.1 to 2.4), independent of histologic type and other standard predictors. For PMFH—the most common radiation-associated sarcoma type—the 5-year disease-specific survival was 44%, compared to 66% for a matched cohort of sporadic PMFH patients ($p = 0.07$).

Given the increased use of radiation therapy as a primary treatment for breast cancer, concern has been expressed that the incidence of sarcoma might increase. In a retrospective review of data from the Surveillance, Epidemiology, and End Results database, Huang and Mackillop[21] analyzed the data on 194,798 women treated for breast cancer between 1973 and 1995. Although follow-up was somewhat short, they demonstrated a 16-fold increase in angiosarcoma in radiotherapy patients versus controls, and a two-fold increase in all soft tissue sarcoma in radiated patients.

Another study cohort included 295,712 patients with primary cancers registered during 1953 to 2000 in the Finnish Cancer Registry.[25] In total, 147 sarcomas were observed (86% of which were soft tissue sarcomas), whereas 88.5 were expected from the national incidence. Among patients with prior breast cancer, 44 sarcomas were observed versus 28.9 expected, a ratio of 1.5 (95% CI = 1.1 to 2.0). After 10 years of follow-up, sarcoma risk was increased among patients who had received neither radiotherapy nor chemotherapy (observed to expected ratio 2.0; 95% CI = 1.3 to 3.0) but was higher in patients who had received chemotherapy and in patients who had received radiotherapy (observed to expected ratio 4.2; 95% CI = 2.9 to 5.8), especially those treated before age 55. These results confirm that the risk of sarcoma is increased after 10 years in tumors other than retinoblastoma but is also independently related to younger age of exposure to radiation, although the risk is also influenced by chemotherapy.[25]

Trauma

Whether trauma is a predisposing factor is controversial. Abdominal desmoid tumors commonly follow parturition and may be located in the bed of a prior surgery. Moreover, desmoids in the extremity, both localized and multifocal, may be associated with antecedent vigorous physical activity.[26] Some authors have speculated that injuries during active sport may predispose to sarcomas in general, and in turn there has been concern that operative trauma, including arthroplasty surgery, may increase soft tissue sarcoma risk. However, Scandinavian studies on more than 100,000 patients who had undergone total hip or knee arthroplasty showed no increased risk of sarcoma, and there were no cases of sarcoma presenting at the site of operation.[27] An injury may merely draw attention to a mass, without being a causative factor.

Chemical Agents

Several chemical carcinogens have an established role in the development of hepatic angiosarcomas: thorotrast, vinyl chloride, and arsenic (including Fowler 1% arsenic solution).[13] The role of other chemical agents in sarcomagenesis remains controversial. Some studies have suggested a link between phenoxy herbicide exposure and development of sarcoma,[28] and soft tissue sarcoma was associated with high occupational exposures in a large industrial cohort.[29,30] However, other studies, including more recent case-control studies, have not confirmed this relationship.[31] Other authors have pointed to the inherent problems in occupational epidemiology in relation to soft tissue sarcoma,

among which are possible recall bias in self-reported exposure data; inconsistent classification of soft tissue sarcomas in the International Classification of Diseases, which is organ based; and, because of the rarity of soft tissue sarcomas, difficulty in assembling a sufficient number of study participants. Exposure to dioxin (contained in Agent Orange) has been suggested as a risk factor for sarcoma[32]; however, none of the reported associations are statistically significant, and several studies found no association.[33–35]

ANATOMIC AND AGE DISTRIBUTION AND PATHOLOGY

Anatomic and Age Distribution

Soft tissue sarcomas can occur in any site throughout the body. A total of 45% are located in the extremities, with 30% of all lesions occurring in the lower limb (most commonly in the thigh); 38% are intra-abdominal, divided between visceral (21%) and retroperitoneal (17%); 10% are truncal; and 5% are head and neck (Fig. 90.1). Soft tissue sarcomas become more common with increased age, and the median age at diagnosis is 65 years. However, the median age varies significantly by histologic type and subtype. In general, the median age of onset tends to be 20 to 50 years in the translocation-associated sarcomas and 50 to 70 years in the complex sarcoma types (Fig. 90.2).

Pathologic Classification and Defining the Biological Potential

Soft tissue tumors, although clinically often nondistinctive, form a varied and complex group that may show a wide range of differentiation[36] (Table 90.1). Their underlying histogenesis has not been clearly defined. Except for subcutaneous lipomas or benign smooth muscle tumors, there is very little evidence that these lesions arise from their mature (differentiated) tissue counterparts. In fact, many liposarcomas arise at sites devoid of adipose tissue, and most rhabdomyosarcomas, which have molecular markers suggesting a myoid origin, develop in locations that lack voluntary muscle.

Soft tissue tumors may be benign, malignant, or borderline. The ratio of benign to malignant tumors is more than 100:1. Soft tissue tumors are notorious for the ease with which benign and malignant cases may be confused, particularly in small biopsy samples. Sarcoma histologic type is generally an important predictor of distinctive patterns of behavior and prognosis. Although many published series have combined all the histologic subtypes of sarcoma, the importance of such subtyping is exemplified by liposarcoma, in which the five histologic subtypes (well differentiated, dedifferentiated, myxoid, round cell, and pleomorphic) have totally different biologies and patterns of behavior.[37–40] A further clear demonstration is the importance in pleomorphic sarcomas of myogenic differentiation, which is associated with a substantially increased risk of metastasis.[41]

As part of the World Health Organization classification of soft tissue tumors, it is now recommended to divide soft tissue tumors into four categories: benign, intermediate (locally aggressive), intermediate (rarely metastasizing), and malignant.[36] Most benign tumors do not recur locally, and those that do recur usually are not locally invasive and can be cured with complete surgical excision. Intermediate, locally aggressive soft tissue tumors often recur locally and are associated with a locally infiltrative growth pattern. Lesions in this category, such as desmoids, do not have any potential to metastasize but typically require wide excision with a margin of normal tissue for good local control. Intermediate rarely metastasizing tumors are often locally aggressive and

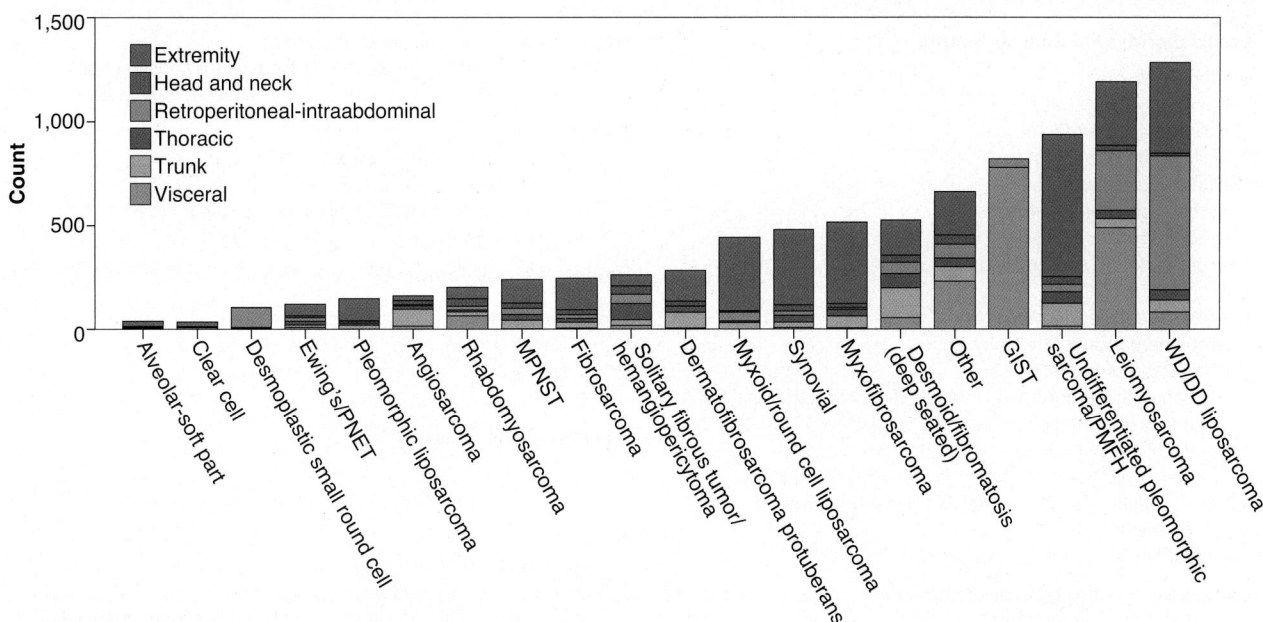

Figure 90.1 Distribution by histologic subtype and site of soft tissue sarcomas in 8,959 patients undergoing surgical resection at Memorial Sloan Kettering Cancer Center from 1982 through 2013. The retroperitoneal/abdominal category excludes visceral sarcomas. PNET, primitive neuroectodermal tumor; MPNST, malignant peripheral nerve sheath tumor; GIST, gastrointestinal stromal tumor; PMFH, pleomorphic malignant fibrous histiocytoma; WD/DD, well-differentiated and dedifferentiated.

occasionally give rise to distant metastases. The risk of metastasis, usually to lymph nodes or lung, is typically <2%, but is not reliably predictable based on histology. Examples of intermediate rarely metastasizing tumors include plexiform fibrohistiocytic tumor and angiomatoid fibrous histiocytoma. Malignant tumors (soft tissue sarcomas), in addition to potential for local invasion and recurrence, have a significant risk of distant metastasis, ranging in most instances from 10% to 100%, depending on histologic type and grade. Some histologically low-grade sarcomas (myxofibrosarcoma, well-differentiated liposarcoma) have a metastatic risk of only 2% to 10%, but these tumor types may progress to more aggressive tumors, acquiring a higher risk of distant spread.

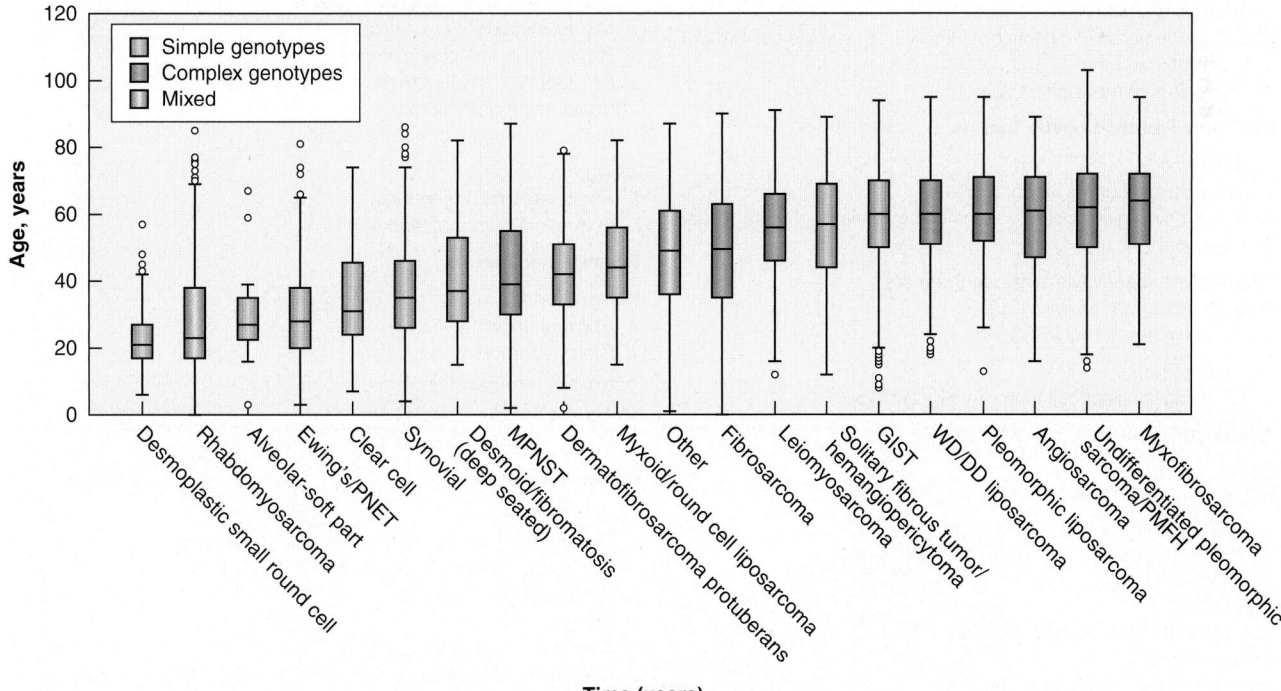

Time (years)

Figure 90.2 Age at diagnosis for sarcoma subtypes. The *boxes* show median and interquartile range, and the *whiskers* show range (with outliers excluded) for 8,959 patients undergoing surgical resection at Memorial Sloan Kettering Cancer Center from 1982 through 2013. Sarcoma subtypes with simple genotypes, shown in *green*, are associated with younger median age at diagnosis than those with complex genotypes, shown in *blue*. PNET, primitive neuroectodermal tumor; MPNST, malignant peripheral nerve sheath tumor; GIST, gastrointestinal stromal tumor; WD/DD, well-differentiated and dedifferentiated; PMFH pleomorphic malignant fibrous histiocytoma.

TABLE 90.1

Histologic Classification of Soft Tissue Tumors

Fibroblastic/Myofibroblastic Tumors

Benign Tumors
- Angiomyofibroblastoma
- Calcifying aponeurotic fibroma
- Calcifying fibrous tumor
- Cellular angiofibroma
- Desmoplastic fibroblastoma
- Elastofibroma
- Fibroma (tendon sheath, nuchal-type)
- Fibromatosis colli
- Fibro-osseous pseudotumor of digits
- Fibrous hamartoma of infancy
- Gardner fibroma
- Inclusion body fibromatosis (Infantile digital fibromatosis)
- Ischemic fasciitis (atypical decubital fibroplasia)
- Juvenile hyaline fibromatosis
- Mammary-type myofibroblastoma
- Myositis ossificans and fibro-osseous pseudotumor of digits
- Nodular fasciitis
- Proliferative fasciitis and myositis

Intermediate (Locally Aggressive) Tumors
- Desmoid-type fibromatoses
- Giant cell angiofibroma
- Lipofibromatosis
- Superficial fibromatoses (palmar and plantar)

Intermediate (Rarely Metastasizing) Tumors
- Dermatofibrosarcoma protuberans (including fibrosarcomatous and pigmented types)
- Infantile fibrosarcoma
- Inflammatory myofibroblastic tumor
- Low-grade myofibroblastic sarcoma
- Myxoinflammatory fibroblastic sarcoma (atypical myxoinflammatory fibroblastic tumor)
- Solitary fibrous tumor (hemangiopericytoma)

Malignant Tumors
- Adult fibrosarcoma
- Low-grade fibromyxoid sarcoma (hyalinizing spindle cell tumor)
- Myxofibrosarcoma
- Sclerosing epithelioid fibrosarcoma

So-Called Fibrohistiocytic Tumors

Benign Tumors
- Deep benign fibrous histiocytoma
- Tenosynovial giant cell tumor (including localized, diffuse types)
- Xanthoma

Intermediate (Rarely Metastasizing) Tumors
- Giant cell tumor of soft tissue
- Plexiform fibrohistiocytic tumor

Malignant Tumors
- Tenosynovial giant cell tumor (malignant type)

Adipocytic Tumors

Benign Tumors
- Lipoma
- Angiolipoma
- Angiomyolipoma
- Chondroid lipoma
- Hibernoma
- Lipoblastoma or lipoblastomatosis
- Lipomatosis
- Lipomatosis of nerve
- Myelolipoma
- Myolipoma
- Spindle cell or pleomorphic lipoma

Intermediate (Locally Aggressive) Tumors
- Atypical lipomatous tumor/well-differentiated liposarcoma (including lipoma-like, sclerosing and inflammatory types)

Malignant Tumors
- Liposarcoma, not otherwise specified
- Dedifferentiated liposarcoma
- Myxoid liposarcoma (including round cell type)
- Pleomorphic liposarcoma

Smooth Muscle Tumors

Benign Tumors
- Deep leiomyoma

Malignant Tumors
- Leiomyosarcoma (excluding skin)

Skeletal Muscle Tumors

Benign Tumors
- Rhabdomyoma (including adult, fetal, and genital types)

Malignant Tumors
- Rhabdomyosarcoma
- Alveolar rhabdomyosarcoma (including solid, anaplastic)
- Embryonal rhabdomyosarcoma (including botryoid, anaplastic)
- Pleomorphic rhabdomyosarcoma
- Spindle cell/sclerosing rhabdomyosarcoma

Vascular Tumors

Benign Tumors
- Angiomatosis
- Hemangioma (including intramuscular, synovial, arteriovenous, and venous types)
- Epithelioid hemangioma
- Lymphangioma

Intermediate (Locally Aggressive) Tumors
- Kaposiform hemangioendothelioma

Intermediate (Rarely Metastasizing) Tumors
- Composite hemangioendothelioma
- Kaposi sarcoma
- Papillary intralymphatic angioendothelioma
- Pseudomyogenic (epithelioid sarcoma-like) hemangioendothelioma
- Retiform hemangioendothelioma

Malignant Tumors
- Angiosarcoma of soft tissue
- Epithelioid hemangioendothelioma

Perivascular Tumors

Benign Tumors
- Angioleiomyoma
- Glomus tumor
- Myopericytoma (including myofibroma and myofibromatosis)

Malignant Tumors
- Malignant glomus tumor (glomangiosarcoma)

Neural Tumors

Benign Tumors
- Benign triton tumor (neuromuscular hamartoma)
- Dermal nerve sheath myxoma
- Ectopic meningioma
- Granular cell tumor
- Hybrid nerve sheath tumor
- Melanotic schwannoma
- Nasal glial heterotopia
- Neurofibroma (diffuse, plexiform, pacinian, epithelioid)
- Perineurioma
- Schwannoma (cellular, plexiform, degenerated)

(continued)

TABLE 90.1

Histologic Classification of Soft Tissue Tumors *(continued)*

Neural Tumors *(continued)*	Intermediate (Rarely Metastasizing) Tumors
	■ Atypical fibroxanthoma
Malignant Tumors	■ Angiomatoid fibrous histiocytoma
■ Malignant granular cell tumor	■ Mixed tumor, not otherwise specified (including malignant type)
■ MPNST (neurofibrosarcoma)	■ Myoepithelioma
■ Epithelioid MPNST	■ Myoepithelial carcinoma
■ Malignant triton tumor (MPNST with rhabdomyosarcoma)	■ Ossifying fibromyxoid tumors (including malignant type)
	■ Phosphaturic mesenchymal tumor (including benign and malignant types)
Extraskeletal Chondro-Osseous Tumors	
	Malignant Tumors
Benign Tumors	■ Alveolar soft part sarcoma
■ Soft tissue chondroma	■ Clear cell sarcoma of soft tissue
	■ Desmoplastic small round cell tumor
Malignant Tumors	■ Epithelioid sarcoma
■ Extraskeletal mesenchymal chondrosarcoma	■ Extrarenal rhabdoid tumor
■ Extraskeletal osteosarcoma	■ Extraskeletal Ewing sarcoma
	■ Extraskeletal myxoid chondrosarcoma
Gastrointestinal Stromal Tumors	■ Intimal sarcoma
	■ Malignant extrarenal rhabdoid tumor
■ Benign gastrointestinal stromal tumor	■ Neoplasms with perivascular epithelioid cell differentiation
■ Gastrointestinal stromal tumor, uncertain malignant potential	(PEComas, including benign and malignant types)
■ Gastrointestinal stromal tumors, malignant	■ Synovial sarcoma (biphasic and spindle cell)
Tumors of Uncertain Differentiation	**Undifferentiated/Unclassified Tumors**
Benign Tumors	Malignant Tumors
■ Acral fibromyxoma	■ Undifferentiated spindle cell sarcoma
■ Deep angiomyxoma	■ Undifferentiated pleomorphic sarcoma
■ Ectopic hamartomatous thymoma	■ Undifferentiated round cell sarcoma
■ Intramuscular myxoma	■ Undifferentiated epithelioid sarcoma
■ Juxta-articular myxoma	■ Undifferentiated sarcoma, not otherwise specified
■ Pleomorphic hyalinizing angiectatic tumor of soft parts	
Intermediate (Locally Aggressive) Tumors	
■ Hemosiderotic fibrolipomatous tumor	

MPNST, malignant peripheral nerve sheath tumor.
Modified from Fletcher CDM, Bridge JA, Hogendoorn P, et al., eds. *WHO Classification of Tumours of Soft Tissue and Bone.* 4th ed. Lyon, France: IARC Press; 2013.

Clinical and Pathologic Features of Specific Soft Tissue Tumor Types

The distribution of adult soft tissue sarcomas by histologic subtype and anatomic site is shown in Fig. 90.1. Overall, the three most common histologic subtypes are liposarcoma, LMS, and UPS/PMFH.

Fibroblastic and Myofibroblastic Tumors

Fibroblastic and myofibroblastic tumors represent a very large subset of mesenchymal tumors. These lesions are generally composed of fibroblasts and myofibroblasts in varying proportions and may be confused with reactive or reparative processes or alternatively with malignant fibrosarcomas. In addition, some fibrous proliferations of infancy and childhood resemble lesions in the adult but have a better prognosis. With improved understanding of the molecular events that lead to formation of fibroblastic and myofibroblastic tumors, both low- and high-grade forms of the lesions have been reproducibly characterized, although a variety of names are still used to designate identical or overlapping entities.[36] Among recent changes in the description of this subset of soft tissue lesions is the inclusion of dermatofibrosarcoma protuberans as a tumor of fibroblastic or myofibroblastic origin. The following sections summarize the features of the most common fibroblastic and myofibroblastic lesions with focus on sarcomas and those that may be mistaken for sarcoma.

Elastofibroma

Elastofibromas are rare, slow-growing benign tumors characteristically arising between the chest wall and the lower part of the

scapula. They may occur bilaterally, and they may grow to large size. Rarely the tumors are observed at the infraolecranon area or near the ischial tuberosities. Elastofibromas have been considered reactive lesions, and they are thought to be associated with repetitive manual tasks. Up to a third of cases are familial, and bilateral subscapular lesions in this context can be diagnosed based on history and imaging alone. For unilateral spontaneous disease, biopsy is commonly employed; histologically, the lesions consist of swollen eosinophilic collagen and elastic fibers with associated fibroblast-like cells. The tumors have copy number alterations in both clonal and nonclonal patterns.[42,43] If the diagnosis of elastofibroma is definitive, surgical resection can be reserved for the symptomatic patient.[44,45]

Fibroma

Fibroma is a nonspecific term usually applied to a group of poorly defined lesions in the skin or soft tissue. Management centers on complete surgical resection. While they can recur locally, metastases are not reported. Fibromas are characterized by a collagenous stroma with fibroblastic and myofibroblastic cells rarely demonstrating signs of atypia. While they can occur in unusual locations such as cardiac ventricle, they are more commonly observed in the skin, on the ovary, or associated with tendon sheaths. Nuchal-type fibromas, most commonly found in the posterior neck, are associated with male sex and diabetes mellitus; unlike common fibromas, nuchal-type fibromas can be infiltrative. Histologically similar are fibromas associated with Gardner syndrome, caused by germline *APC* mutation. These fibromas, which can be found on any area of the body, are commonly associated with metachronous desmoid tumors.

Nodular Fasciitis

Nodular fasciitis is a benign lesion usually seen in adults aged 20 to 40 years. The lesions typically grow rapidly over several weeks and reach 1 to 2 cm but rarely >5 cm. Pain and tenderness are common. The upper extremity is the most common site, especially the volar aspect of the forearm. Nodular fasciitis generally arises in the subcutaneous fascia or the superficial portions of the deep fascia. However, intra-articular fasciitis has been reported. Histologically, the lesions are nodular and nonencapsulated, showing plump mature fibroblasts arranged in short, irregular, or intersecting bundles; some lesions show hyalinization. Over 90% of these tumors have a genomic rearrangement affecting the *USP6* gene, most commonly in the form of a *MYH9-USP6* translocation.[46,47] Because of their high cellular clarity, rapid growth, and high mitotic activity, these lesions are often confused with fibrosarcoma. They are, however, clinically benign; they generally regress spontaneously and recurrence after local excision is uncommon. Computed tomography (CT) and magnetic resonance imaging (MRI) characteristics are not pathognomonic, although they may show either a solid or some partially cystic changes, usually in the subcutaneous tissues.

Myositis Ossificans

Myositis ossificans is usually associated with trauma. The lesion is a benign disorder that histologically is composed of fibrous tissue and bone. Fibro-osseous pseudotumor of the digits may reflect a similar histopathologic entity. Despite its name, myositis ossificans is not necessarily confined to the muscle, nor is inflammation a prominent feature. The condition usually presents in athletic young adults as a tender soft tissue mass. Over a period of weeks, the mass usually becomes firm to hard. Radiographs show calcification several weeks after the lesion appears. Histologically the mass consists of fibroblastic tissue, often with prominent mitotic activity. Nonetheless, this process is benign and may be managed conservatively. It is important to distinguish between myositis ossificans and sarcoma, especially extraskeletal osteosarcoma. In general, myositis ossificans displays a more ordered growth pattern than osteosarcoma with cellular elements found in the center of the tumor and calcified regions almost exclusively in the periphery.

Superficial Fibromatosis

Superficial fibromatoses arise from the fascia or aponeuroses and generally are small and slow growing; they may be more common in patients with diabetes mellitus. Palmar fibromatosis is associated with flexion contractures (Dupuytren contracture) and is by far the most common form, affecting as many as one in five persons aged 65 years and older. This condition is more common in men than in women and tends to be familial. Although benign, these lesions tend to recur after simple excision. Plantar fibromatosis (Ledderhose disease) tends to occur in a somewhat younger age group but may occur with greater frequency in patients with palmar fibromatosis. Much less common is penile fibromatosis (Peyronie disease), which causes pain and curvature of the penis on erection. The fibrous mass in Peyronie disease primarily involves fascial structures, the corpus cavernosum, and rarely the corpus spongiosum. Peyronie disease is more common in men with palmar and plantar fibromatosis than in the general population. Any of the superficial fibromatoses may be managed by surgical excision, though more recently injection with collagenase or treatment with calcium channel blockers has been shown to have efficacy and may reduce the need for surgery.

Desmoid Tumor

Desmoid tumors (deep or aggressive fibromatosis) are rare lesions with an estimated incidence of two to four individuals per million. Histologically, desmoids are bland tumors, with uniform-appearing spindle cells in a densely hyalinized background. On a microscopic level, they are observed to infiltrate into surrounding normal tissues.[48] Desmoids most commonly occur in the abdominal wall

(particularly after pregnancy), in the mesentery of the small bowel, and in the extremity. Multifocal lesions are known to occur in a subset of young patients (often diagnosed between ages 10 to 25).[26,49]

Desmoids do not metastasize, but can be locally aggressive, causing pain, joint contracture, or bowel obstruction. Surgical resection has been the mainstay of therapy. However, compared to other soft tissue sarcomas, desmoids, especially those in the extremities or chest wall, have high local recurrence rates (~15% at 5 years). Nevertheless, individual desmoids exhibit a wide range of behaviors. While some tumors recur after multiple attempts at resection, some never recur, and it is now recognized that some desmoids remain stable in size without any type of intervention. In rare instances, desmoid tumors can cause death, which can result from local compression of vital structures (particularly in the head and neck), fistulization to the bowel by intraabdominal lesions, or injury related to aggressive attempts at resection.

Desmoids, in 85% of cases, have a mutation in exon 3 of the *CTNNB1* gene that activates β-catenin.[50] In a small proportion of desmoids, β-catenin is activated because of germline mutation in the *APC* gene; these desmoids occur in parallel with familial adenomatosis polyposis (classic or attenuated) in Gardner syndrome.[51,52] Presence and site of *CTNNB1* mutation has been reported to be associated with patient outcome,[50] but this has not been validated and its use in prognostication is highly controversial.

Dermatofibrosarcoma Protuberans

Dermatofibrosarcoma protuberans (DFSP) is a generally indolent lesion characterized by translocation of the *COL1A1* and *PDG-FRB* genes.[53] The resultant fusion protein activates platelet-derived growth factor (PDGF) receptor signaling, which likely underlies oncogenesis. The tumor, composed of mononuclear spindle cells, is a relatively monomorphous lesion. It involves both dermis and subcutis. DFSP is histologically similar to benign fibrous histiocytoma but grows in a more infiltrative pattern, spreading along connective tissue septa often with unpredictable radial extensions and multifocal nodules. The center of the tumor consists of uniform plump fibroblasts arranged in a distinct ordered pattern. Unlike fibrous histiocytoma, DFSP stains positive for CD34. Variants with melanin pigmentation (Bednar tumor), prominent myxoid stroma, myoid differentiation, and plaque-like morphology are recognized and may be confused with other types of soft tissue sarcomas.

DFSP is a rare sarcoma, but one of the most common cutaneous forms. This lesion typically presents in early or mid-adult life, beginning as a nodular cutaneous mass anywhere in the body. Growth is usually slow but persistent, and over many years it becomes protuberant and satellite nodules become visible. The gold standard of treatment remains surgery, though the infiltrative nature and multifocality of the lesion have historically led to high rates of local recurrence (up to 50% after simple excision in some series). However, when gross margins of ≥2 cm are planned, most tumors can be completely resected, and in the context of complete microscopic resection, 5-year local recurrence rates are ≤5%.[54–56] Tumors with positive or close surgical margins in anatomically complex sites (e.g., near the brachial plexus) have an elevated risk of local recurrence, which is ameliorated with adjuvant radiotherapy.[57] Postoperative radiotherapy is also indicated in the rare patient who has unresectable macroscopic disease. DFSP is sensitive to imatinib,[58–62] probably because of constitutive activation of the PDGF receptor. The drug is now approved by the US Food and Drug Administration as the first line of treatment for advanced and metastatic disease. Metastasis (to lung or lymph nodes) occurs infrequently and generally only in the context of fibrosarcomatous degeneration, a high-grade form of the cancer.[54,63]

Inflammatory Myofibroblastic Tumor

Inflammatory myofibroblastic tumor (IMT) has gone under the names inflammatory pseudotumor and plasma cell granuloma, among others. Its histology is heterogeneous, with variable grouping of spindle, fibroblastic-myofibroblastic, and inflammatory-type cells. The variable appearance may result from the tumor's genetic heterogeneity. While *ALK* rearrangements are common in the myofibroblastic component of the tumors,[64,65] they occur in <70% of patients (almost exclusively in patients under 40). *ALK* is fused to a range of N-terminal partners, including *RANBP2* and *TPM3*.[66] Rarely, the *HMGA2* gene on chromosome 12 is rearranged.[67] Inflammatory components of the tumor do not have *ALK* fusions.[68,69]

IMT is a locally aggressive process. Many of the tumors occur in the thoracic and abdominal cavities, where they may appear as infiltrative or lobulated lesions on imaging studies.[70,71] Size and location may cause symptoms related to compression of adjacent organs (e.g., bowel obstruction). Diagnosis of IMT is often difficult to confirm preoperatively; therefore, surgical resection may be both diagnostic and therapeutic. When complete resection is possible, it is curative in ~75% of cases. Metastasis is rare (<5%), but local recurrence is more common.[72] Treatment of patients with advanced disease has been guided by the ALK fusions,[73–75] and patients with ALK-positive advanced IMT have responded to crizotinib (according to Response Evaluation Criteria in Solid Tumors [RECIST]).[76,77] In patients without an ALK fusion, treatment for locally aggressive disease is palliative, recognizing that few tumors have metastatic potential and the disease is rarely fatal (5-year survival of 87%). Of note, about 33% of patients with IMT develop a paraneoplastic syndrome including fever, growth failure, malaise, weight loss, anemia, and thrombocytosis.

Solitary Fibrous Tumor/Hemangiopericytoma

Solitary fibrous tumors (SFT) are identified by a prominent hemangiopericytoma-like branching vascular pattern. SFT encompasses fat-forming SFT and those lesions previously called hemangiopericytomas and giant cell angiofibromas, the latter containing giant multinucleated stromal cells and pseudo-vacuolar spaces. SFTs generally appear as slow-growing, well-circumscribed, painless masses. Histologically, they consist of tightly packed cells around thin-walled vascular channels of varying caliber. SFT cells stain for CD34 but not for factor VIII–related antigen. The lesions likely all have a *NAB2-STAT6* fusion protein that results in aberrant activation of EGR1 target genes, including *IGF2* and *FGFR1*.[78,79]

SFT may be found at any location in middle-aged adults (median age, 50). Occasional cases occur in children and adolescents. The adult form is most common in the thorax, pelvis, retroperitoneum, orbit, and lower extremity. Many SFTs are indolent and surgically cured, although some behave like other high-grade sarcomas. Risk factors for metastases include size >10 cm and mitotic rate >4 per 10 high-power fields.[80] Rarely, patients present with a very large SFT and hypoglycemia (Doege-Potter syndrome), which is associated with production of a form of insulin-like growth factor (IGF) 2 by these tumors.[81–84] SFTs are highly resistant to standard doxorubicin-based chemotherapy, but sunitinib and sorafenib have activity.[85,86]

Fibrosarcoma

Adult fibrosarcoma is uncommon (approximately 1% of adult sarcomas).[87] The tumor typically has many copy number alterations, though these do not appear to affect a single driver oncogene or tumor suppressor.[88] Fibrosarcoma is a malignant or intermediate (rarely metastasizing) tumor, composed of relatively homogenous spindle cells with variable collagen production and rare pleomorphism. Classical fibrosarcomas have a herringbone pattern on light microscopy. Like most soft tissue sarcomas with complex karyotypes, fibrosarcomas usually involve the deep tissues of the extremities, trunk, head, and neck of middle-aged and older adults. Some arise in the field of previous radiotherapy. Rarely, fibrosarcomas arise in the ovary or other unusual sites such as the trachea.

Infantile fibrosarcomas mimic the adult form histologically but are characterized by *ETV6-NTRK3* fusion and appear to be more indolent than the adult-type tumor.[89,90]

Myxofibrosarcoma

Myxofibrosarcoma, formerly known as a myxoid variant of malignant fibrous histiocytoma (MFH), is a common type of soft tissue sarcoma. It usually occurs as a painless mass in the limbs and trunk of elderly adults. Histology shows a fibroblastic lesion with pleomorphism, a characteristic curvilinear vascular pattern, and at least a 10% myxoid component.[41,91,92] Local recurrence occurs in up to 50% of cases, and is associated with tumors having a ≥75% myxoid component.[93–96] However, a more recent study that treated 80% of patients with myxofibrosarcoma with adjuvant radiation found only a 14.6% local recurrence rate at 5 years and a 24% 5-year cumulative incidence of distant recurrence.[97]

Low-grade myxofibrosarcoma may progress to high grade in subsequent local recurrences and thus acquire a higher probability for metastatic spread. The most common sites of metastases are lung, bone, and lymph nodes. The overall 5-year survival is 60% to 70%.[93–96] The 5-year disease-specific survival was 80% for patients presenting to Memorial Sloan Kettering Cancer Center (MSKCC) with primary myxofibrosarcoma of the extremity and trunk.

So-Called Fibrohistiocytic Tumors

The concept of fibrohistiocytic differentiation has been challenged, and it is now regarded as a poorly defined morphologic descriptor of histiocytic differentiation. The so-called fibrohistiocytic tumors, originally thought to arise from histiocytes that had fibroblastic potential, are almost certainly fibroblastic in origin. Thus, *fibrohistiocytic* is merely descriptive of their appearance; virtually none of these lesions show true histiocytic differentiation.[98]

Tenosynovial Giant Cell Tumor of Soft Tissue

The tenosynovial giant cell tumors of soft tissue encompasses entities previously called giant cell tumors of the tendon sheath, nodular tenosynovitis, or pigmented villonodular synovitis. These lesions contain multinucleate giant cells, siderophages, foam cells, and inflammatory cells. They are characterized by a t(1;2) translocation involving the colony stimulating factor 1 gene (*CSF1*) and most frequently *COL6A3*. This translocation leads to an increased level of CSF1, which is thought to modulate the inflammatory infiltrate noted in these tumors.[99–101] Three forms of the lesions are recognized: nodular, diffuse, and malignant. Not surprisingly, the form is predictive of biological behavior.[102] The nodular form, which has the greatest abundance of giant cells, is typically a well-circumscribed nodule in the digits. In contrast, the diffuse form has infiltrative borders and most commonly occurs in the large joints (e.g., knee, wrist, foot) or the surrounding soft tissue (e.g., thigh). They can be intra-articular. The malignant-type form demonstrates increased mitotic count and nuclear dysmorphism; these tumors likely have additional molecular alterations (other than *COL6A3-CSF1* translocation) that drive disease progression. Malignant-type tumors may metastasize to lung or lymph nodes.

Surgery is the mainstay of treatment. The recurrence rate is just 10% to 20% for nodular tumors, but 18% to 50% for diffuse-type tumors. With adjuvant radiation, rates of local recurrence may be under 10%.[103,104] Nevertheless, radiation is rarely used because of risk of joint fibrosis and secondary malignancies. Instead, recurrent or unresectable disease can be treated with a trial of imatinib, an inhibitor of the CSF1 receptor.[105] Imatinib treatment results in disease stabilization in approximately 75% of patients. However, imatinib appears less effective in the rare diffuse-type tenosynovial giant cell tumors that have a malignant component.[106] Because of their metastatic potential, malignant-type tumors should be managed aggressively as high-grade sarcomas. Multiple recurrent lesions that threaten limb integrity can be controlled with radiotherapy in both the tendon sheath and intra-articular forms.[103]

Fibrous Histiocytoma

Fibrous histiocytomas are benign tumors that usually present as solitary, slow-growing nodules, although up to one-third are multiple. Histologically, they consist of fibroblastic and histiocytic cells often arranged in a cartwheel or storiform pattern. When such lesions occur in the skin, they are often called *dermatofibromas* or *sclerosing hemangiomas*. Superficial lesions usually are cured by simple excision. Deeper lesions should be resected with a wider margin of normal tissue to prevent local recurrence.

In rare cases, fibrous histiocytomas are aggressive ("malignant dermatofibromas"). These lesions have a propensity for local recurrence, have been reported to metastasize, and, in a few patients, can cause death. Copy number alterations have been detected in these tumors, suggesting an underlying molecular aberrancy resulting in an invasive phenotype.[107]

Xanthoma

Xanthoma refers to a collection of lipid-laden histiocytes and is seen in diseases associated with hyperlipidemia. These lesions are generally cutaneous or subcutaneous but may involve deep soft tissues. Presumably, xanthomas are reactive lesions.

Adipocytic Tumors

Lipoma

Lipomas are the most common benign soft tissue neoplasm. They usually arise in subcutaneous tissue, most frequently in trunk and proximal limbs. Although deep-seated benign lipomas do occur in the mediastinum or retroperitoneum, most fatty neoplasms in the retroperitoneum should be approached surgically as atypical lipomatous tumor/well-differentiated liposarcoma. Most lipomas are soft, painless, slow-growing, and solitary; however, 2% to 3% of patients have multiple lesions that are occasionally seen in a familial pattern. *Lipomatosis* is a term applied to a poorly circumscribed overgrowth of mature adipose tissue that grows in an infiltrating pattern. Solitary lipomas are lobulated lesions composed of fat cells. They are well circumscribed, being demarcated from surrounding fat by a thin, fibrous capsule. Most subcutaneous, solitary lipomas show reproducible cytogenetic aberrations: translocations involving 12q13–15, rearrangements of 13q, or rearrangements involving 6p21–33.[108] In spindle cell lipoma, mature fat is replaced by collagen-forming spindle cells; this lesion typically arises in the posterior neck and shoulder in men between the ages of 45 and 65 years. Spindle cell lipomas show consistent chromosomal aberrations of 13q and 16q.[109] Local excision of lipoma and these variants is generally curative, with local recurrence after simple excision in no more than 1% to 2% of cases.

Intramuscular lipomas differ from their more superficial counterparts by usually being both poorly circumscribed and infiltrative (in ~90% of cases). Intramuscular lipomas typically present in midadult life as slow-growing, deep-seated masses most often located in the thigh or trunk. In a patient with a deep-seated fatty tumor, it is important to exclude atypical lipomatous tumor (see "Liposarcoma"), which tends to be more common than intramuscular lipoma.

Angiolipomas present as subcutaneous nodules, usually in young adults, and in >50% of cases are multiple. The most common site is the upper extremity. Angiolipomas rarely grow >2 cm, but they often are painful, especially during their initial growth period. Microscopically, these tumors consist of adipocytes with interspersed vascular structures. Myxoid and fibroblastic angiolipomas are recognized.

Hibernoma

Hibernoma is a rare, slow-growing, benign neoplasm that resembles the glandular brown fat of hibernating animals. The literature consists primarily of case reports. Most of these tumors arise within the thorax, though hibernomas of the trunk, retroperitoneum, and extremities are also reported. Excision is generally curative.

Angiomyolipoma

The term *angiomyolipoma* is used for a nonmetastasizing renal tumor composed of fat, smooth muscle, and blood vessels. Angiomyolipomas of the liver have also been described. Angiomyolipoma is more common in women than in men and is seen in patients with tuberous sclerosis, caused by germline mutations in *TSC1* or *TSC2*. In addition, sporadic angiomyolipomas sometimes have mutation or loss of TSC1 or TSC2, which function upstream of mammalian target of rapamycin (mTOR) signaling.[110–114] Thus angiomyolipomas may be sensitive to mTOR inhibitors.[110,115–117] Although angiomyolipoma is usually well demarcated from normal kidney, it may extend into the surrounding retroperitoneum. Angiomyolipomas may be solitary or multicentric, and they may produce abdominal pain or hematuria. Wide excision is curative, but tumors that are asymptomatic and not enlarging may be observed.

Liposarcoma

Liposarcoma is primarily a tumor of adults, with a peak incidence between ages 50 and 65 years. It accounts for at least 20% of all soft tissue sarcoma in adults. Liposarcoma may occur anywhere in the body, although the most common sites are thigh and retroperitoneum. Liposarcoma can be divided into three main biological groups: (1) atypical lipomatous tumor/well-differentiated (ALT/WD) liposarcoma and dedifferentiated liposarcoma, (2) myxoid–round cell, and (3) pleomorphic. Each of these groups has distinctive morphology, natural history, and karyotypic and genetic aberrations, which can be of considerable help in diagnosis.

ALT/WD liposarcoma is a locally aggressive, nonmetastasizing, malignant mesenchymal neoplasm composed of proliferating mature adipocytes with significant variation in cell size and nuclear atypia, at least in foci. ALT/WD liposarcoma usually presents as a deep-seated, painless, enlarging mass that over many years can attain a very large size. ALT/WD liposarcomas can be divided into four main morphologic subtypes: adipocytic (lipomalike), sclerosing, inflammatory, and spindle cell. The characteristic cytogenetic abnormality detected in most ALT/WD liposarcomas is supernumerary ring and giant marker chromosomes with amplification of the 12q13–15 region. This region contains the known oncogenes *CDK4*, *MDM2*, and *HMGA2*, which were found amplified in 95%, 87%, and 76% of ALT/WD, respectively.[118] Only 1 of 55 ALT/WD liposarcoma tumors had no 12q amplification. Location is an important predictor of outcome in patients with ALT/WD liposarcoma. Extremity tumors rarely recur and have essentially no mortality. In a series at MSKCC, all cases that recurred did so after 5 years and had a significant component of sclerosing morphology.[119] In contrast, retroperitoneal and mediastinal tumors may recur repeatedly and eventually result in death from uncontrolled local effects; they may also dedifferentiate and metastasize. Dedifferentiation occurs in up to 20% of ALT/WD liposarcomas, with higher risk in deep locations such as the retroperitoneum. In a series of 99 patients with primary retroperitoneal ALT/WD liposarcoma, the 5-year disease-specific survival was 83% and 5-year probability of freedom from local recurrence was 54%.[40]

Dedifferentiated liposarcoma is defined as an ALT/WD liposarcoma, either primary tumor or recurrence, that shows abrupt transition to a region of nonlipogenic sarcoma at least several millimeters in diameter. Radiologic imaging typically shows coexistence of fatty and nonfatty solid components, which in the retroperitoneum may be discontinuous. Macroscopically, dedifferentiated liposarcoma consists of large multinodular yellow masses containing distinct nonlipomatous (dedifferentiated) areas, which are solid and often tan-gray. The dedifferentiated areas may contain areas of necrosis and hemorrhage. Dedifferentiated liposarcoma appears to have a lower risk of distant metastasis than other high-grade pleomorphic sarcomas. Nevertheless, among 65 patients with primary retroperitoneal dedifferentiated liposarcoma, 5-year disease-specific survival was only 20% and 3-year local and distant recurrence-free survival was 17% and 70%, respectively.[40] Dedifferentiated liposarcoma, like ALT/WD, is characterized by ring or giant marker chromosomes and by amplification of the 12q13–15 region. Some other copy number alterations occur at substantially higher frequency in dedifferentiated liposarcoma than in ALT/WD and are thus associated with progression. These include losses centered at 3p14–21, 3q29, 9p22–24, 10p15, 11q23–24, 17q21, and 19q13, and gains at 17p11 and 20q11. Of these progression-associated copy number alterations, the most common, 11q23–24, was noted in 42% of dedifferentiated liposarcoma compared with 4% of ALT/WD. The 11q23–24 loss was associated with genomic complexity and distinct morphology, whereas loss of 19q13 predicted poor prognosis.[118]

Myxoid or round cell liposarcoma accounts for approximately 40% of liposarcomas. The tumor consists of small, evenly dispersed oval or plump cells with little cytoplasm in a myxoid matrix containing a variable number of fat cells. A small number of signet-ring cells and multivacuolated lipoblasts are often present but are not required for diagnosis. The myxoid–round cell subtype usually occurs in the deep soft tissues of the extremities; in >66% of cases it occurs in the thigh musculature.[91] Rarely, myxoid–round cell liposarcoma may arise in the retroperitoneum or in the subcutaneous tissue. More than 90% of myxoid–round cell liposarcomas have a t(12;16)(q13-14;p11) translocation.[120] High histologic grade, defined as ≥5% round cell component, is a predictor of worse outcome in localized myxoid–round cell liposarcoma. Patients with these high-grade lesions have a 5-year survival of 50%.[37,121] In general, pure myxoid lesions (0% to 5% round cell areas) are considered low grade and are associated with a 90% 5-year survival. In contrast to other liposarcoma types, myxoid–round cell liposarcomas tend to metastasize to unusual sites in soft tissue or bone, with multifocal synchronous or metachronous spread to fat pad areas in the retroperitoneum and axilla occurring even in the absence of pulmonary metastasis.[39,121,122] These lesions are also unusual among soft tissue sarcomas in their extraordinarily high response rate to radiotherapy[123] and their substantial sensitivity to ifosfamide[38] and to the DNA minor groove–binding drug trabectedin.[124–126]

Pleomorphic liposarcoma, as the name implies, is a pleomorphic, high-grade, highly malignant sarcoma containing variable numbers of pleomorphic lipoblasts. Mitotic activity is high, and hemorrhage or necrosis is common. Pleomorphic liposarcoma accounts for <5% of all liposarcomas. Most arise in patients older than 50 years and occur in deep soft tissue of the extremities (lower more frequently than upper). Clinically, they metastasize early to lung in >50% of patients, and these patients usually die within a short time. Pleomorphic liposarcomas typically have high chromosome counts, complex structural rearrangements, and multiple regions of significant copy number amplification and deletion.[127] They appear to be somewhat sensitive to gemcitabine-based[128] and ifosfamide-based chemotherapy.[38]

Smooth Muscle Tumors

Leiomyoma

Leiomyomas are benign smooth muscle tumors that are quite common in the uterus and the gastrointestinal (GI) tract. Leiomyoma may also occur deep within the extremities, abdominal cavity, or retroperitoneum. Their histologic appearance is benign, with uniform, spindle-shaped nuclei in cells that appear similar to those of normal smooth muscle. Immunohistochemically, the cells are positive for smooth muscle markers such as smooth muscle actin. Angiomyoma is a histologic subtype of leiomyoma that tends to develop on the extremity at ages 30 to 60. Leiomyomas in women often express estrogen and progesterone receptors, which appear to activate Wnt signaling to promote proliferation of tumor stem cells.[129] These hormone-regulated tumors may regress at

menopause. When they are symptomatic, hormone-regulated tumors can generally be cured by surgical resection; for hormone-receptor–negative tumors, surgery is the treatment of choice.

In three rare clinical scenarios involving symptomatic leiomyomas, management may be difficult. First, cutaneous leiomyoma is a form that arises from the piloerector muscles of the skin. The nodules most often arise on the extensor surfaces of the extremities, and they may follow a dermatomal distribution. Multiple painful tumors may be observed. Although these cutaneous leiomyomas are histologically benign, they frequently recur after surgical excision, and they are often so numerous that excision is not possible. Second, intravenous leiomyomatosis is a rare condition in which nodules of benign smooth muscle tissue grow within the veins of the myometrium and may extend into the uterine and hypogastric veins. Rarely, these tumors extend up the inferior vena cava into the heart. The third management challenge is with diffuse peritoneal leiomyomatosis, which often occurs in association with pregnancy. Compression of adjacent organs may cause obstruction, as in other instances of sarcomatosis.

Leiomyosarcoma

LMSs are malignant lesions that develop from the smooth muscle of blood vessels, visceral structures, or the uterine corpus. Soft tissue LMS usually occurs in middle-aged or older adults and is the predominant sarcoma arising from larger blood vessels. LMSs may arise in any location, but more than half are located in retroperitoneal/intra-abdominal and pelvic sites, most commonly the uterus (see Chapter 73). The tumors are composed of spindle-shaped cells with markers of smooth muscle differentiation such as SMA or desmin. Unlike leiomyoma, however, LMS has many mitotic spindles and may have nuclear and cellular pleomorphism. The LMS genome is characterized by instability and numerous copy number alterations. While most of the copy number alterations are not recurrent, loss of TP53 and PTEN tumors suppressors is common. Recent reports also demonstrate that recurrent mutations in the MED12 oncogene occur in LMS (at least in uterine lesions).[130,131]

LMSs can arise in any vessel and may present insidiously with signs of venous outflow obstruction or pain related to encasement of nearby nerves. LMS of the inferior vena cava can present with the Budd-Chiari syndrome.[132] Treatment of choice is surgical resection. Arterial bypass may be performed. Venous reconstruction, however, is rarely successful, as vein grafts rarely remain patent for prolonged periods. Moreover, patients generally develop collateral veins during the months after resection. Therefore, venous reconstruction can be deferred even in the context of inferior vena cava resection.[132] Tumor grade and size predict risk of disease-related death; retroperitoneal lesions are generally large and high grade, resulting in recurrence risks of >50%.[133] Small LMS-like lesions in the dermis carry no discernable risk of metastasis, and the old term of "cutaneous LMS" has generally been replaced by "atypical intradermal smooth muscle neoplasms."[134]

Skeletal Muscle Tumors

Rhabdomyoma

Nonmalignant tumors of striated muscle—rhabdomyomas—are rare but are clinically benign. They are subdivided into adult, fetal, and genital type lesions; cardiac rhabdomyomas are associated with the tuberous sclerosis syndrome. Adult and fetal rhabdomyomas are most commonly identified in the head and neck. Rhabdomyoma can be distinguished from rhabdomyosarcoma by its lack of nuclear atypia. Pathogenesis appears to be related to activation of the hedgehog pathway; fetal rhabdomyoma may occur in individuals with a germline mutation in the hedgehog inhibitor PTCH1, which is associated with basal cell nevus syndrome. Rhabdomyomas, if symptomatic, are managed with surgical resection.

Rhabdomyosarcomas

Rhabdomyosarcomas (malignant tumors showing skeletal differentiation) are aggressive malignancies that are the most common soft tissue sarcomas of infants and children. Treatment of rhabdomyosarcoma nearly always requires multimodal therapy, typically employing surgery, radiation, and chemotherapy based on a vincristine-dactinomycin-cyclophosphamide backbone.[135,136] The recognized types are embryonal, alveolar, and pleomorphic.

Embryonal Rhabdomyosarcoma. Embryonal rhabdomyosarcoma is a small-cell tumor showing features of embryonic skeletal muscle. It usually arises in the orbit or genitourinary tract in children, though rare cases arise in adolescents and adults. The botryoid type, which frequently originates in mucosa-lined visceral organs such as the vagina and the urinary bladder, generally grows as a polypoid tumor. Genomic analysis demonstrates that these tumors have various copy number alterations that may directly or indirectly affect activity of oncogenes and tumor suppressors such as RB1, p53, RAS, hedgehog, FGFR4, Akt, ALK, Notch, and β-catenin.[137-140] These findings have not yet led to clinically useful targeted therapies, but chemotherapy and radiation are very effective for pediatric embryonal rhabdomyosarcomas, even metastatic cases. Embryonal rhabdomyosarcomas in adults usually regress in response to pediatric chemotherapy regimens, but survival is worse for adults than for children.[141] Factors strongly associated with poor prognosis in adults are metastatic disease at presentation and poor response to chemotherapy.[142]

Alveolar Rhabdomyosarcoma. Unlike the embryonal type, alveolar rhabdomyosarcoma is observed more commonly in adolescents and adults than in younger children. For younger children, alveolar rhabdomyosarcoma appears to have a worse prognosis than embryonal rhabdomyosarcoma. Histologically, the lesion is composed of ill-defined aggregates of poorly differentiated round or oval cells that frequently show central loss of cellular cohesion and formation of irregular "alveolar" spaces. They cytologically resemble lymphoma cells and show partial skeletal differentiation. In most cases, specific translocations create a PAX3-FOXO1 fusion gene (in the majority of patients) or a PAX7-FOXO1 fusion (in a smaller subset); rarely fusion-negative lesions are diagnosed.[143,144] These fusion genes have prognostic significance (see Chapter 89), so fusion gene status, irrespective of histology, is a critical factor in risk stratification.[145,146] Some tumors have amplification of the PAX7-FOXO1 fusion, which is associated with improved outcome though the underlying molecular mechanisms have not been delineated.[147] As in embryonal rhabdomyosarcoma, gene amplifications result in activation of a range of oncogenes. These include FGFR4, ALK, CDK4, and MYCN.[148]

Pleomorphic Rhabdomyosarcoma. Pleomorphic rhabdomyosarcoma is the most common form of rhabdomyosarcoma in adults and can be associated with prior radiation. Histologically, the tumors have pleomorphic round cells and spindle cells with atypical nuclei and markers of skeletal muscle differentiation. They are characterized by complex copy number alterations. The prognosis for these pleomorphic tumors is poor, and in one series, 28 of 38 patients (74%) died of the disease.[149] Treatment is surgical, but, because of the poor prognosis, eligible patients are given adjuvant radiation and chemotherapy. These tumors are less sensitive to systemic therapies than are embryonal or alveolar rhabdomyosarcomas, but some respond to anthracyclines and ifosfamide; in addition, anecdotes indicate some sensitivity to gemcitabine-based chemotherapy.[128]

Vascular Tumors

Hemangioma

Hemangiomas are among the most common soft tissue tumors. Many are present at birth and regress spontaneously; others are noted incidentally on imaging studies. They tend to be asymptomatic; however, some grow rapidly, impinge on vital structures, or cause consumptive thrombocytopenias. Imaging studies generally demonstrate a peripherally enhancing mass with lipomatous regions and spiculated calcium deposits. Management by observation is generally safe. For symptomatic disease, surgical resection is generally curative; sclerotherapy has recently been studied. Diffuse hemangiomatosis in the bone or lungs may be treated effectively with systemic interferon.

Epithelioid Hemangioendothelioma

Epithelioid hemangioendothelioma is a low-grade vascular lesion without structured vessels, but with tumor cells arranged in nests and cords. Epithelioid hemangioendotheliomas occur in the bone and associated soft tissues. In malignant disease, multifocal lesions are often observed, generally within the same limb. Metastases may occur in lung, lymph nodes, and bone.[150] A fusion between the N-terminus of WWTR1 and the C-terminus of CAMTA1 occurs almost uniformly in these lesions, but not other vascular tumors.[151,152] Surgical resection is the treatment of choice; however, multifocal disease often recurs. Nevertheless, <20% of patients die of disease. A phase 2 trial has suggested that treatment with bevacizumab may slow progression or induce partial response in the majority of patients.[153]

Angiosarcoma

Angiosarcoma is a malignant tumor composed of malignant cells that morphologically resemble endothelium to various extents. Angiosarcoma is currently considered to include those tumors previously termed lymphangiosarcoma because of their similarities in histology and outcomes.[36] Most angiosarcomas develop in the skin or superficial soft tissue; <25% are in deep soft tissue.[154] The disease occurs most commonly in the context of lymphedema (Stewart Treves syndrome) or after prior radiation (particularly radiation for breast cancer).[16] Lymphedema-associated angiosarcoma presents difficulties for surgical planning because poor wound healing may compromise the ability to perform limb-sparing procedures. Another challenge is that lymphedema-associated angiosarcoma has high rates of both local and distal recurrence.[155] Multicentric angiosarcomas on the scalp and face of elderly men typically show unrelenting progression, which can cause severe ulceration and infection and eventually metastasis. Features reported to be associated with poor outcome include patient age, tumor depth, and size,[154,156,157] but in general death from disease is common, with the median time to disease-specific death as short as 3 years in some patient subsets. Surgical resection is rarely curative; however, angiosarcomas are relatively sensitive, at least for brief periods of time, to anthracycline-based chemotherapy and taxanes.[158,159] The discovery of KDR mutations and amplification of MYC and FLT4 has led to the investigation of antiangiogenic therapies in this disease.[160,161]

Perivascular Tumors

Glomus Tumor

Glomus tumors are rare soft tissue lesions that are almost always benign.[162] The tumors appear to develop from smooth muscle cells associated with the glomus body, a modified arteriovenous anastomosis in the skin involved in thermal regulation. Unlike most soft tissue tumors, glomus tumors can cause considerable pain. They are most commonly found in the distal extremities (subungual region, hand, wrist, and foot) of young adults, though extradigital lesions are reported.[163] The appropriate treatment is complete local excision. Most patients have sporadic, solitary tumors, for which the underlying genomic alterations are unclear. However, about 10% of patients have multiple lesions, many of them familial. Some of these patients have heterozygous germline mutations in the *GLMN* or *NF1* genes.[164,165]

Neural Tumors

Neurofibroma

Solitary neurofibromas are small, slow-growing cutaneous or subcutaneous nodules that usually arise during the third decade of life. Neurofibromas may occur in unidentifiable cutaneous nerves or in larger trunks. Within an identifiable larger nerve, they expand into a fusiform mass and often extend into soft tissue; they are well defined and they may be nodular. Histologically, they show spindle-shaped cells in a myxoid stroma that contains collagen fibers. Multiple neurofibromas may be associated with NF1 (von Recklinghausen disease), a common genetic disorder caused by an autosomal dominant mutation at the 17q11.2 locus and affecting 1 in 3,000 live births. Clinical features of NF1 include café au lait spots, pigmented hamartomas of the iris, and neurofibromas of several types. Cutaneous neurofibromas arise in the skin in all patients with NF1, with sizes varying from millimeters to centimeters, and some may be painful. Plexiform neurofibromas are larger lesions that affect the large segments of a nerve, thickening and distorting the nerve with greater dysesthetic pain. The difficult distinction is neurofibroma versus MPNST, which may develop in patients with NF1. MPNST is usually distinguished based on rapid growth and increasing symptoms, and is confirmed by biopsy.

Benign Schwannoma

Benign schwannoma, also called neurilemmoma, occurs most commonly in people between the age of 20 and 50 years. Common sites include the head and neck, the flexor surfaces of the extremities, and the paravertebral area of the retroperitoneum. The lesion grows slowly, and if superficial is usually small at the time of diagnosis, but it can reach large size in the retroperitoneum without symptoms. The tumor is usually encapsulated and consists of two components: an ordered cellular region (Antoni A area) and a loose, myxoid component (Antoni B area). Fortunately, diagnosis can often be made by percutaneous core or needle biopsy in patients with lesions in the retroperitoneum, where morbidity of operation is to be avoided. The cellular variant is the lesion most often seen late in life as a painless vertebral mass.[166] Complete resection is curative in most patients.

Granular Cell Tumor

Granular cell tumor is a rare tumor, probably of neural origin. It typically presents in adults as a small, poorly circumscribed subcutaneous mass, commonly seen in the oral cavity, and it is only rarely malignant. Granular cell tumors have been seen in all parts of the body, including the pancreas and bile duct. They can occur in multiple sites. Metastases have been reported in approximately 2% of cases, although most reports are single cases.

Malignant Peripheral Nerve Sheath Tumor

MPNSTs are highly aggressive soft tissue sarcomas that rarely occur sporadically in the general population. They may, however, occur with a lifetime incidence of 8% to 13% in patients with NF1, an autosomal dominant tumor predisposition syndrome caused by germline mutations in the *NF1* gene.[11] Most MPNSTs are associated with major nerves of the body wall and extremities and typically affect adults in the third to fifth decades of life. The lower extremity and the retroperitoneum are the most common sites, but MPNSTs can arise anywhere in the body. These tumors originate from the nerve sheath rather than from the nerve itself. There is also an MPNST with rhabdomyosarcomatous elements, termed a triton tumor, suggesting that the Schwann cell may be the source of a variety of heterologous elements in nerve sheath tumors.[167]

Tumor cells are usually elongated, with frequent mitoses, and are arranged in a hypocellular myxoid stroma; pronounced atypia and epithelioid features are also characteristic. The majority of MPNSTs are high grade and characteristically stain for the S-100 protein. Weak S-100 staining in an MPNST is associated with undifferentiated tumors and a five-fold higher risk of distant metastasis.[168] Tumor size and p53 expression remain the most important independent predictors of disease-specific survival.[168,169] Two recent studies have suggested that patients with NF1-associated MPNST have a worse outcome compared to patients with sporadic MPNST,[170,171] and in one study this outcome difference was independent of tumor size.[171]

Complete surgical resection with or without adjuvant radiotherapy remains the most important treatment for those patients with primary disease. The role of neoadjuvant chemotherapy for patients with large primary and locally recurrent MPNSTs remains controversial. Overall response rates to chemotherapy are 21%, with improved outcomes noted when ifosfamide is added to adriamycin regimens.[172] With an increasing understanding of the signaling pathways activated in MPNSTs, sorafenib, which targets the mitogen-activated protein kinase pathway, has been tested in single cases and in a histology-specific clinical trial.[173,174] Patients with NF1 may be difficult to evaluate, independent of the features of the tumor itself. Staging and follow-up assessments are confounded by the detection of other nodules and masses that, although generally representing benign neurofibromas, need to be distinguished from recurrent local or metastatic disease or a second neurogenic sarcoma.

Extraskeletal Chondro-Osseous Tumors

Extraskeletal Osteosarcoma

Extraskeletal osteosarcomas are rare, high-grade sarcomas defined by production of malignant osteoid and bone. By definition, they are not attached to the skeleton. Unlike typical osteogenic sarcoma of bone, these tumors rarely occur before age 20, and most patients are older than 50 years. Most extraskeletal osteosarcomas arise in the extremities, although they have been reported in other sites, including breast, retroperitoneum, urinary bladder, and other visceral organs. Similar to those osteosarcomas arising from bone, extraskeletal osteosarcomas are highly heterogeneous on the microscopic level. Giant cells are a common feature, but no recurrent genomic events have been characterized. Surgical resection is generally used as single-modality treatment in this disease. Unlike osteogenic sarcoma arising from bone, extraskeletal osteosarcoma is not generally treated with adjuvant chemotherapy, although at least one series indicates a better outcome for patients treated with agents usually employed for classic osteogenic sarcomas.[175]

Tumors of Uncertain Differentiation

For most tumors in this category, there is no clear consensus as to the line of differentiation. However, for some tumors, such as synovial sarcoma and clear cell sarcoma, a line of differentiation can be clearly delineated, but no cellular counterpart in normal mesenchymal tissues can be defined.

Myxoma

Intramuscular myxoma is a rare tumor that occurs in adults, usually in the large muscles of the extremities. Myxomas consist of spindle cells without nuclear atypia. The stroma is composed of abundant myxoid tissue. The tumors are not highly vascular and do not enhance on MRI. Increased cellularity has been noted in a subset of lesions, termed "cellular myxomas."[176] Because of the high myxoid component and subset of cellular lesions, myxomas can appear similar to myxofibrosarcomas on biopsy. An aid to diagnosis is mutations in the *GNAS1* gene, which are common in spontaneous myxoma as compared to myxofibrosarcoma.[177,178]

Multiple intramuscular myxomas occur in association with fibrous dysplasia (Mazabraud syndrome).

Angiomyxoma

Aggressive angiomyxoma is a soft tissue tumor generally identified in the pelvis or perineum of middle aged and older women. The tumors have a highly myxoid stroma with significant vasculature and small spindle or stellate cells without nuclear atypia. Aggressive angiomyxomas typically can slowly grow to large size and generally do not cause obstructive symptoms. Local recurrence is common after surgical resection and can result in considerable morbidity, given the location of these tumors, but distant metastases do not occur. Tumors express high levels of estrogen and progesterone receptors, and advanced disease may be managed with gonadotropin-releasing hormone agonists such as leuprolide. The tumor-initiating cell for angiomyxoma has not been characterized, but rearrangement of *HMGA2* has been observed and appears to be associated with high expression of this oncogene.[179]

Neoplasms with Perivascular Epithelioid Cell Differentiation (PEComas)

The family of tumors known as PEComas are associated with neoplastic cells within the walls of blood vessels in the tumors. PEComas include clear cell "sugar" tumors of the lung, angiomyolipomas, and lymphangioleiomyomatosis (LAM). LAM is characterized by progressive interstitial infiltration of lungs by smooth muscle cells, resulting in cystic changes. It is a rare, progressive cystic lung disease predominantly affecting younger women of reproductive age. In end stages, LAM has been treated by lung transplantation.[180] Angiomyolipomas are benign lesions that may grow quite large, but can safely be observed in most clinical scenarios (see "Adipocytic Tumors"). While angiomyolipomas or LAM do not metastasize, malignant forms of PEComa occur. PEComas such as angiomyolipomas or LAM are found in patients with tuberous sclerosis, and thus it is not surprising that *TSC2* or *TSC1* mutations or deletions are also found in sporadic lesions.[110,113,181,182] Surgical resection may be sufficient to manage isolated tumors, but for metastatic disease or unresectable lesions, inhibitors of mTOR can be an effective treatment.[115,183–185]

Synovial Sarcoma

Synovial sarcoma is a spindle cell tumor with varying extents of epithelial differentiation, including gland formation, and is genetically distinct based on specific chromosomal translocations. Synovial sarcomas may be diagnosed at any age but the majority occur in young adults, between 15 and 35 years of age, and more commonly in males.[186] Over 80% arise in deep soft tissue of the extremities, with about 50% in the lower limbs and most of the remainder in the upper limbs. Synovial sarcoma generally does not originate from synovial tissue, and it may be encountered in regions without apparent relationship to synovial structures, including the head and neck (<10%), thoracic and abdominal wall (<10%), or intrathoracic sites. Synovial sarcoma usually presents as a slow-growing mass with or without pain. Histologically, it may be monophasic or biphasic (i.e., composed of two morphologically distinct types of cells). Biphasic tumors have a characteristic pattern of epithelial cells surrounded by a spindle cell or fibrous component. Monophasic synovial sarcomas may be either fibrous or epithelial type, although the epithelial type is extremely rare. Calcification, with or without ossification, is seen in up to 10% of tumors, and synovial sarcoma may be confused with other calcifying tumors (e.g., thyroid neoplasms, which may exhibit calcification). The spindle cells stain positive for keratin, epithelial membrane antigen, and vimentin. S-100 staining may give positive results.

Nearly all synovial sarcomas contain a chromosomal translocation, t(X;18)(p11.2;q11.2).[187] With the observation that 100% of biphasic and 96% of monophasic synovial sarcomas possess this translocation, it has become the gold standard in diagnosing synovial sarcoma.[188] The translocation fuses the *SS18* (*SYT*) gene with either *SSX1*, *SSX2*, or *SSX4*; the specific *SSX* gene involved may have prognostic significance.[189,190] A recent study has suggested that metastasis in both pediatric and adult synovial sarcoma is strongly associated with genome complexity and with a gene expression signature related to mitotic control.[191]

Extraskeletal Myxoid Chondrosarcoma

Extraskeletal myxoid chondrosarcoma (EMC) is a malignant tumor characterized by a multinodular growth pattern and by chondroblastlike cells arranged in cords, clusters, or delicate networks within an abundant myxoid matrix. It occurs most commonly in the deep soft tissues of the proximal extremities and limb girdles in patients older than 35 years; two-thirds of patients are male. In contrast to the more common skeletal chondrosarcoma of bone, EMC seldom contains mature cartilage, and there is no convincing evidence of cartilaginous differentiation. Ultrastructurally, EMC is characterized by densely packed intracisternal microtubules and prominent mitochondria, whereas these are not apparent in skeletal chondrosarcoma. In addition, a nonrandom reciprocal translocation t(9;22), fusing the *EWSR1* and *NR4A3* genes, is present in about 50% of EMCs[192–194] and is not seen in skeletal chondrosarcoma, which supports the idea that the two diseases have different molecular lineages. A second subgroup of EMC is characterized by a t(9;17) translocation joining *TAF15* and *NR4A3*.[195] EMCs usually grow slowly and long survival is typical, even in patients with metastases, which usually occur in the lung.[196] Nevertheless, with prolonged follow-up, late local recurrence and metastasis are common. EMC is generally resistant to standard chemotherapy,[197] but sunitinib has produced significant tumor regressions in two patients with advanced EMC.[198]

Alveolar Soft Part Sarcoma

Alveolar soft part sarcoma (ASPS) is a rare tumor comprising <1% of soft tissue sarcomas. The tumors are poorly circumscribed lesions that are composed of large epithelioid cells with abundant eosinophilic cytoplasm. The cells are generally arranged in a pseudoalveolar pattern with a highly vascular surrounding stroma. ASPS harbors a t(17-X)(p11.2;q25) translocation, resulting in the highly specific ASPSCR1-TFE3 fusion protein.[199] Like most translocation-associated sarcomas, ASPS is most commonly diagnosed in young adults. Females outnumber males, especially among patients younger than age 20.[200,201]

ASPS often presents in the lower extremities, most commonly the thigh,[201,202] as a painless mass. The tumor grows slowly, and patients may remain asymptomatic over years, even with metastatic disease.[203] Local recurrence after surgery is rare, but ultimate prognosis is poor because ASPS characteristically metastasizes early and is essentially impervious to standard chemotherapy agents. In a large study from MSKCC, the survival rate of patients without metastases at diagnosis was 60% at 5 years, 38% at 10 years, and 15% at 20 years.[201] The ASPSCR1-TFE1 fusion protein activates transcription of the *MET* oncogene, which drives growth of ASPS cells.[204] Ongoing trials are examining the efficacy of MET inhibitors such as crizotinib in this tumor.[205] The tumors also overexpress angiogenic receptor tyrosine kinases, and indeed targeted inhibitors such as sunitinib and bevacizumab have some efficacy for ASPS.[206–208]

Epithelioid Sarcoma

Epithelioid sarcoma, characterized by epithelioid and less commonly spindle-shaped cells, generally arises in the extremities. It occurs in two forms: distal-type (conventional) epithelioid sarcoma, occurring most commonly on the volar aspects of the hands and feet, and proximal-type, occurring most commonly on the perineum, groin, thigh, buttock, or less commonly the axilla. The proximal-type variant consists of large epithelioid carcinoma-like cells with pronounced cytologic atypia and prominent nucleoli frequently exhibiting rhabdoid features.[209] It often grows in a multinodular pattern. Both proximal- and distal-type epithelioid sarcomas often have central regions of necrosis when examined histologically. Tumors located in deep tissue may spread along fascia planes, and thus epithelioid sarcoma requires extensive wide excision for complete tumor removal. Epithelioid sarcoma is also one of the few sarcomas in which lymph node metastases are fairly common, occurring in 20% of patients. Gross nodal disease should be biopsied, and if disease is present but the patient has no apparent distant metastases, a complete lymph node dissection should be considered. The role of sentinel node biopsy is highly debatable, with no proven effect on outcome.

Prognosis for patients with epithelioid sarcoma is generally poor. In a recent series that included 54 patients with localized disease,[210] the 5-year local recurrence–free survival was 54%, distant recurrence–free survival 53%, and overall survival 62%. Independent predictors of worse survival were higher grade and deep location. Epithelioid sarcoma is moderately sensitive to chemotherapy, although responses are typically short lived. Compared with the distal variant, the proximal variant is associated with a more aggressive clinical course, resistance to radiation and chemotherapy, and worse disease-specific survival.[209,211–214] Genetic analysis of epithelioid sarcoma is beginning to define molecular mechanisms for pathogenesis. Aberrations that have been seen include loss of the *SMARCB1* tumor suppressor and upregulation of the epidermal growth factor receptor and mTOR pathways. Combined inhibition of these two pathways inhibited epithelioid sarcoma cell growth in vitro and in a xenograft model.[215,216]

Clear Cell Sarcoma (Melanoma of Soft Parts)

Clear cell sarcoma, initially described by Enzinger,[217] is a sarcoma with melanocytic differentiation, typically involving the tendons and aponeuroses of young adults. The lesions are composed of epithelioid-type cells clustered in nests, each surrounded by collagenous bands. Clear cell sarcoma presents as a slowly growing soft tissue mass. Up to 50% of patients have pain or tenderness. Because its cells contains melanin and it tends to metastasize to regional nodes, clear cell sarcoma is considered to behave more like a melanoma than a soft tissue sarcoma. Genomic profiling and cluster analysis has also grouped these lesions more with melanoma than with sarcomas.[218] However, unlike melanoma, clear cell sarcoma typically has a chromosomal translocation. In >75% of cases, this is t(12;22), fusing the *EWSR1* and *ATF1* genes.[219] The fusion product activates the kinase MET, giving hope that MET inhibitors will have activity against this group of tumors.[220]

The treatment of choice is surgical resection. Gross disease in the lymph node basin is removed in tandem with wide resection of the primary tumor. Given the propensity of this subtype to nodal metastasis, sentinel node biopsy can be considered, though its clinical utility is debated.[221] Size is a prognostic factor in outcome, and the majority of tumors are <5 cm at diagnosis. Metastasis is common, and 5-year survival approaches 50%. Chemotherapy has limited benefit, with platinum-containing regimens offering the most potential benefit, though recent reports suggest that antiangiogenic treatment (e.g., sorafenib and sunitinib) may have activity.[222,223]

Desmoplastic Small Round Cell Tumor

Desmoplastic small round cell tumor is composed of monotonous blue cells as stained on hematoxylin and eosin stain. The cells have little cytoplasm and may be arranged in nests or in an infiltrative pattern within a prominent desmoplastic stroma.[224] The tumors are characterized by a specific t(11;22) translocation, fusing the *EWSRI* and *WT1* genes.[225,226] The disease usually arises in children and young adults, in whom abdominal sarcomatosis is a common presentation. For this reason, prognosis is generally poor and management can be difficult. In a review of 40 histologically proven cases, only 30% of patients were alive at 3 years from diagnosis.[227] Surgical resection is possible for isolated tumors, but more commonly, patients are managed with front-line chemotherapy

followed by debulking. Factors associated with improved overall survival are gross total resection and good responses to chemotherapy agents, such as that used for Ewing sarcoma.[227,228]

Undifferentiated/Unclassified Tumors

High-Grade Undifferentiated Pleomorphic Sarcoma/Pleomorphic Malignant Fibrous Histiocytoma

MFH was originally defined as a malignant pleomorphic spindle cell tumor with fibroblastic and histiocytic differentiation. However, pathologists now agree that this morphology may be shared by a wide range of malignancies.[98] Careful immunohistochemical and histopathologic analysis showed that many sarcomas previously classified as pleomorphic MFH had a specific line of differentiation and could be reclassified as myxofibrosarcoma (30%), myogenic sarcoma (30%), myofibroblastic sarcoma (11%), liposarcoma (4%), soft tissue osteosarcoma (3%), or malignant peripheral nerve sheath tumor (2%), whereas only 16% had no specific line of differentiation.[41] Thus, the term UPS is now reserved for pleomorphic sarcomas that by current technology show no definable line of differentiation.[41,92,98] UPS characteristically is a tumor of later adult life with peak incidence at ages 60 to 70. UPS usually presents as a painless, deep-seated mass; the most common site is the lower extremity, followed by the upper extremity. A subset of UPSs arise at the site of prior radiotherapy[24] and very rare cases arise at the site of chronic ulceration. About 5% of patients present with metastasis, typically to lung. Clinical and pathologic studies have shown a remarkable degree of heterogeneity of morphologic and biological features, prognosis, and treatment response. UPS typically has an aggressive clinical course, with many patients developing metastatic disease within 3 years of diagnosis. The 5-year disease-specific survival was 65% for patients presenting to MSKCC with primary UPS of the extremity and trunk.

Histologic Grading

After establishing the diagnosis of sarcoma, the most critical piece of information the pathologist can provide to the clinician is histologic grade. Grading, based on morphologic features only, evaluates the degree of malignancy and predicts outcomes, mainly the probability of distant relapse. The pathologic features that define grade include mitotic index, necrosis, cellularity, pleomorphism, and histologic type and subtype or differentiation; the two most important factors seem to be the mitotic index and the extent of necrosis.[91,229] Unfortunately, the criteria for grading are neither specific nor standardized, and there is no general consensus on the morphologic criteria to use. Several grading systems are used: a four-grade system (Broders),[230] three-grade systems such as the National Cancer Institute (NCI) grading system[231] and that of the Sarcoma Group of the French Fédération Nationale des Centres de Lutte Contre le Cancer (FNCLCC),[232] and a two-grade system as is used at MSKCC.[233] All of these grading systems have proven to correlate with overall survival and disease-free survival.

In general, the two most widely used grading systems are the NCI system[231] and the FNCLCC system.[234] Both are three-tier systems (high/intermediate/low). A comparative study showed that the prediction of distant metastasis and tumor mortality was slightly better with the FNCLCC system than with the NCI system.[232] However, two studies have evaluated the interobserver reproducibility of the FNCLCC system and showed only 60% to 75% agreement on tumor grade and 61% to 75% agreement on histologic type.[235,236] This high level of disagreement (25% to 40%) even among expert sarcoma pathologists emphasizes the importance of histologic peer review and the need for more objective systems for sarcoma grading and classification.[235–237] In fact, neither the FNCLCC nor NCI system has been formally endorsed by either the World Health Organization[91] or the Association of Directors of Anatomic and Surgical Pathology.[238]

In the MSKCC system, grade is classified as high or low based on the degree of mitotic activity, necrosis, cellularity, and tumor differentiation.[233] Grade in this system has excellent correlation with clinical outcome in many histologic types and has proven to be one of the most important independent predictors of disease-specific survival.[239] In addition, this system avoids the management dilemma of an "intermediate" grade, which in most institutions would be lumped with and treated as high-grade sarcoma, potentially resulting in overtreatment. The authors recognize that in certain situations (approximately 5% to 10% of cases), the distinction between low- and high-grade tumors can be quite difficult, and therefore an intermediate grade would seem the most suitable. These difficult cases can be graded most appropriately by using systematic sampling and thorough examination.

Although there is widespread use of some form of grading system in the diagnosis and management of sarcomas, there is also agreement that no current grading system performs well for every type of sarcoma. For multiple reasons, certain histologic types of sarcoma do not lend themselves well to grading. An example is myxoid/round cell liposarcoma, where round cell histology in just >5% of tumor area is sufficient to predict high-grade behavior, with a >50% risk of distant metastasis.[121] In addition, unequivocal characterization of grade is difficult in large lesions, especially in tumors that can reach 2 or 3 kg.

The lack of standardization on grading has obvious clinical implications. In adjuvant chemotherapy trials, high grade is defined differently at different centers, which makes it hazardous to compare results between trials or to combine results of multiple trials. For example, tumors of 240 patients who participated in the Scandinavian Sarcoma Group adjuvant trial for high-grade extremity sarcoma were reviewed by a panel of reference pathologists. Eligibility was limited to patients with grade 3 or 4 sarcomas in a four-grade system. On review, 5% of the patients were considered ineligible because their tumors were low grade.[235] In addition, the original pathologists and the reference pathologists had considerable discordance with regard to whether a lesion was grade 3 or 4. Although the adjuvant regimen did not affect survival, a difference in survival was noted between patients with tumors of these two grades as assigned by the reference pathologists.

Grading needs to be adapted to the modern management of patients with sarcoma, who often undergo a limited core biopsy rather than an open incisional biopsy. Grading on such limited material needs to be complemented with imaging and molecular data. Extent of necrosis may best be evaluated by imaging studies because they enable macroscopic examination of the entire tumor. Both MRI and magnetic resonance spectroscopy have been used to assess necrosis, chemotherapy response, and grade in sarcoma. Mitotic index is difficult to determine on limited core biopsy material, and MIB-1 (Ki-67) scores of proliferation may be more reproducible[240] and have better predictive value than grading using mitotic index.[241] Other molecular characteristics, such as mutation or nuclear overexpression of TP53 and high Ki-67 proliferation index, are associated with high grade and poor survival.[242] A gene expression signature of 67 genes related to mitosis and chromosome management, the Complexity Index in Sarcomas was an independent predictor of metastasis outcome even adjusting for histologic subtype and FNCLCC grade and is superior to the FNCLCC grading system in determining metastatic outcome for sarcoma patients.[243,244]

DIAGNOSIS AND STAGING

Clinical Features

The presence of soft tissue sarcoma almost invariably is suggested by the development of a mass. This mass is usually large, is often

painless, and may be associated by the patient with an episode of injury. Approximately one-third present with a size <5 cm, one-third with a size 5 to 10 cm, and one-third with a size >10 cm. The focus of the clinical evaluation is to determine the likelihood of a benign or malignant soft tissue tumor, the involvement of muscular or neurovascular structures, and the ease with which biopsy or subsequent excision can be performed. Size becomes an important feature (see "Prognostic Factors"), and definitive diagnosis depends on biopsy results and histologic confirmation.

Differential Diagnosis

The differential diagnosis of a soft tissue mass includes, in addition to sarcoma, a variety of benign lesions, as well as primary or metastatic carcinoma, melanoma, and lymphoma. The major concern when confronted with a soft tissue mass is determining whether the lesion is benign or malignant. In most patients with small lesions, or even on occasion large lesions, the important distinction is lipoma, the most common soft tissue tumor, versus other tumors. Most benign lesions are located in superficial (dermal or subcutaneous) soft tissue. This differentiation may be simple, but it becomes more difficult as the more aggressive and underappreciated inherently benign lesions are considered. Particularly difficult is myositis ossificans. The patient often has a history of trauma and often presents with a large, firm-to-hard lesion that, on plain film, may have intrinsic calcification. However, these signs do not preclude a malignant lesion. With myositis ossificans, Tru-Cut (CareFusion Corporation, San Diego, CA) needle biopsy or open biopsy is often accompanied by aggressive hemorrhage, which suggests a vascular neoplasm. In most cases, diagnosis can be made fairly accurately by either plain film or MRI scan. Certainly, myositis ossificans should be suspected when there is a significant history of trauma and the lesion is particularly hard and has inherent calcification.

For diagnosis to be accurate, the biopsy must be adequate and representative of the tumor, and the tissue must be well fixed and well stained. Antibodies for immunohistochemical staining are available commercially, and this technique is readily applicable to paraffin-embedded tissues. The most useful immunohistochemical markers are the intermediate filaments (e.g., vimentin, keratin, desmin), leukocyte common antigen, and S-100. In addition, the pathologist should be prepared to process tissue from selected cases for electron microscopy, cytogenetic studies, or molecular analysis. This requires that the clinician and pathologist communicate before the biopsy is performed to ensure that the necessary steps are taken in handling the tissue.

Cytogenetic analyses reveal specific clonal chromosomal aberrations, most commonly reciprocal translocations, in the majority of sarcomas.[225,245–248] Among these are 11 different translocations involving the *EWSR1* gene or its family members (*FUS*, *TAF15*) found in five different sarcomas. In a significant subset of sarcomas, translocations can be diagnostically and occasionally prognostically useful. Because conventional cytogenetic analysis is labor intensive and requires short-term culture of the sarcoma cells, molecular genetic techniques (e.g., reverse-transcriptase polymerase chain reaction and fluorescence in situ hybridization [FISH]) may be useful diagnostic adjuncts, particularly for diagnosing and distinguishing among the small cell sarcomas. Oligonucleotide and complementary DNA arrays may eventually add to the sophistication of determining the diagnosis and prognosis of such tumors.[248] FISH testing for specific chromosomal abnormalities is now feasible for routine diagnostic use. FISH is also useful to identify supernumerary ring chromosomes, seen in mesenchymal neoplasms of low or borderline malignancy, such as dermatofibrosarcoma protuberans. Table 89.1 in Chapter 89 ("Molecular Biology of Sarcomas") describes some of the genetic changes identified in soft tissue sarcomas.

As might be expected, there can be considerable disagreement among pathologists on the specific histologic diagnosis in individual cases. When a panel of expert pathologists reviewed pathologic material from 424 patients who entered into Eastern Cooperative Oncology Group sarcoma trials, 10% of cases were rejected as not being sarcoma, and 16% were the subject of disagreement on the histologic subtype.[249] In the Scandinavian Sarcoma Group experience, the specific histologic diagnosis was disputed in 20% of cases.[235] Of 1,463 histologic specimens obtained from patients with connective tissue tumors in France and Italy, grade and histologic subtype were confirmed by an expert pathologist in only 56% of cases. The discordance for 35% of patients was a different characterization of histologic subtype or grade, and in 8% was complete discordance (recharacterized as benign, different histology, or not a sarcoma).[250] With increasing familiarity with the immunohistochemical and genetic studies needed to diagnose soft tissue sarcoma, the rate of this discordance may be decreasing.

Imaging

Imaging studies for soft tissue sarcoma vary, depending to some extent on the site. They involve evaluation of both the primary lesion and the potential site of metastasis. Evaluation of the primary lesion in the extremity and head and neck predominantly is by either CT or MRI. Although MRI provides some increased definition, a Radiology Diagnostic Oncology Group study comparing these modalities showed no benefit of MRI over CT.[251] For the primary sarcoma of intra-abdominal, chest, or retroperitoneal locations, a spiral CT scan is preferable to MRI because air–tissue interface and motion artifacts often degrade MRI quality. In addition, spiral CT allows both the primary and potential for metastasis to be assessed in a single study. What is clear in this era of cost containment is that imaging with multiple modalities, all focusing on the same entity, is not required.

Positron Emission Tomography

Positron emission tomography (PET) has a number of potential uses in sarcoma management, although it has yet to gain universal acceptance. The standard uptake value in ^{18}F-fluorodeoxyglucose (FDG) PET has been associated with histopathologic grade, cellularity, mitotic activity, MIB-1 labeling index, and TP53 over-expression, but it has never been proven to provide independent prognostic information and frequently fails to distinguish benign tumors from low-grade sarcomas.[252–254]

PET may also become useful for determining early responses to systemic therapy for soft tissue sarcoma. Specifically for primary extremity sarcomas, response by FDG-PET was superior to radiologic tumor size changes as a predictor of outcome after treatment with neoadjuvant chemotherapy.[255–258] Similar results have been found for pediatric sarcomas. FDG-PET has been used for the early prediction of chemosensitivity in patients with soft tissue sarcomas who received neoadjuvant chemotherapy; the accuracy was 83% and positive predictive value for responders was 92%.[259] Further studies are needed to determine if FDG-PET is sufficiently specific and accurate in determining chemotherapy response to alter clinical decisions on continuing, discontinuing, or modifying the treatment.

The current role of PET seems to be primarily in the identification of unsuspected sites of metastasis in patients with recurrent high-grade tumors, given the high rate of metastatic disease in this setting.

Imaging Sites of Metastasis

As important as imaging studies of the primary lesion is evaluation of possible sites of metastasis. For patients with extremity lesions, most metastases (70%) go to the lung.[260] For patients with retroperitoneal or visceral lesions, a much more common site for

metastases is the liver, with lung only a secondary site. Nevertheless, no site is immune from soft tissue sarcoma metastasis, and other patterns can be identified (e.g., intra-abdominal soft tissue metastases or pelvic or spinal bony metastases of extremity myxoid or round cell liposarcomas).[122,261]

Lymph node metastases are uncommon, except for certain histologic types usually associated with childhood sarcoma.[262] In the MSKCC experience,[262] 3.7% of 1,066 patients with extremity soft tissue sarcoma had lymph node metastasis. Higher prevalence was seen in epithelioid sarcoma, 3 of 15; rhabdomyosarcoma, 4 of 21; clear cell sarcoma, 2 of 18; and angiosarcoma, 2 of 18. These findings were confirmed by a report from the Royal Marsden Hospital,[263] with 3.4% of 2,127 patients having regional lymph node metastasis. Again, prevalence was higher with rhabdomyosarcoma, epithelioid sarcoma, and angiosarcoma. Thus, for these subtypes, the draining lymph node basin should be subjected to careful clinical examination and complete imaging if indicated.

Patients with visceral and retroperitoneal lesions should have their liver imaged as part of the initial abdominal CT or MRI. For extremity sarcomas, imaging for metastasis is less important for patients with low-grade or small superficial high-grade extremity lesions, and simple chest radiography will suffice. Conversely, for patients with deep or large high-grade extremity lesions, for which the risk of metastatic disease is significant, more extensive evaluation with a CT scan of the chest is often preferred. Although CT is the most commonly used modality to evaluate pulmonary metastases, it is more expensive than radiographs, delivers a higher radiation dose, and may give false-positive results because of small, indeterminate pulmonary nodules. One study correlated thoracotomy with CT and found that only 60% of malignant nodules <6 mm in size were found at thoracotomy.[264] It is unclear if there is a better imaging modality to evaluate metastases of <1 cm. Newer techniques, such as FDG-PET, are being used to evaluate distant metastases and, when combined with CT and conventional imaging, may improve the diagnostic accuracy of preoperative staging. However, overstaging remains a problem in 12% of patients, and PET-CT remains limited in evaluating pulmonary metastases of <1 cm.[265] FDG-PET lacks specificity in its ability to distinguish between low-grade malignancies and benign entities. An additional concern is that many low-grade sarcoma types and several high-grade types, like round cell liposarcoma, do not reliably show uptake for FDG, further limiting its routine use for staging sarcoma patients.

Biopsy

Biopsy can be used to evaluate malignancy, histologic grade, and sometimes histologic type. Precise knowledge of these features enables the treating physician to tailor the treatment plan to the tumor's predicted pattern of local growth, risk of metastasis, and likely sites of distant spread. Either an incisional biopsy or several Tru-Cut core biopsies are required to obtain enough tissue for definitive diagnosis and accurate grading. The biopsy incision or core track should be placed in a location that can be completely excised at the time of definitive resection with minimal sacrifice of overlying skin. Excisional biopsy should be avoided, especially for lesions >3 cm in size, as the contamination of surrounding tissue planes may require the definitive resection to be more extensive.

In general, the important issue with biopsy is the adequacy of the sample. Sufficient viable tissue is required that is both representative of the lesion and available for histopathologic evaluation, immunohistochemistry, and, when necessary, cytogenetics and electron microscopy. As molecular markers become a factor in diagnosis, meticulous attention to the adequacy of biopsy, tissue preservation, and evaluation will be paramount.

Value of Tru-Cut Biopsy

Several studies have examined the value of Tru-Cut biopsy.[266] Its accuracy is lower than for incisional biopsy, though substantially higher than for frozen section, and Tru-Cut biopsy has the advantage that it can be done in an office setting.

Fine Needle Aspiration Cytology

Fine needle aspiration (FNA) cytology has been examined by a number of authors but is usually used only for the confirmation of recurrence rather than for the primary diagnosis. Particular problems with FNA are the limited sampling and lack of tissue architecture, which degrade diagnostic accuracy. In addition, the amount of tissue collected usually does not allow for ancillary molecular diagnostic techniques.

Some authors have argued that biopsy itself is not justified if FNA is available. Rydholm[267] suggested that open biopsy is never indicated, arguing that open biopsy risks local tumor spread and increases both the magnitude of the subsequent operation and the need for adjuvant radiation therapy. Using FNA, the surgeon proceeds directly to open operation. However, this requires referral before antecedent biopsy, a relatively uncontrollable event in the United States. Other authors suggest that this approach results in the referral of 10 patients with benign lesions for every sarcoma patient, certainly an untenable situation under our care system.

The no-biopsy approach presupposes that all that is required is a malignant sarcoma diagnosis and that the type or grade of sarcoma does not determine therapy. The use of FNA in patients with large sarcomas who are candidates for neoadjuvant therapy is also problematic due to difficulty in grading and subtyping these tumors accurately from such small samples. However, proponents argue that immunohistochemistry, electron microscopy, DNA cytology, and chromosomal analysis, all of which can be performed on FNA specimens, will ensure the appropriateness of this approach. However, the authors still favor obtaining adequate tissue from several Tru-Cut cores or an incisional biopsy to determine a definitive histologic diagnosis and grade before initiating treatment.

Frozen Section

In some institutions, frozen section is the diagnostic tool of choice. For diagnosis of malignancy, frozen section is accurate, but for histopathologic subtypes and grade, it is inferior to permanent sections of either Tru-Cut or incisional biopsy.[266]

Sarcoma Staging

The intent of staging systems is to group patients according to their probability of metastasis, disease-specific survival, or overall survival. The major staging used for soft tissue sarcoma is the system developed by the American Joint Committee on Cancer (AJCC). This system, first developed in 1992, has undergone significant changes, based on both histologic and clinical information. The current 2010 AJCC TNM (tumor, node, metastasis) system (Table 90.2) incorporates histologic type, histologic grade, tumor size, depth, regional lymph node involvement, and distant metastasis. It incorporates four major changes compared with the 2002 system. First, it excludes four histologic types: gastrointestinal stromal tumor (GIST), desmoid tumor, Kaposi sarcoma, and infantile fibrosarcoma. Second, it adds three histologic types: angiosarcoma, extraskeletal Ewing sarcoma, and dermatofibrosarcoma protuberans. Third, it reclassifies N1 disease from stage IV to stage III. Fourth, grading has changed from a four-grade to a three-grade system, although it accommodates two-, three-, and four-tiered grading systems.[268]

Analysis of the primary extremity soft tissue sarcomas seen at MSKCC during 1982 to 2009 suggests that the AJCC 2010 staging system nicely discriminates the probability of metastasis and disease-specific survival (Fig. 90.3 and Table 90.2). However, the AJCC staging still has limitations. A recent analysis suggested that risk assessment would be improved by increasing the number of primary tumor size categories from two to four. The analysis also suggested

TABLE 90.2

American Joint Committee on Cancer Staging System (2010)

Stage	Grade	Tumor	Nodes	Metastasis
IA	GX–G1	T1a–1b	N0	M0
IB	GX–G1	T2a–2b	N0	M0
IIA	G2–G3	T1a–1b	N0	M0
IIB	G2	T2a–2b	N0	M0
III	G3	T2a–2b	N0	M0
	G any	T any	N1	M0
IV	G any	T any	N any	M1

From Edge SB, Byrd DR, Compton CC, et al., eds. *The AJCC Cancer Staging Manual.* 7th ed. New York: Springer; 2009.

that patients with N1 M0 disease, whom the AJCC 2010 has moved to stage III, in fact have survival intermediate between that of other stage III patients and the stage IV patients.[269] Unfortunately, this system still fails to adequately account for sarcomas located in the retroperitoneum and may incompletely account for the influence of specific histologic subtypes on outcome. There is as yet no adequate staging system for retroperitoneal or intra-abdominal lesions.

Nomograms

The accuracy of predicting patient outcomes can be increased by integrating multiple clinical and histologic features in a predictive model such as a nomogram. To predict sarcoma-specific survival, MSKCC researchers developed nomograms that integrate information on patient age and tumor size, grade (low versus high), depth, site, and histopathology. Nomograms are available for both primary lesions[270] and locally recurrent[271] lesions. These nomograms can be readily transferred to handheld personal organizers for instant calculation of disease-specific survival probability. Because no current grading system performs well for every histologic type of sarcoma, the authors' groups have recently developed his-

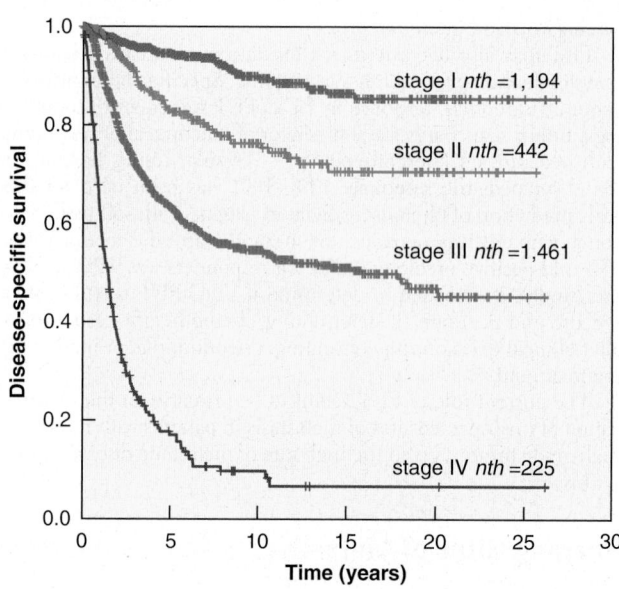

Figure 90.3 Disease-specific survival for patients with extremity soft tissue sarcoma according to the 2010 American Joint Committee on Cancer staging system. The data are for 3,322 patients seen at Memorial Sloan Kettering Cancer Center from 1982 through 2013.

tology-specific nomograms in liposarcoma,[37] synovial sarcoma,[272] and GIST.[273] Site-specific retroperitoneal nomograms have been developed[274–276] as well as a local recurrence nomogram for patients with primary extremity sarcoma to improve selection for adjuvant radiation.[277] As new molecular and genetic biomarkers are discovered and shown to have prognostic value, they can be incorporated into nomograms along with conventional clinical-pathologic variables. This would enable the treating physician to design a treatment strategy tailored to an individual patient's risk of relapse and potential for an aggressive clinical course.

Histologic and Prognostic Factors for Primary Extremity and Truncal Sarcoma

Histopathology is related to anatomic site (see Fig. 90.1), and the common histologic types in the extremities and trunk are liposarcoma, myxofibrosarcoma, UPS/PMFH, and synovial sarcoma. Clinical and pathologic factors that influence outcome were determined from analysis of prospectively collected data from 1,041 patients older than 16 years with localized soft tissue sarcoma of the extremity.[239] The 5-year survival rate was 76%, with a median follow-up of 4 years. Factors that increased risk of local recurrence were age, recurrent disease at presentation, positive margin, and fibrosarcoma or MPNST histology. Factors that increased the risk of disease-specific death were tumor size, depth, and grade, recurrent presentation, positive margin, and MPNST or LMS histology.

Distant recurrence was associated with tumor size, depth, and grade, recurrent presentation, LMS histology, and, to a lesser extent, any nonliposarcoma histology. High-grade lesions have a much greater risk of developing a distant metastasis in the first 30 months. Even low-grade lesions, however, have a slow but inexorable increase in risk of metastasis over the long term.[239] Prognostic factors clearly vary with time. Grade is a dominant factor in early metastasis, but in late recurrence initial size becomes equally important.[278] Postmetastasis survival for most patients is independent of factors involved in the primary presentation, although an association has been found with tumor size.

Bone invasion and neurovascular invasion have historically been considered bad prognostic features. However, bone invasion is relatively uncommon in soft tissue sarcoma, so it has not been uniformly included in any staging system.

Five-year survival does not guarantee cure. An analysis of patients disease-free 5 years after the diagnosis and treatment of extremity lesions showed that 9% would go on to have a recurrence in the next 5 years.[279] Unfortunately, survival has not measurably improved with time when corrected for stage.[280] A review of 1,261 completely resected extremity lesions by 5-year increments for 1982 to 2001 suggested that disease-specific actuarial 5-year survival remained unchanged (approximately 79%) over 20 years. For high-risk patients (those with high-grade, deep tumors of >10 cm), disease-specific survival remains at around 50%.

Site of disease is a clear determinant of outcome and an important prognostic factor. Patients with extremity and superficial trunk lesions certainly do better than patients with retroperitoneal and visceral sarcomas (Fig. 90.4). Death from local recurrence is uncommon in those with extremity lesions but occurs frequently in patients with retroperitoneal liposarcoma.

Innumerable molecular markers have been defined for soft tissue sarcoma—some with prognostic implications—but they have not been included in staging systems. However, the authors expect them to become increasingly important variables.

Diagnostic and Prognostic Factors for Primary Retroperitoneal/Intra-Abdominal Sarcoma

Most patients with retroperitoneal or intra-abdominal sarcoma present with an asymptomatic abdominal mass. On occasion pain

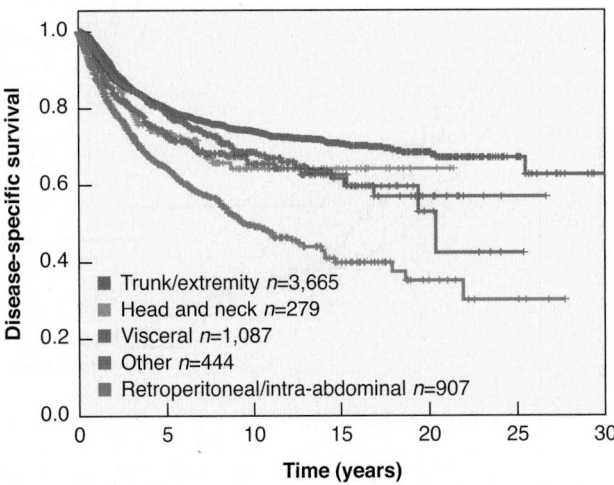

Figure 90.4 Disease-specific survival by site of soft tissue sarcoma. The data are for 6,382 patients admitted to Memorial Sloan Kettering Cancer Center from 1982 through 2013. Patients with retroperitoneal or visceral sarcomas did worse than patients with extremity lesions.

is present, and less common symptoms include GI bleeding, incomplete obstruction, and neurologic symptoms related to retroperitoneal invasion or pressure on neurovascular structures. In one report, only 27% of patients with retroperitoneal sarcoma had neurologic symptoms, which primarily were related to an expanding retroperitoneal mass.[281] Weight loss is uncommon, and incidental diagnosis is the norm. The diagnosis is usually suspected on finding a soft tissue mass on abdominal CT or MRI. Often the diagnosis is clear without biopsy, and many proceed directly to operative resection in the absence of a clinical trial. FNA biopsy or CT-guided core biopsy has a limited role in the routine diagnostic evaluation of these patients. CT-guided core biopsy is indicated if abdominal lymphoma, germ cell tumor, or carcinoma is strongly suspected. Preoperative biopsy is also indicated for patients who present with distant metastasis or advanced local disease that on abdominal or pelvic imaging appears to be difficult to completely remove surgically without substantial morbidity. In most patients, exploratory laparotomy should be performed and the diagnosis made at operation, unless (1) the patient's tumor is clearly unresectable, (2) neoadjuvant chemotherapy or radiotherapy is needed to attempt to make the tumor more resectable, or (3) the patient will be undergoing preoperative investigational treatment.

CT remains the primary modality for evaluation of retroperitoneal and visceral sarcomas. Because the most likely site of visceral metastasis is the liver followed by lung, a CT scan of the chest, abdomen, and pelvis encompasses the primary lesion and the most likely sites of metastasis in a single examination.

Retroperitoneal or intra-abdominal sarcomas (excluding visceral sarcomas such as GIST) account for approximately 15% of all soft tissue sarcomas. The most common histologic types in the retroperitoneum are liposarcoma (60%), LMS (22%), solitary fibrous tumor (5%), and MPNST (2%). Among primary retroperitoneal liposarcomas (excluding pleomorphic liposarcoma and liposarcoma not otherwise specified), about 50% are low grade, with 46% and 3% classified as well differentiated and myxoid, respectively, and 50% are high grade with 49% and 2% classified as dedifferentiated and round cell liposarcoma, respectively.

An analysis of 278 patients with primary retroperitoneal sarcoma[282] showed that grade and completeness of resection were the most important independent prognostic factors for disease-specific survival, with incompletely resected patients having survival similar to that of patients whose disease was unresectable from the outset. In this same study, histology and grade were both significantly associated with local recurrence, with liposarcoma having a 2.6-fold

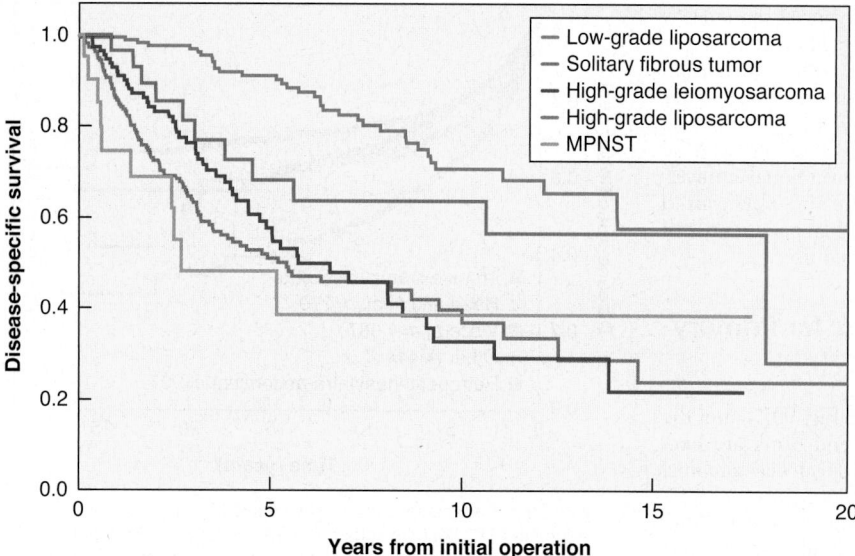

Figure 90.5 Disease-specific survival for patients with primary retroperitoneal/intra-abdominal sarcoma, according to histology. The data are for 632 patients with primary retroperitoneal or intraabdominal sarcoma admitted to Memorial Sloan Kettering Cancer Center from 1982 through 2010. Low-grade liposarcoma consists of well-differentiated and myxoid subtypes. High-grade liposarcoma consists of dedifferentiated, round cell, and pleomorphic subtypes. The most common histologic types vary widely in disease-specific survival ($p < 0.0001$). Disease-specific survival at 5 years was 92% for patients with primary low-grade liposarcoma compared with 50% for patients with primary high-grade liposarcoma. For the group as a whole, disease-specific survival was 69% at 5 years and 55% at 10 years. MPNST, malignant peripheral nerve sheath tumor.

greater risk of local recurrence compared to other histologic types. Other studies have shown that for patients with retroperitoneal or intra-abdominal sarcomas, similar to patients with extremity sarcomas, the histologic type is an important prognostic factor for disease-specific survival, with this outcome worse for patients with MPNST and patients with LMS than for patients with solitary fibrous tumor (Fig. 90.5). Liposarcoma subtype provides additional prognostic information for disease-specific survival (see Fig. 90.5). In a multivariate analysis of liposarcoma, histologic subtype, completeness of resection, age, and contiguous organ resection were all independent predictors of disease-specific survival, with hazard ratios of 6 for subtype and 3.8 for completeness of resection.[40]

MANAGEMENT BY PRESENTATION STATUS, EXTENT OF DISEASE, AND ANATOMIC LOCATION

Management of Extremity and Truncal Sarcoma

Surgical Management of Primary Localized Disease

Although surgery remains the principal therapeutic modality in soft tissue sarcoma, the extent of surgery required, along with the optimum combination of radiotherapy and chemotherapy, remains controversial. The individual patient's clinical and pathologic characteristics—particularly the pattern of spread expected for the patient's histologic subtype—should be used to design the most effective treatment plan. Figure 90.6 shows a suggested algorithm for management of patients with extremity or truncal disease.

Extent of Surgical Resection. The most extensive resection, amputation, should be only rarely indicated for soft tissue sarcoma. At MSKCC, the amputation rate, which was 50% in the late 1960s, is now <5%. Outcomes from amputation versus limb-sparing surgery for extremity lesions were addressed by a prospective, randomized trial with well over 10 years' follow-up. Although local recurrence is greater in those undergoing limb-sparing operation plus irradiation than in those undergoing amputation, disease-free survival is not different.[283] Moreover, the level of handicap can be significantly lower in patients treated with limb-sparing surgery.[284] Amputation should be reserved for tumors that cannot

be resected by any other means, in patients without evidence of metastatic disease and with potential for good long-term functional rehabilitation.

For these reasons, surgery for extremity or truncal tumors most often consists of wide en bloc resection. Historical attempts to resect all muscle bundles from origin to exertion have been supplanted by an encompassing resection, aiming to obtain a 1-cm margin of uninvolved tissue in all directions. Two-centimeter margins are employed for histologic subtypes with infiltrative borders (e.g., DFSP or myxofibrosarcoma). For certain low-grade histologic types, however, even 1-cm margins are not required for excellent local control. For example, well-differentiated liposarcomas of the extremities require only complete excision with a minimal surrounding margin, as the majority of these tumors will not recur, even after a limited or microscopically positive margin excision, as long as the excision is complete. Skin surrounding the biopsy site, tethered to the tumor, or showing neovascularization in association with an underlying lesion should be removed with the specimen; myocutaneous flaps may be considered when a significant defect results or adjuvant radiation will be required. The limiting factor in obtaining wide margins is usually neurovascular or, occasionally, bony juxtaposition. Because very few soft tissue sarcomas invade bone directly, bone rarely needs to be resected; periosteum can be removed to provide an adequate margin when soft tissue sarcoma abuts the bone. Similarly, perineurium can be removed with the tumor to provide margins when the tumor is directly adjacent to a major motor nerve. In rare instances, a major nerve or vascular bundle is encased by a soft tissue sarcoma. Low-grade lesions may be bivalved to preserve the nerve; however, in the case of a high-grade tumor, resection may be required. Vascular bypass can be performed for arterial resections. Bracing can be used to compensate for removal of femoral or sciatic nerves.

Indications for Adjuvant Therapy. As detailed in the next section, radiation therapy should be added to limb-sparing surgery for some high-risk patients. Neoadjuvant chemotherapy or investigational approaches should also be considered for patients with high-grade lesions >10 cm and for those with synovial sarcoma or myxoid/round cell liposarcoma >5 cm (subtypes highly responsive to chemotherapy) (see "Chemotherapy for Primary Localized Extremity/Truncal Sarcoma").

A significant subset of subcutaneous and intramuscular sarcomas can be treated by wide excision alone, with a local recurrence rate of only 8% to 20%.[285–287] For example, in patients with small lesions (<5 cm), complete surgical excision with margins of >1 cm

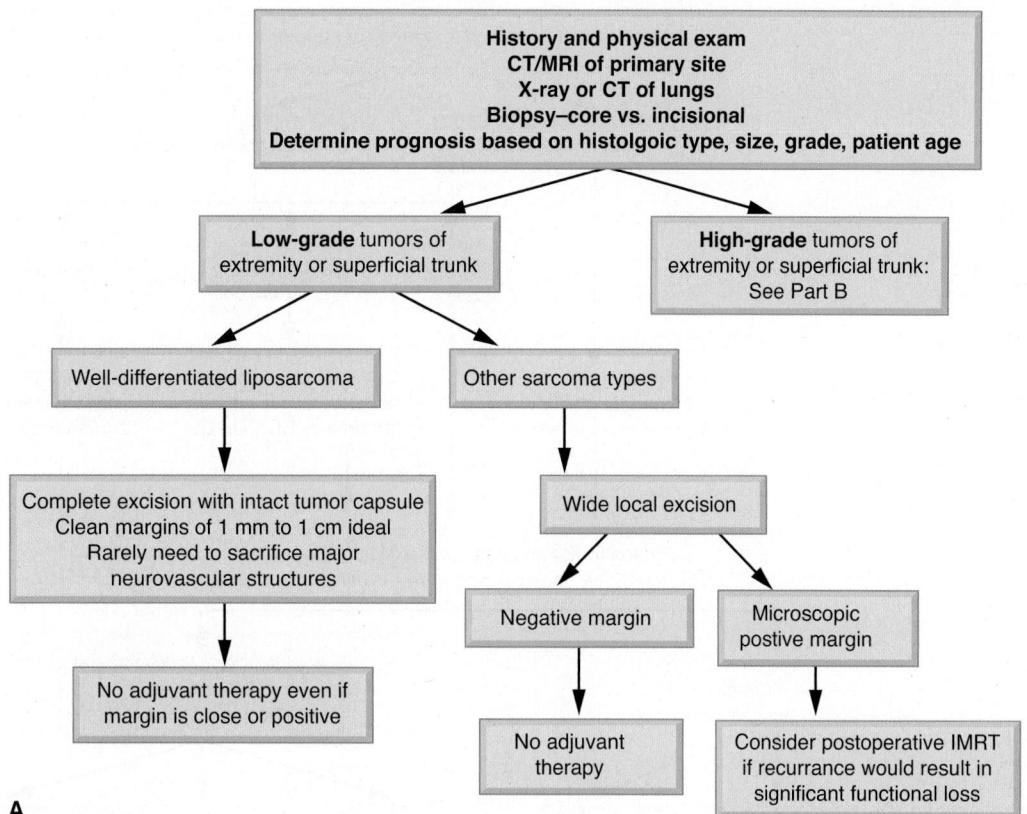

Figure 90.6 Management algorithm for extremity and superficial truncal soft tissue sarcoma. **(A)** Low-grade sarcomas. **(B)** High-grade sarcomas. Note that although postoperative intensity-modulated radiation therapy (IMRT) is mentioned in the algorithm, preoperative IMRT could be used in the same types of patients. CT, computed tomography; MRI, magnetic resonance imaging; RC, round cell; Pleo, pleomorphic; LS, liposarcoma; BRT, brachytherapy. *(continued)*

is usually sufficient without the need for any adjuvant therapy. Indeed, in a group of 159 patients with small primary tumors resected with negative margins, adjuvant radiotherapy showed no benefit: the 5-year local control rate was 77% in those selected to receive adjuvant radiation, compared to 92% in those undergoing surgery alone ($p = 0.08$). If, however, the margin is positive, the authors' policy is to administer radiotherapy to patients with high-grade tumors even if the tumor was $\leq$5 cm. In contrast, patients with large, low-grade lesions such as atypical lipomatous tumors rarely require radiation therapy, as local recurrence rates are low (<10%) in patients treated with surgery alone.[119]

Another factor that should be considered is whether the patient has had a prior unplanned excision (i.e., excision without adequate preoperative staging or consideration of the need to remove normal tissue around tumor). At Princess Margaret Hospital, the rate of local recurrence was significantly higher in patients who were treated after unplanned excision on the outside than in patients who received their treatment at the institution (22% versus 7%; $p = 0.03$).[288] Unplanned excision is very common in community settings when small soft tissue lesions are excised under the presumption that they are benign. In these cases, the authors attempt a re-excision if at all feasible; otherwise, patients are strongly considered for adjuvant irradiation.

Radiation Therapy for Primary Localized Extremity or Truncal Sarcoma

The goals of adjuvant radiotherapy in the management of soft tissue sarcoma are to enhance local control, preserve function, and achieve acceptable cosmesis by contributing to tissue preservation. Adjuvant radiation should be added to the surgical resection for most deep, large (>5 cm), high-grade sarcomas if the excision

margin is close, particularly with extramuscular involvement, or if a local recurrence would necessitate amputation or the sacrifice of a major neurovascular bundle.[289,290] Superficial lesions and smaller contained lesions confined to individual muscles may be managed with surgery alone in expert hands.[257,291] For most other situations, however, evidence strongly suggests that surgery that does not achieve wide clearance through normal tissue has a significantly higher rate of local failure, and even some small lesions may behave adversely.

That adjuvant radiotherapy enhances local control with conservative surgical resection in soft tissue sarcoma overall has been demonstrated in two randomized clinical trials, one using external beam radiation therapy (EBRT) and the other using brachytherapy (BRT).[289,290] However, whether the addition of radiotherapy confers a benefit for small (<5 cm) high-grade lesions is controversial.[292]

The contemporary era has brought newer techniques for radiotherapy planning and delivery that permit unprecedented accuracy in the use of both BRT and EBRT.

External Beam Radiation Therapy. EBRT is the most popular adjuvant radiotherapy approach, perhaps because EBRT relies less than does BRT on special technical and operational requirements. Nevertheless, EBRT requires comprehensive and multidisciplinary pretreatment consultation and accurate pathologic and radiologic assessment.

Postoperative Versus Preoperative External Beam Radiation Therapy. Postoperative EBRT was the first and remains the most widely practiced local adjuvant approach, in part because it does not require that surgery be postponed and because it allows for sterilization of microscopic nests of residual disease. Its use is supported

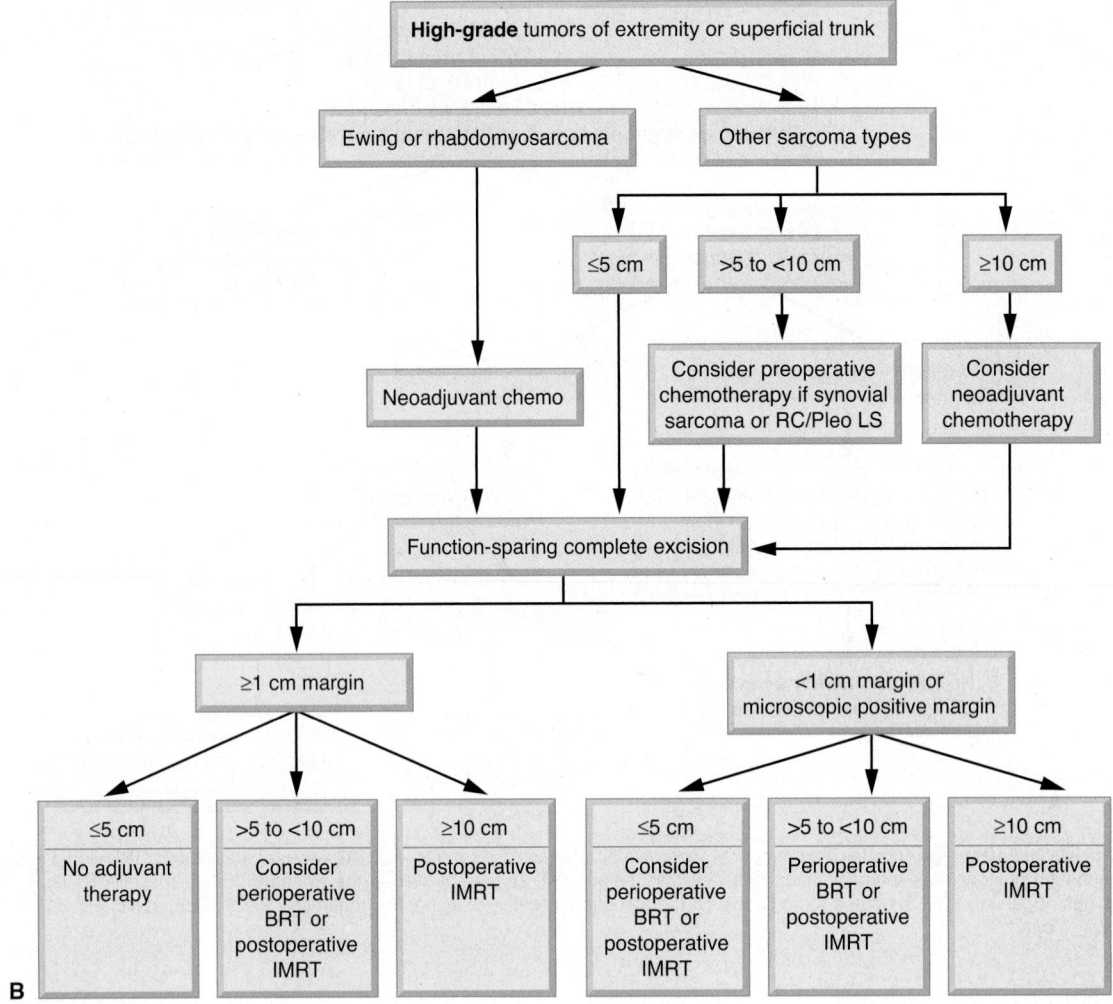

Figure 90.6 *(Continued)*

by numerous single-institution studies and by a randomized trial that showed better local control from conservative surgery followed by EBRT than from surgery alone.[290] Although the postoperative EBRT resulted in significantly worse limb strength, edema, and range of motion, these deficits were often transient and had few measurable effects on activities of daily life or global quality of life.[290] Preoperative EBRT, however, has not been subjected to a randomized comparison against surgery alone.

Both preoperative and postoperative EBRT have their advantages and disadvantages. An advantage of postoperative EBRT is that the entire pathology specimen and final margins are available for pathologic analysis, helping to determine the need for further therapy. A major limitation is that the target is less precisely defined, and therefore volume is larger and dose is higher, resulting in greater late tissue morbidity. With preoperative EBRT, on the other hand, not only is the treatment volume well defined, but the blood supply is intact. The intact vascular supply may reduce the fraction of hypoxic cells particularly at the tumor margins, which under hypoxic conditions tend to be radioresistant, and thus may decrease the dose needed compared to postoperative radiotherapy. Confirmation of this principle, however, remains elusive. The major drawback of preoperative radiotherapy, as detailed subsequently, is that irradiation increases the risk of acute wound complications upon surgery. Which approach is superior remains unclear.

In a trial assessing EBRT sequencing, the Canadian Sarcoma Group randomized 190 patients with extremity soft tissue sarcoma to preoperative or postoperative radiotherapy. Preoperative radiotherapy doubled the risk of early acute wound complication, although this observation seems to apply almost exclusively to lower limb lesions.[293] In the 5-year results from this trial,[294] the preoperative and postoperative arms were nearly identical for local control (93% versus 92%, respectively) and metastatic relapse–free survival (67% versus 69%). In addition, the preoperative and postoperative arms did not differ significantly in overall survival (73% versus 67%; $p = 0.5$) or cause-specific survival (78% versus 73%; $p = 0.6$). Recently, a meta-analysis of pre- versus postoperative radiation in localized resectable soft tissue sarcoma suggested that the risk of local recurrence may be lower after preoperative radiation, and that the risk of metastatic spread is not increased with the delay in surgical resection necessary to complete preoperative radiotherapy.[295]

In the Canadian randomized trial, functional outcomes were collected prospectively.[296] The trial design specified two validated instruments in addition an observer-based instrument.[296] At 6 weeks after surgery, the preoperative group had inferior function, with worse bodily pain scores on all three rating instruments. However, at 3 to 12 months after surgery, the two groups showed no differences in these rating scores.[296] It can be concluded that, for most of the first posttreatment year, the timing of radiotherapy has minimal effect on the function of patients with soft tissue sarcoma. The 2-year function and morbidity results[297] show deteriorating late tissue sequelae (fibrosis and edema) in patients in the postoperative arm, resulting from larger radiotherapy doses and volumes.

Of note, patients with significant fibrosis or edema had significantly lower function scores. In addition, patients who received the higher doses—most of them in the postoperative group—may eventually have a higher rate of bone fractures. These disadvantages of postoperative EBRT may override the higher frequency of acute wound complications with preoperative EBRT, although patients who do experience wound complications continue to experience some impaired function.[298]

Intensity-Modulated Radiation Therapy. The past decade witnessed an unprecedented improvement in delivery of EBRT to complex volumes and shapes. Leading these advances is intensity-modulated radiation therapy (IMRT),[299] which uses computer algorithms for inverse planning and treatment delivery. IMRT may be particularly applicable to complex anatomic volumes such as retroperitoneal sarcoma juxtapositioned to liver or paraspinal lesions, for which conformal avoidance of liver or of kidney and spinal cord is necessary.[300] Avoidance of bone is also possible,[301,302] and the risk of radiation-induced fracture of a weight-bearing bone may be reduced by using specific IMRT dose avoidance objectives (see "Serious Complications of Primary Treatment").

IMRT in the treatment of soft tissue sarcoma appears to enhance normal tissue protection while maintaining oncologic control. Notably, a recent phase 2 trial of preoperative IMRT in lower extremity sarcoma conducted at the Princess Margret Hospital indicated a 5-year local recurrence–free survival of 88% and very favorable doses to bone (mean dose 26.2 Gy, ± 8 Gy) and vulnerable soft tissues, in addition to absence of bone fractures and a reduction in the number and severity of wound complications.[303] IMRT was associated with a similar 5-year local recurrence–free survival (92%) at MSKCC.[304] The local control results for both IMRT studies were also very similar to those with conventional EBRT in both arms of the aforementioned Canadian trial that compared preoperative to postoperative radiotherapy.[294] Taken together, these results indicate that any superiority of IMRT over conventional EBRT is not likely to be based on tumor control but on a reduction in acute and late toxicity. This especially applies to serious problems such as bone fracture.[303,305] Wound complications may also be influenced by reduction in the volume of soft tissue irradiated, especially if the immediate tissues to be used for the wound closure can be spared.[303]

Volume Issues in External Beam Radiation Therapy. Given the generally favorable oncologic results after EBRT, a priority is ameliorating toxicity to normal tissue by exploring reduced treatment intensity, including administered doses or volumes. Prospective assessments of the volumes irradiated in EBRT are emerging, and these results will likely update the guidelines outlining optimal radiotherapy target volumes for EBRT.[301–303]

Targets are defined differently for preoperative versus postoperative radiotherapy. Preoperative radiotherapy can focus on the extent of definable disease (determined using imaging), and the target is based on the anatomic location, containment by barriers to spread (especially intact fascial planes), and allowance for geometric uncertainty related to potential variation in patient setup and physiologic movement. Special situations must also be considered, such as lesions arising in extracompartmental spaces such as the femoral triangle, antecubital space, and popliteal space, because these lesions have the ability to extend considerable distances proximally and distally with less anatomic restraint. Such lesions may spread to the neurovascular bundle early. The radiotherapy margins should reflect this and include undisturbed tissue planes and barriers to tumor incursion.

To cover any microscopic disease, the clinical target volume (CTV) for preoperative radiotherapy generally includes margins amounting to 4 cm longitudinally and 1.5 cm axially. This translates into field coverage approximately 5 cm long, allowing for beam penumbra and treatment uncertainties such as patient movement. Some controversy regarding planning of field coverage

has persisted. A recent Radiation Therapy Oncology Group consensus panel, after reviewing data regarding the local extension of soft tissue sarcomas, set guidelines that included 3-cm longitudinal coverage and 1.5-cm radial coverage.[306] However, these recommendations were not based on outcome efficacy results and conflict slightly with international recommendations provided by members of various cooperative clinical trials groups.[307] The latter recommendations suggest that the 4-cm CTV longitudinal coverage should be maintained until contrary data emerge, as it is based on the only available prospective clinical trial data (the original Canadian preoperative versus postoperative trial), and because histologic assessment of adjacent tissues suggest that microscopic sarcoma cells may be present up to 4 cm away from the gross tumor volume.[293,308] This longitudinal margin was also used in the recent Princess Margaret Hospital phase 2 prospective trial in lower extremity lesions, which is the only prosective outcome data with IMRT at this time.[303]

Postoperative radiotherapy volumes are significantly larger because they ideally encompass all surgically manipulated tissues, with the recognition that this is impossible in some anatomic sites due to the proximity of critical anatomy. In addition, because surgery has disrupted the anatomic planes and they no longer provide containment barriers to tumor growth, the entire CTV extending 4 cm beyond the surgically manipulated tissue must be considered high risk and thus treated for at least the first phase of irradiation (e.g., an appropriate dose is 50 Gy). Subsequently, the volume is reduced to the immediate tumor bed. Alternatively, with a single-phase IMRT approach, a higher dose could be delivered to the small high-risk volume while using a more moderate dose for the more peripheral regions of the CTV.

The international clinical trials group consensus panel mentioned earlier also generally recommended that the CTV extend 4 cm longitudinally beyond the surgically manipulated tissues.[307] Currently, the volume of postoperative radiotherapy is being investigated in a randomized phase 3 trial conducted by the United Kingdom National Cancer Research Network. The trial compares a standard volume (5 cm longitudinal margin to gross tumor volume or 1 cm from the surgical scar, whichever is longer in the cranio–caudal direction and 2 cm axial margin) versus an experimental volume (2 cm longitudinal margin to gross tumor volume and 2 cm axial margin). Patients in both arms of the study will receive 66 Gy over 6.5 weeks; patients in the standard arm, but not the experimental arm, will have a volume reduction after 25 fractions (50 Gy). The goal is to assess if a reduced volume of postoperative radiotherapy will increase limb function without compromising local control.[309]

A final issue concerning choice of irradiation target volume concerns the definition of the areas that may harbor disease and especially whether the risk area should include any peripheral edema that surrounds the tumor. A study noted previously from the Princess Margaret Hospital, which correlated MRI characteristics with pathologic features, suggests that in some cases the edema does harbor sarcoma cells.[308]

Dose Issues in External Beam Radiation Therapy. The dose of radiotherapy represents an additional unexplored area. The preoperative dose used in most institutions is approximately 50 Gy in daily fractions of 1.8 to 2.0 Gy over approximately 5 weeks. Generally, a postoperative boost is administered only if the surgical margins are positive, and the benefit of this boost is unclear. For example, for patients who had positive surgical margins, Delaney et al.[310] reported that the factors associated with local control included total radiotherapy dose >64 Gy (delivered as pre-, post-, or preoperative with a postoperative boost), with the implication that a boost is beneficial following preoperative radiotherapy. A different conclusion was drawn from a retrospective study at the Princess Margaret Hospital of patients with extremity soft tissue sarcoma and positive surgical margins. All patients had been treated with preoperative radiotherapy (50 Gy); 41 received a postoperative boost (typically 16 Gy) and 52 received no other radiotherapy. A common reason for omission of boost was wound complications, which tend to occur in more extensive and adverse cases. Despite this, patients who received a postoperative boost had worse 5-year estimated local recurrence–free survival (74% compared to 90% for preoperative radiotherapy only).[311] This is consistent with recent pooled results from two Harvard groups, which showed no additional benefit to the radiotherapy boost in patients who had a positive surgical margin after preoperative radiotherapy and resection.[312] Consequently at the Princess Margaret Hospital a postoperative boost is not used for patients with microscopically positive resection margins.

Adjuvant Brachytherapy. The fundamental interest in BRT stems from the ability to focus the dose directly on the tumor bed, thereby potentially improving the therapeutic ratio. Very high dose levels in the vicinity of the radioactive sources and the rapid dose fall-off permit dose intensification while protecting the surrounding normal tissue. Therefore, BRT usually spares more normal tissue than EBRT, except when precision techniques such as IMRT are used. Moreover, patients usually complete all their treatment in about 2 weeks compared to 6 to 7 weeks with EBRT, thereby limiting repopulation of residual tumor cells. The technical aspects of BRT differ from those of EBRT, and specific guidelines for its use and technical delivery have been published. BRT, unlike EBRT, requires a specific collaboration between surgical and radiation oncologists. With BRT, unlike in postoperative irradiation, no attempts are made to treat large margins or to include the scar and the drainage site, although it is acknowledged that this approach has not been formally compared with EBRT in similar cases.

The efficacy of BRT was compared to that of IMRT among 134 patients with primary high-grade extremity sarcoma in recent data from MSKCC.[304] The BRT and IMRT groups were similar in terms of traditional prognostic factors, although the IMRT group had a significantly greater proportion of patients with positive or close margins, large tumors, and bone or nerve manipulation. The median follow-up was approximately 4 years. The 5-year local control rate was 92% for the IMRT group compared to 81% for the BRT group ($p = 0.04$). On multivariate analysis, IMRT was the only predictor of improved local control ($p = 0.04$).[304] Earlier evidence from MSKCC suggests that BRT may not provide optimal results in regions unsuited for ideal implant geometry, such as in more proximal regions of the limb.[292]

In patients treated with BRT as the sole radiotherapy, the dose is usually 45 Gy given over 4 to 6 days, and when given as a boost, the dose is usually 15 to 20 Gy from BRT plus 45 to 50 Gy from EBRT. Of importance, the catheters are loaded no sooner than the sixth postoperative day to allow time for wound healing.[313] The most commonly used isotope is low–dose-rate ^{192}Ir; however, high-activity ^{125}I is occasionally used in young patients or to protect the gonads. High–dose-rate ^{192}Ir has been advocated to take advantage of its radiation safety and dose-optimization capabilities.

The BRT CTV may be difficult to define, but in general it is represented by the volume of tissue considered at risk for microscopic extension of tumor and includes the tumor bed visualized on radiographic studies and under direct inspection intraoperatively. The results with adjuvant BRT suggest that radiation treatment directed to the tumor bed plus a 2-cm margin is adequate.[314] Although there is no consensus on the exact size of the margin beyond the tumor bed, generally at least 2 cm longitudinally and 1 cm axially are recommended.[307,315] These volumes would seem to approximate those for preoperative radiotherapy.

Adjuvant BRT has been evaluated in a randomized trial. Patients who underwent complete gross resection were randomly assigned to receive adjuvant BRT ($n = 78$) or no further therapy ($n = 86$). The 10-year actuarial local control rates were 81% in the BRT group and 67% in the no-BRT group ($p = 0.03$). This improvement in local control, however, was limited to patients with histologically high-grade tumors, whose local control was 89%

in the BRT group and 64% in the no-BRT group ($p = 0.001$).[289] The adjuvant BRT did not improve local control in patients with low-grade tumors as the local recurrence rates of 27% (BRT) and 22% (no BRT) were not statistically different.[316] Rigorous psychofunctional testing of 38 long-term survivors in this trial revealed no significant differences in functional outcome between the BRT group and the no-BRT group. The BRT group did, however, have higher levels of anxiety, depression, and appreciation of illness.[317]

BRT is often used in combination with EBRT, but whether all patients need this combination is unclear.[318] An MSKCC study evaluated 105 patients with primary or locally recurrent high-grade soft tissue sarcomas who were treated with wide local excision and radiotherapy: BRT (87 patients) or BRT and EBRT (18 patients). At a median follow-up of 22 months, the two groups had no statistically significant difference in 2-year actuarial local control rate: 82% in the BRT group and 90% in the BRT plus EBRT group ($p = 0.32$).[319] However, case selection was such that the two groups are not completely comparable. Notably, patients were selected for EBRT if they had a positive margin (56%) or if anatomic considerations led to concern about the adequacy of dose coverage with BRT.

BRT is particularly useful when the surgical plan involves resection margins being close. In this situation, if the surgical and pathologic findings are satisfactory, the unused BRT catheters can be removed. Alternatively, BRT allows early delivery of radiation to a reduced and select volume mapped precisely by the intraoperative findings. The American Brachytherapy Society has recommended against BRT as a sole treatment modality in several situations: (1) the CTV cannot be adequately encompassed in the implant geometry, (2) the proximity of critical anatomy is expected to prevent administration of a meaningful dose, (3) the resection margins are positive, and (4) the skin is involved with tumor.[320] In such situations, EBRT may be used alone or with BRT.

High–dose–rate (HDR) BRT has some potential advantages over low–dose–rate BRT, although the experience with HDR BRT for sarcoma is still limited. A typical HDR dose is approximately 36 Gy in 10 fractions using a 6-hour interfraction interval, though some authors have used higher doses.[321] Guided by the more abundant breast cancer experience, a dose of 32 to 34 Gy in twice-daily fractions of 3.4 to 4.0 Gy over 4 to 5 days[322–324] seems useful and safe, though even here there have been reports of fat necrosis in later follow-up.[324] In sarcoma management, authors have observed wound healing complications with HDR BRT.[325,326] In addition, caution should probably be exercised when placing catheters in contact with neurovascular structures, and when such contact cannot be avoided the dose per fraction should probably be curtailed. As yet, no large series evaluating HDR BRT for sarcoma is available, and no studies have directly compared HDR to low–dose–rate BRT. Comparisons are difficult due to nonstandardization of target volumes, dose prescription points, and the delivered dose. However, low–dose–rate BRT may expose the staff caring for patients to radiation, whereas HDR BRT does not. In addition, the HDR approach offers the potential for outpatient delivery.

Sarcomas involving neurovascular structures present a challenge in achieving control while maintaining function. Intraoperative BRT, alone or combined with EBRT, has been used in this setting. A 5-year 69% actuarial survival rate and 90% local relapse–free rate was reported for 79 patients with primary disease. No amputation was required, although 8 of the 79 (10%) had grade 3-4 peripheral neuropathy and fibrosis, and 2 experienced vascular damage. Despite this, the authors considered that intraoperative BRT offers an acceptable conservative option for this particularly adverse presentation.[327]

Intraoperative HDR, a rarely used approach, has been used for the treatment of retroperitoneal sarcoma (see "Retroperitoneal Sarcoma").

Technical Enhancement of Radiotherapy Delivery. IMRT can now be administered very precisely using reference to the position of external surrogate markers or implanted and/or anatomic fiducials to permit the determination of tumor coordinates in all three planes. High-dose, single fraction treatments are often termed stereotactic radiosurgery (SRS), and high-dose, fractionated treatments are variously termed stereotactic radiotherapy or stereotactic body radiotherapy. These approaches are used for very adverse presentations of sarcoma, such as primary spinal sarcoma. Levine et al.[328] used SRS to treat 14 patients with primary spine sarcoma. In seven patients, the treatment was definitive, and all seven had excellent pain relief and were alive with a mean follow-up of 33 months, although two patients had recurrence of tumor and were retreated. Surgery and adjuvant SRS were used in the other seven patients, of whom five remain free from recurrence at a mean follow-up of 43.5 months. Notably, even though the SRS doses were in the mean range of 30 Gy in three fractions, none of these patients had spinal injury from SRS.

High-dose photon/proton radiotherapy has shown promising results. In a phase 2 study, high-dose photon/proton radiotherapy was administered with or without resection for the management of primary, nonmetastatic spine, and paraspinal sarcomas. For 50 patients with a median follow-up of 48 months, the 5-year actuarial rates of local control, recurrence-free survival, and overall survival were 78%, 63%, and 87%, respectively. Three sacral neuropathies appeared after 77.12 to 77.4 Gy equivalents.[329]

Other forms of particle beam radiotherapy are discussed in the "Definitive Radiation" section.

Definitive Radiation. Surgery remains the main treatment for patients with sarcoma of the extremity, and every effort should be made to attempt resection. However, in some patients with unresectable disease or medical contraindications to operation, definitive radiation can be considered for palliation. In a study of 112 patients treated with definitive irradiation to a median total dose of 64 Gy,[330,331] the 5-year rates of local control and overall survival were 45% and 35%, respectively. Local control at 5 years was 51%, 45%, and 9% for tumors <5 cm, 5 to 10 cm, and >10 cm, respectively. Five-year outcomes were worse for patients who received doses of <63 Gy than for those receiving higher doses; local control was 22% versus 60% and overall survival was 14% versus 52%. Complications, however, were more frequent at doses of 68 Gy or more. Thus, the therapeutic window appears to be 63 to 68 Gy.[330]

Similar findings were reported for 57 patients treated with definitive photon beam irradiation to 44 to 88 Gy. The 5-year local control rate was 28%.[332] An additional 15 patients were treated with neutrons without obvious benefit over photons.

Other investigators have considered neutron radiotherapy either alone or in combination with photon beam irradiation. The attraction of neutrons is their high linear energy transfer and lower oxygen enhancement ratio compared to X-rays and the consequent possibility of eliminating hypoxic cells. In addition, neutron irradiation results in less repair of sublethal and potentially lethal damage and less variation in radiosensitivity over the phases of the cell cycle. Unfortunately, all of these biological features also pertain to normal tissue, which implies that late toxicity is likely to be heightened, given the absence of the usual protection afforded by fractionation that occurs with more conventional photon treatment schedules. In a review of the European experience, patients with inoperable tumors or with gross disease after surgery and treated with neutron radiotherapy had a local control rate of 50%, but the rate of severe complications ranged from 6.6% when neutron therapy was used as a boost to 50% when used alone.[333] Schwartz et al.[334] reported a North American experience of fast neutron therapy in a heterogeneous series of bone and in soft tissue sarcomas. Among the 34 patients with unresectable disease, the local relapse–free survival at 1 year was estimated as 62%. Within the entire series of 66 patients, serious chronic radiation-related complications occurred in 10 patients (15%), all of whom had had high neutron doses, large radiotherapy fields, or both.

Another high linear energy transfer method that has been used for the treatment of unresectable soft tissue sarcoma is carbon ion radiotherapy.[335] Although not widely available, this technology has substantially better ability to target tissues safely compared to neutrons because of the enormous energy release at the end of its range. In addition, it offers excellent physical dose distribution and higher relative biological effectiveness. Sugahara et al.[335] described promising results for unresectable sarcomas of both bone and soft tissue with 5-year local control rates of 76% in a small study ($n = 17$, 9 primary and 8 recurrent). Serizawa et al.[336] reported the results of carbon ion radiotherapy for 24 patients with unresectable high-grade retroperitoneal sarcomas, 16 with primary disease, and 8 with recurrent disease. The dose ranged from 52.8 to 73.6 Gy equivalents in 16 fixed fractions over 4 weeks. Overall survival rates were 75% at 2 years and 50% at 5 years. Local control rates were favorably 77% and 69% at 2 and 5 years, respectively. Notably, toxicities were low, with no GI tract complications and no toxicity greater than grade 2. These results suggest that carbon ions may be an alternative to surgery with acceptable morbidity for unresectable sarcomas.

Spot scanning proton beam therapy has been used in the curative treatment of soft tissue sarcomas located in the vicinity of critical structures such as the spinal cord, optic apparatus, bowel, and kidney, with local control comparable to that with EBRT and with acceptable toxicity.[337,338]

Hyperfractionated photon beam radiation has been combined with intravenous iododeoxyuridine as a radiosensitizer. Among 36 patients treated in this fashion, and with a median follow-up of 4 years, the local control rate was 60%.[339]

Definitive radiation combined with chemotherapy is described under "Combined Chemoradiotherapy for Primary Localized Extremity/Truncal Sarcoma."

Chemotherapy for Primary Localized Extremity/Truncal Sarcoma

Surgery and radiation therapy remain the mainstay for local control of soft tissue sarcoma. Because up to half of patients with primary non-GIST sarcomas who achieve adequate local control of disease will develop distant metastasis, it was hoped that adjuvant chemotherapy would help to decrease the frequency of distant metastasis and increase overall survival. Anthracyclines are the agents most active against metastatic sarcoma, so they have been universally employed in adjuvant trials, alone or in combination.

More than 15 studies of adjuvant therapy for soft tissue sarcoma have been performed (Table 90.3), but most of them were small and therefore lack statistical power to detect small changes in overall survival. Among the larger randomized trials, one trial with 104 patients showed some benefit to adjuvant epirubicin (an anthracycline) plus ifosfamide.[340] Overall survival at 5 years was better in the chemotherapy arm ($p = 0.04$), although neither overall survival as a whole nor disease-specific survival was significantly different between arms ($p = 0.05$). Interpretation of the trial was complicated by subtle imbalances in the distribution of patients on the control and treatment arms. Nevertheless, this study has been used as a rationale for adjuvant ifosfamide plus an anthracycline. Another large, randomized trial showed some benefit to adjuvant cyclophosphamide, vincristine, doxorubicin, and dacarbazine (CYVADIC) for patients with sarcoma in the head, neck, or trunk, but not for those with sarcoma in the extremities.[341]

Other randomized trials have shown no benefit to anthracycline-based in the adjuvant[342–344] or neoadjuvant (preoperative)[345] setting. This includes the largest trial to date of adjuvant chemotherapy for patients with sarcoma, which examined adjuvant doxorubicin plus ifosfamide; however, this trial has been criticized for using a low ifosfamide dose and for heterogeneity in tumor site, size, and grade.[344] The trial had nonsignificant improvements in survival outcomes in patients with grade III tumors, limb lesions, and tumors >10 cm; these characteristics continue to be indications for considering adjuvant or neoadjuvant therapy in some specialty centers.

PRACTICE OF ONCOLOGY

1276   **Practice of Oncology** / Sarcomas of Soft Tissue and Bone

TABLE 90.3

Adjuvant Chemotherapy Studies in Soft Tissue Sarcoma

Study	Regimen	Doxorubicin Dose (mg/m²)	No. of Evaluable Patients	Extremity Patients	Median Follow-Up (y)	Reported DFS Control (%)	Reported DFS Treated (%)	Reported OS Control (%)	Reported OS Treated (%)	Ref.
NCI extremity	CAM	50–70	65	65	7.1	**54**	**75**	60	83	506–508
NCI head and neck, trunk, breast	CAM	50–70	31	0	3.0	49	77	58	68	509
NCI retroperitoneal	CAM	50–70	15	0	2.4	84	50	100	47	510
GOG	Dox	60	156	0	NA	47	59	52	60	511
MDA	VACAR	60	47	43	>10	**35**	**55**	57	65	512,513
Mayo Clinic	VCActVAD	50	61	48	5.4	65	83	70	90	349
EORTC	CYVADIC	50	317	216	6.7	**43**	**56**	55	63	341
Intergroup	Dox	70–90	78	50	1.7	55	73	70	91	347,514
ECOG	Dox	70	30	18	>4.9	55	66	52	65	515
Boston	Dox	90	42	25	>3.8	62	67	72	71	516,517
SSG	Dox	60	181	155	3.3	56	62	70	75	342
Rizzoli	Dox	75	77	77	NA	45[a]	73[a]	70[a]	**91[a]**	518,519
UCLA	Dox	90	119	119	2.3	54[a]	58[a]	80[a]	85[a]	520
Fondation Bergonié	CYVADIC	50	59	36	4.4	**32**	**81**	**54**	**87**	521
RPMI	Dox	60–75	19	0	5.0	46	75	36	63	522
ISSG	I/Epi	Epi at 120	104	104	7.5	37	45	43	58	340,523
EORTC/NCIC	Dox/I	50	134	123	7.3	52	56	64	65	345
Austria	AI with DTIC (q 2 wk)	50	58	47	8	56	61	59	61	343,524
Siena	Epi or I/Epi	Various	88	46	7.8	44	69	47	72	525
EORTC 62931	Dox/I	Dox at 75	351	234	8	53	55	68	67	344
SARCGYN	API	50	81	0	4.3	**41**	**55**	55	72	526
1997 meta-analysis	Any	Various	1,568	904	9.4	44	52	53	57	347

DFS, disease-free survival; OS, overall survival; NCI, National Cancer Institute; CAM, cyclophosphamide, doxorubicin, methotrexate; GOG, Gynecologic Oncology Group; Dox, doxorubicin; MDA, MD Anderson Cancer Center; VACAR, vincristine, doxorubicin, cyclophosphamide, dactinomycin; VCActVAD, vincristine, cyclophosphamide, dactinomycin alternating with vincristine, doxorubicin, dacarbazine; EORTC, European Organisation for Research and Treatment of Cancer; CYVADIC, cyclophosphamide, vincristine, doxorubicin, dacarbazine; ECOG, Eastern Cooperative Oncology Group; SSG, Scandinavian Sarcoma Group; NA, not available; UCLA, University of California at Los Angeles; RPMI, Roswell Park Memorial Institute; ISSG, Italian Sarcoma Study Group; I, ifosfamide; Epi, epirubicin; NCIC, National Cancer Institute of Canada; AI, doxorubicin, ifosfamide; DTIC, dacarbazine; API, doxorubicin, cisplatin, ifosfamide.
Note: Significant differences between chemotherapy and control are indicated by **bold type**. DFS and OS are not necessarily indicated at the median follow-up time.
[a] Some patients on the control arm received chemotherapy.

The small size of most adjuvant chemotherapy trials in sarcoma makes interpretation difficult because they lacked statistical power to detect small (e.g., 10% to 20%) changes in overall survival. Therefore, several meta-analyses have been performed,[346] the most rigorous of which was published in 1997,[347] then updated in 2008.[348] Tumor histology for each patient was recorded, but pathology review was not centralized. The 2008 update included 18 trials and 1,953 patients. Chemotherapy was associated with significantly lower risk of local recurrence (odds ratio [OR] = 0.73; 95% CI = 0.56 to 0.94; p = 0.02). Overall survival was not significantly improved with single-agent doxorubicin (OR = 0.84; 95% CI = 0.68 to 1.03; p = 0.09), but it was improved with doxorubicin combined with ifosfamide (OR = 0.56; 95% CI = 0.36 to 0.85; p = 0.01). With the updated data, the absolute risk reduction for death was 5% with adjuvant doxorubicin alone and 11% for doxorubicin combined with ifosfamide.[348]

Note that the adjuvant chemotherapy trials have two possible sources of bias. First, in several of the older studies, a significant proportion of patients were ineligible for analysis. Second, patients who enroll in clinical trials are healthier overall and survive longer than nonrandomized patients, as demonstrated in a study from the Mayo Clinic.[349] In addition, some of the older trials included a number of patients with low-grade or small tumors.

If there is a benefit to adjuvant or neoadjuvant chemotherapy for patients with soft tissue sarcoma overall, it is small. Neoadjuvant chemotherapy has been particularly successful with pediatric sarcomas such as rhabdomyosarcoma and soft tissue Ewing sarcoma, and there is some substantiation of benefit for synovial sarcomas and myxoid–round cell liposarcomas, two subtypes that are chemosensitive in the metastatic setting.[38] The best standard of care that can be offered is a thorough discussion with patients regarding possible options and outcomes.

As previously noted, preoperative chemotherapy has been very successful in the management of predominantly pediatric sarcomas such as Ewing sarcoma and osteosarcoma. This approach has been extended to adult soft tissue sarcomas. Preoperative chemotherapy can make subsequent surgery easier. It also potentially treats micrometastatic disease early, before acquisition of resistance. In addition, before surgery the primary vasculature is still intact for drug delivery. Preoperative chemotherapy can guide postoperative treatment based on pathologic review of the tissue response after chemotherapy. In experimental models, preoperative chemotherapy eliminates a postoperative surge in growth of metastases noted after resection of primary tumors.[298]

Isolated Limb Perfusion. Perfusion of limbs requires isolating the arterial and venous system of the limb by means of a tourniquet and obtaining access to arteries and veins that supply the limb. The arterial and venous supplies of the limb are connected to an extracorporeal circulation system to reoxygenate and circulate the blood. After isolation of the limb, care is taken to ensure that there is no leakage of the circuit into the systemic circulation; technetium-labeled albumin is injected into the circuit, and a probe is used over the heart to ensure isolation of the bypass circuit. Because mild hyperthermia may make chemotherapy more effective in some clinical settings, the blood of the circuit is often warmed to 39°C to 40°C.

Limb perfusion has involved a number of chemotherapeutic agents, such as melphalan, nitrogen mustard, dactinomycin, and doxorubicin. The most effective has been melphalan when given with tumor necrosis factor (TNF). The largest reported series using this technique included 246 patients with primary or recurrent sarcomas that would otherwise require amputation or marked loss of function.[350] These patients were treated with one and occasionally two isolated limb perfusion sessions. After isolation of the extremity, melphalan (10 to 13 mg/L limb volume) was perfused into the limb with a dose of TNF 10 times the lethal dose for humans, under mild hyperthermic conditions. The omission of TNF led to a decrease in tissue dose of melphalan, probably because TNF affects the tumor vasculature. Residual tumor was surgically removed 2 to 4 months after limb perfusion. With a median follow-up of 3 years, 71% of patients had successful limb salvage. Later, a randomized trial demonstrated that lowering the TNF dose to 0.5 mg reduced systemic toxicity without reducing the objective response rate.[351]

It is difficult to compare isolated limb perfusion to standard chemotherapy, given the heterogeneity of patients in the two types of studies. In aggregate, the response rate does appear to be higher in the perfusion studies than in the infusion studies. However, isolated limb perfusion requires substantial expertise and specialized dedicated equipment. Complications of this technique include shock (from systemic leak of TNF); infection; chronic damage to skin, muscles, and nerve; persistent edema; and arterial or venous thrombosis. Experience has led to a decrease in the incidence and severity of complications. Isolated limb perfusion does appear to hold promise for at least a subset of patients who would otherwise require amputation for local control and has been approved for such patients in Europe. Studies are under way to examine the use of regional limb infusion, which would not require bypass machines, as a simplified means of treating otherwise unresectable extremity sarcomas and whether local perfusion may be a viable method for managing patients with pelvic sarcoma.[352]

Combined Chemoradiotherapy for Primary Localized Extremity/Truncal Sarcoma

High-risk soft tissue sarcomas (i.e., those of large size, deep location, and high grade) present a significant dual threat: locally and at distant sites. For this reason, researchers at the Massachusetts General Hospital explored a dose-intense chemoradiation strategy in 48 patients with localized, high-grade, large (>8 cm) soft tissue sarcomas of an extremity.[353] The protocol consisted of three courses of doxorubicin, ifosfamide, mesna, and dacarbazine (MAID) interdigitated with two 22-Gy courses of radiation (11 fractions each). Patients with microscopically positive surgical margins received a 16-Gy boost dose (in eight fractions). Their 7-year actuarial disease-specific survival was 81% and overall survival 79%.[354] Among matched historical controls, survival was significantly lower: 50% and 45%, respectively (p <0.005). As expected, toxicities in the chemoradiation group included significant wound-healing complications in the lower limbs (in 29%).[355] One patient died from late marrow dysfunction attributed to chemotherapy. A multicenter study that included 64 patients treated according to the same protocol also showed significant toxicity, with three patients (5%) having experienced fatal toxicities (myelodysplasia in two and sepsis in one). Moreover, another 53 patients (83%) experienced a variety of grade 4 toxicities, and 5 patients required amputation.[356] At almost 8 years of follow-up, overall survival approximated 70%, which the authors consider compares favorably to expected outcomes for the high-risk cases included in the protocol.[357] Clearly, the use of early neoadjuvant chemoradiotherapy delivered in this fashion is appealing for patients at very highest risk. However, the results require confirmation in prospective trials, especially because of the local and systemic toxicity associated with the protocol.[355]

Multimodal Management of Locally Recurrent Extremity/Truncal Sarcoma

Local recurrence remains a significant factor in long-term morbidity and mortality. Locally recurrent sarcomas are difficult to treat and are more likely to recur, probably as a result of prior contamination of tissue planes as well as intrinsically aggressive tumor biology. Follow-up data confirm that salvage is almost invariably possible, but there is no impact on long-term survival. For patients who undergo resection of their recurrent lesion, important factors in outcome are the size and timing of the recurrence.[358] Patients with a local recurrence that grew to >5 cm in <16 months had a 4-year disease-specific survival of 18%, compared to 81% for patients with a local recurrence of ≤5 cm in >16 months.

Surgery. Repeat resection is the treatment of choice for locally recurrent soft tissue sarcoma in almost any site that is amenable to low-morbidity surgical resection. Repeat resection usually encompasses all palpable tumor and all potential microscopic foci present in adjacent tissues traversed during previous surgical procedures. Assuming the recurrent disease can be surgically resected, adjuvant radiation therapy should be considered for the vast majority of patients.

Radiotherapy. Radiotherapy in the recurrent setting should follow the same principles applicable to the treatment of primary tumors. However, the issues are more complex and often dominated by two confounding issues. First, tissue planes will likely have been disrupted from prior interventions and the true anatomic areas at risk are difficult to define, so there is often need to compromise in the choice of target volumes. Second and more problematic is prior radiotherapy, which results in serious concerns about long-term morbidity, especially affecting bone and neurovascular tissues. The substantial rates of serious complications for salvage reoperation and reirradiation[359] indicate that salvage therapy should be performed cautiously with careful monitoring of side effects.

Torres et al.[360] retrospectively reviewed 62 patients who had undergone prior resection and EBRT, being treated for an isolated first local recurrence of soft tissue sarcoma arising within a previously irradiated field. Local control rates were similar for patients undergoing reirradiation compared to those who did not undergo reirradiation, but complications that required outpatient or surgical management were more common in reirradiated patients (80% versus 17%; $p < 0.001$). The authors have acknowledged that selection for the different treatments may confound interpretation of these results. A study at the Princess Margaret Hospital examined patients with recurrent disease treated with surgery with or without reirradiation (predominantly BRT).[361] The local control rate among 10 reirradiated patients was 100%, compared to only 36% among the 11 patients treated with no further irradiation. However, follow-up was short: median, 24 months. As a general principle, if radiotherapy is used in a previously irradiated field, BRT is often recommended. However, the possibility of complications is real and these decisions must be approached cautiously.[361–363]

When EBRT is used, various strategies can be considered to ameliorate the risk from reirradiation. First, precision techniques such as IMRT should generally be used to optimize volume with exclusion of uninvolved tissues. Second, preoperative, rather than postoperative, radiotherapy may be used to reduce dose and volume to the lowest level possible. Third, treatments may involve a smaller dose per fraction to minimize damage to late responding normal tissues; these fractionation approaches normally require treatment more than once per day. Intraoperative radiotherapy (IORT) has also been considered for salvage therapy, and careful dose limitation to major nerves, ureters, and kidneys may reduce related complications in complex anatomic regions.[364,365] Salvage IORT was analyzed in a multicenter study of 103 patients managed from 1986 to 2012; the 5-year local control was 60%, and 16% of patients had toxicities of grade 3 or greater.[366]

Management of Primary Localized Retroperitoneal Sarcoma

Surgical Management of Primary Localized Retroperitoneal Sarcoma

For retroperitoneal sarcomas, as for extremity or truncal sarcomas, primary surgical resection is the dominant therapeutic modality. A treatment algorithm is shown in Fig. 90.7. Preoperative bowel preparation is important, not because of tumor invasion, but because resection without encompassing the intestine is often technically difficult. For retroperitoneal tumors situated near a

kidney, it is important to evaluate renal function, in particular to establish adequate contralateral renal function, to allow nephrectomy when appropriate.

The major issue in resection of visceral and retroperitoneal lesions is adequate exposure. Thoracoabdominal incisions, rectus-dividing incisions, and incisions extending through the inguinal ligament into the thigh may improve exposure and enhance the ability to achieve a complete resection. The availability of venovenous bypass, adequate and appropriate anesthetic, and blood replacement therapy are all important issues for many of these large lesions.

Although resection of adjacent organs is common,[281] there is only limited evidence that a more extensive resection of adjacent organs affects long-term survival. Two retrospective studies have attempted to examine the role of aggressive surgery with wide margins (including resection of uninvolved adjacent organs) in patients with primary retroperitoneal sarcoma. Both studies show a reduction in the cumulative incidence of local recurrence with aggressive surgery treatment, but no improvement in overall survival, an increase in operative morbidity, and a high (11%) reoperation rate.[367,368] In addition, both these series have significant problems with patient selection bias, unequal follow-up times, and heterogeneous adjuvant radiation and chemotherapy strategies between treatment groups, making interpretation of the local recurrence results difficult. The sacrifice of uninvolved organs beyond what is required to achieve a complete retroperitoneal sarcoma resection should not be performed on a routine basis unless part of a clinical trial, as more extended resections do not seem to improve survival. Further insight into the value of resection of adjacent organs comes from two reviews,[281,369] in which nephrectomy was performed in 46% of cases but the kidney itself was rarely involved. For example, in one of these reviews,[281] only 2 of 30 nephrectomy specimens showed true parenchymal invasion. The resection of a kidney makes little sense when the vena cava is the closest margin. Nevertheless, resection of the kidney is often necessary because of encompassment of the kidney or involvement of the hilar renal vasculature.

The overriding principle is not to be reluctant to resect adjacent organs should they be involved by tumor. Conversely, one should not resect uninvolved organs if they are not the limiting factor for the tumor margin.

The primary factor in outcome is complete surgical resection, followed by the grade of the lesion. Illustrating the importance of complete resection, in a series 693 adult patients with primary retroperitoneal sarcoma resected at MSKCC, the 10-year disease-specific survival for those who had incomplete resection (18%) was substantially worse than that of patients who had complete resection (53% for those with negative margins and 54% for those with positive margins). There is some evidence that incomplete resection is associated with prolonged survival.[370]

Resectability rates vary widely but seem independent of histologic type, grade, or size.[281] The basis for unresectability is usually the presence of peritoneal implants or extensive vascular involvement. Operation should be reserved for those patients for whom complete resection is at least possible, if not probable, and for patients in whom palliation can be achieved. However, it is often difficult to decide how much palliation can be achieved by incomplete removal of tumor.

Retroperitoneal sarcomas remain a major clinical challenge. Most of these tumors are large, making it difficult to obtain adequate margins of resection. Compounding the problem, the proximity of normal organs such as small bowel, large bowel, kidney, and liver makes delivery of therapeutic doses of radiation therapy either difficult or impossible.

Jaques et al.[281] reported the experience with 114 patients at MSKCC from 1982 to 1987. Half of the patients had liposarcoma, whereas 29% had LMS. A total of 65% of patients with primary sarcoma underwent a complete resection; of these, 53% required adjacent organ resection and 40% required resection of more than one adjacent organ. Despite complete resection, local recurrence

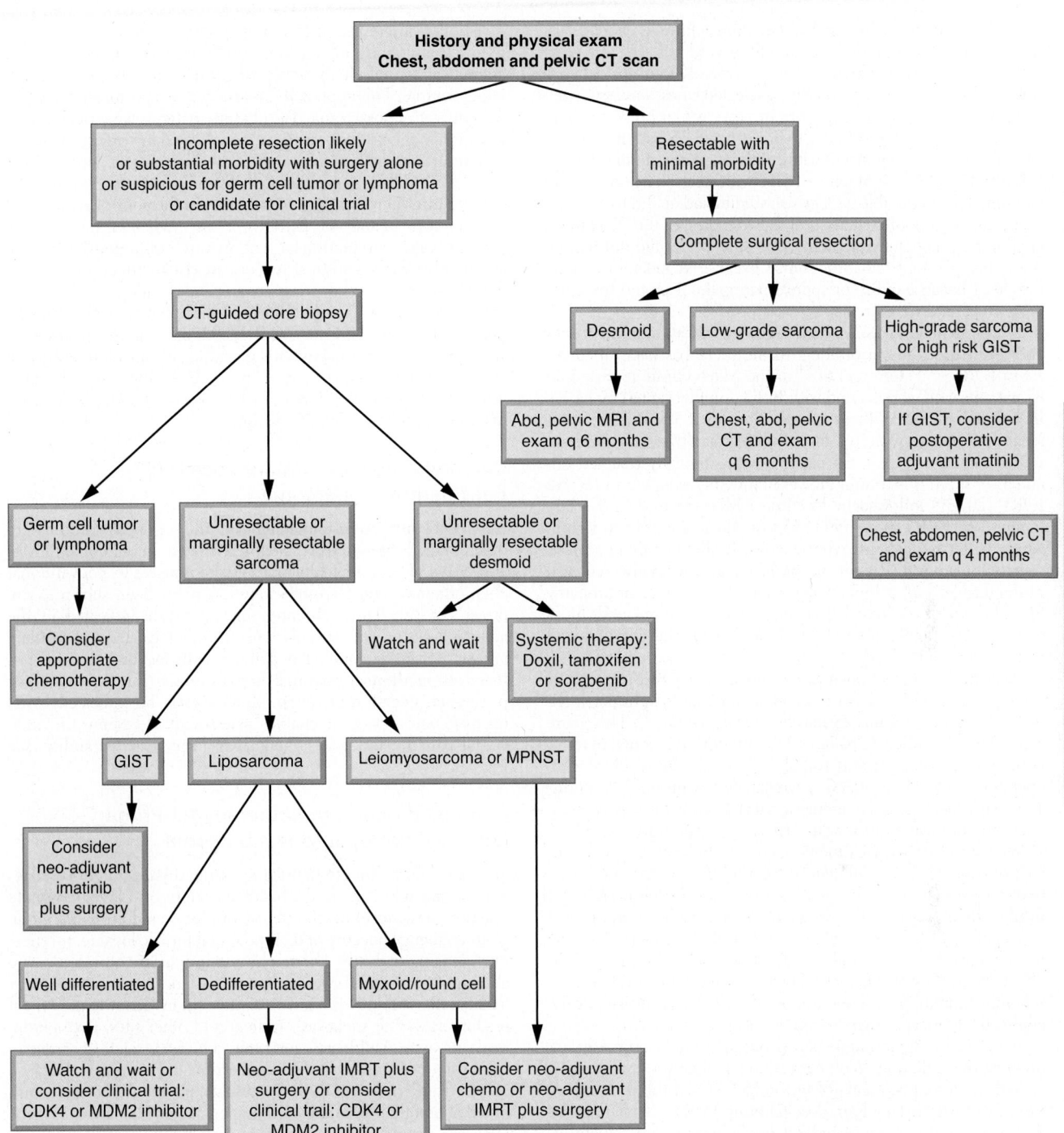

Figure 90.7 Algorithm for the management of retroperitoneal and visceral sarcoma. CT, computed tomography; MRI, magnetic resonance imaging; GIST, gastrointestinal stromal tumor; MPNST, malignant peripheral nerve sheath tumor; IMRT, intensity-modulated radiation therapy.

developed in 40% to 50% of cases. There is a clear need for adjuvant local therapy. Of importance, local recurrence is a problem for both high-grade and low-grade lesions. Jaques et al.[281] reported similar local recurrence rates, but very different times to recurrence: a median of 15 months for high-grade and 42 months for low-grade sarcomas.

Radiation Therapy for Primary Localized Retroperitoneal Sarcoma

The retroperitoneum is a site that may be particularly suited to preoperative radiotherapy for sarcoma, because the tumor has frequently displaced bowel from the target volume. Postoperatively, in contrast, loops of bowel are frequently tethered or fixed within the target area. Postoperative radiation for retroperitoneal sarcoma has high toxicity and unproven efficacy; it can also complicate surgery for later recurrences. Therefore, it is not recommended.

Trials involving preoperative radiotherapy for retroperitoneal sarcoma conducted at the MD Anderson Cancer Center[371] and the Princess Margaret Hospital[372,373] are instructive because the acute toxicity of preoperative radiotherapy was prospectively separated from overall toxicity, and the evidence supports an excellent tolerance profile. In the Princess Margaret Hospital study, 40 patients received median preoperative radiotherapy doses of

45 Gy in 25 fractions; the median radiation volume exceeded 7 L. After 9 years' median follow-up, overall survival was 70% at 5 years and 64% at 10 years, which compares favorably to historical controls.[373] BRT, used postoperatively in selected cases, was associated with toxicity and did not appear to improve tumor outcome. The MD Anderson Cancer Center trial evaluated 35 patients treated with doxorubicin concurrent with escalating doses of radiotherapy (18 to 54 Gy) at 1.8-Gy/fraction; IORT with electron beam was also attempted when feasible.[371] The two studies had qualitatively similar results. In a pooled analysis of these studies, of the 72 patients eligible for preoperative radiotherapy, only 2 (3%) did not receive the entire planned radiation course because of radiation-related toxicity, 1 because of tumor approximating the liver and the other because of grade 3 anorexia.[374]

With the need to deliver higher doses of radiation to the tumor and lower doses to surrounding tissue, there has been an interest in IORT.[375] Petersen et al.[376] at the Mayo Clinic reported on 87 patients who were treated with IORT, supplemented by EBRT in 92% of patients. With a median follow-up of 3 years, the 5-year local control rate was 58% and survival was 50%. In a randomized trial at the NCI,[377] 35 patients with surgically resected sarcomas of the retroperitoneum were randomly assigned to receive IORT (20 Gy) followed by low-dose EBRT (35 to 40 Gy) or to higher-dose EBRT alone (50 to 55 Gy). Local control was significantly better for patients who received IORT, but there was no impact on survival. Patients in the IORT arm, who also received misonidazole, had a higher incidence of peripheral neuropathy than those who received EBRT alone. On the other hand, those who received higher-dose EBRT alone had a higher incidence of radiation enteritis.

At MSKCC, resection was combined with EBRT and HDR intraoperative BRT at 12 to 15 Gy in an attempt to optimize treatment effect and minimize toxicity to critical anatomy.[378] This phase 1 and 2 trial included 32 patients with primary and recurrent retroperitoneal sarcoma. Twenty-five of the patients also received postoperative EBRT (45 to 50.4 Gy). Median follow-up was 33 months, and 5-year local recurrence–free survival was 62%. Five-year actuarial rates of local control were 74% for primary tumors and 54% for recurrent tumors. Treatment-related morbidity was observed in 34% of patients. The most common complication was GI obstruction (six patients, 19%: five grade 3, one grade 5), followed by GI fistula (three patients, 9%: two grade 3, one grade 5). Peripheral neuropathy, a common complication of IORT, developed in only two patients (6%, both grade 2). Treatment-related mortality was 6% ($n = 2$). Given the morbidity associated with IORT and its inherent limitations in large tumor beds, IORT is unlikely to be applicable to most primary retroperitoneal sarcomas.

The ideal radiation approach is one that could dose-escalate preoperative radiation. With conventional radiation, the preoperative dose cannot be escalated beyond 50.4 Gy without incurring excessive toxicity. However, dose-painting IMRT allows targeted dose escalation to areas at highest risk. The posterior structures, where there are no intestines, can receive 60 Gy, while the remaining tumor volume receives 50.4 Gy, thus respecting the tolerance. A report from the University of Alabama showed the feasibility of such an approach.[379] Fourteen patients were treated with preoperative radiation to the whole target volume to 45 Gy, then the area that was judged to be at risk for positive margin was separately boosted with IMRT to bring the total dose to 57.5 Gy. Only one patient experienced grade 3 nausea and vomiting. Eleven patients had complete resection with negative margins. With a median follow-up of 12 months, there was no late toxicity related to radiation. Further dosimetric studies showed the technical feasibility of delivering doses as high as 75.2 to 82.8 Gy using this technique.[379]

On a similar theme, Yoon et al.[380] suggested a coordinated strategy to optimize radiotherapy target coverage without enhancing toxicity by combining advanced radiotherapy techniques, including proton-beam radiotherapy, with aggressive en bloc resection.

Another interesting IMRT strategy for retroperitoneal sarcoma is to focus entirely on the posterior tumor attachment without attempting to include the remaining tumor mass in the irradiated target volume. This approach was assessed in a prospective study of patients with liposarcoma. Twenty-nine patients were treated with radiation to the posterior tumor area followed by surgery; matched patients treated with surgery alone served as controls. Although the tolerance profile was excellent, neither local control nor disease-specific survival was improved over that in the control group.[381]

The true benefit of IMRT—or any radiation therapy—for patients with retroperitoneal sarcoma is continuously debated among physicians who treat this disease. In an attempt to provide definitive guidance, the European Organisation for Research and Treatment of Cancer (EORTC) has opened a randomized, phase 3 trial (EORTC 62092 - 22092) to examine relapse-free survival in patients treated with neoadjuvant radiation compared to those treated with surgery alone.[382] Until the results become available, surgical resection alone remains the standard of care for patients with retroperitoneal sarcoma.

Chemotherapy for Primary Localized Retroperitoneal Sarcoma

The most common histologic types in the retroperitoneum (well-differentiated liposarcoma, dedifferentiated liposarcoma, LMS, and MPNST) are typically not very responsive to conventional chemotherapy, and chemotherapy has never been shown to improve survival. Thus, chemotherapy is rarely indicated in the adjuvant setting for patients with completely resected primary retroperitoneal sarcoma. For patients with locally advanced primary retroperitoneal sarcoma that is unresectable or marginally resectable, neoadjuvant chemotherapy may be indicated based on histologic type as it enables assessment of response in individual patients and occasionally may improve resectability (see Fig. 90.7).

Combined Chemoradiotherapy for Primary Localized Retroperitoneal Sarcoma

One of the difficulties in managing retroperitoneal sarcoma relates to the disparate nature of the histologic subtypes. Large, low-grade liposarcomas constitute about 50% of lesions and present a prodigious challenge because of their potential for late local recurrence, often leading to death. The remaining tumors are of intermediate and high grade, with LMS a frequent histology, and not only recur locally (often rapidly) but have a significant tendency to peritoneal seeding as well as metastasis to liver and other sites. Retroperitoneal sarcomas of all histologies often present as relatively large lesions due to asymptomatic growth within the abdomen. Because of the adverse nature of these sarcomas, a potential strategy is combined chemotherapy and radiotherapy as a neoadjuvant to surgery. However, not many groups have approached this problem specifically, presumably in large part due to the paucity of evidence for a benefit of chemotherapy in these tumors, as outlined previously. Another reason is the wish to minimize toxicity in patients already burdened with medical issues related to the treatment of large tumors.

The feasibility of preoperative combined chemoradiotherapy was demonstrated in a prospective trial from MD Anderson Group.[371] Eligibility was limited to intermediate- and high-grade tumor. Doxorubicin was infused at a low dose (20 mg/m^2 per week for 4 to 5 weeks). Radiation was delivered in escalating doses ranging from 18 Gy to 50.4 Gy total radiation. The protocol also included a 15-Gy electron-beam IORT boost to the bed of the resected tumor. The radiation was very well tolerated, with only 2 (18%) of 11 patients having grade 3 or 4 nausea. These promising feasibility results remain experimental and ideally should prompt the design of randomized trials to address the efficacies of the different elements of the protocol.

Multimodal Management of Locally Recurrent Retroperitoneal Sarcoma

Surgery. Retroperitoneal recurrences are often detected on routine screening with imaging, or patients may present with pain or nonspecific symptoms. After workup to determine the extent of disease, patients with isolated local recurrence should be carefully evaluated to determine feasibility of re-resection. Because current chemotherapy is ineffective for the majority of patients with liposarcoma and because toxicity limits adequate dosing by radiation therapy, complete surgical resection remains the most effective treatment modality. When complete gross resection can be achieved, operation for local recurrence should be attempted. Complete resection is usually possible in 80% of patients presenting with first recurrence and in 60% to 70% of patients presenting with second or subsequent recurrence of their retroperitoneal sarcoma. Surgery may be combined with neoadjuvant systemic therapy or IMRT dependent on the histologic type or subtype, growth rate, and extent of disease.

The most difficult decisions in retroperitoneal liposarcoma are whether a patient is likely to benefit from reoperation and when to perform the reoperation; often a period of monitoring is appropriate. With the aim of informing decisions on the likely benefit from re-resection, an analysis at MSKCC assessed factors that predict survival after re-resection.[383] Of 105 patients who had local recurrence after complete resection of a primary retroperitoneal liposarcoma, 61 underwent complete resection of their first local recurrence. The independent predictors of disease-specific survival were local recurrence size and growth rate and primary histologic variant and grade. Despite aggressive operative management, patients with a local recurrence growth rate >1 cm per month had poor outcomes that were similar to those of patients who were not treated with resection. Only patients with local recurrence growth rates of <0.9 cm per month had improved survival following aggressive resection of the local recurrence. Based on these results, for patients presenting with asymptomatic local recurrence and growth rates ≥1 cm per month, we now recommend treatment with systemic chemotherapy or novel targeted therapy trials. Surgery is considered in this subgroup only if they develop symptoms, such as obstruction or bleeding, that do not respond to medical management. If the local recurrence growth rate is <1 cm per month, immediate surgery is recommended for all symptomatic patients and for asymptomatic patients whose local recurrence is impinging on critical structures (particularly if further growth may result in the need to sacrifice critical organs) or has a solid appearance on CT scan (suspicious for dedifferentiation). Many asymptomatic patients with a well-differentiated–appearing local recurrence that is well away from critical structures may be safely followed off any therapy and monitored to determine if they develop other sites of disease before recommending complete surgical resection. Such an approach can extend the interval between surgical resections, and it enables the surgeon to be more confident that all sites of known disease are encompassed with the planned procedure. Debulking, however, has limited overall value in terms of long-term survival of patients with recurrent lesions.

Radiotherapy. Many variables must be considered in deciding whether to use radiotherapy for locally recurrent retroperitoneal sarcoma. If diffuse intra-abdominal recurrence is present, then an accurate delineation of a target volume is unlikely to be feasible. With each successive recurrence, the situation becomes ever more challenging, and the chances of significant acute and chronic complications from reirradiation increase exponentially. Reirradiation is especially associated with increased morbidity due to adhesions from previous procedures. However, when complete gross resection appears technically feasible and the patient is asymptomatic and otherwise well, the authors favor aggressive treatment, preferably combined with preoperative radiotherapy to a conventional volume if the patient has had no prior radiotherapy.

If prior radiotherapy has been used, subsequent treatment is much more complicated, and alternative strategies may be considered. These need to be determined case by case, but possibilities include using IMRT to a limited region of the retroperitoneum preoperatively. In centers with access to them, IORT or proton beam may provide additional options. In all these deliberations, one needs to recognize that the value of radiotherapy remains unproven and the main motivation to use it is the adverse behavior of the tumor. Most important, attempting to eradicate unresectable gross disease using radiotherapy is generally considered futile, and the dose required to attempt this has real potential to damage critical intra-abdominal structures.

Chemotherapy. Intraperitoneal chemotherapy after debulking of peritoneal metastases has been advocated but remains an investigational approach.

Serious Complications of Primary Treatment

Wound Complications

Wound complications, including infection and dehiscence, are common after resection of extremity sarcomas. Wound complications are exacerbated by adjuvant radiation and chemotherapy, which inhibit wound healing. Early studies on the effects of doxorubicin and X-rays on wound healing in animal models demonstrated that the timing and the combination of antineoplastic agents were critical factors.[384] Radiation or chemotherapy used just before, or in close juxtaposition to, the time of wounding significantly impaired wound healing. This appeared to be due to inhibition of new collagen synthesis.

The influence of preoperative chemotherapy on the risk of wound complications is a complex topic.[385] Perhaps the most comprehensive study is that from the MD Anderson Cancer Center.[386] The authors compared morbidity of radical surgery for soft tissue sarcoma in 104 patients who received induction chemotherapy before surgery and in 204 patients who had surgery first. The most common complications were wound infections and other wound complications; more important, however, the incidence of surgical complications was no different for patients who underwent preoperative chemotherapy than for patients who underwent surgery alone, both for those with sarcomas of the limbs (34% versus 41%) and for those with retroperitoneal or visceral sarcomas (29% versus 34%). Note, however, that the data are sparse and entirely retrospective, and the effects of preoperative chemotherapy are often confounded by concomitant use of preoperative radiotherapy (e.g., in two concurrent radiotherapy plus MAID studies, discussed earlier in this chapter).[356] Preoperative chemotherapy is often delivered by the intra-arterial route, often combined with radiotherapy at the same time, with apparently greater morbidity than when radiotherapy is given alone.[387] Therefore, the risks of intra-arterial preoperative chemotherapy cannot safely be inferred from the results with the "usual" intravenous chemotherapy.

The effects of adjuvant BRT on wound complications have been studied at MSKCC. One finding is that, when radiation delivery via afterloading catheters begins more than 5 days after surgery, the rate of major wound complications falls, approaching that with surgery alone.[313] In the randomized BRT trial,[319] the overall rate of wound complications (wound infection or the need for further operative intervention) in the BRT arm (24%) did not differ significantly from that in the control arm (15%; $p = 0.18$). However, the rate of reoperation was higher in the BRT arm (9% versus 1%; $p = 0.03$). The other covariable that contributed to wound reoperation was the width of the excised skin. If the width was >4 cm, the reoperation rate was 9%, but if the width was ≤4 cm, the rate was 1% ($p = 0.02$).

These types of complications are not unique to BRT but have been shown with external beam irradiation as well.[290,388] In the Canadian trial discussed earlier,[293] which compared preoperative and postoperative irradiation in 190 patients, wound complication was a primary end point of the study. Wound complications were defined as secondary wound surgery, hospital admission for wound care, or need for deep packing or prolonged dressings within 120 days after tumor resection. Patients undergoing preoperative radiation had a significantly higher rate of wound complications than those undergoing postoperative radiation (35% versus 17%; $p = 0.01$).[293] The rates of wound complications in both arms were higher than those in many other studies, most probably because of methods of assessment. In this study, the criteria for an acute wound complication were prospectively applied with a specific requirement for reporting at frequent intervals for the initial 4 months after surgery. In studies using retrospective evaluation, in contrast, complications such as prolonged dressings or packing (often administered to outpatients) may be overlooked.

The rate of wound complications may be reduced by the implementation of IMRT protocols in major referral centers. Careful planning may minimize radiation exposure to planned skin flaps; however, to date outcomes have been variable, and widespread reproducibility of this methodology is difficult.[302] In situations in which wound complications may be anticipated (because of the magnitude of the wound, extent of the resection, prior radiation, and so on), serious consideration should be given to using fresh vascularized tissue in the form of transpositional or free grafts to cover the defect before the placement or delivery of radiation therapy. This approach appears to markedly diminish postoperative morbidity, although the point is difficult to prove because of possible selection bias: nonprimary closure is more common for patients expected to have larger tumors and more problematic resections. In the Canadian trial, the only significant variables associated with wound complication in multivariate analysis were the timing of radiotherapy (i.e., preoperative versus postoperative), the volume of tissue removed at surgery, and the location of the tumor (upper versus lower extremity). The manner of wound closure, comorbidity, age, smoking history, and treatment center had no apparent influence on the risk.[294] Similar observations were made in the MD Anderson Cancer Center study.[389]

Note that the risk of would complications appears to be almost entirely confined to lower-extremity lesions.[293,377,389] This observation implies that, when deciding on the timing of radiotherapy, the risk of wound complications is a less important consideration for sites other than the lower extremities. This may make preoperative radiotherapy advantageous in sites for which restricting radiotherapy dose and volumes may have long-term benefit. Such sites include proximal arm (to protect overlying brachial plexus and lung) and the head and neck (to protect critical anatomy). In the authors' prospective series of patients with head and neck sarcomas treated with preoperative radiotherapy, wound complication rates were relatively low, even in patients with adverse anatomic presentations.[390]

Bone Fracture

Little is known about the impact of adjuvant radiation and chemotherapy on bone fracture. Among 145 patients with soft tissue sarcoma who underwent limb-sparing surgery and postoperative radiation with or without chemotherapy, the fracture rate was 6%.[391] For patients treated with adjuvant BRT in the MSKCC randomized trial, the rate of fracture was 4%, compared to 0% in the control arm, but difference was not statistically significant ($p = 0.2$).[392] A similar fracture risk (7%) was reported for 285 patients with soft tissue tumors treated by radiation and surgery, and that risk of fracture was not related to the dose, timing, and fractionation of radiation therapy.[393] This series had a high rate of complications, including fracture nonunion (45%) and deep infection (20%). These authors suggested that prophylactic intramedullary fixation of the femur should be considered for patients who undergo resection of large tumors in the anterior compartment of the thigh requiring extensive periosteal stripping and adjuvant radiation therapy.

The factors associated with pathological fracture of the femur were analyzed in a study of 205 patients with soft tissue sarcoma of the thigh treated with adjuvant radiation (115 patients with BRT alone, 59 with EBRT alone, and 31 with both).[394] The 5-year actuarial risk was 8.6%. On multivariate analysis, the only variable significantly associated with fracture was periosteal stripping ($p = 0.01$).[394] Other factors were significant in a long-term prospective study from the Princess Margaret Hospital of 364 patients with lower-extremity sarcomas treated with adjuvant EBRT (without adjuvant chemotherapy). The rate of pathological fractures was significantly higher with higher radiotherapy doses (10% for 60 or 66 Gy versus 2% for 50 Gy), and was higher with postoperative than with preoperative radiation therapy.[395]

IMRT dosimetry factors associated with fracture risk were investigated in a case-control study at the Princess Margaret Hospital.[396] The factors that appeared to reduce the risk of radiation-induced fracture were (1) volume of bone irradiated to ≥40 Gy kept below 64%, (2) mean dose to bone <37 Gy, (3) maximum dose anywhere along the length of bone <59 Gy, and perhaps (4) lower mean radiotherapy volume. Knowledge of these types of volumetric dosimetry data should facilitate the planning of dose objectives for IMRT. In fact, in short-term follow-up, patients treated with image-guided IMRT had no fractures in a recently reported series from the Princess Margaret Hospital group.[303]

Other Complications

Another complication encountered with adjuvant radiation is peripheral nerve damage. In the MSKCC randomized trial of BRT, the rate was 9% in the BRT arm compared to 5% in the control arm ($p = 0.5$).[319] In a study of 62 patients treated with postoperative radiation, the rate of peripheral nerve damage was 1.6%.[397] Evolving results suggest that patients treated with postoperative radiotherapy also have worse rates of fibrosis and peripheral edema compared to those receiving preoperative radiotherapy.[297]

A common concern of practitioners is whether postoperative radiotherapy affects the bone and soft tissue grafts used for musculoskeletal reconstructions. Evidence suggests that postoperative radiotherapy can ordinarily be administered 3 to 4 weeks after grafting without detriment to the graft union.[398] Soft tissue reconstruction (e.g., tissue transfer in the form of pedicle flaps, free flaps, or skin grafts) carries a theoretical risk of radiotherapy-related wound breakdown that may require reoperation. This risk has been shown to be very low (5%), and most tissue transfers tolerate subsequent adjuvant radiation therapy well.[399] The authors have observed a higher rate of wound complications that necessitated reoperation in patients who received BRT. It is unclear whether flaps and skin grafts are inherently more susceptible to breakdown in the immediate postoperative period or whether this is a direct result of BRT.

Multimodal Management of Advanced Disease

Control of the primary tumor can be achieved in the vast majority of patients with soft tissue sarcoma, but close to one-half of patients with non-GIST sarcomas succumb to metastatic or locally advanced disease. Median survival from the time metastases are recognized is on the order of 12 months, and 20% to 25% of patients are alive at 2 years. Even the most active chemotherapeutic options are of limited value and are associated with serious and potentially life-threatening toxicity. Newer agents offer at least the hope of less toxicity and greater efficacy than anthracyclines and ifosfamide, at least for selected subtypes.

Outcomes in patients receiving systemic therapy for metastatic sarcoma were quantified in the SArcoma treatment and Burden of Illness in North America and Europe study of 213 patients treated in North America and Europe. Patients were treated with an average of 2.7 lines of chemotherapy. A favorable response was observed in 83% of patients after treatment with first-line chemotherapy (most commonly adriamycin-based), but only 42% and 38% of patients treated with second- and third-line therapies, respectively. Median progression-free survival (PFS) after favorable response was only 8.3 months.[400]

Patients with metastatic sarcoma often feel well at the time that a radiograph or CT reveals metastases and may remain free of symptoms for months or years. Thus, with many patients, alleviation of symptoms is not an immediate concern, although progression is inevitable. Surgical resection can provide selected patients with prolonged periods of freedom from disease, and radiation therapy provides palliation for individual patients who have localized symptomatic metastases. Optimal treatment of patients with unresectable or metastatic soft tissue sarcoma requires an appreciation of the natural history of the disease, close attention to the individual patient, and an understanding of the benefits and limitations of the therapeutic options.

Surgical Resection of Metastatic Disease

Approximately 20% of patients with a soft tissue sarcoma of an extremity or the trunk develop pulmonary metastases, and in the majority, the lung remains the only clinically evident site of metastasis. The histopathology of 1,643 pulmonary metastases has been described.[401] Only 30% of all pulmonary metastases are detected at the time of diagnosis of the primary tumor; among those detected in follow-up, 80% are within 2 years of diagnosis. In retrospective series, 20% to 30% of patients who undergo metastasectomy are alive 5 years later.

In a series of 716 patients with primary extremity sarcoma treated at MSKCC, pulmonary-only metastases occurred in 19%, or 135 patients. Of these, 58% underwent thoracotomy, and 83% of those had a complete resection of their tumors. In the 65 patients who had a complete resection of their tumors, 69% had recurrence with pulmonary metastases as their only site of disease. Median survival time from complete resection was 19 months, and 3-year survival was 11% among all those presenting with lung metastasis only, 23% among those undergoing complete resection, and 0% among those who did not undergo thoracotomy.[260] Incomplete resection was no better than no operation. Chemotherapy had no obvious effect on survival, whether or not the patients underwent thoracotomy. Moreover, at the MD Anderson Cancer Center, response to chemotherapy given before pulmonary resection did not predict improved outcome[402] (in contrast to the experience with chemotherapy for primary sarcoma). After resection of pulmonary metastases with curative intent, 40% to 80% of patients will have recurrence in the lung. Repeat resection is often possible.[403] In a series of 86 patients who underwent repeat resection, predictors of poor survival included more than three lesions, a lesion >2 cm, and high-grade histology. If two or three of these factors were present, disease-specific survival was 10 months.

Histology-Specific Chemotherapy for Advanced Disease

Single Agents. Doxorubicin has been the mainstay of chemotherapy for advanced sarcoma. In recent trials that evaluated doxorubicin (75 mg/m^2) as a front-line treatment, overall response rates were 14% for advanced disease and 20% for metastatic disease, and median PFS rates were 4.6 and 5.2 months, respectively.[404,405] A dose–response relationship has been demonstrated.[406,407] Studies with liposomal doxorubicin showed fewer side effects than those with doxorubicin and similar response rates, despite the fact that the liposomal doxorubicin studies may have had a relatively high proportion of resistant sarcoma subtypes, such as GIST.[408]

Ifosfamide has approximately the same efficacy as doxorubicin. In the past, ifosfamide dosing was limited by severe urothelial toxicity (hemorrhagic cystitis). The uroprotective agent mesna has markedly changed the ability to administer both ifosfamide and cyclophosphamide, and ifosfamide doses as large as 14 to 18 g/m^2 or more over 1 to 2 weeks have been given.[409] Some evidence suggests a dose–response relationship for ifosfamide.[410] This is borne out by the results of the many phase 2 trials examining the use of high-dose ifosfamide in metastatic soft tissue sarcoma. Higher doses of ifosfamide occasionally produce responses in patients who do not respond to lower doses of this or other alkylating agents. Note that synovial sarcoma appears to be particularly responsive to ifosfamide.[411] A new, less toxic metabolite of ifosfamide, TH-302, is under study in phase 3 for patients with metastatic soft tissue sarcomas. TH-302 is a hypoxia-activated prodrug, a bromo-isophosphoramide mustard that is reduced and activated under hypoxic conditions. Although data suggest that TH-302 synergizes with doxorubicin in vitro, it will be up to the randomized study to help determine whether TH-302 and doxorubicin truly have efficacy beyond that of doxorubicin alone or combined with ifosfamide.

A third drug with modest activity in sarcoma is dacarbazine.[412] Dacarbazine has frequently been used in combination chemotherapy with doxorubicin (see "Combination Chemotherapy for Advanced Soft Tissue Sarcoma"). It is given in a variety of schedules, from intravenous continuous infusion as part of the MAID protocol to one large bolus. The major side effects of dacarbazine are nausea and vomiting, which have been substantially reduced with the use of serotonin-antagonist antiemetics. Antiemetic use allows for dacarbazine administration in a single treatment rather than in divided doses. Temozolomide, the oral equivalent of dacarbazine, appears to have some activity against LMSs as well.

Pazopanib, an inhibitor of multiple tyrosine kinases (vascular endothelial growth factors 1, 2, and 3, PDGF receptor A, PDGF receptor B, and KIT), has been evaluated for soft tissue sarcoma. The PALETTE study, a phase 3 randomized trial, enrolled 369 patients with metastatic nonadipocytic soft tissue sarcoma who had been treated with an anthracycline-based regimen. PFS was 4.6 months in patients who received pazopanib versus 1.6 months for those on placebo (p <0.0001). Thus, pazopanib is now a viable systemic treatment for patients with advanced disease.[413] Ongoing studies are evaluating pazopanib in patients with adipocytic sarcomas and chondrosarcoma.

The most significant cytotoxic agent in soft tissue sarcomas is probably trabectedin (ecteinascidin, ET-743), with notable response rates in myxoid–round cell liposarcoma and some responses in LMS. Trabectedin binds the minor groove of DNA and bends the DNA, interfering with transcription and blocking cell cycle progression. Its potency appears to depend on the cell having an intact nucleotide excision repair system. Its toxicity is largely hematologic and hepatic, with significant posttreatment increases in levels of transaminases and occasionally alkaline phosphatase and bilirubin; these toxicities resolve spontaneously and appear to be mitigated with the use of glucocorticoids. In early studies enrolling patients with a variety of sarcoma subtypes, responses were noted in 14 of 189 patients (7%).[414] When tested as first-, second-, or third-line therapy, a 7% minor response rate was also noted.[415] The most exciting recent data regarding trabectedin are its reported activity against myxoid–round cell liposarcoma. In this subtype, the radiologic response rate of single-agent trabectedin is on the order of 50% to 60%—activity as great as that of imatinib in GIST.[124–126,416] Based on these data, trabectedin was approved for use in Europe in 2007.[415,417,418] Although it is not approved in the United States as of 2013, it remains available in an expanded access program. A phase 2 trial of trabectedin in LMS has been reported with response or stable disease in 60% of patients.[419] Trabectedin is also being evaluated in a randomized phase 3 study comparing the efficacy of trabectedin versus dacarbazine in patients with liposarcoma and LMS (NCT01343277) and in combination with doxorubicin in patients with uterine and nonuterine LMS.

As for other single agents, cisplatin and carboplatin have produced occasional responses in phase 2 trials. However, single-agent vincristine, etoposide, and dactinomycin appear to be inactive in adult sarcomas, unlike in pediatric sarcomas. The taxanes also show little activity in sarcomas save for angiosarcoma. More recent data indicate that gemcitabine may have modest activity, dependent on the administration schedule.[420] Few investigational drugs have demonstrated meaningful activity in soft tissue sarcoma, except for epirubicin, a close relative of doxorubicin, now approved for commercial use.

Immunotherapy for sarcoma, which was used in some of the earliest studies in sarcoma adjuvant chemotherapy, is seeing renewed interest, although little success. Cytokines alone appear to be ineffective in sarcoma, as does nonspecific immunotherapy with bacterial cell wall components. Clinical studies at the NCI and elsewhere are beginning to examine vaccines of peptides that represent the fusion proteins observed in specific sarcoma subtypes. Lymphokine-activated killer cell and other T-cell immunotherapy with cytokines was investigated in a very small number of patients at the NCI without any observed responses. Dendritic cell vaccines and other forms of tumor-specific immunotherapy are undergoing investigation and may be relevant to patients with soft tissue sarcoma. The most important development in immunotherapy for soft tissue sarcomas is responses to a T-cell therapy directed against NY-ESO-1, a "cancer–germ cell" antigen found in the majority of synovial sarcomas. Cytotoxic T cells directed against NY-ESO-1 are generated in vitro and used as a therapeutic agent. Among six patients with synovial sarcoma with tumor expression of the NY-ESO-1 protein, 4 (67%) responded to the therapy.[421] This suggests that at least a subset of sarcoma types can be modulated by immunotherapy for patient benefit. A phase 2 study of NY-ESO1-directed T cells is ongoing as of September 2013.[422]

Combination Chemotherapy. A variety of chemotherapy combinations have been developed and examined in phase 2 trials. The typical backbone of combination regimens is doxorubicin (or its analogue epirubicin) with an alkylating agent, with or without other agents. One of the earliest combinations used was doxorubicin and dacarbazine, which has been well studied by the Southwest Oncology Group. Although initial analysis noted a 41% major response rate, a subsequent study of either a bolus or continuous infusion of the same regimen yielded a 17% response rate.[423]

CYVADIC has been widely used for sarcoma therapy in the United States and Europe. Although single-arm studies showed response rates as high as 71%, a randomized trial showed no significant difference in overall survival between patients given CYVADIC and those given doxorubicin as a single agent.[424] The two-drug combinations of ifosfamide with either doxorubicin[424] or epirubicin[425] have consistently given response rates >25%.

MAID was proven effective in metastatic soft tissue sarcoma in a large, randomized phase 2 trial. This trial examined MAID versus doxorubicin and dacarbazine. The study showed an increased response rate in the MAID arm (32% versus 17%; p <0.002).[426] In results that underscore the increased toxicity of aggressive chemotherapy regimens, there were 8 toxicity-related deaths in the study, 7 among the 170 patients treated with 7.5 g/m^2 of ifosfamide per cycle. This dose was decreased to 6 g/m^2 during the course of the study. In a univariate analysis, the two-drug arm showed a survival advantage (13 months versus 12 months for MAID); however, this difference was not significant in a multivariate analysis. As noted later in this chapter under "Dose Intensity," with the introduction of growth factors, the dose intensity of this regimen has become better tolerated.

The combination of cisplatin and mitomycin C with doxorubicin (MAP) yielded a 43% response rate in a study at the Mayo Clinic.[427] The activity of the MAP regimen has been confirmed in a randomized Eastern Cooperative Oncology Group trial.[428]

The response rate is greater for ifosfamide combinations than for regimens without ifosfamide, highlighted in a 2008 meta-analysis.[429] However, 1-year survival was no different with the addition of ifosfamide to other chemotherapy.

A meta-analysis of data from seven large EORTC studies provided a very useful assessment of predictors of outcome after doxorubicin- or epirubicin-containing combination chemotherapy.[430] In multivariate analysis of data for 2,185 patients, whose overall median survival was 51 weeks, the significant predictors of overall survival included good performance status before chemotherapy, lack of liver involvement, low histopathologic grade, long disease-free interval (time since initial sarcoma diagnosis), and young age. The predictors of response to chemotherapy were lack of liver involvement, young age, high grade, and liposarcoma histology (all p <0.01 in a multivariate analysis); LMS histology was not predictive independent of liver metastasis. Although lesions were not stratified by site, these data provide some of the best evidence that response rate does not necessarily correlate with overall survival. Furthermore, these data were collected before GIST was recognized as a distinct sarcoma subtype, and thus the question of liver metastases as a negative prognostic indicator becomes an open question.

Is combination chemotherapy better than single-agent doxorubicin for overall survival for patients with metastatic soft tissue sarcomas? Again, the concept arises that response rates may be dissociated from overall survival rates. Several phase 3 trials have compared combination chemotherapy with single-agent doxorubicin in patients with metastatic disease (Table 90.4), including two trials focused on uterine sarcoma. Several trials had better response rates with combination chemotherapy, but there was no survival advantage over single-agent doxorubicin. Complete responses during these studies were very rare and were not durable. These data argue that single agents are as effective as combination chemotherapy for patients with metastatic disease in terms of overall survival. However, some patients may be eligible for palliative resection of metastatic disease. For these patients, combination chemotherapy, which gives better response rates than single agents, can be considered.

A 2008 meta-analysis confirmed the benefit of combination chemotherapy in terms of response rate and the lack of benefit in terms of 1-year survival.[429] Further confirmation comes from two large international, randomized studies that evaluated the efficacy of single-agent doxorubicin versus doxorubicin plus ifosfamide (EORTC 62012)[404] or doxorubicin plus palifosfamide (PICASSO 3).[405] Both studies were run in the first-line setting in patients with high-grade metastatic soft tissue sarcoma. EORTC 62012 evaluated the efficacy of doxorubicin (75 mg/m^2) versus doxorubicin (75 mg/m^2) plus ifosfamide (10 g/m^2 over 4 days) in 455 patients. At a median follow-up of 56 months, overall survival, the primary end point, was not significantly different: 14.3 months for the combination versus 12.8 months for single-agent doxorubicin. Of note, most of the patients in the doxorubicin arm received ifosfamide (off-study) as a second-line treatment, which may have affected survival results. The objective response rate of the combination was 26.5% versus 13.6% with doxorubicin, and median PFS was 7.4 months versus 4.6 months, respectively (p = 0.002). However, these benefits were achieved at the cost of toxicity, with significantly more grade 3 or greater hematologic toxicity in the combination arm.

PICASSO 3[405] evaluated the efficacy of palifosfamide, a less toxic metabolite of ifosfamide,[431,432] as first-line treatment in patients with intermediate- or high-grade metastatic soft tissue sarcoma. At 113 sites, 447 patients were randomized to doxorubicin (75 mg/m^2) plus palifosfamide (150 mg/m^2 on days 1 to 3 of 21-day cycles) or doxorubicin plus placebo. At a median follow-up of 340 days, the two arms did not differ significantly in the primary endpoint, median PFS (5.98 months for doxorubicin plus palifosfamide versus 5.23 months for doxorubicin plus placebo; p = 0.18), nor did they differ in overall survival (15.9 months versus 16.9 months; p = 0.7). The overall response rate was 28.3% (doxorubicin plus palifosfamide) versus 19.9% (doxorubicin plus placebo).

These data underscore the need to pursue new directions, including seeking synergistic combinations of chemotherapies or

TABLE 90.4

Selected Randomized Trials In Advanced Disease

Group	Regimen	No. of Patients	Response Rate, % (Complete Response Rate, %)	Median Survival (mo)	Ref.
GOG[a]	A	80	16 (6)	7.7	527
	AD	66	24 (10)	7.3	
GOG[a]	A	50	19 (4)	11.6	528
	ACy	54	19 (8)	10.9	
COG	A	41	17 (2)	8.5	529
	ActL	25	4	8.1	
	ActLV	26	0	11.5	
	ActLCyclo	26	0	5.1	
ECOG	A	54	30 (7)	8.6	530
	CyAV	56	21 (5)	7.9	
	CyActV	58	12 (2)	9.5	
ECOG	A	94	18 (5)	8.0	531
	A	88	17 (3)	8.4	
	ADTIC	92	30 (6)	8.0	
ECOG	A	148	17 (4)	9.4	532
	AVD	143	18 (6)	9.0	
ECOG	A	90	20 (2)	<9	428
	AI	88	34 (3)	11	
	MAP	84	32 (7)	9	
EORTC	A	240	23 (4)	12.0	424
	AI	231	28 (5)	12.6	
	CYVADIC	134	28 (8)	11.7	
CALGB/SWOG	AD	170	17 (2)	13.3	426
	AID	170	32 (2)	11.9	
EORTC	A	112	14 (2)	10.4	533
	Epi	111	15 (3)	10.8	
	Epi	111	14 (3)	10.4	
EORTC	A	110	11.8 (NA)	12	534
	I	109	5.5 (NA)	10.9	
	I	107	8.4 (NA)	10.9	
SGRS	A	64	23 (NA)	NA	535
	AI	62	24 (NA)	NA	
EORTC meta-analysis	Any anthracycline-based regimen	2,185	26 (NA)	11.8	430
GOG[b]	I	91	29	8.4	536
	I/Paclitaxel	88	45	13.5	
SGRS	DTIC	52	4 (NA)	8.2	438
	DTIC/Gem	57	12 (NA)	16.8	
SARC	Gem	49	8 (0)	11.5	128
	Gem/Docetaxel	73	16 (3)	17.9	
PALETTE	Placebo	123	0 (0)	10.7	413
	Pazopanib	246	6 (0)	12.5	
SUCCEED	Placebo	364	28.6[c]	19.6	447
	Ridaforolimus	347	40.6[c]	20.9	
GOG[b]	I	91	29	8.4	536
	I/paclitaxel	88	45	13.5	

GOG, Gynecologic Oncology Group; A, doxorubicin; D, dacarbazine; Cy, cyclophosphamide; COG, Central Oncology Group; Act, actinomycin D; L, L-PAM (L-phenylalanine mustard); V, vincristine; Cyclo, cycloleucine; ECOG, Eastern Cooperative Oncology Group; DTIC, dacarbazine; I, ifosfamide; VD, vindesine; M, mitomycin C; P, cisplatin; CALGB, Cancer and Leukemia and Group B; SWOG, Southwest Oncology Group; EORTC, European Organisation for Research and Treatment of Cancer; NA, not available; Epi, epirubicin; SGRS, Spanish Group for Research on Sarcomas; Gem, gemcitabine; SARC, Sarcoma Alliance for Research through Collaboration; PALETTE, Pazopanib Explored in Soft-Tissue Sarcoma Phase 3; SUCCEED, Sarcoma Multicenter Clinical Evaluation of the Efficacy of Ridaforolimus.
[a] Uterine sarcoma only; response rates are only for subset of patients with measurable disease.
[b] Uterine carcinosarcoma only.
[c] Includes stable disease.

PRACTICE OF ONCOLOGY

combinations of standard cytotoxic chemotherapy with immuno-therapeutic approaches or with newer agents that may have more specific targets that would address the heterogeneity of sarcoma.

A combination that does appear to confer a survival benefit over single-agent chemotherapy is gemcitabine with docetaxel. Although as single agents gemcitabine and docetaxel have only borderline activity in sarcoma, the combination yielded a 53% response rate in a phase 2 study of patients with LMS, the great majority of whom had a uterine primary tumor.[433] These data have been confirmed in two other phase 2 studies,[434,435] and in a randomized phase 2 study of gemcitabine versus gemcitabine-docetaxel. In this study, the combination gave a RECIST response rate of 16% (versus 8% for the single agent).[436] More-over, the combination was associated with improved PFS and overall survival, the first such observation for a combination chemotherapy versus single agents. However, the combination was not compared to more standard single agents such as doxo-rubicin. Although other subtypes may respond to this combina-tion, LMS and PMFH were the two subtypes that responded most reproducibly, highlighting the subtype specificity even with standard cytotoxic chemotherapy agents. However, the benefit of the combination of gemcitabine and docetaxel over gemcitabine alone, at least for LMS, has been refuted by a recent study from France of patients with LMS.[437]

A second gemcitabine combination that appears beneficial is gemcitabine plus dacarbazine. A recent phase 2 trial random-ized pretreated patients to dacarbazine alone versus dacarbazine combined with gemcitabine.[438] Stable disease or response was ob-served in 25% versus 49%, respectively ($p = 0.009$), and PFS also favored the combination ($p = 0.005$).

Dose Intensity. A central tenet of oncology is that response to chemotherapy is a function of dose intensity. However, toxicity limits the amount of chemotherapy that can be given in any one cycle. If dose could be increased, responses might be better.

Increases in dose intensity can be facilitated by better support-ive care, such as the use of hematopoietic growth factors. Some of the aggressive regimens for treatment of metastatic sarcoma sat-isfy the American Society of Clinical Oncology guidelines for use of growth factors, given their high rate of associated febrile neu-tropenia.[439] Granulocyte macrophage–colony-stimulating factor (GM-CSF, sargramostim) decreased the myelosuppression seen with combinations such as CYVADIC or MAID[439] and high-dose ifosfamide. GM-CSF allowed for escalation of the dose of doxoru-bicin when given in combination with 5 g/m^2 of ifosfamide, with improvement in response rate.[440] GM-CSF has also been shown to allow increased dose intensity of the MAP combination, allowing addition of ifosfamide.

Similarly, granulocyte colony-stimulating factor (filgrastim) has been widely used to increase dose intensity and decrease myelo-toxicity of aggressive chemotherapeutic regimens such as MAID[441] or dose-escalated doxorubicin and ifosfamide. However, escalated doses (25% increase) in the MAID regimen do not appear to sig-nificantly increase the response rate. There may be other ways to achieve dose intensity. Ifosfamide at low dose over a long term (ap-proximately 2 weeks) showed responses in patients who did not respond to other forms of chemotherapy. However, as mentioned previously, the responsiveness to a particular regimen may not translate into increased survival.

Unfortunately, the cardiac toxicity of doxorubicin and the neph-rotoxicity and central nervous system toxicity of ifosfamide prevent much additional dose escalation. The next logical step is high-dose therapy with stem cell support, which remains investigational for pediatric sarcomas. Such treatment has been associated with long-term disease-free survival for a few patients with Ewing sarcoma, osteosarcoma, or rhabdomyosarcoma. Most of the patients, how-ever, relapsed rapidly, despite the relative chemosensitivity of these sarcoma types. High-dose therapy with stem cell rescue should not be considered for patients with metastatic sarcoma outside the

setting of a clinical trial. Given the poor results of high-dose ther-apy, the pursuit of agents with better activity against specific sar-coma subtypes remains a priority for treatment of relapsed disease.

Protein-Targeted Molecular Therapy for Advanced Disease

With the success of imatinib in GIST and chronic myelogenous leukemia, investigators are examining agents that block specific proteins. Angiogenesis inhibition has emerged as a new frontier for treatment of solid tumors of all types, including sarcoma. However, little efficacy has been seen for interferons, TNP-470 (AGM-1470), or SU5416, a vascular endothelial growth factor pathway inhibitor.[442] Bevacizumab, a recombinant humanized antibody against vascular endothelial growth factor, was studied in patients with angiosarcoma and epithelioid hemangioendothe-lioma.[153] Among 30 evaluable patients, 4 had a partial response and 15 had stable disease with a median time to progression of 26 weeks. This is encouraging and suggests that inhibitors of angiogenesis may have activity in select sarcoma subtypes, spe-cifically those of vascular origin. In addition, ongoing studies are evaluating the efficacy of angiogenesis inhibitors in combination with chemotherapy.

First- and second-generation tyrosine kinase inhibitors have yielded rather disappointing results when employed against non-GIST sarcomas. Imatinib was associated with a very low response rate in a study of 10 sarcoma subtypes.[443] Sorafenib, which tar-gets B-raf and vascular endothelial growth factor receptor-2, showed only minor activity in patients with soft tissue sarcomas, in particular angiosarcoma.[174]

Newer targeted agents are beginning to be assessed, based on the specific biology of sarcoma subtypes. For example, well-differentiated and dedifferentiated liposarcomas demonstrate amplification of *CDK4* and *MDM2* genes on chromosome 12q. The CDK4 inhibitor flavopiridol and the MDM2 inhibi-tor nutlin-3 show antitumor activity in vitro.[444] A CDK4-directed agent that appears active in clinical trials is the specific CDK4/6 inhibitor PD0332991.[445,446] A recent phase 2 trial enrolled patients with well-differentiated and dedifferentiated liposarcoma who were experiencing disease progression.[445] The study was restricted to patients with *CDK4* amplification (assessed by FISH). The median PFS of the trial was 18 weeks, with 66% of the 29 evaluable patients having stable disease at 12 weeks. This greatly exceeded the study's primary endpoint and suggests activity of CDK4/6 inhibitors in patients with well-differentiated and dedifferentiated liposarcomas.

Other targeted agents are under active examination in patients with soft tissue sarcoma. Ridaforolimus, in a phase 3 trial in pa-tients who had reached maximum benefit from other chemother-apy, showed a statistically significant but small benefit: a 3-week improvement in PFS (17.7 weeks versus 14.6 weeks for placebo; $p = 0.01$).[447] Pazopanib, on the other hand, showed a 3-month im-provement in PFS over placebo, leading to its approval by the US Food and Drug Administration for use in patients with advanced soft tissue sarcoma (other than adipocytic subtypes or GIST) after failure of standard systemic therapies.[448] Other new agents are under investigation in specific soft tissue sarcoma subtypes; some of these are discussed subsequently.

Recommendations for Patients with Advanced Disease

Low-grade tumors grow very slowly and may be less responsive to chemotherapy than higher-grade lesions. Accordingly, an asymptomatic patient with stable or only slowly progressive dis-ease can be simply observed. Resection of metastatic disease, in particular lung metastases, provides some patients with long-term survival and can be considered if the lungs are the only site of remaining disease.[260] In patients who present with completely resectable lung metastasis from an extremity primary, perioperative chemotherapy does not appear to be associated with better disease-specific or pulmonary PFS. This suggests that systemic chemotherapy has minimal, if any, long-term impact on the outcome of patients undergoing pulmonary resection for extremity sarcoma metastatic to lung.[449] Histology is of increasing importance in designing effective treatment regimens for patients who present with advanced disease so as to optimize response for the specific soft tissue sarcoma subtype.

Randomized studies have shown that combination chemotherapy can provide a better probability of a response than single-agent doxorubicin. However, overall survival for any combination chemotherapy has not been proven superior to that for single-agent doxorubicin. When a clinical response is needed—for example, before potential surgery for metastases—combinations of agents such as doxorubicin and ifosfamide should be considered, especially for patients with good performance status. For patients with poorer performance status, single-agent doxorubicin remains the standard of care. Pegylated liposomal doxorubicin can be considered in patients who would not tolerate the toxicity of doxorubicin, but the response rate may be lower than that of standard doxorubicin.

If the first-line therapy was doxorubicin alone, the second line can be single-agent ifosfamide or dacarbazine. For LMS, myxofibrosarcoma, PMFH, and perhaps other sarcoma subtypes, gemcitabine either alone or in combinations appears to be an excellent second-line alternative. Ifosfamide is useful against synovial sarcomas and myxoid–round cell and pleomorphic liposarcomas but less useful against LMSs. Dacarbazine has modest activity in soft tissue sarcoma and, with doxorubicin, constitutes a well-studied and well-tolerated combination in metastatic disease. Dacarbazine and temozolomide, an oral version of dacarbazine, show activity against LMS in particular. Patients with angiosarcoma may respond to taxanes, gemcitabine, vinorelbine, pegylated liposomal doxorubicin, sorafenib, as well as standard doxorubicin or ifosfamide chemotherapy. Rhabdomyosarcoma and Ewing sarcoma of soft tissue and bone both respond to single agents and combinations involving topoisomerase 1 inhibitors. Case reports suggest that patients with solitary fibrous tumors and extraskeletal myxoid chondrosarcomas may respond to sunitinib.[198,450] Given the paucity of treatment options and the wide variety of newly available kinase-specific agents, patients with advanced sarcomas are candidates for enrollment in phase 1 and 2 studies of new therapies.

Management of Specific Histologic Subtypes and Sites

Responses of soft tissue sarcoma to chemotherapy differ among the histologic subtypes. Pediatric sarcomas (Ewing sarcoma, osteosarcoma, and rhabdomyosarcoma) are known for their relative sensitivity to chemotherapy. Among adult sarcomas, synovial sarcoma and round cell liposarcoma are generally responsive to chemotherapy. GIST, alveolar soft part sarcoma, and low- to intermediate-grade chondrosarcoma are notorious for their resistance to standard cytotoxic chemotherapy agents. Therefore, an imbalance in the subtypes of sarcoma between patient groups can markedly affect the comparability of the outcomes of those groups.

The site of disease is also an important factor in outcome. Among large, low-grade liposarcomas, those in the extremities are less likely to recur than those in the retroperitoneum. Anatomy of metastatic disease can also affect overall response rates. For example, metastases to liver are less likely to respond to chemotherapy than metastases to another site; however, this may represent the tendency of GISTs, which are relatively chemoresistant, to metastasize to the liver. Variations in the site of disease or metastasis pattern may account at least in part for the different responses noted in randomized trials of chemotherapy for soft tissue sarcoma.

The following subsections give examples of specific sites or subtypes of sarcoma and their characteristics.

Leiomyosarcoma

Insight into the differential response of LMS versus other subtypes such as liposarcoma, synovial sarcoma, or PMFH can be obtained from subset analyses from a variety of randomized studies. Note that subset analyses cannot substitute for primary trials, but they can be useful in generating hypotheses. Doxorubicin appears to be active against LMSs, but ifosfamide appears to add little to the response rate.[428] This finding has been observed in other studies, but there may be contamination of the LMS group with what would today be classified as GISTs. For uterine LMSs, a modest response to ifosfamide was observed in one small study but not in most other studies.

Among the newer agents, trabectedin showed a 6% response rate in a study of LMS and liposarcoma.[451] Gemcitabine and combinations have activity in LMSs as well.[128,433,435,452–456] In a small randomized trial for patients with metastatic or unresectable LMS (uterine and nonuterine), gemcitabine plus docetaxel showed no superiority over docetaxel alone in terms of response rate and PFS.[457] Thus, single-agent gemcitabine may prove to be an option in these clinical scenarios. Other targeted agents have been largely disappointing in patients with LMS.

Treatment of uterine LMS is discussed in greater detail in the section titled "Uterine Sarcoma."

Synovial Sarcoma

Patients with synovial sarcoma have relatively high rates of response to chemotherapy, but this may be due in part to patient factors. Compared to patients with other subtypes, patients with synovial sarcoma tend to be younger and therefore tend to have a better performance status, a positive predictor for response to chemotherapy in the EORTC database. A prognostic nomogram specific to primary synovial sarcoma enables the treating clinician to more precisely assess outcome for the individual patient and to identify those patients most likely to benefit from adjuvant or neoadjuvant chemotherapy.[272]

Ifosfamide-based chemotherapy, in a retrospective study of adult patients with primary extremity synovial sarcoma of ≥5 cm, was independently associated with improved disease-specific survival (hazard ratio = 0.3 compared to no chemotherapy; $p = 0.007$); the 4-year disease-specific survival rates were 88% with chemotherapy 67% with no chemotherapy.[458] Adjuvant or neoadjuvant ifosfamide-based chemotherapy should therefore be considered in the treatment of adult patients with high-risk primary synovial sarcoma of the extremities.

Ifosfamide appears to be active in patients with advanced synovial sarcomas as well. In a study of 13 patients, ifosfamide (at a high dose of 14 to 18 g/m²) had a 100% response rate.

Newer protein-directed therapies have shown only modest activity in synovial sarcoma patients. Pazopanib was associated with an approximate 15% response rate,[459] while its cousin sorafenib had a 0% response rate.[174] Sunitinib, mTOR inhibitors, and other kinase-specific agents are not well examined in synovial sarcoma to date. In the authors' experience, trabectedin has activity against synovial sarcoma. As previously noted, immunotherapy may be appropriate for a subset of patients.[421]

Pediatric Sarcomas in Adult Populations

Adults may develop a number of pediatric sarcomas, including Ewing sarcoma (in soft tissue or bone), rhabdomyosarcoma (usually pleomorphic), and osteosarcoma. These diseases differ from typical adult sarcomas in that they are considered systemic diseases even if they appear to be localized at initial presentation. Ewing sarcoma and rhabdomyosarcoma are typically much more sensitive to chemotherapy than are other adult soft tissue sarcomas.[460]

For adults with rhabdomyosarcoma or Ewing sarcoma, the standard of care is adjuvant (or neoadjuvant) chemotherapy. In osteosarcoma, long-term survival has been achieved in pediatric patients with the use of adjuvant chemotherapy. Unfortunately, adults with osteosarcoma are generally more resistant to chemotherapy than are children. Adults with a typical osteosarcoma of bone should receive neoadjuvant or adjuvant chemotherapy in addition to therapy for local control of the tumor. However, extraskeletal osteosarcoma is treated like other soft tissue sarcomas, largely due to the low response rates to chemotherapy observed in patients with metastatic disease.

Typical regimens for small cell pediatric sarcomas, specifically rhabdomyosarcoma and Ewing sarcoma, include the combination of vincristine, doxorubicin, and cyclophosphamide (dactinomycin, in particular, for rhabdomyosarcoma) and the combination of ifosfamide and etoposide. The MAID regimen also shows activity in pediatric sarcomas. There is debate about whether adults do worse than pediatric patients with the same stage of disease. Adults may present with more advanced-stage disease than do children or adolescents. In addition, adults are less likely than children to tolerate the aggressive regimens of chemotherapy used against these diseases. However, one retrospective study showed that older patients with rhabdomyosarcoma tolerated chemotherapy as well as the pediatric population but fared worse overall.[141] In Ewing sarcoma, the role of age in predicting outcome is controversial.[461] Adults with a sarcoma usually seen in pediatric populations should be included in pediatric protocols whenever feasible to help determine appropriate care for patients with these rare diagnoses.

A new target for therapy in pediatric sarcomas in adults and children alike is IGF 1 receptor (IGF1R), on the basis of the importance of IGF1R in Ewing sarcoma, rhabdomyosarcoma, and osteosarcoma.[462] Unfortunately, response rates for IGF1R antagonists are low, probably well under 20%, for entirely unclear reasons. Patients typically have relatively rapid progression after perceived minor benefits, suggesting that parallel pathways are at least in part to blame for the lack of greater activity of IGF1R antagonists as single agents.

Uterine Sarcoma

Uterine sarcomas are very rare, accounting for 3% to 7% of all uterine malignancies. The uterus is unique in that at least three different sarcomatous entities may arise from this organ: (1) LMS, a tumor of the endometrium; (2) endometrial stromal sarcoma (ESS), the least common type, which usually has very aggressive behavior; and (3) carcinosarcoma (also known as malignant mixed Müllerian tumor [MMMT]), composed of elements of carcinoma and sarcoma. Other uterine sarcomas such as rhabdomyosarcoma are uncommon.

For localized disease, surgery is the main treatment. The use of adjuvant radiation is controversial. Most studies showed some improvement in local control but not in survival. The efficacy of adjuvant radiation may be a function of disease subtype, because spread beyond the uterus (e.g., to lymph nodes) is common in patients with MMMT but less common in patients with LMS. The literature is well represented by EORTC study 55874, which examined radiation therapy versus surgery alone for 224 patients with International Federation of Gynecology and Obstetrics stage I or II uterine sarcoma.[463] Patients who received radiation had a lower risk of local relapse, a benefit observed for patients with MMMT and not LMS.

Uterine Leiomyosarcoma. After resection of a uterine LMS, adjuvant radiation therapy is generally not employed unless there is overt pelvic side-wall involvement with sarcoma. This concept is supported by the negative results for LMS in the phase 3 randomized study from EORTC, although this study was relatively small.[463]

Metastatic uterine LMS is responsive to doxorubicin but less sensitive to ifosfamide and to cisplatin. Uterine LMS is particularly responsive to the combination of gemcitabine and docetaxel,[433] apparently due to the synergy of this combination.[436] This combination was superior to gemcitabine alone in a Bayesian adaptive randomized phase 2 study that examined both LMS and non-LMS sarcomas, but the number of patients with LMS was relatively small, and the number of uterine LMS smaller still.[128] However, a randomized study from France refutes the synergy of gemcitabine and docetaxel, at least for LMS.[437] Another approach for LMS is vinorelbine and gemcitabine, a combination with at least modest activity, though not yet examined in a randomized fashion. Trabectedin has at least some activity in LMS as well.[416] In a phase 2 trial, 60% of patients had response or stable disease when treated with the drug.[419]

Recently, the French Sarcoma Group reported encouraging response rates in uterine LMS to the combination of trabectedin plus doxorubicin.[464] In this phase 2 study, the overall response rate was 55% and the median PFS at 12 weeks was 94%. These are encouraging data that warrant further investigations. Appropriately, a parallel study was performed in nonuterine LMS, recognizing the potential differences between uterine and nonuterine diseases. The results from the nonuterine cohort are forthcoming.

Although uterine LMS often expresses estrogen receptor or progesterone receptor, its rate of response to hormone therapy is very low. In a prospective trial of tamoxifen in treatment of uterine sarcomas, none of the 19 patients with LMS responded.[465]

Endometrial Stromal Sarcoma. The pathologic entity ESS is divided into low-grade ESS and undifferentiated uterine sarcoma (a high-grade lesion). Low-grade ESSs carry a t(7;17)(p15;q21) linking JAZF1 and SUZ12 (JJAZ1),[466] whereas high-grade ESSs have now been linked to an essential translocation involving YWHAE and FAM22A (NUTM2A) or FAM22B (NUTM2B).[467]

Low-grade ESS, but not undifferentiated uterine sarcoma, expresses estrogen and progesterone receptors, and responses to hormonal therapy are seen more in this subtype than in perhaps any other form of sarcoma.

For adjuvant therapy in patients with low-grade ESS, estrogen antagonists may be considered based on small clinical trials[468] but are of unproved benefit. There is no clear standard of care for undifferentiated endometrial sarcomas, although some investigators advocate for adjuvant chemotherapy.

In the recurrent setting, estrogen deprivation is an appropriate first-line therapy for low-grade ESS,[468] and surgical debulking can be considered as well because the disease tends to have an indolent course. For metastatic undifferentiated uterine sarcoma (and recurrent low-grade ESS), ifosfamide is active, as may be doxorubicin.[469]

Desmoid Tumor

Surgery has been considered the gold standard for treatment of desmoid tumors. However, any attempt at complete wide excision must be balanced by consideration for preserving function and the knowledge that local recurrence is common, because there are alternatives for management. Desmoids can be controlled with systemic therapy,[470–476] and they often either remain stable in size or occasionally regress spontaneously. For these reasons, in asymptomatic patients, an initial period of observation is often recommended to determine the biological behavior of the tumor. In a recent series of 142 patients with primary and locally recurrent desmoids, 83 patients were treated with such a "wait and see" policy, whereas 59 were initially offered medical therapy, mainly hormonal therapy and chemotherapy. The 5-year PFS was 50% for the "wait and see" group and 59% for the medically treated patients. This study suggests that many patients with primary and locally recurrent desmoids tumor can be safely managed by observation and thus can avoid the morbidity of surgery or radiotherapy.[477]

However, if a patient is symptomatic or progressing, consideration should be given to systemic therapy, surgery, or rarely radiation to prevent complications from disease progression.

Decisions on which of these modalities to employ can be guided by recent studies that have identified clinical factors predictive of postoperative recurrence. Risk of local recurrence is clearly associated with larger tumor size (>5 cm), site (particularly chest wall and extremity), and younger age at presentation, but not with microscopically positive margins. A nomogram to predict outcomes after resection has been developed and externally validated based data from almost 500 patients.[478,479] Large extremity desmoids in young patients recur in >50% of cases whereas patients with small, abdominal wall tumors have cure rates of >90%.[478] Surgery may, therefore, be employed for patients with small abdominal wall tumors if the tumor is growing or painful, whereas systemic therapy may be a better option for patients with unresectable disease or high risk of recurrence.

A range of systemic therapies has been employed in the management of desmoid tumors. A trial of nonsteroidal anti-inflammatory drugs or hormonal therapy can be considered in most patients. Sulindac and other nonsteroidal anti-inflammatory drugs have produced well-documented responses. There are anecdotal accounts of responses to hormonal manipulation such as tamoxifen, gonadotropin-releasing hormone agonists, or aromatase inhibitors. Responses have also been reported to single-agent doxorubicin and to less toxic liposomal pegylated doxorubicin,[472,480,481] as well as to combination chemotherapy at either standard or relatively low doses.[482] Responses to any of these agents can be slow, with patients needing several months or even 1 to 2 years of therapy to achieve maximum benefit, and therefore therapy should not be abandoned for stable disease, although changes should be made for toxicity. Complete responses to any of these agents are exceptionally rare, and so the timing of discontinuation of therapy in a patient with responding disease remains a difficult question and requires clinical judgment.

Tyrosine kinase inhibitors have been examined in the management of desmoid tumors. The lesions may occasionally respond to imatinib, although, as with other systemic therapy, it remains somewhat unclear whether some of the responses are truly due to treatment.[483,484] PDGF receptors have been identified in desmoid tumors, providing a possible mechanism of action of imatinib. Sorafenib administration has been associated with stable disease in 70% of patients, partial response in 25%, and significant improvement in symptoms in 70%.[485] These responses may occur rapidly, with resolution of symptoms occurring in <2 weeks. In a few instances, patients who experienced a good response to sorafenib have stopped the drug with no evidence of tumor regrowth. The mechanism of response to sorafenib is unclear.

The role of adjuvant radiation in management of desmoid tumors is controversial. Specialists are reluctant to give high doses of radiation to young patients with a disease that may not progress and that will never metastasize. Most authors recommend against postoperative radiation for patients with negative resection margins. Postoperative radiation is, however, more debatable for patients with microscopically positive margins. When such patients are treated with surgery alone, the rates of local control are approximately 56%.[486] Therefore, residual microscopic tumor from a primary lesion does not invariably lead to treatment failure, and adjuvant radiation may be omitted as long as local progression would not cause significant morbidity. The usual dose for adjuvant radiation for primary and most recurrent tumors is around 50 Gy.

Although adjuvant radiation is being used less, definitive radiation is emerging as an alternative to surgery. Ballo et al.[487] reported a 5-year local control rate of 69% for patients treated with radiation for gross disease. Others have reported similar rates.[486] The recommended dose for definitive radiation usually ranges from 56 Gy to 60 Gy. Although radiation is effective, many practitioners remain reluctant to prescribe it, given long-term risk of secondary malignancy and joint fibrosis in this young patient population.

Soft Tissue Sarcomas of the Hands and Feet

Wide local excision is the exception rather than the rule for sarcomas of the hands and feet due to the lack of muscular bulk and the proximity to neurovascular structures and bone. The overall prognosis is inferior to that of tumors at other sites in the extremity. At MSKCC, patients with hand tumors, even those ≤5 cm, had a survival rate significantly lower than that of patients with tumors at other distal extremity sites ($p = 0.0008$).[488]

Although the distal extremities have limited tolerance of radiotherapy, the data suggest that conservative resections with adjuvant radiotherapy should be considered for patients with sarcoma of the hand or foot. Lin et al.[489] reported on 115 patients with soft tissue sarcomas of the hand and foot treated between 1980 and 1998. The majority (95%) were referred after surgery elsewhere. Patients treated with definitive wide re-excision had a 10-year local recurrence–free survival of 88%, which was significantly better than the 58% for patients who did not have re-excision ($p = 0.05$). Radiotherapy improved local control in patients who did not undergo re-excision but did not improve local control in the small number of patients who had definitive re-excision with negative margins. Immediate amputation did not confer a survival benefit. Thus, limb-sparing treatment is possible in many patients with soft tissue sarcomas of the hand and foot. Amputation should be reserved for cases in which the tumor cannot be excised (or re-excised) with adequate margins without sacrifice of functionally significant neurovascular or osseous structures.[489] For patients who undergo adjuvant radiotherapy, special attention needs to be paid to technique to minimize complications and preserve function. Nevertheless, Bray et al.[490] reported good functional outcomes among 20 patients with tumors of the hand and forearm who received adjuvant radiation. At a mean follow-up of 37 months, the local control rate was 88%. Eighty-eight percent of those who survived and did not require amputation were able to return to work and activities of daily living with minimal or no functional limitation.[490]

PALLIATIVE CARE

Surgery

Surgeons have long employed palliative procedures to relieve surgical emergencies such as obstruction, bleeding, and perforation. More recently, attention has been focused on alleviating the more chronic complaints, such as pain, nausea, vomiting, inability to eat, and anemia. The treating surgeon should not allow attempts to improve survival to overshadow the goals of minimizing morbidity and relieving symptoms, so that a terminal patient may die with dignity and without undue suffering and pain.

A prospective analysis of 1,022 palliative procedures from MSKCC[491] demonstrated initial symptom resolution in 80% of patients, although 25% of them required further intervention for recurrent symptoms and 29% for new symptoms. The symptomatic improvements were noted within 30 days. For patients who underwent repair of a pathological fracture, 87% had resolution of bone pain or instability symptoms; for patients undergoing palliative tumor excision, 83% had resolution of wound or tumor hygiene symptoms. For GI symptoms, upper GI obstruction was resolved in 79% of cases, whereas mid- or lower GI obstruction was resolved in 90% of cases. However, palliative procedures were associated with significant morbidity (40%) and mortality (11%) and with limited overall survival (approximately 6 months). Factors associated with poor palliative outcomes were poor performance status, poor nutrition, weight loss, and no previous cancer therapy.

In a retrospective study of patients with intra-abdominal sarcoma who underwent a palliative procedure,[492] 71% of patients had improvement of symptoms at 30 days after the palliative operation, but only 54% of patients remained symptom free after 100 days. Patients with GI tract obstructive symptoms fared worse: 54% had symptomatic relief at 30 days, but only 23% of patients remained symptom free at 100 days. The operative morbidity was 29% overall and almost 50% among patients seeking to palliate GI obstruction. Postoperative mortality was 12%.[492]

In summary, decisions regarding the surgery for the palliation of symptoms from advanced sarcoma require precise surgical judgment that balances the medical prognosis of the sarcoma, the availability and success of nonsurgical treatments, and the individual patient's quality of life and life expectancy. Palliative decision making needs to be individualized and remain flexible as the sarcoma progresses. Decision making is best optimized through effective and frequent communication between the patient, family members, and the surgeon.

Palliative Radiation

Radiotherapy has a limited role in the palliation of soft tissue sarcoma. Notable applications are for relief of bone pain and for cessation of bleeding in fungating tumors; in both cases, response requires only moderate doses of radiation and can be rapid. However, radiotherapy is less effective for mass effects such as obstruction or compression, except for radiosensitive histologies such as rhabdomyosarcoma, myxoid–round cell liposarcoma, or synovial sarcoma. Palliative radiation is most relevant when a lesion lies in direct proximity to critical anatomy such as spine, small bowel, or base of skull and surgery is either impossible or undesirable.

New approaches to palliation that are being explored with promising results include hypofractionated dose schedules[493] and the precision methods SRS[494] and stereotactic body radiation therapy.[495–497]

Chemotherapy

The vast majority of the systemic therapy delivered to patients with metastatic sarcomas is given with palliative intent. Patients with poor performance status are poor candidates for systemic therapy, as they appear to have more adverse events for a given agent or regimen than more fit patients, and appear to benefit less frequently, again with newly diagnosed GIST being perhaps the exception to this rule. When standard chemotherapy agents are exhausted, there are no data that indicate that continuing any sort of systemic therapy is clinically beneficial, with the exception of imatinib in GIST. The means routinely employed to try to relieve symptoms of terminally ill patients include the use of pain medications orally, transdermally, intravenously, or intrathecally; oxygen as needed; and occasionally glucocorticoids. It is also worth emphasizing what is perhaps obvious but often brushed off in the course of a busy day: that even for very ill patients late in the course of their disease, communication with the patient and family will provide a sense of comfort.

FUTURE DIRECTIONS

Although the optimal combination and sequence of surgery, radiation, and chemotherapy remains controversial for sarcoma, optimal treatment increasingly depends on careful stratification of patients by histologic type and subtype and other important prognostic features. New methods for radiation delivery and tumor sensitization as well as continued advances in surgical reconstructive techniques will enable continued improvements in limb preservation and function as well as local control. However, despite these advances, almost 50% of patients with newly diagnosed sarcoma will eventually die from their disease. Metastatic sarcoma, whether

at the time of disease presentation or after local control of primary disease, remains an extremely difficult problem. The search for effective agents will be the focus of continuing research for patients with advanced disease. Outside a few responsive subtypes, the currently available chemotherapies have not improved survival and are associated with significant toxicity. Thus, there is a pressing need to develop new therapies based on selectively targeting the proteins and signaling pathways that drive the survival of specific sarcoma types and subtypes.

There is already a broad movement to identify and test antiangiogenic agents, specific kinase inhibitors, and novel chemotherapeutic agents such as trabectedin in an endeavor to match specific sarcoma subtypes to novel agents. A long effort to understand IGF1R signaling may pay off in the near future for pediatric sarcomas as well as a number of other cancers. Trials targeting the cell cycle (CDK4-RB1) and MDM2-p53 signaling pathways are currently under way in well-differentiated and dedifferentiated liposarcoma. Biological data and preclinical studies support trials using inhibitors of methylation and histone deacetylase in well-differentiated and dedifferentiated liposarcoma,[498] inhibitors of histone deacetylase in synovial sarcoma[499] and Ewing sarcoma,[500] lysine-specific demethylase 1 inhibition strategies in rhabdomyosarcoma, synovial and Ewing sarcoma,[501,502] and inhibitors of Hedgehog and Notch signaling in several sarcoma types.[503,504]

In the longer term, some of the results of gene expression arrays, next-generation sequencing, proteomics, tissue arrays, and mouse models of sarcoma may lead to a more comprehensive and precise determination of key molecular genetic alterations that drive sarcomagenesis for specific sarcoma types and subtypes. This knowledge will improve our ability to design new therapeutics for individual patients and to predict response to such therapy based not only on histologic type and subtype but also on pathway activation in the individual patient.

Because sarcoma is a relatively rare disease, it will be particularly important to conduct clinical trials that select patients based on the upregulation of a particular protein or signaling pathway, as this will increase the chance that the trial will have positive results.

Some biological interventions may have promise, such as inhibitory RNA interference strategies or immunotherapy with vaccines, monoclonal antibodies, dendritic cells, or T cells. Vaccines of the characteristic fusion proteins of sarcomas (or peptides thereof) will be tested in the near future for their effectiveness in the appropriate subtypes of sarcoma, such as many pediatric sarcomas. Vaccines that incorporate dendritic cells appear to be effective immunogens in preclinical studies. Preparations of the immunogenic glycolipids found in sarcoma cell membranes may also provide interesting agents for therapy.

Another emerging new class of therapeutics for cancer is nanoscale particles. Advances in nanotechnology have enabled the design of nanoparticles (in the size range 1 to 100 nm) that can interact with biomolecules on both the cell surface and within the cell.[505] Overexpressed cell-surface markers in sarcomas could be targeted to establish the presence of even single-cell metastases and to deliver high-potency chemotherapeutic or molecular agents to the cancer cell. Such selective nanoparticles could be used in the future to deliver antisense oligonucleotides or small interfering RNAs against cellular protein targets critical for sarcoma cell survival.

With an increasing number of molecular signaling pathways being actively investigated, the many new systemic treatments on the horizon, and the advances in selective radiation, drug, and nanoparticle delivery to sarcoma cells, outcomes for patients with sarcoma are likely to substantially improve in the coming decade.

SELECTED REFERENCES

The full reference list can be accessed at lwwhealthlibrary.com/oncology.

20. Henderson TO, Whitton J, Stovall M, et al. Secondary sarcomas in childhood cancer survivors: a report from the Childhood Cancer Survivor Study. *J Natl Cancer Inst* 2007;99:300–308.

24. Gladdy RA, Qin LX, Moraco N, et al. Do radiation-associated soft tissue sarcomas have the same prognosis as sporadic soft tissue sarcomas? *J Clin Oncol* 2010;28:2064–2069.

37. Dalal KM, Kattan MW, Antonescu CR, et al. Subtype specific prognostic nomogram for patients with primary liposarcoma of the retroperitoneum, extremity, or trunk. *Ann Surg* 2006;244:381–391.

38. Eilber FC, Eilber FR, Eckardt J, et al. The impact of chemotherapy on the survival of patients with high-grade primary extremity liposarcoma. *Ann Surg* 2004;240:686–695.

40. Singer S, Antonescu CR, Riedel E, et al. Histologic subtype and margin of resection predict pattern of recurrence and survival for retroperitoneal liposarcoma. *Ann Surg* 2003;238:358–370.

41. Fletcher CD, Gustafson P, Rydholm A, et al. Clinicopathologic re-evaluation of 100 malignant fibrous histiocytomas: prognostic relevance of subclassification. *J Clin Oncol* 2001;19:3045–3050.

78. Robinson DR, Wu YM, Kalyana-Sundaram S, et al. Identification of recurrent NAB2-STAT6 gene fusions in solitary fibrous tumor by integrative sequencing. *Nat Genet* 2013;45:180–185.

115. Bissler JJ, McCormack FX, Young LR, et al. Sirolimus for angiomyolipoma in tuberous sclerosis complex or lymphangioleiomyomatosis. *N Engl J Med* 2008;358:140–151.

118. Crago AM, Socci ND, DeCarolis P, et al. Copy number losses define subgroups of dedifferentiated liposarcoma with poor prognosis and genomic instability. *Clin Cancer Res* 2012;18:1334–1340.

125. Grosso F, Jones RL, Demetri GD, et al. Efficacy of trabectedin (ecteinascidin-743) in advanced pretreated myxoid liposarcomas: a retrospective study. *Lancet Oncol* 2007;8:595–602.

128. Maki RG, Wathen JK, Patel SR, et al. Randomized phase II study of gemcitabine and docetaxel compared with gemcitabine alone in patients with metastatic soft tissue sarcomas: results of sarcoma alliance for research through collaboration study 002 [corrected]. *J Clin Oncol* 2007;25:2755–2763.

146. Williamson D, Missiaglia E, de Reynies A, et al. Fusion gene-negative alveolar rhabdomyosarcoma is clinically and molecularly indistinguishable from embryonal rhabdomyosarcoma. *J Clin Oncol* 2010;28:2151–2158.

174. Maki RG, D'Adamo DR, Keohan ML, et al. Phase II study of sorafenib in patients with metastatic or recurrent sarcomas. *J Clin Oncol* 2009;27:3133–3140.

184. Wagner AJ, Malinowska-Kolodziej I, Morgan JA, et al. Clinical activity of mTOR inhibition with sirolimus in malignant perivascular epithelioid cell tumors: targeting the pathogenic activation of mTORC1 in tumors. *J Clin Oncol* 2010;28:835–840.

190. Ladanyi M, Antonescu CR, Leung DH, et al. Impact of SYT-SSX fusion type on the clinical behavior of synovial sarcoma: a multi-institutional retrospective study of 243 patients. *Cancer Res* 2002;62:135–140.

232. Guillou L, Coindre JM, Bonichon F, et al. Comparative study of the National Cancer Institute and French Federation of Cancer Centers Sarcoma Group grading systems in a population of 410 adult patients with soft tissue sarcoma. *J Clin Oncol* 1997;15:350–362.

239. Pisters PW, Leung DH, Woodruff J, et al. Analysis of prognostic factors in 1,041 patients with localized soft tissue sarcomas of the extremities. *J Clin Oncol* 1996;14:1679–1689.

270. Kattan MW, Leung DH, Brennan MF. Postoperative nomogram for 12-year sarcoma-specific death. *J Clin Oncol* 2002;20:791–796.

272. Canter RJ, Qin LX, Maki RG, et al. A synovial sarcoma-specific preoperative nomogram supports a survival benefit to ifosfamide-based chemotherapy and improves risk stratification for patients. *Clin Cancer Res* 2008;14:8191–8197.

287. Pisters PW, Pollock RE, Lewis VO, et al. Long-term results of prospective trial of surgery alone with selective use of radiation for patients with T1 extremity and trunk soft tissue sarcomas. *Ann Surg* 2007;246:675–681.

289. Pisters PW, Harrison LB, Leung DH, et al. Long-term results of a prospective randomized trial of adjuvant brachytherapy in soft tissue sarcoma. *J Clin Oncol* 1996;14:859–868.

290. Yang JC, Chang AE, Baker AR, et al. Randomized prospective study of the benefit of adjuvant radiation therapy in the treatment of soft tissue sarcomas of the extremity. *J Clin Oncol* 1998;16:197–203.

293. O'Sullivan B, Davis AM, Turcotte R, et al. Preoperative versus postoperative radiotherapy in soft-tissue sarcoma of the limbs: a randomised trial. *Lancet* 2002;359:2235–2241.

296. Davis AM, O'Sullivan B, Bell RS, et al. Function and health status outcomes in a randomized trial comparing preoperative and postoperative radiotherapy in extremity soft tissue sarcoma. *J Clin Oncol* 2002;20:4472–4477.

329. DeLaney TF, Liebsch NJ, Pedlow FX, et al. Phase II study of high-dose photon/proton radiotherapy in the management of spine sarcomas. *Int J Radiat Oncol Biol Phys* 2009;74:732–739.

347. Adjuvant chemotherapy for localised resectable soft-tissue sarcoma of adults: meta-analysis of individual data. Sarcoma Meta-analysis Collaboration. *Lancet* 1997;350:1647–1654.

350. Eggermont AM, de Wilt JH, ten Hagen TL. Current uses of isolated limb perfusion in the clinic and a model system for new strategies. *Lancet Oncol* 2003;4:429–437.

383. Park JO, Qin LX, Prete FP, et al. Predicting outcome by growth rate of locally recurrent retroperitoneal liposarcoma: the one centimeter per month rule. *Ann Surg* 2009;250:977–982.

437. Pautier P, Bui Nguyen N, Penel N, et al. Final results of a FNCLCC French Sarcoma Group multicenter randomized phase II study of gemcitabine (G) versus gemcitabine and docetaxel (G+D) in patients with metastatic or relapsed leiomyosarcoma (LMS). *J Clin Oncol* 2009;27:(abst 10527).

451. Demetri GD, Chawla SP, von Mehren M, et al. Efficacy and safety of trabectedin in patients with advanced or metastatic liposarcoma or leiomyosarcoma after failure of prior anthracyclines and ifosfamide: results of a randomized phase II study of two different schedules. *J Clin Oncol* 2009;27:4188–4196.

472. Pires de Camargo V, Keohan ML, D'Adamo DR, et al. Clinical outcomes of systemic therapy for patients with deep fibromatosis (desmoid tumor). *Cancer* 2010;116:2258–2265.

523. Frustaci S, Gherlinzoni F, De Paoli A, et al. Adjuvant chemotherapy for adult soft tissue sarcomas of the extremities and girdles: results of the Italian randomized cooperative trial. *J Clin Oncol* 2001;19:1238–1247.

PRACTICE OF ONCOLOGY

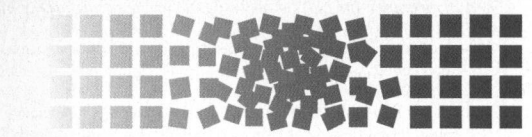

91 Sarcomas of Bone

Richard J. O'Donnell, Steven G. DuBois, and Daphne A. Haas-Kogan

INTRODUCTION

Sarcomas, defined as connective tissue malignancies, can be said to constitute one of the five major oncologic subgroups, together with disorders of the solid organs (carcinomas), the hematologic system, the skin, and the neurologic organs. Of all cancer types, however, sarcomas are the most rare, and in fact, exceedingly so. Furthermore, sarcomas of bone occur at just one-fourth the frequency of sarcomas of soft tissue. However, while soft tissue sarcomas have a multitude of histologic subtypes subject to a variety of grading classification schemes, bone sarcomas have just three distinct categories: chondrosarcoma, Ewing sarcoma, and osteosarcoma. While soft tissue sarcomas are rare in young individuals and occur with increasing frequency as the middle to late decades progress, bone sarcomas, for the most part, are more common in children and young adults, with some exceptions in later years. While the gold standard of treatment for soft tissue sarcomas remains surgery and radiation therapy, with chemotherapy reserved for tumors that are deep, high grade, and large, the management of bone sarcomas varies considerably, according to histology, grade, and stage. Finally, all high-grade sarcomas, whether of bone or soft tissue, share an overall survival rate on the order of 55% to 70%.

In light of their extreme rarity, the varied and complex nature of the care programs often involving national or international protocols, the high stakes nature of limb salvage surgery, and the potential lethality of these tumors, the National Comprehensive Cancer Network (NCCN) has promulgated that, "Primary bone tumors and selected metastatic tumors should be evaluated and treated by a multidisciplinary team of physicians with demonstrated expertise in the management of these tumors."[1] The paramount and central nature of this statement cannot be gainsaid, as judgment regarding management of these uncommon tumors must necessarily be left to the experts. Nonetheless, even the most general reader would err in not seeking a broader fund of knowledge and a higher level of understanding of bone sarcomas, as the hopeful and instructive paradigms offered herein can be of benefit to all oncologic patients, across practice strata. This chapter therefore seeks to be a primer on the diagnosis, staging, treatment, and surveillance of sarcomas of bone, with information ranging from basic principles to detailed descriptions of complex algorithms. After reviewing incidence, etiology, anatomy, pathology, screening, diagnosis, and staging of bone sarcomas, management will be discussed by treatment modality, with attention to stage. Ewing sarcoma, the prototypical high-grade sarcoma presumed to be potentially metastatic at presentation, will be explored first, in terms of the historically agreed-upon gold standards of chemotherapy and radiation therapy. Next, high-grade conventional osteosarcoma will be discussed with regards to universally accepted chemotherapeutic concepts, and occasionally useful radiotherapy options. Surgery for low-grade chondrosarcoma and osteosarcoma lesions will then be undertaken. Limb salvage and amputation approaches for high-grade chondrosarcoma, osteosarcoma, and Ewing sarcoma lesions will be described together, as the local

control decision-making process for these three categories is similar. Finally, continuing care in terms of bone sarcoma surveillance and palliation will be considered.

INCIDENCE AND ETIOLOGY

According to the American Cancer Society, there are estimated to be just 15,040 new cases of sarcoma diagnosed in the United States in 2014.[2] Of these cases, 12,020 will involve the soft tissues, and just 3,020 will involve the bones and joints. This represents an incidence of <1 in 100,000 persons living in the United States per year. The true incidence of some bone malignancies, such as chondrosarcoma, is not well established, as low-grade lesions are relatively common, and no accurate registries exist. For high-grade osteosarcoma and Ewing sarcoma, the incidence is thought to be on the order of one per million.

Another way of illustrating the rarity of these tumors is to consider that bone sarcomas, which result in the third leading cause of cancer death in young individuals, are projected to result in as few as 166 deaths in those <20 years of age in 2014.[3] In part, this remarkable statistic is attributable to the gratifying advances in multidisciplinary management of bone tumors, with 5-year relative survival rates of children up to 14 years of age has increased from 50% in 1978 to 78% in 2008.[3]

The etiology of bone sarcomas is not known with certainty.[4–6] Mutation in the *TP53* gene places patients with Li-Fraumeni syndrome at risk for the development of osteosarcoma.[7–11] Mutation in the *RB1* gene is associated with osteosarcoma in patients with retinoblastoma.[12–15] Rearrangements in the *EWS* and *EFT* genetic loci have been implicated in pathogenesis of Ewing sarcoma.[16–19] The molecular pathogenesis of chondrosarcomas is less well understood, with a variety of genes and signaling pathways having been implicated to date, including *TP53*, hedgehog, insulin-like growth factor, cyclin-dependent kinase 4, hypoxia-inducible factor, matric metalloproteinases, *SRC*, and *AKT*.[20] Other primary bone malignancies associated with mutations, specific translocations, and amplifications/gains include mesencyhmal chondrosarcoma, epithelioid hemangioendothelioma, chordoma, low-grade (parosteal and intramedullary) osteosarcoma, and periosteal chondrosarcoma.[6]

Environmental factors are also known to be involved in the genesis of bone sarcomas. For example, ionizing radiation, either therapeutic or inadvertent, is thought to be responsible for approximately 3% of cases of bone sarcoma.[4,21,22] Independent of radiation exposure, treatment with alkylating agents is known to increase osteosarcoma risk.[4,23]

Some benign bone conditions predispose patients to bone sarcoma development. It is estimated that 0.3% of patients with Paget disease of bone will develop osteosarcoma, most often at an advanced age and with a 5-year survival rate of ≤4%.[24–26] Fibrous dysplasia, including its polyostotic variants, McCune-Albright syndrome and Mazabraud syndrome, can rarely be associated with sarcomatous degeneration, including in less commonly encountered locations such as the ribs, spine, and craniofacial region.[27–31] Individuals with benign cartilage lesions are also subject to chondrosarcoma development. Osteochondromas, whether solitary or in the multiple, autosomal dominant form, are associated with chondrosarcomas that are predominantly low to intermediate grade[32]; on a population level, the incidence of malignant change was estimated to be on the order of 0.9%.[33] Similarly, chondrosarcomas have been described in patients with preexisting solitary enchondromas or polyostotic enchondroma variants (Ollier and Maffucci syndromes).[34] Other benign tumors that can be premalignant include giant cell tumor, osteoblastoma, and synovial chondromatosis.[35] Even nononcologic conditions such as chronic osteomyelitis[36,37] and bone infarcts[38] can evolve into sarcomas (Fig. 91.1).

ANATOMY AND PATHOLOGY

Bone sarcomas can occur through the musculoskeletal system. Osteosarcomas are more prevalent in the appendicular skeleton, with the most prevalent sites being in the distal femur (32%), proximal tibia (15%), proximal humerus (8%), and proximal femur (5%).[39] This distribution corresponds to the relative activity of the physeal plates in the growing skeleton. By contrast, Ewing sarcoma favors the axial skeleton, with the pelvis/sacrum (22%), proximal femur (10%), shoulder girdle (12%), and ribs (8%) being the most common locations, followed by the long bones and sacrum.[39] Chondrosarcoma similarly occurs most frequently in central regions: pelvis/scrum (26%), shoulder girdle (14%), proximal femur (12%), and ribs (11%).[39] When found in the long bones, the epicenter of conventional osteosarcoma lesions tends to be in the metaphysis, with diaphyseal extension, whereas Ewing sarcoma often arises in the diaphysis with metaphyseal extension. Juxtacortical osteosarcoma and chondrosarcoma variants occur on the bone surface.

Some primary bone malignancies manifest in characteristic anatomic locations. Clear cell chondrosarcoma, for instance, most often arises in the femoral head.[40] Parosteal osteosarcoma favors the posterior distal femur.[41] Periosteal osteosarcoma is found in the anterior tibial shaft.[42] Adamantinoma is most frequently encountered in the tibia and/or fibula.[43] Chordoma has a predilection for the sacrum and the clivus.[1,44]

Finally, several histologic equivalents of bone sarcomas can be found in soft tissues and joints. Extraskeletal osteosarcoma is a rare neoplasm that has a median survival of 46 months for patients with localized disease.[45] By contrast, extraosseous Ewing sarcoma has a prognosis similar to its primary bone counterpart.[46] Extraskeletal myxoid chondrosarcoma, also an aggressive soft tissue lesion with high rates of local/distant recurrence and delayed disease-associated death, is a misnomer insofar as the tumor is really of uncertain differentiation with no convincing evidence of cartilaginous differentiation.[47,48] As a rule, it is exceedingly rare for a sarcoma of bone or soft tissue to occur in an intra-articular location, but chondrosarcomas of the synovium, arising de novo or secondary to synovial chondromatosis, have been described.[49]

Gross anatomic pathology varies widely according to histologic subtype, grade, and anatomic location. Although the soft tissue component of many high-grade sarcomas of bone have a characteristic whitish, firm, "fish flesh" appearance, gross findings can run the gamut from heavily ossified areas to myxoid, friable, or frankly necrotic regions, even within the same specimen. As most high-grade bone sarcomas are >5 cm and associated with a soft tissue mass that is extracompartmental to bone, the tumor classification according to the Enneking system[50,51] is most often "T2b."

Microscopic pathology also varies considerably amongst the bone sarcomas. The prototypical bone sarcoma, a conventional high-grade osteosarcoma, consists, in most basic terms, of a spindle

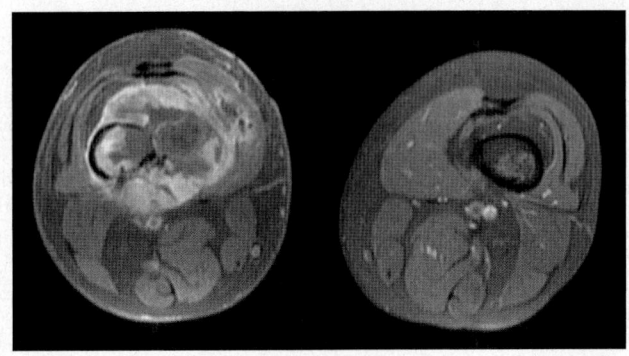

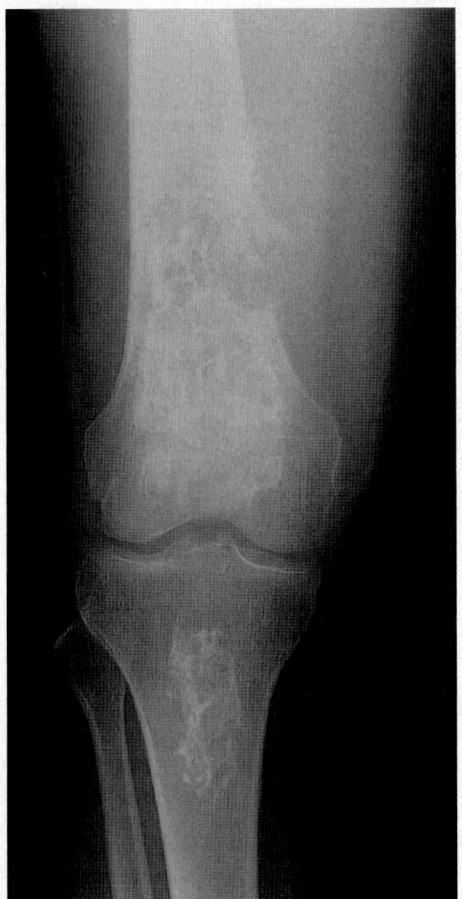

Figure 91.1 (A) Anteroposterior plain radiograph of a 64-year-old man with polyostotic femoral and tibial bone infarcts secondary to alcoholism who developed a destructive distal femoral bone and soft tissue mass. **(B)** Axial T2-weighted magnetic resonance sequence demonstrating a 13 cm distal femoral bone and soft tissue mass with cortical destruction that proved to be a high-grade undifferentiated spindle cell sarcoma. Note the benign bone infarct in contralateral femoral diaphysis.

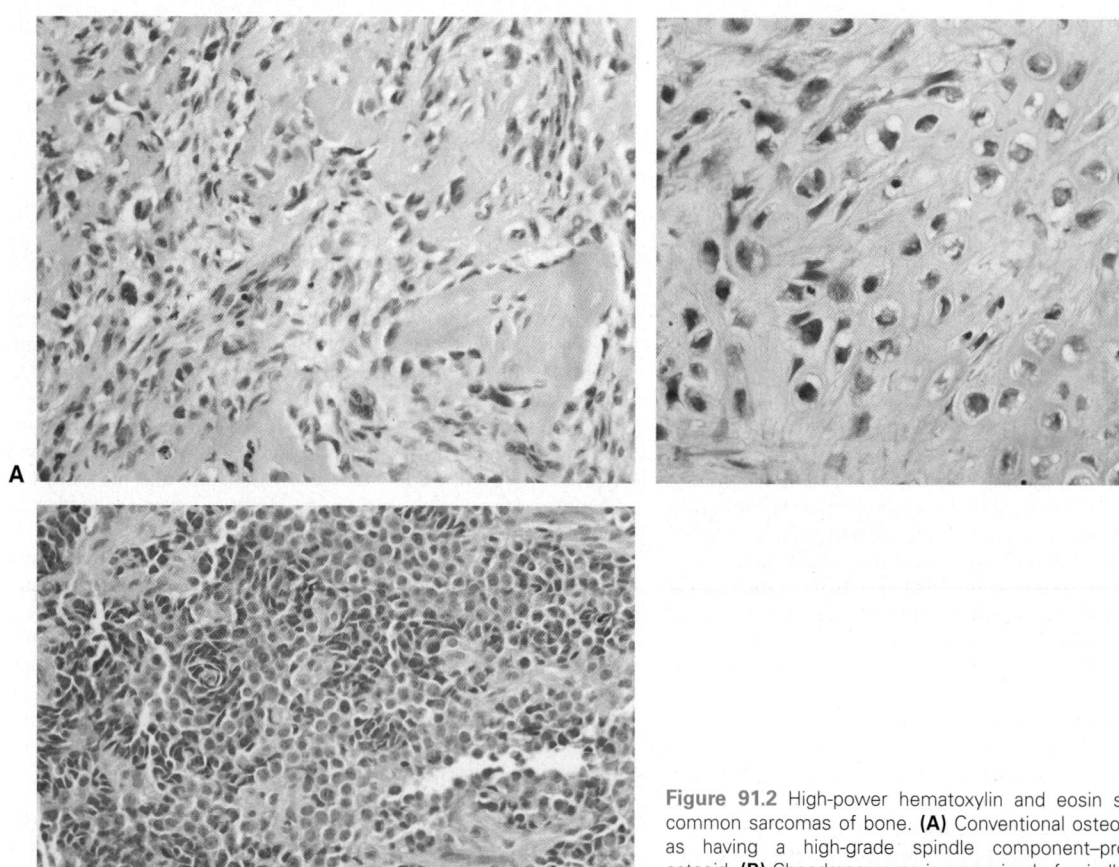

Figure 91.2 High-power hematoxylin and eosin stains of the most common sarcomas of bone. **(A)** Conventional osteosarcoma is defined as having a high-grade spindle component–producing malignant osteoid. **(B)** Chondrosarcoma is comprised of spindle cells and atypical, pleomorphic, hyperchromatic, multinucleated cartilage cells. **(C)** Ewing sarcoma consists of small round blue cells with immunohistochemical and cytogenetic diagnostic confirmation. (Photomicrographs courtesy of Andrew E. Horvai, MD, PhD.)

cell neoplasm that produces osteoid (Fig. 91.2A). A high-grade chondrosarcoma will have a spindle cell component admixed with malignant cartilaginous matrix (Fig. 91.2B). By contrast, Ewing sarcoma is a small round blue cell neoplasm for which the definitive diagnosis is suggested by immunohistochemical staining with CD-99 and confirmed by cytogenetic results of t(11:22) chromosomal translocation (Fig. 91.2C).

From a pathologic standpoint, the World Health Organization recognizes >25 different types of primary bone malignancies.[48] With the exception of plasma cell myeloma, primary non-Hodgkin lymphoma of bone, chondrosarcoma, conventional osteosarcoma, and Ewing sarcoma, the remaining entities are, for the most part, very rare (Table 91.1).

SCREENING

There exist no population-based screening tests applicable to the detection of bone sarcomas. However, a number of syndromic conditions that predispose to the development of primary bone malignancies are known (Table 91.2). Many of the implicated genetic diseases, such as Rothmund-Thomson and Werner syndromes, are exceedingly rare, and no clear algorithms exist for cancer screening. The same is true for more commonly encountered conditions that predispose to bone cancer, such as Li-Fraumeni syndrome, for which a recent workshop concluded, "further tests are needed to test screening protocols . . . which would be aimed at establishing effective screening regimens that take into account the wide diversity of disease phenotypes in *TP53* mutation carriers."[11] For patients with predisposition diagnoses that are

relatively commonly encountered in orthopedic oncology offices, such as hereditary multiple hereditary exostoses, multiple enchondromatoses, polyostotic fibrous dysplasia, and Paget disease, several practical, generalized guidelines can be offered. Plain radiographs of bones that are moderately to severely affected should be obtained yearly. A limited skeletal survey of involved areas (including, as indicated, anteroposterior [AP] and lateral views of the humeri and femora; AP views of the pelvis and distal extremities) should be considered every 2 years. Magnetic resonance (MR), computed axial tomography (CT), and positron emission tomography (PET) screening should be considered based upon a patient's family and personal clinical history. In all circumstances, care should be taken to limit radiation exposure with screening tests. However, as an individual ages, sarcoma risk increases, and so routine surveillance surveys should be offered, especially for deep-seated locations such as the pelvis and shoulder girdle, where most sarcomas in these conditions will become manifest.[33] Because malignancies in these deep-seated areas can become relatively large before symptoms develop, vigilance of occult locations is especially warranted.

DIAGNOSIS

It is nearly universally true of practice patterns within the United States that patients suspected of being at risk for having a bone sarcoma have first had a plain radiographic examination ordered by their initial point of contact within the health-care system. It is also very common for the primary care provider or general orthopedic surgeon to obtain an MR scan of the affected area (Table 91.3).

TABLE 91.1

Primary Bone Malignancies According to World Health Organization Classification

Chondrogenic tumors
  Chondrosarcoma, including primary and secondary variants
    Grade 1
    Grade 2
    Grade 3
    Periosteal
  Dedifferentiated chondrosarcoma
  Mesenchymal chondrosarcoma
  Clear cell chondrosarcoma

Osteogenic tumors
  Low-grade central osteosarcoma
  Conventional osteosarcoma
  Telangiectatic osteosarcoma
  Small cell osteosarcoma
  Parosteal osteosarcoma
  Periosteal osteosarcoma
  High-grade surface osteosarcoma

Fibrogenic tumors
  Fibrosarcoma of bone

Ewing sarcoma

Hematopoietic neoplasms
  Plasma cell myeloma
  Solitary plasmacytoma of bone
  Primary non-Hodgkin lymphoma of bone

Notochordal tumors
  Chordoma

Vascular tumors
  Epitheliod hemangioendothelioma
  Angiosarcoma

Myogenic, lipogenic, and epithelial tumors
  Leiomyosarcoma
  Liposarcoma
  Adamantinoma

Undifferentiated high-grade pleomorphic sarcoma

From Fletcher CDM, Bridge JA, Hogendoorn PCW, et al. *WHO Classification of Tumours of Soft Tissue and Bone*, 4th ed. Lyon: IARC; 2013.

TABLE 91.2

Syndromes Predisposing to Primary Bone Malignancies

Chondrosarcoma
  Enchondromatosis
    Ollier disease
    Maffucci syndrome
  Osteochondromas
    Multiple
    Nonsyndromic
  Tricho-rhino-phalangeal syndrome type 2

Osteosarcoma
  Baller-Gerold syndrome
  Bloom syndrome
  Li-Fraumeni syndrome 1 and 2
  McCune Albright syndrome
  Mazabraud syndrome
  OSLAM syndrome
  Paget disease of bone
  Polyostotic ostelytic dysplasia, hereditary expansile
  RAPADILINO syndrome
  Retinoblastoma
  Rothmund-Thomson syndrome
  Werner syndrome

Undifferentiated pleomorphic sarcoma of bone
  Diaphyseal medullary sclerosis with undifferentiated pleomorphic sarcoma

From Fletcher CDM, Bridge JA, Hogendoorn PCW, et al. *WHO Classification of Tumours of Soft Tissue and Bone*, 4th ed. Lyon: IARC; 2013.

TABLE 91.3

Diagnostic Studies for Sarcomas of the Bone

Laboratory studies
  Serum
    Creatinine, calcium, alkaline phosphatase, lactate dehydrogenase
    Complete blood count, erythrocyte sedimentation rate, C-reactive protein
    Immunoelectrophoresis
  Urine
    Urinalysis
    Immunoelectorphoresis

Radiologic studies
  Plain radiographs
    Orthogonal views
  Nuclear medicine
    Technetium-99m total body bone scan
    [111]Indium-labeled white blood cell scan
  Cross-sectional imaging
    Primary site
      Computed axial tomography with reconstruction images
      Magnetic resonance imaging
    Whole body
      [18]fluorodeoxyglucose positron emission tomography/computed axial tomography

Pathologic studies
  Percutaneous
    Fine needle aspirate
    Core needle
    Image-guided
      Ultrasound
      Computed tomography
  Open (incisional/excisional)

But once concern for the possibility of a bone sarcoma has been raised, further diagnostic tests, many of which are of a specialized nature and involve radiation exposure, should be deferred, and the patient should be immediately referred to a multidisciplinary center skilled in sarcoma management.[1]

History

Good medicine starts with a thorough history. Aggressive bone lesions often give rise to pain before a mass is noted. The nature of the discomfort, in terms of its intensity, frequency, duration, pattern, localization, and aggravating/alleviating factors must be carefully assessed. The patient should be questioned regarding associated symptoms such as numbness, tingling, weakness, stiffness, instability, and gait abnormalities. Documentation of the characteristics of a mass, if present, must be obtained with respect to time course, growth pattern, and presence of localized erythema, warmth, and tenderness. Systemic findings such as fever, sweats, chills, weight loss, and fatigue need to be queried. A past personal and/or family medical history of conditions that predispose to bone malignancies must be explored. In many cases of even high-grade sarcomas, the history is that of an enlarging bone and soft tissue mass that is less painful than might be expected. Knowledge gained regarding history can direct further evaluation away from or toward nonneoplastic, pseudotumorous, aggressive, metabolic, or secondary conditions that can mimic primary bone malignancies, such as osteomyelitis, eosinophilic granuloma, giant cell tumor of bone, osteoblastoma, metastatic disease, or Paget disease (Fig. 91.3).

Physical Examination

Although it may not narrow the differential list considerably, a thorough physical examination remains an essential part of the diagnostic pathway for sarcomas of bone. Café-au-lait spots can signal the presence of fibrous dysplasia; the integrity of the

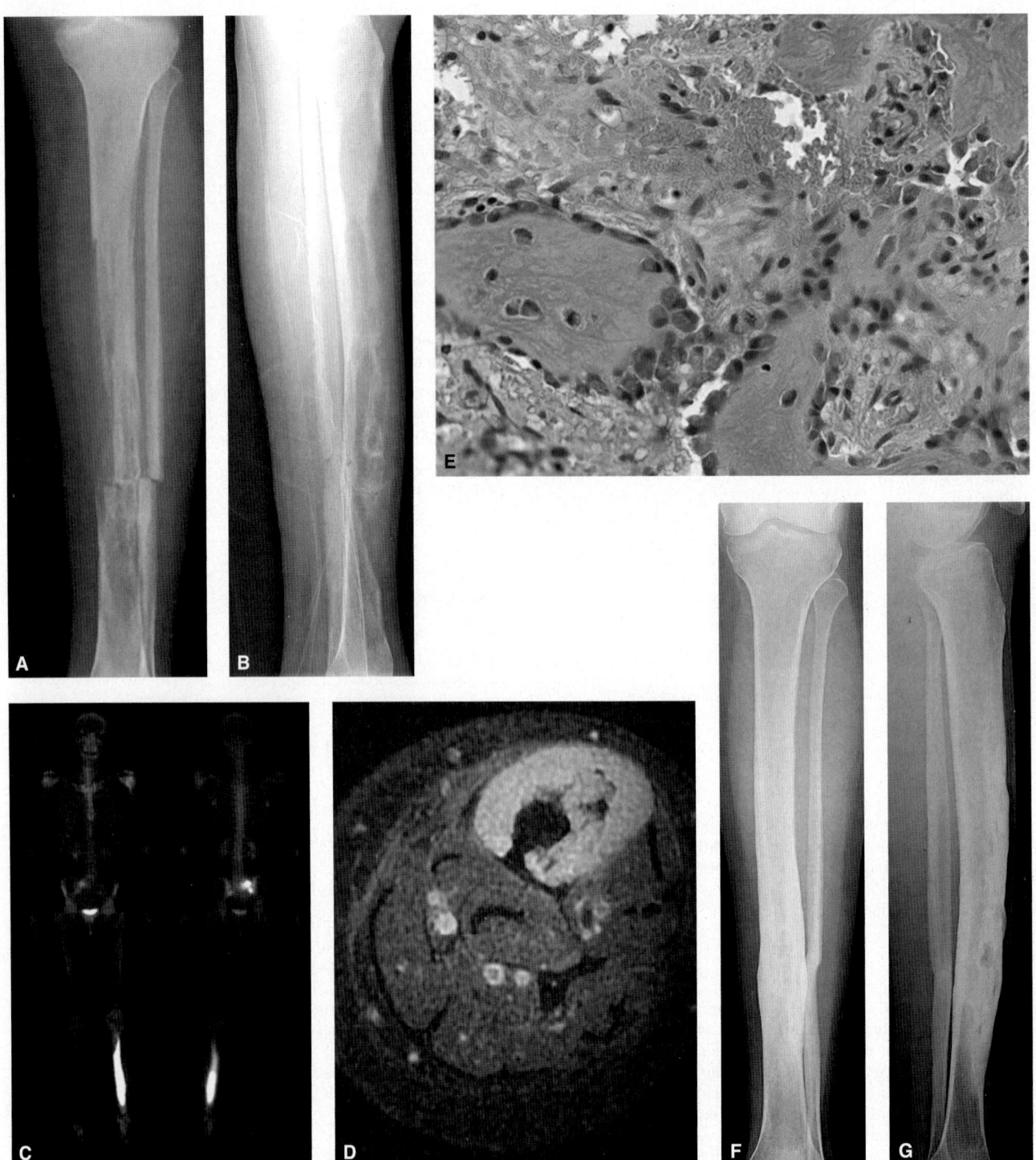

Figure 91.3 A 36-year-old woman presented with lower leg pain and inability to bear weight that developed while jogging. **(A and B)** Plain tibial-fibular radiographs show a transverse distal tibial diaphyseal fracture through a very aggressive bone lesion. **(C)** A total body bone scan revealed intense uptake in the tibial shaft, but also in the ipsilateral sacroiliac region, indicating a polyostotic or metastatic process. **(D)** An axial magnetic resonance scan image documented the presence of a large tibial bone and soft tissue mass. **(E)** The benign diagnosis, which was suggested by the patient's history of familial Paget disease in her grandmother, mother, aunt and uncle, was confirmed by incisional biopsy. **(F and G)** Anteroposterior and lateral radiographs 2 years postfracture showed complete healing; the patient was successfully nonoperatively managed with a long leg cast and subsequent bisphosphonate administration.

integumentary system should be assessed for erythema, warmth, and drainage over the primary site. The size, location, mobility, and consistency of any mass, if present, should be carefully described. The presence of absence of regional lymphadenopathy must be noted. Orthopedic parameters, including limb length, active and passive ranges of motion, joint stability, and gait pattern, need to be reviewed. Finally, a pertinent neurovascular exam must be completed.

Diagnostic Studies

Though neither highly sensitive nor specific, laboratory testing should not be neglected in the evaluation of patients suspected of having a sarcoma of bone. A complete blood count, erythrocyte sedimentation rate, and C-reactive protein level can be helpful in ruling out infection. Alkaline phosphatase and lactic dehydrogenase are sometimes elevated in skeletal sarcomas; creatinine and calcium levels are also useful chemistry tests. Serum and urine immunoelectrophoretic analyses can assist in excluding myeloma, and a basic urinalysis can be used to screen for genitourinary health.

Radiologic imaging represents the bulk of diagnostic studies for aggressive bone conditions. Plain roentgenograms include orthogonal views of the primary skeletal site and two views of chest as an initial assessment of metastatic pulmonary disease. Nuclear medicine tests include technetium-99m total body bone, indium-labeled white blood cell, and PET scans. A bone scan aids in determination of primary site activity, and the presence or absence of polyostotic or metastatic disease. An indium scan can examine the possibility of osteomyelitis. A PET or PET/CT scan quantifies metabolic activity in the primary site and helps to exclude occult metastases. The utility of [F-18]-fluorodeoxy-D-glucose PET/CT scanning in the management of patients with bone sarcoma is well established, and should be considered to be a care standard.[52–58] A dedicated chest CT scan is perhaps the most sensitive way to exclude distant disease in the lungs, which is the most common site of metastatic deposits in patients with sarcoma. CT scanning also has proven utility in studying axial primary sites and juxtacortical lesions, as well as in predicting pathologic fracture risk.[59] Often the best modality for documenting the extent of a primary bone and soft tissue mass is an MR scan, which should include the entire involved bone so as to make sure that skip metastases are not present. Specialized cross-sectional studies, including MR neurograms, MR angiograms, and CT angiograms are sometimes important to assist with surgical planning.

In the case of suspected primary bone malignancy, supreme caution must be taken with respect to the manner in which the biopsy is undertaken. Percutaneous fine needle or core procedures, especially when guided by imaging such as ultrasound, CT, or MR scanning, can be successful in establishing a diagnosis even in deep anatomic locations, especially if a soft tissue mass is present; this method has the advantage maximizing sampling throughout the mass while minimizing contamination.[60–67] As sufficient material must be obtained to perform all histologic, immunohistochemical, cytometric, and cytogenetic studies, thereby allowing an accurate diagnosis, open (incisional) biopsies are often warranted, especially in pediatric cases where multi-institutional protocol studies request centralized pathologic review and other specialized testing. Excisional (resection) biopsy can be considered for smaller lesions that can be completely excised with negative margins and without undue functional compromise; an atypical or low-grade chondrosarcoma arising in an osteochondroma is an example of this type of biopsy procedure. Whenever an open biopsy procedure is chosen, careful attention must be paid to incisional length (short) and placement (in line with the definitive resection procedure), dissection planes (*through* rather than between muscular planes), and avoidance of neurovascular exposure, bleeding, and infection.[68–71] A skilled musculoskeletal pathologist should be immediately available to review the frozen section, confirm the receipt of sufficient biopsy material, and perform direct handling of the specimen.[71] Improperly performed biopsies can delay the start of care, prompt inappropriate treatment, preclude limb salvage by causing infection or contamination, and otherwise result in local recurrence and amputation. The risk of diagnostic errors and complications increases by as much as 12-fold when the biopsy is improperly done.[69] Because of these grave medical and medicolegal concerns, referral to a tertiary center skilled in the multidisciplinary bone sarcoma management *prior* to biopsy is strongly advised.[1]

STAGING

Once all diagnostic studies are complete, formal oncologic staging concludes the pretreatment evaluation process. Staging should be performed according to TNM (tumor, node, metastasis) guidelines with principles set forth by the American Joint Committee on Cancer.[72] For bone sarcomas, staging correlates directly with prognosis, which is of utmost importance when discussing expectations regarding outcomes with patients and families (Table 91.4).

MANAGEMENT BY DIAGNOSIS AND STAGE

Systemic Therapies for Ewing Sarcoma

Chemotherapy for Patients with Newly Diagnosed Ewing Sarcoma

Prior to the routine use of chemotherapy, nearly all patients with newly diagnosed Ewing sarcoma developed distant metastatic disease and ultimately died.[73–75] These observations underscored the nearly universal presence of occult micrometastatic disease in patients with Ewing sarcoma. While local control measures (surgery and/or radiotherapy) are critical to the treatment of patients with Ewing sarcoma, systemic therapy is equally critical to attaining cure.

Early single-institution studies suggested that the regimen of vincristine, doxorubicin, actinomycin-D, and cyclophosphamide (VACA) was active in Ewing sarcoma.[74–76] Follow-up cooperative group trials established the efficacy of VACA and began to refine

TABLE 91.4

American Joint Committee on Cancer Anatomic Stage/Prognostic Groups for Sarcomas of Bone

Stage	Tumor	Nodes	Metastases	Grade
IA	T1	N0	M0	G1,2, low grade, GX
IB	T2	N0	M0	G1,2, low grade, GX
	T3	N0	M0	G1,2, low grade, GX
IIA	T1	N0	M0	G3,4, high grade
IIB	T2	N0	M0	G3,4, high grade
III	T3	N0	M0	G3,4
IVA	Any T	N0	M1a	Any G
IVB	Any T	N1	Any M	Any G
	Any T	Any N	M1b	Any G

From Edge SB, Byrd DR, Compton CC, et al. *AJCC Cancer Staging Manual*, 7th ed. Philadelphia: Lippincott Raven; 2009.

this regimen for Ewing sarcoma. For example, the first North American Intergroup Ewing Sarcoma Study (IESS-I) investigated the role of doxorubicin and whole lung radiation in the context of vincristine, dactinomycin, and cyclophosphamide.[77] Patients with newly diagnosed disease were randomized to one of three arms: vincristine, dactinomycin, and cyclophosphamide (VAC); VAC plus doxorubicin (VACA); or VAC with whole lung radiation. Among 342 eligible patients, patients randomized to VACA had significantly superior relapse-free survival compared to patients randomized to the other two arms. Patients randomized to receive VAC had the worst outcomes, and patients randomized to receive VAC with whole lung radiation had intermediate outcomes. These results definitively established the importance of doxorubicin in the management of Ewing sarcoma, but also demonstrated that whole lung radiation may prevent some cases of relapse even in the absence of documented lung metastasis.

Other national groups adopted the VACA regimen, with largely similar results. For example, the CESS-81 trial was a nonrandomized trial evaluating VACA in patients with localized Ewing sarcoma.[78] This group reported a 5-year disease-free survival rate of 54%. In addition, they identified large tumor size and poor histologic necrosis to neoadjuvant chemotherapy as potential adverse prognostic factors in this setting. The UK Children's Cancer Study Group conducted a similar trial, though the doxorubicin dose intensity was lower than in other trials.[79] They reported a 5-year relapse-free survival rate of 41% and suggested that this inferior outcome may be due to lower doxorubicin dose intensity. The French Society of Pediatric Oncology also treated patients with VACA and reported a 4-year disease-free survival rate of 52%.[80]

Subsequent trials have built upon the success obtained with VACA. Strategies have included changing the dosing strategy in VACA and adding ifosfamide or ifosfamide/etoposide (IE). The French EW88 trial used this first approach to study a more protracted VACA treatment schedule in which cyclophosphamide was delivered daily for 7 days each cycle, with cycles repeated at 2-week intervals.[81] In this nonrandomized trial, outcomes appeared to be superior compared to previous trials, though more intensive local control measures were also prescribed in this trial. Nevertheless, these results suggested that more frequent chemotherapy cycles were beneficial and/or that more protracted cyclophosphamide exposure was beneficial.

The second Intergroup Study (IESS-II) also sought to clarify the optimal mode of administration of VACA.[82] Patients with newly diagnosed localized nonpelvic disease were randomized to one of two different VACA schedules. In the intensive schedule, patients received higher doses of doxorubicin and cyclophosphamide given in cycles administered every 3 weeks. In the protracted schedule, patients received lower doses of these agents and exposure of the cyclophosphamide was distributed across 6 sequential weeks. This design resulted in significantly greater early doxorubicin exposure in the intensive arm as well as a slightly higher cumulative doxorubicin exposure in that arm. Among 214 eligible patients, all outcome measures (relapse-free, disease-free, and overall survival) were superior for patients randomized to the intensive arm. These results emphasized the importance of early doxorubicin intensity and led to adoption of VACA administration in 3-week cycles as a standard approach in subsequent studies.

Based upon response rates of approximately 30% in patients with recurrent Ewing sarcoma, several groups investigated the role of ifosfamide or IE in patients with newly diagnosed disease. The French cooperative group conducted a nonrandomized trial in which ifosfamide replaced cyclophosphamide throughout neoadjuvant and adjuvant chemotherapy that also contained vincristine, doxorubicin, and dactinomycin.[83] Outcomes of the 65 localized patients treated with this strategy were compared to 95 patients treated on a previous French trial in which all patients received cyclophosphamide. Replacing cyclophosphamide with ifosfamide did not appear to improve outcomes compared to historic controls, suggesting that ifosfamide (without etoposide) is not active in this

setting or that eliminating cyclophosphamide exposure altogether was deleterious.

A nonrandomized trial from the UK Children's Cancer Study Group used a similar approach to study ifosfamide, but yielded a different result.[84] A total of 201 patients with localized disease were nonrandomly assigned to receive therapy with ifosfamide replacing cyclophosphamide. Compared to historic controls treated with cyclophosphamide, relapse-free and overall survival appeared more favorable with the use of ifosfamide.

The CESS-86 trial used a similar approach, though in a risk-stratified manner.[85] Patients with small, localized extremity tumors received VACA, whereas patients with either large tumors or axial tumors had ifosfamide substituted for cyclosphosphamide (VAIA). Although patients treated with VAIA were predicted to have inferior outcomes due to adverse baseline risk factors, event-free survival was similar compared to patients with lower risk disease treated with VACA. These results suggested that the use of ifosfamide helped to mitigate the adverse impact of large tumor size and/or axial tumor site.

An Italian Cooperative Group trial nonrandomly evaluated the addition of ifosfamide to VACA in the neoadjuvant setting and the addition of IE in the adjuvant setting.[86] The trial included 160 patients with localized disease. Event-free and overall survival estimates were among the highest reported at that time, suggesting that ifosfamide and/or IE may have improved outcomes in this population.

The most definitive trial on the role of IE was North American Intergroup trial INT-0091.[87] Patients with newly diagnosed Ewing sarcoma were randomized at study entry to receive either standard therapy with vincristine, doxorubicin, and cyclophosphamide (VDC) administered every 3 weeks or VDC cycles alternating every 3 weeks with IE cycles. All patients received the same duration of therapy and the same cumulative dose of doxorubicin, with actinomycin-D substituted once patients received that cumulative doxorubicin dose. A total of 518 eligible patients were randomized, 398 of whom had localized disease at study entry. Among patients with localized disease, there was a statistically significant difference in 5-year event-free survival (54% for patients randomized to VDC versus 69% for patients randomized to VDC/IE). The addition of IE to VDC did not improve outcomes for patients with metastatic disease at initial presentation.[87,88] This result established VDC/IE as a new North American standard of care for patients with newly diagnosed localized Ewing sarcoma.

The next generation of clinical trials from the Children's Oncology Group (COG) has sought to intensify the VDC/IE regimen. Intergroup trial INT-0154 was a randomized trial for patients with newly diagnosed localized Ewing sarcoma.[89] Patients were randomized at study entry to receive standard dose VDC/IE every 3 weeks or higher-dose VDC/IE. Patients in the experimental arm received higher doses of ifosfamide and cyclophosphamide during cycles of chemotherapy. All patients received approximately the same cumulative doses of chemotherapy such that patients on the experimental arm completed therapy earlier than patients on the standard arm. A total of 478 eligible patients were randomized. There was no statistically significant difference in event-free survival between the standard arm and the experimental arm, demonstrating that higher-dose therapy did not improve outcomes.

COG protocol AEWS0031 was also a randomized trial for patients with newly diagnosed localized Ewing sarcoma.[90] This trial sought to intensify therapy not by dose escalation, but rather by decreasing the interval between chemotherapy cycles (interval compression). Patients were randomized at study entry to receive standard therapy with VDC/IE cycles alternating every 3 weeks or to the experimental arm with VDC/IE cycles alternating every 2 weeks. A total of 568 eligible patients were randomized. Patients randomized to the interval-compressed arm had a significantly greater 5-year event-free survival (73% versus 65% for patients randomized to the standard arm). This trial established interval compressed VDC/IE as a new standard approach for patients with localized Ewing sarcoma. Of note, the role of interval compression in patients with newly diagnosed metastatic Ewing sarcoma has not been evaluated.

The European Intergroup Cooperative Ewing's Sarcoma Study (EICESS)-92 trial sought to clarify the role of ifosfamide and etoposide based upon a risk classification strategy in which patients with small, localized tumors were deemed standard risk and patients with large localized tumors or any metastases were deemed high risk.[91] All standard-risk patients received initial therapy with VAIA. These patients were then randomized to receive this same therapy in the adjuvant setting or this same therapy with cyclophosphamide substituting for ifosfamide. Among 155 randomized standard-risk patients, there was no difference in event-free or overall survival between patients who received ifosfamide or cyclophosphamide in the adjuvant setting. These results do not fully clarify the role of ifosfamide in this group as all patients received ifosfamide in the neoadjuvant setting.

High-risk patients in the EICESS-92 trial were randomized at enrollment to receive VAIA or VAIA plus etoposide.[91] Among 492 randomized high-risk patients, there was a trend favoring the addition of etoposide. In particular, patients deemed high-risk due to large localized tumors appeared to benefit from the addition of etoposide, whereas patients with metastatic disease did not appear to benefit from etoposide. These results mirror those obtained from INT-0091 in which the addition of IE benefited patients with localized disease but not patients with metastatic disease.

Based upon this current body of evidence, a standard approach for newly diagnosed patients with localized Ewing sarcoma in North America is to use interval compressed VDC/IE according to AEWS0031. Many clinicians utilize this same regimen for patients with newly diagnosed metastatic disease, though data supporting a benefit of IE or of interval compression are lacking in this population. For both groups, participation in a cooperative group clinical trial should be strongly considered.

Chemotherapy for Patients with Recurrent Ewing Sarcoma

Historically, patients with recurrent Ewing sarcoma had few systemic options. Many such patients were retreated with chemotherapy combinations used as part of initial therapy. One series reported re-responses and durable remissions in patients treated with this strategy at relapse.[92] Additional data suggest that higher dose ifosfamide (15 g/m^2) may be active in patients with recurrent Ewing sarcoma who were treated with lower doses of ifosfamide as part of initial therapy.[93] Given greater options, many clinicians now opt to treat patients with new agents not previously used as part of initial therapy.

Currently, patients with recurrent Ewing sarcoma are candidates for clinical trials of novel agents or may be treated with a number of salvage chemotherapy regimens with documented activity in this setting. The combination of gemcitabine with docetaxel has shown modest activity in patients with recurrent Ewing sarcoma. Two single-institution case series reported no responses among four patients with recurrent Ewing sarcoma.[94,95] A formal phase 2 trial of standard doses of gemcitabine and docetaxel reported 2 patients with partial responses among 14 patients with recurrent Ewing sarcoma.[96] In contrast, another case series reported four of six patients with recurrent Ewing sarcoma with objective responses with the use of higher-dose gemcitabine and docetaxel, suggesting that higher doses of this regimen may have greater activity in this disease.[97] A formal phase 2 trial of higher-dose gemcitabine together with standard-dose docetaxel reported one patient with a partial response among seven patients with recurrent Ewing sarcoma.[98] Taken together, these findings suggest a limited role for this regimen in the management of patients with recurrent Ewing sarcoma.

Campothecin-based regimens are currently the most active available chemotherapy regimens for patients with relapsed Ewing sarcoma. The combination of topotecan with cyclophosphamide has shown activity in this population. A Pediatric Oncology Group (POG) phase 2 trial of this combination included 17 patients with relapsed Ewing sarcoma, 2 with complete response, and 4 with a partial response for an objective response rate of 36%.[99] A retrospective analysis from the German cooperative group included 49 patients with relapsed Ewing sarcoma and disease evaluable for response.[100] On initial response assessment, 16 (33%) had a partial response. Based upon these findings in patients with recurrent Ewing sarcoma, the COG conducted a trial in patients with newly diagnosed metastatic Ewing sarcoma in which patients received an initial window of therapy with either two courses of topotecan monotherapy or topotecan plus cyclophosphamide.[101] Topotecan monotherapy had only modest activity, but two courses of the combination of topotecan plus cyclophosphamide resulted in a response rate of 57%. Based upon these promising results in patients with relapsed or metastatic Ewing sarcoma, the current COG trial for patients with newly diagnosed localized disease (AEWS1031) is a randomized comparison of interval compressed VDC/IE to interval compressed VDC/IE with the addition alternating blocks of topotecan and cyclophosphamide (NCT01231906).

The combination of irinotecan and temozolomide has also shown activity in patients with relapsed Ewing sarcoma. In the initial pediatric phase 1 trial of this regimen, three of seven patients with Ewing sarcoma had objective responses.[102] A multicenter retrospective analysis of 14 patients treated with this regimen showed a response rate of 29%.[103] Follow-up retrospective studies from other institutions reported response rates >60% in this same population.[104,105] This combination is less myelosuppressive than topotecan/cyclophosphamide and may be given as an oral regimen. Given these properties, this combination may serve as a backbone for the development of new regimens that combine chemotherapy with novel agents.

Role of High-Dose Chemotherapy for Patients with Ewing Sarcoma

Given the finding that Ewing sarcoma is a chemosensitive tumor, several groups have evaluated the role of high-dose chemotherapy with autologous stem cell rescue in selected patients with high-risk disease. A single-institution retrospective study reported on the role of this approach in patients with recurrent Ewing sarcoma.[106] On univariate analysis, patients who received high-dose chemotherapy had superior overall survival. In order to try to control for selection bias that may have led to selection of the most favorable patients to receive high-dose chemotherapy, this group performed a multivariate survival analysis. Receipt of high-dose chemotherapy as a component of relapse therapy was associated with improved survival, even after controlling for variables thought to be prognostic at relapse, such as response to salvage therapy and time from diagnosis to relapse.

The majority of studies evaluating this modality have focused on patients with newly diagnosed metastatic Ewing sarcoma. Given the radiosensitivity of Ewing sarcoma, the Children's Cancer Group conducted a trial evaluating high-dose therapy using melphalan, etoposide, and total-body radiation as conditioning.[107] Thirty-two patients with newly diagnosed disease with metastases to the bone and/or bone marrow were nonrandomly assigned to high-dose therapy following induction chemotherapy. Event-free survival was 20% at 2 years and was identical to a historic control group treated with standard-dose chemotherapy, indicating that this regimen did not improve outcomes in this very high-risk patient population.

A series of multicenter trials treated patients with high-dose therapy with busulfan and melphalan conditioning.[108,109] This approach appeared to be feasible following initial induction chemotherapy, though whether outcomes were improved by this approach is not clear in these uncontrolled trials. The Euro-Ewing group applied this approach to a larger group of patients with metastatic disease beyond isolated lung metastases.[110] In this very high-risk patient population, 3-year event-free survival was 27%, suggesting that any improvement in outcome from high-dose therapy was incremental.

One trial has been completed evaluating the role of high-dose chemotherapy in patients with high-risk localized Ewing sarcoma.[111] Patients received a common induction chemotherapy regimen and had response assessed at the time of local control (by histology for patients who underwent surgical local control or by imaging for patients who received radiation for local control). Patients with a poor response to induction chemotherapy were nonrandomly assigned to receive high-dose chemotherapy with busulfan and melphalan conditioning. Only a subset of patients assigned to receive high-dose chemotherapy did so. This selected subset had an event-free survival rate that was similar to patients with a good response who received ongoing standard-dose chemotherapy. Patients with a poor response to induction who did not go on to receive high-dose therapy had significantly inferior outcomes. These results suggest that high-dose therapy may have abrogated the anticipated poor outcomes for patients with a poor response to induction chemotherapy.

A lingering concern and area of controversy in this field is that patients with chemotherapy-responsive disease are both more likely to survive longer and more likely to be candidates for high-dose chemotherapy. In order to circumvent this selection bias, the Euro-Ewing group is conducting the first randomized trial of high-dose chemotherapy in this disease. Patients with newly diagnosed Ewing sarcoma and either isolated lung metastases or localized disease with poor response to initial chemotherapy are eligible. All patients receive induction chemotherapy with vincristine, ifosfamide, doxorubicin, and etoposide.[112] Patients randomized to undergo high-dose chemotherapy receive conditioning with busulfan and melphalan. Patients randomized to receive ongoing chemotherapy receive the combination of vincristine, doxorubicin, and ifosfamide. Until the results of this ongoing randomized trial become available, the role of high-dose chemotherapy for patients with Ewing sarcoma will remain controversial.

Novel Agents for Patients with Ewing Sarcoma

Despite understanding the critical role of *EWSR1* fusion oncogenes in the pathogenesis of Ewing sarcoma, strategies to target *EWSR1* fusion oncogenes and oncoproteins have been difficult to develop. One group used gene expression profiling to identify existing drugs that replicate the gene expression profile associated with *EWSR1/FLI1* knockdown.[113] Cytarabine was one of the most effective drugs in modulating the gene expression profile to emulate that of Ewing sarcoma cells subjected to *EWSR1/FLI1* knockdown. The COG then conducted a phase 2 trial of cytarabine in patients with relapsed Ewing sarcoma, with no responses among 10 patients.[114]

Another novel agent, YK-4-279, was developed to interfere with the interaction of EWS-FLI1 protein and RNA helicase A, an important mediator of EWS-FLI1.[115] This agent has shown preclinical activity against Ewing sarcoma models. Efforts to move this agent or agents with a similar mechanism of action in the clinic are ongoing.

A high-throughput screening study sought to identify existing agents that were able to reduce expression of EWS-FLI1 target genes.[116] Mithramycin was the lead compound emerging from this screen. Follow-up experiments demonstrated preclinical activity against Ewing sarcoma models, leading to an ongoing clinical trial (NCT01610570).

Other novel approaches have tried to exploit additional vulnerabilities identified in laboratory studies of this disease. For example, a large body of literature has suggested that antiangiogenic strategies would be active against Ewing sarcoma.[117] Based on these findings, several trials have been conducted. The COG conducted a trial using VDC/IE together with metronomic vinblastine and celecoxib in patients with newly diagnosed metastatic Ewing sarcoma.[118] This regimen was tolerable, but outcomes did not appear different from previous outcomes reported for this population. A pilot study of bevacizumab added to vincristine, irinotecan, and temozolomide included two patients with Ewing sarcoma, both with objective responses.[119] A nonrandomized multicenter trial of topotecan, cyclophosphamide, and bevacizumab for patients with recurrent Ewing sarcoma is ongoing (NCT01492673).

The insulin-like growth factor 1 receptor (IGF1R) has also been the subject of intense study in preclinical and clinical studies of Ewing sarcoma. The majority of Ewing sarcoma cells and tumor samples express IGF1R.[120] *EWSR1/FLI1* expression reduces the expression of IGF-binding protein 3, an endogenous inhibitor of IGF1R pathway activation.[121] Preclinical studies of IGF1R small molecular inhibitors or inhibitory anti-IGF1R monoclonal antibodies have demonstrated robust activity against Ewing sarcoma models.[122–125] In early phase clinical trials of IGF1R monoclonal antibodies, several patients with recurrent Ewing sarcoma demonstrated objective responses.[126,127] Several phase 2 trials specifically for patients with recurrent Ewing sarcoma were developed, and response rates of approximately 10% were observed without significant single-agent toxicity.[126,128–130] Based upon these promising results in the recurrent setting, the COG is developing a trial of an IGF1R monoclonal antibody together with VDC/IE for patients with newly diagnosed metastatic Ewing sarcoma.

The mammalian target of rapamycin has also been implicated as a potential therapeutic target in Ewing sarcoma. Preclinical studies indicate that rapamycin can reduce levels of EWS/FLI protein and also induce an *EWSR1/FLI1*-inactive gene expression signature.[113,131] In vitro and in vivo studies have shown antitumor activity of rapamycin as a single agent and in combination with cytotoxic chemotherapy.[132,133] To date, no trials of mammalian target of rapamycin inhibition specifically for patients with Ewing sarcoma have been conducted. However, in a phase 1 trial of ridaforolimus, one patient with advanced Ewing sarcoma had a confirmed partial response.[134] One institution is conducting a trial in patients with high-risk Ewing sarcoma in which patients will receive a window of irinotecan, temozolimide, and temsirolimus prior to receiving interval-compressed chemotherapy (NCT01946529).

Most recently, laboratory studies suggest that Ewing sarcoma may be sensitive to inhibition of poly(adenosine diphosphate-ribose) polymerase (PARP). In a large-scale drug screen across myriad cancer histologies, Ewing sarcoma cell lines were found to be uniquely sensitive to the effects of a PARP inhibitor.[135] Another study sought to investigate the mechanism of this observation.[136] They noted that Ewing sarcoma cell lines have evidence of increased DNA damage, an effect that is potentiated in the presence of a PARP inhibitor. The use of a PARP inhibitor together with temozolomide resulted in dramatic preclinical responses compared to temozolomide alone or the PARP inhibitor alone. Based upon these observations, a phase 2 trial of olaparib has been conducted, with results pending (NCT01583543). Other trials of PARP inhibitors as single agents and in combination with other agents are in development.

Radiation Therapy for Patients with Newly Diagnosed Ewing Sarcoma

Advances in radiation delivery and target definition together with improvements in chemotherapy and surgery approaches technique have improved local control for patients with Ewing sarcoma. However, controversy has plagued decisions regarding local control measures particularly for pelvic primaries for which retrospective studies have indicated trends toward better local after surgery compared with radiotherapy, but failed to reach statistical significance. Such studies are fraught with selection bias as patients chosen for radiotherapy rather than resection tend to be those with larger tumors and less robust response to chemotherapy.[137,138] Nonetheless, when feasible, surgery is generally the preferred local therapy modality and radiation is reserved for patients in whom anticipated morbidity from surgery is prohibitive. This leaves approximately 20% of children on COG studies receiving definitive radiation and 15% receiving adjuvant radiation for primary tumor control.

A prospective randomized trial comparing surgery and radiotherapy as local control modality for Ewing sarcoma at any primary site has never occurred and will never take place. Thus we are left with interpretation of data collected for cohorts in which local control decisions are made based on parameters including tumor location, size, response to chemotherapy, patient age, and patient preference based on expected morbidity of each procedure. One such informative study is an analysis of patients with pelvic Ewing sarcomas treated on INT-0091, a randomized controlled study that compared two chemotherapy regimens: VACA and VACA-IE.[139] Treating physicians chose the local control approach, be it surgery, radiation, or both. The authors sought to assess local control modality after adjusting for tumor size and chemotherapy type. Of the 75 studied patients, 12 underwent surgery, 44 received radiotherapy, and 19 received both. Local control rates (80% to 90%) were quite promising even in this group with unfavorable primary site. The 5-year cumulative incidence of local failure was 21% with no significant differences by tumor size or local control modality. However, there was a trend toward benefit in local control with VACA-IE chemotherapy (11% versus 30%; $p = 0.06$). Of note, despite lack of statistical significance, combined surgery and radiotherapy was associated with the lowest rates of local relapse (10.5% for surgery + radiotherapy compared with 25% for either surgery or radiotherapy alone).[139] Similar results, although again, not statistically significant, were reported for the entire cohort of patients, with 2% local recurrence for patients receiving combined modality treatment compared with 5% for surgery and 9% for radiotherapy alone ($p = $ not significant).[89] Not surprisingly, European studies have historically favored combined modality approaches for local control, with 63% of patients treated on EICESS 92 receiving combined surgery and radiation, 19% treated with surgery alone, and 18% with radiotherapy alone. Impressive local control rates were reported, with 95% when surgery was a component of local control compared with 75% when only radiotherapy was used.[140] A dearth of reports describes the durability of local therapy modalities and the functional outcome of each approach. With a particular focus on cure rates, contemporary clinical trials have emphasized event-free survival and overall survival as end points, but better information regarding functional outcomes is critical to informed decisions regarding local therapy modality for individual patients.

Although postoperative radiation has gained favor for patients receiving combined modality therapy for local control, consideration should be given to preoperative radiation for a select group of patients with Ewing sarcoma. For these patients, the goal of preoperative radiotherapy is not to allow an inoperable tumor to become operable, as the data for this approach is lacking for Ewing sarcoma. Rather, in patients for whom the choice of combined modality therapy is made, the rationale for preoperative radiation lies primarily in reducing side effects. Preoperative radiation may allow for smaller fields, less normal tissue exposure, and perhaps lower doses, as has been reported for adults in a prospective, randomized study for adults with soft tissue sarcomas.[141]

Appropriate uses of radiotherapy for patients with newly diagnosed Ewing sarcoma include definitive radiation therapy for unresectable tumors, adjuvant radiation for tumors with incomplete surgical resection or intraoperative spill, chest wall tumors with ipsilateral pleural-based secondary tumor nodules or positive pleural fluid cytology, and pathologically involved lymph nodes. Patients with complete resections (R0) after neoadjuvant chemotherapy with a clear margin (defined as no viable tumor at the cut surface) should not receive radiotherapy; there are some subtle points to be highlighted. These guidelines incorporate not only the traditional factor of extent of surgical resection but also the parameter of percent of tumor necrosis more commonly used in European protocols. Thus, for resected tumors that have >90% necrosis, if the tissue at the margin is bland scar or loose fibrous tissue, margin status should be considered negative and no postoperative radiation should be administered. However, if inflammatory tissue or coagulative tumor necrosis is present at the margin (the cytoarchitecture of the tumor cells is preserved), postoperative radiotherapy is required. In contradistinction, for resected tumors with <90% necrosis, the cut surface of the resected tumor must be normal nonreactive tissue in order to be considered pathologically negative and radiotherapy avoided.

The role of preoperative radiotherapy must be carefully considered. Preoperative radiation should not be undertaken with the goal of rendering an inoperable tumor operable and should be considered only in resectable tumors in select sites such as pelvis and chest wall for which a higher risk of positive microscopic margins is present. Complete surgical excision should be undertaken within 2 weeks of 36 Gy of radiation. Standard radiotherapy doses are 50.4 Gy for microscopic residual and 55.8 Gy for gross residual disease.

One note of caution is in order for the administration of radiation to patients with Ewing sarcoma. High-dose chemotherapy with busulfan/melphalan is now often used for patients with metastatic disease. In late 2003, the pediatric oncology community was alerted to possible severe complications after busulfan/melphalan high-dose chemotherapy and irradiation of the spinal cord.[142] And a subsequent amendment restricted the radiation dose to the spinal cord to 30 Gy after busulfan/melphalan high-dose therapy. To add to these concerns, in 2005, reports from France described severe gastrointestinal toxicities after busulfan/melphalan and pelvic radiotherapy. A detailed analysis of the European Ewing Tumor Working Initiative of National Groups Ewing Tumour Studies-99 study showed further serious toxicities with paraplegias and bowel obstructions leading to deaths.[143] However, in follow-up studies by the German Pediatric Oncology and Hematology Society group, similar severe toxicities were not observed. Although the German group did not confirm such severe toxicities, it must be noted that whereas the median follow-up for gastrointestinal side effects was longer than the longest period for development of radiation associated bowel toxicities in France, the median follow-up for spine toxicities was only 7 months and therefore caution must be exercised. These differing findings may also be the result of lower doses and smaller volumes in the German Pediatric Oncology and Hematology Society group compared to those used in France. Given the critical role of radiotherapy for local control in many patients with Ewing sarcoma, if radiation is anticipated as part of a multimodality approach to local control in patients with axial tumor sites, consideration should be given to avoiding busulfan/melphalan high-dose therapy.[144]

Bone metastases in Ewing sarcoma receive the same dose of 55.8 Gy as does gross disease at the primary site. However, these metastatic sites are often treated at the completion of chemotherapy, months after local control measures, because protracted external beam radiation to such sites might include significant bone marrow volumes and ultimately compromise the ability to administer chemotherapy. Thus a role has emerged for hypofractionated stereotactic body radiotherapy (SBRT) for bone metastases. Safety of administration of such large doses to highly targeted volumes has been aided by improvements in immobilization and image-guidance techniques. Local control rates of 75% to 90% have been achieved by SBRT to spine metastases using 18 to 30 Gy in a single fraction or 24 to 60 Gy in five fractions.[145] In the setting of metastatic bone sarcomas in children, the advantages of SBRT to bone metastases are particularly appealing because completion of the radiation course in one to five fractions with equivalent disease control rates, as conventional fractionation offers the added advantages of minimizing interruptions in systemic therapy and irradiation of smaller volumes.[146]

Systemic Therapies for Osteosarcoma

Chemotherapy for Patients with Newly Diagnosed Osteosarcoma

Chemotherapy plays little role in the management of patients with low-grade or surface osteosarcoma. Historically, there was controversy about the role of chemotherapy in the management of patients with high-grade osteosarcoma. In light of this controversy, the Multi-Institutional Osteosarcoma Study (MIOS) was conducted.[147] Patients with newly diagnosed localized extremity high-grade osteosarcoma were randomized after complete surgical resection to observation or to adjuvant chemotherapy. Chemotherapy consisted of 45 weeks of combination therapy including bleomycin, cyclophosphamide, and actinomycin-D (BCD) cycles, high-dose methotrexate cycles targeted to achieve 1,000 micromolar peak concentration, and cisplatin/doxorubicin cycles. Thirty-six eligible patients were randomized. Of the 18 patients randomized to adjuvant chemotherapy, 6 (33.3%) recurred. Of the 18 patients randomized to observation, 15 (83.3%) recurred and 2 of the 3 patients in this group who did not recur did not accept the outcome of the randomization and were treated with adjuvant chemotherapy. At 2 years from randomization, 66% of the patients randomized to receive adjuvant chemotherapy were relapse-free compared with only 17% of the patients randomized to observation. These results confirmed the significant impact of chemotherapy on outcomes of high-grade osteosarcoma, and this trial established a new standard of care for this disease.

The positive findings from the MIOS trial led to a number of subsequent trials designed to determine the optimal timing and type of chemotherapy. One trial compared adjuvant to neoadjuvant chemotherapy.[148] In this trial (POG-8651), patients with newly diagnosed localized resectable high-grade osteosarcoma were randomized at study entry to undergo immediate surgical resection followed by 42 weeks of adjuvant chemotherapy or to receive 10 weeks of neoadjuvant chemotherapy followed by surgery and then 32 weeks of adjuvant chemotherapy. Aside from the difference in timing of surgical resection, all patients received the same 42 weeks of chemotherapy using a similar regimen to that used in the MIOS trial. A total of 100 eligible patients were randomized. Overall survival, event-free survival, and rates of limb salvage surgery were similar between the two arms of the trial, demonstrating that timing of surgical resection did not impact outcomes. With these results, the use of neoadjuvant chemotherapy became more widespread as this approach allows more time for surgical planning and also allows one to assess the extent of histologic necrosis in response to neoadjuvant chemotherapy.

Two older trials sought to clarify the role and optimal dosing of methotrexate in patients with newly diagnosed localized osteosarcoma. In an Italian trial, patients were randomized to receive methotrexate 200 mg/m^2 or 2 g/m^2 as a component of multiagent adjuvant chemotherapy.[149] Outcomes were equivalent between the two groups. The UK Children's Cancer Study Group conducted a similar trial, though the doses of methotrexate under investigation were 690 mg/m^2 or 7.5 g/m^2.[150] Outcomes were again similar between the randomized groups, suggesting either that methotrexate does not contribute to disease control in osteosarcoma or that lower-dose methotrexate is adequate for efficacy of this agent.

A series of trials from the German/Austrian/Swiss Cooperative Osteosarcoma Study Group (COSS) has clarified the use of cisplatin and doxorubicin in osteosarcoma. In the COSS-80 trial, patients were randomized to chemotherapy with doxorubicin and methotrexate in all patients and either cisplatin or BCD. Outcomes were similar between arms.[151] In the COSS-82 trial, patients were randomized to receive BCD and methotrexate or doxorubicin/cisplatin and methotrexate.[152] Patients with good histologic response at the time of surgery continued to receive that same chemotherapy, whereas patients with poor histologic response received different salvage regimens. A total of 125

evaluable patients were randomized. Patients randomized to the BCD arm with no doxorubicin or cisplatin in the neoadjuvant setting had significantly inferior metastasis-free survival, even though these patients with poor histologic response received doxorubicin and cisplatin in the adjuvant setting. Together with the results of COSS-82, these findings highlighted the importance of early doxorubicin treatment in the management of osteosarcoma.

The European Osteosarcoma Intergroup completed a randomized trial to assess the role of high-dose methotrexate in patients with newly diagnosed localized extremity osteosarcoma.[153] Patients were randomized at study entry to chemotherapy with six cycles of doxorubicin and cisplatin or to that same regimen with a dose of high-dose methotrexate given 10 days prior to each cycle of doxorubicin and cisplatin. Surgical resection was planned at the same time in both arms of the trial such that patients receiving doxorubicin and cisplatin had time to receive three cycles prior to surgery, whereas patients receiving methotrexate had time to receive two cycles prior to surgery. Ninety-nine patients were randomized to each arm of the trial. Disease-free survival was superior for patients randomized to doxorubicin and cisplatin (57% at 5 years compared to 41% for patients randomized to also receive methotrexate). Because all patients received the same planned cumulative dose of doxorubicin and cisplatin, these results highlighted the importance of dose intensity of these agents in the treatment of osteosarcoma. Moreover, these results called into question the role of methotrexate, though the dose used in this trial was lower than used in more recent trials (8 g/m^2 versus 12 g/m^2).

The European Osteosarcoma Intergroup conducted another randomized trial comparing six cycles of doxorubicin and cisplatin to a chemotherapy regimen similar to that used in the MIOS trial.[154] Patients with newly diagnosed localized resectable osteosarcoma were eligible, and 391 eligible patients were randomized. The proportion of patients with a good histologic response to neoadjuvant chemotherapy was similar between randomized groups. Progression-free and overall survival estimates were nearly identical between randomized groups. Based upon these findings, the group concluded that the shorter regimen with doxorubicin and cisplatin is preferable to the more complicated and longer regimen used in the MIOS trial. These results called into question the role of the BCD regimen used in the MIOS trial, which has now largely been abandoned.

This group conducted a subsequent trial evaluating interval compression to dose-intensify the doxorubicin/cisplatin regimen.[155] Patients with newly diagnosed localized osteosarcoma were randomized to receive six cycles of doxorubicin/cisplatin administered either every 3 weeks or every 2 weeks. Surgical resection occurred after two cycles in the every 3-week arm and after three cycles in the every 2-week arm. A total of 497 eligible patients were randomized. Patients in the every 2-week arm had a higher likelihood of achieving a good histologic response, though they had also received an additional cycle of neoadjuvant chemotherapy. Overall survival and progression-free survival were similar between groups, indicating that dose intensification by interval compression did not improve outcomes in this setting.

Based upon promising results in patients with recurrent osteosarcoma (see the following), another series of trials have evaluated the role of ifosfamide or ifosfamide with etoposide in the treatment of patients with osteosarcoma. The POG conducted a trial in patients with newly diagnosed metastatic osteosarcoma in which all patients received a window of therapy with two cycles of high-dose ifosfamide (12 g/m^2 per cycle) prior to surgical resection.[156] Patients then received adjuvant therapy with high-dose methotrexate, doxorubicin/cisplatin, and additional high-dose ifosfamide. Of 27 patients with response-evaluable disease, 8 patients (30%) had an objective radiographic response after the two cycles of window therapy. These results suggested that single-agent ifosfamide is an active regimen in this disease.

The Italian Sarcoma Group conducted a randomized trial evaluating the role of ifosfamide both in neoadjuvant and adjuvant phases of therapy.[157] Patients with localized osteosarcoma were randomized to receive methotrexate, cisplatin, and doxorubicin with or without ifosfamide preoperatively. Patients randomized to not receive ifosfamide preoperatively could have ifosfamide added postoperatively if they had a poor histologic response to neoadjuvant chemotherapy without ifosfamide. Of 246 randomized patients, the proportion of patients with a good histologic response and event-free survival were similar between randomized groups. Given increased hematologic toxicity associated with the ifosfamide arm, the authors concluded that ifosfamide should be reserved for the adjuvant setting in patients with poor histologic response to neoadjuvant therapy without ifosfamide.

North American Intergroup study INT-0133 was a randomized phase 3 trial that included a comparison of patients treated with high-dose methotrexate + cisplatin + doxorubicin (MAP) chemotherapy or MAP plus ifosfamide (9 g/m^2 per course).[158] A total of 677 patients with newly diagnosed localized osteosarcoma were randomized. While the initial analysis of this randomization was complicated by a statistical interaction in the factorial design (described subsequently), a subsequent analysis with longer follow-up determined that the addition of ifosfamide to MAP chemotherapy did not impact the event-free or overall survival.[159]

The POG conducted a trial for patients with newly diagnosed metastatic osteosarcoma in which all patients received two courses of IE prior to surgical resection of the primary tumor.[160] The overall response rate after two courses of IE was 59%. This study design allowed histologic response of the primary tumor to be assessed, with 65% of patients having at least 90% tumor necrosis after two cycles of IE.

The French SFOP OS94 trial sought to determine whether doxorubicin could be replaced by ifosfamide and etoposide in the management of patients with newly diagnosed localized osteosarcoma.[161] Patients were randomized at study entry to receive neoadjuvant chemotherapy with high-dose methotrexate in all patients and either doxorubicin or IE. Adjuvant therapy was determined by histologic response to neoadjuvant chemotherapy. The primary end point was histologic necrosis at the time of surgery. Among 234 evaluable patients, there was a significantly higher rate of good histologic necrosis in patients randomized to IE compared to doxorubicin. These results demonstrate the activity of IE in this setting, though must be viewed in light of the fact that patients in the comparator arm received doxorubicin without cisplatin.

The first European-American osteosarcoma study 1 sought to clarify further the role of IE in patients with newly diagnosed resectable osteosarcoma. All patients received neoadjuvant chemotherapy with MAP, which has become a consensus standard neoadjuvant chemotherapy regimen for patients with newly diagnosed osteosarcoma. Patients with a good histologic response (<10% viable tumor) were eligible for randomization evaluating the role of adjuvant interferon (see the following). Patients without a good histologic response to neoadjuvant chemotherapy (≥10% viable tumor) were eligible to be randomized to receive ongoing adjuvant chemotherapy with MAP or to receive ongoing adjuvant chemotherapy with MAP with the addition of IE. This trial has closed to accrual, but results for this arm of the trial have not yet been reported.

Chemotherapy for Patients with Recurrent Osteosarcoma

Surgical resection of sites of recurrent disease remains a cornerstone of curative therapy at the time of relapse. Chemotherapy options are limited for patients with recurrent osteosarcoma. The combination of IE appears to be among the most active regimens for this population. For example, an initial phase 2 trial of this combination included eight patients with recurrent osteosarcoma, three of whom had an objective response.[162] A follow-up phase 2 trial from the French Society of Pediatric Oncology demonstrated a 48% response rate with this regimen in a population that included largely patients with first recurrent disease.[163]

The combination of gemcitabine and docetaxel has also been investigated for patients with recurrent osteosarcoma. Single-

institution case series have suggested some activity in this setting, mainly with disease stabilization,[95,97] though one group reported objective responses in 3 of 10 patients with recurrent osteosarcoma.[94] Based in part upon these findings, two phase 2 trials have been conducted.[96,164] Sixteen patients with recurrent osteosarcoma enrolled across both trials and only two patients had objective responses (partial response in both). These findings indicate that this regimen has only modest activity in this setting.

Novel Agents for Patients with Osteosarcoma

Multiple groups have attempted to improve outcomes for patients with advanced osteosarcoma by utilizing novel agents. A subgroup of trials has targeted antigens that are overexpressed on some osteosarcomas. Based upon reports of overexpression of human epidermal growth factor receptor 2 (HER2) in a subset of osteosarcoma, the COG conducted a phase 2 trial of trastuzumab together with intensive chemotherapy for patients with newly diagnosed HER2-expressing metastatic osteosarcoma.[165] A total of 41 patients with HER2-expressing tumors were nonrandomly assigned to receive trastuzumab plus chemotherapy, and 55 patients with HER2-negative tumors were nonrandomly assigned to receive chemotherapy. Event-free survival at 30 months was 32% in both cohorts, suggesting little benefit from the addition of trastuzumab.

Osteosarcomas commonly express cell surface disialoganglioside GD2.[166] As such, patients with advanced osteosarcoma have been included in clinical trials of therapeutic monoclonal antibodies targeting GD2. In one phase 1 trial of a murine monoclonal antibody, one of two patients with osteosarcoma had a mixed response.[167] Given high rates of human antimouse antibodies after receipt of the murine monoclonal antibody, a chimeric anti-GD2 antibody was generated and tested in a phase 1 trial.[168] One patient with osteosarcoma was treated and showed clinical evidence of disease stabilization, though ultimately progressed. Based upon these suggestions of clinical activity in osteosarcoma, a trial of a humanized anti-GD2 antibody in patients with advanced GD2-positive osteosarcoma is ongoing (NCT01662804).

Another group of trials has attempted to increase immune clearance of microscopic osteosarcoma cells. The use of muramyl tripeptide phosphatidylethanolamine (MTP-PE) to stimulate antitumor macrophages has been intensely studied in osteosarcoma. In an initial phase 2 trial, patients with recurrent or persistent pulmonary metastatic disease underwent surgical resection and then received adjuvant MTP-PE.[169] Compared to historic controls treated with adjuvant chemotherapy, 24 weeks of MTP-PE prolonged progression-free survival from 4.5 months to 9 months.

These findings stimulated the development of a randomized phase 3 clinical trial of the role of MTP-PE. North American Intergroup Study INT-0133 included 677 patients with localized osteosarcoma randomized to one of four treatment arms, including two arms that included 36 weeks of adjuvant MTP-PE given together with adjuvant chemotherapy.[158] Interpretation of this trial is complicated by the factorial trial design and by the presence of an interaction between the ifosfamide randomization (described previously) and the MTP-PE randomization. Specifically, MTP-PE appeared to prolong event-free survival only among patients also randomized to receive ifosfamide. Post hoc analysis of the trial with additional follow-up was performed. These analyses showed a trend toward prolonged event-free survival as well as a statistically significant increase in overall survival among patients randomized to receive MTP-PE.[159] This result was independent of the results of the ifosfamide randomization. INT-0133 also included a much smaller cohort of patients with newly diagnosed metastatic osteosarcoma. Patients randomized to receive MTP-PE had improved event-free and overall survival rates, though this portion of the trial was not powered to detect statistically significant differences in outcomes between randomized arms.[170] Based in part upon the findings from INT-0133, MTP-PE obtained regulatory approval in Europe for patients with osteosarcoma, though it is not used in North America.

In addition to MTP-PE, interferon has been studied as an immune strategy to reduce the risk of recurrence due to microscopic residual disease. Early results from Sweden demonstrated favorable outcomes in patients who received interferon as an adjuvant therapy following surgical resection of osteosarcoma, even in the absence of chemotherapy.[171] The COSS-80 study included a randomization in which patients received or did not receive interferon in combination with multiagent chemotherapy.[151] There was no difference in outcome according to randomized assignment. Given the results of the Swedish experience and concerns that interferon combined with chemotherapy may blunt the immunostimulatory effects of interferon, the European-American osteosarcoma study 1 trial included another randomized assessment of the role of interferon in patients with newly diagnosed resectable osteosarcoma. Patients with a good histologic response to neoadjuvant chemotherapy were randomized to receive or not receive weekly pegylated interferon-alpha-2b following the completion of all planned chemotherapy. The preliminary results of this randomization have been reported.[172] Among 715 good-responder patients randomized in this portion of the trial, event-free survival was not statistically significantly different for patients randomized to interferon or not. While the final analyses from this trial are still pending, it does not appear as though adjuvant interferon improves outcomes in patients with a good response to neoadjuvant chemotherapy.

A large body of preclinical data demonstrates that bisphosphonates have direct antitumor activity in osteosarcoma.[173] Two studies have investigated the safety of adding a bisphosphonate to standard chemotherapy regimens used in the treatment of osteosarcoma. In one study, monthly pamidronate was administered along with methotrexate, doxorubicin, and cisplatin.[174] The toxicity profile was similar to the expected toxicity profile associated with the chemotherapy backbone and an increased incidence of complications associated with endoprostheses was not observed. In the second study, zoledronic acid was administered every 4 to 6 weeks along with a chemotherapy backbone that included methotrexate, doxorubicin, cisplatin, ifosfamide, and etoposide.[175] Zoledronic acid at standard doses was tolerable together with this intensive backbone. The size of these tolerability studies does not allow one to draw conclusions about the effect of bisphosphonates on event-free survival. An ongoing French randomized phase 3 trial will compare outcomes of patients randomized to treatment with chemotherapy and surgery to patients randomized to treatment with chemotherapy, surgery, and zoledronic acid (NCT00470223). The results of this trial will clarify the role of bisphosphonates in the treatment of newly diagnosed patients with osteosarcoma.

The Italian Sarcoma Group conducted a phase 2 trial of the multitargeted tyrosine kinase inhibitor sorafenib in patients with recurrent osteosarcoma.[176] Thirty-five patients >14 years of age enrolled and received sorafenib 400 mg orally twice daily. Three patients (8%) had confirmed partial responses. The 4-month progression-free survival rate was 46%, suggesting a degree of clinical benefit even in patients without an objective radiographic response.

The lung is the most common site of failure in patients with osteosarcoma. Therefore, strategies to reduce the risk of pulmonary relapse are a high priority in this disease. At least two trials have investigated inhalational therapies specifically to target pulmonary disease in osteosarcoma. The COG conducted a phase 2 trial of inhaled granulocyte macrophage–colony-stimulating factor (GM-CSF).[177] Forty-three patients with first pulmonary relapse of osteosarcoma were treated with inhaled GM-CSF twice daily on alternating weeks. In a subset of patients who had not yet undergone resection of recurrent disease, staged bilateral thoracotomy allowed assessment of the biologic effects of inhaled GM-CSF. Inhaled GM-CSF did not result in significant recruitment of dendritic cells to lung metastases and did not appear to improve event-free survival. Another trial investigated inhaled cisplatin for patients with relapsed osteosarcoma.[178] Nineteen patients with advanced osteosarcoma involving the lung received inhaled cisplatin every 2 weeks. This therapy appeared tolerable, with limited systemic toxicities. One patient had a confirmed partial response, and evaluation of inhaled cisplatin is ongoing as adjuvant therapy in patients with recurrent pulmonary metastatic disease that has been completely resected (NCT01650090).

Radiotherapy for Patients with Osteosarcoma

The mainstay of therapy for osteosarcoma has historically omitted radiation because osteosarcomas were thought to be radioresistant.[179] However, surgery and chemotherapy lead to suboptimal local control in challenging disease sites such as the spine and pelvis. Relatively low doses of 30 to 56 Gy for spine osteosarcomas and 56 to 68 Gy for pelvic disease yielded very disappointing local control rates of <20% in the few patients who were irradiated in the Cooperative Osteosarcoma Study Group.[180,181] However, as higher radiation doses are used, so better local control rates are achieved for unresectable or marginally resectable tumors. Doses of 60 Gy, in 2.5 to 3 Gy once-daily fractions or 1.25 to 1.5 Gy in twice-daily fractions, resulted in local control of 60% in patients with unresectable osteosarcoma.[182] The role of particle radiotherapy for the treatment of unresectable or incompletely resected is promising as well. Kamada et al.[183] reported local control rates of >70% in patients with unresected osteosarcoma treated with carbon ions. Ciernik et al.[184] reported on the Massachusetts General Hospital experience of 55 patients treated with mean dose of 68.4 Gy (standard deviation, 5.4 Gy) for whom 58.2% (range, 11% to 100%) of the dose was delivered using protons. Five-year local control was 72% and five-year overall survival was 67%. Grade 3 to 4 late toxicities were seen in 30.1% of patients, and two died of treatment-related second malignancies.[184] Thus with careful planning and respect for radiation tolerance of adjacent normal structures, radiation therapy can contribute to favorable clinical outcomes in patients with unresectable or marginally resectable osteosarcoma.

Surgical Therapies for Local Control of Sarcomas of Bone

The aforementioned review of systemic chemotherapeutic and local radiotherapeutic management options for bone sarcomas is necessarily directed toward the pediatric population, as this is the most commonly affected population. However, the same principles can and should be applied to adults with Ewing sarcoma, intermediate- to high-grade osteosarcoma, and high-grade and dedifferentiated chondrosarcomas.[185,186] Especially for patients younger than 65 years of age who are in good cardiac health, neoadjuvant chemotherapy offers several potential advantages, including (1) immediate treatment not only of presumed "micrometastatic disease," but also of the primary tumor, so as to make local control easier and/or safer; (2) time for the patient and family to plan and consider various limb salvage versus amputation options; and (3) the opportunity to assess histologic response to chemotherapy, so as to guide adjuvant treatment. For patients with lower-grade chondrosarcoma and osteosarcoma lesions, however, treatment usually consists of surgery only.

Surgery for Patients with Low- to Intermediate-Grade Chondrosarcoma and Osteosarcoma

Enchondromas are benign bone tumors that are exceedingly common, occurring in perhaps as much as 1% of the population. The distal femoral and proximal humeral metaphseyal regions are commonly affected, and patients with periarticular pain are often referred for orthopedic oncologic evaluation. In the vast majority of cases, the cartilage lesions are not thought to be the source of discomfort, and these lesions can be safely followed clinically and radiographically.[187] Subsequent imaging that shows increased plain radiographic lucency, especially if coupled with cortical breakthrough on MR scan, would raise concern that could prompt surgery. The histologic distinctions between a benign enchondroma,

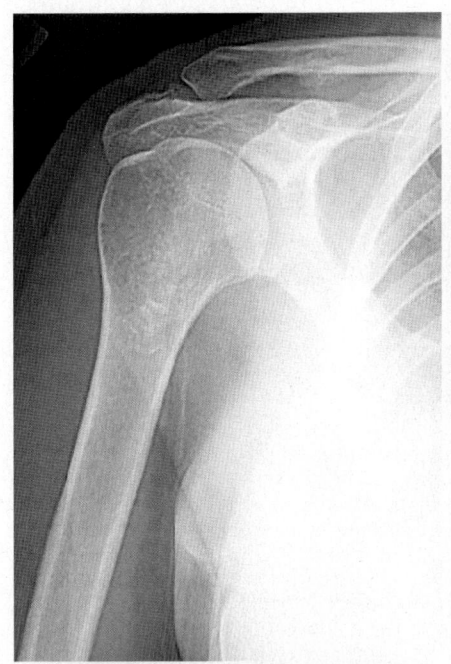

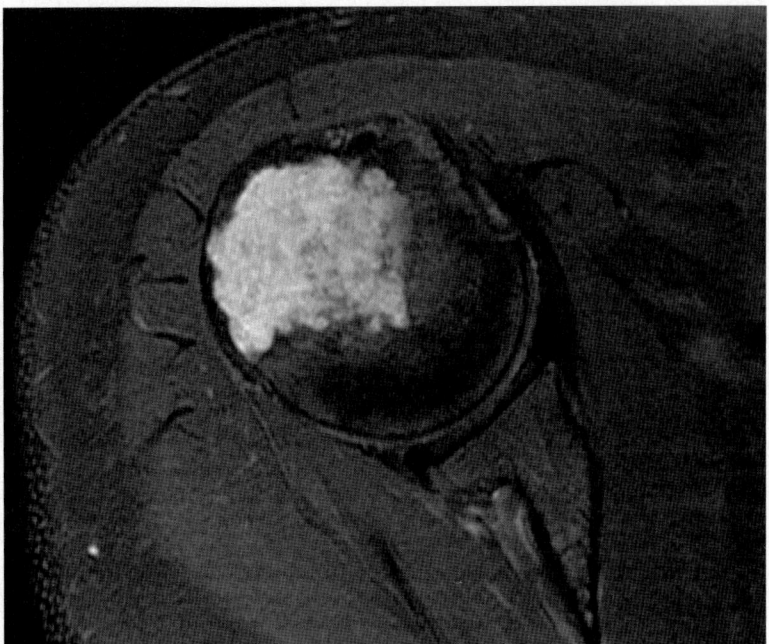

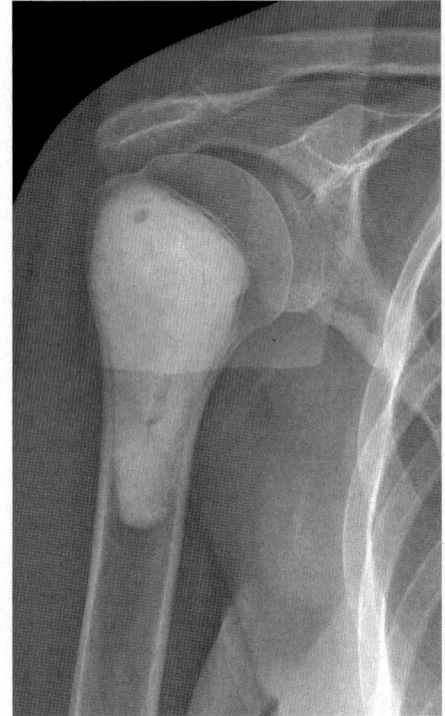

Figure 91.4 A 53-year-old woman presented with a rather subtle plain radiographic finding of a proximal humeral metaphyseal lucency **(A)** after an area of uptake was noted on a screening bone scan obtained for her history of breast cancer. A T2-weighted axial image showed near-perforation of the lateral proximal humeral cortex by a multilobulated cartilage tumor **(B)**. Her computed tomography–guided needle and final pathology were consistent with the diagnosis of an atypical cartilaginous neoplasm/low-grade chondrosarcoma, and she underwent aggressive intralesional treatment consisting of curettage, burring, hydrogen peroxide application, and cement packing. **(C)** Three-year postoperative films showed no sign of local recurrence, and she remained asymptomatic.

an atypical cartilaginous neoplasm, and a low-grade chondrosarcoma are notoriously difficult to establish, but >20% myxoid material and bone permeation are thought to be in keeping with a diagnosis of chondrosarcoma.[188] When this diagnosis is suspected, a PET/CT scan, a preoperative image-guided biopsy, and an intraoperative frozen section can be of assistance in guiding treatment. Localized intraosseous grade 1 chondrosarcoma lesions can be safely and effectively treated with aggressive curettage, burring, and adjuvant application (for instance, hydrogen peroxide washing and argon beam coagulation) prior to cement packing (Fig. 91.4). By contrast, most grade 2 chondrosarcoma lesions are treated, where possible, with resection and reconstruction (Fig. 91.5).

Low-grade osteosarcoma lesions include central and juxtacortical (both parosteal and periosteal) forms. Local control is

accomplished with wide resection with negative margins; reconstruction can generally be accomplished by allografts secured with internal fixation[41] or with endoprostheses. The treatment of grade 2 periosteal chondroblastic osteosarcomas, which often involve the anterior tibial shaft, is controversial as far as chemotherapy is concerned.[42,189,190] Surgery consists of wide resection and reconstruction if possible, although amputation is sometimes necessary for distal lesions (Fig. 91.6).

Surgery for Patients with High-Grade Sarcomas of Bone

As previously mentioned, there exists no randomized study proving the superiority of surgery over radiation therapy for local control

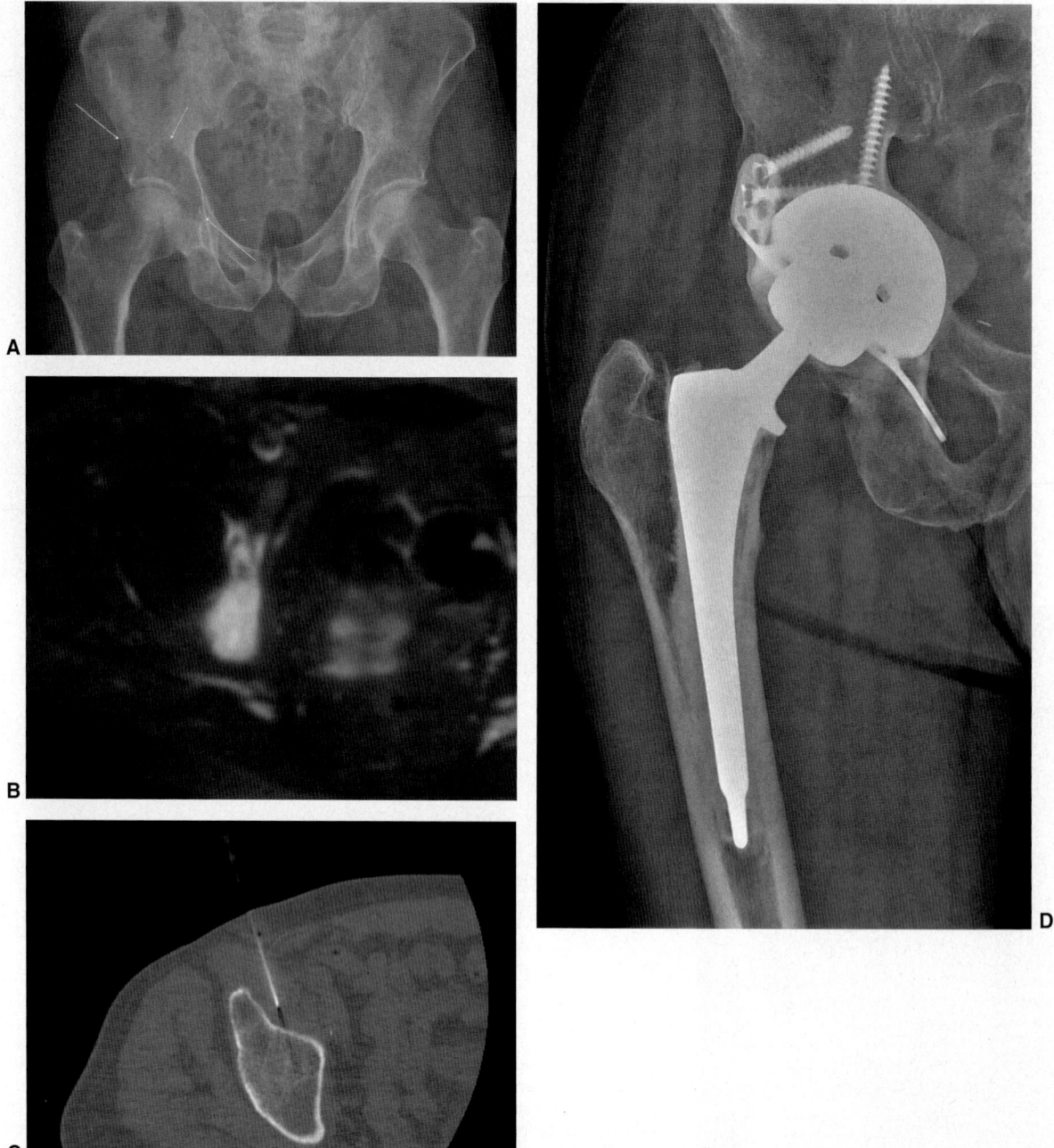

Figure 91.5 A 74-year-old man with a history of left dorsal foot and ankle low-grade myxoid liposarcoma presented nearly 5 years later with a painful right acetabular bone lesion noted on an anteroposterior pelvis radiograph **(A)**. The patient's tumor was evaluated with a magnetic resonance scan **(B)** and a positron emission tomography/computed tomography scan with a maximum standardized uptake value of 5.6. **(C)** His computed tomography–guided biopsy demonstrated an atypical chondrogenic neoplasm, but his final pathology after resection was consistent with a grade II chondrosarcoma. He was reconstructed with a complex cup-cage-cup total hip arthroplasty, and he was without evidence of disease at 1-year follow-up **(D)**.

of Ewing sarcoma. Nonetheless, many patients with Ewing sarcoma, particularly extremity lesions, will undergo surgical resection; if margins are negative, adjuvant radiation can be avoided, thus minimizing the complications of growth arrest, deformity, skin and soft tissue induration, lymphedema, arthrofibrosis, osteonecrosis, fracture, and secondary malignancy. In general, then, surgical local control measures for patients with high-grade sarcomas of bone, whether Ewing sarcoma, chondrosarcoma (grade 3, dedifferentiated, mesenchymal, and clear cell), osteosarcoma (conventional, telangiectatic, small cell, and high-grade surface),

or other subtypes (fibrosarcoma, angiosarcoma, leiomyosarcoma, and undifferentiated pleomorphic) can be considered together. In many respects, the ultimate recommendation of a particular surgical control option rests less on histologic subtype of high-grade sarcoma than on a host of other factors, including patient age, disease stage, anatomic location, expected response to induction therapy, and patient/family socioeconomic and cultural factors, as well as capabilities and biases of the treatment team. Thus, surgical local control planning for each high-grade bone sarcoma patient must be individualized.

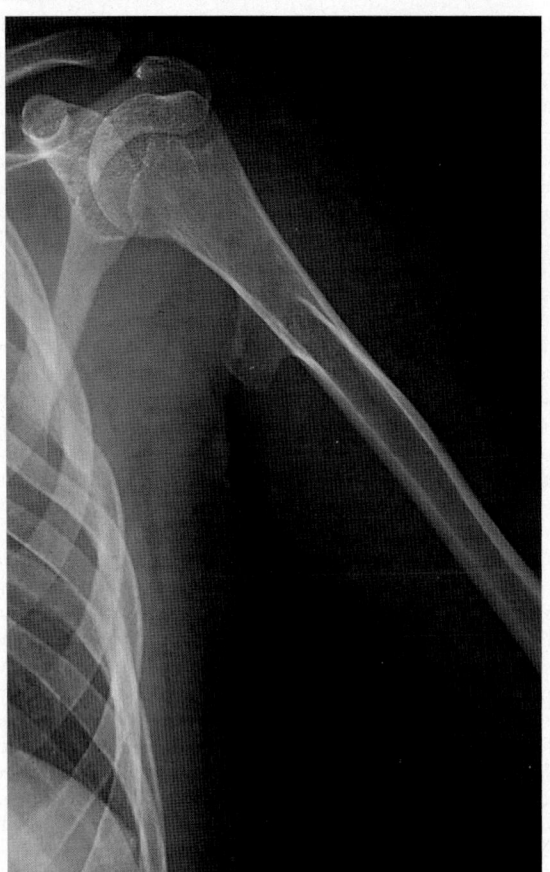

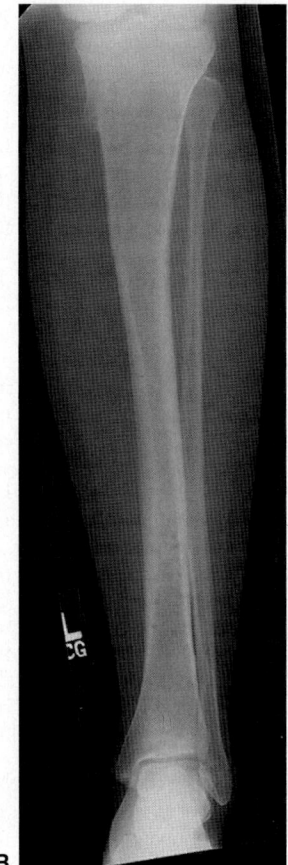

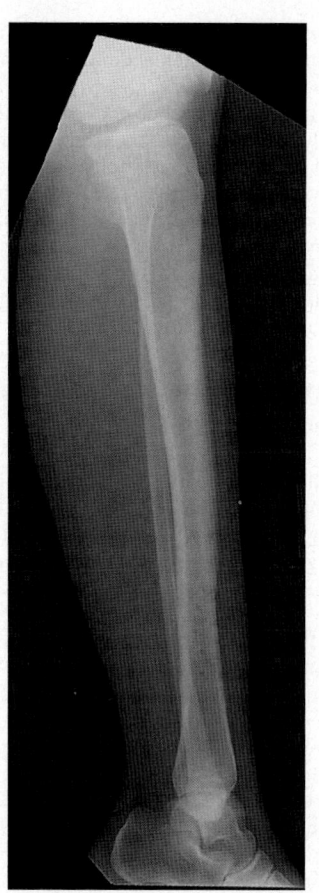

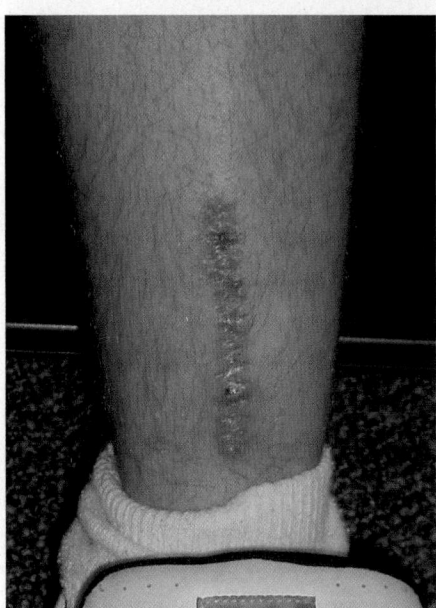

Figure 91.6 A 17-year-old boy presented with a history of multiple exostoses secondary to radiation treatment for severe combined immunodeficiency syndrome as an infant. **(A)** A plain radiograph of the proximal humerus demonstrated a characteristically benign exostosis. **(B–D)** At an outside institution, he underwent intralesional excision of what was thought to be another exostosis involving the anterior distal tibial cortex, as demonstrated in postoperative films and a clinical photo. Histologic review confirmed the diagnosis of grade 2 juxtacortical chondroblastic osteosarcoma. Given the distal location of the tumor, the patient elected to undergo a below knee amputation with curative intent. However, he subsequently developed chest metastases and succumbed to his disease more than 4 years later.

Amputation Versus Limb Salvage

Given the choice, most but not all, patients and families would select limb salvage as a local control option over amputation. With advanced imaging and modern reconstructive techniques, there exist few absolute contraindications to limb salvage. Relative contraindications to a limb salvage effort include major neurovascular involvement, very immature skeletal age, infection, lack of reconstruction (e.g., very distal anatomic location) or soft tissue coverage

options, contamination secondary to biopsy technique and complications, inability to obtain oncologically acceptable margins, and pathologic fracture. The most common reason to recommend amputation is major neurologic involvement by the tumor.

It should be kept in mind by patients, families, and treating physicians that the risk of local recurrence should not preclude a limb salvage effort. While distant metastasis and local recurrence after limb salvage sometimes are diagnosed at the same time, it is crucial to understand that there is no proof that local recurrence *causes* metastasis. Instead, both phenomena are likely related only insofar as they independently confirm the very aggressive nature of a particular tumor. Indeed, studies comparing limb salvage versus amputation have shown no statistically significant differences, not only in terms of local recurrence and overall survival, but also with regards to social, psychological, and functional outcomes.[191–197] Economic analyses have shown that external prosthetic fitting costs more than limb salvage over the long term,[198] and limb salvage is considered by many to be cosmetically superior, but amputee patients have the advantage of needing fewer operations and being able to participate more readily in high impact and endurance type recreational activities.

Amputation: Concepts and Specialized Techniques

Whether involving the upper or lower extremity, amputations should be performed at the most distal level that would assure negative surgical margins while optimizing functional outcome. In general, longer residual limbs offer better biomechanical advantage and more options for prosthetic fitting. However, a through-knee amputation is superior to a very short above knee amputation, as the femoral condyles provide an "end-bearing" residual limb. Major ablative amputations such as hemipelvectomies should be employed only for curative intent, or rarely for palliation when no acceptable alternative exists.[199]

In cases of lower extremity amputation between the midfemoral and midtibial levels, the intraoperative application of an immediate postoperative prosthetic device has proven to effective for enhancing wound healing, decreasing swelling, and allowing immediate 25 lb. partial weight bearing on the first postoperative day, thereby avoiding the medical and psychological adverse effects of recumbency (Fig. 91.7). Although the immediate postoperative prosthetic is not recommended for dysvascular amputees, the technique has proven to be safe for oncology patients, including those receiving chemotherapy.[200–203]

Pediatric high-grade osteosarcoma and Ewing sarcoma commonly occur in the distal femur. For children of very young skeletal age (roughly, girls <8 years old and boys <10 years old), use of expandable endoprostheses is not particularly feasible, because of the number of operations necessary to ensure limb length equality, and the attendant risks of infection, arthrofibrosis, and nerve palsy.[204,205] Because a standard through-femoral amputation in young individuals would result in a very short residual limb, specialized reconstructive techniques have been devised. Rotationplasty utilizes the distal portion of the lower leg, ankle, and foot, with osteosynthesis of the proximal femoral and distal tibial diaphyses occurring after 180-degree rotation around the longitudinal axis.[206–208] Although providing a longer residual limb that is functionally equivalent to a below knee level, roationplasty is not universally accepted in the United States for reasons of cosmesis and prosthetic fitting. An excellent alternative is a turn-up-plasty, in which the osteosynthesis of the proximal tibia and distal femur occurs after 180-degree rotation in the coronal plane.[209,210] This reconstruction preserves the viability of the proximal tibial physis, so that the result is effectively a "growing" end-bearing through knee amputation that is very cosmetically acceptable and easy to fit with an external prosthesis (Fig. 91.8).

One final major advance for amputees is the development of osseointegrated transdermal anchorage systems, which are particularly beneficial for high transfemoral amputees. Though under regulatory review in preparation for clinical trial in the United States, these concepts, which have been successfully employed for more than 20 years by Branemårk and colleagues in Sweden, are gaining increasing acceptance throughout the world.[211,212] By being able to directly secure an external prosthetic device to the limb, patients enjoy a tremendous biomechanical advantage, without the need for conventional socket wear (Fig. 91.9). Prospective studies have demonstrated very good rates of implant retention, with excellent functional outcome in terms of prosthetic usage.[213,214]

Limb Salvage: Options and Recent Advances

As mentioned previously, limb salvage can sometimes be achieved for high-grade bone sarcomas without surgery. This is quite commonly true for Ewing sarcoma, where radiation is used as

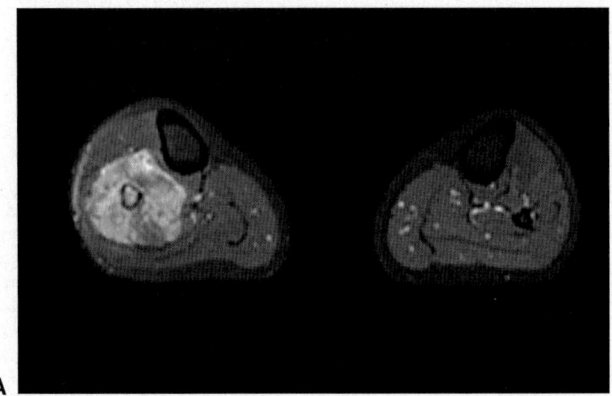
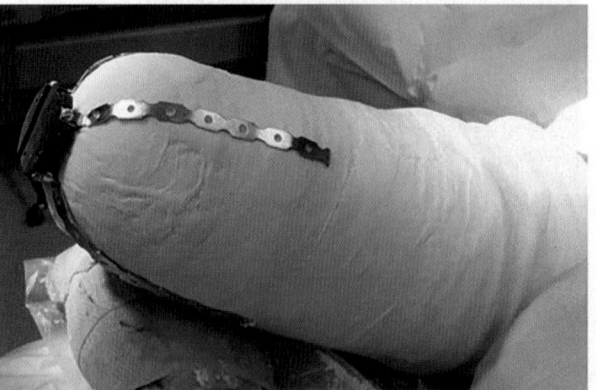
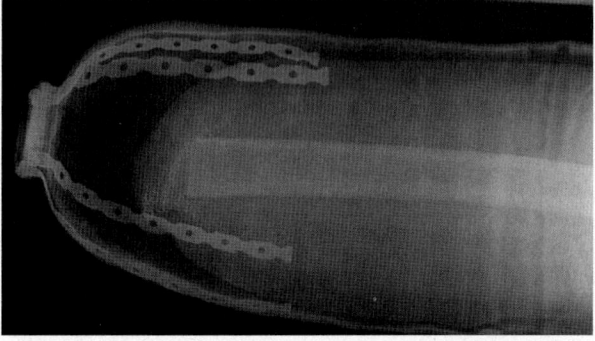

Figure 91.7 An 18-year-old woman presented with a massive extracompartmental proximal fibular osteosarcoma that compromised lower extremity neurovascular structures, as shown in her T2-weighted axial magnetic resonance scan **(A)**. **(B)** After receiving neoadjuvant chemotherapy, she underwent a supracondylar above knee amputation with immediate postoperative prosthetic fitting. **(C)** Radiographic appearance of the immediate postoperative prosthetic, which is ready for fitting with a pylon and prosthetic foot so as to allow ambulation.

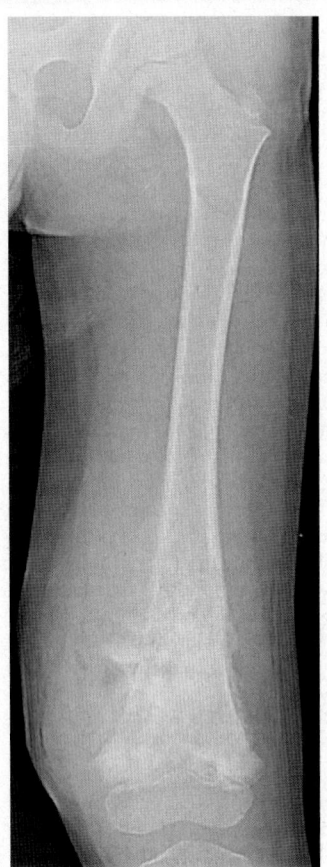
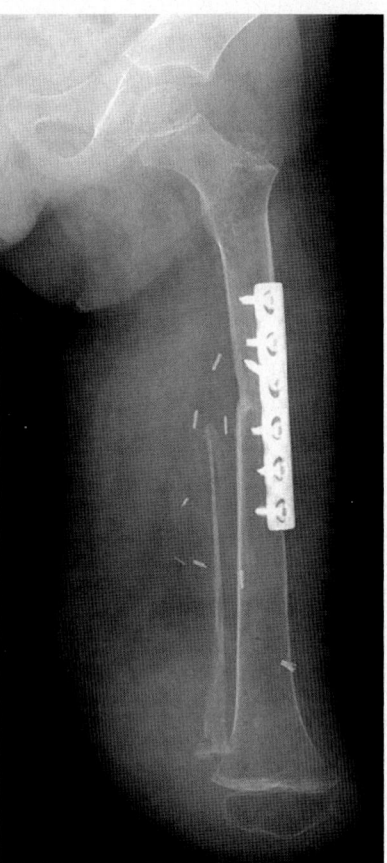

A

B

Figure 91.8 (A) Anteroposterior radiograph of a 3-year-old boy who presented with a large distal femoral high-grade conventional osteosarcoma. After receiving neoadjuvant chemotherapy, the patient underwent tibial turn-up-plasty, with a healed osteosynthesis site and preservation of the proximal tibial physeal plate noted on a 14-month postoperative film **(B)**. The result was functionally equivalent to a "growing" through knee amputation.

monotherapy for local control. Unresectable high-grade osteosarcoma and chondrosarcoma lesions involving the mobile spine, sacrum, and pelvis can also be treated with radiation therapy alone in hopes of achieving palliation, if not local control. For skeletal sarcomas involving "expendable" bones such as the scapula, clavicle, radius, ulna, ribs, iliac wing, and fibula, resection alone (without reconstruction) often results in a successful limb salvage outcome (Fig. 91.10).

In most instances of limb salvage surgery, however, some form of reconstruction needs to be undertaken, and there are myriad methods. Autogenous bone grafts have historically been used for small defects, and in the present day, most commonly for

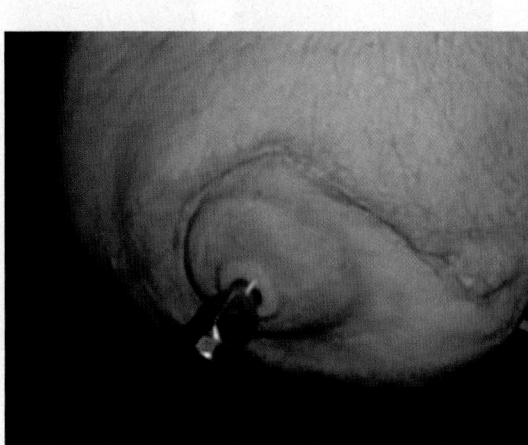
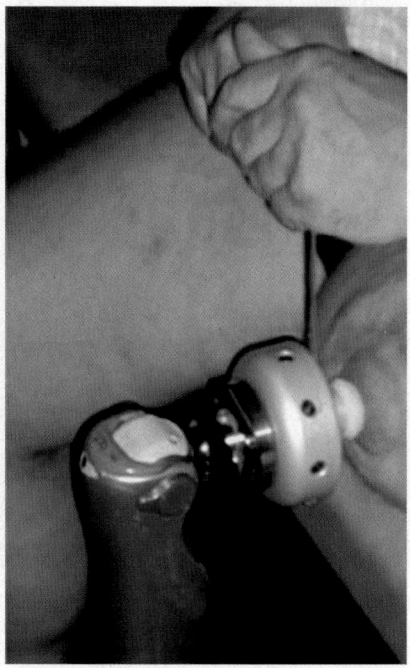

A

B

Figure 91.9 Osseointegrated transdermal anchorage system in a high transfemoral amputee **(A)** allows ease of external prosthetic application and enhanced functional outcome **(B)**.

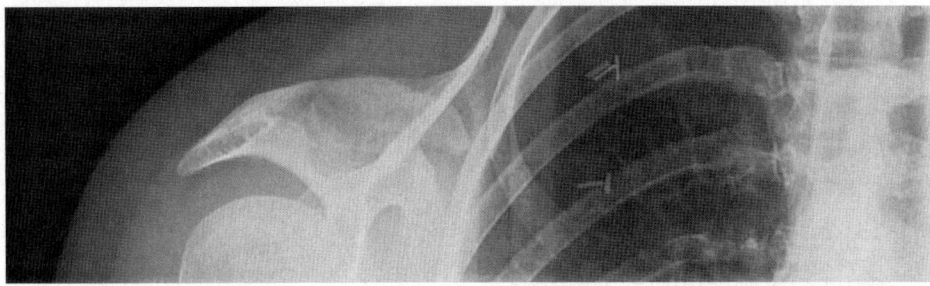

Figure 91.10 Three-year postoperative anteroposterior radiograph demonstrating medial clavicular resection for metastatic high-grade osteosarcoma in a 22-year-old woman with a history of distal femoral osteosarcoma treated 7 years previously.

vascularized fibular transfers, particularly for proximal humeral tumors[215,216] (Fig. 91.11A). Frozen cadaveric osteoarticular and intercalary allografts were in vogue for sarcoma reconstruction in past decades, but complications of nonunion, infection, and fracture have limited their utility.[217–219] Currently, allografts are most often used as part of alloprosthetic composites, principally in the proximal humerus, proximal femur, and proximal tibia.[220]

The majority of extremity limb salvage operations performed for high-grade sarcomas in the Western world are now accomplished with massive metallic endoprosthetic devices. These implants can be fabricated on a custom basis, but more frequently, modular segmental devices are assembled intraoperatively so as to conveniently replicate resection length. Fixation of these megaprostheses has traditionally been accomplished with long cemented or uncemented stems. A recent retrospective review of 2,174 patients who underwent conventional endoprosthetic reconstruction showed a high aseptic complication rate across anatomic sites: soft tissue failure (12%), aseptic loosening (19.1%), structural failure (17.4%), and tumor progression (17.4%).[221] In order to avoid the complications

of aseptic loosening secondary to stress shielding and particle-induced osteolysis, compressive osseointegration technology has been developed to allow stable fixation of endoprostheses to bone by way of an innovative spring-loaded system that applies up to 800 lb of compression force at the bone-prosthetic interface, thereby inducing bone hypertrophy.[222–226] The device also enables salvage of very short metadiaphyseal segments and allows ease of revision in cases of infection, mechanical failure, or infection.[227–230] Reports from several institutions have shown that compressive osseointegration reconstructions are similar or superior to conventional devices at intermediate term follow-up[231–236] (Fig. 91.11B–D).

CONTINUING CARE: SURVEILLANCE AND PALLIATION

In caring for patients with sarcomas of bone, it is important to maintain focus on the overarching priorities: (1) life, (2) limb, (3) limb function, (4) limb length equalization, and (5) cosmesis, in

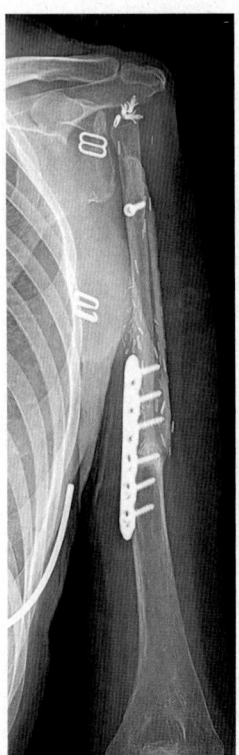 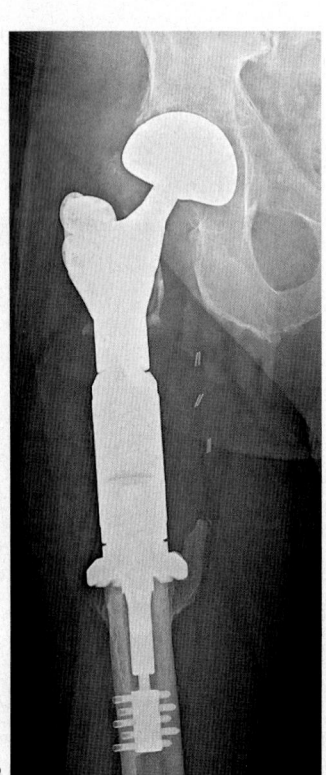 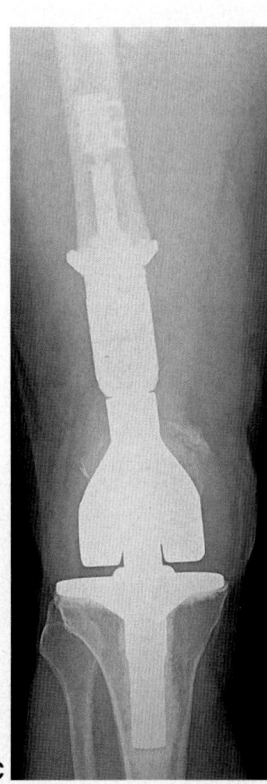 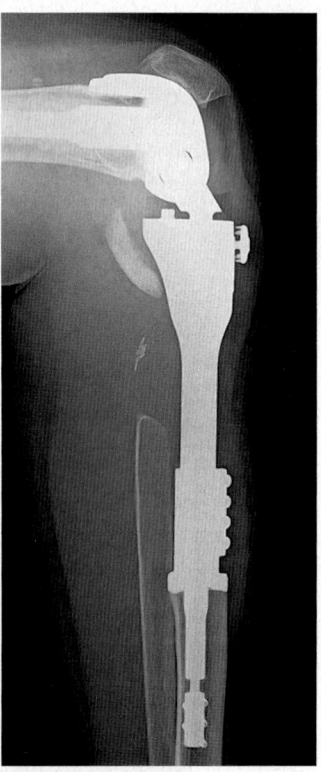

A **B** **C** **D**

Figure 91.11 Examples of extremity limb salvage reconstruction. **(A)** One-year postoperative anteroposterior radiograph of a 30-year-old woman who underwent proximal humeral resection and reconstruction with a double-barreled vascularized fibular autograft for high-grade osteosarcoma. **(B)** Ten-year postoperative anteroposterior film of a man who presented at age 65 with a proximal femoral grade 3 chondrosarcoma, after having undergone resection and compressive osseointegration reconstruction. **(C)** Twelve-year postoperative anteroposterior radiograph of a man who presented at age 53 with a distal femoral grade 2 chondrosarcoma; note the bone hypertrophy at shaft-prosthetic interface. **(D)** Seven-year postoperative lateral radiograph of a woman who presented at age 21 with a high-grade undifferentiated proximal tibial osteosarcoma and underwent compressive osseointegration fixation.

that order.[237] The lion's share of responsibility for overall survival lies with the medical oncology team. The burdens of local control and functional outcome fall mostly to the radiation and orthopedic surgical oncologists. When the "end-of-treatment" occurs, it is essential to remember that the caring continues. Primary physicians are ill-equipped to provide specialized surveillance care for these exceedingly rare tumors. Although increasing conditional survival as the years progress is a cause for optimism,[238] clinical, laboratory, and radiologic parameters need to be followed for a decade or more, given the long tail of these potentially lethal conditions. The NCCN has recommended "physical examination, imaging (radiograph, MR [imaging] with or without CT) of the surgical site as clinically indicated, chest imaging (every 6 months for 5 years

and annually thereafter), and annual cross-sectional abdominal imaging."[1] The evolving importance of PET/CT scan screening for accurate monitoring for local, regional, and distant recurrence has also been pointed out.[239]

When sarcomas of bone are incurable because of progressive metastatic and/or advanced unresectable locoregional disease, selective surgery, standard or experimental chemotherapy, targeted radiation, and expert symptom management must be offered to patients and their families.[240,241] Palliative care should be provided according to NCCN precepts.[242] The authors echo the sentiment of colleagues who have pointed out, "we must always remember that as long as we have something to offer, patients hope for an improvement in their condition. It is this hope that keeps them alive."[240]

SELECTED REFERENCES

The full reference list can be accessed at lwwhealthlibrary.com/oncology.

1. Biermann JS, Adkins DR, Agulnik M, et al. Bone cancer. *J Natl Compr Cancer Netw* 2013;11:688–723.
57. Eary JF, Conrad EU, O'Sullivan J, et al. Sarcoma mid-therapy [F-18]fluorodeoxyglucose positron emission tomography (FDG PET) and patient outcome. *J Bone Joint Surg Am* 2014;96-A:152–158.
66. Virayavanich W, Ringler MD, Chin CT, et al. CT-guided biopsy of bone and soft-tissue lesions: role of on-site immediate cytologic evaluation. *J Vasc Interv Radiol* 2011;22:1024–1030.
69. Mankin HJ, Mankin CJ, Simon MA. The hazards of biopsy, revisited. *J Bone Joint Surg Am* 1996;78-A:656–663.
72. Edge SB, Byrd DR, Compton CC, et al. *AJCC Cancer Staging Manual*, 7th ed. Philadelphia: Lippincott Raven; 2009.
73. Bacci G, Picci P, Gitelis S, et al. The treatment of localized Ewing's sarcoma: the experience at the Istituto Rizzoli in 163 cases treated with and without adjuvant chemotherapy. *Cancer* 1982;49:1561–1570.
74. Chan RC, Sutow WW, Lindberg RD, et al. Management and results of localized Ewing's sarcoma. *Cancer* 1979;43:1001–1006.
75. Zucker JM, Henry-Amar M, Sarrazin D, et al. Intensive systemic chemotherapy in localized Ewing's sarcoma. A historical trial. *Cancer* 1983;52:415–423.
76. Rosen G, Caparros B, Mosende C, et al. Curability of Ewing's sarcoma and considerations for future therapeutic trials. *Cancer* 1978;41:888–899.
77. Nesbit ME Jr, Gehan EA, Burgert EO Jr, et al. Multimodal therapy for the managment of primary, nonmetastatic Ewing's sarcoma of bone: a long-term follow-up of the First Intergroup study. *J Clin Oncol* 1990;8:1664–1674.
78. Jürgens H, Exner U, Gadner H, et al. Multidisciplinary treatment of primary Ewing's sarcoma of bone. A 6-year experience of a European Cooperative Trial. *Cancer* 1988;61:23–32.
79. Craft AW, Cotterill SJ, Bullimore JA, et al. Long-term results from the first UKCCSG Ewing's tumour study (ET-1). *Eur J Cancer* 1997;33:1061–1069.
80. Oberlin O, Patte C, Demeocq F, et al. The response to initial chemotherapy as a prognostic factor in localized Ewing's sarcoma. *Eur J Cancer Clin Oncol* 1985;21:463–467.
81. Oberlin O, Le Deley MC, Bui BN, et al. Prognostic factors in localized Ewing's tumours and peripheral neuroectodermal tumours: the third study of the French Society of Paediatric Oncology (EW88 study). *Br J Cancer* 2001;85:1646–1654.
82. Burgert EO Jr, Nesbit ME, Garnsey LA, et al. Multimodal therapy for the management of nonpelvic, localized Ewing's sarcoma of bone: intergroup Study IESS-II. *J Clin Oncol* 1990;8:1514–1524.
83. Oberlin O, Habrand JL, Zucker JM, et al. No benefit of ifosfamide in Ewing's sarcoma: a nonrandomized study of the French Society of Pediatric Oncology. *J Clin Oncol* 1992;10:1407–1412.
84. Craft A, Cotterill S, Malcolm A, et al. Ifosfamide-containing chemotherapy in Ewing's sarcoma: The Second United Kingdom Children's Cancer Study Group and the Medical Research Council Ewing's Tumor Study. *J Clin Oncol* 1998;16:3628–3633.
85. Paulussen M, Ahrens S, Dunst J, et al. Localized Ewing tumor of bone: final results of the cooperative Ewing's Sarcoma Study CESS 86. *J Clin Oncol* 2001;19:1818–1829.
86. Rosito P, Mancini AF, Rondelli R, et al. Italian Cooperative Study for the treatment of children and young adults with localized Ewing sarcoma of bone: A preliminary report of 6 years of experience. *Cancer* 1999;86:421–428.
87. Grier HE, Krailo MD, Tarbell NJ, et al. Addition of ifosfamide and etoposide to standard chemotherapy for Ewing's sarcoma and primitive neuroectodermal tumor of bone. *N Engl J Med* 2003;348:694–701.
88. Miser JS, Krailo MD, Tarbell NJ, et al. Treatment of metastatic Ewing's sarcoma or primitive neuroectodermal tumor of bone: evaluation of combination ifosfamide and etoposide–a Children's Cancer Group and Pediatric Oncology Group study. *J Clin Oncol* 2004;22:2873–2876.

89. Granowetter L, Womer R, Devidas M, et al. Dose-intensified compared with standard chemotherapy for nonmetastatic Ewing sarcoma family of tumors: a Children's Oncology Group study. *J Clin Oncol* 2009;27:2536–2541.
90. Womer RB, West DC, Krailo MD, et al. Randomized controlled trial of interval-compressed chemotherapy for the treatment of localized Ewing sarcoma: a report from the Children's Oncology Group. *J Clin Oncol* 2012;30:4148–4154.
91. Paulussen M, Craft AW, Lewis I, et al. Results of the EICESS-92 study: two randomized trials of Ewing's sarcoma treatment—cyclophosphamide compared with ifosfamide in standard-risk patients and assessment of benefit of etoposide added to standard treatment in high-risk patients. *J Clin Oncol* 2008;26:4385–4393.
92. Hayes FA, Thompson EI, Kumar M, et al. Long-term survival in patients with Ewing's sarcoma relapsing after completing treatment. *Med Pediatr Oncol* 1987;15:254–256.
93. Ferrari S, Brach del Prever A, Palmerini E, et al. Response to high-dose ifosfamide in patients with advanced/recurrent Ewing sarcoma. *Pediatr Blood Cancer* 2009;52:581–584.
94. Navid F, Reikes Willert J, McCarville MB, et al. Combination of gemcitabine and docetaxel in the treatment of children and young adults with refractory bone sarcoma. *Cancer* 2008;113:419–425.
95. Rapkin L, Qayed M, Brill P, et al. Gemcitabine and docetaxel (GEMDOX) for the treatment of relapsed and refractory pediatric sarcomas. *Pediatr Blood Cancer* 2012;59:854–858.
96. Fox E, Patel S, Wathen JK, et al. Phase II study of sequential gemcitabine followed by docetaxel for recurrent Ewing sarcoma, osteosarcoma, or unresectable or locally recurrent chondrosarcoma: results of the Sarcoma Alliance for Research Through Collaboration study 003. *Oncologist* 2012;17:e321–e329.
97. Mora J, Cruz CO, Parareda A, et al. Treatment of relapsed/refractory pediatric sarcomas with gemcitabine and docetaxel. *J Pediatr Hematol Oncol* 2009;31:723–729.
98. Lee EM, Rha SY, Lee J, et al. Phase II study of weekly docetaxel and fixed dose rate gemcitabine in patients with previously treated advanced soft tissue and bone sarcoma. *Cancer Chemother Pharmacol* 2012;69:635–642.
99. Saylors RL III, Stine KC, Sullivan J, et al. Cyclophosphamide plus topotecan in children with recurrent or refractory solid tumors: A Pediatric Oncology Group Phase II Study. *J Clin Oncol* 2001;19:3463–3469.
100. Hunold A, Weddeling N, Paulussen M, et al. Topotecan and cyclophosphamide in patients with refractory or relapsed Ewing tumors. *Pediatr Blood Cancer* 2006;47:795–800.
101. Bernstein ML, Devidas M, Lafreniere D, et al. Intensive therapy with growth factor support for patients with Ewing tumor metastatic at diagnosis: Pediatric Oncology Group/Children's Cancer Group phase II study 9457–A report from the Children's Oncology Group. *J Clin Oncol* 2006;24:152–159.
102. Wagner LM, Crews KR, Iacono LC, et al. Phase I trial of temozolomide and protracted irinotecan in pediatric patients with refractory solid tumors. *Clin Cancer Res* 2004;10:840–848.
103. Wagner LM, McAllister N, Goldsby RE, et al. Temozolomide and intravenous irinotecan for treatment of advanced Ewing sarcoma. *Pediatr Blood Cancer* 2007;48:132–139.
104. Casey DA, Wexler LH, Merchant MS, et al. Irinotecan and temozolomide for Ewing sarcoma: the Memorial Sloan-Kettering experience. *Pediatr Blood Cancer* 2009;53:1029–1034.
105. Raciborska A, Bilska K, Drabko K, et al. Vincristine, irinotecan, and temozolomide in patients with relapsed and refractory Ewing sarcoma. *Pediatr Blood Cancer* 2013;60:1621–1625.
106. Barker LM, Pendergrass TW, Sanders JE, et al. Survival after recurrence of Ewing's sarcoma family of tumors. *J Clin Oncol* 2005;23:4354–4362.
107. Meyers PA, Krailo MD, Ladanyi M, et al. High-dose melphalan, etoposide, total-body irradiation, and autologous stem-cell reconstitution as consolidation therapy for high-risk Ewing's sarcoma does not improve prognosis. *J Clin Oncol* 2001;19:2812–2820.

108. Luksch R, Tienghi A, Hall KS, et al. Primary metastatic Ewing's family of tumors: results of the Italian Sarcoma Group and Scandinavian Sarcoma Group ISG/SSG IV study including myeloablative chemotherapy and total lung-irradiation. *Ann Oncol* 2012;23:2970–2976.

109. Oberlin O, Rey A, Desfachelles AS, et al. Impact of high-dose busulfan plus melphalan as consolidation in metastatic Ewing tumors: a study by the Société des Cancers de l'Enfant. *J Clin Oncol* 2006;24:3997–4002.

110. Ladenstein R, Pötschger U, Le Deley MC, et al. Primary disseminated multifocal Ewing sarcoma: results of the Euro-EWING 99 trial. *J Clin Oncol* 2010;28:3284–3291.

111. Ferrari S, Sundby Hall K, Luksch R, et al. Nonmetastatic Ewing family tumors: high-dose chemotherapy with stem cell rescue in poor responder patients. Results of the Italian Sarcoma Group/Scandinavian Group III protocol. *Ann Oncol* 2011;22:1221–1227.

112. Juergens C, Weston C, Lewis I, et al. Safety assessment of intensive induction with vincristine, ifosfamide, doxorubicin, and etoposide (VIDE) in the treatment of Ewing tumors in the EURO-E.W.I.N.G. 99 clinical trial. *Pediatr Blood Cancer* 2006;47:22–29.

113. Stegmaier K, Wong JS, Ross KN, et al. Signature-based small molecule screening identifies cytosine arabinoside as an EWS/FLI modulator in Ewing sarcoma. *PLoS Med* 2007;4:e122.

114. DuBois SG, Krailo MD, Lessnick SL, et al. Phase II study of intermediate-dose cytarabine in patients with relapsed or refractory Ewing sarcoma: a report from the Children's Oncology Group. *Pediatr Blood Cancer* 2009;52:324–327.

115. Erkizan H, Kong Y, Merchant M, et al. Small molecule selected to disrupt oncogenic protein EWS-FL1 interaction with RNA Helicase A inhibits Ewing's sarcoma. *Nat Med* 2009;15:750–756.

116. Grohar PJ, Woldemichael GM, Griffin LB, et al. Identification of an inhibitor of the EWS-FLI1 oncogenic transcription factor by high-throughput screening. *J Natl Cancer Inst* 2011;103:962–978.

117. DuBois SG, Marina N, Glade-Bender J. Angiogenesis and vascular targeting in Ewing sarcoma: a review of preclinical and clinical data. *Cancer* 2010;116:749–757.

118. Felgenhauer JL, Nieder ML, Krailo MD, et al. A pilot study of low-dose anti-angiogenesis chemotherapy in combination with standard multiagent chemotherapy for patients with newly-diagnosed metastatic Ewing sarcoma family of tumors: a Children's Oncology Group (COG) phase II study NCT00061893. *Pediatr Blood Cancer* 2013;60:409–414.

119. Wagner L, Turpin B, Nagarajan R, et al. Pilot study of vincristine, oral irinotecan, and temozolomide (VOIT regimen) combined with bevacizumab in pediatric patients with recurrent solid tumors or brain tumors. *Pediatr Blood Cancer* 2013;60:1447–1451.

120. Yee D, Favoni RE, Lebovic GS, et al. Insulin-like growth factor I expression by tumors of neuroectodermal origin with the t(11;22) chromosomal translocation. A potential autocrine growth factor. *J Clin Invest* 1990;86:1806–1814.

121. Prieur A, Tirode F, Cohen P, et al. EWS/FLI-1 silencing and gene profiling of Ewing cells reveal downstream oncogenic pathways and a crucial role for repression of insulin-like growth factor binding protein 3. *Mol Cell Biol* 2004;24:7275–7283.

122. Houghton PJ, Morton CL, Gorlick R, et al. Initial testing of a monoclonal antibody (IMC-A12) against IGF-1R by the Pediatric Preclinical Testing Program. *Pediatr Blood Cancer* 2010;54:921–926.

123. Manara MC, Landuzzi L, Nanni P, et al. Preclinical in vivo study of new insulin-like growth factor-I receptor-specific inhibitor of Ewing's sarcoma. *Clin Cancer Res* 2007;13:1322–1330.

124. Martins AS, Mackintosh C, Herrero Martín D, et al. Insulin-like growth factor I receptor pathway inhibition by ADW742, alone or in combinaton with imatinib, doxorubicin, or vincristine, is a novel therapeutic approach in Ewing sarcoma. *Clin Cancer Res* 2006;12:3532–3540.

125. Scotlandi K, Benini S, Nanni P, et al. Blockage of insulin-like growth factor-I receptor inhibits the growth of Ewing's sarcoma in athymic mice. *Cancer Res* 1998;58:4127–4131.

126. Malempati S, Weigel B, Ingle AM, et al. Phase I/II trial and pharmacokinetic study of cixutumumab in pediatric patients with refractory solid tumors and Ewing sarcoma: a report from the Children's Oncology Group. *J Clin Oncol* 2012;30:256–262.

127. Tolcher AW, Sarantopoulos J, Patnaik A, et al. Phase I, pharmacokinetic, and pharmacodynamic study of AMG 749, a fully human monoclonal antibody to insulin-like growth factor receptor 1. *J Clin Oncol* 2009;27:5800–5807.

128. Juergens H, Daw NC, Geoerger B, et al. Preliminary efficacy of the anti-insulin-like growth factor type I receptor antibody figitumumab in patients with refractory Ewing sarcoma. *J Clin Oncol* 2011;29:4534–4540.

129. Pappo AS, Patel SR, Crowley J, et al. R1507, a monclonal antibody to the insulin-like growth factor 1 receptor, in patients with recurrent or refractory Ewing sarcoma family of tumors: results of a phase II Sarcoma Alliance for Research Through Collaboration study. *J Clin Oncol* 2011;29:4541–4547.

130. Tap WD, Demetri G, Barnette P, et al. Phase II study of ganitumab, a fully human anti-type-1 insulin-like growth factor receptor antibody, in patients with metastatic Ewing family tumors or desmoplastic small round cell tumors. *J Clin Oncol* 2012;30:1849–1856.

131. Mateo-Lozano S, Tirado OM, Notario V. Rapamycin induces the fusion-type independent downregulation of the EWS/FLI-1 proteins and inhibits Ewing's sarcoma cell proliferation. *Oncogene* 2003;22:9282–9287.

132. Houghton PJ, Morton CL, Gorlick R, et al. Stage 2 combination testing of rapamycin with cytotoxic agents by the Pediatric Preclinical Testing Program. *Mol Cancer Ther* 2010;9:101–112.

133. Houghton PJ, Morton CL, Kolb EA, et al. Initial testing (stage 1) of the mTOR inhibitor rapamycin by the Pediatric Preclinical Testing Program. *Pediatr Blood Cancer* 2008;50:799–805.

134. Mita M, Mita AC, Chu QS, et al. Phase I trial of the novel mammalian target of rapamycin inhibitor deforolimus (AP23573; MK-8669) administered intravenously daily for 5 days every 2 weeks to patients with advanced malignancies. *J Clin Oncol* 2008;26:361–367.

135. Garnett MJ, Edelman EJ, Heidorn SJ, et al. Systematic identification of genomic markers of drug sensitivity in cancer cells. *Nature* 2012;483:570–577.

136. Brenner JC, Feng FY, Han S, et al. PARP-1 inhibition as a targeted strategy to treat Ewing's sarcoma. *Cancer Res* 2012;72:1608–1613.

137. Carrie C, Mascard E, Gomez F, et al. Nonmetastatic pelvic Ewing sarcoma: report of the French Society of Pediatric Oncology. *Med Pediatr Oncol* 1999;33:444–449.

138. Wilkins RM, Pritchard DJ, Burgert EO Jr, et al. Ewing's sarcoma of bone. Experience with 140 patients. *Cancer* 1986;58:2551–2555.

139. Yock TI, Krailo M, Fryer CJ, et al. Local control in pelvic Ewing sarcoma: analysis from INT-0091–a report from the Children's Oncology Group. *J Clin Oncol* 2006;24:3838–3843.

140. Dunst J, Schuck A. Role of radiotherapy in Ewing tumors. *Pediatr Blood Cancer* 2004;42:465–470.

141. O'Sullivan B, Davis AM, Turcotte R, et al. Preoperative versus postoperative radiotherapy in soft-tissue sarcoma of the limbs: a randomised trial. *Lancet* 2002;359:2235–2241.

142. Seddon BM, Cassoni AM, Galloway MJ, et al. Fatal radiation myelopathy after high-dose busulfan and melphalan chemotherapy and radiotherapy for Ewing's sarcoma: a review of the literature and implications for practice. *Clin Oncol* 2005;17:385–390.

143. Carrie C, Le Deley MC, Claude L. The radiosensitization effect and toxicity of busulfan containing chemotherapy before radiotherapy for Ewing's sarcomas. *Strahlentherapie Und Onkologie* 2009;185:31.

144. Bölling T, Dirksen U, Ranft A, et al. Radiation toxicity following busulfan/melphalan high-dose chemotherapy in the EURO-EWING-99-trial: review of GPOH data. *Strahlentherapie Und Onkologie* 2009;185:21–22.

145. Lo SS, Sahgal A, Wang JZ, et al. Stereotactic body radiation therapy for spinal metastases. *Discov Med* 2010;9:289–296.

146. Lo SS, Fakiris AJ, Chang EL, et al. Stereotactic body radiation therapy: a novel treatment modality. *Nat Rev Clin Oncol* 2010;7:44–54.

147. Link MP, Goorin AM, Miser AW, et al. The effect of adjuvant chemotherapy on relapse-free survival in patients with osteosarcoma of the extremity. *N Engl J Med* 1986;314:1600–1606.

148. Goorin AM, Schwartzentruber DJ, Devidas M, et al. Presurgical chemotherapy compared with immediate surgery and adjuvant chemotherapy for nonmetastatic osteosarcoma: Pediatric Oncology Group Study POG-8651. *J Clin Oncol* 2003;21:1574–1580.

149. Bacci G, Gherlinzoni F, Picci P, et al. Adriamycin-methotrexate high dose versus adriamycin-methotrexate moderate dose as adjuvant chemotherapy for osteosarcoma of the extremities: a randomized study. *Eur J Cancer Clin Oncol* 1986;22:1337–1345.

150. Krailo MD, Ertel I, Makley J, et al. A randomized study comparing high-dose methotrexate with moderate-dose methotrexate as components of adjuvant chemotherapy in childhood nonmetastatic osteosarcoma: a report from the Childrens Cancer Study Group. *Med Pediatr Oncol* 1987;15:69–77.

151. Winkler K, Beron G, Kotz R, et al. Neoadjuvant chemotherapy for osteogenic sarcoma: results of a Cooperative German/Austrian study. *J Clin Oncol* 1984;2:617–624.

152. Winkler K, Beron G, Delling G, et al. Neoadjuvant chemotherapy of osteosarcoma: results of a randomized cooperative trial (COSS-82) with salvage chemotherapy based on histologic tumor response. *J Clin Oncol* 1988;6:329–337.

153. Bramwell V, Rouesse J, Steward W, et al. Adjuvant CYVADIC chemotherapy for adult soft tissue sarcoma–reduced local recurrence but no improvement in survival: a study of the European Organization for Research and Treatment of Cancer Soft Tissue and Bone Sarcoma Group. *J Clin Oncol* 1994;12:1137–1149.

154. Souhami RL, Craft AW, Van der Eijken J, et al. Randomised trial of two regimens of chemotherapy in operable osteosarcoma: a study of the European Osteosarcoma Intergroup. *Lancet* 1997;350:911–917.

155. Lewis IJ, Nooij MA, Whelan J, et al. Improvement in histologic repsonse but not survival in osteosarcoma patients treated with intensified chemotherapy: a randomized phase III trial of the European Osteosarcoma Intergroup. *J Natl Cancer Inst* 2007;99:112–128.

156. Harris MB, Gieser P, Goorin AM, et al. Treatment of metastatic osteosarcoma at diagnosis: a Pediatric Oncology Group Study. *J Clin Oncol* 1998;16:3641–3648.

157. Ferrari S, Ruggieri P, Cefalo G, et al. Neoadjuvant chemotherapy with methotrexate, cisplatin, and doxorubicin with or without ifosfamide in nonmetastatic osteosarcoma of the extremity: an Italian Sarcoma Group Trial ISG/OS-1. *J Clin Oncol* 2012;30:2112–2118.

158. Meyers PA, Schwartz CL, Krailo M, et al. Osteosarcoma: a randomized, prospective trial of the addition of ifosfamide and/or muramyl tripeptide to cisplatin, doxorubicin, and high-dose methotrexate. *J Clin Oncol* 2005;23:2004–2011.

159. Meyers PA, Schwartz CL, Krailo MD, et al. Osteosarcoma: the addition of muramyl tripeptide to chemotherapy improves overall survival–a report from the Children's Oncology Group. *J Clin Oncol* 2008;26:633–638.

160. Goorin AM, Harris MB, Bernstein M, et al. Phase II/III trial of etoposide and high-dose ifosfamide in newly diagnosed metastatic osteosarcoma: a Pediatric Oncology Group Trial. *J Clin Oncol* 2002;20:426–433.

161. Le Deley MC, Guinebretière JM, Gentet JC, et al. SFOP OS94: a randomised trial comparing preoperative high-dose methotrexate plus doxorubicin to high-dose methotrexate plus etoposide and ifosfamide in osteosarcoma patients. *Eur J Cancer* 2007;43:752–761.

162. Miser JS, Kinsella TJ, Triche TJ, et al. Ifosfamide with mesna uroprotection and etoposide: an effective regimen in the treatment of recurrent sarcomas and other tumors of children and young adults. *J Clin Oncol* 1987;5:1191–1198.

163. Gentet JC, Brunat-Mentigny M, Demaille MC, et al. Ifosfamide and etoposide in childhood osteosarcoma. A phase II study of the French Society of Paediatric Oncology. *Eur J Cancer* 1997;33:232–237.

164. Lee HY, Shin SJ, Kim HS, et al. Weekly gemcitabine and docetaxel in refractory soft tissue sarcoma: A retrospective analysis. *Cancer Treat Res* 2012;44:43–49.

165. Ebb D, Meyers P, Grier H, et al. Phase II trial of trastuzumab in combination with cytotoxic chemotherapy for treatment of metastatic osteosarcoma with human epodermal growth factor receptor 2 overexpression: a report from the Children's Oncology Group. *J Clin Oncol* 2012;30:2545–2551.

166. Heiner JP, Miraldi F, Kallick S, et al. Localization of GD2-specific monoclonal antibody 3F8 in human osteosarcoma. *Cancer Res* 1987;47:5377–5381.

167. Murray JL, Cunningham JE, Brewer H, et al. Phase I trial of murine monoclonal antibody 14G2a administered by prolonged intravenous infusion in patients with neuroectodermal tumors. *J Clin Oncol* 1994;12:184–193.

168. Yu AL, Uttenreuther-Fischer MM, Huang CS, et al. Phase I trial of a human-mouse chimeric anti-disialoganglioside monclonal antibody ch14.18 in patients with refractory neuroblastoma and osteosarcoma. *J Clin Oncol* 1998;16:2169–2180.

169. Kleinerman ES, Gano JB, Johnston DA, et al. Efficacy of liposomal muramyl tripeptide (CGP 19835A) in the treatment of relapsed osteosarcoma. *Am J Clin Oncol* 1995;18:93–99.

170. Chou AJ, Kleinerman ES, Krailo MD, et al. Addition of muramyl tripeptide to chemotherapy for patients with newly diagnosed metastatic osteosarcoma: a report from the Children's Oncology Group. *Cancer* 2009;115:5339–5348.

171. Müller CR, Smeland S, Bauer HC, et al. Interferon-alpha as the only adjuvant treatment in high-grade osteosarcoma: long term results of the Karolinska Hospital series. *Acta Oncol* 2005;44:475–480.

172. Bielack SS, Smeland S, Whelan J, et al. MAP plus maintenance pegylated interferon alpha-2b (MAPIfn) versus MAP alone in patients with resectable high-grade osteosarcoma and good histologic response to preoperative MAP: First results of the EURAMOS-1 "good response" randomization. *J Clin Oncol* 2013;31:LBA10504.

173. Heymann D, Ory B, Gouin F, et al. Bisphosphonates: new therapeutic agents for the treatment of bone tumors. *Trends Mol Med* 2004;10:337–343.

174. Meyers PA, Healey JH, Chou AJ, et al. Addition of pamidronate to chemotherapy for the treatment of osteosarcoma. *Cancer* 2011;117:1736–1744.

175. Goldsby RE, Fan TM, Villaluna D, et al. Feasibility and dose discovery analysis of zolendronic acid with concurrent chemotherapy in the treatment of newly diagnosed metastatic osteosarcoma: a report of the Children's Oncology Group. *Eur J Cancer* 2013;49:2384–2391.

176. Grignani G, Palmerini E, Dileo P, et al. A phase II trial of sorafenib in relapsed and unresectable high-grade ostesarcoma after failure of standard multimodal therapy: an Italian Sarcoma Group study. *Ann Oncol* 2012;23:508–516.

177. Arndt CA, Koshkina NV, Inwards CY, et al. Inhaled granulcoyte-macrophage colony stimulating factor for first pulmonary recurrence of osteosarcoma: effects on disease-free survival and immunomodulation. A report from the Children's Oncology Group. *Clin Cancer Res* 2010;16:4024–4030.

178. Chou AJ, Gupta R, Bell MD, et al. Inhaled lipid cisplatin (ILC) in the treatment of patients with relapsed/progressive osteosarcoma metastatic to the lung. *Pediatr Blood Cancer* 2013;60:580–586.

179. Ogawa Y, Takahashi T, Kobayashi T, et al. Mechanism of apoptotic resistance of human osteosarcoma cell line, HS-Os-1, against irradiation. *Int J Mol Med* 2003;12:453–458.

180. Ozaki T, Flege S, Liljenqvist U, et al. Osteosarcoma of the spine: experience of the Cooperative Osteosarcoma Study Group. *Cancer* 2002;94:1069–1077.

181. Ozaki T, Flege S, Kevric M, et al. Osteosarcoma of the pelvis: experience of the Cooperative Osteosarcoma Study Group. *J Clin Oncol* 2003;21:334–341.

182. Machak GN, Tkachev SI, Solovyev YN, et al. Neoadjuvant chemotherapy and local radiotherapy for high-grade osteosarcoma of the extremities. *Mayo Clin Proc* 2003;78:147–155.

183. Kamada T, Imai R, Serizawa I. Carbon ion radiotherapy in bone and soft tissue sarcoma. Presented at the Proceedings of NRS-MD Anderson Symposium on Clinical Issues for Particle Therapy, 2008.

184. Ciernik IF, Niemierko A, Harmon DC, et al. Proton-based radiotherapy for unresectable or incompletely resected osteosarcoma. *Cancer* 2011;117:4522–4530.

185. Longhi A, Errani C, Gonzales-Arabio D, et al. Osteosarcoma in patients older than 65 years. *J Clin Oncol* 2008;26:5368–5373.

186. Ganjoo KN, Patel S. The treatment outcome for adult patients with Ewing's sarcoma. *Curr Oncol Rep* 2013;15:372–377.

194. Rougraff BT, Simon MA, Kniesl JS, et al. Limb salvage compared with amputation for osteosarcoma of the distal end of the femur. A long-term oncological, functional, and quality-of-life study. *J Bone Joint Surg Am* 1994;76-A:649–656.

195. Davis AM, Devlin M, Griffin AM, et al. Functional outcome in amputation versus limb sparing of patients with lower extremity sarcoma: a matched case-control study. *Arch Phys Med Rehabil* 1999;80:615–618.

196. Refaat Y, Gunnoe J, Hornicek FJ, et al. Comparison of quality of life after amputation or limb salvage. *Clin Orthop Relat Res* 2002;397:298–305.

197. Kong CB, Song WS, Cho WH, et al. Local recurrence has only a small effect of survival in high-risk extremity osteosarcoma. *Clin Orthop Relat Res* 2012;470:1482–1490.

199. O'Donnell RJ, Burch S. Hemipelvectomy and hemicorporectomy: Hindquarter amputation. In: Ames CP, Boriani S, Jandial R, eds. *Spine and Spinal Cord Tumors*. St. Louis, MO: AMP/CRC Press; 2013:759–766.

203. Harrington IJ, Lexier R, Woods JM, et al. A plaster-pylon technique for below-knee amputation. *J Bone Joint Surg Br* 1991;73-B:76–78.

205. Henderson ER, Pepper AM, Marulanda G, et al. Outcome of lower-limb preservation with an expandable endoprosthesis after bone tumor resection in children. *J Bone Joint Surg Am* 2012;94-A:537–547.

210. McDonald DJ, Scott SM, Eckardt JJ. Tibial turn-up for long distal femoral bone loss. *Clin Orthop Relat Res* 2001;383:214–220.

211. Brånemark P-I. *The Osseointegration Book: From Calvarium to Calcaneus*. Berlin: Quintessenz Verlags-GmbH; 2005.

213. Hagberg K, Brånemark R. One hundred patients treated with osseointegrated transfemoral amputation prostheses—rehabilitation perspective. *J Rehabil Res Dev* 2009;46:331–344.

214. Brånemark R, Berlin Ö, Hagberg K, et al. A novel osseointegrated percutaneous prosthetic system for the treatment of patients with transfemoral amputation: a prospective study of 51 patients. *J Bone Joint Surg Br* 2014;96-B:106–113.

216. Ghert M, Colterjohn N, Manfrini M. The use of vascularized fibular grafts in skeletal reconstruction for bone tumors in children. *J Am Acad Orthop Surg* 2007;15:577–587.

219. Ogilvie CM, Crawford EA, Hosalkar HS, et al. Long-term results for limb salvage with osteoarticular allograft reconstruction. *Clin Orthop Relat Res* 2009;467:2685–2690.

221. Henderson ER, Groundland JS, Pala E, et al. Failure mode classification for tumor endoprostheses: retrospective review of five institutions and a literature review. *J Bone Joint Surg Am* 2011;93-A:418–429.

222. Cristofolini L, Bini SA, Toni A. In vitro testing of a novel limb salvage prosthesis for the distal femur. *Clin Biomech (Bristol, Avon)* 1998;13:608–615.

224. Avedian RS, Goldsby RE, Kramer MJ, et al. Effect of chemotherapy on initial compressive osseointegration of tumor endoprostheses. *Clin Orthop Relat Res* 2007;459:48–53.

225. O'Donnell RJ. Compressive osseointegration of modular endoprostheses. *Curr Opin Orthop* 2007;18:590–603.

226. Kramer MJ, Tanner BJ, Horvai AE, et al. Compressive osseointegration promotes viable bone at the endoprosthetic interface: retrieval study of Compress® implants. *Int Orthop* 2008;32:567–571.

227. Tyler WK, Healey JH, Morris CD, et al. Compress® periprosthetic fractures. *Clin Orthop Relat Res* 2009;467:2800–2806.

231. Bhangu AA, Kramer MJ, Grimer RJ, et al. Early distal femoral endoprosthetic survival: cemented stems versus the Compress® implant. *Int Orthop* 2006;30:465–472.

232. O'Donnell RJ. Compressive osseointegration of tibial implants in primary cancer reconstruction. *Clin Orthop Relat Res* 2009;467:2807–2812.

233. Farfalli GL, Boland PJ, Morris CD, et al. Early equivalence of uncemented press-fit and femoral Compress® femoral fixation. *Clin Orthop Relat Res* 2009;467:2792–2799.

234. Pedtke AC, Wustrack RL, Fang AS, et al. Aseptic failure: how does the Compress® implant compare to cemented stems? *Clin Orthop Relat Res* 2011;470:735–742.

235. Healey JH, Morris CD, Athanasian EA, et al. Compress® knee arthroplasty has 80% 10-year survivorship and novel forms of bone failure. *Clin Orthop Relat Res* 2013;471:774–783.

236. Calvert GT, Cummings JE, Bowles AJ, et al. A dual-center review of compressive osseointegration for fixation of massive endoprosthetics: 2- to 9-year followup. *Clin Orthop Relat Res* 2013;472:822–829.

237. Weisstein JS, Goldsby RE, O'Donnell RJ. Oncologic approaches to pediatric limb preservation. *J Am Acad Orthop Surg* 2005;13:544–554.

238. Miller BJ, Lynch CF, Buckwalter JA. Conditional survival is greater than overall survival at diagnosis in patients with osteosarcoma and Ewing's sarcoma. *Clin Orthop Relat Res* 2013;471:3398–3404.

239. Garner HW, Kransdorf MJ, Peterson JJ. Posttherapy imaging of musculoskeletal neoplasms. *Radiol Clin North Am* 2011;49:1307–1323.

240. Merimsky O, Kollender Y, Inbar M, et al. Palliative treatment for advanced or metastatic osteosarcoma. *Isr Med Assoc J* 2004;6:34–38.

241. Errani C, Longhi A, Rossi G, et al. Palliative therapy for osteosarcoma. *Expert Rev Anticancer Ther* 2011;11:217–227.

242. Levy MH, Adolph MD, Back A, et al. Palliative care. *J Natl Compr Cancer Netw* 2012;10:1284–1309.

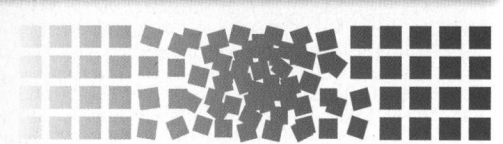

92 Cancer of the Skin

Sean R. Christensen and David J. Leffell

INTRODUCTION

One in five Americans will develop nonmelanoma skin cancer (NMSC) during his or her lifetime. NMSC is the most common human cancer, with an estimated annual incidence of >3 million in 2006 in the United States, higher than the incidence of lung cancer, breast cancer, prostate cancer, and colon cancer combined.[1-3] Despite growing public awareness of the harmful effects of sun and ultraviolet (UV) exposure, the incidence continues to rise. The increasing frequency of NMSC results from the age shift in the population (incidence of NMSC increases with age), high ambient solar irradiance, and increasing leisure time spent with natural or artificial UV exposure. Prognosis depends of biology and location of the lesion, as well as host characteristics.

Economic implications of NMSC are considerable. In the United States alone, Medicare spends $13 billion each year on skin cancer care treatment. Added to this is the cost of treating precancerous lesions such as actinic keratoses (AK), which are increasingly common.

Prevention strategies aimed at reduction of known risk factors, patient education about the importance of early detection and treatment, and the search for more effective and tissue sparing therapies continues.

NONMELANOMA SKIN CANCER

DIAGNOSIS

Although many NMSCs present with classic clinical findings such as nodularity, tissue friability, and erythema, definitive diagnosis can be established only by tissue biopsy. Adequate tissue samples obtained in an atraumatic fashion is critical to histopathologic diagnosis. Skin biopsies may be performed by shave, punch, or fusiform excision. The type of biopsy performed should be based on the morphology of the primary lesion and clinical differential diagnosis. A shave biopsy is usually adequate for raised lesions such as nodular basal cell carcinoma (BCC) and squamous cell carcinoma (SCC), or flat, superficial lesions such as SCC in situ (SCCIS). A punch biopsy is appropriate for lesions with a deeper dermal or subcutaneous extension such as dermatofibrosarcoma protuberans (DFSP). An excisional biopsy may be required for diagnosis of a dermal nodule when morphologic assessment of overall tumor architecture is crucial for proper diagnostic assessment, such as distinguishing between a benign dermatofibroma and a malignant fibrous tumor.

Shave Biopsy

Basic skin biopsy techniques are demonstrated in Fig. 92.1A. A shave biopsy is performed under clean conditions. In the authors' opinion, the use of a sterilized flexible razor blade, which can be precisely manipulated by the operator to adjust the depth of the biopsy, is often superior to the use of a no. 15 scalpel. After the procedure, adequate hemostasis is achieved with topical application of aqueous aluminum chloride (20%), ferric subsulfate (Monsel solution), or electrocautery. Note that ferrous subsulfate may lead to permanent tattooing of the skin so it should not be used on the face unless there is a high likelihood of subsequent definitive surgical treatment.

Punch Biopsy

A punch biopsy is performed under local anesthesia, using a trephine or biopsy punch (Fig. 92.1B). The operator makes a circular incision to the level of the superficial fat, using a rotating or twisting motion of the trephine. Traction applied perpendicularly to the relaxed skin tension lines minimizes redundancy at closure. Hemostasis is achieved by placement of simple, nonabsorbable sutures that can be removed in 7 to 14 days depending on anatomic site. If the punch biopsy is small and not in a cosmetically crucial area, the resulting biopsy wound can often heal very well by second intention.

Excisional Biopsy

After local anesthesia has been achieved under sterile conditions, a scalpel is used to incise an ellipse to the level of the subcutis. Hemostasis is obtained with cautery as needed, and the wound is closed in a layered fashion using absorbable and, if needed removable epidermal sutures.

GENERAL APPROACH TO MANAGEMENT OF SKIN CANCER

The management of skin cancer is guided by the histologic and biologic nature of the tumor, the anatomic site, the underlying medical status of the patient, and whether the tumor is primary or recurrent. Accurate interpretation of the diagnostic biopsy is essential for appropriate clinical management. Depending on the biologic aggressiveness of the tumor, cancers of the skin may be excised or, in some cases of superficial tumors or precancerous lesions, eliminated in a less invasive fashion. Surgical options include conventional excision and Mohs micrographic surgery (MMS). Destructive modalities include curettage and cautery/electrodessication (C&D), cryosurgery, photodynamic therapy (PDT), and laser surgery. Other techniques are topical therapy (e.g., imiquimod, 5-fluorouracil [5-FU]), intralesional interferon, chemotherapy, and radiation therapy (RT). Other than conventional and Mohs surgery, none of these latter techniques provide information about the histologic completeness of the cancer ablation.

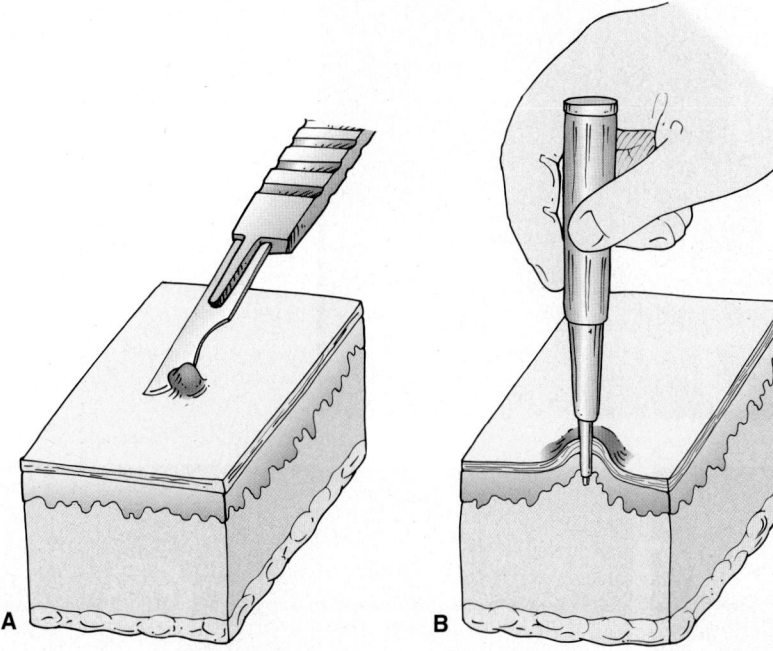

Figure 92.1 Biopsy techniques. Local anesthetic (lidocaine 1% with epinephrine, 1:100,000, unless contraindicated) is injected with a 30-gauge needle. A 30-gauge needle minimizes pain and tissue trauma. Unless otherwise specified, postbiopsy care involves daily cleansing with tap water followed by application of an emollient or an antibiotic ointment and a nonadherent dressing. Although popular in the past, the use of hydrogen peroxide is discouraged because of keratinocyte toxicity. Similarly, triple antibiotic ointments that include Neosporin (Johnson & Johnson, New Brunswick, NJ) or bacitracin may lead to contact dermatitis. For simple skin wounds, petroleum jelly has been shown to be as effective in facilitating healing as antibiotic ointment. **(A)** Shave biopsy. A scalpel blade is manipulated by the operator to adjust the depth of the biopsy. Hemostasis is achieved with topical application of aqueous aluminum chloride, ferrous subsulfate, or electrocautery. **(B)** Punch biopsy. The operator makes a circular incision to the level of the superficial fat, using a rotating or twisting motion of the trephine. Traction applied perpendicularly to the relaxed skin tension lines minimizes redundancy at closure. Hemostasis is commonly achieved by placement of sutures.

Excision

Excisional surgery involves the removal of the cancer and a margin of clinically uninvolved tissue, followed by layered closure or second intention healing. Frozen or permanent sections interpreted by the pathologist determine adequacy of margins. Margins are assessed from representative sections of the specimen in "bread-loaf" fashion, allowing for sampling of the surgical margin. This sampling may occasionally result in a false-negative assessment of clear margins, especially in cases of infiltrating or aggressive-growth cancers. A similar misdiagnosis may occur when one relies on vertically prepared frozen specimens for intraoperative margin control. Excision, especially when performed in a physician's office rather than in a hospital operating room, is effective and cost-efficient for primary, small (<1 cm) NMSCs, without infiltrative or other high-risk features.

Mohs Micrographic Surgery

MMS facilitates optimal margin control and conservation of normal tissue, and it has become the standard of care in a variety of skin cancer subtypes. Individuals trained in the technique perform MMS in the office setting under local anesthesia. After gentle curettage to define the clinical gross margin of the cancer, a 45-degree tangential specimen of tumor with a minimal margin of clinically normal-appearing tissue is excised, precisely mapped in a horizontal fashion, and processed immediately by frozen section for microscopic examination (Fig. 92.2). Optimal margin control is obtained by examination of the entire lateral perimeter of the specimen and contiguous deep margin. Meticulous mapping allows for directed extirpation of any remaining tumor, resulting in a cure rate of >97% to 99% for primary BCC and SCC.[4]

A key defining feature of MMS is that the surgeon excises, maps, and reviews the specimen personally, minimizing the chance of error in tissue interpretation and orientation. MMS has gained acceptance as the treatment of choice for recurrent skin cancers, as well as for primary skin cancers located at anatomic sites that require maximal tissue conservation for preservation of function and cosmesis (Fig. 92.3). Guidelines for the appropriate use of MMS have been published that reinforce the advantages of this technique for selected high-risk tumors.[5] For those tumors with a significant risk of recurrence, MMS is a cost-effective treatment compared with surgical excision when considering associated ambulatory surgery center facility fee and a subsequent re-excision procedure. It is also significantly less expensive than radiotherapy and frozen-section–guided excisional surgery.[6]

Curettage and Cautery/Electrodesiccation

Common methods of treatment of uncomplicated skin cancers on the trunk and extremities and certain facial lesions include C&D and cryotherapy using liquid nitrogen. C&D is performed under clean conditions with local anesthesia. The visible tumor is first removed by curettage, which is extended for a margin of 2 to 4 mm beyond the clinical borders of the cancer. Cautery or electrodesiccation is then performed to destroy another 1 mm of tissue at the lateral and deep margins. C&D can yield satisfactory results after a single cycle of C&D for NMSC tumors <1 cm, especially if the tumor is of the superficial subtype. Salasche[7] recommended that C&D be performed for three cycles to avoid recurrence. The authors believe, based on extensive clinical experience, that if the tumor requires three cycles of C&D, careful consideration should be given to more definitive approaches such as excision or MMS. Detailed reviews of primary BCC treated by C&D revealed 5-year recurrence rates of 8.6% for lesions located on the neck, trunk, and extremities, and between 17.5% and 22% for lesions located on the face.[8]

One potential drawback of C&D is that recurrent tumors following this treatment may be multifocal and develop a more aggressive biologic behavior. C&D is thus reserved for small (<1 cm) superficial or nodular BCCs, AKs, and SCCIS without follicular involvement located on the trunk or extremities.

Cryosurgery

Cryosurgery exposes precancers and NMSCs to destructive sub-zero temperatures. Tissue damage is caused initially by direct effects and subsequently by vascular stasis, ice crystal formation, cell membrane disruption, pH changes, hypertonic damage, and finally thermal shock. Successful cryosurgery requires temperatures reaching −50°C to −60°C at the deep and lateral margins of the tumor. The open-spray technique is used most often and

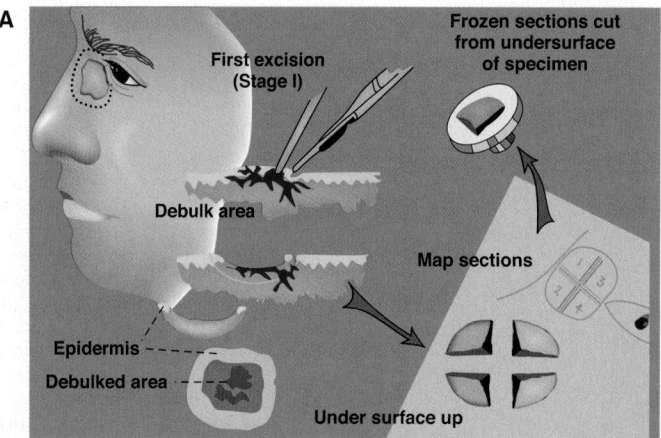

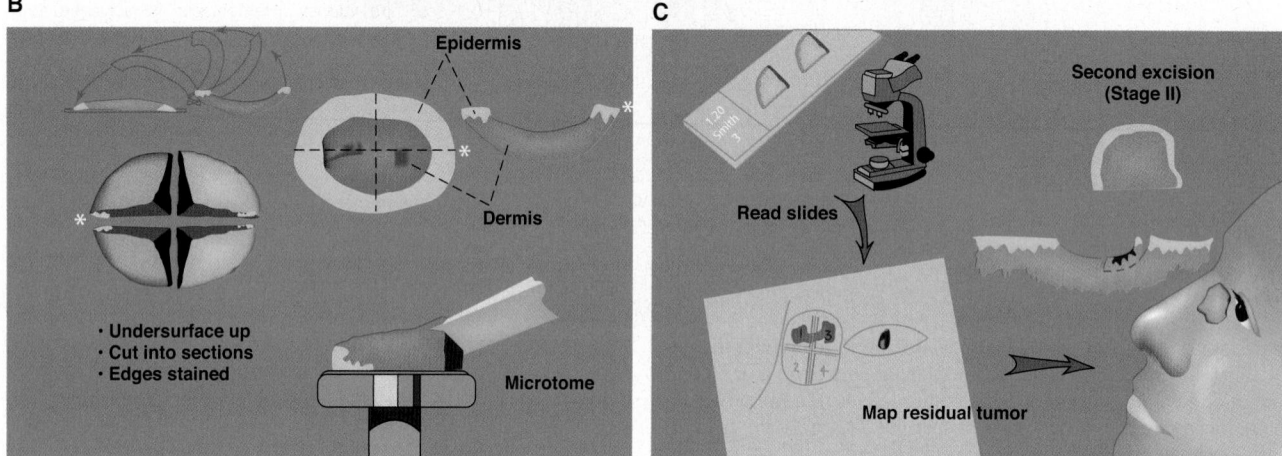

Figure 92.2 Mohs micrographic surgery. **(A–C)** After gentle curettage, a tangential specimen of tumor with a minimal margin of clinically normal-appearing tissue is obtained, precisely mapped, and processed immediately by frozen section for microscopic examination. Superior margin control is obtained through examination of the entire perimeter of the specimen. Precise mapping allows for directed extirpation of any remaining tumor, as shown in **C**. *White asterisks* in panel B track the 3 o'clock position of the lateral margin as the specimen is transected, inverted, and inked. (Courtesy David J. Leffell, MD, and People's Medical Publishing House.)

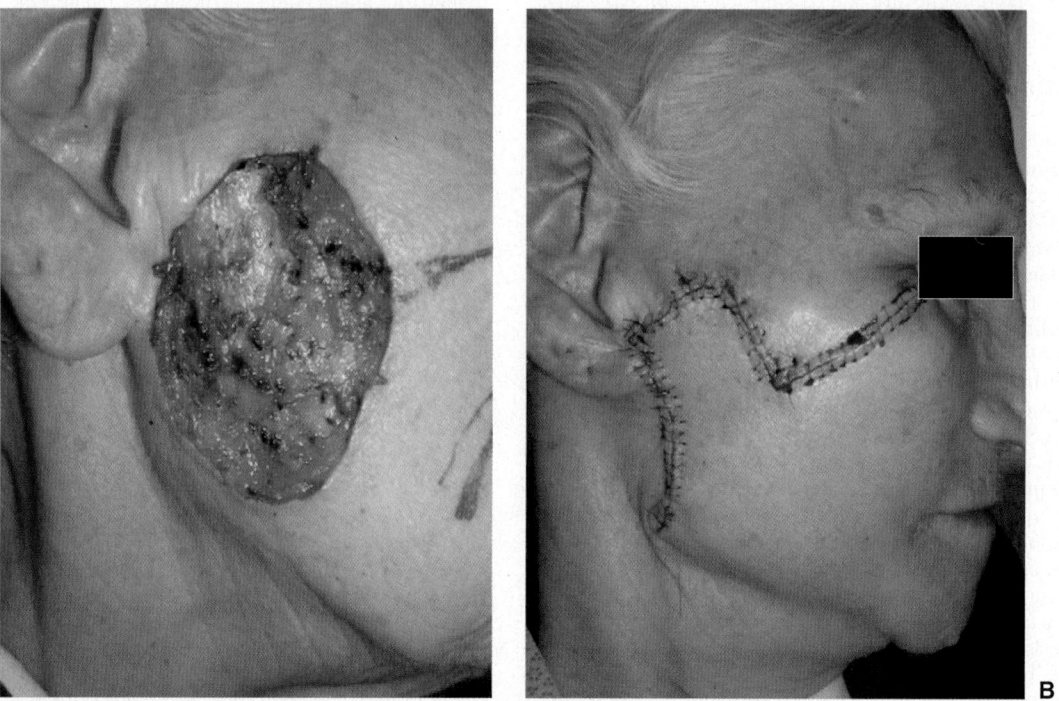

Figure 92.3 (A) Defect resulting from extirpation of basal cell carcinoma by Mohs micrographic surgery. **(B)** Defect repaired with rhomboid transposition flap.

requires pressurized liquid nitrogen spray delivery from a distance of 1 to 3 cm. With the confined-spray technique, liquid nitrogen is delivered through a cone that allows more precise tissue destruction. With the cryoprobe technique, a prechilled metal probe is applied to the tumor. Immediately following cryosurgery, local erythema and edema are apparent. An exudative phase ensues in 24 to 72 hours and is followed by sloughing at approximately day 7. Complete healing is usually seen at 2 to 3 weeks for facial lesions and up to 6 weeks for lesions on the trunk and extremities.

Temporary complications may include extensive drainage, edema, bulla formation, and hypertrophic scarring. Paresthesia may occur with thermal injury to superficial nerves. Other less common side effects may include headache, syncope, febrile reaction, cold urticaria, pyogenic granuloma, delayed hemorrhage, milia formation, or dyschromia (hypo- and hyperpigmentation). Permanent complications may include tissue contraction, hypopigmentation, and scarring.

The clinical usefulness of cryosurgery and C&D is limited by the inability to evaluate treatment margins and therefore thoroughness of tumor eradication. The absence of margin control and a dense postcryosurgery scar, which might obscure recurrence, makes these methods valuable primarily in the care of histologically superficial NMSC.

TOPICAL THERAPY FOR SKIN CANCER

Imiquimod

Imiquimod, an imidazolaquinoline, binds intracellular toll-like receptors 7 and 8 acting as a topical immune-response modifier. Imiquimod promotes a cell-mediated immune response through induction of several cytokines particularly interferon (IFN)-α and IFN-γ and interleukins (IL) 6, 8, and 12 by keratinocytes and peripheral blood mononuclear cells including monocytes, macrophages, and toll-like receptor-7 bearing plasmacytoid dendritic cells.[9–12] The net effect is a T-helper type 1–dominant inflammatory response driven by CD4 T cells. In addition, IFN-γ stimulates cytotoxic T cells to kill virus-infected and tumor cells, facilitating tumor regression. The use of imiquimod is approved by the US Food and Drug Administration (FDA) for treatment of AKs and superficial BCCs on the trunk, neck, or extremities. Studies with topical imiquimod for nodular BCC, SCCIS, and malignant melanoma in situ have shown variable results.[13–15] Imiquimod appears to be effective as monotherapy in carefully selected cases and may have a role postoperatively to decrease the rate of recurrence of certain skin cancers. However, long-term data on cure and recurrence remain to be determined. Close monitoring of the treatment site is essential.

Imiquimod-related adverse events include application site reactions (i.e., erythema, pain, edema, ulceration, bleeding), fatigue, myalgias, fever and chills or flu-like symptoms, headache, diarrhea, nausea, and tender lymphadenopathy.

5-Fluorouracil

5-FU, a chemotherapeutic agent that interferes with DNA synthesis by inhibiting thymidylate synthetase, has been used topically since the 1960s for the treatment of AKs. 5-FU is currently approved by the FDA for the treatment of AKs and superficial BCCs. This drug carries a black box warning urging close supervision by a physician experienced with the administration of antimetabolites. Treatment site reactions following topical 5-FU administration include erythema, edema, and pain. In severe cases, ulcerations and bleeding have been reported. Side effects of 5-FU treatment are exacerbated by prolonged UV radiation (UVR). Poor treatment compliance, due to adverse side effects, is associated with significant failure rates.[11,16]

Diclofenac

Diclofenac is a nonsteroidal anti-inflammatory agent that inhibits cyclooxygenase, the rate-limited enzyme in the synthesis of prostaglandins. Diclofenac has high affinity for cyclooxygenase-2 that is frequently elevated in AKs, melanoma, and NMSC. In addition, diclofenac inhibits prostaglandin-mediated, UV-induced NMSC by decreasing proinflammatory cytokines such as IL-1, tumor necrosis factor–α, and transforming growth factor–β.[17,18] Diclofenac has a modest effect on treatment of AK but has not been shown to be effective in the treatment of NMSC.

Retinoids

Both topically applied and systemic retinoids have consistently been shown to be effective in the prevention and management of NMSCs. The effect of topical retinoids is at best mild, whereas oral retinoids have a different efficacy profile and side effects that frequently limit its usefulness for cancer treatment and prevention. Retinoids downregulate the expression of AP-1 responsive genes, activate transrepression of AP-1, arrest growth, and induce apoptosis and differentiation.[19,20] Retinoids also downregulate the UV-induced overexpression of cyclooxygenase-2, reducing prostaglandins that are normally elevated in AKs and NMSC.[20,21] Isotretinoin at 0.25 to 0.5 mg/kg per day and acitretin at 10 to 20 mg/d are the most common systemic retinoids used for skin cancer chemoprevention, especially in immunocompromised patients.[22] Randomized trials of acitretin for secondary prevention of NMSC have shown a significant benefit in patients of renal transplant and modest benefit that did not reach statistical significance in immunocompetent patients.[23,24] Routine clinical monitoring for signs of retinoid toxicity and laboratory examinations (fasting lipid profile, liver function tests) during systemic therapy are mandatory.

Ingenol Mebutate

Ingenol mebutate is a macrocyclic diterpene ester found in the sap of the *Euphorbia peplus* plant. Ingenol mebutate gel formulations (0.015%, 0.05%) are available for the treatment of AKs. The proposed mechanism of action is induction of apoptosis in proliferating keratinocytes and activation of innate immune effector responses, including rapid release of neutrophil oxidative mediators. Treatment regimens shown to be effective for reduction of AKs include once daily application on three consecutive days to the face or scalp (0.015% gel) or on two consecutive days to the trunk or extremities (0.05% gel).[25]

Photodynamic Therapy

Topical PDT with 5-aminolevulinic acid (ALA) or methylaminolevulinic acid (MAL) is effective in the treatment of certain NMSCs. Following topical application, ALA or MAL accumulates preferentially in malignant and premalignant cells and is metabolized in the intrinsic intracellular heme biosynthesis pathway to protoporphyrin IX. Preferential accumulation of ALA in malignant and premalignant tissues results from the differences in cellular uptake, differential activities of the heme and porphyrin biosynthetic pathways, iron bioavailability, differential properties of stratum corneum, and variable tissue ALA distribution. Protoporphyrin IX is a photoactive intermediate that facilitates the transfer of singlet oxygen species and the generation of free radicals. The reactive oxygen species induce lipid peroxidation, protein cross-linking, and increased membrane permeability. All these processes contribute to irreversible damage and ultimately cell death of malignant and premalignant cells.[26,27]

Both lasers and noncoherent light sources (blue and red light) with wavelengths in a range corresponding to absorption peaks of protoporphyrin IX (from 400 nm to infrared) have been used to activate topically applied ALA and/or MAL.

The use of PDT is currently approved by the FDA for the treatment of AKs. The off-label uses of PDT to treat NMSCs, acne, photodamaged skin, human papillomavirus (HPV)-associated pathologies, lymphocytoma cutis, hidradenitis suppurativa, and other dermatologic conditions are currently under investigation.[28] Scarring and postprocedural dyspigmentation are minimal to nonexisting following PDT.[29] An apparent additional benefit of PDT is photorejuvenation with softening of the appearance of fine lines, rhytids, and acne scars. The mechanism of photorejuvenation is not fully understood, but may relate to increased type I collagen production.[30]

RADIATION THERAPY FOR SKIN CANCER

RT is a treatment option for certain NMSCs, angiosarcoma, Merkel cell carcinoma (MCC), cutaneous lymphomas, some adnexal carcinomas, and other primary and metastatic cutaneous neoplasms. RT, in properly fractionated doses, is indicated when the patient's overall health status (such as elderly patients who are unwilling or unable to undergo surgery) or size of the tumor precludes surgical extirpation. The procedure is also used as an adjuvant treatment of patients with positive surgical margins, perineural invasion (PNI), or local regional nodal metastasis. The effectiveness of RT, however, is limited by the inability to definitively assess and control the tumor margins. In addition, treatment of an excessively large area of normal skin surrounding the tumor may enhance risk of both postradiation dermatitis and future skin cancers. Two modes of RT delivery are electrons and superficially penetrating photons (X-rays).[31] Appropriate radiation margins for clinically visible tumors and/or surgical scars should generally be <3 cm. A protracted fractionation scheme using 2 to 2.5 Gy fractions to a total of 50 to 66 Gy for NMSCs is commonly used to achieve the best chance of durable local control and acceptable late effects.[32] Nonetheless, treatment may be accelerated to a single large fraction (10 to 20 Gy) or three to five fractions of 6 to 7 Gy for patients with significant comorbidities or for smaller lesions in locations with good perfusion where cosmesis is less critical. Accelerated treatment protocols provide excellent local control but have an increased risk of fibrosis, atrophy, telangiectasias, and poor cosmesis. Although a course of RT may be protracted over several weeks, daily treatments last several minutes.

Local control rates for small (<2 cm) BCCs are 90% to 95% with adequate (>90% rated as excellent or good) cosmesis. For larger tumors with bone or cartilage involvement, local control rates decrease to 50% to 75%. These deeply invasive/destructive lesions are best approached with a combined excision and adjuvant RT. In a randomized trial of patients with incompletely excised recurrent BCCs, adjuvant RT improved the 5-year local control rates from 61% to 91%.[33] The 10-year local control rates were similar for both adjuvant RT and repeat surgery (92% versus 90%). The local control for SCC is lower by 10% to 15% compared with equivalent-sized BCCs with RT. For selected cases of small, superficial BCC and SCC, office-based treatment with superficial X-ray therapy was shown in one series to have a favorable recurrence rate of 5.0% at 5 years.[34]

The consideration of acute and permanent tissue effects of RT, such as acute and chronic radiation dermatitis, epidermal atrophy, telangiectasias, altered pigmentation, delayed radiation necrosis, alopecia, and secondary cutaneous malignancies, must be anticipated and managed.[35] Recurrent SCC after RT may be more resistant to treatment than recurrence after surgery alone.[36] The late cosmetic effects are more pronounced with a large dose per fraction (over 3 to 4 Gy), if the total dose is >55 Gy, following treatment to large fields and/or deeply invasive lesions and with continued unprotected sun exposure. RT is most commonly used in the head and neck region,

and treatment of distal extremities should be considered cautiously as poor vascularization and edema increase the risk of posttreatment complications.[33]

ACTINIC KERATOSES

AKs are common cutaneous lesions that occur on sun-exposed areas, particularly in blond or red-haired, fair-skinned individuals with green or blue eyes. They, of course, can occur in patients who do not possess these phenotypic features, and relate most directly to cumulative sun exposure. AKs represent the initial intraepidermal manifestation of abnormal proliferation of keratinocytes and harbor the canonical mutations in tumor suppressor genes (such as $p53$) seen in SCC. As such, AK are precursor lesions with the possibility of progression to SCCIS and invasive SCC.[37]

Clinically, AKs demonstrate one of three behavior patterns: spontaneous regression, persistence, or progression to invasive SCC.[38] The risk of progression of AK to SCC has been calculated between 0.025% and 16% per year, and the calculated total risk of malignant transformation for a patient with AKs followed for a period of 10 years ranges from 6.1% to 10.2%.[39] Approximately 60% to 65% of SCCs arise from prior AKs. Spontaneous regression has been reported in as high as 25.9% of AKs over a 12-month period, although a 15% recurrence rate was noted at follow-up.[37]

PATHOGENESIS OF ACTINIC KERATOSIS

Factors linked to pathogenesis of AKs include (1) exposure to UVB light—UVB causes mutations of the tumor suppressor gene (TSG) $p53$; (2) genetic DNA instability (i.e., xeroderma pigmentosum) or melanin deficiency (albinism); (3) older age; (4) male gender; (5) anatomic location—>80% of AKs are located on the head and neck, dorsal forearms, and hands; and (6) history of immunosuppression—solid organ transplant patients are at significantly increased risk.

Studies of the molecular pathogenesis of AK and SCC have revealed a stepwise progression from normal skin to actinically damaged skin to AK to SCC. Global gene profiling has shown similar patterns of abnormal gene expression in AK and SCC, and the identification of expanded clones of $p53$-mutated keratinocytes in precursor AKs confirms that AKs indeed represent an early stage in the molecular carcinogenesis of NMSC.[40,41] A study of asymptomatic AKs, inflamed AKs, and SCCs similarly showed a stepwise loss of differentiation manifesting as diminishing 27-kD heat-shock protein, an initial increase in lymphocytes suggesting the occurrence of an active inflammatory and immune response, a stepwise increase in the number of cells expressing detectable levels of $p53$ suggesting an increase in DNA damage, decreasing levels of Bcl-2, an apoptosis inhibitor, and loss of Fas antigen, suggesting these cells become less sensitive to FasL-mediated apoptosis as they progress.[42]

CLINICAL FEATURES OF ACTINIC KERATOSIS

AKs are red, pink, or brown papules with a scaly (hyperkeratotic) surface. They occur on sun-exposed areas and are especially common on the balding scalp, forehead, face, dorsal forearms, and hands (Fig. 92.4). Subclinical (nonvisible) AKs are estimated to occur up to 10 times more often than clinically visible AKs, particularly on sun-exposed skin.[37] Actinic cheilitis is a clinical subtype of AK on the lower lip marked by diffuse scaling and erythema or hypopigmentation along the vermilion border. More severe cases may have recurrent erosions or fissures. Although the presentation can be subtle, the elevated risk of mucosal SCC development demands clinical vigilance and warrants treatment of actinic

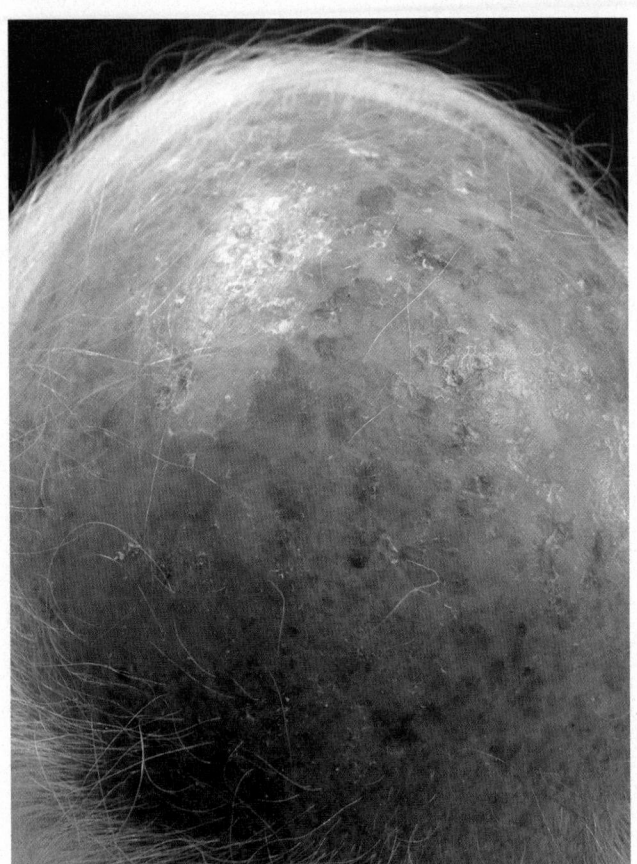

Figure 92.4 Multiple actinic keratoses. Numerous pink thin papules with gritty scale are scattered over the sun-exposed scalp in an elderly man. The lesions are admixed with several tan solar lentigo.

cheilitis, most often with field-directed therapy. Actinic cheilitis is particularly amenable to treatment with PDT, although shorter incubation times must be used on the thin and sensitive skin of the vermilion lip.

The histologic spectrum of AKs includes hyperplastic, atrophic, Bowenoid, acantholytic, and pigmented subtypes.[43] Each subtype is characterized by disordered, atypical keratinocytes with nuclear atypia. In the hyperplastic variant, pronounced hyperkeratosis coexists with parakeratosis. Epidermal hyperplasia and downward displacement without dermal invasion can be noted. A thin epidermis devoid of rete ridges is characteristic of the atrophic variant. Atypical cells predominate in the basal layer. The Bowenoid AK is virtually indistinguishable from BD SCCIS. In the Bowenoid variant, considerable epidermal cell disarray and clumping of nuclei gives a windblown appearance. The presence of suprabasal lacunae is characteristic of acantholytic AK. Excessive melanin is present within the basal layer in the pigmented variant of AK.

TREATMENT OF ACTINIC KERATOSIS

Prevention of disease is always superior and preferable to the need for treatment. Effective preventative measures include avoidance of excessive sun exposure (use of broad-brimmed hats, sun-protective clothing, and sunscreen), patient education, and regular self-examinations to detect the earliest signs of malignant transformation. The effectiveness of topical chemoprevention was demonstrated in a double-blind, randomized clinical trial in which 25 patients applied topical all-trans-retinoic acid (tretinoin) 0.05% cream twice daily for 16 weeks, resulting in a 30.3% reduction in the number of AKs compared with baseline.[44]

Because of their low but real potential to develop into invasive SCC, AK therapy is generally recommended. The management of AK should be based on whether a lesion-directed or field-directed therapy is preferred. Lesion-directed therapy, including ablative and surgical procedures, is reserved for selected cases when only a few clinically visible AKs are present. Field-directed therapy, including ablative, nonablative, and topical treatments, offers the advantage of treating both clinically evident and subclinical lesions that may progress to visible AKs and, potentially, SCC.

Lesion-Directed Therapy

Cryotherapy is the most commonly used lesion-directed treatment modality. Clearance rates range from 39% to 98.8%.[37,45] In a large, multicenter Australian study evaluating the efficacy of cryotherapy for the treatment of AKs on the face and scalp, of the 89 patients and 421 lesions in the intended-to-treat population, there was an average of 67.2% lesion response rate per patient.[46] As mentioned previously, cryotherapy results in the local side effects of pain, erythema, and potentially blistering or crusting, which are generally transient and well-tolerated. Cryotherapy treatment was associated with "good" and "excellent" cosmetic outcomes in 94% of the lesions.

Other lesion-directed treatment options include C&D and surgical excision. Treatment with C&D may require more than one cycle. High cure rates and good cosmetic outcome have been reported, although this treatment is not commonly used for AK. C&D should be generally avoided in recurrent lesions, lesions that have undergone punch biopsy, and lesions in hair-bearing areas.[37]

Field-Directed Therapy

Field-directed treatment modalities include topical pharmacologic therapies including imiquimod, 5-FU, and diclofenac, ablative and nonablative laser resurfacing, PDT, dermabrasion, and deep and medium-depth chemical peels.

5-Fluorouracil

Manufacturer-recommended 5-FU treatment protocol for AKs is twice daily for 2 to 4 weeks. Other protocols proposed in the literature include 5% 5-FU once to twice daily for 2 to 7 weeks; 5% 5-FU once daily, 1 day per week for 12 weeks; and 0.5% 5-FU once or twice daily for 1 to 4 weeks.[37] The literature reports rates of AK resolution with 5-FU that reach 89% with twice-weekly application for 16 weeks, albeit recurrence rates of up to 55% have been reported.[47] In addition, low compliance, because of adverse effects of medication, is associated with significant treatment failure rates.

In a phase 3, double-blind randomized study of 117 patients with at least five AKs treated with 0.5% 5-FU cream once daily, complete clearance rates at 1, 2, and 4 weeks were 26%, 20%, and 48%, respectively.[48] In a large systematic review of 5-FU randomized clinical trials, treatment with 5% 5-FU resulted in an average reduction of 79.5% in the mean number of lesions with clearance rates of 94% and 98% at 2 and 4 weeks, respectively. In comparison, treatment with 0.5% 5-FU resulted in an average reduction in the mean number of lesions of 86.1%. Higher clearance rates with 0.5% 5-FU may represent increased patient medication compliance from lower side effects profile. In the study comparing 0.5% and 5% 5-FU, 85% of patients preferred 0.5% 5-FU.[37]

Imiquimod (Aldara, Medicis Pharmaceutical, Scottsdale, AZ)

The FDA-approved imiquimod treatment protocol for AKs is twice weekly for 16 weeks. Other treatment protocols including more frequent dosing for a shorter time period or pulsed treatment with a 2- to 4-week rest period have been reported with similar efficacy.[37,49] Clearance rates with imiquimod range from 45% to 85%.[50] Reported recurrence rates are 10% and 16% within 1 year and 18 months of treatment, respectively.

Imiquimod is effective and well tolerated for the treatment of AKs in posttransplant, immunosuppressed patients. The safety and efficacy of 5% imiquimod cream for the treatment of AKs in posttransplant patients receiving immunosuppressive therapy within the prior 6 months was evaluated in a multicenter, randomized, placebo-controlled study with reported imiquimod clearance rate of 62.1%.[51] Common reported side effects of imiquimod therapy included site reactions (edema, erythema, vesicles, and erosions/ulcerations), fatigue, headache, diarrhea, nausea, and leucopenia. No serious adverse events were reported.[51] Few randomized trials have directly compared the efficacy of the leading topical treatments for AK, 5-FU, and imiquimod. One study compared 5-FU 5% cream applied twice daily for 2 to 4 weeks with imiquimod 5% cream applied twice daily for 16 weeks in 36 patients with AKs on the face and scalp.[52] At week 24, the total AK count was reduced by 94% and 66% with 5-FU and imiquimod, respectively. Another study randomized patients to either cryotherapy, 5-FU (twice daily for 4 weeks), or imiquimod (three times per week for 4 weeks, repeated if necessary) therapy for multiple AK.[53] Cryotherapy resulted in a 68% initial clinical clearance, compared with 96% for 5-FU and 85% for imiquimod. Sustained clearance at 1 year was greatest in the imiquimod group (73%), compared to 54% for 5-FU and 28% for cryotherapy. Overall, the two topical treatments appear to have similar efficacy, although additional studies are needed to assess whether imiquimod has superior long-term clearance rates.

Photodynamic Therapy with 5-Aminolevulinic Acid. PDT with ALA activated by blue light showed reported overall clearance values for AKs between 50% to 80%.[37] Response rates vary with duration of ALA incubation and thickness of AK lesions. In a randomized, blinded, placebo-controlled study, 243 patients with a total of 1,403 AKs on the scalp and face were treated with ALA (incubation time 14 to 18 hours) and exposure to blue light.[54] At 8 weeks, 30% of patients with partial response were retreated. At 12 weeks, 91% lesion clearance rate was reported. Discomfort was the most commonly reported adverse event.

A randomized study of 36 patients with at least four AKs compared efficacy of two sessions of ALA-PDT or ALA-pulsed dye laser (ALA incubation time, 1 hour) with 0.5% 5-FU cream applied once or twice daily for 4 weeks.[55] At 1 month posttreatment, the overall individual lesion clearance rates for 5-FU, ALA-PDT, and ALA-pulsed dye laser were 70%, 80%, and 50%, respectively. ALA-PDT and ALA-pulsed dye laser were better tolerated than 5-FU. The efficacy of PDT was compared with that of cryotherapy in an open, randomized, controlled study of 202 patients with 732 AKs.[56] Clearance rates for PDT and cryotherapy were 69% and 75%, respectively. Response rates correlated with the lesion thickness, with thinner lesions having higher response rates. Satisfaction with the cosmetic outcomes for PDT and cryotherapy were 96% and 81%, respectively.

Other Field Treatments. Efficacy of topically applied 3% diclofenac gel in 2.5% hyaluronic acid vehicle gel versus vehicle was addressed in a multicenter, randomized, double-blind, placebo-controlled study of 195 patients. Treatment with 3% diclofenac gel twice daily for 30 to 90 days resulted in an improvement of 59% compared with 31% with placebo.[57] As described previously, ingenol mebutate is a recently approved therapy for AK with a simplified dosing regimen that was shown to reduce AK counts by 75% to 83% compared to 0% in patients treated with placebo.[25] Other treatment modalities primarily used for cosmetic procedures, such as chemical peels and ablative and nonablative laser resurfacing, have been reported to be effective

in the treatment of AKs, but high-quality, well-controlled studies of efficacy are lacking.[58]

BASAL CELL CARCINOMA

BCC is a slow-growing neoplasm of nonkeratinizing cells originating from the basal cell layer of the epidermis. BCC is the most common human cancer, accounting for 25% of all human cancers and 75% of skin malignancies diagnosed in the United States.[59] Although BCC rarely metastasizes, it is locally invasive and can result in extensive morbidity through local recurrence and tissue destruction. Typically, BCC develops on sun-exposed areas of lighter-skinned individuals. Approximately 30% of lesions of BCC occur on the nose. Nonetheless, BCC can occur anywhere, including non–sun-exposed areas, and has been reported to occur on the vulva, penis, scrotum, and perianal area. Men are affected slightly more often than are women, and although once rare, before the age of 50 years, BCCs are becoming more common in younger individuals.[1,4]

Intermittent recreational sun exposure, exposure to UVR (UVB confers greater risk than UVA) and sun overexposure (i.e., sunburns), especially in childhood and adolescence, is a significant risk factor for development of BCC. Other factors involved in the pathogenesis include mutations in regulatory TSG, exposure to ionizing radiation, chemicals (e.g., arsenic, polyaromatic hydrocarbons), psoralen plus UVA (PUVA) therapy, and alterations in immune surveillance (i.e., organ transplantation, underlying hematologic malignancy, immunosuppressive medications, or HIV infection).[1]

BCC is substantially more common among survivors of childhood cancers, principally due to previous treatment with ionizing radiation therapy alone or in combination with chemotherapy. In affected individuals with a history of childhood cancers, BCC developed between 20 and 39 years of age, with an increased risk of approximately 40-fold in cancer survivors that had received ≥35 Gy versus those who did not receive radiation therapy.[60]

BCC can be a feature of inherited conditions. Included among these are the nevoid BCC syndrome (NBCCS), Bazex syndrome (X-linked dominant; characterized clinically by follicular atrophoderma, hypotrichosis, hypohidrosis, milia, epidermoid cysts, and facial BCCs), Rombo syndrome (features similar to those of Bazex syndrome with peripheral vasodilation with cyanosis), xeroderma pigmentosum (autosomal recessive disorder in unscheduled DNA repair, clinically characterized by numerous NMSCs and melanomas), and unilateral basal cell nevus syndrome.

NBCCS is a rare autosomal dominant genetic disorder characterized by a mutation in the human patched (*PTCH1*) gene and predisposition to multiple BCC and other tumors, as well as a wide range of developmental defects. Patients with this syndrome may exhibit a broad nasal root, borderline intelligence, odontogenic keratocysts of the jaw, palmar and plantar pits, calcification of the falx cerebri, medulloblastomas, and multiple skeletal abnormalities in addition to a few to thousands of BCCs.[61] Tumor development in patients with NBCCS is related to sun exposure, as BCCs develop most frequently in sun-exposed areas. The clinical course is commonly benign prior to puberty; nonetheless, after puberty individual lesions may progressively enlarge and ulcerate. Individuals with NBCCS are exceedingly sensitive to ionizing radiation. Hundreds of BCCs were reported in children treated with RT for medulloblastoma.

Genomic analysis of patients with NBCCS has elucidated the molecular pathogenesis of BCC. The behavior of neoplasms occurring in NBCCS confirms a classic two-hit model of carcinogenesis—tumors develop in cells sustaining two genetic alterations.[62] The first alteration or hit is inheritance of a mutation in a TSG, and the second is inactivation of the normal homologue by environmental mutagenesis or random genetic rearrangement. Sporadic BCCs would arise in cells that underwent two somatic events, resulting in the inactivation of the NBCCS

TSG *PTCH1*. Studies of BCC have indicated an association with mutations in the *PTCH1* regulatory gene, which maps to chromosome 9q22.3.[63] Loss of heterozygosity at this site is seen in both sporadic and hereditary BCC. Inactivation of the *PTCH1* gene is probably a necessary step for BCC formation. The *PTCH1* protein is part of a receptor complex that regulates the hedgehog signaling pathway, a key regulator of embryonic development and cellular proliferation. The *PTCH1* protein binds to and inhibits *Smoothened*, a transmembrane receptor for the secreted molecule hedgehog. On hedgehog binding, *Smoothened* is released from the inhibitory effects of *PTCH1* and transduces an activating signal via GLI transcription factors.[64,65] Loss of function mutations in *PTCH1* thus permit unopposed *Smoothened* activity and cellular proliferation. This understanding of the molecular pathogenesis of BCC has led to the development of targeted medical therapy for BCC with small molecule inhibitors of *Smoothened*, as discussed subsequently. UV-induced mutations in the *p53* gene, such as cyclobutane pyrimidine dimers (CC → TT) have also been reported in up to 60% of BCCs.[66]

CLINICAL BEHAVIOR OF BASAL CELL CARCINOMA

Although the overall prognosis of the vast majority of BCC is excellent, some tumors exhibit infiltrative growth patterns and extensive subclinical spread. Batra and Kelley[67] looked at risk factors for extensive subclinical spread of more than 1,000 NMSCs treated by MMS. The most significant predictors were anatomic location on the nose of any type of BCC; morpheaform BCC on the cheek; recurrent BCC in men; any tumor located on the neck in men; any tumor located on the ear helix, eyelid, or temple; and increasing preoperative size. Invasive BCC can migrate along the perichondrium, periosteum, fascia, or tarsal plate.[68,69] This type of spread accounts for higher recurrence rates in tumors involving the eyelid, nose, and scalp. Embryonic fusion planes likely offer little resistance and can lead to deep invasion and tumor spread, with very high rates of recurrence. The most susceptible areas include the inner canthus, philtrum, middle to lower chin, nasolabial groove, preauricular area, and the retroauricular sulcus.

PNI is infrequent in BCC and occurs most often in recurrent, clinically aggressive lesions. In a case series, Niazi and Lamberty[70] noted PNI in 0.178% of BCC. In all cases, PNI was associated with recurrent tumors that were most often located in the periauricular and malar areas. Clinically, PNI may present with paresthesia, pain, and weakness or, in some cases, paralysis.

Metastatic BCC is rare, with incidence rates varying from 0.0028% to 0.1%.[71] Interestingly, BCC appears to be uniquely dependent upon surrounding stroma, as experimental transplants of tumors devoid of associated stroma are usually unsuccessful.[72] This concept of stromal dependence may explain the low incidence of metastatic BCC. Metastases, when reported, have involved the lung, lymph nodes, esophagus, oral cavity, and skin. Although long-term survival has been reported, the prognosis for metastatic BCC is generally poor, with an average survival of 8 to 10 months following diagnosis. Platinum-based chemotherapy or molecularly targeted *Smoothened* inhibitors may provide benefit as salvage therapy for metastatic BCC.[72–74]

BASAL CELL CARCINOMA SUBTYPES

Clinical variants of BCC include nodular, micronodular, superficial, infiltrative, morpheaform (also termed *aggressive-growth BCC, fibrosing BCC, sclerosing BCC*), pigmented, cystic BCC, and fibroepithelioma of Pinkus (FEP).[75,76]

Nodular BCC is the most common BCC subtype, accounting for >60% of all tumors. Clinically, it presents as a raised, translucent pearly, skin-toned to pink papule or nodule with prominent

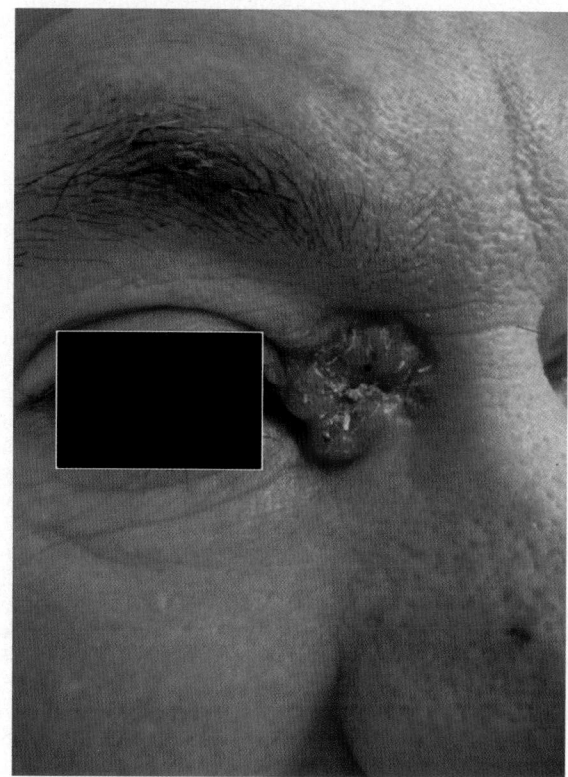

Figure 92.5 Nodular basal cell carcinoma (BCC). A slightly erythematous, pearly nodule with rolled borders is a classic presentation of nodular BCC. Central ulceration is a common feature of nodular BCC.

telangiectasias (Fig. 92.5). Occasionally, the center of the tumor appears depressed or sunken, leaving a rolled, raised border with the classic pearly appearance so-called rodent ulcer. Not infrequently, history of easy bleeding and/or crusting is obtained. Nodular BCC has a propensity for involving sun-exposed areas of the face in individuals over the age of 60. In patients with severe actinic damage, nodular BCCs may appear in the third decade.

Superficial BCC is the second most common subtype of BCC, comprising of up to 15% of all BCCs. It presents in younger patients at a mean age of 57 years. Superficial BCC presents as well-defined, pink to erythematous scaly or eroded macule or plaque commonly with a thin pearly border. It appears predominately on the trunk and may be difficult to differentiate clinically from AK, SCCIS, or an inflammatory lesion.

Infiltrative BCC comprises approximately 5% of all BCCs and develops predominantly in the head and neck region of older adults. Mean age at presentation is 66 years. Clinically, infiltrative BCC most often resembles the nodular form of BCC.

Morpheaform BCC accounts for 3% of all BCCs and commonly develops in the head and neck region of older individuals. It presents as a flat or indurated, slightly firm lesion, without well-demarcated borders, with a white to yellowish hue, and may be difficult to differentiate from a scar. Traction on the skin often highlights the clinical extent of the lesion. Symptoms of bleeding, crusting, and ulceration are often not present in this tumor subtype. The actual size of the cancer is usually much greater than the clinical extent of the tumor. Pigmented BCC is a variant of nodular BCC with clinically visible pigment and may be difficult to differentiate from nodular melanoma. The presence of pigment may be of value in determining adequate excision margins.

FEP, a rare variant of BCC, typically presents on the torso and extremities, but also has been noted on the genitalia, groin, and sole of the foot. Clinically, FEP usually presents as a pink, smooth, dome-shaped, or pedunculated papule, plaque, or nodule.[77] It may be difficult to distinguish clinically from amelanotic melanoma.

HISTOLOGY

Histologic features defining BCC are aggregates of neoplastic basaloid cells stemming from the epidermis or the epithelium of adnexal structures.[75] Aggregates are organized as lobules, islands, nests, or cords of cells that display an orderly arrangement of the basaloid cell nuclei at the periphery, a palisading array. Occasionally, central necrosis or cystic changes are seen within the tumor lobules. Individual tumor cells have uniform, hyperchromatic, round to oval nuclei. Mitotic figures are uncommon, but the presence of apoptotic cells and necrosis is frequently observed. Pleomorphic variant of BCC shows tremendous variability of nuclear size and chromatism, as well as multiple mitoses and multinucleated giant cells. A stromal retraction or clefting around the neoplastic aggregates is commonly seen in the dermis. An accumulation of mucin within and around the tumor lobules may be evident.

Histologic subtypes of BCC include nodular and micronodular, superficial, and infiltrative BCC (Fig. 92.6A,B). Nodular BCC accounts for approximately 50% of all histologic variants of BCCs and exhibits characteristic features as previously described. Superficial multifocal BCC accounts for approximately 15% of BCCs and is a broad lesion characterized by basophilic buds extending from an atrophic epidermis into the papillary dermis. In a two-dimensional view, tumor buds appear to be multifocal, but upon three-dimensional imaging analysis they form a netlike pattern. Retraction artifact is present, as is peripheral palisading within the buds. FEP, which accounts for 1% of BCCs, is characterized by a polypoid lesion in which basaloid cells grow downward from

the surface in a network of anastomoses of cords of cells in loose connective tissue.

The biologic behavior of the micronodular, infiltrating, and morpheaform (sclerosing) subtypes of BCC is more aggressive than that of the nodular and superficial forms. Infiltrative histology is seen in 15% to 20% of BCCs. Individual tumor islands manifest small, irregular outlines with a spiky appearance that invade into and throughout the dermis. Palisading is characteristically absent. The stroma is less myxoid than in the nodular form. In the morpheaform variant, small groups or cords of tumor cells often only one to two cells in thickness infiltrate and dissect a dense, collagenous stroma often parallel to the skin surface. Mixed histology is frequently apparent in BCCs. Areas of follicular, sebaceous, eccrine, or apocrine differentiation may also be seen in some BCCs. BCCs may contain focal areas of squamous differentiation, ranging from individual dyskeratotic cells to keratin pearls. The term *basosquamous (metatypical) carcinoma* denotes BCC with a predominance of mature, atypical keratinizing squamous component. Biologic characteristics of a basosquamous carcinoma are more similar to those of SCC with a possibility for metastasis.

The significance of histologic subtype lies in the correlation with a tumor's biologic aggressiveness. The infiltrative and micronodular types are the most likely to be incompletely removed by conventional wide local excision (WLE). Rates of incomplete excision vary from 5% to 17%.[78] Incompletely excised infiltrative and micronodular BCCs recur at rates of 33% to 39%. Recurrences after RT show a tendency toward infiltrative histology and squamous transformation, and even recurrent BCC after excision or C&D may become metatypical. Although historical reports in the literature suggested that 60% of incompletely excised BCCs will not recur, none of these studies provided an appraisal of recurrence rates as a function of histologic subtype.[68,69] In general, incompletely excised BCCs

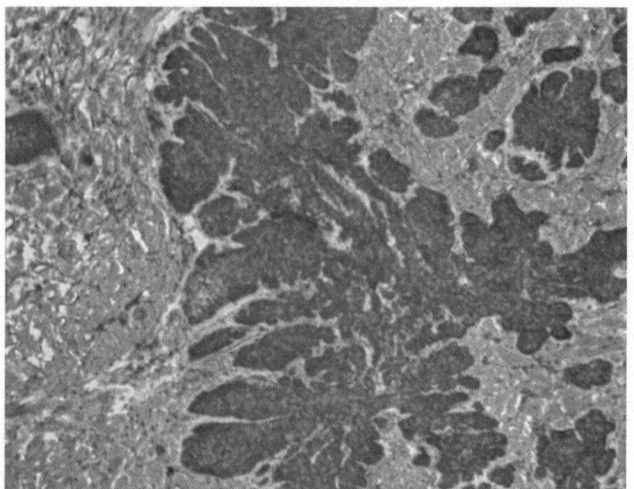

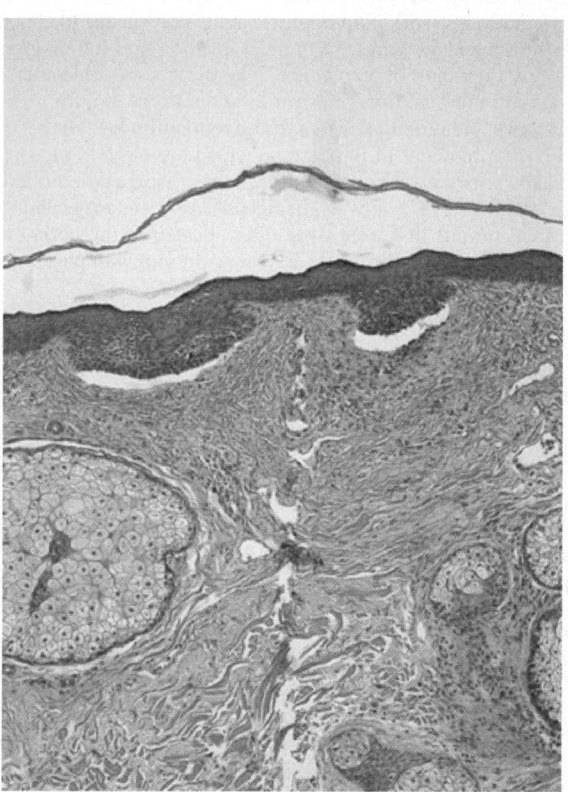

Figure 92.6 (A) Histology of nodular basal cell carcinoma (BCC). Nodular BCC is characterized by the presence of rounded tumor islands extending from the epidermis into the dermis. Peripheral palisading of nuclei is prominent, and surrounding retraction artifact may be present. **(B)** Histology of multifocal superficial BCC. Superficial BCC is characterized by basophilic buds extending from an atrophic epidermis into the papillary dermis. Retraction artifact is present, as is peripheral palisading within the buds.

should be removed completely, preferably by MMS, especially if they occur in anatomically critical areas such as the central zone of the face, retroauricular sulcus, or periocular area.

TREATMENT

Excisional surgery, MMS, and C&D have all been used to treat circumscribed, noninfiltrative BCCs. MMS is the treatment method of choice for all recurrent and infiltrative BCCs, particularly if a tumor is located on the face.[6,79] RT is best suited for poor surgical candidates and patients with extensive lesions not amenable to surgery.[80,81] RT is not indicated for recurrent or morpheaform lesions and in patients with NBCCS.

C&D is frequently used by dermatologists in the treatment of primary BCC. Knox[82] noted cure rates as high as 98.3%. Kopf et al.,[83] in an earlier study, cited a significant difference in the cure rates obtained between patients treated by private practitioners (94.3%) and those treated by trainees in the New York University Skin and Cancer Unit (81.2%). This supports the premise that C&D, although simple and cost-effective, is highly dependent on operator skill. Traditionally, it was recommended that the procedure be repeated for three cycles, but histology, location, and behavior of the tumor should dictate the number of cycles. C&D should be reserved for small or superficial BCCs, not located on the midface, in patients who may not tolerate more extensive surgery.

Surgical excision offers a unique advantage of histologic evaluation of the excised specimen. It has been demonstrated that 4-mm margins are adequate for removal of BCC in 98% of cases of nonmorpheaform BCC of <2 cm in diameter.[78] Extending the excision into subcutaneous fat generally is adequate for a small primary BCC.

MMS permits superior histologic verification of complete removal, allows maximum conservation of tissue, and remains cost-effective as compared with traditional excisional surgery for NMSCs including BCCs.[4,6] In a large study of treatment of primary BCC by Rowe et al.,[84] MMS demonstrated a recurrence rate (RR) of 1% over 5 years. This was superior to all other modalities, including excision (RR = 10%), C&D (RR = 7.7%), RT (RR = 8.7%), and cryotherapy (RR = 7.5%). In a similar study of recurrent BCC, treatment with MMS demonstrated a long-term RR of 5.6%.[85] In that treatment group, MMS was superior to all other modalities, including excision (RR = 17.4%), RT (RR = 9.8%), and C&D (RR = 40%). MMS is the preferred treatment for morpheaform, recurrent, poorly delineated, high-risk, and incompletely removed BCC, and for those sites in which tissue conservation for function and cosmesis is imperative. When the surgical approach is contraindicated, RT is a valid option for management of primary BCC. RT may be indicated postoperatively if margins are ambiguous or involved. Disadvantages of RT include lack of margin control, possible poor cosmesis over time, a drawn-out course of therapy, and increased risk of future skin cancers. The RRs for primary BCC treated by RT range from 5% to 10% over 5 years. Wilder et al.[86] compared local control rates for RT among 85 patients with 115 primary or recurrent biopsy-proven BCCs. A 95% control rate was achieved for primary BCC and a 56% control rate obtained for recurrent BCC at 5 years. Considering cosmesis, RT scars tend to worsen over time, in contrast to surgical scars that tend to improve over time.

Imiquimod is approved by the FDA for the treatment of superficial BCC <2 cm in diameter on the neck, trunk, or extremities. The FDA-recommended regimen is once-daily application 5 days per week for 6 to 12 weeks. Numerous studies evaluated safety and efficacy of imiquimod for superficial BCC.[11,87] Application schedules varied from 2 days per week to twice daily, and the treatment duration ranged from 5 to 15 weeks. Clinical follow-up ranged from 6 months to 5 years. Reported histologic clearance rates ranged from 52% to 81%, albeit high-risk tumors (within 1 cm of the hairline, eyes, nose, mouth, anogenital region, hands, and feet) or tumors >2 cm in diameter regardless of their location

were excluded. Imiquimod has been used off-label for the treatment of nodular and infiltrative BCC.[88,89] Although some studies have shown favorable cure rates, imiquimod treatment of these tumors is generally not recommended as subclinical disease may persist and lead to late recurrence.

The FDA-approved protocol for treating superficial BCC with topical 5-FU is twice-daily application for 3 to 6 weeks irrespective of tumor size or location. Longer treatment protocols with an average 11 weeks are reported in the peer-reviewed literature. In a study of 31 tumors treated twice daily for an average of 11 weeks, a 90% clearance rate was observed histologically 3 weeks posttreatment.[90] Topical PDT has also demonstrated efficacy in the treatment of BCC. Clearance rates for BCC using ALA or MAL PDT range from 76% to 97% for superficial to 64% to 92% for nodular BCC after one to three treatments.[26,28,91] Many studies of PDT for nodular BCC involve curettage of the lesion prior to treatment, however, and it is unclear if the response rate would be as successful without initial curettage. In a well-designed comparative trial, 601 patients with superficial BCC were randomized to treatment with MAL PDT (two treatments given 1 week apart), imiquimod, or 5-FU according to FDA-approved protocols. Complete clinical remission at 1 year was found to be 72.8% for PDT, 83.4% for imiquimod (superior to PDT), and 80.1% for 5-FU (not statistically different from the other treatments). Patients treated with imiquimod or 5-FU were more likely to report bothersome local side effects of the treatment, however.[92]

Historically, systemic therapy for BCC was limited to cytotoxic chemotherapy that was marginally effective as salvage therapy for metastatic disease. Elucidation of the critical role of abnormal hedgehog signaling in BCC, however, has led to development of a novel class of molecularly targeted small molecule inhibitors of *Smoothened*, most notably vismodegib.[74] Based on a seminal trial of 33 patients with metastatic BCC and 63 patients with locally advanced BCC not amenable to surgical therapy, vismodegib was approved (2012) for treatment of advanced BCC (either metastatic or not amenable to surgery or radiation).[73] With once daily oral dosing of 150 mg vismodegib, 30% of patients with metastatic BCC and 43% of patients with locally advanced BCC had an objective response (at least 30% decrease in size of tumors), and 21% of patients with locally advanced BCC had complete clinical resolution of tumors. None of the patients with metastatic BCC had a complete response. Adverse events in the trial were common, including serious adverse events in 25% of patients and fatal adverse events in 7% of patients. Most common adverse events in this and other trials were muscle spasms, alopecia, dysgeusia leading to weight loss, fatigue, diarrhea, and hyponatremia, and between 12% and 54% of patients discontinued therapy because of adverse effects.[73,74,93] Due to the relatively low response rate, the high incidence of adverse events, the potential for resistance with a single mutation,[94] and reports of rapid recurrence of BCC upon discontinuation of the medication,[95] *Smoothened* inhibitors remain a limited, albeit important, addition to our treatment options for BCC. Vismodegib may also be an effective suppressive therapy for select patients with NBCCS, where it was shown to decrease the incidence of new tumors by 93% during an 8-month period.[93]

It is imperative that patients with a history of BCC receive annual full-body skin examinations. Although most recurrences appear within 1 to 5 years, recurrences decades after initial treatment are reported in the literature. Rowe et al.[96,97] found that 30% of recurrences developed within the first year after therapy, 50% within 2 years, and 66% within 3 years. A separate new primary BCC can present at rates of approximately 40% within 3 years, with 20% to 30% within 1 year of treatment of the original lesion.

SQUAMOUS CELL CARCINOMA

SCC is a neoplasm of keratinizing cells that shows malignant characteristics, including anaplasia, rapid growth, local invasion, and metastatic potential. More than 200,000 cases of SCC are diagnosed in the United States each year, making it the second most common human cancer after BCC.[98] People of Celtic descent, individuals with fair complexions, and those with poor tanning ability and predisposition to sunburn are at increased risk for developing SCC. SCC in blacks arises most often on sites of preexisting inflammatory conditions such as burn injuries, scars, or trauma.[99] Patients treated with PUVA or undergoing immunosuppressive therapy following solid-organ transplantation are at increased risk of SCC (see the following).

PATHOGENESIS OF SQUAMOUS CELL CARCINOMA

Major factors involved in the pathogenesis of SCC include cumulative exposure to UVR, genetic mutations, immunosuppression, and viral infections. UVR acts as both a tumor-initiating and a tumor-promoting factor. Both UVA and UVB (UVB more than UVA) contribute to mutagenesis of DNA by inducing UV landmark mutations (two tandem CC:GG to TT:AA and two C:G to T:A transitions at dipyrimidic sites). UV-induced mutations in TSG lead to uncontrolled cell-cycle progression and subsequent transformation of keratinocytes.[100] In addition to direct mutagenesis, exposure to UVB leads to decreased density and antigen-processing capability of Langerhans cells and may suppress production of the T-helper cell type 1 cytokines IL-2 and INF-γ.[101]

Alterations in the TSG *p53* are the most common genetic abnormality found in AK, SCCIS, and invasive SCC. Under normal conditions, UVR induces *p53* gene activity. The amount of p53 protein rapidly increases in keratinocytes after UVR, and drives the expression of downstream genes including *Mdm2*, *GADD45*, and *p21 CIP/WAF1*, leading to cellular arrest in the G1 phase. In cases of squamous dysplasia or SCC, one allele of *p53* contains a missense point mutation with UV signature, while the remaining *p53* allele is often deleted. Based on whole exome sequencing and copy number variation data obtained from cutaneous SCC, it appears that loss of both copies of *p53* is an early event in carcinogenesis, facilitating subsequent clonal expansion and accumulation of many additional point mutations.[102] In this study and in similar studies of SCC of the oropharyngeal mucosa, loss of *p53* was the most common mutation, but inactivating mutations in other TSG were also noted, including *CDKN2A* and *NOTCH1*, which encodes a membrane receptor critical for directing cell fate determination in development.[102–104] Activating mutations or gene amplifications of oncogenes have also been reported in SCC, most notably involving the epidermal growth factor receptor (EGFR) and its downstream signaling components such as *ras*.[40,62,102–105] Although these genome-wide studies highlight the mutational complexity and heterogeneity of SCC, two underlying features emerge. First, that both inactivating mutations in TSGs and activating mutations in oncogenes (often multiple) are required for malignant progression, and second, that loss of functional *p53* is a central feature of SCC pathogenesis observed in a majority of tumors.

Other agents associated with development of SCC include (1) chemical agents (e.g., petroleum, coal tar, soot, arsenic); (2) physical agents (e.g., ionizing radiation); (3) exposure to PUVA: calculated adjusted relative risk for a cumulative exposure of between 100 and 337 treatments is 8.6; (4) HPV, especially important for SCC in the anogenital and periungual regions, in the setting of immunosuppression with HIV and solid-organ transplantation, and in patients with epidermodysplasia verruciformis; and (5) smoking. Development of SCC has also been associated with chronic nonhealing wounds, burn scars, and chronic inflammatory dermatoses (discoid lupus, ulcers, osteomyelitis).[106] Certain cervicofacial regions such as the ear and the lower lip are more prone to developing SCC than BCC. Heritable conditions associated with higher incidence of SCC include xeroderma pigmentosum, dystrophic epidermolysis bullosa, and oculocutaneous albinism.

HPV-16 and -18 are frequently implicated in the pathogenesis of subungual and periungual SCC and SCCIS of the digits.

Immunosuppression, including endogenous (underlying lymphoproliferative disorder) and iatrogenic immunosuppression plays a role in pathogenesis of SCC (see the following). In addition to immunosuppressive agents, other medications may also enhance the risk of SCC. Chronic use of photosensitizing drugs, such as the antifungal agent voriconazole, can facilitate actinic damage and have been implicated in accelerated SCC development, particularly in immunosuppressed patients.[107] Vemurafenib, a tyrosine kinase inhibitor recently approved by the FDA for the treatment of metastatic and unresectable melanomas harboring V600E mutations in the *BRAF* gene, appears to increase the risk of keratoacanthoma and SCC development by directly altering signaling through the Ras-Raf mitogen-activated protein kinase pathway known to be involved in SCC pathogenesis.[108]

CLINICAL FEATURES OF SQUAMOUS CELL CARCINOMA AND ITS VARIANTS

Clinically, SCCIS appears as a discrete solitary, sharply demarcated, scaly pink to red papule or thin plaque (Fig. 92.7). Erythroplasia of Queyrat (SCCIS on the glans of penis of uncircumcised male related to HPV infection) presents as a verrucous or polypoid papule or plaque, often eroded. Invasive SCC appears as a slightly raised papule plaque or nodule that is skin-colored, pink, or red (Fig. 92.8). The surface of the tumor may be smooth, keratotic, or ulcerated. The lesion may also be exophytic or indurated. Rarely, the tumor is symptomatic with pain or pruritus. Bleeding with minimal trauma is common. It can be clinically difficult to distinguish an invasive SCC from a hypertrophic AK, a benign seborrheic keratosis, or a benign inflammatory lesion. An appropriate biopsy should be performed.

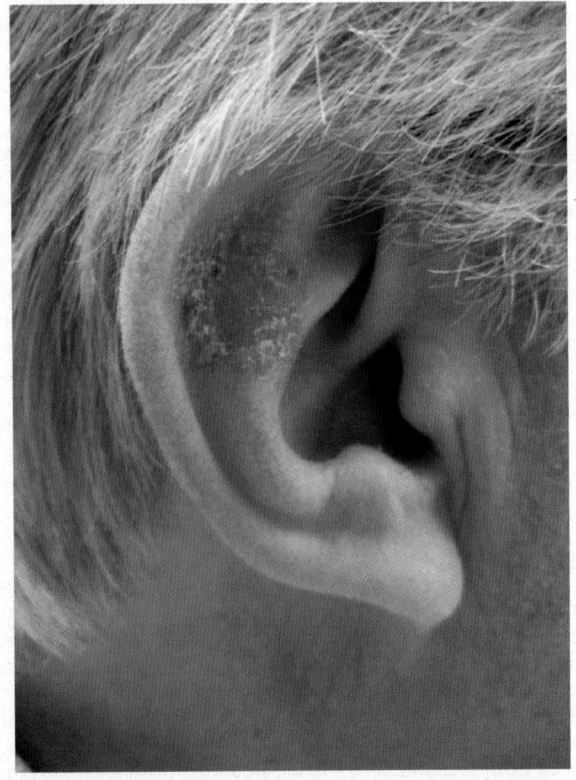

Figure 92.7 Squamous cell carcinoma in situ presents as an erythematous plaque that can be difficult to differentiate from a benign inflammatory process.

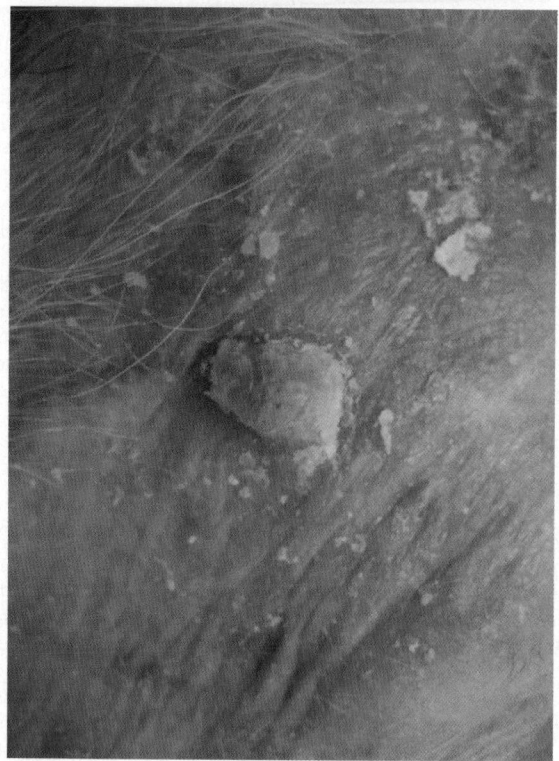
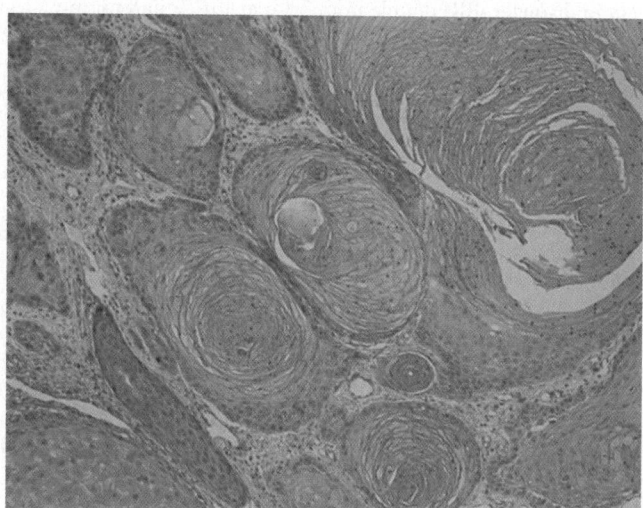

Figure 92.8 (A) Clinical differential diagnosis of cutaneous horn includes squamous cell carcinoma (SCC). Biopsy of the pictured lesion confirmed a clinical diagnosis of SCC. **(B)** Histology of well-differentiated SCC.

Keratoacanthoma (KA) is a variant of SCC defined by a symmetric crateriform architecture and a clinical presentation marked by rapid growth (up to several centimeters) over a period of several weeks. The tumor then typically stabilizes in size and often spontaneously regresses. Although certain KAs may thus behave in a benign fashion, it is impossible to predict which lesions will regress and which will progress. It is thus recommended to treat KAs as a subtype of SCC with appropriate surgical therapy. Verrucous carcinoma, a variant of SCC, includes oral florid papillomatosis, giant condyloma of Buschke-Lowenstein (on the genitalia), and epithelioma cuniculatum (on the plantar foot).[109] Verrucous carcinoma is considered a low-grade carcinoma. It grows slowly and rarely metastasizes, but is frequently deeply invasive into underlying tissue and therefore is difficult to eradicate. Following treatment with RT, verrucous carcinoma may become aggressive or even metastasize.

HISTOLOGY

The histologic criteria defining SCCIS include involvement of the entire thickness of epidermis with pleomorphic keratinocytes and involvement of the adnexal epithelium. The degree of keratinocytes atypia in SCCIS is variable. Marked anaplasia, nuclear crowding, loss of polarity, dysmaturation of the keratinocytes, numerous mitotic figures, including atypical and bizarre forms, and occasional dyskeratotic keratinocytes are seen giving epidermis a "windblown appearance." The epidermis may also be hyperplastic with psoriasiform appearance and broad rete ridges. A pigmented variant of SCCIS has abundant melanin accumulated within keratinocytes and scattered superficial dermal macrophages. The histologic differential diagnosis of SCCIS includes AK, bowenoid papulosis, Paget disease, extramammary Paget disease, and malignant melanoma in situ. Immunostaining may be required for proper diagnostic assessment. Bowenoid papulosis is histologically indistinguishable from SCCIS.

SCC is characterized histologically by its relatively large cellular size, nuclear hyperchromatism, lack of maturation, nuclear atypia, and the presence of mitotic figures. Presence of dermal invasion separates invasive SCC from SCCIS. In well-differentiated SCC, cytoplasmic keratinization is manifested by the presence of keratin pearls (horn cysts) and individual cell dyskeratosis. Invading keratinocytes frequently demonstrate minimal cytologic atypia. In contrast, poorly differentiated or undifferentiated SCC shows decreased evidence of keratinization, higher degree of cytologic atypia, and increased number of mitotic figures. Other histologic subtypes include spindle cell, acantholytic, desmoplastic, and adenosquamous (mucin-producing) SCC, which have all been associated with more invasive tumors and increased risk of recurrence.

CLINICAL BEHAVIOR OF SQUAMOUS CELL CARCINOMA

Cutaneous SCCIS is a full-thickness intraepidermal carcinoma. Most lesions are indolent and enlarge slowly over years, seldom progressing to invasive carcinoma. Retrospective studies suggest that the risk of progression to invasive SCC is approximately 3% to 5%. The risk of progression into invasive disease for genital erythroplasia of Queyrat is approximately 10%.[110] Bowenoid papulosis classically presents as a reddish brown verrucous papule and is associated with HPV-16 and -18. Bowenoid papulosis usually involves the genitals but may be present elsewhere.

While overall the prognosis of cutaneous SCC is good to excellent, it has been estimated that 3% and 2% of patients, respectively, develop nodal metastasis and die from SCC, leading to >4,000 deaths per year in the United States.[98] Several studies have attempted to elucidate which factors define patients at highest risk of disease progression. In a pivotal review of studies of SCCs from 1940 to 1992, Rowe et al.[96] correlated the risk for local recurrence and metastasis with treatment modality, prior treatment, location, size, depth, histologic differentiation, evidence of perineural involvement, precipitating factors other than UVR, and immunosuppression. Tumors arising in areas of chronic inflammation and at mucocutaneous junctions had a 10% to 30% rate of progression to metastatic disease, whereas the incidence of metastasis from SCC arising on sun-exposed skin in the absence of preexisting inflammatory or degenerative conditions varied widely from 0.05% to 16.0%.[96] SCC with perineural involvement exhibited a lower 10-year survival (23% versus 88%) and a higher local RR (47% versus 7.3%) than those without perineural disease. For tumors >2 cm in diameter, RRs double from 7.4% to 15.2%, and for tumors >4 mm in depth, metastasis rates dramatically increase from 6.7% to 45.7%. It was also observed that locally recurrent SCC had an elevated metastasis rate of 30%, particularly when located on the lip and ear (31.5 and 45% metastasis rates, respectively).

Based upon these studies and other retrospective case series, the National Comprehensive Cancer Network identified key clinical and histologic risk factors for recurrence of NMSC,[111] and the American Joint Committee on Cancer (AJCC) developed staging criteria for cutaneous SCC based upon these characteristics in 2011.[112] The AJCC criteria specifically identify four high-risk features: depth >2 mm thickness or Clark level IV or greater, perineural invasion, location on ear or nonglabrous lip, and poor histologic differentiation. Tumors ≤2 cm in diameter with less than two of these high-risk features are classified as T1, whereas tumors >2 cm or any tumor with two or more high-risk features are classified as T2. Immunosuppression is not specifically included in the staging criteria, but the authors acknowledged that this feature is correlated with worse prognosis and must be considered in patient management.[112,113] Tumors with invasion of bone are classified as T3 and T4, depending on whether there is invasion of facial bones (T3) or other skeletal sites (T4).

A critique of the AJCC criteria is that while T3 and T4 are exceedingly rare, T2 tumors comprise a heterogeneous group with anywhere from intermediate to high risk of progression. As such, Schmults and colleagues,[114] based on a restrospective, multivariate analysis of 256 high-risk SCC, proposed an alternative staging system with only four risk factors: tumor diameter ≥2 cm, depth of invasion beyond subcutaneous fat, poor histologic differentiation, and perineural invasion. When tumors with one risk factor were classified as T2a, tumors with two to three risk factors were classified as T2b, and tumors with four risk factors or bone invasion were classified as T3, the authors demonstrated improved prognostication of recurrence or nodal metastasis (<1% for T1, 4% for T2a, 37% for T2b, and >75% for T3 at 5 years). While additional studies are needed to define the optimal tumor staging system, the presence of any of the risk factors discussed here should alert clinicians to the elevated risk of disease progression and the need for appropriate treatment and follow-up.

TREATMENT

Many of the treatments for BCC are also appropriate for SCC. The type of therapy should be selected on the basis of size of the lesion, anatomic location, depth of invasion, degree of cellular differentiation, history of previous treatment, and immune status of the host. There are three general approaches to treatment of SCC: (1) destruction by C&D, (2) removal by excisional surgery or MMS, and (3) radiation therapy.

Cautery/Electrodesiccation

C&D is a simple, cost-effective technique for treating low-risk SCCs. Honeycutt and Jansen[115] reported a 99% cure rate for 281 SCCs after a 4-year follow-up. In this study, two recurrences were noted in lesions <2 cm in diameter. C&D is frequently used for SCCIS; however, as with all forms of destructive therapy, final pathologic review of the tumor is not obtained and clinically

unrecognized foci of invasive tumor are a concern. Although extension of SCCIS down hair follicles has been reported, this appears to be an uncommon phenomenon that has not been systematically assessed. Nevertheless, C&D is generally not indicated for thicker plaques of SCCIS, for tumors in dense hair-bearing areas, or when tumor extends into the subcutaneous layer.

SCCIS may be treated by cryotherapy. As with BCC, two freeze–thaw cycles with a tissue temperature of −50°C are required to destroy the tumor sufficiently. A margin of normal skin also should be frozen to ensure eradication of subclinical disease. Complications include hypertrophic scarring and postinflammatory pigmentary changes, both hypo- and hyperpigmentation. Concealment of recurrence within dense scar tissue presents a danger. Imiquimod has demonstrated efficacy in the treatment of SCCIS, but it is currently not approved by the FDA for the treatment of this neoplasm.[11]

Surgical Modalities

Surgical excision is a well-accepted treatment modality for SCC. Brodland and Zitelli[116] have demonstrated that lesions of <2 cm in diameter can be safely treated by excision, with a 95% confidence interval using margins of 4 mm and 6 mm for low-risk and high-risk tumors, respectively. These investigators defined high risk as a size of ≥2 cm, histologic grade higher than 2, invasion of the subcutaneous tissue, and location in high-risk areas (primarily periorifical central face). Carcinomas of the penis, vulva, and anus are usually treated by excision or MMS. Surgical excision is the treatment of choice for verrucous carcinoma.

MMS is indicated for high-risk SCCs including invasive, poorly differentiated SCCs, and lesions occurring in high-risk anatomic sites or sites in which conservation of normal tissue is essential for preservation of function and/or cosmesis. Recurrence rates with MMS are superior to those obtained with traditional excisional surgery in primary SCC of the ear (3.1% versus 10.9%), primary SCC of the lip (5.8% versus 18.7%), recurrent SCC (10% versus 23.3%), SCC with PNI (0% versus 47%), SCC >2 cm (25.2% versus 41.7%), and poorly differentiated SCC (32.6% versus 53.6%).[109] MMS has proven useful in SCC involving the nail unit and has been used as a limb-sparing procedure in cases of SCC arising in osteomyelitis.

Radiation Therapy

Indications for RT for patients with SCC are similar to those for patients with BCC. The likelihood of cure for early stage lesions is similar for both surgery and RT. Therefore, the decision on which modality to employ depends on other factors, including a patient's underlying medical status, age, expected posttreatment cosmesis, cost, and treatment availability.

In young patients, surgical treatment is a preferable because the late effects of radiation progress gradually with time and, with long-term follow-up, may be associated with a suboptimal cosmetic result compared with surgical resection and reconstruction. In special sites such as lower lip with advanced (over 30% to 50% of the lip involved) SCC, RT allows for excellent maintenance of oral competency with cure rates similar to those of surgical modalities.[33]

Advanced cutaneous cancers may be treated with surgery and adjuvant RT. Adjuvant postoperative RT is added in situations in which the possibility of residual disease is high. In a retrospective study of patients with SCC of the lip, Babington et al.[117] reported a 53% local RR in patients who underwent surgery alone (37% of whom had positive, borderline, or unreported surgical margins) compared with a 6% local RR in the minority of patients treated with surgery and adjuvant RT. In the setting of documented clear surgical margins (such as with MMS), no studies to date have shown a benefit of adjuvant RT,[118] although it has been used anecdotally for tumors deemed particularly high risk. Indications for postsurgical RT include positive margins, PNI (especially if symptomatic), multiple recurrences, and underlying tissue invasion. Advanced unresectable cancers, such as those with marked PNI or with gross disease in the cavernous sinus, may be treated with RT alone.

Management of Regional Lymph Node Metastases

Treatment of nodal disease may involve local RT, lymph node dissection, or a combination of both. Skin cancer metastatic to the parotid nodes is commonly managed with superficial or surgical total parotidectomy followed by adjuvant RT (60 Gy in 30 fractions). Extreme care should be taken to preserve the function of the facial nerve. Nonetheless, in certain cases resection is necessary to achieve a gross total resection. With surgery and adjuvant RT, 5-year disease-free survival ranges from 70% to 75%. Although the risk of subclinical disease in the clinically negative nodes is ≥20%, the ipsilateral neck may be electively irradiated when the parotid is treated postoperatively. RT alone is used for patients with unresectable disease and for those who are medically inoperable. The likelihood of cure is lower with RT-only treatment compared with RT plus surgery, but nodal regression and good palliation are commonly seen. Treatment and palliative doses should be at least 60 to 66 Gy and 40 Gy, respectively.[33]

Cervical node metastases may be managed with neck dissection in patients with a solitary node with no extracapsular extension, and with surgery plus adjuvant RT in patients with more advanced disease.[119] Similar to parotid node metastasis, surgery with adjuvant RT has shown improved 5-year disease-free survival compared to surgery alone (74% versus 34%).[120] Depending on the location of the primary tumor, the probability of subclinical disease in the clinically negative parotid may be high and the parotid nodes should be considered for elective treatment.

Medical Therapy for Advanced Subcutaneous Cell Carcinoma

Apart from surgical therapy or RT, treatment options for SCC are limited. Local, intralesional chemotherapy with methotrexate (one to three injections of 5 to 40 mg each) and 5-FU (up to eight injections of 10 to 150 mg each) have been reported to be up to 100% effective for treatment of KA-type SCC in small case series, although these studies were uncontrolled and this is not a commonly utilized therapy.[121] For typical SCC, intralesional treatment with IFN has been found to be an effective treatment, and may be particularly useful as salvage therapy for advanced or multiply recurrent disease.[122] The largest study to date treated 27 invasive SCC and 7 SCCIS with intralesional IFN-alpha-2b, 1.5 million units three times a week for 3 weeks, and found a 97% cure rate at 3 months, although long-term follow-up was not reported.[123]

The long-term prognosis for metastatic SCC is extremely poor. Treatment of metastatic disease may include systemic chemotherapy or treatment with biologic response modifiers. Although the efficacy of these methods has not been established, the recent development of targeted inhibitors of the EGFR holds promise for treatment of advanced SCC, particularly in light of the known aberrations in EGFR signaling in SCC. Cetuximab is a chimeric monoclonal antibody directed against EGFR that inhibits EGFR signaling; it is approved for treatment of head and neck (mucosal) SCC and has been used off label for cutaneous SCC.[124] The first phase 2 study of monotherapy with weekly cetuximab infusions for unresectable or metastatic cutaneous SCC showed a complete response rate of 6% and a partial response (at least 30% decrease in tumor size) of 22%.[125] Subsequent case reports have shown improved response rates (up to 50% complete response) when cetuximab was combined with adjuvant RT.[124] Although the efficacy of

these investigational treatments is clearly inferior to excisional surgery, it compares favorably to the historical prognosis of advanced SCC, in which 10-year survival rates are <20% for patients with regional lymph node involvement and <10% for patients with distant metastases.[126] While surgical therapy remains the cornerstone of SCC treatment, it is likely that additional molecularly targeted therapeutics will be incorporated as adjuvant or salvage therapy for advanced SCC.

FOLLOW-UP

Invasive SCC can be a potentially lethal neoplasm and warrants close follow-up. A critical review and meta-analysis has found that for people with fewer than three previous NMSCs, the risk of developing another NMSC within the following 3 years is 38%. In people with three to nine previous NMSCs, this risk rises to 93%.[127] In another study, approximately 30% of patients with SCC developed a subsequent SCC, with more than half of these occurring within the first year of follow-up.[128] Thus, it is recommended that patients with SCC be examined every 3 to 6 months during the first 2 years after treatment and at least annually thereafter. Evaluation should include total-body cutaneous examination and palpation of draining lymph nodes. Currently, radiography, magnetic resonance imaging, and computed tomography (CT) play no role in the routine workup of uncomplicated cutaneous SCC.

IMMUNOSUPPRESSION AND NONMELANOMA SKIN CANCER

The role of the immune system in the pathogenesis of skin cancer is still not completely understood. Immunosuppressed patients with lymphoma or leukemia and patients with depressed cellular immunity secondary to HIV infection develop NMSC at a significantly younger age and show a higher frequency of NMSC than the general population.[129] An Italian study of HIV patients found a three-fold increase in the incidence of NMSC over the general population.[130] Incidence of clinically aggressive HPV-related anal SCC is significantly increased in this population, requiring serial examinations and anal cytologies for surveillance.[131]

Solid-organ transplant recipients (e.g., heart, kidney) have a three- to four-fold increased risk over the general population of developing any cancer.[22] These patients experience a marked increase in the incidence of SCCs (40- to 250-fold increase) and BCCs (5- to 10-fold increase). Skin cancers in immunosuppressed patients appear primarily on sun-exposed sites. Incidence of NMSC in renal transplant recipients in Australia increases exponentially over time: 3% within the first year, 25% at 5 years, and 44% at 9 or more years posttransplant.[132] Similar results were observed in heart transplant patients, with an inverted SCC:BCC ratio of 3:1.[133] Furthermore, the SCCs in organ transplant patients occur at a younger age and tend to be more aggressive. There is an increased risk of local recurrence, regional and distant metastasis, and mortality. In case series of renal transplant patients from the United States and Australian heart transplant recipients, SCC-related mortality rates were 5% and 27%, respectively.[133] Although organ transplant recipients have an increased incidence of viral warts, HPV infection does not appear to be the primary cause of skin cancer in this population.[134] Patients who receive hematopoietic transplants do not experience marked increased in skin cancer incidence, presumably because of the shorter duration of immunosuppression.

Cumulative UVR is the primary pathogenic factor for the development of NMSC in solid-organ transplant recipients, but degree, type, duration of immunosuppression, and age at transplantation are also significant.[133] Sirolimus (rapamycin), a bacterial macrolide and antitumor agent, is a newer immunosuppressive agent that shows promise in decreasing incidence and severity of posttransplant NMSCs.[135] Changing immunosuppressive therapy to sirolimus from a standard regimen of calcineurin inhibitors was shown to be effective for secondary prevention of SCC in renal transplant recipients in a randomized trial, decreasing the risk of subsequent SCC by 44%.[136] However, because 23% of patients in the sirolimus group discontinued the medication due to adverse effects (including edema, aphthous ulcers, and pneumonitis), sirolimus is often reserved for use in selected patients with particularly elevated risk of SCC complications. As discussed previously, preventative therapy with systemic retinoids is another viable option for minimizing morbidity from SCC in transplant recipients.[23] Prevention, patient education, aggressive sun protection, and timely and aggressive management of skin cancers as well as altering the degree or type of immunosuppression whenever possible are crucial to reduce the significant risk of NMSC complications in this population.

ANGIOSARCOMA

Angiosarcoma (AS; synonyms are malignant hemangioendothelioma, hemangiosarcoma, and lymphangiosarcoma) is an uncommon, aggressive, usually fatal neoplasm of vascular endothelium origin accounting for <2% of all sarcomas.[137] The overall incidence of this tumor is approximately 0.1 per million per year. Four variants of cutaneous AS currently are recognized and include AS of the "head and neck" (also known as idiopathic AS) accounting for 50% to 60% of all cases, AS in the context of lymphedema (lymphedema-associated AS [LAS]; Stewart-Treves syndrome), radiation-induced AS, and epithelioid AS. Although these variants differ in presentation, they share key features, including clinical appearance of primary lesions, a biologically aggressive nature, and, ultimately, poor outcome.

PATHOGENESIS

Pathogenesis of AS is poorly understood. Approximately 50% of ASs express markers of lymphatic differentiation in addition to vascular endothelium-associated antigens. More recently, AS was found to coexpress podoplanin and podocalyxin, markers of lymphatic and vascular endothelium, respectively.[138] Human herpesvirus-8 etiologic factor in Kaposi sarcoma appears not to be associated with AS. Cumulative sun exposure has not been shown to be a predisposing factor.

CLINICAL PRESENTATION AND PROGNOSIS

Cutaneous AS of the head and scalp usually affects older adults. Approximately 70% of AS occurs in patients over the age of 40 years and the highest incidence of the disease is reported in those over 70 years of age.[137] Men are more commonly affected than women with 1.6 to 3:1 ratio.

Clinically, cutaneous AS presents as a violaceous to red, ill-defined patch on the central face, forehead, or scalp, often initially resembling a bruise.[137] Facial swelling and edema may be present. Differential diagnosis at initial presentation may include benign vascular tumor, hematoma secondary to trauma, or even an inflammatory dermatosis. More advanced lesions are violaceous elevated nodules with propensity to bleed easily. Ulceration may also be present. Satellite lesions are common.

The prognosis of cutaneous AS is poor, with a mortality rate of 50% at 15 months after diagnosis, and the survival rates ranging from 10% to 30% over a 5-year period, with median survival 18 to 28 months.[139,140] Metastatic potential of AS is high. Metastases to lung, liver, lymph nodes, spleen, and brain are common. Prognosis for metastatic disease is poor. Although prognosis does not correlate with degree of cellular differentiation, there appears to be a correlation with lesion size at presentation; increased survival has been demonstrated in lesions <5 cm at time of diagnosis. In a clinical univariate analysis of 69 cases, older age, anatomic site, necrosis, and epithelioid features directly correlated with increased mortality.[141] Other prognostic factors proposed in the literature include depth of invasion >3 mm, mitotic rate, Ki-67 staining, positive surgical margins, and local recurrence.[142]

LAS accounts for about 10% of all cutaneous AS and was first reported by Stewart and Treves[143] in six patients with postmastectomy lymphedema. In each case, AS developed in the ipsilateral arm and occurred several years after mastectomy. Subsequently, LAS was reported after axillary node dissection for melanoma and in the context of congenital lymphedema, filarial lymphedema, and chronic idiopathic lymphedema. The risk for developing LAS 5 years after mastectomy is approximately 5%. The most common site is the medial aspect of the upper arm.

LAS presents as a firm, coalescing violaceous plaque or nodule superimposed on brawny, nonpitting edema. Ulceration may develop rapidly. The duration of lymphedema prior to appearance of AS ranges from 4 to 27 years. The pathogenesis of LAS is incompletely understood and may be related to imbalances in local immune regulation or angiogenesis, leading to proliferation of neoplastic cells. The prognosis is poor, and survival rates are comparable to AS involving the scalp and face. Long-term survival has been reported in isolated cases after amputation of the affected limb.

Radiation-induced AS has been reported to occur after RT for benign or malignant conditions.[137] AS may occur from 4 to 40 years after RT for benign conditions (acne and eczema), or from 4 to 25 years after RT for malignancies. Overall prognosis is poor and comparable to that observed in other forms of AS.

Epithelioid AS is a rare, recently described variant of AS.[144] It tends to involve the lower extremities. On microscopic examination, the tumor may mimic an epithelial neoplasm, with sheets of rounded, epithelioid cells intermingled with irregularly lined vascular channels. Epithelioid AS results in widespread metastases within 1 year of presentation. Prognosis is poor.

HISTOLOGY

Histology of AS, although highly variable in the degree of cellular endothelial differentiation between and within individual tumors, does not vary between individual subtypes.[137] In well-differentiated lesions, an anastomosing network of sinusoidal irregularly dilated vascular channels lined by a single layer of flattened endothelial cells with mild to moderate nuclear atypia is commonly seen. These exhibit a highly infiltrative pattern, splitting collagen bundles and subcutaneous adipose tissue. Less-differentiated tumors show proliferation of atypical, polygonal, or spindle-shaped, pleomorphic endothelial cells with increased mitotic activity and anastomosing vascular channels. In poorly differentiated AS, luminal formation may be no longer apparent and mitotic activity is high. Poorly differentiated AS may mimic other high-grade sarcomas, carcinoma, or even melanoma. The state of cellular differentiation, however, has not been shown to correlate with prognosis.[139] Immunohistochemical analysis may be of value in diagnosis of AS, as cells stain positively for *Ulex europaeus* I lectin and factor VIII–related antigen. *Ulex* I is considered to be more sensitive marker for AS. In addition, AS cells express stem cell antigen CD34 and endothelial cell surface antigen CD31. The majority of AS cases stain positively for vimetin, D2-40, and VEGFR-3.

TREATMENT

Because of the clinical aggressiveness, treatment options for AS are limited. Surgical excision with wide margins is the treatment of choice. Nonetheless, the RRs and possibility of metastatic disease are high even with histologically negative margins and may reflect the tendency for multifocality.[145] Amputation with shoulder disarticulation or hemipelvectomy is recommended for tumors involving the extremities. Because AS tends to extend far beyond clinically appreciated margins, complete surgical removal may be challenging. Several cases of AS have been treated by MMS in an attempt to control margins; however, the difference between AS and normal vasculature may be difficult to interpret on frozen sections, even with the use of immunohistochemical stains.[146] RT and electron beam should be considered postoperatively in an effort to enhance local control.

Patients with isolated lymphatic spread treated with taxol-based chemotherapeutic regimens have a favorable outcome. Both chemotherapy and radical RT are palliative only for metastatic disease and do not improve overall survival.

DERMATOFIBROSARCOMA PROTUBERANS

DFSP is a rare soft tissue sarcoma with aggressive local but low metastatic potential with an annual incidence of approximately 4 per million. DFSP constitutes approximately 1% of all sarcomas and <0.1% of all malignancies.[147] The vast majority, approximately 90% of DFSPs, are low-grade sarcomas, whereas the remainder are classified as intermediate or high grade because of the presence of a high-grade fibrosarcomatous component (DFSP-FS).[148]

DFSP most commonly affects patients in their mid- to late 30s; however, the disease can occur at any age. Childhood and congenital cases of DFSP have been reported.[149] Blacks have slightly higher incidence than whites. Both men and women are equally affected.[150]

PATHOGENESIS

The pathogenesis of DFSP is incompletely understood but may involve factors as diverse as aberrant TSG or a history of local trauma/scarring.[151] More than 90% of DFSP feature a translocation between chromosomes 17 and 22, resulting in the fusion between the collagen type Iα1 gene (COL1A1) and the platelet-derived growth factor (PDGF) β-chain gene (PDGFB). Thus, the growth of DFSP is a result of the deregulation of PDGF β-chain expression and activation of PDGF receptor (PDGFR) protein tyrosine kinase.[151,152]

DFSP classically presents as a solitary, frequently asymptomatic, plaque with violaceous to blue hue. The tumor exhibits slow growth. Most commonly affected sides include trunk and, less frequently, the extremities, head, and neck, but it may occur anywhere.[152] The Bednar tumor is a rare pigmented variant of DFSP.[153] Clinically, it may be difficult to differentiate from a dermatofibroma or a keloid.

HISTOLOGY

Histologically, DFSP arises in the dermis and is composed of monomorphous, dense spindle cells arranged in a storiform pattern and embedded in a sparse to moderately dense fibrous stroma.[154] Irregular projections (tentaclelike) of the tumor are common and may account for the high incidence of local recurrence after excision. The distinction between deep penetrating dermatofibroma (DPDF), which involves the subcutis, and DFSP may be challenging. In most instances, attention to the cytologic constituency of the lesions and the overall architecture is sufficient for differentiation. DPDF is typified by cellular heterogeneity. DPDF includes giant cells and lipidized histiocytes and extends deeply, using the interlobular subcuticular fibrous septa as scaffolds, or is in the form of broad fronts. In contrast, DFSP tends to be monomorphous,

surrounding adipocytes diffusely or extending in stratified horizontal plates. This infiltration is characteristically eccentric, often with long, thin extensions in one direction and not another. Immunostaining for factor XIIIa, CD34, and stromelysin 3 may be helpful in distinguishing DPDF from DFSP. Characteristically, DPDF is diffusely factor XIIIa+, CD34−, and stromelysin 3+, whereas DFSP is factor XIIIa−, CD34+, and stromelysin 3−.[155]

TREATMENT

Treatment options for DFSP include WLE and MMS. Most authors advocate WLE with a minimal margin of at least 3 cm of surrounding skin, including the underlying fascia, without elective lymph node dissection.[156] The likelihood of local recurrence is directly proportional to the adequacy of surgical margins. Conservative resection can lead to RRs of 33% to 60%, whereas wider excision margins (≥2.5 cm) have been reported to reduce the RR to 10%.[157] For well-defined tumors located on trunk or extremities, WLE is likely to achieve tumor clearance with satisfactory cosmetic and functional result. However, extirpation of tumor by MMS, using frozen sections with or without confirmation by examination of paraffin-embedded sections, may be beneficial in sites where maximum conservation of normal tissue is required. Utility of MMS versus WLE was examined in a retrospective review of 48 primary DFSP cases treated at a single institution.[158] Twenty-eight patients underwent WLE and twenty patients underwent MMS. Median WLE margin width was 2 cm. For MMS, the median number of layers required to clear the tumor was two. Positive margins were present in 21.4% (6 of 28) WLE versus 0% MMS. At a median follow-up of 49.9 months for WLE and 40.4 months for MMS, local RRs were 3.6% (1 of 28) and 0%, respectively. The authors concluded that although positive margin resection was more common with WLE, local control was ultimately similar for the two surgical modalities. In a different study, Paradisi et al.[159] compared literature-reported observational data on 41 patients who underwent MMS and 38 who underwent WLE. Recurrence rates were 13.2% and 0% for WLE and MMS at 4.8 and 5.4 years follow-up, respectively. The relative risk of recurrence for WLE versus MMS was 15.9.

In the cases of congenital DFSP treated with MMS, the reported clearance rate was 100% during an average follow-up period of 4.3 years.[160] The clearance rate seen with WLE was 89% with an average follow-up period of 1.9 years. The average margins taken during MMS (1.7 cm) were smaller than those taken with WLE (2.8 cm). Based on superior cure rates and smaller surgical margins, MMS was proposed as first-line treatment for congenital DFSP.

Alternative treatment options for DFSP include RT and chemotherapy. RT was used selectively in a number of cases if surgical resection was not possible or would result in major cosmetic or functional deficit, with good local response.[161,162] A PDGF receptor inhibitor, imatinib, has been used with clinical success in advanced disease.[163,164] In a case series of 10 patients with locally advanced or metastatic disease treated with imatinib, 9 patients showed therapy response.[165] Limited clinical data are available on the use of chemotherapeutic agents such as vinblastine and methotrexate.[161]

RECURRENCE AND METASTATIC POTENTIAL

Patients with DFSP should be followed closely for evidence of local or regional recurrence or metastatic disease. DFSP has a tendency to recur locally. The average time for recurrence is within the first 3 years. DFSP of the head and neck has been reported to have a higher local RR (50% to 75%) than DFSP in other locations and might be related to smaller surgical margins used in cosmetically sensitive areas.[166] Although metastases are rare, multiple local recurrences appear to predispose to distant metastases.[167]

Lymph node metastases occur in approximately 1% of cases, and distant metastases, principally to lung, occur in approximately 4% of DFSP cases. DFSP-associated mortality is low. In a series of 218 patients, the 5- and 10-year mortality rates were 1.5% and 2.8%, respectively.[161]

A fibrosarcomatous variant, DFSP-FS, represents an uncommon form of DFSP that tends to follow a more aggressive clinical course.[168] In a series of 41 patients with DFSP-FS, a mean follow-up period of 90 months revealed a local RR of 58%. Metastatic rate was 14.7%.

MERKEL CELL CARCINOMA

MCC is a rare and aggressive tumor of neuroendocrine cell origin with an estimated annual incidence in the United States of 3 per million people.[169] Incidence of MCC is estimated in men at more than twice that in women, and whites are more than 20 times more likely to develop disease than blacks. The average age at diagnosis is 70 years.[170]

Merkel cells derive from the neural crest and differentiate as a part of the amine precursor uptake and decarboxylation system. Merkel cells function as slowly adapting type I mechanoreceptors.[170]

PATHOGENESIS

The pathogenesis of MCC is incompletely characterized. Given the increased incidence of MCC with increasing age, it is likely that accumulation of oncogenic events plays a role. UVR has been indirectly implicated in the development of MCC. The risk is higher among whites of European ancestry, incidence is inversely related to latitude, and the majority of tumors present on the face (36%), head, extremities, and trunk.[170]

The risk of MCC is particularly high with prior PUVA treatment. A multicenter study of 1,380 patients with psoriasis who were treated with PUVA showed that the incidence of MCC was 100 times higher than expected in the general population.[171] Immunosuppression, whether through iatrogenic means, HIV infection, or neoplasia, may play a role in the development of MCC. Patients with MCC have increased incidence of multiple myeloma, non-Hodgkin lymphoma, and in particular chronic lymphocytic leukemia.[172,173] Rapid progression has been reported in the setting of immunosuppressive therapy after organ transplantation.[174] Numerous chromosomal abnormalities have been described in MCC, but a definite causal relationship has not been established.

Recently, a double-stranded DNA virus, Merkel cell polyomavirus (MCPyV) was elegantly implicated in the pathogenesis of MCC.[175–177] Viral genome was detected in 8 of 10 MCCs and at low levels in 16% of unaffected skin and 8% of tissues from other body sites of patients without MCC. Within MCC substantial variation in the relative number of MCPyV, DNA was noted. Virus-positive MCCs contain between 1 viral DNA copy per 10,000 tumor cells to 10 viral DNA copies per tumor cell. MCPyV was integrated at various locations in the MCC tumor genome in a clonal pattern, suggesting that infection of the cells occurred before their clonal expansion.[177] Increased detection techniques reveal that virtually all MCC contain MCPyV[178] and that both CD4+ and CD8+ antiviral T cells are detectable within tumors and the blood of patients with MCC.[179]

CLINICAL PRESENTATION

Clinically, MCC usually presents as a rapidly growing, firm, flesh-colored or red-violaceous, dome-shaped papule or plaque on sun-exposed skin. Most lesions are <2 cm in diameter at the time of diagnosis. Clinical differential diagnosis often includes leukemia cutis, amelanotic melanoma, metastatic carcinoma, pyogenic granuloma, BCC, and SCC. Regional lymph nodes are involved in up to 30% of patients, and approximately 50% of patients develop systemic disease. Secondary sites of MCC spread include skin (28%), lymph nodes (27%), liver (13%), lung (10%), bone (10%), and brain (6%).[147,180]

HISTOLOGY

Histologic examination of MCC reveals sheets and cords of atypical cells in the dermis extending to the subcutaneous layer that sometimes form an interlacing trabecular or pseudoglandular pattern (Fig. 92.9). Three histologic subtypes have been described: intermediate, trabecular, and small cell. No clinically significant differences between subtypes have been described. A grenz zone separating tumor from epidermis is often present. Individual cell membranes often are indistinct, giving a syncytial appearance. Cells are round to oval and generally noncohesive. Cytoplasm tends to be scant, with round to oval nuclei containing two to three nucleoli. Special stains may prove useful in the histological evaluation of MCC. Cytokeratin-20 staining gives a characteristic parinuclear dot pattern. MCC also stains positively for chromogranin neuron–specific enolase and synaptophysin, and may be weakly

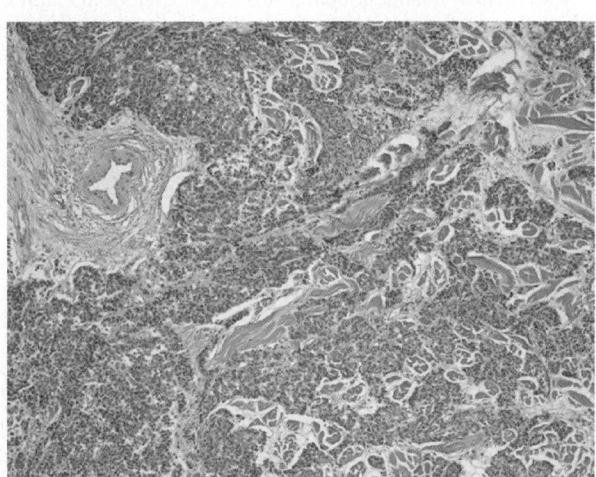
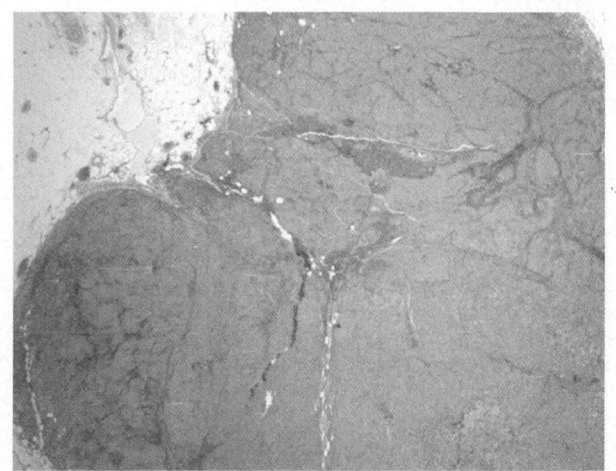

A   **B**

Figure 92.9 (A and B) Histologic examination of cutaneous Merkel cell carcinoma reveals sheets and cords of atypical cells in the dermis extending to the subcutaneous layer that sometimes form an interlacing trabecular or pseudoglandular pattern. Cells are round to oval and generally noncohesive. Cytoplasm tends to be scant, with round to oval nuclei containing two to three nucleoli.

positive for S100 protein.[181] In 2002, it was shown that MCC also stains for the KIT receptor tyrosine kinase (CD117), and perhaps abnormal functioning of the KIT receptor could be involved in the malignant transformation of this tumor.[182]

Histologic differential diagnosis of MCC includes lymphoma, BCC, metastatic oat cell carcinoma, or noncutaneous neuro-endocrine tumors. In contrast to MCC, lymphoma cells are CD45-positive and cytokeratin-20 negative. Melanoma can be differentiated from MCC by strong S100 positivity of melanocytes.

TREATMENT

MCC warrants aggressive therapy. It has a high propensity for local recurrence (20% to 75%), regional (31% to 80%), and distant metastases (26% to 75%). Approximately one-third of patients with MCC eventually die of the disease. Age older than 65 years, male sex, size of primary lesion >2 cm, truncal site, nodal/distant disease at presentation, and duration of disease before presentation (≤3 months) appear to be poor prognostic factors. All patients with histologically confirmed MCC should undergo imaging and laboratory examination to evaluate the full extent of disease. Evaluation must include full-body skin examination with lymph node evaluation, a complete blood cell count, and liver function tests. CT scanning of the chest, pelvis, and abdomen may be indicated to detect distal metastasis.[183] CT scanning of the head and neck may prove valuable in detection of nodal disease. Octreotide scans may be more sensitive than CT scans in diagnosing primary and metastatic MCC.[184] Perianal and vulvar sites have the worst prognosis of all primary sites. Metastases have been noted most commonly in skin and lymph nodes but also in the lung, liver, brain, intestine, bladder, stomach, and abdominal wall.

STAGING

Five competing staging systems have been used to describe MCC. However, these staging systems are highly inconsistent. To address these concerns, a new MCC-specific consensus staging system was developed by the AJCC. Patients with primary MCC with no evidence of regional or distant metastases (either clinically or pathologically) are divided into two stages: stage I for primary tumors no >2 cm in size and stage II for primary tumors >2 cm in size. Stage I and stage II are further divided into A and B substages based on method of nodal evaluation. Patients who have pathologically proven node-negative disease (by microscopic evaluation of their draining lymph nodes) have improved survival (substaged as IIA) compared with those who are evaluated only clinically (substaged as IIB). Stage II has an additional substage (IIC) for tumors with extracutaneous invasion (T4) and negative node status, regardless of whether the negative node status was established microscopically or clinically. Stage III includes patient with nodal disease, either microscopically positive and clinically occult nodes (IIIA) or macroscopic nodes (IIIB). Distant metastases are classified as stage IV MCC.[185]

Before the new AJCC consensus staging system was published, the recent Memorial Sloan Kettering Cancer Center (MSKCC) four-stage system was favored as it was based on the largest number of patients and was the best validated. The stages in the MSKCC system include stage I (primary tumor alone, <2 cm in diameter), stage II (primary tumor alone, >2 cm in diameter), stage III (regional nodal disease), and stage IV (distant metastatic disease).[186]

RECURRENCE AND METASTATIC RISK

MCC has a propensity to recur locally (sometimes with satellite lesions and/or in-transit metastases) following surgical excision. In a review of 18 case series, 279 of 926 patients (30.1%) developed

local recurrence during follow-up. These recurrences have been typically attributed to inadequate surgical margins or possibly a lack of adjuvant radiation therapy.[187] WLE to reduce the risk of local recurrence has been recommended for patients with clinical stage I or stage II disease.

Recommendations about the optimal minimum width and depth of normal tissue margin that should be excised around the primary tumor differ among the various retrospective case series, but this question has not been studied systematically.[180,186,188] No definitive data suggest that extremely wide margins improve overall survival, although some reports suggest that wider margins appear to improve local control.[189]

Recommended management has usually been WLE with 1- to 3-cm margins; however, treatment guidelines are not well defined, owing to the rarity of the tumor, which precludes randomized clinical trials. Recurrence rates after primary therapy for MCC with surgery alone are reported to be within the range of 0% to 50% to 70%. In a single-institution case series of 95 patients with early-stage MCC, a total of 45 (47%) patients relapsed, with 80% of the recurrences occurring within 2 years and 96% within 5 years.[190] Patients with MCC in the head and neck region had a 5-year local-recurrence cumulative incidence of 19% and no distant recurrences, and patients with MCC in the extremity and trunk region had a 5-year local-recurrence cumulative incidence of 2% and a 5-year distant-recurrence cumulative incidence of 22%.[190] MMS has been proposed as being more successful in controlling local disease than WLE, especially in cosmetically sensitive anatomic locations. The relapse rate has been reported to be similar to or better than that of wide excision, but comparatively few cases have been treated in this manner and none in randomized, controlled trials.[188,191,192] In a retrospective review of 38 consecutive patients with MCC of the extremities, WLE and MMS showed similar local RR.[188]

MCC spreads to regional lymph nodes within 2 years in up to 70% of cases. Because of the propensity for early nodal spread and the significant negative impact that nodal disease has on outcome, regional lymph node dissection or sentinel lymph node (SLN) dissection may be advisable. Surgical nodal staging in clinically negative patients has identified positive nodes in at least 25% to 35% of patients.[186] At present, it is questionable whether lymph node dissection has an impact on survival, but it seems to benefit local and regional control. Clinically or radiographically positive nodes should be resected but it is unclear whether elective lymph node dissection provides benefit.

SLN biopsy is a preferred initial alternative to complete elective lymph node dissection for the proper staging of MCC. SLN biopsy is associated with lower morbidity, and in the sites with indeterminate lymphatic drainage, SNL technique can be used to identify the pertinent lymphatic basins. Several reports support the use of SLN biopsy techniques in MCC staging and management.[193–195] One meta-analysis of 10 case series found that SLN positivity strongly predicted a high short-term risk of recurrence and that subsequent therapeutic lymph node dissection was effective in preventing short-term regional nodal recurrence.[195] Another meta-analysis of 12 retrospective case series found that (1) SLN biopsy detected MCC spread in one-third of patients whose tumors would have otherwise been clinically and radiologically understaged, (2) the RR was three times higher in patients with a positive SLN biopsy than in those with a negative SLN biopsy, and (3) the relapse-free survival rate in patients with positive SLN biopsy who did or did not receive additional treatment to the nodes was 51% and 0% at 3 years, respectively.[196] Whether complete dissection of regional nodes following positive SLN biopsy improves definitively survival remains unresolved, however.

Radiation to the primary site has been considered for patients with larger (>2 cm) tumors and locally unresectable tumors, while adjuvant nodal radiation is considered for those with positive regional nodes (stage II).[169,192] Several small retrospective series have shown that radiation plus adequate surgery improves local-regional control compared with surgery alone,[180,196] whereas other series did not show similar results.[186,191] Adjuvant RT offers a substantial benefit in both time to recurrence and disease-free survival, but a survival benefit is yet to be proven.[197] The controversy regarding the utility of adjuvant RT following excision remains.

Chemotherapy is used for nodal, metastatic, and recurrent MCC, but an optimal treatment regimen is yet to be established. From 1997 to 2001, the Trans-Tasman Radiation Oncology Group performed a phase 2 evaluation of 53 patients with MCC with high-risk, local-regional disease. Given the heterogeneity of the population and the nonstandardized surgery, it is difficult to infer a clear treatment benefit of the chemotherapy.[198] Regimens are similar to those used for small cell lung carcinoma. The most commonly used agents are cyclophosphamide, anthracyclines, and cisplatin. In a study by Voog et al.,[199] overall response to first-line chemotherapy for MCC was 61%, with a 57% response in metastatic disease and a 69% response in locally advanced disease. Reported 3-year survival rate was 17% in metastatic disease and 35% in locally advanced disease. Forty-two different regimens were used to treat these 107 reported cases.

PROGNOSIS

The prognosis of MCC is directly correlated with the stage of disease. Reported 5-year survival according to MSKCC classification is 81% for stage I, 67% for stage II, 52% for stage III, and 11% for stage IV.[147] More than 50% of patients experience recurrence with the median time to recurrence of 9 months (range, 2 to 70 months). Ninety-one percent of recurrences occurred within 2 years of diagnosis.[186] Overall survival of head and neck MCC at 5 years postoperatively ranges between 40% and 68%.[200]

MICROCYSTIC ADNEXAL CARCINOMA

Microcystic adnexal carcinoma (MAC) was first described as a distinct entity in 1982 by Goldstein et al.[201] Synonyms quoted in the literature to describe MAC include sclerosing sweat duct carcinoma, malignant syringoma, sweat gland carcinoma with syringomatous features, aggressive trichofolliculoma, and combined adnexal tumor of the skin. MAC originates from pluripotent adnexal keratinocytes capable of both eccrine and follicular differentiation. The pathogenesis of MAC is not completely understood but may involve exposure to ionizing and UVR that may precede development of MAC by as long as 40 years.[202] MAC is an aggressive, locally destructive cutaneous appendageal neoplasm with a high rate of local recurrence but low rate of metastasis. It primarily affects white, middle-aged individuals, although it has been reported in children and blacks. Unlike the other primary cutaneous malignancies, MAC has slight female predominance.

CLINICAL AND HISTOLOGIC FEATURES

MAC classically presents as a smooth-surfaced, nonulcerated, flesh-colored to yellowish asymptomatic nodule, papule, or plaque. When symptomatic, common findings include numbness, tenderness, anesthesia, paresthesia, burning, discomfort, and/or rarely pruritus of the affected site. These symptoms can relate to the frequent PNI of the tumor. MAC is locally aggressive with common perineural invasion and extension to muscle, vascular adventitia, perichondrium, periosteum, and bone marrow. MAC has a clear predilection for the head and neck (86% to 88%), particularly the central face (73%). Other sites include eyelid, scalp, breast/chest, axillae, buttocks, vulva, extremities, and tongue. This tumor is often misdiagnosed clinically and histologically.[202,203]

Histologically, MAC is a tumor of pilar and eccrine differentiation. It may be misdiagnosed as a benign adnexal process. The

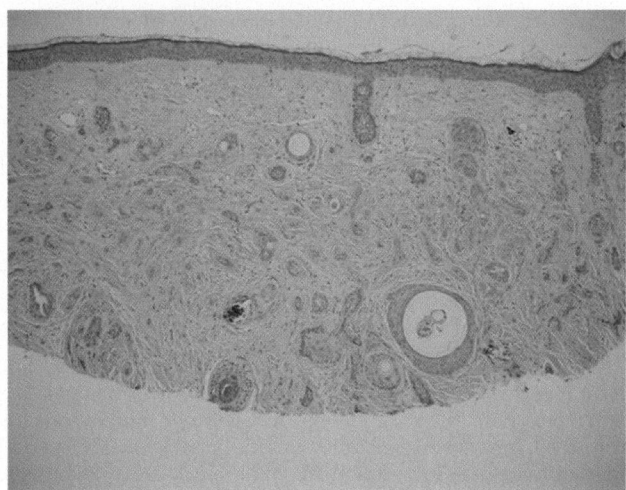

Figure 92.10 Histology of microcystic adnexal carcinoma. The tumor frequently exhibits a stratified appearance with larger keratin horn cysts and epithelial nests, strands, or cords in the superficial dermis and desmoplastic deeper dermis with smaller cysts and more pronounced ductal structures. Horn cysts may contain laminated keratin and/or small vellus hairs. Cysts may be also calcified. Ducts may be well differentiated, with two rows of cuboidal cells, or less differentiated, with single strands without lumina.

tumor frequently exhibits a stratified appearance with larger keratin horn cysts and epithelial nests, strands, or cords in the superficial dermis and desmoplastic features in the deeper dermis with smaller cysts and more pronounced ductal structures (Fig. 92.10). Ducts may be well differentiated, with two rows of cuboidal cells, or less differentiated, with single strands without lumina. Mitotic figures and cytologic atypia are rare. Histologic differential diagnosis of MAC includes desmoplastic trichoepithelioma, benign syringoma, papillary eccrine adenoma, morpheaform BCC, SCC, and metastatic breast carcinoma. Adequately deep biopsy is crucial for correct diagnostic assessment.

TREATMENT AND PROGNOSIS

Current standard of care for MAC is to surgically remove the tumor in its entirety whenever feasible. This task can be challenging in clinical practice because the tumor often extends microscopically centimeters beyond the clinically apparent margins. Margins reported in the literature for WLE vary from a few millimeters to 3 to 5 cm. Extirpation of tumor by MMS may prove beneficial in the management of MAC. Recurrence rates vary significantly between the two surgical techniques with rates after WLE and MMS ranging from 40% to 60%[204] and 0 to 12%,[205] respectively. To date, seven cases of metastases have been reported for a cumulative metastatic rate of <2.1%, although this is likely an overestimate. RT has been used as mono- or adjuvant therapy for MAC with reported success in only one of six case reports, highlighting the tumor's resistance to RT. Patients with MAC should have ongoing examination of the skin and lymph nodes for the remainder of their lifespan, given the potential for late recurrence decades after initial presentation.

SEBACEOUS CARCINOMA

Sebaceous carcinoma (SC) is a malignant adnexal tumor with variable sites of origin, histologic growth patterns, and clinical presentations. About 75% of SCs are periocular in location.[206] Periocular SC may arise from Meibomian glands and, less frequently, from the glands of Zeis. The upper eyelids are most frequently involved.

Approximately 25% of cases of SC involve extraocular sites, which may include head and neck, trunk, salivary glands, and external genitalia.[207] Worldwide, SC affects all races, but Asians are particularly prone to the disease. Women are affected more commonly than men, at a ratio of approximately 2:1. SC classically presents in the seventh to ninth decades.[208] SC is associated with sebaceous adenomas, radiation exposure, and Muir Torre syndrome. Because of the strong association of SC with Muir Torre syndrome, patients presenting with SC should be referred for colonoscopy to assess for occult colon cancer. Routine genetic screening for Muir Torre in the absence of colon lesions is not currently indicated.

CLINICAL AND HISTOLOGIC FEATURES

The most frequent clinical presentation is a slowly growing, painless, subcutaneous nodule. Other presentations include diffuse thickening of the skin, pedunculated papules, or an irregular subcutaneous mass. On the eyelid, SC is most often misdiagnosed as chalazion. It may present as chronic diffuse blepharoconjunctivitis or keratoconjunctivitis, particularly with pagetoid or intraepithelial spread of tumor onto the conjunctival epithelium.[209] SC is the second most common eyelid malignancy after BCC and is the second most lethal after melanoma. Histologically, SCs are classified as well, moderately, or poorly differentiated. Most commonly, lesions have an irregular lobular growth pattern with sebaceous and undifferentiated cells. SC cells exhibit varying degrees of differentiation, nuclear pleomorphism, hyperchromatism, basaloid appearance, and high mitotic activity. Local infiltration of the surrounding tissues and neurovascular spaces can be seen. A known feature of the SC is pagetoid spread, the spread of tumor cells into the overlying epithelium. Special stains, including lipid stains as Oil-Red-O or Sudan IV for fresh tissue, and immunohistochemical stains such as EMA or LeuM1 are also helpful.[210]

TREATMENT AND PROGNOSIS

Treatment options for SC include WLE with 5- to 6-mm margins and extirpation by MMS. The local RR after WLE has been reported to be as high as 36% at 5 years and associated 5-year mortality rate of 18%.[211] In one study of 14 cases of SC excised with frozen-section margin control, five recurrences were observed in cases with surgical margins of 1 to 3 mm, whereas no recurrences were seen with margins of 5 mm.[212] Potential difficulties arise because tumors are often multicentric with discontinuous foci of tumor, and pagetoid spread is difficult to determine even on high-quality, paraffin-embedded sections. Extirpation of SC by MMS has compared favorably to WLE, with local RRs of ≤12% in reported series.[213] A series of poorly differentiated SC successfully treated with RT has also been reported.[214]

SCs have high rates of local recurrence and metastasis, particularly when occurring on the eyelid. SC can spread by lymphatic or hematogenous routes or by direct extension. Distant metastases are reported in up to 20% of cases and may involve the lungs, liver, brain, bones, and lymph nodes. Mortality of SC ranges from 9% to 50%. Extraocular SC has a reported local RR of 29% and metastatic rate of 21%, although there appears to be a reporting bias in the literature for more advanced disease. Small primary lesions <1 cm in diameter may exhibit a more favorable prognosis.

EXTRAMAMMARY PAGET DISEASE

Extramammary Paget disease (EMPD) is a rare cutaneous malignancy of older adults, often on the genitalia, with a mean age of onset of approximately 70 years. While there is a slight female predominance in Caucasian patients, there is a strong 4:1 male predominance in Asians.[215] Although histologically similar to Paget disease of the breast, EMPD is a separate entity with a distinct prognosis and is not related to breast cancer. EMPD is most often a primary intraepidermal malignancy thought to derive from eccrine or apocrine glands. EMPD has been associated with internal malignancy in 15% to 30% of cases, usually colon, bladder, or prostate cancer.[216] These cases of secondary EMPD have a worse prognosis than primary EMPD.

CLINICAL AND HISTOLOGIC FEATURES

EMPD most often presents as a pink to bright red plaque of the genitalia. Scaling, erosion, and maceration are common features. It is usually asymmetric and may extend to the perianal region, inguinal fold, suprapubic region, and medial thigh, but it is classically seen on the scrotum of men or the labia majora of women. Rare cases of primary EMPD have also been described in the axillae.[217] While most cases present as large flat plaques, nodular presentations have been described that portend a worse prognosis, as does clinical lymphadenopathy. Because of its innocuous appearance, EMPD is often misdiagnosed as benign inflammatory conditions such as psoriasis, dermatitis, or superficial fungal infections, and clinicians should have a low threshold for biopsy of suspected inflammatory conditions that do not respond to routine treatment.

Biopsy of EMPD reveals acanthosis with an intraepidermal proliferation of large, pale staining cells with prominent vesicular nuclei. These cells are spread throughout all layers of the epidermis, often forming large clusters just above the basal layer. Mitotic figures may be present. A minority of patients may have extension of EMPD into the superficial or deep dermis, which is associated with decreased survival.[217] Immunohistochemical stains may be helpful in the diagnosis of EMPD. Most cases of EMPD stain with CK7 and GCDFP-15, while CK20 staining may be more common in secondary EMPD.[218]

TREATMENT AND PROGNOSIS

To rule out internal malignancy and secondary EMPD, patients should undergo a colonoscopy and appropriate screening for genitourinary malignancy prior to initiating treatment. Complete surgical excision of EMPD has classically been the standard of care, although local RRs may be as high as 30% to 40%. MMS may be a superior option, with local RRs of 12% to 18% reported in small case series.[215,219] Because of its primarily superficial nature, nonsurgical treatment of primary EMPD has been proposed, with several case reports documenting success (and a few reporting failure) with topical imiquimod therapy.[220,221] In the authors' experience, topical therapy with imiquimod at a variable frequency for up to 12 weeks, titrated to the local inflammatory response, is an effective first-line therapy for primary EMPD. Surgical treatment may be employed for recalcitrant cases, and radiation therapy has also been reported for EMPD with some success.[222] Overall, the prognosis for primary EMPD is good, with a reported 85% overall survival at 5 years.[217] For the majority of patients that present with in situ disease, the prognosis is excellent, while the 14% of patients presenting with deep dermal invasion exhibit a 20-fold increased risk of disease-specific death.

ATYPICAL FIBROXANTHOMA AND MALIGNANT FIBROUS HISTIOCYTOMA

Until recently, atypical fibroxanthoma (AFX) and malignant fibrous histiocytoma were thought to be two distinct presentations of the same malignancy. However, following reclassification of soft tissue sarcomas by the World Health Organization in 2002 that mandated identification of cell line origin in classification of tumors, most cases of malignant fibrous histiocytoma, as previously considered, were found to be merely a morphologic pattern rather than a defined pathologic entity.[223] In a majority of cases, ultrastructural and immunohistochemical examination allowed for reclassification into defined histologic subtypes of sarcomas. Under the new classification, the term *malignant fibrous histiocytoma* is a synonym for undifferentiated pleomorphic sarcoma (UPS) not otherwise specified. UPS is a deep-seated subcutaneous nodule rarely encountered in the skin; it is most often seen on the limbs of elderly patients. UPS is an aggressive tumor with a poor prognosis. Although complete surgical excision is the preferred treatment (often with adjuvant RT), up to 50% of patients may have distant metastasis at the time of initial presentation, with the lung being the most common site.

ATYPICAL FIBROXANTHOMA

AFX is a spindle cell tumor that occurs on the head and neck of sun-exposed individuals and on the trunk and extremities of younger patients. Tumors of the head and neck characteristically present during the eighth decade, whereas tumors involving the extremities often present during the fourth decade. The ratio of affected men to women appears to be equal. A few cases have been reported in children with xeroderma pigmentosum. The pathogenesis of AFX involves exposure to UVR, ionizing radiation, and/or aberrant immune host response. In a series of 10 cases of AFX, 7 cases showed mutation in TSG *p53*, often with UVR signature mutations.[224] Tumors may occur 10 to 15 years after local ionizing radiation. An increased incidence of AFX has been observed in renal transplant patients, and metastatic AFX has been reported in a patient with chronic lymphocytic leukemia.

CLINICAL AND HISTOLOGIC FEATURES

AFX usually presents as an asymptomatic, often rapidly growing, dome-shaped papule or nodule covered by thin epidermis on actinically damaged skin of individuals with a fair complexion. Average size at presentation is 1 to 2 cm. Secondary changes such as serosanguinous crust or ulceration may be present. The clinical appearance is not distinctive, and the clinical differential diagnosis of the lesion often includes pyogenic granuloma, SCC, BCC, amelanotic melanoma, MCC, and cutaneous metastasis. AFX may be found in the setting of other NMSCs.

On microscopic examination, AFX is a dermal or partially exophytic nodule composed of a proliferation of atypical spindle-shaped cells with moderate amounts of cytoplasm and large histiocyte-like atypical cells with abundant pale-staining vacuolated cytoplasm

arranged in haphazard fashion in a collagenous or occasionally myxoid stroma.[225] The neoplastic cells have large, pleomorphic, and heterochromatic "bizarre-looking" nuclei, and some of them are multinucleated. There are numerous typical and atypical mitotic figures. Some cells may contain droplets of lipid. The epidermis overlying the dermal proliferation is commonly ulcerated. Both the spindle-shaped and the histiocyte-like cells stain positively for vimentin, while CD68 and CD10 are often, but not universally, positive in AFX. Stains for HMB-45 and S100, as well as cytokeratin stains, are negative, distinguishing this lesion from spindle cell melanoma and SCC, respectively.[225,226]

TREATMENT AND PROGNOSIS

Treatment of AFX is surgical removal by WLE or MMS. In a large retrospective series of 45 patients comparing WLE with MMS, recurrences were observed during a mean follow-up period of 73.6 months in 12% of 25 cases treated by WLE.[227] Metastatic involvement of the parotid gland occurred in one of these patients, for an overall regional metastatic rate of 4%. In contrast, no recurrences or metastases were observed over a mean follow-up period of 29.6 months in patients treated by MMS. Others have reported similarly favorable outcomes after treatment of AFX by MMS.[228,229] The authors favor the use of MMS for AFX because of the superior margin control and conservation of normal tissue.

Although AFX rarely metastasizes, it is a locally aggressive tumor with metastatic potential. Metastases to the parotid gland, lymph nodes, and lung have been reported. In a series of eight cases of metastatic AFX, poor prognostic indicators included vascular invasion, recurrence, deep-tissue penetration, necrosis, and impaired host resistance.[229,230] Because AFX is often found in the setting of diffuse actinic damage and other NMSCs, close follow-up after complete tumor extirpation is critical.

CARCINOMA METASTATIC TO SKIN

The most frequently observed cutaneous metastatic cancers are breast, colon, and melanoma in women, and lung, colon, and melanoma in men. Cutaneous involvement is also seen in the leukemias, with a wide variation in the morphology of lesions. The scalp is a common site for cutaneous metastatic disease. Immunohistochemical stains may be helpful in determining the site of the primary tumor. The discovery of cutaneous metastatic disease should prompt consultation with an oncologist for staging and management.

SELECTED REFERENCES

The full reference list can be accessed at lwwhealthlibrary.com/oncology.

1. Madan V, Lear JT, Szeimies RM. Non-melanoma skin cancer. *Lancet* 2010;375:673–685.
2. Stern RS. Prevalence of a history of skin cancer in 2007: results of an incidence-based model. *Arch Dermatol* 2010;146:279–282.
3. Rogers HW, Weinstock MA, Harris AR, et al. Incidence estimate of nonmelanoma skin cancer in the United States, 2006. *Arch Dermatol* 2010;146:283–287.
4. Neville JA, Welch E, Leffell DJ. Management of nonmelanoma skin cancer in 2007. *Nat Clin Pract Oncol* 2007;4:462–469.
5. Connolly SM, Baker DR, Coldiron BM, et al. AAD/ACMS/ASDA/ASMS 2012 appropriate use criteria for Mohs micrographic surgery. *J Am Acad Dermatol* 2012;67:531–550.
6. Tierney EP, Hanke CW. Cost effectiveness of Mohs micrographic surgery: review of the literature. *J Drugs Dermatol* 2009;8:914–922.
7. Salasche SJ. Status of curettage and desiccation in the treatment of primary basal cell carcinoma. *J Am Acad Dermatol* 1984;10:285–287.
8. Rodriguez-Vigil T, Vazquez-Lopez F, Perez-Oliva N. Recurrence rates of primary basal cell carcinoma in facial risk areas treated with curettage and electrodesiccation. *J Am Acad Dermatol* 2007;56:91–95.

11. Love WE, Bernhard JD, Bordeaux JS. Topical imiquimod or fluorouracil therapy for basal and squamous cell carcinoma: a systematic review. *Arch Dermatol* 2009;145:1431–1438.
15. Junkins-Hopkins JM. Imiquimod use in the treatment of lentigo maligna. *J Am Acad Dermatol* 2009;61:865–867.
22. Bath-Hextall F, Leonardi-Bee J, Somchand N, et al. Interventions for preventing non-melanoma skin cancers in high-risk groups. *Cochrane Database Syst Rev* 2007;CD005414.
23. Bavinck JN, Tieben LM, Van Der Woude FJ, et al. Prevention of skin cancer and reduction of keratotic skin lesions during acitretin therapy in renal transplant recipients: a double-blind, placebo-controlled study. *J Clin Oncol* 1995;13:1933–1938.
24. Kadakia KC, Barton DL, Loprinzi CL, et al. Randomized controlled trial of acitretin versus placebo in patients at high risk for basal cell or squamous cell carcinoma of the skin. *Cancer* 2012;118:2128–2137.
26. Tierney E, Barker A, Ahdout J, et al. Photodynamic therapy for the treatment of cutaneous neoplasia, inflammatory disorders, and photoaging. *Dermatol Surg* 2009;35:725–746.
27. Lehmann P. Methyl aminolaevulinate-photodynamic therapy: a review of clinical trials in the treatment of actinic keratoses and nonmelanoma skin cancer. *Br J Dermatol* 2007;156:793–801.

32. Halpern JN. Radiation therapy in skin cancer. A historical perspective and current applications. *Dermatol Surg* 1997;23:1089–1093.

34. Cognetta AB, Howard BM, Heaton HP, et al. Superficial x-ray in the treatment of basal and squamous cell carcinomas: a viable option in select patients. *J Am Acad Dermatol* 2012;67:1235–1241.

40. Brash DE, Ziegler A, Jonason AS, et al. Sunlight and sunburn in human skin cancer: p53, apoptosis, and tumor promotion. *J Investig Dermatol Symp Proc* 1996;1:136–142.

41. Padilla RS, Sebastian S, Jiang Z, et al. Gene expression patterns of normal human skin, actinic keratosis, and squamous cell carcinoma. *Arch Dermatol* 2010;146:288–293.

49. Swanson N, Abramovits W, Berman B, et al. Imiquimod 2.5% and 3.75% for the treatment of actinic keratosis: results of two placebo-controlled studies of daily application to the face and balding scalp for two 2-week cycles. *J Am Acad Dermatol* 2010;62:582–590.

51. Ulrich C, Bichel J, Euvrard S, et al. Topical immunomodulation under systemic immunosuppression: results of a multicentre, randomized, placebo-controlled safety and efficacy study of imiquimod 5% cream for the treatment of actinic keratoses in kidney, heart, and liver transplant patients. *Br J Dermatol* 2007;157:25–31.

54. Piacquadio DJ, Chen DM, Farber HF, et al. Photodynamic therapy with aminolevulinic acid topical solution and visible blue light in the treatment of multiple actinic keratoses of the face and scalp: investigator-blinded, phase 3, multicenter trials. *Arch Dermatol* 2004;140:41–46.

59. Kyrgidis A, Vahtsevanos K, Tzellos TG, et al. Clinical, histological and demographic predictors for recurrence and second primary tumours of head and neck basal cell carcinoma. A 1062 patient-cohort study from a tertiary cancer referral hospital. *Eur J Dermatol* 2010;20:276–282.

66. Ziegler A, Leffell DJ, Kunala S, et al. Mutation hotspots due to sunlight in the p53 gene of nonmelanoma skin cancers. *Proc Natl Acad Sci U S A* 1993;90:4216–4220.

67. Batra RS, Kelley LC. Predictors of extensive subclinical spread in nonmelanoma skin cancer treated with Mohs micrographic surgery. *Arch Dermatol* 2002;138:1043–1051.

73. Sekulic A, Migden MR, Oro AE, et al. Efficacy and safety of vismodegib in advanced basal cell carcinoma. *N Engl J Med* 2012;366:2171–2179.

74. Von Hoff DD, LoRusso PM, Rudin C, et al. Inhibition of the hedgehog pathway in advanced basal cell carcinoma. *N Engl J Med* 2009;361:1164–1172.

78. Wolf DJ, Zitelli JA. Surgical margins for basal cell carcinoma. *Arch Dermatol* 1987;123:340–344.

80. Swanson EL, Amdur RJ, Mendenhall WM, et al. Radiotherapy for basal cell carcinoma of the medial canthus region. *Laryngoscope* 2009;119:2366–2368.

81. Mendenhall WM, Amdur RJ, Hinerman RW, et al. Radiotherapy for cutaneous squamous and basal cell carcinomas of the head and neck. *Laryngoscope* 2009;119:1994–1999.

83. Kopf AW, Bart RS, Schrager D, et al. Curettage-electrodesiccation treatment of basal cell carcinomas. *Arch Dermatol* 1977;113:439–443.

85. Rowe DE, Carroll RJ, Day CL Jr. Mohs surgery is the treatment of choice for recurrent (previously treated) basal cell carcinoma. *J Dermatol Surg Oncol* 1989;15:424–431.

87. Marks R, Gebauer K, Shumack S, et al. Imiquimod 5% cream in the treatment of superficial basal cell carcinoma: results of a multicenter 6-week dose-response trial. *J Am Acad Dermatol* 2001;44:807–813.

92. Arits AH, Mosterd K, Essers BA, et al. Photodynamic therapy versus topical imiquimod versus topical fluorouracil for treatment of superficial basal cell carcinoma: a single blind, non-inferiority, randomized controlled trial. *Lancet Oncol* 2013;14:647–654.

93. Tang JY, Mackay-Wiggan JM, Aszterbaum M, et al. Inhibiting the hedgehog pathway in patients with the basal cell nevus syndrome. *N Engl J Med* 2012;366:2180–2188.

96. Rowe DE, Carroll RJ, Day CL Jr. Prognostic factors for local recurrence, metastasis, and survival rates in squamous cell carcinoma of the skin, ear, and lip. Implications for treatment modality selection. *J Am Acad Dermatol* 1992;26:976–990.

98. Karia PS, Han J, Schmults CD. Cutaneous squamous cell carcinoma: estimated incidence of disease, nodal metastasis, and deaths from disease in the United States in 2012. *J Am Acad Dermatol* 2013;68:957–966.

102. Durinck S, Ho C, Wang NJ, et al. Temporal dissection of tumorigenesis in primary cancers. *Cancer Discovery* 2011;1:137–143.

103. Agrawal N, Frederick MJ, Pickering CR, et al. Exome sequencing of head and neck squamous cell carcinoma reveals inactivating mutations in *NOTCH1. Science* 2011;333:1154–1157.

104. Stransky N, Egloff AM, Tward AD, et al. The mutational landscape of head and neck squamous cell carcinoma. *Science* 2011;333:1157–1160.

105. Leemans CR, Braakhuis BJ, Brakenhoff RH. The molecular biology of head and neck cancer. *Nat Rev Cancer* 2011;11:9–22.

111. Miller SJ. The National Comprehensive Cancer Network (NCCN) guidelines of care for nonmelanoma skin cancers. *Dermatol Surg* 2000;26: 289–292.

112. Farasat S, Yu SS, Neel VA, et al. A new American Joint Committee on Cancer staging system for cutaneous squamous cell carcinoma: creation and rationale for inclusion of tumor characteristics. *J Am Acad Dermatol* 2011;64:1051–1059.

113. Brantsch KD, Meisner C, Schonfisch B, et al. Analysis of risk factors determining prognosis of cutaneous squamous cell carcinoma: a prospective study. *Lancet Oncol* 2008;9:713–720.

114. Jambusaria-Pahlajani A, Kanetsky PA, Karia PS, et al. Evaluation of AJCC tumor staging for cutaneous squamous cell carcinoma and a proposed alternative tumor staging sytem. *JAMA Dermatol* 2013;149:402–410.

116. Brodland DG, Zitelli JA. Surgical margins for excision of primary cutaneous squamous cell carcinoma. *J Am Acad Dermatol* 1992;27:241–248.

117. Babington S, Veness MJ, Cakir B, et al. Squamous cell carcinoma of the lip: is there a role for adjuvant radiotherapy in improving local control following incomplete or inadequate excision? *ANZ J Surg* 2003;73:621–625.

118. Jambusaria-Pahlajani A, Miller CJ, Quon H, et al. Surgical monotherapy versus surgery plus adjuvant radiotherapy in high-risk cutaneous squamous cell carcinoma: a systematic review of outcomes. *Dermatol Surg* 2009;35:574–585.

120. Wang JT, Palme CE, Morgan GJ, et al. Predictors of outcome in patients with metastatic cutaneous head and neck squamous cell carcinoma involving cervical lymph nodes: improved survival with the addition of adjuvant radiotherapy. *Head Neck* 2012;34:1524–1528.

121. Kirby JS, Miller CJ. Intralesional chemotherapy for nonmelanoma skin cancer: a practical review. *J Am Acad Dermatol* 2010;63:689–702.

122. Hanlon A, Kim J, Leffell DJ. Intralesional interferon alfa-2b for refractory, recurrent squamous cell carcinoma of the face. *J Am Acad Dermatol* 2013;69:1070–1072.

123. Edwards L, Berman B, Rapini RP, et al. Treatment of cutaneous squamous cell carcinomas by intralesional interferon alfa-2b therapy. *Arch Dermatol* 1992;128:1486–1489.

125. Maubec E, Petrow P, Scheer-Senyarich I, et al. Phase II study of cetuximab as first-line single-drug therapy in patients with unresectable squamous cell carcinoma of the skin. *J Clin Oncol* 2011;29:3419–3426.

126. Cherpelis BS, Marcusen C, Lang PG. Prognostic factors for metastasis in squamous cell carcinoma of the skin. *Dermatol Surg* 2002;28:268–273.

127. Marcil I, Stern RS. Risk of developing a subsequent nonmelanoma skin cancer in patients with a history of nonmelanoma skin cancer: a critical review of the literature and meta-analysis. *Arch Dermatol* 2000;136:1524–1530.

130. Franceschi S, Dal ML, Arniani S, et al. Risk of cancer other than Kaposi's sarcoma and non-Hodgkin's lymphoma in persons with AIDS in Italy. Cancer and AIDS Registry Linkage Study. *Br J Cancer* 1998;78:966–970.

132. Hardie IR, Strong RW, Hartley LC, et al. Skin cancer in Caucasian renal allograft recipients living in a subtropical climate. *Surgery* 1980;87:177–183.

133. Ong CS, Keogh AM, Kossard S, et al. Skin cancer in Australian heart transplant recipients. *J Am Acad Dermatol* 1999;40:27–34.

134. Arron ST, Ruby JG, Dybbro E, et al. Transcriptome sequencing demonstrates that human papillomavirus is not active in cutaneous squamous cell carcinoma. *J Invest Dermatol* 2011;131:1745–1753.

136. Euvrard S, Morelon E, Rostaing L, et al. Sirolimus and secondary skin cancer prevention in kidney transplantation. *N Engl J Med* 2012;367:329–339.

139. Kohler HF, Neves RI, Brechtbuhl ER, et al. Cutaneous angiosarcoma of the head and neck: report of 23 cases from a single institution. *Otolaryngol Head Neck Surg* 2008;139:519–524.

140. Mendenhall WM, Mendenhall CM, Werning JW, et al. Cutaneous angiosarcoma. *Am J Clin Oncol* 2006;29:524–528.

141. Deyrup AT, McKenney JK, Tighiouart M, et al. Sporadic cutaneous angiosarcomas: a proposal for risk stratification based on 69 cases. *Am J Surg Pathol* 2008;32:72–77.

148. Abbott JJ, Oliveira AM, Nascimento AG. The prognostic significance of fibrosarcomatous transformation in dermatofibrosarcoma protuberans. *Am J Surg Pathol* 2006;30:436–443.

150. Monnier D, Vidal C, Martin L, et al. Dermatofibrosarcoma protuberans: a population-based cancer registry descriptive study of 66 consecutive cases diagnosed between 1982 and 2002. *J Eur Acad Dermatol Venereol* 2006;20:1237–1242.

158. Meguerditchian AN, Wang J, Lema B, et al. Wide excision or mohs micrographic surgery for the treatment of primary dermatofibrosarcoma protuberans. *Am J Clin Oncol* 2010;33:300–303.

159. Paradisi A, Abeni D, Rusciani A, et al. Dermatofibrosarcoma protuberans: wide local excision vs. Mohs micrographic surgery. *Cancer Treat Rev* 2008;34:728–736.

161. Fiore M, Miceli R, Mussi C, et al. Dermatofibrosarcoma protuberans treated at a single institution: a surgical disease with a high cure rate. *J Clin Oncol* 2005;23:7669–7675.

168. Mentzel T, Beham A, Katenkamp D, et al. Fibrosarcomatous ("high-grade") dermatofibrosarcoma protuberans: clinicopathologic and immunohistochemical study of a series of 41 cases with emphasis on prognostic significance. *Am J Surg Pathol* 1998;22:576–587.

169. Haag ML, Glass LF, Fenske NA. Merkel cell carcinoma. Diagnosis and treatment. *Dermatol Surg* 1995;21:669–683.

170. Rockville Merkel Cell Carcinoma Group. Merkel cell carcinoma: recent progress and current priorities on etiology, pathogenesis, and clinical management. *J Clin Oncol* 2009;27:4021–4026.

175. Foulongne V, Dereure O, Kluger N, et al. Merkel cell polyomavirus DNA detection in lesional and nonlesional skin from patients with Merkel cell carcinoma or other skin diseases. *Br J Dermatol* 2010;162:59–63.

176. Katano H, Ito H, Suzuki Y, et al. Detection of Merkel cell polyomavirus in Merkel cell carcinoma and Kaposi's sarcoma. *J Med Virol* 2009;81:1951–1958.

185. Merkel cell. In: *American Joint Committee on Cancer: AJCC Cancer Staging Manual*. 7th ed. New York: Springer; 2010:318–319.

190. Bajetta E, Celio L, Platania M, et al. Single-institution series of early-stage Merkel cell carcinoma: long-term outcomes in 95 patients managed with surgery alone. *Ann Surg Oncol* 2009;16:2985–2993.

191. Boyer JD, Zitelli JA, Brodland DG, et al. Local control of primary Merkel cell carcinoma: review of 45 cases treated with Mohs micrographic surgery with and without adjuvant radiation. *J Am Acad Dermatol* 2002;47:885–892.

195. Mehrany K, Otley CC, Weenig RH, et al. A meta-analysis of the prognostic significance of sentinel lymph node status in Merkel cell carcinoma. *Dermatol Surg* 2002;28:113–117.

196. Gupta SG, Wang LC, Penas PF, et al. Sentinel lymph node biopsy for evaluation and treatment of patients with Merkel cell carcinoma: The Dana-Farber experience and meta-analysis of the literature. *Arch Dermatol* 2006;142:685–690.

197. Wilson LD, Gruber SB. Merkel cell carcinoma and the controversial role of adjuvant radiation therapy: clinical choices in the absence of statistical evidence. *J Am Acad Dermatol* 2004;50:435–437.

202. Leibovitch I, Huilgol SC, Selva D, et al. Microcystic adnexal carcinoma: treatment with Mohs micrographic surgery. *J Am Acad Dermatol* 2005;52:295–300.

203. Yu JB, Blitzblau RC, Patel SC, et al. Surveillance, Epidemiology, and End Results (SEER) database analysis of microcystic adnexal carcinoma (aclerosing sweat duct carcinoma) of the skin. *Am J Clin Oncol* 2010;33:125–127.

207. Dasgupta T, Wilson LD, Yu JB. A retrospective review of 1349 cases of sebaceous carcinoma. *Cancer* 2009;115:158–165.

214. Dowd MB, Kumar RJ, Sharma R, et al. Diagnosis and management of sebaceous carcinoma: an Australian experience. *ANZ J Surg* 2008;78:158–163.

215. Lee K, Roh MR, Chung WG, et al. Comparison of Mohs micrographic surgery and wide excision for extramammary Paget's disease: Korean experience. *Dematol Surg* 2009;35:34–40.

217. Hatta N, Yamada M, Hirano T, et al. Extramammary Paget's disease: treatment, prognostic factors and outcome in 76 patients. *Br J Dermatol* 2008;158:313–318.

223. Fletcher CD. The evolving classification of soft tissue tumours: an update based on the new WHO classification. *Histopathology* 2006;48:3–12.

227. Davis JL, Randle HW, Zalla MJ, et al. A comparison of Mohs micrographic surgery and wide excision for the treatment of atypical fibroxanthoma. *Dermatol Surg* 1997;23:105–110.

228. Huether MJ, Zitelli JA, Brodland DG. Mohs micrographic surgery for the treatment of spindle cell tumors of the skin. *J Am Acad Dermatol* 2001;44:656–659.

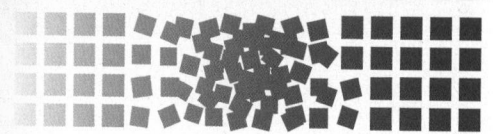

93 Molecular Biology of Cutaneous Melanoma

Michael A. Davies and Levi A. Garraway

INTRODUCTION

The most common forms of skin cancer are basal cell carcinoma, squamous cell carcinoma, and melanoma. While melanoma represents <5% of the cases diagnosed, it is the cause of >70% of the deaths attributable to skin cancer each year. In 2013, an estimated 76,690 new cases of melanoma will be diagnosed, and 9,840 patients will die from this disease.[1] Although the annual incidence and mortality for most major cancers (i.e., lung, colorectal, breast, prostate) are decreasing, the public health burden of melanoma continues to rise. The annual incidence of melanoma has risen steadily at a rate of ~3% per year over the past 25 years.[2–4] As melanoma often strikes individuals who are young and otherwise healthy, it is also a significant financial burden, with an annual estimated cost of $3.5 billion in lost productivity in the United States due to melanoma mortality.[5]

Cutaneous melanoma arises from pigment-producing epidermal melanocytes. Clinically, melanomas are staged using the guidelines established by the American Joint Committee on Cancer.[6] For patients who present with primary tumors only (stage I, stage II), the vertical tumor (Breslow) thickness (in millimeters) and ulceration status are the most powerful indicators of prognosis. Melanoma usually spreads first regionally to draining lymph nodes. For patients with regional disease (stage III), the prognosis is determined by the number of lymph nodes involved, the size of the lymph node metastases (micrometastases versus macrometastases), the pattern of lymph node involvement (lymph nodes, in-transit metastases, or both), and the ulceration status of the primary tumor. Melanoma is also infamous for its ability to metastasize to virtually any distant organ. For patients with distant metastases (stage IV), prognosis is defined by the organ sites involved and the presence or absence of elevated serum lactate dehydrogenase levels. For patients who present with thin primary tumors without high-risk features (stage I), the long-term disease-specific survival is >95%. In contrast, for patients with distant metastases (stage IV), the median survival is 6 to 8 months, and <10% of patients are alive 5 years after diagnosis.

A number of epidemiologic studies have identified a strong link between the risk of cutaneous melanoma and exposure to ultraviolet (UV) radiation.[7,8] This initial insight into the molecular basis of this aggressive disease has expanded tremendously over the last two decades through focused molecular analyses and mechanistic studies in preclinical models. More recently, the development of high-throughput sequencing approaches that allow for exome- and genome-wide assessment of molecular changes have led to a rapid increase in the understanding of the molecular heterogeneity and pathogenesis of melanomas. Notably, these studies have demonstrated that melanomas have one of the highest rates of somatic mutations of all solid tumors (Fig. 93.1). The preponderance of the observed mutations consist of CT or GA substitutions, which are strongly associated with UV radiation–induced DNA damage, and thus confirm at the molecular level the important role of this environmental exposure in this disease.[9] The patterns of somatic

aberrations have also identified a number of key functional pathways that likely contribute to the pathogenesis of this disease. Importantly, many of these findings are rapidly being translated into molecular tests and therapies that are impacting the clinical management and outcomes of patients with this highly aggressive disease.

THE RAS-RAF-MAP KINASE PATHWAY

The RAS-RAF–mitogen-activated protein kinase (MAPK) signaling pathway is a cascade of molecules that is activated by multiple cellular signals and pathways (Fig. 93.2). Signaling through RAS and RAF leads to activation of the ERK1/2 kinases, which regulate a variety of proteins through serine-threonine phosphorylation events and ultimately the transcription of many genes governing cell proliferation, survival, and other critical cellular processes. Examples of transcription factors operant in melanocytes that are regulated by ERK signaling include the microphthalmia-associated transcription factor (MITF, described in detail in the following), various ETS transcription factors, the FOS and JUN immediate early genes, among others.

Extensive genetic and mechanistic studies have unearthed a prevalence of activating MAPK pathway mutations across many tumor types. In particular, activation of this pathway appears to be one of the most frequent and important molecular events in cutaneous melanoma (Fig. 93.3). Toward this end, several MAPK signaling proteins (e.g., RAS and RAF isoforms) are encoded by "classic" oncogenes, and key transcriptional effectors downstream of MAPK also undergo oncogenic dysregulation in melanoma and other cancers. Key MAPK effectors have also been shown to regulate differentiation and senescence in non-transformed melanocytes.

RAS Family GTPases

RAS proteins (H-, K-, and NRAS) are small GTPases that comprise an initial signaling node of the RAS-RAF-MAPK cascade. The discovery of activating mutations in HRAS and KRAS led to investigations that identified mutations in this gene family in multiple cancer types, and thus the significance of this pathway in the pathogenesis of cancer. Activating mutations in NRAS are detected in 20% to 25% of cutaneous melanomas (see Fig. 93.3).[10–12] NRAS mutations are also detected in nevi, particularly congenital nevi.[13] HRAS mutations are uncommon in cutaneous melanomas, but they are detected in Spitz nevi, which are rare, benign lesions most often diagnosed in children and young adults.[14] Despite their high incidence in other cancer types, KRAS mutations are extremely rare in melanocytic lesions.

In mouse models, overexpression of activated HRAS or NRAS on an Ink4a/Arf-null background results in spontaneous melanoma formation.[15,16] However, while HRAS-induced melanomas rarely, if ever, metastasize, NRAS tumors frequently metastasize to draining lymph nodes and distal organs, in line with the apparent selection for NRAS over HRAS mutations in human melanomas.

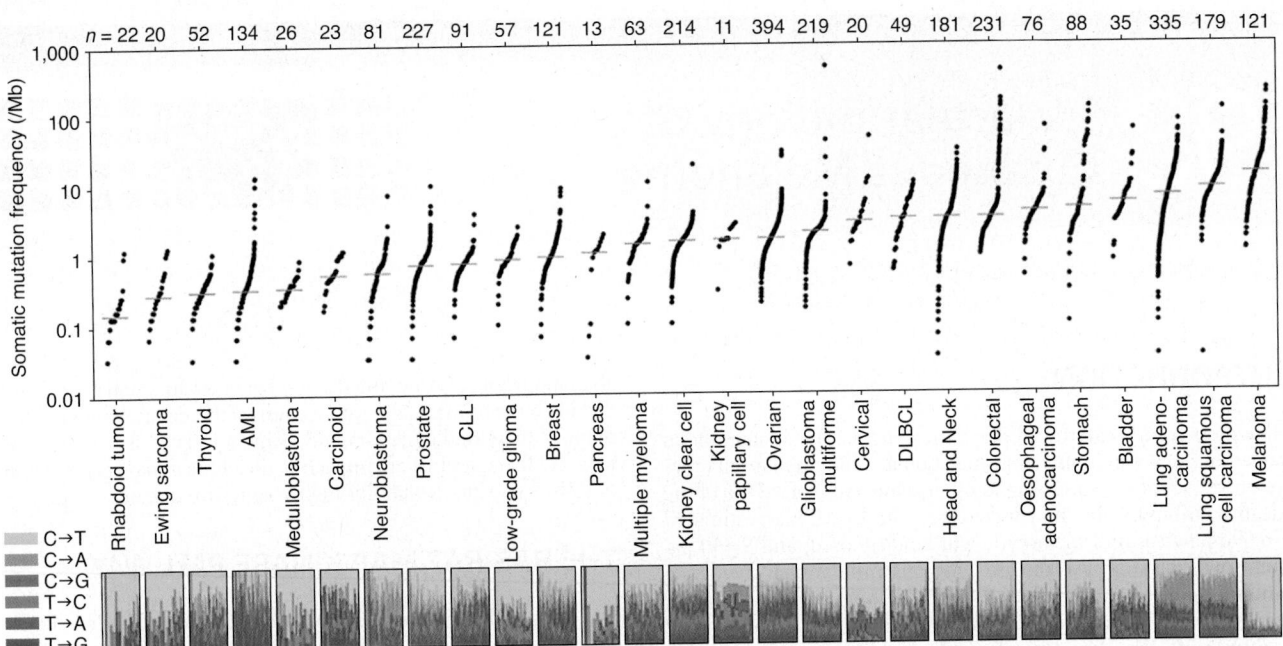

Figure 93.1 The rate of somatic mutations in whole exome sequencing analysis of various types of cancer. Each dot represents the total frequency of mutations (in mutations/Mb) in each exome of the indicated tumor types. Among the 27 tumor types analyzed, melanomas demonstrate the highest median frequency of somatic mutations. AML, acute myeloid leukemia; CLL, chronic lymphocytic leukemia; DLBCL, diffuse large B-cell lymphoma. (Reprinted from Lawrence MS, Stojanov P, Polak P, et al. *Nature.* Vol. 499. London: Nature Publishing Group; 2013:215, with permission.)

Knockdown of *NRAS* in human melanoma cell lines inhibits their viability, indicating dependency on this oncogene for tumorigenicity.[17] Furthermore, shutting off transgene expression in an inducible NRAS model caused regression of melanomas that arose following transgene induction, thereby confirming the RAS oncogene dependency in these tumors.[18]

RAF Kinases

The RAF proteins (ARAF, BRAF, and CRAF) are serine-threonine kinases that comprise critical signaling effectors through the RAS-RAF-MAPK pathway (see Fig. 93.2). While each of these proteins likely plays a role in physiologic signaling, BRAF has a central role in the pathogenesis of melanoma. Somatic hotspot mutations in *BRAF* are detected in 40% to 45% of cutaneous melanoma, making them the most common oncogenic aberration detected in this disease to date.[10] Approximately 95% of these mutations result in substitutions of the valine at the 600 position in the protein. The most common mutation (~70% of *BRAF* mutations) is a T→A transversion, resulting in a valine to glutamate amino acid substitution (V600E). Although the T→A transversion is not classically associated with UV-induced damage, BRAF V600E mutations appear are more common in melanomas arising at sites with intermittent exposure to UV.[19] Other substitutions, particularly the V600K mutation that represents ~20% of *BRAF* mutations in melanoma, are more common in melanomas with evidence of chronic sun damage (CSD), although the overall rate of *BRAF* mutations in those melanomas is lower compared to tumors without CSD.[19–22] BRAF V600 mutations are an early event in melanomas, as they are also present in the majority (~80%) of benign and dysplastic nevi.[23] In addition to mutations affecting V600, somatic events affecting >20 other sites in BRAF have been detected in patients, but overall they are quite rare (total ~5% prevalence).[24]

BRAF is an immediate downstream target of RAS (see Fig. 93.3) in the MAPK pathway. The BRAF(V600E) mutation and other substitutions at the V600 site confer more than 200-fold induction of kinase activity in vitro.[25] Mutations affecting other sites in BRAF can have high, intermediate, or low catalytic activity. However, all

of these mutations cause increased activation of MEK and ERK signaling. This likely occurs in low-activity mutants due to conformational changes that promote heterodimer formation with other RAF isoforms, such as CRAF, in a multiprotein complex with RAS proteins.[24] Notably, while BRAF(V600) mutations and *NRAS* mutations are mutually exclusive in newly diagnosed melanomas, frequent co-occurrence of *NRAS* mutations with nonactivating *BRAF* mutations has been observed.[26,27]

Extensive data suggest that wild-type BRAF operates on a senescence pathway in benign human nevi. Transgenic expression of BRAF(V600E) targeted to melanocytes in zebrafish produced benign nevus-like lesions, whereas invasive melanomas were produced (after extended latency) when crossed into p53-deficient zebrafish.[28] Inducible expression of BRAF(V600E) alone in murine melanocytes resulted in excessive skin pigmentation and the appearance of nevi containing hallmarks of senescence.[29] Human congenital nevi with activating BRAF mutations were shown to express senescence-associated acidic β-galactosidase, the classical senescence-associated marker.[30] This implied that activated BRAF alone is insufficient to induce tumor progression beyond the nevus stage in patients. Interestingly, immunohistochemical staining of nevoid tissues found heterogeneous patterns of INK4A that only partially overlapped with senescence-associated acidic β-galactosidase, suggesting the presence of INK4A-independent pathway(s) operative in oncogene-induced senescence. Expression of BRAF(V600E) in murine melanocytes, in the setting of inactivation of INK4A, caused melanocyte hyperplasia, but no invasive lesions.[31] However, concurrent loss of phosphatase and tensin homolog (PTEN), a negative regulator of the phosphatidylinositol kinase (PI3K) signaling pathway, resulted in 100% penetrance of invasive melanomas that formed spontaneous metastases.

The significance of *BRAF* mutations is now also supported by the functional and clinical effects of inhibiting this target. Early experiments demonstrated that RNAi knockdown of BRAF in human melanoma cells with BRAF(V600E) mutations inhibits ERK activation, induces cell cycle arrest and/or apoptosis, and blunts cell growth.[32,33] These initial results led to the development and testing of potent and selective inhibitors of the BRAF(V600E) protein. Two of these agents (vemurafenib, dabrafenib) have dem-

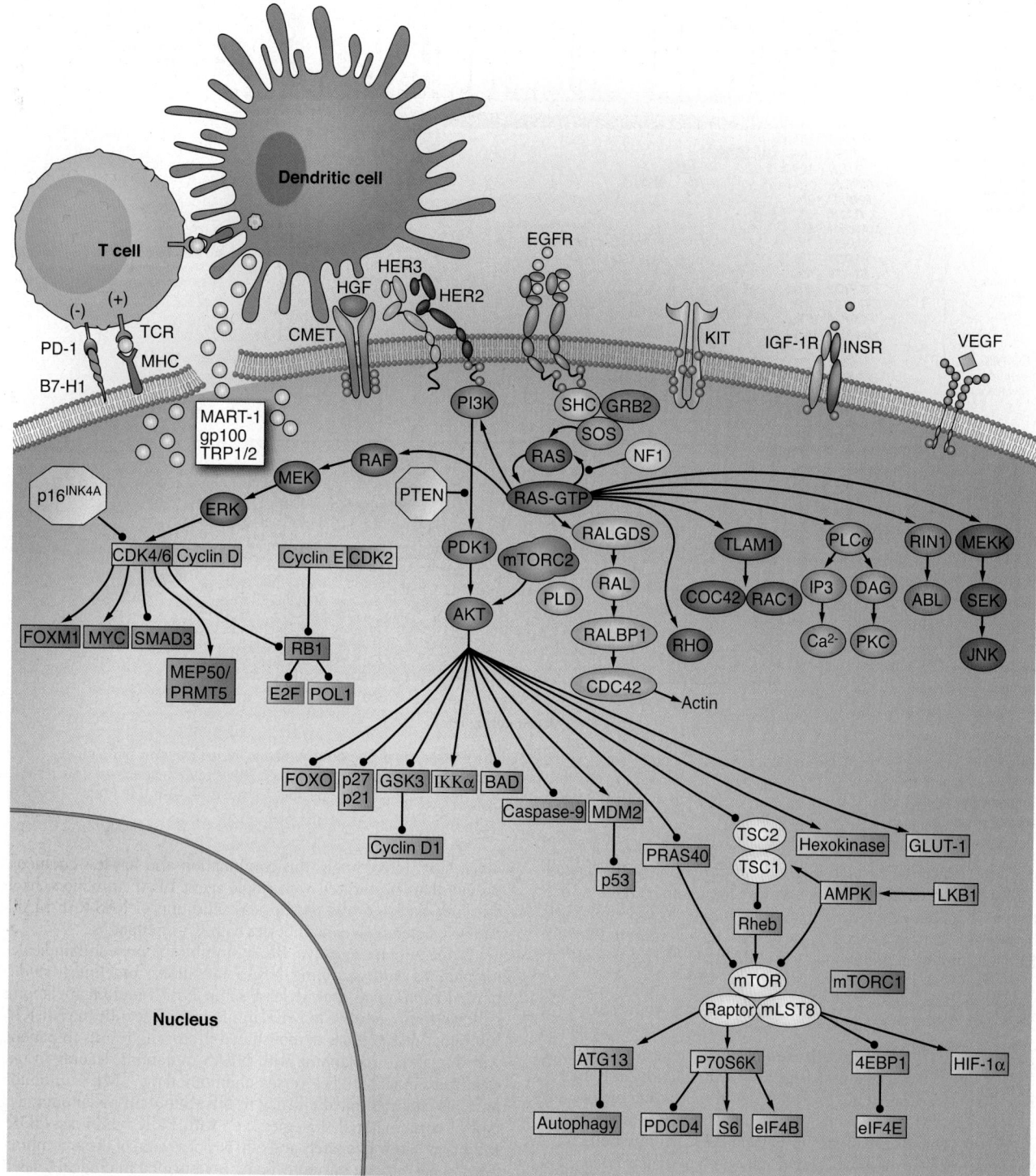

Figure 93.2 Molecular signaling pathways in melanoma. (Reprinted from Sullivan RJ, Lorusso PM, Flaherty KT. *Clinical Cancer Research*. Vol. 19. Philadelphia, PA: American Association for Cancer Research; 2013:5286, with permission.)

onstrated significant improvements in patient outcomes in phase 3 clinical trials, leading to their regulatory approval, while other agents have shown promising results in early testing.[34,35]

Interestingly, use of these selective inhibitors of BRAF(V600E) causes paradoxical activation of the MAPK pathway in melanomas with a wild-type *BRAF*, particularly in those tumors that have an activating *NRAS* mutation.[36,37] This pathway activation causes increased tumor growth in cell lines and xenograft models, and supports the restricted use of these inhibitors to patients with melanoma with activating *BRAF* mutations. This paradoxical signaling

effect also appears to be the underlying mechanism of the proliferative cutaneous lesions (keratoacanthomas and squamous cell carcinomas) that are among the most common toxicities of the selective BRAF inhibitors.[38,39]

While only rarely mutated in melanoma, preclinical studies support the premise that CRAF can also have functional significance in this malignancy.[26] Cells with activating *NRAS* mutations appear to utilize CRAF predominantly to transmit signals to MEK and ERK.[26] While CRAF appears to be largely dispensable in melanomas with BRAF(V600) mutations, it is likely critical for

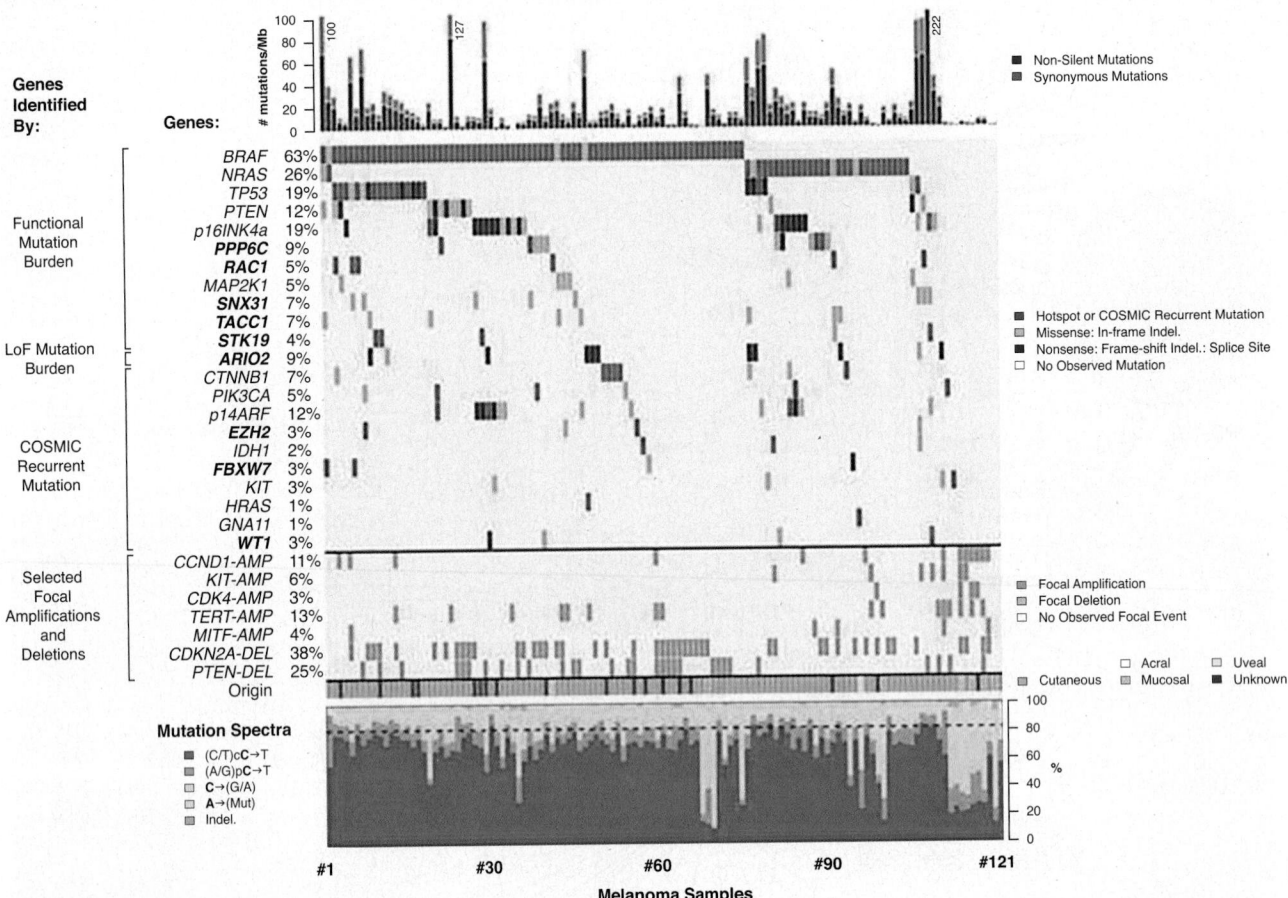

Figure 93.3 A landscape of driver mutations in melanoma. Each *row* indicates the prevalence of somatic mutations, amplifications, or deletions in each indicated gene in the cohort of 121 melanomas. Each *column* indicates the somatic events present in that tumor. The mutation spectra for each tumor is illustrated at the bottom of the figure. (Modified from Hodis E, Watson IR, Kryukov GV, et al. *Cell*. Vol. 150. Cambridge, MA: Cell Press; 2012:259, with permission.)

pathway activation through heterodimer formation with nonactivating BRAF mutations, and it may be a therapeutic target in such tumors.[40] Increased expression and/or signaling by CRAF has also been implicated as a mechanism of resistance to mutant-selective BRAF inhibitors in melanomas with BRAF(V600E) mutations.[41–43]

MEK1/2

Because the MEK1/2 serine-threonine kinases transmit the critical MAPK signal downstream of RAS and RAF, considerable interest has also emerged regarding these kinases in melanoma biology and therapeutics. MEK1/2 mutations are rare in melanoma, and in cancer in general, in contrast to *RAS* and *BRAF* mutations.[11,12,44] Nonetheless, pharmacologic MEK inhibition presents another possible therapeutic strategy for *BRAF*- or *NRAS*-mutant melanomas. Robust preclinical evidence favoring this notion derived from a genetic and pharmacologic analysis showing that various MEK inhibitory compounds demonstrated markedly enhanced potency against BRAF(V600E) cancer cells compared to cell lines lacking oncogenic MAPK pathway mutations.[45] Treatment with the MEK1/2 inhibitor trametinib as a single agent in patients with metastatic melanoma with BRAF(V600E) or BRAF(V600K) mutations resulted in significant improvements in clinical response rates, progression-free survival, and overall survival compared to chemotherapy, leading to its regulatory approval in 2013.[46] In addition, combined treatment with selective RAF inhibitors (i.e., dabrafenib) and MEK inhibitors (i.e., trametinib) significantly improves both the rate and duration of clinical responses.[47] This pivotal observation led to the approval of combined RAF/MEK inhibition for use in BRAF(V600E)-mutant

melanoma. Interestingly, this combination also has less cutaneous toxicity than is observed with single-agent BRAF inhibitors, likely due to blockade of the paradoxical activation of RAS-RAF-MAPK pathway signaling in keratinocytes with RAS mutations.[39]

While mutant-selective BRAF inhibitors are contraindicated for patients with activating *NRAS* mutations, preclinical studies have demonstrated that at least some NRAS-mutant melanoma cells were also sensitive to MEK inhibitors.[45] Recently the MEK1/2 inhibitor MEK162 has demonstrated promising results in patients with metastatic melanoma with NRAS mutations, leading to randomized clinical studies versus chemotherapy.[48] MEK inhibitors have also demonstrated efficacy in NRAS-mutant melanomas as a part of combinatorial strategies (i.e., with PI3K inhibitors, CDK4 inhibitors, etc.). The safety and efficacy of several of these combinations in patients are currently being investigated in clinical trials.[49]

NF1

A small percentage of melanomas lack BRAF or NRAS mutations; however, MAPK signaling is often still operant in this setting. Recent genome characterization efforts have revealed that the tumor suppressor gene *NF1* undergoes inactivating mutations in a substantial proportion of "BRAF/NRAS wild-type" melanomas.[11,12] *NF1* encodes neurofibromin, a so-called RAS-GAP whose normal physiologic role involves negative regulation of RAS signaling effected through cleavage of the RAS-GTP. Consequently, loss of *NF1* leads to dysregualted RAS signaling. *NF1* loss is sufficient to drive melanoma genesis together with other known cancer genes in genetically engineered mouse models of melanoma.[50] Moreover, *NF1* loss has been observed in BRAF-mutant clinical specimens that exhibit resistance to RAF inhibition.[50,51]

THE MEPK PATHWAY AND THERAPEUTIC RESISTANCE

Unfortunately, the impressive clinical effects of RAF and MEK inhibition in BRAF(V600)-mutant melanoma are transient: the vast majority of patients will experience disease progression within one year of treatment (although a subset of patients will enjoy prolonged clinical benefit). Multiple mechanisms of resistance to RAF/MEK inhibition have been described, most of which restore MEK/ERK signaling as the key downstream mechanism. Resistance mechanisms such as *NRAS* mutations[52] or *NF1* inactivation[51] accomplish this by signaling through C-RAF, which is normally inactive in BRAF-mutant melanoma but can be engaged through homo- or heterodimerization in the setting of upstream RAS signaling. An alternative splice isoform of BRAF also acts through RAF-mediated dimerization.[43] Certain receptor tyrosine kinase–driven resistance mechanisms may also work in part by augmenting A- and/or C-RAF activity in a RAS-dependent manner.[42,53] Other resistance effectors may bypass RAF proteins altogether yet still converge on MEK/ERK activation—the kinase COT (encoded by the *MAP3K8* gene) comprises an example of this mechanism.[54] Alternatively, MEK/ERK signaling may be restored through activating somatic mutations in *MAP2K1* or *MAP2K2*, which encode MEK1 and MEK2 kinases, respectively.[55,56] Interestingly, NRAS and MAPK2 mutations have been observed in the setting of resistance to both single-agent RAF inhibition and combined RAF/MEK inhibition,[57] underscoring the importance of sustained ERK signaling as a resistance mechanism to this therapeutic modality.

Although MEK/ERK-independent resistance mechanisms are less well understood, recent data suggest that such effectors may also prove important. For example, a large-scale functional screen for open reading frames whose overexpression produces resistance to MAPK inhibitors identified several dozen genes that can confer resistance to RAF, MEK, and ERK inhibition.[58] Several of these genes encode proteins that may bypass MEK/ERK signaling altogether, whereas others encode transcription factors known to operate downstream of ERK (such as MITF) or that can otherwise substitute for the ERK-driven transcriptional output. As combinatorial MAPK-directed therapy gains traction in BRAF(V600)-mutant melanoma, such ERK-independent resistance mechanisms are likely to become increasingly manifest.

Cell Cycle Regulators

The RB signaling pathway regulates the entry in and progression through the cell cycle. A significant role for this pathway in melanoma was initially implicated by the finding that germline mutations in this pathway (*CDKN2A*, *CDK4*) are the most frequently detected events in familial melanomas (more than three affected family members). Subsequent studies have demonstrated that somatic aberrations in this pathway are ubiquitous in cutaneous melanoma. Functional studies support that dysregulation of cell cycle entry and progression is critical to the pathogenesis of this disease, and potentially contributes to resistance to RAS-RAF-MAPK pathway inhibitors.

The *CDKN2A* Locus

Germline deletions and activating mutations in the *CDKN2A* locus on chromosome 9p21 are the most common event (~40%) prevalent in familial melanoma. Somatic mutations and deletions, or epigenetic silencing, are detected in as many as 70% of cutaneous melanomas.[59,60] Thus, disruption of CDKN2A function

likely plays a central role in melanoma pathogenesis. The CDKN2A locus contains an unusual gene organization, which allows for two separate transcripts and corresponding tumor suppressor gene products to be produced: p16^{INK4A} and p19^{ARF} (see Fig. 93.2). Loss of p16^{INK4A} results in the suppression of retinoblastoma (RB) tumor suppressor activity via increased activation of the CDK4/6-cyclin D1 complex; loss of ARF (p14^{ARF} in human and p19^{ARF} in mouse) downmodulates p53 activity through increased activation of MDM2. Thus, deletion of the entire locus accomplishes the inactivation of two critical tumor suppressor pathways: RB and p53. Homozygous deletion of exons 2 and 3 of the mouse *Cdkn2a* homolog predisposed to a high incidence of melanomas when combined with an activated HRAS transgene in melanocytes.[15] Thus, CDKN2A lesions may "prime" melanocytic tissue for neoplasia.

INK4A

The specific significance of INK4A function is supported by the clinical identification of intragenic mutations of *INK4A* that do not affect the *ARF* coding region that sensitize germline carriers to the development of melanomas.[61] In addition, in familial melanomas that lack CDKN2A aberrations, the most commonly identified genetic event is a point mutation in CDK4 that disrupts the interaction of that protein with INK4A.[62] In a mouse model engineered to be deficient only for Ink4a (with intact ARF), melanoma formation was observed in cooperation with an oncogenic initiating event (activated HRAS), albeit with a longer latency than in mice with deletions affecting the entire locus.[63] Notably, the tumors in these mice were also found to harbor either deletion of ARF or mutation of p53. Therefore, while INK4A is a bona fide tumor suppressor, additional genetic dysregulation of the p53 pathway seems obligatory for melanoma genesis, at least in the mouse.

CDK4

CDK4 is a direct target of inhibition by p16^{INK4A} (see Fig. 93.2) and is a primary regulator of RB activation. As noted previously, germline mutations of *CDK4* that render the protein insensitive to inhibition by INK4A (e.g., Arg24Cys) have been identified in a melanoma-prone kindreds.[61] These tumors retain wild-type INK4A function, suggesting that INK4A is epistatic to CDK4 and that RB pathway deregulation is central to melanoma genesis. Somatic focal amplifications of *CDK4* are also observed (albeit rarely) in sporadic melanomas.[64] Carcinogen treatment induced melanomas in the animals without somatic Ink4a inactivation, similar to the mutual exclusivity observed in familial melanoma.[65] CDK4 interacts with cyclin D proteins (see the following) to drive progression through the G1/S cell cycle checkpoint. Recently, small molecule inhibitors of CDK4 and other CDKs have entered clinical trials in several tumor types, including melanomas. In particular, both tumor genetic data and recent results from genetically engineered mouse models provide a rational basis for combining CDK and MAPK pathway inhibition in NRAS-mutant melanoma.[18]

CCND1

CCND1 encodes the CyclinD1 kinase, which forms a complex with CDK4 or CDK6 to inactivate RB1 (see Fig. 93.2). Amplification of the *CCND1* locus has been identified in relatively rare event in cutaneous melanomas (5% to 10%).[11,66] However, this molecular event is enriched in cutaneous melanomas that do not have mutations in BRAF or NRAS.[11,19] Although it is rare in melanomas with BRAF(V600) mutations, amplification of CyclinD1 has been implicated as predictor of resistance to BRAF inhibitors in preclinical models, and increased copy number of CCND1 correlated with shorter progression-free survival in one study of patients with metastatic melanoma treated with the BRAF inhibitor dabrafenib.[67,68]

RB1

Germline mutations in *RB1* confer predisposition to melanoma in patients who have survived bilateral RB.[69] These melanomas exhibit loss of heterozygosity of the remaining wild-type RB1 allele. In such patients, estimates of increased lifetime risk of melanoma range from 4- to 80-fold. The *RB1* gene locus has been found deleted in some primary cutaneous melanomas,[13] and *RB1* may also be subject to genomic rearrangement in rare instances.[14]

The p53 Pathway

The p53 pathway is critical for maintenance of the normal genome by regulating a multiplicity of mechanisms, including cell cycle checkpoints, DNA damage repair activation, and the appropriate induction of apoptosis. Mutations in the *TP53* gene occur in >50% of all tumors. While initial studies suggested that the *TP53* locus is rarely mutated in human melanomas, whole exome studies have identified mutations in ~20% of tumors, generally in tumors without mutations or deletions affecting *CDKN2A* and P14^ARF [11] Amplification of *MDM2*, which inhibits P53 function, has also been detected in melanomas with intact *CDKN2A*.[64] Functionally, loss of p53 cooperates with activated BRAF in zebrafish, and with activated HRAS in mice, to induce melanomas.[28,70] Thus, while *TP53* is rarely deleted in human melanomas, inactivation of its pathway appears critical for melanomagenesis.

The Phosphatidylinositol 3-Kinase Pathway

The PI3K-AKT pathway is affected by activating oncogenic events more frequently than any other pathway in cancer.[71] PI3K phosphorylates lipids in the cell membrane, causing the recruitment of proteins that have a pleckstrin homology domain. One of the key proteins regulated by PI3K is the serine-threonine kinase AKT. AKT is phosphorylated at two key residues (Ser473 and Thr308) at the cell membrane, activating its catalytic activity. Activated AKT phosphorylates multiple effector proteins, including GSK3, P70S6K, PRAS40, BAD, and more, which regulate cellular processes including proliferation, survival, motility, angiogenesis, and metabolism (see Fig. 93.3). The pathway can be activated genetically in cancer both by activating mutations (i.e., in *PIK3CA*, *AKT1*) and loss of function events (i.e., *PTEN*, *TSC2*) in components of the pathway. The PI3K-AKT pathway is also a critical effector pathway of RAS proteins and many growth factors and their receptors, which are also frequently aberrant in cancer.

As described previously, activation of the RAS-RAF-MAPK pathway is a nearly ubiquitous event in cutaneous melanoma. Overall, genetic events in the PI3K-AKT pathway are less common.[11] However, multiple lines of evidence support that PI3K-AKT signaling functionally complements RAS-RAF-MAPK activation in at least a subset of melanomas. Moreover, recent data indicates that PI3K pathway mutations may arise in the setting of resistance to RAF inhibition.[56,72]

Phosphatase and Tensin Homolog

Of the PI3K pathway mutations that do occur, losses of chromosome 10q encompassing PTEN tumor suppressor is the most frequent, the caveat being that additional tumor suppressor(s) may reside in this region (see the following). PTEN normally downregulates phosphorylated AKT via suppression of the second messenger PIP$_3$ (see Fig. 93.3). Loss of PTEN has been shown to result in increased AKT activity in multiple cancer types, including melanoma. In melanoma, somatic point mutations and homozygous deletions of PTEN are relatively rare. However, although allelic loss of PTEN is observed only in about 20% of melanoma, loss of expression of PTEN is reported to be in the range of 30% to 40% of melanoma tumors.[27,73] In multiple studies, loss of PTEN has shown to occur in melanomas with activating BRAF mutations and in melanomas with wild-type BRAF and NRAS, but it is extremely rare in tumors with NRAS mutations.[74]

As mentioned previously, in a mouse model the presence of simultaneous PTEN loss and oncogenic BRAF induction in melanocytes resulted in 100% penetrance of invasive, metastatic melanomas.[31] Notably, loss of PTEN alone did not cause a melanocytic phenotype. While this complementation of BRAF and PTEN supports the overlap of these alterations that is observed clinically, preclinical models have also demonstrated that loss of PTEN can promote melanoma motility, invasion, and metastasis in the setting of NRAS mutations.[75] However, the significance of this finding is unclear due to the very low prevalence of this occurring naturally. The functional significance of PTEN loss in BRAF/NRAS wild-type melanomas also remains to be elucidated. Functionally, ectopic expression of PTEN in PTEN-deficient melanoma cells can abolish phospho-AKT activity, induce apoptosis, and suppress growth, tumorigenicity, and metastasis.[76] Many different inhibitors of the PI3K-AKT pathway have been developed and are undergoing clinical testing. Previous data suggest that the presence of different molecular mechanisms of PI3K-AKT pathway activation may correlate with activation and functional dependence on different pathway effectors.[77] Preclinical studies support that AKT and PI3K are attractive targets for melanomas with loss of PTEN.[78]

AKT

Loss of PTEN in melanoma tumors and cell lines correlates with markedly increased expression of phospho-AKT (indicative of activation).[73] In addition to loss of PTEN, AKT can be activated by point mutations that affect the pleckstrin homology domain of the proteins. Such mutations of *AKT1* have been detected in multiple tumor types.[79] Analysis of melanoma tumors and cell lines identified the same mutation as a rare event in melanoma (~1% prevalence), but also discovered the analogous mutation in *AKT3*, which has not been reported in other cancers.[80] Each tumor with a mutation in AKT1/3 had a concurrent BRAF(V600) mutation. Copy number gain of the *AKT3* locus has also been detected in melanomas, and functional studies support that metastatic melanomas specifically demonstrate phosphorylation of and functional dependence upon that AKT isoform.[76,81]

Phosphatidylinositol Kinase

Hotspot mutations in PIK3CA, which encodes the predominant catalytic subunit of PI3K, are common in multiple cancer types, including breast, colon, and lung tumors.[82] Mutations in PIK3CA are very rare (<2%) in melanomas, and often affect residues of unknown functional significance.[83] Despite this clinical observation, preclinical studies have shown that the presence of simultaneous activating PI3K and BRAF mutations in melanocytes can induce melanomas in mouse models.[84]

Receptor Tyrosine Kinases

Receptor tyrosine kinsases (RTK) are a diverse family of transmembrane kinases that have been implicated in many neoplasms. Several RTKs map to known regions of recurrent melanoma DNA copy number gain or amplification, with corresponding alterations in their expression levels.

The RTK c-KIT and its ligand (stem cell factor) were both initially shown to play essential roles in melanocyte development. Mutation of either KIT or RTK results in pigmentation deficiencies, and injection of c-Kit blocking antibody in mice was used to identify the presence of melanocyte stem cells within hair follicles.[85] However, numerous immunohistochemical studies linked progressive loss of c-KIT expression with the transition from benign to primary and metastatic melanomas.[86] Thus, at first glance, KIT appeared to be inactivated during melanoma genesis and progression. However, more recently activating mutations and amplification of the *KIT* gene have been identified in cutaneous melanomas with evidence of CSD or that arise on acral surfaces (palms, soles, nail beds).[87] The point mutations in the KIT gene generally occur in the same regions affected in gastrointestinal stromal tumors, where the functional significance of these mutations has been proven by the clinical efficacy of KIT inhibitors for that disease.[86] Functional studies support that KIT mutations can activate multiple signaling pathways, particularly the PI3K-AKT pathway.[88] Inhibition of KIT in melanoma cell lines with recurrent point mutations results in growth inhibition and/or apoptosis.[89] In patients, initial clinical trials of the KIT inhibitor imatinib in populations of patients with KIT mutations and/or amplifications have reported clinical response rates of 10% to 30%.[90,91] This is a much higher response rate than was observed in three previous clinical trials of imatinib in patients with unselected melanoma (~1% response rate), but is much lower than the activity observed in patients with gastrointestinal stromal tumor (>70%).[86] Thus, although many of the clinical responses in patients with KIT mutations have been dramatic and durable, research is ongoing to further understand the significance of KIT mutations, and to develop more effective clinical strategies for patients with melanoma patients with KIT mutations.

Overexpression of the RTK c-MET and its ligand, HGF, is correlated with melanoma progression. Copy gains involving the c-MET locus at 7q33-qter are associated with invasive and metastatic cancers in humans,[92] and elevated MET/HGF expression is correlated with metastatic ability in murine melanoma explants.[47] HGF/SF overexpression in a transgenic mouse model triggered spontaneous melanoma formation after a long latency (up to 2 years); however, time to tumor onset was greatly reduced by exposure to UVB or Ink4a/Arf deficiency.[93] More recently, independent groups of investigators demonstrated that c-MET may be activated by HGF produced by supporting cells in the tumor microenvironment of melanomas.[53,94] This paracrine effect resulted in activation of the PI3K-AKT pathway in the tumor cells and caused resistance to MAPK pathway inhibitors. The clinical utility of c-MET inhibition in melanoma is being tested in ongoing clinical trials.

A sequencing-based study of the tyrosine kinome in melanoma found that *ERBB4* mutations may affect as many as 20% of melanomas.[95] Unlike other well-known oncogene mutations, the *ERBB4* mutations identified in this study were mostly nonrecurrent (e.g., the same amino acid or conserved region was rarely affected). However, *ERBB4* mutations produced increased activation of the receptor itself and PI3K-AKT pathway signaling, as well as dependence upon the corresponding protein for viability. Despite these promising initial findings, the clinical significance of ERBB4 inhibitors in melanoma remains unclear.

MELANIN SYNTHESIS PATHWAY

MITF

MITF encodes a lineage transcription factor whose function is critical to the survival of normal melanocytes. The identification of *MITF* amplification in melanoma defined this transcription factor as a central modifier of melanoma.[96] In so doing, this discovery identified a novel class of oncogenes termed *lineage survival* oncogenes.[97] That is, a tumor may "hijack" extant lineage survival mechanisms in the presence of selective pressures to ensure its own propagation. The elucidation of *MITF* as an oncogene took a cross-tissue approach, wherein the NCI-60 cell line panel representing nine tumor types was subjected to both gene expression and high-density single-nucleotide polymorphism array analysis.[96] A recurrent gain of 3p13–14 significantly segregated

melanoma from other tumor classes, with MITF as the only gene in the region showing maximal amplification and overexpression. MITF amplification was subsequently detected in 10% of primary cutaneous and 15% to 20% of metastatic melanomas by fluorescence in situ hybridization, correlating with decreased survival in Kaplan-Meier analyses of 5-year patient survival. Exogenous MITF showed transforming capabilities in immortalized primary human melanocytes in combination with activated BRAF. Additionally, inhibition of MITF in cell lines showing 3p13–14 amplification reduced growth and survival and conferred sensitivity to certain anticancer drugs. MITF gene disruption leads to coat color defects in mice and pigmentation defects in humans, due to diminished viability of melanocytes. This suggested that MITF was essential for the lineage survival of melanocytes, supporting the contention that it is also critical for the survival of melanomas. More recently, a germline variant (E318K) of MITF has been identified that confers an increased risk of developing melanoma.[98,99]

The downstream elements of the MITF pathway include both pigment enzyme genes as well as genes involved in proliferation, survival, and metabolism.[100,101] MITF intersects with a number of established melanoma pathways, including the transcriptional activation of INK4A, c-Met, and CDK2.[102] Moreover, MITF is regulated by both MAPK signaling and c-KIT.[100,103] Recently, the ETS transcription factor ETV1 was found to positively regulate MITF expression in melanoma, and *ETV1* may function as an amplified melanoma oncogene in its own right.[104] Collectively, these observations place MITF in a central role of melanoma signal integration.

The MC1R Pathway

Pigmentation exerts a major influence on skin tumor susceptibility, as it is well documented that fair skin is more sensitive to UV radiation and melanoma genesis. The mechanism underlying this observation is partially explained by the protective effects of melanin, which is produced by melanocytes and distributed to interfollicular keratinocytes. Genetically, the red hair color/pale skin (RHC) phenotype is linked to variant alleles of the melanocyte-specific melanocortin 1 receptor gene (MC1R), which is central to melanin synthesis.[105] The ligand for the G-protein–coupled MC1R is the MSH peptide, which activates downstream signaling consisting of a cAMP-CREB/ATF1 cascade, culminating in the induced expression of MITF. Not all individuals carrying RHC alleles have identical melanin production, yet increased risk for melanoma genesis remains notable regardless,[106] implying that melanin-independent mechanisms might impact the susceptibility of RHC carriers. One possible node is cAMP, the MC1R as second messenger, which may activate pathways incompletely understood at present, such as MAPK and PI3K.[107]

Experiments have implicated the MSH/MC1R pathway in the normal UV pigmentation (tanning) response in skin, a response that is linked to skin cancer (and melanoma) risk in humans. A "redhead" mouse model (frameshift mutation in *MC1R*) was used to demonstrate that the UV tanning response is dependent on MC1R signaling, because keratinocytes respond to UV by strongly upregulating expression of MSH. The "fairskin" phenotype was rescued by topical administration of a small molecule cAMP agonist.[108] The resulting dark pigmentation in genetically redhead mice was protective against UV-induced skin carcinogenesis. Subsequent analyses revealed that the p53 tumor suppressor protein may function as a "UV sensor" in keratinocytes, translating UV damage into direct transcriptional stimulation of MSH expression.[109]

RAC1

RAC1 is a member of the Rho family of small GTPases that are regulators of cytoskeletal reorganization and cell motility. Recently, two whole exome sequencing studies of >100 melanomas each identified hotspot mutations in *RAC1* that result in a P29S substitution.[11,12] Overall, the mutation was detected in 5% to 10% of samples, making it the third most common gene, after *BRAF* and *NRAS*, to be affected by hotspot mutations in the coding region. Initial characterization of the mutation confirmed that it conferred increased activity to the RAC1 protein, and promoted cell proliferation and motility in vitro. The overall clinical significance of the RAC1 P29S mutation awaits studies determining its clinical associations and functional evaluation of its inhibition.

Telomerase

Telomere stabilization through telomerase dysregulation has long been recognized as a hallmark of carcinogenesis in many cancers. However, the molecular basis for altered telomerase regulation in cancer has remained obscure. Analysis of whole genome sequencing data from a collection of melanoma tumors led to the unexpected discovery of two highly recurrent mutations affecting the promoter of *TERT*, which encodes a key catalytic component of the telomerase enzyme complex.[110,111] Both mutations generate consensus ETS transcription factor binding motifs in the setting of an identical 11-nucleotide stretch, suggesting a gain-of-function effect. Since this index observation, multiple studies have confirmed the high frequency of *TERT* promoter mutations in melanoma and other tumor types, and that the presence of these mutations is associated with enhanced *TERT* expression. Thus, melanoma genetic studies produced the first example of a highly recurrent functional mutation that falls within the regulatory region of a gene.

MOLECULAR GENETICS OF MELANOMA: LOOKING AHEAD

The genetic and molecular understanding of melanoma, and its impact on therapy, is currently in the midst of a transformative era. The last decade witnessed an almost exponential increase in our understanding of the pathogenesis of this disease. Massively parallel sequencing technology has made it possible to obtain the complete sequence of entire cancer genomes or "exomes" (protein coding region of the genome) at ever diminishing costs. Together with developments in computational biology, these advances are rapidly bringing forth new understanding of cancer genome alterations and the tumorigenic mechanisms that result. One of the first cancer genomes to be sequenced was that of a cell line (and its paired normal counterpart) derived from a patient with metastatic melanoma.[112] This effort uncovered more than 33,000 somatic base substitutions, of which 187 were nonsynonymous coding mutations. As expected, most base mutations were C→T transitions indicative of UV exposure.

This initial discovery provided a glimpse into one of the central challenges of melanoma research: to identify which somatic changes are meaningful. The high UV-associated base mutation rate in melanoma suggests that nearly 2% of all genes may harbor nonsynonymous coding mutations in a typical cutaneous melanoma, most of which are likely to be "passenger" events with little biologic consequence to melanoma genesis or progression. Thus, cataloging all significant genomic alterations that might represent "driver" events will require not only sequencing hundreds of tumor specimens but also the principled application of increasingly sophisticated analytical methods for data deconvolution. Initial insights toward this end emerged from a whole-exome sequencing study of melanoma, which utilized a computational algorithm designed to model the effects of evolutionary selection on the cancer genome.[11] This approach facilitated the discovery of several new melanoma genes that might otherwise have been obscured by the high UV-associated mutation rates pervasive in melanoma genomes. Concomitantly, large-scale US (Cancer Genome Atlas) and international efforts (International Cancer Genomic Consortium) have taken on the ambitious goal of comprehensively characterizing the genomes of diverse human tumors including melanomas.[113] Thus, it seems certain that the next decade will witness additional major breakthroughs in melanoma genome characterization that inform the biology and treatment of this malignancy.

While sequencing of large numbers of melanomas will help to identify which mutations are statistically significant, additional approaches are needed to distinguish the complete spectrum of functional "drivers" of melanoma genesis, progression, and maintenance. Such genetic events may confer transforming activity, dictate prognosis, or correlate with responsiveness (or resistance) to emerging targeted therapeutics. While the initial exome sequencing efforts in melanoma have been very informative, they have not included parallel characterization of other molecular characteristics, such as DNA methylation, mRNA and miRNA expression, protein expression and activation, and clinical characteristics and outcomes. The availability of all of these types of data will allow for integrated analysis approaches that will help to elucidate key molecular events and pathways. In addition, hypotheses about critical drivers of melanoma biology will benefit from functional testing. Increasingly, such testing is being performed, at least initially, through the use of high-throughput screening methods using RNAi libraries, collections of small molecules, and/or expression libraries of open reading frames of genes of interest. These approaches allow not only for evaluation of individual genes/targets, but also for more global approaches for data analysis to identify key networks and pathway. Such approaches can help to tailor investigations to focus on individual genes which may be most important functionally or most exploitable clinically.

One challenge in characterizing the molecular biology of melanoma is the recognition that it can be impacted by increasingly effective therapeutics. As noted earlier, multiple studies have been undertaken to characterize the molecular basis of resistance. To date, all studies that have been reported have identified the continued presence of the same mutation in the BRAF gene at the time of disease progression that was present before treatment was started.[114] At the same time, a variety of new genomic features have been identified in the progressing lesions that confirm certain longstanding assumptions while challenging others. As noted earlier, NRAS mutations arise alongside mutated BRAF in the progressing lesions of ~25% of patients.[52] This stands in marked contrast to the mutual exclusivity of these mutations in treatment-naïve tumors, and highlights how such studies must not be constrained by assumptions based on previous observations about the molecular biology of this disease. On the other hand, while some mutations in MEK1/2 cause marked resistance to both BRAF and MEK inhibitors, in other cases the presence of MEK1 mutations does not preclude clinical response to RAF inhibition.[55,115] Thus, not all MEK1 mutations are equivalent, similar to prior findings involving distinct BRAF mutations.[24] The characterization of progressing lesions has also confirmed the molecular heterogeneity of melanoma. Such heterogeneity has been demonstrated by the finding of independent resistance mechanisms within different progressing tumors of individual patients, and within different regions of individual tumors.[72,115,116]

In addition to the aforementioned advances in the field of targeted therapy, melanoma treatment is being revolutionized by improved understanding and targeting of the antitumor immune response. Ipilimumab, an antibody that blocks the inhibitory CTLA4 molecule on the surface of T-cells, was the first therapy to ever demonstrate a survival benefit in a randomized clinical trial in patients with metastatic melanoma, and it gained regulatory approval in 2011.[117] Agents that target other inhibitory molecules, including PD-1 and PD-L1, have recently demonstrated very promising clinical safety and activity in early phase clinical trials.[118,119] While the resistance studies described previously focused on the molecular biology of resistance to MAPK pathway inhibitors, there is also growing evidence that somatic mutations may be critical to the effectiveness of immunotherapy.[120] In addition to creating new antigens that may be recognized by the immune systems, oncogenic signaling pathways in tumors can also influence the antitumor immune response.[121,122]

In the future, integration of melanoma molecular biology with a growing knowledge of the tumor microenvironment and the immune system will likely be needed to propel additional discoveries. While this presently stands as a daunting task, the remarkable progress of the last decade provides a proof-of-concept that advancing our understanding of the molecular basis of this disease will have a tremendous positive impact on the quality of life and survival of patients with this highly aggressive disease.

SELECTED REFERENCES

The full reference list can be accessed at lwwhealthlibrary.com/oncology.

1. Siegel R, Naishadham D, Jemal A. Cancer statistics, 2013. *CA Cancer J Clin* 2013;63:11–30.
3. Jemal A, Saraiya M, Patel P, et al. Recent trends in cutaneous melanoma incidence and death rates in the United States, 1992-2006. *J Am Acad Dermatol* 2011;65:S17–S25.e1–e3.
5. Ekwueme DU, Guy GP Jr, Li C, et al. The health burden and economic costs of cutaneous melanoma mortality by race/ethnicity–United States, 2000 to 2006. *J Am Acad Dermatol* 2011;65:S133–S143.
6. Balch CM, Gershenwald JE, Soong SJ, et al. Final version of 2009 AJCC melanoma staging and classification. *J Clin Oncol* 2009;27:6199–6206.
9. Berger MF, Hodis E, Herrernan TP, et al. Melanoma genome sequencing reveals frequent PREX2 mutations. *Nature* 2012;485:502–506.
10. Hocker T, Tsao H. Ultraviolet radiation and melanoma: a systematic review and analysis of reported sequence variants. *Hum Mutat* 2007;28:578–588.
11. Hodis E, Watson IR, Kryukov GV, et al. A landscape of driver mutations in melanoma. *Cell* 2012;150:251–263.
12. Krauthammer M, Kong Y, Ha BH, et al. Exome sequencing identifies recurrent somatic RAC1 mutations in melanoma. *Nat Genet* 2012;44:1006–1014.
15. Chin L, Pomerantz J, Polsky D, et al. Cooperative effects of INK4a and ras in melanoma susceptibility in vivo. *Genes Dev* 1997;11:2822–2834.
16. Kwong LN, Costello JC, Liu H, et al. Oncogenic NRAS signaling differentially regulates survival and proliferation in melaoma. *Nat Med* 2012;18:1503–1510.
19. Curtin JA, Fridlyand J, Kageshita T, et al. Distinct sets of genetic alterations in melanoma. *N Engl J Med* 2005;353:2135–2147.
23. Pollock PM, Harper UL, Hansen KS, et al. High frequency of BRAF mutations in nevi. *Nat Genet* 2003;33:19–20.
24. Wan PT, Garnett MJ, Roe SM, et al. Mechanism of activation of the RAF-ERK signaling pathway by oncogenic mutations of B-RAF. *Cell* 2004;116:855–867.
25. Davies H, Bignell GR, Cox C, et al. Mutations of the BRAF gene in human cancer. *Nature* 2002;417:949–954.
26. Heidorn SJ, Milagre C, Whittaker S, et al. Kinase-dead BRAF and oncogenic RAS cooperate to drive tumor progression through CRAF. *Cell* 2010;140:209–221.
27. Goel VK, Lazar AJ, Warneke CL, et al. Examination of mutations in BRAF, NRAS, and PTEN in primary cutaneous melanoma. *J Invest Dermatol* 2006;126:154–160.
28. Patton EE, Widlund HR, Kutok JL, et al. BRAF mutations are sufficient to promote nevi formation and cooperate with p53 in the genesis of melanoma. *Curr Biol* 2005;15:249–254.
30. Michaloglou C, Vredeveld LC, Soengas MS, et al. BRAFE600-associated senescence-like cell cycle arrest of human naevi. *Nature* 2005;436:720–724.
31. Dankort D, Curley DP, Cartlidge RA, et al. Braf(V600E) cooperates with Pten loss to induce metastatic melanoma. *Nat Genet* 2009;41:544–552.
34. McArthur GA, Chapman PB, Robert C, et al. Safety and efficacy of vemurafenib in BRAF(V600E) and BRAF(V600K) mutation-positive melanoma (BRIM-3): extended follow-up of a phase 3, randomised, open-label study. *Lancet Oncol* 2014;15:323–332.
35. Hauschild A, Grob JJ, Demidov LV, et al. Dabrafenib in BRAF-mutated metastatic melanoma: a multicentre, open-label, phase 3 randomised controlled trial. *Lancet* 2012;380:358–365.
36. Hatzivassiliou G, Song K, Yen I, et al. RAF inhibitors prime wild-type RAF to activate the MAPK pathway and enhance growth. *Nature* 2010;464:431–435.
39. Su F, Viros A, Milagre C, et al. RAS mutations in cutaneous squamous-cell carcinomas in patients treated with BRAF inhibitors. *N Engl J Med* 2012;366:207–215.
42. Villanueva J, Vultur A, Lee JT, et al. Acquired resistance to BRAF inhibitors mediated by a RAF kinase switch in melanoma can be overcome by cotargeting MEK and IGF-1R/PI3K. *Cancer Cell* 2010;18:683–695.
43. Poulikakos PI, Persaud Y, Janakiraman M, et al. RAF inhibitor resistance is mediated by dimerization of aberrantly spliced BRAF(V600E). *Nature* 2011;480:387–390.
46. Flaherty KT, Robert C, Hersey P, et al. Improved survival with MEK inhibition in BRAF-mutated melanoma. *N Engl J Med* 2012;367:107–114.
47. Flaherty KT, Infante JR, Daud A, et al. Combined BRAF and MEK inhibition in melanoma with BRAF V600 mutations. *N Engl J Med* 2012;367:1694–1703.
48. Ascierto PA, Schadendorf D, Berking C, et al. MEK162 for patients with advanced melanoma harbouring NRAS or Val600 BRAF mutations: a non-randomised, open-label phase 2 study. *Lancet Oncol* 2013;14:249–256.
51. Whittaker SR, Theurillat JP, Van Allen E, et al. A genome-scale RNA interference screen implicates NF1 loss in resistance to RAF inhibition. *Cancer Discov* 2013;3:350–362.
53. Straussman R, Morikawa T, Shee K, et al. Tumour micro-environment elicits innate resistance to RAF inhibitors through HGF secretion. *Nature* 2012;487:500–504.
56. Van Allen EM, Wagle N, Sucker A, et al. The genetic landscape of clinical resistance to RAF inhibition in metastatic melanoma. *Cancer Discov* 2014;4:94–109.
57. Wagle N, Van Allen EM, Treacy DJ, et al. MAP kinase pathway alterations in BRAF-mutant melanoma patients with acquired resistance to combined RAF/MEK inhibition. *Cancer Discov* 2014;4:61–68.
61. FitzGerald MG, Harkin DP, Silva-Arrieta S, et al. Prevalence of germ-line mutations in p16, p19ARF, and CDK4 in familial melanoma: analysis of a clinic-based population. *Proc Natl Acad Sci U S A* 1996;93:8541–8545.
72. Shi H, Hugo W, Kong X, et al. Acquired resistance and clonal evolution in melanoma during BRAF inhibitor therapy. *Cancer Discov* 2014;4:80–93.
73. Davies MA, Stemke-Hale K, Lin E, et al. Integrated molecular and clinical analysis of AKT activation in metastatic melanoma. *Clin Cancer Res* 2009;15:7538–7546.
78. Kwong LN, Davies MA. Navigating the therapeutic complexity of PI3K pathway inhibition in melanoma. *Clin Cancer Res* 2013;19:5310–5319.
86. Woodman SE, Davies MA. Targeting KIT in melanoma: A paradigm of molecular medicine and targeted therapeutics. *Biochem Pharmacol* 2010;80:568–574.
87. Curtin JA, Busam K, Pinkel D, et al. Somatic activation of KIT in distinct subtypes of melanoma. *J Clin Oncol* 2006;24:4340–4346.
90. Carvajal RD, Antonescu CR, Wolchok JD, et al. KIT as a therapeutic target in metastatic melanoma. *JAMA* 2011;305:2327–2334.
91. Hodi FS, Corless CL, Giobbie-Hurder A, et al. Imatinib for melanomas harboring mutationally activated or amplified KIT arising on mucosal, acral, and chronically sun-damaged skin. *J Clin Oncol* 2013;31:3182–3190.
96. Garraway LA, Widlund HR, Rubin MA, et al. Integrative genomic analyses identify MITF as a lineage survival oncogene amplified in malignant melanoma. *Nature* 2005;436:117–122.
98. Yokoyama S, Woods SL, Boyle GM, et al. A novel recurrent mutation in MITF predisposes to familial and sporadic melanoma. *Nature* 2011;480:99–103.
99. Bertolotto C, Lesueur D, Giuliano S, et al. A SUMOylation-defective MITF germline mutation predisposes to melanoma and renal carcinoma. *Nature* 2011;480:94–98.
100. Haq R, Shoag J, Andreu-Perez P, et al. Oncogenic BRAF regulates oxidative metabolism via PGC1alpha and MITF. *Cancer Cell* 2013;23:302–315.
110. Huang FW, Hodis E, Xu MJ, et al. Highly recurrent TERT promoter mutations in human melanoma. *Science* 2013;339:957–959.
111. Horn S, Figl A, Rachakonda PS, et al. TERT promoter mutations in familial and sporadic melanoma. *Science* 2013;339:959–961.
112. Pleasance ED, Cheetham RK, Stephens PJ, et al. A comprehensive catalogue of somatic mutations from a human cancer genome. *Nature* 2010;463:191–196.
115. Trunzer K, Pavlick AC, Schuchter L, et al. Pharmacodynamic effects and mechanisms of resistance to vemurafenib in patients with metastatic melanoma. *J Clin Oncol* 2013;31:1767–1774.
116. Wilmott JS, Tembe V, Howle JR, et al. Intratumoral molecular heterogeneity in a BRAF-mutant, BRAF inhibitor-resistant melanoma: a case illustrating the challenges for personalized medicine. *Mol Cancer Ther* 2012;11:2704–2708.
117. Hodi FS, O'Day SJ, McDermott DF, et al. Improved survival with ipilimumab in patients with metastatic melanoma. *N Engl J Med* 2010;363:711–723.
119. Topalian SL, Hodi FS, Brahmer JR, et al. Safety, activity, and immune correlates of anti–PD-1 antibody in cancer. *N Engl J Med* 2012;366:2443–2454.
121. Boni A, Cogdill AP, Dang P, et al. Selective BRAFV600E inhibition enhances T-cell recognition of melanoma without affecting lymphocyte function. *Cancer Res* 2010;70:5213–5219.

PRACTICE OF ONCOLOGY

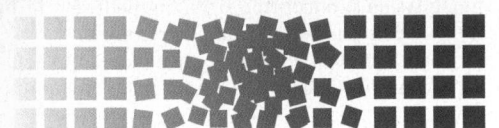

Antoni Ribas, Craig L. Slingluff, Jr., and Steven A. Rosenberg

INTRODUCTION

Melanoma arises from the malignant transformation of the melanocyte, the cell responsible for the production of the pigment melanin. Precursor melanocytes arise in the neural crest and, as the fetus develops, migrate to multiple areas in the body including the skin, meninges, mucous membranes, upper esophagus, and eyes. Melanomas can arise from any of these locations through the malignant transformation of the resident melanocytes. By far the most common location is the hair follicle–bearing skin arising from melanocytes at the dermal/epidermal junction. In the National Cancer Database, 91.2% of melanomas are cutaneous, 5.3% are ocular, 1.3% are mucosal, and 2.2% are of unknown primary site.[1] Each of these types has significant differences in the etiology and genetic makeup, in particular related to the degree of ultraviolet (UV) radiation exposure and their frequency of driver oncogenic mutations. The current understanding of melanoma biology comes from studies of genetic analyses of melanomas correlated with clinicopathologic presentations, which have elucidated two key features of this cancer: (1) cutaneous melanoma, as opposed to mucosal or uveal melanoma, is usually a carcinogen-induced cancer with a high mutational load, demonstrated by the molecular fingerprinting of UV light damage, and (2) the majority of melanomas are dependent on a particular oncogenic signaling pathway, the mitogen-activated protein kinase (MAPK) pathway, through usually mutually exclusive driver mutations in cKit, NRAS, BRAF, GNAQ or GNA11.[2–6] Cutaneous melanomas arising from the trunk and extremities, which are associated with intermittent UV radiation exposure, have high rates of BRAF (50%) or NRAS (20%) mutations.[2,7,8] Mucosal and acrolentigenous melanomas, with low rates of UV radiation exposure, have lower rates of BRAF mutations (5% to 20%) and higher rates of KIT mutations (5% to 10%).[2] The great majority of uveal melanomas have mutually exclusive mutations in the alpha subunits of G-protein–coupled receptors GNAQ and GNA11.[3,4]

The primary focus of this chapter is on cutaneous melanoma, but summary information is presented for the other forms of melanoma, as well as on the subtypes of cutaneous melanoma.

MOLECULAR BIOLOGY OF MELANOMA

Mutational Landscape in Melanoma

Studies of whole exome sequencing (sequencing of the approximately 1.6% of the genome that encodes for expressed proteins) and whole genome sequencing of melanomas compared to matched normal DNA of the same patients are leading to a greatly improved understanding of the genomic alterations in melanoma. The studies of the mutational load of cutaneous melanomas by next generation sequencing demonstrate that melanoma has significantly more sequence variations per megabase of DNA compared to most other cancers. For example, melanomas have 15 times more mutations per megabase of DNA than colorectal cancer and 4 times more than lung cancer.[9] As a high proportion

of these mutations are cytosine to thymine (C>T) substitutions, typical of UV radiation–induced thymine dimmers, it is highly likely that the high rate of sequence variants in melanoma is due to the role of UV as the principal carcinogen in the disease.[10–12]

Two studies have reported on exome sequencing of relative large series of melanomas compared to normal matched DNA. After sequencing the exomes of 147 melanomas, it became evident that sun-exposed melanomas had markedly more UV-like C>T somatic mutations compared to sun-shielded acral, mucosal, and uveal melanomas. These studies confirmed the recurrent mutations in BRAF, NRAS, and cKit. Newly identified recurrently mutated cancer genes included PPP6C, encoding a serine/threonine phosphatase in 12% of sun-exposed melanomas, and were mutually exclusively in tumors with mutations in BRAF or NRAS. Furthermore, an activating mutation in RAC1(P29S) was noted in 9.2% of sun-exposed melanomas.[11] In a similar study, analysis of large-scale melanoma exomes from 121 paired samples[12] also confirmed the recurrent BRAF, NRAS, and cKIT mutations, and discovered six recurrently mutated melanoma genes (PPP6C, RAC1, SNX31, TACC1, STK19, and ARID2), two of which are the same as in the other study. Integration with chromosomal copy number data contextualized the landscape of driver mutations, providing oncogenic insights in BRAF- and NRAS-driven melanoma as well as those without known NRAS/BRAF mutations. In this study, the authors found a higher than expected number of genetic events dysregulating the RB and p53 pathways, which had previously thought to be mostly intact in melanoma.[12]

The first fully sequenced whole genome of any cancer was a melanoma cell line compared to a lymphoblastoid cell line generated from the same patient to provide the comparing source of normal DNA.[10] This study provided the first comprehensive catalogue of somatic mutations from an individual cancer. The dominant mutational signature reflects DNA damage due to UV light exposure. It also revealed an uneven distribution of mutations across the genome, with a lower prevalence in gene footprints, which indicated that DNA repair preferentially functioned in areas with transcribed regions. There are ongoing efforts to perform whole exome sequencing in large panels of melanomas. The largest effort is The Cancer Genome Atlas. It will report on whole exome sequencing on 500 melanoma samples compared to normal exomes, with a subset of cases additionally undergoing whole genome sequencing, DNA methylation studies, RNA sequencing, microRNA sequencing, and reverse phase protein array analysis of phosphorylated proteins.

The studies of whole genome sequencing will be important to understand melanoma genetic alterations in nontranscribed genes since there can also be recurrent mutations in them. This is exemplified by the demonstration of two very common mutations in the promoter of telomerase reverse transcriptase (TERT) by two independent research groups. TERT is the gene coding for the catalytic subunit of telomerase. In one of the studies,[13] mutations in the TERT promoter were reported in 71% of melanomas examined. The mutations increased the transcriptional activity from the TERT promoter by two- to four-fold. This information may be of high relevance beyond melanoma, since examination of 150 cancer cell lines derived from diverse tumor types revealed the same mutations in 24 cases (16%). The other group reached the same conclusion by investigated a melanoma-prone family through linkage analysis and high-throughput sequencing.[14] They identified the same TERT promoter mutations as disease-segregating germline mutations. When they screened TERT promoter mutations in sporadic melanoma, they found them in 74% of human cell lines derived from metastatic melanomas and in 33% of primary melanomas.

Driver Mutations in Melanoma

Melanoma has become a notable example of a cancer histology dependent upon driver oncogenic mutations in the MAPK pathway, with additional genetic alterations in other pathways leading to uncontrolled cell growth and avoidance of apoptosis (Fig. 94.1). There is evidence of MAPK activation by defined point mutations in at least 70% of melanomas, resulting in constitutive signaling leading to oncogenic cell proliferation and escape from apoptosis.[15] The aberrations that lead to MAPK pathway activation in most cutaneous and mucosal melanomas consist in usually mutually exclusive activating mutations in the receptor tyrosine kinase KIT (2% to 3%), the G-protein neuroblastoma RAS viral oncogene homolog (NRAS) (15% to 20%), and the serine-threonine kinase BRAF (40% to 50%).[3–6] Uveal melanomas have a distinct set of driver mutations in GNAQ and GNA11, which are the alpha subunits of G-protein–coupled receptors.[3,4]

Mutations in KIT are found in exons 9, 11, 13, and 17, and there is no one predominant point mutation.[6] Because of this, molecular testing for KIT mutations must evaluate multiple regions of the gene by extended sequencing or multiplexed polymerase chain reaction (PCR) tests. Emerging evidence suggests that not all KIT mutations activate its function, resulting in some mutations being insensitive to KIT inhibitors used for patient treatment.[16] NRAS mutations cluster in the RAS hotspot mutation site Q61, usually Q61L and less frequently Q61R and Q61H. NRAS mutations are more frequent in older individuals and are equally common in melanomas arising from the skin with chronic or intermittent sun damage.[2,17] The vast majority of BRAF mutations in melanoma involve a substitution for valine at the 600th amino acid position to glutamine (V600E).[5,18] The frequency of the BRAF V600E mutation is inversely correlated with age since it is most frequent in melanomas that appear on the skin without chronic sun damage in young adults. BRAF V600K is the second most common variant, which increases in incidence with age. V600D or V600R mutations are much less frequent.[8] Overall, up to 90 different point mutations have been described in BRAF in different cancers, some of which are activating and others are inhibiting its enzymatic activity.[18]

Aberrations in the phosphoinositide 3-kinase (PI3K)/protein kinase B (AKT)/mammalian target of rapamycin pathway, including the phosphatase and tensin homolog (PTEN), are also noted in a significant number of melanomas, but these do not seem to function as true drivers of the malignant phenotype. PTEN alterations include missense mutations, deletions, and insertions, as well as loss of heterozygosity and epigenetic silencing, making interrogation for mutations and genomic rearrangements in PTEN necessary.[19,20] The pathogenesis of melanoma, like most

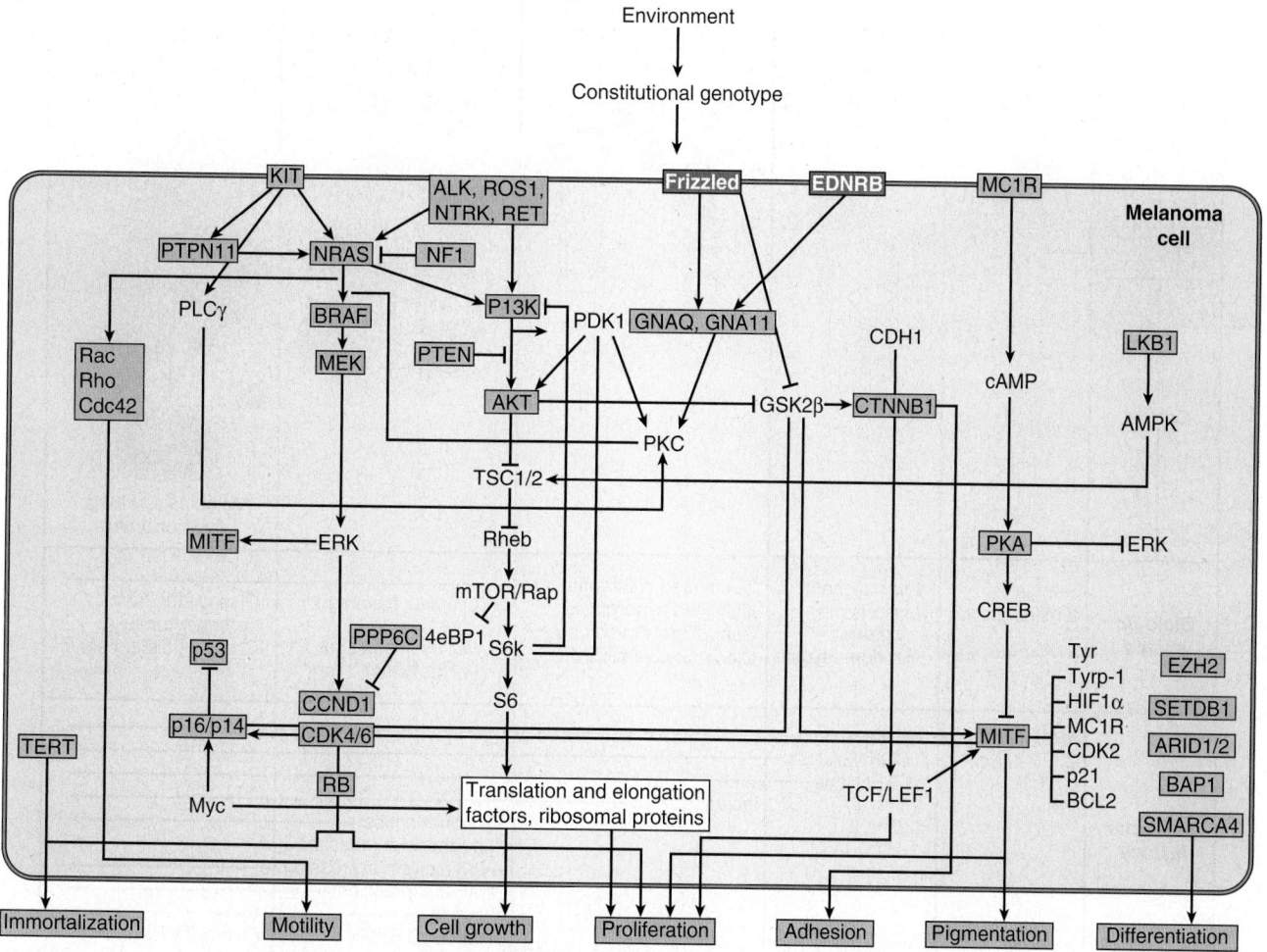

Figure 94.1 Signaling pathways disrupted by genetic alterations and their relationship to the hallmarks of melanoma. Proteins boxed in *red* are affected by gain-of-function mutations; those boxed in *blue* are affected by loss-of-function mutations. (Source: Bastian BC. The molecular pathology of melanoma: an integrated taxonomy of melanocytic neoplasia. *Ann Rev Pathol Mech Dis* 2014;9:239–271.)

other cancers, requires the presence of a driver oncogene and the dysregulation of cell cycle control and apoptosis to provide the full oncogenic signaling and ability to grow autonomously. These happen with the frequent mutations or genetic deletions of CDKN2A, cyclin D1, or the amplification cyclin-dependent kinase 4.[21]

Progression of Melanocytes to Cutaneous Melanoma

Genetic Events in Melanocyte to Melanoma Progression and Oncogene-Induced Senescence

BRAF and NRAS are founding mutations of cutaneous melanoma that are frequently present in benign nevi.[22] Despite of the presence BRAF and NRAS mutations, nevi have an exceedingly low proliferative activity and infrequently progress to melanoma. This is explained because of the phenomenon of oncogene-induced senescence preventing malignant progression to melanoma, where these mutations require functioning with additional genetic events that lead to dysregulation of cell cycle control to result in the development of a progressive melanoma.[15,23] The model for oncogene-induced senescence in melanoma is based on the identity of the main driver mutations (BRAF and RAS) in nevi, the initial phase of proliferative activity they spark, the

formation of a benign nevus in association with the induction of senescence markers (cell cycle arrest, induction of the tumor suppressor p16[INK4a], endoplastic reticulum stress markers and increased SA-βGal activity, and possibly additional senescence biomarkers), and the subsequent cessation of expansion, which is typically maintained for decades.[24]

Cellular Changes in Melanocyte to Melanoma Progression

The transition from melanocyte to metastatic melanoma involves several histologic intermediates, including melanocytic atypia, atypical melanocytic hyperplasia, radial growth phase melanoma, vertical growth phase melanoma, and metastatic melanoma. Atypical melanocytes arising in a preexisting nevus or de novo are very common but rarely progress to melanoma. However, some patients develop confluent atypical melanocytic hyperplasia at the dermal/epidermal junction or nests of atypical melanocytes in the epidermis or at the dermal/epidermal junction. As this process progresses, it reaches a point at which a diagnosis of melanoma is warranted.

Early cutaneous melanomas usually proceed to grow radially, and this is called the *radial growth phase* (RGP) of melanoma, which may continue for years before progressing to the vertical growth phase (VGP) (Figs. 94.2 and 94.3). The RGP of a cutaneous melanoma may include either melanoma in situ or superficial

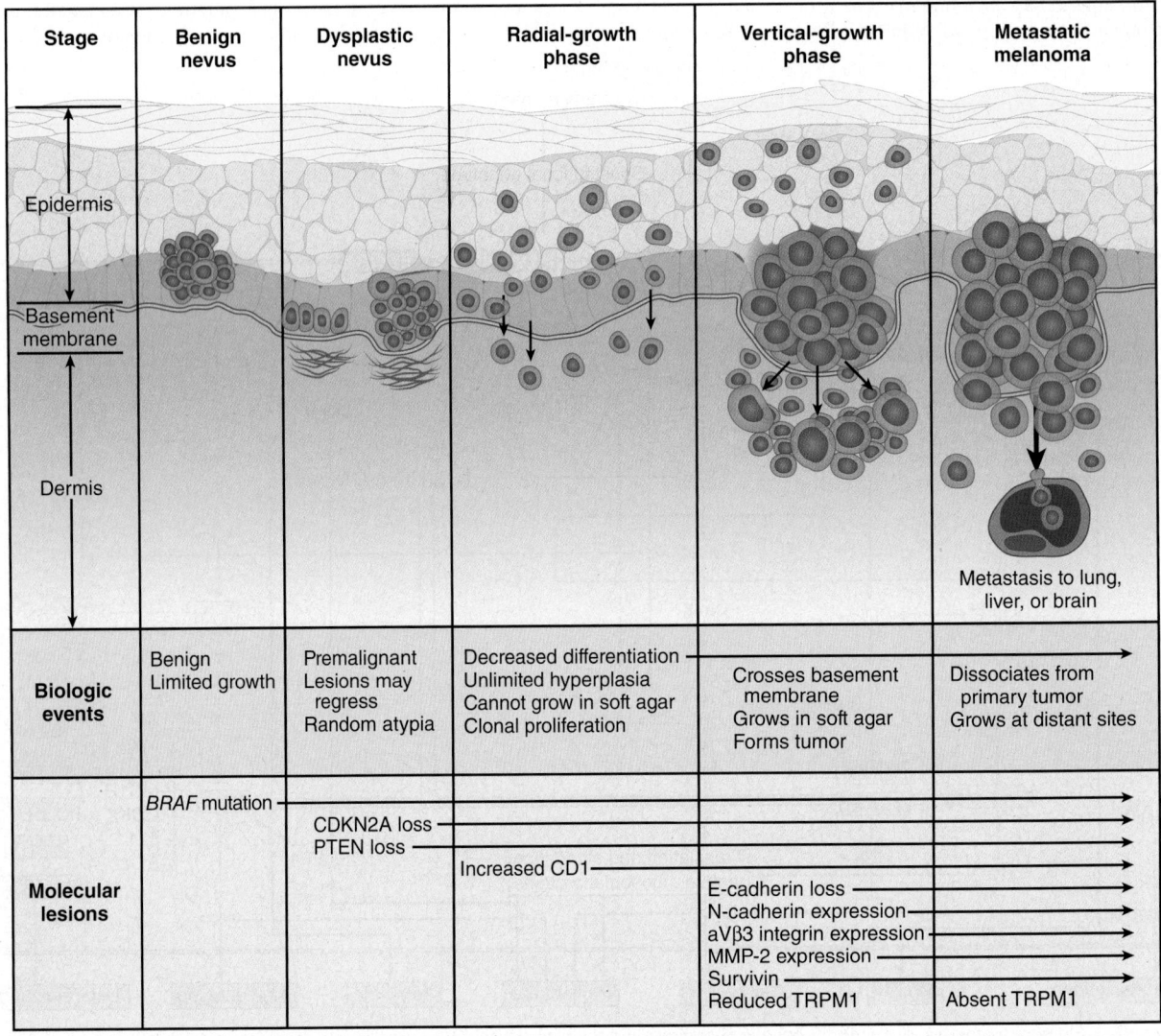

Figure 94.2 Biologic events and molecular changes in the progression of melanoma. (From Miller AJ, Mihm MC Jr. Melanoma. *N Engl J Med* 2006;355:51–65.)

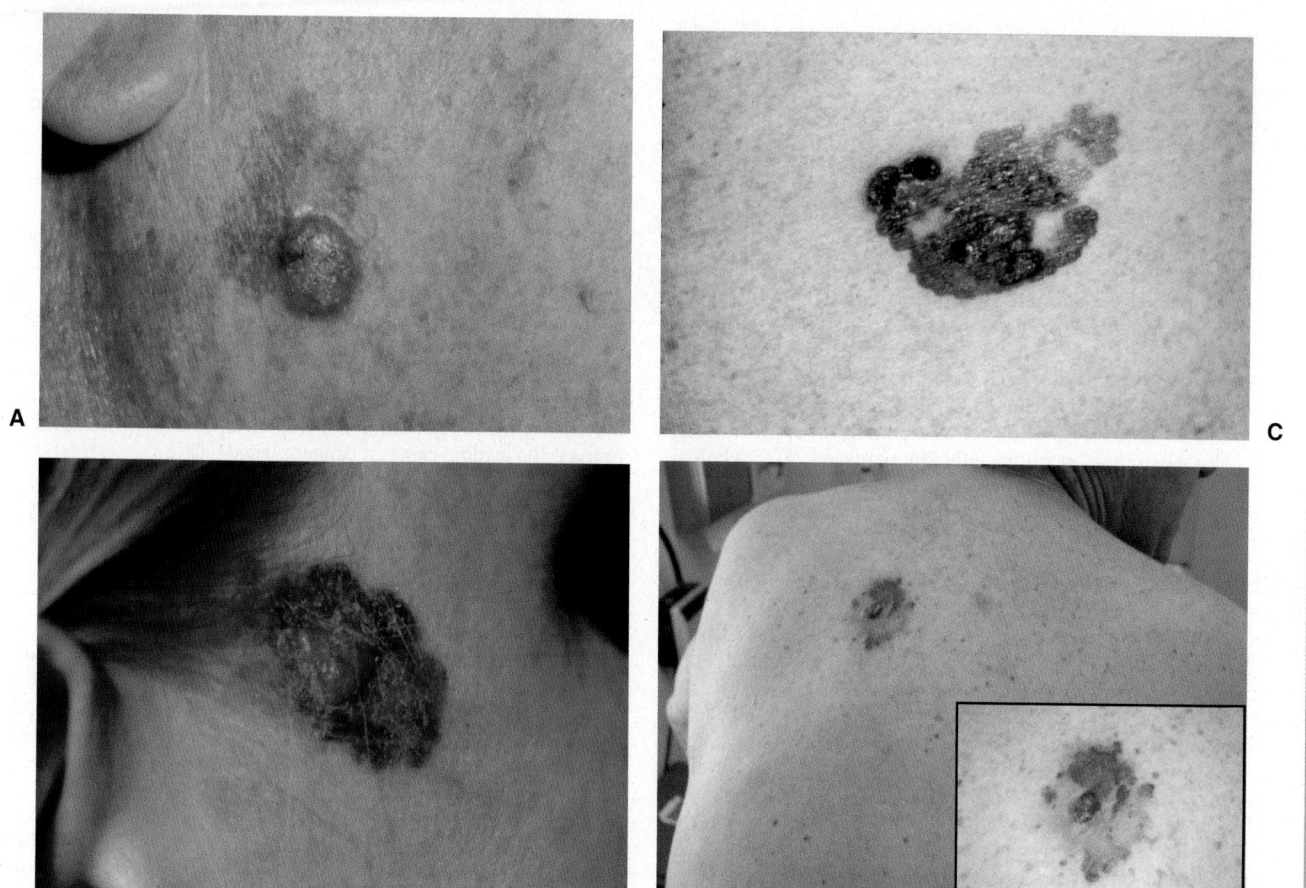

Figure 94.3 (A) A nodule of vertical growth phase melanoma arising from a radial growth phase pigmented macule on the right cheek. **(B)** Superficial spreading melanoma, 2.9 mm thick, arising on the temple of a young woman. There were microscopic satellites, and the patient died of disease within several years. **(C)** Superficial spreading melanoma with all the classic features of the ABCD mnemonic (*a*symmetry, *b*order irregularity, *c*olor variation, and *d*iameter >6 mm). **(D)** Large, ulcerated 2.5 mm superficial spreading melanoma with regression in elderly man.

invasion into the papillary dermis, or both. Melanomas in RGP present clinically as enlarging macules or very minimally raised papular lesions, which are typically (but not always) pigmented. These lesions are rarely symptomatic. If not recognized, these lesions typically progress to the VGP, manifest clinically by a nodular growth of the lesion, often described by the patient as a lesion that began to "raise up." This vertical growth usually arises as a nodule within the RGP component and encompassing only part of the RGP (see Fig. 94.3A,C). Thus, the VGP appears to represent further steps in the process of malignant transformation due to clonal changes in the cells of the RGP.

Some melanomas present as metastatic melanoma in lymph nodes, skin, subcutaneous tissue, or visceral sites without an apparent primary cutaneous site. In some cases, these have been associated with a history of a regressed primary melanocytic lesion. In other cases, such an explanation is less clear. In all of these cases, the prospect of early diagnosis of melanoma is compromised, and the risk of melanoma-associated mortality is increased.

EPIDEMIOLOGY

Malignant melanoma is the sixth most common US cancer diagnosis. The actual incidence of melanoma is increasing more rapidly than that of any other malignancy. It was estimated that 76,690 men and women (45,060 men and 31,630 women) will be diagnosed with and 9,480 men and women will die of melanoma of the skin in 2013.[25] This amounts to 4% of new cancer diagnoses and 1.5% of cancer deaths. In the early part of the 20th century, the lifetime

risk of a white person developing melanoma was approximately 1 in 1,500. Currently, 1 in 49 men and women will be diagnosed with melanoma of the skin during their lifetime. Its incidence is second only to breast cancer for women from birth to age 39 years; similarly, it is the second most common cancer diagnosis for men through age 39 years, slightly less common than leukemia.[26] Overall 5-year survival rates for melanoma have increased from 82% in the late 1970s (1975 to 1977) to 91% in the more recent era (2002 to 2006).[26]

This is a disease that disproportionately affects whites over African Americans, Asians, or Hispanics. In the United States, whites account for 98.2% of cutaneous melanomas reported in the National Cancer Database, with African Americans accounting for 0.7% and Hispanics accounting for 1.1%.[1] This is best explained by a combined effect of UV sunlight exposure and fair skin. It is most striking that the highest per capita incidence of melanoma worldwide is in Australia, and that this high incidence afflicts primarily the Australians of Western European descent who have fair skin, and not the darker-skinned aboriginal population. It is also notable that these fair-skinned European descendants who moved to Australia have much higher incidences of melanoma than the Western European populations that remain in the higher latitudes of Europe. In migrant populations, individuals who move during childhood to areas with greater sun exposure develop melanoma at rates higher than those of their country of origin and similar to those of their adopted country.[27]

In nonwhite populations, there is a much higher proportion of melanomas in acral (subungual, palmar, plantar) and mucosal locations. However, the incidences of those types of melanoma are similar across races. Their higher relative proportion in Asians and African Americans can be best explained by the disproportionate increase in nonacral cutaneous melanomas in fair-skinned whites rather than by an absolute increase in risk of acral and mucosal melanomas in nonwhite populations.

Ocular and nonacral cutaneous melanomas are 50- to 200-fold more likely in white populations than in nonwhite populations, but melanomas in acral and mucosal sites are within twofold of each other across racial groups. Similarly, the increased incidence of melanoma over the last few decades can be explained primarily by increased incidence in white populations, not in nonwhite populations.[28] These observations support the hypothesis that most cutaneous melanomas in white populations are etiologically related to sun exposure but that there may be a baseline risk of melanoma in other locations that is unrelated to sun damage. There are significant molecular differences between acral melanomas and melanomas arising on the skin associated with chronic sun damage, with *B-RAF* and *N-RAS* mutations in approximately 80% of melanomas on chronically sun-damaged skin, whereas those mutations were uncommon in melanomas from acral or mucosal sites or from skin without chronic sun damage.[2]

CHANGES IN INCIDENCE

Data from the Surveillance, Epidemiology, and End Results program reveal an increase in age-adjusted melanoma incidence rates from 8.2 per 100,000 in the 1970s (1974 to 1978) to 18.7 per 100,000 in more recent years (1999 to 2003).[29] From 1990 to 2003, during which there was a 16% decrease in male cancer deaths overall for all cancers, there was a 2% increase in mortality rate from melanoma. From 1991 to 2003, during which there was an 8% decrease in cancer deaths overall for women, there was only a 4% decrease in mortality rate associated with melanoma.[26]

In Australia, and to a lesser extent in the United States, there has been a substantial increase in awareness about melanoma and the value of screening by total-body skin examinations. There also has been a greater proportion of patients diagnosed at earlier and noninvasive stages of disease. Thus, part of the increase in incidence may be explained by increased early diagnosis of lesions with low metastatic potential. However, there has also been a significant increase in mortality from melanoma over the last few decades.[29]

GENDER AND AGE DISTRIBUTION

In the United States and Australia, the gender ratio of melanoma at diagnosis is 2 male to 1 female, but it depends on the age group. Analysis of incidence data for invasive melanoma diagnosed from 1992 to 2006 from 12 cancer registries that participate in the Surveillance, Epidemiology, and End Results program of the National Cancer Institute revealed that, by age, the men-to-women rate ratio ranged from 1.3 (95% confidence interval [CI], 1.2 to 1.3) for ages 40 to 64 years for incidence to 2.6 (2.5 to 2.7) for older than 65 years for both incidence and mortality. However, between the age of 15 and 39 years old, melanoma is more common in females (rate ratio = 0.6).[25] The median age of melanoma patients has increased from 51 years in the 1970s (1974 to 1978) to 57 years in a more recent time period (1999 to 2003). Nonetheless, the median age for diagnosis of melanoma is approximately 10 years lower than the current median age of diagnosis for the more common solid tumors, such as colon, lung, or prostate cancer. The large majority (approximately 80%) of patients with melanoma are diagnosed in the productive years from age 25 to 65 as shown for a representative population from the state of Virginia (Fig. 94.4). Melanoma is common in patients in their 20s and older, but it also is observed in teenagers, and occasionally even in infants and neonates. For women aged 25 to 35 years, melanoma is the leading cause of cancer-related death.

MELANOMA IN CHILDREN, INFANTS, AND NEONATES

Diagnosis and management of melanoma in children, infants, and neonates is complicated by several factors: (1) excisional biopsy of skin lesions often is not feasible under local anesthesia in young children, and (2) pigmented skin lesions with substantial cellular atypia but with structural symmetry may be Spitz nevi, which typically have benign behavior. Thus, some young patients with changing pigmented skin lesions are observed longer than would be advisable because biopsy is more problematic than in most adults. In addition, young patients may undergo incomplete shave biopsy to avoid a full-thickness excision, and information is lost about the architecture of the lesion, leaving a diagnostic dilemma between melanoma and Spitz nevus. Even in the best of circumstances, some melanocytic tumors are difficult to diagnose with certainty. This has led to a formal definition of melanocytic tumors of uncertain malignant potential.[30]

Melanoma deaths in children and young adults have a large effect on total years of life lost because of melanoma. Current recommendations for management of melanoma in children and infants are the same as for adults, and outcomes are generally believed to be comparable.[31]

ANATOMIC DISTRIBUTION

Cutaneous melanoma can occur at any skin site in the body. The most common sites in males are on the back and in the head and neck regions. In women, the most common sites are in the lower

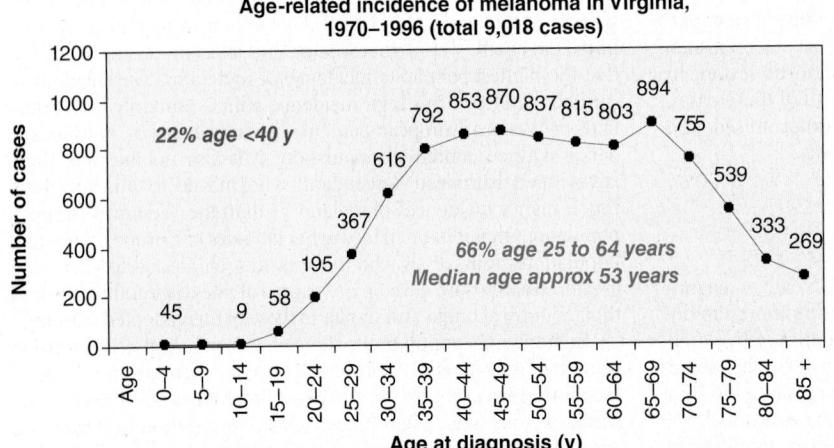

Figure 94.4 Age-related incidence of melanoma in Virginia, 1970 to 1996 (total of 9,018 cases).

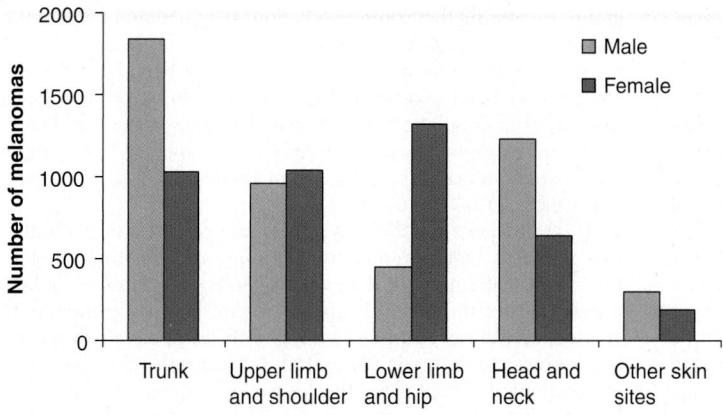

Trunk M:F = 1.8; lower limb M:F = 1/3; headand neck M:F = 1.9

Figure 94.5 Incidence of melanoma in Virginia, 1970 to 1996, by gender.

extremities, commonly below the knee (Fig. 94.5). Lentigo maligna melanoma (LMM) most commonly arises on sun-damaged surfaces of the head and neck in older patients. Acral lentiginous melanoma (ALM) is most common on subungual and other acral locations.

ETIOLOGY AND RISK FACTORS

Ultraviolet Light Exposure

The demographic features of cutaneous melanoma have implicated UV light exposure as a major etiologic factor in the development of melanoma. Multiple studies continue to support an etiologic association between UV irradiation and melanoma.[32] UVC radiation is generally absorbed by the ozone layer. UVB radiation (290 to 320 nm) is associated with sunburn and induction of tanning by melanin pigment production. There are substantial data to support its etiologic role in melanoma.[32] There is also some evidence implicating UVA radiation (320 to 400 nm), although UVA is more associated with chronic sun damage changes.[33] However, the relative role of each type of UV irradiation in melanoma etiology is debated. Animal data suggests that sun exposure early in life increases the risk of melanoma. Human skin grafted on mice will develop nevi and melanomas in the presence of UVB irradiation, further supporting the role of UVB irradiation in melanoma.[34] Similar to the animal modeling, sunburns early in life have been implicated in melanoma incidence.[35] However, chronic sun exposure in individuals who tan well may even be protected against melanoma. The role of sunlight intensity and frequency is debated, but both chronic and intermittent exposure may be relevant.[32] Current data suggest that UV radiation causes melanoma by a combination of DNA damage, inflammation, and immune suppression.[36]

Tanning bed use has been implicated in the etiology of melanoma, in particular tanning bed use in adolescence or early adulthood.[37] Tanning bed use has been formally classified as a carcinogen, and increased awareness of the harmful effects of UV exposure promise to control the increase in melanoma incidence.

Physical Traits

Several physical traits have been linked to increased incidence of cutaneous melanoma. These include blond or red hair, green or blue eyes, presence of multiple (>100) melanocytic nevi, and five or more atypical nevi. A prior diagnosis of melanoma is associated with an eight-fold increased risk of developing a secondary melanoma.

Familial Predisposition

It has been estimated that 5% of melanomas occur in high-risk families with an autosomal dominant inheritance with incomplete penetrance.[38] The most frequent and highest penetrance melanoma susceptibility gene is a germline mutation in CD-KN2A, a tumor suppressor gene that encodes for two different proteins, p16INK4A and p14 ARF.[39] These proteins control cell cycle progression and apoptosis, and have roles in correcting DNA damage and cellular senescence. CDKN2A mutations have been reported in approximately 25% of melanoma-prone families, but this frequency varies highly on the selection criteria used and the region of the world where it is studied. The rare autosomal dominant inherited familial atypical multiple mole melanoma-pancreatic cancer syndrome is associated with CDKN2A mutations, and less frequently to BRCA2 mutations.[40] Another germline mutation linked to familial melanoma is cyclin-dependent kinase 4, which is linked to the function and p16INK4A and controls the retinoblastoma pathway. A germline mutation in microphthalmia-associated transcription factor (*MITF* E318K) represents a medium-penetrance susceptibility gene predisposing to familial melanoma, as well as to sporadic melanoma and renal cell carcinoma.[41,42] The E318K mutation in MITF disrupts sumoylation and enhances transcription of MITF-responsive genes. Other common risk factors include dysplastic nevus syndrome, xeroderma pigmentosum, and a family history of melanoma even without the known genetic traits. The association of melanoma with Li-Fraumeni syndrome, with germline mutations in p53, is currently unclear.[43]

Pregnancy and Estrogen Use

Older literature suggested anecdotally that the incidence of melanoma was higher in pregnant females and that they had a particularly bad outcome. However, multiple systematic and larger studies have shown no evidence of any negative (or positive) impact of prior, concurrent, or subsequent pregnancy on clinical outcome.[44,45] Similarly, there is no clear prognostic relevance for birth control pills or estrogen replacement therapy.[46] The prior sense of an apparent association of pregnancy and melanoma may be due to melanoma being the second most frequent cancer in females of childbearing age. The general recommendation for treatment of women with melanoma diagnosed during pregnancy is to manage them in the same fashion as patients who are not pregnant. Depending on the time during pregnancy at which a melanoma is diagnosed, there can be circumstances in which radiologic imaging may be limited because of concern for the fetus, and major surgery may be delayed until the fetus is at an age when it can survive independently. However, the excision of a primary melanoma certainly can be done in almost any circumstance, under local anesthesia.

The other related question often asked by patients is whether it is advisable to become pregnant and to bear a child after treatment for melanoma. As just stated, there is no evidence that a subsequent pregnancy adversely impacts outcome. However, the more interesting and challenging question is the more personal or social issue of the potential for premature parental death due to melanoma. Thus, it is helpful for patients to understand their risk of future recurrence and melanoma-related mortality because that translates into the risk that the child will grow up losing a parent. Measures of the risk of future disease progression can be defined based on the initial prognosis and the subsequent elapsed time without recurrence, and such information may help to guide patients with this challenging question.[47]

PREVENTION AND SCREENING

Melanomas diagnosed and treated during the RGP have an excellent prognosis. Thus, prevention and early diagnosis can have a great impact on decreasing melanoma morbidity and mortality. The apparent leveling off of melanoma-related mortality rates in Australia and the United States likely is the result of better screening and prevention.

Sun Protection

UV exposure and sunburns, in particular, appear to be etiologic in most melanomas. Thus, protection from UV light, especially in fair-skinned individuals, is believed to have substantial benefit in preventing melanoma.

A clinical trial has provided evidence that regular sunscreen use helps prevent melanoma.[48] This was a randomized trial from March 1992 to August 1996 of 1,621 randomly selected adult residents of a Queensland township in Australia with an initial primary end point testing the prevention of squamous cell and basal cell carcinomas, which the study did demonstrate.[49] Prevention of the development of melanoma was a prespecified secondary end point. Participants were randomly assigned to either a planned sunscreen intervention group or a control group using sunscreen at their discretion. The intervention group received broad-spectrum, sun protection factor (SPF) 16 sunscreen every morning, and was instructed to reapply the sunscreen after a long sun exposure, heavy sweating, or after bathing. After a 10-year follow-up, regular sunscreen use decreased by half the rate of developing new melanomas. This conclusion was based on 11 participants in the intervention group and 22 in the control group being newly diagnosed with either invasive or in situ melanoma ($p = 0.051$). The incidence of invasive melanoma decreased by 73% in the intervention group compared with the control group (3 versus 11 patients, respectively; $p = 0.045$). Therefore, this study provides evidence that use of sunscreen can decrease the incidence of melanoma development.

There are limitations inherent in sunscreen use as the primary means to protecting from UV light damage. One is that certain body sites are not easily covered with sunscreen, such as the scalp. More important, even "waterproof" sunscreens wash off or become less effective with time. Most people also forget to reapply sunscreens frequently enough and may still get burns. There are also sociologic issues, which may differ for different populations and are arguable. However, it is worth considering the provocative findings of a study performed on young adults from Western Europe, who were randomized to receive either SPF10 or SPF30 sunscreen. In a blinded fashion, they were asked to report sun exposure times and sunburns. The number of sunburns was the same in both groups, and sun exposure was greater in the SPF30

group, suggesting that some populations may stay in the sun until they get a burn, and that sunscreen simply helps them to stay in the sun longer.[50] The sun-seeking behavior has been related to an evolutionary need that favored UV exposure to make vitamin D in the skin in populations that migrated to areas of the world with lower sun exposure. In mouse models, the exposure to UV light was linked to increased production of beta-endorphins and recurrent seeking of UV exposure.[51]

It is safe to say that the best protection from the sun is a building, the next best is protective clothing, and the third best is sunscreen. Patients should be advised to use all three. Avoiding midday sun from about 11 a.m. to 3 p.m. by staying indoors is advised, as well as wearing clothing with a thick enough weave that it blocks sunlight, or a formal SPF rating, when possible. Hats are particularly helpful for the face and scalp, which often are highly exposed to sunlight and not so readily covered fully with sunscreen. Otherwise, sunscreen can provide protection to sun-exposed areas when outside.

Screening for Early Diagnosis

Self-Examination

For many patients, they, their spouses, or other family members may be able to screen effectively for new suspicious skin lesions, and this should be encouraged. It is more common for women to detect melanomas than for men to do so, either for themselves or for their partners. In any case, there is value in educating patients about how to detect melanomas if they are at high risk. As many as half of melanomas are identified by the patient or family,[52] and patient self-examination has been associated with diagnosis of thinner melanomas.[53] Teaching aids for patients on how to perform skin self-examination are available from the American Cancer Society and the American Academy of Dermatology. Patients with melanoma or at high risk should be seen regularly by a dermatologist. It is reasonable to suggest that patients perform skin self-examinations more often than their dermatology visits, although there are no proven guidelines. Doing a self-examination once a month may be the easiest for the patient to remember.

The role of skin cancer screening to decrease incidence and mortality from cutaneous melanoma has been prospectively studied in the Schleswig-Holstein project.[54] This was an observational study comparing trends in melanoma mortality in a population-based skin cancer screening project conducted in the northern German region of Schleswig-Holstein, compared to neighboring regions in Germany and Denmark where no such screening was conducted. From July 1, 2003, to June 30, 2004, 360,288 individuals aged 20 years were screened by whole-body examination. They reported that mortality in Schleswig-Holstein melanoma declined by 48% when analyzed using log-linear regression to assess mortality trends. No such change in melanoma mortality rates was noted in the studied adjacent regions. This study provides strong evidence that skin cancer screening programs may reduce melanoma mortality.[54]

Management of the Patient with Numerous Atypical Moles

Some patients have numerous atypical moles. This presentation is commonly described as atypical mole syndrome, dysplastic nevus syndrome, or B-K mole syndrome.[55] These patients have a heightened risk of melanoma, and this is commonly a familial feature. When associated with a family history of melanoma, patients with dysplastic nevus syndrome have a risk of melanoma that may approach 100%. These patients deserve particular attention to melanoma prevention through sun protection and to early diagnosis through aggressive screening. However, the optimal approach for screening is not defined. At a minimum, routine skin examinations by a dermatologist are usually recommended, as often as every 3 months. Visual inspection of the atypical nevi may be augmented by routine digital photography to facilitate detection of subtle changes in radial growth or other changes over time. Although these approaches commonly permit identification of melanomas when they are in situ or thin, it is not known whether they improve survival. In addition, concern remains that visual inspection alone, even for very experienced dermatologists, is inadequate to diagnose all melanomas when they are still curable. Thus, substantial effort is in progress to develop more sensitive and specific diagnostic tools than visual inspection alone. One that is employed routinely in many practices is dermoscopy, also known as epiluminescent microscopy. This involves use of a handheld microscope at the bedside to examine skin lesions in an oil immersion setting. This appears to improve diagnostic accuracy in experienced hands, and increasing experience has made its use more feasible in general practice, especially with considerations for standardization.[56,57] When coupled with the use of a digital camera, the images can be stored and compared over time as well. Computer-assisted digital analysis of these images is also being studied but remains investigational.

Evaluation and management of patients with dysplastic nevus syndrome is complicated by the fact that very few dysplastic nevi will develop into melanoma. Estimates range from a risk of 1 per 1,000 nevi examined in a pigmented lesion clinic being melanoma to 1 per 10,000 nevi becoming melanoma per year.[56,57] Recommendations for management of dysplastic nevi include those from the Melanoma Working Group in the Netherlands and by a National Institutes of Health Consensus Conference.[58]

It is tempting to consider excision of all dysplastic nevi. Although that remains an option, there is no proof that this will decrease risk. Melanomas may arise de novo in 30% to 70% of cases, and so it is not clear that removal of all suspicious nevi will lead to a meaningful improvement in survival. However, it is certainly appropriate to biopsy any nevus that is suspicious, especially one that is changing.

Testing for Genomic Changes in Melanoma

Understanding the genetic makeup of melanoma has become the cornerstone of advances in the management of advanced disease, and it is likely to have an increasing role in the management of earlier stage melanoma. Genetic analyses can be focused on driver oncogenic events or can provide a broader understanding of the genomic aberrations in the cancer. Their study is becoming a standard of care practice in melanoma.

Commercially available tests identifying the BRAF V600E/K mutation have been approved by the U.S. Food and Drug Administration (FDA) and other regulatory bodies as companion diagnostics for the use of novel BRAF and MEK inhibitors. These assays are frequently based on specific PCR probes labeled with fluorescent tags that bind to wild-type and V600E or V600K mutant BRAF sequences. These assays are performed in sections of formalin-fixed paraffin embedded tissue blocks routinely used for pathologic analyses. As with all techniques used to detect somatic mutations, they are limited by the amount of mutant sequence in the initial sample as well as DNA integrity in the sample, and their ability to detect non-V600E BRAF mutations since the primers used are usually restricted to this particular BRAF mutation. Multiplexed single nucleotide extension assays (i.e., Sequenom [San Diego, CA] or SNaPshot [Vanderbilt-Ingram Cancer Center, Nashville, TN]) evaluate a list of specific base mutations of interest, but do not identify mutations outside the interrogated bases. These techniques are designed for simultaneous interrogation of different point mutations. They are particularly suited for the targeted interrogation of known oncogenes that contain mutation hotspots, such as NRAS, BRAF, and GNAQ/GNA11, being relevant for melanoma.[59]

Traditional Sanger sequencing has been the gold standard for the detection of point mutations, but it has been shown to have lower sensitivity than the PCR-based assays, thereby leading to a higher frequency of false negative results. Pyrosequencing provides information from the sequencing 300 and 500 nucleotides at a time, resulting useful for the analysis of mutations clustered in a small gene region. It is a highly sensitive technique, being able to detect mutant DNA when only 5% of the total sample is from the cancer tissue.

Copy number analyses have been very useful in the discovery and description of genes and pathways involved in melanoma pathogenesis. Initially, probe sequences were derived from bacterial artificial chromosomes using array comparative genomic hybridization. More recently, single nucleotide polymorphism–based arrays have been introduced. But currently the approach of choice for the analysis of the DNA alterations in melanoma at the genome level is massively parallel sequencing techniques. These techniques enable the sequencing of exomes and entire genomes of tumor samples (compared to normal DNA from the same patient), with the simultaneous sequencing of a large number of genes and determination of mutations, genetic alterations, and copy number changes. The price and complexity of this type of analysis has rapidly improved, making it feasible to use beyond research studies. Limited panels performing next generation sequencing in what have been called "actionable" genes have been implemented for clinical use. These provide information based on sequencing data of 200 or so genes for which the available literature suggests that they could provide information which may be interpretable to decide on treatment options, in particular in terms of clinical trial participation with new targeted agents.[60]

A clinically applicable approach to genetic testing of melanomas is first performing a targeted testing for the mutation status of BRAF, NRAS, and KIT in cutaneous and mucosal melanoma samples before pursuing alternative mutation interrogation with higher throughput approaches. Next-generation sequencing may be applicable in situations where known mutations are not identified, and the identification of additional genetic mutations is needed.

DIAGNOSIS OF PRIMARY MELANOMA

Characteristics of Primary Melanoma

The classic appearance of primary cutaneous melanoma is summarized by the mnemonic ABCD for asymmetry, border irregularity, color variation, and diameter >6 mm (see Fig. 94.3). Because melanomas arise from melanocytes, which contain the melanin-synthetic pathway, melanomas classically are distinguished by their pigmentation. Melanomas may have shades of brown, black, blue, red, and white. However, there is a wide range in the appearance of melanomas. Some melanomas are pitch black. Others are shades of brown. Some have no visible pigment and appear skin-colored. Still others have a red color only. When melanomas have all of the classic ABCD features, they are typically easy to diagnose. However, those melanomas that lack some of these features can be difficult to diagnose. In addition, in patients with large numbers of atypical nevi, which may also have ABCD features, this mnemonic is often inadequate to aid in early diagnosis. The other important findings that may aid in early diagnosis are a change in a lesion over time or new development of a skin lesion. These warrant evaluation, and in high-risk patients there should be a low threshold for biopsy. In addition, some dermatologists recommend considering the "ugly duckling" sign: A lesion that stands out as different from the patient's other nevi should be evaluated and possibly biopsied.[61] This can be particularly helpful in a patient with a large number of clinically atypical nevi. Both of these approaches may help to identify amelanotic (nonpigmented) melanomas, which often do not meet the ABCD criteria. Some melanomas are not diagnosed until they become symptomatic, and whereas awareness of the symptoms of bleeding, itching, pain, and ulceration are worth noting, these usually connote deep vertical growth and are hallmarks of a late diagnosis, not an early one.

Biopsy

Biopsy of a suspicious skin lesion is necessary for an accurate diagnosis and for optimal staging. The correct way to perform such a biopsy is to make a full-thickness biopsy of the entire lesion, with a narrow (1 to 2 mm) margin of grossly normal skin. The depth of excision should include the full thickness of dermis and thus should extend into the subcutaneous tissue, but it does not need to include all of the subcutaneous tissue except in very thin patients or patients with very thick polypoid lesions that may go deep into the subcutis. This allows assessment of the architecture of the lesion, which is critical for differentiation of melanoma from Spitz nevus, and it permits an accurate measure of tumor thickness, which is critical for prognosis and affects the surgical treatment recommendations. Of importance, desmoplastic melanoma often arises from LMM and is difficult to diagnose both clinically and histologically. Shave biopsies of these lesions can often lead to failure to appreciate the desmoplastic melanoma in the dermis and may substantially delay diagnosis.

For some large lesions (e.g., >2 cm diameter) in cosmetically sensitive locations (e.g., face or genitalia), there may be a rationale for an incisional biopsy, but that also should be performed as a full-thickness skin biopsy. Ideally, it should include the most suspicious area of the lesion and also should include, if possible, a portion of the edge of the lesion where it transitions to normal skin to enable assessment of the junctional change. The incisional biopsy may be an elliptical incision or it may be a full-thickness 4- to 6-mm punch biopsy. Punch biopsies are problematic if too small, if they do not include full-thickness skin, if they are crushed during removal, if they are oriented inaccurately in the paraffin block, or if they are too small to include both the edge of the lesion and the most suspicious or most raised part of the lesion.

Orientation of the incision used for an excisional biopsy should be considered in the context of the prospect for the future need for a wider re-excision. On extremities, the incision and scar should be oriented longitudinally rather than transversely, although some exceptions may be considered near joints to avoid crossing a joint. When in doubt about the optimal orientation, it is very reasonable to perform the excisional biopsy as a simple circular excision, leaving the wound open for secondary or delayed primary closure.

Biopsy of subungual lesions is more challenging. The pigmentary changes seen in patients with subungual melanoma usually extend along the length of the nail, but the lesions usually arise at the proximal end of the nail bed. Access to that location often requires removal of all or a large part of the nail. One or more punch biopsies of the base of the nail bed often constitute the most realistic method for obtaining a biopsy of such lesions, and it may need to be repeated to be diagnostic. A punch biopsy tool can remove a circle of the nail, providing access to the nail bed for punch biopsy of the suspicious area.

Melanoma Subtypes: Histologic Growth Patterns

Classically, four main histologic growth patterns are described for melanomas, but two others are also worth mentioning.

Superficial Spreading Melanoma

The most common type is superficial spreading melanoma, which accounts for about 70% of primary cutaneous melanomas (see Fig. 94.3C). It is typical for the trunk and extremities, except on acral sites. It is associated with pagetoid growth of atypical melanocytes in the epidermis. Superficial spreading melanoma is commonly associated with sun exposure.

Nodular Melanoma

Nodular melanomas lack an RGP, may be nonpigmented, and commonly are diagnosed when relatively thick. Thus, these carry the worst prognosis of the various subtypes of melanoma. They account for about 20% of cutaneous melanomas. By definition, nodular melanomas are in VGP when recognized.

Acral Lentiginous Melanoma

ALMs account for <5% of melanomas.[62] They are typically found on acral sites (subungual, palmar, plantar) and on mucosal surfaces (anorectal, nasopharyngeal, female genital tract). ALM occurs across all races and ethnicities. Its etiology is likely independent of UV light exposure. Because other cutaneous melanomas are uncommon in African, Asian, and Hispanic populations, ALMs on acral sites are proportionally more common in these populations than in fair-skinned whites. ALM is typically associated with a prolonged RGP before vertical growth; however, its locations make it harder to diagnose than other forms of melanoma. Subungual lesions can be detected by linear pigment streaks arising from the base of the nail, but these are not always evident. They can be confused with subungual hematomas, which can lead to diagnostic delay. When there is a question of whether a pigmented subungual lesion may be melanoma or a hematoma, the location of the pigment can be marked and then followed over a short interval (e.g., 3 weeks), during which time a hematoma should move toward the end of the nail, but a melanoma should not.

Subungual melanomas can also present with breakage of the nail or a nonpigmented thickening or drainage, and these are often confused with chronic fungal infections. Any concerning pigmented subungual lesion should be biopsied, but it is sometimes challenging and requires splitting or removing part of the nail. A punch biopsy near the nail bed matrix is often appropriate. In addition, when there is spontaneous chronic inflammation or breakage of the nail, biopsy for melanoma should be considered, even in the absence of pigmentation.

Lentigo Maligna Melanoma

LMMs typically occur in older individuals, in chronically sun-damaged skin, and commonly on the face. They tend to have shades of brown or black, whereas the red and blue colors seen in other melanomas are not typical of LMM. They may also develop areas of regression manifested by depigmentation of part of the lesion. Overall, LMMs account for about 10% to 20% of melanomas in the National Cancer Database experience,[1] 47% of melanomas of the head and neck, and only 2% of melanomas of other regions.[62] LMMs usually have an extensive RGP that extends for many years before developing invasion. When melanoma is just in situ, this RGP portion is called *lentigo maligna* or Hutchinson freckle, as opposed to LMM. These are not to be confused with the benign pigmented macule, lentigo. Lentigo malignas evolve a VGP to become invasive LMMs at a rate estimated to be between 5% and 33%.[63] LMMs are commonly diagnosed as thin lesions. However, more substantial vertical growth can occur, as seen in Figure 94.3A.

Lentiginous Melanoma

Early RGP melanomas sometimes are difficult to classify into the typical patterns of lentigo maligna, superficial spreading melanoma, or ALM. A report defined a distinct entity of lentiginous melanoma. Its features include diameter ≥1 cm, elongated and irregular rete ridges, confluent melanocytic nests and single cells over a broad area of the dermal/epidermal junction, focal pagetoid spread, cytologic atypia, and possible focal dermal fibrosis.[64] Over time, this may represent a growing proportion of melanomas that have traditionally been grouped as superficial spreading melanoma, lentigo maligna, ALM, or unclassified melanomas.

Desmoplastic Melanoma

Desmoplastic melanoma is an uncommon form of melanoma, histologically manifest by dermal melanocytes in a dense stromal response. These lesions are usually nonpigmented and usually have lost the melanin production pathway. They usually stain negative for MART-1/MelanA, gp100, and tyrosinase, but they do stain for S100. The lack of pigmentation and the dense stromal response often interfere with clinical and histologic diagnosis. It occurs most commonly in the head and neck, but it may occur in other body sites.[65] Desmoplastic melanoma may appear de novo as a nonpigmented skin papule or as a dermal/VGP component arising from a preexisting lentigo maligna or other pigmented junctional lesion. Desmoplastic melanomas may have neurotropic features and have been associated with a high rate of local recurrence.[66] However, recent reports suggest that if adequate margins are taken, the risk of local recurrence is low.

The overall mortality risk for desmoplastic melanomas is comparable to that of other invasive melanomas of similar depth of invasion.[67] Multiple studies support the contention that desmoplastic melanomas have a significantly lower risk of nodal metastases than other melanomas,[68–72] with only 1.4% sentinel node positivity among 155 patients with pure desmoplastic melanoma, compared with 18.5% in those with mixed desmoplastic melanoma.[67,68,71,72] There has been a debate about whether to abandon histologic staging of regional nodes in patients with desmoplastic melanoma.[69] It may be appropriate to consider a higher threshold for performing sentinel node biopsy (SNBx) in patients with pure desmoplastic melanoma, but there is no consensus on this question.

Prognostic Factors for Primary Melanomas

The best predictor of metastatic risk is the depth of invasion, measured with an ocular micrometer, from the granular layer of the skin to the base of the primary lesion. This was originally described by Breslow[73] and remains an important factor in staging and prognostic stratification. However, many other histologic and clinical features have relevance for estimating the risk of future metastasis and mortality. These include age, angiolymphatic invasion, mitotic rate, gender, and body site.

Depth of Invasion

Breslow thickness is the depth of invasion measured from the granular layer of the epidermis to the base of the lesion. Melanoma cells involving adnexal structures are considered junctional and are not included in the Breslow depth. The current melanoma staging system of the American Joint Committee on Cancer (AJCC) identifies tumor (T) stage based on Breslow thickness such that T1 lesions are <1 mm thick, T2 lesions are 1 to 2 mm thick, T3 lesions are 2 to 4 mm thick, and T4 lesions are >4 mm thick.[74]

Clark et al.[75] defined depth based on the layer of skin to which the melanoma has invaded. Clark level I melanomas are melanomas in situ, limited to the epidermis or dermal/epidermal junction. Clark level II melanomas invade into the superficial (papillary) dermis, and these are usually RGP lesions. Clark level III melanomas fill the papillary dermis. Clark level IV melanomas invade into the deep (reticular) dermis and have significant metastatic risk. Clark level V melanomas are uncommon and contain invasion into the subcutaneous fat.

It has become apparent that Clark level does not add much additional prognostic value to Breslow thickness and has been removed from the 2010 version of the AJCC staging system.[74] Breslow thickness has an effect on survival, local, regional, and systemic recurrence rates, and that association is continuous, without any apparent breakpoints. Although the staging system requires categorization of thickness ranges, the continuous nature of the risk association should be kept in mind. Thickness is considered in defining the margins of excision for primary melanomas.[76,77]

Ulceration

Ulceration of the primary lesion has been identified as an important negative prognostic feature[76] and is incorporated in the current

staging system such that T1a, T2a, T3a, and T4a melanomas are nonulcerated, and T1b, T2b, T3b, and T4b melanomas are ulcerated. In an analysis of prognostic features in a large multicenter database, the prognosis of an ulcerated lesion was comparable to that of a nonulcerated lesion one T level higher. Thus, the overall stage assignment groups ulcerated lesions with nonulcerated lesions one T level higher (e.g., T2b and T3a are both stage IIA). The staging system is summarized in Tables 94.1 and 94.2 and is described in detail elsewhere.[74]

Patient Gender and Skin Location of Primary Melanoma

The incidence of melanoma is higher for men than women overall, but in adolescents and young adults it is more common in women.[25] Furthermore, for essentially all patient subgroups, the prognosis is better for women than men. Thus, among patients with stage III and IV melanoma, men outnumber women approximately 1.5:1. Women are more likely to have melanomas on the extremities, whereas men are more likely to have melanomas on the trunk and head and neck. The clinical outcome for patients with melanomas on extremities is better than that for patients with truncal or head-and-neck melanomas; thus, the prognostic impact of gender is difficult to distinguish from the impact of tumor location. There may still be, however, a prognostic benefit for female gender independent of tumor location.[76,78] In addition, location of tumors has prognostic relevance in that head-and-neck melanomas have poorer prognosis than trunk or extremity melanomas, and melanomas on acral sites have poorer prognosis than other extremity melanomas.[78,79] A particular location associated with poor prognosis is the mucosal melanoma. Anorectal, female genital, and head-and-neck melanomas of mucosal origin have a mortality risk of 68% to 89% over 5 years.[1,79,80]

Patient Age

The impact of age on prognosis is confusing. There is a greater risk of lymph node metastasis in young patients at the time of SNBx,[81] especially for patients younger than age 35 years, but the melanoma-associated mortality risk increases with age for all thickness ranges.[1,76] This paradox has not been explained. It suggests a possible age-specific curative potential for patients with micrometastatic nodal disease. Alternatively, it is worth considering that the attribution of mortality to melanoma progression is not always straightforward. Older patients have other competing causes for death that could lead to earlier mortality in the presence of metastatic disease. Nonetheless, age does appear to have independent prognostic significance for patients with melanoma.

Growth Pattern

Overall, nodular melanomas have the worst prognosis, associated with their diagnosis at a thicker stage. Lesser risk is associated with ALM, superficial spreading melanoma, and LMM, in that order, all associated with decreasing average Breslow thickness. Generally, the histologic growth pattern of melanoma has little prognostic relevance when Breslow thickness is taken into account. The VGP component appears to be the component of melanoma that determines metastatic risk, and these VGP components are similar, independent of the growth phase in the RGP component. LMMs are a possible exception, in that they appear to have a better prognosis than other histologic types, independent of thickness. Desmoplastic melanoma, superficial spreading melanoma, LMM, and ALM have comparable prognosis, for distant metastases and survival, when stratified by thickness.[68,81]

Mitotic Rate

It is reasonable to expect that the growth rate of melanomas is linked to the rate of tumor cell division. Accordingly, mitotic rate in the dermal component has been identified as a negative

TABLE 94.1

Melanoma Tumor, Node, Metastasis Classification

T Classification	Thickness (mm)	Ulceration Status	Mitotic Rate
TX	Unknown	—	—
T0	No evidence of primary tumor	—	—
Tis	Melanoma in situ	—	—
T1a	≤1.0	No	$<1/mm^2$
T1b	≤1.0	Yes	$≥1/mm^2$
T2a	1.01–2.0	No	Any
T2b	1.01–2.0	Yes	Any
T3a	2.01–4.0	No	Any
T3b	2.01–4.0	Yes	Any
T4a	>4.0	No	Any
T4b	>4.0	Yes	Any

N Classification	No. Nodes with Metastasis	Presentation	In Transit or Satellite Metastasis(es)
NX	Not assessable	—	—
N0	0	—	No
N1a	1	Clinically undetectable[a]	No
N1b	1	Clinically detectable[b]	No
N2a	2–3	Clinically undetectable[a]	No
N2b	2–3	Clinically detectable[b]	No
N2c	0	—	Yes
N3	≥4 or matted	—	—
N3	≥1	Any	Yes

M Classification	Metastatic Site	Serum LDH Level	
M0	None detected	—	
M1a	Distant skin, subcutaneous or node	Normal	
M1b	Lung	Normal	
M1c	All other visceral	Normal	
M1c	Any	Elevated	

LDH, lactate dehydrogenase.
[a] Clinically undetectable nodes are those diagnosed only with sentinel node biopsy or elective lymphadenectomy, and lacking gross extracapsular extension. They are referred to also as micrometastases, but this definition differs from the pathologist's definition of a micrometastasis as one that is <2 mm in diameter.
[b] Clinically detectable nodes are also referred to as macrometastases, but this is a different definition than the pathologist's definition based on a diameter >2 mm. Patients with gross extracapsular extension are also considered to have macrometasetasis.
Modified from Edge S, Byrd DR, Compton CC, et al., (eds.). *AJCC Cancer Staging Manual.* 7th ed. New York: Springer; 2010.

prognostic feature, especially with six or more mitoses per square millimeter.[81,82] Similarly, dermal expression of Ki67, a molecular marker of proliferation, is associated with greater risk of metastasis.[83] For thin melanomas, the presence of any mitotic figures has been associated with metastatic risk, whereas the absence of dermal mitoses is associated with an excellent prognosis.[84] The current staging system incorporates mitotic rate of $≥1/mm^2$ in differentiating low-risk thin melanomas (T1a) from higher-risk thin melanomas (T1b), and data used to define the current staging system identify increasing risk with increasing mitotic rate for all thicknesses.[74] Increased mitotic rate is associated with a poorer prognosis across all thickness ranges, but is not yet incorporated formally in the staging system beyond the current cutoff of $1/mm^2$ for thin lesions.[74,85,86]

Other Prognostic Factors

There is also evidence, and biologic rationale, that angiolymphatic invasion has negative prognostic significance,[81] and that microscopic satellites are associated with poorer prognosis. Satellitosis is incorporated in the current staging system[74] but will be considered separately because it defines the patient as stage III and thus goes beyond assessment of risk factors of the primary lesion alone.

Unresolved Issues in Melanoma Staging

The AJCC staging system is evidence-based and accounts for several important clinical and histopathologic findings. However,

TABLE 94.2

Pathologic Stage Grouping for Cutaneous Melanoma

	Clinical Staging[a]				Pathologic Staging[b]			Five-Year Survival (%)	Ten-Year Survival (%)
0	Tis	N0	M0	0	Tis	N0	M0	>99	>99
IA	T1a	N0	M0	IA	T1a	N0	M0	95	88
IB	T1b	N0	M0	IB	T1b	N0	M0	91	83
	T2a	N0	M0		T2a	N0	M0	89	79
IIA	T2b	N0	M0	IIA	T2b	N0	M0	77	64
	T3a	N0	M0		T3a	N0	M0	79	64
IIB	T3b	N0	M0	IIB	T3b	N0	M0	63	51
	T4a	N0	M0		T4a	N0	M0	67	54
IIC	T4b	N0	M0	IIC	T4b	N0	M0	45	32
III	Any T	N1–3	M0	IIIA	T1a–T4a	N1a	M0	82	63
					T1a–T4a	N2a	M0	73	57
				IIIB	T1b–T4b	N1a	M0	57	38
					T1b–T4b	N2a	M0	54	36
					T1a–T4a	N1b	M0	52	48
					T1a–T4a	N2b	M0	47	39
					T1a–T4a	N2c	M0	N/A	N/A
				IIIC	T1b–T4b	N1b	M0	49	24
					T1b–T4b	N2b	M0	38	15
					T1b–T4b	N2c	M0	N/A	N/A
					Any T	N3	M0	27	18
IV	Any T	Any N	Any M	IV	Any T	Any N	M1a	19	16
					Any T	Any N	M1b	7	3
					Any T	*Any N*	*M1c*	*10*	*6*

N/A, not available.
[a] Clinical staging includes microstaging of the primary melanoma and clinical-radiologic evaluation for metastases. By convention, it should be done after complete excision of the primary melanoma with clinical assessment for regional and distant metastases.
[b] Pathologic staging includes microstaging of the primary melanoma and pathologic information about the regional lymph nodes after partial or complete lymphadenectomy. Pathologic stage 0 or stage IA tumors are the exception; they do not require pathological evaluation of the lymph nodes.
Modified from Edge S, Byrd DR, Compton CC, et al., (eds.). *AJCC Cancer Staging Manual.* 7th ed. New York: Springer; 2010.

several clinical settings are not fully addressed by the AJCC staging system. These include the following.

Positive Deep Margin on Biopsy

When a primary melanoma is diagnosed by shave biopsy, and the tumor extends to the deep margin, it is presumed that the melanoma was deeper than the original measured biopsy depth. Sometimes, on wide local excision there is residual melanoma with a greater depth than on the original biopsy. In that setting, it is appropriate to define the T stage based on the latter depth of invasion. However, in many cases, the wide excision does not reveal any more melanoma, or may reveal tumor that is more superficial. It is generally assumed that in those cases, any residual melanoma at the deep margin may have been destroyed by inflammatory changes after the biopsy. One approach for defining T stage in that setting is to call it TX. The other is to use the T stage of the original depth, even though that is incomplete. The latter has the advantage of distinguishing thin melanomas (e.g., a clinically thin melanoma with thickness <1 mm) from a thick melanoma (e.g., a 5-mm melanoma on shave biopsy, with positive deep margin). Thus, use of TX results in substantial loss of information for patients and their clinicians.

Local Recurrence After Original Incomplete Excision

Some patients present with melanoma after excisional biopsy or destruction (e.g., cryotherapy) of a pigmented skin lesion that was believed to be benign (clinically or histologically) on initial review. When such a lesion recurs and is found to contain melanoma, re-review of the original biopsy is appropriate, if available. Staging of such recurrent melanomas, when the original lesion was not known to be melanoma, is not well addressed.

Skin or Subcutaneous Lesion Without Junctional Involvement and Without Known Primary Melanoma

This is addressed later in this chapter. Cutaneous or subcutaneous nodules that occur in the absence of junctional melanocytic change, and in the absence of any other known primary, are among the most interesting presentations of melanoma. They may be in-transit metastases from primary melanomas that spontaneously regressed (stage IIIB), primary melanomas that arose from dermal nevi or that persisted in the dermis after arising from a partially regressed primary melanoma (stage IIB), or a distant metastasis from an unknown primary melanoma (stage IV, M1a). A review of experience with these lesions at the University of Michigan suggests that they behave more like primary tumors arising in the dermis or subcutaneous tissue.[76] In the current staging system, these are considered stage III.

GENERAL CONSIDERATIONS IN CLINICAL MANAGEMENT OF A NEWLY DIAGNOSED CUTANEOUS MELANOMA (STAGE I–II)

Most melanomas present as clinically localized lesions without clinical or radiologic evidence of metastatic disease. Nonetheless, some of these patients have occult metastases, and the definitive surgical management includes both therapeutic resection and pathologic staging evaluation for regional metastases. The vast majority of primary melanomas are diagnosed on histologic assessment of skin biopsy performed by a dermatologist or a primary care practitioner. The patient then presents to a surgeon or other physician for definitive treatment.

Clinical Evaluation and Radiologic Studies for Patients with Clinical Stage I–II Melanoma

In patients with clinically localized melanoma, there is a wide range of clinical practice in the appropriate radiologic staging studies to be performed. Certainly all patients with such disease should have a complete history and physical examination, with attention to symptoms that may represent metastatic melanoma, including headaches, bone pain, weight loss, gastrointestinal symptoms, and any new physical complaints. Physical examination should carefully assess the site of the primary melanoma for clinical evidence of persistent disease and should evaluate the skin of the entire region (e.g., whole extremity or quadrant of torso, or side of the face) for dermal or subcutaneous nodules that could represent satellite or in-transit metastases. Biopsy should be done for any suspicious lesions and with a very low threshold for biopsy. In addition, physical examination should include thorough evaluation of both the major regional nodal basins (e.g., epitrochlear and axillary for a forearm melanoma) and also any atypical lymph node locations, such as the triangular intermuscular space on the back for upper back primaries.

There is a great deal of uncertainty and debate about appropriate initial staging studies. NCCN Clinical Practice Guidelines in Oncology (NCCN Guidelines®) from 2013 recommend no staging radiographs or blood work for melanoma in situ, and recommend imaging for low-risk thin melanomas (stage IA) "only to evaluate specific signs or symptoms." For clinical stage I–II, no other imaging is recommended. For stage III melanoma, consideration of imaging is recommended, to include chest radiograph (CXR), computed tomography (CT) scans, or positron emission tomography (PET)/CT scans, with consideration of magnetic resonance imaging (MRI) of the brain, and other imaging is suggested only as clinically indicated. More complete staging studies are suggested for stage III melanoma.[87]

CXR for asymptomatic patients with a new diagnosis of clinically localized melanoma yielded suspicious findings in 15% of patients, of whom only 0.1% had a true unsuspected lung metastasis.[88] In a similar study, the yield of true positive CXR was 0% of 248 patients.[89] In patients with stage IIB melanoma, initial staging CT scans identified occult metastasis that changed management in 0.7% of patients.[90] Even in patients with positive SNBx, staging PET scan identified no melanoma metastases in 30 patients, even though there were lymph node metastases in 16% of cases.[91] In patients with clinical T1b–T3b melanomas, true positive rates for all imaging studies was 0.3%, and false-positive rates were 50% to 100% for CXR, 88% for CT and PET/CT scans.[92] Thus, there is a large body of data that argues that

CXR, CT, and PET/CT are all of little or no value in initial staging of melanoma stage 0–IIIA.

PET with fluorodeoxyglucose (FDG) has a role in staging patients with advanced melanoma,[93] but its role in earlier-stage disease is less clear both because it is expensive and because it is associated with substantial radiation exposure. In one study, patients with clinically localized melanomas >1 mm thick, with local recurrence, or solitary in-transit metastases, FDG-PET scanning was performed prior to sentinel node biopsy. Sensitivity for detection of sentinel nodes was only 21%, although specificity was high (97%). In addition, 21% of patients had PET evidence of metastases, but none was confirmed by conventional imaging at that time, and the sensitivity for predicting sites of future disease recurrence was only 11%. Overall sensitivity for detecting occult stage IV disease was only 4%, and this is not recommended for initial staging.[94] These findings are similar to other experiences with PET imaging for intermediate-thickness melanomas.[95,96]

Also, some clinicians send blood for a complete blood count, for serum chemistries, including liver function tests, and for a lactate dehydrogenase (LDH) level, especially as they may be useful prior to surgery under general anesthesia. These also are of low clinical yield in terms of the melanoma but may detect unappreciated concurrent illness that may affect therapeutic decisions, including preoperative assessment. Specifically, if there is microcytic anemia, it should be worked up, with the differential diagnosis to include gastrointestinal metastasis of melanoma. Elevated LDH should prompt a more extensive staging workup, and elevated liver function tests should prompt a hepatobiliary ultrasound or CT scan unless there is another known explanation.

Wide Local Excision for Clinical Stage I–II Melanoma: General Considerations

Wide excision of the primary melanoma is performed to provide local control. Multiple randomized, prospective clinical trials support current recommendations for the extent of the margins of resection. The wide excision also provides an opportunity to evaluate the tissue adjacent to the primary lesion for microscopic satellites, which, if present, have clinical and prognostic significance.

There has been considerable debate about the appropriate margins of excision for primary melanomas, and it is helpful to understand the evolution of thought and data about this topic. In the early 1900s, melanoma was a rare disease, and when it was diagnosed, it was often locally advanced. Surgical resection was often associated with recurrence disease, and there were no guidelines for appropriate and successful surgical management of the primary lesion. In 1907, Handley reported a study that involved histologic examination of tissue sections taken at varied distances from the primary melanoma in a human tissue specimen that he obtained from a patient with a large primary melanoma. In that study, he found microscopic evidence of melanoma cells as far as 5 cm from the primary tumor. He recommended wide re-excision of melanomas with a measured margin of 5 cm from the primary lesion. This recommendation became standard management for melanoma for many decades, with patients typically undergoing radical resections requiring skin grafts ≥10 cm in diameter.

As melanoma became a more frequent diagnosis, there was greater awareness of it, and lesions were often diagnosed at an earlier (thinner) stage. In addition, these large re-excisions usually contained no detectable melanoma cells separate from the primary lesion. These observations, and concern for the morbidity of large resections and skin grafts, led to a questioning of the need for 5-cm margins of resection. It is ironic that the origin of this aggressive resection practice was based on data from a single patient in a single study; however, limiting the margins of excision has required multiple large, randomized, prospective trials. These trials are summarized in Table 94.3 and are detailed in the follow sections.

TABLE 94.3

Prospective Randomized Clinical Trials of Melanoma Excision Margins

Clinical Trial	N	Thickness Ranges (mm)	Margins–Study Groups (cm)	Local Recurrence	Disease-Free Survival	Overall Survival
World Health Organization Melanoma Program Trial No. 10	612	0–2	1 vs. 3–5	None for 0–1 mm with 1 cm margins; for 1–2 mm, more local recurrences with 1 cm margins (NS)	—	No difference
French ■ Cooperative ■ Surgical trial	337	0–2	2 vs. 5		No difference; 10-y DFS 85% and 83%, respectively	No difference; 10-y survival 87% and 86%, respectively
Swedish ■ Cooperative ■ Surgical Trial	989	0.8–2	2 vs. 5	<1% overall	No difference; relative hazard rate for 2 cm margin 1.02 (0.8, 1.3)	No difference; relative hazard rate for 2 cm margin 0.96 (0.75, 1.24)
Intergroup ■ Melanoma trial	740	1–4	2 vs. 4	0.4% (first, recurrence) 0.9% (first recurrence), 2.1% ever for 2 cm margins; 2.6% ever for 4 cm margins	—	10-y disease-specific survival 70% for 2 cm margins; 77% for 4 cm margins (p = 0.074, NS)
British Cooperative ■ Group trial	900	≥2	1 vs. 3	(Locoregional = local + in-transit + nodal) Increase with 1 cm margin (hazard ratio 1.26, p = 0.05)	—	Similar; trend to better survival with 3 cm margins, p >0.1 (NS)

DFS, disease-free survival; NS, not significant.

CLINICAL TRIALS TO DEFINE MARGINS OF EXCISION FOR PRIMARY CUTANEOUS MELANOMAS

The World Health Organization (WHO) Melanoma Program Trial No. 10 randomized 612 melanoma patients with melanomas ≤2 mm in thickness to excision margins of 1 cm versus 3 to 5 cm.[97,98] Patients were stratified into two subgroups: Breslow depth <1 mm versus 1 to 2 mm. There were no differences in survival rates or in rates of distant recurrences with 1-cm margins versus 3- to 5-cm margins with follow-up beyond 15 years.[99] There were more local recurrences for the group with 1-cm margin (eight versus three patients), but this was not a significant difference. There were no local recurrences for melanomas <1 mm thick treated with 1-cm margins. The lack of local recurrences with thin melanomas (<1 mm) after 1-cm margins of excision support this as a standard excision margin for T1 melanomas. The numerically slightly higher (but statistically insignificant) local recurrence risk with thinner margins for T2 melanomas has left questions about the appropriate margin for thicker lesions.

French and Swedish Cooperative Surgical Trials

The French Cooperative Group randomized 337 patients with melanomas up to 2 mm in thickness to 2- or 5-cm margins.[100] Ten-year disease-free survival rates were 85% and 83%, respectively, and ten-year overall survival (OS) rates were 87% and 86%, respectively.[100] The Swedish Melanoma Study Group randomized 989 patients with primary melanoma 0.8 to 2 mm thick on the trunk or extremities to 2- or 5-cm margins. Local recurrences were observed in only eight patients overall (<1%). In a multivariate Cox analysis, estimated hazard rates for OS and recurrence-free survival for those with 2-cm margin were 0.96 (95% CI, 0.75 to 1.24) and 1.02 (95% CI,

0.8 to 1.3), respectively, compared with the 5-cm margins.[101] Both of these studies support 2-cm margins as adequate for melanomas up to 2 mm thick and find no added benefit to 5-cm margins.

Intergroup Melanoma Trial

The Intergroup Melanoma Surgical Trial addressed the question of surgical margins in 740 patients with intermediate-thickness melanomas (1.0 to 4.0 mm thick) randomized to either 2- or 4-cm margins.[102] Patients were stratified by tumor thickness (1 to 2 mm, 2 to 3 mm, and 3 to 4 mm), anatomic site (trunk, head and neck, and extremity), and ulceration (present or absent). Patients with melanomas on the head and neck or distal extremity were not randomized for margin of excision because 4-cm margins are not readily performed in such locations. Thus, 468 patients (group A) were actually randomized for margin of excision. All patients were also randomly assigned to undergo either an elective lymph node dissection (ELND) or observation after wide local excision, and this component of that study is discussed separately.[102]

Among the 468 patients in group A (randomly assigned to excision with 2- versus 4-cm margins), only 3 (0.6%) experienced a local recurrence as the first site of failure, and 11 (2.3%) had local recurrence overall.[102] Among the 272 patients in group B (nonrandomly assigned to excision with a 2-cm margin), a higher rate of local recurrence was observed, with 3.7% having a local recurrence as a first recurrence and 6.2% overall experiencing a local recurrence during the course of their disease.[102] Among these 468 patients in group A, the incidences of local recurrence as first relapse were 0.4% versus 0.9% for 2- and 4-cm margins, respectively, and the incidences of local recurrence at any time were 2.1% versus 2.6%, respectively. In addition, the time to local recurrence and the median survival after local recurrence were unaffected by the extent of the margin. Ten-year disease-specific survival rates for the two groups were 70% and 77% for 2- and 4-cm margins, respectively (p = 0.074, not significant). Thus, this study supports a 2-cm margin as adequate for melanomas 1 to 4 cm thick, and this was associated with rates of local recurrence (as first recurrence) well <1%. Multivariate analysis of data from this study further supported the lack of benefit of wider margin of excision for local control and identified ulceration of the tumor and head-and-neck location only as significant negative prognostic features.

British Cooperative Group Trial

The British randomized trial compared 1- versus 3-cm margins of excision in patients who had cutaneous melanomas ≥2 mm thick (T3, T4).[103] Nine hundred patients with T3 and T4 melanomas were accrued, of whom 25% had T4 melanomas. It is the only randomized trial evaluating margins of excision that included patients with T4 melanomas. Patients with melanoma on head and neck, hands, or feet were excluded. No patients had any surgical procedure to stage the regional nodal basins (sentinel node biopsy or ELND) or systemic adjuvant therapy. The trial was stratified according to tumor thickness (2 to 4 mm versus >4 mm). There were few local recurrences; local recurrences and in-transit metastases were not statistically more frequent in the 1-cm margin group. Locoregional recurrences were defined broadly to include local, in-transit, or regional nodal recurrences. Using that definition, a 1-cm margin of excision was associated with a significantly increased risk of locoregional recurrence (hazard ratio [HR], 1.26; $p = 0.05$). Overall survival was comparable for the two groups ($p = 0.6$); there was a nonsignificant trend toward higher death rate in the group with 1-cm margins (128 versus 105 deaths; HR 1.24, $p = 0.1$). This study has been controversial, and its relevance to current practice is questioned because of the lack of surgical staging of the regional nodes, but it does challenge the safety of 1-cm margins for melanomas >2 mm thick.[103] These results support excision >1 cm for thicker melanomas. The data from the Melanoma Intergroup study support 2-cm margins for melanomas 2 to 4 mm thick. No data have formally compared 2-cm margins with 3-cm margins for T4 melanomas.

SURGICAL STAGING OF REGIONAL NODES

Thin and RGP melanomas are commonly cured by excision alone; however, thicker melanomas may have metastatic potential. Initial management includes an assessment for metastases and consideration of treatment options that may be beneficial in providing regional control and systemic control. Melanoma may metastasize by lymphatic or hematogenous routes. Usually, lymphatic dissemination presents earlier than hematogenous dissemination. Thus, emphasis is placed on staging the regional nodes in patients with melanoma. The finding of lymphatic metastases is associated with a higher risk of systemic disease. Another potential benefit of staging the regional nodes is to select patients for curative resection. There are substantial data on this issue that bear on the current recommendations for surgical staging of nodes, and these are summarized here.

Lymphatic anatomy is variable and is poorly understood in comparison to venous and arterial anatomy. Classic work by Sappey defined aspects of lymphatic drainage patterns from skin and defined the skin regions that typically have lymphatic drainage to major nodal basins. More recently, lymphoscintigraphy has permitted mapping the actual lymphatic drainage patterns from the skin at the site of the primary melanoma. This sometimes identifies lymphatic drainage that differs from Sappey's predictions.

In the past, the standard recommendation was to perform ELNDs for melanomas of intermediate thickness (1 to 4 mm). Despite some retrospective data supporting this approach,[104] subsequent retrospective and prospective studies have failed to show a significant survival advantage to routine ELND.[105–107] In the early 1990s, a new procedure was developed and popularized for surgical staging of node-negative primary melanomas, which is called *intraoperative lymphatic mapping and sentinel lymph node biopsy*. This approach has become routine practice for melanoma management.

The concept and method for SNBx was originally developed by Cabanas[108] for management of penile carcinomas, but it was not pursued extensively. The initial experience with lymphatic mapping and SNBx for melanoma was the work of Morton et al.[109] at the University of California Los Angeles and the John Wayne Cancer Institute. They injected a vital blue dye (isosulfan blue) intradermally and found that this stained the draining lymphatics and stained, in turn, the first node(s) into which these lymphatics empty. This was validated in human clinical experience and it was rapidly adopted as an effective way to identify the first lymph node(s) to which the melanoma drains.[110] The sentinel node(s) serve as sentinels for the remainder of the node basin. Lymphatic mapping permits identification of the specific nodes that drain the relevant area of skin, and so these nodes (typically one or two nodes) can be excised for detailed histopathologic assessment while sparing the remaining nodes in that basin, which are critical for drainage of other skin areas, thus minimizing morbidity, in particular lymphedema.

Lymphoscintigraphy has been coupled with the blue dye injection to support identification of the sentinel node(s), using handheld probes for detection of γ radiation emitted by technetium-99 (^{99}Tc), the radionuclide commonly used in lymphoscintigraphy. Most surgical oncologists performing SNBx use a combination of radionuclide injection several hours preoperatively (in the nuclear medicine suite, up to 1 mCi of ^{99}Tc) and intraoperative intradermal injection of isosulfan blue dye (up to 1 ml) a few minutes prior to the incision. The injection of radiocolloid is shown in Figure 94.6. The sentinel node(s) should be both blue and radioactive ("hot"). However, sometimes the blue dye may fail to enter the node in the short interval before the dissection. Alternatively, if the dissection takes longer than anticipated, the blue dye may transit through the node by the time the node is identified. In addition, technical issues may result in the blue dye and radiocolloid being injected in slightly different areas, such that they identify different nodes. The gamma probe is used to guide the dissection to the sentinel node(s), as suggested in Figure 94.7.

Lymphatic mapping and SNBx using both blue dye and radiocolloid increases sentinel lymph node identification rates to 99% compared with 87% with blue dye ($p < 0.0001$).[111] However, radiocolloid alone has not been formally compared with radiocolloid plus blue dye. There is substantial multicenter and single-center experience with use of radiocolloid alone, which is associated with successful identification of the sentinel node(s) in >99% of patients and with a mean of approximately two sentinel nodes per

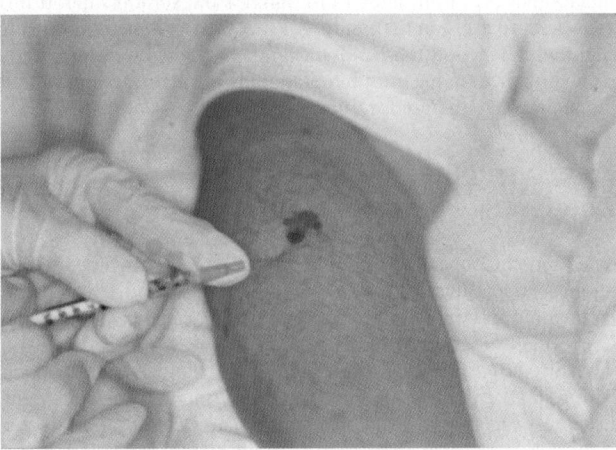

Figure 94.6 Injection of technetium-99 sulfur colloid intradermally near primary melanoma.

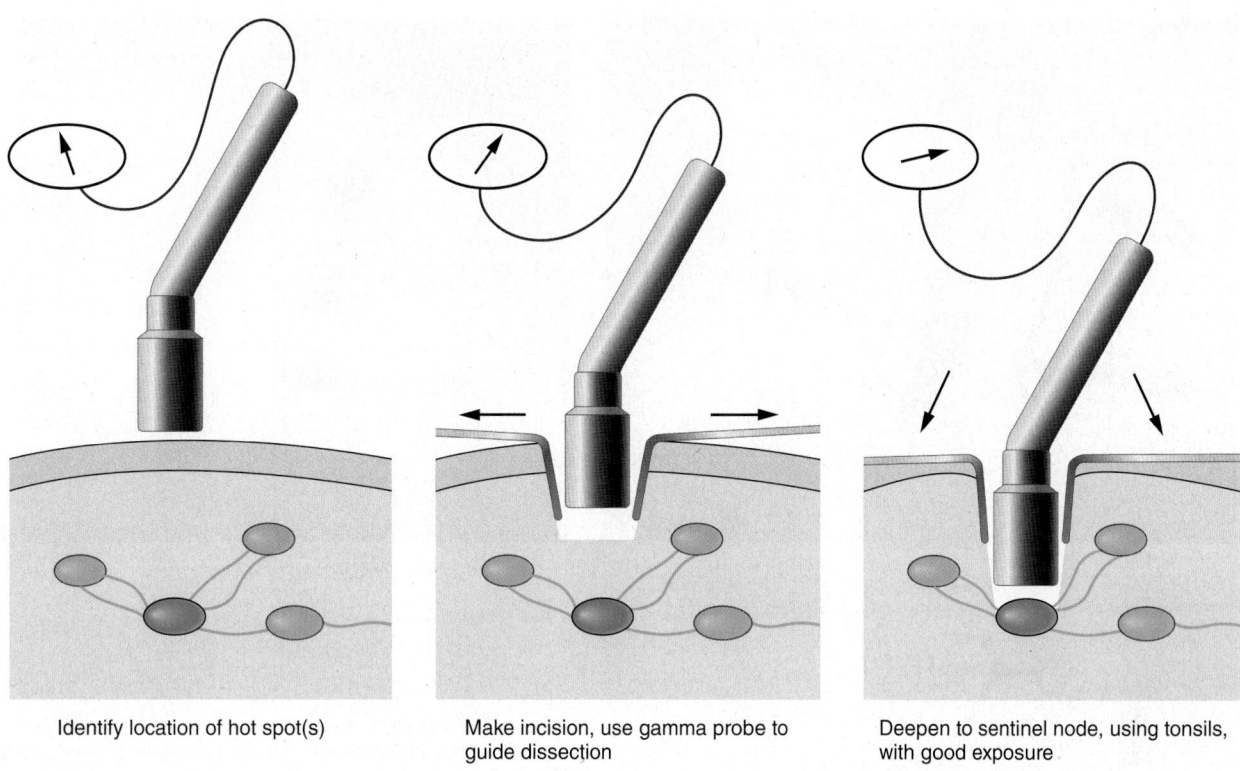

| Identify location of hot spot(s) | Make incision, use gamma probe to guide dissection | Deepen to sentinel node, using tonsils, with good exposure |

Figure 94.7 Schematic of a way to identify and remove the sentinel node using a handheld gamma camera.

patient.[112] The effectiveness of blue dye alone is limited because some patients have drainage to lymph node basins that may not be predicted (e.g., drainage from the right upper back to the left axilla) or drainage to atypical nodal basins (e.g., the triangular intermuscular space on the back, epitrochlear or popliteal nodes, or subcutaneous "in-transit" nodes that are outside a traditional nodal basin).[113,114] Examples of unusual lymph node locations mapped by lymphoscintigraphy are shown in Figure 94.8. Thus, in the large majority of clinical settings, it is most appropriate to perform radiocolloid lymphoscintigraphy in lymphatic mapping for SNBx of melanoma.

In experienced hands, lymphatic mapping should identify a sentinel node in 98% to 100% of cases, and it should be feasible to perform the SNBx with minimal morbidity, on an outpatient basis, and in many cases under local anesthesia with sedation. The early reports of SNBx stress a long learning curve, but as the technology of gamma probes has improved, the technique is less operator dependent. In addition, lymphatic mapping has now been performed long enough that surgical residents trained since the mid-1990s typically have had experience with it for melanoma and for breast cancer. The standard evaluation of a sentinel node includes evaluation of multiple sections of the node, often combined with immunohistochemical staining for melanoma markers (e.g., S100, HMB45, tyrosinase, and/or MART-1/MelanA).

Typical results of SNBx reveal that the rate of positive nodes increases with increasing tumor thickness, as would be expected, from <5% for the thin melanomas that undergo SNBx (e.g., T1b lesions) to approximately 40% for thick melanomas. Current experience with SNBx in most series supports the prognostic value of SNBx in thick melanomas (>4 mm)[115] as well as in thinner lesions. When ELND was performed, it was typically recommended only for melanomas 1.5 to 4 mm thick. However, in the Duke experience, the relative risk of distant versus regional metastases is not dramatically higher for thick melanomas, and this supports a clinical approach that includes the potential for curative resection of regional metastases in these cases.[105] In addition, the low morbidity of SNBx supports a threshold for SNBx in thinner mela-

nomas than the 1.5-mm criterion that was used for performance of ELND.

The overall rate of positive SNBx in most series (typically for melanomas >1 mm) is in the range of 15% to 25%. The percentage of patients with false-negative SNBx in experienced hands and with use of radiocolloid and the handheld gamma probe, with or without blue dye, is typically in the range of 1.9% to 4%.[111] The most rigorous definition of false-negative rate is false negative/(false negative + true positive), and 3% false negative in the setting of 20% true positive represents 13% false-negative rate. False-negative rates have been estimated by seeking nodes containing metastases in the remaining nodal basin after a negative SNBx. In other settings, it is done by defining patients who return with clinically evident nodal metastases after a prior negative SNBx in the same node basin. These may or may not be equivalent. Nonetheless, there is a small percentage of patients who have negative SNBx who later return with nodal metastases in the same nodal basin. Although the procedure is very accurate and does identify the large majority of nodal metastases, it is prudent to follow patients for nodal recurrence even after a negative SNBx.

Lymphatic mapping and SNBx has been applied generally for all cutaneous sites and may also be useful for melanomas of mucous membranes.[116] A challenging area for SNBx is the head and neck. In particular, melanomas of the scalp and of the face may drain to parotid nodes or periparotid nodes, for which SNBx is more complex, more technically challenging, and associated with greater potential morbidity. In addition, false-negative SNBx are more common than in trunk and extremity melanomas, occurring in approximately 10% of patients, for a true false-negative rate that may approach 30%. However, in many cases, it can be performed reliably and still has a place in management.

More recent technology that offers promise for improving sentinel node localization are the development of mobile gamma cameras that can replace the single gamma detector of the gamma probe with an array of hundreds of detectors that permit real-time imaging that rivals that of the fixed gamma camera. This approach has the potential to improve identification of nodes in atypical loca-

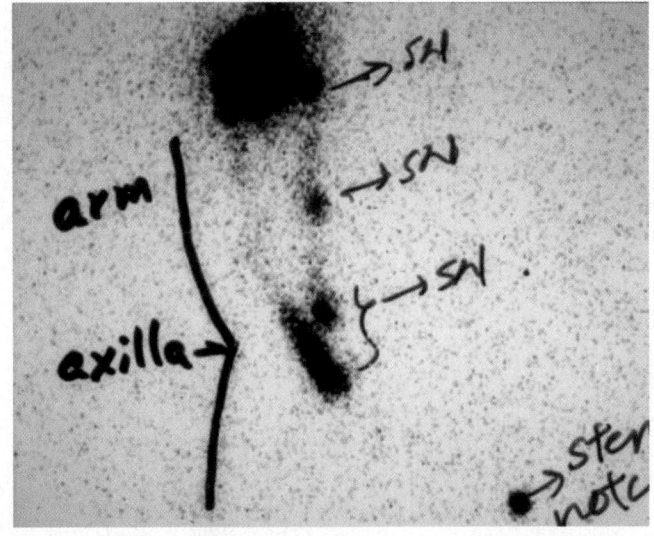

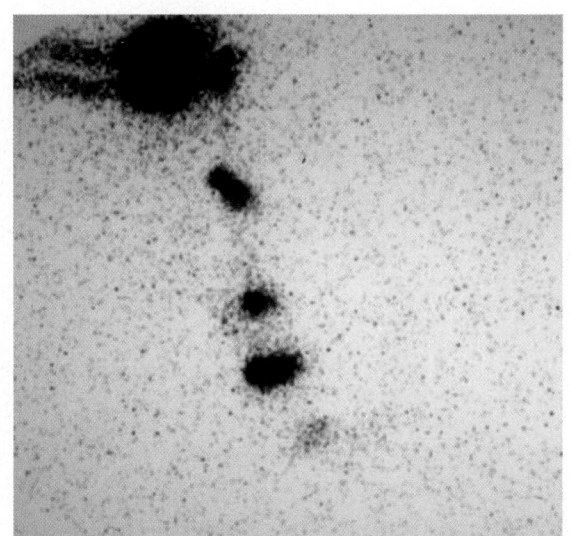

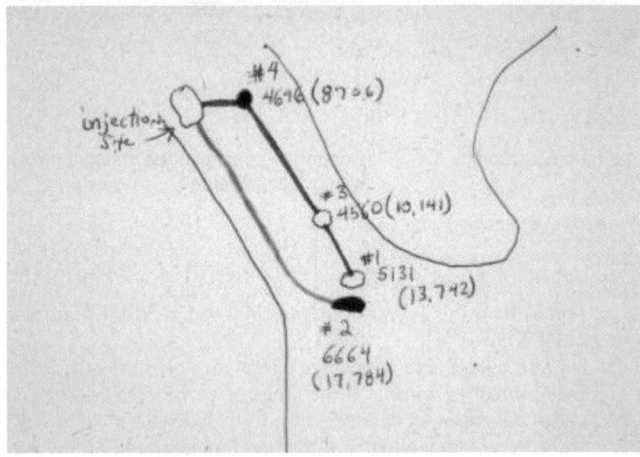

Figure 94.8 Lymphatic mapping from near the elbow along two separate lymphatic channels toward the axilla. An early image **(A)** shows the lymphatic channels clearly. A later image **(B)** shows the sentinel nodes clearly, but the channels are much less evident. One of the sentinel nodes is in subcutaneous tissue near the elbow and is almost missed due to proximity to the injection site (no. 4) **(C)**. The two nodes near the axilla were actually just distal to the true axillary space. One of them was a true sentinel node (no. 2) and contained tumor (designated by the *solid black node*), whereas the other node near it was the third node in that lymphatic channel, so that the first node in that channel was truly sentinel (no. 4) and also contained tumor. The other two nodes downstream from no. 4 were both negative for tumor.

tions and for ensuring adequate clearance of the sentinel nodes.[117] Also promising is single photon-emission computed tomographic/CT imaging, which can provide very discrete localization of sentinel nodes, which may be helpful in selected challenging locations. Despite the high accuracy of SNBx for nodal staging, the false-negative rate may be as high as 10% to 20%,[118] and these new technologies offer a possibility to reduce that false-negative rate.

In performing SNBx, melanoma metastases are sometimes clinically evident in the operating room as small pigmented spots just under the capsule of the node. When these are present, the hottest part of the node is usually precisely at that location (unpublished clinical observations). This may be particularly relevant for some large nodes, where the pathologist can be guided to the portion most at risk of metastasis for detailed histologic assessment (Fig. 94.9). Morton et al.[119] have formalized a technique that may identify the part of the node that is most likely to contain metastases, based on injecting carbon black dye and isosulfan blue dye. This has not yet become standard, but this or other refinements may further increase the accuracy of staging by this procedure.

The Multicenter Sentinel Lymphadenectomy Trial 1 was initially reported in 2006, and updated in 2014, as a randomized, prospective trial of 1,269 patients with melanomas 1 to 4 mm thick who were randomized to SNBx or observation in addition to wide local excision of the primary lesion.[110,120,121] The finding was that there was no difference in 5-year disease-specific survival (87.1% versus 86.6%).[120] Patients who developed clinically positive nodes during follow-up after initial observation of the node basins had worse survival than those with positive nodes found at the time of SNBx; however, this posthoc analysis carries inher-

ent weaknesses.[120] In this trial, patients were randomized 3:2 to wide excision plus SNBx, or wide excision only, respectively. In the group receiving SNBx, 225 of 814 (27.6%) patients underwent early completion lymph node dissection (CLND), compared to 132 of 533 (24.7%) in the control group having delayed CLND. Lymphedema was significantly greater (20.4% versus 12.4%, $p = 0.04$) for those in the observation group who underwent delayed CLND, and hospitalization was longer for delayed

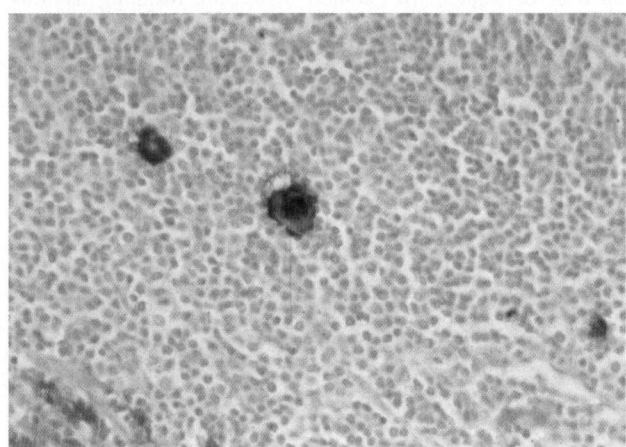

Figure 94.9 Immunohistochemical detection of isolated melanoma cells in a sentinel node when stained for the melanoma marker S100.

CLND.[122] The follow-up results in 2014 supported the conclusion that biopsy-based staging of intermediate-thickness or thick primary melanomas provides important prognostic information and identifies patients with nodal metastases who may benefit from immediate CLND. In this series, SNBx-based management prolonged disease-free survival for all patients and prolonged distant disease-free survival and melanoma-specific survival for patients with nodal metastases from intermediate-thickness melanomas.[121]

One important consideration should be kept in mind, which is often overlooked in considering the potential value of SNBx and subsequent CLND. That consideration is the value to patients of regional control of their tumor, even in the absence of survival benefit. A study evaluating patients' perception of their own utilities for health states suggested that the development of recurrent disease markedly decreases patient perception of their health state, even if it does not impact survival.[123] This study thus suggests that regional tumor control may have value to patients, even in the absence of a survival benefit.

The rationale for performing SNBx for melanoma includes the following: (1) A negative SNBx is a good prognostic indicator that may provide comfort to low-risk patients. (2) A positive SNBx for patients with T1–T3a clinically N0 melanomas (clinical stage I–IIA) renders them candidates for adjuvant high-dose interferon (HDI) therapy, which offers some clinical benefit. (3) Patients with T4 melanomas or with microscopic satellites (N2c, stage IIIB) are further upstaged by the finding of a positive sentinel node, which helps these patients in risk assessment and may make them candidates for selected clinical trials. (4) Many clinical trials require surgical staging of regional nodes, and, thus, sentinel node mapping makes patients candidates for trials that may prove to be of benefit. (5) Identification of melanoma in a sentinel node permits selection of patients for CLND to increase the chance of regional tumor control. (6) Excision of the sentinel node may be curative if there is no tumor beyond the node, even if CLND is not feasible. This hypothesis is being explored explicitly in the Multicenter Selective Lymphadenectomy Trial 2 (MSLT2).

Selection of Patients for Sentinel Node Biopsy

SNBx is generally recommended for patients with melanomas at least 1 mm thick. For thinner melanomas, there is debate about the appropriate criteria for performing SNBx.[81] A common practice is to offer SNBx for thin melanomas with adverse prognostic features, including ulceration. The 2010 staging system also identifies a mitotic rate of ≥ 1 as an adverse prognostic feature, and this is associated with higher risk of sentinel node metastasis. Earlier data also support the relevance of mitotic rate as a prognostic factor in primary melanomas[82] or Clark level IV.[78] There is debate about performing SNBx for thin melanomas that are in VGP, that have dermal mitoses, or that occur in young patients.[81,84] Also, there is rationale for offering SNBx for melanomas <1 mm thick that have a positive deep margin on biopsy and thus are not fully evaluable for depth.

Pure desmoplastic melanomas have a similar overall metastatic and mortality risk as other melanomas, but their risk of regional nodal metastases appears to be lower than that of other melanomas.[67,124] Thus, it may be reasonable to limit SNBx for pure desmoplastic melanomas. However, there is limited experience with managing regional nodes in desmoplastic melanoma, and some desmoplastic melanomas can metastasize to regional nodes.[65]

Sentinel Node Biopsy Subsequent to a Prior Wide Local Excision

SNBx should be performed at the same procedure as wide local excision. However, there are some circumstances in which wide local excision may be performed without SNBx, and there is then a question of whether SNBx can be performed reliably after a prior wide local excision. Such circumstances include a thin melanoma on original biopsy, found to be deeper on re-excision or on second-opinion pathology review. A multicenter experience with 76 patients having SNBx performed after a prior wide local excision revealed a 99% success rate in SNBx, a mean yield of two sentinel nodes per patient, with a 15% overall sentinel node–positive rate, a 4% rate of melanoma recurrence in a negative mapped basin, and only a 1% rate of isolated first recurrence in a node. These and other data support performing SNBx after prior wide local excision, although performing it concurrently with the original wide local excision is preferred.[125]

MANAGEMENT

Clinically Localized Melanoma

Melanoma In Situ (Clinical TISN0M0, Stage 0)

For melanomas confined to the epidermis and epidermal/dermal junction that are diagnosed as melanoma in situ, this is a lesion that is curable in the vast majority of cases by wide excision alone. On initial evaluation, the regional nodes should be examined, as should the skin and subcutaneous tissue between the primary site and these regional node basins. Melanoma in situ by definition is not invasive or metastatic; however, metastatic melanoma to regional nodes has been observed occasionally from melanoma in situ with histologic evidence of regression.[126] Thus, it is prudent to examine the nodes clinically. However, in the absence of clinical evidence of metastasis, there is no need to perform radiologic staging studies. Definitive management involves re-excision with a margin of 5 mm. The standard recommendation is to perform a full-thickness re-excision including underlying subcutaneous tissue, although there are no formal data that a full-thickness skin excision is less adequate for melanoma in situ. However, variation in thickness within the original biopsy specimen may lead to occult invasion that is not observed on the evaluated sections. Thus, it is prudent to perform a full-thickness excision of skin and subcutaneous tissue to the underlying deep fascia. A 5-mm margin is the standard recommendation, but melanoma in situ can extend beyond its visible extent. Thus, if cosmetically acceptable, it is reasonable to obtain a margin of as much as 1 cm, especially if the original biopsy was incomplete. If the margins are positive or close, re-excision to a widely clear margin is recommended. SNBx is not indicated. No adjuvant therapy is needed if the margins are widely clear.

Clinical Follow-Up After Surgical Treatment

Melanomas in situ are curable in the vast majority of cases with surgery alone. However, they rarely may be associated with metastasis, probably attributable either to an invasive component that was not detected because of sampling error, or to an associated regressed invasive component.[126]

Thus, in accord with the NCCN Guidelines®, it is appropriate to follow these patients for local recurrence, in-transit metastasis, or regional node metastasis on an annual basis. The risk of recurrence is not high enough to require specialty follow-up, but a focused physical examination of the patient by the primary care physician is appropriate. More important, patients with melanoma in situ are at increased risk of subsequent primary melanomas, and so close dermatologic follow-up with full-body skin examinations is recommended.

Thin Primary Melanoma (Clinical T1A)

The classic definition of a thin melanoma was based on the original report of Breslow[73] of the association between depth of invasion (Breslow thickness) and subsequent risk of metastasis and death. In that report, patients with melanomas <0.76 mm thick had no

PRACTICE OF ONCOLOGY

TABLE 94.4

Brief Review of Literature on Intratumoral Therapies

Therapy	Regimen	Response Rate Injection Lesions	Response Rate Distant Lesions	Citations
Interferon alpha	10 million IU 3×/wk rec IFNa2b	45% (31% CR, 14% PR)	CR 6%; PR 12% (RR 18%)	Von Wussow, 1988
Rose Bengal (PV-10)	10% PV-10 w/v in saline, 0.5 ml/cc lesion volume	46%	27%	Thompson 2008
Interleukin-2	0.3–6 MIU/lesion, based on size 3 ×/wk	79% (79% CR)	0%	Weide 2010
Electrochemical with bleomycin	Bleomycin (intralesional or IV) plus electrical pulse	96%	New lesions arose soon	Campana 2009, 2012
Imiquimod	Topical daily or BID	Up to 50%	Low	Berman 2002
BCG	Intralesional injection	90%	17%	Morton 1974
Talimogene laherparepvec (T-Vec; HSV-1 encoding GM-CSF)	Intralesional injection	26%	26%	Senzer 2009; Kaufman 2010; Korn 2009; Andtbacka 2013
BCG + imiquimod	BCG then, when inflamed, add imiquimod (n = 9)	67% (56% CR, 11% PR)	—	Kidner 2012
Diphencyprone	Prepared in acetone; administered at increasing doses to cutaneous lesions	100% (57% CR, 43% PR), based on seven patients	Not reported	Damian 2009
2,4-Dinitrochlorobenzene	Intralesional	60%	Not reported	Goodnight 1979

CR, complete response; PR, partial response; RR, response rate; IV, intravenously; BID, twice a day; BCG, Bacillus Calmette–Guérin; HSV-1, herpes simplex virus 1; GM-CSF, granulocyte macrophage–colony-stimulating factor.

subsequent metastasis. Thus, the definition of a thin melanoma had been a melanoma <0.76 mm thick. However, subsequent studies have shown a continuous risk association with increasing thickness, without an absolute "cutoff" at 0.76 mm,[73] and melanomas <0.76 mm in thickness do have approximately a 5% risk of subsequent metastasis.[127] Additional studies have defined additional histopathologic features that affect the prognosis of thin melanomas. The current AJCC staging system addresses several prognostic features of thin melanomas such that T1a melanomas are those <1 mm thick, with less than one mitosis per square millimeter, and without ulceration. In the absence of any clinical evidence of metastasis, these are clinical stage IA melanomas and have a 5-year survival rate of 94%.[74,78]

In most centers, the surgical management of patients with T1a melanomas includes wide excision with a 1-cm margin (including skin and all underlying subcutaneous tissue, to the deep muscle fascia). The margin should be measured from the visible edge of the pigmented lesion or from the biopsy scar, whichever is larger. Excisions of this size can almost always be closed primarily, with exceptions being on the face, palms, and feet, where skin grafts or rotation flaps may be needed.

Surgical Methods in Wide Local Excision (Applies for All Primary Melanoma Thicknesses)

For melanomas of the trunk and proximal extremities, wide local excisions should involve measuring the appropriate margin (usually 1 to 2 cm) around the entire scar from the biopsy, or from the visible edge of residual melanoma, and extending the incision to make an ellipse that is approximately three times as long as it is wide. Ideally, the direction of the scar should be longitudinal on the extremities, occasionally with some modification at joints, and should be along skin lines on the trunk and neck. On the upper back, it is usually best for the scar to run transversely, to minimize tension on it. When the initial biopsy scar is not in the direction that is desired for the final excision, an effective approach is first to mark out the oval shape that is required for the appropri-

ate margins, then rather than extending that to an ellipse that is in the same direction, the ends of that oval can be extended in the desired direction, resulting in a sigmoid-shaped oval, which has two advantages: The closure results in a scar that is more in the desired direction, and the sigmoid shape allows the tension to be distributed in two directions. The excision should include all skin and subcutaneous tissue to the deep fascia, but not including the fascia. When a major cutaneous nerve runs along the deep fascia to innervate distal cutaneous structures, it is appropriate to preserve that nerve. Wide excisions can almost always be performed under local anesthesia, with or without intravenous sedation, in the patient who is thus motivated.

Clinical Follow-Up for Thin Melanomas (Stage IA)

There are no definitive data showing a survival advantage for close follow-up after surgical management of primary or metastatic melanoma; however, there is an expectation from patients for follow-up, and there are treatable recurrences and metastases that can be identified best by physician follow-up. The National Comprehensive Cancer Network® (NCCN®) has issued useful guidelines for treatment and follow-up of melanoma.[128] The risk of metastasis for thin melanomas is in the 5% to 10% range, and less for RGP lesions. In the uncommon case of recurrent thin melanomas, the recurrences usually occur late, often beyond 5 years from diagnosis; the annual risk of recurrence is fairly constant over a long time,[47] so annual follow-up for many years is recommended rather than frequent follow-up in the first few years. Follow-up suggestions are listed in Table 94.7.

Clinical T2A, T2B Melanomas

Melanomas 1 to 2 mm thick, with or without ulceration, should be managed with an initial history and physical examination to elucidate signs or symptoms that could suggest metastatic disease. In the absence of such findings, there is very low yield of additional staging studies, and they are not recommended. In those patients without evidence of metastasis, definitive management includes wide excision with a 1- to 2-cm margin and SNBx. There are definitive data from the Melanoma Intergroup trial that a 2-cm margin is adequate for these patients,[107] and even a 1-cm margin was associated with the same survival as a 3- to 5-cm margin in long follow-up of the WHO Trial 10 (see Table 94.3).[99] However, there has been a slight increase in local recurrence in patients with 1- to 2-mm lesions who had 1-cm margins (versus 3- to 5-cm margins). This is not statistically significant in the patients studied, but it may signal a slight increase in local recurrence risk. When it is feasible to take a 2-cm margin without a skin graft (trunk and proximal extremities in most cases), this is recommended to minimize the chance of local recurrence. However, when the lesion is located on the face or distal extremities, where such a margin may be difficult to achieve without a skin graft, a 1- to 1.5-cm margin is acceptable. If a skin graft will be necessary even to close a 1-cm margin (rare), it is recommended that a 2-cm margin be taken because the morbidity and cost of the skin graft will already be needed. In addition, for lesions that are barely above 1 mm in depth (e.g., 1.03 mm), it certainly is reasonable to use a 1-cm margin.

SNBx is routinely recommended for patients with melanomas 1 to 2 mm thick.[129] If the SNBx is positive, then subsequent management should follow recommendations given later for stage IIIA melanoma (T2a with positive SNBx involving one to three nodes) or stage IIIB melanoma (T2b with positive SNBx involving one to three nodes). However, if the SNBx is negative, then the patient is considered to have been pathologically staged as T2aN0M0 (stage IB) or T2bN0M0 (stage IIA), and no additional surgical management is required and no adjuvant systemic therapy is indicated, other than clinical trials.

Clinical T3A Melanomas (Clinical Stage IIA)

Melanomas 2 to 4 mm thick, without ulceration, represent T3a lesions, and in the absence of metastases, these are clinical stage IIA lesions. They should be managed clinically with a history and physical examination as detailed previously and may be considered for a staging studies and serum LDH level. Definitive management includes wide excision with a 2-cm margin and SNBx for histologic staging of the regional nodes. If the SNBx is negative, then no additional surgical or systemic therapy is indicated other than possible clinical trials. If the SNBx is positive, then management for stage IIIA melanoma should be followed.

Clinical T3B Melanomas (Clinical Stage IIB)

Melanomas 2 to 4 mm thick with ulceration represent T3b lesions and thus are clinical stage IIB melanomas. These are high-risk localized melanomas. Initial management should include a careful history and physical examination. Staging studies are generally of low yield, but in selected high risk cases may be considered, and if there are symptoms suspicious for metastatic disease, there is value in performing indicated imaging studies.[130] Given the higher risk of synchronous metastases that may be detected at diagnosis, systemic staging with CT scans of the chest, abdomen, and pelvis (or PET/CT scan) plus MRI scan of the brain may be indicated if there are symptoms or signs suggestive of systemic metastasis.

In the absence of clinical evidence of metastasis, definitive management is wide excision with a 2-cm margin and an SNBx. If the nodes are negative, the summary stage is IIB (T3bN0M0). For these patients, no additional surgical therapy is needed. However, HDI and pegylated-interferon therapies have been approved for use as postsurgical adjuvant therapy for patients with resected stage IIB-III melanoma. It is worth noting that the randomized clinical trials of adjuvant interferon were performed before the recent revision of the AJCC staging system, when ulceration was not incorporated in the staging system. Thus, the patients with stage IIB in whom interferon was tested did not include the current patients with stage T3bN0. Nonetheless, it is available for such patients,

whose risk is comparable to that of patients with nonulcerated thick melanomas (T4aN0).

Thick Melanomas (T4A, T4B, Greater than 4 mm Thick)

Thick melanomas have been commonly associated with a risk of metastasis and mortality in the range of 50% over 5 to 10 years. Ulceration increases this risk: T4a melanomas are clinical stage IIB, and T4b melanomas are clinical stage IIC. Initial workup should include a history and physical examination, and serum LDH plus more aggressive radiologic imaging as indicated by signs and symptoms. For these high-risk patients, consideration should be given to more complete staging with CT scans of the chest, abdomen, and pelvis plus MRI of the head. Definitive management includes wide excision with at least a 2-cm margin plus SNBx. There are no definitive prospective, randomized data regarding margins for melanomas thicker than 4 mm, but margins of at least 2 cm are recommended. The general experience is that 2-cm margins provide adequate local control for these lesions, suggesting that the strong data supporting the adequacy of 2-cm margins in 1- to 4-mm melanomas may be extrapolated to thicker lesions.[131]

As SNBx has been employed routinely since the early 1990s, most studies show that sentinel node status has independent prognostic value for patients with thick melanomas.[131] Because these patients have a high risk of sentinel node positivity (approximately 35% to 40%), there is a high chance of regional nodal recurrence, and SNBx, followed by CLND, offers the prospect of increasing the chance of regional control. In patients with negative sentinel nodes, adjuvant interferon should be considered because it is approved by the FDA for these patients. This should be discussed in detail with patients.

SPECIAL CONSIDERATIONS IN MANAGEMENT OF PRIMARY MELANOMAS

Primary Melanomas of the Head and Neck

For melanomas on the head and neck, there are important anatomic constraints, and there are times when the optimal margins are not feasible (e.g., a 2-cm margin for a lesion 1 cm below the eye), but to the extent possible, the optimal margins should be obtained and closed with an advancement flap, skin graft, or limited rotation flap. In the unusual circumstance of a large-diameter lentigo maligna on the face that is not amenable to surgical resection because of cosmetic results or comorbid patient conditions, it may be treated with superficial or Grenz X-rays with local control rates reported above 90%.[132] Anecdotal reports of off-label topical treatment with imiquimod ointment have also resulted in effective local control of superficial melanomas.[133,134] This is being used increasingly, with good results in reported experience, but recurrence may occur.[135] Initial experience suggests that imiquimod is not effective at eradicating dysplastic nevi.[136] Desmoplastic melanomas commonly occur in the head and neck region and may have reported local recurrence rates up to 40% to 60% after resection.[137] Other series vary substantially in local recurrence rates of desmoplastic melanomas. One reports local recurrences as first recurrences in 14% of patients, which exceeds that of other histologic types,[69] and another reports no difference in local recurrence rates compared to other melanomas, although the presence of neurotropism was associated with higher risks of local recurrence.[70] An explanation for the high local recurrence rates in some series of desmoplastic melanoma may include inadequate margins of excision because of anatomic constraints in the head and neck. In addition, because desmoplastic melanomas are usually amelanotic, the surgical margins may be underestimated, and the histologic appearance of desmoplastic melanoma can interfere with accurate detection of microscopically positive margins, especially in fibrotic skin. Thus, in patients with desmoplastic melanoma, every effort should be made to obtain adequate margins.[137] If that is not possible, postoperative adjuvant radiation should be considered with 2- to 3-cm margins around the resected lesion because this may reduce subsequent local recurrences.

Neurotropic melanomas of the head and neck have a propensity to recur at the skull base by tracking along cranial nerves, and postoperative adjuvant radiation including the resection bed and the cranial nerve pathway should be considered for this variant.

Primary Melanomas of the Mucous Membranes

Mucosal melanomas of the head and neck, anorectal region, and female genital tract are usually diagnosed when they are thick. They are associated with higher risks of distant metastases and death compared to cutaneous melanoma. They are also associated with higher risks of local recurrence and regional nodal metastases. Staging of these lesions is not addressed completely in the AJCC staging system for cutaneous melanomas, but there are general similarities that can be applied to mucosal melanomas. The depth of invasion is difficult to measure because they are often biopsied in a fragmented way, but they usually are deep lesions, with depths often of ≥1 cm. They should be resected with wide margins if possible. Resection of melanomas of the nasopharynx, oropharynx, and sinuses is limited by the bony structures of the skull and the base of the brain. Vulvovaginal melanomas may be widely resected in many cases but may also be constrained by efforts to preserve urinary and sexual function. They may also be associated with extensive radial growth in addition to the invasive lesion, which can lead to multifocal local recurrences. Anorectal melanoma may usually be resected widely by an abdominoperineal resection, but this morbid operation is not associated with higher survival rates than local excision only.[138] Adjuvant local radiation therapy may be of value when widely clear margins are not feasible.[139] However, no randomized, prospective trials of radiation have been performed in this setting. SNBx has been performed for vulvovaginal melanomas, but its impact on ultimate clinical outcome is not known.[140] It may also be performed for anorectal melanomas,[141] but pelvic and systemic metastases are more concerning for ultimate outcome than the risk of groin metastases. SNBx is not generally feasible for mucous membrane melanomas of the head and neck because of technical considerations.

Mucosal melanomas have not specifically been tested for their response to interferon therapy, but they are considered eligible for interferon, which is reasonable to consider after resection of thick mucosal melanomas with or without lymph node involvement. These patients may also be eligible for clinical trials in the adjuvant setting.

Primary Melanomas of the Fingers and Toes

For melanomas of the plantar aspect of the foot, especially on the anterior weight-bearing surface or on the heel, skin grafts are inadequate for bearing the weight of walking. Thus, it is often effective to rotate the skin of the instep of the foot to cover defects in those areas, with skin grafting of the instep area if needed.

For subungual melanomas of any finger or toe, the appropriate management is amputation at the interphalangeal joint of the toe or just proximal to the distal interphalangeal joint of the finger. Even for subungual melanomas in situ, such an amputation is indicated. These lesions often are found to contain invasion on the final specimen that is not evident on original biopsy, and it is not feasible to resect the entire nail bed with any margin without taking the bone of the distal phalanx because the two are intimately associated. It is important for amputations of the fingers, especially the

thumb, to attach the severed deep flexor tendon to the remaining proximal phalangeal bone, to retain adequate flexor strength after surgery. This can be done by passing a braided multifilament suture through the phalangeal bone and the ligament via holes drilled in the bone in two places. The skin incision for these amputations can be designed by measuring 1 to 2 cm (depending on thickness) from the nail bed and including at least that amount of skin with the amputation. This almost always leaves some skin on the plantar or palmar surface (except when the subungual melanoma has extended well out onto the plantar/palmar surface) that can be used to close the surgical defect and provides a sturdy skin surface.

For melanomas of the proximal toe or finger, the considerations are similar to those for distal and subungual digital melanomas. For melanoma of the toe, amputation of the toe is usually the best choice because the functional morbidity of losing a toe is small. The exception is the great toe, but even amputation of that toe is feasible, although retention of the first metatarsal head is valuable for gait and balance. For small-diameter, thin melanomas proximally located on the fingers, and for toes when appropriate, it occasionally may be feasible to perform a wide excision and skin grafting (rarely primary closure) with preservation of the digit.

SNBx can be performed accurately from these lesions and should usually be performed for melanomas of the fingers or toes if they are at least T1b lesions.

THE ROLE OF RADIATION THERAPY IN THE MANAGEMENT OF PRIMARY MELANOMA LESIONS

The general management of primary melanoma lesions is surgical resection. However, there is a role for definitive or adjuvant radiation therapy in certain histologic variants including lentigo maligna, desmoplastic melanoma, or neurotropic melanoma, and for palliation of unresectable primary disease. Lentigo maligna commonly occurs as a large lesion in the head and neck region of elderly patients. If the patient is medically inoperable or if the proposed resection would result in a poor cosmetic outcome, he or she can be treated with superficial or Grenz X-rays with local control rates above 90%.[132] Desmoplastic melanomas also commonly occur in the head and neck region and have high local recurrence rates. Postoperative adjuvant radiation may be delivered with 2- to 3-cm margins around the resected lesion if margins are inadequate, or following resection of a locally recurrent lesion, and thus as this can substantially reduce subsequent local recurrences.[137] Neurotropic melanomas of the head and neck have a propensity to recur at the skull base by tracking along cranial nerves, and postoperative adjuvant radiation including the resection bed and the cranial nerve pathway should be considered for this variant. Large unresectable primary lesions should be considered for palliative radiation therapy or be enrolled in clinical trials. Of note, the concurrent use of interferon-α2b with radiation or its use 1 month following radiation has been reported to cause increased radiation toxicity and should be used cautiously.[142]

CLINICAL FOLLOW-UP FOR INTERMEDIATE-THICKNESS AND THICK MELANOMAS (STAGE IB–IIC)

Suggestions for follow-up are listed in Table 94.4. For intermediate-thickness melanomas, history and focused physical examination may be done as often as every 3 months and as infrequently as annually, with LDH, and complete blood count at least annually, and other scans done as indicated for symptoms. CT or PET/CT is not likely to have much yield if the other studies and clinical examination are all unremarkable. However, there are circumstances in which they may be useful. Especially for the high-risk primary (e.g., T4b) on the lower extremity, pelvic CT scan or PET/CT may be helpful in identifying iliac nodal recurrences that are difficult to detect on examination. In addition, for high-risk melanomas, brain MRI may be helpful in detecting small brain metastases when they are asymptomatic and amenable to treatment with gamma knife radiation therapy.

Most first recurrences will be in local skin, in-transit skin, or lymph nodes, which can be detected on physical examination and can be treated surgically with some chance of cure. The most common first sites of visceral metastasis are lung and liver. Other frequent sites of metastasis include the gastrointestinal tract, brain, bone, distant skin or nodes, and adrenal glands. Clinical follow-up should elicit any information on headaches, weight loss, change in appetite, bone pain, or other symptoms that could be associated with these metastatic sites. There should be a low threshold for performing radiologic studies to work up such symptoms. However, routine extensive scans have not been shown to improve clinical outcome. In a study of follow-up for patients with stage II-III melanoma, melanoma recurrences were detected based on symptoms in 68%, physical examination findings in 26%, and CXR in 6%.[143] In another study of patients with stage I-II melanoma followed with physical examination, blood tests, and CXR, recurrences were detected by physical examination (72%), patient symptoms (17%), and CXR (11%).[144] The diagnostic yield of laboratory tests is low, but elevations of LDH or other liver function tests may signal a liver metastasis or other new metastasis. New microcytic anemia can be a first sign of gastrointestinal blood loss due to a small bowel metastasis.

REGIONALLY METASTATIC MELANOMA (STAGE III): LYMPH NODE METASTASIS, SATELLITE LESIONS, AND IN-TRANSIT METASTASES

Melanoma has a high propensity to regional metastasis in any of several presentations, all presumably via intralymphatic dissemination. These are the most common first metastases. The presence of regional metastasis is a negative prognostic finding; however, there is some chance of long-term disease-free survival and cure for patients with regional metastases, and they should be managed with curative intent whenever feasible.

There is a wide range of outcomes for patients who develop regional (stage III) metastases. Prognostic features of the primary melanoma have been associated with clinical outcome even after the development of metastases.[145] However, in the assessment of

prognosis of patients with stage III melanoma performed for the current AJCC staging system, only ulceration of the primary lesion had independent prognostic impact,[74,76] and this has been incorporated in the staging system.

Regional metastases are defined as follows:

- *Local recurrence* is best defined as recurrence of melanoma in the scar from the original excision or at the edge of the skin graft if that was used for closure.
- *Satellites metastases* may occur either simultaneously with the original diagnosis or arise subsequent to original excision. Typically, recurrences that are separate from the scar but within 2 to 5 cm of it are considered satellite metastases (Fig. 94.10).
- Regional recurrences beyond 5 cm of the scar but proximal to regional nodes are considered *in-transit metastases* (Fig. 94.11).
- *Regional node metastases* are typically in a draining nodal basin that is near the lesion.

Thus, for example, melanomas of the forearm usually drain to an axillary node. However, the most proximal regional node may be an epitrochlear node or simply a subcutaneous node in an atypical location. With the use of lymphoscintigraphy and SNBx routinely in melanoma, such atypical nodal locations are increasingly defined.[146] It is occasionally difficult to distinguish whether an in-transit metastasis is a regional skin metastasis or a true nodal metastasis.

Management of Local Recurrence

Local recurrence is common after a primary lesion is inadequately excised. This type of local recurrence thus represents a failure of initial surgical management and may not represent the same high risk of distant metastasis and mortality that is associated with local recurrence after what is otherwise considered adequate surgical resection. However, local recurrences after adequate wide excision are associated with a very poor prognosis. In the Intergroup Melanoma trial, local recurrences were associated with 9% to 11% overall 5-year survival rate, as compared with 86% for those without local recurrence.[102]

Despite the bad prognosis associated with local recurrences, some patients either may be cured or may have extended tumor control by surgical resection. It is best to re-resect the entire scar down to the level of fascia, and perhaps including fascia, because there may be more tumor in the scar than is clinically evident, and this type of resection can generally be performed with minimal morbidity. Excision with a 1- to 2-cm margin is reasonable if the recurrences are limited to the scar. In the setting of associated

PRACTICE OF ONCOLOGY

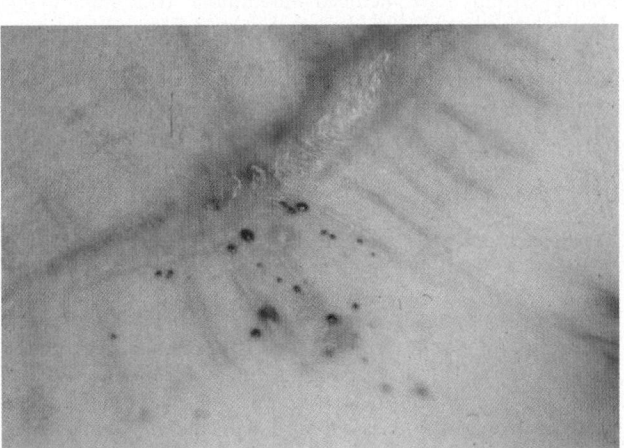

Figure 94.10 Local and satellite metastases after wide excision of melanoma on the chest.

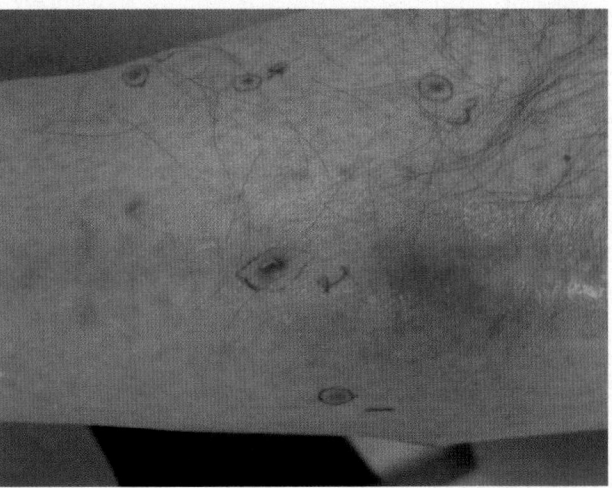

Figure 94.11 Close-up view of in-transit metastases involving the dermis, along the skin of the leg.

satellite metastases, more extensive resection may be appropriate with a skin graft. In patients with concurrent distant disease, a less aggressive approach to the local recurrence may be justified, and simple excision to a clear margin may be acceptable. In addition, it is appropriate to consider SNBx by mapping from the site of the local recurrence.[147] This is usually successful even if there has been a prior SNBx or a prior CLND. This may enable regional control in such high-risk patients in whom the sentinel nodes may be positive in up to 50% of cases.[147] Unresectable recurrent lesions should be considered for palliative radiation therapy.

Management of Satellite and In-Transit Metastases

The presence of in-transit or satellite metastases is a negative prognostic feature, with clinical outcomes similar to those observed for patients with palpable nodal metastases. Satellite and in-transit metastases have comparable biologic and prognostic significance.[148] When a patient presents with a solitary in-transit metastasis or a localized cluster of in-transit metastases, it is reasonable to perform excision of this along with SNBx. The margin of excision should be adequate to obtain free margins. This usually requires a 5- to 10-mm margin. A fairly frequent clinical scenario that is difficult to manage is the patient with multiple in-transit metastases. This most commonly occurs in the lower extremity from primary lesions below the knee, but it may occur in other locations. There is no ideal management for such patients because the natural history almost always involves systemic dissemination of disease, which may occur simultaneously, within a few months, or many years after the in-transit metastases. The large majority of such patients will continue to develop new in-transit metastases over time, and so true control of this process is uncommon. However, there is no reliable systemic therapy for this process; thus, surgery remains the best first option for regional control, when feasible. In some scenarios, surgical management of a symptomatic lesion may be valuable for palliation while addressing the appropriate management of other in-transit disease.

Because these patients typically continue to progress with more in-transit metastases and shorter intervals between metastases, other options for management are needed. Radiation therapy may be considered after surgical resection in this setting. Other regional options include intralesional therapy with interferon-α, interleukin (IL)-2, bacillus Calmette-Guérin (BCG), oncolytic replication competent virus injections and dyes like Rose Bengal[149] or application of diphencyprone,[150] or topical treatment of superficial metastases with imiquimod, all of which can induce responses in the treated lesions and occasionally in untreated lesions.

With the marked improvements in systemic treatments for advanced melanoma the indication for surgical excision of satellite lesions and in-transit melanoma decreases. The presence of these lesions is a hallmark of a melanoma that has ability to metastasize. Therefore, an early systemic intervention with the existing locoregional skin lesions being used as indicators for the effectiveness of the treatment has the potential to change the natural course of that melanoma as opposed to serving as a temporary local therapy. Systemic treatments that could be used in this setting are anti–cytotoxic T-lymphocyte antigen (CTLA4), anti–programmed death 1 PD-1 or anti-PD-L1 antibodies, and the neoadjuvant use of BRAF and other targeted inhibitors.[151]

Isolated Limb Perfusion and Infusion

An option for management of some patients with extensive regional recurrences in an extremity is hyperthermic isolated limb perfusion (ILP) with melphalan or isolated limb infusion. ILP can lead to complete responses in 60% to 90% of patients, with complete responses reported in 25% to 69% of patients.[152,153] Some patients will fail to respond and others may have short-duration responses, but a

subset of patients may have durable complete responses and long-term survival.[153] Retreatment with ILP or isolated limb infusion is feasible with some benefit. There also is some morbidity associated with ILP, including a low risk of limb loss. ILP may also shrink an unresectable recurrence, rendering it resectable. Tumor necrosis factor-α has been explored as a regional therapy agent for use in combination with melphalan in ILP for melanoma, with some encouraging findings in initial assessments. However, a randomized, prospective clinical trial performed through the American College of Surgeons Oncology Group, Z0020, showed no improvement in response rates or clinical outcome with melphalan plus tumor necrosis factor-α compared with melphalan alone.[152]

ILP has also been studied in the adjuvant setting after surgical treatment of a primary melanoma on the extremity, but no benefit was seen with this therapy in the adjuvant setting.[154]

Intratumoral Therapies with Potential Systemic Effects

Intratumoral therapies have been studied to induce regression of injected lesions in patients who are not good candidates for aggressive surgery or in patients with many cutaneous in-transit metastases. Intralesional BCG has been used successfully and occasionally with regression of uninjected lesions as well as injected lesions,[155] A recent randomized phase 3 trial reported clinical responses after intralesional injection of melanoma metastases with an oncolytic herpes virus encoding granulocyte macrophage–colony-stimulating factor (GM-CSF), called talimogene laherparepvec, with improved clinical response rates compared to control patients receiving GM-CSF alone.[156] In that study, there were regressions of treated and untreated lesions, with a 26% response rate (11% complete response) versus 6% with GM-CSF control (1% complete response), with durable response rate of 16% versus 2% ($p < 0.0001$), with a trend to better survival at interim analysis.[156] Review of the literature reveals a range of outcomes with intratumoral injection therapies or topical treatments of cutaneous metastases (see Table 94.4). A general finding is that noninjected lesions regress in some patients, but only if the injected lesions regress.

Other approaches studied for direct treatment of individual metastases, but not included in Table 94.4, include focused radiation therapy, pulsed dye laser therapy, intralesional GM-CSF, electrochemotherapy with cisplatin, or any of several oncolytic viruses administered intralesionally.[157] The German S3 guidelines for melanoma management discuss intralesional medical therapy of local and regional recurrences for melanoma, based on a summary of the literature, and specify that "patients with satellite and in-transit metastases should be treated within the context of clinical studies if possible," and that the highest response rates to intralesional therapy have included intratumoral IL-2, intratumoral electrochemotherapy with bleomycin or cisplatin, or local therapy with diphencyprone. All of these warrant investigation alone or in combination with other active therapies.

Management of Regional Lymph Node Metastases

In patients with metastases to regional nodes, prognosis is related to tumor burden in the nodes and the number of nodes involved with tumor. In numerous studies, the number of metastatic nodes is the dominant prognostic factor in stage III melanoma.[76,158] The extent of lymph node involvement has been studied in various ways. For the current staging system, differentiation was made between clinically occult metastases (sentinel node positive, clinically negative) and clinically positive (palpable) metastatic nodes. This was a significant prognostic distinction.[74,76] Patients with non-ulcerated primary melanomas and one to three positive sentinel nodes are stage IIIA, and 5-year survival probability is significantly better than 50%. However, a palpable node represents stage IIIB disease. Prognosis also is worse for patients with four or more tumor-involved nodes or with satellite or in-transit metastases in addition to nodal metastases (stage IIIC).

Management of Patients After a Positive Sentinel Node Biopsy (Stage IIIa if Nonulcerated Primary Lesion, One to Three Positive Nodes)

The rationale for performing SNBx, when first developed, was to avoid the morbidity of CLND in the 80% to 85% of patients with negative regional nodes, but simultaneously to stage patients accurately and to select those patients with regional nodal metastasis for CLND. However, experience with SNBx for melanoma has been that most patients with positive sentinel nodes have only one positive node, and only about 15% of patients have melanoma metastases identified in CLND specimens.[159] This finding has prompted consideration of abandoning CLND for some patients after positive SNBx. Review of data from the National Cancer Database showed that only about 50% of patients with positive sentinel nodes in the United States undergo CLND.[160] Thus, there is a wide range of practice without clear consensus. Several studies have identified features of the positive sentinel node that predict a low risk of a positive CLND, with the suggestion that CLND may not be necessary in such situations. Features such as the number of positive sentinel nodes, the tumor burden, and the location of tumor in the node plus features of the primary melanoma all are associated with greater risk of positive nonsentinel nodes.[161] However, most clinical experience with SNBx and evaluation of nonsentinel nodes is complicated by the fact that sentinel nodes are evaluated by a much more rigorous histopathologic approach than nonsentinel nodes, and thus the incidence of positive nonsentinel nodes may be greater than the reported 15%. One study used multiantigen reverse transcriptase-PCR to evaluate nonsentinel nodes from patients whose formal pathology report was negative for melanoma and found molecular evidence of melanoma metastases in 54% of these patients.[162] This PCR approach is typically more sensitive than standard histology and may detect positive nodes that have such a low tumor burden as to be clinically insignificant. However, the current limited data suggest that the true rate of positive nonsentinel nodes after a positive SNBx may be somewhere between 15% and 50%.

The standard recommendation has been to perform CLND of any lymph node basin with a positive sentinel node for melanoma.[163] However, some patients refuse to have CLND or are not eligible for it because of medical contraindications. A recent article summarized the combined experience from 16 institutions and reported on the clinical outcome of 134 patients who had positive SNBx but who did not undergo CLND.[164] Their outcomes were compared with a cohort of patients with positive sentinel nodes who did undergo CLND. At a median follow-up of 20 months, 15% of patients had developed recurrent melanoma in lymph nodes as a component of a first recurrence. This was not significantly different from the outcome in patients who underwent CLND.[164] Thus, there is now justification for reconsidering the best surgical management after positive SNBx. Morton and colleagues initiated the MSLT2, which is randomizing patients with positive SNBx to (1) CLND or (2) close observation with lymph node basin ultrasound.[164] This trial will take several years to accrue and additional years for mature data. Until then, there will likely be evolution of perspectives about CLND after SNBx. There is support both for CLND and for close observation after positive SNBx, and thus equipoise exists for the MSLT2 trial. In the midst of this debate, the 2012 joint guidelines from the Society of Surgical Oncology and the American Society of Clinical Oncology recommend CLND for all patients with positive sentinel lymph nodes.[129]

Management of Palpable Metastatic Melanoma in Regional Nodes: Therapeutic or Completion Lymphadenectomy

The other clinical settings for lymphadenectomy include various presentations with clinically evident regional nodes: after a negative SNBx, after observation of a nodal basin, or from an unknown primary melanoma. If lymph node recurrence appears after a prior complete dissection in the same basin, the surgical management may include a repeat node dissection, but if there is confidence that the original dissection was thorough, the repeat procedure may be more limited to the site of evident tumor recurrence.

Metastasis to a regional node represents stage III (A, B, or C) disease and is associated with a subsequent risk of distant metastasis in the range of 40% to 80%. Nonetheless, there is a significant chance of cure after complete lymphadenectomy for stage III melanoma[105,158] with overall 25-year survival rates of 35%.[165] Thus, lymphadenectomy for stage III melanoma is performed with curative intent. However, even if the patient develops distant disease in the future, there is benefit in achieving regional control, which is obtained in about 90% of patients.[105] When regional nodal disease is left in place, it can become extensive, with skin involvement, even ulceration, and with extension to involve major neurovascular structures. An example of extensive axillary recurrence with skin involvement is shown in Figure 94.12. Aggressive surgical management of less extensive disease can avoid these changes in most patients.

There are some specific considerations related to lymph node dissections in different node basins. These are summarized as follows.

Axillary Dissection

Axillary dissection should include all node-bearing tissue in levels I, II, and III. The long thoracic nerve and thoracodorsal neurovascular bundle should be identified and preserved unless involved with tumor. The superior border of dissection should be the axillary vein, anteriorly, which should be skeletonized. However, deep to the axillary vein and plexus, the axillary space extends superiorly and medially substantially above the level of the axillary vein, and that region should be cleared surgically, with careful attention to preservation of the long thoracic nerve, which runs along the chest wall to its origin from spinal nerves. The intercostobrachial nerve and lower intercostal nerves that run through the axillary space may usually be sacrificed. The pectoralis major and minor muscles are usually preserved along with the medial pectoral nerve and vessels, but in reoperative cases or cases with involvement of one or both of

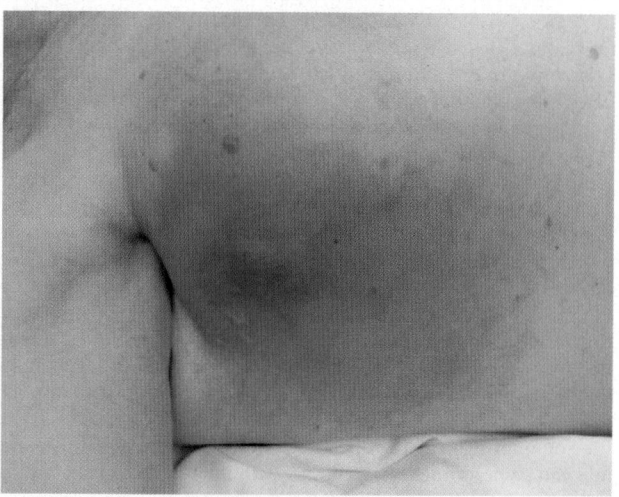

Figure 94.12 Extensive axillary adenopathy before resection.

these muscles, part of all of them may be sacrificed. It is rare for the long thoracic node to be involved with tumor, and it should be preserved because denervation of the serratus anterior muscle leads to "winged scapula" and can be associated with chronic pain related to destabilization of the shoulder. When there is bulky axillary disease, though, it is not uncommon for the thoracodorsal nerve to be involved, and patients usually tolerate sacrifice of that nerve when necessary. However, the possibility of resection of it should be discussed with patients preoperatively, especially when there is bulky adenopathy. In addition, if there is bulky axillary disease, the tumor often abuts or involves the axillary vein. The axillary vein usually consists of more than one vessel running in parallel; thus, sacrifice of the lowest limb of the axillary vein often is accomplished without evident morbidity. Even sacrifice of the entire axillary vein (one or several trunks) is usually tolerated well and can be considered in cases of advanced disease when necessary to enable complete resection of recurrent tumor. A troublesome finding is tumor involvement of the brachial plexus. Definitive therapy of that may require forequarter amputation, which is usually an unappealing option when the risk of systemic recurrence is also likely to be high, as it is in such cases. One alternative is to resect as much as possible while preserving the plexus, followed by adjuvant radiation therapy to the axilla. Another is to resect part of the brachial plexus, which has been reported, and in experienced hands can be done with reasonable outcomes.

In the vast majority of cases, even with some bulky disease, axillary dissection can be performed with minimal morbidity, with full expectation of full range of motion and function after recovery from the surgery over approximately 8 to 12 weeks. Lymphedema is an expected long-term complication, but it is usually a significant clinical issue in only about 10% of patients, and it can often be treated well with compression sleeve and/or manual lymphatic drainage therapy.

Inguinal and Iliac Dissection

For patients with metastatic melanoma to inguinal nodes, complete groin dissection is indicated. The nomenclature and clinical practice patterns vary for this procedure. As described by Spratt et al.,[166] the inguinal region can be defined as including the superficial inguinal region, which is superficial to the fascia that lies immediately superficial to the femoral vessels, and the deep inguinal region, which is deep to that fascia and includes the femoral vessels. The saphenous vein enters the femoral vein in the upper third of the inguinal region and passes through a foramen in the deep fascia. Cloquet node is the deep inguinal node that is classically considered to be the transitional node between the inguinal region and the iliac region. Although it is variable in its location, presence, and size, a superficial groin dissection should include removal of that node and identification of it for histologic evaluation. If that node contains metastatic melanoma, an iliac and obturator dissection is usually indicated. When patients have extensive nodal disease in the inguinal region, a complete inguinal dissection is appropriate, with skeletonization of the femoral artery and vein, often with a Sartorius flap to cover these vessels. However, for completion node dissection after a positive SNBx, a superficial inguinal dissection with excision of Cloquet node may be performed. Cloquet node is accessible through the foramen in which the saphenous bulb is found and is located lateral to the saphenous bulb.

Some surgeons describe the iliac region as the deep groin, but this terminology can lead to ambiguity. An iliac node dissection involves skeletonizing the external iliac vessels and is generally combined with removal of the iliac node-bearing tissue and obturator fat pad (obturator dissection). This dissection extends from the inguinal ligament to the takeoff of the internal iliac vessels and can be performed in continuity with the inguinal dissection or through a separate lower-quadrant abdominal wall incision and a retroperitoneal approach.

Patients with known inguinal metastases should undergo CT scan of the pelvis or PET/CT scan. Clinical evidence of iliac adenopathy or a positive Cloquet node at the time of groin dissection is an indication for iliac and obturator dissection. There is a range of clinical practice; some surgeons perform iliac dissections routinely for patients with extensive inguinal adenopathy.

The risk of lymphedema with inguinal or ilioinguinal dissection is greater than for axillary or cervical node dissections. Although most patients recover well, some degree of lymphedema probably occurs in most patients with this procedure. It may require a fitted compression stocking or massage therapy approaches.

Cervical Dissection

Metastatic melanoma to a cervical node is appropriately managed by complete neck dissection. A modified radical neck dissection should be performed, with preservation of the internal jugular vein, sternocleidomastoid muscle, and spinal accessory nerve. However, if these structures are invaded by tumor or involved with tumor, they can be resected. Sacrifice of the spinal accessory nerve can cause significant morbidity but is occasionally necessary. Melanomas of the face, ear, or anterior scalp often drain to parotid or periparotid nodes. In such cases, superficial parotidectomy is indicated as part of a modified radical neck dissection. In some situations, such as metastases to submental nodes near the midline or very low cervical nodes from a medial shoulder primary, there may be rationale for a neck dissection that is limited based on lymphatic anatomy.

MANAGEMENT OF REGIONAL METASTASES IN PATIENTS WITH VISCERAL OR OTHER DISTANT DISEASE

Regional metastases are common also in patients with advanced distant disease. Management of regional metastases can be important for clinical management even in the setting of distant disease, especially when painful or presenting with skin invasion and impending ulceration.

Melanoma Radiation Therapy

Data exist to support the use of adjuvant radiation to reduce primary and regional nodal recurrences in selected patient populations and for its use for palliation of unresectable primary and nodal recurrences or distant metastases. There is no current consensus regarding the optimal dose fractionation schedule for melanoma. Controversy surrounding the radiosensitivity of melanoma began in the early 1970s when cell survival curves for several human melanoma cell lines were published showing a broad shoulder indicative of high levels of potentially lethal damage repair. This fosters the hypothesis that melanomas were less likely to respond to conventionally fractionated radiation at 2 to 2.5 Gy per fraction and that higher dose per fraction schedules might result in superior clinical outcomes.[167] These studies caused many investigators to adopt high-dose ($\geq$4 Gy per fraction) fractionation schedules for melanoma, and several investigators published improved clinical outcomes with these large fractional doses compared to conventional fractionation.[168] This led the Radiation Therapy Oncology Group (RTOG) to initiate RTOG 83-05, which was a prospective randomized trial comparing the effectiveness of high dose per fraction radiation and conventionally fractionated radiation in the treatment of melanoma. RTOG 83-05 randomized 126 patients with measurable lesions to 8.0 Gy × 4 fractions (32 Gy total) in 21 days delivered once weekly or 2.5 Gy × 20 fractions (50 Gy total) in 26 to 28 days delivered 5 days a week. The study was closed early when interim statistical analysis suggested that further accrual would not reveal a statistical difference between the arms. The 8.0 Gy × 4 fraction arm had a complete remission of 24% and partial remission of 36%, and the 20 × 2.5 Gy arm had a complete remission of 23% and partial remission of 34%.[168] This randomized trial demonstrated that melanoma is a radioresponsive tumor, and conventional and high dose per fraction schedules are equally effective clinically.

Despite the results of this study, many investigators still report that melanoma is a radioresistant histology and most current retrospective clinical reports regarding radiation for melanoma have used a high dose per fraction schedule. Although high dose per fraction treatments can result in increased risk of late radiation toxicity, there are little data to suggest that high dose per fraction schedules such as 30 Gy in five fractions over 2.5 weeks, which is currently commonly used in the adjuvant treatment of nodal basins following lymph node dissection,[169] results in increased late toxicity compared to conventionally fractionated regimens to 50 to 70 Gy. High-dose fractionation schedules are more convenient for the patient, less expensive, allow patients to proceed with systemic therapy sooner, and should be considered as a reasonable option unless critical structures are in the irradiated volume that would be treated above their radiation tolerance or the volume has previously been irradiated. They are particularly appropriate for patients with widespread disease and short life expectancies as they can provide rapid palliation, and late-radiation toxicity is not a concern for this patient population.

The Role of Radiation Therapy in the Management of Regional Nodal Disease

Patients with positive SNBx or palpable regional nodal metastases (stage III disease) are treated with therapeutic inguinal, axillary, or cervical lymph node dissections. Several large retrospective studies have identified lymph node extracapsular extension, large lymph nodes ($\geq$3 cm in diameter), four or more involved lymph nodes, or recurrent disease after previous lymph node dissection as adverse risk factors that increase the risk for nodal basin recurrence following therapeutic nodal dissection to 30% to 50%.[76,170,171] Given the potential morbidity of recurrent unresectable nodal disease with pain, ulceration, bleeding, and lymphedema, these high-risk patients have been treated with high dose per fraction or conventionally fractionated postoperative adjuvant radiation delivered to nodal basins. Retrospective reports from several centers report 5-year locoregional control rates after radiation ranging from 80% to 93%.[169,171] There are no prospective randomized data comparing high dose per fraction schedules to conventional fractionation schedules to compare efficacy or toxicity between these treatment techniques; however, locoregional control rates appear to be equivalent with both schedules, resulting in 87% 5-year locoregional control rate in at least one report.[171]

Despite the improvement in locoregional control, postoperative adjuvant nodal irradiation has not shown a survival benefit. Most reports quote 5-year survival rates of 33% to 0%, which is similar to historic rates of patients not undergoing radiation or patients undergoing radiation following a re-excision of nodal failures, because of high rates of distant metastatic spread in this patient population.[169,171,172] Radiation complication rates in these retrospective studies vary depending on the site irradiated and include lymphedema, fibrosis, nerve plexopathies, and osteonecrosis, with lymphedema of the arm and leg being the major toxicity reported in most series.[169,171,172] Given the retrospective nature of these studies, it is not clear if some of these toxicities are solely attributable to radiation or are related to surgical morbidity or tumor recurrence.

In a multi-institutional report, the outcomes of 615 patients from MD Anderson and Roswell Park Cancer Centers with advanced regional nodal metastatic disease who underwent lymphadenectomy with and without adjuvant radiation were reported retrospectively.[173] On multivariate analysis, the number of positive lymph nodes, the number of lymph nodes removed, and the use of adjuvant radiation were associated with improved regional control. At a median follow-up of 60 months, regional failure occurred in 10% of patients with adjuvant radiation and 41% without adjuvant radiation. Distant metastatic disease developed in 55% of patients treated with adjuvant radiation and 74% of patients treated without adjuvant radiation. On multivariate analysis, disease-specific survival was reported to be significantly improved by the addition of adjuvant radiation.[173] In summary, retrospective data suggest that postoperative adjuvant radiation for patients with stage III disease results in improved locoregional control with reasonable complication rates but with no obvious survival benefit in most reports.

The Trans Tasman Radiation Oncology Group (Study 96.06) is the first prospective single-arm phase 2 study of adjuvant postoperative radiation therapy following lymphadenectomy in malignant melanoma with sufficient statistical power to answer its primary end points of regional in field relapse and late toxicity rates and secondary end points of adjacent relapse, distant relapse, OS, progression-free survival (PFS), and time to in-field recurrence. A total of 234 patients were treated with CLND followed by 48 Gy delivered in 20 fractions with 2.4 Gy per fraction over 4 weeks to the nodal basin using specified treatment guidelines. The reported overall pattern of first relapse showed a regional in-field recurrence rate of 6.8% and a distant relapse rate of 63%. The 5-year OS was 36% and the 5-year regional control rate was 91%. Grade 3 toxicity from axillary and inguinal lymphedema was 9% and 19%, respectively.[174] Burmeister et al.[175] reported results of the first multicenter prospective randomized trial (Trans Tasman Radiation Oncology Group 02.01/ANZMTG 01.02) comparing postoperative adjuvant radiation (48 Gy in 20 fractions) versus observation of patients with high-risk nodal metastatic melanoma (one or more parotid node, two or more cervical or axillary, or three or more groin-positive nodes, extracapsular spread, or $\geq$3 cm diameter cervical or axillary node or $\geq$4 cm groin node) following lymphadenectomy. A total of 250 patients were randomized and 217 were eligible for analysis; with a median follow-up of 27 months, the regional nodal failure rates were 19% for the radiation arm and 31% for the observation arm ($p = 0.041$) and median disease-free survival times and OS times were not significantly different ($p = 0.56$ and 0.12, respectively).[175] This study also found that the extent of extranodal extension (ENE) of melanoma independently predicted in-basin lymph node recurrences (14% for those without ENE, 17% with limited ENE, and 32% with extensive ENE, $p = 0.001$, multivariate).[175] Therefore, adjuvant radiation therapy to a nodal basin in patients with high risk of relapse after surgery improved local control at the expense of increased toxicities, but since the main risk in these patients is systemic relapse, then its use needs to be carefully evaluated in the setting of lack of improvement in PFS and OS.

ADJUVANT SYSTEMIC THERAPY (STAGES IIB, IIC, AND III)

Adjuvant Interferon Therapy

After over 50 years and in excess of 100 randomized clinical trials aimed at decreasing the relapse rate of melanomas at a high risk of relapse after surgery, only interferon-α (in two different formulations) has gained regulatory approval by either the FDA and/or the European Medicines Agency. Interferon-α–based adjuvant therapy has been administered in several variations: (1) HDI-α for 1 month followed by 1 year of intermediate dosing, (2) interferon-α at an intermediate dose administered for 1 or 2 years, (3) interferon-α at a low dose administered for 1 or 3 years, or (4) pegylated interferon administered for a target period of 5 years (Table 94.5). The multiple randomized clinical trials testing the benefits of interferon-α using these different regimens in the adjuvant setting have been subject of metanalysis.[176]

TABLE 94.5

Listing of Major Adjuvant Phase 3 Clinical Trials with Interon Alpha

Study Reference	No. of Patients Eligible for Analysis	TNM Stage	Therapy and IFN Subspecies	IFN Dose and Schedule—Treatment Arm	Median Follow-up at Time of Reporting (y)	DFS	OS	% Node positive
High Dose								
NCCTG 83-7052 Creagan[1]	262	II–III (T2-4N0M0/TanyN+M0)	IFN-α2a vs. observation	IM 20 MU/m² 3×/wk for 4 mo	6.1	NS	NS	61
ECOG E1684 Kirkwood[2]	287	II–III (T4N0M0/TanyN+M0)	IFN-α2b—high dose vs. observation	IV 20 MU/m² 5×/wk for 4 wk → then → SC 10 MU/m² 3×/wk for 48 wk	6.9, 12.1	S	S (S at 6.9 y NS at 12.1 y)	89
ECOG E1690 Kirkwood[3]	642	II–III (T4N0M0/TanyN+M0)	IFN-α2b—high dose vs. low dose vs. observation	High dose: IV 20 MU/m² 5×/wk for 4 wk → then → SC 10 MU/m² 3×/wk for 48 wk; Low dose: SC 3 MU/m² 2×/wk for 2 y	4.3, 6.6	S	NS	75
ECOG E1694 Kirkwood[4]	774	II–III (T4N0M0/TanyN+M0)	IFN-α2b—high dose vs. GMK vaccine	IV 20 MU/m² 5×/wk for 4 wk → then → SC 10 MU/m² 2×/wk for 48 wk	1.3, 2.1	S	S	77
Italian Melanoma Intergroup Chiarion-Sileni[5]	330	III (TanyN1-3M0)	Intensified IFN-α2b every other month vs. IFN-α2b high dose for 1 y	Intensified high dose: IV 20 MU/m² 5×/wk4 wk every other month for four cycles; Standard high dose: IV 20 MU/m² 5×/wk for 4 wk → then → SC 10 MU/m² 3×/wkfor 48 wk	5.0	NS	NS	100
Intermediate Dose								
EORTC 18952 Eggermont[6]	1388	II–III (T4N0M0/TanyN+M0)	IFN-α2b for 1 y vs. 2 y vs. observation	IV 10 MU 5×/wk for 4 wk → then → SC 10 MU 3×/wk for 1 y OR SC 5 MU 3×/wk for 2 y	4.65	NS	NS	74
EORTC 18991 Eggermont[7]	1256	III (TanyN+M0)	PEG IFN-α2b vs. observation	SC 6 µg/kg/wk for 8 wk → then → SC 3 µg/kg/wk for 5 y	3.8	S	NS	100
Low Dose								
AMCG Pehamberger[8]	311	II (T2-4N0M0)	IFN-α2a vs. observation	SC 3 MU 7×/wk for 3 wk → then → SC 3 MU 3×/wk for 1 y	3.4 (mean)	S	NS	0
FCGM Grob[9]	499	II (T2-4N0M0)	IFN-α2a vs. observation	SC 3 MU 3×/wk for 3 y	>3	0.74 (HR), S	0.70 (HR), S	0
WHO-16 Cascinelli[10]	444	III (TanyN+M0)	IFN-α2a vs. observation	SC 3 MU 3×/wk for 3 y	7.3	NS	NS	100

Trial	N	Stage (TNM)	Treatment	Dose/schedule	Median F/U (y)	DFS	OS	%
Scottish Melanoma Cooperative Group Cameron[11]	96	II–III (T3-4N0M0/TanyN+M0)	IFN-α2a vs. observation	SC 3 MU 3×/wk for 6 mo	6.5	NS	NS	Not available
EORTC 18871/ DKG-80 Kleeberg[12]	728	II–III (T3-4N0M0/TanyN+M0)	IFN-α2b vs. IFN-γ vs. ISCADOR M (Weleda, Basel, Switzerland) vs. observation	IFN-α2b: SC 1 MU every other day for 12 mo / IFN-γ: SC 0.2 mg every other day for 12 mo / ISCADOR M	8.2	NS NS NS	NS NS NS	58
UKCCCR/AIM HIGH Hancock[13]	674	II–III (T3-4N0M0/TanyN+M0)	IFN-α2a vs. observation	SC 3 MU 3×/wk for 2 y	3.1	NS	NS	70
DeCOG Hauschild[14]	840	III (T3anyN+M0)	IFN-α2a for 18 mo (A) vs. 3 y (B)	SC 3 MU 3×/wk for 18 mo vs. 3 y	4.3	NS	NS	18
DeCOG Garbe[15]	441	III (TanyN+M0)	IFNα2a (A) vs. IFNα2a + dacarbazine (B) vs. Observation (C)	SC 3 MU 3×/wk for 24 mo (A) vs. SC 3 MU 3×/wk for 24 mo + DTIC 850 mg/m² every 4–8 wk for 24 mo (B) vs.	3.9	S NS	S NS	100%

TNM, tumor, node, metastasis; IFN, interferon; DFS, disease-free survival; OS, overall survival; NCCTG, North Central Cancer Treatment Group; IM, intramuscular; NS, not significant; ECOG, Eastern Cooperative Oncology Group; IV, intravenous; SC, subcutaneous; S, significant; AMCG, Austrian Melanoma Cooperative Group; FCGM, French Melanoma Cooperative Group; HR, hazard ratio; WHO, World Health Organization; EORTC, European Organisation for Research and Treatment of Cancer; UKCCCR, United Kingdom Co-ordinating Committee on Cancer Research; DeCOG, Dermatologic Cooperative Oncology Group.

Provided by Ahmad Tarhini (Adapted from Davar D, Tarhini AA, Kirkwood JM. Adjuvant immunotherapy of melanoma and development of new approaches using the neoadjuvant approach. *Clin Dermatol* 2013;31:237–250).

High Dose
1. Creagan ET, Dalton RJ, Ahmann DL, et al. Randomized, surgical adjuvant clinical trial of recombinant interferon alfa-2a in selected patients with malignant melanoma. *J Clin Oncol* 1995;13:2776–2783.
2. Kirkwood JM, Strawderman MH, Ernstoff MS, et al. Interferon alfa-2b adjuvant therapy of high-risk resected cutaneous melanoma: the Eastern Cooperative Oncology Group Trial EST 1684. *J Clin Oncol* 1996;14:7–17.
3. Kirkwood JM, Ibrahim JG, Sondak VK, et al. High- and low-dose interferon alfa-2b in high-risk melanoma: first analysis of intergroup trial E1690/S9111/C9190. *J Clin Oncol* 2000;18:2444–2458.
4. Kirkwood JM, Ibrahim JG, Sosman JA, et al. High-dose interferon alfa-2b significantly prolongs relapse-free and overall survival compared with the GM2-KLH/QS-21 vaccine in patients with resected stage IIB-III melanoma: results of intergroup trial E1694/S9512/C509801. *J Clin Oncol* 2001;19:2370–2380.
5. Chiarion-Sileni V, Guida M, Romanini A, et al. Intensified high-dose intravenous interferon alpha 2b (IFNa2b) for adjuvant treatment of stage III melanoma: a randomized phase III Italian Melanoma Intergroup (IMI) trial [ISRCTN75125874]. *J Clin Oncol* 2011;29:Abstract 8506.

Intermediate
6. Eggermont AM, Suciu S, MacKie R, et al. Post-surgery adjuvant therapy with intermediate doses of interferon alfa 2b versus observation in patients with stage IIb/III melanoma (EORTC 18952): randomised controlled trial. *Lancet* 2005;366:1189–1196.
7. Bouwhuis MG, Suciu S, Testori A, et al. Phase III trial comparing adjuvant treatment with pegylated interferon Alfa-2b versus observation: prognostic significance of autoantibodies—EORTC 18991. *J Clin Oncol* 2010;28:2460–2466.

Low Dose
8. Pehamberger H, Soyer HP, Steiner A, et al. Adjuvant interferon alfa-2a treatment in resected primary stage II cutaneous melanoma. Austrian Malignant Melanoma Cooperative Group. *J Clin Oncol* 1998;16:1425–1429.
9. Grob JJ, Dreno B, de la Salmonière P, et al. Randomised trial of interferon alpha-2a as adjuvant therapy in resected primary melanoma thicker than 1.5 mm without clinically detectable node metastases. French Cooperative Group on Melanoma. *Lancet* 1998;351:1905–1910.
10. Cascinelli N, Belli F, MacKie RM, et al. Effect of long-term adjuvant therapy with interferon alpha-2a in patients with regional node metastases from cutaneous melanoma: a randomised trial. *Lancet* 2001;358:866–869.
11. Cameron DA, Cornbleet MC, Mackie RM, et al. Adjuvant interferon alpha 2b in high risk melanoma—the Scottish study. *Br J Cancer* 2001;84:1146–1149.
12. Kleeberg UR, Suciu S, Bröcker EB, et al. Final results of the EORTC 18871/DKG 80-1 randomised phase III trial. rIFN-alpha2b versus rIFN-gamma versus ISCADOR M versus observation after surgery in melanoma patients with either high-risk primary (thickness >3 mm) or regional lymph node metastasis. *Eur J Cancer* 2004;40:390–402.
13. Hancock BW, Wheatley K, Harris S, et al. Adjuvant interferon in high-risk melanoma: the AIM HIGH Study—United Kingdom Coordinating Committee on Cancer Research randomized study of adjuvant low-dose extended-duration interferon alfa-2a in high-risk resected malignant melanoma. *J Clin Oncol* 2004;22:53–61.
14. Hauschild A, Weichenthal M, Rass K, et al. Efficacy of low-dose interferon [alpha]2a 18 versus 60 months of treatment in patients with primary melanoma of >= 1.5 mm tumor thickness: results of a randomized phase III DeCOG trial. *J Clin Oncol* 2010;28:841–846.
15. Garbe C, Radny P, Linse R, et al. Adjuvant low-dose interferon [alpha]2a with or without dacarbazine compared with surgery alone: a prospective-randomized phase III DeCOG trial in melanoma patients with regional lymph node metastasis. *Ann Oncol* 2008;19:1195–1201.

PRACTICE OF ONCOLOGY

TABLE 94.6

Summary of Ongoing Phase 2 Adjuvant Trials in High-Risk Melanoma

Study Reference	No. of Patients	TNM Stage	Therapy	Dose and Schedule— Treatment Arm	Primary Endpoint	ClinicalTrials .gov Identifier
EORTC 18071	950	III (T_{any}, N+ except in transit, M0)	Ipilimumab vs. placebo	IV, 10 mg/kg, 4× every 21 d, then starting from week 24 every 12 wk until week 156 or progression, 3 y	RFS	NCT00636168
US Intergroup E1609	1,500	III (IIIB, IIIC), IV (M1a, M1b)	Ipilimumab at 10 mg/kg (Arm A) or 3 mg/kg (Arm C) vs. high-dose interferon-alpha (Arm B)	IV, 10 mg/kg (A) or 3 mg/kg (C), 4× every 21 d, then starting from week 24 every 12 wk, 4× Vs. IV 20 MU/m² 5×/wk for 4 wk, then SC 10 MU/m² 3×/wk for 48 wk	RFS and OS	NCT01274338
COMBI-AD	852	III BRAF V600E/K mutation-positive	Dabrafenib + trametinib vs. placebo	Dabrafenib (150 mg twice daily) and trametinib (2 mg once daily) orally for 12 mo	RFS	NCT01682083
BRIM 8	725	IIC, III BRAF V600 mutation positive by Cobas (Roche, Basel, Switzerland)	Vemurafenib vs. placebo	Vemurafenib 960 mg orally twice daily for 52 wk	DFS	NCT01667419
DERMA	1349	IIIB or IIIC (tumor expression of MAGE-A3 gene)	GSK 2132231A (D1/3-MAGE-3-His fusion protein) vs. placebo	GSK 2132231A IM solution, 13 injections over 27 mo	DFS	NCT00796445

TNM, tumor, node, metastasis; EORTC, European Organisation for Research and Treatment of Cancer; IV, intravenous; RFS, relapse-free survival; OS, overall survival; SC, subcutaneous; DFS, disease-free survival; IM, intramuscular.
Provided by Ahmad Tarhini (Adapted from Davar D, Tarhini AA, Kirkwood JM. Adjuvant immunotherapy of melanoma and development of new approaches using the neoadjuvant approach. *Clin Dermatol* 2013;31:237–250).

Data from a total of 10,499 participants enrolled in 18 randomized clinical trials were reviewed, allowing the evaluation of the therapeutic efficacy of interferon in terms of disease-free survival (17 trials) and OS (15 trials). Adjuvant interferon was associated with significantly improved disease-free survival (HR = 0.83; 95% CI, 0.78 to 0.87, $p < 0.00001$) and OS (HR = 0.91; 95% CI, 0.85 to 0.97; $p = 0.003$). Subgroup analyses failed to detect a significant impact of different regimens of interferon-α administration or patient subgroups with different benefit to this mode of therapy. The use of adjuvant interferon-based therapy has become the standard of care therapy in most melanoma centers and in the community, and it is the basis of most comparator arms in ongoing adjuvant therapy clinical trials (Table 94.6).

High-Dose Interferon-α2B

Adjuvant HDI-α2b was approved by the FDA in 1996 for the treatment of resected stage IIB and stage III melanoma based on the results of the Eastern Cooperative Oncology Group (ECOG) trial E1684.[177] Interferon-α was administered by intravenous infusion, 20 million U/m², for 5 consecutive days every 7 days for 4 weeks during the "induction" phase. For the subsequent 48 weeks, 10 million U/m² were administered by subcutaneous injection on alternate days for a total of three doses every 7 days in the "maintenance" phase. The control arm was observation, which was the standard at the time that the trial was conducted. A total of 287 patients were enrolled, 80% of whom had stage III melanoma; 20% had stage IIB melanoma. Pathologic staging was performed with regional lymph node dissection because SNBx had not yet been introduced. Overall survival was the primary end point, and the trial was designed to detect a 33% improvement. A protocol-specified analysis with median follow-up of 6.9 years revealed a statistically significant 33% improvement

by HR in OS compared to the observation arm after adjusting for other prognostic factors in a multivariate model ($p = 0.012$). Relapse-free survival was also significantly improved (39% improvement by HR compared to observation after adjusting for other prognostic factors; $p = 0.001$). Approximately three-fourths of the interferon-treated patients experiencing grade 3 or 4 toxicities by National Cancer Institute Common Toxicity Criteria. The most common were fatigue, asthenia, fever, depression, and elevated liver transaminases. A subsequent quality-of-life analysis of this trial population suggested that the toxicity associated with this regimen was largely compensated for by the psychological benefit derived from prevention of disease relapse.[178]

Since the reporting of E1684, several other studies of HDI have been conducted. Overall, nearly 2,000 patients with stage IIB and III melanoma have participated in four multicenter, randomized trials, conducted by the US Intergroup, investigating adjuvant HDI-α2b therapy. Data from these E1684, E1690, E1694, and E2696 clinical trials was updated to April 2001.[179] Analysis of treatment effects versus observation was based on data from 713 patients randomized to HDI or observation in trials E1684 and E1690. Overall, this updated analysis confirmed the original conclusions with the extended median follow-up intervals of 2.1 to 12.6 years. Relapse-free survival, but not OS, was significantly prolonged (two-sided log-rank $p = 0.006$) for patients treated with HDI versus observation. Among all patients, ulceration, recurrent disease at entry, enrollment in E1684, and age >49 years significantly negatively impacted relapse-free survival.

The North Central Cancer Treatment Group trial tested a regimen of 20 MU/m² dose of interferon-α2a administered intramuscularly three times per week for 12 weeks for stage II and III disease. This clinical trial demonstrated improvements in median disease-free survival and OS that were nonsignificant, with higher-risk patients appearing to benefit disproportionately.[180]

Several clinical trials have tested a variety of regimens using lower doses of interferon, which have been conducted with the goal of decreasing toxicities while maintain efficacy. EORTC 18871 used a very-low-dose regimen (1 MU subcutaneously every other day), while the low-dose regimen of 3 MU subcutaneously thrice weekly was tested in WHO Melanoma Program Trial 16[181] (stage III), Scottish Melanoma Cooperative Group trial[182] (stage IIB/III), UK Co-ordinating Committee on Cancer Research AIM-High trial[183] (stage IIB/III), E169020 (T4, N1), and the 2010 German Dermatologic Cooperative Oncology Group (DeCOG) study[184] (T3Nx). None of these clinical trials showed a benefit in terms of OS. The 2008 German DeCOG study demonstrated a survival benefit for low-dose interferon but was powered primarily to assess the benefit of combination low-dose irradiation with dacarbazine and not designed to evaluate the low-dose regimen per se.[185] A number of trials have tested intermediate-dose interferon. EORTC 18952 demonstrated a 7.2% increase in distant metastases-free survival in patients with stage IIB/III, which was not statistically significant and no OS benefit was observed.[186]

Shortening the duration of therapy with HDI has also been a focus of clinical testing. The Italian Melanoma Intergroup enrolled 336 patients with stage III disease to receive either standard HDI or an intensified regimen (20 MU/m^2 intravenously 5 days/week for 4 weeks every other month for four cycles). At the 5-year mark, there were no statistically significant differences in either relapse-free survival or OS while toxicities did not increase.[187]

It had been postulated that the first month of intravenous HDI-α2b may be the main component providing benefit in HDI regimens. To test this concept, the ECOG E1697 randomized patients to 4 weeks of intravenous HDI with no maintenance therapy compared to observation. However, the interim analysis of E1697 after 1,150 of an originally planned 1,420 patients led to closing the study for futility.[188]

Pegylated Interferon-α

Pegylated interferon-α2b was approved by the FDA in 2011 for the adjuvant treatment of melanoma with microscopic or gross nodal involvement (stage III) within 84 days of definitive surgical resection including complete lymphadenectomy based on the results of EORTC 18991.[189] This was a randomized clinical trial comparing pegylated interferon-α2b with observation. Pegylation results in substantially slower clearance of interferon after administration. This allows for more stable drug exposure than can be achieved with the shorter-lived conventional interferon-α administered on alternating days by subcutaneous injection. Pegylated interferon can be administered less frequently and at a lower dose per injection but maintaining drug exposure over the course of several days. This results in a lower peak concentration after each dose while increasing the interval during which interferon is at biologically active concentrations in blood. Short-term[189] and long-term follow-up data has been provided on the EORTC 18991 clinical trial.[190] In this study, 1,256 patients with resected stage III melanoma were randomly assigned to observation (n = 629) or pegylated interferon 6 mcg/kg per week for 8 weeks by subcutaneous injection, followed by maintenance at 3 mcg/kg weekly (n = 627) for an intended duration of 5 years. Patients were prospectively stratified according to microscopic (N1) versus macroscopic (N2) nodal involvement, number of positive nodes, ulceration and tumor thickness, sex, and center. The primary end point was recurrence-free survival, and OS was a secondary end point. At 7.6 years of median follow-up, 384 recurrences or deaths had occurred with pegylated interferon versus 406 in the observation group (HR = 0.87; 95% CI, 0.76 to 1.00; p = 0.055); 7-year recurrence-free survival rate was 39% versus 35%. There was no difference in OS (p = 0.57). In stage III-N1 ulcerated melanoma, recurrence-free survival (HR = 0.72; 99% CI, 0.46 to 1.13; p = 0.06), and OS (HR = 0.59; 99% CI, 0.35 to 0.97; p = 0.006) were prolonged with pegylated interferon. Despite the anticipation that

pegylated interferon would be better tolerated than HDI, pegylated interferon was discontinued for toxicity in 37% of patients.

Cytotoxic Chemotherapy and Biochemotherapy in Adjuvant Therapy of Melanoma

There has been a long list of prospective randomized clinical trials testing single-agent or combination-agent chemotherapy in the adjuvant setting, which have been nearly universally negative in terms of providing a clear clinical advantage over the control arm. For example, dacarbazine was not effective in the postoperative setting, whether administered alone or combined with BCG.[99] The only clearly positive clinical trial has been US intergroup study led by SWOG S0008, a phase 3 clinical trial of a biochemotherapy combination compared to standard HDI-α in patients with high-risk melanoma.[191] The investigators sought to determine whether a short course of biochemotherapy would be more effective than HDI as adjuvant treatment in patients with high-risk melanoma. S0008 enrolled patients with stage IIIA-N2a through stage IIIC-N3, who were randomized to either HDI following the E1684 schedule, or biochemotherapy consisting of dacarbazine 800 mg/m^2 on day 1, cisplatin 20 mg/m^2 on days 1 to 4; vinblastine 1.2 mg/m^2 on days 1 to 4; IL-2 9 MU/m^2 per day continuous intravenous administration on days 1 to 4; interferon 5 MU/m^2 per day subcutaneously on days 1 to 4, 8, 10, and 12; and granulocyte–colony-stimulating fator 5 ug/kg per day subcutaneously on days 7 to 16. Biochemotherapy cycles were given every 21 days for three cycles (9 weeks total). Patients were stratified for number of involved nodes (one to three versus four or more), micro- versus macrometastasis, and ulceration of the primary. Coprimary end points were relapse-free survival and OS. Between 2000 and 2007, 432 patients were enrolled. Grade 3-4 adverse events occurred in 64% of patients receiving HDI and 76% of patients randomized to biochemotherapy. At a median follow-up of 7.2 years, biochemotherapy improved relapse-free survival (p = 0.015; HR = 0.75; 95% CI, 0.58 to 0.97), with median relapse-free survival for biochemotherapy of 4.0 years (95% CI, 1.9 years—not reached) versus 1.9 years for HDI (95% CI, 1.2 to 2.8 years), and a 5-year relapse-free survival of 48% versus 39%. However, the OS was not different between the two arms (p = 0.55; HR = 0.98; 95% CI, 0.74 to 1.31), with median OS of 9.9 years (95% CI, 4.62 years—not reached) for biochemotherapy versus 6.7 years (95% CI, 4.5 years—not reached) for HDI, and 5-year OS of 56% for both arms. It was concluded that biochemotherapy could be considered as a shorter alternative to HDI for patients with high-risk melanoma.

Experimental Adjuvant Immunotherapy

There has been a long list of large adjuvant clinical trials with a variety of immunotherapy approaches for melanoma with negative results. The studies used whole tumor cell vaccines like Melacine (Corixa Corporation, Seattle, WA) or Cancervax (Marina del Ray, CA), MAGE-A3 (GlaxoSmithKline, Brentford, UK), ganglioside-based vaccines like GMK (Progenics Pharmaceuticals, Inc., Tarrytown, NY), and smaller studies with melanosomal antigen peptide vaccines. Furthermore, uncontrolled studies in patients with completely surgically resected stage IV (stage IV with no evidence of disease) led to the testing of adjuvant GM-CSF and a multipeptide vaccine in a placebo-controlled, randomized, prospective trial (ECOG E4697). That trial accrued approximately 800 patients but showed no significant beneficial impact of GM-CSF on clinical outcomes.[192] Recent data highlight the critical nature of vaccine adjuvants. Murine and human data suggest that use of incomplete Freund adjuvant with short peptide vaccines may interfere with protective antitumor T-cell responses by recruiting T cells selectively back to the vaccine site rather than to the tumor.[193] On the other hand, vaccines may be made much more effective at inducing T-cell responses in patients by incorporating a toll-like receptor 9 agonist CpG.[194] Thus, new vaccine approaches will explore the value of more optimal adjuvants. Also, the availability now of clinically effective immune therapies for advanced melanoma promises to open the door to new combination immune therapies in the adjuvant setting that will be explored in clinical trials over the next few years (see Table 94.6).

Cytotoxic T-Lymphocyte Antigen 4 and PD-1 Blockade in Adjuvant Therapy

Ipilimumab is a fully human immunoglobulin G1 monoclonal antibody that blocks CTLA4, which has demonstrated improvement in OS in the treatment of metastatic melanoma in two randomized clinical trials.[195,196] This has led to clinical trials investigating the potential for ipilimumab in the adjuvant setting (see Table 94.6). EORTC 18071 is comparing ipilimumab at 10 mg/kg with maintenance therapy against placebo. Accrual is complete and results are pending. E1609 is an accruing clinical trial randomizing patients to ipilimumab at 10 mg/kg or 3 mg/kg for four doses, compared to a control arm receiving standard high-dose adjuvant interferon therapy. Enrollment on the 10 mg/kg arm was put on hold in 2013. Results are not anticipated until 2015. Early evaluation of clinical trials testing anti-PD-1 and anti-PD-L1 antibodies in patients with metastatic melanoma suggest that this class of immune modulating antibodies is likely to provide a high rate of durable tumor responses. S1404 is a planned clinical trial testing the anti-PD-1 IgG4 monoclonal antibody MK-3475 (lambrolizumab) compared to HDI. Results of this trial will take 3 to 4 years.

Neoadjuvant Therapy for Resectable Stage III or IV Melanoma

Neoadjuvant therapy for resectable stage III or stage IV melanoma remains an investigational approach. A study of neoadjuvant interferon for patients with palpable regional lymph node metastases was associated with an objective tumor response rate of 55%.[197] Further studies of this or other neoadjuvant therapies provide opportunities to investigate tumor biology in the tumor microenvironment and may lead to better understanding of the mechanism of antitumor effects of novel therapies.

Clinical Follow-Up for Patients with Regionally Metastatic Melanomas (Stage III)

There is no agreed follow-up plan for surgically resected melanoma. Most studies conducted to date were retrospective analyses of patients diagnosed and relapsing in the era when there were very limited truly active treatment options. Therefore, diagnosing patients at an earlier time point had very little chance of improving outcomes other than resulting in a lead time bias in the assessment of survival. This situation has led to a series of guidelines for follow-up of patients. Such guidelines have been proposed based on an analysis of the site and timing of first relapse in patients with surgically excised stage III melanoma at a single institution.[198] This was based on a review of the clinical records at Memorial Sloan-Kettering Cancer Center between 1992 and 2004 of patients who ultimately relapsed after surgical resection of stage III melanoma. In this group of patients, the overall 5-year relapse-free survival for patients with stage IIIA, IIIB, and IIIC disease was 63%, 32%, and 11%, respectively. Site of first relapse was local/in-transit (28%), regional nodal (21%), or systemic (51%). First relapses were detected by the patient or family in 47% of cases, by the physician in 21%, and by screening radiologic tests in 32%. Based on these observations, the authors proposed that routine physical examinations beyond 3 years for stage IIIA, 2 years for stage IIIB, and 1 year for stage

IIIC; radiologic imaging beyond 3 years for stages IIIA and IIIB; and 2 years for stage IIIC would be expected to detect few first systemic relapses.

National/International Guidelines for Follow-Up

Recommendations for patient follow-up are largely based on the time-dependent risk of recurrence, the likely sites of metastasis, and historical experience with whether recurrences are commonly identified by the patient, the physician, or by imaging or laboratory studies. However, there is also evidence that follow-up is comforting to patients and decreases psychological stress associated with the diagnosis.[199] No studies have shown a clear benefit in terms of survival with closer follow-up, but this could change as there are now effective therapies for advanced melanoma, so that diagnosis of patients when they are well enough to tolerate those therapies may be of clinical value. Thus, routine clinical follow-up continues to be a part of management, but studies of follow-up have mostly been retrospective, and there is a need for more rigorous studies of the global benefit, risk, and cost of follow-up visits, imaging, and serum markers. Two comprehensive guidelines on melanoma management provide guidance on follow-up based on systematic review of the literature, and expert opinion. The NCCN® has been reported in their 2013-14 guidelines,[128] summarized in Table 94.7. Also, evidence-based guidelines were published in 2013 from Germany, from the German Dermatological Society and the DeCOG.[200] These German S3 guidelines are also summarized in the Table 94.6. These two guidelines are very similar, but differ in the extent of cross-sectional imaging recommended, and the use of ultrasound for evaluation of the node basins. The German guidelines also recommend serum S100B levels in follow-up, whereas these are not recommended by the NCCN. Other minor differences are also evident. The NCCN Guidelines also recommend self-exam by patients on a regular basis as well as annual body skin exams for life, for all patients with a history of stage 0-IV melanoma in addition to the recommendations in the table.

Follow-up visits should include history and physical exam, which should focus on skin exam of the primary site, regional nodes, and in-transit sites. Self-examination by the patient is also recommended, which depends on education of the patient and/or family about what findings may signal recurrence. Chest X-rays were not recommended, but there was lower consensus (77%) for this than for most other German S3 recommendations.

MANAGEMENT OF DISTANT METASTASES OF MELANOMA (STAGE IV)

Any patient with distant metastases is considered stage IV. Distant metastases may include skin or soft tissue metastases distant from a known primary site or visceral, bone, or brain metastases. The prognosis is better for skin and subcutaneous tissue metastases, which are considered M1a, than for lung metastases (M1b) or other distant metastases (M1c). In addition, an elevated serum LDH in the setting of distant metastases is associated with a poor prognosis and also is considered M1c disease.[74]

Timing of Distant Metastases

It is uncommon for patients with melanoma to present initially with stage IV disease. Most patients who develop distant metastases do so after an interval from their original management for clinically localized disease or after management for regionally metastatic disease. Often, metastases become evident within 2 to 3 years of diagnosis, but delayed metastasis is also common, and for melanoma, regional and distant metastases have occurred after

TABLE 94.7

Recommendations for Melanoma Follow-Up Adapted from the National Comprehensive Cancer Network V2.2014 and German S3 Guidelines

		Year 1	Year 2	Year 3	Year 4	Year 5	Years 6–10
IA	NCCN	H&P(q6-12)	H&P(q6-12)	H&P(q6-12)	H&P(q6-12)	H&P(q6-12)	[a]
	G-S3	H&P(q6)	H&P(q6)	H&P(q6)	H&P(q12)	H&P(q12)	H&P(q12)
IB-IIA	NCCN	H&P(q6-12)	H&P(q6-12)	H&P(q6-12)	H&P(q6-12)	H&P(q6-12)	[a]
	G-S3	H&P(q3) U/S(q6) S100B(q3)	H&P(q3) U/S(q6)[b] S100B(q3)	H&P(q3) U/S(q6) S100B(q3)	H&P(q6)	H&P(q6)	H&P(q6-12)
IIB	NCCN[d]	H&P(q3-6) Image(q4-12) MRI(q12)	H&P(q3-6) Image(q4-12) MRI(q12)	H&P(q3-12) Image(q4-12) MRI(q12)	H&P(q3-12) Image(q4-12) MRI(q12)	H&P(q3-12) Image(q4-12) MRI(q12)	[a]
	G-S3	H&P(q3) U/S(q6) S100B(q3)	H&P(q3) U/S(q6)[b] S100B(q3)	H&P(q3) U/S(q6) S100B(q3)	H&P(q6)	H&P(q6)	H&P(q6-12)
IIC-IV	NCCN[c,d]	H&P(q3-6) Image(q4-12) MRI(q12)	H&P(q3-6) Image(q4-12) MRI(q12)	H&P(q3-12) Image(q4-12) MRI(q12)	H&P(q3-12) Image(q4-12) MRI(q12)	H&P(q3-12) Image(q4-12) MRI(q12)	[a]
	G-S3	H&P(q3) U/S(q3) S100B(q3) CTs(q6)	H&P(q3) U/S(q3) S100B(q3) CTs(q6)	H&P(q3) U/S(q3) S100B(q3) CTs(q6)	H&P(q3) U/S(q6) S100B(q6)	H&P(q3) U/S(q6a) S100B(q6)	H&P(q6)

NCCN, National Comprehensive Cancer Network; H&P, history and physical exam; U/S, ultrasound exam of draining node basins; S100B = serum S100B level; MRI, magnetic resonance imaging.
[a] In addition, NCCN Guidelines recommend annual physical exams and history on an annual basis, as indicated, after 5 years. The German S3 guidelines extend to 10 years.
[b] Unless no SNBx, then like IIC.
[c] Image = consider chest X-ray, computed tomography, and positron emission tomography/computed tomography.
[d] For imaging in this stage, the NCCN Guidelines specify that imaging should be considered but is not mandatory.

disease-free intervals measured in decades.[201] In general, the interval to detection of distant metastases is shorter for patients who initially present with high-stage disease (e.g., stage IIB–III) and is longest for patients who present with clinically localized thin melanomas (e.g., stage IA).

Patterns of Metastases

Approximately 60% to 80% of first metastases are at local or regional sites including regional nodes. The most common first sites of visceral metastasis are lung and liver (about 10% each), and metastases to distant skin sites are also common. After an initial metastasis, subsequent metastases are more commonly visceral or distant and increasingly become multiple. Common visceral sites of metastasis are lung, liver, brain, gastrointestinal tract (especially small bowel), bone, and adrenal gland.

Prognostic Factors in Distant Metastatic Melanoma (Stage IV)

The new active systemic therapies for advanced melanoma are changing the prognosis of patients. However, no long-term follow-up is available for the most recent trials. Without treatment, or with mostly ineffective therapies, patients with stage IV melanoma were reported to have a median survival of 12 months, with 6 to 9 months for those who presented with visceral metastatic disease (M1c), as long as 15 months for those who presented with skin and lymph node metastases only (M1a), and patients with lung metastases as their only site of visceral organ involvement (M1b) had an intermediate prognosis.[76] Negative prognostic factors in stage IV melanoma also include a large number of metastatic sites, elevated LDH level, and poor performance status.[202]

Clinical Evaluation of Patients with Distant Metastasis (Stage IV)

When a patient is found to have a distant metastasis, the initial steps are to perform full staging studies. This typically should include MRI scan of the brain and either total-body PET/CT scan or CT scans of the chest, abdomen, and pelvis. Other scans or imaging studies (bone scan, soft tissue MRI, ultrasound, or plain films) may be indicated to evaluate known areas of metastasis (e.g., soft tissue masses in extremities) or to evaluate symptoms (e.g., plain films or bone scans for bony symptoms). Melanoma is usually highly avid for FDG uptake due to the strong Warburg effect (aerobic glycolysis even in the presence of sufficient glucose), and therefore metastatic lesions >5 mm are efficiently imaged by PET scans. An exception is uveal melanoma, which has variable FDG uptake even when metastatic. PET/CT scans are helpful in distinguishing tumor from scar in areas of prior surgery, although surgical sites may remain FDG-avid for up to 3 months after surgery. PET is substantially more sensitive for detection of small bowel metastases and lymph node metastases that are borderline in size.[203] PET/CT scan may also be helpful in assessing patients for resectability when there is limited disease on initial assessment.

Histologic or Cytologic Diagnosis

Patients being followed for a history of melanoma may develop new evidence of metastatic disease. In such patients, a new and growing mass in the chest or abdomen is likely to be metastatic melanoma, but tissue confirmation of metastatic melanoma is usually recommended. New masses can represent new primary lung cancers, lymphoma, sarcoid, inflammatory masses, or other changes, and the management and prognosis of these lesions usually differs dramatically from the management and prognosis of stage IV melanoma.

PRACTICE OF ONCOLOGY

If the lesion is in an accessible area of the lung and is about 1 cm in diameter or greater, a CT-guided transthoracic needle biopsy is usually feasible and appropriate for making the diagnosis. If there is a solitary lung mass, and especially if the mass is <1 cm in diameter, then thoracoscopic resection with preoperative localization can be performed with great success and with low morbidity.[204] In the event that the lesion is malignant, then the biopsy may also have some therapeutic value.

Fine needle aspiration biopsy of soft tissue masses or lymph nodes can be rapid and accurate diagnostic approaches either at the bedside or with radiologic localization. Similarly, biopsies of many other tissue lesions can be accomplished by minimally invasive techniques. A fine needle aspirate will be diagnostic in most cases, but a core needle biopsy, when feasible, can improve diagnostic accuracy further. Immunohistochemical stains for S100, HMB45, tyrosinase, and MART-1/MelanA can all be helpful in confirming a diagnosis of melanoma.

Testing for BRAF and Other Genetic Analyses

A major decision point in the management of advanced melanoma is the determination of BRAF mutational status. The clinical development and approval of BRAF and MEK inhibitors has been based on the treatment of a patient population selected based on the expression of mutant BRAF at position V600. This is because preclinical studies predict that BRAF inhibitors are ineffective when BRAF mutations are not present, and there is even data that they may be detrimental by inducing paradoxical MAPK activation (see the following) and increased cancer progression.[205–208] Therefore, the decision to use BRAF inhibitors should be based on a positive testing for a BRAF V600 mutation (either V600E or V600K, with currently less clear benefits in other BRAF mutations).

BRAF mutation needs to be tested from DNA obtained from a melanoma biopsy or resection. It is best to test a metastatic lesion than an archival primary lesion as it cannot be assured that the metastases come from that particular primary lesion. The tumor DNA is usually obtained from formalin-fixed paraffin-embedded tissue blocks, and the assay laboratories usually isolate the genomic DNA from this fixed tissue. The actual BRAF mutation test can be performed using the mutation-specific PCR tests, such as the FDA-approved companion diagnostic assays for the use of vemurafenib, dabrafenib, or trametinib, or by less sensitive Sanger sequencing. In addition, assay panels that provide results from multiple hot-spot single nucleotide mutations have been developed, as well as assays based on next generation sequencing of a panel of several hundred genes that are commonly associated with cancer.[60]

Surgery for Distant Metastases (Stage IV)

Patient Selection and Prognostic Factors

Selected patients may benefit from surgery for distant metastatic (stage IV) melanoma. The benefit can be palliative in some patients and may be curative in rare cases. There are numerous clinical scenarios in which surgery may be considered, and it is not possible to address all of them here. However, it is useful to consider some of them.

Cases in Which the Benefit of Surgery Is Clear

- Anemia due to occult bleeding from intestinal metastasis
- Bowel obstruction due to small bowel metastasis
- Cutaneous or subcutaneous metastasis with ulceration, pain, or impending ulceration
- Lymph node metastasis with neurologic symptoms
- Symptomatic brain metastasis
- Life-threatening hemorrhage from metastasis

Melanoma frequently metastasizes to the gastrointestinal tract. It usually originates as an intramural lesion but grows into the lumen and through the serosa with time. These usually present as anemia due to occult gastrointestinal bleeding or as intermittent small bowel obstruction due to intussusception (Fig. 94.13). They are difficult to diagnose by CT scan in the absence of symptoms. PET/CT is probably the best study now available. However, it may miss small lesions. Nonetheless, when a patient presents with gastrointestinal blood loss or obstruction associated with a small bowel (or other gastrointestinal) metastasis of melanoma, operation is usually indicated. If the tumor involves the mesenteric nodes and is matted, then it may not be feasible or appropriate to resect the entire tumor, but enteroenteric bypass of the obstruction will be palliative. Resection of most or all small bowel metastases can manage bleeding and obstruction effectively. If there is a single small bowel metastasis, then a simple resection and reanastomosis is appropriate (Fig. 94.14). However, if there are numerous small bowel metastases, then excision of large lesions with reanastomosis is appropriate, but small lesions may be excised by partial-diameter excision and stapled (or sewn) closure. If the patient can be rendered surgically free of disease, then there may be long-term survival >5 years in as many as 25% of patients and mean survival >2 years.[209]

Cutaneous, subcutaneous, and nodal metastases are not usually a cause of death, but they can be a cause of substantial morbidity. As they grow, they develop substantial inflammation in the overlying skin (see Fig. 94.12) and without resection may often ulcerate. Because such lesions usually can be resected under local anesthesia with minimal morbidity, it is reasonable to offer resection.

Extensive lymph node metastasis with neurologic symptoms is commonly an issue in the axilla, where tumor growth may compress or invade the brachial plexus and axillary vein. Patients with extensive axillary recurrence with neurologic symptoms and patients with other nodal disease and neurologic symptoms should be considered for radical resection of the involved nodal basin. The morbidity of surgery usually is much less than the morbidity of the tumor left untreated. Major risks of tumor growth include paralysis or major neurologic dysfunction of the extremity, intractable lymphedema, disabling pain, and unresectability.

Brain metastasis is a particularly ominous sign in terms of future survival, which can usually be measured in months. However, some patients with isolated brain metastasis can have long-term control after surgical resection or stereotactic radiation therapy. For patients with symptomatic brain metastases, the presentation with acute cognitive deficits can be dramatic. Steroid therapy should be instituted immediately (4 mg orally every 6 hours per day initially). However, if this fails, or if the presentation is particularly acute with impending herniation, then surgical resection of the brain metastasis can be therapeutic.

Melanoma can metastasize to nodes, adrenal glands, or other sites and then develop spontaneous hemorrhage. Sometimes such bleeding can be trivial, but in some cases, there can be massive hemorrhage into the tissues, with associated hypovolemia. In such cases, resection of the hemorrhagic mass may diminish future risk of bleeding, decrease pain, and delay death.

New effective systemic therapies,[151] including CTLA4 blockade or mutant BRAF inhibition, as well as blockade of PD-1/PD-L1, may be alternatives for managing patients with metastases that are too extensive to resect, but a multidisciplinary team assessment is advised to weigh the short-term risks of delaying surgery against the possibility of major systemic tumor regression with those therapies. In cases where systemic therapy induces partial responses, surgical resection of residual gastrointestinal disease may be feasible to render the patient clinically free of disease.

Cases in Which the Benefit of Surgery Is Likely

- Solitary asymptomatic visceral metastasis resectable with minimal morbidity

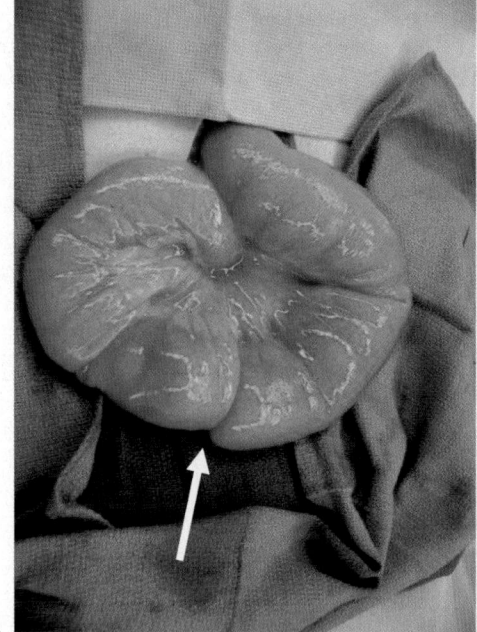

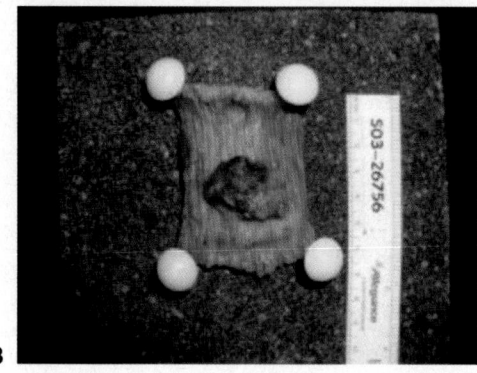

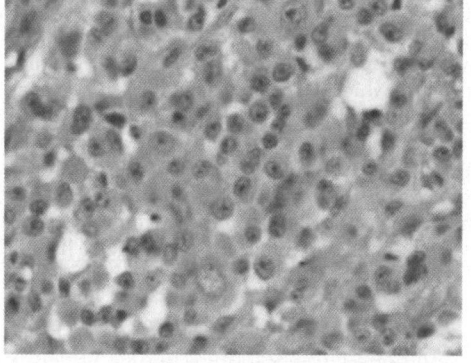

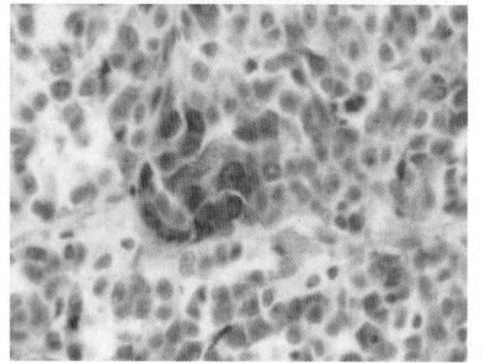

Figure 94.13 Patient presenting with intussusception due to a small bowel metastasis of melanoma. **(A)** The loop of small bowel with intussusception is shown at the time of surgery, prior to enterectomy and reanastomosis. The *arrow* shows the point of intussusception. **(B)** The intraluminal mass is shown with surrounding bowel mucosa. **(C)** Hematoxylin-eosin–stained tissue section of the intussuscepting mass shows melanoma. **(D)** Immunohistochemical stain for a melanoma marker.

■ Bony metastasis with pain or joint involvement, unresponsive to radiation
■ Solitary brain metastasis without symptoms
■ Large, asymptomatic nodal metastasis with concurrent low-volume systemic disease

■ Extensive skin and soft tissue metastases in the absence of visceral metastases
■ Isolated growing metastasis in the setting of stable or regressing metastases after therapy

In general, in a patient with solitary visceral metastasis, if excision can be accomplished with minimal morbidity, the excision can be both therapeutic and diagnostic. The OS for patients with one or several distant metastases resected coupled with experimental melanoma vaccine therapy has been associated with 5-year survival rates in the 40% to 60% range.[210] Another reasonable option for the patient with a single (or few) resectable distant and/or visceral metastases is to enroll in an experimental therapeutic trial or to take an approved systemic therapy in the hope of clinical response but with the additional benefit of having about 3 months of observation time to be sure that no other new visceral lesions appear prior to resection of the lesion in question.

Bone metastases can cause pain and fracture. Radiation therapy is usually the first choice for therapeutic intervention if significant pain exists. If patients are at risk of impending fracture, orthopedic stabilization should be considered before radiation. However, if the lesion does not respond to radiation or is solitary, resection with bone grafting or joint replacement can be considered. Current success rates with such therapy are high, but the period of postoperative recovery can be extended, and so careful patient selection is indicated.

An asymptomatic solitary brain metastasis that is amenable to resection can often be removed surgically with minimal morbidity and often with approximately a 3-day hospital stay. Stereotactic

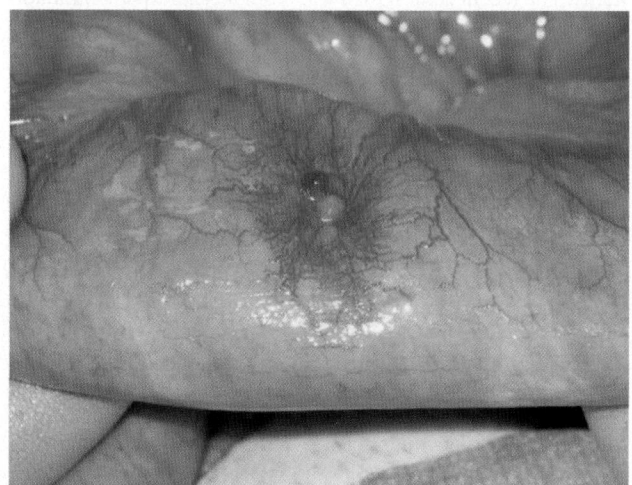

Figure 94.14 Small bowel metastasis of melanoma with extension through the bowel wall and with extensive neovascularity.

radiosurgery (e.g., gamma knife) is often the first choice for treatment of such lesions, but surgery is another reasonable option and probably will have benefit, especially if the solitary brain lesion is >2 to 3 cm diameter, in which case stereotactic radiosurgery may be less effective and surgery may be a preferred option.

In patients with multiple metastases, systemic therapy may be associated with partial clinical responses with progressive growth of one or more lesions while the remainder are stable or shrinking and asymptomatic. In that case, patients may benefit from resecting the one or several tumor deposits that are progressing. This will not be curative, but it may lead to a more prolonged period of good quality of life, with minimal perioperative morbidity.

Cases in Which Some Patients May Benefit from Surgery but Risk and Benefit Are Closely Balanced

- More than one visceral metastasis, without symptoms
- Multiple lung nodules
- Bilateral adrenal metastases
- Extensive skin and soft tissue metastases in the setting of visceral disease

A more difficult decision is whether to treat patients with surgery when they have multiple asymptomatic visceral metastases, such as multiple lung nodules, bilateral adrenal metastases, or extensive skin metastases in the presence of visceral disease. These are generally situations in which surgery is not recommended as the treatment of choice, but there are anecdotes of such patients enjoying prolonged disease-free survival after such surgery, and so it is worth considering in very selected patients. Situations that may push the patient and the clinician toward such an aggressive surgical approach include (1) prior failure of systemic therapy, (2) a young patient for whom perioperative morbidity is not a major concern, and (3) disease sites that are particularly amenable to surgery through limited surgery (e.g., multiple lung nodules amenable to thoracoscopic lobectomy).

Adjuvant Therapy for Resected Stage IV Melanoma

There is no standard adjuvant therapy after resection of metastatic melanoma (stage IV). Interferon has not been thoroughly evaluated in this setting. Therefore, observation remains the standard management of patients in this setting. Investigational vaccines, GM-CSF, CTLA4 blockade, PD-1 blockade, and other experimental therapies are being evaluated for these patients. ECOG 4697, a US intergroup clinical trial testing the potential benefit of GM-CSF as an adjuvant therapy for resected stage IIIB-IV melanoma, demonstrated no impact on survival overall.[192] Several ongoing adjuvant therapy clinical trials for stage III melanoma are open to enrollment to this patient population and are testing the potential benefits of adjuvant therapy with ipilimumab (ECOG 1609), vemurafenib single agent, or dabrafenib and trametinib in combination.

Treatment of Unresectable Metastatic (Stage IV) Melanoma

Progress in Treatment for Metastatic Melanoma

Clinical translation of preclinical scientific knowledge has resulted in the rapid advancement of new therapies active in patients with metastatic melanoma. This contrasts sharply with the lack of significant progress for many years when attempting to treat melanoma with nonspecific agents, in particular chemotherapy, and performing combination studies with low active components. In this context, the OS and PFS was analyzed in 70 US cooperative group single-arm phase 2 clinical trials performed between 1975 and 2005 (termed the Korn meta-analysis) that had been deemed to not be

TABLE 94.8

Summary of Best Clinical Endpoints with Selected Therapies for the Treatment of Advanced Melanoma

Improved overall survival	Ipilimumab (vs. gp100 peptide vaccine) Vemurafenib (vs. dacarbazine) Trametinib (vs. dacarbazine)
Improved progression-free survival	Dabrafenib (vs. dacarbazine) Nab-paclitaxel (vs. dacarbazine) Dabrafenib + trametinib (vs. dabrafenib)
Improved response duration	T-Vec (vs. granulocyte macrophage–colony-stimulating factor)
Validated antitumor activity	High dose interleukin-2 TIL ACT Carboplatin-paclitaxel Dacarbazine Fotemustine
Promising new agents and combinations	Anti-PD-1 antibodies: nivolumab, MK3475, MEDI Anti-PD-L1: BMS559, MPDL8032A BRAF and MEK inhibitor combination Anti-PD-1 and anti-CTLA4 combination
Agents and combinations not supported by data	Nistosurea combination chemotherapy: CVD, biochemotherapy Darmuth regimen and tamoxifen-chemotherapy combinations Thalidomide and thalidomide-chemotherapy combinations Sorafenib and sorafenib-chemotherapy combinations Elesclomol-chemotherapy combinations Peptide vaccines

TIL ACT, tumor infiltrating lymphocyte adoptive cell transfer therapy; PD, programmed death; CTLA, cytotoxic T lymphocyte associated-antigen; CVD, cisplatin-vinblastin-dacarbazine.

promising for further development.[211] From this meta-analysis, individual-level and trial-level data were obtained for patients enrolled onto 42 phase 2 trials. Prognostic factors for OS were performance status, presence of visceral disease, sex, and whether the trial excluded patients with brain metastases. The Korn meta-analysis has provided the minimum benchmarks of OS and PFS at defined time points to compare to new clinical trials in patients with metastatic melanoma. The recent clinical trials with immune checkpoint inhibitors and BRAF inhibitor–based targeted therapies have improved this grim panorama (Table 94.8), and there are reasons to anticipate that treatment options for advanced melanoma will continue to improve. The ability to understand mechanisms of response and resistance to BRAF inhibitor–based therapies and immune checkpoint blockade at a molecular level, and the rapid advancement of the knowledge brought through by the scientific community's renewed interest in melanoma, predicts further improvements in the development of effective therapies for this disease.

Anti–Cytotoxic T-Lymphocyte Antigen 4 Blocking Antibodies

Approaches such as inactivated tumor vaccines, dendritic cell vaccines, or immune-stimulating cytokines like interferon-α and IL-2 are aimed at turning on T cells against cancer. This has led to tumor responses in a minority of patients, but with the remarkable feature that these tumor responses tend to be durable (counted in years) in most cases. This feature, together with the lack of significant activity of standard therapy approaches for melanoma, has maintained the interest in this mode of therapy for advanced

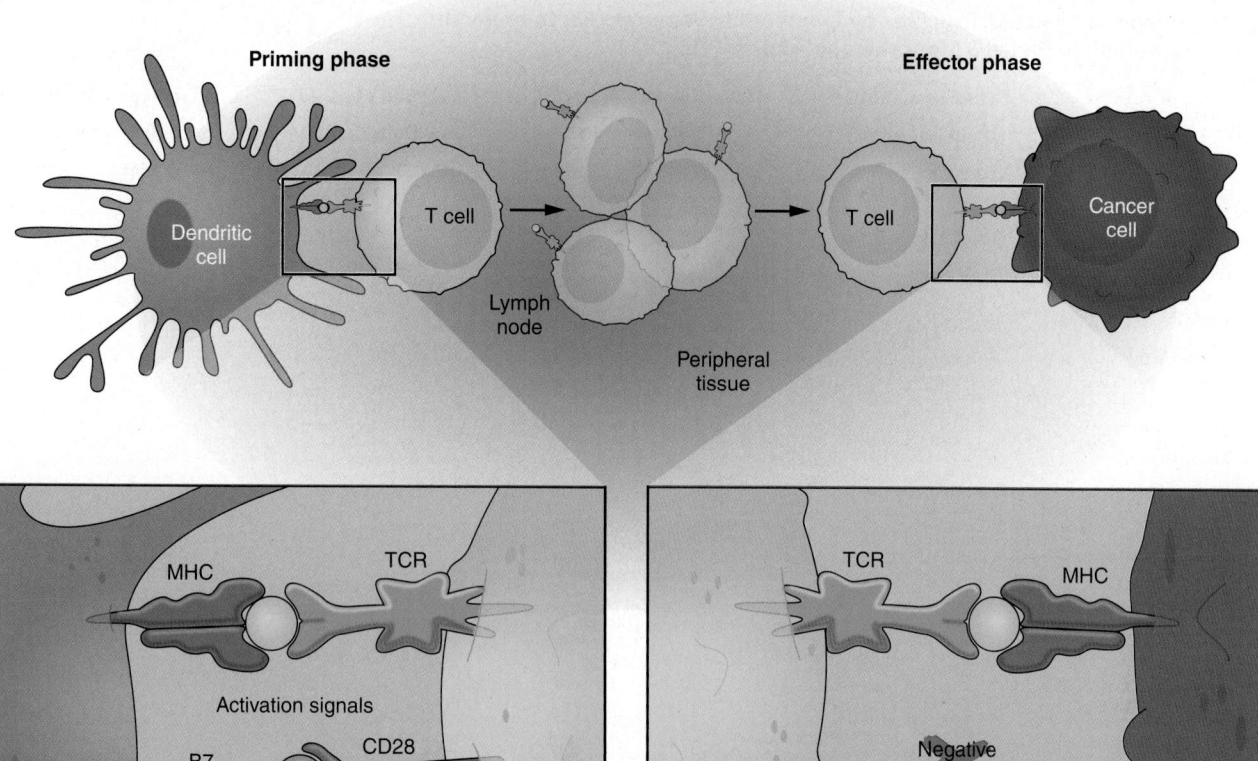

Figure 94.15 Schematic representation of the mechanism of action of anti–cytotoxic T lymphocyte–associated protein 4 (*CTLA-4*) and anti–programmed cell death protein (PD)-1 monoclonal antibodies. Cytotoxic T lymphocyte–associated protein 4 is a negative regulatory signal that limits activation of T cells upon ligation with cluster of differentiation 80 or cluster of differentiation 86 costimulatory molecules expressed by antigen-presenting cells, within the priming phase of a T-cell response in lymph nodes. PD-1 is expressed by T cells upon chronic antigen exposure and results in negative regulation on T cells upon ligation with PD-L1, which is primarily expressed by peripheral tissues including in the tumor microenvironment. The PD-1/PD-L1 interaction happens in the effector phase of a T-cell response. Its blockade with antibodies to PD-1 or PD-L1 results in the preferential activation of T cells with specificity for the cancer. MHC, major histocompatibility complex; TCR, T-cell receptor. (From Ribas A. Tumor immunotherapy directed at PD-1. *N Engl J Med* 2012;366:2517–2519.)

melanoma. Immune responses against cancer are usually kept under negative regulatory control by a series of physiological breaks (checkpoints; Fig. 94.15). Negative immune regulatory checkpoints are induced after T-cell activation. These include CTLA4, which when engaged by the costimulatory molecules B7.1 (CD80) or B7.2 (CD86) results in a dominant negative regulation of T cells by competing with the CD28-positive costimulatory receptor. When an activated T cell arrives to the peripheral tissues, including melanoma metastases, it can be turned off by the PD-1/PD-L1 interaction. PD-1 is a negative regulatory checkpoint receptor that is expressed by T cells upon activation and chronic antigen exposure, as in cancer. Its main peripheral ligand, PD-L1, is expressed by cancer and stromal cells mainly upon exposure to T cell–produced interferons. Therefore, it represents a mechanism of acquired immune resistance that allows melanoma to hide from activated T cells.[212] Release of both the CTLA4 and PD-1 checkpoints has resulted in objective and durable immune-mediated tumor responses in patients with advanced melanoma, and it is an area of active clinical research and drug development.

Ipilimumab (Yervoy, Bristol-Myers Squibb, New York, NY) is a fully human monoclonal antibody (IgG1) that blocks CTLA4. The FDA approved ipilimumab at a dose of 3 mg/kg administered at 3-week intervals for four doses for the treatment of unresectable or metastatic melanoma in 2011. This approval was based on a randomized clinical trial of ipilimumab compared to a gp100 peptide vaccine, or in combination, in patients with previously treated metastatic melanoma.[195] 676 HLA-A*0201–positive patients with unresectable stage III or IV melanoma who had been previously treated with systemic therapy for metastatic disease were randomly assigned, in a 3:1:1 ratio, to ipilimumab plus gp100 (403 patients), ipilimumab alone (137 patients), or gp100 alone (136 patients). Ipilimumab was administered at a dose of 3 mg per kilogram every 3 weeks for up to four treatments (induction). Eligible patients could receive re-induction therapy. The primary end point of median OS with ipilimumab alone was 10.1 months as compared with 6.4 months among patients receiving gp100 alone (HR = 0.66; $p = 0.003$). No difference in OS was detected between the ipilimumab groups (HR with ipilimumab plus gp100 = 1.04; $p = 0.76$),

TABLE 94.9

Comparison of Selected Toxicities by Ipilimumab, Vemurafenib, Dabrafenib, and Trametinib in Phase 3 Monotherapy Trials[16,25,26,41]

| | Hodi et al. 2010[195] | | Chapman et al. 2011[229] | | Hauschild et al. 2012[232] | | Flaherty et al. 2012[236] | |
| | Ipilimumab | | Vemurafenib | | Dabrafenib | | Trametinib | |
Toxicity grades	All grades	Grade 3-4	All grades	Grade 3-4	Grade 2	Grade 3-4	All grades	Grade 3-4
Fatigue	42	5	33	2	5	5	26	4
Pyrexia	12	0	18	0	8	3		
Skin rash	19	1	36	8	NA	NA	57	8
Acneiform dermatitis							19	1
Photosensitivity			30	3				
Pruritus	24	0	22	1				
Palmoplantar disesthesia			7		6	2		
Hyperkeratosis			20	1	12	1		
Alopecia			35	<1			17	<1
cuSCC/KA				18	—	6		
Nausea	35	2	30	7	1	0	18	1
Diarrhea/colitis	29	8	25	<1			43	0
Endocrine	8	2						
Hepatic	4	0						
Arthralgia			49	6	0	1		
Peripheral edema			15				26	1
Hypertension							15	12

NA, not available; cuSCC/KA, cutaneous squamous cell carcinoma and keratoacanthoma.

and the median OS was 10.0 months among patients receiving ipilimumab plus gp100 (HR for death = 0.68; p <0.001). Grade 3-4 immune-related adverse events occurred in 10% to 15% of patients treated with ipilimumab, the most common being colitis, skin rash, and endocrinopathies (Table 94.9). There were 14 deaths related to ipilimumab (2.1%), and 7 were associated with immune-related adverse events. This was the first randomized clinical trial demonstrating an improvement in OS in patients with metastatic melanoma (Table 94.10).

There was a second randomized clinical trial with OS improvement using ipilimumab.[196] This was a frontline trial comparing ipilimumab (10 mg/kg) plus dacarbazine (850 mg/m² of body surface area), or dacarbazine (850 mg/m²) plus placebo, in patients with previously untreated metastatic melanoma. A total of 502 patients were randomized in a 1:1 ratio, with the study drugs given at weeks 1, 4, 7, and 10. Patients with stable disease or an objective response and no dose-limiting toxic effects were eligible to receive ipilimumab every 12 weeks thereafter as maintenance therapy. The primary end point of OS was significantly improved in the group receiving ipilimumab plus dacarbazine compared to dacarbazine plus placebo (11.2 months versus 9.1 months). Survival rates at 1 year (47.3% versus 36.3%), 2 years (28.5% versus

TABLE 94.10

Main Efficacy Endpoints Taking from the Experimental Arm of Randomized Trials Leading to the Approval of Ipilimumab, Vemurafenib, Dabrafenib, and Trametinib

| | Hodi et al. 2010[195,a] | | Chapman et al. 2011[229,b] | | Hauschild et al. 2012[232,b] | | Flaherty et al. 2012[236,b] | |
	Ipilimumab	gp100	Vemurafenib	Dacarbazine	Dabrafenib	Dacarbazine	Trametinib	Dacarbazine or Paclitaxel
Response rate	11%	1.5%	48%	5%	50%	6%	22%	8%
Median PFS	2.9 mo	2.8 mo	5.3 mo	1.6 mo	5.1 mo	2.7 mo	4.8 mo	1.5 mo
HR PFS	0.64		0.26		0.30		0.45	
Median OS	10.1 mo	6.4 mo	NR	NR	NR	NR	NR	NR
HR OS	0.66		0.37		0.61		NR	

PFS, progression-free survival; HR, hazard ratio; OS, overall survival; NR, not reported.
[a] Enrolled previously treated patients with advanced melanoma with no BRAF restriction.
[b] Enrolled patients with BRAF mutant advanced melanoma who had not been previously treated with a systemic therapy.

17.9%), and 3 years (20.8% versus 12.2%) were significantly improved (HR for death = 0.72; p <0.001). Grade 3 or 4 adverse events occurred in 56.3% of patients treated with ipilimumab plus dacarbazine, as compared with 27.5% treated with dacarbazine and placebo (p <0.001). The most frequent toxicities in the experimental combination group were increases in transaminases. No drug-related deaths or gastrointestinal perforations occurred in the ipilimumab–dacarbazine group.

The FDA approval of ipilimumab comes with a black box warning due to the potential for severe and occasionally fatal immune-mediated adverse reactions. The most common are enterocolitis, hepatitis, dermatitis (including toxic epidermal necrolysis), neuropathy, and endocrinopathies like hypophysitis and thyroiditis. The recommendation is to permanently discontinue ipilimumab infusions and initiate systemic high-dose corticosteroid therapy for severe immune-mediated reactions.

Re-induction with ipilimumab after the first four infusions without serious side effects is an option for patients with stable disease sustained for at least 3 months or a prior confirmed partial or complete response. Among 31 patients given re-induction with ipilimumab, a complete or partial response or stable disease was achieved in 13%, 37.5%, and 65.2%, respectively.[213]

Several studies are testing the effects of combinations based on ipilimumab. E1608 is a phase 2 randomized trial that tested the combination of ipilimumab with GM-CSF with the goal of analyzing if this combination improved OS.[214] A total of 245 patients were randomized to ipilimumab (10 mg/kg every 3 weeks intravenously for four courses, then every 12 weeks) plus GM-CSF (250 μg subcutaneously on days 1 to 14 of 21-day cycles) or ipilimumab alone. With a median follow-up of 13.3 months, the response rate and PFS was not different between both arms. In a planned interim analysis, the primary end point of median OS was improved with the combination. One-year OS with the combination was 67.9% (59%, 76%), while it was 51.2% (42.6%, 61.3%) for ipilimumab alone (stratified log rank p_1 = 0.016, p_2 = 0.033; HR = 0.65). Grade 3–5 toxicities were lower with the combination compared to ipilimumab alone (45% compared to 57%, p_2 = 0.078). Therefore, ipilimumab plus GM-CSF may increase OS and decrease toxicities compared to ipilimumab alone. However, this combination remains investigational unless the benefit is confirmed in further clinical trials.

Another anti-CTLA4 antibody has been developed clinically in patients with metastatic melanoma, tremelimumab (by Pfizer and MedImmune-Astra-Zeneca, New York, NY). This fully human IgG2 monoclonal antibody went through phase 1, 2, and 3 testing in melanoma,[215–217] but failed to demonstrate improvement in OS compared to dacarbazine.[216] Potential contributing factors were the study design, the treated population, the dosing regimen, and the postrandomization use of ipilimumab in the control arm.[218]

The main feature of therapy with anti-CTLA4 antibodies is the long durability of tumor responses in patients with an objective tumor response, as exemplified by a patient with metastasis to the lung and liver who initially received ipilimumab and then tremelimumab in May of 2001[219] and continues in response over a decade later. In many instances, it is difficult to assess objective responses as these may appear late after the therapy and go through a process of apparent clinical progression when using standard response evaluation criteria. This has led to the proposal of alternate response evaluation criteria tailored to this mechanism of action, termed the immune-related response criteria.[220,221]

Interleukin-2

The intravenous administration of high-dose IL-2 (aldesleukin) was approved for the treatment of patients with metastatic melanoma in 1998 mainly thanks to its ability to mediate durable complete responses in patients with widespread metastatic disease. The administration of IL-2 represented the first demonstration that purely immunotherapeutic maneuvers could mediate the regression of metastatic cancer.[222,223] IL-2 has no direct effect on cancer

cells, and all of its antitumor activity is a function of its ability to modulate immunologic responses in the host.

The FDA-approved regimen for the treatment of patients with metastatic melanoma using IL-2 involves the use of an intravenous bolus infusion of 600,000 to 720,000 IU/kg every 8 hours to tolerance using two cycles separated by approximately 10 days (maximum of 15 doses per cycle). Results of this treatment are evaluated at 2 months after the first dose, and if tumor is regressing or stable, a second course is then administered.

In the report of the original 270 patients treated at 22 different institutions that was the basis of the approval of IL-2 by the FDA, a 16% objective response rate was obtained, with 17 complete responses (6%) and 26 partial responses (10%).[224] At the last full analysis of these 270 patients, the median duration of response for complete responders had not been reached but exceeded 59 months, and disease progression was not observed in any patient who responded for more than 30 months. An analysis of patients treated from 1988 to 2006 in the Surgery Branch, National Cancer Institute, reported 13 complete responders, only 2 of which had recurred with the remainder ongoing at 1 to 21 years.[225] Thus, IL-2 appears to be one of a very small group of systemic treatments capable of curing patients with a metastatic solid cancer.

Because of the side effects associated with high-dose bolus IL-2 administration, this treatment is generally restricted to patients younger than the age of 70 years with an ECOG performance status of ≤2 and in patients who do not have active systemic infections or other major medical illness of the cardiovascular respiratory or immune system. Because IL-2 often causes transient renal and hepatic toxicity, eligibility criteria generally require normal serum creatinine and serum bilirubin levels. Patients with any history of systemic ischemic heart disease or pulmonary dysfunction should undergo stress testing and pulmonary function tests before initiating therapy, and patients with significant abnormalities should not be included.

The administration of high-dose bolus IL-2 is different than the administration of most cancer therapeutics in that dosing is continued every 8 hours until patients reach grade 3 or 4 toxicity that is not easily reversible by supportive measures. The toxicities of IL-2 administration are transient, with virtually all returning to baseline after IL-2 administration is stopped. Thus, patients are often treated despite creatinine levels that increase to the 2- to 3-mg/dL range because of confidence that renal function will return to normal after cessation of IL-2 administration. Thus, there are no set doses that patients receive, and there is no correlation between the number of doses seen and the likelihood of achieving a response as long as patients receive dosing to tolerance based on physical findings and laboratory measurements.

Administration of Interleukin-2 Plus Vaccine

In 1998, Rosenberg et al.[226] reported an increase in objective response to IL-2 when administered in conjunction with a heteroclitic gp100:209–217(210M) melanoma peptide vaccine. An updated analysis showed a response rate of 12.8% to IL-2 alone compared to a 25.0% response rate to IL-2 plus immunization with this peptide (p = 0.01). A prospective randomized trial in patients with metastatic melanoma of IL-2 alone or in conjunction with this peptide in 185 patients[227] reported centrally reviewed response rates of 6% and 16%, respectively (p = 0.02), with an increase in PFS in the vaccine arm (p = 0.008) and a strong trend toward an increase in survival (17.8 versus 11.1 months, p = 0.06).

BRAF Inhibitors

Vemurafenib (Zelboraf, Roche, Basel, Switzerland) and dabrafenib (Tafinlar, GlaxoSmithKline) are two BRAF inhibitors approved by the FDA, European Medicines Agency, and other regulatory bodies with high antitumor activity in patients with $BRAF^{V600}$ mutant metastatic melanoma mediated by the inhibition of oncogenic MAPK signaling.[151,228] They are both classified as type I BRAF kinase inhibitors because they block the enzymatic activity of BRAF in the activated, mutated conformation, as opposed to type II RAF inhibitors that work only in the inactive conformation, such as sorafenib.[228] In a phase 3 trial in which patients with BRAF[V600E] metastatic melanoma were treated with vemurafenib versus dacarbazine, there was a large early improvement in OS, leading to an early closure of the clinical trial.[229] This was a phase 3 randomized clinical trial comparing vemurafenib (960 mg orally twice daily) with dacarbazine (1,000 mg/m^2 of body surface area intravenously every 3 weeks) in 675 patients with previously untreated, metastatic melanoma with the BRAF[V600E] mutation. A planned interim analysis after 98 deaths led to the closing of this trial. In this interim analysis, vemurafenib was associated with a relative reduction of 63% in the risk of death and 74% in the risk of either death or disease progression, as compared with dacarbazine ($p < 0.001$ for both comparisons). The independent data and safety monitoring board recommended crossover from dacarbazine to vemurafenib for patients under study. Response rates were 48% for vemurafenib and 5% for dacarbazine. At 6 months, OS was 84% (95% CI, 78 to 89) in the vemurafenib group and 64% (95% CI, 56 to 73) in the dacarbazine group. Common adverse events associated with vemurafenib were arthralgia, rash, fatigue, alopecia, keratoacanthoma or squamous cell carcinoma, photosensitivity, nausea, and diarrhea (see Table 94.9); 38% of patients required dose modification because of toxic effects.

Secondary cutaneous squamous cell carcinomas and keratoacanthomas are the most common grade 3-4 toxicities with vemurafenib, which occur in 20% of the patients treated, often with RAS mutations and usually the first 2 to 3 months of therapy.[230] The pathogenesis of their development is due to the inhibition of wild-type BRAF within a dimmer with CRAF, which results in increased MAPK signaling through the paradoxical transactivation of CRAF in the setting of strong RAS-GTP signaling in that cell.[208,231] This is the so-called paradoxical activation of the MAPK pathway with BRAF inhibitors. These skin squamoepithelial proliferative lesions are usually treated with local excision and do not require changing the doses of the BRAF inhibitor.

Dabrafenib was tested in a phase 3 trial in patients with previously untreated stage IV or unresectable stage III BRAF[V600E] mutation–positive metastatic melanoma.[232] Patients were randomly assigned (3:1) to receive dabrafenib (150 mg twice daily, orally) or dacarbazine (1,000 mg/m^2 intravenously every 3 weeks). A total of 250 patients were randomized either to dabrafenib (187 patients) or dacarbazine (63 patients). The primary end point of median PFS was 5.1 months for dabrafenib and 2.7 months for dacarbazine (HR = 0.30; 95% CI, 0.18 to 0.51; $p < 0.0001$) (see Table 94.10). Treatment-related adverse events (grade 2 or higher) occurred in 100 (53%) of the 187 patients who received dabrafenib and in 26 (44%) of the 59 patients who received dacarbazine. The most common adverse events with dabrafenib were skin-related toxic effects, fever, fatigue, arthralgia, and headache (see Table 94.9). An update reported of this phase 3 trial with a longer follow-up showed a median OS in the dabrafenib arm of 18 months compared to 15 months with dacarbazine.[233]

Overall, both vemurafenib and dabrafenib used as single agents showed similar effects in terms of objective response rate and PFS. The incidence of clinically significant photosensitivity is higher with vemurafenib compared to dabrafenib, and the incidence of clinically significant pyrexia is higher with dabrafenib compared to vemurafenib (see Table 94.8).

MEK Inhibitors

MEK inhibitors block signaling in the MAPK pathway downstream from BRAF. These agents effectively inhibit cellular proliferation and tumor growth in BRAF mutant melanoma, although they may also have some activity in NRAS mutant disease.[234,235] Trametinib (Mekinist, GlaxoSmithKline) was approved by the FDA and other regulatory bodies in 2013 based on the results of a phase 3 trial in patients who had metastatic melanoma with a V600E or V600K BRAF mutations.[236] A total of 322 patients were randomly assigned to either trametinib (2 mg orally once daily)

or intravenous dacarbazine (1,000 mg/m^2 of body surface area) or paclitaxel (175 mg/m^2) every 3 weeks. The primary end point of median PFS was 4.8 months in the trametinib group and 1.5 months in the chemotherapy group (HR = 0.45; 95% CI, 0.33 to 0.63; $p < 0.001$) (see Table 94.10). At 6 months, OS was 81% in the trametinib group and 67% in the chemotherapy group despite crossover (HR = 0.54; 95% CI, 0.32 to 0.92; $p = 0.01$). Rash, diarrhea, and peripheral edema were the most common toxic effects in the trametinib group (see Table 94.9) and were managed with dose interruption and dose reduction; asymptomatic and reversible reduction in the cardiac ejection fraction and ocular toxic effects occurred infrequently. Due to the higher incidence of side effects and lower efficacy (see Tables 94.9 and 94.10), the use of BRAF inhibitors is usually preferred over the use of MEK inhibitors for the treatment of patients with BRAF mutant advanced melanoma.

Mechanisms of Resistance to BRAF Inhibitors

Progression on therapy with no evidence of tumor response (innate resistance) to BRAF inhibitors is rare, present in approximately 15% of patients. However, progressive growth after a period of tumor response (acquired resistance) is common with a median PFS of 6 to 7 months. Mechanisms of acquired resistance are diverse and can be categorized between the ones that reactivate the MAPK pathway and the mechanisms that lead to a MAPK pathway–independent signaling that substitutes for the blocked driver oncogenic signal. MAPK reactivating mechanisms are more common and have the common theme of reactivating oncogenic signaling through MEK and ERK. Specific mechanisms reported to date in patient-derived samples include truncations in the BRAF protein resulting in increased kinase activity,[237] amplifications of the mutant BRAF gene,[238] secondary mutations in NRAS or MEK,[239–241] or overexpression of COT.[242] The mechanisms leading to MAPK-redundant pathway activation are less well characterized and most may represent mechanisms of adaptive resistance to provide an alternative survival pathway. These include the overexpression or overactivation of receptor tyrosine kinases like the platelet-derived growth factor receptor beta[239,243] or the insulin-like growth factor receptor 1,[244] leading oncogenic signaling through the PI3K-AKT pathway.

In a study of 100 biopsies taken from patients receiving BRAF inhibitors,[245,246] MAPK reactivation mechanisms were detected among disease progression tissues in 64% of samples; among these, RAS mutations (37%), mutant BRAF amplification (30%), and alternative splicing (20%) were most common. This study also detected genetic alterations in the PI3K-AKT pathway among progressive tissues in 26% of samples. Furthermore, increasing evidence suggests that multiple mechanisms of resistance may develop in the same patient when melanoma relapses after therapy with BRAF inhibitors. In 20% of patients, at least two mechanisms of resistance were detected in the same melanoma in the same or different progressive tumor sites. When studying the genetic features of multiple temporally and geographically distinct baseline and progressive metastatic lesions from an individual patient, it revealed distinct drivers of resistance via both divergent and convergent evolution and evidence of genomic diversification associated with an altered mutational spectra. Therefore, BRAF mutant melanomas acquire BRAF inhibitor resistance via diverse molecular alterations, which indicate MAPK and PI3K-AKT pathway addiction.[246] The finding of multiple genetic mechanisms of escape in the same patient implies that the use of upfront, co-targeting of the escape pathways may be an essential strategy for durable responses.

Combination of Targeted Therapies for BRAF Mutant Melanoma

As the most common core pathway mechanism of resistance to single-agent BRAF inhibitor therapy is mediated by the reactivation of the MAPK pathway through MEK,[246,247] combined therapy with a BRAF and a MEK inhibitor may result in a greater initial tumor response and prevent MAPK-driven acquired resistance mechanisms. A randomized phase 2 trial tested two dosing regimens of combined dabrafenib and trametinib, or dabrafenib alone.[248] The rate of complete or partial response with combination therapy was 76%, as compared with 54% with monotherapy ($p = 0.03$). Median PFS in the combination was 9.4 months, as compared with 5.8 months in the monotherapy group (HR = 0.39; 95% CI, 0.25 to 0.62; $P < 0.001$). Pyrexia was the most common toxicity in the combined therapy group compared with the monotherapy group (71% versus 26%). The combination had the additional benefit of blocking the paradoxical activation of the MAPK pathway induced by BRAF inhibitors, and thus decreasing toxicities compared with BRAF inhibitor monotherapy such as squamous cell carcinomas and hyperkeratotic skin lesions. Other BRAF and MEK inhibitor combinations are being evaluated in clinical trials with promising activity and a distinct safety profile, including the combination of the BRAF inhibitor vemurafenib with the MEK inhibitor cobimetinib, and the BRAF inhibitor LGX818 with the MEK inhibitor MEK162. Several phase 3 trials that compare the BRAF/MEK inhibitor combination with a BRAF inhibitor as monotherapy are ongoing. Therefore, the combination of BRAF and MEK inhibitors is likely to result in improved initial responses through better oncogenic BRAF inhibition, more durable responses by preventing mechanisms of acquired resistance, and decreased toxicities by inhibiting paradoxical MAPK activation with BRAF inhibitors. But the final results of the phase 3 trials will be needed to fully evaluate the benefits of combined therapy compared to single-agent BRAF inhibitors.

When acquired resistance to a BRAF inhibitor has been established, the sequential use of a MEK inhibitor after stopping therapy with the BRAF inhibitor does not result in secondary tumor responses.[249] However, in agreement with preclinical models, there are secondary responses when adding a MEK inhibitor to continued therapy with a BRAF inhibitor in patients progressing on single-agent BRAF inhibitors. In some instances, a secondary response can be achieved with the reintroduction of therapy with a BRAF inhibitor in patients who previously progressed on this therapy and had been off therapy for a period of time.[250]

KIT Inhibitors

Mutations in the KIT receptor occur infrequently (2% to 3% of unselected cases of metastatic melanoma) and are more prevalent in mucosal and acral melanomas.[48] Expression of Kit protein by immunohistochemical staining for CD117 is not sufficient to select for sensitivity to Kit inhibitors, and testing for KIT alterations needs to be performed by DNA sequencing. Imatinib (Gleevec, Novartis, Basel, Switzerland) has modest activity in patients with metastatic melanoma, and KIT mutations in the juxtamembrane domain (L596, V559), as well as K642E, are present.[50,51] The overall durable response rate was 16% (95% CI, 2 to 30) among 51 patients with KIT mutations or genetic amplification, with a median time to progression of 12 weeks.[16] Other drugs such as dasatinib (Sprycel, Bristol-Myer Squibb) and sunitinib (Sutent, Pfizer) also appear to have activity in KIT mutant melanoma.[52–54] Therefore, KIT inhibitors have modest activity in patients with KIT mutant metastatic melanoma.

Single-Agent Chemotherapy

Melanoma is regarded as a relatively chemotherapy-refractory tumor. The specific mechanisms underlying resistance are not well known, but likely derive from the inherent resilience of melanocytes, which have to be naturally resistant to apoptotic death when exposed to UV radiation from the sun. In particular, DNA repair enzymes as well as the expression of efflux pumps for xenobiotics are more highly expressed in melanoma compared with many other cancers.

Dacarbazine, an imidazole carboxamide [5-(3,3-dimethyl-l-triazeno)-imidazole-4-carboxamide], is a classic alkylating agent. It was first evaluated in clinical trials in melanoma in the late 1960s and approved by the FDA for the treatment of metastatic melanoma

in 1974 on the basis of a response rate of approximately 20%,[251] but this response assessment predates modern stringent response evaluation criteria. In the majority of trials, dacarbazine was administered intravenously at daily doses of 200 mg/m^2 for 5 days every 3 or 4 weeks; however, 1,000 mg/m^2 given once every 3 or 4 weeks has been the standard regimen in recent trials. The most common toxicities are myelosuppression and nausea. The severity of myelosuppression rarely requires the use of growth factor support, and the advent of potent antiemetics has significantly improved the tolerability of this agent. Of note, an adequately powered randomized trial of dacarbazine or any other systemic therapy compared with best supportive care has never been undertaken in advanced melanoma.

Temozolomide is an orally available prodrug that is metabolized into the active form MTIC [5-(3-methyltriazen-1-yl) imidazole-4-carboxamide], which is closely related to dacarbazine.[252] MTIC penetrates into the cerebrospinal fluid.[253] Because it is an oral therapy, temozolomide is also more amenable to protracted dosing schedules than dacarbazine, particularly an advantage when combined with fractionated radiation therapy. Single-arm phase 2 trials demonstrated activity in patients with metastatic melanoma, but more modest activity was noted for patients with brain metastases treated with this agent.[254] EORTC 18032 was a phase 3 randomized clinical trial in which a dose-intense schedule of temozolomide was administered (150 mg/m^2 daily for 7 of every 14 days), compared with dacarbazine (1,000 mg/m^2 intravenously every 28 days). This trial randomized 859 patients and sought a 23% improvement in OS as the primary end point. However, OS was not significantly different between the two arms (HR = 1.0; $p = 1.0$). Response rate was superior in the temozolomide group (14.4% versus 9.8%, $p = 0.05$), but PFS was not (HR = 0.92 in favor of temozolomide; $p = 0.092$).[255] Therefore, there is little evidence for the use of temozolomide compared to using dacarbazine in patients with metastatic melanoma.

Fotemustine is a nitrosourea approved by European regulatory bodies for the treatment of advanced melanoma. It is administered by intravenous infusion (100 mg/m^2) weekly for 3 weeks followed by a 4- to 5-week break, with continued administration every 3 weeks for stable or responding patients.[256] A total of 229 patients were randomized to fotemustine or dacarbazine, seeking to demonstrate a 17% absolute difference in objective response rate. The observed difference in response rate (13% for fotemustine versus 6% for dacarbazine) was not statistically significant. Median time to progression was similar for the two arms. Overall survival, a secondary end point, was not significantly improved with fotemustine compared to dacarbazine (median, 7.3 versus 5.6 months).

Nab-paclitaxel is an albumin nanoparticle-bound paclitaxel that was demonstrated to have an improved PFS over dacarbazine in a phase 3 randomized open-label trial in chemotherapy-naïve patients with stage IV metastatic melanoma with no brain metastasis and LDH ≤2 upper limit of normal. Patients received either nab-paclitaxel 150 mg/m^2 on days 1, 8, and 15 every 4 weeks, or dacarbazine 1,000 mg/m^2 every 3 weeks. A total of 529 patients were randomized to nab-paclitaxel ($n = 264$) or dacarbazine ($n = 265$) between April 2009 and June 2011. In the intent-to-treat population, the primary end point of PFS was improved in favor of the nab-paclitaxel group (4.8 and 2.5 median months in the nab-paclitaxel and DTIC arm, respectively; HR = 0.792; 95.1% CI, 0.631 to 0.992; $p = 0.044$). Interim OS was 12.8 with nab-paclitaxel and 10.7 months with dacarbazine (HR = 0.831; 99.9% CI, 0.578 to 1.196; $p = 0.094$). The most common grade 3 or higher treatment-related adverse events was neuropathy with nab-paclitaxel and neutropenia with dacarbazine. The median time to neuropathy improvement was 28 days. Further follow-up to assess potential effects in OS will be needed to determine the role of nab-paclitaxel in patients with advanced melanoma.

Combination Chemotherapy

Over the past 20 years, several uncontrolled clinical trials suggested the benefits of combination chemotherapy regimens, such

PRACTICE OF ONCOLOGY

as cisplatin, vinblastine, and dacarbazine (CVD) and the so-called Dartmouth regimen (cisplatin, carmustine, dacarbazine, and tamoxifen). A phase 3 trial was conducted among 240 patients comparing the Dartmouth regimen with single-agent dacarbazine with the goal of detecting a 50% improvement in OS.[257] The median OS was similar between the two arms (7.7 months for Dartmouth versus 6.3 months for dacarbazine; $p = 0.52$), and 1-year survival rates were also very similar (23% for Dartmouth versus 28% for dacarbazine; $p = 0.38$). The response rate was not significantly higher for the combination regimen (17% for Dartmouth versus 10% for dacarbazine; $p = 0.09$) and was substantially lower than the reported response rate in the smaller, single-institution studies. The Dartmouth regimen was associated with significantly more severe neutropenia, anemia, nausea, and vomiting. In addition, several randomized trials refuted the concept that tamoxifen substantially modulates the efficacy of chemotherapy in metastatic melanoma. CVD was tested in the context of ECOG 3695, in which CVD was the control-arm therapy for 201 patients with metastatic melanoma. The response rate was 12% and median PFS was 3.1 months, suggesting a very low activity.[258] Overall, there is little evidence of benefit with these combination chemotherapy regimens for the treatment of patients with metastatic melanoma.

The combination of carboplatin and paclitaxel has been tested in melanoma, initially as a combination chemotherapy with sorafenib that was then shown to have benefits as a chemotherapy combination without sorafenib. This was based on the results of two randomized clinical trials. E2603 was a US intergroup double-blind, randomized, placebo-controlled phase 3 study that enrolled 823 patients to carboplatin-paclitaxel or the same combination with the addition of sorafenib.[259] At final analysis, the median OS was 11.3 months (95% CI, 9.8 to 12.2 months) for carboplatin-paclitaxel and 11.1 months (95% CI, 10.3 to 12.3 months) for carboplatin-paclitaxel-sorafenib. Median PFS was 4.9 months for carboplatin-paclitaxel-sorafenib and 4.2 months for carboplatin-paclitaxel. Response rate was 20% for carboplatin-paclitaxel-sorafenib and 18% for carboplatin-paclitaxel. This study established a benchmark for the carboplatin-paclitaxel regimen in first-line therapy of metastatic melanoma.

The PRISM study randomized 270 patients with previously treated metastatic melanoma to the same two regimens.[260] The median PFS was 17.9 weeks for carboplatin-paclitaxel and 17.4 weeks for the sorafenib plus carboplatin-paclitaxel arm. Response rate was 11% with carboplatin-paclitaxel versus 12% with the addition of sorafenib. Together, these studies demonstrate that sorafenib has no role in this combination and that carboplatin-paclitaxel has activity in patients with metastatic melanoma.

Biochemotherapy

For most of the 1990s and 2000s, biochemotherapy was considered by many melanoma clinicians as a treatment option due to the lack of other alternatives and the reported high response rates in uncontrolled, mostly single-institution clinical trials. However, over 20 randomized clinical trials have failed to demonstrate an improvement in OS when administering biochemotherapy compared to a control arm, although many have suggested some benefit in terms of PFS or response rate. A meta-analysis of 18 trials involving 2,621 patients provided evidence that biochemotherapy improves response rates over single-agent chemotherapy or cytokine therapy, but this does not appear to translate into a survival benefit.[261] The definitive testing of biochemotherapy has come from two large cooperative group trials.

In E3695, the combination of CVD with interferon and IL-2 administered concurrently was compared with CVD in patients with metastatic melanoma.[258] Accrual was stopped after 416 patients were enrolled because of a preplanned futility analysis. OS was not improved (8.4-month median for biochemotherapy versus 9.1 months for CVD). PFS was superior (5-month median for biochemotherapy versus 3.1 months for CVD) but not significantly

so. Response rate was not significantly higher in the biochemotherapy arm (17% versus 12%).

In EORTC 18951, cisplatin, dacarbazine, and interferon-α were administered to all patients, with "decrescendo" IL-2 administered only to one cohort.[262] A total of 363 patients were accrued, with all receiving dacarbazine 250 mg/m² daily for 3 days, cisplatin 30 mg/m² daily for 3 days, and interferon-α2b, 10 MU/m² daily for 5 days. The experimental arm also received IL-2 for 4 days after completion of the chemotherapy. The dose per day was fixed, but the duration of the infusion was lengthened each day. Survival rate at 2 years was the primary end point, and an improvement from 10% to 20% was sought. The observed difference in 2-year survival (18% for the IL-2–containing arm versus 13% for the arm without IL-2) was not statistically significant. PFS and response rates were not significantly different between the two treatments. In conclusion, there is little supportive evidence to justify the use of biochemotherapy in the management of patients with metastatic melanoma.

EXPERIMENTAL IMMUNOLOGIC THERAPIES FOR METASTATIC MELANOMA

Anti-PD-1 and Anti-PD-L1

Early clinical testing of antibodies blocking PD-1, an inhibitory T-cell receptor belonging to the CD28 superfamily of immune-regulatory receptors, or blocking its main ligand PD-L1 (also known as B7-H1 or CD274), demonstrate a high rate of durable tumor responses.[263–265] PD-1 downregulates T-cell function by blocking T-cell receptor signaling upon binding to its ligands, PD-L1 or PD-L2 (also known as B7-DC or CD273). PD-L1 is expressed by inflamed tissues and cancer mainly in response to interferons, and confers peripheral tolerance from endogenous antigens. PD-L2 is expressed primarily by antigen-presenting cells.[212]

In a phase 1 trial, patients with advanced melanoma, non–small-cell lung cancer, castration-resistant prostate cancer, or renal cell or colorectal cancer were treated with the anti-PD-1 antibody nivolumab at a dose of 0.1 to 10.0 mg/kg of body weight every 2 weeks.[264] Response rate was 28% among patients with melanoma (26 of 94 patients). A maximum tolerated dose was not defined at the range of dosing levels tested. Common treatment-related adverse events included fatigue, rash, diarrhea, pruritus, decreased appetite, and nausea. Overall, grade 3 or 4 treatment-related adverse events were observed in 41 of 296 patients (14%). Drug-related serious adverse events occurred in 32 of 296 patients (11%). Drug-related adverse events of special interest included pneumonitis, vitiligo, colitis, hepatitis, hypophysitis, and thyroiditis. An update analysis of the nivolumab phase 1 clinical trial reported a median OS over 16 months, with more than 40% of patients alive after 3 years of treatment with a long-term favorable safety profile.[266]

In another phase 1 clinical trial, patients with advanced melanoma, with and without prior treatment with ipilimumab, received the anti-PD-1 antibody MK-3475 (transiently known as lambrolizumab) intravenously at 10 mg/kg every 2 or 3 weeks or at 2 mg/kg every 3 weeks.[265] A total of 135 patients with advanced melanoma were treated. The confirmed response rate evaluated by central radiologic review per response evaluation criteria in solid tumors (RECIST) 1.1, across all dose cohorts, was 38% (95% CI, 25 to 44), with the highest confirmed response rate observed in the 10 mg/kg every 2 weeks cohort (52%; 95% CI, 38 to 66). Response rate was not different between patients with and without prior ipilimumab treatment. Responses were durable in the majority of patients. Most adverse events were low grade, and common adverse events attributed to treatment were fatigue, skin rash, pruritus, and diarrhea.

A phase 1 trial has tested the combination of anti-PD-1 therapy with nivolumab with the CTLA4-blocking antibody ipilimumab.[267] Nivolumab and ipilimumab was administered every 3 weeks for four doses followed by nivolumab alone every 3 weeks for four doses to 53 patients with metastatic melanoma. The objective response rate (according to modified WHO criteria) was 40%. At the maximum doses that were associated with an acceptable level of adverse events (nivolumab at a dose of 1 mg/kg of body weight and ipilimumab at a dose of 3 mg/kg), 53% of patients had an objective response. Grade 3 or 4 adverse events related to therapy occurred in 53% of patients, but were qualitatively similar to previous experience with monotherapy and were generally reversible.

Adoptive Cell Transfer Therapy

Adoptive cell transfer (ACT) therapy refers to an immunotherapy approach for the treatment of cancer that involves the infusion to the tumor-bearing host of cells with antitumor activity that can recognize cancer antigens and result in the destruction of cancer cells. Although it is still experimental, ACT has emerged among the most effective treatments for patients with metastatic melanoma; 50% to 70% of patients with metastatic melanoma experience objective cancer regressions by RECIST when treated with ACT.[268,269]

ACT has a variety of advantages compared with other forms of cancer immunotherapy.[270,271] T-lymphocytes, once identified as cancer reactive, can be expanded to large numbers in vitro using cytokine growth factors. Thus, patients can be administered very large numbers of cells, often much larger than can be naturally generated in vivo. These antitumor lymphocytes can be activated in vitro to express appropriate effector functions such as the ability to lyse tumor cells and secrete cytokines. Secreted cytokines can have a variety of secondary antitumor effects at the cancer site such as the destruction of surrounding blood vessels, the direct lysis of tumor cells, and providing chemokine signals to attract additional effector cell types, such as activated macrophages, to the tumor site. Perhaps most important, when using ACT, it is possible to modify the host to enhance the ability of the infused cells to establish, grow, and function in vivo. The ability to immunosuppress the host prior to cell infusion is unique to ACT. Immunosuppression can counteract the impact of T-regulatory cells that can suppress cellular immune reactions as well as remove other endogenous lymphocytes that compete with the infused cells for homeostatic cytokines such as IL-7 and IL-15, which are necessary for antitumor T-cell expansion in vivo.[270]

A critical step in the development of effective ACT for human cancer was the demonstration in 1987 that lymphocytes infiltrating into deposits of human metastatic melanoma could be grown in IL-2. Tumor-infiltrating lymphocytes (TIL) with antitumor activity could be generated from approximately 70% of patients with metastatic melanoma. Using these human TILs, over 50 different antigenic epitopes have been identified in patients with melanoma, including antigens such as MART1 and gp100 that are widely shared among melanomas from different individuals.

The first report of ACT in humans in 1988[271] and extended in 1994[272] used the transfer of autologous TIL followed by the administration of high-dose IL-2. A major improvement in human ACT occurred when immunosuppressive regimens were administered prior to cell infusions, and this change led to a new generation of ACT clinical protocols.[269,273] A schematic of ACT treatment in humans with metastatic melanoma developed in the Surgery Branch of the National Cancer Institute is shown in Figure 94.16,

Adoptive Transfer of Tumor Infiltrating Lymphocytes

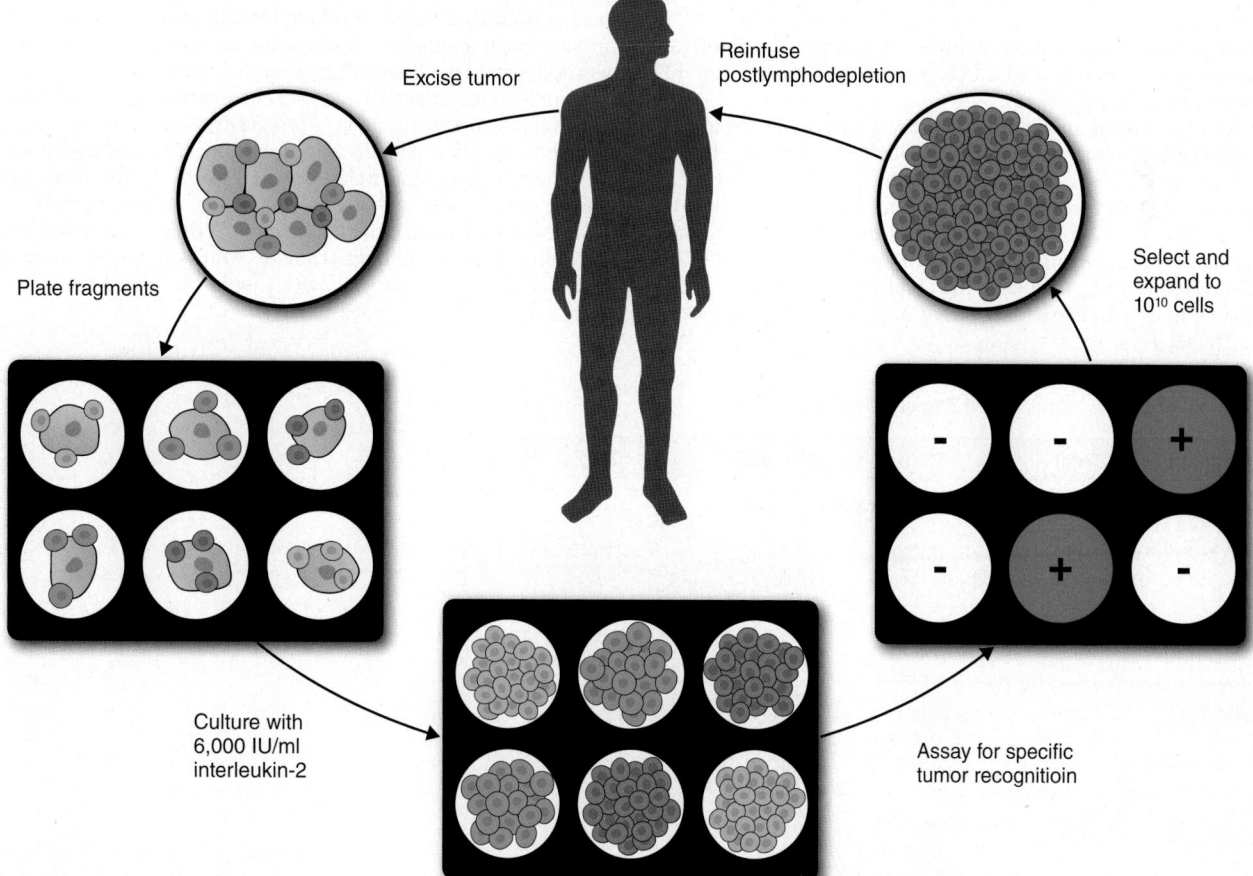

Excise tumor

Reinfuse postlymphodepletion

Plate fragments

Select and expand to 10^{10} cells

Culture with 6,000 IU/ml interleukin-2

Assay for specific tumor recognitioin

Figure 94.16 A schematic representation of the adoptive transfer of tumor-infiltrating lymphocytes into patients following a lymphodepleting preparative regimen.

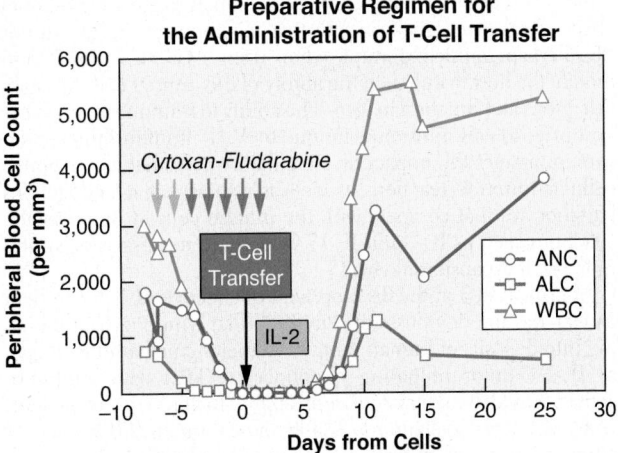

Figure 94.17 The preparative regimen administered prior to the administration of T-cell transfer with typical recovery of neutrophils (*ANC*), lymphocytes (*ALC*), and white blood cells (*WBC*).

and the preparative regimen prior to cell transfer is shown in Figure 94.17. In this treatment, metastatic melanoma deposits are resected and used to generate cultures of TILs with antitumor activity. When cultures reach from 5 to 10 × 10¹⁰ cells, they are infused into patients following an immunosuppressive preparative regimen. The first trial of this approach used a nonmyeloablative preparative regimen consisting of 60 mg/kg of cyclophosphamide for 2 days followed by 5 days of fludarabine at 25 mg/m². On the day following the last dose of fludarabine, the TILs were administered intravenously and IL-2 was then administered for 2 to 3 days at 720,000 IU/kg intravenously every 8 hours. An objective response rate by standard RECIST criteria was seen in 21 of 43 patients (49%)[268] (Fig. 94.18).

Because animal models demonstrated that more profound lymphodepletion was associated with higher antitumor effects, two additional clinical trials were performed in 25 patients each who received this cyclophosphamide–fludarabine chemotherapy plus 2 Gy or 12 Gy of whole-body irradiation. Objective tumor regressions were seen in 13 of 25 (52%) and in 18 of 25 (72%) patients, respectively, including 10 complete regressions (40%) in the latter trial.[268] In these trials, only 1 of 20 complete responders

has recurred, with the others ongoing at 63 to 108 months[269] (Fig. 94.19). These results, although still experimental and available in only a few centers, represent the most effective treatments for patients with metastatic melanoma.[268,269] Factors associated with clinical response included higher telomere lengths, increased numbers of CD27+CD28+ T cells, and increased in vivo persistence at 1 month of the transferred TILs. Among a small subset of 11 patients who had previously been treated with anti-CTLA4, survival and response rate appeared to be higher.

Recent studies using the adoptive transfer of autologous peripheral lymphocytes transduced with genes encoding antitumor T-cell receptors directed against the melanoma/melanocyte antigens MART-1 and gp100 have also shown objective responses in patients with metastatic melanoma,[274,275] though toxicities directed against melanocyte in the eyes and ears limits the application of this gene therapy approach. Analysis of the antigens recognized by TILs associated with complete cancer regression indicate that these transferred cells recognize unique mutations present in each patient's melanoma.[276]

Recently, adoptive transfer of autologous lymphocytes transduced with genes encoding T-cell receptors against the NY-ESO-1 cancer-testis antigen have also mediated regressions in patients with metastatic melanoma.[277]

RADIATION THERAPY FOR METASTATIC MELANOMA (STAGE IV)

The Role of Radiation Therapy in the Management of Distant Metastatic Disease

In general, patients with one to two sites of metastatic melanoma, good performance status, and long interval from diagnosis of the primary lesion should be considered for surgical resection. Patients with widespread metastatic disease may be managed with systemic immunotherapy, targeted therapy, or chemotherapy, with palliative radiation to symptomatic areas of progressive disease. From a radiotherapy perspective, patients with distant metastasis of melanoma are generally managed similar to patients with distant metastases of other solid tumors, with the only main area of controversy being the role of whole-brain radiation therapy (WBRT) for patients with melanoma brain metastases. Patients with widespread systemic disease and short life expectancies should be treated with short courses of high dose per fraction radiation.

Cell Transfer Therapy

Treatment	Total	PR	CR	OR (%)
		Number of patients (duration in months)		
No TBI	43	16 (37%) (84, 36, 29, 28, 14, 12, 11, 7, 7, 7, 7, 4, 4, 2, 2, 2)	5 (12%) (114+, 112+, 111+, 97+, 86+)	21 (49%)
200 TBI	25	8 (32%) (14, 9, 6, 6, 5, 4, 3, 3)	5 (20%) (101+, 98+, 93+, 90+, 70+)	13 (52%)
1200 TBI	25	8 (32%) (21, 13, 7, 6, 6, 5, 3, 2)	10 (40%) (81+, 78+, 77+, 72+, 72+, 71+, 71+, 70+, 70+, 19)	18 (72%)

(20 complete responses: 19 ongoing at 70 to 114 months)

Figure 94.18 The objective response by RECIST criteria of patients receiving cell transfer therapy using either the nonmyeloablative preparative regimen (No TBI) or with addition of 200 or 1,200 cGy total whole body irradiation (TBI). TBI, total body irradiation.

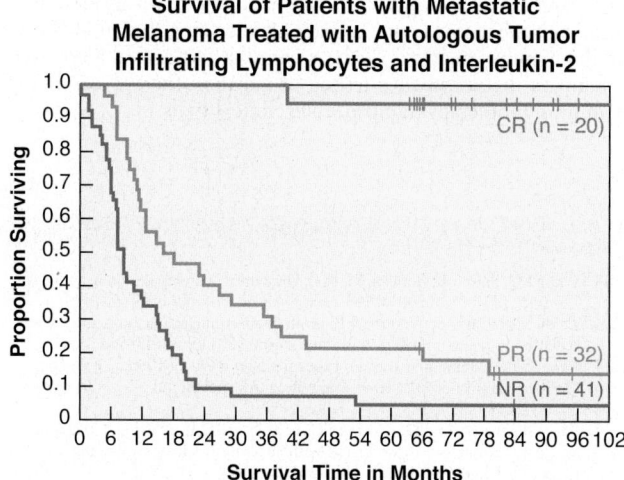

Survival of Patients with Metastatic Melanoma Treated with Autologous Tumor Infiltrating Lymphocytes and Interleukin-2

Figure 94.19 Survival curves of the 93 patients receiving autologous tumor-infiltrating lymphocytes and interleukin-2 following lymphodepleting preparative regimens. Twenty of the ninety-three patients achieved a complete response, and only one has recurred with the remaining complete responders continually disease free beyond 60 months.

Radiation Therapy for Brain Metastases

Carella et al.[278] retrospectively analyzed 60 patients from two RTOG studies performed in the 1970s with cerebral metastases from malignant melanoma to determine the response to whole-brain irradiation and reported that the palliative and survival benefit of WBRT for melanoma patients was comparable to those found for all other primary tumors. However, the median survival times for the two studies were short, only 10 and 14 weeks, and response was measured as symptomatic improvement, which may have been at least partially due to corticosteroids given to reduce cerebral edema. In a retrospective study from the MD Anderson Cancer Center reporting on 87 patients treated for metastatic melanoma to the brain with WBRT with total doses of at least 30 Gy, it was concluded that the frequent use of corticosteroids made it difficult to assess palliative benefit from the radiation, although some patients may have derived benefit as approximately 50% of patients were able to discontinue corticosteroids on the completion of radiation treatments. However, despite this potential benefit, the median survival was only 19 weeks.[279]

Several prospective clinical trials with objective imaging criteria have been conducted to assess tumor response to WBRT alone or with concurrent chemotherapy (temozolomide, fotemustine) in patients with melanoma brain metastases.[254,258,280] These studies suggest that WBRT has limited activity in the treatment of malignant melanoma metastatic to the brain and should be reserved for patients with widespread systemic metastases or diffuse brain metastases that are not amenable to surgical resection or stereotactic radiosurgery.

Stereotactic radiosurgery delivers high doses of radiation in a single fraction to cerebral lesions that are generally <3 cm in diameter and do not involve the brainstem. Yu et al.[281] reported one of the largest retrospective studies to date from the University of California, Los Angeles, consisting of 122 consecutive patients with 332 intracranial melanoma metastases who underwent gamma knife radiosurgery with a median prescribed dose of 20 Gy (range, 14 to 24 Gy). One-third of the patients also received WBRT. The overall median survival was 7 months from radiosurgery and 9.1 months from the onset of brain metastasis. In multivariate analysis, WBRT did not improve survival, and freedom from subsequent brain metastasis depended on intracranial tumor volume.

The RTOG trial 9508 was a phase 3 randomized trial that enrolled 333 patients with one to three brain metastases with multiple histologies (4% of patients had melanoma) to receive WBRT to a total dose of 37.5 Gy in 15 fractions over 3 weeks with and without a radiosurgery boost, with the dose depending on the tumor volume (tumors ≤2 cm received 24 Gy, tumors >2 cm and ≤3 cm received 18 Gy, and tumors >3 cm and ≤4 cm received 15 Gy).[282] Patients with a single brain metastasis had statistically improved survival with a radiosurgical boost compared with those without a boost (6.5 versus 4.9 months, respectively), and the authors concluded that WBRT and stereotactic radiosurgical boost should be the treatment of choice for patients with solitary unresectable brain metastasis. Given the historic data suggesting limited benefit from WBRT for patients with melanoma brain metastasis, the ECOG initiated study E6397, which was a phase 2 trial of radiosurgery for one to three newly diagnosed brain metastases for renal cell carcinoma, melanoma, and sarcoma without WBRT.[283] The dose prescription was based on tumor size and was similar to the RTOG 9508 trial. Thirty-one eligible patients were accrued to this study. The median survival was 8.3 months. The intracranial failure rate in and outside the radiosurgically treated volume at 3 months was 19% and 16%, and at 6 months it was 32% and 32%, respectively. The authors concluded that delaying WBRT may be appropriate for some subgroups of patients with radioresistant tumors, but routine avoidance of WBRT should be approached judiciously given the high intracranial failure rates.

In summary, current data would support the following treatment recommendations for patients with brain metastases from melanoma. All patients with symptomatic cerebral edema should be administered corticosteroids initially. Patients with good performance status and no or minimal systemic disease and a solitary resectable brain lesion should undergo resection. Similar patients with an unresectable brain lesion or up to five small metastatic lesions should be treated with stereotactic radiosurgery, and both groups should be considered for WBRT or close observation with serial imaging. Patients with poor performance status, diffuse systemic disease, and more than five brain lesions have a poor overall prognosis and should be considered for palliative WBRT.

Radiation Therapy for Vertebral Metastases

Patients with vertebral metastases causing spinal cord compression with a reasonable life expectancy of >1 to 2 months should be treated with corticosteroids and surgical decompression if they are operative candidates, with subsequent postoperative radiotherapy as opposed to palliative radiation alone, as this has been shown to result in superior preservation of neurologic function.[284] Patients who are not operative candidates should be considered for radiation therapy. Recent advancements in radiation therapy planning and delivery have led to the development of stereotactic body radiation therapy (SBRT) for lesions in multiple organ sites (lung, liver, and spine). With SBRT, patients are treated with one to five fractions of high-dose and highly conformal radiation isodose distributions.[285] Patients who have limited systemic disease burden who are not considered surgical candidates, or patients with spinal cord compression from disease progression following palliative conventional radiation therapy, should be considered for SBRT.

Current Radiation Research for Melanoma: Interactions with Immune Therapy

Radiation has been reported to have immunomodulatory effects in melanoma animal models thought to be secondary to cell death and inflammation leading to enhanced antigen presentation and antigen-specific cellular immunity, which has been termed the abscopal effect.[286] The two main strategies of integration of radiation into immune-based treatment strategies include local tumor irradiation resulting in enhanced tumor-antigen presentation and antigen-specific cellular immunity,[286,287] and total body irradiation–induced host lymphodepletion resulting in enhanced efficacy of adoptive T-cell transfer-based immunotherapy.[288] Recent

case reports have documented systemic responses triggered after localized radiation therapy in patients receiving the anti-CTLA4 antibody ipilimumab.[289,290] These cases have triggered a renewed interest in the prospective testing of radiation therapy combined with immunotherapy in prospective clinical trials.

REFERENCES

1. Chang AE, Karnell LH, Menck HR. The National Cancer Data Base report on cutaneous and noncutaneous melanoma: a summary of 84,836 cases from the past decade. The American College of Surgeons Commission on Cancer and the American Cancer Society. *Cancer* 1998;83:1664–1678.
2. Curtin JA, Fridlyand J, Kageshita T, et al. Distinct sets of genetic alterations in melanoma. *N Engl J Med* 2005;353:2135–2147.
3. Van Raamsdonk CD, Bezrookove V, Green G, et al. Frequent somatic mutations of GNAQ in uveal melanoma and blue naevi. *Nature* 2009;457:599–602.
4. Van Raamsdonk CD, Griewank KG, Crosby MB, et al. Mutations in GNA11 in uveal melanoma. *N Engl J Med* 2010;363:2191–2199.
5. Davies H, Bignell GR, Cox C, et al. Mutations of the BRAF gene in human cancer. *Nature* 2002;417:949–954.
6. Curtin JA, Busam K, Pinkel D, et al. Somatic activation of KIT in distinct subtypes of melanoma. *J Clin Oncol* 2006;24:4340–4346.
7. Long GV, Menzies AM, Nagrial AM, et al. Prognostic and clinicopathologic associations of oncogenic BRAF in metastatic melanoma. *J Clin Oncol* 2011;29:1239–1246.
8. Menzies AM, Haydu LE, Visintin L, et al. Distinguishing clinicopathologic features of patients with V600E and V600K BRAF-mutant metastatic melanoma. *Clin Cancer Res* 2012;18:3242–3249.
9. Lawrence MS, Stojanov P, Polak P, et al. Mutational heterogeneity in cancer and the search for new cancer-associated genes. *Nature* 2013;499:214–218.
10. Pleasance ED, Cheetham RK, Stephens PJ, et al. A comprehensive catalogue of somatic mutations from a human cancer genome. *Nature* 2010;463:191–196.
11. Krauthammer M, Kong Y, Ha BH, et al. Exome sequencing identifies recurrent somatic RAC1 mutations in melanoma. *Nat Genet* 2012;44:1006–1014.
12. Hodis E, Watson IR, Kryukov GV, et al. A landscape of driver mutations in melanoma. *Cell* 2012;150:251–263.
13. Huang FW, Hodis E, Xu MJ, et al. Highly recurrent TERT promoter mutations in human melanoma. *Science* 2013;339:957–959.
14. Horn S, Figl A, Rachakonda PS, et al. TERT promoter mutations in familial and sporadic melanoma. *Science* 2013;339:959–961.
15. Gray-Schopfer V, Wellbrock C, Marais R. Melanoma biology and new targeted therapy. *Nature* 2007;445:851–857.
16. Carvajal RD, Antonescu CR, Wolchok JD, et al. KIT as a therapeutic target in metastatic melanoma. *JAMA* 2011;305:2327–2334.
17. Viros A, Fridlyand J, Bauer J, et al. Improving melanoma classification by integrating genetic and morphologic features. *PLoS Med* 2008;5:e120.
18. Wan PT, Garnett MJ, Roe SM, et al. Mechanism of activation of the RAF-ERK signaling pathway by oncogenic mutations of B-RAF. *Cell* 2004;116:855–867.
19. Madhunapantula SV, Robertson GP. The PTEN-AKT3 signaling cascade as a therapeutic target in melanoma. *Pigment Cell Melanoma Res* 2009;22:400–419.
20. Kwong LN, Davies MA. Navigating the therapeutic complexity of PI3K pathway inhibition in melanoma. *Clin Cancer Res* 2013;19:5310–5319.
21. Sheppard KE, McArthur GA. The cell-cycle regulator CDK4: an emerging therapeutic target in melanoma. *Clin Cancer Res* 2013;19:5320–5328.
22. Pollock PM, Harper UL, Hansen KS, et al. High frequency of BRAF mutations in nevi. *Nat Genet* 2003;33:19–20.
23. Michaloglou C, Vredeveld LC, Soengas MS, et al. BRAFE600-associated senescence-like cell cycle arrest of human naevi. *Nature* 2005;436:720–724.
24. Mooi WJ, Peeper DS. Oncogene-induced cell senescence—halting on the road to cancer. *N Engl J Med* 2006;355:1037–1046.
25. Jemal A, Saraiya M, Patel P, et al. Recent trends in cutaneous melanoma incidence and death rates in the United States, 1992–2006. *J Am Acad Dermatol* 2011;65:S17–25.e1–e3.
26. Jemal A, Siegel R, Xu J, et al. Cancer statistics, 2010. *CA Cancer J Clin.* 2010;60:277–300.
27. Mack TM, Floderus B. Malignant melanoma risk by nativity, place of residence at diagnosis, and age at migration. *Cancer Causes Control* 1991;2:401–411.
28. Bulliard JL, Cox B. Cutaneous malignant melanoma in New Zealand: trends by anatomical site, 1969–1993. *Int J Epidemiol* 2000;29:416–423.
29. Hayat MJ, Howlader N, Reichman ME, et al. Cancer statistics, trends, and multiple primary cancer analyses from the Surveillance, Epidemiology, and End Results (SEER) Program. *Oncologist* 2007;12:20–37.
30. Elder DE, Xu X. The approach to the patient with a difficult melanocytic lesion. *Pathology* 2004;36:428–434.
31. Shaw HM, Thompson JF. Prognosis in children with melanoma. *N Z Med J* 2001;114:75.
32. Gilchrest BA, Eller MS, Geller AC, et al. The pathogenesis of melanoma induced by ultraviolet radiation. *N Engl J Med* 1999;340:1341–1348.

33. Wang SQ, Setlow R, Berwick M, et al. Ultraviolet A and melanoma: a review. *J Am Acad Dermatol* 2001;44:837–846.
34. Zaidi MR, Davis S, Noonan FP, et al. Interferon-gamma links ultraviolet radiation to melanomagenesis in mice. *Nature* 2011;469:548–553.
35. Elwood JM. Melanoma and sun exposure. *Semin Oncol* 1996;23:650–666.
36. Garibyan L, Fisher DE. How sunlight causes melanoma. *Curr Oncol Rep* 2010;12:319–326.
37. Cust AE, Armstrong BK, Goumas C, et al. Sunbed use during adolescence and early adulthood is associated with increased risk of early-onset melanoma. *Int J Cancer* 2011;128:2425–2435.
38. Badenas C, Aguilera P, Puig-Butille JA, et al. Genetic counseling in melanoma. *Dermatol Ther* 2012;25:397–402.
39. Hussussian CJ, Struewing JP, Goldstein AM, et al. Germline p16 mutations in familial melanoma. *Nat Genet* 1994;8:15–21.
40. Bartsch DK, Langer P, Habbe N, et al. Clinical and genetic analysis of 18 pancreatic carcinoma/melanoma-prone families. *Clin Gen* 2010;77:333–341.
41. Bertolotto C, Lesueur F, Giuliano S, et al. A SUMOylation-defective MITF germline mutation predisposes to melanoma and renal carcinoma. *Nature* 2011;480:94–98.
42. Yokoyama S, Woods SL, Boyle GM, et al. A novel recurrent mutation in MITF predisposes to familial and sporadic melanoma. *Nature* 2011;480:99–103.
43. Curiel-Lewandrowski C, Speetzen LS, Cranmer L, et al. Multiple primary cutaneous melanomas in Li-Fraumeni syndrome. *Arch Dermatol* 2011;147:248–250.
44. Slingluff CL Jr, Reintgen DS, Vollmer RT, et al. Malignant melanoma arising during pregnancy. A study of 100 patients. *Ann Surg* 1990;211:552–557, discussion 558–559.
45. Slingluff CL Jr, Reintgen D. Malignant melanoma and the prognostic implications of pregnancy, oral contraceptives, and exogenous hormones. *Sem Surg Oncol* 1993;9:228–231.
46. MacKie RM. Pregnancy and exogenous hormones in patients with cutaneous malignant melanoma. *Curr Opin Oncol* 1999;11:129–131.
47. Slingluff CL Jr, Dodge RK, Stanley WE, et al. The annual risk of melanoma progression. Implications for the concept of cure. *Cancer* 1992;70:1917–1927.
48. Green AC, Williams GM, Logan V, et al. Reduced melanoma after regular sunscreen use: randomized trial follow-up. *J Clin Oncol* 2011;29:257–263.
49. van der Pols JC, Williams GM, Pandeya N, et al. Prolonged prevention of squamous cell carcinoma of the skin by regular sunscreen use. *Cancer Epidemiol Biomarkers Prev* 2006;15:2546–2548.
50. Autier P, Severi G, Dore JF. Betacarotene and sunscreen use. *Lancet* 1999;354:2163–2164.
51. Mitra D, Luo X, Morgan A, et al. An ultraviolet-radiation-independent pathway to melanoma carcinogenesis in the red hair/fair skin background. *Nature* 2012;491:449–453.
52. Koh HK, Miller DR, Geller AC, et al. Who discovers melanoma? Patterns from a population-based survey. *J Am Acad Dermatol* 1992;26:914–919.
53. Berwick M, Begg CB, Fine JA, et al. Screening for cutaneous melanoma by skin self-examination. *J Natl Cancer Inst.* 1996;88:17–23.
54. Katalinic A, Waldmann A, Weinstock MA, et al. Does skin cancer screening save lives?: an observational study comparing trends in melanoma mortality in regions with and without screening. *Cancer* 2012;118:5395–5402.
55. Clark WH Jr. The dysplastic nevus syndrome. *Arch Dermatol* 1988;124:1207–1210.
56. Naeyaert JM, Brochez L. Clinical practice. Dysplastic nevi. *N Engl J Med* 2003;349:2233–2240.
57. Malvehy J, Puig S, Argenziano G, et al. Dermoscopy report: proposal for standardization. Results of a consensus meeting of the International Dermoscopy Society. *J Am Acad Dermatol* 2007;57:84–95.
58. NIH Consensus Conference. Diagnosis and treatment of early melanoma. *JAMA* 1992;268:1314–1319.
59. Nathanson KL, Martin AM, Wubbenhorst B, et al. Tumor genetic analyses of patients with metastatic melanoma treated with the BRAF inhibitor dabrafenib (GSK2118436). *Clin Cancer Res* 2013;19:4868–4878.
60. Garraway LA, Baselga J. Whole-genome sequencing and cancer therapy: is too much ever enough? *Cancer Discov* 2012;2:766–768.
61. Grob JJ, Bonerandi JJ. The "ugly duckling" sign: identification of the common characteristics of nevi in an individual as a basis for melanoma screening. *Arch Dermatol* 1998;134:103–104.
62. Hoersch B, Leiter U, Garbe C. Is head and neck melanoma a distinct entity? A clinical registry-based comparative study in 5702 patients with melanoma. *Br J Dermatol* 2006;155:771–777.

63. Weinstock MA, Sober AJ. The risk of progression of lentigo maligna to lentigo maligna melanoma. *Br J Dermatol* 1987;116:303–310.
64. King R, Page RN, Googe PB, et al. Lentiginous melanoma: a histologic pattern of melanoma to be distinguished from lentiginous nevus. *Mod Pathol* 2005;18:1397–1401.
65. Murali R, Shaw HM, Lai K, et al. Prognostic factors in cutaneous desmoplastic melanoma: a study of 252 patients. *Cancer* 2010;116:4130–4138.
66. Conley J, Lattes R, Orr W. Desmoplastic malignant melanoma (a rare variant of spindle cell melanoma). *Cancer* 1971;28:914–936.
67. George E, McClain SE, Slingluff CL, et al. Subclassification of desmoplastic melanoma: pure and mixed variants have significantly different capacities for lymph node metastasis. *J Cutan Pathol* 2009;36:425–432.
68. Hawkins WG, Busam KJ, Ben-Porat L, et al. Desmoplastic melanoma: a pathologically and clinically distinct form of cutaneous melanoma. *Ann Surg Oncol* 2005;12:207–213.
69. Posther KE, Selim MA, Mosca PJ, et al. Histopathologic characteristics, recurrence patterns, and survival of 129 patients with desmoplastic melanoma. *Ann Surg Oncol* 2006;13:728–739.
70. Quinn MJ, Crotty KA, Thompson JF, et al. Desmoplastic and desmoplastic neurotropic melanoma: experience with 280 patients. *Cancer* 1998;83:1128–1135.
71. Pawlik TM, Ross MI, Prieto VG, et al. Assessment of the role of sentinel lymph node biopsy for primary cutaneous desmoplastic melanoma. *Cancer* 2006;106:900–906.
72. Han D, Zager JS, Yu D, et al. Desmoplastic melanoma: is there a role for sentinel lymph node biopsy? *Ann Surg Oncol* 2013;20:2345–2351.
73. Breslow A. Thickness, cross-sectional areas and depth of invasion in the prognosis of cutaneous melanoma. *Ann Surg.*1970;172:902–908.
74. Balch CM, Gershenwald JE, Soong SJ, et al. Final version of 2009 AJCC melanoma staging and classification. *J Clin Oncol* 2009;27:6199–6206.
75. Clark WH Jr, From L, Bernardino EA, et al. The histogenesis and biologic behavior of primary human malignant melanomas of the skin. *Cancer Res* 1969;29:705–727.
76. Balch CM, Soong SJ, Gershenwald JE, et al. Prognostic factors analysis of 17,600 melanoma patients: validation of the American Joint Committee on Cancer melanoma staging system. *J Clin Oncol* 2001;19:3622–3634.
77. Day CL Jr, Lew RA, Mihm MC Jr, et al. The natural break points for primary-tumor thickness in clinical Stage I melanoma. *N Engl J Med* 1981;305:1155.
78. Slingluff CL Jr, Vollmer RT, Reintgen DS, et al. Lethal "thin" malignant melanoma. Identifying patients at risk. *Ann Surg* 1988;208:150–161.
79. Slingluff CL Jr, Vollmer R, Seigler HF. Acral melanoma: a review of 185 patients with identification of prognostic variables. *J Surg Oncol* 1990;45:91–98.
80. Yeh JJ, Shia J, Hwu WJ, et al. The role of abdominoperineal resection as surgical therapy for anorectal melanoma. *Ann Surg* 2006;244:1012–1017.
81. Paek SC, Griffith KA, Johnson TM, et al. The impact of factors beyond Breslow depth on predicting sentinel lymph node positivity in melanoma. *Cancer* 2007;109:100–108.
82. Azzola MF, Shaw HM, Thompson JF, et al. Tumor mitotic rate is a more powerful prognostic indicator than ulceration in patients with primary cutaneous melanoma: an analysis of 3661 patients from a single center. *Cancer* 2003;97:1488–1498.
83. Gimotty PA, Van Belle P, Elder DE, et al. Biologic and prognostic significance of dermal Ki67 expression, mitoses, and tumorigenicity in thin invasive cutaneous melanoma. *J Clin Oncol* 2005;23:8048–8056.
84. Gimotty PA, Guerry D, Ming ME, et al. Thin primary cutaneous malignant melanoma: a prognostic tree for 10-year metastasis is more accurate than American Joint Committee on Cancer staging. *J Clin Oncol* 2004;22:3668–3676.
85. Balch CM, Gershenwald JE, Soong SJ, et al. Multivariate analysis of prognostic factors among 2,313 patients with stage III melanoma: comparison of nodal micrometastases versus macrometastases. *J Clin Oncol* 2010;28:2452–2459.
86. Balch CM, Gershenwald JE, Soong SJ, et al. Update on the melanoma staging system: the importance of sentinel node staging and primary tumor mitotic rate. *J Surg Oncol* 2011;104:379–385.
87. Silva E. Adjunct primer for the use of national comprehensive cancer network guidelines for the surgical management of cutaneous malignant melanoma patients. *World J Surg Oncol* 2012;10:54.
88. Terhune MH, Swanson N, Johnson TM. Use of chest radiography in the initial evaluation of patients with localized melanoma. *Arch Dermatol* 1998;134:569–572.
89. Vermeeren L, van der Ent FW, Hulsewe KW. Is there an indication for routine chest X-ray in initial staging of melanoma? *J Surg Res* 2011;166:114–119.
90. Sawyer A, McGoldrick RB, Mackey SP, et al. Does staging computed tomography change management in thick malignant melanoma? *J Plast Reconstr Aesthet Surg* 2009;62:453–456.
91. Constantinidou A, Hofman M, O'Doherty M, et al. Routine positron emission tomography and positron emission tomography/computed tomography in melanoma staging with positive sentinel node biopsy is of limited benefit. *Melanoma Res* 2008;18:56–60.
92. Yancovitz M, Finelt N, Warycha MA, et al. Role of radiologic imaging at the time of initial diagnosis of stage T1b-T3b melanoma. *Cancer* 2007;110:1107–1114.
93. Glaspy JA, Hawkins R, Hoh CK, et al. Use of positron emission tomography in oncology. *Oncology (Williston Park)* 1993;7:41–46, 49–50, discussion 50–52, 55.

94. Wagner JD, Schauwecker D, Davidson D, et al. Inefficacy of F-18 fluorodeoxy-D-glucose-positron emission tomography scans for initial evaluation in early-stage cutaneous melanoma. *Cancer* 2005;104:570–579.
95. Clark PB, Soo V, Kraas J, et al. Futility of fluorodeoxyglucose F 18 positron emission tomography in initial evaluation of patients with T2 to T4 melanoma. *Arch Surg* 2006;141:284–288.
96. Gold JS, Jaques DP, Busam KJ, et al. Yield and predictors of radiologic studies for identifying distant metastases in melanoma patients with a positive sentinel lymph node biopsy. *Ann Surg Oncol* 2007;14:2133–2140.
97. Veronesi U, Cascinelli N. Narrow excision (1-cm margin). A safe procedure for thin cutaneous melanoma. *Arch Surg* 1991;126:438–441.
98. Veronesi U, Cascinelli N, Adamus J, et al. Thin stage I primary cutaneous malignant melanoma. Comparison of excision with margins of 1 or 3 cm. *N Engl J Med* 1988;318:1159–1162.
99. Cascinelli N, Santinami M, Maurichi A, et al. World Health Organization experience in the treatment of melanoma. *Surg Clin North Am* 2003;83:405–416.
100. Khayat D, Rixe O, Martin G, et al. Surgical margins in cutaneous melanoma (2 cm versus 5 cm for lesions measuring less than 2.1-mm thick). *Cancer* 2003;97:1941–1946.
101. Cohn-Cedermark G, Rutqvist LE, Andersson R, et al. Long term results of a randomized study by the Swedish Melanoma Study Group on 2-cm versus 5-cm resection margins for patients with cutaneous melanoma with a tumor thickness of 0.8-2.0 mm. *Cancer* 2000;89:1495–1501.
102. Balch CM, Soong SJ, Smith T, et al. Long-term results of a prospective surgical trial comparing 2 cm vs. 4 cm excision margins for 740 patients with 1-4 mm melanomas. *Ann Surg Oncol* 2001;8:101–108.
103. Thomas JM, Newton-Bishop J, A'Hern R, et al. Excision margins in high-risk malignant melanoma. *N Engl J Med* 2004;350:757–766.
104. Balch CM. The role of elective lymph node dissection in melanoma: rationale, results, and controversies. *J Clin Oncol* 1988;6:163–172.
105. Slingluff CL Jr, Stidham KR, Ricci WM, et al. Surgical management of regional lymph nodes in patients with melanoma. Experience with 4682 patients. *Ann Surg* 1994;219:120–130.
106. Veronesi U, Adamus J, Bandiera DC, et al. Inefficacy of immediate node dissection in stage 1 melanoma of the limbs. *N Engl J Med* 1977;297:627–630.
107. Balch CM, Soong S, Ross MI, et al. Long-term results of a multi-institutional randomized trial comparing prognostic factors and surgical results for intermediate thickness melanomas (1.0 to 4.0 mm). Intergroup Melanoma Surgical Trial. *Ann Surg Oncol* 2000;7:87–97.
108. Cabanas RM. An approach for the treatment of penile carcinoma. *Cancer* 1977;39:456–466.
109. Morton DL, Wen DR, Wong JH, et al. Technical details of intraoperative lymphatic mapping for early stage melanoma. *Arch Surg* 1992;127:392–399.
110. Morton DL, Thompson JF, Essner R, et al. Validation of the accuracy of intraoperative lymphatic mapping and sentinel lymphadenectomy for early-stage melanoma: a multicenter trial. Multicenter Selective Lymphadenectomy Trial Group. *Ann Surg* 1999;230:453–463, discussion 463–465.
111. Gershenwald JE, Colome MI, Lee JE, et al. Patterns of recurrence following a negative sentinel lymph node biopsy in 243 patients with stage I or II melanoma. *J Clin Oncol* 1998;16:2253–2260.
112. Harlow SP, Krag DN, Ashikaga T, et al. Gamma probe guided biopsy of the sentinel node in malignant melanoma: a multicentre study. *Melanoma Res* 2001;11:45–55.
113. Roozendaal GK, de Vries JD, van Poll D, et al. Sentinel nodes outside lymph node basins in patients with melanoma. *Br J Surg* 2001;88:305–308.
114. Gershenwald JE, Thompson W, Mansfield PF, et al. Multi-institutional melanoma lymphatic mapping experience: the prognostic value of sentinel lymph node status in 612 stage I or II melanoma patients. *J Clin Oncol* 1999;17:976–983.
115. Gershenwald JE, Mansfield PF, Lee JE, et al. Role for lymphatic mapping and sentinel lymph node biopsy in patients with thick (> or = 4 mm) primary melanoma. *Ann Surg Oncol* 2000;7:160–165.
116. Morton DL, Cochran AJ, Thompson JF, et al. Sentinel node biopsy for early-stage melanoma: accuracy and morbidity in MSLT-I, an international multicenter trial. *Ann Surg* 2005;242:302–311, discussion 311–313.
117. Vermeeren L, Valdes Olmos RA, Klop WM, et al. A portable gamma-camera for intraoperative detection of sentinel nodes in the head and neck region. *J Nucl Med* 2010;51:700–703.
118. Testori A, De Salvo GL, Montesco MC, et al. Clinical considerations on sentinel node biopsy in melanoma from an Italian multicentric study on 1,313 patients (SOLISM-IMI). *Ann Surg Oncol* 2009;16:2018–2027.
119. Morton DL, Hoon DS, Cochran AJ, et al. Lymphatic mapping and sentinel lymphadenectomy for early-stage melanoma: therapeutic utility and implications of nodal microanatomy and molecular staging for improving the accuracy of detection of nodal micrometastases. *Ann Surg* 2003;238:538–549, discussion 549–550.
120. Morton DL, Thompson JF, Cochran AJ, et al. Sentinel-node biopsy or nodal observation in melanoma. *N Engl J Med* 2006;355:1307–1317.
121. Morton DL, Thompson JF, Cochran AJ, et al. Final trial report of sentinel-node biopsy versus nodal observation in melanoma. *N Engl J Med* 2014;370:599–609.
122. Faries MB, Thompson JF, Cochran A, et al. The impact on morbidity and length of stay of early versus delayed complete lymphadenectomy in mela-

noma: results of the Multicenter Selective Lymphadenectomy Trial (I). *Ann Surg Oncol* 2010;17:3324–3329.

123. Kilbridge KL, Weeks JC, Sober AJ, et al. Patient preferences for adjuvant interferon alfa-2b treatment. *J Clin Oncol* 2001;19:812–823.

124. Gyorki DE, Busam K, Panageas K, et al. Sentinel lymph node biopsy for patients with cutaneous desmoplastic melanoma. *Ann Surg Oncol* 2003;10: 403–407.

125. Gannon CJ, Rousseau DL Jr, Ross MI, et al. Accuracy of lymphatic mapping and sentinel lymph node biopsy after previous wide local excision in patients with primary melanoma. *Cancer* 2006;107:2647–2652.

126. Abramova L, Slingluff CL Jr, Patterson JW. Problems in the interpretation of apparent "radial growth phase" malignant melanomas that metastasize. *J Cutan Pathol* 2002;29:407–414.

127. Slingluff CL Jr, Seigler HF. "Thin" malignant melanoma: risk factors and clinical management. *Ann Plast Surg* 1992;28:89–94.

128. NCCN Clinical Practice Guidelines in Oncology (NCCN Guidelines®) for Melanoma V.2.2014. © National Comprehensive Cancer Network, Inc. 2014. All rights reserved. Accessed April 22, 2014.

129. Wong SL, Balch CM, Hurley P, et al. Sentinel lymph node biopsy for melanoma: American Society of Clinical Oncology and Society of Surgical Oncology joint clinical practice guideline. *J Clin Oncol* 2012;30:2912–2918.

130. Orfaniotis G, Mennie JC, Fairbairn N, et al. Findings of computed tomography in stage IIB and IIC melanoma: a six-year retrospective study in the South-East of Scotland. *J Plast Reconstr Aesthet Surg* 2012;65:1216–1219.

131. Heaton KM, Sussman JJ, Gershenwald JE, et al. Surgical margins and prognostic factors in patients with thick (>4mm) primary melanoma. *Ann Surg Oncol* 1998;5:322–328.

132. Schmid-Wendtner MH, Brunner B, Konz B, et al. Fractionated radiotherapy of lentigo maligna and lentigo maligna melanoma in 64 patients. *J Am Acad Dermatol* 2000;43:477–482.

133. Spenny ML, Walford J, Werchniak AE, et al. Lentigo maligna (melanoma in situ) treated with imiquimod cream 5%: 12 case reports. *Cutis* 2007;79:149–152.

134. Rajpar SF, Marsden JR. Imiquimod in the treatment of lentigo maligna. *Br J Dermatol* 2006;155:653–656.

135. van Meurs T, van Doorn R, Kirtschig G. Recurrence of lentigo maligna after initial complete response to treatment with 5% imiquimod cream. *Dermatol Surg* 2007;33:623–626, discussion 626–627.

136. Somani N, Martinka M, Crawford RI, et al. Treatment of atypical nevi with imiquimod 5% cream. *Arch Dermatol* 2007;143:379–385.

137. Vongtama R, Safa A, Gallardo D, et al. Efficacy of radiation therapy in the local control of desmoplastic malignant melanoma. *Head Neck* 2003;25:423–428.

138. Slingluff CL Jr, Vollmer RT, Seigler HF. Anorectal melanoma: clinical characteristics and results of surgical management in twenty-four patients. *Surgery* 1990;107:1–9.

139. Irvin WP Jr, Bliss SA, Rice LW, et al. Malignant melanoma of the vagina and locoregional control: radical surgery revisited. *Gynecol Oncol* 1998;71: 476–480.

140. Abramova L, Parekh J, Irvin WP Jr, et al. Sentinel node biopsy in vulvar and vaginal melanoma: presentation of six cases and a literature review. *Ann Surg Oncol* 2002;9:840–846.

141. Tien HY, McMasters KM, Edwards MJ, et al. Sentinel lymph node metastasis in anal melanoma: a case report. *Int J Gastrointest Cancer* 2002;32:53–56.

142. Hazard LJ, Sause WT, Noyes RD. Combined adjuvant radiation and interferon-alpha 2B therapy in high-risk melanoma patients: the potential for increased radiation toxicity. *Int J Radiat Oncol Biol Phys* 2002;52:796–800.

143. Weiss M, Loprinzi CL, Creagan ET, et al. Utility of follow-up tests for detecting recurrent disease in patients with malignant melanomas. *JAMA* 1995; 274:1703–1705.

144. Mooney MM, Mettlin C, Michalek AM, et al. Life-long screening of patients with intermediate-thickness cutaneous melanoma for asymptomatic pulmonary recurrences: a cost-effectiveness analysis. *Cancer* 1997;80:1052–1064.

145. Reintgen DS, Cox C, Slingluff CL Jr, et al. Recurrent malignant melanoma: the identification of prognostic factors to predict survival. *Ann Plast Surg* 1992;28:45–49.

146. Thompson JF, Uren RF, Shaw HM, et al. Location of sentinel lymph nodes in patients with cutaneous melanoma: new insights into lymphatic anatomy. *J Am Coll Surg* 1999;189:195–204.

147. Yao KA, Hsueh EC, Essner R, et al. Is sentinel lymph node mapping indicated for isolated local and in-transit recurrent melanoma? *Ann Surg* 2003;238:743–747.

148. Buzaid AC, Ross MI, Balch CM, et al. Critical analysis of the current American Joint Committee on Cancer staging system for cutaneous melanoma and proposal of a new staging system. *J Clin Oncol* 1997;15:1039–1051.

149. Thompson JF, Hersey P, Wachter E. Chemoablation of metastatic melanoma using intralesional Rose Bengal. *Melanoma Res* 2008;18:405–411.

150. Damian DL, Shannon KF, Saw RP, et al. Topical diphencyprone immunotherapy for cutaneous metastatic melanoma. *Australas J Dermatol* 2009; 50:266–271.

151. McArthur GA, Ribas A. Targeting oncogenic drivers and the immune system in melanoma. *J Clin Oncol* 2013;31:499–506.

152. Cornett WR, McCall LM, Petersen RP, et al. Randomized multicenter trial of hyperthermic isolated limb perfusion with melphalan alone compared with melphalan plus tumor necrosis factor: American College of Surgeons Oncology Group Trial Z0020. *J Clin Oncol* 2006;24:4196–4201.

153. Sanki A, Kam PC, Thompson JF. Long-term results of hyperthermic, isolated limb perfusion for melanoma: a reflection of tumor biology. *Ann Surg* 2007; 245:591–596.

154. Lens MB, Dawes M. Isolated limb perfusion with melphalan in the treatment of malignant melanoma of the extremities: a systematic review of randomised controlled trials. *Lancet Oncol* 2003;4:359–364.

155. Morton DL. Cancer immunotherapy: an overview. *Semin Oncol* 1974;1: 297–310.

156. Andtbacka RH, Collichio FA, Amatruda T, et al. OPTiM: A randomized phase III trial of talimogene laherparepvec (T-VEC) versus subcutaneous (SC) granulocyte-macrophage colony-stimulating factor (GM-CSF) for the treatment (tx) of unresected stage IIIB/C and IV melanoma. *J Clin Oncol* 2013;31:Abstr LBA9008.

157. Jahanshahi P, Nasr N, Unger K, et al. Malignant melanoma and radiotherapy: past myths, excellent local control in 146 studied lesions at Georgetown University, and improving future management. *Front Oncol* 2012;2:167.

158. Slingluff CL Jr, Vollmer R, Seigler HF. Stage II malignant melanoma: presentation of a prognostic model and an assessment of specific active immunotherapy in 1,273 patients. *J Surg Oncol* 1988;39:139–147.

159. McMasters KM, Reintgen DS, Ross MI, et al. Sentinel lymph node biopsy for melanoma: controversy despite widespread agreement. *J Clin Oncol* 2001;19:2851–2855.

160. Bilimoria KY, Balch CM, Bentrem DJ, et al. Complete lymph node dissection for sentinel node-positive melanoma: assessment of practice patterns in the United States. *Ann Surg Oncol* 2008;15:1566–1576.

161. Cochran AJ, Wen DR, Huang RR, et al. Prediction of metastatic melanoma in nonsentinel nodes and clinical outcome based on the primary melanoma and the sentinel node. *Mod Pathol* 2004;17:747–755.

162. Wrightson WR, Wong SL, Edwards MJ, et al. Reverse transcriptase-polymerase chain reaction (RT-PCR) analysis of nonsentinel nodes following completion lymphadenectomy for melanoma. *J Surg Res* 2001;98:47–51.

163. McMasters KM, Wong SL, Edwards MJ, et al. Frequency of nonsentinel lymph node metastasis in melanoma. *Ann Surg Oncol* 2002;9:137–141.

164. Wong SL, Morton DL, Thompson JF, et al. Melanoma patients with positive sentinel nodes who did not undergo completion lymphadenectomy: a multi-institutional study. *Ann Surg Oncol* 2006;13:809–816.

165. Faries MB, Morton DL. Surgery and sentinel lymph node biopsy. *Semin Oncol* 2007;34:498–508.

166. Spratt J. Groin dissection. *J Surg Oncol* 2000;73:243–262.

167. Barranco SC, Romsdahl MM, Humphrey RM. The radiation response of human malignant melanoma cells grown in vitro. *Cancer Res* 1971;31:830–833.

168. Katz HR. The results of different fractionation schemes in the palliative irradiation of metastatic melanoma. *Int J Radiat Oncol Biol Phys* 1981;7: 907–911.

169. Ballo MT, Ross MI, Cormier JN, et al. Combined-modality therapy for patients with regional nodal metastases from melanoma. *Int J Radiat Oncol Biol Phys* 2006;64:106–113.

170. Calabro A, Singletary SE, Balch CM. Patterns of relapse in 1001 consecutive patients with melanoma nodal metastases. *Arch Surg* 1989;124:1051–1055.

171. Chang DT, Amdur RJ, Morris CG, et al. Adjuvant radiotherapy for cutaneous melanoma: comparing hypofractionation to conventional fractionation. *Int J Radiat Oncol Biol Phys* 2006;66:1051–1055.

172. Stevens G, Thompson JF, Firth I, et al. Locally advanced melanoma: results of postoperative hypofractionated radiation therapy. *Cancer* 2000;88:88–94.

173. Agrawal S, Kane JM 3rd, Guadagnolo BA, et al. The benefits of adjuvant radiation therapy after therapeutic lymphadenectomy for clinically advanced, high-risk, lymph node-metastatic melanoma. *Cancer* 2009;115:5836–5844.

174. Burmeister BH, Mark Smithers B, Burmeister E, et al. A prospective phase II study of adjuvant postoperative radiation therapy following nodal surgery in malignant melanoma-Trans Tasman Radiation Oncology Group (TROG) Study 96.06. *Radiother Oncol* 2006;81:136–142.

175. Burmeister BH, Henderson MA, Ainslie J, et al. Adjuvant radiotherapy versus observation alone for patients at risk of lymph-node field relapse after therapeutic lymphadenectomy for melanoma: a randomised trial. *Lancet Oncol* 2012;13:589–597.

176. Mocellin S, Lens MB, Pasquali S, et al. Interferon alpha for the adjuvant treatment of cutaneous melanoma. *Cochrane Database Syst Rev* 2013;6:CD008955.

177. Kirkwood JM, Strawderman MH, Ernstoff MS, et al. Interferon alfa-2b adjuvant therapy of high-risk resected cutaneous melanoma: the Eastern Cooperative Oncology Group Trial EST 1684. *J Clin Oncol* 1996;14:7–17.

178. Cole BF, Gelber RD, Kirkwood JM, et al. Quality-of-life-adjusted survival analysis of interferon alfa-2b adjuvant treatment of high-risk resected cutaneous melanoma: an Eastern Cooperative Oncology Group study. *J Clin Oncol* 1996;14:2666–2673.

179. Kirkwood JM, Manola J, Ibrahim J, et al. A pooled analysis of eastern cooperative oncology group and intergroup trials of adjuvant high-dose interferon for melanoma. *Clin Cancer Res* 2004;10:1670–1677.

180. Creagan ET, Dalton RJ, Ahmann DL, et al. Randomized, surgical adjuvant clinical trial of recombinant interferon alfa-2a in selected patients with malignant melanoma. *J Clin Oncol* 1995;13:2776–2783.

181. Cascinelli N, Belli F, MacKie RM, et al. Effect of long-term adjuvant therapy with interferon alpha-2a in patients with regional node metastases from cutaneous melanoma: a randomised trial. *Lancet* 2001;358:866–869.

182. Cameron DA, Cornbleet MC, Mackie RM, et al. Adjuvant interferon alpha 2b in high risk melanoma—the Scottish study. *Br J Cancer* 2001;84:1146–1149.
183. Hancock BW, Wheatley K, Harris S, et al. Adjuvant interferon in high-risk melanoma: the AIM HIGH Study—United Kingdom Coordinating Committee on Cancer Research randomized study of adjuvant low-dose extended-duration interferon Alfa-2a in high-risk resected malignant melanoma. *J Clin Oncol* 2004;22:53–61.
184. Hauschild A, Weichenthal M, Rass K, et al. Efficacy of low-dose interferon {alpha}2a 18 versus 60 months of treatment in patients with primary melanoma of >= 1.5 mm tumor thickness: results of a randomized phase III DeCOG trial. *J Clin Oncol* 2010;28:841–846.
185. Garbe C, Radny P, Linse R, et al. Adjuvant low-dose interferon {alpha}2a with or without dacarbazine compared with surgery alone: a prospective-randomized phase III DeCOG trial in melanoma patients with regional lymph node metastasis. *Ann Oncol* 2008;19:1195–1201.
186. Eggermont AM, Suciu S, MacKie R, et al. Post-surgery adjuvant therapy with intermediate doses of interferon alfa 2b versus observation in patients with stage IIb/III melanoma (EORTC 18952): randomised controlled trial. *Lancet* 2005;366:1189–1196.
187. Ascierto PA, Chiarion-Sileni V, Muggiano A, et al. Interferon alpha for the adjuvant treatment of melanoma: review of international literature and practical recommendations from an expert panel on the use of interferon. *J Chemother* 2013:1973947813Y0000000154.
188. Agarwala SS, Lee SJ, Flaherty LE, et al. Randomized phase III trial of high-dose interferon alfa-2b (HDI) for 4 weeks induction only in patients with intermediate- and high-risk melanoma (Intergroup trial E 1697). *J Clin Oncol* 2011;29:Abstr 8505.
189. Eggermont AM, Suciu S, Santinami M, et al. Adjuvant therapy with pegylated interferon alfa-2b versus observation alone in resected stage III melanoma: final results of EORTC 18991, a randomised phase III trial. *Lancet* 2008;372:117–126.
190. Eggermont AM, Suciu S, Testori A, et al. Long-term results of the randomized phase III trial EORTC 18991 of adjuvant therapy with pegylated interferon alfa-2b versus observation in resected stage III melanoma. *J Clin Oncol* 2012;30:3810–3818.
191. Flaherty LE, Othus M, Atkins MB, et al. Phase III trial of high dose interferon alpha-2b versus cisplatin, vinblastine, DTIC plus IL-2 and interferon in patients with high risk melanoma (SWOG S0008): an intergroup study of CALGB, COG, ECOG and SWOG. *J Clin Oncol* 2012;30:Abstr 8504.
192. Lawson DH, Lee SJ, Tarhini AA, et al. E4697: Phase III cooperative group study of yeast-derived granulocyte macrophage colony-stimulating factor (GM-CSF) versus placebo as adjuvant treatment of patients with completely resected stage III-IV melanoma. *J Clin Oncol* 2010;28:Abstr 8504.
193. Hailemichael Y, Dai Z, Jaffarzad N, et al. Persistent antigen at vaccination sites induces tumor-specific CD8(+) T cell sequestration, dysfunction and deletion. *Nat Med* 2013;19:465–472.
194. Speiser DE, Lienard D, Rufer N, et al. Rapid and strong human CD8+ T cell responses to vaccination with peptide, IFA, and CpG oligodeoxynucleotide 7909. *J Clin Invest* 2005;115:739–746.
195. Hodi FS, O'Day SJ, McDermott DF, et al. Improved survival with ipilimumab in patients with metastatic melanoma. *N Engl J Med* 2010;363:711–723.
196. Robert C, Thomas L, Bondarenko I, et al. Ipilimumab plus dacarbazine for previously untreated metastatic melanoma. *N Engl J Med* 2011;364:2517–2526.
197. Moschos SJ, Edington HD, Land SR, et al. Neoadjuvant treatment of regional stage IIIB melanoma with high-dose interferon alfa-2b induces objective tumor regression in association with modulation of tumor infiltrating host cellular immune responses. *J Clin Oncol* 2006;24:3164–3171.
198. Romano E, Scordo M, Dusza SW, et al. Site and timing of first relapse in stage III melanoma patients: implications for follow-up guidelines. *J Clin Oncol* 2010;28:3042–3047.
199. Dancey A, Rayatt S, Courthold J, et al. Views of UK melanoma patients on routine follow-up care. *Br J Plast Surg* 2005;58:245–250.
200. Pflugfelder A, Kochs C, Blum A, et al. Malignant melanoma S3-guideline "diagnosis, therapy and follow-up of melanoma." *J Dtsch Dermatol Ges* 2013;11:1–116, 1–126.
201. Crowley NJ, Seigler HF. Late recurrence of malignant melanoma. Analysis of 168 patients. *Ann Surg* 1990;212:173–177.
202. Manola J, Atkins M, Ibrahim J, et al. Prognostic factors in metastatic melanoma: a pooled analysis of Eastern Cooperative Oncology Group trials. *J Clin Oncol* 2000;18:3782–3793.
203. Swetter SM, Carroll LA, Johnson DL, et al. Positron emission tomography is superior to computed tomography for metastatic detection in melanoma patients. *Ann Surg Oncol* 2002;9:646–653.
204. Sortini D, Feo CV, Carcoforo P, et al. Thoracoscopic localization techniques for patients with solitary pulmonary nodule and history of malignancy. *Ann Thorac Surg* 2005;79:258–262, discussion 262.
205. Heidorn SJ, Milagre C, Whittaker S, et al. Kinase-dead BRAF and oncogenic RAS cooperate to drive tumor progression through CRAF. *Cell* 2010;140:209–221.
206. Poulikakos PI, Zhang C, Bollag G, et al. RAF inhibitors transactivate RAF dimers and ERK signalling in cells with wild-type BRAF. *Nature* 2010;464:427–430.
207. Halaban R, Zhang W, Bacchiocchi A, et al. PLX4032, a selective BRAF(V600E) kinase inhibitor, activates the ERK pathway and enhances cell migration and proliferation of BRAF melanoma cells. *Pigment Cell Melanoma Res* 2010;23:190–200.
208. Su F, Viros A, Milagre C, et al. RAS mutations in cutaneous squamous-cell carcinomas in patients treated with BRAF inhibitors. *N Engl J Med* 2012;366:207–215.
209. Berger AC, Buell JF, Venzon D, et al. Management of symptomatic malignant melanoma of the gastrointestinal tract. *Ann Surg Oncol* 1999;6:155–160.
210. Tagawa ST, Cheung E, Banta W, et al. Survival analysis after resection of metastatic disease followed by peptide vaccines in patients with Stage IV melanoma. *Cancer* 2006;106:1353–1357.
211. Korn EL, Liu PY, Lee SJ, et al. Meta-analysis of phase II cooperative group trials in metastatic stage IV melanoma to determine progression-free and overall survival benchmarks for future phase II trials. *J Clin Oncol* 2008;26:527–534.
212. Pardoll DM. The blockade of immune checkpoints in cancer immunotherapy. *Nat Rev Cancer* 2012;12:252–264.
213. Margolin KA, Hamid O, Weber JS, et al. Ipilimumab retreatment following induction therapy: The expanded access program (EAP) experience. *J Clin Oncol* 2013;31:Abstr 9041.
214. Hodi FS, Lee SJ, McDermott DF, et al. Multicenter, randomized phase II trial of GM-CSF (GM) plus ipilimumab (Ipi) versus Ipi alone in metastatic melanoma: E1608. *J Clin Oncol* 2013;31:Abstr CRA9007.
215. Ribas A, Camacho LH, Lopez-Berestein G, et al. Antitumor activity in melanoma and anti-self responses in a phase I trial with the anti-cytotoxic T lymphocyte-associated antigen 4 monoclonal antibody CP-675,206. *J Clin Oncol* 2005;23:8968–8977.
216. Ribas A, Kefford R, Marshall MA, et al. Phase III randomized clinical trial comparing tremelimumab with standard-of-care chemotherapy in patients with advanced melanoma. *J Clin Oncol* 2013;31:616–622.
217. Kirkwood JM, Lorigan P, Hersey P, et al. Phase II trial of tremelimumab (CP-675,206) in patients with advanced refractory or relapsed melanoma. *Clin Cancer Res* 2010;16:1042–1048.
218. Ribas A, Hauschild A, Kefford R. Reply to K.S. Wilson et al. *J Clin Oncol* 2013;31:2836–2837.
219. Ribas A, Glaspy JA, Lee Y, et al. Role of dendritic cell phenotype, determinant spreading, and negative costimulatory blockade in dendritic cell-based melanoma immunotherapy. *J Immunother* 2004;27:354–367.
220. Ribas A, Chmielowski B, Glaspy JA. Do we need a different set of response assessment criteria for tumor immunotherapy? *Clin Cancer Res* 2009;15:7116–7118.
221. Wolchok JD, Hoos A, O'Day S, et al. Guidelines for the evaluation of immune therapy activity in solid tumors: immune-related response criteria. *Clin Cancer Res* 2009;15:7412–7420.
222. Rosenberg SA, Lotze MT, Muul LM, et al. Observations on the systemic administration of autologous lymphokine-activated killer cells and recombinant interleukin-2 to patients with metastatic cancer. *N Engl J Med* 1985;313:1485–1492.
223. Lotze MT, Chang AE, Seipp CA, et al. High-dose recombinant interleukin 2 in the treatment of patients with disseminated cancer. Responses, treatment-related morbidity, and histologic findings. *JAMA* 1986;256:3117–3124.
224. Atkins MB, Lotze MT, Dutcher JP, et al. High-dose recombinant interleukin 2 therapy for patients with metastatic melanoma: analysis of 270 patients treated between 1985 and 1993. *J Clin Oncol* 1999;17:2105–2116.
225. Smith FO, Downey SG, Klapper JA, et al. Treatment of metastatic melanoma using interleukin-2 alone or in conjunction with vaccines. *Clin Cancer Res* 2008;14:5610–5618.
226. Rosenberg SA, Yang JC, Schwartzentruber DJ, et al. Immunologic and therapeutic evaluation of a synthetic peptide vaccine for the treatment of patients with metastatic melanoma [see comments]. *Nat Med* 1998;4:321–327.
227. Schwartzentruber DJ, Lawson DH, Richards JM, et al. gp100 peptide vaccine and interleukin-2 in patients with advanced melanoma. *N Engl J Med* 2011;364:2119–2127.
228. Ribas A, Flaherty KT. BRAF targeted therapy changes the treatment paradigm in melanoma. *Nat Rev Clin Oncol* 2011;8:426–433.
229. Chapman PB, Hauschild A, Robert C, et al. Improved survival with vemurafenib in melanoma with BRAF V600E mutation. *N Engl J Med* 2011;364:2507–2516.
230. Sosman JA, Kim KB, Schuchter L, et al. Survival in BRAF V600-mutant advanced melanoma treated with vemurafenib. *N Engl J Med* 2012;366:707–714.
231. Oberholzer PA, Kee D, Dziunycz P, et al. RAS mutations are associated with the development of cutaneous squamous cell tumors in patients treated with RAF inhibitors. *J Clin Oncol* 2012;30:316–321.
232. Hauschild A, Grob JJ, Demidov LV, et al. Dabrafenib in BRAF-mutated metastatic melanoma: a multicentre, open-label, phase 3 randomised controlled trial. *Lancet* 2012;380:358–365.
233. Hauschild A, Grob JJ, Demidov LV, et al. An update on BREAK-3, a phase III, randomized trial: Dabrafenib (DAB) versus dacarbazine (DTIC) in patients with BRAF V600E-positive mutation metastatic melanoma (MM). *J Clin Oncol* 2013;31:Abstract 9013.
234. Solit DB, Garraway LA, Pratilas CA, et al. BRAF mutation predicts sensitivity to MEK inhibition. *Nature* 2006;439:358–362.
235. von Euw E, Atefi M, Attar N, et al. Antitumor effects of the investigational selective MEK inhibitor TAK733 against cutaneous and uveal melanoma cell lines. *Mol Cancer* 2012;11:22.

236. Flaherty KT, Robert C, Hersey P, et al. Improved survival with MEK inhibition in BRAF-mutated melanoma. *N Engl J Med* 2012;367(2):107-114.

237. Poulikakos PI, Persaud Y, Janakiraman M, et al. RAF inhibitor resistance is mediated by dimerization of aberrantly spliced BRAF(V600E). *Nature* 2011;480:387–390.

238. Shi H, Moriceau G, Kong X, et al. Melanoma whole-exome sequencing identifies (V600E)B-RAF amplification-mediated acquired B-RAF inhibitor resistance. *Nat Commun* 2012;3:724.

239. Nazarian R, Shi H, Wang Q, et al. Melanomas acquire resistance to B-RAF(V600E) inhibition by RTK or N-RAS upregulation. *Nature* 2010; 468:973–977.

240. Wagle N, Emery C, Berger MF, et al. Dissecting therapeutic resistance to RAF inhibition in melanoma by tumor genomic profiling. *J Clin Oncol* 2011; 29:3085–3096.

241. Trunzer K, Pavlick AC, Schuchter L, et al. Pharmacodynamic effects and mechanisms of resistance to vemurafenib in patients with metastatic melanoma. *J Clin Oncol* 2013;31:1767–1774.

242. Johannessen CM, Boehm JS, Kim SY, et al. COT drives resistance to RAF inhibition through MAP kinase pathway reactivation. *Nature* 2010;468:968–972.

243. Shi H, Kong X, Ribas A, et al. Combinatorial treatments that overcome PDGFR{beta}-driven resistance of melanoma cells to V600EB-RAF inhibition. *Cancer Res* 2011;71:5067–5074.

244. Villanueva J, Vultur A, Lee JT, et al. Acquired resistance to BRAF inhibitors mediated by a RAF kinase switch in melanoma can be overcome by cotargeting MEK and IGF-1R/PI3K. *Cancer Cell* 2010;18:683–695.

245. Shi H, Hong A, Kong X, et al. A novel AKT1 mutant amplifies an adaptive melanoma response to BRAF inhibition. *Cancer Discov* 201;4:69–79.

246. Shi H, Hugo W, Kong X, et al. Acquired resistance and clonal evolution in melanoma during BRAF inhibitor therapy. *Cancer Discov* 2014;4:80–93.

247. Van Allen EM, Wagle N, Sucker A, et al. The genetic landscape of clinical resistance to RAF inhibition in metastatic melanoma. *Cancer Discov* 2014; 4:94–109.

248. Flaherty KT, Infante JR, Daud A, et al. Combined BRAF and MEK inhibition in melanoma with BRAF V600 mutations. *N Engl J Med* 2012;367: 1694–1703.

249. Kim KB, Kefford R, Pavlick AC, et al. Phase II study of the MEK1/MEK2 inhibitor trametinib in patients with metastatic BRAF-mutant cutaneous melanoma previously treated with or without a BRAF inhibitor. *J Clin Oncol* 2013;31:482–489.

250. Seghers AC, Wilgenhof S, Lebbe C, et al. Successful rechallenge in two patients with BRAF-V600-mutant melanoma who experienced previous progression during treatment with a selective BRAF inhibitor. *Melanoma Res* 2012;22:466–472.

251. Comis RL. DTIC (NSC-45388) in malignant melanoma: a perspective. *Cancer Treat Rep* 1976;60:165–176.

252. Stevens MF, Hickman JA, Langdon SP, et al. Antitumor activity and pharmacokinetics in mice of 8-carbamoyl-3-methyl-imidazo[5,1-d]-1,2,3,5-tetrazin-4(3H)-one (CCRG 81045; M & B 39831), a novel drug with potential as an alternative to dacarbazine. *Cancer Res* 1987;47:5846–5852.

253. Patel M, McCully C, Godwin K, et al. Plasma and cerebrospinal fluid pharmacokinetics of intravenous temozolomide in non-human primates. *J Neurooncol* 2003;61:203–207.

254. Margolin K, Atkins B, Thompson A, et al. Temozolomide and whole brain irradiation in melanoma metastatic to the brain: a phase II trial of the Cytokine Working Group. *J Cancer Res Clin Oncol* 2002;128:214–218.

255. Patel PM, Suciu S, Mortier L, et al. Extended schedule, escalated dose temozolomide versus dacarbazine in stage IV melanoma: final results of a randomised phase III study (EORTC 18032). *Eur J Cancer* 2011;47: 1476–1483.

256. Jacquillat C, Khayat D, Banzet P, et al. Final report of the French multicenter phase II study of the nitrosourea fotemustine in 153 evaluable patients with disseminated malignant melanoma including patients with cerebral metastases. *Cancer* 1990;66:1873–1878.

257. Chapman PB, Einhorn LH, Meyers ML, et al. Phase III multicenter randomized trial of the Dartmouth regimen versus dacarbazine in patients with metastatic melanoma. *J Clin Oncol* 1999;17:2745–2751.

258. Atkins MB, Hsu J, Lee S, et al. Phase III trial comparing concurrent biochemotherapy with cisplatin, vinblastine, dacarbazine, interleukin-2, and interferon alfa-2b with cisplatin, vinblastine, and dacarbazine alone in patients with metastatic malignant melanoma (E3695): a trial coordinated by the Eastern Cooperative Oncology Group. *J Clin Oncol* 2008;26:5748–5754.

259. Flaherty KT, Lee SJ, Zhao F, et al. Phase III trial of carboplatin and paclitaxel with or without sorafenib in metastatic melanoma. *J Clin Oncol* 2013;31:373–379.

260. Hauschild A, Agarwala SS, Trefzer U, et al. Results of a phase III, randomized, placebo-controlled study of sorafenib in combination with carboplatin and paclitaxel as second-line treatment in patients with unresectable stage III or stage IV melanoma. *J Clin Oncol* 2009;27:2823–2830.

261. Ives NJ, Stowe RL, Lorigan P, et al. Chemotherapy compared with biochemotherapy for the treatment of metastatic melanoma: a meta-analysis of 18 trials involving 2,621 patients. *J Clin Oncol* 2007;25:5426–5434.

262. Keilholz U, Punt CJ, Gore M, et al. Dacarbazine, cisplatin, and interferon-alfa-2b with or without interleukin-2 in metastatic melanoma: a randomized phase III trial (18951) of the European Organisation for Research and Treatment of Cancer Melanoma Group. *J Clin Oncol* 2005;23:6747–6755.

263. Brahmer JR, Tykodi SS, Chow LQ, et al. Safety and activity of anti-PD-L1 antibody in patients with advanced cancer. *N Engl J Med* 2012;366:2455–2465.

264. Topalian SL, Hodi FS, Brahmer JR, et al. Safety, activity, and immune correlates of anti-PD-1 antibody in cancer. *N Engl J Med* 2012;366:2443–2454.

265. Hamid O, Robert C, Daud A, et al. Safety and tumor responses with lambrolizumab (anti-PD-1) in melanoma. *N Engl J Med* 2013;369:134–144.

266. Topalian SL, Sznol M, McDermott DF, et al. Survival, durable tumor remission, and long-term safety in patients with advanced melanoma receiving nivolumab. *J Clin Oncol* 2014;32:1020–1030.

267. Wolchok JD, Kluger H, Callahan MK, et al. Nivolumab plus ipilimumab in advanced melanoma. *N Engl J Med* 2013;369:122–133.

268. Rosenberg SA. Cell transfer immunotherapy for metastatic solid cancer—what clinicians need to know. *Nat Rev Clin Oncol* 2011;8:577–585.

269. Rosenberg SA, Yang JC, Sherry RM, et al. Durable complete responses in heavily pretreated patients with metastatic melanoma using T-cell transfer immunotherapy. *Clin Cancer Res* 2011;17:4550–4557.

270. Restifo NP, Dudley ME, Rosenberg SA. Adoptive immunotherapy for cancer: harnessing the T cell response. *Nat Rev Immunol* 2012;12:269–281.

271. Rosenberg SA, Packard BS, Aebersold PM, et al. Use of tumor-infiltrating lymphocytes and interleukin-2 in the immunotherapy of patients with metastatic melanoma. A preliminary report. *N Engl J Med* 1988;319:1676–1680.

272. Rosenberg SA, Yannelli JR, Yang JC, et al. Treatment of patients with metastatic melanoma with autologous tumor-infiltrating lymphocytes and interleukin 2 [see comments]. *J Natl Cancer Inst* 1994;86:1159–1166.

273. Dudley ME, Wunderlich JR, Robbins PF, et al. Cancer regression and autoimmunity in patients after clonal repopulation with antitumor lymphocytes. *Science* 2002;298:850–854.

274. Morgan RA, Dudley ME, Wunderlich JR, et al. Cancer regression in patients after transfer of genetically engineered lymphocytes. *Science* 2006;314:126–129.

275. Johnson LA, Morgan RA, Dudley ME, et al. Gene therapy with human and mouse T-cell receptors mediates cancer regression and targets normal tissues expressing cognate antigen. *Blood* 2009;114:535–546.

276. Robbins PF, Lu YC, El-Gamil M, et al. Mining exomic sequencing data to identify mutated antigens recognized by adoptively transferred tumor-reactive T cells. *Nat Med* 2013;19:747–752.

277. Robbins PF, Morgan RA, Feldman SA, et al. Tumor regression in patients with metastatic synovial cell sarcoma and melanoma using genetically engineered lymphocytes reactive with NY-ESO-1. *J Clin Oncol* 2011;29:917–924.

278. Carella RJ, Gelber R, Hendrickson F, et al. Value of radiation therapy in the management of patients with cerebral metastases from malignant melanoma: Radiation Therapy Oncology Group Brain Metastases Study I and II. *Cancer* 1980;45:679–683.

279. Ellerhorst J, Strom E, Nardone E, et al. Whole brain irradiation for patients with metastatic melanoma: a review of 87 cases. *Int J Radiat Oncol Biol Phys* 2001;49:93–97.

280. Mornex F, Thomas L, Mohr P, et al. [Randomised phase III trial of fotemustine versus fotemustine plus whole brain irradiation in cerebral metastases of melanoma]. *Cancer Radiotherp* 2003;7:1–8.

281. Yu C, Chen JC, Apuzzo ML, et al. Metastatic melanoma to the brain: prognostic factors after gamma knife radiosurgery. *Int J Radiat Oncol Biol Phys* 2002;52:1277–1287.

282. Andrews DW, Scott CB, Sperduto PW, et al. Whole brain radiation therapy with or without stereotactic radiosurgery boost for patients with one to three brain metastases: phase III results of the RTOG 9508 randomised trial. *Lancet* 2004;363:1665–1672.

283. Manon R, O'Neill A, Knisely J, et al. Phase II trial of radiosurgery for one to three newly diagnosed brain metastases from renal cell carcinoma, melanoma, and sarcoma: an Eastern Cooperative Oncology Group study (E 6397). *J Clin Oncol* 2005;23:8870–8876.

284. Patchell RA, Tibbs PA, Regine WF, et al. Direct decompressive surgical resection in the treatment of spinal cord compression caused by metastatic cancer: a randomised trial. *Lancet* 2005;366:643–648.

285. Timmerman RD, Kavanagh BD, Cho LC, et al. Stereotactic body radiation therapy in multiple organ sites. *J Clin Oncol* 2007;25:947–952.

286. Teitz-Tennenbaum S, Li Q, Rynkiewicz S, et al. Radiotherapy potentiates the therapeutic efficacy of intratumoral dendritic cell administration. *Cancer Res* 2003;63:8466–8475.

287. Perez CA, Fu A, Onishko H, et al. Radiation induces an antitumour immune response to mouse melanoma. *Int J Radiat Biol* 2009;85:1126–1136.

288. Wrzesinski C, Paulos CM, Kaiser A, et al. Increased intensity lymphodepletion enhances tumor treatment efficacy of adoptively transferred tumor-specific T cells. *J Immunother* 2010;33:1–7.

289. Postow MA, Callahan MK, Barker CA, et al. Immunologic correlates of the abscopal effect in a patient with melanoma. *N Engl J Med* 2012;366:925–931.

290. Stamell EF, Wolchok JD, Gnjatic S, et al. The abscopal effect associated with a systemic anti-melanoma immune response. *Int J Radiat Oncol Biol Phys* 2013;85:293–295.

95 Genetic Testing in Skin Cancer

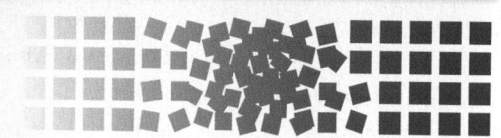

Michele Gabree and Meredith L. Seidel

INTRODUCTION

Many hereditary cancer predisposition syndromes are associated with cutaneous findings. Identification of unique dermatologic features provides an opportunity to distinguish hereditary cancer syndromes with similar associated internal malignancies. Although skin findings are an important diagnostic tool for a number of cancer syndromes, including Cowden syndrome, Birt–Hogg–Dubé, hereditary leiomyomatosis renal cell carcinoma, and others (Table 95.1),[1–18] this section will focus on skin cancer as well as tumor syndromes with cutaneous findings that are not included elsewhere in this book, including hereditary melanoma, basal cell nevus syndrome (BCNS), and neurofibromatosis type 1 (NF1), and neurofibromatosis type 2 (NF2).

The identification of dermatologic abnormalities and their association with internal malignancies often require thorough observation from clinicians. A consultation with a dermatologist may be helpful to identify specific dermatologic abnormalities. In some cases, biopsy and pathology may be necessary for a diagnosis.

GENETIC COUNSELING

Genetic counseling for hereditary skin diseases is similar to the process for other cancer predisposition syndromes. The genetic counseling process generally includes a detailed family and medical history, risk assessment, discussion of benefits, and limitations of available genetic testing, including possible test results, discussion of medical management, and implications for family members.[19] Dermatologic evaluation and review of pathology records pertaining to the cutaneous findings may provide clarification on specific dermatologic observations. Consultation with a dermatologist and/or other specialist who is knowledgeable about hereditary syndromes is often essential to a clinical evaluation. When possible, reviewing the medical records of family members is also helpful to confirm dermatologic diagnoses, as reports of some skin findings in family members may contain some inaccuracies.[20]

HEREDITARY SKIN CANCER AND THE NEUROFIBROMATOSES

In addition to a few known single-gene disorders associated with skin cancers, confounding environmental factors, including solar ultraviolet radiation, as well as other genetic factors also are known to be associated with a varying degree of skin cancer risk. Separately, other hereditary tumor and cancer predisposition syndromes, such as NF1 and NF2, contain benign cutaneous features as common and sometimes predominant findings. General characteristics of a hereditary cancer predisposition syndrome include multiple tumors or cutaneous features in one individual, multiple affected family members, and individuals or families with related tumors, cancers, or unique physical characteristics. In some cases, young age at onset may also suggest a higher likelihood of a hereditary syndrome.

Hereditary Melanoma

Approximately 10% of melanoma cases are attributed to hereditary predisposition. Hereditary melanoma has been associated with mutations in two genes, cyclin-dependent kinase inhibitor 2A (*CDKN2A*) and cyclin-dependent kinase 4 (*CDK4*). Mutations in *CDK4* are rare and have been identified in only a few hereditary melanoma families.[21] Of families with hereditary melanoma, defined as three or more diagnoses of melanoma in one family, approximately 20% to 40% will have a detectable mutation in *CDKN2A*.[22]

CDKN2A and *CDK4* both function as tumor suppressors. *CDKN2A* encodes two transcripts: p16 and p14ARF through alternate reading frames. The majority of *CDKN2A* mutation-carrying families have been found to have mutations that affect the p16 protein. Mutations affecting the function of p14ARF are reportedly rare in cutaneous melanoma families.[23]

Phenotype

Hereditary melanoma has also been referred to as familial atypical mole melanoma syndrome.[24] Although the presence of atypical moles has been associated with an increased risk for melanoma, it has not been identified as a strong predictor of *CDKN2A* mutation status.[25,26]

The penetrance of *CDKN2A* mutations has been observed to be dependent on geography. This is likely due to varying environmental and other genetic factors across geographic regions. A study of *CDKN2A* carriers selected based on positive personal and family history of melanoma observed the melanoma risk for *CDKN2A* mutation carriers to be 58% in Europe, 76% in the United States, and 91% in Australia.[27] In a population-based study of patients with melanoma, the penetrance of *CDNK2A* mutations was observed to be lower (28% risk for melanoma by the age of 80 years).[28] Variants in the melanocortin 1 receptor (*MC1R*) gene have been associated with increased *CDKN2A* penetrance.[29] The prevalence of *MC1R* has been observed to differ with ethnic background and is one example of a genetic factor influencing melanoma risk that varies by geographical region.[30]

In addition to melanoma, other cancers have also been observed in increased frequency in *CDKN2A* mutation carriers. Most notably, an increased risk for pancreatic cancer has been reported in some *CDKN2A* mutation–carrying families.[31] Less commonly, an increased risk for other cancers, including neural system tumors, nonmelanoma skin cancers, uveal melanoma, and head and neck cancers, has also been reported in individuals with *CDKN2A* mutations.[31,32]

In the United States, which is an area of moderate to high melanoma incidence, genetic counseling for hereditary melanoma has been generally recommended in families in which (1) three or more relatives are affected with melanoma, (2) one individual has three or more primary melanomas, or (3) both pancreatic cancer and melanoma are present in one family (Table 95.2).[15] Early age at onset in the absence of a family history of melanoma is not highly suggestive of a *CDKN2A* mutation.[33,34]

Summary of Hereditary Cancer Syndromes with Cutaneous Features

	Cutaneous Features	Internal Tumor Site
Benign cutaneous features prominent		
Cowden syndrome[1,2]	Trichilemmoma, palmoplantar keratoses, oral mucosal papillomas, cutaneous facial papules, lipomas, macular pigmentation of the glans penis	Breast, thyroid, uterus
Birt–Hogg–Dubé[3]	Fibrofolliculomas, trichodiscomas, angiofibromas, perifollicular fibromas, acrochordons	Kidney
Childhood cancer syndrome (homozygous Lynch syndrome)[4]	Neurofibromas, CALMs	Hematologic, neural system, colon, small intestine, urinary tract
Hereditary leiomyomatosis renal cell carcinoma[5]	Cutaneous leiomyomas	Kidney, uterus
Multiple endocrine neoplasia type 2B[6]	Mucosal neuromas of the lips/tongue	Thyroid, adrenal gland, gastrointestinal tract
NF1[7,8]	Neurofibromas (cutaneous and subcutaneous), CALMs, freckling (inguinal, axillary), hypopigmented macules, cutaneous angiomas xanthogranulomas, glomus tumors, hyperpigmentation	Brain, spine, peripheral nervous system, optic pathway, small intestine, neuroendocrine, breast
NF2[7,9]	CALMs (usually one to three), plaque lesions, intradermal schwannomas, subcutaneous schwannomas, cutaneous neurofibromas (uncommon)	Brain, spine, peripheral nervous system, optic pathway
Peutz–Jeghers syndrome[10]	Mucocutaneous pigmentation	Breast, stomach, small intestine, colon, pancreas, ovary, testicle
Tuberous sclerosis complex[11]	Hypomelanotic macules, facial angiofibromas, shagreen patches, fibrous facial plaques, ungual fibromas	Brain, kidney, heart, neuroendocrine
Benign cutaneous features sometimes present		
Multiple endocrine neoplasia type 1[12]	Facial angiofibromas, collagenomas, lipomas	Pituitary, pancreas, parathyroid, gastroenteropancreatic tract
Familial adenomatous polyposis[13]	Lipomas, fibromas, and epidermal cysts	Colon, thyroid, small intestine, liver, brain, pancreas, ampulla of Vater
Skin cancer prominent		
BCNS[14]	Basal cell carcinoma	Brain, ovary, heart
Hereditary melanoma[15]	Melanoma, dysplastic nevi	Pancreas
Xeroderma pigmentosum[16]	Melanoma, basal cell and squamous cell carcinoma, severe sunburn, lentigos, xerosis, erythema, actinic keratoses, poikiloderma	Oral cavity
Skin cancer sometimes present		
Hereditary breast and ovarian cancer syndrome[17]	Melanoma	Breast, ovary, prostate, pancreas
Lynch syndrome[18]	Sebaceous neoplasms, keratoacanthomas	Colon, uterus, stomach, ovary, hepatobiliary tract, urinary tract, small intestine, brain

CALM, café-au-lait macule; NF1, neurofibromatosis type 1; NF2, neurofibromatosis type 2; BCNS, basal cell nevus syndrome.

Referral Criteria for Hereditary Melanoma Genetic Counseling

Three or more relatives on the same side of the family with melanoma
Three or more primary melanomas in one individual
Pancreatic cancer and melanoma on the same side of the family

From Leachman SA, Carucci J, Kohlmann W, et al. Selection criteria for genetic assessment of patients with familial melanoma. *J Am Acad Dermatol* 2009;61:677e1–677e14.

Genetic Testing

Clinical testing for *CDKN2A* and *CDK4* is available in the United States at several commercial laboratories. However, some of the laboratories offering hereditary melanoma testing perform analysis of only *CDKN2A*, given the relatively low-frequency *CDK4* mutations reported.

The utility of genetic testing for *CDKN2A* mutations remains a source of debate. This is partly due to the relatively low frequency of *CDKN2A* mutations in families with melanoma. In addition, many individuals with a personal and/or family history of melanoma are under close surveillance and aware of risk-reduction recommendations; therefore, genetic test results would not alter

TABLE 95.3

CDKN2A Genetic Testing Results and Medical Management Recommendations

Test Result	Medical Management
CDKN2A mutation positive	Melanoma surveillance: ■ Clinical skin examination with dermatologist every 4–6 mo ■ Biopsy should be performed on suspected lesions ■ Avoid prolonged direct sunlight and use sun-protective clothing and sunscreen ■ Monthly self-skin examinations ■ Inform at-risk relatives Pancreatic cancer surveillance[a]: ■ Recommended for individuals with a family history of pancreatic cancer and may be considered in other cases ■ Refer to gastroenterologist for discussion of pancreatic screening options ■ Inform at-risk relatives
CDKN2A variation of unknown significance	Etiology of the melanoma remains unknown: ■ Consider if genetic testing is indicated for other affected relatives ■ Proband and family remain at increased risk for melanoma ■ Screening recommendations should be based on personal and family history
CDKN2A mutation negative	No mutation previously identified in family: ■ Etiology of the melanoma remains unknown ■ Consider if genetic testing is indicated for other affected relatives ■ Proband and family remain at increased risk for melanoma ■ Screening recommendations should be based on personal and family history Mutation previously identified in family: ■ Proband and family remain at increased risk for melanoma, although the risk is lower than for relatives who carry a _CDKN2A_ mutation ■ Screening recommendations should be based on personal and family history

[a] To date, pancreatic cancer surveillance has not been proven to be effective at improving pancreatic cancer outcome.

clinical management.[25] Also, the role of pancreatic cancer surveillance in _CDKN2A_ carriers remains under investigation. Some studies have suggested that knowledge of _CDKN2A_ mutation status improves short-term compliance to risk-reducing behaviors.[35,36] However, information regarding the long-term impact of _CDKN2A_ testing is limited at this time. The possible genetic test results for an individual undergoing _CDKN2A_ genetic testing are shown in Table 95.3.

Individuals with a _CDKN2A_ mutation have a 50% chance of passing the mutation on to their children.

Medical Management

CDKN2A mutation carriers, or individuals at 50% risk to be a carrier, should be monitored carefully for melanoma through clinical and self-examinations (see Table 95.3). In addition, _CDKN2A_ carriers are recommended to avoid prolonged direct sunlight and utilize sun-protective clothing and sunscreen.[25,37]

Individuals who test negative for a familial _CDKN2A_ mutation may also have an increased risk for melanoma. However, this risk has been observed to be lower than the melanoma risk for _CDKN2A_ mutation carriers.[28]

As noted in Table 95.3, _CDKN2A_ mutation carriers, especially those with a family history of pancreatic cancer, are candidates for pancreatic cancer surveillance and should discuss the risks, benefits, and limitations of screening with a gastroenterology specialist.[38] However, to date, the effectiveness of pancreatic surveillance remains under investigation.[39]

Basal Cell Nevus Syndrome

BCNS, also known as Gorlin syndrome or nevoid basal cell carcinoma syndrome, is an autosomal dominant syndrome associated with cutaneous findings, including basal cell carcinoma,

as well as skeletal system, nervous system, and ocular abnormalities.[40] Although BCNS has complete penetrance, the expression is variable.[41]

BCNS is thought to be relatively uncommon, and the incidence of BCNS has been estimated to be 1:30,827 to 1:57,000.[42] The variable expression may cause difficulty in diagnosing BCNS.

BCNS has been associated with mutations in the _patched gene 1_ (_PTCH1_) gene. _PTCH1_ functions as a tumor suppressor in the sonic hedgehog (Shh) pathway, which is also involved in embryonic development.[43] Chromosomal abnormalities of 9q22.3 region, which includes _PTCH1_, have been reported in a few individuals with features of BCNS as well as other features, including short stature, developmental delay, and seizures.[44] Rarely, mutations in other genes, including _SUFU_ and _PTCH2_, have also been reported in individuals with features of BCNS.[45,46]

Phenotype

The phenotype of BCNS is variable, and some characteristics are present at different life stages. Therefore, it is important to obtain a complete medical history, including physical examination and dermatologic, cardiac, and gynecologic examinations as well as radiologic studies to confirm a diagnosis of BCNS.

The clinical manifestations of BCNS include the following.

Skin

Basal Cell Carcinoma. Approximately 50% to 75% of individuals with BCNS will develop basal cell carcinomas.[47] Typically, basal cell carcinomas develop in the late teens through the 30s, but some published reports have indicated the detection of basal cell carcinomas in early childhood in individuals with BCNS. The presence of basal cell carcinomas is also dependent on other factors, including skin type and radiation exposure, including sun exposure.[40,41]

Noncancerous Cutaneous Features. The majority of individuals with BCNS will have multiple nevi present by adulthood.[40] In addition, BCNS is associated with an increased prevalence of facial milia, dermoid cysts, and skin tags. Palmar and plantar pits are also a common feature of BCNS and usually are evident by early adulthood.[40]

Skeletal

Skeletal abnormalities, including rib and spinal abnormalities, are reported with increased frequency in BCNS. The majority of individuals with BCNS are reported to have macrocephaly.[48]

Central Nervous System

Ectopic Calcification. Ectopic calcification, particularly of the falx celebri, has been reported as a common finding in individuals with BCNS.[48]

Brain Tumor. Although other types of brain tumors have been reported in individuals with BCNS, medulloblastoma, typically desmoplastic type, is the most common.[49] Approximately 5% of individuals with BCNS are diagnosed with medulloblastoma, usually around 2 years of age.

Other Features

Jaw Keratocysts. Approximately 75% of affected individuals with BCNS develop multiple jaw keratocysts.[50]

Characteristic Facial Features. Facial features characteristic of BCNS, including macrocephaly, bossing of the forehead, coarse facial features, and facial milia, have been observed in approximately 60% of BCNS cases.[14]

In addition to these features, congenital malformations such as cleft lip/palate, polydactyly, and eye anomalies have also been reported as features of BCNS.[40]

Additional associated tumors including cardiac and ovarian fibromas have also been reported to occur with increased frequency in BCNS.[51,52]

Diagnosis and Genetic Testing

A diagnosis of BCNS was initially based on clinical criteria; however, the availability of molecular testing has identified mutations in individuals with a more variable phenotype. The First International Colloquium on BCNS concluded that the clinical criteria should be used to consider a suspected diagnosis of BCNS rather than as diagnostic criteria.[53] The colloquium recommends that a suspected diagnosis of BCNS be considered in individuals with an identified *PTCH1* mutation and one major clinical criterion, individuals who express two major criteria, and individuals with one major and two minor criteria (Table 95.4).

Genetic testing for the *PTCH1* gene is clinically available. Approximately 50% to 85% of individuals with clinical features of BCNS will have a detectable mutation in the *PTCH1* gene through gene sequencing analysis. Deletions and duplications of the *PTCH1* gene have also been reported.[54]

Approximately 20% to 30% of individuals with BCNS are de novo, meaning that neither parent carries the associated gene mutation.[14] Individuals affected with BCNS have a 50% chance of having an affected child. In cases where a mutation has been identified, testing is an option for at-risk family members. In addition, both preconception genetic diagnosis and prenatal testing are available for known *PTCH1* mutations.

Medical Management

Because of the many variable symptoms of BCNS, individuals with BCNS should be referred to an appropriate specialist depending on the symptoms.

TABLE 95.4

Clinical Criteria for Suspected Diagnosis of Basal Cell Nevus Syndrome

Major criteria
- Early-onset/multiple basal cell carcinoma
- Odontogenic keratocyst of the jaw (<20 y of age)
- Palmaroplantar pitting
- Calcification of the falx cerebri
- Medulloblastoma (usually desmoplastic)
- First-degree relative with BCNS

Minor criteria
- Rib anomalies
- Skeletal malformations and radiologic changes
- Macrocephaly
- Cleft lip/palate
- Ovarian/cardiac fibroma
- Lymphomesenteric cysts
- Ocular abnormalities

BCNS, basal cell nevus syndrome.
From Bree AF, Shah MR. Consensus statement from the first international colloquium on basal cell nevus syndrome (BCNS). *Am J Med Genet A* 2011; 155A:2091–2097.

Basal Cell Carcinoma. Early diagnosis is important for management and to limit cosmetic damage. Surgery, oral retinoids, topical therapies, and photodynamic therapy have all been utilized with varying degrees of success for individuals with BCNS.[47]

Medulloblastoma. Consideration of developmental assessment and physical examination every 6 months is an option for children during infancy and early childhood. Imaging for medulloblastoma surveillance is not currently recommended.[14]

Jaw Keratocysts. Clinical examinations and imaging are recommended for individuals with BCNS, starting during childhood. These tumors may sometimes be detected during routine dental examinations.[55]

Ovarian and Cardiac Fibromas. Affected individuals with cardiac fibromas should be referred to a cardiologist. Ovarian fibromas also warrant a specialty referral and may require surgery, ideally with the aim of preserving fertility.[56]

Radiation Exposure. Given the known increased risk for basal cell carcinoma, it is recommended that individuals with BCNS avoid sun exposure. In addition, it is recommended that other radiation exposure also be avoided if possible, including radiation as treatment for medulloblastoma.[49]

Neurofibromatosis Type 1

NF1 is one of the most common genetic disorders, affecting an estimated 1:2,500 to 1:3,000 individuals at birth.[7] Formerly known as von Recklinghausen disease or peripheral neurofibromatosis, manifestations of the disease affect multiple areas of the body, including, but not limited to, the central and peripheral nervous systems, skin, eyes, skeleton, gastrointestinal system, and the cardiovascular system. Historically, observations of patients with NF1 date back to the 13th century, but the disorder was first formally described in 1882 by Friedrich von Recklinghausen.[7,57,58]

NF1 is a completely penetrant autosomal dominant condition with widely variable expression, both within and between families.[59] No ethnic, racial, or sex predilection has been observed.[57] NF1 is caused by mutations in the NF1 gene on 17q11.2. The protein product of NF1 is neurofibromin, a GTPase-activating protein that is expressed across many tissue types and in particularly high levels within neurocutaneous tissue. It acts as a negative regulator of intracellular Ras signaling pathways involved in cell growth and proliferation.[7,60,61] More recently, NF1 has also been linked to the development of skeletal muscle.[62]

Phenotype

In 1987, the National Institutes of Health developed clinical diagnostic criteria for NF1 (Table 95.5) on which diagnosis of the disease is most often based.[59] The disease usually presents in childhood, beginning with skin findings, which are often present by 1 year of age. In general, the clinical manifestations of NF1 are age dependent: By the age of 6 years, approximately 90% of individuals with NF1 meet diagnostic criteria; by 8 years of age, 97% meet criteria, and virtually all meet the criteria by the time they are 20 years old.[59]

Skin

Among the numerous and variable clinical manifestations of NF1, cutaneous findings feature prominently and can even be the sole basis for a diagnosis of NF1. The following skin findings are hallmark features of NF1, and each is a component of the diagnostic criteria (see Table 95.5).

Café-Au-Lait Macules. Café-au-lait macules (CALM) are the most common and often the earliest presenting feature of NF1. CALMs may be congenital and are observed in almost all patients with NF1 within the first year of life. They often become larger and more numerous through adolescence and may fade as an adult.[57]

Intertriginous Freckling. Skinfold freckling, or Crowe sign, is a cardinal feature of NF1.[59] Freckling occurs most often in the axillary and inguinal regions of the body and is exhibited by up to 90% of patients, usually beginning in childhood. Freckling may also be found in other areas of the body including beneath the breasts in females, on the neck, above the eyelids, around the mouth, and on the trunk in adults.[58]

Neurofibromas. The hallmark feature of NF1, neurofibromas can develop in almost any part of the body, including on or just below the surface of the skin. Cutaneous neurofibromas vary in size (<1 mm to large/disfiguring) and number; they are soft and fleshy, and may be raised or flat, ranging in color from blue/purple to brown to flesh colored. Subcutaneous neurofibromas are firm, tender nodules that are often visible beneath the skin. Cutaneous and/or subcutaneous neurofibromas usually manifest later than CALMs and freckling, either later in childhood or in early adolescence.[58,59]

Less common, nondiagnostic cutaneous features of NF1 include hyperpigmentation, which may be generalized or appearing in conjunction with affected body areas in segmental NF1, glomus tumors, hypopigmented macules (usually on the trunk), xanthogranulomas, cutaneous angiomas, and pruritus.[7,57,60]

Neurologic

Tumors of the central and peripheral nervous systems are prevalent among individuals with NF1. These include spinal neurofibromas, peripheral nerve sheath tumors, plexiform neurofibromas, and astrocytomas. In addition, optic pathway gliomas (OPG) are slow-growing tumors occurring among 15% to 20% of patients, usually by the age of 6 years. OPGs are symptomatic in only 5% of individuals, in which case they are most often diagnosed by the age of 3 years.[7,57,60]

A variety of nontumor neurologic manifestations are reported among individuals with NF1. These include learning disabilities, which occur in 60% or more of children with NF1, decreased IQ (occasionally <70), attention-deficit/hyperactivity disorder, and other behavior difficulties. Unidentified bright objects (UBO) are a characteristic magnetic resonance imaging (MRI) finding in NF1. The clinical significance of UBOs is not known, but some evidence correlates UBO prevalence with severity of cognitive and behavioral difficulties.[58,59] Seizure disorders and multiple sclerosis also occur at a higher frequency in NF1, and Chiari type I malformation, aqueductal stenosis, and macrocephaly have all been reported.[7,59]

Eye

Lisch nodules, or melanocytic iris hamartomas, are asymptomatic eye findings present in most individuals with NF1, usually by the age of 5 to 10 years. Lisch nodules are pathognomonic for NF1 and are most reliably detected by an experienced ophthalmologist by slit-lamp examination.[7,8,60] Glaucoma, choroidal abnormalities, and ptosis are less common but have all been reported in patients with NF1.[7]

Skeletal

Bony growths and other abnormalities of the bone are key features of NF1. Diagnostic bone findings include thinning of the long-bone cortex (with or without pseudoarthrosis) and sphenoid wing dysplasia. In addition, there is an increased frequency of short stature, scoliosis, and, more recently noted, osteopenia and osteoporosis among individuals with NF1.[7,57,60]

Cardiovascular

Cardiovascular complications occur at a higher frequency among patients with NF1 and include congenital heart disease (pulmonary stenosis, coarctation of the aorta), hypertension, cerebrovascular disease, and renal artery stenosis.[7,63] Pulmonary stenosis is more prevalent among patients with classic NF1 but may also be found as part of a variant phenotype that combines features of NF1 and Noonan syndrome.[59]

Other Features

Respiratory Complications. Respiratory complications include restrictive lung disease caused by compression from neurofibroma and metastases from malignant peripheral nerve sheath tumors.[7]

Neurofibromatosis Type 1–Associated Malignancies. The overall increased risk of cancer in NF1 patients is 2.7-fold, and the cumulative risk for patients older than 50 years is 20%.[61] Malignant peripheral nerve sheath tumors are the most common cancerous tumors in NF1. Other malignancies include chronic myelogenous

TABLE 95.5

National Institutes of Health Diagnostic Criteria: Neurofibromatosis Type 1

Clinical diagnosis of NF1 can be made for an individual exhibiting any two (or more) of the following:
- Six or more café-au-lait macules:
  - ≥5 mm prepubertal
  - ≥15 mm postpubertal
- Two or more neurofibromas of any type, or one or more plexiform neurofibromas
- Freckling in the axillary or inguinal region
- Optic glioma
- Two or more Lisch nodules (iris hamartomas)
- A distinctive osseous lesion such as sphenoid dysplasia or tibial pseudoarthrosis
- A first-degree relative with NF1 as defined by the above criteria

NF1, neurofibromatosis type 1.
From Evans DG, Raymond FL, Barwell JG, et al. Genetic testing and screening of individuals at risk of NF2. *Clin Genet* 2012;82:416–424.

leukemia, astrocytoma, rhabdomyosarcoma, gastrointestinal stromal tumors, carcinoid tumors (small intestine), pheochromocytomas (although usually not malignant), and breast carcinoma.[61] There are also a few reports of higher rates of melanoma seen in NF1; however, this association remains controversial.[57]

Diagnosis and Genetic Testing

Up to 50% of individuals with NF1 have no family history and represent de novo mutations. The *NF1* gene has one of the highest spontaneous mutations rates, about 1:10,000, and more than 500 pathogenic mutations have been identified.[61] The reason for the high mutation rate is not fully understood, but may be due in part to the large size of the gene.[59]

Although diagnosis of NF1 is almost always made on a clinical basis using the established criteria, genetic testing is available and can be useful, particularly in certain situations. Mutations are identifiable in 95% of individuals who meet the NF1 clinical diagnostic criteria.[64] In young children with no family history who do not yet meet the diagnostic criteria, genetic testing may aid in differentiating NF1 from other disorders with phenotypic overlap such as Legius syndrome, familial café-au-lait spots, and NF2. Genetic testing may also help identify rare variant forms of the disease that do not satisfy the National Institutes of Health criteria. In families with a previously identified mutation, prenatal diagnosis and prenatal testing are available. A common challenge in prenatal counseling and testing for NF1 arises from the variability and unpredictability of the disease presentation.[7,65]

Given the wide variability in expression of the disease even among members of the same family, it stands to reason that very few genotype–phenotype correlations have been described. It has been noted that individuals carrying a deletion of an entire NF1 allele (approximately 4% to 5% of cases) are likely to exhibit a more severe phenotype, including a greater number of cutaneous neurofibromas, often occurring at younger ages. Cognitive abnormalities are also more frequent and severe, and somatic overgrowth, large hands and feet, and dysmorphic facial features have been reported.[63] In addition, individuals with a three-base-pair in-frame deletion of exon 17 of NF1 may exhibit the common nontumor cutaneous features of NF1, without cutaneous or surface plexiform neurofibromas.[63]

In addition to the high rate of spontaneous mutations, another challenge associated with genetic counseling for NF1 is the high rate of mosaicism. Approximately 40% to 50% of cases are segmental, or mosaic, representing postzygotic NF1 mutations. In these cases, recurrence risks can be difficult to predict; however, they are usually estimated to be <1% unless the germline is affected. Indeed, there are cases of individuals with segmental NF1 bearing children with constitutional disease.[63]

Medical Management

Management of NF1 requires multidisciplinary input and, ideally, should be overseen by practitioners experienced in caring for patients with neurofibromatosis.[58,60]

Recommended surveillance for children with NF1 may vary somewhat by center, but typically includes annual physical and ophthalmologic examination until the age of 8 years. Between the ages of 8 and 18 years, examinations every other year may be sufficient.[58,60,64] Blood pressure monitoring should take place at least annually because of the risk of pheochromocytoma and renal artery stenosis.[58,64] In addition, annual neurologic examinations are advisable, with consideration of neuroimaging in the presence of any abnormal findings.[58] In addition, ongoing developmental and neuropsychological evaluation is recommended to assess cognitive function and to identify learning disabilities.[8,57]

Screening by way of MRI, electroencephalogram, and/or X-ray may be dictated by symptoms, clinical findings, and/or personal and family history. For certain findings, more frequent monitoring may be indicated and, in some cases, treatment may be available.

Plexiform Neurofibroma. Perform MRI every 6 to 12 months to monitor growing lesions. Depending on the location of the lesion, surgical debulking may be possible but is often incomplete, resulting in regrowth.[8,60,64]

Optic Pathway Gliomas. Once identified, MRI is used to monitor OPGs. Quarterly ophthalmologic evaluation is suggested for the first year, followed by annual examination of patients for at least 3 years or until the age of 8 years. Evaluation by endocrinology may be recommended. For symptomatic OPGs, chemotherapy treatment is available, but radiotherapy is not recommended.[8,57]

Malignant Peripheral Nerve Sheath Tumor. Monitor individuals with plexiform neurofibroma for increased size and pain, as well as changes in tumor texture; monitor unexplained neurologic changes. If possible, complete surgical resection is desired, but should be followed by radiation therapy if it is not complete.[8,64]

Cutaneous Neurofibromas. Surgical removal of neurofibromas may be possible when necessary for cosmetic or pain-related reasons.[8,57]

As necessary, referrals should be made to a variety of specialties, including cardiology, nephrology, plastic surgery, otolaryngology, and gastroenterology.

Neurofibromatosis Type 2

NF2 was first described by J. H. Wishart in 1822, at least 50 years prior to von Recklinghausen's description of NF1. Although there is relatively little overlap in the clinical phenotype of the two conditions, NF2 is much less common and was, until relatively recently, often mistaken as a variant form of NF1. It was not until 1987 when linkage studies attributed the conditions to two different genes on different chromosomes that the diseases were formally recognized as separate. Although more common than it was once thought to be, the estimated incidence of NF2 is approximately 1/10 of that of NF1, or 1:30,000 to 1:40,000.[66]

NF2 is inherited in an autosomal dominant manner and is virtually 100% penetrant by the age of 60 years.[9] It is caused by mutations in the NF2 gene on chromosome 22q12. The product of the *NF2* gene is the protein known as merlin (moesin–ezrin–radixin-like protein) or schwannomin, and it is thought to function in cell membrane protein organization, cellular adhesion, and negative regulation of cellular growth, proliferation, and motility.[60,64] The specific mechanism of the tumor suppressor function of merlin has not yet been fully elucidated and is an area of active investigation.[60]

A key difference between NF1 and NF2 relates to cutaneous findings, which, in NF2, may aid in diagnosis but are not diagnostic in and of themselves. The cardinal feature of NF2 is vestibular schwannoma, which arise bilaterally on the eighth cranial nerve in almost all cases of the disease.[7]

Phenotype

Contrary to the name of the disorder, schwannomas and meningiomas, not neurofibromas, are the most prominent tumor types found in NF2.[9,67] Individuals with NF2 most often present between 20 and 30 years of age with hearing loss (frequently unilateral) related to the presence of a vestibular schwannoma. Tinnitus, dizziness, and imbalance are also common adult symptoms at presentation.[9] Although children may also develop similar symptoms, they are more likely to present with less common features of NF2, making examination of other systems the key to accurate diagnosis. In these cases, neurologic examination, eye examination, and careful examination of the skin become crucial.[64] Several sets of NF2 diagnostic criteria exist, and the criteria may still be evolving[68]; however, currently, the most widely used criteria set is the Manchester Diagnostic Criteria, shown in Table 95.6.[60]

TABLE 95.6

Diagnostic Criteria for Neurofibromatosis Type 2

Manchester Diagnostic Criteria for NF2

- Bilateral vestibular schwannoma

  or
- First-degree family member with NF2 and unilateral vestibular schwannoma, or any two of meningioma, glioma, neurofibroma, schwannoma, posterior subcapsular lenticular opacities

  or
- Unilateral vestibular schwannoma and any two of meningioma, glioma, neurofibroma, schwannoma, posterior subcapsular lenticular opacities

  or
- Multiple meningiomas (≥2) and unilateral vestibular schwannoma or any two of glioma, neurofibroma, schwannoma, cataract

NF2, neurofibromatosis type 2.

Skin

Although not hallmarks of the disease, the cutaneous manifestations of NF2 are prevalent and can be detected in up to 70% of cases.[7] As with NF1, skin findings include CALMs; however, when CALMs are present in NF2, it is generally fewer, about one to three per person. Individuals with NF2 may also exhibit plaque lesions on the surface of the skin, intradermal schwannomas, subcutaneous schwannomas, and, very rarely,[7,57,60] cutaneous neurofibromas.[7,9]

Neurologic

Tumors. Bilateral vestibular schwannomas occur in 90% to 95% of patients with NF2.[7] Although malignancy is rare, the location of growth is a common cause of increased morbidity, often causing progressive hearing loss and balance issues.[58] Schwannomas of other cranial nerves are not uncommon among patients with NF2[9]; in addition, spinal and peripheral nerve schwannomas often develop.[64] Meningiomas are the second most common tumor type, found in 58% to 75% of patients with NF2. Both cranial and spinal meningiomas can be found in NF2.[64] More rare, but also observed, are spinal and brainstem ependymomas, as well as spinal and cranial astrocytoma.[7]

Peripheral Neuropathy. The majority of patients with NF2 will develop peripheral neuropathy within their lifetime, often in childhood presenting as a hand or foot drop, or a palsy. Neuropathy is sometimes but not always related to tumor compression.[9]

Eye

Subcapsular lenticular opacities are a key diagnostic feature of NF2. They are found in 60% to 81% of patients and may develop into cataracts.[9,58] Additional ocular findings include epiretinal membranes, or thin translucent or semitranslucent sheets of fibrous tissue, which usually do not decrease visual acuity.[9] In addition, retinal hamartomas appear in 6% to 22% of patients with NF2 and can cause a loss of visual acuity.[9]

Diagnosis and Genetic Testing

In patients with suspected NF2 and a positive family history (two or more family members affected), genetic testing reveals mutations in ≥90%. However, approximately 50% of individuals with NF2 represent de novo mutations in the *NF2* gene. In isolated cases of classic NF2 with no known family history, mutations are identified in approximately 60% to 72%. In families with an identified mutation, presymptomatic genetic testing of at-risk family members is important for management of the disease. Prenatal genetic testing and preimplantation genetic diagnosis are also available.[69]

Somatic mosaicism is observed in roughly 33% of individuals with de novo cases of NF2, and identification of these individuals often relies on confirming the presence of the same mutation in tissue from two distinct NF2-related lesions.[67] Finally, for some mutations, genotype–phenotype correlation data are available.[9]

Medical Management

In general, as with NF1, it is best if patients with NF2 are able to be followed by experienced practitioners in a comprehensive clinic setting. Screening recommendations may include initiation of MRI screening for vestibular schwannomas at the age of 10 years, as symptoms of the tumors are rare in younger patients. When present, growth of vestibular schwannomas is best measured by tumor volume using MRI.[60] Head and spinal MRI is the primary screening tool and should be performed every 2 years for at-risk children younger than 20 years with no symptoms or tumors. After the age of 20 years, the tumors grow slower and screening can be decreased to every 3 to 5 years.[69] Annual ophthalmologic examination is recommended from infancy in at-risk or affected individuals. In addition, the following annual examinations, initiated in infancy, may be recommended: Neurologic examination and audiology with auditory brainstem evoked potentials.[9]

When it is possible, surgery is the primary mode of treatment for NF2 tumors, with the intent of improving quality of life and maintenance of function. Surgery is not always possible and, in some cases, radiation therapy may be used as an alternative. Overall, patients with NF2 have a shorter life expectancy.[60]

CONCLUSION

Dermatologic examinations, when combined with a thorough personal and family medical history, play an important role in the diagnosis of many cancer predisposition syndromes. Although some cutaneous features are strongly indicative of a specific diagnosis, others may be less common or less strongly associated with a particular syndrome; therefore, it remains important to consider these findings in the context of a patient's complete medical and family history. The current availability of molecular testing for many hereditary syndromes has significantly advanced the ability to distinguish and confirm a suspected clinical diagnosis. In addition to the syndromes listed in this chapter, it is important to note that other cancer predisposition syndromes may also have cutaneous components, and with the advancement of molecular testing, additional syndromes are likely to be identified in the future.

REFERENCES

1. Pilarski R. Cowden syndrome: A critical review of the clinical literature. *J Genet Couns* 2009;18:13–27.
2. Hobert JA, Eng C. PTEN hamartoma tumor syndrome: An overview. *Genet Med* 2009;11:687–694.
3. Menko FH, van Steensel MA, Giraud S, et al. Birt-Hogg-Dubé syndrome: Diagnosis and management. *Lancet Oncol* 2009;10:1199–1206.
4. Kruger S, Kinzel M, Walldorf C, et al. Homozygous PMS2 germline mutations in two families with early-onset haematological malignancy, brain tumours, HNPCC-associated tumours, and signs of neurofibromatosis type 1. *Eur J Hum Genet* 2008;16:62–72.
5. Badeloe S, Frank J. Clinical and molecular genetic aspects of hereditary multiple cutaneous leiomyomatosis. *Eur J Dermatol* 2009;19:545–551.

6. Moline J, Eng C. Multiple endocrine neoplasia type 2: An overview. *Genet Med* 2011;13:755–764.
7. Ferner RE. The neurofibromatoses. *Pract Neurol* 2010;10:82–93.
8. Williams VC, Lucas J, Babcock MA, et al. Neurofibromatosis type 1 revisited. *Pediatrics* 2009;123:124–133.
9. Asthagiri AR, Parry DM, Butman JA, et al. Neurofibromatosis type 2. *Lancet* 2009;373:1974–1986.
10. Beggs AD, Latchford AR, Vasen HF, et al. Peutz-Jeghers syndrome: A systematic review and recommendations for management. *Gut* 2010;59: 975–986.
11. Borkowska J, Schwartz RA, Kotulska K, et al. Tuberous sclerosis complex: Tumors and tumorigenesis. *Int J Dermatol* 2011;50:13–20.
12. Winship IM, Dudding TE. Lessons from the skin—cutaneous features of familial cancer. *Lancet Oncol* 2008;9:462–472.
13. Burger B, Cattani N, Trueb S, et al. Prevalence of skin lesions in familial adenomatous polyposis: A marker for presymptomatic diagnosis? *Oncologist* 2011;16:1698–1705.
14. Evans DG, Farndon PA. Nevoid Basal Cell Carcinoma Syndrome. In: Pagon RA, Bird TD, Dolan CR, et al., eds. GeneReviews [Internet]. Seattle, WA: University of Washington, Seattle; 1993. Accessed September 4, 2014.
15. Leachman SA, Carucci J, Kohlmann W, et al. Selection criteria for genetic assessment of patients with familial melanoma. *J Am Acad Dermatol* 2009;61:677e1–677e14.
16. Kremer KH, Di Giovana JJ. Xeroderma Pigmentosum. In: Pagon RA, Bird TD, Dolan CR, et al., eds. GeneReviews [Internet]. Seattle, WA: University of Washington, Seattle; 1993. Accessed September 4, 2014.
17. The Breast Cancer Linkage Consortium. Cancer risks in BRCA2 mutation carriers. *J Natl Cancer Inst* 1999;91:1310–1316.
18. Dores GM, Curtis RE, Toro JR, et al. Incidence of cutaneous sebaceous carcinoma and risk of associated neoplasms: Insight into Muir-Torre syndrome. *Cancer* 2008;113:3372–3381.
19. Robson ME, Storm CD, Weitzel J, et al. American Society of Clinical Oncology policy statement update: Genetic and genomic testing for cancer susceptibility. *J Clin Oncol* 2010;28:893–901.
20. Hemminki K, Eng C. Clinical genetic counselling for familial cancers requires reliable data on familial cancer risks and general action plans. *J Med Genet* 2004;41:801–807.
21. Goldstein AM, Chidambaram A, Halpern A, et al. Rarity of CDK4 germline mutations in familial melanoma. *Melanoma Res* 2002;12:51–55.
22. Hayward NK. Genetics of melanoma predisposition. *Oncogene* 2003;22: 3053–3062.
23. Goldstein AM, Chan M, Harland M, et al. High-risk melanoma susceptibility genes and pancreatic cancer, neural system tumors, and uveal melanoma across GenoMEL. *Cancer Res* 2006;66:9818–9828.
24. Newton Bishop JA, Bataille V, Pinney E, et al. Family studies in melanoma: Identification of the atypical mole syndrome (AMS) phenotype. *Melanoma Res* 1994;4:199–206.
25. Newton Bishop JA, Gruis NA. Genetics: What advice for patients who present with a family history of melanoma? *Semin Oncol* 2007;34:452–459.
26. Bishop JN, Harland M, Randerson-Moor J, et al. Management of familial melanoma. *Lancet Oncol* 2007;8:46–54.
27. Bishop DT, Demenais F, Goldstein AM, et al. Geographical variation in the penetrance of CDKN2A mutations for melanoma. *J Natl Cancer Inst* 2002;94:894–903.
28. Begg CB, Orlow I, Hummer AJ, et al. Lifetime risk of melanoma in CDKN2A mutation carriers in a population-based sample. *J Natl Cancer Inst* 2005;97: 1507–1515.
29. Demenais F, Mohamdi H, Chaudru V, et al. Association of MC1R variants and host phenotypes with melanoma risk in CDKN2A mutation carriers: A GenoMEL study. *J Natl Cancer Inst* 2010;102:1568–1583.
30. Raimondi S, Sera F, Gandini S, et al. MC1R variants, melanoma and red hair color phenotype: A meta-analysis. *Int J Cancer* 2008;122:2753–2760.
31. de Snoo FA, Bishop DT, Bergman W, et al. Increased risk of cancer other than melanoma in CDKN2A founder mutation (p16-Leiden)–positive melanoma families. *Clin Cancer Res* 2008;14:7151–7157.
32. Randerson-Moor JA, Harland M, William S, et al. A germline deletion of p14(ARF) but not CDKN2A in a melanoma-neural system tumour syndrome family. *Hum Mol Genet* 2001;10:55–62.
33. Tsao H, Zhang X, Kwitkiwski K, et al. Low prevalence of germline CDKN2A and CDK4 mutations in patients with early-onset melanoma. *Arch Dermatol* 2000;136:1118–1122.
34. Berg P, Wennberg AM, Tuominen R, et al. Germline CDKN2A mutations are rare in child and adolescent cutaneous melanoma. *Melanoma Res* 2004;14:251–255.
35. Aspinwall LG, Leaf SL, Kohlmann W, et al. Patterns of photoprotection following CDKN2A/p16 genetic test reporting and counseling. *J Am Acad Dermatol* 2009;60:745–757.
36. Aspinwall LG, Leaf SL, Dola ER, et al. CDKN2A/p16 genetic test reporting improves early detection intentions and practices in high-risk melanoma families. *Cancer Epidemiol Biomarkers Prev* 2008;17:1510–1519.
37. Eckerle Mize D, Bishop M, Reese E, et al. Familial Atypical Multiple Mole Melanoma Syndrome. In: Riegert-Johnson DL, Boardman LA, Hefferon T, Roberts M, eds. Cancer Syndromes [Internet]. Bethesda, MD: National Center for Biotechnology Information (US); 2009. Accessed September 3, 2014.
38. Bartsch DK, Sina-Frey M, Lang S, et al. CDKN2A germline mutations in familial pancreatic cancer. *Ann Surg* 2002;236:730–737.
39. Verna EC, Hwang C, Stevens PD, et al. Pancreatic cancer screening in a prospective cohort of high-risk patients: A comprehensive strategy of imaging and genetics. *Clin Cancer Res* 2010;16:5028–5037.
40. Lo Muzio L. Nevoid basal cell carcinoma syndrome (Gorlin syndrome). *Orphanet J Rare Dis* 2008;3:32.
41. Tom WL, Hurley MY, Oliver DS, et al. Features of basal cell carcinomas in basal cell nevus syndrome. *Am J Med Genet A* 2011;155A:2098–2104.
42. Evans DG, Howard E, Giblin C, et al. Birth incidence and prevalence of tumor-prone syndromes: Estimates from a UK family genetic register service. *Am J Med Genet A* 2010;152A:327–332.
43. Lupi O. Correlations between the sonic hedgehog pathway and basal cell carcinoma. *Int J Dermatol* 2007;46:1113–1117.
44. Yamamoto K, Yoshihashi H, Furuya N, et al. Further delineation of 9q22 deletion syndrome associated with basal cell nevus (Gorlin) syndrome: Report of two cases and review of the literature. *Congenit Anom (Kyoto)* 2009; 49:8–14.
45. Pastorino L, Ghiorzo P, Nasti S, et al. Identification of a SUFU germline mutation in a family with Gorlin syndrome. *Am J Med Genet A* 2009;149A: 1539–1543.
46. Fan Z, Li J, Du J, et al. A missense mutation in PTCH2 underlies dominantly inherited NBCCS in a Chinese family. *J Med Genet* 2008;45:303–308.
47. Go JW, Kim SH, Yi SY, et al. Basal cell nevus syndrome showing several histologic types of Basal cell carcinoma. *Ann Dermatol* 2011;23:S36–S40.
48. Kimonis VE, Mehta SG, Digiovanna JJ, et al. Radiological features in 82 patients with nevoid basal cell carcinoma (NBCC or Gorlin) syndrome. *Genet Med* 2004;6:495–502.
49. Amlashi SF, Riffaud L, Brassier G, et al. Nevoid basal cell carcinoma syndrome: Relation with desmoplastic medulloblastoma in infancy. A population-based study and review of the literature. *Cancer* 2003;98:618–624.
50. Mohtasham N, Nemati S, Jamshidi S, et al. Odontogenic keratocysts in nevoid basal cell carcinoma syndrome: A case report. *Cases J* 2009;2:93–99.
51. Ball A, Wenning J, Van Eyk N. Ovarian fibromas in pediatric patients with basal cell nevus (Gorlin) syndrome. *J Pediatr Adolesc Gynecol* 2011;24:e5–e7.
52. Bossert T, Walther T, Vondrys D, et al. Cardiac fibroma as an inherited manifestation of nevoid basal-cell carcinoma syndrome. *Tex Heart Inst J* 2006;33:88–90.
53. Bree AF, Shah MR. Consensus statement from the first international colloquium on basal cell nevus syndrome (BCNS). *Am J Med Genet A* 2011; 155A:2091–2097.
54. Takahashi C, Kanazawa N, Yoshikawa Y, et al. Germline PTCH1 mutations in Japanese basal cell nevus syndrome patients. *J Hum Genet* 2009;54: 403–408.
55. Casaroto AR, Loures DC, Moreschi E, et al. Early diagnosis of Gorlin-Goltz syndrome: Case report. *Head Face Med* 2011;7:2.
56. Morse CB, McLaren JF, Roy D, et al. Ovarian preservation in a young patient with Gorlin syndrome and multiple bilateral ovarian masses. *Fertil Steril* 2011;96:e47–e50.
57. Boyd KP, Korf BR, Theos A. Neurofibromatosis type 1. *J Am Acad Dermatol* 2009;61:1–14.
58. Yohay K. Neurofibromatosis types 1 and 2. *Neurologist* 2006;12:86–93.
59. Radtke HB, Sebold CD, Allison C, et al. Neurofibromatosis type 1 in genetic counseling practice: Recommendations of the National Society of Genetic Counselors. *J Genet Couns* 2007;16:387–407.
60. Ahmad S, ed. *Neurodegenerative Diseases*. Vol. 724. New York: Landes Bioscience and Springer Science+Business Media; 2012.
61. Patil S, Chamberlain RS. Neoplasms associated with germline and somatic NF1 gene mutations. *Oncologist* 2012;17:101–116.
62. Kossler N, Stricker S, Rödelsperger C, et al. Neurofibromin (Nf1) is required for skeletal muscle development. *Hum Mol Genet* 2011;20:2697–2709.
63. Friedman J. Neurofibromatosis 1. June 2, 2009. http://www.ncbi.nlm.nih.gov/books/NBK1109/. Accessed March 6, 2012.
64. Ardern-Holmes SL, North KN. Therapeutics for childhood neurofibromatosis type 1 and type 2. *Curr Treat Options Neurol* 2011;13:529–543.
65. Ponder MMF, Hallowell N, Statham H, et al. Genetic counseling, reproductive behavior and future reproductive intentions of people with neurofibromatosis type 1 (NF1). *J Genet Couns* 1998;7:331–344.
66. Evans DG. Neurofibromatosis type 2 (NF2): A clinical and molecular review. *Orphanet J Rare Dis* 2009;4:16.
67. Goutagny S, Kalamarides M. Meningiomas and neurofibromatosis. *J Neurooncol* 2010;99:341–347.
68. Baser ME, Friedman JM, Joe H, et al. Empirical development of improved diagnostic criteria for neurofibromatosis 2. *Genet Med* 2011;13:576–581.
69. Evans DG, Raymond FL, Barwell JG, et al. Genetic testing and screening of individuals at risk of NF2. *Clin Genet* 2012;82:416–424.

96

Molecular Biology of Central Nervous System Tumors

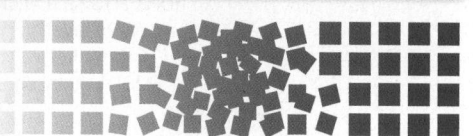

Victoria Clark, Jennifer Moliterno Günel, and Murat Günel

GLIOMAS

Gliomas account for 26.4% of all primary brain tumors, with malignant gliomas (grade III or IV) accounting for 19.9% of all primary brain tumors.[1] The World Health Organization (WHO) classifies gliomas by the cells they morphologically resemble (astrocytes, oligodendrocytes, or a mixture) and groups the tumors into four grades based on histology and aggressiveness.[2] High-grade gliomas (WHO grades III and IV) have a dismal prognosis, with the median survival for grade IV astrocytomas (glioblastoma multiforme [GBM]) less than 15 to 20 months.[3] Low-grade gliomas (WHO grades I and II) are heterogeneous in terms of their prognosis and likelihood to progress to high-grade gliomas.

Adult Low-Grade Gliomas

What drives some adult low-grade gliomas to progression whereas others remain indolent is an area of active investigation. Grade I gliomas, the majority of which are pilocytic astrocytomas, are histologically benign tumors with low potential for malignant progression that primarily occur in the pediatric population and are discussed in detail in the pediatric low-grade glioma section, which follows. Histologically, WHO grade II gliomas can be divided into tumors that arise from astrocytes (diffuse astrocytomas), oligodendrocytes (oligodendrogliomas), or tumors with elements of both cellular populations (oligoastrocytomas).[2] All three histologic subtypes have frequent neomorphic driver mutations affecting the R132 residue of isocitrate dehydrogenase 1 (IDH1),[4] a mutation that generates the oncometabolite 2-hydroxyglutarate (2HG).[5] Ultimately, the IDH1 R132 mutation drives gliomagenesis through epigenetic dysregulation, including DNA CpG hypermethylation (G-CIMP phenotype)[6] and alterations in histone methylation.[7–9] Despite sharing the IDH1 R132 driver mutation, grade II oligodendrogliomas have improved median overall survival (11.6 years for grade II oligodendrogliomas versus 5.6 years for grade II astrocytoma),[10] and a much lower rate of progression to a high-grade glioma (45% for oligodendroglioma versus 74% for astrocytoma).[1] The survival and progression benefit seen in IDH1 mutant grade II gliomas is likely modified by comutations. Oligodendrogliomas commonly have a loss of heterozygosity (LOH) on chromosomes 1p and 19q,[11–13] which is usually the result of a single pericentromeric translocation event.[14] The 1p/19q loss in oligodendrogliomas frequently co-occurs with somatic mutations in capicua transcriptional repressor (CIC, located on chr1) or far upstream element (FUSE) binding protein 1 (FUBP1, located on chr19),[15] and IDH1-CIC/FUBP1-1p/19q loss gliomas have a median survival of 8 years.[16] In contrast, grade II astrocytomas commonly have somatic mutations in the chromatin modifier alpha thalassemia/mental retardation syndrome X-linked (ATRX),[16] mutations in tumor protein p53 (TP53),[4] and LOH at chr17 (where

TP53 is found), and IDH1-ATRX-TP53 gliomas have a median survival of 5 years.[16] This latter group is likely to progress to form secondary GBMs, a process mediated by epigenomic dysregulation and deletion of retinoblastoma 1 (RB1), cyclin-dependent kinase inhibitor 2A (CDKN2A), and phosphatase and tensin homolog (PTEN).[17,18] Oligoastrocytomas have a combination of mutations and chromosomal LOH found in astrocytomas and oligoastrocytomas and a median survival of 6.6 years.[10]

Adult High-Grade Gliomas

Glioblastoma multiforme (WHO grade IV) is the most common malignant brain tumor, accounting for 15.6% of all primary brain tumors and 60% of all gliomas.[1] There are two major routes to GBM formation: de novo formation (primary GBM, 95% of cases), or progression from low-grade glioma (secondary GBM, 5% of cases) (Fig. 96.1).[17] Secondary GBMs occur in younger patients, result in improved survival, and bear IDH1 mutations with common co-mutations in ATRX and TP53 and deletion of RB1, CDKN2A, and PTEN.[16–21] In contrast, primary GBMs occur in older patients, have poor survival, and have dysregulation of three core pathways: p53, retinoblastoma (Rb), and receptor tyrosine kinase/Ras/phosphoinositide 3-kinase (PI3K) signaling (RTK/Ras/PI3K signaling).[17,20,22–24] A recent large-scale GBM next-generation sequencing study by The Cancer Genome Atlas (TCGA) found that the p53 pathway is somatically disrupted in 85.3% of GBMs, through p53 loss (27.9%), homozygous deletion of CDKN2A (57.8%), and amplification of MDM1/2/4 (15.1%).[24] The Rb pathway is also impacted by frequent CDKN2A deletion, and other hits to Rb signaling have been seen via RB1 loss (7.6%) or amplification of cyclin-dependent kinase 4 or 6(CDK4/6) (15.5%), for a total of 78.9% alteration of Rb signaling.[24] Somatic alterations in receptor tyrosine kinases were observed in 67.3% of GBMs, most prominently in epidermal growth factor receptor (EGFR) (57.4%) and platelet-derived growth factor receptor alpha (PDGFRA) (13.1%).[24] Of GBMs showed either PTEN loss or PI3K mutation, and neurofibromin 1 (NF1) loss was seen in 10% of tumors.[24] In combination, the RTK/Ras/PI3K signaling was hit once in 89.6% of tumors and hit multiple times in 39% of tumors.[24] Additionally, 83.3% of GBMs were reported to have recurrent telomerase reverse transcriptase (TERT) promoter mutations (C228T or C250T), and these mutations are mutually exclusive with ATRX mutations.[25]

Based on gene expression profiling, GBMs cluster into four groups: classical (chromosome 7 amplification with chromosome 10 loss, deletion of CDKN2A), mesenchymal (NF1 focal deletions or mutations), proneural (IDH1 mutant or PDGFRA amplification), and neural (EGFR amplification with a neural expression signature).[23] These classifications have a utility for predicting response to therapy; for example, the classical subtype

PRACTICE OF ONCOLOGY

Adult Glioma Formation

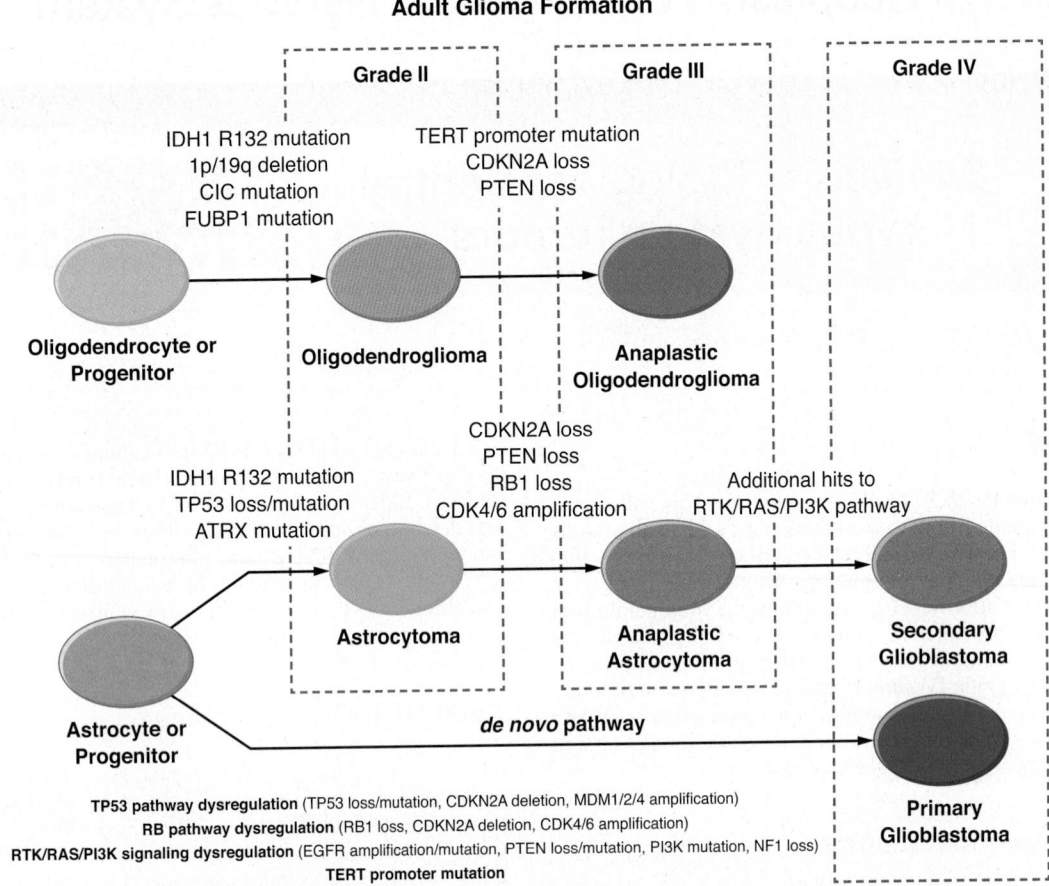

Figure 96.1 Driver events in adult gliomagenesis. Glioblastoma multiforme can either arise from progression of lower grade gliomas (secondary GBM) or de novo (primary GBM). IDH1, isocitrate dehydrogenase 1; CIC, capicua transcriptional repressor; FUBP1, far upstream element (FUSE) binding protein 1; TERT, telomerase reverse transcriptase; CDKN2A, cyclin-dependent kinase inhibitor 2A; PTEN, phosphatase and tensin homolog; TP53, tumor protein p53; ATRX, alpha thalassemia/mental retardation syndrome X-linked; RB1, retinoblastoma 1; CDK4/6, cyclin-dependent kinase 4/6; RTK, receptor tyrosine kinase; PI3K, phosphoinositide 3-kinase; EGFR, epidermal growth factor receptor; NF1, neurofibromin 1.

responds to more intensive therapy whereas the proneural subtype shows no benefit to this regimen.[23] Another prognostic indicator is the CpG island methylator phenotype (G-CIMP) demonstrated in IDH1 mutant proneural tumors, which had a significantly better survival (median of 150 weeks) compared to proneural G-CIMP–negative patients (median survival of 42 weeks) or other GBM subtypes (median survival 54 weeks).[6] Also clinically useful to predict response to therapy is O-6-methylguanine-DNA methyltransferase (MGMT) promoter methylation status,[19,26] because tumors with silenced MGMT are unable to remove the alkyl groups deposited on the O6 position of guanine by alkylating agents such as temozolomide.[27]

Anaplastic (grade III) gliomas, including anaplastic astrocytomas, anaplastic oligoastrocytomas, and anaplastic oligodendrogliomas, are not as well characterized genomically as GBMs. Clinically, they can arise without a prior history of low-grade glioma (presumed de novo) or through progression from low-grade gliomas (secondary anaplastic glioma). Grade III gliomas have a high risk of progression to GBM, although the rate of progression and prognosis varies by histology, with anaplastic astrocytomas having a 5-year overall survival of 26.5% and anaplastic oligodendroglioma having a 5-year overall survival of 50.7%.[1] IDH1 mutations have been observed in 75% to 90% of grade III gliomas.[4,16,28] Anaplastic astrocytomas, accounting for 1.7% of primary brain tumors,[1] commonly have mutations in ATRX, IDH1, and loss of p53 as well as alterations to the Rb pathway (including RB1 loss, CDKN2A deletion, and CDK4/6 amplification).[16,18,28] It is believed that

additional hits in the RTK/Ras/PI3K pathway, including LOH at chr10q, lead to progression to frank glioblastoma.[17,18,21] Anaplastic oligodendrogliomas are rare (0.5% of primary brain tumors),[1] and the progression from grade II oligodendrogliomas (characterized by chr1p/19q loss and IDH1-CIC/FUBP1 mutations) is likely mediated by additional deletion of CDKN2A and PTEN.[13] Like GBMs, recurrent TERT promoter mutations (C288T or C250T) have been identified in anaplastic gliomas, reported in 14.8% of anaplastic astrocytomas, 26.7% of anaplastic oligoastrocytomas, and 88.4% of anaplastic oligodendrogliomas.[25] The differences in TERT promoter mutations between the subtypes is probably due to the higher frequency of ATRX mutations in anaplastic astrocytomas, because TERT promoter mutations are mutually exclusive with ATRX mutations in GBMs and other tumors.[25]

Pediatric Low-Grade Gliomas

Pediatric low-grade gliomas (WHO grade I and II) are the most common brain tumors in children[1] and can be broadly divided into nondiffuse (e.g., pilocytic astrocytomas) and diffuse gliomas. Pilocytic astrocytomas (WHO grade I) are histologically benign tumors with a low probability of malignant progression that are usually pediatric, are primarily found in the cerebellar hemisphere (67%)[10], and are cystic.[2] The mitogen-activated protein kinase/extracellular signal-regulated kinase (MAPK/ERK) pathway was originally implicated in driving the formation of pilocytic astrocytomas through studies of the hereditary tumor syndrome neurofibromatosis type 1, in which ~15% of patients with germline loss-of-function mutations in *NF1*, a negative regulator of Ras signaling, develop pilocytic astrocytomas in addition to café-au-lait spots and cutaneous neurofibromas.[29] Further investigation has revealed that MAPK/ERK pathway activation is crucial to sporadic pilocytic astrocytoma formation, with 90% of cerebellar pilocytic astrocytomas demonstrating a *KIAA1549-BRAF* (B-Raf proto-oncogene, serine/threonine kinase) fusion gene that results in constitutively active BRAF signaling via a truncation of the BRAF autoinhibitory domain.[30–33] Pilocytic astrocytomas can also have constitutive activation of MAPK/ERK through somatic *BRAF V600E* mutations, Kirsten rat sarcoma viral oncogene homolog (*KRAS*) mutations, Raf-1 proto-oncogene, serine/threonine kinase (*RAF1*) fusions, and *NF1* loss-of-function mutations.[32,33] Approximately 20% of noncerebellar pilocytic astrocytomas lack the *KIAA1549-BRAF* fusion, and these fusion-negative tumors have recently been discovered to activate MAPK signaling through additional methods, including fibroblast growth factor receptor 1 (*FGFR1*) alterations (mutations, tyrosine kinase domain [TK] duplications, and gene fusions with transforming, acidic coiled-coil containing protein *1* [*TACC1*]),[32,33] neurotrophic tyrosine kinase, receptor, type 2 (*NTRK2*) fusions resulting in TK truncations that are predicted to induce constitutive dimerization,[33] and protein tyrosine phosphatase, non-receptor type 11 (*PTPN11*) hotspot mutations in tumors co-mutated for *FGFR1*.[33]

Pediatric diffuse gliomas, including diffuse astrocytomas, gangliogliomas, angiocentric gliomas, pleomorphic xanthoastrocytomas, oligodendrogliomas, and oligoastrocytomas,[32,34] differ from pilocytic astrocytomas in their diffuse growth pattern, anatomic location (generally supratentorial), and their propensity for malignant transformation.[2] In a recent study by Zhang et al.,[32] 52% (12 out of 23) of diffuse astrocytomas (WHO grade II) demonstrated ERK/MAPK signaling activation via *FGFR1/3* alterations (fusions or *FGFR1* TK duplication), *BRAF* alterations (*V600E* mutations or fusions), or *KRAS* activating mutation (*Q61H*). This same series identified common, recurrent *FGFR1* alterations in oligodendrogliomas (3 out of 5: *FGFR1* TK duplications) and oligoastrocytomas (6 out of 8, 4 *FGFR1* TK duplications; 1 fusion; 1 mutation).[32] A subset of ERK/MAPK activated diffuse astrocytomas (2 out of 12; 16.67%) had the recurrent H3 histone, family 3A (*H3F3A*) K27M mutation, an alteration that has been frequently described in pediatric glioblastomas.[32]

The majority of other diffuse low-grade gliomas also demonstrate MAPK/ERK activation. Pleomorphic xanthoastrocytomas (WHO grade II) are rare, supratentorial astrocytomas that are found in the pediatric population two-thirds of the time.[35] The 5-year overall survival is 81%, and malignant progression can occur but is generally rare.[36] A recent study showed that 7 out of 10 pleomorphic xanthoastrocytomas had *BRAF V600E* mutations.[32] Similarly, this study found 55.6% (5 out of 9) of gangliogliomas showed ERK/MAPK activation by *BRAF* alterations (*V600E* = 3; *BRAF* fusion production = 2).[32]

In contrast to pilocytic astrocytomas, about one-quarter of pediatric diffuse astrocytomas (6 out of 23; 26%) demonstrated alterations in v-myb avian myeloblastosis viral oncogene homolog (*MYB*), including gene fusion with protocadherin gamma subfamily A, 1 (*PCDHGA1*) or episome formation, and one case of v-myb avian myeloblastosis viral oncogene homolog-like 1 (*MYBL1*) rearrangement.[32] In an independent, copy number alteration study, Ramkissoon et al.[34] identified focal amplification resulting in tandem duplication/truncation of MYBL1 in 28% (5 out of 18) of pediatric diffuse astrocytomas. These MYB/MYBL1 alterations were not observed in pilocytic astrocytomas, although two out of two angiocentric gliomas from Zhang et al.[32] and an additional two angiocentric gliomas from Ramkissoon et al.[34] bore MYB or MYBL1 fusions, providing further implication of this pathway as specific to a subset of diffuse pediatric gliomas.

Pediatric High-Grade Gliomas

Although histologically similar to adult glioblastomas, a subset of pediatric glioblastomas have distinct genomic hits driving tumor formation that implicate epigenetic dysregulation in the formation of these tumors. In a study by Schwartzentruber et al.,[37] recurrent mutations in histone variant H3.3 (H3F3A K27M; G34R/V), commonly co-occurring with damaging mutations in the chromatin remodelers *ATRX* or death-domain associated protein (*DAXX*) and *TP53*, drove pediatric glioblastoma formation in 31% of pediatric GBMs. This percentage may be higher in diffuse intrinsic pontine gliomas (DIPG), where an independent study found that 78% of DIPG contained somatic K27M mutations in *H3F3A* or histone cluster 1, H3b (*HIST1H3B*), whereas *H3F3A* G34R was restricted to non–brain stem pediatric glioblastomas.[38] Recently, H3K27 K27M was characterized to be a dominant-negative mutation that results in a genome-wide reduction of H3K27me3 repressive marks due to altered binding with the polycomb repressive complex 2 (PRC2) and also causes global DNA hypomethylation.[39] In pediatric glioblastomas, these H3.3 mutations were mutually exclusive with the neomorphic IDH1 R132H,[8,37] which was rarely seen in pediatric GBM but has been shown to cause epigenomic dysregulation and DNA hypermethylation (G-CIMP) phenotype.[9] Similar to pediatric low-grade gliomas, the BRAF V600E mutation has been reported in ~10% of pediatric high-grade gliomas[40]; however, unlike the pediatric low-grade gliomas, this mutation commonly co-occurs with homozygous *CDKN2A/B* deletion.[41]

In terms of structural variation, pediatric glioblastomas differ from the classic, primary adult GBM findings of chr7 amplification (74% in adult versus 13% in pediatric) and chr10 loss (80% adult versus 35% pediatric).[42] However, pediatric glioblastomas have more frequent 1q gain (30% in pediatric versus 9% in adult), frequent focal amplification of *PDGFRA* in 12% of tumors, and frequent focal, homozygous deletion of *CDKN2A/B* in 19% of tumors.[42] The driver events for adult and pediatric gliomas are summarized in Table 96.1.

MENINGIOMAS

Meningiomas are the most common primary intracranial tumor, accounting for one-third of all primary brain tumors.[1] Thought to arise from the arachnoid layer of the meninges, meningiomas can be found throughout the neuraxis, and are notable for a wide variety of histologic subtypes (15 according to the 2007 WHO classifications).[43] Although 70% to 80% of meningiomas are benign (WHO grade I), the remaining subset can exhibit more aggressive behavior (WHO grade II and grade III).[43] Recent genomic studies have revealed that 80% of meningiomas can be neatly categorized into three clinically relevant, mutually exclusive genetic groups with differences in histology, anatomic location, and likelihood for malignant progression (Fig. 96.2).[44–46]

The first and largest group, *NF2/chr22 loss* tumors, is characterized by biallelic loss of the tumor suppressor neurofibromin 2 (merlin, NF2). One of the hallmarks of the inherited tumor syndrome neurofibromatosis type II is multiple meningiomas due to germline mutations in the tumor suppressor *NF2*,[47] and biallelic loss of NF2 drives ~50% of sporadic meningioma formation[48] and is a risk factor for malignant transformation. At least 75% of WHO grade II tumors have *NF2/chr22 loss*.[43,44] *NF2/chr22 loss* tumors are more likely to form in the meninges flanking the cerebral convexities, but when they grow in the skull base, the growth is restricted to the posterior and lateral portions of the skull.[44] *NF2/chr22 loss* is also commonly found in spinal meningiomas. Rarely, *NF2/chr22 loss* tumors also have a biallelic loss of the chromatin remodeling gene SWI/SNF related, matrix associated, actin dependent regulator of chromatin, subfamily b, member 1 (*SMARCB1*).[49] Loss of the tumor suppressor SMARCB1, which is also found on chromosome 22, has been reported in various malignant rhabdoid

TABLE 96.1

Summary of Driver Events in Pediatric and Adult Gliomas

WHO Grade	Population	Diagnosis	Pathways Affected	Hallmark Mutations or Structural Abnormalities	Notes
I	Pediatric	Pilocytic astrocytoma	MAPK/ERK pathway	KIAA1549-BRAF fusion (90% of cerebellar)	Single hit to MAPK/ERK signaling
				BRAF V600E	
				KRAS	
				RAF1 fusions	
				NF1 loss of function	
				FGFR1 alterations (mutations, fusion with TACC1), co-mutations in PTPN11 hotspots	
II	Pediatric	Diffuse astrocytoma	MAPK/ERK pathway	FGFR1/3 alterations (fusions or FGFR1 TK duplication)	
				BRAF alterations (V600E mutations or fusions)	
				KRAS activation mutation (Q61H)	
			MYB	MYB, including fusion with PCDHGA1 or episome formation, and 1 case of MYBL1 rearrangement	
II	Adult	Diffuse astrocytoma	Epigenetic dysregulation	IDH1 R132H/C/S	More likely to progress to high grade glioma
			Chromatin remodeling	ATRX	
			TP53 pathway	Mutations in TP53, LOH at chr17	
		Oligodendroglioma	Epigenetic dysregulation	IDH1 R132H/C/S	
			Unknown	1p/19q loss	
				CIC	
				FUBP1	
		Oligoastrocytoma	Epigenetic dysregulation	IDH1 R132H/C/S	
				Combination of genetic events seen in astrocytes and oligodendrocytes	
III	Adult	Anaplastic astrocytoma	Epigenetic dysregulation	IDH1 R132H/C/S	Additional hits in RTK/RAS/P13K pathway drive progression to frank glioblastoma
			Telomere maintenance	TERT promoter mutations	
			Chromatin remodeling	ATRX mutations	
			p53 pathway	TP53 mutations and LOH at chr17	
				CDKN2A loss	
			Rb pathway	RB1 loss	
				CDKN2A loss	
				CDK4/6 amplification	
IV	Pediatric	GBM	Chromatin remodeling	H3F3A K27M; G34R/V	
				ATRX mutations	
				DAXX mutations	
			p53 pathway	TP53	

(continued)

TABLE 96.1

Summary of Driver Events in Pediatric and Adult Gliomas *(continued)*

WHO Grade	Population	Diagnosis	Pathways Affected	Hallmark Mutations or Structural Abnormalities	Notes
IV	Adult	Secondary GBM	Epigenetic dysregulation	IDH1 R132H/C/S	Progressed from lower grade gliomas
			Chromatin remodeling	ATRX mutations	
			p53 pathway	TP53 mutations, LOH at chr17	
			Rb pathway	Loss of RB1	
				Loss of CDKN2A	
			PI3K	Loss of PTEN	
		Primary GBM	TP53 pathway	TP53 loss	
				CDKN2A loss	
				MDM1/2/4 gain	
			RB pathway	CDKN2A loss	
				RB1 loss	
				CDK4/6 amplification	
			Receptor tyrosine kinase	EGFR amplification	
				PDGFRA amplification	
			PI3K	PTEN loss	
				PI3K mutation	
			RAS	NF1 loss	
			Telomere maintenance	TERT	

BRAF, B-Raf proto-oncogene, serine/threonine kinase; KRAS, Kirsten rat sarcoma viral oncogene homolog; RAF1, v-raf-1 murine leukemia viral oncogene homolog 1; TACC1, transforming, acidic coiled-coil containing protein 1; PTPN11, protein tyrosine phosphatase, non-receptor type 11; FGFR1/3, fibroblast growth factor receptor 1/3; TK, tyrosine kinase domain; MYB, v-myb avian myeloblastosis viral oncogene homolog; PCDHGA1, protocadherin gamma subfamily a, 1; MYBL1, v-myb avian myeloblastosis viral oncogene homolog-like 1; IDH1, isocitrate dehydrogenase 1; ATRX, alpha thalassemia/mental retardation syndrome X-linked; TP53, tumor protein p53; CIC, capicua transcriptional repressor; FUBP1, far upstream element (FUSE) binding protein 1; TERT, telomerase reverse transcriptase; CDKN2A, cyclin-dependent kinase inhibitor 2A; RB1, retinoblastoma 1; CDK4/6, cyclin-dependent kinase 4/6; H3F3A, H3 histone, family 3A; DAXX, death-domain associated protein; PTEN, phosphatase and tensin homolog; EGFR, epidermal growth factor receptor; PDGFRA, platelet-derived growth factor receptor alpha; PI3K, phosphoinositide 3-kinase; NF1, neurofibromin 1.

tumors[50,51] as well as in families with multiple meningiomas with schwannomatosis.[52]

The second group of meningiomas, *TRAF7* mutant tumors, have a lower risk of malignant transformation.[44] Somatic mutations in tumor necrosis factor (TNF) receptor-associated factor 7 (*TRAF7*), a proapoptotic N-terminal RING and zinc finger domain protein with E3 ubiquitin ligase activity, have been reported in ~25% of meningiomas (including 27% of grade I tumors). *TRAF7* mutant tumors are commonly comutated for AKT/PI3K/mammalian target of rapamycin (mTOR) pathway members, most notably the recurrent v-akt murine thymoma viral oncogene homolog 1 (AKT1) E17K mutation, which activates PI3K signaling and is reported in 14% of grade I meningiomas.[44,45] A second *TRAF7* subgroup is defined by comutations in the transcription factor Krupple-like factor 4 (KLF4),[44,46] an important regulator of development and one of four Yamanaka factors capable of reprogramming differentiated cells into an induced pluripotent stem cell state.[53] The recurrent KLF4 K409Q mutation, seen in 12% of WHO grade I meningiomas, is in the DNA-binding domain, suggesting that the mutation may alter binding to the consensus sequence.[44,46] Noted for their increased risk of postoperative peritumoral edema[54], 100% of secretory meningiomas are comutated for *KLF4 K409Q* and *TRAF7*[44,46]. *TRAF7* mutant tumors are typically found in the midline of the skull base, especially the anterior skull base, although they can grow in the meninges flanking the frontal lobe.[44]

The third major group of meningiomas is the sonic Hedgehog (SHH) group. Approximately 3% of benign meningiomas have mutations in smoothened, frizzled class (SMO) that activate SHH signaling.[44,45] Interestingly, tumors with *SMO L412F* (n = 5) all localized to the medial anterior fossa.[44] Germline loss-of-function mutations in suppressor of fused homolog (Drosophila) (*SUFU*), which is downstream of SMO and inhibits SHH signaling, have been reported in a family with multiple meningiomas.[55]

MEDULLOBLASTOMAS

Arising in the cerebellum, medulloblastomas (WHO grade IV) are the most common malignant brain tumors in children. These invasive embryonal tumors commonly metastasize to the leptomeninges via the cerebrospinal fluid system, gaining access by extending through the fourth ventricle.[2] The past decade of research has revealed that medulloblastoma is not a homogeneous disease; rather, these tumors can be divided into four subgroups with marked differences in transcriptional profiles, somatic copy number alterations, underlying driver mutations, cell of origin, anatomic location, prognosis, tendency to metastasize, and response to targeted therapies (Fig. 96.3).

The first hints of the existence of different molecular subgroups came from studies of hereditary tumor syndromes. The SHH pathway was implicated in driving medulloblastoma and nevoid basal

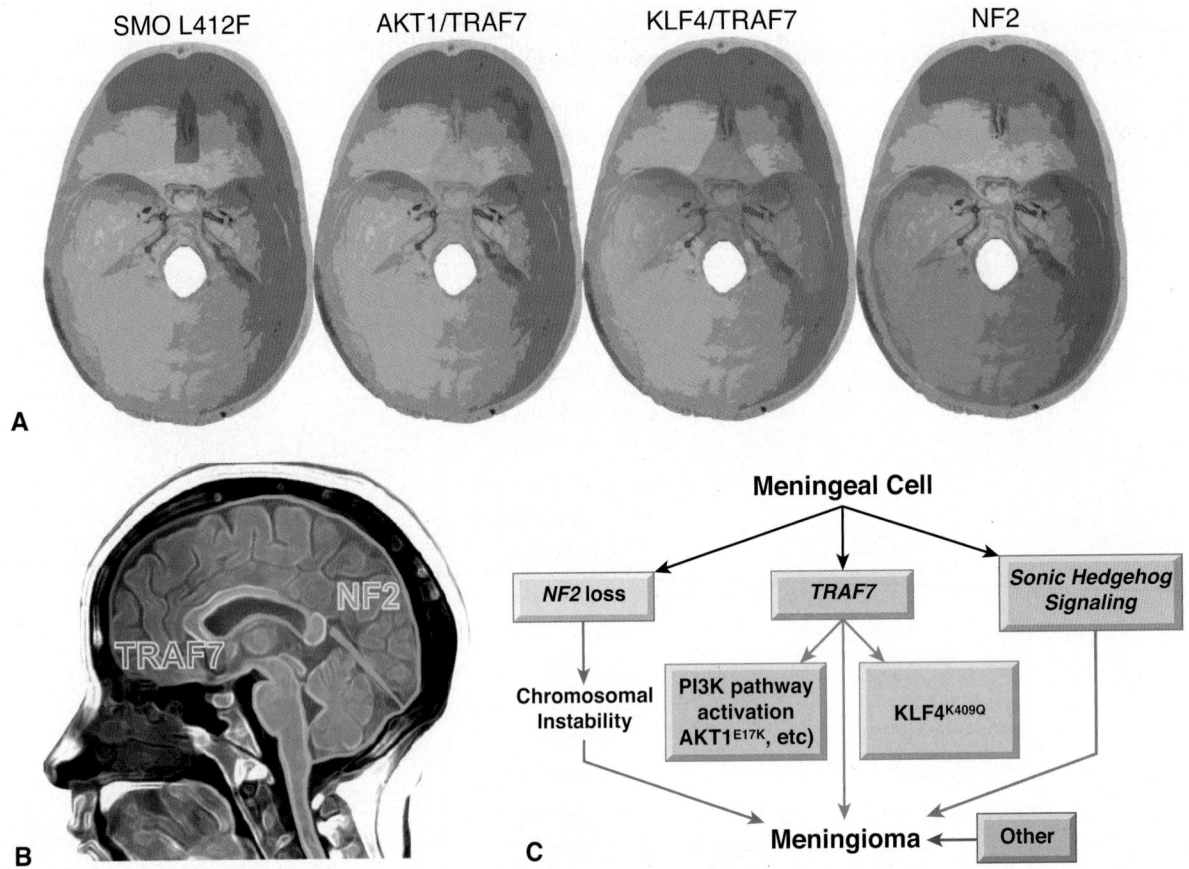

Figure 96.2 Driver events in meningioma formation. **(A)** For grade 1 meningiomas, growth of *NF2/chr22 loss* meningiomas is restricted to the posterior and lateral skull base, whereas non-*NF2* mutant tumors grow in the midline of the skull base. **(B)** For meningiomas flanking the convexities, TRAF7 mutant tumors are found anteriorly. **(C)** Summary of meningioma driver events and known pathway activations. NF2, neurofibromin 2; TRAF7, TNF receptor-associated factor 7; AKT1, v-akt murine thymoma viral oncogene 1; KLF4, Kruppel-like factor 4 (gut); SMO, smoothened, frizzled class receptor.

cell carcinoma formation in patients with Gorlin syndrome, who have activated SHH signaling due to a germline loss of patched 1 (PTCH1).[56,57] The WNT pathway was implicated in driving medulloblastoma formation in patients with Turcot syndrome (now called familial adenomatous polyposis), a subset of whom

had medulloblastomas in addition to inherited colonic polyposis as a result of germline loss-of-function adenomatous polyposis coli (APC) mutations.[58]

Candidate gene studies identified somatic mutations in SHH or WNT pathway genes were found in sporadic medulloblastomas,[59,60]

A

Medullablastoma Subtype Characteristics

Group	Progenitor Cell	Growth	Prognosis	Characteristic mutations	Structural Events
WNT	Lower rhombic lip	4th ventricle, with dorsal brain stem infiltration	Good	*CTNNB1* (91%), *DDX3X, SMARCA4, MLL2, TP53*	Monosomy 6
SHH	Cerebellar granule neuron precursors of the external granule layer	Cerebellar hemispheres	Intermediate	*PTCH1, SUFU, SMO, TP53, MLL2, DDX3X*	Genome instability, including frequent amplification of *MYCN* and *GLI2*, deletion of *PTCH1*
Group 3	Cerebellar granule neuron precursors of the external granule layer, neural stem cells	~30% metastatic at diagnosis (47% for infants)	Poor		Genome instability, including *MYC* amplification, *MYC/PVT1* fusions, somatic copy number alterations in TGFB signaling members including amplification of *OTX2*
Group 4	Unknown	~30% metastatic at diagnosis (36% for infants)	Intermediate	*KDM6A*	Genome instability, including *SNCAIP* tandem duplication, *MYCN* amplification

Figure 96.3 Medulloblastoma subtype characteristics. **(A)** Table summarizing the genomic underpinnings, anatomic location, and presumed progenitor cell for the four medulloblastoma subtypes. **(B)** WNT group medulloblastomas arise in the fourth ventricle, whereas SHH group medulloblastomas arise in the cerebellar hemispheres. CTNNB1, catenin (cadherin-associated protein), beta 1, 88kDa; DDX3X, DEAD (Asp-Glu-Ala-Asp) box helicase 3, X-linked; SMARCA4, SWI/SNF related, matrix associated, actin dependent regulator of chromatin, subfamily a, member 4; MLL2, lysine (K)-specific methyltransferase 2D; TP53, tumor protein p53; PTCH1, patched 1; SUFU, suppressor of fused homolog (*Drosophila*); SMO, smoothened, frizzled class receptor; KDM6A, Lysine (K)-Specific Demethylase 6A; MYCN, v-myc avian myelocytomatosis viral oncogene neuroblastoma derived homolog; GLI2, GLI family zinc finger 2; MYC, v-myc avian myelocytomatosis viral oncogene homolog; OTX2, orthodenticle homeobox 2; SNCAIP, synuclein, alpha interacting protein.

but the development of microarray-based transcriptional profiling and next-generation sequencing have clarified four medulloblastoma subgroups with differential pathway activations and underlying genomic changes. The WNT group (~10% of medulloblastomas), initially identified by unsupervised hierarchical clustering of gene expression profiles,[61] is characterized by somatic activating mutations in beta-catenin (CTNNB1) in 91% of cases.[62–65] CTNNB1 is commonly comutated with DEAD (Asp-Glu-Ala-Asp) box helicase 3, X-linked (DDX3X) in 50% of cases, and this group is also defined by frequent mutations in the chromatin modifier SWI/SNF related, matrix associated, actin dependent regulator of chromatin, subfamily a, member 4 (SMARCA4, 26.3%), lysine (K)-specific methyltransferase 2D (KMT2D or MLL2, 12.5%), and TP53 (12.5%).[62–65] In terms of structural variation, this group has monosomy chromosome 6 but an otherwise stable genome.[66] Elegant mouse modeling experiments have provided compelling evidence that WNT medulloblastomas originate from lower rhombic lip progenitor cells, and WNT subtype medulloblastomas grow within the fourth ventricle and infiltrate the dorsal brain stem.[67] The WNT group has the best prognosis, with a 95% overall 5-year survival.[68] These tumors rarely recur.[69]

The SHH group (~30% of medulloblastomas) shows increased expression of SHH signaling,[70] and commonly bears somatic mutations (PTCH1, SUFU, SMO),[61–64] or somatic copy number alterations (amplification of v-myc avian myelocytomatosis viral oncogene neuroblastoma derived homolog (MYCN) and GLI Family Zinc Finger 2 (GLI2); deletion of PTCH1)[66] impacting SHH pathway members. In addition to Gorlin syndrome, patients with germline TP53 mutations (Li-Fraumeni syndrome) can develop SHH medulloblastomas by chromothripsis-mediated amplification of SHH oncogenes,[71] and TP53 mutations or deletions are seen in 13.6% of SHH tumors.[62,64–66] The subset of SHH medulloblastomas that bear TP53 mutations or deletions, have a particularly a poor prognosis, with a 5-year overall survival of 41% in TP53 mutant SHH cases versus 81% for TP53 wild-type SHH cases.[72] Like the WNT group, the SHH tumors also bear mutations in MLL2 (12.9%) and DDX3X (11.7%).[62–65] However, SHH tumors are more genomically unstable in terms of their structural variation and have frequent focal copy number changes in SHH signaling (18%), p53 signaling (9.4%), and/or RTK/PI3K signaling (10%).[66] In contrast to WNT medulloblastomas, mouse SHH medulloblastomas arise from external granule layer progenitor cells, and in humans are found in the cerebellar hemispheres.[67] SHH tumors have a worse prognosis

than WNT tumors, with a 5-year survival of ~75%.[65,70] They are also more likely to recur than WNT tumors, and the recurrence is generally local (versus metastatic).[73] Clinical use of SHH inhibitors (e.g., SMO inhibitors) has shown initial but transient response.[74,75]

The remaining two groups of medulloblastomas, group 3 and group 4, currently bear generic names while the underlying biology is clarified. Both groups demonstrate genomic instability and tend to present with metastases at diagnosis in ~30% of cases.[70] Group 3 tumors (~25% of medulloblastomas) have high MYC amplification and express a gene signature consistent with photoreceptors/GABAergic (gamma-aminobutyric acid) neurons.[76,77] A recent somatic copy number alterations (SCNA) analysis of >1,000 medulloblastomas revealed that SCNAs found in group 3 are enriched for transforming growth factor beta (TGFB) signaling, including frequent amplification of orthodenticle homeobox 2 (OTX2), which is a TGFB target during neurodevelopment.[66] Mutually exclusive with OTX2 amplification are group 3 tumors with MYC amplification, a large subset of which harbor recurrent MYC/PVT1 gene fusions as a result of chromothripsis on chromosome 8.[66] The 5-year overall survival for group 4 tumors is ~50%.[65,70] Group 4 tumors (~35%) express a neuronal gene signature. Compared to group 3 tumors, group 4 tumors do not have MYC amplification, but have MYCN amplification in 6.3% of tumors (which is also seen in ~8.2% of SHH tumors).[65,66] Damaging mutations in KDM6A, a histone H3K27 demethylase, were restricted to group 4 tumors, but only explain the formation of 12% of tumors.[62–66] Of group 4 tumors, 10.4% had a recurrent synuclein, alpha interacting protein (SNCAIP) tandem duplication, which plays a role in Lewy body formation in Parkinson disease.[66] The 5-year overall survival for group 4 tumors is 75%.[65,70]

EPENDYMAL TUMORS

Ependymomas are glial tumors that arise from cells lining the ventricular system. Interestingly, the anatomic location of ependymoma growth predicts prognosis, with infratentorial ependymomas in children bearing the worst prognosis. Emerging evidence subcategorizing ependymomas by anatomic location has identified differences in age of onset, prognosis, driver mutations, structural variants, and transcriptional profiles (Fig. 96.4). The candidate cancer stem cell of ependymomas is the radial glial cell,[78] which has region-specific patterns of gene expression that

A

Ependymoma Subtype Characteristics

Anatomical Location	Population	Genomic characteristic
Supratentorial	Adult	CDKN2A deletion, amplification of EPHB2
Infratentorial, medial	Pediatric	chr1q gain
Infratentorial, lateral	Young adult	NF2/chr22 loss
Spinal	Adult	NF2/chr22 loss

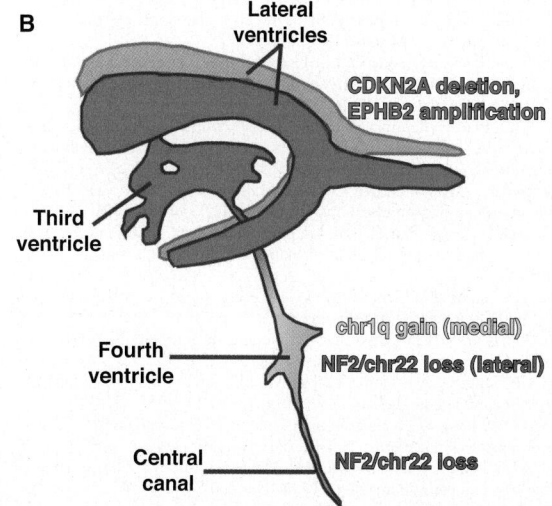

Figure 96.4 Anatomic location correlates with mutation and susceptible population for ependymomas. **(A)** Table summarizing the genomic driver events anatomic location and affected population for ependymomas. **(B)** Spinal ependymomas and lateral infratentorial ependymomas are characterized by NF2/chr22 loss, medial infratentorial ependymomas have chr1q gain, and supratentorial ependymomas have CDKN2A deletion and EPHB2 amplification. NF2, neurofibromin 2; CDKN2A, cyclin-dependent kinase inhibitor 2A; EPHB2, EPH receptor b2.

match the expression profiles of CD133+ ependymal cells harvested from the correlating anatomic compartment (spinal cord versus infratentorial versus supratentorial).[79] For example, patients with the inherited tumor syndrome neurofibromatosis type II frequently have intramedullary spinal ependymomas but not cortical ependymomas, and up to 95% of adult sporadic spinal cord ependymomas have monosomy chr22.[80] In contrast, >90% of supratentorial ependymomas have deletion of *CDKN2A*, frequently with co-occurring focal amplification of EPH Receptor B2 (*Ephb2*). Posterior fossa ependymomas appear to be split into two groups by anatomic location.[81] Lateral posterior fossa tumors are more chromosomally stable, occur in younger patients, have 1q gain, are more likely to recur with metastasis, and have a poor prognosis.[81] In contrast, midline posterior fossa ependymomas have more widespread chromosomal instability, are older, and have chr22 loss.[81]

SUMMARY

In just a few short years, the use of next-generation sequencing technologies has ushered about a golden age of discovery for the molecular pathways driving the formation of central nervous system tumors. Tumors classifications, once based primarily on observable histopathologic findings, are increasingly refined to distinct, clinically relevant entities based on differences in gene mutations, genomic stability, epigenetic changes, differences in gene expression profiles, differences in the anatomic location of growth, differences in response to therapy, and differences in overall survival. The challenge of translating the emerging molecular classifications of brain tumors to successful individualized cancer therapy is daunting, but the major advances brought about by genomic characterization serve as an ideal starting point for hypothesis-driven clinical research.

REFERENCES

1. Ostrom QT, Gittleman H, Farah P, et al. CBTRUS statistical report: primary brain and central nervous system tumors diagnosed in the United States in 2006-2010. *Neuro-oncology* 2013;15:ii1–56.
2. Louis DN, Ohgaki H, Wiestler OD, et al. *The WHO Classification of Tumours of the Central Nervous System*. Geneva, Switzerland: World Health Organization; 2007.
3. Grossman SA, Ye X, Piantadosi S, et al. Survival of patients with newly diagnosed glioblastoma treated with radiation and temozolomide in research studies in the United States. *Clin Cancer Res* 2010;16:2443–2449.
4. Yan H, Parsons DW, Jin G, et al. IDH1 and IDH2 mutations in gliomas. *N Engl J Med* 2009;360(8):765–773.
5. Dang L, White DW, Gross S, et al. Cancer-associated IDH1 mutations produce 2-hydroxyglutarate. *Nature* 2009;462:739–744.
6. Noushmehr H, Weisenberger DJ, Diefes K, et al. Identification of a CpG island methylator phenotype that defines a distinct subgroup of glioma. *Cancer Cell* 2010;17:510–522.
7. Rohle D, Popovici-Muller J, Palaskas N, et al. An inhibitor of mutant IDH1 delays growth and promotes differentiation of glioma cells. *Science* 2013;340:626–630.
8. Sturm D, Witt H, Hovestadt V, et al. Hotspot mutations in H3F3A and IDH1 define distinct epigenetic and biological subgroups of glioblastoma. *Cancer Cell* 2012;22:425–437.
9. Prensner JR, Chinnaiyan AM. Metabolism unhinged: IDH mutations in cancer. *Nature Med* 2011;17:291–293.
10. Ohgaki H, Kleihues P. Population-based studies on incidence, survival rates, and genetic alterations in astrocytic and oligodendroglial gliomas. *J Neuropathol Exp Neurol* 2005;64:479–489.
11. Ransom DT, Ritland SR, Kimmel DW, et al. Cytogenetic and loss of heterozygosity studies in ependymomas, pilocytic astrocytomas, and oligodendrogliomas. *Genes Chromosomes Cancer* 1992;5:348–356.
12. Bello MJ, Vaquero J, de Campos JM, et al. Molecular analysis of chromosome 1 abnormalities in human gliomas reveals frequent loss of 1p in oligodendroglial tumors. *Int J Cancer* 1994;57:172–175.
13. Reifenberger J, Reifenberger G, Liu L, et al. Molecular genetic analysis of oligodendroglial tumors shows preferential allelic deletions on 19q and 1p. *Am J Pathol* 1994;145:1175–1190.
14. Jenkins RB, Blair H, Ballman KV, et al. A t(1;19)(q10;p10) mediates the combined deletions of 1p and 19q and predicts a better prognosis of patients with oligodendroglioma. *Cancer Res* 2006;66:9852–9861.
15. Bettegowda C, Agrawal N, Jiao Y, et al. Mutations in CIC and FUBP1 contribute to human oligodendroglioma. *Science* 2011;333:1453–1455.
16. Jiao Y, Killela PJ, Reitman ZJ, et al. Frequent ATRX, CIC, FUBP1 and IDH1 mutations refine the classification of malignant gliomas. *Oncotarget* 2012; 3:709–722.
17. Ohgaki H, Kleihues P. Genetic pathways to primary and secondary glioblastoma. *Am J Pathol* 2007;170:1445–1453.
18. Dunn GP, Rinne ML, Wykosky J, et al. Emerging insights into the molecular and cellular basis of glioblastoma. *Genes Dev* 2012;26:756–784.
19. Hegi ME, Diserens AC, Gorlia T, et al. MGMT gene silencing and benefit from temozolomide in glioblastoma. *N Engl J Med* 2005;352:997–1003.
20. Parsons DW, Jones S, Zhang X, et al. An integrated genomic analysis of human glioblastoma multiforme. *Science* 2008;321:1807–1812.
21. Furnari FB, Fenton T, Bachoo RM, et al. Malignant astrocytic glioma: genetics, biology, and paths to treatment. *Genes Dev* 2007;21:2683–2710.
22. Cancer Genome Atlas Research Network. Comprehensive genomic characterization defines human glioblastoma genes and core pathways. *Nature* 2008;455:1061–1068.
23. Verhaak RG, Hoadley KA, Purdom E, et al. Integrated genomic analysis identifies clinically relevant subtypes of glioblastoma characterized by abnormalities in PDGFRA, IDH1, EGFR, and NF1. *Cancer Cell* 2010;17:98–110.
24. Brennan CW, Verhaak RG, McKenna A, et al. The somatic genomic landscape of glioblastoma. *Cell* 2013;155:462–477.
25. Killela PJ, Reitman ZJ, Jiao Y, et al. TERT promoter mutations occur frequently in gliomas and a subset of tumors derived from cells with low rates of self-renewal. *Proc Natl Acad Sci U S A* 2013;110:6021–6026.
26. Esteller M, Garcia-Foncillas J, Andion E, et al. Inactivation of the DNA-repair gene MGMT and the clinical response of gliomas to alkylating agents. *N Engl J Med* 2000;343:1350–1354.
27. Erickson LC, Laurent G, Sharkey NA, et al. DNA cross-linking and monoadduct repair in nitrosourea-treated human tumour cells. *Nature* 1980;288: 727–729.
28. Killela PJ, Pirozzi CJ, Reitman ZJ, et al. The genetic landscape of anaplastic astrocytoma. *Oncotarget* 2014;5:1452–1457.
29. Listernick R, Charrow J, Gutmann DH. Intracranial gliomas in neurofibromatosis type 1. *Am J Med Genet* 1999;89:38–44.
30. Jones DT, Kocialkowski S, Liu L, et al. Tandem duplication producing a novel oncogenic BRAF fusion gene defines the majority of pilocytic astrocytomas. *Cancer Res* 2008;68:8673–8677.
31. Forshew T, Tatevossian RG, Lawson AR, et al. Activation of the ERK/MAPK pathway: a signature genetic defect in posterior fossa pilocytic astrocytomas. *J Pathol* 2009;218:172–181.
32. Zhang J, Wu G, Miller CP, et al. Whole-genome sequencing identifies genetic alterations in pediatric low-grade gliomas. *Nat Genet* 2013;45: 602–612.
33. Jones DT, Hutter B, Jager N, et al. Recurrent somatic alterations of FGFR1 and NTRK2 in pilocytic astrocytoma. *Nat Genet* 2013;45:927–932.
34. Ramkissoon LA, Horowitz PM, Craig JM, et al. Genomic analysis of diffuse pediatric low-grade gliomas identifies recurrent oncogenic truncating rearrangements in the transcription factor MYBL1. *Proc Natl Acad Sci U S A* 2013;110:8188–8193.
35. Giannini C, Scheithauer BW. Classification and grading of low-grade astrocytic tumors in children. *Brain Pathol* 1997;7:785–798.
36. Giannini C, Scheithauer BW, Burger PC, et al. Pleomorphic xanthoastrocytoma: what do we really know about it? *Cancer* 1999;85(9):2033–2045.
37. Schwartzentruber J, Korshunov A, Liu XY, et al. Driver mutations in histone H3.3 and chromatin remodelling genes in paediatric glioblastoma. *Nature* 2012;482:226–231.
38. Wu G, Broniscer A, McEachron TA, et al. Somatic histone H3 alterations in pediatric diffuse intrinsic pontine gliomas and non-brainstem glioblastomas. *Nat Genet* 2012;44:251–253.
39. Bender S, Tang Y, Lindroth AM, et al. Reduced H3K27me3 and DNA hypomethylation are major drivers of gene expression in K27M mutant pediatric high-grade gliomas. *Cancer Cell* 2013;24:660–672.
40. Nicolaides TP, Li H, Solomon DA, et al. Targeted therapy for BRAFV600E malignant astrocytoma. *Clin Cancer Res* 2011;17:7595–7604.
41. Schiffman JD, Hodgson JG, VandenBerg SR, et al. Oncogenic BRAF mutation with CDKN2A inactivation is characteristic of a subset of pediatric malignant astrocytomas. *Cancer Res* 2010;70:512–519.
42. Paugh BS, Qu C, Jones C, et al. Integrated molecular genetic profiling of pediatric high-grade gliomas reveals key differences with the adult disease. *J Clin Oncol* 2010;28:3061–3068.
43. Louis DN, Deutsches Krebsforschungszentrum Heidelberg, International Agency for Research on Cancer, et al. *WHO Classification of Tumours of the Central Nervous System*. Geneva, Switzerland: WHO Press; 2007.
44. Clark VE, Erson-Omay EZ, Serin A, et al. Genomic analysis of non-NF2 meningiomas reveals mutations in TRAF7, KLF4, AKT1, and SMO. *Science* 2013;339:1077–1080.
45. Brastianos PK, Horowitz PM, Santagata S, et al. Genomic sequencing of meningiomas identifies oncogenic SMO and AKT1 mutations. *Nat Gen* 2013;45:285–289.

46. Reuss DE, Piro RM, Jones DT, et al. Secretory meningiomas are defined by combined KLF4 K409Q and TRAF7 mutations. *Acta Neuropathol* 2013; 125:351–358.

47. Rouleau GA, Merel P, Lutchman M, et al. Alteration in a new gene encoding a putative membrane-organizing protein causes neuro-fibromatosis type 2. *Nature* 1993;363:515–521.

48. Ruttledge MH, Sarrazin J, Rangaratnam S, et al. Evidence for the complete inactivation of the NF2 gene in the majority of sporadic meningiomas. *Nature Gen* 1994;6:180–184.

49. Schmitz U, Mueller W, Weber M, et al. INI1 mutations in meningiomas at a potential hotspot in exon 9. *Br J Cancer* 2001;84:199–201.

50. Versteege I, Sevenet N, Lange J, et al. Truncating mutations of hSNF5/INI1 in aggressive paediatric cancer. *Nature* 1998;394:203–206.

51. Biegel JA, Zhou JY, Rorke LB, et al. Germ-line and acquired mutations of INI1 in atypical teratoid and rhabdoid tumors. *Cancer Res* 1999;59:74–79.

52. van den Munckhof P, Christiaans I, Kenter SB, et al. Germline SMARCB1 mutation predisposes to multiple meningiomas and schwannomas with preferential location of cranial meningiomas at the falx cerebri. *Neurogenetics* 2012;13:1–7.

53. Takahashi K, Yamanaka S. Induction of pluripotent stem cells from mouse embryonic and adult fibroblast cultures by defined factors. *Cell* 2006;126: 663-676.

54. Regelsberger J, Hagel C, Emami P, et al. Secretory meningiomas: a benign subgroup causing life-threatening complications. *Neuro Oncol* 2009;11: 819–824.

55. Aavikko M, Li SP, Saarinen S, et al. Loss of SUFU function in familial multiple meningioma. *Am J Hum Genet* 2012;91:520–526.

56. Hahn H, Wicking C, Zaphiropoulous PG, et al. Mutations of the human homolog of Drosophila patched in the nevoid basal cell carcinoma syndrome. *Cell* 1996;85:841–851.

57. Johnson RL, Rothman AL, Xie J, et al. Human homolog of patched, a candidate gene for the basal cell nevus syndrome. *Science* 1996;272:1668–1671.

58. Hamilton SR, Liu B, Parsons RE, et al. The molecular basis of Turcot's syndrome. *N Engl J Med* 1995;332(13):839–847.

59. Raffel C, Jenkins RB, Frederick L, et al. Sporadic medulloblastomas contain PTCH mutations. *Cancer Res* 1997;57:842–845.

60. Zurawel RH, Chiappa SA, Allen C, et al. Sporadic medulloblastomas contain oncogenic beta-catenin mutations. *Cancer Res* 1998;58:896–899.

61. Thompson MC, Fuller C, Hogg TL, et al. Genomics identifies medulloblastoma subgroups that are enriched for specific genetic alterations. *J Clin Oncol* 2006;24:1924–1931.

62. Pugh TJ, Weeraratne SD, Archer TC, et al. Medulloblastoma exome sequencing uncovers subtype-specific somatic mutations. *Nature* 2012;488:106–110.

63. Robinson G, Parker M, Kranenburg TA, et al. Novel mutations target distinct subgroups of medulloblastoma. *Nature* 2012;488:43–48.

64. Jones DT, Jager N, Kool M, et al. Dissecting the genomic complexity underlying medulloblastoma. *Nature* 2012;488:100–105.

65. Northcott PA, Jones DT, Kool M, et al. Medulloblastomics: the end of the beginning. *Nat Rev Cancer* 2012;12:818–834.

66. Northcott PA, Shih DJ, Peacock J, et al. Subgroup-specific structural variation across 1,000 medulloblastoma genomes. *Nature* 2012;488:49–56.

67. Gibson P, Tong Y, Robinson G, et al. Subtypes of medulloblastoma have distinct developmental origins. *Nature* 2010;468:1095–1099.

68. Ellison DW, Onilude OE, Lindsey JC, et al. beta-Catenin status predicts a favorable outcome in childhood medulloblastoma: the United Kingdom Children's Cancer Study Group Brain Tumour Committee. *J Clin Oncol* 2005;23(31):7951–7057.

69. Grill J, Dufour C. Neuro-oncology: Stability of medulloblastoma subgroups at tumour recurrence. *Nat Rev Neurol* 2014;10:5–6.

70. Kool M, Korshunov A, Remke M, et al. Molecular subgroups of medulloblastoma: an international meta-analysis of transcriptome, genetic aberrations, and clinical data of WNT, SHH, Group 3, and Group 4 medulloblastomas. *Acta Neuropathol* 2012;123:473–484.

71. Rausch T, Jones DT, Zapatka M, et al. Genome sequencing of pediatric medulloblastoma links catastrophic DNA rearrangements with TP53 mutations. *Cell* 2012;148:59–71.

72. Zhukova N, Ramaswamy V, Remke M, et al. Subgroup-specific prognostic implications of TP53 mutation in medulloblastoma. *J Clin Oncol* 2013;31: 2927–2935.

73. Ramaswamy V, Remke M, Bouffet E, et al. Recurrence patterns across medulloblastoma subgroups: an integrated clinical and molecular analysis. *Lancet Oncol* 2013;14:1200–1207.

74. Rudin CM, Hann CL, Laterra J, et al. Treatment of medulloblastoma with hedgehog pathway inhibitor GDC-0449. *N Engl J Med* 2009;361:1173–1178.

75. Yauch RL, Dijkgraaf GJ, Alicke B, et al. Smoothened mutation confers resistance to a Hedgehog pathway inhibitor in medulloblastoma. *Science* 2009;326:572–574.

76. Cho YJ, Tsherniak A, Tamayo P, et al. Integrative genomic analysis of medulloblastoma identifies a molecular subgroup that drives poor clinical outcome. *J Clin Oncol* 2011;29:1424–1430.

77. Taylor MD, Northcott PA, Korshunov A, et al. Molecular subgroups of medulloblastoma: the current consensus. *Acta Neuropathol* 2012;123:465–472.

78. Taylor MD, Poppleton H, Fuller C, et al. Radial glia cells are candidate stem cells of ependymoma. *Cancer Cell* 2005;8:323–335.

79. Johnson RA, Wright KD, Poppleton H, et al. Cross-species genomics matches driver mutations and cell compartments to model ependymoma. *Nature* 2010; 466:632–636.

80. Ebert C, von Haken M, Meyer-Puttlitz B, et al. Molecular genetic analysis of ependymal tumors. NF2 mutations and chromosome 22q loss occur preferentially in intramedullary spinal ependymomas. *Am J Pathol* 1999;155: 627–632.

81. Witt H, Mack SC, Ryzhova M, et al. Delineation of two clinically and molecularly distinct subgroups of posterior fossa ependymoma. *Cancer Cell* 2011;20:143–157.

PRACTICE OF ONCOLOGY

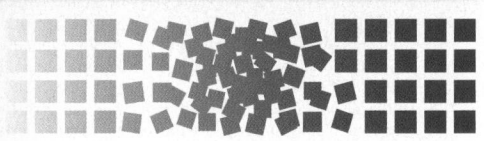

97 Neoplasms of the Central Nervous System

Susan M. Chang, Minesh P. Mehta, Michael A. Vogelbaum, Michael D. Taylor, and Manmeet S. Ahluwalia

EPIDEMIOLOGY OF BRAIN TUMORS

Incidence and Prevalence

The incidence and prevalence of brain and central nervous system (CNS) tumors is imprecisely documented because benign tumors were not required to be reported prior to 2003, and metastatic disease to the brain remains unreported. The major data sources for the United States include the Surveillance, Epidemiology, and End Results (SEER) program and the Central Brain Tumor Registry of the United States (CBTRUS).[1-2] The CBTRUS database from 2006 to 2010 reported 326,711 incident tumors (112,458 malignant and 214,253 nonmalignant), with an overall average annual age-adjusted incidence of 21.03 per 100,000. The overall incidence rate was 5.26 per 100,000 for children 0 to 19 years of age (5.14 per 100,000 for children less than 15 years), and 27.38 per 100,000 for adults (20+ years).[2] The median age at diagnosis is 59 years with approximately 7% of the cases in individuals less than 20 years of age. The distribution patterns of histologies within age groups differ substantially. The most frequently reported histology was nonmalignant meningioma, accounting for about one-third of all tumors. Of all brain and CNS tumors, 42% occurred in males. For the malignant histologies, 55% occurred in males, and in the nonmalignant histologies, 36% occurred in males. The aggregate average annual age-adjusted mortality is 4.25 deaths per 100,000 with considerable variation noted by state. Males were found to have a statistically higher mortality rate for brain and CNS than females in the United States population (5.19 versus 3.46 per 100,000). The estimated total number of new cases is 66,240 (22,810 malignant and 43,430 nonmalignant) for 2014.

In 1993, the World Health Organization (WHO) ratified a new classification, assuming that each tumor results from a specific cell type. Most registries do not contain detailed information regarding the distribution of various CNS tumors, as specified in the WHO classification.[3-4] Many of these tumors are radiographically and clinically diagnosed; examples include infiltrating pontine gliomas, vestibular schwannomas, skull-base meningiomas, and brain metastases. Specific CNS tumor types also differ in incidence based on anatomic location. Figure 97.1 presents a simplified distribution by subtype.

The increased utilization of cranial imaging for headaches, seizures, and trauma has led to an increase in the diagnosis of benign tumors. SEER suggests that between 1975 and 1987, there was a significant increase in the incidence of CNS tumors, which leveled off between 1991 and 2006. Because many patients with CNS tumors survive for several years, the prevalence exceeds the incidence. Overall prevalence rate of individuals with a brain tumor was estimated to be 209 per 100,000 in 2004 and 221.8 per 100,000 in 2010. The female prevalence rate (264.8 per 100,000) was higher than that in males (158.7 per 100,000). The averaged prevalence rate for malignant tumors (42.5 per 100,000) was lower than the prevalence for nonmalignant tumors (166.5 per 100,000). Estimates of the expected number of individuals living with primary brain tumor diagnoses in the United States was 612,770 in 2004 and 688,096 in 2010.[5]

Etiologic Factors

No agent has been definitively implicated in the causation of CNS tumors, and risk factors can be identified only in a minority. Commonly implicated associations described with other malignancies, such as diet, exercise, alcohol, tobacco, and viruses, are generally not considered to be significant for CNS tumors.[6]

Environmental Factors

Farmers and petrochemical workers have been shown to have a higher incidence of primary brain tumors. A variety of chemical exposures have been linked.[7] Ionizing and nonionizing radiation has been implicated, with the clearest association coming from the occurrence of superficial meningiomas in individuals receiving cranial or scalp irradiation, with the association being stronger for young children receiving low doses of irradiation for benign conditions.[8] Exposure to ionizing radiation is a known risk factor for a small percentage of astrocytomas, sarcomas, and other tumors.[9] There is a 2.3% incidence of primary brain tumors in long-term survivors among children given prophylactic cranial irradiation for acute leukemia, a fourfold increase over the expected rate.[10]

In addition, a retrospective study suggests an increased risk for developing gliomas in children undergoing computed tomography (CT) scans.[11] Exposure to dental x-rays performed at a time when radiation exposure was greater than currently used appears to be associated with an increased risk of intracranial meningioma.[12]

There are conflicting reports regarding nonionizing radiation emitted by cellular telephones.[13-19] Several investigators have reported meta-analyses of case control studies evaluating cell phone use and the development of a brain tumor. Kan et al.[16] reviewed nine studies (5,259 cases and 12,074 controls) and showed an overall odds ratio (OR) of 0.90 for cellular phone use and brain tumor development; the OR was 1.25 for long-term users. An OR of 0.98 for developing malignant and benign tumors of the brain as well as the head and neck was reported by Myung et al.[17] when collating 23 case control studies (12,544 cases and 25,572 controls). The International Commission for Non-Ionizing Radiation Protection Standing Committee on Epidemiology reviewed the epidemiologic evidence, and they concluded that there was not a causal association between mobile phone use and malignant gliomas, but for slow-growing tumors, the observation period was too short for conclusive statements.[18] A recent report of the INTERPHONE study, an international, population-based case control study, also did not find an increased risk of gliomas or meningiomas.[19] Glioma incidence has not followed the increase in cell phone use, but because of the potential for a lag in trends, continued surveillance on children who are exposed from an early age is warranted.[15]

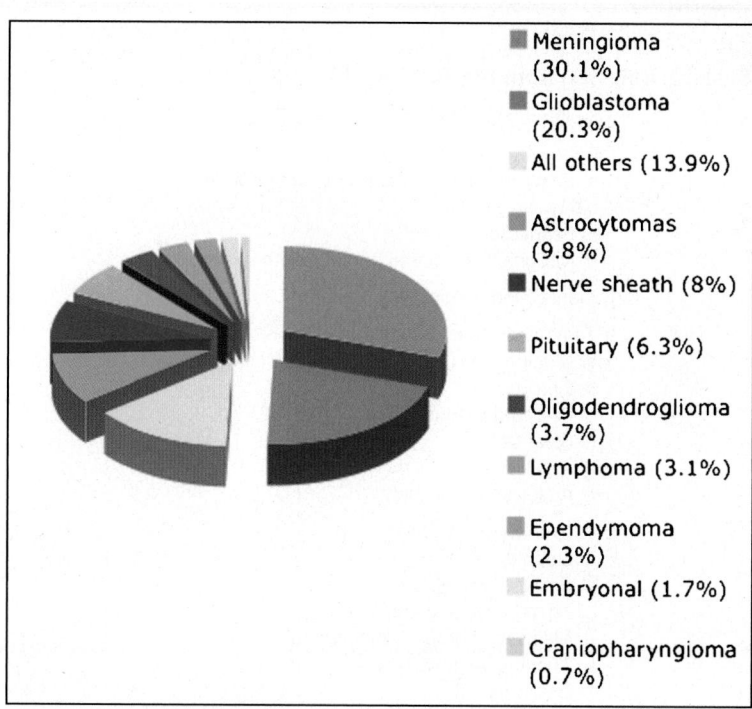

- Meningioma (30.1%)
- Glioblastoma (20.3%)
- All others (13.9%)
- Astrocytomas (9.8%)
- Nerve sheath (8%)
- Pituitary (6.3%)
- Oligodendroglioma (3.7%)
- Lymphoma (3.1%)
- Ependymoma (2.3%)
- Embryonal (1.7%)
- Craniopharyngioma (0.7%)

Figure 97.1 Proportionate distribution of the incidence of central nervous system neoplasms by histopathologic type, based on the Central Brain Tumor Registry of the United States database.

Viral Associations

Although certain canine and feline CNS tumors may have a viral association, the human evidence remains weak. Specifically, no increase in the risk of developing a brain tumor has been associated with previous polio vaccination, which discredits claims that simian virus 40, which contaminated older polio vaccine preparations, caused brain tumors.[20] The exception to this is primary CNS lymphoma, which has been shown to be associated with Epstein-Barr virus.[21] An increase in incidence of primary CNS lymphoma is most likely due to the increasing numbers of immunosuppressed patients in the setting of HIV and posttransplant use of immunosuppressants.[21–22]

The association between human cytomegalovirus (HCMV) infection and glioblastoma was first described by Cobbs et al.[23] in 2002. The presence of HCMV was also demonstrated in glioblastoma and in other gliomas.[24–25] HCMV may have tropism for microglia and CD133-positive glioma cancer stem cells and further work is needed to evaluate the role of this virus.[26]

Hereditary Syndromes

Neurofibromatosis type 1 (NF1) is an autosomal-dominant disorder associated with intra- and extracranial Schwann cell tumors. Optic gliomas, astrocytomas, and meningiomas also occur at higher frequency in NF1. NF2 is characterized by bilateral vestibular schwannomas and meningiomas. Systemic schwannomas also occur in NF2. Subependymal giant cell astrocytoma commonly occur in children with tuberous sclerosis, an autosomal-dominant disorder caused by mutation in the *TSC1* and *TSC2* genes. Other hereditary tumor syndromes affecting the CNS include Li-Fraumeni syndrome (germline mutation in one p53 allele; malignant gliomas); von Hippel-Lindau syndrome (germline mutation of the *VHL* gene; hemangioblastomas), and Turcot syndrome (germline mutations of the adenomatous polyposis gene; medulloblastoma).[27,28] The nevoid basal cell carcinoma syndrome (Gorlin syndrome) is associated with medulloblastomas (and possibly meningiomas) and represents mutations in the *PTCH* suppressor gene or other members of the Sonic hedgehog pathway.[29,30]

Meningiomas and schwannomas are more common in females; gliomas, medulloblastomas, and most other CNS tumors are more common in males. Meningiomas are more common in African Americans and gliomas and medulloblastomas are more common in Caucasians. It has been suggested that there is a lower incidence of meningiomas and a higher incidence of gliomas and vestibular schwannomas in higher socioeconomic groups.[31–34]

CLASSIFICATION

Primary CNS tumors are of ecto- and mesodermal origin and arise from the brain, cranial nerves, meninges, pituitary, pineal, and vascular elements. The WHO classification lists approximately 100 subtypes of CNS malignancies in seven broad categories (Table 97.1).[3,4,35] In spite of the low proliferation rate within the meninges, meningiomas are among the most common CNS tumors. Astrocytes are among the most mitogenically competent cells, and astrocytomas, also referred to interchangeably as *gliomas*, are among the more common primary CNS tumors. The precise cell of origin of gliomas, however, remains unclear.

The WHO classification can be reduced to a simpler working formulation, categorizing the neoplasms into tumors presumably derived from glia, neurons, or from cells that surround the CNS or form specialized anatomic structures. Glial cells are believed to give rise to astrocytomas, oligodendrogliomas, and ependymomas. Neuronal cells are involved in the development of medulloblastoma and primitive neuroectodermal tumors (PNET). In PNETs, anatomic location is pivotal; the transformation of cortical neuroblasts leads to cortical PNETs, retinal neuroblasts form retinoblastoma, and pineal neuroblasts form pineoblastomas. Specialized anatomic structures within the CNS give rise to pituitary adenomas, pineocytomas, chordomas, hemangioblastomas, germ cell tumors, and choroid plexus papillomas and carcinomas.

This working formulation is speculative, based on scant phenotypical and immunohistochemical evidence. For example, oligodendrogliomas are diagnosed based on cellular morphology, including prominent nuclei surrounded by a cytoplasmic halo with a characteristic "fried egg" appearance, and many have codeletions of 1p and 19q. However, no definitive markers for oligodendrogliomas currently exist; these tumors can stain both for glial fibrillary acidic protein, an astrocytic marker, and for synaptophysin, a presumptive neuronal marker.[36] A third of all gliomas have

TABLE 97.1

Classification of Tumors of the Central Nervous System: Selected from the 2007 World Health Organization Classification

1. Neuroepithelial tumors

    Astrocytic tumors
    a. Pilocytic astrocytoma
    b. Subependymal giant cell astrocytoma
    c. Pleomorphic xanthoastrocytoma
    d. Diffuse astrocytoma
        a. Fibrillary astrocytoma
        b. Gemistocytic astrocytoma
        c. Pro-oplasmic astrocytoma
    e. Anaplastic astrocytoma
    f. Glioblastoma
        a. Giant cell glioblastoma
        b. Gliosarcoma
    g. Gliomatosis cerebri

    Oligodendroglial tumors
    a. Oligodendroglioma
    b. Anaplastic oligodendroglioma

    Ependymal tumors
    a. Subependymoma
    b. Myxopapillary ependymoma
    c. Ependymoma
    d. Anaplastic ependymoma

    Choroid plexus tumors
    a. Choroid plexus papilloma
    b. Atypical choroid plexus papilloma
    c. Choroid plexus carcinoma

    Other neuroepithelial tumors
    a. Astroblastoma
    b. Chordoid glioma of the third ventricle
    c. Angiocentric glioma

    Neuronal and mixed neuronal-glial tumors
    a. Dysplastic gangliocytoma of cerebellum (Lhermitte-Duclos)
    b. Desmoplastic infantile astrocytoma/ganglioglioma
    c. Dysembryoplastic neuroepithelial tumor
    d. Gangliocytoma
    e. Ganglioglioma
    f. Anaplastic ganglioglioma
    g. Central neurocytoma
    h. Extraventricular neurocytoma
    i. Cerebellar liponeurocytoma
    j. Papillary glioneuronal tumor
    k. Rosette-forming glioneuronal tumor of the fourth ventricle
    l. Paraganglioma

    Tumors of the pineal region
    a. Pineocytoma
    b. Pineoblastoma

    Embryonal tumors
    a. Medulloblastoma
    b. Primitive neuroectodermal tumors
    c. Atypical teratoid/rhabdoid tumor

2. Tumors of cranial/spinal nerves
    a. Schwannoma (neurilemoma, neurinoma)
    b. Neurofibroma
    c. Perineuroma
    d. Malignant peripheral nerve sheath tumor

3. Tumors of the meninges

    A. Tumors of meningothelial cells
    a. Meningioma
    b. Fibrous
    c. Psammomatous
    d. Clear cell
    e. Atypical
    f. Anaplastic (malignant)

    B. Mesenchymal tumors
    a. Lipoma
    b. Solitary fibrous tumor
    c. Rhabdomyosarcoma
    d. Malignant fibrous histiocytoma
    e. Chondrosarcoma
    f. Osteoma
    g. Hemangioma
    h. Hemangiopericytoma
    i. Kaposi sarcoma

4. Lymphomas and hematopoietic neoplasms
    a. Malignant lymphomas
    b. Plasmacytoma

5. Germ cell tumors
    a. Germinoma
    b. Yolk-sac tumor
    c. Choriocarcinoma
    d. Teratoma
    e. Mixed-germ cell tumors

6. Sellar tumors
    a. Pituitary adenoma
    b. Craniopharyngioma

7. Metastatic tumors

morphologic characteristics of both astrocytoma and oligodendroglioma, leading some to separate gliomas based on their molecular and genetic characteristics.[37] Evidence that suggests that some oligodendrocytes derive from a neuronal lineage, whereas some neuron-derived tumors (embryonal tumors) can show significant areas of glial differentiation, highlights the uncertainty.[38,39] An alternative hypothesis is that all neuroepithelial cells are derived from a common precursor cell (i.e., a multipotent neural stem cell), and hence all neuroepithelial tumors are derived from neural stem cells or their committed progeny.[40] The recent discovery, isolation, and characterization of cancer stem cells from human brain tumors provides supportive evidence.[41] However, more recently it was shown in an animal experiment that gliomas can originate from differentiated cells in the CNS, including cortical neurons.[42]

Approximately 15% of all primary CNS tumors arise in the spinal cord, where the distribution of tumor types is significantly different from that in the brain. Tumors of the lining of the spinal cord and nerve roots predominate (50% to 80% of all spinal tumors); schwannomas and meningiomas are most common, followed by ependymomas. Primary gliomas of the spinal cord are uncommon.[43] In children, three-quarters of tumors are comprised of ependymomas, pilocytic astrocytomas, and other neuroepithelial neoplasms.[2]

ANATOMIC LOCATION AND CLINICAL CONSIDERATIONS

Intracranial Tumors

Intracranial tumors produce five categories of symptoms: those arising from increased intracranial pressure (ICP), seizures, physiologic deficits specific to location, higher order neurocognitive deficits, and endocrinologic dysfunction. A headache arises from irritation of the dura or intracranial vessels or due to elevated ICP from tumor bulk, edema, or obstruction of a cerebrospinal fluid (CSF) pathway. Slow-growing tumors may grow to a remarkably large size without producing headaches, whereas rapidly growing tumors can cause headaches early in their course. Small tumors can cause headaches by growing in an enclosed space that is richly innervated with pain fibers, such as the cavernous sinus, or by causing obstructive hydrocephalus. Nausea and vomiting, gait and balance alterations, personality changes, and slowing of psychomotor function or even somnolence may be present with increased ICP. Because ICP increases with recumbency and hypoventilation during sleep, early-morning headaches that awaken the patient are typical. Sometimes the only presenting symptoms are changes in personality, mood, or mental capacity or slowing of psychomotor activity. Such changes may be confused with depression, especially in older patients. Although fewer than 6% of first seizures result from brain tumors, almost one-half of patients with supratentorial brain tumors present with seizures. An adult with a first seizure that occurs without an obvious precipitating event should undergo magnetic resonance imaging (MRI).

Tumors are sometimes associated with location-specific symptoms. Frontal tumors cause changes in personality, loss of initiative, and abulia (loss of ability to make independent decisions). Posterior frontal tumors can produce contralateral weakness by affecting the motor cortex and expressive aphasia if they involve the dominant (usually the left) frontal lobe. Bifrontal disease, seen with "butterfly" gliomas and lymphomas, may cause memory impairment, labile mood, gait imbalance, and urinary incontinence. These symptoms may be related to alteration of normal cortex and white matter by the tumor itself, or by surrounding tumor-related edema. Improvement of symptoms after a short course of high-dose glucocorticoids is often an indicator of whether the findings are related to tumor-associated edema. In the case of CNS lymphoma, corticosteroids can have a cytotoxic effect also with a reduction in the tumor mass.

Temporal tumors might cause symptoms detectable only on careful testing of perception and spatial judgment, but can also impair memory. Homonymous superior quadrantanopsia, auditory hallucinations, and abnormal behavior can occur with tumors in either temporal lobe. Nondominant temporal tumors can cause minor perceptual problems and spatial disorientation. Dominant temporal lobe tumors can present with dysnomia, impaired perception of verbal commands, and ultimately fluent (Wernicke-like) aphasia. Seizures are more common from tumors in this location.

Parietal tumors affect sensory and perceptual functions. Sensory disorders range from mild sensory extinction or stereognosis, which are observable only by testing, to a more severe sensory loss such as hemianesthesia. Poor proprioception in the affected limb is common and is sometimes associated with gait instability. Homonymous inferior quadrantanopsia, incongruent hemianopsia, or visual inattention may occur. Nondominant parietal tumors may cause contralateral neglect and, in severe cases, anosognosia and apraxia. Dominant parietal tumors lead to alexia, dysgraphia, and certain types of apraxia. Occipital tumors can produce contralateral homonymous hemianopsia or complex visual aberrations, affecting perception of color, size, or location. Bilateral occipital tumors can produce cortical blindness.

Classic corpus callosum disconnection syndromes are rare in brain tumor patients, even though infiltrative gliomas often cross the corpus callosum in the region of the genu or the splenium. Interruption of the anterior corpus callosum can cause a failure of the left hand to carry out spoken commands. Lesions in the posterior corpus callosum interrupt visual fibers that connect the right occipital lobe to the left angular gyrus, causing an inability to read or name colors.

Thalamic tumors can cause local effects and also obstructive hydrocephalus. Either sensory or motor syndromes or, on the dominant side, aphasia is possible. *Thalamic* pain disorders or motor syndromes from basal ganglia involvement may also occur. The most common brainstem tumor is the pontine glioma, which presents most frequently with cranial nerve VI and VII palsies. Long tract signs usually follow, with hemiplegia, unilateral limb ataxia, gait ataxia, paraplegia, hemisensory syndromes, gaze disorders, and occasionally, hiccups. Tectal involvement causes Parinaud syndrome, peduncular lesions cause contralateral motor impairment, and obstruction of the aqueduct causes hydrocephalus.

Tumors in the medulla can have a fulminant course, including dysphagia, dysarthria, and deficits in cranial nerves IX, X, and XII. Involvement of the medullary cardiac and respiratory centers can result in a rapidly fatal course. Fourth ventricular tumors, because of their location, cause symptomatic obstructive hydrocephalus at a relatively small size, with associated disturbances of gait and balance. In addition, nausea and vomiting can be a symptom of a fourth ventricular mass. Rapidly enlarging lesions may end in cerebellar herniation.

Cerebellar tumors have variable localizing presentations. Midline lesions in and around the vermis cause truncal and gait ataxia, whereas more lateral hemispheric lesions lead to unilateral appendicular ataxia, usually worst in the arm. Abnormal head position, with the head tilting back and away from the side of the tumor, is seen often in children but rarely in adults. Mass lesions within or abutting the brain or spinal cord can cause displacement of vital neurologic structures. This can lead, in the brain, to herniation syndromes with respiratory arrest and death and, in the spine, to paraplegia or quadriplegia. A hemorrhage into a tumor can also cause acute neurologic deterioration. This is often associated with iatrogenic coagulopathies such as thrombocytopenia due to chemotherapy or anticoagulation therapy for deep venous thrombosis. Primary tumors that most often bleed de novo are glioblastoma and oligodendrogliomas; of the metastatic tumors, lung cancer, melanoma, renal cell cancer, thyroid cancer, and choriocarcinoma most often show hemorrhage.

Lumbar puncture should not be performed in any of the acute herniation syndromes or when herniation is imminent. In fact, a lumbar puncture should be avoided in the setting of significantly elevated ICP that is directly related to a tumor's mass effect or to obstructive hydrocephalus.

Spinal Axis Tumors

For the clinical presentation of tumors of the spinal axis to be understood, the local anatomy must be appreciated. A spinal tumor can produce local (focal) and distal (remote) symptoms, or both. Local effects indicate the tumor's location along the spinal axis, and distal effects reflect involvement of motor and sensory long tracts within the cord.

Distal symptoms and signs are confined to structures innervated below the level of the tumor. Neurologic manifestations often begin unilaterally, with weakness and spasticity, if the tumor lies above the conus medullaris, or weakness and flaccidity if the tumor is at or below the conus. Impairment of sphincter and sexual function occurs later unless the tumor is in the conus. The upper level of impaired long-tract function usually is several segments below the tumor's actual site. Local manifestations may reflect involvement of bone (with axial pain) or spinal roots, with radicular pain and loss of motor and sensory functions of the root or roots.

NEURODIAGNOSTIC TESTS

Magnetic Resonance Imaging

The imaging modality of choice for most CNS tumors is MRI, which can demonstrate anatomy and pathologic processes in detail.[44] CT is generally reserved for those unable (e.g., because of an implanted pacemaker, metal fragment, or paramagnetic surgical clips) or unwilling (e.g., because of claustrophobia) to undergo MRI. Because of the link of nephrogenic systemic fibrosis to the infusion of gadolinium-based contrast agents, there are new preventative guidelines regarding the administration of gadolinium in patients who may be at high risk.[45]

The most useful imaging studies are T1-weighted sagittal images, gadolinium (Gd)-enhanced and unenhanced T1 axial images, and T2-weighted axial images (Fig. 97.2). Contrast-enhanced MRI provides an improved ability to discern tumors from other pathologic entities, one tumor type from another, and putatively higher from lower grade malignancies. There are, however, limitations in anatomic MRI to definitively diagnose a mass lesion as a tumor.[46] Other confounding diagnoses

include bacterial abscesses, inflammatory disease such as sarcoidosis, tumefactive demyelination, and acute ischemic disease. It is conventionally believed that most low-grade gliomas (except pilocytic astrocytomas and pleomorphic xanthoastrocytoma) do not enhance, but in reviewing imaging studies of patients enrolled in several clinical trials, it is apparent that this may not be so categorical, in that even low-grade gliomas may frequently contain areas of enhancement, raising the concern that these areas might represent high-grade or malignant transformation (Fig. 97.3).[47] In addition, some high-grade lesions may not have contrast enhancement on MRI. Imaging is also unable to discern different histologic subtypes; however, the presence of calcifications is typical of oligodendroglioma.

Neuraxis or Spinal Imaging

In the evaluation of spinal cord tumors, MRI is also the preferred modality, providing superb visualization of the spinal cord contour and (with gadolinium contrast) of most intrinsic tumors (such as ependymomas, astrocytomas, meningiomas, and schwannomas), as well as facilitating the diagnosis of leptomeningeal dissemination. Tumor cysts are readily identified on MRI, and spinal cord tumors can often be distinguished from syringomyelia. Ideally, neuraxis imaging should be performed before surgery. In the immediate postoperative period, spinal MRI scans may be difficult to interpret because arachnoiditis and blood products can mimic leptomeningeal metastasis. Delayed spinal MRI (more than 3 weeks after surgery) combined with an increased dose of gadolinium is a sensitive imaging study for leptomeningeal disease.

Newer Imaging Modalities

Newer MRI techniques include magnetic resonance spectroscopy, dynamic contrast-enhanced MRI, diffusion-perfusion MRI, and functional MRI.[48] In addition, metabolic imaging using positron-emission tomography using various tracers is being explored.[49] These newer techniques remain to be validated as biomarkers of biological behavior or clinical outcome. Posttreatment metabolic scans may help distinguish recurrence from treatment-related

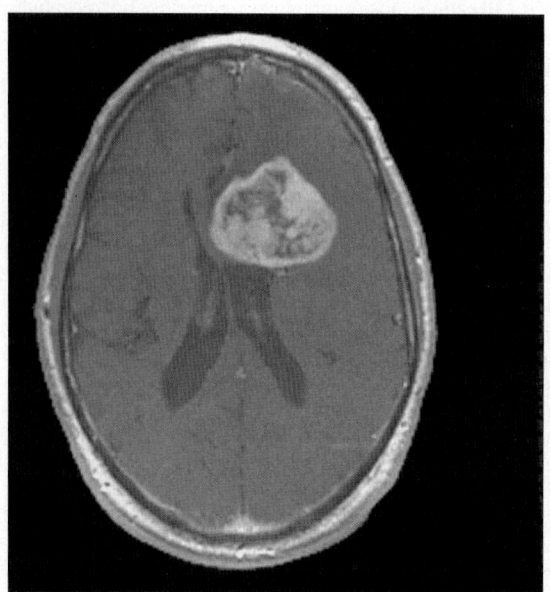
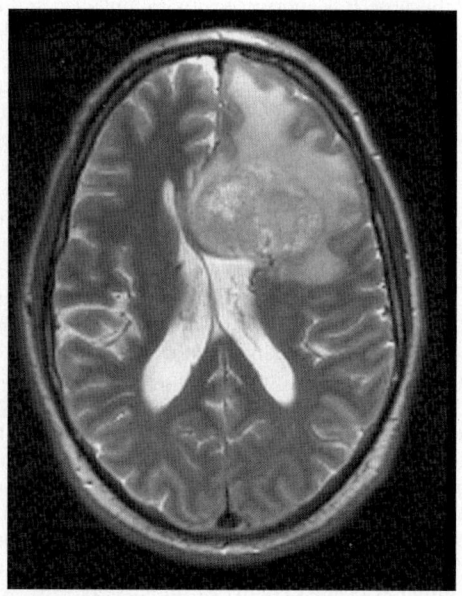

A   **B**

Figure 97.2 Magnetic resonance imaging of a patient with a malignant glioma demonstrates a large mass with heterogenous enhancement **(A)** and significant edema **(B)** on the T2-weighted sequences.

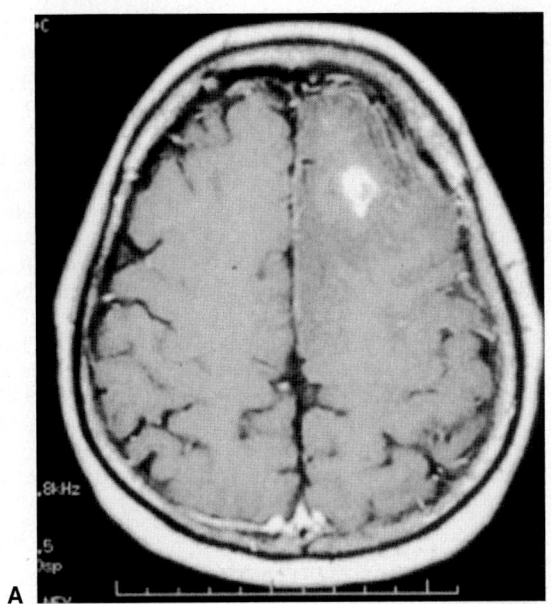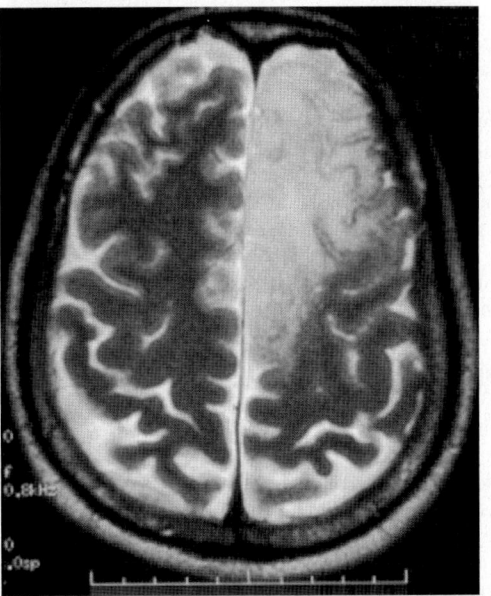

Figure 97.3 A: Low-grade astrocytomas often do not enhance and contrast-enhanced T1-weighted magnetic resonance sequences considerably underestimate the true infiltrative extent of these neoplasms. **B:** The fluid-attenuated inversion recovery (FLAIR) sequence is considerably more useful in appreciating the true extent of such neoplasms.

changes, although most modalities have a relatively high false negative rate. A modification of the standard MRI is quick brain MRI, which uses single-shot, fast-spin echo imaging to allow for adequate demonstration of ventricular anatomy and appropriate evaluation of shunt function.[50]

Pseudoresponse and Pseudoprogression

In malignant gliomas treated with combined modality therapy, it is speculated that 25% to 40% or even more may experience imaging changes relatively early in the course of therapy, usually within a few months, which appears consistent with radiographic progression. However, with time and without any therapy, many of these changes actually improve or even resolve (pseudoprogression), and in patients operated on with a presumptive diagnosis of tumor, the histopathology often reveals large areas of tumor necrosis.[51,52] With the advent of antiangiogenic therapies for malignant gliomas, rapid resolution of tumor enhancement is visualized on MRI, sometimes within days. This is consistent with the traditional definition of response, but in several instances, especially with time, even in the absence of contrast enhancement, tumor progression and clinical deterioration occurs, which is sometimes appreciated as T2 or fluid-attenuated inversion recovery (FLAIR) changes; this phenomenon is labeled as *pseudoresponse*.[53]

Cerebrospinal Fluid Examination

Typically, medulloblastoma, ependymoma, choroid plexus carcinoma, lymphoma, and some embryonal pineal and suprasellar region tumors have a high enough likelihood of spreading to justify CSF examinations to evaluate for malignant cells (cytology) and specific markers, such as human chorionic gonadotropin-β and α-fetoprotein.

CSF spread of a tumor may be associated with several possible findings, including CSF pressure above 150 mm H_2O at the lumbar level in a laterally positioned patient; elevated protein, typically greater than 40 mg/dL; reduced glucose (below 50 mg/mL); and tumor cells by cytologic examination. A high protein concentration with normal glucose levels and normal cytology is also

seen with base of skull tumors, such as vestibular schwannoma, and with spinal cord tumors that obstruct the subarachnoid space and produce stasis of the CSF in the caudal lumbar sac. Sampling of the CSF in the immediate postoperative period may lead to false-positive results, however, and is best done before surgery or more than 3 weeks after surgery, as long as there is no uncontrolled raised intracranial pressure.

SURGERY

Preoperative Considerations

The major objectives of surgery are to maximally remove bulk tumor, reduce tumor-associated mass effect and elevated ICP, and provide tissue for pathologic analysis in a manner that minimizes risk to neurologic functioning. For some tumors, a complete resection can be curative. However, most brain tumors are diffusely infiltrative; for these, surgical cure is rarely possible. Nonetheless, surgery can rapidly reduce tumor bulk with potential benefits in terms of mass effect, edema, and hydrocephalus. Furthermore, there is mostly retrospective evidence for both high-grade and low-grade infiltrative gliomas for which maximizing the extent of bulk tumor removal is associated with a better outcome, albeit so long as new, permanent neurologic deficits are avoided.[54–57] The requirement for histopathologic confirmation of diagnosis is not necessary in certain well-defined situations, but a tissue diagnosis is still required to determine the appropriate treatment course in most circumstances. As molecularly targeted therapies become useful, tissue removal for molecular analysis will become more necessary to guide therapy. Pseudoprogression may make tissue-based confirmation necessary before changes in therapy are instituted.[53] Technologic advances in surgical approaches, techniques, and instrumentation have rendered most tumors amenable to resection; however, for some tumor types or locations, the risk of open operation supports the choice of biopsy for obtaining diagnostic tissue. Biopsy techniques include stereotactic biopsy (with or without a stereotactic frame) using CT, MRI, or both, to choose the target. Metabolic or spectroscopic imaging can be coregistered with anatomic images to choose targets that may be of higher biologic aggressiveness within a tumor that appears homogeneous on standard imaging. In certain settings, an approach using simple ultrasonic guidance can also be considered for obtaining diagnostic tissue.

Unless a lymphoma is being considered, patients are given corticosteroids, usually dexamethasone, immediately preoperatively and often for several days before surgery to reduce cerebral edema and thus minimize secondary brain injury from cerebral retraction. Steroid administration is then continued in the immediate postoperative period and tapered off as quickly as possible. Antibiotics are given just before making the incision to decrease the risk of wound infection.

Anesthesia and Positioning

The routine use of prophylactic anticonvulsants in the perioperative period is a common practice despite recommendations that would seem to discourage that practice.[58,59] Patients with a history of seizures need to have their anticonvulsants maintained at therapeutic dose levels. Under certain circumstances, such as for awake craniotomies with electrocorticography, the use of anticonvulsants for a short time might be warranted.

General Surgical Principles

In the past, localization of the surgical incision and craniotomy were most often performed by a neurosurgeon's understanding of cranial anatomy and an interpretation of preoperative imaging. More recently, image-guided navigation systems have been employed to more effectively localize tumor margins as they project to the cranial surface and thus allow for smaller, precisely positioned craniotomies.[59,60] For tumors not resectable because of their location or diffuseness, a biopsy can be performed stereotactically using frameless or frame-based techniques. Tumors that are limited to the cortical surface may be best sampled with an open biopsy, under direct vision, due to the risk of inadvertent injury to a cortical vessel with a more limited, needle-based approach.

Specialized technology can be used to help define the completeness of a resection. Often, preoperative mapping of functional areas and their connections with MRI-based techniques are used to delineate both cortical areas and important subcortical white matter tracts that subserve speech and motor function.[61] Image-guided navigation systems are almost always employed, but the guidance may lose accuracy over the course of an operation due to brain shift or cyst decompression. Intraoperative imaging with ultrasound, CT, or MRI may be used to determine the extent of residual tumor and to further localize areas where additional tumor may be removed safely.[62] There has been growing use of 5-aminoleuvilinic acid (5-ALA), a prodrug, which is converted by glioma cells into fluorescent porphyrins that can be visualized with an operating microscope equipped with a fluorescent imaging system. The impact of the use of 5-ALA to guide resection of glioblastoma (GBM) on completeness of surgical resection and progression-free survival (PFS) has been demonstrated in a phase III trial.[63] Its use is limited to tumors that enhance with contrast on MRI (or CT), because the conversion of prodrug in low-grade tumors does not produce a sufficient amount of fluorescent porphyrin to be visualized intraoperatively. However, this conversion can be detected with the use of specialized optical instrumentation.[57] Use of 5-ALA in this manner is approved by regulatory authorities in Europe; its use in the United States remains investigational at this time.

Intraoperative cortical-stimulation mapping facilitates the resection of tumors in or adjacent to functionally critical areas. Motor functions can be mapped even under general anesthesia; however, anesthetic agents may increase the threshold to response and hence decrease the sensitivity of mapping. Sensory and speech-associated cortex are typically mapped during an awake craniotomy. Patients are monitored in the specialized care unit overnight after surgery, and an MRI is done within 24 to 48 hours to evaluate the extent of any remaining tumor. It is important that this MRI is done before 72 hours to minimize the appearance of nonspecific contrast enhancement that is related to surgery and might be mistaken for residual tumor.[64,65]

Re-resection of recurrent cerebral astrocytomas can be modestly efficacious.[66] When the initial tumor was low grade, histologic resampling may be necessary to guide further treatment at recurrence. Reoperation offers a chance to implant polymer wafers containing carmustine (bis-chloroethylnitrosourea [BCNU]) or to administer experimental agents, such as gene therapy agents or immunotoxins. A smaller volume of disease at initiation of chemotherapy predicts longer survival; thus, reoperation may improve the efficacy of adjuvant treatment as well as relieve mass effect in some patients.[67] An increasingly important aspect of resection is the need for tumor sampling to allow for a molecular marker analysis, which might provide and aid in assessing the prognosis as well as the probability of benefit from both chemotherapeutic and targeted therapies.

RADIATION THERAPY

General Concepts

Radiation therapy plays an integral role in the treatment of most malignant and many benign primary CNS tumors. It is often employed postoperatively as adjuvant treatment to decrease local failure, to delay recurrence, and to prolong survival in gliomas; as definitive treatment in more radiosensitive diseases such as PNET and germ cell tumors; or as therapy to halt further tumor growth in schwannomas, meningiomas, pituitary tumors, and craniopharyngiomas, and as ablative therapy to abrogate hormonal overproduction in secretory pituitary adenomas. Radiation therapy is also the primary modality in palliating brain metastases, and symptomatic spinal and osseous, as well as soft-tissue skull lesions.

Radiobiologic and Toxicity Considerations

Most neoplasms can potentially be cured if the correct radiation dose can be delivered to the entire tumor and its microscopic extensions. This is not always feasible because the maximum radiation dose deliverable is limited by the tolerance of the surrounding normal tissues, and the identification of regions of microscopic extension remains vague. Radiation tolerance of the CNS depends on several factors, including total dose, fraction size, volume irradiated, underlying comorbidities (particularly hypertension and diabetes), and innate sensitivity. Adverse reactions to cranial irradiation differ in pathogenesis and temporal presentation and are not discussed in detail here.

A major radiobiologic consideration revolves around the selection of total dose and the fractionation schedule. Late or long-term toxicities are generally a function of fraction size (i.e., dose per daily fraction of treatment), and therefore, as the fraction size is increased, such as with radiosurgery, higher late toxicity rates must be anticipated, assuming that normal tissue is encompassed within the high dose field. These late toxicities from larger fraction sizes can be minimized by minimizing the volume irradiated, as is done with radiosurgery, thereby drastically reducing the volume of normal tissues exposed to high doses. Proton and charged particle therapy, such as carbon, etc., are characterized by minimal to no exit dose beyond the target (where the so-called Bragg peak [i.e., the peak region of dose deposition] is placed), thereby sharply targeting the dose, and advantageously sparing tissue distal to the target. For radiosurgery, doses in the order of 12 to 21 Gy in single fractions are often utilized. In conventional radiotherapy, fraction sizes of 2 Gy are routinely utilized and may be lowered to 1.8 Gy per fraction in proximity to the visual apparatus or may be increased to 3 Gy or more per fraction in patients in whom shorter palliative schedules, with lesser concern regarding long-term morbidities, exist. In general, the entire target is treated with a relatively uniform dose, but with the advent of newer delivery methods, it is possible to create dose gradients or dose inhomogeneities within the tumor to match differential radiosensitivity. However, this concept of dose painting remains investigational.

Treatment Planning and Delivery Methods

High-resolution MR fusion with CT planning images has allowed for more precise delineation of targets, although a significant margin, particularly with gliomas, is still necessary to cover microscopic extension.[68] Patient immobilization devices limit intrafraction motion and provide precision in positioning, decreasing the margin required for setup variability. Image-guided radiotherapy (IGRT), using biplanar orthogonal x-ray imaging systems, cone beam CT, megavoltage CT, surface tracking, fiducial monitoring, etc., further improves setup reproducibility and allows for decreased margins. Newer systems in development incorporate on-board MRI, but remain investigational.

IGRT can be incorporated with any radiotherapy method, such as fractionated external-beam radiotherapy and stereotactic radiosurgery (SRS), and is practically mandatory for charged-particle therapy, frameless radiosurgery, fractionated stereotactic radiotherapy (FSRT), and intensity-modulated radiotherapy (IMRT). CT-based three-dimensional conformal radiation (3D-CRT) in which noncoplanar fields with unique entrance and exit pathways can be mapped on the target has improved normal tissue sparing. This allows for avoidance of critical structures, such as the brainstem, optic apparatus, and spinal cord. In IMRT, the photon flux of a beam is modulated in multiple directions during treatment, aimed at mimicking the shape of the target from various viewpoints, thereby producing improved conformality and nonuniform dose distribution. IMRT is increasingly being utilized for CNS tumors, based primarily on dosimetric studies, which suggest superior tumor coverage and reduction in the dose to critical structures (Fig. 97.4).[69] This can be beneficial in specific instances, such as to preserve cochlear function, vision, or pituitary activity.[70]

In FSRT, the concepts of 3D-CRT or IMRT are merged with the accuracy and precision in delivery that characterizes SRS, and, typically, the radiation fraction size is considerably increased, so that the total course of therapy is reduced from the typical 20 to 30 or more fractions to 5 or fewer fractions. Various FSRT systems have been developed, with reported precision between 1 to 3 mm.[71,72] FSRT is often used for larger lesions (e.g., 4 cm or more) and for lesions located in critical regions where single-fraction

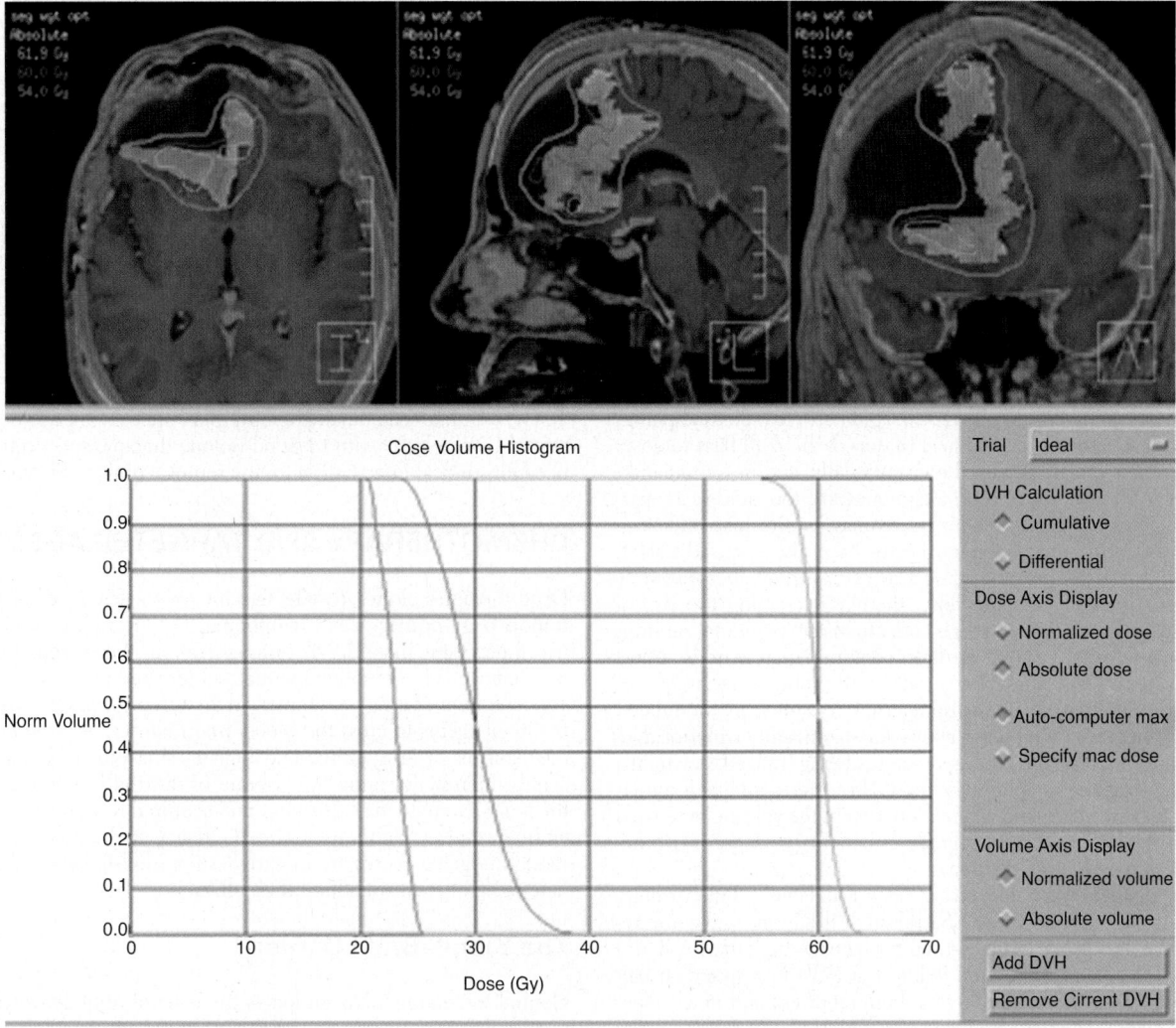

Figure 97.4 Intensity-modulated radiotherapy allows dose shaping to avoid critical structures. In this treatment plan of a right frontal oligodendroglioma (*orange*), tight target coverage and excellent conformal avoidance of the optic chiasm (*red*) and pituitary (*purple*) are achieved, as evidenced by the dose-volume histogram (DVH).

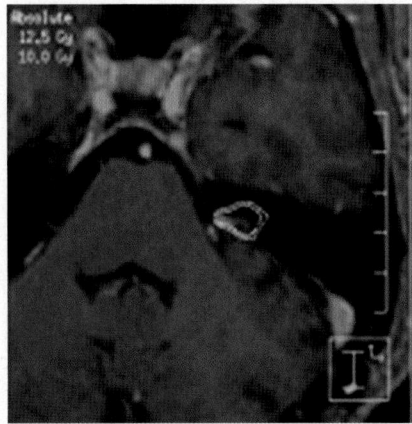 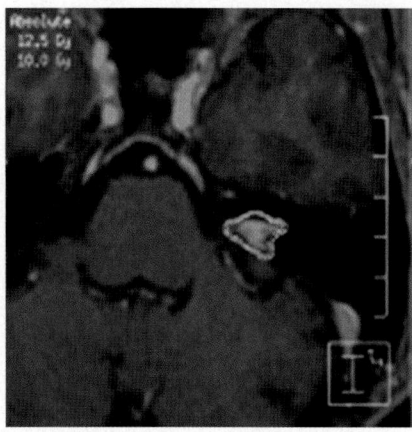 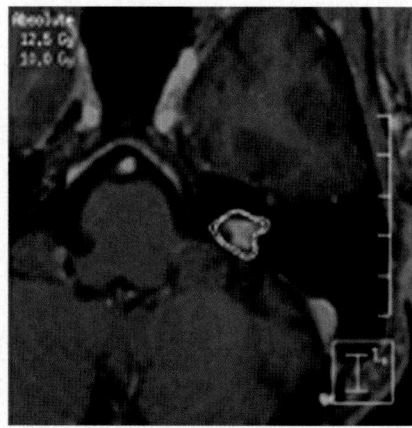

Figure 97.5 Example of radiosurgery dose distribution. This schwannoma is being treated with radiosurgery; the 12.5-Gy prescription isodose line conforms to the lesion.

SRS is disadvantageous because of a higher risk of toxicity, such as larger vestibular schwannomas or meningiomas.

SRS is used to treat a diverse group of lesions. Treatment can be carried out using either a modified or dedicated linear accelerator, cobalt-60 units, or charged particle devices. Several commercial devices have now been developed, each with slightly unique features, including robots that position the linear accelerator at various angles, collimation systems that provide prefixed circular collimators of various sizes or shaped collimated beams, and even intensity-modulated delivery from one or multiple directions, delivered serially, helically, or volumetrically.[73] Radiosurgery plays a dominant role in the treatment of oligometastases to the brain, arteriovenous malformations, schwannomas, and meningiomas and is occasionally used to treat malignant recurrences (Fig. 97.5).

Charged-particle beams, including protons (but not electrons), deposit the majority of their dose at a depth dependent on the initial energy, avoiding the exit dose of photon therapy. This localized dose is known as the *Bragg peak*. Historically, in order to cover larger volumes, proton beams have been modified by passive range modulators that disperse the Bragg peak and broaden the dose deposition, resulting in decreased proximal sparing, while still maintaining distal sparing. Charged-particle radiotherapy has been particularly utilized to treat tumors of the skull base to doses higher than can be achieved conventionally, and in reirradiation settings where conventional techniques are too unsafe. In particular, chordomas and chondrosarcomas require high radiation doses for local control. Proton beams have also been advocated for childhood tumors and tumors in young adults, because they decrease integral radiation dose, thereby decreasing the risk of second malignancies, although concern about incidental neutron production exists.[74,75] The neutron contamination issue is almost nonexistent with approaches similar to the photon technique of intensity modulation, often also referred to as intensity modulated proton therapy (IMPT) and allows for significantly superior *dose sculpting*. Increasingly, this approach is being utilized in patients with lower grade neoplasms of the CNS, where survival is anticipated to be in years, and where reduction in the volume of normal brain irradiated is likely to produce benefits in cognitive, functional, and endocrine domains.

Brachytherapy has historically been widely used, but currently has a limited role in the CNS, although it has enjoyed some resurgence and is occasionally used for recurrent gliomas. A liquid colloid of organically bound iodine-125 (^{125}I) in a spherical balloon continues to be used to treat both recurrent and newly diagnosed malignant gliomas and brain metastases in the postoperative context.[76] At least two randomized trials using seed implants have failed to demonstrate a survival advantage in malignant gliomas. The injection of radioisotopes within the cystic portion of

craniopharyngiomas allows ablation of the secretory lining. A select group of patients with cystic tumors may benefit from the direct instillation of colloidal phosphorus-32 (^{32}P), yttrium-90 (^{90}Y), or gold-198 (^{198}Au).[77,78] This technique will deliver between 200 to 400 Gy to the cyst wall.

Radiolabeled therapy is in the developmental phase. The most commonly used antigenic targets for CNS malignancies are the epidermal growth factor receptor (EGFR), neural cell adhesion molecule (NCAM), tenascin, placental alkaline phosphatase (PLAP), and phosphatidylinositide. Institutions using this technique have utilized murine, chimeric, or humanized monoclonal antibodies attached to ^{131}I, ^{90}Y, rhenium-188 (^{188}Re), and astatine-211 (^{211}At). The evolution of these trials has seen the delivery route move from systemic (intra-arterial or intravenous) to local instillation of the agent into a surgically created resection cavity. Even though the blood–brain barrier is often disrupted by a rapidly growing CNS malignancy, 150 kDa antibodies would still not likely cross to a significant degree.[79] Most of the trials to date are of *dose searching pilot* or phase I design. Using ^{131}I-81C6 (antitenascin monoclonal antibody), a trend toward significant improvement in median survival was shown for patients receiving 40 to 48 Gy versus less than 40 Gy.[80] Unlike seed brachytherapy, there appears to be a very low rate of CNS toxicity with targeted isotope therapy, and a minimal need for surgical intervention for the removal of necrotic regions.

CHEMOTHERAPY AND TARGETED AGENTS

Drug therapies alone are effective for only a few types of CNS tumors (e.g., primary CNS lymphoma) but are useful as adjunctive therapy for many CNS tumors. Among the reasons for the poor efficacy of chemotherapeutic and targeted agents is the low concentration of drug penetration to the tumor because of the difficulty of agents to cross the blood–brain barrier, active transport mechanisms of drug efflux, and high plasma protein binding of agents, thereby lowering the volume of distribution of agents in the brain parenchyma.[81] Intrinsic and acquired resistance remains an important reason for the lowered efficacy of chemotherapy. Although targeted agents are in early testing, multiplicity and alternate signaling pathways limit their efficacy.

The Blood–Brain Barrier

Central to treating CNS tumors is the issue of drug delivery, due to the blood–brain barrier (BBB), a physiologic and functional barrier. The CNS microvasculature has several unique features, including the lack of fenestrations between adjacent endothelial cells and relatively fewer pinocytotic and endocytotic endothelial vesicles. Additionally, adjacent BBB endothelial cells are connected by a continuous extension of tight junctions, which limit passive diffusion between endothelial cells and through capillary structures. Tight junctions within the BBB are also enveloped by astrocytic foot processes, which increase the barrier to passive diffusion across the BBB.

Brain microvasculature selectively transports nutrients through 20 or more active or facilitated carrier transport systems expressed on the endothelial surface.[82] The endothelium is rich with efflux pumps, including the multidrug resistance (MDR) gene–encoded P-glycoprotein that actively removes substrate molecules that may have passed the BBB.[83] There are several methods to disrupt or circumvent the BBB, including the intra-arterial administration of mannitol,[84] which has resulted in significant toxicities and thus have limited its universal use.[85] Noninvasive delivery systems using specialized carriers such as nanosystems (colloidal carriers) with favorable pharmacokinetic and pharmacodynamic properties are being explored.[86,87] Other methods include local administration (Gliadel wafer)[88] or local drug delivery such as convection-enhanced delivery (CED). CED requires the implantation of catheters directly into the brain, followed by continuous infusion of the drug under a constant pressure gradient. Proof of principle for CED has been demonstrated in several studies, but unfortunately, phase III results have been disappointing.[89,90] Another approach is the direct administration of the agent into the CSF. With a few exceptions (e.g., methotrexate, cytarabine, thioTEPA), most compounds cause unacceptable neurologic toxicity, including death, when given into the CSF. Because of this, intrathecal chemotherapy is principally used to treat leptomeningeal metastases and for CNS prophylaxis for high-risk leukemia.

Challenges Specific for Targeted Agents

Despite the availability of targeted agents specific to aberrant signaling pathways in high-grade gliomas, the results of phase II studies of many agents have been disappointing. In addition to the difficulty of delivery of agents across the BBB, there are other challenges that limit the efficacy of these agents. These include accounting for the heterogeneity of tumors, redundancy of pathway interactions, a lack of accurate and reproducible biomarkers to select patients for specific therapies, and difficulty in assessing target modulation.[91–93] Bayesian adaptive randomized designs in clinical trials may allow for more efficient trials compared to those with balanced randomization.[94]

Other Systemic Therapy Considerations

Many antiepileptic agents, including phenytoin, carbamazepine, and phenobarbital, induce the hepatic cytochrome P-450 isoenzyme and glucuronidation drug-elimination systems. The specific isoenzymes induced by these drugs are often capable of metabolizing many agents. For example, standard paclitaxel doses commonly result in subtherapeutic serum levels in patients also using phenytoin.[95] In fact, the maximally tolerated paclitaxel dose in patients using enzyme-inducing P-450 antiepileptics is nearly threefold higher than in patients not using such agents. Similar observations have been made with regard to 9-aminocampothecin, vincristine, teniposide, irinotecan, and targeted agents.[96–99] In addition to different maximal tolerated dose (MTDs) being established depending on the use of enzyme-inducing antiepileptics, the side effect profile and dose-limiting toxicities can also differ.[99,100] Most phase I clinical trials in brain tumor patients now use separate arms for patients who are or are not taking enzyme-inducing antiepileptic drugs or limit enrollment to patients not taking enzyme-inducing antiepileptic drugs. It may be preferable to change to a non–enzyme-inducing antiepileptic agent (e.g., levetiracetam [Keppra]), although it may take days to make the switch and some time for the P-450 enzyme induction to resolve.

SPECIFIC CENTRAL NERVOUS SYSTEM NEOPLASMS

Cerebral Glioma

Pathologic Classification

The histologic subtypes of gliomas include tumors of astrocytic, oligodendroglial, ependymal, and neuroepithelial origin (Table 97.2). Based on the WHO classification,[3] noninfiltrative gliomas are classified as grade I, and infiltrating gliomas are subsequently categorized from grades II to IV. Infiltrative astrocytic tumors are divided into three categories: astrocytoma (including grade II fibrillary, gemistocytic, and protoplasmic), anaplastic astrocytoma (grade III), and glioblastoma (including grade IV giant cell glioblastoma and gliosarcoma). Oligodendrogliomas and ependymomas are either grade II or anaplastic (grade III).

WHO Grade I: Astrocytoma

Low-grade astrocytomas (WHO grade I) such as pilocytic astrocytoma, pleomorphic xanthoastrocytoma, and subependymal giant cell astrocytoma are typically circumscribed and indolent tumors. Missense mutations of the V600E type in the v-RAF murine sarcoma viral oncogene homolog B1 (BRAF) gene were identified

TABLE 97.2

The Variety of Central Nervous System Glial Tumors (Based on 2007 World Health Organization Classification)

Astrocytic tumors
- Pilocytic astrocytoma
- Pilomyxoid astrocytoma
- Subependymal giant cell astrocytoma
- Pleomorphic xanthoastrocytoma
- Fibrillary astrocytoma
- Gemistocytic astrocytoma
- Protoplasmic astrocytoma
- Glioblastoma
- Giant cell glioblastoma
- Gliosarcoma
- Gliomatosis cerebri

Oligodendroglial tumors
- Oligodendroglioma
- Anaplastic oligodendroglioma

Oligoastrocytic tumors
- Oligoastrocytoma
- Anaplastic oligoastrocytoma

Ependymal tumors
- Subependymoma
- Myxopapillary ependymoma
- Ependymoma
- Anaplastic ependymoma

Choroid plexus tumors
- Choroid plexus papilloma
- Choroid plexus carcinoma

Other neuroepithelial tumors
- Astroblastoma
- Anaplastic astroblastoma
- Chordoid glioma of the third ventricle

in these noninfiltrative neoplasms.[101] The highest frequencies were found in pleomorphic xanthoastrocytomas (66%; 65% in its anaplastic variant), gangliogliomas (18%), and pilocytic astrocytomas (9%, especially in tumors with extracerebellar location).[101]

Complete surgical resection, whenever feasible, is the curative mainstay therapy for such tumors. Despite aggressive near total resection, delayed recurrence and eventual malignant transformation are, unfortunately, common. The resection of a low-grade glioma can be difficult in locations such as the optic pathway, hypothalamus, and in those involving deep midline structures. In these instances, asymptomatic patients can be observed carefully for a prolonged period of time and undergo a maximally safe resection only at the time of progression.

In patients who have a recurrent tumor that are not amenable to further resection or who have a residual tumor causing significant morbidity, adjuvant chemotherapy or radiotherapy can improve recurrence-free survival, although the role of chemotherapy in adults remains controversial. Immediate postoperative adjuvant therapies may be appropriate in some cases depending on the location of the tumor, the extent of residual disease, the impracticability of repeated surgical excision, and the availability for follow-up. Generally, radiotherapy is the primary adjuvant treatment used in older children and adults with low-grade gliomas. In young children with unresectable, progressive low-grade gliomas, there is a desire to avoid or delay radiotherapy owing to the long-term radiation-related sequelae; chemotherapy is often utilized here as the initial therapeutic option.[102–105] Some responses from chemotherapy can last for years, and nearly half of all children treated with chemotherapy ultimately require radiotherapy for tumor progression.

In terms of radiotherapy used with a curative intent, in children, the most common situation is with cerebellar and optic-pathway pilocytic astrocytoma, typically after progression on chemotherapy, whereas in adults, this tends to occur most commonly with hypothalamic pilocytic astrocytoma. The typical radiation dose used in this setting is 50.4 to 54.0 Gy, in 1.8 Gy fractions. There is evidence of improved PFS in this situation.[106] Given the young age and long expected survival of these patients, proton beam therapy is often considered for these patients, with the desire to decrease the risk of a second neoplasm, and to treat less normal brain tissue with radiation.[106]

Subependymal giant cell astrocytomas can be effectively treated with everolimus. In a prospective randomized study, 35% of patients in the everolimus group had at least a 50% reduction in the volume of their tumor versus none in the placebo group, although complete responses still remain uncommon, even with this therapy.[107]

WHO Grade II: Low-Grade Glioma

Nonpilocytic or diffusely infiltrating low-grade gliomas are classified as WHO grade II tumors. They may arise from astrocytic, oligodendrocytic, or mixed lineage. Like astrocytomas, oligodendrogliomas display various degrees of clinical aggressiveness. Three common genetic alterations, inactivation of the TP53 tumor suppressor gene, heterozygous point mutations of the isocitrate dehydrogenase-1 (IDH1), and loss of chromosome 22q are involved in the formation of WHO grade II astrocytoma. TP53, located on chromosome 17p, encodes the p53 protein that has an important role in a number of cellular processes, including cell cycle arrest, apoptosis, and response to DNA damage.[108]

Somatic mutations at codon 132 in IDH1 are present in 50% to 80% of WHO grade II and III astrocytic tumors and oligodendroglial tumors, as well as in secondary grade IV glioblastomas.[109,110] These IDH mutations promote the conversion of α-ketoglutarate into D-2-hydroxyglutarate, an oncometabolite that mediates the oncogenic activity of IDH mutations and can be measured by magnetic spectroscopy.[111] Tumors that have IDH mutations carry a better prognosis than do IDH wild-type gliomas of the same histologic grade.[112,113]

An unbalanced t(1;19)(q10;p10) translocation results in a combined loss of chromosomal arms 1p and 19q, which leads to the loss of one hybrid chromosome, and thus, a loss of heterozygosity.[114] This cytogenetic alteration is usually associated with oligodendroglial histology and is rarely found in other tumors. Patients with 1p- and 19q-codeleted tumors have a better prognosis than do histologically similar tumors of the same grade that do not harbor this codeletion.[115]

In addition to histology and molecular characteristics, several variables have been found to be of prognostic importance in low-grade gliomas. Pignatti et al.[116] performed the most comprehensive of these analyses and developed a scoring system to identify patients at varying level of risk for mortality. A multivariate analysis showed that age 40 years or older, astrocytoma histology, maximum diameter 6 cm or greater, tumor crossing the midline, and presence of neurologic deficits negatively impacted survival. Patients with up to two factors were considered low risk (median survival, 7.7 years) and patients with three or more were considered high risk (median survival, 3.2 years). Recently, 339 European Organisation for Research and Treatment of Cancer (EORTC) patients with central-pathology confirmed LGGs were used to develop a new prognostic model for PFS and overall survival (OS).[117] Data from 450 patients with centrally diagnosed LGGs recruited into two large studies conducted by North American cooperative groups were used to validate the models. Both PFS and OS were negatively influenced by the presence of baseline neurologic deficits, a shorter time since first symptoms, an astrocytic tumor type, and tumors larger than 5 cm in diameter.[117]

Surgery for Low-Grade Glioma

Retrospective analyses have suggested that the extent of resection is a significant prognostic variable. The Radiation Therapy Oncology Group (RTOG) performed a prospective evaluation of the natural history of completely resected low-grade gliomas (RTOG-9802), evaluating the recurrence risk in 111 patients with surgeon-defined gross total resections (GTR) and found that the extent of postoperative residual disease was an important variable for time to first relapse.[118] Five-year recurrence rates were 26% versus 68% for patients with less than 1-cm residual tumors versus 1- to 2-cm residual tumors.

Radiation Therapy

The role of radiotherapy—particularly the timing—remains somewhat controversial. Early intervention is indicated for patients with increasing symptoms and radiographic progression. In younger patients (less than 40 years) who have undergone complete resection, observation with imaging is an option. In RTOG-9802, median time to progression in 111 good-risk patients defined as younger than 40 years and with a gross total tumor resection was 5 years.[118] In those who have undergone a subtotal resection or those with high-risk features, postoperative radiotherapy may be recommended, typically 50.4 Gy in 1.8 Gy fractions.

Three phase III trials provide the best evidence with respect to the indications for radiotherapy as well as the dose. In a study by the EORTC (EORTC-22845), 314 patients were randomized to postoperative radiotherapy to 54 Gy (n = 157) or radiotherapy at progression (n = 157).[119] A statistically significant improvement in PFS was associated with early radiotherapy, 5.3 versus 3.4 years (p <0.0001), without a difference in median survival, 7.4 versus 7.2 years.

Two other trials investigated the dose question. In EORTC-22844, 379 patients were randomized to 45 Gy versus 59.4 Gy.[120] With a median follow-up of 74 months, OS (58% versus 59%) and PFS (47% versus 50%) were similar. In an Intergroup study, 203 patients were randomized to 50.4 Gy (n = 101) or 64.8 Gy.[121] There was no significant difference in PFS or OS.

To assess the OS and cause-specific survival (CSS) impact of early adjuvant radiotherapy (EART) following the resection of supratentorial LGG in adults (16 to 65 years), 2,021 patients in the SEER database from 1988 to 2007 were evaluated.[122] Of the 2,021 patients, 871 (43%) received EART, and 1,150 (57%) did not. In the multivariate Cox proportional hazards model, EART was associated with worse OS and CSS. Using a propensity score and instrumental variable analyses to account for known and unknown prognostic factors demonstrated unmeasured confounding variables that may affect this finding.

Consequently, low-dose radiotherapy, 50.4 to 54.0 Gy in 1.8 Gy fractions, has become an accepted practice for selected patients with low-grade gliomas. The target volume is local, with a margin of 2 cm beyond changes demonstrated on traditional MRI sequences. FLAIR images usually show considerable abnormality beyond any enhancing or nonenhancing tumor and whether a smaller margin may be used for planning if FLAIR sequences are utilized is unknown.

Posttreatment cognition remains an important consideration. Brown et al.[123] reviewed the results of the Mini-Mental Status Examination for 203 adults irradiated for low-grade gliomas. Most patients maintained stable neurocognitive status after radiotherapy, and patients with abnormal baseline results were more likely to have improvement in cognitive abilities than to deteriorate after therapy; few patients showed cognitive decline. A more in-depth analysis of formal neurocognitive testing suggest that the tumor itself may have the most deleterious effect on cognitive function.[124] Recognition has been gaining that long-term neurocognitive functional (NCF) impairment following radiotherapy for benign or low-grade adult brain tumors could be associated with hippocampal dose. A dose to 40% of the bilateral hippocampi greater than 7.3 Gy was recently shown to be associated with long-term impairment in list-learning delayed recall.[125] Based on such data, the role of proton therapy as a potential approach to reduce cognitive deficits and other side effects is being explored.

Chemotherapy

Low-grade gliomas have historically been considered chemotherapy resistant. With the recent demonstration of the chemotherapy responsiveness of some low-grade astrocytomas and oligodendrogliomas has renewed interest in investigating chemotherapy for low-grade gliomas.[126,127] It has been demonstrated that some low-grade gliomas, especially optic pathway and hypothalamic tumors, can be responsive to chemotherapy.[31,128] In children, various single and multichemotherapeutic and biological agents are effective at controlling the growth of a low-grade glioma in a setting of a newly progressive lesion, multiply recurrent, or unresectable residual tumors.[102–105,129,130] Platinum-containing regimens result in radiographic response rates greater than 60%.[129] Vinblastine has also demonstrated substantial activity in recurrent low-grade gliomas and is a commonly used second-line agent after treatment failure with vincristine and carboplatin.[131,132] Other second- and third-line therapies for multiply recurrent tumors include thioguanine, procarbazine, lomustine, and vincristine (TPCV) and temozolomide. Irinotecan and bevacizumab are currently being investigated in a multi-institutional phase II trial

for the treatment of progressive low-grade gliomas. Rapamycin, an oral immunosuppressive agent, has been effective at reducing the growth of astrocytomas associated with tuberous sclerosis.[133] Most of the chemotherapy responses seen in children with low-grade gliomas are for contrast-enhancing masses that probably represent pilocytic astrocytomas. Some of these responses can last for years, although nearly half of all children treated with chemotherapy ultimately require radiotherapy. Nonenhancing, diffusely infiltrating astrocytomas in children appear to be much less responsive to chemotherapy. Data on the use of chemotherapy for low-grade glioma in adults are sparse. In a small Southwest Oncology Group trial, adults with incompletely excised low-grade gliomas were randomly assigned to radiation therapy (RT) alone or RT and lomustine ([2-chloroethyl]-3-cyclohexyl]-1-nitrosourea [CCNU]). There was no difference in survival between the two arms.[134] The role of adjuvant procarbazine, CCNU, and vincristine (PCV) for high-risk patients (e.g., less than total resection, age older than 40 years) with low-grade gliomas was evaluated in RTOG-9802. From 1998 to 2002, 251 patients were randomly assigned to RT alone or RT followed by six cycles of PCV. An initial report of this study showed that the 5-year OS rates for RT versus RT/PCV were 7.5 years versus not reached respectively (hazard ratio [HR] = 0.72, 95% confidence interval [CI], 0.47 to 1.10; $p = 0.33$).[135] At the time of that report, however, 65% of the patients were still alive. A recent National Institute of Health press release on more mature results of this study reported significant improvement in OS in the PCV chemotherapy plus RT group (13.3 years) compared to those assigned to RT alone (7.8 years) at a median follow-up of 12 years.[136] Molecular and cytogenetic analyses (isocitrate dehydrogenase mutations and loss of heterozygosity of 1p and 19q, as well as methylation of methylguanine methyltransferase status) and clinical outcome are pending to identify predictive factors for patients with LGG.

Several studies have evaluated PCV in the recurrent setting, and, more recently, temozolomide has also been evaluated (Tables 97.3 and 97.4).[126,127,137–146] In general, approximately half of the patients treated with either temozolomide or PCV experienced imaging stability or improvement of neurologic symptoms. Although results are encouraging, the number of patients treated in these studies was small, and there are questions regarding the criteria used for radiographic response. In the first report of RTOG 0424, the primary endpoint was to compare the 3-year OS of a regimen of concurrent and adjuvant temozolomide and RT in a high-risk low-grade glioma population to the 3-year OS rate of the high-risk EORTC LGG patients reported by Pignatti et al.[116] With a median follow-up time of 4.1 years and a minimum follow-up of 3 years, MST has not yet been reached. The 3-year OS rate was 73.1% (95% CI, 65.3 to 80.8%), significantly improved in comparison to the prespecified historical control with a p value <0.0001.[147] An ongoing intergroup phase III trial is attempting to answer this issue more definitively.

Patients with low-grade oligodendroglial tumors with 1p/19q deletion or t(1p;19q) have longer PFS and OS than those without.[114] Consequently, 1p/19q determination is important in

TABLE 97.3

Procarbazine for Chemotherapy Naive Low-Grade Glioma

Author (Ref.)	Disease	N	Path	Enhancing (%)	Prior RT	RR (%)	1-Y PFS (%)
Stege et al.[140]	Recurrent	5	O, OA	0	Y	60	N/A
	Newly diagnosed	16		0	N	81	N/A
Buckner et al.[142]	Newly diagnosed	28	O, OA	46	N	52	91
Soffieti et al.[139]	Recurrent	26	O, OA	73	Y	62	80
Lebrun et al.[141]	Newly diagnosed	33	O, OA	18	N	27	N/A

CCNU (lomustine), and vincristine; O, oligodendroglioma; OA, oligoastrocytoma; RT, radiotherapy; RR, response rate; PFS, progression-free survival, N/A, not available.

TABLE 97.4						
Temozolomide in Low-Grade Glioma						
Author (Ref.)	**N**	**Path**	**Enhancing (%)**	**Prior RT/ Chemo**	**RR (%)**	**1-Y PFS (%)**
Quinn et al.[127]	46	A, O, AA	70	Y/Y	61	76
Pace et al.[138]	43	A, O, AA	60	Y/Y	47	39
Brada et al.[144]	30	A, O, AA	0	N/N	10	90
Hoang-Xuan et al.[126]	60	O, OA	11	N/N	31	73
Van den Bent et al.[143]	28	O, OA	100	Y/Y	25	11
Pouratian et al.[146]	28	O, OA	24	N/N	52	72
Murphy et al.[145]	13	O, OA	0	N/N	100	N/A
Van den Bent et al.[137]	39	O, OA	100	Y/N	53	40

A, astrocytoma; O, oligodendroglioma; AA, anaplastic astrocytoma; RT, radiotherapy; RR, recurrence rate; PFS, progression-free survival, N/A, not available.

patient counseling and in assessing the results of outcomes in future clinical trials. A randomized phase III EORTC trial stratified patients with low-grade glioma by 1p status prior to randomization to RT versus temozolomide.[148] In the initial results of the trial presented, PFS was not significantly different, and median OS was not reached. 1p deletion was a positive prognostic factor irrespective of treatment (PFS: 0.0003; HR = 0.59; 95% CI, 0.45 to 0.78); OS: 0.002; HR = 0.49; 95% CI, 0.32 to 0.77). First-line treatment with temozolomide compared to radiotherapy did not improve PFS in high-risk LGG patients. A molecular and genetic analysis of LGG has revealed aberrant signaling in the phosphatidylinositol-3-kinase (PI3K)/AKT/mammalian target of rapamycin (mTOR) network; however, a defined role for the inhibition of this pathway in the treatment of LGG remains to be established.[149,150] Targeting this pathway is a therapeutic approach that is being investigated in clinical trials in recurrent LGG patients.

WHO Grade III: Anaplastic Astrocytoma

Prospective and/or randomized evidence indicating that a complete resection of enhancing or an MRI-visible tumor improves survival is lacking, but retrospective analyses reaffirm that this relationship is likely to be present. Nonetheless, almost all of these tumors are characterized by postoperative residual microscopic disease, and radiotherapy is used adjunctively, resulting in a 3-year survival of approximately 55%.[151]

Radiation Therapy

Partial brain fields are used for the treatment of anaplastic astrocytoma; the initial gross tumor volume (GTV) is defined as the T2 or FLAIR abnormality; the boost GTV is defined as the contrast-enhancing volume or the surgical bed; for smaller, nonenhancing tumors, the initial and the boost GTV are often equivalent.[152] The clinical tumor volume (CTV) is defined as an approximately 2-cm margin surrounding the GTV, but not expanding across natural barriers. The initial volume is typically treated to 46 Gy, with the boost volume to 60 Gy. No survival advantage for the use of bromodeoxyuridine as a radiosensitizer was demonstrated.[153] Early versus delayed radiotherapy, utilizing chemotherapy as part of the regimen, was evaluated in a German phase III trial (NOA-04), which is described in the section that follows.

Chemotherapy

The role of chemotherapy remains controversial. Most phase III trials have demonstrated no benefit compared with radiation alone. Both single-agent carmustine and PCV are associated with minimal improvement in survival. Although, for a period of time, PCV was considered the "superior" regimen, database analyses have belied this claim.[151] A meta-analysis by the Glioma Meta-Analysis Trialists' group demonstrated an approximate 6% absolute increase in 1- and 2-year survival for patients who received chemotherapy (2-year survival of 37% versus 31%).[154] A large randomized trial by the Medical Research Council found no benefit of adjuvant PCV compared with RT alone.[155] Although temozolomide is effective for the treatment of recurrent anaplastic astrocytoma, its role as an adjuvant to RT has not been rigorously assessed. Based on these results in recurrent anaplastic astrocytoma, the RTOG initiated a phase III trial (RTOG 9813) to compare radiation with BCNU or CCNU to radiation with temozolomide, and the results are pending.

A comparison of the efficacy and safety of radiotherapy versus chemotherapy with either PCV or temozolomide as initial therapy on patients with newly diagnosed anaplastic glioma showed comparable results in terms of time to treatment failure.[156] Because of the potential prognostic and predictive value of hypermethylation of the O6-methylguanine DNA-methyltransferase (MGMT) promoter and mutations of the *IDH1* gene in malignant gliomas, analyses of these was a correlative part of the study.[110,157,158] Hypermethylation of MGMT promoter and mutations of the *IDH1* gene as well as oligodendroglioma histology reduced the risk of progression. Hypermethylation of MGMT promoter was associated with prolonged PFS in the chemotherapy and RT arms.

Difluoromethylornithine (DFMO), an inhibitor of ornithine decarboxylase, was evaluated in a phase III trial.[159] Of 228 patients, the majority had anaplastic astrocytoma. Following RT, patients were randomized to PCV or PCV plus DFMO. There was a difference in survival during the first 2 years, but this did not continue after 2 years.

Chemotherapy for Recurrent Anaplastic Astrocytomas

Chemotherapy for anaplastic astrocytomas that recur following radiation is of benefit, and both nitrosourea-based regimens and temozolomide have efficacy. The U.S. Food and Drug Administration (FDA) granted accelerated approval for temozolomide on the basis of its activity in recurrent anaplastic astrocytoma; the response rate was 35% for patients who had not received chemotherapy and 20% for patients who had received nitrosourea-based therapy.[160] Many patients are being treated with temozolomide early in the course of their illnesses; therefore, for recurrent anaplastic astrocytoma, nontemozolomide regimens used in glioblastoma are often considered.[161] Several clinical trials to evaluate targeted agents in recurrent malignant glioma often include recurrent grade III histology. Based on documented activity of the antivascular endothelial growth factor antibody in recurrent glioblastoma, this agent has also been used in patients with recurrent anaplastic astrocytoma.[162] A retrospective study reported a 64% radiographic response and a 6-month PFS rate of 60% in 25 patients.[163] Prospective studies are pending.

The NOA-04 phase III trial compared efficacy and safety of RT followed by chemotherapy at progression with the reverse sequence in patients with newly diagnosed anaplastic gliomas.[156] Patients received conventional RT: procarbazine, lomustine (CCNU), and vincristine, or temozolomide at diagnosis. At occurrence of unacceptable toxicity or disease progression, patients in the RT arm were treated with PCV or temozolomide, whereas patients in chemotherapy arms received RT. Median time to failure, PFS, and OS were similar for all arms. Hypermethylation of the MGMT promoter was associated with prolonged PFS in the chemotherapy and RT arm. This study showed that IDH1 mutations are a positive prognostic factor in anaplastic gliomas, with a favorable impact stronger than that of 1p/19q codeletion or MGMT promoter methylation.[156]

WHO Grade III: Anaplastic Oligodendroglioma

Surgery

Surgery retains its role as the principal modality of treatment, as with other glial neoplasms, and the maximum safe resection is considered the standard of care. However, the consideration of risks versus benefits of an aggressive surgical resection should take into account the 1p/19q deletional status of the tumor and the potential for a more favorable natural history and response to medical therapy.

Radiation Therapy

No randomized trials that focus only on these tumors comparing radiation versus no RT have been completed. In general, patients with pure and mixed anaplastic oligodendrogliomas receive postoperative irradiation to 60 Gy in conventional daily fractions of 1.8 to 2.0 Gy using an approach similar to that used for other malignant gliomas. Recent data show a categorical and very large survival benefit for both the 1p19q codeleted and the IDH-mutated anaplastic oligodendrogliomas treated with combination chemoradiotherapy, in comparison to RT alone. Therefore, up-front RT alone should not be the preferred treatment for these good prognosis patients. Conversely, no level 1 data exist to support treating these patients with up-front chemotherapy alone, either, and although this practice is sometimes adopted in practice, it should be subjected to rigorous clinical evaluation, because of the potential for the loss of long-term survivorship in these favorable patients, if either therapy is compromised. These results are described in greater detail in the section that follows.

Chemotherapy

Retrospective series and phase II trials first suggested that oligodendrogliomas are chemosensitive.[137,164,165] In two phase III trials, RT alone was compared with RT plus PCV. In the North American trial (RTOG 9402) patients received PCV for four cycles prior to radiation or no up-front PCV. Survival in the two groups was the same. Patients with 1p and 19q deletions had significantly better outcomes, regardless of treatment.[166] An unprespecified analysis of PFS demonstrated that the benefit from PCV was most notable in patients with 1p and 19q deletions. Long-term results of this study demonstrated that patients with codeleted tumors lived longer than those with non-codeleted tumors irrespective of therapy, and the median survival of those with codeleted tumors treated

with PCV plus RT was twice that of patients receiving RT (14.7 versus 7.3 years).[167] There was no difference in median survival for patients with tumors lacking 1p and 19q deletion.

In the European trial, patients received PCV or no immediate chemotherapy after radiation.[168] PFS was better in the PCV group, but OS was not different. Patients with 1p and 19q deletion had superior survival, regardless of treatment. A further molecular analysis of this cohort demonstrated that MGMT promoter methylation was of prognostic value.[169,170] Long-term follow-up showed that PFS and OS were better in the PCV group, but OS was not different between the two groups (OS in the RT/PCV arm, 42.3 months; in the RT arm, 30.6 months). In patients with a 1p/19q codeletion, there was a trend to more benefit from adjuvant PCV (OS not reached in the RT/PCV group versus 112 months in the RT group).[171] Both trials confirmed the prognostic value of 1p and 19q.

Temozolomide has produced high response rates in patients with anaplastic oligodendroglioma. In 27 newly diagnosed patients treated with temozolomide prior to radiotherapy, the objective response rate was 33% and the 6-month progression rate was 10%.[172]

Chemotherapy for Recurrent Anaplastic Oligodendroglioma

Prospective trials have demonstrated that approximately 50% to 70% of patients with anaplastic oligodendrogliomas that recur after RT respond to chemotherapy.[143] In a study of 48 patients with anaplastic oligodendroglioma/oligoastrocytoma who progressed on PCV, the objective response rate to temozolomide was 44%.[173] Although there is no evidence that the sequence of temozolomide and PCV is superior in terms of efficacy, the absence of cumulative myelosuppression with temozolomide argues for its use initially in the setting of recurrent disease.

Ongoing Clinical Trials for Newly Diagnosed Grade 3 Glioma

Two international trials are being conducted in patients with newly diagnosed grade 3 glioma stratified by 1p 19q status rather than histology. Nondeleted patients are randomized to radiation with or without temozolomide; following RT, there is a second randomization to adjuvant temozolomide or not. Codeleted patients are randomized to three arms, temozolomide alone (phase II group), RT with concomitant and adjuvant temozolomide, or RT with adjuvant PCV (phase III).

WHO Grade IV: Glioblastoma

Surgery

Gliomas are heterogeneous, and therapy is guided by the most aggressive grade in the specimen. Resection provides the best opportunity to obtain an accurate diagnosis. Studies have shown that more complete resections are more likely to provide a high-grade diagnosis and to detect an oligodendroglial component.[174] Two randomized trials of resection of malignant gliomas have been published. In a study by Vuorinen et al.,[175] survival was twice as long with resection compared to biopsy alone. Stummer et al.[63] reported that patients without residual contrast-enhancing tumor had a higher overall median survival time than did those with residual enhancing tumor (17.9 months versus 12.9 months, respectively; $p < 0.001$). Complete resection of an enhancing tumor enhances certain approved or investigational adjuvant therapies (e.g., carmustine wafers, immunotherapy). Resection also is superior to stereotactic biopsy alone for the provision of adequate tissue for the evaluation of molecular and cytogenetic classifications and certain prognostic markers (e.g., MGMT), which may be a requirement for entry into some clinical trials.

There has been extensive work in molecular subtypes of GBM in recent years that include a report of the Cancer Genome Atlas

Research Network[176] and follow-up transcriptome work of glioblastoma provided insights into the major structural and expression alterations that may drive disease pathogenesis and biology in glioblastoma.[177,178] Verhaak et al.[178] proposed a gene expression-based molecular classification of GBM into proneural, neural, classical, and mesenchymal subtypes. Aberrations and gene expression of EGFR, NF1, and platelet-derived growth factor receptor a (PDGFRA)/IDH1 were utilized to define the classical, mesenchymal, and proneural subtypes, respectively. These investigations into the genome and transcriptome reveal GBM as a heterogeneous collection of distinct diseases with multiple dependencies both within and across each particular subtype.[179]

Radiotherapy

Randomized trials have demonstrated a survival benefit with RT.[180] Localized radiation volumes are recommended based on evidence from several sources that GBMs typically recur locally, and the bulk of the infiltrative disease is within a few centimeters of the enhancing rim. However, the wide and somewhat unpredictable degree and direction of dissemination, which is not visualized well with any imaging technique, renders an RT field definition difficult. Outside of clinical trials, consensus regarding the exact field design remains difficult to obtain. In the large randomized trial RTOG 0525 for newly diagnosed GBM, which allowed both a single field treatment or a separate boost field to be utilized, no survival differences were identified, although the number of patients treated with the single field was rather small, in comparison (>80% versus <20%).[181]

Standard therapy uses a total dose of 60 Gy in 30 to 33 fractions based on dose response studies showing a survival improvement for 60 Gy compared to lower doses and without a benefit for higher doses.[182–215] For patients with poor prognostic factors and for those who are not able to tolerate conventional treatment, a shorter course may provide palliation. Older patients (older than 65 years), especially those with poor performance status, have been shown to have limited posttreatment improvement following conventional RT,[183] and several studies have not shown a significant survival difference using shorter courses.[184–218] A number of trials have evaluated the role of temozolomide versus RT in elderly patients with glioblastoma. The German phase III trial (NOA-08) randomized patients 65 years or older with anaplastic astrocytoma or glioblastoma with a minimum karnofsky performance status (KPS) of 60 to either temozolomide or radiotherapy. Of 412 patients who were randomized, 373 received at least one dose of treatment and were included in efficacy analyses. Median survival was 8.6 months in the temozolomide arm compared to 9.6 months with RT. These results met the criteria of "noninferiority" of temozolomide.[185] In an unplanned post hoc analysis, MGMT promoter methylation status was evaluated in 209 patients; promoter methylation was associated with longer OS (11.9 versus 8.2 months). Event-free survival was longer in patients with MGMT methylation who received temozolomide alone versus RT, whereas the opposite was true for patients without MGMT promoter methylation. Therefore, MGMT methylation seems to be a useful predictive biomarker and could aid decision making in elderly patients not fit to receive concurrent chemoradiation.

The Nordic three-arm phase III trial randomized elderly (>60 years) patients with glioblastoma to two different radiotherapy schedules of 60 Gy in 2 Gy per fraction (fxs) over 6 weeks or a hypofractionated schedule of 34 Gy in 3.4 Gy fxs over 2 weeks, versus temozolomide alone.[186] Median survival was significantly longer with temozolomide versus conventional RT (8.3 versus 6.0 months; HR, 0.70; $p = 0.01$), but not hypofractionated radiotherapy (7.5 months; HR, 0.85; $p = 0.24$). This trial suggests that both temozolomide alone and hypofractionated RT alone produce equivalent survival in elderly patients with glioblastoma, and both are superior to standard RT.

These trials did not address the issue of concomitant chemoradiotherapy for the elderly. An ongoing, phase III trial (EORTC

26062-22061 NCIC CTG CE6) compares the OS rates between short-course RT alone and short-course RT given together with temozolomide in newly diagnosed patients with glioblastoma who are older than 65 years of age and who are not fit for standard treatment. This study has completed accrual and results are pending.

Dose Escalation

In the pretemozolomide era, studies evaluating radiosurgery or brachytherapy boosts to conventional RT have not demonstrated a survival advantage.[222–225]

The feasibility and toxicity of dose-escalated photon radiotherapy concurrent with BCNU chemotherapy in patients with supratentorial GBM[187] was the goal of RTOG 9803. There were 209 patients who were enrolled and stratified into two groups based on the size of planned target volume (<75 mL versus ≥75 mL). Within each stratum, four RT dose levels were evaluated: 64, 72, 78, and 84 Gy; all treatments were delivered with a fraction size of 2 Gy. Acute and late grade ≥3 radiotherapy-related toxicities were no more frequent at higher RT doses or with larger tumors. No dose-limiting toxicities were observed at any dose level in either stratum, and as a result, the dose was escalated to 84 Gy in both strata. Median time to RT-related necrosis was 8.8 months (range, 5.1 to 12.5 months). This study demonstrated the feasibility and tolerability of photon dose escalation with an acceptable risk of late CNS toxicity with doses as high as 84 Gy. However, this study was conducted with concurrent BCNU chemotherapy, not the current standard approach of concurrent and adjuvant temozolomide. This chemoradiotherapy regimen has become the backbone of standard postoperative treatment for patients with GBM but has never adequately been tested in a RT dose-escalation or -intensification context. With this standard postoperative chemoradiotherapy regimen, the predominant pattern of failure remains local, highlighting the importance of investigating more intensive local therapies.

Recently, the University of Michigan published results of a clinical trial that escalated dose and dose-per-fraction from 66 Gy to 81 Gy in 30 fractions during chemoradiotherapy with temozolomide for patients with GBM.[188] The maximum tolerated dose with concurrent temozolomide was 75 Gy in 30 fractions (2.5 Gy per fraction). Median survival was 20.1 months, suggesting improved efficacy comparable to other contemporary studies. Interestingly, the probability of in-field failure decreased with increasing dose escalation, setting the stage for more definitive investigations of this approach. Small phase II studies of dose escalation using mixed photon/proton irradiation demonstrated median survival times of 20 to 22 months, and more formal comparative studies need to be performed.[244,245] Alternate particle radiation modalities used in the treatment of gliomas include neutrons, helium ions, other heavy nuclei such as carbon, negative pi-mesons, and thermal neutrons in conjunction with boronated compounds (boron neutron capture therapy). To date, most studies have been designed to determine optimal dose scheduling, efficacy, and safety.

Radiosensitizers and Radioimmunotherapy

Studies using various radiation modifiers such as hyperbaric oxygen, nitroimidazoles and tirapazamine, RSR-13, or carbogen and nicotinamide to overcome the hypoxia present in malignant gliomas have generally yielded disappointing results with no survival advantage.[228,232] Halogenated pyrimidines are incorporated into the DNA of dividing cells due to their biochemical similarity to thymidine. After being incorporated, cells are much more susceptible to single-strand breaks from radiation-induced free radicals and have impaired ability to repair DNA. Prospective clinical studies, however, have not demonstrated a survival advantage.[169] Motexafin gadolinium (MGd) is a redox-active drug that

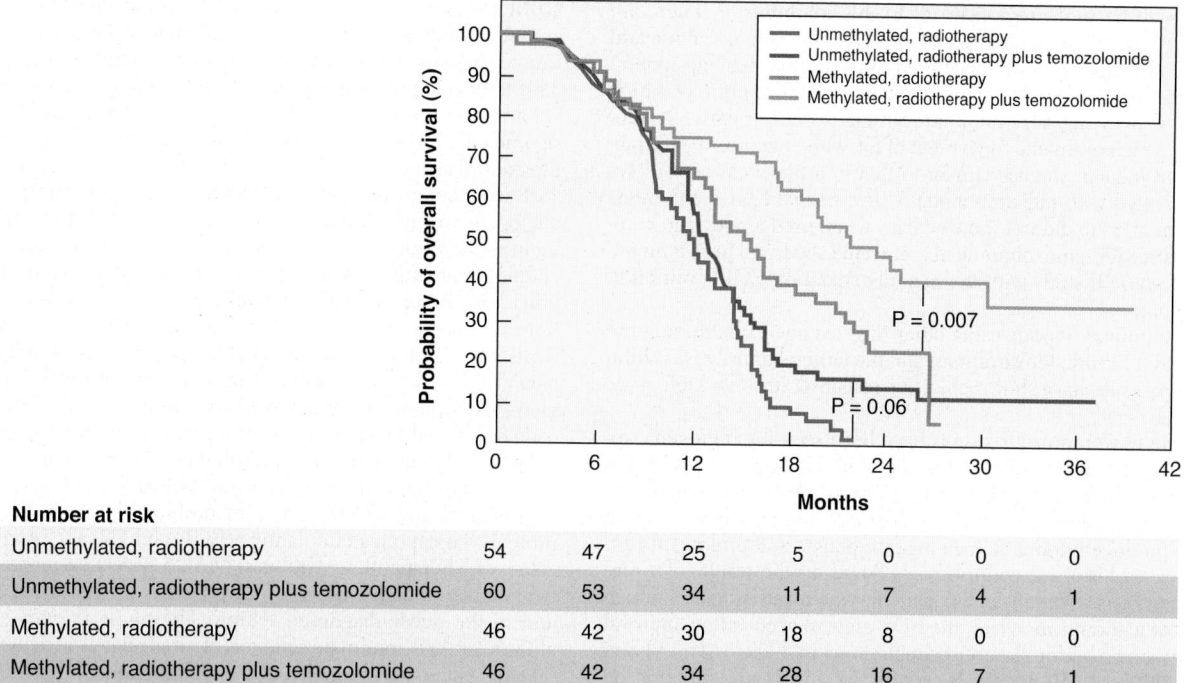

Figure 97.6 Kaplan-Meir survival curves for the two arms of the international glioblastoma trial, demonstrating a significant survival benefit from chemoradiotherapy, compared with radiotherapy. The patients are evaluated by methylguanine DNA-methyltransferase (MGMT) gene promoter methylation status, and the maximum survival benefit is seen in the combination arm when the gene promoter is silenced. (Redrawn from Hegi ME, Diserens AC, Gorlia T, et al. MGMT gene silencing and benefit from temozolomide in glioblastoma. *N Engl J Med* 2005;352:997.)

selectively accumulates in tumor cells. It is thought to sensitize tumors through the production of reactive oxygen species that destabilize cellular metabolism. A phase II RTOG trial did not demonstrate superiority in survival.[189] Studies of radiation synergistic cytotoxics such as the camptothecins or platinum agents also did not demonstrate a survival benefit.[235] Radioimmunotherapy, using various monoclonal antibodies against EGFR or tenascin tagged with ^{125}I have been evaluated.[237,238] These were small studies and demonstrated feasibility; however, randomized controlled studies have not been performed.

Chemotherapy

In a landmark international trial, patients were randomized to RT with or without concurrent and adjuvant temozolomide. Median and 2-year survival were increased by 2.5 months and 16.1%, respectively, in patients receiving temozolomide, and long-term follow-up showed a persistent survival benefit.[190] A companion correlative study demonstrated that methylation of the promoter region of the *MGMT* gene in the tumor was associated with superior survival, regardless of treatment received, but the benefit was maximal for methylated patients.[157] MGMT removes the methyl group from the O6 position of guanine, reversing the cytotoxic effects of methylating agents (such as temozolomide), making the tumor resistant to treatment, while methylation of the promoter region of *MGMT* results in inactivation of *MGMT*. MGMT status was strongly associated with survival (Fig. 97.6). Recognizing that a different schedule of temozolomide may overcome chemotherapy resistance, there have been several studies of alternative dosing of temozolomide both at the time of recurrence and in the newly diagnosed setting.[191,192] A large phase III randomized international study led by the RTOG compared the standard treatment versus a 21- or 28-day adjuvant temozolomide schedule.[181]

Dose-dense temozolomide failed to result in improved efficacy regardless of tumor methylation status but was associated with more profound lymphopenia and fatigue. Strategies to increase the therapeutic ratio of existing chemotherapies, such as the inhibition of DNA repair enzymes (i.e., poly[ADP-ribose] polymerase [PARP]) are being evaluated. These agents are being combined with radiation and chemotherapy to increase the cytotoxicity of the combination approach.[193–195]

Although nitrosourea-based chemotherapy is modestly effective for patients with GBM, its use has been supplanted by temozolomide. There is evidence that carmustine-impregnated wafers implanted into the brain at the time of resection provide modest improvement in outcomes in selected patients compared with patients who received placebo wafers.[196]

Chemotherapy for Recurrent Glioblastoma

Treatment options for recurrent GBM must be tailored to the individual. Few agents have proven activity. A randomized phase II trial of temozolomide versus procarbazine in 225 patients with GBM at first relapse demonstrated that treatment with temozolomide improved median PFS (12.4 weeks versus 8.3 weeks; $p < 0.006$). Radiographic responses were disappointing (5.4% versus 5.3%). Several agents such as the platinoids, taxanes, 5-fluorouracil (5-FU), and irinotecan have been tested, most demonstrating very little activity. In a review of eight clinical trials with 225 recurrent malignant gliomas, the 6-month survival was 15% versus 31% for GBM versus anaplastic astrocytoma.[197]

Targeted Therapies

As the genetic and molecular pathogenesis of gliomas is better understood, new targets are being identified and inhibitors of associated signaling pathways are being developed. One example is EGFR as a frequently deregulated signaling molecule in GBM, prompting phase I and II trials of erlotinib and gefitinib for recurrent high-grade gliomas. Both have shown limited activity[97,198–200] Patients whose tumors demonstrate the variant 3 mutant (EGFR-vIII), with resulting constitutive activation of EGFR tyrosine kinase activity, along with intact phosphatase and tensin analog (PTEN), appear to be more responsive to EGFR inhibitors.[201] There are two reports of the combination of erlotinib with radiation and chemotherapy for newly diagnosed glioblastoma showing modest additional benefit to standard radiochemotherapy, none of which show convincing survival improvement.[202,203] Similarly, RTOG 0211, which evaluated the benefit of RT with concurrent gefitinib, showed median survival similar to that in a historical control cohort treated with radiation alone.[204] Irreversible EGFR inhibitors such as afatinib did not show efficacy when used alone or in combination with temozolomide in recurrent GBM.[205] There is an ongoing phase II study with the second-generation EGFR inhibitor, dacomitinib.

Preliminary reports using other targeted agents, including the mTOR inhibitor, temsirolimus, and the farnesyl transferase inhibitor, tipifarnib, have shown objective responses in a few high-grade gliomas.[206-210]

The most promising results have been seen for angiogenic inhibitors. The most important mediator of angiogenesis in GBM is vascular endothelial growth factor (VEGF). Antiangiogenic therapies such as the anti-VEGF monoclonal antibody bevacizumab have produced dramatic radiologic responses and prolonged PFS relative to historical controls.[211,212] Based on the results of a randomized phase II study of 167 patients who received bevacizumab with or without irinotecan, the FDA granted accelerated approval to bevacizumab for recurrent glioblastoma in 2009.[162] The PFS at 6 months was 43% for single-agent bevacizumab and 50% for the combination arm. The objective response rates were 28% and 38% for the two arms, and median survival times were 9.2 months and 8.7 months, respectively. The most common side effects associated with bevacizumab include fatigue, headache, and hypertension; proteinuria and poor wound healing are also seen. The addition of chemotherapy or targeted therapy to bevacizumab has failed to show any added benefit in recurrent GBM trials, with the exception of the BELOB study, a three-arm multicenter randomized phase II study, in which 148 patients with recurrent glioblastoma were treated with bevacizumab alone, lomustine alone, or the combination of the two. Survival at 9 months was 38%, 43%, and 59%, respectively, and the PFS at 6 months was 16%, 13%, and 41%, respectively, in the three arms.[213] The value of the combination of bevacizumab and lomustine in recurrent GBM is currently being evaluated in EORTC 26101, which was initially a randomized phase II study modified into a two-arm phase III trial to address this question.

There are several reports of small single-arm phase II studies of the combination of bevacizumab with radiation and temozolomide in the newly diagnosed setting.[214] Two large randomized trials evaluated the addition of bevacizumab to the initial combined modality therapy of RT and temozolomide. In RTOG 0825, a randomized, double-blinded, placebo-controlled trial, the addition of bevacizumab to temozolomide and radiation resulted in a longer PFS that did not reach the preset level of significance (10.7 months versus 7.3 months; HR, 0.79). There was no difference in OS between two arms (16.1 versus 15.7 months; HR, 1.13).[215] Another phase III, placebo-controlled randomized trial (AVAglio study) in newly diagnosed glioblastoma showed that the addition of bevacizumab to radiation and temozolomide (experimental arm) significantly prolonged PFS (HR, 0.64; $p < 0.0001$; median, 10.6 versus 6.2 months) as compared to radiation and temozolomide (control arm).[216] However, the median OS was not significantly different in both arms. One-year OS was 72% and 66%, respectively ($p = 0.049$); 2-year OS was 34% and 30%, respectively ($p = 0.24$) in the experimental and control arm. Safety was consistent with known bevacizumab side effects, serious adverse events (AEs) (grade ≥ 3) were 28.7% versus 15.2% grade in the two arms.

As previously discussed, patients with MGMT-nonmethylated GBM have inferior outcomes as compared to those with MGMT-methylated GBM, and temozolomide is less effective in these patients. The open-label GLARIUS trial was a randomized, multicenter study of 170 patients in which MGMT-nonmethylated

GBM patients were randomized (2:1) to radiation with bevacizumab during RT followed by maintenance bevacizumab and irinotecan (experimental arm) compared to standard therapy with daily temozolomide during radiation followed by 6 cycles of temozolomide (control arm).[217] The PFS at 6 months rate of 71.1% was significantly higher in the experimental arm compared to 26.2% in the control arm ($p < 0.0001$ log-rank test).

Recognizing that tumors ultimately evade the effect of antiangiogenic agents through various mechanisms, other strategies include the evaluation of the combination of bevacizumab with chemotherapeutic and targeted agents, and the investigation of other VEGF-targeted agents. Batchelor et al.[218] reported a reduction in contrast enhancement and edema in 12 of 16 GBM patients who received cediranib (AZD2171), an orally administered pan-VEGF receptor inhibitor, with a median PFS of 3.7 months. However, a phase III randomized trial comparing the efficacy of cediranib failed to show any improvement in PFS with cediranib either as monotherapy or in combination with lomustine compared to lomustine alone in recurrent GBM.[219]

VEGF Trap (aflibercept), a recombinantly produced fusion protein that captures circulating VEGF and CT-322 (Angiocept, Adnexus Therapeutics, Waltham, MA), a pegylated recombinant peptide with a high affinity for VEGF was tested in the recurrent and in the newly diagnosed setting. The phase II study showed aflibercept had minimal evidence of single-agent activity in unselected patients with recurrent malignant glioma.[220]

Cilengitide (EMD121974), an integrin inhibitor that showed promise in the recurrent GBM,[221,222] was evaluated in two large, newly diagnosed studies. The first study, CENTRIC, a phase III trial investigated the role of cilengitide combined with the standard treatment for patients with newly diagnosed glioblastoma with MGMT promoter methylation.[223] The study failed to show any additional benefit with cilengitide in this patient population.[223] The other study, CORE, investigated the benefit of cilengitide in the unmethylated MGMT gene promoter in a multicenter, openrandomized phase II trial. There was suggestion of benefit of cilengitide with a median OS of 16.3 months in one of the cilengitide arms compared to the median OS of 13.4 months in the control group (HR: 0.69; $p = 0.033$). However, this drug is not being further developed.

The other antiangiogenic agents that have undergone investigation in recurrent glioblastoma include XL184, a multitargeted tyrosine kinase inhibitor that acts on the VEGFR, hepatocyte growth factor receptor (MET), and c-KIT; and enzastaurin, an inhibitor of protein kinase C-beta that targets VEGF as well as the mTOR pathway.[224] The initial results of these studies have shown similar or inferior outcomes to those reported with other agents.[224-226]

Other mechanisms of cell growth that are being targeted include epigenetic modulation through histone deacetylase inhibitors, the proteasome inhibitor bortezomib, and the glutamate receptor inhibitor talampanel.[227-229]

Gene Therapy Strategies

The efficacy and safety of a locally applied adenovirus-mediated gene therapy with a prodrug-converting enzyme (herpes simplex virus thymidine kinase; sitimagene ceradenovec) followed by intravenous ganciclovir was evaluated in 250 patients with newly diagnosed resectable glioblastoma. Temozolomide was not given in all patients. There was no evidence of a survival advantage to this approach.[230] Previous strategies have similarly been negative, and the challenges of adequate delivery of the virus and gene transduction into the tumor remain paramount.

Immunotherapies

Immunotherapeutic strategies targeting glioblastomas include recombinant immunotoxins, restoration of local and systemic immunosuppression, *one-size-fits-all*, and individualized autologous dendritic cell vaccines.[89,231-233]

Issues in Study Designs for Novel Agents

Several key issues confront the incorporation of new agents in the up-front management of malignant gliomas. First, there is the issue of defining the appropriate end point. In recurrent malignant gliomas, PFS is frequently employed, but because of insufficient evidence linking this to survival in newly diagnosed malignant gliomas, survival remains the gold standard. However, there is considerable heterogeneity in survival outcomes based on clinical and possibly molecular prognostic variables. An adequate staging system has never been developed. The RTOG has analyzed an extensive database of prospectively treated patients (primarily with surgery, radiotherapy, and alkylating chemotherapy), and using a statistical method known as recursive portioning analysis, has developed six prognostic groups, referred to as RTOG recursive portioning analysis classes I to VI. Patients can be segmented into classes using eight variables: age, histology, Karnofsky performance score, mental status, neurologic function, symptom duration, extent of resection, and radiotherapy dose. GBM patients fall in classes III through VI, and their median survival ranges from 4.6 months to 17.9 months (Table 97.5).[234]

GLIOMATOSIS CEREBRI

Gliomatosis cerebri is a rare condition with diffuse involvement of multiple parts of the brain (greater than two lobes). On MRI, there is typically diffuse increased signal on T2-weighted and FLAIR images and a low or absent signal in the affected areas on T1-weighted images (Fig. 97.7). Prognostic factors include age and histology as well as Karnofsky performance score. Treatment remains undefined and includes radiation and chemotherapy.[291–293]

OPTIC, CHIASMAL, AND HYPOTHALAMIC GLIOMAS

Clinical Considerations

Nearly all gliomas of the optic nerve and chiasm are discovered in patients younger than 20 and most occur in those under 10 years of age. Of patients with optic pathway glioma (OPG), 20% to 50% are affected by NF1.[235] Patients with NF1 are more likely to have

TABLE 97.5

Radiation Therapy Oncology Group Recursive Partioning Analysis (RPA) Classification: Survival by Class

RPA Class	Number of Patients	Median Survival (mos)	2-Year Survival (%)
I	139	58.6	76
II	34	37.4	68
III	175	17.9	35
IV	457	11.1	15
V	395	8.9	6
VI	263	4.6	4

lesions involving one or both optic nerves (anterior), whereas chiasmatic or hypothalamic (posterior) involvement is commonly seen among non-NF1 patients (sporadic). Lewis et al.[235] found that gliomas along the anterior visual pathway occurred in 15% of NF1 patients and were occasionally bilateral; 67% of these were neither suspected clinically nor obvious on ophthalmologic examination. In one series, 25% involved the chiasm alone, 33% the chiasm and hypothalamus, and 42% the chiasm and optic nerves or tracts.[236] Clinically, they cause loss of visual acuity (70%), strabismus and nystagmus (33%), visual field impairment (bitemporal hemianopsia, 8%), developmental delay, macrocephaly, ataxia, hemiparesis, proptosis, and precocious puberty. Funduscopic evaluation demonstrates a range of findings from normal optic discs, to venous engorgement, to disc pallor because of atrophy. Chiasmal tumors often grow to involve the hypothalamus, causing a diencephalic syndrome characterized by emaciation (especially in children between 3 months and 2 years of age), motor overactivity, and euphoria. In general, optic nerve gliomas have a better prognosis than those involving the chiasm, and tumors confined to the anterior chiasm have a better outcome than posterior chiasmal tumors.

The natural history of these tumors ranges from indolent growth or spontaneous regression (with NF1) to rapid progression or dissemination (with hypothalamic lesions).[237–239] Generally, the

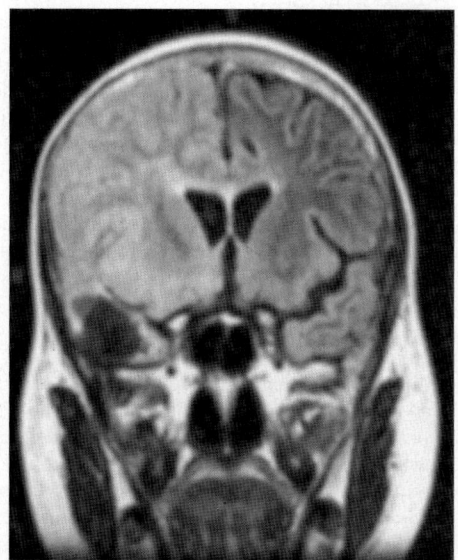
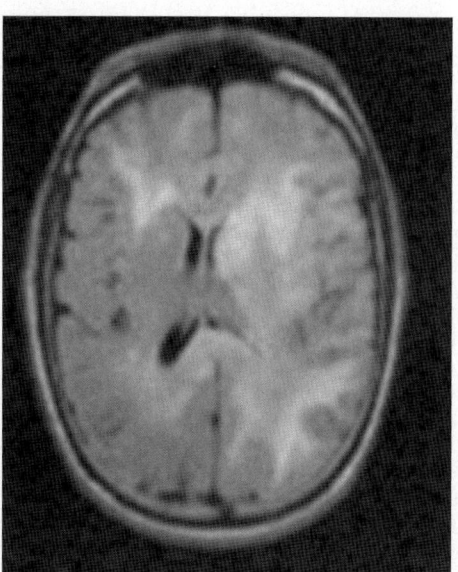

Figure 97.7 Two case examples of gliomatosis cerebri. Note the extensive changes visualized on fluid-attenuated inversion recovery (FLAIR) imaging, involving multiple lobes of the brain, and even an entire hemisphere.

PRACTICE OF ONCOLOGY

prognosis of OPG is good with overall 5-year survival rates ranging between 70% and 90%; however, the long-term morbidity is high.[239–242] NF1 and age less than 5 years at diagnosis have better PFS.[239,243]

Pathologic Considerations

Histopathologically, a majority of these tumors are low-grade gliomas, typically pilocytic or fibrillary astrocytomas. They range from primarily piloid and stellate astrocytes (most common), with or without oligodendroglia, through the gamut of malignant astrocytomas to GBM (rarely). Typically, optic gliomas appear as fusiform expansions of any part of the nerve. They may bridge through the optic foramen and expand as dumbbell tumors. The nerve can be infiltrated by tumor originating in the chiasm, the walls of the third ventricle, or the hypothalamus. A subset of optic pathway tumors can show the more aggressive pathologic variant of *pilomyxoid astrocytoma* as compared to the better known pilocytic astrocytoma.[244]

Imaging Findings

Diagnosis is best made by MRI, which demonstrates enlargement of the affected optic pathway, often with enhancement. The T2 signal may extend posteriorly along the optic tracts as far as the visual cortex, which may represent tumor infiltration or edema. Cysts and calcification are uncommon, but the hypothalamic component can be cystic.

Treatment Decision Making

In general, children with asymptomatic lesions of the optic pathways found by MRI are not treated unless clinical or radiographic progression is documented. Tumors in children with NF1 tend to be more indolent than sporadic tumors. Only one-third to one-half of children with NF1 with asymptomatic optic pathway tumors found on screening MRIs require treatment for increasing visual symptoms.[245] Most children with sporadic tumors undergo imaging because of symptoms and should be treated. Sporadic tumors often present with advanced findings such as hydrocephalus, decreased visual acuity, and endocrinopathies.[246] Rarely, both sporadic and NF-associated optic pathway gliomas can regress spontaneously.[238]

Surgery

Surgery is only rarely indicated for optic pathway gliomas. In appropriate patients, surgery may decrease the recurrence rate and increase the time to recurrence. Patients treated with surgery, followed by radiation and chemotherapy, appear to have the highest long-term control.[247] In patients with progressive symptoms (e.g., severe visual loss and proptosis), unilateral anterior tumors that do not involve the optic chiasm may be resected. Biopsy or subtotal resection can be performed for posterior optic pathway gliomas that involve the hypothalamus and optic tract, particularly if they are symptomatic because of local compression and mass effect. Resection of the chiasm is not indicated due to resultant bilateral blindness.

If the tumor involves the chiasm and the MRI raises suspicion of another tumor type, such as an optic nerve sheath meningioma or another parasellar mass, a confirmatory biopsy can be performed. This is rarely needed in patients with NF1, in whom there is a high index of suspicion for an optic nerve glioma. A subtotal resection is indicated if mass effect produces dysfunction of adjacent structures such as the hypothalamus or the nerve itself. Hydrocephalus can be produced by more posteriorly situated tumors and may be alleviated by debulking. If hydrocephalus persists after debulking, CSF shunting (which may need to be biventricular or require fenestration of the septum) becomes necessary. For unknown reasons, hydrocephalus is often persistent after the CSF pathways have been cleared, requiring the insertion of a CSF diversion device even after tumor removal.

Radiation Therapy

Untreated optic gliomas, especially those involving the chiasm or extending into the hypothalamus or optic tracts, progress locally or are fatal in 75% of patients. Tenny et al.[248] found that only 21% of patients who were followed after biopsy or exploration survived compared with 64% of those who received RT.

Routine postoperative irradiation is not indicated for gliomas confined to the optic nerve, which can be completely resected.[249] RT can prevent tumor progression, improve disease-free survival, and stabilize or improve vision in patients with chiasmal lesions, for whom postoperative residual is the rule. Wong et al.[250] reported that 86% of chiasmal gliomas not treated with RT progressed locally, whereas treatment failure occurred in 45% that underwent RT. Furthermore, control was achieved in 87% of the irradiated patients who received a dose of 50 to 55 Gy compared to 55% of those who received 46 Gy or less.

The prognosis for patients with optic nerve tumors may be better than for those with chiasmal-hypothalamic lesions. In a literature review, local control was found to be achieved for 154 of 189 irradiated anterior chiasmal tumors (81%), whereas 92 of 142 posterior tumors (65%) were controlled. Vision improved in 61 of 210 evaluable patients (29%) and remained stable in 118 of 210 patients (56%).[251] For chiasmal-hypothalamic tumors, RT produced radiographic shrinkage in 11 of 24 (46%) with a median PFS of 70 months compared with 30 months for patients who did not receive RT.[252] Age and tumor location were important prognostic factors, with younger children (less than 3 years), and children with lesions posterior to the chiasm faring less well after radiotherapy.

Three-dimensional conformal radiotherapy, IMRT, and stereotactic techniques are used to minimize the dose to adjacent structures. A report by Debus et al.[253] summarized results in patients treated with fractionated stereotactic radiation therapy (FSRT) (52.2 Gy median dose at 1.8 Gy per day).[253] All patients remained disease free, and no significant complications or marginal failures were seen despite highly conformal radiation fields. Because these tumors are often focal, techniques like FSRT can offer both excellent local control and decreased late effects.

Chemotherapy

In recent years, chemotherapy has played a pivotal role in the management of OPG in young children in order to spare the developing brain from the adverse effects of irradiation.[241,254–257] This is especially important in patients with NF1 who are at significant risk of developing vasculopathy such as moyamoya syndrome and secondary malignancy after receiving radiotherapy.[256,258] Retrospective series suggest that cognitive function is preserved better in children who receive initial chemotherapy compared with RT.[241,259] Although the appropriate agents are still evolving, vincristine plus carboplatin remains the most common first-line regimen.[128] Gnekow et al.[260] reported a 5-year PFS of 73% in 55 patients who were treated with this regimen. The randomized Children's Oncology Group A9952 study showed a 5-year PFS of 35% using carboplatin with vincristine and 48% using thioguanine, procarbazine, lomustine, and vincristine regimen in children with newly diagnosed progressive low-grade glioma.[261] Cisplatin-based regimens have shown responses between 50% and 60% and 5-year PFS of 50%.[262–264] Other studies have shown temozolomide to be effective.[265–267] Vinblastine has also been active in these tumors and is generally a second-line agent.[131,132] Collectively, these data suggest that chemotherapy is helpful in delaying tumor progression in a significant portion of children.

Whether chemotherapy alone can improve vision is controversial. Most studies in the literature lack objective data on visual outcome prior to and after chemotherapy. Moreno et al.[268] conducted a systematic review of eight reports and found only 14.4% of the children treated with chemotherapy had improvement in their vision. Due to the risk of second malignancy, alkylator-based chemotherapies are generally avoided in patients with NF1.

BRAINSTEM GLIOMAS

Clinical and Pathologic Considerations

Brainstem gliomas account for 15% of all pediatric brain tumors but are rare in adults. They can be divided into several distinct types. The diffuse intrinsic pontine gliomas (DIPG) tumors are generally high-grade astrocytomas, either anaplastic astrocytomas or GBM. Completely separate, and clinically distinct are the focal, dorsally exophytic or cervicomedullary lesions that are usually low grade with a better prognosis. Although rare, ependymomas, PNETs, and atypical teratoid-rhabdoid tumors also occur in the brainstem. Nonneoplastic processes that may be confused with a brainstem tumor include neurofibromatosis, demyelinating diseases, arteriovenous malformations, abscess, and encephalitis.

The diagnosis of a DIPG is usually based on a short history of rapidly developing neurologic findings of multiple cranial nerve palsies (most commonly VI and VII), hemiparesis, and ataxia. The initial manifestations of a brainstem glioma are unilateral palsies of cranial nerves VI and VII in approximately 90% of patients. The classic MRI finding is diffuse enlargement of the pons with poorly marginated T2 signal involving 50% or greater of the pons (Fig. 97.8).[269] Most are nonenhancing; in children, enhancing lesions could have either a pilocytic or malignant component; in adults, enhancement is worrisome for a malignant glioma.[270] Cervicomedullary tumors are nonenhancing, well-circumscribed lesions with an exophytic component. Tectal gliomas are nonenhancing and enlarge the tectal plate, often expanding it into the supracerebellar cistern with associated hydrocephalus. Overall, the prognosis is poor for patients with DIPG, with few patients surviving longer than 1 year.[271]

Surgery

Complete resection is almost never possible for the majority if brainstem tumors, and even a biopsy is restricted because of substantial morbidity and mortality.[272,273] In most centers, biopsy of DIPG is not undertaken for very typical cases. Stereotactic needle biopsy can be performed if atypical imaging findings or clinical characteristics suggest another diffuse brainstem disorder. Resection has no place in the treatment of diffuse pontine gliomas in children or adults. For the rare focal astrocytic lesions of the adult or pediatric brainstem, surgery may play a larger role. Tectal gliomas have a typical imaging appearance, and biopsy is neither necessary nor safe. However, the accompanying noncommunicating hydrocephalus (from compression of the aqueduct of Sylvius) can be treated with CSF diversion, either by third ventriculocisternostomy or by ventriculoperitoneal shunting.[274] Dorsally exophytic astrocytomas within the fourth ventricle or at the cervicomedullary junction are often partially resectable with low morbidity and excellent long-term results.[275] These dorsally exophytic brainstem tumors arise from the substance of the pons and are very dangerous to resect in totality. Because many of them will remain indolent after partial resection, complete removal at the first surgery is likely not warranted and associated with severe neurologic deficits. Intrinsic astrocytomas or ependymomas at the cervicomedullary junction can often be completely removed through a posterior midline approach.[276] In a retrospective review of 28 patients with juvenile pilocytic astrocytoma of the brainstem treated with resection in 25 cases and biopsy in 3,[277] the 5- and 10-year PFS rates were 74% and 62%, respectively, after gross total resection or resection with linear enhancement and 19% and 19%, respectively, when solid residual tumor was present, suggesting that long-term survival after resection of these tumors may relate to the extent of initial excision.

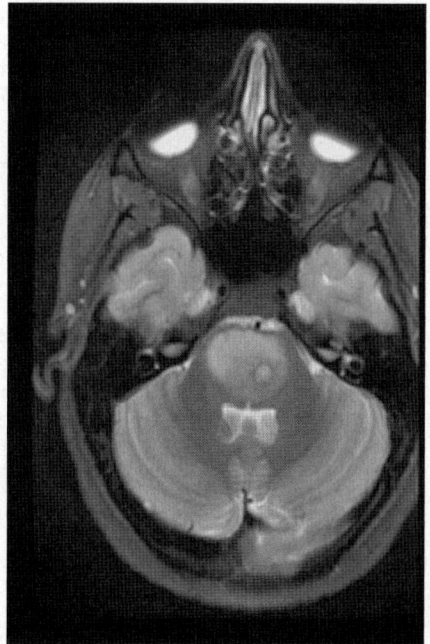
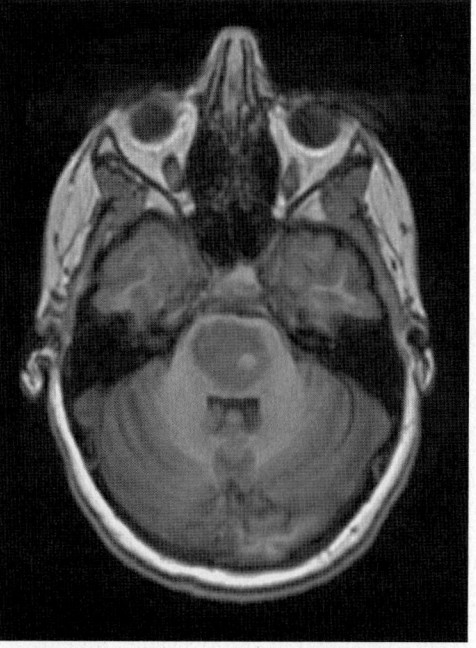

Figure 97.8 Typical magnetic resonance appearance of a diffuse pontine glioma. Diffuse enlargement of the pons is visualized on the T2-weighted image **(A)**; a small amount of hemorrhage is visualized on the noncontrast T1-weighted image **(B)**.

Radiation Therapy

RT, the primary treatment for brainstem tumors, improves survival and can stabilize or reverse neurologic dysfunction in 75% to 90% of patients. The GTV is usually best defined using T2-weighted or FLAIR MRI. A margin of 1.0 to 1.5 cm is added to create a CTV. These lesions should be treated to 54 to 60 Gy using daily fractions of 1.8 to 2.0 Gy. In a multi-institutional survey by Freeman and Suissa,[278] the 1-, 2-, and 5-year survival rates of children treated with conventional RT techniques were 50%, 29%, and 23%, respectively. Hyperfractionation, designed to deliver higher tumor doses, has been evaluated, without a significant survival advantage (median survival, 8.5 months versus 8.0 months for conventional versus hyperfractionated regimens).[279] Several drugs, such as topotecan, and motexafin-gadolinium have been investigated as radiosensitizers, without clear evidence of benefit, and therefore, the role of sensitizers remains investigational.

Fewer data exist with respect to brainstem glioma in adults, but there is some evidence that these tumors may be less aggressive in adults, with OS that ranges from 45% to 66% at 2 to 5 years, perhaps because of a greater frequency of more favorable tumor types.[280] In the series from ANOCEF, 48 adult patients with brainstem gliomas were grouped on the basis of their clinical, radiologic, and histologic features.[270,281] Nearly half had nonenhancing, diffusely infiltrative tumors and had symptoms that were present for longer than 3 months. Eleven of these 22 patients underwent biopsy, and 9 had low-grade histology. Nearly all underwent radiotherapy and had a median survival of 7.3 years. A second group of 15 patients who had presented with rapid progression of symptoms and had contrast enhancement on MRI were described. Fourteen of these patients underwent biopsy, and anaplasia was identified in all 14 specimens. Despite radiotherapy, the median survival in this group was 11.2 months, which approximates the survival in pediatric series.

Chemotherapy

Despite numerous clinical trials, there is no clear evidence to show increased survival for patients with DIPG who receive radiation and chemotherapy as compared to radiation alone. The recent discovery that the majority of DIPGs harbor mutations of lysine 27 (K27) in the histone 3.3 gene (so called K27M mutations) may allow for the development of targeted therapies.[282,283] Similarly, a subset of DIPGs have amplifications of receptor tyrosine kinase family members (i.e., PDGFR-α) suggesting other avenues to targeted therapy.[284] Clinical trials using temozolomide during and after RT have not shown improvement in the outcome.[285–287] Thus, no agent used either during or after radiation treatment has been shown to have benefit over radiation alone.

CEREBELLAR ASTROCYTOMAS

Clinical and Pathologic Considerations

Cerebellar astrocytomas, which occur most often during the first 2 decades of life, arise in the vermis or more laterally in a cerebellar hemisphere. They are usually well circumscribed and can be cystic, solid, or some combination of both. It is not uncommon to have a small tumor (mural nodule) associated with a large cystic cavity.

Histologically, most are low-grade pilocytic astrocytomas that lack anaplastic features. In a series of 451 children, cerebellar astrocytomas accounted for 25% of all posterior fossa tumors, and 89% of the 111 cerebellar astrocytomas were low grade.[288] Approximately 75% of these tumors are located only in the cerebellum, with the remainder involving the brainstem as well. Because these tumors usually arise in the vermis or median cerebellar hemisphere, the clinical presentation is similar to that of medulloblastoma, with

truncal ataxia, headache, nausea, and vomiting. In infants, head enlargement from hydrocephalus is seen. The majority of cerebellar pilocytic astrocytomas have an oncogenic fusion gene (KIAA1549-BRAF) that results in the activation of the BRAF oncogene, and which might be a rational target for future therapy.[289,290]

Surgery

Gross total resection is tantamount to a cure for these lesions.[291,292] In most cases, incomplete removal should be managed by conservative monitoring because the majority of remnants will not grow, will remain low grade, and are easy to remove if they progress in the future.

Radiation Therapy

Nearly all completely resected cerebellar astrocytomas do not require RT. Even when they progress, repeat resection is reasonable if a majority of the tumor can be removed. Only in the most exceptional circumstances would RT be necessary for the treatment of child with a true cerebellar pilocytic astrocytoma.

Chemotherapy

In general, chemotherapy is not indicated. Based on the experience with optic pathway gliomas, several of which have pilocytic features, carboplatin has been used for recurrent tumors.[293,294] There is limited experience with the use of temozolomide in this setting. High-grade gliomas that arise in the cerebellum are treated with regimens identical to their supratentorial counterparts.

GANGLIOGLIOMAS

Clinical and Pathologic Considerations

Gangliogliomas, along with pilocytic astrocytomas, pleomorphic xanthoastrocytomas, and subependymal giant cell astrocytomas, are considered *astroglial variant* forms of low-grade gliomas.[295] They are more circumscribed than diffuse low-grade gliomas, are classified as grade 1 or 2, and do not typically invade the normal brain. Because they less frequently progress to higher grade lesions, surgery alone is often curative. Gangliogliomas are more common in children than adults. They are the most common neoplasms to cause chronic focal epileptic disorders, and they typically arise in the temporal lobe but may also occur in the brainstem, spinal cord, and diencephalon.[296] They may include a cystic component, and the solid portion is free of normal brain parenchyma. Unlike diffuse low-grade gliomas, gangliogliomas enhance on MRI scans. They contain both glial and neuronal elements. The glial elements, which stain for glial fibrillary acidic protein, are almost always astrocytic and often pilocytic, but fibrillary astrocytes are also common. The glial elements dictate whether the lesion is grade 1 or 2. The neurons in the tumor are neoplastic and are characteristically large and relatively mature (i.e., they contain ganglion cells). The presence of neoplastic neurons may be confirmed by immunostaining for neuron-specific enolase and synaptophysin. Grade 2 lesions have rarely been observed to progress to a higher grade.[297,298]

Surgery

Surgical resection is directed at removal of the contrast-enhancing portion of the tumor. Nevertheless, although lesions located within eloquent brain regions are resectable, they may present significant surgical challenges because the boundary between tumor and functional brain may be difficult to define, even with the aid of modern surgical adjuncts (e.g., operating microscope, computer-assisted navigation, functional brain mapping). Although no phase 3 prospective studies have documented the superiority of surgery over other approaches (e.g., radiotherapy), retrospective studies have indicated that complete resection is associated with a very favorable long-term survival.[297–299] Resection of gangliogliomas also can result in seizure control.[300] Grade 2 gangliogliomas may recur, and some patients do poorly. The degree of anaplasia determines the prognosis.

Radiation Therapy

Because resection has the potential to cure most of these lesions, radiotherapy is generally reserved for subtotally resected cases or for recurrences.[301] It is also used for lesions in complex locations where further resection may result in significant morbidity. To determine the optimal strategy for gangliogliomas, Rades et al.[302] conducted a literature-based retrospective study of more than 400 patients treated for ganglioglioma. They examined four different treatment strategies (GTR or subtotal resection [STR] with or without radiotherapy) in 402 patients identified from reports published between 1978 and 2007. Surgery was found to be the mainstay of therapy, with 209 patients undergoing GTR and 193 undergoing STR. Adjuvant radiotherapy was used in 101 patients (20 following GTR and 81 following STR). Patients who underwent GTR had higher rates of OS and PFS than individuals who underwent STR. For patients undergoing GTR, the 10-year rates of local control and OS were 89% and 95%, respectively, better than the 52% and 62% observed for patients undergoing STR. This indirectly indicates that GTR is the most effective treatment strategy for gangliogliomas. For patients undergoing STR followed by postoperative radiotherapy, the 10-year rate of local control was 62%, better than the 52% for patients undergoing STR without postoperative radiotherapy; although the 10-year survival also improved from 65% to 74% with the use of postoperative radiotherapy in patients with subtotally resected tumors, this did not reach statistical significance. For the 40 patients undergoing STR for whom radiotherapy details were known, local recurrence was observed in 6 of 22 (27%) receiving 54 Gy, compared to 7 of 18 (39%) receiving greater than 54 Gy, implying no specific dose–response relationship.

Chemotherapy

Chemotherapy for gangliogliomas is generally reserved for young children who have undergone subtotal resection and who demonstrate disease progression. In older patients, it is typically used as salvage therapy to treat recurrent tumors after the failure of surgery and RT. In general, for astroglial variants such as gangliogliomas, no optimal chemotherapeutic regimens have been defined, and most researchers consider disease stabilization (rather than a complete tumor response) to be a successful outcome.

EPENDYMOMA

Clinical and Pathologic Features

Ependymomas were originally thought to arise from the ependymal cells lining the cerebral ventricles and the vestigial central canal of the spinal cord as they resemble this tissue under the microscope, although more recently it has been accepted that they arise from radial glial cells, a type of CNS stem cell.[303,304] Ependymomas can arise throughout the nervous system, and are usually divided into those from the supratentorial, infratentorial (posterior fossa), and spinal regions. Those in the spinal region are broken down into the intramedullary lesions and the myxopapillary ep-

endymomas of the conus medullaris and cauda equine. Although these tumors look very similar under the microscope (histology), they are demographically, clinically, transcriptionally, and genetically distinct and should not be regarded as the same entity.[304,305] More recently, it has been shown that there are two clear groups of posterior fossa ependymoma, the posterior fossa type A (PFA) tumors and the posterior fossa type B (PFB) tumors.[306,307] PFA tumors occur in young children (infants), are more likely to be lateral (CP angle), and have a terrible prognosis. PFB tumors are diagnosed in older children, found in the midline, and have a much better prognosis than PFA tumors. Figure 97.9 shows the typical magnetic resonance appearance of a midline, the posterior fossa ependymoma. In the past, much was made of the pattern of anaplasia in ependymoma histology, with the diagnosis of anaplasia taking an ependymoma from WHO grade II to WHO grade III. More recently, a number of luminaries in the field of neuro-oncology have shown that the intra- and interobserver reliability in the diagnosis of anaplasia in ependymoma is very high and its clinical utility is, therefore, very limited.[308]

Clinical presentation depends on location. Tumors with ventricular involvement often cause increased ICP and hydrocephalus by obstruction of CSF pathways. Headaches, nausea and vomiting, papilledema, ataxia, and vertigo are frequent. Focal neurologic signs and symptoms are seen with supratentorial ependymomas that involve the parenchyma. The presence of calcification in a fourth ventricular tumor on CT is very suggestive of an ependymoma. Supratentorial parenchymal tumors cannot be readily distinguished from other gliomas by imaging. Posterior fossa tumors in infants that protrude below the foramen magnum are more likely to be ependymomas, as are posterior fossa tumors that cause a head tilt (due to compression of the XIth cranial nerve as it crosses the foramen magnum).

Metastatic dissemination of ependymomas occurs in the leptomeningeal space in a similar pattern to that seen in medulloblastomas, albeit at a much lower rate (<5% of patients at presentation).

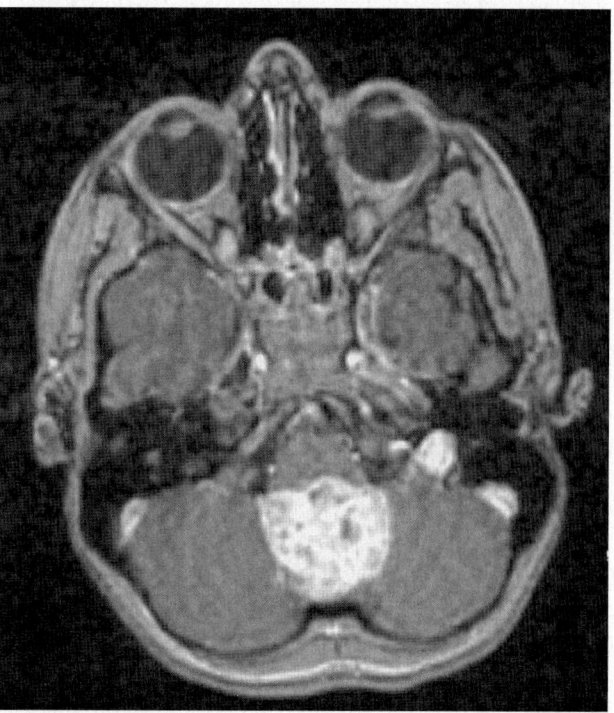

Figure 97.9 Typical magnetic resonance appearance of a posterior fossa ependymoma. The tumor arises from the floor of the fourth ventricle and rapidly expands to occupy it, and compresses the pons/medulla ventrally and the vermis of the cerebellum dorsally. The enhancement is typically heterogenous.

This low rate of observable dissemination at diagnosis has lead to the almost universal use of local, rather than craniospinal radiotherapy at diagnosis for patients with ependymoma.

Subependymomas are benign tumors with an admixture of fibrillary subependymal astrocytes. They are distinct from subependymal giant cell astrocytomas, which occur in the lateral ventricles in tuberous sclerosis. Subependymomas occur most often in the floor or walls of the fourth ventricle in older men. Most are asymptomatic and slow growing, and treatment is rarely needed except for hydrocephalus or demonstrated growth. They are often incidentally found at autopsy.

Surgery

Several retrospective studies support the relationship between postsurgical residual ependymoma and a poorer outcome, and therefore, maximal safe resection is the goal.[309–311] These tumors may also extend through the foramen of Luschka, entangling the cranial nerves in the basal cisterns, which also precludes a complete resection. The less common supratentorial tumors are removed as with any glioma. Avoidance of bleeding into the ventricular system is important to prevent postoperative hydrocephalus.

Radiation Therapy

Postoperative irradiation improves the recurrence-free survival of patients with intracranial ependymomas, and 5-year survival rates with doses of 45 Gy or more range from 40% to 87%.[152] Therapeutic utility of local radiation is established for ependymoma patients, even in infants.[312] Because local failure usually dominates the recurrence patterns, low-grade supratentorial ependymomas are typically treated using partial brain fields with a dose of approximately 54 Gy. Low-grade infratentorial ependymomas are also treated using limited fields. The best survival results in retrospective series have been shown for patients who undergo gross total resection followed by radiotherapy.[374,375] For most patients, a more usual volume consists of the tumor bed and any residual disease plus an anatomically defined margin of 1 to 1.5 cm to create a CTV. Larger margins may be required in areas of infiltration, and special attention must be paid to areas of spread along the cervical spine because 10% to 30% of fourth ventricular tumors extend down through the foramen magnum to the upper cervical spine.[313,314] Patients with neuraxis spread (positive MRI or positive CSF cytology) should receive craniospinal irradiation (40 to 45 Gy) with boosts to the areas of gross disease and to the primary tumor to total doses of 50 to 54 Gy.

Chemotherapy

There is no evidence that any type of chemotherapy improves survival in children with ependymomas.[315] Single-agent carboplatin, cisplatin, and etoposide, as well as multiagent chemotherapy, have been evaluated in small series and, to date, few if any drugs have shown even modest consistent activity in ependymomas.[377–380]

Although a complete removal of the ependymoma has a positive impact on the outcome, a complete resection is achieved in only 40% to 60% of cases.[316,317] Therefore, responsiveness to preirradiation chemotherapy was investigated in a Children's Oncology Group (COG) study where an objective response rate of 58% to preirradiation chemotherapy, consisting of cisplatin, etoposide, cyclophosphamide, and vincristine, in children with incompletely resected ependymoma was seen.[383] The 3-year event-free survival in patients assigned to preirradiation chemotherapy because of incomplete resection was 58% and was comparable to those who had a complete resection and were assigned to irradiation alone. However, 15% of the children who received preirradiation

chemotherapy experienced progression prior to RT. Therefore, a subsequent COG study was carried out that aimed to decrease the progression rate prior to radiotherapy by employing a strategy of *second-look* surgery following the preirradiation chemotherapy in children with residual disease. In this study, patients who had a complete resection of a differentiated supratentorial ependymoma were observed without any further therapy. The results of this study are pending. The recently opened randomized COG study is exploring whether maintenance chemotherapy following radiation will improve event-free survival and OS.

The primary application of chemotherapy, therefore, is investigational, and it is within the realm of neoadjuvant therapy to improve resectability, as primary adjuvant therapy in young children to delay radiotherapy and as possible salvage. In the Baby Pediatric Oncology Group study, a 48% response rate was reported to two cycles of vincristine and cyclophosphamide in 25 children younger than 3 years of age with ependymoma, allowing a delay in radiotherapy by 1 year without impacting the outcome.[318] However, the use of chemotherapy to delay radiotherapy has to be approached cautiously. In a trial of 34 patients with anaplastic ependymoma, 25 patients relapsed relatively rapidly and only 3 patients who did not receive radiotherapy survived.[319]

Despite multimodal therapy, 50% of the patients with ependymoma will experience a relapse. The majority of the recurrences are local, and prognosis is poor after relapse.[320] Resection, reirradiation, and chemotherapy are the common treatment modalities for relapsed ependymoma. Various antineoplastic agents such as etoposide, cyclophosphamide, temozolomide, cisplatin, and irinotecan have failed to improve survival in these patients.[287,321,322] Novel therapies to target molecular pathways are currently under investigation.

MENINGIOMAS

Clinical and Pathologic Considerations

Meningiomas are believed to arise from epithelioid cells on the outer surface of arachnoid villi in the meninges, also known as *arachnoidal cap cells*. The most frequent locations are along the sagittal sinus and over the cerebral convexity (Fig. 97.10). Meningiomas are extra-axial, intracranial, and sometimes intradural—extramedullary spinal tumors that produce symptoms and signs through the compression of adjacent brain tissue and cranial nerves. They often also produce hyperostosis; bony invasion does not indicate malignancy. They rarely metastasize except after multiple resections when they may spread to the lung, where growth is typically slow.

The WHO categorizes this tumor into three grades.[4] Benign (WHO grade I) meningiomas comprise about 70% to 85% of intracranial primaries. With appropriate treatment, approximately 80% of WHO grade I meningiomas remain progression free at 10 or more years.[323] Atypical (WHO grade II) meningiomas account for 15% to 25% of patients. These have greater proliferative capacity, and a seven- to eightfold increased recurrence risk within 5 years.[324] Only about 35% patients with WHO grade II meningiomas remain disease free at 10 years. About 1% to 3% of intracranial meningiomas are anaplastic (WHO grade III). These aggressive malignant tumors have a median OS of less than 2 years.[325]

Surgery

The goal is total resection, including a dural margin, because this is often curative for WHO grade I tumors. The risks of resection must be balanced against the advantages of less-aggressive removal because these tumors are typically slow growing, and the patients are sometimes elderly. Observation is appropriate for some, especially small tumors that are incidentally discovered. In a series of 603 patients who had asymptomatic meningiomas that were

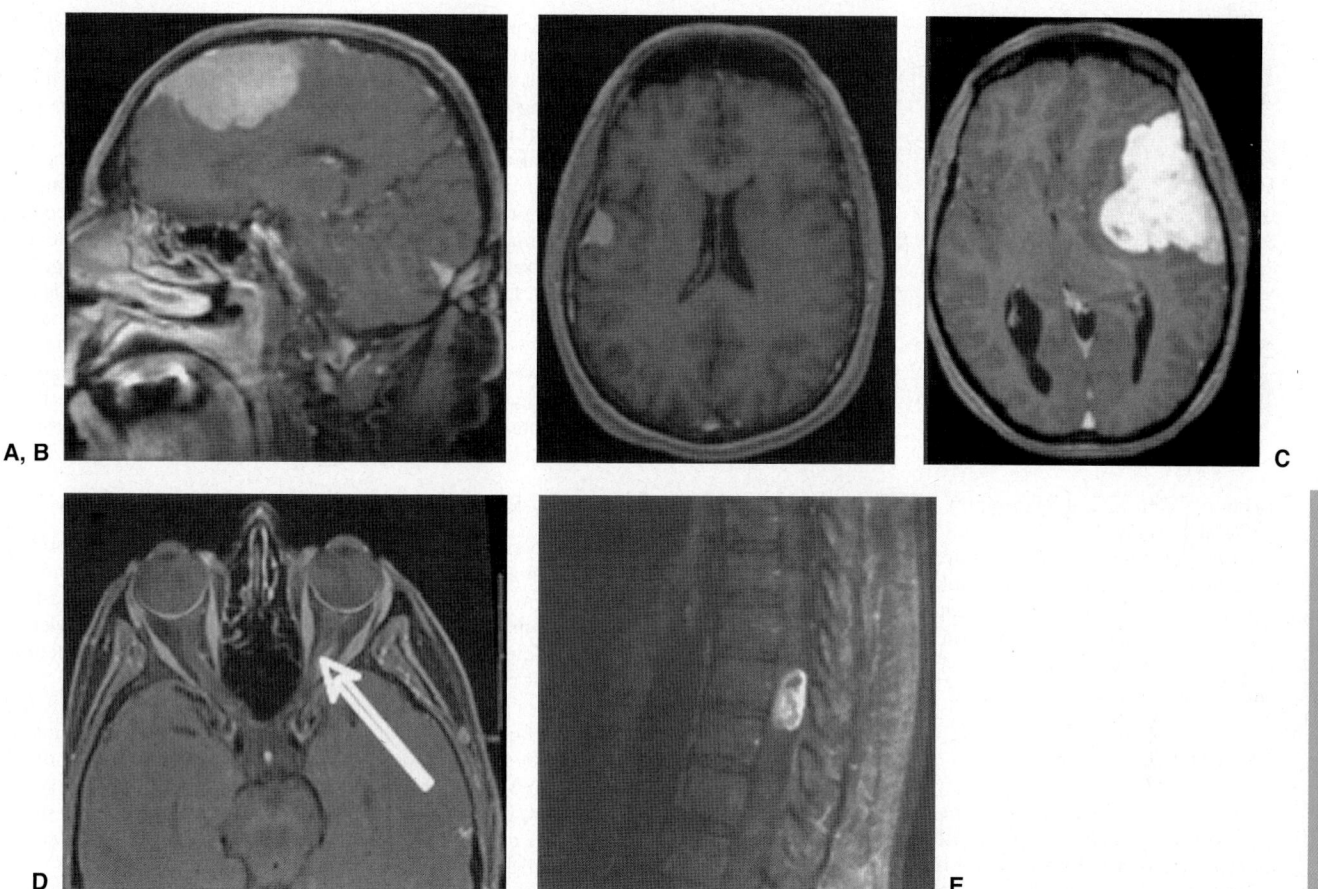

Figure 97.10 These five images show various appearances of meningioma. The most common location is parasagittal **(A)**. Some meningiomas remain small **(B)**, whereas others achieve a massive size with midline shift **(C)**. An optic nerve meningioma (*arrow*) is illustrated in **(D)**, whereas spinal locations are also possible **(E)**.

treated conservatively, Yano and Kuratsu[325] found that approximately 63% exhibited no growth, and only 6% ultimately experienced symptoms. However, a subsequent study of 244 patients with 273 meningiomas indicated that T2 hyperintensity, lack of calcification, size greater than 25 mm, and edema are associated with a shorter time to progression, and those tumors should be followed more closely.[326]

Preoperative Planning

Meningioma surgery requires a detailed knowledge of surgical anatomy. A preoperative angiogram to assess vascularity and to identify or embolize surgically inaccessible feeding arteries is sometimes indicated. Typically, embolization is done within 24 to 96 hours of surgery so that collateral vascular supply to the tumor does not develop. Normally, only the vascular supply from the external carotid artery can be embolized safely. In meningiomas that receive more than 50% of their blood supply from this artery, Kai et al.[327] found the optimum interval between embolization and surgery to be 7 to 9 days, which allowed the greatest degree of tumor softening. For convexity and parafalcine tumors, preoperative imaging may be performed to allow for the use of a neuronavigation system to aid in planning the scalp incision and bony opening.

Simpson Grades of Resection

The completeness of surgical removal is a crucial prognostic factor, and historically, the definitions provided by Donald Simpson have served as a useful guideline.[328] By following 470 patients during a 26-year span, he described five *grades of resection* based on recurrence. A grade 5 resection refers to a biopsy only and is

associated with near-universal progression. A partial tumor resection is labeled Simpson grade 4 and is associated with a recurrence rate of 44%. A Simpson grade 3 resection refers to gross total resection of the tumor, without addressing hyperostotic bone or dural attachments, and is associated with a 29% rate of relapse. A Simpson grade 2 resection includes gross tumor removal, and the dural attachments are either removed or coagulated and the relapse rate drops to 19%; and finally, when hyperostotic bone is also removed for a Simpson grade 1 resection, the relapse rate is 9%.

This definition has subsequently been expanded to include a category referred to as grade 0 resection. Kinjo et al.[329] reported on 37 convexity meningioma patients who underwent gross total resection of the tumor, any hyperostotic bone, and all involved dura with a 2-cm dural margin, and observed no local recurrences, with over half of the patients followed beyond 5 years; this is now widely termed the grade 0 resection. However, apart from convexity primaries, resection to this extent is usually not feasible in other locations.

The likelihood of gross total resection varies considerably among primary sites, with convexity lesions most amenable to complete resection and skull-base lesions least likely to be completely resected. In most surgical series, at least a third of meningiomas reported are not fully resectable.[330]

Recurrence Following Resection

Gross total resection for benign meningiomas remains the preferred treatment and is generally considered definitive. Three large series with extended follow-up are available (Table 97.6). These have remarkably similar rates of local recurrence after gross-total

TABLE 97.6

Recurrence After Gross Total Resection Alone of Meningioma

Study (Ref.)	Number of Patients	Local Recurrence Rate (%)		
		5-Y	10-Y	15-Y
Mirimanoff et al.[330]	145	7	20	32
Stafford et al.[333]	465	12	25	—
Condra et al.[331]	175	7	20	24
Total	**785**	**7–12**	**20–25**	**24–32**

resection: 7% to 12% at 5 years, 20% to 25% at 10 years, and 24% to 32% at 15 years.[330–333]

As expected, recurrence following subtotal resection is more frequent. Outcomes following subtotal resection alone, from four single institutions with up to 20 years of follow-up, are available. Collectively, the rates of progression following subtotal resection at 5, 10, and 15 years are 37% to 47%, 55% to 63%, and 74%, respectively.[330–333]

Radiation Therapy

Given the long natural history of meningiomas and the relatively late recurrences, radiotherapy has not been routinely adopted in the adjuvant context. Further, there is a paucity of clinical trials on which to base recommendations. However, in almost every retrospective series, cohort comparisons suggest that radiotherapy leads to a decrease in recurrence, and some suggest possible survival improvement.

The need for adjunctive RT is determined by the extent of resection, tumor grade, patient age, and performance status. The risk of recurrence following resection has been outlined previously. In general, it is common practice to not use adjunctive radiotherapy after Simpson grade 0, 1, 2, and sometimes 3 resection for grade 1 meningioma.

The risk of relapse after subtotal resection is high.[330–333] Several reports, now numbering over 60, suggest that postoperative irradiation prolongs the time to recurrence. As an illustrative series, Goldsmith et al.[334] reported the results for 140 patients (117 with benign and 23 with malignant tumors) treated with subtotal resection and postoperative irradiation. For patients with benign meningiomas, the 5- and 10-year PFS rates were 89% and 77%, respectively. Patients who received at least 52 Gy had a 20-year PFS rate of greater than 90%. The 5-year PFS of patients treated after 1980 was 98%, compared to 77% for those treated prior to 1980. This improvement was attributed to the availability of cross-sectional imaging for tumor localization and 3-D treatment planning. The size of the residual tumor as well as grade can affect the outcome after radiotherapy. Connell et al.[335] showed that for tumors 5 cm or larger, the 5-year PFS rate was 40%, significantly lower than the 93% observed for smaller tumors. Among patients irradiated for unresectable tumors and in those with residual disease, the volume of visible tumor on imaging studies rarely decreases by more than 15% and often only after many years.

Radiation Therapy for Anaplastic and Malignant Meningioma

Atypical and malignant meningiomas behave more aggressively. Goldsmith et al.[334] reported a 5-year PFS of 48% for 23 patients treated by subtotal resection and irradiation. The recurrence rate among 53 patients with malignant meningiomas collected from six series in the literature was 49%. The recurrence rates were 33% for patients treated with complete resection alone, 12% for those undergoing complete resection and RT, 55% for patients treated by subtotal resection and irradiation, and 100% for those treated by subtotal resection alone.[336] However, other studies in the literature do not categorically support a reduction in local failure with the use of adjuvant radiotherapy for gross totally resected G2 meningioma, and given that the patients referred for this therapy are often selected because of a variety of one or more negative prognostic factors, compared to the cohort of patients that is observed, conclusions regarding the precise value of postoperative radiotherapy for G2 totally resected meningioma remain nonuniform. However, most data suggest that all patients with malignant G3 meningiomas, regardless of the extent of resection, and those with subtotally resected G2 meningioma should be offered postoperative irradiation.[337,338]

Primary Radiotherapy

RT has been used as primary treatment following biopsy or on the basis of imaging findings alone in several small series. An early report from the Royal Marsden Hospital found 47% disease-free survivorship at 15 years in 32 patients.[339] In a recent series, Debus et al.[340] noted no recurrences in patients treated by radiotherapy alone (n = 59).

Optic nerve sheath meningiomas are rare tumors, generally not resected, but treated with radiotherapy as primary management. Narayan et al.[341] found no radiographic progression in any of 14 optic nerve sheath meningioma patients treated with conformal radiotherapy, with more than 5 years of median follow-up. In a study by Turbin et al.,[342] RT alone provided more favorable outcome than observation or surgery alone.

Radiation Dose and Volume Considerations

For benign meningiomas, the planning target volume consists of the residual tumor with a modest margin of normal tissue, defined by MRI and modified by the neurosurgeon's description of the site of residual disease. Extensive tumors of the base of the skull and malignant meningiomas require more generous margins, with special attention to dural extensions toward and through the skull foramina. The preoperative tumor volume is used for planning for completely resected malignant lesions. A dose of 54 Gy in daily fractions of 1.8 Gy is recommended for benign meningiomas, and 60 Gy or higher for atypical and malignant tumors. Complex 3D-CRT treatment planning and delivery techniques and IMRT are used to restrict the dose to normal tissues.

Radiosurgery

Numerous retrospective reports describe the use of radiosurgery for small meningiomas, either residual or progressive after resection, or untreated, skull-base lesions. Local control rates range from 75% to 100% at 5 to 10 years. Complications such as cranial neuropathies, transient neurologic deficits, radiation necrosis, and significant edema have been reported in 6% to 42% of patients treated with radiosurgery.[343,344] Complications are more frequent in patients with large or deep-seated tumors and in those treated with high single doses.[345,346] Fractionated radiotherapy may be preferable for larger tumors.

Chemotherapy

There is currently no defined role for chemotherapy for newly diagnosed or nonirradiated meningiomas. Chemotherapy is generally reserved for recurrent meningioma not amenable to further surgery or radiotherapy. Responses are anecdotal, with no drug or a combination yielding consistent responses. Because many meningiomas express estrogen and progesterone receptors, there have been unsuccessful attempts to use agents such as tamoxifen or antiprogesterones.[347,348] Preliminary data suggest that hydroxyurea[349,350] or interferon-alpha-2B (IFNα-2B)[351] may have activity; however, assessment of efficacy is limited by small numbers of patients treated. Targeted agents such as STI-571 (imatinib), angiogenesis inhibitors such as sunitinib, vatalanib, and EGFR inhibitors have been evaluated, without clear efficacy.[352–355]

PRIMITIVE NEUROECTODERMAL OR EMBRYONAL CENTRAL NERVOUS SYSTEM NEOPLASMS

These tumors of putative embryonal origin predominantly arise in children and include supratentorial PNETs, pineoblastomas, medulloblastomas, ependymoblastomas, and atypical teratoid or rhabdoid tumors. They are characterized by sheets of small, round, blue cells with scant cytoplasm. Historically, small round cell tumors arising in the posterior fossa were called *medulloblastomas*. Given the cytologic similarity between all these tumors regardless of location, it was suggested in the 1980s that they all be designated as PNETs. Although still controversial, the current WHO classification retains medulloblastoma as a distinct type of PNET within the larger group of *embryonal* tumors that includes medulloepitheliomas, neuroblastomas, and ependymoblastomas. Pineoblastomas also retain a separate position within the category of pineal parenchymal tumors. Regardless of formal classification, these tumors are viewed as developmentally aberrant early neural (glial or neuronal or both) progenitor or stem cell neoplasms.

Embryonal tumors with abundant neuropil and true rosettes (ETANTR) are a recently identified variant of PNET and, histologically, have features of ependymoblastomas and neuroblastomas, demonstrating areas of fine fibrillary neuropils intermingled with ependymoblastic rosettes and zones of undifferentiated neuroepithelial cells. ETANTRs are distinguished pathologically from other embryonal tumors by the striking abundance of neuropils.[356]

Recent data have shown quite clearly that medulloblastomas, supratentorial PNETs, atypical teratoid rhabdoid tumor (ATRTs), ETANTRs, and pineoblastomas probably all represent very distinct entities, each with their own biologies and indeed, in many cases, their own biologically important subgroups.[357–363]

Medulloblastoma

Epidemiology

Medulloblastomas comprise 15% to 30% of CNS tumors in children and an estimated 350 to 400 cases are diagnosed in the United States annually.[4] There is a 1.5:1 male-to-female predominance, and 70% are diagnosed by age 20 years. Medulloblastomas become progressively more rare with increasing age, with few cases found in those older than 50 years.[364,365] Gorlin and Turcot syndromes have increased rates of medulloblastoma, but account for only 1% to 2% of medulloblastomas.[29,366]

Pathology

Classically, medulloblastomas have Homer-Wright (neuroblastic) rosettes, although these are found in less than 40% of the cases.[367] Mitoses are frequent, representing a high proliferative index. Immunohistochemical analyses are positive for synaptophysin, which is most prominent in nodules and within the centers of the Homer-Wright rosettes, correlating with a presumed neuronal progenitor origin.[368] According to the last round of WHO classification, medulloblastomas are histologically grade IV and classified into five variants: classical, desmoplastic/nodular, medulloblastoma with extensive nodularity, anaplastic, and large cell.[4] The desmoplastic subtype has collagen bundles interspersed with the densely packed

undifferentiated cells of the classic subtype as well as nodular, reticulin-free "pale islands," or follicles.[369] Medulloblastomas with extensive nodularity are similar to the desmoplastic variant except that the reticulin-free zones are large and rich in neuropil-like tissue. Anaplastic medulloblastomas are relatively rare, accounting for approximately 4% of cases, and have marked nuclear pleomorphism, nuclear moulding, cell-cell wrapping, and high mitotic activity, with a high degree of atypia.

More recently, it has become agreed upon and apparent that, in fact, medulloblastomas are comprised of at least four different molecular subgroups (Wnt, Shh, Group 3, and Group 4), each with their own demographic, clinical, epidemiologic, transcriptional, genetic, and epigenetic features.[359–361,363,370] Because targeted therapies are likely to only be effective within a single subgroup, the next group of clinical trials will likely be subgroup specific.

Radiographic and Clinical Features

Childhood medulloblastomas typically arise within the vermis, expanding into the fourth ventricle. In older patients, tumors in the lateral cerebellar hemispheres are more common (greater than 50% in adults compared with 10% in children).[364]

Clinical signs and symptoms depend on both age, with infants having less specific symptoms, and the anatomic location within posterior fossa. Midline tumors usually present with symptoms of increased intracranial pressure, including nocturnal or morning headaches, nausea and vomiting, irritability, and lethargy—manifestations of progressive hydrocephalus from fourth ventricle compression. Truncal ataxia may be present because of involvement of the vermis, and sixth nerve palsies are the most common nerve deficit. In younger children, a bulging of open fontanelles may occur. Tumors of a lateral origin more frequently have ataxia and unilateral dysmetria. On CT, medulloblastomas are classically discrete vermian masses that are hyperattenuated compared with the adjacent brain and enhance avidly. Imaging variance is common, with frequent cyst formation and calcification (59% and 22% of cases, respectively).[371] MRI is the gold standard. Medulloblastomas are typically iso- to hypointense on T1-weighted images, of variable signal intensity on T2-weighted images, and enhance heterogeneously.[372] MRI provides improved evaluation of foraminal extent beyond the fourth ventricle, invasion of the brainstem, and subarachnoid metastases. Diffusion-weighted images exhibit restriction, allowing PNETs to be distinguished from ependymomas.[373,374]

Staging and Risk Groups

A modified version of the Chang staging system is currently used.[375] T stage has been made less relevant than the extent of residual disease due to advances in neurosurgical techniques. M stage remains crucial. M0 represents no tumor dissemination, whereas M1 represents tumor cells in the CSF. M2 represents presence of gross tumor nodules in the intracranial, subarachnoid, or ventricular space, and M3 represents gross tumor nodules in the spinal subarachnoid space. M4 represents systemic metastasis.

Clinical staging requires the assessment of tumor dissemination and includes CSF cytologic examination. This is frequently not performed prior to surgery because of concern for cerebellar herniation from increased pressure within the posterior fossa. Ventricular fluid is not as sensitive as lumbar fluid in detecting dissemination within the neuraxis.[376] Negative CSF cytology does not preclude more advanced leptomeningeal disease.[377] An MRI examination of the spine has supplanted conventional myelography. CSF dissemination is identified on MRI scans as diffuse enhancement of the thecal sac, nodular enhancement of the spinal cord or nerve roots, or nerve root clumping, predominantly seen along the posterior aspect of the spinal cord based on CSF circulatory patterns.[372] Spine MRI is ideally performed prior to surgery if a medulloblastoma is suspected and the patient is stable; otherwise, 10 to 14 days should elapse after surgery to avoid a potential false positive interpretation from surgical cellular debris and blood products.[378] Metastases outside the CNS are less common and occur in less than 5% of patients and correlate with advanced disease within the neuraxis. Eighty percent of systemic metastases are osseous. A bone scan, chest x-ray, and bilateral marrow biopsies should be routinely performed for M2 and M3 stages.

Patients with medulloblastomas are currently classified as *average* or *high risk* based on age, M stage, extent of residual disease, and pathology. Average-risk patients have M0 stage arising within the posterior fossa, are more than 3 years old, and have less than 1.5-cm tumor residual. Due to the poor prognosis, all patients with anaplastic medulloblastoma are classified as high risk.[379,380] Patients less than 3 years old have particularly poor prognoses. This may represent the presence of more primitive, aggressive tumors, but could also be due to the higher likelihood metastatic disease, subtotal resection, and reduced dose or withholding of radiotherapy. Between 20% and 30% of patients present with neuraxial dissemination, most commonly along the spinal cord. The presence of metastatic disease is prognostically significant, with 5-year PFS rates of 70% for M0 disease, to 57% for M1, and to 40% for M2 or higher in CCG-921.[381] The disease-free survival of high-risk patients treated with craniospinal irradiation (CSI) with or without chemotherapy is 25% to 30%.[401] Historically, average-risk patients have had a 5-year disease-free survival of 66% to 70%, which has increased to 70% to 80% in recent reports.[381,382]

Surgery

In one study, 3-year survival was reduced by 60% in patients who had an incomplete resection of their primary tumor.[383] Although hydrocephalus associated with medulloblastoma obstructing the fourth ventricle can be relieved with a ventriculostomy, ICP may be controlled with corticosteroids, and in most patients, aggressive tumor resection is sufficient to relieve hydrocephalus. Following surgery, gradual weaning of the ventriculostomy is attempted, with internalization 7 or more days after surgery if clamping is untenable. Postoperative shunting for hydrocephalus is necessary in approximately 35% to 40% of patients because of scarring and decreased capacity to resorb CSF.[384] Patients who require long-term shunting are younger and have larger ventricles and a more extensive tumor at presentation.[385] Concern has existed that a ventriculoperitoneal shunting (VP) shunt may cause peritoneal seeding, but this has not been upheld.[386]

With advances in neurosurgical technique, the number of patients not undergoing a gross total or near-total resection is dwindling. MRI should be performed to evaluate the extent of residual disease within 48 to 72 hours following surgery to prevent postsurgical changes from influencing interpretation. Patients with either gross total resection or subtotal resection have better 5-year OS and posterior fossa local control rates than patients who undergo biopsy alone. Although retrospective data infer that a total resection is prognostically favorable, the majority of trials have found that patients who undergo substantial subtotal resection with minimal residual disease treated with both chemotherapy and radiation do just as well as those who undergo total resection.[387] This justifies opting for a near-total resection, particularly when there is invasion of the floor of the fourth ventricle or envelopment of cranial nerves or the posterior inferior cerebellar artery. It is clear, however, that the extent of resection does not impact survival in patients with disseminated disease.[387]

The value of an aggressive resection must be balanced against surgical complications, interchangeably referred to as *posterior fossa syndrome* or *cerebellar mutism syndrome*. These conditions consist of diminished speech and can include emotional lability, hypotonia, long-tract signs, bulbar dysfunction, decreased respiratory drive, urinary retention, and ataxia. These changes can be seen in up to 25% of patients who have undergone a resection of a midline posterior fossa tumor.[388] Although thought to be a temporary, a significant number have persistent deficits.

Radiation Therapy

The aims of radiotherapy are to treat residual posterior fossa disease (or gross deposits of disease anywhere in the craniospinal axis) and also to treat microscopic disease in the craniospinal axis. Historically, CSI has been delivered to 36 Gy with a posterior fossa boost of 54 Gy using conventional fractionation of 1.8 Gy per day.[389] Radiation is typically initially withheld in patients younger than 3 years of age because of the higher risk of neurocognitive damage. Supratentorial PNETs and other embryonal tumors have been treated with the same CSI regimen, with a boost to the tumor bed and residual disease. Supratentorial PNETs treated with an appropriate dose and volume of radiotherapy were found to have a 49% PFS at 3 years compared with 7% with major violations of radiotherapy.[390]

Various alterations to the radiotherapy regimen have been made endeavoring to limit late toxicities. Hyperfractionation has been examined, with one study showing no improvement in survival and an excess of failures outside the primary site, although this was likely attributable to a reduced craniospinal dose of 30 Gy.[391] A recent trial showed that with a reduction in craniospinal dose, adequate disease-free survival with possible preservation of intellectual function is possible.[392] IMRT has been used to provide radiation to the posterior fossa, with a 32% redu. A recent trial showed that with a reduction in craniospinal dose, adequate disease-free survival with possible preservation of intellectual function is possible. p ction in dose to the cochlear apparatus, reducing the risk of grade 3 or 4 hearing loss from 64% to 13%.[70] Improved imaging methods have allowed for more precise delineation of the tumor within the posterior fossa, providing the possibility of avoiding treatment to the entire posterior fossa with the boost dose. Although standard practice has been to boost the entire posterior fossa, retrospective data have shown isolated recurrences outside the tumor bed to be rare.[393,394] Encompassing the tumor bed and a 2-cm margin only for the boost led to less than 5% isolated posterior fossa recurrences.[395]

A combined CCG/Pediatric Oncology Group trial compared standard and reduced dose CSI (36 versus 23.4 Gy) with a posterior fossa boost to 54 Gy in average-risk patients. All patients received concurrent vincristine during radiation with no adjuvant chemotherapy. Patients who received the lower dose had a higher rate of early relapse, lower 5-year event-free survival (67% versus 52%), and lower OS.[396] A comparison of CSI doses of 35 versus 25 Gy in the International Society of Paediatric Oncology (SIOP) II yielded similar results.[397] Further dose reduction is being evaluated in ongoing prospective trials.

Strong advocates for proton therapy have emerged as a result of the sharply diminished exit dose from spinal irradiation and the more conformal treatment of the posterior fossa. A dosimetric analysis that compared photons to protons has demonstrated a decrease in the dose to 50% of the heart volume from 72.2% to 0.5%, and the dose to the cochlea was reduced from 101.2% of the prescribed posterior fossa boost dose to 2.4%.[398] Proton-based radiotherapy also demonstrated a decreased radiation dose to normal tissues compared with IMRT. Overall, a reduction in second malignancies is also anticipated and modeled based on available data, although one controversial report contends that the older generation of proton-beam machines might pose a greater risk of second malignancies because of a higher rate of neutron production and contamination, which is more carcinogenic.[74]

Chemotherapy

Chemotherapy has been used in medulloblastomas with the dual goals of reducing the radiation dose while maintaining optimal disease-free survival rates in average-risk patients and improving disease-free survival in high-risk patients. Tait et al.[399] in SIOP I compared radiotherapy alone versus radiotherapy with concurrent vincristine followed by maintenance vincristine and CCNU. Overall, there was no survival benefit from chemotherapy, but an unprespecified post hoc subgroup analysis identified subgroups that appeared to benefit from chemotherapy, including T3 or T4 disease, and subtotal resection. Similar results were seen in a CCG study.[382] The 5-year disease-free survival rates in the CCG and SIOP studies were 59% and 55%, respectively, for RT plus chemotherapy, and 50% and 43% for RT alone. Based on these results, the routine use of chemotherapy for "high"-risk medulloblastomas has become standard.

For "standard"-risk patients, chemotherapy has been postulated to lead to a reduction in the CSI dose necessary to control microscopic disease. A phase II trial of CCNU, vincristine, and cisplatin for eight cycles following the reduced CSI prescription of 23.4 Gy had a PFS rate of 86% and 79% at 3 and 5 years, respectively.[396] This was superior to historical controls, and CSI to 23.4 Gy with chemotherapy was adopted as the standard of care and reference dose for further trials.

The most recent COG trial for average-risk patients compared cisplatin and vincristine with either CCNU or cyclophosphamide and 23.4 Gy CSI. No differences in outcome were noted, with a 5-year event-free survival and OS rates of 81% and 86%, respectively. The overall outcomes indirectly validated the use of reduced-dose CSI in conjunction with chemotherapy. The ongoing COG trial for average-risk patients is investigating a CSI dose of 18 Gy in patients between 3 to 7 years of age. The 2 × 2 randomization also compares boosting the entire posterior fossa versus a local boost.

Current approaches for high-risk medulloblastomas focus on chemotherapy dose intensification. Vincristine, CCNU, and prednisone had a 63% 5-year PFS rate, better than an 8-in-1 chemotherapy regimen. High-dose cyclophosphamide with autologous stem cell rescue is feasible and provided a 5-year event-free survival of 70% in patients with high-risk disease.[400] In a pilot study involving 57 children, the COG incorporated carboplatin as a radiosensitizer with CSI to 36 Gy and a posterior fossa boost followed by six cycles of maintenance cyclophosphamide, vincristine, and cisplatin. Four-year OS and PFS rates were 81% and 66%, respectively, with an inferior outcome in patients with anaplastic medulloblastoma.

Because the risk of cognitive deficits increases with decreasing patient age, extensive effort has been made to develop regimens that can delay or potentially eliminate the need for radiation in patients younger than 3 years of age. The avoidance of radiation has proved to be more feasible for patients with M0 disease.[401] The addition of intraventricular methotrexate following surgery in a five-drug chemotherapy regimen provided 5-year PFS and OS rates of 58% and 66%, respectively.[383] Although asymptomatic leukoencephalopathy was detected by MRI and mean intelligence quotient (IQ) scores were lower than healthy controls, the mean IQ scores were significantly higher than previous cohorts who had received radiation. A prospective randomized trial of supratentorial PNETs in children younger than 3 years old treated with chemotherapy and omitted or delayed radiation yielded less promising results, with a PFS and OS rates at 3 years of 15% and 17%, respectively. The administration of radiation was the only positive prognostic variable for PFS and OS.[402] The Head Start I trial for young children with localized medulloblastoma consisted of five cycles of cisplatin, vincristine, etoposide, and cyclophosphamide followed by a single high-dose myeloablative chemotherapy regimen of thioTEPA, carboplatin, and etoposide.[403] The 5-year survival was 79%. With the addition of methotrexate, children with disseminated disease had a 5-year PFS of 45% and an OS of 54%.[404]

The addition of conformal RT limited to the posterior fossa and primary site to chemotherapy (cyclophosphamide, vincristine, cisplatin, etoposide) in children between 8 months and 3 years of age with nonmetastatic medulloblastoma increased event-free survival compared with the use of postoperative chemotherapy alone (Children's Oncology Group trial P9934). Neurodevelopmental assessments did not show a decline in cognitive or motor function.[405]

Recurrent medulloblastomas are essentially an incurable and lethal disease. Although it is responsive to a variety of neoplastic

agents, including vincristine, nitrosoureas, procarbazine, cyclophosphamide, etoposide, and cisplatin, with several regimens yielding relatively high response rates, durability is limited. A CCG trial to evaluate carboplatin, thioTEPA, and etoposide with peripheral stem cell rescue showed a 3-year event-free survival and OS of 34% and 46%, respectively.

Long-term effects from treatment can be categorized as neurocognitive, neuropsychiatric, neuroendocrine, and growth retardation. Hypothalamic and pituitary endocrinopathies such as delayed hypothyroidism and decreased growth hormone secretion may occur. Growth retardation can also be secondary to delayed or reduced bone growth, leading to a reduction in sitting height. Neurocognitive deficits have long been recognized secondary to surgery, radiotherapy, and chemotherapy. In one study, 58% of children showed an IQ above 80 at 5 years after treatment, but by 10 years after treatment, only 15% of the patients had an IQ that remained above 80.[406] A prospective study of cognitive function showed an average decline of 14 points in mean IQ, with an average decline of 25 points in patients younger than 7 years of age.[407] Even with risk-adapted RT, patients had a significant yearly decrease in mean IQ, reading, spelling, and math.[408] Psychologic secondary effects are partially attributable to the diminished cognitive function as well as the social challenges caused by the physical manifestations of CSI (e.g., hearing loss, decreased truncal stature, and thin hair) and potential ataxia and abnormal speech patterns. The risk for secondary malignancies also exists. A population-based study tabulated a 5.4-fold increased rate of malignancy when compared with the general population, although this only affected 20 of 1,262 patients at risk.[409]

PINEAL REGION TUMORS AND GERM CELL TUMORS

Clinical and Pathologic Considerations

Pineal and germ cell tumors account for less than 1% of intracranial tumors in adults and 3% to 8% of brain tumors in children.[410] Germinomas are the most common type, accounting for 33% to 50% of pineal tumors. The peak incidence of germ cell tumors is in the 2nd decade, and few present after the 3rd decade. Gliomas are the next most common pineal region tumor (approximately 25%). Pineal parenchymal tumors are nearly as common as glial tumors and are called *pineocytomas* if benign and *pineoblastomas* (a variant of PNET) if malignant; a rare intermediate form also exists.

Germ cell tumors commonly involve the two midline sites, suprasellar and pineal regions, and occasionally are found in other areas such as the basal ganglia, ventricles, cerebral hemispheres, and the spinal cord. Germinomas can occur bifocally or, rarely, even multifocally; the most common bifocal presentation is synchronous involvement of the suprasellar region and the pineal gland.[411] Based on histology and the presence of tumor markers in the serum or CSF, the WHO classification system divides intracranial germ cell tumors into germinomas and nongerminomatous germ cell tumors.[4] Nongerminomatous germ cell tumors are further divided into embryonal carcinomas, yolk sac tumors, choriocarcinomas, and teratomas (mature, immature, or teratoma with malignant transformation). A quarter of the intracranial germ cell tumors have more than one histologic component and are known as mixed germ cell tumors. Alpha-fetoprotein (elevated in yolk sac tumors) and β-human chorionic gonadotropin (elevated in choriocarcinoma, and to a modest extent in germinoma) are generally secreted by these tumors. Mature teratomas do not have elevated tumor markers.

Neurologic signs and symptoms are caused by obstructive hydrocephalus and involvement of ocular pathways. Major symptoms are headache, nausea and vomiting, lethargy, and diplopia. Signs are primarily ocular, but can include ataxia and hemiparesis. The major ocular manifestation is paralysis of conjugate upward gaze (Parinaud syndrome), but pupillary and convergence abnormalities are seen, as are skew deviation and papilledema. Some patients with a pineal germ cell tumor can present with symptoms of diabetes insipidus (DI) without any radiologic evidence of overt suprasellar disease.[412,413]

On CT, these lesions are hyperdense. On MRI, the mass is hypointense on T2-weighted sequences (due to the high cellularity of the mass) and shows enhancement with gadolinium. Calcification and fat may be seen in teratomas or mixed malignant germ cell tumors. Germinomas tend to surround a calcified pineal gland, whereas pineal parenchymal tumors tend to disperse the calcification into multiple small foci. The potential for leptomeningeal dissemination requires imaging of the neuraxis before surgery. Determination of histology, tumor markers, and extent of disease is critical for the optimal management of pineal region tumors. The prognosis varies depending on the histologic type, the size of the tumor, and the extent of disease at presentation.

Surgery

Because pineal tumors are often near the center of the brain, they are among the most difficult brain tumors to remove. Having said that, there is no role for cytoreductive surgery in the treatment of germinoma, which requires only a biopsy from the neurosurgeon followed by radiation, chemotherapy, or both. The application of modern surgical technology with superb illumination, magnification, surgical guidance, and neuroanesthesia has made this region much more accessible. Surgeons can choose from several approaches depending on preference and the tumor's position and extent.[414] The current recommendation is to obtain tissue when a diagnosis cannot be made from serum tumor markers, CSF tumor markers or cytologic examination. Whenever possible, the tumor is completely excised, except when a germinoma is found at open surgery; a biopsy suffices in this situation because germinomas respond well to radiation.[415] Resection is important when tumors are radioresistant or when an excision may be curative (e.g., as in teratomas, arachnoid cysts, and pineal parenchymal tumors).

The place of stereotactic biopsy in the diagnosis of pineal region tumors is unclear. Although biopsies have been described as safe, particularly for large tumors, some avoid it because of the risk of damaging large veins that flank the pineal gland.[416] In addition, there is a risk that tissue sampling of these heterogeneous tumors may not depict the correct histologic nature of all parts of the tumor. Without an accurate diagnosis, treatment planning may be erroneous or inadequate. In favor of biopsy are the advantages of a rapid tissue diagnosis and shortened hospital stay. A transventricular endoscopic biopsy is a much more common clinical scenario currently because it can be performed under direct vision with little risk of damaging deep venous structures. The downside of an endoscopic biopsy is the small size of the biopsy, which can be problematic in the face of a polyphenotypic germ cell tumor.

In patients with a pineal mass and obstructive hydrocephalus from blockage of the aqueduct of Sylvius, endoscopic surgery can play a special role. An endoscopic third ventriculostomy is performed by making a fenestration in the floor of the third ventricle, which relieves hydrocephalus, and the mass in the posterior third ventricle can be viewed and biopsied through a flexible endoscope. A rigid endoscope can also be safely used by placing a second burr hole for the biopsy. CSF for cytology and marker studies can also be obtained, and the walls of the third ventricle inspected for tumor studding. There is a small risk of intraventricular hemorrhage.[417]

Radiation Therapy

With certain exceptions, such as benign teratomas, RT has an established role in the curative treatment of pineal germ cell and parenchymal tumors. The location and infiltrative nature of these lesions often does not allow for a complete resection. In the past, the risk of biopsy or attempted resection often led to the use of RT without histologic confirmation. In such instances, response to low-dose RT, the measurement of α-fetoprotein and human chorionic gonadotropin-β, and CSF cytology were used to provide diagnostic information. There is a tendency to increase the use of biopsy and resection, and treatment without histology is less common.

Five-year survival rates with RT range from 44% to 78% and vary with histology, extent of disease, age, radiation volume, and dose to the primary tumor.[152] In a multi-institutional survey by Wara and Evans,[418] the survival of patients with pineal parenchymal cell tumors or malignant teratomas was 21% (3 of 14) compared with 72% (26 of 36) for those with germinomas. Wolden et al.[419] reported 5-year disease-free survival rates of 91% for germinomas, 63% for unbiopsied tumors, and 60% for nongerminomatous germ cell tumors irradiated to 50 to 54 Gy to the local site with or without treatment to the whole brain or ventricular system. Patients younger than 25 to 30 years old have survival rates of 65% to 80% compared with 35% to 40% for older patients. This may reflect the increased incidence of germinomas in younger patients.

Germinomas are infiltrative tumors that tend to spread along the ventricular walls or throughout the leptomeninges. The incidence of CSF seeding ranges from 7% to 12%. For this reason, fields encompassing the entire ventricular system, the whole brain, and even the entire craniospinal axis have been recommended. The appropriate treatment volume for pineal germinomas was evaluated by Haas-Kogan et al.[420] in 93 patients treated at the University of California–San Francisco (UCSF) or at Stanford. The UCSF group favored whole ventricular irradiation; the Stanford group included CSI. Five-year survival for the combined cohort was 93%, with no difference in survival or distant failure regardless of whether CSI or whole ventricular radiation was given. In some institutions, 25.5 Gy (1.5 Gy per day) whole-brain or whole-ventricular radiation is followed by a boost to the primary site to 45 to 50 Gy. CSI is reserved for patients with disseminated disease at presentation.

Neoadjuvant chemotherapy and low-dose (30 to 40 Gy) focal irradiation is employed by some.[421,422] Chemotherapy might be useful in the young child to defer irradiation. For disseminated or multiple midline germinomas, systemic chemotherapy or CSI is given. CSI doses of 20 to 35 Gy have been used when CSF cytology results are positive. When response to primary chemotherapy is incomplete or the tumor recurs, salvage radiotherapy yields good results.[423]

Nongerminomatous malignant germ cell tumors, whether localized or disseminated, are treated with chemotherapy followed by restaging. After restaging, localized tumors receive focal RT to 54 to 60 Gy, and disseminated tumors receive CSI (54 to 60 Gy to the primary, 45 Gy to the ventricular system [controversial], 35 Gy to the spinal cord, and 45 Gy to localized cord lesions).[419] In a German study, 63 supratentorial PNETs were treated with chemotherapy before or after radiation (35 Gy CSI with a boost to the primary of 54 Gy).[390] The 3-year survival was 49.3% in those for whom treatment was delivered as prescribed, but only 6.7% in those with major protocol violations. This indicates the importance of CSI in pineoblastoma, analogous to the situation with medulloblastoma.

Tumors that tend not to metastasize to the cord, such as teratomas, pineocytomas, and low-grade gliomas, are treated by resection, with localized radiotherapy reserved for patients with residual disease.[424] For selected patients with small residual disease, radiosurgery has been shown to be effective in terms of local control.

Chemotherapy

Chemotherapy for pineal glial neoplasms is similar to that for gliomas elsewhere. Germinomas are chemosensitive and responsive to cisplatin, carboplatin, ifosfamide, cyclophosphamide, bleomycin, and etoposide. Adjuvant multidrug therapy with radiotherapy has produced encouraging disease-free survival and OS. Newly diagnosed germinomas treated with two courses of high-dose cyclophosphamide showed a complete response rate of 91%.[425] Building on this, several studies have reported excellent outcomes with reduced dose radiation combined with chemotherapy.[298,495,499–502]

Given the poor outcome of CNS nongerminomatous germ cell tumors after radiotherapy alone, there is significant interest in the use of chemotherapy. Balmaceda et al.[426] reported the results from using four cycles of carboplatin, etoposide, and bleomycin without radiation. Of 71 patients (45 germinoma and 26 nongerminomatous), 68 were assessable for response; after four cycles, the complete response rate was 57%. The 29 patients with less than a complete response received dose-intensified chemotherapy or surgery, and a further 16 achieved a complete response, for an overall complete response rate of 78%. Despite these high response rates, only 28 of 71 (39%) patients were alive and progression free within 31 months. Subsequently, they treated 20 patients with two cycles of cisplatin, etoposide, cyclophosphamide, and bleomycin, and the 16 patients achieving a complete response received two additional cycles of carboplatin, etoposide, and bleomycin.[427] Nine of the 14 survivors received RT. The chemotherapy response rate was 94%, 5-year OS was 75%, and 36% of patients were event free. Although the complete response rate was high, approximately half the patients developed recurrent disease, suggesting that a multimodal therapeutic approach of surgery, chemotherapy, and radiotherapy is necessary to improve the overall outcome of these tumors. Matsutani et al.[428] analyzed 153 germ cell tumors treated with surgery and RT with or without chemotherapy. The 10-year survival rates for mature and malignant teratomas were 92.9% and 70.7%, respectively. Patients with pure malignant germ cell tumors (embryonal carcinoma, yolk sac tumor, or choriocarcinoma) had a 3-year survival rate of 27.3%. The mixed tumors were divided into three subgroups: (1) mixed germinoma and teratoma; (2) mixed tumors whose predominant characteristics were germinoma or teratoma combined with some elements of pure malignant tumors; and (3) mixed tumors with predominantly pure malignant elements. The 3-year survival rates were 94.1%, 70.0%, and 9.3%, respectively, for the three groups.

High-dose chemotherapy with autologous stem cell rescue has been used for pineoblastoma.[429] Twelve patients were treated with induction chemotherapy followed by CSI with a pineal boost (36 Gy CSI, 59.4 Gy to primary), then with high-dose chemotherapy with stem cell support. Nine of the 12 patients remained disease free, including two infants who never received radiation. The actuarial 4-year PFS and OS were 69% and 71%, respectively. Although still considered investigational, the survival results are impressive. The use of high-dose chemotherapy and autologous bone marrow support has not been as promising for patients with recurrent tumors, although reported data are few.[429]

PITUITARY ADENOMAS

Clinical and Pathologic Considerations

Pituitary tumors are identified incidentally or present through symptoms of local mass effect or as a result of endocrine effects. Pituitary adenomas almost always arise from the anterior pituitary, the adenohypophysis. The tumor initially compresses the gland and, subsequently, the optic chiasm and nerves. Tumors less than 10 mm—microadenomas—rarely compress the optic apparatus. Larger macroadenomas can involve the cavernous sinus bilaterally, the third ventricle (sometimes producing hydrocephalus), and, less commonly, the middle, anterior, or even the posterior fossae. The classic ophthalmologic finding is visual loss, typically starting with bitemporal hemianopsia and loss of color discrimination. Automated visual field testing is more sensitive than simple

confrontation. Occasionally, extraocular palsies can result from the compression or invasion of the nerves in the cavernous sinus. Tumors that present with mass effect are often nonsecreting, but prolactin, growth hormone, thyrotropin, and gonadotropin-producing tumors may also present in this way.

Neuroendocrine abnormalities are usually from tumors that oversecrete hormones but can also result from compression of the pituitary gland and the stalk. The most commonly secreted hormones are prolactin, adrenocorticotropic hormone, or growth hormone. The incidence of the various types of adenoma is variable. In 800 patients operated on at UCSF between 1970 and 1981, 79% were endocrinologically active. Of these, 52% were prolactin secreting, 27% were growth hormone secreting, 20% were corticotropin secreting, and only 0.3% were thyroid-stimulating hormone secreting.[430] Sexual impotence in men and amenorrhea and galactorrhea in women are hallmarks of a prolactin-secreting tumor. Hypogonadism, infertility, and osteopenia are also common.[431] Growth hormone hypersecretion causes acromegaly or, in the rare patient with a tumor occurring before epiphyseal closure, gigantism. The secondary production of insulin-like growth factor-1 (IGF-1; primarily from the liver) or somatomedin C produces skeletal overgrowth changes (e.g., increased hand and foot size, macroglossia, frontal bossing). Soft tissue swelling, peripheral nerve entrapment syndromes, and arthropathies may occur. Hypertension, cardiomyopathy, diabetes, and an increased risk of colon cancer are prevalent with acromegaly. Adrenocorticotropic hormone hypersecretion by a pituitary tumor results in Cushing disease, with weight gain, hypertension, striae, hyperglycemia, infertility, osteoporosis, increased skin pigmentation, and psychiatric symptoms. Rarely, pituitary adenomas can present acutely with headaches, visual loss, and confusion, which can progress to obtundation. This potentially life-threatening condition is termed *pituitary apoplexy.* The etiology of apoplexy is thought to involve tumor infarction due to interruption of its blood supply, but the exact mechanism is not known. Symptomatic pituitary apoplexy is a surgical emergency, and patients need to be carefully medically managed with judicious fluid and salt replacement and administration of high-dose corticosteroids. A need for prolonged hormone replacement therapy is often a consequence of apoplexy.

On MRI, pituitary microadenomas are generally seen within the gland according to the distribution of normal cells. For example, prolactinomas tend to be located laterally within the sella. Microadenomas show subtle hypointensity to the normal gland on T1-weighted sequences and are often more difficult to detect on T2 sequences.[432] Immediately after the administration of contrast, adenomas show less enhancement than adjacent normal glands (Fig. 97.11). On delayed views, the tumor enhances more than the normal gland. Indentation of the sellar floor, stalk deviation, and mass effect on adjacent structures also provide evidence of the presence of tumor.

Surgery

There are two primary goals of surgery for macroadenomas: to decompress the visual pathways by reducing tumor bulk and, for secreting tumors, to normalize hypersecretion, with the preservation of remaining normal pituitary function.

The standard surgical approach for the majority of pituitary tumors is transsphenoidal, which is safer and better tolerated than the transcranial (frontotemporal craniotomy) approach.[433–435] The transsphenoidal approach is used for microadenomas that occupy the sella turcica and for many macroadenomas. Image-guided neuronavigation and intraoperative fluoroscopy are essential to reduce the risk of injury to the carotid arteries. Even when the majority of tumor is actually suprasellar, a transsphenoidal resection can be safely accomplished if the tumor consistency is soft (and tumor aspiration and curettage can thus easily be performed) and if the tumor is situated so that it can drop into the sella with progressive

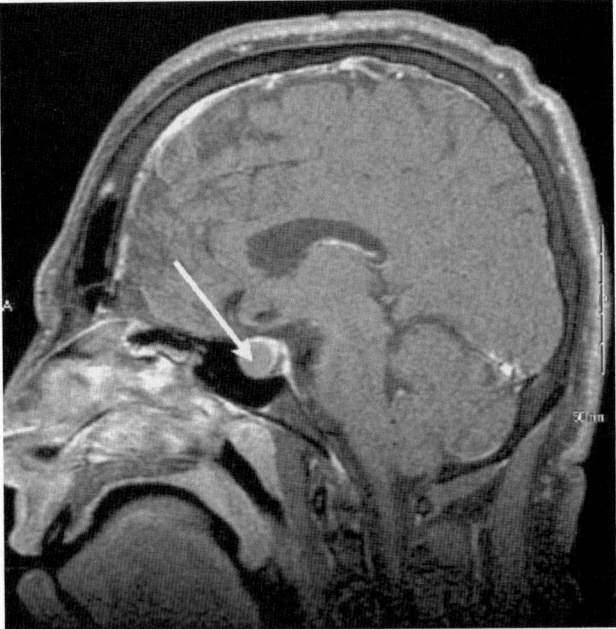

Figure 97.11 Pituitary adenomas are usually isointense to the gland on noncontrast T1-weighted magnetic resonance images; on contrast administration, the normal gland enhances early, as visualized on this sagittal image, whereas the adenoma (*arrow*) continues to remain unenhanced. With late imaging, the adenoma enhances.

resection. Tough, fibrous suprasellar tumors and those that extend laterally into the middle fossa, anteriorly beneath the frontal lobes, or into the posterior fossa may require a craniotomy for resection.[436] A tumor that invades the cavernous sinus is generally not removed. The role of endoscopic transsphenoidal surgery for pituitary adenomas is currently being expanded. Potential advantages include a less invasive surgical approach with a wider field of view and quicker postoperative recovery. Moreover, Cappabianca et al.[436] observed a decreased incidence of complications in a series of 146 consecutively treated patients who underwent an endoscopic endonasal transsphenoidal approach to the sellar region for resection of these tumors, compared with large historical series that employed the traditional microsurgical transsphenoidal approach.

Current surgical cure rates for hormonally active adenomas are 80% to 90% if there is no involvement of the cavernous sinus, suprasellar region, or clivus.[437] Patients with microadenomas have a higher surgical cure rate than patients with macroadenomas.[438] Patients cured of their endocrine disease can expect to have a normal lifespan; however, those with persistent endocrinopathies, and particularly those with acromegaly, may not enjoy a normal lifespan due to the impact of the high hormone levels on multiple organ systems.[437] In patients not biochemically cured with initial surgery, the tumor is often found at the time of second surgery just next to the original site. Patients with persistent acromegaly, however, may not be amenable to biochemical cure with a second surgery because the residual growth hormone secreting cells can be difficult to visualize. Growth through the dura into the adjacent cavernous sinus is often found at repeat surgery even when no tumor is seen preoperatively on MRI.[439] Benveniste et al.[440] found that, although repeated transsphenoidal surgery to treat a recurrent or residual tumor mass was associated with a 93% rate of clinical remission, its use to treat recurrent or persistent hormone hypersecretion produced only a 57% rate of initial endocrinologic remission, with a 37% likelihood of sustaining such remission at a mean of 31 months. Thus, they suggested that for the treatment of residual or recurrent adenomas that cause persistent or recurrent hormone hypersecretion, radiosurgery may be a better option.

Radiation Therapy

RT may be indicated for hormone-secreting adenomas that are not surgically cured and are refractory to pharmacologic management. After subtotal resection of a macroadenoma, more than 50% of patients demonstrate radiographic evidence of progression within 5 years.[441] Younger patients (less than 50 years old) with residual disease have faster tumor regrowth. Ki-67 antigen labeling of more than 1.5% predicts more rapid growth.[442] For these patients, earlier postoperative radiotherapy should be considered.

RT decreases serum growth hormone concentrations to "normal" levels in 80% to 85% of acromegalic patients, but the definition of normalization has varied over time.[443] Growth hormone levels decrease at a rate of 10% to 30% per year, so several years may be required for the levels to normalize.[443] The probability of endocrine cure is highest for tumors with relatively low pre-RT growth hormone elevations (30 to 50 ng/mL); response is less reliable for tumors that produce higher growth hormone levels. In contrast, serum IGF-1 levels remain elevated after radiotherapy, and long-term treatment with somatostatin or its analogs may be required.[444,445] RT controls hypercortisolism in 50% to 75% of adults and 80% of children with Cushing disease. Response occurs within 6 to 9 months of treatment.[446]

Pituitary adenomas may be treated using several different techniques. The most commonly used techniques include 3D-CRT, IMRT, and stereotactic radiotherapy or radiosurgery. Treatment with charged-particle beams has been used at select centers.[447,448] The total dose used for nonfunctioning lesions is 45 to 50 Gy in 25 to 28 fractions of 1.8 Gy. Slightly higher total doses are recommended for secretory lesions. This controls tumor growth in 90% of cases at 10 years.[449–451] Radiation-induced injury to the optic apparatus or adjacent brain with this dose-fractionation scheme is rare, whereas larger fractions or greater total doses lead to a higher incidence of injury. Hypopituitarism may develop, often years after radiation treatment.[451] It is more common in patients who have had both surgery and RT than in those treated with either modality alone. Hypopituitarism is largely correctable by hormone-replacement therapy. One publication suggests that patients treated with surgery and radiation have an elevated risk for late cerebrovascular mortality.[452] Possible contributing factors include hypopituitarism, radiotherapy, and extent of initial surgery. The risk of developing a radiation-induced brain tumor after treatment is 1.3% to 2.7% at 10 years and beyond.[452–454]

Radiosurgery is increasingly being used for treating small residual adenomas.[448,455] In general, patients are eligible for radiosurgery only if the superior extent of the lesions is more than 3 to 5 mm from the optic chiasm. Doses of more than 10 Gy in a single fraction to the optic pathways can cause visual loss.[456] Radiosurgery results in excellent tumor control and appears to cause more rapid biochemical normalization than is seen with conventional RT, with the caveat that it is used primarily for smaller tumors.[457–459] Side effects such as hypopituitarism and cranial nerve injury is also lower with radiosurgery.[460,461]

Reirradiation can be considered for patients with recurrent pituitary adenomas when there has been a long interval after the first course of radiotherapy and other therapeutic methods have been unsuccessful.[462]

Medical Therapy

Medical therapy is very important and effective for patients with secreting pituitary tumors.[463] Dopamine agonists (e.g., bromocriptine or cabergoline) are the most effective therapy for prolactinomas and are often used as primary treatment with definitive treatment reserved for patients who either cannot tolerate or do not respond to a dopamine agonist. Somatostatin analogs (e.g., octreotide and lanreotide) are effective for patients with acromegaly and are usually reserved when there is persistent growth hormone hypersecretion after resection. Control rates with octreotide are approximately 50%; dopamine agonists can control growth hormone production in 10% to 34%.[464] A recently approved growth hormone receptor antagonist (pegvisomant) can be used for patients for whom somatostatin analogs fail. Rates of IGF-1 level normalization as high as 97% have been reported with this agent, but concerns persist that because it acts at the end-organ receptor level, tumor growth may continue in some patients, and the lifetime cost of the agent is prohibitive.[465] Medical therapy for patients with Cushing disease is directed at the adrenal glands to reduce cortisol hypersecretion (ketoconazole). Unfortunately, no known drug effectively reduces pituitary corticotropin production.

CRANIOPHARYNGIOMAS

Clinical and Pathologic Considerations

Craniopharyngiomas are the most common benign nonglial brain tumors in children, occurring primarily in the late 1st and 2nd decades, although they can present at any age.[2,466] Craniopharyngiomas are thought to arise from epithelial cell rests that are remnants of the Rathke pouch at the juncture of the infundibular stalk and the pituitary gland. Most have a significant associated cystic component with only 10% being purely solid. Most craniopharyngiomas become symptomatic because of effects of the combined tumor and cyst on the optic apparatus or hypothalamus or both. They may also compress the pituitary gland or extend superiorly into the third ventricle. Cyst fluid is proteinaceous, and this can be seen on MRI. A CT shows calcification in 30% to 50% of cases.

Common presenting symptoms include headache, visual complaints, nausea, vomiting, and intellectual dysfunction (especially memory loss). Specific visual signs include optic atrophy, papilledema, hemianopsia, unilateral or total blindness, and diplopia with associated cranial nerve palsies. Endocrine abnormalities at presentation can include growth retardation, menstrual abnormalities, and disorders of sexual development or regression of secondary sexual characteristics (or both). DI is uncommon at presentation.[467]

The optimal treatment of any specific patient with a craniopharygioma is complicated, and open to debate. Variables such as patient age, endocrine status, visual status, aeration of the sinuses, extent of solid disease, extent of cystic disease, and involvement of the hypothalamus either unilaterally or bilaterally can all contribute to the decision of optimal therapy. In general, the number of options for therapy for a given patient will vary directly with the number of opinions sought because there are many different approaches and schools of thought as to how best treat this highly variable disease.

Surgery

Craniopharyngiomas are generally resected using a microsurgical subfrontal or pterional approach. More recently, some surgeons have been approaching some lesions using an endoscopic skull base approach from the sphenoid sinus. Larger tumors may require bifrontal or skull-base approaches, including a supraorbital craniotomy. Endoscopically assisted surgery is sometimes used, although outcome advantages have not yet been clearly shown. Although complete resection remains the optimal surgical goal, the risk of devastating long-term effects on hypothalamic function and quality of life cannot be ignored. In some cases, there is no clearly defined plane between tumor and surrounding hypothalamus, which makes aggressive resection dangerous. Aggressive removal is frequently associated with some injury to the pituitary stalk, with subsequent temporary or permanent DI and elements of hypopituitarism.[468–470] These patients require lifelong replacement hormones and inhaled desmopressin acetate spray for the control of

DI. Most patients with preoperative visual loss can expect at least some improvement after surgery. The reported mortality rates for craniopharyngioma resection range from 2% to 43%, with severe morbidity in 12% to 61%.[471] Complications are less likely with experienced surgeons. Alternative approaches include placement of an Ommaya reservoir for largely cystic tumors through which one can instill sclerosing agents (e.g., bleomycin, interferons, or radioisotopes.)

Radiation Therapy

Radioisotope Therapy

Predominantly cystic craniopharyngiomas can be treated with stereotactic or endoscopic instillation of colloidal therapeutic radioisotopes, particularly ^{90}Y or ^{32}P.[469,472] The short penetrance of the beta-particles emitted by these isotopes allows the epithelial cells lining the cyst to be treated without significant dose to neighboring structures. Intracystic therapy may have a role in treating cysts that recur after conventional external-beam irradiation, or even as a primary cyst treatment. Although most cysts shrink with intracystic therapy, one-third of patients require further surgery later.

External-Beam Radiation Therapy

Numerous reports demonstrate that subtotal removal and irradiation produce local tumor control and survival rates comparable to those after radical excision.[473–475] The local control rates after complete resection, subtotal resection alone, and subtotal resection with postoperative irradiation are 70%, 26%, and 75%, respectively. A study from Children's Memorial Hospital in Chicago found a 32% rate of recurrence after complete resection and 0% after subtotal resection and adjuvant radiotherapy.[476] Ten-year survival rates range from 24% to 100% for complete resection, 31% to 52% for subtotal resection, 62% to 86% for incomplete resection and irradiation, and 100% after radiotherapy alone.[471,473,474,476,477] Patients who undergo conservative treatment, including biopsy and cyst drainage and irradiation, appear to enjoy a better quality of life and demonstrate less psychosocial impairment than those initially treated with more extensive resections.[473] Furthermore, conservative therapy is associated with less hypothalamic and pituitary dysfunction and a lower incidence of persistent DI than when a total or near-total excision is attempted. More extensive resections, using a subfrontal approach, may be associated with frontal lobe and visual perceptual dysfunction. The negative impact on IQ is greater in patients treated with aggressive resection than in those treated with conservative surgery and postoperative irradiation.[478]

The radiation treatment volume is based on CT and MRI scans, with relatively small margins. Generally, more sophisticated 3D-CRT and IMRT approaches and stereotactic radiotherapy techniques are increasingly being used to spare surrounding normal tissues.[477] One report showed excellent tumor control (100%) with minimal late toxicity when FSRT (mean dose, 52.2 Gy in 29 fractions) was used.[479] No significant effect on cognition or visual injury was reported. The total dose is 50 to 55 Gy, given in daily 1.8-Gy increments. One review suggested better local control when doses of 55 Gy or more are delivered.[480]

Radiosurgery

The use of radiosurgery is limited by the proximity of most lesions to the optic chiasm and brainstem,[481] and should be reserved for those uncommon tumors confined to the pituitary fossa and away from the chiasm and hypothalamus.[482] Kobayashi et al.[483] reviewed long-term results (follow-up of 65.5 months) of radiosurgical treatment for residual or recurrent craniopharyngiomas after microsurgery in 98 consecutive patients and found only a 20.4% tumor progression rate. They used a tumor margin dose of 11.5 Gy at the retrochiasm and ventral stalk area, which decreased the rate of visual and pituitary function loss so that deterioration both in vision and endocrinologic functions occurred in only six patients (6.1%). Similarly, Albright et al.[469] used radiosurgery as the initial treatment for the solid component of craniopharyngiomas in five children, limiting radiation to the optic chiasm to 8 Gy, and reported no operative morbidity or mortality, whereas 5 of 27 children who underwent microsurgical tumor resection suffered worsened vision postoperatively.

VESTIBULAR SCHWANNOMAS

Clinical and Pathologic Considerations

Schwannomas, also known as *neurilemmomas* or *neurinomas*, are benign neoplasms derived from Schwann cells that show a predilection for sensory nerves. Most intracranial schwannomas arise from the vestibulocochlear nerve, with trigeminal nerves being a distant second in frequency. Previously called *acoustic neuromas*, these neoplasms are more correctly termed *vestibular schwannomas* because they arise from both the superior and inferior portions of the vestibular nerve rather than the cochlear nerve. Vestibular schwannomas are equally common between genders and median age at diagnosis is approximately 50 years, with an overall increased incidence between 45 and 64 years of age. Vestibular schwannomas account for approximately 6% to 8% of intracranial neoplasms. The incidence of vestibular schwannomas is between 0.8 and 1.7 per 100,000, with an increasing incidence since the early 1980s.[484,485] This increased incidence may represent the discovery of asymptomatic lesions by a rising number of cranial imaging studies, predominantly MRI. The rate of incidental vestibular schwannomas detected on MRI ranges from 0.02 to 0.07%.[486,487] More than 90% of vestibular schwannomas are sporadic and unilateral. Bilateral vestibular schwannoma is virtually pathognomonic for NF2 and is one of the key components of the Manchester criteria for the diagnosis of NF2.[488] When associated with NF2, vestibular schwannomas have a significantly earlier disease manifestation and tend to occur in the 2nd or 3rd decade of life.

Vestibular schwannomas arise along the zone of transition between the central and peripheral myelin located near the medial aperture of the internal auditory canal (IAC). Macroscopically, they are typically lobulated, with the eighth cranial nerve located eccentrically along the surface because these tumors grow in an expansile fashion, displacing rather than invading nerves. Vestibular schwannomas in NF2 tend to embed within the seventh and eighth cranial nerve bundles more frequently.[489] As with peripheral schwannomas, a microscopic examination yields Antoni A and B tissue patterns. Vestibular schwannomas are benign, with few case reports of malignant dedifferentiation.

Although vestibular schwannomas arise from the vestibular portion of cranial nerve VIII, cochlear symptoms predominate, with the two most common being hearing loss and tinnitus.[490] Progressive unilateral sensorineural hearing loss is characteristic. An evaluation is typically delayed, with the duration of hypacusis averaging 3.7 years prior to diagnosis. Vertigo and unsteadiness are the most common vestibular symptoms. Facial nerve paresis or spasm may be seen. Large tumors can compress the trigeminal nerve, with paresthesias or neuralgia. Impingement of the brainstem or cerebellum may lead to ataxia and long-tract signs as well as involvement of the lower cranial nerves. Most ominous is the rare patient with nausea and vomiting from fourth ventricular compression and obstructive hydrocephalus.

MRI with thin-section, high-resolution, gadolinium-enhanced T1- and T2-weighted images of the cerebellopontine angle is the study of choice. Vestibular schwannomas typically enhance along the course of the eighth cranial nerve with variable intra- and extracanalicular components. Cystic changes are frequently identified in larger lesions. An MRI allows for the identification of the lesion and potential differentiation from other masses of the cerebellopontine angle such as meningiomas, epidermoid cysts, arachnoid cysts, and, rarely, lipomas. Auditory brainstem response audiometry is less sensitive than MRI.[491] Pure tone and speech audiometry continue to be performed to document hearing loss. Hearing loss is more pronounced at higher frequencies, and the degree of speech discrimination loss is disproportionately worse than the pure tone hearing loss.

Treatment

Treatment revolves around the dual goals of local control and cranial nerve function preservation. Factors that influence treatment choice include tumor size, location, patient age, the presence and degree of symptoms such as tinnitus and vertigo, whether a patient has NF2, the status of contralateral hearing, and patient preference. Consultation with a multidisciplinary team is essential.

Observation

Vestibular schwannomas are typically slow growing, and various studies have shown an increase in size ranging from 0.35 to 2.2 mm per year (mean, 1.42 mm per year).[492] Chalabi et al.[493] reported that with mean follow-up of 4.2 years, 85% of observed vestibular schwannoma were noted to have exhibited measurable growth. Given the slow growth pattern and the recognition that neither surgery nor RT restore hearing lost to a vestibular schwannoma and both pose risks to cranial nerve function, observation is a reasonable choice for some patients. Such an approach requires that the patient be willing to undergo regular annual or semiannual clinical and imaging follow-ups. This course may be selected by many patients with small acoustic neuromas, particularly older patients and patients with multiple medical comorbidities. Patients with functional hearing must understand that further hearing loss, including sudden hearing loss, can occur while under observation.

Surgery

Surgery has the unique advantage of removal of the schwannoma, with a low risk of recurrence following complete resection. Microsurgical resection has been the mainstay of treatment for many years and was previously recommended as the standard of care in a 1991 consensus statement.[494] However, stereotactic radiosurgery has also become accepted as a standard treatment for these tumors.[495] Surgical risks include the inherent risk of general anesthesia, CSF leak, meningitis, headache, hearing loss, and facial nerve paralysis. Hearing preservation is influenced by preoperative hearing acuity, location of the tumor, and size. Loss of facial nerve function is the most significant surgical concern, as well as morbidity. Again, tumor size is a factor, as is the relationship between the facial nerve and tumor. Surgery is made particularly challenging by the increased adherence and infiltration in NF2.[496] The risk of facial nerve injury has decreased since the advent of facial nerve electromyography for intraoperative monitoring. The auditory brainstem response may also be used to evaluate the integrity of the cochlear portion of the eighth cranial nerve intraoperatively, improving the odds of potential avoidance and preservation.

Most modern surgical series achieve complete resection in more than 90% of patients, with some reporting significantly higher rates.[490,497] Subtotal resections are frequently deliberate to preserve hearing or provide emergent, life-saving decompression of the brainstem and fourth ventricle. Results appear to be both surgeon and volume dependent, leading to questions of the widespread applicability of results obtained by subspecialty surgeons in academic institutions.[498] There also appears to be a significant learning curve of 20 to 60 patients with new surgical teams.[499,500] An extensive surgical series of 962 patients undergoing 1,000 vestibular schwannoma operations has been compiled by Samii and Matthies,[490] who reported a 98% complete resection rate with fewer than 1% of non-NF2 patients having a recurrence. The facial and cochlear nerves were preserved in 93% and 68% of patients, respectively, and functional preservation was 39% for patients with intact hearing preoperatively. Mortality was 1.1%, although this included several individuals who were disabled with advanced disease prior to surgery. If hearing is to be preserved, the auditory nerve is also identified and preserved; preservation of hearing is more likely in patients lacking severe adhesion in the interface between the cochlear nerve and the tumor.[501] Life-threatening complications of acoustic neuroma resections are rare except in patients with extremely large tumors.[502] The tendency of postoperative CSF leaks to develop in patients (10% to 13%) is independent of the surgical approach employed and tumor size and may stem from factors such as transient postoperative increases in CSF pressure.[249] Postoperative headaches were a significant morbidity in a cohort of 1,657 patients who underwent surgery for acoustic neuroma.[503] Patients who underwent tumor resection by the retrosigmoid approach (82.3%) were significantly more likely to report their worst postoperative headache as "severe" than those resected using the translabyrinthine (75.2%) or middle fossa approaches (63.3%). In another quality-of-life study, hearing loss was perceived as the most disabling symptom among 386 patients who underwent acoustic neuroma surgery.[504]

Radiosurgery

The most substantial experience in radiation-based treatment is with SRS. Both Gamma Knife units and SRS-compatible linear accelerators may be used to perform SRS. The University of Pittsburgh published a review of 162 consecutive patients treated with SRS to a mean dose of 16 Gy with a tumor control rate of 98%.[505] Subsequent surgical resection was required in four patients. Normal facial function was preserved in 79% and normal trigeminal function was preserved in 73% of patients. Because of the unacceptable cranial nerve morbidity in this and other series, the prescription dose for radiosurgery was lowered to 12 to 13 Gy. Results from the decreased prescription dose have a similarly low rate of recurrence, with 97% tumor control at a mean dose of 13 Gy.[506] The risk of facial nerve weakness dropped to 1%, and hearing preservation improved to 71%. These results were confirmed with longer follow-up.[507] Recently, a prospective cohort study of 82 patients with unilateral vestibular schwannomas smaller than 3 cm compared surgery and SRS and provided level 2 evidence favoring SRS over microscopic surgical resection. Tumor control was not statistically different (100% for surgery versus 96% for SRS). Normal facial movement and preservation of serviceable hearing was more frequent in the SRS group at all time points, and no quality-of-life decline was seen in the SRS group.[508] New incomplete trigeminal and facial cranial neuropathies typically develop at approximately 6 or more months after radiosurgery. These tend to be mild and usually improve within a year after onset. Approximately half of patients with useful hearing before radiosurgery maintain their pretreatment hearing level, and hearing lost before treatment is not regained. The risk of treatment-induced cranial neuropathy is directly related to the volume of the lesion, the dose given, and the length of nerve irradiated.

Fractionated Radiation Therapy

Different fractionation regimens have been tried to capitalize on theoretical radiobiologic differences between the neoplastic vestibular schwannoma and the surrounding normal tissue. Multiple fractions also allow for the treatment of lesions that would otherwise not be amenable to treatment with SRS based on size (more than 3 cm) or location (direct compression of the brainstem). Hypofractionation was examined in a series that compared 25 Gy in five fractions and 30 Gy in 10 fractions. Actuarial hearing preservation rate was 90% at 2 years, and no recurrence or facial nerve weakness occurred.[509] A nonrandomized prospective trial from the Netherlands, however, had a nonstatistically inferior outcome in

hearing preservation when comparing hypofractionation to SRS at 10 to 12 Gy.[510] A comparison of FSRT (50 Gy in 25 fractions) to SRS in a prospective trial showed comparable high control rates and minimal cranial nerve injury, with the exception of retention of useful hearing, which was 81% versus 33% at 1 year (in favor of FSRT) when followed by serial audiometry.[511] Similar rates of tumor control and hearing preservation have been reported by single-institution experiences elsewhere.[512–514]

Several issues confound radiation outcomes assessments for vestibular schwannomas. First, documentation of recurrences can be confounded by inherently slow growth rates and transient post-procedure lesion enlargement.[515,516] Second, ionizing radiation does carry a small inherent risk of inducing secondary neoplasms or malignant transformation of the vestibular schwannoma.[517,518] The risk of a secondary neoplasm can be particularly concerning in tumor-prone genetic conditions such as NF2. However, given the immense number of individuals who have undergone SRS worldwide, the number of presumed radiation-induced malignancies is only a handful and represents, at most, 1 per 1,000 patients. This is substantially lower than the rate of surgery-related mortality. Malignant transformations can also be seen in resected vestibular schwannoma patients who did not receive radiation.[519] Finally, because of increased adherence of the facial nerve to the tumor, eighth nerve preservation rates are lower when the excision is performed for regrowth after radiation when compared to a non-irradiated control group.[520]

Targeted Therapy for Vestibular Schwannoma

There is significant interest in the development of medical therapy for patients with refractory vestibular schwannoma. Aberrant signaling pathways are known to be present, and there are now reports of the use of targeted agents in this disease. In a single patient case report, the EGFR inhibitor erlotinib was associated with radiographic response of the tumor and improved audiologic function.[521] There are also two reports of the use of bevacizumab in the treatment of vestibular schwannoma in the setting of NF1 in patients with a single hearing ear.[522,523] These studies consisted of a small number of patients, but the demonstration of objective regression of tumors and improvement in hearing was impressive, highlighting the need for larger prospective trials of antiangiogenic agents for this disease. There is also a report of using bevacizumab in treating vestibular schwannoma in the patients who have NF2.[522]

GLOMUS JUGULARE TUMORS

Clinical and Pathologic Considerations

Glomus jugulare tumors (paragangliomas) arise from glomus tissue in the adventitia of the jugular bulb (glomus jugulare) or along the Jacobson nerve in the temporal bone, sometimes multifocally. The tumor invades the temporal bone diffusely, but growth is characteristically slow. Sometimes these tumors are endocrine active, with a carcinoid- or pheochromocytoma-like syndrome.[524] Because glomus jugulare tumors occur in the jugular foramen, they commonly cause lower cranial nerve palsies and early symptoms of hoarseness and difficulty swallowing. Facial weakness, hearing loss, and atrophy of the tongue from hypoglossal palsy can follow. Pulsating tinnitus also may be a presenting symptom, and a red pulsating mass is often visible behind the eardrum. A presumptive diagnosis of glomus tumor can be made by CT or MRI scanning, with jugular schwannoma and meningioma being the main differential diagnoses. On CT scans, glomus tumors show a characteristic salt-and-pepper appearance in involved bone; MRI often discloses large blood vessels within the mass. Glomus tumors give positive results on octreotide scintigraphy. These tumors incite a tremendous blood supply, particularly by way of the ascending pharyngeal artery. An angiography provides the definitive diagnosis. Because preoperative tumor embolization is essential to the surgical removal of glomus tumors, the diagnostic angiogram should be taken before surgery. Histopathologically, numerous vascular channels are distinctive. The background is composed of clear cells clumped in a fibrous matrix. A small percentage of glomus tumors are malignant. There is a familial form in which the tumors are multiple.

Surgery

The treatment of glomus jugulare tumors is controversial, with advocates for surgery, RT, radiosurgery, and combined approaches. Although surgery can often provide a cure for these benign tumors, especially for small lesions, RT and radiosurgery avoid the morbidities that may follow surgical removal (e.g., lower cranial nerve and facial palsies). Surgery for glomus tumors is most often jointly performed by a neurosurgeon and an otorhinolaryngologist after preoperative embolization, which may decrease intraoperative blood loss during the resection of these extremely vascular tumors. Complications of this procedure can include swallowing and aspiration problems, CSF leak, and facial palsy.

Radiation Therapy

Even though glomus tumors are histologically benign, RT is effective and has been recommended for symptomatic lesions that cannot be totally resected, even as primary treatment.[525] These tumors regress slowly after irradiation, and the success of RT is measured by the amelioration of symptoms and the absence of disease progression. A review of the literature demonstrated local control rates with radiation in excess of 90% with or without surgery.[526] A dose of 45 to 50 Gy over the course of 5 weeks is recommended.

Radiosurgery

A literature review by Gottfried et al.[527] showed that the use of SRS to treat glomus jugulare tumors has increased. Compared with conventional radiotherapy, radiosurgery involves a shorter treatment time, precise stereotactic localization, and irradiation of a small volume of normal tissue, which results in a reduced incidence of complications. Among 142 patients treated radiosurgically in eight series reviewed by Gottfried et al., tumors diminished in 36.5%, tumor size was unchanged in 61.3%, and subjective or objective improvements occurred in 39%. Although a residual tumor was present in all of these patients, only 2.1% experienced progression, the morbidity rate was 8.5%, and no deaths occurred; however, the incidence of late recurrence is unknown. In another study of eight patients who underwent radiosurgery (median dose of 15 Gy to the tumor margin) for recurrent, residual, or unresectable glomus jugulare tumors, all remained stable without cranial nerve palsies at a median follow-up of 28 months.[528] The authors suggested treatment of small glomus tumors (3 cm or less in average dimension) with radiosurgery and treatment of young patients with large tumors (3 cm or more in average dimension) and patients with symptomatic tumors with surgical resection.

A recent meta-analysis based on data from 19 studies revealed radiosurgical tumor control in 97% of patients. In eight studies with a median follow-up time exceeding 36 months, 96% of patients achieved tumor control.[529]

HEMANGIOBLASTOMAS

Clinical and Pathologic Considerations

Hemangioblastomas account for 1% to 2% of intracranial tumors, arising most often in the cerebellar hemispheres and vermis.

Although usually solitary, these tumors can be multiple and may also occur in the brainstem, spinal cord, and less often, the cerebrum. Cerebellar hemangioblastomas can be sporadic or occur as part of the autosomal-dominant von Hippel-Lindau complex, which is transmitted with more than 90% penetrance.[530] Other entities associated with von Hippel-Lindau disease are retinal angiomatosis, polycystic kidneys, pancreatic cysts, pheochromocytoma, and renal cell carcinoma. Identification of the *VHL* gene on chromosome band 3p25–26 allows individuals who are at risk for the syndrome, or who have some of its components as an apparent sporadic case, to undergo genetic testing with a high degree of accuracy.[531]

Cerebellar hemangioblastomas usually are recognized in the 3rd decade in patients with von Hippel-Lindau disease and in the 4th decade or later in patients with sporadic tumors. These tumors can cause symptoms and signs of cerebellar dysfunction, especially gait disturbance and ataxia, and hydrocephalus from obstruction of CSF pathways. These tumors tend to enlarge slowly, but patients may become symptomatic from tumor cysts, which can grow quickly.[532]

Hemangioblastomas are composed of capillary and sinusoidal channels lined with endothelial cells. Interspersed are groups of polygonal stromal cells with lipid-laden cytoplasm and hyperchromatic nuclei. An immunohistochemical study of these cells shows expression of neuron-specific enolase, vimentin, and S100 protein, but not epithelial membrane antigen or glial fibrillary acidic protein.[533] Grossly, the tumor is often cystic, containing proteinaceous, xanthochromic fluid and with an orange-red, vascular, and firm mural nodule. The cyst wall is a glial nonneoplastic reaction to fluid secreted by the nodule. Some hemangioblastomas lack cysts, especially in the brainstem and spinal cord, but cystic lesions are more often symptomatic, at least in patients with von Hippel-Lindau disease.[532]

The natural history of spinal hemangioblastomas has been described.[532] The authors reviewed the clinical records and MRIs of 160 consecutively treated patients with 331 spinal hemangioblastomas. Most lesions were located in the posterior cord. Cysts were commonly associated with the lesions, often showing faster growth than the solid portion of the tumor. When symptoms appeared, the mass effect derived more from the cyst than from the tumor. These tumors often have alternating periods of tumor growth and stability, and some remain stable in size for many years. These factors have to be considered in the timing and choice of treatment.

Surgery

A complete resection of a hemangioblastoma is often curative. Patients with preoperative hypertension should be evaluated for the presence of a pheochromocytoma, which can be associated with von Hippel-Lindau disease. Hemangioblastomas are very vascular lesions, and a biopsy of a suspected hemangioblastoma, either through an open approach or stereotactically, is usually ill advised because of the high risk of hemorrhage. Surgical resection should be carried out en bloc with avoidance of entry into the lesion, which can result in fierce bleeding reminiscent of an arteriovenous malformation. Preoperative, transarterial embolization is rarely safe because these tumors often receive supply from distal segments of the intra-axial circulation. Fortunately, these hemangioblastomas can be resected with minimal bleeding if resection is carried out entirely in the gliottic plane that surrounds the mass. This is straightforward in most cerebellar tumors, for which a margin of gliottic tissue can be resected with the lesion with little neurologic risk. In contrast, brainstem hemangioblastomas are immediately adjacent to critical structures.[534,535] Sometimes, dissection immediately adjacent to the tumor can cause significant bleeding, with a high risk of inducing neurologic deficits.

These tumors are often associated with significant cysts. Surgery is the optimal treatment for the rapid relief of mass effect.

The cyst wall is not lined with tumor cells, and drainage, rather than excision, of the cyst lining is required. The mural tumor nodule must be entirely resected to avoid cyst recurrence. Cysts can be drained before opening the dura completely to provide brain relaxation, but great care must be taken not to disturb the tumor nodule during this maneuver to avoid inducing significant bleeding. The risk of hemorrhage during the resection is minimized by coagulating and dividing arterial feeders, if they can be visualized, before tumor removal. Finally, hemangioblastomas that occur in patients known to have von Hippel-Lindau disease may not need to be resected or otherwise treated unless they have demonstrated active growth or are symptomatic from mass effect or hydrocephalus. Because many of these patients harbor multiple tumors, other approaches, including radiosurgery, should also be considered, although surgery remains the only option that has a proven benefit.

Radiation Therapy

RT is recommended for patients with unresectable, incompletely excised, and recurrent hemangioblastomas and for those who are medically inoperable. Doses of at least 50 to 55 Gy over the course of 5.5 to 6 weeks appear to be warranted.[536] Because of the noninvasive nature of these lesions, conformal radiotherapy or radiosurgery is indicated.

Radiosurgery should be considered for surgically unresectable hemangioblastomas, as adjuvant treatment for incompletely excised tumors, as definitive treatment for multifocal disease, and as salvage therapy for discrete recurrences after surgery.[100,537] Although SRS treatment of hemangioblastomas in von Hippel-Lindau disease has a low risk for adverse radiation effects, it is associated with diminishing control over a long-term follow-up,[538] and SRS should not be used to prophylactically treat asymptomatic tumors and should be reserved for the treatment of tumors that are not surgically resectable.

Chemotherapy

Because stromal cells in hemangioblastomas secrete VEGF, there is much interest in evaluating small-molecule inhibitors of the vascular endothelial growth factor -2 (VEGF-2) (KDR, FLK-1) receptor as medical management for these tumors, especially for patients with von Hippel-Lindau disease, who routinely harbor multiple hemangioblastomas. Unfortunately, the extreme heterogeneity of tumor growth, with periods of spontaneous stability and a slow overall growth rate, makes it extremely difficult to design trials to rigorously test the efficacy of any systemic therapy. In a small study of sunitinib therapy in 15 patients with von Hippel-Lindau disease–associated tumors, one-third of individuals with renal cell carcinoma achieved a partial response but none with hemangioblastomas.[539]

CHORDOMAS AND CHONDROSARCOMAS

Chordomas and chondrosarcomas are rare, locally destructive, slow-growing, malignant bone tumors. Although skull-base chordomas and chondrosarcomas are sometimes pooled together, recent studies have shown important differences between these entities.

Clinical and Pathologic Considerations

Chordomas arise within aberrant chordal vestiges along the pathway of the primitive notochord that extends from the tip of the dorsum sellae to the coccyx.[540] One-third of chordomas arise cranially, with this location more common in women and younger individuals.[541] Chordomas are extradural, pseudoencapsulated, multilobulated tumors, with a gelatinous consistency centered in

the bone, classically with soft tissue extension. Microscopically, the typical chordoma is characterized by cordlike rows of *physaliferous* cells with multiple round, clear cytoplasmic vacuoles that impart a bubbly appearance to the cytoplasm. Two pathologic variants have been described. The *chondroid chordoma* has areas with cartilaginous features but a genetic profile distinct from chondrosarcomas.[542] The *dedifferentiated chordoma* contains areas of typical chordoma admixed with components that resemble high-grade or poorly differentiated spindle cell sarcoma. In typical chordomas, mitotic figures and atypia are rare; a higher mitotic rate and Ki-67 more than 6% are associated with a shorter doubling time.[543]

Chondrosarcomas are cartilage-producing neoplasm that arise within any of the complex synchondroses in the skull base, with the most common sites of origin being the temporo-occipital synchondrosis (66%), the spheno-occiput synchondrosis (28%), and the sphenoethmoid complex (6%).[544] Thus, chondrosarcomas predominantly originate in more lateral skull-base structures, unlike most chordomas, which originate in the midline. Chondrosarcomas can be difficult to differentiate from chordomas on a pathologic examination. Immunohistochemical advances have improved differentiation between chordomas and chondrosarcomas. In one series of 200 chondrosarcomas, 99% stained positive for S100, 0% for keratin, and epithelial membrane antigen was expressed in 8%.[544] These immunohistochemical studies allow a chondrosarcoma to be differentiated from a chordoma, which is reactive for keratin and epithelial membrane antigen. The same series confirmed the low-grade nature of base of skull chondrosarcomas because a majority were grade 1, with no grade 3 tumors identified. Mesenchymal chondrosarcomas may have a separate, more aggressive natural history.[545]

Symptoms that prompt evaluation are typically cranial nerve deficits with the precise deficit dependent on the location and extent of the tumor. In one series, the most common presentation was headaches with intermittent abducens nerve palsy.[546] Additional symptoms can be caused by intracranial extension with compression of the brainstem, pituitary gland, or optic apparatus. Neck pain may develop in lower clival tumors, possibly the result of pathologic fracture or periosteal expansion.

The differential diagnosis of cranial chordoma and chondrosarcoma includes basal meningioma, schwannoma (neurilemoma), nasopharyngeal carcinoma, pituitary adenoma, and craniopharyngioma. Chondrosarcomas and chordomas cannot be reliably distinguished from each other based on imaging features or location alone.[547] High-resolution CT images with bone and soft tissue algorithms show a discrete, expansile soft tissue mass with extensive bony destruction.[548] On MRI scanning, both chordomas and chondrosarcomas are hyperintense on T2-weighted sequences, with variegated enhancement. The location may be useful in distinguishing chordomas (midline clivus) from chondrosarcomas (petrous apex), although there is considerable overlap. Given the low risk of nodal or hematogenous dissemination, imaging beyond the primary site other than a chest x-ray is typically not indicated unless metastatic disease is suspected clinically.[549] A baseline endocrine evaluation and neuro-ophthalmologic examination are both recommended if diagnostic imaging or symptoms suggest involvement.

Surgery

Surgery for cranial chordomas and chondrosarcomas provides the backbone of treatment and is obligatory to obtain diagnostic tissue, to enhance the effectiveness of subsequent RT, and to improve the patient's clinical condition. An aggressive initial approach may improve overall outcome.[126] Intracranial chordomas occur at the base of the skull, a region relatively remote from surgical access. Approaches to skull-base chordomas and chondrosarcomas often involve teams that include both neurosurgeons and otolaryngologists. There is developing interest in the use of endoscopy for the primary removal of chordomas or to assist in the removal of these tumors via traditional open approaches. Although most series remain small, excellent results have been reported in appropriately selected patients not having extension lateral to the carotid arteries.[550,551] A combination of exposures and procedures can be used for extremely large tumors. One goal of surgery is to remove as much tumor from the optic system and brainstem as possible so that very high doses of radiation can be delivered safely. Optimal treatment of these lesions is complete resection, if possible.

A potentially serious complication of the transsphenoidal, transsphenothmoid, and transoral approaches is CSF leakage into the nose or oropharynx and consequent meningitis. Therefore, every attempt is made to keep the dura intact during these procedures. Because dural invasion by cranial chordomas may occur 50% of the time, dural entry during tumor resection is sometimes unavoidable. Careful intraoperative patching of the leak with fat and muscle grafts followed by postoperative spinal CSF drainage should be undertaken to decrease the risk of infection in these cases. This may be more challenging in the setting of a total endoscopic tumor removal, although some techniques appear to be associated with reasonably low rates of CSF leak. Surgical series have reported gross total resection rates of 43% to 72%, with the most recent series using modern imaging and microsurgical techniques reporting the highest gross total resection rate. In this series, there was a 31% recurrence-free survival at 10 years, which was improved for those without previous intervention, and a 35% recurrence after gross total resection.[552,553] The extent of resection correlated with both recurrence rates and survival. Surgical morbidity can be significant, with Gay et al.[554] reporting a significant transient (53%) and permanent (43%) worsening of the Karnofsky performance score following surgery.

Approaches for chondrosarcomas are different because of the paramedian location of the tumors. Like chordomas, chondrosarcomas begin as extradural tumors, and maintaining the intact dural barrier is paramount. A complete tumor excision, which is paramount in chordoma surgery, is less critical for chondrosarcomas because tumor control rates with adjuvant high-dose radiation are high. Surgery is often tailored to emphasize the removal of tumor portions abutting critical structures such as the chiasm or brainstem to allow adequate radiation treatment. Cranial chordomas often recur after surgery and RT. In this situation, reoperation directed toward symptomatic improvement is the only treatment option. Reoperations are complicated by surgical scarring and tissue compromise from irradiation, and CSF leaks and other complications are more frequent.

Radiation Therapy

A radical excision with negative margins is often not feasible, and even gross excision is often obtained piecemeal with the risk of persistent microscopic disease. Because relentless extension is typical of chordomas and chondrosarcomas and recurrence is a strong predictor of OS, adequate local control is paramount in determining outcome. Radiotherapy is a mainstay of treatment in preventing recurrence or progression of tumor.

Local control of chordomas appears to be dose dependent. Conventional radiation at doses of 50 to 55 Gy does not offer satisfactory local control. A median dose of 50 Gy to chordomas of the skull, sacrum, and mobile spine provided only a 27% local control rate with a median time to progression of 35 months.[549] Durable control was worse in base of skull disease, with only 1 out of 13 clival chordomas remaining disease free. FSRT to 37 spheno-occipital chordomas to a mean dose of 66.6 Gy provided local control rates of 82% at 2 years and 50% at 5 years. Despite a median tumor volume of 55.6 mL, complications were limited with one patient developing a pontine infarct 25 months posttreatment. No instances of optic neuropathy were identified. Chondrosarcomas treated with the same fractionation scheme had 100% 5-year local control.[555]

Radiosurgery

SRS has been used to treat chordomas and chondrosarcomas of the skull base, although its application is limited because of size constraints and proximity to critical structures. In one series, candidates were limited to less than 3 cm in greatest diameter and 5 mm from the optic chiasm, with a mean treatment volume of 4.6 mL and a maximum volume of 10.3 mL.[556] With a mean margin dose of 18 Gy, more than 50% of patients in this mixed series of chondrosarcomas and chordomas had symptomatic improvement and, at a mean follow-up of 40 months, 20% had recurred locally outside of the treatment field. Krishnan et al.[557] reported a similar local control rate (24%) with both in-field and out-of-field recurrences, although no recurrences occurred in patients with chondroid chordomas or chondrosarcomas. The risk of significant radiation-related complications was high at 34%, although complications were seen only in patients who had received prior fractionated radiotherapy.

Particle-Beam Therapy

Charged-particle therapy, because of its innate dose-distribution advantages, has been used for many years to escalate dose to chordomas and chondrosarcomas while minimizing radiation-related side effects. The most extensive experience in treating base of skull chordomas and chondrosarcomas with proton therapy arises from the experience at the Harvard Cyclotron Laboratory. Chordoma relapse-free survival was 59% at 4 years and 44% at 10 years, with similar rates seen in other series.[558–561] Mean dose ranged from 67 to 70.7 cobalt gray equivalent (CGE). Female gender, dose heterogeneity, large tumor size (more than 25 to 75 mL), brainstem invasion, and dose constrained by proximity to critical structures were all associated with higher rates of recurrence.[562] In a study of skull-base chordomas in 73 children and adolescents (mean age, 9.7 years), patients were treated with partial or gross surgical excision and postoperative proton beam irradiation.[559] The mean follow-up period was 7.25 years, and the overall patient survival rate was 81% among 42 patients with conventional chordomas, 17 with chondroid chordomas, and 14 with cellular chordomas, 6 of which were poorly differentiated and highly aggressive. The most recent relatively large proton experience for managing skull-based chordomas comes from the Paul Scherrer Institute (PSI) in Switzerland. They have reported an 81% 5-year local control with surgery plus scanning proton beam therapy in 42 patients, possibly the best data reported in this disease to date. Median total dose for chordomas was 73.5 Gy at 1.8 to 2.0 Gy per fraction. Actuarial 5-year freedom from high-grade toxicity was 94%.[563]

Chondrosarcomas of the skull base had remarkably high local control rates of 99% and 98% at 5 and 10 years, respectively. Pituitary dysfunction and hearing loss were the most common side effects, with depression, memory loss, temporal necrosis, hearing loss, and blindness being less common. Given the relative lack of morbidity and the suboptimal local control for chordomas, dose escalation has been proposed. Recent radiotherapeutic advances include spot-scanning proton radiation.[564] Carbon ion radiotherapy—charged-particle therapy using a heavier ion—has also been used with good local control with a short follow-up and better than expected radiographic responses.[565] Amichetti et al.[566] recently conducted a systematic review of the scientific literature published between 1980 and 2008 on data regarding irradiation of chondrosarcoma of the skull base with proton therapy. From 49 reports retrieved, there were no prospective trials and 9 uncontrolled single-arm studies mainly related to advanced and frequently incompletely resected tumors. According to the inclusion criteria, only four articles, reporting the most recent updated results of the publishing institution, were included in the analysis, providing clinical outcomes for 254 patients. The major findings corroborated the high control rates with low morbidity described previously.

Chemotherapy

In a prospective, phase II clinical study trial, 56 patients with advanced disease were treated with imatinib.[567] In 50 evaluable patients, one partial response (PR) and 35 stable disease (SD, 70%) and a 64% clinical benefit rate (i.e., Response Evaluation Criteria in Sold Tumors [RECIST] complete response + PR + SD ≥6 months) was noted.[567] Patients who have progressed after an initial response to imatinib can respond to combinations of imatinib and sirolimus.[568]

CHOROID PLEXUS TUMORS

Clinical and Pathologic Considerations

Primary tumors of the choroid plexus (CP) are classified according to the WHO as choroid plexus papilloma (CPP, WHO grade I), atypical CPP (grade II), and choroid plexus carcinoma (CPC, grade III).[4] These are rare tumors that occur most often in children younger than 12 years of age. Although the grade might imply a clinical progression, typical CPP are a distinct entity, and almost never progress to CPC. Choroid plexus tumors appear irregular and lobulated, often very red because of underlying vasculature. Histopathologic examinations of papillomas often show an apparently normal choroid plexus, with increased cellular crowding and elongation. CPC show malignant features such as increased cellularity, high mitotic activity, loss of typical cellular architecture, and invasion of the brain parenchyma. Bridging the CPP and CPC is the entity called atypical CPP. Histologically, atypical CPP retains the architecture of the CPP but has high mitotic activity and an increase probability for recurrence after surgical resection. CPCs are commonly seen in families who carry a germline mutation in either the *TP53* gene (Li-Fraumeni syndrome).[569] However, most patients with CPP and sporadic CPC do not harbor a germline TP53 mutation.

In children, CPCs most often occur in the lateral ventricles. In adults, the fourth ventricular papilloma is most common. Third ventricle tumors are exceedingly rare. Because papillomas tend to grow slowly within ventricles, they expand to fill the ventricle and block CSF flow. In addition, papillomas can secrete CSF. CPPs and CPCs can produce hydrocephalus secondary to obstruction of the CSF, CSF overproduction by the tumor, or damage to the CSF resorptive bed from recurrent hemorrhages. As a result, increased ICP without focal findings is the most common presentation. Fourth ventricular tumors can also be associated with focal findings of ataxia and nystagmus. Although CPPS rarely seed throughout the CSF spaces, seeding from carcinomas is frequent and often symptomatic. CPCs will show invasion of the surrounding brain with resultant increased signal on T2-weighted MRI, and signs of rich vascularity (flow voids), often arising medially from the choroidal vessels.

Choroid plexus tumors are seen easily by MRI. Imaging demonstrates a lobulated, well-circumscribed, enhancing, intraventricular lesion, often with associated hydrocephalus. Calcification is not common. Choroid carcinomas may show areas consistent with necrosis and brain invasion.[570]

Surgery

The complete treatment of CPPs is total excision. Hydrocephalus is the rule and simplifies the exposure once the ventricle is opened. Tumor-associated branches of the choroidal vessels are coagulated and divided as early as is feasible in the procedure because this greatly reduces hemorrhaging. Smaller tumors are removed intact and larger tumors are removed piecemeal. Perioperative CSF drainage is used to prevent subdural hygromas. In half of patients, hydrocephalus is relieved by tumor resection, but persistent hydrocephalus requires shunting. The ability to perform a complete resection depends on histologic type, with nearly a 100% complete resection rate for papillomas versus as low as a 33% complete resection rate for CPCs.[571] A meta-analysis of all individual cases of CPC reported as of 2004 (347 patients) showed that in the subgroup of incompletely resected carcinomas, 22.6% of patients required a second surgery.[572] The prognosis for these patients appeared better than for those with incomplete resections who did not undergo a second surgery (2-year OS times were 69% and 30%, respectively).

In the pediatric age group, when the diagnosis of CPC is suspected, the primary tumor resection should not be attempted because these tumors are extremely vascular, leading to the loss of multiple blood volumes and not infrequent intra-operative deaths. Cases of suspected CPC should be treated with an open biopsy, followed by ICE chemotherapy to devascularize the tumor. Subsequent postchemotherapy surgery is much safer and results in a greatly reduced blood loss.

Radiation Therapy

Because CPPs are often cured by a complete resection, radiotherapy is infrequently employed. Further, in a study of 41 patients, Krishnan et al.[573] noted that reoperation for recurrence was required only half the time after the initial subtotal resection, suggesting that adjuvant radiotherapy may not be necessary after the initial subtotal resection in all patients. Because local control outcome at first relapse was poor after the subtotal resection, they concluded that the most reasonable role for RT is after a subtotal resection of a recurrence.

Chemotherapy

Chemotherapy is not used for CPPs, although it has been attempted for CPCs. As with many of the less common CNS tumors, there are no firm guidelines. Anecdotal reports have cited moderate responses to the platinum compounds, as well as to alkylating agents, etoposide, methotrexate, and possibly anthracyclines. A Pediatric Oncology Group study of eight infants with CPC suggests that radiation can be forestalled by using chemotherapy in some infants with these tumors.[574] In a meta-analysis conducted by Wrede et al.,[575] CPCs were analyzed; 104 cases with CPC received chemotherapy and had a statistically better survival than those without chemotherapy.

SPINAL AXIS TUMORS

Clinical and Pathologic Considerations

Most primary spinal axis tumors produce symptoms and signs as a result of cord and nerve root compression rather than parenchymal invasion. The frequency of primary spinal cord tumors is between 10% and 19% of all primary CNS tumors. Parenthetically, the majority of neoplasms that affect the spine are extradural metastases, whereas most primary tumors are intradural. Of the intradural neoplasms, extramedullary schwannomas and meningiomas are the most common. Schwannomas and meningiomas are normally intradural, but occasionally, may present as extradural tumors. Other intradural, extramedullary neoplasms include vascular tumors, chordomas, and epidermoids. Intramedullary tumors include ependymomas, comprising approximately 40% of intramedullary tumors; the remainder are astrocytomas, oligodendrogliomas, gangliogliomas, medulloblastomas, and hemangioblastomas. Approximately half of spinal tumors involve the thoracic spinal canal (the longest spinal segment), 30% involve the lumbosacral spine, and the remainder involve the cervical spine, including the foramen magnum. Schwannomas occur with greatest frequency in the thoracic spine, although they can be found at other levels. They often extend through an intervertebral foramen in a dumbbell configuration. Meningiomas are dural based and arise preferentially at the foramen magnum and in the thoracic spine. Most patients are women. Astrocytomas are distributed throughout the spinal cord, and most ependymomas involve the conus medullaris and the cauda equina. Spinal chordomas are characteristically sacral and only rarely affect the cervical region or the rest of the mobile spine.

Patients may present with a sensorimotor spinal tract syndrome, a painful radicular spinal cord syndrome, or a central syringomyelic syndrome. In the sensorimotor presentation, symptoms and signs reflect compression of the cord. The onset is gradual during weeks to months, initial presentation is asymmetric, and motor weakness predominates. The level of impairment determines the muscle groups involved. Because of external compression, dorsal column involvement results in paresthesia and abnormalities of pain and temperature on the side contralateral to the motor weakness.

Radicular spinal cord syndromes occur because of external compression and infiltration of spinal roots. The main symptom is sharp, radicular pain in the distribution of a sensory nerve root. The intense pain is often of short duration, with pain that is more aching in nature persisting for longer periods. Pain may be exacerbated by coughing and sneezing or other maneuvers that increase ICP. Local paresthesia and numbness are common, as are weakness and muscle wasting. These findings often precede cord compression by months. Often, the pain is difficult for the clinician to differentiate from ordinary musculoskeletal symptoms, which causes diagnostic delay.

Intramedullary tumors, in particular, can give rise to syringomyelic dysfunction by destruction and cavitation within the central gray matter of the cord. This produces lower motor neuron destruction with associated segmental muscle weakness, atrophy, and hyporeflexia. There is also a dissociated sensory loss of pain and temperature sensation with the preservation of touch. As the syrinx increases in size, all sensory modalities are affected.

Surgery

The operating microscope is essential for spinal cord tumor surgery. Ultrasonography can be used to examine the spinal cord through either intact or open dura to find the level of maximum tumor involvement or to differentiate tumor cysts from solid tumors. Intraoperative monitoring of somatosensory-evoked potentials is commonly used, although some surgeons think that changes in somatosensory-evoked potentials may occur only after irretrievable damage has occurred, and this remains a topic of controversy. Motor-evoked potentials are used in some centers to guide resection and have retrospectively been shown by some to decrease long-term motor deficits.

MRI is invaluable for the diagnosis, localization, and characterization of spinal tumors. For extremely vascular tumors—notably, hemangioblastoma—angiography may provide important preoperative delineation of the tumor blood supply. CT scanning is useful for tumors of the bony axis. Determination of the spinal level of the tumor and its exact relation to the cord is important. Corticosteroids are given before, during, and after spinal cord tumor surgery to help control spinal cord edema.

Meningiomas and schwannomas occur in the intradural, extramedullary spinal compartment. Most of these tumors can be completely resected through a laminectomy. They can be easily separated away from the cord, which is displaced but not invaded by tumor. Schwannomas arise most often in the dorsal spinal rootlets, and their removal includes the rootlets involved. They can grow along the nerve root in a dumbbell fashion through a neural foramen. Some of these can be removed by extending the initial laminectomy exposure laterally, whereas others require a separate operation (e.g., a thoracotomy, costotransversectomy, or a retroperitoneal approach). Strictly anteriorly situated cervical tumors can

successfully be removed via an anterior approach using a corpectomy of the appropriate vertebral levels, followed by strut grafting after the tumor resection.

The most common intramedullary tumors are ependymomas and astrocytomas. Except for malignant astrocytomas, resection is the principal treatment for these tumors. Intramedullary tumors are approached through a laminectomy. After dural opening, a longitudinal myelotomy is made, usually in the midline or dorsal root entry zone. The incision is deepened several millimeters to the tumor surface. Dissection planes around the tumor are sought microsurgically and, in the case of ependymomas, usually found and extended gradually around the tumor's surface, whereas removal of the central tumor bulk (by carbon dioxide laser or ultrasonic aspirator) causes the tumor to collapse. Such tumors are usually completely removed, with good long-term outcomes.[576] Some patients later develop a spinal deformity, requiring stabilization procedures.[577] Tumors without clear dissection planes (usually astrocytomas) cannot be removed completely, but bulk reduction can cause long-term palliation. If a frozen-section analysis shows a tumor to be a malignant glioma, a less aggressive surgery is typically performed due to the increased risk of morbidity with little benefit achieved from an extensive debulking procedure.

Radiation Therapy

RT is recommended for unresectable and incompletely resected neoplasms of the spinal axis. In general, doses of 50 to 54 Gy (1.8 Gy per day) are used so that the risk of injury to the cord from radiation is minimized. When lesions involve only the cauda equina or when complete, irreversible myelopathy already has occurred, higher doses are used.

Ependymomas have a longer natural history than astrocytomas. Recurrence of ependymomas may be delayed for as long as 12 years.[578,579] RT is not necessary when ependymomas are removed completely in an en bloc fashion.[576] All nonirradiated patients with incompletely excised lesions reported by Barone and Elvidge[580] and by Shuman et al.[581] experienced recurrence. Postoperative irradiation appears to improve tumor control for incompletely resected ependymomas. Five- and 10-year survival rates in irradiated patients with localized ependymomas range from 60% to 100% and 68% to 95%, respectively, whereas 10-year relapse-free survival rates vary from 43% to 61%.[582] The tumor grade has a significant effect on outcome. Waldron et al.[579] found that for patients with well-differentiated tumors, the 5-year cause-specific survival was 97% compared with 71% for patients with intermediate or poorly differentiated tumors ($p = 0.005$). Myxopapillary ependymomas that arise in the conus medullaris and filum terminale have a better prognosis than the cellular ependymomas that arise in the cord.[583] Local recurrence is the predominant pattern of treatment failure, occurring in 25% of irradiated patients.[579]

The 5- and 10-year survival rates for irradiated patients with low-grade astrocytomas of the spinal cord vary from 60% to 90% and 40% to 90%, respectively; 5- and 10-year relapse-free survival rates range from 66% to 83% and 53% to 83%, respectively.[577,579] Fifty percent to 65% of astrocytomas are controlled locally. Good neurologic condition at the time of irradiation, lower histologic grade, and younger age are favorable factors.[584] Patterns of recurrence for malignant astrocytomas of the spine have been analyzed by MRI.[585] Despite surgery and full-dose radiation, spinal or brain dissemination is the predominant mode of failure.

Chemotherapy

There are no significant controlled clinical trials of chemotherapy for primary spinal axis tumors. Drugs active against intracranial tumors logically may be assumed to be equally efficacious against histologically identical tumors in the spinal cord. Temozolomide is being increasingly used in this setting.

SELECTED REFERENCES

The full reference list can be accessed at lwwhealthlibrary.com/oncology.

1. Pokhrel KP, Vovoras D, Tsokos CP. Histological and demographic characteristics of the distribution of brain and central nervous system tumors' sizes: results from SEER registries using statistical methods. *Int J Biomed Sci* 2012;8:152–162.
2. Ostrom QT, Gittleman H, Farah P, et al. CBTRUS Statistical Report: primary brain and central nervous system tumors diagnosed in the United States in 2006-2010. *Neuro Oncol* 2013;15:ii1–ii56.
3. Kleihues P, Burger PC, Scheithauer BW. The new WHO classification of brain tumours. *Brain Pathol* 1993;3:255–268.
4. Louis DN, Ohgaki H, Wiestler OD, et al. The 2007 WHO classification of tumours of the central nervous system. *Acta Neuropathol* 2007;114:97–109.
6. Bondy ML, Scheurer ME, Malmer B, et al. Brain tumor epidemiology: consensus from the Brain Tumor Epidemiology Consortium. *Cancer* 2008; 113:1953–1968.
8. Sadetzki S, Chetrit A, Freedman L, et al. Long-term follow-up for brain tumor development after childhood exposure to ionizing radiation for tinea capitis. *Radiat Res* 2005;163:424–432.
12. Claus EB, Calvocoressi L, Bondy ML, et al. Dental x-rays and risk of meningioma. *Cancer* 2012;118:4530–4537.
16. Kan P, Simonsen SE, Lyon JL, et al. Cellular phone use and brain tumor: a meta-analysis. *J Neurooncol* 2008;86:71–78.
17. Myung SK, Ju W, McDonnell DD, et al. Mobile phone use and risk of tumors: a meta-analysis. *J Clin Oncol* 2009;27:5565–5572.
19. Samkange-Zeeb F, Schlehofer B, Schuz J, et al. Occupation and risk of glioma, meningioma and acoustic neuroma: results from a German case-control study (interphone study group, Germany). *Cancer Epidemiol* 2010; 34:55–61.
25. Dziurzynski K, Chang SM, Heimberger AB, et al. Consensus on the role of human cytomegalovirus in glioblastoma. *Neuro Oncol* 2012;14:246–255.
28. Gu J, Liu Y, Kyritsis AP, et al. Molecular epidemiology of primary brain tumors. *Neurotherapeutics* 2009;6:427–435.
32. Grayson JK. Radiation exposure, socioeconomic status, and brain tumor risk in the US Air Force: a nested case-control study. *Am J Epidemiol* 1996; 143:480–486.
41. Dirks PB. Cancer: stem cells and brain tumours. *Nature* 2006;444:687–688.
42. Friedmann-Morvinski D, Bushong EA, Ke E, et al. Dedifferentiation of neurons and astrocytes by oncogenes can induce gliomas in mice. *Science* 2012;338:1080–1084.
44. Cha S. Neuroimaging in neuro-oncology. *Neurotherapeutics* 2009;6:465–477.
46. Omuro AM, Leite CC, Mokhtari K, et al. Pitfalls in the diagnosis of brain tumours. *Lancet Neurol* 2006;5:937–948.
47. Price SJ. Advances in imaging low-grade gliomas. *Adv Tech Stand Neurosurg* 2010;35:1–34.
48. Brandao LA, Shiroishi MS, Law M. Brain tumors: a multimodality approach with diffusion-weighted imaging, diffusion tensor imaging, magnetic resonance spectroscopy, dynamic susceptibility contrast and dynamic contrast-enhanced magnetic resonance imaging. *Magn Reson Imaging Clin N Am* 2013;21:199–239.
52. Brandes AA, Franceschi E, Tosoni A, et al. MGMT promoter methylation status can predict the incidence and outcome of pseudoprogression after concomitant radiochemotherapy in newly diagnosed glioblastoma patients. *J Clin Oncol* 2008;26:2192–2197.
53. Wen PY, Macdonald DR, Reardon DA, et al. Updated response assessment criteria for high-grade gliomas: response assessment in neuro-oncology working group. *J Clin Oncol* 2010;28:1963–1972.
55. McGirt MJ, Chaichana KL, Gathinji M, et al. Independent association of extent of resection with survival in patients with malignant brain astrocytoma. *J Neurosurg* 2009;110:156–162.
56. Sanai N, Polley MY, McDermott MW, et al. An extent of resection threshold for newly diagnosed glioblastomas. *J Neurosurg* 2011;115:3–8.
57. Orringer D, Lau D, Khatri S, et al. Extent of resection in patients with glioblastoma: limiting factors, perception of resectability, and effect on survival. *J Neurosurg* 2012;117:851–859.
61. Henry RG, Berman JI, Nagarajan SS, et al. Subcortical pathways serving cortical language sites: initial experience with diffusion tensor imaging fiber tracking combined with intraoperative language mapping. *Neuroimage* 2004;21:616–622.
63. Stummer W, Pichlmeier U, Meinel T, et al. Fluorescence-guided surgery with 5-aminolevulinic acid for resection of malignant glioma: a randomised controlled multicentre phase III trial. *Lancet Oncol* 2006;7:392–401.
64. Vogelbaum MA, Jost S, Aghi MK, et al. Application of novel response/progression measures for surgically delivered therapies for gliomas: Response Assessment in Neuro-Oncology (RANO) Working Group. *Neurosurgery* 2012; 70:234–243.
66. Barker FG 2nd, Chang SM, Gutin PH, et al. Survival and functional status after resection of recurrent glioblastoma multiforme. *Neurosurgery* 1998; 42:709–720.
67. Keles GE, Lamborn KR, Berger MS. Low-grade hemispheric gliomas in adults: a critical review of extent of resection as a factor influencing outcome. *J Neurosurg* 2001;95:735–745.

69. Hermanto U, Frija EK, Lii MJ, et al. Intensity-modulated radiotherapy (IMRT) and conventional three-dimensional conformal radiotherapy for high-grade gliomas: does IMRT increase the integral dose to normal brain? *Int J Radiat Oncol Biol Phys* 2007;67:1135–1144.
70. Huang E, Teh BS, Strother DR, et al. Intensity-modulated radiation therapy for pediatric medulloblastoma: early report on the reduction of ototoxicity. *Int J Radiat Oncol Biol Phys* 2002;52:599–605.
75. Chung CS, Yock TI, Nelson K, et al. Incidence of second malignancies among patients treated with proton versus photon radiation. *Int J Radiat Oncol Biol Phys* 2013;87:46–52.
81. Muldoon LL, Soussain C, Jahnke K, et al. Chemotherapy delivery issues in central nervous system malignancy: a reality check. *J Clin Oncol* 2007; 25:2295–2305.
82. Smith Q, Fisher C, Allen D. The role of plasma protein binding in drug delivery to brain. In: Kobiler D, Lustig S, Shapira S, eds. *Blood–Brain Barrier.* New York: Springer; 2001:311–321.
84. Kroll RA, Neuwelt EA. Outwitting the blood-brain barrier for therapeutic purposes: osmotic opening and other means. *Neurosurgery* 1998;42:1083–1099.
86. Soni V, Kohli DV, Jain SK. Transferrin-conjugated liposomal system for improved delivery of 5-fluorouracil to brain. *J Drug Target* 2008;16:73–78.
88. Brem H, Mahaley MS Jr, Vick NA, et al. Interstitial chemotherapy with drug polymer implants for the treatment of recurrent gliomas. *J Neurosurg* 1991;74:441–446.
89. Kunwar S, Prados MD, Chang SM, et al. Direct intracerebral delivery of cintredekin besudotox (IL13-PE38QQR) in recurrent malignant glioma: a report by the Cintredekin Besudotox Intraparenchymal Study Group. *J Clin Oncol* 2007;25:837–844.
91. Omuro AM, Faivre S, Raymond E. Lessons learned in the development of targeted therapy for malignant gliomas. *Mol Cancer Ther* 2007;6:1909–1919.
92. Chang SM, Lamborn KR, Kuhn JG, et al. Neurooncology clinical trial design for targeted therapies: lessons learned from the North American Brain Tumor Consortium. *Neuro Oncol* 2008;10:631–642.
95. Grossman SA, Hochberg F, Fisher J, et al. Increased 9-aminocamptothecin dose requirements in patients on anticonvulsants. NABTT CNS Consortium. The New Approaches to Brain Tumor Therapy. *Cancer Chemother Pharmacol* 1998;42:118–126.
101. Schindler G, Capper D, Meyer J, et al. Analysis of BRAF V600E mutation in 1,320 nervous system tumors reveals high mutation frequencies in pleomorphic xanthoastrocytoma, ganglioglioma and extra-cerebellar pilocytic astrocytoma. *Acta Neuropathol* 2011;121:397–405.
106. Shaw EG, Daumas-Duport C, Scheithauer BW, et al. Radiation therapy in the management of low-grade supratentorial astrocytomas. *J Neurosurg* 1989;70:853–861.
107. Franz DN, Belousova E, Sparagana S, et al. Efficacy and safety of everolimus for subependymal giant cell astrocytomas associated with tuberous sclerosis complex (EXIST-1): a multicentre, randomised, placebo-controlled phase 3 trial. *Lancet* 2013;381:125–132.
108. Louis DN. Molecular pathology of malignant gliomas. *Annu Rev Pathol* 2006;1:97–117.
110. Yan H, Parsons DW, Jin G, et al. IDH1 and IDH2 mutations in gliomas. *N Engl J Med* 2009;360:765–773.
111. Choi C, Ganji SK, DeBerardinis RJ, et al. 2-hydroxyglutarate detection by magnetic resonance spectroscopy in IDH-mutated patients with gliomas. *Nat Med* 2012;18:624–629.
112. Sanson M, Marie Y, Paris S, et al. Isocitrate dehydrogenase 1 codon 132 mutation is an important prognostic biomarker in gliomas. *J Clin Oncol* 2009;27: 4150–4154.
113. Leu S, von Felten S, Frank S, et al. IDH/MGMT-driven molecular classification of low-grade glioma is a strong predictor for long-term survival. *Neuro Oncol* 2013;15:469–479.
114. Jenkins RB, Blair H, Ballman KV, et al. A t(1;19)(q10;p10) mediates the combined deletions of 1p and 19q and predicts a better prognosis of patients with oligodendroglioma. *Cancer Res* 2006;66:9852–9861.
115. Weiler M, Wick W. Molecular predictors of outcome in low-grade glioma. *Curr Opin Neurol* 2012;25:767–773.
116. Pignatti F, van den Bent M, Curran D, et al. Prognostic factors for survival in adult patients with cerebral low-grade glioma. *J Clin Oncol* 2002;20: 2076–2084.
117. Gorlia T, Wu W, Wang M, et al. New validated prognostic models and prognostic calculators in patients with low-grade gliomas diagnosed by central pathology review: a pooled analysis of EORTC/RTOG/NCCTG phase III clinical trials. *Neuro Oncol* 2013;15:1568–1579.
118. Shaw EG, Berkey B, Coons SW, et al. Recurrence following neurosurgeon-determined gross-total resection of adult supratentorial low-grade glioma: results of a prospective clinical trial. *J Neurosurg* 2008;109:835–841.
119. van den Bent MJ, Afra D, de Witte O, et al. Long-term efficacy of early versus delayed radiotherapy for low-grade astrocytoma and oligodendroglioma in adults: the EORTC 22845 randomised trial. *Lancet* 2005;366:985–990.
120. Karim AB, Maat B, Hatlevoll R, et al. A randomized trial on dose-response in radiation therapy of low-grade cerebral glioma: European Organization for Research and Treatment of Cancer (EORTC) Study 22844. *Int J Radiat Oncol Biol Phys* 1996;36:549–556.

121. Shaw E, Arusell R, Scheithauer B, et al. Prospective randomized trial of low-versus high-dose radiation therapy in adults with supratentorial low-grade glioma: initial report of a North Central Cancer Treatment Group/Radiation Therapy Oncology Group/Eastern Cooperative Oncology Group study. *J Clin Oncol* 2002;20:2267–2276.

123. Brown PD, Buckner JC, Uhm JH, et al. The neurocognitive effects of radiation in adult low-grade glioma patients. *Neuro Oncol* 2003;5:161–167.

125. Gondi V, Hermann BP, Mehta MP, et al. Hippocampal dosimetry predicts neurocognitive function impairment after fractionated stereotactic radiotherapy for benign or low-grade adult brain tumors. *Int J Radiat Oncol Biol Phys* 2013;85:348–354.

126. Hoang-Xuan K, Capelle L, Kujas M, et al. Temozolomide as initial treatment for adults with low-grade oligodendrogliomas or oligoastrocytomas and correlation with chromosome 1p deletions. *J Clin Oncol* 2004;22:3133–3138.

127. Quinn JA, Reardon DA, Friedman AH, et al. Phase II trial of temozolomide in patients with progressive low-grade glioma. *J Clin Oncol* 2003;21:646–651.

130. Packer RJ, Jakacki R, Horn M, et al. Objective response of multiply recurrent low-grade gliomas to bevacizumab and irinotecan. *Pediatr Blood Cancer* 2009;52:791–795.

133. Franz DN, Leonard J, Tudor C, et al. Rapamycin causes regression of astrocytomas in tuberous sclerosis complex. *Ann Neurol* 2006;59:490–498.

134. Shaw EG, Wisoff JH. Prospective clinical trials of intracranial low-grade glioma in adults and children. *Neuro Oncol* 2003;5:153–160.

135. Shaw EG, Wang M, Coons SW, et al. Randomized trial of radiation therapy plus procarbazine, lomustine, and vincristine chemotherapy for supratentorial adult low-grade glioma: initial results of RTOG 9802. *J Clin Oncol* 2012;30:3065–3070.

136. Buckner JC, Pugh SL, Shaw EG, et al. Phase III study of radiation therapy (RT) with or without procarbazine, CCNU, and vincristine (PCV) in low-grade glioma: RTOG 9802 with Alliance, ECOG, and SWOG. *J Clin Oncol* 2014;32:abstract 2000.

137. van den Bent MJ, Taphoorn MJ, Brandes AA, et al. Phase II study of first-line chemotherapy with temozolomide in recurrent oligodendroglial tumors: the European Organization for Research and Treatment of Cancer Brain Tumor Group Study 26971. *J Clin Oncol* 2003;21:2525–2528.

139. Soffietti R, Ruda R, Bradac GB, et al. PCV chemotherapy for recurrent oligodendrogliomas and oligoastrocytomas. *Neurosurgery* 1998;43:1066–1073.

142. Buckner JC, Gesme D Jr, O'Fallon JR, et al. Phase II trial of procarbazine, lomustine, and vincristine as initial therapy for patients with low-grade oligodendroglioma or oligoastrocytoma: efficacy and associations with chromosomal abnormalities. *J Clin Oncol* 2003;21:251–255.

143. van den Bent MJ, Chinot O, Boogerd W, et al. Second-line chemotherapy with temozolomide in recurrent oligodendroglioma after PCV (procarbazine, lomustine and vincristine) chemotherapy: EORTC Brain Tumor Group phase II study 26972. *Ann Oncol* 2003;14:599–602.

144. Brada M, Viviers L, Abson C, et al. Phase II study of primary temozolomide chemotherapy in patients with WHO grade II gliomas. *Ann Oncol* 2003; 14:1715–1721.

149. Wiencke JK, Zheng S, Jelluma N, et al. Methylation of the PTEN promoter defines low-grade gliomas and secondary glioblastoma. *Neuro Oncol* 2007;9:271–279.

151. Prados MD, Scott C, Curran WJ Jr, et al. Procarbazine, lomustine, and vincristine (PCV) chemotherapy for anaplastic astrocytoma: A retrospective review of radiation therapy oncology group protocols comparing survival with carmustine or PCV adjuvant chemotherapy. *J Clin Oncol* 1999;17: 3389–3395.

153. Prados MD, Seiferheld W, Sandler HM, et al. Phase III randomized study of radiotherapy plus procarbazine, lomustine, and vincristine with or without BUdR for treatment of anaplastic astrocytoma: final report of RTOG 9404. *Int J Radiat Oncol Biol Phys* 2004;58:1147–1152.

154. Stewart LA. Chemotherapy in adult high-grade glioma: a systematic review and meta-analysis of individual patient data from 12 randomised trials. *Lancet* 2002;359:1011–1018.

155. Medical Research Council Brain Tumor Working Party. Randomized trial of procarbazine, lomustine, and vincristine in the adjuvant treatment of high-grade astrocytoma: a Medical Research Council trial. *J Clin Oncol* 2001;19: 509–518.

156. Wick W, Hartmann C, Engel C, et al. NOA-04 randomized phase III trial of sequential radiochemotherapy of anaplastic glioma with procarbazine, lomustine, and vincristine or temozolomide. *J Clin Oncol* 2009;27:5874–5880.

157. Hegi ME, Diserens AC, Gorlia T, et al. MGMT gene silencing and benefit from temozolomide in glioblastoma. *N Engl J Med* 2005;352:997–1003.

159. Levin VA, Hess KR, Choucair A, et al. Phase III randomized study of postradiotherapy chemotherapy with combination alpha-difluoromethylornithine-PCV versus PCV for anaplastic gliomas. *Clin Cancer Res* 2003;9:981–990.

160. Yung WK, Prados MD, Yaya-Tur R, et al. Multicenter phase II trial of temozolomide in patients with anaplastic astrocytoma or anaplastic oligoastrocytoma at first relapse. Temodal Brain Tumor Group. *J Clin Oncol* 1999;17:2762–2771.

162. Friedman HS, Prados MD, Wen PY, et al. Bevacizumab alone and in combination with irinotecan in recurrent glioblastoma. *J Clin Oncol* 2009;27:4733–4740.

165. Cairncross G, Macdonald D, Ludwin S, et al. Chemotherapy for anaplastic oligodendroglioma. National Cancer Institute of Canada Clinical Trials Group. *J Clin Oncol* 1994;12:2013–2021.

167. Cairncross G, Wang M, Shaw E, et al. Phase III trial of chemoradiotherapy for anaplastic oligodendroglioma: long-term results of RTOG 9402. *J Clin Oncol* 2013;31:337–343.

168. van den Bent MJ, Carpentier AF, Brandes AA, et al. Adjuvant procarbazine, lomustine, and vincristine improves progression-free survival but not overall survival in newly diagnosed anaplastic oligodendrogliomas and oligoastrocytomas: a randomized European Organisation for Research and Treatment of Cancer phase III trial. *J Clin Oncol* 2006;24:2715–2722.

169. van den Bent MJ, Dubbink HJ, Sanson M, et al. MGMT promoter methylation is prognostic but not predictive for outcome to adjuvant PCV chemotherapy in anaplastic oligodendroglial tumors: a report from EORTC Brain Tumor Group Study 26951. *J Clin Oncol* 2009;27:5881–5886.

171. van den Bent MJ, Brandes AA, Taphoorn MJ, et al. Adjuvant procarbazine, lomustine, and vincristine chemotherapy in newly diagnosed anaplastic oligodendroglioma: long-term follow-up of EORTC brain tumor group study 26951. *J Clin Oncol* 2013;31:344–350.

172. Vogelbaum MA, Berkey B, Peereboom D, et al. Phase II trial of preirradiation and concurrent temozolomide in patients with newly diagnosed anaplastic oligodendrogliomas and mixed anaplastic oligoastrocytomas: RTOG BR0131. *Neuro Oncol* 2009;11:167–175.

173. Chinot OL, Honore S, Dufour H, et al. Safety and efficacy of temozolomide in patients with recurrent anaplastic oligodendrogliomas after standard radiotherapy and chemotherapy. *J Clin Oncol* 2001;19:2449–2455.

177. Phillips HS, Kharbanda S, Chen R, et al. Molecular subclasses of high-grade glioma predict prognosis, delineate a pattern of disease progression, and resemble stages in neurogenesis. *Cancer Cell* 2006;9:157–173.

178. Verhaak RG, Hoadley KA, Purdom E, et al. Integrated genomic analysis identifies clinically relevant subtypes of glioblastoma characterized by abnormalities in PDGFRA, IDH1, EGFR, and NF1. *Cancer Cell* 2010;17: 98–110.

179. Dunn GP, Rinne ML, Wykosky J, et al. Emerging insights into the molecular and cellular basis of glioblastoma. *Genes Dev* 2012;26:756–784.

180. Walker MD, Alexander E Jr, Hunt WE, et al. Evaluation of BCNU and/or radiotherapy in the treatment of anaplastic gliomas. A cooperative clinical trial. *J Neurosurg* 1978;49:333–343.

181. Gilbert MR, Wang M, Aldape KD, et al. Dose-dense temozolomide for newly diagnosed glioblastoma: a randomized phase iii clinical trial. *J Clin Oncol* 2013;31:4085–4091.

182. Walker MD, Strike TA, Sheline GE. An analysis of dose-effect relationship in the radiotherapy of malignant gliomas. *Int J Radiat Oncol Biol Phys* 1979;5:1725–1731.

184. Phillips C, Guiney M, Smith J, et al. A randomized trial comparing 35Gy in ten fractions with 60Gy in 30 fractions of cerebral irradiation for glioblastoma multiforme and older patients with anaplastic astrocytoma. *Radiother Oncol* 2003;68:23–26.

185. Wick W, Platten M, Meisner C, et al. Temozolomide chemotherapy alone versus radiotherapy alone for malignant astrocytoma in the elderly: the NOA-08 randomised, phase 3 trial. *Lancet Oncol* 2012;13:707–715.

186. Malmstrom A, Gronberg BH, Marosi C, et al. Temozolomide versus standard 6-week radiotherapy versus hypofractionated radiotherapy in patients older than 60 years with glioblastoma: the Nordic randomised, phase 3 trial. *Lancet Oncol* 2012;13:916–926.

188. Tsien CI, Brown D, Normolle D, et al. Concurrent temozolomide and dose-escalated intensity-modulated radiation therapy in newly diagnosed glioblastoma. *Clin Cancer Res* 2012;18:273–279.

190. Stupp R, Mason WP, van den Bent MJ, et al. Radiotherapy plus concomitant and adjuvant temozolomide for glioblastoma. *N Engl J Med* 2005;352: 987–996.

191. Clarke JL, Iwamoto FM, Sul J, et al. Randomized phase II trial of chemoradiotherapy followed by either dose-dense or metronomic temozolomide for newly diagnosed glioblastoma. *J Clin Oncol* 2009;27:3861–3867.

192. Perry JR, Belanger K, Mason WP, et al. Phase II trial of continuous dose-intense temozolomide in recurrent malignant glioma: RESCUE study. *J Clin Oncol* 2010;28:2051–2057.

195. Sandhu SK, Yap TA, de Bono JS. Poly(ADP-ribose) polymerase inhibitors in cancer treatment: a clinical perspective. *Eur J Cancer* 2010;46:9–20.

196. Westphal M, Hilt DC, Bortey E, et al. A phase 3 trial of local chemotherapy with biodegradable carmustine (BCNU) wafers (Gliadel wafers) in patients with primary malignant glioma. *Neuro Oncol* 2003;5:79–88.

197. Wong ET, Hess KR, Gleason MJ, et al. Outcomes and prognostic factors in recurrent glioma patients enrolled onto phase II clinical trials. *J Clin Oncol* 1999;17:2572–2578.

200. van den Bent MJ, Brandes AA, Rampling R, et al. Randomized phase II trial of erlotinib versus temozolomide or carmustine in recurrent glioblastoma: EORTC brain tumor group study 26034. *J Clin Oncol* 2009;27:1268–1274.

201. Mellinghoff IK, Wang MY, Vivanco I, et al. Molecular determinants of the response of glioblastomas to EGFR kinase inhibitors. *N Engl J Med* 2005; 353:2012–2024.

206. Chang SM, Wen P, Cloughesy T, et al. Phase II study of CCI-779 in patients with recurrent glioblastoma multiforme. *Invest New Drugs* 2005;23:357–361.

207. Cloughesy TF, Wen PY, Robins HI, et al. Phase II trial of tipifarnib in patients with recurrent malignant glioma either receiving or not receiving enzyme-inducing antiepileptic drugs: a North American Brain Tumor Consortium Study. *J Clin Oncol* 2006;24:3651–3656.

209. Galanis E, Buckner JC, Maurer MJ, et al. Phase II trial of temsirolimus (CCI-779) in recurrent glioblastoma multiforme: a North Central Cancer Treatment Group Study. *J Clin Oncol* 2005;23:5294–5304.

210. Reardon DA, Desjardins A, Vredenburgh JJ, et al. Phase 2 trial of erlotinib plus sirolimus in adults with recurrent glioblastoma. *J Neurooncol* 2010; 96:219–230.

211. Vredenburgh JJ, Desjardins A, Herndon JE 2nd, et al. Phase II trial of bevacizumab and irinotecan in recurrent malignant glioma. *Clin Cancer Res* 2007;13:1253–1259.

212. Kreisl TN, Kim L, Moore K, et al. Phase II trial of single-agent bevacizumab followed by bevacizumab plus irinotecan at tumor progression in recurrent glioblastoma. *J Clin Oncol* 2009;27:740–745.

213. Taal W, Oosterkamp HM, Walenkamp AME, et al. A randomized phase II study of bevacizumab versus bevacizumab plus lomustine versus lomustine single agent in recurrent glioblastoma: The Dutch BELOB study. *J Clin Oncol* 2013;31:2001.

214. Lai A, Filka E, McGibbon B, et al. Phase II pilot study of bevacizumab in combination with temozolomide and regional radiation therapy for upfront treatment of patients with newly diagnosed glioblastoma multiforme: interim analysis of safety and tolerability. *Int J Radiat Oncol Biol Phys* 2008;71:1372–1380.

215. Gilbert MR, Dignam JJ, Armstrong TS, et al. A randomized trial of bevacizumab for newly diagnosed glioblastoma. *N Engl J Med* 2014;370:699–708.

216. Chinot OL, Wick W, Mason W, et al. Bevacizumab plus radiotherapy-temozolomide for newly diagnosed glioblastoma. *N Engl J Med* 2014;370: 709–722.

217. Herrlinger U, Schaefer N, Steinbach JP, et al. Bevacizumab, irinotecan, and radiotherapy versus standard temozolomide and radiotherapy in newly diagnosed, MGMT-nonmethylated glioblastoma patients: First results from the randomized multicenter GLARIUS trial. *J Clin Oncol* 2013;31:LBA2000.

219. Batchelor TT, Mulholland P, Neyns B, et al. Phase III randomized trial comparing the efficacy of cediranib as monotherapy, and in combination with lomustine, versus lomustine alone in patients with recurrent glioblastoma. *J Clin Oncol* 2013;31:3212–3218.

221. Reardon DA, Fink KL, Mikkelsen T, et al. Randomized phase II study of cilengitide, an integrin-targeting arginine-glycine-aspartic acid peptide, in recurrent glioblastoma multiforme. *J Clin Oncol* 2008;26:5610–5617.

223. Stupp R, Hegi ME, Gorlia T, et al. Cilengitide combined with standard treatment for patients with newly diagnosed glioblastoma and methylated O6-methylguanine-DNA methyltransferase (MGMT) gene promoter: Key results of the multicenter, randomized, open-label, controlled, phase III CENTRIC study. *ASCO Meeting Abstracts* 2013;31:LBA2009.

224. Wick W, Puduvalli VK, Chamberlain MC, et al. Phase III study of enzastaurin compared with lomustine in the treatment of recurrent intracranial glioblastoma. *J Clin Oncol* 2010;28:1168–1174.

226. Wick W, Steinbach JP, Platten M, et al. Enzastaurin before and concomitant with radiation therapy, followed by enzastaurin maintenance therapy, in patients with newly diagnosed glioblastoma without MGMT promoter hypermethylation. *Neuro Oncol* 2013;15:1405–1412.

227. Galanis E, Jaeckle KA, Maurer MJ, et al. Phase II trial of vorinostat in recurrent glioblastoma multiforme: a north central cancer treatment group study. *J Clin Oncol* 2009;27:2052–2058.

229. Grossman SA, Ye X, Chamberlain M, et al. Talampanel with standard radiation and temozolomide in patients with newly diagnosed glioblastoma: a multicenter phase II trial. *J Clin Oncol* 2009;27:4155–4161.

230. Westphal M, Yla-Herttuala S, Martin J, et al. Adenovirus-mediated gene therapy with sitimagene ceradenovec followed by intravenous ganciclovir for patients with operable high-grade glioma (ASPECT): a randomised, open-label, phase 3 trial. *Lancet Oncol* 2013;14:823–833.

231. Sampson JH, Heimberger AB, Archer GE, et al. Immunologic escape after prolonged progression-free survival with epidermal growth factor receptor variant III peptide vaccination in patients with newly diagnosed glioblastoma. *J Clin Oncol* 2010;28:4722–4729.

233. Bogdahn U, Hau P, Stockhammer G, et al. Targeted therapy for high-grade glioma with the TGF-beta2 inhibitor trabedersen: results of a randomized and controlled phase IIb study. *Neuro Oncol* 2011;13:132–142.

234. Curran WJ Jr, Scott CB, Horton J, et al. Recursive partitioning analysis of prognostic factors in three Radiation Therapy Oncology Group malignant glioma trials. *J Natl Cancer Inst* 1993;85:704–710.

237. Hernaiz Driever P, von Hornstein S, Pietsch T, et al. Natural history and management of low-grade glioma in NF-1 children. *J Neurooncol* 2010;100: 199–207.

238. Parsa CF, Hoyt CS, Lesser RL, et al. Spontaneous regression of optic gliomas: thirteen cases documented by serial neuroimaging. *Arch Ophthalmol* 2001;119:516–529.

239. Fouladi M, Grant R, Baruchel S, et al. Comparison of survival outcomes in patients with intracranial germinomas treated with radiation alone versus reduced-dose radiation and chemotherapy. *Childs Nerv Syst* 1998;14:596–601.

241. Chan MY, Foong AP, Heisey DM, et al. Potential prognostic factors of relapse-free survival in childhood optic pathway glioma: a multivariate analysis. *Pediatr Neurosurg* 1998;29:23–28.

243. Opocher E, Kremer LC, Da Dalt L, et al. Prognostic factors for progression of childhood optic pathway glioma: a systematic review. *Eur J Cancer* 2006;42:1807–1816.

246. Czyzyk E, Jozwiak S, Roszkowski M, et al. Optic pathway gliomas in children with and without neurofibromatosis 1. *J Child Neurol* 2003;18: 471–478.

248. Tenny RT, Laws ER Jr, Younge BR, et al. The neurosurgical management of optic glioma. Results in 104 patients. *J Neurosurg* 1982;57:452–458.

255. Cappelli C, Grill J, Raquin M, et al. Long-term follow up of 69 patients treated for optic pathway tumours before the chemotherapy era. *Arch Dis Child* 1998;79:334–338.

256. Pierce SM, Barnes PD, Loeffler JS, et al. Definitive radiation therapy in the management of symptomatic patients with optic glioma. Survival and long-term effects. *Cancer* 1990;65:45–52.

257. Donahue B. Short- and long-term complications of radiation therapy for pediatric brain tumors. *Pediatr Neurosurg* 1992;18:207–217.

258. Sharif S, Ferner R, Birch JM, et al. Second primary tumors in neurofibromatosis 1 patients treated for optic glioma: substantial risks after radiotherapy. *J Clin Oncol* 2006;24:2570–2575.

261. Ater J, Holmes E, Zhou T, et al. Results of the COG protocol 9952: a randomized phase 3 study of 2 chemotherapy regimens for incompletely resected low grade glioma in young children. *Neuro-Oncology* 2008;10:452.

265. Kuo DJ, Weiner HL, Wisoff J, et al. Temozolomide is active in childhood, progressive, unresectable, low-grade gliomas. *J Pediatr Hematol Oncol* 2003; 25:372–378.

268. Moreno L, Bautista F, Ashley S, et al. Does chemotherapy affect the visual outcome in children with optic pathway glioma? A systematic review of the evidence. *Eur J Cancer* 2010;46:2253–2259.

269. Donaldson SS, Laningham F, Fisher PG. Advances toward an understanding of brainstem gliomas. *J Clin Oncol* 2006;24:1266–1272.

272. Albright AL. Diffuse brainstem tumors: when is a biopsy necessary? *Pediatr Neurosurg* 1996;24:252–255.

274. Daglioglu E, Cataltepe O, Akalan N. Tectal gliomas in children: the implications for natural history and management strategy. *Pediatr Neurosurg* 2003;38:223–231.

279. Freeman CR, Krischer JP, Sanford RA, et al. Final results of a study of escalating doses of hyperfractionated radiotherapy in brain stem tumors in children: a Pediatric Oncology Group study. *Int J Radiat Oncol Biol Phys* 1993;27:197–206.

282. Khuong-Quang DA, Buczkowicz P, Rakopoulos P, et al. K27M mutation in histone H3.3 defines clinically and biologically distinct subgroups of pediatric diffuse intrinsic pontine gliomas. *Acta Neuropathol* 2012;124: 439–447.

283. Schwartzentruber J, Korshunov A, Liu XY, et al. Driver mutations in histone H3.3 and chromatin remodelling genes in paediatric glioblastoma. *Nature* 2012;482:226–231.

285. Broniscer A, Iacono L, Chintagumpala M, et al. Role of temozolomide after radiotherapy for newly diagnosed diffuse brainstem glioma in children: results of a multiinstitutional study (SJHG-98). *Cancer* 2005;103:133–139.

287. Nicholson HS, Kretschmar CS, Krailo M, et al. Phase 2 study of temozolomide in children and adolescents with recurrent central nervous system tumors: a report from the Children's Oncology Group. *Cancer* 2007;110: 1542–1550.

290. Jones DT, Kocialkowski S, Liu L, et al. Tandem duplication producing a novel oncogenic BRAF fusion gene defines the majority of pilocytic astrocytomas. *Cancer Res* 2008;68:8673–8677.

292. Fernandez C, Figarella-Branger D, Girard N, et al. Pilocytic astrocytomas in children: prognostic factors—a retrospective study of 80 cases. *Neurosurgery* 2003;53:544–553.

294. Mahoney DH Jr, Cohen ME, Friedman HS, et al. Carboplatin is effective therapy for young children with progressive optic pathway tumors: a Pediatric Oncology Group phase II study. *Neuro Oncol* 2000;2:213–220.

298. Luyken C, Blumcke I, Fimmers R, et al. Supratentorial gangliogliomas: histopathologic grading and tumor recurrence in 184 patients with a median follow-up of 8 years. *Cancer* 2004;101:146–155.

299. Compton JJ, Laack NN, Eckel LJ, et al. Long-term outcomes for low-grade intracranial ganglioglioma: 30-year experience from the Mayo Clinic. *J Neurosurg* 2012;117:825–830.

302. Rades D, Zwick L, Leppert J, et al. The role of postoperative radiotherapy for the treatment of gangliogliomas. *Cancer* 2010;116:432–442.

307. Witt H, Mack SC, Ryzhova M, et al. Delineation of two clinically and molecularly distinct subgroups of posterior fossa ependymoma. *Cancer Cell* 2011;20:143–157.

309. Healey EA, Barnes PD, Kupsky WJ, et al. The prognostic significance of postoperative residual tumor in ependymoma. *Neurosurgery* 1991;28:666–671.

310. Jaing TH, Wang HS, Tsay PK, et al. Multivariate analysis of clinical prognostic factors in children with intracranial ependymomas. *J Neurooncol* 2004;68:255–261.

311. Vinchon M, Leblond P, Noudel R, et al. Intracranial ependymomas in childhood: recurrence, reoperation, and outcome. *Childs Nerv Syst* 2005;21: 221–226.

312. Merchant TE, Li C, Xiong X, et al. Conformal radiotherapy after surgery for paediatric ependymoma: a prospective study. *Lancet Oncol* 2009;10: 258–266.

313. Shaw EG, Evans RG, Scheithauer BW, et al. Postoperative radiotherapy of intracranial ependymoma in pediatric and adult patients. *Int J Radiat Oncol Biol Phys* 1987;13:1457–1462.

PRACTICE OF ONCOLOGY

315. Robertson PL, Zeltzer PM, Boyett JM, et al. Survival and prognostic factors following radiation therapy and chemotherapy for ependymomas in children: a report of the Children's Cancer Group. *J Neurosurg* 1998;88:695–703.

317. Pollack IF, Gerszten PC, Martinez AJ, et al. Intracranial ependymomas of childhood: long-term outcome and prognostic factors. *Neurosurgery* 1995; 37:655–666.

320. Bouffet E, Perilongo G, Canete A, et al. Intracranial ependymomas in children: a critical review of prognostic factors and a plea for cooperation. *Med Pediatr Oncol* 1998;30:319–329.

323. Perry A, Stafford SL, Scheithauer BW, et al. Meningioma grading: an analysis of histologic parameters. *Am J Surg Pathol* 1997;21:1455–1465.

326. Oya S, Kim SH, Sade B, et al. The natural history of intracranial meningiomas. *J Neurosurg* 2011;114:1250–1256.

328. Simpson D. The recurrence of intracranial meningiomas after surgical treatment. *J Neurol Neurosurg Psychiatry* 1957;20:22–39.

330. Mirimanoff RO, Dosoretz DE, Linggood RM, et al. Meningioma: analysis of recurrence and progression following neurosurgical resection. *J Neurosurg* 1985;62:18–24.

332. Pollock BE, Stafford SL, Link MJ. Gamma knife radiosurgery for skull base meningiomas. *Neurosurg Clin N Am* 2000;11:659–666.

333. Stafford SL, Perry A, Suman VJ, et al. Primarily resected meningiomas: outcome and prognostic factors in 581 Mayo Clinic patients, 1978 through 1988. *Mayo Clin Proc* 1998;73:936–942.

334. Goldsmith BJ, Wara WM, Wilson CB, et al. Postoperative irradiation for subtotally resected meningiomas. A retrospective analysis of 140 patients treated from 1967 to 1990. *J Neurosurg* 1994;80:195–201.

337. Milosevic MF, Frost PJ, Laperriere NJ, et al. Radiotherapy for atypical or malignant intracranial meningioma. *Int J Radiat Oncol Biol Phys* 1996;34: 817–822.

339. Glaholm J, Bloom HJ, Crow JH. The role of radiotherapy in the management of intracranial meningiomas: the Royal Marsden Hospital experience with 186 patients. *Int J Radiat Oncol Biol Phys* 1990;18:755–761.

340. Debus J, Wuendrich M, Pirzkall A, et al. High efficacy of fractionated stereotactic radiotherapy of large base-of-skull meningiomas: long-term results. *J Clin Oncol* 2001;19:3547–3553.

342. Turbin RE, Thompson CR, Kennerdell JS, et al. A long-term visual outcome comparison in patients with optic nerve sheath meningioma managed with observation, surgery, radiotherapy, or surgery and radiotherapy. *Ophthalmology* 2002;109:890–899.

344. Kondziolka D, Lunsford LD, Coffey RJ, et al. Stereotactic radiosurgery of meningiomas. *J Neurosurg* 1991;74:552–559.

345. Kondziolka D, Nathoo N, Flickinger JC, et al. Long-term results after radiosurgery for benign intracranial tumors. *Neurosurgery* 2003;53:815–821.

359. Northcott PA, Dubuc AM, Pfister S, et al. Molecular subgroups of medulloblastoma. *Expert Rev Neurother* 2012;12:871–884.

361. Northcott PA, Korshunov A, Pfister SM, et al. The clinical implications of medulloblastoma subgroups. *Nat Rev Neurol* 2012;8:340–351.

363. Northcott PA, Korshunov A, Witt H, et al. Medulloblastoma comprises four distinct molecular variants. *J Clin Oncol* 2011;29:1408–1414.

365. Padovani L, Sunyach MP, Perol D, et al. Common strategy for adult and pediatric medulloblastoma: a multicenter series of 253 adults. *Int J Radiat Oncol Biol Phys* 2007;68:433–440.

372. Koeller KK, Rushing EJ. From the archives of the AFIP: medulloblastoma: a comprehensive review with radiologic-pathologic correlation. *Radiographics* 2003;23:1613–1637.

376. Gajjar A, Fouladi M, Walter AW, et al. Comparison of lumbar and shunt cerebrospinal fluid specimens for cytologic detection of leptomeningeal disease in pediatric patients with brain tumors. *J Clin Oncol* 1999;17: 1825–1828.

377. Fouladi M, Gajjar A, Boyett JM, et al. Comparison of CSF cytology and spinal magnetic resonance imaging in the detection of leptomeningeal disease in pediatric medulloblastoma or primitive neuroectodermal tumor. *J Clin Oncol* 1999;17:3234–3237.

378. Kramer ED, Vezina LG, Packer RJ, et al. Staging and surveillance of children with central nervous system neoplasms: recommendations of the Neurology and Tumor Imaging Committees of the Children's Cancer Group. *Pediatr Neurosurg* 1994;20:254–262.

382. Evans AE, Jenkin RD, Sposto R, et al. The treatment of medulloblastoma. Results of a prospective randomized trial of radiation therapy with and without CCNU, vincristine, and prednisone. *J Neurosurg* 1990;72:572–582.

383. Rutkowski S, Bode U, Deinlein F, et al. Treatment of early childhood medulloblastoma by postoperative chemotherapy alone. *N Engl J Med* 2005;352: 978–986.

387. Albright AL, Wisoff JH, Zeltzer PM, et al. Effects of medulloblastoma resections on outcome in children: a report from the Children's Cancer Group. *Neurosurgery* 1996;38:265–271.

388. Robertson PL, Muraszko KM, Holmes EJ, et al. Incidence and severity of postoperative cerebellar mutism syndrome in children with medulloblastoma: a prospective study by the Children's Oncology Group. *J Neurosurg* 2006;105:444–451.

390. Timmermann B, Kortmann RD, Kuhl J, et al. Role of radiotherapy in the treatment of supratentorial primitive neuroectodermal tumors in childhood: results of the prospective German brain tumor trials HIT 88/89 and 91. *J Clin Oncol* 2002;20:842–849.

391. Prados MD, Wara WM, Edwards MS, et al. Hyperfractionated craniospinal radiation therapy for primitive neuroectodermal tumors: early results of a pilot study. *Int J Radiat Oncol Biol Phys* 1994;28:431–438.

392. Carrie C, Muracciole X, Gomez F, et al. Conformal radiotherapy, reduced boost volume, hyperfractionated radiotherapy, and online quality control in standard-risk medulloblastoma without chemotherapy: results of the French M-SFOP 98 protocol. *Int J Radiat Oncol Biol Phys* 2005;63:711–716.

394. Wolden SL, Dunkel IJ, Souweidane MM, et al. Patterns of failure using a conformal radiation therapy tumor bed boost for medulloblastoma. *J Clin Oncol* 2003;21:3079–3083.

395. Gajjar A, Chintagumpala M, Ashley D, et al. Risk-adapted craniospinal radiotherapy followed by high-dose chemotherapy and stem-cell rescue in children with newly diagnosed medulloblastoma (St Jude Medulloblastoma-96): long-term results from a prospective, multicentre trial. *Lancet Oncol* 2006;7: 813–820.

396. Packer RJ, Goldwein J, Nicholson HS, et al. Treatment of children with medulloblastomas with reduced-dose craniospinal radiation therapy and adjuvant chemotherapy: A Children's Cancer Group Study. *J Clin Oncol* 1999;17:2127–2136.

397. Bailey CC, Gnekow A, Wellek S, et al. Prospective randomised trial of chemotherapy given before radiotherapy in childhood medulloblastoma. International Society of Paediatric Oncology (SIOP) and the (German) Society of Paediatric Oncology (GPO): SIOP II. *Med Pediatr Oncol* 1995;25:166–178.

399. Tait DM, Thornton-Jones H, Bloom HJ, et al. Adjuvant chemotherapy for medulloblastoma: the first multi-centre control trial of the International Society of Paediatric Oncology (SIOP I). *Eur J Cancer* 1990;26:464–469.

401. Geyer JR, Sposto R, Jennings M, et al. Multiagent chemotherapy and deferred radiotherapy in infants with malignant brain tumors: a report from the Children's Cancer Group. *J Clin Oncol* 2005;23:7621–7631.

402. Timmermann B, Kortmann RD, Kuhl J, et al. Role of radiotherapy in supratentorial primitive neuroectodermal tumor in young children: results of the German HIT-SKK87 and HIT-SKK92 trials. *J Clin Oncol* 2006;24: 1554–1560.

403. Dhall G, Grodman H, Ji L, et al. Outcome of children less than three years old at diagnosis with non-metastatic medulloblastoma treated with chemotherapy on the "Head Start" I and II protocols. *Pediatr Blood Cancer* 2008;50:1169–1175.

407. Packer RJ, Sutton LN, Atkins TE, et al. A prospective study of cognitive function in children receiving whole-brain radiotherapy and chemotherapy: 2-year results. *J Neurosurg* 1989;70:707–713.

408. Mulhern RK, Palmer SL, Merchant TE, et al. Neurocognitive consequences of risk-adapted therapy for childhood medulloblastoma. *J Clin Oncol* 2005;23:5511–5519.

412. Reddy AT, Wellons JC 3rd, Allen JC, et al. Refining the staging evaluation of pineal region germinoma using neuroendoscopy and the presence of preoperative diabetes insipidus. *Neuro Oncol* 2004;6:127–133.

415. Sawamura Y, de Tribolet N, Ishii N, et al. Management of primary intracranial germinomas: diagnostic surgery or radical resection? *J Neurosurg* 1997; 87:262–266.

416. Regis J, Bouillot P, Rouby-Volot F, et al. Pineal region tumors and the role of stereotactic biopsy: review of the mortality, morbidity, and diagnostic rates in 370 cases. *Neurosurgery* 1996;39:907–912.

417. Pople IK, Athanasiou TC, Sandeman DR, et al. The role of endoscopic biopsy and third ventriculostomy in the management of pineal region tumours. *Br J Neurosurg* 2001;15:305–311.

420. Haas-Kogan DA, Missett BT, Wara WM, et al. Radiation therapy for intracranial germ cell tumors. *Int J Radiat Oncol Biol Phys* 2003;56:511–518.

421. Bouffet E, Baranzelli MC, Patte C, et al. Combined treatment modality for intracranial germinomas: results of a multicentre SFOP experience. Societe Francaise d'Oncologie Pediatrique. *Br J Cancer* 1999;79:1199–1204.

423. Merchant TE, Davis BJ, Sheldon JM, et al. Radiation therapy for relapsed CNS germinoma after primary chemotherapy. *J Clin Oncol* 1998;16:204–209.

425. Allen JC, Kim JH, Packer RJ. Neoadjuvant chemotherapy for newly diagnosed germ-cell tumors of the central nervous system. *J Neurosurg* 1987; 67:65–70.

426. Balmaceda C, Heller G, Rosenblum M, et al. Chemotherapy without irradiation—a novel approach for newly diagnosed CNS germ cell tumors: results of an international cooperative trial. The First International Central Nervous System Germ Cell Tumor Study. *J Clin Oncol* 1996;14:2908–2915.

427. Kellie SJ, Boyce H, Dunkel IJ, et al. Primary chemotherapy for intracranial nongerminomatous germ cell tumors: results of the second international CNS germ cell study group protocol. *J Clin Oncol* 2004;22:846–853.

428. Matsutani M, Sano K, Takakura K, et al. Primary intracranial germ cell tumors: a clinical analysis of 153 histologically verified cases. *J Neurosurg* 1997;86:446–455.

434. Mortini P, Losa M, Barzaghi R, et al. Results of transsphenoidal surgery in a large series of patients with pituitary adenoma. *Neurosurgery* 2005;56: 1222–1233.

435. Nomikos P, Ladar C, Fahlbusch R, et al. Impact of primary surgery on pituitary function in patients with non-functioning pituitary adenomas—a study on 721 patients. *Acta Neurochir (Wien)* 2004;146:27–35.

437. Swearingen B, Biller BM, Barker FG 2nd, et al. Long-term mortality after transsphenoidal surgery for Cushing disease. *Ann Intern Med* 1999;130: 821–824.

446. Jennings AS, Liddle GW, Orth DN. Results of treating childhood Cushing's disease with pituitary irradiation. *N Engl J Med* 1977;297:957–962.

449. McCord MW, Buatti JM, Fennell EM, et al. Radiotherapy for pituitary adenoma: long-term outcome and sequelae. *Int J Radiat Oncol Biol Phys* 1997;39:437–444.

451. Zierhut D, Flentje M, Adolph J, et al. External radiotherapy of pituitary adenomas. *Int J Radiat Oncol Biol Phys* 1995;33:307–314.

459. Kobayashi T, Mori Y, Uchiyama Y, et al. Long-term results of gamma knife surgery for growth hormone-producing pituitary adenoma: is the disease difficult to cure? *J Neurosurg* 2005;102:119–123.

469. Albright AL, Hadjipanayis CG, Lunsford LD, et al. Individualized treatment of pediatric craniopharyngiomas. *Childs Nerv Syst* 2005;21:649–654.

470. Stripp DC, Maity A, Janss AJ, et al. Surgery with or without radiation therapy in the management of craniopharyngiomas in children and young adults. *Int J Radiat Oncol Biol Phys* 2004;58:714–720.

471. Karavitaki N, Brufani C, Warner JT, et al. Craniopharyngiomas in children and adults: systematic analysis of 121 cases with long-term follow-up. *Clin Endocrinol (Oxf)* 2005;62:397–409.

475. Wen BC, Hussey DH, Staples J, et al. A comparison of the roles of surgery and radiation therapy in the management of craniopharyngiomas. *Int J Radiat Oncol Biol Phys* 1989;16:17–24.

477. Hetelekidis S, Barnes PD, Tao ML, et al. 20-year experience in childhood craniopharyngioma. *Int J Radiat Oncol Biol Phys* 1993;27:189–195.

480. Varlotto JM, Flickinger JC, Kondziolka D, et al. External beam irradiation of craniopharyngiomas: long-term analysis of tumor control and morbidity. *Int J Radiat Oncol Biol Phys* 2002;54:492–499.

483. Kobayashi T, Kida Y, Mori Y, et al. Long-term results of gamma knife surgery for the treatment of craniopharyngioma in 98 consecutive cases. *J Neurosurg* 2005;103:482–488.

488. Baser ME, Friedman JM, Wallace AJ, et al. Evaluation of clinical diagnostic criteria for neurofibromatosis 2. *Neurology* 2002;59:1759–1765.

490. Samii M, Matthies C. Management of 1000 vestibular schwannomas (acoustic neuromas): surgical management and results with an emphasis on complications and how to avoid them. *Neurosurgery* 1997;40:11–21.

493. Charabi S, Tos M, Thomsen J, et al. Vestibular schwannoma growth—long-term results. *Acta Otolaryngol Suppl* 2000;543:7–10.

495. Sarmiento JM, Patel S, Mukherjee D, et al. Improving outcomes in patients with vestibular schwannomas: microsurgery versus radiosurgery. *J Neurosurg Sci* 2013;57:23–44.

503. Ryzenman JM, Pensak ML, Tew JM Jr. Headache: a quality of life analysis in a cohort of 1,657 patients undergoing acoustic neuroma surgery, results from the acoustic neuroma association. *Laryngoscope* 2005;115:703–711.

505. Kondziolka D, Lunsford LD, McLaughlin MR, et al. Long-term outcomes after radiosurgery for acoustic neuromas. *N Engl J Med* 1998;339:1426–1433.

508. Pollock BE, Driscoll CL, Foote RL, et al. Patient outcomes after vestibular schwannoma management: a prospective comparison of microsurgical resection and stereotactic radiosurgery. *Neurosurgery* 2006;59:77–85.

511. Andrews DW, Suarez O, Goldman HW, et al. Stereotactic radiosurgery and fractionated stereotactic radiotherapy for the treatment of acoustic schwannomas: comparative observations of 125 patients treated at one institution. *Int J Radiat Oncol Biol Phys* 2001;50:1265–1278.

522. Plotkin SR, Stemmer-Rachamimov AO, Barker FG 2nd, et al. Hearing improvement after bevacizumab in patients with neurofibromatosis type 2. *N Engl J Med* 2009;361:358–367.

527. Gottfried ON, Liu JK, Couldwell WT. Comparison of radiosurgery and conventional surgery for the treatment of glomus jugulare tumors. *Neurosurg Focus* 2004;17:E4.

529. Guss ZD, Batra S, Limb CJ, et al. Radiosurgery of glomus jugulare tumors: a meta-analysis. *Int J Radiat Oncol Biol Phys* 2011;81:e497–e502.

537. Patrice SJ, Sneed PK, Flickinger JC, et al. Radiosurgery for hemangioblastoma: results of a multiinstitutional experience. *Int J Radiat Oncol Biol Phys* 1996;35:493–499.

544. Rosenberg AE, Nielsen GP, Keel SB, et al. Chondrosarcoma of the base of the skull: a clinicopathologic study of 200 cases with emphasis on its distinction from chordoma. *Am J Surg Pathol* 1999;23:1370–1378.

548. Erdem E, Angtuaco EC, Van Hemert R, et al. Comprehensive review of intracranial chordoma. *Radiographics* 2003;23:995–1009.

553. Tzortzidis F, Elahi F, Wright D, et al. Patient outcome at long-term follow-up after aggressive microsurgical resection of cranial base chordomas. *Neurosurgery* 2006;59:230–237.

555. Debus J, Schulz-Ertner D, Schad L, et al. Stereotactic fractionated radiotherapy for chordomas and chondrosarcomas of the skull base. *Int J Radiat Oncol Biol Phys* 2000;47:591–596.

566. Amichetti M, Amelio D, Cianchetti M, et al. A systematic review of proton therapy in the treatment of chondrosarcoma of the skull base. *Neurosurg Rev* 2010;33:155–165.

567. Stacchiotti S, Longhi A, Ferraresi V, et al. Phase II study of imatinib in advanced chordoma. *J Clin Oncol* 2012;30:914–920.

571. McEvoy AW, Harding BN, Phipps KP, et al. Management of choroid plexus tumours in children: 20 years experience at a single neurosurgical centre. *Pediatr Neurosurg* 2000;32:192–199.

574. Duffner PK, Horowitz ME, Krischer JP, et al. Postoperative chemotherapy and delayed radiation in children less than three years of age with malignant brain tumors. *N Engl J Med* 1993;328:1725–1731.

578. Linstadt DE, Wara WM, Leibel SA, et al. Postoperative radiotherapy of primary spinal cord tumors. *Int J Radiat Oncol Biol Phys* 1989;16:1397–1403.

583. Wen BC, Hussey DH, Hitchon PW, et al. The role of radiation therapy in the management of ependymomas of the spinal cord. *Int J Radiat Oncol Biol Phys* 1991;20:781–786.

98 Molecular Biology of Childhood Cancers

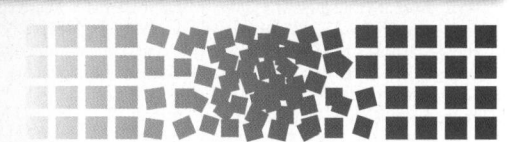

Lee J. Helman and David Malkin

INTRODUCTION

Tumors of childhood are clinically, histopathologically, and biologically distinct from that of adult-onset malignancies. Childhood cancers tend to have short latency periods, are often rapidly growing and aggressively invasive, are rarely associated with exposure to carcinogens, and are generally more responsive to standard modalities of treatment, in particular chemotherapy. Most childhood tumors occur sporadically in families with, at most, a weak history of cancer. In at least 10% to 15% of cases, however, a strong familial association is recognized or the child has a congenital or genetic disorder that imparts a higher likelihood of specific cancer types.[1] Examples of genetic disorders that render a child at increased risk of tumor development include xeroderma pigmentosa, Bloom syndrome, or ataxia telangiectasia, which predispose to skin cancers, leukemias, or lymphoid malignancies, respectively. In all three cases, constitutional gene alterations that disrupt normal mechanisms of genomic DNA repair are blamed for the propensity to cell transformation. Other hereditary disorders, including Beckwith-Wiedemann syndrome (BWS), von Hippel-Lindau disease, Rothmund-Thomson syndrome, and the multiple endocrine neoplasias types 1 and 2, are associated with their respective tumor spectra through constitutional activation of molecular pathways of deregulated cellular growth and proliferation. The cancers that occur in these syndromes are generally secondary phenotypic manifestations of disorders that have distinctive recognizable physical stigmata. On the other hand, some cancer predisposition syndromes are recognized only by their malignant manifestations, with nonmalignant characteristics being virtually absent. These include hereditary retinoblastoma, Li-Fraumeni syndrome (LFS), familial Wilms tumor, and familial adenomatous polyposis coli. Each of these presents with distinct cancer phenotypes and unique molecular defects (Table 98.1). Careful attention to detailed cancer family histories continues to lead to the discovery of new cancer predisposition syndromes and the coincident identification of novel cancer genes.[2]

The study of pediatric cancer and rare hereditary cancer syndromes and associations has led to the identification of numerous cancer genes, including dominant oncogenes, DNA repair genes, and tumor suppressor genes. These genes are important not only in hereditary predisposition, but also in the normal growth, differentiation, and proliferation pathways of all cells. Alterations of these genes have been consistently found in numerous sporadic tumors of childhood and led to studies of their functional role in carcinogenesis. The numerous properties of transformed malignant cells in culture or in vivo can be explained by the complex abnormal interaction of numerous positive and negative growth-regulatory genes. Pediatric cancers offer unique models in which to study these pathways in that they are less likely to be disrupted by nongenetic factors. The embryonic ontogeny of many childhood cancers suggests that better understanding of the nature of the genetic events leading to these cancers will also augment the understanding of normal embryologic growth and development.

This chapter begins with an outline of tumor suppressor genes—the most frequently implicated class of cancer genes in childhood malignancy. This leads into a discussion of molecular features of retinoblastoma, the paradigm of cancer genetics, followed by an analysis of the molecular pathways associated with other common pediatric cancers. Evaluations of the importance of molecular alterations in familial cancers, as well as new approaches in molecular therapeutics are also addressed.

TUMOR SUPPRESSOR GENES

Faulty regulation of cellular growth and differentiation leads to neoplastic transformation and tumor initiation. Many inappropriately activated growth-potentiating genes, or *oncogenes*, have been identified through the study of RNA tumor viruses and the transforming effects of DNA isolated from malignant cells. However, activated dominant oncogenes themselves do not readily explain a variety of phenomena related to transformation and tumor formation. Among these is the suppression of tumorigenicity by the fusion of malignant cells with their normal counterparts. If these malignant cells carried an activated dominant oncogene, it would be expected that such a gene would initiate transformation of the normal cells, likely leading to either embryonic or fetal death. The observation is more readily explained by postulating the existence of a factor in the normal cell that acts to suppress growth of the fused malignant cells. Malignant cells commonly exhibit specific chromosomal deletions (Table 98.2). The best example of this occurs in retinoblastoma, a rare pediatric eye tumor in which a small region of the long arm of chromosome 13 is frequently missing. The presumed loss of genes in specific chromosomal regions argues strongly against the concept of a dominantly acting gene being implicated in the development of the tumor. Comparisons between the frequencies of familial tumors and their sporadic counterparts led Knudson[3] to suggest that the familial forms of some tumors could be explained by constitutional mutations in growth-limiting genes. The resulting inactivation of these genes would facilitate cellular transformation.[4] Such growth-limiting genes were termed *tumor suppressor genes*.

Whereas acquired alterations of dominant oncogenes most commonly occur in somatic cells, mutant tumor suppressor genes may be found either in germ cells or somatic cells. In the former, they may arise de novo or be transmitted from generation to generation within a family. The diversity of functions, cellular locations, and tissue-specific expression of the tumor suppressor genes suggest the existence of a complex, yet coordinated, cellular pathway that limits cell growth by linking nuclear processes with the intra- and extracytoplasmic environment. This discussion is limited to those genes for which pediatric tumors are frequently associated.

TABLE 98.1

Hereditary Syndromes Associated with Childhood Cancer Predisposition

Syndrome	OMIM Entry[a]	Major Tumor Types	Mode of Inheritance	Genes
Hereditary Gastrointestinal Malignancies				
Adenomatous polyposis of the colon	175100	Colon, thyroid, stomach, intestine, hepatoblastoma	Dominant	APC
Juvenile polyposis	174900	Gastrointestinal	Dominant	SMAD4/DPC4
Peutz-Jeghers syndrome	175200	Intestinal, ovarian, pancreatic	Dominant	STK11
Genodermatoses with Cancer Predisposition				
Nevoid basal cell carcinoma syndrome	109400	Skin, medulloblastoma	Dominant	PTCH
Neurofibromatosis type 1	162200	Neurofibroma, optic pathway glioma, peripheral nerve sheath tumor	Dominant	NF1
Neurofibromatosis type 2	101000	Vestibular schwannoma	Dominant	NF2
Tuberous sclerosis	191100	Hamartoma, renal angiomyolipoma, renal cell carcinoma	Dominant	TSC1/TSC2
Xeroderma pigmentosum	278730, 278700, 278720, 278760, 278740, 278780, 278750, 133510	Skin, melanoma, leukemia	Recessive	XPA, B, C, D, E, F, G, POLH
Rothmund-Thomson syndrome	268400	Skin, bone	Recessive	RECQL4
Leukemia/Lymphoma Predisposition Syndromes				
Bloom syndrome	210900	Leukemia, lymphoma, skin	Recessive	BLM
Fanconi anemia	227650	Leukemia, squamous cell carcinoma, gynecologic system	Recessive	FANCA, B, C, D_2, E, F, G
Shwachman-Diamond syndrome	260400	Leukemia/myelodysplasia	Recessive	SBDS
Nijmegen breakage syndrome	251260	Lymphoma, medulloblastoma, glioma	Recessive	NBS1
Ataxia telangiectasia	208900	Leukemia, lymphoma	Recessive	ATM
Genitourinary Cancer Predisposition Syndromes				
Simpson-Golabi-Behmel syndrome	312870	Embryonal tumors, Wilms tumor	X-linked	GPC3
Von Hippel-Lindau syndrome	193300	Retinal and central nervous hemangioblastoma, pheochromocytoma, renal cell carcinoma	Dominant	VHL
Beckwith-Wiedemann syndrome	130650	Wilms tumor, hepatoblastoma, adrenal carcinoma, rhabdomyosarcoma	Dominant	CDKN1C/NSD1
Wilms tumor syndrome	194070	Wilms tumor	Dominant	WT1
WAGR syndrome	194072	Wilms tumor, gonadoblastoma	Dominant	WT1
Costello syndrome	218040	Neuroblastoma, rhabdomyosarcoma, bladder carcinoma	Dominant	H-Ras
Central Nervous System Predisposition Syndromes				
Retinoblastoma	180200	Retinoblastoma, osteosarcoma	Dominant	RB1
Rhabdoid predisposition syndrome	601607	Rhabdoid tumor, medulloblastoma, choroid plexus tumor		SNF5/INI1
Medulloblastoma predisposition	607035	Medulloblastoma	Dominant	SUFU
Sarcoma/Bone Cancer Predisposition Syndromes				
Li-Fraumeni syndrome	151623	Soft tissue sarcoma, osteosarcoma, breast, adrenocortical carcinoma, leukemia, brain tumor	Dominant	TP53
Multiple exostoses	133700, 133701	Chondrosarcoma	Dominant	EXT1/EXT2
Werner syndrome	277700	Osteosarcoma, meningioma	Recessive	WRN
Endocrine Cancer Predisposition Syndromes				
MEN1	131000	Pancreatic islet cell tumor, pituitary adenoma, parathyroid adenoma	Dominant	MEN1
MEN2	171400	Medullary thyroid carcinoma, pheochromocytoma, parathyroid hyperplasia	Dominant	RET

[a] Online Mendelian Inheritance in Man (OMIM), http://omim.org/search/advanced/geneMap.
WAGR, Wilms tumor, aniridia, genitourinary abnormalities, mental retardation; MEN, multiple endocrine neoplasia.
Adapted from Hahn H, Wojnowski L, Zimmer AM, et al. Rhabdomyosarcomas and radiation hypersensitivity in a mouse model of Gorlin syndrome. *Nat Med* 1998;4:619–622.

TABLE 98.2

Common Cytogenetic Rearrangements in Solid Tumors of Childhood

Solid Tumor	Cytogenetic Rearrangement	Genes[a]
Ewing sarcoma	t(11;22) (q24;q12), +8	EWS(22) FLi-1(11)
Neuroblastoma	del1p32–36, DMs, HSRs, +17q21-qter	N-MYC
Retinoblastoma	del13q14	Rb
Wilms tumor	del11p13, t(3;17)	WT1
Synovial sarcoma	t(X;11) (p11;q11)	SSX(X) SYT(18)
Osteogenic sarcoma	del13q14	?
Rhabdomyosarcoma	t(2;13) (q37;q14), t(2;11),3p-,11p-	PAX3(2) FOXO1(13)
Peripheral neuroepithelioma	t(11;22) (q24;q12), +8	EWS(22) FLi-1(11)
Astrocytoma	i(17q)	?
Meningioma	delq22, -22	MN1, NF2, ?
Atypical teratoid/rhabdoid tumor	delq22.11	SNF 5
Germ cell tumor	i(12p)	

[a] Chromosomal location in parentheses.

RETINOBLASTOMA: THE PARADIGM

Retinoblastoma is the prototype cancer caused by mutations of a tumor suppressor gene. It is a malignant tumor of the retina that occurs in infants and young children, with an incidence of approximately 1:20,000.[5] Approximately 40% of retinoblastoma cases are of the heritable form in which the child inherits one mutant allele at the retinoblastoma susceptibility locus (Rb1) through the germ line, and a somatic mutation in a single retinal cell causes loss of function of the remaining normal allele, leading to tumor formation. Tumors are often bilateral and multifocal. The disease is inherited as an autosomal-dominant trait, with a penetrance approaching 100%.[6] The remaining 60% of retinoblastoma cases are sporadic (nonheritable), in which both Rb1 alleles in a single retinal cell are inactivated by somatic mutations. As one can imagine, such an event is rare, and these patients usually have only one tumor that presents itself later than in infants with the heritable form. Fifteen percent of unilateral retinoblastoma is heritable[6] but by chance develops in only one eye. Survivors of heritable retinoblastoma have a several 100-fold increased risk of developing mesenchymal tumors such as osteogenic sarcoma, fibrosarcomas, and melanomas later in life.[7] Several genetic mechanisms have been implicated in elimination of the second wild-type Rb1 allele in an evolving tumor. These include chromosomal duplication or nondisjunction, mitotic recombination, or gene conversion.[8]

The Rb1 gene maps to chromosome 13q14 and encodes a 105kD phosphoprotein.[9,10] The second target gene that led to disease was actually the second copy of the Rb1 locus. Reduction to homozygosity of the mutant allele (or loss of heterozygosity [LOH] of the wild-type allele) would lead to the loss of functional Rb1 and account for tumor development. As well as being altered in retinoblastoma, Rb1 and its protein product are altered in osteosarcomas, small cell lung carcinomas, and bladder, breast, and prostate carcinomas.[10,11] Rb1 plays a central role in the control of cell-cycle regulation, particularly in determining transition from G1 through S (the DNA synthesis) phase in virtually all cell types.

Although it is clear that Rb1 and its protein product play some role in growth regulation, the precise nature of this role remains obscure. In the developing retina, inactivation of the Rb1 gene is necessary but not sufficient for tumor formation.[12] Retinoblastomas develop as a result of a complex interplay of aberrant expression of other cell-cycle control genes. In particular, a tumor surveillance pathway mediated by Arf, MDM2, MDMX, and p53 (see later discussion) is activated after a loss of Rb1 during development of the retina. Rb1-deficient retinoblasts undergo p53-mediated apoptosis and exit the cell cycle. Subsequently, amplification of the MDMX gene and increased expression of MDMX protein are strongly selected for during tumor progression as a mechanism to suppress the p53 response in Rb1-deficient retinal cells.[13] Not only do these observations provide a provocative biologic mechanism for tumor formation in retinoblastoma, but it also offers potential molecular targets for novel therapeutic approaches to this tumor.[14,15] Some Rb1 mutations appear to lead to an attenuated form of the disease, an observation that highlights the variable penetrance in families.[16,17] Outside the retina, Rb1 inactivation is often a rate-limiting step in tumorigenesis generated by multiple genetic events. The molecular characteristics and potential functional activities of Rb1 are outlined in detail elsewhere in this volume.

The patterns of inheritance and presentation of retinoblastoma have been well described and the responsible gene has been identified. The basic mechanisms by which the gene is inactivated are understood, and provocative evidence indicates that the intricate functional interactions of pRB with its binding partners and other cell cycle targets will provide targets for development of novel small molecule therapies.

SDH DEFICIENT GIST

Gastrointestinal stromal tumors (GIST) are the most common mesenchymal tumors found in the gastrointestinal (GI) tract, and occur in both adults and children. Strikingly, unlike most adult GIST tumors that harbor either KIT or platelet-derived growth factor receptor A (PDGFRA) mutations and are susceptible to tyrosine kinase (TK) inhibitors directed against these kinases, 85% of pediatric GIST tumors do not harbor such mutations, and not surprisingly are much less responsive to TK inhibitors. Thus, it appears that a histologically similar tumor in a pediatric population is remarkably biologically distinct from the same tumor in the adult population. It was recently demonstrated that the pediatric-type GIST tumor is characterized by metabolic derangement of the mitochondrial enzyme, succinate dehydrogenase (SDH).[18] Many of these patients have been found to carry germ-line mutations of SDH subunits B, C, or D (SDH$_x$) mutations. These germ-line mutations were first described in Carney-Stratakis syndrome, an inherited predisposition to GIST and paragangliomas.[19] It is noteworthy that these SDH-deficient pediatric predominant GISTs have a marked predilection for gastric location and are more frequent in the female population.[20]

Further characterization of molecular differences between the typical adult GIST, *KIT*, or *PDGFRA* activated tumors and SDH-deficient, pediatric-type GIST tumors revealed marked epigenetic distinctions between these two types of GISTs. Specifically, the SDH-deficient tumors were found to have marked global hypermethylation compared to the TK-mutant GISTs. Of specific note was enrichment for hypermethylation within DNase hypersensitivity sites.[21]

Thus it is clear that most pediatric GISTs are driven by a distinct mechanism related to SDH-deficient function compared to the adult GISTs, which are driven by the mutation activation of KIT or PDGFRA kinases. Furthermore, many of these tumors are associated with germ-line mutations of SDH$_x$, and may or may not be associated with paragangliomas. The finding of global hypermethylation in the pediatric-type GISTs was associated with very stable genomes, suggesting these tumors are epigenetically driven tumors.[21] Overall, these data clearly suggest that despite histologically similar tumors, the GISTs that occur in the younger population have a distinct behavior that will require management that is quite different than the management of adult, TK-mutating GISTs.

NEUROFIBROMATOSES

The neurofibromatoses comprise two similar entities. Neurofibromatosis type 1 (NF1) is one of the most common autosomal-dominantly inherited disorders, affecting about 1 in 3,500 people,[22] half of which arise from new spontaneous mutations. Carriers of mutant NF1 are predisposed to a variety of tumors, including Schwann cell–derived tumors (neurofibromas and malignant peripheral nerve sheath tumors, gliomas including optic nerve gliomas and malignant gliomas, and pheochromocytomas).[23,24] Occurring with less frequency are leukemias, osteosarcomas, rhabdomyosarcomas, GISTs, and Wilms tumors.

Using a standard linkage analysis, the neurofibromatosis type 1 (NF1) gene was mapped to chromosomal band 17q11, and subsequently cloned.[25,26] The NF1 gene is unusual in that it contains three embedded genes, OMGP, EV12A, and EV12B, in a single intron.[27] This gene encodes a 2818 amino acid protein, termed *neurofibromin*, that is ubiquitously expressed. One region of the gene shows extensive structural homology to the GTPase activating domain of mammalian GTP-ase–activating protein (GAP) proteins: loss of the protein's activity results in failure of hydrolysis of GTP to guanosine diphosphate (GDP) by the ras oncoprotein. Loss of neurofibromin function usually results from mutations in one allele of the gene leading to premature truncation of the protein, followed by absence or mutations of the second allele in tumors. This loss of function is thought to lead to elevated levels of the GTP-bound RAS protein that transduces signals for cell division. Downstream modulators of RAS activation in NF1-associated tumors include activation of mammalian target of rapamycin (mTOR) and mitogen activated protein kinase kinase (MEK).[28,29] Thus, although targeting RAS remains elusive, mTOR and MEK inhibitors are currently either available or are being tested in the clinic. Neurofibromatosis type 2 (NF2) is much less frequent than NF1, occurring in only 1 in 1 million persons. Although it is also inherited as an autosomal-dominant disorder with high penetrance, the new mutation rate in NF2 is low.[30] It is clinically characterized by bilateral vestibular schwannomas, spinal nerve root tumors, meningiomas, and ependymomas.

The NF2 locus was mapped to chromosome 22, band q12,[31] and its 69-kDa encoded protein, termed merlin, has been shown to be expressed in various tissues, including the brain, although not as ubiquitously as NF1.[32,33] The mechanism of tumor formation in NF2 appears to be in concordance with the Knudson two-hit model, although the mechanism of action of the NF2 protein has not yet been elucidated. Merlin is a member of the Band 4.1 family of proteins that link cell surface proteins to the cytoskeleton.[34] Merlin has been shown to inhibit the number of signaling pathways critical for normal growth including mTOR, Rac1, and Hippo/YAP, with loss of Merlin leading to activation of these pathways, again suggesting potential therapies aimed at inhibition of these pathways.[34]

NEUROBLASTOMA

Nonrandom chromosomal abnormalities are observed in more than 75% of neuroblastomas.[35] The most common of these is deletion or rearrangement of the short arm of chromosome 1, although loss, gain, and rearrangements of chromosomes 10, 11, 14, 17, and 19 have also been reported. The allelic losses indicate loss of function of as yet unknown tumor suppressor genes in these regions. It is believed that a tumor suppressor gene, such as CHD5 and the kinesin KIF1Bbeta that lies on band p36 of chromosome 1 is critically important in the pathogenesis and aggressive nature of neuroblastoma.[36,37] It has been shown that the loss of chromosome 1p is a strong prognostic factor in patients with neuroblastoma, independent of age and stage.[38] Although it is as yet unclear which gene(s) in this region may be directly implicated in neuroblastoma development, aberrant expression of one candidate—*p73*—which is a member of the *p53* tumor suppressor family, has been suggested to play a role in the neuroblastoma cell growth as well as chemotherapy resistance.[39] *p73* gives rise to multiple functionally distinct protein isoforms as a result of alternative promoter utilization and alternative mRNA splicing.[40,41] Alternative splicing of the *p73* mRNA results in more than seven protein isoforms that differ in the coding sequences of the COOH terminus (TA-p73 α, β, γ, δ, ε, ζ, η).

In addition to these COOH-terminal splice forms, three additional forms, Np73α, ΔNp73β, and ΔNp73γ, are transcribed from an alternative promoter located in intron 3. Higher levels of ΔNp73 are associated with an overall worse clinical prognosis, presumably because of the *antiapoptotic* properties of ΔNp73 and its ability to inactivate both TAp73 and p53.[42,43]

Two other unique cytogenetic rearrangements are highly characteristic of neuroblastomas.[44] These structures, homogeneous staining regions (HSR) and double-minute chromosomes (DM), contain regions of gene amplification. The *N-myc* gene, an oncogene with considerable homology to the cellular protooncogene *c-myc*, is amplified within HSR and DM. Virtually all neuroblastoma tumor cell lines demonstrate amplified and highly expressed *N-myc*,[45] and *N-myc* amplification is thought to be associated with rapid tumor progression. Expression of *N-myc* is increased in undifferentiated tumor cells compared with much lower (or single-copy) levels in more differentiated cells (ganglioneuroblastomas and ganglioneuromas). *N-myc* expression is diminished in association with the in vitro differentiation of neuroblastoma cell lines.[46] This observation formed the basis for current therapeutic trials demonstrating a survival advantage to patients treated with *cis*-retinoic acid.[47] Furthermore, a close correlation exists between *N-myc* amplification and advanced clinical stage.[48]

Neuroblastoma cells that express the high-affinity nerve growth factor receptor trkA[49] can be terminally differentiated by nerve growth factor and may demonstrate morphologic changes typical of ganglionic differentiation. Tumors showing ganglionic differentiation and *trk* gene activation have a favorable prognosis.[49] In contrast, trkB receptor expression is associated with poor-prognosis tumors and appears to mediate resistance to chemotherapy.[50,51] Resistance to multidrug chemotherapeutic regimens (i.e., multidrug resistance) is characteristic of aggressive, poorly responsive *N-myc*–amplified neuroblastomas. It is interesting to note that expression of the multidrug resistance–associated protein, found to confer multidrug resistance in vitro, is increased in neuroblastomas with N-myc amplification, decreased after differentiation of tumor cells in vitro, and associated with poor outcome independent of N-myc amplification.[52] Gain of chromosome segment 17q21-qter, in which BICR5, which encodes Survivin (a member of the apoptosis inhibiting proteins NM23 and PMMID) has been posited as a neuroblastoma-associated candidate gene, has been shown to be the most powerful prognostic factor yet.[53]

A small subset of neuroblastomas is inherited in an autosomal-dominant fashion. Until recently, the only gene definitively associated with neuroblastoma risk was PHOX2B, also linked to central apnea.[54] De novo or inherited missense mutations in the TK domain of the anaplastic lymphoma kinase (ALK) gene on chromosome 2p23 have been observed in the majority of hereditary neuroblastoma families, as well as in somatic tumor cells.[55–58] Current phase I/II clinical trials with ALK inhibitors substantiate the value of such target identification for novel therapies.[59] The role of other molecular alterations in neuroblastoma continues to be elucidated. In addition to chromosomal loss on chromosome 1p36, unbalanced LOH at 11q23 is independently associated with decreased event-free survival. Alterations at 11q23 occur in almost one-third of neuroblastomas, being most commonly associated with stage 4 disease and age at diagnosis greater than 2.5 years. Both 1p36 LOH and 11q23 LOH were independently associated with decreased progression-free survival in patients with low- and intermediate-risk disease.[60]

Yet another valuable biologic marker of clinical significance is telomerase expression and telomere length. In particular, short telomere length is predictive of favorable prognosis, irrespective of disease stage, whereas long or unchanged telomeres are predictive of poor outcome.[61,62] Telomerase expression, as measured by human telomerase reverse transcriptase (hTERT), has been shown to be negative in good-risk neuroblastomas, although it is high in tumors with unfavorable histology.[62] The combined use of these markers—chromosomes 1p and 11q, N-Myc amplification, trkA, and telomerase expression—as prognostic indicators provides a powerful armamentarium with which to develop rational stratified treatment programs for neuroblastomas.

EWING SARCOMA FAMILY OF TUMORS

Ewing sarcoma (ES) is one of the first examples in which the application of molecular diagnostics led to improved tumor classification. ES was first described by James Ewing[63] as a bone tumor characterized by small, blue, round cells and minimal mitotic activity. Turc-Carel et al.[64] identified a recurring reciprocal t(11;22) chromosomal translocation in these tumors in 1983. Investigators subsequently demonstrated a cytogenetically identical t(11;22) in adult neuroblastoma or peripheral primitive neuroectodermal tumor (pPNET), so named because of its histologic similarity to neuroblastoma.[65] Based on the presence of the identical translocation, it was hypothesized that pPNET was related to ES. This translocation breakpoint has been molecularly characterized as an in-frame fusion between a new ES gene, Ewing's sarcoma breakpoint region 1 (EWS), on chromosome 22 and an ETS transcription family member, friend leukemia virus integration 1 (FLI-1), on chromosome 22.[66–68]

In addition to this fusion transcript being identified in pPNET, other variants, notably the chest-wall Askin tumor and soft tissue ES—previously treated as an RMS because of its location in soft tissue—were also shown to bear the identical fusion transcript. In total, five translocations also have been identified, invariably fusing the EWS gene to an ETS family member.[69–72] More than 90% of the ES family of tumors (ESFT) carry the EWS-ETS fusion gene, and a search for EWS-ETS by either reverse transcriptase-polymerase chain reaction or fluorescence in situ hybridization should be considered standard practice in the diagnostic evaluation of suspected ESFTs. Interestingly, although it was suggested that the specific fusion protein expressed in ESFT has prognostic

significance,[73] several prospective studies in the United States and Europe demonstrated no prognostic impact.[74,75] The nature of the novel fusion transcription factor and its downstream targets is currently under intense investigation. One target of the EWS-ETS fusion is repression of the transforming growth factor-β type II receptor,[76] a putative tumor suppressor gene.

Expression profiling analysis has also revealed that p53 is transcriptionally upregulated by the EWS-ETS fusion gene.[77] This is of particular interest because it is now known that expression of EWS-ETS can lead to apoptosis, and that additional alterations such as loss of p53 or p16 signaling, or both, appear to be necessary components of EWS-ETS–induced transformation.[78] Investigators have now taken advantage of RNA interference technology to inhibit EWS–FLI-1 in Ewing cell lines to identify genes regulated by the fusion in the proper context. Using this approach, NKX2.2 and NR0B1 have been found to be a target gene of EWS–FLI-1 that is necessary for oncogenic transformation.[79,80] Recent findings suggest that GGAA microsatellites might mark genes that are upregulated by EWS–FLI-1 binding.[81]

RHABDOMYOSARCOMA

The two major histologic subtypes of RMS, embryonal and alveolar, have both unique histologic appearance as well as distinctive molecular genetic abnormalities, while sharing a common myogenic lineage. Embryonal tumors comprise two-thirds of all RMS, and are histologically characterized by a stroma-rich spindle-cell appearance. Alveolar tumors comprise about one-third of RMS, and are histologically characterized by densely packed small round cells often lining a septation reminiscent of a pulmonary alveolus, giving rise to its name. Both histologic subtypes express muscle-specific proteins, including α-actin, myosin, desmin, and MyoD,[82–84] and they virtually always express high levels of insulin-like growth factor 2 (IGF2).[85,86]

At the molecular level, embryonal tumors are characterized by LOH at the 11p15 locus, which is of particular interest because this region harbors the IGF2 gene.[87,88] The LOH at 11p15 occurs by loss of maternal and duplication of paternal chromosomal material.[89] Although LOH is normally associated with loss of tumor suppressor gene activity, in this instance, LOH with paternal duplication may result in activation of IGF2. This occurs because IGF2 is now known to be normally imprinted; that is, this gene is normally transcriptionally silent at the maternal allele, with only the paternal allele being transcriptionally active.[90,91] Thus, LOH with paternal duplication potentially leads to a twofold gene-dosage effect of the IGF2 locus. Furthermore, in alveolar tumors where LOH does not occur, the normally imprinted maternal allele has been shown to be reexpressed.[92,93] Thus, LOH and loss of imprinting (LOI) may in this case lead to the same functional result—namely, biallelic expression of the normally monoallelically expressed IGF2. However, loss of an as yet unidentified tumor suppressor activity due to LOH also remains a possibility.

Alveolar RMS is characterized by a t(2;13)(q35;q14) chromosomal translocation.[94] Molecular cloning of this translocation has identified the generation of a fusion transcription factor, fusing the 5′ DNA-binding region of PAX-3 on chromosome 2 to the 3′ transactivation domain region of FOXO1 gene on chromosome 13.[95,96] A variant t(1;13)(q36;q14) has been identified in a small number of alveolar RMS tumors that fuses the 5′ DNA-binding region of the PAX-7 gene on chromosome 1 with the identical 3′ transactivation domain of the FOXO1 gene.[97] Fluorescence in situ hybridization (FISH) or reverse transcription polymerase chain reaction (RT-PCR) can be used to identify these PAX3/7-FOXO1 fusions in approximately 90% of tumors, and are diagnostic of alveolar rhabdomyosarcoma (ARMS). As noted previously, the fusion protein generated by the translocation leads to a novel transcription factor.

The recent application of molecular techniques have now clearly shown that PAX3/7-mutation positive RMS is clearly distinct from fusion-negative tumors. At the RNA expression level, fusion-positive tumors cluster together and have an expression profile that is distinct from fusion-negative tumors. Furthermore, the fusion-positive tumors have a much more aggressive clinical behavior.[98] Using current next-generation sequencing techniques, it has now also been shown that the fusion-negative tumors have significantly more mutations per tumor compared to fusion-positive tumors.[99,100] Recurrent mutations identified in fusion-negative RMS included both previously identified (*H, K and NRAS, FGFR4, phosphatidyl–4, 5 bisphosphate 3–kinase catalytic subunit alpha [PIK3CA], and NF1*) as well as a ubiquitin ligase *FBXW7*, and a transcriptional repressor *BCOR*.

Notably, many of the identified mutations in fusion-negative RMS were shown to be transcriptional targets of PAX fusion proteins, suggesting either accumulation of point mutations or upregulation of the same genes by aberrant transcription activation lead to similar tumors. And despite the relative paucity of mutations compared to adult tumors, there is accumulating evidence that targeting members of the RAS/Phosphatidyl – 4, 5 bisphosphate 3 – kinase catalytic subunit alpha (PIC3CA) pathway represents a rational approach to development of new therapeutic approaches to these tumors.[101]

HEREDITARY SYNDROMES ASSOCIATED WITH TUMORS OF CHILDHOOD LI-FRAUMENI SYNDROME

Although a detailed description of the many syndromes that are associated with the development of childhood cancers are beyond the scope of this chapter, several are discussed here to illustrate the breadth of phenotypes and underlying genetic mechanisms that should be considered in their management. A few hereditary cancer syndromes are associated with the occurrence of childhood as well as adult-onset neoplasms. The paradigm LFS cancer was first described in 1969 from an epidemiologic evaluation of more than 600 medical and family history records of patients with childhood sarcomas.[102] The original description of a kindred with a spectrum of tumors that includes soft tissue sarcomas, osteosarcomas, breast cancer, brain tumors, leukemia, and adrenocortical carcinoma (ACC) has been overwhelmingly substantiated by numerous subsequent studies,[103] although other cancers, usually of particularly early age of onset, are also observed.[104] Germ-line alterations of the *TP53* tumor suppressor gene are associated with LFS.[105,106] These are primarily missense mutations that yield a stabilized mutant protein. The spectrum of mutations of *TP53* in the germ line is similar to somatic mutations found in a wide variety of tumors. Carriers are heterozygous for the mutation, and in tumors derived from these individuals, the second (wild-type) allele is frequently deleted or mutated, leading to functional inactivation.[107]

Several comprehensive databases document all reported germ-line (and somatic) *TP53* mutations and are of particular value in evaluating novel mutations as well as phenotype–genotype correlations.[108] Only 60% to 80% of *classic* LFS families have detectable alterations of the gene. It is not yet determined whether the remainder is associated with the presence of modifier genes, promoter defects yielding abnormalities of *TP53* expression, or simply the result of weak genotype–phenotype correlations (i.e., the broad clinical definition encompasses families that are not actual members of LFS). Other candidate predisposition genes, such as *p16, p15, p21, BRCA1, BRCA2,* and *PTEN*, associated with multisite cancer associations have generally been ruled out as potential targets. The role of the hCHK2 checkpoint kinase as an alternative mechanism for functional inactivation of TP53 in LFS has been suggested,[109] although its place as a major contributor to the phenotype has been controversial.[110]

Germ-line *TP53* alterations have also been reported in some patients with cancer phenotypes that resemble the classic LFS phenotype. Between 3% and 10% of children with apparently sporadic RMS or osteosarcoma have been shown to carry germ-line *TP53*

mutations.[111,112] These patients tend to be younger than those who harbor wild-type *TP53*. Germ-line TP53 mutations are observed in more than 60% of children with the anaplastic variant of RMS,[113] and are also overrepresented in children with the Sonic hedgehog (SHH) subgroup of medulloblastomas.[114] It appears as well that more than 75% of children with apparently sporadic ACC carry germ-line *TP53* mutations, although in some of these cases, a family history develops that is not substantially distinct from LFS.[115,116] These important findings indicate a broader spectrum of patients at risk of germ-line *TP53* mutations and refined criteria for *TP53* mutation analyses.[117,118] A striking genotype–phenotype correlation has been observed in a unique subgroup of ACC patients in Brazil in whom the same germ-line *TP53* mutation at codon 337 has been observed in 35 unrelated kindred.[119] The functional integrity of the mutant protein appears to be regulated by alterations in cellular pH,[120] which suggests potential biologic mechanisms in ACC cells by which the *TP53* mutation leads to malignant transformation. All these observations suggest that germ-line *TP53* alterations may be associated with early-onset development of the childhood component tumors of the syndrome.[121] The variability in age of onset and type of cancer among LFS families suggests modifier effects on the underlying mutant *TP53* genotype. An analysis of mutant genotype-to-phenotype correlations reveals intriguing observations. Nonsense, frameshift, and splice mutations yield a truncated or nonfunctional protein commonly associated with early-onset cancers, particularly brain tumors. Missense mutations in the *TP53* DNA-binding domain are frequently observed in the setting of breast and brain tumors, whereas adrenocortical cancers are the only group that is associated with mutations in the non–DNA-binding loops. Age of onset modifiers have also now been established. The protein murine double-minute-2 (MDM2) is a key negative regulator of TP53 and targets TP53 toward proteasomal degradation. The MDM2 single nucleotide polymorphism 309 increases Sp1 transcription factor binding, leading to increased *MDM2* expression levels. Coinheritance of the MDM2 single nucleotide polymorphism 309 T/G isoform is associated with an earlier onset of cancer.[122] The earlier age of onset of cancers with subsequent generations in mutant *TP53* LFS families suggests genetic anticipation. This observation can be partially explained by several molecular mechanisms including accelerated telomere attrition from generation to generation, absence of the PIN3 polymorphism, or excessive DNA copy number variation in *p53* mutation carriers, all of which may be useful predictive markers of tumor age of onset.[122–124] Thus, although germ-line *p53* mutations establish the baseline risk of tumor development in LFS, a complex interplay of modifying genetic cofactors likely defines the specific phenotypes of individual patients.

Beckwith-Wiedemann Syndrome

BWS occurs with a frequency of 1 in 13,700 births. More than 450 cases have been documented since the original reported associations of exomphalos, macroglossia, gigantism, and other congenital anomalies. With increasing age, phenotypic features of BWS become less pronounced. Laboratory findings may include, at birth, hypoglycemia, polycythemia, hypocalcemia, hypertriglyceridemia, hypercholesterolemia, and high serum α-fetoprotein levels. Early diagnosis of the condition is crucial to avoid deleterious neurologic effects of neonatal hypoglycemia and to initiate an appropriate screening protocol for tumor development.[125] The increased risk for tumor formation in BWS patients is estimated at 7.5% and is further increased to 10% if hemihyperplasia is present. Tumors occurring with the highest frequency include Wilms tumor, hepatoblastoma, neuroblastoma, and ACC.[126]

The genetic basis of BWS is complex. Various 11p15 chromosomal or molecular alterations have been associated with the BWS phenotype and its tumors.[127] It is unlikely that a single gene is responsible for the BWS phenotype. Because it appears that

PRACTICE OF ONCOLOGY

abnormalities in the region impact an imprinted domain, it is more likely that normal gene regulation in this part of chromosome 11p15 occurs in a regional manner and may depend on various interdependent factors or genes. These include the paternally expressed genes *IGF2* and *KCNQ10T1* and the maternally expressed genes *H19*, *CDKN1C*, and *KCNQ1*. BWS children who develop rhabdomyosarcoma or hepatoblastoma have epigenetic changes in domain 1, whereas those with Wilms tumor have domain 2 changes or uniparental disomy.[128]

Chromosomal abnormalities associated with BWS are extremely rare, with only 20 cases having been associated with 11p15 translocations or inversions. The chromosomal breakpoint in each of these cases is always found on the maternally derived chromosome 11. This parent-of-origin dependence in BWS suggests that the chromosome translocations disrupt imprinting of a gene in the 11p15 region. On the other hand, BWS-associated 11p15 duplications (approximately 30 reported cases) are always paternally derived, and the duplication breakpoints are heterogeneous.[129] Paternal uniparental disomy, in which two alleles are inherited from one parent (the father), has been reported in approximately 15% of sporadic BWS patients.[130] The insulin/IGF2 region is always represented in the uniparental disomy, although the extent of chromosomal involvement is highly variable. Alterations in allele-specific DNA methylation of *IGF2* and *H19* reflect this paternal imprinting phenomenon.[130] A minority of BWS patients have demonstrable constitutional DNA sequence alterations, the most common of these being *CDKN1C* mutations.[131] Of BWS patients, 25% to 50% exhibit biallelic rather than monoallelic expression of *IGF2*. Another 50% have epigenetic mutations resulting in LOI of *KCNQ10T0*. Of interest, epigenetic changes, such as methylation and chromatin modification, occur in many pediatric and adult cancers,[132] indicating the value of the BWS model in understanding the broad scope of molecular changes in cancer. Despite the associated cytogenetic and molecular findings for some patients, no single diagnostic test exists for BWS. This observation is not unlike that described for LFS, or perhaps for other multisite cancer phenotypes, in which the clarity of the phenotype is often weak, making the genetic link cloudy and the likelihood of multiple pathways to tumor formation strong.

Gorlin Syndrome

Nevoid basal cell carcinoma syndrome, or Gorlin syndrome, is a rare autosomal-dominant disorder characterized by multiple basal cell carcinomas; developmental defects, including bifid ribs and other spine and rib abnormalities; palmar and plantar pits; odontogenic keratocysts; and generalized overgrowth.[133] The SHH signaling pathway directs embryonic development of a spectrum of organisms. Gorlin syndrome appears to be caused by germ-line mutations of the tumor suppressor gene *PTCH*, a receptor for SHH.[134,135] Medulloblastomas develop in approximately 5% of patients with Gorlin syndrome. Furthermore, approximately 10% of patients diagnosed with medulloblastoma by the age of 2 years are found to have other phenotypic features consistent with Gorlin syndrome and also harbor germ-line *PTCH* mutations.[136] Although Gorlin syndrome develops in individuals with germ-line mutations of *PTCH*, a subset of children with medulloblastoma harbor germ-line mutations of another gene, *SUFU*, in the SHH pathway, with accompanying LOH in the tumors. Of further note, mice with heterozygous *PTC* deletions develop RMS.[137] Although RMS is rarely seen with Gorlin syndrome, the mouse studies suggest a possible link between PTC signaling and RMS.[138]

MALIGNANT RHABDOID TUMORS

Malignant rhabdoid tumors are unusual pediatric tumors that occur as primary renal tumors, but have also been described in lung, liver, soft tissues, and the central nervous system, where they are often termed *atypical* and *teratoid rhabdoid tumors*.[139] Recurrent chromosomal translocations of chromosome 22 involving a breakpoint at 22q11.2, as well as complete or partial monosomy 22, have been observed, strongly suggesting the presence of a tumor suppressor gene in this area. The *hSNF5/INI1* gene has been isolated and has been shown to be the target for biallelic, recurrent inactivating mutations.[140] The encoded gene product is thought to be involved in chromatin remodeling. Studies have not only demonstrated the presence of inactivating mutations in the majority of malignant rhabdoid tumors (renal or extrarenal), but also in chronic myelogenous leukemia,[141] as well as in a wide variety of other childhood and adult-onset malignancies.[142] An intriguing feature in some individuals with malignant rhabdoid tumors is the observation of germ-line mutations, suggesting that this family of tumors may occur as a result of a primary inherited defect in one allele of the *INI1* gene.[143] Further studies of the function of this gene will be important in determining its role in tumorigenesis of this wide spectrum of neoplasms.

DICER1 SYNDROME

DICER1 syndrome is a very recently characterized phenotype of distinctive dysontogenetic, hyperplastic, or overtly malignant tumors. The most frequent of these is the rare childhood lung malignancy pleuropulmonary blastoma (PPB). Other manifestations include ovarian Sertoli-Leydig cell tumors (SLCT), nodular thyroid hyperplasia, pituitary blastoma, pineoblastoma, papillary and follicular thyroid carcinoma, cervical rhabdomyosarcoma, cystic nephroma, and possibly, Wilms tumor.[144] Germ-line *DICER1* mutations have been identified in children and young adults affected with one or several of these tumors, and somatic *DICER1* mutations have been found in sporadic component tumors. DICER1 is an endoribonuclease that processes hairpin precursor microRNAs (miRNA) into short, functional miRNAs. Mature 5' miRNAs as well as other components of the RNA-induced silencing complex (RISC) downregulate targeted miRNA.

Unlike the classical Knudson *two-hit* mechanism that inactivates tumor suppressor genes, the effect of DICER1 loss-of-function appears to result from an initial inactivating mutation that reduces by half the amount of wild-type DICER1 protein, followed by a second hit that specifically eliminates production of 5' mature miRNAs. Disease penetrance is highly variable. The risk of potentially lethal tumors such as PPB and pineoblastoma in *DICER1*-mutation carriers indicates a need for clinical surveillance, particularly targeting the lungs, abdomen, and brain.

PREDICTIVE TESTING FOR GERM-LINE MUTATIONS AND CHILDHOOD CANCERS

Several important issues have arisen as a result of the identification of germ-line mutations of tumor suppressor genes in cancer-prone individuals and families. These include ethical questions of predictive testing in such families and in unaffected relatives and the selection of patients to be tested, as well as the development of practical and accurate laboratory techniques, the development of pilot testing programs, and the role of clinical interventions based on test results. This chapter was not meant to discuss these problems in detail, but one would be remiss to ignore their significance.

For several reasons, testing cannot as yet be offered to the general pediatric population, particularly in light of the demonstrably low carrier rate of the abnormal tumor suppressor genes and the general lack of standardized methods of preclinical screening of carriers. Exceptions to these limitations include screening of gene carriers in families with retinoblastoma, BWS, multiple endocrine neoplasia, familial adenomatous polyposis, LFS, hereditary paraganglioma syndromes, and von Hippel-Lindau disease. For some of these diseases, clinical surveillance tools are available, whereas for others, risk-reductive surgery has also been shown to be of value.[145–148] In general, it has been demonstrated that genetic testing does not lead to clinical levels of anxiety, depression, or other markers of psychological distress in children who are tested or their parents.[149,150] However, certain circumstances or personality traits are associated with a greater likelihood of an individual experiencing psychological distress after a positive result.[149] Parents now routinely discuss the options of prenatal diagnosis and preimplantation genetic diagnosis. Multidisciplinary teams must be engaged to provide parents and families the necessary tools with which to approach these ethically challenging decisions.[151,152] The development of screening programs should address aspects of cost, informed consent (particularly where it affects children), socioeconomic impact on the individual tested, consistency in providing results, and counseling. Concerns of risk of employment, health insurance, or life insurance discrimination exist but may be alleviated by congressional legislation to ban such practices.[153]

MOLECULAR THERAPEUTICS

With the identification of alterations in a variety of molecular signaling pathways increasingly identified with application of newer molecular analytic techniques, it has become increasingly apparent that these alterations may potentially represent the *Achilles heel* for these tumors. New agents targeting the TK enzymes as well as agents that alter the epigenetic state of tumors are at various stages of development in early clinical studies of pediatric tumors. A particular issue for the development of targeted therapy for pediatric tumors is the relative effectiveness of standard cytotoxic agents in many tumors. Thus, the identification of single targeted agent activity and the incorporation of such agents into combinations with cytotoxic agents is an important challenge. Ongoing studies incorporating mTOR inhibitors (rhabdomyosarcoma) or IGFIR inhibitors with combination chemotherapy (Ewing sarcoma) will provide important information on whether these approaches will improve outcome. The most important challenge will be to correctly identify the targetable altered pathways that are critical for malignant behavior of specific pediatric tumors and then rapidly test them in a rational approach to improve the outcomes of pediatric cancer patients.

SELECTED REFERENCES

The full reference list can be accessed at lwwhealthlibrary.com/oncology.

2. Choong SC, Priest JR, Foulkes WD. Exploring the endocrine manifestations of DICER1 mutations. *Trends Mol Medicine* 2012;18:503–505.
3. Knudson AG Jr. Mutation and cancer: statistical study of retinoblastoma. *Proc Natl Acad Sci U S A* 1971;68:820–823.
10. Friend SH, Bernards R, Rogelj S, et al. A human DNA segment with properties of the gene that predisposes to retinoblastoma and osteosarcoma. *Nature* 1986;323:643–646.
12. Burkart DL, Sage J. Cellular mechanism of tumor suppression by the retinoblastoma gene. *Nature Rev Cancer* 2008;8:671–682.
18. Janeway KA, Kim SY, Lodish M, et al. Defects in succinate dehydrogenase in gastrointestinal stromal tumors lacking KIT and PDGFRA mutations. *Proc Natl Acad Sci U S A* 2011;108:314–318.
19. McWhinney SR, Pasini B, Stratakis CA. Familial gastrointestinal stromal tumors and germ-line mutations. *N Engl J Med* 2007;357:1054–1056.
21. Killian JK, Kim SY, Miettinen M, et al. Succinate dehydrogenase mutation underlies global epigenomic divergence in gastrointestinal stromal tumor. *Cancer Discovery* 2013;3:648–657.
23. Riccardi VM, Eichner JE. *Neurofibromatosis: Phenotype, Natural History and Pathogenesis.* Baltimore: Johns Hopkins University Press; 1986.
27. Viskochil D, Buchberg AM, Xu G, et al. Deletions and a translocation interrupt a cloned gene at the neurofibromatosis type 1 locus. *Cell* 1990;62:187–192.
29. Jessen WJ, Miller SJ, Jousma E, et al. MEK inhibition exhibits efficacy in human and mouse neurofibromatosis tumors. *J Clin Invest* 2013;123:340–347.
31. Trofatter JA, MacCollin MM, Rutter JL, et al. A novel moesin-, ezrin-, radixin-like gene is a candidate for the neurofibromatosis 2 tumor suppressor. *Cell* 1993;73:791–800.
34. Lin AL, Gutmann DH. Advances in the treatment of neurofibromatosis-associated tumours. *Nat Rev Clin Oncol* 2013;10:616–624.
35. Brodeur GM, Sekhon G, Goldstein MN. Chromosomal aberrations in human neuroblastomas. *Cancer* 1977;40:2256–2263.
36. Fujita T, Igarashi J, Okawa ER, et al. CHD5, a tumor suppressor gene deleted from 1p36 in neuroblastoma. *J Natl Cancer Inst* 2008;100:940–949.
38. Caron H, van Sluis P, de Kraker J, et al. Allelic loss of chromosome 1p as a predictor of unfavorable outcome in patients with neuroblastoma. *N Engl J Med* 1996;334:225–230.
40. Irwin MS, Kaelin WG. p53 family update: p73 and p63 develop their own identities. *Cell Growth Differ* 2001;12:337–349.
41. Melino G, De Laurenzi V, Vousden KH. p73: Friend or foe in tumorigenesis. *Nat Rev Cancer* 2002;2:605–615.
45. Schwab M, Alitalo K, Klempnauer KH, et al. Amplified DNA with limited homology to myc cellular oncogene is shared by human neuroblastoma cell lines and a neuroblastoma tumour. *Nature* 1983;305:245–248.
47. Matthay KK, Villablanca JG, Seeger RC, et al. Treatment of high-risk neuroblastoma with intensive chemotherapy, radiotherapy, autologous bone marrow transplantation, and 13-cis-retinoic acid. Children's Cancer Group. *N Engl J Med* 1999;341:1165–1173.
54. Trochet D, Bourdeaut F, Janoueix-Lerosey I, et al. Germline mutations of the paired-like homeobox 2B (PHOX2B) gene in neuroblastoma. *Am J Hum Genet* 2004;74:761–764.
55. Mosse YP, Laduenslager M, Longo L, et al. Identification of ALK as a major familial neuroblastoma predisposition gene. *Nature* 2008;455:930–935.
59. Mosse YP, Lim MS, Voss SD, et al. Safety and activity of crizotinib for pediatric patients with refractory solid tumors or anaplastic large cell lymphoma: a COG phase I consortium study. *Lancet Oncol* 2013;14:472–480.
63. Ewing J. Classics in oncology. Diffuse endothelioma of bone: proceedings of the New York Pathological Society, 1921. *CA Cancer J Clin* 1972; 22:95–98.
64. Turc-Carel C, Aurias A, Mugneret F, et al. Chromosomes in Ewing's sarcoma. I. An evaluation of 85 cases of remarkable consistency of t(11;22) (q24;q12). *Cancer Genet Cytogenet* 1988;32:229.
66. Delattre O, Zucman J, Ploustagel B, et al. Gene fusion with an ETS DNA binding domain caused by chromosome translocation in human cancers. *Nature* 1992;359:162–165.
74. Le Deley MC, Delattre O, Schaefer KL, et al. Impact of EWS-ETS fusion type on disease progression in Ewing's sarcoma/peripheral primitive neuroectodermal tumor: prospective results from the cooperative Euro-E.W.I.N.G. 99 trial. *J Clin Oncol* 2010;28:1982–1988.
77. Lessnick SL, Dacwag CS, Golub TR. The Ewing's sarcoma oncoprotein EWS/FLI induces a p53-dependent growth arrest in primary human fibroblasts. *Cancer Cell* 2002;1:393–401.
81. Gangwal K, Sankar S, Hollenhorst PC, et al. Microsatellites as EWS/FLI response elements in Ewing's sarcoma. *Proc Natl Acad Sci U S A* 2008;105: 10149–10154.
84. Dias P, Parham DM, Shapiro DN, et al. Myogenic regulatory protein (MyoD1) expression in childhood solid tumors: diagnostic utility in rhabdomyosarcoma. *Am J Pathol* 1990;137:1283–1291.
87. Scrable H, Witte D, Lampkin B, et al. Chromosomal localization of the human rhabdomyosarcoma locus by mitotic recombination mapping. *Nature* 1987;329:645–647.
92. Zhan S, Shapiro DN, Helman LJ. Activation of an imprinted allele of the insulin-like growth factor II gene implicated in rhabdomyosarcoma. *J Clin Invest* 1994;94:445–448.
95. Barr FG, Galili N, Holick J, et al. Rearrangement of the PAX3 paired box gene in the paediatric solid tumour alveolar rhabdomyosarcoma. *Nat Genet* 1993;3:113–117.
99. Chen X, Stewart E, Shelat AA, et al. Targeting oxidative stress in embryonal rhabdomyosarcoma. *Cancer Cell* 2013;24:710–724.
100. Shern JF, Chen L, Chmielecki J, et al. Comprehensive genomic analysis of rhabdomyosarcoma reveals a landscape of alterations affecting a common genetic axis in fusion-positive and fusion-negative tumors. *Cancer Discov* 2014;4: 216–231.
101. Renshaw J, Taylor KR, Bishop R, et al. Dual blockade of the PI3K/AKT/mTOR (AZD8055) and RAS/MEK/ERK (AZD6244) pathways synergistically inhibits rhabdomyosarcoma cell growth in vitro and in vivo. *Clin Cancer Res* 2013;19:5940–5951.
102. Li FP, Fraumeni JF Jr. Rhabdomyosarcoma in children: epidemiologic study and identification of a familial cancer syndrome. *J Natl Cancer Inst* 1969;43:1365–1373.
103. Li FP, Fraumeni JF Jr, Mulvihill JJ, et al. A cancer family syndrome in twenty-four kindreds. *Cancer Res* 1988;48:5358–5362.

105. Malkin D, Li FP, Strong LC, et al. Germ line p53 mutations in a familial syndrome of breast cancer, sarcomas, and other neoplasms. *Science* 1990;250:1233–1238.

108. Leroy B, Fournier JL, Ishioka C, et al. The TP53 website: an integrative resource centre for the TP53 mutation database and TP53 mutant analysis. *Nucl Acids Res* 2013;41:D962–D969.

113. Hettmer S, Archer NM, Somers GR, et al. Anaplastic rhabdomyosarcoma in TP53 germline mutation carriers. *Cancer* 2014;120:1068–1075.

114. Rausch T, Jones DT, Zapatka M, et al. Genome sequencing of pediatric medulloblastoma links catastrophic DNA rearrangements with TP53 mutations. *Cell* 2012;148:59–71.

118. Tinat J, Bougeard G, Baert-Desurmont S, et al. 2009 version of the Chompret criteria for Li-Fraumeni syndrome. *J Clin Oncol* 2009;27:e108–e109.

129. Henry I, Bonaiti-Pellie C, Chehensse V, et al. Uniparental paternal disomy in a genetic cancer-predisposing syndrome. *Nature* 1991;351:665–667.

140. Versteege I, Sevenet N, Lange J, et al. Truncating mutations of hSNF5/INI1 in aggressive paediatric cancer. *Nature* 1998;394:203–206.

146. Villani A, Tabori U, Schiffman JD, et al. Biochemical and imaging surveillance in TP53 mutation carriers with Li-Fraumeni syndrome: a prospective observational study. *Lancet Oncology* 2011;12:559–567.

147. Jasperson KW, Kohlmann W, Gammon A, et al. Role of rapid sequence whole body MRI screening in SDH-associated hereditary paraganglioma families. *Fam Cancer* 2013;13:257–265.

151. Lammens C, Bleiker Aaronson N, Aaronson N, et al. Attitudes towards preimplantation genetic diagnosis for hereditary cancer. *Fam Cancer* 2009;8: 457–464.

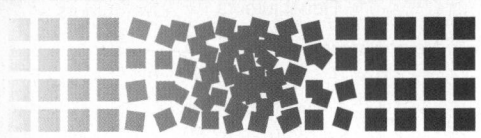

99 Solid Tumors of Childhood

Alberto S. Pappo, Fariba Navid, Rachel C. Brennan, Matthew J. Krasin,
Andrew M. Davidoff, and Wayne L. Furman

INTRODUCTION

Solid tumors account for about one-third of the estimated 14,000 cases of cancer diagnosed each year in patients under 20 years in the United States (Fig. 99.1).[1]

Since 1975, the overall mortality rates for childhood cancer have decreased by 50% and survival rates for childhood cancer now exceed 80%; however, this progress has been most evident for children with hematologic malignancies, and mortality rates for children affected by some of the most common pediatric solid tumors such as neuroblastoma and sarcomas have remained virtually unchanged over the past 20 years.[2] The reasons for the lack of progress in patients with solid tumors when compared to those with hematologic malignances is unclear but might be related to the relatively limited numbers of patients available to conduct randomized trials and the scarcity of recurrent and actionable genetic aberrations reported to date.[2,3]

MULTIDISCIPLINARY CARE IS ESSENTIAL FOR CHILDREN AND ADOLESCENTS WITH SOLID TUMORS

The management of pediatric solid tumors is complex and requires a coordinated multidisciplinary approach that incorporates multiple subspecialties including surgery, radiology, pathology, radiotherapy, oncology, and physical therapy.[4]

Local control of the tumor may be achieved with the use of surgery, radiation therapy, or both. The use of neoadjuvant chemotherapy offers the theoretical advantage of decreasing the risk of micrometastatic dissemination as well as primary tumor size and, therefore, limiting the extent of surgery and the radiation doses.[4] In addition, the administration of preoperative chemotherapy fa- ·cilitates the evaluation of histologic response in the resected surgical specimen providing important prognostic and therapeutic information.[5]

Surgery plays a dual role in the management of pediatric solid tumors because it provides tissue for diagnosis and biologic studies as well as a mechanism for removing the primary tumor. The role of debulking surgery is controversial.[6,7] Surgery can also be used later in the course of treatment to remove residual tumor, and the results of the surgery may provide important information regarding the need for additional radiotherapy or chemotherapy.[8–10]

The radiation oncologist should evaluate the patient prior to the initiation of any therapy and to help select the radiation plan and optimal treatment modality. The patient's age, extent of disease, and disease status all play a role in selecting the appropriate radiotherapeutic approach from the available techniques including intensity modulated radiation therapy (IMRT), three-dimensional (3D) conformal radiotherapy, proton beam radiation therapy (PBRT), and brachytherapy.

NEUROBLASTOMA

Neuroblastomic tumors comprise a spectrum of tumors that arise from primitive sympathetic ganglion cells and include neuroblastomas, ganglioneuroblastomas, and ganglioneuromas (Fig. 99.2). They can originate anywhere along the sympathetic ganglia; about half arise in the adrenal medulla. This group of tumors is known for a broad spectrum of clinical behaviors ranging from a completely benign mass to spontaneous regression to widely disseminated, aggressive, and often fatal disease.[11–14] Tumors can be subdivided into distinct risk categories based on clinical and biologic features.[11,15] Historically, treatment has been tailored based on determination of the risk of recurrence for a given patient. A combination of clinical and biologic features of disease have been used to classify patients as low, intermediate, and high risk.[11,15]

Epidemiology

Neuroblastoma is the third most common childhood cancer after leukemia and brain tumors. From 2006 to 2010, the age-adjusted incidence of neuroblastoma was 10.1 per 1 million children aged 0 to 14 years.[1,16] During the first year of life, neuroblastoma accounts for the majority of cancer cases with an incidence almost double that of leukemia; 16% of infant neuroblastomas are diagnosed during the first month of life.[16]

There are approximately 650 children diagnosed each year with neuroblastoma in the United States[16] and their median age at diagnosis is 19.1 months (573 days).[17] Neuroblastoma is slightly more common in Caucasians and males, with the greatest sex-specific incidence difference occurring during infancy.[16]

The majority of neuroblastomas are sporadic. About 1% to 2% of cases are associated with a history of neuroblastoma in immediate or extended family members.[18–23] An early analysis of these family pedigrees suggests an autosomal-dominant mode of inheritance with incomplete penetrance.[24] Although many of these familial neuroblastoma patients present before 1 year of age, and more frequently have multifocal primaries,[14,25] there is also great clinical and biologic heterogeneity among patients in the same kindred.[19–21,26] Recently, germ-line mutations in the anaplastic lymphoma kinase (ALK) gene were identified as the cause of most cases of hereditary neuroblastomas.[25,27–30] Another less common cause of hereditary neuroblastoma involves germ-line mutations of the pairedlike homeobox 2B (PHOX2B) gene.[31–33] These children often have concomitant neural crest disorders (neurocristopathies),[34] including Hirschsprung disease,[32,34,35] and congenital hypoventilation syndrome.[33,34,36] Other genetic conditions that may predispose for the development of neuroblastoma include neurofibromatosis,[32,37,38] Turner syndrome,[39] and Beckwith-Wiedemann syndrome.[40]

Pathology

Neuroblastic tumors, which include ganglioneuromas, ganglioneuroblastomas, and neuroblastomas (see Fig. 99.2), are derived

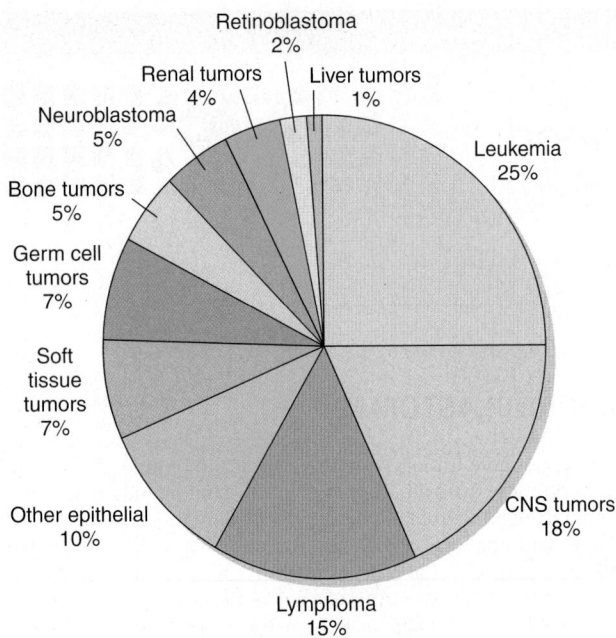

Figure 99.1 Age adjusted Surveillance, Epidemiology, and End Results (SEER) Cancer Incidence rates by the International Classification of Childhood Cancer category 0–19 years of age, all races, both sexes, SEER 2002–2010. CNS, central nervous system.

from primitive cells involved in the development of the sympathetic nervous system.[41] The most undifferentiated neuroblastic tumors are composed of neuroblasts with very few schwannian (stromal) cells. Immunohistochemistry may be useful in distinguishing neuroblastoma from other small round blue cell tumors, and immunoreactivity is commonly observed to neuron-specific enolase, synaptophysin, chromogranin A, NB84, and S100. As tumors become more differentiated, the ratio of Schwann to neuroblastoma cells increases, and the neuroblasts appear more mature. Ganglioneuroblastoma can be subdivided into either a stroma-rich, intermixed variant, or nodular variant. Ganglioneuroma is predominantly composed of Schwann cells studded with maturing or fully mature ganglion cells and is considered a benign tumor. These tumors were originally classified according to an "age-linked" classification system by Shimada et al.,[42] which was subsequently clarified and adopted for international use by the International Neuroblastoma Pathology Committee (INPC).[43–45] These tumors are morphologically classified into four histologic subtypes according to the balance between neural-type cells (primitive neuroblasts, maturing neuroblasts, and ganglion cells) and the Schwann-type cells (Schwannian blasts and mature Schwann cells) and the degree of surrounding Schwannian stroma: (1) neuroblastoma (Schwannian stroma-poor), undifferentiated, poorly differentiated, and differentiating; (2) ganglioneuroblastoma, intermixed (Schwannian stroma-rich); (3) ganglioneuroma (Schwannian stroma dominant), maturing and mature; and (4) ganglioneuroblastoma, nodular (composite Schwannian stroma rich/stoma dominant and stroma poor).[43] The grade of neuroblastic differentiation and mitosis-karyorrhexis index (MKI; defined as the number of tumor cells in mitosis and in the process of karyorrhexis) and age of patient are then used to assign to either a *favorable* or *unfavorable* prognostic group (Fig. 99.3).[44]

Neuroblastoma tumors are classified into favorable histology (FH) and unfavorable histology (UH) lesions based on the degree of stromal development, morphology, MKI, and age.

The INPC system's prognostic significance was confirmed in a retrospective review of two Children's Cancer Group (CCG) protocols that demonstrated a threefold difference in the 5-year event-free survival (EFS) for patients with FH versus UH features.[46]

Molecular Biology

Amplified segments of DNA in the form of homogeneously staining regions of chromosomes (HSR) or extrachromosomal DNA called double-minute chromosomes (DMs) are often found in neuroblastomas (Fig. 99.4). The gene that was consistently amplified in these segments was identified by Schwab and colleagues[47] as a myc-related gene, which was eventually called MYCN (v-myc avian myelocytomatosis viral oncogene neuroblastoma-derived homolog). Amplification of MYCN is predominantly associated with advanced stage disease, rapid tumor progression, and poor prognosis.[48,49] A 5- to 500-fold amplification of the MYCN gene is found in about 22% of all patients with neuroblastoma,[11] and in approximately 30% to 40% of patients with advanced stage disease (see Fig. 99.4).[48,49] Amplification (increased gene copy number) results in persistently high levels of the MYCN protein, a DNA-binding transcription factor known to cause malignant transformation in tumor models. The negative prognostic significance of MYCN amplification (>10 copies per haploid genome) is independent of age, stage, or other genetic alterations and remains an important part of the current international risk group classification system.[50,51]

The DNA content (ploidy) of tumors is either near diploid or hyperdiploid.[50,52] Near-diploid tumors in patients less than 18 to 24 months of age are associated with an adverse prognosis, whereas hyperdiploid tumors in this age group are associated with low-stage disease and a favorable outcome.[53,54] In the new International Risk Group pretreatment classification system, ploidy is only used to stratify patients less than 18 months old with metastatic disease who do not have MYCN-amplified tumors.[51]

Chromosomal deletions or gains are also frequently identified. Loss of heterozygosity (LOH; loss of one allele) at chromosome 1p36 and 11q occurs in 23% and 34% of tumors respectively.[55] A gain of chromosome 17 or 17q is present in 50% to 60% of neuroblastomas and is associated with an aggressive phenotype.[56] Trk, a family of neurotropin receptors, is important in the development of the central and peripheral nervous system. Elevated expression of TrkA or TrkC is seen in favorable, low-stage tumors. Low expression of TrkA or elevated expression of full-length TrkB is seen in advanced-stage MYCN-amplified tumors.[57] Additionally, TrkB expression has been linked to chemotherapeutic resistance.[57,58] Among the most common mutations in sporadic neuroblastoma is in the α-thalassemia/mental retardation syndrome X-linked (ATRX) gene, which is seen in children over 12 years of age (44%).[59] The evaluation of a chromosomal translocation in a neuroblastoma patient led to the identification of a family of genes on chromosome 1, now called neuroblastoma breakpoint family (NBPF).[60] Copy number variation in this region (1q21.1) has also been shown to be highly associated with neuroblastoma, probably through disruption of one of the NBPF genes, NBPF23.[61] A number of technologic advances have enabled the analysis of whole genome or exomes of tumors to provide insight into the pathogenesis of neuroblastoma and are under investigation to refine risk assignment.[62–68] For example, risk polymorphisms at 6p22, identified by genome-wide association studies (GWAS), have been associated with sporadic neuroblastoma, and homozygosity for any of these alleles is associated with high-risk features.[69] Similarly, common variations in the BRCA1-associated RING domain 1 (BARD1) gene have been implicated in the development of high-risk disease.[70] By expanding these GWAS studies, this same group also identified risk alleles within the LMO1 (LIM domain only 1) gene at 11p15.4 that were more common in tumors with high-risk disease (p <0.0001), suggesting that LMO1 may be a neuroblastoma oncogene.[71]

Diagnosis

About two-thirds of neuroblastomas originate in the abdomen, with 50% beginning in the adrenal gland. Other common sites include the chest (16%), neck (3%), and pelvic sympathetic ganglia (3%). Approximately 50% of tumors have spread to the bone or bone

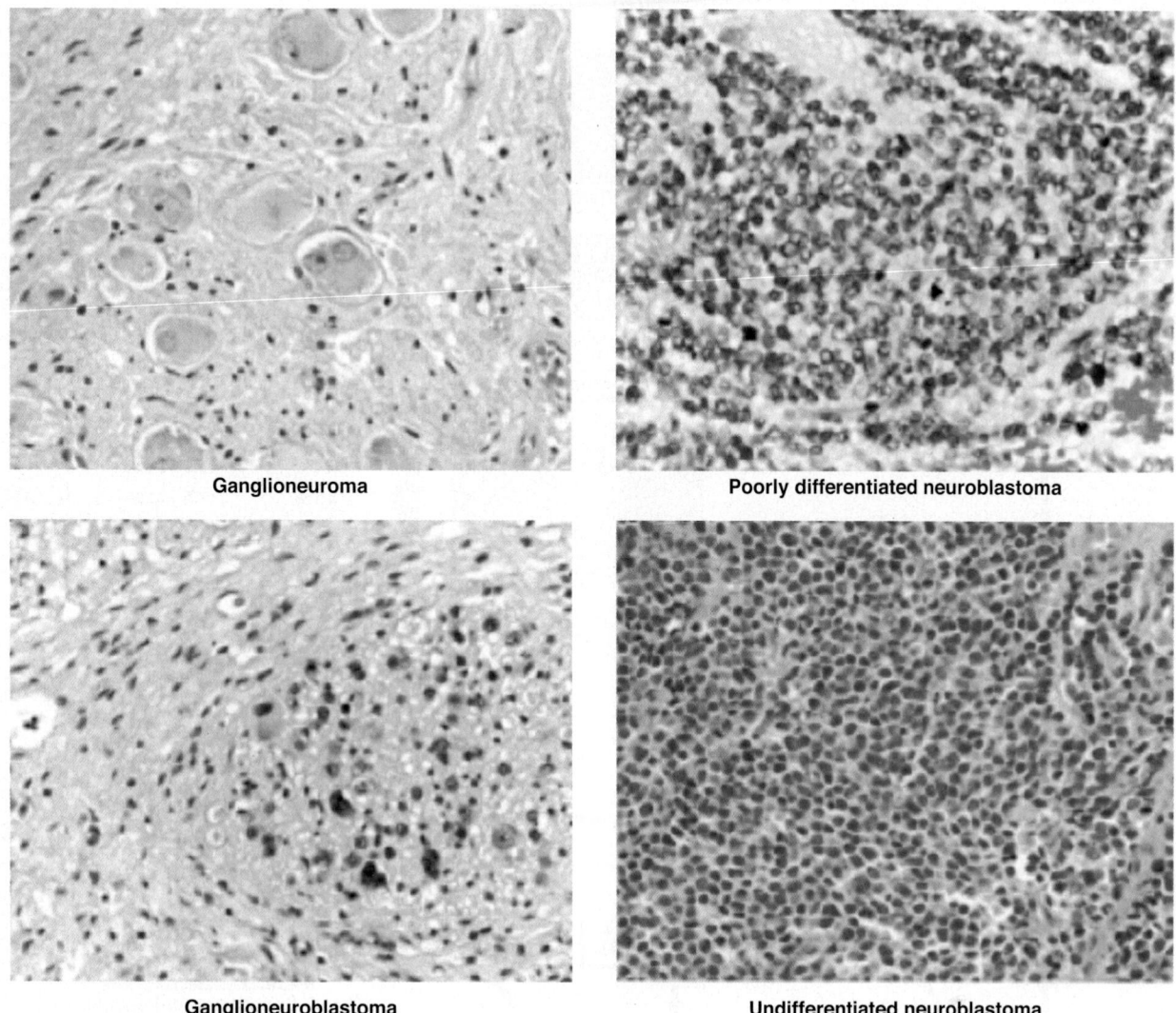

Ganglioneuroma

Poorly differentiated neuroblastoma

Ganglioneuroblastoma

Undifferentiated neuroblastoma

Figure 99.2 The principal histopathologic subtypes of neuroblastoma (hematoxylin and eosin). (Courtesy of Dr. Jesse Jenkins, Department of Pathology, St. Jude Children's Research Hospital.)

marrow at presentation.[51] The pattern of metastatic spread varies with age and histology of the tumor. Infants with favorable histologies are more likely to have liver and skin metastases. Unfavorable histology tumors are more likely to spread to the bone marrow and bones.[72] At presentation, abdominal tumors can cause increased abdominal girth, a palpable mass, diarrhea, or constipation. Many thoracic tumors are detected incidentally; however, large thoracic or cervical tumors can cause Horner syndrome, superior vena cava syndrome, or mechanical airway obstruction. Children with bone metastases may have a limp, complain of pain, or develop periorbital swelling, ecchymoses, or proptosis. Fever and hypertension are often present.

The evaluation of a child suspected of having neuroblastoma begins with a careful history and physical examination. A detailed head and neck exam, looking for skull metastases; "raccoon eyes,"[73] proptosis, or other eye abnormalities; and Horner syndrome should be performed. Attention to neurologic function is critical due to the paraspinal location of many tumors, which can result in spinal cord compression and permanent loss of function if not treated expeditiously.[74] Similarly, blindness has developed in children with periorbital disease while staging evaluations were being completed.[75] In infants, the examination must include a search for skin and subcutaneous metastases that appear

as reddish-purple, raised lesions.[76] Because neuroblastomas produce catecholamine metabolites, the measurement of these can often help narrow the diagnosis.[77,78] Urine samples for quantitative excretion of vanillylmandelic acid (VMA) and homovanillic acid (HVA) are elevated in more than 80% of patients[79] and should be part of the diagnostic evaluation for every patient. These markers are also useful to evaluate the effectiveness of therapy and to monitor for disease recurrence.[80] Ultrasound is often the initial radiologic study to identify the tumor. However, magnetic resonance imaging (MRI) or computerized tomography (CT) of the chest, abdomen, and pelvis is required to clearly define the location and extent of the primary tumor. Radiographically, a neuroblastoma typically appears as a heterogeneous mass with calcifications. Adrenal and retroperitoneal tumors characteristically involve and displace the major vessels.

Patients with paraspinal primary tumors may have asymptomatic extension through the spinal foramina. Due to the increased risk of neurologic compromise, these patients should undergo further imaging of the spinal canal using MRI with contrast. Imaging of the head should be considered in any child with palpable skull lesions, ptosis, or orbital ecchymosis.[75]

Tumors can secrete a vasoactive intestinal polypeptide resulting in intractable diarrhea and abdominal distention that resolves after

PRACTICE OF ONCOLOGY

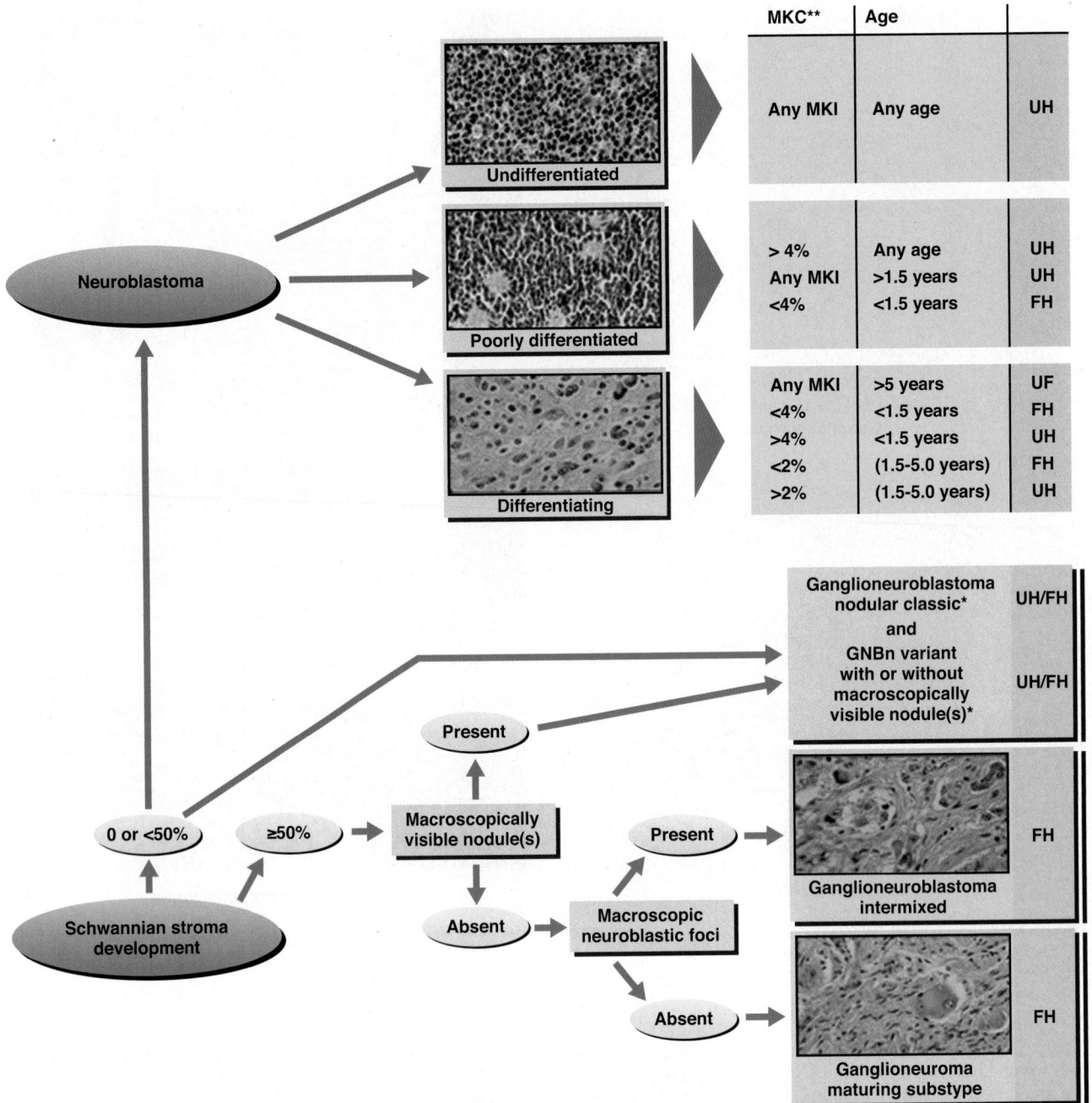

Figure 99.3 The International Neuroblastoma Pathology classification schema. Neuroblastoma tumors are classified into favorable (FH) and unfavorable (UH) histology lesions based on degree of stromal development, morphology, mitosis-karyorrhexis index (MKI), and age. GNBn, ganglioneuroblastoma. (From Park JR, Eggert A, Caron H. Neuroblastoma: biology, prognosis, and treatment. *Hematol Oncol Clin North Am* 2010;24:65–86, with permission.)

resection. In the largest review of 22 patients, most presented with significant weight loss and metabolic abnormalities, and 16 out of 22 had 1 to 21 months of gastrointestinal (GI) symptoms prior to the diagnosis of neuroblastoma. Although usually associated with differentiating tumors of low stage, 6 of these 22 were high-risk patients who developed diarrhea upon initiation of chemotherapy.[81] Opsoclonus-myoclonus-ataxia (OMA) syndrome, often called *dancing eyes*,[82] *dancing feet* is seen in up to 3% of children with neuroblastoma and presents with chaotic, multidirectional eye movements, spontaneous limb jerking, and ataxia. Many patients also have significant behavioral problems, sleep disturbances, and learning defects.[83,84] Although this process is thought to arise as a consequence of immune-mediated cross-reactivity between neuroblasts and the central nervous system, no specific antibody

or lymphocyte marker has been identified.[85] The tumors associated with OMA patients typically are of favorable biology and limited stage, and thus, patients with this condition have an excellent cancer prognosis.[86,87] Although the movements may resolve over time, most children have persistent neurologic deficits, including speech and cognitive delays and behavioral problems.[88,89]

Spinal cord involvement with infiltration of the intervertebral foramina is often seen in the initial evaluation of neuroblastoma[90]; however, only about 5% of children at the time of diagnosis develop symptoms related to spinal cord compression.[74,91] Spinal cord compression is considered an oncologic emergency because prolonged compression of the spinal cord can lead to irreversible loss of function. This can be treated with urgent radiation therapy, neurosurgery, or chemotherapy. Although there is no current

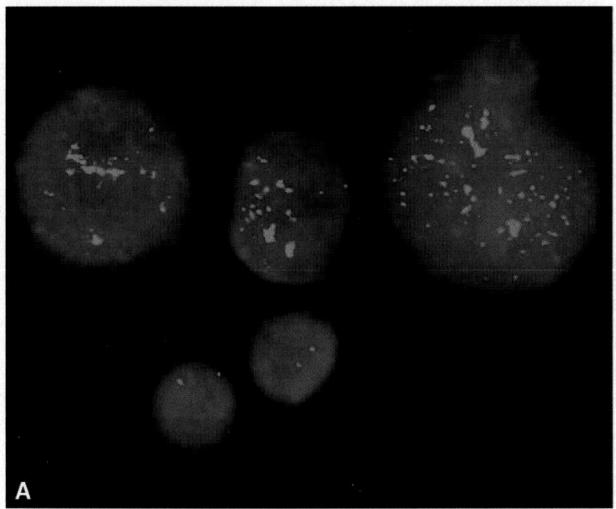
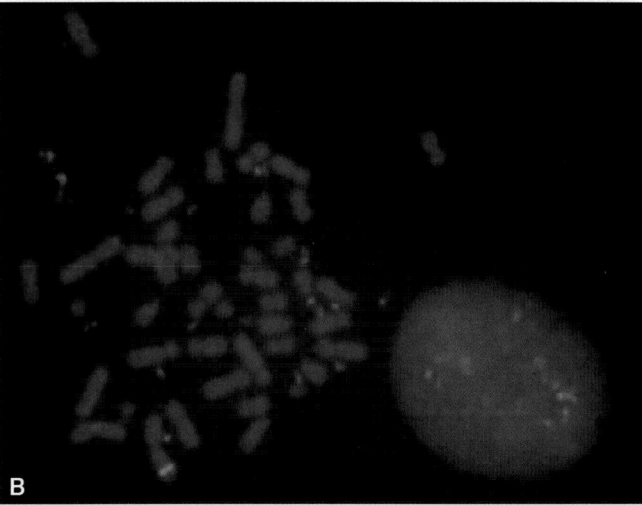

Figure 99.4 (A) shows upper three cells with MYCN amplification, having likely both, homogeneously stained regions (HSR) and double minutes (DM); the lower cells are normal with two copies each of the MYCN signals. **(B)** shows a metaphase plate with DM scattered outside the chromosomes. (Courtesy of Dr. Susana Raimondi, Department of Pathology, St. Jude Children's Research Hospital.)

consensus as to the best initial treatment,[92] a retrospective analysis suggests that each of these modalities are equally effective in the short term. However, there are significant differences in late effects.[90,93–95] The management of this rare presentation requires an experienced multidisciplinary team and the treatment recommendations should be made on a case-by-case basis specific to the severity and duration of symptoms and an assessment of the anticipated short- and long-term risks of the specific intervention.[90,92]

Metaiodobenzylguanidine (MIBG) is an analog of norepinephrine and is taken up by tissues that express the norepinephrine transport protein, which includes almost 90% of neuroblastomas.[96,97] With a sensitivity of about 90% and a specificity of 100%, MIBG has replaced technetium-99m bone scans and has been recommended as a standard agent for staging patients with neuroblastoma[96,98,99] because of its sensitivity and specificity; all patients should undergo MIBG scans at the time of diagnosis and at subsequent intervals after the start of treatment to assess response. In the 10% of patients who have negative MIBG scans, fludeoxyglucose (^{18}F-FDG) positron-emission tomography (PET) scans can be considered.[98] Newer PET agents, such as fluorine-18-L-dihydroxyphenylalanine (^{18}F-Dopa) are also under investigation.[100] Bone marrow involvement should be further evaluated by bilateral aspiration and a biopsy.[99,101]

Other malignancies for which neuroblastoma can occasionally be confused include other *small, round, blue cell* tumors such as rhabdomyosarcoma, the Ewing sarcoma family of tumors, non-Hodgkin lymphoma, and acute leukemia. If the diagnosis is to be based on material from bone marrow, it is recommended that these cells be confirmed to be neuroblasts by immunohistochemistry staining with synaptophysin[102] or chromogranin[103] and that urine HVA and/or VMA be >3.0 SD above mean per milligram creatinine for age.[99]

Screening

Because infants have the best prognosis and because more than 80% of patients with neuroblastoma have elevated catecholamine markers that can be easily measured, screening infants was thought to be a promising approach.[104] Unfortunately, two carefully controlled trials definitively demonstrated that screening did not reduce mortality and, in fact, because many infant neuroblastomas spontaneously regress, led to over diagnosis and treatment of patients that needed no intervention.[105–108]

Staging

The International Neuroblastoma Staging System (INSS), developed in 1988[109] and revised in 1993[99] (Table 99.1) was developed to facilitate comparison among trials and is the current staging system used in North American and European cooperative group trials. This system is a postsurgical staging system, in that it uses the extent of initial surgical resection to stage patients. The INSS is significantly affected by the experience of the surgeon, leading to variability in stage assignments. To better define homogenous pretreatment patient cohorts and compare trials conducted in different regions of the world, another staging system, based on preoperative, image-defined risk factors (Tables 99.2A and 99.2B), called the International Risk Group classification system.[110] The predictive prognostic significance of this system will be tested in future prospective clinical trials.

Management by Risk Group

The treatment of neuroblastoma incorporates a number of clinical and biologic variables, in addition to the stage of disease, to evaluate the risk of recurrence and to thus determine the intensity of treatment. The Children's Oncology Group's (COG) risk categories incorporate the patient's age at presentation, stage of the tumor, histologic appearance, quantitative DNA content, and presence or absence of *MYCN* amplification within the tumor cells (Table 99.3).

The age at presentation is an important prognostic factor, because infants tend to have tumors with more favorable features, including stage and histology. A multivariate analysis of 3,666 patients enrolled in cooperative group studies demonstrated 82% 4-year EFS for children less than 18 months versus 42% for those more than 18 months.[17] Adolescents and young adults rarely present with neuroblastoma, but their tumors tend to be indolent and fatal.[110–112]

The variables selected by other pediatric oncology cooperative groups to define the risk categories have not been uniform. To be able to compare trials worldwide, an international conference developed a consensus approach to pretreatment risk stratification, now called the International Neuroblastoma Risk Group (INRG) Classification System (see Tables 99.2A and 99.2B).[51] This new classification system is different than that of the COG in that it

International Neuroblastoma Staging System Criteria[99]

Stage	Definition
1	Localized tumor with complete gross excision, with or without microscopic residual disease; representative ipsilateral lymph nodes negative for tumor microscopically (nodes attached to and removed with the primary tumor may be positive)
2A	Localized tumor with incomplete gross excision; representative ipsilateral nonadherent lymph nodes negative for tumor microscopically
2B	Localized tumor with or without complete gross excision, with ipsilateral nonadherent lymph nodes positive for tumor; enlarged contralateral lymph nodes must be negative microscopically
3	Unresectable unilateral tumor infiltrating across the midline[a] with or without regional lymph node involvement; or localized unilateral tumor with contralateral regional lymph node involvement; or midline tumor with bilateral extension by infiltration (unresectable) or by lymph node involvement[b]
4	Any primary tumor with dissemination to distant lymph nodes, bone, bone marrow, liver, skin, and/or other organs (except as defined for stage 4S)
4S	Localized primary tumor (as defined for stage 1, 2A, or 2B), with dissemination limited to skin, liver, and/or bone marrow[c] (<10% involvement) (limited to infants <1 year of age)

Note: Multifocal primary tumors should be staged according to the greatest extent of disease and followed by the subscript "M."
[a] The midline is defined as the vertebral column. Tumors originating on one side and crossing the midline must infiltrate to or beyond the opposite side of the vertebral column.
[b] Patients are upstaged to International Neuroblastoma Staging System stage 3 if there is proven malignant effusion within the abdominal cavity or bilateral thoracic cavity.
[c] Marrow involvement in stage 4S should be minimal (i.e., <10%) of total nucleated cells identified as malignant on bone marrow biopsy or on marrow aspirate. More extensive marrow involvement would be considered to be stage 4. The metaiodobenzylguanidine (MIBG) scan, if performed, should be negative in the marrow. From Brodeur GM, Prichard J, Berthold F, et al. Revisions of the international criteria for neuroblastoma diagnosis, staging, and response to treatment. *J Clin Oncol* 1993;11:1466–1477.

uses the new INRG staging system,[113] and adds the presence/absence of 11q aberrations. As new trials are developed, the value of this new risk group classification system will be validated.

Low Risk

Children with low-risk neuroblastomas generally include patients of any age with localized, resectable tumors (Table 99.4). Low-risk tumors comprise about 50% of all neuroblastomas. Surgery is the primary treatment, and overall survival rates are greater than 90%.[114–116] Recently, a prospective study of 87 infants less than 6 months of age and with small (volume ≤16 mL) isolated adrenal masses who were observed only showed that 81% (67 out of 83) were spared surgery with a median follow-up of 3.2 years and an overall survival at 3 years of 100%.[117] Thus, expectant observation without surgery in this subgroup of patients should be considered standard treatment and, in fact, the authors recommend extending this approach to "all localized noninfiltrative neuroblastoma tumors [corresponding to the International Neuroblastoma Risk

International Neuroblastoma Risk Group (INRG) Staging System[113]

Stage	Description
L1	Localized tumor not involving vital structures as defined by the list of Image Defined Risk Factors and confined to one body compartment
L2	Local–regional tumor with presence of one or more Image Defined Risk Factors
M	Distant metastatic disease (except Stage MS)
MS	Metastatic disease in children <18 months with metastases confined to skin, liver, and/or bone marrow

Group Staging System stage L1; see Table 99.2][113] in infants less than 1 year of age."[117]

A 4S neuroblastoma is a *special*[118] entity because the high rate of spontaneous regression allows for a delay or elimination of chemotherapy for up to 80% of children.[119,120] Two subsets are more likely to require chemotherapy: those tumors with unfavorable biologic features (i.e., *MYCN* amplification) and tumors in infants younger than 2 months who have extensive liver disease. Untreated, the latter case leads to a higher incidence of mortality, because massive hepatomegaly prevents adequate chest wall expansion.[120,121] These children should receive chemotherapy or low-dose radiation (4.5 to 6 Gy in three to four fractions) to decrease tumor size.

Intermediate Risk

Children with intermediate-risk tumors comprise 10% to 15% of new cases and are defined as: infants (<365 days old) with INSS 3 or 4 tumors without *MYCN* amplification and favorable histology, children (≥365 days old) with INSS 3 tumors without *MYCN* amplification and favorable histology, or INSS 4 with unfavorable histology and/or diploid DNA (Table 99.5).[122] Surgery is an important component of treatment, as is the addition of moderately intensive chemotherapy (i.e., carboplatin, etoposide, adriamycin, cyclophosphamide). Radiotherapy is reserved for children with progression or those who have unresectable tumors after chemotherapy. This approach has led to excellent survival of 50% to 100%, depending on the clinical and biologic characteristics.[123–125] In a recent report from the COG, 479 children were treated according to a biologically based risk assignment system. Of these, 323 with favorable biologic characteristics received four courses of chemotherapy and 141 children with unfavorable biology received eight courses. This approach resulted in a 3-year EFS of 88±2% and 3-years overall survival of 96±1%.[122]

High Risk

Approximately 50% to 60% of children present with metastatic disease at diagnosis and the vast majority of these are classified as

TABLE 99.2B

International Neuroblastoma Risk Group (INRG) Consensus Pretreatment Classification System.[51]

INRG Stage	Age (months)	Histologic Category	Grade of Tumor Differentiation	MYCN	11q Aberration	Ploidy	Pretreatment Risk Group
L1/L2		GN maturing; GNB intermixed					A Very low
L1		Any, except GN maturing or GNB intermixed		N/A Amplified			B Very low K High
L2	<18	Any, except GN maturing or GNB intermixed		 N/A	No Yes		D Low G Intermediate
	≥18	GNB nodular; neuroblastoma	Differentiating Poorly differentiated or undifferentiated	N/A N/A Amplified	No Yes		E Low H Intermediate N High
M	<18 <12 12–<18 <18 ≥18			N/A N/A N/A Amplified		Hyperdiploid Diploid Diploid	F Low I Intermediate J Intermediate O High P High
MS	<18			 NA Amplified	No Yes		C Very low Q High R High

GNB, ganglioneuroblastoma; GN, ganglioneuroma; N/A, not applicable.

high-risk patients.[126] As seen in Table 99.6, children with high-risk disease predominantly include children more than 18 months of age with INSS 4 disease. Other subsets of high-risk patients include children of any age with INSS 2a/b or 3 disease and *MYCN* amplification, children ≥18 months with INSS 3 and unfavorable histology, and infants (<1 year of age) with *MYCN* amplification. The treatment consists of four general components: (1) induction chemotherapy, (2) surgical resection of all gross disease, (3) consolidation, which generally includes myeloablative chemotherapy with stem-cell rescue and radiation therapy to the tumor bed, and then (4) treatment of minimal residual disease (MRD). Despite this intensive therapy, almost half of all high-risk patients eventually relapse and die of their disease.[126]

Induction Chemotherapy. Standard chemotherapy regimens for high-risk disease include combinations of the epipodophyllotoxins etoposide or teniposide, platinum-based agents, cyclophosphamide, and doxorubicin; other active agents such as ifosfamide and topotecan have also been included in some regimens.[127–134] A retrospective analysis in 1991 of 44 published clinical trials showed a convincing correlation between dose intensity and response and progression-free survival, particularly with cisplatin and teniposide.[135] Although a later review did not corroborate these findings,[136] the general approach worldwide has been to increase the intensity of induction chemotherapy. In the only recent randomized trial comparing induction regimens, 262 patients were assigned to either rapid treatment (N = 130) with cisplatin (C), vincristine (O), carboplatin (J), etoposide (E), and cyclophosphamide (C) (COJEC), or standard treatment (N = 132) with vincristine, cisplatin (P), etoposide, cyclophosphamide (OPEC) alternating with vincristine, carboplatin, etoposide, cyclophosphamide (OJEC). The rapid regimen was given every 10 days and the standard regimen was given every 21 days. The same cumulative doses of each drug, except vincristine, were administered and the relative dose-intensity of the rapid regimen was 1.94 compared to the standard regimen.[137] There was no difference in the overall survival (OS) at 5 and 10 years, although the EFS at 5 years

was significantly better in the rapid group (30.2% versus 18.2%; p = 0.022). Also, patients progressed to consolidation a median of 55 days earlier, prompting the authors to speculate that this might have contributed to the better outcome in the rapid group.[137] The lack of difference in OS and relatively inferior outcomes, compared to other induction regimens,[133] make interpretation of these results difficult. What is clear is that response, as measured by MIBG scans at the end of induction, strongly correlate with overall outcome[138–140] and that further refinement in induction therapy may focus on those *ultra* high-risk patients who have inferior early response as measured by MIBG or more sensitive quantitative methods.[141,142]

Surgery. The role and timing of surgery in the management of children with high-risk neuroblastoma is uncertain.[143] Although some reports of patients with stage 3 or 4 disease have found that gross total resection of the primary tumor and metastatic local–regional disease has been associated with improved local tumor control and increased overall patient survival,[144–147] other reports have not.[7,148,149] Nevertheless, the COG as well the major European cooperative group, SIOPEN,[137] currently recommend gross total resection of the primary tumor and regional disease in patients with high-risk neuroblastoma. The resection is often delayed until near the end of induction, even though tumor volume reduction appears to plateau after the second or third course of chemotherapy,[150] and there are some data that early resection may provide a survival benefit.[151] The goal of surgical local control is to remove all visible tumors without jeopardizing vital organs or delaying chemotherapy; however, most primary tumors invade local structures and surround major blood vessels, making resection difficult. Complete removal at the time of diagnosis is possible for less than 20% of patients.[146,152] Resection of invasive tumor is associated with complications, including the removal of normal organs, hemorrhage, renal injury,[153] vascular injury, chylous ascites and chronic diarrhea. After treatment with chemotherapy, complete removal becomes possible in more than 50%.[7]

TABLE 99.3

Children's Oncology Group Risk Categories for Neuroblastoma

INSS Stage	Age	MYCN	INPC Histology	Ploidy	Other	Risk Group Assignment
1	Any	Any	Any	Any		Low
2A/2B	Any	Not amp	Any	Any	Resection ≥50%, asymptomatic	Low
2A/2B	Any	Not amp	Any	Any	Resection ≥50% symptomatic	Intermediate
2A/2B	Any	Not amp	Any	Any	Resection <50%	Intermediate
2A/2B	Any	Not amp	Any	Any	Biopsy only	Intermediate
2A/2B	Any	Amp	Any	Any	Any degree of resection	High
3	<547 d	Not amp	Any	Any		Intermediate
3	≥547 d	Not amp	Favorable	Any		Intermediate
3	Any	Amp	Any	Any		High
3	≥547 d	Not amp	Unfavorable	Any		High
4	<365 d	Amp	Any	Any		High
4	<365 d	Not amp	Any	Any		Intermediate
4	365–<547 d	Amp	Any	Any		High
4	365–<547 d	Any	Any	DI = 1		High
4	365–<547 d	Any	Unfavorable	Any		High
4	365–<547 d	Not amp	Favorable	DI > 1		Intermediate
4	≥547 d	Any	Any	Any		High
4S	<365 d	Not amp	Favorable	DI > 1	Asymptomatic	Low
4S	<365 d	Not amp	Any	DI = 1	Asymptomatic or symptomatic	Intermediate
4S	<365 d	Missing	Missing	Missing	Too sick for biopsy	Intermediate
4S	<365 d	Not amp	Any	Any	Symptomatic	Intermediate
4S	<365 d	Not amp	Unfavorable	Any	Asymptomatic or symptomatic	Intermediate
4S	<365 d	Amp	Any	Any	Asymptomatic or symptomatic	High

Amp, amplified; DI, DNA Index.

Consolidation. Early studies using high-dose chemotherapy showed a strong correlation of increasing dose intensity with progression-free survival in metastatic neuroblastoma.[135,154] The critical importance of dose intensity ultimately led to the integration of high-dose chemotherapy and autologous stem cell transplant (ASCT) into modern treatment regimens for high-risk

TABLE 99.4

Children's Oncology Group Definition of Low-Risk Neuroblastoma

Stage	Age	MYCN	Ploidy	INPC Histology	Other
1	Any	Any	Any	Any	
2A/B	Any	Not amplified	Any	Any	Resection ≥50%; asymptomatic
4s	<365 d	Not amplified	DI>1	Favorable	asymptomatic

neuroblastoma.[155–157] Although with it comes unique challenges and risks, the use of myeloablative ASCT allows for the delivery of chemotherapeutic doses not usually feasible due to the dose-limiting toxicity of myelosuppression. Although there is no consensus on the optimal conditioning regimen, many nonrandomized studies supported the use of ASCT as consolidation[158] and several randomized trials have subsequently made ASCT following intensive induction chemotherapy part of the *standard of care* in the treatment of children with high-risk neuroblastoma.[129,158–160]

One of the most common myeloablative regimens used worldwide is a combination of busulfan and melphalan (BuMel). A recent retrospective analysis of nearly 3 decades of European experience with ASCT for neuroblastoma revealed a survival benefit for BuMel over other melphalan-based conditioning regimens.[161] The 343 patients treated with this regimen in first remission had a 5-year OS rate of 48%.[162] Specifics regarding transplant-related complications were not reported. A recent, smaller retrospective study from Spain using a BuMel conditioning reported a progression-free survival of 57% among 36 patients at a mean follow-up of 55 months.[162] There were no toxic deaths reported and no reported veno-occlusive disease (VOD). Risk of complications from this regimen may be age dependent; a report of infants treated with a busulfan-melphalan regimen (with or

PRACTICE OF ONCOLOGY

TABLE 99.5

Children's Oncology Group Definition of Intermediate-Risk Neuroblastoma

Stage	Age	MYCN	Ploidy	INPC Histology	Other
2A/B	Any	Not amplified	Any	Any	Resection ≥50%; symptomatic
2A/B	Any	Not amplified	Any	Any	Resection <50%
2A/B	Any	Not amplified	Any	Any	Biopsy only
3	<547 d	Not amplified	Any	Any	
3	≥547 d	Not amplified	Any	Favorable	
4	<365 d	Not amplified	Any	Any	
4	365–<547 d	Not amplified	DI > 1	Favorable	
4s	<365 d	Not amplified	DI = 1	Any	With or without symptoms
4s	<365 d	Missing	Missing	Missing	Too ill for biopsy
4s	<365 d	Not amplified	Any	Any	Symptomatic
4s	<365 d	Not amplified	Any	Unfavorable	With or without symptoms

DI, DNA Index.

without cyclophosphamide) reported VOD in 9 of 12 children treated, including one death.[163] However, this regimen utilized oral busulfan, which has been shown to have a higher risk of complications.

Another common myeloablative regimen is a combination of carboplatin or cisplatin, etoposide, and melphalan (CEM), and it has been used in some of the largest reported US trials.[160] The SIOP Europe Neuroblastoma Group (SIOPEN) randomized patients to receive BuMel or CEM in the HR-NBL1 trial with the primary aim to demonstrate superiority based on EFS. This randomization was closed early due to superiority of the BuMel regimen. A significant difference in EFS in favor of BuMel (3-years EFS 49% versus 33%) was observed as well as for OS (3-years OS 60% versus 48%; p = 0.004). This difference was mainly related to the relapse and progression incidence, which was significantly (p =0.001) lower with BuMel (48% versus 60%).[164] Although these data clearly show the superiority of the BuMel conditioning regimen over CEM when used with the Rapid COJEC induction regimen of HR-NBL1,[137] it remains to be demonstrated if this would hold true if BuMel were used after other induction regimens.

TABLE 99.6

Children's Oncology Group Definition of High-Risk Neuroblastoma

Stage	Age	MYCN	Ploidy	INPC Histology
2A/B	Any	Amplified	Any	Any
3	Any	Amplified	Any	Any
3	≥547 d	Not amplified	Any	Unfavorable
4	<365 d	Amplified	Any	Any
4	365–<547 d	Amplified	Any	Any
4	365–<547 d	Any	DI = 1	Any
4	365–<547 d	Any	Any	Unfavorable
4	≥547 d	Any	Any	Any

Because undetected neuroblastoma cells present in autologous bone marrow can contribute to relapse,[165] the COG evaluated the role of purging stem cell products with a cocktail of five monoclonal antibodies targeting neuroblasts, attached to magnetic beads. All children received identical induction chemotherapy and myeloablation. Enrollees were randomly assigned to receive nonpurged peripheral blood stem cells (PBSC; N = 243) or purged PBSC (N = 243); 192 from the nonpurged and 180 from the purged group received ASCT. The 5-year EFS was 36% in the unpurged group (95% confidence interval [CI] 30 to 42) and 40% (33 to 46) in the group who received purged PBSCs (p = 0.77).[166] Thus nonpurged PBSCs are acceptable for support of children receiving myeloablation during consolidation.

Based on improvements in EFS seen in patients treated with myeloablative consolidation and ASCT, several nonrandomized studies, which were further dose intensified using tandem, nonoverlapping myeloablative conditioning regimens. suggested this approach may further improve outcome.[167–172] A pilot study of tandem transplant following intensive induction chemotherapy was developed by COG (ANBL00P1) to test the feasibility and toxicity for use as one of the arms of a randomized phase III study.[172] Patients received the first consolidation with thioTEPA and cyclophosphamide and, upon recovery, received a second ABMT with carboplatin, etoposide phosphate, and melphalan. Forty-one patients were enrolled; eight did not receive any ASCT. Of the 33 who received the first ASCT, 26 went on to receive the second. The 3-year EFS was 44.8±9.5% and this tandem ASCT combination was used as the experimental arm in a randomized phase III trial comparing single versus tandem ASCT (ANBL0532).[172] This trial completed accrual in February of 2012 and results are still pending.

Radiation Therapy. ASCT for neuroblastoma has been performed using various combinations of chemotherapy with and without total body irradiation (TBI). Although the optimum chemotherapeutic combination has not been conclusively demonstrated, the incorporation of TBI has not improved survival, but rather increases transplant-related complications.[161,173] However, because primary site failure persists as a component of tumor progression, primary site irradiation has been used as part of consolidation therapy for patients with high-risk neuroblastoma,[129,174–177] including those enrolled on the recent COG ANBL0532 study.[178] In the setting of recurrent or incurable disease, radiotherapy can also be used to treat bone and soft tissue metastasis to control pain and to prevent a loss of organ function.[179]

Treatment of Minimal Residual Disease. Finally, additional treatment with biologics (i.e., 13-*cis*-retinoic acid) in the setting of minimal residual disease appears to improve survival. CCG randomized children after consolidation with high-dose chemotherapy and ASCT to receive 6 months of *cis*-retinoic acid. The 3-year EFS was significantly better among those who received *cis*-retinoic acid than those assigned to receive no further therapy (46% versus 29%, respectively; p = 0.027).[129] Targeted immunotherapy, using a chimeric monoclonal antibody, ch14.18, against the tumor-associated disialoganglioside, GD2, has been ongoing for more than 2 decades. A recent randomized study from the COG found that the administration of ch14.18, in combination with interleukin-2, granulocyte macrophage colony stimulating factor, and *cis*-retinoic acid following recovery from consolidation was associated with an improved 2-year EFS (66±5% versus 46±5%) and OS (86±4% versus 75±5%) (p = 0.02).[180] This study has established a new standard of care for all children with high-risk disease in the future.

WILMS TUMOR

Wilms tumor is the most common primary malignant renal tumor of childhood. Advances in therapy since the inception of the prospective randomized trials conducted by various multi-institutional cooperative groups have led to an OS rate of 90%, although success has been achieved at a cost of serious chronic health conditions 25 years after diagnosis in 25% of survivors.[181]

Epidemiology and Genetics

Among North American children less than 15 years of age, the incidence of Wilms tumor is 1 in 10,000 children, or approximately 500 new cases per year.[182] Wilms tumor accounts for 6% of all childhood tumors, but more than 90% of all renal cancers in patients under the age of 20 years.[183] The risk for developing Wilms tumor is higher in African Americans and lower among Asian populations.[183] Although unilateral disease is more common, with males presenting at a slightly earlier age (37 months) than females (43 months), approximately 6% of patients harbor bilateral disease at diagnosis, with males presenting slightly earlier (24 months) than females (31 months).[184]

A variety of syndromes and congenital abnormalities are associated with the development of Wilms tumor. A deletion of chromosome 11p13 that encompasses the *WT1* and *PAX6* gene results in Wilms tumor, aniridia, genitourinary anomalies, and mental retardation (WAGR syndrome), whereas *WT1* point mutations at 11p13 are implicated in Denys-Drash syndrome (DDS), and Frasier syndrome.[185–187] A second Wilms tumor locus, *WT2*, is located at 11p15 and has been linked to an increased incidence of Wilms tumor in Beckwith-Wiedemann syndrome (BWS).[186,188] Specific to the *WT2* locus, at least 10 imprinted genes that have preferential expression by the maternal or paternal allele have been identified, including *IGF2*, *H19*, *p57*, and *LIT1*.[186] Other overgrowth syndromes associated with an increased susceptibility for the development of Wilms tumor include Simpson-Golabi-Behmel syndrome, Sotos syndrome, and Perlman syndrome. Patients with isolated hemihypertrophy, aniridia, Bloom syndrome, Alagille syndrome, trisomy 18, or Li-Fraumeni syndrome are also at risk for developing Wilms tumor.[186,189,190] Familial predisposition accounts for 1% to 2% of cases, and putative familial Wilms tumor genes have been mapped to 17q12-21 (*FWT1*) and 19q13.4 (*FWT2*).[185] Children with hereditary syndromes that predispose to the development of Wilms tumor should receive abdominal screening ultrasounds every 3 months until 8 years of age.[190] Although they

appear to respond to treatment similarly as other children, patients with a predisposition (*WT1* mutation) and Wilms tumor have a higher incidence of bilateral disease, intralobar nephrogenic rests, and end-stage renal disease.[187]

Pathology

Most Wilms tumors are solitary and composed of varying proportions of blastemal, stromal, and epithelial cells that recapitulate normal kidney development. Anaplasia, either *focal* or *diffuse*, is characterized by the presence of large nuclei, irregular mitotic features, and hyperplasia and is associated with adverse clinical outcomes.[191,192] In focal anaplasia, cells with anaplastic nuclear changes are confined to sharply restricted foci within the primary tumor.[192] A recent analysis has demonstrated that the presence of anaplasia even in stage I disease adversely affects clinical outcome.[193]

Wilms tumor must be distinguished histologically from other pediatric renal tumors, including renal cell carcinoma,[194] clear cell sarcoma,[195] and rhabdoid tumor of the kidney,[196] as well as neuroblastoma. Clear cell sarcoma and malignant rhabdoid tumor of the kidney were previously considered to belong to the *unfavorable histology* group of Wilms tumors, but are now considered to be distinct categories of renal tumors. Rhabdoid tumor of the kidney tends to metastasize to the lung and brain. Primary rhabdoid tumors of the kidney and brain (atypical teratoid or rhabdoid tumors) share deletions of chromosome band 22q11.2, the site of *SMARCB1* (also known as *INI1*, *BAF47*, and *SNF5*), a putative tumor suppressor gene.[197,198] Another important renal neoplasm, congenital mesoblastic nephroma, is important to recognize because it is usually curable by nephrectomy alone. These tumors are typically identified in the first months of life, with a median age at diagnosis of 2 months.[199] They are associated with the t(12;15) translocation that produces the *ETV6-NTRK3* fusion gene product.[200]

Precursor lesions, or nephrogenic rests, have been identified in the renal parenchyma of approximately 36% of patients with Wilms tumor.[201,202] Nephroblastomatosis is a term that describes kidneys with multifocal or diffuse nephrogenic rests. Perilobar rests, located along the perimeter of a renal lobe, are strongly associated with synchronous bilateral Wilms tumors, BWS, and hemihyperplasia, whereas intralobar rests (within the renal lobe) show a strong association with metachronous tumors and WAGR and DDS.[203] Children with nephroblastomatosis have an increased risk of developing Wilms tumor and require close monitoring.[204]

Biologic prognostic factors, such as gain of 1q, LOH at chromosomal regions 1p and 16q, supplement stage, and histology when assigning risk. Gain of 1q is associated with increased risk of relapse in patients with favorable histology Wilms tumor.[205] LOH of chromosomes 1p and 16q is present in approximately 5% of favorable histology tumors and is associated with increased risk of relapse and mortality.[206] The recently closed COG trial incorporated these factors prospectively into treatment decisions with augmented therapy for patients with LOH and favorable histology; a data analysis is pending. In a retrospective analysis of patients with very low risk disease (stage 1, FH, <550 g, <24 months of age) who were treated with surgery alone, *WT1* mutations, and 11p15 LOH were associated with a higher risk of relapse.[207]

Clinical Presentation and Natural History

Most children with Wilms tumor come to medical attention because of abdominal swelling or the presence of an abdominal mass that may be noted by the caregiver during bathing or dressing the child. Abdominal pain, gross hematuria, and fever may be present at diagnosis.[208] Hypertension is present in approximately 20% of cases.[209]

Clinical Evaluation and Staging

With gentle palpation to maintain tumor capsule integrity, location and size of the abdominal mass and its movement with respiration should be noted. A varicocele may be associated with the presence of a tumor thrombus in the renal vein or inferior vena cava.[210] An evaluation for signs of associated syndromes, such as aniridia, hemihypertrophy, and genitourinary abnormalities, is mandatory. Laboratory studies should include a complete blood cell count, liver function tests, renal function tests, serum chemistries including calcium, and a urinalysis.

Diagnostic Imaging

Imaging should define the local and distant extent of the tumor, evaluate the renal veins and surrounding vessels to detect the presence of a tumor thrombus, and assess the contralateral kidney to rule out bilateral lesions, all of which are important prior to surgery.

The initial radiographic study is often an abdominal ultrasound examination to determine the consistency of the mass and the organ of origin, and to assess patency of the inferior vena cava. CT or MRI is appropriate for imaging of the primary tumor and to provide adequate visualization of the contralateral kidney, liver, and abdomen to define metachronous and metastatic tumors in the abdomen and pelvis. MRI may be superior to other imaging modalities in delineating nephroblastomatosis.[211]

Both plain radiographs of the chest (chest x-ray) and a chest CT should be performed to determine the presence of pulmonary metastases. In many cases, nodules detected by more sensitive CT scans do not necessarily represent a metastatic tumor, and current studies focused on determining which patients truly require intensified therapy with radiation.[212] Imaging of the brain or skeleton is usually reserved for patients with rhabdoid tumors of the kidney and clear cell sarcoma of the kidney.

Staging

The staging criteria developed by the National Wilms Tumor Study Group (NWTSG) is shown in Table 99.7. The NWTSG approach allows for an adequate assessment of the extent of disease and histologic characteristics of the tumor and facilitates the collection of tumor tissue for biologic studies prior to therapy. In contrast, the SIOP approach (staging not shown) uses preoperative chemotherapy, decreasing the volume of tumor, and thereby decreasing the perioperative risk of tumor spillage. As a result of these treatment philosophies, children enrolled on NWTSG trials receive radiation therapy more often, whereas patients on the SIOP trials receive more cumulative doses of anthracyclines.[213–215]

Treatment

Tumor stage and histology are the main prognostic indicators that determine the treatment regimen for Wilms tumor, whereas patient age at presentation and biologic factors (LOH 1p and 16q) were tested prospectively in the most recent COG (NWTS) trials (results pending). Surgery and chemotherapy comprise the main therapy for Wilms tumors, with the addition of radiation for metastatic or histologically aggressive tumors.

Surgery

Surgical resection is the primary method for achieving local control and is usually performed at the time of diagnosis in North American studies (COG/NWTS). A review of children treated on the NWTS-IV demonstrated an increased incidence of local recurrence in those cases in which lymph node biopsies were not

TABLE 99.7

National Wilms Tumor Study Group Staging for Renal Tumors

Stage	Description
I	a. Tumor is limited to the kidney and completely excised b. The tumor was not ruptured before or during removal c. The vessels of the renal sinus are not involved beyond 2 mm d. There is no residual tumor apparent beyond the margins of excision
II	a. Tumor extends beyond the kidney but is completely excised b. No residual tumor is apparent at or beyond the margins of excision c. Tumor thrombus in vessels outside the kidney is stage II if the thrombus is removed en bloc with the tumor
III	Residual tumor confined to the abdomen: a. Lymph nodes in the renal hilum, the periaortic chains, or beyond are found to contain tumor b. Diffuse peritoneal contamination by the tumor c. Implants are found in the peritoneal surfaces d. Tumor extends beyond the surgical margins either microscopically or grossly e. Tumor is not completely resectable because of local infiltration into vital structures
IV	Presence of hematogenous metastases or metastases to distant lymph nodes
V	Bilateral renal involvement at the time of initial diagnosis

From Metzger ML, Dome JS. Current therapy for Wilms' tumor. *Oncologist* 2005;10:815–826, with permission.

obtained.[216] Presumably, these children were understaged and thus undertreated. Additionally, this review clearly demonstrated that operative rupture, whether localized to the renal fossa or diffusely spread within the peritoneal cavity, was associated with an increased incidence of local recurrence.[216]

Routine exploration of the contralateral kidney is not necessary if imaging is satisfactory and does not suggest a bilateral process.[217,218] Nephrectomy alone followed by observation for patients less than 2 years of age with stage I favorable histology tumors that weigh less than 550 g resulted in only an 85% EFS, and even though the study was stopped early, the OS was still 100% for this group of patients.[219,220] Further analysis identified a WT1 mutation and an 11p15 LOH as risk factors associated with relapse in this patient group.[207] Prenephrectomy chemotherapy and nephron sparing techniques may benefit patients with bilateral disease at diagnosis.[221] Children with syndromic, unilateral Wilms tumor who have an increased risk of late renal failure (i.e., DDS or WAGR) may also benefit from partial nephrectomy or nephron sparing surgery.[222,223] Preoperative treatment of Wilms tumor should be considered in children with a solitary kidney, bilateral renal tumors, tumor in a horseshoe kidney, tumor thrombus in the inferior vena cava above the level of the hepatic veins,[224,225] and respiratory distress as a result of extensive metastatic disease.[226] In children with bilateral disease or involvement of a solitary kidney, preoperative chemotherapy is intended to permit maximal conservation of uninvolved renal parenchyma. In the current COG renal tumor protocol, children who present with bilateral renal masses receive two to four cycles of chemotherapy without biopsy

(COG-AREN0534, NCT00945009). A biopsy is reserved for those patients whose tumors do not show appropriate volume reduction. Definitive surgery should be performed by week 12.

The role of surgical resection in the management of solitary pulmonary metastases was evaluated by the NWTSG in 211 patients with no therapeutic benefit identified when surgical resection was added to pulmonary radiotherapy and chemotherapy.[227] Four-year survival rates were identical in the two groups.

Chemotherapy

Vincristine and dactinomycin, with the addition of doxorubicin for more advanced disease, form the backbone of most combinations for the treatment of Wilms tumor.[213] The recommended standard drug regimens and duration of therapy according to stage and intergroup studies are listed in Table 99.8. The five consecutive NWTSG studies have provided the foundation for current care in North America and the results of various US and European trials are depicted in Table 99.9.[222,228–233,236,237]

NWTS-1 documented that postoperative radiation therapy is not required for children with stage I/II favorable histology or stage I anaplastic histology tumors when postnephrectomy chemotherapy with vincristine and dactinomycin is administered; NWTS-2 showed that doxorubicin improved relapse-free survival for group II through IV patients, NWTS-3 upstaged all patients with lymph node involvement to stage III, and provided evidence that patients with stage III favorable histology who receive adjuvant chemotherapy and radiation require augmented therapy with either doxorubicin or higher radiation therapy dose (20 Gy) for successful outcomes. Concerns about late effects of radiation resulted in the selection of the three-drug regimen (vincristine, dactinomycin, and doxorubicin) with lower radiation therapy dose (10 Gy) as standard therapy in this group.[234,235] Furthermore, this trial showed that the addition of cyclophosphamide to the standard three-drug regimen (vincristine, dactinomycin, and doxorubicin) does not improve the outcome of patients with stage IV/favorable histology tumors, but was potentially useful in patients with anaplastic tumors. In NWTS-4, the addition of cyclophosphamide proved to benefit patients with stage II through IV anaplastic tumors. In addition, therapy was reduced for low-risk patients, and *pulse-intensive* regimens were shown to maintain excellent survival with less toxicity than previous regimens.[236] Anaplasia, either diffuse or focal, adversely affects the outcome even after the administration of conventional chemotherapy with vincristine, dactinomycin, and doxorubicin. Cyclophosphamide and etoposide, when added to vincristine, dactinomycin, and doxorubicin, improved the survival of patients with stage II through IV diffuse anaplasia in NWTS-5.[193] A trial incorporating carboplatin to improve outcomes was stopped early due to toxicity of this regimen (UH1). Results of NWTS-5 indicate that patients with stage I anaplasia had lower than expected survival and will require augmented therapy in upcoming studies.

Salvage therapy is successful in up to 80% of patients with low-stage favorable histology tumors initially treated with vincristine, dactinomycin, and no radiotherapy.[237] Late recurrence more than 5 years after the diagnosis is rare, but is associated with a similar outcome to earlier recurrence.[238] At the time of relapse, approximately 50% of unilateral Wilms tumor patients who have received standard chemotherapy, three-drug chemotherapy, and radiation can be successfully re-treated.[239–241] Alternating cyclophosphamide/etoposide and carboplatin/etoposide, surgery and radiation led to 48% OS in high-risk patients with 53% OS in high-risk patients with lung-only relapse on the NWTS-5 relapse protocol.[239] The benefit of high-dose chemotherapy with autologous stem cell rescue (single or tandem transplants) is uncertain,[242] although it has been shown that patients with residual disease do not do as well.[243] Alternative agents, including topotecan[244] and irinotecan,[245] have shown some promising antitumor activity in phase 1/2 studies and require further evaluation in clinical trials.

Radiation Therapy

Successive NWTSG trials refined the dosages and indications to decrease radiation exposure while maintaining local control and control of metastatic pulmonary lesions (see Table 99.7). Patients with stage I and II favorable histology tumors do not require abdominal radiotherapy, whereas those with stage III favorable histology or stages I to III focal or diffuse anaplastic disease require adjuvant radiotherapy to the flank or abdomen. The tumor and renal beds with a 1- to 2-cm margin are treated in cases of positive resection margins, nodal involvement, or local spillage during surgery. Care must be taken to provide a uniform dosage to the vertebral column to limit the risk of scoliosis. Whole-abdominal radiotherapy is used for patients with preoperative rupture, diffuse spill during surgery, or when peritoneal metastasis is present. A dose of 10.8 Gy is sufficient for local control in stage III favorable histology patients if they also received chemotherapy with vincristine, dactinomycin, and doxorubicin.[246] Most patients receive radiotherapy within 8 to 12 days of nephrectomy without compromise in local–regional control.[247] Currently, it is recommended that radiotherapy start within 14 days of a nephrectomy.

Whole-lung irradiation (12 Gy) has been recommended for patients who present with pulmonary metastases, which has

---

TABLE 99.8

Treatment Regimens for Wilms Tumor with Favorable or Standard Histologic Features from Recently Completed NWTSG and SIOP Studies

| Stage | NWTS-5 | | SIOP93-01 | | |
| | Chemotherapy | Radiation Therapy | Chemotherapy | | Radiation Therapy |
			Preoperative	Postoperative	
I	VA × 18 weeks	—	VA × 4 weeks	VA × 4 weeks	—
II	VA × 18 weeks	—	VA × 4 weeks	VDA × 27 weeks	Node negative: none Node positive: 15 Gy
III	VDA × 24 weeks	10.8 Gy	VA × 4 weeks	VDA × 27 weeks	15 Gy
IV	VDA × 24 weeks	12 Gy lung (if lung metastasis) 10.8 Gy flank (if local stage III)	VDA × 6 weeks	CR after 9 weeks: VCA × 27 weeks	None if lung lesions disappear by week 9, otherwise 12 Gy No CR after 9 weeks: ICED × 34 weeks

V, vincristine; A, dactinomycin; D, doxorubicin; CR, complete remission; I, ifosfamide; C, carboplatin; E, etoposide.
From Metzger ML, Dome JS. Current therapy for Wilms' tumor. *Oncologist* 2005;10: 815–826, with permission.

TABLE 99.9

Summary of Patient Outcomes from Recently Reported Large Studies of Wilms Tumor

Study	Stage	Relapse-Free Survival/ Event-Free Survival (%)	Overall Survival (%)	Reference
NWTS-3		16 yr:	16 yr:	237
	I	92.5	97.6	
	II	89.6	92.9	
	III	80.4	86.2	
	IV	76.5	79.5	
NWTS-4	I	94.9 (2 yr)	98.7 (2 yr)	238,234
	II	83.6 (8 yr)	93.8 (8 yr)	
	III	88.9 (8 yr)	93 (8 yr)	
	IV	80.6 (2 yr)	89.5 (2 yr)	
	V (synchronous, FH)	74 (8 yr)	89 (8 yr)	223
	V (synchronous, AH)	40 (8 yr)	45 (8 yr)	223
NWTS-5		4 yr:	4 yr:	235
	I (age <24 mos, tumor weight <550 g)	84	98	
	I/II, no LOH	91	98	
	I/II, LOH 1p and 16q	75	91	
	III/IV, no LOH	83	92	
	III/IV, LOH 1p and 16q	66	78	
	V, any LOH	61	81	
	I, diffuse anaplasia	68	79	
	II, diffuse anaplasia	83	82	
	III, diffuse anaplasia	65	67	
	IV, diffuse anaplasia	33	33	
	V, diffuse anaplasia	25	42	
SIOP-9		2 yr:	5 yr:	230
	I (FH)	100	100	
	I (includes AH)	88	93	
	II N0	84	88	
	II N1 and III	71	85	
	Unfavorable (AH, WT, CCSK, and rhabdoid)	71	71	
SIOP93-01	Nonanaplastic	5 yr:	5 yr:	
	I	88.3	97	231
	II	91.9 (5 yr)	96.7 (5 yr)	232
	III	84.3 (5 yr)	91.5 (5 yr)	232
UKW3	Nonanaplastic	5 yr:	5 yr:	
	I	85.7	96.4	233
	II	83.3	93.8	
	III	79.6	89.9	
	IV	71.7	81.1	
	V	70.8	78.6	

FH, favorable histology; AH, anaplastic histology; N0, no lymph node involvement; N1, lymph node involvement; WT, Wilms tumor; CCSK, clear cell sarcoma of kidney; UKW, United Kingdom Children's Cancer Study Group Wilms Tumor trial.

historically been defined by the presence of nodules on chest x-ray. However, CT now allows for the identification of much smaller lesions. Ehrlich et al.[212] found that, in those patients whose pulmonary lesions were biopsied, only 82% of isolated lesions and 69% of multiple pulmonary lesions were actually tumor. Review of NWTS-4 and -5 identified patients with favorable histology and CT-only pulmonary lesions treated with standard three-drug therapy demonstrated no difference in EFS with or without the addition of radiation.[248] For the SIOP 93-01 study, pulmonary radiation was successfully limited to those patients with unresectable, persistent nodules or high-risk primary tumor histology after receiving prenephrectomy chemotherapy for 6 weeks and postnephrectomy chemotherapy for 9 weeks.[249] To develop a response-based approach to

pulmonary radiation therapy, a recently closed COG trial evaluated the feasibility of eliminating radiotherapy in children whose chest CT scans demonstrated complete resolution of pulmonary nodules at week 6 of therapy. The results of this strategy are pending.

RETINOBLASTOMA

Retinoblastoma is a rare childhood cancer of the developing retina that often presents with leukocoria and is fatal if untreated. Early detection and judicious therapy based on laterality and stage of disease has resulted in survival rates exceeding 90% in the United States for localized (intraocular) disease.

Epidemiology

The incidence rate in the United States for the period 1975 to 1995 is estimated at 3.7 cases per million (about 300 new cases per year) with no racial predilection or significant difference between males and females.[183] Worldwide, approximately 9,000 new cases are diagnosed each year.[250] Over 85% of patients in the United States present with localized intraocular disease at diagnosis. Two-thirds of cases are diagnosed before 2 years of age and 95% before age 5 years. For unilateral disease, the median age at diagnosis is 2 years; for bilateral disease, the median age at diagnosis is less than 12 months. Approximately one-quarter of cases are bilateral and, therefore, have the heritable form of the disease (either sporadic or familial). In the remaining 75% of cases (unilateral), 10% to 15% of patients are found to have the heritable form of the disease. Parents and siblings of patients with retinoblastoma should undergo a thorough ophthalmoscopic examination while genetic testing is pending.

Biology and Genetics

Retinoblastoma is caused by the biallelic inactivation of the retinoblastoma gene, *RB1*, a tumor suppressor gene that is located on the long arm of chromosome 13 (13q14).[251] Mutations in the *RB1* gene are transmitted as a highly penetrant, autosomal-dominant trait.[252] Patients with 13q- syndrome may have other associated abnormalities, such as distinct facial features, mental retardation, and growth failure.[253] Additionally, these patients have more episodes of neutropenia and GI toxicity than other children with retinoblastoma when receiving systemic chemotherapy (Brennan, unpublished). Recently, rare cases of MYCN-amplified retinoblastoma without *RB1* mutation have been reported.[254] Despite the loss of a tumor suppressor gene, the retinoblastoma genome is relatively stable, with epigenetic dysregulation of cancer pathways, including upregulation of the proto-oncogene SYK, driving further tumorigenesis.[255] Regardless of therapy, patients with heritable retinoblastoma are at an increased risk of developing secondary malignancies, particularly sarcomas, brain cancer, and melanoma[256,257]; those with familial, heritable retinoblastoma may be at an even higher risk.[258] The cumulative incidence of secondary malignancies 50 years after diagnosis in a large US cohort was 36% for hereditary retinoblastoma survivors and 5.7% for nonhereditary survivors; however, the mortality was 25.5% for hereditary retinoblastoma survivors and 1.0% for nonhereditary survivors.[259]

Pathology

Retinoblastoma is composed of uniform small, round, or polygonal cells, which have a scanty, poorly staining cytoplasm. The sparse cytoplasm is located at one side of the cell, suggesting the appearance of an embryonal retinal cell. The nucleus is large and deeply staining, giving the characteristic *small, round, blue cell* appearance. Three types of cellular arrangements may be identified: the Homer-Wright rosette, the Flexner-Wintersteiner rosette, and the fleurette. Calcification and necrosis are often observed.[260]

Clinical Presentation

Leukocoria, an abnormal white reflection from the retina compared with the normal *red reflex*, is the most common presenting sign of retinoblastoma.[261] Strabismus, conjunctival erythema, and decreased visual acuity are other common presenting complaints. Esotropia or exotropia may be present on examination, with decreased visual acuity as a result of involvement of the macula by the tumor or the presence of tumor cells and debris in the vitreous.[262] The eye may be red and painful because of uveitis after spontaneous necrosis of a retinal tumor or from neovascular glaucoma.

Evaluation

The diagnosis of retinoblastoma is based on clinical history (including family history) and results of examination of both eyes under general anesthesia. Once confirmed, the staging evaluation of a child with retinoblastoma should include an ultrasound of the orbits and MRI of the brain and orbits.[263,264] An MRI is useful to evaluate the extent of extraocular (orbital or pineal gland) disease. Although optic nerve enhancement may be concerning for the extraorbital spread of disease, pathology (enucleation) remains the gold standard.[265] Retinoblastoma may metastasize to the central nervous system, bones, or bone marrow.[266,267] A further evaluation for metastatic disease with lumbar puncture, bone marrow aspiration/biopsy, and bone scan is reserved for patients with involvement of extraretinal structures, including the orbit or optic nerve, or when symptoms, signs, pathology, or diagnostic imaging studies suggest the involvement of distant sites.[268,269]

Staging

The patient is staged according to the burden of local and metastatic disease, whereas the eye is *grouped* according to the extent of intraocular disease present. Martin and Reese[270] first proposed a staging system for patients with retinoblastoma in 1942. Two decades later, the Reese and Ellsworth[271] grouping (R-E) attempted to predict the risk of enucleation with external-beam radiotherapy alone (Group Ia through Vb; Table 99.10). Although the R-E group (per eye) is still widely referenced today, the clinical value of utilizing a radiation-based system in an era of multimodal therapy that does not account for the presence of subretinal seeds and was developed before the introduction of indirect ophthalmoscopy is unclear. In 2001, the COG incorporated a new classification system (Group A through E) for grouping intraocular retinoblastoma that could be utilized among all institutions participating

TABLE 99.10

Reese-Ellsworth Grouping System for Retinoblastoma

Group	Description
Group I	
A	Solitary tumor, <4 disc diameters in size, at or behind the equator
B	Multiple tumors, <4 disc diameters in size, all at or behind the equator
Group II	
A	Solitary tumor, 4–10 disc diameters in size, at or behind the equator
B	Multiple tumors, 4–10 disc diameters in size, behind the equator
Group III	
A	Any lesion anterior to the equator
B	Solitary tumors >10 disc diameters behind the equator
Group IV	
A	Multiple tumors, some >10 disc diameters
B	Any lesion extending anteriorly to the ora serrata
Group V	
A	Massive tumors involving more than one-half the retina
B	Vitreous seeding

Adapted from Stannard C, Lipper S, Sealy R, Sevel D. Retinoblastoma: correlation of invasion of the optic nerve and choroid with prognosis and metastases. *Br J Ophthalmol* 1979;63:560–570.

TABLE 99.11

International Classification System for Intraocular Retinoblastoma

Group	Defining Features
Group A *Small tumors away from fovea and disk*	■ Tumors <3 mm and ■ Located at least 3 mm from fovea and 1.5 mm from the optic disc
Group B *All remaining tumors confined to the retina*	■ All other tumors confined to retina not in Group A ■ Subretinal fluid <3 mm from the base of tumor
Group C *Local subretinal fluid or seeding*	■ Local subretinal fluid alone >3 mm to <6 mm from tumor ■ Vitreous seeding or subretinal seeding 3 mm from the tumor
Group D *Diffuse subretinal fluid or seeding*	■ Subretinal fluid alone >6 mm from tumor ■ Vitreous seeding or subretinal seeding >3 mm from tumor
Group E *Presence of poor prognosis features*	■ More than two-thirds of globe filled with tumor ■ Tumor in anterior segment or the ciliary body ■ Iris neovascularization, neovascular glaucoma ■ Tumor necrosis, phthisis bulbi

in clinical trials (Table 99.11). This classification system, which identifies the likelihood of treatment failure requiring enucleation or EBRT (group A = very low risk; group E = very high risk), was originally developed at Children's Hospital Los Angeles and is now used internationally.[272] The St. Jude Children's Research Hospital developed a staging system that is defined by the extent of tumor involving the retina and globe, or by the presence of extrachoroidal disease.[273] Another staging system developed by Chantada et al.[274] provides a common international classification for patients with extraocular retinoblastoma.

Treatment

Patients with suspected retinoblastoma should be referred to a pediatric ophthalmologist with expertise in the management of intraocular tumors and a pediatric oncologist experienced in the treatment of retinoblastoma. Treatment aims to preserve life and useful vision and is based on laterality and the stage of disease. Protective eyewear is recommended for all patients. With the high percentage of survivors, treatment decisions must carefully weigh

the functional outcome and potential long-term sequelae of local and systemic therapies.[275]

Enucleation

In view of the excellent response of this tumor to globe-sparing interventions, enucleation is considered in selective situations. Recently, more aggressive attempts at ocular salvage, regardless of visual potential, are being attempted (see the following). However, the most strongly considered indications for enucleation include (1) a unilateral retinoblastoma that completely fills the globe or that has damaged and disrupted the retina or vitreous so extensively that restoration of useful vision is not possible (and attempts at ocular salvage may place the patient at risk for metastatic disease); (2) a tumor that is present in the anterior chamber; (3) a painful glaucoma with a loss of vision after rubeosis iridis; (4) a progressive retinoblastoma disease unresponsive to all other forms of local therapy; and (5) cases with permanent vision loss in which extraocular tumor is suspected. The standard surgical technique is modified to allow excision of the longest possible segment of optic nerve in continuity with the globe.[276] After removal, the globe and optic nerve are inspected for evidence of extraocular extension of the tumor. A hydroxyapatite implant is placed in the muscle funnel, which improves the cosmetic result and the promotion of normal development of the bony orbit.[277]

Local Therapies

When combined with chemoreduction, local therapies, including laser, cryotherapy, and radioactive plaque brachytherapy, consolidate treatment and improve disease control for patients with R-E group I through IV disease.[278,279] Patients with R-E group V disease may require additional therapy, including external-beam radiation.[280]

Laser is useful for tumors ≤2.5 mm in thickness and ≤4.5 mm in diameter (<4 disc diameters).[278] Like laser therapy, cryotherapy produces an avascular scar, but is more often utilized for tumors 2.5 mm in diameter and 1.0 mm thick located anterior to the equator and confined to the sensory retina.[281] Radioactive plaque brachytherapy using iodine-125 radiation may be utilized for tumor consolidation, but is more commonly used in the setting of localized recurrence for tumor control or for salvage.[282,283] Plaque brachytherapy does not appear to have the risk of secondary malignancies seen in external-beam radiation.[283]

Radiation Therapy

External-beam radiation therapy is indicated for patients with advanced disease that has not responded adequately to chemotherapy and local treatments but who has useful vision, or patients with extraorbital extension of disease, usually after enucleation. Patients requiring radiation receive doses between 40 and 45 Gy, depending on tumor size, patient age, and the presence of vitreous seeding.[284] Modern radiotherapy uses megavoltage accelerators and CT- and MRI-based treatment planning to allow for sparing of the lens and bony orbits. Together with daily image guidance for field placement, these techniques may further reduce known radiotherapy-related late effects to surrounding structures.[285] Proton therapy can potentially decrease dosage to the surrounding bony orbits by more than 60% and avoid significant dosage to the hypothalamus compared with intensity-modulated radiotherapy, with equivalent target coverage.[286]

The preservation of some useful vision in these patients is an obvious advantage of such a treatment approach, but the risk of secondary malignancies after external-beam radiation in young children is well defined.[259,287] Kleinerman et al.[288] published long-term results of 1,601 survivors of retinoblastoma and reported a 3.1-fold increase in the risk of secondary cancers for hereditary retinoblastoma survivors who received radiation therapy. Among hereditary retinoblastoma survivors, radiation therapy increased the cumulative incidence of second malignancies to 38% in patients who received radiation compared with 21% of hereditary patients without radiation. The authors also found the risk of osteosarcomas was higher in patients who received chemotherapy with radiation, compared with radiation alone.

After enucleation, local irradiation to include the orbit and the optic nerve up the chiasm is recommended for all patients with extension of retinoblastoma into the orbit. Presentation with exophthalmos, inability to retain the prosthesis, or a palpable mass through the eyelids suggests the presence of orbital extension of the tumor. The identification of an extraocular mass, histologic confirmation of tumor cells at the cut end of the optic nerve at the time of enucleation, or rupture of the globe during removal is associated with orbital contamination with the tumor.

Chemotherapy

The use of neoadjuvant chemotherapy in treating retinoblastoma was prompted by success in salvaging patients with recurrent extraocular disease.[289,290] Since the 1990s, there have been a series of studies documenting promising rates of vision-sparing therapy without external-beam radiotherapy in intraocular disease.[280,291,292] Most chemoreduction regimens are platinum based and utilize carboplatin over cisplatin (due to reduced ototoxicity). Other active agents include vincristine, etoposide, cyclophosphamide, doxorubicin, and topotecan.[291,293–297] Cyclosporin A has also been used as a multidrug-resistant reversal agent.[298] Despite the initial response, which is most pronounced in patients with R-E group I through IV tumors, chemotherapy alone rarely achieves durable disease control and is, therefore, paired with local therapies, as described previously. Patients with R-E group V disease, especially those with vitreous seeds, are at highest risk for chemoreduction failure and tumor recurrence/resistance.

Because tumor shrinkage may prevent enucleation, patients with bilateral disease are candidates for conservative treatment with chemoreduction. Indeed, in bilateral retinoblastoma cases, the assessment of which eye is most likely to be capable of functional vision is difficult until a response to chemotherapy is determined. Adjuvant chemotherapy is utilized after enucleation in patients who have high-risk histologic features, including invasion of the choroid (massive), anterior chamber, or ciliary body/iris, postlaminar optic nerve involvement with concomitant invasion of the choroid, or involvement of sclera or tumor present at the cut end of the optic nerve.[295,299]

Other recent areas of clinical investigation include locally delivered chemotherapeutic agents to increase drug concentration within the eye such as periocular chemotherapy (subconjunctival or subtenon injection),[300] supraselective intra-arterial chemotherapy,[301,302] and intravitreal chemotherapy.[303] Because several reports have shown promising results, the techniques of intra-arterial and intravitreal chemotherapy will be prospectively evaluated in upcoming COG clinical trials to carefully evaluate the feasibility and toxicity of each regimen. At the same time, preclinical retinoblastoma research is providing novel therapies that target key pathways in retinoblastoma tumorigenesis.[255,304,305] Pairing the right drug and delivery technique will translate into therapy that can save globes and vision while reducing the long-term effects of radiation and chemotherapy.

Metastatic Disease

Although most patients in the United States present with localized (intraocular) disease, 10% to 15% of patients will have evidence of extraocular spread at diagnosis. Patients with heritable disease (RB1 mutation) have a 3% to 9% risk of developing trilateral disease, or disease invading the pineal gland, although this may be lower in this era of improved MRI (tumor versus cyst of pineal gland) and systemic chemotherapy.[264]

Therapy for patients with metastatic disease requires a multimodal approach with intensive systemic chemotherapy, external beam radiation, and, for patients with distant systemic or central nervous system (CNS) metastatic disease, autologous bone marrow transplantation.[289,306–308] Despite aggressive therapy, survival for patients with metastatic retinoblastoma outside of the CNS is 50%, with survival decreasing to <10% for those with CNS metastatic disease.

Late Effects and Long Term Follow-Up

Although patients treated for intraocular retinoblastomas have an excellent prognosis, those with germ-line RBI mutations remain at risk for secondary malignancies. Patients treated with chemotherapy are at risk for late effects, including secondary leukemia with exposure to etoposide[309,310] and ototoxicity with exposure to carboplatin.[311,312] There is also a growing awareness of the other long-term consequences that reach beyond the genetic and physical effects of therapy, such as health-related quality of life and neurocognitive and psychosocial outcomes.[313,314] Further investigation through COG and other large retinoblastoma treatment centers is underway.

PEDIATRIC BONE SARCOMAS: OSTEOSARCOMA AND EWING SARCOMA

Osteosarcoma and Ewing sarcoma account for approximately 5% of all pediatric malignancies.[183,315,316] Although the biologic properties of these tumors are distinct, their treatment principles are quite similar.[317] Osteosarcoma has a bimodal age distribution, with the first peak in the 2nd decade of life and the second peak occurring in older adults over the age of 65 years. A comprehensive discussion of osteosarcoma is provided in Chapter 91. This section will focus on the main features of osteosarcoma in the younger population, including its unique molecular, genetic, and cytogenetic features.

Osteosarcoma

Epidemiology

Osteosarcoma is the most common primary, malignant bone tumor in children and adolescents, accounting for 4% of all childhood cancers. In the United States, approximately 400 new cases are diagnosed in those younger than 20 years of age.[183] The peak age of incidence corresponds with the time of most rapid bone growth, 16 years in boys and 12 years in girls.[318] The disease is slightly more prevalent in males and in African Americans.[318]

Biology and Molecular Genetics

The majority of osteosarcomas are sporadic. However, certain conditions, such as previous exposure to ionizing radiation[319] and alkylating agents,[320] predispose individuals to the development of osteosarcoma. Additionally, a large proportion of patients older than 40 years who develop osteosarcoma also have Paget disease of bone.[321] Osteosarcoma is also associated with several cancer-predisposition syndromes, including hereditary retinoblastoma, Li-Fraumeni syndrome (LFS), and Rothmund-Thomson syndrome (RTS).

Patients with hereditary retinoblastoma have germ-line mutations in the *RB1* gene and somatic mutations in retinal cells, resulting in retinoblastoma. The majority of secondary nonocular malignancies in these patients are sarcomas, and more than a third of these are osteosarcomas, half of which occur within a previously irradiated field.[257,287,322] LFS is a familial cancer syndrome in which affected family members have a wide spectrum of cancers, including osteosarcoma.[323] Many of these patients carry germ-line mutations in the *p53* tumor suppressor gene.[324,325] Screening of a large series of children with osteosarcoma showed that approximately 3% to 4% carried constitutional germ-line mutations in *p53*.[326] RTS is an autosomal-recessive condition characterized by a distinctive rash (poikiloderma), small stature, skeletal anomalies, sparse hair, and increased risk for OS. In a cross-sectional study of 41 patients with RTS, 13 patients (30%) had osteosarcoma.[327] Two-thirds of patients had constitutional mutations in the *RECQL4* gene, and the presence of mutations correlated with osteosarcoma risk.[328] Because these genetic conditions are known to predispose individuals to osteosarcoma, careful detailing of family history in a patient with newly diagnosed osteosarcoma is important to identify underlying genetic risk and for genetic counseling of family members.

In view of these genetic predisposition syndromes, it is not surprising that the *RB1* and *p53* genes are also frequently altered in sporadic osteosarcoma tumors. Approximately 70% of primary osteosarcoma tumors have alterations in the *RB1* gene.[329–331] Regulators of the *RB1* pathway, including cyclin-dependent kinases 4 and 6, cyclin D1, and p16[INK4a], are also altered in some cases of osteosarcoma.[332–334] Inactivating mutations of the *p53* gene occur in approximately 50% of all sporadic cancers. The overall frequency of *p53* mutations in osteosarcoma ranges from 15% to 30% depending on the detection methods used.[335] Other members of the *p53* pathway, including p14[ARF] and MDM2, are altered in

some cases of sporadic osteosarcoma.[336,337] Unlike *p53* and *RB1*, the *RECQL4* gene has not been found to be mutated in cases of sporadic osteosarcoma.[338]

Clinical Presentation and Natural History

Most patients with osteosarcoma present with pain and soft-tissue swelling. Approximately 5% to 10% may present with a pathologic fracture of the affected bone.[339,340] Systemic symptoms such as fever, weight loss, and malaise are generally absent. A physical examination usually demonstrates a firm, tender mass and restricted range of motion in the affected extremity. Laboratory evaluation results are usually normal except for elevated alkaline phosphatase (in approximately 40%),[341] elevated lactate dehydrogenase (in approximately 30%),[342] and elevated erythrocyte sedimentation rate, none of which are specific for osteosarcoma.

Osteosarcoma in the pediatric population preferentially involves the metaphyseal region of the long bones, in contrast to Ewing sarcoma, which typically arises in the diaphyseal region of the long bones. The primary site of disease in 80% of patients with osteosarcoma is an extremity, most commonly (in descending order) the distal femur, proximal tibia, and proximal humerus. Unlike Ewing sarcoma, osteosarcoma rarely affects the axial skeleton.[343] Approximately 20% of patients with osteosarcoma present with clinically detectable metastatic disease, most frequently to the lungs and less often to bones.

Diagnostic and Staging Evaluation

The initial evaluation of a suspected bone tumor involves obtaining a patient's complete history and performing a physical examination. Radiographic studies allow for an assessment of the anatomic site, the extent of local invasion, and the pattern of extension.[344] If the tumor involves an extremity, then plain radiographs should encompass both proximal and distal joint regions, and they should be taken in two planes. Characteristic findings suggestive of osteosarcoma on a radiograph include a mixed lytic and sclerotic appearance, periosteal new bone formation with lifting of the cortex and the formation of the Codman triangle, and ossification of the soft tissue in a radial or *sunburst* pattern (Fig. 99.5).[343] Even if the plain radiographs are classic for osteosarcoma, further imaging of the primary tumor by MRI or CT is required to evaluate the extent of the tumor for surgery-planning purposes. The imaging should include the entire tumor-bearing bone in order to assess for skip metastases (i.e., isolated tumor foci within the same bone as the primary tumor). Although both CT and MRI are equally accurate for local staging of tumors, an MRI is preferable for evaluating soft-tissue extension and joint and marrow involvement.[344]

Because patients with metastatic disease at presentation have a significantly worse outcome than do patients with localized disease, a thorough search for sites of metastases is imperative. Staging workup for osteosarcoma includes a technetium-99 bone scan to evaluate the involvement of other bones and a chest CT to detect pulmonary metastases. Studies evaluating the utility of FDG PET/CT in osteosarcoma staging show that FDG PET/CT may be more sensitive and accurate than a bone scan in detecting bone metastases.[345,346] Furthermore, the results of several studies suggest that changes in the metabolic tumor activity as assessed by PET/CT during therapy correlate with the percentage of tumor necrosis at the time of definitive surgery.[347,348] A histologic confirmation is indicated in pulmonary lesion(s) that cannot be unequivocally defined as being a metastatic disease. Finding one or more pulmonary (or pleural) nodules of at least 1-cm diameter *or* three or more nodules of at least 0.5-cm diameter generally indicates definite pulmonary metastases and may not require a biopsy. Fewer or smaller lesions may or may not represent metastatic disease; therefore, confirmation by resection may be indicated.[344] There are no laboratory studies that are diagnostic or prognostic

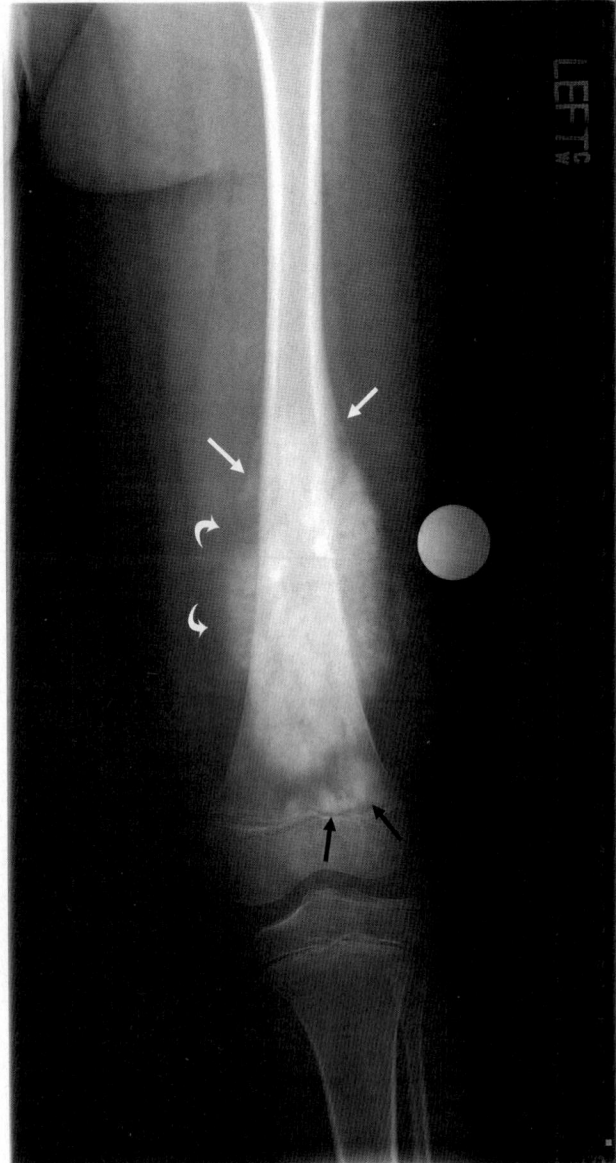

Figure 99.5 Radiographic appearance of osteosarcoma involving the distal femoral diaphysis and metaphysis, with Codman triangles at the proximal end of the tumor *(white arrows)* and an associated sunburst periosteal reaction *(curved arrows)*. Skip metastases are suggested by the presence of round sclerotic foci abutting the growth plate *(black arrows)*.

for osteosarcoma.[349] General laboratory tests such as a complete blood count; electrolyte counts including calcium, magnesium, and phosphorus; liver and renal function tests; and alkaline phosphatase and lactate dehydrogenase (LDH) measurements should be performed to obtain baseline values.[349]

Pathology

None of the radiographic features described previously are pathognomonic for osteosarcoma; therefore, a tissue biopsy is required to make a definitive diagnosis. The differential diagnosis for a bone lesion with aggressive features (e.g., the presence of a Codman triangle, associated soft-tissue mass, permeative appearance) on imaging studies includes Ewing sarcoma, lymphoma, and metastatic tumor. It may also occasionally include benign bone lesions, such as osteochondroma and giant cell tumor, and nonneoplastic

conditions, such as osteomyelitis, eosinophilic granuloma, and aneurysmal bone cyst. The biopsy should be performed by an orthopedic surgeon experienced in the management of malignant bone tumors, ideally by the same surgeon who will perform the definitive surgery. Proper planning of the biopsy with careful consideration of the future definitive surgery is important so as not to jeopardize the subsequent treatment, particularly in the case of a limb-salvage procedure.[350]

Osteosarcoma is thought to be derived from primitive bone-forming mesenchymal cells.[135] The histologic diagnosis is based on the presence of a malignant sarcomatous stroma associated with the production of *tumor* osteoid or immature bone.[351] Several types of osteosarcomas have been identified based on histologic, clinical, and radiographic features including conventional osteosarcoma (80%), which is the type most frequently encountered in children and adolescents. Conventional osteosarcomas are further subdivided into osteoblastic (50% of conventional OS), fibroblastic (25%), and chondroblastic (25%) variants depending on the presence of the predominant type of matrix.[352] The main feature that distinguishes these tumors from the malignant fibrosarcomas and chondrosarcomas, which also arise from primitive mesenchymal cells, is the production of osteoid.[351]

Other variants of osteosarcoma include parosteal, telangiectatic, small-cell, periosteal, low-grade central, and high-grade surface.[353,354] All variants are considered to be high-grade tumors except for low-grade central and parosteal osteosarcomas, which are considered to be low-grade tumors, and periosteal osteosarcoma, which is thought to be intermediate grade.[354,355] Small-cell osteosarcoma can be histologically confused with other small, round cell tumors, especially Ewing sarcoma.[356] The tumors may stain positive for CD99 and may contain the Ewing sarcoma breakpoint region 1 (EWSR1) gene rearrangement.[357] Two other distinct variants of osteosarcoma have been described, osteosarcoma of the jaw and extraosseous osteosarcoma. Osteosarcoma of the jaw tends to occur in older patients, has an indolent course, and is more often associated with local recurrences than with distant metastases. Extraosseous osteosarcoma is rarely encountered and usually occurs after exposure to radiation.[358]

In contrast to other pediatric sarcomas, osteosarcomas do not have any specific translocations or other molecular genetic abnormalities that can serve as diagnostic or tumor-specific markers of disease. Cytogenetically, osteosarcoma tumors have complex numerical and structural chromosomal abnormalities with significant cell-to-cell variation and heterogeneity, highlighting the complexity and instability of the genetic makeup of osteosarcoma.[359–363]

Treatment

The mainstays of therapy for osteosarcoma are surgery and chemotherapy. The outcome of patients with nonmetastatic osteosarcoma has improved dramatically during the past 3 to 4 decades from an EFS rate of 10% to 20% to one of 65% to 70%, mostly because of the addition of adjuvant chemotherapy as well as improvements in surgical and diagnostic imaging techniques.[343,364–366] The care of patients with osteosarcoma requires a team approach involving oncologists, orthopedic surgeons, pathologists, oncology nurses, physical therapists, social workers, and child life specialists.

Chemotherapy

Localized Disease. Because of current combinations of surgery and chemotherapy, long-term disease-free survival and OS rates for osteosarcoma are greater than 60%. Based on the results of cooperative group trials over the past years (Table 99.12), the current standard three-drug chemotherapy regimen for patients with localized disease includes doxorubicin, cisplatin, and high-dose methotrexate (MAP). Patients receive neoadjuvant chemotherapy with these drugs for approximately 10 weeks and then undergo

TABLE 99.12

Treatment Results in Selected Cooperative Group Studies of Localized Osteosarcoma

Study (Reference)	Study Duration	Number of Patients	Chemotherapy	Event-Free Survival	Comment
INT 0133[407]	1993–1997	172 168 167 170	MAP MAP + MTP-PE MAPI MAPI + MTP-PE	6-yr 64% 6-yr 63% 6-yr 58% 6-yr 71%	No significant difference in EFS between groups
P9754[663]	1999–2002	111 54 56	MA (600 mg/m^2) P MA (600 mg/m^2) PI MAPIE	2-yr 69%	No significant difference in EFS between groups
POG-8651[369]	1986–1993	55 45	MAP/surgery wk 0 MAP/surgery wk 10	5-yr 69% 5-yr 61%	No significant difference in EFS between groups
ISG/SSG I[371]	1997–2000	182	MAPI (15 g/m^2)	5-yr 64%	Outcome similar to studies using standard dose ifosfamide
COSS 86[664]	1986–1988	56 72 41	MAPI + ia (HR) MAPI (HR) MAP (LR)	10-yr 63% 10-yr 70% 10-yr 66%	No difference in EFS between groups
EOI[665]	1993–2002	250 254	AP q3wk AP q2wk	5-yr 39% 5-yr 41%	Improved histologic response in interval compressed arm, but no difference in EFS
EURAMOS1[374]	2005–2011	358 357 N/A N/A	MAP (GR) MAP + INF (GR) MAP (PR) MAPIE (PR)	3-yr 74% 3-yr 77% N/A N/A	No significant difference in EFS between groups

M, methotrexate; A, doxorubicin; P, cisplatin; MTP-PE, muramyl tripeptide-phosphatidyl ethanolamine; I, ifosfamide; E, etoposide; ISG/SSG, Italian Sarcoma Group and Scandinavian Sarcoma Group; ia, intra-arterial cisplatin; COSS, Cooperative German-Austrian-Swiss Osteosarcoma Study Group; HR, high risk; LR, low risk; EOI, European Osteosarcoma Intergroup; GR, good responder; INF, interferon; EURAMOS1, European and American Osteosarcoma Study; PR, poor responder; N/A, not available.

definitive surgery, which is followed by adjuvant chemotherapy for approximately 20 weeks. The exceptions to this therapy scheme in localized disease are low-grade central and parosteal osteosarcomas and some periosteal osteosarcomas without high-grade features; these variants are traditionally treated with surgery alone.[354]

The benefit of adjuvant chemotherapy in the treatment of osteosarcoma was clearly demonstrated in two prospective trials that randomly assigned patients to observation or chemotherapy following surgery.[342,365,367] The concept of *neoadjuvant* or *induction* chemotherapy (i.e., chemotherapy given before definitive surgical resection) was prompted by the development of techniques for limb-sparing procedures and the need to control disease while the prosthesis was being constructed.[368] In a prospective randomized trial by the Pediatric Oncology Group (POG) of neoadjuvant chemotherapy versus primary surgery followed by adjuvant chemotherapy[369] outcomes were similar between the two groups, with 5-year EFS rates of approximately 61% and 69% (p = 0.8), respectively. Subsequent trials examining whether intensifying or adding other chemotherapy agents have not resulted in substantial improvements in OS for patients with osteosarcoma.[370,371]

The use of immunostimulatory agents in the treatment of osteosarcoma was tested in a joint POG and CCG randomized study (INT-0133).[5] The aim of this study was to determine whether adding the macrophage-activating agent MTP-PE (muramyl tripeptide phosphatidylethanolamine; mifamurtide) to chemotherapy would enhance survival in patients with newly diagnosed osteosarcoma. The study also evaluated whether adding ifosfamide to the standard three-drug MAP regimen improved survival. Initial results suggested that there may be some modest benefit to patients treated with MTP-PE, and with additional follow-up of patients treated on this study show that adding MTP-PE had an improved 6-year OS rate from 70% to 78%. The drug is not available in the United States for clinical use.

The most recent study, an international trial (EURAMOS 1) for patients with resectable localized or metastatic osteosarcoma,

has completed accrual. All patients were initially treated with standard three-drug induction with MAP. Those whose disease was classified as having a good response (>90% tumor necrosis) after induction chemotherapy continued with the same chemotherapy but were randomized to receive pegylated interferon α-2b, an immune-modulating cytokine that some Scandinavian studies have shown to have activity against osteosarcoma.[372,373] Patients whose disease had poor histologic responses were randomized to receive high-dose ifosfamide and etoposide in addition to the standard three drugs. Preliminary results of the cohort of patients who experienced good responses to induction MAP chemotherapy showed no improvement in EFS rates of patients who received interferon α-2b versus those that received MAP alone; however, only 75% of patients who were randomized to receive interferon actually started the drug, and of those, only 55% completed all specified therapies.[374]

Metastatic Disease. The presence of metastatic disease at presentation is associated with a poor prognosis. In the absence of an available clinical trial, most patients with metastatic disease receive MAP chemotherapy with high-dose ifosfamide with or without etoposide.[369,375,376]

The ability to control all foci of macroscopic disease is essential in managing metastatic osteosarcoma. Patients with pulmonary metastatic disease have a survival rate of 30% to 50%, whereas patients with bone metastases have a worse prognosis.[377,378] Similarly, patients with multifocal osteosarcoma have a dismal prognosis.

Multiple studies have demonstrated that the removal of all sites of metastatic or recurrent disease (e.g., pulmonary lesions), even after completion of chemotherapy, can result in long-term survival.[379–381] In a large analysis of the Cooperative Osteosarcoma Study Group, which included more than 1,700 consecutively treated patients, the 10-year survival probability was 40%

for metastatic patients who had all sites of metastatic disease resected.[382] However, patients with extrapulmonary metastases (e.g., bone metastases) are less likely to be cured, particularly those with multifocal disease.[383] Ongoing strategies to improve the outcome of patients with metastatic osteosarcoma include the use of MTP-PE,[384] bisphosphonates,[385,386] and molecularly targeted agents such as those against vascular endothelial growth factor (VEGF) and platelet-derived growth factor (PDGF) receptors, mammalian target of rapamycin (mTOR), and Src kinase.[387]

Local Control. Osteosarcoma is relatively radioresistant; therefore, surgery alone is the mainstay of local control. The choice of limb salvage versus amputation for extremity tumors depends on the location and extent of the tumor, the ability to achieve good surgical margins, and proximity to the joints and neurovascular bundle. As long as the tumor is removed in its entirety with disease-free margins, then the type of surgery—limb salvage versus amputation—does not seem to influence outcome.[388] On the basis of the results of studies assessing quality of life and functional measures, most patients who undergo limb salvage procedures report an improved quality of life and demonstrate better functional ability than do those who have amputations.[389,390]

Pelvic Tumors and Unresectable Disease. Patients with primary tumors of the axial skeleton generally have poor outcomes because surgery does not provide adequate local control. In some pelvic and most vertebral primary tumors, complete resection often is not possible. Most pelvic osteosarcomas can be treated by hemipelvectomy; however, more centrally located pelvic tumors, especially those involving the sacrum, are unresectable. Only a few pelvic osteosarcomas can be treated by limb-sparing resection (i.e., internal hemipelvectomy). Contraindications to resection are unusually large extraosseous extensions with sacral plexus or major vascular involvement. In general, these tumors cannot be resected with negative margins and are best treated by chemotherapy and radiotherapy.

Radiation Therapy. Historically, osteosarcoma has been considered to be relatively radioresistant; therefore, radiation therapy is generally not used as a definitive primary treatment of this disease. Radiation may be used in patients with microscopic positive margins of resection in doses of 55 to 68 Gy with local control rates ranging between 67% and 78%.[391] Patients with gross residual or unresected disease have been treated to doses of 70 Gy or higher. Treatment volumes have consisted of the gross residual disease or tumor bed plus a 1- to 2-cm clinical margin. In the setting of metastatic or unresectable osteosarcoma, radiotherapy may also be of benefit by improving pain in up to 76% of cases.[392] Despite the relative rarity of patients with osteosarcomas requiring radiation, its use can be of benefit in the management of both local and metastatic sites of disease.

Recurrent Disease. Outcomes for patients with local or distant relapse are poor.[393–395] Effective therapy for these patients is challenging and is limited by the paucity of salvage chemotherapeutic agents active against this disease. Chemotherapy agents that have been used in the relapse setting include high-dose ifosfamide,[396] gemcitabine and docetaxel,[397–399] cyclophosphamide, and etoposide.[400] More recently, targeted agents such as sorafenib have been used.[401] Isolated pulmonary disease with a single unilateral lung lesion is more likely to result in long-term disease-free survival than is bilateral pulmonary disease or bony metastasis. A longer disease-free interval (>12 to 24 months) from initial therapy is associated with longer disease-free survival.[394,402,403]

Prognostic Factors

The most important prognostic factors for survival in patients with osteosarcoma are the presence of metastatic disease and the extent of tumor necrosis following induction chemotherapy, with more than 90% necrosis (i.e., grades 3 or 4) being favorable and less than 90% (i.e., grades 1 or 2) necrosis being less favorable.[370,404–407] Other prognostic variables have been less definitive in predicting outcomes. Some of these factors include age, tumor size, and tumor location.[382] Location is important because axial tumors, such as those of the pelvis, skull, or vertebrae, fare worse because of the difficulty in achieving a complete surgical resection with disease-free margins.

Ewing Sarcoma

Epidemiology

The term Ewing sarcoma was previously used to refer to the least-differentiated of a group of small, round cell tumors that share a recurring chromosomal translocation (discussed in detail in the following paragraphs). Over the years, this group of tumors became designated as the Ewing sarcoma family of tumors and includes Askin tumors (Ewing sarcoma arising in the chest wall) and the more histologically differentiated peripheral primitive neuroectodermal tumors. The 2013 World Health Organization classification proposed that the phrase *Ewing sarcoma* be used to refer to this family of tumors.[408] We will follow this recommendation in this section.

Ewing sarcoma is the second most common primary bone tumor in pediatric patients after osteosarcoma, accounting for approximately 2% of childhood malignancies. About 200 cases of Ewing sarcoma are diagnosed in the United States per year.[183] Most of these tumors arise in the 2nd decade of life. There is a slight male predominance, and African and Asian children are rarely affected by this cancer.[183] Ewing sarcoma can arise in bone and, less commonly (about 30%), in the soft tissue (i.e., extraosseous) anywhere in the body.[409]

Biology and Molecular Genetics

The cell-of-origin of Ewing sarcoma is unknown but is presumed to arise from a mesenchymal stem cell.[410–413] These tumors characteristically have recurrent chromosomal translocations that, in almost all cases, involve the *EWSR1* gene on chromosome 22 and a member of the ETS family of transcription factors.[414,415] Of Ewing sarcoma tumors, 85% harbor t(11;22) (q24;q12), resulting in the fusion of the *EWSR1* and *FLI1* genes. Another 10% to 15% of tumors are associated with t(21;22) (q22;q12), which generates the *EWSR1-ERG* fusion gene. Less commonly, EWS, or the related protein FUS, is fused to another ETS family transcription factor (i.e., ETV1, EIAF, FEV, or ETV4), resulting in the same Ewing phenotype.[416]

Heterogeneity in the *EWSR1-FLI1* fusion gene is based on the location of the chromosomal breakpoint. The most common rearrangement, designated type 1, consists of the first seven exons of *EWSR1* fused to exons six to nine of *FLI1*. This fusion gene accounts for over half of all cases. The type 2 rearrangement, accounting for about 25% of cases, fuses *EWSR1* to exon 5 of *FLI1*. There is no prognostic significance based on the type of fusion protein.[417,418] As a chimeric transcription factor, EWS-FLI1 is believed to regulate a number of critical downstream target genes that have been implicated in tumor biology, including members of the Sonic Hedgehog and GLI1 pathways.[419,420]

Evidence shows that directly inhibiting EWS-FLI1's oncogenic activity by altering its interaction with critical binding partners such as RNA helicase A (RHA) significantly alters tumor biology. A small-molecule inhibitor that disrupts the EWS-FLI1/RHA interaction decreases xenograft growth and increases tumor cell apoptosis.[421] Additional evidence suggests that several intracellular signal transduction pathways are significantly altered in these tumors, including insulin-like growth factor receptor 1 (IGF-1R) and the phosphatidylinositol-3 kinase (PI3K)–mTOR pathway.[422] Drugs targeting these pathways are being explored as possible new therapeutic agents for Ewing sarcoma, including anti–IGF-1R antibodies and mTOR inhibitors.[423–426]

Clinical Presentation and Natural History

Patients with osseous Ewing sarcoma typically present with localized pain and swelling in the affected bone and may have other nonspecific symptoms such as fever, decreased appetite, and weight loss, which are usually seen in advanced disease.[427,428] In contrast to osteosarcoma, Ewing sarcoma is equally distributed between extremity and axial sites. The lower extremity—primarily, the femur—is the most common site of disease, followed by the pelvis and the chest wall.[429] Ewing sarcoma can also affect nonosseous structures, and this usually occurs in the soft tissues, but it can also arise in the GI tract, the kidneys, the adrenal gland, the lung, and other rare sites. The presenting symptom in these cases is site specific.

Metastatic disease is present in approximately 25% of patients at the initial diagnosis.[430] The most frequent site of metastases is the lungs, followed by the bones, and bone marrow.[429] Other sites of metastases, such as the lymph nodes, the liver, or the brain, are relatively rare unless in end-stage disease.

There is no specific blood or urine test to diagnose Ewing sarcoma. Abnormal laboratory findings at the time of diagnosis may include elevated LDH and alkaline phosphatase levels. LDH is useful as a gauge of tumor burden and usually falls with effective therapy and rises with disease recurrence.[431]

Diagnostic Staging Evaluation

An evaluation of suspected Ewing sarcoma includes a radiographic examination of the primary tumor site and documentation of the presence or absence of distant metastases. Plain radiographs and MRI or CT scans should be initially obtained to characterize and define the local extent of the primary tumor. An MRI provides the most precise definition of the extent of the tumor and its relation to nearby nerves and vessels. Lesions that originate in the long bones characteristically involve the diaphyses, with extension toward the metaphyses. On plain films, a lytic or mixed lytic–sclerotic lesion is usually identified in the bone. A multilamellar periosteal reaction (i.e., onion skin appearance [Fig. 99.6]) and lifting of the periosteum (i.e., Codman triangle), or less frequently, radiating bone spicules, may be present. The lesion is usually poorly marginated and has a permeative and destructive pattern.

CT scans of the chest should be obtained to evaluate for pulmonary metastases. A biopsy of solitary pulmonary nodules should be strongly considered before classifying the disease as being metastatic. A technetium-99m whole-body radionuclide bone scan should be obtained to detect bone metastases. FDG PET/CT is highly sensitive in screening for bone metastases Ewing sarcoma[432–434] and may be a useful predictor of outcome, similar to histologic response, after induction chemotherapy.[435] Bilateral bone marrow sampling is required to complete the staging of all patients regardless of primary site or tumor size. Microscopically detectable bone marrow metastases occur in less than 10% of patients and are associated with a poor prognosis.[436]

Pathology

A biopsy of the tumor and an histopathologic examination are required for diagnosis. It is critical for the surgeon performing the diagnostic biopsy to place the incision appropriately to avoid complicating future resection. Under light microscopy, Ewing sarcoma falls under the category of small, round, blue cell tumors that includes neuroblastomas, rhabdomyosarcomas, lymphoblastic

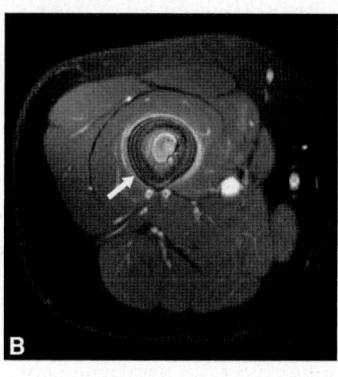
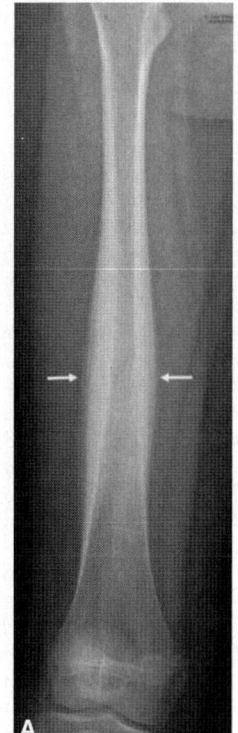

Figure 99.6 Multilamellar periosteal reaction (*arrows*) in a plain radiograph **(A)** and MRI axial T2-weighted image **(B)** of the femur of a young girl who presented with intermittent leg pain. Diagnostic considerations included Ewing sarcoma, osteomyelitis, osteosarcoma, and Langerhans cell histiocytosis. Open biopsy of the lesion revealed Ewing sarcoma.

lymphomas, and, less commonly, histiocytosis and small-cell osteosarcomas. Ewing cells have a high nuclear-to-cytoplasmic ratio and appear homogenous, with uniform round nuclei that contain evenly distributed chromatin and little mitotic activity.[415] The cytoplasm is typically scant and weakly eosinophilic; however, intracellular accumulation of glycogen may confer a positive periodic acid–Schiff test. Some tumors may demonstrate neuroectodermal differentiation. These tumors typically have Homer-Wright pseudorosettes on light microscopy and positive immunohistochemical staining for synaptophysin, neuron-specific enolase, S100, and CD57.[415] More than 95% of Ewing sarcomas express CD99 (encoded by the *MIC2* gene) on their cell membranes.[429] Although CD99 staining of the cell membranes in a honeycomb pattern is suggestive of Ewing sarcoma, it is not pathognomonic and may be seen in a variety of tumors, including synovial sarcoma, mesenchymal chondrosarcoma, and B-cell and T-cell leukemia/lymphoma.[437–440]

The rapid identification of *EWSR1* gene rearrangements by performing reverse transcription–polymerase chain reaction assays or fluorescence in situ hybridization assays on fresh, frozen, or paraffin-embedded specimens is useful for expeditiously discriminating between Ewing sarcoma and other morphologically similar small round cell tumors.[414]

Treatment

Chemotherapy. Ewing sarcoma is a very chemotherapy-sensitive tumor, and the outcome of patients with this disease has greatly improved as a result of intensifying systemic multiagent chemotherapy, particularly that of anthracycline and alkylating agents, as well as improvements in surgical and radiation techniques and supportive care (e.g., use of hematopoietic growth factors). Using current treatment strategies, over 70% of patients who present with localized disease are cured of their disease. However, the prognosis of patients with metastatic or recurrent disease remains poor, with a long-term survival rate of less than 30%.[441]

Localized Disease. Results of the major treatment trials for localized Ewing sarcoma are summarized in Table 99.13.[411,442–454] Early cooperative group studies using adjuvant chemotherapy documented the efficacy of a four-drug regimen with vincristine (V), actinomycin D (A), cyclophosphamide (C), and doxorubicin (D) in combination with local control measures. By using these strategies, survival rates were improved from less than 20% to more than 40%.[448,449] The next generation of studies confirmed the benefit of the addition of ifosfamide and etoposide in the treatment of Ewing sarcoma. A randomized phase III study conducted by the first American Intergroup Ewing trial (INT-0091/POG-8850/CCG-7881) demonstrated a superior outcome in patients with localized disease treated with VD(A)C alternating with ifosfamide (I) and etoposide (E) compared to VD(A)C alone (5-year EFS, 69% ± 3% versus 54 % ± 4% respectively, p = 0.005).[447] Similar improvements in survival with the addition of ifosfamide have been reported in studies by the National Cancer Institute and multiple European cooperative groups.[444,455,456]

Dose intensification of the VDC-IE regimen in a second intergroup POG-CCG study (CCG-7942/POG-9354) of nonmetastatic Ewing sarcoma showed that a dose-intensified 30-week treatment schedule did not improve EFS beyond that of the standard 48-week schedule.[446] However, a strategy of interval compression delivering the five-drug standard therapy (VDC-IE) in 30 weeks (chemotherapy every 14 days versus every 21 days) led to improved survival rates, with a median 5-year EFS rate of 73% for the compressed cohort and 65% for the patients treated every 21 days (see Table 99.13).[454]

In Europe, the collaborative study EURO-Ewing 99 is using risk-based stratification to assign patients into three risk groups based on tumor volume, presence, and pattern of metastatic disease, and histologic response to six cycles of four-drug induction chemotherapy (VIDE).[429,457] After induction therapy, the study includes two randomized comparisons: patients with localized disease having a good response (i.e., less than 10% viable tumor after VIDE) continue therapy with either VAC or VAI; patients with either large tumors (i.e., more than 200 mL) or tumors having a poor response (i.e., more than 10% viable tumor after VIDE) receive VAI or busulfan–melphalan megatherapy. This study is nearing completion of accrual (see Table 99.13).

Metastatic Disease. The treatment for patients who present with metastatic Ewing sarcoma is challenging. In contrast to the improvement in survival for patients with nonmetastatic disease, no comparable benefit from the addition of IE has been demonstrated for patients who present with metastatic disease. In the first CCG-POG intergroup study (INT-0091), 120 patients with metastatic disease were evaluated using treatment regimens similar to those previously described for nonmetastatic patients. The addition of ifosfamide and etoposide in the metastatic group provided no survival advantage for those who did or did not receive IE.[458] Results of studies testing dose-intensification strategies, including the use of total body irradiation and myeloablative chemotherapy followed by autologous stem cell rescue, have been disappointing.[436,459–463] The EURO-Ewing 99 study described previously had an additional arm (R3) for patients with newly diagnosed primary disseminated disease. Two-hundred and eighty-one patients were treated with six cycles of VIDE, one cycle of VAI, and then surgery and/or radiation followed by high-dose busulfan–melphalan and autologous stem cell transplant. The 3-year EFS rate of these patients was 27% ± 3%.[461] Poor prognostic factors included age of 14 years or older, tumor volume of 200 mL or more, increased number of bone metastases, and bone marrow and bone involvement.

Recurrent Disease. Although most patients with Ewing sarcoma can experience a complete response to multimodal therapy,

about 30% of patients with localized disease and more than 70% of those with metastatic disease at initial presentation experience recurrent disease. The median time to relapse in most studies is approximately 16 to 21 months from diagnosis.[464–466] The overall prognosis for these patients is dismal, with less than 20% survival. However, patients with early relapse (i.e., less than 2 years from diagnosis) fare worse than do those with late relapse (i.e., less than 10% survival).[464–466] In terms of long-term follow-up surveillance and counseling, it is important to recognize that recurrences of Ewing sarcoma can occur very late, more than 5 years from diagnosis.[467]

There is no established salvage regimen for patients with recurrent disease. Combination chemotherapy regimens of cyclophosphamide and topotecan[468–470]; irinotecan and temozolomide[471,472]; ifosfamide, carboplatin, and etoposide[473–475]; and gemcitabine and docetaxel[476] have demonstrated antitumor activity in the relapse setting. Myeloablative chemotherapy and, in some cases, total body irradiation have been attempted in an effort to improve the prognosis for patients with high-risk or relapsed disease, with only modest improvement in outcome and at the cost of significant toxicity.[477,478]

Local Control. Local control with surgical resection or high-dose radiotherapy in addition to chemotherapy is imperative for curative therapy in Ewing sarcoma. The inclusion of 12 to 15 weeks of systemic chemotherapy before the introduction of local control measures has become standard practice, regardless of tumor size, location, or stage, unless the tumor causes an immediate threat to survival, such as spinal cord compression or cardiopulmonary compromise. As of 2013, there has been no randomized trial to determine whether surgery or radiotherapy is superior in achieving local control. For decades, radiotherapy was the standard local treatment modality, but surgery is now the preferred modality if a complete resection is feasible.[479] In prospective but nonrandomized trials, the improved survival in the surgical resection group has generally been attributed to the allocation of larger tumors with a correspondingly poorer prognosis to the radiation group. In some situations, particularly in patients who are at high risk for local treatment failure after resection, a combination of surgery and radiation is warranted. Decisions about local control should take into account resectability, functional outcome, long-term morbidity, the risk of late-onset secondary malignancies in tissues exposed to high-dose radiotherapy, and patient preference. Factors that influence the success of local control include the initial location of the primary tumor, with central disease having a poorer prognosis, and initial tumor response to chemotherapy as shown by the percentage of tumor necrosis.[237]

Surgery. In general, patients with resectable primary tumors receive induction chemotherapy followed by definitive surgery alone. For extremity tumors, limb salvage is preferred; however, if limb salvage or irradiation are not feasible, then amputation is warranted. Central pelvic or spinal lesions are frequently treated with radiation alone because surgery with negative margins is often not feasible. Chest wall lesions often present as large tumors extending into the thoracic cavity. Preoperative chemotherapy can greatly reduce the size, vascularity, and friability of the tumor, facilitating resection and decreasing the risk of intraoperative tumor rupture.[480–482] Because surgical outcome is improved in patients receiving preoperative chemotherapy, they are less likely to require postoperative chest wall radiotherapy, which has well-established risks of cardiac and pulmonary damage and radiation-induced second malignancies.[483]

Radiation Therapy. Radiation therapy is delivered in either the adjuvant or definitive setting based on the finding of involved surgical margins or unresectable disease. The selection of patients for radiation therapy should be made by a multidisciplinary team involving orthopedic oncologists, pediatric oncologists, and pediatric

TABLE 99.13

Treatment Results in Selected Clinical Studies of Localized Ewing Sarcoma

Study (Reference)	Study Duration	Schedule	Patients	5-Year Event-Free Survival (%)[a]	p Value[a]	Comments
IESS Studies						
IESS-I[449]	1973–1978	VAC / VAC + WLI / VACD	342	24 / 44 / 60	VAC vs VAC + WLI, 0.001 / VAC vs VACD, 0.001 / VAC + WLI vs VACD, 0.05	Value of D; Benefit of WLI?
IESS-II[443]	1978–1982	VACD-HD / VACD-MD	214	68 / 48	0.03	Value of aggressive cytoreduction
INT-0091(POG-8850/CCG-7881)[447]	1988–1993	VACD / VACD + IE	200 / 198	54 / 69	0.005	Value of addition of IE
CCG-7942/POG-9354[446]	1995–1998	VDC + IE 48 wks / VDC + IE 30 wks	492	72 / 70	0.57	No benefit from dose escalation of alkylating agents
AEWS0031[454]	2001–2005	VDC + IE every 3 wks / VDC + IE every 2 wks	568	65 / 73	0.48	Value of interval compressed therapy
ROI, Bologna, Italy						
REN-3[442]	1991–1997	VDC + VIA + IE	157	71		Surgery in 78% of patients
SFOP, France						
EW-88[450]	1988–1991	VD + VD/VA	141	58		Histologic response better predictor of outcome than tumor volume
EW-93[453]	1993–1999	SR: VACD / IR: VACD + IE / HR: VD + IE + BuMel/ASCT	214	70 / 54 / 48		No advantage of IE in the IR group; potential benefit of BuMel/ASCT for HR group
UKCCSG/MRC Studies						
ET-1[445]	1978–1986	VACD	120	41: extremity, 52; axial, 38; pelvic, 13		Tumor site as the most important prognostic factor
ET-2[444]	1987–1993	VAID	201	62: extremity, 73; axial, 55; pelvic, 41		Importance of the administration of high-dose alkylating agents (I)
CESS Studies						
CESS-81[448]	1981–1985	VACD	93	55: <100 mL, 80; ≥100 mL 31 (both 3 yr) / Viable tumor <10, 79; >.10, 31 (both 3 yr)		Tumor volume (< or ≥100 mL) and histologic response are prognostic factors
CESS-86[451]	1986–1991	SR: VACD / HR: VAID	301	52 (10 yr) / 51 (10 yr)		Benefit of intensive treatment with I for high-risk patients (≥100 mL or central axis)
EICESS Studies (CESS + UKCCSG)						
EICESS-92[666]	1992–1999	SR: VAID vs VACD / HR: VAID vs EVAID	155 / 326	68 vs 67 / 51 vs 61	0.8406 / 0.2141	Randomized comparisons not significant; suggestion that addition of etoposide increased survival in HR group

IESS, Intergroup Ewing Sarcoma Study; V, vincristine; A, actinomycin D; C, cyclophosphamide; D, doxorubicin; WLI, whole-lung irradiation; HD, high dose; MD, moderate dose; I, ifosfamide; E, etoposide; SR, standard risk; IR, intermediate risk; HR, high risk; ASCT, autologous stem cell transplant; ROI, Rizzoli Orthopaedic Institute; SFOP, French Society of Paediatric Oncology; CESS, Cooperative Ewing Sarcoma Studies; UKCCSG, United Kingdom Children's Cancer Study Group; MRC, Medical Research Council; EICESS, European Intergroup Cooperative Ewing Sarcoma Studies.

[a] P values are given only for trials comparing randomized treatment arms. Values are for 5-year survival unless otherwise noted.

PRACTICE OF ONCOLOGY

radiation oncologists in order to best select a local control approach that maximizes the potential for high rates of local control with minimal toxicity. Modern radiation treatment techniques are now used that rely on CT simulation, target delineation, and treatment techniques, including conformal radiation therapy, intensity modulated radiation therapy, and proton beam radiation therapy.

The dose of radiation prescribed is dependent on the volume of the disease. Patients undergoing surgical resection with microscopically involved surgical margins (either after induction chemotherapy or at diagnosis) should receive adjuvant radiation therapy to the tumor bed to a dose of 50.4 Gy at 1.8 Gy per treatment fraction daily. Patients with gross disease present at the time of radiation therapy should be treated to doses of 55.8 Gy at 1.8 Gy per treatment fraction. Patients with no tumor present at the surgical margin but a poor histologic response to preoperative chemotherapy may also benefit from adjuvant radiation therapy.[484] Other primary site prognostic factors that negatively impact local or overall disease control include the size of the tumor (≥8 cm) and the pelvic site of the disease.[485–487] Patients with these prognostic factors that place them at high risk for local failure are candidates for more aggressive surgical resections and radiation dose escalation on clinical trials.

Ewing sarcoma was historically treated with large radiation portals and POG prospectively evaluated whole-bone (i.e., conventional) irradiation compared with tailored treatment fields, and a published analysis of this trial supports the efficacy of a more limited treatment volume as defined by prechemotherapy tumor extent.[488] Modern treatment volumes for patients requiring radiation include all areas of gross disease, including areas the tumor initially infiltrated at diagnosis and the initially involved bone. Patients undergoing surgical resection, but still requiring adjuvant radiation should have the tumor bed or surgical cavity targeted. These target volumes should be expanded by 1 to 1.5 cm to account for microscopic spread of disease and treated to the doses indicated previously. The timing of radiation therapy usually occurs after the initial 12 weeks of chemotherapy. The risk of secondary sarcomas arising in irradiated bone is reported as being from 5% to 10% at 20 years from diagnosis. In patients treated with doses of 60 Gy or more, a significant excess risk of secondary bone sarcomas has been reported compared to the risk in those patients treated with doses below 48 Gy.[489]

Ewing sarcoma is one of few diseases in which radiation therapy is used curatively for metastatic disease. Whole-lung irradiation has proven effective for the consolidation of lung metastases after chemotherapy. Multiple trials have demonstrated superior EFS and OS rates when whole-lung radiation is given.[479] Paulussen et al.[490] analyzed patients in three cooperative Ewing sarcoma studies and found that the EFS rate was significantly higher for patients who received whole-lung irradiation. Whole-lung doses between 15 and 18 Gy are used with minimal acute toxicity to treat patients after initial chemotherapy.

Prognostic Factors

The most important prognostic factor for outcome still remains the presence of metastatic disease at diagnosis. Patients with isolated pulmonary metastases do better (about 30% disease-free survival) than those with bone or bone marrow metastases (about 20% disease-free survival), but all fare worse than patients with nonmetastatic disease.[447,491,492] Large tumor size and volume and high serum LDH levels at diagnosis correlate with an adverse outcome in some studies.[430,431,487] Children with nonmetastatic pelvic primary sites also have a poorer prognosis than children with primary tumors of the extremities, although this difference may be related to the larger size and more difficult resectability of pelvic tumors.[491]

Although not a prognostic factor assessable at the time of diagnosis, the histologic response to chemotherapy appears to be a strong predictor of treatment outcome. Poor histologic response (<90% tumor necrosis) correlates with a poor prognosis, whereas complete or near complete tumor necrosis correlates with good outcome, with a 5-year EFS rate of 84% to 95%.[493,494]

As understanding of the molecular pathogenesis of Ewing sarcoma continues to increase, other prognostic markers, such as those derived from genetic expression analyses of primary and metastatic tumors, may identify genetic signatures that allow for the stratification of disease into low- and high-risk subgroups.[495,496] These studies may also provide clues as to which patients may benefit from various targeted therapies.

RHABDOMYOSARCOMA

Epidemiology and Genetics

Rhabdomyosarcoma is the most common soft tissue sarcoma in children, accounting for 3% to 4% of all cases of childhood cancer and for approximately 350 new cancer cases each year in patients younger than 20 years of age.[1,182,183] Rhabdomyosarcoma is more common in males and Caucasians, and two-thirds of cases occur in patients under the age of 10 years with a median age at diagnosis of 5 years.[497] Although most cases of rhabdomyosarcoma are sporadic, there are several genetic and environmental factors that have been associated with a heightened risk of developing the disease, including:

- Germ-line P53 mutations[498]
- Costello syndrome[499]
- Beckwith-Wiedemann syndrome[500]
- Neurofibromatosis type I[501]
- Germ-line DICER1 mutations[502]
- Parental use of cocaine and marijuana[503]
- Birthing order and accelerated in utero growth[504,505]

Although rhabdomyosarcoma can arise in multiple sites of the body, the most common sites in decreasing order of frequency include the head and neck (including the orbit and parameningeal areas [35%]), the genitourinary tract (including the bladder, prostate, vagina, vulva, uterus, and paratesticular area [26%]), and extremities (19%).[10] Only about 20% of children with rhabdomyosarcoma present with disseminated disease, which most commonly involves the lung.[506]

Pathology and Molecular Biology

The International Classification of Rhabdomyosarcoma recognizes three main categories of rhabdomyosarcoma:[507]

1. Superior prognosis (both are variants of embryonal rhabdomyosarcoma):
   a. Botryoid
   b. Spindle cell
2. Intermediate prognosis
   a. Embryonal rhabdomyosarcoma
3. Poorer prognosis
   a. Alveolar rhabdomyosarcoma
   b. Undifferentiated sarcoma

In contrast, the World Health Organization recognizes four variants of rhabdomyosarcoma and these subtypes, including embryonal, alveolar, pleomorphic, and spindle cell/sclerosing rhabdomyosarcoma.[508] The presence of focal and diffuse anaplasia can be documented in about 13% of cases of rhabdomyosarcoma, and its presence may be of prognostic significance in patients with intermediate-risk embryonal rhabdomyosarcoma.[509] In children and adolescents, the two most common types of rhabdomyosarcoma are the embryonal (65%) and alveolar (25%) subtypes and each of these entities have unique clinical and biologic features that will be described in more detail.[510,511]

Embryonal tumors have a more favorable clinical outcome, often affect younger male patients, and most commonly arise in the head, neck, and genitourinary regions (Fig. 99.7).[497,507,512] The botryoid variant of rhabdomyosarcoma resembles a bunch of grapes and characteristically arises in hollow organs such as the bladder, the biliary tract, the vagina, and occasionally, the conjunctiva and ear.[507,513] In children, spindle cell tumors most commonly arise in the paratesticular area, whereas the sclerosing variant has been reported to more commonly affect the extremities and the head and neck region.[508,514] Embryonal tumors are characterized by a loss of heterozygosity at the imprinted 11p15 locus, resulting in a loss of the maternal allele and duplication of the paternal allele that encodes the IGF-2 growth factor and is believed to participate in rhabdomyosarcoma tumorigenesis. This loss of imprinting also suggest that inactivation of a tumor suppressor gene at the maternal locus may promote tumorigenesis.[515,516] Embryonal tumors are characterized by a high background mutation rate and overall number of single-nucleotide variants (see Fig. 99.7) as well a multiple chromosomal gains and losses most often involving chromosome 8 gains (74% of cases). Gains of chromosomes 2, 7, 11, 12, 13q21, and 20 as well as losses of 1p36, 6, 9q22,14q21, and 17 have been reported.[517,518] Activating RAS pathway mutations involving KRAS, NRAS, and HRAS have been documented in 42% of cases of embryonal rhabdomyosarcoma.[519] Mutations involving the FGFR4, ALK, BRAF, CTNNB1, PIK3CA, and PTPN11 genes have been described less frequently.[520,521] Embryonal tumors have also been reported to have MDM2 amplification,[517] loss of PTEN, BCL2L1 amplification, homozygous deletions of CDKN2B, increased GLI expression, NF1 deletions, and ALK copy number gains.[519,521] In contrast to patients with embryonal tumors, children with alveolar tumors have a worse clinical outcome and their tumors more commonly arise in the trunk and extremities (see Fig. 99.7).[512,522] Genomically, these tumors are characterized by a t(2;13) (q35;q14) or t(1;13) (p36;q14), in which the PAX3 gene on the long arm of chromosome 2 or the PAX7 gene in chromosome

1 is fused with the FOXO1 gene on the long arm of chromosome 13 (see Fig. 99.7).[523] In addition, ALK gene copy number gains are seen in the majority of cases of alveolar rhabdomyosarcoma, and copy number gains and overexpression of MYCN have been associated with an adverse clinical outcome in this disease.[521,524] Approximately 18% of alveolar rhabdomyosarcomas lack FOXO1 rearrangements[510] and are termed fusion-negative alveolar rhabdomyosarcomas. These patients clinically behave more like patients with embryonal tumors, suggesting that the presence of a PAX/FOXO1 fusion is a key determinant of clinical behavior and should be incorporated into the risk stratification of the disease.[517,525]

Diagnosis and Staging

Given the heterogeneous location of this tumor, rhabdomyosarcoma can cause a variety of signs and symptoms. Head and neck tumors, which comprise about one-third of all cases of rhabdomyosarcoma, can present with proptosis, ophthalmoplegia, nasal drainage, and obstruction, headache, cranial nerve palsies, dysphonia, dysphagia, and palpable adenopathy.[526] Patients with genitourinary tumors, which account for 25% of cases of rhabdomyosarcoma, can present with hematuria, dysuria, hydronephrosis palpable abdominal mass, vaginal discharge, and palpable painless masses.[526] Tumors in the extremities, which account for about 20% of cases of rhabdomyosarcoma, can present with swelling, palpable adenopathy, and pain.[526] Tumors on the trunk, pelvis, and abdomen can present with nerve root compression, palpable mass or adenopathy, jaundice (biliary tract tumors), and perirectal pain and swelling.[526,527]

A staging evaluation should include a complete blood count, serum chemistries, bone or PET scan, bilateral bone marrow aspirates and biopsies, CT of the chest, CT or MRI of the primary tumor, and CT or MRI of abdomen and pelvis for abdominal, pelvic, and lower extremity tumors. A recent report from the COG

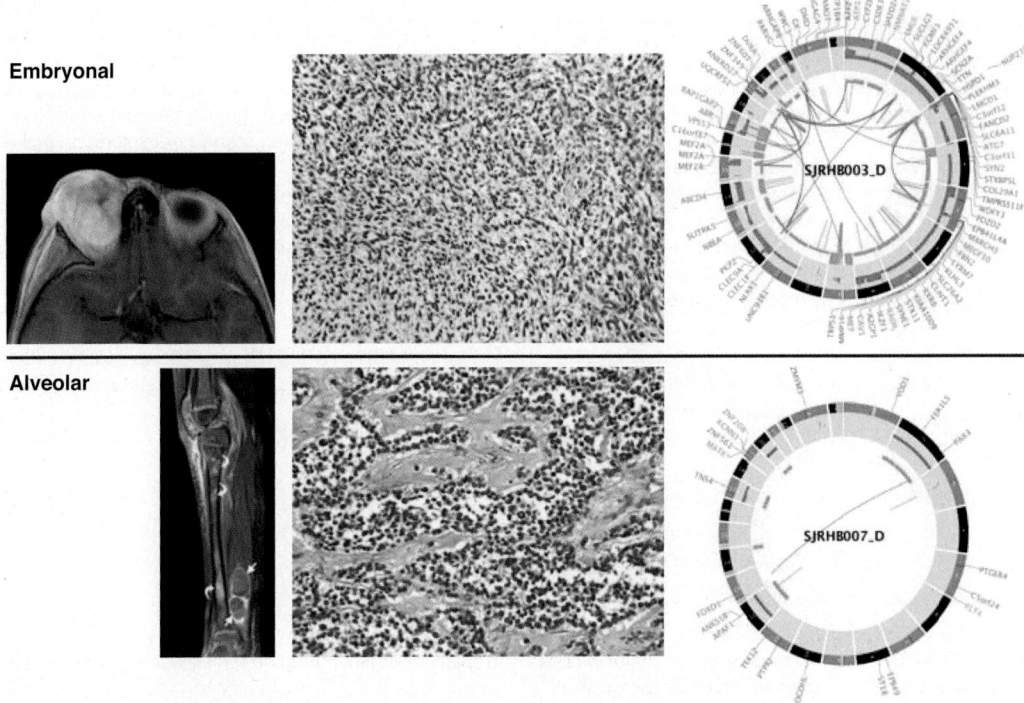

Figure 99.7 Clinical, histologic, and genomic features of embryonal and alveolar rhabdomyosarcoma.

suggests that up to one-third of patients with rhabdomyosarcoma, specifically those with embryonal noninvasive node-negative disease can be spared an extensive metastatic evaluation that includes a bone marrow examination and a bone scan.[528] Studies investigating the role of PET scan in initial staging and as a predictor of clinical outcome in pediatric rhabdomyosarcoma are ongoing.[529,530] Routine cranial imaging is not indicated unless there is evidence of spinal involvement and cerebrospinal fluid examination should be reserved for patients with parameningeal primaries.[531] Following a biopsy, a routine evaluation of regional nodes should be reserved for patients with extremity tumors and those with paratesticular tumors who are older than 10 years of age.[532] Sentinel node biopsy is increasingly being used to assess nodal involvement in patients with extremity tumors.[533]

Patients with rhabdomyosarcoma are staged using a surgicopathologic grouping system as well as a pretreatment staging system as shown in Tables 99.14 and 99.15.[534,535] About 16% of patients have group I disease (completely resected), 20% have group II disease (microscopic residual), 48% have group III disease (incompletely resected), and 16% present with group IV disease (metastatic).[536] In addition, all patients should be staged using the pretreatment tumor, regional nodes, metastasis (TNM) staging system, which stratifies patients into four different categories based on the site of the primary tumor, tumor size, presence or absence of nodal and distant disease, and invasiveness. Using both

systems in addition to histologic subtype, pediatric rhabdomyosarcoma can be classified into three distinct risk groups (Table 99.16). Patients with low-risk disease, which account for about one-third of cases can be further subdivided into two subsets as shown in Table 99.16.[537] Patients with intermediate risk account for about 50% of cases, and those with high-risk disease account for about 16% of cases (see Table 99.16).

Prognostic Factors

Clinical group, stage, histologic subtype, age, and treatment (see Table 99.16) are the most important predictors of outcome in childhood rhabdomyosarcoma.[538] Patients with low-risk disease (embryonal tumors stage 1 through 3 group I, II and stage 1 group III) are expected to have a 5-year OS rate in excess of 95%.[539] Patients with intermediate-risk disease (stage 2, 3 group III embryonal and stage 1 through 3 group I through III alveolar) have an estimated 4-year EFS of about 70% and the outcome of these patients has not changed significantly over time.[540] Certain subsets of patients with intermediate-risk embryonal tumors such as those with T2 tumors, extremity primaries, and age <1 year and ≥10 years have a poorer clinical outcome.[538] Similarly, patients with intermediate-risk alveolar tumors who present with stage 3 group III N1 disease have a particularly poor prognosis.[538] Patients with high-risk disease

---

TABLE 99.14

Intergroup Rhabdomyosarcoma Study (IRS) Clinical Grouping Classification

Group I: Localized disease, completely resected

(Regional nodes not involved: Lymph node biopsy or dissection is required except for head and neck lesions)
(a) Confined to muscle or organ of origin.
(b) Contiguous involvement; infiltration outside the muscle or organ of origin, as through fascial planes.

NOTATION: This includes both gross inspection and microscopic confirmation of complete resection. Any nodes that may be inadvertently taken with the specimen must be negative. If the latter should be involved microscopically, then the patient is placed in the Group IIb or IIc (see the following).

Group II: Total gross resection with evidence of regional spread

(a) Grossly resected tumor with microscopic residual disease.
(Surgeon believes that he has removed all of the tumor, but the pathologist finds tumor at the margin of resection and additional resection to achieve clean margin is not feasible.) No evidence of gross residual tumor. No evidence of regional node involvement. Once radiotherapy and/or chemotherapy have been started, reexploration and removal of the area of microscopic residual does not change the patient's group.
(b) Regional disease with involved nodes, completely resected with no microscopic residual.

NOTATION: Complete resection with microscopic confirmation of no residual disease makes this different from Groups IIa and IIc. Additionally, in contrast to Group IIa, regional nodes (which are completely resected, however) are involved, but the most distal node is histologically negative.

(c) Regional disease with involved nodes, grossly resected, but with evidence of microscopic residual and/or histologic involvement of the most distal regional node (from the primary site) in the dissection.

NOTATION: The presence of microscopic residual disease makes this group different from 2b, and nodal involvement makes this group different from Group 2a.

Group III: Incomplete resection with gross residual disease

(a) After biopsy only
(b) After gross or major resection of the primary (>50%)

Group IV: Distant metastatic disease present at onset

(Lung, liver, bones, bone marrow, brain, and distant muscle and nodes)
NOTATION: The previous excludes regional nodes and adjacent organ infiltration which places the patient in a more favorable grouping (as noted under Group II).

Note: The presence of positive cytology in cerebrospinal fluid (CSF), pleural or abdominal fluids, as well as implants on pleural or peritoneal surfaces are regarded as indications for placing the patient in Group IV.

TABLE 99.15

Tumor, Regional Nodes, Metastasis Pretreatment Staging Classification for Rhabdomyosarcoma

Stage	Sites	Tumor	Size	Node	Metastasis
1	Orbit Head and neck (excluding parameningeal) GU, nonbladder/nonprostate biliary tract	T_1 or T_2	a or b	N_0 or N_1 or N_x	M_0
2	Bladder/prostate, extremity, cranial parameningeal, other (includes trunk, retroperitoneum, etc.) (excludes biliary tract)	T_1 or T_2	a	N_0 or N_x	M_0
3	Bladder/prostate, extremity, cranial parameningeal, other (includes trunk, retroperitoneum, etc.) (excludes biliary tract)	T_1 or T_2	a b	N_1 N_0 or N_1 or N_x	M_0 M_0
4	All	T_1 or T_2	a or b	N_0 or N_1	M_1

Definitions:

Tumor	T(site)$_1$	Confirmed to anatomic site of origin (a) ≤5 cm in diameter in size (b) >5 cm in diameter in size
	T(site)$_2$	Extension and/or fixative to surrounding tissue (a) ≤5 cm in diameter in size (b) >5 cm in diameter in size
Regional Nodes	N_0	Regional nodes not clinically involved
	N_1	Regional nodes clinically involved by neoplasm
	N_x	Clinical status of regional nodes unknown (especially sites that preclude lymph node evaluation)
Metastasis	M_0	No distant metastasis
	M_1	Metastasis present

GU, Genitourinary.

continue to fare poorly with less than 30% of patients expected to be disease-free at 3 years following diagnosis.[541] Children with high-risk disease who are between 1 and 9 years of age, present with a favorable primary tumor, have less than three metastatic sites, and no evidence of bone or bone marrow disease have an expected 5-year failure-free survival of about 50%.[541] Recent studies have confirmed that the presence of PAX/FOXO1 fusions are the main determinant of clinical outcome and that previously identified metagene sets derived from gene-expression profiles were largely dominated by the effect of fusion status.[525] Several reports suggest that the presence of a PAX7/FOXO1 rearrangement is associated with a better clinical outcome, but these findings need to be confirmed in larger prospective studies.[525,542]

Management

Principles of Therapy

As previously mentioned, the management of rhabdomyosarcoma requires a multidisciplinary team, and current therapy is assigned according to three distinct risk groups (low, intermediate, and high) that incorporate information regarding stage, clinical group, and histology of the tumor (see Table 99.16)[537].

Local Therapy

Surgical considerations for the treatment of rhabdomyosarcoma are site specific, and given the high degree of chemosensitivity of these tumors, extensive surgeries in certain sites such as the orbit, the bladder, the vagina, and the biliary tract are unwarranted.[527] When feasible, reexcision of positive margins in patients with extremity and trunk primaries is associated with improved survival.[543] Second-look surgeries in selected patients may help identify and resect the residual viable tumor and convert patients with a partial or minor radiographic response into a complete response either reducing or eliminating the need for radiotherapy.[8,537,544] It is estimated that about 60% of patients with residual radiographic abnormalities will have evidence of a viable tumor at the time of second-look surgery, and this finding is associated with an inferior failure-free survival, particularly if microscopic or gross residual disease is left behind.[8] In addition, the results of second-look procedures can

TABLE 99.16

Risk Subgroups of Rhabdomyosarcoma

Risk	Proportion of Patients	Stage	Group	Histology	5-Year Event-Free Survival	Therapy
Low subset 1	30%	1,2	I–II III orbit	Embryonal	90%	VA ± C ± RT
Low subset 2	30%	1 3	III nonorbit I,II	Embryonal	87%	VA ± C ± RT
Intermediate	55%	2,3 1,2,3	III I–III	Embryonal Alveolar	65%–73%	VAC ± other agent + RT
High	15%	4	IV	Embryonal and alveolar	<30%	VAC ± other agents + RT

V, vincristine; A, actinomycin D; C, cyclophosphamide; RT, Radiotherapy.

help tailor the dose or eliminate the use of radiotherapy in selected cases.[8,537,542] The use of debulking procedures has a very limited role in the management of rhabdomyosarcoma, although one report suggests that patients with debulking may improve the survival of patients with embryonal retroperitoneal tumors.[6,545]

Radiotherapy should be administered to all children with the exception of those with group I embryonal tumors. A recent report also suggests that patients with stage 1, 2 group I alveolar tumors can be spared the use of radiotherapy.[546] The use of conformal radiotherapy or hyperfractionated radiotherapy does not improve local control.[547,548] The recommended doses for node-negative microscopic residual disease are 36 Gy and 41.4 Gy for those with microscopic disease and pathologically proven but grossly negative nodal disease. For a gross residual tumor, the recommended dose is 45 Gy for orbital and 50.4 Gy for nonorbital primary sites. The selection of reduced doses of radiation for patients with orbital sites of involvement is supported by the D9602 trial where the use of reduced doses of radiotherapy without an alkylating agent in patients with embryonal group IIA and orbital group III tumors did not compromise local control rates (~15% local failure).[549] The treatment volumes for patients requiring radiation include all areas of gross disease, including areas the tumor initially infiltrated at diagnosis. Patients undergoing surgical resection, but still necessitating adjuvant radiation should have the tumor bed or surgical cavity targeted. These target volumes should be expanded by 1 cm to account for the microscopic spread of disease and treated to the doses indicated previously. The timing of radiation therapy usually occurs after the initial 12 or 18 weeks of chemotherapy based on whether that patient has localized or metastatic disease. Several attempts have been made to eliminate the need for radiation therapy in very young patients due to the risks of late toxicity from radiation. Although a delay of radiation therapy in very young patients may be considered if the patient's clinical response is acceptable (both maximizing the age of the patient at the time of radiation and minimizing the volume of the radiation targets), the elimination of radiation altogether based on a complete chemotherapeutic response should not be considered outside of a clinical trial. In the D9602 trial, patients with group III vaginal tumors experienced unacceptably high local failure rates in excess of 60% when they followed a response-based approach that attempted to eliminate radiation therapy without the use of higher dose cyclophosphamide.[550]

Systemic Therapy

Chemotherapy

All children with rhabdomyosarcoma should receive chemotherapy. The most common regimen used in North America consists of vincristine, actinomycin D, and cyclophosphamide (VAC); ifosfamide is preferentially used in the European trials.[512,551] Other agents such as topotecan, melphalan, methotrexate, ifosfamide, etoposide, irinotecan, and doxorubicin have also proven active, but their addition to VAC regimens failed to improve outcomes in intermediate and high risk patients.[552] See Table 99.16 for the current outcomes and treatment recommendations for patients with low-, intermediate-, and high-risk tumors.[537] For low-risk patients, who account for one-third of all cases of rhabdomyosarcoma, the administration of VA or VAC with or without radiotherapy is associated with survival rates in excess of 90%. Because of the excellent prognosis, the recently completed trial ARST 0331 for low-risk patients examined the feasibility of limiting the duration of therapy and the exposure to alkylating agents; preliminary results are only available in abstract form. Patients with intermediate-risk disease comprise about half of all patients with rhabdomyosarcoma and their survival depending on stage, group, and histology ranges from 59% to 83%.[540] The use of alternating drug combinations with VAC and irinotecan is currently being investigated in the D9803 COG trial. Despite marked improvements in survival of nonmetastatic patients, survival for the remaining 16% of high-risk patients who present with metastatic disease has remained unchanged during the past 30 years. End intensification with high-dose chemotherapy, dose intensification of alkylating agents, and integration of novel agents has failed to improve survival in these patients.[552,553] The Soft Tissue Sarcoma Committee of COG has relied on preclinical xenograft models to identify potentially active agents and to translate these findings into frontline window studies for children with previously untreated poor prognosis rhabdomyosarcoma, and the current high-risk trial is investigating the addition of temozolomide and IGF-1R inhibitors to standard chemotherapy.[554,555]

Less than one-third of children who develop a recurrence of rhabdomyosarcoma are expected to survive long term; however, patients who had stage 1 group I embryonal tumors at diagnosis and experienced a localized relapse >18 months from diagnosis have a higher likelihood of cure.[556,557]

HEPATOBLASTOMA

Epidemiology

Approximately two-thirds of primary liver tumors in children are malignant, and they account for 1.1% of all cancers in children less than 20 years old (see Fig. 99.1).[183]

Hepatoblastoma is the most common, accounting for two-thirds of all pediatric liver cancers, with hepatocellular carcinoma accounting for the vast majority of the remaining cases.[558] The incidence rates for hepatoblastoma have steadily increased over time, doubling from 0.8 per million from 1975 to 1979 to 1.5 per million from 1990 to 1995, and more recently, increasing at a rate of 4.3% (95% CI, 0.2% to 8.7%) annually.[558,559] In contrast, the incidence of hepatocellular carcinoma (HCC) has decreased from 0.6 per million to 0.2 per million.[1]

Hepatoblastoma accounts for over 90% of all malignant liver tumors in children under the age of 5 years, and is slightly more common in males (1.2:1) and Caucasian children.[558,560,561] The median age at presentation is 16 to 18 months.[562,563] The most common risk factors for the development of hepatoblastoma include low birth weight,[564,565] familial adenomatous polyposis coli (FAP),[566,567] BWS,[40] and hemihypertrophy.[568] There are also several case reports suggesting a predisposition for hepatoblastoma in children with trisomy 18.[569,570]

Genetic Abnormalities

Most cases of hepatoblastoma are sporadic. Only about 15% of hepatoblastoma patients have genetic syndromes, the most common of these being FAP.[571] The risk for developing hepatoblastoma in FAP families is up to 800 times higher than that of the general population[566,572] and, in two studies, up to 10% of patients with sporadic hepatoblastoma had germ-line mutations of the APC gene.[566,573] Thus, screening of all families of hepatoblastoma patients for FAP may be appropriate.[567,573] Other common recurring genetic changes in hepatoblastoma include gains of whole chromosomes, particularly 2, 8 and 20,[571,574] and up to 18% have unbalanced translocations involving chromosome 1.[574-576]

Prematurity has been increasingly recognized as a risk factor for the development of hepatoblastoma, and in one Japanese study, hepatoblastoma accounted for nearly 60% of all cancers seen in premature babies weighing less than 1,000 g at birth.[577] In another study, a clear correlation between a rising rate in hepatoblastoma and the percentage of low- and very low-birth-weight newborns was documented.[578] A case-controlled study is currently being conducted by the COG to better delineate the role of prematurity and other factors in the development of hepatoblastoma.

Pathology

Hepatoblastoma is an embryonal tumor that is thought to arise from a liver stem cell.[579,580] Thus, tumors have various combinations of epithelial, mesenchymal, embryonal, macrotrabecular, and undifferentiated cells.[581] Although there is no consensus classification system, two pathologic subtypes have been identified with very different prognoses: (1) pure fetal histology and (2) small cell undifferentiated (SCU). Pure fetal tumors are composed of sheets of cells that resemble fetal hepatocytes, have minimal mitotic activity (<2/10 high-power × 400 microscopic fields) and commonly contain clusters of hematopoietic precursors.[581] These tumors are curable with surgery alone.[582] At the other end of the spectrum are SCU tumors, accounting for less than 5% of all hepatoblastomas.[581] These tumors are often associated with low alpha-fetoprotein (AFP) at diagnosis (<100 ng/mL)[583] and may lack SMARCB1/INI1 nuclear expression,[584] suggesting that a subset of these tumors may be malignant rhabdoid tumors, rather than hepatoblastomas.

Clinical Presentation

Patients most commonly present with a palpable asymptomatic abdominal mass. Other common symptoms include nausea, vomiting, anorexia, and weight loss; jaundice is uncommon. Patients presenting with fatigue may also be anemic, and acute abdominal pain may indicate tumor rupture. Hepatoblastoma patients can present with isosexual precocity, as a consequence of elevations of β-human chorionic gonadotropin (HCG), and hemihypertrophy can be seen in up to 10% of patients.[585] The presenting physical findings in children with HCC are similar to those encountered in patients with hepatoblastoma.

Evaluation and Staging

A laboratory evaluation should include a complete blood count, tests of renal and hepatic function, and urinalysis. Thrombocytosis is not uncommon in children presenting with hepatoblastoma, presumably a result of thrombopoietin production by the tumor.[586,587] The serum levels of total bilirubin, alkaline phosphatase, and alanine aminotransferase and aspartate aminotransferase are not generally useful for the differential diagnosis of malignant hepatic tumors in children. Serum levels of AFP are elevated in approximately 90% of patients with hepatoblastoma and in 67% (29 out of 43) of children with HCC in the last COG trial[588] and 70% (28 out of 40) of children with HCC in SIOPEL1.[563,589] A very low or high value (<100 ng/L or >1,000,000 ng/L) at diagnosis as well as a low early decline (<1 log) prior to definitive surgery has been associated with poor prognosis in hepatoblastoma.[590,591] If the diagnosis of HCC is established, testing for hepatitis B surface antigen, hepatitis B antibody, serum iron, total iron-binding capacity, serum ferritin, and α_1-antitrypsin should be performed. The initial radiographic evaluation often is with an abdominal ultrasound. However, a CT and/or an MRI are required for a definitive evaluation of the mass. A multiphase CT may ultimately be obtained to further define the anatomic relationship of the tumor to adjacent blood vessels—information that may be critical in surgical planning. In addition, this type of study may further suggest the most likely tumor histology. PET/CT may also be a useful modality.[592] The evaluation should also include a CT of the chest to search for metastases.[593]

The staging system used in therapeutic studies of hepatic tumors conducted by the COG segregates patients according to the resectability of the primary tumor and the presence or absence of metastatic disease.[594,595]

The European SIOP Liver Tumor Study Group (SIOPEL) uses a pretreatment extent of disease (PRETEXT) staging system (Fig. 99.8).[596,597]

This preoperative classification scheme identifies four PRETEXT categories reflecting the number of sections of the liver free of tumor and describes extension of disease into portal and hepatic veins, the vena cava, or intra-abdominal extrahepatic sites. A recent study comparing both staging systems suggests that the PRETEXT and COG systems can accurately predict survival in patients who might benefit from upfront surgical resection and reduced therapy

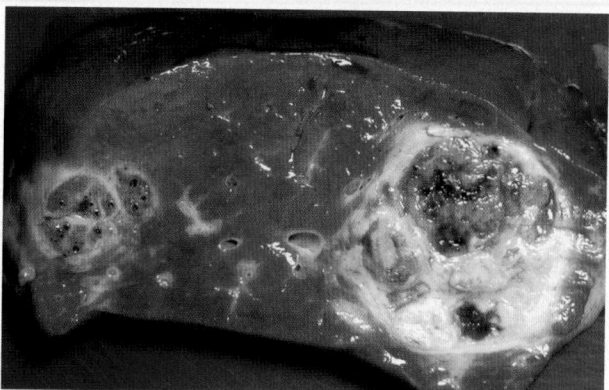

Figure 99.8 Liver resection of a patient with pretreatment extent of disease (PRETEXT) stage IV disease who underwent a successful liver transplant. The resected specimen shows multiple areas of viable tumor.

as well as patients with unresectable disease who are at increased risk of death.[595]

Prognostic Factors

The initial extent of disease (Staging; COG or SIOPEL)[595,598] and tumor resectability[599] as well as AFP values at diagnosis (less than 100 ng/L[583,600] or >1,000,000 ng/mL[591]), histology (pure fetal[582] or small cell undifferentiated histology[601]) are the main predictors of outcome in hepatoblastomas.[595] The presence of vascular involvement by the tumor is an additional adverse factor that has been used by the SIOPEL to classify patients as high risk. However, in a multivariate analysis, this did not hold up, perhaps because these patients often also have higher PRETEXT stage and/or metastatic disease.[600] In children with HCC, tumor resectability is essentially the only prognostic factor.[588,589] In adult patients, other important prognostic factors include cirrhosis, tumor size, the presence of metastases, satellite lesions, vascular invasion, or invasion of the tumor capsule.[602,603]

Treatment

Surgery

Complete tumor resection is essential for a cure.[599,604–607] Unfortunately, fewer than half of patients with hepatoblastoma[594] and less than 20% of children with HCC have resectable disease at the time of diagnosis.[588,589,608] Among the factors that render a liver tumor unresectable include invasion or close proximity to major vessels or involvement of both lobes.[604] Treatment with chemotherapy before definitive surgery has allowed for complete tumor resection in more than two-thirds of children whose hepatoblastomas were initially deemed unresectable.[594,609,610] In contrast, HCC is much less responsive to chemotherapy, limiting the effectiveness of preoperative pharmacologic intervention. In the SIOPEL report, all but two patients received preoperative chemotherapy and 36% (14 out of 40) eventually had gross total resection.[589] When feasible, aggressive attempts at the initial resection of HCC should be pursued.

Liver transplantation has been used by several centers for children with unresectable hepatoblastoma, with 10-year survival rates in excess of 80% for those who underwent this procedure as "primary" surgical therapy.[611–613]

This approach has also been used for patients with HCC.[589,614–619] Chemoembolization and/or radiofrequency ablation of hepatic malignancies has been increasingly used in adults with HCC.[620] Their overall role in the treatment of pediatric HCC remains to be defined.[621–623]

Radiation Therapy

Traditionally, radiation therapy has had a limited role in the treatment of hepatoblastoma or HCC given the low tolerance that the normal liver has for radiation. In the era of image-guided radiotherapy, radiation may be delivered to liver tumors with less hepatotoxicity.[624,625] Not much information is available in children regarding the use of radiotherapy in hepatoblastoma or HCC. In one report, doses of 25 to 45 Gy were associated with six of eight children with incompletely resected hepatoblastomas surviving after multimodality treatment.[626]

Chemotherapy

Before the identification of active chemotherapy, more than half of all children with hepatoblastoma were not amenable to surgical resection because of either extensive intrahepatic disease or the presence of extrahepatic metastases. Chemotherapy has enabled the successful surgical resection of many of these patients, resulting in cure rates approaching 80% in patients who have successful complete resections.[627–629] Thus, the role of chemotherapy in the treatment of hepatoblastoma is well established.[594,627,629–632] The most active agent is cisplatin.[627] Other active agents include doxorubicin, vincristine, 5-fluorouricil, carboplatin, etoposide and ifosfamide,[594,632–636] and more recently, irinotecan.[637,638] A randomized study using cisplatin-based chemotherapy demonstrated that the combination of doxorubicin and cisplatin was equivalent to the combination of cisplatin, vincristine, and 5-fluorouracil (CFV),

but the latter triplet was associated with less myelosuppression, toxic deaths, and a decreased need for prolonged hyperalimentation.[594] Thus, the latter regimen has become the standard for treating patients in North America. In Europe, SIOPEL preferentially used a cisplatin–doxorubicin-containing regimen (Table 99.17).[598]

A recent SIOPEL prospective randomized trial suggests, however, that patients with localized hepatoblastoma who have three or less liver sectors involved can be successfully treated with single-agent cisplatin.[627] A significantly worse outcome was recently reported by investigators of the COG when carboplatin and cisplatin were alternated in newly diagnosed patients with advanced-stage disease (see Table 99.17), suggesting that platinum intensification in this manner was ineffective.[639] The primary role of cisplatin in the treatment of hepatoblastoma was further corroborated by the recent SIOPEL report in which dose-intensive single-agent cisplatin (given every 2 weeks) was as effective as the combination of cisplatin and doxorubicin in children younger than 16 years of age with standard-risk hepatoblastoma.[627]

The 5-year EFS for patients with hepatoblastoma using cisplatin-containing regimens is about 70%, but survival is closely dependent on the tumor stage at diagnosis: $91 \pm 4\%$ for stage I, 100% for stage II, $64 \pm 5\%$ for stage III, and $25 \pm 7\%$ for stage IV.[594] Similar 5-yr EFS results based on PRETEXT staging have been published by SIOPEL investigators: 100%, 83%, 56%, and 46%, respectively, for patients with PRETEXT stages I through IV.[609] Patients with metastatic disease continue to fare poorly regardless

---

TABLE 99.17

Results of Intergroup Studies (Children's Oncology Group and SIOP Liver Tumor Study Group) for the Treatment of Hepatoblastoma

Study (Reference)	Number of Patients	Treatment	Outcome	Comments
POG/CCG[594]	173	CDDP–V–5-FU vs CDDP–Dox	5-yr S 69% 5-yr S 72% (p = 0.88)	Regimen without doxorubicin less toxic with similar survival
COG P 9645[639]	53 56	CDDP–V–5-FU vs CBDCA–CDDP	1-yr EFS 57% 1-yr EFS 37% (p = 0.017)	Intensified platinum regimens increase the probability of adverse outcomes in children with hepatoblastoma
SIOPEL I[609]	154	CDDP–Dox	5-yr S 75%	138 received preoperative chemotherapy only, and of these 72% had a complete resection
SIOPEL 2[610]	67 58	Standard risk (PRETEXT I, II, III) CDDP only HR–CDDP–CBDCA–Dox	3-yr S 91 ± 7% 3-yr S 53 ± 13%	97% of SR had complete tumor resections Results led to randomized comparison of CDDP vs. PLADO for SR (SIOPEL 3)
SIOPEL 3[627]	126 129	CDDP only CDDP–Dox	3-yr S 95% 3-yr S 93%	Dox can be safely omitted from treatment of SR patients
SIOPEL-3HR[628]	151	High risk (PRETEXT IV, P+, V+, E+, metastases, AFP <100 ng/mL) CDDP/Dox/CBDCA	3-yrs EFS 65%; 3-yr OS 69%	70% (106/151) achieved complete resection of tumor lesions, including metastases
SIOPEL-4[629]	62	High risk (PRETEXT IV, P+, V+, E+, metastases, AFP <100 ng/mL, or tumor rupture) CDDP/Dox/CBDCA	3-yr EFS 76%; 3-yr OS 83%	Increased dose-intensity of CDDP; GTR of all tumor achieved in 46/62 (74%) high-risk patients
HB 89[634]	72	Ifos–CDDP–Dox	"Long-term" EFS 75%	GTR in 92%
HB 94[591]	69	Ifos–CDDP–Dox	3-yr S 77%	GTR 86% (54/63) Long-term EFS of 95% in those with GTR
JPLT-1[667]	134	CDDP–pirarubicin	3-yr S 77.8%	GTR 72%
JPLT-2[668]	212	CDDP–pirarubicin Ifos–pirarubicin–etop-CBDCA	3-yr S 82.4%	GTR 82%; 3-yr S 88%. Macroscopic disease /unresectable 3-yr S 56% (p <0.001)

CDDP, cisplatin; V, vincristine; 5-FU, 5-fluorouracil; S, survival; Dox, doxorubicin; CBDCA, carboplatin; HR, high risk; PLADO, cisplatin + doxorubicin; SR, standard risk; GTR, gross total resection; Ifos, ifosfamide; etop, etoposide.

of the regimen used, and their survival is less than 30%. Nearly one-third of patients who relapse following therapy with CFV can be salvaged with further surgery and a doxorubicin-based regimen.[640]

Currently, the COG study for patients with newly diagnosed hepatoblastoma (AHEP0731) is assigning treatment based on an assessment of risk. The factors incorporated in the risk group assignment include: COG stage, histology (pure fetal or SCU) and AFP. Very low-risk patients are defined as those with stage I tumors, pure fetal histology (PFH), and AFPs >100 ng/mL and are treated with surgery alone; those with low-risk disease are those with grossly resected tumors (stages I or II), AFPs >100 ng/mL, and who do not have SCU histology. These patients are treated with two courses of CFV chemotherapy. Intermediate-risk patients are defined as those with stage III tumors or those with stage I/II tumors with any SCU elements, as long as AFP is greater than 100 ng/mL. These patients receive six cycles of CFV with doxorubicin added to each cycle. Finally high-risk patients, defined as those with metastatic disease or AFP <100 ng/mL, regardless of stage, will receive an initial two courses of irinotecan/vincristine, followed by courses of CFV with doxorubicin.

In conclusion, although hepatoblastoma is a rare childhood cancer, cooperative group trials have enabled significant improvements in treatment. Because of the success of these trials and the rarity of these tumors, additional progress will require further international collaboration. Planning is ongoing for an international trial (Pediatric Hepatoblastoma International Therapeutic Trial [PHITT]), including all of the worldwide pediatric liver tumor cooperative groups from the United States, Europe, and Japan to evaluate what is the best chemotherapy for these children.

GERM CELL TUMORS

Epidemiology

Germ cell tumors account for 3.5% of cases of cancer in children under 15 years of age but for 16% of all cancers in those who are 15 to 19 years of age.[183] In pediatrics, germ cell tumors have a bimodal age distribution with peaks during infancy and puberty.[641] In boys under 4 years, gonadal and extragonadal tumors are evenly represented and teratomas and yolk sac carcinomas predominate, whereas most of the tumors in patients older than 10 years are located in the testis and are of nonseminomatous histology (teratoma, embryonal carcinoma, mixed). In girls, the majority of tumors in patients younger than 4 years of age are extragonadal, whereas germinomas and teratomas affecting the ovary are most commonly seen in patients over 10 years of age.[641] Sacrococcygeal tumors account for 40% of all childhood germ cell tumors and 78% of all extragonadal tumors[642]; less common extragonadal sites include the mediastinum, the retroperitoneum, the vagina, and the pineal region. Predisposing conditions for the development of pediatric germ cell tumors include cryptorchidism, Turner syndrome, Klinefelter syndrome, and androgen insensitivity syndromes.[642,643]

Pathology

Pediatric germ cell tumors comprise a diverse group of histologies reflecting the pluripotent nature of the primordial germ cells. There are several subtypes of germ cell tumors, the most common being teratomas (37%), yolk sac tumors (27%), germinomas (18%), mixed (12%), embryonal carcinomas (2%), and choriocarcinomas (2%).[644]

Laboratory Markers

AFP and the β subunit of HCG (β-HCG) are oncofetoproteins, which are elevated in the serum of patients with a variety of germ cell tumors. AFP reaches peak concentrations at 12 to 14 weeks and declines to levels of less than 10 ng/L by 1 year of age. The

half-life of AFP is 5 to 7 days. AFP is elevated in patients with yolk sac and embryonal carcinomas.[642]

β-HCG is a glycoprotein secreted by the placenta, and its half-life is only 26 to 36 hours. Elevated levels in patients with germ cell tumors implies the presence of syncytiotrophoblastic cells, which are seen in germinomas, embryonal carcinomas, and choriocarcinomas.[642]

Clinical Presentation, Staging, and Treatment

The following section briefly summarizes the clinical presentation and treatment recommendations for germ cell tumors in specific anatomic areas. In general, pediatric patients with germ cell tumors can be divided into three risk categories that determine the type of therapy they receive (Table 99.18). A recent study suggests

TABLE 99.18

Staging of Pediatric Germ Cell Tumors

Stage	Extent of Disease
Testicular Germ Cell Tumors	
I	Limited to testis (testes), completely resected by high inguinal orchiectomy; no clinical, radiographic, or histologic evidence of disease beyond the testes. Patients with normal or unknown tumor markers at diagnosis must have a negative ipsilateral retroperitoneal node sampling to confirm stage I disease if radiographic studies demonstrate lymph nodes >2 cm.
II	Transscrotal biopsy; microscopic disease in scrotum or high in spermatic cord (≤5 cm from proximal end). Failure of tumor markers to normalize or decrease with an appropriate half-life.
III	Retroperitoneal lymph node involvement, but no visceral or extra-abdominal involvement. Lymph nodes >4 cm by CT or >2 cm, and <4 cm with biopsy proof.
IV	Distant metastases, including liver.
Ovarian Germ Cell Tumors	
I	Limited to ovary (peritoneal evaluation should be negative). No clinical, radiographic, or histologic evidence of disease beyond the ovaries. (Note: The presence of gliomatosis peritonei does not result in changing stage I disease to a higher stage).
II	Microscopic residual; peritoneal evaluation negative. (Note: The presence of gliomatosis peritonei does not result in changing stage II disease to a higher stage). Failure of tumor markers to normalize or decrease with an appropriate half-life.
III	Lymph node involvement (metastatic nodule); gross residual or biopsy only; contiguous visceral involvement (omentum, intestine, bladder); peritoneal evaluation positive for malignancy.
IV	Distant metastases, including liver.
Extragonadal Germ Cell Tumors	
I	Complete resection at any site, coccygectomy for sacrococcygeal site, negative tumor margins.
II	Microscopic residual; lymph nodes negative.
III	Lymph node involvement with metastatic disease. Gross residual or biopsy only; retroperitoneal nodes negative or positive.
IV	Distant metastases, including liver.

PRACTICE OF ONCOLOGY

that the addition of other prognostic factors that include age, LDH and AFP levels, and the presence of a mediastinal primary tumor may help refine the risk stratification of patients with pediatric germ cell tumors.[645]

In general, following surgical resection, patients with mature and immature teratomas as well as patients with stage I gonadal tumors (see the following section) can be observed and chemotherapy can be reserved to salvage patients who recur. For patients with more advanced stage disease, the use of cisplatin-based regimens has dramatically improved the outcome of patients with germ cell tumors, and with current regimens, over 80% of children with disseminated disease and over 90% of those with localized disease can be cured.[646–648] The administration of higher doses of cisplatin may benefit subsets of patients with stage III/IV extragonadal tumors; however, this treatment is associated with significant ototoxicity.[648] Attempts to reduce the rates of ototoxicity by adding amifostine to high-dose platinum were unsuccessful in one COG trial.[649] In another trial, the addition of high-dose cyclophosphamide to standard-dose platinum proved to be feasible, but its benefit could not be adequately assessed given the low numbers of patients enrolled.[650]

Extragonadal Germ Cell Tumors

Sacrococcygeal teratoma occur in 1 in 35,000 live births, are the most common germ cell tumors in infants and newborns, and more commonly affect girls.[651] Approximately 80% of these tumors are diagnosed within the first month of life.

Four types of sacrococcygeal teratomas have been defined on the basis of the abdominopelvic extent and the presence or absence of external extension (Fig. 99.9).[651] The frequency of malignancy is closely associated with the type of teratoma and the age

at presentation; girls and boys older than 2 months of age have a malignancy rate of 48% and 67%, respectively.[652] Surgery is the mainstay of therapy for sacrococcygeal tumors and should include the removal of the coccyx to minimize local recurrence. Surgical sequelae that affect bowel and bladder control are reported in 11% to 41% of survivors.[651] Children with benign sacrococcygeal tumors have an excellent outcome with surgery alone, but recurrences that often contain a yolk sac component are seen in 11% of patients with mature teratomas and in 4% of patients with immature teratomas.[653] This finding argues in favor of close follow-up of these patients for 3 years following resection.[651] Patients with malignant yolk sac tumors located in the abdomen and pelvis are highly responsive to chemotherapy and have an excellent survival (approximately 90%) when treated with platinum-containing regimens.[654]

Mediastinal Germ Cell Tumors

These tumors more commonly affect adolescent males and are associated with Klinefelter syndrome. In the first year of life, teratomas predominate, whereas older patients have yolk sac or mixed germ cell tumors. Patients may be asymptomatic or present with respiratory symptoms such as cough and dyspnea; infants and toddlers more often present with respiratory symptoms that may also include hemoptysis and upper airway obstruction.[642] The diagnosis is established by biopsy of the primary tumor or an involved supraclavicular lymph node. Staging studies should include serum chemistries; a complete blood count; tumor marker studies; a CT of the chest, abdomen, and pelvis; an MRI of the brain if clinically symptomatic; and a bone scan if metastases are evident at diagnosis in other sites such as the lung.

The use of cisplatin-containing regimens has dramatically improved the outcome for children with malignant mediastinal germ

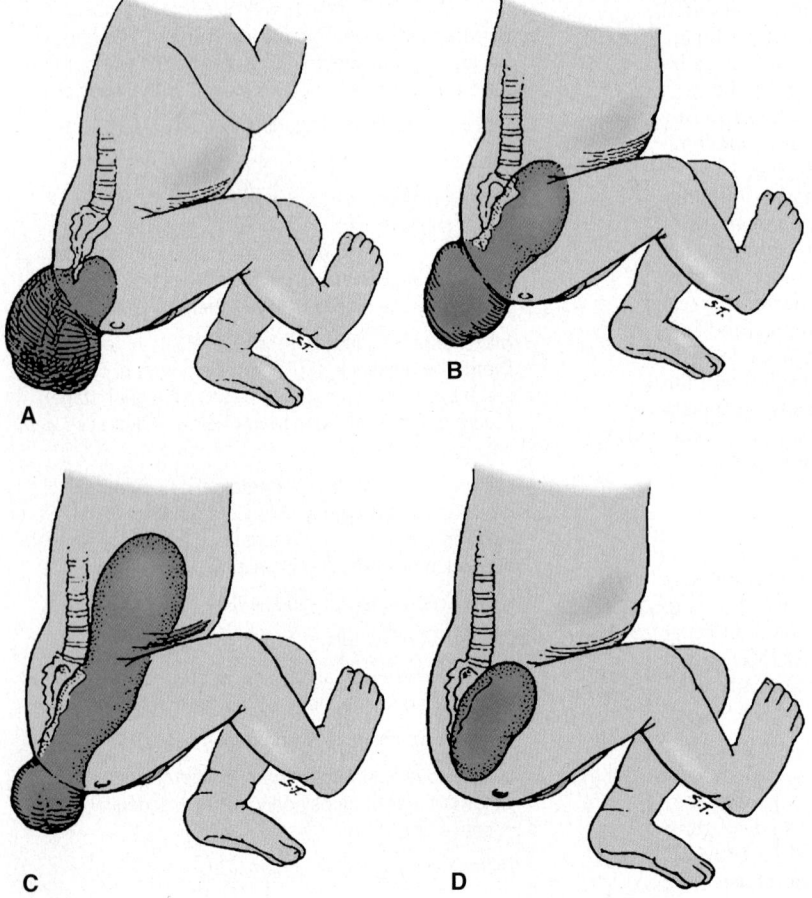

Figure 99.9 Types of sacrococcygeal teratoma. **A:** Type I predominantly external, **B:** Type II external and intrapelvic, **C:** Type III predominantly pelvic, **D:** Type IV presacral. (From Rescorla FJ, Breitfeld PP. Pediatric germ cell tumors. *Curr Probl Cancer* 1999;23(6):257, with permission from Elsevier.)

cell tumors, but patients who are ≥12 years of age have a sixfold increased risk of death (survival <50%) compared to younger patients with tumors located in other sites.[655] The use of a high-dose platinum regimen in one trial was not associated with a significant difference in clinical outcome.[655]

Gonadal Tumors

Testicular tumors make up approximately 17% of all pediatric germ cell tumors. About 75% of testicular tumors in children are of germ cell origin; in prepubertal males, teratomas and yolk sac carcinomas are the most common histologies, whereas mixed germ cell tumors are seen in older patients.[644] Children with primary testicular tumors often present with painless testicular enlargement, and in about 20% of cases, they are associated with hydroceles or inguinal hernias.[642] The preoperative evaluation should include an ultrasound, a complete blood count, a chest radiograph, and serum chemistries, including AFP and β-HCG levels. After the diagnosis is established, the metastatic evaluation should include CT scans of the chest, abdomen, and pelvis. A bone scintigraphy should be performed in all patients with advanced stage disease, and brain imaging should be obtained when clinically indicated.

All scrotal masses should be explored through an inguinal incision. If the AFP is elevated and a malignancy is suspected, a radical orchiectomy with control of the vessels at the internal ring should be performed. If a benign lesion with a normal AFP is being considered as a diagnostic possibility, an enucleation of the mass following opening of the tunica can be performed after mobilizing the testicle and controlling the cord.[651]

Patients with nonseminomatous stage I germ cell tumors (completely resected tumors) can be treated with radical orchiectomy alone, reserving the use of chemotherapy for relapse (Table 99.19).[656,657] Children with more advanced stage disease (intermediate-risk disease; see Table 99.19) should be treated with standard courses of cisplatin, etoposide, and bleomycin and are expected to have a 6-year survival in excess of 90%.[648]

Ovarian tumors account for approximately 29% of all pediatric germ cell tumors and the incidence of this tumor increases with a peak at 18 years of age. Teratomas are the most common germ cell tumor of the ovary in children and adolescents, and dysgerminoma is the most common malignant germ cell tumor of the ovary in this patient population. Presenting symptoms include pain, abdominal distension, and acute abdomen, which may result from tumor hemorrhage, rupture, or torsion. Other less common symptoms include vaginal bleeding or precocious puberty (mostly in patients with sex-cord stromal tumors).[651] The initial work-up should include a complete blood count and serum chemistries, including

TABLE 99.19

Treatment of Pediatric Germ Cell Tumors

Risk	Treatment	5-Year Survival (%)
Low Risk Stage 1 testicular Stage 1 ovarian	Surgery only	<95
Intermediate Risk Stage II–IV ovary Stage II–IV testes Stage I–II extragonadal	PEB × 3 or 4	<90
High Risk Stage II–IV extragonadal Stage IV ovary	PEB × 4	70–75

PEB, cisplatin, etoposide, bleomycin.

AFP and β-HCG. The preoperative radiographic evaluation should include an abdominal ultrasonography and CT scans of the abdomen and pelvis. Once the tissue diagnosis is established, a metastatic evaluation that includes a CT of the chest and a bone scintigraphy (for advanced cases) should be performed. Surgical exploration should be performed through a laparotomy, and the following additional samples should be obtained: peritoneal washings, an examination of omentum with resection of adherent or abnormal areas, an exploration of retroperitoneal nodes with resection of abnormal nodes, and an inspection of the contralateral ovary with a biopsy of abnormal areas.[658] Every attempt should be made to spare uninvolved fallopian tubes and the uterus to preserve fertility. Ovarian tumors are staged using the POG/CCG staging system, which represents a simplified version of the International Federation of Gynecology and Obstetrics staging system.

Surgery alone is sufficient for a cure in patients with mature and immature teratomas, and the presence of gliomatosis elements does not affect the prognosis.[642,659,660] For patients with stage 1 seminomatous (dysgerminoma) and nonseminomatous malignant germ cell tumors, European and North American trials including a recently completed COG trial demonstrate that close observation following surgery is a reasonable strategy; although one-third of patients recur, more than 95% can be successfully salvaged and cured with chemotherapy at the time of relapse.[657,661,662] Current pediatric regimens for the treatment of stages II through IV ovarian germ cell tumors use a combination of standard-dose cisplatin, etoposide, and bleomycin with 6-year event-free survival and OS rates in excess of 86% and 93%, respectively (see Tables 99.18 and 99.19).[648]

SELECTED REFERENCES

The full reference list can be accessed at lwwhealthlibrary.com/oncology.

1. Howlader N, Noone AM, Krapcho M, et al., eds. *SEER Cancer Statistics Review, 1975-2010.* Bethesda, MD: National Cancer Institute; 2013.
11. Brodeur GM. Neuroblastoma: biological insights into a clinical enigma. *Nat Rev Cancer* 2003;3:203–216.
12. Maris JM, Hogarty MD, Bagatell R, et al. Neuroblastoma. *Lancet* 2007; 369:2106–2120.
13. Maris JM. Recent advances in neuroblastoma. *N Engl J Med* 2010;362: 2202–2211.
14. Park JR, Eggert A, Caron H. Neuroblastoma: biology, prognosis, and treatment. *Hematol Oncol Clin North Am* 2010;24:65–86.
15. Maris JM. The biologic basis for neuroblastoma heterogeneity and risk stratification. *Curr Opin Pediatr* 2005;17:7–13.
17. London WB, Castleberry RP, Matthay KK, et al. Evidence for an age cutoff greater than 365 days for neuroblastoma risk group stratification in the Children's Oncology Group. *J Clin Oncol* 2005;23:6459–6465.
47. Schwab M, Alitalo K, Klempnauer KH, et al. Amplified DNA with limited homology to myc cellular oncogene is shared by human neuroblastoma cell lines and a neuroblastoma tumour. *Nature* 1983;305:245–248.

48. Brodeur GM, Seeger RC, Schwab M, et al. Amplification of N-myc in untreated human neuroblastomas correlates with advanced disease stage. *Science* 1984;224:1121–1124.
51. Cohn SL, Pearson AD, London WB, et al. The International Neuroblastoma Risk Group (INRG) classification system: an INRG Task Force report. *J Clin Oncol* 2009;27:289–297.
99. Brodeur GM, Pritchard J, Berthold F, et al. Revisions of the international criteria for neuroblastoma diagnosis, staging, and response to treatment. *J Clin Oncol* 1993;11:1466–1477.
106. Woods WG, Gao RN, Shuster JJ, et al. Screening of infants and mortality due to neuroblastoma. *N Engl J Med* 2002;346:1041–1046.
113. Monclair T, Brodeur GM, Ambros PF, et al. The International Neuroblastoma Risk Group (INRG) staging system: an INRG Task Force report. *J Clin Oncol* 2009;27:298–303.
122. Baker DL, Schmidt ML, Cohn SI, et al. Outcome after reduced chemotherapy for intermediate-risk neuroblastoma. *N Engl J Med* 2010;363:1313–1323.
129. Matthay KK, Villablanca JG, Seeger RC, et al. Treatment of high-risk neuroblastoma with intensive chemotherapy, radiotherapy, autologous bone marrow transplantation, and 13-cis-retinoic acid. Children's Cancer Group. *N Engl J Med* 1999;341:1165–1173.

PRACTICE OF ONCOLOGY

135. Cheung NV, Heller G. Chemotherapy dose intensity correlates strongly with response, median survival, and median progression-free survival in metastatic neuroblastoma. *J Clin Oncol* 1991;9:1050–1058.

180. Yu AL, Gilman AL, Ozkaynak MF, et al. Anti-GD2 antibody with GM-CSF, interleukin-2, and isotretinoin for neuroblastoma. *N Engl J Med* 2010;363:1324–1334.

190. Scott RH, Walker L, Olsen OE, et al. Surveillance for Wilms tumour in at-risk children: pragmatic recommendations for best practice. *Arch Dis Child* 2006;91:995–999.

193. Dome JS, Cotton CA, Perlman EJ, et al. Treatment of anaplastic histology Wilms' tumor: results from the fifth National Wilms' Tumor Study. *J Clin Oncol* 2006;24:2352–2358.

206. Grundy PE, Breslow NE, Li S, et al. Loss of heterozygosity for chromosomes 1p and 16q is an adverse prognostic factor in favorable-histology Wilms tumor: a report from the National Wilms Tumor Study Group. *J Clin Oncol* 2005;23:7312–7321.

207. Perlman EJ, Grundy PE, Anderson JR, et al. WT1 mutation and 11P15 loss of heterozygosity predict relapse in very low-risk wilms tumors treated with surgery alone: a children's oncology group study. *J Clin Oncol* 2011;29:698–703.

213. Metzger ML, Dome JS. Current therapy for Wilms' tumor. *Oncologist* 2005;10:815–826.

214. Green DM. Controversies in the management of Wilms tumour - immediate nephrectomy or delayed nephrectomy? *Eur J Cancer* 2007;43:2453–2456.

220. Shamberger RC, Anderson JR, Breslow NE, et al. Long-term outcomes for infants with very low risk Wilms tumor treated with surgery alone in National Wilms Tumor Study-5. *Ann Surg* 2010;251:555–558.

221. Hamilton TE, Ritchey ML, Haase GM, et al. The management of synchronous bilateral Wilms tumor: a report from the National Wilms Tumor Study Group. *Ann Surg* 2011;253:1004–1010.

235. Green DM. The treatment of stages I-IV favorable histology Wilms' tumor. *J Clin Oncol* 2004;22:1366–1372.

237. Green DM, Cotton CA, Malogolowkin M, et al. Treatment of Wilms tumor relapsing after initial treatment with vincristine and actinomycin D: a report from the National Wilms Tumor Study Group. *Pediatr Blood Cancer* 2007;48:493–499.

239. Malogolowkin M, Cotton CA, Green DM, et al. Treatment of Wilms tumor relapsing after initial treatment with vincristine, actinomycin D, and doxorubicin. A report from the National Wilms Tumor Study Group. *Pediatr Blood Cancer* 2008;50:236–241.

248. Grundy PE, Green DM, Dirks AC, et al. Clinical significance of pulmonary nodules detected by CT and Not CXR in patients treated for favorable histology Wilms tumor on national Wilms tumor studies-4 and -5: a report from the Children's Oncology Group. *Pediatr Blood Cancer* 2012;59:631–635.

249. Verschuur A, Van Tinteren H, Graf N, et al. Treatment of pulmonary metastases in children with stage IV nephroblastoma with risk-based use of pulmonary radiotherapy. *J Clin Oncol* 2012;30:3533–3539.

251. Friend SH, Bernards R, Rogelj S, et al. A human DNA segment with properties of the gene that predisposes to retinoblastoma and osteosarcoma. *Nature* 1986;323:643–646.

254. Rushlow DE, Mol BM, Kennett JY, et al. Characterisation of retinoblastomas without RB1 mutations: genomic, gene expression, and clinical studies. *Lancet Oncol* 2013;14:327–334.

255. Zhang J, Benavente CA, McEvoy J, et al. A novel retinoblastoma therapy from genomic and epigenetic analyses. *Nature* 2012;481:329–334.

268. Pratt CB, Meyer D, Chenaille P, et al. The use of bone marrow aspirations and lumbar punctures at the time of diagnosis of retinoblastoma. *J Clin Oncol* 1989;7:140–143.

272. Linn Murphree A. Intraocular retinoblastoma: the case for a new group classification. *Ophthalmol Clin North Am* 2005;18:41–53.

279. Wilson MW, Haik BG, Liu T, et al. Effect on ocular survival of adding early intensive focal treatments to a two-drug chemotherapy regimen in patients with retinoblastoma. *Am J Ophthalmol* 2005;140:397–406.

280. Shields CL, Honavar SG, Meadows AT, et al. Chemoreduction plus focal therapy for retinoblastoma: factors predictive of need for treatment with external beam radiotherapy or enucleation. *Am J Ophthalmol* 2002;133:657–664.

283. Shields CL, Shields JA, Cater J, et al. Plaque radiotherapy for retinoblastoma: long-term tumor control and treatment complications in 208 tumors. *Ophthalmology* 2001;108:2116–2121.

287. Marees T, Moll AC, Imhof SM, et al. Risk of second malignancies in survivors of retinoblastoma: more than 40 years of follow-up. *J Natl Cancer Inst* 2008;100:1771–1779.

288. Kleinerman RA, Tucker MA, Tarone RE, et al. Risk of new cancers after radiotherapy in long-term survivors of retinoblastoma: an extended follow-up. *J Clin Oncol* 2005;23:2272–2279.

291. Friedman DL, Himelstein B, Shields CL, et al. Chemoreduction and local ophthalmic therapy for intraocular retinoblastoma. *J Clin Oncol* 2000;18:12–17.

293. Qaddoumi I, Billups CA, Tagen M, et al. Topotecan and vincristine combination is effective against advanced bilateral intraocular retinoblastoma and has manageable toxicity. *Cancer* 2012;118:5663–5670.

299. Chantada GL, Dunkel IJ, de Davila MT, et al. Retinoblastoma patients with high risk ocular pathological features: who needs adjuvant therapy? *Br J Ophthalmol* 2004;88:1069–1073.

306. Rodriguez-Galindo C, Wilson MW, Haik BG, et al. Treatment of metastatic retinoblastoma. *Ophthalmology* 2003;110:1237–1240.

318. Mirabello L, Troisi RJ, Savage SA. Osteosarcoma incidence and survival rates from 1973 to 2004: data from the Surveillance, Epidemiology, and End Results Program. *Cancer* 2009;115:1531–1543.

340. Bacci G, Longhi A, Versari M, et al. Prognostic factors for osteosarcoma of the extremity treated with neoadjuvant chemotherapy: 15-year experience in 789 patients treated at a single institution. *Cancer* 2006;106:1154–1161.

369. Goorin AM, Schwartzentruber DJ, Devidas M, et al. Presurgical chemotherapy compared with immediate surgery and adjuvant chemotherapy for nonmetastatic osteosarcoma: Pediatric Oncology Group Study POG-8651. *J Clin Oncol* 2003;21:1574–1580.

373. Whelan J, Patterson D, Perisoglou M, et al. The role of interferons in the treatment of osteosarcoma. *Pediatr Blood Cancer* 2010;54:350–354.

382. Bielack SS, Kempf-Bielack B, Delling G, et al. Prognostic factors in high-grade osteosarcoma of the extremities or trunk: an analysis of 1,702 patients treated on neoadjuvant cooperative osteosarcoma study group protocols. *J Clin Oncol* 2002;20:776–790.

392. Mahajan A, Woo SY, Kornguth DG, et al. Multimodality treatment of osteosarcoma: radiation in a high-risk cohort. *Pediatr Blood Cancer* 2008;50:976–982.

407. Meyers PA, Schwartz CL, Krailo MD, et al. Osteosarcoma: the addition of muramyl tripeptide to chemotherapy improves overall survival—a report from the Children's Oncology Group. *J Clin Oncol* 2008;26:633–638.

408. de Alava E, Lessnick SL, Sorensen PH. In: Fletcher CDM, Bridge JA, Hogendoorn PC, et al., eds. *WHO Classification of Tumours of Soft Tissue and Bone*. Lyon: International Agency of Research on Cancer; 2013: 305–309.

416. Sankar S, Lessnick SL. Promiscuous partnerships in Ewing's sarcoma. *Cancer Genet* 2011;204:351–365.

441. Balamuth NJ, Womer RB. Ewing's sarcoma. *Lancet Oncol* 2010;11:184–192.

447. Grier HE, Krailo MD, Tarbell NJ, et al. Addition of ifosfamide and etoposide to standard chemotherapy for Ewing's sarcoma and primitive neuroectodermal tumor of bone. *N Engl J Med* 2003;348:694–701.

454. Womer RB, West DC, Krailo MD, et al. Randomized controlled trial of interval-compressed chemotherapy for the treatment of localized Ewing sarcoma: a report from the Children's Oncology Group. *J Clin Oncol* 2012;30:4148–4154.

458. Miser JS, Goldsby RE, Chen Z, et al. Treatment of metastatic Ewing sarcoma/primitive neuroectodermal tumor of bone: evaluation of increasing the dose intensity of chemotherapy—a report from the Children's Oncology Group. *Pediatr Blood Cancer* 2007;49:894–900.

461. Ladenstein R, Potschger U, Le Deley MC, et al. Primary disseminated multifocal Ewing sarcoma: results of the Euro-EWING 99 trial. *J Clin Oncol* 2010;28:3284–3291.

479. Dunst J, Schuck A. Role of radiotherapy in Ewing tumors. *Pediatr Blood Cancer* 2004;42:465–470.

491. Cotterill SJ, Ahrens S, Paulussen M, et al. Prognostic factors in Ewing's tumor of bone: analysis of 975 patients from the European Intergroup Cooperative Ewing's Sarcoma Study Group. *J Clin Oncol* 2000;18:3108–3114.

497. Ognjanovic S, Linabery AM, Charbonneau B, et al. Trends in childhood rhabdomyosarcoma incidence and survival in the United States, 1975-2005. *Cancer* 2009;115:4218–4226.

506. Breneman JC, Lyden E, Pappo AS, et al. Prognostic factors and clinical outcomes in children and adolescents with metastatic rhabdomyosarcoma—a report from the Intergroup Rhabdomyosarcoma Study IV. *J Clin Oncol* 2003;21:78–84.

511. Pappo AS, Shapiro DN, Crist WM, et al. Biology and therapy of pediatric rhabdomyosarcoma. *J Clin Oncol* 1995;13:2123–2139.

512. Crist WM, Anderson JR, Meza JL, et al. Intergroup rhabdomyosarcoma study-IV: results for patients with nonmetastatic disease. *J Clin Oncol* 2001;19:3091–3102.

517. Williamson, D, Missiaglia E, de Reynies A, et al. Fusion gene-negative alveolar rhabdomyosarcoma is clinically and molecularly indistinguishable from embryonal rhabdomyosarcoma. *J Clin Oncol* 2010;28:2151–2158.

520. Shukla N, Ameur N, Yilmaz I, et al. Oncogene mutation profiling of pediatric solid tumors reveals significant subsets of embryonal rhabdomyosarcoma and neuroblastoma with mutated genes in growth signaling pathways. *Clin Cancer Res* 2012;18:748–757.

525. Missiaglia E, Williamson D, Chisholm J, et al. PAX3/FOXO1 fusion gene status is the key prognostic molecular marker in rhabdomyosarcoma and significantly improves current risk stratification. *J Clin Oncol* 2012;30:1670–1677.

536. Wexler LH, Meyer WH, Helman LJ. Rhabdomyosarcoma. In: Poplack DG, PIzzo PA, eds. *Principles and Practice of Pediatric Oncology*. Philadelphia: Lippincott Williams and Wilkins; 2011: 923–953.

537. Malempati S, Hawkins DS. Rhabdomyosarcoma: review of the Children's Oncology Group (COG) Soft-Tissue Sarcoma Committee experience and rationale for current COG studies. *Pediatr Blood Cancer* 2012;59:5–10.

538. Meza JL, Anderson J, Pappo AS, et al. Analysis of prognostic factors in patients with nonmetastatic rhabdomyosarcoma treated on intergroup rhabdomyosarcoma studies III and IV: the Children's Oncology Group. *J Clin Oncol* 2006;24:3844–3851.

539. Raney RB, Walterhouse DO, Meza JL, et al. Results of the Intergroup Rhabdomyosarcoma Study Group D9602 protocol, using vincristine and dactinomycin with or without cyclophosphamide and radiation therapy, for newly diagnosed patients with low-risk embryonal rhabdomyosarcoma: a report from the Soft Tissue Sarcoma Committee of the Children's Oncology Group. *J Clin Oncol* 2011;29:1312–1318.

541. Oberlin O, Rey A, Lyden E, et al. Prognostic factors in metastatic rhabdomyosarcomas: results of a pooled analysis from United States and European Cooperative Groups. *J Clin Oncol* 2008;26:2384–2389.

547. Lin C, Donaldson SS, Meza JL, et al. Effect of radiotherapy techniques (IMRT vs. 3D-CRT) on outcome in patients with intermediate-risk rhabdomyosarcoma enrolled in COG D9803—a report from the Children's Oncology Group. *Int J Radiat Oncol Biol Phys* 2012;82:1764–1770.

552. Lager JJ, Lyden ER, Anderson JR, et al. Pooled analysis of phase II window studies in children with contemporary high-risk metastatic rhabdomyosarcoma: a report from the Soft Tissue Sarcoma Committee of the Children's Oncology Group. *J Clin Oncol* 2006;24:3415–3422.

557. Pappo AS, Anderson JR, Crist WM, et al. Survival after relapse in children and adolescents with rhabdomyosarcoma: A report from the Intergroup Rhabdomyosarcoma Study Group. *J Clin Oncol* 1999;17:3487–3493.

563. Litten JB, Tomlinson GE. Liver tumors in children. *Oncologist* 2008;13: 812–820.

581. Lopez-Terrada D, Alaggio R, de Davila MT, et al. Towards an international pediatric liver tumor consensus classification: proceedings of the Los Angeles COG liver tumors symposium. *Mod Pathol* 2014;27:472–291.

582. Malogolowkin MH, Katzenstein HM, Meyers RL, et al. Complete surgical resection is curative for children with hepatoblastoma with pure fetal histology: a report from the Children's Oncology Group. *J Clin Oncol* 2011;29:3301–3306.

583. De Ioris M, Brugieres L, Zimmermann A, et al. Hepatoblastoma with a low serum alpha-fetoprotein level at diagnosis: the SIOPEL group experience. *Eur J Cancer* 2008;44:545–550.

589. Czauderna P, Mackinlay G, Perilongo G, et al. Hepatocellular carcinoma in children: results of the first prospective study of the International Society of Pediatric Oncology group. *J Clin Oncol* 2002;20:2798–2804.

594. Ortega JA, Douglass EC, Feusner JH, et al. Randomized comparison of cisplatin/vincristine/fluorouracil and cisplatin/continuous infusion doxorubicin for treatment of pediatric hepatoblastoma: a report from the Children's Cancer Group and the Pediatric Oncology Group. *J Clin Oncol* 2000;18:2665–2675.

609. Pritchard J, Brown J, Shafford E, et al. Cisplatin, doxorubicin, and delayed surgery for childhood hepatoblastoma: a successful approach—results of the first prospective study of the International Society of Pediatric Oncology. *J Clin Oncol* 2000;18:3819–3828.

610. Perilongo G, Shafford E, Maibach R, et al. Risk-adapted treatment for childhood hepatoblastoma. Final report of the second study of the International Society of Paediatric Oncology—SIOPEL 2. *Eur J Cancer* 2004;40:411–421.

611. Otte JB, Pritchard J, Aronson DC, et al. Liver transplantation for hepatoblastoma: results from the International Society of Pediatric Oncology (SIOP) study SIOPEL-1 and review of the world experience. *Pediatr Blood Cancer* 2004;42:74–83.

627. Perilongo G, Maibach R, Shafford E, et al. Cisplatin versus cisplatin plus doxorubicin for standard-risk hepatoblastoma. *N Engl J Med* 2009;361:1662–1670.

628. Zsiros J, Maibach R, Shafford E, et al. Successful treatment of childhood high-risk hepatoblastoma with dose-intensive multiagent chemotherapy and surgery: final results of the SIOPEL-3HR study. *J Clin Oncol* 2010;28: 2584–2590.

629. Zsiros J, Brugieres L, Brock P, et al. Dose-dense cisplatin-based chemotherapy and surgery for children with high-risk hepatoblastoma (SIOPEL-4): a prospective, single-arm, feasibility study. *Lancet Oncol* 2013;14:834–842.

630. Perilongo G, Shafford E, Plaschkes J. SIOPEL trials using preoperative chemotherapy in hepatoblastoma. *Lancet Oncol* 2000;1:94–100.

632. Douglass EC, Reynolds M, Finegold M, et al. Cisplatin, vincristine, and fluorouracil therapy for hepatoblastoma: a Pediatric Oncology Group study. *J Clin Oncol* 1993;11:96–99.

634. von Schweinitz D, Byrd DJ, Hecker H, et al. Efficiency and toxicity of ifosfamide, cisplatin and doxorubicin in the treatment of childhood hepatoblastoma. Study Committee of the Cooperative Paediatric Liver Tumour Study HB89 of the German Society for Paediatric Oncology and Haematology. *Eur J Cancer* 1997;33:1243–1249.

641. Poynter JN, Amatruda JF, Ross JA. Trends in incidence and survival of pediatric and adolescent patients with germ cell tumors in the United States, 1975 to 2006. *Cancer* 2010;116:4882–4891.

642. Olson TA, Schneider D, Perlman EJ. Germ cell tumors. In: Pizzo PA, Poplack DG, eds. *Principles and Practice of Pediatric Oncology.* Philadelphia: Lippincott Williams and Wilkins; 2011: 1045–1067.

645. Frazier AL, Rumcheva P, Olson T, et al. Application of the adult international germ cell classification system to pediatric malignant non-seminomatous germ cell tumors: a report from the Children's Oncology Group. *Pediatr Blood Cancer* 2008;50:746–751.

648. Cushing B, Giller R, Cullen JW, et al. Randomized comparison of combination chemotherapy with etoposide, bleomycin, and either high-dose or standard-dose cisplatin in children and adolescents with high-risk malignant germ cell tumors: a pediatric intergroup study—Pediatric Oncology Group 9049 and Children's Cancer Group 8882. *J Clin Oncol* 2004;22: 2691–2700.

650. Malogolowkin MH, Krailo M, Marina N, et al. Pilot study of cisplatin, etoposide, bleomycin, and escalating dose cyclophosphamide therapy for children with high risk germ cell tumors: A report of the children's oncology group (COG). *Pediatr Blood Cancer* 2013;60:1602–1605.

651. Rescorla FJ. Pediatric germ cell tumors. *Semin Pediatr Surg* 2012;21:51–60.

655. Marina N, London WB, Frazier AL, et al. Prognostic factors in children with extragonadal malignant germ cell tumors: a pediatric intergroup study. *J Clin Oncol* 2006;24:2544–2548.

657. Rodriguez-Galindo C, Frailo M, Frazier L, et al. Children's Oncology Group's 2013 blueprint for research: rare tumors. *Pediatr Blood Cancer* 2013;60:1016–1021.

659. Cushing B, Giller R, Ablin A, et al. Surgical resection alone is effective treatment for ovarian immature teratoma in children and adolescents: a report of the pediatric oncology group and the children's cancer group. *Am J Obstet Gynecol* 1999;181:353–358.

660. Mann JR, Gray ES, Thornton C, et al. Mature and immature extracranial teratomas in children: the UK Children's Cancer Study Group Experience. *J Clin Oncol* 2008;26:3590–3597.

PRACTICE OF ONCOLOGY

100 Leukemias and Lymphomas of Childhood

Karen R. Rabin, Judith F. Margolin, Kala Y. Kamdar, and David G. Poplack

INTRODUCTION

The cure rates seen in pediatric oncology are some of the best in modern oncology. These are largely related to the remarkable progress in the treatment of leukemias and lymphomas, where cure rates have improved from less than 10% to 80% to 95%.[1-4] Cure rates for pediatric myeloid leukemia are lower, in the 60% to 70% range.[5,6] The improvement in outcomes for all of pediatric cancer are the result of the successful implementation of cooperative group clinical trials at the national and even international level.[7] Currently, more than two-thirds of children with cancer in the United States are treated in clinical trials.[7] Although there are many similarities in treating children and adults with these diseases, there are also differences that pertain to development and growth, drug metabolism, and psychosocial issues.

LEUKEMIAS

Incidence, Histology, and General Outcomes

Acute lymphoblastic leukemia (ALL), the most common malignancy of childhood, accounts for 75% of leukemias and is curable in 80% to 95% of cases.[8] Figure 100.1 demonstrates the improvement in survival in pediatric ALL on successive cooperative group trials from 1968 to 2005.[1] Although there are variations with age, sex, and ethnicity, the majority of ALL cases have pre–B immunophenotype and FAB L1 histology (80% of cases); 20% are of T-cell origin. The peak incidence of pediatric ALL is between ages 2 and 5 years. ALL is slightly more common in American Caucasians than in African Americans, and there is a slightly increased incidence in male patients.[9] Approximately 5,000 children are diagnosed with ALL each year in the United States, with an incidence of 29.2 per million.[9] The Surveillance, Epidemiology, and End Results (SEER) program data show that the incidence of ALL has been climbing slowly. Controversy exists concerning whether and how incidence and outcomes differ between racial and ethnic groups. Studies from the 1990s suggest that Caucasians have slightly higher survival rates than those of African ancestry and Hispanics, although this is confounded in part by the fact that those of African ancestry and Hispanics more often develop high-risk forms of ALL.[10-12] Racial and ethnic disparities in access to care and adherence to treatment may also have an adverse impact on survival.[13,14]

Acute myeloid leukemia (AML) accounts for approximately 15% to 20% of childhood leukemias, chronic myelogenous leukemia (CML) accounts for 3% to 4%, and juvenile myelomonocytic leukemia (JMML) and other rarer histologies account for less than 1%. The incidence of AML is currently estimated to be 5 to 7 cases per million in the United States.[15] Myelodysplastic syndrome (MDS) is a relatively rare diagnosis in childhood, generally progresses to AML, and is treated with similar regimens (including bone marrow transplant) as AML.[16] AML incidence is slightly higher in African Americans and Hispanics in the United States,

and survival is slightly lower.[17,18] Because of intrinsic differences in drug sensitivity between ALL and AML cells, progress in treating AML has been less dramatic than that of ALL. Nevertheless, current cure rates in AML have risen to approximately 45% to 65% with the advent of more intensive conventional chemotherapy and bone marrow transplant (BMT) (Fig. 100.2).[19,20]

Etiology

Environmental Factors

There is extensive literature and a continued interest in exploring possible relationships between infectious or environmental exposures and increased risk of childhood leukemia. However, most studies show weak or no correlation of these factors with the incidence of leukemia.[21-23] Electromagnetic fields have not been found to be significant in pediatric malignancies.[24-26] There is an emerging body of evidence from population-based studies of polymorphisms of drug-metabolizing genes, such as *NQO1* and *GST* polymorphisms, that may be associated with an increase or decrease in an individual's risk for developing leukemia based on exposures to particular environmental toxins like benzene and other organic solvents, quinine-containing substances, and flavonoids.[27]

Genetics

There is significant evidence that genetic factors play a role in the etiology of pediatric leukemia. Within the leukemic blasts themselves, there are characteristic cytogenetic changes (Table 100.1), many of which have prognostic significance (see later discussion). Key genetic changes found in childhood leukemia (especially in younger patients) may occur in utero or very early in life.[28,29] Evidence includes the detection of cells bearing these changes in neonatal blood spots[30] and transmission of leukemia by twin–twin transfusion.[31] The *delayed infection* hypothesis holds that children in developed countries are spared the frequent early infections that are necessary for normal development of the immune system. An infection occurring at a later time is then hypothesized to elicit a pathologic, myelosuppressive response, providing a selective growth advantage to the preleukemic clone, leading to development of overt leukemia.[32]

In most cases, leukemia appears to result from a complex interplay between environmental and genetic factors. Recently, genome-wide association studies have identified several constitutional genetic variations with moderate but statistically significant effects on the relative risk of ALL.[33-36] Collectively, variants in *IKZF1*, *ARID5B*, *CEBPE*, and *CDKN2A* may account for up to 80% of the attributable risk of developing ALL in Europeans.[35] *ARID5B* and *GATA3* polymorphisms have been identified as associated with both ALL susceptibility and relapse hazard, and may contribute to racial disparities in outcome, because high-risk alleles occurred more frequently in subjects with a greater degree of Native American ancestry.[37]

In addition to somatic and germ-line genetic changes associated with leukemia, there are well-described cases of familial

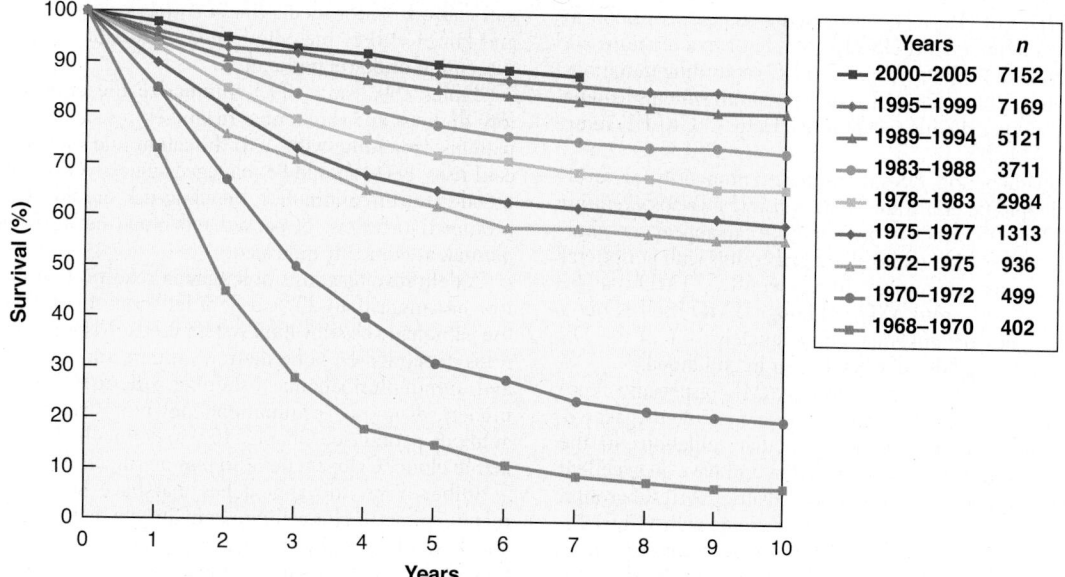

Figure 100.1 Improvement in survival of children with acute lymphoblastic leukemia. Overall survival probability by treatment era for 29,287 children with ALL who enrolled in trials from 1968 to 2005 conducted by the Children's Oncology Group (COG), the Pediatric Oncology Group (POG), and the Children's Cancer Group (CCG). The 2000 to 2005 curve includes CCG, POG, and COG. The 1995 to 1999 curve includes CCG and POG. All other curves are CCG. (Adapted from Hunger SP, Lu X, Devidas M, et al. Improved survival for children and adolescents with acute lymphoblastic leukemia between 1990 and 2005: a report from the children's oncology group. *J Clin Oncol* 2012;30:1663–1669.)

leukemia, including recently described mutations in the hematopoietic transcription factor *PAX5*,[38] as well as strong associations between leukemia risk and immunodeficiency and several somatic genetic disorders (e.g., Down syndrome [DS], Bloom syndrome, ataxia telangiectasia, Shwachman-Diamond syndrome, Noonan syndrome, neurofibromatosis).[8] Recently, a new association has been described between Li-Fraumeni syndrome, a well-known cancer predisposition syndrome, and hypodiploid ALL.[39]

Patients with DS have a 10- to 20-fold increased risk of developing leukemia.[40] The occurrence of leukemia in DS patients appears to be unrelated to the other congenital abnormalities and

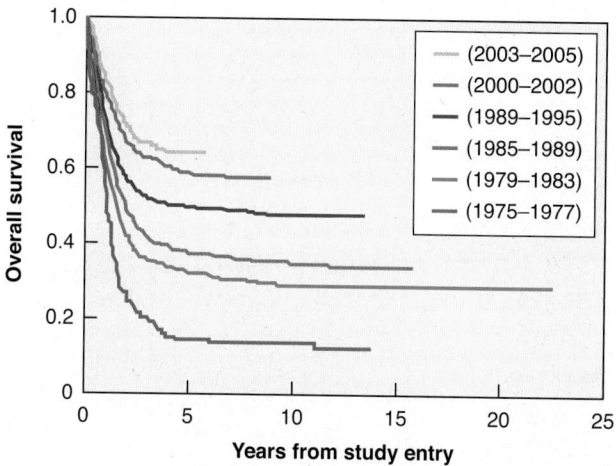

Figure 100.2 Improvement in survival of children with acute myeloid leukemia. Incremental improvements in overall survival in Children's Oncology Group and legacy trials in de novo childhood AML during the years indicated. (From Gamis AS, Alonzo TA, Perentesis JP, et al. Children's Oncology Group's 2013 blueprint for research: acute myeloid leukemia. *Pediatr Blood Cancer* 2013;60:964–971.)

TABLE 100.1

Acute Leukemia: Favorable and Unfavorable Prognostic Factors

Acute Lymphoblastic Leukemia

Favorable	Unfavorable
■ Age, 1–9 years	■ Age, <1 or ≥10 years
■ White blood cell count <50,000/mcL	■ White blood cell count ≥50,000/mcL
■ High hyperdiploidy (DNA index >1.16; and especially trisomies of chromosomes 4 and 10)	■ Hypodiploidy (DNA index <0.81 or <44 chromosomes)
■ Chromosomal translocation t(12;21) or *ETV6-RUNX1*	■ Chromosomal alterations t(9;22) or *BCR-ABL1* *MLL* gene rearrangement iAMP21 (intrachromosomal amplification of chromosome 21)
■ CNS-1	■ *IKZF1* gene deletion or mutation
■ Rapid response to induction chemotherapy	■ Ph-like gene expression profile
	■ Extramedullary disease
	■ Slow response to induction chemotherapy

Acute Myeloid Leukemia

Favorable	Unfavorable
■ Core binding factor transcription complex, t(8;21) or inv(16)	■ Monosomy 5, 5q deletion
■ Acute promyelocytic leukemia t(15;17)	■ Monosomy 7
■ Down syndrome	■ FLT3 internal tandem duplication
■ Rapid response to induction chemotherapy	■ Secondary AML/ myelodysplastic syndrome
	■ Slow response to induction chemotherapy

CNS, central nervous system.

medical problems of DS.[41] The cytogenetic changes common in ALL occur less frequently in DS-ALL,[42–45] but two alterations are markedly enriched: (1) Janus kinase 2 (*JAK2*) activating mutations in approximately 20% of DS-ALL, and (2) rearrangements leading to overexpression of cytokine receptor-like factor 2 (*CRLF2*) in up to 50% of DS-ALL.[46–48]

In the neonatal period, DS patients have a propensity for developing a nonneoplastic entity known as *transient myeloproliferative disease* (TMD) of DS, which at presentation, can appear very similar to AML (i.e., very high white blood cell counts with peripheral myeloblasts), but usually resolves spontaneously.[49] TMD may be difficult to distinguish from AML. Although TMD itself is not a form of malignancy or leukemia, approximately 30% of the DS patients with TMD will develop AML later in childhood.[49]

When patients with DS do develop AML (especially those younger than age 2 years), they tend to develop acute megakaryoblastic leukemia (AMKL), display particular mutations in the *GATA-1* hematopoietic transcription factor, and have an excellent prognosis compared to other adult and pediatric AML subgroups. The disease-free survival (DFS) for DS patients with *GATA-1*+ AMKL is over 90%, with regimens significantly less intensive than those required for other AML cases.[50] The reasons behind the increased risk of leukemia in DS remain unknown.

Clonal Nature of Lymphoid Cancers

Lymphoid malignancies appear to have derived from an original abnormal progenitor that lost the ability to fully differentiate and formed a *clone* of leukemic blast cells. ALL blasts are characterized by early cytoplasmic and surface lymphoid antigens (detectable by flow cytometry), as well as incomplete immunoglobulin (Ig) and T-cell receptor (TCR) gene rearrangements, suggesting they arise from a precursor T- or B-lymphoid progenitor. AML may arise from a multipotent or committed myeloid progenitor. Persistence of subclinical amounts of leukemia during or after therapy is called minimal residual disease (MRD).[51] MRD may be detected by flow cytometry or polymerase chain reaction (PCR)-based detection of Ig/TCR rearrangements or chromosomal translocations.[52] Use of high-throughput sequencing technologies for MRD detection is being undertaken on a research basis and may hold promise as a future clinical test with even higher sensitivity and precision.[53]

Diagnosis

The presenting signs and symptoms of a child with leukemia reflect the impact of bone marrow infiltration, the extent of extramedullary disease spread, and problems arising from changes in blood viscosity and chemistry related to the size, number, and breakdown products of leukemic blasts (tumor lysis).[12] Leukostasis from high white blood cell (WBC) counts may cause signs and symptoms ranging from mild respiratory symptoms and pulmonary infiltrates, to stroke, cranial or peripheral neuropathies, hematuria, renal failure, and ocular findings.[8] AML blasts are larger, less flexible, and contain granules that can cause inflammation and clotting. Thus, AML has a higher risk of serious systemic problems then ALL for a given high WBC (e.g., >100,000/mm[3]). Gingival infiltration and orbital and periorbital soft tissue masses (chloromas) are often seen in AML.[54] AML FAB subtypes 4 and 5 have a tendency to present with chloromas.

Central nervous system (CNS) involvement is more common in ALL but is also possible with AML.[55,56] CNS involvement is most often meningeal involvement, but may manifest as cranial nerve involvement, and occasionally, frank leukemic infiltrates in the parenchyma of the brain. CNS involvement may be asymptomatic or manifest as cranial nerve palsies, seizures, or focal neurologic findings. Testicular involvement generally manifests as a painless, palpable mass. Hepatosplenomegaly is common in both ALL and AML, and may compromise respiration in small children. Lymphomatous involvement of nodes or extranodal tissue

can cause superior mediastinal or superior vena cava syndromes, and bowel wall or mesenteric node infiltrations can cause intussusception or bowel perforation.

Tables 100.2 and 100.3 summarize the clinical and laboratory findings and differential diagnosis, respectively, for pediatric patients presenting with ALL. Infection and bleeding are significant risks. Fever should be managed aggressively with intravenous broad-spectrum antibiotics. Bleeding risk should be addressed by prompt transfusions of packed red blood cells, platelets, and/or plasma, as clinically indicated.

A definitive diagnosis of leukemia requires that the bone marrow has more than 20% to 25% leukemic blasts (depending on the pathologic classification system used).[57] Traditionally, the diagnosis depended on bone marrow aspirate and biopsy morphology and immunohistochemical staining patterns. The cornerstone of modern diagnosis is immunophenotyping, using flow cytometry antibody panels (see Chapter 107) to define the lineage of the leukemic clone. Cytogenetics also play a critical role.

Other diagnostic approaches that have become standard in many centers include fluorescent in situ hybridization (FISH), and PCR (to identify specific fusion proteins arising from chromosomal rearrangements). Finally, several techniques are used primarily on a research basis, such as RNA expression arrays, DNA copy number and single-nucleotide polymorphism (SNP) arrays, and whole-genome and whole-exome sequencing.[58–61] These techniques will be used increasingly for clinical decision making as well, such as to identify cryptic, actionable mutations[62] or to predict susceptibility to targeted therapy.[63,64]

TABLE 100.2

Clinical and Laboratory Features at Diagnosis in Children with Acute Lymphoblastic Leukemia

Clinical and Laboratory Features	Percentage of Patients
Symptoms and Physical Findings	
Fever	61
Bleeding (e.g., petechiae or purpura)	48
Bone pain	23
Lymphadenopathy	50
Splenomegaly	63
Hepatosplenomegaly	68
Laboratory Features	
Leukocyte count (mm[3])	
<10,000	53
10,000–49,000	30
>50,000	17
Hemoglobin (g/dL)	
<7.0	43
7.0–11.0	45
>11.0	12
Platelet count (mm[3])	
<20,000	28
20,000–99,000	47
>100,000	25
Lymphoblast morphology	
L1	84
L2	15
L3	1

TABLE 100.3

Differential Diagnosis in Childhood Acute Lymphoblastic Leukemia

- Nonmalignant conditions
  - Juvenile rheumatoid arthritis
  - Infectious mononucleosis
  - Idiopathic thrombocytopenic purpura
  - Pertussis; parapertussis
  - Aplastic anemia
  - Acute infectious lymphocytosis
- Malignancies
  - Neuroblastoma
  - Retinoblastoma
  - Rhabdomyosarcoma
- Unusual presentations
  - Hypereosinophilic syndrome

TABLE 100.4

Definitions of Central Nervous System Disease Status at Diagnosis of Acute Lymphoblastic Leukemia Based on Cerebrospinal Fluid Findings[65]

Status	Cerebrospinal Fluid Findings
CNS-1	No lymphoblasts
CNS-2	<5 WBCs/mcL with definable blasts on cytocentrifuge examination
CNS-3	≥5 WBCs/mcL with blast cells (or cranial nerve palsy)

Management

Prognostic Factors in Management of Pediatric Acute Lymphoblastic Leukemia

As outcomes with modern therapy in pediatric ALL have improved, many factors previously shown to be important for predicting a prognosis have lost statistical significance. Five factors have retained prognostic significance and constitute the basis on which patients are stratified in most treatment protocols. These factors are (1) age at presentation, (2) WBC at presentation, (3) specific cytogenetic abnormalities, (4) presence or absence of CNS involvement (Table 100.4), and (5) rapidity of initial response to chemotherapy.[8] The 1996 National Cancer Institute (NCI) consensus criteria standardized definitions of age, initial WBC, and CNS involvement to facilitate a comparison of clinical trial results between groups.[65] Cooperative groups differ in incorporation of cytogenetics and response to therapy. General principles of

modern ALL protocols include treatment of low-risk disease with less-intensive chemotherapy to minimize toxicity while maintaining excellent overall survival (OS) (90% to 95%), whereas high-risk disease (OS, 40% to 85%) is treated with more intensive therapy.[8]

The age-determined risk groups are less than 1 year (infant ALL), 1.0 to 9.99 years (standard risk ALL), and ≥10 years (high-risk ALL). Infants constitute a very high-risk group. *MLL* (11q23) rearrangements are frequent, especially t(4;11)(q21;q23), and are associated with hyperleukocytosis, extramedullary disease, and common acute lymphoblastic leukemia antigen (CALLA) (CD10) negativity.[66,67] Cure rates on current infant protocols have improved modestly to approximately 50%.[68,69] Results are poorest in infants under 3 months of age with *MLL* rearrangement. Unlike for some other high-risk ALL subgroups, current evidence does not suggest a benefit of stem cell transplant.[69]

Adolescents and young adults have also traditionally demonstrated lower cure rates, although survival has improved significantly with early intensive postinduction therapy.[12,70] In B-lineage ALL, presenting with a WBC count more than 50,000/mcL, and particularly over 100,000/mcL, is associated with a high risk of relapse.

Blast cell cytogenetics and ploidy have a significant prognostic impact in ALL (Fig. 100.3). High hyperdiploidy (≥50 chromosomes or DNA index >1.16) is associated with good prognosis, particularly with trisomies of chromosomes 4 and 10.[71–73] Hypodiploidy (<45 chromosomes) and especially haploidy

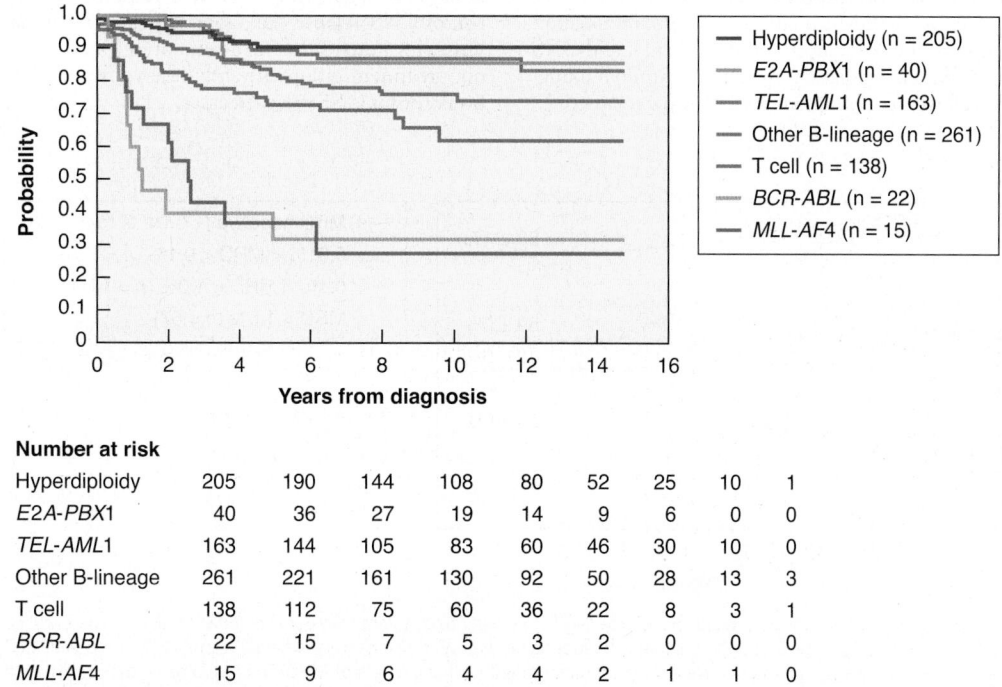

Number at risk

Hyperdiploidy	205	190	144	108	80	52	25	10	1
*E2A-PBX*1	40	36	27	19	14	9	6	0	0
*TEL-AML*1	163	144	105	83	60	46	30	10	0
Other B-lineage	261	221	161	130	92	50	28	13	3
T cell	138	112	75	60	36	22	8	3	1
BCR-ABL	22	15	7	5	3	2	0	0	0
*MLL-AF*4	15	9	6	4	4	2	1	1	0

Figure 100.3 Kaplan-Meier analysis of event-free survival according to biologic subtype of leukemia. (From Pui CH, Robison LL, Look AT. Acute lymphoblastic leukaemia. *Lancet* 2008;371:1030–1043.)

(23 chromosomes) are associated with a poor prognosis.[72,74] Two other recently identified unfavorable abnormalities are *IKZF1* alterations[75] and intrachromosomal amplification of chromosome 21 (iAMP21).[76] *CRLF2* overexpression has been found to have an independent adverse prognostic impact in some studies, but not others.[77,78]

The most common translocation in pediatric ALL is t(12;21) (p12;q22), forming the *ETV6-RUNX1* (also known as *TEL-AML1*) fusion. This cryptic translocation occurs in 25% of US pediatric ALL cases, less frequently in other geographic and ethnically defined populations, and is associated with a favorable prognosis.[79,80] The Philadelphia chromosome (Ph+) refers to the t(9;22) (9q34;q11) translocation, forming the *BCR-ABL1* fusion. Ph+ ALL is less prevalent in children than adults and was historically associated with a dismal prognosis. Treatment of Ph+ ALL and CML were revolutionized by imatinib mesylate, a selective tyrosine kinase inhibitor active against the *BCR-ABL1* fusion. The addition of imatinib to conventional chemotherapy has improved survival from approximately 30% to 40% to 80%, and hematopoietic stem cell transplant (HSCT) in first remission is no longer considered as the standard of care.[81–83] Ongoing studies are investigating the efficacy of later generation tyrosine kinase inhibitors such as dasatinib.[84]

Numerous translocations occur in T-lineage ALL, but they are not generally associated with a prognosis. Activating *NOTCH1* mutations occur in over 50% of T-ALL cases, and are associated with a favorable prognosis.[85,86] Because mutated *NOTCH1* activity depends on γ-secretase activity, γ-secretase inhibitors are being investigated as a novel therapeutic approach. Early T-cell precursor (ETP) is a very unfavorable prognostic subgroup identified based on a distinctive immunophenotype, constituting approximately 10% of T-lineage ALL, which bears a gene expression signature and mutational profile similar to myeloid leukemia.[61,87]

CNS and testicular involvement are unfavorable prognostic signs, for which therapy is intensified.[56] The CNS is considered a sanctuary site because many systemic treatments do not adequately penetrate the blood–brain barrier, so CNS preventive therapy is required in all patients to prevent eventual CNS relapse. CNS prophylaxis is usually achieved through systemic and intrathecal chemotherapy. Although CNS involvement at diagnosis has generally been treated in the past with the addition of radiation to intensive chemotherapy, some advocate for reserving CNS radiation for use only in the case of CNS relapse.[88] Both testicular and CNS relapses require site-directed radiation as well as systemic reinduction due to increased risk of subsequent bone marrow relapse.[12,89]

All modern pediatric ALL treatment protocols use the prognostic factors outlined here, in varying ways, to stratify patients into different risk groups that receive treatment of different intensity. The first phase of treatment (*induction*) lasts 4 to 6 weeks and includes a glucocorticoid, vincristine (VCR), asparaginase, and for high-risk patients, an anthracycline (usually daunomycin).[12] The Berlin-Frankfurt-Munster group begins induction with a *steroid window*, and the degree of cytoreduction during this window is used in risk assessments.[90] Some groups intensify induction with additional medications. Rapid response to induction is an important prognostic variable (Fig. 100.4).[8,73] Induction failure (≥25% marrow blasts at the end of induction) is rare (2% to 5% of cases) and generally associated with a poor prognosis, although a recent large retrospective analysis reported an unexpected heterogeneity in survival, ranging from 10% to 70%, depending on age, cytogenetics, and B- versus T-lineage disease.[91]

Induction is usually followed by a *consolidation phase* to reinforce the bone marrow remission and to administer CNS prophylaxis. Subsequent intensive phases may be termed *intensification*, *delayed intensification*, or *reinduction/reconsolidation*, with the intensity depending on the risk group.[12,92,93] These intensive courses are generally delivered within the first 6 to 12 months of treatment, followed by a *maintenance* or *continuation* phase lasting 2 to 3 years, which consists of antimetabolite treatment (usually consisting of methotrexate weekly and 6-mercaptopurine daily), periodic intrathecal (IT) treatments, and periodic *pulses* of VCR and oral glucocorticoids with the frequency of these pulses varying by protocol and treatment group. To minimize and avoid treatment-related toxicities, strict supportive care guidelines are employed. Therapy-related mortality on frontline pediatric ALL protocols is generally under 2% to 3%. Overall treatment duration is usually between 2 and 3.5 years. On current Children's Oncology Group regimens, boys receive an additional year of maintenance, but many other cooperative study groups treat both genders for approximately 2 years.

CNS-directed therapy is usually present in all phases, but is most intensive during the first several months. CNS therapy uses intrathecal chemotherapy, high-dose systemic chemotherapy (principally, higher dose methotrexate or cytarabine), and/or cranial radiation.[56,94] Because it is often associated with neurocognitive deficits, endocrine, and growth abnormalities, cranial radiation has generally been reserved only for patients at highest risk of CNS relapse (i.e., approximately 5% of patients who present with initial CNS involvement or T-cell disease), but at least one treatment group currently reserves the use of cranial irradiation only for CNS-relapsed cases.[88] Through the years, the doses of

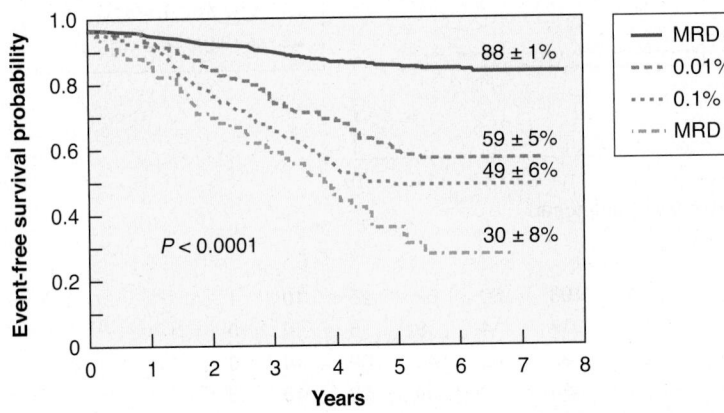
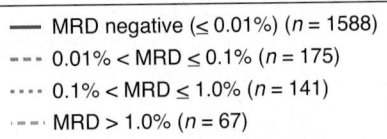

Figure 100.4 Effect of minimal residual disease (MRD) on prognosis. Event-free survival (EFS) of all patients enrolled on the Pediatric Oncology Group 9900 series therapeutic studies with satisfactory end-induction MRD. The 5-year EFS values plus or minus standard error are shown for patients with varying levels of MRD. The outcome of those with high levels of MRD is very poor, but even those with 0.01% to 0.1% MRD have only a 59% ± 5% 5-year EFS. (From Borowitz MJ, Devidas M, Hunger SP, et al. Clinical significance of minimal residual disease in childhood acute lymphoblastic leukemia and its relationship to other prognostic factors: a Children's Oncology Group study. *Blood* 2008;111:5477–5485.)

cranial radiation have decreased from the 24- to 36-Gy range that was used on early protocols to 18 Gy for treatment and 12 Gy on some CNS preventive therapy regimens.[56]

Therapy for relapsed ALL depends on the location of relapse (isolated extramedullary, bone marrow, or combined) and the duration of initial remission. Extramedullary relapse generally has a better prognosis than bone marrow relapse, but requires localized in addition to systemic chemotherapy.[12] For testicular relapse, local therapy involves orchiectomy, followed by irradiation of the remaining testicle and scrotal area.[12,95] Fertility will be compromised (so postpubertal males should be offered sperm banking), and hormonal supplements should be offered as needed. Prognosis after a testicular relapse remains quite good. For CNS relapse, local therapy involves intensified intrathecal therapy, varying regimens of high-dose systemic therapy, and the addition of cranial and/or craniospinal radiation.

All relapse types have a worse prognosis if they occur during therapy or within 6 months of completing therapy.[96] Interestingly, a recent study indicated that postrelapse survival does not differ according to the intensity of chemotherapy received prior to relapse.[97] Multiple medications and regimens are being tested for induction in relapsed and refractory leukemia. A common approach is to administer several intensive blocks of conventional chemotherapy agents, with or without a concomitant novel investigational agent.[98] Promising results have been recently obtained with clofarabine and clofarabine-containing regimens.[99–101] Blinatumomab, a CD19/CD3-bispecific T-cell engaging (BiTE) antibody, has shown promising response rates and prolonged survival in relapsed B-lineage ALL in adults, and is currently in a phase II international trial in pediatrics.[102,103] Promising recent results have been obtained using chimeric antigen receptor-modified T cells with specificity for CD19, termed CTL019 cells.[104] The most recent update on this trial reported that among 20 patients (including 16 pediatric) with treatment refractory CD19+ ALL, 14 patients (82%) achieved complete remission, with robust in vivo expansion of CTL019 cells, and 11 of 17 evaluable patients maintained an ongoing CR during median follow-up of 2.6 months.[105]

The decision between chemotherapy and HSCT for second complete remission has been controversial. HSCT is usually used for relapse within 6 months of the completion of initial treatment (CR1 <30 months), but the decision also depends on suitable donor availability, the difficulty (number and intensity of induction attempts needed to achieve CR2), and the overall health of the recipient.[106] Prior to HSCT, patients with relapsed ALL typically receive induction and consolidative chemotherapy, because the chances of success with HSCT are extremely low in the setting of continued active disease. Autologous BMT in ALL is no longer recommended.

Prognostic Factors and Management of Pediatric Acute Myeloid Leukemia

In contrast with ALL, there are fewer standard clinical or laboratory-based factors in AML that consistently relate to prognosis. Table 100.1 reviews prognostic factors in pediatric ALL and AML. Poor prognostic factors that predict lower remission rates and/or decreased event-free survival (EFS) include blast cytogenetics with monosomy 5 or 7, 5q deletion, FLT3/ITD, and secondary AML/MDS.[19,107–109] Adolescents and young adults have an increased risk of treatment-related mortality, but no significant difference in OS.[110] A swift response to induction chemotherapy (i.e., remission after one cycle of chemotherapy), favorable cytogenetics, and DS (with FAB M7) are predictive of better outcomes.[108] Favorable cytogenetics in AML include core binding factor alterations (the t[8;21] *AML1/ETO* fusion and inv[16]), and the t(15;17) *PML/RARα* fusion seen in acute promyelocytic leukemia (APL) (see Chapter 107). Two other recently identified favorable cytogenetic alterations (CCAAT) are mutations in *NPM1*[111] and CCAAT/enhancer-binding protein alpha (*CEBP*).[112] In addition to genetic

alterations, MRD is being integrated into current AML studies as an important prognostic marker.[113] Although many findings in AML are similar between adults and children, important biologic and therapeutic differences are emerging. An example of this is that mutations of the *KIT* receptor tyrosine kinase have a similar frequency in pediatric core binding factor AML as those found in adult AML, but lack the poor prognosis seen in adults.[109]

There have been incremental improvements in AML outcomes over recent decades, with current overall survival in the 60% to 70% range (see Fig. 100.2). These improvements have come through increased intensity of therapy and improved supportive care.[114,115] The inherent drug resistance of AML cells poses challenges because the intensification of therapy required is associated with significant treatment-related toxicity, particularly infections.[19]

With the exception of DS patients with FAB M7 AML and patients with APL, most pediatric AML induction therapies include two cycles of ara-C and daunomycin, with or without thioguanine and/or etoposide. Studies have shown that the intensity of induction therapy is important for OS.[19] In the Children's Cancer Group 2891 protocol, intensively timed induction (starting the second cycle on day 14 regardless of count recovery) did not change the induction (CR1) rate, but it did have a profound effect on eventual cure rate.[116] Although fewer than 5% of pediatric AML patients present with CNS disease, as many as 20% will suffer an isolated CNS relapse.[55] Intrathecal chemotherapy (usually ara-C) has been found by several groups to effectively reduce the risk of CNS relapse.[19]

Conventional postinduction consolidative chemotherapy in pediatric AML usually involves two to three cycles of high-dose ara-C–based combinations, to which anthracycline, etoposide, or ifosfamide/cyclophosphamide may be added. There is no proven benefit to maintenance chemotherapy, so conventional treatment is rarely more than four to eight cycles.[19,117]

Gemtuzumab ozogamicin (GO), a newer agent consisting of an antibody to CD33 coupled to calicheamicin (a toxic antitumor antibiotic), has shown some promise in relapsed AML and was recently tested in a randomized, prospective trial for frontline disease by the Children's Oncology Group.[118] GO was significantly associated with improved EFS, but not OS. Other adult and pediatric trials of GO in AML have yielded mixed results, and at present, it has been voluntarily withdrawn from the commercial market and its role in AML therapy remains to be determined. Two promising novel biologic agents, the proteasome inhibitor bortezomib[119] and the kinase inhibitor sorafenib (which inhibits FLT3)[120] are currently being tested for efficacy in combination with frontline conventional chemotherapy. The indications for HSCT in pediatric AML, preparative regimens, timing (CR1 or later), and type of donor are the focus of intensive ongoing controversy and research.[116,121,122]

Pediatric APL has among the highest cure rates in pediatric AML. These patients should receive all-*trans*-retinoic acid (ATRA), which directly binds to the t(15;17) translocation, which forms a fusion protein combining the promyelocytic leukemia (*PML*) gene with the retinoic acid receptor alpha (*RARα*) gene, which is causative for this form of AML.[123] They should also receive conventional chemotherapy during both induction and consolidation phases. Patients who respond to this therapy have an 80% to 85% survival rate and should not be subjected to HSCT.[124] Similar to adult therapies for APL (see Chapter 107), arsenic trioxide, found to be useful for salvage in patients who became resistant to ATRA, is currently being tested in upfront pediatric APL regimens (both alone and in combination with ATRA and conventional chemotherapy) in an effort to improve DFS in CR1.[125] Rapid initiation of therapy is particularly important in APL due to the risk of severe bleeding complications in untreated disease. Early deaths from bleeding are often not captured on clinical trials, but population-based studies indicate that they are a significant cause of mortality.[126] Despite the remarkable successes with ATRA and arsenic trioxide with and without conventional chemotherapy, there remain patients with APL with relapsed and refractory disease, and many of these can still be cured with HSCT.[127]

DS patients with AMKL (see earlier discussion) do well with lower dose ara-C regimens and standard timing of their induction cycles. Current results in DS AMKL are the best of any AML subgroup outside of APL, with 70% to 85% EFS, with patients under 2 years showing the best results, and thus not requiring intensive chemotherapy or HSCT.[128–130]

The prognosis for pediatric patients who relapse after either conventional or HSCT therapy for AML is poor. A second CR can be obtained using similar ara-C and anthracycline-containing regimens in 20% to 70% of patients, but the likelihood of obtaining a cure is approximately half the rate for de novo AML.[131] Clofarabine alone and in combination (see ALL relapse discussion) with other chemotherapeutic agents also shows some efficacy.[100,101] HSCT in early relapse or CR2 for AML patients who were previously transplanted in CR1 is a strategy that has had some success.[131–133] Other novel therapies, including FLT3 inhibitors and hypomethylating agents, are currently being studied.[134]

Rarer Forms of Leukemia in Children

Chronic leukemias, with the exception of CML, do not occur in children. Ph+ CML is rare in childhood (<1% to 2% of all pediatric leukemia cases).[135] When it does occur, it typically presents in adolescents and is in the chronic phase. Therapy is similar to that recommended in adults, with imatinib (along with hydroxyurea if the initial counts are high, and/or the patient presents with a high degree of hepatosplenomegaly) as the mainstay of induction and maintenance therapy. The use of alternative tyrosine kinase inhibitors such as dasatinib and nilotinib are being investigated in children as well as adults.[136] Because there is no clear end point for when or whether any of these tyrosine kinase inhibitors can be safely discontinued, many pediatric oncologists continue to consider hematopoietic stem cell transplantation in remission.

JMML, a myeloproliferative disorder unique to childhood, is characterized by extreme monocytosis, hepatosplenomegaly, thrombocytopenia, and increased fetal hemoglobin.[137] Bone marrow morphology is often consistent with myelodysplasia as well as myeloproliferation, and cytogenetics frequently reveals a monosomy 7 clone. Mutations in *PTN11*, *CBL*, and other *RAS* pathway genes have also been noted.[138,139] Although the clinical course can be indolent (requiring only intermittent blood product and antibiotic support), JMML patients often progress to frank marrow failure. Neither aggressive AML-type chemotherapy nor splenectomy has been shown to significantly prolong survival, so these approaches are starting to be reserved for those patients who are symptomatic. The most definitive therapy in JMML is an allogeneic BMT.[140] Overall

DFS with BMT in JMML has been in the 40% to 55% range, with relapse the major reason for failure. Novel therapies targeting the rat sarcoma (*RAS*), rapidly accelerated fibrosarcoma (*RAF*), mitogen activated protein kinase (*MEK*), mammalian target of rapamycin (mTOR), signal transducer and activator of transcription 5 (*STAT5*), and other signaling pathways are currently under investigation.[137]

Mixed phenotype acute leukemia (MPAL) is a new designation established by the World Health Organization (WHO) 2008 classification, replacing the prior diagnosis of biphenotypic acute leukemia, which was based on the European Group for the Immunological Classification of Leukemias (EGIL) and the WHO 2001 classification.[141] MPALs constitute only approximately 0.5% to 1% of acute leukemias, with combined lineage differentiation that is most often B- and myeloid, followed by T- and myeloid, and rarely B- and T- or trilineage. The WHO classification recognizes two specific subgroups, characterized by a *BCR-ABL* rearrangement and *MLL* rearrangement, as well as a subgroup for the remainder of cases, which have other nonspecific chromosomal abnormalities. There are little systematic data about this rare form of leukemia, but outcomes are generally poor. Some data suggest that ALL-directed therapy may be more effective than AML-directed therapy. Allogeneic stem cell transplant is frequently employed.

LYMPHOMAS

Lymphomas constitute approximately 10% of cancer in children, and are the third most common pediatric malignancy (behind leukemias and brain tumors).[142] Two-thirds of lymphomas in children are a heterogeneous group of lymphomas categorized as non-Hodgkin lymphomas (NHL), and the remainder are Hodgkin lymphomas (HL). Table 100.5 compares the differences in presenting and staging features between pediatric NHL and HL. The histology, biology, and management of lymphoma differs in children compared to adults. For example, the indolent, low-grade lymphomas seen in adults are rarely seen in children. Additionally, radiation and certain types of chemotherapy are minimized when possible to reduce detrimental effects on growth and development and other late effects of therapy such as second malignancies.

Non-Hodgkin Lymphoma

The Revised European–American Classification of Lymphoid Neoplasms (REAL) classification, which has served as the basis for the WHO classification of hematopoietic and lymphoid tumors, categorizes lymphomas according to phenotype and differentiation.[143]

TABLE 100.5

Comparison of Hodgkin Lymphoma and Non-Hodgkin Lymphoma in Pediatric Patients

Feature	Hodgkin Lymphoma	Non-Hodgkin Lymphoma
Age	Mostly >10 y	Any age in children
Stage at diagnosis	Mostly localized	Commonly widespread
Constitutional symptoms	Alter prognosis	Do not affect prognosis
CNS involvement	Rare	Occurrence increases with AIDS
Mediastinal involvement	Most common with nodular sclerosing Hodgkin lymphoma	Most common with lymphoblastic lymphoma
Gastrointestinal involvement	Rare	Occurs
Abdominal nodal involvement	Can be small or large, mesenteric rare	Usually enlarged, mesenteric common
Bone involvement	Rare	Occurs
Marrow involvement	Rare	Common

Adapted from Rademaker, J. Hodgkin's and non-Hodgkin's lymphomas. *Radiol Clin North Am* 2007;45:69–83.

Pediatric NHLs appear in four major categories: (1) precursor T- and, less commonly, precursor B-lymphoblastic lymphoma (30% of pediatric NHLs), (2) Burkitt and Burkitt-like lymphoma (40% to 50%), (3) diffuse large B-cell lymphoma (15%), and (4) anaplastic large cell lymphoma (10%).[142] These subtypes are high-grade, acute diseases and, rarely, truly localized diseases. Major improvement in the survival of children with NHL has occurred during the past 20 years, correlating with the advent of systemic multiagent chemotherapy regimens, as opposed to a reliance on localized therapies such as surgery and radiation.

The Cotswold revision of the Ann Arbor NHL staging and classification system used in adult NHLs has mostly been replaced in pediatrics by the St. Jude's Research Hospital staging system outlined in Table 100.6, which incorporates common presentations of pediatric NHL including increased extranodal involvement, bone marrow and CNS involvement, and on contiguous spread of disease.[144] Surgical/pathologic staging is no longer carried out in either pediatric NHL or HL cases. Diagnosis generally relies on biopsy and radiologic scans, usually a combination of computed tomography (CT) and nuclear medicine scans and, occasionally, magnetic resonance imaging.[145] The current 5-year EFS rates for early low-stage disease are in the 90% to 95% range and from 70% to 90% for the higher stage presentations.[4,142]

Unlike ALL or HL, there is no sharp age peak for the occurrence of NHL in children. There is a marked imbalance in the male to female incidence, which approaches a 3:1 ratio.[142,146] With the exception of children with rare, inherited, or acquired immunodeficiency syndromes (e.g., Wiskott-Aldrich syndrome, common variable immune deficiency, ataxia–telangiectasia, X-linked lymphoproliferative syndrome, HIV/AIDS, or exposure to immunosuppressive drugs after solid organ or bone marrow transplants), most children who develop NHL have a history of normal health and no known risk factors. The main exception to this concerns the possible etiologic role of the Epstein-Barr virus (EBV). EBV is strongly associated with lymphomas in HIV patients, lymphoproliferative diseases found in posttransplant patients, and endemic Burkitt lymphoma, and it is found in many cases of HL (see later discussion) in otherwise healthy children.[147,148]

Lymphoblastic lymphomas share many molecular, biologic, cytogenetic, and therapeutic characteristics with ALL, and are now treated with similar chemotherapy protocols.[12,146] The distinction between ALL and lymphoblastic lymphoma is somewhat arbitrary because those patients with more than 25% lymphoblasts in their bone marrow at diagnosis (despite the existence of a large lymphomatous mass elsewhere in the body) are designated as having ALL. Morphologically, the cells are indistinguishable, and the immunophenotypes generally overlap.[146,149] In contrast to ALL however, precursor T-lymphoblastic lymphoma is more common than precursor B-lymphoblastic lymphoma, with more than 75% of lymphoblastic lymphoma cases demonstrating precursor T-cell immunophenotype.

The typical presentation of children with lymphoblastic lymphoma is that of a patient with rapidly enlarging neck and mediastinal lymphadenopathy. Particular attention needs to be paid to hydration status, kidney function, and whether the kidneys are directly involved with the disease. CT and positron-emission tomography (PET) are helpful for assessing the degree of organ involvement, but care must be taken in requiring children with mediastinal masses to lie supine (which can compress both central blood vessels and airways) or undergo sedation (which causes vasodilation and decreased blood return to the heart).[150] A histologic diagnosis should be sought in the least invasive way possible. Prebiopsy steroids or *postage stamp irradiation* (use of a small radiation field to emergently relieve airway compression) can be done, but the steroids may jeopardize obtaining the histologic diagnosis or accurate staging. CNS status should be assessed prior to systemic chemotherapy, and prophylactic intrathecal chemotherapy should be administered early.[146] Prognostic factors include the level of bone marrow involvement at diagnosis and CNS involvement at diagnosis.

Primary therapy for lymphoblastic lymphoma (of either B- or T-cell histology) consists of multiagent chemotherapy without radiation. Stage I lymphoblastic cases do very well with short treatments (three to five cycles) of cyclophosphamide, doxorubicin, vincristine, and prednisone (CHOP regimen or similar), and a relatively short (24 weeks versus 2 to 3 years with ALL) maintenance phase of antimetabolite (6-mercaptopurine daily and weekly oral methotrexate).[142,146] Higher stage (stages II, III, and IV) lymphoblastic cases require more intensive regimens and a prolonged maintenance phase such as that used for ALL. The benefit of high-dose methotrexate and cranial radiation remain controversial in lymphoblastic lymphoma.[151–153] Nelarabine is a novel nucleoside analog with preferential cytotoxicity in T-lineage lymphoid malignancies that is being studied in current protocols.[154] Because activating NOTCH1 mutations are found in the majority of T-cell

TABLE 100.6

St. Jude Children's Research Hospital Staging System for Pediatric Non-Hodgkin Lymphoma

Stage	Description
I	A single tumor (extranodal) or single anatomic area (nodal), with the exclusion of mediastinum or abdomen
II	A single tumor (extranodal) with regional node involvement Two or more nodal areas on the same side of the diaphragm Two single (extranodal) tumors with or without regional node involvement on the same side of the diaphragm A primary gastrointestinal tract tumor, usually in the ileocecal area, with or without involvement of associated mesenteric nodes only[a]
III	Two single tumors (extranodal) on opposite sides of the diaphragm Two or more nodal areas above and below the diaphragm All the primary intrathoracic tumors (mediastinal, pleural, thymic) All extensive primary intra-abdominal disease[a] All paraspinal or epidural tumors, regardless of other tumor sites
IV	Any of the previous with initial central nervous system or bone marrow involvement[b]

[a] Stage II abdominal disease typically is limited to a segment (usually distal ileum) of the gut plus or minus the associated mesenteric nodes only, and the primary tumor can be completely removed grossly by segmental excision. Stage III abdominal disease typically exhibits spread to para-aortic and retroperitoneal areas by implants and plaques in mesentery or peritoneum, or by direct infiltration of structures adjacent to the primary tumor. Ascites may be present, and the complete resection of all gross tumor is not possible.

[b] If bone marrow involvement is present at diagnosis, the percentage of blasts or abnormal cells must be 25% or less to be classified as stage IV non-Hodgkin lymphoma. If there are more than 25% blasts, the patient is classified as having acute leukemia (either precursor B- or T-acute lymphoblastic leukemia or L3 acute lymphoblastic leukemia).

leukemias, gamma-secretase inhibitors that block Notch 1 signaling are another class of agents whose role in treatment regimens is being assessed.[155,156] Relapse in lymphoblastic lymphoma is, fortunately, an uncommon problem, but when it does occur it happens either during or shortly after completion of therapy. Relapse of low-stage disease can frequently be salvaged using the more intensive chemotherapy designed for high-stage disease.[157] Lymphoblastic lymphoma patients who relapse after higher stage treatment have a poor prognosis and are candidates for nelarabine, phase I agents and/or BMT if response is obtained to salvage therapy.[157] Radiation to areas of bulk disease and total-body irradiation are incorporated into the transplant regimens, but, in general, radiation does not have a role in primary treatment or reinduction at relapse.

Burkitt and Burkitt-like lymphoma are mature B-cell lymphomas. Endemic Burkitt lymphoma (usually presenting with localized head and neck masses—most frequently, the jaw) in Africa is quite common (100 cases per million children), and 95% are associated with EBV. Sporadic Burkitt lymphoma, as seen in the United States, typically presents with an abdominal mass, occurs in 1 to 2 cases per million children, and only 15% are associated with EBV.[158] The most common presentation in the United States is of a boy age 5 to 10 years, with a right lower quadrant mass and/or acute abdomen secondary to an ileocecal intussusception. If the tumor is limited to the distal ileum or cecum, it should be completely excised along with its associated mesentery, and the bowel repaired with an end-to-end anastomosis.[159] These children have low-stage disease, require less chemotherapy, and have an excellent outcome. More frequently, the abdominal involvement is much more diffuse.

Burkitt lymphoma cells have a mature B-cell immunophenotype (expressing cell surface immunoglobulin, usually IgM) and are characterized morphologically by homogeneous round-to-oval nuclei, multiple nucleoli, and intensely basophilic cytoplasm with large vacuolated areas containing fat. Burkitt-like lymphoma shares pathologic and molecular features with diffuse large B-cell lymphoma and responds to similar chemotherapy as Burkitt lymphoma. The majority of Burkitt lymphoma cases display the t(8;14) (q24;q32) translocation in which c-myc from chromosome 8 is translocated to the Ig heavy-chain locus on chromosome 14. In this translocation and in two less common variants, t(2;8) (p12;q24) and t(8;22) (q24;q11), the c-myc oncogene is overexpressed because of the influence of Ig regulatory regions (enhancers).[160]

The diagnosis of Burkitt lymphoma must be done very expeditiously as these tumors grow swiftly and patients are at high risk of intestinal obstruction (from intussusception) and metabolic problems related to tumor lysis syndrome. Tumor lysis often begins even before chemotherapy. Special attention must be paid to serum electrolyte balance (including calcium/phosphate balance), and vigorous intravenous hydration and alkalinization to improve uric acid excretion is essential. Allopurinol or recombinant urate oxidase, rasburicase, is used to block uric acid production. Occasionally, the lysis syndrome can be severe enough to cause acute renal failure, and dialysis must be used to maintain fluid and reestablish electrolyte balance.

Children with low-stage, African-endemic Burkitt lymphoma have been successfully treated with single or multiple doses of cyclophosphamide. Therapies as brief as 4 weeks have been successfully employed.[161] These strategies result in lower cure rates, but they make it feasible to treat large numbers of children with lower toxic death and complication rates in resource-poor settings.[162] Higher stage Burkitt lymphoma (stages 3 and 4) requires significantly more intensive chemotherapy, involving much higher doses of cyclophosphamide, and the addition of an anthracycline, high-dose ara-C, methotrexate, and VP-16 to the CHOP schemas. Many current high-stage Burkitt lymphoma protocols use hematopoietic growth factor support to enhance bone marrow recovery in order to allow intensive cycles to be given approximately every 3 weeks. These protocols are intensive, but they are usually of a short (6- to 8-month) duration. There have been some efforts to reduce chemotherapy and to add biologic agents like rituximab (anti-CD20 antibody) to reduce

toxicity of treatment in patients who have HIV or other medical problems.[163,164] Currently, the efficacy of the addition of rituximab to advanced stage Burkitt lymphoma protocols is being investigated.[165] The cure rate for pediatric patients with higher stage (stage III and IV) Burkitt lymphoma is now 80% to 90%.[166] The management of relapsed Burkitt lymphoma is problematic. Relapses usually occur during therapy or shortly after the cessation of therapy. Low-stage patients can sometimes be effectively treated using a high-stage primary protocol. Higher stage relapsed patients may try a salvage therapy such as R-ICE (rituximab, ifosfamide, carboplatin, etoposide) or phase I therapies, and BMT should be considered if a response is achieved.[167]

The workup and staging of large cell lymphomas are similar to that described for other forms of NHL. Diffuse large B cell lymphoma (DLBCL) tends to present with large mediastinal masses, but bone, lymph node, and abdominal presentations are also seen. Bone marrow and CNS involvement are not common. Combination chemotherapy is effective against DLBCL, and radiation does not have a role in therapy for most cases. DLBCL and anaplastic large cell lymphoma (ALCL) used to be treated similarly as large cell lymphomas, the mature B-cell lymphomas (DLBCL and Burkitt lymphoma) are now grouped together on contemporary treatment protocols. However, it is not clear that DLBCL requires as much CNS-directed therapy as Burkitt lymphoma because CNS involvement is less common for DLBCL. Primary mediastinal B-cell lymphoma (PMBL) is a subtype of DLBCL that often presents with sclerosis and has a less favorable prognosis. PMBL shares some biologic features with Hodgkin lymphoma, and alternate treatment regimens are being investigated for PMBL based on differences in biology and prognosis.[168]

ALCL tends to present with involvement of lymph nodes and extranodal sites including the skin, the lung, other soft tissues, and bone. Bone marrow and CNS involvement are uncommon. The majority of ALCL cases have T-cell immunophenotype. ALCL is also known for cytogenetically presenting with the t(2;5) (p23;q35) translocation, which fuses nucleophosmin with a transmembrane tyrosine-specific protein kinase known as anaplastic lymphoma kinase. Three to five cycles of CHOP or APO (adriamycin, prednisone, Oncovin/VCR) have been used, and more recently, Associazione Italiana Ematologia Oncologia Pediatrica (AIEOP) ALCL-99 with EFS that ranges from 70% to 85%.[169] Targeted therapy with crizotinib, an inhibitor of the anaplastic lymphoma kinase (ALK), a tyrosine kinase, has produced promising responses in early studies in relapsed ALK-positive ALCL.[170] Another targeted therapy demonstrating promising activity against both ALCL and Hodgkin lymphoma is brentuximab vedotin, an anti-CD30 directed monoclonal antibody conjugated to a microtubule-disrupting agent.[171]

Hodgkin Lymphoma

The natural history and outcome of treatment in HL is similar in young children and adults, but treatment decisions (and regimens) are different in children based on the need for attention to late effects of therapy. Risk-adapted therapy seeks to maintain excellent cure rates of 80% to 90%, whereas limiting radiation and certain types of chemotherapy that may cause long-term organ damage, growth problems, infertility, and second malignancies.[5,172] HL is rare below the age of 5 years, with the majority of pediatric cases presenting in children older than 11 years. Young patients (<10 years) have a 3:1 male to female ratio. This imbalance returns to the approximately equal male to female ratio seen in adult disease as the age of presentation climbs. The age of HL incidence in industrialized countries is bimodal, with the first peak in adults 20 to 30 years of age and the second peak occurring much later in adulthood.[173]

The etiology of HL is unknown, but EBV is found in up to 40% of cases.[174] There are also familial and geographic clusters that suggest an inherited, environmental, or infectious contribution to etiology.[174] Most children (90%) present with painless adenopathy in the neck, and 60% have involvement of anterior mediastinum, paratracheal, or hilar lymph nodes. The Cotswold modification of the Ann Arbor Staging System (described in Chapter 103) is used for all ages. B symptoms (defined as in adults) include unexplained fever (more than 38°C [100.4°F]), drenching night sweats, and more than 10% weight loss. B symptoms are present in approximately 30% of newly diagnosed pediatric HL cases.[175] The process of clinical staging includes both site of involvement and the presence of B symptoms and is described in detail for adult patients in Chapter 102. There is no longer any role for staging laparotomy, because localized radiation is no longer used as a sole treatment modality in pediatric HL. Increasingly, PET scans are being used to assess staging and early response and to guide further treatment, as opposed to exclusive reliance on CT.[176]

The malignant cells in HL constitute a minority (estimated at 0.1% to 10%) of the cell population of the discernible tumor.[177] Inflammatory cells (histiocytes, plasma cells, lymphocytes, eosinophils, and neutrophils) make up the bulk of the tumor. The malignant cells are actually malignant lymphocytes with specific, characterized immunophenotypes. The WHO classifies four subtypes of classic HL: (1) nodular sclerosing, (2) mixed cellularity, (3) lymphocyte rich, and (4) lymphocyte depleted. Nodular lymphocyte-predominant HL (NLPHL) is another important subtype of HL.

The most common presenting histology in pediatric HL is nodular sclerosing type, which accounts for more than 50% of the cases (40% of the younger patients but 70% of the adolescents).[173] It is characterized by bands of fibrosis and a thickened lymph node capsule that are discernible even in a gross pathologic section. These nodes and masses tend to form scars that can lead to residual masses, which appear as opacified lesions on radiologic studies for years after a full clinical response. Mixed cellularity is responsible for approximately 30% of pediatric cases. It is commonly seen in children less than 10 years of age and is highly associated with EBV positivity. The lymphocyte-depleted form of HL is quite rare, except in children with HIV. The lymphocyte-rich variant is quite rare in children (approximately 5% of the cases), has a high incidence of mediastinal masses and stage III disease, but has an older average age of presentation (32 years).[173]

With the exception of NLPHL, treatment for all of the various HL histologies is the same and is based on staging. Risk-adapted therapy in pediatric HL is composed of three to six cycles of combination chemotherapy followed by involved field radiation therapy (IFRT) for higher risk patients. The composition of the chemotherapy regimens has varied during the years, but combinations of vinca alkaloids, alkylating agents (cyclophosphamide commonly used now), steroids, anthracyclines, and bleomycin have been used. Current therapies for low-risk HL attempt to reduce exposure to alkylators, anthracyclines, and bleomycin and IFRT to reduce the risk of late effects.

Therapy for higher risk HL (higher stage at presentation or slow response to therapy) currently involves additional cycles of higher dose combination chemotherapy and IFRT, with EFS rates still in the 80% to 90% range when risk-adapted therapy is given.[3] Targeted therapy such as brentuximab vedotin, discussed previously, will be studied in frontline therapy regimens. Treatment for relapsed or refractory pediatric HL is beyond the scope of this chapter, but the medications (e.g., ifosfamide and vinorelbine) and approaches (e.g., BMT) are usually similar to those used in adults (see Chapter 102). Novel therapies under investigation include antibodies targeting CD30 (brentuximab vedotin), CD25, and other antigens; the proteasome inhibitor bortezomib; and histone deacetylase inhibitors; as well as cytotoxic T-cell based therapies directed against both EBV-associated and EBV-negative lymphomas.[3]

NLPHL disease affects 10% to 15% of pediatric patients, is more common among male and younger patients, and is usually clinically localized (low stage). Stage I patients do well with surgical resection only (no chemotherapy or radiotherapy) and close follow-up.[178] For stage II/III, most would be treated with several cycles of relatively low-dose chemotherapy (i.e., avoiding the use of alkylators, topoisomerase inhibitors) and radiation therapy. Preliminary evidence suggests that this approach for NLPHL leads

to an overall survival close to 100%, and should decrease the late effects of secondary malignancy and infertility.[179] Many current study protocols would forgo even low-dose IFRT for these young patients who achieve a complete response with low-dose chemotherapy, but this should still be considered an experimental approach because combination low-dose chemotherapy and IFRT has been the standard of care, and there are reports of relapse after chemotherapy-only treatments.

SUPPORTIVE CARE

There is no question that a large part of the success of modern leukemia and lymphoma treatment is related to the major improvements in supportive care that coincided with improvements in chemotherapy. These advances have included improved blood products, antibiotics, antifungals, and better intensive care unit support of critically ill pediatric patients. Erythropoietin has been used sparingly in pediatric oncology, and is not generally incorporated in frontline therapies for any of the lymphoid cancers. Leukocyte growth factors (granulocyte colony-stimulating factor, granulocyte-macrophage colony-stimulating factor, and PEGylated forms, such as pegfilgrastim) are used sparingly in pediatric leukemia and lymphoma therapies for multiple reasons, including (1) concerns (mostly not substantiated in the literature) that these factors may stimulate the growth of these diseases, (2) multiple studies that show no changes in overall outcome when these factors are used, (3) financial burden, and (4) the addition of needle sticks and/or the increased infection risk from entering central lines daily. Growth factors are, however, used routinely in many relapse and higher stage lymphoma protocols to enable a dose-intensive chemotherapy schedule and avoid long periods of profound neutropenia.

LONG-TERM, PALLIATIVE, AND HOSPICE CARE IN PEDIATRIC ONCOLOGY

The survivors of current lower risk (less intensively treated) forms of ALL, NHL, and HL in childhood can now expect prolonged DFS, intact fertility, lesser cognitive and social disruption, and an easier integration into standard medical and social environments than in the past. Survivors from higher doses and larger radiation fields used in the 1960s and 1970s, as well as from regimens involving higher cumulative doses of chemotherapy, continue to have an increased risk of important long-term toxicities, including endocrine, growth, fertility, and learning disabilities, along with cardiac, renal, liver, and other end-organ toxicities.[180] Second malignancies are another serious problem, arising from carcinogenic exposures to chemotherapy and radiotherapy, as well as possibly an innate propensity to develop cancer.[181] It has been estimated that pediatric cancer survivors will soon represent as many as 1 in 250 adult Americans in the 15- to 45-year-old population.[182] Reducing late effects of therapy while preserving cure rates is a crucial goal in improving outcomes in childhood leukemia and lymphoma.[183]

Even with cure rates that reach, in many categories of disease, into the over 90% region, a substantial number of children still die of leukemia and lymphoma. A small number die after failing their first regimens, but many succumb after alternately succeeding and then failing several attempts at cure. A discussion of hospice and palliative care for these children and support for their families is beyond the scope of this chapter, but this is an area of active interest and involvement in most pediatric oncology programs. Hospice and palliative care treatments in pediatrics share some of the same concerns, goals, and methods as programs for adults. However, the unique requirements of psychosocial support in children, and the impact of a possible death of a child on a family, lead most experts to guide these patients to pediatric centers.

SELECTED REFERENCES

The full reference list can be accessed at lwwhealthlibrary.com/oncology.

1. Hunger SP, Lu X, Devidas M, et al. Improved survival for children and adolescents with acute lymphoblastic leukemia between 1990 and 2005: a report from the Children's Oncology Group. *J Clin Oncol* 2012;30:1663–1669.
2. Inaba H, Greaves M, Mullighan CG. Acute lymphoblastic leukaemia. *Lancet* 2013;381:1943–1955.
3. Freed J, Kelly KM. Current approaches to the management of pediatric Hodgkin lymphoma. *Paediatr Drugs* 2010;12:85–98.
4. Reiter A. Non-Hodgkin lymphoma in children and adolescents. *Klin Padiatr* 2013;225:S87–S93.
5. Creutzig U, van den Heuvel-Eibrink MM, Gibson B, et al. Diagnosis and management of acute myeloid leukemia in children and adolescents: recommendations from an international expert panel. *Blood* 2012;120:3187–3205.
6. Rubnitz JE, Gibson B, Smith FO. Acute myeloid leukemia. *Hematol Oncol Clin North Am* 2010;24:35–63.
8. Pui CH, Robison LL, Look AT. Acute lymphoblastic leukaemia. *Lancet* 2008;371:1030–1043.
10. Bhatia S, Sather HN, Heerema NA, et al. Racial and ethnic differences in survival of children with acute lymphoblastic leukemia. *Blood* 2002;100:1957–1964.
13. Pui CH, Pei D, Pappo AS, et al. Treatment outcomes in black and white children with cancer: results from the SEER database and St Jude Children's Research Hospital, 1992 through 2007. *J Clin Oncol* 2012;30:2005–2012.
14. Bhatia S, Landier W, Shangguan M, et al. Nonadherence to oral mercaptopurine and risk of relapse in Hispanic and non-Hispanic white children with acute lymphoblastic leukemia: a report from the children's oncology group. *J Clin Oncol* 2012;30:2094–2101.
18. Children's Oncology Group, Aplenc R, Alonzo TA, et al. Ethnicity and survival in childhood acute myeloid leukemia: a report from the Children's Oncology Group. *Blood* 2006;108:74–80.
22. McNally RJ, Eden TO. An infectious aetiology for childhood acute leukaemia: a review of the evidence. *Br J Haematol* 2004;127:243–263.
32. Greaves M. Infection, immune responses and the aetiology of childhood leukaemia. *Nat Rev Cancer* 2006;6:193–203.
33. Trevino LR, Yang W, French D, et al. Germline genomic variants associated with childhood acute lymphoblastic leukemia. *Nat Genet* 2009;41:1001–1005.
39. Holmfeldt L, Wei L, Diaz-Flores E, et al. The genomic landscape of hypodiploid acute lymphoblastic leukemia. *Nat Genet* 2013;45:242–252.
40. Zwaan MC, Reinhardt D, Hitzler J, et al. Acute leukemias in children with Down syndrome. *Pediatr Clin North Am* 2008;55:53–70.
46. Bercovich D, Ganmore I, Scott LM, et al. Mutations of JAK2 in acute lymphoblastic leukaemias associated with Down's syndrome. *Lancet* 2008;372:1484–1492.
47. Russell LJ, Capasso M, Vater I, et al. Deregulated expression of cytokine receptor gene, CRLF2, is involved in lymphoid transformation in B cell precursor acute lymphoblastic leukemia. *Blood* 2009;114:2688–2698.
48. Mullighan CG, Collins-Underwood JR, Phillips LA, et al. Rearrangement of CRLF2 in B-progenitor- and Down syndrome-associated acute lymphoblastic leukemia. *Nat Genet* 2009;41:1243–1246.
49. Massey GV, Zipursky A, Chang MN, et al. A prospective study of the natural history of transient leukemia (TL) in neonates with Down syndrome (DS): Children's Oncology Group (COG) study POG-9481. *Blood* 2006;107:4606–4613.
52. Campana D. Minimal residual disease in acute lymphoblastic leukemia. *Semin Hematol* 2009;46:100–106.
56. Pui CH, Howard SC. Current management and challenges of malignant disease in the CNS in paediatric leukaemia. *Lancet Oncol* 2008;9:257–268.
60. Mullighan CG, Goorha S, Radtke I, et al. Genome-wide analysis of genetic alterations in acute lymphoblastic leukaemia. *Nature* 2007;446:758–764.
61. Zhang J, Ding L, Holmfeldt L, et al. The genetic basis of early T-cell precursor acute lymphoblastic leukaemia. *Nature* 2012;481:157–163.
64. Roberts KG, Morin RD, Zhang J, et al. Genetic alterations activating kinase and cytokine receptor signaling in high-risk acute lymphoblastic leukemia. *Cancer Cell* 2012;22:153–166.
65. Smith M, Arthur D, Camitta B, et al. Uniform approach to risk classification and treatment assignment for children with acute lymphoblastic leukemia. *J Clin Oncol* 1996;14:18–24.
70. Nachman JB, La MK, Hunger SP, et al. 2009. Young adults with acute lymphoblastic leukemia have an excellent outcome with chemotherapy alone and benefit from intensive postinduction treatment: a report from the Children's Oncology Group. *J Clin Oncol* 27:5189–5194.
73. Borowitz MJ, Devidas M, Hunger SP, et al. Clinical significance of minimal residual disease in childhood acute lymphoblastic leukemia and its relationship to other prognostic factors: a Children's Oncology Group study. *Blood* 2008;111:5477–5485.
74. Nachman JB, Heerema NA, Sather H, et al. Outcome of treatment in children with hypodiploid acute lymphoblastic leukemia. *Blood* 2007;110:1112–1115.
75. Mullighan CG, Su X, Zhang J, et al. Deletion of IKZF1 and prognosis in acute lymphoblastic leukemia. *N Engl J Med* 2009;360:470–480.
76. Rand V, Parker H, Russell LJ, et al. Genomic characterization implicates iAMP21 as a likely primary genetic event in childhood B-cell precursor acute lymphoblastic leukemia. *Blood* 2011;117:6848–6855.
79. Rubnitz JE, Wichlan D, Devidas M, et al. Prospective analysis of TEL gene rearrangements in childhood acute lymphoblastic leukemia: a Children's Oncology Group study. *J Clin Oncol* 2008;26:2186–2191.

83. Schultz KR, Bowman WP, Aledo A, et al. Improved early event-free survival with imatinib in Philadelphia chromosome-positive acute lymphoblastic leukemia: a Children's Oncology Group study. *J Clin Oncol* 2009;27:5175–5181.
86. Weng AP, Ferrando AA, Lee W, et al. Activating mutations of NOTCH1 in human T cell acute lymphoblastic leukemia. *Science* 2004;306:269–271.
87. Coustan-Smith E, Mullighan CG, Onciu M, et al. Early T-cell precursor leukaemia: a subtype of very high-risk acute lymphoblastic leukaemia. *Lancet Oncol* 2009;10:147–156.
88. Pui CH, Campana D, Pei D, et al. Treating childhood acute lymphoblastic leukemia without cranial irradiation. *N Engl J Med* 2009;360:2730–2741.
91. Schrappe M, Hunger SP, Pui CH, et al. Outcomes after induction failure in childhood acute lymphoblastic leukemia. *N Engl J Med* 2012;366:1371–1381.
96. Nguyen K, Devidas M, Cheng SC, et al. Factors influencing survival after relapse from acute lymphoblastic leukemia: a Children's Oncology Group study. *Leukemia* 2008;22:2142–2150.
97. Freyer DR, Devidas M, La M, et al. Postrelapse survival in childhood acute lymphoblastic leukemia is independent of initial treatment intensity: a report from the Children's Oncology Group. *Blood* 2011;117:3010–3015.
98. Raetz EA, Borowitz MJ, Devidas M, et al. Reinduction platform for children with first marrow relapse of acute lymphoblastic leukemia: a Children's Oncology Group Study [corrected]. *J Clin Oncol* 2008;26:3971–3978.
101. Hijiya N, Gaynon P, Barry E, et al. A multi-center phase I study of clofarabine, etoposide and cyclophosphamide in combination in pediatric patients with refractory or relapsed acute leukemia. *Leukemia* 2009;23:2259–2264.
102. Topp MS, Kufer P, Gokbuget N, et al. Targeted therapy with the T-cell-engaging antibody blinatumomab of chemotherapy-refractory minimal residual disease in B-lineage acute lymphoblastic leukemia patients results in high response rate and prolonged leukemia-free survival. *J Clin Oncol* 2011;29:2493–2498.
104. Grupp SA, Kalos M, Barrett D, et al. Chimeric antigen receptor-modified T cells for acute lymphoid leukemia. *N Engl J Med* 2013;368:1509–1518.
106. Mehta PA, Davies SM. Allogeneic transplantation for childhood ALL. *Bone Marrow Transplant* 2008;41:133–139.
107. Kaspers GJ, Zwaan CM. Pediatric acute myeloid leukemia: towards high-quality cure of all patients. *Haematologica* 2007;92:1519–1532.
110. Canner J, Alonzo TA, Franklin J, et al. Differences in outcomes of newly diagnosed acute myeloid leukemia for adolescent/young adult and younger patients: a report from the Children's Oncology Group. *Cancer* 2013;119:4162–4169.
121. Bunin NJ, Davies SM, Aplenc R, et al. Unrelated donor bone marrow transplantation for children with acute myeloid leukemia beyond first remission or refractory to chemotherapy. *J Clin Oncol* 2008;26:4326–4332.
124. Ribeiro R. Update on the management of pediatric acute promyelocytic leukemia. *Clin Adv Hematol Oncol* 2006;4:263–265.
134. Moore AS, Kearns PR, Knapper S, et al. Novel therapies for children with acute myeloid leukaemia. *Leukemia* 2013;27:1451–1460.
136. Suttorp M, Eckardt L, Tauer JT, et al. Management of chronic myeloid leukemia in childhood. *Curr Hematol Malig Rep* 2012;7:116–124.
137. Loh ML. Recent advances in the pathogenesis and treatment of juvenile myelomonocytic leukaemia. *Br J Haematol* 2011;152:677–687.
141. Matutes E, Pickl WF, Van't Veer M, et al. Mixed-phenotype acute leukemia: clinical and laboratory features and outcome in 100 patients defined according to the WHO 2008 classification. *Blood* 2011;117:3163–3171.
142. Shukla NN, Trippett TM. Non-Hodgkin's lymphoma in children and adolescents. *Curr Oncol Rep* 2006;8:387–394.
151. Asselin BL, Devidas M, Wang C, et al. Effectiveness of high-dose methotrexate in T-cell lymphoblastic leukemia and advanced-stage lymphoblastic lymphoma: a randomized study by the Children's Oncology Group (POG 9404). *Blood* 2011;118:874–883.
154. DeAngelo DJ. Nelarabine for the treatment of patients with relapsed or refractory T-cell acute lymphoblastic leukemia or lymphoblastic lymphoma. *Hematol Oncol Clin North Am* 2009;23:1121–1135.
156. Real PJ, Ferrando AA. NOTCH inhibition and glucocorticoid therapy in T-cell acute lymphoblastic leukemia. *Leukemia* 2009;23:1374–1377.
160. Molyneux EM, Rochford R, Griffin B, et al. Burkitt's lymphoma. *Lancet* 2012;379:1234–1244.
163. Patte C, Auperin A, Gerrard M, et al. Results of the randomized international FAB/LMB96 trial for intermediate risk B-cell non-Hodgkin lymphoma in children and adolescents: it is possible to reduce treatment for the early responding patients. *Blood* 2007;109:2773–2780.
166. Harris NL, Jaffe ES, Stein H, et al. A revised European-American classification of lymphoid neoplasms: a proposal from the International Lymphoma Study Group. *Blood* 1994;84:1361–1392.
170. Gambacorti-Passerini C, Messa C, Pogliani EM. Crizotinib in anaplastic large-cell lymphoma. *N Engl J Med* 2011;364:775–776.
171. Younes A, Gopal AK, Smith SE, et al. Results of a pivotal phase II study of brentuximab vedotin for patients with relapsed or refractory Hodgkin's lymphoma. *J Clin Oncol* 2012;30:2183–2189.
172. Sandlund JT, Hudson MM. Hematology: Treatment strategies for pediatric Hodgkin lymphoma. *Nat Rev Clin Oncol* 2010;7:243–244.
181. Mody R, Li S, Dover DC, et al. Twenty-five-year follow-up among survivors of childhood acute lymphoblastic leukemia: a report from the Childhood Cancer Survivor Study. *Blood* 2008;111:5515–5523.
183. Robison LL. Late effects of acute lymphoblastic leukemia therapy in patients diagnosed at 0-20 years of age. *Hematology Am Soc Hematol Educ Program* 2011:238–242.

101 Molecular Biology of Lymphomas

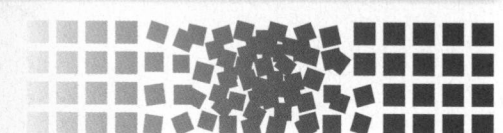

Laura Pasqualucci and Riccardo Dalla-Favera

PRACTICE OF ONCOLOGY

INTRODUCTION

The term lymphoma identifies a heterogeneous group of biologically and clinically distinct neoplasms that originate from cells in the lymphoid organs and have been historically divided into two distinct categories: non-Hodgkin lymphoma (NHL) and Hodgkin lymphoma (HL).[1] During the past few decades, significant progress has been made in elucidating the molecular pathogenesis of lymphoid malignancies as a clonal expansion of B cells (in the majority of cases) or T cells. The molecular characterization of the most frequent genetic abnormalities associated with lymphoma has led to the identification of multiple proto-oncogenes and tumor suppressor genes, whose abnormal functioning contributes to lymphoma pathogenesis. Relatively less is known about the pathogenesis of T-cell NHL (T-NHL) and HL. This chapter will focus on the molecular pathogenesis of the most common and well-characterized types of lymphoma, including B-cell NHL (B-NHL), T-NHL, HL, and chronic lymphocytic leukemia (CLL), which also derives from mature B cells. Emphasis will be given to the mechanisms of genetic lesion and the nature of the involved genes in relationship to the normal biology of lymphocytes.

THE CELL OF ORIGIN OF LYMPHOMA

The number of B and T cells in the adult are not significantly different; however, 85% of lymphomas originate from mature B cells, whereas only 10% to 15% derive from the T-cell lineage. This bias may be explained in part by the unique DNA modification events that take place in normal B lymphocytes in order to enable the production of highly efficient neutralizing antibodies and that are mechanistically more complex than those utilized by T cells to encode T-cell receptors. The biology of these processes thus represents a key concept for the understanding of lymphomagenesis.

B-Cell Development and the Dynamics of the Germinal Center Reaction

B lymphocytes are generated from a common pluripotent stem cell in the bone marrow, where precursor B cells first assemble their immunoglobulin heavy chain locus (*IGH*) followed by the light chain loci (*IGL*) through a site-specific process of cleavage and rejoining, known as V(D)J recombination.[2] Cells that fail to express a functional (and nonautoreactive) antigen receptor are eliminated within the bone marrow, whereas B-cell precursors that have successfully rearranged their antibody genes are positively selected to migrate into peripheral lymphoid organs as mature, naïve B cells.[3] In most B cells, the subsequent maturation steps are linked to the histologic structure of the germinal center (GC), a specialized microenvironment that forms following the

encounter of naïve B cells with a foreign antigen, in the context of signals delivered by CD4+ T cells and antigen-presenting cells (Fig. 101.1).[3–5]

GCs are highly dynamic structures in which B cells transit back and forth between two zones that are conserved across several species: the dark zone (DZ), which consists of rapidly proliferating centroblasts (CB) (doubling time: 6 to 12 hours), and the light zone (LZ), which consists of more quiescent cells termed centrocytes (CC), amidst a network of resident accessory cells (follicular dendritic cells [FDC] and human T follicular helper [Tfh] cells).[6–9] According to currently accepted models, the DZ is the site where GC B cells modify the variable region of their *IG* genes (IgV) by the process of somatic hypermutation (SHM), which introduces mostly single nucleotide substitutions with few deletions and duplications in order to change their affinity for the antigen.[3,5,10–12] Conversely, the LZ is the site of selection based on affinity to the antigen. A critical regulator of the GC reaction is BCL6,[13,14] a transcriptional repressor[15] that negatively modulates the expression of a broad set of genes, including those involved in B-cell receptor (BCR) and CD40 signaling,[16,17] T-cell mediated B-cell activation,[16] induction of apoptosis,[16,18] response to DNA damage (by modulation of genes involved in the sensing and execution of DNA damage responses),[19–22] various cytokine and chemokine signaling pathways (e.g., those triggered by interferon and transforming growth factor beta [TGFβ]),[16,18] and plasma cell differentiation, via suppression of the PRDM1/BLIMP1 master regulator.[23–26] This transcriptional program suggests that BCL6 is critical to establish the proliferative status of CBs and to allow the execution of antigen-specific DNA modification processes (SHM and class-switch recombination) without eliciting responses to DNA damage; furthermore, BCL6 keeps in check a variety of signaling pathways that could lead to premature activation and differentiation prior to the selection for the survival of cells producing high affinity antibodies.

CBs are then believed to cease proliferation and shuttle to the LZ, where they are rechallenged by the antigen through the interaction with CD4+ T cells and FDCs.[3,4,7,8] CCs expressing a BCR with reduced affinity for the antigen will be eliminated by apoptosis, whereas a few cells with greater affinity will be selected for survival and differentiation into memory cells and plasma cells,[4] or reenter the DZ following stimulation by a variety of different signals.[9] Iterative rounds of mutations and selections lead to affinity maturation at the population level. In the GC, CCs also undergo class-switch recombination (CSR), a DNA remodeling event that confers distinct effector functions to antibodies with identical specificities.[27] SHM and CSR represent B-cell–specific functions that modify the genome of B cells via mechanisms involving single- or double-strand breaks and which depend on the activity of the activation-induced cytidine deaminase (AID) enzyme,[28–30] a notion that will become important in the understanding of the mechanisms generating genetic alterations in B-NHL.

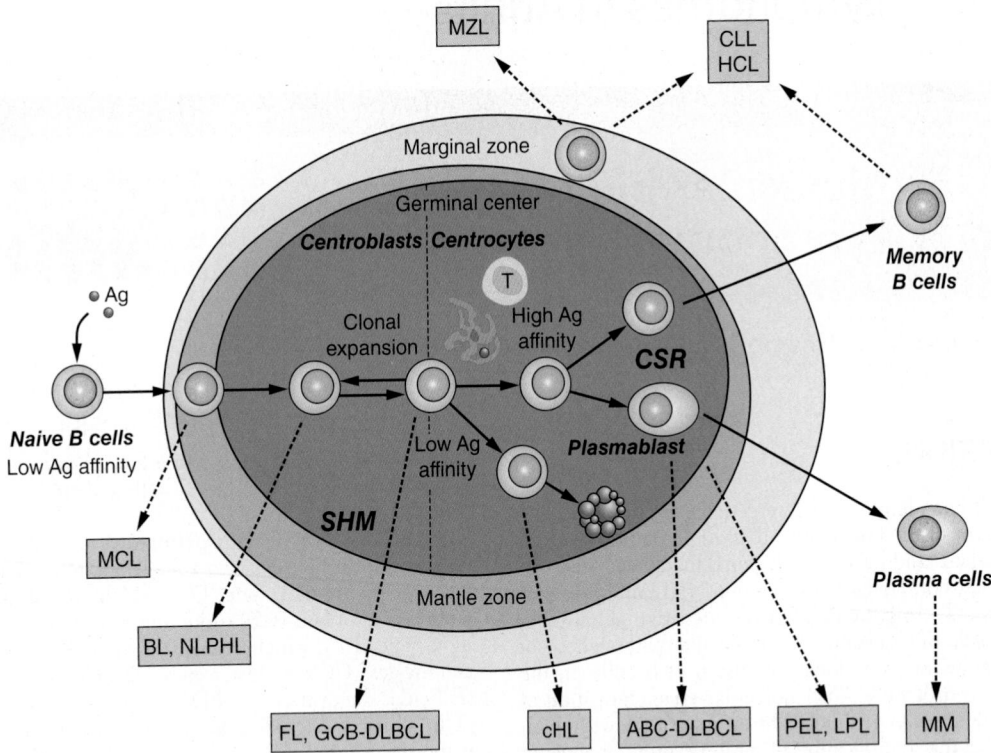

Figure 101.1 Normal B-cell development and lymphomagenesis. Schematic representation of a lymphoid follicle, constituted by the germinal center (GC), the mantle zone, and the surrounding marginal zone. B cells that have successfully rearranged their *IG* genes in the bone marrow move to peripheral lymphoid organs as naïve B cells. Upon encounter with a T-cell dependent antigen, B cells become proliferating centroblasts in the GC and eventually transition into centrocytes, which shuttle back and forth between the dark and light zone while undergoing iterative rounds of SHM and selection. Only GC B cells with high affinity for the antigen will be positively selected to exit the GC and further differentiate into plasma cells or memory B cells, whereas low-affinity clones are eliminated by apoptosis. *Dotted arrows* link various lymphoma types to their putative normal counterpart, identified based on the presence of somatically mutated IgV genes, as well as on distinctive phenotypic features. CSR, class-switch recombination; SHM, somatic hypermutation; MCL, mantle-cell lymphoma; FL, follicular lymphoma; BL, Burkitt lymphoma; GCB-DLBCL, germinal center B cell-like diffuse large B-cell lymphoma; ABC-DLBCL, activated B cell-like diffuse large B-cell lymphoma; PEL, primary effusion lymphoma; LPL, lymphoplasmacytic lymphoma; NLPHL, nodular lymphocyte predominance Hodgkin lymphoma; cHL, classical Hodgkin lymphoma; MZL, marginal zone lymphoma; HCL, hairy cell leukemia; CLL, chronic lymphocytic leukemia; MM, multiple myeloma.

Once these processes are completed, two critical signals for licensing GC exit are represented by engagement of the BCR by the antigen and activation of the CD40 receptor by the CD40 ligand present on CD4+ T cells. These signals induce the downregulation of BCL6 at the translational and transcriptional level, respectively, thus restoring DNA damage responses, as well as activation and differentiation capabilities.

Although oversimplified, this schematic description of the GC reaction is useful to introduce two basic concepts for the understanding of B-NHL pathogenesis. First, the activity of SHM, which introduces irreversible DNA changes in the genome, allowed for the conclusion that most B-NHL types, with the exception of most mantle-cell lymphoma (MCL), derive from GC-experienced B cells that underwent clonal expansion within the GC, because the malignant clones harbor hypermutated IgV sequences containing largely identical mutations, suggesting the derivation from a single founder cell.[31] Second, two common mechanisms of oncogenic lesions in B-NHL—namely, chromosomal translocations and aberrant somatic hypermutation (ASHM)—result from mistakes in the machinery that normally diversifies the Ig genes during B lymphocytes differentiation, further supporting the GC origin of most B-NHL (Fig. 101.2).[32] Finally, the definition of two distinct phases during GC development reflects different transient states within the same B-cell developmental step, which can be recognized in different B-NHL subtypes to some extent.

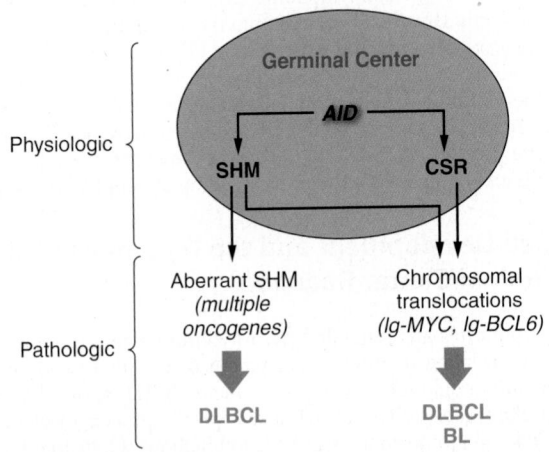

Figure 101.2 Model for the initiation of chromosomal translocations and ASHM during lymphomagenesis. B-NHL–associated genetic lesions are favored by mistakes occurring during the physiologic processes of SHM and CSR in the highly proliferative environment of the GC *(top)*. These events lead to chromosomal translocations, which in most cases juxtapose the *IG* genes to one of several proto-oncogenes (e.g., *BCL2* or *MYC*), and ASHM of multiple target genes, thus contributing to the pathogenesis of lymphoma. DLBCL, diffuse large B-cell lymphoma; BL, Burkitt lymphoma.

T-Cell Development

The process of T-cell development proceeds through sequential stages defined according to the expression of the molecules CD4 and CD8. Committed lymphoid progenitors exit the bone marrow and migrate to the thymus as early T-cell progenitors or double negative 1 (DN1) cells, which lack the expression of both CD4 and CD8 and harbor unrearranged T-cell receptor (TCR) genes.[33] In the thymic cortex, T cells advance through the double negative stages DN2, DN3, and DN4, while undergoing specific rearrangements at the TCRβ locus in order to acquire expression of the pre-TCR.[33] Those thymocytes that have successfully recombined the pre-TCR will be selected to further differentiate into double positive cells (CD4+CD8+), which express a complete surface TCR and can then enter a process of positive and negative selection in the medulla, before exiting the thymus as single positive T cells.[33] The end result of this process is a pool of mature T cells that exhibit coordinated TCR and coreceptor specificities, as required for effective immune responses to foreign antigens. Most mature T-NHLs arise from postthymic T cells in the lymphoid organs.

GENERAL MECHANISMS OF GENETIC LESIONS IN LYMPHOMA

Analogous to other cancers, lymphoma represents a multistep process deriving from the accumulation of multiple genetic lesions affecting oncogenes and tumor suppressor genes, including chromosomal translocations, point mutations, genomic deletions, and copy number (CN) gains/amplifications.

Chromosomal Translocations

Although also found in nonlymphoid tumors, chromosomal translocations represent the genetic hallmark of malignancies derived from the hematopoietic system. These events are generated through the reciprocal and balanced recombination of two specific chromosomes and are often recurrently associated with a given tumor type, where they are clonally represented in each tumor case.

The precise molecular mechanisms underlying the generation of translocations remain partially unclear; however, significant advances have been made in our understanding of the events that are required for their initiation.[34] It has been documented that

chromosomal translocations occur at least in part as a consequence of mistakes during *Ig* and TCR gene rearrangements in B and T cells, respectively, and, based on the characteristics of the chromosomal breakpoint, can be broadly divided into three groups: (1) translocations derived from mistakes of the recombination activating gene RAG-mediated V(D)J recombination process, as is the case for translocations involving *IGH* and *CCND1* in MCL or *IGH* and *BCL2* in follicular lymphoma (FL)[34–36]; (2) translocations mediated by errors in the AID dependent CSR process, such as those involving the *Ig* genes and *MYC* in sporadic Burkitt lymphoma (BL)[34]; (3) translocations occurring as by-products of the AID-mediated SHM mechanism, which also generates DNA breaks, such as those joining the *Ig* and *MYC* loci in endemic BL.[34] Conclusive experimental evidence for the involvement of antibody-associated remodeling events has been provided through in vivo studies performed in lymphoma-prone mouse models, where the removal of the AID enzyme was sufficient to abrogate the generation of *MYC-IGH* translocations in normal B cells undergoing CSR[37,38] and to prevent the development of GC-derived B-NHL.[39]

The common feature of all NHL-associated chromosomal translocations is the presence of a proto-oncogene in the proximity of the chromosomal recombination sites. In most lymphoma types, and in contrast with acute leukemias, the coding domain of the oncogene is not affected by the translocation, but its pattern of expression is altered as a consequence of the juxtaposition of heterologous regulatory sequences derived from the partner chromosome (proto-oncogene deregulation) (Fig. 101.3). This process of proto-oncogene deregulation is defined as homotopic if a proto-oncogene whose expression is tightly regulated in the normal tumor counterpart becomes constitutively expressed in the lymphoma cell, and heterotopic when the proto-oncogene is not expressed in the putative normal counterpart of the tumor cell and undergoes ectopic expression in the lymphoma. In most types of NHL-associated translocations, the heterologous regulatory sequences responsible for proto-oncogene deregulation are derived from antigen receptor loci, which are expressed at high levels in the target tissue.[34] However, in certain translocations, such as the ones involving *BCL6* in diffuse large B-cell lymphoma (DLBCL), different promoter regions from distinct chromosomal sites can be found juxtaposed to the proto-oncogene in individual tumor cases, a concept known as *promiscuous translocations*.[40–47]

Less commonly, B-NHL associated chromosomal translocations juxtapose the coding regions of the two involved genes to form a chimeric unit that encodes for a novel fusion protein, an outcome typically observed in chromosomal translocation

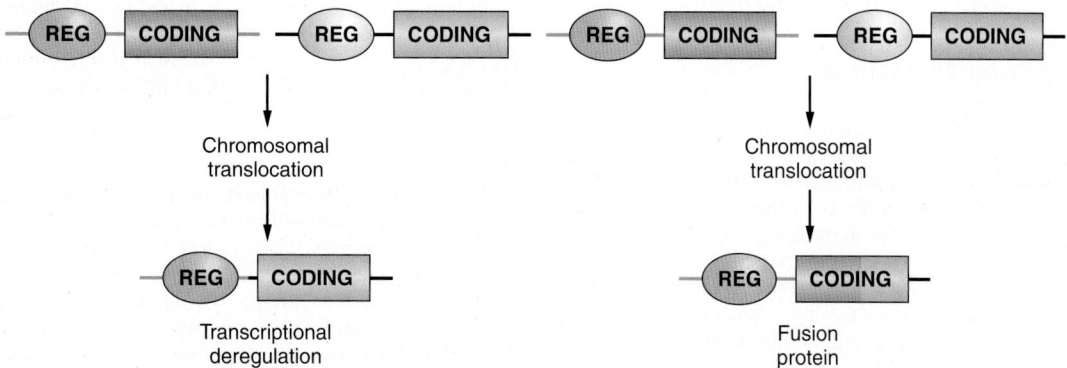

Figure 101.3 Molecular consequences of chromosomal translocations. *Top panel*: The two genes involved in prototypic chromosomal translocations are graphically represented, with their regulatory (REG) and coding sequences. Only one side of the balanced, reciprocal translocations is indicated in the figure. *Bottom panel*: Distinct outcomes of chromosomal translocations. In the case of transcriptional deregulation *(left scheme)*, the normal regulatory sequences of the proto-oncogene are substituted with regulatory sequences derived from the partner chromosome, leading to deregulated expression of the proto-oncogene. In most B-NHLs, the heterologous regulatory regions derive from the *IG* loci. In the case of fusion proteins *(right scheme)*, the coding sequences of the two involved genes are joined in frame into a chimeric transcriptional unit that encodes for a novel fusion protein, characterized by novel biochemical and functional properties.

associated with acute leukemia (see Fig. 101.3). Examples are the t(11;18) of mucosa-associated lymphoid tissue (MALT) lymphoma and the t(2;5) of anaplastic large-cell lymphoma (ALCL). The molecular cloning of the genetic loci involved in most recurrent translocations has led to the identification of a number of proto-oncogenes involved in lymphomagenesis.

Aberrant Somatic Hypermutation

The term aberrant somatic hypermutation defines a mechanism of genetic lesion that appears to derive from a malfunction in the physiologic SHM process, leading to the mutation of multiple non-Ig genes.[48] This phenomenon is uniquely associated with B-NHL and particularly with DLBCL, where over 10% of actively transcribed genes have been found mutated as a consequence of ASHM.

In GC B cells, SHM is tightly regulated both spatially and temporally to introduce mutations only in the rearranged *IgV* genes[49] as well as in the 5′ region of a few other genes, including *BCL6* and the *CD79* components of the B-cell receptor,[50–53] although the functional role of mutations found in these other genes remains obscure. On the contrary, multiple mutational events were found to affect numerous loci have been found mutated in over half of DLBCL cases and, at lower frequencies, in few other lymphoma types.[54–58] The identified target loci include several well known proto-oncogenes such as *PIM1*, *PAX5*, and *MYC*, one of the most frequently altered human oncogenes.[48] These mutations are typically distributed within ~2 kb from the transcription initiation site (i.e., the hypermutable domain in the Ig locus)[59] and, depending on the genomic configuration of the target gene, may affect nontranslated as well as coding regions, thus holding the potential of altering the response to factors that normally regulate their expression or changing key structural and functional properties.[48] This is the case of *MYC*, where a significant number of amino acid substitutions have proven functional consequences in activating its oncogenic potential. Nonetheless, a comprehensive characterization of the potentially extensive genetic damage caused by ASHM is still lacking, and the mechanism involved in this malfunction has not been elucidated.

Copy Number Gains and Amplifications

In addition to chromosomal translocations and ASHM, the structure of proto-oncogenes and their pattern of expression can be altered by CN gains and amplifications, leading to overexpression of an intact protein. Compared to epithelial cancer, only a few genes have been identified so far as specific targets of amplification in B-NHL, as exemplified by *REL* and *BCL2* in DLBCL[60–63] and by the genes encoding for programmed cell death 1 PD-1 ligands in primary mediastinal B-cell lymphoma (PMBCL).[64,65]

Activating Point Mutations

Somatic point mutations in the coding sequence of a target proto-oncogene may alter the biologic properties of its protein product, leading to its stabilization or constitutive activation. Over the past few years, the use of genomewide, high throughput sequencing technologies has allowed for the identification of numerous previously unsuspected targets of somatic mutations in cancer, including lymphoid malignancies. These genes will be discussed in individual disease sections. Of note, mutations of the *RAS* genes, a very frequent proto-oncogene alteration in human neoplasia, are rare in lymphomas.[66]

Inactivating Mutations and Deletions

Until recently, the *TP53* gene, possibly the most common target of genetic alteration in human cancer,[67] remained one of few bona fide tumor suppressor genes involved in the pathogenesis of NHL, although at generally low frequencies and restricted to specific

disease subtypes, such as BL and DLBCL derived from the transformation of FL or CLL.[68,69] The mechanism of *TP53* inactivation in NHL is analogous to the one observed in human neoplasia in general, entailing a point mutation of one allele and a chromosomal deletion or mutation of the second allele. However, recent efforts taking advantage of genomewide technologies revealed several additional candidate tumor suppressor genes that are lost in B-NHL through specific chromosomal deletions and/or deleterious mutations. Two such genes lie on the long arm of chromosome 6 (6q), a region long known to be deleted in a large percentage of aggressive lymphomas associated with poor prognoses.[70,71] The *PRDM1/BLIMP1* gene on 6q21 is biallelically inactivated in ~25% of ABC-DLBCL cases,[72–74] and the gene encoding for the negative nuclear factor kappa B (NF-κB) regulator A20 on chromosome 6q23 is commonly lost in ABC-DLBCL, PMBCL, and subtypes of marginal zone lymphoma and HL.[75–78] Monoallelic inactivating mutations and deletions were found to affect the acetyltransferase genes *CREBBP* and *EP300* in a significant proportion of DLBCL and FL, suggesting a role as haploinsufficient tumor suppressors.[79] These two lymphoma types also harbor truncating mutations of *MLL2*,[80] which is emerging as one of the most commonly mutated genes in cancer. Among the tumor suppressors preferentially inactivated by CN losses, it is important to mention the *DLEU2/miR15-a/16.1* cluster on chromosome 13q14.3, the most frequent alteration in CLL (>50% of cases),[81] and *CDKN2A/B (p16/INK4a)*, which is inactivated by focal homozygous deletions in transformed FL (tFL), Richter syndrome (RS), and ABC-DLBCL,[82–84] and less frequently, by epigenetic transcriptional silencing in various B-NHL.[85]

Infectious Agents

Viral and bacterial infections have both been implicated in the pathogenesis of lymphoma. At least three viruses are associated with specific NHL subtypes: the Epstein-Barr virus (EBV), the human herpesvirus-8/Kaposi sarcoma–associated herpesvirus (HHV-8/KSHV), and the human T-lymphotropic virus type 1 (HTLV-1). Other infectious agents, including HIV, hepatitis C virus (HCV), *Helicobacter pylori*, and *Chlamydophila psittaci* have an indirect role in NHL pathogenesis by either impairing the immune system and/or providing chronic antigenic stimulation.

EBV was initially identified in cases of endemic African BL,[86,87] and was subsequently also detected in a fraction of sporadic BL, HIV-related lymphomas, and primary effusion lymphomas (PEL).[88–92] Upon infection, the EBV genome is transported into the nucleus of the B lymphocyte, where it exists predominantly as an extrachromosomal circular molecule (episome).[93] The formation of circular episomes is mediated by the cohesive terminal repeats, which are represented by a variable number of tandem repeats (VNTR) sequence.[93,94] Because of this termini heterogeneity, the number of VNTR sequences enclosed in newly formed episomes may differ considerably, thus representing a clonal marker of a single infected cell.[94] Evidence for a pathogenetic role of the virus in NHL infected by EBV is at least twofold. First, it is well recognized that EBV is able to significantly alter the growth of B cells.[93] Secondly, EBV-infected lymphomas usually display a single form of fused EBV termini, suggesting that the lymphoma cell population represents the clonally expanded progeny of a single infected cell.[88,89] Nonetheless, the role of EBV in lymphomagenesis is still unclear, because the virus infects virtually all humans during their lifetime and its transforming genes are commonly not expressed in the tumor cells of BL.

HHV-8 is a gammaherpesvirus initially identified in tissues of HIV-related Kaposi sarcoma[95] and subsequently found to infect PEL cells as well as a substantial fraction of multicentric Castleman disease.[96–98] Phylogenetic analysis has shown that the closest relative of HHV-8 is herpesvirus saimiri (HVS), a gamma-2 herpesvirus of primates associated with T-cell lymphoproliferative disorders.[99] Like other gammaherpesviruses, HHV-8 is also lymphotropic, and infect lymphocytes both in vitro and in vivo.[95,97,98] Lymphoma cells naturally infected by HHV-8 harbor the viral genome in its episomal configuration and display a marked restriction of viral gene expression, suggesting a pattern of latent infection.[99]

The HTLV-1 RNA retrovirus was first isolated from a cell line established from an adult T-cell leukemia/lymphoma (ATLL) patient.[100] Unlike acutely transforming retroviruses, the HTLV-1 genome does not encode a viral oncogene nor does it transform T cells by cis-activation of an adjacent cellular proto-oncogene, because the provirus appears to integrate randomly within the host genome.[101–103] The pathogenetic effect of HTLV-1 was initially attributed to the viral production of a trans-regulatory protein (HTLV-1 tax) that can activate the transcription of several host genes.[104–110] However, Tax expression is suppressed in vivo, most likely to allow for an immune escape of the infected cells, questioning its role in transformation. More recently, a viral factor has been identified, which is thought to be involved in cell proliferation and viral replication and which may be responsible for HTLV-1–mediated lymphomagenesis.

An association between B-NHL and infection by HCV, a single stranded RNA virus of the Flaviviridae family, has been proposed based on the increased risk of developing lymphoproliferative disorders observed among HCV-positive patients[111] and also on the results of interventional studies demonstrating that eradication of HCV with antiviral treatment could directly induce lymphoma regression in seropositive patients affected by indolent NHL.[112] Although the underlying mechanisms remain unclear, current models suggest that chronic B-cell stimulation by antigens associated with HCV infection may induce nonmalignant B-cell expansion, which subsequently evolves into B-NHL by accumulating additional genetic lesions.

The causative link between antigen stimulation by *H. pylori* and MALT lymphoma originating in the stomach is documented by the observation that *H. pylori* can be found in the vast majority of the lymphoma specimens,[113–115] and eradication of infection with antibiotics leads to long-term complete regression in 70% of cases.[116] However, cases with t(11;18)(q21;21) respond poorly to antibiotic eradication,[117] suggesting additional players.

C. psittaci, an obligate intracellular bacterium, was recently linked to the development of ocular adnexal marginal zone B-cell lymphoma (MZL), although variations in prevalence among different geographical areas remain a major investigational issue.[118,119] In this indolent lymphoma, *C. psittaci* causes both local and systemic persistent infection, and presumably contributes to lymphomagenesis through its mitogenic activity and its ability to promote polyclonal cell proliferation and resistance to apoptosis in the infected cells in vivo. Notably, bacterial eradication with antibiotic therapy is often followed by lymphoma regression.[120]

MOLECULAR PATHOGENESIS OF B-NHL

The following section will focus on well-characterized genetic lesions that are associated with the most common types of B-NHL, classified according to the World Health Organization (WHO) classification of lymphoid neoplasia.[1] The molecular pathogenesis of HIV-related NHL will also be addressed, whereas the pathogenesis of other B-cell NHLs remains far less understood. Lymphoblastic lymphoma, which is considered the same disease as T- and B-acute lymphoblastic leukemia, will not be covered in this chapter.

Mantle Cell Lymphoma

Cell of Origin

Mantle cell lymphoma is an aggressive disease representing ~5% of all NHL diagnoses and generally regarded as incurable.[1] Based on immunophenotype, gene expression profile, and molecular features, such as the presence of unmutated IgV genes in the vast

majority of cases, MCL has been historically considered as derived from naïve, pre-GC peripheral B cells located in the inner mantle zone of secondary follicles (see Fig. 101.1).[121] More recently, the observation of BCR diversity, including *IGHV* hypermutation, in a subset of tumor cases (15% to 40%) has shifted this paradigm, suggesting the existence of distinct molecular subtypes, including one influenced by the CG environment.

Genetic Lesions

MCL is typically associated with the t(11;14)(q13;q32) translocation, that juxtaposes the *IGH* gene at 14q32 to a region containing the *CCND1* gene (also known as *BCL1*) on chromosome 11q13.[122–124] The translocation consistently leads to homotopic deregulation and overexpression of cyclin D1, a member of the D-type G1 cyclins that regulates the early phases of the cell cycle and is normally not expressed in resting B cells.[125–127] By deregulating cyclin D1, t(11;14) is thought to contribute to malignant transformation by perturbing the G1-S phase transition of the cell cycle.[121] Importantly, the frequency and specificity of this genetic lesion, together with the expression of cyclin D1 in the tumor cells, provides an excellent marker for MCL diagnosis.[1]

In addition to t(11;14), up to 10% of MCLs overexpress aberrant or shorter cyclin D1 transcripts, as a consequence of secondary rearrangements, microdeletions, or point mutations in the gene 3' untranslated region.[128–130] These alterations lead to cyclin D1 overexpression through the removal of destabilizing sequences and the consequent increase in the mRNA half-life, and are more commonly observed in cases characterized by high proliferative activity and a more aggressive clinical course. The pathogenic role of cyclin D1 deregulation in human neoplasia is suggested by the ability of the overexpressed protein to transform cells in vitro and to promote B-cell lymphomagenesis in transgenic mice, although only when combined to other oncogenic events[131,132]; however, an animal model that faithfully recapitulates the features of the human MCL is still lacking.

Other genetic alterations involved in MCL include biallelic inactivation of the *ATM* gene by genomic deletions and mutations,[133] loss of *TP53* (20% of patients, where it represents a marker of poor prognosis),[134] and inactivation of the *CDKN2A* gene by deletions, point mutations, or promoter hypermethylation (approximately half of the cases belonging to the MCL variant characterized by a blastoid cell morphology).[135] Also associated with aggressive tumors are mutations activating the Notch signaling pathway, including *NOTCH1* (12% of clinical samples) and *NOTCH2* (5% of samples); these lesions, which are mutually exclusive, mostly consist of truncating events that remove the PEST sequences required for NOTCH protein degradation and, thus, lead to protein stabilization.[136,137] Other recurrent mutations were reported in genes encoding the antiapoptotic protein BIRC3, the Toll-like receptor 2 (TLR2), the chromatin modifiers WHSC1 and MLL2, and the MEF2B transcription factor.[136] In a small number of cases, *BMI1* is amplified and/or overexpressed, possibly as an alternative mechanism to the loss of *CDKN2A*.[138,139]

Burkitt Lymphoma

Cell of Origin

BL is an aggressive lymphoma comprising three clinical variants, namely sporadic BL (sBL), endemic BL (eBL), and HIV-associated BL, often diagnosed as the initial manifestation of AIDS.[1] In all variants, the presence of highly mutated IgV sequences[140–143] and the expression of a distinct transcriptional signature[144,145] unequivocally confirm the derivation from a GC B cell.

Genetic Lesions

All BL cases, including the leukemic variants, share a virtually obligatory genetic lesion (i.e., chromosomal translocations involving the *MYC* gene on region 8q24 and one of the *Ig* loci on the partner chromosome).[146,147] In ~80% of cases, this is represented by the *IGH* locus, leading to t(8;14)(q24;q32), whereas in the remaining 20% of cases, either *IGκ* (2p12) or *IGλ*(22q11) are involved.[146–149] Although fairly homogeneous at the microscopic level, these translocations display a high degree of molecular heterogeneity, the breakpoints being located 5′ and centromeric to *MYC* in t(8;14), but mapping 3′ to *MYC* in t(2;8) and t(8;22).[146–150] Further molecular heterogeneity derives from the exact breakpoint sites observed on chromosomes 8 and 14 in t(8;14): Translocations of eBL tend to involve sequences at an undefined distance (>1,000 kb) 5′ to *MYC* on chromosome 8 and sequences within or in proximity to the *IGHJ* region on chromosome 14.[151,152] In sBL, t(8;14) preferentially involves sequences within or immediately 5′ to *MYC* (<3 kb) on chromosome 8 and within the *IGH* switch regions on chromosome 14.[151,152]

The common consequence of t(8;14), t(2;8) and t(8;22) is the ectopic and constitutive overexpression of the MYC proto-oncogene,[153–155] which is normally absent in the majority of proliferating GC B cells,[13] in part due to BCL6-mediated transcriptional repression.[156] Oncogenic activation of MYC in BL is mediated by at least three distinct mechanisms: (1) juxtaposition of the *MYC* coding sequences to heterologous enhancers derived from the *Ig* loci;[153–155] (2) structural alterations of the gene 5′ regulatory sequences, which affect the responsiveness to cellular factors controlling its expression[157]—in particular, the *MYC* exon 1/intron 1 junction encompasses critical regulatory elements that are either decapitated by the translocation or mutated in the translocated alleles; and (3) amino acid substitutions within the gene exon 2, encoding for the protein transactivation domain.[158,159] These mutations can abolish the ability of *p107*, a nuclear protein related to *RB1*, to suppress *MYC* activity[160] or increase protein stability.[161,162]

MYC is a nuclear phosphoprotein that functions as a sequence-specific DNA-binding transcriptional regulator controlling proliferation, cell growth, differentiation, and apoptosis, all of which are implicated in carcinogenesis.[163] In addition, MYC controls DNA replication independent of its transcriptional activity, a property that may promote genomic instability by inducing replication stress.[164] Consistent with its involvement in multiple cellular processes, the MYC target gene network is estimated to include ~15% of all protein-coding genes as well as noncoding RNAs.[163,165] In vivo, MYC is found mainly in heterodimeric complexes with the related protein MAX, and such interaction is required for MYC-induced stimulation of transcription and cell proliferation.[166–172] In NHL carrying *MYC* translocations, constitutive expression of MYC induces the transcription of target genes with diverse roles in regulating cell growth by affecting DNA replication, energy metabolism, protein synthesis, and telomere elongation.[163,172,173] Furthermore, deregulated MYC expression is thought to cause genomic instability, and thus contributes to tumor progression by facilitating the occurrence of additional genetic lesions.[174] Dysregulation of MYC expression in a number of transgenic mouse models leads to the development of aggressive B-cell lymphomas with high penetrance and short latency.[162,175,176] These mouse models confirm the pathogenetic role of deregulated MYC in B cells, although the resulting tumors tend to be more immature than the human BL, most likely due to the early activation of the promoter sequences used for the expression of the MYC transgene.

More recently, the application of new genomics technologies revealed additional oncogenic mechanisms that cooperate with MYC in the development of this aggressive lymphoma. Mutations of the transcription factor 3 (TCF3) (10% to 25%) and its negative regulator ID3 (35% to 58%) are highly recurrent in all three subtypes of BL, where they promote tonic (antigen-independent) BCR signaling and sustain survival of the tumor cell by engaging the phosphoinositide 3-kinase (PI3K) pathway (Fig. 101.4).[177] In addition, TCF3 can promote cell-cycle progres-

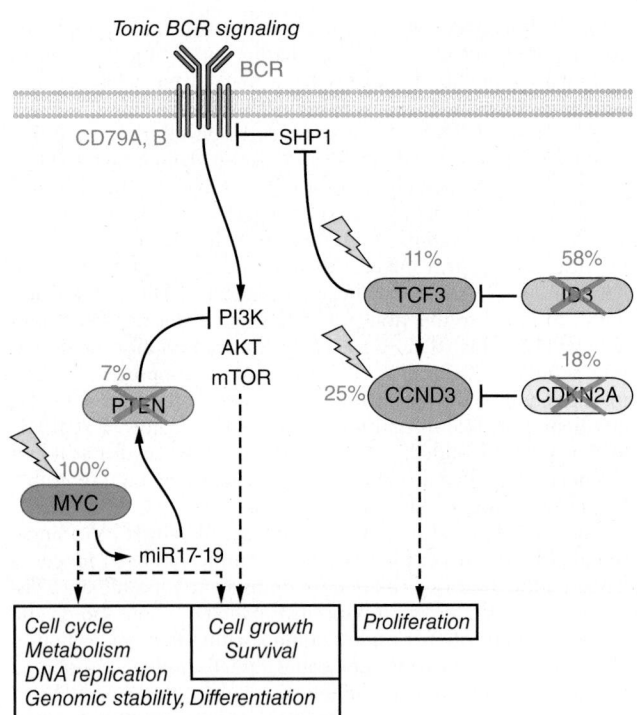

Figure 101.4 Most common genetic lesions identified in BL. *Lightning bolts* indicate activating mutations and *crosses* denote inactivating events. mTOR, mammalian target of rapamycin.

sion by transactivating CCND3. Notably, *CCND3* is itself a target of gain-of-function mutations in 38% of sBL, where these events affect conserved residues in the carboxyl terminus of this D-type cyclin, which are implicated in the control of protein stability, leading to higher expression levels. Interestingly, *CCND3* mutations occur in only 2.6% of eBL, suggesting alternative oncogenic mechanisms in this subtype.[177] Other common genetic lesions include the loss of *TP53* by mutation and/or deletion (35% of both sBL and eBL cases),[68] inactivation of *CDKN2B* by deletion or hypermethylation (17% of samples),[85] and deletions of 6q, detected in ~30% of cases, independent of the clinical variant.[70] Finally, one contributing factor to the development of BL is monoclonal EBV infection, present in virtually all cases of eBL and in ~30% of sBL.[86,88,178,179] The consistent expression of EBER, a class of small RNA molecules, has been proposed to mediate the transforming potential of EBV in BL.[180] However, EBV infection in BL displays a peculiar latent infection phenotype characterized by negativity of both EBV-transforming antigens LMP1 and EBNA2; thus, the precise pathogenetic role of this virus has remained elusive.[181]

Follicular Lymphoma

FL represents the second most common type of B-NHL (~20% of diagnoses) and the most common low-grade B-NHL.[1] It is an indolent but largely incurable disease, characterized by a continuous pattern of progression and relapses that often culminates in its histologic transformation to an aggressive lymphoma with a diffuse large cell architecture and a dismal prognosis (20% to 30% of cases).[182,183]

Cell of Origin

The ontogeny of FL from a GC B cell is supported by the expression of specific GC B-cell markers such as BCL6 and CD10, together with the presence of somatically mutated Ig genes showing evidence of ongoing SHM activity.[1]

Genetic Lesions

The genetic hallmark of FL is represented by chromosomal translocations affecting the *BCL2* gene on chromosome band 18q21, which are detected in 80% to 90% of cases independent of cytologic subtype, although less frequent in grade 3 FL.[184–187] These rearrangements join the 3' untranslated region of *BCL2* to an *IG* J_H segment, resulting in the ectopic expression of BCL2 in GC B cells,[184,185,188–192] where its transcription is normally repressed by BCL6.[18,193] Approximately 70% of the breakpoints on chromosome 18 cluster within the major breakpoint region, whereas the remaining 5% to 25% map to the more distant minor cluster region, located ~20 kb downstream of the *BCL2* gene.[184,185,188,189] Rearrangements involving the 5' flanking region of *BCL2* have been described in a minority of cases.[194] The *BCL2* gene encodes a 26-kd integral membrane protein that controls the cell apoptotic threshold by preventing programmed cell death and, thus, may contribute to lymphomagenesis by inducing apoptosis resistance in tumor cells independent of antigen selection. Nevertheless, additional genetic aberrations are required for malignant transformation. Most prominent among them are mutations in multiple epigenetic modifiers, including the methyltransferase *MLL2* (80% to 90% of cases),[80] the polycomb-group oncogene *EZH2* (7% of patients),[195] the acetyltransferases *CREBBP* and *EP300* (40% of cases),[79,80] and multiple core histones,[196] which may all contribute to transformation by remodeling the epigenetic landscape of the precursor tumor cell. A major role is also played by chronic antigen stimulation.[197,198]

Whole-exome sequencing and CN analysis of sequential, clonally related FL and tFL biopsies has recently provided the ability to characterize the molecular events that are specifically acquired during histologic progression to DLBCL, and thus presumably play a major role in conferring this more aggressive phenotype. tFL-specific lesions include inactivation of *CDKN2A/B* through deletion, mutation, and hypermethylation (one-third of patients),[84,136,199] rearrangements and amplifications of *MYC*,[84,200] *TP53* mutations/deletions (25% to 30% of cases),[69,201–203] loss of chromosome 6 (20%),[70] ASHM, and although larger cohorts of patients will need to be studied, biallelic loss of the immune regulator *B2M*.[84] Chromosomal translocations of the *BCL6* gene are detected in 6% to 14% of all FL cases, and were shown to have a significantly higher prevalence in the group of patients that undergo transformation into aggressive DLBCL.[204–207]

Diffuse Large B-Cell Lymphoma

DLBCL is the most common form of B-NHL, accounting for ~40% of all new diagnoses in adulthood and including cases that arise de novo, as well as cases that derive from the clinical evolution of various, less aggressive B-NHL types (i.e., FL and CLL).[1,208]

Cell of Origin

Based on gene expression profile analysis, at least three well-characterized molecular subtypes have been recognized within this diagnostic entity, which reflect the derivation from B cells at various developmental stages. Germinal center B-cell–like (GCB) DLBCL appears to derive from proliferating GC cells; ABC-DLBCL shows a transcriptional signature related to BCR-activated B cells or to B cells committed to plasmablastic differentiation; and PMBCL is postulated to arise from post-GC thymic B cells. The remaining 15% to 30% of cases remain unclassified.[209–212] Stratification according to gene expression profiles has prognostic value, because patients diagnosed with GCB-DLBCL display better overall survival compared to ABC-DLBCL,[63] but is imperfectly replicated by immunophenotyping or morphology and does not presently inform differential therapy[213,214]; thus, it is not officially incorporated into the WHO classification. A separate classification schema identified three discrete subsets defined by the expression of genes involved in oxidative phosphorylation, B-cell receptor/

proliferation, and tumor microenvironment/host inflammatory response.[215]

Genetic Lesions

The heterogeneity of DLBCL is reflected in the catalog of genetic lesions that are associated with its pathogenesis, and include balanced reciprocal translocations, gene amplifications, chromosomal deletions, single point mutations, and relatively unique among all NHL, ASHM. During the past few years, the application of genomewide approaches such as whole-exome/transcriptome/genome sequencing and single nucleotide polymorphism (SNP) array analysis have provided a comprehensive picture of the DLBCL genomic landscape. One important finding of these studies is that, compared to other B-cell malignancies, DLBCL shows a significantly higher degree of genomic complexity, harboring on average 50 to more than 100 lesions per case, with great diversity across patients.[80,216,217] Although many of the identified lesions can be variably found in both molecular subtypes of the disease, consistent with a general role during transformation, others appear to be preferentially or exclusively associated with individual DLBCL subtypes, indicating that GCB and ABC-DLBCL utilize distinct oncogenic pathways (Fig. 101.5).

GCB and ABC Shared Lesions. The most prominent program disrupted in DLBCL, independent of subtype, is represented by epigenetic regulation of chromatin due to mutations in the *CREBBP/EP300* acetyltransferase genes (35% of cases) and the *MLL2* H3K4 trimethyltransferase (~30% of cases).[79,80,217] These lesions may favor tumor development by reprogramming the cancer epigenome and, in the case of *CREBBP/EP300*, by altering the balance between the activity of the BCL6 oncogene, which is typically inactivated by acetylation, and the tumor suppressor p53, which requires acetylation at specific residues for its function.[79]

Deregulated activity of the BCL6 oncoprotein due to a multitude of genetic lesions is also a major contributor to DLBCL pathogenesis, in both GCB and ABC-DLBCL. Chromosomal rearrangements of the *BCL6* gene at band 3q27 are observed in up to 35% of cases,[71,205,218] although with a twofold higher frequency in the ABC-DLBCL subtype (see Fig. 101.4).[219] These rearrangements juxtapose the intact coding domain of *BCL6* downstream and in the same transcriptional orientation to heterologous sequences derived from the partner chromosome, including *IGH* (14q23), *IGκ* (2p12), *IGλ* (22q11), and at least 20 other chromosomal sites unrelated to the *IG* loci.[40–47] The majority of these translocations result in a fusion transcript in which the promoter region and the first noncoding exon of *BCL6* are replaced by sequences derived from the partner gene.[41,220] Because the common denominator of these promoters is a broader spectrum of activity throughout B-cell development, including expression in the post-GC differentiation stage, the translocation is thought to prevent the downregulation of BCL6 expression that is normally associated with differentiation into post-GC cells. Deregulated expression of an intact BCL6 gene product is also sustained by a variety of indirect mechanisms, including gain-of-function mutations in its positive regulator MEF2B (~11% of cases),[221] inactivating mutations/deletions of *CREBBP/EP300*,[79] and mutations/deletions of *FBXO11* (~5%),[222] which encodes a ubiquitin ligase involved in the control of BCL6 protein degradation. These lesions play a critical role in lymphomagenesis by enforcing the proliferative phenotype typical of GC cells, while suppressing proper DNA damage responses; moreover, constitutive expression of BCL6 blocks terminal differentiation, as confirmed by a mouse model in which deregulated BCL6 expression causes DLBCL.[223]

DLBCL cells have also acquired the ability to escape both arms of immune surveillance, including cytotoxic T lymphocytes (CTL)-mediated cytotoxicity (through genetic loss of the *B2M/* human leukocyte antigen class I [*HLA-I*] genes) and natural killer (NK) cell–mediated death (through genetic loss of the CD58 molecule).[224] Analogous effects may be achieved in PMBCL by disruption of the major histocompatibility complex class II

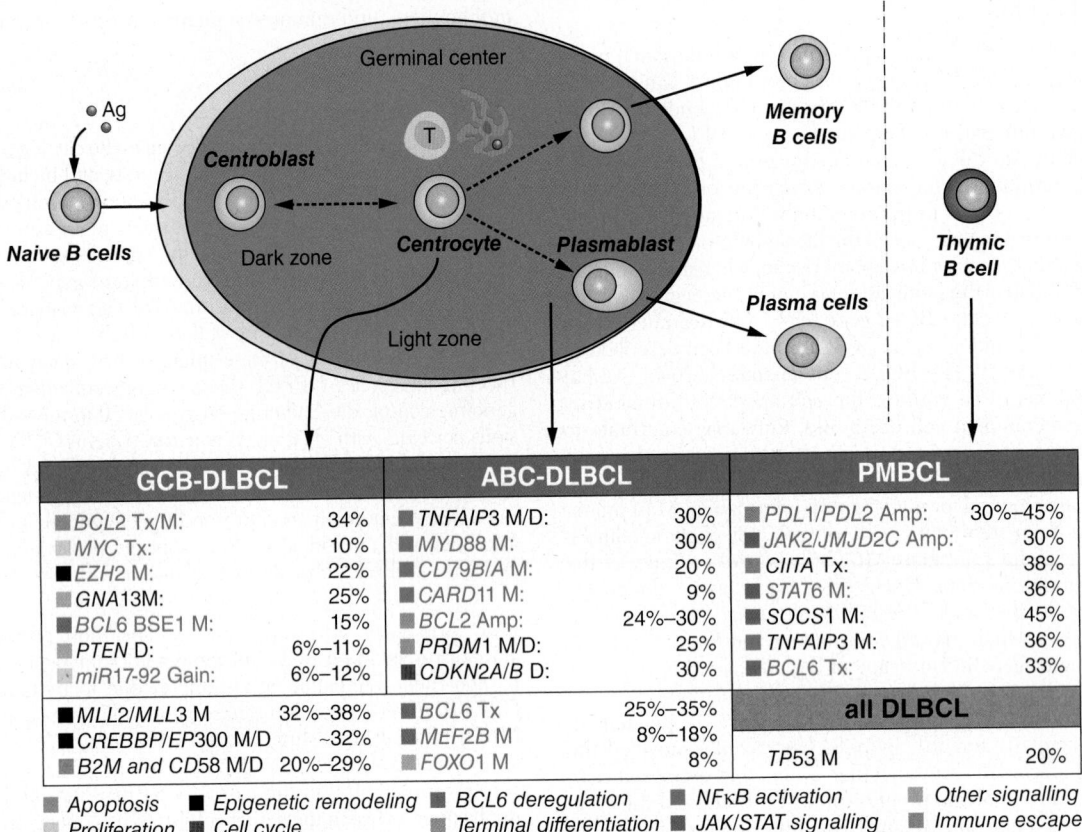

Figure 101.5 Genetic lesions associated with DLBCL. Most common genetic lesions identified in the three major DLBCL subtypes, including lesions that are shared between GCB- and ABC-DLBCL and lesions that are preferentially segregating with individual molecular subtypes. Loss-of-function alterations are in *black* and gain-of-function events are in *red. Color-coded squares* denote the biologic function/signaling pathway affected by the alteration.

(MHC-II) transactivator class II major histocompatibility complex transactivator (CIITA) and amplification of the genes encoding for the immunomodulatory proteins *PDL1/PDL2*.

Finally, approximately 50% of all DLBCL are associated with ASHM.[48] The number and identity of the genes that accumulate mutations in their coding and noncoding regions due to this mechanism varies in different cases and is still largely undefined. However, preferential targeting of individual genes has been observed in the two main DLBCL subtypes, with mutations of *MYC* and *BCL2* being found at significantly higher frequencies in GCB-DLBCL, and mutations of *PIM1* almost exclusively observed in ABC-DLBCL. ASHM may, therefore, contribute to the heterogeneity of DLBCL via the alteration of different cellular pathways in different cases. Mutations and deletions of the *TP53* tumor suppressor gene are detectable in ~20% of cases, including those that originate from the transformation of FL, and are more often associated with chromosomal translocations involving *BCL2*.[69]

GCB-DLBCL. Genetic lesions specific to GCB-DLBCL include the t(14;18) and t(8;14) translocations, which deregulate the BCL2 and MYC oncogenes in 34% and 10% of cases, respectively.[63,193,225,226] Also exquisitely restricted to this subtype are mutations of the *EZH2* gene,[195] which encodes a histone methyltransferase responsible for trimethylating Lys27 of histone H3 (H3K27), mutations of the S1PR2 adaptor protein GNA13, mutations affecting an autoregulatory domain within the BCL6 5′ untranslated exon 1,[219,227,228] and deletions of the tumor suppressor *PTEN*.[83,229]

Somatic mutations of the BCL6 5′ regulatory sequences are detected in up to 75% of DLBCL cases[52,230,231] and reflect the activity of the physiologic SHM mechanism that operates in normal GC B cells.[52,53] However, a functional analysis of numerous mutated

BCL6 alleles uncovered a subset of mutations that are specifically associated with GCB-DLBCL and that are not observed in normal GC cells or in other B-cell malignancies.[227] These mutations deregulate BCL6 transcription by disrupting an autoregulatory circuit through which the BCL6 protein controls its own expression levels via binding to the promoter region of the gene[227,228] or by preventing CD40-induced BCL6 downregulation in post-GC B cells.[232] Because the full extent of mutations deregulating BCL6 expression has not been characterized, the fraction of DLBCL cases carrying abnormalities in BCL6 cannot be determined.

ABC-DLBCL. Several genetic abnormalities are observed almost exclusively in ABC-DLBCL, including amplifications of the *BCL2* locus on 18q24[233,234]; mutations within the NF-κB (*CARD11, TNFAIP3/A20*),[75,235] B-cell receptor (*CD79B*),[236] and TLR (*MYD88*)[237] signaling pathways; inactivating mutations and deletions of *BLIMP1*[72–74]; chromosomal translocations deregulating the BCL6 oncogene; and deletion or lack of expression of the p16 tumor suppressor. Mutations of the *ATM* gene have been reported in a small subset of cases.[238]

A predominant feature of ABC-DLBCL is the constitutive activation of the NF-κB signaling pathway, initially evidenced by the selective expression of a signature enriched in NF-κB target genes, and by the requirement of NF-κB for proliferation and survival of ABC-DLBCL cell lines. This phenotype is sustained by a variety of alterations affecting positive and negative regulators of NF-κB, as well as other adaptor molecules converging on activation of NF-κB, specifically in this disease subtype. In up to 30% of cases, the *TNFAIP3* gene, encoding for the negative regulator A20, is biallelically inactivated by mutations and/or deletions, thus preventing termination of NF-κB responses.[75,76] The tumor suppressor role of A20 was documented by the observation that reconstitution of A20 knockout cell lines with a wild-type protein induces apoptosis and blocks proliferation, in part due to suppression of NF-κB activity.[75,76] In an additional ~10% of ABC-DLBCL, the *CARD11* gene is targeted by oncogenic mutations clustering in the protein coiled-coil domain and enhancing its ability to transactivate NF-κB target genes.[235] Less commonly, mutations were found in a variety of other genes encoding for NF-κB components, overall accounting for over half of all ABC-DLBCL[75] and suggesting that yet unidentified lesions may be responsible for the NF-κB activity in the remaining fraction of cases.

In addition to constitutive NF-κB activity, ABC-DLBCLs display evidence of chronic active BCR signaling, which is associated with somatic mutations affecting the immunoreceptor tyrosine-based activation motif (ITAM) signaling modules of *CD79B* and *CD79A* in 10% of ABC-DLBCL biopsy samples, but rarely in other DLBCLs.[236] Moreover, silencing several BCR proximal and distal subunits is toxic to ABC-DLBCL. These findings provided genetic evidence in support of the development of therapies targeting BCR signaling,[236] and indeed, kinase inhibitors that interfere with this signaling pathway are emerging as a new treatment paradigm for ABC-DLBCL.

Approximately 30% of ABC-DLBCL patients harbor a recurrent change in the intracellular Toll/interleukin-1 receptor domain of the MYD88 adaptor molecule, which has the potential to activate NF-κB as well as JAK/STAT3 transcriptional responses.[237] Although the relationship between *MYD88* mutations and TLR signaling has not been studied, MYD88 was shown to be required for the survival of ABC-DLBCLs, indicating a pathogenic role for TLR in this disease type.

A second important program that is disrupted by genetic lesions in ABC-DLBCL includes terminal B-cell differentiation. In up to 25% of ABC-DLBCL cases, the *PRDM1* gene is inactivated by biallelic truncating or missense mutations and/or genomic deletions, as well as by transcriptional repression through constitutively active, translocated BCL6 alleles.[72–74] The *PRDM1* gene encodes for a zinc finger transcriptional repressor that is expressed in a subset of GC B cells undergoing plasma cell differentiation and in all plasma cells,[239,240] and is an essential requirement for terminal B-cell differentiation.[241] Thus, BLIMP1 inactivation contributes to lymphomagenesis by blocking post-GC B-cell differentiation. Consistently, translocations deregulating the *BCL6* gene are exceedingly rare in *BLIMP1* mutated DLBCLs, suggesting that BCL6 deregulation and BLIMP1 inactivation represent alternative oncogenic mechanisms converging on the same pathway (Fig. 101.6).

PMBCL. PMBCL is a tumor observed most commonly in young female adults, which involves the mediastinum and displays a distinct gene expression profile, largely similar to HL.[211,212] A genetic hallmark of both PMBCL and HL is the amplification of chromosomal region 9q24, detected in nearly 50% of patients.[83,242] This relatively large interval encompasses multiple genes of possible pathogenetic significance, including the gene encoding for the *JAK2* tyrosine kinase and the *PDL1/PDL2* genes, which encode for inhibitors of T-cell responses[64,83,242] and have been linked to impaired antitumor immune responses in several cancers. Other lesions affecting regulators of immune responses in PMBCL include genomic breakpoints and mutations of the MHC class II transactivator gene *CIITA*, which may reduce tumor cell immunogenicity by downregulating surface HLA class II expression.[64,65,243] The ability of the previously mentioned lesions to interfere with the interaction between the lymphoma cells and the microenvironment suggests a central role for escape from immuno-surveillance mechanisms. Besides contributing to lymphomagenesis, elevated expression levels of these genes may, in part, explain the unique features of these lymphoma types, which are characterized by a significant inflammatory infiltrate. PMBCL also shares with HL the presence of genetic lesions affecting the NF-κB pathway and

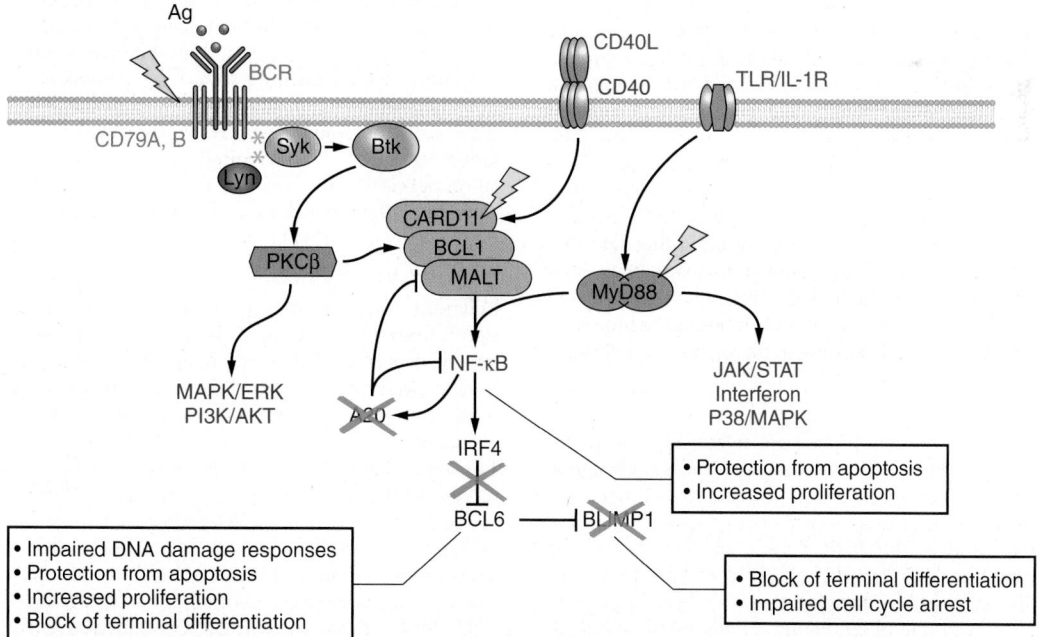

Figure 101.6 Pathway lesions in ABC-DLBCL. Schematic representation of a germinal center centrocyte, expressing a functional surface BCR, a CD40 receptor and a TLR. In normal B cells, engagement of the BCR by the antigen *(spheres)*, interaction of the CD40 receptor with the CD40L presented by T-cells, and activation of the TLR converge on activation of the NF-κB pathway, including its targets IRF4 and A20 among others. IRF4, in turn, downregulates BCL6 expression, allowing the release of BLIMP1 expression, a master plasma cell regulator required for terminal differentiation. In ABC-DLBCL, multiple genetic lesions disrupt this pathway at multiple levels in different cases (percentages as indicated); these lesions contribute to lymphomagenesis by favoring the antiapoptotic and pro-proliferative function of NF-κB, as well as chronic active BCR and JAK/STAT3 signaling, while blocking terminal B-cell differentiation through mutually exclusive deregulation of BCL6 and inactivation of BLIMP1.

the deregulated expression of receptor tyrosine kinases.[78,244–246] In particular, mutations of the transcription factor STAT6, amplifications/overexpression of JAK2 (which promote STAT6 activation via interleukin 3 (IL-3)/IL-4), and inactivating mutations of its negative regulator SOCS1 are highly recurrent in PMBCL, pointing to the JAK/STAT signaling pathway as a major disease contributor.

DLBCL Derived from CLL and FL Transformation. Recently, exome sequencing studies examining sequential biopsies of CLL/RS or FL/tFL have provided insights onto the molecular mechanisms that drive the transformation process. These analyses extended the set of genetic lesions that are specifically acquired during transformation and include CDKN2A/B loss, TP53 loss, and MYC translocations (in both conditions), along with ASHM and B2M inactivation in tFL, or NOTCH1 mutations in RS.[82,84] They also allowed for reconstruction of the evolutionary history of the dominant tumor clone during transformation, revealing that FL and tFL derive from a common ancestor mutated clone through divergent evolution, as opposed to RS, which, analogous to CLL progression,[247] arises from the predominant CLL clone through a linear pattern. Finally, comparison with de novo DLBCL showed that, despite their morphologic resemblance, the genomic landscapes of RS and tFL are largely unique in that they are characterized by distinct combinations of alterations otherwise not commonly observed in de novo DLBCL/NOS.[82,84]

Extranodal Marginal Zone Lymphoma of Mucosa-associated Lymphoid Tissue (MALT)

Cell of Origin

Mucosa-associated lymphoid tissue (MALT) lymphoma represents the third most common form of NHL,[1] and has steadily risen in incidence over the last 2 decades.[248] The presence of rearranged and somatically mutated IgV genes,[31,249] together with the architectural relationship with MALT,[1] indicate the post-GC origin of these tumors, possibly from a marginal zone memory B cell (see Fig. 101.1). A number of observations support a critical role for antigen stimulation, particularly in the pathogenesis of gastric MALT lymphoma: (1) This disease is associated with chronic infection of the gastric mucosa by H. pylori in virtually all cases[113–115]; (2) eradication of H. pylori by antibiotic treatment can lead to tumor regression in ~70% of cases[116,250]; and (3) MALT lymphoma cells express autoreactive BCR, in particular to rheumatoid factors.[251,252] Whether the development of MALT lymphoma arising in body sites other than the stomach also depends on antigen stimulation remains an open question. In this respect, it is remarkable that salivary gland and thyroid MALT lymphoma are generally a sequela of autoimmune processes, namely Sjögren syndrome and Hashimoto thyroiditis, respectively.

Genetic Lesions

Most of the structural aberrations that are selectively and recurrently associated with MALT lymphoma target the NF-κB signaling pathway, suggesting a critical role in the disease pathogenesis. The most common among these lesions is the t(11;18)(2;33) translocation, which involves the BIRC3 gene on 11q21 and the MALT1 gene on 18q21,[253,254] and is observed in 25% to 40% of gastric and pulmonary MALT lymphomas.[255–257] BIRC3 plays an evolutionary conserved role in regulating programmed cell death in diverse species, whereas MALT1, together with BCL10 and CARD11, is a component of the ternary complex that plays a central role in BCR and NF-κB signaling activation.[258] Notably, the wild-type proteins encoded by these two genes are incapable of activating NF-κB, in contrast to the BIRC3/MALT1 fusion protein, suggesting that the translocation confer a survival advantage to the tumor by leading to inhibition of apoptosis and constitutive NF-κB activation without the need for upstream signaling.[253,254,259] In an additional 15% to 20% of cases, MALT1 is translocated to the

IGH locus as a consequence of t(14;18)(q32;q21),[260,261] whereas ~5% of patients harbor abnormalities of chromosomal band 1p22, generally represented by t(1;14)(p22;q32); the latter deregulates the expression of BCL10, a cellular homolog of the equine herpesvirus-2 E10 gene, which contains an amino-terminal caspase recruitment domain (CARD) homologous to that found in several apoptotic molecules.[262,263] BCL10, however, does not have proapoptotic activity in vivo, where it functions as a positive regulator of antigen-induced activation of NF-κB.[258,264,265] Thus, the translocation may provide both antiapoptotic and proliferative signals mediated via NF-κB transcriptional targets.

A more recently identified translocation associated, although not restricted to, MALT lymphoma is t(3;14)(p13;q32),[266,267] which leads to the deregulated expression of FOXP1, a member of the Forkhead box family of winged-helix transcription factors involved in the regulation of Rag1 and Rag2 and essential for B-cell development.[268] Finally, homozygous or hemizygous loss of TNFAIP3 due to mutations and/or deletions has been reported in 20% of MALT lymphoma patients, typically in a mutually exclusive pattern with other alterations leading to NF-κB activation.[77] Other recurrent genetic lesions in this disease include trisomy 3,[269,270] BCL6 alterations, and TP53 mutations.[271–273]

Chronic Lymphocytic Leukemia

Cell of Origin

CLL is a malignancy of mature, resting B lymphocytes that originates from the oncogenic transformation of a common precursor resembling an antigen-experienced B cell.[274] This notion was conclusively demonstrated when gene expression profile studies revealed that, although CLL can express somatically mutated or unmutated IgV genes at approximately equal percentages,[275,276] all cases share a homogeneous signature more related to that of CD27+ memory and marginal zone B cells.[277,278] Moreover, an analysis of the Ig gene repertoire in these patients indicates very similar, at times almost identical, antigen receptors among different individuals.[279–284] This finding, known as stereotypy, strongly supports a role for the antigen in CLL pathogenesis. The histogenetic heterogeneity of CLL carries prognostic relevance, because cases with mutated Ig genes are associated with a significantly longer survival.[285,286] Intriguingly, 6% of the normal elderly population develops a monoclonal B-cell lymphocytosis (MBL) that is considered the precursor to CLL in 1% to 2% of cases.[287]

Genetic Lesions

Different from most mature B-NHL and consistent with the derivation from a post-GC or GC-independent B cell, CLL cases are largely devoid of balanced, reciprocal chromosomal translocations.[81] On the contrary, CLL is recurrently associated with several numerical abnormalities, including trisomy 12 and monoallelic or biallelic deletion/inactivation of chromosomal regions 17p, 11q, and 13q14 (Table 101.1).[81] Of these, the deletion of 13q14 represents the most frequent chromosomal aberration, being observed in up to 76% of cases as a monoallelic event, and in 24% of cases as a biallelic event. Interestingly, this same deletion is also found in subjects with MBL.[287] In all affected cases, the minimal deleted region (MDR) encompasses a long noncoding RNA (DLEU2) and two microRNAs expressed as a cluster, namely miR-15a and miR-16-1.[288–290] The causal involvement of 13q14–MDR-encoded tumor suppressor genes in CLL pathogenesis was demonstrated in vivo in two animal models, which developed clonal lymphoproliferative diseases with features of MBL, CLL, and DLBCL at 25% to 40% penetrance.[291] Trisomy 12 is found in approximately 16% of patients evaluated by interphase fluorescent in situ hybridization and correlates with poor survival, but no specific gene(s) have been identified.[292–294] Deletions of chromosomal region 11q22-23 (18% of cases) almost invariably encompass the

TABLE 101.1

Most Common Genetic Lesions Associated with Non-Hodgkin Lymphoma

NHL Subtype	Genetic Abnormality	Cases Affected (%)	Involved Gene	Functional Consequences	Gene Function
Mantle cell lymphoma	t(11;14)(q13;q32)	95	CCND1	Transcriptional deregulation	Cell-cycle regulation
Burkitt lymphoma	t(8;14)(q24;q32) t(2;8)(p11;q24) t(8;22)(q24;q11)	80 15 5	MYC MYC MYC	Transcriptional deregulation Transcriptional deregulation Transcriptional deregulation	Control of proliferation and growth
Follicular lymphoma	t(14;18)(q32;q21) t(2;18)(p11;q21) t(18;22)(q21;q11)	90 Rare Rare	BCL2 BCL2 BCL2	Transcriptional deregulation Transcriptional deregulation Transcriptional deregulation	Antiapoptosis
Diffuse large B-cell lymphoma (GCB)	t(8;14)(q24;q32) t(14;18)(q32;q21) t(3;other)(q27;other) EZH2 M	10 30 15 20	MYC BCL2 BCL6 EZH2	Transcriptional deregulation Transcriptional deregulation Transcriptional deregulation Unknown	Proliferation and growth Antiapoptosis Master regulator of GC responses Chromatin remodeling
Diffuse large B-cell lymphoma (ABC)	t(3;other)(q27;other) TNFAIP3 M/D PRDM1 M/D CD79B M CARD11 M 18q21 amplification	25 20 20 18 9 30	BCL6 TNFAIP3 PRDM1 CD79B CARD11 BCL2	Transcriptional deregulation Loss of function Loss of function Gain of function Gain of function Increased gene dosage	Master regulator of GC responses Negative NF-κB regulator Terminal B-cell differentiation Activation of BCR signaling Positive NF-κB regulator Antiapoptosis
Primary mediastinal B-cell lymphoma	9p24.1 amplification	50	JAK2 PDL1, PDL2	Increased gene dosage Increased gene dosage	JAK/STAT pathway regulation Immunomodulatory responses
Mucosa-associated lymphoid tissue (MALT) lymphoma	t(11;18)(q21;q21) t(14;18)(q32;q21) t(3;14)(p13;q32) t(1;14)(p22;q32)	30 15–20 10 5	API2-MALT1 MALT1 FOXP1 BCL10	Fusion protein Transcriptional deregulation Transcriptional deregulation Transcriptional deregulation	Positive NF-κB regulator Positive NF-κB regulator Transcription factor Positive NF-κB regulator
Lymphoplasmacytic lymphoma	t(9;14)(p13;q32)	50	PAX5	Transcriptional deregulation	B-cell proliferation and differentiation
Anaplastic large cell lymphoma	t(2;5)(p23;q35)	60[a]	NPM/ALK	Fusion protein	Tyrosine kinase
Classic Hodgkin lymphoma	TNFAIP3 M/D SOCS1 M/D 2p13 amplification 9p24.1 amplification	40[b] 45 50 50	TNFAIP3 SOCS1 REL JAK2 PDL1, PDL2	Loss of function Loss of function Increased gene dosage Increased gene dosage Increased gene dosage	Negative NF-κB regulator Inhibition of JAK-STAT pathway Positive NF-κB regulator Inhibition of JAK/STAT pathway Immunomodulatory responses

GCB, germinal center B-cell–like; ABC, activated B-cell-like; M, mutation; D, deletion. See also Fig. 101.5 for a more complete list of the recurrent genetic lesions in DLBCL.
[a] In the adult population; 85% in childhood.
[b] Sixty percent in Epstein-Barr Virus-negative cases.

ATM gene and may thus promote genomic instability.[295–297] These lesions can be observed in the patient germ line, and may thus account, at least in part, for the familial form of the disease. Another important target within the 11q22-23 deleted region is the BIRC3 gene, encoding for a negative regulator of NF-κB.[298] The identification of inactivating mutations and the evidence of constitutive NF-κB activation in these cases suggests that NF-κB could serve as a therapeutic target in this poor prognosis category of patients. Deletions of 17p13, which include the TP53 tumor suppressor and which are frequently accompanied by a mutation of the second allele,[68,299] are observed in ~7% of CLL at diagnosis but are enriched in cases that underwent transformation to RS, a highly aggressive lymphoma with poor clinical outcome.[82] More recently, gain-of-function mutations of NOTCH1 and mutations of SF3B1 were discovered in 5% to 10% of diagnostic CLL samples,[300–303]

where they seem to predict an adverse outcome, as supported by their preferential enrichment in RS (30% of cases) and fludarabine refractory cases (25%), respectively (Fig. 101.7).[82,300–304]

HIV-Related Non-Hodgkin Lymphoma

The association between an immunodeficiency state and the development of lymphoma has been recognized in several clinical conditions, including congenital (e.g., Wiskott-Aldrich syndrome), iatrogenic (e.g., treatment with immunosuppressive agents), and viral-induced (e.g., AIDS) immunodeficiencies. Detailed investigations have been conducted on the molecular pathophysiology of HIV-related NHL, which are primarily classified into three clinico-pathologic categories: BL, DLBCL, and PEL.[1,305,306] Based

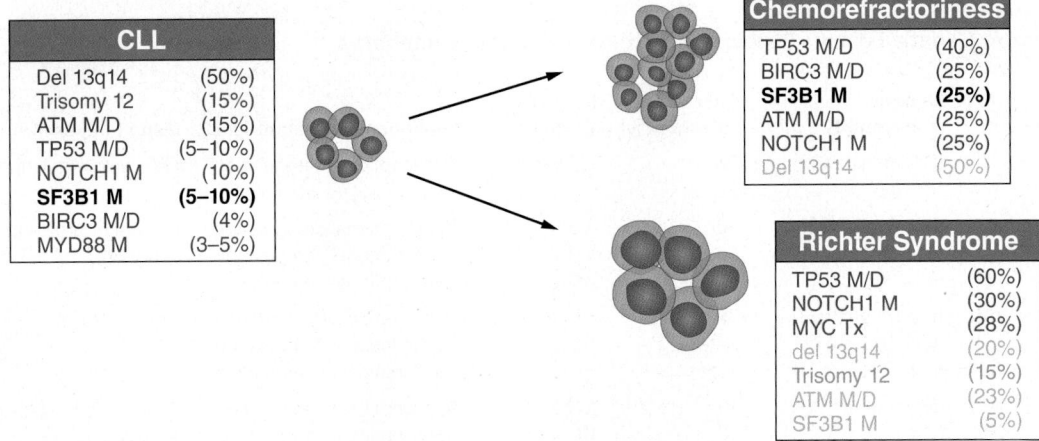

Figure 101.7 Genetic lesions associated with CLL. Frequency of common genetic alterations observed in unselected CLL cases at diagnosis, fludarabine-resistant CLL and RS. Blue, loss of function mutations; Red, gain-of-function mutations.

on the site of origin, HIV-related NHLs are generally grouped into systemic HIV-related NHL (i.e., DLBCL and BL) and HIV-related PCNSL, which is characterized by a uniform morphology consistent with a diffuse architecture of large cells.[1,305,306]

Cell of Origin

HIV-related NHLs invariably derive from B cells that have experienced the GC reaction, as indicated by the presence of somatic mutations in the IG and BCL6 genes, as well as by several phenotypic and transcriptional features.[305–307] Based on the presence or absence of immunoblastic features and on the expression pattern of BCL6, CD138, and the EBV-encoded LMP1, both HIV-related DLBCL and PCNSL can be segregated into two distinct histogenetic categories. Cases displaying the BCL6+/CD138−/LMP1− phenotype closely resemble the phenotype of GC B cells, whereas BCL6−/CD138+/LMP1+ cases are morphologically consistent with immunoblastic lymphoma, plasmacytoid, and reflect a post-GC stage of B-cell differentiation.[305,306] PEL consistently derives from B cells, reflecting a preterminal stage of differentiation.[97,308–310]

Genetic Lesions. The three categories of HIV-related NHL associate with distinctive molecular pathways. HIV-related BLs consistently displays activation of MYC due to chromosomal translocations that are structurally similar to those found in sBL, whereas rearrangements of BCL6 are always absent.[307] HIV-related BLs also frequently harbor mutations in TP53 (60%), BCL6 5′ noncoding sequences (60%), and, in 30% of cases, infection of the tumor clone by EBV, although the EBV-encoded antigens LMP1 and EBNA2 are not expressed.[311,312] Stimulation and selection by antigens, frequently represented by autoantigens, appear to be a prominent feature.[142,313]

Different from BL, the most frequent genetic alteration detected in HIV-related DLBCL is infection by EBV, which occurs in approximately 60% to 70% of cases and is frequently, although not always, associated with the expression of LMP1.[89,91,312] Moreover, HIV-related DLBCLs carry BCL6 rearrangements in 20% of cases,[314] and mutations of the BCL6 5′ noncoding region in 70% of cases.[315]

All HIV-related PCNSLs show evidence of EBV infection.[316] However, only the subset with immunoblastic morphology expresses the LMP1 transforming protein.[317] These tumors display ASHM[57] and harbor oncogenic mutations in the CARD11 gene (16% of cases),[318] which may explain, in part, the constitutive NF-κB activity previously recognized in this lymphoma subtype. Although some reports have suggested that HHV-8 may be related to PCNSL pathogenesis in immunocompromised patients, extensive analyses have unequivocally ruled out this hypothesis.[319,320]

The last type of HIV-related NHL that has been characterized at the molecular level is PEL, also known as body cavity–based lymphoma.[97,308,309] This entity is associated with HHV-8 infection in 100% of cases and clinically presents as effusions in the serosal cavities of the body (pleura, pericardium, peritoneum) in the absence of solid tumor masses.[97,308,309] In addition to HHV-8, PEL cases frequently show coinfection of the tumor clone by EBV.[90,92,97,308,309]

MOLECULAR PATHOGENESIS OF T-CELL NON-HODGKIN LYMPHOMA

Peripheral T-cell lymphoma (PTCL) encompasses a highly heterogeneous and relatively uncommon group of diseases representing 5% to 10% of all NHLs worldwide, with significant geographical variation in both incidence and relative prevalence.[1] PTCLs arise from mature post-thymic T cells and, according to the clinical presentation of the disease, are listed as leukemic or disseminated, predominantly extranodal, cutaneous, and predominantly nodal.[1] Although the study of T-cell neoplasms is hampered by the rarity of these diseases and the difficulty of collecting homogeneous sample series, significant advances were made over the past decades in our understanding of their biology, classification, and prognosis.

Adult T-Cell Lymphoma/Leukemia (HTLV-1 Positive)

Cell of Origin

The term ATLL identifies a spectrum of lymphoproliferative diseases associated with HTLV-I infection that is mainly restricted to southwestern Japan and the Caribbean basin.[1,321] The United States and Europe are considered low-risk areas, because less than 1% of the population are HTLV-I carriers[322] and only 2% to 4% of seropositive individuals eventually develop ATLL.[1,101,102] Clonal rearrangement of the TCR is evident in all cases, and clonal integration of the virus has been observed.[323,324]

Genetic Lesions

Compared to other mature T-cell tumors, the molecular pathogenesis of ATLL has been elucidated to a wider extent. Particularly, the role of HTLV-I has been linked to the production of a transregulatory protein (HTLV-1 tax), that markedly increases expression of all viral gene products and transcriptionally activates the expression of certain host genes, including IL-2, CD25, c-sis, c-fos, and granulocyte-macrophage colony-stimulating factor (GM-CSF).[104–106,107,108] Indeed, a property of ATLL cells is the constitutively high expression of the IL-2 receptor. The central role of these genes in normal T-cell activation and growth, together with the results of in vitro studies, support the notion that tax-mediated activation of these host genes represents an important mechanism by which HTLV-1 initiates T-cell transformation.[104] In addition, tax interferes with DNA damage repair functions and with mitotic checkpoints,[109,110,325] which is consistent with the fact that ATLL cells harbor a high frequency of karyotypic abnormalities.

The long period of clinical latency that precedes the development of ATLL (usually 10 to 30 years), the small percentage of infected patients that develop this malignancy, and the observation that leukemic cells from ATLL are monoclonal suggest that HTLV-1 is not sufficient to cause the full malignant phenotype.[101–103] A model for ATLL, therefore, implies an early period of tax-induced polyclonal T-cell proliferation that, in turn, would facilitate the occurrence of additional genetic events leading to the monoclonal outgrowth of a fully transformed cell. In this respect, a recurrent genetic lesion in ATLL is represented by mutations of the *TP53* tumor suppressor gene, which is inactivated in 40% of cases.[326,327]

Peripheral T-Cell Lymphoma, Not Otherwise Specified

This category represents the largest and most heterogeneous group of PTCLs, and includes all cases that lack specific features allowing classification within another entity. The majority of these cases derive from αβ CD4+ T cells and show aberrant defective expression of one or several T-cell–associated antigens.[328] Based on gene expression profiling, peripheral T cell lymphoma/not otherwise specified (PTCL/NOS) as a group appears to be most closely related to activated T cells than to resting T cells and can be segregated according to similarities with the transcriptional signature of CD4+ and CD8+ T cells. However, no correlation is observed between gene expression profiles (GEP) and immunophenotype, likely reflecting the variable detection of T-cell antigens in the disease.

Genetic Lesions

Clonal numerical and structural aberrations are found in most PTCL/NOS by conventional cytogenetics and in all cases by more sensitive approaches such as array-based methods. For a few loci, the correlation between gene CN and expression has been confirmed, suggesting a pathogenetic role. Candidate genes include *CDK6* on chromosome 7q, *MYC* on chromosome 8, and the NF-κB regulator *CARD11* at 7p22, whereas losses of 9p21 are associated with a reduced expression of *CDKN2A/B*.[329] Chromosomal translocations involving the *TCR* loci have been reported in rare cases and remain poorly understood, because the identity of the translocation partner has not been identified, with few exceptions: the *BCL3* gene, the poliovirus receptor-related 2 (*PVRL2*) gene found in the t(14;19)(q11;q13) translocation, and the *IRF4* gene, which is cloned in two cases.[330–332] More recently, whole-exome sequencing studies revealed the presence of recurrent heterozygous mutations in the *RHOA* small GTPase gene (18% of patients), including a hot-spot Gly17Val substitution that was shown to have inhibitory effects in the Rho-signaling pathway, potentially via the sequestration of GEP proteins.[333,334] These mutations appear to segregate with a subset of Tfh-like PTCL/NOS, characterized by the expression of CD10 and PD-1, the proliferation of CD21+FDCs, and EBER positivity. In a smaller number of cases, mutations were also found in *TET2*, *DNM3TA*, *IDH2*, *TET3*, *FYN*, and *B2M*.[333,334]

Angioimmunoblastic T-Cell Lymphoma

Cell of Origin

Angioimmunoblastic T-cell lymphoma (AITL) is an aggressive disease of the elderly and accounts for about one-third of all PTCL cases in Western countries.[335] The tumor cells display a mature CD4+CD8- T-cell phenotype, with frequent aberrant loss of one or several T-cell markers and coexpression of BCL6 and CD10 in at least a fraction of cells. Gene expression profile studies have conclusively established the cellular derivation of AITL from follicular helper T cells,[336] as initially suspected based on the expression of single markers.[337]

Genetic Lesions

Until recently, the scarce number of genetic studies had failed to provide any significant clues regarding the oncogenic pathways involved in AITL. However, a major discovery emerged in 2013 from two whole-exome sequencing studies that identified highly recurrent mutations of *RHOA* in 67% of all AITL cases.[333,334] These mutations are analogous to those observed in PTCL/NOS, but are not found in other mature B- and T-cell neoplasms, strongly suggesting a role for the disruption of the RHO-signaling pathway in the pathogenesis of this disease. Additional clonal aberrations have been reported in up to 90% of AITL patients and include chromosomal imbalances as well as mutations in *TET2*, *IDH2*, and *DNMT3A*, which are common to various hematologic malignancies, whereas chromosomal translocations affecting the TCR loci are extremely rare.[329,333,334]

Cutaneous T-Cell Lymphoma

Genetic lesions are involved in a limited but significant fraction of primary CTCLs showing a molecular marker of clonality. Most notable among them are rearrangements of the *NFKB2* gene at 10q24, leading to a chimeric protein that retains the rel effector domain and can bind κB sequences in vitro,[338,339] but that lacks the ankyrin regulatory domain required for regulating the physiologic nuclear/cytoplasm distribution. The translocation may thus contribute to lymphoma development by causing constitutive activation of the NF-κB pathway.

Anaplastic Large Cell Lymphoma

Cell of Origin

ALCL is a distinct subset of T-NHL (~12% of cases), whose normal cellular counterpart has not yet been established.[1,321] The tumor is composed of large pleomorphic cells that exhibit a unique phenotype characterized by positivity for the CD30 antigen and the loss of most T-cell markers.[1,340] Based on the expression of a chimeric protein containing the cytoplasmic portion of anaplastic lymphoma kinase (ALK) (see the following), ALCL may be subdivided in two groups, displaying distinct transcriptional signatures[341]: The most common and curable is ALK-positive ALCL, and the more aggressive is ALK-negative ALCL.[1,342–344] However, the identification of a common 30-genes predictor that can discriminate ALCL from other T-NHL, independent of ALK status, suggests that these two subgroups are closely related and may derive from a common precursor.[345]

Genetic Lesions

The genetic hallmark of ALK+ALCL is a chromosomal translocation involving band 2p23 and a variety of chromosomal partners, with t(2;5)(p23;q35) accounting for 70% to 80% of the cases.[1,346] Cloning of the translocation breakpoint in t(2;5) demonstrated the involvement of the *ALK* gene on 2p23 and the nucleophosmin (*NPM1*) gene on 5q35.[347] As a consequence, the aminoterminus of NPM is linked in frame to the catalytic domain of ALK, driving transformation through multiple molecular mechanisms[347]: (1) the *ALK* gene, which is not expressed in normal T-lymphocytes, becomes inappropriately expressed in lymphoma cells, conceivably because of its juxtaposition to the promoter sequences of *NPM*, which are physiologically expressed in T cells; and (2) all translocations involving *ALK* produce proteins with constitutive tyrosine activity, due in most cases to spontaneous dimerization induced by the various fusion partners.[346] Constitutive ALK activity, in turn, results in the activation of several downstream signaling cascades, with the JAK/STAT and PI3K/AKT pathways playing central roles.[348–351] The transforming ability of the chimeric NPM/ALK protein has been proven both in vitro and in vivo in transgenic mouse models.[352–354]

In a minority of cases, fusions other than NPM/ALK cause the abnormal subcellular localization of the corresponding chimeric ALK proteins and the constitutive activation of ALK. Among these alternative rearrangements, the most frequent involve TPM3/TPM4, TRK-fused genes,[355] ATIC,[356,357] CLTCL1, and MSN. The diversity of known ALK fusion partners was further expanded by the recent identification of a novel TRAF1/ALK fusion transcript leading to constitutive NF-κB expression.[358] No recurrent cytogenetic abnormality has been described in ALK-negative ALCL, leaving the molecular events responsible for this disease subtype largely unknown.

MOLECULAR PATHOGENESIS OF HODGKIN LYMPHOMA

HL is a B-lymphoid malignancy characterized by the presence of scattered large atypical cells—the mononucleated Hodgkin cells and the multinucleated Reed-Sternberg cells (HRS)—residing in a complex admixture of inflammatory cells.[1,359] Based on the morphology and phenotype of the neoplastic cells, as well as on the composition of the infiltrate, HL is segregated in two major subgroups: nodular lymphocyte-predominant HL (NLPHL) (~5% of cases) and classic HL (cHL), comprising the nodular sclerosis, mixed cellularity, lymphocyte-depleted, and lymphocyte-rich variants. Until recently, molecular studies of HL have been hampered by the paucity of the tumor cells in the biopsy (typically less than 1%, although occasional cases can present more than 10% HRS cells). However, the introduction of sophisticated laboratory techniques allowing for the isolation and enrichment of neoplastic cells has markedly improved our understanding of HL histogenesis.

Cell of Origin

Despite the fact that HRS of cHL cells have lost the expression of nearly all B-cell–specific genes,[360–362] both HL types represent clonal populations of B cells, as revealed by the presence of clonally rearranged and somatically mutated Ig genes.[363,364] In about 25% of cHL cases, nonsense mutations disrupt originally in-frame IGHV gene rearrangements (crippling mutations), thereby preventing antigen selection. These data suggest that HRS cells of cHL have escaped apoptosis through a mechanism not linked to antigen stimulation.[364]

Genetic Lesions

A number of structural alterations lead to the constitutive activation of NF-κB in cHL. Nearly half of the cases display amplification of REL, which is associated with increased protein expression levels[365,366]; gains or translocations of the positive NF-κB regulator BCL3 were also reported.[330] More recently, a number of inactivating mutations were found in genes coding for negative regulators of NF-κB, including NFKBIA (20% of cases), NFKBIE (15%), and TNFAIP3 (40%), among others.[78,367–369] Notably, TNFAIP3-mutated cases are invariably EBV negative, suggesting that EBV infection may substitute, in part, for the pathogenic function of its protein product A20 in causing NF-κB constitutive activation.[78,369] In the past few years, genetic aberrations that modulate the tumor microenvironment have been uncovered using massively parallel DNA sequencing techniques, including genomic gains of PD-L1 (CD274) and PD-L2 (CD273) and translocations of CIITA.[64,65,243] Amplification of JAK2, mutations of STAT6, and inactivating mutations of SOCS1, a negative regulator of the JAK/STAT signaling pathway, are often found in NLPHL[242,246]; in an additional large fraction of cases, constitutive JAK/STAT activity is sustained by autocrine and paracrine signals.[359] BCL6 translocations have been reported in the lymphocytic and histiocytic (L&H) cells of NLPHL, but only rarely in cHL,[370,371] and translocations of BCL2 or mutations in positive or negative regulators of apoptosis (e.g., TP53, FAS, BAD, and ATM) are virtually absent.[369] As mentioned, an important pathogenic cofactor in cHL, but not NLPHL, is represented by monoclonal EBV infection, which occurs in approximately 40% of cHLs and up to 90% of HIV-related HLs, suggesting that infection precedes clonal expansion.[359] Of the viral proteins encoded by the EBV genome, infected HRS cells most commonly express LMP1, LMP2, and EBNA1, but not EBNA2.[359]

SELECTED REFERENCES

The full reference list can be accessed at lwwhealthlibrary.com/oncology.

1. Swerdlow SH, Campo E, Harris NL, et al., eds. WHO Classification of Tumours of Haematopoietic and Lymphoid Tissues. Lyon: International Agency for Research on Cancer; 2008.
3. Rajewsky K. Clonal selection and learning in the antibody system. Nature 1996;381:751–758.
4. Klein U, Dalla-Favera R. Germinal centres: role in B-cell physiology and malignancy. Nat Rev Immunol 2008;8:22–33.
9. Victora GD, Schqickert TA, Fooksman DR, et al. Germinal center dynamics revealed by multiphoton microscopy with a photoactivatable fluorescent reporter. Cell 2010;143:592–605.
10. Di Noia JM, Neuberger MS. Molecular mechanisms of antibody somatic hypermutation. Annu Rev Biochem 2007;76:1–22.
19. Phan RT, Dalla-Favera R. The BCL6 proto-oncogene suppresses p53 expression in germinal-centre B cells. Nature 2004;432:635–639.
27. Honjo T, Kinoshita K, Muramatsu M. Molecular mechanism of class switch recombination: linkage with somatic hypermutation. Annu Rev Immunol 2002;20:165–196.
29. Muramatsu M, Kinoshita K, Fagarasan S, et al. Class switch recombination and hypermutation require activation-induced cytidine deaminase (AID), a potential RNA editing enzyme. Cell 2000;102:553–563.
30. Revy P, Muto T, Levy Y, et al. Activation-induced cytidine deaminase (AID) deficiency causes the autosomal recessive form of the Hyper-IgM syndrome (HIGM2). Cell 2000;102:565–575.
34. Kuppers R, Dalla-Favera R. Mechanisms of chromosomal translocations in B cell lymphomas. Oncogene 2001;20:5580–5594.
37. Ramiro AR, Jankovic M, Eisenreich T, et al. AID is required for c-myc/IgH chromosome translocations in vivo. Cell 2004;118:431–438.

38. Robbiani DF, Bothmer A, Callen E, et al. AID is required for the chromosomal breaks in c-myc that lead to c-myc/IgH translocations. Cell 2008;135:1028–1038.
39. Pasqualucci L, Bhagat G, Jankovic M, et al. AID is required for germinal center-derived lymphomagenesis. Nat Genet 2008;40:108–112.
42. Ye BH, Lista F, Lo Coco F, et al. Alterations of a zinc finger-encoding gene, BCL-6, in diffuse large- cell lymphoma. Science 1993;262:747–750.
48. Pasqualucci L, Neumeister P, Goossens T, et al. Hypermutation of multiple proto-oncogenes in B-cell diffuse large-cell lymphomas. Nature 2001;412:341–346.
52. Pasqualucci L, Migliazza A, Fracchiolla N, et al. BCL-6 mutations in normal germinal center B cells: evidence of somatic hypermutation acting outside Ig loci. Proc Natl Acad Sci U S A 1998;95:11816–11821.
53. Shen HM, Peters A, Baron B, et al. Mutation of BCL-6 gene in normal B cells by the process of somatic hypermutation of Ig genes. Science 1998;280:1750–1752.
68. Gaidano G, Ballerini P, Gong JZ, et al. p53 mutations in human lymphoid malignancies: association with Burkitt lymphoma and chronic lymphocytic leukemia. Proc Natl Acad Sci U S A 1991;88:5413–5417.
72. Mandelbaum J, Bhagat G, Tang H, et al. BLIMP1 is a tumor suppressor gene frequently disrupted in activated B cell-like diffuse large B cell lymphoma. Cancer Cell 2010;18:568–579.
75. Compagno M, Lim WK, Grunn A, et al. Mutations of multiple genes cause deregulation of NF-kappaB in diffuse large B-cell lymphoma. Nature 2009;459:717–721.
76. Kato M, Sanada M, Kato I, et al. Frequent inactivation of A20 in B-cell lymphomas. Nature 2009;459:712–716.
78. Schmitz R, Hansmann ML, Bohle V, et al. TNFAIP3 (A20) is a tumor suppressor gene in Hodgkin lymphoma and primary mediastinal B cell lymphoma. J Exp Med 2009;206:981–989.

79. Pasqualucci L, Dominguez-Sola D, Chiarenza A, et al. Inactivating mutations of acetyltransferase genes in B-cell lymphoma. *Nature* 2011;471: 189–195.

80. Morin RD, Mendez-LAgo M, Mungall AJ, et al. Frequent mutation of histone-modifying genes in non-Hodgkin lymphoma. *Nature* 2011;476: 298–303.

81. Dohner H, Stilgenbauer S, Benner A, et al. Genomic aberrations and survival in chronic lymphocytic leukemia. *N Engl J Med* 2000;343:1910–1916.

84. Pasqualucci L, Khiabanian H, Fangazio M, et al. Genetics of follicular lymphoma transformation. *Cell Rep* 2014;6:130–140.

95. Chang Y, Cesarman E, Pessin MS, et al. Identification of herpesvirus-like DNA sequences in AIDS-associated Kaposi's sarcoma. *Science* 1994;266:1865–1869.

97. Cesarman E, Chang Y, Moore PS, et al. Kaposi's sarcoma-associated herpesvirus-like DNA sequences in AIDS-related body-cavity-based lymphomas. *N Engl J Med* 1995;332:1186–1191.

112. Hermine O, et al. Regression of splenic lymphoma with villous lymphocytes after treatment of hepatitis C virus infection. *N Engl J Med* 2002;347:89–94.

115. Parsonnet J, Hansen S, Rodriguez L, et al. Helicobacter pylori infection and gastric lymphoma. *N Engl J Med* 1994;330:1267–1271.

116. Wotherspoon AC, Doglioni C, Diss TC, et al. Regression of primary low-grade B-cell gastric lymphoma of mucosa-associated lymphoid tissue type after eradication of Helicobacter pylori. *Lancet* 1993;342:575–577.

125. Motokura T, Bloom T, Kim HG, et al. A novel cyclin encoded by a bcl1-linked candidate oncogene. *Nature* 1991;350:512–515.

147. Dalla-Favera R, Martinotti S, Gallo RC, et al. Translocation and rearrangements of the c-myc oncogene locus in human undifferentiated B-cell lymphomas. *Science* 1983;219:963–967.

156. Dominguez-Sola D, Victora GD, Ying CY, et al. The proto-oncogene MYC is required for selection in the germinal center and cyclic reentry. *Nature immunology* 2012;13:1083–1091.

163. Meyer N, Penn LZ. Reflecting on 25 years with MYC. *Nat Rev Cancer* 2008;8:976–990.

164. Dominguez-Sola D, Ying CY, Grandori C, et al. Non-transcriptional control of DNA replication by c-Myc. *Nature* 2007;448:445–451.

177. Schmitz R, Young RM, Ceribelli M, et al. Burkitt lymphoma pathogenesis and therapeutic targets from structural and functional genomics. *Nature* 2012;490:116–120.

186. Cleary ML, Smith SD, Sklar J. Cloning and structural analysis of cDNAs for bcl-2 and a hybrid bcl-2/immunoglobulin transcript resulting from the t(14;18) translocation. *Cell* 1986;47:19–28.

196. Okosun J, Bodor C, Wang J, et al. Integrated genomic analysis identifies recurrent mutations and evolution patterns driving the initiation and progression of follicular lymphoma. *Nat Genet* 2014;46:176–181.

209. Alizadeh AA, Eisen MB, Davis RE, et al. Distinct types of diffuse large B-cell lymphoma identified by gene expression profiling. *Nature* 2000;403: 503–511.

211. Savage KJ, Monti S, Kutok JL, et al. The molecular signature of mediastinal large B-cell lymphoma differs from that of other diffuse large B-cell lymphomas and shares features with classical Hodgkin lymphoma. *Blood* 2003;102:3871–3879.

212. Rosenwald A, Wright G, Leroy K, et al. Molecular diagnosis of primary mediastinal B cell lymphoma identifies a clinically favorable subgroup of diffuse large B cell lymphoma related to Hodgkin lymphoma. *J Exp Med* 2003;198:851–862.

217. Pasqualucci L, Trifonov V, Fabbri G, et al. Analysis of the coding genome of diffuse large B-cell lymphoma. *Nat Genet* 2011;43:830–837.

221. Ying CY, Dominguez-Sola D, Fabi M, et al. MEF2B mutations lead to deregulated expression of the oncogene BCL6 in diffuse large B cell lymphoma. *Nat Immunol* 2013;14:1084–1092.

223. Cattoretti G, Pasqualucci L, Ballon G, et al. Deregulated BCL6 expression recapitulates the pathogenesis of human diffuse large B cell lymphomas in mice. *Cancer Cell* 2005;7:445–455.

232. Saito M, Gao J, Basso K, et al. A signaling pathway mediating downregulation of BCL6 in germinal center B cells is blocked by BCL6 gene alterations in B cell lymphoma. *Cancer Cell* 2007;12:280–292.

235. Lenz G, Davis RE, Ngo VN, et al. Oncogenic CARD11 mutations in human diffuse large B cell lymphoma. *Science* 2008;319:1676–1679.

236. Davis RE, Ngo VN, Lenz G, et al. Chronic active B-cell-receptor signalling in diffuse large B-cell lymphoma. *Nature* 2010;463:88–92.

237. Ngo VN, Young RM, Schmitz R, et al. Oncogenically active MYD88 mutations in human lymphoma. *Nature* 2011470:115–119.

241. Shapiro-Shelef M, Lin KI, McHeyzer-Williams LJ, et al. Blimp-1 is required for the formation of immunoglobulin secreting plasma cells and pre-plasma memory B cells. *Immunity* 2003;19:607–620.

243. Steidl C, Shah SP, Woolcock BW, et al. MHC class II transactivator CIITA is a recurrent gene fusion partner in lymphoid cancers. *Nature* 2011;471: 377–381.

277. Klein U, Tu Y, Stolovitzky GA, et al. Gene expression profiling of B cell chronic lymphocytic leukemia reveals a homogeneous phenotype related to memory B cells. *J Exp Med* 2001;194:1625–1638.

278. Rosenwald A, Alizadeh AA, Widhopf G, et al. Relation of gene expression phenotype to immunoglobulin mutation genotype in B cell chronic lymphocytic leukemia. *J Exp Med* 2001;194:1639–1647.

287. Rawstron AC, Bennett FL, O'Connor SJ, et al. Monoclonal B-cell lymphocytosis and chronic lymphocytic leukemia. *N Engl J Med* 2008;359:575–583.

288. Calin GA, Dumitru CD, Shimizu M, et al. Frequent deletions and down-regulation of micro- RNA genes miR15 and miR16 at 13q14 in chronic lymphocytic leukemia. *Proc Natl Acad Sci U S A* 2002;99:15524–15529.

291. Klein U, Lia M, Crespo M, et al. The DLEU2/miR-15a/16-1 cluster controls B cell proliferation and its deletion leads to chronic lymphocytic leukemia. *Cancer Cell* 2010;17:28–40.

300. Fabbri G, Rasi S, Rossi D, et al. Analysis of the chronic lymphocytic leukemia coding genome: role of NOTCH1 mutational activation. *J Exp Med* 2011;208:1389–1401.

301. Puente XS, Pinyol M, Quesada V, et al. Whole-genome sequencing identifies recurrent mutations in chronic lymphocytic leukaemia. *Nature* 2011;475:101–105.

303. Wang L, Lawrence MS, Wan Y, et al. SF3B1 and other novel cancer genes in chronic lymphocytic leukemia. *N Engl J Med* 2011;365:2497–2506.

321. de Leval L, Bisig B, Thielen C, et al. Molecular classification of T-cell lymphomas. *Crit Rev Oncol Hematol* 2009;72:125–143.

333. Palomero T, Couronne L, Khiabanian H, et al. Recurrent mutations in epigenetic regulators, RHOA and FYN kinase in peripheral T cell lymphomas. *Nat Genet* 2014;46:166–170.

334. Sakata-Yanagimoto M, Enami T, Yoshida K, et al. Somatic RHOA mutation in angioimmunoblastic T cell lymphoma. *Nat Genet* 2014;46:171–175.

346. Chiarle R, Voena C, Ambrogio C, et al. The anaplastic lymphoma kinase in the pathogenesis of cancer. *Nat Rev Cancer* 2008;8:11–23.

347. Morris SW, Kirstein MN, Valentine MB, et al. Fusion of a kinase gene, ALK, to a nucleolar protein gene, NPM, in non- Hodgkin's lymphoma. *Science* 1994;263:1281–1284.

359. Kuppers R. The biology of Hodgkin's lymphoma. *Nat Rev Cancer* 2009;9: 15–27.

PRACTICE OF ONCOLOGY

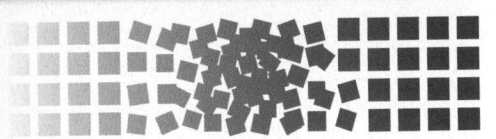

102 Hodgkin's Lymphoma

Anas Younes, Antonino Carbone, Peter Johnson, Bouthaina Dabaja, Stephen Ansell, and John Kuruvilla

INTRODUCTION

Although a relatively rare type of cancer, with an estimated 8,000 new cases per year in the United States, Hodgkin's lymphoma (HL) have fascinated scientists and clinicians for more than a century.[1,2] Remarkably, before the cell of origin and the biology of HL were elucidated, it became one of the earliest human cancers to be cured with multiagent chemotherapy.[1,3] Over the past 50 years, a significant progress has been made toward our understanding of HL biology, cell of origin, pathology, and treatment options. Therefore, many seminal observations that were made during the past few decades are now considered of historical value. For example, HL histologic classification evolved through multiple systems, starting from the initial histologic classification by Jackson and Parker in 1944, to the current system which is based on the World Health Organization (WHO) classification (Fig. 102.1).[4,5]

BIOLOGY OF HODGKIN'S LYMPHOMA

Cell of Origin

Molecular studies of isolated tumor cells have demonstrated that lymphocyte-predominant (LP) cells of nodular lymphocyte-predominant Hodgkin's lymphoma (NLPHL) are derived from antigen-selected germinal center (GC) B cells, whereas Reed-Sternberg (RS) cells in classic HL (cHL) appear to be derived from preapoptotic *crippled* GC B cells (Table 102.1).[6–9] Molecular features of LP cells include the presence of clonally rearranged and somatically mutated immunoglobulin (Ig)V gene cells, with signs of ongoing somatic hypermutation in a fraction of cases (see Table 102.1). These data linked the origin of LP cells in NLPHL to GC B cells. Another important feature supporting this linking was the immunohistochemical expression of BCL6 (a typical GC B-cell marker) in LP cells (Table 102.2).[10,11] Accordingly, LP cells can morphologically be observed in an environmental architecture resembling the structure of a secondary follicle, which contains a reactive GC. In fact, in the early phases of NLPHL, LP cells can be found in follicular structures in association with follicular dendritic cells (FDC) and GC type T-helper cells, in this regard resembling GC.[12]

The derivation of NLPHL from GCs is supported by the following features: (1) the expression of the BCL6 gene product and CD40 by LP cells[13,14]; (2) the occurrence of numerous CD4+/CD57+/PD1 T cells surrounding the LP cells, as seen in normal GCs and progressively transformed GCs (PTGC)[6]; (3) the presence of an FDC meshwork (CD21+/CD35+) within the tumor nodules[15]; and (4) the global gene expression profile.[16] Conversely, molecular features of RS cells in cHL demonstrate that they are probably derived from GC B cells that have acquired disadvantageous immunoglobulin variable chain gene mutations and normally would have undergone apoptosis.[6–8] In parallel to molecular investigations, biologic markers identifying distinct subsets of *mature* B cells have been used to study the cell of origin (see Table 102.2). According to the differential expression of these markers, LP and RS cells resemble *mature* B cells deriving from different stages of B-cell differentiation (i.e., GC and post-GC, respectively).

Reed-Sternberg Cells Lack Common B-Cell Markers

The loss of the B-cell phenotype in RS cells is unique among human lymphomas in the extent to which the lymphoma cells have undergone reprogramming of gene expression. As shown in gene expression profiling (GEP) studies, RS cells have lost the expression of most B-cell–typical genes and acquired expression of multiple genes that are typical for other types of cells in the immune system. Moreover, RS cell gene expression is most similar to that of Epstein-Barr virus (EBV)-transformed B cells, and cell lines derived from diffuse large-cell lymphomas showing features of in vitro activated B cells.[17]

The deregulated expression of inhibitors of B-cell molecules (inhibitor of differentiation and DNA binding 2 [ID2], activated B-cell factor 1 [ABF1], and notch 1), the downregulation of B-cell transcription factors (OCT2, BOB1, and PU.1), and the epigenetic silencing of B-cell genes (CD19 and immunoglobulin H [IgH]) all seem to be involved in the loss of the B-cell phenotype in RS cells.[17,18]

Multiple Signaling Pathways and Transcription Factors Have Deregulated Activity in Reed-Sternberg Cells

Very recently, biologic studies on HL cell lines using new technologies have shown that multiple signaling pathways and transcription factors have deregulated activity in RS cells. Involved pathways and transcription factors included nuclear factor kappa B (NF-κB), Janus kinase/signal transducers and activators of transcription (Jak-Stat), phosphoinositide 3-kinase (PI3K)–Akt, extracellular signal-regulated kinase (ERK), activating protein-1 (AP-1), notch 1, and receptor tyrosine kinases.[7,19] Functional studies have shown that in normal B GC cells, the activation of the CD40 receptor leads to NF-κB–mediated induction of the interferon regulatory factor 4/multiple myeloma oncogene 1 (IRF4/MUM1) transcription factor. CD40 engagement in HL cell lines by both soluble (s) CD40L and membrane-bound (mb) CD40L upregulates IRF4/MUM1 expression by HL cells.[20] CD40 engagement in HL cells by both sCD40L and mbCD40L enhances both clonogenic capacity and colony cell survival of HL cell lines, stimulates proliferation and rescue from apoptosis, mediates in vitro rosetting of activated CD4+ T cells to HL cells, and increases ERK phosphorylation and cell survival.[14,21]

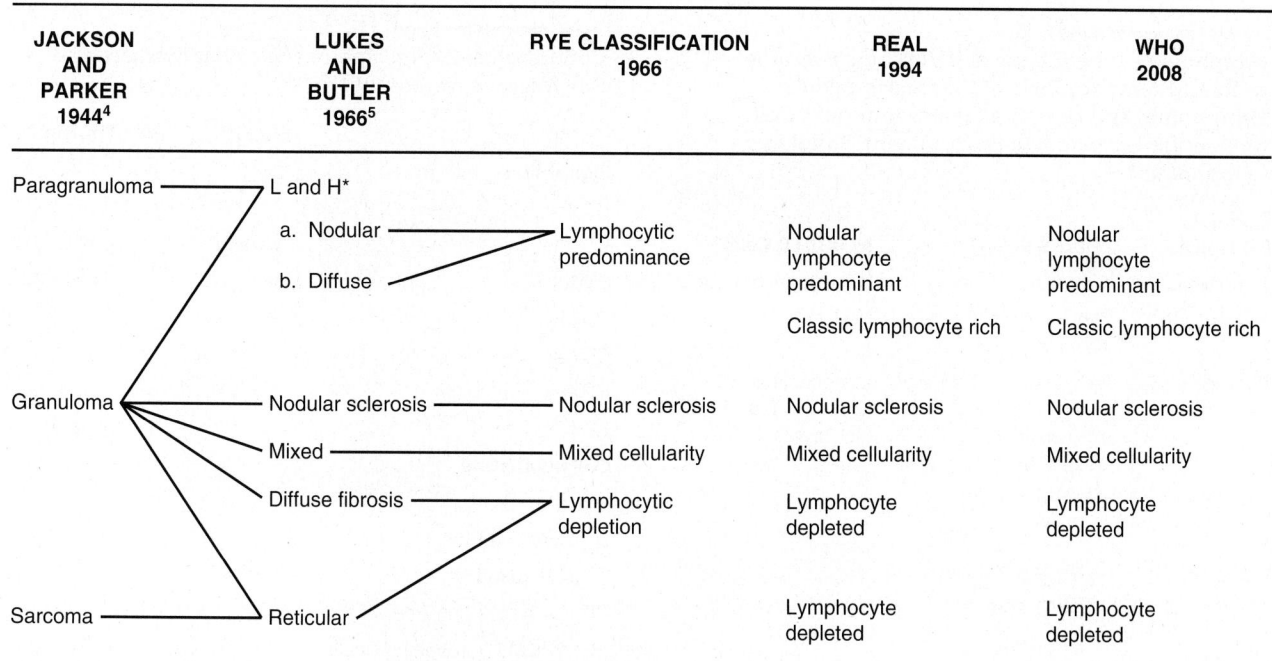

Figure 102.1 Comparison of classifications of Hodgkin's lymphoma.
*Lymphocytic and histiocytic

PATHOLOGY OF HODGKIN'S LYMPHOMA

The REAL Classification and the WHO Proposal

The most recent contribution is provided by the Revised European American Lymphoma (REAL) classification[22] and the WHO proposal, which, on the basis of a combination of phenotypic and morphologic features, subdivided HL into two distinct pathologic and biologic entities: NLPHL and cHL. cHL includes four subtypes (see Table 102.2) (see the following). LP cells of NLPHL

and RS cells of cHL have different morphology, different phenotype, and different infection pattern with the EBV.[22] LP cells express CD20, CD45, and epithelial membrane antigen (EMA) antigens, whereas RS cells display CD15-positive, CD30-positive, and CD45-negative phenotypes. EBV infection is usually present only in the RS cells of cHL, which express EBV encoded latent membrane protein 1 (LMP1) (Table 102.3).[22,23]

Nodular Lymphocyte-Predominant Hodgkin's Lymphoma

Morphology

NLPHL is characterized by a nodular, or a nodular and diffuse, proliferation of RS cell variants known as LP cells. LP cells are large and usually have one large multilobated nucleus and scant cytoplasm. The nucleoli are usually multiple, basophilic, and smaller than those seen in classical RS cells.

TABLE 102.1

Cell of Origin and Cell Lineage of Hodgkin's Lymphoma

Feature[1-3]/ Expression[5,6]	RS Cells of cHL	LP Cells of NLPHL
Proposed cellular origin	Preapoptotic GC B cell	Ag-selected, mutating GC B cell
Ig gene (single-cell PCR)	Rearranged, clonal, mutated, "crippled"	Rearranged, clonal, mutated ongoing
Somatically mutated Ig VAR genes	Yes	Yes
Presence of destructive somatic mutation	Yes (25%)	No
BCR	No	Yes
B-cell specific transcription factors (OCT-2, BOB1, PU1)	Very rarely	Yes
B-lineage commitment and maintenance factor PAX-5	Yes (low level)	Yes

PCR, polymerase chain reaction; Ig, immunoglobulin; VAR, variable; BCR, B-cell receptor.

TABLE 102.2

Expression of Molecular Markers in Hodgkin's Lymphoma

Expression[5,6]	RS Cells of cHL	LP Cells of NLPHL
B-cell markers (CD20, CD79)	Rarely	Yes
GC B-cell markers (BCL6, AID)	Rarely	Yes
Plasma cell markers (MUM1, CD138)	Often	No
Molecules involved in Ag presentation (MHC class II, CD40, CD80, CD86)	Yes	Yes
Markers for non–B cells (e.g., TARC, granzyme B, perforin)	Yes (variably)	No
T-cell markers	Yes (rarely)	No

AID, activation-induced cytidine deaminase; MUM1, multiple myeloma oncogene 1; Ag, antigen; MHC, major histocompatibility complex; TARC, thymus and activation-regulated chemokine.

Morphologic, Phenotypic and Virologic Features of Reed-Sternberg Cells of Classic Hodgkin's Lymphoma, and Lymphocyte-Predominant Cells of Nodular Lymphocyte Predominant Hodgkin's Lymphoma[25]

Features/ Expression	cHL/RS Cells	NLPHL LP Cells
Tumor cells	Diagnostic RS cells	LP or "popcorn" cells
Pattern	Diffuse, interfollicular, nodular	Nodular
Background	Lymphocytes, (T cells > B cells) histiocytes, eosinophils, plasma cells	Lymphocytes, (B cells > T cells) histiocytes
Fibrosis	Common	Rare
CD15	+	−
CD19	+ (20%–30%)	+
CD20	+ (20%–30%)	+
CD22	+ (20%–30%)	−
CD30	+	−
CD40	+	+
CD45	−	+
EMA	−	+
IRF4/MUM1	+	+
BCL6	+ (30%)	+
EBV infection	+ (30%–40%)	−

Comparative Expression of Molecular Markers and Cell Microenvironment[10,11,15,26,27]

	NLPHL	THCRBCL
Expression		
CD15	−	−
CD30	Usually −	− or +
EMA	+	Usually +
CD20	+	+
CD79a	+	+
IRF4	+	− or +
EBV	−	Usually −
Cell population		
T cells	v or +	+
B cells/B and T cells	+	−
CD57 + rosetting T cells	+ or −	−
CD40L + rosetting T cells	−	−
IRF4/MUM1 + rosetting T cells	+	−
Histiocytes	− or +	+
DRCs meshworks	+	−

THCRBCL, T/histiocyte cell–rich B-cell lymphoma; DRCs, dendritic reticulum cells.

Phenotype

LP cells are positive for CD20, CD79a, CD75, BCL6, and CD45 and epithelial membrane antigen in nearly all cases (see Table 102.3).[11,19] CD75, formerly LN1, is superior to CD20 and CD79a in detecting LP cells. LP cells express CD75 strongly, whereas small reactive B cells in the background show weak cytoplasmic positivity in the Golgi area but no membranous staining, in accordance with their mantle cell phenotype. CD20 is expressed in LP cells equally or less than in the small reactive B cells in the background. CD79a is even worse than CD20 in detecting LP cells because preferentially stains of small reactive B cells. The OCT2, BOB1, PAX5, and PU.1 B-cell transcription factors and the activation-induced deaminase enzyme (which is involved in somatic hypermutation and class switch recombination mechanisms in Ig genes), are consistently coexpressed (see Table 102.1).[11,19]

Microenvironment

The LP cells reside within nodules consisting of spherical meshworks of FDCs that are filled with nonneoplastic inflammatory cells. Inflammatory cells include small B cells, T cells that specifically express CD3 and CD4, and histiocytes. Furthermore, the inflammatory cells of nodules of NLPHL are characterized by an increase in GC-derived CD57+, IRF4/MUM1+, and PD-1+ T cells (see Table 102.3). Tia1 and CD40L-positive CD3/CD4 positive T cells are absent. PD1 ringing is a feature commonly seen in NLPHL.[15,19,24,25]

In conclusion, LP cells of NLPHL clearly resemble GC B cells in many phenotypic and genetic aspects, and proliferate in association with a cellular microenvironment that retains key features of a normal GC environment. Although LP cells are found to be even more similar to diffuse large B-cell lymphoma (including T-cell/histiocyte-rich large B-cell lymphoma) in terms of phenotypic and gene expression aspects, the environmental characteristics discriminate between these lymphomas (Table 102.4).

Microenvironment and Histologic Patterns

Well-recognized morphologic features of NLPHL include a nodular, or a nodular and diffuse, proliferation of scattered LP tumor cells, set against a background of reactive lymphocytes reminiscent of a primary follicle. Different patterns are recognizable in NLPHL on morphologic and immunohistologic grounds. Fan and colleagues[26] identified six distinct immunoarchitectural patterns (*classical* nodular, serpiginous/interconnected nodular, nodular with prominent extranodular LP cells, T-cell–rich nodular, diffuse with a T-cell–rich background, and diffuse, B-cell–rich pattern) and two variant patterns (presence of small GCs within the nodules and the presence of prominent sclerosis) (Fig. 102.2). In the nodular pattern originally described by Fan and colleagues[26] as pattern A, rare LP cells are seen outside of the nodule. In other patterns, however, increasing numbers of LP cells extend outside of the neoplastic nodules and infiltrate the perinodular space (see Fig. 102.2).[26]

A recent study recognized an additional nodular pattern of NLPHL in which LP cells reside in an environment reminiscent of lymphoid follicles and do not invade the extranodular space (Fig. 102.3).[12,27] The recognition of this pattern primarily relies on the identification within the nodules of BCL6+ and CD20+ LP cells, surrounded by rosetting PD1+ T cells. CD23 and CD21 immunostaining usually detects meshworks of FDCs, which entrap the LP cells and the surrounding T-cell rosettes. LP tumor cells are localized within an environment reminiscent of a secondary follicle or, more frequently, within neoplastic nodules reminiscent of a primary follicle without residual GCs (see Fig. 102.3).

Regarding the relationship of these histopathologic patterns to the clinical course of the disease, the pattern A of Fan and colleagues was usually seen in those patients presenting with earlier

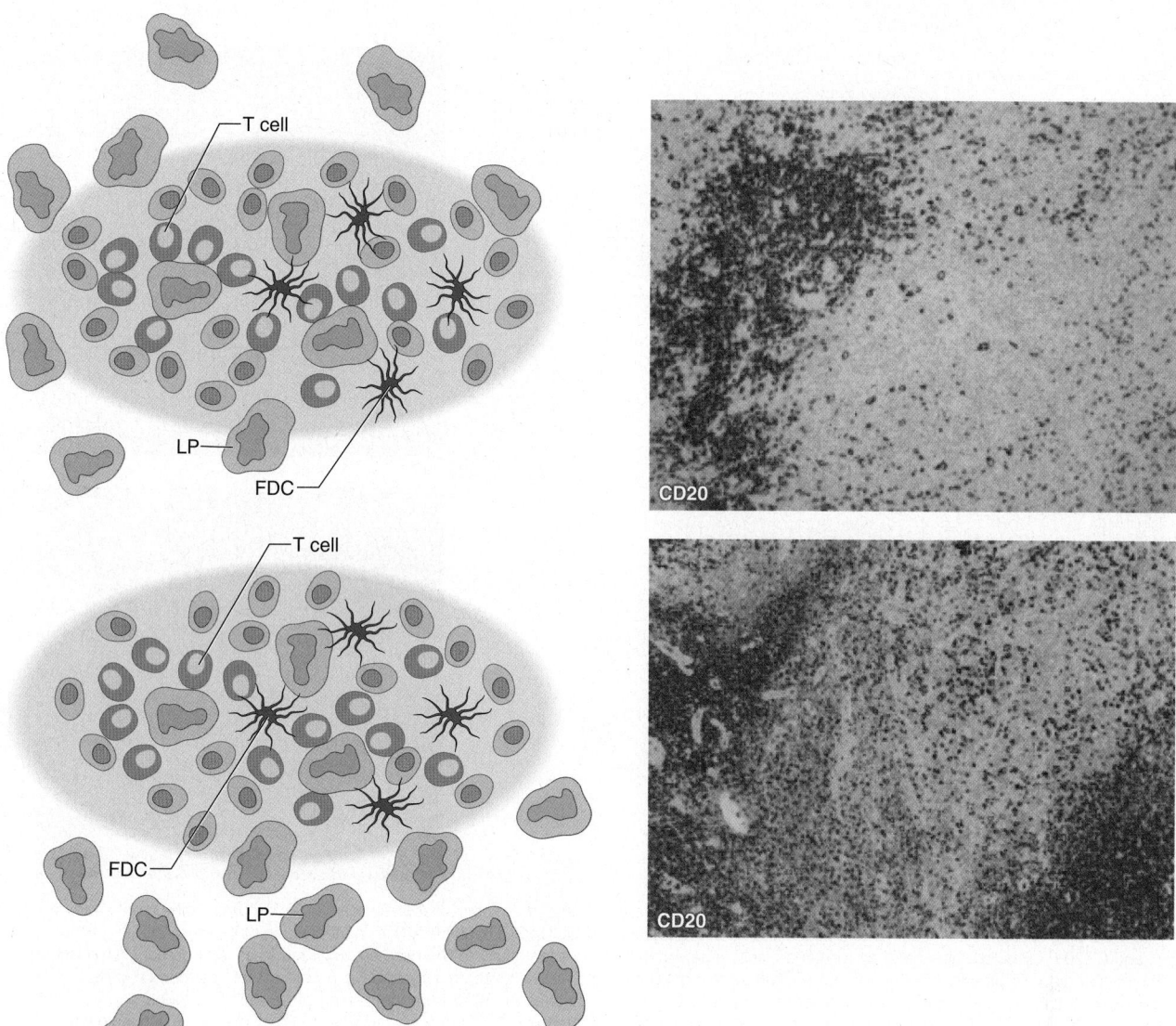

Figure 102.2 Major patterns on nodular lymphocyte predominate Hodgkin's lymphoma, as described by Fan and colleagues. Schematic representation *(to the left)*, microphotographs of CD20 immunostaining of LP cells *(to the right)*. *(Top)* Pattern A of Fan and colleagues.[26] *Classical* nodular pattern with rare extranodular LP cells. *(Top left)* In the *classical* nodular pattern, described by Fan and colleagues, the *B-cell–rich* nodules usually contain a prominent FDC meshwork that encompasses the LP cells. In these cases, the neoplastic LP cells are found to be located predominantly within the nodular structures, but rare LP cells extend outside of the nodule. *(Top right) Classical* nodular pattern. The pattern is characterized by scattered CD20+ LP cells within a nodular, reactive background dominated by small IgD+ B cells (not shown). The nodules contain a prominent CD23+ positive FDC meshwork that encompasses the LP cells (not shown). Rare LP cells can be found outside of the nodules. *(Bottom)* Pattern C of Fan and colleagues.[26] Nodular pattern with prominent extranodular LP cells. *(Bottom left)* During the progression of the disease, more LP cells extend outside of the nodules and infiltrate the perinodular space. Importantly, the presence of numerous LP cells outside the nodules may predict for progression to a diffuse pattern. The presence of many extranodular LP cells may characterize the pattern described by Fan and colleagues as "nodular with prominent extranodular LP cells". *(Bottom right)* Microphotograph of CD20 immunostaining of LP cells. This pattern shows more CD20+ LP cells *(at the center)* extending outside of the nodules. The extranodular LP cells are set in a background of reactive T cells and are not associated with FDC meshworks (not shown). Images were acquired with the Olympus dotSlide Virtual microscopy system using an Olympus BX51 microscopy equipped with PLAN APO 2×/0.08 and UPLAN SApo 40×/0.95 objectives.

clinical stage NLPHL. In general, the clinical impact of the different histopathologic patterns is still uncertain. Understanding this issue is difficult, because more than one pattern is frequently present at the same time.[28]

Classic Hodgkin's Lymphoma

Morphology

The so-called RS cell is the diagnostic key for this lymphoma because of its typical morphology: a giant cell with bi- or multinucleation and huge nucleoli. The typical morphology of binucleated

and multinucleated RS cells and their mononuclear variant, the so-called Hodgkin's cell, are not specific to cHL, because they can also be observed in B-NHL (especially in diffuse large B-cell lymphoma [DLBCL] of the anaplastic variant), but they are pathognomonic for cHL in conjunction with an abundant cellular background composed of a varying spectrum of nonneoplastic inflammatory cells.[5]

Based on the characteristics of the reactive infiltrate, four histologic subtypes have been distinguished: lymphocyte-rich cHL (LRCHL), nodular sclerosis (NS) cHL, mixed cellularity (MC) cHL, and lymphocyte depletion (LD) cHL. LRCHL accounts for only a small fraction (3% to 5%) of all HLs. Most LRCHLs

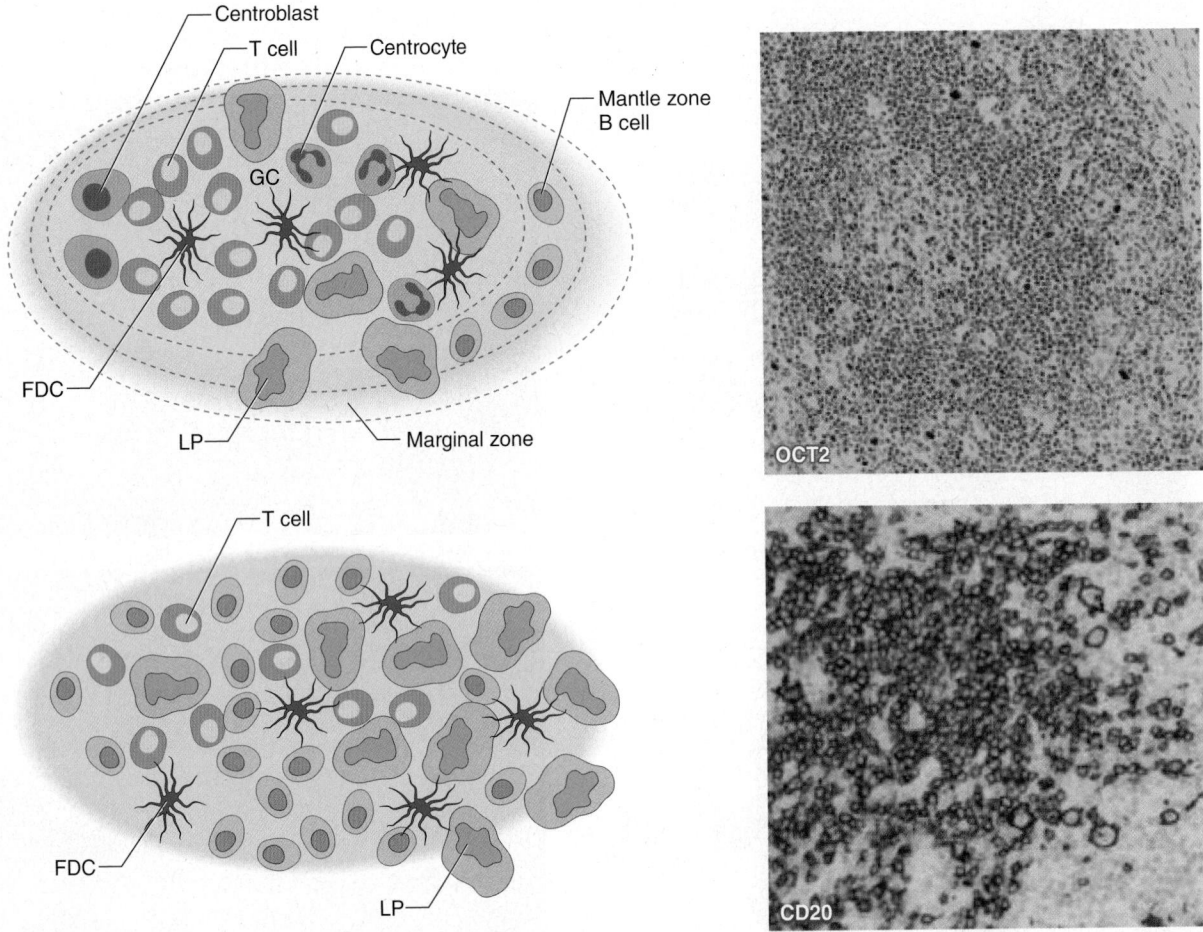

Figure 102.3 Nodular lymphocyte-predominant Hodgkin's lymphoma (NLPHL) may show a nodular pattern in which tumor cells do not invade the surrounding spaces. Schematic representation and microphotographs of OCT2, BCL6, and CD20 immunostaining of LP cells. OCT-2+, BCL6+, and CD20+ LP cells, surrounded by rosetting T cells (see schematic representation, *to the left*), are localized in an environment reminiscent of lymphoid follicles with (*Top*) or without (*Bottom*) a recognizable germinal center containing reactive B cells. In this pattern, LP cells do not extend outside of the nodules. *Top:* A schematic figure and microphotographs of OCT2 immunostaining of LP cells located in a follicle with recognizable germinal center. *Bottom:* A schematic figure and microphotograph of CD20 immunostainings of LP cells located in a nodule without a recognizable germinal center. Images were acquired with the Olympus dotSlide Virtual microscopy system using an Olympus BX51 microscopy equipped with PLAN APO 2×/0.08 and UPLAN SApo 40×/0.95 objectives.

have a better prognosis than do other cHLs and are characterized histologically by a small number of RS cells expressing a cHL immunophenotype. Based on these histologic and clinical features, there is no clear consensus on whether LRCHL represents a distinct disorder or just an early presentation of cHL. On the other hand, LRCHL cases display features intermediate between those of cHL and NLPHL.[11,19]

Phenotype

Phenotypically, RS cells of cHL are consistently positive for CD30, CD15, CD40, and IRF4/MUM1 (see Table 102.3).[23]

Microenvironment

cHL is a lymphoid neoplasm, derived from B cells, composed of mononuclear Hodgkin's cells and multinucleated RS cells residing in an abundant cellular microenvironment. In cHL, microenvironmental cell types include T- and B-reactive lymphocytes, eosinophils, mast cells, histiocytes/macrophages, plasma cells, and granulocytes (Fig. 102.4).[25,29–33] In addition, a great number of fibroblast-like cells and interdigitating/reticulum cells are detectable, often in association with RS cells, within the collagen bands of NS cHL. Fibrosis—considered a common morphologic feature

of HL lesions—is found more frequently in cHL subtypes than in NLPHL. An abnormal network of cytokines and chemokines and/or their receptors in RS cells is involved in the attraction of many of the microenvironmental cells into the lymphoma background (see Fig. 102.4).[8,34]

Nonmalignant inflammatory/immune cellular components of the HL microenvironment express molecules involved in cancer cell growth and survival, such as CD30L or CD40L, or in immune escape, such as programmed death 1 (PD-1). For example, CD30L+ eosinophils and mast cells, and proliferation-inducing ligand (APRIL)+ neutrophils, are consistently admixed to RS cells, whereas CD40L-expressing CD4+ T lymphocytes rosette RS cells. A considerable fraction of infiltrating CD4+ T cells are regulatory T (Treg) cells. Treg cells and PD-1+ T cells also interact with RS cells, which produce the Treg attractant galectin-1 and the PD-1 ligand (PDL-1).[7,25,29] The nonmalignant cells that compose most of the cellular background of cHL are recruited and/or induced to proliferate by tumor cells. They in turn produce soluble or membrane-bound molecules involved in tumor cell growth and survival. Numerous molecules are involved directly or indirectly in the recruitment and/or proliferation of cells constituting the cHL microenvironment. Normal cells may be recruited by cytokines/chemokines produced by RS cells or by T cells and

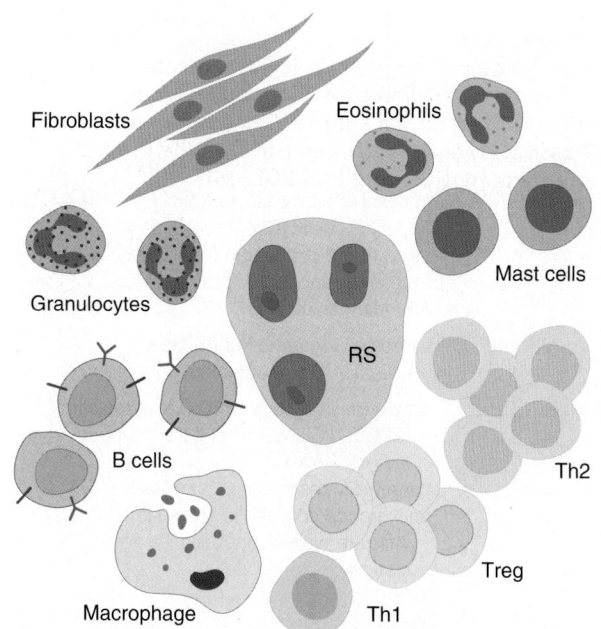

Figure 102.4 Reed-Sternberg (RS) cell and its microenvironment. An RS cell is shown within a rich, polymorphic cellular microenvironment that expresses members of the TNFR family protein and is embedded in a network of cytokines and chemokines. Treg, regulatory T cell; Th1, T-helper cell type 1); Th2, T-helper cell type 2.

fibroblasts activated by RS cells. RS cells produce molecules capable of inducing proliferation and/or differentiation of eosinophils, Treg cells, and fibroblasts.[29]

Epstein-Barr Virus Infection

Generally, in the different histologic subtypes of cHL, the immunophenotypic and genetic features of RS cells are identical, whereas their association with EBV shows differences. EBV is found in RS cells in about 40% of cHL cases in the Western world, mostly in cases of MC and LD HL, and less frequently in NS and LRCHL. Conversely, EBV is found in RS cells in nearly all cases of HL occurring in patients infected with HIV.[35] Independent studies have recently demonstrated that EBV can transform antigen receptor–deficient GC B cells, which enables their escape from apoptosis. The continued survival of the *rescued* preapoptotic B cells allows their proliferation. The EBV-encoded latent membrane protein (LMP) 2A is likely to function as the surrogate receptor through which B-cell signaling is triggered. This mechanism of EBV/LMP2A-induced the escape of antigen receptor-deficient GC B cells from apoptosis offers an intriguing model of lymphomagenesis. EBV infection might also affect the microenvironment composition by increasing the production of molecules involved in immune escape and T-cell recruitment, such as interleukin 10 (IL-10), CCL5, CCL20, and CXCL10.[36] LMP1 could have an interacting role with the microenvironment. Recent evidence indicates that EBV can manipulate the tumor microenvironment through the secretion of specific viral and cellular components into exosomes, small endocytically derived vesicles that are released from cells.[37,38] Exosomes produced by tumor cells from EBV-infected nasopharyngeal carcinoma contain LMP1, which can activate critical signaling pathways in uninfected neighboring cells, suggesting messenger functions of virus-modified exosomes.[37] Moreover, in B-cell lines, EBV-modified exosomes would activate cellular signaling mediated through integrins, actin, interferon, and NF-κB.[38] Further insights in these mechanisms are emerging from

the understanding of the capability of EBV to modulate the (tumor-like) microenvironment.

DIFFERENTIAL DIAGNOSIS

Pathologically, HL subtypes should be distinguished from other B-cell lymphomas showing large and CD30 expressing tumor cells. Figure 102.5 shows B-cell lymphomas, which can be differentiated from NLPHL and cHL on immunophenotypic grounds. The figure also includes lymphomas that have overlapping features with cHL or NLPHL. Most importantly, NLPHL should be differentiated from T-cell/histiocyte-rich large B-cell lymphoma (THRLBCL), a DLBCL subtype, and from the rare cHL variant termed lymphocyte-rich cHL.[11,19]

Nodular Lymphocyte-Predominant Hodgkin's Lymphoma

According to current criteria, the detection of one nodule showing the typical features of NLPHL in an otherwise diffuse growth pattern is sufficient to exclude the diagnosis of primary THRLBCL. NLPHL may mimic THRLBCL in a subset of cases in which T cells, rather than B cells, are predominant. This typically occurs in older lesions in which T cells have infiltrated the nodules of B cells and disrupted the nodular architecture.[11] This finding was previously termed NLPHL with diffuse areas; the current preferred term is NLPHL, THRLBCL-like. These kinds of lesions have not been associated with aggressive clinical behavior. The presence of small B-cells and CD4+/CD57+ T cells points to a NLPHL diagnosis, whereas the absence of small B-cells, and the presence of CD8+ cells and TIA1+ cells points to primary

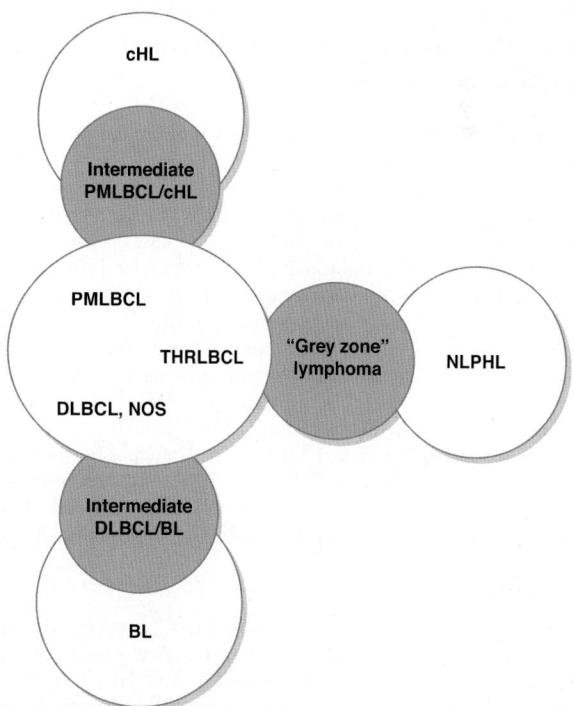

Figure 102.5 Provisional borderline categories for B-cell lymphomas that do not clearly fit into one entity. They include the intermediate PMLBCL/cHL category and a "grey zone" lymphoma between THRLBCL and NLPHL. PMLBCL, primary mediastinal large B-cell lymphoma; THRLBCL, T-cell/histiocyte-rich large B-cell lymphoma; NOS, not otherwise specified.

THRLBCL (see Table 102.4). However, there may be a morphologic and phenotypic gray area between THRLBCL and NLPHL. CD4+/CD57+/PD1 small lymphocytes resetting around typical CD20+/BCL6+ LP cells are useful for the differential diagnosis with PTGC, LRCHL, and THRLBCL. In addition, staining for OCT2, PAX5, and PU1 should be considered as an important diagnostic tool. Interestingly, IgD identifies a subgroup of cases (10% to 20%) with peculiar phenotypical and clinical features.

LRCHL is the most difficult cHL subtype to differentiate from NLPHL, and misclassification has frequently been found in retrospective studies. RS cells in LRCHL can resemble LP cells morphologically; but, immunophenotypically RS cells in LRCHL are positive for CD30 and often express CD15. CD20 can be expressed but is typically weaker and less uniform than CD30 expression. NLPHL is PAX5+, OCT2+, and PU.1+, whereas cHL, including LRCHL, is PAX5+/−, OCT2−, and PU.1−. The distinction between NLPHL and LRCHL is essential, owing to therapeutic and prognostic differences.

cHL

cHL variants should be distinguished from DLBCL subtypes or DLBCL NOS variants that express CD30 (see Fig. 102.5), despite the fact that RS cells have lost much of the B-cell–specific markers. Most or all RS cells also lack the transcription factors OCT2, BOB.1, and PU.1. Instead, RS cells display, in varying frequency, molecules not normally expressed by B cells and B-NHL, such as CD30, CD15, CD70, thymus and activation-regulated chemokine (TARC), A20, fascin, and RANTES.

Finally, cHL cases rich in neoplastic cells may resemble, in particular, large B-cell lymphoma displaying anaplastic morphology and expressing CD30 or primary mediastinal large B-cell lymphoma (PMBCL). There is also a true morphologic and biologic overlap between PMBCL and cHL cases (see Fig. 102.5).

Overlapping Features of PMLBCL with cHL: The So-Called Mediastinal Gray Zone Lymphoma

Mediastinal B-cell lymphomas are mostly represented by NS cHL and PMLBCL. Although PMLBCL and NS cHL have several distinctive pathologic features (Table 102.5),[39–42] these entities exhibit strikingly similar clinical presentations (young women with an anterior mediastinal mass) and, in some cases, show overlap in pathologic, genetic, and molecular features (see Table 102.5). A provisional category, designated *B-cell lymphoma, unclassifiable, with features intermediate between DLBCL and cHL* has been introduced in the WHO proposal to encompass such cases. Table 102.5 shows the main morphologic, phenotypic, and genetic features that may be useful in distinguishing PMLBCL, cHL, and the provisional intermediate category PMLBCL/cHL.

Variant sharing features of DLBCL with anaplastic morphology and cHL may also occur. This shows an expression of CD30, CD15, surface markers, and transcription factors of B cells, commonly absent from RS cells (CD45RB, CD20, CD79, and OCT2).

Molecular Features

In accordance with overlapping phenotypes between cHL and B-cell lymphomas, these lymphomas have a gene expression profile that is intermediate between DLBCL and HL, but closely resembles PMLBCL. Activation of the NF-κB pathway, known to enhance the survival of RS cells, is also a feature of PMLBCL and may represent a survival pathway shared by both neoplasms, likely through the activation of antiapoptotic genes. Activation of the PI3K/AKT pathway were recently identified as a further shared pathogenic mechanism between PMLBCL and cHL. Taken together, molecular features that are common to both lymphoma

TABLE 102.5	
Morphologic and Phenotypic Features that may be Useful in a Differential Diagnosis among Primary Mediastinal Large B-Cell Lymphoma, Classical Hodgkin's Lymphoma, and the Provisional Intermediate Category PMLBCL/cHL[23,43–48]	
cHL	Typical RS cells (CD30+, CD15+) Background containing T cells, B cells, plasma cells, eosinophils, fibroblasts Abundant sclerosis
Intermediate	Large cells resembling RS cells (CD20+, B-cell transcription factors +)
PMLBCL/cHL	Admixed large cells with clear cytoplasm (CD20−, CD15−, B-cell transcription factors + weak) Large cells resembling centroblasts Background containing sparse inflammatory infiltrate with eosinophils, plasma cells, histiocytes, and T cells Sclerosis (variable) Necrosis (frequent)
PMLBCL	Large cells with clear cytoplasm, multilobated nuclei, large cells with RS-like morphology (CD30+, CD15−, CD20+, B-cell transcription factors +). Diminished background containing eosinophils, plasma cells, T cells Fine compartmentalizing sclerosis

entities include a decrease of BCR pathway signaling, constitutive NF-κB activation, activation of the cytokine–JAK-STAT pathway, and aberrant activation of the PI3K/AKT pathway. The identification of molecular links between PMLBCL and cHL supports the hypothesis that there may be some pathogenetic overlap between the two entities and that these diseases may in fact represent opposite ends of a continuum.[39–42]

HIV-Associated Hodgkin's Lymphoma

The Pre-Highly Active Antiretroviral Therapy Era

In the first years of the AIDS epidemic, HIV-associated HL displayed clinical, pathologic, and biologic peculiarities when compared with HL in people uninfected with HIV. First, HIV-associated HL exhibited unusually aggressive clinical behavior, which mandated the use of specific therapeutic strategies, and it was associated with a poor prognosis. Second, the pathologic spectrum of HIV-associated HL differed markedly from that of HL in people uninfected with HIV. In particular, the aggressive histologic subtypes of cHL, namely MC and LD, predominated among HIV-associated HL.[43] Tumor tissue was characterized by an unusually large proportion of RS cells infected by EBV. The fact that LMP1 was expressed in virtually all HIV-associated HL cases suggested that EBV plays an etiologic role in the pathogenesis of HIV-associated HL.

The Highly Active Antiretroviral Therapy Era

People with HIV/AIDS (PWHA) seem to be at increased risk of HL than in first years of the epidemic. HL is presently the most common non–AIDS-defining cancer. Patients infected with HIV, who are modestly immunocompromised due to the improvement in CD4 counts associated with this treatment, are more at risk for the development of the nodular sclerosis subtype.[44] In this regard, it has been postulated that with increasing CD4+ T cells resulting from highly active antiretroviral therapy (HAART), the appropriate cellular milieu of cHL, surrounding the RS cells, may again be available. In PWHA with improved immunity, CD4+ T cells provide adequate antiapoptotic pathways and mechanisms for immune escape by tumor cells allowing, in this way, the expansion and maintenance of full expression of the disease, as occurs in cHL among people without AIDS.[35,45–47] Alternatively, HL may arise as part of an immune reconstitution syndrome. Hypothetically, RS cell may already be present in severe immunosuppressed patients, and partial restoration may allow for the recruitment of surrounding immune cells and the manifestation of the tumor.[48,49] A recent study evaluating the effect of immune reconstitution on HL incidence among a cohort of male veterans infected with HIV ever receiving combination antiretroviral therapy (cART) highlighted that immunosuppression and poor viral control may increase HL risk, specifically during immune reconstitution in the interval post-cART initiation. These findings further suggested an immune reconstitution–type mechanism in HIV-related HL development.[50]

EARLY-STAGE HODGKIN'S LYMPHOMA

The management of early-stage Hodgkin's lymphoma exemplifies several important principles of oncology. These include the progressive improvement of cure rates through careful clinical research; the identification of prognostic features and new markers of optimal response; the refinement of treatment by the exploration of multimodality approaches; the vital importance of long-term follow-up; and a holistic analysis of the outcomes of treatment. Overall, this is one of the success stories of modern oncology, with modern treatment achieving high initial cure rates (up to 90% with the first-line of therapy) and good overall survival at around 95% after 5 years or more. Because it most often affects younger people in the 2nd to 4th decade of life, this has important implications for the goals of treatment, which must include not only the maximization of initial tumor control but also the avoidance of preventable long-term side effects.

Prognostic Features

The relatively orderly progression of cHL has long been recognized.[51] It generally develops through involvement of adjacent nodes in the same anatomical site, then in adjacent nodal areas,

and it is extremely rare to find isolated deposits in two distant nodes. The same is not true for nodular lymphocyte-predominant disease, which, in this respect, more closely resembles a low-grade non-Hodgkin's lymphoma: It often presents with a single isolated node in the neck, but if it does progress, the dissemination is often to distant sites without intervening nodal involvement.

The predictable spread of cHL has allowed for the construction of a staging system based on anatomical extent, so that early-stage disease is defined by involvement of nodal groups on one side of the diaphragm only, more usually the thorax. Stage I disease is confined to a single anatomical nodal group (cervical, supraclavicular, axillary, anterior mediastinal, etc.), whereas a disease affecting more than one such group is stage II.

Beyond this division on the basis of nodal involvement, many studies have identified further prognostic features through retrospective analyses of large series of patients in clinical trials, mostly treated with extended field radiotherapy. This has allowed for the subdivision of early-stage disease into favorable and unfavorable categories. These do not represent biologically distinct processes, but act as a useful indicator of the severity of the illness and its optimum management, even though the current approaches to treatment are different to those in use when the factors were identified. Although a variety of stratification systems have been devised, common features include the presence of bulky disease (usually in the mediastinum), more advanced age (with a cutoff of 40 or 50 years of age), elevated erythrocyte sedimentation rate (ESR), systemic symptoms, and multiple or extranodal sites of involvement (Table 102.6).

Radiation Therapy

The effective treatment of HL by radiotherapy began with the work of Gilbert in the 1920s.[52] He introduced the rationale for treating both the evident sites of nodal involvement and adjacent but clinically uninvolved lymph nodes, on the basis that these were likely to contain microscopic disease. Peters[53] took the same approach at the Princess Margaret Hospital in the 1940s, publishing a landmark paper in the *American Journal of Roentgenology* in 1950, which described the cure of limited HL by high-dose, fractionated radiation. She reported 5- and 10-year survival rates of 88% and 79%, respectively, for patients with stage I disease, which transformed the outlook for an illness previously thought to have no long-term survivors.

In the early days, radiation therapy utilized fields that included the entire lymphatic system, total lymphoid irradiation (TLI), to

PRACTICE OF ONCOLOGY

TABLE 102.6

Criteria Used to Stratify Early-Stage Hodgkin's Lymphoma

	EORTC	GHSG	NCIC/ECOG	NCCN 2010
Risk factors	a) Large mediastinal mass (>1/3) b) Age ≥50 years c) ESR ≥50 without B symptoms or ≥30 with B symptoms d) ≥4 nodal areas	a) Large mediastinal mass b) Extranodal disease c) ESR ≥50 without B symptoms or ≥30 with B symptoms d) ≥3 nodal areas	a) Histology other than LP/NS b) Age ≥40 years c) ESR ≥50 d) ≥4 nodal areas	a) Large mediastinal mass (>1/3) or >10 cm b) ESR ≥50 or any B symptoms c) ≥3 nodal areas d) >1 extranodal lesion
Favorable	CS I–II (supradiaphragmatic without risk factors	CS I–II without risk factors	CS I–II without risk factors	CS I–II without risk factors
Unfavorable	CS I–II (supradiaphragmatic with ≥1 risk factors	CS I or CS IIA with ≥1 risk factors CS IIB with c) or d) but without a) and b)	CS I–II with ≥1 risk factors	CS I–II with ≥1 risk factors (differentiating between bulky disease and other risk factors for treatment guidelines)

EORTC, European Organisation for Research and Treatment of Cancer; GHSG, German Hodgkin's Lymphoma Study Group; NCIC, National Cancer Institute of Canada; CS, Clinical stage.

relatively higher biologic radiation dosages compared to contemporary treatment. Extended field radiation therapy (EFRT) included all nodal sites using three radiation fields classically known as mantle, para-aortic–spleen, and inverted Y. A variation of EFRT was also used known as subtotal nodal irradiation (STNI).[54] This was effective, and in many cases curative, but was accompanied by important long-term toxicities, especially the induction of second malignancies and accelerated cardiovascular disease.[55–60] It remained the principal approach to treatment of early disease until clinical trials demonstrated that a combination strategy with chemotherapy could produce superior cure rates with much less irradiation, leading to a reduction of the irradiated field size to only the involved field (IF); the latter was based on a series of studies aimed at minimizing the toxicity of radiation therapy treatment. The German Hodgkin's Lymphoma Study Group (GHSG) HD8 showed in a randomized trial that reducing the treatment volume from EFRT to involved field radiation therapy (IFRT), when combined with chemotherapy, is equally effective. The European Organisation for Research and Treatment of Cancer (EORTC) H7 showed a similar outcome comparing IFRT to STNI.[61,62]

The developments in functional imaging, treatment planning, and image-guided radiation therapy have made it possible to better define and further decrease the radiation fields. Thus, IFRT, which is based on anatomic landmarks and encompassing adjacent uninvolved nodal stations, is no longer appropriate. Based on the fact that most recurrences occur in the original nodal sites, involved node irradiation therapy (INRT) was suggested; the field, in this case, is confined to the macroscopically involved nodes on imaging studies at diagnosis. Although this requires a significant margin around the node to allow and ensure adequate coverage, it can still result in significantly lower exposure to adjacent critical structures.[63] No formal comparison has been made to the results with IFRT, but multiple studies have shown no loss of efficacy with INRT (Fig. 102.6).[64,65]

Using INRT requires acquiring images at diagnosis in treatment positions and prior to the start of chemotherapy to minimize anatomic position variations between diagnostic and radiation

treatment planning imaging. Because that is not practical in most cases, new guidelines defining involved site radiation therapy (ISRT) has been introduced by the International Lymphoma Radiation Oncology Group (ILROG). The new standard of care represents a significant reduction in the volume included in the previously used IFRT by using modern imaging and radiation planning techniques to limit the amount of normal tissue being irradiated.

Combined Modality Therapy

The recognition that HL is highly sensitive to cytotoxic chemotherapy led to the testing of systemic treatment in early stage disease. By administering limited doses of chemotherapy, it has been shown possible to reduce both the extent and dose of radiotherapy, while still maintaining high cure rates.[66–68] The success of this approach has depended on the different treatment of favorable and unfavorable disease, with results in favorable groups excellent even after low impact chemotherapy, such as two cycles of doxorubicin, bleomycin, vinblastine, and dacarbazine (ABVD) or the attenuated EBVP regimen. The EORTC H7-F study compared STNI to six cycles of EBVP followed by IFRT (36 to 40 Gy), with better results from the combined modality treatment: 10-year event-free survival was 88% versus 78%, and overall survival was 92% in both arms.[62] The GHSG HD10 study in favorable early disease compared results in a 2 × 2 randomization between two or four cycles of ABVD and 20 or 30 Gy of IFRT. All four groups had very high cure rates, with progression-free survival of 92% and overall survival of 97% at 5 years,[69] suggesting that two cycles of ABVD and 20 Gy of IFRT is sufficient treatment for carefully selected favorable disease.

A slightly different picture has emerged from studies of unfavorable early disease, where many patients present with bulky mediastinal nodes. Here, there is a threshold of treatment intensity below which the results become less favorable, with an apparent interaction between the efficacy of chemotherapy and the dose of irradiation used. Attenuated use of either modality can be compensated by the other, but if both elements are reduced too far, the freedom from treatment failure is lowered as the result of the excess of early recurrences. The EORTC H8-U trial showed the equivalence of either six or four cycles of MOPP-ABV when given before IFRT (36 to 40 Gy), or four cycles of MOPP-ABV before STNI, with 5-year event-free survivals of 84%, 88%, and 87%, respectively, and 10-year overall survival estimates of 88%, 85%, and 84%, respectively, indicating that treatment more intensive than four cycles of MOPP-ABV and IFRT was unnecessary, and that less toxic treatment might be possible.[70] More recently, the GHSG HD11 study has tested a 2 × 2 randomization between four cycles of ABVD and four cycles of the baseline bleomycin, etoposide, doxorubicin, cyclophosphamide, vincristine, procarbazine, and prednisone (BEACOPP) regimen before either 20 Gy or 30 Gy IFRT. The least intensive arm, four cycles of ABVD and 20 Gy, showed inferior 5-year progression-free survival at 82%, compared to 87%, although overall survival was unaffected, at 94.5%.[71] This suggests that for the unfavorable early-stage group, it may hazardous to reduce treatment below a threshold of four cycles of ABVD and 30 Gy IFRT, unless some means can be found to select those patients for whom further deintensification can be attempted, such as the use of functional imaging.

Chemotherapy Alone

Recognition of the long-term toxicity of extended field irradiation has led many investigators to test approaches by which radiotherapy may be omitted altogether from the treatment of early HL.[72,73] Two large randomized trials have been performed, in pediatric and adult patients, respectively, and both demonstrated that the omission of radiotherapy slightly reduced control of the disease,

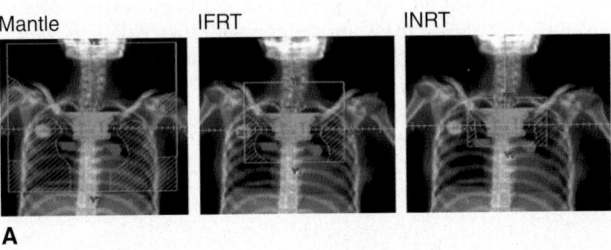

A

Mantle · IFRT · INRT

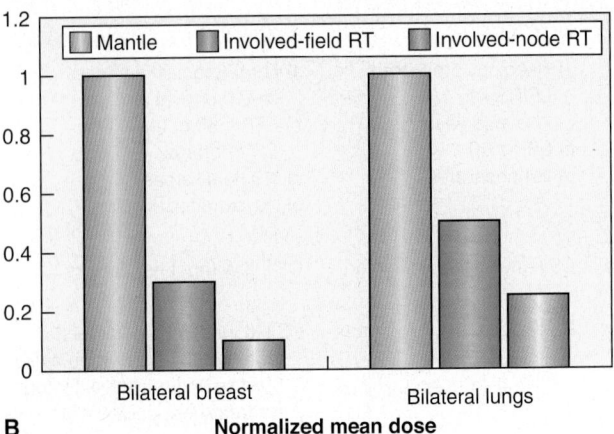

B Normalized mean dose

Mantle · Involved-field RT · Involved-node RT

Bilateral breast · Bilateral lungs

Figure 102.6 Differing radiation volumes in Hodgkin's lymphoma.

reflected in lower progression-free survival, but had no adverse impact on overall survival.

The North American Children's Oncology Group study CCG 5942, tested the omission of low-dose IFRT (21 Gy) for those in complete remission after four cycles of COPP-ABV chemotherapy. The study was closed prematurely when an interim analysis showed a difference in the progression rates in the two arms. With a median 7.7 years follow-up, the event-free survival favored the radiotherapy group (93% versus 83%; $p = 0.004$), with most recurrences in the chemotherapy-alone group seen at the sites of original disease. There was, however, no difference in overall survival, estimated at 97% at 10 years[74].

In adults with early-stage nonbulky disease, the intergroup Eastern Oncology Cooperative Group (ECOG)/National Cancer Institute of Canada (NCIC) study tested treatment with ABVD alone to either 35 Gy STNI in favorable disease, or two cycles of ABVD followed by STNI in unfavorable cases. The first report of this study, with a median follow-up of 4.2 years, showed inferior freedom from progression in the chemotherapy-alone arms (87% versus 93%), with the unfavorable group particularly disadvantaged by the omission of radiotherapy.[75] The initial analysis showed no difference in overall survival, but with longer follow-up, a different picture emerged, with inferior 10-year survival among the patients who had received radiotherapy (87% versus 94%, respectively; $p = 0.04$). The risk of death from lymphoma was not different between the arms, but the risk of death from other causes was more than three-fold higher among those treated with radiotherapy, and much of the excess was due to second cancers.[76] It is important to note, however, that this protocol involved much more extensive irradiation than is currently in use, making extrapolation of the results difficult.

In the absence of direct comparative trials between modern combined modality therapy and chemotherapy alone, a meta-analysis was performed using the intergroup study ABVD-alone group and the comparable patients from the GHSG HD10 and HD 11 studies who received ABVD and IFRT. This showed that the short-term disease control was inferior with ABVD alone, reflected in worse 8-year time to progression (93% versus 87%; hazard ratio [HR], 0.44; 95% confidence interval [CI], 0.24 to 0.78), but that overall survival was not adversely affected in these groups, with 95% alive in the long-term follow-up.[77] The impact of combined modality treatment was particularly apparent among patients who showed less than complete remission after chemotherapy, suggesting that some means of selecting those with chemosensitive disease for deescalation of therapy would be attractive, and might allow radiotherapy to be omitted without a loss of disease control.

Response-Adapted Treatment

Much interest has been generated in the possible use of functional imaging to give an early indication of chemosensitivity in HL. The technique most widely tested is 2-(18F)fluoro-2-deoxy-D-glucose positron emission tomography (FDG-PET), the application of which as an interim readout of efficacy has been enhanced by the development of a highly reproducible five-point scale for reporting the results (Table 102.7).[78] This approach appears to improve the sensitivity for the detection of residual active lymphoma when compared to conventional computed tomography,[79] but the data from prospective randomized studies using it as a guide to therapy are not yet mature enough for firm conclusions, and it is clear that there is a small but definite false-negative rate for FDG-PET, probably of the order of 5% to 10%.

Two studies have reported early results, with broadly similar outcomes (Table 102.8). The United Kingdom National Cancer Research Institute RAPID study randomized patients with nonbulky early-stage disease who had an interim PET score of 1 or 2 after three cycles of ABVD to either 30 Gy IFRT or no further therapy, and found that the 3-year progression-free survival and overall survival

TABLE 102.7

Five-Point Scale for the Interpretation of Interim FDG-PET Scanning

Score	PET/CT Result
1	No uptake above background
2	Uptake ≤ mediastinum
3	Uptake > mediastinum but ≤ liver
4	Uptake moderately increased compared to the liver at any site
5	Uptake markedly increased compared to the liver at any site
X	New areas of uptake unlikely to be related to lymphoma

were not significantly different.[80] There was, however, a trend toward inferior disease control, which became significant when patients who did not receive the radiotherapy as allocated were excluded (97% versus 90.7%; HR, 2.39; $p = 0.003$). Similarly, the EORTC H10 study compared two strategies of therapy: standard treatment with ABVD and IFRT, stratified according to baseline prognostic factors, versus a nonradiotherapy approach, but using further chemotherapy, for those with negative FDG-PET scans after two cycles of ABVD.[81] The results with a short follow-up suggested inferior disease control in the experimental PET-directed arms, although the number of progressions was small and a much longer follow-up will be required to determine whether there is any detrimental effect on survival.

Taken overall, the evidence suggests that for early HL, the use of combined modality treatment produces optimum results in terms of disease control, with a very high expectation of cure from the initial therapy. There is, however, a large proportion of patients (around 90%) who will be curable with chemotherapy alone, and the number needed to treat with radiation in order to achieve 1 extra cured patient is between 15 and 30 according to these trials. Given these figures and the perceived risks of late toxicity from radiotherapy, many patients may prefer the slightly higher risk of recurrent lymphoma to the potential for longer term morbidity. This will, of course, be subject to other variables such as their age, the sites of involvement (and thus the radiotherapy fields), and their baseline risk category. In general, the results of treatment from either approach are very good, and it is reassuring that in almost all the trials carried out, a small reduction in disease control does not have any detrimental effect on overall survival, thanks to the excellent results of second-line therapy, when it is required.

ADVANCED-STAGE HODGKIN'S LYMPHOMA

In patients with advanced-stage HL (stages IIB to IV), the introduction of more effective and less toxic front-line treatment regimens during the last few decades has steadily improved the prognosis. However, complete remissions after initial therapy are not achieved in approximately 20% of patients with stage III to IV disease, eventually leading to disease progression. The current clinical challenge in patients with advanced stage disease is to increase the number of patients with durable remissions and a favorable outcome after initial treatment, while decreasing the incidence of long-term toxicities. The identification of poor prognostic features may allow for a risk-adapted approach to therapy to potentially increase the likelihood of cure and also to minimize side effects.

TABLE 102.8

TABLE 102.8

Response-Adapted Clinical Trials for Early-Stage Hodgkin's Lymphoma

Trial	Eligibility	Treatment Regimens	N	Outcome	Reference
RAPID	Nonbulky Stage I/II Favorable and Unfavorable	ABVD × 3 cycles PET positive: A: ABVD + IFRT 30 Gy	A: 145	A: OS at 3 years = 93.9% PFS at 3 years = 85.9%	80
		PET negative: B: IFRT 30 Gy C: Observation	B: 209 C: 211	B: OS at 3 years = 97% PFS at 3 years = 93.8% C: OS at 3 years = 99.5% PFS at 3 years = 90.7%	
EORTC H10	Favorable Stage I/II	ABVD × 3 + INRT 20 Gy A: PET positive B: PET negative	A: 33 B: 188	A: Data not available B: PFS at 1 year = 100%	81
		ABVD × 2 C: PET positive: Esc BEACOPP × 2 + INRT 30 Gy D: PET negative: ABVD × 2	C: 27 D: 193	C: Data not available D: PFS at 1 year = 94.9%	
EORTC H10	Unfavorable Stage I/II	ABVD × 4 + INRT 30 Gy A: PET positive B: PET negative	A: 88 B: 251	A: Data not available B: PFS at 1 year = 97.3%	81
		ABVD × 2 C: PET positive: Esc BEACOPP × 2, INRT 30 Gy D: PET negative: ABVD × 4	C: 76 D: 268	C: Data not available D: PFS at 1 year = 94.7%	

OS: Overall survival; PFS: Progression free survival.

In general, ABVD chemotherapy remains the most widely used treatment for newly diagnosed patients with advanced-stage HL in the United States. Dose-intense regimens such as escalated BEACOPP are more commonly used in Europe, but are also considered in North America in patients with multiple poor prognostic factors. The future management of advanced-stage HL patients, however, is being shaped by PET-directed approaches and the incorporation of novel agents into these standard combinations.

Prognostic Factors in Advanced Disease

The presence of adverse prognostic factors at diagnosis is one of the methods used to select therapy in HL and the International Prognostic Score (IPS) is an established risk stratification system for advanced disease patients (Table 102.9).[82] This prognostic

TABLE 102.9

International Prognostic Score (IPS)[82]

Adverse Prognostic Factors for Advanced Hodgkin's Lymphoma

≥45 years
Stage IV
Male
WBC ≥ 15,000 cells/μl
Lymphocytes < 600 cells/μl or <8% of WBC count, or both
Albumin < 4.0 g/dL
Hemoglobin < 10.5 g/dL

WBC, white blood cell count.

model was constructed using seven factors associated with a poor outcome (serum albumin less than 4 g per deciliter, hemoglobin less than 10.5 g per deciliter, male sex, age 45 years or older, stage IV disease, leukocytosis of at least 15,000 per cubic millimeter, and lymphocytopenia of less than 600 per cubic millimeter or less than 8% of the white cell count). Although the IPS is highly predictive of freedom from disease progression, it does have limitations. The IPS does not adequately define the truly high-risk patients, because only 7% of the patients in the original study were in the high-risk group and their failure-free survival (FFS) at 5 years was still quite reasonable at 42%.[82] Furthermore, treatment strategies and supportive care have changed since the development of this prognostic model, and although the IPS is still clearly predictive of outcome, its performance may not be as good as originally described.[83–85]

Therefore, efforts have been made to improve the prognostication of the IPS by the incorporation of additional clinical prognostic factors,[86,87] the inclusion of biologic parameters,[88–99] or the addition of an early disease response assessment.[100,101] Biologic factors that have been studied include molecular profiling of the tumor and the RS cells[88,93–95]; the measurement of circulating cytokines or receptors including IL-10, CCL17, or soluble CD30[89–92,98]; and the enumeration of immune cells such as macrophages in the tumor microenvironment.[96,97,99] Although many of the biologic factors have prognostic significance independent of the IPS, they have not been adopted in everyday practice due to issues of reproducibility and a lack of prospective validation. On the other hand, an early response assessment as measured by an interim PET/computed tomography (PET/CT) scan has been shown to be a very powerful prognostic tool that is independent of clinical and biologic prognostic factors, including the IPS.[100–102] Interim PET/CT scanning has been introduced into standard clinical practice and is also being utilized as a method to direct treatment choices.

Choice of Initial Therapy

Combination chemotherapy forms the basis of treatment for patients with advanced-stage HL (Table 102.10). Initially, the MOPP regimen (nitrogen mustard, vincristine, procarbazine, and prednisone) was developed for previously untreated patients with very advanced HL, and a long-term follow-up of patients treated with the MOPP regime has confirmed that this combination can cure advanced HL. MOPP resulted in a freedom from progression rate of 54% and an overall survival of 48 % at 20 and now 40 years.[103] Although the MOPP regimen had a significant impact on the survival of patients who may previously have died of progressive disease, at least one-third of patients relapsed after MOPP chemotherapy and long-term complications were frequently seen in patients who received the combination.

To improve patient outcomes and decrease toxicity, other chemotherapy combinations such as ABVD were developed. An initial randomized trial compared alternating cycles of ABVD and MOPP chemotherapy to a dose and scheduled modified MOPP chemotherapy, and the alternating regimen was found to be superior in respect to the complete remission rate, freedom from progression, and overall survival.[104] Subsequently, a number of randomized trials were performed using ABVD in combination with MOPP chemotherapy or using ABVD alone. MOPP, ABVD, and MOPP alternating with ABVD were compared and the complete response rate and freedom from progression was initially found to be superior in patients receiving ABVD or the alternating program, but subsequent follow-up reports of the study show no difference in disease-free or overall survival when compared to a MOPP program also given at reduced doses.[105] Two further studies compared the MOPP/ABVD hybrid regimen to MOPP alternating with ABVD, and the regimens were found to be equivalent.[106,107] When the MOPP/ABV hybrid regimen was compared to ABVD, ABVD chemotherapy was found to be superior with less toxicity.[83] The results of these trials led to ABVD chemotherapy being regarded as a standard of care for patients with advanced HL based on the clinical efficacy of the combination, the ease of administration, and the acceptable toxicity profile.

As an alternative to ABVD, the Stanford V regimen was developed as a short duration regimen combined with radiation therapy.[108] The initial single institution results with the regimen showed excellent results with a 5-year freedom from progression of 89% and an overall survival of 96%. These promising results were confirmed in a multi-institutional study.[109] The Stanford V regimen has subsequently been compared to ABVD in a number of randomized trials. Initial studies suggested that ABVD might be superior to Stanford V with a 10-year failure-free survival that was superior in ABVD treated patients; however, it has been argued that the differences in outcome may be due to the fact that radiotherapy in the Stanford V arm was administered differently from what was originally described.[110] Two subsequent randomized trials comparing ABVD to Stanford V have found no difference in response rate, failure-free survival, or overall survival between the regimens.[111,112] Overall, ABVD is felt to be superior to Stanford V in patients with advanced disease.

The GHSG also developed new regimens for patients with advanced HL, particularly standard dose and dose-escalated BEACOPP.[113] A randomized trial comparing COPP (cyclophosphamide, vincristine, procarbazine, and prednisone) alternating with ABVD to escalated or standard BEACOPP showed that patients receiving escalated BEACOPP had improved disease control and overall survival.[114] The improvement in outcome for patients treated with escalated BEACOPP was sustained with long-term follow-up.[115] Although these results were encouraging, long-term complications including acute myeloid leukemia

or myelodysplastic syndrome appeared to be more frequent in patients treated with escalated BEACOPP. A similar Italian study compared six cycles of ABVD to four cycles of escalated BEACOPP followed by two cycles of standard BEACOPP and to six cycles of a multidrug intensive regimen. When the results from the ABVD arm were compared the BEACOPP arm, there was an improved progression-free survival with BEACOPP, but the overall survival was not different. Although more toxicity was seen in the BEACOPP-treated patients, poor-risk patients tended to benefit most when treated with BEACOPP.[116]

Since these initial studies, a number of randomized studies have been performed to determine the optimal number of cycles of BEACOPP needed to maintain the clinical benefit but potentially decrease toxicity, and also to define the subgroup of patients most likely to benefit from a more intensive treatment approach. In a study restricted to those younger than 60 years of age, the GHSG found that six cycles of escalated BEACOPP followed by radiotherapy to PET-positive masses was more effective in terms of freedom from treatment failure and less toxic than eight cycles of the same regimen.[117] This led the GHSG to conclude that six cycles of escalated BEACOPP is their standard for advanced HL. To determine whether the high-risk group of patients are those who benefit most from escalated BEACOPP, the EORTC 20012 trial randomized advanced-stage Hodgkin patients with an IPS ≥3 to either eight cycles of ABVD or four cycles of escalated BEACOPP followed by four cycles of standard or baseline BEACOPP.[118] At a median follow-up of 3.9 years, event-free survival, which was the primary endpoint, was similar between treatment arms. Although more relapses were observed with ABVD treatment, early discontinuations were more common in BEACOPP-treated patients. In this high-risk group of patients, however, overall survival was not significantly improved with the use of BEACOPP.

Treating physicians who favor using escalated BEACOPP as initial therapy for advanced-stage HL have pointed to the high response rate and improved event-free survival as the reason to use this combination. In contrast, those who favor using ABVD as initial therapy have cited the complication rate with escalated BEACOPP, as well as the ability to salvage relapsing patients with stem cell transplantation, as reasons to use a less intensive treatment first. To compare these approaches, a randomized comparison of ABVD and escalated BEACOPP was reported, but the analysis included second-line therapy if administered.[119] Patients with residual or progressive disease after initial ABVD or escalated BEACOPP were treated with salvage therapy, including stem cell transplantation. The authors analyzed the outcome after initial therapy, but also analyzed the outcome after salvage therapy. The freedom from first progression significantly favored patients receiving escalated BEACOPP when compared to patients treated with ABVD (85% compared to 73%; $p = 0.004$). However, after completion of all planned therapy including salvage therapy for those with residual or progressive disease, the 7-year rate of freedom from second progression was not significantly different (88% in the escalated BEACOPP group and 82% in the ABVD group; $p = 0.12$) and the 7-year overall survival rate was 89% and 84%, respectively ($p = 0.39$). Severe adverse events were more commonly seen in patients receiving escalated BEACOPP. These results have led some to suggest that initial therapy may not need to be highly aggressive in all patients due to the fact that relapsing patients may be salvaged with subsequent intensive therapy.[120] Others have pointed out that overall survival was a secondary endpoint in this study and that the study was small compared to other similar trials.[121] In an attempt to clarify whether a survival difference exists, a meta-analysis was performed that suggested that six cycles of escalated BEACOPP may well improve overall survival when compared to ABVD.[122]

Overall, it is clear that escalated BEACOPP has greater efficacy than ABVD in patients up to 60 years of age, although escalated BEACOPP-treated patients experience more toxicity, particularly if they are in the upper segment of this age range. Acute and long-term toxicity may, however, be improved by the use of six

TABLE 102.10

Frontline Regimens Commonly Used for Newly Diagnosed Patients with Hodgkin's Lymphoma

Regimen/Drug	Dose	Route	Schedule (Day)	Cycle Length (Days)	Reference
ABVD				28	105
Doxorubicin (adriamycin)	25 mg/m^2	IV	1, 15		
Bleomycin	10 units/m^2	IV	1, 15		
Vinblastine	6 mg/m^2	IV	1, 15		
Dacarbazine	375 mg/m^2	IV	1, 15		
BEACOPP (baseline)				21	113
Etoposide	100 mg/m^2, 200 mg/m^2 if PO	IV	1–3, or PO days 2–3		
Doxorubicin	25 mg/m^2	IV	1		
Cyclophosphamide	650 mg/m^2	IV	1		
Vincristine	1.4 mg/m^2 (cap at 2 mg/m^2)	IV	8		
Bleomycin	10 units/m^2	IV	8		
Procarbazine	100 mg/m^2	PO	1–7		
Prednisone	40 mg/m^2	PO	1–14		
Escalated BEACOPP				21	243
Etoposide	200 mg/m^2	IV	1–3		
Doxorubicin	35 mg/m^2	IV	1		
Cyclophosphamide	1250 mg/m^2	IV	1		
Vincristine	1.4 mg/m^2 (cap at 2 mg/m^2)	IV	8		
Bleomycin	10 units/m^2	IV	8		
Procarbazine	100 mg/m^2	PO	1–7		
Prednisone	40 mg/m^2	PO	1–14		
COPP				28	114
Cyclophosphamide	650 mg/m^2	IV	1, 8		
Vincristine	1.4 mg/m^2 (cap at 2 mg/m^2)	IV	1, 8		
Procarbazine	100 mg/m^2	PO	1–14		
Prednisone	40 mg/m^2	PO	1–14		
MOPP				28	105
Mechlorethamine	6 mg/m^2	IV	1, 8		
Vincristine	1.4 mg/m^2 (cap at 2 mg/m^2)	IV	1, 8		
Procarbazine	100 mg/m^2	PO	1–14		
Prednisone	40 mg/m^2	PO	1–14		
Stanford V				28	108
Mechlorethamine	6 mg/m^2	IV	1		
Doxorubicin	25 mg/m^2	IV	1, 15		
Vinblastine	6 mg/m^2	IV	1, 15		
Vincristine	1.4 mg/m^2 (cap at 2 mg/m^2)	IV	8, 22		
Bleomycin	5 units/m^2	IV	8, 22		
Etoposide	60 mg/m^2	IV	15		
Etoposide	120 mg/m^2 or 60 mg/m^2 IV	PO	16		
Prednisone	40 mg/m^2	PO	Every other day Start taper day 10		
VEPEMB				28	244
Vinblastine	6 mg/m^2	IV	1		
Cyclophosphamide	500 mg/m^2	IV	1		
Procarbazine	100 mg/m^2	PO	1–5		
Prednisone	30 mg/m^2	PO	1–5		
Etoposide	60 mg/m^2	PO	15–19		
Mitoxantrone	6 mg/m^2	IV	15		
Bleomycin	10 mg/m^2	IV	15		
VBM				21–28	245
Vinblastine	6 mg/m^2	IV	1, 8		
Bleomycin	10 mg/m^2	IV	1, 8		
Methotrexate	30 mg/m^2	IV	1, 8		

IV, intravenous; PO, by mouth.

rather than eight cycles of escalated BEACOPP. It is also clear that approximately two-thirds of patients with advanced HL may not need intensive therapy such as escalated BEACOPP, because they will be cured with ABVD. Clinical risk factors, treatment burden and cost, fertility issues, the risk of long-term relapses, as well as potential short- and long-term complications should be considered as physicians and patients decide which regimen to use as initial treatment for advanced-stage HL.

Positron-Emission Tomography–Directed Approaches

A strategy to potentially optimize therapy for HL, by possibly increasing efficacy and decreasing toxicity, is to utilize PET scans during treatment. Because changes in glucose metabolism precede changes in tumor size, responses can be assessed earlier during treatment with PET scans than with CT. Early interim PET scan imaging after chemotherapy for HL has been shown to be a sensitive prognostic indicator of outcome in patients with advanced disease.[123] In prospective studies, interim PET scans after two cycles of ABVD chemotherapy was a significant predictor of progression-free or event-free survival in patients with advanced-stage disease.[101,102] Similar findings were reported for patients treated with Stanford V or escalated BEACOPP.[124,125] Current clinical trials are now testing whether patient outcomes can be improved by modifying treatment based on the interim PET scan results. In patients who have an inadequate response based on the interim PET scan, treatment is either intensified or salvage therapy is contemplated.

Initial studies testing whether deescalation to less intense or abbreviated therapy maintains efficacy in patients who have a complete response by the interim PET scan suggest that this approach is feasible. Avigdor et al.[126] treated advanced-stage HL patients with two cycles of escalated BEACOPP and deescalated to ABVD chemotherapy for four cycles if the PET scan after the initial two cycles was negative. Patients who did not achieve a negative scan were removed from the study and considered for salvage therapy followed by high-dose chemotherapy and autologous stem-cell transplantation. Seventy-two percent of patients had a negative scan, and deescalation to ABVD resulted in a 4-year progression-free survival of 87%.[126] In a similar fashion, the GHSG HD18 trial is testing whether the number of cycles of escalated BEACOPP can be reduced from six to four in patients with a negative interim PET scan.

An alternative approach is to intensify therapy in patients who do not have a negative interim PET scan. Initial studies have explored whether patients can start treatment with two cycles of ABVD and escalate to BEACOPP if the interim scan is positive.[127,128] Initial reports suggest that this strategy, with BEACOPP intensification only in interim PET-positive patients, showed better results than ABVD-treated historic controls, and spared BEACOPP toxicity in the majority of patients.[127] A similar strategy is being prospectively explored in the UK National Cancer Research Institute Response Adapted Therapy using FDG-PET imaging in the advanced HL (RATHL) trial. In this study, all patients receive two courses of ABVD chemotherapy, and PET-negative patients are randomized between ABVD and AVD, to test whether the omission of bleomycin reduces lung toxicity while achieving an equivalent outcome. Patients who remain PET positive undergo treatment escalation with BEACOPP, thereby attempting to improve remission rates. These studies are still in progress.

Consolidation Radiotherapy

An alternative strategy to modifying the initial treatment for advanced-stage HL is to attempt to consolidate the response following initial chemotherapy. Radiotherapy is commonly used as consolidation following primary chemotherapy, with the goal of improving responses or preventing progression in patients with residual masses.

The precise subgroup of patients with advanced-stage HL who benefit from consolidative radiotherapy has changed over time with the use of different chemotherapy regimens and the routine use of PET scans in clinical practice. For patients treated with standard anthracycline-based chemotherapy, those with only a partial response to treatment as determined by conventional restaging may convert to complete remissions after consolidation radiotherapy. Patients with a complete response to initial treatment, however, do not appear to benefit from consolidation radiotherapy.[129]

As more intensive regimens have been used, resulting in more complete responses, the need for consolidation radiotherapy has decreased. This may be particularly true when intensive approaches are coupled with a PET-based evaluation of residual masses to confirm a complete response. In three successive GHSG trials for advanced HL, the use of radiotherapy was reduced in each study as treatment was intensified and a PET scan analysis was included. In the HD9 trial, two-thirds of patients treated with COPP/ABVD or BEACOPP received radiotherapy. In contrast, in the HD15 trial where PET scans guided the decision, only 11% of patients were treated with radiotherapy after escalated BEACOPP without compromising patient outcome.[117] These studies suggest that the use of radiotherapy can possibly be restricted to patients with PET-positive residual masses after escalated BEACOPP treatment; however, the exact role of radiotherapy in ABVD-treated patients in the era of PET scans is not well defined.

Incorporating Novel Agents into Frontline Therapy

Previous strategies to improve the outcome of patients with advanced-stage HL have largely focused on the intensification of therapy. This has resulted in trials becoming focused on younger patients who are in good health and has also resulted in increased toxicity of therapy. However, not all newly diagnosed patients with HL are young with a good performance score. Also, patients and physicians are concerned about toxicity associated with treatment and want to minimize complications. New treatment approaches that benefit a greater proportion of patients and that are associated with less toxicity are, therefore, needed. The most promising strategy to achieve this may be to add novel agents to less intense chemotherapy regimens. Novel agents currently being used in combination with chemotherapy in the frontline setting include brentuximab vedotin, rituximab, and lenalidomide.

The use of brentuximab vedotin is currently attracting substantial interest, and this agent is being combined with modified forms of the ABVD and BEACOPP combinations. Brentuximab vedotin was initially combined with ABVD, and then substituted for bleomycin in a phase 1 study.[130] In this study, complete responses after the conclusion of front-line therapy were achieved in 95% of the 22 patients receiving ABVD plus brentuximab and in 96% of the 25 receiving AVD plus brentuximab. Significant pulmonary toxicity, however, was seen when brentuximab vedotin was given with the bleomycin-containing regimen, resulting in the concurrent use of bleomycin and brentuximab vedotin being contraindicated. Based on the very high response rate, and the fact that brentuximab vedotin when given with AVD was well tolerated, a randomized phase 3 trial comparing ABVD and AVD plus brentuximab vedotin (ECHELON-1 trial) has been initiated.

The GHSG is also exploring the use of brentuximab in combination with BEACOPP variants, namely a more conservative variant BrECAPP (brentuximab vedotin, etoposide, cyclophosphamide, doxorubicin, procarbazine, and prednisone) and a more aggressive variant BrECADD (brentuximab vedotin, etoposide, cyclophosphamide, doxorubicin, dacarbazine, and dexamethasone). The interim results of a randomized phase 2 trial suggest that use of these anti-CD30 targeted BEACOPP variants is feasible without compromising the efficacy associated with escalated BEACOPP.[131]

Two clinical trials have added rituximab to ABVD chemotherapy to deplete intratumoral B cells and that express CD20 and which may support the growth and survival of the malignant cells. Both studies demonstrated high complete response rates, and the event-free survival in both studies suggested promising activity of the combination. Furthermore, the combination was also effective in patients with high IPS scores. However, the efficacy of this combination will need to be confirmed in a randomized trial.[132,133]

A further strategy being evaluated by the GHSG is the addition of lenalidomide to moderate-dose chemotherapy for newly diagnosed advanced-stage patients. In a recent phase 1/2 study, the efficacy and safety of four to eight cycles of AVD chemotherapy plus lenalidomide at doses of 5 to 35 mg per day, followed by radiotherapy, was tested in elderly patients.[134] The regimen was well tolerated and the preliminary response results were encouraging, suggesting that adding new drugs to modified chemotherapy regimens holds significant promise for the future.

Complications of Treatment

The initial treatment of patients with HL with chemotherapy, often in combination with radiotherapy, results in a significant proportion of patients who are cured of their disease. The toxicity of treatment, however, is a significant limitation to its use. Although early toxicities of therapy are commonly manageable and of short duration, late toxicities are often irreversible and may result in life-threatening complications. The late effects of treatment determine the long-term morbidity, mortality, and quality of life of patients with HL. In the first 10 years after treatment, most deaths are due to disease progression or relapse, but beyond this time point, deaths due to late effects predominate.[135]

Acute hematologic toxicity, with possible infectious complications and treatment-related mortality, is associated with the intensity of the treatment combination, the age of the patient, and their comorbid conditions.[136,137] These toxicities are commonly managed by dose modifications and growth factor support. For patients receiving bleomycin, pulmonary toxicity is a concern. Bleomycin lung toxicity is a potentially life-threatening complication and may be more prevalent in patients receiving ABVD chemotherapy.[138]

A significant complication after treatment is the development of second malignancies. These can involve solid organs (most commonly lung, skin, breast, or gastrointestinal) or be hematologic (leukemia, myelodysplasia, or secondary lymphomas).[139] The risk of second malignancies is highest after treatment for childhood HL.[140,141] In those patients treated for HL before adulthood, the risk of developing a second malignant disease has been estimated to be almost 20 times greater than the general population, with a 30-year cumulative risk of 18% for male patients and 26% for female patients.[141] The most common second malignancy in female patients is breast cancer. Important risk factors for therapy-associated breast cancer are age of younger than 20 years at the time of treatment and treatment with extended field radiotherapy that includes the mediastinum.[142,143] The risk of breast cancer is estimated to be approximately 30% in patients who received 40 Gy to the mediastinum before 25 years of age.[144]

Chemotherapy drugs, especially alkylating agents, contribute to the risk of hematologic malignancies, particularly acute myeloid leukemia (AML) and myelodysplasia. The cumulative risk of developing AML is approximately 1.5% for patients treated for advanced stage Hodgkin lymphoma with chemotherapy regimens such as ABVD.[145] There may be an increase in the incidence of myelodysplasia and AML when more intensive regimens such as escalated BEACOPP are used. The overall rate of other second malignancies, however, appears similar when more intensive and less intensive chemotherapy regimens are compared.[115]

Other late effects include infertility, cardiac effects, endocrine dysfunction, peripheral neuropathy, and local effects from radiotherapy. Alkylating agents may induce male and female sterility, but

this is far less frequent in patients treated with ABVD-like regimens than alkylating-containing regimens such as BEACOPP.[146–149] An increase in myocardial infarction, congestive cardiac failure, asymptomatic coronary disease, valvular dysfunction, and stroke have been recorded after treatment for HL, and the risk of cardiac mortality may persist for many years after completing therapy.[150]

SPECIAL CIRCUMSTANCES

Elderly Patients

Elderly patients with HL are a heterogeneous population, particularly when life expectancy, comorbidities, and functional status are considered. Patients older than 65 years constitute approximately 20% of the HL population, but less than 10% of patients included in clinical trials are >60 years. The results of clinical trials are, therefore, not broadly applicable to the elderly who often have difficultly tolerating aggressive treatment approaches. Elderly patients may even have difficulty tolerating ABVD chemotherapy, and response rates to ABVD in elderly patients are typically lower than those seen in younger patients. Older patients often have a poorer event-free survival after ABVD treatment when compared to younger patients.[151]

One reason for the relatively poor outcome in elderly patients is their susceptibility to the toxic effects of intensive therapy, and many have coexisting conditions that affect their ability to tolerate standard treatments. Although fit elderly patients can be treated with curative intent using the same therapeutic regimens as used in younger patients, toxicities and complications are more frequent.[151,152] For more frail elderly patients or those with significant comorbidities, alternative regimens such as VEPEMB (vinblastine, cyclophosphamide, procarbazine, prednisolone, etoposide, mitoxantrone, and bleomycin) or VBM (vinblastine, bleomycin, and methotrexate) could be considered.[153–155] New targeted agents such as brentuximab vedotin, alone or in combination with less toxic agents, are being studied in the treatment of elderly patients with HL.

Pregnancy

HL is one of the most common cancers in pregnant patients, with concurrent pregnancy reported in approximately 3% of all patients.[156,157] Overall, the prognosis and clinical course of HL diagnosed in pregnant women are similar to other patients.[158]

If possible, treatment of asymptomatic, early-stage, pregnant patients should be delayed until after the second trimester or until they complete their pregnancy. If treatment is required, it may be possible to control the disease with single-agent vinblastine to allow the pregnancy to go to term.[156,158,159] Patients who progress while receiving vinblastine can be treated with ABVD chemotherapy during the second or third trimester. Although radiotherapy should be generally avoided during pregnancy, advances in radiotherapy techniques have significantly reduced the risk of fetal complications and radiotherapy could be used if needed.[160] Treatment should not be delayed if the patient has symptomatic, advanced-stage, or progressive HL. If treatment is required and the patient does not want a therapeutic abortion, the successful completion of pregnancy without fetal malformation is possible with the use of ABVD or similar regimens.[161]

Salvage Chemotherapy and Stem Cell Transplantation

Salvage chemotherapy followed by autologous stem cell transplantation (ASCT) has become the treatment of choice in patients with relapsed HL or if the disease is refractory to initial chemotherapy.[162,165] Two randomized phase 3 clinical trials showed improved progression-free survival in patients receiving high-dose chemotherapy (HDCT), compared to those treated with standard-dose salvage chemotherapy, although there was no statistically significant difference in overall survival.[164,165]

Although these randomized controlled trials form the basis for the management of patients with relapsed or refractory HL (RR-HL), the challenge to clinicians remains how best to apply these data to patients as primary treatment strategies evolve. Improvements in the management of patients undergoing ASCT (the use of peripheral blood stem cells [PBSC] and modern supportive care) and allogeneic stem cell transplantation (alloSCT; the use of nonmyeloablative or reduced-intensity conditioning techniques and increased experience with matched unrelated and alternative donor stem cell sources) have led to improved safety, increasing age, and comorbidity cutoffs for transplant patients. These technical advances have granted further accessibility to stem cell transplant therapies. With the advent of active novel agents, the role of stem cell transplantation in the management of HL may need to be addressed again in randomized controlled trials.

Prognostic Factors in Relapsed/Refractory Hodgkin's Lymphoma

Multiple studies have identified prognostic factors in RR-HL who undergo salvage chemotherapy and ASCT. The largest studies of prognostic factors in patients not specifically selected for ASCT have been performed by the GHSG. Separate studies have examined prognostic factors in primary refractory HL (defined as progressing while on primary treatment or within 3 months of completion) and the second paper examined patients who relapsed beyond 3 months after completion of primary therapy. In the primary treatment setting, 206 patients were identified with the significant adverse prognostic factors identified from multivariate analysis being poor performance status (ECOG >0), age >50 years, and failure to obtain a temporary remission to initial therapy.[166] In the relapse setting, 422 patients were studied and the significant adverse prognostic factors for overall survival identified in multivariate analysis were anemia (hemoglobin <120 in males, <105 in females), advanced clinical stage (III or IV), and time to treatment failure of <12 months.[167]

In summary, other series and institutional reviews generally confirm that that time to relapse after initial therapy along with advanced stage and poor performance status at relapse are consistent predictors of poor outcome. Time to relapse is of clinical significance because the GHSG primary refractory series had a 5-year OS of 26% compared to 46% for early relapsers after chemotherapy (3 to 12 months) and 71% for late relapsers (after 12 months) in their series studying relapsers.[16,18] Prospective validation of the predictors of outcome identified by Josting et al.[16,18] have yet to be performed.

TREATMENT

Salvage Chemotherapy Prior to Autologous Stem Cell Transplantation and Peripheral Blood Stem Cell Mobilization

Despite a multitude of published phase 2 studies reporting results of salvage regimens for RR-HL,[168–178] Randomized control trial (RCTs) of second-line regimens have not been performed and, thus, there is no obvious *standard of care* regimen. The published RCTs of ASCT for RR-HL employed mini-BEAM or dexa-BEAM and the control arm of the most recent GHSG trial used dexamethasone, cytarabine, and cisplatin (DHAP), so these regimens can be considered as *standard* regimens in this setting.[164,165,179] Because the goal of salvage chemotherapy is to enable patients to proceed to ASCT, the ideal regimen should have a high response rate with minimal toxicity, and not impair the collection of peripheral blood stem cells for ASCT. Although the RCTs of ASCT support the use

of multidrug regimens including carmustine (BCNU), etoposide, cytarabine, and melphalan (mini-BEAM), these regimens have significant hematologic toxicity, requiring frequent hospitalization for febrile neutropenia, and a high incidence of transfusion support (Table 102.11). Stem cell mobilization appears to be compromised following treatment with mini-BEAM.[180]

Given the multicenter experience with DHAP reported by the GHSG, a platinum-based regimen such as DHAP is a reasonable choice given comparable response rates and less toxicity.[179] When given prior to randomization in the HD-R2 study, DHAP lead to complete response (CR)/complete response unconfirmed (CRu) in 24%, PR in 46%, and SD in 20%. As the trial allowed patients to proceed to randomization as long as they did not have PD, 90% of patients proceeded toward transplant. Several published and widely used salvage chemotherapy regimens are summarized in Figure 102.1. These trials report similar response rates to DHAP, and there is no evidence to demonstrate that one is superior over others. Although the dexa-BEAM regimen had an overall response rate (ORR) of 81% in the GHSG/EBMT phase 3 ASCT trial, treatment related mortality (TRM) from salvage chemotherapy in that study was 5%. Other trials have reported a lower TRM between zero to 2%, a more acceptable level given the typically young age and lack of comorbidity typical of patients in this setting. Although the optimal number of cycles of salvage chemotherapy is unknown, two to three cycles of treatment are usually given by convention with a need to balance optimizing response and the risk of further toxicity.

The available institutional series reporting response rates to salvage chemotherapy often include a mixture of patients with primary refractory and relapsed disease with most series likely unable to demonstrate differences due to a lack of statistical power. Patients with primary refractory HL have an inferior response rate to second-line chemotherapy (51% versus 83%; p <0.0001),[181] which highlights the unique and inferior biology in this group of patients. The proportion of primary refractory patients in reported series along with other imbalances of prognostic factors and typically small sample sizes in these series likely explain any potential variation in reported response rates.[163,166,176,182–184]

Despite aggressive combination chemotherapy, between 10% to 40% of patients do not achieve a response to salvage chemotherapy and there are no RCT data supporting ASCT in nonresponders. Courses of alternative salvage chemotherapy have been given in an attempt to demonstrate chemosensitive disease prior to transplant. Studies have largely assessed responses using CT scan–based criteria. These series have largely reported selected patient populations and are characterized by small numbers, although the goal of achieving a response and proceeding to ASCT occurs in approximately half of the patients.[185–188]

An important issue related to salvage chemotherapy is the potential for second-line therapy to impair the ability to mobilize peripheral blood stem cells to support potentially curative high-dose chemotherapy. The efficacy of salvage chemotherapy for HL must be balanced by toxicity and the impact on subsequent PBSC mobilization. Success rates for PBSC mobilization have not been consistently reported in the RCTs or trials assessing the efficacy of salvage therapy. Some studies report that regimens containing melphalan, such as dexa-BEAM or mini-BEAM, may result in reduced stem cell mobilization.[189–191] Available results for commonly employed regimens demonstrate that at least 80% of patients undergoing PBSC mobilization reach a minimum threshold of 2.0×10^6 CD34 cells per kilogram.[180,192]

The Role of Functional Imaging in Response Assessment Prior to Autologous Stem Cell Transplantation

The use of FDG-PET in response assessment postsalvage chemotherapy and prior to ASCT is increasing despite a lack of large prospective data. Outside of response assessment, FDG-PET

TABLE 102.11

Salvage Regimens Commonly Used for the Treatment of Relapsed and Refractory Hodgkin's Lymphoma

Regimen/Drug	Dose	Route	Schedule (Day)	Cycle Length (Days)	Reference
GVD				21	246
Gemcitabine	1,000 mg/m²	IV	1, 8		
Vinorelbine	20 mg/m²	IV	1, 8		
Liposomal doxorubicin	15 mg/m²	IV	1, 8		
IGEV				21	247
Vinorelbine	20 mg/m²	IV	1		
Gemcitabine	800 mg/m²	IV	1, 4		
Ifosfamide	2,000 mg/m²	IV	1–4		
Prednisone	100 mg	PO	1–4		
MESNA	1,200 mg/m²	IV	1–4, 30 min prior then at 4 and 8 h		
DHAP				14–21	248
Cisplatin	100 mg/m²	IV	1		
Cytarabine	2,000 mg/m²	IV	Day 2, Q12 h × 2 doses		
Prednisone	40 mg	IV	1–4		
ICE				14	249
Ifosfamide	5,000 mg/m²	IV	2		
Carboplatin	AUC5	IV	2		
Etoposide	100 mg/m²	IV	1–3		
MESNA	5,000 mg/m²	IV	2		
Augmented ICE				14	195
Ifosfamide	5,000 mg/m²	IV	1, 2		
Carboplatin	AUC5	IV	3		
Etoposide	200 mg/m²	IV	Day 1, Q12 hours × 3 doses		
MESNA	5,000 mg/m²	IV	1, 2		
Brentuximab vedotin	1.8 mg/kg	IV	1	21	229
Dexa-BEAM				28	168, 250
Dexamethasone	8 mg	PO	Day 1–10, Q8 hour		
Carmustine	60 mg/m²	IV	2		
Etoposide	75–150 mg/m²	IV	4–7		
Cytarabine	100 mg/m²	IV	Day 4–7, Q12 hour × 8 doses		
Melphalan	20 mg/m²	IV	3		
Mini-BEAM				28	164, 169
Carmustine	60 mg/m²	IV	1		
Etoposide	75 mg/m²	IV	2–5		
Cytarabine	100 mg/m²	IV	Day 2–5, Q12 hour × 8 doses		
Melphalan	30 mg/m²	IV	6		
ASHAP				21	171
Doxorubicin	10 mg/m²	IV, continuous infusion	1–4		
Cisplatin	25 mg/m²	IV, continuous infusion	1–4		
Cytarabine	1,500 mg/m²	IV	5		
Methylprednisolone	500 mg	IV	1–5		
VIP				28	172
Etoposide	75 mg/m²	IV	1–5		
Ifosfamide	1,200 mg/m²	IV	1–5		
Cisplatin	20 mg/m²	IV	1–5		
GDP				21	174
Gemcitabine	1,000 mg/m²	IV	1, 8		
Dexamethasone	40 mg	PO	1–4		
Cisplatin	75 mg/m²	IV	1		

(continued)

TABLE 102.11

Salvage Regimens Commonly Used for the Treatment of Relapsed and Refractory Hodgkin's Lymphoma *(continued)*

Regimen/Drug	Dose	Route	Schedule (Day)	Cycle Length (Days)	Reference
GEM-P				28	175
Gemcitabine	1,000 mg/m^2	IV	1, 8		
Methylprednisolone	1,000 mg	PO or IV	1–5		
Cisplatin	75 mg/m^2	IV	15		
MINE				28	176
Mitoguazone	500 mg/m^2	IV	1, 5		
Ifosfamide	1,500 mg/m^2	IV	1–5		
Vinorelbine	15 mg/m^2	IV	1, 5		
Etoposide	150 mg/m^2	IV	1–3		
IVE				21	251
Epirubicin	50 mg/m^2	IV	1		
Etoposide	200 mg/m^2	IV	1–3		
Ifosfamide	3,000 mg/m^2	IV	1–3		
MESNA	3,000 mg/m^2	IV	1–3		

IV, intravenous; PO, by mouth.

scanning can also be viewed as a biomarker with a positive test after salvage therapy, suggesting a higher rate of relapse post-ASCT (whether this is due to tumor-related or other factors in the FDG-PET avid lesion remains to be elucidated). Retrospective institutional series suggest that abnormal functional imaging (FI; either gallium or FDG-PET scan) after salvage therapy and prior to ASCT are predictive of poor outcome (3-year OS of 58% versus 87% if negative FI). In particular, patients who had achieved a PR with CT imaging could be discriminated by FI; in those with negative FI, outcome was similar to patients in CR (3-year OS of 90% in CR, 80% in PR with negative functional imaging) but significantly inferior if positive (65%).[193] A large series studying FI after ifosfamide, carboplatin, etoposide (ICE) chemotherapy reported similar results with a 5-year event-free survival (EFS) of 31% for FI-positive disease compared to 75% if negative.[194]

The group at MSKCC has reported results of a prospective study that tested the strategy of attempting to achieve a negative FDG-PET scan prior to ASCT.[195] In patients that had a positive FDG-PET scan following ICE salvage chemotherapy, a non–cross-resistant chemotherapy regimen to ICE (GVD [gemcitabine, vinorelbine, and liposomal doxorubicin]) was given as a second-line salvage chemotherapy regimen. A positive FDG-PET scan was seen in 38% of cases post-ICE; 26 of 33 patients that received GVD achieved a response (CR, PR, or MR) and went onto transplant. Of these 33 patients, a negative FDG-PET scan was achieved in 52% and their outcome appeared similar to the patients who were FDG-PET negative after ICE. These data demonstrate that the goal of FDG-PET negativity prior to autograft is likely of value and that the use of a non–cross-resistant regimen can be successful in approximately half of patients. Unfortunately, the outcome of FDG-PET–avid patients that were transplanted remains poor with an EFS of 25% at a median follow-up beyond 4 years. Validation of this observation in other series and with other commonly used regimens would help to confirm this treatment approach.

Autologous Stem Cell Transplantation High-Dose Therapy Regimens and Strategies

The role of ASCT in HL has been defined by two published phase 3 RCTs.[164,165] The GHSG/EBMT assigned 161 patients with relapsed HL to receive two cycles of dexa-BEAM chemotherapy, and randomized responding patients to either two additional

cycles of dexa-BEAM or high-dose therapy and ASCT. Freedom from treatment failure at 3 years was significantly improved in the ASCT group (55 versus 34%; p = 0.02), although there was no difference in overall survival.[165] These trials of ASCT did not include chemorefractory patients; only cohort and registry data address the benefit of ASCT in these patients.[162,163,166]

The role of ASCT in lymphoma overtly refractory to chemotherapy has not been well defined in the modern literature. The Seattle group reported the outcome of 64 chemoresistant (defined as less than a partial remission) HL patients who were transplanted on protocols conducted between 1986 and 2005. At a median follow-up of 4.2 years post-ASCT, 5-year PFS and OS were 17% and 31%, respectively, suggesting inferior outcomes when compared to ASCT in chemosensitive patients.

The two randomized trials of ASCT for RR-HL used BCNU, etoposide, Ara-C, melphalan (BEAM) HDCT. Other single institution studies report outcomes with diverse regimens.[50,196–200] The lack of randomized comparisons of HDCT regimens makes it difficult to conclude that there is an optimum regimen in terms of toxicity and efficacy. Late effects including second primary malignancies, cognitive deficits, and chronic fatigue are important considerations, but the impact of HDCT on these outcomes and if they vary between regimens remain unclear.

Further intensification of high-dose regimens has not been a successful strategy in RR-HL,[50] but single-arm studies augmented-dose mobilization regimens,[47] or additional therapy after stem cell collection[52] have been reported to improve outcomes. The Cologne high-dose sequential (HDS) protocol begins with an induction phase of two cycles of DHAP chemotherapy followed by response assessment. Responders proceed to HDS, which consists of 4g/m^2 of cyclophosphamide followed by G-CSF and subsequent PBSC collection, 8 g/m^2 of methotrexate with vincristine 1.4 mg/m^2, etoposide 2 g/m^2 with G-CSF and an optional second PBSC collection, and finally, BEAM HDCT and ASCT. Based on a multicenter phase 2 pilot trial showing HDS to be feasible with acceptable toxicity, the GHSG subsequently led an RCT.[201] The HD-R2 trial, a randomized comparison of HDS therapy followed by ASCT to standard DHAP and ASCT failed to show any benefit for the experimental HDS arm over the standard arm with no significant differences in freedom from treatment failure, progression-free, or overall survival were observed.[202]

An alternative intensification strategy that has been tested is the use of tandem autologous transplants.[203] This approach was prospectively tested in a large GELA cohort study. The multicenter

GELA-led H96 trial tested a risk-adapted approach in which patients were assigned to a single or tandem autograft based on the presence of risk factors at the initiation of savage therapy. Patients with primary refractory disease or at least two poor risk factors (time to relapse <12 months, relapse in a prior radiation field, or stage III/IV disease at the time of relapse) were considered high risk and planned to receive tandem ASCT, whereas patients with standard risk received a single autograft.[204] With an acceptable TRM of 6% and a 5-year OS of 46% in the poor-risk group, this trial demonstrated feasibility, but it does not address the benefit of this strategy in a controlled trial.

Consolidation Strategies: Radiation Postautograft and Maintenance

Many transplant centers use radiation therapy (RT) peri- and post-ASCT in order to maximize treatment because autograft remains the last standard curative treatment option in RR-HL. Unfortunately, the role of radiation around ASCT has not been evaluated in prospective randomized trials. In the GHSG randomized study of ASCT versus dexa-BEAM, 11 of the randomized patients (approximately 10% of the patients on trial) received radiation (6 in the ASCT arm) for what was felt to be residual disease.[165] In the HD-R2 study, consolidative IFRT of 30 Gy was given per protocol in patients who had a >1.5 cm lesion on CT scan at day 100 post-BEAM HDCT and ASCT.[179] In total, 25 of 241 patients randomized (10%) received radiation for residual CT findings.

Outside of the RCT setting, institutional practice incorporating RT varies substantially. The transplant regimens used at MSKCC employ either subtotal or total lymphoid irradiation (STLI or TLI) to 18 Gy, accelerated involved field radiation (IFRT to 18-Gy total given as twice per day fractions for 5 days) or IFT with a total dose of 18 36 Gy in patients who have received prior radiation or had a contraindication to TLI. Thus, effectively all patients receive some radiation as part of their salvage therapy.[195] In contrast, patients at Princess Margaret would receive IFRT if they had a localized recurrence prior to salvage therapy or the presence of a lesion >5 cm if technically feasible. This policy led to the use of posttransplant radiation in 26% of patients.[205]

In contrast, maintenance therapy has been tested in two RCTs, although there are no data currently unavailable. The histone deacetylase inhibitor panobinostat was tested in patients post-ASCT with the trial terminated early and without meaningful numbers to report. The other study tested brentuximab vedotin (an antibody-drug conjugate targeting CD30) against placebo in a large RCT. Results are expected in 2014.

Allogeneic Stem Cell Transplants

AlloSCT continues to be emphasized as a treatment option in advanced HL due to the young age and lack of comorbidity in many patients. Historically, myeloablative alloSCT has been employed in advanced phases of the disease but with poor results because NRM often exceeded 50% and relapses were not uncommon.[206–209] The role of myeloablative alloSCT in HL appeared limited; although dose intensity can be delivered in the context of a myeloablative allograft and donor stem cells are free of tumor cell contamination, the presence of a clinically significant graft-versus-Hodgkin's lymphoma (GVHL) effect has not been clearly demonstrated.

More recently, reports have demonstrated signs of GVHL following donor lymphocyte infusion (DLI).[210–213] In addition to this antitumor effect, the safety of allogeneic transplantation has improved with the use of reduced intensity allogeneic stem cell transplantation (RIC-allo). These approaches have become increasingly popular due to decreased rates of early treatment-related

mortality.[214–217] Despite early favorable outcomes, mature results of RIC-allo available in the literature consistently demonstrate a lack of long-term disease control with progression-free survival estimates of approximately 25% to 30% and overall survival estimates of 35% to 60% at least 2 years post-SCT.[212,214–217]

The Grupo Español de Linfomas/Trasplante Autólogo de Médula Ósea (GEL/TAMO) and EBMT have reported the results of a large prospective study of RIC-allo in RR-HL.[218] Although the trial was incompletely accrued over 7 years, 78 patients ultimately proceeded through a RIC-allo transplant with a preparative regimen consisting of fludarabine 150 mg/m^2, melphalan 140 mg/m^2, and Graft versus host disease (GVHD) prophylaxis of cyclosporine and short-course methotrexate. With a median follow-up of 38 months, 3-year outcomes included a relapse rate of 59%, PFS of 25%, and OS of 43%. Although post-SCT outcomes were similar in matched sibling and unrelated donors, patients with chemorefractory disease had an inferior PFS (25% versus 64% at 1 year). Chronic GVHD was associated with a reduced rate of relapse posttransplant. In patients with relapse after allo-SCT, DLI alone generate an overall response rate of 40%. These results suggest the presence of a GVHL effect in a prospective multicenter trial, but highlight the high relapse rate and not insignificant toxicity even with RIC-allo approaches.

Given the increasing usage of unrelated and alternative donors for allografts, it becomes critical to review disease-specific results in homogeneous patient populations because there are few prospective or multicenter trials. The M.D. Anderson Cancer Center has reported a prospective trial of RIC-allo in both sibling and matched unrelated donor (MUD) using fludarabine-based regimens with the majority accrued onto the fludarabine-melphalan 140 mg/m^2 arm.[219] The 2-year OS and PFS were reported at 64% and 32%, respectively, with no differences in OS, PFS, or relapse between related and MUD transplants. The study is limited by sample size, with 58 patients in total, although the majority (33) received MUD allografts. In a series from the United Kingdom, investigators reported the outcome of RIC-allo in 49 patients (31 related, 18 MUD) who underwent transplants using a regimen consisting of fludarabine-melphalan 140 mg/m^2 and alemtuzumab.[211] Although OS and PFS were not statistically significantly different, nonrelapse mortality was significantly inferior in MUD transplants (34.1% versus 7.2%). Four-year OS and PFS estimates were 55.7% and 39%, respectively.

Retrospective institutional and registry series have also been published. The Center for International Blood and Marrow Transplant Research (CIBMTR) reviewed 143 allografts from matched unrelated donors using reduced intensity or nonmyeloablative regimens reported between 1999 and 2004.[220] The results demonstrate feasibility with a 2-year TRM of 33% and 2-year OS and PFS of 37% and 20%, respectively. Reduced intensity and nonmyeloablative transplants did not differ significantly in outcome. Another large study reported the outcome of 90 nonmyeloablative transplants from related (n = 38), MUD (n = 24), or haploidentical (n = 28) donors at the Baltimore and Seattle programs.[215] A multivariate analysis did not demonstrate any differences in OS between the three donor sources; however, significantly improved PFS (HR, 0.3) was found in haploidentical transplants compared to related or unrelated transplants. Matched related and unrelated donors had similar PFS. NRM was also significantly lower for haploidentical recipients (HR, 0.14) compared to related recipients. An interpretation of this result is difficult given the patient inclusion from two centers and how biases may influence the prognostic factors in patients undergoing allograft from these varied donor sources.

Finally, the outcome of umbilical cord blood transplants (UCBT) has also been reported in RR-HL. The Minnesota group reported their results in lymphoma in which 23 patients received cord blood transplants for HL; the TRM was 13%, the cumulative relapse rate was 43%, PFS was 33%, and the OS at 3 years was 43%.

The age range for the entire lymphoma cohort was 6 to 68 years of age (median of 46 years of age), and 86% of patients received double cord transplants.[221] A slightly larger series of 29 UCBT patients older than 15 years was reported by Eurocord-Netcord with the Lymphoma Working Party of the EBMT. At 1-year posttransplant, PFS was 30%; OS, NRM, and relapse rates were not reported for the HL subgroup.[222]

In summary, the available data regarding allo-SCT in HL only confirms the feasibility of the procedure. In the datasets that present homogeneous patient populations, it appears that there are signs of reasonable efficacy, although the relapse rates remain troubling and few studies are being performed to address this issue. Given advances in the field of alternative donor transplantation, it is reasonable to consider MUD, haploidentical, and UCBT in the management of patients with RR-HL. Unfortunately, prospective trials have done little more than demonstrate a potential role for these procedures in the management of the disease; they have not established the optimal timing of RIC-allo, and these series include a heterogeneous patient population, including patients who have not received an autograft. Given the evidence and lack of toxicity with ASCT, it becomes difficult to justify the toxicity and mortality of an allograft from any donor source prior to an autograft regardless of the perceived risk of the disease without high quality data.

The role of allograft is best established in patients who have failed an autograft. There are many possible options for treatment in this setting, which include conventional cytotoxics, radiation therapy, and investigational agents. In the absence of randomized comparisons with standard therapy, RIC-allo transplant has been compared to retrospective cohorts by two groups.[223,224] Both the UK and Italian reports demonstrated an overall survival advantage favoring allografting. Unfortunately, both studies suffer from the standard issues surrounding retrospective cohort comparisons and relatively small sample sizes. These results can only remain hypothesis generating. Patient selection remains a potential confounding issue in all allo-SCT reports (particularly in retrospective institutional or registry reviews), and the benefit of RIC-allo to patients with RR-HL remains open to debate.

Second Autologous Stem Cell Transplants

A second autograft has been considered an option for patients who relapse after a prior ASCT. In such cases, stem cells must be available from the initial procedure or need to be collected a second time. There are limited institutional and registry data to support such a strategy and such cases are obviously highly selected. The CIBMTR reported a series that included 21 HL patients who underwent a second autograft.[225] With day 100 TRM of 11%, 5-year PFS and OS were 30% for the entire cohort, with no difference in outcome between NHL and HL cases. Outcomes were inferior in patients who were retransplanted within 1 year of the initial autograft (5-year PFS of zero versus 32%; p = 0.001).

The role of a second autograft remains unclear but can be considered in patients with a time to relapse of greater than 1 year after the initial transplant. Integrating the data regarding second autografts, allografts along with the increasing number of targeted therapies, conventional palliative systemic approaches, and radiation becomes more challenging as options continue to increase.

The challenge remains how best to manage patients who progress or relapse after ASCT given the variety of standard treatment options (single and multiagent chemotherapy, radiation therapy), intensive treatment strategies (second autografts, RIC-allo transplants) or drug development trials that are currently available. Because no comparative prospective data are available to inform this decision, clinicians and patients will have to make careful choices.

Management of Patients with Relapsed Hodgkin's Lymphoma After Stem Cell Transplant

Approximately 20% of patients with HL will not be cured with currently available first-line and second-line treatment modalities, and will require additional therapy. Patients with relapsed or refractory HL after receiving ASCT have unmet medical needs, and are considered candidates for drug development. The median survival following relapse from ASCT is estimated to be only 2.4 years, which is even shorter for those whose disease relapsed within 1 year from the transplant.[226] Because of the poor prognosis, several novel agents are being evaluated in this patient population, but brentuximab vedotin remains the only drug approved by the U.S. Food and Drug Administration (FDA) for this indication.

Brentuximab Vedotin

Since its initial identification as a possible Hodgkin's and Reed-Sternberg (HRS)-associated antigen, CD30 became a widely sought after target for novel therapy of patients with HL. In the following 3 decades, the expression and function of CD30 were further clarified by several independent groups. CD30 is a member of the tumor necrosis factor cell receptor superfamily. CD30 is highly expressed in HRS cells, but is also expressed by the malignant cells of anaplastic large cell lymphoma, peripheral T-cell lymphoma, primary mediastinal diffuse large B-cell lymphoma, and other uncommon solid tumors. Several attempts to develop naked anti-CD30 antibody therapy failed to produce meaningful clinical responses. In contrast, major clinical responses were achieved by conjugating the naked anti-CD30 antibody SGN30 to antitubulin monomethyl auristatin E (MMAE), to generate the antibody drug-conjugate (ADC) brentuximab vedotin.

Based on promising preclinical activity, a first-in-man phase 1 study of brentuximab vedotin was initiated to evaluate its safety. The study rapidly enrolled 45 patients with relapsed or refractory CD30-positive HL (93%) and anaplastic large cell lymphoma, of whom 73% received prior ASCT.[227] Escalating doses of brentuximab vedotin (from 0.1 mg per kg to 3.6 mg per kg) were administered intravenously every 3 weeks. Treatment was very well tolerated, but rare dose-limiting toxicities were observed, including grade 4 thrombocytopenia, grade 3 hyperglycemia, and febrile neutropenia. The recommended phase 2 dose was established as 1.8 mg per kg every 3 weeks. Although the study primary objective was to evaluate the safety of brentuximab vedotin, 86% of the patients had tumor reductions, and 17 patients achieved complete or partial remissions. A second phase 1 study investigated the safety and tolerability of brentuximab vedotin administered on a weekly schedule for 3 weeks, followed by 1 week of rest.[228] A total of 37 patients (31 had HL) were enrolled and treated, of whom 62% previously received an ASCT. The dose-limiting toxicities were grade 3 diarrhea and/or vomiting and grade 4 hyperglycemia. Complete and partial clinical remissions were observed in 46% of the patients. Collectively, these two phase 1 studies demonstrated the safety of brentuximab vedotin, and provided valuable information on the potential clinical efficacy in patients with relapsed and refractory HL.

In a follow-up pivotal phase 2 clinical trial, 102 patients with relapsed HL after receiving ASCT were treated with 1.8 mg per kilogram brentuximab vedotin given every 3 weeks.[229] Of 102 patients, 76 (75%) achieved partial or complete remissions (34% CRs). The median duration of response in patients who achieved complete remissions was approximately 2 years. The most common treatment-related side effects were peripheral neuropathy (42%), nausea (35%), and fatigue (34%). Grade 3 or higher neuropathy was seen in 8% of patients and was the most common reason for the discontinuation of brentuximab vedotin. Results of this study lead to the approval of brentuximab vedotin by the FDA in 2011.

Current strategies are aiming at incorporating brentuximab vedotin in front-line and second-line chemotherapy regimens. In the front-line setting, brentuximab vedotin was initially combined with standard ABVD in patients with advanced stage HL. In this phase 1 study, 51 patients with newly diagnosed patients with advanced stage HL were treated with brentuximab vedotin administered every 2 weeks on the same day of each ABVD therapy. The phase 2 recommended dose was established at 1.2 mg per kilogram of brentuximab vedotin given with standard dose and the schedule of ABVD. However, this combination was associated with an unexpected increase in pulmonary toxicity that was similar to bleomycin lung toxicity. Subsequently, an additional cohort of patients was treated without bleomycin (brentuximab vedotin + AVD), which resulted in a similar high response rate, but with no pulmonary toxicity. Of 22 patients, 21 (95%) patients given brentuximab vedotin and ABVD achieved complete remission, as did 24 (96%) of 25 patients given brentuximab vedotin and AVD. Based on these data, an international randomized study comparing standard ABVD with AVD plus brentuximab vedotin was initiated. In the second-line setting, a sequential therapy of brentuximab vedotin followed by ICE chemotherapy is currently being investigated in transplant-eligible patients with relapsed and refractory HL.

Investigational Agents

Histone Deacetylase Inhibitors

Histone deacetylase (HDAC) inhibitors are good candidates for HL therapy due to their unique mechanisms of action. HDAC inhibitors have been shown to have a direct antitumor effect by activating the intrinsic caspase pathway and downregulating antiapoptotic proteins, in addition to an indirect effect by disrupting the favorable microenvironment and activating the immune response.[230] For example, HDAC inhibitors can alter the phenotype and function of T cells in the HL microenvironment by decreasing the expression of the chemotaxis chemokine CCL17 (TARC).[230,231] Furthermore, HDAC inhibitors may restore antitumor immunity by upregulating OX40L.[232]

Several HDAC inhibitors have recently been evaluated for the treatment of relapsed HL with variable results. Vorinostat demonstrated the weakest clinical activity, with only 1 of 25 patients achieving a partial remission.[233] On the other hand, panobinostat and mocetinostat demonstrated higher response rates, but also more toxic effects. Mocetinostat (MGCD0103) is an oral non-hydroxamate HDAC inhibitor that preferentially inhibits HDAC class I and IV.[234,235] In a phase 2 study, 51 patients with relapsed or refractory HL were treated with 110 mg or 85 mg of mocetinostat three times a week.[236] Approximately 60% of patients had a reduction in their tumor measurements, with 24% achieving partial remissions. Toxicities include thrombocytopenia, fatigue, pneumonia, anemia, and pericardial effusion.[236] Panobinostat, a pan HDAC inhibitor, also demonstrated a promising clinical activity in patients with relapsed HL. In a phase 2 study, 129 patients were treated with 40 mg panobinostat and 27% achieved partial or complete remissions.[237]

PI3K/AKT/mTOR Pathway Inhibitors

The PI3K signaling pathway regulates a wide variety of essential cellular functions, including glucose metabolism, cell survival, and proliferation.[238–240] The PI3K signaling pathway is activated in many malignancies, including in Hodgkin's and non-Hodgkin's lymphomas, making it an appealing target for therapeutic intervention. There are four isoforms of PI3K (α, β, γ, and δ) that can be selectively inhibited by a variety of small molecules. Idelalisib (GS-1101 or CAL101) is an oral PI3K-δ–selective small molecule inhibitor that demonstrated promising clinical activity in a variety of B-cell malignancies, but it showed a limited clinical activity in patients with relapsed HL.[241] In a different study, the dual PI3K-δ/γ inhibitor IPI-145 produced a 33% response rate in an ongoing phase 1 clinical trial. Targeting the downstream mammalian target of rapamycin (mTOR) kinase also demonstrated promising clinical activity in patients with relapsed HL. For example, everolimus produced an overall response rate of 42% of patients.[242]

REFERENCES

1. Canellos GP, Rosenberg SA, Friedberg JW, et al. Treatment of Hodgkin lymphoma: a 50-year perspective. *J Clin Oncol* 2014;32:163–168.
2. Siegel R, Naishadham D, Jemal A. Cancer statistics, 2013. *CA Cancer J Clin* 2013;63:11–30.
3. Re D, Thomas RK, Behringer K, et al. From Hodgkin disease to Hodgkin lymphoma: biologic insights and therapeutic potential. *Blood* 2005;105:4553–4560.
4. Jackson H Jr, Parker F Jr. Hodgkin's disease. *N Engl J Med* 1944;230:1–8.
5. Lukes RJ, Butler JJ. The pathology and nomenclature of Hodgkin's disease. *Cancer Res* 1966;26:1063–1083.
6. Kuppers R, Rajewsky K. The origin of Hodgkin and Reed/Sternberg cells in Hodgkin's disease. *Annu Rev Immunol* 1998;16:471–493.
7. Kuppers R. The biology of Hodgkin's lymphoma. *Nat Rev Cancer* 2009;9:15–27.
8. Re D, Kuppers R, Diehl V. Molecular pathogenesis of Hodgkin's lymphoma. *J Clin Oncol* 2005;23:6379–6386.
9. Kuppers R, Rajewsky K, Zhao M, et al. Hodgkin disease: Hodgkin and Reed-Sternberg cells picked from histological sections show clonal immunoglobulin gene rearrangements and appear to be derived from B cells at various stages of development. *Proc Natl Acad Sci U S A* 1994;91:10962–10966.
10. Eberle FC, Mani H, Jaffe ES. Histopathology of Hodgkin's lymphoma. *Cancer J* 2009;15:129–137.
11. Smith LB. Nodular lymphocyte predominant Hodgkin lymphoma: diagnostic pearls and pitfalls. *Arch Pathol Lab Med* 2010;134:1434–1439.
12. Carbone A, Gloghini A. "Intrafollicular neoplasia" of nodular lymphocyte predominant Hodgkin lymphoma: description of a hypothetic early step of the disease. *Hum Pathol* 2012;43:619–628.
13. Falini B, Bigerna B, Pasqualucci L, et al. Distinctive expression pattern of the BCL-6 protein in nodular lymphocyte predominance Hodgkin's disease. *Blood* 1996;87:465–471.
14. Carbone A, Gloghini A, Gattei V, et al. Expression of functional CD40 antigen on Reed-Sternberg cells and Hodgkin's disease cell lines. *Blood* 1995;85:780–789.
15. Mason DY, Banks PM, Chan J, et al. Nodular lymphocyte predominance Hodgkin's disease. A distinct clinicopathological entity. *Am J Surg Pathol* 1994;18:526–530.
16. Brune V, Tiacci E, Pfeil I, et al. Origin and pathogenesis of nodular lymphocyte-predominant Hodgkin lymphoma as revealed by global gene expression analysis. *J Exp Med* 2008;205:2251–2268.
17. Schwering I, Brauninger A, Klein U, et al. Loss of the B-lineage-specific gene expression program in Hodgkin and Reed-Sternberg cells of Hodgkin lymphoma. *Blood* 2003;101:1505–1512.
18. Stein H, Marafioti T, Foss HD, et al. Down-regulation of BOB.1/OBF.1 and Oct2 in classical Hodgkin disease but not in lymphocyte predominant Hodgkin disease correlates with immunoglobulin transcription. *Blood* 2001;97:496–501.
19. Stein H, Bob R. Is Hodgkin lymphoma just another B-cell lymphoma? *Curr Hematol Malig Rep* 2009;4:125–128.
20. Aldinucci D, Rapana B, Olivo K, et al. IRF4 is modulated by CD40L and by apoptotic and anti-proliferative signals in Hodgkin lymphoma. *Br J Haematol* 2010;148:115–118.
21. Zheng B, Fiumara P, Li YV, et al. MEK/ERK pathway is aberrantly active in Hodgkin disease: a signaling pathway shared by CD30, CD40, and RANK that regulates cell proliferation and survival. *Blood* 2003;102:1019–1027.
22. Harris NL, Jaffe ES, Stein H, et al. A revised European-American classification of lymphoid neoplasms: a proposal from the International Lymphoma Study Group. *Blood* 1994;84:1361–1392.
23. Younes A, Carbone A. Clinicopathologic and molecular features of Hodgkin's lymphoma. *Cancer Biol Ther* 2003;2:500–507.

24. Carbone A, Gloghini A, Aldinucci D, et al. Expression pattern of MUM1/IRF4 in the spectrum of pathology of Hodgkin's disease. *Br J Haematol* 2002;117:366–372.

25. Carbone A, Gloghini A, Cabras A, et al. The Germinal centre-derived lymphomas seen through their cellular microenvironment. *Br J Haematol* 2009;145:468–480.

26. Fan Z, Natkunam Y, Bair E, et al. Characterization of variant patterns of nodular lymphocyte predominant hodgkin lymphoma with immunohistologic and clinical correlation. *Am J Surg Pathol* 2003;27:1346–1356.

27. Carbone A, Gloghini A. Nodular lymphocyte predominant Hodgkin lymphoma may show a nodular pattern in which tumour cells do not invade the surrounding spaces. *Br J Haematol* 2013;163:537–538.

28. Carbone A, Spina M, Gloghini A, et al. Nodular lymphocyte predominant Hodgkin lymphoma with non-invasive or early invasive growth pattern suggests an early step of the disease with a highly favorable outcome. *Am J Hematol* 2013;88:161–162.

29. Aldinucci D, Gloghini A, Pinto A, et al. The classical Hodgkin's lymphoma microenvironment and its role in promoting tumour growth and immune escape. *J Pathol* 2010;221:248–263.

30. Poppema S, van den Berg A. Interaction between host T cells and Reed-Sternberg cells in Hodgkin lymphomas. *Semin Cancer Biol* 2000;10:345–350.

31. Carbone A, Gloghini A, Gruss HJ, et al. CD40 ligand is constitutively expressed in a subset of T cell lymphomas and on the microenvironmental reactive T cells of follicular lymphomas and Hodgkin's disease. *Am J Pathol* 1995;147:912–922.

32. Steidl C, Lee T, Shah SP, et al. Tumor-associated macrophages and survival in classic Hodgkin's lymphoma. *N Engl J Med* 2010;362:875–885.

33. Ma Y, Visser L, Roelofsen H, et al. Proteomics analysis of Hodgkin lymphoma: identification of new players involved in the cross-talk between HRS cells and infiltrating lymphocytes. *Blood* 2008;111:2339–2346.

34. Skinnider BF, Mak TW. The role of cytokines in classical Hodgkin lymphoma. *Blood* 2002;99:4283–4297.

35. Carbone A, Gloghini A, Serraino D, et al. HIV-associated Hodgkin lymphoma. *Curr Opin HIV AIDS* 2009;4:3–10.

36. Aldinucci D, Gloghini A, Pinto A, et al. The role of CD40/CD40L and interferon regulatory factor 4 in Hodgkin lymphoma microenvironment. *Leuk Lymphoma* 2012;53:195–201.

37. Meckes DG Jr, Shair KH, Marquitz AR, et al. Human tumor virus utilizes exosomes for intercellular communication. *Proc Natl Acad Sci U S A* 2010;107:20370–20375.

38. Meckes DG Jr, Gunawardena HP, Dekroon RM, et al. Modulation of B-cell exosome proteins by gamma herpesvirus infection. *Proc Natl Acad Sci U S A* 2013;110:E2925–2933.

39. Carbone A, Gloghini A, Aiello A, et al. B-cell lymphomas with features intermediate between distinct pathologic entities. From pathogenesis to pathology. *Hum Pathol* 2010;41:621–631.

40. Rosenwald A, Wright G, Leroy K, et al. Molecular diagnosis of primary mediastinal B cell lymphoma identifies a clinically favorable subgroup of diffuse large B cell lymphoma related to Hodgkin lymphoma. *J Exp Med* 2003;198:851–862.

41. Savage KJ, Monti S, Kutok JL, et al. The molecular signature of mediastinal large B-cell lymphoma differs from that of other diffuse large B-cell lymphomas and shares features with classical Hodgkin lymphoma. *Blood* 2003;102:3871–3879.

42. Gualco G, Natkunam Y, Bacchi CE. The spectrum of B-cell lymphoma, unclassifiable, with features intermediate between diffuse large B-cell lymphoma and classical Hodgkin lymphoma: a description of 10 cases. *Mod Pathol* 2012;25:661–674.

43. Tirelli U, Errante D, Dolcetti R, et al. Hodgkin's disease and human immunodeficiency virus infection: clinicopathologic and virologic features of 114 patients from the Italian Cooperative Group on AIDS and Tumors. *J Clin Oncol* 1995;13:1758–1767.

44. Biggar RJ, Jaffe ES, Goedert JJ, et al. Hodgkin lymphoma and immunodeficiency in persons with HIV/AIDS. *Blood* 2006;108:3786–3791.

45. Gloghini A, Carbone A. Why would the incidence of HIV-associated Hodgkin lymphoma increase in the setting of improved immunity? *Int J Cancer* 2007;120:2753–2754.

46. Deeken JF, Tjen ALA, Rudek MA, et al. The rising challenge of non-AIDS-defining cancers in HIV-infected patients. *Clin Infect Dis* 2012;55:1228–1235.

47. Engels EA. Non-AIDS-defining malignancies in HIV-infected persons: etiologic puzzles, epidemiologic perils, prevention opportunities. *AIDS* 2009;23:875–885.

48. Novak RM, Richardson JT, Buchacz K, et al. Immune reconstitution inflammatory syndrome: incidence and implications for mortality. *AIDS* 2012;26:721–730.

49. Rajasuriar R, Khoury G, Kamarulzaman A, et al. Persistent immune activation in chronic HIV infection: do any interventions work? *AIDS* 2013;27:1199–1208.

50. Kowalkowski MA, Mims MP, Amiran ES, et al. Effect of immune reconstitution on the incidence of HIV-related Hodgkin lymphoma. *PLoS One* 2013;8:e77409.

51. Rosenberg SA, Kaplan HS. Evidence for an orderly progression in the spread of Hodgkin's disease. *Cancer Res* 1966;26:1225–1231.

52. Gilbert R. Radiotherapy in Hodgkin's disease (malignant granulomatosis): anatomic and clinical foundations; governing principles; results. *Am J Roentgenol Radium Ther Nucl Med* 1939;41:198–241.

53. Peters MV. A study of survivals in Hodgkin's disease treated radiologically. *Am J Roentgenol Radium Ther Nucl Med* 1950;63:299–311.

54. Kaplan HS. Clinical evaluation and radiotherapeutic management of Hodgkin's disease and the malignant lymphomas. *N Engl J Med* 1968;278:892–899.

55. Bowers DC, McNeil DE, Liu Y, et al. Stroke as a late treatment effect of Hodgkin's Disease: a report from the Childhood Cancer Survivor Study. *J Clin Oncol* 2005;23:6508–6515.

56. Franklin J, Pluetschow A, Paus M, et al. Second malignancy risk associated with treatment of Hodgkin's lymphoma: meta-analysis of the randomised trials. *Ann Oncol* 2006;17:1749–1760.

57. Hancock SL, Tucker MA, Hoppe RT. Factors affecting late mortality from heart disease after treatment of Hodgkin's disease. *JAMA* 1993;270:1949–1955.

58. Mulrooney DA, Yeazel MW, Kawashima T, et al. Cardiac outcomes in a cohort of adult survivors of childhood and adolescent cancer: retrospective analysis of the Childhood Cancer Survivor Study cohort. *BMJ* 2009;339:b4606.

59. Travis LB, Hill D, Dores GM, et al. Cumulative absolute breast cancer risk for young women treated for Hodgkin lymphoma. *J Natl Cancer Inst* 2005;97:1428–1437.

60. Swerdlow AJ, Cooke R, Bates A, et al. Breast cancer risk after supradiaphragmatic radiotherapy for Hodgkin's lymphoma in England and Wales: a National Cohort Study. *J Clin Oncol* 2012;30:2745–2752.

61. Engert A, Schiller P, Josting A, et al. Involved-field radiotherapy is equally effective and less toxic compared with extended-field radiotherapy after four cycles of chemotherapy in patients with early-stage unfavorable Hodgkin's lymphoma: results of the HD8 trial of the German Hodgkin's Lymphoma Study Group. *J Clin Oncol* 2003;21:3601–3608.

62. Noordijk EM, Carde P, Dupouy N, et al. Combined-modality therapy for clinical stage I or II Hodgkin's lymphoma: long-term results of the European Organisation for Research and Treatment of Cancer H7 randomized controlled trials. *J Clin Oncol* 2006;24:3128–3135.

63. Girinsky T, Specht L, Ghalibafian M, et al. The conundrum of Hodgkin lymphoma nodes: to be or not to be included in the involved node radiation fields. The EORTC-GELA lymphoma group guidelines. *Radiother Oncol* 2008;88:202–210.

64. Campbell BA, Voss N, Pickles T, et al. Involved-nodal radiation therapy as a component of combination therapy for limited-stage Hodgkin's lymphoma: a question of field size. *J Clin Oncol* 2008;26:5170–5174.

65. Paumier A, Ghalibafian M, Beaudre A, et al. Involved-node radiotherapy and modern radiation treatment techniques in patients with Hodgkin lymphoma. *Int J Radiat Oncol Biol Phys* 2011;80:199–205.

66. Bonadonna G, Bonfante V, Viviani S, et al. ABVD plus subtotal nodal versus involved-field radiotherapy in early-stage Hodgkin's disease: long-term results. *J Clin Oncol* 2004;22:2835–2841.

67. Hoskin PJ, Smith P, Maughan TS. Long-term results of a randomised trial of involved field radiotherapy vs extended field radiotherapy in stage I and II Hodgkin lymphoma. *Clin Oncol* 2005;17:47–53.

68. Sasse S, Klimm B, Gorgen H, et al. Comparing long-term toxicity and efficacy of combined modality treatment including extended- or involved-field radiotherapy in early-stage Hodgkin's lymphoma. *Ann Oncol* 2012;23:2953–2959.

69. Engert A, Plutschow A, Eich HT, et al. Reduced treatment intensity in patients with early-stage Hodgkin's lymphoma. *N Engl J Med* 2010;363:640–652.

70. Fermé C, Eghbali H, Meerwaldt JH, et al. Chemotherapy plus involved-field radiation in early-stage Hodgkin's disease. *N Engl J Med*. 2007;357(19):1916-1927.

71. Eich HT, Diehl V, Görgen H, et al. Intensified chemotherapy and dose-reduced involved-field radiotherapy in patients with early unfavorable Hodgkin's lymphoma: final analysis of the German Hodgkin Study Group HD11 trial. *J Clin Oncol* 2010;28:4199–4206.

72. Canellos GP, Abramson JS, Fisher DC, et al. Treatment of favorable, limited-stage Hodgkin's lymphoma with chemotherapy without consolidation by radiation therapy. *J Clin Oncol* 2010;28:1611–1615.

73. Straus DJ, Portlock CS, Qin J, et al. Results of a prospective randomized clinical trial of doxorubicin, bleomycin, vinblastine, and dacarbazine (ABVD) followed by radiation therapy (RT) versus ABVD alone for stages I, II, and IIIA nonbulky Hodgkin disease. *Blood* 2004;104:3483–3489.

74. Wolden SL, Chen L, Kelly KM, et al. Long-term results of CCG 5942: a randomized comparison of chemotherapy with and without radiotherapy for children with Hodgkin's lymphoma—a report from the Children's Oncology Group. *J Clin Oncol* 2012;30:3174–3180.

75. Meyer RM, Gospodarowicz MK, Connors JM, et al. Randomized comparison of ABVD chemotherapy with a strategy that includes radiation therapy in patients with limited-stage Hodgkin's lymphoma: National Cancer Institute of Canada Clinical Trials Group and the Eastern Cooperative Oncology Group. *J Clin Oncol* 2005;23:4634–4642.

76. Meyer RM, Gospodarowicz MK, Connors JM, et al. ABVD alone versus radiation-based therapy in limited-stage Hodgkin's lymphoma. *N Engl J Med* 2012;366:399–408.

77. Hay AE, Klimm B, Chen BE, et al. An individual patient-data comparison of combined modality therapy and ABVD alone for patients with limited-stage Hodgkin lymphoma. *Ann Oncol* 2013;24:3065–3069.

PRACTICE OF ONCOLOGY

78. Barrington SF, Qian W, Somer EJ, et al. Concordance between four European centres of PET reporting criteria designed for use in multicentre trials in Hodgkin lymphoma. *Eur J Nucl Med Mol Imaging* 2010;37:1824–1833.

79. Hutchings M, Loft A, Hansen M, et al. FDG-PET after two cycles of chemotherapy predicts treatment failure and progression-free survival in Hodgkin lymphoma. *Blood* 2006;107:52–59.

80. Radford J, Barrington S, Counsell N, et al. Involved field radiotherapy versus no further treatment in patients with clinical stages IA and IIA Hodgkin lymphoma and a 'negative' PET scan after 3 cycles ABVD. Results of the UK NCRI RAPID Trial. *ASH Annual Meeting Abstracts* 2012; 120:a547.

81. Andre M, Reman O, Federico M, et al. Interim analysis of the randomized EORTC/LYSA/FIL intergroup H10 trial on early PET-scan driven treatment adaptation in stage I/II Hodgkin lymphoma. *ASH Annual Meeting Abstracts* 2012;120:a549.

82. Hasenclever D, Diehl V. A prognostic score for advanced Hodgkin's disease. International Prognostic Factors Project on Advanced Hodgkin's Disease. *N Engl J Med* 1998;339:1506–1514.

83. Duggan DB, Petroni GR, Johnson JL, et al. Randomized comparison of ABVD and MOPP/ABV hybrid for the treatment of advanced Hodgkin's disease: report of an intergroup trial. *J Clin Oncol* 2003;21:607–614.

84. Guisado-Vasco P, Arranz-Saez R, Canales M, et al. Stage IV and age over 45 years are the only prognostic factors of the International Prognostic Score for the outcome of advanced Hodgkin lymphoma in the Spanish Hodgkin Lymphoma Study Group series. *Leuk Lymphoma* 2012;53:812–819.

85. Moccia AA, Donaldson J, Chhanabhai M, et al. International Prognostic Score in advanced-stage Hodgkin's lymphoma: altered utility in the modern era. *J Clin Oncol* 2012;30:3383–3388.

86. Gobbi PG, Ghirardelli ML, Solcia M, et al. Image-aided estimate of tumor burden in Hodgkin's disease: evidence of its primary prognostic importance. *J Clin Oncol* 2001;19:1388–1394.

87. Vassilakopoulos TP, Angelopoulou MK, Siakantaris MP, et al. Prognostic factors in advanced stage Hodgkin's lymphoma: the significance of the number of involved anatomic sites. *Eur J Haematol* 2001;67:279–288.

88. Scott DW, Chan FC, Hong F, et al. Gene expression-based model using formalin-fixed paraffin-embedded biopsies predicts overall survival in advanced-stage classical Hodgkin lymphoma. *J Clin Oncol* 2013;31:692–700.

89. Sarris AH, Kliche KO, Pethambaram P, et al. Interleukin-10 levels are often elevated in serum of adults with Hodgkin's disease and are associated with inferior failure-free survival. *Ann Oncol* 1999;10:433–440.

90. Vassilakopoulos TP, Nadali G, Angelopoulou MK, et al. Serum interleukin-10 levels are an independent prognostic factor for patients with Hodgkin's lymphoma. *Haematologica* 2001;86:274–281.

91. Visco C, Nadali G, Vassilakopoulos TP, et al. Very high levels of soluble CD30 recognize the patients with classical Hodgkin's lymphoma retaining a very poor prognosis. *Eur J Haematol* 2006;77:387–394.

92. Casasnovas RO, Mounier N, Brice P, et al. Plasma cytokine and soluble receptor signature predicts outcome of patients with classical Hodgkin's lymphoma: a study from the Groupe d'Etude des Lymphomes de l'Adulte. *J Clin Oncol* 2007;25:1732–1740.

93. Rassidakis GZ, Medeiros LJ, Vassilakopoulos TP, et al. BCL-2 expression in Hodgkin and Reed-Sternberg cells of classical Hodgkin disease predicts a poorer prognosis in patients treated with ABVD or equivalent regimens. *Blood* 2002;100:3935–3941.

94. Sanchez-Espiridion B, Montalban C, Lopez A, et al. A molecular risk score based on 4 functional pathways for advanced classical Hodgkin lymphoma. *Blood* 2010;116:e12–e17.

95. Chetaille B, Bertucci F, Finetti P, et al. Molecular profiling of classical Hodgkin lymphoma tissues uncovers variations in the tumor microenvironment and correlations with EBV infection and outcome. *Blood* 2009;113: 2765–3775.

96. Steidl C, Lee T, Shah SP, et al. Tumor-associated macrophages and survival in classic Hodgkin's lymphoma. *N Engl J Med* 2010;362:875–885.

97. Steidl C, Connors JM, Gascoyne RD. Molecular pathogenesis of Hodgkin's lymphoma: increasing evidence of the importance of the microenvironment. *J Clin Oncol* 2011;29:1812–1826.

98. Sauer M, Plutschow A, Jachimowicz RD, et al. Baseline serum TARC levels predict therapy outcome in patients with Hodgkin lymphoma. *Am J Hematol* 2013;88:113–115.

99. His ED. Biologic features of Hodgkin lymphoma and the development of biologic prognostic factors in Hodgkin lymphoma: tumor and microenvironment. *Leuk Lymphoma* 2008;49:1668–1680.

100. Hutchings M, Loft A, Hansen M, et al. FDG-PET after two cycles of chemotherapy predicts treatment failure and progression-free survival in Hodgkin lymphoma. *Blood* 2006;107:52–59.

101. Gallamini A, Hutchings M, Rigacci L, et al. Early interim 2-[18F]fluoro-2-deoxy-D-glucose positron emission tomography is prognostically superior to international prognostic score in advanced-stage Hodgkin's lymphoma: a report from a joint Italian-Danish study. *J Clin Oncol* 2007;25:3746–3752.

102. Cerci JJ, Pracchia LF, Linardi CC, et al. 18F-FDG PET after 2 cycles of ABVD predicts event-free survival in early and advanced Hodgkin lymphoma. *J Nucl Med* 2010;51:1337–1343.

103. Longo DL, Young RC, Wesley M, et al. Twenty years of MOPP therapy for Hodgkin's disease. *J Clin Oncol* 1986;4:1295–1306.

104. Bonadonna G, Valagussa P, Santoro A. Alternating non-cross-resistant combination chemotherapy or MOPP in stage IV Hodgkin's disease. A report of 8-year results. *Ann Intern Med* 1986;104:739–746.

105. Canellos GP, Anderson JR, Propert KJ, et al. Chemotherapy of advanced Hodgkin's disease with MOPP, ABVD, or MOPP alternating with ABVD. *N Engl J Med* 1992;327:1478–1484.

106. Viviani S, Bonadonna G, Santoro A, et al. Alternating versus hybrid MOPP and ABVD combinations in advanced Hodgkin's disease: ten-year results. *J Clin Oncol* 1996;14:1421–1430.

107. Connors JM, Klimo P, Adams G, et al. Treatment of advanced Hodgkin's disease with chemotherapy—comparison of MOPP/ABV hybrid regimen with alternating courses of MOPP and ABVD: a report from the National Cancer Institute of Canada clinical trials group. *J Clin Oncol* 1997;15:1638–1645.

108. Bartlett NL, Rosenberg SA, Hoppe RT, et al. Brief chemotherapy, Stanford V, and adjuvant radiotherapy for bulky or advanced-stage Hodgkin's disease: a preliminary report. *J Clin Oncol* 1995;13:1080–1088.

109. Horning SJ, Williams J, Bartlett NL, et al. Assessment of the stanford V regimen and consolidative radiotherapy for bulky and advanced Hodgkin's disease: Eastern Cooperative Oncology Group pilot study E1492. *J Clin Oncol* 2000;18:972–980.

110. Chisesi T, Bellei M, Luminari S, et al. Long-term follow-up analysis of HD9601 trial comparing ABVD versus Stanford V versus MOPP/EBV/CAD in patients with newly diagnosed advanced-stage Hodgkin's lymphoma: a study from the Intergruppo Italiano Linfomi. *J Clin Oncol* 2011;29: 4227–4233.

111. Hoskin PJ, Lowry L, Horwich A, et al. Randomized comparison of the stanford V regimen and ABVD in the treatment of advanced Hodgkin's Lymphoma: United Kingdom National Cancer Research Institute Lymphoma Group Study ISRCTN 64141244. *J Clin Oncol* 2009;27:5390–5396.

112. Gordon LI, Hong F, Fisher RI, et al. Randomized phase III trial of ABVD versus Stanford V with or without radiation therapy in locally extensive and advanced-stage Hodgkin lymphoma: an intergroup study coordinated by the Eastern Cooperative Oncology Group (E2496). *J Clin Oncol* 2013;31: 684–691.

113. Diehl V, Sieber M, Ruffer U, et al. BEACOPP: an intensified chemotherapy regimen in advanced Hodgkin's disease. The German Hodgkin's Lymphoma Study Group. *Ann Oncol* 1997;8:143–148.

114. Diehl V, Franklin J, Pfreundschuh M, et al. Standard and increased-dose BEACOPP chemotherapy compared with COPP-ABVD for advanced Hodgkin's disease. *N Engl J Med* 2003;348:2386–2395.

115. Engert A, Diehl V, Franklin J, et al. Escalated-dose BEACOPP in the treatment of patients with advanced-stage Hodgkin's lymphoma: 10 years of follow-up of the GHSG HD9 study. *J Clin Oncol* 2009;27:4548–4554.

116. Federico M, Luminari S, Iannitto E, et al. ABVD compared with BEACOPP compared with CEC for the initial treatment of patients with advanced Hodgkin's lymphoma: results from the HD2000 Gruppo Italiano per lo Studio dei Linfomi Trial. *J Clin Oncol* 2009;27:805–811.

117. Engert A, Haverkamp H, Kobe C, et al. Reduced-intensity chemotherapy and PET-guided radiotherapy in patients with advanced stage Hodgkin's lymphoma (HD15 trial): a randomised, open-label, phase 3 non-inferiority trial. *Lancet* 2012;379:1791–1799.

118. Carde PP, Karrasch M, Fortpied C, et al. ABVD (8 cycles) versus BEACOPP (4 escalated cycles => 4 baseline) in stage III-IV high-risk Hodgkin lymphoma (HL): First results of EORTC 20012 Intergroup randomized phase III clinical trial. *ASCO Meeting Abstracts* 2012;30:8002.

119. Viviani S, Zinzani PL, Rambaldi A, et al. ABVD versus BEACOPP for Hodgkin's lymphoma when high-dose salvage is planned. *N Engl J Med* 2011;365:203–212.

120. Connors JM. Hodgkin's lymphoma—the great teacher. *N Engl J Med* 2011;365:264–265.

121. Tam CS, Herschtal A, Seymour JF. ABVD versus BEACOPP for Hodgkin's lymphoma. *N Engl J Med* 2011;365:1544–1545.

122. Skoetz N, Trelle S, Rancea M, et al. Effect of initial treatment strategy on survival of patients with advanced-stage Hodgkin's lymphoma: a systematic review and network meta-analysis. *Lancet Oncol* 2013;14:943–952.

123. Terasawa T, Lau J, Bardet S, et al. Fluorine-18-fluorodeoxyglucose positron emission tomography for interim response assessment of advanced-stage Hodgkin's lymphoma and diffuse large B-cell lymphoma: a systematic review. *J Clin Oncol* 2009;27:1906–1914.

124. Advani R, Maeda L, Lavori P, et al. Impact of positive positron emission tomography on prediction of freedom from progression after Stanford V chemotherapy in Hodgkin's disease. *J Clin Oncol* 2007;25:3902–3907.

125. Markova J, Kahraman D, Kobe C, et al. Role of [18F]-fluoro-2-deoxy-D-glucose positron emission tomography in early and late therapy assessment of patients with advanced Hodgkin lymphoma treated with bleomycin, etoposide, adriamycin, cyclophosphamide, vincristine, procarbazine and prednisone. *Leuk Lymphoma* 2012;53:64–70.

126. Avigdor A, Bulvik S, Levi I, et al. Two cycles of escalated BEACOPP followed by four cycles of ABVD utilizing early-interim PET/CT scan is an effective regimen for advanced high-risk Hodgkin's lymphoma. *Ann Oncol* 2010;21:126–132.

127. Gallamini A, Patti C, Viviani S, et al. Early chemotherapy intensification with BEACOPP in advanced-stage Hodgkin lymphoma patients with a interim-PET positive after two ABVD courses. *Br J Haematol* 2011;152:551–560.

128. Gallamini A, Rossi A, Patti C, et al. Early Treatment Intensification in Advanced-Stage High-Risk Hodgkin Lymphoma (HL) Patients, with a Positive FDG-PET Scan After Two ABVD Courses – First Interim Analysis of the GITIL/FIL HD0607 Clinical Trial. *Blood* 2012;120:550.

129. Aleman BM, Raemaekers JM, Tirelli U, et al. Involved-field radiotherapy for advanced Hodgkin's lymphoma. *N Engl J Med* 2003;348:2396–2406.

130. Younes A, Connors JM, Park SI, et al. Brentuximab vedotin combined with ABVD or AVD for patients with newly diagnosed Hodgkin's lymphoma: a phase 1, open-label, dose-escalation study. *Lancet Oncol* 2013;14: 1348–1356.

131. Borchmann P, Eichenauer DA, Plütschow A, et al. Targeted beacopp variants in patients with newly diagnosed advanced stage classical hodgkin lymphoma: interim results of a randomized phase II study. *Blood* 2013; Abst# 4344.

132. Kasamon YL, Jacene HA, Gocke CD, et al. Phase 2 study of rituximab-ABVD in classical Hodgkin lymphoma. *Blood* 2012;119:4129–4132.

133. Younes A, Oki Y, McLaughlin P, et al. Phase 2 study of rituximab plus ABVD in patients with newly diagnosed classical Hodgkin lymphoma. *Blood* 2012;119:4123–4128.

134. Böll B, Plütschow A, Fuchs M, et al. German Hodgkin Study Group Phase I trial of doxorubicin, vinblastine, dacarbazine, and lenalidomide (AVD-Rev) for older Hodgkin lymphoma patients. *Blood* 2013;Abst# 3054.

135. Ng AK, Bernardo MP, Weller E, et al. Long-term survival and competing causes of death in patients with early-stage Hodgkin's disease treated at age 50 or younger. *J Clin Oncol* 2002;20:2101–2108.

136. Boll B, Gorgen H, Fuchs M, et al. ABVD in older patients with early-stage Hodgkin lymphoma treated within the German Hodgkin Study Group HD10 and HD11 trials. *J Clin Oncol* 2013;31:1522–1529.

137. Wongso D, Fuchs M, Plutschow A, et al. Treatment-related mortality in patients with advanced-stage Hodgkin lymphoma: an analysis of the German Hodgkin Study Group. *J Clin Oncol* 2013;31:2819–2824.

138. Martin WG, Ristow KM, Habermann TM, et al. Bleomycin pulmonary toxicity has a negative impact on the outcome of patients with Hodgkin's lymphoma. *J Clin Oncol* 2005;23:7614–7620.

139. Cote GM, Canellos GP. Can low-risk, early-stage patients with Hodgkin lymphoma be spared radiotherapy? *Curr Hematol Malig Rep* 2011;6:180–186.

140. Bhatia S, Yasui Y, Robison LL, et al. High risk of subsequent neoplasms continues with extended follow-up of childhood Hodgkin's disease: report from the Late Effects Study Group. *J Clin Oncol* 2003;21:4386–4394.

141. Hodgson DC, Gilbert ES, Dores GM, et al. Long-term solid cancer risk among 5-year survivors of Hodgkin's lymphoma. *J Clin Oncol* 2007;25:1489–1497.

142. Franklin J, Pluetschow A, Paus M, et al. Second malignancy risk associated with treatment of Hodgkin's lymphoma: meta-analysis of the randomised trials. *Ann Oncol* 2006;17:1749–1760.

143. Baxi SS, Matasar MJ. State-of-the-art issues in Hodgkin's lymphoma survivorship. *Curr Oncol Rep* 2010;12:366–373.

144. Travis LB, Hill D, Dores GM, et al. Cumulative absolute breast cancer risk for young women treated for Hodgkin lymphoma. *J Natl Cancer Inst* 2005;97:1428–1437.

145. Scholz M, Engert A, Franklin J, et al. Impact of first- and second-line treatment for Hodgkin's lymphoma on the incidence of AML/MDS and NHL—experience of the German Hodgkin's Lymphoma Study Group analyzed by a parametric model of carcinogenesis. *Ann Oncol* 2011;22:681–688.

146. Behringer K, Breuer K, Reineke T, et al. Secondary amenorrhea after Hodgkin's lymphoma is influenced by age at treatment, stage of disease, chemotherapy regimen, and the use of oral contraceptives during therapy: a report from the German Hodgkin's Lymphoma Study Group. *J Clin Oncol* 2005;23:7555–7564.

147. Sieniawski M, Reineke T, Josting A, et al. Assessment of male fertility in patients with Hodgkin's lymphoma treated in the German Hodgkin Study Group (GHSG) clinical trials. *Ann Oncol* 2008;19:1795–1801.

148. Hodgson DC, Pintilie M, Gitterman L, et al. Fertility among female hodgkin lymphoma survivors attempting pregnancy following ABVD chemotherapy. *Hematol Oncol* 2007;25:11–15.

149. Kulkarni SS, Sastry PS, Saikia TK, et al. Gonadal function following ABVD therapy for Hodgkin's disease. *Am J Clin Oncol.* 1997;20:354–357.

150. Swerdlow AJ, Higgins CD, Smith P, et al. Myocardial infarction mortality risk after treatment for Hodgkin disease: a collaborative British cohort study. *J Natl Cancer Inst* 2007;99:206–214.

151. Evens AM, Hong F, Gordon LI, et al. The efficacy and tolerability of adriamycin, bleomycin, vinblastine, dacarbazine and Stanford V in older Hodgkin lymphoma patients: a comprehensive analysis from the North American intergroup trial E2496. *Br J Haematol* 2013;161:76–86.

152. Evens AM, Sweetenham JW, Horning SJ. Hodgkin lymphoma in older patients: an uncommon disease in need of study. *Oncology* 2008;22:1369–1379.

153. Gobbi PG, Federico M. What has happened to VBM (vinblastine, bleomycin, and methotrexate) chemotherapy for early-stage Hodgkin lymphoma? *Crit Rev Oncol Hematol* 2012;82:18–24.

154. Levis A, Anselmo AP, Ambrosetti A, et al. VEPEMB in elderly Hodgkin's lymphoma patients. Results from an Intergruppo Italiano Linfomi (IIL) study. *Ann Oncol* 2004;15:123–128.

155. Proctor SJ, Wilkinson J, Jones G, et al. Evaluation of treatment outcome in 175 patients with Hodgkin lymphoma aged 60 years or over: the SHIELD study. *Blood* 2012;119:6005–6015.

156. Pereg D, Koren G, Lishner M. The treatment of Hodgkin's and non-Hodgkin's lymphoma in pregnancy. *Haematologica* 2007;92:1230–1237.

157. Woo SY, Fuller LM, Cundiff JH, et al. Radiotherapy during pregnancy for clinical stages IA-IIA Hodgkin's disease. *Int J Radiat Oncol Biol Phys* 1992;23:407–412.

158. Yahalom J. Treatment options for Hodgkin's disease during pregnancy. *Leuk Lymphoma* 1990;2:151.

159. Connors JM. Challenging problems: coincident pregnancy, HIV infection, and older age. *Hematology Am Soc Hematol Educ Program* 2008: 334–339.

160. Kal HB, Struikmans H. Radiotherapy during pregnancy: fact and fiction. *Lancet Oncol.* 2005;6:328–333.

161. Rizack T, Mega A, Legare R, et al. Management of hematological malignancies during pregnancy. *Am J Hematol* 2009;84:830–841.

162. Lazarus HM, Rowlings PA, Zhang MJ, et al. Autotransplants for Hodgkin's disease in patients never achieving remission: a report from the Autologous Blood and Marrow Transplant Registry. *J Clin Oncol* 1999;17:534–545.

163. André M, Henry-Amar M, Pico JL, et al. Comparison of high-dose therapy and autologous stem-cell transplantation with conventional therapy for Hodgkin's disease induction failure: a case-control study. *J Clin Oncol* 1999;17:222.

164. Linch DC, Winfield D, Goldstone AH, et al. Dose intensification with autologous bone-marrow transplantation in relapsed and resistant Hodgkin's disease: results of a BNLI randomised trial. *Lancet* 1993;341:1051–1054.

165. Schmitz N, Pfistner B, Sextro M, et al. Aggressive conventional chemotherapy compared with high-dose chemotherapy with autologous haemopoietic stem-cell transplantation for relapsed chemosensitive Hodgkin's disease: a randomised trial. *Lancet* 2002;359:2065–2071.

166. Josting A, Rueffer U, Franklin J, et al. Prognostic factors and treatment outcome in primary progressive Hodgkin lymphoma: a report from the German Hodgkin Lymphoma Study Group. *Blood* 2000;96:1280–1286.

167. Josting A, Franklin J, May M, et al. New prognostic score based on treatment outcome of patients with relapsed Hodgkin's lymphoma registered in the database of the German Hodgkin's lymphoma study group. *J Clin Oncol* 2002;20:221–230.

168. Pfreundschuh MG, Rueffer U, Lathan B, et al. Dexa-BEAM in patients with Hodgkin's disease refractory to multidrug chemotherapy regimens: a trial of the German Hodgkin's Disease Study Group. *J Clin Oncol* 1994;12: 580–586.

169. Colwill R, Crump M, Couture F, et al. Mini-BEAM as salvage therapy for relapsed or refractory Hodgkin's disease before intensive therapy and autologous bone marrow transplantation. *J Clin Oncol* 1995;13:396–402.

170. Martin A, Fernandez-Jimenez MC, Caballero MD, et al. Long-term follow-up in patients treated with Mini-BEAM as salvage therapy for relapsed or refractory Hodgkin's disease. *Br J Haematol* 2001;113:161–171.

171. Rodriguez J, Rodriguez MA, Fayad L, et al. ASHAP: a regimen for cytoreduction of refractory or recurrent Hodgkin's disease. *Blood* 1999;93:3632–3636.

172. Ribrag V, Nasr F, Bouhris JH, et al. VIP (etoposide, ifosfamide and cisplatinum) as a salvage intensification program in relapsed or refractory Hodgkin's disease. *Bone Marrow Transplant* 1998;21:969–974.

173. Josting A, Rudolph C, Reiser M, et al. Time-intensified dexamethasone/cisplatin/cytarabine: an effective salvage therapy with low toxicity in patients with relapsed and refractory Hodgkin's disease. *Ann Oncol* 2002;13: 1628–1635.

174. Baetz T, Belch A, Couban S, et al. Gemcitabine, dexamethasone and cisplatin is an active and non-toxic chemotherapy regimen in relapsed or refractory Hodgkin's disease: a phase II study by the National Cancer Institute of Canada Clinical Trials Group. *Ann Oncol* 2003;14:1762–1767.

175. Chau I, Harries M, Cunningham D, et al. Gemcitabine, cisplatin and methylprednisolone chemotherapy (GEM-P) is an effective regimen in patients with poor prognostic primary progressive or multiply relapsed Hodgkin's and non-Hodgkin's lymphoma. *Br J Haematol* 2003;120:970–977.

176. Ferme C, Mounier N, Divine M, et al. Intensive salvage therapy with high-dose chemotherapy for patients with advanced Hodgkin's disease in relapse or failure after initial chemotherapy: results of the Groupe d'Etudes des Lymphomes de l'Adulte H89 Trial. *J Clin Oncol* 2002;20:467–475.

177. Proctor SJ, Jackson GH, Lennard A, et al. Strategic approach to the management of Hodgkin's disease incorporating salvage therapy with high-dose ifosfamide, etoposide and epirubicin: a Northern Region Lymphoma Group study (UK). *Ann Oncol* 2003;14:i47–i50.

178. Bonfante V, Viviani S, Devizzi L, et al. High-dose ifosfamide and vinorelbine as salvage therapy for relapsed or refractory Hodgkin's disease. *Eur J Haematol Suppl* 2001;64:51–55.

179. Josting A, Müller H, Borchmann P, et al. Dose intensity of chemotherapy in patients with relapsed Hodgkin's lymphoma. *J Clin Oncol* 2010;28: 5074–5080.

180. Kuruvilla J, Nagy T, Pintilie M, et al. Similar response rates and superior early progression-free survival with gemcitabine, dexamethasone, and cisplatin salvage therapy compared with carmustine, etoposide, cytarabine, and melphalan salvage therapy prior to autologous stem cell transplantation for recurrent or refractory Hodgkin lymphoma. *Cancer* 2006;106:353–360.

181. Puig N, Pintilie M, Seshadri T, et al. Different response to salvage chemotherapy but similar post-transplant outcomes in patients with relapsed and refractory Hodgkin's lymphoma. *Haematologica* 2010;95:1496–1502.

PRACTICE OF ONCOLOGY

182. Moskowitz CH, Kewalramani T, Nimer SD, et al. Effectiveness of high dose chemoradiotherapy and autologous stem cell transplantation for patients with biopsy-proven primary refractory Hodgkin's disease. *Br J Haematol* 2004;124:645–652.

183. Akhtar S, El Weshi A, Abdelsalam M, et al. Primary refractory Hodgkin's lymphoma: outcome after high-dose chemotherapy and autologous SCT and impact of various prognostic factors on overall and event-free survival. A single institution result of 66 patients. *Bone Marrow Transplant* 2007;40:651–658.

184. Czyz J, Szydlo R, Knopinska-Posluszny W, et al. Treatment for primary refractory Hodgkin's disease: a comparison of high-dose chemotherapy followed by ASCT with conventional therapy. *Bone Marrow Transplant* 2004;33:1225–1229.

185. Brandwein JM, Callum J, Sutcliffe SB, et al. Evaluation of cytoreductive therapy prior to high dose treatment with autologous bone marrow transplantation in relapsed and refractory Hodgkin's disease. *Bone Marrow Transplant* 1990;5:99–103.

186. Stewart AK, Brandwein JM, Sutcliffe SB, et al. Mini-beam as Salvage Chemotherapy for Refractory Hodgkin's Disease and Non-Hodgkin's Lymphoma. *Leuk Lymphoma* 1991;5:111–115.

187. Ardeshna KM, Kakouros N, Qian W, et al. Conventional second-line salvage chemotherapy regimens are not warranted in patients with malignant lymphomas who have progressive disease after first-line salvage therapy regimens. *Br J Haematol* 2005;130:363–372.

188. Villa D, Seshadri T, Puig N, et al. Second-line salvage chemotherapy for transplant-eligible patients with Hodgkin's lymphoma resistant to platinum-containing first-line salvage chemotherapy. *Haematologica* 2012;97:751–757.

189. Dreger P, Kloss M, Petersen B, et al. Autologous progenitor cell transplantation: prior exposure to stem cell-toxic drugs determines yield and engraftment of peripheral blood progenitor cell but not of bone marrow grafts. *Blood* 1995;86:3970–3978.

190. Watts MJ, Sullivan AM, Jamieson E, et al. Progenitor-cell mobilization after low-dose cyclophosphamide and granulocyte colony-stimulating factor: an analysis of progenitor-cell quantity and quality and factors predicting for these parameters in 101 pretreated patients with malignant lymphoma. *J Clin Oncol* 1997;15:535–546.

191. Weaver CH, Zhen B, Buckner CD. Treatment of patients with malignant lymphoma with Mini-BEAM reduces the yield of CD34+ peripheral blood stem cells. *Bone Marrow Transplant* 1998;21:1169–1170.

192. Moskowitz CH, Nimer SD, Zelenetz AD, et al. A 2-step comprehensive high-dose chemoradiotherapy second-line program for relapsed and refractory Hodgkin disease: analysis by intent to treat and development of a prognostic model. *Blood* 2001;97:616–623.

193. Jabbour E, Hosing C, Ayers G, et al. Pretransplant positive positron emission tomography/gallium scans predict poor outcome in patients with recurrent/refractory Hodgkin lymphoma. *Cancer* 2007;109:2481–2489.

194. Moskowitz AJ, Yahalom J, Kewalramani T, et al. Pre-transplant functional imaging predicts outcome following autologous stem cell transplant for relapsed and refractory Hodgkin lymphoma. *Blood* 2010;116:4934–4937.

195. Moskowitz CH, Matasar MJ, Zelenetz AD, et al. Normalization of pre-ASCT, FDG-PET imaging with second-line, non-cross-resistant, chemotherapy programs improves event-free survival in patients with Hodgkin lymphoma. *Blood* 2012;119:1665–1670.

196. Crump M, Smith AM, Brandwein J, et al. High-dose etoposide and melphalan, and autologous bone marrow transplantation for patients with advanced Hodgkin's disease: importance of disease status at transplant. *J Clin Oncol* 1993;11:704–711.

197. Stewart DA, Guo D, Gluck S, et al. Double high-dose therapy for Hodgkin's disease with dose-intensive cyclophosphamide, etoposide, and cisplatin (DICEP) prior to high-dose melphalan and autologous stem cell transplantation. *Bone Marrow Transplant* 2000;26:383–388.

198. Stuart MJ, Chao NS, Horning SJ, et al. Efficacy and toxicity of a CCNU-containing high-dose chemotherapy regimen followed by autologous hematopoietic cell transplantation in relapsed or refractory Hodgkin's disease. *Biol Blood Marrow Transplant* 2001;7:552–560.

199. Evens A, Altman J, Mittal B, et al. Phase I/II trial of total lymphoid irradiation and high-dose chemotherapy with autologous stem-cell transplantation for relapsed and refractory Hodgkin's lymphoma. *Ann Oncol* 2007;18:679–688.

200. Bains T, Chen AI, Lemieux A, et al. Improved outcome with busulfan, melphalan and thiotepa conditioning in autologous hematopoietic stem cell transplant for relapsed/refractory Hodgkin lymphoma. *Leuk Lymphoma* 2014;55:583–587.

201. Josting A, Rudolph C, Mapara M, et al. Cologne high-dose sequential chemotherapy in relapsed and refractory Hodgkin lymphoma: results of a large multicenter study of the German Hodgkin Lymphoma Study Group (GHSG). *Ann Oncol* 2005;16:116–123.

202. Josting A, Muller H, Borchmann P, et al. Dose intensity of chemotherapy in patients with relapsed Hodgkin's lymphoma. *J Clin Oncol* 2010;28:5074–5080.

203. Fung HC, Stiff P, Schriber J, et al. Tandem autologous stem cell transplantation for patients with primary refractory or poor risk recurrent Hodgkin lymphoma. *Biol Blood Marrow Transplant* 2007;13:594–600.

204. Morschhauser F, Brice P, Ferme C, et al. Risk-adapted salvage treatment with single or tandem autologous stem-cell transplantation for first relapse/refractory Hodgkin's lymphoma: results of the prospective multicenter h96 trial by the GELA/SFGM study group. *J Clin Oncol* 2008;26:5980–5987.

205. Puig N, Pintilie M, Seshadri T, et al. Different response to salvage chemotherapy but similar post-transplant outcomes in patients with relapsed and refractory Hodgkin's lymphoma. *Haematologica* 2010;95:1496–1502.

206. Gajewski JL, Phillips GL, Sobocinski KA, et al. Bone marrow transplants from HLA-identical siblings in advanced Hodgkin's disease. *J Clin Oncol* 1996;14:572–578.

207. Peniket AJ, Ruiz de Elvira MC, Taghipour G, et al. An EBMT registry matched study of allogeneic stem cell transplants for lymphoma: allogeneic transplantation is associated with a lower relapse rate but a higher procedure-related mortality rate than autologous transplantation. *Bone Marrow Transplant* 2003;31:667–678.

208. Anderson JE, Litzow MR, Appelbaum FR, et al. Allogeneic, syngeneic, and autologous marrow transplantation for Hodgkin's disease: the 21-year Seattle experience. *J Clin Oncol* 1993;11:2342–2350.

209. Akpek G, Ambinder RF, Piantadosi S, et al. Long-term results of blood and marrow transplantation for Hodgkin's lymphoma. *J Clin Oncol* 2001;19:4314–4321.

210. Anderlini P, Acholonu SA, Okoroji GJ, et al. Donor leukocyte infusions in relapsed Hodgkin's lymphoma following allogeneic stem cell transplantation: CD3+ cell dose, GVHD and disease response. *Bone Marrow Transplant* 2004;34:511–514.

211. Peggs KS, Hunter A, Chopra R, et al. Clinical evidence of a graft-versus-Hodgkin's-lymphoma effect after reduced-intensity allogeneic transplantation. *Lancet* 2005;365:1934–1941.

212. Peggs KS, Sureda A, Qian W, et al. Reduced-intensity conditioning for allogeneic haematopoietic stem cell transplantation in relapsed and refractory Hodgkin lymphoma: impact of alemtuzumab and donor lymphocyte infusions on long-term outcomes. *Br J Haematol* 2007;139:70–80.

213. Alvarez I, Sureda A, Caballero MD, et al. Nonmyeloablative stem cell transplantation is an effective therapy for refractory or relapsed hodgkin lymphoma: results of a Spanish prospective cooperative protocol. *Biol Blood Marrow Transplant* 2006;12:172–183.

214. Burroughs LM, O'Donnell PV, Sandmaier BM, et al. Fludarabine-melphalan as a preparative regimen for reduced-intensity conditioning allogeneic stem cell transplantation in relapsed and refractory Hodgkin's lymphoma: the updated M.D. Anderson Cancer Center experience. *Haematologica* 2008;93:257–264.

215. Burroughs LM, O'Donnell PV, Sandmaier BM, et al. Comparison of outcomes of HLA-matched related, unrelated, or HLA-haploidentical related hematopoietic cell transplantation following nonmyeloablative conditioning for relapsed or refractory Hodgkin lymphoma. *Biol Blood Marrow Transplant* 2008;14:1279–1287.

216. Marcel PD, Parameswaran NH, Jeanette C, et al. Unrelated donor reduced-intensity allogeneic hematopoietic stem cell transplantation for relapsed and refractory Hodgkin lymphoma. *Biol Blood Marrow Transplant* 2009;15:109–117.

217. Sureda A, Robinson S, Canals C, et al. Reduced-intensity conditioning compared with conventional allogeneic stem-cell transplantation in relapsed or refractory Hodgkin's lymphoma: an analysis from the Lymphoma Working Party of the European Group for Blood and Marrow Transplantation. *J Clin Oncol* 2008;26:455–462.

218. Sureda A, Canals C, Arranz R, et al. Allogeneic stem cell transplantation after reduced intensity conditioning in patients with relapsed or refractory Hodgkin's lymphoma. Results of the HDR-ALLO study - a prospective clinical trial by the Grupo Espanol de Linfomas/Trasplante de Medula Osea (GEL/TAMO) and the Lymphoma Working Party of the European Group for Blood and Marrow Transplantation. *Haematologica* 2012;97:310–317.

219. Anderlini P, Saliba R, Acholonu S, et al. Fludarabine-melphalan as a preparative regimen for reduced-intensity conditioning allogeneic stem cell transplantation in relapsed and refractory Hodgkin's lymphoma: the updated M.D. Anderson Cancer Center experience. *Haematologica* 2008;93:257–264.

220. Devetten MP, Hari PN, Carreras J, et al. Unrelated donor reduced-intensity allogeneic hematopoietic stem cell transplantation for relapsed and refractory Hodgkin lymphoma. *Biol Blood Marrow Transplant* 2009;15:109–117.

221. Brunstein CG, Cantero S, Cao Q, et al. Promising progression-free survival for patients low and intermediate grade lymphoid malignancies after nonmyeloablative umbilical cord blood transplantation. *Biol Blood Marrow Transplant* 2009;15:214–222.

222. Rodrigues CA, Sanz G, Brunstein CG, et al. Analysis of risk factors for outcomes after unrelated cord blood transplantation in adults with lymphoid malignancies: a study by the Eurocord-Netcord and lymphoma working party of the European group for blood and marrow transplantation. *J Clin Oncol* 2009;27:256–263.

223. Thomson KJ, Peggs KS, Smith P, et al. Improved outcome following reduced intensity allogeneic transplantation in Hodgkin's lymphoma relapsing post-autologous transplantation. *Blood* 2005;106:abstract 657.

224. Castagna L, Sarina B, Todisco E, et al. Allogeneic stem cell transplantation compared with chemotherapy for poor-risk Hodgkin lymphoma. *Biol Blood Marrow Transplant* 2009;15:432–438.

225. Smith SM, van Besien K, Carreras J, et al. Second autologous stem cell transplantation for relapsed lymphoma after a prior autologous transplant. *Biol Blood Marrow Transplant* 2008;14:904–912.

226. Arai S, Fanale M, Devos S, et al. Defining a Hodgkin lymphoma population for novel therapeutics after relapse from autologous hematopoietic cell transplantation. *Leuk Lymphoma* 2013;54:2531–2533.

227. Younes A, Bartlett NL, Leonard JP, et al. Brentuximab vedotin (SGN-35) for relapsed CD30-positive lymphomas. *N Engl J Med* 2010;363:1812–1821.

228. Fanale MA, Forero-Torres A, Rosenblatt JD, et al. A phase I weekly dosing study of brentuximab vedotin in patients with relapsed/refractory CD30-positive hematologic malignancies. *Clin Cancer Res* 2012;18:248–255.

229. Younes A, Gopal AK, Smith SE, et al. Results of a pivotal phase II study of brentuximab vedotin for patients with relapsed or refractory Hodgkin's lymphoma. *J Clin Oncol* 2012;30:2183–2189.

230. Buglio D, Georgakis GV, Hanabuchi S, et al. Vorinostat inhibits STAT6-mediated TH2 cytokine and TARC production and induces cell death in Hodgkin lymphoma cell lines. *Blood* 2008;112:1424–1433.

231. Buglio D, Mamidipudi V, Khaskhely NM, et al. The class-I HDAC inhibitor MGCD0103 induces apoptosis in Hodgkin lymphoma cell lines and synergizes with proteasome inhibitors by an HDAC6-independent mechanism. *Br J Haematol* 2010;151:387–396.

232. Sharpe AH, Wherry EJ, Ahmed R, et al. The function of programmed cell death 1 and its ligands in regulating autoimmunity and infection. *Nat Immunol* 2007;8:239–245.

233. Kirschbaum MH, Goldman BH, Zain JM, et al. A phase 2 study of vorinostat for treatment of relapsed or refractory Hodgkin lymphoma: Southwest Oncology Group Study S0517. *Leuk Lymphoma* 2012;53:259–262.

234. Zhou N, Moradei O, Raeppel S, et al. Discovery of N-(2-aminophenyl)-4-[(4-pyridin-3-ylpyrimidin-2-ylamino)methyl]benzamide (MGCD0103), an orally active histone deacetylase inhibitor. *J Med Chem* 2008;51:4072–4075.

235. Fournel M, Bonfils C, Hou Y, et al. MGCD0103, a novel isotype-selective histone deacetylase inhibitor, has broad spectrum antitumor activity in vitro and in vivo. *Mol Cancer Ther* 2008;7:759–768.

236. Younes A, Oki Y, Bociek RG, et al. Mocetinostat for relapsed classical Hodgkin's lymphoma: an open-label, single-arm, phase 2 trial. *Lancet Oncol* 2011;12:1222–1228.

237. Younes A, Sureda A, Ben-Yehuda D, et al. Panobinostat in patients with relapsed/refractory Hodgkin's lymphoma after autologous stem-cell transplantation: results of a phase II study. *J Clin Oncol* 2012;30:2197–2203.

238. Engelman JA. Targeting PI3K signalling in cancer: opportunities, challenges and limitations. *Nat Rev Cancer* 2009;9:550–562.

239. Yuan TL, Cantley LC. PI3K pathway alterations in cancer: variations on a theme. *Oncogene* 2008;27:5497–5510.

240. Hennessy BT, Smith DL, Ram PT, et al. Exploiting the PI3K/AKT pathway for cancer drug discovery. *Nat Rev Drug Discov* 2005;4:988–1004.

241. Meadows SA, Vega F, Kashishian A, et al. PI3Kdelta inhibitor, GS-1101 (CAL-101), attenuates pathway signaling, induces apoptosis, and overcomes signals from the microenvironment in cellular models of Hodgkin lymphoma. *Blood* 2012;119:1897–1900.

242. Johnston PB, Pinter-Brown L, Rogerio J, et al. Everolimus for relapsed/refractory classical Hodgkin lymphoma: multicenter, open-label, single-arm, phase 2 study. *54th ASH Annual Meeting* 2012;Abstract 2740.

243. von Tresckow B, Plütschow A, Fuchs M, et al. Dose-intensification in early unfavorable Hodgkin's lymphoma: final analysis of the German Hodgkin Study Group HD14 trial. *J Clin Oncol* 2012;30:907–913.

244. Levis A, Anselmo AP, Ambrosetti A, et al. VEPEMB in elderly Hodgkin's lymphoma patients. Results from an Intergruppo Italiano Linfomi (IIL) study. *Ann Oncol* 2004;15:123–128.

245. Gobbi PG, Federico M. What has happened to VBM (vinblastine, bleomycin, and methotrexate) chemotherapy for early-stage Hodgkin lymphoma? *Crit Rev Oncol Hematol* 2012;82:18–24.

246. Bartlett NL, Niedzwiecki D, Johnson JL, et al. Gemcitabine, vinorelbine, and pegylated liposomal doxorubicin (GVD), a salvage regimen in relapsed Hodgkin's lymphoma: CALGB 59804. *Ann Oncol* 2007;18:1071–1079.

247. Santoro A, Magagnoli M, Spina M, et al. Ifosfamide, gemcitabine, and vinorelbine: a new induction regimen for refractory and relapsed Hodgkin's lymphoma. *Haematologica* 2007;92:35–41.

248. Josting A, Rudolph C, Reiser M, et al. Time-intensified dexamethasone/cisplatin/cytarabine: an effective salvage therapy with low toxicity in patients with relapsed and refractory Hodgkin's disease. *Ann Oncol* 2002;13:1628–1635.

249. Moskowitz CH, Bertino JR, Glassman JR, et al. Ifosfamide, carboplatin, and etoposide: a highly effective cytoreduction and peripheral-blood progenitor-cell mobilization regimen for transplant-eligible patients with non-Hodgkin's lymphoma. *J Clin Oncol* 1999;17:3776–3785.

250. Schmitz N, Pfistner B, Sextro M, et al. Aggressive conventional chemotherapy compared with high-dose chemotherapy with autologous haemopoietic stem-cell transplantation for relapsed chemosensitive Hodgkin's disease: a randomised trial. *Lancet* 2002;359:2065–2071.

251. Proctor SJ, Jackson GH, Lennard A, et al. Strategic approach to the management of Hodgkin's disease incorporating salvage therapy with high-dose ifosfamide, etoposide and epirubicin: a Northern Region Lymphoma Group study (UK). *Ann Oncol* 2003;14:i47–i50.

PRACTICE OF ONCOLOGY

103 Non-Hodgkin's Lymphoma

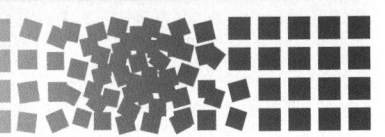

Arnold S. Freedman, Caron A. Jacobson, Peter Mauch, and Jon C. Aster

INTRODUCTION

Non-Hodgkin's lymphomas (NHL) are neoplastic transformations of mature B, T, and natural killer (NK) cells. Although NHLs and Hodgkin's lymphoma (HL) both infiltrate lymphohematopoietic tissues, their biologic and clinical behaviors are distinct. And although both are among the most sensitive malignancies to radiation and cytotoxic therapy, their cure rates differ. HLs are cured in about 80% of all patients employing both conventional and salvage treatment strategies, whereas NHLs are cured in less than 50% of patients.

EPIDEMIOLOGY AND ETIOLOGY

In 2014, there were an estimated 70,890 new cases of NHL in the United States, which constituted 4% of all new cancers in both males and females.[1] This is more than seven times the incidence of HL. There is a slight male-to-female predominance and a higher incidence for Caucasians than for African Americans. The incidence rises steadily with age, especially after age 40. Lymphomas are among the most common malignancies in patients between the ages of 20 and 40 years. Moreover, the incidence of NHL nearly doubled between 1970 and 1995. Although the rate of increase has slowed since the mid 1990s the incidence has continued to rise by 1.5% to 2% each year. NHL ranks as the ninth most common cause of cancer-related death in men in the United States and eighth in women. In 2014, 18,990 deaths from NHL were predicted. The 5-year survival rates for NHL is 72% for Caucasians and 63% for African Americans.

There are striking differences in the age-dependent incidence of NHL by histologic subtype. In children, diffuse large B-cell lymphoma (DLBCL), Burkitt's lymphoma (BL), and lymphoblastic lymphoma are most common. Although DLBCL is also the most common histologic subtypes in adults, the indolent lymphomas (small lymphocytic and follicular lymphomas [FL]) are extremely rare in children.

Exposures and Diseases Associated with Non-Hodgkin's Lymphoma

Infectious agents are involved in the pathogenesis of some NHLs. Epstein-Barr virus (EBV) is most commonly associated with a variety of B-cell NHLs, including endemic, sporadic, and AIDS-associated BL, lymphomas that arise in the setting of immunosuppression, including after organ transplantation and treatment of autoimmune diseases, in the setting of HIV infection, and a subset of lymphomas that arise in otherwise normal elderly individuals (Table 103.1).[2] EBV infection is also implicated in extranodal NK cell and T-cell lymphomas that involve the upper aerodigestive tract as well as other extranodal sites, as well as a small number of other unusual and uncommon T-cell malignancies.[3] Infection with human T-lymphotropic virus type 1 (HTLV-1) has been implicated in adult T-cell leukemia-lymphoma (ATLL) seen in the Caribbean and Japan.[4] Human herpes virus 8 (HHV-8) infection is associated with primary effusion lymphoma, where the viral genome is found within tumor cells in virtually 100% of cases.[5] Chronic hepatitis B infection has also been associated with an increased risk of NHL.[6] The marginal zone lymphomas (MZL) have been linked to many infectious agents. The gastric extra-nodal MZLs are associated with Helicobacter pylori infection.[7] Splenic MZL has been associated with hepatitis C infections.[8] The ocular adnexal MZL has been linked with Chlamydia psittaci infections,[9] and immunoproliferative small intestinal disease (Mediterranean lymphoma, alpha heavy chain disease) has been associated with Campylobacter jejuni.[10] Borrelia burgdorferi infection has been associated with extranodal MZLs of the skin in cases from Europe.[11]

An increased risk of NHL has been associated with a number of environmental exposures and/or disease states (see Table 103.1).[12,13] There is controversial evidence that certain chemical exposures, specifically the herbicide phenoxyacetic acid, increase the risk of NHL.[14] Other potential environmental associations include exposure to arsenic, pesticides, fungicides, chlorophenols, or organic solvents, halomethane, lead, vinyl chloride, or asbestos.[15,16] Occupational exposures associated with an increased risk include agricultural work, welding, and work in the lumber industry.[17] NHL has been observed as a late complication of prior chemotherapy and/or radiation therapy. Specifically, patients with HL treated with radiation therapy and chemotherapy exhibit an increased risk of developing secondary DLBCL.[18]

Diseases of inherited and acquired immunodeficiency as well as autoimmune diseases are associated with an increased incidence of lymphoma (see Table 103.1). The association between immunosuppression and induction of NHLs is compelling because, if the immunosuppression can be reversed, a percentage of these lymphomas regress spontaneously.[19] The incidence of NHL is nearly 100-fold increased for patients undergoing organ transplantation necessitating chronic immunosuppression, and is greatest in the first year posttransplant. About 30% of these arise as a polyclonal B-cell proliferation that evolves into a clonal B-cell malignancy. The NHLs that occur in the context of immunosuppression or immunodeficiency, including human immunodeficiency virus 1 (HIV-1) infection, are frequently associated with EBV.[20] Histologically, DLBCLs are most frequently associated with immunosuppression and autoimmune diseases, although almost all histologies can be seen. The rare inherited immunodeficiency diseases (X-linked lymphoproliferative syndrome, Wiskott-Aldrich syndrome, Chédiak-Higashi syndrome, ataxia telangiectasia, and common variable immunodeficiency syndrome) are complicated by highly aggressive lymphomas. The elevated incidence of lymphoma in iatrogenic immunosuppression, AIDS, and autoimmune disease argues strongly for immune dysregulation contributing in the pathogenesis of some lymphomas.[21,22] An increased risk of NHL has been observed in first-degree relatives with NHL, HL, or chronic lymphocytic leukemia (CLL). In large databases studies, about 9% of patients with lymphoma or CLL have a first-degree relative with a lymphoproliferative disorder.[23,24]

TABLE 103.1

Conditions Associated with the Development of Lymphoma

Inherited Immunodeficiency States	Acquired Immunodeficiency States	Autoimmune and Inflammatory Disorders	Chemicals and Drugs	Infectious Agents (Other than HIV)
Klinefelter's syndrome	Acquired agammaglobulinemia	Rheumatoid arthritis	Phenytoin	Epstein-Barr virus
Chédiak-Higashi syndrome	HIV-1 infection	Autoimmune hemolytic anemia	Dioxin, agent orange, pesticides	HTLV-1
Ataxia telangiectasia	Iatrogenic	Systemic lupus erythematosus	Ionizing radiation	HHV-8
Wiskott-Aldrich syndrome	Multicentric Castleman's disease	Sjögren's syndrome	Chemotherapy, radiation therapy	*Helicobacter pylori*
Common variable immunodeficiency		Hashimoto's thyroiditis	Tumor necrosis factor agonists	*Campylobacter jejuni*
X-linked lymphoproliferative disease		Acquired angioedema	Hair dyes	*Chlamydia psittaci*
Autoimmune lymphoproliferative disease		Inflammatory bowel disease		*Borrelia afzelii*
Bloom syndrome		Celiac disease		HCV
				MTB

HIV-1, human immunodeficiency virus-1; HTLV-1, human T cell lymphotropic virus-1; HHV-8, human herpes virus-8; HCV, hepatitis C virus; MTB, *Mycobacterium tuberculosis*.

BIOLOGIC BACKGROUND FOR CLASSIFICATION OF LYMPHOID NEOPLASMS

Current lymphoma classification systems divide the lymphomas into different entities based, in part, on their perceived cell of origin (Fig. 103.1, Table 103.2). During embryogenesis, hematopoietic stem cells (HSC) from the liver and the placenta give rise to progenitor cells that migrate to the thymus and bone marrow where they undergo a program of antigen-independent differentiation into T- and B-cell lineage precursor cells, directed largely by the microenvironment.[25] Postnatally, all lymphoid cells are derived from bone marrow HSCs, which give rise to very early lymphoid progenitors with B, T, and NK lymphocyte potential. These cells, in turn, yield B-cell progenitors in the marrow, the site of early stages of B-cell differentiation, as well as other progenitors that migrate to the thymus and undergo T-cell differentiation.

B-Cell Development

The initial commitment to B-cell differentiation by lymphoid progenitors in the bone marrow requires the expression of the master B lineage transcription factor PAX5, which directly upregulates the expression of early B lineage markers such as CD19.[26] Subsequent precursor B-cell development depends on a transcriptional program that is driven by PAX5 and downstream transcription factors and prosurvival signals produced by stepwise rearrangement of immunoglobulin (Ig) genes, which requires the lymphoid-specific recombination factors RAG1 and RAG2 and also involves the specialized DNA polymerase terminal deoxynucleotidyl transferase (TdT).[27] During development, pre-B cells pass through checkpoints that correspond to specific stages of Ig gene assembly, beginning with rearrangement of the Ig heavy chain locus (*IgH*).[28] Productive (in-frame) rearrangement of *IgH* leads to the expression of IgM heavy chain, which combines with a lambdalike polypeptide to enable the assembly of pre–B-cell receptors. The pre–B-cell receptor generates signals that prevent apoptosis, turns off further *IgH* gene rearrangement (contributing to allelic exclusion, the

expression of only a single IgH in each B-cell clone), and turns on rearrangements of the Ig light chain loci, first the kappa loci and, if these rearrangements are nonproductive, then the lambda light chain loci. During the period of Ig gene rearrangement, pre-B cells lack complete surface Ig and express CD19 and CD10, the common acute lymphoblastic leukemia antigen.[29] Precursor B cells that productively rearrange one or another light chain locus express the surface Ig receptor (sometimes referred to as the B-cell receptor [BCR]), which also transmits key survival signals that prevent apoptosis. Cells that express surface Ig upregulate additional B-cell markers such as CD79a, cytoplasmic and surface CD22, and CD20, as well as prosurvival factors such as BCL2, and downregulate CD10 and TdT emerging from the process as mature, immunologically naïve B cells.

In mice, two major types of naïve B cells have been defined. Roughly 90% of circulating and tissue-based B cells fall into the B2 class. B2 cells are widely distributed and largely respond to antigens in a T-cell–dependent fashion, a process that yields class-switched plasma cells expressing high-affinity Ig. B1 cells can be further subdivided into those that do or do not express the antigen CD5.[30] CD5+ B1a cells produce broadly reactive natural IgM, whereas CD5− B1b cells can generate T-independent, long-lasting memory-type IgM responses to some infectious pathogens. Whether B1 cells exist as a distinct B-cell lineage in humans has been (and remains) controversial, but it is notable that some human B-cell tumors, particularly CLL, is comprised of cells bearing some similarity to murine B1 cells.

From the marrow, naïve B cells migrate through the blood and extravasate into secondary lymphoid tissues, such as the spleen, the lymph nodes, and mucosa-associated lymphoid tissues in the gut. Homing of B cells to specific tissues appears to be controlled largely by chemokines that activate chemokine receptors expressed on B cells.[31] Upon encountering an antigen in peripheral tissues, B cells may either be induced to differentiate directly into short-lived IgM secreting plasma cells or may migrate to B-cell follicles. Antigen-mediated B-cell activation requires the transcription factor MYC and is accompanied by an increase in cell size and entry into cell cycle.[32,33] Once in follicles, the B cells downregulate MYC and BCL2 and upregulate the transcriptional repressor

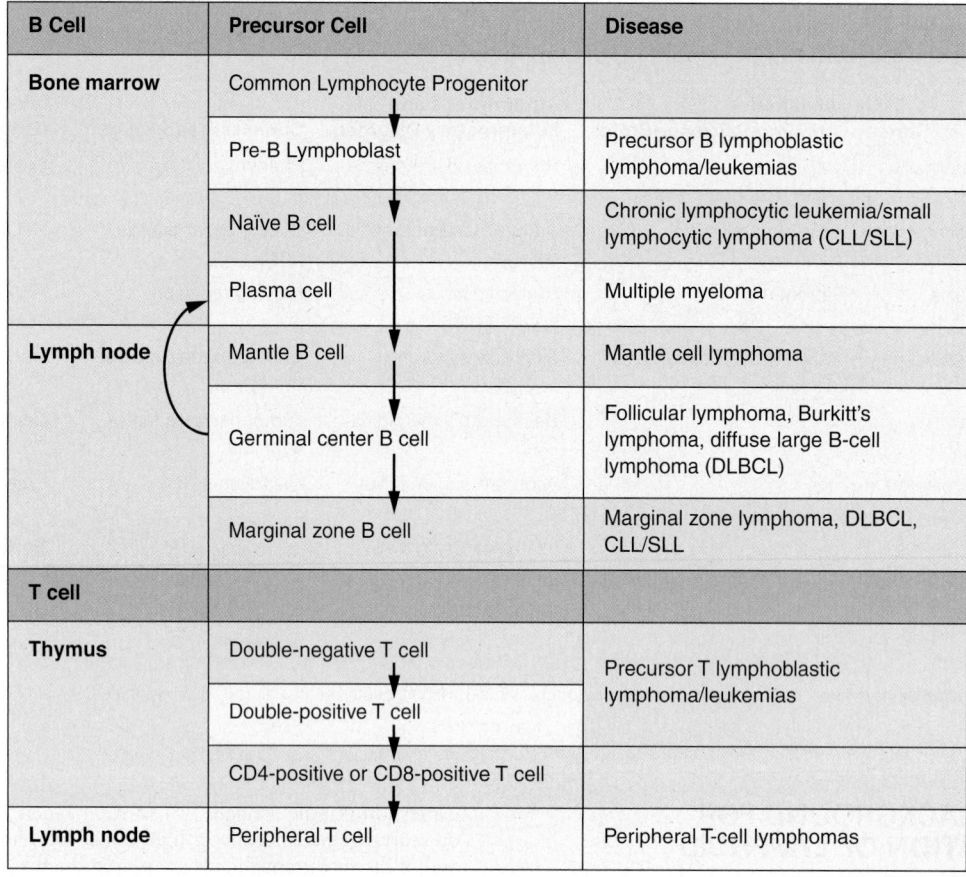

Figure 103.1 B- and T-cell development and cell of origin of lymphomas.

B Cell	Precursor Cell	Disease
Bone marrow	Common Lymphocyte Progenitor	
	Pre-B Lymphoblast	Precursor B lymphoblastic lymphoma/leukemias
	Naïve B cell	Chronic lymphocytic leukemia/small lymphocytic lymphoma (CLL/SLL)
	Plasma cell	Multiple myeloma
Lymph node	Mantle B cell	Mantle cell lymphoma
	Germinal center B cell	Follicular lymphoma, Burkitt's lymphoma, diffuse large B-cell lymphoma (DLBCL)
	Marginal zone B cell	Marginal zone lymphoma, DLBCL, CLL/SLL
T cell		
Thymus	Double-negative T cell	Precursor T lymphoblastic lymphoma/leukemias
	Double-positive T cell	
	CD4-positive or CD8-positive T cell	
Lymph node	Peripheral T cell	Peripheral T-cell lymphomas

TABLE 103.2

Cluster Designations (CD) of Antigens Useful in Non-Hodgkin Lymphoma Classification

CD	Normal Lymphocyte Expression	Neoplastic Lymphocyte Expression
1a	Cortical thymocytes; Langerhans cells	Precursor T-lymphoblastic lymphoma/leukemia; Langerhans cell neoplasms
2	T and NK cells	T- and NK cell lymphomas
3	T (cytoplasmic and surface) and NK (cytoplasmic only) cells	T- and NK cell lymphomas
4	T and NK cells	T- and NK cell lymphomas
5	T cells, naïve B cells	Chronic lymphocytic leukemia/small lymphocytic lymphoma (CLL/SLL); mantle cell lymphoma; T-cell neoplasms
7	T and NK cells	T and NK cell lymphomas
8	T- and NK cell subsets	Some T and NK cell lymphomas
10	Precursor and germinal center B cells	Precursor B and T lymphoblastic lymphoma/leukemia; follicular lymphoma; Burkitt's lymphoma; diffuse large B cell lymphoma (DLBCL)
11c	B cell subset; CD8 T cells; NK cells	Hairy cell leukemia; splenic marginal zone lymphoma; CLL/SLL
16	NK cells	NK cell and some T-cell lymphomas
19	B cells	B-cell lymphomas
20	Mature B cells (except plasma cells)	Mature B-cell lymphomas
23	Activated B cells, follicular dendritic cells	CLL/SLL
25	Activated T and B cells	Hairy cell leukemia; adult T-cell leukemia/lymphoma
30	Activated lymphocytes (B, T, and NK cells)	Anaplastic large cell lymphoma (ALCL)
56	NK and activated T cells	NK and T-cell lymphomas; plasma cell neoplasms
57	NK and T-cell subsets	NK and T-cell lymphomas
103	Mucosal intraepithelial lymphocytes	Hairy cell leukemia; enteropathy-type T-cell lymphoma
138	Plasma cells	Plasma cell neoplasms; plasmablastic lymphoma

BCL6, which, like MYC, is essential for secondary B-cell follicle formation; secondary follicles are also known as germinal centers.[34] Downregulation of BCL2 may permit the elimination of B cells making low affinity antibodies, and in fact, most B cells entering into the germinal centers undergo apoptosis and are phagocytosed by resident macrophages (often referred to as tingible body macrophages because they contain a readily visible nuclear fragment derived from defunct B cells). The key roles of MYC, BCL2, and BCL6 in this process explain why the genes encoding these factors are commonly mutated in B-cell lymphomas (discussed later). Follicular B cells also upregulate the expression of activation-induced cytosine deaminase (AID), a gene product required for both somatic hypermutation and Ig class switching. Cells that by chance acquire mutations that increase Ig affinity for an antigen survive thanks to signals transmitted through the Ig receptor and go on to undergo class-switching, a process that is regulated by cytokines.[35] The germinal center reaction also requires follicular dendritic cells and a special class of CD4-positive follicular T cells that express the CD40 ligand.[36] B cells that survive this process may leave the germinal centers to take up residence in surrounding marginal zones to become long-lived memory B cells, or may terminally differentiate into plasma cells, which may take up residence in the medulla of the lymph nodes or the red pulp of the spleen, or home back to the bone marrow.

It is notable that the most common human lymphomas are B-cell tumors composed of lymphocytes with somatically mutated Ig genes, an alteration that marks these tumors as having arisen from cells that have experienced a germinal center reaction. Many of these same tumors also have mutations that bear the molecular hallmarks of mistakes that occurred during attempted somatic hypermutation or class-switching in germinal centers; indeed, mutations involving MYC, BCL2, and BCL6 identical to those found in lymphomas are also found at a low frequency in normal germinal center B cells obtained from both children and adults. Thus, the relatively high frequency of tumors derived from germinal center B cells likely reflects the error-prone nature of the molecular events that permit antibody class-switching and affinity maturation.

T-Cell Development

Progenitors from the bone marrow that travel to the thymus become committed to T-cell differentiation via interactions with thymic epithelial cells (TEC) (see Fig. 103.1). TECs express ligands for Notch receptors such as DLL4, leading to activation of the receptor NOTCH1, which is essential for early stages of T-cell development.[37] As during early B-cell development, early T-cell development is controlled by a transcriptional program induced by a master transcription factor (NOTCH1) and by survival signals mediated by complexes containing components of the T-cell receptor (TCR).[38] In most developing T cells, this begins with rearrangement of the TCRβ genes, which (as in B cells) requires RAG1 and RAG2 and involves the participation of TdT. Productive, in-frame rearrangement of the TCRβ gene permits expression of the TCRβ polypeptide, which pairs with pre-Tα polypeptides and assembles into the pre–T-cell receptor. Prosurvival signals transmitted by pre-Tα allow cells to go on to rearrange the TCRα genes, and cells with productive TCRα rearrangements express TCRαβ receptors on their cell surfaces in complex with CD3 polypeptides. Surviving cells also upregulate the CD4 and CD8 coreceptors and proceed through both negative and positive antigenic selection, during which cells expressing autoreactive TCRs or TCRs that fail to recognize antigen in the context of major histocompatibility complex (MHC) antigens are eliminated by apoptosis.[39] Cells emerging from the thymus as naïve T cells express either CD4, a coreceptor for MHC class II antigens, or CD8, a coreceptor for MHC class I antigens. A much smaller subset of thymic T-cell progenitors productively rearrange their δ and γ TCR genes, and emerge from the thymus as naïve γδ-TCR–expressing T cells.

Like naïve B cells, naïve T cells home to peripheral tissues under the influence of chemokines, with most γδ T cells homing to gut and skin, and αβ T cells homing much more widely to secondary lymphoid tissues and other sites. γδ T cells are considered to be relative primitive cells that contribute to *natural* immunity, whereas αβ T cells can differentiate further into a number of different types of effector cells, depending on the dose, timing, and context of subsequent antigenic exposures. αβ T cells recognize antigen when it is presented in the context of an MHC molecule. CD4+ T cells, or T-helper cells, bind to and recognize an antigen presented by MHC class II molecules, whereas CD8+ T cells or cytotoxic T cells bind to and recognize antigen presented by MHC class I molecules. Activation also requires CD40 and CD40L interaction and CD28/CTLA4 and B7 interaction between the T cell and the antigen presenting cell (APC).[40] Antigen stimulation of CD8-positive T cells may give rise to CD8-positive effector cytotoxic cells or to long-lived CD8-positive memory cells. By contrast, antigen stimulation of CD4-positive cells can produce a number of CD4-positive effector cell types, including: T helper 1 (Th1) cells, which activate macrophages and cytotoxic T cells through their production of interleukin 2 (IL-2) and interferon gamma; T helper 2 (Th2) cells, which activate B cells through their production of IL-4, -5, -6, and -13[41,42]; T helper 17 (Th17) cells, which stimulate neutrophils through production of IL-17 and IL-22; and regulatory T cells (Treg), which produce immunosuppressive cytokines such as IL-10. Finally, follicular helper T cells are CD4+ T cells that home to the germinal center via CXCR5 and CXCL13 interactions and play a role in B-cell Ig class switching and Ig production.[43]

Natural Killer Cells

There is a third class of lymphocytes that can kill targets without MHC restriction, namely NK cells, which are a component of the innate host immune system. NK cells recognize and kill cells that lack MHC class I molecules (including virally infected cells and malignant cells), as well as antibody-coated targets through interactions with Fc receptors on the NK cell surface. NK cells lack surface CD3 and do not have rearranged TCR genes. Morphologically, these cells are slightly larger than resting T and B cells and have paler cytoplasm that contains azurophilic granules, an appearance similar to that of activated cytotoxic T cells.

Immunophenotyping of Lymphoid Cells

As has been alluded to, lymphocytes at various stages in ontologic development can be defined and differentiated by the detection of certain antigens on the cell surface (see Table 103.2). This antigen footprint is referred to as the immunophenotype of the cell. It can be detected by a flow cytometric analysis of single cell suspensions from whole blood, bone marrow, body fluid, or disaggregated tissue using fluorescently labeled antibodies against these antigens or by immunohistochemistry, which involves the incubation of paraffin-embedded tissue sections with enzyme-linked antibodies against these antigens followed by a colorimetric reaction. These techniques have become vital in diagnosing and monitoring lymphomas, and have provided insight into the normal counterparts of the malignant lymphocyte.

Chromosomal Translocations and Oncogene Rearrangements

Given the mechanism of Ig and TCR gene rearrangements in lymphoid cells—namely, the formation of DNA breaks with the joining of new pieces of DNA—it is not surprising that lymphomas are frequently found to have chromosomal translocations that involve the activation of an oncogene or inactivation of a tumor suppressor

TABLE 103.3

Genetic Features of B- and T-Cell Lymphomas

Genetic Feature	Genes	Lymphoma
t(8;14) t(2;8) t(8;22)	MYC/IgH MYC/Igκ MYC/Igλ	Burkitt's lymphoma
t(11;14)	BCL1 (CCND1)/IgH	Mantle cell lymphoma; multiple myeloma
t(14;18) t(3;14)	BCL2/IgH BCL6/IgH	Follicular lymphoma; diffuse large B-cell lymphoma (DLBCL)
t(11;18) t(1;14) t(14;18) t(3;14)	API2/MALT1 BCL10/IgH MALT1/IgH FOXP1/IgH	MALT lymphoma
Trisomy 3 7q21 deletion	Unknown CDK6	Splenic marginal zone lymphoma
11q23 deletion 13q14 deletion 17p13 deletion Trisomy 12	ATM Unknown TP53 Unknown	Chronic lymphocytic leukemia/small lymphocytic lymphoma (CLL/SLL); del(17p) and del(13q) also in multiple myeloma; del(11q) also in T-cell prolymphocytic leukemia (T-PLL)
t(9;14) 6q21 deletion	PAX5/IgH Unknown	Lymphoplasmacytic lymphoma
9p gain	JAK2, PDL1, PDL2	Mediastinal large B-cell lymphoma
inv(14) t(14;14)	TCRα/TCL1	Peripheral T-cell lymphoma, NOS; T-PLL
t(2;5) t(1;2) t(2;3) t(2;17) inv(2)	NPM1/ALK TPM3/ALK TFG/ALK CTLC/ALK ATIC/ALK	Anaplastic large cell lymphoma (ALCL)
Trisomy 3 Trisomy 5	Unknown Unknown	Angioimmunoblastic T-cell lymphoma
Isochromosome 7q	Unknown	Hepatosplenic T-cell lymphoma

MALT, mucosa-associated lymphoid tissue; CTLC, clathrin heavy chain 1.

gene (Table 103.3). The former is more common, whereby a proto-oncogene is brought under the control of a constitutively active promoter. The resulting overexpression of the involved gene (now called an oncogene) conveys oncogenic properties on the gene and its protein product, which is responsible for induction and/or maintenance of some aspect of the transformed phenotype. Examples of this type of event include the (8;14)(q24;q32) translocation in BL, involving the MYC proto-oncogene and the IgH gene; the (14;18)(q32;q32) translocation in follicular lymphoma, involving the BCL2 proto-oncogene and the IgH gene; and the (11;14) (q13;q32) translocation in mantle cell lymphoma, involving the gene encoding cyclin D1 (CCDN1) and the IgH gene. Less commonly, chromosomal translocations produce fusion genes that encode chimeric oncogenic proteins. Examples of this include the (2;5)(p23;q35) translocation involving the ALK and NPM1 genes in anaplastic large cell lymphoma (ALCL) and the t(11;18)(q21;q21) translocation involving the API2 and MLT genes in mucosa-associated lymphoid tissue (MALT) lymphoma. These translocations and rearrangements can be detected by polymerase chain reaction (PCR) using probes that span the chromosomal breakpoints, reverse transcriptase PCR (RT-PCR) to detect the RNA product of the fusion gene, or fluorescence in situ hybridization (FISH) using probes to specific chromosomal segments. In cases where the translocation results in the expression of a protein or portion of a protein that is never expressed in normal lymphocytes (e.g., anaplastic lymphoma kinase [ALK]

kinase), immunohistochemistry can be used to detect the protein and infer the presence of a rearrangement involving the gene that encodes that protein.

LYMPHOMA CLASSIFICATION: THE PRINCIPLES OF THE WORLD HEALTH ORGANIZATION (WHO) CLASSIFICATION OF LYMPHOID NEOPLASMS

In 2001, the World Health Organization (WHO) published a new classification of tumors of the hematopoietic and lymphoid tissues (Table 103.4).[44] It was the end result of a project that began in 1995 with 10 committees of pathologists and a Clinical Advisory Committee of international experts to ensure the clinical utility of the classification system. It incorporated, with minor edits, the 1994 consensus by the International Lymphoma Study Group regarding a list of lymphoid neoplasms that were distinct and recognizable by pathologists called the Revised European and American Lymphoma (REAL) classification.[45] The principle behind the classification system is to use and integrate all of the relevant information, including morphology, immunophenotype, genetics, and clinical features, to define disease entities with the relative importance of each type of information varying from disease to disease. The WHO classification system was recently updated and diseases were

> **TABLE 103.4**

World Health Organization Classification of Lymphoid Neoplasms 2008

Precursor B- and T-Cell Neoplasms
Precursor B-lymphoblastic leukemia/lymphoma
Precursor T-lymphoblastic leukemia/lymphoma

Mature B-Cell Neoplasms
Chronic lymphocytic leukemia/small lymphocytic lymphoma
B-cell prolymphocytic leukemia
Lymphoplasmacytic lymphoma
Splenic marginal zone lymphoma
Hairy cell leukemia
Splenic B-cell lymphoma, unclassifiable
    Splenic diffuse red pulp small B-cell lymphoma
    Hairy cell leukemia – variant
Plasma cell neoplasms
    Monoclonal gammopathy of undetermined significance (MGUS)
    Plasma cell myeloma
    Solitary plasmacytoma of bone
    Extraosseous plasmacytoma
    Monoclonal immunoglobulin deposition disease
Extranodal marginal zone lymphoma
Nodal marginal zone lymphoma
Follicular lymphoma
Primary cutaneous follicle center lymphoma
Mantle cell lymphoma
Diffuse large B-cell lymphoma (DLBCL)
    T cell/histiocyte-rich large B-cell lymphoma
    Primary DLBCL of the central nervous system
    Primary cutaneous DLBCL, leg type
    EBV-positive DLBCL of the elderly
DLBCL associated with chronic inflammation
Lymphomatoid granulomatosis
Primary mediastinal large B-cell lymphoma
Intravascular large B-cell lymphoma
ALK-positive large B-cell lymphoma
Plasmablastic lymphoma
Large B-cell lymphoma arising in HHV-8–associated multicentric
    Castleman's disease
Burkitt's lymphoma (BL)
B-cell lymphoma, unclassifiable, with features intermediate
    between DLBCL and BL
B-cell lymphoma, unclassifiable, with features intermediate
    between DLBCL and HL

Mature T- and NK Cell Neoplasms
T-cell prolymphocytic leukemia
T-cell large granular lymphocytic leukemia
Chronic lymphoproliferative disorder of NK cells
Aggressive NK cell leukemia
EBV-positive T-cell lymphoproliferative diseases of childhood
    Systemic EBV+ T-cell lymphoproliferative disease of childhood
    Hydroa vaccinforme-like lymphoma
Adult T-cell leukemia/lymphoma
Extranodal NK/T-cell lymphoma, nasal type
Enteropathy-type T-cell lymphoma
Hepatosplenic T-cell lymphoma
Subcutaneous panniculitis-like T-cell lymphoma
Mycosis fungoides
Sézary's syndrome
Primary cutaneous CD30+ T-cell lymphoproliferative disorders
    Primary cutaneous anaplastic large cell lymphoma
    Lymphomatoid papulosis
Primary cutaneous peripheral T-cell lymphomas, rare subtypes
    Primary cutaneous γ-δ T-cell lymphoma
    Primary cutaneous CD8+ aggressive epidermotropic cytotoxic
        T-cell lymphoma
    Primary cutaneous CD4+ small/medium T-cell lymphoma
Peripheral T-cell lymphoma, not otherwise specified
Angioimmunoblastic T-cell lymphoma
Anaplastic large cell lymphoma, ALK+
Anaplastic large cell lymphoma, ALK–

Immunodeficiency-Associated Lymphoproliferative Disorders
Lymphoproliferative diseases associated with primary immune
    disorders
Lymphomas associated with HIV infection
Posttransplant lymphoproliferative disorders (PTLD)
    Plasmacytic hyperplasia and infectious mononucleosis-like PTLD
    Polymorphic PTLD
    Monomorphic PTLD
    Classical HL-type PTLD
Other iatrogenic immunodeficiency-associated lymphoproliferative
    disorders

reclassified in 2008 based on new and evolving information with regard to each of these disease characteristics.

Categories of Lymphoid Neoplasms

There are five main categories of lymphoid neoplasms defined by the WHO: precursor B- and T-cell neoplasms, mature B-cell neoplasms, mature T/NK cell neoplasms, HL, and immunodeficiency-associated lymphoproliferative disorders (see Table 103.4). Each category is a set of distinct diagnoses that are not further classified or grouped by grade, prognosis, or clinical behavior but instead are considered unique entities. In 2001, there were 48 such entities plus additional variants. In 2008, several additions were made, and several provisional diagnostic categories were created that reflect the additional information being gleaned from technology, such as gene expression profiling (GEP) and the consequent recognition of heterogeneity within existing disease entities. For example, within DLBCL, GEP can differentiate between two broad categories of disease, namely the germinal center B-cell type (GCB) and the activated B-cell type (ABC), with different prognoses.[46]

These categories have not yet been adopted into the WHO because they are not yet relevant to differential treatment strategies, but new treatments are being developed with these GEPs in mind, and treatment effect is being stratified by DLBCL subtype in ongoing clinical trials, and this will likely become clinically relevant in the near future. Furthermore, disease location is being recognized as important in distinguishing one DLBCL from another, with DLBCL of certain locations like the central nervous system (CNS) or primary cutaneous DLBCL, leg type, having unique clinical presentations, clinical behavior, and GEPs compared with nodal DLBCL; these have been added as distinct entities to the 2008 WHO. The microenvironment is another important defining feature of some lymphomas and, as such, T-cell/histiocyte–rich large B-cell lymphoma was added to the updated classification. Finally, two provisional categories have been created to recognize lymphomas that have features intermediate between two types of lymphoma, the so-called gray zone lymphomas: B-cell lymphoma unclassifiable (BCLU) with features intermediate between BL and DLBCL (BCLU-BL/DLBCL) and BCLU with features intermediate between HL and DLBCL (BCLU-HL/DLBCL). These categories were created recognizing that they are likely a heterogenous group of disease, with some most closely resembling BL or HL, some most closely resembling DLBCL, and some belonging to distinct entities, helping to create a more systematic approach to their study and classification.

PRINCIPLES OF MANAGEMENT OF NON-HODGKIN'S LYMPHOMA

Differential Diagnosis and Sites of Disease at Presentation

More than two-thirds of patients with NHL present with persistent painless peripheral lymphadenopathy. At the time of presentation, a differential diagnosis of generalized lymphadenopathy necessitates the exclusion of infectious etiologies such as bacteria (including mycobacteria), viruses (e.g., infectious mononucleosis, cytomegalovirus, hepatitis B, HIV), and parasites (toxoplasmosis) as well as inflammatory and autoimmune diseases, and metastatic malignancies. It is generally agreed that a lymph node larger than 1.5×1.5 cm that is not associated with a documented infection and that persists longer than 4 weeks should be considered for a biopsy.[47] A biopsy should be performed immediately for patients with other findings suggesting malignancy (e.g., systemic complaints or B symptoms, such as fever, night sweats, weight loss). However, lymph nodes in several histopathologic subtypes of NHLs frequently wax and wane. In teenagers and young adults, infectious mononucleosis and HL should be placed high in the differential diagnosis. Involvement of Waldeyer's ring, epitrochlear, and mesenteric nodes are more frequently observed in patients with NHL than in patients with HL. About 40% of all patients with NHL present with systemic complaints. B symptoms are more common in patients with aggressive histologies approaching 50%. Less frequent presenting symptoms, occurring in less than 20% of patients, include fatigue, malaise, and pruritus.

NHLs also present with thoracic, abdominal, and/or extranodal symptoms. Although much less common than with HL, approximately 20% of patients with NHL have mediastinal adenopathy. These patients most frequently present with persistent cough, chest discomfort, or without clinical symptoms but have an abnormal chest radiograph. Occasionally, a superior vena cava syndrome accompanies presentation. A differential diagnosis of mediastinal presentation includes infections (e.g., histoplasmosis, tuberculosis, infectious mononucleosis), sarcoidosis, HL, as well as other malignancies. Involvement of retroperitoneal, mesenteric, and pelvic nodes is common in most histologic subtypes of NHL. Unless massive or leading to obstruction, nodal enlargement in these sites often does not produce symptoms. In contrast, patients with an abdominal mass, massive splenomegaly, or primary gastrointestinal (GI) lymphoma present with complaints similar to those caused by other space-occupying lesions. These complaints include chronic pain, abdominal fullness, and early satiety, symptoms associated with visceral obstruction or even acute perforation and GI hemorrhage. Rarely, patients present with symptoms of unexplained anemia. Those with aggressive NHLs can present with primary cutaneous lesions, testicular masses, acute spinal cord compression, solitary bone lesions, and rarely, lymphomatous meningitis. Symptoms of primary NHL of the CNS include headache, lethargy, focal neurologic symptoms, seizures, and paralysis.

When NHL involves an extranodal site, the differential diagnosis is more difficult. NHL uncommonly presents in the lungs as bronchovascular, lymphangitic, nodular, or alveolar patterns of involvement.[48] Between 25% and 50% of patients with NHLs present with hepatic infiltration, although relatively few present with large hepatic masses. Of the advanced-stage indolent lymphomas, nearly 75% of patients have microscopic hepatic infiltration at presentation. In contrast, primary hepatic lymphoma is rare and is nearly always an aggressive histology. Primary lymphoma of bone

is another uncommon extranodal site, occurring in less than 5% of patients and often presenting as bone pain. Most frequently, lytic lesions are observed on standard radiographs. The most common sites of primary lymphoma of bone include the femur, the pelvis, and the vertebrae. Approximately 5% of NHLs are primary GI lymphomas. These tumors are often associated with hemorrhage, pain, or obstruction. The stomach is most frequently involved, followed by the small intestine, and the colon. Most GI lymphomas are of the diffuse aggressive histologies, specifically DLBCL, mantle cell lymphoma (MCL), and intestinal T-cell lymphoma. The most common site for extranodal MZLs is the stomach. A subset of MCLs presents as multiple intestinal polyposis, which may arise at any site in the GI tract. An uncommon presentation (2% to 14%) of NHL is renal infiltration, and even less common is localized presentation in the prostate, testis, or ovary. The typical histologic subtypes of these sites are DLBCL, BL, and gray zone tumors with features intermediate between DLBCL and BL. Rare sites of primary lymphoma include the orbit, heart, breast, salivary glands, the thyroid, and the adrenal gland.

Diagnosis and Initial Management

After the initial biopsy, a careful history and physical exam should be done to help assess the extent and pace of disease. Attention should be paid to the duration of symptoms and pace of symptomatic progression, whether symptoms associated with a poorer prognosis, such as fevers, night sweats, or unexplained weight loss are present, and to localizing symptoms that may point toward lymphomatous involvement of specific sites, such as the chest, abdomen, or CNS. Concurrent illness that may impact therapy or monitoring on therapy should be ascertained, including a history of diabetes or congestive heart failure. A physical exam should pay close attention to all the peripherally accessible sites of lymph nodes; the liver and spleen size; Waldeyer's ring; whether there is a pleural or pericardial effusion or abdominal ascites; whether there is an abdominal, testicular or breast mass; and whether there is cutaneous involvement because all of these findings may influence further evaluation and disease management.

Laboratory studies should be obtained, including complete blood count, routine chemistries, liver function tests, and serum protein electrophoresis to document the presence of circulating monoclonal paraproteins. The serum beta-2 microglobulin level and serum lactate dehydrogenase (LDH) are important independent prognostic factors in NHL. A bone marrow biopsy should be considered for staging and prognostic purposes depending on the disease histology and the results of other laboratory and staging studies. An evaluation of the cerebrospinal fluid (CSF) for lymphomatous involvement may be indicated in the setting of concerning neurologic signs or symptoms or a disease that has a high propensity to spread to the CNS. The latter includes a disease involving the paranasal sinuses, testes, and epidural space, as well as highly aggressive histologies like BL.

Imaging studies depend on the histology of the lymphoma as well as the clinical presentation. Chest, abdominal, and pelvic computed tomography (CT) scans are essential for accurate staging to assess lymphadenopathy for indolent lymphomas. Radionuclide scans have clinical utility as diagnostic and monitoring studies. [67]Gallium scanning, used based on the ability of this isotope to bind transferrin receptors on tumor cells, has been replaced by positron-emission tomography (PET) using ^{18}F-fluorodeoxyglucose (FDG). FDG-PET scanning is highly sensitive for detecting both nodal and extranodal sites involved by NHL. PET scanning is particularly useful for the histologically aggressive lymphomas, including BL, DLBCL, plasmablastic lymphoma, and the aggressive T-cell lymphomas, but is less reliable in lower grade histologies like MZLs.[49] The intensity of FDG avidity, or standardized uptake value (SUV), correlates with histologic aggressiveness.[50,51] PET scanning detects an actively metabolizing tumor in residual masses following or during chemotherapy, and persistent abnormal uptake predicts for early relapse and/or reduced survival.[52] It is more accurate than the detection of a residual mass on CT scans, which can often be a false positive. Consensus recommendations regarding PET scanning were published as a result of an International Harmonization Project. Among the recommendations are that PET only be used for DLBCL and HL, scanning during therapy be only part of clinical trials, and the scan after all therapy is completed should be done at least 3 but preferably 6 to 8 weeks after chemotherapy and 8 to 12 weeks after radiation or chemoradiotherapy. There is no evidence that a long-term follow up should include PET scanning.[53] Finally, magnetic resonance imaging (MRI) is useful in detecting bone, bone marrow, and CNS disease in the brain and spinal cord.

Staging and Prognostic Systems

The Ann Arbor staging system developed in 1971 for HL was adapted for staging NHLs (Table 103.5).[54] This staging system focuses on the number of tumor sites (nodal and extranodal), the location, and the presence or absence of systemic, or B, symptoms. Table 103.5 summarizes the essential features of the Ann Arbor system.

The concept of staging has less impact in NHL than in HL. Only a minority of patients with both indolent and aggressive NHL have localized disease at diagnosis, and there is little therapeutic benefit to distinguish between stage III and stage IV disease because the treatment options are identical. The prognosis is more dependent on histology and clinical parameters than the stage at presentation. Staging in NHLs, therefore, is done to identify the minority of patients who can be treated with local therapy or combined modality treatment and to stratify within histologic subtypes to determine the prognosis and to assess the impact of treatment.

Probably more important than staging is the International Prognostic Index (IPI), which provides risk stratification (Table 103.6).[55] The IPI was developed based on an analysis of over 2,000 patients with diffuse aggressive NHLs treated with an anthracycline-containing regimen. This analysis identified age (≤60 years versus >60 years); serum LDH (≤ normal versus > normal); performance status (0 or 1 versus 2 to 4); stage (I or II versus III or IV); and extranodal involvement (≤ one site versus > one site) to be independently prognostic for overall survival. Four risk groups were identified based on the number of risk factors: low risk (0 or 1); low intermediate (2); high intermediate (3); and high (4 to 5). The

TABLE 103.6

International Prognostic Index (IPI)

Age >60 years
LDH > upper limit normal
ECOG Performance Status ≥2
Ann Arbor Stage III or IV
Number of extranodal disease sites >1

# of Factors	Risk Group	3-year EFS (%)	3-year PFS (%)	3-year OS (%)
0–1	Low	81	87	91
2	Low Intermediate	69	75	81
3	High Intermediate	53	59	65
4–5	High	50	50	59

ECOG, Eastern Cooperative Oncology Group; EFS, event-free survival; PFS, progression-free survival; OS, overall survival.
Adapted from Ziepert M, Hasenclever D, Kuhnt E, et al. Standard International Prognostic Index remains a valid predictor of outcome for patients with aggressive CD20+ B-cell lymphoma in the rituximab era. *J Clin Oncol* 2010;28:2373–2380.

5-year overall survival rates for patients with scores of 0 to 1, 2, 3, and 4 to 5 were 73%, 51%, 43%, and 26%, respectively. For the patients aged 60 years or less, only stage, LDH, and performance status were of prognostic significance. Patients ≤60 years with zero, one, two, or three risk factors had 5-year survival rates of 83%, 69%, 46%, and 32%, respectively. Survival rates for those age >60 years with the same scores were 56%, 44%, 37%, and 21%, respectively. The IPI has been adapted following treatment with cyclophosphamide, adriamycin, vincristine, and prednisone plus rituximab (CHOP-R) therapy for DLBCL. Within that model, the 4-year progression-free survival is 94%, 80%, and 53% for zero and one, two, or three or more risk factors, respectively.[56]

A similar predictive model has been developed for follicular lymphoma based on the analysis of over 4,000 patients with follicular NHL, known as the follicular lymphoma IPI or FLIPI (Table 103.7).[57] This study identified the following prognostic

TABLE 103.5

Ann Arbor Staging for Lymphoma

Stage	Description
I	Involvement of a single lymph node region (I) or single extranodal site (IE)
II	Involvement of two or more lymph node regions or lymphatic structures on the same side of the diaphragm alone (II) or with involvement of limited, contiguous, extralymphatic organ or tissue (IIE)
III	Involvement of lymph node regions on both sides of the diaphragm (III), which may include the spleen (IIIS), or limited, contiguous, extralymphatic organ or tissue (IIIE), or both (IIIES)
IV	Diffuse or disseminated foci of involvement of one or more extralymphatic organs or tissues, with or without associated lymphatic involvement

Note: All stages are further subdivided according to the absence (A) or presence (B) of systemic B symptoms including fevers, night sweats, and/or weight loss (>10% of body weight over 6 months prior to diagnosis).

TABLE 103.7

Follicular Lymphoma International Prognostic Index (FL-IPI)

Age >60 years
LDH > upper limit normal
Hgb <12 g/dL
Ann Arbor Stage III or IV
Number of involved nodal areas >4

# of Factors	Risk Group	5-year OS (%)	10-year OS (%)
0–1	Low	91	71
2	Intermediate	78	51
3–5	High	52	59

LDH, lactate dehydrogenase; Hgb, hemoglobin; OS, overall survival.
Adapted from Solal-Celigny P, Roy P, Colombat P, et al. Follicular lymphoma international prognostic index. *Blood* 2004;104:1258.

factors: age >60 years, stage III/IV, more than four nodal sites, elevated serum LDH concentration, and hemoglobin less than 12. The 10-year survival rates for patients with zero to one (low risk), two (intermediate risk), or three or more (high risk) of these adverse factors averaged 71%, 51%, and 36%, respectively. Similar disease-specific IPIs have been developed for mantle cell lymphoma and peripheral T-cell lymphoma as well. These prognostic indices take into account the proliferative index and cell surface markers, respectively.[58,59]

More recently, as discussed in the section on the 2008 update to the WHO, GEP has been used to examine DLBCL to identify patients with different prognoses.[46] Based on gene expression, DLBCLs have been subclassified into GCB or ABC types. Patients with GCB-like DLBCL had significantly better overall survival than those with the ABC-like variant. Based on findings from GEP, immunohistochemical staining of a limited number of proteins has been proposed as an alternative method for subtyping of DLBCL and prognostication.[60] Germinal center and nongerminal center B-cell derivation can be determined by the expression of markers such as CD10, B cell lymphoma–6 protein (BCL-6), and multiple myeloma oncogene 1 (MUM1). Based on immunohistochemistry, it is estimated that approximately 40% of DLBCLs are of the GCB subtype, with the remainder falling into the non-GCB group.

Restaging after treatment is typically done 6 to 8 weeks following the completion of chemotherapy (or chemoimmunotherapy), or 8 to 12 weeks after the completion of radiotherapy or combination chemotherapy and radiotherapy, to assess for disease response to treatment. The most important prognostic factor is the achievement of a complete response to therapy. Restaging at the completion of treatment is often with the repetition of studies that were abnormal at diagnosis. It should be noted that patients with certain lymphomas or bulky disease may not have complete regression of their lymphadenopathy despite there not being any remaining active lymphoma. Nuclear studies, like PET/CT scans, and/or rebiopsy can be helpful in differentiating residual fibrotic tissue from active lymphoma.

SPECIFIC DISEASE ENTITIES

Precursor B-Cell and T-Cell Leukemia/ Lymphoma

Lymphoblastic lymphoma and acute lymphoblastic leukemia appear to be different manifestations of the same disease entity (see Chapter 110). Cytologically, both are composed of blasts with a high nuclear-to-cytoplasmic ratio, scant cytoplasm, and nuclei with slightly coarse chromatin with multiple small nucleoli. The nuclei may be oval, but more often are folded or convoluted. The blasts are usually intermediate in size, but they may be large, or in unusual cases, so small that there may be confusion morphologically with CLL. When lymph nodes are involved, they are diffusely effaced by blasts. Mitotic figures are usually frequent, and (as with all high-grade lymphomas) some cases contain frequent tingible body macrophages, producing a starry-sky appearance that mimics BL.

Approximately 85% to 90% of lymphoblastic lymphomas are of the T-cell lineage, with the remainder being of the B-cell type. Both are comprised of tumor cells with immunophenotypes that correspond to stages of pre-T and pre-B–cell development, respectively. B-lymphoblastic tumors express CD19 and are variably positive for other B lineage markers and negative in most cases for surface immunoglobulin. T lymphoblastic tumors usually express cytoplasmic CD3 but may be surface CD3 negative, and show variable expression of other T-cell markers. Most lymphoblastic tumors are positive for TdT, a specific marker of immature lymphoid cells that can be detected by flow cytometry or immunohistochemistry.

Although lymphoblastic lymphomas represent a major subgroup of childhood NHLs, they are unusual in adults (2% of adult NHLs). Patients are usually adolescent or young adult males who present with lymphadenopathy in cervical, supraclavicular, and axillary regions (50%) or with a mediastinal mass (50% to 75%). These masses can be associated with superior vena cava syndrome, tracheal obstruction, and pericardial effusions. Less commonly, patients present with extranodal disease (skin, testicular, or bony involvement). More than 80% of patients present with stage III or stage IV disease, almost 50% have B symptoms, and the majority has an elevated LDH. Although the bone marrow can be uninvolved at presentation, virtually all patients develop bone marrow infiltration and a subsequent leukemic phase indistinguishable from T-cell acute lymphoblastic leukemia. Patients with bone marrow involvement have a very high incidence of CNS infiltration. B-cell lymphoblastic lymphoma is a very rare entity, with patients having a median age of 39 years.[61] B-cell lymphoblastic lymphomas present without a mediastinal mass but instead involve lymph nodes and extranodal sites.

The treatment of precursor B-cell and T-cell lymphoblastic leukemia/lymphoma is detailed in Chapter 110.

Follicular Lymphoma

Introduction

FL is the second most common lymphoma diagnosed in the United States and western Europe, making up approximately 20% of all NHLs, and 70% of indolent lymphomas.[62] The median age at diagnosis is 60 years, and there is a slight female predominance.[63,64] The incidence is increased among relatives of persons with FL.[65]

Pathology

FLs are malignant counterparts of normal germinal center B cells.[44] FL recapitulates the architecture of normal germinal centers (GC) of secondary lymphoid follicles.[44] The neoplastic cells consist of a mixture of centrocytes (small- to medium-sized cells with irregular or cleaved nuclei and scant cytoplasm) and centroblast (large cells with oval nuclei, several nucleoli, and moderate amounts of cytoplasm). The clinical aggressiveness of the tumor correlates with the number of centroblasts that are present. The WHO classification[44] adopted grading from 1 to 3 based on the number of centroblasts counted per high power field (hpf): Grade I, 0 to 5 centroblasts/hpf; Grade II, 6 to 15 centroblasts/hpf; Grade III, more than 15 centroblasts/hpf. Grade III has been subdivided into grade IIIa, in which centrocytes predominate, and grade IIIb, in which there are sheets of centroblasts.[66] Although the grading system remains in place, clinically, grade I and II and many cases of grade IIIa FLs are approached similarly. Akin to normal GCs, small numbers of T cells and follicular dendritic cells are present in the malignant follicles; however, tingible body macrophages, cells that have ingested apoptotic cells that are common in reactive GCs, are not observed. Involvement of the peripheral blood with malignant cells is commonly seen, and morphologically, these cells have notches and have been referred to as *buttock cells*. FL grade IIIb is an aggressive disease grouped with diffuse large B-cell lymphoma. Bone marrow involvement is exceedingly common in FL patients, usually taking the form of paratrabecular lymphoid aggregates.[44]

Immunophenotype and Genetics

FL cells express monoclonal immunoglobulin light chain, CD19, CD20, CD10, and BCL6 and are negative for CD5 and CD23. In virtually all cases, FL cells overexpress BCL-2. Clonal Ig gene rearrangements are present and, in most cases, the Ig loci have extensive somatic mutations, further supporting a GC origin. Approximately 85% of FLs have the t(14;18), which drives overexpression of BCL-2, a member of a family of proteins that blocks apoptosis. However, multiple genetic events are required for the development of FL, because the t(14;18) can be identified in a small fraction of normal B cells in most normal children and adults. Deep sequencing studies have established that the most common mutations in FL (90% of tumors) involve mixed-lineage leukemia 2 protein (*MLL2*), a gene encoding a histone H3 methylase.[67,68] Less common recurrent mutations involve other genes involving epigenetic modifying genes, such as *EZH2*, *CREBBP*, and *EP300*, indicating that genetically determined alterations in the epigenome contribute to FL in ways that remain to be defined. Other recent studies suggest that reactive cells within the malignant microenvironment also contribute to the pathobiology of FL, based on evidence that immune signatures of T cell and macrophage infiltration defined by gene expression profiling are predictive of outcome.[69]

Clinical Features

Patients with FL generally present with asymptomatic lymphadenopathy, which often waxes and wanes over the course of years. Bone marrow involvement is present in 70% of patients, whereas involvement of other nonlymphoid organs is uncommon. Less than 20% of patients present with B symptoms or an increased serum LDH. In a small subset of patients, the disease presents in the intestine; such patients usually have an early stage and a favorable prognosis.[70] Histologic transformation of FL to DLBCL occurs in 10% to 70% of patients over time, with a risk of about 2% to 3% per year[71–73] and is associated with the rapid progression of lymphadenopathy, extranodal disease (besides the marrow), B symptoms, elevated serum LDH, and calcium.

Prognosis

Measures of outcome include the FLIPI (see Table 103.7) and tumor grade.[74] A modified version of this score, the FLIPI2, evaluated five parameters, with some overlap of the FLIPI.[75] The utility of the FLIPI2 model remains uncertain. Since the incorporation of rituximab into the mainstream therapy of FL, the FLIPI has continued to be a useful prognostic model.[76]

FL tumors are graded from 1 to 3 and this grade has some prognostic utility. There has generally been suboptimal consensus of pathologists on grading FL. There is no evidence to support a different treatment approach between grade I and grade II FL. Differences in molecular genetics as well as clinical behavior suggest that FL grade IIIa is more commonly an indolent disease, whereas grade IIIb is an aggressive disease.[44,77]

The investigation of the cellular microenvironment of FL has provided interesting insights into prognosis.[78–87] It has been suggested that FL is an immunologically functional disease in which an interaction between the tumor cells and the microenvironment modulates clinical behavior. These studies, which have observed an impact on the prognosis of reactive macrophages and T cells, need additional study in larger data sets and a prospective design with uniformly treated patient populations.

Treatment of Early Stage Disease

Less than 10% of patients with FL have stage I/II disease.[88] Radiation therapy is the treatment of choice for limited stage FL and results in a 5-, 10-, and 15-year freedom from treatment failure of 72%, 46%, and 39%, and an overall 5-, 10-, and 15-year survival rates of 93%, 75%, and 62%, respectively, with a median survival of approximately 19 years.[89] A dose of 24 to 30 Gy appears to be highly effective, with no evidence of benefit for higher doses.[90] However, most patients with stage I disease treated in the United States do not receive radiation therapy.[88] This is surprising given a large study of over 6,000 patients with stage I or stage II FL diagnosed from 1973 to 2004, 34% of whom were initially treated with RT, where patients who received initial radiation therapy (RT) had higher rates of disease-specific survival at 5 years (90% versus 81%), 10 years (79% versus 66%), 15 years (68% versus 57%), and 20 years (63% versus 51%).[91]

In pre-rituximab era studies, adjuvant chemotherapy probably does not add additional benefit after local RT.[92] A recent retrospective analysis suggested an improved progression-free survival (PFS) outcome with chemoimmunotherapy or systemic therapy plus RT as compared to RT alone, with no impact on overall survival (OS).[93] This will require additional study. If significant morbidity is possible from RT based on the location of the disease area or if the patient chooses to not receive RT, observation may be a reasonable alternative, especially for stage II patients.[94] In this report, the median OS of selected untreated patients was 19 years. At a median follow-up of 7 years, 63% of patients had not required treatment.

Treatment of Advanced Stage Disease

The overwhelming majority of patients have advanced stage disease at diagnosis. Patients with asymptomatic FL do not require immediate treatment unless they have symptomatic nodal disease, compromised end organ function, B symptoms, symptomatic extranodal disease, or cytopenias. This approach is supported by randomized prospective trials of observation versus immediate treatment. One of the largest trials compared immediate treatment with chlorambucil to observation.[95] At a median follow-up of 16 years, no difference in OS and cause-specific survival was seen between the two approaches. Similar results have been noted in other prospective trials of initial treatment versus observation.[96]

A major question is whether rituximab might change this approach in early treatment in asymptomatic patients. A retrospective analysis of good risk patients who were either observed or received single-agent rituximab[97] found no negative impact of watchful waiting. A prospective study compared observation to rituximab alone or rituximab followed by maintenance in previously untreated FL. The median time to next treatment was 34 months in the watch and wait patient but was not reached in the rituximab-treatment arm. The 3-year PFS was 33%, 80%, and 90% of the observed, rituximab, or rituximab followed by maintenance patients, respectively, with 95% OS in all three groups. The important issues of time to second therapy, quality of life, impact on histologic transformation, cost, toxicity, and future responses to rituximab are not yet addressed.[98]

Rituximab has changed the paradigm of treating FL. The recent improvement in survival of patients with FL is largely due to the use of anti-CD20 monoclonal antibody-based therapy.[99] The benefit of adding rituximab to combination chemotherapy for the initial treatment has been demonstrated in multiple randomized trials of chemotherapy with or without rituximab (see Table 103.2).[100–104] All of these trials have demonstrated improved response rates and time to progression in the rituximab plus chemotherapy arms, as well as improvement in OS. FDG-PET scanning has been employed to evaluate responses to CHOP-R in previously untreated patients. PET scanning was predictive when performed after four cycles and at the end of therapy. The 2-year PFS was significantly higher for PET-negative than PET-positive patients when employed as an interim or end of therapy scan. The 2-year OS was also significantly higher for PET-negative than PET-positive patients. This will require further study but may change management in the future.[105]

Other chemotherapy drugs plus rituximab have also been used for the initial therapy of FL. Bendamustine plus rituximab (BR) has been compared to CHOP-R in a randomized phase III trial with bendamustine (90 mg/m^2 days 1 and 2) plus rituximab (375 mg/m^2 day 1) in 513 patients with advanced follicular, marginal zone, lymphoplasmacytic, and mantle cell lymphoma.[106] In this study, a superior median PFS in favor of BR versus CHOP-R was seen (69.5 versus 31.2 months) at 45 months. Moreover with BR, less toxicity, including lower rates of grade 3 and 4 neutropenia and leukopenia were observed. There was no difference in OS at a median follow-up of 45 months. Intensifying the schedule of CHOP-R from every 21 to every 14 days was also of no benefit.[107] Fludarabine plus rituximab[108] and fludarabine, mitoxantrone, dexamethasone, and rituximab[109] both showed response rates of over 90% in previously untreated patients. However, significant neutropenia and opportunistic infections were observed with these regimens. A randomized phase III trial compared three regimens in previously untreated stage II to IV FL patients: CHOP-R; cyclophosphamide, vincristine, prednisone, and rituximab (CVP-R); or rituximab, fludarabine, and mitoxantrone (R-FM). Both R-FM and CHOP-R were superior to CVP-R in 3-year PFS and time to treatment failure (TTF), but there was no difference in OS.[110] The current impact of this study is uncertain given the favorable results and lower toxicity seen with BR.

Rituximab alone has been used as the first therapy in patients with FL, with overall response rates of around 70% and complete response (CR) rates of over 30% reported.[111–113] The most favorable data of single-agent rituximab is the recent update of the swiss group for clinical cancer research (SAKK) trial.[114] Patients received four weekly doses, and then patients with stable disease or better were randomized to observation or four doses of maintenance therapy, one dose every 2 months. In this study, 202 patients with previously untreated or relapsed/refractory FL administered four weekly doses of single-agent rituximab has been reported. The 151 patients with responding or stable disease at week 12 were randomized to no further treatment or prolonged rituximab maintenance every 2 months for four doses. At a median follow-up of 35 months, patients who received the prolonged rituximab maintenance had a twofold increase in event-free-survival (23 months versus 12 months). With a longer follow-up, 45% of newly diagnosed patients in this study were in remission at 8 years with the addition of maintenance rituximab.

Maintenance rituximab has also been shown to benefit patients who received chemotherapy without rituximab as part of the initial treatment. A randomized trial of maintenance rituximab versus observation after CVP with the majority having FL reported that patients who received maintenance rituximab had improved rates of 3-year PFS (68% versus 33%). Survival rates were similar between the two groups.[115] With the current paradigm of treating patients with concurrent chemotherapy plus rituximab, this study has less applicability.

The use of maintenance rituximab after chemoimmunotherapy in patients with FL has been examined in a large randomized trial.[116] Although maintenance rituximab appears to improve PFS rates, toxicities, albeit tolerable, are increased and the effect on OS is, to date, unclear. The Primary Rituximab and Maintenance (PRIMA) phase III intergroup trial randomly assigned 1,018 patients with previously untreated FL that responded to chemoimmunotherapy (CVP-R, CHOP-R, or fludarabine, cyclophosphamide, mitoxantrone, and rituximab [FCM-R]) maintenance with rituximab (375 mg/m^2 every 8 weeks for 24 months) or placebo.[116] At a median follow-up of 36 months from randomization, patients assigned to rituximab maintenance had a higher rate of PFS (75% versus 58%). A higher percentage of patients in complete response/complete response, unconfirmed (CRu) at 24 months (72% versus 52%) was also seen 2 years postrandomization in patients receiving maintenance rituximab. There was a significantly higher percentage of patients with grade III/IV adverse events and infections in the rituximab maintenance group. At this time, OS is the same in both groups.

Radioimmunotherapy alone has been used as the initial treatment in a limited number of patients with FL. [131]Itositumomab was given to 76 previously untreated patients with FL leading to overall and complete response rates of 95% and 75%, respectively, and, at 5-years, OS and PFS rates of 89% and 59%, respectively.[117] [131]I tositumomab is no longer commercially available. [90]Yttrium ([90]Yi)-ibritumomab tiuxetan has also been studied as sole initial therapy with excellent results with limited follow-up.[118]

Radioimmunotherapy has also been used as consolidation following conventional chemotherapy induction in patients with FL. Both [90]Yi-ibritumomab tiuxetan and ^{131}I-tositumomab have been studied. This approach has been associated with very high response rates, conversions of partial response (PR) to CR, and well-maintained responses.[119–121] A phase III trial compared [90]Yi-ibritumomab tiuxetan

to observation following a CR or PR to induction chemotherapy for treatment-naïve patients with FL.[122] Of note, the majority of patients did not receive rituximab along with the induction chemotherapy. At 8 years, both the PR and CR patients who received [90]Yi-ibritumomab tiuxetan had significantly longer median PFS with improvement of about 36 months. In contrast to this study, a randomized trial of CHOP plus rituximab to CHOP followed by [131]Itositumomab did not see any differences in PFS between the two arms.[123]

High-dose therapy and autologous stem cell transplantation (ASCT) has been used to consolidate first remission for patients with FL. These studies generally preceded the widespread use of rituximab. With ASCT in first remission, about 50% of patients are disease free at 10 years and beyond following ASCT, but an increased risk of second malignancies, including myelodysplastic syndrome (MDS), acute myelogenous leukemia (AML), and solid tumors, has been observed with long follow-ups of these patients. Several randomized trials have examined the role of ASCT in previously untreated patients with FL following an induction therapy.[124–129] The majority of these studies have demonstrated a significant improvement in PFS, but no impact on OS.[130] One reason for the lack of impact on OS has been the excess number of second malignancies.

Although allogeneic stem cell transplantation (alloSCT) can potentially lead to a cure for patients with FL due to the significant treatment related mortality, this is largely reserved for patients with relapsed and more refractory disease.

Treatment of Relapsed FL

When patients with relapsed FL require treatment, there are many options, ranging from rituximab alone to combination chemotherapy plus rituximab, radioimmunotherapy, and for selected patients, stem cell transplantation.

A recent update of single-agent rituximab therapy in patients with relapsed FL is from the randomized SAKK trial.[114] With a long follow-up, 35% of responders remain in remission at 8 years. However, in the context of current induction therapy that includes chemotherapy and rituximab in the majority of patients, it is uncertain if the response data to single-agent rituximab is as high or durable as in patients who received chemotherapy without rituximab as induction therapy. There is a evidence, however, that retreatment with rituximab in patients with relapsed, largely FL, who had previously responded to rituximab had a response rate of 40% with a median time to progression of 18 months following retreatment.[131]

The combination of chemotherapy and rituximab has enhanced the efficacy of treatment of relapsed FL. Probably the largest study treated selected patients with relapsed FL who were previously not treated with an anthracycline- or rituximab-containing regimen.[132] Patients were randomized to CHOP or CHOP-R and responding patients were randomized to 2 years of maintenance rituximab or observation. The overall and CR rates were significantly improved in the CHOP-R group, and the median PFS was improved by approximately 12 months. An update of this study with a median follow-up of 6 years reported that maintenance rituximab also improved median PFS by 2.4 years. The OS at 5 years following maintenance was 74% versus 64% with observation alone. Given the current paradigm of chemoimmunotherapy and maintenance, the applicability of these data to presently treated patients is uncertain.

Another regimen in which a benefit for the addition of rituximab was seen for relapsed disease in a randomized trial employing FCM.[133] A number of phase 2 trials of other agents plus rituximab associated with quite high response rates included BR with 90% response rate (RR) and median PFS of 2 years.[134–136] Single-agent bendamustine has an overall RR of 77% with a median response duration of 6.7 months.[134] With more widespread use of BR as initial therapy, BR will be employed less for recurrent disease. The regimen FCR has a similarly high response rate but with significant myelosuppression.[137] Phase 2 studies employing bortezomib and rituximab and bortezomib, rituximab, and bendamustine have reported RRs of approximately 50% and 93%, respectively.[138,139]

The anti-CD20 radioimmunotherapy agents have been employed for treatment of patients with relapsed and refractory FL.[140] The RRs in this patient population are similar with both agents, with 60% to 80% of patients responding. The median PFS is about 12 months, although the approximately 20% to 37% of patients who achieve a CR have a median time to progression of approximately 4 years.[141,142] A randomized trial compared single-agent rituximab to [90]Yi-ibritumomab in patients with relapsed indolent (predominantly FL).[143] The overall and CR rates were significantly higher with radioimmunotherapy (RIT), but no difference in time to progression or OS was observed. Retreatment with these agents remains controversial, with uncertainty of delivery of full dose and concerns of second malignancies.[144]

FL is extremely responsive to RT; low-dose RT (e.g., total dose of 4 Gy, given as two consecutive daily 2-Gy fractions) can be used for the palliation of patients who have symptoms related to a single disease site, with CR rates of 57% and overall RRs of 82%.[145] Patients who go into CR have long, durable local control rates. There are no significant side effects of treatment, even in the head and neck region where higher doses would cause xerostomia and mucositis.

The use of either ASCT or alloSCT in FL is controversial and the subject of numerous clinical trials.[146] A large number of phase 2 studies prior to the availability of rituximab, involving high-dose therapy and autologous hematopoietic stem cell transplantation (HCT) have shown that approximately 40% of patients with good performance status and chemosensitive relapsed disease may experience prolonged PFS and OS.[147–151] Prior to the widespread use of rituximab for in vivo purging, many strategies were taken to render the autologous stem cell collections free of lymphoma cells. Although single institution studies suggested that reinfusion of tumor-free stem cells led to a decreased relapse rate, it remains controversial as to whether there is a benefit, particularly now with rituximab treatment. The only phase 3 randomized trial (the chemotherapy, unpurged stem cell transplantation, purged stem cell transplantation [CUP] trial) comparing ASCT to conventional chemotherapy in relapsed FL patients demonstrated a higher PFS and OS for ASCT, and no benefit for purging the stem cell graft.[152] A retrospective analysis of patients undergoing ASCT following rituximab-based salvage therapy did not suggest a benefit of ASCT as compared to conventional therapy. Unfortunately, as has been seen in ASCT in first remission, second malignancies—both solid tumors and MDS and AML—are reported following ASCT.

Phase 2 studies have looked at the use of in vivo purging pre-ASCT and maintenance therapy with rituximab following ASCT in patients with relapsed FL. These suggest an improvement in PFS, similar to what has been seen following conventional chemotherapy and chemoimmunotherapy. A phase 3 trial in patients with relapsed FL has investigated the inclusion of rituximab for in vivo purging pre-ASCT and 2 years of maintenance post-ASCT.[153] There was an improvement in PFS for patients receiving rituximab for in vivo purging, maintenance, and the combination of both as compared to no rituximab, but no OS benefit.

AlloSCT has been investigated in patients with relapsed FL. Both myeloablative and reduced intensity conditioning (RIC) approaches have been employed. Unfortunately, myeloablative conditioning has a treatment related mortality of up to 40%; however, the relapse rate is less than 20%.[154] There is enthusiasm for RIC alloSCT because it has lower treatment-related mortality,[155–157] but some reports suggest that the relapse rate may be higher than conventional myeloablative conditioning. The role of alloSCT versus ASCT for FL remains uncertain. A recent National Comprehensive Cancer Network (NCCN) database retrospective analysis found significantly higher 3-year OS for ASCT versus alloSCT (87% versus 61%).[158] Certainly, for younger patients with more resistant disease, alloSCT remains a potentially curative option for relapsed FL.

Histologic Transformation

Part of the natural history of any indolent B-cell NHLs is progression to a higher grade histologic subtype, most commonly DLBCL, but much less commonly, BL or even HL can be seen.[71,159] Histologic transformation (HT) is most commonly seen in FL, but is also seen in patients with MZL, lymphoplasmacytic lymphoma, and small lymphocytic lymphoma/CLL (where this is referred to as a Richter transformation), and a biopsy is critical in order to demonstrate transformation. HT occurs at a rate of approximately 2% to 3% per year.[72] The clinical presentation of HT includes rapid growing masses, extranodal disease, B symptoms, hypercalcemia, and elevated serum LDH. *TP53* mutations and translocations or amplifications of *MYC* are the most common genetic abnormalities seen in HT.

Historically, HT to DLBCL has been associated with a very poor prognosis. In a series from Stanford, previously untreated patients and patients with limited disease and no prior therapy at transformation had improved prognoses.[160] Although the median survival for all patients with transformation was only 22 months, those who achieved a CR to combination chemotherapy had an actuarial survival of 75% at 5 years. More recent studies suggest that CHOP-R may improve OS for patients with transformed disease. Patients who have not previously received an anthracycline-containing regimen should be treated with CHOP-R and, assuming a CR is obtained, monitored. For previously treated patients, high-dose therapy and ASCT should be considered assuming the patient has chemosensitive disease. Patients with histologic transformation can have later relapses with indolent lymphoma.

Newer Agents

There are a multitude of new approaches that have been studied in patients with FL. This includes monoclonal antibodies, idiotype vaccines, immunomodulatory agents, and novel drugs such as kinase inhibitors.

Monoclonal antibodies directed against other B-cell–associated antigens as well as new anti-CD20 monoclonal antibodies (mAb) are being investigated in FL. These have included anti-CD80,[161,162] anti-CD22 mAbs,[163,164] and anti-CD40.[165] Several new anti-CD20 monoclonal antibodies are being evaluated in patients with FL who are refractory to rituximab. These include several humanized antibodies that are designed to have less infusion toxicity and a better antibody-dependent cell-mediated cytotoxicity effector function.[166–168] The other mAb of interest is obinutuzumab, the first type II, glycoengineered, and humanized monoclonal anti-CD20 antibody.[169] In rituximab-refractory patients in the high-dose cohort, the RR was 55% with a median PFS of 11.9 months. Studies of obinutuzumab in combination with chemotherapy have shown 93% to 98% RRs in relapsed and refractory FL patients.[170]

A number of immunostimulatory agents have been studied to enhance the activity of rituximab. These include cytokines such as IL-2 and immunostimulatory DNA sequences known as CpGs.[171] To date, although having immunomodulatory effects, the impact on enhancing the therapeutic effect of rituximab has been limited. A phase 2 study of lenalidomide plus rituximab has reported high RRS, but a phase 3 study will be needed to demonstrate superiority over rituximab alone.[172]

The other area of interest has been in active immunization, focusing largely on the idiotype protein as the antigen. To date, there have been three randomized studies employing idiotype proteins coupled to a protein called keyhole limpet hemocyanin (KLH) following the induction of remission in patients with FL. The Favrille trial used rituximab for induction therapy. The median time to progression (TTP) was 9 months for the idiotype-KLH (Id-KLH) vaccinated patients and 12.6 months in the control group (p = 0.019).[173] However, this difference was attributed to more patients with high-risk FLIPI scores in the Id-KLH arm. The Biovax study reported showing a 14-month improvement in PFS for the Id-KLH vaccinated patients as compared to control; however, the induction chemotherapy was intense and remissions had to be sustained for 12 months prior to the initiation of vaccination.[174] The trial using the MyVax Id-KLH conjugate following CVP chemotherapy failed to show any PFS advantage. Based on these studies, it is unlikely at the present time that idiotype vaccinations will be pursued in FL.

B-cell kinases are logical targets for therapy in FL. To date, three kinase inhibitors, idelalisib, ibrutinib, and fostamatinib, which target the phosphoinositide 3-kinase (PI3k) p110δ, Bruton's tyrosine kinase (BTK), and spleen tyrosine kinase (SYK), respectively, have been tested. In relapsed and refractory FL patients, the response rates to idelalisib,[175] ibrutinib,[176] and fostamatinib[177] were 62% (including other indolent NHLs besides FL), 27%, and 10%, respectively. These agents are undergoing additional study, in combination with chemotherapy and as maintenance following remission induction, to better define their role.

Follicular Lymphoma Grade III

FL grade III has been historically referred to as follicular large cell lymphoma. It is histologically defined by the presence of more than 15 centroblasts per hpf. It is further subdivided into grade IIIa, where centrocytes are present, and grade IIIb, where there are sheets of centroblasts. These are further differentiated by the presence of *BCL6* rearrangements in a high fraction of grade IIIb cases. Because many studies likely include both grade IIIa and IIIB, this heterogeneity may affect an interpretation of the outcomes. Although the follicular architecture is intact, the clinical presentation, behavior, and outcome with treatment in many patients with FL grade IIIb more closely approximates that of DLBCL.[178–180] In contrast to DLBCL, the relapse rate of FL grade IIIb is higher in some series, but survival is longer.[181] A recent series suggested similar outcomes of grade IIIa and IIIB cases and no benefit for the inclusion of anthracyclines in the treatment regimen.[182]

Small Lymphocytic Lymphoma/B-Cell Chronic Lymphocytic Leukemia

Introduction

Small lymphocytic lymphoma (SLL) is a mature (peripheral) B-cell malignancy. It is synonymous with CLL. The malignant cells in SLL and CLL are morphologically, immunophenotypically, and genetically identical. The difference between these two diagnoses is the clinical presentation, with a nonleukemic presentation in SLL. The diagnosis is made by an examination of involved tissue, such as the lymph node or bone marrow.

SLL represents less than 5% of all NHLs. CLL/SLL comprises 90% of chronic lymphocytic leukemias in Western countries. Less than 10% of patients present with only nodal involvement (i.e., SLL). However, most patients with SLL at presentation ultimately develop bone marrow and blood infiltration. The median age at diagnosis is 65 years.[63] At least 80% have stage IV disease due to bone marrow involvement at diagnosis.

Pathology

The cells within lymphoid tissues in CLL/SLL are small lymphocytes with condensed chromatin, round nuclei, and occasionally, a small nucleolus.[44] Larger lymphoid cells with prominent nucleoli and dispersed chromatin are also seen. These larger lymphoid cells are usually clustered together in so-called proliferation centers, which are pathognomonic. Roughly 60% of SLL/CLLs have Ig genes that show evidence of *significant* somatic mutation, defined as a rearranged Ig heavy-chain gene with a sequence that differs from germ-line position at 2% or more of the Ig V region nucleotides, which is taken as evidence of origin from an antigen-stimulated B cell.[183]

Immunophenotype and Genetics

SLL/CLL cells express low-level monoclonal surface Ig, usually IgM or IgM and IgD. They also express human leukocyte antigen-DR (HLA-DR) and the B-cell antigens CD19, CD20, and CD23, and are characteristically CD5 positive. About 40% of cases express CD38. Expression of the tyrosine kinase ZAP70 is also observed in a subset of cases and correlates with a more aggressive clinical course.[184]

Immunoglobulin genes are clonally rearranged, with IgV region somatic mutations in up to 60% of patients. Cytogenetic abnormalities include trisomy 12, which is present in about 40% of cases, as well as 13q deletions (45% to 55% of cases), 11q deletions (17% to 20% of cases), and 17p deletions (7% to 10% of cases). Cases with 13q deletions have the most favorable prognosis, whereas those with del(11q) or del(17p) have an unfavorable prognosis.[185] The t(11;14) involving the cyclin D1 (*CCDN1*) gene has been described, but many of these cases are believed to be leukemic variants of mantle cell lymphoma. Deep sequencing studies of CLL have revealed a number of recurrent mutations, the most common of which involve the *NOTCH1*, *MYD88*, and *SF3B1* genes.[186]

Clinical Presentation

Most patients with SLL present with painless generalized lymphadenopathy, which has frequently been present for several years. B symptoms are rare. Hepatosplenomegaly is present in less than 50% of patients. The peripheral blood in patients with SLL may be normal or reveal only a mild lymphocytosis; by definition, patients with SLL have an absolute lymphocyte count of $<5,000/\mu L$ at the time of diagnosis. A serum paraprotein is found in about 20% of cases, and hypogammaglobulinemia is present in about 40%. Both CLL and SLL patients may develop autoimmune hemolytic anemia, pure red cell aplasia, and autoimmune thrombocytopenia. Elevated serum LDH is uncommon, whereas increased levels of serum beta-2 microglobulin are more frequently seen and can be a marker disease burden. SLL/CLL can transform to DLBCL (Richter syndrome), an event that is associated with a short survival.[187] These patients present with rapidly growing masses, elevated serum LDH, and B symptoms. Rarely, transformation can be to B-cell prolymphocytic leukemia (B-PLL), which is characterized by high white cell counts and splenomegaly. It also has a poor prognosis.

Treatment of Small Lymphocytic Lymphoma

Patients with stage I SLL should be treated with involved field radiation, and not combined modality therapy or chemotherapy alone. In one limited series of 14 patients with stage I or II disease treated with 40 to 44 Gy, the 10-year freedom from relapse rates were 80% and 62% for stage I and stage II disease, respectively. Generally, patients with stage II or more advanced SLL are treated with chemotherapy regimens used for CLL (see Chapter 110). For patients with advanced stage disease who do not need systemic therapy but have one site causing symptoms, low-dose radiation (200 cGy for two fractions) can provide reasonable palliation, although the local control rates are not as high as seen with FL.[145]

Lymphoplasmacytic Lymphoma

Lymphoplasmacytic lymphoma represents about 1% of all NHLs. In some cases, patients present with mixed cryoglobulinemia, possibly related to concurrent hepatitis C virus infection.[188,189]

Pathology

Lymphoplasmacytic lymphoma is an indolent lymphoma composed of a diffuse proliferation comprised of a mixture of small lymphocytes, lymphoplasmacytic cells, and plasma cells.[190] Immunoglobulin inclusions in the cytoplasm (Russell bodies) or invaginating into the nucleus (Dutcher bodies) are commonly seen. Unlike multiple myeloma, amyloidosis is rare. Occasional cases may also contain frequent larger immunoblast-like cells.

Immunophenotype and Genetics

Monoclonal cytoplasmic immunoglobulin is seen within the plasmacytoid cells and plasma cells by immunohistochemistry. The admixed lymphoid cells express B-cell antigens CD19, CD20, and surface IgM, and in general, do not express CD10 or CD23. A minor subset of cases is positive for CD5. Waldenström macroglobulinemia is an entity caused by high levels of monoclonal IgM that is generally associated with lymphoplasmacytic lymphoma (LPL). Deletions of 6q21 have been identified in 40% to 60% of patients with Waldenström macroglobulinemia. Activating mutations in *MYD88*, an adaptor protein that appears to function in signaling pathways downstream of the Ig receptor that lead to activation of the transcription factor nuclear factor kappa B (NF-κB) activation, are highly associated with LPL, being present in close to 100% of cases. However, mutations of *MYD88* are not specific for LPL, because they are also seen less commonly in DLBCL and other low-grade B-cell NHLs.

Clinical Presentation

Clinically, this disease is similar to small lymphocytic lymphoma. The median age is early 60s, and nearly all patients have stage IV disease by virtue of bone marrow involvement. B symptoms and elevated serum LDH are uncommon. Lymph node and splenic involvement are common. In the WHO clinical study, 5-year OS (58%) and failure-free survival (25%) were similar to SLL.

Treatment

At least 25% of patients with LPL/waldenstrom's macroglobulinemia (WM) have no indications for therapy at initial presentation. The indications for treatment include constitutional symptoms, cytopenias, or less commonly, symptomatic lymphadenopathy or splenomegaly. Other reasons for treatment are hyperviscosity related to the elevated serum IgM and paraneoplastic neuropathy.

Analogous to other indolent B-cell NHLs, rituximab plays a significant role in the therapy of LPL. Single-agent rituximab is indicated for minimally symptomatic patients. Approximately half of patients will have a partial response to single-agent rituximab.[191] One can see transient increases in serum IgM levels after rituximab that can cause or exacerbate hyperviscosity.

Chemoimmunotherapy has largely replaced single agents for the treatment of LPL. Commonly used regimens include: dexamethasone, rituximab, cyclophosphamide (DRC)[192]; bortezomib plus rituximab with or without dexamethasone (BRD)[193]; or thalidomide plus rituximab.[194] The latter two have limitations due to neuropathy. For DRC, the overall and complete response rates were 83% and 7%, respectively, and 2-year OS and PFS rates were 81% and 67%, respectively. Bortezomib and rituximab and thalidomide-rituximab have similar response rates. Alkylating agents, including chlorambucil and bendamustine, have RRs in excess of 80%. Purine analogs are active agents; however, stem cell toxicity can be an issue with purine analogs as well as chlorambucil.[195] For recurrent disease, one can often utilize agents that were previously used. For patients with more refractory LPL, the mammalian target of rapamycin (mTOR) inhibitor everolimus, anti-CD52 mAb, and the oral Bruton's tyrosine-kinase inhibitor, ibrutinib, are active. Selected patients with relapsed disease are considered for high-dose therapy with ASCT or alloSCT. The results seen are similar to that of other indolent lymphomas.

There are rare patients who have stage IE disease with this histology (i.e., renal involvement). In this case, modest dose RT (12 to 18 Gy) within the organ tolerance can provide long-term control and, occasionally, a cure.

Marginal Zone Lymphomas

MZLs are indolent NHLs that include three diseases arising from post-GC marginal zone B cells: splenic marginal zone B-cell lymphoma (± villous lymphocytes); extranodal marginal zone B-cell lymphoma of mucosa-associated lymphoid tissue (MALT) type (MALT-type lymphoma, or MALT lymphoma); and nodal marginal zone B-cell lymphoma.[196,197]

Nodal MZL

Nodal MZLs constitute less than 1% of all NHLs. These lymphomas are primarily nodal diseases without evidence of extranodal involvement.

Pathology

Within lymph nodes, there are collections of B cells in a parafollicular, perivascular, and perisinusoidal distribution that often bear a monocytoid appearance, having folded nuclear contours and moderate abundant pale cytoplasm. These cells may surround reactive-appearing GCs and mantle zones. A subset of cases is also associated with variable degrees of plasmacytoid differentiation.

Immunophenotype and Genetics

Cells express monoclonal surface immunoglobulin (IgM > IgG > IgA) as well as CD19, CD20, CD79a, and are negative for CD10 and CD23. A minor subset of cases may be CD5 positive. Cases with plasmacytoid differentiation may show monoclonal expression of cytoplasmic kappa or lambda light chain by immunohistochemistry. Such cases may be associated with small monoclonal immunoglobulin spikes, but these are generally under 0.5 g/dL and are not associated with hyperviscosity. A subset of cases expresses surface IgD, analogous to splenic MZL. Immunoglobulin genes are rearranged with evidence of somatic mutation, implying a post-GC origin. There are no known chromosomal abnormalities specific to nodal MZL.

Clinical Features

Over 70% of patients present with stage III/IV disease, and the majority are asymptomatic. Bone marrow involvement is less common (45%) than in most indolent lymphomas. The 5-year survival for patients with nodal MZL is 55% to 79%. Similar to other indolent lymphomas, histologic transformation can occur with nodal MZL.

Treatment

The optimal therapy for patients with nodal MZL is not known. Patients are frequently treated with chemoimmunotherapy, typically either alkylating agents or purine analogs plus rituximab, which produce RRs in excess of 80%. A recent phase III study comparing CHOP-R to BR included 67 patients with MZL not otherwise specified.[106] There was no difference (p < 0.32) in median PFS between CHOP-R (47 months) and BR (57 months). For now, patients should be offered either clinical trials or treated with regimens used for FL.

Splenic Marginal Zone Lymphoma (± Villous Lymphocytes)

Splenic MZL (± villous lymphocytes) constitutes less than 1% of all NHLs, with a median age of 65 to 70 years and uncommon before the age of 50 years.[63] It is more common in Caucasians, with no gender predominance. Splenic MZL has been associated with viral infections, specifically hepatitis C and Kaposi's sarcoma–associated herpesvirus (KSHV). In one study, treatment of hepatitis C induced regression of the lymphoma.

Pathology

In splenic MZL, there is an expansion of marginal zones in the spleen. Plasma cell differentiation may be seen in a subset of cases, but as in nodal MZL, monoclonal spikes, if present, are less than 0.5 mg/dL. Bone marrow, lymph nodes, and peripheral blood involvement (referred to as splenic lymphoma with villous or nonvillous lymphocytes) can also be present. Generally, cells have small nuclei, but in the peripheral blood, they typically have abundant cytoplasm with "shaggy" or villous projections.

Immunophenotype and Genetics

Splenic MZL cells express monoclonal surface IgM, IgD, CD19, and CD20. The tumor cells generally lack CD5 and CD10, helping to distinguish this tumor from SLL/CLL, MCL, and FL. They also typically are negative for CD25, CD103, and annexin A1, which helps to distinguish splenic MZL from hairy cell leukemia. Ig genes have evidence for somatic hypermutation in about half the cases. In splenic MZL, trisomy 3 is present in 39% of cases, which is found in other MZLs. Abnormalities of chromosome 7q are also frequently seen. Deep sequencing identified recurrent somatic mutations in genes involved in the NOTCH, NF-κB, and B-cell receptor pathways, as well as mutations in *TP53*.[198] *NOTCH2* mutations have been reported in 21% to 25% of cases, and were associated with a poor prognosis.

Clinical Features

Patients typically present with splenomegaly, lymphocytosis, and cytopenias, with lymphadenopathy being a much less common feature. B symptoms and elevated LDH are uncommon. Because of marrow and peripheral blood involvement, over 90% of cases have stage IV disease at diagnosis. IgM monoclonal gammopathies and mixed cryoglobulinemia can be seen, especially with a hepatitis C infection. Acquired C1 esterase deficiency seen in many B-cell lymphoproliferative disorders and can be a feature of splenic MZL.[199] The survival of patients is in excess of 70% at 10 years. A prognostic model based on three risk factors—hemoglobin less than 12 g/dL, LDH level greater than normal, and albumin level less than 3.5 g/dL—could identify patients with 5-year cause-specific survivals of 88% for patients with zero risk factors, 73% for patients with one factor, and 50% for patients with two or three factors.[200]

Therapy

Similar to other indolent NHLs, many patients with splenic MZL do not require immediate therapy. Asymptomatic patients without splenomegaly or cytopenias can be observed. Patients with symptomatic splenomegaly and or significant cytopenias merit treatment. Those uncommon patients who also have hepatitis C may benefit from treatment of the infection, suggesting that tumor growth and survival is promoted by factors or signals elaborated in response to hepatitis C antigens. Splenectomy is reasonable for selected patients with excellent relief of symptoms and cytopenias. Splenectomy was associated with an overall response rate of 85% and an estimated PFS and OS at 5 years of 58% and 77%, respectively. For patients who are not surgical candidates, splenic radiation has some utility. In general, 150 cGy is given to the entire spleen three times per week. The total dose must remain under renal tolerance because the left kidney is almost always in the field. Single-agent rituximab can improve splenomegaly and cytopenias in over 90% of patients.[201] In a study of induction with weekly rituximab followed by maintenance, the RR was 95%, with OS and PFS at 5 years of 92% and 73%, respectively.[202] Other options for therapy at relapse are similar to those used for FL, and include retreatment with rituximab, alkylating agents, and purine analogs in combination with rituximab.

Extranodal Marginal Zone Lymphoma

MALT lymphoma is a subtype of MZL involving extranodal tissues. The most common site is the stomach, but MALT lymphoma has been described in a number of different organs and tissues including the skin, salivary glands, the lung, the small bowel, ocular adnexa, the breasts, the bladder, the thyroid, the dura, and the synovium. It has been associated with a variety of chronic inflammatory and infectious conditions, including autoimmune diseases such as Sjögren's syndrome and Hashimoto's thyroiditis, and infections with *Helicobacter pylori* (*H. pylori*), *Borrelia burgdorferi* (*B. burgdorferi*), *Chlamydophila psittaci* (*C. psittaci*), *Campylobacter jejuni* (*C. jejuni*), and hepatitis C virus (HCV).[203–206] MALT lymphoma behaves indolently and is principally observed until symptoms related to organ impairment become evident; however, in many cases, early stage disease treatment with radiation therapy or antibiotic therapy appears to be curative. There are few dedicated studies of MALT lymphoma outside of early stage disease and much of the management of advanced stage disease is extrapolated from the FL literature, which often includes a small number of MZL patients.

Epidemiology

MALT lymphomas account for approximately 5% to 8% of all NHLs, but represent 50% to 70% of all MZLs.[63,207] It is the third most common subtype of NHL after DLBCL and FL. The median age at diagnosis is 60 years, with incidence nearly equal in men and women. Two-thirds of patients present with stage I/II disease, with a minority of patients having more advanced disease at diagnosis. B symptoms and bone marrow involvement are rare. MALT lymphomas can transform into a more aggressive lymphoma, but this occurs rarely. The most common transformation is into an activated B-cell–like DLBCL.[208] Nearly half of all MALT lymphomas involve the gastric mucosa, where over 60% are associated with an *H. pylori* infection.

Pathology

MALT lymphomas are malignancies of antigen-stimulated B cells, which normally reside in lymph nodes within the marginal zone that is found outside the mantle zones of B-cell follicles.[197] Histologically, they are characterized by a monoclonal infiltrate of small- to medium-sized cells with abundant cytoplasm and irregular nuclear contours. Variable numbers of larger centroblast-like cells may also be present, and a subset of cases exhibit plasmacytic differentiation. An essential pathologic feature is the presence of lymphoepithelial lesions created by the invasion of mucosal glands and crypts by aggregates of lymphoma cells, producing an appearance that resembles the lymphocyte M-cell structures found in normal Peyer patches.

Immunophenotype and Genetics

MALT lymphomas are surface Ig positive, and are also positive for B-cell markers (CD19, CD20, CD79a, and CD22), and negative for CD5, CD10, CD23, and cyclin D1.[44] Uncommonly, MALT lymphomas are CD5 positive and this is associated with a worse prognosis; these lymphomas may have cytogenetic changes such as trisomy 3 and del7q.[209] Distinguishing MALT lymphomas from benign reactive lymphoid infiltrates may be difficult; in this circumstance, light chain restriction by flow cytometry or immunoglobulin heavy chain gene rearrangement studies by PCR can be helpful.

Other cytogenetic abnormalities that have been reported in MALT lymphomas include t(11;18), t(14;18), t(1;14), t(3;14), and trisomy 8. The t(11;18) is the most common; it occurs in 18% to 53% of MALT lymphomas of any site and is associated with a low-grade histology.[210,211] It produces the fusion of the apoptosis inhibitor 2 (*API2*) gene and the *MALT1* gene. The resulting fusion gene encodes a chimeric protein that stimulates the activation of NF-κB, a transcription factor that turns on a number of genes that promote proliferation and inhibit apoptosis.[212] The t(11;18) translocation predicts for a poor response to *H. pylori*–directed therapies in gastric MALT lymphoma.[213] A substantial proportion of malignant B cells in MALT lymphomas express B-cell receptors with strong homology to rheumatoid factors, and this appears to be mutually exclusive with the presence of the t(11;18) translocation.[214] This suggests that t(11;18)-negative MALT lymphomas are driven by the stimulation of high-affinity B-cell receptors by antibody–antigen immune complexes and activated T cells, whereas t(11;18)-positive MALT lymphomas are not dependent on B-cell receptor signaling, but instead are driven by constitutive activation of NF-κB. The t(14;18), which pairs the *MALT1* gene with the IgH gene and drives overexpression of MALT1 protein, is more common in nongastric MALT lymphomas.[215] The t(1;14), which results in the overexpression of BCL10, is rarer overall but more frequent in gastric and pulmonary MALT lymphomas. The t(3;14) translocation is present in 10% of thyroid, ocular adnexal, and cutaneous MALT lymphomas.[216] This translocation involves the IgH and *FOXP1* genes and drives overexpression of the FOXP1 transcription factor. Of note, overexpression of MALT1, BCL10, and FOXP1 are all believed to result in NF-κB hyperactivation, making this a common feature of genetically diverse MALT lymphomas. MALT lymphomas are also more often associated with gains at chromosomes 3p, 6p, and 18p, and del(6q23) than the other subtypes of MZL.[217]

Clinical Presentation

The clinical presentation of MALT lymphoma depends in large part on the site of disease. Gastric and intestinal MALT lymphomas may present with symptoms of dyspepsia and abdominal pain, sometimes with signs and symptoms of bowel obstruction, but rarely with bleeding. These lymphomas are diagnosed on endoscopy with biopsies from multiple areas of endoscopically abnormal tissue as well as random sampling of macroscopically uninvolved mucosa. Involvement of the salivary and lacrimal glands, on the other hand, can result in Sjögren's-like syndromes of dry eyes and mouth. MALT lymphomas involving the ocular adnexa typically present with painless conjunctival injection and photophobia, resembling allergic conjunctivitis. Patients with bronchus-associated lymphoid tissue (BALT) lymphomas typically are older men and can have symptoms including cough, fever, and/or weight loss.[218] Other sites of disease often present with an obstructing mass. Some patients are diagnosed incidentally, either because of imaging studies or an exam of the eye or GI track done for another reason or as part of an evaluation for a monoclonal gammopathy, which is present in approximately 25% to 35% of MALT lymphoma patients; this feature is generally associated with plasmacytoid differentiation.[219] B symptoms are rare in this disease.[63] Bone marrow involvement is present in a minority of patients; therefore, cytopenias are rare, as is disease in the peripheral blood.

In addition to the blood tests that are standard for patients with NHL at diagnosis, patients with MALT lymphomas should have a few additional tests. HCV testing should be performed given its association with MALT lymphoma; an HIV virus test is advised. Additional laboratory studies to consider include a β$_2$-microglobulin, serum protein electrophoresis and immunofixation, and serum light chains. Staging is done with CT scans of the chest, abdomen, and pelvis, as well as imaging of the neck, including the parotids and salivary glands, and orbits with CT or MRI. A bone marrow biopsy should be considered for patients with multifocal disease, and an evaluation of the gastric mucosa is reasonable for all patients with nongastric MALT lymphoma given the documented high rate of gastric involvement in these patients.[220]

Treatment

Management of MALT lymphoma depends both on stage and site of disease. As an indolent lymphoma with a long OS, close observation at diagnosis until the development of signs, symptoms, or organ function impairment as a result of the disease is appropriate for patients with advanced stage disease. An exception is patients with advanced stage MALT lymphoma and concomitant HCV infection; a trial of anti-HCV antiviral therapy in these patients may result in regression of their lymphoma. For patients with early stage and localized disease, however, treatment with radiation therapy or treatment with antibiotics, such as for *H. pylori*–positive gastric MALT lymphoma, has been associated with high RRs and durable responses, many of which may represent cures.

Treatment of symptomatic or organ impairing relapsed, refractory, or advanced stage disease is similar to approaches used in FL with chemotherapy, immunotherapy, or chemoimmunotherapy.

Gastric MALT lymphoma represents a paradigm for treating early stage, localized MALT lymphomas. For those associated with an *H. pylori* infection that do not harbor a t(11;18) translocation, eradication of *H. pylori* is effective treatment and results in good long-term disease control and OS.[221–223] In patients with *H. pylori*–negative lymphomas, MALT lymphomas with a t(11;18) translocation, or lymphomas that fail to respond to *H. pylori* therapy, RT is the preferred treatment modality.[224] Chemotherapy, immunotherapy, or chemoimmunotherapy is active in this disease but is generally reserved for patients with relapsed or refractory disease to antibiotic therapy or RT, or patients with more advanced stage or aggressive disease.[225,226] Similarly, MALT lymphoma of the ocular adnexa is primarily treated with RT.[227] However, given the association described by some groups between *C. psittaci* infection and MALT lymphoma in this area, antibiotic therapy with doxycycline has been studied.[228] The RR of single-agent doxycycline for MALT lymphoma of the ocular adnexa was 83%, with two-thirds of patients having partial responses. The 2-year PFS was 55%.

For relapsed or refractory disease or disease that is more extensive at presentation, agents that have been used and reported include single-agent therapy with alkylating agents such as chlorambucil or cyclophosphamide, purine analogs such as cladribine, bortezomib, and rituximab, and occasionally, multiagent anthracycline-based chemotherapy for younger patients with more aggressive disease. The use of single-agent, continuous, low-dose oral chlorambucil or cyclophosphamide in patients with early or advanced stage disease yielded CR rates of 75% and a relapse rate of 21% during the 8 year follow-up.[229] Single-agent rituximab in patients with stage I through IV MALT lymphoma (15 gastric, 10 nongastric) who were either chemotherapy naïve or who had progressed following chemotherapy resulted in an overall response rate of 73% and was better for chemotherapy-naïve patients than for previously treated patients (87% versus 45%).[225] Duration of response was short, however, with 36% of responders progressing at a median of 10.5 months. Combination chemoimmunotherapy with rituximab and fludarabine results in response rates of 85% to 100% and 2- to 3-year PFS of 80% to 100% at the expense, however, of significantly greater toxicity.[230] MALT lymphoma is extremely sensitive to radiation therapy, and this modality has a role in the palliation of patients with advanced disease.

Mantle Cell Lymphoma

MCL is a malignancy of monomorphous small- to medium-sized B cells with the characteristic t(11;14) leading to overexpression of the cyclin D1 cell cycle regulator in the majority of cases.

Pathology

MCLs are neoplastic counterparts of naïve "mantle zone" B cells. Morphologically, MCL can have either diffuse architecture, or a vaguely nodular appearance, occasionally growing predominantly in expanded mantle zones around reactive GCs. Cytologically, in most cases, the neoplastic cells are small- to medium-sized and have irregular nuclei and scant cytoplasm. Some cases of MCL have a predominance of intermediate-size cells with more open "blastic" chromatin; such blastic variants are associated with a high mitotic rate. Other cases are comprised of a spectrum of cells, including large cells (pleomorphic variant).

Immunophenotype and Genetics

MCLs express B-cell antigens, surface IgM (usually together with surface IgD), CD5, and CD43 and usually lack CD10 and CD23. Overexpression of cyclin D1 further distinguishes these tumors from most other entities. IgH variable gene segments lack a somatic mutation in 84% of cases (pre-GC), with the remainder being mutated.[231] By FISH, greater than 90% of MCLs have the t(11;14) associated with the rearrangement of the cyclin D1 gene (CCDN1). The remaining cases do not overexpress cyclin D1, but instead usually overexpress cyclin D2, cyclin D3, or cyclin E due to the presence of translocations involving these genes and the IgH locus.[232] Cyclin D1–negative cases are similar clinically to cyclin D1–positive cases[233] and have a similar gene expression profile. Deep sequencing[234] has identified NOTCH1 mutations in a minority of cases, which may be associated with a poor prognosis. SOX11 overexpression is also associated with a worse prognosis.[232,235]

Clinical Features. MCL constitutes about 7% of all NHLs. About 75% of patients are males, with a median age of 63 years. Approximately 70% of patients have stage IV disease, and B symptoms are observed in approximately one-third of patients. Typical sites of involvement are the lymph nodes, the spleen, the liver, Waldeyer's ring, and bone marrow. Peripheral blood involvement is present in 25% to 50% of patients at presentation. MCL can involve any region of the GI tract (88% lower tract, 43% upper tract by endoscopy), occasionally presenting as multiple intestinal polyposis.[236] CNS involvement is rare and is usually associated with a leukemic phase.

The median survival of patients with MCL is 4 to 5 years and improving. Approximately 10% to 15% of patients have a disease with a more indolent disease, with minimal lymphadenopathy, mild splenomegaly, and a proliferation index measured by Ki-67 staining of around 10%.[237] These patients have a disease that behaves more like an indolent NHL, where a *watchful waiting* approach does not compromise response to therapy or survival. In contrast, patients with the blastic variant at diagnosis have a median survival of 18 months. Blastic transformation occurs in 35% of patients, with a risk of 42% at 4 years, and once occurring, the median survival is 3.8 months.[238]

Prognostic models have been employed for patients with MCL. The IPI developed for diffuse aggressive NHLs provides stratification of patients. Attempts to improve on the IPI include the mantle cell lymphoma International Prognostic Index (MIPI), which includes age, performance status (PS), LDH, and white blood cell count (WBC)[58] as prognostic factors, and several reports show that the MIPI is better than the IPI at stratifying patients.[239] The proliferation index alone and also when incorporated into the MIPI provides additional predictive power.[240] Gene expression profiling has been examined in MCL patients. In those studies, the proliferation signature and high expression of cyclin D1 were associated with an unfavorable prognosis.[241] Mutations and deletions of p53 are also associated with a worse prognosis.[242]

Treatment. The majority of patients with MCL have a disseminated disease requiring treatment. An indolent behaving disease is seen in 10% to 15% of patients, where a delay of initiation of treatment was not deleterious.[241] The treatment of MCL historically involved single alkylating agents as well as combination chemotherapy (CVP, CHOP) to which 30% to 50% of patients had a CR, with a median duration of 1 to 3 years.[243] In a meta-analysis, single alkylating agents offered results similar to combination chemotherapy.[244] A small number of patients with MCL will present with stage I to II disease. These patients are potentially curable with combined chemotherapy and involved field radiation (30 Gy). Chemoimmunotherapy has shown a significant impact in the treatment of MCL. A meta analysis of 638 patients with MCL showed that rituximab-containing regimens significantly increased median survival (37 versus 27 months)[245] as compared to chemotherapy alone. One of the mainstays of chemoimmunotherapy for the initial treatment of MCL is CHOP-R. However, results of a randomized trial comparing CHOP-R to BR reported superior PFS with BR with less toxicity.[106] In patients with a median age of 70 years, the median PFS for BR was 35 months, compared to 22 months with

CHOP-R. One other randomized study compared CHOP-R to the fludarabine, cyclophosphamide, rituximab (FCR) regimen. In that study, for patients over age 60 years, CHOP-R and FCR had similar CR rates, but CHOP-R had less toxicity, and the OS at 4 years was 62% versus 47% in favor of CHOP-R.[246] This study included a second randomization of maintenance with interferon-α or rituximab until progression. For the patients who received CHOP-R, a significant survival benefit from maintenance rituximab was observed, with an estimated 4-year OS rate of 87% versus 63%.

More aggressive approaches for the initial treatment of MCL have been the rituximab, hyperfractionated cyclophosphamide, vincristine, doxorubicin, dexamethasone (R-HyperCVAD) regimen or the consolidation of first remission following chemoimmunotherapy with high-dose therapy and ASCT. The most recent update from the M.D. Anderson Cancer Center of R-HyperCVAD reported a median OS not reached at 8 years, and a median time to failure of 4.6 years.[247] A multi-institution SWOG phase 2 trial of R-HyperCVAD reported median PFS and OS of 4.8 and 6.8 years, respectively. However, 39% of patients were unable to complete the planned treatment.[248] A similar issue was found in a report from academic centers in Italy, where, despite excellent disease control with R-HyperCVAD, with OS and FFS of 86% and 61%, respectively, 63% of patients were unable to complete the planned treatment course with the most common reason being treatment-related toxicity.[249] There has been only one randomized trial comparing ASCT to conventional therapy, and this was in the pre-rituximab era. Autologous transplant for patients younger than 65 years, in first CR or PR, demonstrated improvements in PFS as compared to interferon-α maintenance, but a nonstatistically significant improvement in OS.[250] Many phase 2 studies have intensified the induction therapy prior to ASCT in an attempt to improve outcomes. The Nordic regimen (CHOP-R + high-dose cytarabine [HiDAC] and ASCT for mantle cell lymphoma)[251] has yielded excellent results, with median OS and response duration longer than 10 years, and a median event-free survival (EFS) of 7.4 years. An analysis of outcome by MIPI score found that, at 10 years, 70% of patients with low-intermediate MIPI-B were alive, but only 23% of the patients were still alive with high MIPI-B.

The majority of patients with MCL relapse from primary therapy. Three agents are U.S. Food and Drug Administration (FDA) approved for relapsed MCL: bortezomib, lenalidomide, and ibrutinib. Bortezomib has a 29% overall RR, and a 5% CR/Cru with a median duration of 7 months.[252] Lenalidomide is FDA approved for bortezomib failures, with a 26% RR (CR, 7%), and a median duration of response of 17 months.[253,254] Ibrutinib has a 68% RR, with a 21% CR, and a median duration of 17.5 months.[255] Another oral kinase inhibitor targeting CDK4/6 is under investigation for relapsed patients.[256] Conventional chemotherapy agents, including purine analogs and bendamustine, are active in relapsed patients.[135] For patients with localized progression, local RT can provide reasonable palliation.[257] MCL is one of the most sensitive tumors to RT, and modest doses of radiation (20 Gy) can shrink even large masses and, therefore, should be considered in chemorefractory patients.

SCT for relapsed MCL patients has been of limited benefit. With long follow-ups, patients undergoing ASCT have a high relapse rate.[258] There is interest in nonmyeloablative alloSCT for select patients with relapsed disease. The 3-year PFS and OS are 30% and 40%, respectively.[259] Given the poor prognosis for patients with relapsed MCL, clinical trials should be explored for these patients.

Diffuse Large B-Cell Lymphoma

DLBCL constitutes 31% of all NHLs, and is the most common histologic subtype. Although, in the past, DLBCL was considered one disease, in the 2008 WHO classification, DLBCL is recognized to encompass many entities (see Table 103.4). Caucasian Americans have a higher incidence of DLBCL than African Americans, Asian Americans, and Native or Alaskan Native Americans. There is a slight male predominance, and the median age is 64 years. There is a familial component in some cases, with about a 3.5-fold increased risk in relatives of probands with DLBCL. Patients with congenital or acquired immunodeficiency, patients on immunosuppression, and patients with autoimmune disorders have a higher risk of developing DLBCL, often EBV related. This implicated immune dysfunction is a risk factor for the disease. DLBCL can arise as a histologic transformation from any indolent B-cell NHL or CLL.

Pathology

DLBCLs consist of a diffuse proliferation of large cells that have a high mitotic rate. The only unifying feature is the large size of the tumor cells, which may have centroblastic, immunoblastic, plasmablastic, or anaplastic morphologies. In a subset of cases, classified as T-cell/histiocyte-rich large B-cell lymphoma, there are only scattered large tumor cells in a background of abundant small T cells and epithelioid histiocytes.[260]

Immunophenotype and Genetics

The normal cellular counterparts for DLBCL are GC and post-GC activated B cells. Tumor cells generally express B-cell antigens (CD19, CD20, CD79a), monoclonal sIgM, and occasionally, other heavy chain isotypes. CD5-positive cases are uncommon and may have a worse prognosis.[261] CD10 and BCL6 expression typifies tumors of GC origin (GCB), whereas expression of MUM1 favors a non-GC, activated B-cell type origin (ABC). Of DLBCLs, 25% to 80% are reported to express BCL2, whereas approximately 70% express BCL6.[44,262] CD30 positivity (14% of cases) is associated with better survival.[263]

Several chromosomal abnormalities have been observed in DLBCL. Rearrangements of BCL6 are found in a small proportion of FLs (6% to 13%), but occur in about 30% of DLBCLs.[264] Many different *BCL6* translocations have been described, all of which replace the *BCL6* promoter with the promoter of another gene that is highly expressed in GC B cells, thus driving the overexpression of BCL6. Other tumors have point mutations in the BCL6 promoter that prevent BCL6 (a transcriptional repressor) from negatively regulating its own expression.[265] BCL6 overexpression leads to increased proliferation and survival of GC B cells, and also blocks differentiation into plasma cells by interfering with the activity of the transcription factor PRDM1 (also known as BLIMP1).[266] Another 20% to 30% of DLBCLs are associated with the t(14;18). Surprisingly, the t(14;18) is not always associated with BCL2 protein overexpression by immunohistochemistry.[267] Ig genes consistently show somatic mutations in the Ig variable region genes.[268] By GEP, the GCB type is often associated with the t(14;18) and amplifications of the *REL* oncogene on chromosome 2. In contrast, the ABC type is associated with a loss of 6q21 and trisomy 3, gains of 3q and 18q21-22, and mutations of *EZH2*.[269,270] The involved area on 6q includes PRDM1 (*BLIMP1*), reinforcing the idea that PRDM1, a master regulator of plasma cell differentiation, functions as a tumor suppressor in B cells.[271] ABC cases also have a high level activation of NF-κB, a transcription factor implicated in the B-cell receptor signaling pathway that supports B-cell proliferation and survival.[272] Recently, there has been great interest in the clinical implications of *MYC* rearrangements and overexpression in DLBCL. *MYC* is rearranged in 10% of DLBCLs, with the partner gene being one of the Ig genes in 60% of cases and some other gene in 40% of cases. Approximately 20% of *MYC*-rearranged cases have concurrent *BCL2* or *BCL6* rearrangements, a combination referred to as *double hit lymphoma*.[273] Amplification and/or overexpression of MYC independent of rearrangements or amplification has also been described and is also associated with a poor prognosis.[274,275] Deep sequencing of DLBCL samples have found extensive mutations, especially in the same histone-modifying genes implicated in FL—the histone acetyltransferases *EP300* and *CREBP* and the histone methyltransferase *MLL2*. Thus, like FL, epigenetic changes are likely to have a central pathogenic role in DLBCL.[276]

Clinical Features

Patients have a median of age 64 years, although younger in African Americans versus Caucasians.[277] Patients present with rapidly enlarging masses, either nodal enlargement or extranodal disease. DLBCL presents as stage I or IE disease approximately 20% of the time. The disease is confined to one side of the diaphragm (stage I or II) in approximately 30% to 40% of patients. Stage IV disease is seen in approximately 40% of patients. B symptoms occur in 30% of patients, and serum LDH is elevated in over half the patients. Extranodal sites are common, occurring in 40% of cases, including the GI tract, the testis,[278] the bone, the thyroid, the skin, the CNS, and bone marrow. DLBCL is highly invasive, with local compression of blood vessels, airways, involvement of peripheral nerves, and destruction of bone. Bone marrow involvement initially is found in only 10% to 20% of patients and has a strong correlation with the risk of spread to the CNS.[279] Other sites of extranodal disease, specifically testicular, paranasal sinus, epidural, and the presence of multiple extranodal sites, are other risks for CNS dissemination.

Therapy of Early Stage Diffuse Large B-Cell Lymphoma

Less than 20% of patients with DLBCL have localized disease. The recommended treatment for localized disease outside of clinical trials is abbreviated, combination chemoimmunotherapy plus involved field radiotherapy, or combination chemoimmunotherapy alone. The benefit of adding radiotherapy to 6 to 8 cycles of chemotherapy remains unclear. The SWOG randomized trial from the pre-rituximab era in patients with localized diffuse aggressive lymphoma compared eight cycles of CHOP to three cycles of CHOP plus involved field radiotherapy.[280] Patients treated with three cycles of CHOP plus radiotherapy had a significantly better 5-year PFS and OS than patients treated with eight cycles of CHOP (77% versus 64% for PFS, 82% versus 72% for OS). Overall life-threatening toxicity and cardiac toxicity were significantly higher in the patients receiving CHOP alone. The benefit of attenuated chemotherapy was largely found in patients over the age of 60 years. Although there is no analogous randomized trial that incudes rituximab, there is a phase II trial of patients with early stage DLBCL employing three cycles of CHOP-R followed by involved field RT.[281] Patients had at least one adverse risk factor for early stage disease specifically: age >60 years, increased serum LDH, stage II disease, or performance status ≥1. The PFS and OS at 2 and 4 years was 93% and 88%, and 95% and 92%, respectively.

In the pre-rituximab era, another randomized trial compared eight courses of CHOP with or without involved field radiotherapy in patients with previously untreated bulky or extranodal stage I or stage II diffuse aggressive NHL. The disease-free survival was greater for CR patients who received radiotherapy (73% versus 56%), although 10-year OS was similar in the two treatment arms (68% versus 65%).[282] The role of RT remains uncertain in patients with stage I or II disease. In patients aged 60 years or younger with low-risk disease, an aggressive regimen (rituximab, doxorubicin, cyclophosphamide, vindesine, bleomycin, and prednisone [ACVBP]) was superior to CHOP plus radiation.[283] Similarly, in patients over age 60 years, the addition of RT did not improve DFS or OS for patients who received four cycles of CHOP alone.[284] A phase III study in patients age 60 years or under with IPI score of 0 or 1 compared six cycles of CHOP to CHOP-R, with all patients with bulk disease (masses greater than 7.5 cm) or extranodal sites receiving involved field radiation. If one looks at the patients with an IPI score of 0 with no bulk, which includes early stage patients, the 5-year EFS is approximately 90% with CHOP-R alone. This supports the notion that chemoimmunotherapy alone is a reasonable option for early stage disease. However, in patients with bulk disease often defined as masses greater than 7.5 cm, the outcome is worse than for patients without bulk. In the randomized MabThera International Trial (MInT) trial of CHOP versus CHOP-R, all patients (IPI 0 or IPI 1) with masses >7.5 cm received 30 to 40 Gy of involved field radiation to those sites. Those patients with IPI of 0 and bulk disease had a 10% to 15% lower PFS than patients without bulk.[285] A randomized trial of a similar patient population is examining whether involved field radiation impacts outcomes for patients with bulk disease or extranodal disease (the UNFOLDER trial). Early data in this trial suggests a benefit for RT after chemotherapy. Presently, the most appropriate management of patients with early stage DLBCL with bulk disease remains controversial.

Therapy of Advanced Stage Diffuse Large B-Cell Lymphoma

If a clinical trial is not available, the current recommendation for the treatment of advanced stage DLBCL is combination chemotherapy with CHOP-R for patients both under age 60 years as well as over age 60 years. Questions that have been addressed in trials has been the number of cycles, the interval for those cycles, and whether more intensive therapy including high-dose therapy and stem cell support has a significant impact on outcome.

In patients with DLBCL ages 60 to 80 years, the Groupe d'Etude des Lymphomes de l'Adulte (GELA) group reported that eight cycles of CHOP-R was superior to CHOP alone in terms of PFS, disease-free survival (DFS), and OS with no added toxicity.[286,287] A U.S. Intergroup study compared in a similar population administering CHOP or CHOP-R given on a different schedule.[288] Responding patients were randomly assigned to receive either rituximab maintenance therapy or no maintenance. A beneficial impact of rituximab added to CHOP chemotherapy on EFS and OS was observed; however, no benefit was seen for maintenance rituximab following CHOP-R induction. Similarly, in patients less than 60 years of age, with an IPI of 0 and 1, the addition of rituximab to CHOP improved time to treatment failure and OS compared to CHOP alone.[285]

The number of cycles of therapy has been examined in the rituximab with CHOP over age 60 years (RICOVER-60) trial, in patients over age 60 years. This study compared six to eight cycles of CHOP or CHOP-R administered every 14 days (CHOP-R 14). CHOP-R was superior to CHOP given for six or eight cycles (70% versus 57%), and there was no benefit of eight cycles of CHOP-R over six cycles (with two additional doses of rituximab).[289] In another study, CHOP-R given every 21 days (CHOP-R 21) for eight cycles was compared to six cycles of CHOP-R 14.[290] More grade III/IV neutropenia was seen in the CHOP-R 21 (57%/31%) treated patients, whereas more thrombocytopenia occurred in the CHOP-R 14–treated patients. With a median follow-up of 40 months, there was no difference in PFS or OS. Another study from the GELA trial did not find an improvement in outcome with CHOP-R 14. This supports the notion that CHOP-R 21 for six to eight cycles is the standard of care.

Attempts to intensify therapy have included alternative regimens and ASCT. The GELA group treated patients under age 60 years with IPI of 1 with the more aggressive regimen R-ACVBP followed by consolidation with methotrexate and leucovorin.[291] When compared to CHOP-R plus intrathecal methotrexate, R-ACVBP plus methotrexate and leucovorin led to higher PFS and OS. Several studies have examined the role of high-dose therapy and ASCT in first CR/PR for patients with aggressive NHL prior to the addition of rituximab to combination chemotherapy. In the pre-rituximab era, the overall benefit of ASCT in first remission for patients with DLBCL remains uncertain despite many randomized trials. A meta-analysis of 3,079 patients treated on 15 randomized trials with either conventional therapy or ASCT

in first CR, showed no difference in EFS, OS, or treatment-related mortality.[292] Two recent studies in the rituximab era have not resolved this issue of ASCT in first CR. R-CHOEP (rituximab, cyclophosphamide, adriamycin, vincristine, etoposide, and prednisone) was compared to R-MegaCHOEP, sequential high-dose therapy with stem cell support, for high-intermediate or high-risk age adjusted IPI score patients. There was more hematologic toxicity with R-MegaCHOEP. With a median follow-up of 42 months, no statistical difference was seen in 3-year EFS (70% versus 61%) or OS (74% versus 70%).[293] More recently, a US intergroup trial treated patients with age-adjusted high-intermediate and high-risk IPI scores with at least a PR after five cycles of CHOP-based therapy (CHOP or CHOP-R), to a total of six cycles of CHOP-based therapy followed by ASCT versus a total of eight cycles of CHOP-based therapy alone.[294] Patients who relapsed after chemotherapy alone could undergo ASCT as salvage therapy. After a median follow-up of 6.3 years, ASCT was associated with a higher PFS at 2 years (69 versus 55%; hazard ratio [HR] 1.72; 95% confidence interval [CI], 0.82 to 1.94) but no difference in OS (74 versus 71%; HR 1.26; 95% CI, 0.82 to 1.94). To date, the data do not support ASCT as a consolidation for first remission.

Treatment of Relapsed or Refractory Diffuse Large B-Cell Lymphoma

The majority of relapses from CHOP-R therapy are seen within the first 2 years after the completion of treatment. However, 18% of relapses occur greater than 5 years after the initial treatment.[295] The failure of primary therapy to induce a CR or early relapse within the first few months of completing treatment is associated with a particularly poor prognosis. We generally recommend that patients who relapse after a CR be rebiopsied, because a subset will have FL.

Once relapse or refractory disease has been determined, the next issue to resolve is whether the goal is potential curative therapy or palliation. For patients with poor performance status, particularly elderly patients, the goal is often palliation. Local radiation can provide transient palliation. Other chemotherapy agents, including single agents such as cytarabine[296] or bendamustine,[297] are associated with overall RRs of 50% to 63%, a CR rate of 37%, and a median PFS of approximately 6 months.[298] The all oral-agent regimen PEPC (prednisone, etoposide, cyclophosphamide, and procarbazine) can induce remission in over 50% of patients.[299] Clinical trials may be an option for some of these patients depending on eligibility criteria.

The majority of patients with relapsed and refractory DLBCL receive combination chemotherapy, often with rituximab. Various combinations of drugs, including ifosfamide, carboplatin, etoposide, cytarabine, gemcitabine, and cisplatin, have been utilized for relapsed disease. The goal is to identify patients with chemosensitive disease who have the greatest likelihood of benefiting from high-dose therapy and ASCT, which leads to a higher long-term DFS and OS for relapsed DLBCL. A major question has been whether one second-line regimen is superior. The collaborative trial in relapsed aggressive lymphoma (CORAL) study compared R-ICE (rituximab, ifosfamide, carboplatin, and etoposide) to R-DHAP (rituximab, dexamethasone, high-dose cytarabine, and cisplatin), followed by ASCT.[300,301] No difference in overall RR, EFS, or OS was seen between the two regimens, with approximately 60% of patients responding. A subset analysis suggested that patients with a GCB DLBCL may have a better treatment outcome with R-DHAP versus R-ICE. The ultimate goal of salvage therapy is to achieve disease control to proceed to ASCT. It has been known since 1987 that disease sensitivity is the best determinant of outcome with high-dose therapy and ASCT. Three patient groups were identified based on the response to most recent treatment. Patients with chemosensitive disease have 30% to 50% long-terms DFS, those with chemorefractory disease have 10% to 15% long-term DFS and those with primary refractory disease have essentially no benefit from ASCT.[302] A major question was whether patients with chemosensitive disease benefit from ASCT or simply continuing salvage chemotherapy. The Parma study addressed this question, where 109 patients who had relapsed after having achieved a CR and responded to two cycles of DHAP were randomized to high-dose therapy and ASCT or four additional cycles of DHAP. ASCT was associated with a superior failure-free survival (51% versus 12% at 5 years) and OS (53% versus 32% at 5 years).[303] In the rituximab era, the long-term results of ASCT are less favorable than reported in the Parma trial, with about 30% long-term survivors in remission. Investigators have, to date, failed to improve on these results with the addition of maintenance therapy posttransplant with rituximab,[304] an anti-CD19 immunotoxin, or the oral kinase inhibitor enzastaurin, or adding radioimmunotherapy to the conditioning regimen. For patients with relapsed or refractory DLBCL, high-dose therapy and ASCT remain the treatments of choice for patients with chemosensitive disease. If the recurrence is localized, adjuvant RT either before or after high-dose therapy and ASCT may be beneficial. For patients with chemorefractory disease, clinical trials or palliative therapy should be considered. Several new agents have shown some promise in patients with relapsed DLBCL, including ibrutinib, particularly in the ABC cell of origin subtype, lenalidomide[253] and everolimus.[305]

Allogeneic bone marrow transplantation is generally not the favored approach for relapsed DLBCL patients. Although highly selected patients can have prolonged remission, this is at the expense of a high treatment-related mortality. Overall, there is no advantage for alloSCT. Patients with recurrent disease following ASCT who have good performance status and chemosensitive disease are now considered for alloSCT usually with reduced intensity conditioning, rather than ablative alloSCT where morbidity and mortality are exceedingly high. Studies have reported a 40% to 60% year PFS with this approach, but with a treatment-related mortality of 20% for RIC alloSCT and up to 40% for myeloablative transplants.[306,307]

Chimeric antigen receptor T (CAR-T) cells are another investigational immunotherapy approach to treating malignancies that have had some early success in CLL and B-cell acute lymphoblastic leukemia.[308–310] This strategy uses T cells collected from a patient that are genetically modified to express a receptor that will bind to a surface antigen expressed on the patient's own tumor cells. In the case of B-cell malignancies, this antigen has been CD19. After infusion, autologous CAR-T cells home to sites of disease and also persist over time. The CARs consist of an extracellular antigen recognition domain (typically a single chain Fv variable fragment from a monoclonal antibody) linked via a transmembrane domain to an intracellular signaling domain (usually the CD3ζ endodomain), resulting in the redirection of T-cell specificity toward target antigen-positive cells, and one or more costimulatory domains including CD28, 4-1BB, or OX40 to enhance cytokine secretion and effector cell expansion, and prevent activation-induced apoptosis and immune suppression by tumor-related metabolites.[311] Eight patients with DLBCL and/or primary mediastinal large B-cell lymphoma (PMLBCL) who have been treated with anti-CD19 CAR-T cells have been reported.[312] Five of these patients had a CR (2) or PR (3) that persisted for up to 19 months following therapy.

Other Large B-Cell Lymphomas

Intravascular Large B-Cell Lymphoma

Intravascular large B-cell lymphoma (ILCL) is a rare subtype in which lymphoma cells proliferate within small blood vessels without producing a tumor mass or detectable circulating tumor cells.[313–315] The tumor cells resemble centroblasts or immunoblasts, express B-cell–associated antigens, and are usually CD10 negative and MUM1 positive. Patients present with a variety of symptoms caused by the occlusion of small vessels. These include B symptoms, rapidly progressive neurologic signs (dementia, cerebral vascular accident, and/or peripheral neuropathy), and skin lesions imitating an inflammatory rash. Western and Asian subtypes have

been identified, with less frequent CNS and skin involvement in the former. Laboratory abnormalities include elevated serum LDH and anemia. The diagnosis is made by demonstrating large lymphoma cells within small to medium blood vessels. The diagnosis can be difficult, but if the disease is suspected, a *blind* biopsy of normal-appearing skin can be diagnostic. If this is not informative, a biopsy of other sites of suspected involvement may necessary. The treatment of patients with ILBL includes both systemic chemoimmuno-therapy and therapy for the CNS. Prior to rituximab, the prognosis for these patients was poor, with less than 10% long-term survivors. With an earlier diagnosis and therapy with CHOP-R, the 2-year PFS and OS have been reported to be 56% and 66%, respectively. CNS prophylaxis with either intrathecal or high-dose systemic methotrexate is recommended. Patients with secondary involvement of the brain or spinal cord at diagnosis, depending on the clinical situation, may need intrathecal chemotherapy, systemic high-dose methotrexate, and/or radiation to the sites of involvement.

T-Cell Histiocyte-Rich Large B-Cell Lymphoma

In this uncommon subtype of DLBCL, the majority of the tumor cell mass is comprised of nonneoplastic T cells and/or histiocytes, with malignant B cells making up less than 10% of the cellularity.[316] The lymphoma cells express CD20 but lack CD5, CD10, and CD138. An IPI of 2 or greater was reported in one series in a majority (77%) of patients, often with spleen, liver, and marrow involvement. The outcome of treatment is controversial, with one large series showing a less favorable prognosis, and a second suggesting a similar outcome to other forms of DLBCL when matched for risk factors.

EBV-Positive DLBCL of the Elderly. EBV-positive DLBCL of the elderly is a provisional entity in the 2008 WHO classification. It is seen in patients greater than age 50 years, without known immunodeficiency or prior lymphoma. In Asian countries, this accounts for 8% to 10% of DLBCL in patients without a known immunodeficiency.[317,318] It is less common in Western countries. Patients often present with extranodal disease in addition to lymph nodes. Due to older age, frequent extranodal disease, and poor performance status, these patients often have a poor prognosis.

ALK-Positive Large B-Cell Lymphoma. These are rare variants of large B-cell lymphomas that expresses CD30 and ALK kinase, usually due to a t(2;17) that fuses *ALK* to the clathrin heavy chain 1 gene (*CTLC*). These tumors often have a plasmablastic appearance and have been reported to have a poor prognosis.[319]

Special Situations

Testicular Diffuse Large B-Cell Lymphoma

DLBCL presenting in the testis is the most common malignant tumor in that site in men over 60 years of age, and constitute 1% of all lymphomas.[278,320] Other less common histologies include BL in children and, rarely, FL. Historically, the long-term results of treatment are worse for these patients than predicted by the IPI. Despite therapy, patients are at risk for relapse systemically, in the CNS, and in the contralateral testis. Therefore, following orchiectomy, patients require systemic therapy, and strong consideration should be given to CNS prophylaxis with either systemic or intrathecal methotrexate, as well as prophylactic radiation to the contralateral testis. Much of the data for treating this condition is from small series without randomized trials to address management issues. A recent international prospective trial of 53 patients with untreated stage I or II primary testicular lymphoma treated with six to eight cycles of CHOP-R 21, four weekly doses of intrathecal methotrexate (12 mg), and RT to the contralateral testis (30 Gy) for all patients and (30 to 36 Gy) to regional nodes for patients with stage II disease.[278] With a median follow-up of 65 months, the OS and

PFS at 5 years was 85% and 74%, respectively. Only three relapses were seen in the CNS. This study defines the current standard of care with chemoimmunotherapy, CNS prophylaxis, and radiation to the contralateral testis.

Treatment of the Aggressive Non-Hodgkin's Lymphoma in the Elderly

Lymphoma occurs at a higher incidence with increasing age.[321–323] Patients over age 60 years as shown in the IPI have a lower CR rate, PFS, and OS than patients 60 years of age or less. The reasons are probably a combination of increased treatment-related mortality and comorbidities. Biologically, the disease may also be different in older individuals, which may account, in part, for the higher IPI scores that have been reported in elderly patients. Dose reductions in these patients may also explain the less favorable outcome. The SWOG reported a CR rate of 37% in patients 65 years of age and older who received initial 50% dose reductions of cyclophosphamide and doxorubicin. Complete remission rates were 52%, a rate similar to those of younger patients, when full-dose chemotherapy was used.

Randomized trials have clearly demonstrated a significant survival benefit for the addition of rituximab to combination chemotherapy for DLBCL in patients over age 60 years.[289,321–323,324] In light of the concerns of increased toxicity of treatment in elderly patients, several regimens have been reported with this in mind. A recent report of 149 patients age 80 years or older, employed reduced doses of cyclophosphamide, adriamycin, and vincristine at about 50% of standard dosing of CHOP-R (R-mini CHOP).[325] Grade 3/4 neutropenia and thrombocytopenia was seen in 39% and 7% of patients, respectively, and 12 toxic deaths were seen. The 2-year OS and PFS were 59% and 47%, respectively. For patients who are not considered candidates for standard-dose or reduced-dose chemoimmunotherapy, regimens such as PEPC or BR[326] can be useful for palliation in elderly patients, with over 50% RRs and a median PFS of over 6 months.

The approach toward elderly patients with aggressive lymphoma should be similar to patients age 60 years or younger, with curative intent. Supportive care measures with hematopoietic growth factors can be considered, albeit controversially, as well as prophylactic antibiotics. Analogous to younger patients, elderly patients should be considered for clinical trials if eligible and feasible.

Primary Mediastinal Large B-Cell Lymphoma

Within the category of DLBCL is a distinct clinical entity known as PMLBCL, representing 2.4% of all NHLs and 7% of all cases of DLBCL.[327]

Pathology

Histologically, the large tumor cells often have finer nuclear membranes and smaller nucleoli than other subtypes of DLBCL, sometimes making it difficult to distinguish the tumor cells from reactive macrophages in small biopsies. Not infrequently, a few multinucleated cells reminiscent of Reed-Sternberg variants may be admixed with more typical tumor cells. The tumor cells diffusely infiltrate the mediastinum and often elicit dense fibrosis, another feature that may render biopsies difficult to interpret.

Immunophenotype and Genetics

PMLBCLs express B-cell antigens CD19, CD20, CD22, TRAF1, and c-Rel, but lack sIg and CD5.[323] Unlike other DLBCLs, a low level expression of CD30 is seen in most cases, and a high fraction of tumors expresses TRAF1 and have nuclear REL. *BCL2* and *BCL6* rearrangements are absent. Translocations of the *CIITA* (major histocompatibility complex class II transactivator) gene are noted in about 40% of cases. Copy number gains in the region on chromosome 9p containing the genes for janus kinase 2 (*JAK2*) and programmed cell death ligand 1 and 2 (*PDL1* and *PDL2*) are

common. PDL1 and PDL2 are ligands for the programmed cell death receptor 1 (PD-1), which has a role in suppressing T-cell function.[269] PMLBCL resembles classical Hodgkin's disease (HD) by GEP,[329] because one-third of the most highly expressed genes in PMLBCLs are also expressed in the Reed-Sternberg cells of HL.

Clinical Features

PMLBCLs have a female predominance, with median age of 40 years. Over 70% of these patients present with stage I/II bulky disease involving the mediastinum, with pleural and pericardial effusions in about 50% of the patients. Superior vena cava syndrome is frequently seen in these patients. An elevated LDH (77%) and B symptoms (47%) are common. Relapses occur locally or in extranodal sites, including the liver, the GI tract, the kidneys, the ovaries, and the CNS.

Treatment

The general approach toward patients with PMLBCL has been similar to patients with localized DLBCL, with the majority of patients receiving combined modality therapy. The most recent results with chemoimmunotherapy demonstrate a 3-year OS of 89% with CHOP-R therapy. In the MInT trial, 87 patients with PMLBCL[330] received six cycles of CHOP-R, 75% of whom also received RT; only 7% of patients who received radiation subsequently progressed or relapsed. A recent study of 51 patients treated with dose-adjusted etoposide, prednisone, vincristine, cyclophosphamide, doxorubicin (EPOCH) plus rituximab (DA-EPOCH-R), and no radiotherapy, reported an outstanding PFS (93%) and OS (100%). The two failures received radiation and were rendered disease free.[331] These studies suggest that six cycles of CHOP-R followed by RT, or six to eight cycles of DA-EPOCH-R and no RT gives excellent results in PMBCL.

Grey Zone Lymphoma

In 2008, the WHO created provisional diagnoses to capture B-cell lymphomas with features between two established diagnoses: BL and DLBCL, and classical Hodgkin's lymphoma (cHL) and DLBCL.[332] These lymphomas constitute the grey zone lymphomas.

B-Cell Lymphoma, Unclassifiable, with Features Intermediate Between B-Cell Lymphoma and Diffuse Large B-Cell Lymphoma

These lymphomas differ morphologically from DLBCL in that the neoplastic cells often range from intermediate to large in size, may have a very high Ki-67 index, and are uniformly CD10 positive. They differ from BL in that the cells are more variable in size, are often BCL2 positive, may be BCL6 negative, and may have a Ki-67 index lower than 100%. Although defined by morphologic features, GEP has, likewise, identified a group of lymphomas with a GEP between that of BL and DLBCL.[333] This group is not synonymous with B-cell lymphoma, unclassifiable (B-UNC)/BL/DLBCL but the two overlap, suggesting B-UNC/BL/DLBCL is not a unique entity but rather a group of distinct lymphomas, including true BL, DLBCL, and unclassifiable lymphomas, which require further characterization.

Although potentially heterogeneous, these lymphomas carry a poor prognosis and are associated with high IPIs and frequent extranodal sites; this trend may be driven by inclusion of a subset of tumors with a particularly poor prognosis.[334,335] Although the IPI remains the most powerful prognostic tool we have for DLBCL, certain genetic events are being recognized as indicators of particularly high-risk disease. Most notably, the presence of multiple concurrent chromosomal translocations, commonly involving *MYC* and *BCL2*, defines a group with an extraordinarily poor prognosis.[273] This was first noted in Burkitt-like lymphoma, many of which were B-UNC/BL/DLBCL. No patients with these *double-hit* lymphomas were alive at 1 year. In DLBCL, dual translocations are present in 12% to 14% of cases and are similarly associated with a poor prognosis.[336] B-UNC/BL/DLBCL is enriched for these *double-hit* lymphomas, with 30% to 45% harboring both *MYC* and *BCL2* translocations. Although the majority of double-hit lymphomas fall into this diagnostic category, not all B-UNC/BL/DLBCLs are double-hit lymphomas. Double-hit lymphomas with this histology, however, appear to have a particularly poor prognosis, with a median OS of 4 months compared to 3 years in double-hit DLBCL with typical morphologic features.[337]

Although the prognosis for this group as a whole is poor, there has been no systematic investigation of the treatment of B-UNC/BL/DLBCL, and thus, no prospective evidence supporting the intensification of therapy over CHOP-R. However, three groups have retrospectively looked at the impact of intensified chemotherapy on outcomes for B-UNC/BL/DLBCL.[343,338] These analyses are limited in that they are retrospective, small, and likely included patients without B-UNC/BL/DLBCL. However, each showed that intensive regimens such as a modified Magrath regimen with cyclophosphamide, vincristine, doxorubicine, methotrexate/ifosphamide, etoposide, cytarabine (CODox-M/IVAC), HyperCVAD, and DA-EPOCH-R had better outcomes over CHOP-R (overall response rate [ORR] 86% versus 57%, 4-year PFS approximately 50% to 65% versus 0% to 30%). Another group retrospectively examined the outcomes following intensive therapy compared with CHOP-R in 53 patients with aggressive B-cell lymphoma with high-grade features with or without an *MYC* translocation.[335] Notably, patients in this study had a lower risk than is typical for B-UNC/BL/DLBCL. Amongst all patients, there was no improvement in OS with intensive regimens (4-year OS of 50% to 60%); this relatively good OS is widely different from previous reports and perhaps reflects the good risk profile of this cohort. However, among patients with an *MYC* translocation, intensive regimens resulted in a significantly longer PFS and a trend toward longer OS over CHOP-R, and, for double-hit lymphomas in this category, there was a nonsignificant trend toward a shorter PFS and OS compared with patients with an isolated MYC translocation. This suggests that perhaps it is the double-hit lymphomas within the category of B-UNC/BL/DLBCL that drives their poor prognosis, and these are patients that might benefit from intensive chemotherapy like modified Magrath or DA-EPOCH-R. Data from patients with MYC translocation-positive DLBCL treated with DA-EPOCH-R by the National Cancer Institute phase 2 studies are promising; nine patients (8%) harbored an *MYC* translocation and had a 4-year EFS of 83%.[339] This regimen is currently being explored further in BL and MYC translocation-positive DLBCL in a multicenter trial.

At the present time, there is not sufficient evidence to suggest that all patients with B-UNC/BL/DLBCL should be treated with regimens more intense than CHOP-R. This is a heterogenous group of patients with varied prognoses and natural histories, some of whom may do well with standard CHOP-R. However, for double-hit lymphomas, many of which are B-UNC/BL/DLBCL, CHOP-R is insufficient. These patients should be encouraged to participate in clinical trials. In the absence of a trial, intensified regimens of DA-EPOCH-R or modified Magrath, with or without an ASCT or alloSCT, can be considered. Agents that target BCL2 and an MYC-driven protein, aurora A kinase, are currently in development and may prove useful in these lymphomas; these patients should be considered for clinical trials when available.

B-Cell Lymphoma, Unclassifiable, with Features Intermediate Between DLBCL and Classical Hodgkin's Lymphoma

An overlap between the clinical and pathologic features of PMLBCL and cHL has been recognized for some time. Both typically occur in younger female patients, involve contiguous nodal stations, and on biopsy, demonstrate a variable number of malignant B cells within a fibrotic inflammatory infiltrate. In 2003, two groups explored GEPs of newly diagnosed PMLBCL, DLBCL, and cHL and found that the GEP of PMLBCL more closely resembled cHL than DLBCL.[329,340] Specifically, PMLBCL had a low expression of genes involved in B-cell receptor signaling but a high expression of genes involved in IL-13 receptor signaling as well as immunomodulatory genes such as *PDL1* and *PDL2*. In addition, both cHL and PMLBCL are associated with amplification of 9p24.1, which contains the genes for *JAK2* and *PDL1*, and this correlated with increased PD-L1 expression.[341] The recognition of some lymphomas with features intermediate between PMLBCL and cHL, or B-UNC/cHL/DLBCL, further supports the pathologic relationship between these two malignancies.

Among patients with B-UNC/cHL/DLBCL, the majority are men, with presentations in the mediastinum. Histopathologically, one sees pleomorphic tumor cells resembling both the Hodgkin Reed-Sternberg (HRS) cell of cHL and the large, atypical B cell of DLBCL or PMLBCL. These cells appear in sheets, separated by fibrotic stroma with an associated inflammatory infiltrate. Immunohistochemical profiles of the malignant cells demonstrate frequent positivity for CD45, CD20, CD79a, and CD30, but are often CD15 negative; other B-cell markers like PAX5, organic cation transporter 2 (OCT-2), and BOB1 are often positive. Methylation profiling reveals a profile intermediate between that of PMLBCL and cHL, corroborating that it is distinct, perhaps on a continuum between the two.[342] Interestingly, patients can have composite lymphomas in which DLBCL and cHL present sequentially; whether these lymphomas relate to B-UNC/cHL/DLBCL is unknown. However, the methylation profiles of both components of a single case of a composite lymphoma were most similar to that of B-UNC/cHL/DLBCL, suggesting that they are related.

The prognosis is notably poorer in B-UNC/cHL/DLBCL than in cHL or PMLBCL.[343] This is partly due to differences in pathobiology, but may also result from not knowing whether to treat with an NHL or a cHL regimen. There are no large prospective studies, but consensus has favored treating like NHL. There are single-arm studies demonstrating good activity of CHOP in HL, making CHOP-R an acceptable first-line therapy.[344,345] More recently, 16 patients with B-UNC/cHL/DLBCL were treated with DA-EPOCH-R, and 4-year EFS and OS was only 45% and 75%, respectively.[339] This regimen, however, was more effective in PMLBCL, where the 5-year EFS and OS were 93% and 97%, respectively.[331] Following combination chemotherapy, the role of involved field radiation therapy (IFRT) in both cHL and PMLBCL is debated. Despite frequently presenting with bulky mediastinal disease, patients with PMLBCL enjoy a favorable prognosis, with a 5-year OS >80% following CHOP-R and 97% following DA-EPOCH-R. Whether to radiate patients who achieve a complete metabolic response following CHOP-R is uncertain, but radiation was omitted in such cases in the DA-EPOCH-R series. The only published randomized trial of radiotherapy for this disease was stopped early due to increased relapses in the nonradiated group at the interim analysis; all patients on this study had a complete response to CHOP-R.[346] A large randomized clinical trial is ongoing in Europe to decidedly answer this question. Despite the lack of evidence supporting RT in patients who have a complete response to chemotherapy with B-UNC/cHL/DLBCL, many are referred for radiation given their worse prognosis.

Burkitt's Lymphoma

Burkitt's lymphoma is a rare disease in adults, comprising less than 1% of adult NHLs, whereas BL constitutes 30% of nonendemic pediatric lymphomas.[347]

Pathology

BL cells resemble the small noncleaved cells within normal GCs of secondary lymphoid follicles. The mitotic rate is high, and analogous to normal GCs, frequent tingible body macrophages are seen, producing the classical *starry sky* appearance. The fraction of Ki-67 positive (proliferating cells) in BL is typically 99% or greater.[64]

Immunophenotype and Genetics

BL is a tumor of B-lineage derivation identified by the expression of CD19, CD20, sIgM, CD10, and BCL6, but not BCL2.[348] Endemic BLs are EBV positive, whereas the majority of non-endemic BLs are EBV negative. BL is associated with a translocation involving *MYC* on chromosome 8q24 in over 95% of the cases. The most common partners are chromosomes 14, 2, or 22, rearrangements that produce fusions of MYC with either the *IgH* (80%), kappa (15%), or lambda (5%) light chain genes. The breakpoints in *MYC* and *IgH* differ in endemic versus sporadic BL. MYC translocation is absent in <5% of cases, so-called atypical BL.[44] These cases are otherwise typical of BL, and share a characteristic GEP with cases of BL that are associated with MYC rearrangements.[333,349,350]

Clinical Features

BL is, in general, a pediatric tumor that has three major clinical presentations. The endemic (African) form presents as a jaw or facial bone tumor that spreads to extranodal sites, including the ovary, the testis, the kidney, the breast, and especially to the bone marrow and meninges. The nonendemic form has an abdominal presentation with massive disease, ascites, and renal, testis, and/or ovarian involvement, and, like the endemic form, also spreads to the bone marrow and CNS. Immunodeficiency-related cases more often involve lymph nodes and may present as acute leukemia. BL has a male predominance and is typically seen in patients less than 35 years of age.

Treatment

BL in adults has been similarly treated with regimens designed for pediatric populations. CHOP with intrathecal methotrexate should be considered insufficient treatment. Short, intensive therapy with CNS prophylaxis is the standard approach.[338,351] The original Magrath regimen (CODOX-M/IVAC) had a 92% 2-year OS.[352] Other, more recent series with this regimen in older patients have reported a 2-year OS of 82% for low-risk patients and 70% for high-risk patients.[353,354] Similar results have been seen with HyperCVAD rituximab-methotrexate-cytarabine.[355] A recent study of DA-EPOCH-R for six to eight cycles (two cycles past complete response) reported outstanding results with freedom from progression (FFP) of 95% and OS of 100% at a median follow-up of 86 months.[356] There is presently no evidence that first remission autologous transplant is indicated for adult BL.[357] The outcome for relapsed patients is dismal, with adults rarely cured with ASCT.[358]

MATURE T-CELL AND NATURAL KILLER CELL NEOPLASMS

Mycosis Fungoides

For a discussion of mycosis fungoides, see Chapter 104.

Peripheral T-Cell Lymphomas, Not Otherwise Specified

Peripheral T-cell lymphomas (PTCL) includes a number of entities, which constitute 15% of all NHLs in adults.[359] PTCL, not otherwise specified (NOS), comprising 6% of all NHLs, is the term used for cases that are not other entities defined in the WHO classification (e.g., ALCL).

Pathology

Features of PTCL, NOS vary widely and lack findings typical of other specific subtypes of PTCL. Lymph nodes are diffusely effaced by atypical lymphoid cells, which may include a spectrum of cell sizes or may be comprised mainly of large cells. The tumor cells may induce some degree of vascular proliferation and may be associated with varied stromal and host cell responses, sometimes including prominent infiltrates composed of eosinophils and/or macrophages. Mitoses, apoptosis, and geographic necrosis may also be seen.

Immunophenotype and Genetics

In contrast to B-cell lymphomas, the pattern of expression of T-cell surface antigens is variable. The normal cellular counterparts of PTCL NOS are mature peripheral T cells. T-cell-associated antigens are expressed (CD3+/−, CD2+/−).[360] CD4 is more often more expressed than CD8 and tumors may be CD4-/CD8-. In most cases, one or more "mature" T-cell antigens are lost, such as CD5 or CD7. TCR genes are usually rearranged. The most common translocations are t(7;14), t(11;14), inv(14), and t(14;14)—translocations that involve TCR genes.

Clinical Features

Peripheral T-cell lymphoma NOS[326] are aggressive NHLs, presenting with a median age of 65 years, with 69% of patients having stage III/IV disease. Both nodal and extranodal sites are common, including the skin, the liver, the spleen, and other viscera. B symptoms and pruritus are commonly seen. Laboratory abnormalities, including eosinophilia and hemophagocytic syndrome, are features of PTCL NOS.

Treatment

For PTCL NOS, most studies failed to show any advantage for regimens other than CHOP. A retrospective subset analysis of a phase 3 study in PTCL patients of CHOP versus CHOEP showed a significant improvement in EFS for PTCL patients younger than age 60 years with a normal LDH at diagnosis, but there was no difference in OS.[361] Various prognostic models for PTCL NOS have evolved, but generally, the IPI provides a reasonable stratification of outcome, with low-risk patients having a 55% 2-year OS and high-risk patients having a less than 15% 2-year OS.[361] ASCT has been applied to patients with PTCL NOS in first remission with approximately 50% 3- to 5-year PFS and OS. Given the generally unfavorable outcome for patients with PTCL NOS, clinical trials should be considered.

Recurrent disease is associated with very poor prognosis, with the median second PFS and OS after relapse of 4.6 and 6.7 months, respectively.[362] Conventional agents such as gemcitabine have limited activity.[363] Several FDA-approved drugs for relapsed PTCL, including the antifolate agent pralatrexate and HDAC inhibitors romidepsin and belinostat, all of which have a 25% to 30% RR with median durations of response of less than 18 months.[364,365] Nonmyeloablative alloSCT has a role for selected patients with 5-year OS and PFS of 50% and 40%, respectively, and nonrelapsed mortality of 12%.[366]

Angioimmunoblastic T-Cell Lymphoma

Angioimmunoblastic T-cell lymphoma (AITL) constitutes 4% of all NHLs and about 20% all T-cell NHLs.

Pathology and Genetics

Lymph nodes are diffusely effaced by a polymorphous population of lymphocytes of varying size, shape, and immunoblasts. Stains for CD21, CD23, and CD35 reveal an expanded network of follicular dendritic cells, which often surround tumor cells with moderately abundant clear cytoplasm. The neoplastic cells resemble normal CD4-positive follicular T cells, and in addition to expression of pan–T-cell markers such as CD3, often express CXCL13, PD-1, CD10, and BCL6. Immunoblasts in the background are often EBV-positive B cells, which expand in this disease and may give rise to secondary EBV-positive B-cell lymphomas. Trisomy 3 and/or 5 may occur.[367] Deep sequencing has revealed mutations in about 50% of cases in ten-eleven translocation 2 (*TET2*), an epigenetic modifier previously implicated in myelodysplastic syndromes.[368] Around 33% of PCTL NOS were also found to have *TET2* mutations in the same study; many of these tumors had some features reminiscent of AITL, suggesting that there is an overlap between these two disease categories.

Clinical Features

AITL presents in patients with a median age of 62 years. Often, there is acute onset of generalized lymphadenopathy, hepatomegaly, fever, B symptoms, skin rash with a lymphohistiocytic infiltrate, and autoimmune phenomenon, including polyarthritis, thyroid dysfunction, and hemolytic anemia. Laboratory study abnormalities include eosinophilia, polyclonal hypergammaglobulinemia, elevated serum LDH, anemia, and a positive Coombs test. Bone marrow involvement is common, with over 80% of patients having stage III or IV disease. The median survival ranges from 15 to 36 months, with patients dying of relapse, secondary EBV-positive DLBCL, or opportunistic infection.

Treatment

Up to one-third of patients with AITL can have spontaneous remissions or initial remissions to corticosteroids alone. AITL is approached similarly to PTCL NOS, with combination chemotherapy with 5-year OS and failure-free survival of 32% and 18%, respectively.[369] ASCT in first remission is an option for younger patients based on phase 2 studies. For relapsed disease, the options are similar to PTCL NOS, except few responses to pralatrexate were seen.

Enteropathy-Associated T-Cell Lymphoma

Enteropathy-associated T-cell lymphoma (EATL) is a rare aggressive disease of intraepithelial T cells that is often associated with a history of gluten enteropathy.[370,371] The more common type 1 is associated with clinical or serologic evidence of celiac disease and HLADQA1*0501, DQB1*0201 genotype.[372] Treatment of celiac disease with a gluten-free diet prevents the development of lymphoma.[370] Type II EATL is not associated celiac disease and is now considered not to be an EATL.

Pathology

Two variants have been described: type I and type II. Type I EATL is grossly characterized by diffuse infiltration of the bowel wall by an atypical lymphoid infiltrate that often produces mucosal ulcerations, sometimes accompanied by tumorous masses. The morphology of the tumor cells varies, but often they are large and have anaplastic features. In cases associated with celiac sprue, adjacent mucosa may show a dense infiltrate of small intraepithelial lymphocytes associated with villous atrophy. These cells may have the same TCR rearrangement as the large tumor cell population, suggesting that they represent a precursor lesion to EATL that arises in the setting of long-standing celiac disease. Type II EATL is not associated with celiac disease and may represent a different entity.

Immunophenotype and Genetics

Type I EATL cells express CD3 and CD103, an integrin expressed on intestinal lymphocytes. The tumor cells may be CD4 positive (11%), CD8 positive (43%), or CD4/CD8 double negative, and some cases are CD30 positive as well. Type II EATL cells are positive for CD8 and CD56.[373] Of type I and II cases, 50% to 60% have am-

plifications of the 9q31.3 region. A distinct feature of type II EATL is amplification of *MYC* due to copy gains of chromosome 8q24.

Clinical Features and Therapy

Patients with EATL present with intestinal obstruction, perforation, and bleeding. In some patients, there is a brief history of gluten sensitivity or worsening gluten enteropathy. Uncommonly, there is extraintestinal disease with dissemination to the lungs or skin. The small bowel is the most common site of disease, with the stomach or colon affected less often, whereas other viscera, the lung, the skin, or soft tissues may also be involved.[371] These patients have a very poor prognosis, with a median survival of 10 months. Surgery for limited-stage disease cures a small number of patients. Intensive induction with combination chemotherapy, including high-dose methotrexate, and autologous SCT in first remission, may yield better outcomes than chemotherapy alone.[374]

Anaplastic Large-Cell Lymphoma

ALCL constitutes 2% of all NHLs, but is the third most common T-cell NHL. ALCL is more frequent in children, representing 10% of all pediatric lymphomas. It is a heterogeneous disease category with several molecular and clinicopathologic subtypes. One of these unusual forms arises within the breast in association with breast implants.[375]

Pathology

Several morphologic variants of ALCL are recognized. The most common (80%) are cases composed of large cells with round or pleomorphic, often horseshoe-shaped or *embryoid* nuclei with multiple (or single) prominent nucleoli, which are referred to as *hallmark* cells. These cells have abundant cytoplasm, which gives them an epithelioid or histiocyte-like appearance. The remaining morphologies, which are most commonly seen in children, are the small-cell, lymphohistiocytic, and monomorphic variants. Tumor cells may preferentially localize within the sinuses of lymph nodes, producing an appearance that can be mistaken for metastatic solid tumors.

Immunophenotype and Genetics

Virtually all cases are CD30 positive. Over 60% of cases express CD3, CD25, CD43, or CD45RO, and many cases are CD4 positive. Unlike classical HL, ALCL cells usually lack CD15. A minority do not express B- or T-cell antigens, and up to 40% of cases may fail to express the common leukocyte antigen (CD45). TCR genes are clonally rearranged in most cases, but some tumors (particularly those that fail to express T-cell markers) apparently lack TCR rearrangements. Rearrangements involving the *ALK* gene are present in 40% to 60% of cases, more commonly in children and younger adults. The most common rearrangement is the t(2;5), which fuses a portion of the nucleolar protein nucleophosmin-1 (*NPM1*) gene on chromosome 5q35 to a portion of *ALK* on chromosome 2p23.[376] The resulting fusion gene encodes a chimeric NPM–ALK fusion protein with constitutive tyrosine-kinase activity. Immunohistochemistry for ALK can be used to reliably identify cases associated with *ALK* gene rearrangements.

Clinical Features

ALCL encompasses at least three distinct clinicopathologic entities: primary systemic ALCL, ALK positive; primary systemic ALCL, ALK negative; and primary cutaneous ALCL. Systemic ALCL, regardless of ALK status, may present in lymph nodes or extranodal sites, including but not limited to the skin. Primary cutaneous ALCL is morphologically similar to systemic ALCL but lacks ALK expression or rearrangements, and is by definition restricted to the skin at diagnosis (see Chapter 104). ALCL has a male predominance, with a median age of 34 years for ALK-positive disease, and 58 years for ALK-negative disease.[377] Except for age, there is no difference in clinical presentations of ALK-positive and ALK-negative systemic disease. Patients with systemic disease often present with B symptoms, peripheral and retroperitoneal adenopathy, and skin involvement (25% of patients). Although marrow involvement is infrequent, 60% of patients have stage III or IV disease.

Treatment

Generally, ALCL has been treated with combination chemotherapy, largely CHOP. A subset analysis of the randomized CHOP versus CHOEP trial in patients less than age 60 years with normal LDH, found superior outcome with CHOEP (90% versus 55% OS).[361] Compared to other peripheral T-cell NHLs, ALCL has the highest 5-year OS, driven by the IPI score and the expression of ALK, with ALK-positive disease associated with a favorable prognosis,[378,379] with 8-year OS of 82% versus only 49% in ALK disease. The major impact of ALK expression was seen in patients age 40 years or greater.[380] For relapsed patients, options include SCT following reinduction therapy. The anti-CD30 antibody drug conjugate brentuximab vedotin (anti-CD30 monomethyl auristatin E [MMAE] antitubulin conjugate) is highly active,[381] with an overall RR of 86%, and a CR rate of 57%, with the median duration of CR of 13 months. Brentuximab is being examined in the initial treatment of ALCL. Crizotinib, an inhibitor of the ALK tyrosine kinase, has reported activity in relapsed disease.[382]

Hepatosplenic T-Cell Lymphoma

Hepatosplenic T-cell lymphoma is an extremely rare disease of cytotoxic T cells.

Pathology

The tumor cells infiltrate the red pulp of the spleen and liver sinusoids as well as the bone marrow, although this can be subtle. Cells are medium sized with round nuclei, moderately condensed chromatin, and moderately abundant pale cytoplasm.

Immunophenotype and Genetics

The tumor cells are CD2+, CD3+, variably CD8+, CD7+, and CD56+. In contrast to most PTCL, which generally express the $\alpha\beta$ T-cell receptor, these tumors commonly express $\gamma\delta$ T-cell receptor. Isochromosome 7q and trisomy 8 have been reported in many cases, and these tumors are genetically distinct from other PTCL.[383]

Clinical Features and Treatment

Hepatosplenic T-cell lymphoma is an extremely rare disease presenting in adolescents and young adults, with a male predominance. Features include marked hepatosplenomegaly, often with marrow involvement, and occasionally, peripheral blood involvement and pancytopenia.[384,385] Of patients, 10% to 20% occur in immunosuppressed, solid-organ allograft recipients and in patients with Crohn's disease on thiopurines.[386] This is an aggressive disease, which usually relapses after the initial response to chemotherapy. The median survival is 1 to 2 years, with rare patients being long-term survivors after alloSCT.

Subcutaneous Panniculitis-Like T-Cell Lymphoma

Subcutaneous panniculitis-like T-cell lymphoma is a rare T-cell NHL of cytotoxic CD8+ T cells presenting with subcutaneous nodules.[387] This entity represents less than 1% of all NHLs.

Pathology

The cellular infiltrates are found in the subcutaneous fat and generally spare the overlying skin. This consists of an infiltrate of small, medium, and large atypical lymphocytes that infiltrate fat lobules, often forming rims around individual adipocytes. Cells express CD3 and CD8, and are usually negative for CD4 and CD56. Cytotoxic granules containing granzyme B, T cell intercellular antigen 1 (TIA-1) and perforin are also present. Most cases express $\alpha\beta$ TCRs, but a subset expresses $\gamma\delta$ TCRs instead. Like other PTCLs, there is often an aberrant immunophenotype marked by loss of one or more T-cell antigens (e.g., CD2, CD5, CD7). Clonal T-cell receptor rearrangements are present, but no specific cytogenetic abnormalities for this disease have been reported.

Clinical Features

This disease affects females more than males, with an age ranging from 40 to 60 years. The disease is localized to the skin with extremely uncommon involvement of other sites, including lymph nodes or bone marrow. The disease can wax and wane, and many patients' disease behaves like cutaneous T-cell NHLs, with a 5-year OS of 82%. Hemophagocytic lymphohistiocytosis (HLH) is reported in 17% of patients, and is associated with much lower 5-year survival (46 versus 91%). Patients with HLH merit combination chemotherapy and should be considered for SCT.

Extranodal Natural Killer/T-Cell Lymphomas, Nasal Type

Extranodal NK/T-cell lymphoma, nasal type, is an extranodal lymphoma usually presenting in the upper aerodigestive tract with occasional extranodal sites. This is a malignancy of NK cells that is generally EBV positive, with some cases of cytotoxic T-cell origin. This disease is rare in the United States and Europe, but is much more common in Asia (Hong Kong) and native populations in Peru.[388]

Pathology

Extranodal NK/T-cell lymphoma, nasal type, has widely varying cytologic features, but usually consists of a proliferation of a mixture of small and atypical lymphoid cells. The most characteristic features are prominent vascular invasion associated with fibrinoid necrosis of vessels walls and infarction of surrounding tissues.[3,389] In touch preparations, cytoplasmic azurophilic granules may be seen in the neoplastic cells.

Immunophenotype and Genetics

The cells express CD2, CD56, and cytoplasmic CD3 and are generally negative for CD4, CD8, TCR, and surface CD3. The T-cell receptor and Ig genes are usually germ line. EBV genomes are present in virtually all cases. There is loss of heterozygosity at 6q and 13q, with frequent overexpression of p53 and/or TP53 mutations.

Clinical Features

The extranodal NK/T-cell lymphomas, nasal type are rare, typically presenting in males with an average age of 60 years. The vast majority of patients have localized disease with nasal obstruction and a destructive mass involving the nose sinuses and palate. Stage I disease is present in 81% of patients, and stage II disease in 17% of patients.[390] B symptoms are uncommon. Although uncommon, other extranasal sites include: the intestines (37%), the skin (26%), the testis (17%), the lung (14%), the eye or soft tissue (9% each), the adrenal gland (6%), the brain (6%), and the breast or tongue (3% each). Patients with extranasal disease have higher stage, elevated LDH, bulky disease, and a poor performance status. Extranasal disease is associated with a worse prognosis than the nasal subtype for both early and late stage disease.[390] A prognostic index for NK/T-cell lymphoma has been developed with the factors including B symptoms, stage III or IV disease, elevated LDH, and lymph node involvement.[391] CNS risk is increased in patients with three or four factors (10%) compared with less than 2% of those with one or two features.[392] The EBV viral load at diagnosis and end of therapy is predictive of PFS and OS.[393]

Treatment

Overall, patients with stage IE/IIE have a 5-year DFS of 59%. The 5-year OS and PFS for patients with stage IE disease is 78% and 63%, respectively, and for stage IIE, the OS and PFS is 46% and 40%, respectively. In this series, there was no difference between combined modality and RT alone.[390,395] For patients with stage IE/IIE, early use of radiotherapy (50 to 55 Gy) is critical to optimal treatment. This is usually delivered with IMRT, a technique that allows for a reduction of dose to critical organs such as the eyes. This technique often uses treatment planning that fuses the MRI with the planning CT scan for optimal delineation of the tumor volume. Patients who received initial treatment with RT followed by chemotherapy had superior CR and OS rates as compared to patients who received chemotherapy before RT. Patients with stage II to IV disease generally have a very poor prognosis with relapses in other extranodal sites. More recent studies suggest that combined modality treatment may yield more favorable results. Phase 2 trials of concurrent RT and weekly cisplatin followed by three cycles of etoposide, ifosfamide, cisplatin, and dexamethasone reported overall RR of 83% and 3-year PFS and OS of 85% and 86%, respectively.[396–399] For disseminated NK/T-cell lymphoma, only 30% of patients achieve a CR with CHOP chemotherapy with median OS of 4.3 months.[390] Regimens with L-asparaginase have shown promising results in relapsed disease.[400,401] The regimen SMILE (dexamethasone, methotrexate, ifosfamide, L-asparaginase, and etoposide) in disseminated disease has an ORR of 79%, with 45% CRs. The 1-year PFS and OS of 53% and 55%, respectively, have been reported.[402]

Adult T-Cell Leukemia/Lymphoma

ATLL is a highly aggressive disease that is associated with infection by the HTLV-1 in 100% of cases.[403–405] This virus is endemic in southern Japan, the Caribbean basin, western Africa, the Southeastern United States and northeast Iran. The virus predominantly spreads by breast milk, and may be transmitted through sexual exposure and/or blood transfusion. The disease has a long clinical latency period, suggesting that HTLV-1 may not be sufficient for disease. The risk of developing ATLL following infection with HTLV-1 is estimated to be 4%. HTLV-1 causes an ATLL-like disease in severe combined immune deficiency (SCID) mice.[406]

Pathology

Lymph nodes are diffusely effaced by an atypical lymphoid infiltrate that preferentially involves T-cell zones and the medulla. The most characteristic morphologic feature is seen in the peripheral blood, where the circulating tumor cells often have multilobated nuclear contours, referred to as a *sunflower* or *starburst* appearance.

Immunophenotype and Genetics

ATLL is a tumor of CD4+ T cell, expressing CD2, CD3, CD5, CD25, but lacking CD7. The uniformly high levels of CD25 and variable expression of the transcription factor FOXO1 has led to the suggestion that this may be a tumor of Tregs. Deletions at 6q, trisomy 3, and monosomy X and Y are common, but key genetic events associated with ATLL development are largely unknown.

Clinical Features

The median age of ATLL patients is 60 years, with a male predominance.[406,407] There are several variants of the disease: acute (60% of patients), lymphomatous (20% of patients), chronic (15% of patients), and smoldering (5% of patients), with median survivals of 6 months, 10 months, 24 months, and not yet reached, respectively.[408] The chronic form can evolve into the acute type. Patients present with bone marrow and peripheral blood involvement, high white blood cell count, hypercalcemia (due to parathyroid hormone [PTH]-related protein, transforming growth factor beta [TGF-β], and receptor activator of NF-κB [RANK] ligand), lytic bone lesions, lymphadenopathy, hepatosplenomegaly, skin lesions resembling cutaneous T-cell lymphoma, and interstitial pulmonary infiltrates. Opportunistic infections can also accompany the clinical presentation, including pneumocystis, cryptococcus meningitis, strongyloides, and disseminated herpes zoster.[409]

Therapy

ATLL is generally approached with intensive multiagent chemotherapy regimens.[410,411] Antiviral therapy with zidovudine and interferon-α should be considered upfront for the smoldering, chronic subtype. A retrospective analysis of 116 patients suggested an improved survival with interferon-α and zidovudine antiviral therapy for acute, chronic, and smoldering subtypes, whereas patients with the lymphomatous type experienced a better outcome with first-line chemotherapy.[411,412] For the acute leukemia lymphoma type, a phase 3 randomized trial of 118 patients[413] reported that an intensive regimen vincristine, cyclophosphamide, doxorubicin, and prednisone, VCAP; doxorubicin, ranimustine, and prednisone, AMP; and vindesine, etoposide, carboplatin, and prednisone, VECP (VCAP-AMP-VECP) had a significantly higher CR rate but no difference in overall RR than CHOP-14 with intrathecal methotrexate. The 3-year OS was 24% with VCAP-AMP-VECP, but only 13% with CHOP. Based on expression of the CCR4 chemokine receptor on ATLL cells, mogamulizumab, an anti-CCR4 mAb is being investigated in combination with chemotherapy.[414] With the poor results of chemotherapy, both myeloablative and reduced intensity alloSCT has been applied to ATLL, with limited success.[415–417]

Primary Central Nervous System Lymphoma

Primary CNS lymphoma is the subject of Chapter 105.

Central Nervous System Prophylaxis for Aggressive Lymphomas

Prophylaxis for the development of CNS disease in DLBCL is highly controversial. Several sites of disease, including the testis, the ovary, bone marrow, the breast, the epidural space, and paranasal sinuses, have been reported to be associated with a high risk of CNS dissemination. A high-intermediate or high IPI score and multiple extranodal sites are also risk factors. Patients with BCLU-BL/DLBCL, as well as patients with *double-hit* cytogenetics, are at increased risk. In a retrospective analysis of aggressive NHLs, in the pre-rituximab era, the cumulative risk of CNS involvement was 2.8%. Intraparenchymal and intraspinal disease occurred in 66%, whereas isolated leptomeningeal disease was seen in only 26%. Eighty percent of CNS relapses occurred on or within 6 months of completing chemotherapy, suggesting a subclinical disease at diagnosis. In the current period of chemoimmunotherapy, it remains controversial if the addition of rituximab lowers the risk of CNS disease.[418] With the significant number of parenchymal relapses, intrathecal chemotherapy alone may be inadequate prophylaxis, making high-dose methotrexate a potentially more effective therapy. However, there is no compelling evidence that high-dose methotrexate is superior to the intrathecal route.

Lymphoma in Children

See Chapter 100 for a discussion of lymphomas in children.

Posttransplant Lymphoproliferative Disorders

Posttransplant lymphoproliferative disorders (PTLD) are a common and significant complication following solid organ transplantation, occurring in up to 10% of adult patients.[419] PTLD is less commonly seen after alloSCT. They constitute a heterogeneous collection of diagnoses ranging from early lesions, with reactive plasmacytic hyperplasia, to polymorphic PTLD, with polyclonal or monoclonal expansion of atypical lymphoid cells, to monomorphic PTLD, with lymphoma histopathology and immunophenotype.[332] They differ from nontransplant-related adult lymphomas in that they tend to be extranodal, high grade, and have an aggressive clinical course with a mortality often exceeding 50%.

PTLD following hematopoietic SCT is usually a malignancy of donor lymphoid cells, whereas PTLD following solid organ transplantation is traditionally thought to be of recipient origin in the majority of cases, although donor-derived cases have been reported and typically involve the grafted organ. In both PTLD following hematopoietic and solid organ transplantation, over 80% of PTLDs are of B-cell origin.[420] PTLD following solid organ transplantation can occur early, within the first year following transplant, or late, at 1 year or greater from transplantation. Early PTLD is much more common, with an incidence of 224 per 100,000 that falls to 54 per 100,000 by the second year. Over 90% of early onset B-cell PTLDs are EBV positive, whereas over 50% of late onset B-cell PTLD are EBV negative.[421] Immunosuppression following solid organ transplantation, however, results in a loss of EBV-specific cytotoxic T cells allowing for growth and acquisition of additional mutations in EBV-transformed B cells, such as alterations in *MYC*, *BCL6*, *TP53*, and DNA hypermethylation.[422]

EBV serologic status before transplant, as well as the degree and type of immunosuppression following transplant, are risks of developing PTLD. EBV-naïve patients pretransplant and younger patients have higher risk of PTLD.[423] The nature of immunosuppression is also related to risk. The use of anti–T-cell mAbs, tacrolimus, and multiple immunosuppressive agents are associated with increased risk.

The incidence of PTLD varies with the type of organ being transplanted; in adult patients, this ranges from 1% to 3% of kidney and liver transplants, from 1% to 6% of heart transplants, from 2% to 6% of heart–lung transplants, from 4% to 10% of lung transplants, and up to 20% of small bowel transplants.[424]

Antiviral agents have been studied in both the treatment and prophylaxis settings. For treatment, no study has demonstrated a clear benefit, although they may have some efficacy in early or polymorphic disease.[19] Antiviral therapy (ganciclovir) may decrease PTLD in high-risk EBV-seronegative patients.[425] The other strategy for early intervention is to monitor EBV viral load. EBV viral load has been shown to be significantly increased in patients who develop PTLD.[426] The use of a rising or increased viral load to alter clinical practice has been investigated following hematopoietic SCT, with a reduction in immunosuppression and/or preemptive therapy with rituximab or EBV cytotoxic T cells.[427] But this has not yet translated into studies investigating preemptive changes in clinical management in the solid organ transplant setting.

Pathology

The histologic appearance of PTLD is highly variable. The WHO classification system includes the following categories: (1) early lesions, reactive plasmacytic hyperplasia, and infectious mononucleosis-like; (2) polymorphic PTLD, infectious mononucleosis-like appearance with architectural effacement and tissue destruction; (3) monomorphic PTLD (classified according to lymphoma classification schemes), including DLBCL, BL, multiple myeloma, plasmacytoma, PTCL NOS, other types of T-cell lymphoma; and HL and Hodgkin's-like lymphomas.[44]

Clinical Presentation and Prognosis

PTLDs present as both nodal and extranodal disease. CNS involvement was reported in 22% of PTLDs. Other common extranodal sites include the lung and GI tract, which may be associated with a better prognosis. In solid organ transplants of the heart, lung, and liver, the allograft is reported to be the site of disease in 22% of cases. Survival statistics in PTLD are variable, owing to the heterogeneity of the diagnosis, ranging from early lesions to monomorphic PTLD, and to advances in therapy. Median 1-year and 5-year survival are approximately 50% to 60% and 30% to 40%, respectively, depending on the type of organ transplanted. Reported median OS is 20 to 30 months.[428,429] The IPI for aggressive NHLs has been applied to PTLD with limited utility. Other prognostic models for PTLD have been developed with risk factors being age ≥60 years, eastern cooperative oncology group (ECOG) PS ≥2, and elevated LDH.[430] Low (zero risk factors), intermediate (one risk factor), and high-risk (two to three risk factors) groups had 2-year OS rates of 88%, 50%, and 0%, respectively.

Therapy

There are no established treatment recommendations for PTLD given the heterogeneity of the diagnosis, from pathology to prognosis, and the general lack of prospective, randomized studies in the field. As we have learned more about the varied natural history of the different diseases and their risk and prognostic factors, therapy can now be better tailored to the individual patient. For instance, a stepwise approach to therapy is often indicated for patients with either early lesions or polymorphic disease, starting with a reduction in immunosuppression with or without the addition of antiviral therapy, to single-agent rituximab, to chemoimmunotherapy if indicated. This typically involves a 25% to 50% reduction in cyclosporine and tacrolimus and discontinuation of azathioprine and mycophenolate mofetil.[431]

For patients with monomorphic disease, the initial reduction in immunosuppression is typically accompanied by the addition of rituximab with or without chemotherapy, depending on the aggressiveness and histopathology of the disease.[432] RRs to rituximab alone range from 44% to 79%.[433] The PFS and OS at a follow-up of 27.5 months in these studies range from 42% to 47%, respectively. Patients with higher risk, more aggressive monomorphic disease are treated with sequentially dosed rituximab followed by CHOP with encouraging results with an overall RR of 90% (68% complete).[434,435]

Antiviral therapy has been investigated in more resistant disease. The combination of arginine butyrate, an activator of latently infected lymphoma cells via the induction of EBV thymidine kinase, has been combined with ganciclovir with encouraging results in limited number of patients treated. SCT has anecdotal experience in refractory patients. EBV-specific allogeneic T-cell lines may also have a role in refractory disease.[436]

HIV–Associated Non-Hodgkin's Lymphoma

Aggressive NHLs are AIDS-defining malignancies. The diagnosis and management is detailed in Chapter 117. AIDS-related NHL occurs in three broad categories: systemic lymphoma, which represents about 85% of all lymphomas; primary CNS lymphoma, accounting for 15% of all lymphomas; and primary effusion or body cavity lymphomas, which are rare.[44] The breakdown of histologic subtypes includes DLBCL (75%); BL (20%); plasmablastic lymphoma (less than 5%); T-cell lymphoma (1% to 3 %); and indolent B-cell lymphomas (less than 10%). About 30% of AIDS-related lymphomas have deregulation of the bcl-6 gene and a similar number have c-myc abnormalities. Approximately 60% of cases have abnormalities of p53.[437] The pathogenesis is analogous to PTLD, with EBV infection playing a major role in HIV-associated NHLs.[438] An HHV-8 infection is associated with primary effusion lymphoma.[5] The risk factors for developing lymphoma include depressed CD4 count, high HIV viral load, and a lack of effective antiretroviral therapy. Other risks include a lack of the *CCR5-32* deletion.

Systemic AIDS-related NHLs are generally highly aggressive diseases.[439] Besides nodal disease, extranodal disease is exceedingly common, with GI tract, skin and soft tissues, liver, lung, heart, as well as bone marrow and CNS involvement (in 5% to 20% of cases). B symptoms are also common presenting symptoms.

Plasmablastic lymphoma is a rare subtype of large B-cell NHL.[440] The cells have plasmacytoid cytoplasmic features like plasma cells, but often have large nuclei with large single nucleoli. The malignant cells express plasma cell markers (e.g., CD38, CD138, MUM1) and often lack pan–B-cell markers (e.g., CD20, CD79a). This disease was originally described as oropharyngeal plasmablastic lymphomas that occur most frequently in HIV-positive individuals and are often EBV positive. An identical tumor can also occur in other immunodeficiency states. Plasmablastic lymphoma is a very aggressive disease with a poor prognosis.

Primary effusion lymphomas (PEL) present in fluid collections in the pleura, the peritoneum, or the pericardium, or, more rarely, in the CSF.[441] Solid tumor variants of PEL occur rarely in the GI tract. The PEL cells are large and pleomorphic, often lack CD20 and CD19, but may be CD79a+ and CD45+; they also often express CD30 and CD138. They are uniformly associated with Kaposi's sarcoma herpesvirus/HHV-8, and most tumors are coinfected with HHV-8 and EBV. Both plasmablastic lymphomas and PELs rarely occur in nonimmunocompromised hosts.

Presently, more than 50% of patients with AIDS-related lymphoma have long-term DFS. By histology, patients with HL have about a 70% long-term OS, patients with DLBCL and BL around 50%, and patients with primary CNS lymphoma the lowest at 20% to 25%.[351] Treatment for AIDS-related DLBCL with CD4 count that is 50 or greater should be CHOP-R. There is controversy concerning the inclusion of rituximab if the CD4 count is less than 50.[442] For plasmablastic lymphoma or if the Ki-67 staining is greater than 80%, we consider DA-EPOCH, adding rituximab if the patient is CD20 positive. Examination of the CSF is considered for all patients, as is prophylaxis against *Pneumocystis jiroveci* pneumonia, herpes zoster, and Candida as well as continuation of antiretroviral therapy, if tolerated. For BL histology, we consider CODOX-M/IVAC rather than CHOP-R.[443] Based on a recent report in both patients who are HIV positive and patients who are HIV negative, DA-EPOCH-R is an alternative choice.[356]

SELECTED REFERENCES

The full reference list can be accessed at lwwhealthlibrary.com/oncology.

1. Siegel R, Ma J, Zou Z, et al. Cancer statistics, 2014. *CA Cancer J Clin* 2014;64:9–29.
2. Kuppers R. Mechanisms of B-cell lymphoma pathogenesis. *Nat Rev Cancer* 2005;5:251–262.
17. Persson B, Fredriksson M, Olsen K, et al. Some occupational exposures as risk factors for malignant lymphomas. *Cancer* 1993;72:1773–1778.
21. Smedby KE, Hjalgrim H, Askling J, et al. Autoimmune and chronic inflammatory disorders and risk of non-Hodgkin lymphoma by subtype. *J Natl Cancer Inst* 2006;98:51–60.
23. Wang SS, Slager SL, Brennan P, et al. Family history of hematopoietic malignancies and risk of non-Hodgkin lymphoma (NHL): a pooled analysis of 10 211 cases and 11 905 controls from the International Lymphoma Epidemiology Consortium (InterLymph). *Blood* 2007;109:3479–3488.
24. Brown JR, Neuberg D, Phillips K, et al. Prevalence of familial malignancy in a prospectively screened cohort of patients with lymphoproliferative disorders. *Br J Haematol* 2008;143:361–368.
25. Orkin SH, Zon LI. Hematopoiesis: an evolving paradigm for stem cell biology. *Cell* 2008;132:631–644.
26. Busslinger M. Transcriptional control of early B cell development. *Ann Rev Immunol* 2004;22:55–79.
27. Chen J, Alt FW. Gene rearrangement and B-cell development. *Curr Opin Immunol* 1993;5:194–200.
28. Korsmeyer SJ, Hieter PA, Ravetch JV, et al. Developmental hierarchy of immunoglobulin gene rearrangements in human leukemic pre-B-cells. *Proc Natl Acad Sci U S A* 1981;78:7096–7100.
31. Campbell JJ, Butcher EC. Chemokines in tissue-specific and microenvironment-specific lymphocyte homing. *Curr Opin Immunol* 2000;12:336–341.
32. Calado DP, Sasaki Y, Godinho SA, et al. The cell-cycle regulator c-Myc is essential for the formation and maintenance of germinal centers. *Nat Immunol* 2012;13:1092–1100.
34. Fukuda T, Yoshida T, Okada S, et al. Disruption of the Bcl6 gene results in an impaired germinal center formation. *J Exp Med* 1997;186:439–448.
35. Muramatsu M, Kinoshita K, Fagarasan S, et al. Class switch recombination and hypermutation require activation-induced cytidine deaminase (AID), a potential RNA editing enzyme. *Cell* 2000;102:553–563.
37. Radtke F, Fasnacht N, Macdonald HR. Notch signaling in the immune system. *Immunity* 2010;32:14–27.
39. Klein L, Hinterberger M, Wirnsberger G, et al. Antigen presentation in the thymus for positive selection and central tolerance induction. *Nat Rev Immunol* 2009;9:833–844.
41. Delves PJ, Roitt IM. The immune system. Second of two parts. *N Engl J Med* 2000;343:108–117.
42. Delves PJ, Roitt IM. The immune system. First of two parts. *N Engl J Med* 2000;343:37–49.
44. Swedlow SH, Campo E, Harris NL, et al., eds. *WHO Classification of Tumours of Haematopoietic and Lymphoid Tissues.* Lyon, France: IARC; 2008.
45. Harris NL, Jaffe ES, Stein H, et al. A revised European-American classification of lymphoid neoplasms: a proposal from the International Lymphoma Study Group. *Blood* 1994;84:1361–1392.
46. Rosenwald A, Wright G, Chan WC, et al. The use of molecular profiling to predict survival after chemotherapy for diffuse large-B-cell lymphoma. *N Engl J Med* 2002;346:1937–1947.

49. Elstrom R, Guan L, Baker G, et al. Utility of FDG-PET scanning in lymphoma by WHO classification. *Blood* 2003;101:3875–3876.
50. Schoder H, Noy A, Gonen M, et al. Intensity of 18fluorodeoxyglucose uptake in positron emission tomography distinguishes between indolent and aggressive non-Hodgkin's lymphoma. *J Clin Oncol* 2005;23:4643–4651.
51. Juweid ME, Wiseman GA, Vose JM, et al. Response assessment of aggressive non-Hodgkin's lymphoma by integrated International Workshop Criteria and fluorine-18-fluorodeoxyglucose positron emission tomography. *J Clin Oncol* 2005;23:4652–4661.
52. Zinzani PL, Fanti S, Battista G, et al. Predictive role of positron emission tomography (PET) in the outcome of lymphoma patients. *Br J Cancer* 2004;91:850–854.
53. Juweid ME, Stroobants S, Hoekstra OS, et al. Use of positron emission tomography for response assessment of lymphoma: consensus of the Imaging Subcommittee of International Harmonization Project in Lymphoma. *J Clin Oncol* 2007;25:571–578.
54. Rosenberg SA. Validity of the Ann Arbor staging classification for the non-Hodgkin's lymphomas. *Cancer Treat Rep* 1977;61:1023–1027.
55. A predictive model for aggressive non-Hodgkin's lymphoma. The International Non-Hodgkin's Lymphoma Prognostic Factors Project. *N Engl J Med* 1993;329:987–994.
56. Sehn LH, Berry B, Chhanabhai M, et al. The revised International Prognostic Index (R-IPI) is a better predictor of outcome than the standard IPI for patients with diffuse large B-cell lymphoma treated with R-CHOP. *Blood* 2007;109:1857–1861.
57. Solal-Celigny P, Roy P, Colombat P, et al. Follicular lymphoma international prognostic index. *Blood* 2004;104:1258–1265.
58. Hoster E, Dreyling M, Klapper W, et al. A new prognostic index (MIPI) for patients with advanced-stage mantle cell lymphoma. *Blood* 2008;111:558–565.
59. Gallamini A, Stelitano C, Calvi R, et al. Peripheral T-cell lymphoma unspecified (PTCL-U): a new prognostic model from a retrospective multicentric clinical study. *Blood* 2004;103:2474–2479.
60. Hans CP, Weisenburger DD, Greiner TC, et al. Confirmation of the molecular classification of diffuse large B-cell lymphoma by immunohistochemistry using a tissue microarray. *Blood* 2004;103:275–282.
63. Armitage JO, Weisenburger DD. New approach to classifying non-Hodgkin's lymphomas: clinical features of the major histologic subtypes. Non-Hodgkin's Lymphoma Classification Project. *J Clin Oncol* 1998;16:2780–2795.
66. Ott G, Katzenberger T, Lohr A, et al. Cytomorphologic, immunohistochemical, and cytogenetic profiles of follicular lymphoma: 2 types of follicular lymphoma grade 3. *Blood* 2002;99:3806–3812.
68. Pasqualucci L, Trifonov V, Fabbri G, et al. Analysis of the coding genome of diffuse large B-cell lymphoma. *Nat Genet* 2011;43:830–837.
69. Kridel R, Sehn LH, Gascoyne RD. Pathogenesis of follicular lymphoma. *J Clin Invest* 2012;122:3424–3431.
72. Link BK, Maurer MJ, Nowakowski GS, et al. Rates and outcomes of follicular lymphoma transformation in the immunochemotherapy era: a report from the University of Iowa/MayoClinic Specialized Program of Research Excellence Molecular Epidemiology Resource. *J Clin Oncol* 2013;31: 3272–3278.
73. Montoto S, Davies AJ, Matthews J, et al. Risk and clinical implications of transformation of follicular lymphoma to diffuse large B-cell lymphoma. *J Clin Oncol* 2007;25:2426–2433.

74. Relander T, Johnson NA, Farinha P, et al. Prognostic factors in follicular lymphoma. *J Clin Oncol* 2010;28:2902–2913.

75. Federico M, Bellei M, Marcheselli L, et al. Follicular lymphoma international prognostic index 2: a new prognostic index for follicular lymphoma developed by the international follicular lymphoma prognostic factor project. *J Clin Oncol* 2009;27:4555–4562.

76. Buske C, Hoster E, Dreyling M, et al. The Follicular Lymphoma International Prognostic Index (FLIPI) separates high-risk from intermediate- or low-risk patients with advanced-stage follicular lymphoma treated front-line with rituximab and the combination of cyclophosphamide, doxorubicin, vincristine, and prednisone (R-CHOP) with respect to treatment outcome. *Blood* 2006;108:1504–1508.

77. Wahlin BE, Yri OE, Kimby E, et al. Clinical significance of the WHO grades of follicular lymphoma in a population-based cohort of 505 patients with long follow-up times. *Br J Haematol* 2012;156:225–233.

79. Canioni D, Salles G, Mounier N, et al. High numbers of tumor-associated macrophages have an adverse prognostic value that can be circumvented by rituximab in patients with follicular lymphoma enrolled onto the GELA-GOELAMS FL-2000 trial. *J Clin Oncol* 2008;26:440–446.

83. Glas AM, Knoops L, Delahaye L, et al. Gene-expression and immunohistochemical study of specific T-cell subsets and accessory cell types in the transformation and prognosis of follicular lymphoma. *J Clin Oncol* 2007;25:390–398.

85. Kuppers R. Prognosis in follicular lymphoma—it's in the microenvironment. *N Engl J Med* 2004;351:2152–2153.

88. Friedberg J, Huang J, Dillon H, et al. Initial therapeutic strategy in follicular lymphoma: an analysis from the National LymphoCare Study. *J Clin Oncol* 2006;24: 428s.

89. Guadagnolo BA, Li S, Neuberg D, et al. Long-term outcome and mortality trends in early-stage, Grade 1-2 follicular lymphoma treated with radiation therapy. *Int J Radiat Oncol Biol Phys* 2006;64:928–934.

90. Lowry L, Smith P, Qian W, et al. Reduced dose radiotherapy for local control in non-Hodgkin lymphoma: a randomised phase III trial. *Radiother Oncol* 2011;100:86–92.

92. Kelsey SM, Newland AC, Hudson GV, et al. A British National Lymphoma Investigation randomised trial of single agent chlorambucil plus radiotherapy versus radiotherapy alone in low grade, localised non-Hodgkins lymphoma. *Med Oncol* 1994;11:19–25.

93. Friedberg JW, Byrtek M, Link BK, et al. Effectiveness of first-line management strategies for stage I follicular lymphoma: analysis of the National LymphoCare Study. *J Clin Oncol* 2012;30:3368–3375.

94. Advani R, Rosenberg SA, Horning SJ. Stage I and II follicular non-Hodgkin's lymphoma: long-term follow-up of no initial therapy. *J Clin Oncol* 2004;22:1454–1459.

95. Ardeshna KM, Smith P, Norton A, et al. Long-term effect of a watch and wait policy versus immediate systemic treatment for asymptomatic advanced-stage non-Hodgkin lymphoma: a randomised controlled trial. *Lancet* 2003;362:516–522.

97. Solal-Celigny P, Bellei M, Marcheselli L, et al. Watchful waiting in low-tumor burden follicular lymphoma in the rituximab era: results of an F2-study database. *J Clin Oncol* 2012;30:3848–3853.

101. Hiddemann W, Kneba M, Dreyling M, et al. Frontline therapy with rituximab added to the combination of cyclophosphamide, doxorubicin, vincristine, and prednisone (CHOP) significantly improves the outcome for patients with advanced-stage follicular lymphoma compared with therapy with CHOP alone: results of a prospective randomized study of the German Low-Grade Lymphoma Study Group. *Blood* 2005;106:3725–3732.

102. Marcus R, Imrie K, Belch A, et al. CVP chemotherapy plus rituximab compared with CVP as first-line treatment for advanced follicular lymphoma. *Blood* 2005;105:1417–1423.

103. Marcus R, Imrie K, Solal-Celigny P, et al. Phase III study of R-CVP compared with cyclophosphamide, vincristine, and prednisone alone in patients with previously untreated advanced follicular lymphoma. *J Clin Oncol* 2008;26:4579–4586.

104. Salles G, Mounier N, de Guibert S, et al. Rituximab combined with chemotherapy and interferon in follicular lymphoma patients: results of the GELA-GOELAMS FL2000 study. *Blood* 2008;112:4824–4831.

106. Rummel MJ, Niederle N, Maschmeyer G, et al. Bendamustine plus rituximab versus CHOP plus rituximab as first-line treatment for patients with indolent and mantle-cell lymphomas: an open-label, multicentre, randomised, phase 3 non-inferiority trial. *Lancet* 2013;381:1203–1210.

111. Colombat P, Salles G, Brousse N, et al. Rituximab (anti-CD20 monoclonal antibody) as single first-line therapy for patients with follicular lymphoma with a low tumor burden: clinical and molecular evaluation. *Blood* 2001;97:101–106.

113. Witzig TE, Vukov AM, Habermann TM, et al. Rituximab therapy for patients with newly diagnosed, advanced-stage, follicular grade I non-Hodgkin's lymphoma: a phase II trial in the North Central Cancer Treatment Group. *J Clin Oncol* 2005;23:1103–1108.

114. Martinelli G, Schmitz SF, Utiger U, et al. Long-term follow-up of patients with follicular lymphoma receiving single-agent rituximab at two different schedules in trial SAKK 35/98. *J Clin Oncol* 2010;28:4480–4484.

115. Hochster H, Weller E, Gascoyne RD, et al. Maintenance rituximab after cyclophosphamide, vincristine, and prednisone prolongs progression-free survival in advanced indolent lymphoma: results of the randomized phase III ECOG1496 Study. *J Clin Oncol* 2009;27:1607–1614.

116. Salles G, Seymour JF, Offner F, et al. Rituximab maintenance for 2 years in patients with high tumour burden follicular lymphoma responding to rituximab plus chemotherapy (PRIMA): a phase 3, randomised controlled trial. *Lancet* 2011;377:42–51.

118. Scholz CW, Pinto A, Linkesch W, et al. (90)Yttrium-ibritumomab-tiuxetan as first-line treatment for follicular lymphoma: 30 months of follow-up data from an international multicenter phase II clinical trial. *J Clin Oncol* 2013;31:308–313.

122. Morschhauser F, Radford J, Van Hoof A, et al. Phase III trial of consolidation therapy with yttrium-90-ibritumomab tiuxetan compared with no additional therapy after first remission in advanced follicular lymphoma. *J Clin Oncol* 2008;26:5156–5164.

123. Press OW, Unger JM, Rimsza LM, et al. Phase III randomized intergroup trial of CHOP plus rituximab compared with CHOP chemotherapy plus (131)iodine-tositumomab for previously untreated follicular non-Hodgkin lymphoma: SWOG S0016. *J Clin Oncol* 2013;31:314–320.

124. Brown JR, Feng Y, Gribben JG, et al. Long-term survival after autologous bone marrow transplantation for follicular lymphoma in first remission. *Biol Blood Marrow Transplant* 2007;13:1057–1065.

125. Deconinck E, Foussard C, Milpied N, et al. High-dose therapy followed by autologous purged stem-cell transplantation and doxorubicin-based chemotherapy in patients with advanced follicular lymphoma: a randomized multicenter study by GOELAMS. *Blood* 2005;105:3817–3823.

126. Lenz G, Dreyling M, Schiegnitz E, et al. Myeloablative radiochemotherapy followed by autologous stem cell transplantation in first remission prolongs progression-free survival in follicular lymphoma: results of a prospective, randomized trial of the German Low-Grade Lymphoma Study Group. *Blood* 2004;104:2667–2674.

127. Sebban C, Mounier N, Brousse N, et al. Standard chemotherapy with interferon compared with CHOP followed by high-dose therapy with autologous stem cell transplantation in untreated patients with advanced follicular lymphoma: the GELF-94 randomized study from the Groupe d'Etude des Lymphomes de l'Adulte (GELA). *Blood* 2006;108:2540–2544.

128. Ladetto M, De Marco F, Benedetti F, et al. Prospective, multicenter randomized GITMO/IIL trial comparing intensive (R-HDS) versus conventional (CHOP-R) chemoimmunotherapy in high-risk follicular lymphoma at diagnosis: the superior disease control of R-HDS does not translate into an overall survival advantage. *Blood* 2008;111:4004–4013.

129. Gyan E, Foussard C, Bertrand P, et al. High-dose therapy followed by autologous purged stem cell transplantation and doxorubicin-based chemotherapy in patients with advanced follicular lymphoma: a randomized multicenter study by the GOELAMS with final results after a median follow-up of 9 years. *Blood* 2009;113:995–1001.

130. Al-Khabori M, de Almeida JR, Guyatt GH, et al. Autologous stem cell transplantation in follicular lymphoma: a systematic review and meta-analysis. *J Natl Cancer Inst* 2012;104:18–28.

132. van Oers MH, Van Glabbeke M, Giurgea L, et al. Rituximab maintenance treatment of relapsed/resistant follicular non-Hodgkin's lymphoma: long-term outcome of the EORTC 20981 phase III randomized intergroup study. *J Clin Oncol* 2010;28:2853–2858.

135. Robinson KS, Williams ME, van der Jagt RH, et al. Phase II multicenter study of bendamustine plus rituximab in patients with relapsed indolent B-cell and mantle cell non-Hodgkin's lymphoma. *J Clin Oncol* 2008;26:4473–4479.

138. de Vos S, Goy A, Dakhil SR, et al. Multicenter randomized phase II study of weekly or twice-weekly bortezomib plus rituximab in patients with relapsed or refractory follicular or marginal-zone B-cell lymphoma. *J Clin Oncol* 2009;27:5023–5030.

141. Fisher RI, Kaminski MS, Wahl RL, et al. Tositumomab and iodine-131 tositumomab produces durable complete remissions in a subset of heavily pretreated patients with low-grade and transformed non-Hodgkin's lymphomas. *J Clin Oncol* 2005;23:7565–7573.

145. Russo AL, Chen YH, Martin NE, et al. Low-dose involved-field radiation in the treatment of non-hodgkin lymphoma: predictors of response and treatment failure. *Int J Radiat Oncol Biol Phys* 2013;86:121–127.

146. Montoto S, Corradini P, Dreyling M, et al. Indications for hematopoietic stem cell transplantation in patients with follicular lymphoma: a consensus project of the EBMT-Lymphoma Working Party. *Haematologica* 2013;98:1014–1021.

147. Rohatiner AZ, Nadler L, Davies AJ, et al. Myeloablative therapy with autologous bone marrow transplantation for follicular lymphoma at the time of second or subsequent remission: long-term follow-up. *J Clin Oncol* 2007;25:2554–2559.

152. Schouten HC, Qian W, Kvaloy S, et al. High-dose therapy improves progression-free survival and survival in relapsed follicular non-Hodgkin's lymphoma: results from the randomized European CUP trial. *J Clin Oncol* 2003;21:3918–3927.

153. Pettengell R, Schmitz N, Gisselbrecht C, et al. Rituximab purging and/or maintenance in patients undergoing autologous transplantation for relapsed follicular lymphoma: a prospective randomized trial from the lymphoma working party of the European group for blood and marrow transplantation. *J Clin Oncol* 2013;31:1624–1630.

154. van Besien K, Loberiza FR Jr, Bajorunaite R, et al. Comparison of autologous and allogeneic hematopoietic stem cell transplantation for follicular lymphoma. *Blood* 2003;102:3521–3529.
155. Khouri IF, McLaughlin P, Saliba RM, et al. Eight-year experience with allogeneic stem cell transplantation for relapsed follicular lymphoma after nonmyeloablative conditioning with fludarabine, cyclophosphamide, and rituximab. *Blood* 2008;111:5530–5536.
157. Tomblyn MR, Ewell M, Bredeson C, et al. Autologous versus reduced-intensity allogeneic hematopoietic cell transplantation for patients with chemosensitive follicular non-Hodgkin lymphoma beyond first complete response or first partial response. *Biol Blood Marrow Transplant* 2011;17:1051–1057.
158. Evens AM, Vanderplas A, LaCasce AS, et al. Stem cell transplantation for follicular lymphoma relapsed/refractory after prior rituximab: a comprehensive analysis from the NCCN lymphoma outcomes project. *Cancer* 2013;119:3662–3671.
166. Hagenbeek A, Gadeberg O, Johnson P, et al. First clinical use of ofatumumab, a novel fully human anti-CD20 monoclonal antibody in relapsed or refractory follicular lymphoma: results of a phase 1/2 trial. *Blood* 2008;111:5486–5495.
169. Salles GA, Morschhauser F, Solal-Celigny P, et al. Obinutuzumab (GA101) in patients with relapsed/refractory indolent non-Hodgkin lymphoma: results from the phase II GAUGUIN study. *J Clin Oncol* 2013;31:2920–2926.
170. Radford J, Davies A, Cartron G, et al. Obinutuzumab (GA101) plus CHOP or FC in relapsed/refractory follicular lymphoma: results of the GAUDI study (BO21000). *Blood* 2013;122:1137–1143.
173. Freedman A, Neelapu SS, Nichols C, et al. Placebo-controlled phase III trial of patient-specific immunotherapy with mitumprotimut-T and granulocyte-macrophage colony-stimulating factor after rituximab in patients with follicular lymphoma. *J Clin Oncol* 2009;27:3036–3043.
175. Kahl B, Byrd J, Flinn I, et al. Clinical safety and activity in a phase 1 study of CAL-101, an isoform-selective inhibitor of phosphatidylinositol 3-kinase P110δ, in patients with relapsed or refractory non-Hodgkin lymphoma. *Blood* 2010;116:abstract 1777.
176. Fowler F, Porte Sharman J, Smith S, et al. The Btk Inhibitor, PCI-32765, induces durable responses with minimal toxicity in patients with relapsed/refractory B-cell malignancies: results from a phase I study. *Blood* 2010;116:abstract 964.
184. Rassenti LZ, Jain S, Keating MJ, et al. Relative value of ZAP-70, CD38, and immunoglobulin mutation status in predicting aggressive disease in chronic lymphocytic leukemia. *Blood* 2008;112:1923–1930.
192. Dimopoulos MA, Anagnostopoulos A, Kyrtsonis MC, et al. Primary treatment of Waldenstrom macroglobulinemia with dexamethasone, rituximab, and cyclophosphamide. *J Clin Oncol* 2007;25:3344–3349.
193. Treon SP, Ioakimidis L, Soumerai JD, et al. Primary therapy of Waldenstrom macroglobulinemia with bortezomib, dexamethasone, and rituximab: WMCTG clinical trial 05-180. *J Clin Oncol* 2009;27:3830–3835.
201. Else M, Marin-Niebla A, de la Cruz F, et al. Rituximab, used alone or in combination, is superior to other treatment modalities in splenic marginal zone lymphoma. *Br J Haematol* 2012;159:322–328.
202. Kalpadakis C, Pangalis GA, Angelopoulou MK, et al. Treatment of splenic marginal zone lymphoma with rituximab monotherapy: progress report and comparison with splenectomy. *Oncologist* 2013;18:190–197.
210. Auer IA, Gascoyne RD, Connors JM, et al. t(11;18)(q21;q21) is the most common translocation in MALT lymphomas. *Ann Oncol* 1997;8:979–985.
221. Wundisch T, Thiede C, Morgner A, et al. Long-term follow-up of gastric MALT lymphoma after Helicobacter pylori eradication. *J Clin Oncol* 2005;23:8018–8024.
224. Tsang RW, Gospodarowicz MK, Pintilie M, et al. Localized mucosa-associated lymphoid tissue lymphoma treated with radiation therapy has excellent clinical outcome. *J Clin Oncol* 2003;21:4157–4164.
225. Conconi A, Martinelli G, Thieblemont C, et al. Clinical activity of rituximab in extranodal marginal zone B-cell lymphoma of MALT type. *Blood* 2003;102:2741–2745.
227. Uno T, Isobe K, Shikama N, et al. Radiotherapy for extranodal, marginal zone, B-cell lymphoma of mucosa-associated lymphoid tissue originating in the ocular adnexa: a multiinstitutional, retrospective review of 50 patients. *Cancer* 2003;98:865–871.
228. Govi S, Dolcetti R, Ponzoni M, et al. Final results of a multicenter phase II trial with translational elements to investigate the possible infective causes of ocular adnexal marginal zone B-cell lymphoma (OAMZL) with particular reference to chlamydia species and the efficacy of doxycycline as first-line lymphoma treatment (the IELSG#27 TRIAL). *Blood* 2011;118:a267.
229. Hammel P, Haioun C, Chaumette MT, et al. Efficacy of single-agent chemotherapy in low-grade B-cell mucosa-associated lymphoid tissue lymphoma with prominent gastric expression. *J Clin Oncol* 1995;13:2524–2529.
230. Brown JR, Friedberg JW, Feng Y, et al. A phase 2 study of concurrent fludarabine and rituximab for the treatment of marginal zone lymphomas. *Br J Haematol* 2009;145:741–748.
233. Salaverria I, Zettl A, Bea S, et al. Specific secondary genetic alterations in mantle cell lymphoma provide prognostic information independent of the gene expression-based proliferation signature. *J Clin Oncol* 2007;25:1216–1222.
235. Nygren L, Baumgartner Wennerholm S, Klimkowska M, et al. Prognostic role of SOX11 in a population-based cohort of mantle cell lymphoma. *Blood* 2012;119:4215–4223.
237. Martin P, Chadburn A, Christos P, et al. Outcome of deferred initial therapy in mantle-cell lymphoma. *J Clin Oncol* 2009;27:1209–1213.
239. Geisler CH, Kolstad A, Laurell A, et al. The Mantle Cell Lymphoma International Prognostic Index (MIPI) is superior to the International Prognostic Index (IPI) in predicting survival following intensive first-line immunochemotherapy and autologous stem cell transplantation (ASCT). *Blood* 2010;115:1530–1533.
240. Determann O, Hoster E, Ott G, et al. Ki-67 predicts outcome in advanced-stage mantle cell lymphoma patients treated with anti-CD20 immunochemotherapy: results from randomized trials of the European MCL Network and the German Low Grade Lymphoma Study Group. *Blood* 2008;111:2385–2387.
241. Fernandez V, Salamero O, Espinet B, et al. Genomic and gene expression profiling defines indolent forms of mantle cell lymphoma. *Cancer Res* 2010;70:1408–1418.
245. Griffiths R, Mikhael J, Gleeson M, et al. Addition of rituximab to chemotherapy alone as first-line therapy improves overall survival in elderly patients with mantle cell lymphoma. *Blood* 2011;118:4808–4816.
246. Kluin-Nelemans HC, Hoster E, Hermine O, et al. Treatment of older patients with mantle-cell lymphoma. *N Engl J Med* 2012;367:520–531.
248. Bernstein SH, Epner E, Unger JM, et al. A phase II multicenter trial of hyperCVAD MTX/Ara-C and rituximab in patients with previously untreated mantle cell lymphoma: SWOG 0213. *Ann Oncol* 2013;24:1587–1593.
250. Dreyling M, Lenz G, Hoster E, et al. Early consolidation by myeloablative radiochemotherapy followed by autologous stem cell transplantation in first remission significantly prolongs progression-free survival in mantle-cell lymphoma: results of a prospective randomized trial of the European MCL Network. *Blood* 2005;105:2677–2684.
251. Geisler CH, Kolstad A, Laurell A, et al. Nordic MCL2 trial update: six-year follow-up after intensive immunochemotherapy for untreated mantle cell lymphoma followed by BEAM or BEAC + autologous stem-cell support: still very long survival but late relapses do occur. *Br J Haematol* 2012;158:355–362.
252. O'Connor OA, Moskowitz C, Portlock C, et al. Patients with chemotherapy-refractory mantle cell lymphoma experience high response rates and identical progression-free survivals compared with patients with relapsed disease following treatment with single agent bortezomib: results of a multicentre Phase 2 clinical trial. *Br J Haematol* 2009;145:34–39.
253. Witzig TE, Vose JM, Zinzani PL, et al. An international phase II trial of single-agent lenalidomide for relapsed or refractory aggressive B-cell non-Hodgkin's lymphoma. *Ann Oncol* 2011;22:1622–1627.
255. Wang ML, Rule S, Martin P, et al. Targeting BTK with ibrutinib in relapsed or refractory mantle-cell lymphoma. *N Engl J Med* 2013;369:507–516.
257. Rosenbluth BD, Yahalom J. Highly effective local control and palliation of mantle cell lymphoma with involved-field radiation therapy (IFRT). *Int J Radiat Oncol Biol Phys* 2006;65:1185–1191.
259. Le Gouill S, Kroger N, Dhedin N, et al. Reduced-intensity conditioning allogeneic stem cell transplantation for relapsed/refractory mantle cell lymphoma: a multicenter experience. *Ann Oncol* 2012;23:2695–2703.
260. Abramson JS. T-cell/histiocyte-rich B-cell lymphoma: biology, diagnosis, and management. *Oncologist* 2006;11:384–392.
263. Hu S, Xu-Monette ZY, Balasubramanyam A, et al. CD30 expression defines a novel subgroup of diffuse large B-cell lymphoma with favorable prognosis and distinct gene expression signature: a report from the International DLBCL Rituximab-CHOP Consortium Program Study. *Blood* 2013;121:2715–2724.
273. Aukema SM, Siebert R, Schuuring E, et al. Double-hit B-cell lymphomas. *Blood* 2011;117:2319–2331.
274. Barrans S, Crouch S, Smith A, et al. Rearrangement of MYC is associated with poor prognosis in patients with diffuse large B-cell lymphoma treated in the era of rituximab. *J Clin Oncol* 2010;28:3360–3365.
277. Shenoy PJ, Malik N, Nooka A, et al. Racial differences in the presentation and outcomes of diffuse large B-cell lymphoma in the United States. *Cancer* 2011;117:2530–2540.
278. Vitolo U, Chiappella A, Ferreri AJ, et al. First-line treatment for primary testicular diffuse large B-cell lymphoma with rituximab-CHOP, CNS prophylaxis, and contralateral testis irradiation: final results of an international phase II trial. *J Clin Oncol* 2011;29:2766–2772.
279. van Besien K, Ha CS, Murphy S, et al. Risk factors, treatment, and outcome of central nervous system recurrence in adults with intermediate-grade and immunoblastic lymphoma. *Blood* 1998;91:1178–1184.
280. Miller TP, Dahlberg S, Cassady JR, et al. Chemotherapy alone compared with chemotherapy plus radiotherapy for localized intermediate- and high-grade non-Hodgkin's lymphoma. *N Engl J Med* 1998;339:21–26.
281. Persky DO, Unger JM, Spier CM, et al. Phase II study of rituximab plus three cycles of CHOP and involved-field radiotherapy for patients with limited-stage aggressive B-cell lymphoma: Southwest Oncology Group study 0014. *J Clin Oncol* 2008;26:2258–2263.
285. Pfreundschuh M, Trumper L, Osterborg A, et al. CHOP-like chemotherapy plus rituximab versus CHOP-like chemotherapy alone in young patients with good-prognosis diffuse large-B-cell lymphoma: a randomised controlled trial by the MabThera International Trial (MInT) Group. *Lancet Oncol* 2006;7:379–391.
286. Coiffier B, Lepage E, Briere J, et al. CHOP chemotherapy plus rituximab compared with CHOP alone in elderly patients with diffuse large-B-cell lymphoma. *N Engl J Med* 2002;346:235–242.

PRACTICE OF ONCOLOGY

289. Pfreundschuh M, Schubert J, Ziepert M, et al. Six versus eight cycles of bi-weekly CHOP-14 with or without rituximab in elderly patients with aggressive CD20+ B-cell lymphomas: a randomised controlled trial (RICOVER-60). *Lancet Oncol* 2008;9:105–116.

290. Cunningham D, Hawkes EA, Jack A, et al. Rituximab plus cyclophosphamide, doxorubicin, vincristine, and prednisolone in patients with newly diagnosed diffuse large B-cell non-Hodgkin lymphoma: a phase 3 comparison of dose intensification with 14-day versus 21-day cycles. *Lancet* 2013;381: 1817–1826.

292. Greb A, Bohlius J, Schiefer D, et al. High-dose chemotherapy with autologous stem cell transplantation in the first line treatment of aggressive non-Hodgkin lymphoma (NHL) in adults. *Cochrane Database Syst Rev* 2008;23(1):CD004024.

294. Stiff PJ, Unger JM, Cook JR, et al. Autologous transplantation as consolidation for aggressive non-Hodgkin's lymphoma. *N Engl J Med* 2013;369: 1681–1690.

297. Ohmachi K, Niitsu N, Uchida T, et al. Multicenter phase II study of bendamustine plus rituximab in patients with relapsed or refractory diffuse large B-cell lymphoma. *J Clin Oncol.* 2013;31:2103–2109.

299. Ruan J, Martin P, Coleman M, et al. Durable responses with the metronomic rituximab and thalidomide plus prednisone, etoposide, procarbazine, and cyclophosphamide regimen in elderly patients with recurrent mantle cell lymphoma. *Cancer* 2010;116:2655–2664.

300. Gisselbrecht C, Glass B, Mounier N, et al. R-ICE versus R-DHAP in relapsed patients with CD20 diffuse large B-cell lymphoma (DLBCL) followed by autologous stem cell transplantation: CORAL study. *J Clin Oncol* 2009;27:8509.

301. Gisselbrecht C, Glass B, Mounier N, et al. Salvage regimens with autologous transplantation for relapsed large B-cell lymphoma in the rituximab era. *J Clin Oncol* 2010;28:4184–4190.

303. Philip T, Guglielmi C, Hagenbeek A, et al. Autologous bone marrow transplantation as compared with salvage chemotherapy in relapses of chemotherapy-sensitive non-Hodgkin's lymphoma. *N Engl J Med* 1995;333: 1540–1545.

304. Gisselbrecht C, Schmitz N, Mounier N, et al. Rituximab maintenance therapy after autologous stem-cell transplantation in patients with relapsed CD20(+) diffuse large B-cell lymphoma: final analysis of the collaborative trial in relapsed aggressive lymphoma. *J Clin Oncol* 2013;31:1662–1668.

306. Salit RB, Fowler DH, Wilson WH, et al. Dose-adjusted EPOCH-rituximab combined with fludarabine provides an effective bridge to reduced-intensity allogeneic hematopoietic stem-cell transplantation in patients with lymphoid malignancies. *J Clin Oncol* 2012;30:830–836.

307. van Kampen RJ, Canals C, Schouten HC, et al. Allogeneic stem-cell transplantation as salvage therapy for patients with diffuse large B-cell non-Hodgkin's lymphoma relapsing after an autologous stem-cell transplantation: an analysis of the European Group for Blood and Marrow Transplantation Registry. *J Clin Oncol* 2011;29:1342–1348.

314. Ponzoni M, Ferreri AJ, Campo E, et al. Definition, diagnosis, and management of intravascular large B-cell lymphoma: proposals and perspectives from an international consensus meeting. *J Clin Oncol* 2007;25:3168–3173.

315. Shimada K, Matsue K, Yamamoto K, et al. Retrospective analysis of intravascular large B-cell lymphoma treated with rituximab-containing chemotherapy as reported by the IVL study group in Japan. *J Clin Oncol* 2008;26: 3189–3195.

316. Achten R, Verhoef G, Vanuytsel L, et al. T-cell/histiocyte-rich large B-cell lymphoma: a distinct clinicopathologic entity. *J Clin Oncol* 2002; 20:1269–1277.

322. Fields PA, Linch DC. Treatment of the elderly patient with diffuse large B cell lymphoma. *Br J Haematol* 2012;157:159–170.

325. Peyrade F, Jardin F, Thieblemont C, et al. Attenuated immunochemotherapy regimen (R-miniCHOP) in elderly patients older than 80 years with diffuse large B-cell lymphoma: a multicentre, single-arm, phase 2 trial. *Lancet Oncol* 2011;12:460–468.

326. Weisenburger DD, Savage KJ, Harris NL, et al. Peripheral T-cell lymphoma, not otherwise specified: a report of 340 cases from the International Peripheral T-cell Lymphoma Project. *Blood* 2011;117:3402–3408.

330. Rieger M, Osterborg A, Pettengell R, et al. Primary mediastinal B-cell lymphoma treated with CHOP-like chemotherapy with or without rituximab: results of the Mabthera International Trial Group study. *Ann Oncol* 2011; 22:664–670.

331. Dunleavy K, Pittaluga S, Maeda LS, et al. Dose-adjusted EPOCH-rituximab therapy in primary mediastinal B-cell lymphoma. *N Engl J Med* 2013; 368:1408–1416.

336. Savage KJ, Johnson NA, Ben-Neriah S, et al. MYC gene rearrangements are associated with a poor prognosis in diffuse large B-cell lymphoma patients treated with R-CHOP chemotherapy. *Blood* 2009;114:3533–3557.

337. Johnson NA, Slack GW, Savage KJ, et al. Concurrent expression of MYC and BCL2 in diffuse large B-cell lymphoma treated with rituximab plus cyclophosphamide, doxorubicin, vincristine, and prednisone. *J Clin Oncol* 2012; 30:3452–3459.

340. Savage KJ, Monti S, Kutok JL, et al. The molecular signature of mediastinal large B-cell lymphoma differs from that of other diffuse large B-cell lymphomas and shares features with classical Hodgkin lymphoma. *Blood* 2003;102:3871–3879.

341. Green MR, Monti S, Rodig SJ, et al. Integrative analysis reveals selective 9p24.1 amplification, increased PD-1 ligand expression, and further induction via JAK2 in nodular sclerosing Hodgkin lymphoma and primary mediastinal large B-cell lymphoma. *Blood* 2010;116:3268–3277.

346. Aviles A, Neri N, Fernandez R, et al. Randomized clinical trial to assess the efficacy of radiotherapy in primary mediastinal large B-lymphoma. *Int J Radiat Oncol Biol Phys* 2012;83:1227–1231.

349. Dave SS, Fu K, Wright GW, et al. Molecular diagnosis of Burkitt's lymphoma. *N Engl J Med* 2006;354:2431–2442.

351. Ribera JM, Garcia O, Grande C, et al. Dose-intensive chemotherapy including rituximab in Burkitt's leukemia or lymphoma regardless of human immunodeficiency virus infection status: final results of a phase 2 study (Burkimab). *Cancer* 2013;119:1660–1668.

352. Magrath I, Adde M, Shad A, et al. Adults and children with small non-cleaved-cell lymphoma have a similar excellent outcome when treated with the same chemotherapy regimen. *J Clin Oncol* 1996;14:925–934.

353. Lacasce A, Howard O, Lib S, et al. Modified magrath regimens for adults with Burkitt and Burkitt-like lymphomas: preserved efficacy with decreased toxicity. *Leuk Lymphoma* 2004;45:761–767.

355. Thomas DA, Faderl S, O'Brien S, et al. Chemoimmunotherapy with hyper-CVAD plus rituximab for the treatment of adult Burkitt and Burkitt-type lymphoma or acute lymphoblastic leukemia. *Cancer* 2006;106:1569–1580.

356. Dunleavy K, Pittaluga S, Shovlin M, et al. Low-intensity therapy in adults with Burkitt's lymphoma. *N Engl J Med* 2013;369:1915–1925.

362. Mak V, Hamm J, Chhanabhai M, et al. Survival of patients with peripheral T-cell lymphoma after first relapse or progression: spectrum of disease and rare long-term survivors. *J Clin Oncol* 2013;31:1970–1976.

363. Zinzani PL, Venturini F, Stefoni V, et al. Gemcitabine as single agent in pretreated T-cell lymphoma patients: evaluation of the long-term outcome. *Ann Oncol* 2010;21:860–863.

364. Malik SM, Liu K, Qiang X, et al. Folotyn (pralatrexate injection) for the treatment of patients with relapsed or refractory peripheral T-cell lymphoma: U.S. Food and Drug Administration drug approval summary. *Clin Cancer Res* 2011;16:4921–4927.

365. Coiffier B, Pro B, Prince HM, et al. Results from a pivotal, open-label, phase II study of romidepsin in relapsed or refractory peripheral T-cell lymphoma after prior systemic therapy. *J Clin Oncol* 2012;30:631–636.

366. Dodero A, Spina F, Narni F, et al. Allogeneic transplantation following a reduced-intensity conditioning regimen in relapsed/refractory peripheral T-cell lymphomas: long-term remissions and response to donor lymphocyte infusions support the role of a graft-versus-lymphoma effect. *Leukemia* 2012;26(3):520–526.

369. Federico M, Rudiger T, Bellei M, et al. Clinicopathologic characteristics of angioimmunoblastic T-cell lymphoma: analysis of the international peripheral T-cell lymphoma project. *J Clin Oncol* 2013;31:240–246.

374. Sieniawski M, Angamuthu N, Boyd K, et al. Evaluation of enteropathy-associated T-cell lymphoma comparing standard therapies with a novel regimen including autologous stem cell transplantation. *Blood* 2010;115:3664–3670.

378. Sonnen R, Schmidt WP, Muller-Hermelink HK, et al. The International Prognostic Index determines the outcome of patients with nodal mature T-cell lymphomas. *Br J Haematol* 2005;129:366–372.

379. Gascoyne RD, Aoun P, Wu D, et al. Prognostic significance of anaplastic lymphoma kinase (ALK) protein expression in adults with anaplastic large cell lymphoma. *Blood* 1999;93:3913–3921.

381. Pro B, Advani R, Brice P, et al. Brentuximab vedotin (SGN-35) in patients with relapsed or refractory systemic anaplastic large-cell lymphoma: results of a phase II study. *J Clin Oncol* 2012;30:2190–2196.

382. Gambacorti-Passerini C, Messa C, Pogliani EM. Crizotinib in anaplastic large-cell lymphoma. *N Engl J Med* 2011;364:775–776.

384. Belhadj K, Reyes F, Farcet JP, et al. Hepatosplenic gammadelta T-cell lymphoma is a rare clinicopathologic entity with poor outcome: report on a series of 21 patients. *Blood* 2003;102:4261–4269.

387. Willemze R, Jansen PM, Cerroni L, et al. Subcutaneous panniculitis-like T-cell lymphoma: definition, classification, and prognostic factors: an EORTC Cutaneous Lymphoma Group Study of 83 cases. *Blood* 2008;111:838–845.

389. Chim CS, Ma SY, Au WY, et al. Primary nasal natural killer cell lymphoma: long-term treatment outcome and relationship with the International Prognostic Index. *Blood* 2004;103:216–221.

394. Huang MJ, Jiang Y, Liu WP, et al. Early or up-front radiotherapy improved survival of localized extranodal NK/T-cell lymphoma, nasal-type in the upper aerodigestive tract. *Int J Radiat Oncol Biol Phys* 2008;70:166–174.

398. Yamaguchi M, Tobinai K, Oguchi M, et al. Concurrent chemoradiotherapy for localized nasal natural killer/T-cell lymphoma: an updated analysis of the Japan clinical oncology group study JCOG0211. *J Clin Oncol* 2012;30:4044–4046.

402. Yamaguchi M, Kwong YL, Kim WS, et al. Phase II study of SMILE chemotherapy for newly diagnosed stage IV, relapsed, or refractory extranodal natural killer (NK)/T-cell lymphoma, nasal type: the NK-Cell Tumor Study Group study. *J Clin Oncol* 2011;29:4410–4416.

405. Tsukasaki K, Hermine O, Bazarbachi A, et al. Definition, prognostic factors, treatment, and response criteria of adult T-cell leukemia-lymphoma: a proposal from an international consensus meeting. *J Clin Oncol* 2009;27:453–459.

412. Bazarbachi A, Plumelle Y, Carlos Ramos J, et al. Meta-analysis on the use of zidovudine and interferon-alfa in adult T-cell leukemia/lymphoma showing improved survival in the leukemic subtypes. *J Clin Oncol* 2010;28:4177–4183.

417. Ishida T, Hishizawa M, Kato K, et al. Allogeneic hematopoietic stem cell transplantation for adult T-cell leukemia-lymphoma with special emphasis on preconditioning regimen: a nationwide retrospective study. *Blood* 2012;120:1734–1741.

418. Boehme V, Schmitz N, Zeynalova S, et al. CNS events in elderly patients with aggressive lymphoma treated with modern chemotherapy (CHOP-14) with or without rituximab: an analysis of patients treated in the RICOVER-60 trial of the German High-Grade Non-Hodgkin Lymphoma Study Group (DSHNHL). *Blood* 2009;113:3896–3902.

419. Opelz G, Dohler B. Lymphomas after solid organ transplantation: a collaborative transplant study report. *Am J Transplant* 2004;4:222–230.

426. Riddler SA, Breinig MC, McKnight JL. Increased levels of circulating Epstein-Barr virus (EBV)-infected lymphocytes and decreased EBV nuclear antigen antibody responses are associated with the development of posttransplant lymphoproliferative disease in solid-organ transplant recipients. *Blood* 1994;84(3):972–984.

430. Choquet S, Oertel S, LeBlond V, et al. Rituximab in the management of post-transplantation lymphoproliferative disorder after solid organ transplantation: proceed with caution. *Ann Hematol* 2007;86:599–607.

433. Evens AM, David KA, Helenowski I, et al. Multicenter analysis of 80 solid organ transplantation recipients with post-transplantation lymphoproliferative disease: outcomes and prognostic factors in the modern era. *J Clin Oncol* 2010;28:1038–1046.

434. Gonzalez-Barca E, Domingo-Domenech E, Capote FJ, et al. Prospective phase II trial of extended treatment with rituximab in patients with B-cell post-transplant lymphoproliferative disease. *Haematologica* 2007;92:1489–1494.

435. Trappe R, Oertel S, Leblond V, et al. Sequential treatment with rituximab followed by CHOP chemotherapy in adult B-cell post-transplant lymphoproliferative disorder (PTLD): the prospective international multicentre phase 2 PTLD-1 trial. *Lancet Oncol* 2012;13:196–206.

436. Bollard CM, Rooney CM, Heslop HE. T-cell therapy in the treatment of post-transplant lymphoproliferative disease. *Nat Rev Clin Oncol* 2012;9:510–519.

440. Castillo JJ, Furman M, Beltran BE, et al. Human immunodeficiency virus-associated plasmablastic lymphoma: poor prognosis in the era of highly active antiretroviral therapy. *Cancer* 2012;118:5270–5277.

441. Simonelli C, Spina M, Cinelli R, et al. Clinical features and outcome of primary effusion lymphoma in HIV-infected patients: a single-institution study. *J Clin Oncol* 2003;21:3948–3954.

442. Barta SK, Xue X, Wang D, et al. Treatment factors affecting outcomes in HIV-associated non-Hodgkin lymphomas: a pooled analysis of 1546 patients. *Blood* 2013;122:3251–3262.

PRACTICE OF ONCOLOGY

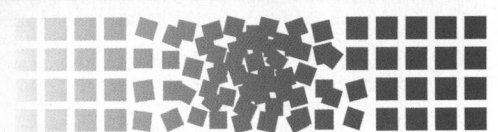

104 Cutaneous Lymphomas

Francine M. Foss, Juliet F. Gibson, Richard L. Edelson, and Lynn D. Wilson

INTRODUCTION

The cutaneous lymphomas comprise a heterogeneous group of malignancies of both T and B lymphocytes that localize to the skin. According to Surveillance, Epidemiology, and End Results (SEER) data, the skin is the second most common site of extranodal non-Hodgkin's lymphoma, with an estimated annual incidence of 1:100.000.[1] The Dutch and Austrian Cutaneous Lymphoma registries report that more than 70% of all cutaneous lymphomas are of T-cell origin, and 22% are of B-cell origin.[2] The term *cutaneous T-cell lymphoma* (CTCL) was formally adopted in 1979 at a conference sponsored by the National Cancer Institute (NCI) to describe a heterogeneous group of malignant T-cell lymphomas with primary manifestations in the skin. The World Health Organization and European Organization for Research and Treatment of Cancer (WHO–EORTC) classification of primary cutaneous lymphomas (Table 104.1, 104.2) defines three groups of cutaneous lymphomas: the cutaneous T-cell and natural killer (NK) lymphomas, the cutaneous B-cell lymphomas, and the precursor hematologic neoplasms.[2]

Further subgrouping based on clinical outcomes has been proposed for the cutaneous T-cell entities.[2,3] The entities with indolent clinical behavior include mycosis fungoides (MF) and its variants, the cutaneous CD30+ entities, subcutaneous panniculitis-like T-cell lymphoma, and the primary cutaneous CD4+ small-/medium-sized pleomorphic T-cell lymphoma. Included in the aggressive group are Sézary syndrome (SS), the NK/T-cell disorders, gamma-delta positive disorders, CD8+ cutaneous diseases, and primary cutaneous peripheral T-cell lymphoma (PTCL). A similar classification for the cutaneous B-cell lymphomas has been proposed based on the histology (follicular or large cell type) and site of disease, with favorable outcomes seen in disease of the head or upper trunk and an unfavorable prognosis seen with either disseminated lesions or disease in the lower extremities (Table 104.3).

MYCOSIS FUNGOIDES AND THE SÉZARY SYNDROME

MF was first reported by Alibert in 1806 as a common epidermotropic lymphoma with an indolent evolution characterized by cutaneous lesions in the forms of patches, plaques, or skin tumors. In 1980, Bunn et al.[4] reported the presence of Sézary cells in the blood of patients with MF, and the Sézary syndrome (diffuse erythroderma, circulating Sézary cells, and involvement of lymph nodes and bone marrow) was thus identified.[5–7] The International Society of Cutaneous Lymphoma (ISCL) established criteria for the diagnosis of SS, which include an absolute Sézary count of at least 1,000 cells/mm^3 in the blood, immunophenotypic abnormalities (expanded CD4+ populations and/or loss of antigens such as CD2, CD3, CD5, or CD4), or the presence of a T-cell clone in the blood.[8]

Epidemiology and Etiology

According to SEER data, the incidence of MF–CTCL had increased 3.2-fold between 1973 and 1984. The overall incidence rate is approximately 4 per 1 million, with an incidence of 1,500 cases per year. The actual incidence rate may be an order of magnitude higher, given possible underreporting and the difficulty and confusion in making the diagnosis. The incidence of MF rises with age such that the majority of patients are between 40 and 60 years. The disease is 2.2 times more common in men than in women, and incidence rates are somewhat higher in African Americans than in Caucasians.

One hypothesis regarding the etiology of MF/SS is that it may possibly represent a clonal evolution from a chronic antigenic stimulus. Associations with exposure to occupational chemicals or pesticides have been proposed but not definitely demonstrated in epidemiologic studies.[5,6] In other studies, an association with a *Chlamydia* infection of keratinocytes has been proposed, but data demonstrating *Chlamydia* proteins in affected skin lesions are equivocal.[9,10] The association between human T-cell leukemia virus (HTLV) type 1 infection and adult T-cell leukemia-lymphoma (ATLL) or Epstein-Barr virus in conjunction with nasal NK/T-cell lymphoma is not reflected in the epidemiology of MF–CTCL, but there are reports of the detection of HTLV-like viral particles in affected skin lesions and antibodies to HTLV-1 tax protein in patients with MF/SS.[11–14] These results suggest the association of perhaps a yet unknown retrovirus in some cases of MF/SS. Although there is no known geographical clustering and no evidence of maternal transmission of the disease, there are reports of multiple cases of MF/SS in a small number of families.

Pathobiology

The immunophenotypic profile of MF is one of clonal mature CD4+ CD45RO+ T cells with a marked homing capacity for the papillary dermis and epidermis. Some CTCL variants are CD8+ and different subtypes have distinct prognoses. Antigen loss is characteristic of the disease, with a loss of CD7, CD5, or CD2 and dim staining for CD3. Sézary cells express a TH2 phenotype, with secretion of interleukin (IL)-4, IL-5, IL-6, IL-10, and IL-13. The pruritus characteristic of the disease is related to secretion of IL-5 as well as other chemokines. One characteristic of the disease, even at its earliest stages, is profound immunosuppression with aberrant T-cell repertoires, cutaneous anergy, and increased susceptibility to bacterial and opportunistic infections.[15,16]

The homing to skin by CTCL cells appears to be mediated in part by expression of the surface glycoprotein cutaneous lymphoid antigen (CLA), an antigen whose expression is low or absent on normal infiltrating T cells.[17,18] CLA mediates binding to E-selectin on endothelial cells of cutaneous venules, thereby facilitating their exit from the circulation and into the skin. CLA is the physiologic ligand of endothelial cell E-selectin, a cell adhesion molecule

TABLE 104.1

World Health Organization–European Organisation for Research and Treatment of Cancer Classification of Cutaneous Lymphomas with Primary Cutaneous Manifestations

Cutaneous T-cell and NK-cell lymphomas

  Mycosis fungoides

  MF variants and subtypes

    Folliculotropic MF

    Pagetoid reticulosis

    Granulomatous slack skin

  Sézary syndrome

  Adult T-cell leukemia/lymphoma

  Primary cutaneous CD30+ lymphoproliferative disorders

    Primary cutaneous anaplastic large cell lymphoma

    Lymphomatoid papulosis

  Subcutaneous panniculitis-like T-cell lymphoma

  Extranodal NK/T-cell lymphoma, nasal type

  Primary cutaneous peripheral T-cell lymphoma, unspecified

    Primary cutaneous aggressive epidermotropic CD8+ T-cell lymphoma (provisional)

  Cutaneous gamma/delta T-cell lymphoma (provisional)

  Primary cutaneous CD4+ small-/medium-sized pleomorphic T-cell lymphoma (provisional)

Cutaneous B-cell lymphomas

  Primary cutaneous marginal zone B-cell lymphoma

  Primary cutaneous follicle center lymphoma

  Primary cutaneous diffuse large B-cell lymphoma, leg type

  Primary cutaneous diffuse large B-cell lymphoma, other

    Intravascular large B-cell lymphoma

Precursor hematologic neoplasm

  CD4+/CD56+ hematodermic neoplasm (blastic NK-cell lymphoma)

NK, natural killer; MF, mycosis fungoides.
From Willemze R, Jaffe ES, Burg G, et al. WHO-EORTC classification for cutaneous lymphomas. *Blood* 2005;105:3768–3785, with permission.

TABLE 104.2

Clinical Outcomes Based on World Health Organization–European Organisation for Research and Treatment of Cancer Classification for Cutaneous T-Cell Lymphomas

WHO–EORTC Classification	Frequency (%)	Disease-Specific 5-year Survival (%)
Indolent behavior		
Mycosis fungoides and its variants	50	88–100
Primary cutaneous ALCL	8	95
Lymphomatoid papulosis	12	100
Subcutaneous panniculitis like	1	82
Primary CD4+ small/medium pleomorphic	2	75
Aggressive behavior		
Sézary syndrome	3	24
NK/T nasal type	<1	–
Primary cutaneous CD8+ lymphoma	<1	18
Primary cutaneous gamma/ delta T-cell lymphoma	<1	–
Primary cutaneous peripheral T-cell lymphoma unspecified	2	16

ALCL, anaplastic large-cell lymphoma.
From Willemze R, Jaffe ES, Burg G, et al. WHO-EORTC classification for cutaneous lymphomas. *Blood* 2005;105:3768–3785; Willemze R, Meijer CJ. Classification of cutaneous T-cell lymphoma: from Alibert to WHO-EORTC. *J Cutan Pathol* 2006;33:18–26, with permission.

expressed on the surface of endothelial cells of cutaneous venules during chronic inflammation.[19] Chemokine receptor CCR4 expressed by cells binds chemokine CCL17 that has adhered to the luminal side of the endothelium, facilitating T-cell leukocyte function antigen-1 binding to endothelial cell intracellular adhesion molecule-1 and fostering extravasation into the dermis.[4]

One of the most striking features of MF/SS is epidermotropism, or infiltration of the epidermis by malignant T cells.

TABLE 104.3

Cutaneous B-Cell Lymphoma Prognostic Index

CBCL-PI Group	Histology	Site	Overall Survival	Relative Survival	HR	95% CL	p
IA	Any indolent[a]	Any	81	94	1.0		
IB	Diffuse large B cell	Favorable[b]	72	86	1.3	0.99–1.7	0.06
II	Diffuse large B cell	Unfavorable[c]	48	60	2.1	1.6–2.7	<0.0001
	Immunoblastic diffuse large B cell	Favorable					
III	Immunoblastic diffuse large B cell	Unfavorable	27	34	4.5	2.8–7.2	<0.0001

Note: Model is adjusted for age; sex; race; year of diagnosis; confirmed B-cell lineage; Surveillance, Epidemiology, and End Results historic stage; and treatment with radiation.
[a] Indolent histologies include follicular, marginal zone, small lymphocyte not otherwise specified, and lymphoplasmacytic.
[b] Favorable skin sites include the head/neck and arm.
[c] Unfavorable skin sites include the trunk, leg, and disseminated.
CBCL-PI, cutaneous B-cell lymphoma prognostic index; HR, hazard ratio; CL, confidence limit.
From Smith BD, Smith GL, Cooper DL, et al. The cutaneous B-cell lymphoma prognostic index: a novel prognostic index derived from a population-based registry. *J Clin Oncol* 2005;23:3390–3395.

The pathognomonic feature of MF is the Pautrier's microabscess, a collection of clonal malignant cells within the epidermis. The Pautrier's microabscesses may be a consequence of the expression of intracellular adhesion molecule-1 (ICAM-1) on keratinocytes. ICAM expression is induced by interferon (IFN), which is produced by infiltrating T cells and is a ligand for leukocyte function antigen-1.[20,21] In advanced disease or SS, the keratinocytes lose the ability to express ICAM-1 due to low levels of IFN-γ production, resulting in loss of epidermotropism.[21] Although specimens from early lesions of MF have lymphocytes in both the epidermis and dermis, clonality studies on dissected cells demonstrated that virtually all of the lymphocytes found in the epidermis belong to the malignant clone, whereas the dermis contains a predominance of inflammatory cells and nonmalignant lymphocytes.

Although there is no characteristic chromosomal translocation in patients with MF and SS, significant chromosomal instability is noted and losses on 1p, 10q, 13q, and 17p and gains of 4, 17q, and 18 are commonly observed.[22,23] Genetic instability is also evidenced by significant copy number alterations even in early disease.[24] Recent studies have shown a high prevalence of deletions or translocations involving a gene, NAV3, at 12q2, which has helicase-like activity and might therefore contribute to genomic instability.[25] Chromosomal amplification of JunB at 19p12 has also been detected in MF/SS and is thought to be contributory to the TH2 cytokine profile characteristic of Sézary cells.[26] In Lin et al.,[24] 21 regions of amplification and 42 regions of deletion were identified, with significant amplifications of 8q (MYC) and 17q (signal transducer and activator of transcription 3 [STAT3]) and deletions of 17p (TP53) and 10 (phosphatase and tension homologue [PTEN], FAS).[24]

DIAGNOSIS AND STAGING

The diagnosis of MF depends on both clinical and histopathologic criteria. The skin manifestations can be in the form of patches, plaques, erythroderma, cutaneous tumors, or ulcers. Early patch and plaque lesions may be indistinguishable from those of benign dermatoses, including psoriasis, eczema, large plaque parapsoriasis, or drug eruptions. The distribution of the lesions favors non–sun-exposed areas such as the *bathing trunk* distribution. An early diagnosis can be difficult and may rely on multiple biopsies obtained from different lesions over time. The ISCL has developed criteria for the diagnosis of early-stage MF that relies on clinical, histopathologic, immunopathologic, and molecular criteria[27] (Table 104.4). Of note, T-cell receptor clonality can be found in benign dermatoses and in lymphomatoid papulosis and pityriasis lichenoides (clonal dermatitis).[28,29] Long-term follow-up of patients with clonal dermatitis reveals a significant risk of progression to overt MF, suggesting careful follow-up.

Early lesions of MF may be asymptomatic, such as scaling erythematous macular eruptions often in sun-shielded areas (Fig. 104.1). A patch is defined as a lesion that is not elevated or indurated and that may be hyper- or hypopigmented. A plaque is raised or indurated and may be associated with scaling, crusting, or ulceration. A tumor is a lesion that is more than 1 cm with evidence of depth or vertical growth. Erythroderma is defined as diffuse erythema involving more than 80% of the skin surface with or without scaling.[8]

Painful and/or pruritic erythroderma may arise de novo or during any of the earlier described phases and is not always associated with frank T-cell leukemia (as in SS). Infrequently, MF presents with cutaneous tumor nodules in the absence of patches or plaques (as in *tumor d'emblée*). Patients may also present with or progress to involvement of visceral organs.

The Sézary Syndrome

The diagnostic criteria for SS are dependent on the presence of a circulating Sézary cell count of at least 1,000 cells/mm³. The phenotype is typically that of a mature, memory CD4+ T

TABLE 104.4

International Society for Cutaneous Lymphomas Algorithm for the Diagnosis of Early-Stage Mycosis Fungoides

Criteria	Major (2 Points)	Minor (1 Point)
Clinical		
Persistent and/or progressive patches and plaques plus	Any 2	Any 1
1. Non–sun-exposed location		
2. Size/shape variation		
3. Poikiloderma		
Histopathologic		
Superficial lymphoid infiltrate plus	Both	Either
1. Epidermotropism		
2. Atypia		
Molecular/Biologic		
Clonal *TCR* gene rearrangement	–	Present
Immunopathologic		
1. CD2, 3, 5 <59% of T cells	–	Any 1
2. CD7 <10% of T cells		
3. Epidermal discordance from expression of CD2, 3, 5, and 7 on dermal T cells		

From Pimpinelli N, Olsen EA, Santucci M, et al. Defining early mycosis fungoides. *J Am Acad Dermatol* 2005;53:1053–1063, with permission.

cell with a frequent loss of normal T-cell antigens (CD3, CD5, CD2, CD7, and CD26).[8] The CD4/CD8 ratio is elevated, usually more than 10, and a T-cell clone is detected in the blood by polymerase chain reaction (PCR). The presence of more than 1,000 Sézary cells/mm³ is not absolutely diagnostic of SS in the absence of other clinical features of the disease, because these cells may be seen in about 5% of patients with benign dermatoses manifested by erythroderma.[30,31] Histopathologic features in skin biopsies of patients with SS can be nonspecific, and there is a loss of epidermotropism in up to 70% of cases. Cytogenetic studies demonstrate unbalanced translocations and deletions, often involving 1p, 10q, 14q, and 15q, with evidence of clonal evolution and chromosomal instability over time.[32] A differential diagnosis includes viral or drug-induced exanthems, atopic dermatitis, or psoriasis.

Clinical features of the SS include extensive skin involvement with erythroderma, which may progress to lichenification, palmoplantar hyperkeratosis, and diffuse exfoliation. Skin edema, hypoalbuminemia due to insensible fluid loss related to impaired skin integument, and intense pruritus are frequently observed in patients with advanced disease. Lymphadenopathy, histopathologically effaced nodes, and bone marrow involvement are common. Significant immunosuppression occurs related to impaired T-helper function as well as T-cell repertoire skewing, leading to a high incidence of infections, particularly related to indwelling intravenous catheters. The overall prognosis is poor, with a median survival of 2 to 4 years.[33]

Staging and Prognosis of Mycosis Fungoides and the Sézary Syndrome

Staging systems for MF have been developed based on clinical features of skin involvement as well as infiltration of lymph nodes

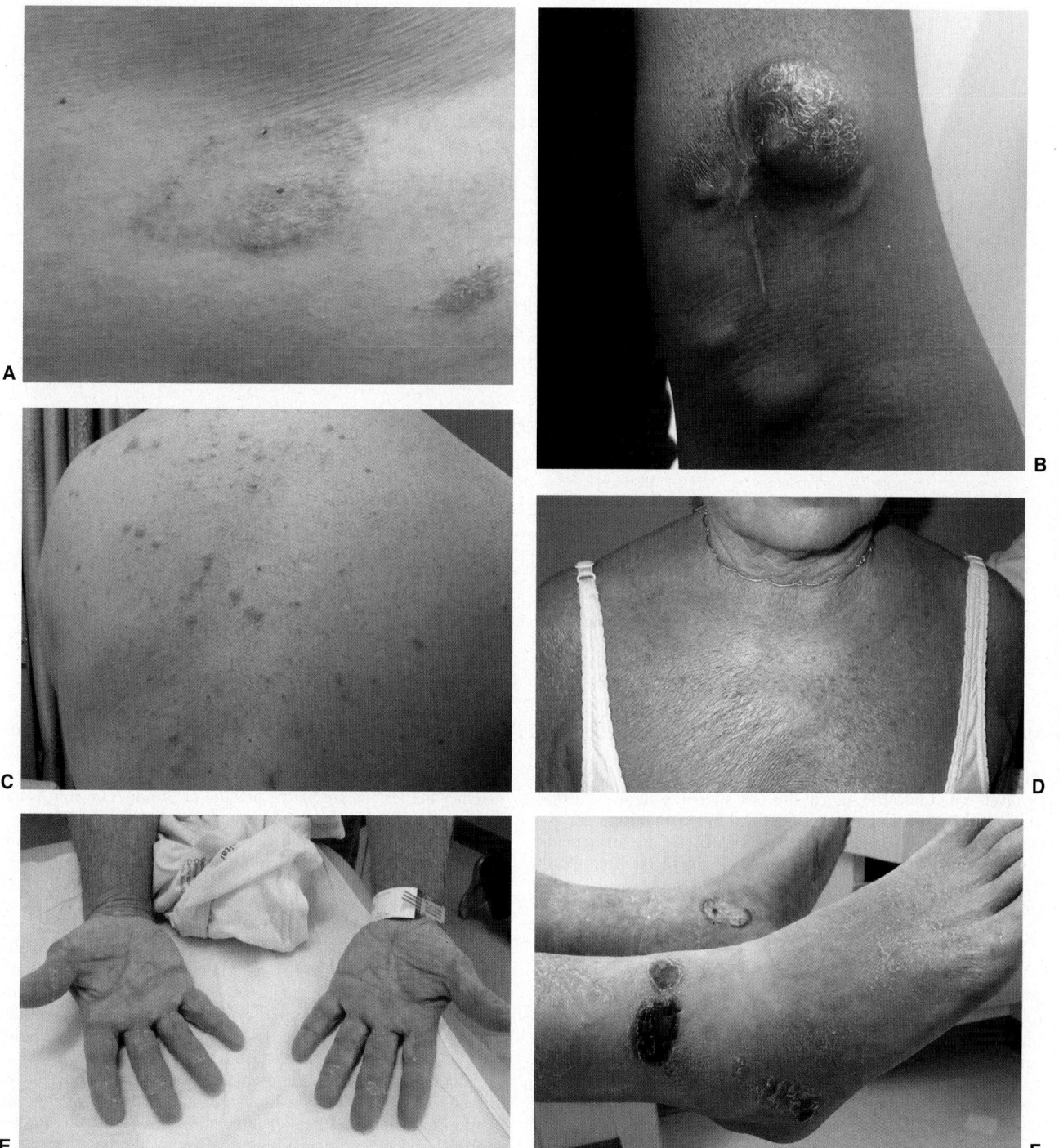

Figure 104.1 Mycosis fungoides and the Sézary syndrome. **(A)** Mycosis fungoides cutaneous plaque. **(B)** Cutaneous tumor. **(C)** Folliculotropic mycosis fungiodes. **(D)** Sézary syndrome with diffuse erythroderma. **(E)** Hyperkeratosis and involvement of palms with Sézary syndrome. **(F)** CD8+ cytotoxic T-cell lymphoma of the skin.

and viscera. Skin involvement is defined on the basis of the type of lesions and extent. T1 and T2 diseases are patches or plaques involving less than or more than 10% of the skin surface, respectively. T3 disease is the presence of at least one cutaneous tumor. T4 disease is erythroderma. Lymph node involvement has been classified based on the degree of infiltration with malignant cells. The dermatopathic node demonstrates typically many atypical lymphocytes in three to six cell clusters (LN2) or larger aggregates of atypical lymphocytes with nodal architecture preserved (LN3) clusters of T cells often with expansion of the parafollicular

zones. LN4 nodes are effaced by tumor cells, and typically such effacement is by atypical lymphocytes or neoplastic cells.[5] T-cell receptor rearrangement (TCRR) is found in half of patients with LN3 nodes and rarely in those with LN2 histology.[34] Bone marrow involvement has been shown to have prognostic significance based on the degree of involvement, with cytologically atypical lymphoid aggregates and infiltrative disease associated with inferior survival.[35] In retrospective studies, bone marrow involvement was associated with blood involvement and advanced lymph node disease.[7,36–38]

PRACTICE OF ONCOLOGY

TABLE 104.5

Staging Systems for Mycosis Fungoides

MF Cooperative Group 1979[a]				ISCL Group 2007[b]				
Stage	T	N	M	Stage	T	N	M	B
IA	1	0	0	IA	1	0	0	0, 1
IB	2	0	0	IB	2	0	0	0, 1
IIA	1–2	1	0	II	1–2	1–2	0	0, 1
IIB	3	0, 1	0	IIB	3	0–2	0	0, 1
III	4	0, 1	0	III	4	0–2	0	0–1
				IIIA	4	0–2	0	0
				IIIB	4	0–2	0	1
IVA	1–4	2–3	0	IVA₁	1–4	0–2	0	2
IVB	1–4	2–3	1	IVA₂	1–4	3	0	0–2
				IVA₃		0–3	1	0–2

Note: T1 patches or plaques. <10% bovine serum albumin (BSA); T2 patches or plaques, >10% BSA; T3, cutaneous tumors; T4, erythroderma; N1 = LN 0–2; N2 = LN 3; N3 = LN 4; B0, <5% of lymphocytes are atypical; B1, >5% of lymphocytes are atypical; B2, >1,000 Sézary cells/mm³ with positive clone.
[a] Data derived from Agar NS, Wedgeworth E, Crichton S, et al. Survival outcomes and prognostic factors in mycosis fungoides/Sezary syndrome: validation of the revised International Society for Cutaneous Lymphomas/European Organisation for Research and Treatment of Cancer staging proposal. *J Clin Oncol* 2010;28:4730–4739.
[b] Proposed modifications to the staging system by the International Society of Cutaneous Lymphoma (ISCL). Olsen E, Vonderheid E, Piminelli N, et al. Revisions to the staging and classification of mycosis fungoides and Sezary syndrome: a proposal of the International Society for Cutaneous Lymphomas (ISCL) and the cutaneous lymphoma task force of the European Organization of Research and Treatment of Cancer (EORTC). *Blood* 2007;110:1713.

The initial staging system for MF/SS was proposed by the MF Cooperative Group in 1979 and was based on skin involvement, palpable nodes, and visceral involvement.[39] More recently, the ISCL further stratifies patients based on the extent of blood involvement (Table 104.5).[40] In this new system, patients with significant blood involvement are identified in the erythroderma, or stage III group, and patients with stage IVA disease are further categorized based on the degree of lymph node and blood infiltration. Early stage (TI/T2) disease has been proposed to be divided into patch alone versus both patch and plaque disease. These changes have been validated by Agar et al.,[41] who analyzed the outcome of 1,502 MF/SS patients at their institution.

Overall outcome in MF/SS is correlated with clinical stage, and retrospective studies have identified the extent of skin involvement as well as visceral disease as the most important prognostic factors.[7,14,38] Patients with limited patch/plaque disease covering less than 10% of their skin surface have a prognosis indistinguishable from that of age-, sex-, and race-matched controls.[42] The 10-year disease-specific survival for patients with more extensive skin involvement with patches or plaques is 83%, whereas those with tumors or histologically documented lymph node involvement had survivals of 42% or 20%, respectively.[38] Patients with effaced lymph nodes or the presence of large cell transformation had a uniformly poor prognosis.[43,44] Other poor prognostic factors include blood involvement and loss of T-cell markers CD5 and CD7.[45] Even in patients with B0 disease, the presence of T-cell clonality has been shown to portend a worse prognosis.[41]

CLINICAL EVALUATION OF PATIENTS WITH CUTANEOUS LYMPHOMA

An initial evaluation should include a careful assessment of the number and distribution of each type of skin lesion. The Skin Weighted Assessment Tool divides the body surface into areas that are assigned a value based on the percent of total body surface area represented.[46] The observer then estimates the percent of each body area involved with disease based on the estimation that the palm of the hand is 1%. The involvement is weighted based on whether the lesions are patch, plaque, or tumor. The sum is the skin score, which can be recorded and monitored during therapy.

Skin biopsies at multiple sites may be necessary to establish the diagnosis because lesion morphology varies even for different lesions from the same patient and the quality and quantity of infiltrating cells may be affected by topical therapies, including topical steroids. In addition, most of the cells in the underlying, often much more impressive dermal infiltrate are nonneoplastic reactive CD4+ and CD8+ T lymphocytes. Features of pleomorphism and the presence of large cells should be noted. Transformation to a large cell phenotype in patients with MF/SS is associated with a poor prognosis. Immunophenotyping and molecular studies for TCRR should be performed on skin biopsies.

Laboratory studies should include flow cytometry to detect circulating neoplastic cells. In investigational settings, it is possible to use monoclonal antibodies directed against TCR-Vb families to detect and precisely quantitate the levels of circulating leukemia cells. In most instances, the level of circulating CTCL cells is actually much higher than estimated by less-sensitive techniques such as by evaluation of the peripheral smear for atypical cells.[21] In many patients, the expansion of the neoplastic T-cell clone is accompanied by depression of normal T cells to levels comparable with those observed in advanced AIDS. Such a de facto T-cell deficiency may both explain the susceptibility of erythrodermic CTCL patients to infection by bacterial, viral, and fungal pathogens and contribute to the progression of the disease, which is often held in check by host immune mechanisms.[47]

Flow cytometry should be performed with antibodies to the CD4, CD8, CD3, CD45R0, and CD26 antigens. The ratio of CD4+ to CD8+ cells is normally 0.5:3.5; elevations in this ratio correlate with total leukocyte count and with extent of skin disease in CTCL patients. An elevated ratio of CD4+ to CD8+

cells above 4.5:1.0 strongly suggests significant levels of circulating CTCL cells. Dual color staining with CD4 and other antigens can detect low or absent expression of CD3, CD7, or CD26 as a feature of Sézary cells.

Imaging studies (computed tomography scan or magnetic resonance imaging) are recommended at the initial evaluation, especially for those with advanced disease, as well as during follow-up, to detect enlargement of thoracic, abdominal, or pelvic nodes. Positron emission tomography has been performed for patients with CTCL, but there is not enough experience to reliably determine the sensitivity and specificity in cutaneous lymphoma.[48,49] Pathologically enlarged lymph nodes should be biopsied at the initial staging and subsequently if enlargement is detected on the physical examination or imaging studies because a proportion of patients with CTCL may have other lymphomas (B or T cell; e.g., Hodgkin's) concurrently. A bone marrow biopsy should be obtained in patients with advanced disease, including those with SS, as well as in patients with compromised hematologic function. Biopsies of visceral organs such as the liver should be dictated based on clinical indication or to confirm findings on imaging studies.

PRINCIPLES OF THERAPY OF MYCOSIS FUNGOIDES AND THE SÉZARY SYNDROME

Treatment approaches for MF/SS depend on the clinical stage of disease. Early-stage disease that is localized to the skin (patch or plaque disease) has an excellent chance of cure or long-term control with therapies directed to the skin alone. In contrast, tumor stage disease, extensive plaque stage disease that is refractory to topical therapies, and nodal or visceral disease can be palliated but rarely cured. Over the past 15 years, a number of novel agents have shown activity in MF/SS (Table 104.6). Because MF/SS is immunosuppressive and an immunologically responsive disease, initial therapies for many patients involve cutaneous and biologic approaches, which act directly on CTCL cells (e.g., they are directly cytotoxic) but also have indirect effects (e.g., alter the cutaneous environment) that may play a role in disease control.[50]

Skin-Directed Therapy

Skin-directed modalities include those for localized disease (radiotherapy, bexarotene, and carmustine) and those applicable to total skin therapy (topical chemotherapy with nitrogen mustard [NM], phototherapy, and total skin electron-beam therapy [TSEBT]; Table 104.6). All skin-directed therapies exert their primary effects on disease confined to the skin by inducing apoptosis of tumor cells and interfering with the local production of cytokines by epithelial and stromal cells necessary for neoplastic T-cell survival and proliferation.[51]

Approximately 7% of patients with stage I disease present with a solitary cutaneous lesion or several in proximity. Wilson et al.[52] found that the rate of clinical remission after local external-beam radiotherapy is very high (approximately 95%) in these patients and may be the treatment of choice. In one study, a total of 21 patients were treated with electron-beam radiation to a median dose of 20 Gy. With a median follow-up of 36 months, the actuarial disease-free survival rates at 5 and 10 years were 75% and 64%, respectively, with a local control rate of 83% at 10 years.

Topical Chemotherapies

Topical NM is one of the first treatments for cutaneous manifestations of MF. The NM liquid can be applied to the skin as an aqueous solution of 10 mg/dL or applied in an ointment base. Long-term effects include induction of second cutaneous malignancies (e.g., squamous cell carcinomas) and hyperpigmentation

and hypopigmentation. Between 64% and 90% of NM-treated patients with T1 and T2 CTCL can achieve a complete response to therapy.

Topical Bexarotene Gel

Bexarotene (Targretin) is a novel RXR retinoid (retinoid X receptor) that has been shown to be effective both systemically and topically for patients with MF/SS. The overall response rate to topical bexarotene in clinical trials was 44%. The drug is not absorbed to any significant levels. The irritant dermatitis induced by the retinoid limits the use of the gel to patients with body surface area (BSA) of less than 15% because of discomfort. In many cases, topical bexarotene gel is used, alternating with topical steroids to minimize the irritant effect.

Phototherapy

Phototherapy has been effective for patients with MF/SS because keratinocytes are resistant to ultraviolet (UV) light–induced injuries, whereas lymphocytes are extremely sensitive to light in the form of either UVA (320 to 400 nm), UVB (290 to 320 nm), or narrow-band UVB (311 nm). Currently, narrow-band UVB is used most commonly because of the low risk of secondary skin neoplasms. Patients typically are treated three to four times per week for approximately 30 to 40 treatments to achieve a remission, and then treatment frequency is decreased to a maintenance schedule at weekly intervals. Broad-band UVB has the same treatment schedule.

Photochemotherapy with orally administered PUVA (ultraviolet A light with oral methoxypsoralen) has been an effective therapy for patients with patch and plaque stage MF. The intensity of the light and frequency of administration are titrated based on patient response and tolerability. Maintenance treatment is often necessary to prevent disease recurrence.

Combination Regimens Involving PUVA Photochemotherapy

Several well-conducted trials have assessed the role of PUVA in combination with various systemic agents, notably IFN-α and retinoids. Phase I and II studies of PUVA (three times weekly) combined with variable doses of IFN-α (maximum tolerated dose of 12 MU/m² three times weekly) in 39 patients with MF (all stages) and SS have reported an overall response rate of 100%.[53] The median duration of response (DOR) was 28 months, with a median survival of 62 months.

A randomized controlled trial compared PUVA (two to five times weekly) plus IFN-α (9 MU three times weekly) with IFN-α plus a retinoic acid receptor (RAR) retinoid, acitretin (25 to 50 mg per day), in 98 patients with a maximum duration of treatment in both groups of 48 weeks.[54] In 82 patients with stage I/II diseases, complete response rates were 70% in the PUVA/IFN group compared with 38% in the IFN/acitretin group. Time to response was 18.6 weeks in the PUVA/IFN group, compared with 21.8 weeks in the IFN/acitretin group.

Total Skin Electron-Beam Therapy

Total skin electron-bean therapy (TSEB) involves the use of electrons ranging in energy between 4 and 7 MeV applied homogeneously to the skin surface.[55] Structures below the deep dermis are relatively spared because most of the dose (80%) is typically administered within the first 10 mm of depth, and less than 5% beyond 20 mm depth. Generally, doses to skin target are in the range of 30 to 36 Gy. Blood and superficial lymph nodes may receive 20% to 40% of the skin surface dose, and this may be clinically important.

TSEBT may be administered as just one in a sequence of treatments for CTCL in a particular patient. For example, TSEBT

TABLE 104.6

Treatments for Mycosis Fungoides/Sézary Syndrome

Therapy	Response (%)	Toxicities
Topical Agents		
Mechlorethamine or carmustine	CRR Stage I: 76–86 Stage IIA: 55 Stage III: 22–49	Contact dermatitis, secondary cutaneous malignancies
Bexarotene	Stage IA–IIA: 21 CR, 42 PR	Contact dermatitis
Phototherapy		
UVB	CRR Stage IA/IB: 75–83	Erythema, pruritus
PUVA	CRR Stage IA: 79–88 Stage IB: 52–59 Stage IIA: 83 Stage III: 46	Nausea, phototoxic reactions, secondary cutaneous malignancies
PUVA plus IFN-α (1) vs. acitretin plus IFN-α (2)	CRR Stage I/II: 70 (1) vs. 38 (2)	Flulike symptoms
Immunotherapy		
IFN-α	ORR IA–IV: 40–80	Flulike syndrome, hematologic toxicity, nausea, fatigue
ECP	ORR III–IV: 31–86	Hypotension, fever
Radiotherapy		
Total skin electron-beam therapy	CRR Stage IA–IIA: 96 Stage IIB: 36 Stage III: 60	Secondary cutaneous malignancies, pigmentation, anhidrosis, pruritus, alopecia, xerosis, telangiectasia
Cytotoxic Chemotherapy		
EPOCH	ORR Stage IIB–IV: 80	Myelosuppression
Pentostatin	ORR Stage IIB: 75 Stage III: 58 Stage IV: 50	Lymphopenia
Fludarabine plus IFN-α	ORR Stage IIA–IVA: 58 Stage IVB: 40	Neutropenia
Gemcitabine	ORR Stage IIB/III: 70	Neutropenia
Pegylated liposomal doxorubicin	ORR Stage IA–IV: 88	Infusion-related events
Novel Targeted Strategies		
Bexarotene	ORR Stage IA/IIA: 20–67 Stage IIB–IV: 49	Hypertriglyceridemia hyperlipidemia, hypothyroidism
Vorinostat	ORR: 29 Stage IA/IIA: 20–31 Stage IIB–IV: 25–30	Diarrhea, nausea, vomiting, fatigue
Romidepsin	ORR: 34–38 Stage IB/IIA: 25–66 Stage IIB–IVA: 29–38	Nausea, vomiting, anorexia, diarrhea, headache, ageusia
Denileukin diftitox	Stage I/IIA: 37 Stage IIB–IV: 24 Stages II–IV (less heavily pretreated) 62	Flulike symptoms, infusion-related events, vascular leak syndrome

(continued)

TABLE 104.6

Treatments for Mycosis Fungoides/Sézary Syndrome *(continued)*

Therapy	Response (%)	Toxicities
Novel Targeted Strategies (continued)		
Denileukin diftitox + bexarotene	ORR: 72	Lymphopenia, leukopenia
Alemtuzumab	ORR III–IV: 86–100	Infusion reaction, immunosuppression
Zanolimumab	ORR: 56 IA–IIA: 34 IIB–IVB: 22	Low-grade infection, eczematous dermatitis
Mogamulizumab	ORR: 37 MF: 29 SS: 47	Infusion reaction, skin rash
Brentuximab vedotin	ORR: 71 MF: 50 LyP and pc-ALCL: 100	Peripheral neuropathy, drug rash, diarrhea, fatigue

CRR, complete response rate; CR, complete response; PR, partial response; UVB, ultraviolet B; PUVA, ultraviolet A light with oral methoxypsoralen; ORR, overall response rate; ECP, extracorporeal photochemotherapy; EPOCH, etoposide, vincristine, doxorubicin, cyclophosphamide, and prednisone; SS, Sézary syndrome; LyP, lymphomatoid papulosis; pc-ALCL, primary cutaneous anaplastic large-cell lymphoma.

is excellent treatment for patients with diffuse involvement with thick plaques or cutaneous tumors and is also suitable for patients with symptomatic erythroderma–T4 disease.[56] TSEBT is also an excellent alternative for patients with extensive patches or thin plaques refractory to PUVA or other skin-directed therapies.[57] Subsequently, TSEBT may be administered to a patient several times using a variety of dose schedules, as clinically required to help control progressive disease.

Clinical complete response rates for patients with T1 or T2 (patch or plaque) disease range from 71% to 98% and are higher in patients with less-extensive disease. Patients with T1 and T2 disease treated with TSEBT have disease-free and overall survivals of 50% to 65% and 80% to 90%, respectively, at 5 years, although patients with antecedent or coexisting lymphomatoid papulosis or alopecia mucinosa–follicular mucinosis appear to have a shorter disease-free survival after TSEBT than those who do not. Patients with more advanced T3 and T4 disease fare significantly worse, with 5-year disease-free and overall survivals of approximately 20% and 50%, respectively. However, those T3 patients with less than 10% of the total skin surface involved by CTCL have significantly better disease-free and overall survival after TSEBT than those with more extensive disease. For patients with erythrodermic MF (T4) who are managed with TSEBT alone (32 to 40 Gy), without concomitant or neoadjuvant therapy, the complete response rate is approximately 70%. The 5-year progression-free, cause-specific, and overall survivals are 26%, 52%, and 38%, respectively.[56] Based on data from Stanford lower dose TSEBT can also be considered. Overall response rates were in excess of 90% in thoise T2-T4 disease receiving 5–19 Gy. For those who received 1–<20 gy and 20 to <30 Gy, overall response was in excess of 95%.[58]

Palliation of adenopathy or visceral involvement in patients with N3 disease can be accomplished by the use of appropriate high-energy orthovoltage or megavoltage photons to doses of 20 to 30 Gy. Even 6 to 8 Gy in three fractions are sufficient (e.g., when combined with TSEBT). Combinations of TSEBT with total nodal radiation have been investigated. Although feasible, such combinations do not appear to prolong survival and may be associated with hematologic toxicities not observed with TSEBT alone. TSEBT is well tolerated by most patients; acute sequelae either during or within the initial 6 months after treatment may include pruritus, desquamation, alopecia, epilation, hypohidrosis, xerosis, erythema, lower extremity edema, bullae of the feet, and onychoptosis. Chronic changes can include atrophy of the

skin, telangiectasia, alopecia, hypohidrosis, and xerosis. Second malignancies such as squamous and basal cell carcinomas, as well as malignant melanomas, have been observed in patients treated with TSEBT, particularly in patients exposed to multiple therapies that are themselves known to be mutagenic, such as PUVA and mechlorethamine.[57,59]

For patients who suffer diffuse cutaneous recurrences after TSEBT not amenable to other skin-directed therapies, a second course of TSEBT is both feasible and worthwhile. At Yale University, a total of 14 patients have received two courses and 5 patients received three courses of TSEBT. The median total dose after these additional courses was 57 Gy, and 86% of the patients achieved a complete response after the second course, with a median disease-free interval of 11.5 months. The median dose was 36 Gy for the first course, 18 Gy for the second, and 12 Gy for the third.[60] A similar experience was reported from Stanford University, where 15 patients were identified who had been treated with a second course of TSEBT (median dose of 20 Gy), with a complete response rate of 40%.[61] Nine of these patients had a partial response to therapy, and the median total dose for the entire group was 56 Gy. In both series, repeat courses were relatively well tolerated, and sequelae were similar to those observed during and after the first course of therapy.

Combined and Sequential Therapy

The adjuvant use of PUVA after TSEBT in patients with T1 and T2 disease significantly decreased cutaneous relapse. Patients treated with adjuvant PUVA after TSEBT had a 5-year disease-free survival of 85%, compared with 50% for those not receiving PUVA ($p < 0.02$). The median disease-free survival for the T1 patients receiving adjuvant PUVA was not reached at 103 months, versus 66 months for the non-PUVA group ($p < 0.01$). For those with T2 disease, the disease-free survival figures were 60 and 20 months, respectively ($p < 0.03$).[62] Adjuvant topical NM also appears able to delay cutaneous recurrence after TSEBT. In 1999, Chinn et al.[63] from Stanford University showed that TSEBT with or without NM provided improved response rates compared with mustard alone for those patients with T2 and T3 level disease (76% versus 39%, $p < 0.03$ for T2; 44% versus 8%, $p < 0.05$ for T3).[63] For those with patch/plaque (T2), adjuvant mustard offered improved freedom from relapse after TSEBT compared with no adjuvant treatment. No significant survival differences were noted between the groups.

PRACTICE OF ONCOLOGY

The combination of extracorporeal photochemotherapy (ECP) administered during and after TSEBT may improve survival (p <0.06) for patients with T3 or T4 disease who have achieved a complete response to TSEBT; however, the group of treated patients was small, and the data are retrospective.[64] Wilson et al.[65] identified a significant improvement in cause-specific survival for erythrodermic patients (blood status both B0 and B1) treated with the combination of TSEBT and ECP compared with those not treated with ECP. The 2-year progression-free, cause-specific, and overall survivals for those receiving TSEBT/ECP were 66%, 100%, and 88%, respectively, compared with 36%, 69%, and 63%, respectively, for those not managed with the combination.

SYSTEMIC THERAPY FOR MYCOSIS FUNGOIDES AND THE SÉZARY SYNDROME

Biologic Therapies

IFN-α has been demonstrated in a number of studies to be a highly active agent in CTCL with response rates ranging from 40% to 80%.[66] Doses have ranged from 1 to 18 mU administered subcutaneously on a number of schedules, the most common being three times a week. IFN-γ has also demonstrated activity but is not as widely used. Constitutional symptoms and bone marrow suppression have limited aggressive and long-term use of interferons for many patients. Early studies with high-dose IL-2 has demonstrated activity in relapsed CTCL but with significant toxicity. In a recent study of intermediate-dose IL-2, 11 patients (median age, 60 years) with advanced or refractory CTCL underwent 8-week cycles of daily subcutaneous injections of 11 mIU, 4 days per week for 6 weeks, followed by 2 weeks off of therapy. This dose was well tolerated, and there were four partial responses, three of which were sustained.[67] IL-12 has also demonstrated activity in early and advanced MF. A phase 2 study demonstrated responses in 43% of the patients, with response durations ranging from 3 to 45 weeks.[68]

Extracorporeal Photochemotherapy

ECP, or photopheresis, involves a leukapheresis to isolate mononuclear cells that are exposed ex vivo to UVA in the presence of methoxypsoralen and then reinfused back into the patient. Methoxypsoralen incorporates into DNA and, in the presence of UV light, induces strand breaks and, subsequently, apoptosis. Circulating T cells and Sézary leukemia cells are more susceptible to UVA-induced apoptosis than are monocytes. The mechanism of action of ECP is believed to be related to the induction of apoptosis in clonal Sézary T cells, leading to uptake and processing of tumor antigens by immature dendritic cells generated from the effects of the ECP process on circulating monocytoid precursors.[69,70] The process of ECP has been shown to induce a cell-mediated antitumor response. Clinical improvement with ECP has been demonstrated in both patients with SS and in patients with tumor and plaque-stage CTCL.

In a study of ECP in erythrodermic CTCL, Edelson et al. demonstrated an overall response rate of 83%. Since then, studies have reported a range of overall response rates from 31% to 86% and vary in their definition of response (50% clearing or 25% clearing).[45,71–73] There is some evidence that ECP may be advantageous even in early stage disease (stage T1/T2) when there is any blood involvement.[74] Immune adjuvant therapies have been combined with ECP and have shortened the time to response.[75–78] Duvic et al.[79] compared treatment of stage III and IV MF/SS patients with ECP alone or ECP in combination with IFN-α, bexarotene, or granulocyte monocyte colony–stimulating factor and found a 57% response rate in the group undergoing combination therapy as compared to 40% in those undergoing ECP alone.

Bexarotene (Retinoid Therapy)

Bexarotene (Targretin) is an oral RXR selective retinoid that has been shown to alter T-cell trafficking through downregulation of CCR4 and E-selectin.[81] It is active both topically and orally. In a clinical trial of heavily pretreated refractory CTCL, oral monotherapy with bexarotene had a response rate of 54% in early-stage and 45% in advanced-stage CTCL patients. The median response duration was 299 days with continuous dosing at a dose of 300 mg/m^2 per day, and responses occurred in all groups of patients (57% at stage IIB, 32% at stage III, 44% at stage IVA, and 40% at stage IVB) including those with large-cell transformation. Pruritus decreased significantly in the treated patients and led to overall improvement in quality-of-life indices.[82] The major toxicities of bexarotene included elevations in serum lipids and cholesterol and suppression of thyroid function.

Bexarotene combination therapy has been studied extensively but has yielded limited additional benefit. Straus et al.[83] demonstrated that bexarotene in combination with IFN-α-2b did not have an increased response rate as compared to bexarotene alone. In the EORTC task force's phase 3 randomized clinical trial investigating PUVA and bexarotene, there also was no significant difference between groups.[84] A phase 2 clinical trial (GEMBEX) of gemcitabine and bexarotene showed lower response rates than those for gemcitabine monotherapy. Another phase 2 trial investigating liposomal doxorubicin and bexarotene found no added benefit of bexarotene.[85] A clinical trial of pralatrexate and bexarotene is ongoing.

Histone Deacetylase Inhibitors

Histone deacetylase (HDAC) inhibitors modulate gene expression by inhibiting the deacetylation of histone proteins associated with DNA, thereby permitting expression of a number of genes. HDAC inhibition has been shown to induce histone acetylation, cell cycle arrest, and apoptosis in leukemia and lymphoma cell lines. The HDAC inhibitor romidepsin was tested in clinical trials at the NCI, and responses were seen in patients with T-cell lymphomas who received 14 mg/m^2 given intravenously on days 1, 8, and 15 of a 21-day cycle.[86] Two multicenter phase 2 trials of romidepsin have been completed and have led to U.S. Food and Drug Administration (FDA) approval for romidepsin in CTCL.[86,87] In these trials, the overall response rate in 167 patients with advanced or refractory CTCL was 35%, with 6% achieving a clinical complete response. The median response duration was 11 and 14 months in the NCI and the sponsor phase 2 studies, respectively. The most frequent adverse events (all grades) were nausea, constitutional symptoms, thrombocytopenia, and reversible ST-T segment changes.

Vorinostat (Zolinza, suberoylanilide hydroxamic acid), an orally bioavailable HDAC inhibitor, was explored in a phase 1/2 study and showed activity in CTCL.[88] In a subsequent phase 2 study, vorinostat administered at 400 mg daily was associated with a 29% response rate in 74 patients with refractory CTCL, including 61 with stage IIB or higher disease. The response durations ranged from 34 to 441+ days.[89] Overall, 32% of patients had relief of pruritus. Panobinostat is an oral HDAC inhibitor that has been shown to have activity in CTCL. Of 139 patients enrolled in a phase 2 trial of panobinostat 20 mg three times a week, the response rate was 17.3%.[91]

Denileukin Diftitox

Denileukin diftitox is a fusion protein consisting of the IL-2 gene joined to the active and membrane-translocating domains of diphtheria toxin. In the pivotal trial that led to FDA approval of denileukin diftitox, the drug was administered at a dose of either 9 mg per kilogram or 18 mg per kilogram, for 5 days every 21 days, in 71 patients with relapsed or refractory CTCL.[92] The median number of prior therapies in this study was five. The overall response rate was similar for both dose groups and was 30% overall, with

10% complete responses (7 patients) and 20% partial responses (14 patients).[92] The median response duration was 6.9 months. The major toxicities included a reversible elevation of hepatic transaminases, a hypersensitivity syndrome associated with drug infusion, and a mild vascular leak syndrome, all of which were alleviated in part by steroid pretreatment.[93]

A randomized, placebo-controlled phase 3 trial has been completed comparing denileukin diftitox at doses of 9 and 18 ug per kilogram daily for 5 days on a 21 day schedule in patients with earlier stage CTCL who have had fewer prior therapies.[94] Of 144 patients treated, the overall response rates were 46%, 37%, and 15% for the 18 ug, 9 ug, and placebo arms, respectively. A combination study of bexarotene (75 to 300 mg) and denileukin diftitox (18 μg per kilogram for 3 days every 21 days)[95] reported an overall response rate of 70%, with four complete responses (35%) and four partial responses (35%). This study demonstrated that doses of bexarotene greater than 150 mg per day were capable of in vivo upregulation of CD25 (IL-2) expression and may enhance the efficacy of denileukin diftitox.

Monoclonal Antibodies

Alemtuzumab, a humanized monoclonal antibody that targets the CD52 antigen, has been shown to be active in relapsed or refractory T-cell lymphomas. Recent studies with lower doses of alemtuzumab (10 mg three times per week) have reported responses in 6 of 10 patients, including 2 complete responses and 4 partial responses, with minimal immunosuppression.[96,97]

Zanolimumab a high-affinity, fully humanized monoclonal antibody that targets the CD4 receptor.[98] It has shown promising results in 49 patients with biopsy-proven CD4+ CTCL, including 23 patients with advanced-stage disease.[99] Partial remissions were reported in 16 of 36 (44%) evaluable patients overall, including 3 of 6 with advanced disease at 980 mg per week.

Mogamulizumab (KW-0761) is a humanized anti-CCR4 antibody that enhances antibody-dependent cellular cytotoxicity against malignant T cells. CCR4 has been shown to have increased expression in a subset of patients with MF.[100] The overall response rate in a phase 2 trial of mogamulizumab in relapsed/refractory CTCL patients was 37% (29% in MF, 47% in SS).[101] Phase 2 studies are ongoing in CTCL, PTCL, and ATLL.

Brentuximab vedotin is a CD30-targeted antibody conjugated to an auristatin (monomethyl auristatin E [MMAE]), an antitubulin agent. After binding to CD30, the molecule is internalized and MMAE is released and binds to tubulin, leading to cell cycle arrest. In a phase 2 open label trial of 48 patients with CD30+ lymphoproliferative disorders including lymphomatoid papulosis (LyP) and primary cutaneous anaplastic large-cell lymphoma (pc-ALCL) or CD30+ MF, brentuximab demonstrated an overall response rate of 71% (34 out of 48), with 35% of patients achieving a complete remission (17 out of 48). Interestingly, it showed a 50% overall response rate in MF irrespective of the level of CD30 expression.[102]

Cytotoxic Chemotherapy

Combination chemotherapy regimens have produced higher responses in patients with advanced refractory CTCL, but these responses have not been durable. A study of infusional EPOCH (etoposide, vincristine, doxorubicin, bolus cyclophosphamide, and oral prednisone) in advanced refractory CTCL demonstrated an overall response rate of 80% (12 patients), with 4 (27%) complete responses but a response duration of 8 months.[103] Treatment-related toxicity was significant, with 61% of the patients experiencing grade 3/4 myelosuppression. Because of the high risk of infection and myelosuppression and modest response durations with combination chemotherapy, single-agent therapies are preferred except in patients who are refractory or who present with extensive adenopathy and/or visceral involvement and require immediate palliation.

Purine Analogs

Response rates up to 70% have been reported for single-agent pentostatin in refractory patients. Investigators at the M.D. Anderson Cancer Center reported a response rate of 56% for dose-escalated pentostatin (3 to 5 mg/m^2 per day for 3 days on a 21-day schedule) in 42 patients with CTCL.[104] The failure-free survival was 2.1 months. Grade 3/4 neutropenia occurred in 21% of patients. The incidence of infectious complications with pentostatin was initially high but was subsequently reduced by prophylactic trimethoprim and antiviral therapies. In a combination study of pentostatin at 4 mg/m^2 per day for 3 days with intermediate-dose IFN-α, the overall response rate was similar, but the median progression-free survival was improved to 13.1 months.[105]

Fludarabine and cladribine have demonstrated more modest single-agent activity in MF/SS. The combination of fludarabine with IFN-α had greater efficacy with an overall response rate of 51% (4 complete responses, 14 partial responses) with a median progression-free survival of 5.9 months and an overall survival of 19.6 months.[106] Similarly, a combination of fludarabine (18 mg/m^2) and cyclophosphamide (250 mg/m^2) for 3 days monthly was associated with a DOR of 10 months but with significant hematologic toxicity.[107]

Gemcitabine has demonstrated impressive clinical activity in advanced and refractory CTCL. In a study of chemotherapy-naïve patients treated with 1,200 mg/m^2, the response rate was 75%, with 22% complete response rate.[108]

Liposomal Doxorubicin

Pegylated liposomal doxorubicin is an active agent in Kaposi's sarcoma and has been shown to accumulate in involved skin lesions. In patients with advanced MF, response rates of 80% have been reported. In one small prospective multicenter study investigating liposomal doxorubicin monotherapy in 25 patients, 5 complete responses and 9 partial responses were reported.[109] In a larger phase 2 trial carried out at the EORTC of 49 patients with stage IIB, IVA, or IVB MF, 3 patients experienced a complete response and 17 experienced a partial response with a median duration of response of 6 months and a median time to progression of 7.4 months.[110] With the exception of infusion related events, liposomal doxorubicin was well tolerated with no grade 3 or 4 adverse events (AEs).

Pralatrexate

Pralatrexate is a promising new folate antagonist with activity in patients with T-cell lymphoma that has been approved for patients with aggressive peripheral T-cell lymphoma and MF with large cell transformation. In preclinical studies, pralatrexate has been shown to be more potent than methotrexate.[111] In the PROPEL study, 111 patients with relapsed or refractory PTCL were treated with pralatrexate. The overall response rate was 29%, with a median duration of response of 10.1 months.[112] In an open label phase 1 clinical trial including 54 CTCL patients who failed at least one systemic therapy, pralatrexate was given at a dose of 15 mg/m^2 for 3 to 4 weeks, and the overall response rate was 41% (35% partial response, 6% complete response).[113] Grade 3/4 adverse events were mucositis and leukopenia. In patients with transformed MF in the PROPEL study, the overall response rate was 25% (n = 3), demonstrating efficacy in a group that is largely refractory to therapy.

Autologous and Allogeneic Bone Marrow Transplantation

Results with autologous stem cell transplantation have not been promising in patients with MF/SS. One major issue in many studies is eradication of disease prior to transplant, and most patients have undergone extensive prior therapy. Molina et al.[114] reported successful outcomes with donor transplants in six of eight refractory CTCL patients. All achieved a complete remission; however, two died from transplant-related complications. Paralkar[115] reported results using reduced intensity conditioning regimens in 12 refractory CTCL patients. Six patients (50%) achieved complete remission and the median duration of response was 22 months. In a retrospective analysis of allogeneic transplant for MF and SS, in a group of 60 patients where 44 underwent reduced intensity conditioning (RIC), patients with RIC had a 1- and 3-year overall survival of 73% and 63%, respectively, supporting a significant graft versus lymphoma effect.[116]

OTHER CUTANEOUS LYMPHOMAS

Primary CD30+ Lymphoproliferative Disorders

The primary CD30+ lymphomas comprise a spectrum of disease, with LyP being a clonal but nonmalignant variant and cutaneous ALCL (C-ALCL) resembling its systemic counterpart. Clinically and histopathologically, LyP and C-ALCL may be indistinguishable. The classic presentation of LyP is papular, papulonodular, or papulonecrotic skin lesions at different stages of development with a waxing and waning course. The lesions often disappear within 12 weeks and often leave a scar. The median patient age is 45 years, but the disease does occur in children; the male to female ratio is 1.5:1. Three histologic subtypes have been identified, all demonstrating large CD30+ cells with (type A) or without (type C) infiltrating inflammatory cells.[117] In some cases (type B), there is infiltration of the epidermis, similar to MF. Up to 60% of cases demonstrate clonality for T-cell receptor (TCR), but the (2;5) (p23;q35) translocation characteristic of alk+ ALCL is not present. Up to 20% of cases may be preceded by or follow another lymphoma, including MF, ALCL, or Hodgkin's lymphoma. For most patients, the prognosis is excellent, and the disease is managed either with no treatment, low doses of oral methotrexate, or PUVA. In a series of 118 isolated cases of LyP, only 4% of patients developed systemic lymphoma.

C-ALCL is similar to systemic ALCL except for the cutaneous presentation and the absence of systemic disease. All patients with C-ALCL should undergo careful staging to rule out systemic involvement before being classified as C-ALCL. Most patients present with solitary nodules, tumors, or ulcerating lesions that may spontaneously regress, but multifocal disease has been observed in up to 20% of patients. The histopathologic features of the disease include the presence of large, anaplastic cells that express CD30 antigen in more than 70% of the tumor cells. The tumor cells demonstrate clonality for TCRR, an activated CD4 phenotype with loss of other T-cell antigens and frequent expression of cytotoxic proteins (granzyme B, T-cell intracellular antigen-1 [TIA-1], perforin). The (2;5) (p23;q35) alk translocation that is frequently seen in systemic ALCL is uncommonly observed in C-ALCL. In addition, the systemic ALCL expresses epithelial membrane antigen, which is absent in C-ALCL. The overall prognosis is excellent and most patients are treated by surgical excision and/or local radiotherapy to the lesions. For recurrent disease, low doses of methotrexate or other cytotoxic agents may be used. A new family of humanized anti-CD30 antibodies has been developed and has shown efficacy in both systemic and cutaneous ALCL.

Subcutaneous Panniculitis-like T-Cell Lymphoma and Cutaneous Peripheral T-Cell Lymphoma Unspecified

Subcutaneous panniculitis-like T-cell lymphoma (SPTL) and cutaneous peripheral T-cell lymphomas have distinct clinicopathologic features and outcomes. SPTCL is comprised of two subtypes, the alpha/beta and the gamma/delta, and both are characterized

by subcutaneous masses or flat plaques that mainly involve the legs but may be generalized. Often, patients present with B symptoms such as fever, fatigue, and weight loss. The WHO–EORTC classification has separated these phenotypes because of their disparate outcomes.[2] The alpha/beta SPTCL is characterized by subcutaneous infiltrates that spare the epidermis and dermis and rim individual fat cells. In early stages, the tumor cells may lack significant atypia and an inflammatory infiltrate may be present, leading to a diagnosis of inflammatory panniculitis. The phenotype of the malignant lymphocytes is CD3+, CD4−, and CD8+ with an expression of cytotoxic proteins. The outcome for the alpha/beta type of SPCL is excellent, with an 80% 5-year survival. Treatments include corticosteroids, single-agent chemotherapy, and radiotherapy. The cutaneous gamma/delta T-cell lymphomas are characterized by disseminated disease with frequent mucosal and extranodal involvement. Hemophagocytic syndrome may occur. Histopathologic features include involvement of the dermis, epidermis, and fat with rimming of fat globules and angioinvasion. The phenotype of the cells is CD3+, CD2+−, CD8+, and CD56+ beta F1− with a lack of expression of either CD4 or CD8. Most patients have a poor outcome despite aggressive chemotherapy, with a median survival of 15 months reported in one series of 33 patients.

Primary cutaneous PTCL unspecified is characterized by infiltration of the dermis by CD3+ CD4+ or CD3+ CD8+ pleomorphic small- and medium-sized cells, in many cases with an admixture of reactive lymphocytes. Most cases demonstrate a loss of T-cell markers and are CD30 negative and rarely CD56+. The clinical features are plaques or tumors, often on the face, neck, or upper trunk. The estimated 5-year survival of the CD4+ types is 80% and the preferred treatments are surgery, radiation, or single-agent chemotherapy. The CD8+ variants often express cytotoxic phenotypes (granzyme B+, perforin+, TIA-1+) and are characterized by ulcerative or necrotic tumor or plaques with frequent dissemination to visceral sites but rarely to lymph nodes. The median survival for this group of patients is 32 months despite aggressive systemic chemotherapy.

The Cutaneous Natural Killer Lymphomas

Extranodal NK/T-cell lymphoma is an Epstein-Barr virus–positive lymphoma with an NK or cytotoxic T-cell phenotype most commonly found in South America, South Asia, and Central America. The skin is the second most common site of involvement after the nasal cavity and sinuses. Skin manifestations include ulcerative or necrotic skin lesions characterized histopathologically by angiodestruction and extensive necrosis. The neoplastic cells express CD2, CD56, and cytotoxic proteins but lack surface CD3. The TCR is often germ line, and Epstein-Barr virus is almost always expressed. The median survival for disease presenting in the skin alone is 27 months, and 5 months for those presenting with other sites of disease.

Another variant of cutaneous NK lymphoma, the blastic NK lymphoma, has been recently reclassified by the WHO–EORTC as CD4+/CD56+ hematodermic neoplasm because recent studies have demonstrated a plasmacytoid dendritic cell derivation. This neoplasm commonly presents in the skin with solitary or multiple tumors or nodules. Most patients who present with skin involvement only rapidly develop widespread disease in multiple visceral sites. The infiltrates are CD4+ CD56+, and CD45RA+ cells, which lack CD3 and cytotoxic proteins and express CD123 and TCL 1, which are characteristic of plasmacytoid dendritic cells. The differential diagnosis is myelomonocytic or lymphocytic leukemia cutis, which can be distinguished by staining for myeloperoxidase and CD3, respectively. The skin biopsy is notable for a diffuse nonepidermotropic infiltration of the dermis by intermediate-sized blastlike cells with frequent mitoses. The prognosis is poor, with a median survival of 14 months. Initial therapy is often with acute myeloid leukemia type of regimens, which induce brief initial responses.

Cutaneous B-Cell Lymphoma

The primary cutaneous B-cell lymphomas (PCBCL) are 1.4 times more common in men than women, and more common in Caucasians.[118] The etiology of PCBCL is also unclear, and the pathogenesis not well understood, but *Borrelia* has been identified in a small percentage of patients presenting with PCBCL. For PCBCL, nodal classification systems have been used, but given the different natural history of such lesions, specific classification and prognostic systems are necessary. In addition to the WHO–EORTC classification system for both T- and B-cell cutaneous lymphomas, other prognostic systems have been developed that take the location and histology of the lesion into account.[119]

Types of Primary Cutaneous B-Cell Lymphomas

The histologic subtypes of PCBCLs include marginal zone, follicular center cell type, and diffuse large cell (see Table 104.1). Mucosa-associated lymphoid tissue can be found in a variety of anatomic locations, and marginal zone lymphoma of the skin is the cutaneous counterpart. Small lymphocytes and reactive germinal centers are frequently appreciated in conjunction with marginal zone cells. The expression of CD20, CD79, and, commonly, bcl-2 but not bcl-6 has been identified in addition to the identification of the *IHG* and *MLT* genes of chromosomes 14 and 18, respectively. Follicle center cell cutaneous lymphomas often spare the epidermis and may consist of centrocytes, germinal centers, and reactive T cells. A follicular pattern is common and the expression of CD20 and CD79 is often noted. The expression of bcl-2 and MUM-1 is typically absent. The t(14:18) translocation, which is often seen in the nodal counterpart, is absent in the cutaneous presentation.

Cutaneous plasmacytoma consists of a cutaneous infiltrate of plasma cells without bone marrow involvement. This presentation of PCBCL is quite rare and may present as papules, plaques, or tumors/nodules. Typically, the dermis is occupied by mononuclear cells, and amyloid deposition is often identified within the infiltrate. Immunoglobulins are often present, and cells may express CD38.

Diffuse large B-cell type is distinguished based on whether it occurs on the leg and whether it is intravascular type. Expression of CD20 and CD79 may be seen, and lesions identified on the lower extremity may express bcl-2, bcl-6, and MUM-1. Lesions that are found in other cutaneous locations may also express these markers, but more typically they are found on the lower extremities. Inactivation of p16 suppressor genes, additions for 18q and 7p, and loss of 6q may be noted with cutaneous diffuse large B-cell lymphoma.[120]

Treatment for PCBCL depends on the histopathologic subtype. More indolent forms of PCBCL, such as marginal zone or follicle center cell, tend to be bothersome to the patient, but rarely follow an aggressive clinical course. Radiotherapy, surgical excision, and observation are options for such patients. Radiotherapy for PCBCL is very much the same as that described for MF–CTCL. The technical aspects of the treatment delivery are quite similar, as are the side effects. Patients who present with diffuse large cell leg-type histology are typically treated more aggressively, given the relatively poor outcomes with radiotherapy alone. Combined modality therapy is often considered for this group of patients, and therapeutic courses tend to follow those used in nodal lymphomas of similar histology. If the histology is diffuse large cell, but not of the leg type, consideration can be given to the use of radiotherapy alone as the sole therapeutic modality. Rituximab has been used in the management of patients with PCBCL and in those with widespread disease, but the evidence regarding efficacy and outcomes is anecdotal, and series are small. For patients with localized CBCL, the complete response rates approach 100%, with 5-year disease-free survivals of approximately 50%.[118,121–125]

SELECTED REFERENCES

The full reference list can be accessed at lwwhealthlibrary.com/oncology.

2. Willemze R, Jaffe ES, Burg G, et al. WHO-EORTC classification for cutaneous lymphomas. *Blood* 2005;105:3768–3785.
3. Willemze R, Meijer CJ. Classification of cutaneous T-cell lymphoma: from Alibert to WHO-EORTC. *J Cutan Pathol* 2006;33:18–26.
4. Bunn PA Jr, Huberman MS, Whang-Peng J, et al. Prospective staging evaluation of patients with cutaneous T-cell lymphomas. Demonstration of a high frequency of extracutaneous dissemination. *Ann Intern Med* 1980;93:223–230.
5. Sausville EA, Worsham GF, Matthews MJ, et al. Histologic assessment of lymph nodes in mycosis fungoides/Sezary syndrome (cutaneous T-cell lymphoma): clinical correlations and prognostic import of a new classification system. *Hum Pathol* 1985;16:1098–1109.
6. Schechter GP, Bunn PA, Fischmann AB, et al. Blood and lymph node T lymphocytes in cutaneous T cell lymphoma: evaluation by light microscopy. *Cancer Treat Rep* 1979;63:571–574.
8. Vonderheid EC, Bernengo MG, Burg G, et al. Update on erythrodermic cutaneous T-cell lymphoma: report of the International Society for Cutaneous Lymphomas. *J Am Acad Dermatol* 2002;46:95–106.
11. Pancake BA, Wassef EH, Zucker-Franklin D. Demonstration of antibodies to human T-cell lymphotropic virus-I tax in patients with the cutaneous T-cell lymphoma, mycosis fungoides, who are seronegative for antibodies to the structural proteins of the virus. *Blood* 1996;88:3004–3009.
18. Picker LJ, Kishimoto TK, Smith CW, et al. ELAM-1 is an adhesion molecule for skin-homing T cells. *Nature* 1991;349:796–799.
20. Nickoloff BJ, Griffiths CE. T lymphocytes and monocytes bind to keratinocytes in frozen sections of biopsy specimens of normal skin treated with gamma interferon. *J Am Acad Dermatol* 1989;20:736–743.
21. Nickoloff BJ, Griffiths CE, Baadsgaard O, et al. Markedly diminished epidermal keratinocyte expression of intercellular adhesion molecule-1 (ICAM-1) in Sezary syndrome. *JAMA* 1989;261:2217–2221.
22. Mao X, Orchard G, Lillington DM, et al. Amplification and overexpression of JUNB is associated with primary cutaneous T-cell lymphomas. *Blood* 2003;101:1513–1519.

23. Scarisbrick JJ, Woolford AJ, Russell-Jones R, et al. Loss of heterozygosity on 10q and microsatellite instability in advanced stages of primary cutaneous T-cell lymphoma and possible association with homozygous deletion of PTEN. *Blood* 2000;95:2937–2942.
24. Lin WM, Lewis JM, Filler RB, et al. Characterization of the DNA copy-number genome in the blood of cutaneous T-cell lymphoma patients. *J Invest Dermatol* 2012;132:188–197.
25. Karenko L, Hahtola S, Paivinen S, et al. Primary cutaneous T-cell lymphomas show a deletion or translocation affecting NAV3, the human UNC-53 homologue. *Cancer Res* 2005;65:8101–8110.
27. Pimpinelli N, Olsen EA, Santucci M, et al. Defining early mycosis fungoides. *J Am Acad Dermatol* 2005;53:1053–1063.
32. Mao X, Lillington D, Scarisbrick JJ, et al. Molecular cytogenetic analysis of cutaneous T-cell lymphomas: identification of common genetic alterations in Sezary syndrome and mycosis fungoides. *Br J Dermatol* 2002;147:464–475.
33. Scarisbrick JJ, Whittaker S, Evans AV, et al. Prognostic significance of tumor burden in the blood of patients with erythrodermic primary cutaneous T-cell lymphoma. *Blood* 2001;97:624–630.
35. Graham SJ, Sharpe RW, Steinberg SM, et al. Prognostic implications of a bone marrow histopathologic classification system in mycosis fungoides and the Sezary syndrome. *Cancer* 1993;72:726–734.
36. Diamandidou E, Colome M, Fayad L, et al. Prognostic factor analysis in mycosis fungoides/Sezary syndrome. *J Am Acad Dermatol* 1999;40:914–924.
38. Sausville EA, Eddy JL, Makuch RW, et al. Histopathologic staging at initial diagnosis of mycosis fungoides and the Sezary syndrome. Definition of three distinctive prognostic groups. *Ann Intern Med* 1988;109:372–382.
40. Olsen E, Vonderheid E, Pimpinelli N, et al. Revisions to the staging and classification of mycosis fungoides and Sezary syndrome: a proposal of the International Society for Cutaneous Lymphomas (ISCL) and the cutaneous lymphoma task force of the European Organization of Research and Treatment of Cancer (EORTC). *Blood* 2007;110:1713–1722.
41. Agar NS, Wedgeworth E, Crichton S, et al. Survival outcomes and prognostic factors in mycosis fungoides/Sezary syndrome: validation of the revised International Society for Cutaneous Lymphomas/European Organisation for Research and Treatment of Cancer staging proposal. *J Clin Oncol* 2010;28:4730–4739.

42. Kim YH, Bishop K, Varghese A, et al. Prognostic factors in erythrodermic mycosis fungoides and the Sezary syndrome. *Arch Dermatol* 1995;131:1003–1008.

43. Diamandidou E, Colome-Grimmer M, Fayad L, et al. Transformation of mycosis fungoides/Sezary syndrome: clinical characteristics and prognosis. *Blood* 1998;92:1150–1159.

44. Dmitrovsky E, Matthews MJ, Bunn PA, et al. Cytologic transformation in cutaneous T cell lymphoma: a clinicopathologic entity associated with poor prognosis. *J Clin Oncol* 1987;5:208–215.

45. Olsen EA, Rook AH, Zic J, et al. Sezary syndrome: immunopathogenesis, literature review of therapeutic options, and recommendations for therapy by the United States Cutaneous Lymphoma Consortium (USCLC). *J Am Acad Dermatol* 2011;64:352–404.

46. Stevens SR, Ke MS, Parry EJ, et al. Quantifying skin disease burden in mycosis fungoides-type cutaneous T-cell lymphomas: the severity-weighted assessment tool (SWAT). *Arch Dermatol* 2002;138:42–48.

48. Kumar R, Xiu Y, Zhuang HM, et al. 18F-fluorodeoxyglucose-positron emission tomography in evaluation of primary cutaneous lymphoma. *Br J Dermatol* 2006;155:357–363.

49. Tsai EY, Taur A, Espinosa L, et al. Staging accuracy in mycosis fungoides and sezary syndrome using integrated positron emission tomography and computed tomography. *Arch Dermatol* 2006;142:577–584.

50. Kim YH, Liu HL, Mraz-Gernhard S, et al. Long-term outcome of 525 patients with mycosis fungoides and Sezary syndrome: clinical prognostic factors and risk for disease progression. *Arch Dermatol* 2003;139:857–866.

52. Wilson LD, Kacinski BM, Jones GW. Local superficial radiotherapy in the management of minimal stage IA cutaneous T-cell lymphoma (Mycosis Fungoides). *Int J Radiat Oncol Biol Phys* 1998;40:109–115.

53. Kuzel TM, Roenigk HH Jr, Samuelson E, et al. Effectiveness of interferon alfa-2a combined with phototherapy for mycosis fungoides and the Sezary syndrome. *J Clin Oncol* 1995;13:257–263.

55. Jones GW, Kacinski BM, Wilson LD, et al. Total skin electron radiation in the management of mycosis fungoides: Consensus of the European Organization for Research and Treatment of Cancer (EORTC) Cutaneous Lymphoma Project Group. *J Am Acad Dermatol* 2002;47:364–370.

57. Jones G, Wilson LD, Fox-Goguen L. Total skin electron beam radiotherapy for patients who have mycosis fungoides. *Hematol Oncol Clin North Am* 2003;17:1421–1434.

59. Licata AG, Wilson LD, Braverman IM, et al. Malignant melanoma and other second cutaneous malignancies in cutaneous T-cell lymphoma. The influence of additional therapy after total skin electron beam radiation. *Arch Dermatol* 1995;131:432–435.

60. Wilson LD, Quiros PA, Kolenik SA, et al. Additional courses of total skin electron beam therapy in the treatment of patients with recurrent cutaneous T-cell lymphoma. *J Am Acad Dermatol* 1996;35:69–73.

62. Quiros PA, Jones GW, Kacinski BM, et al. Total skin electron beam therapy followed by adjuvant psoralen/ultraviolet-A light in the management of patients with T1 and T2 cutaneous T-cell lymphoma (mycosis fungoides). *Int J Radiat Oncol Biol Phys* 1997;38:1027–1035.

63. Chinn DM, Chow S, Kim YH, et al. Total skin electron beam therapy with or without adjuvant topical nitrogen mustard or nitrogen mustard alone as initial treatment of T2 and T3 mycosis fungoides. *Int J Radiat Oncol Biol Phys* 1999;43:951–958.

65. Wilson LD, Jones GW, Kim D, et al. Experience with total skin electron beam therapy in combination with extracorporeal photopheresis in the management of patients with erythrodermic (T4) mycosis fungoides. *J Am Acad Dermatol* 2000;43:54–60.

66. Olsen EA, Bunn PA. Interferon in the treatment of cutaneous T-cell lymphoma. *Hematol Oncol Clin North Am* 1995;9:1089–1107.

67. Foss FM, Higgins B. Intermediate dose interleukin-2 demonstrates activity in patients with relapsed or refractory cutaneous T-cell lymphoma. *Blood* 2004;104:2642.

68. Duvic M, Sherman ML, Wood GS, et al. A phase II open-label study of recombinant human interleukin-12 in patients with stage IA, IB, or IIA mycosis fungoides. *J Am Acad Dermatol* 2006;55:807–813.

69. Berger CL, Xu AL, Hanlon D, et al. Induction of human tumor-loaded dendritic cells. *Int J Cancer* 2001;91:438–447.

75. Suchin KR, Cucchiara AJ, Gottleib SL, et al. Treatment of cutaneous T-cell lymphoma with combined immunomodulatory therapy: a 14-year experience at a single institution. *Arch Dermatol* 2002;138:1054–1060.

77. Bisaccia E, Gonzalez J, Palangio M, et al. Extracorporeal photochemotherapy alone or with adjuvant therapy in the treatment of cutaneous T-cell lymphoma: a 9-year retrospective study at a single institution. *J Am Acad Dermatol* 2000;43:263–271.

79. Duvic M, Chiao N, Talpur R. Extracorporeal photopheresis for the treatment of cutaneous T-cell lymphoma. *J Cutan Med Surg* 2003;7:3–7.

82. Duvic M, Hymes K, Heald P, et al. Bexarotene is effective and safe for treatment of refractory advanced-stage cutaneous T-cell lymphoma: multinational phase II-III trial results. *J Clin Oncol* 2001;19:2456–2471.

83. Straus DJ, Duvic M, Kuzel T, et al. Results of a phase II trial of oral bexarotene (Targretin) combined with interferon alfa-2b (Intron-A) for patients with cutaneous T-cell lymphoma. *Cancer* 2007;109:1799–1803.

84. Whittaker S, Ortiz P, Dummer R, et al. Efficacy and safety of bexarotene combined with psoralen-ultraviolet A (PUVA) compared with PUVA treatment alone in stage IB-IIA mycosis fungoides: final results from the EORTC Cutaneous Lymphoma Task Force phase III randomized clinical trial (NCT00056056). *Br J Dermatol* 2012;167:678–687.

85. Straus DJ, Duvic M, Horwitz SM, et al. Final results of phase II trial of doxorubicin HCl liposome injection followed by bexarotene in advanced cutaneous T-cell lymphoma. *Ann Oncol* 2014;25:206–210.

86. Piekarz RL, Frye R, Turner M, et al. Phase II multi-institutional trial of the histone deacetylase inhibitor romidepsin as monotherapy for patients with cutaneous T-cell lymphoma. *J Clin Oncol* 2009;27:5410–5417.

87. Whittaker SJ, Demierre MF, Kim EJ, et al. Final results from a multicenter, international, pivotal study of romidepsin in refractory cutaneous T-cell lymphoma. *J Clin Oncol* 2010;28:4485–4491.

88. Duvic M, Talpur R, Ni X, et al. Phase 2 trial of oral vorinostat (suberoylanilide hydroxamic acid, SAHA) for refractory cutaneous T-cell lymphoma (CTCL). *Blood* 2007;109:31–39.

89. Olsen EA, Kim YH, Kuzel TM, et al. Phase IIb multicenter trial of vorinostat in patients with persistent, progressive, or treatment refractory cutaneous T-cell lymphoma. *J Clin Oncol* 2007;25:3109–3115.

90. Pohlman B, Advani R, Duvic M, et al. Final results of a phase II trial of belinostat (PXD101) in patients with recurrent or refractory peripheral or cutaneous T-cell lymphoma. *Blood* 2009;Abstract 920.

91. Duvic M, Dummer R, Becker JC, et al. Panobinostat activity in both bexarotene-exposed and -naive patients with refractory cutaneous T-cell lymphoma: results of a phase II trial. *Eur J Cancer* 2013;49:386–394.

92. Olsen E, Duvic M, Frankel A, et al. Pivotal phase III trial of two dose levels of denileukin diftitox for the treatment of cutaneous T-cell lymphoma. *J Clin Oncol* 2001;19:376–388.

93. Foss FM, Bacha P, Osann KE, et al. Biological correlates of acute hypersensitivity events with DAB(389)IL-2 (denileukin diftitox, ONTAK) in cutaneous T-cell lymphoma: decreased frequency and severity with steroid premedication. *Clin Lymphoma* 2001;1:298–302.

94. Negro-Vilar A, Prince H, Duvic M, et al. Efficacy and safety of denileukin diftitox (Dd) in cutaneous T-cell lymphoma (CTCL) patients: Integrated analysis of three large phase III trials. *J Clin Oncol* 2008;26:8551.

95. Foss F, Demierre MF, DiVenuti G. A phase-1 trial of bexarotene and denileukin diftitox in patients with relapsed or refractory cutaneous T-cell lymphoma. *Blood* 2005;106:454–457.

96. Kennedy GA, Seymour JF, Wolf M, et al. Treatment of patients with advanced mycosis fungoides and Sezary syndrome with alemtuzumab. *Eur J Haematol* 2003;71:250–256.

97. Lundin J, Hagberg H, Repp R, et al. Phase 2 study of alemtuzumab (anti-CD52 monoclonal antibody) in patients with advanced mycosis fungoides/Sezary syndrome. *Blood* 2003;101:4267–4272.

108. Marchi E, Alinari L, Tani M, et al. Gemcitabine as frontline treatment for cutaneous T-cell lymphoma: phase II study of 32 patients. *Cancer* 2005;104:2437–2441.

109. Quereux G, Marques S, Nguyen JM, et al. Prospective multicenter study of pegylated liposomal doxorubicin treatment in patients with advanced or refractory mycosis fungoides or Sezary syndrome. *Arch Dermatol* 2008;144:727–733.

110. Dummer R, Quaglino P, Becker JC, et al. Prospective international multicenter phase II trial of intravenous pegylated liposomal doxorubicin monochemotherapy in patients with stage IIB, IVA, or IVB advanced mycosis fungoides: final results from EORTC 21012. *J Clin Oncol* 2012;30:4091–4097.

112. O'Connor OA, Pro B, Pinter-Brown L, et al. Pralatrexate in patients with relapsed or refractory peripheral T-cell lymphoma: results from the pivotal PROPEL study. *J Clin Oncol* 2011;29:1182–1189.

113. Horwitz SM, Kim YH, Foss F, et al. Identification of an active, well-tolerated dose of pralatrexate in patients with relapsed or refractory cutaneous T-cell lymphoma. *Blood* 2012;119:4115–4122.

115. Paralkar VR, Nasta SD, Morrissey K, et al. Allogeneic hematopoietic SCT for primary cutaneous T cell lymphomas. *Bone Marrow Transplant* 2012;47:940–945.

117. Kadin ME. Pathobiology of CD30+ cutaneous T-cell lymphomas. *J Cutan Pathol* 2006;33:10–17.

118. Smith BD, Glusac EJ, McNiff JM, et al. Primary cutaneous B-cell lymphoma treated with radiotherapy: a comparison of the European Organization for Research and Treatment of Cancer and the WHO classification systems. *J Clin Oncol* 2004;22:634–639.

121. Eich HT, Eich D, Micke O, et al. Long-term efficacy, curative potential, and prognostic factors of radiotherapy in primary cutaneous B-cell lymphoma. *Int J Radiat Oncol Biol Phys* 2003;55:899–906.

124. Piccinno R, Caccialanza M, Berti E, et al. Radiotherapy of cutaneous B cell lymphomas: our experience in 31 cases. *Int J Radiat Oncol Biol Phys* 1993;27:385–389.

125. Rijlaarsdam JU, Toonstra J, Meijer OW, et al. Treatment of primary cutaneous B-cell lymphomas of follicle center cell origin: a clinical follow-up study of 55 patients treated with radiotherapy or polychemotherapy. *J Clin Oncol* 1996;14:549–555.

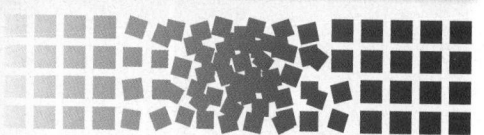

105 Primary Central Nervous System Lymphoma

Tracy T. Batchelor

EPIDEMIOLOGY

Primary central nervous system lymphoma (PCNSL) is an extranodal non-Hodgkin lymphoma (NHL) confined to the brain, leptomeninges, eyes, or spinal cord. PCNSL accounts for approximately 2% of all primary central nervous system (CNS) tumors, with a median age of 65 years at diagnosis.[1] The annual incidence rate is 0.47 cases per 100,000 person-years.[1,2] Since 2000, there has been an increase in the overall incidence of PCNSL, especially in the elderly.

PATHOLOGY

Approximately 90% of PCNSL cases are diffuse large B-cell lymphomas (DLBCL), with the remainder consisting of T-cell lymphomas, poorly characterized low-grade lymphomas, or Burkitt lymphomas.[3] Primary CNS DLBCL is composed of centroblasts or immunoblasts clustered in the perivascular space, with reactive lymphocytes, macrophages, and activated microglial cells intermixed with the tumor cells. Most tumors express pan–B-cell markers, including CD19, CD20, CD22, and CD79a. The molecular mechanisms underlying transformation and localization to the CNS are poorly understood.[4] Limitations in molecular studies of PCNSL include the rarity of the disease and the limited availability of tissue because the diagnosis is most often made with stereotactic needle biopsy. Like systemic DLBCL, PCNSL harbors chromosomal translocations of the BCL6 gene, deletions in 6q, and aberrant somatic hypermutation in proto-oncogenes including MYC and PAX5. Inactivation of CDKN2A is also commonly observed in both entities. Also like DLBCL, PCNSL can be classified into three molecular subclasses by gene expression profiling: type 3 large B-cell lymphoma, germinal center B cell, and activated B-cell lymphoma. However, certain molecular features distinguish primary CNS DLBCL from systemic DLBCL. Gene expression profiles demonstrate that PCNSL is characterized by differential expression of genes related to adhesion and the extracellular matrix pathways, including MUM1, CXCL13, and CHI3L1. The ongoing somatic hypermutation with biased use of V_H gene segments that has been observed in PCNSL is suggestive of an antigen-dependent proliferation. These observations are consistent with the hypothesis that PCNSL is secondary to antigen-dependent activation of circulating B cells, which subsequently localize to the CNS by expression of various adhesion and extracellular matrix–related genes. However, further molecular studies to investigate the transforming events and the subsequent events responsible for CNS tropism in PCNSL are needed. Insights into the molecular pathogenesis of PCNSL may allow for the development of targeted therapeutic approaches for tumors.[4]

DIAGNOSIS AND PROGNOSTIC FACTORS

Neurocognitive symptoms are the most common presenting clinical features of PCNSL. The International PCNSL Collaborative Group (IPCG) has developed guidelines to determine the extent of disease.[5] A gadolinium-enhanced brain magnetic resonance imaging (MRI) scan is the most sensitive radiographic study for the detection of PCNSL (Fig. 105.1). Most PCNSL patients present with a single brain mass. The mass is typically isointense to hyperintense on T2-weighted MRI sequences and homogeneously enhancing on postcontrast images. The diagnosis of PCNSL is typically made by stereotactic brain biopsy, cerebrospinal fluid (CSF) analysis, or by analysis of vitreous aspirate in patients with ocular involvement. Given the possible delay in diagnosis and treatment with the latter two methods, prompt stereotactic biopsy is advised in almost all cases that are surgically accessible. Secondary CSF and ocular involvement occurs in approximately 15% to 20% and 5% to 20% of PCNSL patients, respectively. Presenting symptoms of ocular involvement include eye pain, blurred vision, and floaters.[6] B symptoms such as weight loss, fevers, and night sweats are infrequent in PCNSL. A thorough diagnostic evaluation is needed to establish the extent of the lymphoma and to confirm localization to the CNS. Physical examination should consist of a lymph node examination, a testicular examination in men, and a comprehensive neurologic examination. A lumbar puncture should be performed if not contraindicated, and CSF should be assessed by flow cytometry, cytology, and immunoglobulin heavy-chain gene rearrangement. Because extraneural disease must be excluded to establish a diagnosis of *primary* CNS lymphoma, CT or CT/positron-emission tomography (PET) scans of the chest, abdomen, and pelvis, and a bone marrow biopsy and aspirate should be performed to exclude occult systemic disease. Involvement of the optic nerve, retina, or vitreous humor should be excluded with a comprehensive eye evaluation by an ophthalmologist that includes a slit-lamp examination. Blood tests should include a complete blood count, a basic metabolic panel, serum lactate dehydrogenase, and HIV serology.[5]

Two prognostic scoring systems have been developed specifically for PCNSL.[7,8] In a retrospective review of 105 PCNSL patients, the International Extranodal Lymphoma Study Group (IELSG) identified age >60 years, Eastern Cooperative Oncology Group (ECOG) performance status >1, elevated serum lactate dehydrogenase (LDH) level, elevated CSF protein concentration, and involvement of deep regions of the brain as independent predictors of poor prognosis. In patients with 0 to 1 factors, 2 to 3 factors, and 4 to 5 factors, the 2-year survival proportions were 80%, 48%, and 15%, respectively. In another prognostic model, PCNSL patients were divided into three groups based on age and performance status: (1) <50 years old, (2) ≥50 years old with a Karnofsky Performance Scale (KPS) ≥70, and (3) ≥50 years old with a KPS <70. Based on these three divisions, significant differences in overall and failure-free survival were observed.

STAGING

There is no staging system that correlates with prognosis or response to treatment in PCNSL. However, because PCNSL is a

PRACTICE OF ONCOLOGY

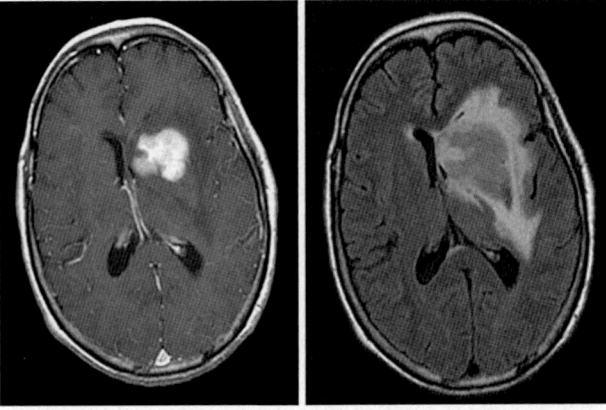

Figure 105.1 Magnetic resonance images from a patient with PCNSL. A T1-weighted, postcontrast, sequence *(left)* demonstrates intense, homogenous enhancement of the tumor in the region of the left caudate nuclear. A T2/fluid attenuated inversion recovery (FLAIR) sequence *(right)* demonstrates hyperintense signal surrounding the tumor, reflecting a vasogenic cerebral edema. (Courtesy of Priscilla Brastianos, MD.)

multicompartmental disease potentially involving the brain, spinal cord, eyes, and CSF, the IPCG recommends an extent of disease evaluation, as noted previously, which will enable clinicians to follow the response to therapy.[5]

TREATMENT

Defining a response to treatment in PCNSL requires an assessment of all sites involved by the disease. The IPCG has established response criteria that have been adopted into most prospective clinical trials (Table 105.1).[5]

Corticosteroids decrease tumor-associated edema and may result in partial radiographic regression of the tumor. An initial response to corticosteroids is associated with a favorable outcome in PCNSL.[9] However, after an initial response to corticosteroids,

almost all patients quickly relapse. Corticosteroids should be avoided if possible prior to a biopsy, given the risk of disrupting cellular morphology, resulting in a nondiagnostic pathologic specimen.

Surgical resection is not part of the standard treatment approach for PCNSL given the multifocal nature of this tumor.[10] The role of neurosurgery in PCNSL is to establish a diagnosis via a stereotactic biopsy.

Standardized induction and consolidation treatment for PCNSL has yet to be defined. Historically, PCNSL was treated only with whole brain radiation (WBRT) at doses ranging from 36 to 45 Gy, which resulted not only in a high proportion of radiographic responses, but also in rapid relapse. In a multicenter, phase II trial, 41 patients were treated with WBRT to 40 Gy plus a 20 Gy tumor boost and achieved a median overall survival (OS) of only 12 months.[11] Given the lack of durable responses to radiation and the risk of neurotoxicity associated with this modality of therapy, WBRT alone is no longer a recommended treatment for most patients with PCNSL. Moreover, because PCNSL is an infiltrative, multifocal disease, focal radiation or radiosurgery is not recommended. The most effective treatment for PCNSL is intravenous, high-dose methotrexate (HD-MTX) at variable doses (1 to 8 g/m^2), typically utilized in combination with other chemotherapeutic agents and/or WBRT. However, there is no consensus on the optimal dose of HD-MTX or on the role of radiation in combination with methotrexate in the management of PCNSL. A number of randomized trials are ongoing to address these issues. Doses of methotrexate ≥ 3 g/m^2 result in therapeutic concentrations in the brain parenchyma and CSF, and when combined with WBRT, lead to more durable treatment responses.[12–14] In a phase II trial, 79 PCNSL patients were randomized to receive either HD-MTX (3.5 g/m^2, day 1 *or* HD-MTX (3.5 g/m^2, day 1) + cytarabine (2 g/m^2 twice per day, days 2 to 3). Each chemotherapy cycle was 21 days. All patients underwent consolidative WBRT after induction chemotherapy. The HD-MTX + cytarabine arm had a higher proportion of complete radiographic responses and a superior 3-year OS.[14] However, it is now widely recognized that there is a high incidence of neurotoxicity with combined modality treatment that includes WBRT.[15] The latter observation prompted studies utilizing *lower doses* of WBRT. In a

---

TABLE 105.1

International PCNSL Collaborative Group Consensus Guidelines for the Assessment of Response in PCNSL

Response	Brain Imaging	Steroid Dose	Ophthalmologic Examination	Cerebrospinal Fluid Cytology
Complete response	No contrast enhancing disease	None	Normal	Negative
Unconfirmed complete response	No contrast enhancing disease	Any	Normal	Negative
	Minimal enhancing disease	Any	Minor RPE abnormality	Negative
Partial response	50% decrease in enhancement	N/A	Normal or minor RPE abnormality	Negative
	No contrast enhancing disease	N/A	Decrease in vitreous cells or retinal infiltrate	Persistent or suspicious
Progressive disease	25% increase in enhancing disease	N/A	Recurrent or new disease	Recurrent or positive
	Any new site of disease			
Stable disease	All scenarios not covered by responses above			

RPE, retinal pigment epithelium.
Abrey LE, Batchelor TT, Ferreri AJ, et al. Report of an international workshop to standardize baseline evaluation and response criteria for primary CNS lymphoma. *J Clin Oncol* 2005;23:5034–5043.

multicenter, phase II study, no significant neurocognitive decline was observed after consolidative reduced dose WBRT (23.4 Gy) and cytarabine in patients who had achieved a complete response to induction chemotherapy including HD-MTX.[16] However, further study and longer neuropsychological follow-up of these patients is necessary to definitively assess the safety of this regimen because numerous studies have demonstrated the delayed neurotoxic effects of WBRT in the PCNSL population and the reduced risk of neurotoxicity in regimens consisting of chemotherapy alone.[17,18] Given the risk of clinical neurotoxicity, other studies have assessed whether WBRT can be *eliminated* from the initial management of PCNSL. In a multicenter, phase III trial, patients were randomized to receive HD-MTX–based chemotherapy with or without WBRT.[19] Five hundred and fifty-one patients were enrolled, of whom 318 were treated per protocol. The intent to treat analysis revealed that patients treated in the combined modality arm (chemotherapy + WBRT) achieved prolonged progression-free survival (PFS) but no improvement in OS, demonstrating that the elimination of WBRT from the treatment regimen did not compromise OS. This has led to deferral of WBRT and chemotherapy-alone approaches for newly diagnosed PCNSL patients. These approaches are based on a foundation of HD-MTX. Variable doses and schedules of HD-MTX have been utilized, but in general, doses ≥ 3 g/m^2 delivered as an initial bolus followed by an infusion over 3 hours administered every 10 to 21 days is recommended for optimal outcomes and adequate CSF concentrations.[20] Multiple, phase II studies have demonstrated the safety, efficacy, and relatively preserved cognition of HD-MTX–based chemotherapy regimens.[21,22] Moreover, longer duration of induction chemotherapy with HD-MTX (>six cycles) results in higher complete response proportions.[16,21]

Several first-generation chemotherapy regimens for PCNSL included intrathecal chemotherapy. However, a number of nonrandomized studies that included intrathecal chemotherapy did not improve outcomes in PCNSL relative to regimens that did not include intrathecal injections of chemotherapy.[23,24] Moreover, the ability to consistently achieve micromolar concentrations of MTX in the CSF at a dose of 8 g/m^2 has led to the elimination of intrathecal chemotherapy from most of the chemotherapy regimens currently in use. However, the question regarding the role of intrathecal chemotherapy in the management of PCNSL should ultimately be addressed in a randomized trial.

Rituximab, a chimeric monoclonal antibody targeting the CD20 antigen on B lymphocytes, is being incorporated in combination regimens for PCNSL. When rituximab is administered intravenously at doses of 375 to 800 mg/m^2, CSF levels from 0.1% to 4.4% of serum levels are achieved. Despite limited CSF penetration, radiographic responses have been observed in relapsed PCNSL patients treated with rituximab monotherapy, and this antibody has been incorporated into contemporary regimens for PCNSL.[25] In a cooperative group, phase II study, 44 PCNSL patients were treated with induction chemotherapy consisting of HD-MTX at 8 g/m^2 (day 1), rituximab at 375 mg/m^2 (day 3), and temozolomide at 150 mg/m^2 (days 7 through 11), all of which are drugs with demonstrated efficacy as monotherapy in PCNSL.[22] This induction chemotherapy was followed by consolidation chemotherapy consisting of intravenous etoposide 5 mg/kg as a continuous infusion over 96 hours and cytarabine at 2 g/m^2 every 12 hours for 8 doses. Of these patients, 68% achieved complete response, median PFS of the entire group was 4 years, and median OS was not observed at the time of publication. These results are comparable to any regimen that *includes* WBRT. It is noteworthy that PFS was shorter in PCNSL patients in whom chemotherapy was delayed >1 month after diagnosis compared to those patients who promptly initiated chemotherapy (3-year PFS of 20% versus 59%; p = 0.05). This observation highlights the importance of prompt biopsy and early initiation of chemotherapy in this patient population.

Given the limited durability of responses observed in many studies of PCNSL, there is increasing interest in high-dose chemotherapy (HDT) followed by autologous stem cell transplantation (ASCT) as first-line, consolidative therapy for PCNSL. Conditioning regimens including thioTEPA have demonstrated the most encouraging results. In a multicenter, phase II study, 79 patients were treated with induction HD-MTX, cytarabine, rituximab, and thioTEPA, followed by carmustine and thioTEPA conditioning prior to ASCT. The overall radiographic response (ORR) was 91%, 2-year OS was 87%, and treatment-related deaths occurred in <10% of enrolled patients. The toxicities, mostly cytopenias, were manageable.[26] There are three ongoing, multicenter, randomized trials comparing the efficacy of consolidative HDT/ASCT versus chemotherapy or WBRT for newly diagnosed PCNSL (Table 105.2).

Treatment in the Elderly

Elderly patients account for more than half of all the subjects diagnosed with PCNSL.[27] The risk of neurotoxicity is highest in this population and, in general, chemotherapy alone is the preferred option for this subgroup. The majority of PCNSL patients >60 years of age develop clinical neurotoxicity after treatment with a WBRT-containing regimen, and some of these patients die of treatment-related complications, rather than recurrent disease.[28] Several studies have indicated that HD-MTX at doses of 3.5 to 8 g/m^2 is well tolerated in elderly patients with manageable grade 3 or 4 renal and hematologic toxicity.[29,30] In a multicenter, randomized, phase II trial of chemotherapy alone in elderly patients with PCNSL, 98 patients were randomized to receive three cycles of either MPV-A (methotrexate 3.5 g/m^2, days 1 and 15; procarbazine 100 mg/m^2, days 1 through 7; vincristine 1.4 mg/m^2, days 1 and 15) or MT (methotrexate 3.5 g/m^2, days 1 and 15; temozolomide 100 to 150 mg/m^2, days 1 through 5 and 15 through 19) with one additional cycle of cytarabine (3 g/m^2 per day for 2 consecutive days) in the MPV arm only. Although trends favored the MPV-A regimen over the simpler, less toxic MT regimen with respect to complete response rate, PFS, and OS, none of these differences reached statistical difference.[31] Subsequent studies suggest that the addition of rituximab to both MPV and MT could increase the radiographic response rate. Both of these chemotherapy regimens are options in elderly PCNSL patients.

Salvage Treatment

Despite high initial response rates with HD-MTX–based induction therapy, most patients with PCNSL relapse. Moreover, there is a small subset of patients who have HD-MTX–refractory disease. Prognosis of progressive or relapsed PCNSL is poor, with a limited number of prospective, phase II studies for guidance on management. Rechallenge with HD-MTX has been shown to be effective in patients who had previously responded to this agent. In a multicenter, retrospective study of 22 relapsed PCNSL patients, 91% had a radiographic response to the first salvage treatment with HD-MTX, and 100% to second salvage. The median OS from the first salvage was 61.9 months.[32] In a phase II trial of 43 patients with relapsed or refractory PCNSL, salvage therapy with high-dose cytarabine and etoposide was followed by HDT/ASCT with a conditioning regimen consisting of thioTEPA, busulfan, cyclophosphamide. There were 27 patients who ultimately proceeded to transplantation. Of 27 patients, 26 had a CR and the median PFS and OS in this group were 41.1 and 58.6 months, respectively.[33] In patients who were not initially treated with HDT/ASCT, this strategy remains an option. It is noteworthy that in a small series of patients with relapsed PCNSL after initial HDT/ASCT, a second autotransplantation was successful as salvage treatment.[34] Finally, WBRT in patients who have not received it as a part of their initial

TABLE 105.2

TABLE 105.2

Randomized Trials in Primary Central Nervous System Lymphoma

Induction	Consolidation
Completed Trials	*Completed Trials*
Medical Research Council Phase II, n = 53 (stopped early) CHOP versus WBRT followed by CHOP[39]	**G-PCNSL-SG-1 – NCT00153530** Phase III, n = 551, age ≥18 y Arm 1: Methotrexate ± ifosfamide → WBRT Arm 2: Methotrexate ± ifosfamide[19]
IELSG 20 – NCT00210314 Phase II; n = 79, Ages 18–75 y Induction Arm 1: Methotrexate + Cytarabine → WBRT Induction Arm 2: Methotrexate → WBRT[14]	
ANOCEF-GOELAMS – NCT00503594 Phase II, n = 95, age ≥60 y Arm 1: Methotrexate, procarbazine, vincristine, cytarabine Arm 2: Methotrexate, temozolomide[31]	
Ongoing Trials	*Ongoing Trials*
IESLG 32 - NCT01011920 Phase II, n = 200, Ages 18–70 y Induction Arm 1: Methotrexate, cytarabine Induction Arm 2: Methotrexate, cytarabine, rituximab Induction Arm 3: Methotrexate, cytarabine, rituximab, thioTEPA	**IESLG 32 - NCT01011920** Phase II, n = 104, Ages 18–70 y Consolidation Arm 1: WBRT Consolidation Arm 1: HDT/ASCT
ALLG/HOVON – EudraCT 2009-014722-42 Phase III, n = 200, Ages 18–70 y Arm 1: Methotrexate, BCNU, teniposide, prednisone → Cytarabine, WBRT Arm 2: Methotrexate, BCNU, teniposide, prednisone → Cytarabine, WBRT	**ANOCEF-GOELAMS - NCT00863460** Phase II, n = 100, Ages 18–60 y R-MBVP → Consolidation Arm 1: HDT/ASCT Consolidation Arm 2: WBRT
	RTOG 1114 - NCT01399372 Phase II, n = 84, Age ≥18 y Methotrexate, procarbazine, vincristine, rituximab → Consolidation Arm 1: WBRT (lower dose) → cytarabine Consolidation Arm 2: Cytarabine
	Alliance 51101 - NCT01511562 Phase II, n = 160, Ages 18–75 y Methotrexate, temozolomide, rituximab, cytarabine → Consolidation Arm 1: HDT/ASCT Consolidation Arm 2: Etoposide, cytarabine

CHOP, cyclophosphamide, hydroxydaunorubicin, oncovin (vincristine), prednisone; ANOCEF, Association des Neuro-Oncologue d'Expression Française; GOELAMS, Groupe Ouest Est d'Etude des Leucémies et Autres Maladies du Sang; G-PCNSL-SG, German Primary CNS Lymphoma Study Group; ALLG, Australasian Leukaemia and Lymphoma Group; HOVON, Stichting Hemato-Oncologie voor Volwassenen Nederland (Dutch-Belgian Cooperative Trial Group for Hematology Oncology); BCNU, bischloroethylnitrosourea; IELSG, International Extranodal Lymphoma Study Group; NCT, national clinical trial; R-MBVP, rituximab, methotrexate, BCNU, VP-16 (etoposide), prednisone; RTOG, Radiation Therapy Oncology Group.

treatment is an effective option in the relapsed PCNSL setting, although the risk of neurotoxicity remains.[35,36] Many clinicians reserve WBRT for those patients with chemotherapy-refractory disease or at the time of relapse. In a series of 27 relapsed or refractory PCNSL patients treated with WBRT (median dose: 36 Gy), 74% achieved an ORR and the median OS was 10.6 months. Delayed neurotoxicity rates of 15% were noted at doses >36 Gy, even in the setting of short survival.[35] Novel therapeutics currently under study for systemic DLBCL have entered early phase clinical trials in primary CNS DLBCL and include bendamustine, lenalidomide, pomalidomide, everolimus, and pemetrexed.[4]

Neurotoxicity

The most frequent complication in long-term PCNSL survivors is delayed neurotoxicity. The exact incidence of delayed neurotoxicity is unclear, because earlier studies did not systematically assess neurocognitive function with serial neuropsychological testing. The elderly are at highest risk for this complication, with nearly all patients over the age of 60 developing clinical neurotoxicity following combined modality therapy. Treatment with WBRT has been identified as the major risk factor for the development of late neurotoxicity. Common symptoms and signs include deficits in attention, memory, executive function, gait ataxia, and incontinence. These deficits have a detrimental impact on quality of life. Radiographic findings include periventricular white matter changes, ventricular enlargement, and cortical atrophy. Pathologic studies reveal demyelination, hippocampal neuronal loss, and large-vessel atherosclerosis.[37] Although the pathophysiology is unclear and likely multifactorial, damage to neural progenitor cells has been implicated to play an important role in radiation-related neurotoxicity.[38] Currently, there are no treatments to reverse these delayed neurotoxic effects. It is critical that serial neuropsychological assessments are incorporated into the management of patients with PCNSL, because cognitive outcome is a critical end point. The IPCG has developed an instrument for this purpose, which is composed of quality of life questionnaires and standardized neuropsychological tests that include an assessment of executive function, attention, memory, and psychomotor speed.[15]

SELECTED REFERENCES

The full reference list can be accessed at lwwhealthlibrary.com/oncology.

1. Dolecek TA, Propp JM, Stroup NE, et al. CBTRUS statistical report: primary brain and central nervous system tumors diagnosed in the United States in 2005–2009. *Neuro Oncol* 2012;14:v1–v49.

2. Villano JL, Koshy M, Shaikh H, et al. Age, gender, and racial differences in incidence and survival in primary CNS lymphoma. *Br J Cancer* 2011;105: 1414–1418.

3. Swerdlow SH, Campo E, Harris NL, et al., eds. *WHO Classification of Tumours of the Haematopoietic and Lymphoid Tissues.* Lyon, France: International Agency for Research on Cancer; 2008.

4. Ponzoni M, Issa S, Batchelor TT, et al. Beyond high-dose methotrexate and brain radiotherapy: novel targets and agents for primary CNS lymphoma. *Ann Oncol* 2014;25:316–322.

5. Abrey LE, Batchelor TT, Ferreri AJ, et al. Report of an international workshop to standardize baseline evaluation and response criteria for primary CNS lymphoma. *J Clin Oncol* 2005;23:5034–5043.

6. Chan CC, Rubenstein JL, Coupland SE, et al. Primary vitreoretinal lymphoma: a report from an International Primary Central Nervous System Lymphoma Collaborative Group symposium. *Oncologist* 2011;16:1589–1599.

11. Nelson DF, Martz KL, Bonner H, et al. Non-Hodgkin's lymphoma of the brain: can high dose, large volume radiation therapy improve survival? Report on a prospective trial by the Radiation Therapy Oncology Group (RTOG): RTOG 8315. *Int J Radiat Oncol Biol Phys* 1992;23:9–17.

13. DeAngelis LM, Seiferheld W, Schold SC, et al. Combination chemotherapy and radiotherapy for primary central nervous system lymphoma: Radiation Therapy Oncology Group Study 93-10. *J Clin Oncol* 2002;20:4643–4648.

14. Ferreri AJ, Reni M, Foppoli M, et al. High-dose cytarabine plus high-dose methotrexate versus high-dose methotrexate alone in patients with primary CNS lymphoma: a randomised phase 2 trial. *Lancet* 2009;374:1512–1520.

15. Correa DD, Maron L, Harder H, et al. Cognitive functions in primary central nervous system lymphoma: literature review and assessment guidelines. *Ann Oncol* 2007;18:1145–1151.

16. Morris PG, Correa DD, Yahalom J, et al. Rituximab, methotrexate, procarbazine and vincristine followed by consolidation reduced-dose whole-brain radiotherapy and cytarabine in newly diagnosed primary CNS lymphoma: final results and long-term outcome. *J Clin Oncol* 2013;31:3971–3979.

17. Doolittle ND, Korfel A, Lubow MA, et al. Long-term cognitive function, neuroimaging and quality of life in primary CNS lymphoma. *Neurology* 2013;81:84–92.

18. Juergens A, Pels H, Rogowski S, et al. Long-term survival with favorable cognitive outcome after chemotherapy in primary central nervous system lymphoma. *Ann Neurol* 2010;67:182–189.

19. Thiel E, Korfel A, Martus P, et al. High-dose methotrexate with or without whole brain radiotherapy for primary CNS lymphoma (G-PCNSL-SG-1): a phase 3, randomised, non-inferiority trial. *Lancet Oncol* 2010;11:1036–1047.

20. Ferreri AJ, Guerra E, Regazzi M, et al. Area under the curve of methotrexate and creatinine clearance are outcome-determining factors in primary CNS lymphomas. *Br J Cancer* 2004;90:353–358.

21. Batchelor T, Carson K, O'Neill A, et al. Treatment of primary CNS lymphoma with methotrexate and deferred radiotherapy: a report of NABTT 96-07. *J Clin Oncol* 2003;21:1044–1049.

22. Rubenstein JL, Hsi ED, Johnson JL, et al. Intensive chemotherapy and immunotherapy in patients with newly diagnosed primary CNS lymphoma: CALGB 50202 (Alliance 50202). *J Clin Oncol* 2013;31:3061–3068.

25. Batchelor TT, Grossman SA, Mikkelsen T, et al. Rituximab monotherapy for patients with recurrent primary CNS lymphoma. *Neurology* 2011;76: 929–930.

26. Illerhaus G, Fritsch K, Egerer G, et al. Sequential high dose immunochemotherapy followed by autologous peripheral blood stem cell transplantation for patients with untreated primary central nervous system lymphoma—a multicentre study by the Collaborative PCNSL Study Group Freiburg. Presented at: 2012 American Society of Hematology Annual Meeting; 2012; Atlanta, GA.

29. Jahnke K, Korfel A, Martus P, et al. High-dose methotrexate toxicity in elderly patients with primary central nervous system lymphoma. *Ann Oncol* 2005;16: 445–449.

30. Zhu JJ, Gerstner ER, Engler DA, et al. High-dose methotrexate for elderly patients with primary CNS lymphoma. *Neuro Oncol* 2009;11:211–215.

31. Omuro A, Chinot O, Taillandier L, et al. Multicenter randomized phase II trial of methotrexate (MTX) and temozolomide (TMZ) versus MTX, procarbazine, vincristine, and cytarabine for primary CNS lymphoma (PCNSL) in the elderly: an Anocef and Goelams Intergroup study. Presented at: 2013 American Society of Clinical Oncology Annual Meeting; 2013; Chicago, IL.

32. Plotkin SR, Betensky RA, Hochberg FH, et al. Treatment of relapsed central nervous system lymphoma with high-dose methotrexate. *Clin Cancer Res* 2004;10:5643–5646.

33. Soussain C, Hoang-Xuan K, Taillandier L, et al. Intensive chemotherapy followed by hematopoietic stem-cell rescue for refractory and recurrent primary CNS and intraocular lymphoma: Societe Francaise de Greffe de Moelle Osseuse-Therapie Cellulaire. *J Clin Oncol* 2008;26: 2512–2518.

35. Nguyen PL, Chakravarti A, Finkelstein DM, et al. Results of whole-brain radiation as salvage of methotrexate failure for immunocompetent patients with primary CNS lymphoma. *J Clin Oncol* 2005;23:1507–1513.

37. Lai R, Abrey LE, Rosenblum MK, et al. Treatment-induced leukoencephalopathy in primary CNS lymphoma: a clinical and autopsy study. *Neurology* 2004;62:451–456.

38. Monje ML, Vogel H, Masek M, et al. Impaired hippocampal neurogenesis after treatment for central nervous system malignancies. *Ann Neurol* 2007;62:515–520.

106 Molecular Biology of Acute Leukemias

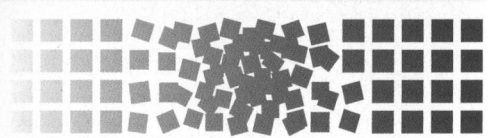

Glen D. Raffel and Jan Cerny

INTRODUCTION

Our understanding of the molecular genetics of acute leukemias has improved dramatically over the past decade. Fueled in part by the availability of the complete sequence of the human genome, more than 100 different mutations have been identified that can be causally implicated in the pathogenesis of acute leukemias (Table 106.1). At first glance, the plethora of mutations presents a discouraging prospect for the development of molecular-targeted therapies. However, far more mutations are identified than there are phenotypes of acute leukemia, and a theme is developed in this chapter that many of these mutations must target similar signal transduction or transcriptional pathways. Thus, it is plausible to consider therapeutic approaches that target these shared pathways of transformation. Although many mutations remain to be identified, those observed thus far have provided critical insights into the pathophysiology of leukemia and the development of novel therapeutic targets.

LEUKEMIC STEM CELL

An important emerging concept in the pathobiology of leukemia is the existence of a *leukemic stem cell*. In normal hematopoietic development, there is a rare population of hematopoietic stem cells that have self-renewal capacity and that give rise to multipotent hematopoietic progenitors. These multipotent myeloid or lymphoid progenitors do not have a self-renewal capacity but mature into normal terminally differentiated cells in the peripheral blood. It is hypothesized that there is a leukemic stem cell that has limitless self-renewal capacity and that gives rise to clonogenic leukemic progenitors that do not have self-renewal capacity but are incapable of normal hematopoietic differentiation. Hypothesized functional differences between the rare leukemic stem cells and the bulk of derived leukemic progeny such as increased quiescence or engagement within a protective niche are believed to provide an intrinsic chemoresistance.

The first convincing evidence in support of the existence of a leukemic stem cell was derived from experiments in which human leukemic cells were injected into immunodeficient nonobese diabetic mice with severe combined immunodeficiency disease (NOD-SCID) mice.[1,2] These data show that the resultant leukemias are derived from as few as 1:1000 to 1:10,000 cells, indicating that there is a rare population of human leukemic cells that have self-renewal capacity in this assay. These cells have similar immunophenotypes to normal self-renewing hematopoietic progenitors and suggest that the leukemogenic mutation occurs in a hematopoietic stem cell. In support of this hypothesis, clonal cytogenetic abnormalities, such as the t(9;22), have been detected in primitive hematopoietic progenitors such as CD34+CD38– cells.[3]

However, this paradigm has been recently challenged and revised. First, new protocols that enhance engraftment of human leukemia in the xenotransplant setting have been described, suggesting the importance of homing and the role of the microenvironment.[4] Data also show that it may be the leukemic oncogenes themselves that confer properties of self-renewal. In a murine system, transduction of the leukemia oncogenes mixed-lineage leukemia 1/eleven nineteen leukemia *(MLL/ENL)*, monocytic leukemia zinc finger protein/transcriptional intermediary factor 2 *(MOZ/TIF2)* or *MLL/ALL1* fused gene from chromosome 9 protein *(AF9)* can confer properties of self-renewal to purified committed hematopoietic progenitors that have no capacity for self-renewal.[5,6] *HOX* family and *NOTCH* genes, frequent mutational targets in acute leukemia as discussed later in this chapter, have been found to have significant roles in hematopoietic stem cell self-renewal.[7] Secondary mutations may also enable activation of similar self-renewal pathways. For example, an analysis of cells from acute myeloid leukemia (AML) blast crisis in chronic myeloid leukemia (CML) shows a shift in the leukemic stem cell to an immunophenotype of a committed myeloid progenitor and concurrent nuclear localization of β-catenin, a process thought to increase stem cell self-renewal.[8] One of the major goals is the identification of transcriptional programs, genes, and pathways that confer limitless self-renewal and may be targets for therapeutic intervention.

ELUCIDATION OF GENETIC EVENTS IN ACUTE LEUKEMIA

The search for causative mutations in acute leukemia has accelerated in recent years due to the availability of new means for evaluating genome integrity in leukemic cells. The bulk of known translocations and deletions were found by analyzing conventionally stained chromosomal banding patterns of karyotypes. The classical karyotypic analysis is able to identify lesions with a resolution of 5 to 10 Mb. These include balanced reciprocal chromosomal translocations, such as t(8;21)(q22;q22) or t(15;17)(q22;q21); internal deletions of single chromosomes, such as 5q- or 7q-; gain or loss of whole chromosomes (+8 or −7); or chromosome inversions, such as inv(3), inv(16), or inv(8). Array-based technologies such as comparative genomic hybridization (CGH) and single-nucleotide polymorphism (SNP) arrays allow detailed (<35 kb) mapping of unbalanced insertions or deletions.[9,10] Array CGH determines DNA copy gain or loss by comparing the hybridization of sample DNA to a series of clones or oligonucleotides from regions throughout the genome bound to a chip with a normal reference DNA sample. SNP arrays differ in that oligomers of SNP sequences representing known alleles throughout the genome are used in the array to measure changes in expected genotype and copy number. Finally, low-cost high-throughput sequencing and

TABLE 106.1

Selected Examples of Cytogenetic and Molecular Abnormalities in Leukemia

Lesion	Genes Involved	Derivation of Abbreviation	Protein Characterization	Disease
Mutations Involving the Core-Binding Factors (CBFS)				
t(8;21)(q22;q22)	*ETO (CBFA2T1)* (8q22)	Eight twenty-one	Zinc finger protein	AML
AML1/ETO	*AML1 (RUNX1)* (21q22)	Acute myeloid leukemia 1	α subunit of CBF complex	
inv(16)(p13q22)	*MYH11 (SMMHC)* (16p13)	Myosin heavy chain 11	Smooth muscle myosin heavy chain	AML
CBFβ/MYH11	*CBFB/CBFβ* (16q22)	Core-binding factor-β	β subunit of CBF complex	
t(3;21)(q26;q22)	*EVI1* (3q26)	Ecotropic virus integration site 1	Multiple zinc fingers	MDS, AML
AML1/EVI1	*AML1 (RUNX1)* (21q22)	Acute myeloid leukemia 1	α subunit of CBF complex	CML-BC
t(12;21)(p13;q22)	*TEL (ETV6)* (12p13)	Translocation ETS leukemia	ETS-related transcription factor	ALL
TEL/AML1	*AML1 (RUNX1)* (21q22)	Acute myeloid leukemia 1	α subunit of CBF complex	
AML1 deletion/truncation	*AML1 (RUNX1)*	Acute myeloid leukemia 1	α subunit of CBF complex	FDP/AML
Fusions Involving MLL				
t(4;11)(q21;q23)	*AF4* (4q21)	*ALL1* fused chromosome 4	Transactivator	ALL, AML
MLL/AF4	*MLL* (11q23)	Mixed-lineage leukemia	*Drosophila* trithorax homolog	
t(11;19)(q23;p13.3)	*MLL* (11q23)	Mixed-lineage leukemia	*Drosophila* trithorax homolog	AML, ALL
MLL/ENL	*ENL* (19p13.3)	Eleven nineteen leukemia	Transcription factor	
t(9;11)(p22;q23)	*AF9* (9p22)	*ALL1* fused chromosome 9	Nuclear protein, ENL homology	AML, ALL
MLL/AF9	*MLL* (11q23)	Mixed-lineage leukemia	*Drosophila* trithorax homolog	
t(1;11)(q21;q23)	*AF1q* (1q21)	*ALL1* fused chromosome 1q	No homology to any known protein	AML
MLL/AF1	*MLL* (11q23)	Mixed-lineage leukemia	*Drosophila* trithorax homolog	
MLL partial tandem duplication	*MLL* (11q23)	Mixed-lineage leukemia	*Drosophila* trithorax homolog	AML
Fusions Involving RAR-α				
t(15;17)(q22;q12-21)	*PML* (15q21)	Promyelocytic leukemia	Zinc finger protein	APL
PML/RARα	*RAR-α* (17q21)	Retinoic acid receptor-α	Retinoic acid receptor-α	
t(11;17)(q23;q21)	*PLZF* (11q23)	Promyelocytic leukemia zinc finger	Zinc finger protein	APL
PLZF/RARα	*RAR-α* (17q21)	Retinoic acid receptor-α	Retinoic acid receptor-α	
T(5;17)(q32;q21)	*NPM1*	Nucleophosmin	Chaperone	APL
NPM1/RARα	*RAR-α* (17q21)	Retinoic acid receptor-α	Retinoic acid receptor-α	
Mutations Involving Lymphoid Differentiation Factors				
dic(9;12)(p13;p13)	*PAX5* (9p13)	Paired box 5	Transcription factor	B-ALL
PAX5/TEL	*TEL (ETV6)* (12p13)	Translocation ETS leukemia	Transcription factor	
PAX5 loss of function	*PAX5* (9p13)	Paired box 5	Transcription factor	B-ALL
EBF1 loss of function	*EBF1*	Early B-cell factor 1	Transcription factor	B-ALL
IKZF1 loss of function/DN	*IKZF1*	IKAROS family zinc finger 1	Transcription factor	B-ALL
LEF1 loss of function	*LEF1*	Lymphoid enhancer binding factor 1	Transcription factor	ALL
t(17;19)(q22;p13.3)	*HLF* (17q22)	Hepatic leukemia factor	Leucine zipper	B-ALL
TCF3/HLF	*TCF3 (E2A)* (19p13.3)	Transcription factor 3	bHLH transcription factor	
Mutations Involving Hox Genes				
t(7;11)(p15;p15)	*HOXA9* (7p15)	Homeobox A9	Homeobox protein	AML/MDS
NUP98/HOXA9	*NUP98* (11p15)	Nuclear pore 98	Nucleoporin	AML
t(12;13)(p13;q12)	*TEL (ETV6)*	Ten-eleven translocation	Transcription factor	AML
TEL/CDX2	*CDX2*	Caudal type homeobox 2	Homeobox protein	
t(1;19)(q23;p13)	*TCF3 (E2A)*	Transcription factor 3	Transcription factor	B-ALL
TCF3/PBX1	*PBX1*	Pre–B-cell leukemia homeobox 1	Homeobox protein	

(continued)

TABLE 106.1

Selected Examples of Cytogenetic and Molecular Abnormalities in Leukemia *(continued)*

Lesion	Genes Involved	Derivation of Abbreviation	Protein Characterization	Disease
Other Transcription Factors				
t(1;22)(p13;q13) OTT1/MAL	*OTT1 (RBM15)* (1p13) *MAL (MKL1)* (22q13)	One twenty-two Megakaryocytic acute leukemia	*Spen* homolog Serum response cofactor	AMKL
GATA1s truncation	*GATA1*	GATA binding protein 1	Transcription factor	AMKL
CEBPA truncation	*CEBPA*	CCAAT/enhancer binding protein-α	Transcription factor	AML
NOTCH1 PEST/HD point mutations	*NOTCH1*	Notch 1 (*Drosophila* wing phenotype)	Transcription factor	T-ALL
t(6;9)(p23;q34) DEK/NUP214	*DEK* (6p23) *NUP214 (CAN)* (9q34)	Not relevant to molecule Nuclear pore 214	Transcription factor Nucleoporin	AML
Translocations Involving the Immunoglobulin Enhancer Loci				
t(8;14)(q24;q32)	*MYC* (8q24) *IGH* (14q32)	Myelocytomatosis virus Immunoglobulin heavy chain	bHLH/bZIP transcription factor Ig heavy chain promoter	B-ALL
t(2;8)(p12;q24)	*IGK* (2p12) *MYC* (8q24)	Immunoglobulin κ-chain Myelocytomatosis virus	Igκ-chain promoter bHLH/bZIP transcription factor	B-ALL
t(8;22)(q24;q11)	*MYC* (8q24) *IGL* (22q11)	Myelocytomatosis virus Immunoglobulin λ-chain	bHLH/bZIP transcription factor Igλ-chain promoter	B-ALL
t(X;14)(p22;q32) &	*IGH* (14q32)	Immunoglobulin heavy chain	Ig heavy chain promoter	B-ALL
t(Y;14)(p11;q32)	*CRLF2* (Xp22)/(Yp11)	Cytokine receptor-like 2	Extracellular receptor	
Translocations Involving the T-Cell Receptor Genes				
t(1;14)(p32;q11)	*TAL1/SCL* (1p33) *TCRα/δ* (14q11)	T-cell acute leukemia 1/stem cell leukemia T-cell receptor-α/δ	bHLH transcription factor T-cell receptor promoter	T-ALL
t(1;7)(p32;q34)	*TAL1/SCL* (1p32) *TCRβ* (7q34)	T-cell acute leukemia 1/stem cell leukemia T-cell receptor-β	bHLH transcription factor T-cell receptor promoter	T-ALL
t(7;9)(q34;q34)	*TCRβ* (7q34) *TAL2/SCL2* (9q34)	T-cell receptor-β T-cell acute leukemia 2/stem cell leukemia	T-cell receptor promoter bHLH transcription factor	T-ALL
t(7;19)(q34;p13)	*TCRβ* (7q34) *LYL1* (19p13)	T-cell receptor-β Lymphoid leukemia 1	T-cell receptor promoter bHLH transcription factor	T-ALL
t(8;14)(q24;q11)	*MYC* (8q24) *TCRα/δ* (14q11)	Myelocytomatosis virus T-cell receptor-α/δ	bHLH/bZIP transcription factor T-cell receptor promoter	T-ALL
t(11;14)(p15;q11)	*LMO1* (11p15) *TCRα/δ* (14q11)	LIM only 1 T-cell receptor-α/δ	Zinc finger T-cell receptor promoter	T-ALL
t(11;14)(p13;q11)	*LMO2* (11p13) *TCRα/δ* (14q11)	LIM only 2 T-cell receptor-α/δ	Zinc finger T-cell receptor promoter	T-ALL
t(7;10)(q34;q24)	*TCRβ* (7q34) *HOX11* (10q24)	T-cell receptor-β Homeobox 11	T-cell receptor promoter Homeobox gene	T-ALL
t(7;9)(q34;q34.3)	*TCRβ* (7q34) *NOTCH1* (9q34.3)	T-cell receptor-β Notch 1 (drosophila wing)	T-cell receptor promoter Transcription factor	T-ALL
Receptors and Signaling Molecules				
t(9;22)(q34;q11) BCR/ABL1	*BCR* *ABL1*	Breakpoint cluster region c-Abl oncogene 1	S/T kinase, GTPase activating Nonreceptor tyrosine kinase	AML, ALL
FLT3 ITD and activating loop mutation	*FLT3R*	FMS-like tyrosine kinase	Receptor tyrosine kinase	AML
NRAS activating mutation	*NRAS*	Neuroblastoma rat sarcoma viral oncogene homolog	Small GTPase	AML, ALL
KRAS activating mutation	*KRAS*	Kirsten rat sarcoma viral oncogene homolog	Small GTPase	AML, ALL

(continued)

TABLE 106.1

Selected Examples of Cytogenetic and Molecular Abnormalities in Leukemia *(continued)*

Lesion	Genes Involved	Derivation of Abbreviation	Protein Characterization	Disease
Receptors and Signaling Molecules				
KIT activating mutation	*KIT*	v-Kit feline sarcoma viral oncoprotein	Receptor tyrosine kinase	AML
JAK2, JAK3 activating mutation	*JAK2, JAK3*	Janus kinase 2, 3	Nonreceptor tyrosine kinase	AMKL
MPL activating mutation	*MPL*	Myeloproliferative leukemia virus oncogene	Thrombopoietin receptor	AMKL
Epigenetic Modifiers				
inv8(p11q13)	*MOZ*	Monocytic leukemia zinc finger protein	K(lysine) acetyltransferase	AML
MOZ/TIF2	*TIF2*	Transcriptional intermediary factor 2	Nuclear receptor coactivator	
TET2 LOH4q24, loss of function	*TET2*	Ten-eleven translocation 2	Methylcytosine dioxygenase	AML, MDS, MPN
IDH1/2 activating mutation	*IDH1/IDH2*	Isocitrate dehydrogenase 1 and 2	Isocitrate dehydrogenase	AML, MDS, MPN
DNMT3 loss of function	*DNMT3*	DNA methyltransferase 3	Cytosine-5-methyltransferase	AML
EZH2 loss of function	*EZH2*	Enhancer of zeste homolog 2	Histone methyltransferase	MDS, MPN, AML
Tumor Suppressors				
WT1 loss of function	*WT1*	Wilms tumor 1	Transcriptional regulator	AML
TP53 deletion (−17p)	*TP53*	Tumor protein p53 kDa	Transcription factor	AML, ALL

AML, acute myeloid leukemia; CBF, core-binding factor; MDS, myelodysplastic syndrome; CML, chronic myeloid leukemia; ETS, E twenty-six retrovirus; ALL, acute lymphoblastic leukemia; ENL, eleven-nineteen leukemia; MLL, mixed-lineage leukemia; APL, acute promyelocytic leukemia; B-ALL, B lineage acute lymphoblastic leukemia; AMKL, acute megakaryocytic leukemia; bHLH, basic helix–loop–helix; T-ALL, T lineage acute lymphoblastic leukemia; bZIP, basic region/leucine zipper; Ig, immunoglobulin; LIM, Lin-11, Isl-2, Mec-3 homeodomain; MPN, myeloproliferative neoplasia; LOH, loss of heterozygosity.

microarray-based resequencing techniques have allowed for the identification of new somatic mutations at the single-nucleotide level and are making enormous inroads into the pathogenesis, prognosis, and classification of leukemias with *normal* cytogenetics. Worldwide initiatives to sequence large numbers of cancer genomes, including leukemia subtypes, are being coordinated and cataloged through the International Cancer Genome Consortium (http://www.icgc.org) and the Cancer Genome Atlas (TCGA) (https://tcga-data.nci.nih.gov/tcga).[12]

Although intensive effort has focused on chromosomal translocations in leukemia, in part because of their high frequency in various kinds of leukemia, it has become increasingly clear that point mutations play an important role in a spectrum of leukemias. Ongoing high-throughput sequencing initiatives have identified numerous solitary and recurring somatic point mutations within the various leukemic subtypes. The interpretation of this sequencing data requires the identification of *driver* versus *passenger* mutations. *Driver* mutations cause genetic alterations contributing to leukemic pathophysiology, whereas *passenger* mutations occur in leukemia cells and are propagated but are not etiologic to the disease.[13] It is, therefore, essential that newly discovered somatic mutations in leukemia undergo subsequent biologic validation through sequencing studies in an experimental model system.

MUTATIONS THAT TARGET CORE-BINDING FACTOR

Core-binding factor (CBF) is targeted by more than a dozen different chromosomal translocations in acute leukemias, including the t(8;21) or inv(16), observed in approximately 20% of AMLs,

and the t(12;21), present in approximately 25% of patients with pediatric B-lineage acute lymphoblastic leukemia (ALL).[14] Adult patients with CBF leukemias have a favorable prognosis and the *translocation ETS leukemia (TEL)/AML1* fusion that is expressed as a consequence of t(12;21) in children confers a favorable prognosis among B-cell ALL.[15] CBF is a heterodimeric transcription factor composed of the AML1 (also known as RUNX1 or CBFA2) and CBFβ proteins that is critical for normal hematopoietic development. Loss of function of either subunit results in a complete lack of definitive hematopoiesis.[16,17] The AML1 subunit of CBF contacts DNA but only weakly transactivates target genes as a monomer. When bound to its heterodimeric partner CBFβ, which does not itself contact DNA, transactivation of CBF target genes is dramatically enhanced.[15,18,19] CBF transactivates a spectrum of target genes that are important in normal myeloid development, including transcription factors (e.g., *PU.1, CEBP/A* and *GATA1*), cytokines (e.g., granulocyte-macrophage colony-stimulating factor [GM-CSF]) and cytokine receptors (such as macrophage-colony stimulating factor [M-CSF] receptor), as well as in lymphoid development, such as the T-cell receptor beta (TCRβ) enhancer and the immunoglobulin (Ig) heavy-chain loci.[18–21] Because CBF targets genes that are important for normal hematopoietic development, a mutation or gene rearrangement that resulted in loss of function of either AML1 or CBFβ might be expected to impair hematopoietic differentiation.[15,18,19]

In addition to frequent involvement of *AML1* as a consequence of chromosomal translocations, it has been determined that loss-of-function mutations in *AML1* are responsible for the inherited leukemia syndrome familial platelet disorder with propensity to develop AML (FPD/AML).[22,23] Approximately 3% to 5% of sporadic cases of AML harbor loss-of-function mutations in *AML1*,[22,24] with a higher frequency in M0 AML (25%) and in AML or myelodysplastic syndrome (MDS) with trisomy 21. AML1 loss-of-function mutations are associated with poor rather than good prognosis subgroups such as acute myeloid leukemia 1/eight twenty-one (AML1/ETO); however, this may be a result of occurring in the context of myelodysplasia or mixed lineage leukemias.[19]

Compelling evidence has been shown that translocations that target CBF result in a loss of function through dominant negative inhibition. The AML1/ETO fusion associated with t(8;21) and the CBFβ/MYH11 (aka CBFβ/SMMHC) fusion associated with inv(16) are dominant negative inhibitors of CBF and impair hematopoietic differentiation. The expression of either the AML1/ETO or CBFβ/MYH11 fusion genes from their endogenous promoter in mice completely inhibits the function of the residual AML1 or CBFβ alleles, resulting in a lack of definitive hematopoiesis and resultant embryonic lethality.[16,17] The phenotype observed is the same as that seen in AML1–/– or CBFβ–/– mice, indicating that the AML1/ETO or CBFβ/MYH11 fusions, respectively, act as potent dominant negative inhibitors of the native proteins.[25,26] However, AML1/ETO and CBFβ/MYH11 have been shown to confer novel contributory gain-of-function effects beyond those involving CBF transcriptional targets. For example, AML1/ETO blocks the tumor suppressors p14ARF and nuclear factor 1 (NF1), whereas CBFβ/MYH11 blocks the expression of p15INK4B.[27,28] AML1/ETO downregulates DNA-repair genes, perhaps enhancing genomic instability.[29] Histone deacetylases (HDAC) and DNA-methyltransferases (DNMT) associated with AML1/ETO alter the epigenetic profile of normal and leukemic cells to generate global changes in gene expression, which may be integral to leukemogenesis.[30,31] Respective inhibitors such as suberanilohydroxamic acid (SAHA) and azacytidine may, therefore, have therapeutic value in CBF leukemias.[18]

Although the expression of AML1/ETO leads to alterations of gene expression and hematopoietic cell proliferation leukemia and confers the ability to serially replate in methylcellulose culture (a measure of self-renewal potential), this does not result in the development of leukemia in an animal model. However, co-expression of an alternatively spliced isoform of the AML1/ETO transcript, AML1/ETO9a, which includes an extra exon, exon 9a, of the ETO gene (AML1/ETO9a encodes a C-terminally truncated AML1-ETO protein of 575 amino acids) leads to a rapid development of leukemia in a mouse retroviral transduction–transplantation model.[32] The presence of AML1/ETO9a closely correlates with the presence of activating c-KIT mutations in humans, conferring a poor prognosis.[33] Similarly, the expression of CBFβ/MYH11 in adult hematopoietic cells results in leukemia only after a markedly prolonged latency; this latency can be shortened using mutagenesis strategies.[26] In summary, translocations that target CBF impair hematopoietic differentiation and confer certain properties of leukemic stem cells, such as the ability to serially replate, but are not sufficient to cause leukemia.

In pediatric B-ALL, 25% of cases have t(12;21)(p13;q13) in which the TEL (aka ETV6) gene translocates into AML1, thus allowing the production of a chimeric protein, TEL/AML1 (aka ETV6/RUNX1).[34,35] TEL is a transcriptional repressor mediated through associated HDACs and, like AML1, has requirements in fetal and definitive hematopoiesis.[30,34,36] TEL has 30 known fusion partners of different functional classes, including tyrosine kinases such as in TEL/platelet-derived growth factor receptor (PDGFR) and HOX genes such as in PAX5/TEL, although TEL/AML1 is the most common.[34] The fusion protein preserves the central repressor domain in TEL and contains almost the entire AML1 protein sequence. TEL/AML1 has the ability to bind to AML1 consensus sequences but now brings an HDAC-dependent repressor function to AML1-responsive promoter elements, thereby suppressing AML1 targets.[34] In addition, physiologic TEL function may be dysregulated by the fusion through heterodimerization via TEL helix–loop–helix domains.[34] TEL/AML1 is often found in conjunction with

deletions in the pre-B receptor, VPREB, and the tumor suppressor gene, CDKN2A.[37]

CHROMOSOMAL TRANSLOCATIONS THAT TARGET THE RETINOIC ACID RECEPTOR ALPHA GENE

The empiric observation that all-trans-retinoic acid (ATRA) induces complete responses in patients with acute promyelocytic leukemia (APL) drove the subsequent cloning of the t(15;17)(q22;q21) fusion gene involving the RARα locus. Several groups demonstrated at approximately the same time that the RARα gene on chromosome 17 was fused to a novel partner that was eventually identified as the promyelocytic leukemia (PML) gene.[38–40] Two reciprocal fusion RNA species are produced as a consequence of the translocation, RARα/PML and PML/RARα. The PML/RAR-α fusion protein contains the zinc finger of PML fused to the DNA- and protein-binding domains of RAR-α. Several other chromosomal translocations target the RARα locus and are associated with an APL phenotype. The best studied of these is the promyelocytic leukemia zinc finger (PLZF/RAR-α) fusion, which also aberrantly recruits the nuclear corepressor complex. However, in contrast with the PML/RAR-α fusion, ATRA is not able to relieve corepression mediated by the PLZF/RAR-α fusion and thus is not effective in patients who harbor the t(11;17) associated with this fusion gene.[41]

The PML gene has a broad, although incompletely understood role in the homeostasis of nuclear proteins as an organizing component of nuclear bodies (PML-NB) responsible for nuclear structure and shuttling.[42,43] Recently, an important independent cytoplasmic role for PML as a tumor suppressor has been uncovered, whereby PML localized to the contact points between the endoplasmic reticulum and mitochondrial-associated membranes controls calcium transport and apoptosis.[44] PML is essential for maintaining self-renewal in hematopoietic stem cells (HSC) as shown by a mouse knockout model of PML, which demonstrated increased proliferation and premature exhaustion in the HSC compartment.[45] The PML region of PML-RARα was also identified as the target for arsenic trioxide therapy. The binding of arsenic increases PML oligomerization followed by SUMOylation, which in turn, causes PML/RARα degradation.[46]

RARα possesses a DNA-binding domain, a hormone-binding domain, and a retinoid X receptor (RXR)–binding domain, all of which are included within the PML/RARα chimeric protein. RARα transactivates multiple genes involved in myeloid differentiation.[47] PML/RARα homodimers, enabled via a coiled coil domain in the PML portion, bind to RAR sites and repress genes important for granulocytic differentiation in part through HDAC and corepressor recruitment.[47] PML/RARα, however, does not have effects solely through dominant inhibition of RARα/RXR binding sites. PML/RARα was shown to have an extended repertoire of DNA consensus binding sites beyond those found for RARα.[48] PML/RARα appears to extensively modify histone-acetylation and methylation marks in expressing cells in an ATRA-dependent manner, likely through recruitment of HDACs and histone methyltransferases and demethylases within the PML-RARα complex.[48,49] Drug targeting of PML/RARα-associated epigenetic modifying proteins may, therefore, provide effective adjuncts to ATRA-based therapies.

The transforming properties of the PML/RARα fusion gene have been tested in murine models. Expression of PML/RAR-α in transgenic mice from promoters that direct expression to the promyelocyte compartment result in an APL-like phenotype.[50–52] However, there is approximately a 6-month lag before the development of leukemia, incomplete penetrance of approximately 15% to 30%, and acquired karyotypic abnormalities, all suggesting that second mutations are required for induction of leukemia.

In at least some cases, activating mutations in FLT3 may be the additional mutation required. ATRA is efficacious in leukemic animals expressing both PML/RAR-α and activated FLT3, and this model has allowed for the preclinical testing of newer agents such as arsenic trioxide.[53]

MUTATIONS THAT TARGET HOX FAMILY MEMBERS

HOX genes are homeodomain-containing transcription factors important in patterning in vertebrate development and in hematopoietic development.[54,55] *HOX* genes are clustered in four genomic loci *HOXA-D*, although additional *orphan HOX* genes occur elsewhere in the genome. Transactivation by HOX genes is potentiated by cofactors such as pre–B cell leukemia (PBX1) and myeloid ecotropic insertion site (Meis1). NUP98, a nuclear transport protein, is a fusion partner to at least eight different HOX genes in AML as well as numerous other genes.[56] *HOX* gene expression is tightly regulated during hematopoietic development. HOXA9, for example, is expressed in early hematopoietic progenitor cells but is downregulated during hematopoietic differentiation and is undetectable in terminally differentiated cells. The expression of NUP98/HOXA9 results in derepression of *HOXA* cluster genes, several of which promote HSC self-renewal.[54,56]

The contribution of the NUP98 moiety to leukemic transformation is not fully understood. NUP98 is normally a component of the nuclear pore complex and is constitutively and ubiquitously expressed. However, several lines of evidence suggest that NUP98 contributes more than a constitutively activated promoter. For example, NUP98 motifs known as *FG repeats* are essential for transformation and may serve to recruit transcriptional coactivators, such as CBP/p300, to HOXA9 DNA-binding sites.[57] In murine models of leukemia, overexpression of HOXA9 alone is not sufficient to cause AML, but coexpression of HOXA9 with transcriptional cofactors, such as MEIS1, results in efficient induction of AML.[58] Thus, the NUP98 moiety in the context of the NUP98/HOXA9 fusion may serve multiple functions, including provision of an active promoter, and recruitment of transcriptional coactivators such as CBP/p300 that subserve the function of other cofactors such as MEIS1. Epidemiologic evidence that the NUP98 moiety contributes to leukemogenesis includes the observation that there are now a spectrum of fusion proteins involving components of the nuclear pore that are targeted by chromosomal translocations in acute leukemias. These include *NUP98* and *NUP214* fused to a diverse group of partners, including *HOXA9* and *HOXD13*, and the *DDX10*, *PMX1*, *DEK*, and *ABL1* genes, respectively.

Dysregulated *HOX* gene expression may be important in leukemias that do not directly target HOX family members. Several proteins that are upstream of HOX expression have been observed as fusion genes associated with AML, the most frequent of these are *MLL* gene rearrangements. More than 40 chromosomal translocations target *MLL* and result in fusions of *MLL* with a broad spectrum of partners. In addition, dysregulation of HOX genes by an enhancer effect, which occurs in t(7;10)(q34;q24), where the TCRβ translocates into the HOX11 locus, is an important contributor to T cell acute lymphoid leukemia (T-ALL) leukemogenesis.[59] However, a common biologic feature of all of these may be their ability to dysregulate *HOX* gene expression during hematopoietic development. For example, t(12;13) associated with AML results in the expression of high levels of CDX2 from the *TEL* locus.[60] CDX2 is a homeotic protein that regulates the expression of HOX family members in the colonic epithelium. As in hematopoietic development, *HOX* gene expression is highest in colonic stem cells in the colonic crypts and is downregulated with maturation. It has been shown that CDX2 and CDX4 can dysregulate HOX expression in hematopoietic progenitors and can result in leukemia.[58,60] Evidence to support this includes the ability of CDX2 to induce leukemia in murine retroviral transduction models.[58,60]

Taken together, these data indicate that the NUP98/HOXA9 fusion transforms hematopoietic progenitors in part through dysregulated overexpression and by transactivation mediated through the NUP98 transactivation domain that recruits CBP. However, like other gene rearrangements involving hematopoietic transcription factors, expression of NUP98/HOXA9 alone is not sufficient to cause leukemia. In murine bone marrow transplant models, NUP98/HOXA9 induces AML only after markedly prolonged latencies indicative of a requirement for second mutation. Coexpression of Meis1 or FLT3ITD with NUP98/HOXA9 in mice significantly shortens the latency; however, these mutations are not present in all human cases, suggesting that additional cooperating pathways exist.[61,62]

CHROMOSOMAL TRANSLOCATIONS THAT TARGET THE *MLL* GENE

The *MLL* locus is involved in more than 80 different chromosomal translocations with a remarkably diverse group of fusion partners[63,64] and are associated with mostly French-American-British (FAB) subtype M4 or M5, and fewer with M2 AML. Patients who have received prior chemotherapy for cancer and develop AML (therapy-related MDS/therapy-related AML [t-AML]) often have abnormalities in 11q23, especially those patients treated with topoisomerase inhibitors such as etoposide or topotecan. Chromosomal translocations involving band 11q23 result in the expression of a fusion gene containing amino-terminal *MLL* sequences fused to a wide variety of partners. There has been no common functional motif or activity ascribed to all partners; however, specific fusions may be associated with specific leukemic phenotypes. The MLL/AF4 fusion associated with t(4;11) is frequently observed in infant leukemias and is associated with an ALL phenotype in more than 90% of cases, whereas the MLL/AF9 fusion associated with the t(9;11) is almost exclusively associated with AML. Certain MLL fusion genes also have prognostic significance. For example, patients with t(9;11)(p22;q23) have a better outcome than those with other translocations involving 11q23.

The MLL gene encodes a large, ubiquitously expressed protein. The *Drosophila* protein trithorax, a homolog of *MLL*, regulates patterning and *HOX* gene expression during development. It has been hypothesized, in part based on these observations, that MLL might be required for maintenance of *HOX* gene expression.[65] Mice that have homozygous deficiency for *MLL* have an embryonic lethal phenotype at postconception day 10.5. Even heterozygous animals have developmental anomalies in the axial skeleton and hematopoietic deficits, including anemia.[66] Thus, as for other genes targeted by chromosomal translocations, *MLL* is important for normal hematopoietic development.

Major advances have been made recently regarding the mechanisms underlying MLL and MLL-fusion gene function. MLL binds a broad cohort of epigenetic regulators including bromodomain-containing 3 and 4 (BRD3 and BRD4); the H3K79 histone methyl transferase, DOT1; the lysine-specific demethylase, KDM1A; and the polycomb-repressive complex 2 (PRC2). Although MLL possesses a Su(var)3-9, enhancer-of-zeste and trithorax (SET) homology H3K4 histone methyl-transferase, it is not retained in MLL-fusion proteins. MLL and MLL fusions also require complex formation with menin (MEN1) and lens epithelium–derived growth factor (LEDGF) to be able to interact with DNA and activate target genes.[67,68] MLL fusions have been shown to affect transcriptional *poising* at target genes as part of a larger super elongation complex (SEC).[69] The control of RNA polymerase II elongation after recruitment to promoter sites provides an additional layer of regulation to target genes such as *HOXA9*.[69,70] MLL fusions also form a complex known as *DotCom*, which, via associated DOT1 activity, yields H3K79 di/trimethylation marks, thus altering expression at affected genes.[69] MLL-fusion/DotCom interaction allows binding and transcription at target genes of the

Wnt/β-catenin pathway via binding of nuclear-localized β-catenin. The Wnt pathway is essential for fetal HSC self-renewal, and aberrant activation of its downstream targets mediated by MLL-fusions is hypothesized to confer self-renewal properties to leukemic stem cells (LSCs).[71]

Although various MLL fusions have similar transforming properties in vitro, there are distinctive differences in disease penetrance and latency in the murine models depending on the fusion partner. It is possible that the *MLL* gene rearrangement may be critical for transformation, whereas the fusion partners confer properties related to disease phenotype. The long latency of disease in murine models supports the hypothesis that MLL fusions, like the PML/RAR-α and CBF-related fusion proteins, require second mutations to cause leukemia.

As noted previously in the section Leukemic Stem Cell, data indicate that certain *MLL* fusion genes may also confer properties of self-renewal to hematopoietic progenitors. MLL/ENL expression in common myeloid progenitors or granulocyte-monocyte progenitors in a murine system conferred properties of self-renewal, including the ability to serially replate in methylcellulose cultures and to engender a transplantable AML phenotype in recipient animals.[5] Similarly, in a mouse model of *MLL/AF9* oncogene-induced leukemia, up to a quarter of the leukemic cells exhibited stem cell behavior.[72] Furthermore, the *MLL/AF9*-positive LSC are heterogeneous as they give rise to ALL when injected into immunodeficient mice. The same cells cause AML when injected into immunodeficient mice that are transgenic for the human genes stem cell factor (SCF), GM-CSF, and interleukin 3 (IL-3).[73] These data indicate that leukemogenic mutations may occur in cells that have no intrinsic self-renewal capacity and yet confer these properties by activation of specific transcriptional programs, which may be further modified by clues from the microenvironment.

MUTATION OF *C/EBP*α

C/EBPα is a 42-kDa hematopoietic transcription factor that is required for normal myeloid lineage differentiation and that inhibits proliferation.[74] C/EBPα is downregulated in 50% of AML, often through methylation of its promoter region.[75] Therefore, loss of C/EBPα function in leukemia likely impairs myeloid differentiation and removes a block on proliferation.[76] Two major types of C/EBPα point mutations have been described in AML—short frameshifting mutations in the region encoding the amino-terminus, causing the expression of a shortened 30-kDa protein with dominant negative activity, and in-frame insertions or deletions in the region of the carboxy-terminus, which alter the DNA-binding or dimerization domains, causing a loss of function.[77] Two-thirds of C/EBPα-mutated leukemias have both N- and C-terminal mutations on each allele.[76] Although the bulk of C/EBPα mutations occur in patients with normal cytogenetics, overall and progression-free survival is more favorable; therefore, C/EBPα status is an important prognostic determinant.[78] In contrast to AML, 2% of pre–B-ALL has been shown to have an upregulation of C/EBPα or family members through enhancer effects of IgH locus translocation into the C/EBPα locus as seen in t(14;19)(q32;q13).[79,80]

MUTATION OF GATA-1

GATA-1 mutations are associated with a subset of acute megakaryocytic leukemias (AMKL) (FAB M7), in particular leukemias arising in patients with Down syndrome (constitutional trisomy 21).[81] GATA-1 is a transcription factor promoting erythroid and megakaryocytic development.[82,83] GATA-1 mutations result in the early termination of the full-length GATA-1 protein; however, translation of a short-form (GATA-1s) from an alternate initiation codon occurs. GATA-1s is theorized to function as either a hypomorphic

or dominant negative allele, and dysregulation of GATA-1 pathways are thought to contribute to leukemogenesis.[84,85] GATA-1 mutations are often seen in a transient myeloproliferative disorder (TMD), which precedes Down syndrome–associated AMKL, suggesting that a GATA-1 mutation is an early event cooperating with germ-line trisomy 21.[84] GATA-1 mutations have been noted in Down syndrome fetal livers, and GATA-1s expression in a mouse model causes hyperproliferation of fetal liver megakaryocytes, supporting the hypothesis of an in utero origin of the disease.[86] Current efforts to identify the critical cooperating genes dysregulated in trisomy 21 are utilizing mouse models possessing trisomies syntenic with the 8.35-Mb Down syndrome critical region to identify candidate genes.[87]

t(1;22) TRANSLOCATION ASSOCIATED WITH INFANT AMKL

The t(1;22)(p13;q13) is associated with the majority of non–Down syndrome AMKL in infants and results in the expression of the *OTT1/MAL* (aka *RBM15/MKL1*) fusion gene.[88,89] OTT1 (RBM15) contains three amino-terminal RNA recognition motifs and a Spen paralog and ortholog C-terminal motif that is a transcriptional activator/repressor. *Ott1* deletion in mice reveals multiple hematopoietic roles, including megakaryocyte growth and hematopoietic stem cell function.[90,91] The MAL (MKL1) gene is a Rho-GTPase–regulated cofactor for serum response factor (SRF) and controls megakaryocyte development.[92,93] A knockin mouse model expressing OTT1/MAL is able to recapitulate AMKL and demonstrated constitutive transcriptional activation from recombination signal binding protein for immunoglobulin kappa J (RBPJκ) binding sites, including Notch1 downstream targets, which is essential for its pathogenesis.[94]

MUTATIONS OF EPIGENETIC MODIFIERS

Several translocations associated with leukemia involve transcriptional coactivators and chromatin modifying proteins that have no apparent DNA-binding specificity. These include the mixed-lineage leukemia/ CREB-binding protein (MLL/CBP) and MOZ/CBP fusions that involve the transcriptional coactivator CBP and the MLL/p300 and MOZ/TIF2 fusions, which involve the coactivators p300 and TIF2, respectively.[95,96] Although TIF2 itself is not known to have histone acetylase transferase (HAT) activity, a hallmark of the coactivators CBP and p300, it has a well-characterized CBP interaction domain that serves to recruit CBP into a complex with MOZ/TIF2.[97] Thus, recruitment of CBP/p300 is a shared theme among this group of fusion genes.

The transcriptional targets and transformation properties of this class of fusion proteins are not fully understood. Transduction of MLL/CBP into primary murine bone marrow cells followed by transplantation results in a long-latency AML, suggesting the need for secondary mutations.[98] MOZ/TIF2 also results in leukemia in a similar model system. MOZ is a HAT protein that contains a nucleosome-binding domain and an acetyl–coenzyme A–binding catalytic domain. A mutational analysis shows that leukemogenic activity requires MOZ nucleosome-binding activity and CBP recruitment activity, but the MOZ HAT activity is dispensable. These data would be consistent with a CBP gain-of-function in which CBP is recruited to MOZ nucleosome-binding sites.[97] However, it has also been hypothesized that the leukemogenic potential of this class of fusions may be related to dominant negative interference with CBP/p300 or that the translocation leads to simple loss of function of CBP expressed from one allele. In support of this hypothesis, loss of a single allele of CBP/p300 in the human Rubinstein-Taybi syndrome increases predisposition to malignancies, including colon cancer and mice that are heterozygous for CBP that develop hematopoietic tumors.[99]

The *TET2* gene located on 4q24 belongs to the ten-eleven translocation (TET) family (*TET1, TET2, TET3*), which converts 5-methylcytosine (5-mC) to hydroxymethylcytosine (5-hmC), the initial step in DNA demethylation. Mutations of the *TET2* gene have been found in 8% to 27% of AML cases, in 20% to 25% of MDS cases, and in 4% to 13% of myeloproliferative neoplasms (MPN) cases. TET2 mutations are mono-allelic loss of function in most cases, including missense, frameshift, and nonsense mutations. The presence of the mutant *TET2* is associated with superior survival in MDS and inferior survival in AML and chronic myelomonocytic leukemia (CMML).[100] TET2 mutations are almost mutually exclusive with isocitrate dehydrogenase (IDH1/2) mutations, suggesting a similar epigenetic defect as IDH1/2 mutations.[101] In vivo, TET2 inactivation induced both myeloid and also lymphoid malignancies. The precise mechanisms and downstream effects of TET2 are as yet unknown.[102]

Mutations in the gene encoding *IDH1/2* functionally overlap with TET2 mutations, resulting in hypermethylation of leukemia cells, disruption of TET2 function, and impaired hematopoietic differentiation. IDH1 and IDH2 are nicotinamide adenine dinucleotide phosphate (NADP)-dependent IDHs that catalyze isocitrate to alpha-ketoglutarate (α-KG) in the tricarboxylic acid (TCA) cycle.[103] IDH1/2 mutations are detected in 15% to 33% of AML, mostly in normal karyotype AML, in 3.5% of MDS, in 2% to 5% of MPN, and also in glioma.[103] The mutations have been shown to exhibit a gain of function, leading to an aberrant accumulation of 2-hydroxyglutarate (2-HG). 2-HG is an oncometabolite, which inhibits an enzymatic activity of TET2 and stimulates hypoxia-inducible factor 1-alpha (HIF1α), leading to the initiation and promotion of cancer.[104] The impact of IDH mutations on the survival of AML patients is unclear. Some studies have observed no difference in outcome with respect to the IDH mutation status, whereas others have demonstrated a poor prognostic impact in certain AML subgroups.

Mammalian DNMTs catalyze the transfer of a methyl group onto the 5'-position of cytosine at CpG dinucleotides. DNMT3A and DNMT3B catalyze de novo DNA methylation, whereas DNMT1 is primarily responsible for maintenance methylation. Recurrent *DNMT3A* mutations at multiple sites were recently detected in a large cohort (22%) of patients with AML. Several different loss-of-function mutations have been found in all exons of DNMT3A, whereas a missense point mutation at amino acid R882, which decreases catalytic activity and DNA binding affinity, is most frequently identified.[105] DNMT3A-null hematopoietic stem cells have increased self-renewal capacity and lose their differentiation potential, which was accompanied by an aberrant methylation pattern implicated in leukemogenesis.[106] However, knockout of DNMT3A alone was not sufficient to initiate leukemia. DNMT3A mutations were reported to occur more frequently in AML with a normal karyotype and associated with FAB M5 morphology. The association with *NPM1* and *FLT3* mutations, unique DNA methylation and gene expression profiles, as well as unfavorable prognoses were observed in conjunction with *DNMT3A* mutations.[105]

EZH2 is a H3K27 methyltransferase, which is one of the components of PRC2, required for silencing target genes and maintaining the *stemness* in stem cells. EZH2 augments leukemogenesis by the inhibition of differentiation programs in leukemic stem cells.[107] EZH2 mutations were found 6% of MDS cases and in 3% to 13% of MPN cases, but rarely in AML.[108]

CHROMOSOMAL TRANSLOCATIONS THAT RESULT IN OVEREXPRESSION OF c-MYC

The chromosomal translocations described thus far result in the expression of aberrant fusion genes. Chromosomal translocations may also result in the overexpression of otherwise normal genes as a result of juxtaposition of a gene not normally expressed in adult hematopoietic tissues adjacent to an active promoter or enhancer. Most of those identified thus far involve the Ig or TCR enhancer loci, and thus most of these are associated with lymphoid malignancies; however, alternative mechanisms resulting in MYC overexpression have been shown to be important in AML or CML blast crisis.[109]

The prototypical example of juxtaposition of an Ig enhancer locus to an oncogene resulting in B-cell leukemia and lymphoma is the t(8;14)(q24;q32), resulting in overexpression of the MYC basic helix–loop–helix/basic region/leucine zipper (bHLH/bZIP) transcription factor on chromosome 8 due to juxtaposition to the Ig heavy-chain enhancer on chromosome 14.[110] Similar phenotypes ensue from juxtaposition to other Ig enhancers in the human genome, such as the Igκ locus on chromosome 2 or the Igλ locus on chromosome 22, and are characterized as B-ALL or lymphoma. Overexpression of MYC from Ig enhancers in murine models results in B-cell leukemias and lymphomas, confirming a central role for MYC overexpression in transformation. MYC is fully active as a transcription factor when heterodimerized with MAX. MAX is normally a homodimer, or a heterodimer complexed with MAD, which represses transcription. Overexpression of MYC is thought to shift the equilibrium in favor of an MYC-MAX homodimer that transactivates a wide range of target genes, including those involved in metabolism, cell cycle, and apoptosis and those contributing to leukemogenesis.[111]

CHROMOSOMAL TRANSLOCATIONS INVOLVING THE T-CELL RECEPTOR

T-cell leukemias are often associated with overexpression of a number of genes due to juxtaposition to the *TCR* enhancer loci (*TCRβ* at chromosome 7q34 or *TCRα/δ* at chromosome 14q11). Overexpression is thus associated with T-cell phenotypes, including T-cell ALL and lymphoma. For example, T-cell ALL may be associated with overexpression of bHLH family members that include T-cell acute leukemia 1/stem cell leukemia (TAL1/SCL), TAL2/SCL2, LYL1, homeo-box 11 (HOX11), HOX11L2, LIM only 2 (LMO2), LMO1, and MYC.[110,112] In addition to the minority of T-ALL cases with gene rearrangements involving these loci, it has been demonstrated that many patients without evident cytogenetic abnormalities overexpress TAL1, LMO2, HOX11, or HOX11L2.

POINT MUTATIONS IN ACUTE LEUKEMIA

Oncogenic RAS Mutations

Activating mutations in RAS may be associated with AML, ALL, and MDS, typically at codons 12, 13, or 61 in N- or K-RAS. The reported incidence varies widely between studies from 25% to 44%, and RAS mutations may confer a worse prognosis.[113,114] RAS mediates signals from upstream receptors through multiple downstream effectors including phosphoinositol 3' kinase (PI3K) and the rapidly accelerated fibrosarcoma/mitogen activated protein kinase kinase/extracellular signal-regulated kinase (RAF/MEK/ERK) pathways.[114,115] Considerable effort has been devoted to developing small-molecule inhibitors of RAS activation, with a focus on prenylation inhibitors, including farnesyl transferase and geranylgeranylation inhibitors that preclude appropriate targeting of activated RAS to the plasma membrane.[115,116] Specifically targeting activated RAS mutants remains an attractive option, and prenyltransferase inhibitors appear to have activity in AML. However, clinical activity is not correlated with the presence of activating mutations in RAS or even with inhibition of the target farnesyl transferase itself.[116,117] Several possible interpretations can be made of these observations, including the possibility that

RAS is activated by mechanisms other than intrinsic point mutations (e.g., constitutively activated tyrosine kinases such as FLT3), that other proteins that are targets of prenylation are important in leukemia pathogenesis, or that farnesyl transferase inhibitors have off-target effects. Additional efforts have focused on inhibiting the downstream effectors instead including PI3K and RAF/MEK/MAPK.[115]

Activating Mutations in Tyrosine Kinases and Associated Receptors

The identification and characterization of activating mutations in hematopoietic tyrosine kinases has been one of the exciting developments in the pathogenesis of AML. Substantial evidence has been shown that chromosomal translocations that activate tyrosine kinases can contribute to the pathogenesis of CML and other MPNs. The most common of these is the *BCR/ABL* gene rearrangement, but other examples include the TEL/ABL, TEL/PDGFβR, TEL/Janus kinase 2 (JAK2), H4/PDGFβR, FIP1/PDGFβR, and rabaptin/PDGFβR fusion proteins. However, these fusion genes are only rarely encountered in AMLs. Approximately 1% to 2% of cases of de novo AML have the *BCR/abelson (ABL)* gene rearrangement, whereas *BCR/ABL* gene rearrangement is present in 20% to 30% of adult ALL[118] and in 2% to 3% of children with ALL.[119] The Philadelphia chromosome[120] is a translocation between the *ABL1* oncogene on the long arm of chromosome 9 and a breakpoint cluster region (*BCR*) on the long arm of chromosome 22, t(9:22), resulting in a fusion gene,[121] *BCR/ABL1*, that encodes an oncogenic protein with constitutively active tyrosine kinase activity. The molecular weight of this protein depends on the precise chromosome breakpoint. Most patients with ALL express a 190-kDa protein (p190), and the remainder express a 210-kDa oncoprotein (p210), which is also commonly found in CML. Although *BCR/ABL* may be necessary and sufficient for the development CML, this is not the case for Ph+ ALL. *SRC* kinases are required for the development of Ph+ ALL.[122] There are many additional epigenetic changes, copy number abnormalities, and mutations downstream of *BCR-ABL* that contribute to the very aggressive clinical course. In addition, very rare cases of disease progression from CML to AML are associated with the acquisition of second mutations such as the *NUP98/HOXA9, AML1/ETO,* or *AML1/EVI1* rearrangement.

Point mutations in the tyrosine kinase activation loop and juxtamembrane (JM) mutations that activate *FLT3* and *c-KIT*, receptor tyrosine kinases normally expressed on hematopoietic progenitors, have been identified in a significant proportion of AML cases. These findings may have important therapeutic implications with the demonstration of the efficacy of molecular targeting of the ABL kinase in BCR/ABL-positive CML and CML blast crisis with imatinib.[123] Activating mutations in *FLT3* have been reported in approximately 30% to 35% of cases of AML.[124] In 20% to 25% of cases, internal tandem duplications (ITD) within the JM domain result in constitutive activation of FLT3. These can range in size from a few to more than 50 amino acids and are always in frame. Because of the extensive variability in size and exact position of the repeats within the JM domain, it has been hypothesized that these mutations impair an autoinhibitory domain, resulting in constitutive kinase activation in the absence of ligand. In support of this, the crystallographic structure of FLT3 demonstrates a seven amino acid extension of the JM domain that intercalates into the catalytic domain, thereby precluding kinase activation.[125] It is likely that ITD mutations in this region would disrupt the structure of the autoinhibitory domain, resulting in kinase activation.

Large studies have confirmed the frequency of these mutations in adult and pediatric AML populations and that mutations in *FLT3* appear to confer a poor prognosis.[126–128] In an additional 5% to 10% of cases, so-called activating loop mutations occur near position D835 in the tyrosine kinase.[129] When these mutations (D835 position) develop during treatment with a FLT3 inhibitor, they confer resistance to this inhibitor.[130] High throughput sequencing of AML patient samples lacking known FLT3 mutations revealed nine novel acquired mutations resulting in amino acid changes within the extracellular, JM, and activation domains; however, only four of the nine changes were *driver* mutations capable of kinase activation and conferring growth factor independence, thus emphasizing the need for biologic validation of sequencing data.[131] *FLT3* mutations may occur in conjunction with known gene rearrangements, such as *AML1/ETO, PML/RARα,* CBFβ/MYH11, or MLL. Analogous activating loop mutations at position D816 have also been reported in *C-KIT* in approximately 5% of cases of AML. Activating mutations in the thrombopoietin receptor, MPLW515L, originally identified in myelofibrosis with myeloid metaplasia (MMM), and MPLT487A have been observed in both primary cases of AMKL and those secondary to MMM.[132–134]

The JAK1 through 3 family of nonreceptor tyrosine kinases, in addition to involvement in translocation-derived fusions such as TEL/JAK2, have been found to contain activating point mutations. JAK kinases are important signaling intermediaries of multiple hematopoietic cytokine receptors and downstream effectors such as signal transducer and activator of transcription (STAT) proteins.[135] JAKV617F, originally identified as a causative mutation in *polycythemia vera,* is also seen in 8% de novo AML and up to 77% of AML cases transformed from MPN.[136,137] Additional mutations in JAK2 and JAK3 have been isolated in AMKL.[134,138] Mutations in JAK1, 2, or 3 are found in approximately 11% of BCR/ABL-negative childhood acute lymphoid leukemia and were often concurrent with deletion of the IKAROS lymphoid-specific transcription factor and the CDKN2A/B tumor suppressor.[139] Activating phosphorylation of STAT3 and STAT5a/b has been reported in a substantial proportion (44% to 76%) of AML patients[136] and confers a poor prognosis.[140,141]

A recently described subtype of precursor ALL is characterized by *cytokine receptor-like factor 2 (CRLF2)* alterations, which occur in about 5% to 7% of pediatric ALL, but in a significantly higher proportion of ALL with Down syndrome (~50%). Overexpression of CRLF2 is associated with activation of the JAK-STAT pathway. The mechanism involves translocation of *CRLF2* and the *immunoglobulin heavy chain (IGH@)* locus or a deletion juxtaposing *CRLF2* with the *P2RY8* promoter. The P2RY8/CRLF2 fusion appears to be the most relevant prognostic factor independent of CRLF2 overexpression for poor outcome and high risk of relapse.[142]

As sequencing efforts continue, it is likely that the list of activating kinase mutations will continue to increase. Because kinases are proving to be relatively amenable to targeted therapy, the opportunities for treatment tailored to these activated kinases should likewise expand.

MUTATIONS IN TUMOR SUPPRESSOR GENES

The Wilms tumor gene was originally described as a tumor suppressor gene in patients with Wilms tumor, aniridia, genitourinary anomalies, and mental retardation (WAGR).[143] *WT1* is found in adult tumors from different origins, and these tumors arise in tissues that normally do not express *WT1*; therefore, it has been suggested that the expression of *WT1* might play an oncogenic role in these tumors.[144] *WT1* is located at the chromosome 11p and encodes for a transcription factor with N-terminal transcriptional regulatory domain and C-terminal zinc finger domain (exon 7 to 10). The expression of *WT1* inversely correlates with the degree of differentiation in the hematopoietic system because it is present in CD34+ cells and absent in mature leukocytes.[144,145] *WT1* functions as a potent transcription regulator of genes important for cell survival and cell differentiation. The disruption of *WT1* function promotes stem cell proliferation and hampers differentiation.[144] Although the precise role of *WT1* in normal and malignant hematopoiesis remains to be further elucidated, it seems to have a dual role in leukemia.[146]

The wild-type form of *WT1* is highly (75% to 100%) expressed in a variety of acute leukemias.[147] Consistent with the function of an oncogene is the pattern of *WT1* expression in CML, where low levels are found in the chronic phase, but are frequently increased in the accelerated and blast crisis phase.[148] High levels of *WT1* in patients after chemotherapy is associated with a poor prognosis.

WT1 can act as a tumor suppressor in mice.[149] Mutation of the *WT1* gene can be detected in approximately 10% of normal karyotype AMLs.[150,151] Mutations that cluster to exon 7 (mostly frameshift mutations resulting from insertions and deletions) and exon 9 (mostly substitutions) are associated with a poor clinical outcome.[151–153] These data are examples of *WT1* as a tumor suppressor. On the other hand, a recent study analyzed mutations within the entire *WT1* coding sequence in a very large cohort of young adults with normal karyotype AML. Contrary to the previous observations,[151–153] *WT1* mutations had no prognostic impact.[154] The different results from these large studies could be explained by the variable biologic role of *WT1* in AML, possible differences in therapy, and other patient characteristics. Therefore, it is desirable that testing for *WT1* mutations becomes part of the risk assessment in future clinical trials to resolve these discrepancies.

TP53 is a tumor suppressor that induces cell-cycle arrest in a response to apoptotic cell death or DNA repair due to genotoxic substances, oncogenes, hypoxia, DNA damage, or ribonucleotide depletion.[155] Inactivation of *TP53* plays an important role during neoplastic transformation in solid tumors and also during progression of hematologic malignancies.[156–158] Animal experiments suggest that the loss of one *TP53* allele could be sufficient for tumorigenesis.[159] This could be relevant for the development of leukemia in patients with a single *TP53* deletion. The loss of 17p in AML is often accompanied by a *TP53* mutation resulting in a loss of heterozygosity.[160,161] Another possibility is the inactivation of downstream mediators of *TP53*, which affect not only cell-cycle arrest, but also DNA repair and apoptosis. Alternatively, overexpression of genes inhibiting or promoting degradation of TP53 can be considered—for instance, MDM2 gene amplifications have been detected in B-CLL.[162] *TP53* deletion can be present as a loss of 17p as a part of a complex aberrant karyotype or as a single chromosomal aberration, both resulting in a poor clinical outcome.[163–166] The incidence of *TP53* aberrations is high in AML with a complex aberrant karyotype (up to 70%),[163] but relatively rare in other AML groups (2% to 9%),[128,163,167] and *TP53* mutations without cytogenetic alteration are a rare event.[161,168] Low-risk AML t(8;21) or inv(16) are not associated with *TP53* deletion. There is significant positive association between *TP53* deletion and other high-risk chromosomal aberrations such as del(5q) and monosomy 5 and 7.[20,166] Molecular risk factors *FLT3-ITD* and *NPM1* mutation do not seem to cluster with the *TP53* deletion in complex karyotype patients.[166] *TP53*-deleted cells have greater resistance to various conventional antileukemic drugs.[169] However, published data of multidrug-resistance gene expression showed a negative influence on therapy response in complex aberrant patients.[170] The association of *TP53* deletion and *MDR1* expression has been confirmed for CML, but not for AML.[171] Hence, an independent mechanism of resistance needs to be considered.[166] Taken together, *TP53* deletion is a high-risk factor conveying a poor outcome, and further studies are necessary to provide and evaluate alternative therapies.

ACTIVATING MUTATIONS OF NOTCH

NOTCH1 is a component of an evolutionarily conserved pathway shown to direct T-cell lineage determination in early and late stages of lymphocyte development as well as play a role in hematopoietic

stem cell self-renewal.[172,173] NOTCH1 is a heterodimeric transmembrane receptor. Ligand binding to NOTCH1 allows proteolytic cleavage of the heterodimerization domain (HD) by adamalysin (ADAM)-type protease and γ-secretase of the C-terminal intracellular domain (ICD), which then localizes to the nucleus to function as a transactivator. Involvement of NOTCH1 in T-ALL had been observed with the rare t(7;9)(q34;q34.3) in which translocation of TCRβ locus into the *NOTCH1* gene results in the expression of the truncated, transcriptionally active ICD. A series of point mutations in NOTCH1 were identified in over half of all T-ALL cases.[112,174] These mutations clustered in two primary locations, the HD and the proline-, glutamate-, serine-, and threonine-rich (PEST) domain. The missense mutations within the HD domain make NOTCH1 more amenable to γ-secretase–mediated cleavage, thus enhancing activation. The PEST domain controls the rate of degradation of the activated ICN. PEST domain mutants are primarily small insertions/deletions into the reading frame, causing a deletion of all or part of the domain and extending the half-life of the activated ICN. An alternative mechanism for NOTCH1 activation are inactivating mutations of the F Box protein, FBXW7, which is a component of the ubiquitin ligase complex that targets the NOTCH1 ICN as well as MYC for degradation and which occurs in ~15% of T-ALL.[110,175]

Fortuitously, γ-secretase inhibitors (GSI) had already undergone significant clinical development due to the involvement of γ-secretase in processing the pathogenic β-amyloid peptide associated with Alzheimer's dementia. Initial clinical trials of GSIs in T-ALL have shown minimal effects on disease and significant gastrointestinal toxicity.[176] Use of GSIs in combination with agents affecting alternative pathways may provide synergism and improve efficacy. Treatment of a mouse model of T-ALL with GSIs and corticosteroids has demonstrated that GSIs are capable of abrogating corticosteroid resistance in established cell lines as well as limiting GSI-mediated gut toxicity.[177]

MUTATIONS ALTERING LOCALIZATION OF NPM1

Nucleophosmin (NPM1) encodes a protein that acts as a molecular chaperone between the nucleus and cytoplasm. It is involved in multiple cellular processes, including the regulation of TP53/ARF pathways, ribosome biogenesis, and the duplication of centrosomes.[178] *NPM1* had been previously identified in acute leukemias as a translocation fusion partner with *RAR* and *MLF* as well as with *ALK* in anaplastic large cell lymphoma. Aberrant cytoplasmic localization of *NPM1* has been observed in 25% to 30% of adult AML and is associated with point mutations within exon 12, which are hypothesized to enhance a nuclear export motif within the expressed protein.[179] The mechanism by which mutated *NPM1* causes leukemia is not clear; however, the cytoplasmic localization of NPM1 is thought to be intrinsic to its altered function.[180] *NPM1* mutations are found more frequently in AML with normal karyotypes (50% to 60%) and more apt to have *FLT3-ITD* mutations as well. Among normal cytogenetic AMLs, the presence of cytoplasmic *NPM1* in the absence of the *FLT3-ITD* is associated with a more favorable prognosis.[180]

MUTATION OF LYMPHOID DEVELOPMENT GENES IN ACUTE LYMPHOID LEUKEMIA

An important mechanism underlying the pathogenesis of B-lineage ALL is the mutation of transcription factors essential for B-cell commitment and differentiation.[181] Due to the requirement of these factors for normal early to late precursor B development, the immunophenotypic stage most closely related to the leukemias, it is hypothesized that the loss of normal expression levels leads to a block in differentiation, a critical step in leukemogenesis.[182]

Although translocations involving these genes had been identified in a smaller percentage of B-cell ALLs, earlier, high-resolution SNP arrays and genomic sequencing of disease samples has actually demonstrated that frequent microdeletions and point mutations are extremely common.[181] PAX5 is a master regulator of B-cell development at the pro– and pre–B-cell stage, the immunophenotypic stage most closely related to many B-ALLs.[37] PAX5 is a DNA-binding protein capable of interaction with corepressors, chromatin remodeling proteins, and other transcription factors such as erythroblastosis virus E26 oncogene homolog-1 (ETS1) and myeloblastosis (MYB).[37] The dual role of PAX5 is to simultaneously transactivate downstream factors promoting B-cell development and repress genes of alternative lineages such as *NOTCH1* and *CSFR1*.[183] Deletion of *Pax5* in mice yields early B cells that are not completely committed to B differentiation and can be trans-differentiated through the use of cytokines into other lineages.[183] Several rare translocations have been identified involving *PAX5*, including dic(9;12)(p13;p13), generating the PAX5/ETV6 fusion protein, which functions as a dominant negative.[184] In actuality, 30% of B-ALLs possess monoallelic loss-of-function mutations when examined by sequencing.[182] How PAX5 haploinsufficiency contributes to B-ALL leukemogenesis is not entirely clear, and PAX5 mutational status does not appear to influence prognosis.[181]

IKAROS family members (IKZF1–3) are also frequently mutated in B-ALL.[185] IKZF1 is essential for hematopoietic stem cell function and lymphoid commitment.[186,187] IKZF1 possesses zinc finger domains important for DNA-binding domains and homo/heterodimerization. Like PAX5, IKZF1 both activates lymphoid-specific genes such as IL-7R and represses genes, such as PU.1, required for alternative lineages. The function of IKZF1 as a transcriptional activator may be modulated through inherent mechanisms of chromatin remodeling and transcriptional elongation.[188] Approximately 15% of pediatric B-ALL patients have deletions or point mutations in IKZF1 leading to loss of function or dominant negative activity and correlating with a poor prognosis.[185] Interestingly, IKZF1 mutations are more frequently associated with mutations in tyrosine kinases such as BCR/ABL1 and JAK2 and cytokine receptors such as IL7R and CRLF2.[37] Furthermore, IKZF1 mutations appear in 20% of lymphoid blast crises evolving from chronic myelogenous leukemia.[189]

Other recurrent mutations have been found, to a lesser frequency, in a large number of lymphoid-specific transcription factors, including, for example, E2A, encoded by the *transcription factor 3 (TCF3)* gene, EBF1, and LEF1. The most common mutation in TCF3 in B-ALL is the translocation, t(1;19)(q23;p13), encoding the fusion product, TCF3/PBX1, which is postulated to dysregulate both B-cell and HOX-associated pathways.[190] EBF1 has reported monoallelic loss-of-function mutations in B-ALL, whereas *LEF1* has been observed with mono- and biallelic deletions in both T- and B- ALL.[182] The common feature of these genetic lesions are their requirement in normal lymphopoiesis, and deciphering the pathophysiologic effect of each mutation, particularly with regard to haploinsufficiency, will guide future therapeutic efforts.

MUTATIONAL COMPLEMENTATION GROUPS IN ACUTE LEUKEMIAS

Several lines of evidence indicate that more than one mutation is necessary for the pathogenesis of acute leukemia. First, there is evidence for the acquisition of additional cytogenetic abnormalities with disease progression from CML to AML (i.e., CML blast crisis). Published examples of progression in BCR/ABL-positive CML include the acquisition of t(3;21) AML1/EVI1, t(8;21) AML1/ETO, or t(7;11) NUP98/HOXA9 gene rearrangements. Progression of chronic myelomonocytic leukemia to AML in a patient with the *TEL/PDGFβR* gene rearrangement was associated with acquisition of a t(8;21) AML1/ETO gene rearrangement.[191] Second, expression of the AML1/ETO or CBFβ/MYH11 fusion proteins in murine models is not sufficient to cause AML.[26,192] Chemical mutagens

must be used in these contexts to generate second mutations that cause the AML phenotype. Third, evidence indicates that in some cases the *TEL/AML1* gene rearrangement associated with pediatric ALL may be acquired in utero, but ALL does not develop until years later, indicating a requirement for a second mutation.[193] Fourth, AML develops in transgenic mice that express the PML/RAR-α fusion protein only after a long latency of 3 to 6 months, with incomplete penetrance, indicating a need for a second mutation.[50–52]

The genetic epidemiology of AML provides important clues to the nature of the collaborating mutations. One broad complementation group in AML is comprised of mutations that activate signal transduction pathways. These include activating mutations in FLT3, RAS, and KIT, and more rarely, the BCR/ABL and TEL/PDGFβR fusion associated with disease progression in CML. These can be viewed as a complementation group because, although they are collectively present in approximately 50% of cases of AML, they rarely, if ever, occur together in the same patient.

A second complementation group, typified by translocations involving hematopoietic transcription factors, includes *AML1/ETO, CBFβ/SMMHC, PML/RARα, NUP98/HOXA9, MLL* gene rearrangements, and *MOZ/TIF2* and they are never observed together in the same leukemia. In general, this second class of mutations impair hematopoietic differentiation and may confer properties of self-renewal to the leukemic stem cell but are not sufficient to cause leukemia when expressed alone. However, one mutation from each of these two complementation groups often coexists in the same leukemia. For example, activating mutations in FLT3 or RAS have been observed in association with virtually all of the fusion genes in the second class described earlier.[194]

These findings suggest a hypothesis for pathogenesis of AML in which there are two broad classes of cooperating mutations (Fig. 106.1A).[194] One class, exemplified by activating mutations in *FLT3* or *RAS*, confers either a proliferative or survival advantage, or both, to hematopoietic progenitors but do not affect differentiation. These mutations do not confer self-renewal capacity as assessed in part by the ability to serially replate in culture or to serially transplant disease in murine models.[195,196] A second class of mutations, exemplified by *AML1/ETO, CBFβ/SMMHC, PML/RARα, NUP98/HOXA9, MLL* gene rearrangements, and *MOZ/TIF2* serve primarily to impair hematopoietic differentiation and confer properties of self-renewal. Together, these cooperating mutations induce the AML phenotype characterized by enhanced proliferative and survival advantage, impaired differentiation, and limitless self-renewal capacity. Although the two class model holds for a limited number of mutational combinations, it likely broadly simplifies the interplay between genetic lesions, because many have dual pleotropic effects on proliferation and differentiation.

Deeper insight into the cooperativity of different mutations has been aided by whole-genome or whole-exome sequencing of DNA samples. The Cancer Genome Atlas Consortium recently published the results of sequencing 200 individual AML samples along with matched epigenetic and RNA expression analysis.[12] Only an average of 13 coding mutations/genomes were uncovered, less than observed for most solid tumors. Mutations were grouped into the functional classes: transcription factor fusions, NPM1 related, tumor suppressors, DNA methylation related, signaling, chromatin modifying, myeloid transcription factor, cohesion complex, and spliceosome complex related. Certain mutational groups are mutually exclusive of each other, indicating possible convergent downstream pathways. For example, mutations in cohesion, spliceosome, signaling, and histone modification pathways do not usually occur in the same patient (Fig. 106.1B).[12,197] Experimental validation of these novel individual mutations alone or in conjunction with suspected cooperating lesions is an important focus to identify driver versus passenger mutations and clinical significance. In addition, sequencing of a population, which allows for the quantification of mutational frequency in subclones in consecutive patient samples during the diagnosis, treatment, and relapse, identifies the mutations important for leukemia, initiation, progression, and resistance.[198]

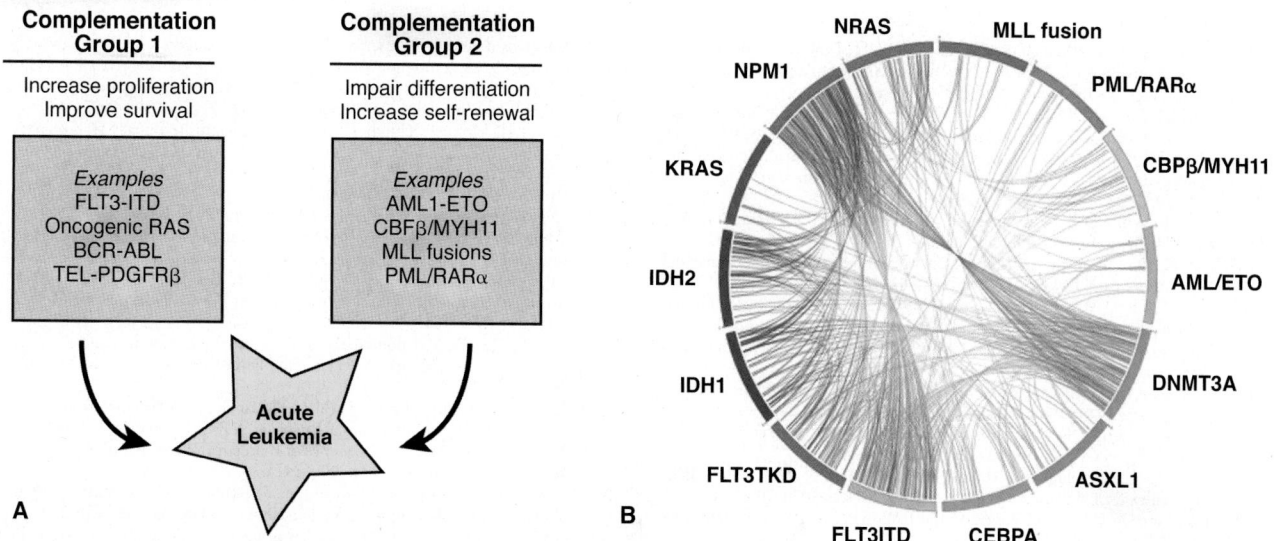

Figure 106.1 Cooperating mutations in acute leukemia. **A:** A classic model of leukemogenesis, composed of two broad complementation groups, is defined by a lack of concurrence of any two mutations in the same complementation group in the same patient. One group is characterized by activating mutations in signal transduction pathways. When expressed alone, these mutations confer a proliferative or survival advantage, or both, but do not affect differentiation. The second group is associated with impaired differentiation and the ability to confer properties of self-renewal to hematopoietic progenitors. Together, the complementation groups collaborate to engender the acute leukemia phenotype. **B:** Circos plot showing concurrent mutational groups in 498 cases of AML. Each connecting line represents simultaneous mutations in an AML sample and demonstrates the how high resolution analysis of AML genomes can establish complementation groups for recurrent mutations. (Modified from Sanders MA, Valk PJ. The evolving molecular genetic landscape in acute myeloid leukaemia. *Curr Opin Hematol* 2013;20:79–85.)

CONCLUSION

The quest to elucidate the essential pathophysiologic changes involved in leukemogenesis has been accelerated with the usage of newer technologies, such as high resolution mapping and high throughput sequencing. It is now possible to identify specific molecular pathways complementing known recurrent translocations as well as gaining insight into the mechanisms underlying normal karyotype leukemias. Not only can these novel mutations be used for more accurate prognostication, but they can also provide an opportunity for drug development, targeting the essential pathways dysregulated in leukemia. As the availability of pathway-targeted therapeutics increases, interrogation of a patient's leukemia for alterations at the genomic level may allow for individualized therapy addressing the pathways responsible for leukemic cell survival, proliferation, and differentiation, which ideally would improve treatment efficacy and reduce therapy-related morbidity and mortality.

SELECTED REFERENCES

The full reference list can be accessed at lwwhealthlibrary.com/oncology.

1. Lapidot T, Sirard C, Vormoor J, et al. A cell initiating human acute myeloid leukaemia after transplantation into SCID mice. *Nature.* 1994;367:645–648.
2. Bonnet D, Dick JE. Human acute myeloid leukemia is organized as a hierarchy that originates from a primitive hematopoietic cell. *Nat Med* 1997;3:730–737.
3. Buss EC, Ho AD. Leukemia stem cells. *Int J Cancer* 2011;129:2328–2336.
6. Huntly BJ, Shigematsu H, Deguchi K, et al. MOZ-TIF2, but not BCR-ABL, confers properties of leukemic stem cells to committed murine hematopoietic progenitors. *Cancer Cell* 2004;6:587–596.
9. Speicher MR, Carter NP. The new cytogenetics: blurring the boundaries with molecular biology. *Nat Rev Genet* 2005;6:782–792.
11. International Cancer Genome Consortium, Hudson TJ, Anderson W, et al. International network of cancer genome projects. *Nature* 2010;464:993–998.
12. Cancer Genome Atlas Research Network. Genomic and epigenomic landscapes of adult de novo acute myeloid leukemia. *N Engl J Med* 2013;368:2059–2074.
13. Stratton MR, Campbell PJ, Futreal PA. The cancer genome. *Nature* 2009;458:719–724.
14. Koschmieder S, Halmos B, Levantini E, et al. Dysregulation of the C/EBPalpha differentiation pathway in human cancer. *J Clin Oncol* 2009;27:619–628.
19. Ichikawa M, Yoshimi A, Nakagawa M, et al. A role for RUNX1 in hematopoiesis and myeloid leukemia. *Int J Hematol* 2013;97:726–734.
26. Castilla LH, Garrett L, Adya N, et al. The fusion gene Cbfb-MYH11 blocks myeloid differentiation and predisposes mice to acute myelomonocytic leukaemia. *Nat Genet* 1999;23:144–146.
34. De Braekeleer E, Douet-Guilbert N, Morel F, et al. ETV6 fusion genes in hematological malignancies: a review. *Leuk Res* 2012;36:945–961.
35. Mulligan CG. Genomic characterization of childhood acute lymphoblastic leukemia. *Semin Hematol* 2013;50:314–324.
37. Tijchon E, Havinga J, van Leeuwen FN, et al. B-lineage transcription factors and cooperating gene lesions required for leukemia development. *Leukemia* 2013;27:541–552.
39. Kakizuka A, Miller WH Jr, Umesono K, et al. Chromosomal translocation t(15;17) in human acute promyelocytic leukemia fuses RAR alpha with a novel putative transcription factor, PML. *Cell* 1991;66:663–674.
46. Zhang XW, Yan XJ, Zhou ZR, et al. Arsenic trioxide controls the fate of the PML-RARalpha oncoprotein by directly binding PML. *Science* 2010;328:240–243.
47. de Thé H, Chen Z. Acute promyelocytic leukaemia: novel insights into the mechanisms of cure. *Nat Rev Cancer* 2010;10:775–783.
54. Alharbi RA, Pettengell R, Pandha HS, et al. The role of HOX genes in normal hematopoiesis and acute leukemia. *Leukemia* 2013;27:1000–1008.
64. Slany RK. The molecular biology of mixed lineage leukemia. *Haematologica* 2009;94:984–993.
69. Mohan M, Lin C, Guest E, et al. Licensed to elongate: a molecular mechanism for MLL-based leukaemogenesis. *Nat Rev Cancer* 2010;10:721–728.
72. Somervaille TC, Cleary ML. Identification and characterization of leukemia stem cells in murine MLL-AF9 acute myeloid leukemia. *Cancer Cell* 2006;10:257–268.
76. Paz-Priel I, Friedman A. C/EBPalpha dysregulation in AML and ALL. *Crit Rev Oncog* 2011;16:93–102.
83. Bresnick EH, Katsumura KR, Lee HY, et al. Master regulatory GATA transcription factors: mechanistic principles and emerging links to hematologic malignancies. *Nucleic Acids Res* 2012;40:5819–5831.
84. Wechsler J, Greene M, McDevitt MA, et al. Acquired mutations in GATA1 in the megakaryoblastic leukemia of Down syndrome. *Nat Genet* 2002;32:148–152.
85. Malinge S, Izraeli S, Crispino JD. Insights into the manifestations, outcomes, and mechanisms of leukemogenesis in Down syndrome. *Blood* 2009;113:2619–2628.

PRACTICE OF ONCOLOGY

97. Deguchi K, Ayton PM, Carapeti M, et al. MOZ-TIF2-induced acute myeloid leukemia requires the MOZ nucleosome binding motif and TIF2-mediated recruitment of CBP. *Cancer Cell* 2003;3:259–271.

101. Patel JP, Gonen M, Figueroa ME, et al. Prognostic relevance of integrated genetic profiling in acute myeloid leukemia. *N Engl J Med* 2012;366:1079–1089.

102. Moran-Crusio K, Reavie L, Shih A, et al. Tet2 loss leads to increased hematopoietic stem cell self-renewal and myeloid transformation. *Cancer Cell* 2011;20:11–24.

104. Dang L, White DW, Gross S, et al. Cancer-associated IDH1 mutations produce 2-hydroxyglutarate. *Nature* 2009;462:739–744.

105. Ley TJ, Ding L, Walter MJ, et al. DNMT3A mutations in acute myeloid leukemia. *N Engl J Med* 2010;363:2424–2433.

108. Ernst T, Chase AJ, Score J, et al. Inactivating mutations of the histone methyltransferase gene EZH2 in myeloid disorders. *Nat Genet* 2010;42:722–726.

109. Delgado MD, Albajar M, Gomez-Casares MT, et al. MYC oncogene in myeloid neoplasias. *Clin Transl Oncol* 2013;15:87–94.

110. O'Neil J, Look AT. Mechanisms of transcription factor deregulation in lymphoid cell transformation. *Oncogene* 2007;26:6838–6849.

112. Van Vlierberghe P, Ferrando A. The molecular basis of T cell acute lymphoblastic leukemia. *J Clin Invest* 2012;122:3398–3406.

113. Steelman LS, Franklin RA, Abrams SL, et al. Roles of the Ras/Raf/MEK/ERK pathway in leukemia therapy. *Leukemia* 2011;25:1080–1094.

115. Takashima A, Faller DV. Targeting the RAS oncogene. *Expert Opin Ther Targets* 2013;17:507–531.

121. Rowley JD. Letter: A new consistent chromosomal abnormality in chronic myelogenous leukaemia identified by quinacrine fluorescence and Giemsa staining. *Nature* 1973;243:290–293.

122. Hu Y, Liu Y, Pelletier S, et al. Requirement of Src kinases Lyn, Hck and Fgr for BCR-ABL1-induced B-lymphoblastic leukemia but not chronic myeloid leukemia. *Nat Genet* 2004;36:453–461.

131. Frohling S, Scholl C, Levine RL, et al. Identification of driver and passenger mutations of FLT3 by high-throughput DNA sequence analysis and functional assessment of candidate alleles. *Cancer Cell* 2007;12:501–513.

137. Frohling S, Lipka DB, Kayser S, et al. Rare occurrence of the JAK2 V617F mutation in AML subtypes M5, M6, and M7. *Blood* 2006;107:1242–1243.

138. Walters DK, Mercher T, Gu TL, et al. Activating alleles of JAK3 in acute megakaryoblastic leukemia. *Cancer Cell* 2006;10:65–75.

150. King-Underwood L, Renshaw J, Pritchard-Jones K. Mutations in the Wilms' tumor gene WT1 in leukemias. *Blood* 1996;87:2171–2179.

152. Virappane P, Gale R, Hills R, et al. Mutation of the Wilms' tumor 1 gene is a poor prognostic factor associated with chemotherapy resistance in normal karyotype acute myeloid leukemia: the United Kingdom Medical Research Council Adult Leukaemia Working Party. *J Clin Oncol* 2008;26:5429–5435.

161. Fenaux P, Jonveaux P, Quiquandon I, et al. P53 gene mutations in acute myeloid leukemia with 17p monosomy. *Blood* 1991;78:1652–1657.

166. Seifert H, Mohr B, Thiede C, et al. The prognostic impact of 17p (p53) deletion in 2272 adults with acute myeloid leukemia. *Leukemia* 2009;23:656–663.

173. Pancewicz J, Nicot C. Current views on the role of Notch signaling and the pathogenesis of human leukemia. *BMC Cancer* 2011;11:502.

174. Weng AP, Ferrando AA, Lee W, et al. Activating mutations of NOTCH1 in human T cell acute lymphoblastic leukemia. *Science* 2004;306:269–271.

175. Thompson BJ, Buonamici S, Sulis ML, et al. The SCFFBW7 ubiquitin ligase complex as a tumor suppressor in T cell leukemia. *J Exp Med* 2007;204:1825–1835.

177. Real PJ, Tosello V, Palomero T, et al. Gamma-secretase inhibitors reverse glucocorticoid resistance in T cell acute lymphoblastic leukemia. *Nat Med* 2009;15:50–58.

179. Falini B, Mecucci C, Tiacci E, et al. Cytoplasmic nucleophosmin in acute myelogenous leukemia with a normal karyotype. *N Engl J Med* 2005;352:254–266.

181. Mulligan CG. Molecular genetics of B-precursor acute lymphoblastic leukemia. *J Clin Invest* 2012;122:3407–3415.

182. Mulligan CG, Goorha S, Radtke I, et al. Genome-wide analysis of genetic alterations in acute lymphoblastic leukaemia. *Nature* 2007;446:758–764.

183. Nutt SL, Heavey B, Rolink AG, Busslinger M. Commitment to the B-lymphoid lineage depends on the transcription factor Pax5. *Nature* 1999;401:556–562.

185. Mulligan CG, Su X, Zhang J, et al. Deletion of IKZF1 and prognosis in acute lymphoblastic leukemia. *N Engl J Med* 2009;360:470–480.

186. Georgopoulos K, Bigby M, Wang JH, et al. The Ikaros gene is required for the development of all lymphoid lineages. *Cell* 1994;79:143–156.

189. Mulligan CG, Miller CB, Radtke I, et al. BCR-ABL1 lymphoblastic leukaemia is characterized by the deletion of Ikaros. *Nature* 2008;453:110–114.

191. Golub TR, Barker GF, Lovett M, et al. Fusion of PDGF receptor beta to a novel ets-like gene, tel, in chronic myelomonocytic leukemia with t(5;12) chromosomal translocation. *Cell* 1994;77:307–316.

193. Wiemels JL, Cazzaniga G, Daniotti M, et al. Prenatal origin of acute lymphoblastic leukaemia in children. *Lancet* 1999;354:1499–1503.

197. Sanders MA, Valk PJ. The evolving molecular genetic landscape in acute myeloid leukemia. *Curr Opin Hematol* 2013;20:79–85.

198. Welch JS, Ley TJ, Link DC, et al. The origin and evolution of mutations in acute myeloid leukemia. *Cell* 2012;150:264–278.

107 Management of Acute Leukemias

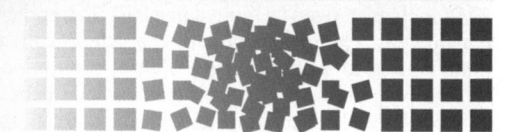

Partow Kebriaei, Marcos de Lima, Elihu H. Estey, and Richard Champlin

INTRODUCTION

Acute leukemias result from malignant transformation of immature hematopoietic cells followed by clonal proliferation and accumulation of the transformed cells. The pathogenesis of leukemia transformation is incompletely defined but is likely to be a multistep process.[1] Acute leukemias are characterized by aberrant differentiation and maturation of the malignant cells, with a maturation arrest and accumulation of leukemic blasts in the bone marrow. Acute leukemias are categorized according to their differentiation along the myeloid or lymphoid lineage. In 10% to 20% of patients, the leukemic cells have characteristics of both myeloid and lymphoid cells. Typically myeloid and lymphoid markers are found on the same cell. Less often, separate myeloid and lymphoid populations are present.

Hematopoietic cells are derived from stem cells and progenitors giving rise to the myeloid and lymphoid system. Stem cells have the fundamental properties of self-renewal and differentiation into distinct lineages. Hematopoietic stem cells and progenitors are resident in the bone marrow where they are supported and regulated through interactions with the local microenvironment. Leukemia likely develops after transformation of a hematopoietic stem cell or progenitor, which acquires stem cell–like properties of unlimited self-renewal.[2] The malignant stem cells represent a small fraction of the leukemia. The bulk of leukemic cells are the differentiated progeny that undergo limited maturation along the myeloid or lymphoid lineage. Leukemia chemotherapy must eradicate the disease while sparing normal hematopoietic stem cells. Treatments that eradicate the differentiated leukemia cells typically do not eradicate the malignant stem cells; consequently, relapse of the leukemia commonly occurs.[3] High-dose, stem cell–toxic therapies may be used if followed by hematopoietic stem cell transplantation (HSCT) to restore normal hematopoiesis, and HSCT is an important modality of treatment for acute leukemias. However, a significant antileukemia effect mediated by donor T and natural killer (NK) cells also plays an important role in allogeneic transplantation, particularly for acute myelogenous leukemia (AML). A better understanding of the biology of normal and malignant stem cells and the marrow microenvironment is required for development of more effective therapies.

Although the cause of acute leukemias is unknown, malignant transformation is unlikely to be the result of a single event. Rather, it is likely caused by the culmination of multiple processes that produce genetic damage secondary to physical or chemical exposure in susceptible progenitor cells. Genomic analyses indicate that AML has fewer mutations than all solid tumors studied to date, with an average of 13 coding mutations per patient, of which only an average of 5 (and on occasion as few as 2) are recurrently mutated (*driver*) mutations; among the latter aberrations in DNA (cytosine-5)-methyltransferase 3A (*DNMT3a*), isocitrate dehydrogenase (*IDH*), tet methylcytosine dioxygenase 2 (*TET2*), or nucleophosmin (*NPM1*) contribute to the establishment of a founding AML clone and in FMS-like tyrosine kinase 3 (*FLT3*) to progression to the clinically apparent disease. The nonrecurrent *passenger* mutations appear to represent mutations that occur during the life span of normal hematopoietic progenitors and are retained when a malignant mutation(s) occurs. Over time, subclones arise characterized by other mutations that contribute to resistance.[4,5] Leukemia may occur following exposure to a number of carcinogens, such as benzene or radiation exposure. Acute leukemias may occur following chemotherapy, such as alkylators or topoisomerase II inhibitors, or radiation therapy given for another malignancy.[6,7] These secondary leukemias typically have a high risk of cytogenetic abnormalities and have a poor prognosis. Other acquired factors include infectious agents and environmental toxins. Among infectious causes, the Epstein-Barr virus is associated with mature B-cell or Burkitt's acute lymphoblastic leukemia (ALL). Inherited genetic abnormalities that predispose to leukemia include ataxia telangiectasia, Down syndrome, and certain polymorphisms in Methylenetetrahydrofolate Reductase (*MTHFR*) (a gene involved in the folate metabolism).[8]

The presenting clinical symptoms are a result of bone marrow failure or the effects of tissue infiltration or circulating leukemia cells. Patients commonly complain of fatigue or spontaneous bleeding. Weight loss, fever, night sweats, and lethargy may also be present. Infections related to neutropenia may occur. Central nervous system (CNS) involvement is more common in ALL than AML. Bone and testicular involvement is also more commonly seen in ALL, and most commonly in children rather than adults.[9] On physical examination, pallor and signs associated with thrombocytopenia may be present, such as gingival bleeding, epistaxis, petechiae, ecchymoses, or fundal hemorrhages. Less commonly, generalized lymphadenopathy, hepatosplenomegaly, or dermal involvement by leukemia cutis may be present. T-lineage ALL may commonly present with a mediastinal mass.

The diagnosis of acute leukemias requires morphologic identification of malignant blasts in the blood and bone marrow.[10] This requires an evaluation of peripheral blood and bone marrow aspirate smears, phenotypic analysis of the blasts by cytochemical studies and flow cytometry, or immunohistochemistry with an appropriate panel of surface and cytoplasmic markers. Acute leukemias are classified according to their differentiation into the myeloid or lymphoid lineage, although some cases appear biphenotypic. The French–American–British Group (FAB) described a widely utilized classification system[11] that has been largely replaced by the World Health Organization's (WHO) classification system.[12] Cytospin slides made from cerebrospinal fluid (CSF) are used to diagnose CNS involvement. The current definition of CNS involvement used by the Children's Cancer Group (CCG) is greater than five white blood cells (WBC) per microliter of CSF plus unequivocal blasts identified on the cytospin.[13] However, the risk for CNS relapse and the need for additional CNS-directed therapy is controversial when there are less than WBC per microliter of CSF, but blasts are present. Some studies suggest that the presence of blasts, even in the absence of pleocytosis, requires additional CNS-directed therapy,[14] whereas others do not. A related concern is the prognostic significance of a traumatic lumbar puncture at diagnosis. Most studies concur that the presence of blasts in a traumatic lumbar puncture is associated with an inferior outcome.[15]

PRACTICE OF ONCOLOGY

ACUTE MYELOGENOUS LEUKEMIA

AML is characterized by limited myeloid differentiation of the malignant cells. The malignant cells characteristically undergo maturation arrest at the level of the blast or promyelocyte, although varying proportions of mature hematopoietic cells are leukemia derived. The cells display myeloid specific markers, including Auer rods (aberrant primary granules), cytochemistry (Sudan black, myeloperoxidase, or nonspecific esterase), and cell surface antigens.[11] The WHO classification system's criterion for a diagnosis of AML is >20% blasts in marrow or blood, with patients having <20% blasts said most often to have a myelodysplastic syndrome (MDS). However, this distinction is purely arbitrary. And, indeed, the natural history of patients with 10% to 19% blasts (high-risk MDS) frequently bears more resemblance to that of AML than to that of patients with <10% blasts. Furthermore, the outcome of AML *therapy* is often similar in patients with high-risk MDS as in those with AML.

Management Options for Acute Myelogenous Leukemia

Broadly speaking, there are three management options for AML: supportive care only, supportive care plus standard anti-AML therapy, or supportive care plus investigational anti-AML therapy. When the disease was first systematically described 50 years ago, few patients lived more than 4 to 6 months after diagnosis. Today, with the advent of better antibiotics and transfusion practices, the natural history is almost certainly better, particularly in patients with WBC <25,000 to 50,000/μL. Nonetheless, it is safe to say that patients will, on average, lose >90% of their remaining life expectancy if given supportive care only. Furthermore, quality of life suffers dominated by time spent waiting for frequent transfusions and hospital admissions for infections, which ultimately lead to death. For these reasons, patients presenting to academic medical centers are generally interested in treatment beyond supportive care. This leads to a decision between standard and investigational therapies. The results of the latter are, by definition, unknown. It follows that the decision must rest on the likely outcome of standard therapy. The worse the outcome, the more likely appropriately informed patients select a clinical trial. Hence, the topic of prognostic factors with standard therapies is fundamental to the management of AML. Here, standard induction therapies will refer to (1) 3 days of an anthracycline, usually daunorubicin or idarubicin (days 1 through 3), plus 7 days of ara-C (100 to 200 mg/m² days 1 through 7), (2) decitabine or azacitidine, or (3) a lower dose of ara-C and standard postremission therapies of the previous, including ara-C at doses of 0.5 to 3.0 g/m².

Prognostic Factors in Acute Myelogenous Leukemia

There are two types of prognostic factors: those associated with treatment-related mortality (TRM) and those associated with resistance to therapy. Although there is considerable overlap between these two, TRM is often defined as death occurring within the first 28 days of initial therapy or occurring in patients in remission. Patients dying within the first 28 days appear to be a qualitatively distinct group. Resistance then may be considered as failure to enter remission despite not incurring TRM or as relapse from remission. Although considerable attention is often devoted to TRM and associated morbidity, there is little doubt that even in patients in their 70s, resistance is a more frequent cause of failure to enter complete remission (CR), and that relapse is at least threefold more common than death in CR.

Predictors of Treatment-Related Mortality

Although it is commonly believed that age is the principal covariate associated with TRM, Walter et al.[16] found that performance status is more important than age and that both interact with lower albumin and platelet count, higher creatinine, WBC and percentage of blood blasts, and secondary AML. These were all used to compute a TRM score following the use of 3+7 as given in the Southwest Oncology Group (SWOG) or higher doses of ara-C as given at M. D. Anderson Cancer Center (MDACC). As such, they defined a group of patients who might be candidates for *less intense* therapies. However, this possibility needs to account for decreasing TRM rates, as noted by Othus et al.[17] In SWOG, these declined from 18% in 1991 through 1995 to 3% in 2006 through 2009. Analogous figures at MDACC were 16% and 4%. The decline was independent of covariates such as those considered in the TRM score. The possibility that this reflected a tendency in recent years to give less intense drugs, such as azacitidine or decitabine rather than 3+7, to older patients at high risk of TRM who thus would be excluded from analyses seems unlikely because the same temporal trend in TRM was found in both younger and older patients; it seems improbable that the former were more likely to receive less intense therapy in recent years. Othus et al.'s data emphasize that the main problem in AML therapy is resistance. Hence, merely decreasing intensity is unlikely to result in improved outcomes unless efficacy is improved in parallel.

Predictors of Resistance to Standard Therapy

Cytogenetics. Various means to classify pretreatment AML cytogenetics have been proposed (Table 107.1 and 107.2), and generally separate patients into three to four distinct prognostic groups.

Favorable Group. The core binding factor (CBF)–related AMLs have the most favorable prognosis and constitute 10% to 15% of cases in patients under age 60 years.[18] CBFs regulate the transcription of genes involved in the differentiation of normal blasts into mature progeny. CBFs contain a β unit (*CBFB*, located on the long arm of chromosome 16) and an α unit, one of which is known as *RUNX1* (formerly *AML1* and located on chromosome 21). The CBF AMLs result from translocations involving *RUNX1* or *CBFB*. Specifically, in t(8;21) *RUNX1* is fused with *RUNX1T1* (formerly *ETO*) located on chromosome 8, whereas in inv(16), *CBFB* is linked with the *MYH11* gene located on the short arm of chromosome 16. These abnormal CBFs exert a *dominant negative* effect over normal CBFs, leading to differentiation block and, in the presence of other genetic aberrations that promote survival of the affected stem cells, to AML. It is important to distinguish deletion of the long arm of chromosome 16(del16q), which does not affect *CBFB*, from translocation between the two chromosome 16s, t(16;16), which is quite rare but does disrupt *CBFB* and, unlike del16q, behaves clinically like inv(16). Eighty-five percent of cases of inv(16) or t(8;21) AML are found in those under age 60 years. Although inv(16) is most frequently associated with the FAB subtype M4Eo, 40% of the 145 cases of inv(16) AML seen at MDACC over the past 25 years have had less than 5% eosinophils. Similarly, although t(8;21) AML is most often seen in the FAB subtype M2, 30% of the 124 cases at MDACC were seen in association with other FAB subtypes.

Inv(16) AML and t(8;21) AML differ in several ways. For example, t(8;21) tends to present with lower WBC counts and is frequently accompanied by the loss of a sex chromosome (particularly the Y) or a deletion (del) of the long arm (q) of chromosome 9(del9q), whereas inv(16) is often accompanied by trisomy (+) 22 (+22), +(8), or +(21). Although both inv(16) and t(8;21) are distinguished by CR rates of approximately 90% and long remissions and survival, inv(16) AML is more apt to respond once relapse occurs; as a result, patients with inv(16) tend to live longer

TABLE 107.1

Acute Myeloid Leukemia Prognostic Index

Group	NCRI (formerly MRC)	SWOG/ECOG	CALGB
Best	inv(16); t(8;21)	inv(16); t(8;21) w/o del (9q) or complex changes	inv(16); t(8;21)
Intermediate	Normal; 11q abnormalities[a]; +8; Others not in favorable or unfavorable groups	Normal; +8; Others not in favorable or unfavorable groups	Normal; t(9;11); +8 (for relapse); del(5q); Loss of 7q
Worst	−5/−7; Complex (≥5 chromosomes involved)	−5/−7; Complex (≥3 chromosomes involved); 11q abnormalities[a]; inv(3q); del(20q); t(6;9); abnormal 17p	Complex (≥3 chromosomes involved); −7; +8 (for survival); inv(3)

NCRI, National Cancer Research Institute; MRC, Medical Research Center; SWOG, Southwest Oncology Group; ECOG, Eastern Cooperative Oncology Group; CALGB, Cancer and Leukemia Group B.
[a] Patients with t(9;11) may fall into the intermediate group and patients with other 11q abnormalities into the unfavorable group.

than those with t(8;21). The prognosis of CBF AML is quite variable (although not as variable as normal karyotype AML). Thus, long-term remissions occur in only 25% to 30% of patients aged >65 years or with high levels of mutant tyrosine-protein kinase (*C-KIT*) alleles.[19]

Worst Group. There is some debate as to the placement of patients with other abnormal karyotypes. Thus, for example, both the Medical Research Council (MRC) and SWOG cytogenetic classification systems include patients with +8,−Y in an *intermediate* prognostic group together with normal cytogenetic (NC)-AML (see Table 107.1). However, although the MRC considers del20q or t(6;9) AML in its intermediate group, the SWOG places these in its *worst* group, and other differences exist (see Table 107.1). However, there is very little debate about the great bulk of patients

in the worst group: those with monosomy of chromosome 5 (−5), and/or 7 (−7), deletions (del) of the long arms of chromosomes 5 (del 5q) or 7 (del 7q) and with abnormalities of 3q. Particularly poor prognoses have been associated with *complex* abnormalities involving at least three to four distinct changes. In the last 5 years, some of the prognostic import of complex cytogenetics has been attributed to an association with a *monosomal karyotype* (MK+) defined by the presence of two or more autosomal monosomies (i.e., not involving the X or Y chromosome) or by the presence of one autosomal monosomy and a structural change, which is a translocation but no addition. MK+ patients are largely incurable with standard therapy, with median survivals of approximately 6 months. Now it appears that alterations in the tumor suppressor gene TP53, located on the short arm(p) of chromosome 17, underlie the prognostic effect of MK.

TABLE 107.2

European Leukemia Net Classification System

Prognostic Group	Proportion of De Novo Patients in Group by Age <60 years, Age ≥60 years	Subsets
Favorable	41%, 20%	Inv (16), t(16;16), t(8;21) NC with NPM mutation (NPM+) but no FLT3 ITD (ITD−) NC with mutated CEBPA
Intermediate 1	18%, 19%	NPM− ITD− NPM+ ITD+ NPM− ITD+
Intermediate 2	19%, 30%	Cytogenetic abnormalities (including t9;11) not considered best or worst
Adverse	22%, 31%	3q abnormalities, t(6;9), −7,−5, del 5q, abnormal 11q (other than t9;11), abnormal 17p, complex abnormalities

NC, normal cytogenetics; FLT3, FMS-like tyrosine kinase 3; ITD, internal tandem duplication; NPM, nucleophosmin; CEBPA, CCAAT enhancer binding protein alpha.

PRACTICE OF ONCOLOGY

Intermediate Group. Criteria for intermediate cytogenetics differ (see Table 107.1). However, there is agreement that patients with NC-AML are the lynchpin of this group. NC-AML occurs in 25% to 40% of patients depending on age (less frequent with increasing age) and type of AML (less frequent with therapy related AML [t-AML]). As might be expected from the term *intermediate cytogenetics* and the frequency of NC-AML, NC-AML is associated with greater variation in outcome than any other single cytogenetic group.

NPM, FLT3 ITD, and CEBPA. Recent years have shown the ability of molecular biology to dissect this heterogeneity. Today, patients with NC-AML should routinely be tested for internal tandem duplications (ITD) in the *FLT3* gene, mutations in the nucleophosmin gene (*NPM1*), and in the CCAAT enhancer-binding protein alpha (*CEBPA*) gene. Most cost effectively, this would be done once a diagnosis of NC-AML is established (the prognostic relevance of *NPM*, *FLT3*, and *CEBPA* being less in other patients than in those with NC-AML), and *CEBPA* testing would only be carried out in patients who were negative for *FLT3*, *ITD*, and *NPM1*. NC-AML patients with *NPM1* mutations but without *FLT3* ITDs and patients with a double *CEBPA* mutation have a prognosis with standard therapy essentially equivalent to patients with best cytogenetics. In contrast, patients with *FLT3* ITDs have a prognosis more closely resembling that of patients with the worst cytogenetics. This has been codified in the widely employed four-group European Leukemia Net (ELN) Classification system (see Table 107.2). The system has been tested in patients with de novo AML that did not contribute to its development; treatment was standard. Each of the four groups were relevant in patients age <60 years, whereas the two intermediate groups were difficult to distinguish prognostically in older patients.

Secondary AML. Although many studies detailing effects of various molecular markers include only patients with de novo AML, there is little doubt that t-AML or AML following a documented abnormality in blood count for 1 to 3 months before the diagnosis of AML, often called an antecedent hematologic disorder (AHD), is associated with resistance. T-AML and AML after an AHD are collectively known as secondary AML. The association between resistance and secondary AML is independent of the tendency of patients with secondary AML to have the worst group cytogenetics (see previously). The relative effects of an AHD and t-AML remain to be established, although it has been suggested that the latter is more important.

Age. Although much of the association between older age and resistance reflects an association with the worst group cytogenetics (see previously) and/or with secondary AML, age per se probably predisposes to resistance.

Mutations Other than *NPM, FLT3* ITD, and *CEBPA*. The ability of cytogenetics, *NPM*, and *FLT3* ITD, along with older age and secondary AML to predict resistance has been studied using areas under receiver operating characteristic curves (AUC). An AUC of 1.0 indicates perfect prediction, an AUC of 0.5 is a coin flip (sensitivity = specificity), and an AUC of 0.6 to 0.69, 0.70 to 79, and 0.80 to 0.89 is often taken as denoting poor, fair, and good predictive ability, respectively. Walter et al.[16] defined resistance in several ways: (1) no CR despite no death within 28 days of starting therapy (TRM), (2) as in 1 plus relapse within 3 months, (3) as in 1 plus relapse within 6 months, and (4) as in 1 plus relapse within 1 year. They used data from 4,565 patients treated on trials of the national cooperative groups of the UK (MRC/National Cancer Research Institute [NCRI]) and the Netherlands (HOVON) and on trials of the SWOG and MDACC in the United States. Age, performance status, WBC count, secondary disease, cytogenetic risk, and *FLT3-ITD/NPM1* mutation status were each independently associated with failure to achieve CR despite no early death (*primary refractoriness*). However, the AUC of a bootstrap-corrected multivariate model predicting this outcome was only 0.78, indicating fair predictive ability. Removal of *FLT3*-ITD and *NPM1* information slightly decreased the AUC (0.76). The prediction of therapeutic resistance, defined as primary refractoriness or early treatment failure as indicated by short relapse-free survival (RFS), was more difficult, with AUCs for models predicting primary refractory disease or RFS of ≤3, ≤6, or ≤12 months of 0.75/0.73 (with/without inclusion of *FLT3*-ITD/ *NPM1* data), 0.76/0.73, and 0.75/0.71, respectively.[16] These data indicate that our ability to forecast resistance based on routinely available clinical covariates is limited and argues for the integration of additional disease characteristics to optimize outcome projection in AML.

Minimal Residual Disease

Although the incorporation of the pretreatment molecular information described previously will likely improve prognostic accuracy, the information obtained posttreatment will almost certainly also be relevant. Of particular note are assessments of minimal residual disease (MRD) in patients in CR by standard criteria. Given that AML relapses in most patients, such patients presumably have residual AML (MRD) even in CR. Quantification of MRD would allow broad recommendations for postremission therapy. In particular, patients with low levels of MRD that remain stable or decrease might continue on their initial therapy. In contrast, therapy might be changed in patients with high or rising MRD levels, in an effort to possibly avert subsequent hematologic relapse. Because relapse can only be diagnosed when more than 5% blasts are present in the marrow, the sensitivity of morphologic examination of the marrow for the detection of relapse is only 1 in 20. In contrast, if 30 metaphases are examined, a cytogenetic examination has a sensitivity of 1 in 30, whereas fluorescence in situ hybridization (FISH) typically has a sensitivity of 1 in 500.

MRD can be determined by polymerase chain reaction (PCR) to detect (1) leukemia fusion genes (such as those characteristic of inv 16, t(8;21), or t(15;17)); (2) mutations (e.g., in *NPM1*); or (3) overexpression of genes such as Wilms tumor 1 (*WT1*). PCR techniques generally have sensitivities of 1 in 10 (−4). An MRD can also be examined by multiparameter flow cytometry (MPFC), which relies on the identification of patterns of cell surface antigens characteristic of the patient's AML. The sensitivity is 1 in 10 (−3)−10 (−4). Buccisano et al.[20] have shown that patients with *good* (inv 16, t8;21) or intermediate karyotypes who have MRD detected by MPFC (MRD+) at the end of postremission therapy have outcomes resembling those in patients with *FLT3* ITD+ or unfavorable karyotype AML. In turn, patients who are *FLT3* ITD+ but without MRD fare better than those who are *FLT3* ITD+ with MRD. In patients where both MPFC and PCR are applicable, data suggest PCR is more sensitive and specific. It remains to be established whether blood can be used rather than bone marrow, whether MRD should be assessed at multiple time points (e.g., CR, immediately after completion of post remission therapy and beyond), what levels of MRD should motivate a change in therapy and whether these levels are reproducible at different centers, and critically, whether a reduction in MRD will lead to better relapse-free or overall survival rather than MRD merely being a surrogate of refractory AML.

Treatment of Newly Diagnosed Acute Myelogenous Leukemia

Treatment of AML begins with induction chemotherapy, with the goal of achieving CR with a resolution of morphologically detectable disease and the restoration of normal blood counts. This is followed by postremission therapy to eradicate MRD. Both chemotherapy and HSCT have been utilized, and each approach has a major role in the treatment of this disease. An AML cure occurs in only a minority of patients with available forms of chemotherapy. HSCT has a greater antileukemia effect but is associated with higher TRM.

Regardless of a patient's age, the initial goal in treating AML is to produce a CR, defined as a marrow with less than 5% myeloblasts, a neutrophil count greater than 1,000/μL, and a platelet count greater than 100,000/μL.[21,22] When successful, induction therapy preferentially targets AML blasts, thus allowing normal blasts to resume control of hematopoiesis. Obtaining CR is critical because, at least in the past, only patients who do so have a chance of potential cure. An operational definition of potential cure is a remission lasting 2 to 3 years, after which the risk of relapse declines sharply to less than 10%.[23] Responses less than CR are now recognized: CRp for which the criteria are the same as CR except that the platelet count can be <100,000/μL, although platelet transfusions are not being given,[21] and CRi for which no blood count minima are specified, however, the marrow must be reasonably cellular (e.g., least 200 cells must be counted)[21] because if such were not the case, a CRi could be produced in any patient by simply rendering the marrow hypoplastic with high doses of cytotoxic chemotherapy. It remains unclear whether CRp or CRi will prolong survival to the same extent as CR.[24] It is known that CRp and CRi are more likely to be associated with MRD than CR.[25] However, following treatments where CR is perhaps more likely to be associated with MRD (e.g., after use of lower intensity treatments such as azacitidine or decitabine), there may be less value to obtaining a CR.[25]

Prolongation of the initial response has traditionally entailed further chemotherapy, typically two to four courses of *consolidation* with or without subsequent prolonged lower dose *maintenance*. However, several randomized studies suggest that maintenance chemotherapy, although occasionally prolonging remissions, does not lengthen survival.[26] These results have spurred interest in development of new approaches. In particular, recent years have seen the advent of targeted therapy. Although, as described previously, successful chemotherapy is itself selectively toxic to AML blasts, targeted therapy is taken to mean therapy that, although perhaps less toxic to AML blasts than chemotherapy, is much less toxic than chemotherapy to normal blasts and to gastrointestinal epithelium, damage to which can lead to sepsis and death. However, as noted previously, the main problem in AML is overcoming resistance, even in patients in their 70s.[27,28] It is axiomatic that therapy depends on the prognosis. Accordingly, we will discuss induction and postremission therapy according to the patient's prognostic group with standard therapy, as determined by the ELN classification system (see Table 107.2) and within each group note modifications that might be made for patients whose prognosis might differ from that of the group as a whole (e.g., older patients). The focus will be on the choice between standard therapy, now including decitabine and azacitidine, which are widely used in the treatment of older patients, and investigational treatment.

European Leukemia Net Favorable Prognosis Patients

Remission induction should typically consist of 3 days (days 1 through 3) of drugs, such as daunorubicin or idarubicin, that interact with the enzyme topoisomerase 2 (topo II) and 7 days (days 1 through 7) of the pyrimidine analog cytarabine (ara-C) at 100 mg/m² daily; such combinations are called 3+7. A bone marrow aspiration is typically obtained approximately 14 days after the initiation of 3+7. If the marrow shows less than 10% blasts or is hypocellular, marrows are repeated, usually weekly, until it is clear that either a CR has occurred or that there has been a reappearance of AML, often best assessed using MPFC, which can distinguish an excess of normal blasts often seen during marrow recovery from chemotherapy from an excess of AML blasts.

Retreatment usually takes the form of either another course of 3+7, the administration of high-dose ara-C, or of an investigational salvage regimen. SWOG data indicate a CR rate of 40% with a second course of 3+7, which competes favorably with previous investigational *salvage* regimens.[29,30] Furthermore, the SWOG analysis could not identify patients more or less likely to respond to a second 3+7 course.[29,30]

Two randomized trials have shown that a daily daunorubicin dose of 90 mg/m² in 3+7 is superior to a daily dose of 45 mg/m² in patients up to age 65 years, particularly in patients with CBF AML.[31,32] A French retrospective study suggested that 90 mg/m² might be superior to 60 mg/m² in patients with CBF AML.[33] The MRC/NCRI in the United Kingdom is currently randomizing patients between these two doses. Although a French trial suggests that idarubicin at 12 mg/m² daily for 3 days is superior to daunorubicin at 80 mg/m² daily for 3 days,[34] there have often been greater differences between separate randomized trials examining this issue than between daunorubicin and idarubicin in a given study. As a result, there is a consensus that these drugs are interchangeable in 3+7, with idarubicin (12 mg/m² daily, days 1 through 3) and daunorubicin (60 mg/m² daily, days 1 through 3) used most frequently.

The ara-C dose to be used during induction has also been the subject of debate.[35] The HOVON/SAKK group randomized 431 adults age <60 years to ara-C at a daily dose 200 mg/m² for 7 days (previously shown equivalent to 100 mg/m² daily for 7 days[36]) during cycle 1 of induction therapy and 1 g/m² twice daily on days 1 through 5 during cycle 2 of induction therapy and 429 similar patients to 1 g/m² every 12 hours on days 1 through 6 in cycle 1 and 2 g/m² twice daily on days 1, 2, 4, and 6 in cycle 2. Idarubicin 12 mg/m² daily for 3 days was given during cycle 1 and amsacrine, analogous to idarubicin/daunorubicin, was given during cycle 2.[5] Subsequently, patients with CBF AML in remission received 1 cycle of mitoxantrone + etoposide, whereas patients with other cytogenetic findings received an autologous or allogeneic transplant. With a median follow-up of 5 years, there was no difference between the two regimens in CR rate (80% to 82%) and, at 5 years, the cumulative incidences of relapse, relapse-free survival, event-free survival (34% to 35%), and overall survival (40% to 42%) were similar between the two regimens. Furthermore, there was no suggestion that any cytogenetic group benefited more from the higher dose ara-C regimen; in particular, 5-year survival rates were 64% to 67% in patients with CBF AML. The latter results seem equivalent to those using ara-C doses of 3 g/m² twice daily on days 1, 3, and 5 during postremission therapy as is often done in the United States. Othus et al. have recently not found an advantage in patients with NC-AML who were *NPM*+/*FLT3* ITD negative according to whether they received during induction standard 3+7 (in SWOG) or idarubicin + ara-C at 1.5 g/m² daily for 3 to 4 days (at MDACC). Both groups received intermediate (1 g/m² per dose) and high (2 to 3 g/m² per dose) doses during postremission therapy.[37] The HOVON and SWOG/M. D. Anderson results seem to indicate that there is no benefit for intermediate- or high-dose ara-C during induction. However, as indicated by a randomized Cancer and Leukemia Group B (CALGB) study, there is a benefit for higher doses of ara-C during postremission therapy after 3+7 induction in CBF AML (3 g/m² twice daily on days 1, 3, and 5 versus 400 mg/m² or, particularly, 100 mg/m² daily for 5 days) or in NC-AML (with the 3 g/m² and 400 mg/m² doses being equivalent and both superior to the 100 mg/m²,[38] although as noted in MRC's AML 15 trial, the 3 g/m² dose can be replaced by 1.5 g/m².[39]

The duration of postremission therapy is also uncertain, although it seems that between two (based on HOVON data[5]) and four cycles (based on MRC/NCRI data[39]) are sufficient. It is likely that determinations of MRD (e.g., using PCR in CBF and *NPM*+/*FLT3* ITD–negative AML[40,41]) will be important here. For example, in patients with CBF, AML MRC/NCRI randomized data suggest that a fifth cycle might be useful in patients who are MRD negative after the fourth cycle, but not in patients who are MRD positive after the fourth cycle. Patients who are MRD positive after the completion of planned postremission therapy might be candidates for further therapy. Given their low risk of relapse relative to the risk of nonrelapse mortality following allogeneic HSCT, a general consensus is that the average patient with CBF, *NPM+/FLT3* ITD–negative AML, or *CEBPA+* AML is not a candidate for HSCT in CR1,[42] although recent data suggest that HSCT is indicated in patients with double *CEBPA* mutations.[43]

There are clearly patients in the best prognosis group who have worse prognoses than the averages reported on trials. These include CBF AML patients age 60 to 65 years,[19] and those with high levels of mutant *CKIT* alleles.[19] Reduced-intensity HSCT is an alternative in the former. A randomized American–German trial is examining dasatinib in CBF AML based on the drug's ability to inhibit *CKIT*, which is mutated in 20% to 25% of these patients and overexpressed in others.[44] Finally, meta-analyses of several trials randomizing patients to 3+7+/– gemtuzumab ozogamicin (GO) 3 to 6 mg/m² once during remission induction have indicated unequivocal survival benefit due to a lower incidence of relapse in patients with CBF (and many with NC-AML) leading to attempts to reintroduce this drug into clinical practice.[45,46] Fludarabine as given in FLAG-ida therapy also appears to be useful as induction and postremission therapy in CBF AML.[39]

European Leukemia Net Intermediate 2 and Worst Prognosis Groups

Even patients age <60 years in the intermediate 2 group have 5-year survival rates of only 20% to 25% and median survivals of less than 2 years, recalling that the ELN prognostic system does not account for the unfavorable effect of secondary AML.[22] Hence, these patients, particularly those in the worst group, are considered prime candidates for clinical trials.[22] Although it is not unreasonable to use 3+7 for induction and to begin the trial once in CR, it is noteworthy that differences in induction therapy can affect relapse[45–47] and, accordingly, survival rates; furthermore, CR rates in the worst groups are generally <50%.[27] Here, we will describe therapies that, although not likely better than standard, are in common clinical use.

Dose Intensification

Generally, intensification of an ara-C dose (e.g., to 3 g/m² every 12 hours on days 1, 3, and 5) during postremission therapy has not improved outcomes in intermediate 2 or the worst patients,[38] or if improving it "statistically," it has improved it only minimally (e.g., *p* = 0.02, but from zero to only 13% 5-year survival in the HOVON trial).[5]

Clofarabine, Cladribine, and Fludarabine

The MRC/NCRI group has conducted two randomized trials involving clofarabine. Older patients considered fit for intensive therapy had similar outcomes whether given clofarabine + daunorubicin or daunorubicin + 10 days of standard dose ara-C.[48] Older patients not considered fit for intensive therapy had higher CR rates but similar survival when given clofarabine rather than low-dose ara-C.[49] A multicenter trial randomizing patients with relapsed AML also found higher CR rates but similar survival with clofarabine + high-dose ara-C compared with high-dose ara-C alone, largely due to more TRM in the clofarabine arm.[50] The Polish Acute Leukemia Group reported longer survival in adults age <60 years with either de novo or secondary AML randomized to daunorubicin, ara-C (DA) + cladribine (DAC) rather than to standard induction DA.[4] In contrast, a randomized MRC/NCRI trial in adult patients age <60 years found that FLAG-ida given for induction and one postremission course was associated with longer event-free survival

and fewer relapses than daunorubicin + ara-C, although survival was similar due to more deaths in CR with FLAG-ida.[39]

Azacitidine and Decitabine

The majority of patients in the intermediate 2 and worst prognostic groups are aged >65 years. It is in these groups that azacitidine and decitabine have found greatest use. It is becoming apparent that results with these drugs used alone rival those with *more intense* therapies, at least in older patients. For example, Quintas-Cardama et al.[51] found similar overall survival (OS) among 557 patients aged >65 years given regimens generally containing ara-C at 1 to 2 g/m² daily and idarubicin or fludarabine +/– other agents and 114 patients given decitabine (n = 67) or azacitidine (n = 57) despite higher CR rates with the more intense therapies.[51] An international study randomizing 485 patients age >65 years, one-third of whom had the worst prognosis cytogenetics and one-third of whom had secondary AML, found median survivals of 7.7 months for decitabine at 20 mg/m² daily for 5 days versus 5.0 months for standard treatment (88% low-dose ara-C, 12% supportive care only).[52] A focus on whether the difference is *statistically significant* (p = 0.037) loses sight of the unsatisfactory results in both arms, with patients losing >90% of their normally remaining life expectancy. An analogous trial involving azacitidine leads to the same conclusion.[53] Thus, a fundamental question is whether results with either drug can be improved. One possibility is identifying patients more likely to respond either based on molecular characteristics or less active disease. Examples of the latter are patients in CR, although use of decitabine to delay relapse appears to have been unsuccessful,[54] or patients with MRD after HSCT.[55] A second possibility is a combination with other active drugs. A combination of decitabine with deoxyguanosine (SGI-110) increases exposure to decitabine but has not obviously improved outcomes to date.[56] More fundamentally, it remains unclear whether azacitidine or decitabine, although known as hypomethylating agents, actually exert their effects via hypomethylation.[57]

Gemtuzumab Ozogamicin

In contrast to its utility in patients with CBF AML, meta-analyses have not indicated a role for this drug in combination in ELN intermediate 2 and the worst prognosis patients.[45]

Hematopoietic Stem Cell Transplantation

It is generally recommended that patients in ELN intermediate 2 or the worst prognosis groups receive HSCT in CR1 as detailed in the transplant section that follows.

ELN Intermediate 1 Prognosis Group

Here, the decision between the relatively standard approaches discussed for the favorable group and the emphasis on clinical trials stressed in the last section is more difficult. It is perhaps, at times, best to defer this decision to the patient; experience suggests that given the same prognostic data following use of standard therapies, some patients will prefer these, whereas others prefer a trial. Here, the need for new prognostic information is most acute and there might be great use in incorporating posttreatment information into the decision; examples include time or courses to CR,[58] achievement of CRp/CRi rather than CR,[24] or MRD measured by MPFC[20] or PCR for *NPM1*[41] or *WT1*.[59] The use of FLAG-ida might be considered because its ability to decrease high relapse rates relative to CBF AML might justify the increased incidence of death in CR associated with its use.[39] Transplantation in CR1 is often suggested, although it is possible that, provided CR rates after relapse are in the 50% range (much more likely than in the ELN intermediate 2 and the worst groups), a strategy of delaying HSCT until the second CR may be reasonable.[60]

Although their prognosis is, on average, worse than others in the ELN intermediate 1 group, patients with *FLT3* ITDs are currently included in this group (see Table 107.2). They often present with a high WBC count, usually have NC-AML, although t(6;9) AML is very specific for *FLT3* ITDs, and, although having CR rates similar to others with NC-AML, are prone to relapse.[61] The abnormal tyrosine kinase activity associated with *FLT3* ITDs can be inhibited by various drugs (tyrosine-kinase inhibitors [TKI]). Used alone, *FLT3* inhibitors have limited activity in relapsed/refractory AML, with quizartinib being the most effective, producing *composite CR* rates of about 50%, with >90% of the responses being CRi rather than CR or CRp. However, this response rate has allowed 25% to 35% of patients given quizartinib to subsequently receive HSCT.[62] It is uncertain whether the failure of count recovery, and hence, the lack of CRs reflects concomitant quizartinib-induced inhibition of *CKIT* or the presence of other aberrations in the blasts that are not affected by *FLT3* inhibitors. However, the latter possibility has motivated the addition of chemotherapy to quizartinib.[63] Sorafenib, a commercially available *FLT3* inhibitor, has been combined with 3+7 and compared with 3+7 alone in two randomized studies. In patients aged >60 years the combination produced only increased toxicity,[64] but in younger patients, it was associated with longer event-free but not overall survival. In neither study were effects different in patients with or without *FLT3* ITDs,[65] indicating that sorafenib's relevant mechanism of action may be independent of *FLT3* inhibition and perhaps prefiguring a more general use of chemotherapy–sorafenib combinations. Even quizartinib, presumed to be a much more selective *FLT3* inhibitor than sorafenib, may also have activity in patients without *FLT3* ITDs.[62] As predicted by various genomic studies, resistance to quizartinib is associated with the emergence of new subclones: In the case of quizartinib these contain *FLT3* point mutations whose abnormal TK activity might be decreased by crenolanib, another *FLT3* inhibitor.[66] Although it is generally accepted that patients with FLT3 ITDs should receive HSCT in CR1, *FLT3* ITDs predict for relapse even after HSCT. Accordingly, another potential role for quizartinib, and by extension other targeted agents, is the prevention of relapse after HSCT or even in patients who cannot receive HSCT.

Summary of Treatment Recommendations

Patients with favorable prognoses as specified by the ELN[22] can be treated with standard therapy emphasizing higher doses of ara-C post-CR (HiDAC), although it remains unknown if the same is true in patients considered at best risk based on *NPM1*+/ *FLT3* ITD–status rather than cytogenetics. Older patients with CBF AML and CBF patients with multiple alleles affected by *CKIT* mutations have worse prognoses than average CBF and thus might be candidates for (reduced intensity) HSCT or for clinical trials with dasatinib. The choice of 3+7 rather than a clinical trial for induction in the ELN intermediate 1 group depends on whether patients see their prognosis with the former as good enough to be reluctant to undertake a clinical trial, which might produce a worse outcome. FLAG-ida might be useful as induction and postremission therapy in the intermediate 1 and CBF groups and the availability of gemtuzumab ozogamicin (GO) as part of induction therapy would be useful because the drug clearly prolongs survival in CBF and in many intermediate 1 patients.[46] In contrast, CR rates are often <50% in the ELN intermediate 2 and adverse groups with standard therapy making a clinical trial particularly important, recalling that the choice of induction therapy can affect the relapse rate. The general consensus is that patients in the intermediate 1, 2, and adverse groups should receive HSCT in the first CR. Results with HSCT are still sufficiently poor that clinical trials involving new transplant preparative regimens or the means to prevent post-HSCT relapse should be considered in these groups, as discussed later in this chapter. Given that many older patients will fall into the intermediate 2 or the worst ELN prognostic categories and have particularly poor outcomes with standard therapy, most such patients are candidates for clinical trials, as suggested by both ELN[22] and National Comprehensive Cancer Network (NCCN)[67] guidelines. It is important to recall that the major cause of treatment failure in older patients is resistance to therapy, not TRM. Thus, the use of less intense therapy is appropriate only if the chosen therapy is plausibly more effective, and not merely less toxic, than standard therapy. These recommendations are summarized in Table 107.3. Regardless of specific recommendations, any choice of therapy in older patients must refer to the observations of Sekeres et al.[68] that 74% of older patients estimated that their chances of cure with 3+7 were at least 50%; in contrast, 85% of their physicians estimated this chance to be less than 10%. Although the most plausible cause of this discrepancy is a patient's natural tendency to hope for a favorable outcome, there may also be gaps in communication between physicians and patients.

Acute Promyelocytic Leukemia

Acute promyelocytic leukemia (APL) has a unique pathophysiology and requires special considerations for treatment. In more than 95% of cases, APL results from a chromosomal translocation, t(15;17). This translocation results in a fusion protein

PRACTICE OF ONCOLOGY

TABLE 107.3

Treatment Recommendations According to European Leukemia Net Prognostic Group

ELN Group (see Table 107.2)	Induction	Postremission	Other Considerations
Best	3+7; consider FLAG-ida if CBF	1 cycle of idarubicin + ara-C 1g/m² BID × 5 days; then 1–3 cycles with ara-C as above; consider 1 cycle FLAG-ida particularly if CBF	(a) Dose reductions if treatment-related mortality (TRM) scores > 10–20 and clinical trials if TRM scores > 20; (b) Reduced-intensity HSCT for older CBF patients or those with high levels of CKIT mutation; (c) Trials of dasatinib for the latter
Intermediate 1	3+7, FLAG-ida, or clinical trial	If high level FLT3 ITD HSCT in CR1 using related donor or unrelated donor; if not, using related donor or postremission therapy as in ELN best group	If high level FLT3 ITD (a) clinical trial combining 3+7 and newer FLT3 inhibitors quizartinib, crenolanib, or (b) 3+7 + sorafenib if age <60 years
Intermediate 2 or worst	Clinical trial	HSCT in CR1 using related or unrelated donors	(a) Trials testing means to decrease relapse post-HSCT (b) Supportive care only if TRM score > 20–30

PML/retinoic acid receptor alpha (RARα), the gene for *PML* being located on chromosome 15 and the gene for *RAR*α on chromosome 17. The PML-RARα protein, an aberrant form of the normal RAR, recruits corepressor complexes that inhibit transcription of genes involved in promyelocytic differentiation.[69] Predictors of APL in patients with AML are younger age, Hispanic ethnicity, and obesity.[70] Although it typically has a distinctive morphology characterized by abnormal granules and multiple Auer rods, a microgranular variant exists. The possibility of this variant must be borne in mind in patients who present without morphologically typical APL but with the coagulopathy that is the clinical hallmark of the disease. The diagnosis of APL requires proof of the PML-RARα rearrangement. Although this can be obtained by demonstration of the presence of t(15;17), at least 2 to 3 days are required for test results. Immediate confirmation of the diagnosis can be made by using immunohistochemistry to demonstrate an abnormal pattern of anti-PML antibody nuclear staining consequent to the formation of PML-RARα (the PML oncogenic domains test). If doubt remains about the diagnosis, all-transretinoic acid (ATRA) should be added to 3+7.[69]

APL is very sensitive to daunorubicin or idarubicin and is uniquely sensitive to ATRA and arsenic trioxide. The responsiveness to the anthracyclines may reflect the absence of multidrug resistance gene (*MDR1*) in APL cells,[71] whereas pharmacologic doses of ATRA release corepressor complexes and lead to degradation of PML-RARα.[69] For many years, the initial treatment of APL has consisted of idarubicin 12 mg/m² daily for 4 to 5 days and ATRA 45 mg/m² until CR (AIDA regimen).[69] Use of transfusions to maintain the platelet count above 30,000/μL, serum fibrinogen above 150 mg/mL, and the international normalized ratio (INR) below 1.5 is mandatory. Ten percent to 25% of patients will develop the APL differentiation syndrome (APLDS) characterized by fever, weight gain/edema, pleural effusions, and pulmonary infiltrates; the WBC is often elevated. Steroids (e.g., methylprednisolone 45 mg intravenous (IV) daily with subsequent tapering) are effective for the treatment of APLDS. The principal prognostic factor in untreated APL is initial WBC. Patients with WBC less than 10,000/μL will have CR rates greater than 90% with idarubicin plus ATRA, whereas patients with higher WBC counts will have CR rates of 80% to 85%. Almost all patients who fail to achieve CR die, which is usually related to bleeding in the brain or lung before treatment begins or in the first few days thereafter. Once in CR, patients typically receive three courses of consolidation with idarubicin 12 mg/m² daily for 3 days and ATRA 45 mg/m² daily on a 2-week on, 2-week off basis. With this treatment, at least 90% of patients should test negative using PCR to detect residual PML-RARα transcripts after completion of consolidation therapy; patients who are not have a 50% chance of relapse versus 5% for patients who are PCR negative. The former should receive arsenic trioxide (ATO) with or without GO[72] and an allogeneic stem cell transplant if these measures do not produce PCR negativity. Although many protocols omit ara-C, allowing for the administration of higher doses of idarubicin or daunorubicin, a French trial found superior results in patients randomized to receive ara-C in addition to ATRA and daunorubicin.[73] It has been suggested, however, that this outcome reflected the use of relatively low doses of daunorubicin.

Recent developments have highlighted the use of ATO for newly diagnosed rather than purely for relapsed APL. The use of ATO during consolidation in patients treated with AIDA has largely obviated the need for maintenance therapy.[74] After demonstration by Estey et al.[75] that ATRA + ATO could be used without the addition of chemotherapy to cure patients presenting with WBC <10,000/μL, LoCoco et al.[75] randomized patients age less than 70 years old with WBC <10,000/μL between ATRA/idarubicin (AIDA) as conventionally given and ATO/ATRA as described by Estey et al.[75] With a median follow-up of 34 months, 2-year event-free survival was 87% with AIDA and 96% with ATO + ATRA (*p* = 0.02 for superiority) and 2-year survival was also better with ATO + ATRA (*p* = 0.02).[76] Fever, prolonged myelosuppression, and early deaths were more common with AIDA and clinically insignificant hepatotoxicity with ATO + ATRA. It is likely that ATO + ATRA will become the new standard for treatment of APL with WBC <10,000/μL. The relapse rate appears so low that there is probably no need to routinely monitor patients with PCR testing. Similarly, Australasian Leukemia Study Group data suggest that the addition of ATO to AIDA induction will improve outcomes in patients presenting with WBC >10,000/μL.[77] In these patients, however, PCR monitoring in CR probably remains necessary for 2 years. Attention in APL currently focuses on the discrepancy between results, such as those described previously, in academic centers and the poorer results noted in population-based studies[78]; it has been proposed that the initiation of ATRA upon suspicion of a diagnosis of APL might reduce this discrepancy.[78]

Salvage Therapy

Salvage therapy refers to treatment given for relapsed AML or AML that has never gone into CR (primary refractory). As usual, it is critical to assess a patient's chance for success following the administration of standard salvage therapy, using regimens such as FLAG + ida or mitoxantrone + etoposide + ara-C (2 g/m² daily for 5 days) (MEC). A principal predictor of response to first salvage therapy is the duration of first remission; this has been true even when the therapy used for salvage contained no drugs used initially. As is often the case, consideration of several covariates to assess prognosis is useful.[79] Data presented in the section on transplantation suggest that HSCT should be the first option for such patients, although the possibility of selection bias contributing to results with HSCT needs to be kept in mind. There is also uncertainty as to whether those patients in whom a donor is available should receive investigational chemotherapy before HSCT. If HSCT is unavailable or while a search for a donor is ongoing, patients should receive investigational treatments, including or not including conventional agents.

Hematopoietic Stem Cell Transplantation for Acute Myelogenous Leukemia

Stem cell transplantation provides the possibility of cure for a significant fraction of patients with AML. The approach utilizes a preparative regimen of chemotherapy or radiation with the goal of eradicating the leukemia and providing sufficient immunosuppression of the recipient to prevent rejection of the transplant. There is also an allogeneic graft-versus-leukemia (GVL) effect in which donor T and NK cells act to eradicate malignant cells that survive the preparative regimen.[80] Autologous transplants can be done. Patients initially have their own hematopoietic cells collected and cryopreserved; these cells are then reinfused after high-dose therapy to restore hematopoiesis. Improvements in supportive care, histocompatibility, and tissue matching and development of less toxic preparative regimens have all increased the likelihood of success with autologous or allogeneic transplantation. This section reviews the role of HSCT in the treatment of AML in adults.

Prognostic Factors and Indications for Transplant

Outcomes of HSCT are improved if the transplant is performed earlier in the disease course, preferably in CR, due to less chemo-refractoriness and the lower likelihood of infectious or chemotherapy-related side effects. The major prognosticator is disease status at transplant (Fig. 107.1). Prognostics of patients in CR are significantly better than for those with active disease at the time of HSCT. Similarly, most of the covariates discussed in the previous paragraphs retain their influence in the setting of HSCT, such as cytogenetics and FLT3 mutational status (Fig. 107.2).[81] Secondary

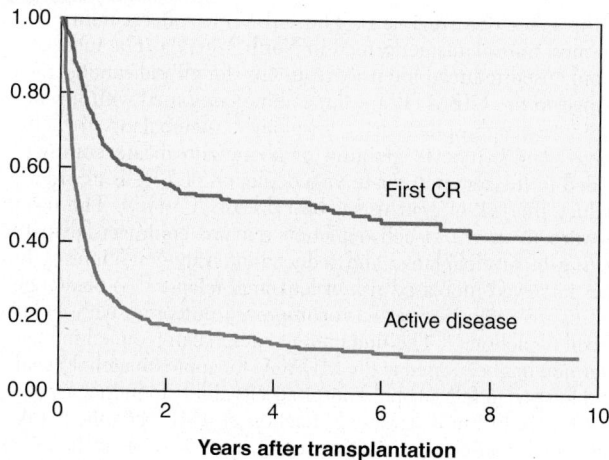

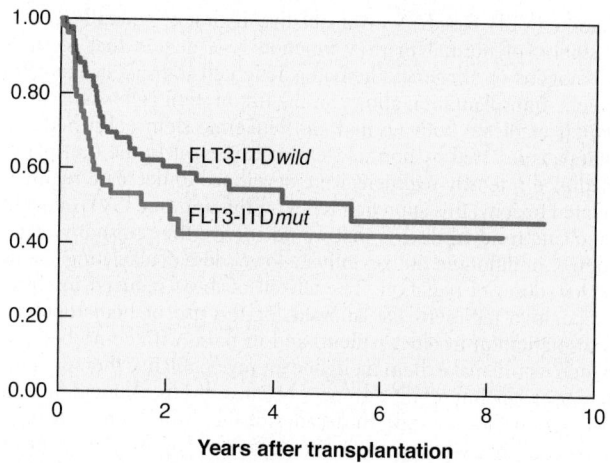

Figure 107.1 Disease status at transplantation is the major determinant of survival after allogeneic hematopoietic stem cell transplantation (HSCT) for acute myelogenous leukemia (AML). Leukemia-free survival (LFS) of 773 AML patients (379 were in first complete remission and 394 had active disease at HSCT) who underwent first allogeneic HSCT using matched related, matched unrelated, and mismatched donors between 2001 through 2012. Three-year LFS were 52.2% and 15.6% for CR1 and active disease patients, respectively. (Data courtesy of Dr. Betul Oran.)

Figure 107.2 The influence of FLT3-ITD mutational status on survival is illustrated here. Leukemia-free survival of 227 AML patients that underwent first allogeneic hematopoietic stem cell transplantation (HSCT) in first complete remission and FLT3-ITD mutation at diagnosis were evaluable. Donors included matched related, matched unrelated, and mismatched. Three-year LFS after HSCT were 56.9% and 42.6% for patient with FLT3-ITDwild and FLT3-ITDmut at diagnosis, respectively. (Data courtesy of Dr. Betul Oran.)

AMLs are considered high risk and the outcome without allogeneic HSCT is generally poor.[82] The presence of MRD is also a negative prognosticator prior to HSCT.[83–85] A large retrospective registry study investigated outcomes of AML patients transplanted with active disease. The authors found that five adverse pretransplant variables significantly influenced survival: the presence of circulating blasts, the first CR duration less than 6 months, the use of a donor other than a human leukocyte antigen (HLA)-identical sibling, a Karnofsky score less than 90, and poor risk cytogenetics.[86] It is generally accepted that fit patients with disease that is primarily refractory to chemotherapy or that has relapsed are eligible for allogeneic or autologous HSCT, as will be discussed. There is, however, controversy surrounding HSCT in first CR. Table 107.4 lists indications for allogeneic HSCT in AML.

Preparative Regimens and Regimen Intensity

The preparative regimen (chemotherapy with or without radiation therapy that precedes the infusion of hematopoietic progenitor cells) provides treatment for AML and the necessary immunosuppression to prevent graft rejection of an allogeneic transplant. Preparative regimens may be chemotherapy or total body irra-

---

TABLE 107.4

Indications for Allogeneic Transplant in Acute Myelogenous Leukemia

Disease Stage	Cytogenetics[a]	Mutations
First remission	Diploid: presence of mutations may dictate decision to transplant	FLT3 ITD FLT3 TKD NPM with FLT3 or ERG mutation MLL PTD Overexpression of BAALC Overexpression of ERG
First remission	Complex; del 5, del 7	
First remission, age > 50–55 years	Diploid cytogenetics: controversial	
First remission, therapy-related or secondary disease[b]	All eligible	All eligible
Primary induction failure	All eligible	All eligible
Second or subsequent remission	All eligible	All eligible
Relapsed, active disease	All eligible	All eligible

ITD, internal tandem duplication; NPM, nucleophosmin; ETS-related gene; FLT3, FMS-like tyrosine kinase 3; TDK, tyrosine-kinase domain.
[a] There is variability in the definition of high-risk cytogenetics depending on the classification used. There is also some controversy surrounding the influence of chromosomal abnormalities involving the *MLL* gene located at 11q23, such as in t(9;11), t(6;11), and t(11;19). Some authors will classify patients with these abnormalities as intermediate-risk disease, as opposed to granting them high-risk status. Presence of 9q and 11q abnormalities may also place patients in first complete remission in a higher than desired risk of relapse.
[b] Secondary disease: preceding myelodysplastic syndrome or chemo- or radiation-therapy induced.

diation (TBI) based. A myeloablative regimen generally causes cessation of normal marrow function to a degree that requires autologous or allogeneic hematopoietic cell transplant. Hematopoietic transplantation allows for the use of stem cell toxic agents, which eradicate both normal and leukemic stem cells; hematopoiesis is restored by normal stem cells present in the transplant. Reduced intensity regimens were developed to decrease regimen related toxicity; this approach relies on the immune GVL effect to eradicate residual disease that would survive the preparative regimen. Conditioning utilizes either a lower dose of alkylating agents or low doses of radiation. The advent of these reduced intensity preparative regimens has allowed for the use of hematopoietic transplantation in older patients and in those with comorbidities, which would make them ineligible for myeloablative therapy. This has been an important advance, because the peak incidence of AML is in the 6th and 7th decades of life. Still, there is controversy regarding which patients should receive myeloablative versus reduced-intensity preparative regimens. The safety of myeloablative regimens is improving, and their use for *fit* patients aged 55 to 65 years is now an attainable goal. Randomized clinical trials will be necessary to resolve this question of regimen choice and intensity. It is recommended that older patients with AML be treated within clinical trials.

Myeloablative Regimens.
The most commonly used myeloablative regimens are cyclophosphamide-TBI (Cy-TBI),[87] busulfan-cyclophosphamide (BuCy),[88] and, more recently, busulfan and fludarabine.[89] The development of BuCy as an alternative to TBI-containing regimens led to ongoing debates as to which conditioning regimen is the best for the treatment of myeloid leukemias with HSCT. Two randomized studies were performed. The Nordic group compared Cy-TBI to BuCy in a heterogeneous group of patients with AML, lymphoid malignancies, and CML receiving allogeneic HSCT.[90] Results indicated improved Disease free survival (DFS) among advanced stage disease patients treated with Cy-TBI, along with an increased rate of long-term complications for recipients of BuCy. Similarly, Blaise et al.[91] studied young patients with AML in first CRs and concluded that Cy-TBI and allogeneic HSCT produced better disease-free and overall survival than BuCy. The major pitfall of these reports is the use of the oral busulfan formulation, which results in unpredictable plasma levels. The Center for International Bone Marrow Transplant Research (CIBMTR) compared the use of oral or intravenous (IV) BuCy and Cy-TBI in 1,230 AML patients who received allogeneic transplantation in first remission. There was less nonrelapse mortality and relapse 1 year after transplant, and improved leukemia free survival (LFS) in recipients of IV busulfan compared to TBI regimens.[92] A prospective cohort study tested the hypothesis of noninferiority of survival after IV busulfan ablative regimens, compared to TBI-based regimens for myeloid leukemia patients (n = 1,025 versus n = 458, respectively). Two-year probability of survival was better after IV busulfan treatment (56% versus 48%; $p = 0.03$).[93] Another retrospective registry analysis performed with the European Cooperative Group for Bone Marrow Transplantation (EBMT) database found IV BuCy to lead to similar outcomes to CyTBI for the treatment of AML in first CRs.[94] Exchanging cyclophosphamide for the nucleoside analog fludarabine may increase the safety margin of the regimen.[95] Fludarabine appears to increase alkylator-induced cell killing by inhibiting DNA-damage repair and is highly immunosuppressive. A preparative regimen using fludarabine and single daily dosing of IV busulfan has been studied in multiple centers and appears to be effective and potentially less toxic than the commonly used BuCy regimen.

Reduced Intensity Conditioning Regimens.
Given the relative insensitivity of AML to the GVL effect, chemotherapy or radiation intensity is an important component of HSCT. There is a trade-off between nonrelapse mortality (NRM) and dose intensity, which may negate the decrease in relapse rates associated with higher dose regimens. The CIBMTR collects information on most transplants performed in North America. The most commonly used reduced-intensity regimens (for all indications) as reported to the CIBMTR are fludarabine combined with low-dose TBI,[96] cyclophosphamide,[97] busulfan,[98] melphalan,[99] or other drugs. Antithymocyte globulin or alemtuzumab are commonly added to the regimen for in vivo depletion of T cells in order to reduce the risk of graft versus host disease (GVHD). The use of in vitro or in vivo T-cell depletion remains controversial in the setting of myeloablative and reduced-intensity conditioning, but the perceived increased risk of leukemia relapse[100] is challenged by reports indicating similar or improved outcomes with ex vivo T-cell depletion.[101] The fludarabine–melphalan reduced-intensity regimen has been used at the MDACC for approximately 15 years, and long-term follow-up demonstrates its ability to induce durable disease control in a significant fraction of AML patients.[102] Likewise, the Seattle group experience of treating AML in first CRs (median age of 59 years) with a nonmyeloablative, low-dose TBI-based regimen achieved a low TRM rate.[103]

Transplants for AML in First Complete Remission.
Although multiple phase 2 studies have indicated that both allogeneic and autologous transplants benefit subsets of patients with AML in first CRs, the conclusions from randomized trials are less clear.[104–107] The majority of studies indicate that allogeneic and autologous transplants are associated with lower relapse rates but also with higher mortality rates in CR (especially allogeneic HSCT). Nonrelapse mortality (death of all causes for patients in CRs) traditionally has reduced the benefit of less relapses after allogeneic HSCT, and most randomized studies did not show statistically significant advantage in survival (Table 107.5). The debate is far from resolved, given that newer preparative regimens (as discussed previously) and improvements in supportive care are reducing nonrelapse mortality significantly. A common feature of these large clinical trials is the fact that, although most patients assigned to chemotherapy will complete the intended treatment, a significant minority of those assigned will not receive an allogeneic or autologous HSCT.

Most studies indicate that the use of consolidation chemotherapy prior to myeloablative or reduced intensity allogeneic HSCT in first remission does not influence survival after transplant.[108]. In the autologous HSCT setting, however, another retrospective registry analysis concluded that consolidation may improve transplant outcomes. Leukemia-free and overall survival rates were improved for those who received consolidation, but the number of consolidation cycles (one versus two) and the cytarabine dose did not significantly affect transplantation outcomes.[109]

The European Organization of Research and Treatment of Cancer—Leukemia Group/ Gruppo Italiano Malattie EMatologiche dell'Adulto (EORTC-LG/GIMEMA) AML-10 trial set out to compare autologous and allogeneic HSCT for patients in first CRs.[107] After one course of consolidation chemotherapy, patients younger than 46 years with an HLA-identical sibling donor were assigned to undergo allogeneic HSCT, whereas all others were to undergo autologous HSCT. In the donor group, 68.9% received an allogeneic HSCT, whereas in the no-donor subset, an autologous transplant was performed in 55.8% of those eligible. DFS was improved in the former group, whereas the death rate in first CR was decreased in the latter (17.4% versus 5.3%). OS was similar, but DFS was improved for patients with poor prognosis cytogenetics after allogeneic HSCT, especially for patients aged 15 to 35 years. Instead, however, the MRC study indicated an advantage in survival for allogeneic transplanted recipients with intermediate-risk disease.[105] In both the EORTC/GIMENA AML-8 and the MRC AML-10 trials, the relapse-free survival was improved with autologous HSCT when compared to chemotherapy alone, without an OS benefit. The likelihood of achieving another remission after relapse was higher in the chemotherapy arms, which led to the similar survival.

TABLE 107.5

Acute Myeloid Leukemia in First Complete Remission: Studies Comparing Allogeneic and Autologous Hematopoietic Stem Cell Transplantation to Chemotherapy

Clinical Study/Type (Ref.)	No. of Patients and Age	Treatment Assignment	Proportion Completing Assigned Treatment	Risk of Relapse	Actuarial Progression-Free Survival	Preparative Regimen	Treatment-related Mortality	Actuarial Survival
United Kingdom Medical Research Council Acute Myeloid Leukemia 10 trial Prospective, genetic randomization[252]	N = 1,602 in CR1 <56 years Tissue typed = n = 1,063	**Donor** n = 419 **No donor** n = 868	61% (n = 257) (allogeneic HSCT) 93% (chemotherapy) 66% (autologous HSCT)	Donor vs. no donor 36% vs. 52% (**p = 0.001**) Auto vs. chemo only 37% vs. 58% (**p = 0.0007**)	Benefit for allogeneic HSCT in intermediate risk cytogenetics 50% vs. 39% (**p = 0.004**)	Cy-TBI for both autologous and allogeneic HSCT(BuCy in 43 patients)	**Donor:** allogeneic = 24% Chemo = 11% **No donor:** autologous[a] = 12% Chemo = 8%	Donor × no donor 55% × 50% (**p = 0.1**) Benefit for allogeneic HSCT in intermediate risk cytogenetics 55% × 44% (**p = 0.02**) Autologous × chemo 7-year: 57% × 45% (**p = 0.2**)
The European Organisation for Research and Treatment of Cancer Leukemia Group and Gruppo Italiano Malattie Ematologiche dell' Adulto (EORTC-LG/GIMEMA) Prospective, genetic randomization[107]	N = 734 in CR1 that received a single intensive consolidation chemotherapy <46 years	**Donor** n = 293 **No donor** n = 441	55.8% (autologous HSCT) 68.9% (allogeneic HSCT)	Donor vs. no donor 30% vs. 52% (**p <0.0001**) **Poor risk cytogenetics:43% vs. 18% (p = NS)**	4-year Donor vs. no donor 52% vs. 42% (**p = 0.44**)	Cy-TBI or BuCy	Death in CR1: Donor × no donor 17% × 5% (**p <0.0001**)	Donor × no donor 58% × 51% (**p = 0.18**)
Dutch-Belgian Hemato-Oncology Cooperative Group (HOVON) and the Swiss Group for Cancer Research (SAKK) Retrospective analysis of three prospective studies conducted from 1987 to 2004. Genetic randomization[111]	N = 1,032 patients in CR after two chemotherapy cycles Consolidation: either third cycle of chemotherapy, auto or allo-HSCT Age <55 years Median follow-up from diagnosis is 63 months	**Donor** n = 326 patients (32%) **No donor** n = 706 (68%)	82% (n = 268) (allogeneic HSCT) 28% (n = 165) (autologous HSCT) No donor group: 8% received allogeneic HSCT from other donors, 65% went to receive a 3rd chemo cycle	Donor vs. no donor 32% vs. 59% (**p <0.001**) **Reduction in risk of relapse was observed in all cytogenetics categories, including poor risk group**	Donor vs. no donor 48% vs. 27%, HR 0.7, 95% CI, 0.59–0.84 (**p <0.001**) Improved DFS was observed in all cytogenetics categories, but was only significant in the intermediate and poor risk groups Age <40 years (HR 0.59, 95% CI, 0.46–0.77; p <0.001) Age <40 years: HR 0.83, 95% CI, 0.64–1.07; p = NS)	BuCy	Death in CR1: Donor × no donor 21% × 4% (**p <0.001**)	Donor × no donor 4-year survival 54% × 46%(HR 0.85, CI 0.70–1.03; **p = 0.09**)

NS, not statistically significant; HR, hazard ratio; CI, confidence interval; CR, complete remission; DFS, disease-free survival; HSCT, hematopoietic stem cell transplant; Cy-TBI, cyclophosphamide and total-body irradiation; BuCy, busulfan and cyclophosphamide.
[a] Two patients died after unrelated donor transplant.

PRACTICE OF ONCOLOGY

Jourdan et al.[110] reported the long-term follow-up results of four studies investigating postremission consolidation strategies conducted by the Bordeaux Grenoble Marseille Toulouse (BGMT) cooperative group in Europe. The donor group (i.e., with the HLA-identical sibling) comprised 182 patients (38% of those who had achieved a first CR); allogeneic HSCT was performed in 171 patients (94%). The no-donor group had 290 patients, of which 62% received an autologous HSCT. The intent-to-treat analysis (donor versus no donor) showed a statistically nonsignificant advantage in overall 10-year survival probability of 51% versus 43% for the donor group. Patients were stratified using the covariates WBC count at diagnosis, the FAB subtype, the cytogenetic risk, and the number of induction courses to achieve a CR. An intermediate risk group benefited from allogeneic HSCT, with longer survival, whereas small numbers precluded definitive conclusions in other subgroups.

Cornelissen et al.[111] updated the follow-up and consolidated the results of three consecutive studies sponsored by the Dutch-Belgian Hemato-Oncology Cooperative Group (HOVON) and the Swiss Group for Cancer Research (SAKK) between 1987 and 2004. These studies investigated myeloablative allogeneic HSCT for young patients with AML in first CR, comparing results in patients with a transplant donor identified versus those with no donor who received conventional chemotherapy. Subsets of patients in the no-donor subgroup were eligible to receive autologous HSCT. The initial sample size was 2,287 patients. Patients younger than 55 years, without FAB M3 disease, who achieved a first CR after a maximum of two cycles of chemotherapy and then received consolidation treatment were considered eligible for allogeneic HSCT (n = 1,032, 45% of the cohort). The donor group comprised 326 patients (32%), and the no-donor group comprised 599 patients (58%). In the donor group, 82% went on to an allogeneic transplant. Patients in the donor group had fewer relapses and longer DFS. Patients with a donor younger than 40 years of age and with an intermediate- or poor-risk profile had statistically significantly improved DFS.

It is likely that some subsets of patients in first CR will benefit more from HSCT than others. Patients older than 55 years have an extremely poor outcome with conventional chemotherapy. Historically, they have not been eligible for myeloablative allogeneic transplantation because of concern for toxicities, but this group may benefit from nonmyeloablative allogeneic HSCT. A feasibility study demonstrated a marked improvement in relapse-free survival with nonablative allogeneic transplants in elderly patients with AML in first CR compared to patients without a donor who received standard chemotherapy.[112] The incorporation of comorbidity indexes to estimate NRM risk have contributed to patient selection as well, and the proportion of patients ultimately receiving allogeneic HSCT is increasing, especially in reference centers.[113,114]

High-dose ara-C–containing chemotherapy regimens, on the other hand, have improved the outcome of young patients, particularly for patients with good risk cytogenetics (t[8;21] and inv16); the consensus is to not perform allogeneic HSCT in these patients while in first CR. An HLA-compatible family donor (an HLA-identical sibling or a one-antigen mismatch relative) is available in less than 35% of the cases. Unrelated donor transplants that are HLA matched using high resolution methods for the HLA-A, -B, -C, and -DR loci fare comparably with matched sibling donors.[115] Interestingly, in the unrelated donor setting, it is possible that donor-derived NK cell reactivity could reduce relapse rates. A study of 1,277 patients with AML that received unrelated donor HSCT indicated that the activating KIR2DS1 gene provided an HLA-C–dependent prevention of relapse, whereas the donor KIR3DS1 gene was correlated with reduced mortality. This information may guide donor choice aiming at relapse prevention.[116]

Autologous HSCT has been proposed and extensively investigated as an option for first CR consolidation (see Table 107.5). The role of autologous HSCT in first CR, however, remains controversial. Phase 2 and 3 studies demonstrate that some subgroups of AML patients may benefit from autologous HSCT, with a reduction in relapse and improvement in leukemia-free survival. Patients with unfavorable cytogenetics do not appear to benefit, and allogeneic transplant is their preferred option. AML patients, however, are very often poor mobilizers of stem cells, possibly due to AML and treatment-related changes on the normal stem cell pool. Reinfusion of leukemia stem cells contained in the autologous graft is a possibility, and gene marking studies have demonstrated that malignant cells contained in the autograft may contribute to systemic relapse.[117] *Purging* describes the various ex vivo procedures that have been used to eliminate these residual leukemic cells from the graft.[118] Preclinical studies have suggested that this strategy significantly reduces the number of clonogenic progenitors. Chemotherapeutic agents have been extensively used for ex vivo purging, but none of the purging techniques have been tested in a randomized fashion, and conclusive evidence of a benefit for purged grafts is lacking.

Most studies of autologous HSCT enrolled patients younger than 50 years old. However, autologous HSCT transplants have also been investigated for patients older than 60 years. The EORTC-GIMEMA AML-13 trial proposed the collection of peripheral blood stem cells after induction therapy with mitoxantrone, cytarabine, and etoposide (MICE) with or without G-CSF, and consolidation chemotherapy with idarubicin, cytarabine, and etoposide (mini-ICE). Patients aged 61 to 70 years with good performance status were eligible. Of 61 patients, 54 (88%) had peripheral blood stem cells harvested, but only 35 patients received autologous HSCT (57%). The 3-year disease-free and overall survival rates were 21% and 32%, respectively. The authors considered this a negative study that exemplified the limitations of dose intensification for patients with AML in this age range.[119] An updated analysis of the multicenter European AML96 trial (n = 586 patients) suggested a role for autologous transplants for AML in first CR. Patients were to be consolidated with allogeneic or autologous transplantation, or with chemotherapy. Patient risk was estimated based on age, percentage of CD34-positive blasts, FLT3-ITD mutant–to–wild-type ratio, cytogenetic risk, and de novo or secondary AML. Allogeneic improved survival in the favorable subgroup, and autologous transplants improved survival in the intermediate-risk group.[120] It is possible that new molecularly defined subgroups of AML patients in first CR might benefit from autologous transplantation, but clear recommendations will have to await analysis of larger patient cohorts and/or historic databases and correlative samples.[43]

A meta-analysis of 24 trials comparing chemotherapy to autologous and allogeneic HSCT that involved 6,007 patients (3,638 patients with cytogenetics information), remission-free survival benefit was observed for poor-risk (hazard ratio [HR], 0.69; 95% confidence interval [CI], 0.57 to 0.84) and intermediate-risk AML (HR, 0.76; 95% CI, 0.68 to 0.85) but not for good-risk disease (HR 1.06; 95% CI, 0.80 to 1.42). Similar results were obtained in the OS analysis. Allogeneic HSCT improved survival for poor-risk (HR 0.73; 95% CI, 0.59 to 0.90) and intermediate-risk AML (HR 0.83; 95% CI, 0.74 to 0.93) but not for good-risk AML (HR 1.07; 95% CI, 0.83 to 1.38). The use of autologous HSCT was not associated with improved outcomes.[121] Therefore, considering that TRM has decreased substantially in the context of allogeneic HSCT, this approach is considered in all adult patients up to age 75 years in first CR who do not have good risk cytogenetics if a sibling or a molecularly matched unrelated donor (HLA-A, -B, -C, -DRB1, -DQB1) is available (see Table 107.5). The decision to proceed to HSCT in first CR should take into account disease and patient-related factors, as well as donor source and expected TRM. It has been proposed that allogeneic HSCT should be considered in situations where DFS is expected to be improved by at least 10%.[122]

Transplantation for Acute Myelogenous Leukemia in Relapse and Primary Induction Failure. Outcomes of relapsing AML patients are influenced to a large extent by the duration of the first CR. First remissions shorter than 6 months and failure to achieve a CR with initial therapy (primary induction failure) are associated with a likelihood of CR of less than 10% to 20%. Patients relapsing within the first year of remission that fail to respond to the first salvage attempt are, for practical purposes, incurable with standard chemotherapy regimens. Autologous HSCT has been used to treat relapsed and refractory patients, but with poor results. Allogeneic HSCT is considered the treatment of choice for AML in primary induction failure or beyond the first CR, resulting in long-term disease-free survival in 20% to 40% of patients.[123] Results of allogeneic and autologous HSCT are generally better if performed in the second CR as opposed to during an active relapse. However, results were comparable in patients in early relapse versus second remission if one can proceed promptly with HSCT.[124]

Armistead et al.[125] performed a retrospective review to evaluate all relapsed AML patients treated at MDACC between 1995 and 2004. Median age was 58 years, and 59% of the patients had poor risk cytogenetics. After removing patients who died from their initial salvage therapy or who received a stem cell transplant as their first salvage regimen, the survival outcomes from 490 patients (130 of whom were transplanted) were analyzed. This cohort was divided into the 113 patients who achieved a second CR and the 377 who did not. In both groups, the patients who underwent allogeneic HSCT had a statistically significant survival benefit compared to those who did not. In patients who achieved a second CR, 2-year overall survival was 45% versus 20% for patients who did not undergo transplant after achieving a second CR ($p = 0.005$). For the relapsed refractory group, 2-year OS in the transplant cohort was 13% versus zero for the nontransplanted patients ($p < 0.001$).[125]

The value of salvage chemotherapy prior to transplant is controversial. As indicated previously, patients in second CR have a better prognosis after HSCT than those transplanted in relapse in most studies. On the other hand, early and more indolent relapses should probably be treated with allogeneic transplantation as soon as possible, assuming that an acceptable donor is readily available. A patient who had a remission duration of 6 months or less is unlikely to enter second remission with chemotherapy, which may be needed, however, given the speed of progression or other problems that may preclude allogeneic HSCT in a timely fashion. Patients transplanted in second CR will have long-term disease control in 20% to 60% of the cases with HSCT, whereas patients transplanted in primary induction failure will benefit in 10% to 30% of the cases. The cure rate for patients in first and subsequent relapses is in the 10% to 30% range and, as expected, refractory relapses comprise the worse subgroup.

Alternative Donor Transplantation. As discussed previously, many patients lack an HLA-compatible related or unrelated donor. It is often necessary to proceed to transplantation urgently, and unrelated donor searches typically require several months to identify a donor. Therefore, alternative approaches have been studied, including unrelated umbilical cord blood (CB) transplants or related haploidentical grafts.

Cord blood is a rich source of hematopoietic stem cells for transplantation. The number of cells is approximately 1 log fewer than in a typical bone marrow harvest, but CB transplants are associated with less severe GVHD. This has allowed for the successful use of cord blood transplants from donors mismatched for up to two of the HLA-A and -B (intermediate resolution) and -DR loci (high-resolution typing). As the number of transplants reported to the international registries increases, the importance of high-resolution typing for class I HLA genes is also becoming clearer.[126] Given the lower cell dose, cord blood transplants are associated with slower engraftment, particularly in adults. Results of retrospective studies are similar to those with unrelated donor bone marrow transplants in selected patient populations.[127,128] Although outcomes are better in pediatric patients, cord blood transplants have been used successfully in patients in the 6th and 7th decades of life.[129,130]

A variety of approaches are under investigation aiming at expediting CB engraftment in adults, including ex vivo expansion.[131,132]

Individuals inherit one HLA haplotype from each parent, so almost all patients will have a haploidentical relative available. Haploidentical transplants are associated with a high risk of graft rejection and GVHD. The *classic* approach utilized extensive ex vivo T-lymphocyte depletion in order to prevent GVHD. Engraftment is enhanced by transplantation of large numbers of CD34+ cells. This labor-intensive approach is linked to delayed immune recovery posttransplant.[133] Another approach is the use of T-cell replete hematopoietic stem cell grafts followed by two doses of posttransplant cyclophosphamide, with or without additional immunosuppression.[134] There is increasing preclinical and clinical evidence that NK cells mediate a potent antileukemia effect. Donor versus host NK-cell reactivity can thus be predicted by *KIR* gene expression in the donor and the absence of inhibitory KIR ligands in the recipient (HLA BW4 and C alleles). AML patients who receive haploidentical HSCT in which donor NK cells were predicted to be alloreactive had significantly lower relapse rates and improved leukemia-free survival.[135]

Treatment and Prevention of Relapse after Allogeneic Transplantation. AML recurrence is a major cause of treatment failure. A reduction of early TRM, leading to higher overall survivorship rates, and transplantation of patients at high risk for relapse have led to an increase in the number of recurrences after allogeneic HSCT. There is no homogeneity or consensus regarding treatment of this difficult clinical scenario. Donor lymphocyte infusion, second transplant, chemotherapy, and immunosuppression withdrawal are commonly used with low success rates. CR duration after HSCT is a major determinant of salvage success, as is response to treatment of relapse.[136] The biology of disease relapse is complex, and this is an area of active basic and clinical research.[137,138] The prevention of relapse may include immunologic or pharmacologic interventions, such as the use of leukemia-specific cytotoxic T lymphocytes or the maintenance of remission with 5-azacitidine or other drugs, such as FLT3 inhibitors for patients harboring the mutation. Low-dose azacitidine maintenance of remission is currently under investigation in a randomized trial.[55,139–143]

ACUTE LYMPHOBLASTIC LEUKEMIA

ALL is a heterogeneous disease with distinct biologic and prognostic groupings. Considerable progress has been made in understanding the biology of ALL, which has led to more precise disease prognostication and treatment strategies tailored to specific disease subgroups. This has resulted in dramatic improvements in the outcomes of children with ALL, with cure rates up to 80%. The therapeutic approach for adult ALL is modeled on pediatric regimens, and although initial remission rates range between 80% to 90%, only 25% to 50% of adults achieve long-term disease-free survival. This stark difference in outcome for adults as compared to children has been variously attributed to the greater incidence of adverse cytogenetic subgroups found in adults and possibly poorer tolerance and compliance of adults with intensive therapies required for the successful treatment of ALL. Continued research into the biology of this heterogeneous disease and further development of targeted therapies used in a risk-stratified manner will hopefully lead to comparable survival rates in the near future.

Epidemiology

ALL accounts for approximately 20% of acute leukemias in adults, with increasing incidence above 50 years of age. The incidence of ALL is more common in Caucasians compared with African Americans, with an age-adjusted overall incidence in the United States of 1.5 per 100,000 in Caucasians and 0.8 per 100,000 in African Americans.[144] A higher incidence of ALL has been reported in industrialized countries and urban areas. Finally, ALL is slightly more common among men than among women (1.3 to 1.0).

Diagnosis and Evaluation

Historically, the FAB classification system distinguished three subtypes of ALL based on cell morphology.[11] L1 lymphoblasts, which were small to intermediate in size, were the most common, followed by L2, which defined slightly larger sized blasts, and finally L3, which defined large blasts, described as having a *starry sky* appearance, which were seen in Burkitt's leukemia or lymphoma. This classification system has been replaced by the WHO system, which is based on immunophenotypic, cytogenetic, and molecular information, and consequently provides more precise and clinically relevant disease subgroupings.[12]

Of all cases of ALL, 85% are of B-cell lineage, and the most common form is the precursor B phenotype (also called common precursor-B ALL or early precursor-B ALL); these cells express a B-cell immunophenotype (CD19, CD22), TdT, cytoplasmic CD79A, CD34, CD10 (CALLA), and lack cytoplasmic μ and surface immunoglobulin (sIg). It is found frequently in patients with the Philadelphia chromosome, t(9;22)(q34;q11). A less common type, termed pro-B ALL, lacks CD10 expression and may represent an earlier level of B-cell maturation. Mature B-cell lineage ALL has the immunophenotype of mature B cells with sIg expression and is seen with Burkitt's leukemia or lymphoma. T-lineage ALL accounts for 15% to 20% of cases. This *common thymocyte* type expresses pan T-cell markers, CD2, cytoplasmic CD3 (cCD3), CD7, CD5, and distinctively shows coexpression of CD4 and CD8 and expression of CD1a. A more primitive type called *prothymocyte* or *immature thymocyte* type has TdT, cCD3, and variable expression of CD5, CD2, and CD7, but lacks CD4, CD8, and CD1a.

More recently, using molecular profiling, a distinct subset within the immature thymocyte group has been identified as early T-cell precursor (ETP) with very poor prognosis.[145] These leukemias express one or more myeloid or stem cell markers (CD117, CD34, HLA-DR, CD13, CD33, CD11b, or CD65) in addition to the immature thymocyte markers.[145] The mature T-lineage phenotype expresses the pan T-cell markers, variable TdT, but lacks CD1a.

Cytogenetic and Molecular Abnormalities

Specific and well-characterized recurring chromosomal abnormalities facilitate diagnosis, confirm subtype classification, and have major prognostic value for treatment planning. Abnormalities in chromosome number or structure are found in approximately 90% of children and 70% of adult ALL patients.[146–150] Differences in the frequency at which good- and poor-risk prognosis cytogenetic abnormalities occur in children versus adults may partially explain the differences in treatment outcomes between childhood and adult ALL. These cytogenetic abnormalities are acquired somatic mutations that frequently result from translocations of chromosomal DNA and lead to new aberrant protein products presumed to be responsible for the cellular dysregulation that leads to the malignant state. Deletions or loss of DNA may eliminate genes that have tumor suppressor functions. Gains of additional chromosomes may lead to gene dosage effects that provide transformed cells with survival advantages. As in AML, cytogenetic abnormalities in ALL define unique prognostic groups, as listed in Table 107.6.

Molecular methods are increasingly used to better understand the genetic consequences of these cytogenetic abnormalities intrinsic to the pathophysiology of ALL, as well as to refine prognosis and identify novel therapeutic targets in ALL. Quantitative reverse transcription polymerase chain reaction technology (RT-PCR) allows for quantification of MRD, which is an independent

TABLE 107.6

Common Karyotypic Abnormalities in Pediatric and Acute Lymphoblastic Leukemia

Phenotype	Karyotype	Genes Involved	Function of Fusion Protein	Frequency (%) in ALL		Overall Survival (%) at 3–5 Years	
				Children	Adults	Children	Adults
Pro-B	t(4;11) (q21;q23)	MLL, AF4	Alters HOX gene expression	5–8	3–6	<10	10–24
Pre-B	t(1;19) (q23;p13)	E2A, PBX1	Transcription factor; induction of cell differentiation arrest	5–6	1–3	70–80	30–60
B lineage	t(9;22) (q34;q11)	BCR, ABL	Tyrosine kinase	2–3	15–36	30–80[a]	45–75[a]
B lineage	t(12;21) (p13;q22) or del 12p	ETV6-RUNX1	Alters HOX gene expression	20–25	1–3	85–90	40
T lineage	14q11, 7q35, 7p14-15	Translocation of oncogenes to T-cell receptor genes	Overexpression of respective proteins	40–50	<5	65–75	30–60
B or T lineage	t(8;14), t(8;22), t(2;8)	c-MYC	MYC overexpression	2–5	3–7	75–85	20–45
B or T lineage	del 9p/9p abnormality	MTAP, CDKN2, CDKN2B	Tumor suppressor genes	10	<10	60	40–60
B or T lineage	del 6q	?	Tumor suppressor genes?	5	<10	>70	30–40
B or T lineage	<45 chromosomes			5–7	4–10	25–50	10–20
B or T lineage	>50 chromosomes			25–38	2–10	80–90	40–50

[a] These results include the use of imatinib with average 3-year follow-up.

prognostic factor in both pediatric and adult ALL.[151,152] High-resolution genomic profiling has revealed distinct gene-expression patterns in subtypes of ALL, which may be used to yield insights into the biology of ALL and identify new therapeutic targets[153-159] as well as further refine disease-risk stratification[160,161] and identify genetic markers associated with drug sensitivity and resistance pathways.[162] For example, alterations in the lymphoid transcription factor gene IKZF1 (IKAROS), are present in 70% of patients with BCR-ABL ALL, and some patients without the BCR-ABL translocation; both the BCR-ABL–positive and BCR-ABL–negative patients behave similarly with poor outcome.[163] Importantly, patients with the IKAROS gene profile harbor novel kinase-activating mutations[164] and xenograft models show evidence for response to TKIs.[165] Additionally, activating NOTCH1 mutations are present in up to 50% of T-ALL cases, and the signaling pathways and target genes responsible for Notch1-induced neoplastic transformation are currently under investigation; the nuclear factor kappa B (NF-κB) pathway appears to be one of the major mediators, suggesting that the use of gamma-secretase inhibitors used in combination with NF-κB inhibitors, such as bortezomib, may have synergistic effects.[166]

Mechanisms for drug resistance are also affected by pharmacogenomics, which is the study of how genetic variation among individuals contributes to interindividual differences in efficacy and toxicity of drugs.[167,168,169] For example, hyperdiploid cells accumulate more methotrexate polyglutamates because they possess extra copies of the gene-encoding reduced folate carrier, an active transporter of methotrexate.[170] Associations also have been identified between germ-line genetic characteristics (genes that encode drug-metabolizing enzymes, transporters, and drug targets) and drug metabolism and sensitivity to chemotherapy. Rocha et al.[171] studied 16 genetic polymorphisms that affected the pharmacodynamics of antileukemic agents and observed that, among 130 children with high-risk disease, the glutathione S-transferase μl (GSTM1) nonnull genotype was associated with a higher risk of recurrence, which was increased further by the thymidylate synthetase (TYMS) 3/3 genotype.

Finally, epigenetic changes, including hypermethylation of tumor-suppressor genes or microRNA genes, and hypomethylation of oncogenes have been identified in up to 80% of patients with ALL,[172,173] and insights into these mechanisms provide another area for therapeutic development.[174]

Therapy for Acute Lymphoblastic Leukemia

Treatment for adult ALL is modeled on therapy developed for childhood ALL and consists of remission induction, consolidation, and maintenance therapy and CNS prophylaxis, using a risk-stratified approach. Selecting therapy based on patient- and disease-specific prognostic factors has led to a significant improvement in outcomes for childhood ALL, and the adoption of this approach for adults has had a similarly favorable impact.

Prognostic Factors and Risk Assessment

Classic evaluations of prognostic features in adult ALL have led to five widely accepted features: age, WBC count, leukemic cell immunophenotype, cytogenetic subtype, and time to achieve CR.[175] The presence of recurring molecular abnormalities and detection of MRD are more recently used prognostic features based on increasing data supporting their predictive value (Table 107.7).[176] The presence of any of these features portends a high risk for relapse following standard ALL therapy, and the remaining patients are considered standard risk. Up to 75% of adults with ALL are considered to be poor-risk patients, with an expected DFS rate of 25%, and 25% of adults with ALL constitute standard-risk patients, with a projected DFS rate of greater than 50%.[177] Age, WBC count, and treatment response during induction therapy remain classic prognostic features.

TABLE 107.7

Unfavorable Prognostic Features in Adult Acute Lymphoblastic Leukemia

Characteristic	High-Risk Factor(s)
Clinical Factors	
Age	>35 years
Leukocytosis	>30 × 10⁹/L (B lineage); >100 × 10⁹/L (T lineage)
Immunophenotype	Early T-cell precursor
Karyotype	t(9;22)(q24;q11.2), t(4;11)(q21;q23), t(8;14) (q24.1;q32), complex, low hypodiploidy
Molecular profile	IKZF1, CRLF2, TP53, LYL1
Treatment Related	
Therapy response	Time to morphologic CR >4 weeks
	Persistent MRD

CR, complete response; MRD, minimal residual disease.

Age is a continuous variable with OS, decreasing with increasing age; OS ranges from 34% to 57% for patients younger than 30 years compared with only 15% to 17% for patients older than 50 years.[178] A high WBC count is also a continuous variable; generally, a WBC count greater than 30,000/μL or 50,000/μL for B-lineage ALL and greater than 100,000/μL for T-lineage ALL predict for poor prognosis. Of note, while an increased WBC count holds prognostic significance independently as a measure of tumor burden, a high WBC count may be also associated with increased risk of complications during induction therapy, increased risk of CNS relapse, and association with poor-risk cytogenetic subgroups (e.g., t[4;11] and t[9;22]). Finally, the achievement of CR and time to CR after induction therapy carry significant prognostic implications, with patients who require more than 4 weeks to achieve a CR having a lower likelihood of being cured. The emergence of MRD monitoring provides an even more accurate assessment of disease response. In contrast to children, a decrease in MRD burden occurs more slowly in adults.[151] In general, the presence of MRD, defined as 10^{-4} at any time after the start of consolidation is associated with an increased relapse risk, and the predictive value increases at later time points.[151] Patel et al.[152] prospectively analyzed MRD samples following induction, consolidation, and maintenance of 161 patients with non–T-lineage, Ph negative, ALL treated on the international MRC UKALL XII/ECOG 2993 trial. MRD status best discriminated outcome after 10 weeks of therapy, when the relative risk of relapse was 8.95-fold higher in MRD-positive patients and the 5-year relapse-free survival was 15% compared to 71% in MRD-negative patients. The predictive value of MRD depends on the technical quality of the assay and the frequency of monitoring. There is not yet consensus on the clinically relevant time points to measure MRD or the standard methodology to measure MRD.

Specific cytogenetic abnormalities have a major impact on prognosis. The presence of the Ph chromosome and t(4;11) (q21;q23) has been associated with inferior survival in multiple large series.[150,177,179] Additionally, the presence of the t(8;14) (q24.1;q32) complex karyotype, defined as *five or more* chromosomal abnormalities or low hypodiploidy or near triploidy, was noted to result in poor survival in the analysis of patients treated on the UKALL XII/ECOG 2993 trial; in contrast, the presence of hyperdiploidy or del(9p) indicated a good prognosis.[179] Of note, the t(8;14) associated with a mature B ALL phenotype has a poor prognosis when treated with standard ALL regimens. However, modified ALL regimens, incorporating

CD20-targeted therapy, now result in significantly better survival for this group.[180] Similarly, although the Ph chromosome has traditionally been considered a marker of high-risk disease, the outcome for this subset of patients has greatly changed with the incorporation of TKIs into classic ALL therapy. Reports from studies incorporating TKI into their regimens show a greater proportion achieving CR and MRD negativity, and thus suggesting a better prognosis.[181–183] Finally, patients with early T-cell precursor ALL form a distinct subset of patients with T lineage with inferior CR rates and increased rates of relapse.[145]

Remission Induction

In the remission-induction phase of therapy, the goals are to eradicate 99% of the initial tumor burden and to restore normal hematopoiesis and performance status. Current induction regimens for adults consist of at least a glucocorticoid (prednisone, prednisolone, or dexamethasone), vincristine, and an anthracycline, with expected remission rates of 72% to 92% and a median remission duration of 18 months (Table 107.8). Dexamethasone has replaced prednisone based on better in vitro antileukemic activity and higher drug levels in the CSF.[184] The German multicenter study group for ALL (GMALL) noted decreased early mortality when dexamethasone was given in an interrupted schedule rather than continuously.[185] The most commonly used anthracycline is daunorubicin, and attempts have been made to increase the dosage, with no clear benefit noted, possibly due to the increased hematologic toxicity.[186] Intensification of the induction regimen has been attempted with the addition of cyclophosphamide, asparaginase, or cytarabine. Although no clear improvement in CR rates have been noted,[187,188] remission duration may be improved in some ALL subtypes (e.g., cytarabine in T-ALL, cyclophosphamide in mature B ALL). Additionally, treatment intensification specifically for patients in the adolescent age range (e.g., 15 to 20 years old) appears to result in better outcomes with survival rates nearing those of pediatric patients.[189] The use of targeted therapies during induction (e.g., rituximab for mature B ALL and imatinib for Ph + ALL) has improved CR rates for these subtypes of ALL. Finally, supportive care is of great importance during this period. Treatment-related early deaths occur in up to 10% of patients,

and significant comorbidities, such fungal infections, occur as a consequence of prolonged cytopenia. The use of growth factors lessens the regimen-induced myelosuppression and may allow for the timely administration of treatment. In a randomized trial, the use of G-CSF during induction was associated with faster recovery of neutrophils and decreased hospital stay.[190] In the G-CSF treated group, the CR rate was higher (90% versus 81%; $p = 0.10$), and the rate of induction deaths was lower (4% versus 11%; $p = 0.04$).

Consolidation Therapy

Once in remission, the consolidation is administered at a relatively higher level of intensity in efforts to further reduce the leukemic burden and decrease the likelihood of relapse. Consolidation may include rotational consolidation programs, modified induction regimens, or HSCT. Most regimens include methotrexate, cytarabine, cyclophosphamide, and asparaginase. But it is difficult to compare regimens as the number and schedule of the chemotherapy agents used vary. Results from the UKALL XA, GIMEMA ALL 0288, and PETHEMA (Programa para el Estudio de la Terapéutica en Hemopatía Maligna) ALL-89 multicenter randomized trials failed to demonstrate a benefit for intensification in terms of prolonging OS and DFS.[186,191,192] However, more recent nonrandomized studies and regimens using a risk-adapted strategy indicate that intensive consolidation may improve outcome.

In the CALGB 8811 study, the induction course consisted of a five-drug combination and was followed by early and late intensification courses with eight drugs.[193] This regimen improved the median duration of CR and median survival to 29 and 36 months, respectively—considerably better than results with earlier trials.[193] A dose-intense regimen of hyperfractionated cyclophosphamide, vincristine, doxorubicin, and dexamethasone (hyper-CVAD), alternating with high doses of cytarabine and methotrexate, led to significantly higher CR rates and survival ($p < 0.01$)[187] when compared to the less-intense vincristine, doxorubicin, dexamethasone (VAD) regimen,[194] with an OS of 38% at 5 years.

Finally, the GMALL 05/93 study intensified consolidation in a subtype-specific manner. High-dose methotrexate was used in standard-risk B-lineage ALL, high-dose methotrexate, and

---

> ### TABLE 107.8
>
> **Selected Prospective Trials in Adult Acute Lymphoblastic Leukemia**

Study (Ref.)	Year	N	Median Age (Range)	SCT	CR (%)	Early Death (%)	Survival (%)
CALGB 8811, USA[193]	1995	197	32 (16–80)	–	85	9	50 (3 yr)
CALGB 9111, USA[190]	1998	198	35 (16–83)	Ph+	82	8	43 (3 yr)
LALA 87, France[197]	2000	572	33 (15–60)	D	76	9	27 (10 yr)
GMALL 05/93, Germany[195]	2001	1,163	35 (15–65)	R	83	NR	35 (5 yr)
JALSG-ALL93, Japan[201]	2002	263	31 (15–59)	D	78	6	33 (6 yr)
GIMEMA 0288, Italy[186]	2002	778	28 (12–60)	–	82	11	27 (9 yr)
M. D. Anderson Cancer Center, USA[253]	2004	288	40 (15–92)	Ph+	92	5	38 (5 yr)
EORTC ALL-3, Europe[202]	2004	340	33 (14–79)	D	74	NR	36 (6 yr)
LALA 94, France[198]	2004	922	33 (15–55)	R	84	5	36 (5 yr)
Pethema ALL-93, Spain[203]	2005	222	27 (15–50)	HR	82	6	34 (5 yr)
MRC XII/ECOG E 2993, UK-USA[199]	2008	1,913	31 (15–65)	D	91	NR	39 (5 yr)
Hovon, Netherlands[200]	2009	433	29 (15–55)	D	89	7	40 (5 yr)

SCT, stem cell transplant; HSCT, hematopoietic stem cell transplantation; ALL, acute lymphoblastic leukemia; Ph+, HSCT in Philadelphia–positive ALL; D, prospective HSCT in all patients with donor; R, HSCT according to prospective risk model; HR, prospective HSCT in high-risk patients only; NR, not reported.
[a] Median survival in months.

high-dose cytarabine in high-risk B-linage ALL, and cyclophosphamide and cytarabine in T-linage ALL. The CR rate was 87% in standard-risk patients, with a 5-year OS of 55%.[195] Intensified induction and consolidation improved the CR and DFS rates in a subset of high-risk patients with the pro–B ALL immunophenotype, in whom a continuous CR rate of 41% was achieved as compared to 19% for the others.[195]

Hematopoietic Stem Cell Transplantation for Acute Lymphoblastic Leukemia in First Remission

Allogeneic hematopoietic transplantation has a major role in the treatment of ALL, particularly in patients who have recurrent disease or high-risk features (NCCN guidelines). The role of allogeneic HSCT for ALL patients in first CR is controversial. A review of a number of small, phase 2 trials in high-risk adult ALL who underwent allogeneic HSCT in first CR suggests a higher DFS when compared with historic controls based on conventional chemotherapy, ranging broadly from 21% to 71%.[196] Several multicenter, randomized, prospective studies have been conducted (see Table 107.8). To minimize patient selection bias, these trials employed a "genetic" randomization method, offering allogeneic HSCT in first CR to all patients with a sibling donor and chemotherapy or autologous HSCT to patients without a donor. Results were then analyzed using intent-to-treat methods that compared patients with or without donors.

The multicenter French study group Leucemie Aigue Lymphoblastique de l'Adulte completed two large studies between 1986 and 1991 (LALA-87)[197] and 1994 and 2002 (LALA-94).[198] Using an intent-to-treat analysis, a significant DFS and OS benefit was observed for allogeneic HSCT in high-risk patients in both trials. High-risk was defined as having one or more of the following factors: presence of the Ph chromosome, null ALL, age older than 35 years, WBC count greater than 30×10^9/L, or time to CR greater than 4 weeks. The international MRC UKALL XII/ECOG E2993 trial also noted significantly improved survival (53% versus 45%) for patients who received an allogeneic HSCT in first CR as compared to chemotherapy or autologous HSCT.[199] However, in contrast to the LALA studies, this advantage was confined to the standard-risk patient subset (OS 63% versus 51%) due to the high TRM observed in the high-risk group (39%) as compared to the standard-risk group (20%). Of note, high risk in this study was defined as age older than 35 years or a high WBC (greater than 30,000 for B-lineage or greater than 100,000 for T-ALL); Ph+ patients were excluded in this analysis. Similarly, the advantage of SCT was confined to standard-risk ALL in a similar study by the Dutch Cooperative Trials group.[200] In contrast to these studies, no survival advantage was noted for allogeneic HSCT in first CR in three other multicenter, prospective studies.[201–203] In the EORTC ALL-3 trial, although the donor group had a lower relapse rate (38% versus 56%; $p = 0.001$), it also had a higher cumulative incidence of death in CR (23% versus 7%; $p = 0.0004$), resulting in similar survival rates (41% versus 39%).[202] Finally, no survival advantage has ever been shown for autologous HSCT as compared to chemotherapy for patients who do not have a matched related donor.[197–199,202,203]

In addition to the transplant donor, the transplant preparative regimen, source of stem cells, and immunosuppression prophylaxis all impact treatment outcome. TBI remains the standard backbone for myeloablative ALL transplant preparative regimens. The most widely used regimen remains the combination of TBI and cyclophosphamide, although a retrospective analysis of registry data from the CIBMTR suggests that the combination of TBI and etoposide may afford better survival for patients in second CR when compared to cyclophosphamide and TBI.[204] Nonradiation-containing regimens, most commonly busulfan and cyclophosphamide, have been investigated in hopes of decreasing radiation-related complications, with no significant differences noted in outcome.[205,206]

As illustrated in the MRC UKALL XII/ECOG 2993 study, an increasing TRM rate with age compromises the antileukemia benefit for older patients.[199] Because the incidence of ALL increases in adults over age 50 years, transplant approaches with reduced TRM are needed. Reduced-intensity preparative regimens are under evaluation with a goal to reduce toxicity.

The EBMT reported results from the largest series of 97 adult patients with ALL treated with reduced-intensity conditioning (RIC) HSCT and confirmed the benefit of RIC for patients in remission, with a 2-year OS of 52% versus 27% for patients transplanted with advanced disease.[207] Smaller studies have corroborated the benefit for RIC transplantation for older patients with early stage ALL.[208–210] Marks et al.[206] compared transplant conditioning regimen intensity, myeloablative versus RIC, within the limitations of a retrospective analysis in patients with Ph-ALL receiving an allogeneic HSCT in first CR and second CR. Although regimen intensity did not impact TRM or relapse risk in a multivariate analysis, a significantly older patient population was able to tolerate RIC versus myeloablative conditioning (median age 45 years versus 28 years; $p < 0.001$). Thus, RIC merits further investigation in prospective studies.

Maintenance Therapy

Maintenance therapy is administered to patients in remission after consolidation therapy at a low level of intensity, but for a protracted period of time. It has experienced the least modification over time. It consists of a backbone of daily 6-mercaptopurine, weekly methotrexate, and monthly pulses of vincristine and prednisone, generally administered for 2 to 3 years.[211] Attempts to omit maintenance, or shorten its duration to 12 to 18 months, have led to inferior results.[175] However, maintenance therapy is not necessary in mature B ALL, in which a high cure rate is achieved with short-term, dose-intense regimens. The best maintenance regimen for Ph+ patients is not clear but should include a TKI, and is also recommended after transplant,[212] although the duration post-SCT is not clear. Many investigators recommend maintaining the WBC count below 3,000/μL during maintenance. Transaminitis is commonly observed during this period and appears to be caused by the methylated metabolites of mercaptopurine. It is not necessary to alter the regimen because of liver enzyme elevation, because the transaminitis promptly resolves with completion of therapy.

Central Nervous System Prophylaxis

CNS prophylaxis can consist of intrathecal (IT) chemotherapy (methotrexate, cytarabine, corticosteroids), high-dose systemic chemotherapy (methotrexate, cytarabine, L-asparaginase), and CNS irradiation. Despite aggressive systemic therapy, the CNS remains a sanctuary site, and without specific meningeal-directed therapy, CNS disease will develop in up to 50% of adult patients.[14] Risk factors for CNS disease include elevated WBC or lactate dehydrogenase (LDH) at diagnosis, traumatic lumbar puncture, and T-lineage ALL phenotypes. Although some trials still rely on CNS irradiation, most treatment regimens are adopting a risk-adapted approach[213] and attempting to omit CNS irradiation[175] due to its many acute and late complications, including endocrinopathy, neurocognitive deficits, and secondary cancers.

Treatment of Specific Acute Lymphoblastic Leukemia Subgroups

Philadelphia Chromosome–Positive Acute Lymphoblastic Leukemia

Historically, patients with Ph+ ALL have had a poor prognosis, with long-term DFS rates of 10% to 20%.[214] Allogeneic transplantation from a related or unrelated donor was widely used for consolidation, with 30% to 65% long-term survival for patients receiving HSCT in first CR.[215–217] Beyond first remission, HSCT was curative in only a small fraction of patients, with DFS ranging between 5% and 17%.[218]

However, the development of potent TKI of the tyrosine kinase activity of the BCR-ABL fusion product, resulting from the Philadelphia chromosome translocation, has revolutionized therapy for Ph-associated leukemias. Imatinib mesylate was the first TKI to demonstrate significant activity in patients with CML and Ph+ ALL,[219] although response duration in Ph+ ALL was short, with a median time to progression and median OS of 2.2 and 4.9 months, respectively. However, synergistic effects have been observed in vitro when imatinib has been combined with commonly used chemotherapy agents, and a number of studies have investigated the benefit of concurrent or sequential administration of imatinib with chemotherapy. Results from these trials suggest that the incorporation of imatinib into standard ALL therapy results in significantly improved remission induction rates, more patients being able to receive transplant in first remission, and ultimately, better OS rates ranging from 52% to 78%.[181–183,220] Whether consolidation with HSCT in first CR will remain the standard of care for these patients will depend on the durability of the remission inductions, which is currently under investigation. Long-term follow-up of the GRAAPH-2003 study, which incorporated imatinib into its remission and consolidation treatment, resulted in a 50% 4-year OS for patients receiving allogeneic SCT compared with 33% at for those not transplanted.[221] A national multicenter trial is currently in progress in which patients with Ph+ ALL were prospectively randomized to continued chemotherapy or allogeneic transplants in an effort to determine the best route of consolidation for these patients.

The role of imatinib in the treatment of elderly patients with Ph+ ALL is of particular interest. This is a group with a historically poor outcome due to poor tolerance of the standard chemotherapy regimens and disease resistance. Several trials have examined various approaches in this population. Use of imatinib and methylprednisolone alternated with chemotherapy improved the CR rate and OS at 1 year in 30 patients older than 55 years as compared to historical controls (72% versus 29% and 66% versus 44%, respectively).[222] More impressive was a 100% CR noted among 29 patients, with median age 60 years, ranging from 61 to 83 years, who were treated with a combination of imatinib and prednisone only. The median survival from diagnosis was 20 months.[223] Finally, Ottmann et al.[224] conducted a randomized trial of imatinib monotherapy versus standard induction therapy followed by imatinib plus standard consolidation chemotherapy for all patients. Fifty-five patients with a median age of 67 years were treated. The imatinib-treated arm had a significantly higher CR rate (96% versus 50%) with less regimen-related toxicity as compared to the standard induction arm; however, there was no significant difference in OS between the two arms (42% at 2 years).

The development of resistance to imatinib has led to the search for alternative, second-generation TKI such as dasatinib and nilotinib.[225,226] Dasatinib is a dual Src and Abl kinase inhibitor that has shown significant activity in patients with imatinib-resistant disease.[227–229] The significant activity of dasatinib has prompted investigation of its use in front-line regimens. Early response rates suggest a higher and faster rate of molecular remissions when compared to imatinib.[230,231]

Mature B-Lineage Acute Lymphoblastic Leukemia

Treatment of Burkitt's leukemia or lymphoma with the conventional ALL regimens have been disappointing. Short-duration, intensive regimens that maintain serum drug concentrations and minimize treatment delays have demonstrated the greatest efficacy in this disease, mainly due to its high-growth fraction.[232] These regimens incorporate strategies such as the use of fractionated cyclophosphamide, alternation of non–cross-resistant cytotoxic agents between treatment cycles, and aggressive CNS prophylaxis.[233] More recently, the addition of the anti-CD20 monoclonal antibody rituximab has further improved the outcome of patients with Burkitt's leukemia or lymphoma. Thomas et al.[234] administered rituximab in addition to the hyper-CVAD regimen and reported a CR rate of 86%, with 3-year OS of 89%. This was significantly better than the 19% 3-year survival reported for hyper-CVAD alone.

T-Cell Acute Lymphoblastic Leukemia and T-Lymphoblastic Lymphoma

The survival of patients with T-cell ALL and T-lymphoblastic lymphoma (T-LBL) has improved significantly using the regimens designed for ALL, with OS ranging from 50% to 70%.[235] Use of mediastinal radiation given after chemotherapy appears to reduce mediastinal relapse. A proportion of patients with relapsed disease can achieve a second CR and long-term survival with allogeneic stem cell transplant. Compared to patients with B-lineage ALL, the spectrum of genetic abnormalities in T-cell ALL is less well characterized; FISH or PCR testing is required to detect the higher rate of cryptic chromosomal translocations and gene mutations in T-cell ALL. Subset analysis of T-cell ALL patients treated on the MRC/UKALL trial revealed complex cytogenetics, CD13 positivity, and CD1a negativity to be associated with poorer outcome.[236] Greater understanding of the molecular pathogenesis of this subset of ALL has led to the development of novel therapies, such as nelarabine and forodesine,[237] developed specifically towards neoplastic T cells, and gamma-secretase and TKIs developed specifically toward aberrant pathways.[156,158] In CALBG study 19801, 26 patients with relapsed T-cell ALL received nelarabine at 1.5 g/m^2 per day on days 1, 3, and 5 repeated every 22 days, with a median number of two courses administered.[238] A relatively high CR rate of 31% was noted in this heavily treated group of patients, suggesting that nelarabine induces cytotoxicity through therapeutic pathways different from that of currently used standard drugs. Furthermore, the median DFS was 20 weeks, which should allow sufficient time for a select group of patients with a preserved performance status to proceed to transplant (approximately one-third of patients progressed to transplant in this study). These findings were corroborated in a recent German study in which 126 patients with relapsed/refractory T-ALL or LBL received single-agent nelarabine and 36% of patients achieved CR. Eighty percent of the patients in CR subsequently received SCT, with a 3-year OS of 31% for the transplanted patients.[239] The most common nonhematologic toxicity noted in the study was reversible peripheral sensory and motor neuropathy.[238] Nelarabine is also being combined with standard combination chemotherapy to improve long-term outcome in higher risk T-ALL.[240] Unfortunately, many of the commonly used agents for ALL therapy, such as vincristine and methotrexate, also have neuropathic toxicities, so nelarabine use remains limited. Newer strategies, including long continuous infusions of nelarabine, are currently being explored to reduce dose-limiting neurotoxicity.

Treatment of Primary Refractory or Relapsed Adult Acute Lymphoblastic Leukemia

Most current induction regimens obtain complete responses in 72% to 92% of newly diagnosed patients. Early deaths account for some of the induction failures, but in most studies, 5% to 10% of patients have disease that is resistant to the remission induction regimen. These patients often have poor prognostic factors at presentation, and additional attempts at induction chemotherapy may be unsuccessful. Several studies suggest that patients with an HLA-identical sibling benefit if they proceed directly to allogeneic transplantation without undergoing a second attempt at induction therapy.[123,241] In the largest of these studies, approximately 35% of these patients with primary refractory disease became long-term disease-free survivors.[242]

In addition to primary refractory patients, 60% to 70% of patients who achieve a complete response eventually relapse. Numerous regimens have been reported in the setting of relapsed ALL. These can be divided into two main groups: those that repeat the regimens used for newly diagnosed patients and those that involve high-dose, typically cytarabine-based regimens, with no superior reinduction therapy identified. Cytarabine has been used in combination with L-asparaginase, anthracyclines, or mitoxantrone, with responses as high as 72%.[243,244] However, these are transient, short-lived responses, and allogeneic HSCT remains the most effective modality for achieving durable remissions for patients in or beyond second CR. Two large multicenter trials have best characterized prognosis and outcome following relapse. The outcome of 609 adults with relapsed ALL, all of whom were previously treated on the MRC UKALL12/ECOG 2993 study, was investigated.[245] The survival at 5 years after relapse was 7%. Factors predicting a good outcome after salvage therapy were young age (OS 12% for patients older than 20 years versus 3% for patients older than 50 years) and duration of first remission greater than 2 years (OS 11% versus 5%). When survival was evaluated based on treatment strategy, survival following HSCT ranged from 15% to 23% depending on donor type (15% for autograft, 16% for matched unrelated donor, 23% for matched related donor), and was significantly better than chemotherapy only at 4% ($p < 0.00005$).[245] Oriol et al.[246] reported on the outcome of 263 adults with relapsed ALL, all of whom were previously treated on four consecutive PETHEMA trials with similar induction therapies. OS at 5 years was 10%. Factors predicting a good outcome were identical to the prior study: age less than 30 years (OS 21% versus 10%) and duration of first remission greater than 2 years (OS 36% versus 17%). Forty-five percent of patients achieved a second remission, with better outcomes noted in the group who then proceeded to transplant. The best outcome was noted for patients younger than 30 years old with a long first remission duration transplanted in second CR, with an OS of 38% at 5 years. TRM was higher for patients who had received a prior transplant during first remission (TRM 45% versus 23%), but there was no difference in OS. Similar long-term leukemia-free survival rates of 14% to 43% have been

reported from other small series for patients who received HSCT in second CR. As expected, the primary cause of failure is relapse (greater than 50%).

CNS relapse occurs in approximately 2% to 10% of patients who have received appropriate prophylaxis. In the majority of patients, concurrent bone marrow relapse can be documented. Occasionally, CNS relapse may occur without demonstrable systemic relapse; however, this event almost always predicts subsequent bone marrow relapse, and patients with isolated CNS relapse should first receive CNS-directed therapy and then systemic reinduction chemotherapy. Long-term outcome is poor, with zero to 6% OS at 4 years.[245] Intensive treatment, with a combination of intrathecal or radiotherapy and systemic chemotherapy, followed by consolidation with HSCT may improve results.

Several new agents are being investigated in the treatment of acute lymphoblastic leukemia. Among the more successful approaches has been the use of novel monoclonal antibodies alone and in combination with chemotherapy. The anti-CD20 monoclonal antibody rituximab has already been successfully implemented in the treatment of CD20+ and Burkitt's leukemia. A new anti-CD20 antibody, ofatumumab is currently under investigation. Inotuzumab ozogamicin, a novel anti-CD22 antibody conjugated to calicheamicin is also being developed in the treatment of B-ALL and has shown promise. In a phase 2 study of 49 patients with relapsed and refractory B-ALL with a median age of 36 years, the OR rate was 57%.[247] Further single-agent and combination studies are ongoing. A novel T-cell engaging CD19/CD3 bispecific antibody, blinatumomab, has also shown impressive activity in patients with previously treated ALL. In a phase 2 trial of blinatumomab in patients with MRD or persistent disease after induction/consolidation for B-ALL, 16 out of 21 (76%) patients became MRD negative, with a relapse-free survival of 78% at a median of 405 days.[248] Further studies of blinatumomab in the relapsed setting are ongoing. Further investigation into the genetic basis of ALL continues to uncover pathogenic driver mutations and activated signaling pathways that could potentially be therapeutically targeted.[249] Finally, cellular therapy in the form of T-cell therapy is showing great promise in patients with advanced ALL. Patients with multiply-relapsed ALL are showing dramatic responses to treatment with chimeric antigen receptor–modified, CD19-directed T-cell therapy.[250] This approach is being used as a bridge to transplant,[251] and has been evaluated in the adjuvant setting in the form of a preemptive donor lymphocyte infusion (DLI).[252]

SELECTED REFERENCES

The full reference list can be accessed at lwwhealthlibrary.com/oncology.

1. Fialkow PJ, Janssen J, Bartram CR. Clonal remissions in acute nonlymphocytic leukemia: evidence for a multistep pathogenesis of the malignancy. *Blood* 1991;77:1415–1417.
2. Reya T, Morrison SJ, Clarke MF, et al. Stem cells, cancer, and cancer stem cells. *Nature* 2001;414:105–111.
6. Pui CH, Ribeiro RC, Hancock ML, et al. Acute myeloid leukemia in children treated with epipodophyllotoxins for acute lymphoblastic leukemia. *N Engl J Med* 1991;325:1682–1687.
10. Cheson BD, Cassileth PA, Head DR, et al. Report of the National Cancer Institute-sponsored workshop on definitions of diagnosis and response in acute myeloid leukemia. *J Clin Oncol* 1990;8:813–819.
12. Harris NL, Jaffe ES, Diebold J, et al. World Health Organization classification of neoplastic diseases of the hematopoietic and lymphoid tissues: report of the Clinical Advisory Committee meeting-Airlie House, Virginia, November 1997. *J Clin Oncol* 1999;17:3835–3849.
16. Walter RB, Othus M, Borthakur G, et al. Prediction of early death after induction therapy for newly diagnosed acute myeloid leukemia with pretreatment risk scores: a novel paradigm for treatment assignment. *J Clin Oncol* 2011;29:4417–4423.

17. Othus M, Kantarjian H, Petersdorf S, et al. Declining rates of treatment-related mortality in patients with newly diagnosed AML given 'intense' induction regimens: a report from SWOG and MD Anderson. *Leukemia* 2014;28:289–292.
18. Downing JR. The core-binding factor leukemias: lessons learned from murine models. *Curr Opin Genet Dev* 2003;13:48–54.
20. Buccisano F, Maurillo L, Spagnoli A, et al. Cytogenetic and molecular diagnostic characterization combined to postconsolidation minimal residual disease assessment by flow cytometry improves risk stratification in adult acute myeloid leukemia. *Blood* 2010;116:2295–2303.
21. Cheson BD, Bennett JM, Kopecky KJ, et al. Revised recommendations of the international working group for diagnosis, standardization of response criteria, treatment outcomes, and reporting standards for therapeutic trials in acute myeloid leukemia. *J Clin Oncol* 2003;21:4642–4649.
22. Dohner H, Estey EH, Amadori S, et al. Diagnosis and management of acute myeloid leukemia in adults: recommendations from an international expert panel, on behalf of the European LeukemiaNet. *Blood* 2010;115:453–474.
24. Walter RB, Kantarjian HM, Huang X, et al. Effect of complete remission and responses less than complete remission on survival in acute myeloid leukemia: a combined Eastern Cooperative Oncology Group, Southwest Oncology Group, and M. D. Anderson Cancer Center Study. *J Clin Oncol* 2010;28:1766–1771.

PRACTICE OF ONCOLOGY

29. Sudipto M, Sekeres MA, Godwin J, et al. Prediction of CR on reinduction in patients with newly diagnosed acute myeloid leukemia given intensive induction regimens: a report from SWOG and Cleveland Clinic. *Blood* 2013;122:3924.

30. Appelbaum FR, Petersdorf S, Erba HP, et al. Evaluation of which patients get a second course of 3+7 on cooperative group trials for newly diagnosed acute myeloid leukemia: a report from SWOG. *Blood* 2013;122:3925.

31. Fernandez HF, Sun Z, Yao X, et al. Anthracycline dose intensification in acute myeloid leukemia. *N Engl J Med* 2009;361:1249–1259.

32. Löwenberg B, Ossenkoppele GJ, van Putten W, et al. High-dose daunorubicin in older patients with acute myeloid leukemia. *N Engl J Med* 2009;361:1235–1248.

33. Bertoli S, Delabesse E, Mozzicoonacci M-J, et al. Impact of anthracycline dose intensification on minimal residual disease and outcome of core binding factors acute myeloid leukemias. *Blood* 2013;122:2681.

37. Othus M, Faderl SH, Stirewalt DL, et al. Impact of cytarabine dose in the induction regimen on the outcome of patients with newly diagnosed acute myeloid leukemia with or without NPM1 and/Or FLT3 mutations: a SWOG and MD Anderson Cancer Center Report. *Blood* 2013;122:2686.

39. Burnett AK, Russell NH, Hills RK, et al. Optimization of chemotherapy for younger patients with acute myeloid leukemia: results of the medical research council AML15 trial. *J Clin Oncol* 2013;31:3360–3368.

40. Yin JA, O'Brien MA, Hills RK, et al. Minimal residual disease monitoring by quantitative RT-PCR in core binding factor AML allows risk stratification and predicts relapse: results of the United Kingdom MRC AML-15 trial. *Blood* 2012;120:2826–2835.

42. Koreth J, Schlenk R, Kopecky KJ, et al. Allogeneic stem cell transplantation for acute myeloid leukemia in first complete remission: systematic review and meta-analysis of prospective clinical trials. *JAMA* 2009;301:2349–2361.

43. Schlenk RF, Taskesen E, van Norden Y, et al. The value of allogeneic and autologous hematopoietic stem cell transplantation in prognostically favorable acute myeloid leukemia with double mutant CEBPA. *Blood* 2013;122:1576–1582.

44. Geyer S, Zhao J, Caroll AJ, et al. Adding the KIT inhibitor dasatinib (DAS) to standard induction and consolidation therapy for newly diagnosed patients (pts) with core binding factor (CBF) acute myeloid leukemia (AML): initial results of the CALGB 10801 (Alliance) study. *Blood* 2013;122:357.

45. Petersdorf S, Estey EH, Othus M, et al. The addition of gemtuzumab ozogamicin (GO) to induction chemotherapy reduces relapse and improves survival in patients without adverse risk karyotype: results of an individual patient meta-analysis of the five randomised trials. *Blood* 2013;122:356.

46. Ravandi F, Estey EH, Appelbaum FR, et al. Gemtuzumab ozogamicin: time to resurrect? *J Clin Oncol* 2012;30:3921–3923.

48. Burnett AK, Russell NH, Kell J, et al. A comparison of daunorubicin/Ara-C (DA) versus daunorubicin/clofarabine (DClo) and two versus three courses of total treatment for older patients with AML and high risk MDS: results of the UK NCRI AML16 trial. *ASH Annual Meeting Abstracts* 2012;120:892.

51. Quintas-Cardama A, Ravandi F, Liu-Dumlao T, et al. Epigenetic therapy is associated with similar survival compared with intensive chemotherapy in older patients with newly diagnosed acute myeloid leukemia. *Blood* 2012;120:4840–4845.

52. Kantarjian HM, Thomas XG, Dmoszynska A, et al. Multicenter, randomized, open-label, phase III trial of decitabine versus patient choice, with physician advice, of either supportive care or low-dose cytarabine for the treatment of older patients with newly diagnosed acute myeloid leukemia. *J Clin Oncol* 2012;30:2670–2677.

53. Fenaux P, Mufti GJ, Hellstrom-Lindberg E, et al. Azacitidine prolongs overall survival compared with conventional care regimens in elderly patients with low bone marrow blast count acute myeloid leukemia. *J Clin Oncol* 2010;28:562–569.

55. de Lima M, Giralt S, Thall PF, et al. Maintenance therapy with low-dose azacitidine after allogeneic hematopoietic stem cell transplantation for recurrent acute myelogenous leukemia or myelodysplastic syndrome: a dose and schedule finding study. *Cancer* 2010;116:5420–5431.

57. Estey EH. Epigenetics in clinical practice: the examples of azacitidine and decitabine in myelodysplasia and acute myeloid leukemia. *Leukemia* 2013;27:1803–1812.

60. Burnett AK, Goldstone A, Hills RK, et al. Curability of patients with acute myeloid leukemia who did not undergo transplantation in first remission. *J Clin Oncol* 2013;31(10):1293–301.

61. Gale RE, Green C, Allen C, et al. The impact of FLT3 internal tandem duplication mutant level, number, size, and interaction with NPM1 mutations in a large cohort of young adult patients with acute myeloid leukemia. *Blood* 2008;111:2776–2784.

68. Sekeres MA, Stone RM, Zahrieh D, et al. Decision-making and quality of life in older adults with acute myeloid leukemia or advanced myelodysplastic syndrome. *Leukemia* 2004;18:809–816.

69. Sanz MA, Grimwade D, Tallman MS, et al. Management of acute promyelocytic leukemia: recommendations from an expert panel on behalf of the European LeukemiaNet. *Blood* 2009;113:1875–1891.

75. Estey E, Garcia-Manero G, Ferrajoli A, et al. Use of all-trans retinoic acid plus arsenic trioxide as an alternative to chemotherapy in untreated acute promyelocytic leukemia. *Blood* 2006;107:3469–3473.

76. Lo-Coco F, Avvisati G, Vignetti M, et al. Retinoic acid and arsenic trioxide for acute promyelocytic leukemia. *N Engl J Med* 2013;369:111–121.

79. Breems DA, Van Putten WL, Huijgens PC, et al. Prognostic index for adult patients with acute myeloid leukemia in first relapse. *J Clin Oncol* 2005;23:1969–1978.

80. Horowitz MM, Gale RP, Sondel PM, et al. Graft-versus-leukemia reactions after bone marrow transplantation. *Blood* 1990;75:555–562.

81. Schlenk RF, Döhner K, Krauter J, et al. Mutations and treatment outcome in cytogenetically normal acute myeloid leukemia. *N Engl J Med* 2008;358:1909–1918.

83. Walter RB, Gooley TA, Wood BL, et al. Impact of pretransplantation minimal residual disease, as detected by multiparametric flow cytometry, on outcome of myeloablative hematopoietic cell transplantation for acute myeloid leukemia. *J Clin Oncol* 2011;29:1190–1197.

85. Walter RB, Buckley SA, Pagel JM, et al. Significance of minimal residual disease before myeloablative allogeneic hematopoietic cell transplantation for AML in first and second complete remission. *Blood* 2013;122:1813–1821.

86. Duval M, Klein JP, He W, et al. Hematopoietic stem-cell transplantation for acute leukemia in relapse or primary induction failure. *J Clin Oncol* 2010;28:3730–3738.

87. Thomas ED, Buckner CD, Banaji M, et al. One hundred patients with acute leukemia treated by chemotherapy, total body irradiation, and allogeneic marrow transplantation. *Blood* 1977;49:511–533.

89. Andersson BS, de Lima M, Thall PF, et al. Once daily iv busulfan and fludarabine (iv Bu-Flu) compares favorably with iv busulfan and cyclophosphamide (iv BuCy2) as pretransplant conditioning therapy in AML/MDS. *Biol Blood Marrow Transplant* 2008;14:672–684.

92. Copelan EA, Hamilton BK, Avalos B, et al. Better leukemia-free and overall survival in AML in first remission following cyclophosphamide in combination with busulfan compared with TBI. *Blood* 2013;122:3863–3870.

93. Bredeson C, Lerademacher J, Kato K, et al. Prospective cohort study comparing intravenous busulfan to total body irradiation in hematopoietic cell transplantation. *Blood* 2013;122:3871–3878.

94. Nagler A, Rocha V, Labopin M, et al. Allogeneic hematopoietic stem-cell transplantation for acute myeloid leukemia in remission: comparison of intravenous busulfan plus cyclophosphamide (Cy) versus total-body irradiation plus Cy as conditioning regimen—a report from the acute leukemia working party of the European group for blood and marrow transplantation. *J Clin Oncol* 2013;31:3549–3556.

95. de Lima M, Anagnostopoulos A, Munsell M, et al. Nonablative versus reduced-intensity conditioning regimens in the treatment of acute myeloid leukemia and high-risk myelodysplastic syndrome: dose is relevant for long-term disease control after allogeneic hematopoietic stem cell transplantation. *Blood* 2004;104:865–872.

96. Baron F, Maris MB, Sandmaier BM, et al. Graft-versus-tumor effects after allogeneic hematopoietic cell transplantation with nonmyeloablative conditioning. *J Clin Oncol* 2005;23:1993–2003.

98. Slavin S, Nagler A, Naparstek E, et al. Nonmyeloablative stem cell transplantation and cell therapy as an alternative to conventional bone marrow transplantation with lethal cytoreduction for the treatment of malignant and nonmalignant hematologic diseases. *Blood* 1998;91:756–763.

99. Giralt S, Thall PF, Khouri I, et al. Melphalan and purine analog–containing preparative regimens: reduced-intensity conditioning for patients with hematologic malignancies undergoing allogeneic progenitor cell transplantation. *Blood* 2001;97:631–637.

102. Oran B, Giralt S, Saliba R, et al. Allogeneic hematopoietic stem cell transplantation for the treatment of high-risk acute myelogenous leukemia and myelodysplastic syndrome using reduced-intensity conditioning with fludarabine and melphalan. *Biol Blood Marrow Transplant* 2007;13:454–462.

105. Burnett AK, Wheatley K, Goldstone AH, et al. The value of allogeneic bone marrow transplant in patients with acute myeloid leukaemia at differing risk of relapse: results of the UK MRC AML 10 trial. *Br J Haematol* 2002;118:385–400.

106. Zittoun RA, Mandelli F, Willemze R, et al. Autologous or allogeneic bone marrow transplantation compared with intensive chemotherapy in acute myelogenous leukemia. European Organization for Research and Treatment of Cancer (EORTC) and the Gruppo Italiano Malattie Ematologiche Maligne dell'Adulto (GIMEMA) Leukemia Cooperative Groups. *N Engl J Med* 1995;332:217–223.

107. Suciu S, Mandelli F, de Witte T, et al. Allogeneic compared with autologous stem cell transplantation in the treatment of patients younger than 46 years with acute myeloid leukemia (AML) in first complete remission (CR1): an intention-to-treat analysis of the EORTC/GIMEMAAML-10 trial. *Blood* 2003;102:1232–1240.

110. Jourdan E, Boiron JM, Dastugue N, et al. Early allogeneic stem-cell transplantation for young adults with acute myeloblastic leukemia in first complete remission: an intent-to-treat long-term analysis of the BGMT experience. *J Clin Oncol* 2005;23:7676–7684.

111. Cornelissen JJ, van Putten WL, Verdonck LF, et al. Results of a HOVON/SAKK donor versus no-donor analysis of myeloablative HLA-identical sibling stem cell transplantation in first remission acute myeloid leukemia in young and middle-aged adults: benefits for whom? *Blood* 2007;109:3658–3666.

112. Estey E, de Lima M, Tibes R, et al. Prospective feasibility analysis of reduced-intensity conditioning (RIC) regimens for hematopoietic stem cell transplantation (HSCT) in elderly patients with acute myeloid leukemia (AML) and high-risk myelodysplastic syndrome (MDS). *Blood* 2007;109:1395–1400.

113. Sorror ML, Appelbaum FR. Risk assessment before allogeneic hematopoietic cell transplantation for older adults with acute myeloid leukemia. *Expert Rev Hematol* 2013;6:547–562.

114. Mawad R, Gooley TA, Sandhu V, et al. Frequency of allogeneic hematopoietic cell transplantation among patients with high- or intermediate-risk acute myeloid leukemia in first complete remission. *J Clin Oncol* 2013;31:3883–3888.

115. Flomenberg N, Baxter-Lowe LA, Confer D, et al. Impact of HLA class I and class II high-resolution matching on outcomes of unrelated donor bone marrow transplantation: HLA-C mismatching is associated with a strong adverse effect on transplantation outcome. *Blood* 2004;104:1923–1930.

122. Cornelissen JJ, Gratwohl A, Schlenk RF, et al. The European LeukemiaNet AML Working Party consensus statement on allogeneic HSCT for patients with AML in remission: an integrated-risk adapted approach. *Nat Rev Clin Oncol* 2012;9:579–90.

125. Armistead PM, de Lima M, Pierce S, et al. Quantifying the survival benefit for allogeneic hematopoietic stem cell transplantation in relapsed acute myelogenous leukemia. *Biol Blood Marrow Transplant* 2009;15:1431–1438.

126. Eapen M, Klein JP, Ruggeri A, et al. Impact of allele-level HLA matching on outcomes after myeloablative single unit umbilical cord blood transplantation for hematologic malignancy. *Blood* 2014;123:133–140.

127. Rocha V, Labopin M, Sanz G, et al. Transplants of umbilical-cord blood or bone marrow from unrelated donors in adults with acute leukemia. *N Engl J Med* 2004;351:2276–2285.

130. Eapen M, Klein JP, Sanz GF, et al. Effect of donor-recipient HLA matching at HLA A, B, C, and DRB1 on outcomes after umbilical-cord blood transplantation for leukaemia and myelodysplastic syndrome: a retrospective analysis. *Lancet Oncol* 2011;12:1214–1221.

131. Metheny L, Caimi P, de Lima M. Cord blood transplantation: can we make it better? *Front Oncol* 2013;3:238.

132. de Lima M, McNiece I, Robinson SN, et al. Cord-blood engraftment with ex vivo mesenchymal-cell coculture. *N Engl J Med* 2012;367:2305–2315.

133. Aversa F, Tabilio A, Velardi A, et al. Treatment of high-risk acute leukemia with T-cell–depleted stem cells from related donors with one fully mismatched HLA haplotype. *N Engl J Med* 1998;339:1186–1193.

134. Luznik L, Fuchs EJ. High-dose, post-transplantation cyclophosphamide to promote graft-host tolerance after allogeneic hematopoietic stem cell transplantation. *Immunol Res* 2010;47:65–77.

135. Ruggeri L, Capanni M, Mancusi A, et al. Natural killer cell alloreactivity in haploidentical hematopoietic stem cell transplantation. *Int J Hematol* 2005;81:13–17.

136. Oran B, Giralt S, Couriel D, et al. Treatment of AML and MDS relapsing after reduced-intensity conditioning and allogeneic hematopoietic stem cell transplantation. *Leukemia* 2007;21:2540–2544.

137. Vago L, Perna SK, Zanussi M, et al. Loss of mismatched HLA in leukemia after stem-cell transplantation. *N Engl J Med* 2009;361:478–488.

143. de Lima M, Porter DL, Battiwalla M, et al. Proceedings from the National Cancer Institute's Second International Workshop on the Biology, Prevention, and Treatment of Relapse after Hematopoietic Stem Cell Transplantation: Part III. Prevention and Treatment of Relapse after Allogeneic Transplantation. *Biol Blood Marrow Transplant* 2014;20:4–13.

145. Coustan-Smith E, Mullighan CG, Onciu M, et al. Early T-cell precursor leukaemia: a subtype of very high-risk acute lymphoblastic leukaemia. *Lancet Oncol* 2009;10:147–156.

146. Faderl S, Kantarjian HM, Talpaz M, et al. Clinical significance of cytogenetic abnormalities in adult acute lymphoblastic leukemia. *Blood* 1998;91:3995–4019.

147. Szczepański T, Harrison CJ, van Dongen JJ. Genetic aberrations in paediatric acute leukaemias and implications for management of patients. *Lancet Oncol* 2010;11:880–889.

149. Moorman AV, Harrison CJ, Buck GA, et al. Karyotype is an independent prognostic factor in adult acute lymphoblastic leukemia (ALL): analysis of cytogenetic data from patients treated on the Medical Research Council (MRC) UKALLXII/Eastern Cooperative Oncology Group (ECOG) 2993 trial. *Blood* 2007;109:3189–3197.

151. Brüggemann M, Raff T, Flohr T, et al. Clinical significance of minimal residual disease quantification in adult patients with standard-risk acute lymphoblastic leukemia. *Blood* 2006;107:1116–1123.

152. Patel B, Rai L, Buck G, et al. Minimal residual disease is a significant predictor of treatment failure in non T-lineage adult acute lymphoblastic leukaemia: final results of the international trial UKALL XII/ECOG2993. *Br J Haematol* 2010;148:80–89.

155. Mullighan CG, Goorha S, Radtke I, et al. Genome-wide analysis of genetic alterations in acute lymphoblastic leukaemia. *Nature* 2007;446:758–764.

159. Grabher C, Harald von Boehmer A. Notch 1 activation in the molecular pathogenesis of T-cell acute lymphoblastic leukaemia. *Nat Rev Cancer* 2006;6:347–359.

160. Mullighan CG, Su X, Zhang J, et al. Deletion of IKZF1 and prognosis in acute lymphoblastic leukemia. *N Engl J Med* 2009;360:470–480.

162. Holleman A, Cheok MH, den Boer ML, et al. Gene-expression patterns in drug-resistant acute lymphoblastic leukemia cells and response to treatment. *N Engl J Med* 2004;351:533–542.

163. Mullighan CG, Miller CB, Radtke I, et al. BCR-ABL1 lymphoblastic leukaemia is characterized by the deletion of Ikaros. *Nature* 2008;453:110–114.

164. Roberts KG, Morin RD, Zhang J, et al. Genetic alterations activating kinase and cytokine receptor signaling in high-risk acute lymphoblastic leukemia. *Cancer Cell* 2012;22:153–166.

168. Evans WE, Relling MV. Moving towards individualized medicine with pharmacogenomics. *Nature* 2004;429:464–468.

169. Relling MV, Ramsey LB. Pharmacogenomics of acute lymphoid leukemia: new insights into treatment toxicity and efficacy. *Hematology Am Soc Hematol Educ Program* 2013;2013:126–130.

175. Pui CH, Evans WE. Treatment of acute lymphoblastic leukemia. *N Engl J Med* 2006;354:166–178.

176. Rowe JM. Prognostic factors in adult acute lymphoblastic leukaemia. *Br J Haematol* 2010;150:389–405.

180. Thomas DA, O'Brien S, Kantarjian HM. Monoclonal antibody therapy with rituximab for acute lymphoblastic leukemia. *Hematol Oncol Clin North Am* 2009;23:949–971.

182. Thomas DA, Faderl S, Cortes J, et al. Treatment of Philadelphia chromosome–positive acute lymphocytic leukemia with hyper-CVAD and imatinib mesylate. *Blood* 2004;103:4396–4407.

183. de Labarthe A, Rousselot P, Huguet-Rigal F, et al. Imatinib combined with induction or consolidation chemotherapy in patients with de novo Philadelphia chromosome–positive acute lymphoblastic leukemia: results of the GRAAPH-2003 study. *Blood* 2007;109:1408–1413.

184. Rowe JM, Buck G, Burnett AK, et al. Induction therapy for adults with acute lymphoblastic leukemia: results of more than 1500 patients from the international ALL trial: MRC UKALL XII/ECOG E2993. *Blood* 2005;106:3760–3767.

199. Goldstone AH, Richards SM, Lazarus HM, et al. In adults with standard-risk acute lymphoblastic leukemia, the greatest benefit is achieved from a matched sibling allogeneic transplantation in first complete remission, and an autologous transplantation is less effective than conventional consolidation/maintenance chemotherapy in all patients: final results of the International ALL Trial (MRC UKALL XII/ECOG E2993). *Blood* 2008;111:1827–1833.

202. Labar B, Suciu S, Zittoun R, et al. Allogeneic stem cell transplantation in acute lymphoblastic leukemia and non-Hodgkin's lymphoma for patients < or = 50 years old in first complete remission: results of the EORTC ALL-3 trial. *Haematologica* 2004;89:809–817.

203. Ribera JM, Oriol A, Bethencourt C, et al. Comparison of intensive chemotherapy, allogeneic or autologous stem cell transplantation as post-remission treatment for adult patients with high-risk acute lymphoblastic leukemia. Results of the PETHEMA ALL-93 trial. *Haematologica* 2005;90:1346–1356.

204. Marks DI, Forman SJ, Blume KG, et al. A comparison of cyclophosphamide and total body irradiation with etoposide and total body irradiation as conditioning regimens for patients undergoing sibling allografting for acute lymphoblastic leukemia in first or second complete remission. *Biol Blood Marrow Transplant* 2006;12:438–453.

206. Marks DI, Wang T, Pérez WS, et al. The outcome of full-intensity and reduced-intensity conditioning matched sibling or unrelated donor transplantation in adults with Philadelphia chromosome–negative acute lymphoblastic leukemia in first and second complete remission. *Blood* 2010;116:366–374.

207. Mohty M, Labopin M, Tabrizzi R, et al. Reduced intensity conditioning allogeneic stem cell transplantation for adult patients with acute lymphoblastic leukemia: a retrospective study from the European Group for Blood and Marrow Transplantation. *Haematologica* 2008;93:303–306.

212. Pfeifer H, Wassmann B, Bethge W, et al. Randomized comparison of prophylactic and minimal residual disease-triggered imatinib after allogeneic stem cell transplantation for BCR-ABL1-positive acute lymphoblastic leukemia. *Leukemia* 2013;27:1254–1262.

213. Cortes J, O'Brien SM, Pierce S, et al. The value of high-dose systemic chemotherapy and intrathecal therapy for central nervous system prophylaxis in different risk groups of adult acute lymphoblastic leukemia. *Blood* 1995;86:2091–2097.

214. Wetzler M, Dodge RK, Mrozek K, et al. Prospective karyotype analysis in adult acute lymphoblastic leukemia: the cancer and leukemia Group B experience. *Blood* 1999;93:3983–3993.

215. Laport GG, Alvarnas JC, Palmer JM, et al. Long-term remission of Philadelphia chromosome–positive acute lymphoblastic leukemia after allogeneic hematopoietic cell transplantation from matched sibling donors: a 20-year experience with the fractionated total body irradiation–etoposide regimen. *Blood* 2008;112:903–909.

217. Fielding AK, Rowe JM, Richards SM, et al. Prospective outcome data on 267 unselected adult patients with Philadelphia chromosome–positive acute lymphoblastic leukemia confirms superiority of allogeneic transplantation over chemotherapy in the pre-imatinib era: results from the International ALL Trial MRC UKALLXII/ECOG2993. *Blood* 2009;113:4489–4496.

221. Tanguy-Schmidt A, Rousselot P, Chalandon Y, et al. Long-term follow-up of the imatinib GRAAPH-2003 study in newly diagnosed patients with de novo Philadelphia chromosome-positive acute lymphoblastic leukemia: a GRAALL study. *Biol Blood Marrow Transplant* 2013;19:150–155.

230. Ravandi F, O'Brien S, Thomas D, et al. First report of phase 2 study of dasatinib with hyper-CVAD for the frontline treatment of patients with Philadelphia chromosome–positive (Ph+) acute lymphoblastic leukemia. *Blood* 2010;116:2070–2077.

231. Ravandi F, Jorgensen JL, Thomas DA, et al. Detection of MRD may predict the outcome of patients with Philadelphia chromosome-positive ALL

treated with tyrosine kinase inhibitors plus chemotherapy. *Blood* 2013;122:1214–1221.

236. Marks DI, Paietta EM, Moorman AV, et al. T-cell acute lymphoblastic leukemia in adults: clinical features, immunophenotype, cytogenetics, and outcome from the large randomized prospective trial (UKALL XII/ECOG 2993). *Blood* 2009;114:5136–5145.

241. Terwey T, Massenkeil G, Tamm I, et al. Allogeneic SCT in refractory or relapsed adult ALL is effective without prior reinduction chemotherapy. *Bone Marrow Transplant* 2008;42:791–798.

245. Fielding AK, Richards SM, Chopra R, et al. Outcome of 609 adults after relapse of acute lymphoblastic leukemia (ALL); an MRC UKALL12/ECOG 2993 study. *Blood* 2007;109:944–950.

247. Kantarjian H, Thomas D, Jorgensen J, et al. Inotuzumab ozogamicin, an anti-CD22-calecheamicin conjugate, for refractory and relapsed acute lymphocytic leukaemia: a phase 2 study. *Lancet Oncol* 2012;13:403–411.

248. Topp MS, Kufer P, Gokbuget N, et al. Targeted therapy with the T-cell-engaging antibody blinatumomab of chemotherapy-refractory minimal residual disease in B-lineage acute lymphoblastic leukemia patients results in high response rate and prolonged leukemia-free survival. *J Clin Oncol* 2011;29:2493–2498.

250. Grupp SA, Kalos M, Barrett D, et al. Chimeric antigen receptor-modified T cells for acute lymphoid leukemia. *N Engl J Med* 2013;368:1509–1518.

251. Brentjens RJ, Davila ML, Riviere I, et al. CD19-targeted T cells rapidly induce molecular remissions in adults with chemotherapy-refractory acute lymphoblastic leukemia. *Sci Transl Med* 2013;5:177ra38.

252. Kebriaei P, Huls H, Singh H, et al. First clinical trials employing *Sleeping Beauty* gene transfer system and artificial antigen presenting cells to generate and infuse t cells expressing CD19-specific chimeric antigen receptor. *ASH Annual Meeting Abstracts* 2013:166a.

108 Molecular Biology of Chronic Leukemias

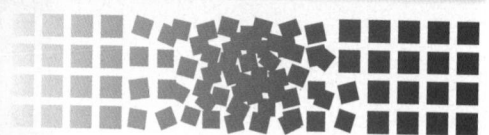

James S. Blachly*, Christopher A. Eide*, John C. Byrd, and Anupriya Agarwal

INTRODUCTION

Chronic myeloid leukemia (CML) and chronic lymphocytic leukemia (CLL) are very different diseases and yet share important clinical features. Both are usually diagnosed in an indolent stage characterized by the expansion of differentiating cells that can last for several, sometimes many years. In both, the acquisition of additional mutations promotes progression to advanced therapy-refractory disease and both are incurable with currently available drug therapy. In this chapter, we will discuss the key pathogenetic mechanisms of CML and CLL, with an emphasis on recent data and potential therapeutic implications.

CHRONIC MYELOID LEUKEMIA

CML is caused by the constitutively active tyrosine kinase BCR-ABL1 generated as the result of a reciprocal translocation between chromosomes 9 and 22. The annual incidence of CML is 1.3 to 1.5 per 10^5, with a slight male preponderance, but no significant differences across ethnicities. The only established CML risk factor is exposure to ionizing radiation, evident from studies in survivors of the nuclear explosions in Japan and patients exposed to Thorotrast or radiotherapy. During the initial chronic phase (CP), cellular differentiation and function are largely maintained, therapy is effective, and mortality is low. Without effective treatment, the disease invariably progresses to a rapidly fatal blastic phase (BP) of myeloid or lymphoid nature.

Pathogenesis

The first cases of what was probably CML were described by Bennett and Virchow in the mid 1840s. In 1960, Philadelphia cytogeneticists Nowell and Hungerford[1] described a "minute" chromosome 22 in CML cells that became known as the Philadelphia (Ph) chromosome. In 1973, the work of another cytogeneticist, Janet Rowley,[2] revealed that this abnormality is, in fact, the result of a reciprocal translocation between chromosomes 9 and 22 (t[9;22] [q34;q11]). The genes juxtaposed by the translocation were subsequently identified as *ABL1* (Abelson) on 9q34 and breakpoint cluster region (*BCR*) on chromosome 22q11 (Fig. 108.1A). As a result of the (9;22) translocation, the *BCR-ABL1* fusion gene is formed on the derivative of chromosome 22 (22q−, Ph), whereas the reciprocal *ABL1-BCR* resides on the derivative of 9q+. A series of seminal studies demonstrated that the constitutive tyrosine kinase activity of BCR-ABL1 is required for cellular transformation and that the clinical disease was reproducible in a murine model.[3] According to the World Health Organization, the presence of *BCR-ABL1* in the context of a myeloproliferative neoplasm is diagnostic of CML, although the translocation is also found in a subset of patients with acute lymphoblastic leukemia (ALL) and rare cases of acute myeloid leukemia (AML).

Molecular Anatomy of the BCR-ABL1 Junction

The breakpoints within *ABL1* occur upstream of exon 1b, downstream of exon 1a, or more frequently, between the two. Regardless of the exact breakpoint location, splicing of the primary transcript yields an mRNA in which *BCR* sequences are fused to *ABL1* exon a2. Breakpoints within *BCR* localize to one of three breakpoint cluster regions. More than 90% of CML patients and one-third of Ph+ ALL patients express the 210-kDa isoform of BCR-ABL1, in which the break occurs in the 5.8-kb major breakpoint cluster region (M-*bcr*), which spans exons e12-e16 (formerly exons b1-b5). Alternative splicing gives rise to either b2a2 (e13a2) or b3a2 (e14a2) transcripts,[4] which are mutually exclusive and present in 36% and 64% of patients, respectively. Patients with b3a2 rearrangements are, on average, older than patients with b2a2 transcripts and have elevated platelet levels.[5] The remainder of Ph+ ALL patients and rare CML cases harbor breakpoints further upstream in the 54.4-kb minor breakpoint cluster region (m-*bcr*), generating an e1a2 transcript that is translated into p190$^{BCR-ABL1}$.[6] A third breakpoint downstream of exon 19 in the micro breakpoint cluster region (μ-*bcr*) gives rise to an e19a2 *BCR-ABL1* mRNA and p230$^{BCR-ABL1}$ and is associated with neutrophilia. The reciprocal *ABL1-BCR* transcript, although detectable in approximately two-thirds of patients, does not seem to play any significant role in pathogenesis.[7]

Functional Domains of BCR-ABL1 and Kinase Activation

p210$^{BCR-ABL1}$ contains several distinct domains (Fig. 108.1B).[8] The N-terminal coiled-coil domain of BCR allows BCR-ABL1 dimerization, which is critical for kinase activation. The p210$^{BCR-ABL1}$ protein also retains the serine/threonine kinase and Rho guanine nucleotide exchange factor homology (Rho-GEF) domains of BCR, which are deleted in p190$^{BCR-ABL1}$, which may explain differences in disease phenotype associated with the two variants. In contrast to BCR, the ABL1 sequence is almost completely retained, including SRC homology domains 2 and 3, the tyrosine–kinase domain, a proline-rich sequence, and a large C terminus with nuclear localization signal, DNA-binding, and actin-binding domains. The N-terminal "cap" region of ABL1, which is lost in the BCR-ABL1 fusion, negatively regulates kinase activity by binding to a hydrophobic pocket at the base of the kinase domain, which, in the 1b isoform, is mediated by N-terminal myristoylation.

Signal Transduction

Numerous substrates and binding partners of BCR-ABL1 have been identified (see Fig. 108.1B) that contribute to increased proliferation, decreased apoptosis, defective adhesion to bone marrow stroma, and genetic instability.[9] Because a comprehensive review of the multiple implicated pathways is beyond the scope of this chapter, we will focus on those for which strong evidence supports a rate-limiting role in disease pathogenesis.

*Share equal contribution.

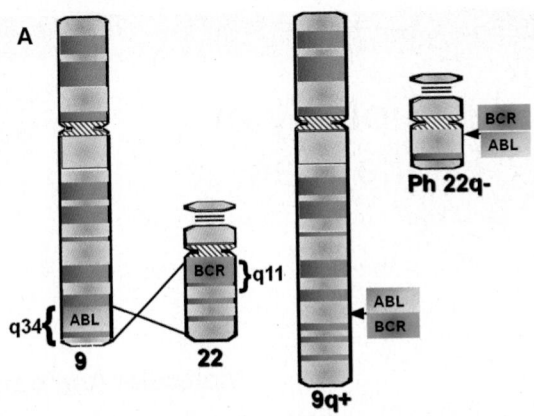

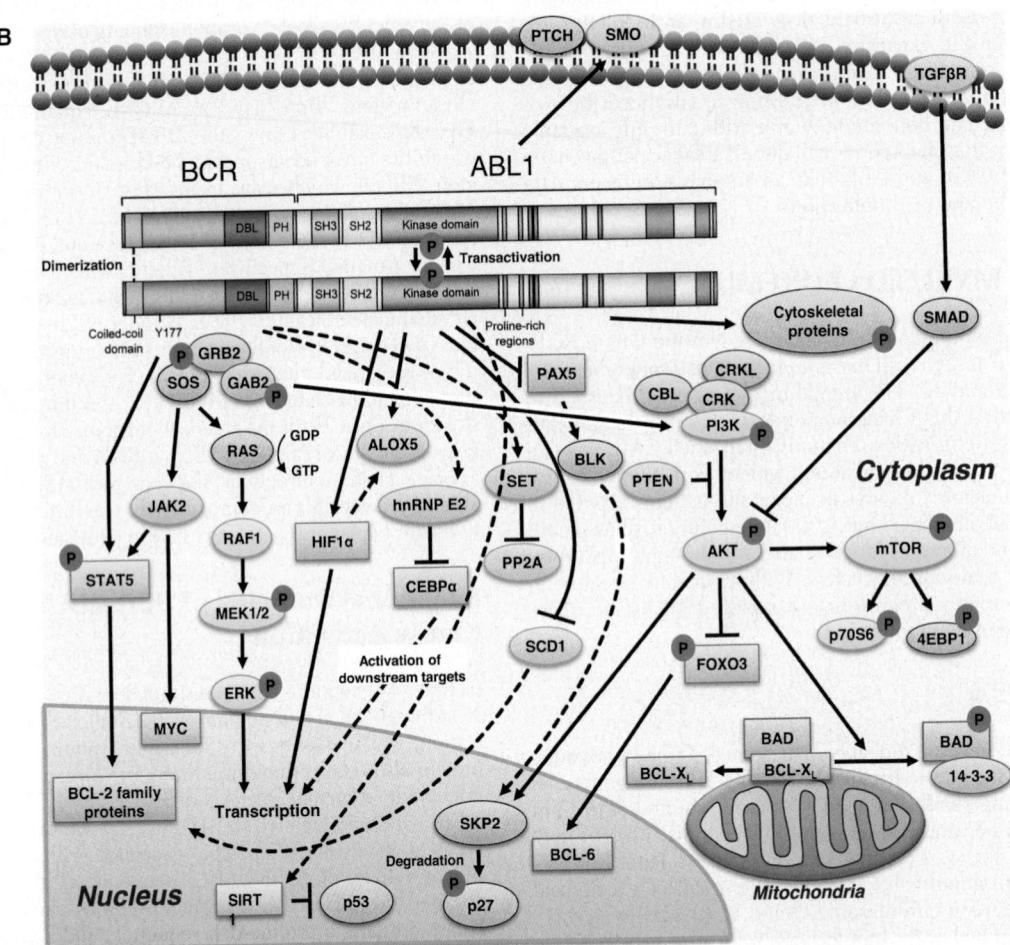

Figure 108.1 (A) A Schematic representation of the t(9;22)(q34;q11) translocation that creates the Philadelphia (Ph) chromosome. The *ABL1* and *BCR* genes reside on the long arms of chromosome 9 and 22, respectively. As a result of the (9;22) translocation, the *BCR-ABL1* gene is formed on the derivative of chromosome of 22 (22q−, Ph chromosome), whereas the reciprocal *ABL1-BCR* resides on the derivative of 9q+. **(B)** The BCR-ABL1 domain structure and simplified representation of molecular signaling pathways activated in CML cells. Following dimerization of BCR-ABL1, autophosphorylation generates docking sites on BCR-ABL1 that facilitate interaction with intermediary adapter proteins *(purple)* such as GRB2. CRKL and CBL are also direct substrates of BCR-ABL1 that are part of a multimeric complex. These BCR-ABL1–dependent signaling complexes in turn lead to activation of multiple pathways whose net result is enhanced survival, inhibition of apoptosis, and perturbation of cell adhesion and migration. A subset of these pathways and their constituent transcription factors *(blue)*, serine/threonine-specific kinases *(green)*, and apoptosis-related proteins *(red)* are shown. Also included are a few pathways that have been more recently implicated in CML stem cell maintenance and BCR-ABL1–mediated disease transformation *(orange)*. However, it is important to note that this is a simplified diagram and that many more associations between BCR-ABL1 and signaling proteins have been reported. DBL, diffuse poorly-differentiated B-cell lymphoma; SH3, Src homology 3; SH2, Src homology 2; GRB2, growth factor receptor-bound protein 2; SOS, son of sevenless; PI3K, phosphatidylinositol-3 kinase; JAK2, janus kinase; RAS-GTP, rat sarcoma-guanosine triphosphate; RAS-GDP, rat sarcoma-guanosine diphosphate; hnRNP E2, heterogeneous nuclear ribonucleoprotein E2; AKT, RAC-alpha serine/threonine-protein kinase; mTOR, mammalian target of rapamycin; STAT5, signal transducer and activator of transcription 5; MEK1/2, mitogen-activated protein kinase 1/2; CEBPa, CCAAT/enhancer binding protein alpha; PP2A, protein phosphatase 2A; ERK, extracellular signal-regulated kinase; FOXO3, forhead O transcription factor; SKP2, S-phase kinase-associated protein 2; BAD, BCL2-associated agonist of cell death.

Phosphatidylinositol-3 Kinase

Phosphatidylinositol-3 kinase (PI3K) is activated by autophosphorylation of tyrosine 177, which generates a high-affinity docking site for the GRB2 adapter, which in turn recruits GAB2 into a complex that activates PI3K. Consistent with a critical role of the Y177/GRB2/GAB2 axis, a mutation of this critical tyrosine to phenylalanine or a lack of GAB2 abrogates myeloid leukemia.[10] An alternative pathway of PI3K activation is a complex formation between its p85 regulatory subunit, CBL, and CrkL, which bind to the SH2 and proline-rich domains of BCR-ABL1.[11] PI3K activates the serine/threonine kinase AKT, which suppresses the activity of the forkhead O transcription factors (FOXO), thereby promoting survival.[12] Additionally, PI3K enhances cell proliferation by promoting proteasomal degradation of p27 through upregulation of S-phase kinase-associated protein 2 (SKP2), the F-Box recognition protein of the SCF^{SKP2} E3 ubiquitin ligase.[13] Another important outlet of PI3K signaling is the AKT-dependent activation of mammalian target of rapamycin (mTOR), which enhances protein translation and cell proliferation.[14]

Rat Sarcoma/Mitogen-Activated Protein Kinase Pathways

GRB2-mediated recruitment and activation of son of sevenless (SOS) promotes exchange of guanosine triphosphate (GTP) for GDP on rat sarcoma (RAS).[15] GTP-RAS activates mitogen-activated protein kinase (MAPK), promoting proliferation. Signaling from RAS to MAPK involves the serine/threonine kinase RAF-1[16] and ras-related C3 botulinum toxin substrate (RAC), another GTP–GDP exchange factor.[17] A crucial role for the latter is supported by the fact that a lack of RAC1/2 delays BCR-ABL1–driven leukemia in a murine model.

Janus Kinase/Signal Transducer and Activator of Transcription Pathway

BCR-ABL1 activates signal transducer and activator of transcription 5 (STAT5) through direct phosphorylation or indirectly through phosphorylation by hematopoietic cell kinase (HCK), a SRC family kinase, or janus kinase 2 (JAK2).[18] Active STAT5 induces the transcription of antiapoptotic proteins like myeloid cell leukemia 1 (MCL-1) and B-cell lymphoma-extra large (Bcl-xL).[19] JAK2 has been shown to play a central role in the cytokine signaling machinery that enables survival of CML stem cells in the presence of BCR-ABL1 tyrosine kinase inhibitors. Recent studies have also shown that the complete lack of STAT5 abrogates both myeloid and lymphoid leukemogenesis, implicating it as a potential target for the elimination leukemic stem cells.[20–22]

Cytoskeletal Proteins

BCR-ABL1 phosphorylates several proteins involved in adhesion and migration, including focal adhesion kinase (FAK), paxillin, p130 CrK-associated substrate (p130CAS), and human enhancer of filamentation 1 (HEF1). This and the activation of RAS[23] are thought to impair integrin-mediated adhesion of CML progenitors to stroma and the extracellular matrix, causing premature circulation as well as abnormal proliferation of Ph+ progenitors.[24] A novel adaptor protein pathway in which BCR-ABL1 interaction with Grb2-related adaptor downstream of Shc (GADS)/SH2 domain containing leukocyte protein of 76kDa (SLP-76)/non-catalytic region of tyrosine kinase adaptor protein 1 (NCK1) regulates the actin cytoskeleton and nonapoptotic membrane blebbing was also recently described.[25]

DNA Repair

BCR-ABL1 impairs DNA damage surveillance by various mechanisms. For example, BCR-ABL1 has been shown to suppress checkpoint kinase 1 (CHK1) through the inhibition of ataxia telangiectasia and Rad3-related protein (ATR)[26] or the downregulation of breast cancer 1, early onset (BRCA1), a substrate of ataxia telangiectasia mutated (ATM).[27] Nonhomologous end joining and homologous recombination, both critical double-strand break repair pathways, are defective in CML. BCR-ABL1 also upregulates RAD51, inducing rapid but low-fidelity double-strand break repairs on challenge with cytotoxic agents and inducing reactive oxygen species (ROS) that promote chronic oxidative DNA damage, double-strand breaks, and point mutations. It has been demonstrated that BCR-ABL1 kinase inhibits the activity of uracil-DNA glycosylase (UNG2), which leads to the accumulation of uracil derivatives in genomic DNA and contributes to increased point mutations.[28] Lastly, telomere length decreases with disease progression from CP to BP.[29]

Although significant progress has been made to understand the extraordinary complexity of CML biology, a complete picture is still elusive. To overcome the limitations of investigating single pathways, quantitative proteomics[30] and whole transcriptome analyses[31] are being used to establish a comprehensive picture of BCR-ABL1 signaling. These results suggest that cellular processes in CML, rather than relying on a single pathway, use integrated networks to fully realize their leukemogenic potential.

Murine Models of Chronic Myeloid Leukemia

The most commonly used murine model of CML is the retroviral expression of BCR-ABL1 in bone marrow followed by transplantation into lethally irradiated syngeneic recipients, which develop a CML-like myeloproliferative neoplasm.[32] Recently, an inducible transgenic mouse model has been developed, in which conditional BCR-ABL1 expression is under the control of the three enhancers of the murine stem cell leukemia (SCL) gene. This model serves as a promising new tool for studying leukemogenic mechanisms in hematopoietic stem cells during disease initiation and progression.[33] Lastly, xenograft models use various strains of immunodeficient mice for engraftment of primary CML cells.[34] A limitation of xenograft models is low engraftment of CML CP cells, probably because of their compromised interactions with the microenvironment as a result of species differences in cytokines and adhesion molecules. Promising results have been obtained by injecting CML cells directly into the livers of newborn mice.[35]

Chronic Myeloid Leukemia Stem Cells

The origin of CML in a pluripotent hematopoietic stem cell (HSC) was elegantly demonstrated in the late 1970s.[36] BCR-ABL1 does not confer self-renewal, implying that it must be acquired by an HSC already endowed with this capacity.[37] For unknown reasons, the main cellular expansion occurs in the progenitor cell compartment, while, at least initially, the majority of HSCs are Ph negative.[38] Serial xenograft studies have shown that CML leukemia stem cells (LSC) reside within the quiescent CD34+38− fraction of bone marrow cells. Significant progress has recently been made by the identification of the interleukin 1 (IL-1) receptor–associated protein (IL-1RAP) as a surface marker specifically expressed on CD34+38− CML LSC.[39] Several genes were shown to have a critical role for LSC maintenance in CML, including promyelocytic leukemia (PML),[40] Rac2 GTPase,[41] smoothened (SMO)/hedgehog (Hh),[42] Wnt/β-catenin,[43,44] phosphatase and tensin homolog (PTEN),[45] hypoxia-inducible factor 1 (HIF-1),[46] B lymphoid kinase (BLK),[47] stearoyl-CoA desaturase1 (SCD1),[48] transforming growth factor beta (TGF-β), and FOXO3a.[12] Additionally, BCL6 was reported to be required for the maintenance of LSCs in CML and contribute to drug resistance.[49] BCL6 expression in these cells is regulated in a PTEN/AKT/FOXO-dependent manner. Recently, an interesting new role of lipid metabolism has emerged in CML stem cell maintenance due to the increased expression of arachidonate 5-lipoxygenase (ALOX5). Alox5 knockout mice fail to develop CML, suggesting a critical role of ALOX5 in CML leukemogenesis.[50] Sirtuin 1 (SIRT1), a nicotinamide adenine dinucleotide–dependent protein deacetylase that promotes cell survival under metabolic, oxidative, and genotoxic stresses through deacetylation of multiple substrates including p53, Ku70, and FOXO, is also transcriptionally activated by BCR-ABL1. SIRT1 knockdown or inhibition by a small-molecule inhibitor effectively suppresses the development of CML-like myeloproliferative disease in mice.[51] Importantly, it has been shown that CML stem cell survival may be independent of BCR-ABL1 kinase activity.[52] A number of studies further suggest that the bone marrow microenvironment provides survival signals to LSCs by involving a number of mechanisms such as chemokine (C-X-C motif) receptor 4 (CXCR4)/stromal cell-derived factor 1 (SDF-1),[53,54] N-cadherin, and Wnt/β-catenin.[55] However, the fact that many of these genes are also critical for maintenance and self-renewal of normal HSCs may be an obstacle to exploiting them as therapeutic targets.

Progression to Blastic Phase

Disease progression is believed to be due to the accumulation of molecular abnormalities that lead to a loss of terminal differentiation capacity of the leukemic clone, which continues to depend on BCR-ABL1 activity. BCR-ABL1 mRNA and protein levels are higher in CML-BP than in CP cells, including CD34+ granulocyte macrophage progenitors (GMP), which are expanded in BP.[56] One of the mechanisms that enhances BCR-ABL1 activity in BP is inactivation of the phosphatase protein phosphatase 2A (PP2A) through upregulation of SET.[57,58] Constitutive BCR-ABL1 activity has also been shown to perturb the CML transcriptome,[59] resulting in altered expression of genes implicated in BP (e.g., preferentially expressed antigen in melanoma [PRAME], myeloid zinc finger 1 [MZF1], ecotropic virus integration site 1 [EVI-1], Wilms tumor 1 [WT1], and JUN-B). Interestingly, a six-gene signature (NIN1/RPN12 binding protein 1 homolog [S. cerevisiae] [NOB1], DEAD [Asp-Glu-Ala-Asp] box polypeptide 47 [DDX47], immunoglobulin superfamily member 2 [IGSF2], lymphotoxin beta receptor 4 [LTBR4], scavenger receptor class B, member 1 [SCARB1], and solute carrier family 25 member A [SLC25A3]) was recently found to accurately discriminate early from late CP, CP from AP, and CP from BP[60]; however, the biologic role of these genes in disease progression is still unknown.

CML-BP patients also harbor various additional genetic lesions such as additional chromosomes, gene insertions and deletions, and/or point mutations. A deep-sequencing study of a small cohort of CML-BP patients detected mutations in 76.9% of cases.[61] The most common mutations (other than those in the BCR-ABL1 kinase domain) occur at the loci of the runt-related transcription factor (RUNX1),[62] the additional sex combs like 1 (ASXL1), WT1, and the tumor suppressor gene TP53[63] in myeloid BP and in cyclin-dependent kinase inhibitor 2A/2B (CDKN2A/B), and the Ikaros transcription factor (IKZF1) in lymphoid BP.[64]

The most striking feature of BP, the loss of differentiation capacity, suggests that the function of key myeloid transcription factors must be compromised. Occasionally, the differentiation block can be ascribed to mutations that result in the formation of dominant-negative transcription factors such as runt-related transcription factor 1- ecotropic virus integration site 1 (AML1-EVI-1) or nucleoporin 98kDa-homeobox A9 (NUP98-HOXA9), which block differentiation or favor preferential growth of immature precursors.[65,66] Isolated cases of myeloid transformation have been associated with the acquisition of core binding factor mutations typical of AML. A more universal mechanism appears to be the BCR-ABL1–induced downregulation of CCAAT/enhancer binding protein-α (CEBPα) through the stabilization of the translational regulator heterogeneous nuclear ribonucleoprotein E2 (hnRNP E2), which is low or undetectable in CP but readily detectable in CML-BP.[67]

Aberrant Wnt/β-catenin activation cooperates with interferon-regulatory factor 8 (Irf8)[68] to contribute to CML progression by conferring self-renewal capacity to GMPs.[69] The acquisition of self-renewal by GMPs is expected to greatly increase the pool of LSCs in BP. Recently, a crucial role of the RNA-binding protein Musashi2 (MSI2) was shown in CML progression to BP, where MSI2 represses the expression of Numb, a protein that impairs the development and propagation of BP.[70] Interestingly, expression microarray studies have implicated a few genes such as β-catenin not only in disease progression, but also in resistance to tyrosine–kinase inhibitors, supporting the view that drug resistance and disease progression share a common genetic basis.[71] This has implications for prognostication as well as for the development of strategies to prevent progression and overcome resistance.

Conclusions

BCR-ABL1 orchestrates an integrated network of signaling pathways that upend the physiologic control of proliferation, cell death, DNA repair, and microenvironment interaction and lead to the clinical phenotype of CML. Cooperation with additional genetic events that accumulate over time inevitably leads to BP and drug resistance. Although significant progress has been made toward understanding transformation and disease progression, much remains to be learned. Efforts toward determining the molecular pathways critical for the maintenance of these cells, and to develop better and faster techniques to differentiate the LSC from the normal HSC, have been intensified in the last decade. The availability of genomewide scanning tools has undoubtedly accelerated this process. This knowledge has been used to design new strategies to target LSCs and hopefully lead to the discovery of new therapeutic targets to eliminate CML stem cells, overcome drug resistance unless effective therapy is initiated early on, and improve the prognosis of patients whose disease has progressed on therapy.

CHRONIC LYMPHOCYTIC LEUKEMIA

CLL is one of the most common leukemias in adults and has a relatively consistent immunophenotype, including dim surface immunoglobulin expression, CD19, CD20, CD23, along with the pan T-cell marker CD5.[72] The impact on overall survival in both young and elderly patients with CLL is substantial: patients diagnosed under the age of 50 have a median expected life span of 12.3 years, compared to 31.2 years in an age-matched control group.[73] Although younger patients have poor outcomes and shortened survival with CLL, several studies have also identified elderly patients as a high-risk group for poor survival following treatment.[74–77] A subset of CLL patients have indolent disease for many years and do not require therapy. Improving our understanding of the origin, biology, and progression of CLL will improve risk stratification and will help identify new treatments for this disease.

Origin of Chronic Lymphocytic Leukemia

The identification of a normal B-cell counterpart remains controversial.[78–80] Unlike most other B-cell lymphomas and leukemias (with the notable exception of mantle cell lymphoma), CLL coexpresses typical mature B-cell markers with CD5. This prompted many to hypothesize that CLL may be derived from CD5+ B cells whose immunoglobulin (Ig) V_H is unmutated. However, the overall phenotype of CLL with expression of CD5, CD23, and CD19, and low levels of surface IgM or IgD is not observed in any normal B-cell counterpart. Additionally, investigators identified that approximately 40% of CLL cases have an unmutated IGHV locus, whereas the remainder are mutated.[81,82] These two groups were also shown to have distinct clinical features, prompting the hypothesis that CLL may represent two distinct diseases.[81,82]

In contrast, two seminal articles examining gene expression profiling in CLL and normal B cells provided findings suggesting that CLL is in fact one disease with a common CLL gene signature.[83,84] The first, by Klein et al.,[83] examined mRNA profiles derived from *IGHV* unmutated, *IGHV* mutated, and normal B cells from different stages of differentiation. An unsupervised analysis of gene expression profiles demonstrated that *IGHV* mutated and unmutated CLL cases were not distinguished in any manner among a common profile typical of CLL. This CLL profile in the majority of samples most resembled postgerminal center memory B cells and lacked any similarity to naïve B cells, CD5+ B cells, or germinal center centroblasts. A supervised analysis of *IGHV*-unmutated and -mutated CLL did, however, demonstrate distinct genes that could separate these two clinical subsets of CLL.

A second article, published concurrently by Rosenwald et al.,[84] demonstrated similar findings of a common CLL profile described by Klein et al., as compared with other normal B cells and B-cell malignancies. In particular, the CLL gene phenotype was not shared by CD5+ normal B cells, thereby providing corroborating evidence that this is likely not the CLL cell of origin. In an unsupervised analysis of CLL samples, *IGHV*-unmutated and -mutated samples were intermingled. However, a supervised analysis of *IGHV*-unmutated and -mutated CLL again identified a number of genes differentially expressed in the former group related to B-cell receptor signaling and proliferation. In particular, ZAP70 (zeta-chain associated protein kinase) was overexpressed in *IGHV*-unmutated CLL as compared with *IGHV*-mutated CLL.[85–88]

Subsequent studies have suggested that ZAP-70 expression may partly explain why *IGHV*-unmutated CLL patients show more B-cell receptor signaling activity upon ligation of the B-cell receptor.[89–91] Multiple studies confirming both the clinical prognostic significance of *IGHV* mutational status and/or ZAP-70 expression have subsequently been reported. *IGHV* status and/or ZAP70 represent very strong independent variables in predicting early disease progression, treatment remission duration, and survival of CLL patients. The variability in direct measurement of ZAP-70 among investigators has limited the application of this biomarker clinically, but more recently, *ZAP70* methylation status has been demonstrated to be a clinically relevant surrogate.[92] In the future, the assessment of methylation may supplant the direct measurement of ZAP-70.

Chromosomal Abnormalities in the Pathogenesis of Chronic Lymphocytic Leukemia

In CLL, conventional metaphase cytogenetics can identify chromosomal aberrations in only 20% to 50% of cases because of the low in vitro mitotic activity of CLL tumor cells.[93] Early unstimulated metaphase karyotype studies of CLL demonstrated abnormalities, including trisomy 12, deletions at 13q14, structural aberrations of 14q32, and deletions of 11q, 17p, and 6q in descending frequency of occurrence.[94] In addition, complex karyotype (three or more abnormalities) occurs in approximately 15% of patients and was noted in these early studies to predict for rapid disease progression, Richter's transformation, and inferior survival.[95–97] A stimulated metaphase analysis has also been reported with the identification of translocations in 33 of 96 patients (34%) that were both balanced and unbalanced, which is associated with significantly shorter median time from diagnosis to requiring therapy and overall survival.[98] Subsequent comparative genomic hybridization (CGH) and global single nucleotide polymorphism (SNP) array studies in CLL have confirmed these and other chromosomal deletions in CLL.[99–101] Increasing aberrations in these same studies of CGH or SNP arrays have been associated with more aggressive disease.

Given the limitation of standard or stimulated karyotype analysis, interphase cytogenetics of known abnormalities are used to identify common, clinically significant aberrations in CLL. The largest study of interphase cytogenetics resulted in improved sensitivity to detect partial trisomies (12q12, 3q27, 8q24), deletions (13q14, 11q22-23, 6q21, 6q27, 17p13), and translocations (band 14q32) in more than 80% of all cases. In a large study of 325 patients by Döhner et al.,[102] a hierarchical model consisting of five genetic subgroups was constructed on the basis of regression analysis of CLL patients with chromosomal aberrations. The patients with a 17p deletion had a median survival time of 32 months and the shortest treatment-free interval (TFI) of 9 months, whereas patients with an 11q deletion followed closely with 79 months and 13 months, respectively.[102] The favorable 13q14 deletion group had a long TFI of 92 months and a median survival of 133 months, whereas the group without detectable chromosomal anomalies and those with trisomy 12 fell into the intermediate group with median survival of 111 and 114 months, respectively. Their TFI was 33 and 49 months, respectively. Based on this pivotal study, CLL patients are prioritized in a hierarchical order (deletion 17p13 > deletion 11q22-q23 > trisomy 12 > no aberration > deletion 13q14).[102] Interestingly, patients with high-risk interphase cytogenetics or other complex abnormalities almost always have *IGHV* unmutated or ZAP-70–positive CLL.[103]

The frequency of recurrent deletions in CLL suggests the possibility of unique tumor suppressor genes in these lost regions. In particular, attention to coding genes within the 13q14 region failed to identify a viable tumor suppressor gene candidate for many years of investigation to the frustration of multiple investigators. However, in 2002, Croce and colleagues[104] identified miR-15 and miR-16, two noncoding microRNAs, in the deleted region of 13q14. MicroRNAs range in size from 21 to 25 nucleotides and represent a newly recognized class of gene products whose function is to silence genes through binding to the 3′-untranslated region of specific genes to inhibit translation. When near compatible hybridization of the noncoding RNA exists, RNA transcription can also be antagonized. This same group later showed that miR-16 regulates the expression of bcl-2, which is overexpressed in CLL and other B-cell lymphoproliferative disorders.[105] Multiple different studies have associated specific miR expression with rapid disease progression, fludarabine resistance, and poor prognosis. In addition, miR-34a has been directly related to the adverse outcome associated with p53 dysfunction.[106,107] At the time of writing this chapter, several reports are coming forth in CLL and other types of cancer about the role of miRs in cell-to-cell communication via exosomes. Further study of miRs in CLL is under way to elucidate their full role in the pathogenesis and progression of CLL. In addition, other conserved, larger noncoding RNAs with different siRNA and epigenetic silencing roles have been recently identified to have a significant role in CLL.

Recurrent Mutations in Chronic Lymphocytic Leukemia

Several groups have recently used next-generation sequencing to demonstrate a number of recurrent mutations in CLL, including known and novel mutations in over two dozen genes with functions as diverse as cell cycle control (*ATM, TP53*), histones (*HISTH1E*), inflammation (*MYD88, DDX3X, MAPK1*), Notch signaling (*FBXW7, NOTCH1*), general signal transduction (*BRAF, KRAS, PRKD3*), gene transcription (*SMARCA2, NFKBIE*), and RNA processing (*SF3B1, XPO1*).[108–111] These mutations are seen in select genetic subtypes—for instance, NOTCH1 in patients with trisomy 12,[112] MyD88 among *IGHV*-mutated patients,[110] and SF3B1 in del(11q22.3) patients.[108] Although the disease potential of alterations in, for example, *TP53, ATM*, or even the very rare *BRAF* mutation may be clear, the pathogenesis of most of these recurrently mutated genes or pathways remain yet to be worked out and is a promising area for investigation, particularly if experimental therapeutics could be targeted to patients according to their specific genomic alterations. Additionally, several of these genes, including NOTCH1[110,113] and SF3B1,[108] also appear to impact the prognosis of CLL, providing justification for potentially assessing mutational status to predict disease outcome.

Progression of Chronic Lymphocytic Leukemia: The Role of Genomic Instability and Clonal Evolution

Several studies have been examined for features associated with clonal evolution and have noted this to be more frequent in patients with IGHV-unmutated status[114] or those expressing the surrogate marker for IGHV-mutational status, ZAP-70.[115] In another study, patients with long telomere length were more likely to have IGHV-mutated disease and del(13q14), whereas those with del(11q22.3), del(17p13.1), complex karyotype (more than abnormalities), and IGHV-unmutated disease were likely to have extended telomeres.[116] Furthermore, one small study suggested long telomere length among patients with IGHV-unmutated disease could identify patients with an expected extended progression-free survival.[117] More recently, Landau et al.[118] examined the role of intratumoral heterogeneity and the presence of subclonal driver mutations in the progression of CLL. Using sequencing and copy number analysis at multiple time points, early events (del(13q), +12, MYD88 mutation) could be delineated from later events (e.g., SF3B1, TP53 mutation), and the development of mutations or expansion in preexisting subclones could be related to the administration of chemotherapy. In addition, the presence of subclonal driver mutations early in the disease was an independent adverse prognostic factor. The contributions of telomere length, global hypomethylation, and subclonal driver mutations' clonal expansion to CLL progression still require further study.

Chronic Lymphocytic Leukemia and Proliferation

For decades, CLL was viewed as a nonproliferating leukemia driven solely by disrupted apoptosis and extended tumor cell survival. This paradigm was, in part, perpetuated based on the nonproliferating blood compartment. However, it has been recognized that, as with normal B cells, CLL cell proliferation likely occurs in sites where microenvironment stimulation can occur, such as the lymph node and bone marrow. In such sites, proliferation centers are observed with a high proportion of dividing CLL cells that are often surrounded by either T cells or accessory stromal cells capable of providing cytokine costimulation.[119,120] In patients, all body compartments can now be accurately measured with the oral intake of heavy water, and the birth rate of CLL tumor cells can thereby be assessed in vivo.[121] These studies have demonstrated a broad range of proliferation of CLL cells, varying by disease state and IGHV-mutational status.[122,123] As one might expect, this proliferation rate identified through heavy water studies in CLL was shown to be predictive of disease progression. Collectively, these studies have at least partially discredited the theory that CLL is purely an accumulative disease and have focused the study on specific body compartments that have very different biologic features of proliferation.

Chronic Lymphocytic Leukemia and Disrupted Apoptosis

Because the normal counterpart to CLL is unknown, it is quite difficult to directly compare differences in spontaneous apoptosis. However, several studies derived from CLL do provide evidence that apoptosis is disrupted. Despite the rarity of BCL2

gene rearrangement in CLL, overexpression of BCL2 mRNA and Bcl-2 protein is common and has been shown to contribute to both disrupted spontaneous apoptosis and also ex vivo drug resistance.[124–128] Similarly, other antiapoptotic Bcl-2 family member proteins including MCL-1, A1, and Bcl-xL have also been shown to be elevated either in resting CLL or in CLL cells exposed to soluble and contact factors present in the microenvironment; these factors also contribute to drug resistance.[129–131]

Finally, a host of transcription factors involving the nuclear factor kappa B (NF-κB),[132] WNT,[133] Hedgehog,[134] and JAK/STAT[135] signaling pathway have been shown to be constitutively active and also to contribute to disrupted apoptosis and drug resistance in CLL. In particular, differential activation of NF-κB in CLL[136–140] versus normal resting B cells, its prognostic significance[141–143] with respect to predicting outcome, and also its positive role in regulating many of the antiapoptotic genes upregulated in CLL has generated particular interest.

B-Cell Receptor Signaling in Chronic Lymphocytic Leukemia

The identification of the divergent natural history of CLL based on IGHV-mutational status, ZAP-70 expression, and associated enhanced B-cell receptor signaling has raised interest in this pathway's role in the pathogenesis of CLL.[89–91,144] Why the BCR is constitutively active in CLL is not yet clear, but current theories include stimulation by self- or ubiquitous environmental antigens as well as tonic BCR self-transactivation. Downstream, activation of the proximal lyn and syk kinases, and Bruton's tyrosine kinase (BTK), in turn, has been demonstrated in CLL.[145–149] Additionally, increased activity of the PI3K pathway has been reported.[150–152] Complementing this, a study demonstrated that mature memory B-cell development was, in great part, dependent on the PI3K pathway.[152] A study of the isoform-specific inhibitor of PI3K-δ demonstrated that much of the survival protection generated by the microenvironment from stromal cells, cytokines (CD40L, IL-6, tumor necrosis factor alpha [TNF-α]), and fibronectin contact is mediated via PI3K-δ isoform signaling.[153] Moving inhibitors of B-cell receptor kinase pathway inhibitors into clinical trials has been of great interest. Here, syk, PI3K-δ isoform inhibitors, and BTK inhibitors have demonstrated dramatic and often rapid clinical responses with relatively favorable toxicity profile in CLL patients.[154] The success of such therapeutics further emphasizes the importance of BCR signaling in the pathogenesis of CLL.

Conclusion

Data concerning the pathogenesis of CLL continue to accumulate. Emerging from such work is the importance of epigenetics in the progression of CLL from normal B cells, the presence of recurrent genetic mutations, and the critical role of enhanced B-cell receptor signaling. Mouse models have demonstrated the importance of NF-κB, Bcl-2, Tcl1, and loss of miR-15, miR-16, and DLEU2 in the pathogenesis of CLL. The application of these principles (e.g., ibrutinib to quench tonic BCR signaling) in human trials is already yielding dramatic changes in the treatment of patients with CLL.[154] It is likely that current investigations, combined with whole-transcriptome sequencing, global proteomic assessment, and miR profiling, will lead to further advances in risk stratification and treatments for CLL.

ACKNOWLEDGMENTS

We thank Dr. Michael Deininger to help us in preparation of the 9th edition of this chapter, which served as a scaffold for the 10th edition.

SELECTED REFERENCES

The full reference list can be accessed at lwwhealthlibrary.com/oncology.

1. Nowell PC, Hungerford DA. Chromosome studies on normal and leukemic human leukocytes. *J Natl Cancer Inst* 1960;25:85–109.
2. Rowley JD. Letter: A new consistent chromosomal abnormality in chronic myelogenous leukaemia identified by quinacrine fluorescence and Giemsa staining. *Nature* 1973;243:290–293.
3. Daley GQ, Van Etten RA, Baltimore D. Induction of chronic myelogenous leukemia in mice by the P210bcr/abl gene of the Philadelphia chromosome. *Science* 1990;247:824–830.
7. Melo JV, Gordon DE, Cross NC, et al. The ABL-BCR fusion gene is expressed in chronic myeloid leukemia. *Blood* 1993;81:158–165.
9. Quintás-Cardama A, Cortes J. Molecular biology of bcr-abl1-positive chronic myeloid leukemia. *Blood* 2009;113:1619–1630.
13. Agarwal A, Bumm TG, Corbin AS, et al. Absence of SKP2 expression attenuates BCR-ABL-induced myeloproliferative disease. *Blood* 2008;112: 1960–1970.
18. Ilaria RL Jr, Van Etten RA. P210 and P190(BCR/ABL) induce the tyrosine phosphorylation and DNA binding activity of multiple specific STAT family members. *J Biol Chem* 1996;271:31704–31710.
26. Melo JV, Barnes DJ. Chronic myeloid leukaemia as a model of disease evolution in human cancer. *Nat Rev Cancer* 2007;7:441–453.
30. Brehme M, Hantschel O, Colinge J, et al. Charting the molecular network of the drug target Bcr-Abl. *Proc Natl Acad Sci U S A* 2009;106:7414–7419.
31. Gerber JM, Gucwa JL, Esopi D, et al. Genome-wide comparison of the transcriptomes of highly enriched normal and chronic myeloid leukemia stem and progenitor cell populations. *Oncotarget* 2013;4:715–728.
32. Pear WS, Miller JP, Xu L, et al. Efficient and rapid induction of a chronic myelogenous leukemia-like myeloproliferative disease in mice receiving P210 bcr/abl-transduced bone marrow. *Blood* 1998;92:3780–3792.
52. Corbin AS, Agarwal A, Loriaux M, et al. Human chronic myeloid leukemia stem cells are insensitive to imatinib despite inhibition of BCR-ABL activity. *J Clin Invest* 2011;121:396–409.
53. Agarwal A, Fleischman AG, Petersen CL, et al. Effects of plerixafor in combination with BCR-ABL kinase inhibition in a murine model of CML. *Blood* 2012;120:2658–2668.
58. Agarwal A, MacKenzie R, Oddo J, et al. A novel SET antagonist (OP449) is cytotoxic to CML cells, including the highly-resistant BCR-ABLT315I mutant, and demonstrates enhanced efficacy in combination with ABL tyrosine kinase inhibitors. *Am Soc Hematol* 2011;118:3757.
61. Grossmann V, Kohlmann A, Zenger M, et al. A deep-sequencing study of chronic myeloid leukemia patients in blast crisis (BC-CML) detects mutations in 76.9% of cases. *Leukemia* 2011;25:557–560.
69. Jamieson CH, Ailles LE, Dylla SJ, et al. Granulocyte-macrophage progenitors as candidate leukemic stem cells in blast-crisis CML. *N Engl J Med* 2004;351:657–667.
70. Ito T, Kwon HY, Zimdahl B, et al. Regulation of myeloid leukaemia by the cell-fate determinant Musashi. *Nature* 2010;466:765–768.
81. Hamblin TJ, Davis Z, Gardiner A, et al. Unmutated Ig V(H) genes are associated with a more aggressive form of chronic lymphocytic leukemia. *Blood* 1999;94:1848–1854.

82. Damle RN, Wasil T, Fais F, et al. Ig V gene mutation status and CD38 expression as novel prognostic indicators in chronic lymphocytic leukemia. *Blood* 1999;94:1840–1847.
83. Klein U, Tu Y, Stolovitzky GA, et al. Gene expression profiling of B cell chronic lymphocytic leukemia reveals a homogeneous phenotype related to memory B cells. *J Exp Med* 2001;194:1625–1638.
84. Rosenwald A, Alizadeh AA, Widhopf G, et al. Relation of gene expression phenotype to immunoglobulin mutation genotype in B cell chronic lymphocytic leukemia. *J Exp Med* 2001;194:1639–1647.
87. Rassenti LZ, Huynh L, Toy TL, et al. ZAP-70 compared with immunoglobulin heavy-chain gene mutation status as a predictor of disease progression in chronic lymphocytic leukemia. *N Engl J Med* 2004;351:893–901.
91. Chen L, Huynh L, Apgar J, et al. ZAP-70 enhances IgM signaling independent of its kinase activity in chronic lymphocytic leukemia. *Blood* 2008; 111:2685–2692.
92. Claus R, Lucas DM, Stilgenbauer S, et al. Quantitative DNA methylation analysis identifies a single CpG dinucleotide important for ZAP-70 expression and predictive of prognosis in chronic lymphocytic leukemia. *J Clin Oncol* 2012;30:2483–2491.
98. Mayr C, Speicher MR, Kofler DM, et al. Chromosomal translocations are associated with poor prognosis in chronic lymphocytic leukemia. *Blood* 2006; 107:742–751.
102. Döhner H, Stilgenbauer S, Benner A, et al. Genomic aberrations and survival in chronic lymphocytic leukemia. *N Engl J Med* 2000;343: 1910–1916.
104. Calin GA, Dumitru CD, Shimizu M, et al. Frequent deletions and down-regulation of micro- RNA genes miR15 and miR16 at 13q14 in chronic lymphocytic leukemia. *Proc Natl Acad Sci U S A* 2002;99:15524–15529.
108. Wang L, Lawrence MS, Wan Y, et al. SF3B1 and other novel cancer genes in chronic lymphocytic leukemia. *N Engl J Med* 2011;365:2497–2506.
115. Shanafelt TD, Witzig TE, Fink SR, et al. Prospective evaluation of clonal evolution during long-term follow-up of patients with untreated early-stage chronic lymphocytic leukemia. *J Clin Oncol* 2006;24:4634–4641.
118. Landau Dan A, Carter Scott L, Stojanov P, et al. Evolution and impact of subclonal mutations in chronic lymphocytic leukemia. *Cell* 2013;152: 714–726.
123. Messmer BT, Messmer D, Allen SL, et al. In vivo measurements document the dynamic cellular kinetics of chronic lymphocytic leukemia B cells. *J Clin Invest* 2005;115:755–764.
132. Furman RR, Asgary Z, Mascarenhas JO, et al. Modulation of NF-kappa B activity and apoptosis in chronic lymphocytic leukemia B cells. *J Immunol* 2000;164:2200–2206.
136. Chen SS, Raval A, Johnson AJ, et al. Epigenetic changes during disease progression in a murine model of human chronic lymphocytic leukemia. *Proc Natl Acad Sci U S A* 2009;106:13433–13438.
153. Herman SE, Gordon AL, Wagner AJ, et al. Phosphatidylinositol 3-kinase-δ inhibitor CAL-101 shows promising preclinical activity in chronic lymphocytic leukemia by antagonizing intrinsic and extrinsic cellular survival signals. *Blood* 2010;116:2078–2088.
154. Byrd JC, Furman RR, Coutre SE, et al. Targeting BTK with ibrutinib in relapsed Chronic lymphocytic leukemia. *N Engl J Med* 2013;369:32–42.

PRACTICE OF ONCOLOGY

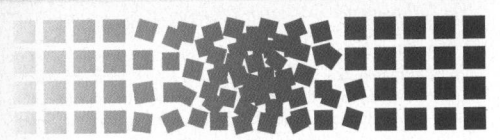

109 Chronic Myelogenous Leukemia

Brian J. Druker and David Marin

INTRODUCTION

Chronic myelogenous leukemia (CML; also called *chronic myeloid leukemia*) is a clonal hematopoietic disorder caused by an acquired genetic defect in a pluripotent stem cell. CML is a bi- or triphasic illness, with most patients diagnosed in a relatively indolent chronic or stable phase that is characterized by excessive numbers of myeloid lineage cells that fully mature. The disease has the capacity to progress to a more aggressive leukemia as a malignant clone loses the capacity for terminal differentiation. This more aggressive or advanced phase can be further subdivided into an accelerated phase and a blastic phase, with the blastic phase being akin to an acute leukemia and having a dismal prognosis.[1]

CML has become a paradigm for targeted drug development based on an understanding of the molecular pathogenesis of a disease. A series of discoveries led to the recognition that the BCR-ABL protein, which results from a reciprocal translocation involving chromosomes 9 and 22, has a central role in the pathogenesis of CML. The BCR-ABL protein functions as a constitutively activated tyrosine kinase and this knowledge led to the development of imatinib (Gleevec, Glivec), a drug that specifically inhibits the BCR-ABL tyrosine kinase.[2] Other tyrosine-kinase inhibitors (TKI) with improved potency have been developed, and BCR-ABL TKIs are now the standard therapy for newly diagnosed patients with CML. Allogeneic hematopoietic cell transplantation (HCT), which was the preferred therapy prior the advent of targeted therapy, is now reserved for patients with resistance to TKIs or for patients with advanced phase disease.

EPIDEMIOLOGY

CML accounts for approximately 15% of all leukemias, with 4,000 to 5,000 new cases diagnosed in the United States annually. The incidence of CML is 1.6 to 2.0 cases per 100,000 persons per year, and the incidence is similar in all countries worldwide.[3] Although CML occurs in all age groups, its incidence increases with each decade of life, making it mainly a disease of adults. According to the Surveillance, Epidemiology, and End Results (SEER) program, the median age at diagnosis is 66 years, which is much higher than that reported in single-institutional series and clinical trials.[3] The disease has a slight male predominance (2.2:1.3).[3]

The only known risk factor for the development of CML is exposure to radiation at high doses. This is evident from studies of survivors of the atom bomb explosions in Japan in 1945 and from follow-ups of patients treated with radiation for ankylosing spondylitis and cervical cancer.[4–6] No known association has been found between CML and infectious agents or chemical exposures, and no familial predisposition has been implicated in CML.

PATHOGENESIS

The discovery of the Philadelphia (Ph) chromosome in 1960 made CML the first human neoplasm to be characterized by a consistent cytogenetic marker.[7] In 1973, the Ph chromosome, a shortened chromosome 22 (22q-), was shown to be the result of a balanced, reciprocal translocation between the long arms of chromosomes 9 and 22, t(9;22) (q34;q11) (Fig. 109.1).[8] In the 1980s, the *BCR-ABL* chimeric gene and protein formed as a result of the (9;22) translocation was characterized and its central role in the pathogenesis of CML was established.[9,10] The Ph chromosome and *BCR-ABL* are found in cells of the myeloid, erythroid, and megakaryocytic lineages, some B cells, and a small proportion of T cells, but not in other cells of the body, establishing CML as a clonal disorder that originates in a pluripotent hematopoietic stem cell.

The (9;22) translocation transposes the *ABL* (Abelson) proto-oncogene from chromosome 9 into a relatively small, 5.8-kb genomic region on chromosome 22 named the *breakpoint cluster region (bcr)*.[11] Although the genomic breakpoints in the *ABL* gene are highly variable, they almost always occur upstream of the second exon (a2), resulting in translocation of all but exon 1 of *ABL*. Two slightly different chimeric *BCR-ABL* genes are present in most patients with CML, depending on the precise location of the breakpoint in the *BCR* gene. Breaks can occur between exon e13 (also known as b2) and exon e14 (b3), yielding an e13a2 fusion messenger RNA (mRNA), whereas a break occurring between exons 14 and 15 produces an e14a2 fusion mRNA (Fig. 109.2).[9] In the majority of patients, either e13a2 or e14a2 transcripts are present, but occasionally, patients have both transcripts in their leukemia cells. Although the e14a2 mRNA encodes a BCR-ABL protein that is 25 amino acids larger than that encoded by the e13a2 transcript, both are referred to as *p210BCR-ABL*. Patients with e13a2 or e14a2 transcripts have similar prognoses. In 5% of the patients, the breakpoint occurs in other regions of the BCR gene resulting in the so-called *rare transcripts*; these transcripts have the same biological activity as the more common ones.[1,9] It is important, however, to identify patients harboring these rare transcripts because molecular monitoring may otherwise prove impossible.

The BCR-ABL fusion protein resides in the cytoplasm and has constitutive tyrosine kinase activity compared to the tightly regulated activity of the normal *ABL* product (p145).[12,13] The BCR-ABL tyrosine kinase binds to and phosphorylates numerous intracellular proteins. The net effect of this is to induce all of the phenotypic abnormalities observed in patients with CML.[9] These include increased proliferation or decreased apoptosis of hematopoietic stem or progenitor cells leading to a massive increase in myeloid cell numbers and the premature release of immature myeloid cells into the circulation, postulated to be due to a defect in adherence of myeloid progenitors to marrow stroma and genetic instability resulting in disease progression. Despite the complexity of BCR-ABL signal transduction, all of the transforming functions of BCR-ABL depend on its tyrosine kinase activity, making this disease an ideal candidate for therapy directed against this activity.

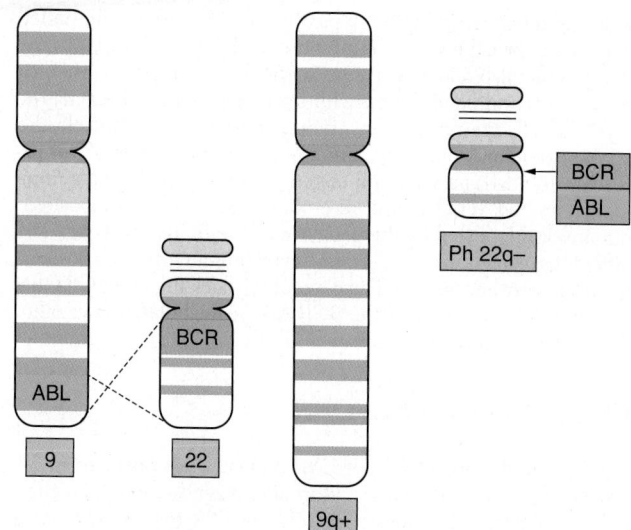

Figure 109.1 Diagrammatic representation of the formation of the Philadelphia (Ph) chromosome. The normal chromosomes 9 and 22 are shown, along with the derivative chromosomes 9q+ and 22q- (Ph). The approximate positions of the normal *ABL* gene at 9q34 and *BCR* at 22q11 and the *BCR-ABL* fusion gene formed as a result of the translocation are shown.

DIAGNOSIS

Clinical Manifestations

Of patients with CML, 90% are diagnosed in the chronic or stable phase. Of patients in older studies, 10% to 20% and as many as 50% in more recent series present without symptoms and are diagnosed as a result of finding an elevated white blood count on routine blood sampling. The most common presenting symptoms of CML are related to anemia, splenomegaly, and increased cell turnover. These symptoms include fatigue, left upper quadrant pain, abdominal distention or discomfort, early satiety, weight loss, and night sweats.[14]

Occasionally, patients may present with a hyperviscosity syndrome, which requires leukapheresis, with manifestations such as stroke, priapism, stupor, or visual changes caused by retinal hemorrhage. The most common physical finding is splenomegaly, its magnitude correlating with the degree of leukocytosis. Ecchymoses are frequently observed, but spontaneous bleeding is uncommon. A lymphadenopathy is not usually seen in the chronic phase.

Laboratory Tests

Peripheral Blood and Bone Marrow

The diagnosis of CML is frequently suspected from an examination of the peripheral blood and bone marrow. The white blood cell (WBC) count in the chronic phase of CML usually exceeds 50×10^9/L at the time of diagnosis and can range up to 800×10^9/L. During the chronic phase, leukemic WBCs differentiate and function normally. The peripheral blood smear shows a full spectrum of myeloid cells from blasts to neutrophils, with blasts comprising less than 15% and usually less than 5% of the WBC differential. Basophilia is invariably present, and its absence should prompt consideration of other myeloproliferative disorders. Eosinophilia is also commonly present. The majority of patients have thrombocytosis and, on occasion, the platelet count may be more than 1000×10^9/L. Most patients with CML have a normochromic, normocytic anemia that is inversely proportional to the degree of leukocytosis.

The bone marrow in patients with chronic phase CML is markedly hypercellular, with a predominance of myeloid cells with full maturation. Blasts are fewer than 15% and most commonly fewer than 5%, and basophilia is also present. Megakaryocytes are usually increased in number, are characteristically small, are hypo- or monolobated, and have a tendency to cluster. Erythroid hypoplasia is frequently present and may seem exaggerated because of the increased myeloid-to-erythroid ratio. Erythroid precursors are otherwise morphologically unremarkable. Reticulin fibrosis is usually absent or mild but may become more prominent with disease progression.[15]

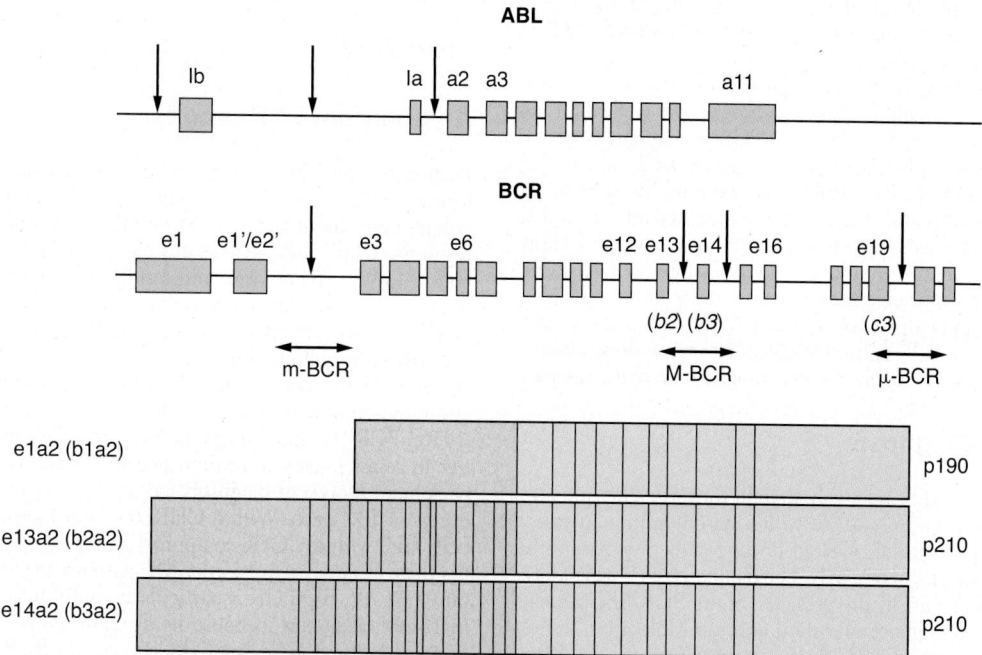

Figure 109.2 Schematic representation of the genomic structure of the normal *ABL* and *BCR* genes (*top*) and various fusion transcripts generated by the different *BCR-ABL* fusion genes (*bottom*). The b2a2 or the b3a2 transcript is found in the majority of patients with chronic myelogenous leukemia. See text for details.

Cytogenetics

A cytogenetic analysis of 20 bone marrow metaphases has been the standard method to detect the Ph chromosome, which is present in the majority of cells at diagnosis. Although most patients have a typical t(9;22)(q34;q11), approximately 5% have variant translocations that have no impact on prognosis.[16] These variant translocations may be simple, involving chromosome 22 and a chromosome other than chromosome 9, or they may be complex, involving one or more other chromosomes in addition to chromosomes 9 and 22.[17] Clonal cytogenetic abnormalities in addition to the Ph chromosome are present at diagnosis in approximately 5% of patients diagnosed in chronic phase.[18,19] The most common are duplication of the Ph chromosome and trisomy 8, iso-17q, and trisomy 19.[18,19] These abnormalities have only a small adverse prognostic impact when identified at diagnosis.[19]

Molecular Testing

The diagnosis of CML requires the presence of BCR-ABL. In 95% of patients, its presence can be inferred by the detection of the Ph chromosome using standard cytogenetics. Another 5% of patients with a hematologic picture resembling CML who lack a detectable Ph chromosome will have a BCR-ABL fusion gene detectable by fluorescence in situ hybridization (FISH) or reverse transcription–polymerase chain reaction (RT-PCR). These Ph chromosome–negative, BCR-ABL–positive patients have a clinical course that is indistinguishable from that of Ph chromosome–positive, BCR-ABL–positive patients.[20] Patients with a hematologic picture resembling CML, but who are Ph chromosome negative and BCR-ABL negative, are classified within the myeloproliferative neoplasm group.[21] Some of these patients have mutations in the SETBP1[22] or CSF3R[23] genes, whereas others remain genetically unclassified.

FISH detects the colocalization of large, fluorescently labeled genomic probes specific to the BCR and ABL genes. FISH can be performed on metaphase or interphase cells and on peripheral blood. At diagnosis, when typically 90% of cells are BCR-ABL positive, FISH is a highly accurate diagnostic test, because false-negative results are uncommon.[24] However, because of the random colocalization of the signals from the BCR and ABL probes, 8% to 10% of normal cells score positive, making FISH less useful at low disease burdens. A lower false-positive rate can be obtained with dual-FISH (D-FISH), which uses probes that span the breakpoint region.[25]

RT-PCR to amplify the unique sequences created by the fusion of BCR and ABL is a highly sensitive technique that is ideal for the detection of minimal residual disease.[24] PCR testing can either be qualitative, providing information as to the presence or absence of the BCR-ABL transcript, or quantitative, assessing the amount of BCR-ABL message. Quantitative RT-PCR is preferred for monitoring and may allow for the early detection of resistance to therapy.[26] False-positive and false-negative results are both possible with RT-PCR, and rigorous controls are required to detect these instances. False-negative results can be due to poor quality RNA, failure of the reaction or failure of the PCR primers to detect rare transcripts, whereas false-positive results are usually due to contamination of the sample.

Differential Diagnosis

The diagnosis of CML is relatively straight forward. The presence of a WBC count over 50×10^9/L with a peripheral blood smear showing a full spectrum of myeloid lineage cells plus basophilia should raise the suspicion of CML. The diagnosis of chronic phase CML can be confirmed by the presence of the BCR-ABL gene as described in the Cytogenetics section and the Molecular Testing section and by the absence of advanced phase features described later in Advanced Phase Disease.

The main differential diagnosis includes a leukemoid reaction and other myeloproliferative neoplasms. In patients with a leukemoid reaction, which is typically seen in patients with underlying infections, the WBC count is usually less than 50×10^9/L and the peripheral blood smear consists predominantly of segmented neutrophils and bands, often with toxic granulations. Less mature myeloid cells are rarely seen; there is no basophilia; and the Ph chromosome and BCR-ABL are absent. Approximately 5% of patients with CML present with extreme thrombocytosis and a minimally elevated WBC count, resembling essential thrombocytosis, but are distinguished by the presence of the BCR-ABL gene. The differential diagnosis with other myeloproliferative neoplasm is relatively easy because the latter frequently lack the basophilia that is seen with CML and lack the BCR-ABL gene, but may have other molecular abnormalities such as SETBP1 or CSF3R mutations.

PROGNOSTIC FACTORS

Historically, the progression of CML to blast crisis occurred in 5% to 10% of patients in the first 2 years after diagnosis and, thereafter, the annual progression rate increased from 20% to 25%. The Sokal score was developed to predict the probability of disease progression, but this and a variety of other factors are now being used to predict the probability of optimal response to therapy. The Sokal score was developed to predict the probability of disease progression.[27] Despite it being developed in a pre-TKI era and as a predictor for disease progression, it has been found useful to predict the probability of achieving an optimal response to imatinib.[28,29]; however, it has been less useful for predicting responses to newer TKIs.[30,31] The Sokal score is a numerical value that is calculated from a complex equation that takes into account four factors at diagnosis: the percentage of blasts in peripheral blood, platelet count, spleen size (centimeters below the costal margin) and age of the patient.[27] Patients then were divided according to their individual numerical value into three risk groups: low, intermediate, and high, risk of progression, with median survivals of 5, 4, and 3 years, respectively. Many of these patients received therapies not currently in use, such as busulfan and hydroxyurea; however, the Sokal score remains useful to predict the response of patients treated with imatinib, but less so with newer TKIs.[28,31] Other variables closely related with the Sokal score such as hemoglobin and white blood count at diagnosis also have prognostic value.[29,32,33]

THERAPY

Assessment of Response

Response to therapy in patients with CML is assessed by the monitoring of blood counts, cytogenetics, and real-time quantitative polymerase chain reaction (RQ-PCR). A complete hematologic response (CHR) indicates the normalization of the complete blood count (CBC), spleen size, and resolution of symptoms related to the CML. A partial cytogenetic response corresponds to 1% to 35% of Ph-positive metaphases and a complete cytogenetic response (CCyR) is the absence of the Ph chromosome on conventional cytogenetic analysis; a major cytogenetic response (MCyR) is the combination of partial and CCyR.

RQ-PCR has emerged as the most effective and efficient manner to assess leukemic burden because it can easily be done on peripheral blood. At diagnosis, an untreated patient may have in excess of 10^{12} cells. With a CHR, this falls to approximately 10^{11} cells and, with a CCyR, to approximately 10^{10} cells. Because the majority of newly diagnosed CML patients treated with TKIs obtain a CCyR, RQ-PCR is particularly useful for monitoring minimal residual disease because its dynamic range extends two-logs or more below a CCyR. RQ-PCR measure BCR-ABL transcripts in relation to a control gene such as normal ABL or GUSB, and can be expressed as the absolute ratio or as log reductions from the 100% value. In an attempt to introduce some level of uniformity, many laboratories are using the International Scale (IS), whereby values are *corrected* to those obtained in a reference laboratory.[34] It is generally accepted that CCyR corresponds to an approximately 2-log reduction in transcript levels or 1% IS.[35] Major molecular response (MR3) is defined as a 3-log reduction in transcript levels or 0.1% IS, and this should correspond to a leukemia burden of approximately 10^9 cells. Similarly, MR4 is defined as a 4-log reduction (0.01% IS, or 10^8 leukemic cells). A complete molecular response (CMR) is generally defined as the absence of detectable BCR-ABL transcripts, a status that depends on the technology and criteria for negativity employed, with the limits of technology being somewhere between MR4 and MR5.

Treatment of Chronic Phase Disease

BCR-ABL TKIs are the standard frontline therapy for newly diagnosed patients with chronic phase CML. Hydroxyurea, a well-tolerated oral agent that inhibits DNA synthesis by inhibiting ribonucleotide reductase, remains in use as an initial therapy to control blood counts pending definitive diagnosis and therapy. Allogeneic HCT, although curative, is typically reserved for patients with resistance to TKI therapy or in the management of advanced phase disease due to its morbidity and mortality. Interferon-α, a previous mainstay of therapy, has been supplanted by TKIs, and has been used with variable results in clinical trials attempting to improve molecular responses to TKIs.

BCR-ABL Tyrosine-Kinase Inhibitors

BCR-ABL TKIs inhibit the BCR-ABL tyrosine kinase by competing with ATP binding to the kinase. The first drug of this class was imatinib, which rapidly became the treatment of choice for patients with chronic phase CML after it was approved by the U.S. Food and Drug Administration (FDA) in 2001.[2] Today, imatinib, nilotinib, dasatinib, bosutinib and ponatinib are licensed for use in CML. They differ in their respective affinity for the ABL-binding pocket—for example, imatinib has a BCR-ABL IC50 of 221 nM, whereas ponatinib has an IC50 of 0.37 nM and respective half-lives, ranging from 13 hours for imatinib to 4 hours for dasatinib. They also differ in their ability to inhibit other tyrosine kinases, with ponatinib, dasatinib, and bosutinib being the most promiscuous, whereas imatinib and nilotinib are the most specific. Other kinases inhibited by imatinib and nilotinib include the platelet-derived growth factor receptors KIT, and ARG (*ABL*-related gene), whereas the other drugs inhibit SRC family members amongst many others. These differences explain, at least in part, the different toxicity profiles of the various drugs.[36–40] Despite that, it is possible to define a drug class side effect profile that includes myelosuppression, fatigue, gastrointestinal disturbances, hepatotoxicity, myalgias, arthralgias, and skin rashes.[41] All five drugs can cause these side effects, but the relative frequency of the individual side effect differs for each drug. Common toxicities observed are listed in Table 109.1.

TABLE 109.1

Comparison of Side Effects (All Grades) Reported in More Than 10% of the Patients Between Imatinib 400 mg Per Day, Nilotinib 300 mg Twice Per Day, Dasatinib 100 mg Per Day, and Bosutinib 500 mg Per Day

| Side Effect | Percentage (%) | | Clinical Trial |
	Imatinib	Alternative TKI	
Peripheral edema	14	5	ENESTnd (Nilotinib)
	38	11	DASISION (Dasatinib)
	38	11	BELA (Bosutinib)
Pleural effusion	Rare	Rare	ENESTnd (Nilotinib)
	0	14	DASISION (Dasatinib)
	Rare	Rare	BELA (Bosutinib)
Skin rash	11	31	ENESTnd (Nilotinib)
	17	11	DASISION (Dasatinib)
	15	20	BELA (Bosutinib)
Nausea	31	11	ENESTnd (Nilotinib)
	23	10	DASISION (Dasatinib)
	35	31	BELA (Bosutinib)
Vomiting	14	5	ENESTnd (Nilotinib)
	10	5	DASISION (Dasatinib)
	13	32	BELA (Bosutinib)
Diarrhea	21	8	ENESTnd (Nilotinib)
	21	19	DASISION (Dasatinib)
	21	68	BELA (Bosutinib)
Fatigue	8	11	ENESTnd (Nilotinib)
	11	9	DASISION (Dasatinib)
	12	11	BELA (Bosutinib)
Musculoskeletal pain or muscle spasm	24	7	ENESTnd (Nilotinib)
	39	22	DASISION (Dasatinib)
	20	2	BELA (Bosutinib)
Headache	8	14	ENESTnd (Nilotinib)
	11	13	DASISION (Dasatinib)
	8	10	BELA (Bosutinib)

Based on data from the ENESTnd, DASISION, and BELA trials.[50,51,61,110,111]

Imatinib

With over 15 years of experience and hundreds of thousands of patients using imatinib as first-line therapy, the side effects are well understood and there are no apparent long-term safety concerns. Approximately 70% of patients that receive imatinib as first-line therapy will achieve CCyR by 12 months, and 80% will have done so by 5 years.[28,29] The 8-year survival for 553 patients treated with imatinib as part of a randomized trial comparing imatinib to interferon plus Ara-C was 85%, or 93% if only CML-related deaths were considered. This high survival rate has been confirmed in additional single-center studies.[42] Imatinib is given once daily, normally with food (in order to prevent nausea). The current standard dose of imatinib is 400 mg per day. Several randomized studies comparing 400 mg per day to 800 mg per day in newly diagnosed patients revealed more rapid responses with the higher doses; however, one-third of patients required dose reduction due to greater toxicity. With longer follow-up, the response rates to 400 mg per day and higher doses are similar. Progression-free survival (PFS) was not impacted by the higher doses, although a recent study from Germany has suggested that deeper molecular remissions that are more frequently obtained with higher doses of imatinib may translate into a trend toward improved PFS.[43–45]

Nilotinib

Nilotinib is a BCR-ABL inhibitor that was rationally designed to be more potent and selective than imatinib. Until recently, it had been used as a second-line agent at a dose of 400 mg twice daily. At this dose, it induces CCyR in 30% to 40% of the patients who are resistant to imatinib, and most interestingly, there is no cross-intolerance with imatinib.[46–48] Nilotinib obtained a license for first-line use in 2010. The first-line dose is 300 mg twice daily. Nilotinib is administered twice daily in a fasting state because food increases absorption and may lead to increased side effects, particularly the prolongation of Qtc intervals. Overall, nilotinib is well tolerated and causes less nausea, myalgia, arthralgia, and fluid retention than imatinib. On the other hand, it produces skin rashes or pruritus in the majority of patients; in most cases, these can be easily controlled with antihistamines. Nilotinib induces hyperglycemia in approximately 40% of patients; it also causes increases in cholesterol and triglyceride levels. Hepatotoxicity is frequent, although this is normally limited to mild increases in transaminases that do not require action. A severe toxic hepatitis occurs rarely. Similarly, nilotinib causes an increase in the bilirubin level in the majority of patients, but this seldom necessitates any modification of therapy. Nilotinib has also been associated with progressive peripheral arterial occlusive disease,[49] although the incidence of this complication is not yet clear.

Dasatinib

Dasatinib is a multitarget kinase inhibitor that is more than 300 times more potent than imatinib in inhibiting the BCR-ABL oncoprotein in vitro.[50,51] As with nilotinib, most of the experience to date has been using dasatinib in patients who are resistant to imatinib. Initially, dasatinib was used at a dose of 70 mg twice daily due to its short half-life, but a large randomized study comparing several schedules of dasatinib in patients with imatinib resistance showed that 100 mg once daily was equally efficacious to the 70 mg twice daily or 140 mg once daily schedules, but with significantly less toxicity for chronic phase patients.[52] Dasatinib induces CCyR in 30% to 40% of patients with imatinib resistance.[48,53,54] Dasatinib was also approved for first-line use in chronic phase CML patients at a dose of 100 mg per day. Dasatinib is generally well tolerated. Pleural effusions are the main complication of dasatinib therapy. Most

studies report an incidence below 25%, although rates as high as 54% have been reported.[51,55–58] Pleural effusions can occur at any time during therapy and often recur despite a dose reduction. Diagnostic thoracocentesis is not usually required and, in practice, the effusion nearly always resolves on discontinuing the drug. Resolution of the pleural effusion can be accelerated by using 0.5 mg per kilogram of prednisolone for 1 or 2 weeks. Dasatinib has been associated with pulmonary hypertension. The incidence of this complication is not clearly established, and it may be at least partially reversible on discontinuation of the drug.[59]

Bosutinib

Bosutinib is a dual SRC and ABL TKI, which is currently licensed only for second-line use. Similarly to nilotinib and dasatinib, bosutinib induces CCyR in 30% to 40% of the patients who are resistant to at least one prior TKI therapy.[60] Bosutinib has also been evaluated in newly diagnosed patients, but it did not meet its primary endpoint of improved rates of CCyR at 1 year.[61] The drug is well tolerated. Its main side effect is diarrhea, which can easily be managed symptomatically.[60–62] Bosutinib has also been found to cause pleural effusions and pulmonary hypertension, although the incidence of both complications appears to be lower than with dasatinib.

Ponatinib

Ponatinib is the latest addition to the TKI armamentarium. It has been licensed for the management of patients who are resistant to at least two prior TKIs or who harbor the kinase domain mutation T315I. This mutation confers resistance to all the other TKIs discussed in this chapter. The peculiar chemical structure of ponatinib allows it to overcome the steric hindrance caused by the substitution of a threonine by isoleucine in position 315 of the kinase domain.[63] The efficacy of ponatinib has been explored in the PACE study where approximately 200 chronic phase patients who were resistant or intolerant to either dasatinib or nilotinib (the majority of these patients had failed at least three prior TKI lines) and 64 chronic phase patients with the T315I mutation were treated with 45 mg daily. The CCyR rate was 46% with a higher response rate in patients with the T315I mutation.[64–66] The main side effects are skin rash, pancreatitis, and hepatotoxicity. Various cardiac, cerebral, and peripheral vascular thrombotic events have been reported in patients on ponatinib. These have occurred in up to 27% of patients treated with ponatinib and have included fatal myocardial infarction and stroke. These vascular side effects led to the early termination of the phase 3 trial comparing ponatinib with imatinib as frontline therapy and a recommendation that lower doses of ponatinib be used—30 mg in patients initially and 15 mg after patients achieve a MR3. To date, strategies combining ponatinib with antithrombotic agents have not been formally reported.

Choice of Initial Therapy for the Newly Diagnosed Patient in Chronic Phase

Imatinib, nilotinib, and dasatinib are licensed for first-line use. Four randomized studies have been conducted comparing imatinib to newer TKIs, one each comparing imatinib to nilotinib or bosutinb, and two comparing imatinib to dasatinib. Data from these studies are summarized in Table 109.2. A few generalities emerge from these studies. All therapies are extremely effective with excellent PFS. The newer, more potent TKIs induce faster cytogenetic and molecular responses, but in only the imatinib versus nilotinib study has this translated into a significant difference in PFS at 3 years. In the other studies, there was either

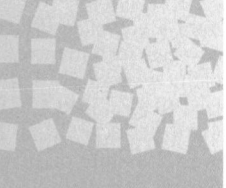

TABLE 109.2

Comparison of the Efficacy Profiles of Imatinib, Nilotinib, Dasatinib, and Bosutinib as Front-line Therapy for Chronic Phase Patients Using Results of the Randomized Trials Comparing Nilotinib 300 mg Twice Daily Versus Imatinib 400 mg Daily (Enestnd),[110,111] Dasatinib 100 mg Once Daily Versus Imatinib 400 mg Daily (Dasision),[50,51] Dasatinib 100 mg Daily Versus Imatinib 400 mg Daily (North America Cooperative Group),[112] and Bosutinib 500 mg Once Daily Versus Imatinib 400 mg Once Daily (Bela)[61]

	ENESTnd		DASISION		North America Cooperative Group		BELA	
	Imatinib	Nilotinib	Imatinib	Dasatinib	Imatinib	Dasatinib	Imatinib	Bosutinib
Number	283	282	260	259	123	123		
CCyR at 12 months	65%*	80%*	73%*	85%*	72%	83%	68%	70%
CCyR at 24 months	77%*	87%*	82%	85%			81%*	87%*
MR3 at 12 months	27%*	55%*	28%*	46%*	33%	47%	27%*	41%*
MR3 at 24 months	44%*	71%*	46%*	64%*			52%*	67%*
MR4.5 at 24 months	9%*	25%*	8%	17%				
PFS at 24 months	95.2%	98.0%	92.1%	93.7%				
OS at 24 months	96.3	97.4%	95.2%	95.3%	97% (at 3 years)	97% (at 3 years)	95%	97%
Patients still on therapy at 24 months	67%	74%	75%	77%			71%*	63%*

The rates of response (CCyR, MR3, and MR4.5) are given as cumulative incidences. Progression free-survival (PFS) and overall survival (OS) are expressed as 2-year probabilities. Patients still on therapy at 24 months are expressed as proportions. Asterisks indicate that the difference is statistically significant (p <0.05).

no difference or a trend to improved PFS, but no studies have shown a significant difference in overall survival (OS). With most relapses on imatinib occuring in the first 3 years, it is unlikely that additional follow-up will lead to significant changes in this data.

Imatinib is still the first-line TKI for many clinicians because its long-term side effect profile is well understood. Further, in most health systems, it is significantly cheaper than dasatinib or nilotinib. The main arguments in favor of using nilotinib or dasatinib as first-line therapies are that they induce deep molecular responses in a higher proportion of patients and that this may impact PFS. With optimal responses to imatinib being highly dependent on the Sokal score, it would be reasonable to choose nilotinib or dasatinib for patients with higher risk Sokal scores.

Another consideration for the selection of initial therapy is comorbid conditions based on the side effect profiles described in Table 109.1. For example, nilotinib can increase the glucose level and serum lipids in a significant proportion of patients; therefore, clinicians may want to avoid nilotinib when treating a patient with diabetes or a dyslipidemia. Similarly, it has been suggested that patients with cardiovascular risk factors should not receive nilotinib because of the risk of developing peripheral arterial occlusive disease. It also should be avoided in patients with a history of pancreatitis. Dasatinib has been shown to inhibit platelet function and has been associated with hemorrhages, so one would favor the use of other TKIs in patients with platelet or clotting disorders. Patients of advanced age and patients with a history of autoimmune disease have a higher risk of developing pleural effusions on dasatinib. Other patients with preexisting pulmonary disease should not receive dasatinib because of the risk of developing pleural effusions, although there is no evidence that patients with pulmonary disease are more likely to develop pleural effusions. The major limitation of this strategy is that it only can be used in the proportion of patients with the relevant comorbidities. In addition, there are no specific circumstances where imatinib should be avoided in preference to other TKIs.

Management of Chronic Phase Patients on Tyrosine Kinase Inhibitor Therapy

TKI therapy can be started as soon as the definitive diagnosis of CML is made. Hydroxyurea may be used to control the peripheral counts while awaiting the results of diagnostic testing. Hydroxyurea can be stopped as soon as patients start on TKI therapy or may be continued for 1 or 2 weeks in cases where the WBC or platelet count is very high. Concomitant therapy with allopurinol is recommended until the WBC is consistently in the normal range. Tumor lysis syndrome is exceedingly rare even in patients with advanced phase disease. After initiating therapy, the WBC count should begin to fall within the first 2 weeks and usually normalizes within 6 weeks. The normalization of the platelet count is commonly delayed by 1 to 3 weeks.[28,67] Myelosuppression occurs in about 10% to 25% of patients. It may occur at any time, but it is more frequent within the first 2 to 6 weeks. Patients should have complete blood counts checked weekly to every other week during the first 2 months of therapy. In the absence of significant myelosuppression, the frequency of hematologic monitoring can be reduced. It is advisable to monitor electrolytes, calcium, magnesium levels, and hepatic and renal function at the same time as the CBC because liver toxicity, hypocalcemia, hypomagnesia, and changes in electrolytes levels are relatively common. Nonhematologic toxicity is normally managed with supportive measures or by interrupting the TKI therapy until resolution of side effects and then by the reintroduction the TKI at the same or at a reduced dose depending on the nature and the severity of the specific side effects. Because there is very little cross-intolerance between the various TKIs, it is advisable to switch TKIs for potentially dangerous or recurrent side effects with the exception of myelosuppression, which is more likely related to the underlying disease.

Bone marrow cytogenetics should be monitored every 6 months until a complete cytogenetic response CCyR is obtained. Some advocate for a marrow at 3 months, but the prognostic significance of this is less clear. With the wider availability of RQ-PCR standardized to the IS, RQ-PCR may replace the necessity of performing marrows. RQ-PCR for BCR-ABL transcripts should be performed every 3 months on peripheral blood for at least the first 2 years on therapy and, depending on response and stability, may be monitored every 4 to 6 months.

Relapse on therapy is defined as a loss of a previously obtained response, such as a loss of CHR, loss of CCyR, or increase in RQ-PCR transcript level. Relapses can be due to a number of factors such as the development of resistance or poor adherence to therapy. Adherence to therapy should be discussed with all patients on a regular basis.[33] Increases in the BCR-ABL transcript level are not always easy to interpret because the accuracy of the test varies substantially depending on the depth of response. It is important to confirm an increase in the transcript level with a second test before altering TKI therapy. Small increases in the transcript numbers are frequent. In general, increases by a factor of two or three on the IS are common and can be ignored because they seldom reflect resistance. At lower transcript levels, increases greater than 5-fold are common and in most cases can be dismissed. The magnitude of the increases is more critical than the loss of MR3, MR4, or CMR, which do not have clinical relevance. Repeated increases beyond interassay variability or confirmed increases consistent with loss of CCyR are should be taken seriously.

Prognostic Landmarks on Therapy

Patient responses are normally assessed at 3, 6, and 12 months. Failure to achieve a CHR at 3 months is rare, and these patients have a poor prognosis.[68] Cytogenetic and molecular response have been evaluated for prognostic significance. One of the most widely accepted landmarks is the achievement of a CCyR at 12 months,[28,29,48,69–72] and many other parameters are based on the likelihood of obtaining this response. For example, for patients who do not achieve an MCyR by 6 months, the chances of obtaining a CCyR at 12 months is 50% or less.[29,68]

Another parameter that is gaining acceptance as having prognostic significance is the BCR-ABL transcript ratio at 3 months. Several studies have shown that patients with a BCR-ABL transcript ratio greater than 10% on the IS have a significantly higher PFS and lower cumulative incidence of CCyR and deep molecular responses (MR3 or higher).[42,73] Similar results have been obtained

for patients treated with dasatinib or nilotinib.[48] One possible limitation to the use of this parameter is the lack of availability of standardized molecular testing.

A third parameter that has been analyzed for prognostic significance is the achievement of a MR3. An analysis of the phase 3 randomized clinical trial comparing imatinib to interferon-α plus Ara-C reported that patients who had achieved MR3 by 12 months had a superior PFS than the patients who were in CCyR but not in MR3.[74] These results were not confirmed by a subsequent analysis.[28] Other groups have also failed to confirm a PFS or OS benefit in patients who achieve MR3,[68,75] whereas a recent update from a German CML study suggested that OS is improved in patients who achieve a MR3 at 12 months. Others have suggested that achieving MR3 represents a safe haven with a low risk of disease progression or relapse. Patients in CCyR who have not achieved MR3 were shown in one study to be more likely to lose their CCyR,[68] but this has not been confirmed in subsequent studies. In most patients who achieve a CCyR, the BCR-ABL transcript level declines over time, which means that a sizable proportion of patients who have failed to achieve MR3 will still do so at a later time without further intervention. Whether achieving even deeper responses will impact PFS, OS, or allow treatment to be discontinued is the focus of future investigations.

Management of Hematologic Toxicity on Tyrosine Kinase Inhibitors

Grade 3 or 4 myelosuppression is relatively common at the onset of TKI therapy and probably reflects the elimination of hematopoiesis from Ph chromosome–positive stem cells before Ph-negative hematopoiesis can be adequately expanded. In the randomized studies comparing imatinib to nilotinib and imatinib to dasatinib, it appears that dasatinib is the most myelosuppressive, followed by imatinib, with nilotinib at 300 mg twice daily being the least myelosuppressive (Table 109.3). Even with nilotinib at 300 mg twice per day, 10% of patients will develop grade 3 or 4 myelosuppression. Although dasatinib may suppress normal hematopoiesis, the suppression of normal hematopoiesis by imatinib and nilotinib is relatively minimal; thus, dose reductions of imatinib and nilotinib are unlikely to expedite the recovery of normal blood counts. In the case of imatinib, doses lower than 300 mg per day may allow for the emergence of resistant leukemic clones, but the minimum adequate doses of dasatinib and nilotinib have not been established. For chronic phase patients, treatment should only be interrupted for an absolute neutrophil count of less than 1.0×10^9/L and a platelet count less than 50×10^9/L. These parameters can

TABLE 109.3

Comparison of Grade 3/4 Myelosuppression Between Imatinib 400 mg Per Day, Nilotinib 300 mg Twice Per Day, Dasatinib 100 mg Per Day, and Bosutinib 500 mg Per Day

	Percentage (%)		
	Imatinib	**Alternative TKI**	**Clinical Trial**
Anemia	5	3	ENESTnd (Nilotinib)
	8	11	DASISION (Dasatinib)
	7	6	BELA (Bosutinib)
Neutropenia	20	12	ENESTnd (Nilotinib)
	21	24	DASISION (Dasatinib)
	24	11	BELA (Bosutinib)
Thrombocytopenia	9	10	ENESTnd (Nilotinib)
	11	19	DASISION (Dasatinib)
	14	14	BELA (Bosutinib)

Based on data from the ENESTnd, DASISION, and BELA trials.[50,51,61,111,112]

be modified for patients with more advanced disease. The use of myeloid or erythroid growth factors while continuing therapy with imatinib appears to be safe. For patients with recurrent myelosuppression, the ability to obtain optimal responses may be compromised; thus, these patients may be candidates for more aggressive therapy. Recurrent pancytopenia is associated with primary cytogenetic resistance in spite of dose reduction or change of TKI therapy. This cohort of patients has a poor prognosis. One possible explanation for this phenomena is that hematologic toxicity is linked to a lack of an expandable Ph-negative stem cell population that can restore effective Ph-negative hematopoiesis, and; therefore, these patients are intrinsically unable to respond adequately to TKI therapy.[29,30]

Management of Primary Treatment Resistance or Relapse

A loss of disease control in the first 5 years of therapy occurs in approximately 15% of chronic phase patients treated with imatinib. Point mutations in the BCR-ABL kinase domain that render the kinase less sensitive to imatinib are observed in approximately 40% of patients who relapse on therapy, but only in a minority of patients with primary resistance (defined as an inability to reach the landmarks defined in Prognostic Landmarks on Therapy). Regardless, all patients being considered for a change in therapy should have the ABL kinase domain sequenced because this may influence the choice of therapy. The point mutations that mediate resistance are scattered throughout the ABL kinase domain and disrupt critical contact points between imatinib and the BCR-ABL protein or induce structural alterations that prevent TKI binding.[2,76] Other mechanisms of resistance include BCR-ABL amplification, drug efflux, and BCR-ABL–independent mechanisms, such as clonal evolution.[77]

Given that the majority of patients who relapse have disease that remains dependent on the BCR-ABL kinase, it was logical to develop novel agents that inhibit imatinib-resistant mutations. As noted previously, dasatinib, nilotinib, bosutinib, and ponatinib were initially developed for patients with imatinib resistance or intolerance. All of these compounds inhibit the majority of imatinib-resistant mutations other than T315I, which is only inhibited by ponatinib.[36,37,78,79] The potency of the various drugs against kinase mutations varies. Some mutations are less sensitive to nilotinib (Y253H, E255K/V, and F359V/C), whereas others are less sensitive to dasatinib (F317L and V299L), bosutinib (F317L and V299L), or ponatinib (E255V).[80] T315I is the most common mutation that emerges in patients with resistance to dasatinib, bosutinib, and nilotinib, but this is rare (<2%) in patients not exposed to these drugs. Highly drug resistant compound mutations have been seen on occasion.[81]

If a patient becomes resistant or intolerant to a first-line therapy, second-line therapy should be started without delay. Patients who require second-line therapy because of nonhematologic toxicity and those with secondary cytogenetic resistance (loss of CCyR) to first-line TKI therapy have a 50% to 90% probability of achieving stable CCyR on second-line therapy.[31,48] Patients with primary cytogenetic resistance, particularly when associated with recurrent pancytopenia, constitute a poor risk group.[42,48] There are no randomized studies comparing the efficacy of the various drugs, and the various single-arm phase 2 studies report similar efficacy for all the drugs. Importantly, most of the published experience is based on the use of nilotinib, dasatinib, and bosutinib in patients who have failed imatinib. Limited data exists on the efficacy of these drugs on patients who have failed nilotinib or dasatinib. None exists on the use of imatinib after failure of other TKIs. The choice of second-line therapy may be guided by mutational analysis or potential toxicities. Once the new therapy is started, patients receiving second-line therapy should be managed and assessed for response as described in the first-line section. Responses

to second-line TKIs are as durable as first-line responses; therefore, responding patients do not necessarily need to be considered for allogeneic HCT.[48]

Hematopoietic Cell Transplantation

Until 1999, CML was the leading indication for allogeneic HCT, but with the widespread availability of imatinib and the other TKIs, HCT rates for CML have fallen.[82] However, the proportion of patients with advanced stage CML who proceed to HCT has increased.[83] HCT remains an effective therapy for patients who are resistant to TKIs and remain in chronic phase and for patients with advanced phase disease whose leukemia can be restored to the chronic phase.

If transplantation is performed with myeloablative conditioning during chronic phase using an HLA-identical sibling donor, 5-year survival rates are 60% to 80%, with a 10-year disease-free survival of 50% to 60%, and a 20-year survival of 38%.[84] Survival estimates roughly halve as the disease progresses from chronic phase to accelerated phase to blast crisis. For younger patients, HCT performed using unrelated donors yields results similar to those obtained with HLA-matched siblings.[85]

Reduced-intensity conditioning regimens, otherwise known as *nonmyeloablative regimens*, emphasize immunosuppression rather than myeloablation to facilitate engraftment, and can be performed in the outpatient setting. The cure relies on immune reconstitution from the donor, with or without additional lymphocyte infusions, to eradicate residual disease. Common preparative regimens include combinations of fludarabine, busulfan, low-dose total body irradiation, T-cell antibodies, and other immunosuppressive drugs. The reduced-intensity conditioning regimens avoid the high early mortality associated with myeloablative conditioning and prolonged neutropenia. Reduced intensity conditioning have shown to be superior to myeloablative HCT in patients over 60 years of age.[86] However, infections and acute and chronic graft versus host disease remain significant problems. Disease-free survival ranges from 40% to 85% at 3 to 5 years.[87,88] Imatinib has been used after HCT for prophylaxis against relapse. Small studies suggest that imatinib can be safely administered from the time of engraftment through the first post-HCT year in patients at high risk of post-transplant relapse.[89,90] Dasatinib and nilotinib post-HCT have also been used in a small number of patients.[91] These small numbers do not allow for an assessment of the effectiveness of this approach in increasing long-term disease-free survival rates.

Relapse after HCT is a common problem, particularly if T-cell depletion is used. Imatinib as the initial treatment for patients who relapse into the chronic phase after allogeneic HCT restores CMR in 83% of patients in molecular relapse and 58% of those in cytogenetic relapse.[92] Approximately 10% to 25% of patients attaining complete molecular remissions are able to discontinue imatinib after 6 to 24 months and remain in remission, whereas the others require either reinstitution of imatinib or donor lymphocyte infusions.[93] Lower and less durable responses to imatinib are seen in patients relapsing into the accelerated phase or blast crisis.[94] Early studies with dasatinib and nilotinib confirm their efficacy in this situation, but the number of patients studied is too small to draw firm conclusions.[91,95] Patients who relapse cytogenetically or hematologically into the chronic phase can also be treated with donor lymphocyte infusions, with 60% to 80% achieving durable remissions and a 5-year disease-free survival rate of approximately 50%.[96–98] In contrast, patients in the accelerated phase and blast crisis are much less responsive to immune manipulations. The risks of donor lymphocyte infusions are significant and result in a treatment-related mortality of 8% to 20%.[99] To date, formal comparison of donor lymphocyte infusions versus TKIs has been undertaken. In addition, strategies need to be developed for using TKIs plus donor lymphocyte infusions for the treatment of relapse after HCT.

ADVANCED PHASE DISEASE

The transformation to advanced phase typically occurs gradually, with the disease becoming more difficult to control with medical therapy. In other patients, the disease transforms abruptly into an acute leukemia, also known as *blast crisis*. Approximately 65% of patients evolve to blast crisis with myeloid lineage blasts; 30% have blasts of pre–B-lymphoid origin; and 5% have undifferentiated or T-cell blasts. On occasion, an isolated blast phase of extramedullary origin may occur while the patient's blood and marrow still meet the criteria for chronic phase disease.

The intermediate period, during which the patient is no longer in the chronic phase but is not yet in blastic transformation, has been termed the *accelerated phase*. Currently accepted criteria for accelerated phase include: (1) progressive splenomegaly and myelofibrosis; (2) bone marrow or peripheral blood blasts ≥15% but <30%; (3) bone marrow or peripheral blood blasts plus promyelocytes ≥30%; (4) bone marrow or peripheral blood basophils ≥20%; (5) platelet count <100 × 10^9/L unrelated to therapy; and (6) clonal evolution in a Ph-chromosome–positive clone.[100] The blastic phase is defined as bone marrow or peripheral blood blast ≥30% or the presence of extramedullary blast infiltrates.

Clonal cytogenetic abnormalities besides a single Ph chromosome may be acquired in patients with CML as their disease progresses, and up to 80% of patients with overt blastic transformation have additional cytogenetic abnormalities. The molecular basis of disease progression is poorly defined, but point mutations or deletions in the *p53* tumor suppressor gene have been observed in up to 25% of patients with myeloid blast crisis, and as many as 50% of patients with lymphoid transformation show a homozygous deletion in the *p16* tumor suppressor gene.[101]

Therapy of Advanced Phase Disease

The prognosis for patients in advanced phase remains poor. Although TKIs induce CCyR in 10% to 45% of patients treated with these drugs, remissions are typically short lasting.[102,103] For example, dasatinib as monotherapy for patients in blast crisis induces a CCyR in 20% to 40% of the patients,[103,104] but a majority of the patients relapse within 1 year, and the median survival is 8 months.[105] Conventional chemotherapy regimens such as a combination of fludarabine, cytarabine, idarubicin and filgrastim (FLAG-IDA) can induce CCyR in 30% to 40% of patients who have progressed to the blastic phase, but again, the majority of patients relapse within 6 months, and the survival is poor.[105] Currently, the standard therapy for patients who present with blast crisis or who have progressed to this phase on TKI

therapy consists of two or three courses of conventional acute leukemia-like chemotherapy or a TKI in monotherapy followed by stem cell transplantation in eligible patients. With this approach, only 20% of the patients are alive at 5 years[84] (<20% at 2 years for patients who are not candidates for allogeneic HCT[105]). Because TKIs have been used successfully in combination with conventional chemotherapy for the therapy of Ph-positive acute lymphoblastic leukemia (ALL),[106] clinical trials are currently exploring the combination of chemotherapy with TKIs for patients in blast crisis.

The accelerated phase is a heterogeneous entity, and there are no large studies dissecting the prognosis of patients according to the different accelerated phase criteria. Most investigators consider patients in the accelerated phase due to a high percentage of blasts to have a similar prognosis to patients in the blastic phase. One of the major limitations of TKI therapy in accelerated phase patients is that the majority of these patients have also already received a TKI. Dasatinib induces a 20% to 30% CCyR rate in patients who have progressed to the accelerated phase on imatinib.[107] Because relapses in these patients are common, HCT should remain a consideration for eligible patients whose disease can be returned to the chronic phase and for patients who fail to achieve an MCyR by 3 months or a CCyR by 6 months.

FUTURE DIRECTIONS

There are now numerous treatment options available for patients with CML. While long-term disease control appears possible with current therapies, disease is not eradicated. Therefore, the most critical area for future development is minimal residual disease. Although the molecular basis of disease persistence is poorly understood, studies of the mechanism are ongoing. Meanwhile, a variety of therapies based on the manipulation of the immunologic system and signal transduction pathways are being investigated for their ability to impact CML stem cells, although it is not clear that it is necessary to eradicate every CML stem cell in order to achieve a cure. Several groups have discontinued imatinib in patients with a consistently negative RQ-PCR for BCR-ABL transcripts using a sensitive assay (>4.5 logs). In these studies, up to 40% of patients have maintained their PCR undetectable status with the majority of molecular relapses occurring within the first 6 months off of therapy.[108,109] With newer TKIs potentially achieving deeper molecular remissions, studies have commenced on the discontinuation of these drugs to see if a larger percentage of patients can discontinue therapy. If a larger percentage of patients achieve a molecular remission and a similar or greater percentage are able to discontinue therapy, the goal of achieving molecular remission may become a goal of treatment guidelines.

SELECTED REFERENCES

The full reference list can be accessed at lwwhealthlibrary.com/oncology.

7. Nowell PC, Hungerford DA. A minute chromosome in human chronic granulocytic leukemia. *Science* 1960;132:1497.
8. Rowley JD. A new consistent chromosomal abnormality in chronic myelogenous leukaemia identified by quinacrine fluorescence and Giemsa staining. *Nature* 1973;243:290–293.
9. Deininger MW, Goldman JM, Melo JV. The molecular biology of chronic myeloid leukemia. *Blood* 2000;96:3343–3356.
10. de Klein A, van Kessel AG, Grosveld G, et al. A cellular oncogene is translocated to the Philadelphia chromosome in chronic myelocytic leukaemia. *Nature* 1982;300:765–767.
11. Groffen J, Stephenson JR, Heisterkamp N, et al. Philadelphia chromosomal breakpoints are clustered within a limited region, *bcr*, on chromosome 22. *Cell* 1984;36:93–99.
12. Konopka JB, Watanabe SM, Witte ON. An alteration of the human c-abl protein in K562 leukemia cells unmasks associated tyrosine kinase activity. *Cell* 1984;37:1035–1042.
13. Lugo TG, Pendergast AM, Muller AJ, et al. Tyrosine kinase activity and transformation potency of bcr-abl oncogene products. *Science* 1990;247:1079–1082.

14. Savage DG, Szydlo RM, Goldman JM. Clinical features at diagnosis in 430 patients with chronic myeloid leukaemia seen at a referral centre over a 16-year period. *Br J Haematol* 1997;96:111–116.
26. Cross NC. Quantitative PCR techniques and applications. *Br J Haematol* 1995;89:693–697.
27. Sokal JE, Cox EB, Baccarani M, et al. Prognostic discrimination in "good-risk" chronic granulocytic leukemia. *Blood* 1984;63:789–799.
28. Druker B, Guilhot F, O'Brien S, et al. Five-year follow-up of imatinib therapy for newly diagnosed chronic myelogenous leukemia in chronic-phase shows sustained responses and high overall survival. *N Engl J Med* 2006;355:2408–2417.
29. de Lavallade H, Apperley JF, Khorashad JS, et al. Imatinib for newly diagnosed patients with chronic myeloid leukaemia: incidence of sustained responses in an intention-to-treat analysis. *J Clin Oncol* 2008;26:3358–3363.
31. Milojkovic D, Nicholson E, Apperley JF, et al. Early prediction of success or failure using second generation tyrosine kinase inhibitors for chronic myeloid leukemia. *Haematologica* 2010;92:224–231.
32. Sokal JE, Baccarani M, Tura S, et al. Prognostic discrimination among younger patients with chronic granulocytic leukemia: relevance to bone marrow transplantation. *Blood* 1985;66:1352–1357.

33. Marin D, Bazeos A, Mahon FX, et al. Adherence is the critical factor for achieving molecular responses in chronic myeloid leukemia patients who achieve complete cytogenetic responses on imatinib. *J Clin Oncol* 2010;24: 2381–2388.

34. Cross NC, White HE, Muller MC, et al. Standardized definitions of molecular response in chronic myeloid leukemia. *Leukemia* 2012;26:2172–2175.

36. Weisberg E, Manley PW, Breitenstein W, et al. Characterization of AMN107, a selective inhibitor of native and mutant Bcr-Abl. *Cancer Cell* 2005;7:129–141.

37. O'Hare T, Shakespeare WC, Zhu X, et al. AP24534, a pan-BCR-ABL inhibitor for chronic myeloid leukemia, potently inhibits the T315I mutant and overcomes mutation-based resistance. *Cancer Cell* 2009;16:401–412.

38. Remsing Rix LL, Rix U, Colinge J, et al. Global target profile of the kinase inhibitor bosutinib in primary chronic myeloid leukemia cells. *Leukemia* 2009;23:477–485.

41. Marin D. Initial choice of therapy among plenty for newly diagnosed chronic myeloid leukemia. *Hematology Am Soc Hematol Educ Program* 2012;2012:115–121.

42. Marin D, Ibrahim AR, Lucas CM, et al. Assessment of BCR-ABL1 transcript levels at 3 months is the only requirement for predicting outcome for patients with chronic myeloid leukemia treated with tyrosine kinase inhibitors. *J Clin Oncol* 2012;30:232–238.

43. Cortes JE, Baccarani M, Guilhot F, et al. Phase III, randomized, open-label study of daily imatinib mesylate 400 mg versus 800 mg in patients with newly diagnosed, previously untreated chronic myeloid leukemia in chronic phase using molecular end points: tyrosine kinase inhibitor optimization and selectivity study. *J Clin Oncol* 2010;28:424–430.

44. Baccarani M, Rosti G, Castagnetti F, et al. Comparison of imatinib 400 mg and 800 mg daily in the front-line treatment of high-risk, Philadelphia-positive chronic myeloid leukemia: a European LeukemiaNet Study. *Blood* 2009;113:4497–4504.

45. Hehlmann R, Müller MC, Lauseker M, et al. Deep molecular response is reached by the majority of patients treated with imatinib, predicts survival, and is achieved more quickly by optimized high-dose imatinib: results from the randomized CML-Study IV. *J Clin Oncol* 2014;32:415–423.

46. Kantarjian H, Giles F, Wunderle L, et al. Nilotinib in imatinib-resistant CML and Philadelphia chromosome-positive ALL. *N Engl J Med* 2006;354: 2542–2551.

47. Kantarjian HM, Giles FJ, Bhalla KN, et al. Nilotinib is effective in patients with chronic myeloid leukemia in chronic phase after imatinib resistance or intolerance: 24-month follow-up results. *Blood* 2011;117:1141–1145.

48. Milojkovic D, Apperley JF, Gerrard G, et al. Responses to second line tyrosine kinase inhibitors are durable: an intention to treat analysis in chronic myeloid leukemia patients. *Blood* 2012;119:1838–1843.

50. Kantarjian H, Shah NP, Hochhaus A, et al. Dasatinib versus imatinib in newly diagnosed chronic-phase chronic myeloid leukemia. *N Engl J Med* 2010;362:2260–2270.

51. Kantarjian HM, Shah NP, Cortes JE, et al. Dasatinib or imatinib in newly diagnosed chronic-phase chronic myeloid leukemia: 2-year follow-up from a randomized phase 3 trial (DASISION). *Blood* 2012;119:1123–1129.

52. Shah NP, Kantarjian HM, Kim DW, et al. Intermittent target inhibition with dasatinib 100 mg once daily preserves efficacy and improves tolerability in imatinib-resistant and -intolerant chronic-phase chronic myeloid leukemia. *J Clin Oncol* 2008;26:3204–3212.

53. Talpaz M, Shah NP, Kantarjian H, et al. Dasatinib in imatinib-resistant Philadelphia chromosome-positive leukemias. *N Engl J Med* 2006;354: 2531–2541.

58. Porkka K, Khoury HJ, Paquette RL, et al. Dasatinib 100 mg once daily minimizes the occurrence of pleural effusion in patients with chronic myeloid leukemia in chronic phase and efficacy is unaffected in patients who develop pleural effusion. *Cancer* 2010;116:377–386.

60. Cortes JE, Kantarjian HM, Brummendorf TH, et al. Safety and efficacy of bosutinib (SKI-606) in chronic phase Philadelphia chromosome positive CML patients with resistance or intolerance to imatinib. *Blood* 2011;118: 4567–4576.

61. Cortes JE, Kim DW, Kantarjian HM, et al. Bosutinib versus imatinib in newly diagnosed chronic-phase chronic myeloid leukemia: results from the BELA trial. *J Clin Oncol* 2012;30:3486–3492.

63. Cortes JE, Kantarjian H, Shah NP, et al. Ponatinib in refractory Philadelphia chromosome-positive leukemias. *N Engl J Med* 2012;367:2075–2088.

67. O'Brien SG, Guilhot F, Larson RA, et al. Imatinib compared with interferon and low-dose cytarabine for newly diagnosed chronic-phase chronic myeloid leukemia. *N Engl J Med* 2003;348:994–1004.

68. Marin D, Milojkovic D, Olavarria E, et al. European LeukemiaNet criteria for failure or sub-optimal response reliably identify patients with CML in early chronic phase treated with imatinib whose eventual outcome is poor. *Blood* 2008;112:4437–4444.

71. Jabbour E, Kantarjian H, O'Brien S, et al. The achievement of an early complete cytogenetic response is a major determinant for outcome in patients with early chronic phase chronic myeloid leukemia treated with tyrosine kinase inhibitors. *Blood* 2011;118:4541–4546.

72. Quintas-Cardama A, Kantarjian H, Jones D, et al. Delayed achievement of cytogenetic and molecular response is associated with increased risk of progression among patients with chronic myeloid leukemia in early chronic phase receiving high-dose or standard-dose imatinib therapy. *Blood* 2009;113: 6315–6321.

74. Hughes TP, Kaeda J, Branford S, et al. Frequency of major molecular responses to imatinib or interferon alfa plus cytarabine in newly diagnosed chronic myeloid leukemia. *N Engl J Med* 2003;349:1423–1432.

76. Shah N, Nicoll J, Nagar B, et al. Multiple BCR-ABL kinase domain mutations confer polyclonal resistance to the tyrosine kinase inhibitor imatinib (STI571) in chronic phase and blast crisis chronic myeloid leukemia. *Cancer Cell* 2002;2:117–223.

78. Shah NP, Tran C, Lee FY, et al. Overriding imatinib resistance with a novel ABL kinase inhibitor. *Science* 2004;305:399–401.

81. Shah NP, Skaggs BJ, Branford S, et al. Sequential ABL kinase inhibitor therapy selects for compound drug-resistant BCR-ABL mutations with altered oncogenic potency. *J Clin Invest* 2007;117:2562–2569.

82. Gratwohl A, Schwendener A, Baldomero H, et al. Changes in the use of hematopoietic stem cell transplantation: a model for diffusion of medical technology. *Haematologica* 2010;95:637–643.

83. Giralt SA, Arora M, Goldman JM, et al. Impact of imatinib therapy on the use of allogeneic haematopoietic progenitor cell transplantation for the treatment of chronic myeloid leukaemia. *Br J Haematol* 2007;137: 461–467.

84. Pavlu J, Szydlo RM, Goldman JM, et al. Three decades of transplantation for chronic myeloid leukemia: what have we learned? *Blood* 2011; 117:755–763.

95. Wright MP, Shepherd JD, Barnett MJ, et al. Response to tyrosine kinase inhibitor therapy in patients with chronic myelogenous leukemia relapsing in chronic and advanced phase following allogeneic hematopoietic stem cell transplantation. *Biol Blood Marrow Transplant* 2010;16:639–646.

101. Calabretta B, Perrotti D. The biology of CML blast crisis. *Blood* 2004;103: 4010–4022.

102. Druker BJ, Sawyers CL, Kantarjian H, et al. Activity of a specific inhibitor of the BCR-ABL tyrosine kinase in the blast crisis of chronic myeloid leukemia and acute lymphoblastic leukemia with the Philadelphia chromosome. *N Engl J Med* 2001;344:1038–1042.

107. Kantarjian H, Cortes J, Kim DW, et al. Phase 3 study of dasatinib 140 mg once daily versus 70 mg twice daily in patients with chronic myeloid leukemia in accelerated phase resistant or intolerant to imatinib: 15-month median follow-up. *Blood* 2009;113:6322–6329.

108. Rousselot P, Huguet F, Rea D, et al. Imatinib mesylate discontinuation in patients with chronic myelogenous leukemia in complete molecular remission for more than 2 years. *Blood* 2007;109:58–60.

109. Mahon FX, Rea D, Guilhot J, et al. Discontinuation of imatinib in patients with chronic myeloid leukaemia who have maintained complete molecular remission for at least 2 years: the prospective, multicentre Stop Imatinib (STIM) trial. *Lancet Oncol* 2010;11:1029–1035.

110. Saglio G, Kim DW, Issaragrisil S, et al. Nilotinib versus imatinib for newly diagnosed chronic myeloid leukemia. *N Engl J Med* 2010;362:2251–2259.

111. Kantarjian HM, Hochhaus A, Saglio G, et al. Nilotinib versus imatinib for the treatment of patients with newly diagnosed chronic phase, Philadelphia chromosome-positive, chronic myeloid leukaemia: 24-month minimum follow-up of the phase 3 randomised ENESTnd trial. *Lancet Oncol* 2011;12: 841–851.

112. Radich JP, Kopecky KJ, Appelbaum FR, et al. A randomized trial of dasatinib 100 mg versus imatinib 400 mg in newly diagnosed chronic-phase chronic myeloid leukemia. *Blood* 2012;120:3898–3905.

PRACTICE OF ONCOLOGY

Chronic Lymphocytic Leukemias

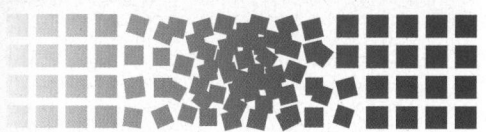

William G. Wierda and Susan M. O'Brien

INTRODUCTION

Chronic lymphocytic leukemia (CLL) is a monoclonal hematopoietic disorder characterized by progressive expansion of B lymphocytes. These small, mature-appearing lymphocytes accumulate in the blood, bone marrow, lymph nodes, liver, and spleen. CLL is the most common leukemia in the Western world, accounting for 25% to 30% of all adult leukemias.[1]

The estimated number of new CLL cases for 2014 was 15,720, with 9,100 men and 6,620 women affected; the median age at diagnosis was 72 years, and incidence increases with increasing age. During the same year, the estimated number of deaths was 4,600, with 2,800 men and 1,800 women; the median age at death was 79.[2,3] The majority of patients have significant comorbidities, which are associated with advanced age. As a result, they tend to have health, geographic, and access limitations. Patients with CLL seen at academic centers and enrolled in clinical trials tend to be younger, with a median age of 58 to 62 years, thereby limiting the ability to generalize results from such trials to community practice.

In Asian countries, CLL represents only 5% of leukemias, with T-cell phenotype predominating. Geographic and ethnic differences in incidence are most likely the result of genetic factors, as Japanese who settled in Hawaii do not have a higher incidence of CLL than native Japanese.[4] Population studies did not link CLL diagnosis to known occupational or environmental risk factors.[5] CLL has a strong familial aggregation, with a two- to seven-fold higher prevalence among family clusters than in the general population.[6]

MOLECULAR BIOLOGY

Immunophenotype

Clonality of CLL is confirmed by restricted expression of either kappa or lambda immunoglobulin light chain on the cell surface membrane.[1] Immunoglobulin gene rearrangement and usage is clonal; therefore, the CLL cells possess a unique idiotypic specificity and often have cytogenetic or molecular abnormalities.[7] With the use of sensitive techniques, monoclonal immunoglobulin can be detected in the serum of some patients, although only 5% to 10% of patients produce large enough quantities to be detected by serum electrophoresis. CLL cells express the B-cell markers CD19, CD20, CD21, CD23, and CD24; most CLL cells are also positive for major histocompatibility complex class II (DR and DQ), Fc receptors, and have receptors for mouse erythrocytes (Table 110.1).[8] Some surface markers that are usually found on normal B cells, including CD22, are infrequently found on CLL cells. CLL cells characteristically express CD5, an antigen normally found on T cells. Small numbers of normal polyclonal B cells can express CD5 and are predominantly in fetal circulation or in tonsils of normal adults. They usually are not detected in peripheral blood using standard immunophenotyping techniques.

Unexpectedly, as high as 3.5% of otherwise normal individuals over age 40 may harbor a population of clonal (by light chain analysis) CD5+/19+/23+ B cells.[9] These asymptomatic individuals do not have an absolute lymphocytosis, lymphadenopathy, or other clinical evidence of CLL and are referred to as having monoclonal B lymphocytosis (MBL). Furthermore, as many as 13% of family members of patients with familial CLL harbor a population of cells with an immunophenotype consistent with CLL, but do not fulfill CLL diagnostic criteria. Therefore, the prevalence of a monoclonal lymphoproliferative process is potentially much higher than previously appreciated. It is estimated that the rate of progression from MBL to CLL is 1 to 2% per year.[10] Currently, there is no indication to perform screening for MBL.

Immunoglobulin Heavy Chain Variable Gene (*IGHV*) Mutation Status

Because CD5+ B cells are found in fetal spleen and because surface immunoglobulin D is present on cells that have not encountered antigen in the germinal center, it was long thought that CLL cells were derived from naïve B cells. Normal B-cell development involves an antigen-independent phase and an antigen-dependent phase. During the antigen-independent phase, B cells undergo rearrangement of the V, D, and J genes in the bone marrow. Somatic mutation of the heavy- and light-chain variable gene occurs after encounter with antigen in the germinal center. Somatic mutation has occurred when there is <98% sequence homology with the germline gene. The figure of 98% is used because polymorphisms may account for lesser degrees of disparity.[11]

In the 1990s, data emerged that a significant percentage of patients had mutation of the immunoglobulin heavy chain variable gene (*IGHV*) in their CLL cells. Subsequently, it was confirmed that approximately 50% of patients have a mutated *IGHV* and that this provided prognostic information; patients with an unmutated *IGHV* have significantly shorter survival.[12,13] Characterization of the *IGHV* sequence is labor-intensive and has not been readily exportable to clinical laboratories. Thus, correlates with mutation status that may be more easily identified may be more accessible. A correlation between expression of CD38 and lack of somatic mutation was described.[12] Although the correlation is significant and the presence of CD38, irrespective of mutation status, is associated with inferior survival, a significant minority of patients have mutated *IGHV* and yet express CD38, and vice versa. These patients may have an intermediate prognosis. Also, there is variation in CD38 expression over time and by disease site (e.g., blood versus bone marrow) in some patients.

It was hypothesized that as patients with CLL can be segregated into two distinct prognostic categories based on *IGHV* mutation status, CLL may represent two separate disease entities, one derived from a naïve B cell that expressed unmutated *IGHV* and the other derived from a memory B cell that had been exposed to antigen and displayed a mutated *IGHV*. This hypothesis has been examined using gene expression profiling.[14] Investigators found that

TABLE 110.1

Immunophenotyping in Chronic B-Cell Leukemias

Disease	sIg	CD5	CD23	FMC7	CD22	CD79b	CD10
CLL	Weak	++	++	−/+	Weak/−	Weak/−	−
B-PLL	Strong	−/+	−/+	++	+	++	−
HCL	Strong	−	−	++	++	+	−
SLVL	Strong	−/+	−/+	++	++	++	−
FL	Strong	−	−	++	++	++	++
MCL	Strong	++	−/+	++	++	++	−/+

sIg, surface immunoglobulin; CLL, chronic lymphocytic leukemia; +, present; −, not present; B-PLL, B-cell prolymphocytic leukemia; HCL, hairy cell leukemia; SLVL, splenic lymphoma with villous lymphocytes; FL, follicular lymphoma; MCL, mantle cell lymphoma.

mutated and unmutated CLLs show a common gene expression pattern that is clearly distinguishable from that of other lymphomas, as well as normal B cells. Nevertheless, although the overall profile was similar, there were differentially expressed genes between the two groups. The gene that was most differentially expressed in one series was zeta-associated protein 70 (ZAP-70), with unmutated cases having significant expression of ZAP-70. Interestingly, ZAP-70 is normally found in T cells, where it functions as an intracellular signal–transduction molecule for the T-cell receptor. It was subsequently shown that ligation of the B-cell receptor (BCR) in CLL cells that expressed ZAP-70 produced greater tyrosine phosphorylation of cytosolic proteins than did stimulation of CLL cells that did not express ZAP-70; therefore, it may

function in activating CLL cells. Expression of ZAP-70 was analyzed in 56 patients with CLL and was correlated with mutational status, disease progression, and survival in retrospective analyses (Fig. 110.1).[15]

Molecular Abnormalities

Conventional chromosome banding identified cytogenetic abnormalities in 40% to 50% of CLL cases; trisomy 12 was most common. This technique is hampered by the low mitotic activity of CLL cells. Fluorescence in situ hybridization (FISH), using genomic DNA probes to detect aberrations in interphase

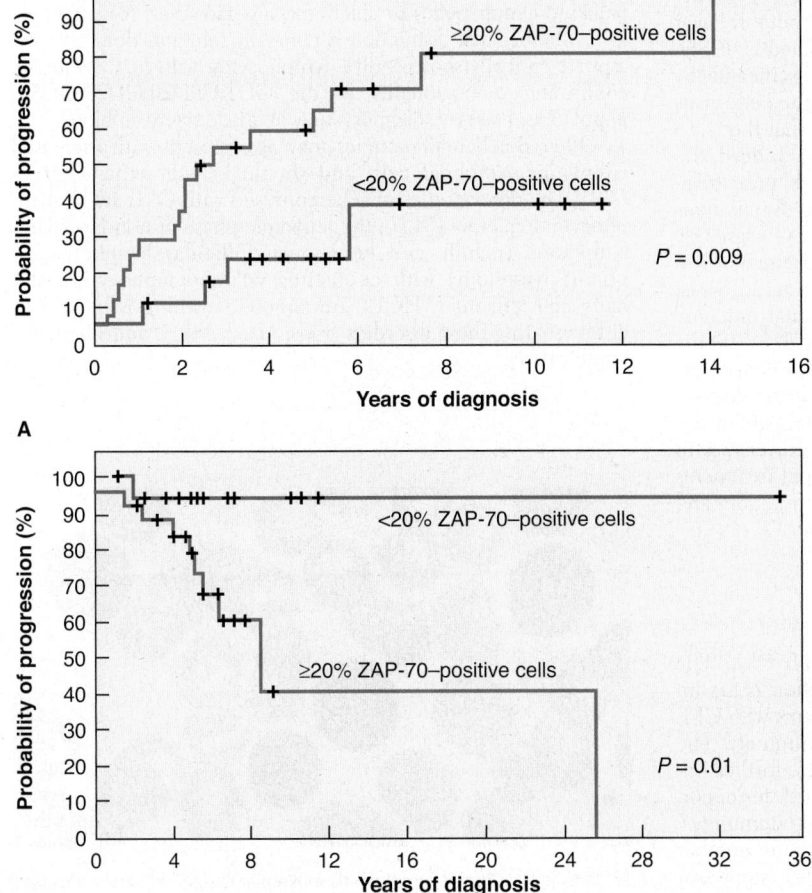

Figure 110.1 Kaplan-Meier estimates of the actuarial risk of disease progression **(A)** and the likelihood of survival **(B)** among patients with Binet stage A chronic lymphocytic leukemia, according to the level of expression of zeta-associated protein 70 (ZAP-70).

cells, enhanced the ability to detect molecular abnormalities in CLL. FISH has shown molecular abnormalities in over 80% of CLL cases.[7]

Deletion 13q [del(13q)] is the most common genetic aberration in CLL; it is found by FISH as a sole abnormality in 55% of cases, followed by 11q deletion (18%) [del(11q)], 12q trisomy (16%), and 17p deletion (7%) [del(17p)].[7] Prognosis in CLL has been correlated with the presence of these chromosomal abnormalities. When divided into five hierarchical prognostic categories in order of highest risk—del(17p), del(11q), 12q trisomy, no abnormalities, and del(13q) (sole abnormality)—the survival times were 32 months, 79 months, 114 months, 111 months, and 133 months, respectively. Patients with del(17p) or del(11q) had more advanced disease with extensive lymphadenopathy. With hierarchical categorization, patients are assigned according to their highest-risk abnormality, including when multiple abnormalities are present. Clonal evolution can occur over time, particularly in the setting of cytotoxic treatment; therefore, repeated FISH assessment is important with changes in clinical status, such as in patients needing retreatment.

The frequency of del(13q) led to a search for a potentially new tumor suppressor gene in that location. At least eight genes were identified and screened for alterations at the DNA or RNA level, or both, but studies failed to find consistent involvement of any of those genes. However, two potentially relevant microRNA (miR) genes, miR15 and miR16, were identified in the critical minimal deleted region of del(13q) and were noted to be deleted or downregulated in more than two-thirds of all CLL cases.[16] MicroRNAs are nontranslated small RNAs that function to regulate gene expression. Both miR15 and miR16 negatively regulate *BCL-2* transcript level; the absence of miR15 and miR16 in cases with del(13q) may lead to Bcl-2 overexpression and resultant resistance to apoptosis.

Whole-exome sequencing of CLL cases identified mutated genes that may contribute to the pathogenesis and biology of the disease.[17–19] The frequency of mutated genes appears notably lower than the occurrence of cytogenetic abnormalities noted by FISH. Mutations are mostly private, and frequencies vary significantly by the patient population being characterized (e.g., untreated versus relapsed or refractory CLL). It is therefore unlikely that there is a single driver mutation that accounts for the disease. Indeed, the limited number of cases sequenced, the diversity in prior treatments among cases, and the relatively low frequency of mutations likely relate to the diversity in reported mutations. Consistently reported genes reported as mutated, albeit at low frequency, include *NOTCH1*, *SF3B1*, *TP53*, *MYD88*, *XPO1*, and *ATM*. Some of these mutations have been associated with clinical outcome such as *TP53*, *SF3B1*, *NOTCH1*, *ATM*, and *BIRC3*.[18–20] Some mutations may result in decreased protein level or function, others may result in activation or increased protein levels, depending on the gene and mutation. Serial sampling of individual patients for whole-exome sequencing is leading to insights into diversities in clonal evolution and an appreciation for how different treatments may impact the emergence, frequency, and type of mutations and loss of others through the course of a patient's disease.[21–23]

IMMUNE ABNORMALITIES

CLL cells disrupt immune function in patients with CLL. The most prominent manifestation of immune dysfunction is the increased risk and frequency of infections. Many patients with CLL succumb to infection or ineffectively treated autoimmunity. The treatments used for CLL, such as purine analogues, further immunosuppress patients and put them at increased risk for opportunistic infections and may exacerbate or unmask autoimmunity.

Early in the disease, in untreated CLL, the absolute number of T cells is increased with inversion of the T helper–T suppressor cell ratio.[24,25] The CD4 to CD8 ratio continues to drop with disease progression or after therapy with nucleoside analogues or alemtuzumab. Qualitative functional assessment of T cells has been inconclusive. Normal and decreased CD4-cell function has been reported. Similarly, decreased, normal, or excessive CD8-cell function has been reported. Others have shown that T-cell functions may be impaired by immunosuppressive factors produced by CLL cells.[24] Hypogammaglobulinemia is a common and progressive immune defect in patients with CLL and is another factor that increases the risk for infection. The pathogenesis of hypogammaglobulinemia in CLL is poorly understood. Impaired B-cell function and regulatory abnormalities of T cells, including the reversal of the normal helper–suppressor cell ratio, may play roles. In addition, CLL-derived natural killer (NK) cells have been shown to suppress immunoglobulin secretion by normal B cells in vitro.

DIAGNOSIS

The International Workshop on CLL (IWCLL) in 2008[26] updated the National Cancer Institute Working Group 1996 guidelines[27] for diagnostic criteria and treatment for CLL.

International Workshop on Chronic Lymphocytic Leukemia Revised Diagnostic Criteria

1. A blood monoclonal B lymphocyte count $>5 \times 10^9$/L, with <55% of the cells being atypical (prolymphocytes).
2. B-lymphocyte monoclonality should be demonstrated with cells expressing B-cell surface antigens (CD19, CD20, CD23), low-density surface immunoglobulin (M or D), and CD5.

A monoclonal B cell count $>5 \times 10^9$/L was specified to distinguish CLL from small lymphocytic lymphoma in patients with palpable lymph nodes or splenomegaly. However, it is arguable as to whether that distinction is clinically relevant. Bone marrow aspirate typically shows >30% lymphocytes, with flow cytometry confirming monoclonality in the CD19/CD20/CD23/CD5+ population; however, diagnosis may be made solely on blood.

Other B-cell malignancies may also present with increased circulating lymphoid cells and should be differentiated from CLL. The diseases that may be confused with CLL are prolymphocytic leukemia (PLL), the leukemic phase of non-Hodgkin's lymphoma (mantle cell lymphoma, follicular lymphoma, or splenic lymphoma with circulating villous lymphocytes), and hairy cell leukemia (HCL). Immunophenotyping is helpful in differentiating these disorders (Figs. 110.2, 110.3, and 110.4; see Table 110.1).

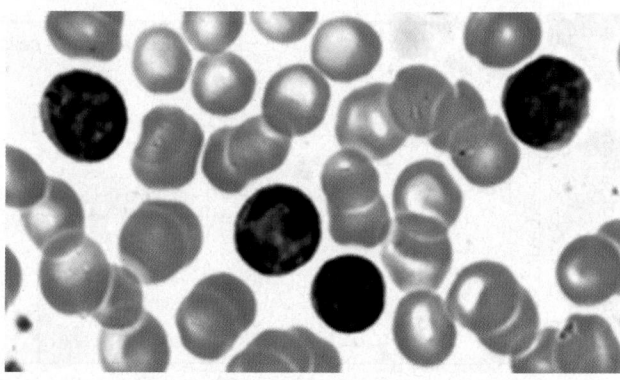

Figure 110.2 Chronic lymphocytic leukemia. Peripheral smear showing mature-appearing lymphocytes.

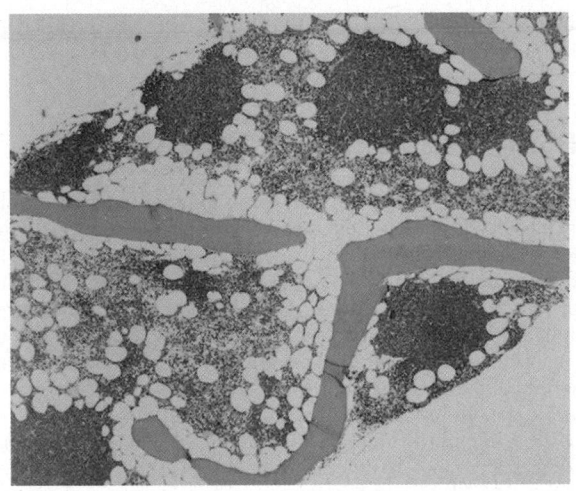 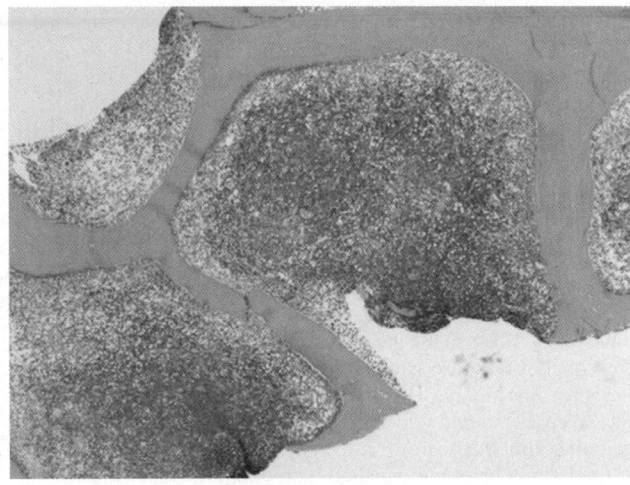

A   B

Figure 110.3 Chronic lymphocytic leukemia. Bone marrow infiltration may range from nodular/focal **(A)** to diffuse **(B)**.

PRACTICE OF ONCOLOGY

Clinical Manifestations

The majority of individuals diagnosed with CLL are asymptomatic and initially identified on routine blood count. Some patients remain asymptomatic for a long period of time. In patients presenting with symptoms, the most common is fatigue, which is generally mild. Sometimes, enlarged lymph nodes or the development of an infection is the initial manifestation of disease. Bacterial infections, such as pneumonia, are more common in patients who present with advanced-stage disease. Infections secondary to opportunistic organisms, particularly herpes zoster, may occur. Exaggerated skin reaction to a bee sting or an insect bite (Wells' syndrome) is frequent in CLL. In contrast to the situation in lymphoma, fever in the absence of infection is rare in CLL. Lymph nodes, when enlarged, are usually discrete, freely movable, and nontender. Splenomegaly may occur, but massive splenomegaly is usually seen in patients with advanced disease. Splenic infarction is rare. Hepatomegaly occurs less frequently than splenomegaly. Skin involvement occurs in <5% of cases. Leptomeningeal leukemia is rare and, if present, is usually seen

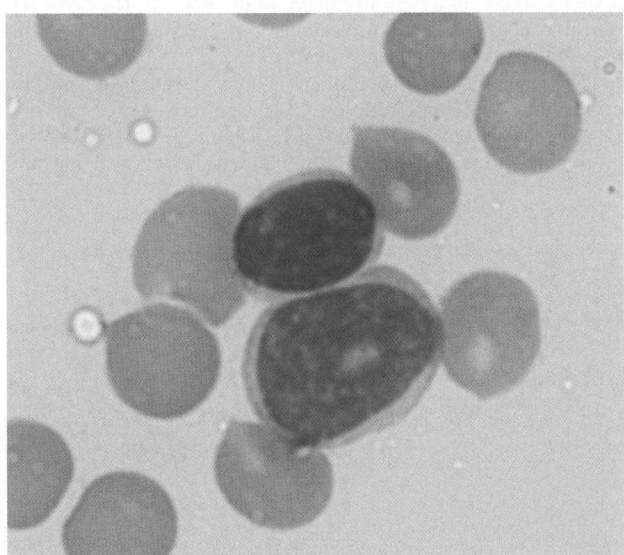

Figure 110.4 Prolymphocyte juxtaposed with a mature-appearing lymphocyte. Note larger size, less-condensed chromatin, and prominent nucleolus.

in patients with refractory disease. Malignant pleural effusions are also rare, and when present, are associated with aggressive disease and poor prognosis.

Laboratory Findings

Absolute lymphocyte counts range from 5×10^9/L to over 500×10^9/L. Leukostasis is uncommon in CLL, probably because of the small size and pliability of the leukemia cells. The lymphocyte count usually increases over time, but fluctuations in the absolute lymphocyte count of untreated patients may occur, particularly in the setting of infection. The lymphocytes are typically small and mature appearing, but there may be variations in cell morphology, with some lymphocytes being larger or atypical, whereas others may be plasmacytoid or cleaved or there may be prolymphocytes. Ruptured lymphocytes or "smudge" cells are commonly seen in the peripheral smear, reflecting fragility and distortion during preparation of the peripheral smear on the glass slide. Marrow infiltration by lymphocytes is universal, affecting from 30% to 100% of the cellularity, with overall increased marrow cellularity. The patterns of lymphoid infiltration of the marrow seen in biopsy specimens include nodular, interstitial, diffuse, or a combination. Patients with diffuse infiltration typically have advanced disease and a worse prognosis. Nodular and interstitial or "nondiffuse" patterns are associated with less advanced disease and better outcome.

Anemia (hemoglobin <11 g/dl) and thrombocytopenia (platelet count <100×10^9/L) are found in a minority of patients at diagnosis but develop with disease progression. A positive direct antiglobulin (Coombs') test is seen in approximately 25% of cases, but overt autoimmune hemolytic anemia (AIHA) occurs less frequently. The incidence of a positive Coombs' test increases significantly with clinical stage.[28] Immune thrombocytopenia is usually diagnosed on the basis of a low platelet count in the presence of adequate numbers of megakaryocytes in the bone marrow. Neutropenia may also be encountered. These cytopenias may be the result of bone marrow failure due to "packed" marrow by CLL or occur as a result of an immune-mediated process or hypersplenism. Hypogammaglobulinemia occurs in approximately 50% of patients with CLL. At diagnosis, it may be noted in <10% of patients, but its incidence increases significantly with disease progression. Usually, all three immunoglobin classes (G, A, and M) are decreased, but in some patients, only one or two may be low. Significant hypogammaglobulinemia and neutropenia potentially result in increased susceptibility to bacterial infections.

Autoimmune Complications

When autoantibodies occur in CLL, they are usually targeted against hematopoietic cells, resulting in AIHA, immune thrombocytopenia, immune-mediated granulocytopenia, or pure red cell aplasia; AIHA is the most frequent.[29] The autoantibodies are typically polyclonal and usually immunoglobulin G, indicating that they are not produced by the leukemic clone.[30] The severity of the autoimmune phenomenon does not necessarily correlate with the severity of CLL, and such events may develop in patients whose disease is responding to therapy. Prednisone is the most commonly used treatment for autoimmune complications, with high initial response rates. It is usually given at a dose of 1 mg/kg orally and tapered once a response is noted. Relapses are not uncommon. Cyclosporin A is another effective therapy and can produce good results, even in steroid-refractory patients.[31] CD20 and CD52 monoclonal antibodies (mAb) rituximab and alemtuzumab have been used alone or in combination with chemotherapy in some patients in whom standard therapy fails.[32,33] Splenectomy is also a viable therapeutic option for refractory cases.[28,34]

Staging

The clinical course for individuals with CLL is variable; survival times range from 2 to over 20 years from diagnosis. In 1975, Rai et al.[35] developed a staging system consisting of five stages (Rai 0 to IV) based on Dameshek's model of orderly disease progression in CLL (Table 110.2). The Rai staging system was later modified into a three-stage system: low-risk (Rai 0), intermediate-risk (Rai I, II), and high-risk (Rai III, IV). A similar staging system was developed in Europe by Binet et al.[36] Both classifications reflect bulk of disease and extent of marrow compromise (i.e., anemia, thrombocytopenia). Both staging systems have been recognized as simple and reliable predictors of survival (see Table 110.2). Although most patients in the high-risk group (Rai III, IV; Binet C) have a progressive clinical course and shortened survival, the course of the disease is not uniform. Patients in the low- and intermediate-risk groups may have an indolent disease course that spans years or even decades, or the course may be progressive and associated with a shortened survival. Thus, it is helpful to have prognostic factors associated with clinical outcomes particularly for the low-risk group. Several prognostic factors have been associated with shortened survival in CLL. These include a short lymphocyte doubling time (<6 months), a diffuse pattern of bone marrow infiltration, advanced age and male gender, abnormal karyotype, high serum levels of β_2-microglobulin and soluble CD23, and a CLL-PLL category (11% to 54% prolymphocytes in the blood).[37] Newer prognostic factors in CLL include *IGHV* mutation status, expression of CD38 and ZAP-70, and gene mutations. A prognostic model integrating cytogenetic abnormalities identified by FISH with

mutated *NOTCH1*, *SF3B1*, *BIRC3*, and *TP53* was proposed as a dynamic prognostic algorithm for overall survival (OS).[20]

TREATMENT AND RESPONSE CRITERIA

An unusual feature of CLL compared to other leukemias is that making the diagnosis is not necessarily an indication to initiate treatment. This is true for several reasons. CLL is a disease of the older population; it may be diagnosed in an asymptomatic patient and have a prolonged course; CLL is not curable with current standard treatment approaches; and a survival advantage was not demonstrated in clinical trials of early intervention. Given that the majority of patients are older than 70 years, may have serious comorbid conditions associated with aging, and may have indolent disease, a significant fraction of patients will die of other causes and may never require therapy for their CLL.

The IWCLL revised criteria for active disease, an indication to initiate treatment,[26] include constitutional symptoms attributable to CLL: weight loss (>10% of baseline weight within the preceding 6 months), extreme fatigue (Eastern Cooperative Oncology Group performance status 2 or higher), fever (temperature higher than 38°C or 100.5°F for at least 2 weeks) or night sweats without evidence of infection; evidence of progressive bone marrow failure characterized by the development of or worsening of anemia, thrombocytopenia, or both; AIHA or autoimmune thrombocytopenia, or both, poorly responsive to corticosteroid therapy; massive (>6 cm below the left costal margin) or progressive splenomegaly; massive (>10 cm in longest diameter) or progressive lymphadenopathy; and progressive lymphocytosis defined as an increase in the absolute lymphocyte count by >50% over a 2-month period, or a doubling time predicted to be <6 months. Hypogammaglobulinemia or monoclonal gammopathy alone are not sufficient criteria to initiate therapy.

Several European groups conducted trials in the 1980s to evaluate whether immediate treatment in patients with early stage disease could improve survival.[38] These large randomized trials of immediate chlorambucil (CLB) therapy versus watch-and-wait were consistent in showing no survival benefit with early treatment. However, given significantly better current therapies, this question has been raised again. A limitation of randomizing all early stage patients is that approximately one-third of them may never require therapy for their disease, thus reducing the potential benefit of early treatment. Furthermore, the discovery of prognostic factors that identify early stage patients with a high likelihood of developing progressive disease may allow for randomized trials to more directly address this question of the benefit of early treatment.

The response criteria published in 1988[39] by the National Cancer Institute Working Group on CLL were revised in 1996[27] and most recently updated by the IWCLL (Table 110.3).[26] Updated recommendations made were that patients treated on clinical trial have

---

TABLE 110.2

Staging of Chronic Lymphocytic Leukemia

Rai Stage	Modified Rai Stage	Description	Binet Stage	Description
0	Low risk	Lymphocytosis only	A	Two or fewer lymphoid-bearing areas
I	Intermediate risk	Lymphocytosis and lymphadenopathy	B	Three or more lymphoid-bearing areas
II	Intermediate risk	Lymphocytosis and splenomegaly with/without lymphadenopathy	—	—
III	High risk	Lymphocytosis and anemia (hemoglobin, <11 g/dl)	C	Anemia (hemoglobin, <10 g/dl) or thrombocytopenia (platelets, 100 × 10⁶/dl)
IV	High risk	Lymphocytosis and thrombocytopenia (platelets, <100 × 10⁶/dl)	—	—

TABLE 110.3

2008 International Workshop on Chronic Lymphocytic Leukemia Revised National Cancer Institute–Sponsored Working Group Response Criteria for Chronic Lymphocytic Leukemia

Parameter[a]	CR (all required)	PR
Lymphocytes	≤4,000/μl[b]	≥50% ↓[c]
LNs	No palpable disease (LN <1.5 cm)[d]	≥50% ↓[c]
Splenomegaly	None	≥50% ↓[c]
Hepatomegaly	None	≥50% ↓[c]
Bone marrow	<30% lymphocytes, no nodules[e]	NA
Constitutional symptoms	None	Variable
Neutrophils	≥1,500/μl	≥1,500/μl or ≥50% improvement[f]
Platelets	>100,000/μl	>100,000/μl or ≥50% improvement[f]
Hemoglobin	>11 g/dl (untransfused)	>11 g/dl or ≥50% improvement[f]

CR, complete response; PR, partial response; ↓, decrease; LN, lymph node; NA, not applicable.
[a] Assessed at least 2 months after completion of therapy.
[b] Include minimal residual disease assessed for clinical trials with reported sensitivity of method.
[c] Must achieve at least two parameters.
[d] Computed tomography scan of chest, abdomen, and pelvis desired for patients to confirm for patients on clinical trial.
[e] Less than 30% lymphocytes in marrow with residual nodules should have immunohistochemistry to characterize nodules.
[f] Must achieve at least one parameter.

evaluation of the blood or bone marrow by sensitive tests for minimal residual disease (MRD) such as multicolor flow cytometry or allele-specific polymerase chain reaction (PCR) for the *IGHV* gene and have confirmation of nodal response by computed tomography scan. In some patients who achieve complete remission by IWCLL criteria, one or both of these methods can demonstrate residual disease, referred to as MRD. Patients free of MRD following treatment have a longer remission duration and longer survival.[40,41] Therefore, in addition to improving complete remission rates, investigators are focusing on eliminating MRD to improve treatment outcomes.

A sensitive four-color flow cytometry assay was developed to differentiate CLL cells (CD5/CD19 with CD20/CD38, CD81/CD22, and CD79b/CD43) from normal B cells.[42] The assay can detect one CLL cell in 10^4 to 10^5 leukocytes. PCR techniques can also be used to assess MRD. Consensus primers for *IGHV* can be used in 70% to 80% of patients and may detect 1 in 10^4 residual cells. Allele-specific oligonucleotide primers generated for individual patients are more sensitive, detecting 1 in 10^5 CLL cells. Development of quantitative PCR techniques may aid in following patients over time but are technically complicated and therefore not available for routine clinical use.

Alkylating Agent-Based Treatments

For decades, the mainstay of therapy for CLL was alkylating agents, CLB and cyclophosphamide (CTX). These alkylating agents were given with or without corticosteroids. Various doses and schedules of oral CLB have been used. CLB is usually administered for several months, and the dose is adjusted to avoid its primary toxicity, myelosuppression. The overall response rate with either CLB or CTX monotherapy is approximately 40% to 60%, with 3% to 5% complete remission. Alkylating agents were combined with steroids to improve response rates.[43] Alkylating agent–based combinations have also included an anthracycline. No superior alkylating-agent combination has been identified.

Purine Analogues

Purine analogues, including fludarabine monophosphate, 2-chlorodeoxyadenosine (2-CdA), and pentostatin (deoxycoformycin), all have activity in treating patients with CLL.[43]

In a phase 2 trial conducted at MD Anderson Cancer Center, fludarabine was given at a dose of 30 mg/m² per day for 5 days every 4 weeks. A response rate of 59% was observed in 68 previously treated patients, with 15% achieving complete remission. A subsequent study explored the combination of fludarabine and prednisone. Response rates were identical to those seen with fludarabine monotherapy, but the addition of prednisone was associated with increased incidence of *Pneumocystis jiroveci* and *Listeria monocytogenes* infections. The major side effects associated with fludarabine were myelosuppression and immunosuppression, with low CD4 counts lasting for many months to years after completion of treatment.[43]

Single-arm studies evaluated fludarabine in previously untreated patients. Overall response rates were higher at 70% to 80%, and complete remission was seen in 10% to 25%.[43] An oral formulation of fludarabine was evaluated in relapsed patients with CLL. Seventy-eight patients received oral fludarabine 40 mg/m² per day for 5 days every 4 weeks for six to eight courses. The overall response rate was 51%, which was almost identical to prior trials using the intravenous formulation as a salvage regimen. Furthermore, oral fludarabine was used in the first-line Leukemia Research Foundation CLL4 trial[44] comparing fludarabine plus CTX versus fludarabine versus CLB, demonstrating efficacy and tolerability with the oral formulation, which is now approved by the US Food and Drug Administration (FDA).

Comparative Studies

A randomized European trial compared six courses of fludarabine versus six courses of CTX, doxorubicin, and prednisone (CAP) in 196 patients with Binet stage B or C CLL (Table 110.4).[45] In previously treated patients, a significantly higher overall response rate was observed with fludarabine compared to CAP. In previously untreated patients (see Table 110.4), the response rates with fludarabine were similar to those with CAP, but the duration of response was significantly longer with fludarabine. The French Cooperative Group on CLL randomized nearly 1,000 previously untreated patients to one of three treatment regimens: fludarabine, CTX, doxorubicin, prednisone, and vincristine, or CAP.[46] Higher overall response rate and longer time to progression were seen with fludarabine. Infection rates were similar, but extramedullary toxicity was less with fludarabine.

Randomized Trials of Monotherapy or Alkylating Agent–Based Combinations as Initial Treatment for Chronic Lymphocytic Leukemia

Study (Ref.)	Agent	No. of Patients	CR (%)	OR (%)	Median RD	Median OS (mo)
Leporrier et al.[46]	Fludarabine vs.	341	40	71	32 mo (TTP)	69
	CAP vs.	240	15	58	28 mo (TTP)	70
	CHOP	357	30	72	30 mo (TTP)	67
Rai et al.[47]	Fludarabine + chlorambucil vs.	123	20	61	NR	55
	Fludarabine vs.	170	20	63	25 mo (TTP)	66
	Chlorambucil	181	4	37	14 mo (TTP)	56
Johnson et al.[45]	Fludarabine vs.	52	23	71	NR	60% at 4 y
	CAP	48	17	60	7	60% at 4 y
GCLLSG CLL5[49,a]	Fludarabine vs.	87	7	72	19 (PFS)	46
	Chlorambucil	98	0	51	18 (PFS)	64
Knauf et al.[50]	Bendamustine vs.	162	31	68	21.6 (PFS)	NR
	Chlorambucil	157	2	31	8.3 (PFS)	NR
Hillmen et al.[76]	Alemtuzumab vs.	149	24	83	14.6	NR
	Chlorambucil	148	2	55	11.7	NR

CR, complete remission; OR, overall response; RD, remission duration; OS, overall survival; CAP, cyclophosphamide, doxorubicin, prednisone; CHOP, cyclophosphamide, doxorubicin, prednisone, vincristine; TTP, time-to-progression; NR, not reached; GCLLSG, German Chronic Lymphocytic Leukemia Study Group; PFS, progression-free survival.
[a] Age 65 years and older.

Results from an Intergroup trial with 509 previously untreated patients with CLL showed significantly higher complete and overall remission rates in patients treated with fludarabine versus those given CLB (see Table 110.4).[47] A third arm, fludarabine plus CLB, was closed early because of infection-related toxicity. Crossover was allowed for patients with no response or relapse. Half the patients who failed to respond to CLB responded to fludarabine, including a 14% complete remission rate. In contrast, only 7% of patients who failed to respond to fludarabine achieved partial response with CLB. Although longer response duration and improved progression-free survival (PFS) were noted in patients treated with fludarabine, no difference in OS was found between the two groups in the initial report. However, updated data, with significantly longer follow-up, reported improved OS for patients treated initially with fludarabine; this difference in the survival curves emerged after 6 years follow-up.[48] The German CLL Study Group (GCLLSG) CLL5 evaluated fludarabine versus CLB monotherapy as initial treatment for patients older than 65 years (see Table 110.4).[49] Surprisingly, while treatment with fludarabine was associated with superior complete (7% versus 0%) and overall (72% versus 51%) response rates, there was no associated improvement in PFS or OS for these "elderly" patients. Thus, standard first-line treatment of the elderly does not require fludarabine.

Bendamustine has a benzimidazole (purinelike) ring structure with an alkylating group and has potent alkylating agent activity, inducing intra- and interstrand DNA crosslinks. Bendamustine was compared to CLB in a randomized phase 3 trial for previously untreated patients with CLL (see Table 110.4).[50] Treatment with bendamustine was associated with superior PFS (21.6 months versus 8.3 months), and complete (31% versus 2%) and overall (68% versus 31%) response rates; this was the basis for FDA approval of this agent. Myelosuppression was mild but more frequent with bendamustine; this did not result in an increased infection rate.

Fludarabine inhibits excision repair of DNA interstrand crosslinks induced by CTX, thereby potentiating activity and providing a rationale for combining these agents.[51] Phase 2 trials, which combined fludarabine and CTX (FC), suggested increased efficacy compared to that seen in historical patients treated with fludarabine monotherapy.[52–54] Three large randomized trials evaluated the efficacy of FC versus fludarabine monotherapy in previously untreated patients (Table 110.5). In the GCLLSG CLL4 trial, previously untreated patients younger than 65 with indications for treatment were randomized to receive six courses of FC or fludarabine.[55] The U.S. Intergroup E2997 trial[56] randomized previously untreated patients to receive FC or fludarabine and the UK Leukemia Research Foundation CLL4 trial[44] randomized patients to FC, fludarabine, or CLB in a 1:1:2 randomization. All three trials demonstrated superior PFS with FC treatment over fludarabine or CLB, and this was associated with superior complete and overall response rates. There was more myelosuppression with the combination, yet there was no difference in the incidence of infections in any of the trials. None of these trials showed a difference in OS with the follow-up available. Patients with del(17p) were confirmed to be high-risk with lower response rates and shorter survival compared to patients with other chromosome abnormalities, regardless of treatment. Patients with del(11q) were high-risk, but there appeared to be a large benefit for those patients treated with an alkylating agent combined with fludarabine. Patients with an unmutated *IGHV* gene had similar response rates to those with a mutated *IGHV*; however, their PFS and OS was shorter for those with an unmutated *IGHV* gene.

Cladribine (2-CdA) and pentostatin (2-deoxycoformyin) have activity in treating CLL.[57] There are no head-to-head comparisons available for purine analogue monotherapy. The large randomized Polish Adult Leukemia Group (PALG)-CLL2 trial compared cladribine monotherapy, cladribine with CTX, versus cladribine with CTX and mitoxantrone (CMC) as initial therapy and demonstrated a higher complete response rate for CMC compared to the other treatments (see Table 110.5).[58] Neutropenia was more common with CMC, as was infection. There were no significant differences in PFS or OS rates among the three arms. The PALG-CLL3 phase 3 trial demonstrated equivalent efficacy with cladribine

TABLE 110.5

Randomized Trials of Purine Analog Monotherapy versus Combinations as Initial Treatment for Chronic Lymphocytic Leukemia

Study (Ref.)	Agent	No. of Patients	CR (%)	OR (%)	Median PFS (mo)
GCLLSG CLL4[55]	FC vs.	164	24	95	48
	Fludarabine	164	7	83	20
E2997[56]	FC vs.	137	23	74	32
	Fludarabine	132	6	60	19
LRF CLL4[44]	FC vs.	196	38	94	43
	Fludarabine vs.	194	15	80	23
	Chlorambucil	387	7	72	20
PALG CLL2[58]	CMC vs.	151	36	80	24
	CC vs.	162	29	83	22
	Cladribine	166	21	77	24
PALG CLL3[59]	CC vs.	211	47	88	28
	FC	212	46	82	27

CR, complete remission; OR, overall response; PFS, median progression-free survival; GCLLSG, German Chronic Lymphocytic Leukemia Study Group; FC, fludarabine + cyclophosphamide; LRF, Leukemia Research Foundation; PALG, Polish Adult Leukemia Group; CMC, cladribine + mitoxantrone + cyclophosphamide; CC, cladribine + cyclophosphamide.

with CTX and FC for previously untreated patients with CLL (see Table 110.5).[59] Patients with del(17p) had poor outcomes with either treatment.

Monoclonal Antibodies

Alemtuzumab is a humanized mAb targeting CD52, an antigen that is highly expressed on CLL cells and normal T and B lymphocytes. Alemtuzumab was originally approved by the FDA based on the pivotal trial that demonstrated monotherapy activity in fludarabine-refractory patients with CLL (Table 110.6).[60–74] Complete and partial remissions were noted in 2% and 31% of 93 treated patients, respectively; 55 (59%) had stable disease. Similar results were reported in a trial with a similar patient population treated with the same dose and duration of alemtuzumab administered subcutaneously.[75] Subcutaneous administration eliminates the infusion-related side effects, although local injection site reactions occur. Alemtuzumab was very effective at eliminating disease in the peripheral blood and bone marrow; bulky lymphadenopathy was less effectively treated, a pattern observed in other studies with alemtuzumab. The T-cell suppression that occurred with this agent has been concerning. As a consequence, a significant incidence of infections (including cytomegalovirus reactivation) is associated with therapy. Antibacterial and antiviral prophylaxis should always be used with alemtuzumab. Other studies confirmed the activity of alemtuzumab in less heavily pretreated patients (see Table 110.6). A randomized first-line trial demonstrated superior PFS associated with alemtuzumab monotherapy compared to CLB, as well as higher complete and overall response rates (see Table 110.4).[76]

The mechanism of action for alemtuzumab is independent of p53. TP53 is a gene deleted in patients who have loss of chromosome 17p. Loss of p53 function by deletion or mutation confers resistance to treatment with standard chemotherapy such as CLB and purine analogues. Alemtuzumab was reported to have activity in patients with leukemia cells that lack p53 function.[77] Despite treatment with alemtuzumab, patients with del(17p) have short remission duration and OS. Alemtuzumab was also combined with high-dose methylprednisolone for previously treated and treatment-naïve patients with better results, although there is concern for immunosuppression and risk for infection (see Table 110.6).

Rituximab is a chimeric immunoglobulin G1 CD20 mAb; CD20 is expressed on malignant and normal B cells.[78] Relatively low levels of CD20 are expressed on CLL cells compared to normal B or neoplastic B cells of other lymphomas. In addition, circulating CD20 was demonstrated in the plasma of patients with CLL; this may inhibit the capacity of rituximab to bind to CLL cells, resulting in rapid clearance and negatively affecting pharmacokinetics.[79] Rituximab binds to the large-loop domain of CD20 and mediates antileukemic activity predominantly through antibody-dependent cellular cytotoxicity and complement-dependent cytotoxicity (CDC) (type I CD20 mAb). Standard-dose rituximab monotherapy has limited activity in treating CLL (see Table 110.6). Dose-intense[80] and dose-dense[81] rituximab monotherapy increased efficacy (see Table 110.6). In addition, greater efficacy was seen when rituximab was used as first-line therapy (see Table 110.6).[82] Maintenance rituximab is not routine practice for patients with CLL.

The primary toxicity seen with rituximab is usually with the initial infusion and is predominantly fever and chills. These symptoms are generally mild to moderate, subside with completion or discontinuation of the infusion, and abate with subsequent infusions. Although normal B cells are also targeted by rituximab, trials to date have shown no significant decrease in immunoglobulin levels, and infection rates are low.

Rituximab was combined with alemtuzumab based on the rationale of targeting two distinct antigens expressed on CLL cells as well as the differential effectiveness by disease site; rituximab has activity in treating lymph node disease, and alemtuzumab is highly effective at clearing blood and bone marrow. Efficacy and tolerability were demonstrated in both untreated and previously treated CLL (see Table 110.6). In addition, rituximab was combined with high-dose methylprednisolone in an active regimen for untreated and previously treated patients (see Table 110.6). Immunosuppression was seen with this combination, owing to the use of high-dose steroids, and was effectively managed with prophylactic antibiotics.

Ofatumumab is a fully human immunoglobulin G1 CD20 mAb that binds to an epitope encompassing both large- and small-loop domains of CD20 and is highly effective at CDC (type I CD20 mAb). Ofatumumab monotherapy was first evaluated in phase 1 and 2 trials of escalating doses of four weekly infusions

TABLE 110.6

Monocloncal Antibody–Based Therapy for Chronic Lymphocytic Leukemia

Study (Ref.)	Monoclonal Antibody	Prior Rx	No. Patients Evaluable	CR (%)	OR (%)	Median PFS (mo)
Alemtuzumab						
Keating et al.[60]	30 mg IV TIW × 12 wk	Yes[a]	93	2	33	9
Osterborg et al.[61]	30 mg IV TIW × 12 wk	Yes	29	4	42	12
Rai et al.[62]	30 mg IV TIW × 16 wk	Yes	24	0	33	19.6
Ferrajoli et al.[63]	30 mg IV TIW × 12 wk	Yes	42	5	31	NA
Moreton et al.[40]	30 mg IV TIW × 16 wk	Yes	91	35	54	NA
Lundin et al.[64]	30 mg SC TIW × 18 wk	No	41	19	87	NR
Stilgenbauer et al.[75]	30 mg SC TIW × 12 wk	Yes[a]	103	4	34	7.7
NCRI-CLL206[65]	30 mg IV TIW × 16 wk + HDMP 1 gm/m^2 daily × 5, c1–4	No/Yes[b]	39	36	85	11.8
Rituximab						
McLaughlin et al.[66]	375 mg/m^2 IV weekly × 4	Yes	30	0	13	NA
Huhn et al.[67]	375 mg/m^2 IV weekly × 4	Yes	28	0	25	5
O'Brien et al.[80,c]	500–825 mg/m^2 IV weekly × 4	Yes	24	0	21	—
	1,000–1,500 mg/m^2 IV weekly × 4	Yes	7	0	43	8
	2,250 mg/m^2 IV weekly × 4	Yes	8	0	75	
Byrd et al.[81,d]	375 mg/m^2 IV TIW × 4 wk	No/Yes	29	4	52	11
Hainsworth[68]	375 mg/m^2 IV weekly × 4 then q 6 mo for 2 y	No	43	9	58	19
Ferrajoli[69]	375 mg/m^2 IV weekly × 4 GM-CSF 25 mcg SC TIW × 8	Yes	118	9	65	NA
Castro et al.[70]	375 mg/m^2 IV weekly × 4 + HDMP 1 gm/m^2 d1–5	Yes[a]	14	36	93	15
Bowen et al.[71]	375 mg/m^2 IV weekly × 4 + HDMP 1 gm/m^2 d1–5	Yes	37	22	78	21
Castro et al.[72]	375 mg/m^2 IV weekly × 4 + HDMP 1 gm/m^2 d1–3	No	28	32	96	30
Alemtuzumab + Rituximab						
Faderl et al.[73]	A-30 mg IV TIW × 4 wk + R-375 mg/m^2 IV weekly × 4	Yes	48	8	52	6
Zent et al.[74]	A-30 mg SC TIW × 4 wk + R-375 mg/m^2 IV weekly × 4	No	30	37	90	12.5
Ofatumumab						
Coiffier et al.[83]	2,000 mg IV weekly × 4	Yes	26	0	50	NA
Wierda et al.[84]	2,000 mg IV weekly × 8, then monthly × 4	FA-ref	59	0	58	5.7
		BF-ref	79	1	47	5.9

Rx, treatment; CR, complete remission; OR, overall response; PFS, progression-free survival; IV, intravenous; TIW, thrice weekly; NA, not available; SC, subcutaneous; NR, not reached; NCRI, National Cancer Research Institute; HDMP, high-dose methylprednisolone; GM-CSF, granulocyte macrophage–colony-stimulating factor; FA-ref, refractory to both fludarabine and alemtuzumab; BF-ref, refractory to fludarabine with bulky (>5 cm) adenopathy.
[a] Fludarabine refractory.
[b] All patients had del(17p).
[c] Dose-intense regimen.
[d] Dose-dense regimen.

(see Table 110.6).[83] The pivotal trial that led to FDA approval of ofatumumab enrolled patients who were refractory to fludarabine and alemtuzumab (FA-ref) as well as fludarabine-refractory patients with bulky (>5 cm) lymph nodes (and therefore poor candidates for treatment with alemtuzumab) (BF-ref); regulatory approval was based on outcome for the FA-ref group. Patients received ofatumumab 2,000 mg intravenously weekly for 8 weeks, then monthly for 4 months. The overall response rate was 58% and 47% for the FA-ref and BF-ref group, respectively. The median PFS and OS were 5.7 months and 13.7 months, respectively, in the FA-ref and 5.9 months and 15.4 months, respectively, in the BF-ref group, representing clinical benefit for these patients compared to historic outcomes with available treatment (see Table 110.6).[84] First infusion-associated toxicity was most common and effectively managed with premedication. Infection was seen, but expected in these highly refractory, heavily pretreated patients. Response rates, median survival, and adverse effects were similar between rituximab-treated, rituximab-refractory, and rituximab-naïve patients.[85]

Chemoimmunotherapy

In vitro data demonstrate synergy between fludarabine and rituximab. Rituximab downmodulates levels of the antiapoptotic protein bcl-2 and may sensitize leukemia cells to fludarabine-induced apoptosis. Furthermore, fludarabine downmodulates expression of complement-resistance proteins, CD46, CD55, and CD59 on malignant B cells and renders them more susceptible to rituximab-induced CDC. The randomized phase 2 multi-institutional Cancer and Leukemia Group B (CALGB) 9712 trial evaluated the activity of concurrent versus sequential fludarabine and rituximab as first-line treatment (Table 110.7).[86–90] All patients in this study

TABLE 110.7

Chemoimmunotherapy for Patients with Chronic Lymphocytic Leukemia

Study (Ref.)	Treatment	Prior Rx	No. Evaluable	CR (%)	OR (%)	Median PFS (mo)
FluCam[87]	F: 30 mg/m² IV d1–3, c1–6 A: 30 mg IV d1–3, c1–6	Yes	36	30	83	13 (TTP)
Mauro et al.[88]	F: 30 mg/m² IV d1–3, c1–4 A: 30 mg IV d1–3, c1–4	No (Age ≤60)	45	24	76	3-y PFS 42.5%
Elter et al.[107]	Randomized (phase 3) F: 25 mg/m² IV d1–5, c1–6 vs. F: 30 mg/m² IV d1–3, c1–6 A: 30 mg IV d1–3, c1–6	Yes Yes	167 168	4 13	75 82	17 24
Hillmen et al.[89]	Chl: 10 mg/m²/d PO d1–7, c1–6 R: 375–500 mg/m² IV d1, c1–6	No	100	10	84	24
Foa et al.[90]	Chl: 8 mg/m²/d PO d1–7, c1–8 R: 375–500 mg/m² IV d1, c3–8 Maintenance: R: 375 mg/m² IV q 8 wk × 12	No (Age >65)	85	17	82	35
GCLLSG CLL11[108]	Randomized (phase 3) Chl: 0.5 mg/kg PO d1,15, c1–6 vs. Chl: 0.5 mg/kg PO d1,15, c1–6 R: 375–500 mg/m² IV d1, c1–6 vs. Chl: 0.5 mg/kg PO d1,15, c1–6 Ob: 1000 mg IV d1,8,15, c1; d1, c2–6	(CIRS >6) No No No	118 330 333	0 7 21	31 65 78	11 15 27
CALGB 9712[86]	Randomized (phase 2) Concurrent F: 25 mg/m² IV d1–5, c1–6 R: 375 mg/m² IV d1,4, c1; d1, c2–6 2 mo observation then R: 375 mg/m² IV weekly × 4 vs. Sequential F: 25 mg/m² IV d1–5, c1–6 2 mo observation then R: 375 mg/m² IV weekly × 4	No No	51 53	47 28	90 77	2-y PFS 70% 2-y PFS 70%
MDACC-FCR[92–95]	F: 25 mg/m² IV d2–4, c1; d1–3, c2–6 C: 250 mg/m² IV d2–4, c1; d1–3, c2–6 R: 375–500 mg/m² IV d1, c1–6	No[92,94] Yes[93,95]	300 177	72 25	95 73	80 28
Foon et al.[101]	F: 20 mg/m² IV d2–4, c1; d2–3, c2–6 C: 150 mg/m² IV d2–4, c1; d2–3, c2–6 R: 375 mg/m² IV d1, c1; 500 mg/m² d14, c1; 500 mg/m² d1, c2–6; then 500 mg/m² q 3 mo	No	63	73	94	70
Bosch et al.[98]	F: 25 mg/m² IV d1–3, c1–6 C: 250 mg/m² IV d1–3, c1–6 M: 6 mg/m² IV d1, c1–6 R: 375–500 mg/m² IV d1, c1–6	No	71	83	96	NR
Faderl et al.[99]	F: 25 mg/m² IV d2–4, c1; d1–3, c2–6 C: 250 mg/m² IV d2–4, c1; d1–3, c2–6 M: 6 mg/m² IV d1, c1–6 R: 375–500 mg/m² IV d1, c1–6	No	30	83	96	NR
Hillmen et al.[100]	Randomized (phase 2) F: 24 mg/m²/d PO d1–5, c1–6 C: 150 mg/m²/d PO d1–5, c1–6 M: 6 mg/m² IV d1, c1–6 vs. F: 24 mg/m²/d PO d1–5, c1–6 C: 150 mg/m²/d PO d1–5, c1–6 M: 6 mg/m² IV d1, c1–6 R: 375–500 mg/m² IV d1, c1–6	Yes Yes	26 26	8 15	58 65	18 18
Kay et al.[103]	P: 2 mg/m² IV d1, c1–6 C: 600 mg/m² IV d1, c1–6 R: 375 mg/m² IV d1, c2–6	No	64	41	91	33

(continued)

TABLE 110.7

Chemoimmunotherapy for Patients with Chronic Lymphocytic Leukemia *(continued)*

Study (Ref.)	Treatment	Prior Rx	No. Evaluable	CR (%)	OR (%)	Median PFS (mo)
Shanafelt et al.[104]	P: 2 mg/m^2 IV d1, c1–6 C: 600 mg/m^2 IV d1, c1–6 Of: 300–1,000 mg IV d1, c1–6	No	48	46	96	NR
Lamanna et al.[102]	P: 4 mg/m^2 IV d1, c1–6 C: 600 mg/m^2 IV d1, c1–6 R: 375 mg/m^2 IV d1, c2–6	Yes	32	25	75	40 (TTF)
Fischer et al.[106]	B: 70 mg/m^2 IV d1,2, c1–6 R: 375–500 mg/m^2 IV d1, c1–6	Yes	78	9	59	14 (EFS)
Fischer et al.[105]	B: 90 mg/m^2 IV d1,2, c1–6 R: 375–500 mg/m^2 IV d1, c1–6	No	117	23	88	34 (EFS)
GCLLSG CLL8[96]	Randomized (phase 3) F: 25 mg/m^2 IV d2–4, c1; d1–3, c2–6 C-250 mg/m^2 IV d2–4, c1; d1–3, c2–6 R: 375–500 mg/m^2 IV d1, c1–6 vs. F: 25 mg/m^2 IV d2–4, c1; d1–3, c2–6 C: 250 mg/m^2 IV d2–4, c1; d1–3, c2–6	(CIRS ≤6) No No	409 408	44 22	90 80	52 33
REACH[97]	Randomized (phase 3) F: 25 mg/m^2 IV d2–4, c1; d1–3, c2–6 C: 250 mg/m^2 IV d2–4, c1; d1–3, c2–6 R: 375–500 mg/m^2 IV d1, c1–6 vs. F: 25 mg/m^2 IV d1–3, c1–6 C: 250 mg/m^2 IV d1–3, c1–6	Yes Yes	276 276	24 13	70 58	30.6 20.6

Rx, treatment; CR, complete remission; OR, overall response; PFS, progression-free survival; F, fludarabine; IV, intravenous; c, course; A, alemtuzumab; TTP, time to progression; Chl, chlorambucil; R, rituximab; PO, by mouth; GCLLSG, German Chronic Lymphocytic Leukemia Study Group; Ob, obinutuzumab; CIRS, cumulative illness rating scale; CALGB, Cancer and Leukemia Group B; MDACC, MD Anderson Cancer Center; C, cyclophosphamide; M, mitoxantrone; NR, not reported; P, pentostatin; Of, ofatumumab; TTF, time to treatment failure; B, bendamustine; EFS, event-free survival.

received rituximab; the concurrent group received 2.5 times the cumulative dose given to the sequential group. This trial achieved the primary end point of demonstrating a significantly higher complete remission rate of 47% in the concurrent group versus 28% in the sequential group. The overall response rate and PFS were not significantly different between the two groups. Shorter PFS was noted for patients with unmutated *IGHV*; shorter PFS and OS were noted for patients with del(17p) or del(11q) by FISH. Notably, the incidence of grade 3 to 4 neutropenia was higher in patients who received concurrent fludarabine and rituximab (77%), compared to sequential (41%) treatment. No significant difference was seen in the incidence of infection between the two arms. Subsequently, an analysis comparing patients treated on the CALGB 9712 trial versus a historical group of patients treated first-line with fludarabine monotherapy in the randomized CALGB 9011 trial (no rituximab) demonstrated a statistically significantly higher complete remission rate, overall response rate, 2-year disease-free survival, and 2-year OS, favoring patients who received fludarabine and rituximab.[91]

The combination of fludarabine, CTX, and rituximab (FCR) was initially evaluated in phase 2 trials in previously treated and chemotherapy-naive patients with CLL (see Table 110.7).[92–95] In 300 previously untreated patients with CLL, the complete remission rate with FCR was 72% and the overall response rate was 95%, with most patients having no detectable disease by two-color flow cytometry evaluation of the bone marrow at the end of therapy.[92] Over 40% of complete responders tested were free of disease in the bone marrow by PCR for *IGHV*. This was the highest response rate reported for any regimen in previously untreated patients with CLL. The estimated median PFS was 80 months.

The GCLLSG CLL8 trial was a randomized multicenter phase 3 clinical trial of FCR versus FC for previously untreated patients (see Table 110.7).[96] This trial clearly demonstrated superior median PFS

associated with FCR (52 months) versus FC (33 months) as well as superior complete and overall response rates at 44% and 95% versus 22% and 88%, respectively. FCR treatment was also associated with a higher incidence of grade 3 or 4 neutropenia (33.7% versus 21%; $p <0.0001$); however, there was no difference in the incidence of grade 3 or 4 infection (18.8% versus 14.9%; $p = 0.14$). Most importantly, this trial demonstrated superior OS associated with first-line treatment with FCR (84% alive) versus FC (79% alive) at 38 months ($p = 0.01$). The largest benefit was seen for patients with Binet stage A and B disease and patients younger than 70.

The REACH trial was an international randomized phase 3 trial with identical treatment arms as CLL8 and enrolled previously treated patients (see Table 110.7).[97] Eligible patients could only have had one prior treatment that did not include rituximab or FC. The conclusions of this trial were consistent with those of CLL8: superior PFS associated with superior complete and overall response rate for FCR versus FC. Thus far, no difference in OS between treatment arms has been observed in the REACH trial.

Efforts to improve the efficacy of the FCR regimen have included adding mitoxantrone to the regimen in clinical trial (see Table 110.7).[98–100] There was no evidence that this addition produced a marked improvement over FCR. In addition, in an effort to reduce the myelosuppression of FCR and make the regimen more tolerable, a phase 2 trial was conducted with reduced doses of fludarabine and CTX and with the addition of maintenance rituximab, referred to as "FCR-lite" (see Table 110.7).[101] Impressive response rates, with a high complete response rate of 73%, and durable remissions were reported. Rituximab or ofatumumab was combined with pentostatin and CTX for previously treated and chemotherapy-naive patients with CLL (see Table 110.7).[102–104] Both studies demonstrated that this regimen was active and well tolerated; the most common toxicity was myelosuppression, and nausea and vomiting were the most common nonhematologic toxicities.

Results from a variety of clinical trials with chemoimmunotherapy regimens for CLL and non-Hodgkin's lymphomas generally indicate synergy between the mAbs and chemotherapy. Indeed, rituximab was also combined with bendamustine and evaluated in phase 2 trials for previously treated and chemotherapy-naïve patients with CLL (see Table 110.7).[105,106] Efficacy and tolerability were demonstrated with this regimen. Furthermore, fludarabine was combined with alemtuzumab for untreated and previously treated patients with CLL; superior efficacy over fludarabine monotherapy and safety were also demonstrated for this combination (see Table 110.7). In a randomized phase 3 trial of previously treated patients with CLL, fludarabine plus alemtuzumab prolonged PFS and OS, albeit with an increase in serious adverse events in the combination treatment group.[107]

Older (age ≥65 years) individuals and those with comorbidities have difficulty tolerating regimens that are more myelosuppressive such as FC or FCR. Furthermore, a randomized trial did not show benefit with fludarabine in first-line treatment for these individuals. Therefore, there have been several clinical trials combining CLB with a CD20 mAb aimed at developing an active and effective chemoimmunotherapy regimen that could be tolerated by this population, with less myelosuppression (see Table 110.7). CLB was combined with rituximab, giving encouraging preliminary results. Obinutuzumab is a type II CD20 mAb, resulting in potent direct induction of apoptosis, and is glycoengineered to enhance antibody-dependent cellular cytotoxicity. The GCLLSG conducted a three-arm, phase 3 trial (CLL11) of CLB monotherapy versus CLB with rituximab versus CLB with obinutuzumab (see Table 110.7).[108] This trial demonstrated superior PFS and OS with obinutuzumab and CLB over CLB monotherapy and demonstrated superior PFS with obinutuzumab over rituximab when combined with CLB. Treatment was well tolerated in these patients with comorbidities, and these trial results led the FDA to approve of obinutuzumab in this setting.

Eliminating Minimal Residual Disease

The clinical benefit of eliminating MRD was suggested in a report of 91 previously treated patients with CLL who received alemtuzumab; 20% had eradication of MRD in the blood and bone marrow evaluated by four-color flow cytometry.[40] MRD-free status was associated with longer PFS and OS. Clinical trials focused on prospectively evaluating the impact of eliminating MRD on PFS and OS are ongoing.

For patients with residual disease after purine analogue–based therapy, the marrow is the usual site of involvement. Because alemtuzumab has significant activity in clearing blood and bone marrow, it was evaluated in trials to eliminate MRD following chemotherapy.[109,110] These studies demonstrated the ability to improve responses and achieve MRD-free status in a percentage of patients treated with alemtuzumab, with anticipated associated risk for infection. However, studies reported unacceptable toxicity with this strategy.[111–113]

B-Cell Signaling Pathway Inhibitors for Treatment of Chronic Lymphocytic Leukemia

CLL cells receive stimulation, including growth and survival signals, from the microenvironment of bone marrow, lymph nodes, and spleen. The microenvironment provides signals directing CLL cell proliferation and survival through binding and ligation of surface receptors and soluble factors such as cytokines and chemokines. Bruton's tyrosine kinase (BTK) has emerged as a central intracellular signal transduction molecule in CLL cell interactions with the microenvironment and for survival.[114] BTK is a central molecule in signal transduction for the BCR as well as CD19, CD38, CD40, CXCR4 chemokine receptor, tumor necrosis factor receptors, and toll-like receptors. BCR signaling and interaction of CLL cells with the microenvironment involve complex biochemical cascades and protein interactions for intracellular signaling. Other key signal transduction molecules include phosphoinositide 3-kinase (PI3K) and spleen tyrosine kinase. These molecules are being targeted for inhibition with small molecules as a therapeutic strategy. The furthest along in clinical development is ibrutinib, an orally administered irreversible inhibitor of BTK recently approved by the FDA for patients with relapsed CLL. Idelalisib is an oral reversible inhibitor of PI3K, and there are spleen tyrosine kinase inhibitors in clinical development.

Bruton's Tyrosine Kinase Inhibitors

X-linked agammaglobulinemia results from mutation in BTK, leading to lack of mature B cells. BTK is essential in the Akt, extracellular signal-regulated protein kinase, and nuclear factor-κB signaling pathways of B cells. BTK inhibition occurs following covalent binding of ibrutinib to cysteine-481. Preclinical studies with ibrutinib demonstrated inhibition of BCR-stimulated activation of nuclear factor-κB and extracellular signal-regulated protein kinase, resulting in death of malignant B cells; antitumor activity was also seen in animal models of B-cell malignancies. A phase 1/2 clinical trial was reported with ibrutinib administered to 85 previously treated patients with CLL demonstrating durable disease control with continuous 420 mg or 840 mg daily monotherapy.[115] There were no dose-limiting toxicities, and target inhibition was associated with clinical reductions in tumor bulk. There was not a difference in activity between the two dose levels; 420 mg once daily is the recommended dose. The overall response rate was 71% (2 complete responses; 58 partial responses) by standard response criteria. Similar responses were noted across risk categories, including for high-risk del(17p), heavily pretreated, and advanced-stage disease. Best response was typically achieved by 1 year on treatment, with lymph node responses occurring rapidly, and lymphocytosis requiring longer time to improve. Most patients had transiently increased lymphocytosis upon initiating treatment, which likely represents egress of leukemia cells from lymph nodes and other protective niches. The 2-year PFS rate was 75% and OS rate was 83%, indicating durable responses with limited follow-up. Grade 3–4 treatment-related toxicity was rare. The most common toxicity was diarrhea, occurring in 49% of patients, 95% of which were grade 1–2. Ibrutinib monotherapy was evaluated as first-line treatment in 31 patients 65 years old or older.[116] The most common toxicities were diarrhea and nausea, occurring in 68% and 48% of patients, respectively; nearly all were grade 1–2. This was a very well-tolerated treatment, and the overall response rate was 71%, with 13% complete response and 58% partial response, with durable remissions although limited follow-up.

Ibrutinib was evaluated against ofatumumab monotherapy in 391 patients with relapsed CLL in an international randomized phase 3 clinical trial.[117,118] Treatment consisted of either ibrutinib 420 mg orally daily until progression or ofatumumab 300 mg first dose then 2,000 mg for seven weekly followed by four monthly doses. The primary end point was reached with an impressive improvement in PFS for ibrutinib (ibrutinib hazard ratio = 0.22; $p <0.001$), with a relatively short overall median follow-up time of 9.4 months. Remarkably, there was a significant improvement in OS for those patients treated with ibrutinib (hazard ratio for death = 0.43; $p = 0.005$). Similarly improved outcomes were seen for high-risk patients, including those with del(17p) and those with fludarabine-refractory CLL. Diarrhea, fatigue, fever, and nausea were the most commonly reported adverse effects experienced by the patients treated with ibrutinib and were mild. According to early reports, mechanisms of ibrutinib resistance appear to include mutation of BTK at cysteine-481 (C481S) and gain-of-function mutations in PLCγ2, a signaling molecule immediately downstream of BTK.[119]

Phosphoinositide 3-Kinase Inhibitor

There are four class I PI3K isoforms; PI3K-delta is expressed by leukocytes and participates in B cell development, signaling, and survival. PI3K mediates downstream signaling for the BCR as well as CXCR4, CD40, and CD49d. Idelalisib is an orally bioavailable, reversible small molecule inhibitor of p110δ of the PI3K complex; it produces no significant inhibition of other class I isoforms and no significant off-target inhibition of PI3K class II or III isoforms, mammalian target of rapamycin, or DNA protein kinases.

A phase 1 trial of idelalisib was conducted in relapsed and refractory patients with low-grade lymphoproliferative diseases, including CLL.[120] Idelalisib was well tolerated; elevated liver enzymes was the most frequent toxicity, and treatment resulted in a 30% response rate in relapsed patients with CLL.[120] There was rapid and marked reduction in lymph node size and an initial increase followed by decrease in circulating leukemia cells, indicating an initial redistribution of cells followed by cell death. A phase 3 clinical trial evaluated the activity of idelalisib in combination with rituximab versus rituximab with placebo as treatment for patients with relapsed CLL in 220 frail individuals with comorbidities or cytopenias.[121] Idelalisib 150 mg was dosed twice daily continuously in 110 patients. Rituximab was administered to all patients at 375 mg/m² first dose, 500 mg/m² every 2 weeks for four doses, then every 4 weeks for three doses (eight total doses). This trial demonstrated superior efficacy for combined idelalisib and rituximab over rituximab and placebo with a hazard ratio for PFS of 0.15 (p <0.001) and hazard ratio for OS of 0.28 (p = 0.02); serious adverse events occurred in 40% and 35%, respectively this led to FDA approval of the combination.

NEW AND NOVEL TREATMENTS FOR CHRONIC LYMPHOCYTIC LEUKEMIA

A number of new therapeutic approaches are under development for patients with CLL. Important novel strategies or novel targets and pathways include targeting Bcl-2 family members for inhibition with BH3-mimetics, immune-modulating agents such as lenalidomide, and cellular therapy strategies.

Bcl-2 Inhibitors

CLL cells express high levels of antiapoptotic proteins of the Bcl-2 family, rendering them long-lived and resistant to senescence and death. Small molecule inhibitors of Bcl-2 family members are in therapeutic development. Navitoclax (ABT-263) is an orally administered small molecule inhibitor of Bcl-2, Bcl-w, and Bcl-xL. In vitro treatment of CLL cells with navitoclax induced cell death. A phase 1/2 trial of orally administered navitoclax was conducted and generated promising results. The majority of patients treated in the study had >50% reduction in leukemia counts, and some patients experienced reduction in lymph node size.[122] The dose-limiting toxicity was thrombocytopenia secondary to accelerated platelet senescence from inhibition of Bcl-xL in platelets. Given this activity, ABT-199 was designed as a molecule with greater affinity for Bcl-2 and reduced affinity for Bcl-xL.[123] A phase 1 trial is ongoing with ABT-199 monotherapy[124] and in combination with CD20 mAb.

Immunemodulation

Lenalidomide, a thalidomide analogue, has immunomodulatory and antiangiogenic activities. The mechanisms of action and effects on the microenvironment are not well understood. Lenalidomide monotherapy was initially studied in relapsed CLL. Phase 2 clinical trials in relapsed or refractory patients with CLL evaluated continuous and interrupted (21 of 28 days) administration of up to 25 mg daily and reported overall response rates of 32% to 47%

with 7% to 9% achieving complete remission, including patients who achieved MRD-free status.[125,126] Furthermore, responses were noted in patients with high-risk features including del(11q) and del(17p). Subsequently, trials evaluated first-line monotherapy, demonstrating tolerability, good responses, and durable disease control.[127,128] In a study of 60 symptomatic patients with untreated CLL age 65 years or older, lenalidomide at an initial dose of 5 mg/d (and titrated up) was well tolerated and resulted in a 65% response rate.[128,129] Improvement in hypogammaglobulinemia and T-cell counts were noted in this setting, suggesting immune restoration. Subsequently, lenalidomide was evaluated in combination with rituximab for previously treated CLL.[130] The addition of CD20 mAb appeared to improve outcomes compared to monotherapy for relapsed disease.

Lenalidomide safety and toxicity concerns have been tumor lysis syndrome and tumor flare reaction, which occur upon initiation of treatment, as well as myelosuppression, which can be dose-limiting and occurs while patients are on treatment. Tumor lysis syndrome and tumor flare reaction have been minimized by initiating lenalidomide at low dose (2.5 mg to 5 mg daily), and by initiating CD20 mAb prior to lenalidomide in patients receiving the combination. Lenalidomide remains a promising agent with unique properties and is being studied earlier in treatment, in combinations and as maintenance therapy in CLL.

Cellular Therapy for Chronic Lymphocytic Leukemia

Chimeric Antigen Receptor–Bearing T-Cell Therapy

Immune-based cellular therapy takes advantage of the ability of the immune system to seek out and eliminate malignant cells in the body. It potentially provides a mechanism of surveillance to prevent recurrence of disease. Allogeneic stem cell transplant is a form of immune cellular therapy, which is curative for some patients with CLL. Another strategy of immune cellular therapy is being developed, based on T-cell expression of chimeric antigen receptors (CARs).[131–134] CARs are engineered immune receptors introduced ex vivo into T cells, usually autologous, that redirect these cells to react against CLL cells. Graft-versus-host reactions are avoided with autologous T cells, while inducing and enhancing a graft-versus-leukemia effect. The CAR is a recombinant protein composed of an antigen-binding domain derived from single-chain immunoglobulin variable genes, hinge-stalk-transmembrane domain, derived on CD8, constant domain of immunoglobulin or other molecule, and intracellular signaling domains derived from CD3ζ and costimulatory domains derived from CD28 and/or CD137. The engineered gene is transduced into autologous T cells and expressed on the surface where it can bind to target antigen and induce T-cell activation, cytokine production, proliferation, and killing of cells expressing the target antigen. CD19 is expressed by malignant B cells, including CLL, as well as normal B cells and has been targeted with CARs. On-target effects include a leukemia-specific reaction as well as elimination of normal B cells, resulting in hypogammaglobulinemia. While very robust treatment effects were reported, including durable complete remissions, infusion-related side effects, and more notably, cytokine-release syndrome have been challenging. Hypogammaglobulinemia has inspired a search for better and more specific leukemia-associated or leukemia-specific antigens. This strategy is in early phase trials and appears promising.

Allogeneic Stem Cell Transplantation

Myeloablative allogeneic stem cell transplantation was not a viable option in CLL in the past because of the prohibitive toxicity of this approach in older patients. Autologous bone marrow transplantation has been evaluated for CLL,[135,136] but does not appear to have a role. Reduced-intensity conditioning has made allogeneic stem cell transplant (allo-SCT) available for significantly more patients with CLL. While allo-SCT was associated with long-term remissions and possible cure, there is patient selection and reporting bias in these data. Early data with nonmyeloablative allogeneic transplant indicated almost universal engraftment, although the development of chimerism was slower than with myeloablative transplants. Patients with sensitive disease who were transplanted had a better outcome than those who had resistant disease.[137] Long-term follow-up data have been reported showing a 5-year OS rate of 50%.[138,139] Notably, immune manipulation by withdrawal of immunosuppression or donor lymphocyte infusions enhanced clinical responses, indicating that CLL is a disease vulnerable to immune-mediated elimination and control. A 6-year OS rate of 58% was reported in a series of 90 previously treated patients who underwent reduced-intensity conditioning and allo-SCT, with an event-free survival of 38% for the same period.[140] Furthermore, no association was noted between the presence of mutations in *TP53*, *SF3B1*, or *NOTCH1* and OS or EFS, indicating efficacy for patients with high-risk features. Smaller series reported similar outcomes.[141–143] A single-center retrospective study of outcomes for individuals with relapsed CLL who had a matched allogeneic donor versus no donor showed improved survival for individuals who had a matched donor in landmark analysis starting 3 months after donor search was initiated. These data indicate that allo-SCT may improve survival for patients with relapsed high-risk CLL.[144]

Splenectomy

Studies suggest hematologic and survival benefits from splenectomy in patients with CLL. Splenectomy may be beneficial in individuals with immune-mediated cytopenias such as AIHA and immune thrombocytopenia purpura after corticosteroid failure or in improving blood counts in patients with hypersplenism. In a study from MD Anderson Cancer Center,[34] perioperative mortality among 55 patients was 9%, mostly related to poor preoperative performance status. Improvements in the platelet count, neutrophil count, and hemoglobin occurred in 81%, 59%, and 33% of patients, respectively. Among patients with Rai stage IV disease, a trend for improved survival was observed using case-control analysis.

Therapeutic Considerations for Specific Problems in Patients with Chronic Lymphocytic Leukemia

The most common cause of morbidity in patients with CLL is infection. Because hypogammaglobulinemia is a contributing factor to patients' increased susceptibility to infections, a randomized double-blind study evaluated the use of intravenous immunoglobulin, 400 mg/kg, versus placebo given every 3 weeks for 1 year to 84 patients with CLL.[145,146] A significant reduction in bacterial infections was seen in the group treated with intravenous immunoglobulin, but no statistically significant difference was observed in the number of life-threatening infections or nonbacterial infections. Because of the high cost of this therapy, monthly intravenous immunoglobulin therapy is best used in patients with hypogammaglobulinemia who experience repeated bacterial infections.[147,148]

SECOND MALIGNANCIES AND TRANSFORMATION

Approximately 25% of patients with CLL develop second neoplasms, the most common being skin cancer. Second neoplasm is the cause of death in 7% to 10% of patients. In approximately 2% to 6% of patients, CLL may evolve into a high-grade lymphoma

of the diffuse large-cell type (Richter's transformation); less commonly Hodgkin's histology is diagnosed. Richter's transformation may arise from the original CLL clone, and its onset is heralded by fever, weight loss, a rising lactate dehydrogenase, and an asymmetric rapid lymph node enlargement.[149] Because the lymphoma may be patchy, a gallium or positron emission tomography scan, usually negative in CLL, may aid in identifying a "hot" lymph node that can be targeted for biopsy. Transformation must be diagnosed by histology. The prognosis of Richter's transformation is poor, with a median survival of only 6 months. Prolymphocytic transformation develops in approximately 2% to 5% of patients with CLL. This transformation is different immunophenotypically and clinically from primary or de novo PLL. Secondary PLL is marked by development of refractory anemia and thrombocytopenia, progressive splenomegaly, and an increase in the percentage of prolymphocytes to >30% of the leukemia cells. As with Richter's transformation, PLL transformation portends a poor prognosis despite aggressive therapy.

Therapy-related myeloid neoplasia (myelodysplasia or acute myeloid leukemia) is also a concern in CLL. In long-term follow-up of the US Intergroup Study E2997, 4.7% of patients developed therapy-related myeloid neoplasia at a median of 5 years from initial therapy.[150]

PROLYMPHOCYTIC LEUKEMIA

PLL is characterized by a high number of circulating prolymphocytes, splenomegaly, minimal lymphadenopathy, and a median survival of <3 years. This leukemia can be present at diagnosis or evolve from CLL.[151] Prolymphocytes are larger and less homogeneous than CLL cells and have abundant clear cytoplasm, clumped chromatin, and a prominent nucleolus. Prolymphocytes can be of either B- or T-cell type. B-PLL cells usually do not express CD5 but stain strongly for surface immunoglobulin and FMC7 (see Table 110.1). In 20% of cases of PLL, T-cell markers are expressed.

Splenectomy and lymphomalike regimens have been used to treat PLL without much success. Nucleoside analogue–based regimens appear to be the most effective, and alemtuzumab has shown promising activity in T-PLL.[152]

LARGE GRANULAR LYMPHOCYTE LEUKEMIA

Large granular lymphocytes (LGLs) are larger than normal lymphocytes and contain azurophilic granules in their cytoplasm. LGLs comprise 10% to 15% of peripheral blood mononuclear cells and are predominantly of NK-cell phenotype, a smaller fraction being of T-cell phenotype. There are generally four lymphoproliferative disorders of LGL: reactive/transient LGL expansion, chronic LGL lymphocytosis, indolent LGL leukemia, and aggressive LGL leukemia.[153] Clonal expansion of LGL can be of NK-cell or T-cell phenotype; the T-cell phenotype comprises 80% of LGL leukemias. T-LGL cells have a CD3+/CD57+/CD56− immunophenotype, and NK-LGL express CD3−/CD56+/CD57−. Clonality in T-LGL leukemia may be established by T-cell receptor gene rearrangement studies. T-LGL leukemia is usually indolent. Patients present with cytopenias, including neutropenia with accompanying infections, pure red cell aplasia, thrombocytopenia, and anemia. Serologic abnormalities, such as the presence of rheumatoid factor or antinuclear antibody, or both, hypergammaglobulinemia, and high β_2-microglobin are frequent. A small percentage of LGL leukemias have a more aggressive course, and these cases tend to have an NK-cell phenotype. Because lymphocyte counts are usually not elevated, diagnosis requires a high degree of suspicion and a careful examination of the peripheral blood smear and bone marrow. Although the disease may be indolent, most patients

PRACTICE OF ONCOLOGY

require treatment for cytopenias. Various therapies, including low-dose methotrexate (10 mg/m^2 orally once weekly), cyclosporine (2 mg/kg orally every 12 hours), or CTX (100 mg orally daily) with or without oral prednisone (1 mg/kg orally daily) have all been effective. Complete remissions may be seen in up to 50% of cases. Lymphoma-type regimens, such as CTX, doxorubicin, prednisone, and vincristine, have not been effective for aggressive disease.

HAIRY CELL LEUKEMIA

HCL is a rare B-cell lymphoproliferative disorder that affects adults and represents 2% of all leukemias. It has a marked preponderance in men. Most patients have cytopenias; splenomegaly is also frequent.[154] Hairy cells can be seen in the peripheral blood, but at low frequency, and therefore are easily missed. These cells are twice as large as normal lymphocytes, with the nuclei showing a loose chromatin pattern and villi-like cytoplasmic projections (best viewed under phase contrast microscopy). Hairy cells infiltrate the bone marrow in an interstitial or focal pattern, with clear zones in between cells ("fried egg appearance"). Marrow reticulin is increased, and aspirates may result in a dry tap. Immunophenotypic analysis of hairy cells shows the presence of CD19, CD20, CD22, CD25, and CD103, and, in contrast to CLL, hairy cells are negative for CD5 and CD23. Hairy cells also stain strongly for surface immunoglobulin and FMC7. Use of the CD103 antibody, which stains tartrate-resistant acid phosphatase, has obviated the need for cytochemical staining for tartrate-resistant acid phosphatase.

The BRAF V600E mutation was recently found to be present in all patients with HCL, a finding that is likely to have an impact on the diagnosis and possibly the treatment of this disease.[155,156] Vemurafenib is a BRAF inhibitor[157] currently in clinical trials as therapy for relapsed or refractory HCL.

HCL has no staging system. For many years, the only effective therapy was splenectomy.

Treatments for Hairy Cell Leukemia

Nucleoside Analogues

Pentostatin (2′ deoxycoformycin) and cladribine (2-CdA) are the nucleoside analogues that are the mainstay of treatment of HCL.[158] Pentostatin is administered at 4 mg/m^2 every 2 weeks until maximum response, and cladribine is given at 0.1 mg/kg per day as a continuous intravenous infusion for 7 days; the same total dose can be administered as a 2-hour infusion over 5 days. Because cladribine involves a single course of therapy and produces remission rates comparable to those of pentostatin, cladribine is used more frequently in the United States for the treatment of HCL. Multiple series have reported high response rates, with patients remaining in remission for many years. The majority of relapsed patients achieve second remission when retreated with pentostatin or cladribine. The choice of agent may depend on the duration of the first remission: if <3 years, an alternate agent should be used; if >5 years, the same agent may be given. The role of interferon-alpha is currently limited to patients who are unresponsive to nucleoside analogues.

Monoclonal Antibody-Drug Conjugate

A percentage of patients may relapse with cladribine-resistant disease. In addition, 10% to 20% of patients have a variant form of HCL with high numbers of circulating hairy cells and a poor response to nucleoside analogues. Classic and variant hairy cells strongly express CD22, a B-cell adhesion molecule. Data suggest marked efficacy of a recombinant immunotoxin, BL22, in the treatment of chemotherapy-resistant HCL.[159] This immunotoxin contains the variable domain of the anti-CD22 mAb RFB4, which is fused to a fragment of *Pseudomonas* exotoxin called *PE38* that lacks the domain necessary for cell binding and contains only the domain responsible for cell death. The phase 1 trial of BL22 included 16 cladribine-resistant patients with HCL; 11 achieved complete remission and 2 partial remissions were reported. Side effects included transient hypoalbuminemia, elevated aminotransferase levels and in 2 of 16 patients, a reversible hemolytic-uremic syndrome developed. A phase 2 trial was conducted with BL22 in 36 patients with relapsed or refractory HCL.[160] Overall, 47% achieved complete response and 25% partial response; 2 (6%) patients experienced reversible hemolytic-uremic syndrome. Patients with smaller spleen were more likely to achieve complete response. Neutralizing antibodies were identified in four (11%) patients, which prevented retreatment. Moxetumomab pasudotox (HA22 or CAT-8015) is derived from BL22, selected for high-affinity for CD22. A phase 1 trial of moxetumomab pasudotox was performed in 28 patients with chemotherapy-resistant HCL.[161] Doses included 5 mcg/kg to 50 mcg/kg intravenously every other day for three doses for each course, with up to 16 courses repeated every 4 weeks. The median number of courses given was four, and no dose-limiting toxicity was observed up to the highest dose tested. The overall response rate was 86% and 46% achieved CR; these responses were durable.

SELECTED REFERENCES

The full reference list can be accessed at lwwhealthlibrary.com/oncology.

2. Jemal A, Siegel R, Xu J, et al. Cancer statistics, 2010. *CA Cancer J Clin* 2010;60:277–300.
3. Siegel R, Ma J, Zou Z, et al. Cancer statistics, 2014. *CA Cancer J Clin* 2014;64:9–29.
9. Rawstron AC, Green MJ, Kuzmicki A, et al. Monoclonal B lymphocytes with the characteristics of "indolent" chronic lymphocytic leukemia are present in 3.5% of adults with normal blood counts. *Blood* 2002;100:635–639.
10. Rawstron AC, Bennett FL, O'Connor SJ, et al. Monoclonal B-cell lymphocytosis and chronic lymphocytic leukemia. *N Engl J Med* 2008;359:575–583.
12. Damle RN, Wasil T, Fais F, et al. Ig V gene mutation status and CD38 expression as novel prognostic indicators in chronic lymphocytic leukemia. *Blood* 1999;94:1840–1847.
13. Hamblin TJ, Davis Z, Gardiner A, et al. Unmutated Ig V(H) genes are associated with a more aggressive form of chronic lymphocytic leukemia. *Blood* 1999;94:1848–1854.
14. Rosenwald A, Alizadeh AA, Widhopf G, et al. Relation of gene expression phenotype to immunoglobulin mutation genotype in B cell chronic lymphocytic leukemia. *J Exp Med* 2001;194:1639–1647.
15. Crespo M, Bosch F, Villamor N, et al. ZAP-70 expression as a surrogate for immunoglobulin-variable-region mutations in chronic lymphocytic leukemia. *N Engl J Med* 2003;348:1764–1775.
16. Calin GA, Dumitru CD, Shimizu M, et al. Frequent deletions and down-regulation of micro- RNA genes miR15 and miR16 at 13q14 in chronic lymphocytic leukemia. *Proc Natl Acad Sci U S A* 2002;99:15524–15529.
18. Quesada V, Conde L, Villamor N, et al. Exome sequencing identifies recurrent mutations of the splicing factor SF3B1 gene in chronic lymphocytic leukemia. *Nat Genet* 2012;44:47–52.
19. Wang L, Lawrence MS, Wan Y, et al. SF3B1 and other novel cancer genes in chronic lymphocytic leukemia. *N Engl J Med* 2011;365:2497–2506.
20. Rossi D, Rasi S, Spina V, et al. Integrated mutational and cytogenetic analysis identifies new prognostic subgroups in chronic lymphocytic leukemia. *Blood* 2013;121:1403–1412.
21. Landau DA, Carter SL, Stojanov P, et al. Evolution and impact of subclonal mutations in chronic lymphocytic leukemia. *Cell* 2013;152:714–726.
22. Ouillette P, Saiya-Cork K, Seymour E, et al. Clonal evolution, genomic drivers, and effects of therapy in chronic lymphocytic leukemia. *Clin Cancer Res* 2013;19:2893–2904.
23. Schuh A, Becq J, Humphray S, et al. Monitoring chronic lymphocytic leukemia progression by whole genome sequencing reveals heterogeneous clonal evolution patterns. *Blood* 2012;120:4191–4196.
26. Hallek M, Cheson BD, Catovsky D, et al. Guidelines for the diagnosis and treatment of chronic lymphocytic leukemia: a report from the International Workshop on Chronic Lymphocytic Leukemia updating the National Cancer Institute-Working Group 1996 guidelines. *Blood* 2008;111:5446–5456.

31. Cortes J, O'Brien S, Loscertales J, et al. Cyclosporin A for the treatment of cytopenia associated with chronic lymphocytic leukemia. *Cancer* 2001; 92:2016–2022.
35. Rai KR, Sawitsky A, Cronkite EP, et al. Clinical staging of chronic lymphocytic leukemia. *Blood* 1975;46:219–234.
36. Binet JL, Auquier A, Dighiero G, et al. A new prognostic classification of chronic lymphocytic leukemia derived from a multivariate survival analysis. *Cancer* 1981;48:198–206.
40. Moreton P, Kennedy B, Lucas G, et al. Eradication of minimal residual disease in B-cell chronic lymphocytic leukemia after alemtuzumab therapy is associated with prolonged survival. *J Clin Oncol* 2005;23:2971–2979.
41. Bottcher S, Ritgen M, Fischer K, et al. Minimal residual disease quantification is an independent predictor of progression-free and overall survival in chronic lymphocytic leukemia: a multivariate analysis from the randomized GCLLSG CLL8 trial. *J Clin Oncol* 2012;30:980–988.
47. Rai KR, Peterson BL, Appelbaum FR, et al. Fludarabine compared with chlorambucil as primary therapy for chronic lymphocytic leukemia. *N Engl J Med* 2000;343:1750–1757.
49. Eichhorst BF, Busch R, Stilgenbauer S, et al. First-line therapy with fludarabine compared with chlorambucil does not result in a major benefit for elderly patients with advanced chronic lymphocytic leukemia. *Blood* 2009; 114:3382–3391.
50. Knauf WU, Lissichkov T, Aldaoud A, et al. Phase III randomized study of bendamustine compared with chlorambucil in previously untreated patients with chronic lymphocytic leukemia. *J Clin Oncol* 2009;27:4378–4384.
55. Eichhorst BF, Busch R, Hopfinger G, et al. Fludarabine plus cyclophosphamide versus fludarabine alone in first-line therapy of younger patients with chronic lymphocytic leukemia. *Blood* 2006;107:885–891.
56. Flinn IW, Neuberg DS, Grever MR, et al. Phase III trial of fludarabine plus cyclophosphamide compared with fludarabine for patients with previously untreated chronic lymphocytic leukemia: US Intergroup Trial E2997. *J Clin Oncol* 2007;25:793–798.
58. Robak T, Blonski JZ, Gora-Tybor J, et al. Cladribine alone and in combination with cyclophosphamide or cyclophosphamide plus mitoxantrone in the treatment of progressive chronic lymphocytic leukemia: report of a prospective, multicenter, randomized trial of the Polish Adult Leukemia Group (PALG CLL2). *Blood* 2006;108:473–479.
60. Keating MJ, Flinn I, Jain V, et al. Therapeutic role of alemtuzumab (Campath-1H) in patients who have failed fludarabine: results of a large international study. *Blood* 2002;99:3554–3561.
61. Osterborg A, Dyer MJ, Bunjes D, et al. Phase II multicenter study of human CD52 antibody in previously treated chronic lymphocytic leukemia. European Study Group of CAMPATH-1H Treatment in Chronic Lymphocytic Leukemia. *J Clin Oncol* 1997;15:1567–1574.
64. Lundin J, Kimby E, Bjorkholm M, et al. Phase II trial of subcutaneous anti-CD52 monoclonal antibody alemtuzumab (Campath-1H) as first-line treatment for patients with B-cell chronic lymphocytic leukemia (B-CLL). *Blood* 2002;100:768–773.
65. Pettitt AR, Jackson R, Carruthers S, et al. Alemtuzumab in combination with methylprednisolone is a highly effective induction regimen for patients with chronic lymphocytic leukemia and deletion of TP53: final results of the national cancer research institute CLL206 trial. *J Clin Oncol* 2012;30:1647–1655.
66. McLaughlin P, Grillo-Lopez AJ, Link BK, et al. Rituximab chimeric anti-CD20 monoclonal antibody therapy for relapsed indolent lymphoma: half of patients respond to a four-dose treatment program. *J Clin Oncol* 1998;16:2825–2833.
70. Castro JE, Sandoval-Sus JD, Bole J, et al. Rituximab in combination with high-dose methylprednisolone for the treatment of fludarabine refractory high-risk chronic lymphocytic leukemia. *Leukemia* 2008;22:2048–2053.
72. Castro JE, James DF, Sandoval-Sus JD, et al. Rituximab in combination with high-dose methylprednisolone for the treatment of chronic lymphocytic leukemia. *Leukemia* 2009;23:1779–1789.
73. Faderl S, Thomas DA, O'Brien S, et al. Experience with alemtuzumab plus rituximab in patients with relapsed and refractory lymphoid malignancies. *Blood* 2003;101:3413–3415.
74. Zent CS, Call TG, Shanafelt TD, et al. Early treatment of high-risk chronic lymphocytic leukemia with alemtuzumab and rituximab. *Cancer* 2008; 113:2110–2118.
75. Stilgenbauer S, Zenz T, Winkler D, et al. Subcutaneous alemtuzumab in fludarabine-refractory chronic lymphocytic leukemia: clinical results and prognostic marker analyses from the CLL2H study of the German Chronic Lymphocytic Leukemia Study Group. *J Clin Oncol* 2009;27:3994–4001.
76. Hillmen P, Skotnicki AB, Robak T, et al. Alemtuzumab compared with chlorambucil as first-line therapy for chronic lymphocytic leukemia. *J Clin Oncol* 2007;25:5616–5623.
80. O'Brien SM, Kantarjian H, Thomas DA, et al. Rituximab dose-escalation trial in chronic lymphocytic leukemia. *J Clin Oncol* 2001;19:2165–2170.
81. Byrd JC, Murphy T, Howard RS, et al. Rituximab using a thrice weekly dosing schedule in B-cell chronic lymphocytic leukemia and small lymphocytic lymphoma demonstrates clinical activity and acceptable toxicity. *J Clin Oncol* 2001;19:2153–2164.
83. Coiffier B, Lepretre S, Pedersen LM, et al. Safety and efficacy of ofatumumab, a fully human monoclonal anti-CD20 antibody, in patients with relapsed or refractory B-cell chronic lymphocytic leukemia: a phase 1–2 study. *Blood* 2008;111:1094–1100.
84. Wierda WG, Kipps TJ, Mayer J, et al. Ofatumumab as single-agent CD20 immunotherapy in fludarabine-refractory chronic lymphocytic leukemia. *J Clin Oncol* 2010;28:1749–1755.
85. Wierda WG, Padmanabhan S, Chan GW, et al. Ofatumumab is active in patients with fludarabine-refractory CLL irrespective of prior rituximab: results from the phase 2 international study. *Blood* 2011;118:5126–5129.
86. Byrd JC, Peterson BL, Morrison VA, et al. Randomized phase 2 study of fludarabine with concurrent versus sequential treatment with rituximab in symptomatic, untreated patients with B-cell chronic lymphocytic leukemia: results from Cancer and Leukemia Group B 9712 (CALGB 9712). *Blood* 2003;101:6–14.
88. Mauro FR, Molica S, Laurenti L, et al. Fludarabine plus alemtuzumab (FA) front-line treatment in young patients with chronic lymphocytic leukemia (CLL) and an adverse biologic profile. *Leuk Res* 2014;38:198–203.
89. Hillmen P, Gribben JG, Follows GA, et al. Rituximab plus chlorambucil as first-line treatment for chronic lymphocytic leukemia: Final analysis of an open-label phase II study. *J Clin Oncol* 2014;32:1236–1241.
90. Foa R, Del Giudice I, Cuneo A, et al. Chlorambucil plus rituximab with or without maintenance rituximab as first-line treatment for elderly chronic lymphocytic leukemia patients. *Am J Hematol* 2014;89:480–486.
91. Byrd JC, Rai K, Peterson BL, et al. Addition of rituximab to fludarabine may prolong progression-free survival and overall survival in patients with previously untreated chronic lymphocytic leukemia: an updated retrospective comparative analysis of CALGB 9712 and CALGB 9011. *Blood* 2005;105:49–53.
92. Keating MJ, O'Brien S, Albitar M, et al. Early results of a chemoimmunotherapy regimen of fludarabine, cyclophosphamide, and rituximab as initial therapy for chronic lymphocytic leukemia. *J Clin Oncol* 2005;23: 4079–4088.
93. Wierda W, O'Brien S, Wen S, et al. Chemoimmunotherapy with fludarabine, cyclophosphamide, and rituximab for relapsed and refractory chronic lymphocytic leukemia. *J Clin Oncol* 2005;23:4070–4078.
94. Tam CS, O'Brien S, Wierda W, et al. Long-term results of the fludarabine, cyclophosphamide, and rituximab regimen as initial therapy of chronic lymphocytic leukemia. *Blood* 2008;112:975–980.
95. Badoux XC, Keating MJ, Wang X, et al. Fludarabine, cyclophosphamide, and rituximab chemoimmunotherapy is highly effective treatment for relapsed patients with CLL. *Blood* 2011;117:3016–3024.
97. Robak T, Dmoszynska A, Solal-Celigny P, et al. Rituximab plus fludarabine and cyclophosphamide prolongs progression-free survival compared with fludarabine and cyclophosphamide alone in previously treated chronic lymphocytic leukemia. *J Clin Oncol* 2010;28:1756–1765.
100. Hillmen P, Cohen DR, Cocks K, et al. A randomized phase II trial of fludarabine, cyclophosphamide and mitoxantrone (FCM) with or without rituximab in previously treated chronic lymphocytic leukaemia. *Br J Haematol* 2011;152:570–578.
101. Foon KA, Mehta D, Lentzsch S, et al. Long-term results of chemoimmunotherapy with low-dose fludarabine, cyclophosphamide and high-dose rituximab as initial treatment for patients with chronic lymphocytic leukemia. *Blood* 2012;119:3184–3185.
102. Lamanna N, Kalaycio M, Maslak P, et al. Pentostatin, cyclophosphamide, and rituximab is an active, well-tolerated regimen for patients with previously treated chronic lymphocytic leukemia. *J Clin Oncol* 2006;24:1575–1581.
103. Kay NE, Geyer SM, Call TG, et al. Combination chemoimmunotherapy with pentostatin, cyclophosphamide, and rituximab shows significant clinical activity with low accompanying toxicity in previously untreated B chronic lymphocytic leukemia. *Blood* 2007;109:405–411.
104. Shanafelt T, Lanasa MC, Call TG, et al. Ofatumumab-based chemoimmunotherapy is effective and well tolerated in patients with previously untreated chronic lymphocytic leukemia (CLL). *Cancer* 2013;119: 3788–3796.
105. Fischer K, Cramer P, Busch R, et al. Bendamustine in combination with rituximab for previously untreated patients with chronic lymphocytic leukemia: a multicenter phase II trial of the German Chronic Lymphocytic Leukemia Study Group. *J Clin Oncol* 2012;30:3209–3216.
106. Fischer K, Cramer P, Busch R, et al. Bendamustine combined with rituximab in patients with relapsed and/or refractory chronic lymphocytic leukemia: a multicenter phase II trial of the German Chronic Lymphocytic Leukemia Study Group. *J Clin Oncol* 2011;29:3559–3566.
107. Elter T, Gercheva-Kyuchukova L, Pylylpenko H, et al. Fludarabine plus alemtuzumab versus fludarabine alone in patients with previously treated chronic lymphocytic leukaemia: a randomised phase 3 trial. *Lancet Oncol* 2011;12:1204–1213.
108. Goede V, Fischer K, Busch R, et al. Obinutuzumab plus chlorambucil in patients with CLL and coexisting conditions. *N Engl J Med* 2014;370: 1101–1110.
110. O'Brien SM, Kantarjian HM, Thomas DA, et al. Alemtuzumab as treatment for residual disease after chemotherapy in patients with chronic lymphocytic leukemia. *Cancer* 2003;98:2657–2663.
112. Schweighofer CD, Ritgen M, Eichhorst BF, et al. Consolidation with alemtuzumab improves progression-free survival in patients with chronic lymphocytic leukaemia (CLL) in first remission: long-term follow-up of a randomized phase III trial of the German CLL Study Group (GCLLSG). *Br J Haematol* 2009;144:95–98.

113. Jones JA, Ruppert AS, Zhao W, et al. Patients with chronic lymphocytic leukemia with high-risk genomic features have inferior outcome on successive Cancer and Leukemia Group B trials with alemtuzumab consolidation: subgroup analysis from CALGB 19901 and CALGB 10101. *Leuk Lymphoma* 2013;54:2654–2659.

114. Ponader S, Burger JA. Bruton's tyrosine kinase: from X-linked agammaglobulinemia toward targeted therapy for B-cell malignancies. *J Clin Oncol* 2014;32:1830–1839.

115. Byrd JC, Furman RR, Coutre SE, et al. Targeting BTK with ibrutinib in relapsed chronic lymphocytic leukemia. *N Engl J Med* 2013;369:32–42.

117. Byrd JC, Brown JR, O'Brien S, et al. Ibrutinib versus ofatumumab in previously treated chronic lymphoid leukemia. *N Engl J Med* 2014;371:213–223.

118. Byrd JC, Brown JR, O'Brien SM, et al. Randomized comparison of ibrutinib versus ofatumumab in relapsed or refractory (R/R) chronic lymphocytic leukemia/small lymphocytic lymphoma: Results from the phase III RESONATE trial. *J Clin Oncol* 2014;32:Abstr LBA7008.

119. Woyach JA, Furman RR, Liu TM, et al. Resistance mechanisms for the Bruton's tyrosine kinase inhibitor ibrutinib. *N Engl J Med* 2014;370:2286–2294.

120. Brown JR, Byrd JC, Coutre SE, et al. Idelalisib, an inhibitor of phosphatidylinositol 3 kinase p110delta, for relapsed/refractory chronic lymphocytic leukemia. *Blood* 2014;123:3390–3397.

122. Roberts AW, Seymour JF, Brown JR, et al. Substantial susceptibility of chronic lymphocytic leukemia to BCL2 inhibition: results of a phase I study of navitoclax in patients with relapsed or refractory disease. *J Clin Oncol* 2012;30:488–496.

123. Souers AJ, Leverson JD, Boghaert ER, et al. ABT-199, a potent and selective BCL-2 inhibitor, achieves antitumor activity while sparing platelets. *Nat Med* 2013;19:202–208.

124. Seymour JF, Davids MS, Pagel JM, et al. Bcl-2 inhibitor ABT-199 (GDC-0199) monotherapy shows anti-tumor activity including complete remissions in high-risk relapsed/refractory (R/R) chronic lymphocytic leukemia (CLL) and small lymphocytic lymphoma (SLL). *Blood* 2013;122:Abstr 872.

125. Chanan-Khan A, Miller KC, Musial L, et al. Clinical efficacy of lenalidomide in patients with relapsed or refractory chronic lymphocytic leukemia: results of a phase II study. *J Clin Oncol* 2006;24:5343–5349.

126. Ferrajoli A, Lee BN, Schlette EJ, et al. Lenalidomide induces complete and partial remissions in patients with relapsed and refractory chronic lymphocytic leukemia. *Blood* 2008;111:5291–5297.

127. Chen CI, Bergsagel PL, Paul H, et al. Single-agent lenalidomide in the treatment of previously untreated chronic lymphocytic leukemia. *J Clin Oncol* 2011;29:1175–1181.

128. Badoux XC, Keating MJ, Wen S, et al. Lenalidomide as initial therapy of elderly patients with chronic lymphocytic leukemia. *Blood* 2011;118:3489–3498.

129. Strati P, Keating MJ, Wierda WG, et al. Lenalidomide induces long-lasting responses in elderly patients with chronic lymphocytic leukemia. *Blood* 2013;122:734–737.

130. Badoux XC, Keating MJ, Wen S, et al. Phase II study of lenalidomide and rituximab as salvage therapy for patients with relapsed or refractory chronic lymphocytic leukemia. *J Clin Oncol* 2013;31:584–591.

131. Brentjens RJ, Riviere I, Park JH, et al. Safety and persistence of adoptively transferred autologous CD19-targeted T cells in patients with relapsed or chemotherapy refractory B-cell leukemias. *Blood* 2011;118:4817–4828.

132. Grupp SA, Kalos M, Barrett D, et al. Chimeric antigen receptor-modified T cells for acute lymphoid leukemia. *N Engl J Med* 2013;368:1509–1518.

133. Kalos M, Levine BL, Porter DL, et al. T cells with chimeric antigen receptors have potent antitumor effects and can establish memory in patients with advanced leukemia. *Sci Transl Med* 2011;3:95ra73.

134. Porter DL, Levine BL, Kalos M, et al. Chimeric antigen receptor-modified T cells in chronic lymphoid leukemia. *N Engl J Med* 2011;365:725–733.

139. Khouri IF, Bassett R, Poindexter N, et al. Nonmyeloablative allogeneic stem cell transplantation in relapsed/refractory chronic lymphocytic leukemia: long-term follow-up, prognostic factors, and effect of human leukocyte histocompatibility antigen subtype on outcome. *Cancer* 2011;117:4679–4688.

140. Dreger P, Schnaiter A, Zenz T, et al. TP53, SF3B1, and NOTCH1 mutations and outcome of allotransplantation for chronic lymphocytic leukemia: six-year follow-up of the GCLLSG CLL3X trial. *Blood* 2013;121:3284–3288.

142. Michallet M, Socie G, Mohty M, et al. Rituximab, fludarabine, and total body irradiation as conditioning regimen before allogeneic hematopoietic stem cell transplantation for advanced chronic lymphocytic leukemia: long-term prospective multicenter study. *Exp Hematol* 2013;41:127–133.

143. Richardson SE, Khan I, Rawstron A, et al. Risk-stratified adoptive cellular therapy following allogeneic hematopoietic stem cell transplantation for advanced chronic lymphocytic leukaemia. *Br J Haematol* 2013;160:640–648.

144. Herth I, Dietrich S, Benner A, et al. The impact of allogeneic stem cell transplantation on the natural course of poor-risk chronic lymphocytic leukemia as defined by the EBMT consensus criteria: a retrospective donor versus no donor comparison. *Ann Oncol* 2014;25:200–206.

150. Smith MR, Neuberg D, Flinn IW, et al. Incidence of therapy-related myeloid neoplasia after initial therapy for chronic lymphocytic leukemia with fludarabine-cyclophosphamide versus fludarabine: long-term follow-up of US Intergroup Study E2997. *Blood* 2011;118:3525–3527.

155. Arcaini L, Zibellini S, Boveri E, et al. The BRAF V600E mutation in hairy cell leukemia and other mature B-cell neoplasms. *Blood* 2012;119:188–191.

156. Tiacci E, Trifonov V, Schiavoni G, et al. BRAF mutations in hairy-cell leukemia. *N Engl J Med* 2011;364:2305–2315.

157. Dietrich S, Glimm H, Andrulis M, et al. BRAF inhibition in refractory hairy-cell leukemia. *N Engl J Med* 2012;366:2038–2040.

161. Kreitman RJ, Tallman MS, Robak T, et al. Phase I trial of anti-CD22 recombinant immunotoxin moxetumomab pasudotox (CAT-8015 or HA22) in patients with hairy cell leukemia. *J Clin Oncol* 2012;30:1822–1828.

111 Myelodysplastic Syndromes

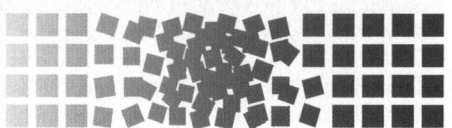

Rami S. Komrokji, Eric Padron, and Alan F. List

INTRODUCTION

The myelodysplastic syndromes (MDS) represent a spectrum of hematopoietic stem cell malignancies that share morphologic features of dysplasia, ineffective hematopoiesis, and a risk for leukemia evolution. The hallmark of early disease is accelerated apoptosis and proliferation of bone marrow precursors that drives increased marrow cellularity and peripheral cytopenias. In advanced disease, increasing maturation impairment is accompanied by the acquisition of survival signals that leads to increasing proportions of myeloblasts. MDS are clonal stem cell neoplasms that arise from interplay of genetic and epigenetics events with altered microenvironmental pressures that are senescence dependent. Although the risk of progression to acute myeloid leukemia (AML) varies, the majority of patients succumb to complications related to cytopenias.[1]

HISTORICAL PERSPECTIVE

The description of MDS dates back to early 1900s when reference was first made to a group of patients with a form of anemia refractory to available treatments. The term *anemia pseudoaplastica* was one of the earliest descriptions of MDS.[2] In the late 1940s, it was thought that the disease progresses to leukemia and, hence, the term *preleukemia* was applied.[3] The definition was expanded to include peripheral blood descriptors such as neutropenia and thrombocytopenia in the early 1950s.[4] The French-American-British (FAB) group coined the term *myelodysplastic syndromes* in a series of proposals on acute leukemias in 1976 and later expanded the FAB classification in 1980s.[5,6] The original FAB classification included only two categories: refractory anemia with excess blasts (RAEB) and chronic myelomonocytic leukemia (CMML), to which others were added in 1982. In 1997, the International Prognostic Scoring System (IPSS) was introduced.[7] Under the auspices of the World Health Organization (WHO), the pathologic classification of MDS was refined and later revised in 2008.[7,8,9] New prognostic models were later introduced, such as the WHO Prognostic Scoring System (WPSS), the Global M.D. Anderson Risk Model, the Lower Risk M.D. Anderson Model, and more recently, the revised-IPSS (IPSS-R).[10–13]

Recent years witnessed an acceleration in understanding the disease biology and associated molecular genetics events. Today, molecular abnormalities are demonstrable in more than 80% of MDS patients. Finally, in the past decade, three medications were approved specifically for the treatment of MDS: azacitidine, decitabine, and lenalidomide.

EPIDEMIOLOGY

MDS is one of the most common hematologic malignancies. According to the Surveillance, Epidemiology, and End Results (SEER): the United States cancer surveillance program 2006 to 2010 statistics, the age-adjusted incidence rate of MDS was 4.8 per 100,000 and 0.4 per 100,000 for CMML.[14] MDS was more common in males (6.5 per 100,000) than in females (3.7 per 100,000). MDS is a disease of the elderly (median age at diagnosis is 72 years); the incidence rate was highest among 80 years and older (20 per 100,000).[14] SEER/North American Association of Central Cancer Registries (NAACCR) reported a similar MDS annual age-adjusted incidence rate of 3.27 per 100,000.[15] The incidence rate among the Medicare population (age >65 years) was 162 per 100,000, which translates to approximately 45,000 newly diagnosed cases per year.[16] Recent data suggest a high rate of uncaptured MDS cases among hospital cancer registries.[17] The incidence of MDS reported from Europe is similar to that observed in the United States, ranging from 3.2 to 8.1 per 100,000.[18] Interestingly, a lower incidence, younger age, and different spectrum of pathologic subtypes have been reported in Asia.[19]

ETIOLOGY

For the vast majority of cases, senescence per se is the highest risk factor for MDS development. Familial/genetic predisposition contributes to a small proportion of MDS cases.[20] There is an increased risk of MDS among inherited bone marrow failure syndromes (BMFS), such as Fanconi anemia, dyskeratosis congenita, severe congenital neutropenia, and Shwachman–Diamond syndrome.[20] Familial cases of MDS beyond BMFS are well recognized and molecularly distinct. Two important familial syndromes are the familial platelet disorder with a propensity to myeloid malignancy, arising from an autosomal-dominant *RUNX-1* germ-line gene mutation that results in thrombocytopenia with a corresponding frequency of MDS/AML in carriers that approaches 50%[21] and familial MDS/AML with *GATA2* mutation, which is also autosomal dominant but with variable penetrance.[22]

Benzene exposure is a well-recognized environmental exposure linked to AML/MDS.[23] The risk of MDS but not AML was increased among petroleum distribution workers at relatively lower levels of exposure in a dose-dependent manner.[24] Cigarette smoking had also been associated with an increased risk of developing MDS. In a meta-analysis, current and former smokers had increased risks of MDS, with an odds ratio (OR) of 1.81 (95% confidence interval [CI], 1.24 to 2.66) and 1.67 (95% CI, 1.42 to 1.96), respectively.[25] A population-based study from Sweden suggested that a prior history of infection (OR, 1.3; 95% CI, 1.1 to 1.5) or autoimmune disease (OR 2.1-fold; 95% CI, 1.7 to 2.6) significantly increased the probability of developing MDS.[26]

A case-control study was conducted to investigate associations between lifestyle characteristics and MDS risk.[27] A family history of hematopoietic cancer (OR = 1.92), smoking (OR = 1.65), and exposure to agricultural chemicals (OR = 4.55) or solvents (OR = 2.05) were associated with MDS. The highest risk was among smokers exposed to solvents/agricultural chemicals (OR = 3.22).

In the context of successful chemotherapeutic treatment of other hematologic malignancies and solid tumors, a growing percentage of MDS cases are considered secondary or arising from prior radiation or chemotherapy. Treatment-related MDS (t-MDS) accounts for 10% to 20% of all MDS cases. It is generally characterized by a high rate of unfavorable cytogenetics and poor outcome. Chemotherapy and, to a lesser extent, radiotherapy are associated with an increased the risk of developing AML/MDS.[28,29] The risk of t-MDS varies from less than 1% (adjuvant breast cancer chemotherapy studies) to 15% (heavily treated lymphoma patients). Two types of t-MDS are recognized: Type I is related to alkylating agent exposure where MDS occurs after a latency period of 3 to 5 years in which monosomy 5 or 7 are cytogenetic characteristics of the disease; and type II t-MDS is related to treatment with topoisomerase II inhibitors, which generally arises after a short interval from chemotherapy exposure and rapidly progresses to AML. Chromosome 11q23 abnormalities that involve the *MLL* gene are characteristic of this type.[30] Radiation-related MDS have a prognosis similar to de novo MDS.[31]

PATHOLOGY

The diagnosis of MDS requires the presence of persistent cytopenia(s) in the absence of hematinic deficiencies such as vitamin B12 or folic acid, and one of the following: (1) demonstration of cytologic dysplasia in ≥10% of cells in a given lineage, (2) demonstration of increased myeloblasts (5% to 19%) (Fig. 111.1),[32] or (3) a specific cytogenetic abnormality detected in the setting of sustained unexplained cytopenia ("presumptive MDS" by WHO 2008 criteria). In certain cases, the diagnosis of MDS can be made without clear evidence of morphologic dysplasia, such as CMML if monocytes are persistently elevated.

A 500 cell count differential is recommended, with exclusion of lymphocytes and plasma cells. Cytologic dysplasia must exceed 10% of cells in any lineage and the percentage of myeloblasts calculated. If the absolute percentage of erythroid precursors is 50% or greater, the percentage of myeloblasts is estimated among nonerythroid precursors. Iron stains are essential to address the percentage of ring sideroblasts. The bone marrow core biopsy could complement the bone marrow aspirate in several aspects,[30] namely, cellularity, dysmegakaryopoiesis, and identifying clusters of abnormal localization of immature precursors (ALIP), which are immature cells/myeloblasts or promyelocytes that are displaced from the paratrabecular area to the intertrabecular areas often corresponding to the vascular niche. In addition, the reticulin stain provides information regarding medullary fibrosis, which can add prognostic information.[33,34]

The French-British-American Classification

The original FAB classification (Table 111.1) included only two of the subtypes.[5] In 1982, a revision to the FAB classification expanded that to five subgroups: refractory anemia (RA), refractory anemia with ring sideroblasts (RARS), RAEB, RAEB in transformation (RAEB-t), and CMML.[6]

The World Health Organization Classification

The WHO classification was proposed to address some of the FAB shortcomings.[35,36] WHO distinguishes between single lineage and multilineage dysplasia: Categories of refractory cytopenia with multilineage dysplasia (RCMD) and RCMD with ring sideroblasts (RCMD-RS) were added, capturing those cases with dysplastic changes in either myeloid or megakaryocytic lineages in addition to erythroid dysplasia. The 5q- syndrome was recognized as a distinct subset, with an isolated cytogenetic abnormality involving del(5q) and less than 5% myeloblasts. RAEB was divided into RAEB I with 5% to 9% blasts and RAEB II with 10% to 19% blasts.[35,37] RAEB-t was omitted and the blast threshold for AML diagnosis lowered

to 20% rather than 30%.[35,37,38] Finally, WHO recognizes MDS/myeloproliferative neoplasms (MPN). This includes diseases such as CMML, juvenile myelomonocytic leukemia (JMML), and atypical chronic myeloid leukemia (aCML).[35,37,38] CMML is further classified based on the percentage of bone marrow blasts, where CMML type 1 includes 0% to 4% blasts and/or promonocytes on peripheral blood or <10% in the bone marrow, and type 2 includes 5% to 19% blasts and promonocytes in the peripheral blood or <20% in the bone marrow.[8]

The WHO classification was revised in 2008,[39,40] adding the category of refractory cytopenia with unilineage dysplasia (RCUD) that include RA, refractory neutropenia (RN) and refractory thrombocytopenia (RT). The patients may have a corresponding cytopenia but not pancytopenia. Patients with pancytopenia and unilineage dysplasia, patients with no overt dysplasia but cytogenetic evidence of MDS, and cases of RCUD or RCMD with peripheral blood (PB) blasts of 1% are categorized as MDS unclassified (MDS-U). RAEB-1 includes 2% to 4 % peripheral blood blasts and RAEB-II includes 5% to 19% peripheral blood blasts. The presence of Auer rods regardless of blast percentage qualifies as RAEB-II or CMML-2.[41] A provisional entity of refractory anemia with ring sideroblasts and thrombocytosis (RARS-T) was proposed in which there is a sustained thrombocytosis of 450,000/mm^3 or greater.[42] Up to 50% of RARS-T patients harbor a gain-of-function mutation involving the Janus kinase 2 (*JAK2*) gene. A subset of patients with CMML and eosinophilia with accompanying genetic abnormalities involving the platelet-derived growth factor receptor alpha (PDGFRα) or PDGFRβ were reclassified as myeloid neoplasms with eosinophilia.[43]

Hypocellular MDS (or *hypoplastic* MDS) is not recognized as a distinct entity with the WHO classification. It accounts for 10% to 20% of MDS cases. The challenge on diagnosis is to distinguish those cases from aplastic anemia.[44] Although not part of the WHO classification, the term idiopathic cytopenia of unknown significance (ICUS) was proposed for those cases with persistent cytopenia(s) unrelated to nutritional deficiency that have dysplasia in less than 10% of cells in any lineage and that lack cytogenetic abnormalities. Many of those patients may develop MDS over time. Whether the latter cases can be distinguished a priori by the presence of gene mutations is under investigation. Some cases may also demonstrate dysplasia below the 10% WHO cutoff with no cytopenia, referred to as idiopathic dysplasia of unknown significance (IDUS).[45]

PATHOGENESIS

MDS is a clonal disease driven by acquisition and expansion of genetic alterations (Fig. 111.2). The clonal nature of many MDS cases was first apparent by the conventional metaphase karyotype analysis. Studies leveraging restriction fragment length polymorphisms (RFLP) of X-chromosome genes in females, single nucleotide polymorphism (SNP) arrays, and glucose-6-phosphate dehydrogenase (G6PD) analyses confirmed that hematopoiesis is clonal across all subtypes of MDS.[46–49] The two most comprehensive studies demonstrating the frequency and nature of chromosome abnormalities in MDS confirmed that approximately 50% of patients with MDS harbor a chromosome abnormality.[50,51] The most common recurrent abnormalities were del(5q) (30%), −7 or 7q− (21%), and +8 (16%). Deletion of genes encoded within the commonly deleted region (CDR) of human del(5q) MDS is sufficient to induce an MDS phenotype, indicating that these recurrent genetic lesions are critical to the development of the disease.[52]

In addition to large chromosomal deletions or duplications, DNA sequencing technology has uncovered gene mutations that aggregate within pathways previously unrecognized to be important in MDS pathogenesis. These include mutations predicted to result in deregulation of genes involved in signaling pathways and epigenetic control, RNA splicing, and transcription factors.[53]

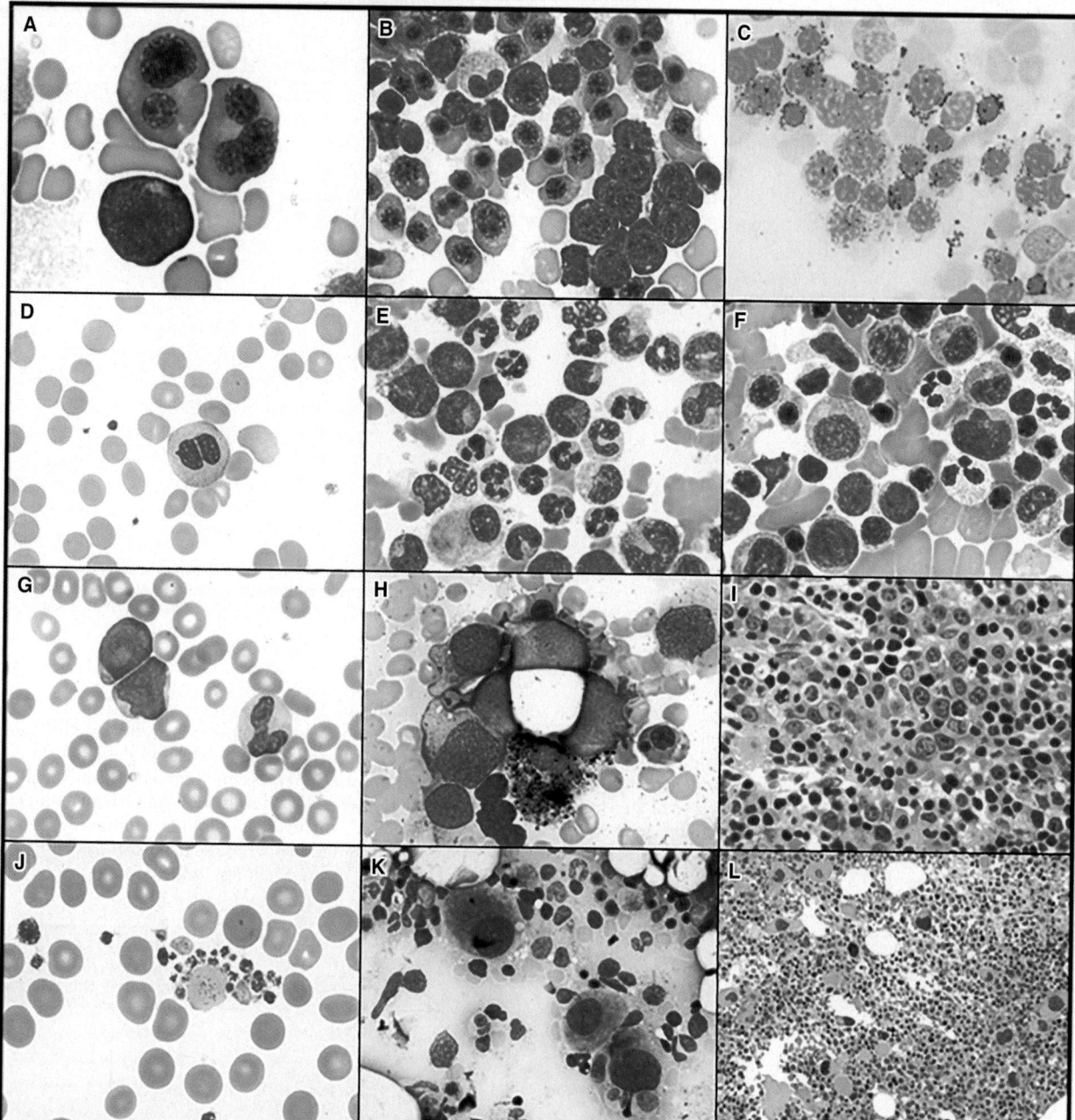

Figure 111.1 Morphologic findings of myelodysplasia in peripheral blood and bone marrow. **A:** Erythroid precursors displaying cytoplasmic to nuclear maturation asynchrony and multinucleation in bone marrow aspirate smear (Wright Giemsa stain). **B:** Bone marrow aspirate with erythroid hyperplasia, left shifted and megaloblastoid maturation, occasional nuclear budding and binucleation (Wright Giemsa strain). **C:** Numerous ringed-sideroblasts are highlighted by Prussian-blue iron stain in bone marrow aspirate. **D:** Circulating granulocytes showing pseudo-Pelger-Huet change with hyposegmentation and hypogranulation in cytoplasm in peripheral blood smear (May-Grünwald-Giemsa stain). **E:** Abnormal distribution of cytoplasmic granules or patch loss of granules in eosinophilic precursors as well as abnormal lobation of neutrophils are present in the peripheral blood of a MDS patient (May-Grünwald-Giemsa stain). **F:** Predominant myeloid dysplasia including marked hypogranulation, cytoplasmic to nuclear maturation asynchrony with increased immature precursors/myeloblasts noted in bone marrow aspirate (Wright Giemsa stain). **G:** Circulating blasts with round to oval nucleus, lacy chromatin, one to more than one very prominent nucleoli and a small amount of cytoplasm are identified in peripheral blood smear (May-Grünwald-Giemsa stain). There is a single Auer rod noted in the cytoplasm of one blast, and a background of hypogranulated granulocytes is present (May-Grünwald-Giemsa stain). **H:** Bone marrow aspirate containing small to large blasts with fine chromatin, visible to prominent nucleoli and scant to some amount of basophilic cytoplasm admixed with dysplastic polychromatic normoblasts showing nuclear budding (Wright Giemsa stain). **I:** Bone marrow core biopsy showing non–paratrabecular-located immature myeloid precursors in cluster; abnormal localization of immature precursors (ALIPs) (hematoxylin and eosin [H&E] stain). **J:** Dysplastic platelets displaying variable in size and shape including giant hypogranulated platelets. **K:** Medium-sized megakaryocytes with single lobated nucleus characterized in 5q- syndrome, subtype of myelodysplastic syndrome. **L:** Representative bone marrow core biopsy of 5q- syndrome with moderately increased in single or hypolobated megakaryocytes (H&E stain).

TABLE 111.1

Gene Mutations in MDS

FAB	WHO	WHO 2008	Dysplasia	BM Blast (%)	PB Blasts (%)
RA	■ RA ■ MDS-U ■ RCMD ■ Del(5q) MDS	■ RCUD RA RN, RT ■ RCMD ■ Isolated del(5q) ■ MDS-U	Erythroid Nonerythroid Erythroid + other Erythroid + mega Unilineage + pancytopenia or RCMD/RCUD with 1% PB blasts	<5 <5 <5 <5 <5	<1 <1 <1 <1 1
RARS	■ RARS ■ RCMD-RS	■ RARS ■ RCMD-RS	Erythroid only Erythroid + other (all >15% ring sideroblasts)	<5 <5	<1 <1
RAEB	■ RAEB-1 ■ RAEB-2	■ RAEB-1 ■ RAEB-2	>1 lineage >1 lineage	5–9 10–19	2–4[a] 5–19[a] Auer rods[a]
RAEB-t	■ AML	■ AML	Myeloid + other	>20	
CMML	■ MDS/MPD CMML JMML aCML MDS/MPD-U	■ MDS/MPN CMML JMML BCR/Abl neg CML MDS/MPD-U	Variable >1 × 10⁹/L monocytosis	<20	

BM, bone marrow; PB, peripheral blood; RA, refractory anemia; MDS-U, MDS unclassified; RCMD, refractory cytopenia with multilineage dysplasia; RCUD, refractory cytopenia with unilineage dysplasia; RN, refractory anemia; RT, refractory thrombocytopenia; mega, megakaryocyte; RARS, refractory anemia with ring sideroblasts; RCMD-RS, RCMD with ring sideroblasts; RAEB-t, RAEB in transformation; MPD, myeloproliferative disease; JMML, juvenile myelomonocytic leukemia; MPD-U, MPD unclassified; CML, chronic myeloid leukemia.
[a] Diagnosis and Classification of MDS.

Mutations are common in MDS, because targeted sequencing of select genes can identify at least one event (average: three events per sample) in approximately 80% of cases.[54] Although there are no MDS-defining mutations, a *genomic fingerprint*, which is characteristic of MDS is materializing as a result of several large-scale gene sequencing efforts. Among the most common gene mutations in MDS is that involving the gene, ten-eleven-translocation-2 (*TET2*).[55] Inactivating *TET2* mutations, which disrupt TET2

enzymatic activity, are frequently observed in MDS. TET2 catalyzes the conversion of methyl cytosine to hydroxymethylcytosine (5-hmC), thereby inducing subsequent DNA demethylation and the release of epigenetic repression.[56] Patients with *TET2* gene mutations have lower DNA levels of 5-hmC with consequent increased genomic methylation. Other commonly mutated epigenetic modifiers include the associated sex-linked combs like 1 (*ASLX1*) gene.[57–60] *ASXL1* belongs to the polycomb gene family

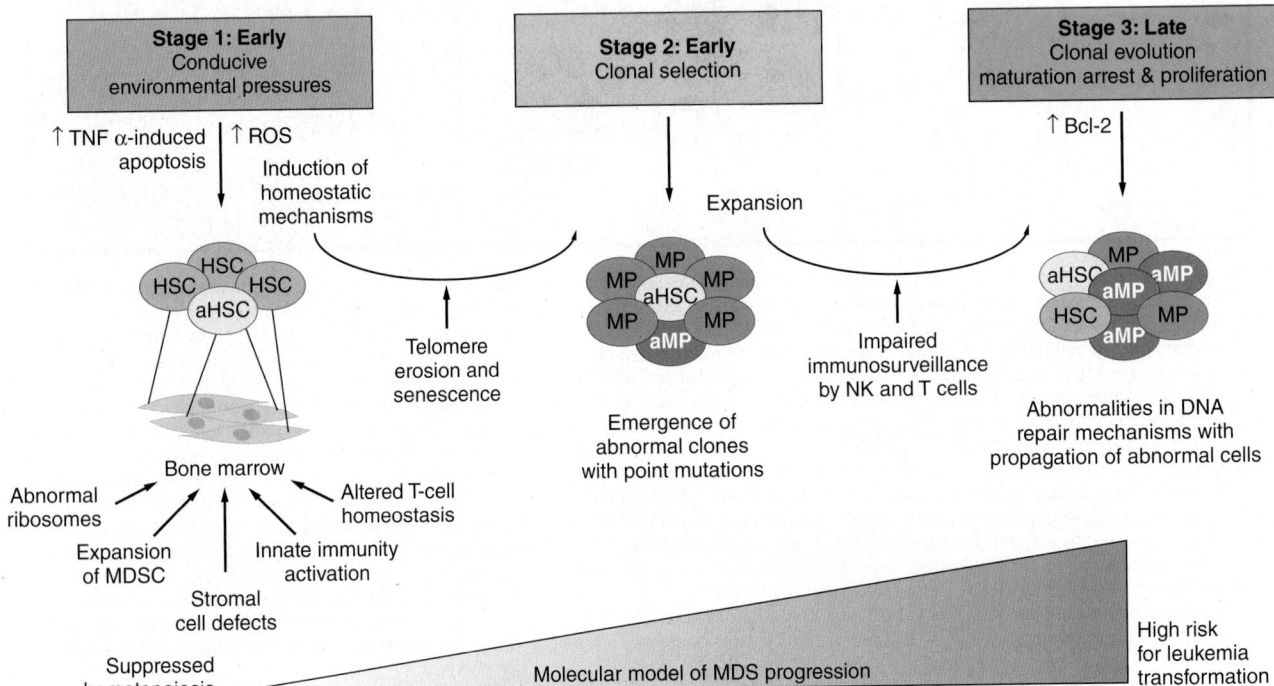

Figure 111.2 Model of MDS progression. TNFα, tumor necrosis factor apha; ROS, ; HSC, hematopoietic stem cell; aHSC, abnormal hematopoeitic stem cell; MDSC, myeloid derived suppressor cells; MP, myeloid progenitors; aMP, abnormal myeloid progenitor; NK, natural killer. (Modified from Epling-Burnette PK, List AF. Advancements in the molecular pathogenesis of myelodysplastic syndrome. *Curr Opin Hematol* 2009;16:70–76.)

and is an essential component of chromatin remodeling through its interaction with the polycomb repressive complex 2 (PRC2).[61,62] Deletion and conditional knock-in murine models for both *TET2* and *ASXL1* demonstrate that these lesions are sufficient to induce a myeloid neoplasm akin to MDS.[61,63,64]

Next-generation sequencing of MDS genomes recently identified genes involved in the regulation of alternative gene splicing.[65] Subsequent studies have shown that they are among the most common gene mutations in MDS.[53,54] They appear to occur early in disease pathogenesis, alter RNA splicing, and are prognostically relevant.[66–68] Interestingly, the two most common mutations involving the splicing factor 3b subunit 1 (*SF3B1*) and serine/arginine-rich splicing factor 2 (*SRSF2*) genes have strong phenotypic linkage with ringed sideroblasts and monocyte expansion (CMML), respectively.[67,69]

Lastly, the specific type and number of gene mutations directly impacts clinical behavior and risk of progression to AML. Elegant work using whole-genome sequencing to reconstruct the clonal architecture of MDS cases that transform to AML at sequential time points demonstrates that this transformation is associated with the acquisition and expansion of distinct genetic events.[70] Emerging data, however, suggest that these events do not display complete fidelity. That is, the same genetic events can be responsible for disease initiation, and therefore, disease founding in one case while representing a secondary event in another case with the same diagnosis. Collectively, these and other gene mutations described in Table 111.2 demonstrate that distinct genetic events can result in MDS and are likely the major drivers of the disease and its behavior.

Dysregulation of Immunity as a Driver in MDS

The environmental cues that are conducive to emergence of the genetic events that lead to MDS are unknown. Bone marrow stromal alterations have been implicated, but an intriguing emerging hypothesis that immune dysregulation and associated chronic inflammatory changes may be a critical environmental pressure in MDS pathogenesis. Clinical and laboratory evidence suggests that both adaptive and innate immunity is altered and potentially contributory to MDS pathogenesis. It is this inflammation that could represent the nidus for mutational acquisition in some patients, or these inflammatory changes are induced by an expanded clone. A recent population-based study demonstrated a strong linkage between chronic immune stimulation and autoimmune disorders with MDS predisposition.[26] Several studies confirmed the higher than expected association between MDS and autoimmune disease.[26,71–73]

Impaired T-cell homeostasis and early senescence is a feature of patients with MDS.[74] Indeed, up to 50% of T cells are clonal and even more appear to have intrinsic defects in telomerase function, perhaps accounting for their premature senescence.[75,76] In addition to expansion and senescence, the T-cell receptor (TCR) repertoire appears to be augmented and hematopoietic inhibitory capacity appears to be increased.[77] Lastly, T-cell characteristics can mark clinical parameters in MDS. For instance, the expansion of effector memory T-regulator cells (T_{regs}) is associated anemia and increased blast percentage, and represents an unfavorable prognostic biomarker.[78]

Activation of innate immunity with consequent nuclear factor kappa B (NF-κB) induction contributes to the inflammatory microenvironment in MDS.[79,80] Haplodeficiency of two microRNA genes, *miR-145* and *miR-146a*, located within the distal commonly deleted region of chromosome 5q at 5q32, results in constitutive activation of Toll-like receptor (TLR) signaling in del(5q) MDS. Toll-interleukin 1 receptor domain–containing adapter protein (*TIRAP*) and tumor necrosis factor receptor–associated factor-6 (*TRAF6*), which encode key intermediates involved in the MyD88-dependent TLR-signaling pathway, are targets of miR-145 and miR-146a, thereby upregulating their expression with allelic insufficiency. Myeloid-derived suppressor cells (MDSC), potent effectors of innate immunity, are recently recognized as critical cellular effectors involved in the pathogenesis of MDS. MDSCs are markedly expanded in the bone marrow of MDS patients and promote ineffective hematopoiesis. These MDSCs are genetically distinct from the MDS clone, overproduce hematopoietic suppressive cytokines, and also act as potent effectors of apoptosis that target autologous hematopoietic progenitors. MDSC expansion is driven by excess generation of the proinflammatory molecule S100A9, which is a ligand for TLR4. Moreover, a transgenic S100A9 mouse model phenocopies human MDS, displaying bone marrow accumulation of MDSC accompanied by progressive age-dependent multilineage cytopenias and cytologic dysplasia.[81]

The 5q Minus Syndrome

The hematologic and pathologic phenotype of the 5q- syndrome is now recognized to be a product of haploinsufficiency of several genes located within the CDR at 5q32.[82] Among 40 genes residing in the CDR, only inactivation of *RPS14* impaired erythroblast proliferation and viability, whereas corresponding overexpression of *RPS14* was sufficient to rescue erythropoiesis in primary del(5q) MDS specimens.[83] Haploinsufficiency for *RPS14* disrupts ribosome assembly, leading to nucleolar stress and sequestration of the human homolog of the mouse double minute 2 protein (MDM2) by free ribosomal proteins, thereby triggering its degradation and p53 stabilization.[84] A murine model of the human 5q− syndrome generated by allelic deletion of the genes in the human CDR showed that p53 inactivation rescues the hematologic features.[52] Gene dosage of two dual specificity phosphatases encoded within or adjacent to the proximal CDR at 5q31 (i.e., cell division cycle 25C [Cdc25C] and protein phosphatases 2A catalytic domain alpha [PP2Aca]), underlies the selective suppression of del(5q) clones.[85]

CLINICAL PRESENTATION

The most common clinical presentation of MDS is sustained and progressive cytopenia with corresponding symptoms and complications. Macrocytic anemia is the most common hematologic

TABLE 111.2

Spectrum of Genetic Alterations in Myelodysplastic Syndromes

Gene Symbol	Molecular Pathway Affected	Incidence in MDS (%)
ASXL1	Epigenetics	20–25
TET2	Epigenetics	30–35
IDH2	Epigenetics	1–5
EZH2	Epigenetics	5
DNMT3a	Epigenetics	10–15
BCOR	Epigenetics	1–5
STAG2	Cohesin	5–10
TP53	Genome stability	5
SRSF2	Splicing	15–20
U2AF1	Splicing	5–10
ZRSR2	Splicing	5–10
SF3B1	Splicing	30–35
NRAS	Signaling	1–5
CBL	Signaling	5
RUNX1	Signaling	10
JAK2	Signaling	5

feature, mandating the exclusion of common causes of anemia and nutritional deficiencies. In one analysis, MDS was the fifth most common cause of anemia in elderly patients after iron deficiency, bleeding, renal insufficiency, and anemia of chronic disease.[30,86] Thrombocytopenia and/or platelet dysfunction are common in MDS patients, with an overall prevalence ranging from 40% to 65%. Thrombocytopenia is more common in higher risk diseases, but occurs in lower risk patients and can be exacerbated by therapy. The frequency of hemorrhagic death ranges from 14% to 24%.[87] Bleeding can occur even in the absence of thrombocytopenia attributable to platelet dysfunction as evidenced by a prolonged bleeding time corresponding to an increase in atypical megakaryocytes.[88]

Among all patients with MDS, over one-third will undergo transformation into AML. In the remaining patients, the majority will succumb to infection, in part from neutropenia, iron overload, and granulocyte dysfunction illustrated by impaired phagocytic adhesion, chemotaxis, and microcidal killing.[89] Bacterial pneumonias and skin abscesses are most common, but unusual/opportunistic infections such as disseminated *Mycobacterium avium-intracellulare*,[90] *Aeromonas hydrophila* endocarditis,[91] bacterial thyroiditis,[92] and Epstein-Barr virus hepatitis may arise.[92]

MDS patients can also manifest a wide range of autoimmune phenomena such as cutaneous vasculitis, polymyalgia rheumatica, necrotizing panniculitis, Coombs-positive autoimmune hemolytic anemia, sweet syndrome, and an seronegative arthritis.[93–96]

In patients with MDS/MPN such as CMML, hepatosplenomegaly, lymphadenopathy, and pleural effusion are manifestations attributed to the proliferative nature of this group.[97] In patients with RARS-T, the risk of thrombotic events is similar to essential thrombocytosis.[98]

RISK ASSESSMENT AND PROGNOSIS

Risk stratification and prognostic assessment represent a critical first step in the management of MDS (Table 111.3). It provides useful information for the patients as to "the disease forecast" and, more importantly, allows physicians to tailor therapy accordingly. For patients with a higher risk, the goal of therapy is to alter the natural history of the disease and to extend survival. The goal of therapy in lower risk MDS is to alleviate symptomatic cytopenias using treatments that may restore effective hematopoiesis and lessen associated complications. The prognosis will depend on the inherent disease's specific features and host-related features. Risk models in MDS are constructed by incorporating several validated prognostic variables in a weighted scoring system, permitting patients to be divided into defined risk groups.

The International Prognostic Scoring System

The IPSS remains the most widely used staging system in MDS.[7] It has been embraced by community oncologists, adopted in clinical trials, and forms the basis of determining the time table for allogeneic hematopoietic cell transplantation in decision models. However, IPSS has several shortcomings. It was not developed as a dynamic system. It does not account for severity of cytopenias, and it overlooks two-thirds of the cytogenetic abnormalities encountered. Moreover, the IPSS is not applicable to patients with MDS/MPN or t-MDS.

The Revised IPSS

The IPSS-R was proposed as a refinement to adjust for those deficiencies of the original IPSS.[13] The major changes include the incorporation of less common karyotype abnormalities, the prognostic relevance of which was discerned from the larger patient cohort, and the weighing of the severity of each lineage of cytopenia. Several groups have validated the new prognostic system.[99,100]

The Global M.D. Anderson Scoring System

The Global M.D. Anderson Scoring System (MDAS) incorporates host factors such as age and performance status,[11] as well as anemia, transfusion burden, karyotype, and most importantly, the severity of thrombocytopenia. It captures the prognostic impact of leukocytosis for MDS/MPN. This model further refines IPSS. The MDAS upstaged 25% of patients to a higher risk category.[101] It can be applied for MDS/MPN cases, as well as t-MDS.

Other risk models that had been utilized and validated include the *Lower Risk M.D. Anderson Scoring System (LR-MDAS)*,[102] and the *WPSS*, which is more widely used in Europe.[10] For MDS/MPN subtypes, only the MDAS, discussed previously, can be applied. Several other models have been developed specifically for CMML (Table 111.4).

Five gene mutations independently predicted overall survival in a large cohort of MDS patients after adjusting for age and IPSS score.[103] These five genes include mutations involving TP53 (hazard ratio [HR], 2.48), EZH2 (HR, 2.13), ETV6 (HR, 2.04), RUNX1 (HR, 1.47), and ASXL1 (HR, 1.38). In lower risk MDS, EZH2, NRAS, and ASXL1 gene mutations upstaged 21% of low/intermediate 1 (int-1) IPSS risk MDS patients.[104] Only the EZH2 mutation provided additional risk discrimination to upstage 8% of the patients classified by LR-MDAS.[104]

The causes of death in MDS include AML transformation in 30% to 40% of all patients (10% to 20% of lower risk MDS patients), whereas the vast majority, unfortunately, succumb due to complications secondary to the disease, namely infection and bleeding.[105] Other important prognostic factors in MDS include red blood cell (RBC) transfusion dependence[106] and elevated serum ferritin >1,000 ng/mL, which is associated with both inferior overall survival and time to AML transformation.[107] Bone marrow fibrosis in MDS is typically associated with a higher risk disease, increased myeloblasts, or complex cytogenetics, and worse outcome. Patients with bone marrow fibrosis are often categorized morphologically as MDS-U or MDS with fibrosis (MDS-F).[34]

Patients with MDS often suffer from other medical comorbidities that may impact survival, affect performance status, and limit therapeutic options. Using the ACE-27 comorbidity index, the median survival was 31.8, 16.8, 15.2, and 9.7 months for those with none, mild, moderate, and severe comorbidities, respectively ($p < 0.001$). A prognostic model including age, IPSS, and comorbidity score predicted median survival.[108] The Italian group added further refinement by developing an MDS-specific comorbidity index (MDS-CI). Cardiac disease, moderate to severe liver disease, severe pulmonary disease, renal disease, and history of solid tumors were found to independently affect the risk of nonleukemic death, whereas diabetes and cerebrovascular disease did not.[109]

MANAGEMENT OF MYELODYSPLASTIC SYNDROMES

Erythropoiesis-Stimulating Agents

More than 90% of MDS patients have anemia, and 30% to 50% are transfusion dependent.[110] Erythropoiesis-stimulating agents (ESA) are the most widely used treatment for anemia in lower risk MDS; more than 50% of newly diagnosed and established patients in the United States receive ESA. Response rates range from 15% to 20% in unselected patients receiving doses equivalent to 40,000 to 60,000 U of epoetin alpha weekly.[111] Treatment lasting 8 to 12 weeks provides an adequate trial to assess ESA responsiveness, with median duration of responses ranging from 12 to 24 months.[112] Case-matching studies suggest a survival advantage among erythroid responders.[112] Darbepoetin is at least as effective as epoetin alfa.[113] Patient selection improves response probability to ESAs and conserves resources. Using a simple model based on

TABLE 111.3

Risk Stratification Models in Myelodysplastic Syndromes

IPSS

Variable	Score
Bone Marrow Blasts (%)	
<5	0
5–10	0.5
11–20	1.5
21–30	2.0
Karyotype[a]	
Good	0
Intermediate	0.5
Poor	1.0
Cytopenia[c]	
0/1	0
2/3	0.5

Risk Group	Sum Score	OS (y)
Low	0	5.7
Int-1	0.5–1	3.5
Int-2	1.5–2.0	1.1
High	≥2.5	0.4

IPSS-R

Variable	Score
Bone Marrow Blasts (%)	
<2	0
>2–<5	1
5–10	2
>10	3
Karyotype[b]	
Very good	0
Good	1
Intermediate	2
Poor	3
Very poor	4
Hgb ≥10 g/dL	0
8–<10 g/dL	1
<8 g/dL	1.5
ANC ≤0.8	0.5
Platelets ≥100	0
50–100	0.5
<50	1

Risk Group	Sum Score	OS (y)
Very good	0–2	8.8
Good	3–5	5.3
Int	6–7	3.0
Poor	8–9	1.6
Very poor	10–18	0.8

WPSS

Variable	Score
WHO Category	
RA, RARS, Del(5q)	0
RCMD, RCMD-RS	1
RAEB-I	2
RAEB-II	3
Karyotype[a]	
Good	0
Intermediate	1
Poor	2.0
Transfusion[d]	
Yes	1
No	0

Risk Group	Sum Score	OS (mos)
Very Low	0	141
Low	1	66
Intermediate	2	48
High	3–4	26
Very High	5–6	9

Global MDAS

Variable	Score
PS >2	2
Age (y)	
60–64	1
≥65	2
Platelets (× 10⁹/L)	
<30	3
30–49	2
50–199	1
Hgb <12 g/dL	2
BM blasts (%)	
5–10	1
11–29	2
WBC >20 × 10⁹/L	2
Karyotype	
Chromosome 7 Abn or complex ≥3 Abns	3
Transfusion	1

Risk Group	Sum Score	OS (mos)
Low	0–4	54
Int-1	5–6	25
Int-2	7–8	14
High	≥9	6

LR-MDAS

Variable	Score
Unfavorable cytogenetics[e]	1
Age ≥60 y	2
Hb <10 g/dL	1
Plt <50 × 10⁹/L	2
50–200 × 10⁹/L	1
BM blasts ≥4%	1

Risk Group	Sum Score	OS (mos)
Cat-1	0–2	80
Cat-2	3–4	27
Cat-3	≥5	14

MDAS, M.D. Anderson Scoring System; LR-MDAS, Lower Risk M.D. Anderson Scoring System; Hb, hemoglobin; Plt, platelet; BM, bone marrow; Hgb, hemoglobin; WBC, white blood cell count; ANC, absolute neutrophil count; Abn, abnormality.

[a] Good is normal, –Y, del(5q), del(20q). Intermediate is other karyotypic abnormalities. Poor is complex (≥three abnormalities) or chromosome 7 abnormalities.

[b] Very good –Y, del(11q). Good is normal, single del(5q), del(12p), del(20q), or double including del(5q). Intermediate includes single del(7q), +8, i(17q), +19, or any double not including del(5q). Poor includes der(3q). monosomy 7, double including –7/7q, or three abnormalities. Very poor is more than three abnormalities.

[c] Hb <10 g/dL; ANC <1,800/μL; platelets <100,000/μL.

[d] RBC transfusion dependence was defined as having at least one RBC transfusion every 8 weeks over a period of 4 mos

[e] In this analysis, diploid and 5q were favorable cytogenetics, all others were considered as unfavorable cytogenetics.

PRACTICE OF ONCOLOGY

TABLE 111.4

Prognostic Models in Chronic Myelomonocytic Leukemia

Score	Blast	IMP	NOC	DOC	LDH	Karyotype	Lymph	WBC	PS	Age	Mol
Bournemouth[a]	X		X								
Dusseldorf[b]	X		X		X						
IPSS[7]	X		X			X					
MDAPS[c]	X	X					X				
Spanish[d]	X				X			X			
MDASC[e]	X			X		X		X	X	X	
IPSS-R[13]	X			X		X				X	
Mayo[f]		X		X				X			
GFM[68]				X				X		X	X

Blast, myeloblast and promonocyte percentage in the bone marrow; IMP, immature myeloid precursor (represent the sum of peripheral blasts, promyelocytes, myelocytes, and metamyelocytes); NOC, number of cytopenias; DOC, duration of cytopenias; LDH, lactate dehydrogenase; lymph, lymphocyte count; WBC, white blood cell count; PS, Eastern Cooperative Oncology Group performance status; Mol, molecular profiling; MDAPS, MD Anderson Score from Prognostication in CMML; MDASC, Global MD Anderson Scoring System; GFM, Groupe Francias des Myelodysplasia.
[a] Worsley A, Oscier DG, Stevens J, et al. Prognostic features of chronic myelomonocytic leukaemia: a modified Bournemouth score gives the best prediction of survival. *Br J Haematol* 1988;68:17–21.
[b] Aul C, Gattermann N, Heyll A, et al. Primary myelodysplastic syndromes: analysis of prognostic factors in 235 patients and proposals for an improved scoring system. *Leukemia* 1992;6:52–59.
[c] Onida F, Kantarjian HM, Smith TL, et al. Prognostic factors and scoring systems in chronic myelomonocytic leukemia: a retrospective analysis of 213 patients. *Blood* 2002;99:840–849.
[d] Such E, Germing U, Malcovati L, et al. Development and validation of a prognostic scoring system for patients with chronic myelomonocytic leukemia. *Blood* 2013;121:3005–3015.
[e] Kantarjian H, O'Brien S, Ravandi F, et al. Proposal for a new risk model in myelodysplastic syndrome that accounts for events not considered in the original International Prognostic Scoring System. *Cancer* 2008;113:1351–1361.
[f] Patnaik MM, Padron E, Laborde RR, et al. Mayo prognostic model for WHO-defined chronic myelomonocytic leukemia: ASXL1 and spliceosome component mutations and outcomes. *Leukemia* 2013;27:1504–1510.

pretreatment endogenous serum erythropoietin (EPO) concentration (<100, 100 to 500, or >500 U per liter) and RBC transfusion burden ($<$ or ≥ 2 U per month one would distinguish three response categories: high probability of erythroid response (74%), intermediate (23%), and low (7%).[114]

Lenalidomide

Lenalidomide is approved by the U.S. Food and Drug Administration (FDA) for the treatment of transfusion-dependent anemia in lower risk MDS patients with a chromosome 5q deletion (del[5q]) with or without additional cytogenetic abnormalities. In the lenalidomide registration (MDS-003) phase II clinical trial, the overall transfusion response rate was 76%, with 67% achieving transfusion independence.[115] The median time to response was 4.6 weeks, accompanied by a median rise in hemoglobin (Hgb) of 5.4 g/dL. Median duration of response exceeded 2 years and is longer in patients with isolate del(5q). Lenalidomide was administered at a dose of 10 mg daily either continuously or for 21 days every 4 weeks. Cytogenetic response and hematologic improvement were the strongest independent covariates for overall survival (OS) (HR, 5.295; $p < 0.001$).[116,117] Recent studies indicate that *TP53* gene mutations are demonstrable in approximately 20% of del(5q) MDS patients, expand over time, and are associated with a higher risk of disease progression and a lower frequency of cytogenetic response to lenalidomide.[118–120]

The most commonly observed adverse event was early myelosuppression, generally occurring in the first 8 weeks of treatment (62%). More than half of the patients (55%) experienced neutropenia, and 44% had thrombocytopenia. Dose reduction or treatment interruption for hematologic adverse events was necessary in the majority (84%) of patients. The median time to first dose reduction was 22 days. At week 24, only 32% of patients were receiving a 10-mg dose. Early cytopenias with lenalidomide treatment correlated with the probability of achieving RBC transfusion

independence.[121] Non–hematologic-adverse events include dry skin, rash and pruritus, itching of the scalp, and diarrhea. Hypothyroidism has been reported in approximately 7% of patients.[122,123] Patients with renal insufficiency were excluded. In such patients, it is prudent to adjust the dosage based on creatinine clearance given the renal excretion of lenalidomide.[124] The incidence of venous thromboembolic events (VTE) in MDS patients treated with lenalidomide monotherapy was low, with VTE reported in 3% of the del(5q) patients.

A subsequent phase III, placebo-controlled study (MDS-004) compared two different doses and schedules of lenalidomide in the same del(5q) MDS population.[125] Two hundred and five patients were randomized to receive treatment with either lenalidomide 10 mg daily for 21 days every 4 weeks, continuous treatment with lenalidomide 5 mg daily, or placebo. The rates of sustained transfusion independence (>24 weeks) were 53.6%, 33.3%, and 6%, respectively ($p < 0.001$). Cytogenetic response rates were also highest in the 10-mg arm. The median rise in hemoglobin was highest in patients treated with the 10-mg lenalidomide dose. No difference was observed in the frequency or magnitude of myelosuppression between the two lenalidomide doses, nor was there a difference in the rate of AML transformation.

The use of lenalidomide in lower risk non-del(5q) MDS was explored in a phase II study (MDS-002), which enrolled 214 non-del(5q) patients.[126] Based on the International Working Group 2000 (IWG 2000) response criteria, 26% patients achieved transfusion independence. Median rise in hemoglobin was 3.2 g/dL, and median duration of response was 41 weeks. Attempts to improve the activity of lenalidomide in non-del(5q) patients include biomarker-guided patient selection and combination strategies with an ESA.[127,128] Preliminary results of a randomized phase II clinical trial comparing lenalidomide to a lenalidomide/ESA combination yielded higher erythroid response rates with the combination treatment: 23% versus 40%, respectively ($p = 0.043$).

Lenalidomide's mechanism of action in MDS is karyotype specific. In del(5q) MDS, lenalidomide relieves p53 arrest by stabilizing MDM2 to permit cell cycle reentry by inhibiting the haplodeficient PP2A. The resulting hyperphosphorylation of inhibitory serine/threonine residues on MDM2 suppresses its autologous ubiquitination, thereby stabilizing the protein and, in turn, promoting the proteasomal degradation of p53.[84] In non-del(5q) MDS, lenalidomide enhances erythroid receptor signaling. The inhibition of PP2A promotes coalescence of lipid rafts with attendant incorporation of the erythropoietin receptor along with its signaling intermediates to yield a more efficient receptor signaling platform.[129]

The use of lenalidomide in higher risk MDS patients remains investigational. Several studies reported modest response rates and rates of transfusion independence.[130–132] A high rate of complete response have been reported when combining azacitidine and lenalidomide in higher risk MDS in a phase I/II trial, which is the subject of an ongoing intergroup randomized phase II clinical study.[133] Use of lenalidomide in the treatment of MDS/MPN subtypes is often extrapolated from its use in MDS. Nonproliferative lower risk CMML patients were included in the studies summarized previously. Anecdotal case reports suggest lenalidomide activity in patient with the RARS-T subtype.[134]

Azanucleosides

Azacitidine and decitabine are azanucleoside analogs with varied capacity to act as hypomethylating agents (HMA) to reverse epigenetic gene repression. Covalent bonds formed between deoxycytidine nucleotides and DNA methyltransferase deplete the enzyme and, as a consequence, promotes demethylation of silenced genes. These agents also are cytotoxic as DNA interactive nucleoside analogs and, in the case of azacitidine, which is incorporated largely into RNA, by inhibiting RNA translation and protein synthesis.

Azacitidine was the first FDA-approved drug for the treatment of all FAB MDS subtypes.[135] The overall CR+partial response (PR) rate was 23% (CR, 7%; PR, 16%), with a corresponding extension in median time to AML transformation from 12 to 21 months. The subsequent AZA-001 trial was the first study to demonstrate a survival advantage for any treatment in higher risks MDS.[136] Patients with intermediate 2 (Int-2) or high-risk MDS (n = 358) were randomized to treatment with either azacitidine or conventional care regimens (CCR) that included either best supportive care (BSC) alone, low-dose cytarabine, or intensive AML-type induction chemotherapy. The median OS was significantly extended in the azacitidine group compared to CCR: 24.5 months versus 15 months, respectively ($p = 0.0001$). AML progression was delayed by more than 14 months with the azacitidine treatment. Hematologic response rates also favored azacitidine, with 45% achieving RBC transfusion independence compared to 11% with CCR. The OS benefit with azacitidine treatment extended to those patients with AML according to the WHO classification (myeloblasts: 20% to 30%). A landmark analysis at cycle four revealed that patients who achieve hematologic improvement (HI) or better response according to IWG criteria experienced a survival advantage.[137] The probability of HI response, and therefore the potential for survival improvement, diminish with time, reaching less than 15% after 6 months of treatment.[138] Poor-risk cytogenetics, increased myeloblasts, and prior treatment with low-dose cytarabine are predictive variables for a lower response rate.[139] The loss of function mutations involving the *TET2* gene is associated with a higher rate of response to azacitidine.[140] In lower risk MDS, nearly 50% of patients achieve HI and/or RBC transfusion independence (TI). The HI rate with treatment with a 5-day regimen appears equivalent to 5-2-2 or 5-2-5 regimens with less toxicity; however, its impact, if any, on OS is unknown.[141]

Decitabine was FDA approved based on a phase III trial in the United States comparing 15 mg/m^2 intravenously (IV) administered over 3 hours every 8 hours for 3 consecutive days to BSC in patients with INT-1, -2, and HR MDS.[142] The overall response

rate was 30% with decitabine (9% CR, 8% PR, and 13% HI). Kantarjian et al.[143] compared three decitabine schedules using a reduced cumulative dosing schedule in a similar population. This study identified 20 mg/m^2 IV daily for 5 days as the preferred schedule, where the CR rate was 39%. The ADOPT trial was a multicenter validation study involving 99 MDS patients treated with the 20 mg/m^2 5-day regimen; the study reported 17% CR with a corresponding median OS of 19.4 month.[144] A subsequent phase III study compared the effects of the FDA-approved decitabine regimen to supportive care in Int-2 and high-risk MDS.[145] The OS and the median time to AML transformation or death were not significantly different from the supportive care (SC) arm.

Outcomes after azanucleoside failure is poor, with median OS ranging from 4 to 8 months, and a 12-month survival of approximately 30%.[146–148] CR rates with standard intensive chemotherapy are 20% or less. Treatment of patients who fail azanucleosides represent an unmet need. Recent data suggest that outcomes are poor after azanucleoside failure in lower risk MDS as well.[149]

Small numbers of MDS/MPN patients, namely CMML, were included in the original azanucleoside clinical trials. Large retrospective series suggest similar response rates, but probably an inferior effect on OS. Splenomegaly and leukocytosis are predictors for worse outcomes among CMML patients treated with azacitidine.[150]

Immunosuppressive Therapy

HI is observed in approximately one-third of unselected MDS patients treated with antithymocyte globulin (ATG) with or without cyclosporine. Age is the strongest covariate for hematologic response. In a multivariate analysis age, the duration of RBC TD and the presence of a human leukocyte antigen DR15 were independent response variables.[151] Other retrospective studies identified bone marrow hypocellularity and the presence of a paroxysmal nocturnal hemoglobinuria clone as covariates for response to immunosuppressive therapy (IST). Rabbit ATG offers comparable effectiveness in treating MDS patients.[152] Alemtuzumab was reported to yield high response rates in preselected patients with the previously described features associated with the probability for response to IST.[153]

Allogeneic Hematopoietic Cell Transplantation

Allogeneic hematopoietic cell transplantation (AHCT) remains the only known curative treatment for patients with MDS. Unfortunately, the majority of MDS patients are not candidates for the procedure due to advanced age or comorbidities, and the procedure itself carries significant morbidity and mortality. With the decision of Medicare to provide coverage with evidence development for the AHCT in MDS patients in 2008, the number of procedures performed in the United States for patients with MDS, particularly those older than 60 years, has significantly increased over the past decade.

Using a markovian decision analysis model, early AHCT is recommended for higher risk MDS patients to maximize survival potential, whereas for lower risk patients, delaying AHCT until disease progression is a strategy that offered best overall survival.[154] A subsequent decision model in the azanucleoside era utilizing data from reduced intensity AHCT and predominantly in elderly patients (60 to 70 years) confirmed the recommendation of early AHCT for higher risk MDS and delayed AHCT for those with a lower risk.[155] No randomized controlled trials, evaluating AHCT versus nontransplant strategies, are available.

The most important predictors of outcome after AHCT are disease status (myeloblasts >5% and poor risk cytogenetics), but not age.[156] A study reported experience involving 1,333 MDS patients >50 years (449 patients >60 years) who underwent HCT. Four-year OS estimates for the 50 to 60 year olds and the <60 years cohort was 34% and 27%, respectively.

The question of therapy prior to AHCT remains controversial. Earlier studies did not show a convincing advantage for induction

PRACTICE OF ONCOLOGY

chemotherapy prior to AHCT; however, those studies were not randomized and were subject to selection bias by treating higher risk patients with chemotherapy. Among patients who receive intensive chemotherapy, those who achieved CR prior to AHCT had a better outcome. A phase II study evaluated 265 consecutive patients who received an AHCT. There was no difference in 3-year OS whether patients received azacitidine, intensive chemotherapy, or azacitidine preceded or followed by intensive chemotherapy (55% versus 48% versus 32%, respectively; p = 0.07).[157] Azanucleosides may also play a role as a maintenance strategy post-HCT. de Lima et al.[158] demonstrated that maintenance therapy with low-dose azacitidine (32 mg/m^2 for four cycles) is feasible in the post-AHCT setting for recurrent AML or MDS. This strategy is the subject of a prospective randomized clinical trial.[158] An analysis of 435 patients with higher risk MDS who had failed treatment with azanucleosides showed that patients who proceeded to AHCT or investigational agents had better survival compared to those offered supportive care or conventional chemotherapy, whether a low or an intensive dose.[147]

Iron Chelation Therapy

Several groups reported that iron overload and elevated serum ferritin in MDS patients is associated with inferior OS and higher rate of leukemia evolution.[107] Nonrandomized studies suggest that iron chelation therapy (ICT) impacts outcomes in lower risk MDS.[159,160] Two studies showed that the oral iron chelator deferasirox (Exjade) effectively lowered serum ferritin and labile plasma iron concentration in lower risk MDS.[161,162] Adverse effects from deferasirox may include renal failure, diarrhea, hepatic failure, and gastrointestinal hemorrhage. Deferasirox is contraindicated in patients with a creatinine clearance less than 40 mL per minute, higher risk MDS patients, and in patients with platelet count less than 50 $\times$ 10^9/L. Deferiprone (Ferriprox) is another oral iron chelator approved in the United States. The adverse effect of greatest concern is agranulocytosis, but it has less renal toxicity.[163] The MDS foundation recommends the consideration of ICT in transfusion-dependent lower risk MDS patients with serum ferritin persistently >1,000 ng/mL, whereas the National Comprehensive Cancer Network (NCCN) guidelines use a >2,500 ng/mL threshold. An ongoing randomized phase III, placebo-controlled study (TELESTO) is intended to address the potential clinical benefit of deferasirox chelation therapy.

How Do I Treat MDS Patients?

The first step in the management of MDS requires confirming the diagnosis, which in many instances, may require a hematopathologist's experienced eyes.[164] After establishing a diagnosis, risk stratification is critical for management decisions. We complement the standard IPSS risk model by newer clinical risk models such as IPSS-R and MDAS (or CMML-specific models in cases of CMML), and a molecular profile to more precisely delineate the disease risk category.[7,11,13,165]

For higher risk patients, we initiate treatment with azacitidine 75 mg/m^2 SC for 7 days every 28 days and assess patients for hematopoeitic stem cell transplant (HCT) in the absence of major comorbidities and a good performance status.[155] For patients who do not proceed to AHCT, we continue treatment until disease progression or loss of response. The response to azacitidine is evaluated after 4 to 6 cycles. If the disease is stable or better, treatment is continued. Experience from the AZA-001 trial tells us that hematologic improvement is predictive for improved overall survival.[136,166] In patients with baseline thrombocytopenia and neutropenia, we do not delay therapy or reduce dose, but rather provide more focused supportive care with close hematologic monitoring. We avoid the use of granulocyte-colony stimulating factor (G-CSF) or GM-CSF except in the setting of febrile neutropenia. Combination strategies adding to the backbone of azacitidine are being explored in clinical trials such as the combinations with lenalidomide, vorinostat, or pracinostat.[167–169] Crossing over to the alternate azanucleoside is generally minimally effective.[170] We consider a clinical trial or AHCT for those patients after azanucleoside failure.[147] Several agents are under investigation in patients after azanucleoside failure. A phase III trial with rigosertib, a multikinase inhibitor, recently completed accrual.[171] In cases of secondary AML, response rates to standard 3 + 7 induction chemotherapy is disappointing, with short OS. In this setting, we offer patients intensive chemotherapy, preferably in the context of a clinical trial such as the phase III randomized study comparing CPX-351 (liposomal formulation of a 5:1 molar ratio of cytarabine and daunorubicin), which demonstrated promising efficacy in a phase II randomized study.[172] Outside the context of a clinical trial, we favor the use the cladribine, cytarabine, G-CSF, and mitoxantrone (CLAG-M) regimen for induction in secondary AML after azacitidine failure, for which we previously reported a >50% complete response rate.[173]

In lower risk MDS, anemia remains the most common indication for therapy. In patients with a low endogenous serum erythropoietin level (<500 mU/mL) and low transfusion burden, we begin treatment with an ESA. An 8- to 12-week minimum trial of epoetin alfa is started at a dose of 40,000 to 60,000 U weekly or darbepoetin alfa dose equivalence as sufficient. In the absence of response, and particularly for patients with RARS, we consider the addition of G-CSF.[111] Subsequent treatment alternatives are guided by the type and severity of additional cytopenias, and include lenalidomide or azacitidine. For non-del(5q) lower risk MDS, lenalidomide may be considered in patients with isolated anemia and adequate platelets and neutrophils.[126] Use of lenalidomide prior to azanucleosides may yield higher response rates.[174] Lenalidomide in combination with ESA is currently under investigation with promising higher responses than lenalidomide alone.[127,128] Azacitidine is also used for lower risk MDS patients. We commonly use azacitidine at a dose of 75 mg/m^2 for 5 days in lower risk patients.[141] For MDS patients younger than 60 years of age with a short duration of transfusion dependence, a cluster of differentiation 4 cells (CD4):CD8 ratio <2.0 or those with trisomy 8, immunosuppressive therapy is a reasonable treatment strategy. For lower risk MDS patients with thrombocytopenia or neutropenia, particularly if the goal of treatment is to improve thrombocytopenia, azanucleosides are the treatment of choice or IST if there is a high chance of response. In del(5q) lower risk MDS patients who either failed or are not a candidate for treatment with an ESA, lenalidomide is the treatment of choice in the presence of adequate neutrophil and platelet counts.[115] Lenalidomide is administered daily at a dose of 10 mg orally. Complete blood counts are monitored weekly during the first 8 weeks. The vast majority of patients will need dose interruption after 2 to 3 weeks, with resumption of lenalidomide treatment upon hematologic recovery at the next lower dose level. In selected patients with lower risk MDS who are younger and who have no major comorbidities, AHCT may be discussed after failure of standard therapy. In our opinion, clinical trials remain the standard of care for treating MDS patients and should be considered whenever available.

SELECTED REFERENCES

The full reference list can be accessed at lwwhealthlibrary.com/oncology.

1. Vardiman JW, Thiele J, Arber DA, et al. The 2008 revision of the World Health Organization (WHO) classification of myeloid neoplasms and acute leukemia: rationale and important changes. *Blood* 2009;114:937–951.

6. Bennett JM, Catovsky D, Daniel MT, et al. Proposals for the classification of the myelodysplastic syndromes. *Br J Haematol* 1982;51:189–199.

7. Greenberg P, Cox C, LeBeau MM, et al. International scoring system for evaluating prognosis in myelodysplastic syndromes. *Blood* 1997;89:2079–2088.

10. Malcovati L, Germing U, Kuendgen A, et al. Time-dependent prognostic scoring system for predicting survival and leukemic evolution in myelodysplastic syndromes. *J Clin Oncol* 2007;25:3503–3510.

11. Kantarjian H, O'Brien S, Ravandi F, et al. Proposal for a new risk model in myelodysplastic syndrome that accounts for events not considered in the original International Prognostic Scoring System. *Cancer* 2008;113:1351–1361.

13. Greenberg PL, Tuechler H, Schanz J, et al. Revised International Prognostic Scoring System for myelodysplastic syndromes. *Blood* 2012;120:2454–2465.

15. Rollison DE, Howlader N, Smith MT, et al. Epidemiology of myelodysplastic syndromes and chronic myeloproliferative disorders in the United States, 2001–2004, using data from the NAACCR and SEER programs. *Blood* 2008;112:45–52.

16. Goldberg SL, Chen E, Corral M, et al. Incidence and clinical complications of myelodysplastic syndromes among United States Medicare beneficiaries. *J Clin Oncol* 2010;28:2847–2852.

20. Churpek JE, Lorenz R, Nedumgottil S, et al. Proposal for the clinical detection and management of patients and their family members with familial myelodysplastic syndrome/acute leukemia predisposition syndromes. *Leuk Lymphoma* 2013;54:28–35.

26. Kristinsson SY, Björkholm M, Hultcrantz M, et al. Chronic immune stimulation might act as a trigger for the development of acute myeloid leukemia or myelodysplastic syndromes. *J Clin Oncol* 2011;29:2897–2903.

34. Della Porta MG, Malcovati L, Boveri E, et al. Clinical relevance of bone marrow fibrosis and CD34-positive cell clusters in primary myelodysplastic syndromes. *J Clin Oncol* 2009;27:754–762.

51. Haase D, Germing U, Schanz J, et al. New insights into the prognostic impact of the karyotype in MDS and correlation with subtypes: evidence from a core dataset of 2124 patients. *Blood* 2007;110:4385–4395.

52. Barlow JL, Drynan LF, Hewett DR, et al. A p53-dependent mechanism underlies macrocytic anemia in a mouse model of human 5q- syndrome. *Nat Med* 2010;16:59–66.

53. Papaemmanuil E, Gerstung M, Malcovati L, et al. Clinical and biological implications of driver mutations in myelodysplastic syndromes. *Blood* 2013;122:3616–3627.

54. Haferlach T, Nagata Y, Grossmann V, et al. Landscape of genetic lesions in 944 patients with myelodysplastic syndromes. *Leukemia* 2014;28:241–247.

59. Bejar R, Stevenson K, Abdel-Wahab O, et al. Clinical effect of point mutations in myelodysplastic syndromes. *N Engl J Med* 2011;364:2496–2506.

65. Yoshida K, Sanada M, Shiraishi Y, et al. Frequent pathway mutations of splicing machinery in myelodysplasia. *Nature* 2011;478:64–69.

68. Itzykson R, Kosmider O, Renneville A, et al. Prognostic score including gene mutations in chronic myelomonocytic leukemia. *J Clin Oncol* 2013;31:2428–2436.

79. Wei Y, Dimicoli S, Bueso-Ramos C, et al. Toll-like receptor alterations in myelodysplastic syndrome. *Leukemia* 2013;27:1832–1840.

83. Ebert BL, Pretz J, Bosco J, et al. Identification of RPS14 as a 5q− syndrome gene by RNA interference screen. *Nature* 2008;451:335–339.

84. Wei S, Chen X, McGraw K, et al. Lenalidomide promotes p53 degradation by inhibiting MDM2 auto-ubiquitination in myelodysplastic syndrome with chromosome 5q deletion. *Oncogene* 2013;32:1110–1120.

104. Bejar R, Stevenson KE, Caughey BA, et al. Validation of a prognostic model and the impact of mutations in patients with lower-risk myelodysplastic syndromes. *J Clin Oncol* 2012;30(27):3376–3382.

106. Malcovati L, Porta MG, Pascutto C, et al. Prognostic factors and life expectancy in myelodysplastic syndromes classified according to WHO criteria: a basis for clinical decision making. *J Clin Oncol* 2005;23:7594–7603.

107. Sanz G, Nomdedeu B, Such E, et al. Independent impact of iron overload and transfusion dependency on survival and leukemic evolution in patients with myelodysplastic syndrome. *ASH Annual Meeting Abstracts* 2008;112:(abstract 640).

114. Hellstrom-Lindberg E, Gulbrandsen N, Lindberg G, et al. A validated decision model for treating the anaemia of myelodysplastic syndromes with erythropoietin + granulocyte colony-stimulating factor: significant effects on quality of life. *Br J Haematol* 2003;120:1037–1046.

115. List A, Dewald G, Bennett J, et al. Lenalidomide in the myelodysplastic syndrome with chromosome 5q deletion. *N Engl J Med* 2006;355:1456–1465.

116. List A, Dewald G, Bennett J, et al. Cytogenetic response to lenalidomide is associated with improved survival in patients with chromosome 5q deletion. *Leuk Res* 2007;31:s38.

119. Jadersten M, Saft L, Smith A, et al. TP53 mutations in low-risk myelodysplastic syndromes with del(5q) predict disease progression. *J Clin Oncol* 2011;29:1971–1979.

125. Fenaux P, Giagounidis A, Selleslag D, et al. A randomized phase 3 study of lenalidomide versus placebo in RBC transfusion-dependent patients with low-/intermediate-1-risk myelodysplastic syndromes with del5q. *Blood* 2011;118:3765–3776.

126. Raza A, Reeves JA, Feldman EJ, et al. Phase 2 study of lenalidomide in transfusion-dependent, low-risk, and intermediate-1 risk myelodysplastic syndromes with karyotypes other than deletion 5q. *Blood* 2008;111:86–93.

133. Sekeres MA, Tiu RV, Komrokji R, et al. Phase 2 study of the lenalidomide and azacitidine combination in patients with higher-risk myelodysplastic syndromes. *Blood* 2012;120:4945–4951.

135. Silverman LR, Demakos EP, Peterson BL, et al. Randomized controlled trial of azacitidine in patients with the myelodysplastic syndrome: a study of the cancer and leukemia group B. *J Clin Oncol* 2002;20:2429–2440.

136. Fenaux P, Mufti GJ, Hellstrom-Lindberg E, et al. Efficacy of azacitidine compared with that of conventional care regimens in the treatment of higher-risk myelodysplastic syndromes: a randomised, open-label, phase III study. *Lancet Oncol* 2009;10:223–232.

141. Lyons RM, Cosgriff TM, Modi SS, et al. Hematologic response to three alternative dosing schedules of azacitidine in patients with myelodysplastic syndromes. *J Clin Oncol* 2009;27:1850–1856.

143. Kantarjian H, Oki Y, Garcia-Manero G, et al. Results of a randomized study of 3 schedules of low-dose decitabine in higher-risk myelodysplastic syndrome and chronic myelomonocytic leukemia. *Blood* 2007;109:52–57.

144. Steensma DP, Baer MR, Slack JL, et al. Multicenter study of decitabine administered daily for 5 days every 4 weeks to adults with myelodysplastic syndromes: the alternative dosing for outpatient treatment (ADOPT) trial. *J Clin Oncol* 2009;27:3842–3848.

145. Lubbert M, Suciu S, Baila L, et al. Low-dose decitabine versus best supportive care in elderly patients with intermediate- or high-risk myelodysplastic syndrome (MDS) ineligible for intensive chemotherapy: final results of the randomized phase III study of the European Organisation for Research and Treatment of Cancer Leukemia Group and the German MDS Study Group. *J Clin Oncol* 2011;29:1987–1996.

147. Prebet T, Gore SD, Esterni B, et al. Outcome of high-risk myelodysplastic syndrome after azacitidine treatment failure. *J Clin Oncol* 2011;29:3322–3327.

151. Sloand EM, Wu CO, Greenberg P, et al. Factors affecting response and survival in patients with myelodysplasia treated with immunosuppressive therapy. *J Clin Oncol* 2008;26:2505–2511.

154. Cutler CS, Lee SJ, Greenberg P, et al. A decision analysis of allogeneic bone marrow transplantation for the myelodysplastic syndromes: delayed transplantation for low-risk myelodysplasia is associated with improved outcome. *Blood* 2004;104:579–585.

155. Koreth J, Pidala J, Perez WS, et al. Role of reduced-intensity conditioning allogeneic hematopoietic stem-cell transplantation in older patients with de novo myelodysplastic syndromes: an international collaborative decision analysis. *J Clin Oncol* 2013;31:2662–2670.

157. Damaj G, Duhamel A, Robin M, et al. Impact of azacitidine before allogeneic stem-cell transplantation for myelodysplastic syndromes: a study by the Société Française de Greffe de Moelle et de Thérapie-Cellulaire and the Groupe-Francophone des Myélodysplasies. *J Clin Oncol* 2012;30(36):4533–4540.

158. de Lima M, Giralt S, Thall PF, et al. Maintenance therapy with low-dose azacitidine after allogeneic hematopoietic stem cell transplantation for recurrent acute myelogenous leukemia or myelodysplastic syndrome: a dose and schedule finding study. *Cancer* 2010;116:5420–5431.

160. Rose C, Brechignac S, Vassilief D, et al. Does iron chelation therapy improve survival in regularly transfused lower risk MDS patients? A multicenter study by the GFM (Groupe Francophone des Myelodysplasies). *Leuk Res* 2010;34:864–870.

161. List AF, Baer MR, Steensma D, et al. Deferasirox (ICL670; Exjade(R)) reduces serum ferritin (SF) and labile plasma iron (LPI) in patients with myelodysplastic syndromes (MDS). *ASH Annual Meeting Abstracts* 2007;110:(abstract 1470).

162. Gattermann N, Schmid M, Porta MD, et al. Efficacy and safety of deferasirox (Exjade(R)) during 1 year of treatment in transfusion-dependent patients with myelodysplastic syndromes: results from EPIC Trial. *ASH Annual Meeting Abstracts* 2008;112:(abstract 633).

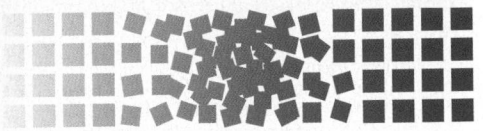

112 Plasma Cell Neoplasms

Nikhil C. Munshi and Kenneth C. Anderson

INTRODUCTION

Plasma cell neoplasms represent a spectrum of diseases characterized by clonal proliferation and the accumulation of immunoglobulin-producing terminally differentiated B cells. The spectrum includes clinically benign common conditions, such as monoclonal gammopathy of unknown significance (MGUS), as well as rare disorders such as Castleman's disease and α heavy chain disease; indolent conditions such as Waldenström's macroglobulinemia; the more common malignant entity, plasma cell myeloma; and a more aggressive form, plasma cell leukemia, with circulating malignant plasma cells in the blood. All of these disorders share common features of plasma cell morphology, production of immunoglobulin molecules, and immune dysfunction. A plasma cell neoplasm is considered to originate from a single B cell, with resultant monoclonal protein secretion that characterizes its type. Occasional oligoclonal or polyclonal protein abnormalities are observed in conditions such as Castleman's disease.

There are five major classes of immunoglobulin (Ig) synthesized by normal B cells and plasma cells: IgG, IgA, IgM, IgD, and IgE. The dysfunctional plasma cells secrete one of these intact immunoglobulin molecules; however, there may be a discrepancy in the production of the heavy and light chains leading to an imbalance with an excess of κ or λ light chain that is excreted in the urine (Bence Jones proteinuria), or in some instances, a production of only excess κ or λ light chain molecules. Occasionally, plasma cells do not secrete any paraproteins (nonsecretory type myeloma); however, they usually have cytoplasmic immunoglobulin and produce low levels of immunoglobulins undetectable by current methods. Although myeloma can be associated with any of the immunoglobulin subtypes, the IgM type is predominately associated with other malignant conditions such as Waldenström's macroglobulinemia and chronic lymphocytic leukemia (CLL).

HISTORY

The earliest evidence of myeloma has been reported from Egyptian mummies; however, the first published clinical description of the disease was reported in 1850 in England. A patient, Thomas Alexander McBean, presented to Dr. William Macintrye of London in 1845 with symptoms of episodic fatigue, diffuse bone pain, and urinary frequency. The urinalysis detected a urinary protein with a peculiar heat property, and McIntyre called it *mollities and fragilitas ossium* due to the patient's bony symptoms.[1] Later that year, Dr. Henry Bence Jones also tested urine specimens provided by Macintyre and corroborated the heat properties of urinary light chains. Bence Jones thought that the protein was the *hydrated deuteroxide of albumin* (now called Bence Jones proteins) and published his findings several years before Macintyre published his case report.[2] After the patient died in 1846, a surgeon, Dr. John Dalrymple, examined several bones, and his gross and microscopic observations are consistent with morphology of myeloma cells.

The term *multiple myeloma* was coined by Rustizky in 1873 following his independent observation in a similar patient with multiple bone lesions. Kahler, in 1889, published a review on this condition and the disease became known, particularly in Europe, as Kahler's disease.[3] Ellinger, in 1899, described the increased serum proteins and sedimentation rate in myeloma. In 1900, Wright described the involvement of plasma cells in this neoplasm and, for the first time, he described roentgenographic abnormalities in myeloma, which to date remain a hallmark of this disease.

The development of bone marrow aspiration in 1929,[4] electrophoresis to separate serum proteins in 1937,[5] and a later report of a specific spike in the γ globulin region, enhanced the diagnosis and understanding of myeloma. Identification of the heavy and light chains in the monoclonal protein by immunoelectrophoresis was described by Grabar in 1953, confirming the monoclonality of immunoglobulin in this disease. Other developments in recent times include understanding of the role of the bone marrow microenvironment in myeloma cell growth, survival, and development of drug resistance through cell–cell interactions and activation of cytokine networks.[6,7] The significance of chromosomal translocations in myeloma pathobiology, and more recently, the use of gene expression profiling and whole genome sequencing, are providing insights into the molecular pathogenesis of the disease.

No effective systemic therapy existed before 1947, when urethane was reported to show an effect in a few patients. However, a subsequent randomized trial indicated that the survival of patients receiving urethane was inferior to that observed with a placebo.[8] The first successful use of chemotherapeutic agent in myeloma was reported in 1958 by Blokhin and colleagues with the use of a racemic mixture of D-and L-phenylalanine mustards (Sarcolysine). Subsequently, the D- and L-isomers of phenylalanine mustard were tested separately, and the antimyeloma activity was found to reside in the L-isomer, melphalan. In 1962, Bergsagel and colleagues from the Southwest Oncology Group reported remissions in about one-third of myeloma patients treated with melphalan.[9] The administration of high doses of glucocorticoid was first reported to induce remissions in relapsing or refractory myeloma in 1967.[10] The use of melphalan in combination with prednisone was then studied extensively.[11] The role of high-dose therapy was investigated by McElwain in 1983, and the addition of bone marrow and, subsequently, stem cell transplantation improved safety and allowed for further dose escalation.[12] In the last 10 years, an elucidation of the genomic changes driving the disease process, coupled with improved understanding of the role of the bone marrow microenvironment in myeloma biology and the development of drug resistance, has led to the identification of novel targets and directed agents including immunomodulatory drugs, thalidomide, lenalidomide, and pomalidomide; proteasome inhibitors, bortezomib and carfilzomib; inhibitors directed at histone deacetylases, phosphoinositide 3-kinase (PI3K)/Akt signaling; as well as antibodies targeting CS1, CD138, and CD38.

EPIDEMIOLOGY

According to the most recent data from the Surveillance, Epidemiology, and End Results (SEER) program, multiple myeloma (MM) is a relatively uncommon malignancy in the United States, representing 1.4% of all malignancies in Caucasians and 2.0% in African Americans. Among hematologic malignancies, it constitutes 10% of the tumors and ranks as the second most frequently occurring hematologic cancer in the United States after non-Hodgkin's lymphoma. The prevalence of myeloma in the United States in 2011 was over 83,367 and estimated new cases in 2014 are approximately 24,050; 11,090 patients are expected to die from myeloma in 2014. The disease is more common in men and has an average annual age-adjusted (1970 US standard) incidence rate per 100,000 among Caucasians of 7.2 in men and 4.3 in women, whereas for African Americans, the incidence is 14.7 in men and 10.5 in women. The increased incidence in African Americans is not explained by factors such as social or economic condition, household size, or family income.[13] A study in the African population from Ghana has demonstrated an incidence of MGUS similar to the African American population, possibly implicating genetic risk factors.[14] The incidence rates for other ethnic groups including Asian/Pacific islanders, American Indians, and Alaskan natives are also lower relative to US Caucasians. The Chinese and Japanese populations similarly have a lower incidence than Caucasians. A recent survey of MGUS in 12,481 US patients showed significantly higher (p <0.001) prevalence of MGUS in African Americans (3.7%) compared with Caucasians (2.3%) (p = 0.001) or Hispanics (1.8%).[15] The incidence of multiple myeloma has slowly increased in the US Caucasian population since 1970; however, the incidence among African Americans has increased more prominently during the 1970s to 1990s. These observed differences in the prevalence have not been associated with any difference in the disease characteristics, response to therapy, and prognosis of myeloma worldwide.

The incidence of myeloma and other plasma cell disorders increases with advancing age. The median age at diagnosis is 69 years. The mortality pattern also closely follows the incidence curves for age distribution, with a median age at death of 75 years. The proportion of patients surviving at 5 years in 2010 was 45%. As seen in Figure 112.1, fewer than 2% of patients are younger than 40 years, whereas almost 50% patients are older than 70 years. A similar age distribution is also observed in other related plasma cell disorders including MGUS and Waldenström's macroglobulinemia.

ETIOLOGY

Environmental Exposure

Exposure to ionizing radiation is the strongest single factor linked to an increased risk of multiple myeloma.[16] This has been documented in atomic bomb survivors who have a five times greater incidence than a control group with a latent period of approximately 20 years from exposure.[17] People exposed to low levels of radiation also demonstrate an increased incidence of myeloma, including radiologists, employees in the nuclear industry, or those handling radioactive materials. An association between exposure to various chemicals and the risk of multiple myeloma remains ill defined. Exposure to metals, especially nickel; agricultural chemicals; benzene and petroleum products; other aromatic hydrocarbons; agent orange; and silicon have been considered as potential risk factors.[16,18–20] In contrast, alcohol and tobacco consumption has not been clearly linked to myeloma. Among medications, only mineral oil used as a laxative has been reported to be associated with an increased risk of multiple myeloma in some patients.[21,22]

Hereditary and genetic factors may predispose patients to myeloma development.[23,24] Among 37 families with at least two family members who had myeloma, occurrence among siblings was reported in 25 of the families. However, direct genetic linkage has not been established. Myeloma risk also appears to be enhanced by the presence of HLA-Cw2 in both African American and Caucasian populations. In a study in 917 Ghanaian men, the prevalence of MGUS was twice that in Caucasian men, implicating race-related genetic susceptibility in the higher rates of MGUS in African populations.[14] More recently, high throughput genomic studies have identified various novel genomic changes in myeloma with significant clinical implications. A meta-analysis of two genome-wide association studies in myeloma (N = 1,661) showed that the t(11;14)(q13;q32) translocation, in which CCND1 is placed under the control of the immunoglobulin heavy chain enhancer, was strongly associated with the CCND1 c.870G>A polymorphism (p = 7.96 × 10[−11]), suggesting a model where a specific chromosomal translocation is associated with a constitutive genetic factor.[25] Recently, Genome Wide Association Studies (GWAS) have identified common single nucleotide polymorphisms (SNP) at 2p23.3(rs6746082), 3p22.1(rs1052501), 3q26.2(rs10936599), 6p21.33(rs2285803), 7p15.3(rs4487645), 17p11.2(rs4273077), and 22q13.1(rs877529) to influence MM risk; the same SNPs were also evaluated for MGUS risk and four of these SNPs (rs1052501,

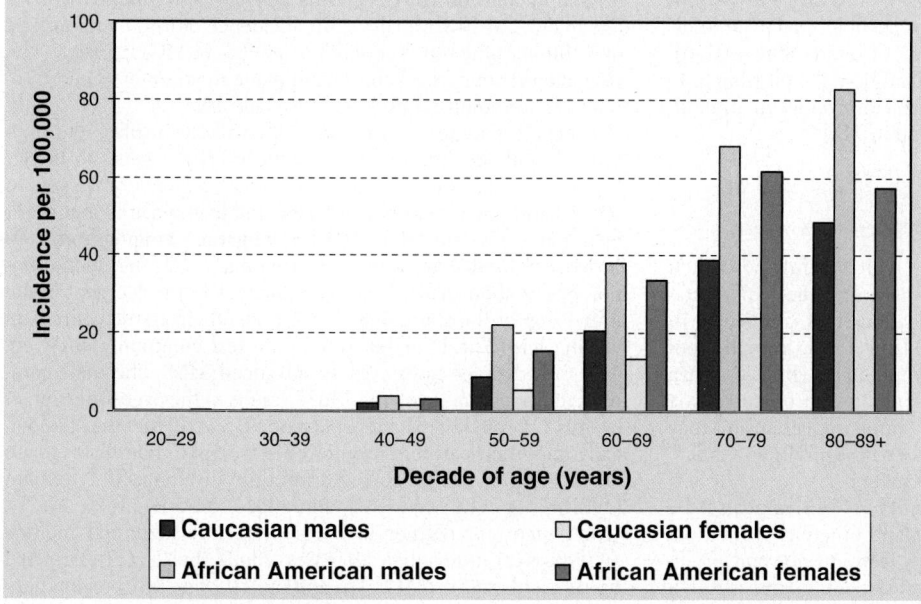

Figure 112.1 Multiple myeloma averages for age-, sex-, and race-specific incidence per 100,000 in United States, 1996 to 2000. An increase in incidence is noted with advancing age, and a higher incidence is observed in males than females and in the African American than in the Caucasian population.

rs2285803, rs4487645, and rs4273077) independently also influenced the development of MGUS. Collectively, these data support the view that genetic variation predisposes one to MGUS, thereby influencing the risk of developing MM.[26]

MGUS has been considered to be a premalignant condition; however, the rate of conversion to myeloma remains extremely low and is often associated with additional genetic changes.[27,28] Repeated infections or antigenic stimulation of the plasma cell compartment has also been proposed as a possible predisposing condition for developing myeloma. In one interesting patient report in the literature, a prior therapy with horse antiserum against tetanus led to a subsequent development of MGUS that lasted for 3 decades before conversion to MM. At the time of myeloma diagnosis, the serum IgG component was found to react specifically against horse α-2 macroglobulin.[29] This report suggests an initial antigen-driven stimulation of monoclonal protein-producing plasma cells, which eventually became malignant after acquiring additional genetic alterations. MGUS has been observed in mice dependent on strain of mice, age, preexisting immune status, and antigenic stimulation. MGUS has been associated with immune disorders and infectious diseases. In one report of 57 patients with MGUS who had undergone an evaluation for *Helicobacter pylori* infection for various gastrointestinal (GI) symptoms, 39 (68%) had evidence of *H. pylori* infection and 11 of these 39 patients (28%) had normalization of the serum paraproteins following eradication of this infection.[30] Seroprevalence of *H. pylori*, however, has not been consistently correlated with MGUS.[31] Development of MGUS has also been reported with T-cell deficiency disorders as in AIDS.[32] Importantly, a recent study indicates that the diagnosis of symptomatic MM is always preceded by MGUS by 2 or more years.[33]

Although epidemiologic studies have not been able to conclusively establish an association between MM and infectious or autoimmune diseases, a recent retrospective cohort study in US veterans demonstrated significantly elevated risks of MM in patients with a history of autoimmune, infectious, and inflammatory disorders. Risks for MGUS were generally of similar magnitude. These results indicate that various types of immune-mediated conditions might act as triggers for MM/MGUS development.[34] Although an initial report suggested the presence of the human herpes virus 8 (HHV8; Kaposi's sarcoma herpes virus) in the bone marrow dendritic cells of the majority of patients with MM,[35] analogous to its association with other lymphoproliferative diseases such as Castleman's disease,[36] body-cavity lymphoma,[37] and Kaposi's sarcoma,[38] other investigators have failed to identify HHV8 in myeloma cells or dendritic cells from various sources including mobilized peripheral blood stem cells.[39–42] Because HHV8 produces unique gene products, including possible growth promoting factors for myeloma such as analogs of interleukin 6 (IL-6), insulin-like growth factor 1 (IGF-1), and an IL-8, the possible linkage of HHV8 to myeloma was intriguing. However, even antibodies against HHV8 have not been observed in MM.[43]

PATHOGENESIS

MM is a germinal center–derived tumor with a mainly postswitch B-cell phenotype characterized by extensive Ig gene hypermutation in a pattern suggesting antigen selection. This is reflected in the exceedingly rare occurrence of IgM myeloma. Somatic mutations of other loci, such as B-cell lymphoma 6 (BCL-6), have also been reported in myeloma B cells, along with characteristic immunoglobulin gene rearrangement.[44] Similar mechanisms may be affecting other cell-cycle control genes whose products regulate cell proliferation and malignant transformation.

As in most malignancies, the pathogenesis of MM appears to be associated with dysregulated expression and function of multiple key cellular genes controlling apoptosis, cell growth, and proliferation. Understanding the evolution of myeloma from MGUS

has provided a background for a multistep process involving alterations in various oncogenes and tumor suppressor genes.[45] In one study, the presence of 14q32 abnormalities were reported in patients with MGUS, and the addition of chromosome 13 change was associated with a transformation to overt MM.[46] This led to a theory that a subset of myeloma may derive from prior MGUS with a high incidence of monosomy 13, versus a second group of de novo myeloma in which other genetic abnormalities may be involved.[46] However, two recent reports suggest that all myelomas are preceded by MGUS[33,47] and that a small subset of MGUS carry del(13) along with t(4;14), which is not associated with an increased rate of progression to myeloma.[48,49] In one study in patients with smoldering myeloma, high-risk chromosomal aberrations (del(17p13), t(4;14), and +1q21) were observed in 35.9% of patients and predicted adverse prognostic factors for the progression to active myeloma, independent of tumor mass. Moreover, hyperdiploidy, which in myeloma is considered to be a low-risk feature, was present in 43.3% of smoldering and indolent multiple myeloma (SMM) patients and was an adverse prognostic factor.[50]

Myeloma occurs not only in humans, but also in mice, canines, and hamsters. In fact, genetic susceptibility to plasma cell tumors has been demonstrated in an inbred strain of mice. A common factor in various species has been the prevalence of endogenous retroviruses.[51,52] Animal models are now providing a basis for understanding the role of activation of oncogenes and tumor suppressor genes, cytokines, and the role of the bone marrow microenvironment in promoting and sustaining myeloma cell growth.

Cytogenetic and Molecular Genetic Alterations

Myeloma karyotypes are complex, with an average of 11 numeric and structural abnormalities per cell.[53] The relative incidence of gain or loss of various chromosomes with involved p and q arms are shown in Figure 112.2. The low proliferative activity of the tumor cells and possible clonal evolution have been obstacles to the identification of specific chromosomal and molecular changes in myeloma. The frequency and complexity of the chromosomal aberrations increases with advanced disease, and is uniformly abnormal in plasma cell leukemia. The detection of a complex karyotype predicts for poor prognosis. The newer techniques of multicolor fluorescent in situ hybridization (FISH) and spectral karyotyping, along with refined G-banding techniques, have identified many nonrandom changes in a large number of patients.[54–56] Using these techniques, over 90% of patients have involvement of at least one chromosome. A substantial fraction of MGUS plasma cells are also reported to have aneuploidy. By FISH analysis, the incidence of trisomy for at least one chromosome was reported in over 40% of MGUS cells.[57] The characteristic numerical abnormalities are monosomy 13 and trisomies of chromosome 3, 5, 7, 9, 11, 15, and 19.

The most frequent structural abnormality involves chromosome 1 and the immunoglobulin heavy chain gene at 14q32. By conventional cytogenetics, the 14q32 region is involved in translocation in 20% to 40% of cases, and by molecular and FISH techniques it is detectable at higher frequency, ranging from 50% in MGUS to 90% in advanced myeloma.[53,58,59] The demonstration of this abnormality in MGUS suggests its involvement in the initial step of transformation.[46,60,61] Light-chain translocations involving Igλ (22q11) or Igκ (2p12) are less commonly observed, with only 20% of cases even in advanced MM. The most common translocation involving 14q32 results in the overexpression of cyclins D1 (on 11q13) and D3 (on 6p21).[58,62] The other biologically important partner chromosomes are 4p16 (fibroblast growth factor receptor 3 [FGFR3] and multiple myeloma SET domain [MMSET]), 16q23 (c-MAF), and 20q11 (MAFB) (Table 112.1). Other recurrent partner loci less frequently identified include 8q24 (c-myc) in less than 5% cases, 18q21 (bcl-2), (11q23 mixed lineage leukemia 1 [MLL-1]), and 6p21.1. The 4p16 region con-

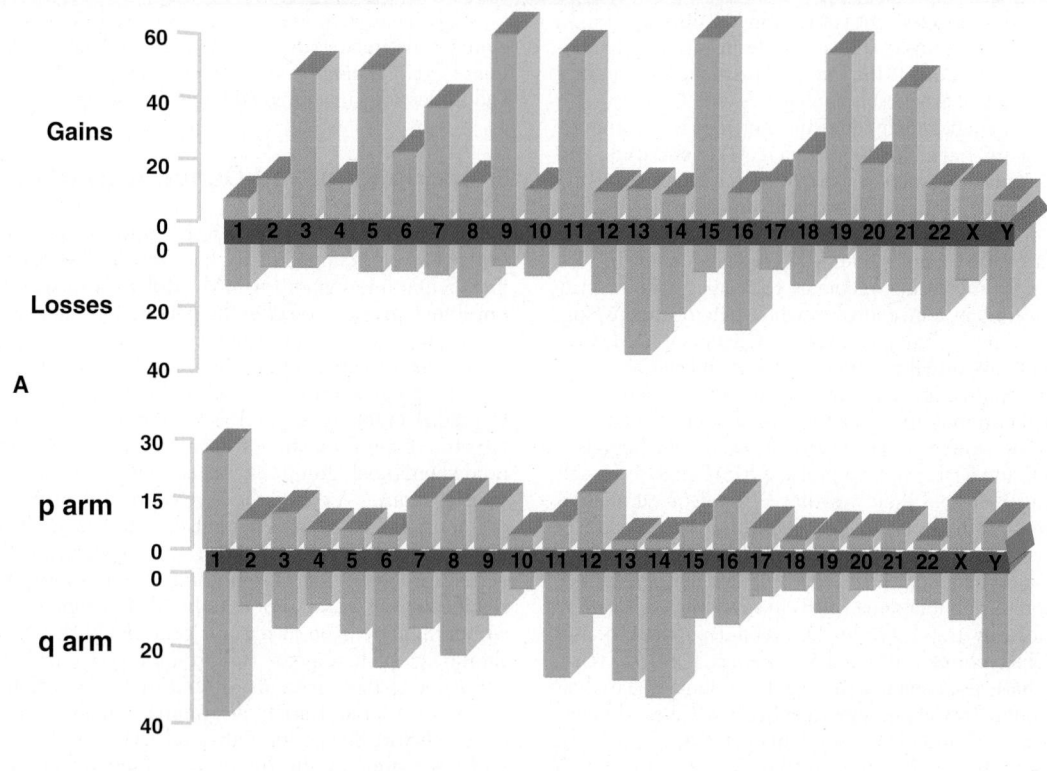

Avg. 11 Events/Karyotype

Figure 112.2 Summary karyotypic abnormalities in 158 patients with evaluable abnormal cytogenetics from a study of 492 patients demonstrating *chromosomal chaos*. **A:** Numeric changes with trisomies (gain) and monosomies (loss). **B:** Structural changes involving the short (p) and long (q) arm. (Courtesy of J. R. Sawyer.)

tains FGFR3 and MMSET genes. FGFR3 and its activating mutations trigger mitogen-activated protein (MAP) kinase signaling and growth of myeloma cells.[63] Mutated FGFR3 also confers resistance to caspase 3–related apoptosis.[64–66] This translocation also activates the *MMSET* gene, a homolog of *MLL1*, which is also independently involved in 11q23 translocation. With the enhanced sensitivity of spectral karyotyping, a nonrandom involvement of

t(14:16) (q32:q22-23) has been described. A molecular analysis of the locus at chromosome 16q22 shows fusion of the immunoglobulin heavy chain with the sequence near the c-MAF oncogene, a b-ZIP transcription factor.[67] Additionally, translocation partners t(9;14) involving the paired box gene 5 (PAX-5) and t(6;14) involving interferon regulatory factor 4 (IRF4) gene have been described.[68,69] In the majority of cases, however, the translocating

TABLE 112.1

Recurrent Chromosomal Aberrations

Nonimmunoglobulin Sites for Illegitimate Switch Recombination in Multiple Myeloma

Chromosome	Frequency % Patients	Gene(s)	Function
11q13	30	Cyclin D1	Induces growth
4p16	25	FGFR3, MMSET	Growth factor
8q24	5	c-myc	Growth/apoptosis
16q23	1	c-maf	Transcription factor
6p25	<1	IRF4 transcription factor	Differentiation and growth
9p13	1	PAX-5	Transcription factor
20q12	1	MAFB	Transcription factor
18q21	1	Bcl-2	Antiapoptosis
Structural Chromosomal Aberrations			
del 17p13	15	p53 ?	
del 13	40–55	?	
Hypodiploidy	20–30	–	
Hyperdiploidy	45–50	–	

partner chromosome locus is not yet identified. Although 14q32 is one of the common translocations, its role in myeloma pathogenesis remains unclear due to the variety of partner chromosomes involved and its lack of prognostic significance.

Standard cytogenetics techniques did not identify rearrangements involving 8q24, which contains the c-MYC oncogene and is commonly involved in murine plasmacytoma. However, FISH analyses in one study identified karyotypic abnormalities that involve c-MYC in 45% cases of advanced myeloma.[70] Another study using interphase FISH confirmed c-MYC rearrangement in 15% of MM cases, with increasing frequency correlating with severity of disease. Interestingly, c-myc involvement is heterogeneous, suggesting its role in the evolution of disease.[71] Changes in c-MYC in the form of either abnormal size transcript or high level of expression have been reported in a majority of patients in one study.[72,73]

A deletion of chromosome 13 or 13q arm identified by conventional karyotyping confers a poor prognosis, even after high-dose therapy.[74] Using the RB1 gene as a probe, a FISH analysis reveals RB1 deletion in >40% of these patients.[75] In a detailed analysis of the 13q chromosome using an 11 probe FISH panel, >80% of 50 patients showed molecular deletions, with 13q14 representing a critical region most frequently involved.[76] Additionally, constitutive phosphorylation of retiniblastoma (pRB) in myeloma cells can be further enhanced by IL-6.[77] Cyclin D, cyclin-dependent kinases (CDK), and CDK inhibitors p15 and p16 (ink), p21 and p27 (cip), and p57 (kip), have also been investigated in myeloma due to their effect on pRB phosphorylation. Abnormalities in p16 and p15 have been reported in 75% and 67% of myeloma patients, respectively, suggesting an important defect in the pRB regulatory pathway.[78–80]

Mutations involving Ras are observed in about 39% of newly diagnosed MM patients, and are more frequently observed following progressive disease. Activating mutations of the ras oncogenes may also result in growth factor independence and the suppression of apoptosis in MM. One of the commonly altered genes in many malignancies is p53. In myeloma, abnormalities in p53 are detected in less than 10% of patients with early stage disease.[81,82]; however, p53 abnormalities represent an important late event associated with progression to an aggressive form of the disease. A study of p53 gene mutations in 52 patients with myeloma showed 7 of 52 patients to have p53 abnormalities, all with a clinically advanced and aggressive acute/leukemic stage of MM.[81] Murine double minute 2 (MDM2), an important inhibitor of p53 function, is overexpressed in the majority of myeloma cell lines; however, increased MDM2 expression is infrequently observed in primary myeloma cells.[83]

An important antiapoptotic gene, BCL-2, is uniformly overexpressed in low-grade non-Hodgkin's lymphoma. In this family of genes, BCL-2 and BCL-XL are antiapoptotic genes, whereas BAX, BAD, and BCL_{XS} are proapoptotic genes. A balance between these genes determines cell survival. The t(14:18) translocation involving the BCL-2 gene is quite rare (2% to 3%) in myeloma. However, numerous myeloma cells lines as well as primary cells, express high levels of BCL-2.[84,85] Its relationship to development of drug resistance, as well as radiation resistance in myeloma cells is also well described.[86,87] One study in 63 patients showed a significant correlation between BCL-2 expression and resistance to therapy with interferon, but not melphalan and prednisone.[88] The association of BCL-2 expression with prognosis remains controversial, as one small study failed to show a correlation with short survival. BCL-XL is upregulated in myeloma cells as a consequence of IL-6–induced activation of signal transducers and activators of transcription 3 (STAT-3).[89] It confers a drug-resistant phenotype and, in conjunction with bcl- 2, leads to increased genetic instability. Mcl-1, another antiapoptotic gene, is overexpressed in MM and is upregulated by IL-6. Its overexpression mediates potent resistance to apoptosis, and conversely, its downregulation by antisense oligonucleotide triggers apoptosis. Finally, Bcl-6 expression in MM cells is induced by its interaction with BMSC and is modulated, at least in part, via Janus kinase (JAK)/STAT-3 and canonical nuclear factor kappa B (NF-κB) pathways, and targeting Bcl-6, either directly or via these cascades, inhibits MM cell growth in the bone marrow (BM) milieu.[90]

High telomerase activity has also been demonstrated in myeloma cells, relative to normal cells and other malignant cell lines.[91] Telomerase activity confers growth and survival in MM, and is therefore an additional target for therapeutic intervention.

Transcriptional and Genomic Studies

Gene expression profiling, as well as studies focused on relative gains or loss of genomic DNA, have provided both prognostic and therapeutic information in MM. Molecular diagnostic tools and novel therapeutics now offer the potential for more accurate prognosis and personalized treatment.

The expression profiling studies in MM have provided insight into the progression of MGUS to MM, and provided the basis to predict outcome, as well as to identify potential therapeutic targets.[45] Expression studies have identified subtypes within the nonhyperdiploid group associated with specific chromosomal translocations.[92] A comprehensive expression profiling the survey of uniformly treated MM patients has identified 70 genes predictive of early disease-related death. Interestingly, one-third of these genes are located on chromosome 1, confirming the potential significance of chromosome 1 in MM pathobiology.[93] Patients with a high risk score using this gene signature had significantly shorter complete response (CR) duration (20% patients at 3 years) compared to those patients without such high risk features (60% at 5 years). A multivariate discriminant analysis identified a 17-gene signature that performed as well as the 70-gene model. A second large study by the Intergroupe Francophone du Myelome (IFM) group studied gene expression profiles in 182 newly diagnosed patients and developed a 15-gene model to calculate a risk score associated with overall survival. In this study, the high-risk group had an overexpression of cell cycle progression and its surveillance-related genes, whereas a hyperdiploid signature and heterogeneous gene expression characterized low-risk patients. Overall survival at 3 years in the low-risk group was 91% versus only 47% in the high-risk group, and these results were independent of traditional prognostic factors.[94] In a recent study in 320 newly diagnosed myeloma patients from the Dutch–Belgian/German HOVON-65/GMMG-HD4 trial, gene expression profiling identified a 92-gene signature and 10 subgroups in MM, which may represent unique diagnostic entities with potential novel therapeutic targets.[95] Additional expression profile studies have begun to define subtypes of myeloma with different prognostic significance following various therapies. An apparent lack of uniformity in the genes identified by these investigations suggests that therapy-related factors may determine the influence of different classes of genes in MM. Based on cytogenetics as well as expression data, cyclin D dysregulation occurs in the early pathogenesis of MM.

A high-resolution analysis of recurrent copy number alterations, coupled with expression analyses in MM cell lines and primary MM cells using array comparative genomic hybridization (aCGH), has identified distinct genomic subtypes. Additionally, this study has defined 87 discrete minimal common regions that have identified gene candidates for targeted drug discovery, improved the understanding of MM initiation and progression, and improved the prediction of clinical outcomes (Fig. 112.3). A high-density, SNP array analysis of myeloma cells from 192 newly diagnosed patients identified genomic copy number alteration in 98% of patients.[96] Amplifications in 1q and deletions in 1p, 12p, 14q, 16q, and 22q were the most frequent lesions associated with adverse prognosis, whereas amplifications of chromosomes 5, 9, 11, 15, and 19 were linked to a favorable prognosis. Amp(1q23.3), amp(5q31.3), and del(12p13.31) have been identified in a multivariate analysis to be independent prognostic factors. This prognostic model was validated in an independent validation cohort of 273 patients with myeloma, and identified patients with amp(5q31.3) alone and low serum beta-2-M to have an excellent prognosis (5-year overall survival, 87%) versus patients with del(12p13.31)

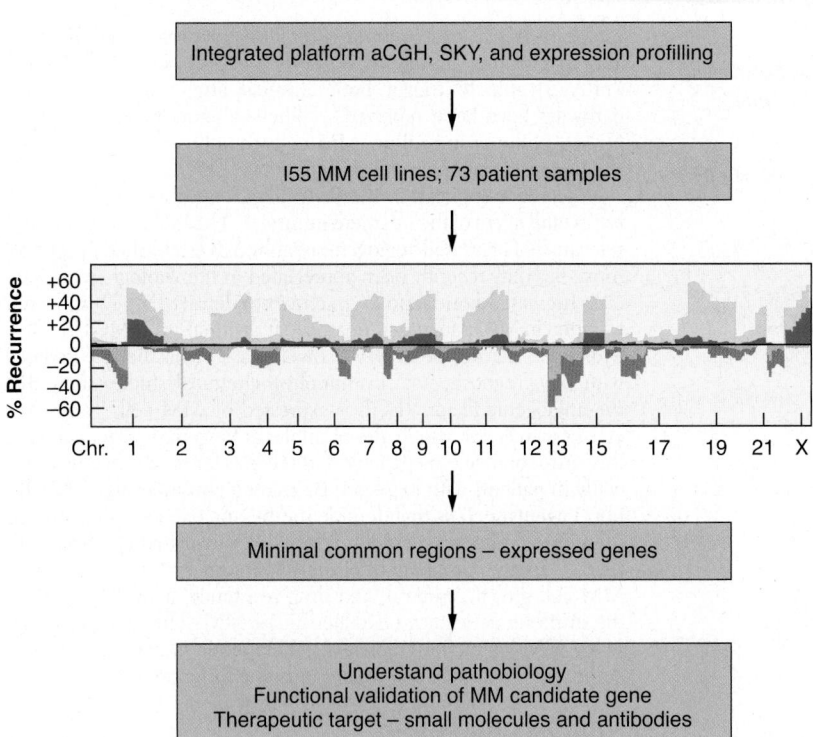

Figure 112.3 An array-based comparative genomic hybridization analysis evaluating 55 cell lines and 73 patient samples identified recurrent areas of gains and losses in multiple myeloma (MM) with the potential for understanding biology and validating target genes, which will then be potential therapeutic targets.

PRACTICE OF ONCOLOGY

alone or amp(5q31.3) and del(12p13.31) and high serum beta-2-M with a poor outcome (5-year overall survival, 20%).

Epigenetic changes modulating myeloma cell growth and survival genes are also reported. For example, methylation of *p16*, a negative cell cycle regulator, is common and reported to be an early event even in MGUS. However, p16 methylation was not predictive of overall survival in a single large cohort study. The acetyl-lysine recognition domains (bromodomains) of putative coactivator proteins have been shown to play a significant role in transcriptional initiation and elongation as well as chromatin-dependent signal transduction. The bromodomain and extra-terminal (BET) bromodomain proteins have been identified as regulatory factors for c-Myc expression in myeloma, and their inhibition induces antiproliferative effects associated with cell-cycle arrest and cellular senescence in both in vitro and in vivo models.[97] A recent global methylation analysis (N = 159) of purified myeloma cells has identified prognostically important, epigenetically inactivated tumor suppressor genes. In this analysis, the combination of DNA methylation and gene expression profile identified hypermethylated GPX3, RBP1, SPARC, and TGFBI genes to be associated with significantly shorter overall survival, independent of other high-risk features such as International Staging System (ISS) stage or adverse cytogenetics.[98]

A role of microRNAs (miR) and potential therapeutic targeting of multiple mRNAs has recently been described in myeloma. miRNA expression profiling of MM and MGUS cells compared to normal donor plasma cells identified the overexpression of miR-21, miR-106b, and miR-181a and b in MM and MGUS samples, as well as selective upregulation of miR-32 and miR-17-92 in MM, but not in MGUS.[99] Another study analyzed the expression level of miRs and the gene expression profile in 60 newly diagnosed myeloma patients, and identified significantly dysregulated miRs expression in cytogenetically distinct subtypes.[100] The putative targets and their function are now being defined (e.g., miR-192, 194, and 215), which are downregulated in a subset of newly diagnosed myeloma, are transcriptionally activated by p53 and then modulate MDM2 expression. In addition, miR-192 and 215 target the IGF pathway, prevent the enhanced migration of plasma cells into bone marrow, and are positive regulators of p53, suggesting that their downregulation plays a key role in myeloma pathogenesis.[101] Recently, a role for miR-21,[102] miR-29,[103] and miR-34a[104] in

supporting myeloma cell growth and survival have been defined, suggesting their potential as novel therapeutic targets.

Mutational changes in myeloma have now been evaluated using whole genome sequencing. An initial report using massively parallel sequencing of 38 tumor genomes and their comparison to matched normal DNAs identified several new oncogenic mechanisms based on the pattern of somatic mutations across the data set. These include mutations of genes involved in protein translation (seen in nearly half of the patients), histone methylation, and blood coagulation as well as NF-κB signaling, evidenced by mutations in 11 members of the NF-κB pathway.[105]

Using high-resolution SNP arrays (N = 24), clonal content and evolution was evaluated in myeloma. This analysis suggested selection and growth of genetically distinct subclones, which were not initially competitive against the dominant population but survived following therapy, with new acquired anomalies and subsequent outgrowth. These data point to the need to target and eradicate even a minor clone.[106] Recently, whole exome sequencing, copy number profiling, and a cytogenetics analysis performed in 84 myeloma samples have identified new candidate genes, including truncations of SP140, Lymphotoxin-beta (LTB), roundabout, axon guidance receptor, homolog 1 (ROBO1), and clustered missense mutations in early growth response protein 1 (EGR1). A further analysis revealed a complex subclonal structure including subclonal driver mutations. Serial sampling was performed in 15 patients, which revealed diverse patterns of clonal evolution: linear evolution, differential clonal response, and branching evolution. Diverse processes contributing to the mutational repertoire including kataegis and somatic hypermutation have been identified, and their relative contribution changed over time. This study demonstrates that the myeloma genome is heterogeneous, with clonal diversity at diagnosis and further evolution over time.[107]

Microenvironment and Cell Signaling

Myeloma cells express adhesion molecules that mediate interaction with the microenvironment, including both bone marrow stromal cell elements and extracellular matrix proteins (Table 112.2). These adhesion molecules mediate both homotypic and heterotypic adhesion. Adhesion not only plays a role in migration and

TABLE 112.2

Adhesion Molecule Expression on Normal Plasma Cells, Multiple Myeloma, and Plasma Cell Leukemia Cells

Adhesion Molecule	Normal Plasma Cell	MM Cell	PCL Cell
CD11a	+	−	−
CD11b	−	−	+
CD44	+	+	+
CD54	+	+	+
CD56	−	+	−
CD58	−	+	ND
LFA-1	−	−/+	+
VLA-4	+	−/+	ND
VLA-5	+	+	−
MPC-1	+	+	−
RHAMM	−	+	−/+
Syndecan-1	+	+	−
Surface Molecules			
CD19	+	−	−
CD28	−	+	+
CD38	+	+	+
CD40	+	+	+[a]
CD45	+	−[b]	−

PCL, plasma cell leukemia.
[a] CD40 expression is enhanced on PCL cells relative to normal plasma cells and MM cells.
[b] CD45 on immature myeloma cells.

localization of myeloma cells in the bone marrow, but also induces tumor cell growth and survival. For example, syndecan-1, a cell surface transmembrane heparan sulfate proteoglycan present on MM cells, interacts with type I collagen, and regulates growth of MM cells; it also mediates increased osteoclast activity.[108,109] Elevated levels of syndecan-1 shed into serum correlate with increased tumor mass, decreased matrix metalloproteinase-9 activity in the serum, and a poor prognosis.[108]

The BM microenvironment consists of a variety of cell types including stromal cells (BMSC), endothelial cells, osteoclasts, osteoblasts, as well as immune cells. The physical interaction between myeloma cells and these cells in the BM milieu plays a crucial role in MM pathogenesis both by direct adhesion-mediated signaling, as well as by secretion of factors such as IL-6, IGF-1, vascular endothelial growth factor (VEGF), B-cell activating factor (BAFF), fibroblast growth factor (FGF), stromal cell–derived factor (SDF) 1α, and tumor necrosis factor alpha (TNF-α), which mediate tumor cell growth, survival, drug resistance, and migration.[110–114] These interactions lead to the activation of several proliferative/antiapoptotic signaling cascades in MM cells: PI3K/Akt, Ras/Raf/mitogen-activated protein kinase (MAPK) kinase (MEK)/extracellular signal-related kinase (ERK), JAK 2/ STAT-3, and NF-κB pathways. These pathways lead to MM cell growth, survival, antiapoptosis, migration, and development of drug resistance. Additionally, adhesion as well as cytokines secreted from MM cells and accessory cells in turn further augment cytokine secretion from these cells.

Activation of NF-κB has been noted in myeloma cells, especially following their interaction with BMSC. A number of abnormalities contributing to the dysregulation of NF-κB and constitutive activation of the noncanonical NF-κB pathway have recently been described.[115] Elevated expression of NF-κB-inducing

kinase (NIK) due to genomic alterations or protein stabilization, and inactivating mutations of TNF receptor-associated factor 3 (TRAF3) able to trigger both classical and alternative NF-κB pathways have been reported.[116] These alterations activating the NF-κB pathway may allow MM cells to achieve autonomy from the bone marrow microenvironment.[117]

Each accessory cell in the BM milieu contributes differently to the overall effect of the microenvironment. The biologic and clinical relevance of increased angiogenesis, although established in solid tumors, has only recently been appreciated in hematologic malignancies. Increased bone marrow microvessel density (MVD) has been reported in MM patients compared to individuals with MGUS.[118–120] Moreover, the degree of MVD myeloma BM has been correlated with the prognosis.[121,122] Immunohistochemical studies show that the angiogenic factor VEGF is expressed by MM cells.[123] Hepatocyte growth factor, which also promotes angiogenesis, is increased in the serum of myeloma patients and predicts for poor outcome, especially in patients with increased β2 microglobulin levels.[124] Finally, novel agents such as thalidomide inhibit angiogenesis and can also overcome drug resistance in myeloma. Plasmacytoid dendritic cells (pDC), another component of the BM microenvironment, support MM cell growth, survival, and drug resistance, as well as mediate the immune deficiency characteristic of MM. Therefore, targeting pDC–MM interactions represent a therapeutic strategy to both overcome drug resistance and restore immune function in MM.[125]

Role of Cytokines

Myeloma cells and BMSCs produce cytokines including IL-6,[110] IGF-1,[114] VEGF,[112] SDF-1,[113] TNF-α,[111] TGF-β,[126] IL-21,[127] and others that mediate tumor cell growth, survival, antiapoptosis, migration, and the development of drug resistance.

Interleukin 6

IL-6 is an essential growth and survival factor for myeloma. The IL-6 receptor expressed by myeloma cells is composed of two polypeptide components: the α chain (gp80, IL-6Rα) and the signal transducing β chain (gp130). The gp130 component is shared by a family of cytokines including oncostatin M and leukemia inhibitory factor. The interaction of IL-6 with its receptor activates Ras/RAF/MEK/ERK, JAK/STAT, and PI3K/Akt signaling pathways, mediating growth, survival, and drug resistance (Fig. 112.4). IL-6 is mainly produced by stromal cells following the binding of myeloma cells and is also triggered by other cytokines including TNF-α,[111] IL-1β VEGF, and IL-17 in the BM milieu.[112] IL-6 mediates both autocrine and paracrine growth of myeloma cells. It increases the proportion of cells in S phase, prevents apoptosis of malignant plasma cells, and confers resistance to antitumor agents such as dexamethasone (Dex). Soluble IL-6Rα, shed by myeloma cells into the serum, can amplify the response of myeloma cells to IL-6; both high serum IL-6Rα levels and high serum IL-6 levels portend a poor prognosis. IL-6 and soluble IL-6Rα also mediate enhanced bone resorption by osteoclasts. To date, IL-6 has been targeted therapeutically using antibodies specific for IL-6 or its receptor. However, these treatment approaches have produced only transient responses in a small number of patients.

Insulin-like Growth Factor 1

IGF-1 is a growth and survival factor for human MM, which activates PI3K and MAPK signaling pathways mediating proliferation and antiapoptosis.[128,129] It induces more potent protection against Dex than does IL-6. IGF-1 upregulates FLICE-like inhibitory protein (FLIP), X-linked inhibitor of apoptosis (XIAP), and Bcl-2-related protein A1 (A1/Bfl1),[128] and increases telomerase activity, thereby further enhancing tumor cell growth and survival.[130] IGF-1 also mediates the adhesion and migration of myeloma cells via β1-integrin.[114] These studies have identified IGF-1 as a novel therapeutic target; both antibodies and small molecule inhibitors against IGF-1 have been investigated in preclinical studies.

Growth of the MM cell in the BM microenvironment

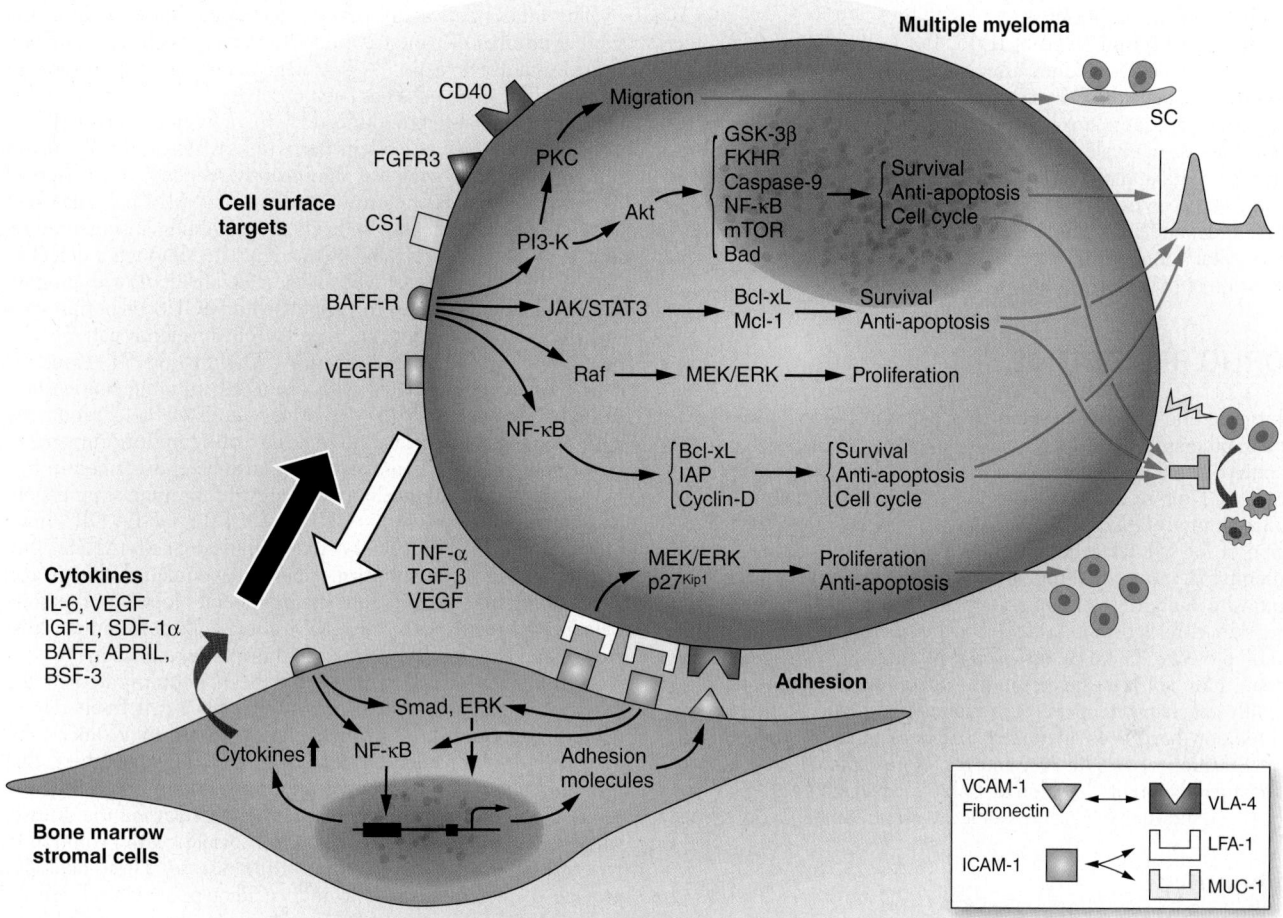

Figure 112.4 The interaction and adhesion of multiple myeloma (MM) cells to the bone marrow (BM) stromal cells (BMSCs) leads to adhesion- and cytokine-mediated signaling. MM cell binding to BMSCs induces the activation of p42/44 mitogen-activated protein kinase (MAPK) and nuclear factor kappa B (NF-κB) in BMSCs. The activation of NF-κB upregulates adhesion molecules on BMSCs. Cytokines secreted through this interaction includes interleukin-6 (IL-6) secretion, tumor necrosis factor α (TNF-α), and vascular endothelial growth factor (VEGF) to activate the main signaling pathways (p42/44 MAPK, Janus kinase (JAK)/signal transducer and activator of transcription 3 (STAT3) and/or phosphatidylinositol 3-kinase (PI3K)/Akt and their downstream targets, which triggers MM cell growth, survival, and migration.

The RAS/RAF/MAPK kinase (MEK)/MAPK pathway mediates the proliferation of MM. JAK/ STAT3 along with upregulation of BCL-X$_L$ and MCL1 mediates survival. PI3K/Akt through downstream activation of BAD and NF-κB, and/or inactivation of caspase-9 mediates antiapoptosis. NF-κB and forkhead in rhabdomyosarcoma (FKHR) modulate cyclin D and KIP1, thereby regulating cell-cycle progression. Signaling through PI3K induces downstream protein kinase C (PKC) activity and MM cell migration. ICAM1; intercellular adhesion molecule 1; LFA1, lymphocyte function-associated antigen 1; muc1, mucin 1; VCAM1, vascular cell adhesion molecule 1; VLA4, very-late antigen 4; IGF1, insulin-like growth factor-1; IL, interleukin; SDF-1α, stromal-cell-derived factor-1α. (Adapted from Hideshima T, Mitsiades C, Tonon G, et al. Understanding multiple myeloma pathogenesis in the bone marrow to identify new therapeutic targets. *Nat Rev Cancer* 2007;7:585.)

Vascular Endothelial Growth Factor

VEGF has only modest proliferative effects on myeloma cells; however, it plays a more important role in triggering tumor cell migration and angiogenesis.[131,132] Its production in the BM milieu is upregulated both by myeloma cell adhesion to BMSCs and by IL-6.[133] Because it is a specific endothelial cell mitogen, elevated levels in myeloma may account, at least in part, for increased angiogenesis.[123] Myeloma cells express fms-related tyrosine kinase 1 (FLT1), and VEGF triggers its phosphorylation and activation of downstream MEK and protein kinase C (PKC) signaling. These data have provided the preclinical rationale to evaluate VEGF as a therapeutic target. Although PTK787, a potent inhibitor of VEGF receptor, has shown antimyeloma activity in vitro,[134] it has not shown clinical activity.

Other Cytokines

TNF-α is secreted by myeloma cells and does not have any significant direct effect on myeloma cell growth and survival; however, it induces the secretion of IL-6 by BMSCs. It is also a strong inducer of NF-κB activation, thereby upregulating adhesion molecules, with resultant binding of myeloma cells to BM and cell adhesion–mediated drug resistance (CAMDR). Although specific antibody inhibitors of TNF-α have not shown a clinical response, thalidomide and its immunomodulatpry drug (IMiD) analogs have potent anti-TNF-α activity and can overcome CAMDR.

SDF-1 is expressed by BMSCs, and its receptor CXCR4 is expressed by myeloma cells. It induces only a minimal proliferative effect; however, it plays a more important role mediating migration.

PRACTICE OF ONCOLOGY

TGF-β is produced by MM cells and induces the secretion of IL-6 by BMSCs; it also contributes to immunosuppression, which is characteristic of myeloma.

Increased serum levels of IL-17, IL-21, IL-22, and IL-23, the proinflammatory cytokines associated with Th17 cells, are also observed in myeloma. IL-17 promotes myeloma cell growth and adhesion to bone marrow stromal cells, as well as contributes to bone disease in myeloma. In combination with IL-22, it also inhibits the production of Th1-mediated cytokines including interferon gamma (IFN-γ).[135] IL-21 induces proliferation and inhibits apoptosis independent of IL-6 signaling. It triggers phosphorylation of Jak1, Stat3, and Erk1/2 (p44/42 MAPK). TNF-α upregulates expression of both IL-21 and IL-21 receptor (IL-21R).

DRUG RESISTANCE

Intrinsic and acquired resistance of plasma cells to conventional chemotherapy is common, and as a result, only 50% of patients achieve a partial response, with few complete responses to melphalan. Drug resistance is mediated by several mechanisms.[136] An altered intracellular drug concentration may be due to overexpression of the MDR1 gene, encoding for P-glycoprotein, an integral membrane protein that functions as an ATP-dependent drug efflux pump, a multidrug resistance–associated protein (MRP), and a lung resistance–related protein (LRP), a member of the class of major vault proteins.[137] To date, however, strategies targeting these mechanisms have not been successful in overcoming drug resistance. Recently, mechanisms operative in inducing resistance to proteasome inhibition have been identified that have included upregulation or activation of Hsp90, Akt, and aggresomal protein degradation. Downregulation of Cereblon or lack of degradation of IKZF1 or 3 has been shown to mediate resistance to immunomodulatory agents.

Phenotype

Myeloma cells display heterogeneous cell surface phenotypes, with differences both between different patients and within the same patient at different disease stages. In general, all myeloma cells express high levels of CD38, with immature plasma cells additionally expressing CD45 and the IL-6 receptor.[138–140] More mature myeloma cells do not express CD45 and lack IL-6 receptor expression.[141] A subpopulation of myeloma cells may also express CD10, CD56, or CD49e (very late activation antigen 5 [VLA5]).[141–143] CD28 expression is associated with more aggressive disease[144]; CD20 expression is present on 20% to 30% of myeloma patients, and can be further upregulated with IFN-α.[145] The identity of the myeloma stem cell still remains an enigma. B cells expressing CD19 and CD11b can be induced to mature on stromal cells into monotypic plasma cells, suggesting that this cellular compartment may contain myeloma cell progenitors.[146,147] Using allele-specific oligonucleotide polymerase chain reaction (PCR) and the severe combined immunodeficiency (SCID)-hu model, the myeloma stem cell will be better defined in the future. These cell surface characteristics have also allowed for the development of eight color flow cytometries to measure minimal residual disease.

Immune Status

Myeloma patients present with suppressed immune function due to a variety of factors. Most significant is the suppression of uninvolved immunoglobulins (e.g., in patients with IgG myeloma, there is suppression of serum IgA and IgM levels).[148] The factors causing this suppression include a direct effect of monoclonal immunoglobulin, increased soluble Fc receptor or Fc expressing cells, suppression of helper cell functions, monoclonal Ig, and macrophage-related factors that affect B-cell maturation to plasma cells.[149] The recovery of uninvolved immunoglobulins to normal

levels following effective therapy has been associated with both improved survival and protection from infectious complications.

The total T-cell count may be decreased; however, in a substantial number of patients, it may be normal, with no significant changes in CD8 cells.[150–152] A stage-dependent suppression of natural killer (NK) cells has been observed.[153] Deficiency of CD4 helper cells is also pronounced.[154] In one study, the proliferation and frequency of Epstein Barr virus (EBV)- and influenza A (inf A)- specific T cells was significantly reduced in a cohort of 24 newly diagnosed or conventionally treated MM patients when compared with 19 healthy individuals, suggesting an impaired response of CD8+ T cells in MM patients.[155] Although a defect in NK T-cell function has also been detected in patients with progressive myeloma compared to patients with MGUS or nonprogressive disease,[156] invariant NK T cells from myeloma patients can be activated and expanded in vitro.[157] Dysfunctional T regulatory cells have been associated with disturbed immune homeostasis in both MGUS and MM.[158] Elevated levels of IL-17 producing Th17 cells, possibly related to high IL-6 and transforming growth factor beta (TGF-β) expression, have also been described in myeloma, and promote myeloma cell growth, immune suppression, and osteoclast function.[135] CD11b(+)CD14(–)HLA-DR(–/low) CD33(+)CD15(+) myeloid-derived suppressor cells (MDSC) are a heterogeneous, immature myeloid cell population that is also significantly increased in both the peripheral blood and the bone marrow of patients with active MM; these cells both induce MM growth and suppress T-cell–mediated immune responses.[159]

Anti-idiotype T-cell response has been demonstrated in the majority of patients, with higher Id-specific T-cell frequency in MGUS and early stages of myeloma compared to advanced disease.[160] This observation has lead to a provocative hypothesis that immunologic response plays an important role in controlling the proliferation of the malignant clone in early stages of the disease, whereas loss of immune regulation is associated with evolution to an overt or more aggressive form of the disease. These data also provide the scientific basis to induce idiotype-specific T-cell responses for therapeutic application through either vaccination in vivo or the production of idiotype- or myeloma-specific cytotoxic T lymphocytes (CTL) in vitro.[161]

Murine Models

Three different models of murine myeloma have been described to study myeloma pathogenesis. In an inbred C57BL/Ka strain of mice, 16% spontaneously developed monoclonal gammopathies without tumor formation by 2 years.[51,52,162] In another model, BALB/c mice with a low spontaneous incidence of monoclonal gammopathies, the induction of plasmacytoma or myeloma is observed after the intraperitoneal injection of mineral oil or pristane.[51] Plasmacytomas, which develop within the oil, or other foreign body–mediated granulomas and lymphoplasmacytic infiltration can be blocked by the administration of indomethacin and accelerated by subsequent infection of the mice with Abelson's virus. Interestingly, however, the C57BL/Ka strain, with a high incidence of spontaneous monoclonal gammopathies, is relatively resistant to the induction of plasmacytoma by mineral oil. Plasmacytoma progression is associated with the dysregulated expression of c-myc as a result of translocation analogous to t(8;14) in humans. These plasmacytomas produce IgA immunoglobulins, and a growth factor present in the peritoneal fluid has been confirmed to be IL-6. Additionally, when animals are raised in a germfree environment, the incidence of myeloma after mineral oil stimulation is markedly reduced, whereas that of other lymphoid neoplasms increases.[51] These studies suggest an important role of immune stimulation in myeloma development. A third model uses subcutaneous growth of murine plasmacytoma cell lines such as MOPC11 in immunocompetent mice, which allows for the study of immune modulation.

Human myeloma cell lines can grow and disseminate in a SCID mouse model, providing a unique opportunity to study this disease in an in vivo setting.[163] The introduction of fetal human bone into SCID mice (SCID-hu) has allowed for the engraftment and proliferation of the stromal cell–dependent human myeloma cell line[164] as well as primary human myeloma cells[165,166] in >80% mice and the monitoring of tumor burden by the detection of human myeloma–specific protein (soluble IL-6 receptor) or human Ig and light chains in murine blood samples, respectively. In this murine model of primary human disease, the fetal bone undergoes osteoporotic and osteolytic change as a consequence of clonotypic plasma cell proliferation and production of human cytokines. This model provides a unique opportunity to study the importance of stromal cell–myeloma cell interactions, as well as genetic and molecular mechanisms critical for myeloma growth and dissemination in vivo, and may provide clues to the origin of myeloma stem cells, thereby providing the opportunity to evaluate new treatment approaches targeting the myeloma cell and its microenvironment and bone disease in myeloma. A transgenic Eu-directed X-box Binding Protein-1 (XBP-1) spliced isoform mouse model has been generated in which mice develop features of MGUS and progress to MM.[167] XBP-1 is a transcription factor that is required for plasma cell differentiation, which is expressed at high levels in MM cells versus normal plasma cells.[168] This model provides a unique opportunity to study the biology of human myeloma and assess novel therapies in vivo. Recently, conditional MYC transgene expression has been demonstrated in Vk*MYC mice, which eventually develop an indolent multiple myeloma with features characteristic of human disease. This model serves to highlight the role of myc in myeloma and provides a unique animal model to test therapeutic or preventative strategies in myeloma.[169]

CLINICAL MANIFESTATIONS

Patients with MM may be entirely asymptomatic and diagnosed on routine blood work or may present with a myriad of symptoms such as hematologic manifestations, bone-related problems, infections, various organ dysfunctions, neurologic complaints, or bleeding tendencies (Table 112.3). These signs and symptoms result from direct tumor involvement in BM or extramedullary plasmacytomas, the effect of the protein produced by the tumor cells deposited in various organs, the production of cytokines by the tumor cells or by the BM microenvironment, and effects on the immune system.

TABLE 112.3

Clinical Features of Multiple Myeloma

Symptoms	Common Cause
Bone pain	Pathologic fracture
Easy fatigue	Anemia, high serum IL-6, therapy
Nausea and vomiting	Renal failure, hypercalcemia
Recurrent infections	Low uninvolved Ig, T cell dysfunction, therapy
Paraplegia	Cord compression
Confusion and CNS symptoms	Hyperviscosity or hypercalcemia
Peripheral neuropathy	Nerve compression, amyloidosis, POEMS, immune-mediated effects, therapy induced

CNS, central nervous system; Ig, immunoglobulin; POEMS, polyneuropathy, organomegaly, endocrinopathy, monoclonal gammopathy, and skin changes.

Anemia

A normochromic normocytic anemia is usually observed in myeloma patients due to tumor cell involvement of the marrow as well as inadequate erythropoietin responsiveness. The suppressive effects of various cytokines on erythropoiesis and the effect of renal dysfunction on erythropoietin production are also contributing factors. High immunoglobulin levels exacerbate the anemia due to dilutional effects. Anemia gives rise to fatigue, weakness, and occasionally, shortness of breath. Erythropoietin (Epo) administration is, therefore, an important supportive care therapy for patients with symptomatic anemia. In one study, improvement in hemoglobin by more than 2 g per deciliter was observed in 60% of treated patients, and responses were more frequent in patients with low Epo levels than in patients with normal or high levels (72% versus 20%).

Renal Failure

Nephropathy is one of the serious adverse complications that can be observed at the time of clinical presentation. The etiology of renal failure can be multifactorial. The most common cause is the development of light chain tubular casts leading to interstitial nephritis (myeloma kidney).[170] Another common cause of renal dysfunction is hypercalcemia leading to osmotic diuresis, volume depletion, and prerenal azotemia. Other modes of kidney involvement in myeloma include light chain deposition disease, which is more commonly associated with kappa light chain proteins and impaired glomerular filtration; AL amyloidosis, which is more frequently associated with lambda light chain (especially lambda light chain subtype VI) and may have an initial presentation as nephrotic range proteinuria; and renal calcium deposition, leading to interstitial nephritis.[171–173] The presence of lambda light chains in the urine is also more commonly associated with myeloma kidney. Bence Jones proteins bind to a common peptide segment of Tom-Horsfall glycoprotein to promote heterotypic aggregation and deposition in the kidney.[174] Additional factors exacerbating renal failure in myeloma patients include the use of nonsteroidal anti-inflammatory drugs for pain control, hyperuricemia, nephrotoxic chemotherapeutic agents, intravenous contrast for radiographic studies, bisphosphonate therapy, as well as calcium deposition and stones in the kidney. The proteinuria observed in patients with amyloidosis is more often nonspecific, which can help to differentiate it from typical myeloma-related kidney disease characterized by excessive light chain excretion.[175] Pathologic renal changes similar to human myeloma–related nephropathy develop in IL-6 transgenic mice expressing IL-6 under metallothionein-1 promoter, indicating a relationship between constitutive high IL-6 expression in the liver, dysproteinemia and long acute-phase response, and renal changes.[176]

Hypercalcemia and Bone Disease

The mechanism of bone abnormalities in myeloma, especially destruction, is an unbalanced process of increased osteoclast activity and suppressed osteoblast activity. These changes are due to an increase in osteoclast-activating factors produced predominantly by the BM microenvironment and also by myeloma cells.[177,178] These factors include IL-1β, TNF-β (lymphotoxin), IL-6, and macrophage inflammatory proteins-1 (MIP-1) alpha.[179–182] The receptor activator of nuclear factor kappa B ligand (RANKL) plays an important role in osteoclast differentiation via its receptor located on the osteoclast membrane. A member of the TNF family, it was originally described as a factor secreted by T cells, which induces maturation of dendritic cells. RANKL is also secreted by stromal cells and osteoblasts and induces differentiation and maturation of osteoclast progenitors. Moreover, its production is elicited by factors such as parathyroid hormone (PTH), PTH-related peptide (PTHrP), and OAFs.[178,183] Osteoprotegerin (OPG) acts as a decoy receptor for RANKL,[184,185] and has been implicated in the development of bone changes in myeloma. Additionally, a recently identified soluble factor produced by myeloma cells, DKK-1, inhibits osteoblast activity and is being therapeutically targeted.[186,187] Similarly, activin A, a TGF-β family member that induces osteolysis by inhibiting osteoblast differentiation via SMAD2-dependent distal-less homeobox-5 downregulation, is now being targeted therapeutically.[188]

All of these factors contribute to the development of osteoporosis and lytic bone lesions. Radiographic findings of such destruction are shown in Figure 112.5. These bone changes frequently involve the vertebral column and result in compression fractures, lytic bone lesions, and related pain.

A new onset of back pain or other bone pain is a frequent presenting symptom in myeloma patients. Changes in the cytokine milieu and bone destruction may also lead to the development of hypercalcemia, which is observed in approximately 25% of patients at some stage of the disease. Symptoms of high calcium include mental status changes, lethargy, constipation, and vomiting. High paraprotein levels, low albumin levels, or both are commonly observed in patients with myeloma, and require measurement of ionized calcium. Hypercalcemia may also contribute to renal failure and should, therefore, be considered an oncologic emergency requiring prompt intervention.

Infections

Myeloma patients are at risk for developing recurrent bacterial infections due to deficiencies in both humoral and cellular immunity.[149,189,190] Various factors including high monoclonal immunoglobulin levels, soluble Fc receptor in serum, and TGF-β lead to the suppression of B-cell function, which in turn leads to depressed uninvolved immunoglobulins.[126,191] This impairment in the patients' ability to mount humoral responses predisposes patients to infections with bacteria that are ordinarily opsonized by antibodies against bacterial antigens. Patients also have profound T-cell dysfunction due to various immunosuppressive cytokines such as TGF-β and IL-6 secreted by the microenvironment and fas ligand, which is present on the membrane of myeloma cells. Additional causes of immune suppression include programmed death-ligand 1 (PD-L1) and programmed cell death protein 1 (PD-1) expression on MM cells and MM T cells, respectively, as well as increased T-regulatory cells in MM. The therapy for myeloma, especially high-dose corticosteroids, increases infection-related risks in these patients. Therapy with bortezomib is also associated with a higher frequency of herpes zoster.[192] The highest risk of infection is within the first 2 months of initiation of therapy, as well as in patients with renal failure and in those with relapsed and refractory disease. Recurrent bacterial, fungal, and viral infections in myeloma require prompt diagnosis and treatment with additional prophylactic measures while receiving immunosuppressive therapy. Infections are an important cause of morbidity and the most common cause of death in patients with myeloma.[193]

Neurologic Symptoms

The most common cause of neurologic abnormalities is related to a tumor mass effect, especially compression of the spinal cord or cranial or spinal nerves. This may present as motor or, less frequently, sensory neuropathy. An interesting constellation of symptoms described as POEMS syndrome (polyneuropathy, organomegaly, endocrinopathy, monoclonal gammopathy, and skin changes) is observed in osteosclerotic myeloma with prominent

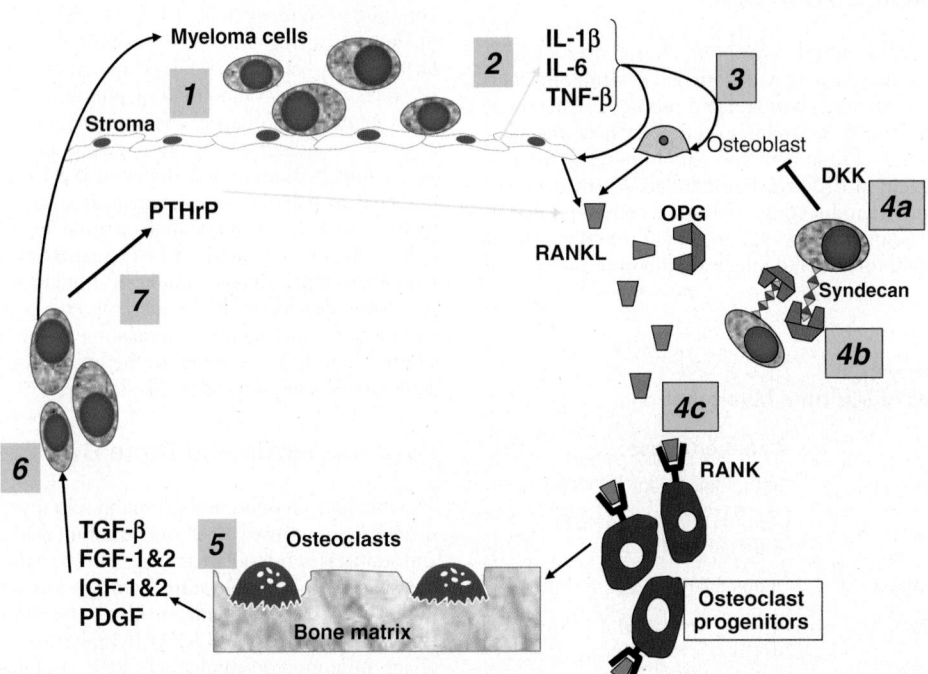

Figure 112.5 The biology of bone destruction in multiple myeloma (MM): **1.** MM cells adhere to stroma. **2.** Stromal cells secrete osteoclast activating factors (OAFs). **3.** OAFs elicit stroma and osteoblasts to secrete receptor activator of NF-κB ligand (RANKL). **4a.** DKK-1 produced y myeloma cells blocks osteoblast activity. **4b.** RANKL is blocked by osteoprotegerin (OPG); OPG levels are reduced in MM due to syndecan trapping OPG. **4c.** Excess RANKL is available to stimulate osteoclast differentiation and maturation. **5.** Increased osteoclastic activity leads to increased cytokine release from the bone matrix. **6.** These cytokines stimulate MM cell growth, which increases process number 1. **7.** These cytokines also cause a release of parathyroid hormone–related protein (PTHrP) from MM cells, which activate stromal cells to secrete additional RANKL. TGF, tumor growth factor; FGF, fibroblast growth factor; IGF, insulin-like growth factor; PDGF, platelet-derived growth factor; IL, interleukin; TNF, tumor necrosis factor.

sensory neuropathy.[194–197] The biologic and cellular basis of these manifestations is not yet well understood. Additionally, neurologic symptoms may occur as a consequence of hypercalcemia or hyperviscosity. Leptomeningeal involvement in myeloma with manifestations involving the central nervous system (CNS) has been described, usually in the late phase of the disease and associated with high-risk chromosomal abnormalities, plasmablastic morphology, and extramedullary manifestations.[198,199] Paraneoplastic CNS syndromes have also been described, possibly related to an immune mechanism directed at proteins present in the CNS, including the cerebellum. Peripheral neuropathy in myeloma may be due to an infiltrative process associated with the deposition of amyloid protein in the paraneural or *vasa nervorum*; due to a metabolic abnormality such as hypercalcemia, uremia, or hyperviscosity; or mediated by an autoimmune process or cytokines.[200] Peripheral neuropathy is also observed in patients with MGUS and more frequently associated with IgM paraprotein. More recently, peripheral neuropathy has been observed frequently with therapeutics, including thalidomide and bortezomib, especially with their prolonged use.

Hyperviscosity

The M components in myeloma can cause hyperviscosity and compromise circulation when the serum immunoglobulin levels exceed certain levels. The incidence is highest in Waldenström's macroglobulinemia with IgM, followed by IgA myeloma (25% patients), and is least common in IgG myeloma (<10% patients).[201–203] It can also be observed when immunoglobulins have a self-aggregating property leading to increased viscosity—for example, the IgG3 subclass is more commonly associated with hyperviscosity.[204] The syndrome is usually observed when serum viscosity exceeds 4.0 centipoise (cP) units relative to normal serum and manifests with circulatory compromise involving the CNS, the kidneys, and the lungs; it may also be associated with bleeding complications. Due to varying characteristics of idiotypes, the same level of increased viscosity may produce different severities of symptoms in individual patients. A high level of suspicion for this syndrome is important in any patient with paraproteinemia and either mental status changes or pulmonary distress, because prompt plasmapheresis can alleviate symptoms and avoid irreversible organ damage.

Coagulopathy

Myeloma patients may acquire coagulation abnormalities related to a high level of paraprotein interfering with the normal coagulation cascade or exhibit specific antibody activity leading to a clinical syndrome similar to acquired deficiency of factor VIII.[205,206] Additional factors, such as thrombosis in capillary circulation associated with hyperviscosity and anoxia, may lead to coagulation-related complications in 15% of patients with IgG myeloma and in more than 33% of patients with IgA myeloma. Although platelet counts are not suppressed in the early stages of myeloma, functional abnormalities of platelets have been described and may also contribute to bleeding.

Acquired activated protein C resistance is reported as a common single transitory baseline coagulation abnormality associated with venous thrombo embolism (VTE) in myeloma patients.[207] Additionally, patients may also present in a hypercoagulable state related to acquired deficiencies in protein S, or lupus anticoagulants leading to thromboembolic complications.[208] The fab fragment of the myeloma protein binds to fibrin and may prevent its aggregation.[209] Factor X deficiency is reported in patients with systemic AL amyloidosis[210]; however, an inhibitor has not been demonstrated in vitro to account for this manifestation.

Therapy may also increase the hypercoagulable state in myeloma. An increased incidence of deep venous thrombosis (12% to 24%) is observed in patients taking thalidomide and lenalidomide,

especially along with dexamethasone or other combination chemotherapies. In one study, 12 out of 50 patients (24%) receiving thalidomide developed deep vein thrombosis (DVT), compared to 2 out of 50 (4%) patients receiving identical therapy without thalidomide.[211] Activated protein C resistance in the absence of factor V Leiden mutation and high serum homocysteine levels are associated with an increased risk of thrombotic complications with thalidomide.[212]

Extramedullary Disease

Extramedullary disease manifestations are uncommon in patients with myeloma at presentation. However, such manifestations have been observed more frequently in the setting of advanced stage disease or relapse following allogeneic transplantation. In a large study of 1,965 patients, primary extramedullary plasmacytoma was detected in 66 patients and secondary plasmacytoma was detected in 35 patients. The most common sites for extramedullary disease at diagnosis were the skin and soft tissues, whereas liver involvement was most prominent at relapse or progression. Extramedullary involvement may be suspected in patients who have more aggressive features of myeloma, including high lactate dehydrogenase levels, immunoblastic morphology, high tumor cell labeling index, and complex karyotypic features.[213] In the 70- and 80-gene risk models, it is associated with high-risk features and shorter survival.[214]

Diagnosis

As myeloma patients present with a variety of symptoms not specific to the disease, the diagnosis of myeloma is quite often delayed. An older patient with a new onset of unexplained back pain or bone pain, recurrent infection, anemia, or renal insufficiency should be screened for myeloma. Additional findings, including hyperproteinemia or proteinuria, anemia, hypoalbuminemia, low immunoglobulin levels, or marked elevation of erythrocyte sedimentation rate, should prompt for a further complete evaluation for a diagnosis of plasma cell myeloma.

The first step in the evaluation includes tests to confirm the presence, type, and quantity of monoclonal protein, as well as the detection and quantification of clonal plasma cells (Table 112.4). The second component to differentiate MGUS, SMM versus symptomatic myeloma is to identify end organ damage by performing a hemogram to detect anemia, a complete skeletal radiographic survey to detect bone lesions, and a chemistry profile to detect renal dysfunction and hypercalcemia. The diagnostic criteria for MGUS, SMM, and active MM are shown in Table 112.5.[215] A third component in the investigative workup involves an evaluation of prognostic variables including markers of tumor burden, genomic profiles, and therapy-related changes. Guidelines by the International Myeloma Workshop and National Comprehensive Cancer Center Network summarizes the standard investigative workup in myeloma.[216,217]

Protein Electrophoresis

Among patients with myeloma, 70% have IgG, 20% have IgA, and 5% to 10% have production of monoclonal light chains only. A small proportion (less than 1%) of patients produce monoclonal IgD, IgE, IgM, or have nonsecretory myeloma. The suppression of uninvolved immunoglobulins (e.g., IgM and IgA in IgG myeloma) is present in a majority of the patients at diagnosis. Suppression of all three major classes of immunoglobulins should raise the possibility that the patient may have light chain–only disease, IgD or IgE myeloma, or nonsecretory disease. Patients producing intact immunoglobulin can also have excess light chain production and excretion in the urine (Fig. 112.6). The distribution of κ and λ light chains in the majority of myeloma cases is similar, except in

TABLE 112.4

Patient Evaluation

Presence and Characterization of Monoclonal Protein

Serum protein electrophoresis

Quantitative immunoglobulin

24-hour urine: total protein and Bence Jones protein

Immunofixation of urine and serum

Serum free light chain and ratio

Detection of Clonal Plasma Cells

Bone Marrow

Aspirate and biopsy

– Histology

– Clonality by immunostaining: kappa/lambda

– Flow cytometry

– Cytogenetics and fluorescent in situ hybridization (FISH)

Laboratory Evaluation

Chemistry panel (renal, calcium, albumin, uric acid, LDH)

Beta-2 microglobulin, C-reactive protein

Radiologic Evaluation

Skeletal Survey

MRI with STIR images

Bone densitometry

Evaluation of Prognostic Factors

Cytogenetics (metaphase karyotype and FISH)

Serum B2 microglobulin and serum albumin

Serum lactate dehydrogenase

Specialized Studies for Selected Patients

Abdominal fat pad or rectal biopsy for amyloid

Solitary lytic lesion biopsy

Serum viscosity if IgM component or high IgA levels or serum M-component >7 g/dL

Immunofixation for IgD or IgE in select cases

MRI, magnetic resonance imaging; STIR, short tau inversion recovery; CBC, complete blood cell count; LDH, lactate dehydrogenase; Ig, immunoglobulin.

IgD myeloma in which the λ light chain is more common. Currently, there is no difference in therapeutic approach between the different types of myeloma; however, patients with IgA myeloma, despite a higher initial response rate, have inferior survival.

Myeloma plasma cells usually produce a single, abnormal, and unique monoclonal antibody with a constant isotype and light-chain restriction. Rare occurrences of biclonal and triclonal cases have been reported at the time of diagnosis.[218] Occurrence of isotype switch and the appearance of abnormal protein bands have been reported in myeloma patients after treatment, especially high-dose therapy,[219] which appears to be related to the recovery of normal immunoglobulin production rather than alteration in disease biology. This change is also associated with improved survival. Occasionally, patients with initial intact Ig production relapse with only Bence Jones proteinuria (light chain escape) or nonsecretory disease, and this change has been correlated with more aggressive disease.[220]

A further analysis of a unique variable region in the myeloma-related idiotype (e.g., CDRIII) provides information on the monoclonal nature of the protein and also provides a tool to investigate minimal residual disease.[221]

Serum Free Light and Heavy/Light Chain

The measurement of serum free light chain (FLC) concentration has become an important tool to diagnose and follow the disease process, including response to therapy. It is especially useful in patients with light chain–only disease, oligo or nonsecretory myeloma, renal disease, amyloidosis, and as a prognostic marker, in MGUS and SMM, where an abnormal kappa/lambda free light chain ratio predicts a higher likelihood of progression to active myeloma.[222–226] Recently, a novel heavy/light chain (HLC) assay has been developed to quantitate the different light chain types of each immunoglobulin class (e.g., IgGκ, IgGλ, IgAκ, and IgAλ), which has been applied for both response assessments[227] and for prognostication.[228] For example, in a study where both HLC and FLC testing was utilized in 156 patients with IgG or IgA myeloma, the HLC ratio identified the presence of disease in 8 out of 31 patients with CR by conventional criteria.

Bone Marrow Examination

Various degrees of BM infiltration are observed in myeloma, with the majority of patients having an excess number of plasma cells. The pattern of BM involvement (diffuse versus nodular) is important, because patients with nodular disease seem to have poorer outcomes (in contrast to CLL).[229] The morphology of the plasma cell seems to be an important factor determining the severity of the disease. This is based on a histologic examination (Bartl grade) in which grade I suggests a slow growing disease, whereas grade III represents plasmablastic disease with an aggressive course.[230] There is also an increased incidence of cytogenetic abnormalities in patients with higher grade disease. Plasma cells contain cytoplasmic immunoglobulins with a constant heavy and light chain, which can be evaluated by a flow cytometric analysis or immunohistochemical staining of plasma cells.[231] When coupled with DNA staining using propidium iodide, a two-parameter analysis can detect changes in DNA content in myeloma cells (Fig. 112.7). DNA aneuploidy is observed in the BM of more than 80% patients, suggesting the existence of chromosomal abnormalities in the majority of patients.[231] This analysis also provides an objective marker to evaluate the response to therapy and to distinguish reactive from clonal plasmacytosis, especially in nonsecretory disease. A hypodiploid tumor cell has also been associated with refractoriness to standard-dose therapy.

Radiographic Evaluation

The radiographic survey of bone still remains a standard diagnostic evaluation, which shows osteopenia in an early phase of the disease and lytic punched out lesions associated with increasing tumor burden (Fig. 112.8). Osteosclerotic lesions are observed in POEMS syndrome.[194,196] Due to the predominant osteoclastic activity with osteoblastic inactivity, bone scans are seldom positive and are therefore not useful in the diagnosis of MM.

As demineralization of bone (osteoporosis) is one of the common manifestations of myeloma, measurement of bone mineral density (BMD) by dual-energy X-ray absorptiometry (DEXA) is an important evaluation at diagnosis.[232] In a study of 66 patients at diagnosis, the majority of the patients had decreased BMD with lumbar mean BMD value (Z score) $-1.24 +/- 1.45$. Following standard-dose therapy, lumbar BMD increased by 0.7%, whereas, in a group treated with high-dose therapy, the improvement was by 4.6% (p = 0.02).[233] Similar improvements in BMD have also been noted in patients undergoing high-dose therapy with the addition of bisphosphonates.[234] Differential effects of pamidronate on cortical and cancellous bone have been described in patients with myeloma undergoing autotransplants.[233,234]

TABLE 112.5

Diagnostic Criteria for Multiple Myeloma, Myeloma Variants, and Monoclonal Gammopathy of Unknown Significance[215]

Monoclonal Gammopathy of Undetermined Significance (MGUS) or Monoclonal Gammopathy, Unattributed/Unassociated (MG[u])

M protein in serum <30 g/L

Bone marrow clonal plasma cells <10%

No evidence of other B-cell proliferative disorders

No myeloma related organ or tissue impairment (no end organ damage, including bone lesions)

Asymptomatic Myeloma (Smoldering Myeloma)

M protein in serum >30 g/L and/or

Bone marrow clonal plasma cell ≥10%

No related organ or tissue impairment (no end organ damage, including bone lesions) or symptoms

Symptomatic Multiple Myeloma

M protein in serum and/or urine*

Bone marrow (clonal) plasma cells* or plasmacytoma

Related organ or tissue impairment (end organ damage, including bone lesions)

*If flow cytometry is performed, most plasma cells (>90%) will show a neoplastic phenotype.

Solitary Plasmacytoma of Bone

No M protein in serum and/or urine*

Single area of bone destruction due to clonal plasma cells

Bone marrow not consistent with multiple myeloma

Normal skeletal survey (and MRI of spine and pelvis if done)

No related organ or tissue impairment (no end organ damage other than solitary bone lesion)*

*A small M component may sometimes be present

Nonsecretory Myeloma

No M protein in serum and/or urine with immunofixation

Bone marrow clonal plasmacytosis ≥10% or plasmacytoma

Related organ or tissue impairment (end organ damage, including bone lesions)

Extramedullary Plasmacytoma

No M protein in serum and/or urine*

Extramedullary tumor of clonal plasma cells

Normal bone marrow

Normal skeletal survey

No related organ or tissue impairment (end organ damage including bone lesions)

*A small M component may sometimes be present.

Multiple Solitary Plasmacytomas (± Recurrent)

No M protein in serum and/or urine*

More than one localized area of bone destruction or extramedullary tumor of clonal plasma cells, which may be recurrent

Normal bone marrow

Normal skeletal survey and MRI of spine and pelvis if done

No related organ or tissue impairment (no end organ damage other than the localized bone lesions)

*A small M component may sometimes be present.

Myeloma-Related Organ or Tissue Impairment (End Organ Damage) (ROTI)

Calcium levels increased: serum calcium >0–25 mmol/L above the upper limit of normal or >2–75 mmol/L

Renal insufficiency: creatinine >173 mmol/L

Anemia: hemoglobin 2 g/dL below the lower limit of normal or hemoglobin <10 g/dL

Bone lesions: lytic lesions or osteoporosis with compression fractures (MRI or CT may clarify)

Other: symptomatic hyperviscosity, amyloidosis, recurrent bacterial infections (more than two episodes in 12 months)

MRI, magnetic resonance imaging; CT, computed tomography.

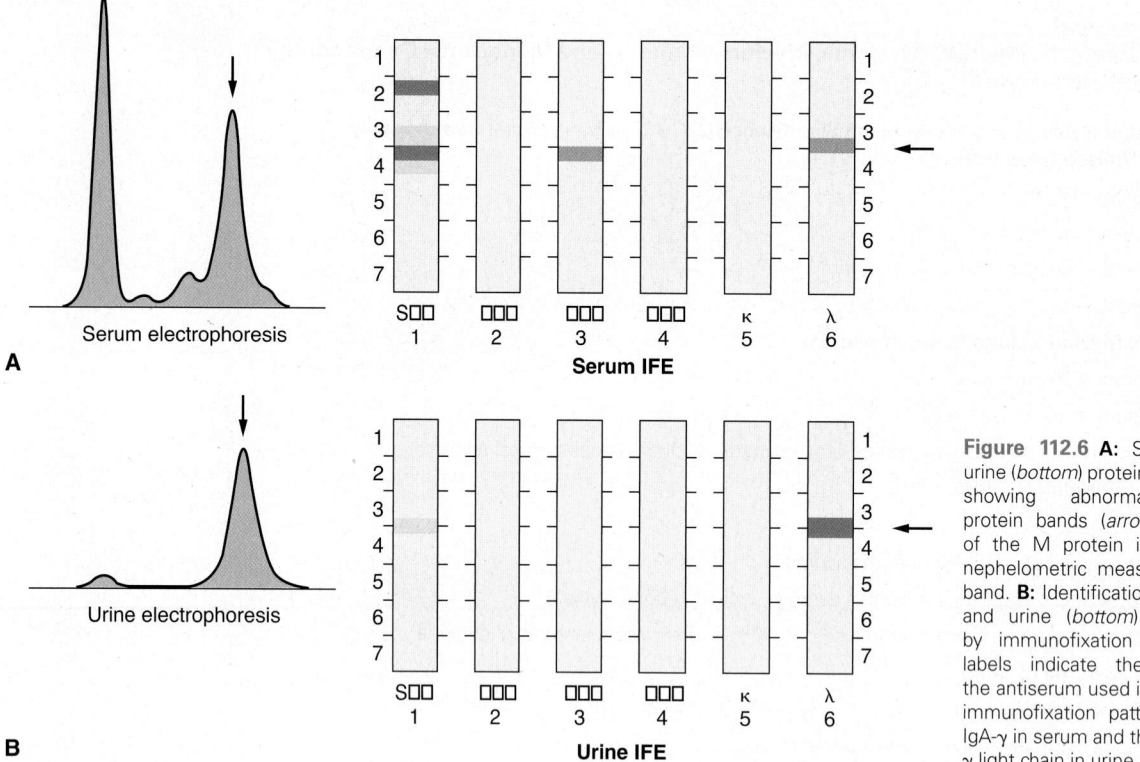

Figure 112.6 A: Serum (*top*) and urine (*bottom*) protein electrophoresis showing abnormal monoclonal protein bands (*arrow*). Quantitation of the M protein is performed by nephelometric measurement of the band. **B:** Identification of serum (*top*) and urine (*bottom*) M component by immunofixation technique. The labels indicate the specificity of the antiserum used in developing the immunofixation pattern. The top is IgA-γ in serum and the bottom is free γ light chain in urine

Magnetic resonance imaging (MRI) of bone marrow provides a better assessment of tumor burden. More than 95% of myeloma patients have MRI abnormalities: one-third each have diffuse involvement of the bone marrow, focal lesions, or heterogeneous focal and diffused marrow involvement (Fig. 112.9A). Because myeloma is a macrofocal disease, random BM sampling may not

be diagnostic or predictive of disease status, and MRI short tau inversion recovery images (STIR) may provide a better assessment of bone marrow involvement in myeloma.[235-237] An MRI of the spine and pelvis is required in all patients with a solitary plasmacytoma and SMM, both to detect occult lesions and to predict progression. In symptomatic myeloma, an MRI can be considered as a

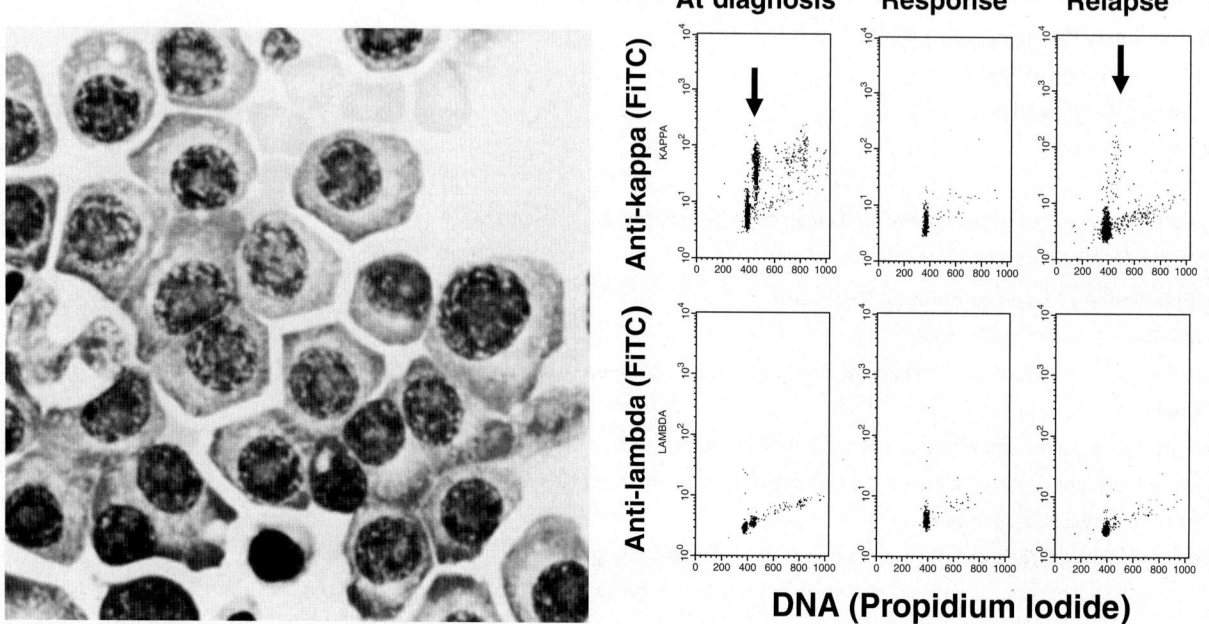

Figure 112.7 A: Bone marrow plasma cells in a patient with IgG myeloma showing neoplastic plasma cells at various stages of differentiation. **B:** Two parameter flow cytometry of DNA content of bone marrow cells; abscissa (propidium iodide) and cytoplasmic immunoglobulin (ordinate, anti-κ or anti-γ fluorescein isothiocyanate [FiTC]). At diagnosis, approximately 45% hyperdiploid tumor cells show κ light chain restriction (*left panel*); at the time of maximal response, no hyperdiploid light chain restricted cells are seen (*middle panel*); at the time of early relapse, the reappearance of small hyperdiploid and κ light chain restricted population (<1%) is indicative of reemergence of small number of clonal cells, which may not yet be apparent on cytological examination of the bone marrow (*right panel*). A population of κ restricted but diploid cell population (*small arrow*) may represent a second clone.

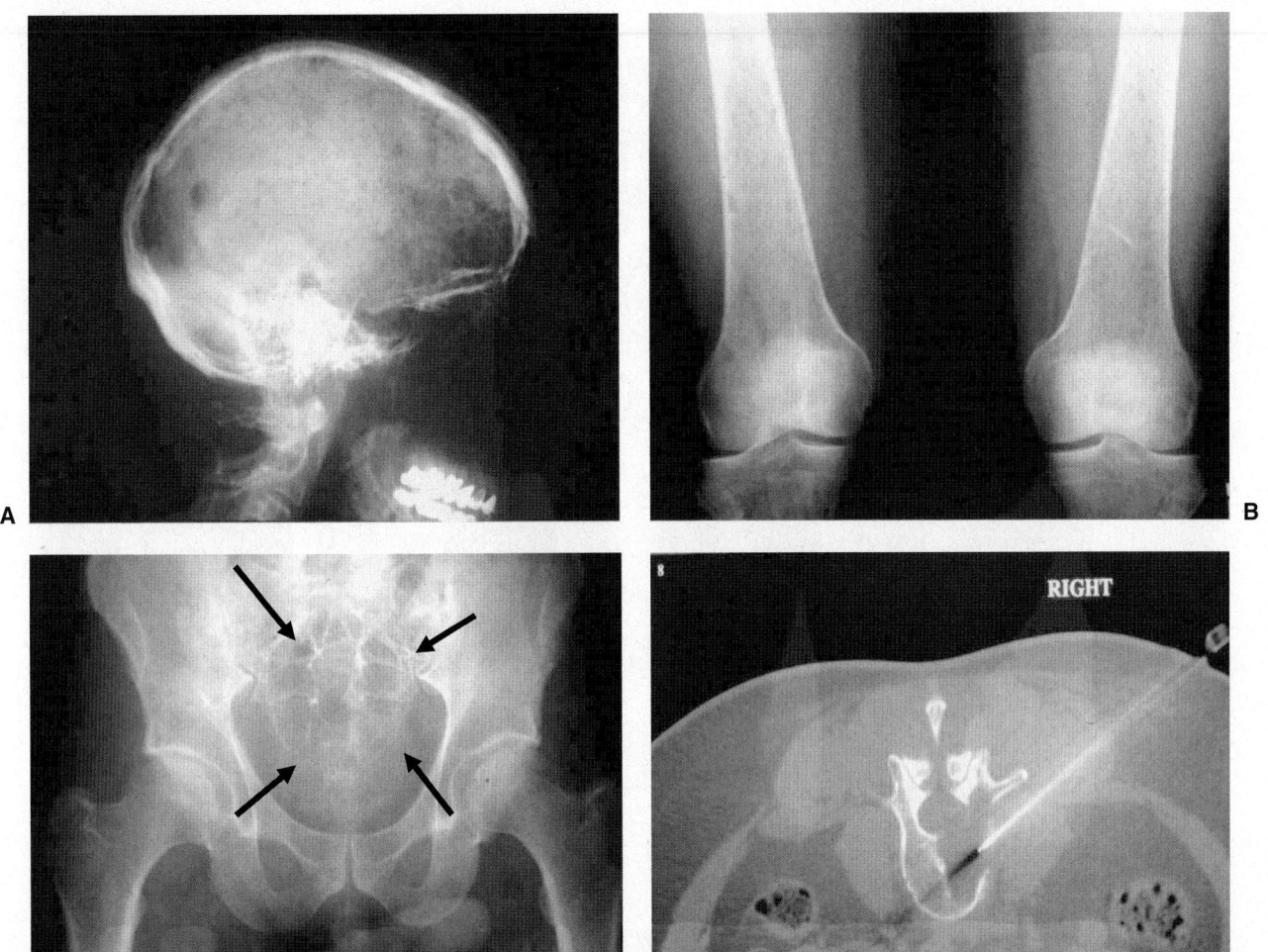

Figure 112.8 Typical skeletal changes on roentgenogram. **A:** Example of "punched-out" lytic lesions in skull. **B:** Small lytic lesions in the left femur. **C:** Large lytic lesion in sacrum. **D:** Fine-needle aspiration biopsy of the vertebral lesion. (Courtesy of Hemendra Shah.)

routine evaluation to detect unsuspected focal lesions and plasmacytomas involving the spine and pelvis, to define patterns of bone marrow involvement (i.e., diffuse pattern or a high number of focal lesions), to obtain a detailed evaluation of a painful area of the skeleton, and to investigate suspicion of cord compression.[238,239] A focal marrow plasmacytoma can be further analyzed through computerized tomography (CT)-guided fine needle aspiration (see Fig. 112.8), allowing for cytologic diagnosis. With effective therapy, the MRI pattern may change (Fig. 112.9B): Diffuse involvement of the marrow may evolve into focal disease, and normalization of MRI abnormalities may provide a better definition of complete responses.[237] Positron-emission tomography (PET) scanning has also been evaluated in a small number of studies and may provide a better functional definition of lesions observed on MRI or CT scans, as well as allowing for the selection of lesions for biopsy.[237,240] The PET–CT scan is utilized for the detection of extraosseous soft tissue masses, as well as for the evaluation of rib and appendicular bone lesions. A combination of PET–CT and MRI scans may improve the diagnostic accuracy for solitary plasmacytoma.[238] A recent study has identified the independent predictive value of baseline fludeoxyglucose (FDG)-PET/CT and of FDG suppression before high-dose therapy.[241]

Differential Diagnosis

In the presence of end organ damage associated with monoclonal protein and clonal plasma cells in bone marrow, the distinction of active myeloma from SMM and MGUS can be readily established (see Table 112.5). Patients with nonsecretory myeloma are diagnosed based on marrow plasmacytosis and the presence of bone lesions. MRI abnormalities and CT- or MRI-guided fine-needle aspiration biopsy of involved anatomic sites are important for the follow-up of the disease.

The diagnosis of solitary plasmacytoma of bone or soft tissue requires intense investigation to rule out systemic disease. Bone marrow examination in a true solitary lesion is normal, with no evidence of a clonal cell population. An MRI evaluation for myelomatous involvement of the BM helps detect early lesions before their detection by standard roentgenographic examination. The detection of such lesions and cytologic confirmation through CT- or MRI-guided fine-needle aspiration biopsy may help confirm a solitary plasmacytoma and its genetic makeup. In an individual with MGUS, such detection may change the diagnosis to solitary plasmacytoma or MM. It is important to note that patients with MGUS or solitary plasmacytoma seldom have suppression of uninvolved immunoglobulins. Conventional cytogenetic results are usually normal in MGUS; however, monoclonal plasma cells in some individuals with MGUS may be aneuploidy, and chromosomal abnormalities including IgH translocations and chromosome 13 deletions of unclear prognostic significance have been reported in MGUS.

Besides plasma cell neoplasms, various other conditions can present with monoclonal immunoglobulin secretion. These conditions include other B-cell neoplasms including CLL and B-cell non-Hodgkin's lymphoma; autoimmune conditions such as cold

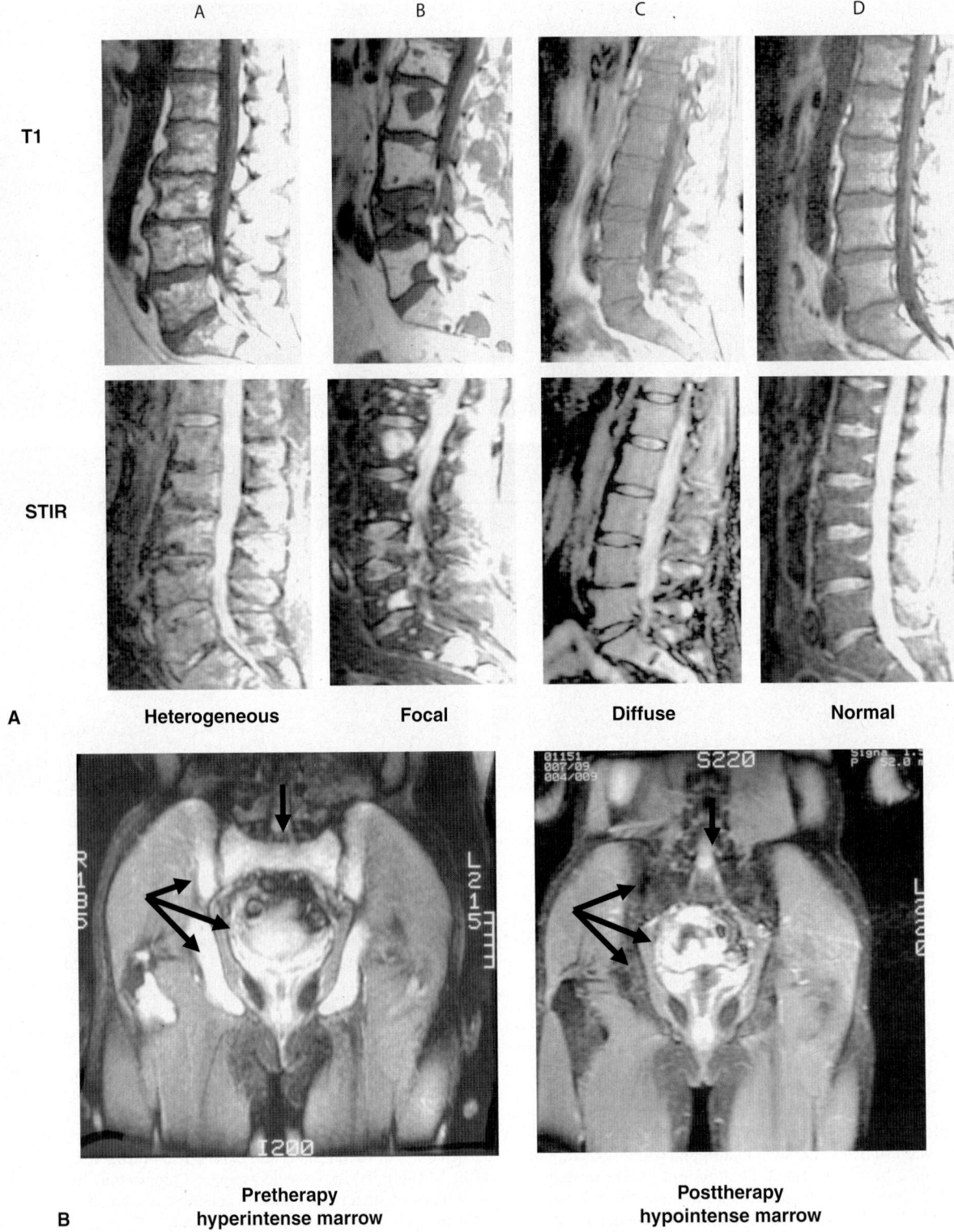

Figure 112. 9 **A:** Magnetic resonance imaging (MRI) pattern in multiple myeloma at diagnosis: T1-weighted and STIR (short inversion-time inversion recovery) imaging shows approximately one-third of patients each presenting with heterogeneous pattern (*panel 1*), focal plasmacytoma lesions (*panel 2*), or diffuse homogeneous hyperintense marrow pattern (*panel 3*). Hyperintensity of marrow on STIR image is suggestive of uniform marrow involvement by myeloma. Few patients have a hypointense and homogenous pattern also seen in normal individuals (*panel 4*). **B:** The hyperintense marrow pattern suggestive of extensive marrow involvement pretherapy (*left; arrows*) changes to hypointense pattern following complete response and normalization of marrow (*right, arrows*); fine-needle aspiration examination in 72 patients with MRI-focal disease showed a tumor in 92%, indicating that minimal response focal lesions in myeloma represent a tumor.

agglutinin diseases, mixed cryoglobulinemia, hypergammaglobulinemia, and Sjögren's syndrome; inflammatory or storage diseases such as lichen myxedema, Gaucher's disease, sarcoidosis, and cirrhosis; and rarely, other malignancies such as chronic myeloid leukemia as well as colon, breast, or prostate cancer.

Protein deposition disease involving various organs requires additional special diagnostic procedures. Deposition of amyloid protein (amyloidosis) can be clinically suspected based on macroglossia, vascular fragility (raccoon's eyes, periorbital subcutaneous hemorrhages), carpal tunnel syndrome, organomegaly, nephropathy, and cardiomegaly with arrhythmia. The detection of Congo red-positive amyloid with classic apple-green birefringence when visualized under polarized light in perivascular areas and subcutaneous fat, as well as bone marrow or rectal biopsy specimens, are diagnostic of AL amyloid. Electrocardiography may reveal low voltage, and an echocardiographic evaluation shows thickening of the interventricular septum or classic speckled pattern in the myocardium. Endomyocardial biopsy may establish the diagnosis of cardiac amyloid, which is usually associated with elevated serum brain natriuretic peptide (BNP) levels. Another manifestation of amyloid deposition includes autonomic dysfunction due to amyloid deposition in the vasa nervorum of the autonomic nerves, leading to orthostatic hypotension. Amyloid deposition in adrenal glands leads to hypoadrenalism; in the spleen, it may lead to hyposplenism with thrombocytosis; in the liver, it may be suspected based on elevated alkaline phosphatase and γ-glutamyl transpeptidase; and in the gastrointestinal tract, it may lead to malabsorption syndrome. Renal dysfunction must be further investigated with a renal biopsy, because light chain cast nephropathy or light chain deposition disease may be reversible following aggressive therapy, whereas deposition of amyloid requires a different therapeutic approach. As the deposition of immunoglobulin and light chain can mimic many manifestations of AL amyloid, an immunofluorescence analysis of unfixed tissue is important for a diagnosis.

Staging and Risk Assessment

Following the diagnostic investigation, more detailed cellular and molecular studies are required to stage myeloma and evaluate prognostic variables that determine the patient's probable outcome.

Patients with MM have variable disease courses, with survival ranging from less than 1 year with high-risk aggressive disease to more than 10 years with indolent presentation or sensitive disease. Various characteristics have been identified to predict the possible course of the disease. An evaluation of prognostic factors is important to define therapeutic strategies, permit comparison of clinical trial results, and predict life expectancy after diagnosis. The current risk stratification is applicable to newly diagnosed patients using parameters obtained at the diagnosis. On relapse, there is often an acquisition of additional or new risk features in which case patients should be reclassified as having high-risk disease. As shown in Table 112.6, prognostic factors are related to the tumor burden, the intrinsic property of the tumor, host and microenvironmental influences, and treatment/intervention-related factors.

A clinical staging system for MM using a standard laboratory measurement was developed by Durie and Salmon, which was predictive of clinical outcomes after standard-dose chemotherapy.[242] However, this staging system is not predictive of outcomes in patients undergoing high-dose chemotherapy as well as novel agents-based therapy and is no longer used clinically.

β2-microglobulin (β2M) has been identified as one of the most consistent predictors of survival in plasma cell myeloma. β2M, the light chain gene of the class I histocompatibility antigens expressed on the surface of all nucleated cells, is shed into the blood. Its renal excretion explains its elevation in renal failure. In MM, β2M, therefore, reflects both tumor burden and renal function.[243,244] High β2M (>2.5 mg per liter) levels carry a poor

TABLE 112.6
Prognostic Variable
Tumor-Burden Related Factors
β-2 microglobulin
>3 lytic bone lesions
Hemoglobin
Serum calcium
Tumor-Biology Related Factors
Cytogenetic/FISH abnormality (t(4;14), t(14;16), del17p-); hypodiploidy
Gene expression profile pattern
Plasma cell labeling index
Bartl grade
Mitotic activity
IgA myeloma
C-reactive protein (CRP)
LDH
Soluble IL-6 receptor
Renal failure
Tumor Microenvironment-Related Factors
Bone marrow microvessel density
Serum syndecan-1 levels
MMP-9 levels
Soluble CD16
Treatment-Related Factors
Tandem transplant
Achieving complete response or very good partial response
Patient-Related Factors
Age
Albumin
Performance status
Other organ problems not related to myeloma or amyloid deposits

Ig, immunoglobulin; LDH, lactate dehydrogenase; MMP-9, Matrix metallopeptidase 9.

prognosis for treatment with both standard-dose and high-dose therapy.[245] The combination of serum β2M along with serum albumin has been proposed as a three-stage ISS (Table 112.7). Although this system predicts for outcome following both high-dose therapy as well as novel agents-based treatment, it lacks consideration of tumor biology–related factors, such as cytogenetics or molecular markers.

Cytogenetics

Because the myeloma cell represents a mature differentiated cell with low proliferative activity, cytogenetic abnormalities are not frequently detected. Abnormalities are observed in only one-third of the patients at the time of diagnosis; however, a repeated analysis increases the yield to almost one-half of patients. The normal karyotypic pattern observed in the remaining half most likely originates from dividing normal hematopoietic cells.[53]

Cytogenetic abnormalities have been identified as a major prognostic factor in plasma cell myeloma. Although the detection

TABLE 112.7

International Staging System

Stage	Criteria	Median Survival (mo)
I	Serum β₂ microglobulin <3.5 mg/L Serum albumin ≥3.5 g/dL	62
II	Not stage I or III	44
III	Serum β₂ microglobulin ≥5.5 mg/L	29

There are two categories for stage II: serum β₂ microglobulin <3.5 mg/L but serum albumin <3.5 g/dL; or serum β₂ microglobulin 3.5 to <5.5 mg/L irrespective of the serum albumin level.

of any cytogenetic abnormality is considered to suggest a higher risk disease, the specific abnormalities considered as poor risk are cytogenetically detected chromosomal 13 or 13q deletion and detection by FISH of t(4;14); t(14;16) and del17p. Del13 or 13q-detected only by FISH and in the absence of other abnormality does not carry significantly higher risk, whereas t(11;14) does not predict superior outcome. The cytogenetic and interphase FISH analysis has identified numeric aberrations involving trisomies of chromosomes 3, 5, 7, 9, 11, 15, 19, and 21, which predict for favorable outcomes.[55] Limited studies have shown that 1q34+, and del1p may have clinical significance as a poor risk feature. Importantly, both bortezomib and lenalidomide are able to overcome adverse outcomes associated with chromosome 13 deletion and, to a lesser extent, t(4;14).[246]

Other independent factors associated with poor prognosis include elevated C-reactive protein (CRP), elevated serum lactate dehydrogenase (LDH) with extramedullary disease, serum IL-6, serum soluble IL-6 receptor, and IgA isotype.[247] Because CRP levels reflect IL-6 activity and elevated CRP levels can be associated with acute-phase reactions including inflammation and infections, the predictive value of elevated CRP in myeloma is important only when other possible causes for its elevation are ruled out. BM plasmacytosis reflects tumor burden, but does not predict survival. Peripheral blood monoclonal plasma cells predict for survival in myeloma: In a study of 254 patients, blood monoclonal plasma cell counts ≥4% in 57% patients were associated with a median survival of 2.4 years compared with 4.4 years in patients with less than 4% circulating plasma cells.[248]

Among the various other disease biology–related variables, plasma cell proliferation rate, as measured by the labeling index (LI), is a valuable prognostic factor: Early in the disease, the proportion of myeloma cells in the cell cycle is small; bromodeoxyuridine or tritiated thymidine methods show a median of 1% cycling cells at the diagnosis. With progressive disease, the LI increases, suggesting a more proliferative phenotype. The LI has important prognostic significance, because patients with more than 1% cells in the S-phase in BM have worse outcomes[231,249,250]; however, the lack of standardized reproducible methods to measure the LI has limited its use as a prognostic marker. One study combining β2M and LI identified a low-risk group with both parameters low, an intermediate-risk group with one parameter high, and a high-risk group with both parameters high to have median survivals of 71 months, 40 months, and 15 months, respectively.[250] Additional tumor-related factors predictive of inferior survival include an increased soluble IL-6 receptor level, elevated serum LDH with extramedullary disease, and increased tumor cell mitotic activity (greater than 1 per high power field).

Among the microenvironment-related factors, BM MVD has been identified as an important prognosticator. High MVD in BM (≥4 per high power field) at the diagnosis confers shorter event-free survival (EFS; 2.7 versus 4.3 years; p = 0.03) and overall survival (OS; 7.9+ versus 4.3 years; p = 0.006) after high-dose

chemotherapy.[251] An increased level of serum syndecan-1, as well as reduced levels of soluble CD16, have been described to portend a poor prognosis.[252]

Among therapy- and intervention-related prognostic factors, the type of response and length of response to prior therapy are additional risk stratification criteria; progression while on therapy and a short duration of response to prior therapy are poor risk features. The speed of response does not suggest poor overall outcomes with newer agents.

The risk stratification is applicable to newly diagnosed patients. However, the myeloma cell can acquire new changes over time, acquiring the same genomic abnormalities at relapse that are predictive of poor outcomes at diagnosis. Thus, in good-risk patients, it is necessary to evaluate for high-risk features at relapse. There is also a consensus that the high-risk features will change in the future, with the introduction of other new agents or possibly new combinations.[253]

An analysis of genome-wide copy number alterations (CNA) in 192 newly diagnosed, uniformly treated patients with MM using high-density SNP array suggested global genomic instability in MM.[96] One of three distinct patterns of CNAs are present in 98% of cases. A multivariate analysis identified a prognostic model that includes amp(1q23.3), amp(5q31.3), and del(12p13.31) as the most powerful independent adverse markers (p <0.0001). The availability of larger scale expression profiling data in uniformly treated patient populations has provided the basis for RNA-based prognostic classification systems.[92] Three large studies have evaluated the prognostic significance of gene expression profiling to identify poor-risk patient populations; the UAMS 70-gene model,[93] the 15-gene IFM model,[94] and the 92-gene HOVON model.[95] Interestingly, these studies identified patients with a short survival, but were not designed to select patients with very good risk. It is intriguing that none of these models share common genes, highlighting the redundancy in the genes and pathways that control growth, proliferation, and survival; differences in the treatment used to define the patient population; and the complexity of tumor cell biology. These initial attempts at molecular classification and prognostication will need further validation and incorporation into more commonly available methods for larger application. Moreover, the high-risk features identified previously are highly dependent on the therapeutic intervention used. For example, the newer biologically based therapies such as lenalidomide and bortezomib are able to overcome drug resistance, and some traditional adverse prognostic factors are no longer predictive of survival. Additional molecular studies with FISH analysis, as well as proteomic and genomic analyses, including SNP, may identify future uniformly applicable prognostic systems.

TREATMENT

The therapeutic intervention in plasma cell disorders is dependent on the presenting condition. For example, individuals with the diagnosis of MGUS do not require immediate treatment. Patients with solitary plasmacytomas can be treated with local therapy only, whereas those with indolent asymptomatic myeloma can smolder for a long period of time prior to becoming symptomatic and requiring treatment.

Solitary Plasmacytoma

Solitary plasmacytoma requires specialized techniques for accurate staging, including a CT scan and MRI to exclude more disseminated disease. Solitary plasmacytomas of the bone involve vertebral bodies in one-third of patients and frequently affect men (70%) at a younger age (median 56 years).[254] A monoclonal protein in the serum is observed in 24% to 54% of patients, but no detectable monoclonal protein is observed, even on immunofixation, in the remaining cases. Extramedullary plasmacytomas are diagnosed less frequently and require a workup including MRI and PET scanning to rule out additional sites or disseminated disease. The optimal therapy for true solitary plasmacytoma is curative-dose (4,000 to 5,000 cGy) radiotherapy.[255,256] With this dose, local tumor recurrence rates have been less than 10%; 30% of patients with solitary osseous plasmacytomas versus more than 70% of patients with solitary extramedullary plasmacytomas achieve long disease-free survival.[257,258] Monoclonal protein disappears after radiotherapy in 25% to 50% of patients, suggesting a possible eradication of the disease; conversely, the reappearance of monoclonal protein predicts for recurrence of the disease. With better staging using MRI, true solitary plasmacytoma of bone can be cured in a high proportion of patients.

Monoclonal Gammopathy of Unknown Significance and Smoldering Myeloma

Patents with MGUS or smoldering myeloma have a low tumor mass and indolent disease course presenting without specific symptoms. Such patients do not have end organ damage. In patients with indolent light chain disease, Bence Jones proteinuria does not exceed >10 g per day. About 1% patients with MGUS per year progress to symptomatic myeloma. Non-IgG subtype, abnormal kappa/lambda free light chain ratio, and serum M protein more than 1.5 g per deciliter are associated with higher incidences of progression from MGUS to myeloma. Patients with none of these risk features have a 5% chance of progression, whereas those with all three features have a 60% chance of progression to myeloma in 20 years. The features responsible for the higher risk of progression from smoldering myeloma to active MM are bone marrow plasmacytosis >30%, abnormal kappa/lambda free light chain ratio, and serum M protein >30 g per liter (3.0 g per deciliter). Patients with all three adverse features have a nearly 50% chance of progression in 2 years.[259,260] Typically, patients with MGUS require no therapy. Similarly, patients with smoldering myeloma are also not treated routinely until disease progression or the appearance of end organ damage, such as the development of bone lesions or anemia. However, ongoing clinical trials have focused on evaluating the role of early intervention to prevent the progression of smoldering to symptomatic myeloma. For example, an evaluation of thalidomide in 31 patients with indolent myeloma showed responses in 66% of patients, with the potential to delay the progression to symptomatic disease.[261] In a recent phase 3 randomized, open-label, trial, 119 high-risk smoldering myeloma patients were assigned to treatment (lenalidomide at a dose of 25 mg per day on days 1 to 21, plus dexamethasone at a dose of 20 mg per day on days 1 to 4 and days 12 to 15, at 4-week intervals for nine cycles) or observation.[262] Patients in the treatment group received a maintenance regimen (lenalidomide at a dose of 10 mg per day on days 1 to 21 of each 28-day cycle for 2 years) after completing induction treatment. After the induction phase, a partial response or better was achieved in 79% of patients in the treatment group, which increased to 90% during the maintenance phase. With a median follow-up of 40 months, the median time to progression was significantly longer in the treatment group compared to the observation group (median not reached versus 21 months, respectively; p < 0.001). Importantly, the 3-year overall survival rate was also significantly higher in the treatment compared to the control group (94% versus 80%; p = 0.03). The treatment was well tolerated. This study for the first time suggests that an early intervention in patients with high-risk smoldering myeloma may provide survival benefit. However, further investigations are necessary to establish an optimal patient population and directed intervention that may help with the prevention of progression of SMM to active MM and may prolong overall survival.

Symptomatic Multiple Myeloma

Standard-Dose ConventionalTherapy

Oral melphalan and prednisone was the first successful combination chemotherapy for myeloma; subsequently, various other single agents and combinations, as well as high-dose chemotherapy regimens, have been investigated and reported to have significant antimyeloma activity.

Melphalan and Prednisone. Treatment with oral melphalan and prednisone (MP) achieves a partial response (PR) in 50% to 60% of patients, with 3% to 5% of patients achieving a CR, and provides symptomatic relief as well as tumor mass reduction.[263] The median response duration is 18 months, and OS is 24 to 36 months. The absorption of oral melphalan is unpredictable, requiring its ingestion on an empty stomach and an increase in dose if the patient does not develop cytopenia.[264] With the availability of an intravenous formulation, dose and pharmacokinetics are now predictable. Frequent complications after MP therapy include the development of cytopenia and, with chronic administration, myelodysplastic changes in the marrow. MP in any combination should not be used as induction therapy in patients eligible for high-dose therapy and stem cell transplant because melphalan damages stem cells and compromises the ability to mobilize adequate numbers of stem cells. As described as follows, MP is now combined with one of the novel agents.

VAD and Alkylating Agent-Based Combinations. Various chemotherapeutic combinations have been investigated in myeloma, including vincristine (V), cyclophosphamide (C), BCNU (B), melphalan (M), adriamycin (A), and prednisone (P). Commonly used combinations in the past include VBMCP or VMCP/VBAP.[265,266] These combinations are no longer utilized. Similarly, high-dose dexamethasone (40 mg orally on days 1 through 4, 9 through 12, and 17 through 20) in combination with 24-hour continuous infusion of vincristine (0.25 mg/m^2) and adriamycin (9 mg/m^2) (VAD) for 4 days[267] was once a preferred induction regimen achieving a nearly 50% response rate; however, with the availability of novel agent-based combinations, VAD is no longer used as an induction regimen.[268] Although effective, high-dose dexamethasone used in various dosages (20 to 40 mg) and schedules (once a week, 4 days every 2 weeks to a 4 days on and 4 days off regimen) have been associated with predisposition to systemic infections, as well as insomnia, hyperactivity, hyperglycemia, and psychiatric problems. An Eastern Co-operative Oncology Group study suggests that dexamethasone once a week in combination with lenalidomide may be less toxic and more effective than a high-dose dexamethasone regimen.[269] Glucocorticoids downregulate IL-6 production and induce apoptosis in vitro; conversely, myeloma cells can be rescued from glucocorticoid-mediated killing by the addition of IL-6 to in vitro cultures or by coculturing them with bone marrow stromal cells, which are a source of IL-6 in vivo.

Interferon. Interferon causes direct growth inhibition, as well as antiangiogenic and immunomodulatory activity. Although it has been one of the most investigated agents in myeloma especially in maintenance settings, it has not demonstrated significant beneficial effects.[270,271] A meta-analysis of eight trials involving 929 patients showed prolongation of relapse-free survival by 7 months and OS by 5 months in patients receiving IFN. However, a large US intergroup study failed to show a benefit of IFN maintenance after high-dose therapy.[272] IFN is associated with flulike symptoms, weight loss, impotence, depression, mental status changes, and cytopenias; in addition, its prolonged use has been associated with inability to mobilize stem cells, therefore, it is no longer utilized.

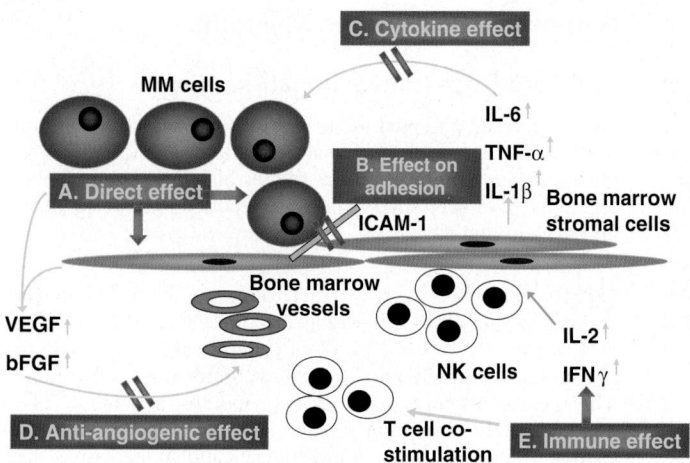

Figure 112.10 Potential mechanisms of action of thalidomide and its analogs. **A:** Direct effect on the myeloma cells. **B:** Inhibition of MM cell–BMSC adhesion. **C:** Inhibition of cytokine production in the microenvironment. **D:** Antiangiogenic effects through inhibition of the proangiogenic cytokines. **E:** Modulation of immune function, especially NK cells and T cells. MM, multiple myeloma; BMSC, bone marrow stromal cells; ICAM, intracellular adhesion molecule; IL, interleukin; TNF, tumor necrosis factor; VEGF, vascular endothelial growth factor; bFGF, basic fibroblast growth factor; IFN, interferon; NK, natural killer.

Radiation Therapy

Radiation therapy was considered the mainstay of treatment for myeloma prior to the availability of chemotherapeutic options. However, with more effective therapy, the role of radiation has now been limited.[273] A definitive role remains in patients with solitary bone and extramedullary plasmacytoma. Importantly, patients with solitary bone plasmacytoma treated with definitive radiation therapy (4,000 to 5,000 cGy) have progression-free survival of 30%, compared to 70% in those with extramedullary plasmacytomas.[255–258,274] The indication for radiation therapy in MM remains palliation in cases of impending pathologic fracture and to treat spinal cord compression. In patients with bone pain or symptomatic soft tissue masses, radiation is only considered when patients have failed chemotherapeutic options.[275,276] Radiation to BM-containing areas, such as the pelvic bone, should be used judiciously if there is a need for the collection of stem cells. The dose of palliative radiation therapy ranges from 1,500 to 2,500 cGy. Studies to date have failed to show any benefit of hemibody radiation in MM. However, total body radiation has been used prior to allogeneic and autologous transplantation. More recent studies have demonstrated that total body radiation does not provide additional cytoreductive potential; moreover, when combined with high-dose melphalan conditioning, it increases treatment-related morbidity and mortality, as well as delays immune recovery compared to high dose melphalan alone. Recent studies with nonmyeloablative regimens followed by allogeneic stem cell transplantation use low-dose radiation and achieve adequate engraftment, avoiding myeloablation and attendant toxicity of total body irradiation.

Novel Biologically Based Agents

Novel therapeutic agents specifically targeting the mechanisms whereby myeloma cells grow and survive in the BM milieu can overcome resistance to standard-dose and high-dose therapies. The immunomodulatory agents thalidomide and its analog lenalidomide, as well as the proteasome inhibitor bortezomib, are agents that have demonstrated efficacy in both relapsed and newly diagnosed myeloma and have now been integrated into standard algorithms for myeloma management.

Thalidomide. The initial rationale for use of thalidomide in myeloma was its known antiangiogenic activity, coupled with reports of increased angiogenesis in MM BM. Further investigations have shown that besides their direct effect on MM cells, thalidomide and other immunomodulatory agents (lenalidomide and pomalidomide) abrogate the adhesion of MM cells to BMSCs and block the secretion of MM growth and survival factors such as IL-6, TNF-α, VEGF, and FGF triggered by the binding of MM cells to BMSCs.[277] Additionally, these agents significantly modulate immune responses by expanding the number and function of NK cells, improving DC function, and enhancing T-cell function by providing T-cell costimulatory signals through the B7-CD28 pathway.[277] Importantly, two recent studies have shown that lenalidomide binds to cereblon (CRBN), the substrate-recognition subunit of a ubiquitin ligase complex. This in turn leads to specific ubiquitination and, subsequently, degradation of two related transcription factors, Ikaros family zinc finger 1 (IKZF1) and Aiolos IKZF3, with essential roles in B- and T-cell differentiation, as well as myeloma cell survival (Fig. 112.10).[278,279] A glutamine residue within the second zinc finger of IKZF1 and IKZF3 seems to provide the specificity of this interaction, because its absence in the highly homologous Ikaros family members IKZF2 and IKZF4 makes then resistant to lenalidomide. Importantly, the expression of IKZF1 or IKZF3 mutants lacking the key glutamine residue in the CRBN degron sequence or knockdown of CRBN conferred lenalidomide resistance. These results now provide a unique molecular understanding of lenalidomide activity, as a single agent or in combination.

Thalidomide was initially evaluated in a phase 2 study in 169 posttransplant-relapsed MM patients in incremental doses of 200 mg to 800 mg. A partial response was observed in 26% patients, with an overall response rate of 34%.[280,281] Subsequently, the efficacy of thalidomide alone and in combination has been confirmed in several phase 2 and 3 studies in MM (Table 112.8A). In combination with dexamethasone, it achieved >50% responses in relapsed MM patients and 70% responses in newly diagnosed patients. Additional combinations of thalidomide with MP have improved overall response, as well as both EFS and OS, in newly diagnosed patients over the age of 65 years (Table 112.8B). The major toxicities of thalidomide are somnolence, constipation, and neurologic symptoms, including neuropathy, fatigue, and DVT.[211] Due to the significant risk of DVT and pulmonary embolism when thalidomide is used in combination with dexamethasone, a prophylaxis against clotting is warranted in all patients. Although aspirin has been used as prophylaxis in patients at a low risk of DVT, either standard-dose Coumadin or low–molecular-weight heparin is indicated in patients at a higher risk of DVT.[282]

Lenalidomide. Lenalidomide, a more potent analog of thalidomide, in a phase 1 clinical trial, achieved at least a minimal response (at least a 25% reduction in paraproteins) in 15 of 24 (63%) patients, including in 11 patients who had received prior thalidomide.[283] A subsequent randomized study in patients with at least one prior therapy of lenalidomide and dexamethasone versus dexamethasone alone achieved PR or better rate (61% versus 20%; p <0.001); CR rate (14% versus 0.6%; p <0.001); a median time to progression (11.1 months versus 4.7 months;

TABLE 112.8A

Thalidomide Regimens in Relapsed/Refractory Multiple Myeloma

Study	Phase	N	Regimen	Media # of Prior Tx	Median TTP (mo)	CR/VGPR (%)	CR + PR (%)	Reference
Singhal	II	84	Thal	N/R	3.0 (EFS)	17	25	N Engl J Med 1999
Barlogie	II	169	Thal	N/R	~5 (EFS)	20	30	Blood 2001
Palumbo	II	77	Thal + Dex	2	12	18	41	Haematol 2001
Dimopoulos	II	44	Thal + Dex	3	4.2	30	55	Ann Oncol 2001
Terpos	II	50	MD-T	2	21.2	10 (CR)	62	Hematologica 2006

Tx, treatment; TTP, time to progression; CR, complete response; VGPR, very good partial response; PR, partial response; Thal, thalidomide; N/R, not reported; EFS, event-free survival; Dex, dexamethasone; MD-T, melphalan, dex, thalidomide.

p <0.001); and median overall survival (29.6 versus 20.2 months; p <0.001). In newly diagnosed patients, lenalidomide combined with dexamethasone achieves PR or better in over 90% of patients.[284] A similar study in Europe had almost identical results. Recently, lenalidomide and low-dose dexamethasone (Rd) versus melphalan, prednisone, and thalidomide (MPT) have been compared in a multicenter, open-label, phase 3 trial in newly diagnosed transplant-ineligible MM patients ≥65 years of age. A total of 1,623 patients (median age, 73 years) were randomized to one of three arms: Rd in 28-day cycles until disease progression (Arm A); Rd in 28-day cycles for 72 weeks (18 cycles, Arm B); or MPT in 42-day cycles for 72 weeks (12 cycles, Arm C). Overall response was 75%, 72%, and 62%, for Arms A, B, and C, respectively (p <0.00001). Continuous treatment with Rd (Arm A) had a 28% reduction in the risk of progression or death (hazard ratio [HR] = 0.72; p = 0.00006), with a 22% reduction in risk of death in favor of Arm A versus Arm C (HR = 0.78; p = 0.01685). All other secondary end points also showed an improvement in favor of Arm A versus Arm C; DOR (HR = 0.63; p <0.00001), and PFS2 (HR = 0.78; p = 0.0051). In Arm A versus Arm C

grade 3/4 neutropenia was 28% versus 45% and neuropathy 5% versus 15%. This study establishes Rd with continuous treatment until progression as a standard of care in newly diagnosed MM in older individuals.[285] Tables 112.9A and B list selected major studies demonstrating the activity of lenalidomide in both relapsed and newly diagnosed myeloma. Importantly, no significant somnolence, constipation, or neuropathy is observed with lenalidomide. However, myelosuppression was the dose-limiting toxicity and requires monitoring during therapy. Similar to thalidomide, it is associated with an increased incidence of DVT and requires concurrent prophylactic measures for its prevention.[282] Due to its renal excretion, a dose modification is necessary when used in patients with renal dysfunction.

Bortezomib. Bortezomib is the first-in-class proteasome inhibitor originally used in MM due to its blockade of NF-κB activation and related paracrine IL-6 production by BMSCs. Bortezomib has been subsequently demonstrated to act directly on MM cells to induce apoptosis through both caspase 8 and 9 activation, to overcome the protective effects of IL-6, and to add to the anti-MM

TABLE 112.8B

Thalidomide Regimens in Newly Diagnosed Multiple Myeloma

Study	Phase	N	Regimen	CR/VGPR (%)	CR + PR (%)	1-yr Survival (%)	Reference
Rajkumar (Mayo)	II	50	Thal + Dex	N/R	64	N/R	JCO 2002
Cavo	II	71	Thal + Dex	17	66	N/R	Hematologica 2004
Rajkumar, E1A00	III	103	Thal + Dex	4 (CR)	63	80	JCO 2006
Rajkumar, MM003	III	470	Thal + Dex	44	69	80	ASH 2006
Palumbo	III	129	MP-T	36	76	87	Lancet 2006
Facon	III	124	MP-T	50	81	88	ASCO 2006
Barlogie	III	323	TT2 + Thal	69	83	92	N Engl J Med 2006
Goldschmidt	III	203	TAD	7	80	N/R	ASH 2005
Wang	II	36	Thal + Bort + Dex (VTD)	19	92	N/R	ASH 2005

CR, complete response; VGPR, very good partial response; PR, partial response; Thal, thalidomide; Dex, dexamethasone; N/R, not reported; MP-T, melphalan, prednisone, thalidomide; TT2, total therapy 2; TAD, thalidomide, adriamycin, dex; Bort, bortezomib.

TABLE 112.9A

Lenalidomide Regimens in Relapsed/Refractory Multiple Myeloma

Study	Phase	N	Regimen	Median # of Prior Tx	Median TTP (mo)	CR/VGPR (%)	CR + PR (%)	Reference
Richardson	I/II	24	Len	3	N/R	13	30	*Blood* 2002
Richardson	II	102	Len	>3	4.6	4	17	*Blood* 2006
Weber	III	171	Len + Dex	3	11.1	13	59	*ASCO* 2006
Dimopoulos	III	176	Len + Dex	3	11.3	15	59	*ASCO* 2006
Richardson	I	36	Len + Bort	5	N/R	6	39	*ASH* 2006
Richardson	I/II	28	Len + Bort + Dex	5	N/R	6	31	*ASH* 2006
Baz	I/II	52	Len + DVD (Len + PLD + Bort)	3	12	29	75	*Ann Oncol* 2006

Tx, treatment; TTP, time to progress; CR, complete response; VGPR, very good PR; PR, partial response; Len, lenalidomide; N/R, not reported; Dex, dexamethasone; Bort, bortezomib PLD, liposomal doxorubicin.

effects of Dex. Importantly, it acts in the microenvironment to inhibit the binding of MM cells to BMSCs, the secretion of MM growth promoting cytokines, and BM angiogenesis.[286–289] Based on its efficacy and safety profile in a phase 1 study, a multicenter phase 2 trial in 193 evaluable patients showed a 35% PR or greater response.[290] The median duration of response was 12 months, and the median OS was 16 months. Grade 3 adverse events included thrombocytopenia (28%), fatigue (12%), peripheral neuropathy (12%), and neutropenia (11%). The addition of Dex in this study improved responses in 19% patients, confirming synergism between these two agents. A subsequent randomized study in 669 patients with relapsed myeloma comparing bortezomib versus Dex reported a higher response rate (38% versus 18% respectively; p <0.001), a longer time to progression (6.22 months versus 3.49 months, respectively; p <0.001), and a longer survival (1-year survival rate 80% versus 66%, respectively; p = 0.003).[291] Tables 112.10A and B list selected major studies demonstrating its activity in both relapsed and newly diagnosed myeloma. In a randomized multicenter international study, the combination of bortezomib and pegylated liposomal doxorubicin was shown to be superior to bortezomib alone for both overall response (50% versus 42% respectively; p = 0.05) and time to progression (9.3 months versus 6.5 months respectively; p <0.0001), leading to U.S. Food and Drug Administration (FDA) approval of this combination in relapsed MM.[292] Bortezomib has been shown to overcome the adverse outcome associated with t(4;14),[293] can be given safely in patients with renal failure,[294] and improves osteoblastic activity.[295] The major toxicities include fatigue, diarrhea, reversible thrombocytopenia, and peripheral neuropathy. In a randomized phase 3 study of 222 relapsed MM patients, the subcutaneous administration of bortezomib was compared with traditional intravenous administration. overall response rates (ORR) after four cycles was 42% in both groups, and no significant differences in time to progression (median 10.4 months versus 9.4 months; p = 0.387) and 1-year OS (72.6% versus 76.7%; p = 0.504) were observed. Importantly, toxicity profiles were improved with the subcutaneous versus intravenous administration, including peripheral neuropathy of any grade (38% versus 53%; p = 0.044) and grade 2 or worse (24% versus 41%; p = 0.012), making subcutaneous administration a preferred route of administration.[296]

Induction Therapy in the Newly Diagnosed Patient

Decision about the induction regimen and its dose and schedule in newly diagnosed MM is partly influenced by the patient's age and comorbidities. Importantly, in a transplant-eligible patient, alkylating agents should be avoided because these agents may compromise stem cell collection. In newly diagnosed patients, thalidomide and dexamethasone have been demonstrated to be superior to dexamethasone alone (ORR 63% versus 41%, respectively; p = 0.0017).[297] Based on this data, thalidomide and dexamethasone is approved by the FDA as an induction regimen. With the availability of lenalidomide and bortezomib, alternative combinations have been investigated and are now preferred. The Southwest Oncology Group (SWOG) compared lenalidomide plus dexamethasone (LD) (n = 97) to placebo plus high-dose

TABLE 112.9B

Lenalidomide Regimens in Newly Diagnosed Multiple Myeloma

Study	Phase	N	Regimen	CR/VGPR (%)	CR + PR (%)	1-yr Survival Rate (%)	Reference
Rajkumar; Lacy	II	34	Len + Dex	56	91	90	*Blood* 2005
Niesvizky	II	42	Len + Dex + clarithro	51	94	86	*ASCO* 2006
Rajkumar, E4A03 Arm A	III	223	Len + standard-dose Dex	N/A	N/A	87	*Lancet Oncol.* 2007
Rajkumar, E4A03 Arm B	III	222	Len + low-dose Dex	N/A	N/A	96	*Lancet Oncol.* 2007
Palumbo	I/II	21	Len + MP (MP-R)	48	81	100	*EHA* 2007

CR, complete response; VGPR, very good PR; PR, partial response; Len, lenalidomide; Dex, dexamethasone; clarithro, clarithromycin; N/A, not available; MP, melphalan, prednisone; MP-R, MP+lenalidomide.

TABLE 112.10A

Bortezomib Regimens in Relapsed/Refractory Multiple Myeloma

Study	Phase	N	Regimen	Median # of Prior Tx	Median TTP (mo)	CR/VGPR (%)	CR + PR (%)	Reference
Richardson	II	188	Bort	>3	~7	10	27	*N Engl J Med* 2003
Richardson	III	333	Bort	2	6.2	4	43	*N Engl J Med* 2005
Richardson	I/II	28	Len + Bort + Dex	5	N/R	6	31	*ASH* 2006
Harrousseau	III	324	Bort + PLD	≥2	9.3	36	48	*ASH* 2006; *ASCO* 2007
Terpos	II	53	VMDT (Bort + Mel + Thal + Dex)	2	9.5	37	60	*ASH* 2006
Palumbo	I/II	30	Bort + MPT (VMPT)	3	N/R	43	67	*ASH* 2006

Tx, treatment; TTP, time to progress; CR, complete response; VGPR, verygood PR; PR, partial response; Bort, bortizomib; Len, lenalidomide; N/R, not reported; Dex, dexamethasone; Mel, melphalan; PLD, liposomal doxorubicin; Thal, thalidomide; VMDT, bortezomib, melphalan, dex, thalidomide; MPT, melphalan, prednisone, thalidomide.

dexamethasone (D) (n = 95) in newly diagnosed myeloma in a randomized study.[298] Overall response rate and 1-year progression-free survival were superior with LD (78% versus 48%; p <0.001 and 78% versus 52%; p = 0.002, respectively), whereas 1-year OS was similar (94% versus 88%; p = 0.25). Toxicities were more pronounced with LD (neutropenia grade 3 to 4: 21% versus 5%; p ≤0.001 and DVT despite aspirin prophylaxis: 23.5% versus 5%; p ≤0.001). A randomized study performed by ECOG compared lenalidomide at 25 mg daily for 3 weeks out of 4 along with high-dose Dex (40 mg days 1 through 4, 9 through 12, and 17 through 20) versus lenalidomide with low-dose Dex (40 mg once a week).[269] With 445 patients randomized, 79% patients receiving high-dose and 68% patients on low-dose dexamethasone had CR or PR within four cycles (p = 0.008). However, OS at 1 year was 96% versus 87% in favor of the low-dose dexamethasone group (p = 0.0002); and toxicity was also higher in the high-dose versus low-dose dexamethasone group (any grade 3 or 4 toxicity 52% versus 35%, respectively, p = 0.0001; early mortality 5.4% versus 0.5% respectively, p = 0.003 and DVT 26% versus 12% respectively, p = 0.0003). Bortezomib-containing regimens have also been evaluated in newly diagnosed patients. Jagannath et al.[299] have reported 18% CR and 88% overall response rates in a phase 2 study using a combination of bortezomib and Dex in newly diagnosed patients.

The IFM group has randomized 242 newly diagnosed patients to VAD or bortezomib plus dexamethasone (VD) followed by dexamethasone, cyclophosphamide, etoposide, cis-platinum (DCEP) consolidation and autologous stem-cell transplantation.[300] CR/nCR (15% versus 6%), at least VGPR (38% versus 15%), and overall response (79% versus 63%) rates after four cycles of induction therapy were significantly higher with VD compared to VAD. Interestingly, the superior response after induction also translated into significantly improved response after transplant with CR/nCR (35% versus 18%) and at least VGPR (54% versus 37%) rates in favor of VD compared to the VAD group. Median progression-free survival (PFS) was 36.0 months versus 29.7 months (p = 0.064) with VD versus VAD. The incidence of severe adverse events appeared similar between the groups. A short-term bortezomib induction has been reported to improve outcomes of patients with t(4;14) but not del(17p).[301] The recently approved proteasome inhibitor carfilzomib has also been evaluated in newly diagnosed patients. In combination with lenalidomide and dexamethasone, it achieves 94% overall response and 80% CR/nCR after 12 cycles. In a phase 1/2 study in patients with newly diagnosed MM (n = 53) after a median of 12 cycles of carfilzomib, lenalidomide, dexamethasone (CRd) (range, 1 to 25), 62% patients achieved at least a near CR and 42% stringent CR. In 36 patients completing eight

TABLE 112.10B

Bortezomib Regimens in Newly Diagnosed Multiple Myeloma

Study	Phase	N	Regimen	CR/VGPR (%)	CR + PR (%)	1-yr Survival (%)	Reference
Richardson	II	63	Bort	10	40	N/R	*ASCO* 2006
Jagannath	II	48	Bort ± Dex	19	90	80	*BrJH* 2005
Harousseau	II	48	Bort + Dex	31	66	N/R	*Haem* 2006
Harousseau	III	79	Bort + Dex	43	82	N/R	*ASH* 2006
Rosinol	II	40	Alternating Bort/Dex	22	64	N/R	*ASCO* 2007
Mateos	I/II	60	MP-V	43	89	87	*Blood* 2006
Oakervee	II	21	PAD	29	95	N/R	*BrJH* 2005
Orlowski	II	29	Bort + PLD	28	79	N/R	*ASH* 2006
Barlogie	II	303	TT3 with Bort	80	90	92	*ASCO* 2007

CR, complete response; VGPR, very good PR; PR, partial response; Bort (V), bortizomib; Dex (D), dexamethasone; N/R, not reported; Thal (T), thalidomide; MP, melphalan, prednisone; PAD, bortezomib, adriamycin, dex; PLD, liposomal doxorubicin; TT3, total therapy 3.

or more cycles, 78% patients reached at least a near CR and 61% achieved a stringent CR. With a median follow-up of 13 months (range, 4 to 25 months), the 24-month PFS estimate was 92%. Thus, CRd is well tolerated with exceptional response rates.[302]

With the success of two-drug combinations, three-drug combinations have been investigated with demonstrated high response rates. Bortezomib and dexamethasone have been combined with thalidomide (VTD: CR 32%, VGPR: 62%, and ORR: 94%), doxorubicin (VDD CR/nCR: 31%, VGPR: 42%, and ORR: 83%), cyclophosphamide[303] (VCD CR/nCR: 39%, VGPR: 61%, and ORR: 88%), and lenalidomide[304] (VRD CR/nCR: 52%, VGPR: 74%, and PR: 100%). A four-drug combination combining VRD with cyclophosphamide has not shown a clear benefit. These novel agent combinations have progressively improved both frequency and depth of responses in newly diagnosed patients with myeloma (Fig. 112.11).

For patients who are not transplant candidates, the same regimen described previously can be utilized. In addition, MP in combination with novel agents has significantly improved outcomes. Five randomized studies have compared MP with thalidomide (MPT) versus MP (Table 112.11) and demonstrated both superior overall response and complete response rate, as well as event-free survival (four out of five studies) and OS (two out of five studies), suggesting MPT as an active regimen in this patient population. The combination of bortezomib with MP (VMP) has been compared with MP in a randomized study,[305] which demonstrated superior CR and PR rates for the VMP regimen (71% versus 35% and 30% versus 4% respectively; p <0.001). The time to progression for the VMP group was 24.0 months, as compared with 16.6 months for the MP cohort (p <0.001). The combination of lenalidomide with MP followed by lenalidomide maintenance (MPRR) has been compared with

MP and demonstrated higher response rates (CR 18% versus 5% and ORR 76% versus 49%; p <0.001) and PFS (not reached versus 13.2 months; p = 0.002). A four-drug combination combining MPT with bortezomib has not shown significant further improvements.

High-Dose Therapy with Peripheral Blood Stem Cell Support

To overcome resistance to standard-dose therapy, a pilot study by the late Tim McElwain and his colleagues at the Royal Marsden Hospital evaluated the role of melphalan dose escalation (140 mg/m^2). They reported complete remissions in refractory patients[12]; however, treatment-related mortality was high due to BM toxicity. Bone marrow support in subsequent studies improved the treatment-related mortality, and dose escalation of melphalan to 200 mg/m^2 further improved response.

Transplant in Newly Diagnosed Patients

The initial demonstration of activity of high-dose melphalan therapy lead to series of evaluations of the role of high-dose therapy with stem cell support in myeloma. These studies reported complete remissions in up to 50% of patients, with prolongation of EFS and OS to more than 3 years and more than 5 to 6 years, respectively.[306–310]

The superiority of high-dose chemotherapy with autologous BM support was confirmed in a randomized trial conducted by IFM. The response rate (≥50% reduction in myeloma protein) in 100 patients receiving high-dose therapy (Mel-140 + TBI) was 81% (22% complete remission) compared with 57% (5% complete

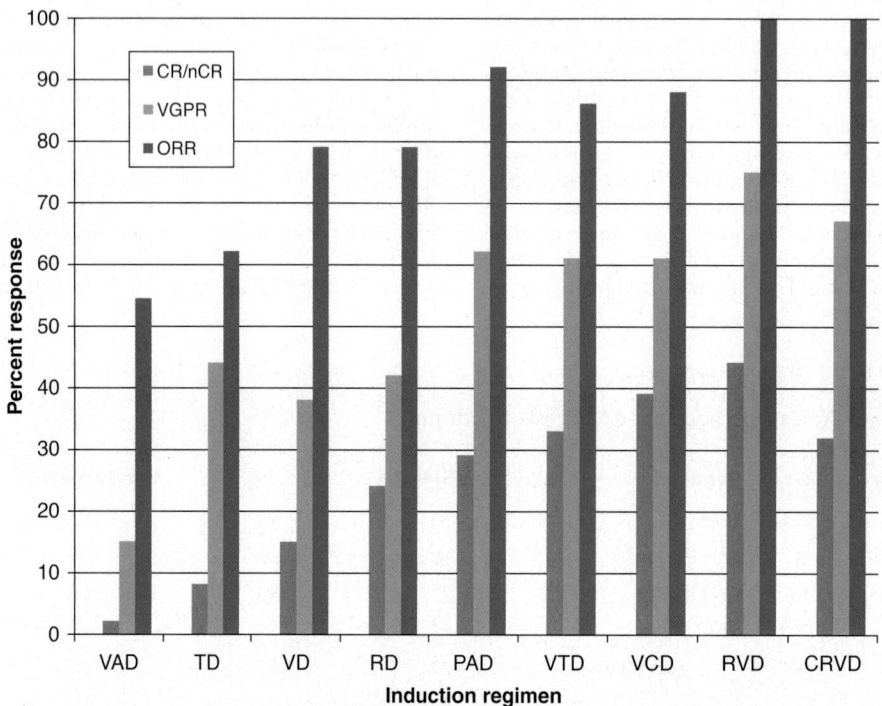

Figure 112.11 Progressive improvement in response to combination therapies incorporating newer agents. The nCR/CR, VGPR, and ORR rates following induction therapy of newly diagnosed multiple myeloma patients is plotted for common novel agent combinations selected from larger phase III and II studies and compared with VAD regimen. VAD, vincristine, adriamycin, and dexamethasone; T, thalidomide; D, dexamethasone; R, Lenalidomide; P, bortezomib; V, bortezomib (except in VAD); A, adriamycin; C, cyclophosphamide. CR/nCR, complete response/near CR; VGPR, very good partial response; ORR, overall response rate.

TABLE 112.11

Randomized Studies Comparing Mp-Related Regimens: Results

Authors/Study	Regimen	Complete Response	Partial Response	PFS (median months)	OS (median months)
Palumbo et al./GIMEMA[402]	MPT vs MP	16% vs 4% (p <0.001)	69% vs 48% (p <0.0001)	21.8 vs 14.5 (p = 0.0004)	45 vs 47.6 (p value NS)
Facon et al./IFM 99-06[403]	MPT vs MP	13% vs 2% (p = 0.0008)	76% vs 35% (p <0.0001)	27.5 vs 18 (p <0.0001)	51.5 vs 33 (p = 0.006)
Hulin et al./IFM 01-01[404]	MPT vs MP	7% vs 1% (p <0.001)	62% vs 31% (p <0.001)	24 vs 18.5 (p = 0.001)	44 vs 29 (p = 0.028)
Wijermans et al./HOVON[405]	MPT vs MP	2% vs 2%	66% vs 45% (p <0.001)	13 vs 9 (p <0.001)	40 vs 32 (p = 0.05)
Waage et al./NMSG[406]	MPT vs MP	–	57% vs 40% (p <0.0001)	15 vs 14 (p value NS)	29 vs 32 (p value NS)
San Miguel et al./VISTA[305]	MPV vs MP	30% vs 4% (p <0.001)	71% vs 35% (p <0.001)	24 vs 16.6[a] (p <0.001)	Not reached vs 43
Palumbo et al.[407]	MPRR vs MP	18% vs 5% (p <0.001)	77% vs 49% (p <0.001)	Not reached vs 13 (p = 0.002)	Not reached

MP, melphalan, prednisone; PFS, progression-free survival; OS, overall survival; NS, significant difference.
[a] TTP, time to progression.

remission) in a similar number of patients receiving standard-dose chemotherapy consisting of VMCP (vincristine, melphalan, cyclophosphamide, and prednisone) alternating with a BVAP (carmustine, vincristine, doxorubicin, and prednisone) regimen (p <0.001). Significantly longer event-free (median, 28 versus 18 months) and overall (median, 57 versus 42 months) survivals were reported after high-dose therapy (Fig. 112.12). The projected 5-year EFS and OS were 28% and 52% after high-dose therapy compared to 10% and 12% following standard-dose therapy, respectively.[311]

A similar response and survival benefit has been reported from the Medical Research Council (MRC)-VII trial, which randomized 407 patients to either standard-dose chemotherapy or HDT with transplantation.[312] A Spanish trial of 164 patients treated with HDT versus conventional therapy also showed a superior CR rate in the HDT arm, with a trend for prolonged EFS and OS in the HDT arm (Table 112.12).[313] In contrast, the Myeloma Autogreffe Group (MAG) trial by Fermand et al.[314] in 190 newly diagnosed MM pa-

tients failed to show superiority of HDT. The US intergroup study, which randomized patients between HDT versus conventional therapy followed by delayed HDT at relapse, failed to show superiority of HDT for either achievement of CR or OS; EFS benefit was modest (4 months) in the high-dose therapy cohort.[272] A meta-analysis combining nine studies comprising 2,411 patients reported a combined hazard of death with HDT of 0.92 (95% confidence interval [CI], 0.74 to 1.13) and a combined hazard of progression with HDT of 0.75 (95% CI, 0.59 to 0.96). The analysis of the randomized data indicated PFS benefit, but not OS benefit, for HDT with single autologous transplantation in multiple myeloma.[315]

Although the responses to induction therapy have now significantly improved with the use of novel agent combination therapies (see Fig. 112.11), some recent studies have indicated that HDT is able to further improve the depth of response (Fig. 112.13). These observations have raised questions about the role of HDT in newly diagnosed patients with myeloma receiving novel agent

PRACTICE OF ONCOLOGY

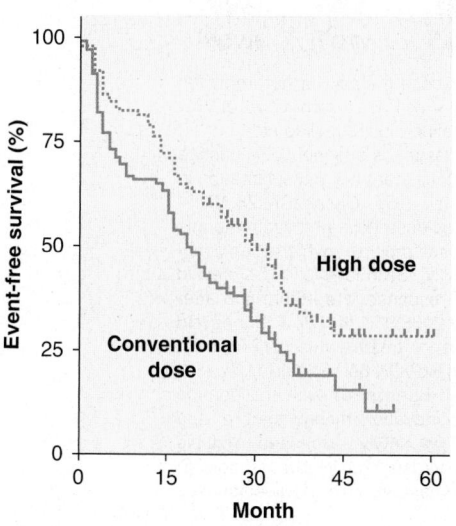
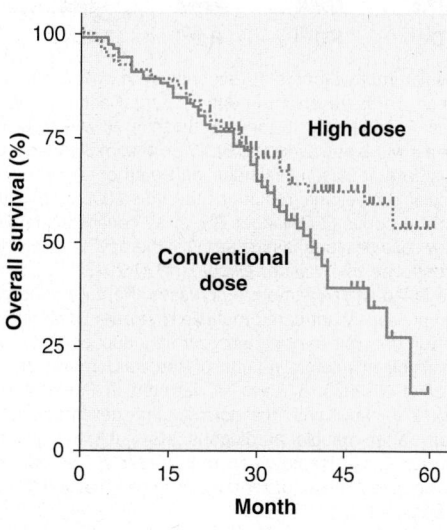

Figure 112.12 Comparative trials of high-dose therapy (HDT) versus standard-dose chemotherapy (SDT). IFM-90 (Intergroupe Francais de Myelome) randomized trial with 100 patients accrued to each arm comparing SDT with VMCP-VBAP and HDT with melphalan 140 mg/m² plus total body irradiation (800 cGy). Higher complete remission rates and significantly longer event-free and overall survival were noted with HDT. (From Harousseau JL, Attal M, Divine M, et al. Autologous stem cell transplantation after first remission induction treatment in multiple myeloma. A report of the French Registry on Autologous Transplantation in Multiple Myeloma. *Stem Cells* 1995;13:132–139, with permission.)

TABLE 112.12

Results of Large Randomized Study Comparing Standard Dose Therapy Versus High-Dose Therapy

Authors		No. of Patients (n)	CR (%)	EFS (median months)	OS (median months)
Attal et al.[311]	Conventional	100	5[b]	18[b]	37[b]
	HDT	100	22	27	52
Fermand et al.[314]	Conventional	96	–	18.7[b]	50.4[a]
	HDT	94	–	24.3	55.3
Blade et al.[313]	Conventional	83	11[b]	34.3[b]	66.9[a]
	HDT	81	30	42.5	67.4
Child et al.[312]	Conventional	200	8.5[b]	19.6[b]	42.3[b]
	HDT	201	44	31.6	54.8
Barlogie et al.[272]	Conventional	255	15[a]	21[a]	53[a]
	HDT	261	17	25	58

CR; complete remission; EFS, event-free survival; OS, overall survival; HDT, high-dose therapy.
[a] No significant difference.
[b] Significant difference.

combination therapy. Two recent studies have reconfirmed the role of high-dose therapy in myeloma. In one study, patients received four cycles of lenalidomide and dexamethasone and were then randomized to either Cytoxan, lenalidomide, and dexamethasone (CRD) for six cycles or HDT with melphalan 200 mg/m² (Mel200) with transplant. PFS with Mel200 was significantly longer than after CRD: 27 months versus not reached (p = 0.012). A second study compared MPR versus Mel200 after Rd induction therapy and reported superior PFS (24 versus 36 months respectively (p <0.0001) with a trend in improved 5-year OS, 62 versus

71% (p = 0.27) in favor of Mel200. An ongoing study is evaluating the role of transplant in patients receiving RVD combination.

Tandem Transplants

Attempts to further improve the results of autotransplantation have included intensification with tandem transplants. Harousseau et al.[316] were the first to report feasibility of tandem autologous BM transplantation, with a 69% CR rate in a small select group of patients. Barlogie et al.[317] investigated a sequential non–cross-resistant

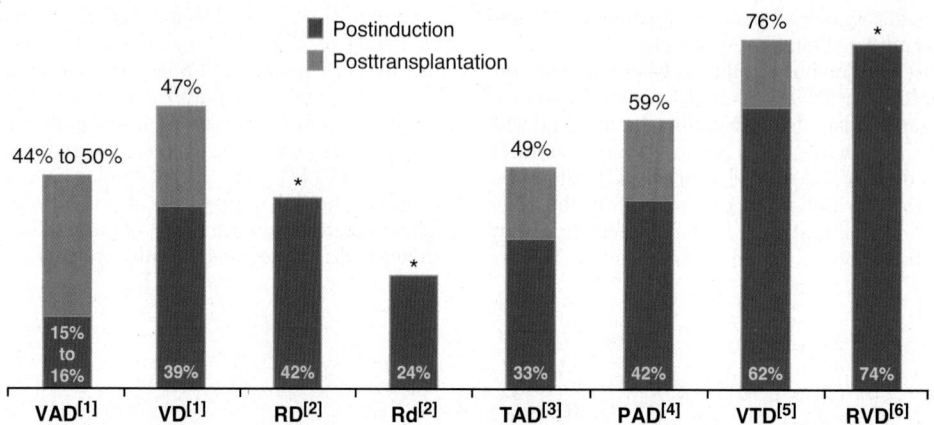

Figure 112.13 Despite improvements in response with novel agents, high-dose therapy further improves the depth of response. * Posttransplant intention-to-treat data not available. V or P, bortezomib except VAD where V is vincristine; A, Adriamycin; D, dexamethasone; d, weekly D; R, lenalidomide; T, thalidomide.
1. Harousseau JL, Attal M, Avet-Loiseau H, et al. Bortezomib plus dexamethasone is superior to vincristine plus doxorubicin plus dexamethasone as induction treatment prior to autologous stem-cell transplantation in newly diagnosed multiple myeloma: results of the IFM 2005-01 phase III trial. *J Clin Oncol* 2010;28:4621–4629. 2. Rajkumar SV, Jacobus S, Callander NS, et al. Lenalidomide plus high-dose dexamethasone versus lenalidomide plus low-dose dexamethasone as initial therapy for newly diagnosed multiple myeloma: an open-label randomised controlled trial. *Lancet Oncol* 2010;11:29–37. 3. Lokhorst HM, Schmidt-Wolf I, Sonneveld P, et al. Thalidomide in induction treatment increases the very good partial response rate before and after high-dose therapy in previously untreated multiple myeloma. *Haematologica* 2008;93:124–127. 4. Sonneveld P, Schmidt-Wolf IG, van der Holt B, et al. Bortezomib induction and maintenance treatment in patients with newly diagnosed multiple myeloma: results of the randomized phase III HOVON-65/ GMMG-HD4 trial. *J Clin Oncol* 2012;30:2946–2955. 5. Cavo M, Tacchetti P, Patriarca F, et al. Bortezomib with thalidomide plus dexamethasone compared with thalidomide plus dexamethasone as induction therapy before, and consolidation therapy after, double autologous stem-cell transplantation in newly diagnosed multiple myeloma: a randomised phase 3 study. *Lancet* 2010;376:2075–2085. 6. Richardson PG, Weller E, Lonial S, et al. Lenalidomide, bortezomib, and dexamethasone combination therapy in patients with newly diagnosed multiple myeloma. *Blood* 2010;116:679–686.

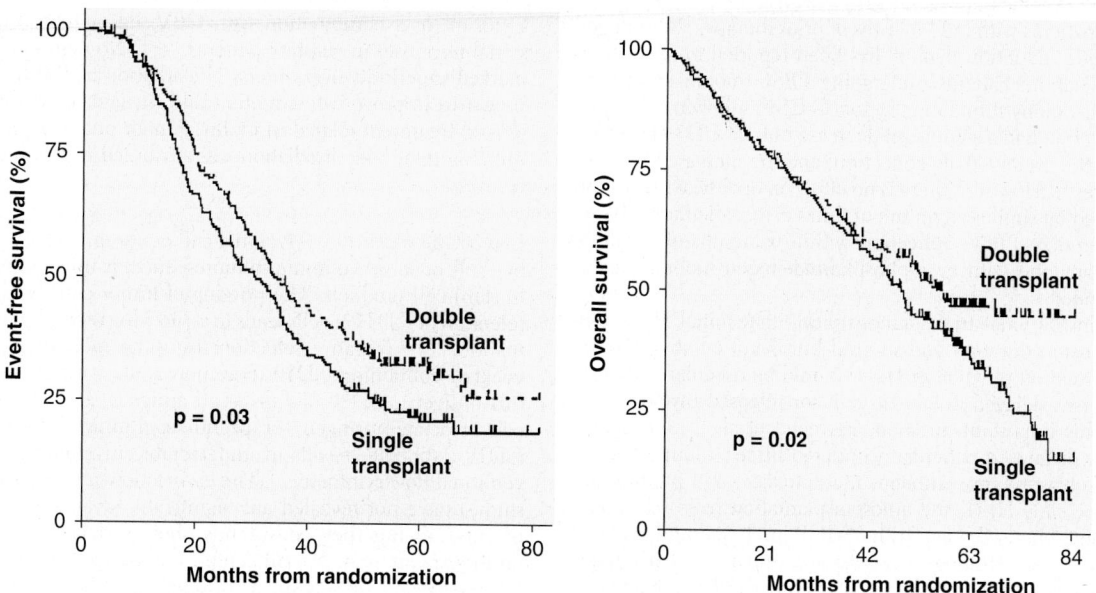

Figure 112.14 Comparative trial of single versus double high-dose therapy (HDT). IFM 94 trial with 399 patients randomized to a single HDT with melphalan 140 mg/m² plus total body irradiation (800 cGy) versus first HDT with melphalan 140 mg/m² and subsequent second HDT with melphalan 140 mg/m² plus total body irradiation (800 cGy). Superior event-free and overall survival was noted with double HDT. (From Attal M, Harousseau JL, Facon T, et al. Single versus double autologous stem-cell transplantation for multiple myeloma. *N Engl J Med* 2003;349:2495–2502, with permission.)

remission induction regimen followed by tandem autologous transplantations (*total therapy*) in 231 newly diagnosed patients: 41% of patients achieved CR after two transplants, and the median EFS and OS times were 43 months and 68 months, respectively.

Attal et al.[245] (IFM-94) reported a randomized comparison of single HDT (melphalan [140 mg/m²] and TBI [8 Gy]) versus double HDT (melphalan [200 mg/m²], followed by melphalan [140 mg/m²] and TBI [8 Gy]) in 399 newly diagnosed patients. This study reported no significant improvement in CR or very good PR rate between the two arms (42% versus 50% respectively; p = 0.10); however, there was a significant improvement in the double HDT arm in probability of EFS at 7 years (10% versus 20%; p = 0.03) and estimated OS at 7 years (21% versus 42%; p = 0.01) (Fig. 112.14). A similar study by the Dutch-Belgian Hematology-Oncology Cooperative Group (HOVON) (n = 255) showed a su-

perior CR rate (13 versus 28%) and EFS (20 versus 22 months) in favor of tandem transplants; however, it failed to show OS benefit. The MAG (n = 193) and Bologna (n = 178) trials, with a median follow-up of 27 to 30 months, have not yet shown a significant benefit for tandem transplantation (Table 112.13).

Various factors need special consideration in the management of myeloma with high-dose chemotherapy. These factors include a source of stem cells, the conditioning regimen, the timing of transplant, and tumor-cell purging.

Timing of High-Dose Therapy. To obtain high-quality hematopoietic stem cells, the ideal timing for stem cell collection is early in the course of the induction treatment. The ability to collect adequate stem cells (≥2 × 10⁶ CD34+ cells per kilogram) in patients with less than 12 months of prior therapy is 86% compared

TABLE 112.13

Single Versus Double ASCT for Newly Diagnosed Multiple Myeloma

Study	ASCT	No. of Patients	CR (%)[a]	Median EFS (mo)	Median OS (mo)
Attal et al.[245] (IFM94)	Single	199	42[b] (p = NS)	25 (p = 0.03)	48 (p = 0.01)
	Double	200	50[b]	30	58
Fermand et al.[314] (MAG95)	Single	94	42[a] (p = NS)	No difference	No difference
	Double	99	37[a]		
Sonneveld et al.[408] (HOVON24)	Single	148	13 (p = 0.002)	20 (p = 0.02)	55 (p = NS)
	Double	155	28	22	50
Cavo et al.[409] (Bologna 96)	Single	115	35 (p = NS)	Significant prolongation of EFS with double SCT	59 (p = NS)
	Double	113	48		73

ASCT, autologous stem cell transplantation; CR, complete remission; EFS, event-free survival; OS, overall survival; SCT, stem cell transplant.
[a] CR + minimum residual disease.
[b] CR + VGPR.

to 48% in patients with >24 months of prior therapy.[318] Prolonged lenalidomide induction therapy has been reported to affect stem cell mobilization. Patients undergoing PBSC mobilization with granulocyte-colony stimulating factor (G-CSF) following lenalidomide induction had a significant decrease in total CD34 (+) cells collected, the average daily collection, and the increased number of aphereses.[319] However, there is no effect on quality of PBSC collected based on similar engraftment times across all groups. Based on these studies, PBSC collection within 6 months of lenalidomide therapy and with cyclophosphamide-based mobilization is recommended.[320,321]

Multi-institutional trials demonstrating that initial HDT prolongs remission duration and survival but is not curative has led to the exploration of whether HDT should be used early after diagnosis versus delayed as a treatment for relapsed myeloma. To evaluate this important question, Fermand et al.[314] randomized 185 newly diagnosed patients to undergo three to four cycles of VAMP (vinblastine, doxorubicin, methotrexate, and prednisone) followed by early HDT and autotransplantation (n = 91) versus conventional chemotherapy with VMCP for 1 year and HDT at relapse (n = 94). Although patients who underwent early transplantation had significantly longer EFS times (39 months versus 13 months), OS was identical in both arms (median, 64.6 and 64 months). Importantly, the time without symptoms and toxicity analysis reflecting quality of life (mean, 27.8 versus 22.3 months) showed superior results for the early HDT arm (Table 112.14). Vesole et al.[322] have confirmed effectiveness of high-dose chemotherapy as a salvage therapy achieving EFS and OS times of 21 and >43 months, respectively, in 135 patients with advanced refractory MM. In this study, patients with primary unresponsive disease had superior outcomes to patients with resistant relapse (progression on last-salvage chemotherapy), with EFS of 37 months versus 17 months, respectively (p = 0.0004), and OS of 43 months versus 21 months, respectively (p = 0.0003). Gertz et al.,[323] from the Mayo clinic, have also reported a similar experience in 64 patients undergoing elective delayed transplant at the time of progression following standard therapy. Finally, the Intergroup trial in the United States randomizing patients to up-front high-dose therapy or standard therapy with high-dose therapy as a salvage treatment also confirms a similar modest EFS benefit for early versus late transplants.[272]

High-Dose Regimen. High-dose melphalan (140 to 200 mg/m^2), with or without total body irradiation, is the most common conditioning regimen used in myeloma.[324-326] Melphalan's predominant myelotoxicity and metabolism independent of renal function is ideal for MM patients who commonly have renal function abnormalities. Melphalan seems to be superior to thioTEPA when given with total body irradiation, with patients achieving longer relapse-free and overall survival duration.[326] A combination regimen containing high-dose carboplatin with etoposide and

Cytoxan, or a combination with CBV, has achieved only occasional responses in resistant patients.[327,328] No regimen has shown marked superiority over others. The addition of TBI has not been shown to improve cytoreduction and, in fact, increases morbidity and treatment-related mortality. A poor outcome in one study utilizing total body irradiation was attributed to delayed immune recovery.

Stem Cell Purging. Myeloma cell contamination, as evaluated by PCR or sensitive immunofluorescence, is universally observed in stem cell products. The purging of tumor cells by the positive selection of CD34+ cells leads to a 3 to 5 log reduction in contamination.[329,330] Negative selection using the monoclonal antibody cocktail containing CD10 (common acute lymphoblastic leukemia antigen); CD20 (a pan B-cell antigen); and PCA-1 (plasma cell–associated antigen) or peanut agglutinin (PNA) and anti-CD19 antibodies results in undetectable myeloma cells by conventional flow cytometry.[309] The early follow-up results from these studies have not revealed any significant advantage in responses or survival, but they consistently show a delay in engraftment posttransplantation. A multicenter, randomized study comparing CD34-selected PBSCs versus unselected PBSCs in 131 patients failed to show any significant difference in EFS or OS time.[331] Even when cells were purged using FACS sorting of very early hematopoietic stem cells (CD34$^+$, Thy1$^+$, and Lin), relapses were frequent and patients had delayed hematopoietic engraftment and suppressed immune status for prolonged periods of time.[332,333] Due to these data, emphasis is now on strategies to improve responses to HDT, rather than on purging autografts.

Hematopoietic Stem Cell Source. Mobilized PBSCs provide for more rapid engraftment compared to BM. Myeloma patients with less than 1 year of prior therapy had faster granulocyte and platelet recovery after peripheral blood stem cell transplants compared with BM autografts.[334] The duration of prior chemotherapy, especially with stem-cell–damaging agents (melphalan, BCNU, and high-doses of cyclophosphamide) along with radiation to BM-containing areas, significantly affects the ability to procure adequate quantities of PBSCs and engraftment kinetics posttransplant.[335] After mobilization with cyclophosphamide and GM-CSF, normal PBSCs are mobilized during the first 3 days of leukapheresis, whereas peak levels of contaminating myeloma cells are present on subsequent days. These myeloma cells show a higher LI and a more immature phenotype (CD19$^+$).[336]

Management of Older Patients

Unlike in the past, melphalan and prednisone is no longer a standard of care for older adults with myeloma. The two- and three-drug combinations of novel agents described previously for newly diagnosed patients remains an important option. In this age group, which most of the time is not considered eligible for transplant, the combination of bortezomib, or lenalidomide, or both with dexamethasone is considered the preferred option. However, MP in combination with these novel agents also achieves high levels of response and can be considered an alternative (see Fig. 112.11). A recent study showing superiority and decreased secondary malignancy risk of continuous Rd combination over MPT suggests that future utilization of MP based therapy will decrease in newly diagnosed older individuals with myeloma. To manage toxicity, the dose of therapeutic agents, including dexamethasone, needs to be reduced in patients >75 years of age.[337] The presence of comorbidities, frailty, and disabilities needs to be assessed and considered in the selection of agents and dose modifications.[338] As the incidence of myeloma increases with age, the role of HDT has also been evaluated in patients >65 years old. Older age does not impact stem cell mobilization or engraftment.[339] The feasibility and efficacy of HDT with PBSC transplant has been evaluated

TABLE 112.14

Stem Cell Transplantation as Upfront Versus Rescue Treatment: Results of a Randomized Study

	Early Transplant N = 91	Late Transplant N = 94
CR	19%	5%
Med EFS	39 mo	13 mo
Med OS	64.6 mo	64 mo
TWISTT	27.8 mo	22.3 mo

Note: Median f/u 58 months.
CR, complete remission; EFS, event-free survival; TWISTT, time without symptoms or treatment toxicity.
[a] Significant difference.

in patients 70 years old (median age, 72 years of age; range, 70 to 83 years of age) treated with melphalan (200 mg/m^2 or 140 mg/m^2).[340] Of note, treatment-related mortality was higher (16%) in the initial 25 patients receiving melphalan at 200 mg/m^2. CR was achieved in 27% patients, but median CR duration was only 1.5 years, with 3-year EFS and OS rates projected at 20% and 31%, respectively. Although this study confirms the feasibility of HDT in older patients with MM, it also indicates a higher risk in this patient population. High response rates using the novel agent combinations are decreasing the consideration of HDT in this elderly population.

Management of Patients with Renal Dysfunction

One-third of patients with overt MM present with renal insufficiency. With hydration, control of hypercalcemia, and effective therapy, it is reversible in 50% cases. Renal dysfunction of <6 months duration and the rapid initiation of therapy with a reduction in monoclonal protein are associated with a higher likelihood of improvement in renal function. Improved renal function is observed mainly in patients with light chain cast nephropathy and light chain deposition disease; therefore, renal biopsy is used to identify these reversible conditions and the need for aggressive treatment. A number of agents can be safely used in patients with renal dysfunction. This includes steroids, melphalan,[341] cyclophosphamide, bortezomib,[294,342] and thalidomide. Ease of administration, limited toxicity, and effectiveness make these novel agents the primary modes of therapy for myeloma patients with renal failure. In one retrospective analysis, 24 patients on dialysis were treated with bortezomib or bortezomib-based combinations. Of 20 patients with available response data, 75% patients achieved at least PRs, with 30% patients achieving CRs + near CRs. One patient was spared dialysis, and three other patients became independent of dialysis following bortezomib-based treatment.[294,342] Lenalidomide has predominant renal excretion and requires dose modification if used in patients with renal failure based on creatinine clearance.[342] However, pomalidomide can be safely administered in these patients. Because the pharmacokinetics of melphalan are unaltered by renal failure, such patients have been previously considered as potential candidates for high-dose therapy.[341] In one study, high-dose melphalan and PBSC transplantation was used to treat 81 patients with MM and renal dysfunction (creatinine >2 mg per deciliter).[343] Although renal failure had no impact on the quality of stem cell collection and/or engraftment, treatment-related mortality rates were 6% and 13% after the first and second autologous SCTs, respectively, and melphalan at 200 mg/m^2 caused excessive toxicity. Complete remission was achieved in 31 patients (38%) after tandem SCT, and the probabilities of EFS and OS at 3 years were 48% and 55%, respectively. Dose reduction and close monitoring are therefore needed to ensure the safety of the procedure, and the role of transplantation in the setting of renal failure remains investigational.

Maintenance Therapy

Despite improvements in remission rates, there is no clear plateau in the survival curves following conventional or HDT. Although the proportion of patients achieving complete responses has increased, all patients eventually relapse. Various maintenance therapies have been evaluated in MM in an effort to sustain remission. IFN-α is the most widely evaluated agent as maintenance therapy; however, randomized studies have only demonstrated modest improvements in EFS and OS times (5 to 12 months) in patients achieving remission with standard-dose therapy, and its role following HDT has not been confirmed.[344] Low-dose prednisone administered on alternate days has prolonged remission duration following standard-dose therapy in a single randomized study.[345] In the last few years, many studies have evaluated novel agent-based maintenance regimens (Table 112.15). Attal and his

TABLE 112.15

Randomized Studies Comparing Maintenance Therapy in Myeloma

Authors/ Study	Regimen	PFS (median months)	OS (median months)
Spencer et al.[410]	Control vs thalidomide/ prednisone	23 vs 42 (p <0.001)	75 vs 86 (p = 0.004)
Barlogie et al.[411]	Control vs thalidomide	44% vs 57% (p = 0.01)[a]	Not reached
Attal et al.[346]	Control vs thalidomide + pamidronate	36 vs 52 (p = 0.009)	77 vs 87 (p = 0.04)
Attal et al.[347]	Control vs lenalidomide	24 vs Not reached (p <0.0001)	80% vs 88%[b]
Palumbo et al.[348]	MPRR vs MPR	Not reached vs 13.2 (p = 0.002)	Not reached
McCarthy et al.[349]	Control vs lenalidomide	Not reached vs 25.5 (p <0.001)[c]	Not reached
Mateos et al.[351]	VP vs VT	32 vs 24 (p = 0.01)	Not reached

PFS, progression-free survival; OS, overall survival; NA, not accessed; M, melphalan; P, prednisone; R, lenalidomide; RR lenalidomide with maintenance; V, bortezomib; T, thalidomide.
[a] Five-year PFS rates.
[b] Survival after 3 years.
[c] TTP, time to progression.

colleagues from the IFM group reported improved probability of EFS and OS at 3 years in patients receiving thalidomide and pamidronate compared to the patient cohorts receiving either pamidronate alone or no maintenance therapy following high-dose therapy (PFS 52%, 37%, and 36%, respectively; p <0.009; OS 87%, 74%, and 77%, respectively; p <0.04).[346] In this study, patients had not received thalidomide prior to its evaluation as maintenance therapy, and the benefit was observed in those patients who had further evidence of response to thalidomide. The prolonged use of thalidomide leads to the development of neuropathy, and more recently, lenalidomide, which has a more favorable toxicity profile, has been evaluated as maintenance therapy in the dose of 10 to 15 mg daily for 21 out of a 28-day cycle in three different studies: two posttransplantations and one following standard-dose MPR therapy.[347–349] All three studies show clear evidence of benefit, evidenced by the prolongation of PFS. One of the studies (CALGB 100104) has now shown OS benefit with lenalidomide maintenance, whereas two other studies with limited follow-ups are yet to observe an OS improvement. Importantly, all three studies show a small increased incidence of second primary malignancy in the arms receiving lenalidomide compared to placebo. This has prompted a careful evaluation and discussion with the patient of the benefit of lenalidomide maintenance. Because of its significant benefit, lenalidomide is considered the standard of care for maintenance therapy in myeloma. The HOVON trial has compared vincristine, adriamycin, and dexamethasone induction followed by high-dose melphalan and transplantation with Velcade maintenance versus Velcade, adriamycin, and dexamethasone induction high-dose melphalan and transplantation followed by thalidomide maintenance. With a 5-year follow-up, there is a PFS and OS benefit in the Velcade arm, including patients with high-risk (p17 deleted) MM.[350] In the nontransplant population, a recent study has also highlighted the use of a Velcade-based maintenance regimen especially in combination with low-dose thalidomide.[351] Additional immune manipulations, such as idiotype vaccinations, protein-pulsed dendritic cell–based vaccinations, dendritic cell–MM cell fusion vaccinations, and/or PD-1 checkpoint blockades are all strategies under evaluation as maintenance treatments to prolong EFS and OS in patients with myeloma.[352,353]

Minimal Residual Disease

Due to improvements in therapies, higher frequencies and depth of responses are being observed. There is emerging data that patients achieving CRs have superior survival outcomes compared to those achieving partial responses or no responses. This has now led to the investigation of methods to refine CR definition. The current definition includes the absence of paraprotein in the urine and serum by immunofixation and the disappearance of clonal plasma cells in the bone marrow using cytologic examination; stringent CR in addition requires normalization of the kappa/lambda free light chain ratio. The newer sensitive seven-color flow cytometric immunophenotypic assays can detect 1 clonal cell in 10^4 normal cells, and a molecular method that incorporates allele-specific oligonucleotide PCR (ASO-PCR) can detect up to 1 clonal cell in 10^{5-6} normal cells, each enhancing the ability to detect greater depth of response. To obviate the need for patient-specific customization, a sequencing-based molecular method is now being developed that identifies clonal gene rearrangements using consensus primers to universally amplify rearranged IgH and k gene segments, followed by high-throughput sequencing to quantify these rearrangements in follow-up minimal residual disease (MRD) samples.[354] In early studies using multiparameter flow cytometry, the prognostic value of MRD was assessed: in 378 patients after induction therapy and at day 100 after autologous stem cell transplantation (ASCT) and in 245 patients at the end of induction therapy in nontransplant patients. In patients undergoing ASCT, the absence of MRD at day 100 after ASCT was highly predictive of a favorable outcome (PFS, $p < 0.001$; OS, $p = 0.0183$), including in patients achieving immunofixation-negative CR ($p = 0.0068$). An MRD assessment after induction therapy in the non–intensive-pathway patients was not predictive of outcome (PFS, $p = 0.1$). This and other emerging data highlight the need to measure and achieve molecular CR in myeloma.[355] Similarly, in a study using a multiparameter flow cytometry method to detect MRD in 241 patients in CR at day +100 after ASCT, the detection of persistent MRD after ASCT was the only independent factor (HR, 8.0; $p = 0.005$), besides high-risk cytogenetics, that predicted for unsustained CR and a poor outcome.[356]

Allogeneic Transplantation

Syngeneic Transplantation

Bensinger et al.[357] have reported their experience with 11 patients receiving syngeneic transplants: Five patients achieved CR and three achieved PR, with one patient from both groups alive at 9 and 15 years after transplantation, respectively. A larger experience from the European bone marrow transplant (EBMT) Registry compared 25 patients undergoing syngeneic transplants with 125 case-matched patients undergoing autotransplantation or allogeneic transplantation.[358] The complete remission rate was not significantly different between the three grafts (twin: 68%, autologous: 48%, and allogeneic: 58%). However, patients undergoing syngeneic transplantation had significantly superior median survival time compared with autologous (72 months versus 25 months; $p = 0.009$) or allogeneic (72 months versus 16 months; $p = 0.008$) transplant recipients.

Allogeneic Transplantation

Allogeneic transplantation has remained a difficult procedure in myeloma. An elder age population with limited donor availability coupled with frequent renal impairment has restricted the use of

---

TABLE 112.16

Studies of Allogeneic Transplantation for Newly Diagnosed Myeloma

Authors	No. of Patients	TRM (%)	CR (%)	OS (actuarial, months)	EFS (actuarial, months)
Gahrton et al.	162	41	44	28% at 84	45% at 60
Bensinger et al.	80	44	36	20% at 54	24% at 54
Alyea et al.	61[a]	5	28	40% at 36	20% at 38

TRM, treatment-related mortality; CR, complete remission; OS, overall survival; EFS, event-free survival.
[a] T-cell depleted.

matched sibling transplantation in MM. Additionally, almost 50% 1-year mortality has limited use of this procedure to only a high-risk patient population. Importantly, the allogeneic graft versus myeloma (GVM) effect may result in a favorable long-term outcome after allogeneic transplantation. Results of three large studies are listed in Table 112.16. A retrospective analysis of a case-matched analysis of EBMT registry data compared 189 patients receiving allografts with an equal number of patients from the same time period receiving autotransplants. This study showed a superior median survival outcome for patients undergoing autotransplants compared to allogeneic transplants (34 versus 18 months, respectively).[359] The 1-year treatment-related mortality was significantly higher following allogeneic transplantation (41% with allotransplants and 13% with autotransplants). However, patients undergoing allogeneic transplantation and surviving the 1st year had a tendency for better PFS and OS.

A very low transplant-related mortality of 10% has been reported from a single-center experience from the Dana-Farber Cancer Institute due to the selective depletion of CD6$^+$ T cells as the sole form of a graft versus host disease (GvHD) prophylaxis.[360] However, the median PFS time was 12 months, and the median OS time was 22 months, a result inferior to their previous experience of autologous transplantation. Case-matched comparative studies from other single institutions have also failed to show a survival advantage for allotransplants.[361]

Donor Lymphocyte Infusions

A GVM effect has been demonstrated by the induction of CR with donor lymphocyte infusion (DLI) following relapse after allogeneic transplantation.[362] In a large study, Lokhorst et al.[363] have reported 6 CR and 8 PR following DLI in 27 patients after allotransplant. Five of these patients remained disease free >30 months after DLI. However, DLI was associated with acute GvHD in 55% and chronic GvHD in 26% of patients. Five patients experienced BM aplasia, which was fatal in two cases. A similar DLI experience has been reported by Salama et al.[364] Several strategies have been explored to reduce GvHD after DLI,[365,366] including lowering the number of T cells infused, the selective depletion of CD8$^+$ T cells, and the use of herpes simplex virus (HSV) thymidine kinase gene transduction of DLI to allow for use of ganciclovir to deplete T cells if significant GvHD develops. Immunizing donors with an idiotype vaccine may allow for the selective transfer of T cells specific for GVM without increasing the incidence of GvHD.

Nonmyeloablative Transplants

Studies in a canine model showed that a nonmyeloablative dose of TBI could lead to successful engraftment when used in conjunction with a combination of cyclosporine and

TABLE 112.17

Representative Studies of Miniallogeneic Transplantation in Myeloma

Authors	Conditioning	No. of Patients	TRM at 1 year (%)	Response (%)	Acute Grade II–IV GVHD (%)	Chronic Extensive GVHD (%)	PFS/EFS/DFS	OS
Lee et al.[412]	Mel or Mel/ TBI/Flu	45	36	CR 64	36	36	3-y EFS 13%	Median 14 mo 2 y 74%
Maloney et al.[370]	PBSCT + TBI/ MMF/cvc	54	7	CR 57 PR 26	39	46	2-y PFS 55%	18 mo 78%
Bruno et al.[371]	PBSCT + TBI/ MMF/Cyc	58	7	CR 55 PR 31	43	36	Median 43 mo	Median >46 mo

TRM, treatment-related mortality; GVHD, graft versus host disease; PFS, progression free survival; EFS, event-free survival; DFS, disease-free survival; OS, overall survival; Mel, melphalan; TBI, total body irradiation; Flu, fludarabine; CR, complete response; PR, partial response; PBSCT, peripheral blood stem cell transplant; Cyc, cyclosporine.

mycophenolate mofetil.[367] This animal experience, coupled with reduced day 100 transplant-related mortality in pilot studies in patients, has allowed for allogeneic-matched sibling transplantation in patients who were otherwise considered poor risk for the standard allogeneic preparative regimen. Results from larger published studies evaluating nonmyeloablative regimens with allogeneic transplantation are listed in Table 112.17. Badros et al.[368] first reported on 31 patients undergoing allogeneic transplants following nonmyeloablative conditioning with melphalan (100 mg/m²). Transplant-related mortality in the first 120 days was low (10%). Nineteen (61%) patients achieved CR or near CR; however, acute GvHD developed in 18 patients (58%), and chronic GvHD was seen in 10 patients (35%).[368] Giralt et al.[369] have used reduced intensity conditioning with fludarabine and melphalan in 16 patients; successful engraftment was observed in all patients; however, the 100-day mortality rate was 20% and the 1-year mortality rate was 40%, with only six patients alive after a median follow-up period of 15 months. Maloney et al.[370] have evaluated the combination of initial autotransplantation for tumor cytoreduction followed by nonmyeloablative matched-sibling transplantation in 54 patients. The treatment was performed in an outpatient setting with a low 100-day mortality (2%). The overall response rate was 83%, with 53% achieving CRs. With a median follow-up of 552 days after allografting, OS is 78%. However, GvHD continues to be a problem; 38% of patients developed acute GvHD and 46% developing chronic GvHD requiring therapy.

In a more recent clinical study, 162 consecutive patients with newly diagnosed myeloma who were less than 65 years of age received induction therapy with VAD, followed by either nonmyeloablative total-body irradiation and stem cells from the HLA-identical sibling after an initial autograft (n = 80) or two consecutive myeloablative doses of melphalan, each of which was followed by autologous stem-cell rescue if an HLA-identical donor was not available (n = 82). After a median follow-up of 45 months (range, 21 to 90), the median OS (80 months versus 54 months; p = 0.01) and event-free survival (35 months versus 29 months; p = 0.02) were longer in the patients with HLA-identical siblings than in the patients without HLA-identical siblings. Treatment-related mortality did not differ significantly between the two groups, (p = 0.09) but disease-related mortality was significantly higher in the double-autologous transplant group (43% versus 7%; p <0.001). The cumulative incidence rates of > grades I and grade IV GvHD were 43% and 4%, respectively. These results suggest a role for allografting, especially in patients with high-risk disease where improvement in long-term outcome has been limited.[371] Although the early clinical results with nonmyeloablative transplants are encouraging, this

strategy is associated with significant morbidity due to acute and chronic GvHD and a mortality rate of 10% to 20% at 1 year. Another study by Risonol et al.[372] reported on 110 patients with MM undergoing ASCT, who either received a second ASCT (85 patients) or a reduced-intensity conditioning allograft (allo-RIC; 25 patients), depending on the HLA-matched sibling donor availability. Although there was a trend toward a longer PFS (median, 31 months versus not reached; p = 0.08) in favor of allo-RIC, it was associated with a trend toward a higher transplantation-related mortality (16% versus 5%; p = 0.07), and there was no statistical difference in event-free survival and overall survivals.[372] It should, therefore, only be utilized in the context of clinical trials attempting to improve patient outcome by both enhancing efficacy and reducing toxicity.[373] The CTN most recently compared single autografts followed by nonmyeloablative allografts if a matched donor was available versus a second autograft in the absence of an appropriate donor and found that the outcome was similar in both arms.[374] Due to attendant toxicity in all allografting studies, including nonmyeloablative regimens, allotransplant is recommended primarily in the context of a clinical trial to exploit the graft versus MM immune effect while avoiding attendant toxicity.

Bisphosphonates

The second- and third-generation bisphosphonates, pamidronate and zoledronate, reduce skeletal complications and bone pain in myeloma (Table 112.18).[375,376] Their mechanism of action includes the downregulation of osteoclast activity, decreased IL-6 production, the activation of gamma/delta T cells with antimyeloma activity, and the induction of apoptosis of osteoclasts through the inhibition of farnesyl and geranylgeranyl transferase activity.[377,378] Besides reducing bone-related problems, the continued administration of pamidronate over 21 months showed some survival advantage (21 versus 14 months; p = 0.041) in patients receiving salvage chemotherapy and pamidronate versus chemotherapy alone.[375,379] In vitro cytotoxic effects of bisphosphonates have been observed in myeloma cell lines[380,381] and patient cells in vitro, as well as in patient tumor specimens in the SCID-hu in vivo model. Preliminary reports of pamidronate administered alone frequently (every 2 weeks) have shown a response or delay in disease progression in occasional patients.[382] Pamidronate 90 mg and zoledronic acid 4 mg are equipotent in reducing bone-related problems in myeloma; the infusion time for zoledronic acid is 15 minutes compared to 1 to 2 hours for pamidronate.

The role of zoledronic acid was confirmed by the MRC Myeloma IX study, in which 1960 patients were randomized to

TABLE 112.18

Summary of Published Placebo-Controlled Trials of Bisphosphonates in Patients with Multiple Myeloma

	Belch et al.[413]	Lahtinen et al.[414]	Berenson et al.[375]
No. of Evaluable Patients	166	336	377
Bisphosphonate Therapy	Etidronate 5 mg/kg daily (oral)	Clondronate 2.4 g/d (oral) for 24 months	Pamidronate 90 mg (IV q 4 weeks × 9 cycles)
Lytic Bone Lesions	0	+	0
Pathologic Fractures	0	0	+
Radiation Therapy	NA	NA	+
Bone Pain	0	0	+
Hypercalcemia	0	0	+
Survival	−	0	+

0, no effect; +, beneficial effect; −, negative effect; NA, not assessed.

intravenous zoledronic acid or oral clodronic acid (1,600 mg per day): There was a significantly lower incidence of skeletal-related events with zoledronic acid (27% versus 35%, respectively; p = 0.0004) both in patients with and without bone lesions at baseline.[383] The results of this study support the early use of zoledronic acid in newly diagnosed MM, irrespective of bone disease status. A further analysis of this data suggested that its continued use beyond 2 years was beneficial. Interestingly, the study also showed that zoledronic acid reduced mortality by 16% versus clodronic acid (p = 0.0118), and extended median OS by 5.5 months (50.0 months versus 44.5 months; p = 0.04). Zoledronic acid also significantly improved PFS by 12% (95% CI, 2 to 20) versus clodronic acid (p = 0.0179), for the first time confirming antimyeloma activity of bisphosphonates. Rates of complete, very good partial, or partial response did not differ significantly between the zoledronic acid and clodronic acid groups.[384] Patients on long-term bisphosphonates should be monitored for development of renal toxicity. Renal dysfunction induced by pamidronate affects mainly tubules and manifests first as proteinuria followed by a rise in creatinine, whereas zoledronic acid affects glomeruli and manifests as a rise in creatinine without proteinuria. Even mild renal dysfunction requires bisphosphonate dose adjustment, and renal effects of bisphosphonates can be partly prevented by extending the duration of infusion. Osteonecrosis of the jaw (ONJ) is another complication of prolonged bisphosphonate therapy, which is observed in patients with dental procedures and in relationship to dental infection. In one study, 11 of 292 patients with MM (3.8%) had ONJ.[385] There is also some association between prolonged use and development of ONJ. Due to the increased detection of this complication, a prophylactic dental checkup and follow-up is recommended. After 2 years of administration, the frequency of administration of bisphosphonate may be modified in patients achieving VGPR or CR.[386] In a large phase 3 study, the antimyeloma activity of zoledronic acid has been described. Multiple agents directed at novel bone-directed targets are under investigation. The efficacy of denosumab, a RANKL-targeting antibody, has been confirmed in a phase 3 study in myeloma and breast cancer. An antibody targeting DKK-1 (BHQ-880), which improves osteoblastic activity, and a chimeric protein targeting

activin A (ACE-011), are currently under evaluation in phase 1/2 clinical studies.

Therapy in Relapsed Patients

The options and therapeutic strategies for relapsed MM patients depend on the induction regimen used and whether the patients have undergone high-dose therapy and stem cell transplant. With the availability of multiple novel agents that have been approved for clinical use in MM— bortezomib, lenalidomide/dexamethasone, bortezomib and liposomal doxorubicin, pomalidomide, and carfilzomib—the choice will partly depend on the agent or combination not used as an induction and on the presence of existing toxicity such as neuropathy, cytopenias, or DVT.

The results of the international randomized phase III trial of bortezomib (1.3 mg/m^2 intravenously [IV] on days 1, 4, 8, and 11 every 3 weeks for eight cycles) have demonstrated its superiority over dexamethasone alone (40 mg by mouth [PO] on days 1 through 4, 9 through 12, and 17 through 20 every 5 weeks for four cycles) in terms of response rates (38% versus 18%, respectively; p <0.001), median time to progression (6.22 months versus 3.49 months respectively; p <0.001) and survival (1-year survival 80% versus 66%, respectively; p = 0.003) in 669 relapsed patients with MM who had received one to three prior therapies.[291] Another open label study has further confirmed the ability of added dexamethasone to improve response in relapsed patients. Various combinations of bortezomib with other agents such as doxorubicin, cyclophosphamide, and melphalan have been used to treat patients with MM, and results of larger representative studies are shown in Table 112.10B. For example, a randomized phase 3 multicenter international study has confirmed that the combination of bortezomib and pegylated liposomal doxorubicin is superior to bortezomib alone for both overall response (50% versus 42% respectively; p = 0.05), and time to progression (9.3 months versus 6.5 months, respectively; p <0.0001) in relapsed MM patients. Additionally, a combination of oral cyclophosphamide, dexamethasone, and bortezomib in 50 patients with relapsed/refractory MM has been reported to achieve ORR in 88% of patients, with a median event-free survival of 10 months and median overall survival not yet reached. The broader clinical benefit of other regimens remains to be determined.

Lenalidomide has been evaluated in two large phase 3 studies comparing it in combination with dexamethasone to high-dose dexamethasone and placebo. The combination of lenalidomide and dexamethasone showed significant advantages in the response rate (CR + PR: 56% versus 24%, respectively; p <0.001) and in time to progression (14 versus 5 months, respectively; p <0.01), as well as OS (30 versus 20 months, respectively; p <0.01). Lenalidomide was equally active in patients with or without previous exposure to bortezomib or thalidomide. However, lenalidomide in combination with high-dose dexamethasone had significantly higher rates of DVT (14% versus 5%, respectively; p <0.01). Lenalidomide has also been assessed in combination with bortezomib and dexamethasone in a phase 1/2 trial in patients with relapsed or refractory MM.

A pilot phase 1/2 study in relapsed refractory myeloma has evaluated the combination of lenalidomide and bortezomib in 38 patients. A 61% minimal response or better was observed, and 83% patients achieved stable disease or better when dexamethasone was added, including patients whose MM was resistant to either agent alone. Thalidomide has also been an active agent, both alone and in combination with dexamethasone in relapsed patients (see Table 112.8B). Although lenalidomide activity has been demonstrated in patients relapsing after thalidomide, it is unclear whether patients relapsing after lenalidomide will respond to thalidomide. A combination of bortezomib (1.0 to

1.3 mg/m²), thalidomide (50 to 200 mg per day) and dexametha-sone (40 mg for 4 days) has been evaluated by Zangari et al.: In 83 patients with relapsed/refractory disease (over 70% patients having previously received thalidomide), 80% overall response with 16% CRs was reported. In relapsed MM, the combina-tion of conventional chemotherapy not previously used with or without novel agents can be effective. Four-drug combinations such as DCEP (dexamethasone, cyclophosphamide, etoposide, and cis-platinum), have been reported to achieve high response rates in relapsed patients, especially with aggressive disease. A regimen incorporating thalidomide + adriamycin with DCEP (DTPACE) for relapsed/refractory MM (n = 236) prior to HDT/SCT achieved 32% PR after two cycles of DTPACE, with 16% attaining a CR or nCR.[387]

A number of newer agents have been investigated in relapsed and/or refractory myeloma. In 2013, two novel agents, carfilzomib and pomalidomide, have been approved by the FDA for use in relapsed/refractory patients with myeloma. Carfilzomib, a second-generation proteasome inhibitor that selectively and irreversibly binds its target, has demonstrated single-agent and combination activity in relapsed and refractory patients with MM. In patients with relapsed MM after ≥ two previous therapies including bort-ezomib and an immunomodulatory agent and refractory to the last treatment (n = 42), the best ORR was 16.7%, and the median duration of response was 7.2 months.[388] In another phase 2, open-label, multicenter clinical trial (n = 35), patients with relapsed and/or refractory MM following one to three prior therapies in-cluding at least one bortezomib-based regimen, the best ORR was 17.1%, the median duration of response was > 10.6 months, and the median time to progression was 4.6 months.[389] In an ex-panded single-arm phase 2 study, patients received single-agent carfilzomib 20 mg/m² intravenously twice weekly for 3 of 4 weeks in cycle 1, then 27 mg/m² for ≤12 cycles. In this study, 95% of 266 patients were refractory to their last therapy and 80% refrac-tory or intolerant to both bortezomib and lenalidomide. In this study, ORR was 23.7%, with a median duration of response of 7.8 months, and median OS was 15.6 months.[390] Based on results of these studies, carfilzomib is now FDA approved for the treat-ment of relapsed myeloma. In another study in 129 bortezomib-naive patients with relapsed MM, ORR was 42.4% in Cohort 1 and 52.2% in Cohort 2, in which patients received an increased dose of 27 mg/m² after the first cycle.[391] A low incidence of pe-ripheral neuropathy (17.1% overall; one grade 3; no grade 4) was observed in these bortezomib-naive patients. Notably, in all stud-ies, peripheral neuropathy and neuropathy-related AEs were gen-erally mild and infrequent. An analysis of response and survival data from the PX-171-03 study (n = 229) identified 62 patients (27.1%) with high-risk cytogenetics profiles (del[17p]13, t[4;14] or t[14;16] by FISH or deletion 13 or hypodiploidy by metaphase cy-togenetics) versus 167 patients (72.9%) with standard risk. Overall response was comparable between these two groups (25.8% versus 24.6%, respectively), but there was a trend in high-risk patients for a shorter median duration of response (5.6 months versus 8.3 months, respectively) and OS (9.3 months versus 19.0 months, respectively; p = 0.0003). This study suggests that single-agent carfilzomib is efficacious and has the potential to at least partially overcome the impact of high-risk cytogenetics in heavily pre-treated MM.[392]

Pomalidomide, a more potent immunomodulatory drug, has demonstrated activity even in patients with MM resistant to le-nalidomide. Pomalidomide at doses of 2 or 4 mg per day with weekly dexamethasone at 40 mg has demonstrated excellent activ-ity in patients with MM. A phase 2 study (n = 35) confirmed re-sponses in the 2-mg cohort (14% VGPR, 11% PR, and 23% MR), with an overall response rate (ORR) of 49%; and in the 4-mg co-hort (3% CR, 9% VGPR, 17% PR and 14% MR), with an ORR of 43%. Overall survival at 6 months was 78% and 67% in the 2- and 4-mg cohort, respectively. Myelosuppression was the most common toxicity.[393] In another study (n = 60), pomalidomide 2 mg daily with Dex 40 mg orally on days 1, 8, 15, and 22 of each cycle in relapsed or refractory MM achieved a 63% response, including 5% CR and 28% VGPR. Responses were observed in 40% patients with lenalidomide-refractory MM. The median PFS was 11.6 months.[394] A phase 1 dose-escalation study determined the maximum tolerated dose (MTD) of oral pomalidomide 4 mg to be administered on days 1 to 21 of each 28-day cycle in pa-tients with relapsed and refractory MM, with Dex added if no response occurred after four cycles. Among the 38 patients en-rolled (including 22 with added dexamethasone), 42% achieved a partial response or better, and 3% achieved a complete response or better. The median dura-tion of response, PFS, and OS were 4.6, 4.6, and 18.3 months, respectively.[395] IFM conducted a phase 2 randomized study com-paring pomalidomide (4 mg) on days 1 to 21 (n = 43) or con-tinuously (n = 41) over a 28-day cycle, plus dexamethasone given weekly, and reported similar response rates (35% versus 34%); time to progression (5.8 versus 4.8 months) and OS (14.9 versus 14.8 months); along with a similar toxicity profile, primarily my-elosuppression, in both groups.[396] These studies have established pomalidomide 4 mg per day on days 1 to 21 of a 28-day cycle with 40-mg weekly dexamethasone as a standard for future studies. A phase 3, multicenter, randomized, open-label study of pomalido-mide in combination with low-dose dexamethasone demonstrated a significant PFS and OS advantage over dexamethasone alone in patients with relapsed/refractory MM.[397] In a recent phase 1 study combining pomalidomide with bortezomib and dexamethasone in patients with relapsed/refractory MM showed 73% ORR and 27% VGPR, including 73% patients whose disease progressed on lenalidomide.[398]

Based on preclinical synergistic activity and phase 2 studies showing the ability of HDAC inhibitors (vorinostat and pano-binostat) to overcome bortezomib resistance, ongoing phase 3 studies comparing bortezomib with combination of bortezomib with vorinostat and with panobinostat have been completed. Al-though increased responses were noted in relapsed MM treated with bortezomib and vorinostat versus vorinostat, alone, the PFS advantage was only one month, with treatment limited by diarrhea, thrombocytopenia, and fatigue.[399] The more selective HDAC inhibitor ricolinostat has been combined with bortezo-mib, as well as with lenalidomide/dexamethasone[400] and has achieved responses with a more favorable side effect profile. The combination of bortezomib and Akt inhibitor perifosine is able to overcome bortezomib resistance.[401] Finally, an antibody target-ing CS-1 cell surface molecule (elotuzumab) has been shown to achieve over 80% response when combined with lenalidomide/dexamethasone in relapsed MM, and anti-CD38 monoclonal an-tibodies (daratumumab) are similarly achieving responses, even in high-risk relapsed MM.

Other Potential Agents and Future Direction

Both in vitro systems and in vivo animal models have been de-veloped to characterize mechanisms of MM cell homing to BM, as well as factors (MM cell–BM stromal cell interactions, cyto-kines, angiogenesis) promoting MM cell growth, survival, drug resistance, and migration in the BM milieu. These model systems have allowed for the development of several promising biologically based therapies including the previously mentioned anti-CS1 an-tibody elotuzumab, the anti-CD38 antibody daratumumab, the HDAC6 inhibitor ricolinostat, as well as heat shock protein 90 inhibitor (AUY 922) and telomerase inhibitor GRN 163L, among many others (Fig. 112.15). Detailed oncogenomic studies are identifying novel targets and pathways operative in myeloma, and ongoing studies are determining mechanisms of action of novel agents at a gene and protein level in order to provide the frame-work for rational combination clinical trials that will overcome drug resistance and improve patient outcomes.

SELECTED REFERENCES

The full reference list can be accessed at lwwhealthlibrary.com/oncology.

2. Bence J. On a new substance occurring in the urine of a patient with mollities and fragilis ossium. *Phil Trans R Soc Lond* 1848;55:673.

6. Chauhan D, Uchiyama H, Akbarali Y, et al. Multiple myeloma cell adhesion-induced interleukin-6 expression in bone marrow stromal cells involves activation of NF-kappa B. *Blood* 1996;87:1104–1112.

8. Holland JF, Hosley H, Scharlau C, et al. A controlled trial of urethane treatment in multiple myeloma. *Blood* 1966;27:328–342.

13. Cohen HJ, Crawford J, Rao MK, et al. Racial differences in the prevalence of monoclonal gammopathy in a community-based sample of the elderly. *Am J Med* 1998;104:439–444.

14. Landgren O, Katzmann JA, Hsing AW, et al. Prevalence of monoclonal gammopathy of undetermined significance among men in Ghana. *Mayo Clin Proc* 2007;82:1468–1473.

25. Weinhold N, Johnson DC, Chubb D, et al. The CCND1 c.870G>A polymorphism is a risk factor for t(11;14)(q13;q32) multiple myeloma. *Nat Genet* 2013;45:522–525.

27. Kyle RA, Therneau TM, Rajkumar SV, et al. A long-term study of prognosis in monoclonal gammopathy of undetermined significance. *N Engl J Med* 2002;346:564–569.

28. Avet-Loiseau H, Facon T, Daviet A, et al. 14q32 translocations and monosomy 13 observed in monoclonal gammopathy of undetermined significance delineate a multistep process for the oncogenesis of multiple myeloma. Intergroupe Francophone du Myelome. *Cancer Res* 1999;59:4546–4550.

30. Malik AA, Ganti AK, Potti A, et al. Role of Helicobacter pylori infection in the incidence and clinical course of monoclonal gammopathy of undetermined significance. *Am J Gastroenterol* 2002;97:1371–1374.

33. Landgren O, Kyle RA, Pfeiffer RM, et al. Monoclonal gammopathy of undetermined significance (MGUS) consistently precedes multiple myeloma: a prospective study. *Blood* 2009;113:5412–5417.

34. Brown LM, Gridley G, Check D, et al. Risk of multiple myeloma and monoclonal gammopathy of undetermined significance among white and black male United States veterans with prior autoimmune, infectious, inflammatory, and allergic disorders. *Blood* 2008;111:3388–3394.

45. Davies FE, Dring AM, Li C, et al. Insights into the multistep transformation of MGUS to myeloma using microarray expression analysis. *Blood* 2003;102:4504–4511.

46. Avet-Loiseau H, Li JY, Morineau N, et al. Monosomy 13 is associated with the transition of monoclonal gammopathy of undetermined significance to multiple myeloma. Intergroupe Francophone du Myelome. *Blood* 1999;94:2583–2589.

47. Weiss BM, Abadie J, Verma P, et al. A monoclonal gammopathy precedes multiple myeloma in most patients. *Blood* 2009;113:5418–5422.

49. Kaufmann H, Ackermann J, Baldia C, et al. Both IGH translocations and chromosome 13q deletions are early events in monoclonal gammopathy of undetermined significance and do not evolve during transition to multiple myeloma. *Leukemia* 2004;18:1879–1882.

50. Neben K, Jauch A, Hielscher T, et al. Progression in smoldering myeloma is independently determined by the chromosomal abnormalities del(17p), t(4;14), gain 1q, hyperdiploidy, and tumor load. *J Clin Oncol* 2013;31:4325–4332.

58. Hallek M, Bergsagel LP, Anderson KD. Multiple myeloma: increasing evidence for a multistep transformation process. *Blood* 1998;91:3–21.

62. Chesi M, Bergsagel PL, Brents LA, et al. Dysregulation of cyclin D1 by translocation into an IgH gamma switch region in two multiple myeloma cell lines [see comments]. *Blood* 1996;88:674–681.

64. Chesi M, Nardini E, Brents LA, et al. Frequent translocation t(4;14)(p16.3;q32.3) in multiple myeloma is associated with increased expression and activating mutations of fibroblast growth factor receptor 3. *Nat Genet* 1997;16:260–264.

65. Chesi M, Brents LA, Ely SA, et al. Activated fibroblast growth factor receptor 3 is an oncogene that contributes to tumor progression in multiple myeloma. *Blood* 2001;97:729–736.

70. Shou Y, Martelli ML, Gabrea A, et al. Diverse karyotypic abnormalities of the c-myc locus associated with c-myc dysregulation and tumor progression in multiple myeloma. *Proc Natl Acad Sci U S A* 2000;97:228–233.

71. Avet-Loiseau H, Gerson F, Magrangeas F, et al. Rearrangements of the c-myc oncogene are present in 15% of primary human multiple myeloma tumors. *Blood* 2001;98:3082–3086.

91. Shammas MA, Shmookler Reis RJ, Akiyama M, et al. Telomerase inhibition and cell growth arrest by G-quadruplex interactive agent in multiple myeloma. *Mol Cancer Ther* 2003;2:825–833.

93. Shaughnessy JD Jr, Zhan F, Burington BE, et al. A validated gene expression model of high-risk multiple myeloma is defined by deregulated expression of genes mapping to chromosome 1. *Blood* 2007;109:2276–2284.

94. Decaux O, Lode L, Magrangeas F, et al. Prediction of survival in multiple myeloma based on gene expression profiles reveals cell cycle and chromosomal instability signatures in high-risk patients and hyperdiploid signatures in low-risk patients: a study of the Intergroupe Francophone du Myelome. *J Clin Oncol* 2008;26:4798–4805.

95. Broyl A, Hose D, Lokhorst H, et al. Gene expression profiling for molecular classification of multiple myeloma in newly diagnosed patients. *Blood* 2010;116:2543–2553.

96. Avet-Loiseau H, Li C, Magrangeas F, et al. Prognostic significance of copy-number alterations in multiple myeloma. *J Clin Oncol* 2009;27:4585–4590.

97. Delmore JE, Issa GC, Lemieux ME, et al. BET bromodomain inhibition as a therapeutic strategy to target c-Myc. *Cell* 2011;146:904–917.

99. Pichiorri F, Suh SS, Ladetto M, et al. MicroRNAs regulate critical genes associated with multiple myeloma pathogenesis. *Proc Natl Acad Sci U S A* 2008;105:12885–12890.

100. Gutierrez NC, Sarasquete ME, Misiewicz-Krzeminska I, et al. Deregulation of microRNA expression in the different genetic subtypes of multiple myeloma and correlation with gene expression profiling. *Leukemia* 2010;24:629–637.

105. Chapman MA, Lawrence MS, Keats JJ, et al. Initial genome sequencing and analysis of multiple myeloma. *Nature* 2011;471:467–472.

106. Magrangeas F, Avet-Loiseau H, Gouraud W, et al. Minor clone provides a reservoir for relapse in multiple myeloma. *Leukemia* 2013;27:473–481.

107. Bolli N, Avet-Loiseau H, Wedge DC, et al. Heterogeneity of genomic evolution and mutational profiles in multiple myeloma. *Nat Commun* 2014;5:2997.

115. Keats JJ, Fonseca R, Chesi M, et al. Promiscuous mutations activate the noncanonical NF-kappaB pathway in multiple myeloma. *Cancer Cell* 2007;12:131–144.

116. Annunziata CM, Davis RE, Demchenko Y, et al. Frequent engagement of the classical and alternative NF-kappaB pathways by diverse genetic abnormalities in multiple myeloma. *Cancer Cell* 2007;12:115–130.

120. Rajkumar SV, Mesa RA, Fonseca R, et al. Bone marrow angiogenesis in 400 patients with monoclonal gammopathy of undetermined significance, multiple myeloma, and primary amyloidosis. *Clin Cancer Res* 2002;8:2210–2216.

121. Munshi NC, Wilson C. Increased bone marrow microvessel density in newly diagnosed multiple myeloma carries a poor prognosis. *Semin Oncol* 2001;28:565–569.

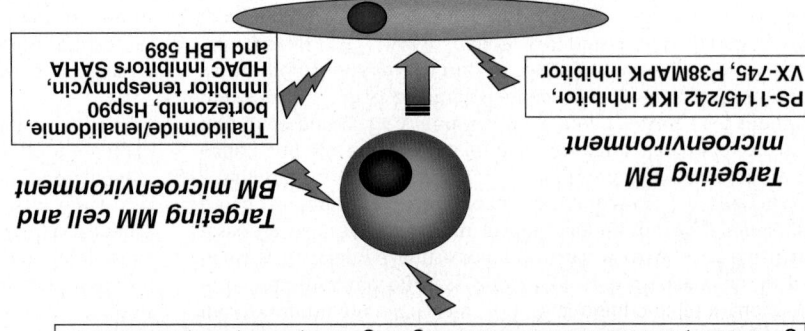

Targeting MM cell

Telomerase inhibitor GRN 163L, IGF1R inhibitor, AKT inhibitor perifosine liposomal doxorubicin, epothilone B, farnesyltransferase inhibitor, trial genasense, monoclonal antibodies targeting CD40, CD56, CS1, vaccination

Targeting MM cell and BM microenvironment

Thalidomide/lenalidomide, bortezomib, Hsp90 inhibitor tenespimycin, HDAC inhibitors SAHA and LBH 589

Targeting BM microenvironment

PS-1145/242 IKK inhibitor, VX-745, P38MAPK inhibitor

Figure 112.15 Novel therapies in preclinical or clinical development targeting the myeloma cells or their microenvironment or both.

125. Chauhan D, Singh AV, Brahmandam M, et al. Functional interaction of plasmacytoid dendritic cells with multiple myeloma cells: a therapeutic target. Cancer Cell 2009;16:309–323.

131. Podar K, Tai YT, Davies FE, et al. Vascular endothelial growth factor triggers signaling cascades mediating multiple myeloma cell growth and migration. Blood 2001;98:428–435.

135. Prabhala RH, Pelluru D, Fulciniti M, et al. Elevated IL-17 produced by TH17 cells promotes myeloma cell growth and inhibits immune function in multiple myeloma. Blood 2010;115:5385–5392.

155. Maecker HT, Anderson KS, von Bergwelt-Baildon MS, et al. Viral antigen-specific CD8+ T-cell responses are impaired in multiple myeloma. Br J Haematol 2003;121:842–848.

158. Prabhala RH, Neri P, Bae JE, et al. Dysfunctional T regulatory cells in multiple myeloma. Blood 2006;107:301–304.

160. Yi Q, Osterborg A, Bergenbrant S, et al. Idiotype-reactive T-cell subsets and tumor load in monoclonal gammopathies. Blood 1995;86:3043–3049.

164. Tassone P, Neri P, Carrasco DR, et al. A clinically relevant SCID-hu in vivo model of human multiple myeloma. Blood 2005;106:713–716.

167. Carrasco DR, Sukhdeo K, Protopopova M, et al. The differentiation and stress response factor XBP-1 drives multiple myeloma pathogenesis. Cancer Cell 2007;11:349–360.

183. Tricot G. New insights into role of microenvironment in multiple myeloma. Lancet 2000;355:248–250.

186. Tian E, Zhan F, Walker R, et al. The role of the Wnt-signaling antagonist DKK1 in the development of osteolytic lesions in multiple myeloma. N Engl J Med 2003;349:2483–2494.

189. Broder S, Humphrey R, Durm M, et al. Impaired synthesis of polyclonal (non-paraprotein) immunoglobulins by circulating lymphocytes from patients with multiple myeloma Role of suppressor cells. N Engl J Med 1975;293:887–892.

210. Furie BC, Furie B. Syndrome of acquired factor X deficiency and systemic amyloidosis in vivo studies of the metabolic fate of factor X. N Engl J Med 1977;297:81–85.

211. Zangari M, Anaissie E, Barlogie B, et al. Increased risk of deep-vein thrombosis in patients with multiple myeloma receiving thalidomide and chemotherapy. Blood 2001;98:1614–1615.

213. Barlogie B, Smallwood L, Smith T, et al. High serum levels of lactic dehydrogenase identify a high-grade lymphoma-like myeloma. Ann Intern Med 1989;110:521–525.

214. Usmani SZ, Heuck C, Mitchell A, et al. Extramedullary disease portends poor prognosis in multiple myeloma and is over-represented in high-risk disease even in the era of novel agents. Haematologica 2012;97:1761–1767.

216. Dimopoulos M, Kyle R, Fermand JP, et al. Consensus recommendations for standard investigative workup: report of the International Myeloma Workshop Consensus Panel 3. Blood 2011;117:4701–4705.

219. Zent CS, Wilson CS, Tricot G, et al. Oligoclonal protein bands and Ig isotype switching in multiple myeloma treated with high-dose therapy and hematopoietic cell transplantation. Blood 1998;91:3518–3523.

221. Martinez-Lopez J, Lahuerta JJ, Pepin F, et al. Prognostic value of deep sequencing method for minimal residual disease detection in multiple myeloma. Blood 2014;123:3073–3079.

222. Rajkumar SV, Kyle RA, Therneau TM, et al. Serum free light chain ratio is an independent risk factor for progression in monoclonal gammopathy of undetermined significance. Blood 2005;106:812–817.

223. Dispenzieri A, Lacy MQ, Katzmann JA, et al. Absolute values of immunoglobulin free light chains are prognostic in patients with primary systemic amyloidosis undergoing peripheral blood stem cell transplantation. Blood 2006;107:3378–3383.

224. Mead GP, Carr-Smith HD, Drayson MT, et al. Serum free light chains for monitoring multiple myeloma. Br J Haematol 2004;126:348–354.

226. van Rhee F, Bolejack V, Hollmig K, et al. High serum free-light chain levels and their rapid reduction in response to therapy define an aggressive multiple myeloma subtype with poor prognosis. Blood 2007;110:827–832.

227. Ludwig H, Milosavljevic D, Zojer N, et al. Immunoglobulin heavy/light chain ratios improve paraprotein detection and monitoring, identify residual disease and correlate with survival in multiple myeloma patients. Leukemia 2013;27:213–219.

235. Moulopoulos LA, Dimopoulos MA, Smith T, et al. Prognostic significance of magnetic resonance imaging in patients with asymptomatic multiple myeloma. J Clin Oncol 1995;13:251–256.

237. Walker R, Barlogie B, Haessler J, et al. Magnetic resonance imaging in multiple myeloma: diagnostic and clinical implications. J Clin Oncol 2007;25:1121–1128.

238. Bartel TB, Haessler J, Brown TL, et al. F18-Fluorodeoxyglucose positron emission tomography in the context of other imaging techniques and prognostic factors in multiple myeloma. Blood 2009;114:2068–2076.

239. Dimopoulos M, Terpos E, Comenzo RL, et al. International myeloma working group consensus statement and guidelines regarding the current role of imaging techniques in the diagnosis and monitoring of multiple myeloma. Leukemia 2009;23:1545–1556.

241. Zamagni E, Nanni C, Patriarca F, et al. A prospective comparison of 18F-fluorodeoxyglucose positron emission tomography-computed tomography, magnetic resonance imaging and whole-body planar radiographs in the

245. Attal M, Harousseau JL, Facon T, et al. Single versus double autologous stem-cell transplantation for multiple myeloma. N Engl J Med 2003;349:2495–2502.

246. Avet-Loiseau H, Daviet A, Brigaudeau C, et al. Cytogenetic, interphase, and multicolor fluorescence in situ hybridization analyses in primary plasma cell leukemia: a study of 40 patients at diagnosis, on behalf of the Intergroupe Francophone du Myelome and the Groupe Francais de Cytogenetique Hematologique. Blood 2001;97:822–825.

247. Vesole DH, Tricot G, Jagannath S, et al. Autotransplants in multiple myeloma: what have we learned? Blood 1996;88:838–847.

248. Witzig TE, Gertz MA, Lust JA, et al. Peripheral blood monoclonal plasma cells as a predictor of survival in patients with multiple myeloma [see comments]. Blood 1996;88:1780–1787.

249. Witzig TE, Kimlinger NJ, Katzmann JA, et al. Peripheral blood B cell labeling indices are a measure of disease activity in patients with monoclonal gammopathies. J Clin Oncol 1988;6:1041–1046.

251. Munshi N, Wilson C, Penn J, et al. Angiogenesis in newly diagnosed multiple myeloma (MM): poor prognosis with increased microvessel density (MVD) in bone marrow biopsies (BMBX). Blood 1998;92:98a.

253. Munshi NC, Anderson KC, Bergsagel PL, et al. Consensus recommendations for risk stratification in multiple myeloma: report of the International Myeloma Workshop Consensus Panel 2. Blood 2011;117:4696–4700.

254. Dimopoulos MA, Moulopoulos LA, Delasalle K, et al. Solitary plasmacytoma of bone and asymptomatic multiple myeloma. Hematol Oncol Clin North Am 1992;6:359–369.

256. Liebross RH, Ha CS, Cox JD, et al. Solitary bone plasmacytoma: outcome and prognostic factors following radiotherapy. Int J Radiat Oncol Biol Phys 1998;41:1063–1067.

257. Corwin J, Lindberg RD. Solitary plasmacytoma of bone vs. extramedullary plasmacytoma. Cancer 1979;43:1007–1013.

259. Kyle RA, Remstein ED, Therneau TM, et al. Clinical course and prognosis of smoldering (asymptomatic) multiple myeloma. N Engl J Med 2007;356:2582–2590.

260. Dispenzieri A, Kyle RA, Katzmann JA, et al. Immunoglobulin free light chain ratio is an independent risk factor for progression of smoldering (asymptomatic) multiple myeloma. Blood 2008;111:785–789.

261. Rajkumar SV, Gertz MA, Lacy MQ, et al. Thalidomide as initial therapy for early-stage myeloma. Leukemia 2003;17:775–779.

262. Mateos MV, San Miguel JF. Treatment for high-risk smoldering myeloma. N Engl J Med 2013;369:1764–1765.

264. Alexanian R, Haut A, Khan AU, et al. Treatment for multiple myeloma. Combination chemotherapy with different melphalan dose regimens. JAMA 1969;208:1680–1685.

268. Cavo M, Zamagni E, Tosi P, et al. Superiority of thalidomide and dexamethasone over vincristine-doxorubicindexamethasone (VAD) as primary therapy in preparation for autologous transplantation for multiple myeloma. Blood 2005;106:35–39.

269. Rajkumar SV, Jacobus S, Callander NS, et al. Lenalidomide plus high-dose dexamethasone versus lenalidomide plus low-dose dexamethasone as initial therapy for newly diagnosed multiple myeloma: an open-label randomised controlled trial. Lancet Oncol 2010;11:29–37.

272. Barlogie B, Kyle RA, Anderson KC, et al. Standard chemotherapy compared with high-dose chemoradiotherapy for multiple myeloma: final results of phase III US Intergroup Trial S9321. J Clin Oncol 2006;24:929–936.

277. Raje N, Anderson K. Thalidomide—a revival story [editorial; comment]. New Engl J Med 1999;341:1606–1609.

278. Kronke J, Udeshi ND, Narla A, et al. Lenalidomide causes selective degradation of IKZF1 and IKZF3 in multiple myeloma cells. Science 2014;343:301–305.

279. Lu G, Middleton RE, Sun H, et al. The myeloma drug lenalidomide promotes the cereblon-dependent destruction of Ikaros proteins. Science 2014;343:305–309.

280. Barlogie B, Desikan R, Eddlemon P, et al. Extended survival in advanced and refractory multiple myeloma after single-agent thalidomide: identification of prognostic factors in a phase 2 study of 169 patients. Blood 2001;98:492–494.

281. Singhal S, Mehta J, Desikan R, et al. Antitumor activity of thalidomide in refractory multiple myeloma [see comments]. N Engl J Med 1999;341:1565–1571.

282. Palumbo A, Rajkumar SV, Dimopoulos MA, et al. Prevention of thalidomide- and lenalidomide-associated thrombosis in myeloma. Leukemia 2008;22:414–423.

283. Richardson PG, Schlossman RL, Weller E, et al. Immunomodulatory drug CC-5013 overcomes drug resistance and is well tolerated in patients with relapsed multiple myeloma. Blood 2002;100:3063–3067.

284. Weber DM, Chen C, Niesvizky R, et al. Lenalidomide plus dexamethasone for relapsed multiple myeloma in North America. N Engl J Med 2007;357:2133–2142.

286. Hideshima T, Anderson KC. Molecular mechanisms of novel therapeutic approaches for multiple myeloma. Nat Rev Cancer 2002;2:927–937.

288. Hideshima T, Richardson P, Chauhan D, et al. The proteasome inhibitor PS-341 inhibits growth, induces apoptosis, and overcomes drug resistance in human multiple myeloma cells. Cancer Res 2001;61:3071–3076.

289. Mitsiades CS, Poulaki V, et al. Molecular sequelae of proteasome inhibition in human multiple myeloma cells. Proc Natl Acad Sci U S A 2002;99:14374–14379.

290. Richardson PG, Barlogie B, Berenson J, et al. A phase 2 study of bortezomib in relapsed, refractory myeloma. N Engl J Med 2003;348:2609–2617.

291. Richardson PG, Sonneveld P, Schuster MW, et al. Bortezomib or high-dose dexamethasone for relapsed multiple myeloma. N Engl J Med 2005;352:2487–2498.

292. Orlowski RZ, Zhuang SH, Parekh T, et al. The combination of pegylated liposomal doxorubicin and bortezomib significantly improves time to progression of patients with relapsed/refractory multiple myeloma compared with bortezomib alone: results from a planned interim analysis of a randomized phase III study. Blood 2006;108:404a.

293. Jagannath S, Richardson PG, Sonneveld P, et al. Bortezomib appears to overcome the poor prognosis conferred by chromosome 13 deletion in phase 2 and 3 trials. Leukemia 2007;21:151–157.

294. Chanan-Khan AA, Mehta J, et al. Activity and safety of bortezomib in multiple myeloma patients with advanced renal failure: a multicenter retrospective study. Blood 2007;109:2604–2606.

295. Zangari M, Esseltine D, Lee CK, et al. Response to bortezomib is associated to osteoblastic activation in patients with multiple myeloma. Br J Haematol 2005;131:71–73.

296. Moreau P, Pylypenko H, Grosicki S, et al. Subcutaneous versus intravenous administration of bortezomib in patients with relapsed multiple myeloma: a randomised, phase 3, non-inferiority study. Lancet Oncol 2011;12:431–440.

297. Rajkumar SV, Blood E, Vesole D, et al. Phase III clinical trial of thalidomide plus dexamethasone compared with dexamethasone alone in newly diagnosed multiple myeloma: a clinical trial coordinated by the Eastern Cooperative Oncology Group. J Clin Oncol 2006;24:431–436.

298. Zonder JA, Crowley J, Hussein MA, et al. Lenalidomide and high-dose dexamethasone compared with dexamethasone as initial therapy for multiple myeloma: a randomized Southwest Oncology Group trial (S0232). Blood 2010;116:5838–5841.

300. Harousseau JL, Attal M, Avet-Loiseau H, et al. Bortezomib plus dexamethasone is superior to vincristine plus doxorubicin plus dexamethasone as induction treatment prior to autologous stem-cell transplantation in newly diagnosed multiple myeloma: results of the IFM 2005-01 phase III trial. J Clin Oncol 2010;28:4621–4629.

301. Avet-Loiseau H, Leleu X, Roussel M, et al. Bortezomib plus dexamethasone induction improves outcome of patients with t(4;14) myeloma but not outcome of patients with del(17p). J Clin Oncol 2010;28:4630–4634.

302. Jakubowiak AJ, Dytfeld D, Griffith KA, et al. A phase 1/2 study of carfilzomib in combination with lenalidomide and low-dose dexamethasone as a frontline treatment for multiple myeloma. Blood 2012;120:1801–1809.

304. Richardson PG, Weller E, Lonial S, et al. Lenalidomide, bortezomib, and dexamethasone combination therapy in patients with newly diagnosed multiple myeloma. Blood 2010;116:679–686.

305. San Miguel JF, Schlag R, Khuageva NK, et al. Bortezomib plus melphalan and prednisone for initial treatment of multiple myeloma. N Engl J Med 2008;359:906–917.

308. Fermand JP, Ravaud P, Chevret S, et al. High-dose therapy and autologous blood stem cell transplantation in multiple myeloma: preliminary results of a randomized trial involving 167 patients. Stem Cells 1995;13:156–159.

309. Anderson KC, Andersen J, Soiffer R, et al. Monoclonal antibody-purged bone marrow transplantation therapy for multiple myeloma. Blood 1993;82:2568–2576.

310. Harousseau JL, Attal M, Divine M, et al. Autologous stem cell transplantation after first remission induction treatment in multiple myeloma. A report of the French Registry on Autologous Transplantation in Multiple Myeloma. Stem Cells 1995;13:132–139.

311. Attal M, Harousseau JL, Stoppa AM, et al. A prospective, randomized trial of autologous bone marrow transplantation and chemotherapy in multiple myeloma. Intergroupe Francais du Myelome. N Engl J Med 1996;335:91–97.

312. Child JA, Morgan GJ, Davies FE, et al. High-dose chemotherapy with hematopoietic stem-cell rescue for multiple myeloma. N Engl J Med 2003;348:1875–1883.

313. Bladé J, Sureda A, Diaz-Mediavilla J, et al. High-dose therapy autotransplantation/intensification vs continued conventional chemotherapy in multiple myeloma patients responding to initial treatment chemotherapy. Results of a prospective randomized trial from the Spanish Cooperative group PET. HEMA. Blood 2001;98:815a.

314. Fermand JP, Ravaud P, Chevret S, et al. High-dose therapy and autologous peripheral blood stem cell transplantation in multiple myeloma: up-front or rescue treatment? Results of a multicenter sequential randomized clinical trial. Blood 1998;92:3131–3136.

315. Koreth J, Cutler CS, Djulbegovic B, et al. High-dose therapy with single autologous transplantation versus chemotherapy for newly diagnosed multiple myeloma: A systematic review and meta-analysis of randomized controlled trials. Biol Blood Marrow Transplant 2007;13:183–196.

316. Harousseau JL, Laporte JP, et al. Double-intensive therapy in high-risk multiple myeloma. Blood 1992;79:2827–2833.

317. Barlogie B, Jagannath S, Desikan KR, et al. Total therapy with tandem transplants for newly diagnosed multiple myeloma. Blood 1999;93:55–65.

320. Mark T, Stern J, Furst JR, et al. Stem cell mobilization with cyclophosphamide overcomes the suppressive effect of lenalidomide therapy on stem cell collection in multiple myeloma. Biol Blood Marrow Transplant 2008;14:795–798.

325. Desikan KR, Fassas A, Siegel D, et al. Superior outcome with melphalan 200 mg/m² (MEL 200) for scheduled second autotransplant compared to MEL+TBI or CTX for myeloma (MM) in pre-tx-2 PR. Blood 1997;90:231a.

330. Schiller G, Vescio R, Freytes C, et al. Transplantation of CD34+ peripheral blood progenitor cells after high-dose chemotherapy for patients with advanced multiple myeloma. Blood 1995;86:390–397.

331. Stewart AK, Vescio R, Schiller G, et al. Purging of autologous peripheral-blood stem cells using CD34 selection does not improve overall or progression-free survival after high-dose chemotherapy for multiple myeloma: results of a multicenter randomized controlled trial. J Clin Oncol 2001;19:3771–3779.

333. Tricot G, Gazitt Y, Leemhuis T, et al. Collection, tumor contamination, and engraftment kinetics of highly purified hematopoietic progenitor cells to support high dose therapy in multiple myeloma. Blood 1998;91:4489–4495.

334. Harousseau JL, Attal M, Divine M, et al. Comparison of autologous bone marrow transplantation and peripheral blood stem cell transplantation after first remission induction treatment in multiple myeloma. Bone Marrow Transplant 1995;15:963–969.

336. Gazitt Y, Tian E, Barlogie B, et al. Differential mobilization of myeloma cells and normal hematopoietic stem cells in multiple myeloma after treatment with cyclophosphamide and granulocyte-macrophage colony-stimulating factor. Blood 1996;87:805–811.

337. Palumbo A, Anderson K. Multiple myeloma. N Engl J Med 2011;364:1046–1060.

338. Palumbo A, Rajkumar SV, San Miguel JF, et al. International Myeloma Working Group consensus statement for the management, treatment, and supportive care of patients with myeloma not eligible for standard autologous stem-cell transplantation. J Clin Oncol 2014;32:587–600.

340. Badros A, Barlogie B, Siegel E, et al. Autologous stem cell transplantation in elderly multiple myeloma patients over the age of 70 years. Br J Haematol 2001;114:600–607.

341. Tricot G, Alberts DS, Johnson C, et al. Safety of autotransplants with high-dose melphalan in renal failure: a pharmacokinetic and toxicity study. Clin Cancer Res 1996;2:947–952.

342. Dimopoulos MA, Terpos E, Chanan-Khan A, et al. Renal impairment in patients with multiple myeloma: a consensus statement on behalf of the International Myeloma Working Group. J Clin Oncol 2010;30:4976–4984.

344. Browman G, Bergsagel D, Sicheri D, et al. Randomized trial of interferon maintenance in multiple myeloma: a study of the National Cancer Institute of Canada Clinical Trials Group. J Clin Oncol 1995;13:2354–2360.

345. Berenson JR, Crowley JJ, Grogan TM, et al. Maintenance therapy with alternate-day prednisone improves survival in multiple myeloma patients. Blood 2002;99:3163–3168.

346. Attal M, Harousseau JL, Leyvraz S, et al. Maintenance therapy with thalidomide improves survival in patients with multiple myeloma. Blood 2006;108:3289–3294.

347. Attal M, Lauwers-Cances V, Marit G, et al. Lenalidomide maintenance after stem-cell transplantation for multiple myeloma. N Engl J Med 2012;366:1782–1791.

348. McCarthy PL, Owzar K, Hofmeister CC, et al. Lenalidomide after stem-cell transplantation for multiple myeloma. N Engl J Med 2012;366:1770–1781.

349. Palumbo A, Hajek R, Delforge M, et al. Continuous lenalidomide treatment for newly diagnosed multiple myeloma. N Engl J Med 2012;366:1759–1769.

350. Sonneveld P, Schmidt-Wolf IG, van der Holt B, et al. Bortezomib induction and maintenance treatment in patients with newly diagnosed multiple myeloma: results of the randomized phase III HOVON-65/GMMG-HD4 trial. J Clin Oncol 2012;30:2946–2955.

351. Mateos MV, Oriol A, Martinez-Lopez J, et al. Bortezomib, melphalan, and prednisone versus bortezomib, thalidomide, and prednisone as induction therapy followed by maintenance treatment with bortezomib and thalidomide versus bortezomib and prednisone in elderly patients with untreated multiple myeloma: a randomised trial. Lancet Oncol 2010;11:934–941.

353. Rosenblatt J, Avivi I, Vasir B, et al. Vaccination with dendritic cell/tumor fusions following autologous stem cell transplant induces immunologic and clinical responses in multiple myeloma patients. Clin Cancer Res 2013;19:3640–3648.

354. Munshi NC, Anderson KC. Minimal residual disease in multiple myeloma. J Clin Oncol 2013;31:2523–2526.

356. Paiva B, Gutierrez NC, Rosinol L, et al. High-risk cytogenetics and persistent minimal residual disease by multiparameter flow cytometry predict unsustained complete response after autologous stem cell transplantation in multiple myeloma. Blood 2012;119:687–691.

358. Gahrton G, Svensson H, Bjorkstrand B, et al. Syngeneic transplantation in multiple myeloma—a case matched comparison with autologous and allogeneic transplantation. Bone Marrow Transpl 1999;24:741–745.

360. Alyea EP, Anderson KC. Allotransplantation for multiple myeloma. Cancer J 2001;7:166–174.

362. Tricot G, Vesole DH, Jagannath S, et al. Graft-versus-myeloma effect: proof of principle. Blood 1996;87:1196–1198.

363. Lokhorst HM, Schattenberg A, Cornelissen JJ, et al. Donor lymphocyte infusions for relapsed multiple myeloma after allogeneic stem-cell transplantation: predictive factors for response and long-term outcome. Blood 2000;18:3031–3037.

365. Munshi NC, Govindarajan R, Drake R, et al. Thymidine kinase (TK) gene-transduced human lymphocytes can be highly purified, remain fully functional and are killed efficiently with ganciclovir. *Blood* 1997;89:1334–1340.

368. Badros A, Barlogie B, Siegel E, et al. Improved outcome of allogeneic transplantation in high-risk multiple myeloma patients after nonmyeloablative conditioning. *J Clin Oncol* 2002;20:1295–1303.

369. Giralt S, Aleman A, Anagnostopoulos A, et al. Fludarabine/melphalan conditioning for allogeneic transplantation in patients with multiple myeloma. *Bone Marrow Transplant* 2002;30:367–373.

371. Bruno B, Rotta M, Patriarca F, et al. A comparison of allografting with autografting for newly diagnosed myeloma. *N Engl J Med* 2007;356:1110–1120.

372. Rosinol L, Perez-Simon JA, Sureda A, et al. A prospective PETHEMA study of tandem autologous transplantation versus autograft followed by reduced-intensity conditioning allogeneic transplantation in newly diagnosed multiple myeloma. *Blood* 2008;112:3591–3593.

374. Krishnan A, Pasquini MC, Logan B, et al. Autologous haemopoietic stem-cell transplantation followed by allogeneic or autologous haemopoietic stem-cell transplantation in patients with multiple myeloma (BMT CTN 0102): a phase 3 biological assignment trial. *Lancet Oncol* 2011;12:1195–1203.

375. Berenson JR, Lichtenstein A, Porter L, et al. Efficacy of pamidronate in reducing skeletal events in patients with advanced multiple myeloma. *N Engl J Med* 1996;334:488–493.

379. Berenson JR, Lichtenstein A, Porter L, et al. Long-term pamidronate treatment of advanced multiple myeloma patients reduces skeletal events. *J Clin Oncol* 1998;16:593–602.

383. Morgan GJ, Child JA, Gregory WM, et al. Effects of zoledronic acid versus clodronic acid on skeletal morbidity in patients with newly diagnosed multiple myeloma (MRC Myeloma IX): secondary outcomes from a randomised controlled trial. *Lancet Oncol* 2011;12:743–752.

384. Morgan GJ, Davies FE, Gregory WM, et al. First-line treatment with zoledronic acid as compared with clodronic acid in multiple myeloma (MRC Myeloma IX): a randomised controlled trial. *Lancet* 2010;376:1989–1999.

385. Wang EP, Kaban LB, Strewler GJ, et al. Incidence of osteonecrosis of the jaw in patients with multiple myeloma and breast or prostate cancer on intravenous bisphosphonate therapy. *J Oral Maxillofac Surg* 2007;65:1328–1331.

386. Kyle RA, Yee GC, Somerfield MR, et al. American Society of Clinical Oncology 2007 clinical practice guideline update on the role of bisphosphonates in multiple myeloma. *J Clin Oncol* 2007;25:2464–2472.

387. Lee CK, Barlogie B, Munshi N, et al. DTPACE: an effective, novel combination chemotherapy with thalidomide for previously treated patients with myeloma. *J Clin Oncol* 2003;21:2732–2739.

388. Jagannath S, Vij R, Stewart AK, et al. An open-label single-arm pilot phase II study (PX-171-003-A0) of low-dose, single-agent carfilzomib in patients with relapsed and refractory multiple myeloma. *Clin Lymphoma Myeloma Leuk* 2012;12:310–318.

389. Vij R, Siegel DS, Jagannath S, et al. An open-label, single-arm, phase 2 study of single-agent carfilzomib in patients with relapsed and/or refractory multiple myeloma who have been previously treated with bortezomib. *Br J Haematol* 2012;158:739–748.

392. Jakubowiak AJ, Siegel DS, Martin T, et al. Treatment outcomes in patients with relapsed and refractory multiple myeloma and high-risk cytogenetics receiving single-agent carfilzomib in the PX-171-003-A1 study. *Leukemia* 2013;27:2351–2356.

394. Lacy MQ, Hayman SR, Gertz MA, et al. Pomalidomide (CC4047) plus low-dose dexamethasone as therapy for relapsed multiple myeloma. *J Clin Oncol* 2009;27:5008–5014.

395. Richardson PG, Siegel D, Baz R, et al. Phase 1 study of pomalidomide MTD, safety, and efficacy in patients with refractory multiple myeloma who have received lenalidomide and bortezomib. *Blood* 2013;121:1961–1967.

396. Leleu X, Attal M, Arnulf B, et al. Pomalidomide plus low-dose dexamethasone is active and well tolerated in bortezomib and lenalidomide-refractory multiple myeloma: Intergroupe Francophone du Myelome 2009-02. *Blood* 2013;121:1968–1975.

397. San Miguel J, Weisel K, Moreau P, et al. Pomalidomide plus low-dose dexamethasone versus high-dose dexamethasone alone for patients with relapsed and refractory multiple myeloma (MM-003): a randomised, open-label, phase 3 trial. *Lancet Oncol* 2013;14:1055–1066.

399. Dimopoulos M, Siegel DS, Lonial S, et al. Vorinostat or placebo in combination with bortezomib in patients with multiple myeloma (VANTAGE 088): a multicentre, randomised, double-blind study. *Lancet Oncol* 2013;14:1129–1140.

400. Santo L, Hideshima T, Kung AL, et al. Preclinical activity, pharmacodynamic, and pharmacokinetic properties of a selective HDAC6 inhibitor, ACY-1215, in combination with bortezomib in multiple myeloma. *Blood* 2012;119:2579–2589.

113 Cancer of Unknown Primary Site

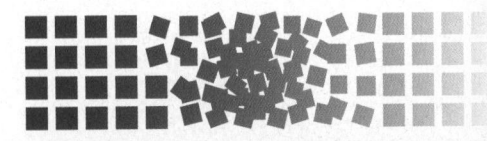

F. Anthony Greco and John D. Hainsworth

INTRODUCTION

Cancer of unknown primary (CUP) site is a clinical syndrome that includes many types of advanced cancers. Patients are considered to have CUP if no anatomical primary site is identified after clinical evaluation. As diagnostic techniques improve, the spectrum of patients with CUP continues to evolve.

Patients with CUP are common. The exact incidence is unknown because many of these patients are assigned other diagnoses and therefore are not accurately represented in tumor registries. Nonetheless, in the United States, CUP accounted for approximately 2% of all cancer diagnoses reported by Surveillance, Epidemiology, and End Results (SEER) registries.[1] International registries from seven other countries have reported incidences ranging from 2.3% to 7.8%.[2] The authors believe a more realistic estimate of the incidence of these patients is 5% of all invasive cancers, or approximately 80,000 to 90,000 patients per year in the United States.

Patients in this heterogeneous group have a wide variety of clinical presentations and histologic tumor types. Most patients have metastatic carcinoma; however, many neoplasms have categorize using histologic features alone. At autopsy, primary sites (usually <2 cm in size) can be located in the majority of patients; the molecular basis of this unusual biologic behavior is undefined. The preponderance of poorly treated tumor types in autopsy series (lung, pancreas, stomach, colon, liver) has led to negativity surrounding the diagnosis of CUP.[3]

Until recently, the major advance in the management of CUP was the recognition of several important patient subsets, identified by clinical and/or pathologic features and shown to benefit from specific first-line therapy. For the remainder of CUP patients (about 80%), empiric chemotherapy regimens were developed and resulted in modest benefit. At the time these regimens were developed, most types of solid tumors were poorly treated, and considerable overlap existed in the chemotherapy regimens used to treat sensitive tumor types. In this context, the possibility of developing a broad-spectrum chemotherapy regimen to adequately treat most of the treatable tumor types within the CUP population seemed feasible. However, during the last 20 years, treatments have not only improved for many tumor types, but have also become more site specific. Therefore, the idea of providing optimal treatment to patients with a diverse group of solid tumors using a single chemotherapy regimen is no longer feasible.

An accurate prediction of the tissue of origin is now possible for the majority of patients with CUP, using either improved panels of immunohistochemical (IHC) stains or molecular gene expression tumor profiling (MTP). Although the anatomical primary sites cannot be found in most patients even after the tissue of origin is predicted, increasing clinical experience confirms that these predictions can effectively guide site-specific therapy for patients with CUP.

This chapter is divided into three major sections. The first section reviews the pathologic evaluation of patients with CUP. New information regarding the emerging and important role of MTP assays is included. In the second section, the clinical evaluation of CUP patients is summarized. Situations in which clinical results from the pathologic evaluation direct the clinical evaluation are addressed. Finally, the treatment of patients with CUP is discussed, with an emphasis on the favorable prognostic subsets and the new paradigm of site-specific therapy directed at the tissue of origin.

PATHOLOGIC EVALUATION

Histologic examination by hematoxylin and eosin (H&E) staining of a biopsy tumor specimen remains the gold standard for the initial evaluation and provides a practical classification system on which to base a subsequent evaluation. In the broad category of CUP, there are five major light microscopic histologic diagnoses: (1) poorly differentiated neoplasm, (2) poorly differentiated carcinoma (with or without features of adenocarcinoma), (3) well-differentiated and moderately well-differentiated adenocarcinoma, (4) squamous cell carcinoma, and (5) neuroendocrine carcinoma. Sarcoma and melanoma are also occasionally diagnosed without an obvious primary tumor site, and management of these patients follows established guidelines. These histologic diagnoses define patient groups that vary to some extent with respect to clinical characteristics, a recommended diagnostic evaluation, treatment, and prognosis (Fig. 113.1). Because a histologic examination rarely allows for the identification of the site of tumor origin, an additional pathologic evaluation is important in almost every patient with CUP. A fine-needle aspiration biopsy usually does not contain enough of a biopsy specimen for the necessary pathologic evaluation, and should not be performed as the initial diagnostic procedure. Close communication between the oncologist and pathologist is critical to ensure that the most important diagnostic studies are obtained with the available biopsy material.

Poorly Differentiated Neoplasms of Unknown Primary Site

If the pathologist cannot differentiate a general category of neoplasm (e.g., carcinoma, lymphoma, melanoma, sarcoma), the tumor is designated a poorly differentiated neoplasm. A more precise diagnosis is essential because many patients in this category have responsive tumors. Approximately 5% of all patients with CUP (4,000 patients annually) present with this diagnosis after a standard histologic evaluation. However, only a few remain without a defined lineage after specialized pathologic studies including IHC staining, electron microscopy, and, recently, MTP.[4-7] (These techniques are discussed separately.) In reported series, 35% to 65%

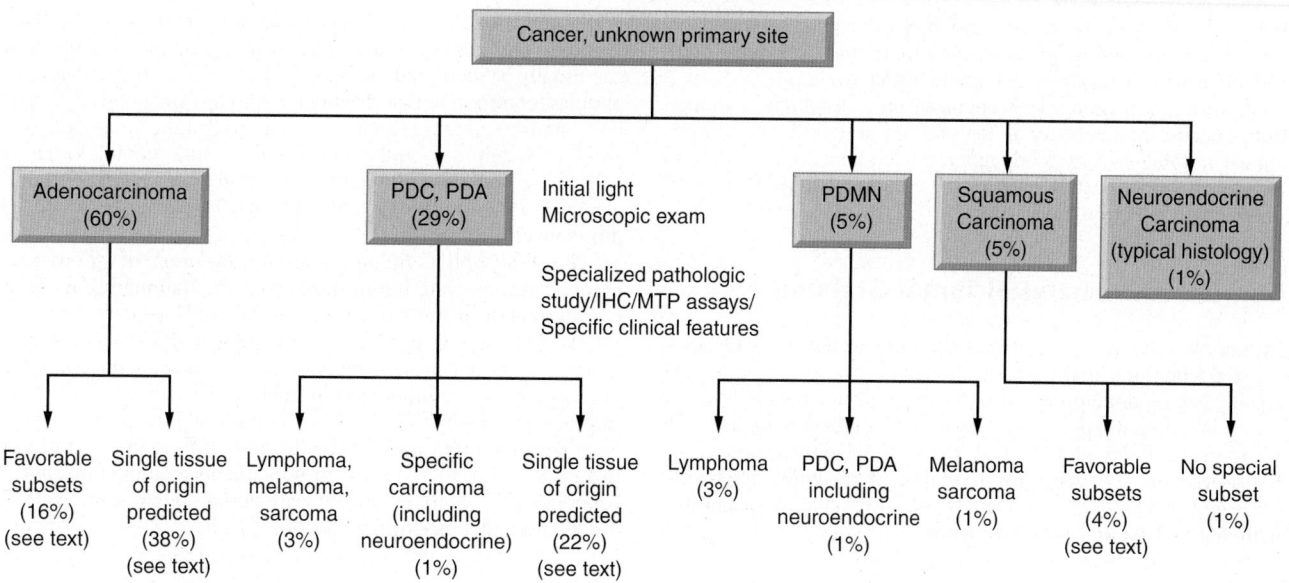

Figure 113.1 Relative size of various subgroups of patients as determined by clinical, specialized pathologic, and molecular evaluations. PDC, poorly differentiated carcinoma; PDA, poorly differentiated adenocarcinoma; IHC, immunohistochemistry; MTP, molecular tumor profiling; PDMN, poorly differentiated malignant neoplasm.

of poorly differentiated neoplasms were found to be lymphomas, which were highly responsive to specific therapy.[4,5] Most of the remaining tumors were carcinomas, including poorly differentiated neuroendocrine tumors. Melanoma and sarcoma together account for less than 15% of all patients.

Poorly Differentiated Carcinoma

Poorly differentiated carcinomas (PDC) account for approximately 30% of CUP (about 25,000 patients annually). In approximately one-third of these patients, some features of adenocarcinomatous differentiation can be identified (poorly differentiated adenocarcinoma). Some patients have extremely responsive neoplasms, and therefore, a careful pathologic evaluation is crucial.

Histopathologic features that can differentiate chemotherapy-responsive tumors from nonresponsive tumors have not been identified.[8] Even with a careful retrospective review of these tumors, responsive tumors of well-defined types (e.g., germ cell tumor, lymphoma) are only rarely identified.

All PDCs should undergo additional pathologic study for the purposes of (1) identifying other tumor types (e.g., lymphoma, sarcoma, melanoma) occasionally mistaken for carcinoma, (2) identifying neuroendocrine tumors, and (3) to determine the tissue of origin. Additional pathologic studies should include IHC stains, an MTP assay, and occasionally, electron microscopy and a karyotypic/cytogenetic analysis.

Adenocarcinoma

Well-differentiated and moderately differentiated adenocarcinomas are the most common tumors identified by light microscopy and account for 60% of CUP diagnoses (about 50,000 patients annually). These are the patients that many physicians associate with the entity of CUP. Typically, patients are elderly and have metastatic tumors at multiple sites. The sites of metastasis frequently determine the clinical presentation; common metastatic sites include the lymph nodes, the liver, the lung, and the bone.

The diagnosis of adenocarcinoma is based on light microscopic features, particularly the formation of glandular structures by neoplastic cells. All adenocarcinomas share histologic features, and the primary tumor site usually cannot be determined by a

histologic examination. Certain histologic features are typically associated with a particular tumor type (e.g., papillary serous features with ovarian cancer and signet ring cells with gastric cancer). However, these features are not specific enough to be used as definitive evidence of their origin.

The identification of relatively cell-specific proteins by IHC staining has improved the ability to predict the tissue of origin in CUP patients.[7,9,10] Panels of IHC stains are most useful and are often directed by clinical features (e.g., sites of metastases, gender). Molecular tumor profiling assays are relatively accurate and often provide additional diagnostic information. Both of these diagnostic modalities should be utilized in the pathologic evaluation of adenocarcinoma of unknown primary site.

Squamous Carcinoma

Squamous carcinoma represents approximately 5% of patients with CUP (about 4,000 patients annually). Approximately 90% of these patients have specific clinical syndromes for which effective treatment is available; therefore, an appropriate clinical evaluation is important.

A definitive diagnosis of squamous carcinoma is usually made by a histologic examination. On occasion, an MTP assay may diagnose the tissue of origin. An additional pathologic study with IHC and MTP should be considered in patients with poorly differentiated squamous carcinoma, particularly if the clinical presentation is atypical.

Neuroendocrine Carcinoma

Neuroendocrine carcinoma with widely varying clinical and histologic features account for approximately 3% of all CUP (about 3,500 patients annually). Improved pathologic methods for diagnosing neuroendocrine tumors have resulted in the recognition of an increased incidence and wider spectrum of these neoplasms.[11]

Two general subgroups can be routinely recognized by histologic features. Low-grade tumors share the same histologic features as carcinoids and islet cell tumors and may secrete bioactive substances. An MTP assay may point to the tissue of origin[12,13]; in some instances (e.g., pancreatic origin), defining the site of origin carries treatment implications. A second histologic group

PRACTICE OF ONCOLOGY

(variously described as small-cell carcinoma, atypical carcinoid, or poorly differentiated neuroendocrine carcinoma) has typical neuroendocrine features and a high-grade histology.

A third group cannot be recognized on a histologic examination, because neuroendocrine features are absent. These tumors appear histologically as poorly differentiated neoplasms or PDCs; an accurate identification requires IHC staining, an MTP assay, or occasionally, electron microscopy.

Immunohistochemical Tumor Staining

Immunohistochemical staining is the most widely available specialized technique for the classification of neoplasms.[7,9–22] Staining usually can be done on formalin-fixed, paraffin-embedded tissue, which broadens its applicability. Most IHC antibodies are directed at normal cellular proteins that are retained during neoplastic transformation. The ongoing development of antibodies to increasingly tissue-specific proteins makes this area of diagnostic pathology a dynamic and evolving field.

Several important questions can usually be answered by IHC staining. The correct lineage of poorly differentiated neoplasms can usually be identified (Table 113.1).[7,9,10,14–16] In particular, lymphomas (common leukocyte antigen staining) and poorly differentiated neuroendocrine carcinomas (chromogranin, synaptophysin, and CD56 staining) can be recognized,[10,15] and staining for germ cell tumors (octamer-binding transcription factor 4 [OCT4], placental alkaline phosphatase [PLAP]) may be diagnostic in an appropriate clinical situation.

The ability of IHC staining to identify the origin of various neoplasms has improved, but in most cases, the staining results must be interpreted in the context of clinical and histologic features. An exception is the prostate-specific antigen (PSA) stain, which is very specific for prostate carcinoma.[7] Stains suggestive of other primary sites are summarized in Table 113.1. The use of panels improves specificity[7,9,10,19–22]; several classic staining patterns have been described that are usually diagnostic of the tissue of origin (e.g., CK7+/CK20–/TTF-1+ in lung adenocarcinoma or CK7–/CK20+/CDX2+ in colorectal carcinoma). Four stains (CK7, CK20, thyroid transcription factor-1 [TTF1], CDX2) form the

TABLE 113.1

Immunohistochemical Tumor Staining Patterns in the Differential Diagnosis of Cancer of Unknown Primary[a]

Tumor Type	Immunohistochemical Staining
Carcinomas	Pan-cytokeratin AE1/3 (+), EMA (+), S100 (–), CLA (–), vimentin (–), CK7, 20 (variable)
Lymphomas	CLA (+), pan-cytokeratin AE1/3 (–), EMA (–), S100 (–)
Melanoma	S100 (+), HMB45 (+), melan-A (+) (all variable), pan-cytokeratin (–), CLA (–)
Sarcoma	Vimentin (+), desmin (+), CD117 (+), myogen (+), factor VIII antigen (+) (all variable), pan-cytokeratin AE1/3 (usually –), S100 (usually –), CLA (–), HMB45 (–), melan-A (–)
Neuroendocrine	Epithelial stains (+), chromogranin (+), synaptophysin (+), CD56 (+) (all variable)
Specific Sarcomas	
Gastrointestinal stromal tumor	CD117 (+), CD34 (+), DOG1 (+)
Mesothelioma	Calretinin (+), CD5/6 (+), WT1 (+), mesothelin (+)
Specific Carcinomas	
Colorectal	CK20 (+), CK7 (–), CDX2 (+)
Lung: adenocarcinoma	CK7(+), CK20 (–), TTF1 (+), napsin A (+)
Lung: squamous	CK7 (+), CK20 (–), P63 (+), CK5/6 (+)
Lung: neuroendocrine (small cell/large cell)	TTF1 (+), chromogranin (+), synaptophysin (+), CD56 (+)
Breast	CK7 (+), ER (+), PR (+), GCDFP-15 (+), Her2/neu (+), mammaglobin (+), GATA3 (+) (all variable)
Ovary	CK7 (+), ER(+), WT1 (+), PAX8 (+), mesothelin (+) (all variable)
Bladder (transitional cell)	CK20 (+), CK5/6 (+), p63(+), GATA3 (+), urothelin (+) (all variable)
Prostate	PSA (+), CK7 (–), CK20 (–)
Pancreas	CK7 (+), Ca19-9 (+), mesothelin (+)
Renal	RCC (+), PAX8 (+), CD10 (+), pan-cytokeratin AE 1/3 (+) (all variable)
Liver	Hepar1 (+), CD10 (+)
Adrenocortical	Alpha-inhibin (+), melan-A (+), CK7(–), CK20(–)
Germ cell	PLAP (+), OCT4 (+)
Thyroid/follicular/papillary	Thyroglobulin (+), TTF1 (+), PAX8 (+)

[a]Derived from references 7, 9, 10, and 14–23.
EMA, epithelial membrane antigen; S100, calcium-binding protein expressed in melanocytes; CD56, neural cell adhesion molecule; CLA, common leukocyte antigen; CK, cytokeratin; HMB-45, anti-human melanosome antibody; melan-A, melanoma antigen; CD34, cluster of differentiation molecule; CD117, tyrosine kinase receptor (c-kit); CDX2, intestinal specific transcription factor; DOG1, calcium dependent chloride channel; Napsin A, novel aspartic proteinase of the pepsin family; TTF1, thyroid transcription factor 1; ER, estrogen receptor; PR, progesterone receptor; GCDFP-15, gross cystic fluid protein 15; GATA3, zinc finger transcription factor family; WT1, Wilms' tumor transcription factor; PAX8, paired box gene 8; p63, tumor suppression gene protein; PSA, prostate specific antigen; RCC, brush border of proximal kidney tubule antibody; CD10, common acute lymphocytic leukemia antigen; hepar1, hepatocyte paraffin 1 marker; PLAP, placental alkaline phosphatase; OCT4, octamer-binding transcription factor 4.

basis of several diagnostic patterns or suggest other possibilities and are appropriate initial stains on most CUP biopsies.

Several problems are associated with the IHC stains. Technical expertise is required to perform these tests accurately; interpretation is subjective and requires an experienced pathologist. False-positive and false-negative results can occur with any of these stains. For example, some carcinomas stain with vimentin, some sarcomas stain with cytokeratins, and a wide variety of carcinomas do not always stain in the expected patterns.[7,22] Some classic staining patterns (see Table 113.1) can overlap with staining patterns of other carcinomas, forcing the pathologist to consider two or three possible primary sites. It is not feasible to routinely perform multiple unselected stains on biopsy specimens, and management of the tissue is becoming extremely important. Consideration of the clinical setting helps to direct the selection of stains and may narrow the spectrum of possibilities if patterns are not completely specific. For example, in a patient with mucin-positive adenocarcinoma and metastases to the liver, a CK20+/CK7–/CDX-2+ staining pattern provides strong evidence for colorectal carcinoma. The IHC findings may lead to additional diagnostic procedures; in the previous example, a colonoscopy should be performed and may identify the anatomical primary site.

In many cases, a single tissue of origin site cannot be identified with certainty even after an histologic examination, IHC staining, and correlation with clinical features. An electron microscopy or karyotypic analysis is occasionally helpful in this setting. However, the use of MTP assays allows for the identification of the tissue of origin in many cases where IHC is nondiagnostic.

Electron Microscopy

A diagnosis can be made by electron microscopy in some poorly differentiated neoplasms, but should be reserved for the study of neoplasms whose lineage is unclear after a routine light microscopy, IHC staining, and an MTP assay. Electron microscopy may be useful in undifferentiated sarcoma. Ultrastructural features such as neurosecretory granules (neuroendocrine tumors) or premelanosomes (melanoma) can suggest a particular tumor. Undifferentiated tumors can lose these specific ultrastructural features; therefore, the absence of a particular ultrastructural finding cannot be used to rule out a specific diagnosis. Electron microscopy is not able to distinguish among various adenocarcinomas and cannot usually identify a tissue of origin.

Karyotypic or Cytogenetic Analysis

The existence of specific chromosomal abnormalities is well characterized in several neoplasms. Most B-cell non-Hodgkin's lymphomas are associated with tumor-specific immunoglobulin gene rearrangements, and typical chromosomal changes have been identified in some B-cell and T-cell lymphomas and in Hodgkin's lymphoma.[23,24] In rare instances, these studies or an MTP assay is necessary when a diagnosis of lymphoma cannot otherwise be established.

The recognition of specific chromosome 12 abnormalities in germ cell tumors (e.g., i[12p], del[12p], multiple copies of 12p) occasionally allowed for the identification of extragonadal germ cell tumors in young men with poorly differentiated carcinoma of unknown origin. Motzer et al.[25] performed a karyotypic analysis on tumors in 40 young men with the extragonadal germ cell syndrome or midline carcinomas of uncertain histogenesis. In 12 of the 40 patients, abnormalities of chromosome 12 (e.g., i[12p]; del [12p]; multiple copies of 12 p) were diagnostic of a germ cell tumor. Other specific abnormalities were diagnostic of melanoma (two patients) and one patient each with lymphoma, peripheral neuroepithelioma, and desmoplastic small cell tumor. Of the germ cell tumors diagnosed on the basis of genetic analysis, five patients achieved a complete response to cisplatin-based chemotherapy.

These data confirm the authors' previously formulated hypothesis that some of these patients have histologically atypical germ cell tumors.

A few other nonrandom chromosomal rearrangements have been identified and occasionally can be useful in the diagnosis of CUP. Some examples include: t(11:22) in peripheral neuroepitheliomas, desmoplastic small round cell tumors, and Ewing's tumor[26–28]; t(15:19) in children and young adults with carcinoma of midline structures of uncertain histogenesis[29]; chromosome 12 abnormalities in germ cell tumors[30–32]; t(2:13) in alveolar rhabdomyosarcoma; 3p deletion in small-cell lung cancer; 1p deletion in neuroblastoma; t(X:18) in synovial sarcoma; and 11p deletion in Wilms' tumor. Epstein-Barr viral genomes in the tumor cells of CUP patients with cervical node metastases highly suggest nasopharyngeal primaries.[33,34]

However, most of these neoplasms can now be identified using methods that are more widely available (IHC, MTP assays), and karyotypic analyses should be reserved for patients with the histologic diagnoses of poorly differentiated neoplasm or PDC, in whom other studies fail to narrow the diagnostic spectrum.

Molecular Tumor Profiling Assays and Cancer Classification

Gene expression or molecular profiling of human neoplasms arose from a DNA microarray analysis described about 20 years ago,[35,36] and subsequent studies have expanded genomic understanding of neoplasms.[37–45] A pivotal study in cancer classification was reported by Golub et al.,[37] and demonstrated for the first time that patterns of gene expression alone could discriminate acute myeloid leukemia from acute lymphoblastic leukemia. Other investigators demonstrated that numerous cancer types could be classified accurately by measuring the differential expression of specific gene sets.[41–61] The basis of molecular profiling in recognizing specific cancer types is the identification of the genes responsible for the synthesis of proteins required for specific normal cellular functions or relatively specific cytoplasmic microRNAs in the many different normal cell types in humans. Cancer cells often retain some of the functional characteristics specific to their tissues of origin, and can be recognized by their gene expression profiles.[59] Therefore, molecular profiling assays designed to determine the type of cancer measure gene expression dynamics in relation to cell lineage, rather than cancer-specific molecular abnormalities.

Patients with CUP represent a large heterogeneous group with clinically undefined anatomical primary tumor site and are ideal candidates for classification by molecular profiling.[38] Several MTP assays (molecular cancer classifiers) have been validated in the identification of known cancers and studied in CUP.

Two such assays are commercially available.[59,61] One of these is a 92-gene reverse transcription polymerase chain reaction (RT-PCR) mRNA assay[59] (Cancer TYPE ID; bioTheranostics, Inc.), whereas the other uses microarray methodology[61] to measure tissue-specific microRNAs (Cancer of Origin Test, Rosetta Genomics). A third microarray mRNA assay was previously also offered (Tissue of Origin Test), but is no longer available.[49]

Two studies of more than 100 tumors each have compared the accuracy of IHC and MTP assays in determining the tissue of origin of known primary cancers.[62,63] These blinded studies usually had generous amounts of tissue to test and allowed the participating pathologists to do numerous IHC stains. The MTP assay diagnostic accuracy was superior to IHC, particularly when tumors were poorly differentiated, or when the IHC diagnosis was unclear following the first round of IHC stains. In addition, the molecular diagnosis required much less tumor tissue (two to three unstained slides). These data support a further evaluation of MTP assays in CUP, particularly when IHC staining is inconclusive or when limited biopsy tissue is available.

STUDIES OF MOLECULAR GENE EXPRESSION TUMOR PROFILING ASSAYS IN CANCER OF UNKNOWN PRIMARY DIAGNOSIS

Accuracy in Tissue of Origin Diagnosis

The determination of the tissue of origin in CUP patients has fundamental importance and has always been the goal of their evaluation. Improved IHC and MTP assays have the potential, when used in conjunction with other clinicopathologic data, to determine the tissue of origin in most CUP patients. However, in order to feel confident in the use of an MTP assay, three questions needed to be addressed: (1) Are they accurate in diagnosing known primary cancers? (2) Are they accurate in diagnosing the tissue of origin in CUP? (3) Are the outcomes of CUP patients improved by site-specific therapies directed by MTP diagnoses? Substantial evidence supports the accuracy of MTP in diagnosing known cancers and CUP, and some of these data are reviewed here. The third question has also been addressed and is discussed in a later section (see Site-Specific Treatment Directed by Results of Molecular Gene Expression Tumor Profiling Assays).

When applied to biopsy specimens from metastatic sites or primary tumors of known cancers, various MTP assays have correctly predicted the tissues of origins and/or primary sites in about 85% of patients.[46–51,59–61] All these studies were blinded and used the known cancer type as the reference. The accuracy of the various MTP assays has not been directly compared.

Accurate identification of the tissue of origin in CUP by MTP is difficult to validate, because the anatomical primary tumor site is unknown and only rarely becomes apparent during the subsequent clinical course of these patients. It would seem reasonable to assume that these assays have a similar accuracy rate in CUP because they have previously demonstrated in metastatic cancers of known types. This assumption is supported by the results of several studies in CUP patients (Table 113.2).[46,47,53–58,64–68] Most studies of the accuracy of MTP assay diagnoses have been indirect, based on the correlation of the assay diagnosis with clinical features and other pathology studies (particularly IHC). In these studies, the MTP predictions correlated closely with the diagnoses suspected on the basis of standard clinical/pathologic findings. In a total of 698 CUP patients from a dozen studies using various MTP assays/platforms, an average of 80% of the molecular diagnoses were consistent with one of the suspected tissues of origin.[46,47,53–58,64–68]

The authors and associates have studied the initial version of the 92-gene RT-PCR MTP assay in CUP patients to determine the accuracy and ability to complement standard pathology.[69] Three methods were used to assess the accuracy of the MTP assay, including a direct validation (gold standard reference) in patients who had their anatomical primary sites (latent primaries) found months to years after their initial CUP diagnoses. Two other indirect methods were used: (1) a comparison of the MTP and IHC diagnoses when IHC was able to predict a single tissue of origin, and (2) additional supportive directed IHC and clinical/histologic findings obtained after the MTP assay diagnoses.

A total of 171 CUP patients were evaluated: 151 prospectively seen from 2008 through 2010, and 20 others with latent primaries identified retrospectively from 501 patients seen from 2001 through 2008. The molecular diagnoses of these patients are listed in Table 113.2. Although the assay requires only 300 to 500 tumor cells, there was insufficient biopsy remaining (RNA) to perform the assay in 22 patients (12.9%). In 5 others (3%), the assay results were unclassifiable or not diagnostic of a single site. Of the 149 patients with sufficient tumor specimens, 144 (96%) were diagnosed with a single tissue of origin (23 tumor types).

Twenty-four patients (20 from retrospective group,[58] and 4 from prospective group) had their latent primary sites detected at a median time of 12 months (range: 2.2 to 78.5 months) after their

TABLE 113.2

Molecular Gene Expression Tumor Profiling Assay Diagnoses

Site	Number	%
Insufficient tumor	22	12.9
Unclassifiable	5	3
Lung/adeno, large cell	18	10.5
Colorectal	26	15.2
Lung/small cell	6	3.5
Lung/squamous cell	1	0.6
Hepatocellular	10	5.8
Breast	15	8.8
Pancreas	9	5.2
Ovary	9	5.2
Bladder	7	4
Kidney	7	4
Gallbladder	6	3.5
Melanoma	5	3
Skin/squamous	5	3
Endometrium	3	1.7
Sarcoma	4	2.3
Testicle	3	1.7
Stomach	2	1.2
Thyroid	2	1.2
Mesothelioma	2	1.2
Others	4	2.4

Note: N = 171.
Adapted from Greco FA, Lennington WJ, Spigel DR, et al. Molecular profiling diagnosis in unknown primary cancer; accuracy and ability to complement standard pathology. *J Natl Cancer Inst* 2013;105:782–790.

initial diagnosis/evaluation of CUP. In 75% (18 of 24 patients), the MTP assay diagnosis of their initial biopsies matched the latent primary tumor sites. In contrast, the IHC evaluation was successful in identifying the site of tumor origin in only 6 of 24 patients (25%).

The second method to assess the accuracy of MTP involved a comparison with IHC predictions in the 52 cases (30%) in which IHC suggested a single tissue of origin (Table 113.3). In 40 of these 52 patients (77%), the MTP and IHC diagnoses were identical. Others have reported similar results from five studies in a total of 65 patients (78% with identical IHC and MTP assay diagnoses) using various assays.[54,55,57,67,70]

The third method to access MTP assay accuracy involved performing additional directed diagnostic studies not included in the initial evaluation (IHC studies, clinical testing, histology review) to support the MTP assay diagnoses. Fifty-four patients (32%) had MTP assay diagnoses that did not match any of the suggested IHC diagnoses; 35 of these patients had remaining biopsy specimens available for additional studies. In 74% of these patients (26 of 35), additional findings supported the accuracy of the MTP assay diagnoses (Table 113.4).

All three methods used in this study support the accuracy (75% to 80%) of the 92-gene RT-PCR assay in determining the tissue of origin in CUP. The accuracy is similar to that seen with MTP assays when tested in known cancer types. The aggregate data from many other studies in patients with CUP[46,47,53–58,64–68] provide additional support of the value of molecular diagnoses. Molecular tumor profiling complements IHC, and usually provides a single

TABLE 113.3

Comparison of MTP Assay Diagnosis with IHC in Tumors with a Single Site Predicted by IHC

Diagnosis	Single Diagnosis by IHC Staining	IHC Staining Pattern	Agreement of MTP Assay Diagnoses with IHC Diagnoses	% Agreement
Colorectal	16	CK20+, CK7–, CDX-2+	15	93
Lung/adeno/large cell	19	CK20–, CK7+, TTF-1+	14	74
Lung/neuroendocrine	3	CK7+, TTF1+, chromogranin+ or synaptophysin+ or CD56+	2	66
Breast	5	CK20–, CK7+, mammaglobin+ or ER+ or GCDFP-15+	5	100
Melanoma	3	S100+, Melan-A+ or HMB45+	2	66
Germ cell	2	PLAP+ or OCT4+	1	50
Ovary	1	CK20–, CK7+, CA125+, WT1+, ER+	0	0
Hepatocellular	1	CD10+, Hepar-1+	1	100
Sarcoma	1	Vimentin+, CK7–, S100–, desmin+, CK20–	0	0
Prostate	1	CK20–, CK7–, PSA+	0	0
Total	52		40	77

Note: N = 52.
CK, cytokeratin; CDX-2; intestinal specific transcription factor 2; S100, calcium-binding protein expressed in melanocytes; ER, estrogen receptor; GCDFP-15, gross cystic disease fluid protein 15; CA125, cancer antigen 125; WT1, Wilms' tumor transcription factor; hepar-1, hepatocyte paraffin 1 marker.
Adapted from Greco FA, Lennington WJ, Spigel DR, et al. Molecular profiling diagnosis in unknown primary cancer; accuracy and ability to complement standard pathology. *J Natl Cancer Inst* 2013;105:782–790.

diagnosis when IHC is inconclusive. When IHC predicted a single tissue of origin (as in 33% of patients in our series) the MTP assay prediction has high concordance and is probably not necessary.

As MTP is incorporated into the diagnostic evaluation of CUP patients, several potential pitfalls should be considered.[69] First, tumor biopsy specimens are often small, and the medical oncologist and pathologist should use available tissue judiciously. Performing multiple IHC stains in a tumor that is difficult to classify can deplete the biopsy and preclude MTP. In some cases, a repeat biopsy should be considered. Second, MTP assay diagnoses are not 100% accurate, even in the identification of known cancer types. MTP predictions should always be considered in context with clinical features and results of other pathologic studies. If the MTP diagnosis is inconsistent with other findings, additional directed IHC stains or a clinical evaluation may help to support the diagnosis. Third, several neoplasms have overlapping gene expressions, and a misdiagnosis may occur in these circumstances (e.g., breast, salivary gland, and skin adnexal tumors have similar gene expression profiles). Fourth, any tumor types that are not included in the MTP assay panel cannot be diagnosed, and may be considered unclassifiable or misdiagnosed as a cancer with an overlapping gene expression profile.

Diagnosis in Poorly Differentiated Neoplasms

The use of modern IHC staining is usually effective at defining the tumor lineage in CUP patients with poorly differentiated neoplasms. In the uncommon tumor that defies classification, MTP usually clarifies the lineage and, in some cases, can identify the tissue of origin.[71]

From 2000 through 2012, 751 CUP patients were seen at the authors' referral center,[71] and 30 (4%) had no definitive lineage determined after extensive IHC (median of 18 stains; range: 9 to 51). The archival biopsies were tested with the 92-gene RT-PCR assay and when feasible, the additional evaluation was performed to support the molecular diagnoses (e.g., directed IHC not previously done, fluorescence in situ hybridization (FISH) for specific molecular abnormalities, gene sequencing, repeat biopsies, and correlation with clinical features). Four tumors were unclassifiable by

MTP, and one additional tumor had insufficient biopsy material available (17%). A lineage diagnosis was made in 25 of 30 patients (83%), including carcinoma in 10 (germ cell: 3, neuroendocrine: 2, others: 5), sarcoma in 8 (mesothelioma: 3, primitive neuroectodermal tumor [PNET]: 1, others: 5), melanoma in 5, and hematopoietic neoplasm in 2 (lymphoma: 2). Additional directed IHC, genetic testing (BRAF, i12p), or repeat biopsies done after MTP confirmed the MTP diagnoses in 11 of 15 patients (73%). Earlier use of MTP in the diagnosis of these difficult cases would have resulted in the expedited identification of tumor lineage in almost all patients, and often in a prediction of the specific tissue of origin. Because this group of tumors contains germ cell tumors, lymphoma, neuroendocrine tumors, and melanomas, an accurate diagnosis is critical. Molecular tumor profiling appears superior to IHC in the diagnosis of these undifferentiated cancers.

Diagnosis of the Cancer of Unknown Primary Renal Cell Carcinoma Subset

The renal carcinoma subset of CUP has not been previously systematically addressed. A few CUP cases have been reported[72,73] after recognition by pathologic features or MTP. The diagnosis of renal carcinoma is of practical importance, because these tumors are usually insensitive to cytotoxic chemotherapy, yet may often be treated with good control by a number of approved targeted/biologic drugs. When clear cell histology is seen in a CUP biopsy, the possibility of renal carcinoma is considered, and IHC may be diagnostic. However, histologies of adenocarcinoma or poorly differentiated carcinoma may not suggest renal carcinoma, and IHC stains to support the diagnosis of renal carcinoma may not be done.

In order to further characterize the renal cancer subset, 488 CUP patients seen from 2008 to 2012 had MTP of their biopsies using the 92-gene RT-PCR assay.[74] In many of these patients, MTP results were available for patient management. A renal carcinoma diagnosis was made in 22 patients (4.5%), including the subtypes papillary in 8, clear cell in 7 and unknown in 7. None of these patients had a primary site detected by abdominal computed tomography, and the metastatic sites most often included retroperitoneal nodes (63%), mediastinal nodes (31%), lung (22%), and bone

TABLE 113.4

Results of Additional IHC Stains and/or Clinicopathologic Studies Performed to Support MTP Assay Diagnoses in Tumors with Uncertain Initial IHC Diagnoses

MTP Assay Diagnoses (All with Uncertain IHC Diagnoses)	Additional Subsequent IHC and/or Clinicopathologic Findings
1. Kidney	CD10+, CA-9+, vimentin+
2. Kidney	RCC+
3. Kidney	Histologic review: scattered papillary and chromophobe features, vimentin+
4. Kidney	CD10+, CA-9+
5. Hepatocellular	Serum α-fetoprotein 5259, reticulin stain+
6. Hepatocellular	Serum α-fetoprotein 1326
7. Hepatocellular	Serum α-fetoprotein 649, Hepar1+
8. Hepatocellular	Serum α-fetoprotein 810
9. Hepatocellular	Serum α-fetoprotein 501
10. Ovary/serous	ER+, PR+, WT1+
11. Ovary/clear cell	New ascites, WT1+
12. Mesothelioma	Abdominal and pelvic masses, calretinin+
13. Mesothelioma	Abdominal mass, calretinin+
14. Sarcoma	CK7−, CK20−, S100−, LCA−, vimentin+, isolated bone/soft tissue lesion
15. Sarcoma	Desmin+, vimentin+, rapid growth chest wall and lung masses
16. Skin/squamous (also breast signature) suggests skin adnexal carcinoma	Isolated epidermal lesion (primary adnexal skin adenocarcinoma); initially felt to be metastatic
17. Skin/squamous (also breast signature) suggests skin adnexal carcinoma	Isolated epidermal lesion (primary adnexal skin adenocarcinoma); initially felt to be metastatic
18. Lung/neuroendocrine	Synaptophysin+
19. Lung/neuroendocrine	Chromogranin+, synaptophysin+
20. Endometrium	Pelvic mass, PR+, ER+
21. Intestine/carcinoid	CK20+, synaptophysin+, CDX2+
22. Bladder	CK7−, CK20−, p63+, histologic review: areas of transitional cell carcinoma
23. Breast	ER+
24. Intestinal	CDX2+
25. Seminoma	CK7−, CK20−, PLAP+
26. Prostate	Developed sclerotic bone lesions, serum PSA 32 (initially normal)
27–35. Various diagnoses	No additional supportive data found

Note: N = 35.
CD10, common acute lymphocytic leukemia antigen; CA-9, cancer antigen 9; cancer antigen 9; RCC, brush border of proximal kidney tubule antibody; hepar1, hepatocyte paraffin 1 marker; ER, estrogen receptor; PR, progesterone receptor; WT1, Wilms' tumor transcription factor; CK, cytokeratin; S100, calcium-binding protein expressed in melanocytes; LCA, leukocyte common antigen; CDX2, intestinal specific transcription factor.
Adapted from Greco FA, Lennington WJ, Spigel DR, et al. Molecular profiling diagnosis in unknown primary cancer; accuracy and ability to complement standard pathology. *J Natl Cancer Inst* 2013;105:782–790.

(18%). Only 1 biopsy had clear cell histology; 15 were PDC and 6 were adenocarcinomas (4 with papillary features). Because the histology did not suggest renal carcinoma in most patients, only three tumors (14%) had renal directed IHC (RCC, PAX8 stains) performed. However, additional IHCs performed to support the MTP assay diagnoses were typical of a renal origin in seven of nine tumors where a remaining biopsy was available. Sixteen patients received first-line treatment for advanced renal carcinoma; the objective response was 18% and the median survival was 13.4 months.

Renal cell carcinoma is a subset of CUP, which can be diagnosed by MTP assay and/or IHC. When the histologic examination does not identify clear cell features, the diagnosis of renal carcinoma may not be considered, and IHC staining for renal cancer may not be done. Papillary renal carcinoma was a relatively common subtype in the group studied. These patients are important to identify because they may benefit from renal cell–directed targeted drugs but not from empiric chemotherapy.

Diagnosis of the Cancer of Unknown Primary Colorectal Subset

These patients have been characterized recently and are a favorable subset. These data are discussed later (see section Treatment: Favorable Subsets: Colorectal Profile).

Summary

Molecular tumor profiling can predict the tissue of origin in a majority (about 95%) of patients with CUP when there is sufficient biopsy material available. These predictions are accurate in 75% to 80% of patients, as determined by several methods, including an evaluation of CUP patients who developed latent primaries. The correlation between IHC and MTP diagnoses is good (about 80%) when IHC predicts a specific tissue of origin; in patients with diagnostic IHC, MTP is not necessary. However, in the majority of patients, IHC is inconclusive and MTP provides valuable additional diagnostic information. The optimal identification and evaluation of several subgroups of potential therapeutic importance, including colorectal, renal cell, and poorly differentiated neoplasms now requires the use of MTP in conjunction with a standard pathologic evaluation. A specific diagnosis of some tissues of origin by MTP should trigger additional molecular analysis, because effective targeted therapy for patient subsets is becoming common. For example, a prediction of non–small-cell lung cancer, should prompt an analysis for treatable molecular alterations, including epidermal growth factor receptor (EGFR)-activating mutations and anaplastic lymphoma kinase (ALK) or ROS1 rearrangements.

CLINICAL FEATURES AND EVALUATION

Most patients with CUP develop signs or symptoms at the site of a metastatic lesion and are diagnosed with advanced cancer. The subsequent clinical course is usually dominated by symptoms related to metastases; a latent primary site becomes obvious in about 5% of patients during their lifetime. At autopsy, a primary site is identified in about 75% of patients.[3,6] Primary sites in the pancreas, lung, colon/rectum, and liver account for approximately 60% of those identified. Primary sites in the breast, ovary, and prostate are uncommon in autopsy series, but data from MTP assay series suggest that the biliary tract, the urothelial tract, the breast, and the ovarian tissues of origin are more common than previously recognized.[6,52]

Although some clinical differences exist, there is substantial overlap between the clinical features of patients with adenocarcinoma and PDC. Patients with PDC have a somewhat younger median age and usually exhibit rapid tumor growth. These patients may also have a more frequent location of dominant metastatic sites in the mediastinum, retroperitoneum, and peripheral lymph nodes. The clinical evaluation of patients with these histologies should follow the same guidelines. Patients with neuroendocrine carcinoma and squamous carcinoma are discussed separately.

TABLE 113.5

Initial Diagnostic Evaluation

- Complete history: including detailed review of systems
- Complete physical examination: including pelvic examination, stool for occult blood
- Complete blood cell count, comprehensive metabolic panel, lactate dehydrogenase, urinalysis
- Computed tomography scans of chest, abdomen, and pelvis
- Mammography in women
- Serum prostate-specific antigen in men
- Positron emission tomography scan in selected patients
- Pathology: including screening immunohistochemistry marker stains (CK7, CK20, TTF-1, CDX2)
- MTP assay if small biopsy specimen

Clinical Evaluation

The recommended clinical evaluation for all patients is summarized in Table 113.5. In actuality, many of these procedures are usually done in the process of diagnosing CUP. The goal is to find the anatomical primary site or, if not possible, the tissue of origin. Although positron-emission tomography (PET) scanning may be useful in some patients,[57] it should not be considered routine in the initial CUP evaluation; definitive data in large numbers of patients have not been published[75] and PET was not superior to computed tomography (CT) in finding a primary site in one comparative study.[76]

A further evaluation of patients should be directed by results of the initial clinical and pathologic evaluations. A focused evaluation may: (1) identify an anatomical primary site, (2) narrow the spectrum of possible tissues of origin, (3) identify specific favorable subsets of patients, or (4) identify the tissue of origin even if the anatomical primary site is undetectable.

Table 113.6 summarizes the additional evaluation indicated for several common clinical presentations. An additional focused

TABLE 113.6

Focused Diagnostic Evaluation of Patient Subsets Defined by Initial Clinicopathologic Evaluation

Initial Evaluation	Additional Evaluation
Women with features of possible breast cancer (bone, lung, liver metastases, CK7+)	Breast magnetic resonance imaging ER, GCDFP-15, GATA3 stains, FISH for HER2 (MTP assay if necessary)
Women with features of possible ovarian cancer (pelvic/peritoneal metastases; CK7+)	Pelvic/intravaginal ultrasound WT1, PAX8 stains (MTP assay if necessary)
Mediastinal/retroperitoneal mass	Testicular ultrasound Serum HCG, AFP PLAP, OCT4 stains; FISH for i(12p) (MTP assay if necessary)
Features of lung cancer (hilar/mediastinal adenopathy; CK7+, TTF1+, Napsin A+)	Bronchoscopy (MTP assay if necessary), Genetic studies for EGFR mutations, ALK/ROS1 rearrangements
Features of colon cancer (liver/peritoneal metastases; CK20+/CK7−, CDX2+)	Colonoscopy (MTP assay if necessary), Genetic study for KRAS mutation
Poorly differentiated carcinoma, with or without clear cell features	Stains for chromogranin, synaptophysin, RCC, hepar-1, HMB-45, Melan-A (If melanoma stains +, genetic study for BRAF mutation; if hepar-1+, obtain serum AFP; if neuroendocrine stains +, obtain octreotide scan (MTP assay if necessary)

CK, cytokeratin; ER, estrogen receptor; GCDFP-15, gross cystic fluid protein 15; GATA3, zinc finger transcription factor family; WT1, Wilms' tumor transcription factor; PAX8, paired box gene 8; HCG, human chorionic gonadotropin; AFP, α-fetoprotein; OCT4, octamen-binding transcription factor 4; HMB-45, anti-human melanoma antibody 45.

PRACTICE OF ONCOLOGY

evaluation should be triggered by either clinical findings or IHC results during the initial evaluation. An MTP assay is indicated when IHC or other testing is not conclusive. Panels of IHC stains and an MTP assay are complementary and when considered in conjunction with all other data provide a tissue of origin diagnosis in the majority of CUP patients.

Neuroendocrine Carcinoma

Although the initial clinical evaluation is the same (see Table 113.5), patients with neuroendocrine carcinoma require special consideration in determining appropriate treatment. Of major importance is the separation of this group into tumors with low-grade histology (classic carcinoid) and indolent clinical course versus those with high-grade histology (small or large cell with neuroendocrine features) and an aggressive clinical course. Some of the high-grade carcinomas may not be recognized as neuroendocrine by H&E staining, but are usually diagnosed by IHC or MTP assay.

Low-grade neuroendocrine carcinomas, when presenting with an unknown primary site, most frequently involve the liver. Other metastatic sites include the lymph nodes (usually abdominal or mediastinal) and bone. Some are associated with various syndromes caused by the secretion of bioactive peptides (carcinoid syndrome, glucagonoma syndrome, VIPomas, Zollinger-Ellison syndrome). An additional clinical evaluation in these patients should include serum or urine screening for these substances. In addition to the evaluation listed in Table 113.5, an octreotide scan as well as an upper and lower gastrointestinal endoscopy should be performed, because some of these patients have detectable primary sites in the gastrointestinal tract. An MTP assay may diagnose the tissue of origin in some patients[12,13]; the identification of a pancreatic site of origin is potentially important because targeted drugs (sunitinib, everolimus) are useful in this setting.

High-grade neuroendocrine carcinomas of unknown primary site are usually found in multiple metastatic sites and rarely secrete bioactive peptides. Patients with small- or large-cell histology and a history of cigarette smoking should be suspected of having an occult lung primary and a fiber optic bronchoscopy should be considered. Patients with a positive tumor cell IHC stain for TTF1 should also be considered for a bronchoscopy. Extrapulmonary small-cell carcinomas arising from a variety of other primary sites (salivary glands, paranasal sinuses, esophagus, pancreas, colon/rectum, bladder, prostate, uterus, cervix) have been described and are occasionally identified during a clinical evaluation. A colonoscopy should be considered in patients with tumor IHC staining positive for CDX2.

The origin of these high-grade neuroendocrine carcinomas remains unclear. The tissue of origin may be determined in some patients by an MTP assay, but this knowledge now usually does not change therapy for most patients. Some patients with small-cell histology may have occult small-cell lung cancer. However, more than half of these patients have no smoking history, which makes this diagnosis unlikely. It has been speculated that these undifferentiated tumors share the same origin as the low-grade neuroendocrine tumors, and are at opposite ends of a *spectrum* of tumor biology. However, it now seems more likely that these high-grade neuroendocrine tumors have a different oncogenesis; many share the chromosomal abnormalities commonly seen in small-cell lung cancer (deletions of chromosomes 3p, 5q, 10q, and 17p), whereas no shared molecular abnormalities have been found with indolent carcinoid-type tumors.[77,78]

Anaplastic or atypical carcinoid tumors arising in the gastrointestinal tract are responsive to platinum-based chemotherapy, whereas carcinoid tumors with typical histology are usually resistant.[79] A few reports of patients with extrapulmonary small-cell carcinomas of unknown primary site have also documented chemotherapy responsiveness and occasional long-term survival after systemic therapy.[80,81] However, the term *extrapulmonary small-cell carcinoma* implies the existence of a known primary site; some

CUP neuroendocrine tumors may have arisen from an occult extrapulmonary site, but are aptly described as neuroendocrine carcinoma of unknown primary site.

Squamous Carcinoma

Squamous carcinoma, as opposed to other histologies, often presents with isolated metastases in the cervical or inguinal lymph nodes. The cervical nodes are the most common metastatic site. Patients are usually middle aged or elderly, and frequently, they have abused tobacco or alcohol, although recently it has also been associated with human papilloma virus infection. When the upper or middle cervical nodes are involved, a primary tumor in the head and neck region should be suspected. The clinical evaluation should include an examination of the oropharynx, hypopharynx, nasopharynx, larynx, and upper esophagus by direct endoscopy, with a biopsy of any suspicious areas. CT of the neck better defines the disease in the neck and occasionally identifies a primary site. PET scanning in this subset is indicated, because it can frequently identify primary tumor sites.[82] Detection of Epstein-Barr virus genome in the tumor tissue is highly suggestive of a nasopharyngeal primary site,[33,34,83] particularly in poorly differentiated carcinomas. When the lower cervical or supraclavicular nodes are involved, a primary lung cancer should be suspected. A fiber optic bronchoscopy may identify a lung primary if other evaluations are unrevealing.[84]

An ipsilateral or bilateral tonsillectomy has been advocated as a diagnostic modality in patients with single nodal or bilateral nodal involvement, respectively.[85] In one series of 87 patients who had tonsillectomy as part of their workup for cervical node presentations, 26% had a tonsillar primary identified.[86] The identification of the primary site has several advantages in this group of patients, including the ability to develop a specific treatment plan, a reduction of the radiation therapy fields, more accurate assessment of prognosis, and easier follow-up.

Most patients with involvement of inguinal nodes have a detectable primary site in the anogenital area. Careful examination of the anal canal, vulva, vagina, uterine cervix, penis, and scrotum is important, with biopsy of any suspicious areas. The identification of a primary site in these patients is consequential because curative therapy is available for carcinomas of the vulva, vagina, cervix, and anus, even after it has spread to regional nodes.

Metastatic squamous carcinoma in areas other than the cervical or inguinal nodes usually represents metastasis from an occult lung cancer, but metastases from several other sites (the esophagus, skin, uterine cervix, and anal canal) are also possible. An MTP assay may be useful in the diagnosis of the tissue of origin and provides the basis of site-specific therapy.

TREATMENT

The heterogeneous group of patients with CUP contains some patients who experience long-term survival after appropriate treatment and others for whom treatment makes little or no impact. Patients who have an anatomical primary site defined during their clinical evaluation do not have CUP and should be treated appropriately for their defined tumor type. A second group of patients can be identified as having favorable subsets and, in most, their tissues of origin may be presumed, even when the anatomical primary site is not identified (Table 113.7). The management of these subsets is detailed in this section. Most CUP patients (approximately 80%) do not fit into a favorable subset, even after an appropriate clinical and pathologic evaluation. Empiric chemotherapy has been the treatment standard for many years, and will be briefly reviewed. However, there is now ample evidence to support the use of site-specific therapy for most patients, guided by IHC and MTP predictions of the tissue of origin. These new data will also be reviewed.

TABLE 113.7

Carcinoma of Unknown Primary Site: Summary of Evaluation and Therapy of Favorable Subsets

Carcinoma	Clinical Evaluation[a]	Special Studies	Subsets	Therapy	Prognosis
Adenocarcinoma (well-differentiated or moderately differentiated)[b]	Chest, abdominal CT scan; PET scan Men: Serum PSA Women: Mammogram Additional studies to evaluate symptoms, signs	Men: PSA stain Women: ER, PR, Other IHC (see text) MTP assay (see text)	1. Women, axillary node involvement[b] 2. Women, peritoneal carcinomatosis[b] 3. Men, blastic bone metastases, high serum PSA, or PSA tumor staining 4. Single metastatic site[b] 5. Colon cancer profile	1. Treat as primary breast cancer 2. Surgical cytoreduction plus chemotherapy 3. Hormonal therapy for prostate cancer 4. Resection and/or radiotherapy 5. Treat as metastatic colon cancer	Survival improved with specific therapy
Squamous carcinoma	Cervical node presentation[b] Panendoscopy PET scan Supraclavicular presentation[b] Bronchoscopy PET scan Inguinal presentation[b] Pelvic, rectal examinations, anoscopy, PET scan	Genetic analysis including MTP assay (see text)	1. Cervical adenopathy; nasopharyngeal cancer identified by PCR for Epstein-Barr viral genes 2. Supraclavicular 3. Inguinal adenopathy	1. Radiation therapy, neck dissection, chemotherapy 2. Radiation therapy, chemotherapy 3. Inguinal node dissection, radiation therapy, chemotherapy	Survival improved 1. 25%–50% 5-y survival 2. 5%–15% 5-y survival 3. 15%–20% 5-y survival
Poorly differentiated carcinoma, poorly differentiated adenocarcinoma	Chest, abdominal CT scans, serum HCG, AFP; PET scan; additional studies to evaluate symptoms, signs	IHC; electron microscopy; genetic analysis; MTP assay (see text)	1. Atypical germ cell tumors (identified by chromosome 12 abnormalities) 2. Extragonadal germ cell syndrome (two features) 3. Lymph node–predominant tumors (mediastinum, retroperitoneum, peripheral nodes) 4. Gastrointestinal stromal tumors (identified by CD117 stain) 5. Other groups (see text)	1. Treatment for germ cell tumor 2. Cisplatin/etoposide 3. Treat with site-specific therapy (see text) 4. Imatinib 5. Treat with site-specific therapy (see text)	1. 40%–50% cure rate 2. Survival improved (10%–20% cured) 3. Survival improved 4. Survival improved 5. Survival improved
Neuroendocrine carcinoma	Chest, abdominal CT	IHC, Electron microscopy Genetic analysis including MTP assay (see text)	1. Low-grade 2. Small-cell carcinoma (or Ewing's family of tumors) 3. Poorly differentiated	1. Treat as advanced carcinoid 2, 3. Carboplatin/ etoposide or platinum/etoposide (or other)	1. Indolent biology/ long survival 2, 3. High response rate, survival improved; rarely cured

PSA, prostate-specific antigen; ER, estrogen receptor; PR, progesterone receptor; HCG, human chorionic gonadotropin; AFP, α-fetoprotein.
[a] In addition to history, physical examination, routine laboratory tests, and chest x-ray films.
[b] May also present with poorly differentiated carcinoma, and management and outcome are similar.

Favorable Subsets

Women with Peritoneal Carcinomatosis

Adenocarcinoma, particularly serous adenocarcinoma, causing diffuse peritoneal involvement, is typical of ovarian carcinoma, although carcinomas from the gastrointestinal tract, lung, or breast can occasionally produce this clinical syndrome. On occasion, women with diffuse peritoneal carcinomatosis have no primary site found in the ovaries or elsewhere in the abdomen at the time of laparotomy. These patients frequently have histologic features typical of ovarian carcinoma, such as papillary serous configuration or psammoma bodies, and also share clinical features, such as elevated serum cancer antigen 125 (CA-125) levels. These tumors are more common in women with a family history of ovarian cancer, and prophylactic oophorectomy does not always protect them from this tumor.[87] Like ovarian carcinoma, the incidence of primary peritoneal carcinoma is increased in women with *BRCA1/2* mutations.[88]

It is now clear that many of these carcinomas arise from the peritoneal surface (primary peritoneal carcinoma) or from the fimbriated end of the fallopian tubes.[89,90] Many of these tumors have characteristic IHC findings (ovary pattern) or diagnostic MTP assays. Carcinomas arising from the peritoneal (mesothelial) surface or the uterine tubes share a common lineage (müllerian derivation) and biology with ovarian carcinoma. Support for this hypothesis has been strengthened by the demonstration of gene expression profiles nearly identical to ovarian carcinoma.[58] Treatment of these women with standard ovarian carcinoma regimens (surgical cytoreduction followed by taxane/platinum chemotherapy) produces results similar to those seen in ovarian cancer.[91–93] This entity has very rarely been seen in men.[94]

Women with Axillary Lymph Node Metastases

Breast cancer should be suspected in women who have metastatic carcinoma in an axillary lymph node.[95] Men with occult breast cancer can present in this fashion, but these are very rare. The initial lymph node biopsy should be stained for IHC breast markers. When positive, these findings provide strong support of the diagnosis.[96] An MTP assay may also be diagnostic in this setting.

If no other metastases are identified, these patients may have stage II breast cancer with an occult primary, which is potentially curable with appropriate therapy. Magnetic resonance imaging and PET have occasionally identified primary breast cancer even with normal mammography.[97–99] A modified radical mastectomy has been recommended, even when physical examination and mammography are normal. An invasive breast primary has been identified after mastectomy in 44% to 80% of patients. Primary tumors are usually less than 2 cm in diameter and may measure only a few millimeters; occasionally in patients, only a noninvasive tumor is identified in the breast. Prognosis after primary therapy is similar to that of other patients with stage II breast cancer.[95] Radiation therapy to the breast after axillary lymph node sampling and chemotherapy represents a reasonable alternative primary therapy.[100] Either neoadjuvant or adjuvant systemic therapy is indicated in this setting, following guidelines established for the treatment of stage II breast cancer.

Women with metastatic sites in addition to the axillary lymph nodes, particularly when supported by IHC and/or a MTP assay diagnosis, should be managed as metastatic breast cancer. Hormone receptor and *HER2* status are of particular importance in these patients because they may derive major benefit from hormonal therapy, chemotherapy, or HER2-targeted agents.

Men with Elevated Serum Prostate-Specific Antigen or Prostate-Specific Antigen Tumor Staining

Serum prostate-specific antigen (PSA) concentrations should be measured in men with adenocarcinoma of unknown primary site. These tumors can also be stained for PSA. Even when clinical features (i.e., metastatic pattern) do not suggest prostate cancer, a positive PSA (serum or tumor stain) is reason for a trial of androgen deprivation.[101,102] In some of these patients, a needle biopsy of the prostate might confirm the primary site but may not be necessary for optimal clinical management. Osteoblastic bone metastases in the absence of a defined origin and other metastatic sites are also an indication for an empiric hormone trial, regardless of the PSA findings. Although IHC is usually diagnostic, an MTP assay may also provide a definitive diagnosis.

Extragonadal Germ Cell Cancer Syndrome

The extragonadal germ cell cancer syndrome was first described in 1979.[103–105] The full syndrome, which is seen in only a minority of patients, has the following features: (1) occurrence in men less than 50 years of age; (2) predominant tumor location in the midline (mediastinum, retroperitoneum) or multiple pulmonary nodules; (3) short duration of symptoms (less than 3 months) and a history of rapid tumor growth; (4) elevated serum levels of human chorionic gonadotropin (HCG), α-fetoprotein (AFP), or both; and (5) good response to previously administered radiation therapy or chemotherapy. These tumors may be definitively diagnosed by IHC and/or an MTP assay or by testing for specific chromosome 12 abnormalities. If the diagnosis remains uncertain, patients with this syndrome may still have atypical germ cell tumors, and treatment with cisplatin-based chemotherapy is recommended.

Single Site of Neoplasm

When only one site of neoplasm is identified (e.g., one node group, one mass), the possibility of an unusual primary tumor mimicking metastatic disease should be considered. Several unusual tumors could present in this fashion, including Merkel-cell neuroendocrine tumors, skin adnexal tumors (e.g., apocrine, eccrine, and sebaceous carcinomas), sarcomas, melanomas, or lymphomas that are mistakenly interpreted as metastatic carcinoma. Patients with a clinically detectable single metastasis (brain, liver, adrenal, subcutaneous tissue, bone, intestine, lymph node, skin, or other sites) usually have other undetectable sites. Some of these patients may have a primary tumor at the single site that developed from embryonic rest cells or adult stem cells. A PET scan may be helpful to exclude other unsuspected metastatic sites.[106]

These patients without other documented metastasis should be treated with aggressive local therapy because a minority enjoy long-term, disease-free survival. If their tissue of origin is determined by IHC or MTP, site-specific systemic chemotherapy should be considered in either the neoadjuvant or adjuvant setting.

Patients with a single small site of metastasis frequently survive 1 year or longer, regardless of their tissue of origin, and thus represent a favorable prognostic subset. In a reported group of patients presenting with single brain metastasis of unknown primary site, 15% remained progression free 5 years after definitive therapy.[107] The authors have treated and followed 36 patients with single site metastases (unpublished observations). All patients had local therapy (resection with or without radiotherapy) and most also received empiric chemotherapy regimens. The median survival in this group is 17 months; 1-, 2-, and 3-year survivals are 65%, 40%, and 28%, respectively. These overall results may be improved with site-specific systemic therapy.

Squamous Carcinoma Involving Cervical or Supraclavicular Lymph Nodes

Squamous carcinoma most frequently presents with unilateral involvement of the cervical lymph nodes. The recommended clinical evaluation (previously described) results in the identification of a head and neck primary site in almost 85% of patients. In those without a defined anatomical primary site, an occult primary site in the head and neck may be presumed.

When no primary site is identified, local treatment should be given to the involved neck. Results have been reviewed in more than 1,400 patients, derived primarily from retrospective single-institution experiences and treated with a variety of local treatment modalities.[108] In many of these series, a large minority of patients had PDC or adenocarcinoma. Long-term, disease-free survival was achieved in 30% to 40% of patients following treatment with local modalities. The results obtained using radical neck dissection, high-dose radiation therapy, or a combination of these modalities have been similar. The volume of tumor in the involved neck influences outcome, with N1 or N2 disease having a significantly higher cure rate than N3 or massive neck involvement.[109] Poorly differentiated carcinoma also represents a poor prognostic factor in these patients. When resection is used alone, a primary tumor in the head and neck subsequently becomes apparent in 20% to 40% of patients. Primary tumors surface less commonly when radiation therapy is used, presumably because of the eradication of occult head and neck primary sites within the radiation field. Radiation therapy dosages and techniques should be similar to those used in patients with primary head and neck cancer, and the nasopharynx, oropharynx, and hypopharynx may be included in the irradiated field.

The role of chemotherapy for carcinoma in cervical lymph nodes is now generally accepted. No randomized studies have been performed, but a nonrandomized comparison favored chemotherapy plus radiotherapy versus local therapy[110] (median survival: 37 months versus 24 months). Concurrent treatment with chemotherapy and radiotherapy is now standard in locally advanced head and neck carcinoma, and should be the treatment of choice for squamous cell carcinoma in cervical lymph nodes.

Patients with low cervical and supraclavicular nodes do not do as well because lung cancer is a frequent site of occult primary tumors, although the skin, uterine cervix, esophagus, and anus are also possible primary sites. Molecular assays may be helpful in predicting the primary site. Patients with no detectable disease below the clavicle should be treated with aggressive local therapy, and 10% to 15% have long-term, disease-free survival. Concurrent chemotherapy should also be considered for these patients.

Squamous Carcinoma Involving Inguinal Lymph Nodes

Most patients with squamous carcinoma involving inguinal lymph nodes have a detectable primary site in the anogenital areas. For the unusual patient in whom no primary site is identified, inguinal lymph node dissection with or without radiation therapy to the inguinal area sometimes results in long-term survival.[111] An MTP assay may diagnose the tissue of origin and suggests appropriate therapy. These patients should also be considered for neoadjuvant or adjuvant chemotherapy, because occult primaries from the uterine cervix and anal canal are likely to be responsive to chemotherapy.

Low-Grade Neuroendocrine Carcinoma

These tumors usually exhibit an indolent biology, and slow progression over the years is likely. Management should follow guidelines established for metastatic carcinoid or islet cell tumors from known primary sites. Treatment with octreotide long-acting release (LAR) results in an increase in time to tumor progression with low toxicity.[112] Depending on the clinical situation, appropriate management may also include local therapy (resection of isolated metastasis, hepatic artery ligation or embolization, cryotherapy, radiofrequency ablation). Several cytotoxic agents have some activity (streptozotocin, doxorubicin, 5-fluorouracil, capecitabine, temozolomide), and results with targeted agents (sunitinib, everolimus) from pancreatic primaries are promising. These neoplasms are usually refractory to intensive systemic chemotherapy, and cisplatin-based chemotherapy produces low response rates.[104]

High-Grade Neuroendocrine Carcinomas

Patients with aggressive neuroendocrine carcinomas are those with either small-cell carcinoma or PDC (often large cell) with neuroendocrine staining by IHC or a diagnosis by MTP assay. Tumors with these histologies are initially responsive to combination chemotherapy, and patients should be considered for a trial of treatment.

The initial report of 29 patients with poorly differentiated neuroendocrine tumors[113] was updated to include 99 patients, with 94 treated with combination chemotherapy.[108] These patients had clinical evidence of rapid tumor growth and multiple metastases. Of 87 assessable patients, 59 (68%) responded to a platinum-based combination regimen. Nineteen patients (22%) had complete responses, and 13 remained continuously disease free more than 2 years after the completion of therapy.

The results of a prospective trial using the combination of paclitaxel, carboplatin, and oral etoposide in 48 patients (of the 99 previously listed) have been reported.[114] The majority of these

cancers were initially called PDC (about 20% were small-cell carcinoma) and were later defined as neuroendocrine by IHC staining or electron microscopy. These patients usually had several sites of metastasis, often with a predominant tumor in the bones, liver, and nodes (particularly retroperitoneum and mediastinum). The overall response rate was 55%, with six complete responses (13%). The median survival was 14 months and 10 patients survived beyond 2 years (range: 2 to 6 years).

Data remain limited in this uncommon group of patients; however, current first-line chemotherapy should include the platinum-based regimens used for small-cell lung cancer. In the uncommon patient with a single site of involvement, radiation therapy with or without resection should be added to combination chemotherapy.

In some of these patients, MTP assays may diagnose the tissue of origin,[12,13] but it remains uncertain if this knowledge can be applied to improve therapies in the high-grade tumors, although the gastrointestinal primaries may respond to site-specific regimens such as folinic acid, fluorouracil, and oxaliplatin (FOLFOX).

Poorly Differentiated Carcinoma

Although patients with PDC form a large and heterogeneous group, the inclusion of patients with highly treatable neoplasms within this group has been recognized since the late 1970s.[103–105] At that time, several young men with mediastinal tumors were reported who had complete responses to combination chemotherapy. Elevated serum levels of HCG or AFP were common in these young men. Although the histology was not diagnostic, these patients were thought to have histologically atypical extragonadal germ cell tumors. Several other specific cancers have also subsequently been identified in some of these patients (i.e., thymic neoplasms, neuroendocrine tumors, midline carcinoma with t[15;19], sarcomas, melanomas, lymphomas), but others defy precise classification.

Further evidence for the responsiveness of tumors in many other patients has accumulated over the years. Based on the encouraging results in a few patients treated from 1976 to 1978, the authors prospectively studied the role of cisplatin-based therapy. In a series of reports, the authors documented a high overall response rate and long-term disease-free survival in a minority of these patients[115–118]; a small cohort (5% to 10%) were long-term disease-free survivors. Other investigators also demonstrated the responsiveness of selected patients with PDCs.[119–124]

Several years ago, many PDC patients included in these reports had neoplasms that are now identifiable and included either in the favorable subsets already discussed or other recognized responsive neoplasms. These patient subsets included (1) the extragonadal germ cell syndrome, (2) poorly differentiated neoplasms otherwise not specified, (3) anaplastic lymphomas misdiagnosed as carcinoma, (4) thymic carcinomas, (5) primary peritoneal carcinomas, (6) poorly differentiated neuroendocrine carcinomas, and (7) carcinomas with metastases predominantly involving the retroperitoneum, mediastinum, and peripheral lymph nodes. If a patient has PDC, the diagnostic evaluation should target these possibilities. After these subgroups are excluded, the remaining patients have a similar prognosis to the large majority of the adenocarcinoma group. These patients should be evaluated in the same fashion as those with adenocarcinomas, with particular attention given to determining the site of origin using IHC and/or MTP.

Colorectal Cancer Profile

With the introduction of more effective cytotoxic agents and targeted therapies, the median survival of patients with metastatic colorectal carcinoma has increased from 8 to about 24 months.[125,126] It is therefore important to identify the subset of CUP patients with colorectal cancer in order to administer appropriate therapies. The improved specificity of IHC staining for colorectal cancer, coupled with the recent availability of MTP assays, facilitates the identification of this patient subset. The outcome data in these patients treated with colorectal chemotherapy are similar to known advanced colorectal cancer; therefore, this subset merits inclusion as a CUP favorable subset.

Patients with typical clinical features (liver, peritoneal metastases), histology compatible with a lower gastrointestinal primary, and typical IHC staining (CDX2+ and/or CK20+/CK7−) have been defined as having the *colon cancer profile*. Several such patients described by Varadhachary et al.[127,128] had excellent responses and survival when treated with colorectal cancer regimens.

Substantial data now indicate that CUP patients with a colorectal tissue of origin can be accurately identified using IHC stains and/or MTP.[53,127–131] A total of 172 CUP patients with colorectal profiles have been treated with site-specific colorectal regimens. The objective response rates were usually above 50%, and the combined median survival of all these patients was 26 months.

Although these data are largely retrospective, the outcome results are far superior than expected from empiric chemotherapy in CUP (ineffective in colorectal carcinoma) and similar to those achieved in patients with known metastatic colorectal cancer. Further prospective studies may confirm these results. In the meantime, these data are sufficient to recommend treatment with colorectal cancer regimens for CUP patients with either an IHC or MTP colorectal profile.

Empiric Therapy for CUP

Chemotherapy

Approximately 80% of CUP patients are not represented in any of the favorable prognostic clinical subsets (see Table 113.7). In the past, empiric chemotherapy was used for most of these patients because their tissue of origin could not be determined. The history and more recent results of empiric chemotherapy have been reviewed previously.[132–134] and will be briefly discussed here.

Several reports of survival in large groups of patients with CUP[135–142] help to establish a historical control and define the natural history of this syndrome. These historical series included a total of 31,419 patients. Because these reports were retrospective, treatments were not uniform, and some patients received no systemic therapy. The median survival was 5 months, with a 1-year survival of 22% and 5-year survival of 5%. Most patients who survived for 1 year or longer had clinical features now known to be associated with a favorable prognosis. Squamous cell carcinoma (usually in neck nodes) and well-differentiated neuroendocrine carcinoma (carcinoid, islet cell–type histology) reported from some of these series (N = 2,971) had median, 1-year, and 5-year survivals of 20 months, 66%, and 30%, respectively.

Between 1990 and 2000, the introduction of several new drugs with rather broad-spectrum antineoplastic activity improved treatments and prognoses for patients with several common epithelial cancers, and also resulted in a modest improvement in the empiric treatment of CUP.[143] A number of combinations containing these new drugs (taxanes, gemcitabine, vinorelbine, irinotecan, topotecan, oxaliplatin), often combined with a platinum agent, had modest activity in CUP patients and became standard regimens.

The Minnie Pearl Cancer Research Network/Sarah Cannon Oncology Research Consortium (MPCRN/SCORC) completed 10 sequential prospective trials[144–153] (nine phase 2 with 692 patients and one phase 3 with 198 patients), often incorporating platinums with paclitaxel,[144,145] docetaxel,[145,146] gemcitabine,[147,148] gemcitabine/irinotecan,[149,150] bevacizumab/erlotinib,[151] and oxaliplatin[152] into the first-line or second-line therapy for 890 patients with unfavorable prognostic features. The median survival of the 692 first-line patients was 9.2 months and the 1-, 2-, 3-, 4-, 5-, 8-, and 10-year survivals were 39%, 20%, 12%, 11%, 9%, 8%, and 8%, respectively.

Several trials of empiric chemotherapy reported by others over the past 15 years[119–124,132–134,154–164] revealed similar results. The primary end points of 12 of these trials were response rate or median survival.[133] The median survival of all these patients was 9.1 months. The 1-year survival (reported in 12 trials) ranged from 25% to 52% (mean: 34.4%), and at 2 years, survival (reported in 8 trials) ranged from 5% to 18% (mean: 12.3%). Only one study reported a 3-year survival rate (11%). These survival results are very similar to the 692 patients reported by the MPCRN/SCORC studies,[144–153] and superior to historical survival data and to the combined data from multiple prospective clinical trials reported from 1964 to 2002.[2,108] It is of note that in all studies of 100 or more patients, the median survival following empiric regimens is about 9 months.[134,147,150,153,157] The survival curve has been shifted to the right, and the survival at 2 years is comparable to the 1-year survival of historical control patients. Comparison of the existing trials does not allow for the definition of an optimum regimen; several two-drug combinations appear similar.

The era of empiric chemotherapy for most patients with CUP is nearing its end. Improved IHC stains and MTP assays accurately identify the tissue of origin in most patients and provide a more rational framework for decisions regarding therapy. The advantages of site-specific therapy are supported by an increasing amount of clinical data. In the small minority of CUP patients that remain without a defined tissue of origin, empiric chemotherapy remains the standard approach.

Targeted Therapy

A number of agents broadly targeting pathways critical to some cancers (i.e., vascular endothelial growth factor [VEGF] and EGFR inhibitors) have been incorporated into the standard therapy of various solid tumors. It is likely that some patients in the heterogeneous CUP group would also benefit from these targeted agents. Although there has been limited clinical experience with targeted agents, definite activity has been documented.

The combination of bevacizumab and erlotinib was evaluated in a group of 51 patients[151] with very poor prognostic features and the majority in the second-line setting. The median survival was 7.4 months with 33% of patients alive at 1 year and 18% at 2 years. Survival seemed superior to second-line chemotherapy previously reported and was similar to results of many first-line chemotherapy trials.

This trial was followed by a first-line phase 2 study evaluating standard empiric chemotherapy (paclitaxel and carboplatin) plus bevacizumab and erlotinib.[165] Sixty patients with good performance status were treated. The median survival was 12.6 months, and the 2-year survival was 27%. In neither trial were patients selected on the basis of molecular tumor abnormalities predictive of response to the study targeted therapy.

Future development of targeted therapy in CUP will depend on the documentation of molecular targets for which drugs are available. The genomic analysis of biopsy samples, particularly with next-generation sequencing technologies, has opened the door to this potential in many cancers. Because CUP represents many types of metastatic cancer, there is an opportunity to find a variety of actionable genetic alterations. A few CUP patients with EGFR-activating mutations or ALK rearrangements have responded to treatment with inhibitors of these targets.[166,167] Recently, a preliminary report[168] reviewed 1,350 biopsies of CUP patients who had molecular profiling by a number of techniques and several *actionable* biomarkers were identified, including targeted protein overexpression (steroid receptors, MET), activating mutations (BRAF, EGFR, PIK3CA), protein loss (PTEN), and gene copy number variations (HER2, TOP2A, MET amplification) in a large number of these specimens.

Although the therapeutic implications of these findings are largely unexplored, the identification of the tissue of origin should lead to a focused search for tumor-specific molecular abnormalities. Examples include BRAF in melanoma, EGFR and ALK/ROS1 in lung adenocarcinoma, HER2 in breast/gastric/gastroesophageal cancers, and KRAS in colorectal cancer. The identification of these abnormalities should guide patient management and provide additional effective treatment options. The role of genomic testing in advanced cancer is rapidly evolving and is likely to play a larger role in the near future.

Prognostic Factors

The identification of prognostic factors in patients with CUP continues to evolve as the group is divided into an increasing number of subsets. By definition, patients who fit into the favorable subsets have better prognoses compared to the remaining patients. As new treatable subsets are identified, the clinicopathologic features of the remaining patients can be expected to change. The ability to determine the tissue of origin in most patients will make the specific type of cancer in each patient one of the most important prognostic factors. Therefore, results of previous analyses of prognostic factors, conducted primarily in CUP patients receiving empiric chemotherapy, may no longer be relevant to the current population.

Several investigators have analyzed prognostic factors and proposed models.[118,132,169-173] These patients had unfavorable prognostic features and most received empiric chemotherapy regimens. Liver metastasis, poor performance status, elevated serum lactate dehydrogenase and/or alkaline phosphatase levels, hypoalbuminemia, multiple visceral metastasis, lymphopenia, and male gender were negative factors.

Prognostic factors that have been repeatedly identified are related to tumor location, extent of tumor, performance status, and measures of general health status. None of these features is surprising, because most have been repeatedly identified as prognostic factors in patients with various known solid tumors. The tissues of origin in CUP can now usually be determined, and further study is necessary to see if prognoses are similar to their counterparts with known cancers after appropriate site-directed therapies.

Site-Specific Treatment Directed by Results of Molecular Gene Expression Tumor Profiling Assays

Because the tissue of origin can now be accurately predicted in most patients with CUP, the assumption that this information should result in better treatment seems reasonable. However, clinical data confirming this assumption have developed only recently, and some skepticism still remains. One cause for concern is the unique biology of CUP (evidenced by the fact that the primary site does not become apparent); it has been speculated that these cancers, regardless of their origins, will respond differently to treatment. If so, the ability to identify the tissue of origin may not lead to improved therapy.

At present, clinical data suggest that CUP represents a collection of cancer types, which, if identified, will respond to site-specific therapy in a predictable way. The largest experience comes from the treatment of patients in several of the favorable CUP subsets, where treatment follows guidelines for a specific cancer type based on a presumed (but unidentified) site of origin. Examples include women with serous adenocarcinoma involving the peritoneum who are treated for ovarian cancer, women with isolated axillary adenocarcinoma who are treated for breast cancer, and patients with squamous carcinoma involving cervical lymph nodes who are treated for head and neck cancer. In all of these subsets, treatment results are similar to results for the corresponding cancer types. Recently, CUP patients identified by IHC or MTP as having a colorectal site of origin (but with no identifiable colon anatomical primary site) have been demonstrated to respond well to treatment for advanced colorectal cancer.

A prospective evaluation of site-specific therapy selected on the basis of an MTP assay diagnoses has recently been published.[131] In this large prospective phase 2 multicenter study, CUP patients had their biopsies tested with the 92-gene RT-PCR assay and were treated with standard site-specific therapies based on the assay diagnoses of the tissues of origin. Of the 253 patients with successful assays performed, 242 (98%) had a single tissue of origin predicted. Twenty-six different tissues of origin were diagnosed. Assay-directed standard therapies were administered to these patients, and the median survival was 12.5 months, comparing favorably to the median 9-month survival expected with empiric chemotherapy.

Various patient subsets also had outcomes that supported the accuracy of the MTP predictions and the efficacy of assay-directed therapy. In 115 patients, the assay predicted tumor types relatively responsive to standard therapies (colorectal, breast, ovary, kidney, prostate, bladder, lung, germ cell, high-grade neuroendocrine, and lymphoma); this group of patients had a median survival of 13.4 months. When the assay predicted less responsive tumor types in 79 patients (biliary tract, pancreas, gastroesophageal, liver, sarcoma, uterine cervix, endometrium, mesothelioma, melanoma, skin, thyroid, head/neck, and adrenal) the median survival was only 7.6 months (p = 0.04) (Fig. 113.2). In addition, groups of

PRACTICE OF ONCOLOGY

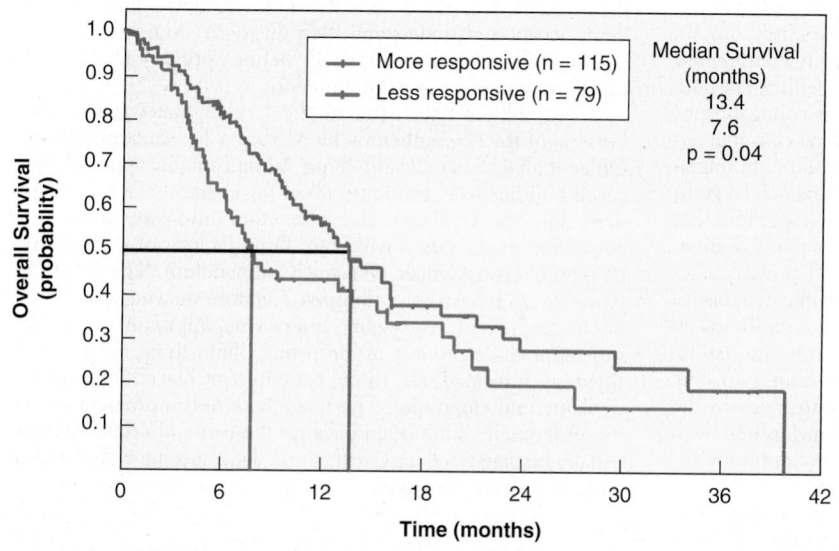

Figure 113.2 Survival of CUP patients after site-specific treatment directed by MTP assay: responsive tumor types versus less responsive tumor types. Median survival 13.4 versus 7.6 months (p = 0.04). NSCLC, non–small-cell lung cancer; SCLC, small-cell lung cancer. (Adapted from Hainsworth JD, Rubin MS, Spigel DR, et al. Molecular gene expression profiling to predict the tissue of origin and direct site-specific therapy in patients with carcinoma of unknown primary site: a prospective trial of the Sarah Cannon Research Institute. *J Clin Oncol* 2012;31:217–223.)

patients with individual cancer types were assessed. Although the groups were small, the median survivals were generally within the range expected for these cancer types (median survival months: breast, 28; ovary, 30; non–small-cell lung, 15.9; colorectal, 12.5; pancreas, 8.2; biliary tract, 6.8).

These results are consistent with those from retrospective studies and provide evidence that site-specific therapy improves the efficacy of treatment for patients with CUP. As expected, patients with more responsive tumor types have greater benefit. Given the heterogeneity of CUP (at least 26 cancer types in the previous study and many more subtypes), it would be extremely challenging to perform a phase 3 randomized study comparing empiric chemotherapy to assay-directed site-specific therapy and difficult to interpret the results if it were accomplished. The varieties of cancers within CUP are diverging along different treatment pathways on the basis of their origin and knowledge of specific treatable molecular alterations, and there is no longer any reason to consider these diverse cancers for treatment with the same empiric chemotherapy regimen.

A sizable minority of patients with CUP will not currently benefit much, if at all, from site-specific therapies because therapy for their tumor types is relatively ineffective. Confidence in the tissue of origin diagnoses by IHC and/or MTP will allow these patients to receive more effective therapy once therapy for their tumor types improves.

SPECIAL ISSUES IN CARCINOMA OF UNKNOWN PRIMARY SITE

Biology of the Primary Tumor

The biology of the primary tumor in CUP remains an enigma. Most patients harbor a clinically undetectable anatomical primary tumor site, as demonstrated by autopsy series.[3,6] It is remarkable that many of these invasive primary tumors measure less than 1 cm. The mechanism explaining clinically occult invasive primary tumor sites remains unknown, but almost certainly will be clarified by a better understanding of the molecular mechanisms controlling primary tumor growth and metastasis. These mechanisms may be different than those found in their easily detected cognate primary cancers.

There are several other potential explanations for the apparent absence of a primary cancer in some of these patients. First, the primary cancers may inexplicably regress or involute entirely, despite the fact that metastasis already occurred. This theory is supported by the scarring seen occasionally in the testicle with metastatic germ cell neoplasms (i.e., *burned-out primary*). Second, the primary may have arisen from embryonic epithelial *rest cells* that are fully differentiated but did not complete their appropriate migration in utero to their designated tissue or organ. Extragonadal germ cell tumors with primaries in the mediastinum, retroperitoneum, or undescended testicle are known examples of this phenomenon. Third, some of these patients have unrecognized primary neoplasms, such as extragonadal germ cell tumors, thymic neoplasms, lymphomas, melanomas, or sarcomas, which arise from these cellular lineages virtually anywhere in the body. Fourth, the pathogenesis of some of these carcinomas may result from a specific germ line genetic lesion present in all cells, as is suggested by the unusual occurrence of CUP in monozygotic twin brothers with primary immunodeficiency disorder (X-linked hyperimmunoglobulin M syndrome).[174]

Finally, some of these neoplasms may arise from adult stem cells with an ability to differentiate to multiple lineages.[175–179] Hematopoietic stem cells appear to be able to give rise to or transform into liver cells as well as muscle, gastrointestinal, skin, and brain cells.[175] Reserve precursor stem cells exist within the connective tissue compartments throughout postnatal life[178] and can form any

lineage in any tissue if they undergo neoplastic transformation. Therefore, some tumors might continue to reflect the differentiation or transformation of adult stem cells and may be *tumors of adult stem cells*. For example, seemingly metastatic adenocarcinoma in bone, liver, lymph node, or elsewhere may, in fact, arise in these sites from an adult stem cell with the capacity to become any type of cell and to develop as a *primary* neoplasm in any of these tissues.[176]

Although CUPs share a metastatic phenotype, it is currently unknown whether these tumors share specific unique molecular abnormalities. A genomic analysis of CUP demonstrates multiple abnormalities, but these are not unique and are shared with many advanced known solid tumors (e.g., various chromosomal 1p abnormalities).[180] Similarly, the expression of p53, bcl-2, cMYCc, RAS, NOTCH1-3, JAGGED1, phosphoMAPK, PTEN, pAKT, cMET, HER2, hypoxia-related protein, and MET mutations have been observed in some CUP tumors, but are not specific.[168,181–188] Although the search for a CUP-specific gene signature continues, none has yet been identified. At present, most evidence suggests that CUP retains typical site-specific markers and can often be identified by IHC and/or MTP assays; however, this does not preclude the coexistence of CUP group-specific molecular abnormalities. Techniques are now available to study the CUP genome (next-generation sequencing technologies, proteomics, and metabolomics), and the pathogenesis of this syndrome may be eventually explained by specific genetic/epigenetic alterations.

Carcinoma of Unknown Primary Site as a Distinct Clinical Syndrome

The authors have found it amazing over the past 3 decades how often patients and their referring physicians are frustrated by CUP. Physicians are often somewhat obsessed with finding the anatomical primary site or at least with giving the patient a site diagnosis. There are many reasons underlying these feelings. Some patients think their oncologist may not be a very good diagnostician and seek the advice of others. Some oncologists feel relatively inadequate and wonder what other test(s) they might order; some have been relatively tentative, not feeling confident in recommending therapy. With improved ability to accurately predict the tissue of origin, most of these issues should be alleviated. Patients are better served, and physicians eventually feel more comfortable, and therefore manage these patients more effectively once their patients accept and understand their diagnosis. Nonetheless, these patients will still lack anatomically defined primary sites and will therefore remain a distinct population.

A second practical issue in the United States is the reimbursement for chemotherapy by Medicare for cancer diagnoses. Other than U.S. Food and Drug Administration approval for a specific tumor type, reimbursement for chemotherapy is usually determined by Medicare (and some other third-party insurers) by consulting compendia—Medicare Drug Policies or the National Comprehensive Cancer Network Compendium. The list of *approved* drugs is based on published literature showing *effectiveness* or clinical benefit in a specific tumor type. For many years, CUP was not included in any of the listings. Four drugs are currently listed as indicated for these patients (paclitaxel, carboplatin, cisplatin, and etoposide). The magnitude of this problem should be substantially diminished because the tissue of origin can now usually be diagnosed and, with these data, specific coded cancer diagnoses can be recorded.

Isolated Pleural and/or Pericardial Effusion

An isolated malignant pleural and/or pericardial effusion is most frequently a manifestation of a peripheral lung adenocarcinoma.

The diagnosis of mesothelioma or a metastatic tumor from other sites (breast, ovary, primary peritoneal, others) should also be considered. In a series of 42 patients, a primary lung cancer was eventually found in 15 patients (36%).[189] The primary may not be apparent even after chest tube drainage. Cytology usually shows adenocarcinoma; positive TTF1 and CK7 stains support a diagnosis of lung carcinoma. Other IHC stains (i.e., calretinin in mesothelioma) or an MTP assay may also assist in defining a primary site. An MTP assay may be successfully performed on small numbers of cancer cells, and in these circumstances should be a preferred test.

In one small series of patients,[189] empiric chemotherapy produced symptomatic improvement in 29 of 37 patients, and 30 of 37 patients had their pleural effusion reduced by chemotherapy; median survival was 12 months (range: 3 to 60 months).

Germ Cell Tumors with Metastases of Other Histologies

On occasion, patients with germ cell tumors, particularly extragonadal primaries, may have a metastatic lesion that consists of only somatic tumor cells. This is particularly true for neuroendocrine or sarcomatous differentiation, but can include any histology. Therefore, patients may be diagnosed as having a neuroendocrine tumor or sarcoma. In these rare instances, a primary germ cell tumor (usually extragonadal) is present elsewhere and subsequently becomes clinically apparent. It is difficult to make the diagnosis initially. An elevated plasma alpha-fetoprotein (AFP) or human chorionic gonadotropin (HCG) level and/or the presence of a mediastinal and/or retroperitoneal lesions supports this possibility. Chromosomal analysis, IHC staining, or an MTP assay may confirm the diagnosis of germ cell tumor. The treatment of choice is cisplatin-based chemotherapy. Surgical resection should be pursued later if feasible. These patients have a worse prognosis than those with typical germ cell tumors, probably because the somatic cell tumors are less sensitive to chemotherapy.

Melanoma and Amelanotic Melanoma

Approximately 10% to 15% of all melanomas that present with an unknown primary site are believed to be amelanotic. This diagnosis should be viewed with skepticism. At times, the only reason for the pathologic diagnosis is the similarity of the histologic pattern to melanoma, even though no pigment is demonstrated. Detailed pathologic and molecular study has occasionally revealed a group of other specific diagnoses, including lymphomas, neuroendocrine tumors, germ cell tumors, sarcomas, and PDC (not otherwise specified).

Melanosomes or premelanosomes seen on electron micrographs have been considered diagnostic of melanoma, but on rare occasions, these structures are seen in other tumors. Some believe amelanotic melanomas do not always form premelanosomes, raising the question as to whether they are really melanomas. Immunohistochemical panels and an MTP assay are also useful in supporting the diagnosis.

The history of a resected, abraded, or frozen pigmented skin lesion would favor melanoma. In addition, the rare primary visceral melanoma should be considered (e.g., eye, adrenal, bowel, anus, others) as the source of the disease in questionable cases. For patients with the diagnosis of amelanotic melanoma, particularly without diagnostic IHC stains, an MTP assay, or a BRAF mutation, an alternative diagnosis should be considered. Mutations of BRAF have been found in approximately 50% of melanomas, and if present, would also support a presumptive diagnosis of melanoma and consideration of therapy with a BRAF inhibitor.

UNKNOWN PRIMARY CANCER IN CHILDREN

There are limited data in children, and as expected, many of these neoplasms represent embryonal malignancies.[190] They are exceedingly rare. In patients with carcinoma, not otherwise specified, the authors favor following the same management plan as for adults.

Midline Carcinoma in Young Adults and Children with t(15;19) and *BRD4-NUT* Oncogene

A few young patients have been described with carcinomas arising from midline locations and an associated chromosomal translocation t(15;19) (q13,p13.1).[29,191] Patients with this syndrome are usually children or young adults; most have poorly differentiated carcinoma and widespread metastasis. The primary tumor site is difficult to identify in many patients. The *NUT* (nuclear protein in testes) oncogene is common to all these tumors and supports their possible origin from a specific cell type, perhaps an early epithelial progenitor cell that is more common in the first 2 or 3 decades of life. Perhaps these tumors are an example of *stem cell tumors* (see section Biology of the Primary Tumor in Special Issues in Carcinoma of Unknown Primary Site).

A recent review of 54 patients[191] revealed poor median survival (6.7 months) and 2-year survival of 19% despite surgery and radiation therapy when feasible and intensive chemotherapies. These patients are clinically similar to the extragonadal germ cell cancer syndrome and, without a positive t(15;19), some of these patients could be included in that clinical syndrome and vice versa. Further knowledge of these *NUT*-rearranged carcinomas and improved targeted therapies for these patients are likely to follow with their more broad recognition.

NEW TREATMENT PARADIGM

As described in this chapter, improved diagnostic methods have changed the clinical evaluation and therapy for most CUP patients. A change from empiric chemotherapy to site-specific therapy based on tissue of origin diagnosis is now indicated for the majority of patients, as we recently reviewed.[192]

In Figure 113.3, we summarize the management approach. After standard initial clinical and pathologic evaluations, selected patients should have an additional directed clinical evaluation, IHC staining, and/or an MTP assay of the tumor specimen. Patients with an identified anatomical primary site should be treated accordingly, and patients who fit into an identified favorable subset should receive appropriate subset-specific therapy (see section Favorable Subsets). Patients who have their tissue of origin diagnosed by IHC should receive site-specific therapy. Patients in neither of these categories should have MTP; site-specific therapy should then be based on the tissue of origin diagnosis. Diagnoses made by IHC and/or MTP should be interpreted in conjunction with clinical features and pathologic results. Empiric chemotherapy is indicated for the small minority without a defined tissue of origin, and clinical trials should always be considered.

Some may now think that CUP will be a rare entity once most patients are assigned a tissue of origin and become a subset or member of a recognized cancer type, albeit without a defined anatomical primary site. This may be a clinical reality once it is agreed upon that the survival of CUP patients with defined origins are similar to the patients with anatomically defined primary sites. However, the syndrome persists and the biologic phenomenon explaining CUP for now remains a mystery. Further knowledge of the genetic/epigenetic mechanisms may eventually explain CUP

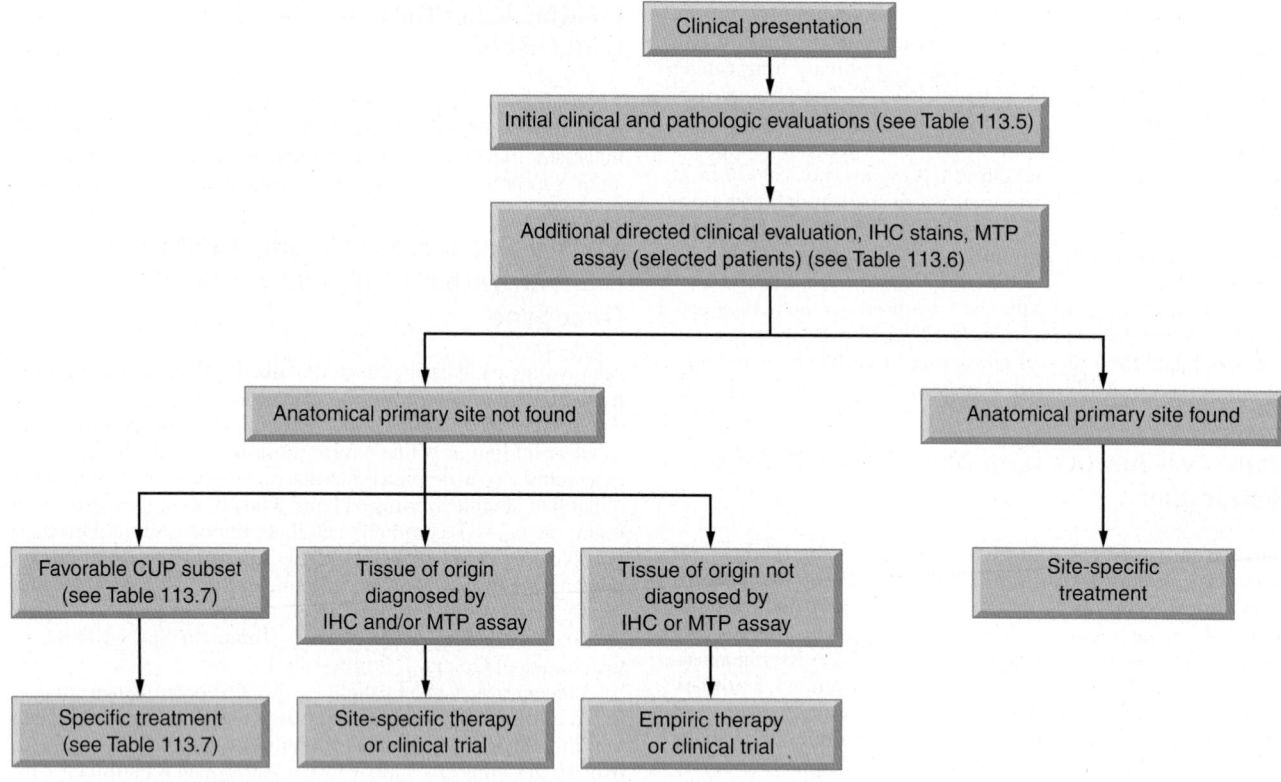

Figure 113.3 New management paradigm for the CUP patient.

and lead to new targeted therapies for patients with this enigmatic syndrome and perhaps for other patients with metastatic cancers.

The evolution of improved, more personalized therapies for CUP patients is linked to the wave of precision therapies for many types of known cancer types based on genomic understanding; in addition, the dawn of clinically impressive and beneficial immunotherapy (such as CTLA-4, PD-1, PDL-1 inhibitors, and genetically engineered T cells) for many common solid tumor patients is here. There is no other reasonable option now but to further define in

each patient the type and subtype of neoplasm he or she harbors within the CUP syndrome before planning definitive therapy.

The integration of molecular diagnostics into CUP patient management is already supported by clinical data, but continued investigation is necessary to further refine management recommendations. Even with the ability to identify the tissue of origin, further improvements in the treatment of many of these patients are dependent on the development of improved treatments for advanced solid tumors.

SELECTED REFERENCES

The full reference list can be accessed at lwwhealthlibrary.com/oncology.

2. Pavlidis N, Briasoulis E, Hainsworth J, Greco FA. Diagnostic and therapeutic management of cancer of an unknown primary. *Eur J Cancer* 2003;39: 1990–2005.
5. Horning SJ, Carrier EK, Rouse RV, et al. Lymphomas presenting as histologically unclassified neoplasms: characteristics and response to treatment. *J Clin Oncol* 1989;7:1281–1287.
7. Owen KA. Pathologic evaluation of unknown primary cancer. *Semin Oncol* 2009;36:8–37.
10. Oien KA, Dennis JL. Diagnostic work-up of carcinoma of unknown primary: from immunohistochemistry to molecular profiling. *Ann Oncol* 2012;23:271–277.
11. Stoyianni A, Pentheroudakis G, Pavlidis, N. Neuroendocrine carcinoma of unknown primary: a systematic review of the literature and a comparative study with other neuroendocrine tumors. *Cancer Treat Rev* 2011;37:358–365.
12. Kerr SE, Schnabel CA, Sullivan PS, et al. A 92-gene cancer classifier predicts the site of origin for neuroendocrine tumors. *Modern Pathology* 2014;27: 44–54.
22. Anderson GG, Weiss LM. Determining tissue if origin for metastatic cancers: meta-analysis and literature review of immunohistochemistry performance. *Appl Immunohistochem Mol Morphol* 2010;18:3–8.
25. Motzer RJ, Rodriguez E, Reuter VE, et al. Molecular and cytogenic studies in the diagnosis of patients with midline carcinomas of unknown primary site. *J Clin Oncol* 1995;13:274–282.

29. French CA, Kutok JL, Faquin WC, et al. Midline carcinoma of children and young adults with NUT rearrangement. *J Clin Oncol* 2004;22: 4135–4139.
32. Summersgill B, Goker H, Osin P, et al. Establishing germ cell origin of undifferentiated tumors by identifying gain of 12p material using comparative genomic hybridization analysis of paraffin-embedded samples. *Diagn Mol Pathol* 1998;7:260–266.
37. Golub TR, Slonim DK, Tamayo P, et al. Molecular classification of cancer: class discovery and class prediction by gene expression monitoring. *Science* 1999; 286:531–537.
38. Greco FA, Erlander MG. Molecular classification of unknown primary cancer site. *Mol Diagn Ther* 2009;13:367–373.
40. Sotiriou C, Piccart MJ. Taking gene-expression profiling to the clinic: when will molecular signatures become relevant to patient care? *Nature Rev Cancer* 2007;7:545–553.
41. Ramaswamy S, Tamayo P, Rifkin R, et al. Multiclass cancer diagnosis using tumor gene expression signatures. *Proc Natl Acad Sci U S A* 2001;98: 15149–15154.
42. MacConaill LE. Existing and emerging technologies for genomic profiling. *J Clin Oncol* 2013;31:1815–1824.
43. Abaan OD, Polley EC, Davis SR, et al. The exomes of the NCI-60 panel: a genomic resource for cancer biology and systems pharmacology. *Cancer Res* 2013;73:4372–4382.
45. Bloom G, Yang IV, Boulware D, et al. Multi-platform, multi-site, microarray-based human tumor classification. *Am J Path* 2004;164:9–16.

48. Rosenfeld N, Aharonov R, Meiril E, et al. MicroRNAs accurately identify cancer tissue origin. *Nature Biotech* 2008;26:462–469.

49. Monzon FA, Lyons-Weiler M, Buturovic LJ, et al. Multicenter validation of a 1,550-gene expression profile for identification of tumor tissue of origin. *J Clin Oncol* 2009;27:2503–2508.

50. Ma X-J, Pate R, Wang X, et al. Molecular classification of human cancers using a 92-gene real-time quantitative polymerase chain reaction array. *Arch Path Lab Med* 2006;130:465–473.

51. Pillai R, Deeter R, Rigl CT, et al. Validation of a microarray-based gene expression test for tumors with uncertain origins using formalin-fixed paraffin-embedded (FFPE) specimens. *J Mol Diagn* 2011;13:48–56.

53. Varadhachary G, Talantov D, Raber M, et al. Molecular profiling of carcinoma of unknown primary and correlation with clinical evaluation. *J Clin Oncol* 2008;26:4442–4448.

55. Horlings HM, van Laar RK, Kerst JM, et al. Gene expression profiling to identify the histogenetic origin of metastatic adenocarcinomas of unknown primary. *J Clin Oncol* 2008;26:4435–4441.

58. Greco FA, Spigel DR, Yardley DA, et al. Molecular profiling in unknown primary cancer: tissue of origin prediction. *Oncologist* 2010;15:500–506.

59. Erlander MG, Ma XJ, Kesty NC, et al. Performance and clinical evaluation of the 92-gene real-time PCR assay for tumor classification. *J Mol Diagn* 2011;13:493–503.

60. Kerr SE, Schnabel CA, Sullivan PS, et al. Multisite validation study to determine performance characteristics of a 92-gene molecular cancer classifier. *Clin Cancer Res* 2012;18:3952–3960.

61. Meiri E, Mueller WC, Rosenwald S, et al. A second-generation microRNA-based assay for diagnosing tumor tissue origin. *The Oncologist* 2012;17:801–812.

62. Weiss LM, Cha PG, Schroeder BE, et al. Blinded comparator study of immunohistochemistry analysis versus 92-gene cancer classifier in the diagnosis of the primary site in metastatic tumors. *J Molecular Diagn.* 2013;15:263–269.

63. Handorf CR, Kulkarni A, Grenut JD, et al. A multisite study comparing the diagnostic accuracy of the gene expression profiling and immunohistochemistry for primary site identification in metastatic tumors. *Am J Surg Pathol.* 2013;37:1067–1075.

65. Pentheroudakis G, Pavlidis N, Fountzilas G, et al. Novel microRNA-based assay demonstrates 92% agreement with diagnosis based on clinicopathologic and management data in a cohort of patients with carcinoma of unknown primary. *Mol Cancer* 2013;12:57.

67. Varadhachary Gr, Spector Y, Abbruzzese JL, et al. Propective gene signature study using microRNA to identify the tissue of origin in patients with carcinoma of unknown primary. *Clin Cancer Res* 2011;17:4063–4070.

68. Ferracin M, Pedriali M, Veronese A, et al. Micro RNA profiling for the identification of cancers with unknown primary tissue of origin. *J Pathol* 2011;225:43–53.

69. Greco FA, Lennington WJ, Spigel DR, et al. Molecular profiling diagnosis in unknown primary cancer; accuracy and ability to complement standard pathology. *J Natl Cancer Inst* 2013;105:782–790.

71. Greco FA, Spigel DR, Hainsworth JD. Molecular tumor profiling of poorly differentiated neoplasms of unknown primary site. *J Clin Oncol* 2013;31:217–223.

72. Sorscher SM, Greco FA. Papillary renal carcinoma presenting as a cancer of unknown primary and diagnosed through gene expression profiling. *Case Rep Oncol* 2012;5:229–232.

74. Hainsworth JD, Spigel DR, Greco FA. Renal cell carcinoma presenting as cancer of unknown primary: diagnosis by molecular tumor profiling. *J Clin Oncol* 2013;31:abstract e15501.

76. Moller AK, Loft A, Berthelsen AK, et al. A prospective comparison of 18F-FDG PET/CT and CT as diagnostic tools to identify the primary tumor site in patients with extracervical cancer of unknown primary site. *Oncologist* 2012;17:1146–1154.

82. Rusthoven KE, Koshy M, Pauline AC. The role of fluorodeoxyglucose positron emission tomography in cervical lymph node metastases from an unknown primary tumor. *Cancer* 2004;101:2641–2649.

85. Varadhachary GR, Abbruzzese JL, Lenzi R. Diagnostic strategies for unknown primary cancer. *Cancer* 2004;100:1776–1785.

93. Pentheroudakis G, Pavidis N. Serous papillary peritoneal carcinoma: unknown primary tumor ovarian cancer counterpart or a distinct entity? A systematic review. *Crit Rev Oncol Hematol* 2010;75:27–42.

95. Pentheroudakis G, Lazaridis G, Pavlidis N. Axillary nodal metastases from carcinoma of unknown primary (CUPAx): a systematic review of published evidence. *Breast Cancer Res Treat* 2010;119:1–11.

108. Greco FA, Hainsworth JD. Cancer of unknown primary site. In: DeVita VT, Lawrence TS, Rosenberg SA, eds. *Cancer Principles and Practice of Oncology.* 8th ed. Philadelphia: Lippincott Williams & Wilkins; 2008:2363.

110. De Braud F, Heilbrun LK, Ahmed K, et al. Metastatic squamous cell carcinoma of an unknown primary localized to the neck: advantages of an aggressive treatment. *Cancer* 1989;64:510–515.

112. Rinke A, Muller HH, Schade-Brittinger C, et al. Placebo-controlled double-blind, prospective, randomized study of the effect of octreotide LAR in the control of tumor growth in patients with metastatic neuroendocrine midgut tumors: a report from the PROMID Study Group. *J Clin Oncol* 2009;27:4656–4663.

113. Hainsworth JD, Johnson DH, Greco FA. Poorly differentiated neuroendocrine carcinoma of unknown primary site: a newly recognized clinicopathologic entity. *Ann Intern Med* 1988;109:364–371.

114. Hainsworth JD, Spigel DR, Litchy S, et al. Phase II trial of paclitaxel, carboplatin, and etoposide in advanced poorly differentiated neuroendocrine carcinoma: a Minnie Pearl Cancer Research Network Study. *J Clin Oncol* 2006;24:3548–3554.

115. Richardson RL, Schoumacher RA, Fer MF, et al. The unrecognized extragonadal germ cell cancer syndrome. *Ann Intern Med* 1981;94:181–186.

116. Greco FA, Vaughn WK, Hainsworth JD. Advanced poorly differentiated carcinoma of unknown primary site: recognition of a treatable syndrome. *Ann Intern Med* 1986;104:547–553.

117. Hainsworth JD, Greco FA. Treatment of patients with cancer of an unknown primary site. *N Engl J Med* 1995;329:257–263.

118. Hainsworth JD, Johnson DH, Greco FA. Cisplatin-based combination chemotherapy in the treatment of poorly differentiated carcinoma and poorly differentiated adenocarcinoma of unknown primary site: results of a 12 year experience at a single institution. *J Clin Oncol* 1992;10:912–922.

127. Varadhachary GR, Raber MN, Matamoros A, et al. Carcinoma of unknown primary with a colon cancer-profile changing paradigm and emerging definitions. *Lancet Oncol* 2008;9:596–599.

128. Varadhachary GR, Karanth S, Qiao W, et al. Carcinoma of unknown primary with gastrointestinal profile: immunohistochemistry and survival data for this favorable subset. *In J Clin Oncol* 2014;19:479–484.

129. Greco FA, Lennington WJ, Spigel DR, et al. Carcinoma of unknown primary site: outcomes in patients with colorectal profile treated with site-specific chemotherapy. *J Cancer Ther* 2012;3:37–43.

130. Hainsworth JD, Schnabel CA, Erlander MG, et al. A retrospective study of treatment outcomes in patients with carcinoma of unknown primary site and a colorectal cancer molecular profile. *Clin Colorectal Cancer* 2012;11:112–118.

131. Hainsworth JD, Rubin MS, Spigel DR, et al. Molecular gene expression profiling to predict the tissue of origin and direct site-specific therapy in patients with carcinoma of unknown primary site: a prospective trial of the Sarah Cannon Research Institute. *J Clin Oncol* 2012; 31:217–223.

132. Greco FA, Hainsworth JD. Cancer of unknown primary site. In: DeVita VT, Lawrence TS, Rosenberg SA, eds, *Cancer Principles and Practice of Oncology.* 9th ed. Philadelphia: Lippincott Williams and Wilkins; 2011:2033.

133. Greco FA, Pavlidis N. Treatment for patients with unknown primary carcinoma and unfavorable prognostic factors. *Semin Oncol* 2009;36:65–74.

143. Greco FA. Therapy of adenocarcinoma of unknown primary: are we making progress? *J Natl Compr Conc Netw* 2008;6:1061–1067.

144. Hainsworth JD, Erland JB, Kalman CA, et al. Carcinoma of unknown primary site: treatment with one-hour paclitaxel, carboplatin and extended schedule etoposide. *J Clin Oncol* 1997;15:2385–2393.

151. Hainsworth JD, Spigel DR, Farley C, et al. Bevacizumab and erlotinib in the treatment of patients with carcinoma of unknown primary site: a phase II trial of the Minnie Pearl Cancer Research Network. *J Clin Oncol* 2007;25:1747–1752.

153. Hainsworth JD, Spigel DR, Clark BL, et al. Paclitaxel/carboplatin/etoposide versus gemcitabine/irinotecan in the first-line treatment of patients with carcinoma of unknown primary site: a randomized, phase III Sarah Cannon Oncology Research Consortium Trial. *Cancer J* 2010;16:70–75.

165. Hainsworth JD, Spigel DR, Thompson DS, et al. Paclitaxel/carboplatin plus bevacizumab/erlotinib in the first-line treatment of patients with carcinoma of unknown primary site. *Oncologist* 2009;14:1189–1197.

167. Penley WC, Spigel Dr, Greco FA, et al. Confirmation of non-small cell lung cancer diagnosis using ALK testing and genetic profiling in patients presenting with carcinoma of unknown primary site. *J Clin Oncol* 2013;31:abstract e115004.

176. McCulloch EA. Stem cells and diversity. *Leukemia* 2003;17:1042–1048.

191. Bauer DE, Mitchell CM, Strait KM, et al. Clinicopathologic features and long-term outcomes of NUT midline carcinoma. *Clin Cancer Res* 2012;18: 5773–5779.

192. Hainsworth JD, Greco FA. Gene expression profiling in patient with carcinoma of unknown primary site. From transnational research to standard of care. *Virchows Arch* 2014;464:393–402.

PRACTICE OF ONCOLOGY

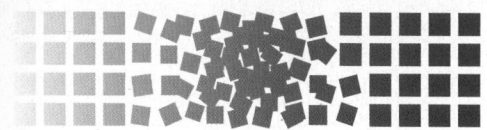

114 Benign and Malignant Mesothelioma

Harvey I. Pass, Michele Carbone, Lee M. Krug, and Kenneth E. Rosenzweig

INTRODUCTION

Malignant mesotheliomas (MM) are highly aggressive neoplasms that arise primarily from the surface serosal cells of the pleural, peritoneal, and pericardial cavities. The disease is characterized by a long latency from the time of exposure to asbestos to the onset of disease, suggesting that multiple somatic genetic events are required for tumorigenic conversion of a normal mesothelial cell.

MECHANISM OF ASBESTOS CARCINOGENESIS

There are six types of asbestos: amosite, crocidolite, anthophyllite, actinolite, tremolite, and chrysotile.[1] The five types other than chrysotile are termed *amphibole asbestos*. Several nonasbestos minerals (e.g., erionite, wincherite) are very similar to asbestos structurally and chemically and are also capable of causing mesothelioma in humans. The mechanisms responsible for asbestos carcinogenicity are linked to the secretion of tumor necrosis factor (TNF)-alpha by mesothelial cells and macrophages exposed to asbestos that in turn leads to NFκB activation.[2] The activation of the NFκB pathway in mesothelial cells allows them to survive the toxic insult and the genetic damage caused by asbestos, and these damaged but viable cells may proliferate into a mesothelioma.[2]

Animal Models of Asbestos Carcinogenicity

Mesotheliomas and sarcomas are induced in a dose-dependent fashion after intrapleural and intraperitoneal injection of asbestos into animals.[3-5] Chronic inhalational studies are thought to be the best representation of asbestos carcinogenicity. Because of the cost of these experiments, however, very few have been performed.

Asbestos Carcinogenicity in Humans

Although injection and inhalation studies in animals suggest that all forms of asbestos are equally carcinogenic and that there is a clear dose-response relationship between asbestos exposure and mesothelioma risk, epidemiologic studies in humans do not support these observations. The proportion of mesotheliomas that are thought to be associated with asbestos varies in the literature from 16% to 90%.[1] Although this wide range may reflect the distinct populations studied, it is more likely a result of the different methodologies used to determine exposure rates.[1] Most human studies have indicated that amosite and crocidolite exposure carry a much greater risk than exposure to chrysotile.[6,7] Chrysotile, however, is frequently combined with tremolite, an amphibole, that may instead be responsible for mesothelioma development.[8]

In humans, there is no clear dose-response curve to asbestos, and a threshold level below which mesotheliomas do not develop has not been determined, although it is generally accepted in the scientific community that background levels of exposure, such as those found in the lungs of almost all individuals, do not increase the risk of mesothelioma. It is estimated that <5% of asbestos miners exposed to high levels of asbestos develop mesotheliomas[1]; however, wives of some of these workers have developed mesotheliomas after they were presumably exposed to lower levels of asbestos compared to their husbands while washing their clothes.[9,10] Similarly, mesothelioma development commonly occurs in workers in occupations in which asbestos exposure is higher than in the general population, but much lower than in asbestos miners. The carpenters, electricians, and construction workers who have developed mesotheliomas are a reflection of this.[11] These data suggest that high levels of exposure are not necessarily correlated with increased risk of malignancy compared to moderate asbestos exposure, arguing against a classic dose-response relationship.[1]

Mechanism of Asbestos Pathogenicity

It is thought that when fibers reach the alveoli after inhalation, smaller fibers are phagocytized and efficiently removed from the lung. Larger fibers are not easily engulfed and can usually only be removed if solubilized. However, amphiboles are not soluble and thus remain in the lung. These fibers may eventually reach the pleura via the lymphatics or direct extension, where they may lead to pleural plaques, fibrosis, and mesothelioma. In the pleura, asbestos fibers may cause mutagenic changes through hydroxy radical and superoxide anion production during phagocytosis, leading to DNA strand breaks and deletions. Most recently, data implicating necrosis in the genesis of mesothelioma have been reported in which the release of HMGB1 is necessary as a critical initial step in the pathogenesis of asbestos-related disease and provides a mechanistic link between asbestos-induced cell death, chronic inflammation, and mesothelial carcinogenesis.[12] Inflammation due to asbestos deposition contributes to asbestos carcinogenesis.[2,13,14] Phagocytic macrophages at these sites of inflammation internalize asbestos and release mutagenic reactive oxygen species and numerous cytokines including TNF-α and interleukin (IL)-1, which have been linked to asbestos-related carcinogenesis.[2,15] By inducing cell necrosis, asbestos causes the release of HMGB1,[12] a typical damage-associated molecular pattern[16,17] and a key mediator of inflammation.[18] Activation of Nalp3 inflammasome ensues with subsequent IL-1β secretion, a process that is enhanced by asbestos-induced production of reactive oxygen species.[19,20] Additionally, HMGB1 is released by reactive macrophages, other inflammatory cells, and human mesothelial cells (HMC[12]) upon exposure to asbestos. HMGB1 is a critical regulator in the initiation of asbestos-mediated inflammation leading to the release of TNF-α and subsequent NF-κB signaling[12] (Fig. 114.1). During programmed necrosis, HMGB1 translocates from the nucleus to the cytosol and the extracellular space, where it binds several pro-inflammatory molecules and triggers the inflammatory responses that distinguish this type of cell death from apoptosis. Secreted

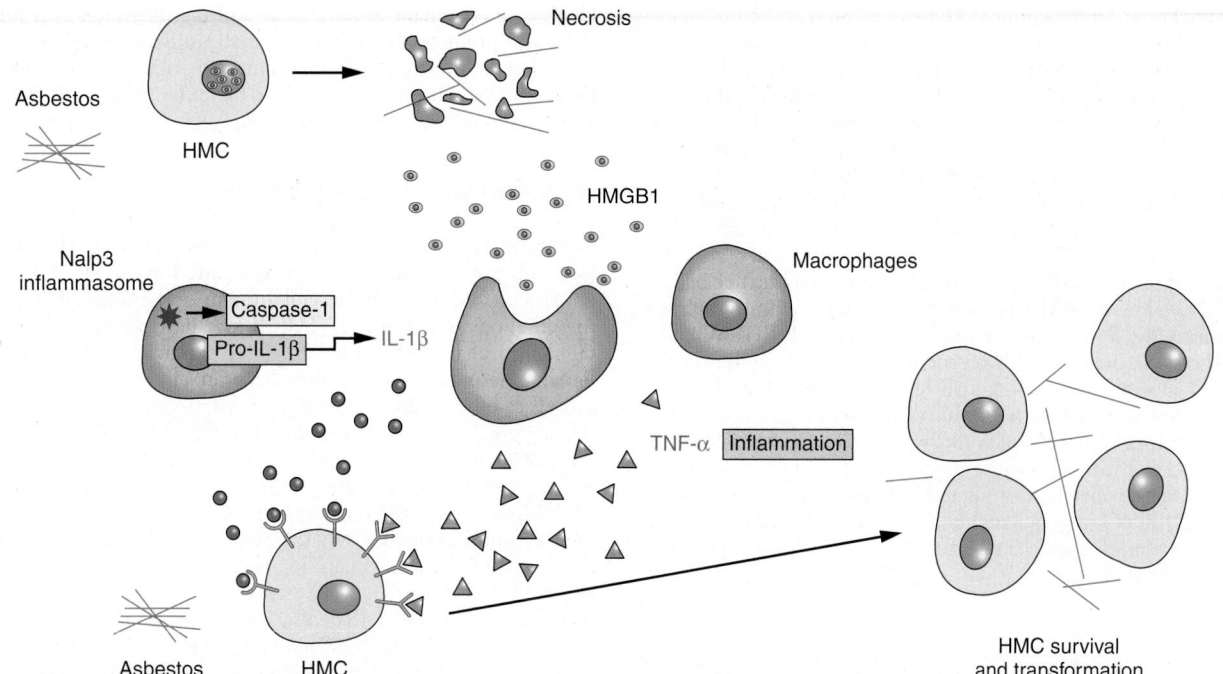

Figure 114.1 Working hypothesis for mesothelioma carcinogenesis. Asbestos causes necrotic human mesothelial cell (*HMC*) death, leading to the release of HMGB1 into the extracellular space. As a typical damage-associated molecular pattern and a key mediator of inflammation, HMGB can induce activation of Nalp3 inflammasome and subsequent interleukin (*IL*)-1β secretion, as well as eliciting macrophage accumulation and triggering the inflammatory response and tumor necrosis factor–α secretion, which increases the survival of asbestos-damaged HMCs. This allows key genetic alterations to accumulate within HMCs that sustain asbestos-induced DNA damage, leading to the initiation of mesothelioma.

HMGB1 stimulates RAGE, TLR2, and TLR4 (the three main HMGB1 receptors) expressed on neighboring inflammatory cells such as macrophages and induces the release of several inflammatory cytokines, including TNF-α and IL-1β. TNF-α–induced NF-κB signaling has been shown to be a critical link between inflammation and carcinogenesis in multiple cancer models, including mesothelioma.[2] Specifically, asbestos-mediated TNF-α signaling induces the activation of NF-κB–dependent mechanisms, promoting the survival of HMCs after asbestos exposure,[2] and thus allowing HMCs with accumulated asbestos-induced genetic damage to survive, divide, and propagate genetic aberrations in premalignant cells that can give rise to a malignant clone. In addition, HMGB1 enhances the activity of NF-κB, which promotes tumor formation, progression, and metastasis.[21] An investigation into the targeting of extracellular HMGB1 as a novel strategy for mesothelioma prevention and/or therapy is currently under way.[22]

It is difficult to reconcile what is known about the carcinogenic actions of asbestos and the long latency period between asbestos exposure and mesothelioma development. Lanphear and Buncher[23] reviewed 21 studies of 1,690 mesotheliomas and found that 96% occurred at least 20 years after exposure; the mean latency was 32 years. Several theories have been postulated to describe what happens during this latency period.[24] It is widely believed that asbestos induces genetic alterations in mesothelial cells over a long period that eventually lead to malignant cells. This may occur if a key regulatory gene, such as the *INK4a/ARF* locus, is deleted or silenced. With loss of key regulatory genes, additional mutations could accumulate rapidly. INK4a/ARF codes for p16 (a cyclin-dependent kinase inhibitor) and for p14ARF, which promotes murine double minute-2 degradation, preventing murine double minute-2 from neutralizing p53. Both p16 and p14ARF are often deleted in MM (see "Alterations of Specific Tumor Suppressor Genes in Mesothelioma"). This process may allow enough mutations to accumulate to lead to malignancy. Cell growth from this point would be rapid, leading to a clinically detectable tumor.[1]

OVERVIEW OF MOLECULAR MECHANISMS IN MESOTHELIOMA

Cytogenetic Assessment of Malignant Mesotheliomas

Deletions of specific chromosomal sites in the short (p) arms of chromosomes 1, 3, and 9, and long (q) arm of 6 are repeatedly observed in these tumors. Using newer molecular platforms including array comparative genomic hybridization and representational oligonucleotide microarray analysis, deletions in chromosomes 22q12.2, 19q13.32, and 17p13.1 appear to be the most frequent events (55% to 74%), followed by deletions in 1p, 9p, 9q, 4p, and 3p, and gains in 5p, 18q, 8q, and 17q (23% to 55%). Increasing numbers of copy number abnormalities in mesothelioma are associated with poor prognosis, especially when associated with deletions in 9p21.3 encompassing CDKN2A/ARF and CDKN2B, as detailed later.[24] Analysis of the minimal common areas of frequent gains and losses has pointed to novel potential tumor suppressor genes (TSG) including OSM (22q12.2), FUS1, PL6 (3p21.3), DNAJA1 (9p21.1), and CDH2 (18q11.2–q12.3).[25]

Alterations of Specific Tumor Suppressor Genes in Mesothelioma

p16

Cheng et al.[26] reported homozygous deletions of one or more of the three *p16* exons in 34 of 40 (85%) malignant mesothelioma cell lines and a point mutation in one cell line. Downregulation of *p16* was observed in four of the remaining cell lines. Homozygous deletions of *p16* were identified in 5 of 23 (22%) malignant mesothelioma tumor samples. Downregulation of *p16* in malignant mesothelioma cells may result from 5′CpG island hypermethylation, as has been demonstrated in other types of cancer. *P16* inactivation by homozygous deletions or methylation is a frequent event in Japanese patients with malignant pleural mesotheliomas (MPM).[27] Homozygous deletion is the major cause of the *P16* inactivation,[28] but methylation also leads to the inactivation of *P16* when the *P16* alleles are retained.[27] Homozygous deletions at this locus can lead to the inactivation of another putative TSG, *p14*ARF, because *p16* and *p14*ARF share exons 2 and 3 although their reading frames differ.[29,30] The prognostic significance of p16/CDKN2A loss in MM has been defined both by immunohistochemistry and fluorescence in situ hybridization (FISH). With the FISH analysis of primary MM tissue samples or MM cells from the pleural effusion, over 70% of cases showed homozygous deletions of the *CDKN2A/ARF* locus. Both loss of p16 protein expression by immunohistochemistry and homozygous deletion of p16 by FISH are associated with an adverse prognosis.[31] Loss of p15 is also associated with codeletion of microRNA (miR)-31.[32] Protein phosphatase (PPP6C), upregulated in MPM, is a target of mir-31, and reintroduction of miR-31 in mesothelioma cells has a suppressive effect on MM cells.[32]

p53

Cell lines derived from murine models of asbestos-induced mesothelioma have reduced or absent expression of p53 messenger RNA (mRNA) compared to the RNA from nontumorigenic cell lines or reactive mesothelial cells.[33] In human cell lines derived from patients with malignant mesothelioma, attention has turned to specific mutations or genetic abnormalities in *p53*. In general, mutational analyses of *p53* in mesothelioma have not revealed reasons for its inactivation.

Wilms Tumor Gene

The detection of Wilms tumor gene (*WT1*) mRNA or protein provides a specific molecular or immunohistochemical marker for differentiation of mesothelioma from other pleural tumors, in particular adenocarcinoma.[34] Vaccination protocols that exploit the selective presence of *WT1* in mesothelioma are under way at selected institutions.[35]

Neurofibromatosis Gene

The tumor suppressor merlin is encoded by the neurofibromatosis type 2 gene (*NF2*), which is located on chromosome 22q12, and mutations in this gene have been found in 40% of mesothelioma and 50% of malignant mesothelioma cell lines.[36,37] Mutations including deletions and insertions lead to truncated and inactivated merlin. Experimental animal models indicate that disruption of the *NF2* signaling pathway, together with a deficiency in *ink4a*, is essential for mesothelioma development.[38]

ALTERATIONS OF ONCOGENES IN MESOTHELIOMA

C-sis (Platelet-Derived Growth Factor)

Malignant mesothelioma cell lines produce numerous growth factors and cytokines, possibly as a consequence of altered oncogene status. One of the more intriguing oncogenes in malignant mesothelioma is C-sis, which codes for one of the two chains (alpha and beta) of platelet-derived growth factor (PDGF). Gerwin et al.[39] were the first to describe elevation of RNA levels for both chains of PDGF in mesothelioma cell lines and correlated the increase with PDGF-like activity secreted by the cells. It is of interest that overexpression of A chain transforms human mesothelial cells to the tumorigenic phenotype in vitro and that the use of antisense

ODN to the A chain inhibits growth of mesothelioma cell lines. PDGF-D promotes mesothelioma cell proliferation by targeting ROCK or MAP kinase through autocrine activation of PDGF-beta receptor[40]; however, in general, therapies targeting PDGF in mesothelioma have been unsuccessful.[41]

Transforming Growth Factor

Transforming growth factor-B (TGF-B) is another growth-regulatory and immunomodulatory cytokine, and high levels of TGF-B have been described in several human and mouse malignant mesothelioma cell lines.[42,43] TGF-B may have a potential role in regulation of the differential PDGF receptor expression in malignant mesothelioma and thus have an effect on proliferation as well as other events. TGF-B production by tumors plays a significant role in blocking immune response by preventing T-cell infiltration into tumors, inhibition of T-cell activation/function, and mediation of T regulatory cell–induced immunosuppression. TGF-blockers (soluble receptors/antibodies) and receptor inhibitors have antitumor effects that, in several models, are due primarily to immunologic mechanisms. TGF blockade had antitumor effects that were CD8+ T-cell dependent in a murine malignant mesothelioma model.[44] Recently, it was reported that a combined triple treatment of anti-CD25 monoclonal antibody, anti–cytotoxic T-lymphocyte antigen-4 monoclonal antibody and TGF-beta soluble receptor resulted in long-term clearance of MPM tumors and memory against tumor rechallenge.[45]

Insulin Growth Factor

Insulin growth factor (IGF) is another of the important autocrine loops in mesothelioma.[46] The IGF receptor-1 pathway is a significant regulator of mesothelioma growth acting through downstream kinases such as Akt. In humans, both normal mesothelium and mesothelioma cell lines express IGF-1 and IGF-1R RNAs (by Northern blot or reverse transcriptase polymerase chain reaction), and IGF-1 protein is detected in their conditioned media. These studies suggest that mesothelioma growth, both in human and animal models for the disease, may involve the IGFs, and trials using anti-IGF-1R antibodies or small-molecule IGF blockade are being formulated for mesothelioma.[47] Cixutumumab, a humanized monoclonal antibody to IGF-IR, has been investigated using early passage tumor cells and an in vivo human mesothelioma tumor xenograft model. Cixutumumab induced antibody-dependent cell-mediated toxicity and in vivo, cixutumumab treatment delayed growth of H226 mesothelioma tumor xenografts in mice and improved the overall survival of these mice compared to controls.[48] A phase 2 clinical trial of cixutumumab is currently ongoing for the treatment of patients with mesothelioma.

Angiogenic Mechanisms in Mesothelioma

The most relevant cytokines and growth factors in angiogenic pathways involve the ILs (specifically IL-6 and IL-8), fibroblast growth factors (FGF), vascular endothelial growth factors (VEGF), platelet-derived endothelial growth factors, and IGFs. Moreover, mutational or posttranslational silencing of TSGs or their products, particularly *p53* and *p16*, has also been associated with increased angiogenic mechanisms.

IL-6 levels are elevated in the serum and pleural effusions of patients with mesothelioma, and there have been correlations seen between the IL-6 level and the degree of thrombocytosis in these patients.[49] IL-6 expression is elevated in tissues undergoing angiogenesis, but by itself it has a limited role in proliferation of endothelial cells. IL-6, however, induces angiogenesis by elevating the expression of VEGF, a specific mitogen for vascular endothelial cells. Serum VEGF and IL-6 levels are elevated in patients with mesothelioma, and their levels each correlate with platelet count.[50] IL-8 is also an important angiogenic factor for the development of new capillaries in vivo and has direct growth-potentiating activity in mesothelioma. Pleural fluid from patients with mesothelioma has significantly higher IL-8 levels by enzyme-linked assay compared to patients with other malignant effusions.[51] Mesotheliomas present with a high intratumoral vessel density that also have prognostic relevance,[42,52,53] and immuno-histochemically, VEGF, FGF-1 and -2, and TGF-B immunoreactivity are present in 81%, 67%, 92%, and 96%, respectively, of mesotheliomas, and in 20%, 50%, 40%, and 10%, respectively, of samples of the nonneoplastic mesothelium. Depending on the study, high immunohistochemical FGF-2 expression[53] or VEGF expression by reverse transcriptase polymerase chain reaction correlate with more tumor aggressiveness and worse prognosis for mesothelioma.[52,54]

Simian Virus 40

SV40 is a DNA tumor virus that has been associated with the development of malignant mesothelioma.[55] Although this virus is endogenous in rhesus monkeys, epidemiologic studies have shown that it is also widespread among the human population. The mode by which the virus was transferred from monkey to human is uncertain, but the bulk of this transfer may have occurred from 1954 to 1963 through SV40-contaminated polio vaccines administered worldwide. Moreover, polio vaccines produced in the former Union of Soviet Socialist Republics remained contaminated with infectious SV40 at least until 1978.[56]

The association of SV40 with mesothelioma started with the observation that when hamsters were injected with SV40 into the pleural space, all of the animals developed mesotheliomas within 6 months. This finding prompted investigations into the possibility that some mesotheliomas in humans could be attributed to SV40 infection directly or with SV40 acting as a cocarcinogen with asbestos. Mesothelioma samples studied in 1994 showed that 60% of the samples contained SV40 DNA and expressed the SV40 large T antigen. The results were confirmed by numerous laboratories using a variety of techniques such as PCR, FISH, Western blot, immunohistochemistry, and laser dissection/PCR, but the percentage of positive samples varied from 6% to 83%, and a few studies were completely negative. Technical and geographical differences may account for these variances.

Although the epidemiologic data are not available, mechanistic experiments in human mesothelial cells[57,58] and animal experiments[59] strongly support a pathogenic role of SV40 in mesothelioma. It is unlikely, however, that SV40 acts alone in mesothelioma development, as most cancers are multifactorial, and most mesotheliomas occur in asbestos-exposed individuals. SV40 has been shown to be a cocarcinogen in causing mesothelioma in animals and malignant transformation of mesothelial cells in tissue culture.[60,61] It is safe to say that a definitive role for the virus in human mesothelioma has not been unequivocally demonstrated but ongoing debate regarding its role will continue.

Radiation and Mesothelioma

In the literature, there are a few studies reporting mesothelioma development in patients exposed to thorotrast (intravenously) or who had received radiation to the chest and abdomen.[1] In some of these cases, asbestos exposure could not be ruled out, and SV40 status was not investigated. However, in a few cases in which mesotheliomas developed in young adults who received radiotherapy (RT) because of Wilms tumor, radiation was the only likely causative factor. Studies in rats support a role for radiation as a causative factor. Although it appears that radiation may cause mesotheliomas, the number of mesotheliomas for which it is responsible is probably small.

Carbon Nanoparticles

Engineered single-wall carbon nanotubes (SWCNT) are a class of nanoparticles being actively evaluated for myriad industrial and biomedical applications.[62] Preliminary cellular and animal exposure investigations on the toxicity and pathogenicity of SWCNTs have demonstrated biologic interactions, including toxicity, inflammatory reactions, oxidative stress, and fibroproliferative response.[63–65] SWCNTs are biopersistent and have the ability to distribute to subpleural areas after pharyngeal aspiration. Reports have described the induction of mesothelioma in p53+/− mice by multiwall carbon nanotubes.[66,67] These investigations compelled the present studies of potential interactions of SWCNTs with mesothelial cells. Exposure to SWCNTs induced reactive oxygen species generation, increased cell death, enhanced DNA damage and H2AX phosphorylation, and activated poly(adenosine diphosphate-ribose) polymerase, AP-1, NFκB, p38, and Akt in a dose-dependent manner. These events recapitulate some of the key molecular events involved in mesothelioma development associated with asbestos exposure.[68,69] In addition, nickel nanoparticles enhance the in vitro activity of PDGF in regulating chemokine production in rat mesothelial cells through a mechanism involving reactive oxygen species generation and prolonged activation of ERK-1.[70]

Genetic Predisposition to Mesothelioma: Erionite and BAP1

Recent evidence indicates that genetic predisposition plays an important role in determining individual susceptibility to mineral fiber carcinogenesis and to the development of mesothelioma. In the villages of Karain (population ~600), Tuzkoy (population ~1,400), and Sarihidir (this village was abandoned) in Cappadocia, a region in Central Anatolia, Turkey, ≥50% of deaths are caused by malignant mesothelioma.[71] This epidemic has been linked to exposure to a mineral fiber called *erionite*, one of the most potent mineral fibers in causing mesothelioma. However, mesothelioma was more frequent in certain families than others, leading to observations that some families in Turkey were unusually susceptible to erionite carcinogenesis.[71] Erionite is present in many parts of the world, including western American states such as North Dakota,[72,73] but so far the contribution of erionite to the increased incidence of mesothelioma has not been studied except in Turkey.

Similar families have also been identified in other parts of the world[74] and in the United States, where they appear to be unusually susceptible to asbestos carcinogenesis. Recently, BRCA-associated protein 1 (BAP1) has been identified as a novel MPM TSG. BAP1 is located at the 3p21, a region frequently deleted in MM, and encodes for a deubiquitinase enzyme known to target histones and other proteins. BAP1 appears to exert its antitumor activities mainly in a BRCA-independent manner,[75] with regulation of the cell epigenome, via modulation of histone H2A ubiquitination and chromatin accessibility.[76] However, the relevance of BAP1 to the biology of normal and cancer cells remains largely unexplained; in fact, manipulation of BAP1 in cancer cells has often yielded unexpected or even contradictory results. For example, silencing of BAP1 in MM and uveal melanoma cell lines resulted in reduced cell growth.[77,78]

Bott et al.[77] originally described the association of somatic mutations of BAP1 in 23% of mesothelioma samples. In a larger series of patients, the same group confirmed that somatic BAP1 mutations occur in about 20% of pleural MM and reported that the only clinical variable significantly different among those with and without BAP1 mutations was smoking (former or current), with BAP1 mutations more prevalent among smokers (75% versus 42%).[79] A Japanese study reported BAP1 gene alterations (either deletions or sequence-level mutations) in 61% of their 23 MM samples.[80] Whether this discrepancy results from the different methodologies

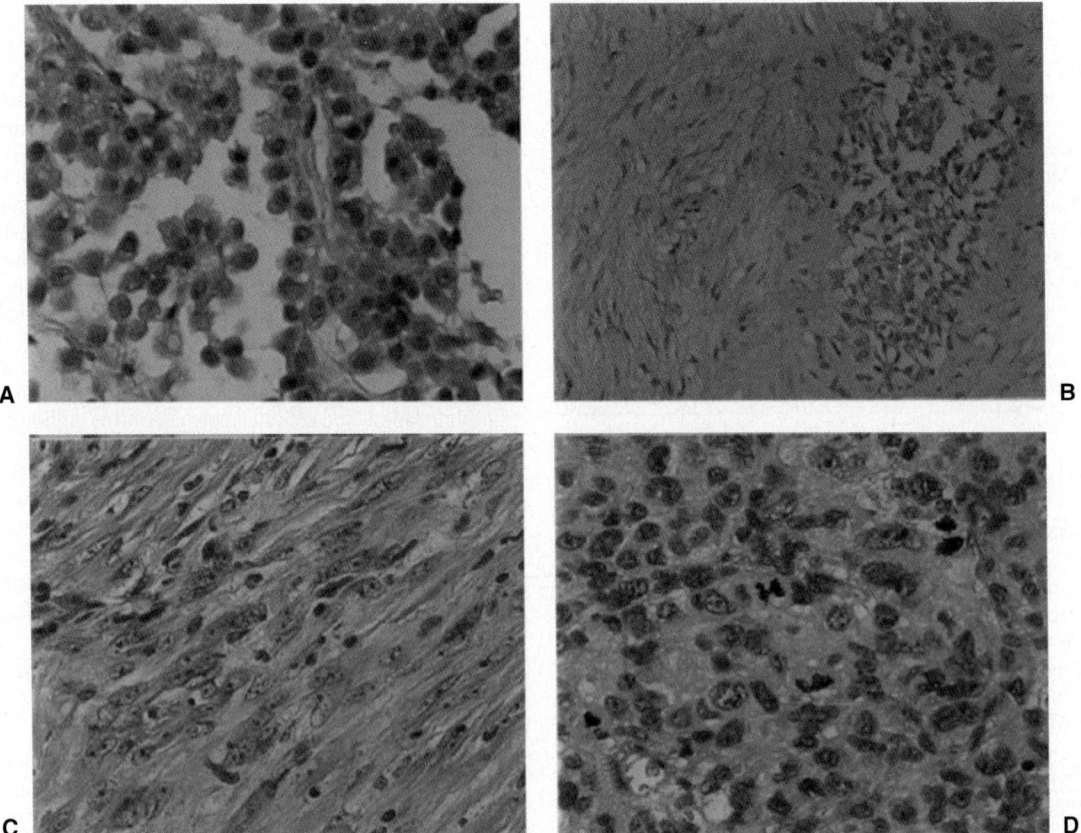

Figure 114.2 Histology of mesothelioma. **(A)** Epithelioid mesothelioma. Note tubular structures and malignant mesothelioma cells showing a hobnail morphology with bland nuclei and abundant cytoplasm. **(B)** Biphasic malignant mesothelioma, showing a nest of mesothelioma cells with epithelial differentiation within the sarcomatoid component. **(C)** Sarcomatoid mesothelioma, positivity for pankeratin, and rare foci of cells suggestive of epithelioid differentiation indicated the diagnosis. **(D)** High-grade sarcoma, a highly aggressive tumor that is vimentin-positive but vimentin-negative over 15 different immunostains for other markers and without distinctive electron microscopic features. In this case, the diagnosis of mesothelioma could not be confirmed. Original magnification: **A**, **C**, and **D**, × 400; **B**, × 200.

in sample preparation and detection of BAP1 mutations or it is an intrinsic difference between the two populations (e.g., due to ethnicity) has still to be determined. A third recent study from Arzt et al.,[81] with a separate cohort of 52 pleural MM, reported absence of BAP1 IHC staining in 60% of pleural MM, confirming previous results. Moreover, there was no correlation between BAP1 expression and asbestos exposure, and it was suggested that expression of BAP1 in tumor samples is inversely correlated to survival.

Germline BAP1 mutations were reported by Testa and Carbone[82] in two US families having a high frequency of MPMs. In the same study, 22% sporadic MM tumors harbored somatic BAP1 mutations. These findings have promoted speculation that BAP1 germline mutations can cause a novel cancer syndrome characterized by a significant excess of both pleural and peritoneal MM, uveal and cutaneous melanoma, and possibly other tumors.

PATHOLOGY OF MESOTHELIOMA

Benign Mesotheliomas

There are a number of benign mesothelial proliferations that must be distinguished from malignant mesothelioma including multicystic mesothelioma (*multilocular peritoneal inclusion cyst*), adenomatoid mesotheliomas, and well-differentiated papillary mesothelioma. Localized mesothelioma, better referred to as *localized fibrous tumor of the pleura* (FTP), is similar to other fibrous tumors found elsewhere in the body. The tumor

cells have a benign appearance and are usually immersed in a fibrous and characteristically vascular stroma. FTPs are characteristically negative for cytokeratin (a marker of mesothelial cells) and positive for CD34, which suggests that these cells are not of mesothelial origin. The most important predictive factor in the prognosis of FTP is whether the tumor can be completely resected. Pedunculated tumors have a much better prognosis than tumors that grow over a broad pleural area.[83–85] Surgical resection (Fig. 114.2) is the treatment of choice, with complete resection of the tumor and its pedunculated portion along with the site of origin. Five-year survival rates as high as 97% have been reported. En bloc resection of the lung, chest wall, or diaphragm may be necessary. For recurrences, re-excision is the treatment of choice. Long-term survival with re-excision is possible, but with incomplete resection or malignant transformation the median survival is 24 to 36 months.

Malignant Mesothelioma

Histologically, malignant mesothelioma can show an epithelial morphology (malignant mesothelioma epithelial type), a fibrous morphology (malignant mesothelioma fibrous type, also called sarcomatoid type), or a combination of both (mixed type or biphasic malignant mesothelioma) (Fig. 114.3). Most MM (50% to 60%) are of the epithelial type, approximately 10% are sarcomatoid, and the remainder are biphasic MM.

The diagnosis of malignant mesothelioma is usually straightforward, in contrast to common belief, provided that the pathologist

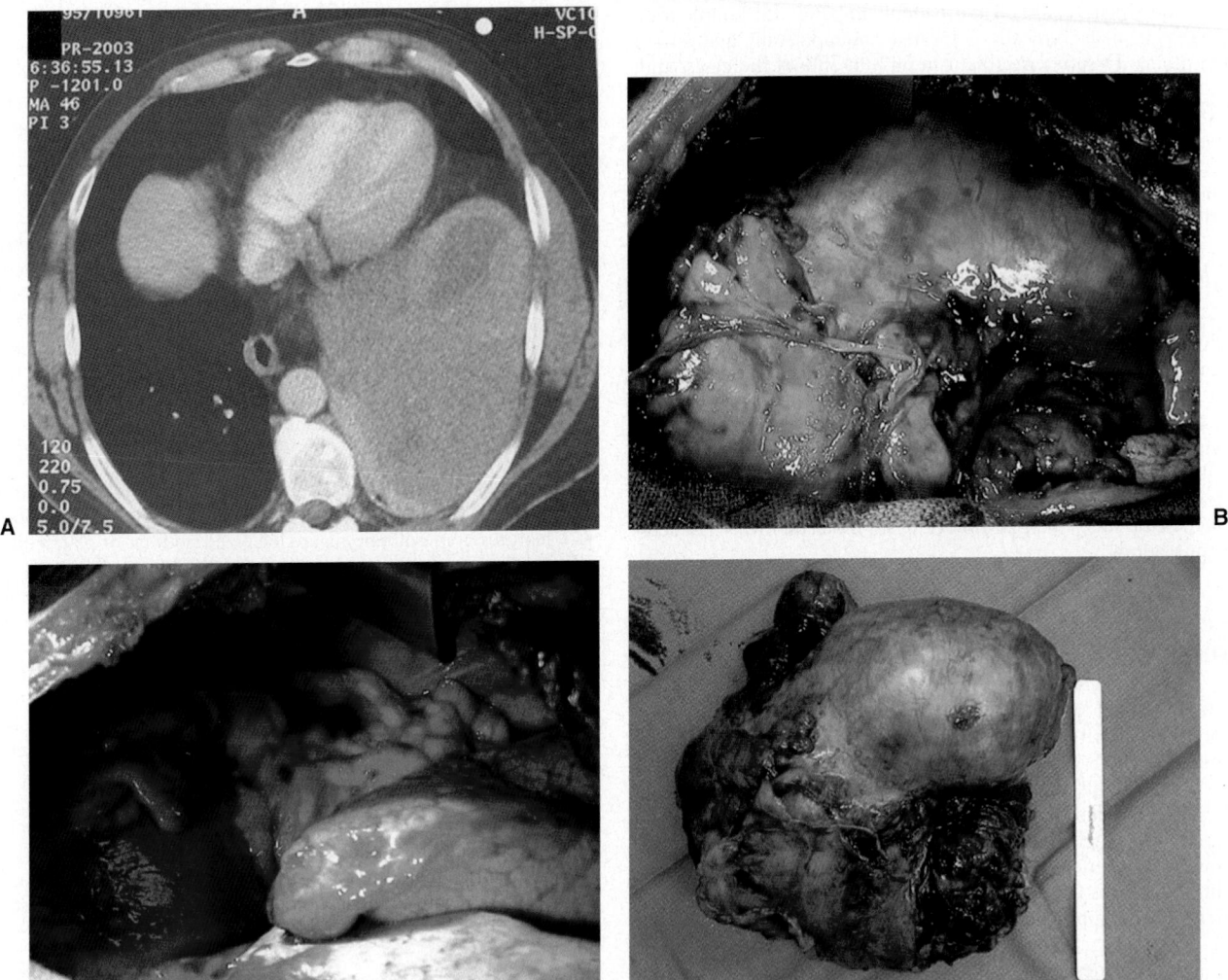

Figure 114.3 Fibrous tumor of pleura. **(A)** Computed tomography reveals a large mass compressing the lower lobe of the lung. **(B)** Intraoperative photograph. Tumor arose from a wide stalk on the diaphragm. **(C)** Intraoperative photograph after resection of the mass revealing expansion of the lung and no other disease. **(D)** Resected specimen.

has extensive experience with this malignancy. Some epithelial mesotheliomas grow forming sheets of epithelioid cells. To rule out mimics of mesothelioma, the diagnosis should be confirmed by immunohistochemistry, which shows that the tumor cells are diffusely positive for pankeratin, keratin 5/6, calretinin, and WT-1, and negative for the epithelial markers such as CEA, CD15, Ber-EP4, Moc-31, TTF-1, and B72.3. For epithelial mesotheliomas, positive stainings for pankeratin and calretinin and negative stainings for three epithelial markers are considered sufficient for diagnosis.

Biphasic mesotheliomas can be distinguished from carcinosarcomas metastasizing from various organs and from biphasic synovial sarcomas by using either electron microscopy or molecular testing for the X;18 translocation that is diagnostic of synovial sarcoma.[86]

Newer methods are under development for distinguishing mesothelioma from adenocarcinoma and include microRNA profiling of the tumors. Gee et al.[87] have described the use of seven miRNAs (miR-200c, miR-141, miR-200b, miR-200a, miR-429, miR-203, and miR-205) to distinguish lung adenocarcinoma from mesothelioma with a 10% misclassification error. Others have described a three microRNA profile (mir-205, mir-193a-3p, and mir-192) for the differential diagnosis of mesothelioma from colon, renal, lung, and breast cancer with a 95% specificity and 96% sensitivity.[88]

EPIDEMIOLOGY AND CLINICAL PRESENTATION

The death rates for mesothelioma parallel the consumption of asbestos by individual countries. When one considers mesothelioma death rates from 2000 to 2004 as a function of asbestos usage in the 1960s, Australia has the highest death rate for the disease in the world.[89] It is predicted that between 2000 and 2049, over 400,000 lives will be lost in those countries from the disease.[90] In the United States, there have been 2,500 deaths per year from the disease since 1999, with workers with industrial exposures in construction and shipbuilding being at highest risk, followed by plumbers, pipe fitters, and steamers. Mesothelioma affects men in their 50s, 60s, and 70s due to the aforementioned 25- to 40-year latency period between occupational asbestos exposure and the development of the tumor.[91] Women and children can have the disease, but the male-to-female ratio is approximately 4.5:1.[92]

Symptoms

As many as 25% of patients with the disease have symptoms for ≥6 months before seeking medical attention. The right side is affected more than the left side (60% versus 40%), most likely because of the right side's greater volume.

Approximately 60% of the patients present with nonpleuritic chest pain that classically is located posterolaterally and low in the thorax. Dyspnea is present in 50% to 70% of the cases, and, indeed, 80% of the patients present with dyspnea and effusion. The presence of a pleural effusion is documented at some time in the course of the disease in 95% of patients with MPM. With the increasing use of positron emission tomography for pretreatment planning, between 5% and 25% of patients are found to have metastatic disease at presentation.[93]

Physical Examination

Physical examination reveals decreased breath sounds, dullness to percussion, or decreased motion of the involved chest wall. Failure to significantly relieve the dyspnea after thoracentesis may indicate that the lung is "trapped." In the late stages of the disease, there is often dramatic cachexia, marked contraction of the involved chest with narrowed interspaces, and hypertrophy of the contralateral hemithorax. A chest wall mass occurs in up to 25% of patients, often at the site(s) of prior thoracentesis, thoracotomy, or thoracoscopy wounds.

Laboratory Examination and Blood Biomarkers

Mesothelioma patients have nonspecific laboratory findings, including hypergammaglobulinemia, eosinophilia, and/or anemia of chronic disease. It has been recently noted that 14% to 15% of patients have elevated homocysteine levels, reflecting folic acid deficiency; 17% have biochemical evidence of vitamin B_{12} deficiency; and 32% have biochemical signs of vitamin B_6 deficiency.[94] The most striking laboratory abnormality is thrombocytosis (>400,000), which is seen in 60% to 90% of patients,[95] and approximately 15% of patients have platelet counts >1,000,000.

Soluble mesothelin-related peptide (SMRP), osteopontin (OPN), and megakaryocyte potentiating factor are presently under investigation as early detection or therapy monitoring markers. Robinson et al.[96] reported that determination of SMRP in serum is a marker of mesothelioma with a sensitivity of 83% and specificity of 95% in the first 48 patients with MPM tested. These data have been validated by other laboratories in the United States[97,98] and internationally.[99] Changes in serum SMRP levels parallel clinical course/tumor size, and SMRP was elevated in 75% of patients at diagnosis.[100] Studies using SMRP in an attempt to diagnose early mesothelioma in high-risk cohorts have so far been disappointing, but follow-up is still short.[101,102]

OPN is a glycoprotein that mediates cell-matrix interactions and is regulated by proteins in cell-signaling pathways that have been associated with asbestos-induced carcinogenesis.[103] In a study that compared serum OPN levels of patients with MPM to those of asbestos-exposed individuals without cancer, serum OPN levels rose with duration of asbestos exposure and degree of radiographic abnormality (plaques and fibrosis versus other lesser findings[104]), and using a cutpoint of 48.3 ng of OPN per milliliter resulted in 77.6% sensitivity and 85.5% specificity when comparing the group exposed to asbestos with the group with mesothelioma. Follow-up studies have demonstrated that serum OPN is not reliable because of the presence of a thrombin cleavage site, which causes degradation of the marker.[105] Plasma OPN,[106] although not specific to mesothelioma, is being evaluated in the disease for both prognosis and early detection utility. A blinded validation of plasma fibulin 3 confirmed excellent discrimination between MPM plasma and all non-MPM cohorts including those with benign or malignant effusions. Pleural effusion fibulin 3 was also discriminatory between MPM effusions and non-MPM effusions.[107]

Radiologic Examination

Malignant mesothelioma can have a diverse radiographic appearance. Many of the early changes are associated with a previous exposure to asbestos, consisting both of pleural and parenchymal changes, including pleural plaques or parenchymal pulmonary fibrosis.

Chest Radiography

The most common chest radiography features associated with mesothelioma progression and symptoms include the presence of a pleural effusion, diffuse pleural thickening, and nodularity. The involved hemithorax can eventually have smooth, lobular pleural masses that infiltrate the pleural space and fissures[108–110] in 45% to 60% of patients with contraction and fixation of the chest (Fig. 114.4). The lung becomes encased, and the mediastinum shifts because of volume loss.

Chest Tomography

Pleural changes on chest tomography (CT) include pleural plaques, diffuse pleural thickening, and pleural effusion. Additional CT features of mesothelioma are localized nodular or plaque-like pleural thickening, possibly associated with pleural effusion. The lobulated pleural encasement frequently causes lower lobe collapse (Fig. 114.5). Intrapulmonary nodules can occur in 60% of patients, and infiltration into fissures along with enlarged hilar and mediastinal lymph nodes may be seen. The CT allows a better view of the involved pericardium, which is irregularly thickened and associated with infiltration to the pericardial fat pad. A clear fat plane between the inferior diaphragmatic surface and the adjacent abdominal organs as well as a smooth inferior diaphragmatic contour may imply resectability.[111] CT may reveal a hemidiaphragm encased by a mass or poor definition between the liver, stomach, and inferior diaphragmatic surface.

Volumetric measurements using CT have recently been studied with regard to their prognostic capability (see "Prognostic Indicators").

Magnetic Resonance Imaging

Studies have suggested that gadolinium contrast enhancement magnetic resonance imaging can improve mesothelioma staging (Fig. 114.6). Detection of diaphragm invasion and invasion of endothoracic fascia or a single chest wall focus may be better with magnetic resonance imaging compared with CT.[111]

Positron Emission Tomography Imaging

There are a number of studies of positron emission tomography (PET) and the radionuclide imaging agent [18F]fluorodeoxyglucose (FDG) in mesothelioma (Fig. 114.7). Early studies reported that FDG-PET was accurate in the diagnosis of pleural malignancies, specifically mesothelioma.[112–116] Recent studies have concentrated on the accuracy of PET in defining nodal and extrathoracic metastases prior to surgical therapy.[93,112] Because of false-positive results in patients with FDG-avid pleural inflammatory/infectious etiologies, all FDG-avid extrathoracic sites should be histologically confirmed in patients with MPM being considered for extrapleural pneumonectomy (EPP).

DIAGNOSTIC APPROACH FOR PRESUMED MESOTHELIOMA

Thoracentesis and Closed Pleural Biopsy

Patients who present with a large, unexplained pleural effusion and minimal or moderate evidence of pleural thickening should have initial thoracentesis and pleural biopsy, especially if a history of asbestos exposure or mesothelioma in a family member is elicited. By preserving a cell block from the pleural fluid and using both histochemical

Second-Line Therapy

No standard of care regimen for patients with previously treated malignant mesothelioma exists, and there are no clear data confirming that second-line therapy increases overall survival. Best supportive care, local RT, and pain medications should be given to patients when required, and chemotherapy may also be considered. Only one phase 3 trial has been conducted in this setting, but it included patients who did not receive a pemetrexed-based regimen as first-line therapy.[195,197] In this study, 243 patients were treated with single-agent pemetrexed and supportive care, or supportive care alone. Treatment with pemetrexed increased the response rate (18.7% versus 1.7%; $p < .0001$) and disease control rate (59.3% versus 19.2%; $p < 0.0001$), though overall survival was not improved because a significant number of patients in the supportive care arm ended up receiving chemotherapy. Treatment with pemetrexed or pemetrexed plus cisplatin also yielded high disease control rates in previously treated patients in the Expanded Access Trial.[195,198] However, the current widespread use of pemetrexed/cisplatin as first-line therapy makes these findings mostly irrelevant.

Patients who receive pemetrexed combinations as first-line therapy may derive further benefit from being retreated with pemetrexed, particularly if there is a long interval before progression. In a retrospective analysis of second-line therapy, 42 patients who had been pretreated with pemetrexed were rechallenged, and this resulted in a higher disease control rate, longer progression-free survival, and longer overall survival as compared to treatment with a different agent.[199]

The data supporting the use of other second-line therapies is similarly lacking. A multiple regression analysis that adjusted for baseline prognostic factors found that patients enrolled in the phase 3 trial comparing pemetrexed/cisplatin to cisplatin alone had a longer survival if they received poststudy chemotherapy which primarily consisted of either gemcitabine or vinorelbine.[200] As treatment with single-agent vinorelbine trended toward improving survival in the Medical Research Council phase 3 three-arm trial, it seems a reasonable option for second-line therapy. Stebbing et al.[201] conducted a phase 2 trial with vinorelbine given at a dose of 30mg/m^2 weekly and found a 16% response rate and overall survival of 9.6 months. Only a fraction of the patients in that trial were previously treated with pemetrexed and cisplatin, however. In a retrospective analysis including 56 evaluable patients who had mostly received pemetrexed-based first-line therapy and were treated with vinorelbine or gemcitabine as second- or third-line therapy, there was 1 partial response (with gemcitabine) giving a response rate of 2% (95% CI = 0% to 5%). Forty-six percent of patients had stable disease. Median progression free survival was 1.4 months for both vinorelbine and gemcitabine, while overall median survival was 5.4 months and 4.7 months, respectively. Given the unclear benefit of further chemotherapy, these patients should ideally be enrolled in a clinical trial if available.

NOVEL THERAPEUTIC APPROACHES

Angiogenesis Inhibition

Several lines of evidence support angiogenesis inhibition as a potential therapeutic strategy in mesothelioma. VEGF induces proliferation of mesothelial cells in culture, and the addition of VEGF-neutralizing antibodies inhibits this effect.[52,202] Mesothelioma tumor specimens express VEGF and its receptors.[203,204] High levels of VEGF have also been detected in the serum and pleural effusions of patients with mesothelioma and correlate with poorer survival.[203,205]

The VEGF monoclonal antibody bevacizumab has been extensively studied in mesothelioma. In a randomized phase 2 trial, 106 patients received six cycles of gemcitabine and cisplatin combined with bevacizumab or placebo followed by maintenance therapy with bevacizumab or placebo.[206] No improvement in response rate, progression-free survival, or overall survival was seen with the addition of bevacizumab. A subgroup analysis noted that higher baseline plasma VEGF levels were correlated with a shorter progression-free and overall survival, and that patients with VEGF levels less than the median had longer progression-free and overall survival when treated with bevacizumab. Other studies have explored bevacizumab in combination with pemetrexed and cisplatin. In a single-arm, phase 2 trial with this regimen, 53 patients enrolled at four US centers achieved a progression-free survival of 6.9 months, a disease control rate of 75%, and a median overall survival of 14.8 months; these results compare favorably with historical controls.[207] A French Intergroup study is currently testing pemetrexed/cisplatin plus bevacizumab versus placebo in a definitive randomized phase 2/3 design.

Thalidomide, a drug with a checkered past due to its teratogenic effects, but effective and approved for use in multiple myeloma, has a putative mechanism of action of antiangiogenesis. A phase 1/2 study of thalidomide identified a suitable dose of 200 mg daily and demonstrated 28% disease stabilization for >6 months.[208] However, a phase 3 trial conducted in the Netherlands that randomized 222 patients to maintenance thalidomide versus observation after completion of platinum-based chemotherapy did not demonstrate any benefit in progression-free survival (3.6 months versus 3.5 months; HR = 0.95).[209]

A number of VEGF receptor multikinase inhibitors have been tested in mesothelioma, and they demonstrate a consistent low level of activity (Table 114.7). Most of these drugs also inhibit other growth signaling pathways including PDGF receptors and c-KIT which are also relevant in MPM.[210,211] The first agent in this class to be tested was SU5416, which yielded responses in 11% of patients, but clinical development for this drug was subsequently halted.[212] A CALGB study with sorafenib highlights the issues of patient selection when studying novel agents in mesothelioma.[213] In this trial, patients could receive sorafenib as first- or second-line therapy. Patients who had received previous chemotherapy survived for a median of 13.2 months, compared with 5 months for chemonaïve patients, though this large difference was not statistically significant ($p = 0.3$). One-year survival was also greater in the previously treated patients compared with those who were chemonaïve (57% versus 30%). This suggests that the patients treated as first-line may have been poor candidates for standard chemotherapy, while the patients treated as second-line had maintained a good performance status after chemotherapy. Sunitinib malate was tested in two phase 2 trials. In the Australian study,[214] 53 patients received sunitinib as second-line therapy at a dose of 50 mg on an intermittent schedule of 28 out of every 42 days. The confirmed response rate was 12%, but 65% had stable disease including many patients with some degree of tumor shrinkage. That response rate could not be confirmed, however, in a Canadian trial,[215] which noted only one response in an untreated patient and none in the cohort of previously treated patients. Survival rates were generally poor in both studies. The sum of these trials suggests that these agents may have limited activity, but perhaps should optimally be combined with chemotherapy. This concept is being tested in a Southwest Oncology Group randomized phase 2 trial of pemetrexed/cisplatin with or without cederinib.

Histone Deacetylase Inhibitors

In addition to directly regulating transcription through changes in chromatin structure, histone deacetylase inhibitors modulate the acetylation of transcription factors and other nonhistone proteins. This leads to a range of biologic effects that have shown relevance to MPM in preclinical studies.[216] Vorinostat is an oral agent that binds to the catalytic site of histone deacetylase subtypes 1, 2, 3, and 6 thereby inhibiting their activity.[217] In a phase 1 trial of

TABLE 114.7

Phase 2 Studies with Multikinase Inhibitors of Vascular Endothelial Growth Factor Receptor

Agent	Line of Therapy	N	Overall Response Rate (%)	Stable Disease Rate (%)	Progression-Free Survival (mo)	Overall Survival (mo)
SU5416[212]	Second	23	11	38	2	12.4
Cediranib[299]	First or second	51	10	34	1.8	4.4
Cediranib[300]	Second	54	9	34	2.6	9.5
Pazopanib[301]	First or second	34	NR	56	4.4	11.1
Sorafenib[213]	First or second	51	6	54	3.6	9.7
Sunitinib[302]	Second	53	12	65	3.5	6.1
Sunitinib[303]	First or second	35	3	60	2.7	7.5
Vatalanib[41]	First	47	6	72	4.1	10.0

NR, not reported.

vorinostat, two unconfirmed partial responses were observed in the 13 patients with mesothelioma, and several others had prolonged disease stabilization.[218] These data led to the largest phase 3 trial in mesothelioma in which 661 patients previously treated with one or two prior chemotherapy regimens were randomized 1:1 to vorinostat or placebo. However, vorinostat did not impact overall survival; the median overall survival for vorinostat versus placebo was 30.7 weeks versus 27.1 weeks with a HR of 0.98.[219]

Mammalian Target of Rapamycin Inhibitors

The neurofibromatosis-2 (NF2) gene is mutated in 50% to 60% of MM resulting in loss of the protein Merlin. Merlin mediates contact-dependent inhibition of cell proliferation in normal cells, primarily through inhibition of mammalian target of rapamycin (mTOR).[220] In knockout models of Merlin, mTOR activity becomes unregulated, and this leads to increased cell proliferation that can be abrogated by mTOR inhibition. In mesothelioma cell lines, Merlin loss activates mTORC1 signaling, and cells with NF2 mutations are selectively sensitive to drugs targeting mTORC1.[221] These data provide the rationale for studying the mTOR inhibitors in patients with mesothelioma. However, a Southwest Oncology Group phase 2 study with everolimus in previously treated patients failed to reach its predefined 4-month progression-free survival end point.[222] Agents that also block phosphoinositide-3-kinase along with mTOR appear to have greater efficacy in early trials, though. In an expansion cohort of a phase 1 trial with GDC0980, four patients achieved a partial response, including one patient at 50 mg, one patient with the PIK3CA mutation R88Q at 8 mg, and two at the recommended phase 2 dose of 30 mg. Furthermore, 11 (41%) patients remained on study for >6 months, and 2 (7%) remained on study >12 months.[223]

Mesothelin-Directed Therapy

Mesothelin is an immunogenic cell surface antigen[224,225] involved in cell proliferation, cell signaling, adhesion, and metastases.[226–228] In normal tissues, it is expressed only in the pleura, pericardium, and peritoneum at low levels,[225,229] and it is expressed in essentially all MPM tumors.[98,224,230–232] Several therapeutic approaches targeting mesothelin have shown promise. Amatuximab (MORAb-009) is a chimeric IgG1 antibody tested in a single-arm phase 2 trial in combination with standard chemotherapy for patients with advanced MPM. Although progression-free survival did not differ from historical control and thus the trial did not meet its predefined primary end point, 90% of patients had a radiographic response or stable disease, and overall survival was significantly greater than

anticipated with a number of patients remaining on maintenance antibody treatment for an extended time. A follow-up randomized trial with that agent is planned. A mesothelin immunoconjugate, SS1P, consisting of antimesothelin Fv fused to Pseudomonas exotoxin A, demonstrated minor activity in phase 1 trials; however, efficacy was hampered by the development of neutralizing antibodies.[229,233] However, when SS1P was administered along with immunosuppressive agents pentostatin and cyclosphosphamide, dramatic tumor regressions were observed in 3 out of 10 patients, and 2 other patients had major responses to chemotherapy following that therapy.[234] The group at the University of Pennsylvania has begun treating patients with genetically engineered T cells targeting mesothelin and have reported on one patient having a minor response after recovery from a severe infusion reaction.

RADIOTHERAPY FOR MESOTHELIOMA

Curative Radiation Therapy as a Single Modality

The limitation of potentially "curative" RT for treatment of MPM is the inability to treat a large volume of disease in the chest with a curative radiation dose (>60 Gy) because of the risks of severe damage to normal tissue. Previous studies from the 1980s administered approximately 50 Gy to the pleural space with most studies demonstrating a median overall survival ranging from 3 to 10 months. Patients who received treatment had an improved outcome than those who did not receive treatment, although this is likely the result of a selection bias, with those fit enough to undergo a full course of radiation likely to have a greater survival regardless of treatment given.[123,235–239] RT as a sole therapy should be used rarely and only in the setting of patients who are unable to tolerate any form of systemic chemotherapy.

Combined Chemotherapy and Definitive Radiotherapy

The poor results reported for definitive RT alone have led to studies evaluating the combination of chemotherapy and radiation. Both Ruffie et al.[236] and Linden et al.[240] have reported that the median survival is increased in patients treated with combined modality therapy compared with RT alone. Some investigators have evaluated the addition of radiation sensitizers to definitive RT. Herscher et al.[241] from the National Cancer Institute studied the use of a 5-day continuous infusion of paclitaxel with radical RT in patients with mesothelioma and non–small-cell lung cancer. In patients with mesothelioma, the hemithoracic radiation was delivered before the chemotherapy. Chen et al.[242] reported a 12% complete response rate and an 88% partial response rate when pulsed paclitaxel was delivered during RT in a phase 1 trial. Although these combination approaches are interesting, it is not likely that the addition of radiation sensitizers to radical RT will be curative, and as such, definitive chemoradiotherapy should be considered experimental for patients with mesothelioma.

Combined Surgical Resection and Definitive Radiotherapy

RT can be used as an adjuvant treatment after EPP or P/D. After an EPP, radical RT can be administered without concern for damage to the underlying ipsilateral lung because it has been removed surgically. However, radical RT after a P/D continues to place the intact ipsilateral lung at risk for substantial loss of function and toxicity.

Rusch et al.[140,243] at Memorial Sloan Kettering Cancer Center completed a phase 2 trial of EPP followed by postoperative radiation in patients with pleural mesothelioma. Eighty-eight patients with biopsy-confirmed mesothelioma were treated. Twenty-one patients were unresectable and taken off the study. The majority of patients ($n = 62$) underwent an EPP followed by 54 Gy delivered through anterior and posterior fields in 30 fractions of 1.8 Gy. Five patients were treated with a pleurectomy (PL), which was followed by intraoperative RT to a dose of 15 Gy using a high-dose iridium applicator. This was followed by 54 Gy to the hemithorax via anterior and posterior fields in the same fractionation schedule as those who underwent EPP. There were seven postoperative deaths, all primarily related to pulmonary complications in patients who had undergone an EPP. A total of 33 patients had some complications, with the most common being atrial arrhythmias (17 patients), respiratory failure (6 patients), pneumonia (5 patients), and empyema (5 patients). Only the patients who underwent EPP were considered for survival analysis. The median survival was 17 months, with an overall survival of 27% at 3 years. Only 13% had locoregional recurrence, with the majority of patients failing to respond and having distant metastases. The authors concluded that their approach of aggressive surgery with EPP followed by high-dose radiation to the entire hemithorax provided a favorable outcome for those patients who were able to complete the therapy when compared to historical data.

Intensity-modulated RT (IMRT) offers the potential for administering higher doses of RT with better target coverage to the hemithorax while minimizing normal tissue toxicities. IMRT is a highly conformal radiation technique that allows more effective sparing of normal tissues, providing an opportunity for safer, less toxic treatments and increased efficacy by enabling higher radiation doses to the tumor. It comes with a much higher level of dosimetric control and certainty leading to better target coverage than conventional techniques.[244] Areas of dose inhomogeneity are readily recognizable and can be corrected. Rice et al.[245] and Forster et al.[246] at the MD Anderson Cancer Center treated patients with MPM with IMRT after EPP. Recent data in 100 patients who underwent EPP, 63 of whom were treated with IMRT, reveal a median survival of 14.2 months and 3-year survival of 20% for patients with IMRT. Recurrences in the irradiated field occurred in only three patients, and distant disease observed in 54% of patients was the major pattern of failure. Liver injury has been documented after hemithoracic IMRT.[247] However, pulmonary toxicity appears to be the most significant late toxicity observed in patients with MPM after IMRT.[248–250] Allen et al.[248] reported fatal pulmonary complications in 6 of 13 patients with MPM treated with IMRT to a dose of 54 Gy to the clinical target volume. The median time from completion of IMRT to the onset of radiation pneumonitis was 30 days (range, 5 to 57 days). Recent data from Kristensen et

al.[250] showed fatal pulmonary toxicity in 4 of 26 (15%) of patients with MPM treated with induction chemotherapy, EPP, and postoperative IMRT to a pleural surface dose of 50 Gy. These reports of pulmonary toxicity emphasize that care should be taken when planning and delivering IMRT to the hemithorax. An alternative technique using electrons and IMRT has been reported as an alternative to IMRT alone. However, it appears that better coverage of the target volume is achieved with IMRT.[251,252] If the use of IMRT after EPP is planned, doses of 45 to 50 Gy in 1.8 to 2.0 Gy fractions are typically recommended. In addition to other standard normal tissue constraints, a mean lung dose of ≤9 Gy and a V5 (volume of lung receiving ≥5 Gy) of ≤65% should be used during the planning process.

Gomez et al.[253] retrospectively analyzed 86 patients who underwent hemithoracic IMRT after EPP at MD Anderson Cancer Center. Grade 3 or worse pulmonary toxicity occurred in 11.6% of patients. There were five fatal cases of pulmonary toxicity: three from radiation pneumonitis and two from bronchopleural fistula. At 2 years, the rates of overall survival, local control, and distant control were 32%, 55%, and 40% respectively. Fourteen patients (16%) experienced local failure and only two of these patients had local failure alone. Fifty-one patients (59%) had distant metastases, which included failures in the contralateral hemithorax and the abdomen.

A retrospective review from the University of North Carolina examined 30 patients who received IMRT following EPP.[254] The median dose to the ipsilateral hemithorax was 45 Gy with an 8 to 25 Gy boost in nine patients. Two-year local control, disease-free survival, and overall survival rates were 47%, 34%, and 50%, respectively. Four patients (13%) developed radiation pneumonitis, including one fatality (3%).

Radiation after Lung Sparing

In a retrospective review of patients having P/D at Memorial Sloan Kettering Cancer Center from 1974 to 2003, 123 patients received external-beam RT (median dose, 42.5 Gy; range, 7.2 to 67.8 Gy) to the ipsilateral hemithorax postoperatively. The median and 2-year overall survival for all patients was 13.5 months (range, 1 to 199 months) and 23%, respectively. Multivariate analysis for overall survival revealed a radiation dose <40 Gy ($p = 0.001$), nonepithelioid histology ($p = 0.002$), left-sided disease ($p = 0.01$), and the use of an implant ($p = 0.02$) to be unfavorable. These data reinforce the concept that residual disease cannot be eradicated with external RT with or without brachytherapy and that a more extensive surgery followed by external RT might be required to improve local control and overall survival.[255] Moreover, intraoperative RT for mesothelioma is associated with toxicity and failure to prolong survival.[256]

An experience with pleural IMRT in 36 patients with two intact lungs has recently been reported.[257] All patients were planned with a PET/CT scan to aid target delineation. With a median dose of 46.8 Gy, 1- and 2- year survival was 75% and 53%, respectively, with a median survival of 26 months in patients who underwent P/D. Seven (20%) patients experienced grade 3 or 4 pneumonitis. A typical treatment plan is presented in Figure 114.10.

A prospective study from Aviano, Italy, reported on 28 patients who were treated with helical tomotherapy after P/D or biopsy alone.[258] All patients had FDG-PET scans after surgery for staging and were treated to an intended dose of 50 to 60 Gy. Five patients (18%) had respiratory toxicity, but only two were grade 3 (7%); none were grade 5. The contralateral lung dose was strongly correlated with the risk of pneumonitis.

Prevention of Scar Recurrences

Malignant seeding in approximately 20% to 50% of patients with mesothelioma along thoracentesis tracts, biopsy tracts, chest

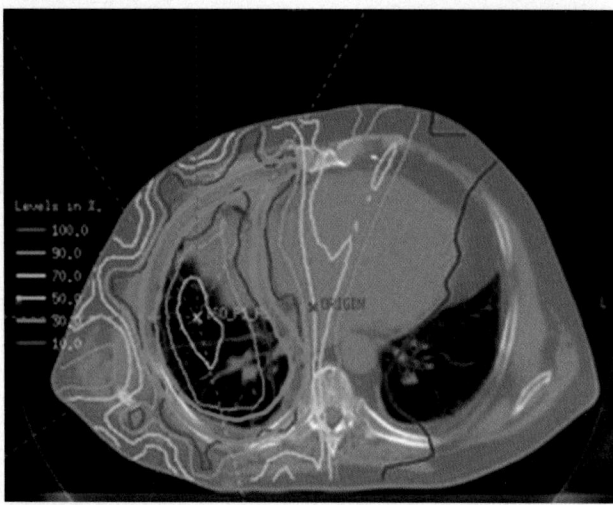

Figure 114.10 Radiation therapy after pleurectomy decortication. Isodense beam distribution showing example of typical isodose distribution using eight angles equally spaced over the 200-degree to 240-degree sector encompassing the ipsilateral lung. Area within *green lines* depicts target volume. (Color version of figure is available online at http://www.semthorcardiovascsurg.com). (Reprinted from Rosenzweig KE, Zauderer MG, Laser B, et al. Pleural intensity-modulated radiotherapy for malignant pleural mesothelioma. *Int J Radiat Oncol Biol Phys* 2012;83:1278–1283, Copyright (2012), with permission from Elsevier.)

tube sites, and surgical incisions is a common complication of procedures in these patients.[119,259] Boutin et al.[119] randomized 40 patients after an invasive diagnostic procedure to either RT (7 Gy × three fractions) or no treatment. No patient in the radiation treatment group developed subcutaneous nodules. Alternatively, 8 of 20 patients in the untreated group developed metastases. Two additional small randomized trials have suggested that the use of short-course RT does not reduce the frequency of cutaneous seeding after invasive procedures.[121,260] These data are inconclusive, and reviews of contemporary practice patterns suggest that radiation is commonly used to prevent scar recurrences.[261,262]

Palliation Using Radiation Therapy

RT is commonly used to palliate pain in patients with advanced mesothelioma,[157] and investigators from the Netherlands have reported using palliative RT to treat painful chest wall metastases in patients with mesothelioma. Ball and Cruickshank[237] reported a 72% rate of symptom improvement using palliative courses of RT. Ruffie et al.[263] and Davis et al.[264] reported the results of palliative RT in patients with mesothelioma. When doses >45 Gy were used, pain relief was attained in >50% of the cases.

More recently, some centers have investigated the use of IMRT for unresectable patients. Treatment techniques prior to the advent of IMRT would have necessitated significant dose inhomogeneity in the setting of intact lung. Palliative RT to the entire hemithorax should only be considered when first-line and second-line chemotherapeutic options have been exhausted.

Proton Beam Radiation

The widespread interest in proton RT has begun to carry over to MPM. To date, two theoretical planning studies have been published that suggest that proton therapy allows better sparing of normal organs at risk while providing better target coverage in patients after EPP.[265,266] However, many uncertainties regarding the feasibility of proton therapy in thoracic RT remain, given the significant impact of respiratory motion and stark tissue density variation in the thorax on accurate proton dosimetry. Clinical validation of proton therapy for MPM remains to be shown.

SELECTED REFERENCES

The full reference list can be accessed at lwwhealthlibrary.com/oncology.

1. Carbone M, Kratzke RA, Testa JR. The pathogenesis of mesothelioma. *Semin Oncol* 2002;29:2–17.
2. Yang H, Bocchetta M, Kroczynska B, et al. TNF-alpha inhibits asbestos-induced cytotoxicity via a NF-kappaB-dependent pathway, a possible mechanism for asbestos-induced oncogenesis. *Proc Natl Acad Sci U S A* 2006;103:10397–10402.
3. Altomare DA, Vaslet CA, Skele KL, et al. A mouse model recapitulating molecular features of human mesothelioma. *Cancer Res* 2005;65:8090–8095.
4. Wagner JC, Berry G, Timbrell V. Mesotheliomata in rats after inoculation with asbestos and other materials. *Br J Cancer* 1973;28:173–185.
12. Yang H, Rivera Z, Jube S, et al. Programmed necrosis induced by asbestos in human mesothelial cells causes high-mobility group box 1 protein release and resultant inflammation. *Proc Natl Acad Sci U S A* 2010;107:12611–12616.
13. Carbone M, Ly BH, Dodson RF, et al. Malignant mesothelioma: facts, myths, and hypotheses. *J Cell Physiol* 2012;227:44–58.
14. Hillegass JM, Shukla A, Lathrop SA, et al. Inflammation precedes the development of human malignant mesotheliomas in a SCID mouse xenograft model. *Ann N Y Acad Sci* 2010;1203:7–14.
18. Bianchi ME. DAMPs, PAMPs and alarmins: all we need to know about danger. *J Leukoc Biol* 2007;81:1–5.
19. Dostert C, Petrilli V, Van Bruggen R, et al. Innate immune activation through Nalp3 inflammasome sensing of asbestos and silica. *Science* 2008;320:674–677.
22. Jube S, Rivera ZS, Bianchi ME, et al. Cancer cell secretion of the DAMP protein HMGB1 supports progression in malignant mesothelioma. *Cancer Res* 2012;72:3290–3301.
25. Ivanov SV, Miller J, Lucito R, et al. Genomic events associated with progression of pleural malignant mesothelioma. *Int J Cancer* 2009;124:589–599.
28. Altomare DA, Menges CW, Xu J, et al. Losses of both products of the Cdkn2a/Arf locus contribute to asbestos-induced mesothelioma development and cooperate to accelerate tumorigenesis. *PLoS One* 2011;6:e18828.
29. Yang CT, You L, Uematsu K, et al. p14(ARF) modulates the cytolytic effect of ONYX-015 in mesothelioma cells with wild-type p53. *Cancer Res* 2001;61:5959–5963.
31. Dacic S, Kothmaier H, Land S, et al. Prognostic significance of p16/cdkn2a loss in pleural malignant mesotheliomas. *Virchows Arch* 2008;453:627–635.
34. Amin KM, Litzky LA, Smythe WR, et al. Wilms' tumor 1 susceptibility (WT1) gene products are selectively expressed in malignant mesothelioma. *Am J Pathol* 1995;146:344–356.
35. Zauderer MG, Krug LM. Novel therapies in phase II and III trials for malignant pleural mesothelioma. *J Natl Compr Canc Netw* 2012;10:42–47.
36. Cheng JQ, Lee WC, Klein MA, et al. Frequent mutations of NF2 and allelic loss from chromosome band 22q12 in malignant mesothelioma: evidence for a two-hit mechanism of NF2 inactivation. *Genes Chromosomes Cancer* 1999;24:238–242.
39. Gerwin BI, Lechner JF, Reddel RR, et al. Comparison of production of transforming growth factor-beta and platelet-derived growth factor by normal human mesothelial cells and mesothelioma cell lines. *Cancer Res* 1987;47:6180–6184.
42. Kumar-Singh S, Weyler J, Martin MJ, et al. Angiogenic cytokines in mesothelioma: a study of VEGF, FGF-1 and -2, and TGF beta expression. *J Pathol* 1999;189:72–78.
47. Pass HI, Mew DJ, Carbone M, et al. The effect of an antisense expression plasmid to the IGF-1 receptor on hamster mesothelioma proliferation. *Dev Biol Stand* 1998;94:321–328.
52. Ohta Y, Shridhar V, Bright RK, et al. VEGF and VEGF type C play an important role in angiogenesis and lymphangiogenesis in human malignant mesothelioma tumours. *Br J Cancer* 1999;81:54–61.
56. Carbone M, Pass HI. Evolving aspects of mesothelioma carcinogenesis: SV40 and genetic predisposition. *J Thorac Oncol* 2006;1:169–171.
68. Pacurari M, Castranova V, Vallyathan V. Single- and multi-wall carbon nanotubes versus asbestos: are the carbon nanotubes a new health risk to humans? *J Toxicol Environ Health A* 2010;73:378–395.

71. Carbone M, Emri S, Dogan AU, et al. A mesothelioma epidemic in Cappadocia: scientific developments and unexpected social outcomes. *Nat Rev Cancer* 2007;7:147–154.

75. Carbone M, Yang H, Pass HI, et al. BAP1 and cancer. *Nat Rev Cancer* 2013;13:153–159.

79. Zauderer MG, Bott M, McMillan R, et al. Clinical characteristics of patients with malignant pleural mesothelioma harboring somatic BAP1 mutations. *J Thorac Oncol* 2013;8:1430–1433.

94. Vogelzang NJ, Rusthoven JJ, Symanowski J, et al. Phase III study of pemetrexed in combination with cisplatin versus cisplatin alone in patients with malignant pleural mesothelioma. *J Clin Oncol* 2003;21:2636–2644.

96. Robinson BW, Creaney J, Lake R, et al. Mesothelin-family proteins and diagnosis of mesothelioma. *Lancet* 2003;362:1612–1616.

97. Beyer HL, Geschwindt RD, Glover CL, et al. MESOMARK: a potential test for malignant pleural mesothelioma. *Clin Chem* 2007;53:666–672.

98. Pass HI, Wali A, Tang N, et al. Soluble mesothelin-related peptide level elevation in mesothelioma serum and pleural effusions. *Ann Thorac Surg* 2008;85:265–272.

99. Hollevoet K, Reitsma JB, Creaney J, et al. Serum mesothelin for diagnosing-malignant pleural mesothelioma: an individual patient data meta-analysis. *J Clin Oncol* 2012;30:1541–1549.

100. Creaney J, Robinson BW. Detection of malignant mesothelioma in asbestos-exposed individuals: the potential role of soluble mesothelin-related protein. *Hematol Oncol Clin North Am* 2005;19:1025–1040, v.

104. Pass HI, Lott D, Lonardo F, et al. Asbestos exposure, pleural mesothelioma, and serum osteopontin levels. *N Engl J Med* 2005;353:1564–1573.

119. Boutin C, Rey F, Viallat JR. Prevention of malignant seeding after invasive diagnostic procedures in patients with pleural mesothelioma. A randomized trial of local radiotherapy. *Chest* 1995;108:754–758.

126. Curran D, Sahmoud T, Therasse P, et al. Prognostic factors in patients with pleural mesothelioma: the European Organization for Research and Treatment of Cancer experience. *J Clin Oncol* 1998;16:145–152.

127. Fennell DA, Parmar A, Shamash J, et al. Statistical validation of the EORTC prognostic model for malignant pleural mesothelioma based on three consecutive phase II trials. *J Clin Oncol* 2005;23:184–189.

128. Edwards JG, Abrams KR, Leverment JN, et al. Prognostic factors for malignant mesothelioma in 142 patients: validation of CALGB and EORTC prognostic scoring systems. *Thorax* 2000;55:731–735.

132. Meniawy TM, Creaney J, Lake RA, et al. Existing models, but not neutrophil-to-lymphocyte ratio, are prognostic in malignant mesothelioma. *Br J Cancer* 2013;109:1813–1820.

133. Gordon GJ, Jensen RV, Hsiao LL, et al. Using gene expression ratios to predict outcome among patients with mesothelioma. *J Natl Cancer Inst* 2003;95:598–605.

136. Pass HI, Goparaju C, Ivanov S, et al. hsa-miR-29c* is linked to the prognosis of malignant pleural mesothelioma. *Cancer Res* 2010;70:1916–1924.

138. Hollevoet K, Nackaerts K, Gosselin R, et al. Soluble mesothelin, megakaryocyte potentiating factor, and osteopontin as markers of patient response and outcome in mesothelioma. *J Thorac Oncol* 2011;6:1930–1937.

139. Cappia S, Righi L, Mirabelli D, et al. Prognostic role of osteopontin expression in malignant pleural mesothelioma. *Am J Clin Pathol* 2008;130:58–64.

140. Ivanova AV, Goparaju CM, Ivanov SV, et al. Protumorigenic role of HAPLN1 and its IgV domain in malignant pleural mesothelioma. *Clin Cancer Res* 2009;15:2602–2611.

145. Butchart EG, Ashcroft T, Barnsley WC, et al. Pleuropneumonectomy in the management of diffuse malignant mesothelioma of the pleura. Experience with 29 patients. *Thorax* 1976;31:15–24.

146. Rusch VW. A proposed new international TNM staging system for malignant pleural mesothelioma. From the International Mesothelioma Interest Group. *Chest* 1995;108:1122–1128.

149. Richards WG, Godleski JJ, Yeap BY, et al. Proposed adjustments to pathologic staging of epithelial malignant pleural mesothelioma based on analysis of 354 cases. *Cancer* 2010;116:1510–1517.

150. Pass HI, Temeck BK, Kranda K, et al. Preoperative tumor volume is associated with outcome in malignant pleural mesothelioma. *J Thorac Cardiovasc Surg* 1998;115:310–317.

151. Gill RR, Richards WG, Yeap BY, et al. Epithelial malignant pleural mesothelioma after extrapleural pneumonectomy: stratification of survival with CT-derived tumor volume. *AJR Am J Roentgenol* 2012;198:359–363.

163. Rice D, Rusch V, Pass H, et al. Recommendations for uniform definitions of surgical techniques for malignant pleural mesothelioma: a consensus report of the international association for the study of lung cancer international staging committee and the international mesothelioma interest group. *J Thorac Oncol* 2011;6:1304–1312.

164. Cao CQ, Yan TD, Bannon PG, et al. A systematic review of extrapleural pneumonectomy for malignant pleural mesothelioma. *J Thorac Oncol* 2010;5:1692–1703.

166. Sugarbaker DJ, Jaklitsch MT, Bueno R, et al. Prevention, early detection, and management of complications after 328 consecutive extrapleural pneumonectomies. *J Thorac Cardiovasc Surg* 2004;128:138–146.

169. Vogelzang NJ, Rusthoven JJ, Symanowski J, et al. Phase III study of pemetrexed in combination with cisplatin versus cisplatin alone in patients with malignant pleural mesothelioma. *J Clin Oncol* 2003;21:2636–2644.

173. Weder W, Stahel RA, Baas P, et al. The MARS feasibility trial: conclusions not supported by data. *Lancet Oncol* 2011;12:1093–1094.

179. Krug LM. An overview of chemotherapy for mesothelioma. *Hematol Oncol Clin North Am* 2005;19:1117–1136, vii.

182. Nowak AK, Byrne MJ, Williamson R, et al. A multicentre phase II study of cisplatin and gemcitabine for malignant pleural mesothelioma. *Br J Cancer* 2002;87:491–496.

191. Van Meerbeeck JP, Gaafar R, Manegold C, et al. Randomized phase III study of cisplatin with or without raltitrexed in patients with malignant pleural mesothelioma: an intergroup study of the European Organisation for Research and Treatment of Cancer Lung Cancer Group and the National Cancer Institute of Canada. *J Clin Oncol* 2005;23:6881–6889.

195. Taylor P, Castagneto B, Dark G, et al. Single-agent pemetrexed for chemonaive and pretreated patients with malignant pleural mesothelioma: results of an International Expanded Access Program. *J Thorac Oncol* 2008;3:764–771.

200. Manegold C, Symanowski J, Gatzemeier U, et al. Second-line (post-study) chemotherapy received by patients treated in the phase III trial of pemetrexed plus cisplatin versus cisplatin alone in malignant pleural mesothelioma. *Ann Oncol* 2005;16:923–927.

206. Kindler HL, Karrison TG, Gandara DR, et al. Multicenter, double-blind, placebo-controlled, randomized phase II trial of gemcitabine/cisplatin plus bevacizumab or placebo in patients with malignant mesothelioma. *J Clin Oncol* 2012;30:2509–2515.

216. Paik PK, Krug LM. Histone deacetylase inhibitors in malignant pleural mesothelioma: preclinical rationale and clinical trials. *J Thorac Oncol* 2010;5:275–279.

218. Krug LM, Curley T, Schwartz L, et al. Potential role of histone deacetylase inhibitors in mesothelioma: clinical experience with suberoylanilide hydroxamic acid. *Clin Lung Cancer* 2006;7:257–261.

219. Krug L, Kindler H, Calvert AH. VANTAGE 014: Vorinostat in patients with advanced malignant pleural mesothelioma who have failed prior pemetrexed and etiehr cisplain or carboplatin therapy: a phase III, randomized, double-blind, placebo-controlled trial. *Eur J Cancer* 2011;1:2–3.

224. Hassan R, Ho M. Mesothelin targeted cancer immunotherapy. *Eur J Cancer* 2008;44:46–53.

229. Hassan R, Bullock S, Premkumar A, et al. Phase I study of SS1P, a recombinant anti-mesothelin immunotoxin given as a bolus I.V. infusion to patients with mesothelin-expressing mesothelioma, ovarian, and pancreatic cancers. *Clin Cancer Res* 2007;13:5144–5149.

233. Kreitman RJ, Hassan R, FitzGerald DJ, et al. Phase I trial of continuous infusion anti-mesothelin recombinant immunotoxin SS1P. *Clin Cancer Res* 2009;15:5274–5279.

234. Hassan R, Miller AC, Sharon E, et al. Major cancer regressions in mesothelioma after treatment with an anti-mesothelin immunotoxin and immune suppression. *Sci Transl Med* 2013;5:208ra147.

237. Ball DL, Cruickshank DG. The treatment of malignant mesothelioma of the pleura: review of a 5-year experience, with special reference to radiotherapy. *Am J Clin Oncol* 1990;13:4–9.

243. Rusch VW, Rosenzweig K, Venkatraman E, et al. A phase II trial of surgical resection and adjuvant high-dose hemithoracic radiation for malignant pleural mesothelioma. *J Thorac Cardiovasc Surg* 2001;122:788–795.

244. Krayenbuehl J, Oertel S, Davis JB, et al. Combined photon and electron three-dimensional conformal versus intensity-modulated radiotherapy with integrated boost for adjuvant treatment of malignant pleural mesothelioma after pleuropneumonectomy. *Int J Radiat Oncol Biol Phys* 2007;69:1593–1599.

245. Rice DC, Smythe WR, Liao Z, et al. Dose-dependent pulmonary toxicity after postoperative intensity-modulated radiotherapy for malignant pleural mesothelioma. *Int J Radiat Oncol Biol Phys* 2007;69:350–357.

248. Allen AM, Czerminska M, Janne PA, et al. Fatal pneumonitis associated with intensity-modulated radiation therapy for mesothelioma. *Int J Radiat Oncol Biol Phys* 2006;65:640–645.

252. Gupta V, Krug LM, Laser B, et al. Patterns of local and nodal failure in malignant pleural mesothelioma after extrapleural pneumonectomy and photon-electron radiotherapy. *J Thorac Oncol* 2009;4:746–750.

254. Gupta V, Mychalczak B, Krug L, et al. Hemithoracic radiation therapy after pleurectomy/decortication for malignant pleural mesothelioma. *Int J Radiat Oncol Biol Phys* 2005;63:1045–1052.

256. Rosenzweig KE, Fox JL, Zelefsky MJ, et al. A pilot trial of high-dose-rate intraoperative radiation therapy for malignant pleural mesothelioma. *Brachytherapy* 2005;4:30–33.

257. Rosenzweig KE, Zauderer MG, Laser B, et al. Pleural intensity-modulated radiotherapy for malignant pleural mesothelioma. *Int J Radiat Oncol Biol Phys* 2012;83:1278–1283.

265. Krayenbuehl J, Hartmann M, Lomax AJ, et al. Proton therapy for malignant pleural mesothelioma after extrapleural pleuropneumonectomy. *Int J Radiat Oncol Biol Phys* 2010;78:628–634.

266. Lorentini S, Amichetti M, Spiazzi L, et al. Adjuvant intensity-modulated proton therapy in malignant pleural mesothelioma. A comparison with intensity-modulated radiotherapy and a spot size variation assessment. *Strahlenther Onkol* 2012;188:216–225.

275. Pass HI. Biomarkers and prognostic factors for mesothelioma. *Ann Cardiothorac Surg* 2012;1:449–456.

277. Weder W, Kestenholz P, Taverna C, et al. Neoadjuvant chemotherapy followed by extrapleural pneumonectomy in malignant pleural mesothelioma. *J Clin Oncol* 2004;22:3451–3457.

278. Weder W, Stahel RA, Bernhard J, et al. Multicenter trial of neo-adjuvant chemotherapy followed by extrapleural pneumonectomy in malignant pleural mesothelioma. *Ann Oncol* 2007;18:1196–1202.

284. Krug LM, Pass HI, Rusch VW, et al. Multicenter phase II trial of neoadjuvant pemetrexed plus cisplatin followed by extrapleural pneumonectomy and radiation for malignant pleural mesothelioma. *J Clin Oncol* 2009;27:3007–3013.

285. Van Schil PE, Baas P, Gaafar R, et al. Trimodality therapy for malignant pleural mesothelioma: results from an EORTC phase II multicentre trial. *Eur Respir J* 2010;36:1362–1369.

291. Bolukbas S. Long-term outcome after radical pleurectomy followed by chemoradiation for malignant pleural mesothelioma: a 10-year single center experience. 11th International Conference of the International Mesothelioma Interest Group. 2012. Abstract.

295. Lang-Lazdunski L, Bille A, Lal R, et al. Pleurectomy/decortication is superior to extrapleural pneumonectomy in the multimodality management of patients with malignant pleural mesothelioma. *J Thorac Oncol* 2012;7:737–743.

296. Rena O, Casadio C. Extrapleural pneumonectomy for early stage malignant pleural mesothelioma: a harmful procedure. *Lung Cancer* 2012;77:151–155.

297. Sorensen JB, Ravn J, Krisetensen C. Two simultaneous consecutive nonrandomized cohorts of operable patients with MPM receiving induction therapy followed either by EPP and postoperative radiotherapy or pleurectomy decortication alone. 2012. Presented at International Mesothelioma Interest Group Meeting, October 2012, Boston, MA.

298. Pass H. Mesothelioma revisited: a multidisciplinary approach. Presented at International Mesothelioma Interest Group Meeting, October 2012, Boston, MA.

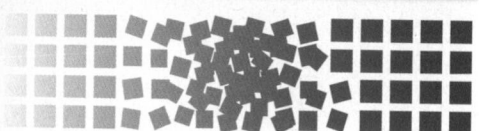

115 Peritoneal Metastases and Peritoneal Mesothelioma

Marcello Deraco, Dominique M. Elias, Olivier Glehen, C. Wiliam Helm, Paul H. Sugarbaker, and Vic J. Verwaal

INTRODUCTION

Peritoneal carcinomatosis, mesothelioma, and sarcomatosis are included in the group of diseases collectively referred to, in this chapter, as peritoneal metastases. Over the past three decades, there has emerged an increasing optimism concerning an individualized management plan for cancer dissemination within the abdomen and pelvis. The clinical problem was originally defined by several important clinical studies that established the natural history of peritoneal surface malignancy.[1–3]

Concomitant with these manuscripts that identified the dismal prognosis of patients with peritoneal metastases, isolated reports appeared concerning an emerging technology that described a new approach to management. This alternative treatment plan had two essential components. First, cytoreductive surgery (CRS) was used in an attempt to resect all visible implants within the abdomen and pelvis. Peritonectomy along with visceral resections was developed to surgically eradicate cancer on peritoneal surfaces.[4] The second component was local-regional chemotherapy (intraperitoneal chemotherapy) used in the operating room or within the early postoperative period before adhesions develop. Chemotherapy used in the operating room with moderate heat has been referred to as hyperthermic intraperitoneal chemotherapy (HIPEC)[5]; chemotherapy used within the early postoperative period has been referred to as early postoperative intraperitoneal chemotherapy (EPIC).[6] The chemotherapy is used in an attempt to eradicate free cancer cells and minute attached nodules that remain following surgery.[7]

The unique aspect of this new combination of treatments was the perioperative timing of the chemotherapy. Currently, the perioperative chemotherapy may be both intravenous and intraperitoneal, and may be administered in the operating room or in the early postoperative period. HIPEC now abbreviates the term hyperthermic perioperative chemotherapy and includes all perioperative chemotherapy regimens. It is not adjuvant chemotherapy and it is not neoadjuvant chemotherapy; it is chemotherapy used simultaneously with a major cytoreductive surgical procedure. Of course, all efforts to maintain benefits from systemic chemotherapy in patients with peritoneal metastases or mesothelioma must continue. Patients with peritoneal surface malignancy are required to be a focus of the multidisciplinary team (MDT).

NATURAL HISTORY STUDIES DOCUMENT THE IMPORTANCE OF LOCAL-REGIONAL PROGRESSION

A strong rationale for the emergence of CRS and HIPEC as a valid treatment option comes from natural history studies. In a proportion of patients, recurrence of the primary cancer isolated to the surfaces of the abdomen and pelvis is a reality. Primary or recurrent disease at the resection site and on peritoneal surfaces in the absence of hepatic metastases or systemic metastases does occur; these patients are appropriate for treatment by CRS and HIPEC. Isolated peritoneal surface progression of abdominal or pelvic malignancy is not unusual.[8–12]

To fully understand the importance of cancer cells that gain access to the peritoneal space prior to or at the time of a cancer resection, one must appreciate the pathophysiology of disease. Figure 115.1 illustrates the mechanism of local-regional progression. Cancer cells at low density result in peritoneal metastases at a distance from the primary cancer resection. Cancer cells at higher density become trapped within raw tissue surfaces at the resection site. A fusiform layer of cancer that conforms to the anatomic structures within the bed of the primary resection site results from high-density seeding.[13] The progression of cancer implants within the resection site and on peritoneal surfaces in the absence of liver metastases or systemic disease presents a major rationale for comprehensive local-regional treatments.[14]

PATIENT SELECTION USING QUANTITATIVE PROGNOSTIC INDICATORS

A second factor strongly recommending CRS and HIPEC as a valid treatment option comes from well-established selection factors applied to this patient population. With some variations between diseases, the same group of quantitative prognostic indicators operates for all patients with peritoneal surface malignancy. Now, prognostic indicators are used to refine the selection of patients to those most likely to benefit and to exclude those who are unlikely to benefit.[15,16] Histopathology, the peritoneal cancer index (PCI), the completeness of cytoreduction score (CC), radiologic imaging by computed tomography (CT), and TNM (tumor, node, metastasis) stage with peritoneal cytology play a central role in patient selection.

Biologic Aggressiveness as Measured by Histopathology for Epithelial Appendiceal Neoplasms and Peritoneal Mesothelioma

Mucinous appendiceal neoplasms have a broad spectrum of aggressiveness, and the histologic type of the appendiceal neoplasm has a profound effect on survival following treatment by CRS and HIPEC.[17] Patients with adenomucinosis obtain maximal survival benefit, while those with mucinous carcinoma show survivals similar to that for peritoneal metastases of colorectal origin.[18]

Seven different histologic patterns of peritoneal mesothelioma contribute to three distinct histologic groups that have a very different prognosis following treatment with CRS and HIPEC: poor prognosis for sarcomatoid, deciduoid, or biphasic types; intermediate prognosis for papillary and epithelial types; and excellent prognosis for low-grade or multicystic types.[19,20]

Intraoperative dissemination of gastric cancer

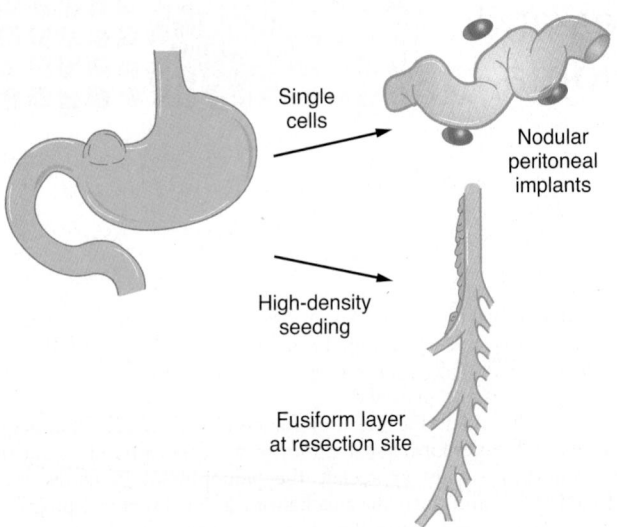

Single cells

Nodular peritoneal implants

High-density seeding

Fusiform layer at resection site

Figure 115.1 Intraoperative dissemination of gastric cancer cells. If cancer cells gain access to the peritoneal space either prior to or at the time of gastrectomy, two patterns of dissemination are observed. Low density of cancer cells into the free peritoneal space results in nodules as peritoneal implants. A high density of cancer cells dropped into the cancer resection site results in a layering of cancer.

Extent of Disease as Measured by the Peritoneal Cancer Index

The PCI is an assessment combining lesion size (0 to 3) with tumor distribution (abdominopelvic regions 0 to 12) to estimate the ex-tent of disease within the abdomen and pelvis as a numerical score (Fig. 115.2).[21] It is calculated from observations obtained at the time of surgical exploration of the abdomen and pelvis, and should be recorded by the surgeon before leaving the operating room. The higher the PCI, the less likely CRS and HIPEC will result in long-term survival for all the peritoneal surface malignancies discussed in this chapter.

The Completeness of Cytoreduction Score Performed after the Resection

The size of residual tumor nodules visually determined after CRS has been completed has a profound effect on outcome. The new definition of complete cytoreduction is no visible evidence of cancer or only minute nodules reliably penetrated by HIPEC, a completeness of cytoreduction score of 0 (CC-0) or CC-1, respec-tively. With few exceptions, a CC-0 or CC-1 score is necessary for long-term benefit with CRS and HIPEC.[21]

Preoperative Radiologic Imaging by Computed Tomography

CT of the chest, abdomen, and pelvis is an essential tool in the selection of patients for CRS with HIPEC. Systemic metastases and spread to pleural surfaces can be identified. The location and quantity of mucinous carcinoma within the peritoneal cavity can be accurately determined.[22,23] Unfortunately, nonmucinous peri-toneal metastases may be greatly underestimated by CT.[24] If the small bowel and its mesentery are layered by tumor or a large mass of cancer occupies the epigastric region, the likelihood of achiev-ing complete cytoreduction is small. The CT should be performed with maximal intravenous and oral contrast in order to identify pa-tients who have small bowel compartmentalization versus diffuse involvement of the small bowel and its mesentery.

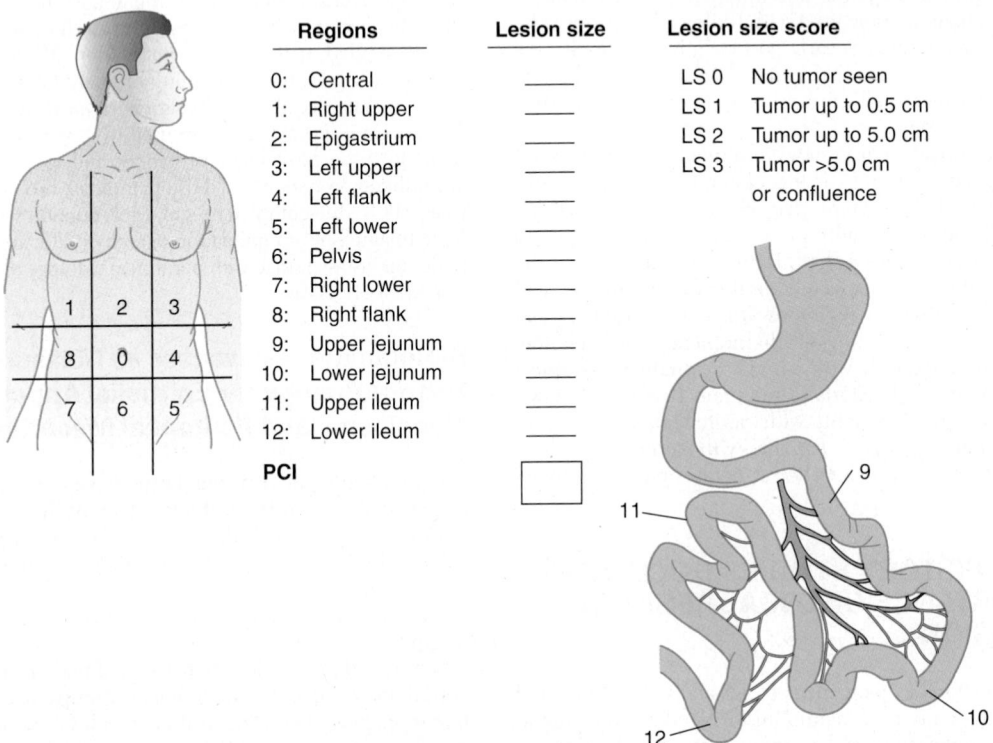

Regions		Lesion size	Lesion size score	
0:	Central	_____	LS 0	No tumor seen
1:	Right upper	_____	LS 1	Tumor up to 0.5 cm
2:	Epigastrium	_____	LS 2	Tumor up to 5.0 cm
3:	Left upper	_____	LS 3	Tumor >5.0 cm
4:	Left flank	_____		or confluence
5:	Left lower	_____		
6:	Pelvis	_____		
7:	Right lower	_____		
8:	Right flank	_____		
9:	Upper jejunum	_____		
10:	Lower jejunum	_____		
11:	Upper ileum	_____		
12:	Lower ileum	_____		
PCI		☐		

Figure 115.2 The peritoneal cancer index (*PCI*). This index combines a size and a distribution parameter to achieve a numerical score. The lesion size (*LS*) is used to quantitate the size of peritoneal nodules. The distribution of tumor is determined within the 13 abdominopelvic regions.

Tumor, Node, Metastasis Stage, Peritoneal Cytology, and Clinical Features of the Primary Cancer

A careful survey of the peritoneal surfaces at the time of primary gastrointestinal cancer resection combined with a knowledgeable and timely gross and histopathologic assessment of the resected specimen can accurately predict the incidence of peritoneal metastases that will occur in follow-up. Also, in advanced gastrointestinal cancers, peritoneal cytology provides important prognostic information. This information should be used by the MDT to consider proactive treatment with CRS and HIPEC. It is possible to prevent peritoneal metastases in high-risk groups or treat peritoneal metastases by second-look surgery in patients with documented disease.[25–30] The fast pace at which peritoneal metastases progress and the profound effect of extent of disease (PCI) on outcome indicate this approach. Table 115.1 presents the clinical features that should alert the MDT to a high risk for peritoneal metastases.[31,32]

Pharmacokinetic Advantage of Perioperative Chemotherapy

Another argument in favor of CRS and HIPEC as a treatment option for peritoneal surface malignancy is a well-studied pharmacologic rationale. As determined by physical properties, some chemotherapy agents are especially appropriate for hyperthermic use in the peritoneal cavity after CRS has been completed. Other cell cycle–specific chemotherapy agents are more appropriate for EPIC. As experience with different perioperative chemotherapy regimens has accumulated, the use of multiple-agent chemotherapy given both intravenously and intraperitoneally has evolved and promises to be increasingly effective. Heat targeting of both intravenous and intraperitoneal chemotherapy to the peritoneal surface cancer nodule is a goal of treatment.

Combined Use of Cytoreductive Surgery and Perioperative Chemotherapy as a Standard of Care in Selected Patients

A final argument for use of CRS and HIPEC as a treatment option for peritoneal surface malignancy concerns the well-defined management parameters that are currently in practice at experienced treatment centers. A standardized cytoreductive surgical procedure involves visceral resections and peritonectomy procedures in an attempt to leave the abdomen visibly free of cancer. After the CRS is complete, tubes and drains are positioned to facilitate inflow and outflow of the chemotherapy solution. The chemotherapy solution circulates through roller pumps and a heat exchanger to maintain moderate hyperthermia (42°C/109°F) within the abdomen and pelvis. The skin edges are elevated on a self-retaining retractor (open method) or the skin closed (closed method) in order to create a reservoir for the hyperthermic chemotherapy solution.

The sequence of cancer resection, intraoperative chemotherapy washing, and then intestinal reconstruction may be important to optimize the destruction of small volumes of cancer cells and prevent tumor cell entrapment in adhesions, suture lines, and the abdominal incision. During the peritonectomy and visceral resections, large volumes of cancer are removed; however, residual cancer cells remain and must be eradicated.

A review of the important recent contributions to the literature that critically assesses the benefits of CRS and HIPEC in different disease states constitutes the remainder of this chapter.

APPENDICEAL MALIGNANCY

Natural History

Although similarities exist, there are unique features of appendiceal malignancies as compared to colorectal adenocarcinoma. The first and probably the most obvious difference between the colon and the appendix malignancies is the diameter of the bowel lumen involved. A colon tumor grows as an intraluminal mass in the bowel and will invade through the wall. The intraluminal growth pattern causes the primary cancer to reach the serosa in a late stage. In contrast, the appendix is a small organ, up to 1 cm in diameter, with a thin wall. A tumor may obliterate the appendix lumen in an early stage. This may cause a rupture of the wall of the appendix, allowing a spreading of tumor cells into the abdominal and pelvic cavity. Early in the natural history of the disease, these neoplastic cells implant with a high efficiency throughout the peritoneal cavity and progress as peritoneal metastases.[33,34]

Histologic Classification

The biology of appendiceal malignancies varies from simple mucinous adenoma to solid intestinal type adenocarcinoma. The histology of the peritoneal metastases from the primary tumor itself has a major influence on the outcome of the treatment by CRS and HIPEC. Ronnett et al.[35] and Bruin et al.[36] described three different types in their analyses of appendiceal malignancies. Metastases

TABLE 115.1

Tumor, Node, Metastasis Stage, Peritoneal Cytology, and Clinical Features of the Primary Cancer as an Estimate of the Incidence of Subsequent Peritoneal Metastases to Guide Proactive Treatment Strategies

Clinical Feature	Incidence of Peritoneal Metastases Observed in Follow-up (%)	
	Colorectal Cancer	Gastric Cancer
Peritoneal nodules detected with primary cancer resection	70[a]	100
Ovarian metastases	60[a]	100
Perforation through the primary cancer	50[a]	75[b]
Positive margin of resection (R-1 resection)	70	70
Positive peritoneal cytology before or after resection	40[a]	80
Adjacent organ or structure invasion	20[a]	40
T3	20	60
T4	20	75
T3/T4 mucinous cancer	40[a]	NA
Signet ring histomorphology	20	70
Fistula formation	20	NA
Obstruction of primary cancer	20	60

NA, not applicable.
[a] Data from Honore C, Goere D, Souadka A, et al. Definition of patients presenting a high risk of developing peritoneal carcinomatosis after curative surgery for colorectal cancer: a systematic review. *Ann Surg Oncol* 2013;20:183–192.
[b] Data from Tsujimoto H, Hiraki S, Sakamoto N, et al. Outcome after emergency surgery in patients with a free perforation caused by gastric cancer. *Exp Ther Med* 2010;1:199–203.

PRACTICE OF ONCOLOGY

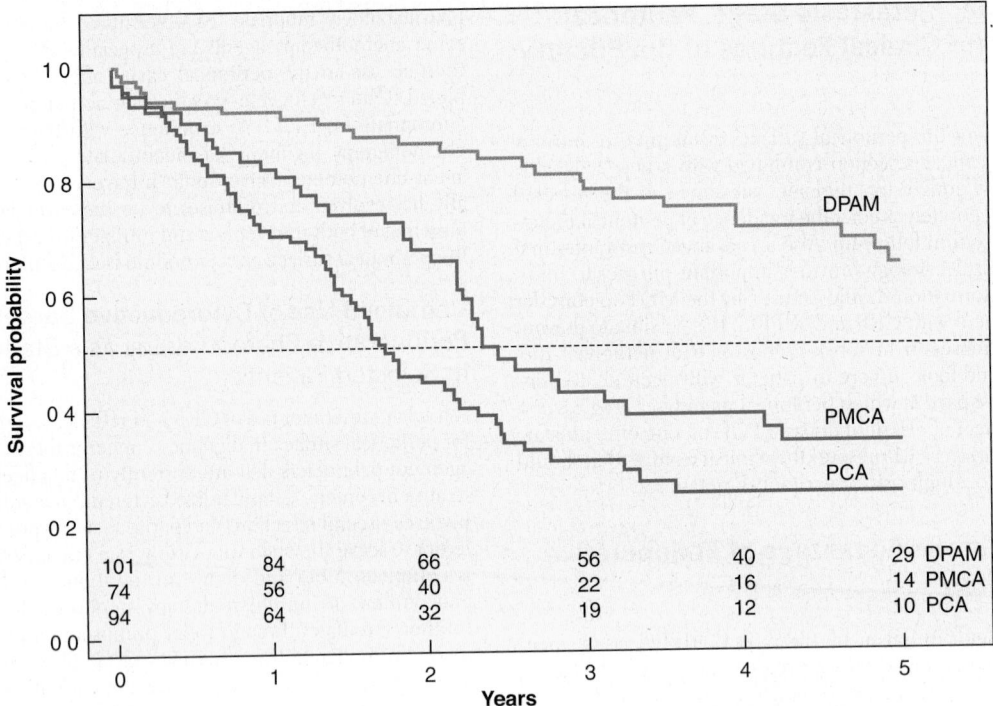

Figure 115.3 Survival of 269 patients with peritoneal metastases of an appendiceal neoplasm by histologic classification. DPAM, disseminated peritoneal adenomucinosis; PMCA, peritoneal mucinous carcinoma; PCA, peritoneal carcinoma. (From Bruin S, Verwaal VJ, Vincent A, et al. A clinicopathologic analysis of peritoneal metastases from colorectal and appendiceal origin. *Ann Surg Oncol* 2010;17:2330–2340.)

with >90% mucus, flat epithelial cells, no atypia, and no mitoses had a good prognosis despite a high PCI. At the other end of the spectrum, peritoneal metastases with much atypia, abundant mitoses, and <50% mucus has a prognosis similar to colorectal carcinomatosis and is referred to as peritoneal carcinoma.

Outcome of Treatment of Peritoneal Dissemination by Cytoreductive Surgery Followed by Hyperthermic Perioperative Chemotherapy

The survival outcome with peritoneal dissemination of appendiceal origin neoplasms is shown in Figure 115.3. The overall survival is shown according to the histologic classification. For the least aggressive form (disseminated peritoneal adenomucinosis), the median survival is not reached within 5 years.[36] Those patients who were affected by peritoneal carcinoma had a much poorer prognosis. The median survival was only 14 months in these patients. These survival data compare with the median survival of peritoneal metastases of colorectal origin treated with cytoreduction followed by HIPEC. Accepting the fact that complete resection is always the goal of CRS, these data document that survival with peritoneal metastases from appendiceal malignancies is highly dependent upon the histopathologic characteristics of the tumor.

Success in the treatment of recurrence after primary treatment with CRS followed by HIPEC is a unique feature of appendiceal peritoneal metastases. Benefit depends largely on the number and location of tumor masses. With a limited number of locations, the first choice is resection; if more diffuse disease is present and CRS is complete, a second HIPEC can be performed.[37,38] In patients in whom the pathology is more aggressive, definitive treatment with systemic chemotherapy, with all it limitations, should be considered by the MDT.

Surgical Learning Curve

Cytoreduction followed by HIPEC is a complex treatment that demonstrates a surgical learning curve.[39,40] The peak of the learning curve in the study of Smeenk et al.[31] was reached after approximately 130 procedures. Surgical skill is undoubtedly the main component of this learning process, but modified treatment strategies for an individual patient and experience in handling complications by the entire medical team has contributed to a decreased morbidity and mortality.[41,42]

COLORECTAL PERITONEAL METASTASES: CURATIVE TREATMENT AND PREVENTION

Stage IV colorectal cancer is a very morbid disease, with a 5-year survival rate of 10% and a median survival of 14.4 months. The prognosis is significantly worse when peritoneal metastases are present, with a median survival of 6.7 months versus 18.1 months without peritoneal metastases ($p < 0.01$).[43] When colorectal peritoneal metastases are diagnosed, the crucial question for the MDT is whether curative (complete CRS with HIPEC) or palliative therapy (systemic chemotherapy) should be the goal of treatment.

Incidence of the Disease and Incidence of Peritoneal Metastases

At the initial diagnosis of colon cancer, the peritoneal surface is involved with tumor in 10% to 15% of patients.[11,44] Besides the liver, the peritoneal surfaces are the most common sites of cancer recurrence after "curative" colorectal cancer resections. Unfortunately, cancer progression occurs in as many as 50% of patients who have an R0 resection. In 10% to 35% of patients with recurrent disease, the anatomic site of treatment failure is confined to the peritoneal surface.[11,44] With recurrent disease, when peritoneal metastases are of limited extent (low PCI), potentially curative treatment options should be considered.

Useful Prognostic Indicators for the Disease

Contraindications for this combined treatment are the presence of metastases at another site (although, up to three easily resectable liver metastases is not an absolute contraindication),[45] a poor general status (the combined treatment is rather aggressive), and extensive peritoneal metastases (PCI >20). Extensive disease is likely to be unresectable in its entirety. Also, even when a complete cytoreduction is possible, the prognosis is poor. Most of the series using complete CRS with HIPEC report a poor survival rate when the PCI is higher than 20.[46,47]

Results of Treatment

Figure 115.4 reports the survival rates according to the completeness of surgery in the 523 patients collected by the Association Française de Chirurgie.[47] Five years after surgery, no patient was alive if the size of the residual tumor nodules exceeded 2.5 mm after surgery, whereas 30% of the patients were alive if complete CRS was possible (p <0.0001). These data are confirmed in the Dutch HIPEC study, which included 960 patients.[48]

A crucial role for hyperthermia for HIPEC is currently unknown for humans. In a randomized trial in rats, those treated with HIPEC survived longer than those treated with intraperitoneal chemotherapy alone or with intraperitoneal hyperthermia alone.[49] A recent retrospective study compared similar patients (all of whom underwent a laparotomy) with resectable peritoneal metastases treated with complete CRS and HIPEC to patients who received standard systemic chemotherapy. Median survival was 63 months in the complete CRS with HIPEC group versus 24 months in the systemic chemotherapy group.[50]

Summary of Important Results from Other Institutions

This combined treatment (complete CRS and HIPEC) is effective. Benefits were definitively demonstrated by the randomized study of the Amsterdam group: 105 patients who presented with colorectal peritoneal metastases were randomized between surgery with HIPEC and systemic chemotherapy versus systemic chemotherapy alone.[51] In this study, close to 50% of the patients in

the experimental arm were at presentation not good candidates for HIPEC because their peritoneal metastases could not be completely resected. Despite this bias, the reported median survival was 22 months in the experimental arm versus 13 months in the control group (p = 0.032). At eight years the benefit persisted.[52]

The results obtained with complete CRS with HIPEC in the Association Française de Chirurgie study showed a 5-year overall survival of 30%.[47] This result accepts clinical data over an 18-year interval and includes the learning curves of 28 different centers. It is the least favorable data ever to be reported by the authors' group. The results of experienced centers concerning patients who underwent complete CRS and HIPEC show 5-year overall survival rates close to 40%. It was 32% for the 70 patients in the study by da Silva et al.,[46] 43% for the 59 patients in the Verwaal et al.[51] study, and 48% for the 30 patients treated by Elias et al.[53] Such a survival rate has never been published before for colorectal peritoneal metastases, even if the report includes only selected patients.

Furthermore, these results in the treatment of peritoneal metastases are similar to those obtained with hepatectomy for liver metastases. Selected patients with peritoneal metastases should be treated with this combined therapy just as selected patients with liver metastases should be treated with hepatectomy given that similar results are achieved in terms of survival.[54]

Prevention of Peritoneal Metastases in Patients at High Risk for Progression

Unfortunately, early diagnosis of peritoneal metastases is not possible with radiologic imaging, but only with a laparotomy. This is why the authors proposed second-look surgery plus HIPEC in asymptomatic patients who presented with a primary exhibiting a high risk of developing peritoneal metastases.[28,55] High-risk patients were those who presented with a few (resected) peritoneal implants, ovarian metastases, or perforated tumors. Second-look surgery was performed 6 months after the end of the classic 6 months of systemic adjuvant chemotherapy. Among 47 patients, macroscopic peritoneal metastases was found and treated in 50% of them. In the remaining patients with no macroscopic peritoneal metastases, peritoneal recurrence occurred frequently in those who did not receive HIPEC, but rarely in those who did receive HIPEC (p = 0.02). Finally, only 17% of the patients treated at the time of second-look surgery with HIPEC developed a peritoneal recurrence.[28]

Reports of complete CRS and HIPEC being used to simultaneously treat the primary colorectal cancer and the peritoneal metastases have appeared.[25-27] Also, patients without established peritoneal disease but at high risk for subsequent peritoneal progression are being treated with HIPEC during the same procedure used to resect the primary tumor.[26] The rationale for this proactive approach is three-fold: First, after the primary cancer resection and complete CRS, the PCI was maximally low. Second, reliable radiologic tests to detect the progression of a low volume of peritoneal metastases do not exist. And third, this proactive approach does not require a second-look surgery. With rectal cancer, a second-look approach with CRS and HIPEC may rarely, if ever, be curative.[46,56]

DIFFUSE MALIGNANT PERITONEAL MESOTHELIOMA

Clinical Presentation and Diagnosis

Diffuse malignant peritoneal mesothelioma (DMPM) is characterized by progressive peritoneal seeding, eventually leading to the patient's death due to tumor layering on peritoneal surfaces, bowel obstruction, and intractable malignant ascites. Patients are usually diagnosed with presenting signs and symptoms of advanced disease. In a recently published series of 81 patients with DMPM reported

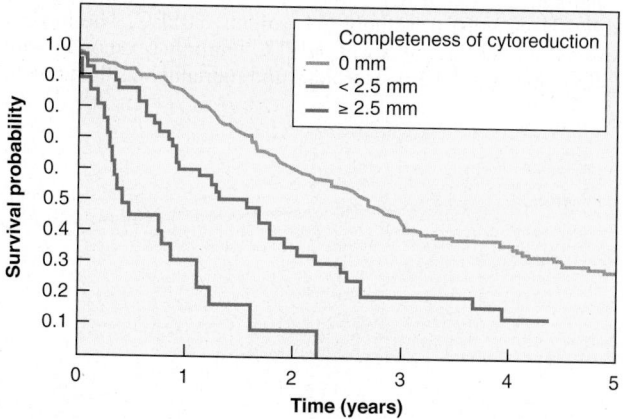

Figure 115.4 Overall survival according to the completeness of cytoreduction after cytoreductive surgery and hyperthermic perioperative chemotherapy for peritoneal metastases. (Elias D, Gilly F, Boutitie F, et al. Peritoneal colorectal carcinomatosis treated with surgery and perioperative intraperitoneal chemotherapy: retrospective analysis of 523 patients from a multicentric French study. *J Clin Oncol* 2010:28:63–68.)

by an Italian group, ascites, abdominal pain, and asthenia were the most frequent symptoms present on 77%, 69%, and 43% of patients, respectively. CT scan shows ascites, peritoneal thickening, abdominal mass, and mesenteric thickening, respectively, on 80%, 63%, 32%, and 29% of cases.[57] CT scan is used as an accurate prognostic radiologic test for patient selection for comprehensive treatment.[23]

Cytologic diagnosis of ascitic fluid is often inconclusive, as cells frequently resemble elements with mesothelial hyperplasia. In the series of the Washington Cancer Institute, diagnosis was made by fluid sampling in 0 of 68 patients. Laparotomy was required in 44% of patients, laparoscopy in 52%, and ultrasound/CT-guided biopsy in 4%.[58] Recently, refined cytological and ultrastructural methods have enhanced the diagnostic accuracy of cytologic assessment.[56]

Treatment and Results with Systemic Chemotherapy

Numerous single-drug and combination regimens have been tested over the past decades with modest results. Preliminary data also suggest a possible survival advantage for a combination of cisplatin and pemetrexed as compared to cisplatin alone. Other cytotoxic agents that have shown to be active in this setting include vinorelbine and gemcitabine, either alone or combined with platinum compounds. In historical case series, standard therapy with palliative surgery and systemic or intraperitoneal chemotherapy is associated with a median survival of about 1 year, ranging from 9 to 15 months.[59,60]

The combined approach consisting of CRS and HIPEC modified the natural history of DMPM with a dramatic improvement in outcomes in multiple single institution studies and in a multi-institutional registry series.[9,19,61–64] Median survival grew from 12 months with a systemic chemotherapy treatment to 53 months with CRS with HIPEC, with 50% 5-year overall survival.[65]

GASTRIC CANCER

Treatment and Prevention of Peritoneal Metastases

Peritoneal dissemination is the most frequent pattern of metastasis and recurrence with gastric cancer. Also, it occurs in 5% to 20% of patients being explored for potentially curative resection.[66] In the past, gastric cancer peritoneal metastases was regarded as a terminal disease, only to be palliated. Over the past two decades, novel therapeutic approaches have emerged, combining gastrectomy and peritonectomy procedures with perioperative chemotherapy.[67] Because of the aggressive nature of gastric cancer, the question regarding the efficiency of this combined procedure remains controversial.

Natural History and Palliative Treatment

The studies that prospectively evaluated patients with peritoneal dissemination of gastric cancer indicated median survival of not more than 6 months.[2] Despite improvements in systemic chemotherapy with encouraging tumor response rates, there has been no improvement in survival.[68] Positive effects of palliative gastric cancer resection have been recently reported in patients with peritoneal metastases but without any long-term survivors.[66]

Curative Treatment: Cytoreductive Surgery and Hyperthermic Perioperative Chemotherapy

The experience of a few single institution phase 2 studies showed encouraging survival results following treatment of peritoneal metastases along with primary gastric cancer.[69–74] Recently, a collaborative effort of French institutions collected data from 159 patients and represents the largest experience with treatment of peritoneal metastases of gastric origin.[72] With a median follow-up of 20.4 months, the overall median survival was only 9.2 months but the 5-year survival rate was 13%, with some long-term survivors. These survival results are less encouraging than those obtained for other peritoneal surface malignancies, reflecting a more aggressive disease process, less response to this combined treatment modality, and the need for more strict patient selection. But the combination of CRS with HIPEC was the only therapeutic strategy that reported survivors at 5 years. In the recent French study, a 5-year survival of 23% and a median survival of 15 months were obtained in patients treated with complete macroscopic resection (Fig. 115.5).[72]

Primary gastric cancer with localized and small peritoneal nodules seems to be the best indication for this combined procedure. In the French study, in patients who had undergone complete CRS, the extent of peritoneal metastases measured by PCI represented the only strong prognostic factor.[72] When the PCI was >12, despite a complete CRS, no patient was alive at 3 years. The institution in which the procedure was performed played an important role in the postoperative course and in survival, suggesting the importance of a learning curve.[41,42,75,76] The high rates of morbidity and mortality reported may reach 60% and 6.5%, respectively.[72] These high rates of morbidity and mortality emphasize the necessity for patient selection using strict criteria regarding physiologic age and general status.

Important data regarding the treatment of peritoneal metastases from gastric cancer was provided by Yang and colleagues.[77] In a randomized trial, patients were treated by cytoreductive surgery with (34 patients) or without (34 patients) HIPEC. The median survival was 11.9 months with HIPEC but only 6.5 months with CRS alone ($p = 0.046$). Morbidity and mortality was the same in

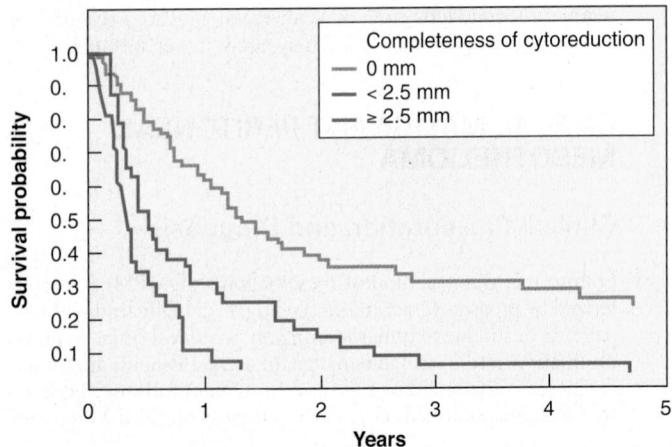

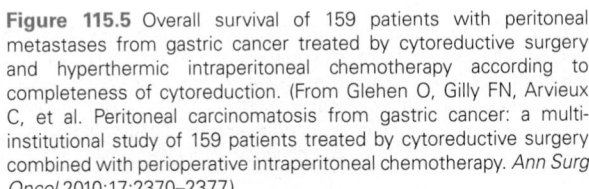

Figure 115.5 Overall survival of 159 patients with peritoneal metastases from gastric cancer treated by cytoreductive surgery and hyperthermic intraperitoneal chemotherapy according to completeness of cytoreduction. (From Glehen O, Gilly FN, Arvieux C, et al. Peritoneal carcinomatosis from gastric cancer: a multi-institutional study of 159 patients treated by cytoreductive surgery combined with perioperative intraperitoneal chemotherapy. *Ann Surg Oncol* 2010;17:2370–2377.)

both groups. Limited but real benefits for HIPEC were demonstrated. Currently, Rau and colleagues in Germany are conducting a similar phase 3 trial, the GASTRIPEC study.[78]

Prevention of Gastric Cancer Peritoneal Metastases

For many Korean and Japanese researchers, HIPEC has been performed in an adjuvant setting in phase 3 trials. Most of them demonstrated the benefit of HIPEC, especially for T3, T4, and lymph node–positive gastric tumors.[79–82] In Western countries, some small experiences also suggested the benefit of using HIPEC as adjuvant treatment for primary gastric cancer presenting with peritoneal metastases.[83,84] Yan and coworkers in a meta-analysis showed that HIPEC with or without EPIC after resection of advanced gastric primary cancer is associated with improved overall survival. However, increased risk of intra-abdominal abscess and neutropenia were also demonstrated.[85] Xu et al., in their meta-analysis, reported similar results.[86] Currently, a prospective randomized trial is being performed in France to test adjuvant HIPEC in gastric cancer.[87]

PERITONEAL METASTASES IN OVARIAN CANCER

Cytoreductive Surgery and Hyperthermic Perioperative Chemotherapy in Epithelial Ovarian Cancer

There is emerging data helping to define the potential role of HIPEC for epithelial ovarian cancer. A registry for patients with ovarian cancer was initiated to collect data from many centers in a format that allowed analysis for factors such as prognostic indicators, variations in technique, and outcomes.[88] Patient eligibility included epithelial ovarian, fallopian tube, or primary peritoneal carcinoma treated with HIPEC at some point in the natural history of the disease. Each participating institution used its own HIPEC technology regarding chemotherapy solutions, duration of perfusion, temperature, and technique of open or closed peritoneal lavage. In the initial report, 141 women were analyzed who had been treated with either frontline ($n = 26$), at interval debulking ($n = 19$), for consolidation ($n = 12$), or for recurrence ($n = 83$). The median overall survival was 30.3 months. In multivariable analysis, the factors significant for increased survival were sensitivity to platinum response ($p = 0.048$), completeness of cytoreduction score of 1 or 0 ($p = 0.025$), carboplatin alone or combination ($p = 0.011$), and duration of hospital stays of ≤ 10 days ($p = 0.021$).

Ceelen and coworkers reported on 42 women treated for recurrent heavily pretreated ovarian cancer with extensive CRS and HIPEC.[89] In multivariate analysis, overall survival was influenced by completeness of cytoreduction, type of chemoperfusion drug, nodal status, and tumor grade. In a Cox regression model, only completeness of cytoreduction (hazard ratio = 0.06 to 0.8; $p = 0.022$) and tumor grade (hazard ratio = 1.23 to 12.6; $p = 0.021$) were independent predictors of overall survival.

Bakrin et al.[90] reported a French multicenter prospective study of 246 women with recurrent or persistent ovarian cancer treated by CRS and HIPEC. The effects of PCI, CC score, and platinum sensitivity versus resistance are shown in Figure 115.6. They conclude that salvage therapy combining optimal CRS and HIPEC is feasible and may achieve long-term survival in highly selected patients with recurrent ovarian carcinoma, including those with platinum-resistant disease, with acceptable morbidity. Into their updated experience on 566 patients, they underlined the role of PCI in patient selection because of its major and independent prognostic impact for advanced and recurrent ovarian cancer.[91]

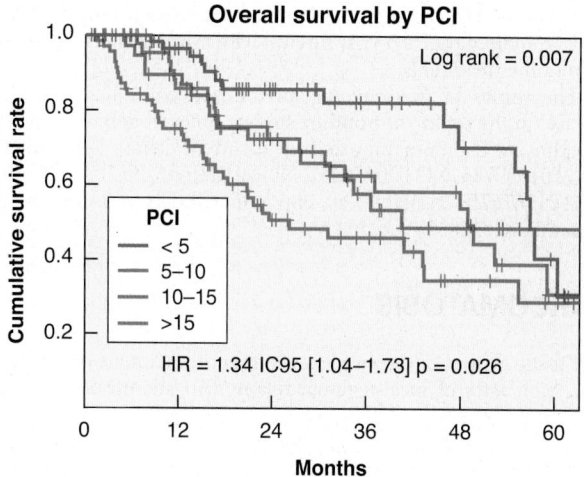

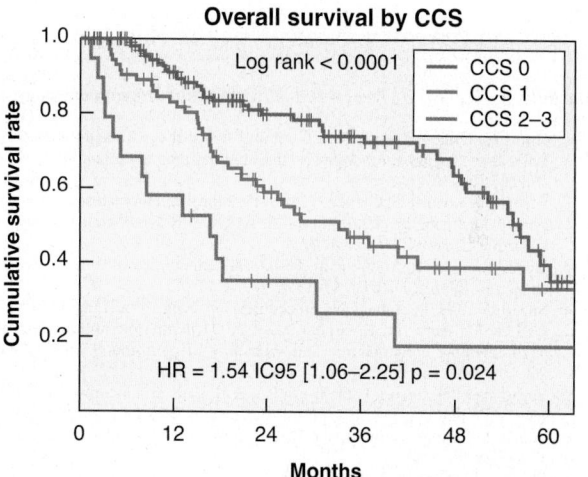

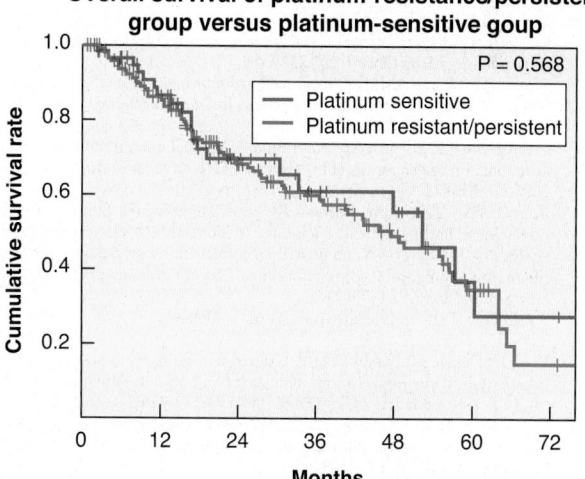

Figure 115.6 Overall survival of 246 patients with recurrent or persistent ovarian cancer by (*top*) peritoneal cancer index (*PCI*), (*middle*) completeness of cytoreduction (*CCS*), (*bottom*) platinum-resistant/persistent group versus platinum-sensitive group. HR, hazard ratio. (From Bakrin N, Cotte E, Golfier F, et al. Cytoreductive surgery and hyperthermic intraperitoneal chemotherapy (HIPEC) for persistent and recurrent advanced ovarian carcinoma: A multicenter, prospective study of 246 patients. *Ann Surg Oncol* 2012;19:4052–4058.)

In a case-control study, Fagotti et al.[92] reported significantly better 5-year survival of 68.4% versus 42.7% ($p = 0.017$) for 30 cases of platinum-sensitive recurrent ovarian cancer undergoing CRS and HIPEC versus 37 control patients who underwent either

CRS without HIPEC and/or systemic chemotherapy only. Deraco et al.[93] reported 60.7% 5-year survival with CRS and HIPEC used as frontline treatments.

The results of five ongoing randomized controlled trials of HIPEC in the setting of frontline surgery, interval debulking after neoadjuvant chemotherapy and for recurrent disease are awaited (NCT01539785, NCT00426257, NCT01091636, NCT01628380, NCT01767675: available at http://clinicaltrials.gov/. Accessed November 27, 2013).

SARCOMATOSIS

Soft tissue tumors of the viscera or retroperitoneum are associated with high rates of local-regional relapse. An attempt to achieve adequate margins of excision may be impossible because of anatomic constraints. Cancer cell seeding into the peritoneal cavity either prior to or at the time of sarcoma resection combined with positive or narrow margins of excision result in this high likelihood of local-regional recurrence.[94] In patients with local-regional disease progression or sarcomatosis, the survival is limited to approximately 2 years.

If CRS is performed in this group of patients and combined with HIPEC, the median survival is extended past 2 years. In four of the five studies referenced, an overall 5-year survival was >30%.[95–99] Unusually large benefits with CRS and HIPEC in patients with uterine sarcomatosis have been reported.[100] The mechanical removal of sarcoma peritoneal metastases that occurs with HIPEC may be as important or even more important than the cytotoxic effects. A consensus statement has been published.[101]

SELECTED REFERENCES

The full reference list can be accessed at lwwhealthlibrary.com/oncology.

1. Chu DZ, Lang NP, Thompson C, et al. Peritoneal carcinomatosis in non-gynecologic malignancy. A prospective study of prognostic factors. *Cancer* 1989;63:364–367.
2. Sadeghi B, Arvieux C, Glehen O, et al. Peritoneal carcinomatosis from non-gynecologic malignancies: results of the EVOCAPE 1 multicentric prospective study. *Cancer* 2000;88:358–363.
3. Jayne DG, Fook S, Loi C, et al. Peritoneal carcinomatosis from colorectal cancer. *Br J Surg* 2002;89:1545–1550.
4. Sugarbaker PH. Peritonectomy procedures. *Ann Surg* 1995;221:29–42.
5. Glehen O, Cotte E, Kusamura S, et al. Hyperthermic intraperitoneal chemotherapy: nomenclature and modalities of perfusion. *J Surg Oncol* 2008;98:242–246.
6. Sugarbaker PH, Graves T, DeBruijn EA, et al. Early postoperative intraperitoneal chemotherapy as an adjuvant therapy to surgery for peritoneal carcinomatosis from gastrointestinal cancer: pharmacological studies. *Cancer Res* 1990;50:5790–5794.
8. Segelman J, Granath F, Holm T, et al. Incidence, prevalence and risk factors for peritoneal carcinomatosis from colorectal cancer. *Br J Surg* 2012;99:699–705.
11. Dawson LE, Russell AH, Tong D, et al. Adenocarcinoma of the sigmoid colon: sites of initial dissemination and clinical patterns of recurrence following surgery alone. *J Surg Oncol* 1983;22:95–99.
12. Brodsky JT, Cohen AM. Peritoneal seeding following potentially curative resection of colonic carcinoma: implications for adjuvant therapy. *Dis Colon Rectum* 1991;34:723–727.
13. Carmignani CP, Sugarbaker TA, Bromley CM, et al. Intraperitoneal cancer dissemination: mechanisms of the patterns of spread. *Cancer Metastasis Rev* 2003;22:465–472.
17. Ronnett BM, Zahn CM, Kurman RJ, et al. Disseminated peritoneal adenomucinosis and peritoneal mucinous carcinomatosis. A clinicopathologic analysis of 109 cases with emphasis on distinguishing pathologic features, site of origin, prognosis, and relationship to "pseudomyxoma peritonei." *Am J Surg Pathol* 1995;19:1390–1408.
18. Sugarbaker PH. Epithelial appendiceal neoplasms. *Cancer J* 2009;15:225–235.
19. Yan TD, Deraco M, Baratti D, et al. Cytoreductive surgery and hyperthermic intraperitoneal chemotherapy for malignant peritoneal mesothelioma: multi-institutional experience. *J Clin Oncol* 2009;27:6237–6242.
20. Cerruto CA, Brun EA, Chang D, et al. Prognostic significance of histomorphologic parameters in diffuse malignant peritoneal mesothelioma. *Arch Pathol Lab Med* 2006;130:1654–1661.
25. Pestieau SR, Sugarbaker PH. Treatment of primary colon cancer with peritoneal carcinomatosis: comparison of concomitant vs. delayed management. *Dis Colon Rectum* 2000;43:1341–1346, discussion 1347–1348.
26. Sammartino P, Sibio S, Biacchi D, et al. Prevention of peritoneal metastases from colon cancer in high-risk patients: Preliminary results of surgery plus prophylactic HIPEC. *Gastroenterol Res Pract* 2012;2012:141585.
27. Braam HJ, Boerma D, Wiezer MJ, et al. Hyperthermic perioperative chemotherapy during primary tumour resection limits extent of bowel resection compared to two-stage treatment. *Eur J Surg Oncol* 2013;39:988–993.
28. Elias D, Goere D, Di Pietrantonio D, et al. Results of systematic second-look surgery in patients at high risk of developing colorectal peritoneal carcinomatosis. *Ann Surg* 2008;247:445–450.
30. Delhorme JB, Triki E, Zeca I, et al. Mandatory second-look surgery after surgical treatment of peritoneal carcinomatosis of colonic origin. (personal communication)

31. Honore C, Goere D, Souadka A, et al. Definition of patients presenting a high risk of developing peritoneal carcinomatosis after curative surgery for colorectal cancer: a systematic review. *Ann Surg Oncol* 2013;20:183–192.
38. Yan TD, Bijelic L, Sugarbaker PH. Critical analysis of treatment failure after complete cytoreductive surgery and perioperative intraperitoneal chemotherapy for peritoneal dissemination from appendiceal mucinous neoplasms. *Ann Surg Oncol* 2007;14:2289–2299.
40. Verwaal VJ, van Tinteren H, Ruth SV, et al. Toxicity of cytoreductive surgery and hyperthermic intra-peritoneal chemotherapy. *J Surg Oncol* 2004;85:61–67.
42. Smeenk RM, Verwaal VJ, Zoetmulder FA. Learning curve of combined modality treatment in peritoneal surface disease. *Br J Surg* 2007;94:1408–1414.
43. Rosen SA, Buell JF, Yohida A, et al. Initial presentation with stage IV colorectal cancer. *Arch Surg* 2000;135:530–534.
45. Elias D, Benizri E, Pocard M, et al. Treatment of synchronous peritoneal carcinomatosis and liver metastases from colorectal cancer. *Eur J Surg Oncol* 2006;32:632–636.
46. da Silva RG, Sugarbaker PH. Analysis of prognostic factors in seventy patients having a complete cytoreduction plus perioperative intraperitoneal chemotherapy for carcinomatosis from colorectal cancer. *J Am Coll Surg* 2006;203:878–886.
47. Elias D, Gilly F, Boutitie F, et al. Peritoneal colorectal carcinomatosis treated with surgery and perioperative intraperitoneal chemotherapy: retrospective analysis of 523 patients from a multicentric French study. *J Clin Oncol* 2010;28:63–68.
49. Koga S, Hamazoe R, Maeta M, et al. Treatment of implanted peritoneal cancer in rats by continuous hyperthermic peritoneal perfusion in combination with an anticancer drug. *Cancer Res* 1984;44:1840–1842.
50. Elias D, Lefevre JH, Chevalier J, et al. Complete cytoreductive surgery plus intraperitoneal chemohyperthermia with oxaliplatin for peritoneal carcinomatosis of colorectal origin. *J Clin Oncol* 2009;27:681–685.
54. Elias D. Peritoneal carcinomatosis or liver metastases from colorectal cancer: similar standards for a curative surgery? *Ann Surg Oncol* 2004;11:122–123.
55. Sugarbaker PH. Second-look surgery for colorectal cancer: revised selection factors and new treatment options for greater success. *Int J Surg Oncol* 2011;2011:915078.
57. de Pangher Manzini V, Recchia L, Cafferata M, et al. Malignant peritoneal mesothelioma: a multicenter study on 81 cases. *Ann Oncol* 2010;21:348–353.
62. Sugarbaker PH, Yan TD, Stuart OA, et al. Comprehensive management of diffuse malignant peritoneal mesothelioma. *Eur J Surg Oncol* 2006;32:686–691.
65. Deraco M, Bartlett D, Kusamura S, et al. Consensus statement on peritoneal mesothelioma. *J Surg Oncol* 2008;98:268–272.
66. Hioki M, Gotohda N, Konishi M, et al. Predictive factors improving survival after gastrectomy in gastric cancer patients with peritoneal carcinomatosis. *World J Surg* 2010;34:555–562.
68. Boku N, Gastrointestinal Oncology Study Group of Japan Clinical Oncology Group. Chemotherapy for metastatic disease: review from JCOG trials. *Int J Clin Oncol* 2008;13:196–200.
69. Yonemura Y, Kawamura T, Bandou E, et al. Treatment of peritoneal dissemination from gastric cancer by peritonectomy and chemohyperthermic peritoneal perfusion. *Br J Surg* 2005;92:370–375.
71. Fujimoto S, Takahashi M, Mutou T, et al. Improved mortality rate of gastric carcinoma patients with peritoneal carcinomatosis treated with intraperitoneal hyperthermic chemoperfusion combined with surgery. *Cancer* 1997;79:884–891.

76. Yan TD, Links M, Fransi S, et al. Learning curve for cytoreductive surgery and perioperative intraperitoneal chemotherapy for peritoneal surface malignancy—a journey to becoming a Nationally Funded Peritonectomy Center. *Ann Surg Oncol* 2007;14:2270–2280.

78. Prospektive multizentrische Phase III-Studie zur zytoreduktiven Chirurgie mit hyperthermer intraperitonealer Chemoperfusion nach präoperativer Chemotherapie beim Magenkarzinom inkl. AEG mit primärer peritonealer Metastasierung (Gastripec I). EudraCT-Number: 2006-006088-22 Phase III-Trial.

84. De Roover A, Detroz B, Detry O, et al. Adjuvant hyperthermic intraperitoneal preoperative chemotherapy (HIPEC) associated with curative surgery for locally advanced gastric carcinoma. An initial experience. *Acta Chir Belg* 2006;106:297–301.

89. Ceelen WP, VanNieuwenhove Y, Van Belle S, et al. Cytoreduction and hyperthermic intraperitoneal chemoperfusion in women with heavily pretreated recurrent ovarian cancer. *Ann Surg Oncol* 2012;19:2352–2359.

92. Fagotti A, Costantini B, Petrillo M, et al. Cytoreductive surgery plus HIPEC in platinum-sensitive recurrent ovarian cancer patients: a case-control study on survival in patients with two year follow-up. *Gynecol Oncol* 2012;127:502–505.

94. Karakousis CP, Kontzoglou K, Driscoll DL. Intraperitoneal chemotherapy in disseminated abdominal sarcoma. *Ann Surg Oncol* 1997;4:496–498.

95. Bilimoria MM, Holtz DJ, Mirza NQ, et al. Tumor volume as a prognostic factor for sarcomatosis. *Cancer* 2002;94:2441–2446.

Intraocular Melanoma

Paul T. Finger

INTRODUCTION

Metastatic choroidal melanoma patients rarely present with the classic "distended abdomen and a glass eye." Though metastases occur in up to 50% of cases, most do not cause symptoms having been discovered by periodic hepatic screening.[1,2] The rationale for early detection is that it allows for palliative treatment, enrollment in clinical trials, and end-of-life planning.[3]

Prosthetic eyes are less commonly required after uveal melanoma treatment. This is because fewer patients with uveal melanoma are being treated by removal of the eye (enucleation). For example, at The New York Eye Cancer Center, <10% of patients with uveal melanoma typically require enucleation. This trend toward eye preservation can be related to early detection, referral of smaller more treatable uveal melanoma, and the widespread belief that radiation is equivalent to enucleation for the prevention of metastases.[4] Confronted with the choice between enucleation and eye-sparing radiation therapy, patients prefer to keep their eye.

Vision-sparing radiation therapy techniques are widely used around the world. For example, 47 eye cancer specialists from 10 countries participated in a committee to create the American Brachytherapy Society Ophthalmic Oncology Task Force guidelines for plaque radiation therapy.[5] In these guidelines, enucleation was recommended in cases of American Joint Committee on Cancer (AJCC) stage T4e uveal melanomas, tumors with basal dimensions that exceed the limits of irradiation; blind painful eyes and those with no light perception vision. Thus multicenter, international consensus allows for eye and vision-sparing plaque brachytherapy for almost all patients.[5] This shift toward eye preservation has been augmented by the advent of postradiation, eye- and vision-preserving laser photocoagulation as well as antivascular endothelial growth factor (anti-VEGF) treatment. In 2007, radiation maculopathy and radiation optic neuropathy were first suppressed by periodic intraocular injections of bevacizumab (Avastin, Genentech, South San Francisco, CA).[6–8] Since that time, centers around the world have used anti-VEGF treatment to preserve vision, eyes, and quality of life for most patients.

In the modern era, patients with metastatic uveal melanoma are likely to present with a normal abdominal examination, their natural globe, and binocular vision.

INCIDENCE AND ETIOLOGY

Uveal melanomas are the most common primary intraocular malignancy in adults and account for 5% of all melanomas.[9] As compared to Caucasians, uveal melanoma is progressively less likely to occur in Hispanics, Asians, and Africans.[10] The incidence of ocular melanomas for whites in the United States (Surveillance, Epidemiology, and End Results program) was 0.69 per 100,000 person-years for males and 0.54 for females.[11,12] The Collaborative Ocular Melanoma Study (COMS) found the mean age of enrolled patients was 60.[13] Patients with dysplastic nevus syndrome, ocular

melanosis, and the nevus of Ota have been found to be at greater risk to develop uveal melanoma.[14]

Environmental causes are less clear.[9,15] While a 2011 multicenter, international study of biopsy-proven iris melanomas found that most occurred on the lower, more sun-exposed iris, others have suggest no correlation to ultraviolet light.[9,16] Though specific genetic defects have been found within choroidal melanoma cells, there is no clear mode of inheritance.[17,18]

ANATOMY AND PATHOLOGY

The uvea is the primary vascular matrix of the eye. It is continuous within the iris, ciliary body, and choroid. Melanocytes within any of these structures can transform. However, intraocular melanoma location affects tumor size at diagnosis, prognosis for vision, and risk for metastasis.

Iris melanomas are the most easily visible. They tend to be the smallest at diagnosis, spindle cell type, and least likely to metastasize.[16] In contrast, ciliary body melanomas are the least visible as they are hidden behind the iris, typically discovered as larger, and more likely to have metastasized.[19]

Choroidal melanomas are located posterior to the ciliary body. Often asymptomatic, they are commonly found during routine periodic ophthalmic examination. Thus, choroidal melanomas are typically small to medium-sized tumors. When symptomatic, choroidal melanomas can induce early changes in vision and/or symptoms of "flashing lights" due to tumor-induced exudative retinal detachment. A subset termed "subfoveal choroidal melanomas" are located beneath the center of vision and are recognized earlier due to visual symptoms and are thus smaller and less likely to have metastasized.[20]

Therefore, unless a melanoma is large enough to be visible, extend into the visual axis, tilt the natural lens, induce a symptomatic exudative retinal detachment, or displace the fovea, they are discovered during routine eye examination.

Histology

In 1931, Callender recognized distinct types of melanocytes within uveal melanomas.[21–23] His subsequent cytology-based tumor staging system "The Callender Classification" divided uveal melanoma into three categories:

1. Spindle cell melanomas (spindle A, spindle B, or both)
2. Mixed-cell melanomas, when less than half of the cells are composed of epithelioid cells
3. Epithelioid cell melanomas, greater than half are composed of epithelioid cells

While there is general agreement that epithelioid cell melanomas are more aggressive, there exists great variation among pathologists' diagnosis of cell types, the number of sections required for review, and the quantity of epithelioid cells required to make the diagnosis of an "epithelioid cell melanoma."[24]

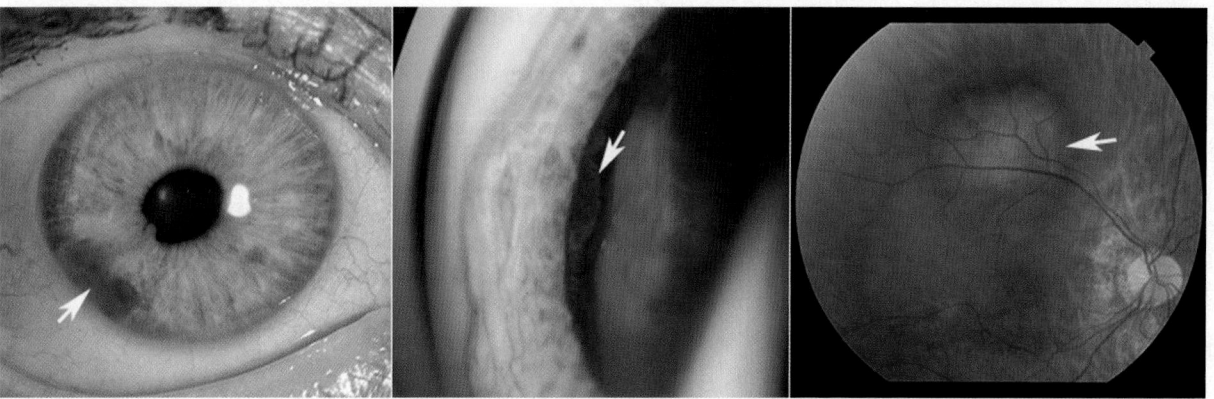

Figure 116.1 *Left*, iris melanoma (*arrow*) in inferior quadrant demonstrates corectopia, ectropion uvea, and intrinsic vascularity (at pupillary margin). *Middle*, a pigmented ciliary body melanoma (*arrow*) causing anterior iris displacement and a sector cataract of the adjacent lens. *Right*, a posterior choroidal melanoma demonstrating MOST (Melanoma = Orange pigment, Subretinal fluid and Thickness ≥2 mm).

Intraocular Tumor Growth Patterns

Uveal melanomas either grow from a preexisting nevus or de novo. However, there are uveal-location specific patterns of tumor growth:

Iris Melanoma

Iris melanomas typically originate in the iris stroma. While growing, they can displace, erode, or consume the underlying iris pigment epithelium.[25] Along its posterior margin, it may invade the trabecular meshwork gaining egress to the episcleral aqueous veins and or grow into the adjacent ciliary body. When discohesive, tumor-cell dispersion can induce secondary glaucoma.[26] Other signs that suggest malignancy include iris dysfunction such as corectopia (irregular pupil) or dysmorphisms such as ectropion uveae and tumor neovascularization (Fig. 116.1, left). Additional tumor-associated vasculopathies include dilated iris feeder vessels and adjacent episcleral hypervascularity.

Ciliary Body Melanoma

Ciliary body melanomas arise immediately posterior to the iris and are more likely to indent the adjacent lens and cause lenticular astigmatism and cataract (Fig. 116.1, middle). They can infiltrate along ciliary vessels and nerves to form nodules of epibulbar extrascleral extension (Fig. 116.2, left). The sclera above the tumor may exhibit recruited "sentinel" blood vessels. As ciliary body melanomas enlarge, they may find resistance at the iris root, leading to a circumferential growth pattern as to form an intraocular "ring" melanoma. Alternatively, they can erode through and displace the iris root into the anterior chamber.

Choroidal Melanoma

Choroidal melanomas arise posterior to the ciliary body (Fig. 116.1, right). As a choroidal melanoma grows, it typically displaces the overlying retina inwards toward the vitreous humor to form a dome shape.[27] High interstitial tumor pressure, leakage, and tumor invasion combine to obliterate, erode, and weaken the overlying tissues. In 25% of cases, the choroidal melanoma breaks though its overlying Bruch's membrane and mushrooms beneath the retina.[27] A rare, alternative growth pattern is "diffuse melanoma." This tumor is low-lying, more superficial spreading, and causes less uveal thickening.

Extrascleral Extension

Extrascleral tumor extension can occur with any size uveal melanoma (Fig. 116.2). However, it is more common with tumors located in the ciliary body, larger choroidal melanomas, or after sclera weakening by laser thermotherapy. Less common paths of extraocular and orbital extension include through the emissary vortex veins and into the optic nerve.

OPHTHALMIC DIAGNOSIS

Finger's "MOST" Mnemonic

There is consensus that, when seen together, the most common characteristics of choroidal melanoma are diagnostic. As a choroidal melanoma invades and destroys the overlying retinal pigment

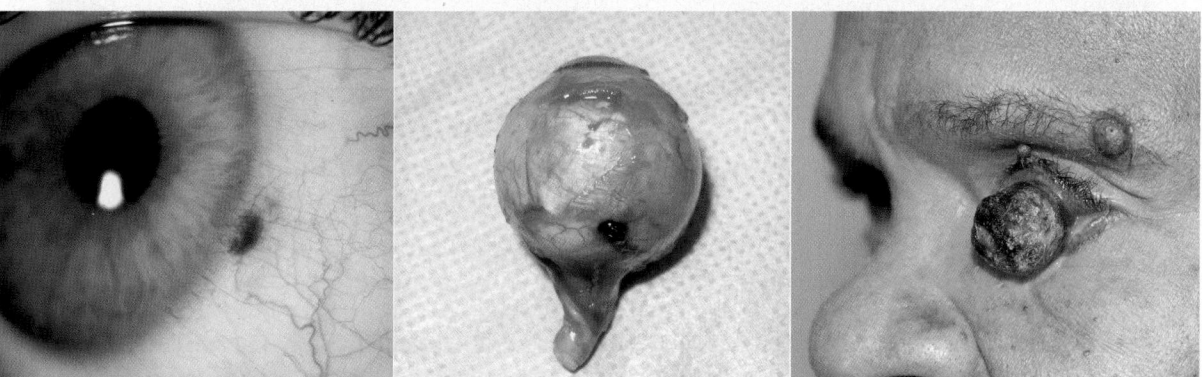

Figure 116.2 *Left*, minimal extrascleral extension as seen before plaque radiation therapy. *Middle*, a nodule of moderate extrascleral melanoma seen after enucleation. *Right*, in this case, massive orbital recurrence is seen 16 months after enucleation surgery. (Reprinted from Finger PT, Tena LB, Semenova E, et al. Extrascleral extension of choroidal melanoma: post-enucleation high-dose-rate interstitial brachytherapy of the orbit. *Brachytherapy*. 2014;13:275–280, with permission from Elsevier.)

epithelium, accumulations of orange pigment (lipofuscin and melanolipofuscin) can be visualized on the surface of a choroidal melanoma (Fig. 116.3, top left). Choroidal melanoma–associated incontinent tumor blood vessels leak serum beneath the retina, seen as overlying retinal pigment epithelial detachments or subretinal fluid. Lastly, choroidal melanomas are typically ≥2 mm thick. Therefore, Dr. Finger created the mnemonic MOST where Melanoma = Orange pigment + Subretinal fluid + Thickness of ≥2 mm. That said, not all choroidal melanomas will exhibit all three findings. However, MOST is diagnostic when all three are present.

Ophthalmic Examination

The clinical diagnosis of iris, ciliary body, and choroidal melanomas has reached a high degree of accuracy.[22] In the modern era, multimodality tumor imaging can be used to clinically diagnose almost all uveal melanomas. Office-based imaging techniques range from photography, intraocular angiography, fundus autofluorescent imaging, optical coherence tomography, transillumination, and ultrasound imaging. Select cases may require orbital radiographic imaging (magnetic resonance imaging [MRI], computed tomography [CT], or positron emission tomography [PET]/CT). Biopsy is rarely required for diagnosis.[22]

Ophthalmic Photography and Angiography

Photographic techniques include slit-lamp, gonioscopy for iris and ciliary body tumors, as well as fundus photography for choroidal melanoma. Photography documents the current state of the affected eye, facilitates observations of tumor characteristics, and plays an important role in the diagnosis of tumor growth, posttreatment tumor response, and normal tissue side effects.

Fundus Autofluorescent Imaging

Light (500 to 750 nm, peak 630) is used to induce hyperautofluoresence from orange pigment lipofuscin.[28] Thus, fundus autofluorescence can be used to detect and document one of the most important diagnostic characteristics of choroidal melanoma (Fig. 116.3, top right).

Intraocular Angiography

Angiographic photography is used to evaluate tumor microcirculation. Though some choroidal melanomas may demonstrate a pathognomonic choroidal "double circulation" pattern and/or late diffuse microaneurysms, many merely show diffuse or focal hyper-

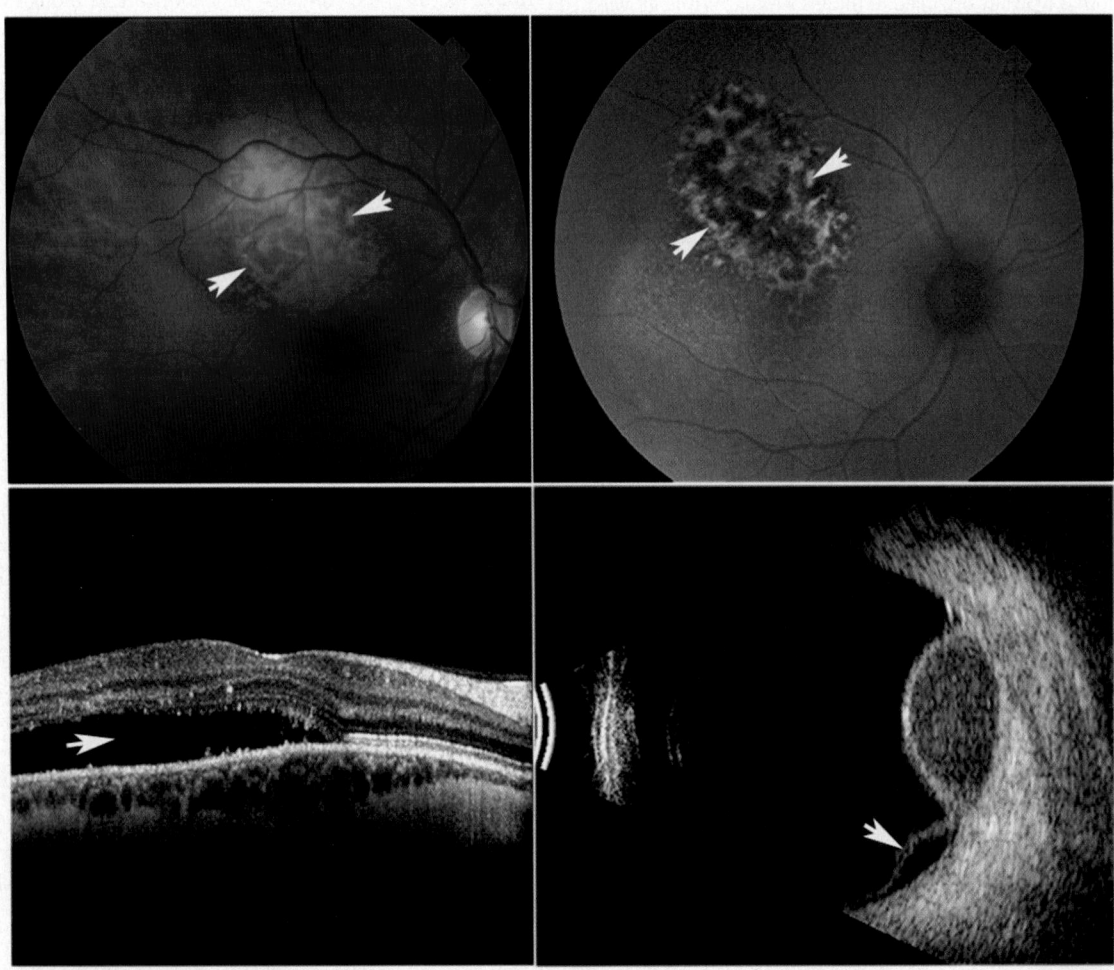

Figure 116.3 *Top left,* fundus photograph demonstrates orange pigment lipofuscin deposition (*arrows*) on the surface of the choroidal melanoma, subretinal fluid extending into the macula, and thickness ≥2 mm seen on ultrasound imaging. *Top right,* fundus autofluorescence imaging reveals orange pigment lipofuscin hyperautofluorescence (*arrows*). *Bottom left,* optical coherence tomography reveals exudative subretinal fluid (*arrow*) from the melanoma. *Bottom right,* 20 MHz B-scan ultrasound imaging reveals a typical dome-shaped, medium-reflective choroidal melanoma with a secondary exudative retinal detachment (*arrow*).

fluorescence. However, these findings can be used to distinguish between the hypofluorescence of choroidal hemorrhage, the coarse vascular pattern of choroidal hemangioma, or the plethora of subretinal hyperfluorescent microaneurysms seen with angiography of choroidal metastasis.

Optical Coherence Tomography

Optical coherence tomography is a laser light-based computerized imaging system used to create tomographic slices and three-dimensional volumes of the retina, choroid, and sclera. Tumor associated subretinal and intraretinal fluid are best seen with optical coherence tomography (Fig. 116.3, bottom left).

Ophthalmic Ultrasound Imaging

Ultrasound imaging offers 0.1 mm resolution of intraocular tissues. Ultrasound imaging of choroidal melanoma typically reveals low to moderate internal tumor reflectivity, a dome shape, and/or secondary exudative retinal detachment (Fig. 116.3, bottom right).[27] Less common ultrasound-imaged tumor characteristics include a mushroom shape, choroidal excavation, and extrascleral extension, as well as internal vascularity on dynamic examination. Alternative tumor-specific ultrasonographic diagnostic findings of choroidal hemangioma, osteoma, hemorrhage, or metastasis help differentiate these tumors.

High-frequency (20 to 50 MHz) ultrasonography also called ultrasound biomicroscopy (UBM) has allowed almost histopathology quality imaging of iris melanoma capable of viewing extension into the underlying pigment epithelium or adjacent ciliary body.[29] Smaller ciliary body melanomas have been detected by ultrasound biomicroscopy, saving both vision and life.

Ultrasound imaging is commonly used to measure the height and basal dimensions of all uveal melanomas.[27,29] Tumor measurements have been used to detect tumor growth, facilitate radiation therapy (plaque brachytherapy and proton beam), and to monitor posttreatment tumor regression.

Intraocular Tumor Biopsy

Unlike cutaneous melanoma, biopsy of uveal melanoma is controversial. With the exception of transcorneal biopsy of iris melanomas, transvitreal and transscleral biopsy requires a conjunctival and scleral incision. Discohesive tumor cells are liberated within the eye and exit through the sclerostomy into the orbit. Though no one has proved a metastatic risk associated with choroidal melanoma biopsy, known risks include vitreous hemorrhage, retinal tear, retinal detachment, infection, and cataract. Consensus indications for uveal tumor biopsy include atypical tumors, metastatic tumors, when patients require a pathology diagnosis, and for genetic/molecular analysis.[30]

The recent advent of genetic/molecular analysis of choroidal melanoma, its resultant prognostic information, and evolving systemic treatment protocols have prompted eye cancer specialists to recommended biopsy.[31] However, the risks of biopsy must be weighed against the accuracy of clinical diagnosis and the lack of an effective treatment for metastatic disease.

UNIVERSAL STAGING AND UVEAL MELANOMA

The American Joint Committee on Cancer–International Union for Cancer Control Ophthalmic Oncology Task Force

The AJCC and The Eye Cancer Foundation sponsored The AJCC Ophthalmic Oncology Task Force with a directive to include

members of the International Union for Cancer Control (UICC).[32] Thus the seventh edition AJCC eye cancer staging system was created by 46 eye cancer specialists from 11 countries (France, England, Sweden, Finland, the United States of America, Canada, India, Japan, The Netherlands, Hungary, and Germany).[32] These included experienced specialists in medical oncology, pediatric oncology, radiation oncology, medical physics, radiology, ocular plastic surgery, orbit, pathology, and ophthalmic oncology.

As a result, the seventh edition AJCC-UICC staging for uveal melanoma has become widely accepted.[5,33–35] Most ophthalmic journals now either require or suggest authors use the seventh edition AJCC staging system in manuscript preparation. Adopted by the UICC, world cancer agencies use AJCC staging for uveal melanoma (Table 116.1). Universal staging has allowed us to better categorize and understand medical information.[34,36,37] The AJCC staging system for uveal melanoma has been validated by a large single-center study and is currently being evaluated within a second large multicenter, retrospective database study (http://www.eyecancer.com/research/bioinformatics-grid-big).[34,58]

MANAGEMENT OF THE PRIMARY UVEAL MELANOMA

The Case for Observation of Small T1 Uveal Melanomas

Eye cancer specialists may observe small choroidal melanomas for evidence of tumor growth prior to treatment. This is because current belief is that "small choroidal melanomas" carry a low risk ($\approx$11%) for metastases and that most current treatments risk severe vision loss. In addition, observation of small choroidal melanomas has been justified by the concept that "tumor growth demonstrates malignancy." In practice, documented tumor growth both reassures the doctor that the tumor is malignant and reassures the patient that treatment is indicated. Specifically, the risk of treatment-related loss of vision is more than offset by a reduction in the probability of metastasis and tumor-induced vision loss.

This is particularly true for patients with small choroidal melanomas close to the fovea, monocular patients, or systemically ill patients. In these cases, serial observation may allow for years of useful vision prior to treatment. For all patients, the case for observation of small melanoma growth has been governed by the potential benefit of vision preservation (in the affected eye).

The Case Against Observation of Small T1 Uveal Melanomas

Once the eye cancer specialist is convinced that a tumor is a malignant (albeit small) choroidal melanoma, treatment becomes the most reasonable choice. In support of this approach, one can cite multiple studies that show increased tumor size (specifically largest tumor diameter) is associated with an increased risk of metastatic death.[4,38,39] Therefore, it is reasonable to assume that such observations of malignant melanoma growth increase (albeit marginally) a patient's risk for metastatic disease.

Currently, all patients with small choroidal melanoma can be offered effective eye- and vision-sparing treatments.[40] They typically require particularly small radiation treatment volumes that can be associated with less vision loss. Should radiation retinopathy and optic neuropathy occur, they are treatable with intravitreal anti-VEGF medications.[6–8,41]

In 2013, researchers at The New York Eye Cancer Center analyzed the results of 72 small melanomas treated with palladium-103 plaque brachytherapy and followed for a mean 54 months.[40] The authors noted that almost half of the eyes developed radiation maculopathy and almost 20% developed radiation optic neuropathy.

TABLE 116.1

American Joint Committee on Cancer Tumor, Node, Metastasis–Based Classification System Tumor Staging

Thickness (mm)

	≤3.0	3.1–6.0	6.1–9.0	9.1–12.0	12.1–15.0	15.1–18.0	>18.0
>15.0					4	4	4
12.1–15.0				3	3	4	4
9.1–12.0		3	3	3	3	3	4
6.1–9.0	2	2	2	2	3	3	4
3.1–6.0	1	1	1	2	2	3	4
≤3.0	1	1	1	1	2	2	4

Largest basal diameter (mm)

Primary tumor: uveal melanoma
TX Primary tumor cannot be assessed
T0 No evidence of primary tumor

Iris
T1 Tumor limited to the iris
T1a Tumor limited to the iris not >3 clock hours in size
T1b Tumor limited to the iris >3 clock hours in size
T1c Tumor limited to the iris with pigmentary glaucoma
T2 Tumor confluent with or extending into the ciliary body, choroid, or both
T2a Tumor confluent with or extending into the ciliary body, choroid, or both, with pigmentary glaucoma
T3 Tumor confluent with or extending into the ciliary body, choroid, or both, with scleral extension
T3a Tumor confluent with or extending into the ciliary body, choroid, or both, with scleral extension and pigmentary glaucoma
T4 Tumor with extrascleral extension
T4a Tumor with extrascleral extension <5 mm in diameter
T4b Tumor with extrascleral extension >5 mm in diameter

Ciliary Body and Choroid
T1 Tumor size category 1
T1a Tumor size category 1 without ciliary body involvement and extraocular extension
T1b Tumor size category 1 with ciliary body involvement
T1c Tumor size category ≤1 without ciliary body involvement but with extraocular extension <5 mm in diameter

T1d Tumor size category 1 with ciliary body involvement and extraocular extension >5 mm in diameter
T2 Tumor size category 2
T2a Tumor size category 2 without ciliary body involvement and extraocular extension
T2b Tumor size category 2 with ciliary body involvement
T2c Tumor size category 2 without ciliary body involvement but with extraocular extension ≤5 mm in diameter
T2d Tumor size category 2 with ciliary body involvement and extraocular extension ≤5 mm in diameter
T3 Tumor size category 3
T3a Tumor size category 3 without ciliary body involvement and extraocular extension
T3b Tumor size category 3 with ciliary body involvement
T3c Tumor size category 3 without ciliary body involvement but with extraocular extension ≤5 mm in diameter
T3d Tumor size category 3 with ciliary body involvement and extraocular extension ≤5 mm in diameter
T4 Tumor size category 4
T4a Tumor size category 4 without ciliary body involvement and extraocular extension
T4b Tumor size category 4 with ciliary body involvement
T4c Tumor size category 4 with ciliary body involvement but with extraocular extension ≤5 mm in diameter
T4d Tumor size category 4 with ciliary body involvement and extraocular extension ≤5 mm in diameter
T4e Any tumor size category with extraocular extension >5 mm in diameter

However, since the advent of intravitreal anti-VEGF therapy for radiation retinopathy and optic neuropathy, only 19% or 4 of 21 affected patients lost more than two lines on the visual acuity chart. Clearly, the clinical decision "to treat or not to treat a small choroidal melanoma" is both complex and controversial (http://www.eyecancer.com/research/article/12).

Overview: Treatment of Uveal Melanoma

Fewer patients must lose their eye due to choroidal melanoma. This shift has been partly related to the COMS finding that (in treatment of select medium-sized melanomas) plaque radiation therapy was equivalent to enucleation for survival.[4] This resulted in a shift toward the use of eye and vision-sparing treatments within subspecialty eye cancer centers.[5]

Radiation therapy is presently the most widely used eye-sparing treatment. Methods include brachytherapy plaque techniques and external beam radiation using photons, charged particles, stereotactic radiosurgery, or multisource cobalt units.[5,35] The techniques with the most widely reported clinical experience are plaque brachytherapy and proton beam. A comparison of clinical outcomes is given in Table 116.2.[4,37,42–49]

Episcleral Plaque Radiation Therapy

Low energy plaques (iodine-125 [^{125}I] or palladium-103 [^{103}Pd]) are bowl-shaped devices constructed to house rice-sized radioactive sources (or seeds).[35] Ruthenium-106 (^{106}Ru) plaques are solid disc-shaped electron-emitting sources where the beta-radionuclide is covered by a 0.1 mm thick layer of silver at its episcleral aperture.[35]

TABLE 116.2

Radiation Therapy for Choroidal Melanoma[a]

Authors	Radiation	Study Group Size	Mean Dose (Gy)	Mean Follow-up (mo)	Recurrence (%)	Secondary Enucleation (%)	Neovascular Glaucoma (%)	Metastasis (%)	Visual Acuity
COMS[4,42,43]	I-125	657	≥85 Gy to 5 mm	60	10	13	N/A	10 (5-y) 18 (10-y)	57% >20/200 at 3 y
Packer et al.[44]	I-125	64	91	64	7.8	17.2	10.9	15.6	45% better or 20/100 at 5.3 y
Fontanesi et al.[45]	I-125	144	79	46	2.3	9.7	5.5	5.5	41% better or 20/200 at 3.9 y
Lommatzsch[46]	Ru-106	205	100	80	15	26	1.3	20	N/A
Char, Kroll, and Castro[47]	Helium	218	70	110	5	22	35	18.6 (5-y) 23.6 (10-y)	33% better or 20/200 at 10 y
Brovkina and Zarubei[48]	Proton	63	100–125	34	19	25	N/A	6	N/A
Gragoudas et al.[49]	Proton	128	70	64	3	6	N/A	20.5	42% better than 20/200 at 5.3 y
Mean		**211**	**87**	**65**	**9**	**17**	**11.7**	**13.7**	**46% better or 20/200 at 5.5 y**
Present study Finger et al.[37]	Pd-103	400	73	51	3%	3.5%	2.5%	6% 7.3 (5-y) 13.4 (10-y)	79% better or 20/200 at 5 y 69% better or 20/200 at 10 y

Gy, Gray; COMS, Collaborative Ocular Melanoma Study; I-125, iodine-125; N/A, data not available; Ru-106, ruthenium-106; Pd-103, palladium 103.
[a] Large-scale, single modality series with similar follow-up.
Used with permission of the journal, *Ophthalmology.* The original source for this material is Finger PT, Chin KJ, Duball G, et al. Palladium-103 ophthalmic plaque radiation therapy for choroidal melanoma: 400 treated patients. *Ophthalmology* 2009;116:790–796.

Low-energy plaque construction and dosimetry requires a multispecialty team that integrates information about each tumor size and location from data derived from clinical examination, photography, and ultrasound imaging.[35,50] The plaque is temporarily sutured to the sclera overlying the tumor, left in place for 5 to 7 days, and then surgically removed.[5]

Recent research suggests that dose to the fovea and lens can be correlated to the incidence of radiation maculopathy and cataract, respectively.[51,52] However, each type of plaque has characteristic patterns of dose distribution within the eye. For example, [106]Ru plaques emit electrons with limited intraocular penetration and less side-scatter penumbra (compared to [103]Pd or ^{125}I). Conversely, [103]Pd and ^{125}I offer greater intraocular penetration and more side scatter. All these characteristics must be taken into account when choosing a radionuclide source and plaque size.[35,50] Lastly, it is important to consider dose to normal ocular structures, because side effects may be predicted based on these measurements.[20,51–53]

The 2014 American Brachytherapy Society (ABS) guidelines for ophthalmic plaque radiation therapy include potential methods to decrease ocular morbidity and patient mortality.[5] Specifically, that ophthalmic radiation therapy should be performed in subspecialty eye cancer referral centers, that radiation oncologists and medical physicists follow the American Association of Physicists in Medicine–ABS guidelines for plaque construction, dosimetry, and quality assurance, that preoperative comparative dosimetry of available radiation sources be considered prior to treatment and that centers use the seventh edition AJCC staging system to periodically report clinical outcomes.[5,33,35,50]

Proton Beam

Proton beam for uveal melanoma is available at 13 institutions around the world. Pioneered at Harvard University, typical treatment involves surgical placement of metallic markers on the episclera around the tumor's base.[49] Then protons are administered over 4 consecutive days and thus four high-dose-rate treatment fractions to a prescription dose of 60 Gy. Proton therapy has been effective for local tumor control, preservation of the globe, and functional vision (see Table 116.2).

However, in contrast to low-energy plaque therapy, proton beam typically requires an anterior entrance dose resulting in more commonly reported lash loss, dry eye, neovascular glaucoma, and cataract.[54] Also unlike plaques, proton treatment can be confounded by eye movement leading to a mobile target volume.[54]

Two clinical studies compared plaque versus proton.[55,56] Both reported that charged particles offered local tumor control and reasonable vision retention compared to plaque brachytherapy. However, anterior segment complications, particularly iris neovascularization, glaucoma, and secondary enucleation, were higher after proton beam therapy.[57]

TREATMENT FOR SPECIAL CASES

Iris and Iridociliary Melanoma

The overall 5-year risk for iris melanoma metastasis is 10.7%.[16] However, small iris melanomas are often observed for growth prior to treatment. Surgical iridectomy or iridocyclectomy used to be the most common treatment. However, there has been a transition to relatively safe, tissue-sparing radiation therapy techniques.[58–60] For example, plaque brachytherapy avoids the uncommon risks of intraocular surgery: infection, hemorrhage, acute cataract, and retinal detachment. Radiation treatment offers iris retention, retained iris function, and relatively large treatment margins. With long-term follow-up, epicorneal [103]Pd plaque brachytherapy has been associated with excellent local control, a high-risk of radiation cataract formation, and almost no risk for radiation-related keratopathy, retinopathy, or optic neuropathy.[53]

Choroidal Melanomas that Touch or Surround the Optic Disc

Standard plaque placement covers the tumor plus a 2- to 3-mm surrounding margin.[5,35] However, obtaining standard plaque placement becomes difficult when choroidal melanoma margins are near, touch, or surround the optic disc. Ophthalmoscopy typically reveals a 1.75-mm optic disc diameter, with its edge located 3.4 mm nasal to the fovea. However, just behind the eye, the optic nerve is enveloped by a 5-mm diameter optic nerve sheath.[61] Therefore, with a plaque placed against the retrobulbar optic nerve sheath, it cannot advance closer than 1.5 mm from the intraocular optic disc. When a choroidal melanoma touches or surrounds the optic disc, standard plaque positioning is impossible.

In 2005, 8-mm wide, variable depth slots were cut into standard COMS-type plaques.[62] This allowed the optic nerve sheath to enter the plaque, thus overcome the optic nerve sheath obstruction. This normalized the plaque's position and thus the treatment volume. The slot, however, presents additional medical physics challenges. The radioactive seeds must be affixed in nonstandard patterns around the slot, to fill in the treatment volume, and provide improved local control.[63]

Large T3 and T4 Choroidal Melanomas

Large tumor size is not necessarily a contraindication for eye sparing radiation therapy (see Table 116.1). For example, the 2014 ABS Ophthalmic Oncology Task Force Guidelines suggest that contraindications for plaque therapy be related to extraocular extension, basal diameters that exceed the limits of brachytherapy, blind painful eyes, and those with no light perception vision.[5] With these parameters, enucleation is generally reserved for those rare melanomas >20 mm in diameter, >16 mm thick, suspected optic nerve invasion, with multifocal recurrence, and at the patient's request.[5,40]

Extrascleral Tumor Extension

Extrascleral extension has been functionally defined as minimal (microscopic or encapsulated), moderate (localized unencapsulated nodule), or massive that fills most or part of the orbit (see Fig. 116.2).[64] In clinical practice, minimal extension may be included within the irradiated zone; moderate and select massive extrascleral extension can be removed by enucleation with local orbital resection to a point where there is no residual visible tumor. Subsequent external beam radiation therapy (50 Gy) would be employed to treat the presumed residua of subclinical orbital melanoma.[64]

Otherwise unresectable, massive extrascleral extension typically requires orbital exenteration with postoperative radiation therapy. Though postresection radiation typically involves 6 MV photons from a linear accelerator, this treatment is associated with significant loss of hair (eyelash and brow), dry sunken sockets, and poor cosmetic results. High-dose-rate interstitial brachytherapy has been recently reported to improve cosmesis without sacrificing local control.[64]

The Collaborative Ocular Melanoma Study

The COMS was the largest multicenter, prospective randomized clinical trial on treatment of choroidal melanoma. The COMS medium-sized choroidal melanoma trial compared the efficacy of enucleation versus ^{125}I plaque radiotherapy for the prevention of metastasis. It consisted of 1,317 patients from 43 centers in the United States and Canada randomly assigned to enucleation or ^{125}I plaque brachytherapy. At 12 years, 471 of 1,317 patients had died. The 12-year all-cause mortality rate was 43% in the ^{125}I brachytherapy arm and 41% among those enucleated. Thus, the COMS found no statistically significant difference in survival.[4]

The COMS large-sized choroidal melanoma trial enrolled tumors that were ≥16 mm in basal dimension or >10 mm in height. In order to determine if enucleation induced metastases, these tumors were randomized to receive 20 Gy (4 Gy in five daily fractions) versus no radiation prior to enucleation. At 12-years follow-up, the COMS found no survival advantage attributable to pre-enucleation radiation, effectively ending this practice.[13]

QUALITY OF LIFE

The COMS group interviewed 209 patients from the medium-sized tumor study.[65] They found those who had brachytherapy initially noted significantly better visual function than those treated with enucleation. Select parameters included ability to drive and peripheral vision, for up to 2 years following treatment. However, after 3 to 5 years after treatment, those differences diminished along with visual function. In addition, patients treated with plaque brachytherapy experienced more symptoms of anxiety than patients treated by enucleation.[65]

In consideration of the advent and evolution of vision sparing anti-VEGF medication therapy for radiation maculopathy and optic neuropathy, it may be reasonable to assume that current patients are benefiting from more long-lasting functional vision and improved quality of life.[41,66]

DIAGNOSIS OF UVEAL MELANOMA METASTASIS

History and Physical

Not all eye cancer specialists are located in subspecialty centers. Therefore, each eye cancer specialist (often without medical oncology guidance) typically determines how patients will be initially staged and subsequently screened for metastatic disease. Worldwide patterns are largely dependent on social and economic conditions as well as the availability of radiographic imaging.

That said, when medical oncologists are referred patients with a history of uveal melanoma, the initial TNM (tumor, node, metastasis) staging (seventh edition, AJCC) should be used to help determine their metastatic risk (see Table 116.1).[33] A history of weight loss, subcutaneous nodularity, or abdominal pain should raise suspicion. Signs or symptoms of radicular or focal bone pain suggest possible osseous disease. The choroidal melanoma specific physical examination should focus on subcutaneous nodularity (subcutaneous nodules can be normal or have a dark blue color), focal back pain, hepatomegaly, or ascites.[39]

Systemic Surveys

Before Treatment

Liver enzymes assays have proved very specific but not sensitive for hepatic metastases.[2] Thus, the COMS surveillance protocol led to late discovery of patients with advanced metastatic disease. In contrast, periodic hepatic radiographic imaging typically provides early detection of asymptomatic liver metastases.

At The New York Eye Cancer Center, initial uveal melanoma systemic screening is performed utilizing a physical examination, a hematologic survey, and a total body PET/CT. These PET/CT surveys have revealed that when patients were discovered with metastasis, 100% had hepatic and 75% had multiorgan disease (mostly subcutaneous and osseous).[67–69] Almost all had larger T3- or T4-sized tumors. An additional non–tumor-size-dependent finding was that 3.3% had second nonocular primary cancers.[68,70,71] Further, in evaluation of the primary intraocular melanoma, PET/CT specific uptake values (>4) were associated with metastasis. After treatment, specific uptake value has been used to evaluate uveal melanoma viability.[72,73]

After Treatment

In consideration of the incidence of metastasis after local treatment, I currently recommend that follow-up staging include abdominal imaging every 6 months for 4 years and then annually for at least 6 additional years (Fig. 116.4).[2,34,37,74–78] In consideration of both preference and efficacy, abdominal MRI and CT are preferred over ultrasound imaging.

In sum, PET/CT allows for whole body scanning and staging with remarkably high positive predictive values. In addition to staging, PET/CT is used to clarify the nature of suspicious MRI, CT, or ultrasonographic findings. Also consider that, whole body imaging offers patients piece of mind, particularly those at high risk for metastatic disease.

The Incidence of Metastasis

Multiple large and several statistically significant studies have found that largest tumor diameter can be used to predict risk for metastasis.[4,13,39] In addition, a relatively recent European based multicenter, international study found intraocular melanoma size was predictive for metastatic disease, This study was used as a framework component of the 7th edition AJCC uveal melanoma staging system (see Table 116.1).[19,33,38] Additional risk factors for metastasis were ciliary body and extrascleral extension.

Management of Patients with Metastatic Disease

Though the liver is the most commonly discovered site of metastatic uveal melanoma spread, most are found to have multifocal hepatic or multiorgan disease. Therefore, when hepatic metastases are suspected or confirmed systemic staging is warranted.[3]

In cases where metastases are limited to the liver, or when the liver must be treated, local control or palliation of liver metastases can be achieved with a wide range of procedures. The literature contains reports of hepatic artery chemoembolization, hepatic perfusion, or radiofrequency ablation.[79,80] In these cases, procedure selection is made in consideration of the extent of hepatic disease, the location of the tumors, the patient's performance status, and the institution's interventional capability. Relatively rare cases of solitary, slow-growing hepatic or extrahepatic metastasis, typically found 5 or more years after treatment of their primary uveal melanoma, have been treated by local metastasectomy.[80–82]

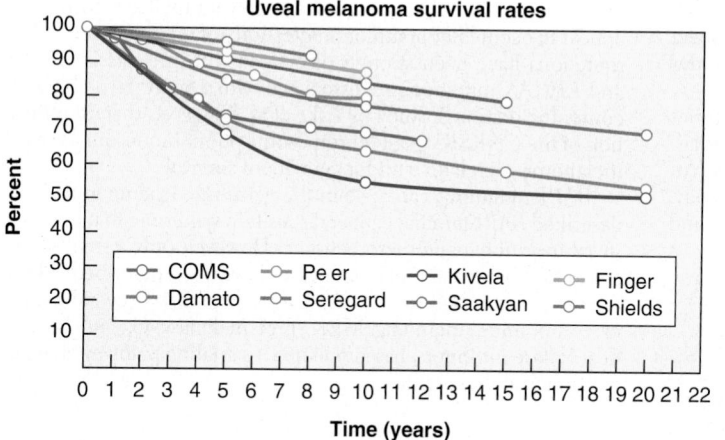

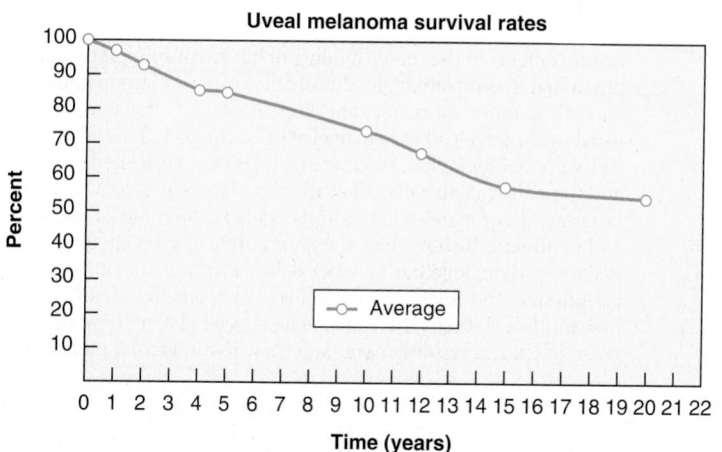

Figure 116.4 Metastatic death from uveal melanoma. COMS, Diener-West et al.[2]; Damato, Damato[74]; Pe'er, Kaiserman et al.[75]; Seregard, Bergman et al.[76]; Kivela, Kujala et al.[77]; Saakyan, Saakyan et al.[78]; Finger, Finger, et al.[37]; Shields, Shields et al.[34] Table courtesy of Ekaterina Semenova, MD. The data used to make these graphs was culled from the published literature.

In that there is no accepted treatment, patients with metastatic uveal melanoma should be treated within clinical trials (http://www.cancer.gov/clinicaltrials/search/results?protocolsearchid =7978738&vers=1). In addition, registration of ongoing studies offers the best chance to avoid duplication of nonfunctional studies.[3]

Clinical Trials for Systemic Metastases

Systemic chemotherapy, cytokine therapy with interleukin-2 and interferon-γ has been ineffective. However, new insights regarding biomarkers, genetic targets expressed by tumor cells, as well as antiangiogenic drugs are leading innovative treatment strategies.[83]

Genetic tumor typing offers the potential to identify high-risk patients for treatment of presumed subclinical metastatic disease. Conversely, lower-risk patients may not need as rigorous periodic surveillance. Should a functional genetic pathway be identified and a pharmaceutical blockade initiated, metastatic uveal melanoma may become manageable.

BIOMARKERS: PROGNOSTIC AND PREDICTIVE FACTORS

Clinical Prognostic Factors

Tumor Size and Location

Uveal melanoma size or largest tumor dimension has been the most reproducible biomarker for choroidal melanoma metastasis. It is also useful, because tumor measurements are typically available at the time of diagnosis. Utilizing the COMS data, Diener-West et al.[39] performed a meta-analysis of 5-year mortality among enucleated patients, providing weighted estimates of 5-year mortality after enucleation: 16% for small tumors, 32% for medium-sized tumors, and 53% for large tumors. This analysis also found older patient age was a significant risk factor for metastasis.[39]

Iris melanomas tend to be smaller and carry a four to five times lower (10.7%, 5-year) mortality rate than other uveal melanomas. Risk factors for iris melanoma metastasis include tumors >5 mm in largest diameter and or those were confluent with the ciliary body. In contrast, ciliary body melanomas are typically hidden behind the iris and can develop large "ring melanoma" configurations with a 5-year mortality of 53%. Extrascleral extension (orbital invasion) is also a risk factor for metastasis.[64]

Diffuse Growth Pattern

Choroidal melanomas are typically dome or mushroom shaped, but 5% grow in a diffuse pattern.[84] These diffuse melanomas are low-lying tumors often with indistinct or irregular margins that are more difficult to treat. Iris melanomas can also occur as the diffuse variant, starting as a solitary tumor then evolving to multifocal lesions after treatment.[85]

Histopathologic, Physiologic, Genetic, and Molecular Prognostic Factors

Tumor-Infiltrating Lymphocytes and Macrophages

Uveal melanomas have been noted to contain lymphocytes, thought to represent an important component of the host's immune response to the tumor. In several studies, both T- and B-lymphocyte infiltration were associated with higher mortality. In addition, tumor-infiltrating macrophages (CD68+ cells) are an independent prognostic factor with regard to survival.[86]

Genetics and Molecular Biology

Of the cytogenetic and molecular genetic changes within uveal melanoma, it is the partial or complete loss of one chromosome 3 that is most widely described.[43,87–90] It has not only been associated with aggressive features such as greater tumor size, ciliary body involvement, the presence of epithelioid cells, and closed loop vasculogenic mimicry, but is also considered a biomarker for metastasis.

Gene expression profiling involves the simultaneous measurement of mRNA expression of multiple genes in order obtain a real-time view of tumor biology. Three gene expression profiling subgroups have been identified and related to risk for metastatic disease.[91]

Earlier studies of molecular deregulation provided interesting insights into the molecular pathogenesis of uveal melanoma. For example, Rb protein is expressed in virtually all melanomas, indicating a lack of *Rb* gene mutation.[92] A combination of microarray gene expression profiling and comparative genomic hybridization showed that gain of chromosome 8q correlates strongly with expression of *DDEF1*, a gene located at 8q24.[93] Therefore, *DDEF1* overexpression might be a pathogenetically relevant consequence of chromosome 8q amplification associated with aggression of uveal melanoma.[93]

Individual gene mutations have improved our understanding of the etiology of uveal melanoma. Mutation of the G-protein α subunits GNAQ and GNA11 are mutually exclusive and represent early or initiating events that constitutively activate the mitogen-activated protein kinase pathway in around 85%. Mutations in BRCA1-associated protein-1 (*BAP1*), splicing factor 3B subunit 1 (*SF3B1*), and *EIF1AX* appear to be largely mutually exclusive and appear to occur later in tumor progression. Of interest, while *BAP1* mutations have been strongly associated with metastasis, *SF3B1* and *EIF1AX* mutations are associated with a more favorable outcome. In addition, a study by Lake et al.[94] suggests that amplification of the *CNKSR3* gene (chromosome 6q) in monosomy 3 uveal melanoma correlates with longer patient survival.[91]

BAP1 mutations can arise in the germline, leading to a newly described *BAP1* familial cancer disposition syndrome that includes uveal melanoma and mesothelioma. However, only a small number of familial uveal melanoma cases have been described. These discoveries have led to new clinical trials to assess several classes of compounds, including MEK, protein kinase C, and histone deacetylase inhibitors, based on known signaling pathway changes within uveal melanomas.[17]

SUMMARY

Improvements in the understanding of the environmental, clinical, physiologic, cytopathologic, histopathologic, immunopathologic, as well as more recent genetic and molecular characteristics of uveal melanoma lead us to marvel at its complexity. This chapter reviews the demographic, physiologic, treatment-associated, genetic, and molecular factors that allow uveal melanomas to grow and metastasize. It compares and contrasts available methods of diagnosis and treatment. It shows how the community of eye cancer specialists are working together to better define our nomenclature, medical physics, and treatment guidelines. This chapter clearly shows how multidisciplinary eye cancer care is needed to achieve the best possible clinical results for our patients with intraocular melanoma.

SELECTED REFERENCES

The full reference list can be accessed at lwwhealthlibrary.com/oncology.

2. Diener-West M, Reynolds SM, Agugliaro DJ, et al. Screening for metastasis from choroidal melanoma: the Collaborative Ocular Melanoma Study Group Report 23. *J Clin Oncol* 2004;22:2438–2444.

4. Collaborative Ocular Melanoma Study Group. The COMS randomized trial of iodine 125 brachytherapy for choroidal melanoma: V. Twelve-year mortality rates and prognostic factors: COMS report No. 28. *Arch Ophthalmol* 2006;124:1684–1693.

7. Finger PT, Chin K. Anti-vascular endothelial growth factor bevacizumab (avastin) for radiation retinopathy. *Arch Ophthalmol* 2007;125:751–756.

13. Hawkins BS, Collaborative Ocular Melanoma Study Group. The Collaborative Ocular Melanoma Study (COMS) randomized trial of pre-enucleation radiation of large choroidal melanoma: IV. Ten-year mortality findings and prognostic factors. COMS report number 24. *Am J Ophthalmol* 2004;138:936–951.

16. Khan S, Finger PT, Yu GP, et al. Clinical and pathologic characteristics of biopsy-proven iris melanoma: a multicenter international study. *Arch Ophthalmol* 2012;130:57–64.

17. Harbour JW. The genetics of uveal melanoma: an emerging framework for targeted therapy. *Pigment Cell Melanoma Res* 2012;25:171–181.

22. Accuracy of diagnosis of choroidal melanomas in the Collaborative Ocular Melanoma Study. COMS report no. 1. *Arch Ophthalmol* 1990;108:1268–1273.

23. Albert DM, Ruzzo MA, McLaughlin MA, et al. Establishment of cell lines of uveal melanoma. Methodology and characteristics. *Invest Ophthalmol Vis Sci* 1984;25:1284–1299.

26. Radcliffe NM, Finger PT. Eye cancer related glaucoma: current concepts. *Surv Ophthalmol* 2009;54:47–73.

27. Collaborative Ocular Melanoma Study Group, Boldt HC, Byrne SF, et al. Baseline echographic characteristics of tumors in eyes of patients enrolled in the Collaborative Ocular Melanoma Study: COMS report no. 29. *Ophthalmology* 2008;115:1390–1397, 1397.e1-e2.

30. Augsburger JJ, Shields JA. Fine needle aspiration biopsy of solid intraocular tumors: indications, instrumentation and techniques. *Ophthalmic Surg* 1984;15:34–40.

32. Finger PT, 7th Edition, AJCC-UICC Ophthalmic Oncology Task Force. The 7th edition AJCC staging system for eye cancer: an international language for ophthalmic oncology. *Arch Pathol Lab Med* 2009;133:1197–1198.

33. The 7th Edition AJCC-OOTF. Malignant melanoma of the uvea. In: Edge SE, Byrd Dr, Compton CA, Fritz AG, et al., ed. *AJCC Cancer Staging Manual*. Vol X. 7th ed. New York, NY: Springer; 2009:547–559.

34. Shields CL, Kaliki S, Furuta M, et al. American Joint Committee on Cancer classification of posterior uveal melanoma (tumor size category) predicts prognosis in 7731 patients. *Ophthalmology* 2013;120:2066–2071.

35. Chiu-Tsao ST, Astrahan MA, Finger PT, et al. Dosimetry of (125)I and (103) Pd COMS eye plaques for intraocular tumors: report of Task Group 129 by the AAPM and ABS. *Med Phys* 2012;39:6161–6184.

36. Finger PT. Do you speak ocular tumor? *Ophthalmology* 2003;110:13–14.

37. Finger PT, Chin KJ, Duvall G, et al. Palladium-103 ophthalmic plaque radiation therapy for choroidal melanoma: 400 treated patients. *Ophthalmology* 2009;116:790–796, 796.e1.

38. Kujala E, Damato B, Coupland SE, et al. Staging of ciliary body and choroidal melanomas based on anatomic extent. *J Clin Oncol* 2013;31:2825–2831.

39. Diener-West M, Reynolds SM, Agugliaro DJ, et al. Development of metastatic disease after enrollment in the COMS trials for treatment of choroidal melanoma: Collaborative Ocular Melanoma Study Group Report No. 26. *Arch Ophthalmol* 2005;123:1639–1643.

43. Jampol LM, Moy CS, Murray TG, et al. The COMS randomized trial of iodine 125 brachytherapy for choroidal melanoma: IV. Local treatment failure and enucleation in the first 5 years after brachytherapy. COMS report no. 19. *Ophthalmology* 2002;109:2197–2206.

50. Rivard MJ, Chiu-Tsao ST, Finger PT, et al. Comparison of dose calculation methods for brachytherapy of intraocular tumors. *Med Phys* 2011;38:306–316.

53. Yousef YA, Finger PT. Lack of radiation maculopathy after palladium-103 plaque radiotherapy for iris melanoma. *Int J Radiat Oncol Biol Phys* 2012;83:1107–1112.

54. Finger PT. Radiation therapy for choroidal melanoma. *Surv Ophthalmol* 1997;42:215–232.

55. Wilson MW, Hungerford JL. Comparison of episcleral plaque and proton beam radiation therapy for the treatment of choroidal melanoma. *Ophthalmology* 1999;106:1579–1587.

56. Char DH, Quivey JM, Castro JR, et al. Helium ions versus iodine 125 brachytherapy in the management of uveal melanoma. A prospective, randomized, dynamically balanced trial. *Ophthalmology* 1993;100:1547–1554.

57. Hungerford JL, Foss AJ, Whelahan I, et al. Side effects of photon and proton radiotherapy for ocular melanoma. *Front Radiat Ther Oncol* 1997;30:287–293.

59. Finger PT. Plaque radiation therapy for malignant melanoma of the iris and ciliary body. *Am J Ophthalmol* 2001;132:328–335.

63. Finger PT, Chin KJ, Tena LB. A five-year study of slotted eye plaque radiation therapy for choroidal melanoma: near, touching, or surrounding the optic nerve. *Ophthalmology* 2012;119:415–422.

64. Finger PT, Tena LB, Semenova E, et al. Extrascleral extension of choroidal melanoma: Post-enucleation high-dose-rate interstitial brachytherapy of the orbit. *Brachytherapy* 2014;13:275–280.

65. Melia M, Moy CS, Reynolds SM, et al. Quality of life after iodine 125 brachytherapy vs enucleation for choroidal melanoma: 5-year results from the Collaborative Ocular Melanoma Study: COMS QOLS Report No. 3. *Arch Ophthalmol* 2006;124:226–238.

68. Freton A, Chin KJ, Raut R, et al. Initial PET/CT staging for choroidal melanoma: AJCC correlation and second nonocular primaries in 333 patients. *Eur J Ophthalmol* 2012;22:236–243.

71. Diener-West M, Reynolds SM, Agugliaro DJ, et al. Second primary cancers after enrollment in the COMS trials for treatment of choroidal melanoma: COMS Report No. 25. *Arch Ophthalmol* 2005;123:601–604.

72. Finger PT, Chin K, Iacob CE. 18-Fluorine-labelled 2-deoxy-2-fluoro-D-glucose positron emission tomography/computed tomography standardised uptake values: a non-invasive biomarker for the risk of metastasis from choroidal melanoma. *Br J Ophthalmol* 2006;90:1263–1266.

73. Finger PT, Chin KJ. [(18)F]Fluorodeoxyglucose positron emission tomography/computed tomography (PET/CT) physiologic imaging of choroidal melanoma: before and after ophthalmic plaque radiation therapy. *Int J Radiat Oncol Biol Phys* 2011;79:137–142.

77. Kujala E, Makitie T, Kivela T. Very long-term prognosis of patients with malignant uveal melanoma. *Invest Ophthalmol Vis Sci* 2003;44:4651–4659.

79. Feldman ED, Pingpank JF, Alexander HR Jr. Regional treatment options for patients with ocular melanoma metastatic to the liver. *Ann Surg Oncol* 2004;11:290–297.

80. Sato T. Locoregional management of hepatic metastasis from primary uveal melanoma. *Semin Oncol* 2010;37:127–138.

81. Helton WS. Ocular melanoma metastatic to the liver: the role of surgery in multimodality therapy. *Ann Surg Oncol* 2004;11:242–244.

83. Triozzi PL, Eng C, Singh AD. Targeted therapy for uveal melanoma. *Cancer Treat Rev* 2008;34:247–258.

86. Makitie T, Summanen P, Tarkkanen A, et al. Tumor-infiltrating macrophages (CD68(+) cells) and prognosis in malignant uveal melanoma. *Invest Ophthalmol Vis Sci* 2001;42:1414–1421.

87. Prescher G, Bornfeld N, Hirche H, et al. Prognostic implications of monosomy 3 in uveal melanoma. *Lancet* 1996;347:1222–1225.

89. Sandinha MT, Farquharson MA, McKay IC, et al. Monosomy 3 predicts death but not time until death in choroidal melanoma. *Invest Ophthalmol Vis Sci* 2005;46:3497–3501.

91. Harbour JW. Molecular prognostic testing and individualized patient care in uveal melanoma. *Am J Ophthalmol* 2009;148:823–829.e1.

PRACTICE OF ONCOLOGY

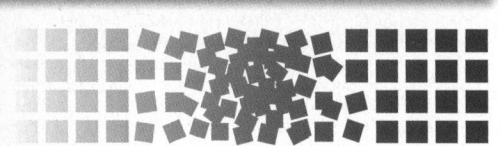

117 HIV-Associated Malignancies

Robert Yarchoan, Thomas S. Uldrick, Mark N. Polizzotto, and Richard F. Little

INTRODUCTION

In 1981, the US Centers for Disease Control and Prevention (CDC) reported the first cases of Kaposi sarcoma (KS) and *Pneumocystis jiroveci* pneumonia (PCP) that heralded a pandemic now known as AIDS. AIDS was subsequently found to be caused by a novel retrovirus, HIV. During the initial decade of the epidemic, patients often manifested KS or aggressive B-cell non-Hodgkin lymphoma (NHL). Before effective HIV therapy was developed, these patients had a high mortality. Since 1993, three tumors have been considered AIDS-defining in the context of HIV: KS, certain NHL (Table 117.1), and invasive cervical cancer.[1]

With the development first of nucleoside reverse transcriptase inhibitors starting in the mid-1980s[2] and subsequently of protease inhibitors and nonnucleoside reverse transcriptase inhibitors, combination antiretroviral therapy (cART) involving three or more drugs became broadly available in 1996.[3] There are now 30+ antiretroviral agents approved that target one of several stages of the HIV lifecycle.[4] HIV suppression with cART leads to increases in CD4 lymphocyte counts, improved immune function, decreased immune activation, decreased infectious complications, decreased mortality, and decreased infectivity,[5–10] transforming HIV infection into a manageable chronic disease.

The availability of cART has also transformed cancer epidemiology in people with HIV. Although AIDS-defining tumors remain the most common cancers, the incidence of KS and NHL decreased after cART became widely available in the United States and other developed countries.[11] Additionally, over the past 15+ years, therapy for major AIDS-associated cancers has also improved.[12] At the same time, the number of persons with HIV in the United States has increased by >50% due to an estimated 40,000 to 50,000 new HIV infections each year[11,13] and a decrease in infectious deaths. Worldwide, >30 million people are infected with HIV. With HIV-infected individuals living longer, the population at risk for malignant complications has increased and is aging.[14] In addition to AIDS-defining malignancies, patients infected with HIV are at increased risk of certain other cancers, including classical Hodgkin lymphoma (cHL), lung, anal, head and neck, liver, and nonmelanoma skin cancer.[15] Other common cancers such as breast or colon cancer are not more frequent in patients infected with HIV; even so, the burden of these cancers is increasing as the HIV-infected population ages. As such, the cumulative risk of developing *non-AIDS defining malignancies* (NADM) (Table 117.2) is an increasing public health concern.[7,16–19] Until there are improved HIV prevention strategies[10,20] or a broadly available HIV cure,[21] cancer burden will likely continue to increase substantially. Given these epidemiologic trends, oncologists will be called on to manage more cancer in people with HIV.

CANCER AND HIV: INCIDENCE AND ETIOLOGY

Epidemiologic studies have led to important discoveries regarding pathogenesis of HIV-associated tumors. KS in AIDS had a different natural history than the form in elderly men described by Moritz Kaposi in 1872[22] and occurred in a specific subpopulation of patients with AIDS: young men who had sex with other men (MSM).[23,24] MSM without HIV also occasionally developed KS. This suggested that KS had an infectious cause other than HIV itself, and ultimately a novel gamma-herpesvirus, *KS-associated herpes virus* (KSHV) or *human herpes virus (HHV)-8*, was discovered in 1994.[25] KSHV is an essential causative agent for all epidemiologic forms of KS. Seroprevalence of KSHV parallels geographic incidence of KS.[26] In the United States, KSHV seroprevalence is high in MSM but is <10% in the general population.[27]

KS epidemiology has evolved with the changing AIDS epidemic. In the United States prior to 1985, KS was the initial manifestation of AIDS in approximately 30% of cases.[28] However, after peaking in the early 1990s, its incidence declined in developed countries with the introduction of nucleoside antiretrovirals and then cART. In the United States, the incidence of AIDS-associated KS decreased by 84% in the period 1996 to 2002 compared with 1990 to 1995.[29] Further declines since 2002 have been more modest, with incidence relatively stable at about 62 cases per 100,000 person years in recent years.[11] It remains the second most common tumor in people with HIV/AIDS in the United States,[11,18] In regions such as sub-Saharan Africa, where KSHV and HIV infection are each highly prevalent, KS is a substantial public health burden.[30,31] In parts of sub-Saharan Africa, KS has been reported to be the most common tumor in men, representing almost half of all cancers, and also the second most frequent tumor in women.[31–33] Increasing access to cART via programs such as the Joint United Nations Programme on HIV/AIDS and the US President's Emergency Plan for AIDS Relief appears to be decreasing KS incidence in parts of sub-Saharan Africa,[34] but the extent of this change remains to be defined.

Excess cases of NHL were also noted early in the AIDS epidemic, and certain NHLs were included in the 1985 AIDS case definition.[35] In the CDC 1993 definition of AIDS, three NHLs were considered AIDS-defining: Burkitt (or equivalent), immunoblastic (or equivalent), or primary brain.[1] This terminology is now dated; however, several lymphomas remain strongly associated with HIV. In this chapter, we use the term AIDS-related lymphoma (ARL) when referring to epidemiologic data that does not segregate the various lymphoid tumors (see Table 117.1).[36] However, ARL is no longer a clinically useful term, and lymphomas should be classified using current World Health Organization criteria.[36] For AIDS-defining lymphomas, risk in patients infected with HIV in the pre-cART era was more than 250-fold greater than the general population. Most lymphomas that occur in patients

TABLE 117.1

HIV-Associated Lymphomas[a]

Lymphomas also occurring in immunocompetent patients
  Burkitt lymphoma
  Diffuse large B-cell lymphoma
    Germinal center subtype
    Activated B-cell subtype
  Extranodal marginal zone B-cell lymphoma of mucosa-
    associated lymphoid tissue type (rare, mainly in pediatric
    patients)
  Classic Hodgkin lymphoma (commonly mixed cellularity or
    lymphocyte depleted forms)[b]

Lymphomas occurring more specifically in HIV-positive patients
  Primary effusion lymphoma
  Large B-cell lymphoma arising in human herpes virus-8
    associated multicentric Castleman disease
  Plasmablastic lymphoma
  Primary diffuse large B-cell lymphoma of the central nervous
    system (in patients with AIDS, >95% Epstein-Barr virus
    associated)

Lymphomas also occurring in other immunodeficiency states
  Polymorphic B-cell lymphoma (post-transplant
    lymphoproliferative disorder–like)

[a] Adapted from the most current lymphoma nomenclature from (The 2008 *World Health Organization Classification of Tumours of Haematopoietic and Lymphoid Tissues*[36]).
The Centers for Disease Control and Prevention definition of AIDS-defining lymphoma in 1993 as Burkitt (or equivalent term), immunoblastic (or equivalent term), and primary brain lymphoma is based on older terminology.
[b] In this chapter, as in general usage, Hodgkin lymphoma will be considered as a separate entity and will not be encompassed in the term *AIDS-related lymphoma*.

TABLE 117.2

Risks of Various Malignant Conditions in Patients with AIDS[a]

	Tumor	Standard Incidence Ratio	
		Pre-cART (1980–1989)	cART (1996–2002)
AIDS-Defining	Kaposi sarcoma	52,900	3,640
	Non-Hodgkin lymphoma	79.8	49.5
	Burkitt lymphoma	57.4	49.5
	DLBCL	98.1	29.6
	Immunoblastic	140.5	59.5
	Primary diffuse large B-cell lymphoma of the CNS	5,000	1,020
	Cervix	7.7	5.3
Non–AIDS-Defining	Hodgkin lymphoma	7.0	13.6
	Oral cavity and pharynx	1.2 (NS)	2.1
	Anus	18.3	19.6
	Lung	2.5	2.6
	Vagina and vulva	0 (NS)	4.4 (NS)
	Seminoma	2.6	0.8 (NS)
	Penis	0 (NS)	8.0
	Renal cell carcinoma	0.8 (NS)	1.9
	Liver	2.4 (NS)	3.3
	Myeloma	2.7 (NS)	2.2
	Breast	0	0.8 (NS)
	Colon	0.9 (NS)	1.0 (NS)
	Prostate	0.9 (NS)	0.5

cART, combination antiretroviral therapy; DLBCL, diffuse large B-cell lymphoma; CNS, central nervous system; NS, not significant.
[a] Identification of cancers in people with AIDS based on matches to the cancer registries in patients grouped according to AIDS onset as either prior to development of combination antiretroviral therapy (1980–1989) or following cART (1996–2002). Cancer risk was described using the standardized incidence ratio, which compares incidence to that in the general population. All standardized incidence ratios in table are significant (*p* <0.05) unless noted.
From Engels EA, Pfeiffer RM, Goedert JJ, et al. Trends in cancer risk among people with AIDS in the United States 1980-2002. *AIDS* 2006;20:1645–1654, with permission.

infected with HIV are high-grade mature B-cell lymphomas,[37] including diffuse large B-cell lymphoma (DLBCL) with either centroblastic (germinal center [GC]) or immunoblastic (activated B-cell [ABC]) phenotypes,[38] Burkitt lymphoma (BL), plasmablastic lymphoma (PBL), primary diffuse large B-cell lymphoma of the central nervous system (PCNSL), and primary effusion lymphoma (PEL). By contrast, these histologies make up 25% of NHL in the general population.[39] ARL risk increases with the degree and duration of immunosuppression, and is inversely related to CD4 count.[40] Inflammation[41–44] and uncontrolled HIV viremia[45–48] also contribute to lymphoma risk. Since the advent of cART, NHL incidence has decreased by 50%.[49] Overall, populations on cART have improved immune status and CD4 counts at levels where lymphoma standardized risk ratio is lower. Still, within any CD4 cell strata, the standardized risk ratio for lymphoma remains elevated in individuals infected with HIV and comparable between pre-cART and early cART eras.[49] Indeed, changes in NHL incidence partially reflect changes in the proportion living with a certain CD4+ cell level. Despite a decrease in incidence, with an estimated incidence of 97 per 100,000 person-years in the cART era, NHL is the commonest malignancy in individuals infected with HIV in the United States.[18] ARL is an increasing public health problem in areas of sub-Saharan African with high HIV prevalence.[50,51]

With cART, epidemiologic and clinical patterns of ARL have changed. In the United States, ARL survival has increased since introduction of cART by nearly two-fold,[12,29,52] due in part to the effect of cART on AIDS and its infectious complications, as well as a shift away from poor-prognosis histologies that tend to occur with advanced AIDS.[53] This is most remarkable for PCNSL, which generally occurs in patients with <50 CD4 cells/mm[3], and whose incidence has fallen 80%.[29] For systemic ARL, immunoblastic subtypes predominated in the pre-cART era, but the predominant subtypes emerging in areas where cART is widely available are those with the GC phenotype of DLBCL and BL,[49,54–56] which are

associated with longer survival.[57] Lymphoma therapeutic advances also contribute to improved survival. With current regimens, prognosis for the most common HIV-associated lymphomas approach that of the general population. This is particularly apparent for the GC phenotype of DLBCL[55] and BL.[52] Outcomes in PCNSL remain poor,[53,58] in part due to difficulty in diagnosis, neurologic comorbidities, lack of standardized therapy, and delayed or inadequate treatment of lymphoma.[59]

While the incidence of ARL and KS has decreased, the incidence of certain NADMs has increased. Where cART is widely available, NADMs now occur as frequently as AIDS-defining malignancies.[19,60] Furthermore, cancer has emerged as the leading cause of death in people with HIV,[7,58,60–62] with about half of cancer-associated deaths caused by AIDS-defining malignancies and half by NADM.[7,63] Excess risk of certain NADMs is partly attributable to patients infected with HIV having increased infection with, and in some cases, poor immunologic control of oncogenic pathogens, such as *human papillomavirus* (HPV), *Epstein-Barr virus* (EBV), *hepatitis B virus* (HBV), and *hepatitis C virus*. It is possible that additional infectious agents will be discovered and found responsible for some of these tumors. For example, a novel virus, *Merkel cell polyomavirus*, was recently identified as the etiologic agent for Merkel cell carcinoma,[64] a rare skin cancer that occurs with increased frequency in immunosuppressed individuals, including those with HIV.[65] Other risk factors for certain of these tumors are more common in patients with HIV, including cigarette smoking and alcohol use. For many of these tumors, there is evidence that HIV also plays a pathogenic role, although the mechanisms may be complex or indirect. For example, a nearly five-fold excessive lung cancer risk in HIV appears related to age and cART use, but not CD4 cell count, and the risk remains approximately two-fold greater than that of the general population even when adjusted for smoking.[66,67] A contributing factor increasing the risk of lung cancer in people with HIV may be recurrent lung infections.[67,68]

KAPOSI SARCOMA

Pathophysiology

KS is a multifocal angioproliferative tumor caused by KSHV. Its characteristic purplish lesions are found histologically to have proliferating spindle cells with markers of lymphatic endothelial cells, leaky vascular slits, and an inflammatory infiltrate.[69–71] KS spindle cells are generally considered polyclonal or oligoclonal, although advanced lesions may have elements of monoclonality.[72,73] The lesions are most commonly cutaneous, but may involve internal organs including the lungs, lymphatic system, and gastrointestinal tract (Fig. 117.1).

KSHV is a necessary cause of KS. In the absence of cofactors such as HIV or iatrogenic immunosuppression, the risk of KS among individuals infected with KSHV is relatively low. KS was initially categorized based on epidemiologic characteristics. As first described by Moritz Kaposi in 1872,[22] KS was an indolent tumor usually seen in elderly Mediterranean men (now called *classical* KS). KS also exists in parts of Africa, where KSHV seroprevalence is 40% to 80% (*endemic* KS, seen in men, women, and occasionally young patients), in immunosuppressed populations (i.e., transplant recipients [*iatrogenic* KS]), and persons with HIV (*epidemic* KS). Clinical behavior varies between epidemiologic subtypes and

may be related to etiology of underlying immunodeficiency and presence of other KSHV-associated diseases.

Hyperproliferation of KSHV-infected spindle cells is the hallmark of KS.[74–76] KSHV modifies host cellular pathways by multiple mechanisms, in part through expression of KSHV-encoded mimics of human genes, viral microRNA, and activation of cellular genes.[77] Through these mechanisms, KSHV activates prosurvival and proangiogenic pathways. In particular, a KSHV-encoded G-protein–coupled receptor (vGPCR, also known as ORF74) induces production of vascular endothelial growth factor (VEGF) and other angiogenic factors.[75,78–80] Other important viral proteins include homologues of a macrophage inhibitory protein with angiogenic activity[74,81] and a viral interleukin (IL)-6 (vIL-6) with inflammatory and prosurvival effects. KSHV also induces c-Kit and endothelial-to-mesenchymal transformation.[82,83] These and overproduction of human cytokines and growth factors such as VEGF and platelet derived growth factor by KSHV-infected cells contribute to spindle cell proliferation and angiogenesis.

The marked elevation in KS in immunosuppressed individuals suggests an important role for defective immune surveillance of KSHV in risk of KS pathogenesis.[84,85] Decreasing CD4 cell count is associated with increasing risk of KS in both AIDS-associated and classic KS.[86,87] In patients with controlled HIV, KS is associated with a T-cell immunosenescense phenotype marked by increased CD57+ and decreased CD28+ T cells.[88] Patients with KS have decreased KSHV-specific CD4 responses compared to HIV/KSHV co-infected individuals without KS.[85] KS response to immune modulation is associated with increases in absolute CD4 count and/or KSHV-specific T-cell responses in patients infected with HIV on cART and organ transplant recipients after reduction in immunosuppression.[89–91] HIV may promote KS by other mechanisms as well. For example, the Tat protein of HIV can enhance infection of target cells by KSHV.[92]

Staging and Prognosis

KS is a multifocal tumor without evidence of clonal expansion and dissemination. KS can arise simultaneously at multiple sites (see Fig. 117.1) but should not be described as metastatic. Standard oncologic staging and response criteria are not applicable. The most widely used staging system for KS is the AIDS Clinical Trials

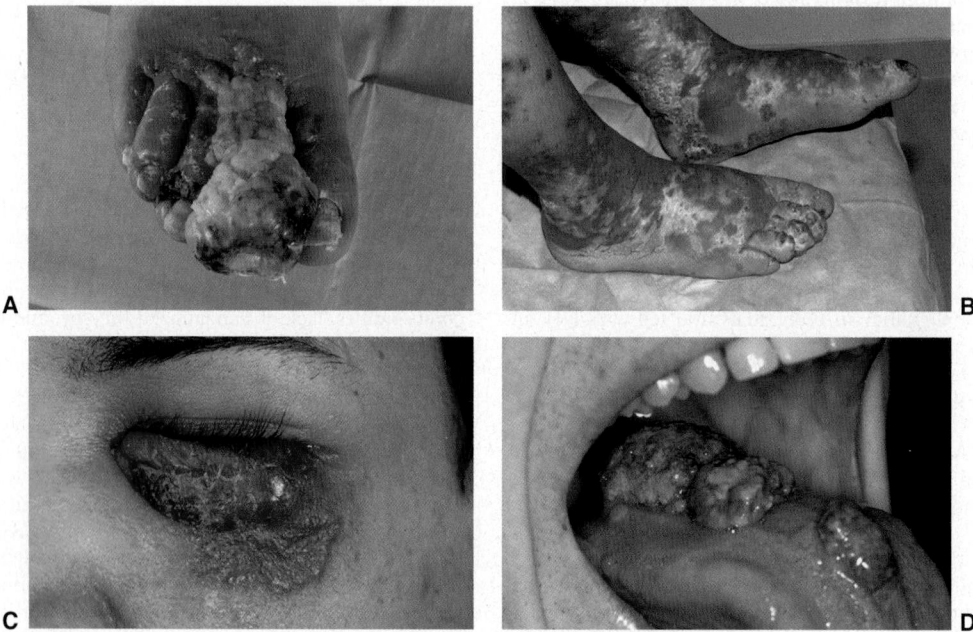

Figure 117.1 (A–B) Mucocutaneous manifestations of AIDS-Kaposi sarcoma observed in the era of combination antiretroviral therapy.

TABLE 117.3

Revised and Proposed AIDS Clinical Trials Group Staging Classification for Kaposi Sarcoma[a]

Stage	Good Risk (0) (All of the Following)	Poor Risk (1) (Any of the Following)
Tumor (T)	Confined to skin and/or lymph nodes and/or nonnodular oral disease confined to the palate	Tumor-associated edema or ulceration Extensive oral KS Gastrointestinal KS KS in other nonnodal viscera
Immune system (I) (not included if HIV-sensitive to cART[49])	CD4 cells $<150/mm^3$	CD4 cells $<150/mm^3$
Systemic illness (S)	No history of opportunistic infection or thrush	History of opportunistic infections and/or thrush; "B" symptoms present
	No B symptoms (unexplained fever, night sweats, $>10\%$ involuntary weight loss, or diarrhea) persisting more than 2 weeks	Performance status <70
	Other HIV-related illness (e.g., neurologic disease, lymphoma)	Performance status <70 (Karnofsky)

KS, Kaposi sarcoma; cART, combination antiretroviral therapy.

[a] Based on Krown et al.[93] and Nasti et al.[94] The revised CD4 cutoff of 150 cells/mm^3 [93] is lower than the original proposal of 200 cells/mm^3. However, in the cART era, CD4 cells do not appear to confer prognostic information. Example of staging: in the pre-cART era, a patient with KS restricted to the skin, CD4 count of 10 cells/mm^3, and a history of *Pneumocystis jiroveci* pneumonia would be $T_0I_1S_1$, and would be considered poor risk.[30] Suggested revision since cART would be staged as T_0S_1, and would be considered good risk.[94]

Group Oncology Committee TIS staging system[93,94] (Table 117.3). Risk stratification is based on tumor burden ($T_{0\ or\ 1}$), immune status ($I_{0\ or\ 1}$), and presence of any systemic illness ($S_{0\ or\ 1}$). For each category, poor risk (subscript 1) is defined respectively by the presence or extensive cutaneous or oral disease, tumor-associated edema, ulceration, or visceral disease (T_1); CD4 <150 cells/mm^3 (I_1); and the presence of other opportunistic infections, constitutional symptoms, or poor performance status (S_1). Before cART, poor risk in one or more categories was considered poor risk. In the cART era, a baseline CD4 cutoff of 150 cells/mm^3 is not as important prognostically,[95] and two main risk categories have been defined: good risk (T_0S_0, T_1S_0, or T_0S_1) and poor risk (T_1S_1). Notably, pulmonary involvement carries a particularly elevated risk of death.[96] Also, women who develop HIV-associated KS have a worse prognosis independent of other TIS risk factors.[95,97,98]

In assessing KS response to therapy, most clinical trials use some modification of criteria established by the AIDS Clinical Trials Group Oncology Committee.[99] Criteria for a partial response include 50% decrease in the total number of prespecified indicator lesions, 50% decrease in the area of measured cutaneous lesions, or flattening of 50% of nodular indicator lesions in the absence of progressive disease. Complete response requires resolution of all measurable disease, although residual skin hyperpigmentation is common. Outside of the research setting, KS is commonly treated to a symptomatic endpoint or response plateau.

Treatment

Treatment with cART is fundamental to therapy of HIV-associated KS, and generally should be the first therapeutic maneuver. Drugs associated with iatrogenic KS, such as steroids, cyclosporine, and rituximab, should be avoided or minimized.[100,101] KS-specific therapy is reserved for select cases, in particular patients with advanced (T_1) KS who generally will not have adequate and timely responses to cART alone or patients who have some other need for a rapid response. In patients with pulmonary KS, chemotherapy may be required urgently. Also, specific KS therapy is used in patients with KS unrelated to HIV that requires therapy, or transplant patients that do not respond to changes in the immunosuppressive regimen.

Regression of KS with cART alone has been documented in up to 80% of cART-naïve patients with early disease (T_0).[95,102,103] Control of HIV viremia and immune reconstitution are key

determinants of the anti-KS effect of cART. Some laboratory studies have suggested that HIV protease inhibitors may have specific KS activity,[104] but clinical trials have generally not shown any such benefit of protease inhibitor-based cART in preventing or treating KS.[103,105,106] The time to partial response or better with cART alone is commonly 6 to 12 months, and many responses are incomplete. In a randomized trial in South Africa of cART versus cART with early chemotherapy in treatment-naïve patients with largely T_1 disease, the group randomized to chemotherapy showed a significantly higher KS response at 12 months (39% versus 66%), supporting a role for KS-specific therapy in patients with KS-associated morbidity. Overall, however, survival was similar in both arms.[95] Patients infected with HIV occasionally demonstrate new KS or KS progression soon after cART initiation. It has been suggested that an immune reconstitution inflammatory syndrome may be contributing to the KS progression.[107,108] However, the pathogenesis of worsening or initial development of KS in the setting of initiation of cART remains unclear. Such patients should be considered for additional anti-KS therapy.

Localized therapies are generally of limited utility in KS and can be associated with troublesome toxicity. However, for patients with symptomatic disease in a highly restricted area, a number of approaches have activity. While a biopsy is needed to confirm the diagnosis of KS, surgical resection is otherwise rarely indicated. Also, clear surgical margins do not suggest cure and KS can even develop in the site of a surgical scar.[109] Topical 9-*cis*-retinoic acid (Panretin gel; Eisai Inc., Woodcliff Lake, NJ) is approved by the US Food and Drug Administration (FDA) for use in KS. While response in up to 45% of treated lesions are reported, local inflammation is common and the cosmetic result may also be inadequate.[110–112] Intralesional injection or iontophoresis of low-dose vinblastine (0.1 mL of 0.1 mg/mL) or 3% sodium tetradodecyl sulfate injection (0.1 to 0.3 mL), as well as laser therapy and cryotherapy[113] have also been described. Again, these local therapies can be painful, cosmetic results may be unsatisfactory, and disease progression outside of treatment site is common. Radiation therapy is effective, though progression outside the treated area is common. Local toxicities can include radiation dermatitis or ulceration. Over the longer term, induration and fibrosis may develop. For these reasons, it is generally reserved for disease that is quite limited, yet causing severe pain or distress. Dosing is individualized, ranging from an 8 Gy single dose to fractionated therapy to a total of 16 to 30 Gy.

Indications for systemic therapy in HIV-associated KS are imprecise and should be individualized. Strong indications include KS that is life threatening, symptomatic visceral or substantial pulmonary disease, and cutaneous disease that is extensive, ulcerating, or associated with edema or pain. In such cases, it should be initiated as soon as possible. Systemic therapy is also justified in more limited disease where response to cART alone is unlikely to be sufficient or timely from a symptomatic perspective, or where worsening KS would not be tolerated. It may also be justified when KS impairs quality of life due to social withdrawal or psychological distress. Although complete and long-lasting resolution of evident disease can be realized, this outcome does not imply cure. Treatment is aimed at decreasing tumor burden and symptom palliation, which may require chronic intermittent administration.

Several cytotoxic agents have activity in KS. The most commonly used agents are liposomal doxorubicin and paclitaxel. Liposomal doxorubicin is approved by the FDA for KS and has become the standard-of-care first-line chemotherapy, generally at the dose of 20 mg/m^2 every 3 weeks.[102] In the cART era, response rates of 45% to 80% may be anticipated.[114,115] Liposomal daunorubicin is also approved for advanced KS, though less commonly used. An important consideration with anthracyclines is the risk of cumulative cardiotoxicity; the FDA warns against cumulative lifetime doses exceeding 550 mg/m^2. While the risk appears to be lower with liposomal formulations than with bolus nonliposomal anthracyclines, this dose should not be exceeded without cardiac monitoring and individualized risk-benefit analysis. Paclitaxel is approved by the FDA as second-line therapy for KS, with responses ranging from 59% to 71% demonstrated in phase 2 trials conducted prior to the use of cART.[116,117] A randomized trial comparing liposomal doxorubicin 20 mg/m^2 every 3 weeks with paclitaxel 100 mg/m^2 every 2 weeks in subjects with advanced KS showed comparable efficacy, but increased hematologic and neurologic toxicity in the paclitaxel arm.[115] Symptomatic progression after ceasing therapy was common, and overall progression-free survival at 12 months was approximately 70%.[115]

Other agents with demonstrated KS activity include vincristine, vinblastine, doxorubicin, etoposide, and bleomycin. Oral etoposide 50 mg/day on days 1 through 7 of a 14-day cycle is active, with an overall response rate of 36% in previously treated patients, the majority of whom were not receiving cART.[118] This approach may be useful in resource-limited settings, although the risk of secondary myeloid leukemia raises concerns with long-term administration. Early in the AIDS epidemic, high response rates were obtained with combination regimens of doxorubicin, bleomycin, and vinblastine or vincristine, although toxicity was often substantial.[119] This regimen has been largely replaced by liposomal doxorubicin, which was shown in a randomized trial to be more effective and less toxic.[120]

A further systemic option is interferon (IFN)-α, a cytokine with immune modulatory and antiangiogenic activity. In HIV-associated KS, it is most active in patients with limited disease and preserved CD4 counts.[121,122] Unfortunately, systemic side effects limit tolerability for many patients. Constitutional symptoms, cytopenias, mood disturbances including major depression, and hypothyroidism are common and may be severe. Most practitioners begin with IFN-α 1 to 5 × 10^6 units subcutaneous injection daily and gradually increase the dose as tolerated. IFN-α should be used in combination with cART in HIV-associated KS.[123]

A general strategy is to treat patients with KS until a response plateau or remission is attained. The number of cycles of chemotherapy required is variable. Patients with good immune reconstitution on cART are more likely to be able to stop chemotherapy after an early response, with maintained or even improved KS response with cART continuation. However, some patients require ongoing or periodic antitumor therapy in addition to cART. In cases of advanced immune suppression or uncontrolled HIV, KS may progress shortly after discontinuing therapy, and close observation is required. Growth of KS after therapy with a given chemotherapy

does not necessarily imply tumor resistance, and a previously effective agent can often be used again.

There is a substantial unmet clinical need for novel, less toxic agents for KS. Established therapies have important limitations. In particular, there are few effective oral agents, and the most useful cytotoxic agents often are associated with neutropenia. The risk of cumulative anthracycline cardiotoxicity can limit use of liposomal anthracyclines, making them less favorable in heavily pretreated patients and patients with coexisting cardiovascular disease. Also, delivery of the most effective agents within existing health infrastructure is impracticable and/or unaffordable in resource-limited settings. Development of effective oral anti-KS agents could assist in addressing this significant global health problem.[30,124]

Oral agents that interfere with KSHV replication have been shown to prevent KS in patients with AIDS; a randomized clinical trial of ganciclovir for *cytomegalovirus* infections showed systemic administration was associated with a lower rate of KS development.[125] However, the risk/benefit ratio of antiherpetic agents in preventing KS has not been evaluated and may be unfavorable. Furthermore, targeting KSHV replication with antiviral drugs has shown little utility in treating established KS. Ganiclovir and cidofovir have been evaluated in small studies, but not found to have meaningful activity in either classic or HIV-associated KS.[126,127]

Given the angiogenic nature of KS and its sensitivity to changes in immune status, both immune-modulating and antiangiogenic therapies have been explored in clinical trials. The cytokine IL-12 showed promising results alone and in combination with chemotherapy.[128,129] Thalidomide, an oral agent with immune modulatory and antiangiogenic effects, has shown activity in two phase 2 studies, though its use is limited by toxicity.[130,131] Studies are under way of thalidomide analogs. Targeted inhibition of angiogenesis with the monocolonal antibody to VEGF, bevacizumab,[132] and imatinib,[133] an inhibitor of c-kit and the platelet-derived growth factor receptor, have shown activity in phase 2 studies. Interestingly, in renal transplant–associated KS, modification of immunosuppression from cyclosporine to the mammalian target of rapamycin inhibitor sirolimus leads to tumor regression.[134] However, in a study of sirolimus in HIV-associated KS, responses were limited and drug interactions with the antiretroviral drug ritonavir complicated dosing.[135] Ongoing clinical studies will help define the role of additional novel agents in KS.

Kaposi Sarcoma Herpes Virus–Associated Multicentric Castleman Disease

The term Castleman disease is used to describe a group of related lymphoproliferative disorders. There are several forms of idiopathic Castleman disease that can be classified either anatomically (unicentric or multicentric) or by morphology (hyaline-vascular, plasma cell, or mixed histology). With the discovery of KSHV, it was recognized that this virus causes a plasmablastic variant of multicentric Castleman disease (MCD).[136] Nearly all Castleman disease arising in the setting of HIV infection is KSHV-associated MCD (KSHV-MCD). This polyclonal[137] hyperproliferative B-cell disorder is considered rare, although its incidence is not well defined. Unlike KS, KSHV-MCD may be more common since the advent of cART.[138]

KSHV-MCD is characterized by intermittent flares of inflammatory symptoms, including fevers, fatigue, cachexia, and edema, together with lymphadenopathy and splenomegaly. Gastrointestinal and respiratory symptoms are common, and rheumatologic, neurologic, and dermatologic manifestations may also be present. Laboratory abnormalities include anemia, thrombocytopenia, hypoalbuminemia, hyponatremia, and elevated C-reactive protein.[139,140] The clinical course may wax and wane, but untreated, it is frequently fatal, with patients succumbing to inflammatory manifestations or progressing to large cell lymphoma.[141]

The symptoms of KSHV-MCD, while potentially severe, are nonspecific. KSHV-MCD should be considered in the differential diagnosis of patients with HIV and unexplained lymphadenopathy, splenomegaly, and/or inflammatory symptoms or autoimmune phenomena, particularly anemia or thrombocytopenia. Diagnosis generally requires excisional lymph node biopsy and demonstration of KSHV-infected plasmablasts. There is no validated staging or prognostic system, although definitions of symptomatic disease[142] and National Cancer Institute (NCI) response criteria have been defined for clinical studies.[139] These criteria rely on evaluation of clinical signs and common laboratory abnormalities. Symptomatic KSHV-MCD is associated with an elevated circulating KSHV viral load and associated cytokine dysregulation. In particular, viral IL-6 production and induction of human IL-6 and IL-10 are implicated as pathogenic factors.[92,140,141] KSHV viral load decreases with effective therapy.[139,140]

There is no standard therapy for KSHV-MCD. However, based on an appreciation of the viral etiology and pathogenic mechanisms of KSHV-MCD, new therapeutic modalities are being developed that can control disease activity,[101,139,142] improve overall survival,[143] and may reduce the risk of KSHV-associated lymphoma.[144] Best studied is the anti-CD20 monoclonal antibody rituximab.[101,142] Most patients respond initially to rituximab-containing regimens. However, rituximab monotherapy may be insufficient in advanced disease, and it has been associated with exacerbation of concurrent KS. Approximately 30% of patients will relapse within 1 year.[101,142] Rituximab combined with liposomal doxorubicin (in part to control KS) appears promising in preliminary reports.[145] Zidovudine and ganciclovir are activated to toxic moieties by KSHV-encoded enzymes; based on this observation, high-dose zidovudine combined with ganciclovir has been tested and found to be active, although not as effective as rituximab in patients with severe inflammatory symptoms.[139] Historically, chemotherapy regimens used in NHL[141] and/or splenectomy[141,146] have sometimes been used; however, recent studies suggest these can often be replaced by targeted approaches, sparing patients unnecessary toxicities and long-term infectious risks associated with splenectomy.[147] Patients infected with HIV should receive cART, although intolerance to a number of drugs, including antiretrovirals, may occur until MCD is controlled. Given the many uncertainties in managing patients with KSHV-MCD, including length of treatment, role of maintenance therapy, and evaluation and management of concurrent malignancies, consideration should be given to referral to a clinical trial.

Inflammatory symptoms similar to those in KSHV-MCD have been described in patients infected with KSHV without pathologic evidence of KSHV-MCD.[148] These patients presented with a constellation of fevers, cachexia, and laboratory abnormalities including cytopenias, hypoalbuminemia, and elevated C-reactive protein. Patients had elevated KSHV viral loads and disturbances of vIL-6 and human IL-6 and IL-10 similar to those seen in KSHV-MCD. However, splenomegaly, and lymphadenopathy were not prominent, and pathologic evidence of KSHV-MCD was not demonstrable. This syndrome has been provisionally named KSHV inflammatory cytokine syndrome, and a working case definition has been proposed.[149] KSHV inflammatory cytokine syndrome may accompany KSHV-associated tumors (KS or PEL) or occur in their absence. Its pathophysiology, clinical outcomes, and relationship to KSHV-MCD are being evaluated.

LYMPHOID TUMORS IN PATIENTS WITH HIV

Overview

Lymphoid tumors (see Table 117.1) in individuals infected with HIV represent a range of histologies and include lymphomas seen in immunocompetent patients as well as lymphomas more specifically associated with HIV infection. Risk for individual tumors vary based on the underlying HIV disease status, while outcomes are largely defined by the natural history of a specific tumor as well as choice of an appropriate therapeutic approach for a given tumor. The most common tumors, DLBCL, BL, and cHL, generally occur among patients infected with HIV with relatively preserved immune function. Treatment options for these tumors are informed by clinical studies, and they are highly curable, highlighting the importance of accurate diagnosis of HIV disease status. Less common tumors include PCNSL, systemic DLBCL with immunoblastic phenotype, plasmablastic lymphoma, PEL, and KSHV-MCD (previously discussed with KS). These tumors continue to represent a clinical challenge due to lack of prospective clinical studies, but should also generally be approached with curative intent.

Prior to the cART era, prognosis for patients with HIV with lymphoid tumors was determined primarily by CD4 cell count.[150] Systemic ARLs were often treated as a single disease entity, often with reduced dose chemotherapy regimens, and outcomes were generally poor. However, clinical trials performed in the cART era demonstrate that standard-dose chemotherapy regimens can be administered and improve survival. While baseline CD4 cell count remains important prognostically, lymphoma-specific features[49,52,55,151] and treatment related factors are now critical, especially in patients with CD4 cell counts >100/mm[3].

Clinical decision making must be based both on lymphoma classification and assessment of the immune status and possible AIDS-related comorbidities. The clinical status of patients with HIV infection ranges from healthy with preserved immunity to immunosuppressed with multiple comorbidies. An individualized clinical approach must take this potential spectrum into account. For healthier patients, treatment is similar to the HIV-unrelated counterpart. However, patients with advanced AIDS may not tolerate therapy as well, and close coordination of chemotherapy with HIV management and supportive care is critical. Importantly, poor performance status is often due to the underlying malignancy or treatable opportunistic infections, and even patients with poor performance status should be considered for full-dose curative therapies in most instances. With a shift in demographics of HIV infection to communities with less access to medical care, patients continue to present with lymphoma as the initial manifestation of HIV. These cART-naïve patients usually have HIV that can be rapidly suppressed, and with effective lymphoma treatment and access to cART, they generally have favorable long-term survival. Effective cancer therapy in these patients is therefore essential.

Pathophysiology

HIV-related lymphomagenesis depends on numerous factors, including the degree of immune suppression (discussed with each specific tumor type) and cumulative time with uncontrolled HIV viremia.[47] The pathogenesis is related to B-cell immune activation. Elevated serum cytokines including IL-6, IL-10,[42,152] and tumor necrosis factor-β, as well as the activation marker, soluble CD30,[153] are detectable prior to ARL diagnosis. Several genetic polymorphisms related to B-cell activation are also associated with ARL risk, including the 3'A variant of stromal cell–derived factor 1[154] and -592C/C IL-10 promoter.[42] The HIV coreceptor CCR5 deletion variant CCR5-Δ32 also confers protection against NHL, independent of its HIV protective effect.[155] In the setting of HIV, B-cell activation in EBV-infected cells may be increased in part due to expression of a virally encoded CD40-like latent membrane protein.[156] Activation also occurs also in EBV-uninfected B-cells through other inflammatory stimuli[44,48] and perhaps direct interactions with HIV itself.[157,158]

Regardless of the nature of immune activation, translocations and aberrant somatic hypermutation are common features of many ARL,[159] including DLBCL and BL. For most ARL, B-cell activation leads to upregulation of activation-induced cytidine deaminase,[160] an enzyme required for GC class switch recombination and somatic hypermutation. However, activation-induced cytidine deaminase also can induce mutations and pathogenic translocations,[161] which is a critical step in lymphomagenesis. Translocation of *c-myc/Ig* are seen in not only in BL, but are also present in DLBCL in patients infected with HIV at a higher frequency than observed in HIV-uninfected cases,[162] and a majority of EBV+ plasmablastic lymphomas.[163]

Clinical Presentation, Staging, and Approach to Treatment

Lymphoid malignancy can be the initial presenting illness in HIV,[164,165] and HIV testing should be performed in patients with aggressive B-cell lymphomas or cHL. ARL frequently presents with either a rapidly growing mass or "B" symptoms (fever, night sweats, or weight loss in excess of 10% of the normal body weight). Extranodal involvement of bone marrow, gastrointestinal tract, and central nervous system (CNS) is common.[37] Staging should include computed tomography of neck, chest, abdomen, and pelvis; fluorodeoxyglucose ([18]FDG)-positron emission tomography (PET); lactate dehydrogenase; complete blood count with differential; bone marrow biopsy; and lumbar puncture with evaluation of cerebral spinal fluid (CSF) by cytology and flow cytometry. Evaluation of cardiac function is recommended. CNS imaging, generally with magnetic resonance imaging (MRI) with gadolinium, should be performed to evaluate for CNS involvement in patients with NHL, particularly BL. CNS imaging is not standard for cHL or KSHV-MCD, although in rare cases, cHL in patients with HIV can involve the CNS. Baseline HIV viral load, CD4 count, HBV core antibody and surface antigen, and hepatitis C virus serology should be evaluated. Patients with detectable HBV core antibody or surface antigen should be screened for quantitative HBV viral load.

A high percentage (12% to 57%) of patients with ARL, especially BL, have CNS involvement at presentation.[37,54,55] Routine CNS prophylaxis is generally used, although some favor stratifying patients based on extranodal disease. Prophylaxis has varied between studies, but generally includes intrathecal methotrexate (12 mg) and/or cytosine arabinoside (50 mg) for a total of four to eight doses. CNS involvement by DLBCL confers a poor prognosis. Several intensive intraventricular and intrathecal methotrexate schedules have shown activity. Most commonly, therapy is administered using an Ommaya reservoir twice weekly until 2 weeks after negative CSF flow cytometry is documented (for a minimum of eight doses), and then continued weekly for 6 to 8 weeks, then monthly for 6 months.[55,56]

Supportive care and use of cART during lymphoma therapy deserves special consideration. While effective cART has reduced the incidence of HIV-associated lymphoid tumors and has improved survival, no randomized trial exists to clarify the utility of cART during chemotherapy. On one hand, earlier control of HIV viremia and immune reconstitution may improve long-term infectious outcomes, especially in patients with low CD4 counts. However, there are important potential pharmacokinetic and toxicity interactions between cART and chemotherapeutic agents. As a class, protease inhibitors (especially ritonavir) inhibit CYP3A4 and have potential interactions with other drugs, such as cyclophosphamide.[166–168] Additionally, zidovudine should generally be avoided because of additive hematotoxicity, and renal function should be monitored in patients on tenofovir. Nonetheless, substantial data from phase 2 studies that have included cART suggest that chemotherapy and cART can be concomitantly administered,[169] usually with growth factor support. However, use of cART during chemotherapy for DLBCL and BL is not essential, and phase 2 studies of dose-adjusted etoposide, doxorubicin, and vincristine with oral prednisone and bolus cyclophosphamide (DA-EPOCH; both with

and without rituximab) demonstrated excellent results while withholding cART during lymphoma treatment.[54,55] More recently, pooled data from 19 trials with varied approaches to cART suggests that after correction for CD4 count and other prognostic and treatment-related factors, concurrent cART may be associated with improved response rates and a trend toward improved overall survival.[170] While these studies suggest an advantage for concurrent cART, it is important that in the face of toxicity-limiting ability to administer curative-intent therapy, suspension of nonessential drugs, including cART, is a reasonable first maneuver, especially in patients with CD4 counts >100 cells/mm³. When cART is discontinued, it should be resumed promptly after completion of therapy. Often, physicians who treat patients infected with HIV who have lymphoid tumors, continue cART, preferably with a protease inhibitor–sparing regimen. Additionally, newer antiretroviral drugs to avoid during chemotherapy are class-combination formulations that contain potent pharmacologic boosters such as cobicistat, which may have substantial effects on the chemotherapy. It is also reasonable to defer cART initiation in patients not on therapy until after initiating chemotherapy.

Given risk of infections both during and after completion of chemotherapy, especially in patients with CD4 counts <100 cells/mm³, attention to supportive care is critically important. All patients infected with HIV being treated for lymphoma, regardless of baseline CD4 count, should receive prophylaxis against PCP, preferably with trimethoprim-sulfamethoxazole. Patients with a CD4 count <50 to 100 cells/mm³ also require azithromycin 1,200 mg weekly as prophylaxis against atypical mycobacterial infections. Prophylaxis against herpes simplex virus reactivation using valacyclovir should be strongly considered. Patients with detectable hepatitis B viremia require antiviral therapy for HBV. Care is required to ensure that therapy of intercurrent HBV avoids compromising HIV control, as single-agent therapy for HBV will increase the likelihood of a specific HIV mutation, M184V, which renders patients resistant to several important antiretroviral agents. Patients with mucosal *Candida* infections should not receive azoles concurrently with chemotherapy.

Diffuse Large B-Cell Lymphoma

The majority of NHL occurring in patients with HIV are large B-cell lymphomas or BL. With more sophisticated molecular categorization, DLBCL itself is increasingly recognized as a constellation of genetically unique diseases. In the setting of HIV, various large B-cell lymphoma subtypes are associated with the degree of immune suppression and in some cases dysregulated control of oncogenic herpesviruses.

Immunohistochemical (IHC) markers are helpful in categorizing DLBCL subtypes (Table 117.4) and may provide important diagnostic and prognostic information.[57,171–173] However, DLBCL seen in HIV is often categorized as DLBCL, not otherwise specified, because it does not meet the criteria of the other more highly specified DLBCL types. Although many cases are DLBCL, not otherwise specified, phenotypic characterization as centroblastic (associated with higher CD4 cells and with GC phenotype) and the immunoblastic variant (associated with lower CD4 cells and the ABC phenotype) remains useful.[55] Gene expression profiling (GEP) is the gold standard for distinguishing GC from ABC DLBCL in patients not infected with HIV. However, gene expression profiling and associated IHC algorithms were not developed or validated in the setting of HIV-associated DLBCL. Identification of DLBCL subtypes by ICH does not consistently segregate the biologic entities into the GEP-defined prognostic groups, regardless of HIV status.[174] However, assessment of GEP in HIV DLBCL is needed to insure that there are no major differences in ABC and GBC DLBCL subtypes based on HIV status. A combination of IHC for B-cell lineage markers and the KSHV protein, latency-associated nuclear antigen, in situ hydridization for

TABLE 117.4

Comparison of HIV-Associated Lymphomas

Histogenetic Origin	Histology	Viral Associations (%)		Histogenetic Markers (%)			Pathobiologic Markers (%)				CD4 Cells	Prospects for Chemosensitivity	Prognosis in cART Era
		EBV	KSHV	MUM1	Syn-1	BCL-2	BCL-6	P53	c-MYC			
Germinal center	Burkitt lymphoma	<50	0	<15	0	0	100	60	100	May be relatively well preserved	Favorable	Excellent
	DLBCL–GC	<30	0	<30	0	0	>75	Rare	0–50	Variable	Favorable	Excellent
Postgerminal center	DLBCL–ABC	>50	Rare	100	>50	30	0	0	0–20	Usually low	Intermediate	Relatively poor
	PCNSL	>95	0	>50	<60	90	<50	0	0	<50/mm^3	Unknown	Poor
	Primary effusion lymphoma	>80	100	100	>90	0	0	0	0	Variable	Unknown	Poor
	Plasmablastic lymphoma	>70	Rare	100	100	0	0	Rare	0	Variable	Unknown	Poor

EBV, Epstein-Barr virus; KSHV, Kaposi sarcoma–associated herpes virus; MUM1, multiple myeloma-1; cART, combination antiretroviral therapy; DLBCL, diffuse large B-cell lymphoma; GC, germinal center subtype; ABC, activated B-cell subtype; PCNSL, primary diffuse large B-cell lymphoma of the central nervous system.

EBV-encoded small RNAs, and evaluation for *c-myc/Ig* transloca- tions is warranted, and is generally necessary to categorize the rarer large B-cell lymphoma subtypes such as PBL and PEL. Determi- nation of B-cell clonality by polymerase chain reaction (PCR) evaluation of immunoglobulin genes is sometime helpful, and additional molecular diagnostic biomarkers are likely to become increasingly important. Given development of novel agents such as lenalidomide and ibrutinib in HIV-unrelated DLBCL, it will become increasingly important to determine DLBCL subtypes in the setting of HIV, as these agents appear particularly active in ABC DLBCL. In anticipation of these advances, the NCI- sponsored AIDS-Malignancy Consortium (AMC) is conducting trials to determine safety and dosing considerations of novel agents in conjunction with the various classes of cART.

Therapy with curative intent is indicated for nearly all patients with HIV and lymphoid malignancies. This is particularly true for the commonest and best-studied tumor, DLBCL. DA-EPOCH-R (rituximab, 96-hour continuous infusion etoposide, doxorubicin, and vincristine with oral prednisone and bolus cyclophospha- mide, followed by filgrastim, dose-adjusted for tolerance), short- course DA-EPOCH with dose-dense rituximab (SC-EPOCH-RR), R-CHOP (rituximab, cyclophosphamide, doxorubicin, vincristine, and prednisone), and R-CDE (rituximab, 96-hour continuous in- fusion cyclophosphamide, doxorubicin, and etoposide, followed by filgrastim) have all been evaluated prospectively (Table 117.5). Studies have enrolled populations with varying HIV-related and other characteristics, as well as differing disease subtypes, includ- ing in some cases BL and unclassifiable NHL, as well as a varying or unknown proportion of GC and immunoblastic phenotypes of DLBCL. They have also used different approaches to cART and varying numbers of chemotherapy cycles. Given the impact of these factors, comparison of studies is difficult. Nonetheless, re- cent studies have clarified the role of rituximab, provided evidence that patients can tolerate full-dose regimens, and demonstrated that patients with GC DLBCL and BL generally have excellent outcomes when treated with SC-EPOCH-RR.[55,170,175,176] Recently, pooled data from 1,546 patients in 19 ARL prospective trials was analyzed for treatment factors affecting outcomes. It demon- strated that after correcting for established prognostic factors and intensity of chemotherapy, compared to CHOP, infusional che- motherapy resulted in decreased treatment-related mortality and progressive disease, as well as improved overall survival for patients with DLBCL.[170] This should be viewed as the strongest level of evidence data supporting infusional chemotherapy over standard bolus R-CHOP in HIV-related DLBCL.

The majority of ARLs express CD20, and consensus exists that rituximab, an anti-CD20 monoclonal antibody, should be used in CD20-expressing lymphomas in the setting of HIV. The pooled ARL prospective trial data[170] showed rituximab conferred a remark- able overall survival benefit with a hazard ratio of 0.51 ($p < 0.0001$) after correcting for established prognostic factors and intensity of chemotherapy. Some of the major studies included in this pooled analysis are discussed in the following, and this pooled data should be viewed as the strongest evidence level to support use of ritux- imab in patients with HIV and CD20+ lymphoma. These results are important, because early in the cART era, a randomized phase 3

TABLE 117.5

Selected Regimens and Outcomes for AIDS-Associated Non-Hodgkin Lymphoma

Regimen	Evaluable Patients/ Total Patients	Median Baseline CD4 cells/mm³	Complete Response Rate (%)	Percent Progression-Free 1 y	Percent Progression-Free 2 y	Study (Ref.)
Infusional CDE (cART-era patients only)	55/55	227	44		36	Sparano et al.[256]
Three pooled phase II trials of R-CDE	74/74	161	70		59	Spina et al.[179]
Dose-adjusted EPOCH (cART deferment until chemotherapy completion)	39/39	198	74		73	Little et al.[54]
Randomized						Sparano et al.[176]
R-DA-EPOCH	48/54	181	73	78	66	
vs. DA-EPOCH followed by rituximab	53/56	194	55	66	63	
Short-course dose-adjusted EPOCH-RR (cART deferment until chemotherapy completion)						
Diffuse large B-cell lymphoma	33/33	208	91		84	Dunleavy et al.[55]
Subgroup analysis, GC	21			96		
Subgroup analysis, non-GC	8			38		
Burkitt lymphoma	11/11	322	100	100	100	Dunleavy et al.[56]
Randomized						Kaplan et al.[178]
R-CHOP	99/99	130	57.6	50	34	
vs. CHOP	50/51	147	47	48	38	
Phase 2 R-CHOP						
High-risk patients excluded	52/61	172	77	69		Boue et al.[167]
No exclusion of high-risk patients	80/86	158	69	55		Ribera et al.[168]

CDE, cyclophosphamide, doxorubicin, and etoposide; cART, combination antiretroviral therapy; R-CDE, rituximab with CDE; EPOCH, etoposide, doxorubicin, and vincristine with oral prednisone and bolus cyclophosphamide; R-DA-EPOCH, rituximab (R) with dose-adjusted (DA) EPOCH; R-CHOP, rituximab with cyclophosphamide, doxorubicin, vincristine, and prednisone (CHOP).
Patients enrolled in the short-course DA-EPOCH-RR study received cyclophosphamide 750 mg/m² compared to lower doses adjusted to CD4 counts in the other DA-EPOCH studies, as well as additional rituximab 375 mg/m² on day 6 of therapy. Only the studies in Dunleavey et al.[55] and Ribera et al.[168] were limited to diffuse large B-cell lymphoma.

trial comparing CHOP with R-CHOP found insufficient evidence of a rituximab benefit. The study showed evidence of rituximab activity; complete response rate was 22% higher in the R-CHOP arm, and only 8% of the group receiving R-CHOP had disease progression, compared with 21.6% of those receiving CHOP alone, consistent with expectations of rituximab benefit in the non-HIV setting.[177] However, the trial was not powered to be statistically significant at this level of difference. Additionally, 14% of patients receiving rituximab died of treatment-related infections, annulling any survival advantage.[178] Importantly, the majority of deaths were attributed to infections in patients with <50 CD4 cells/mm^3 at entry. Two subsequent phase 2 trials of R-CHOP in ARL have demonstrated a complete response rate of 69% to 75%.[167,168] In one trial that excluded high-risk patients with CD4 <100 cells/mm^3, prior AIDS-defining illnesses, or Eastern Cooperative Oncology Group performance status <2, no excess in infectious deaths were observed.[167] These findings emphasize the importance of detailed attention to management of AIDS, including antibiotic prophylaxis and surveillance for infections, in patients with <50 CD4+ cells/mm^3 undergoing immunochemotherapy.

Rituximab has also been evaluated in combination with infusional regimens in HIV-associated lymphomas. An early phase 2 trial of DA-EPOCH with suspension of cART reported a complete response rate of 74% and a disease-free and overall survival of 92% and 60%, respectively, at a median follow-up of 53 months.[54] Two follow-up studies evaluated rituximab combined with DA-EPOCH. The first was an AMC-sponsored multicenter randomized phase 2 study of DA-EPOCH with concurrent versus sequential rituximab. Cyclophosphamide dosing was based on CD4 count, and cART was continued in 71% of patients. Therapeutic benefit of rituximab was suggested, with a 73% complete response rate in the concurrent rituximab arm compared with 55% in the sequential rituximab arm.[176] In a study performed by the NCI intramural program, SC-EPOCH-RR with suspension of cART during therapy and no decrease in cyclophosphamide dosing based on CD4 count was evaluated in patients with DLBCL.[55] The number of cycles administered was adapted to response, with patients receiving one cycle beyond stable radiographic and negative ^{18}FDG-PET scans. Patients received a median of three cycles (range, three to five cycles). Complete response rate was 91%, and with 5-year median follow-up, progression-free and overall survival were 85% and 68%, respectively. Tumor histogenesis was important prognostically: 95% of patients with GC phenotype were progression-free, compared with <40% with ABC phenotype. Additional studies to evaluate the generalizability of interim ^{18}FDG-PET in determining the number of cycles are required. The third rituximab-based regimen is R-CDE. In a pooled analysis from three phase 2 studies of R-CDE every 4 weeks for six cycles, and with 76% of patients receiving concurrent cART, the complete response rate was 70% and both disease-free and overall survival were 55% at a median follow-up of 23 months.[179] There was a 3% infection-related death rate during treatment, and additional deaths due to opportunistic infections following treatment.

Primary Diffuse Large B-Cell Lymphoma of the Central Nervous System

AIDS-related PCNSL almost always occurs in patients with a CD4 count of <50 cells/mm^3. Contrast computed tomography or MRI usually demonstrates single or multiple contrast-enhancing masses that are not reliably distinguishable from toxoplasmosis or other CNS processes. Definitive diagnosis requires stereotactic biopsy. In the pre-cART era, patients with AIDS and PCNSL rarely survived more than 6 months, regardless of treatment.[180,181] Despite cART, outcomes in AR-PCNSL remain poor.[53,58] Factors associated with improved survival include receiving lymphoma-directed therapy, availability of cART, and lack of a diagnosis of CNS infection prior to PCNSL diagnosis.[59] For patients with AIDS and

ring-enhancing brain masses, optimal outcome is predicated on initiation of cART and timely institution of appropriate therapy for the brain lesions. Treatment delays increase the likelihood of permanent residual neurologic disability. Historically, this patient population was treated with empiric antibiotics for possible toxoplasmosis with a 2-week watch-and-wait period; however, this approach is no longer justified. Neurologic impairment with a brain mass should be viewed as a medical urgency requiring appropriate diagnostic evaluations and prompt treatment.

A major advance in diagnosis of CNS masses in patients with AIDS was the incorporation of relatively noninvasive diagnostic methods.[182,183] Essentially, all AIDS-PCNSL is EBV-related,[183] and detection of EBV DNA by PCR in the CSF combined with positive brain ^{201}Tl single-photon emission computed tomography (^{201}Tl-SPECT) has been shown to reliably predict the presence of PCNSL.[184] Increased ^{201}Tl-SPECT uptake combined with positive EBV-DNA had 100% sensitivity and 100% positive predictive value for PCNSL, whereas if both tests have negative results, negative predictive value is 100%. ^{18}FDG-PET is also highly specific for malignancy and can also be used in combination with evaluation of CSF for EBV in patients with <50 CD4 cells/mm^3.[185,186] These diagnostic modalities should be incorporated in upfront evaluation of patients with AIDS and CNS masses. However, it should be noted that CSF evaluation of EBV-PCR is not specific for PCNSL.[187,188] Also, brain ^{18}FDG-PET can detect other malignancies, and evaluation must take into account the possibility of CNS involvement of systemic NHL or metastatic NADM. Ideally, PCNSL requires tissue diagnosis. Nonetheless, in the context of CD4 count <50 cells/mm^3, the combination of a high EBV viral load in the CSF, a ring-enhancing brain mass on MRI, and a positive ^{201}Tl-SPECT or ^{18}FDG-PET may be considered highly suggestive of AIDS-PCNSL, and if a tissue diagnosis cannot be obtained, it can be used as a basis to institute therapy for presumptive AIDS-related PCNSL.

There is no standard therapy for AIDS-related PCNSL, and patients should be considered for referral to a clinical trial. Treatment should include initiation of cART, which has been shown in retrospective studies to improve overall survival.[181,189] AIDS-PCNSL is highly responsive to whole-brain irradiation, and most patients can be expected to have initial clinical improvement. Early in the cART era, the 1-year overall survival with whole-brain irradiation and cART was only 20%.[181] In a subsequent Japanese report, the estimated 3-year overall survival in patients receiving >30 Gy whole-brain irradiation (57% received focal boost) combined with cART was 64%.[190] However, given improved survival of patients with AIDS with the availability of cART and the risk of devastating late neurotoxicity from radiation therapy to the CNS, especially when combined with chemotherapy,[54,191] radiation-sparing approaches may be preferable. The best therapeutic approach in such patients may be shown to be institution of cART to achieve rapid immune reconstitution and control the EBV-related lymphoproliferative process, along with immunochemotherapy for the lymphoma. Intriguingly, reports of sustained complete responses in select patients with posttransplant primary CNS EBV-associated lymphoproliferative disorder treated with rituximab alone have been reported.[192] Ongoing clinical trials are investigating the incorporation of rituximab into chemotherapy-based PCNSL treatments, and preliminary data suggest this to be useful.[193,194]

Lymphomas Found More Specifically in HIV: Plasmablastic Lymphoma and Primary Effusion Lymphoma

A number of rare lymphomas can develop in patients infected with HIV. Two recently recognized large B-cell lymphomas are of special interest given their strong association with both HIV and gamma-herpes viruses. PBL is an EBV-associated B-cell NHL proposed as a new entity in 1997.[140] Although most common in the setting of HIV, PBL also occurs in organ transplantation patients and elderly individuals.[195–197] It often presents in the oral cavity, but may occur at other extranodal or nodal sites. A retrospective review of 112 published cases summarized the spectrum of clinical presentations.[198] HIV-associated PBL was found to usually present as either stage I or stage IV disease and to have a 7:1 male:female predominance. The median CD4 count at diagnosis was 178 cells/mm³. Ann Arbor staging did not appear prognostic, and patients with stage I disease should be treated the same as those with systemic disease. PBL is characterized by a high proliferative index and aggressive clinical course, perhaps due to c-*myc*/*Ig* translocations that are seen in 74% of EBV-associated plasmablastic lymphomas.[163] Historically, prognosis has been poor, with median survival <2 years. Outcomes are poor with CHOP.[199] However, retrospective data suggest outcomes for PBL in patients infected with HIV may be improved in the cART era.[200] In 17 patients infected with HIV with PBL, 1-year overall survival was 67% with a number of patients alive at several years. As a rare disease, additional studies are required to better define optimal therapy. Currently, treatment with regimens effective in tumors with high proliferative rates, such as DA-EPOCH, is recommended, preferably within the setting of a clinical trial.

PEL is a rare KSHV-associated aggressive mature B-cell lymphoma that usually presents as a lymphomatous effusion; patients are at risk for other KSHV-associated malignancies. Patients often present with inflammatory syndromes, hypoalbuminemia, thrombocytopenia, anemia, and associated elevated IL-6 and circulating KSHV viral load.[201] Pleural, peritoneal, pericardial, and leptomeningeal presentations can be seen. Extracavitary PEL has phenotypic and molecular similarities to PEL[202] and may present in a variety of locations, including lymph nodes, the gastrointestinal tract, or cutaneous tissues. Diagnosis of PEL depends on the demonstration of KSHV infection of tumor cells. In >70% of cases, tumor cells are co-infected with EBV. Common B-cell surface markers (CD19, CD20, CD79a) are absent, while activation markers (CD30, CD38, CD71, CD138) are often present; immunoglobulin gene rearrangements confirm B-cell monoclonality. Evaluation of the extent of disease should be performed following the guidelines for NHL staging. There are few data to guide therapy in PEL, and the outcome is generally poor, with a median survival of <6 months in most case series.[203] However, there are a few case reports of patients having long-term remissions. Patients should ideally be treated within clinical studies if possible.

Burkitt Lymphoma

BL often occurs in patients with relatively preserved immune status and makes up 17% of HIV-associated lymphomas in the cART era.[53] Until recently, clinical trials of ARL generally included both DLBCL and BL. It is now appreciated that just as in the HIV-unrelated setting, BL requires specialized curative intent therapy. CHOP-based therapy results in poor outcomes in HIV-associated BL,[52] and increasing evidence supports short course intense therapy or short course low-intensity therapy with EPOCH-R. Studies of BL in the adult setting are mainly comprised of relatively small phase 2 studies, and randomized data does not exist to inform standard treatment, therefore the phase 2 data presented is the best evidence available. Additionally, the pooled data analysis from 19 ARL studies had an insufficient number of BL cases to form firm conclusions.

Importantly, excellent 90% long-term overall survival was recently reported for BL in 11 patients infected with HIV treated with SC-EPOCH-R with cART deferred until after treatment.[56] This study treated 30 patients overall, and the HIV-positive and HIV-unrelated patients all did equally well. A prospective NCI sponsored study with participation by the US Cooperative Groups is under way to further evaluate DA-EPOCH-R in BL. An important advantage to EPOCH-R in this setting is its favorable toxicity profile. Most cycles can often be given as an outpatient.

The more conventional short course high-intensity BL regimens have also been studied in HIV and are feasible to administer. However, they are toxic regimens requiring hospitalization in most cases and have some treatment-related mortality. CODOX-M/IVAC (cyclophosphamide, vincristine, doxorubicin, methotrexate plus ifosfamide, etoposide, and cytarabine)[204] is one such regimen.[205,206] A 70% complete response rate was seen in retrospective studies in HIV-associated BL; however, treatment-related mortality was 30%.[206] Evaluation of a prospective AMC–sponsored phase 2 study of 34 patients treated with modified CODOX-M/IVAC combined with rituximab is ongoing. Preliminary results demonstrated 1-year overall survival of 83% and 9% treatment-related mortality.[207] HyperCVAD (cyclophosphamide, vincristine, doxorubicin, dexamethasone, cytarabine, mesba, methotrexate, leucovorin) has also been reported in 13 patients with a 2-year overall survival of 48%.[208] Inclusion of rituximab in whatever regimen is used is recommended. DA-EPOCH-R with full-dose cyclophosphamide and intrathecal methotrexate should be strongly considered for patients with AIDS-BL, preferably within the ongoing NCI-sponsored national clinical trial.

Hodgkin Lymphoma

cHL[209] occurs with a markedly increased frequency in people infected with HIV; it is categorized as an NADM. EBV-associated mixed cellularity histology is most common, while nodular sclerosis histology is most common in patients who are HIV-negative.[210,212] The association between cHL and CD4 cell count is complex. In general, cHL occurs when the CD4 cells are relatively intact. Often, the diagnosis is made shortly after the diagnosis of HIV and median CD4 count is at diagnosis is >200 cells/mm³.[210,212] Declining CD4 counts are sometimes noted before diagnosis and later attributed to cHL itself.[213] There is uncertainty as to why there is excess risk of cHL in the first year of cART therapy, but it has been speculated that disease manifestations may be related to an immune reconstitution phenomena. Interestingly, a precipitous drop in CD4 cells in the year before cHL diagnosis may be a heralding event.[165,213] Patients with HIV-associated Hodgkin lymphoma are generally older and present with higher-stage disease. They present less frequently with mediastinal involvement as noted in the nodular sclerosing subtype, and more frequent involvement of extranodal sites of disease, and more frequent "B" symptoms compared to patients with cHL and without HIV. Bone marrow involvement is common, and 20% of cases of hemophagocytic syndrome in patients with HIV may be attributed to cHL.[214]

In the cART era, treatment outcome for cHL in patients infected with HIV is comparable to the HIV-unrelated counterpart.[215] Conventional chemotherapy regimens such as ABVD (doxorubicin, bleomycin, vinblastine, and dacarbazine)[216] or risk-adapted combined-modality therapy are often used.[212] In a prospective German multicenter study, 108 patients with HIV-associated cHL were treated with risk and stage-adapted therapy. Patients with early stage disease were treated with two to four cycles of ABVD and involved–field radiation, while those with unfavorable disease were treated with six to eight cycles of BEACOPP (bleomycin, etoposide, cyclophosphamide, vincristine, procarbazine and prednisone), unless they had advanced HIV infection, in which case they were treated with ABVD. Patients received concurrent cART. The 2-year progression-free survival was 95% to 100% for early stage disease and 89% for advanced-stage disease. Two-year overall survival in the entire cohort was 90.7%. Although toxicities were manageable in this study, severe hematotoxity and neurotoxicity due to drug-drug interactions between vinblastine and protease inhibitors have been observed, and as with ARL, protease inhibitor–based regimens should generally be avoided.[217] A clinical trial sponsored by the AMC is currently evaluating the anti-CD30-immunotoxin brentuximab in combination with doxorubicin, vincristine, and dacarbazine in HIV-associated cHL.

Relapsed and Refractory Lymphoma in Patients Infected with HIV

Outside the setting of HIV infection, high-dose chemotherapy with autologous peripheral stem cell transplant (HDT-PBSCT) is sometimes used for patients with relapsed DLBCL or cHL. HDT-PBSCT is feasible in patients infected with HIV.[218–221] Across several conditioning regimens, treatment-related mortality is 3% to 5%, and outcomes are generally comparable to HIV-negative patients.[218–221] There is the risk of secondary myelodysplastic syndrome.[221] In a retrospective series across AMC sites, 88 patients with refractory lymphoma were treated with curative intent second-line therapy with regimens such as DA-EPOCH; ifosfamide, carboplatin, etoposide; and etoposide, methylprednisolone, cytarabine, and cisplatin. A total of 32 patients (36%) had a response to second-line therapy (21 complete responses), and 10 went on to HDT-PBSCT. However, there was no difference in survival amongst those who went on to transplant compared to those who did not, with estimated 1-year survival in responding patients of approximately 70%.[222] These results suggest that HDT-PBSCT transplant outcomes in DLBCL and HL are comparable with results in HIV-negative patients, but that durable responses may be achievable with second-line therapy alone in some cases.

Allogeneic transplant has also been explored in a limited number of patients with ARL. In one case where a patient infected with HIV with refractory leukemia received a matched unrelated donor transplant, the use of a donor with a Δ32 CCR5 mutation that makes the cells resistant to infection with CCR5 strains of HIV appears to have resulted in the eradication of HIV infection.[223] However, two other cases of allogeneic transplantation in which the donor did not have the Δ32 mutation failed to achieve such eradication, even though cART was continued throughout therapy. Future studies will be needed to clarify the role of allogeneic transplantation in the treatment of refractory lymphoma as well as its potential role in eradicating HIV.

HUMAN PAPILLOMAVIRUS–ASSOCIATED CANCER IN HIV INFECTION

Patients infected with HIV have an increased incidence of several cancers caused by HPV, including cancer of the cervix, anus, penis, vulva, oral pharynx, and tonsil.[224,225] Of these, only cancer of the cervix is considered AIDS-defining.[1] Women infected with HIV have about a five-fold increased incidence of cervical cancer as compared with women not infected with HIV.[225] The increase in all these cancers is related both to an increased exposure to oncogenic strains of HPV and an impaired ability to clear these strains attributed to HIV-associated immunodeficiency. Women infected with HIV also have an increased risk of premalignant cervical,[226] vulvovaginal, and anal intraepithelial neoplasia.[227] Compared to women not on cART, women on cART have a decreased incidence of precancerous cervical lesions, increased regression of existing precancerous lesions, and increased clearance of oncogenic HPV.[228–230] Although not AIDS-defining, people with HIV, especially women and MSM, have a markedly increased risk of anal cancer. The annual incidence of anal cancer in patients with HIV in the United States, estimated at 80 per 100,000 individuals, is much higher than that of the general population, and is increasing.[225] Smoking and lower CD4 nadir are associated with increased risk of development of anal cancer.[231,232] Other HPV-associated cancers, especially cancers of the oral pharynx and tonsil, have also increased in the past decade in individuals infected with HIV.

Cervical Cancer

Prevention of cervical cancer is an important part of care for women with HIV. In the United States, cervical cancer screening guidelines are based largely on regular periodic cervical Papanicolaou (Pap) testing.[233] The CDC and the US Preventative Services Task Force recommend cytologic screening as part of the initial evaluation when HIV is diagnosed.[234] Pap smears showing severe inflammation with reactive squamous cellular changes should be repeated within 3 months. If the initial Pap smear is normal, additional evaluation should be repeated within 6 months. Subsequent monitoring guidelines vary. Additional evaluation of HPV DNA, with a subsequent screening frequency of 6 months in women with detectable high-risk subtypes of HPV and yearly in those without high-risk HPV has been proposed.[235] High-risk women with normal PAP smears should be re-evaluated at least annually, whereas approaches used in women not infected with HIV have been advocated for women on effective cART, relatively preserved CD4 counts, no evidence of oncogenic HPV, and negative Pap smears.

If a Pap smear shows squamous intraepithelial lesions or atypical squamous cells of undetermined significance, cervical colposcopic examination with directed biopsies of mucosal abnormalities is indicated. Management of premalignant cervical lesions in woman with HIV, especially those with low CD4 counts, is more complicated than that in women not infected with HIV because of higher rates of positive margins and recurrent cervical intraepithelial neoplasia (CIN).[236,237] Low-grade lesions (CIN1) are generally observed, and higher-grade lesions (CIN2-3) are generally treated. Initiation of cART and associated immune reconstitution has been associated with regression of lesions over time and may decrease the risk of recurrence.[228] Treatment options for CIN include ablative therapy, loop excision of the transformation zone, or conization procedures, and should be individualized based on lesion size and location. In resource-limited settings, cervical cancer is a leading cause of cancer-related mortality in women. In this setting, development of cervical cancer screening programs that are less technologically intensive and do not depend on cytopathology are underway. Programs based on cervical visual inspection with acetic acid and immediate cryotherapy (a "screen and treat" approach) as well as rapid HPV testing and treating are being scaled-up and evaluated.[238–241]

Invasive cervical cancer should largely be approached using principles of oncologic management that guide treatment in HIV-negative patients. The International Federation of Gynecology and Obstetrics staging system, used for patients not infected with HIV, is used in this population as well. More recently, [18]FDG-PET has been incorporated in the initial assessment of women with cervical cancer to evaluate para-aortic lymph nodes. However, in women with HIV and cervical cancer, results should be interpreted with the understanding that uncontrolled HIV viremia is associated with generalized lymph node [18]FDG avidity.[242] Treatment is based on clinical stage. There are no clinical trials specific to women infected with HIV with cervical cancer, and HIV-positive women with cervical cancer should be treated in the same manner as those without HIV infection, with cART integrated into the overall treatment plan.

Anal Cancer

Given biologic similarities to cervical cancer and the effectiveness of cervical cancer screening, some experts have suggested that routine periodic cytologic examination of the anal mucosa should also be considered in high-risk individuals.[243] Programs to screen men and women infected with HIV for anal intraepithelial neoplasia and to treat high-grade lesions have been developed. This approach has the potential to prevent anal cancer by detecting and treating premalignant lesions.[244] The primary tool to screen for anal cancer is cytology of the anal epithelium. Most practitioners recommend that abnormal cytology should be followed up with high-resolution anoscopy. Treatment decisions are based on the grade of the lesion. Current options for high-grade anal intraepithelial neoplasia include local treatment with topical immune modulators (e.g., imiquimod)[245,246] or antiviral agents (e.g., cidofovir),[247] electrocautery, laser or infrared coagulation,[248,249] and surgery. It should be noted, however, that while plausible, treatment of anal dysplasia has not been shown to prevent anal cancer. Also, a major difference between anal and cervical cancer prevention is the greater difficulty and morbidity in surgical resection of precancerous lesions of the anus and a high rate of recurrence. An NCI-funded prospective study is planned to determine the effect of treatment of precancerous lesions on subsequent development of anal cancer.

The standard of care for stages I–III anal cancer is concurrent chemoradiation, and patients with HIV should receive standard regimens. In the pre-cART era, patients with CD4 counts <200 cells/mm[3] were more likely to suffer treatment-related toxicity including cytopenias, intractable diarrhea, moist desquamation requiring hospitalization, or a colostomy either for a therapy-related complication or for salvage, whereas patients with ≥200 CD4 cells/mm[3] appeared to have better disease control with acceptable morbidity.[250] However, with the availability of cART, as well as increasing use of intensity-modulated radiation therapy in the treatment of anal cancer over the past decade, toxicities associated with concurrent chemoradiation in this patient population may have decreased. Outcomes in patients with HIV receiving concurrent chemoradiation, including mitomycin-C–based therapy, appear comparable to that of the general population.[251] Surgical abdominoperineal resection is an option for patients with poor performance status and those who do not wish to undergo concurrent chemoradiation. Patients are left with a permanent colostomy, and therefore surgery is generally employed only for the management of locoregional recurrence.

FUTURE DIRECTIONS

Many HIV-associated cancers are associated with oncogenic viruses. In this regard, HIV can play a varied role. HIV-induced immunosuppression can lead to an environment where oncogenic viral infection and opportunistic neoplasia can develop relatively unchecked. HIV can also stimulate immune system cytokine production that promotes cellular proliferation and oligoclonal expansions of premalignant cells. There are thus opportunities to reduce the risk of various HIV-associated cancers by preventing or treating either HIV or the specific oncogenic virus. The HBV and HPV vaccines, for example, hold the potential to dramatically reduce the incidence of hepatocellular, anogenital, and oropharyngeal cancers. Also, studies of the biology of the oncogenic viruses may lead to more targeted treatment or prevention strategies.

In the cART era, NADMs are an increasingly important cause of morbidity and mortality.[19,61] For some NADM, there are biologic differences between those that arise in patients infected with HIV compared to patients not infected with HIV. In cHL, for example, patients infected with HIV are more likely than the general population to develop mixed cellularity and lymphocyte-depleted subtypes. However, in other cancers, such biologic differences have not been established. There is an NCI initiative to encourage enrollment of patients infected with HIV on NCI-funded cancer trials whenever possible. In the absence of evidence for specialized cancer treatment regimens in patients with HIV, standard therapeutic approaches should be strongly considered, especially in patients with good performance status and who are free of other HIV infectious comorbidities.

With the availability of cART, many patients infected with HIV are now able to tolerate standard cancer therapy, including allogeneic stem cell transplantation.[252] Special considerations in treating patients with HIV and cancer include whether to modify the standard treatment for the cancer, whether to continue or start cART, and whether prophylaxis is required for herpes simplex virus, PCP, or *Mycobacterium avium*-intracellulare. Special attention should be paid to potential drug-drug interactions between antiretroviral agents and chemotherapeutic agents. Furthermore, protease inhibitors, especially nelfinavir, may have radiosensitizing effects. Pharmacokinetic studies evaluating the effect of commonly used antiretroviral agents on chemotherapeutic agents are warranted.[253,254]

Although increased knowledge about treatment outcomes for patients with HIV and cancer are required, it appears that with the better-studied tumors, treatment outcomes for HIV-related malignancies that are equivalent to those obtained in HIV-seronegative patients may be attainable.[55,251] In order to promote the oncologic care of patients with HIV/AIDS, it will be important for clinical trials to increasingly include or focus on this population.[255]

SELECTED REFERENCES

The full reference list can be accessed at lwwhealthlibrary.com/oncology.

1. 1993 revised classification system for HIV infection and expanded surveillance case definition for AIDS among adolescents and adults. *MMWR Recomm Rep* 1992;41:1–19.
2. Yarchoan R, Mitsuya H, Myers CE, et al. Clinical pharmacology of 3'-azido-2',3'-dideoxythymidine (zidovudine) and related dideoxynucleosides. *N Engl J Med* 1989;321:726–738.
7. Bonnet F, Burty C, Lewden C, et al. Changes in cancer mortality among HIV-infected patients: the Mortalite 2005 Survey. *Clin Infect Dis* 2009;48:633–639.
11. Shiels MS, Pfeiffer RM, Gail MH, et al. Cancer burden in the HIV-infected population in the United States. *J Natl Cancer Inst* 2011;103:753–762.
14. Yarchoan R, Tosato G, Little RF. Therapy insight: AIDS-related malignancies—the influence of antiviral therapy on pathogenesis and management. *Nat Clin Pract Oncol* 2005;2:406–415.
18. Engels EA, Biggar RJ, Hall HI, et al. Cancer risk in people infected with human immunodeficiency virus in the United States. *Int J Cancer* 2008;123:187–194.
19. Silverberg MJ, Abrams DI. AIDS-defining and non-AIDS-defining malignancies: cancer occurrence in the antiretroviral therapy era. *Curr Opin Oncol* 2007;19:446–451.
25. Chang Y, Cesarman E, Pessin MS, et al. Identification of herpesvirus-like DNA sequences in AIDS-associated Kaposi's sarcoma. *Science* 1994;266:1865–1869.
42. Breen EC, Boscardin WJ, Detels R, et al. Non-Hodgkin's B cell lymphoma in persons with acquired immunodeficiency syndrome is associated with increased serum levels of IL10, or the IL10 promoter -592 C/C genotype. *Clin Immunol* 2003;109:119–129.

54. Little RF, Pittaluga S, Grant N, et al. Highly effective treatment of acquired immunodeficiency syndrome-related lymphoma with dose-adjusted EPOCH: impact of antiretroviral therapy suspension and tumor biology. *Blood* 2003;101:4653–4659.
55. Dunleavy K, Little RF, Pittaluga S, et al. The role of tumor histogenesis, FDG-PET, and short course EPOCH with dose-dense rituximab (SC-EPOCH-RR) in HIV-associated diffuse large B-cell lymphoma. *Blood* 2010;115:3017–3024.
56. Dunleavy K, Pittaluga S, Shovlin M, et al. Low-intensity therapy in adults with Burkitt's lymphoma. *N Engl J Med* 2013;369:1915–1925.
59. Uldrick TS, Pipkin S, Scheer S, et al. Factors associated with survival among patients with AIDS-related primary central nervous system lymphoma. *AIDS* 2014;28(3):397–405.
64. Feng H, Shuda M, Chang Y, et al. Clonal integration of a polyomavirus in human Merkel cell carcinoma. *Science* 2008;319:1096–1100.
74. Boshoff C, Endo Y, Collins PD, et al. Angiogenic and HIV-inhibitory functions of KSHV-encoded chemokines. *Science* 1997;278:290–294.
81. Moore PS, Boshoff C, Weiss RA, et al. Molecular mimicry of human cytokine and cytokine response pathway genes by KSHV. *Science* 1996;274:1739–1744.
87. Brown EE, Whitby D, Vitale F, et al. Virologic, hematologic, and immunologic risk factors for classic Kaposi sarcoma. *Cancer* 2006;107:2282–2290.
92. Aoki Y, Tosato G. HIV-1 Tat enhances Kaposi sarcoma-associated herpesvirus (KSHV) infectivity. *Blood* 2004;104:810–814.
93. Krown SE, Testa MA, Huang J. AIDS-related Kaposi's sarcoma: prospective validation of the AIDS Clinical Trials Group staging classification. AIDS Clinical Trials Group Oncology Committee. *J Clin Oncol* 1997;15:3085–3092.

94. Nasti G, Talamini R, Antinori A, et al. AIDS-related Kaposi's sarcoma: evaluation of potential new prognostic factors and assessment of the AIDS Clinical Trial Group Staging System in the Haart Era—the Italian Cooperative Group on AIDS and Tumors and the Italian Cohort of Patients Naive From Antiretrovirals. *J Clin Oncol* 2003;21:2876–2882.

95. Mosam A, Shaik F, Uldrick TS, et al. A randomized controlled trial of highly active antiretroviral therapy versus highly active antiretroviral therapy and chemotherapy in therapy-naive patients with HIV-associated Kaposi sarcoma in South Africa. *J Acquir Immune Defic Syndr* 2012;60:150–157.

99. Krown SE, Metroka C, Wernz JC. Kaposi's sarcoma in the acquired immune deficiency syndrome: a proposal for uniform evaluation, response, and staging criteria. AIDS Clinical Trials Group Oncology Committee. *J Clin Oncol* 1989;7:1201–1207.

102. Krown SE. Highly active antiretroviral therapy in AIDS-associated Kaposi's sarcoma: implications for the design of therapeutic trials in patients with advanced, symptomatic Kaposi's sarcoma. *J Clin Oncol* 2004;22:399–402.

103. Bower M, Weir J, Francis N, et al. The effect of HAART in 254 consecutive patients with AIDS-related Kaposi's sarcoma. *AIDS* 2009;23:1701–1706.

106. Martinez V, Caumes E, Gambotti L, et al. Remission from Kaposi's sarcoma on HAART is associated with suppression of HIV replication and is independent of protease inhibitor therapy. *Br J Cancer* 2006;94:1000–1006.

107. Bower M, Nelson M, Young AM, et al. Immune reconstitution inflammatory syndrome associated with Kaposi's sarcoma. *J Clin Oncol* 2005;23:5224–5228.

115. Cianfrocca M, Lee S, Von Roenn J, et al. Randomized trial of paclitaxel versus pegylated liposomal doxorubicin for advanced human immunodeficiency virus-associated Kaposi sarcoma: evidence of symptom palliation from chemotherapy. *Cancer* 2010;116:3969–3977.

116. Welles L, Saville MW, Lietzau J, et al. Phase II trial with dose titration of paclitaxel for the therapy of human immunodeficiency virus-associated Kaposi's sarcoma. *J Clin Oncol* 1998;16:1112–1121.

120. Northfelt DW, Dezube BJ, Thommes JA, et al. Pegylated-liposomal doxorubicin versus doxorubicin, bleomycin, and vincristine in the treatment of AIDS-related Kaposi's sarcoma: results of a randomized phase III clinical trial. *J Clin Oncol* 1998;16:2445–2451.

125. Martin DF, Kuppermann BD, Wolitz RA, et al. Oral ganciclovir for patients with cytomegalovirus retinitis treated with a ganciclovir implant. Roche Ganciclovir Study Group. *N Engl J Med* 1999;340:1063–1070.

131. Little RF, Wyvill KM, Pluda JM, et al. Activity of thalidomide in AIDS-related Kaposi's sarcoma. *J Clin Oncol* 2000;18:2593–2602.

133. Koon HB, Honda K, Lee JY, et al. Phase II AIDS Malignancy Consortium (AMC) trial of imatinib in AIDS-associated Kaposi's sarcoma (KS). *12th International Conference on Malignancies in AIDS and Other Acquired Immunodeficiencies*. Bethesda, MD: Infectious Agents and Cancer; 2010:5:A61.

135. Krown SE, Roy D, Lee JY, et al. Rapamycin with antiretroviral therapy in AIDS-associated Kaposi sarcoma: an AIDS Malignancy Consortium study. *J Acquir Immune Defic Syndr* 2012;59:447–454.

136. Soulier J, Grollet L, Oksenhendler E, et al. Kaposi's sarcoma-associated herpesvirus-like DNA sequences in multicentric Castleman's disease. *Blood* 1995;86:1276–1280.

139. Uldrick TS, Polizzotto MN, Aleman K, et al. High-dose zidovudine plus valganciclovir for Kaposi sarcoma herpesvirus-associated multicentric Castleman disease: a pilot study of virus-activated cytotoxic therapy. *Blood* 2011;117:6977–6986.

140. Polizzotto MN, Uldrick TS, Wang V, et al. Human and viral interleukin-6 and other cytokines in Kaposi sarcoma herpesvirus-associated multicentric Castleman disease. *Blood* 2013;122:4189–4198.

142. Gerard L, Berezne A, Galicier L, et al. Prospective study of rituximab in chemotherapy-dependent human immunodeficiency virus associated multicentric Castleman's disease: ANRS 117 CastlemaB Trial. *J Clin Oncol* 2007;25:3350–3356.

143. Hoffmann C, Schmid H, Muller M, et al. Improved outcome with rituximab in patients with HIV-associated multicentric Castleman disease. *Blood* 2011;118:3499–3503.

148. Uldrick TS, Wang V, O'Mahony D, et al. An interleukin-6-related systemic inflammatory syndrome in patients co-infected with Kaposi sarcoma-associated herpesvirus and HIV but without Multicentric Castleman disease. *Clin Infect Dis* 2010;51:350–358.

166. Ratner L, Lee J, Tang S, et al. Chemotherapy for human immunodeficiency virus-associated non-Hodgkin's lymphoma in combination with highly active antiretroviral therapy. *J Clin Oncol* 2001;19:2171–2178.

170. Barta SK, Xue X, Wang D, et al. Treatment factors affecting outcomes in HIV-associated non-Hodgkin lymphomas: a pooled analysis of 1546 patients. *Blood* 2013;122:3251–3262.

175. Levine AM. HIV-associated lymphoma. *Blood* 2010;115:2986–2987.

176. Sparano JA, Lee JY, Kaplan LD, et al. Rituximab plus concurrent infusional EPOCH chemotherapy is highly effective in HIV-associated B-cell non-Hodgkin lymphoma. *Blood* 2010;115:3008–3016.

178. Kaplan LD, Lee JY, Ambinder RF, et al. Rituximab does not improve clinical outcome in a randomized phase III trial of CHOP with or without rituximab in patients with HIV-associated non-Hodgkin's lymphoma: AIDS-malignancies consortium trial 010. *Blood* 2005;106:1538–1543.

179. Spina M, Jaeger U, Sparano JA, et al. Rituximab plus infusional cyclophosphamide, doxorubicin, and etoposide in HIV-associated non-Hodgkin lymphoma: pooled results from 3 phase 2 trials. *Blood* 2005;105:1891–1897.

187. Cingolani A, Gastaldi R, Fassone L, et al. Epstein-Barr virus infection is predictive of CNS involvement in systemic AIDS-related non-Hodgkin's lymphomas. *J Clin Oncol* 2000;18:3325–3330.

198. Castillo J, Pantanowitz L, Dezube BJ. HIV-associated plasmablastic lymphoma: lessons learned from 112 published cases. *Am J Hematol* 2008;83:804–809.

202. Carbone A, Gloghini A, Vaccher E, et al. Kaposi's sarcoma-associated herpesvirus/human herpesvirus type 8-positive solid lymphomas: a tissue-based variant of primary effusion lymphoma. *J Mol Diagn* 2005;7:17–27.

205. Wang ES, Straus DJ, Teruya-Feldstein J, et al. Intensive chemotherapy with cyclophosphamide, doxorubicin, high-dose methotrexate/ifosfamide, etoposide, and high-dose cytarabine (CODOX-M/IVAC) for human immunodeficiency virus-associated Burkitt lymphoma. *Cancer* 2003;98:1196–1205.

210. Tirelli U, Errante D, Dolcetti R, et al. Hodgkin's disease and human immunodeficiency virus infection: clinicopathologic and virologic features of 114 patients from the Italian Cooperative Group on AIDS and Tumors. *J Clin Oncol* 1995;13:1758–1767.

211. Hoffmann C, Chow KU, Wolf E, et al. Strong impact of highly active antiretroviral therapy on survival in patients with human immunodeficiency virus-associated Hodgkin's disease. *Br J Haematol* 2004;125:455–462.

214. Fardet L, Lambotte O, Meynard JL, et al. Reactive haemophagocytic syndrome in 58 HIV-1-infected patients: clinical features, underlying diseases and prognosis. *AIDS* 2010;24:1299–1306.

220. Re A, Michieli M, Casari S, et al. High-dose therapy and autologous peripheral blood stem cell transplantation as salvage treatment for AIDS-related lymphoma: long-term results of the Italian Cooperative Group on AIDS and Tumors (GICAT) study with analysis of prognostic factors. *Blood* 2009;114:1306–1313.

223. Hutter G, Nowak D, Mossner M, et al. Long-term control of HIV by CCR5 Delta32/Delta32 stem-cell transplantation. *N Engl J Med* 2009;360:692–698.

232. Guiguet M, Boue F, Cadranel J, et al. Effect of immunodeficiency, HIV viral load, and antiretroviral therapy on the risk of individual malignancies (FHDH-ANRS CO4): a prospective cohort study. *Lancet Oncol* 2009;10:1152–1159.

234. Workowski KA, Berman SM. Sexually transmitted diseases treatment guidelines, 2006. *MMWR Recomm Rep* 2006;55:1–94.

236. Maiman M, Fruchter RG, Serur E, et al. Recurrent cervical intraepithelial neoplasia in human immunodeficiency virus-seropositive women. *Obstet Gynecol* 1993;82:170–174.

238. Denny L, Kuhn L, Hu CC, et al. Human papillomavirus-based cervical cancer prevention: long-term results of a randomized screening trial. *J Natl Cancer Inst* 2010;102:1557–1567.

240. Sahasrabuddhe VV, Parham GP, Mwanahamuntu MH, et al. Cervical cancer prevention in low- and middle-income countries: feasible, affordable, essential. *Cancer Prev Res* 2012;5:11–17.

243. Palefsky JM. Anal cancer prevention in HIV-positive men and women. *Curr Opin Oncol* 2009;21:433–438.

244. Goldie SJ, Kuntz KM, Weinstein MC, et al. The clinical effectiveness and cost-effectiveness of screening for anal squamous intraepithelial lesions in homosexual and bisexual HIV-positive men. *JAMA* 1999;281:1822–1829.

247. Stier EA, Goldstone SE, Einstein MH, et al. Safety and efficacy of topical cidofovir to treat of high-grade perianal and vulvar intraepithelial neoplasia in HIV-positive men and women. *AIDS* 2013;27:545–551.

253. Deeken JF, Pantanowitz L, Dezube BJ. Targeted therapies to treat non-AIDS-defining cancers in patients with HIV on HAART therapy: treatment considerations and research outlook. *Curr Opin Oncol* 2009;21:445–454.

255. Persad GC, Little RF, Grady C. Including persons with HIV infection in cancer clinical trials. *J Clin Oncol* 2008;26:1027–1032.

256. Sparano JA, Lee S, Chen MG, et al. Phase II trial of infusional cyclophosphamide, doxorubicin, and etoposide in patients with HIV-associated non-Hodgkin's lymphoma: an Eastern Cooperative Oncology Group Trial (E1494). *J Clin Oncol* 2004;22:1491–1500.

PRACTICE OF ONCOLOGY

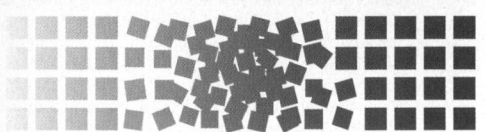

118 Transplantation-Related Malignancies

Smita Bhatia and Ravi Bhatia

INTRODUCTION

An important and potentially devastating complication of hematopoietic cell transplantation (HCT) is the occurrence of subsequent malignant neoplasms (SMN).[1–11] The magnitude of risk of SMNs after HCT ranges from 8-fold to 11-fold that of the general population (Table 118.1).

Several host and clinical factors are associated with an increased risk of SMNs after HCT. These include age at HCT, exposure to chemotherapy and radiation prior to HCT, use of total-body irradiation (TBI) and high-dose chemotherapy for myeloablation, infection with viruses such as Epstein-Barr virus (EBV) and hepatitis B and C viruses, type of transplantation (autologous versus allogeneic), and immunodeficiency after HCT aggravated by the use of immunosuppressive drugs for prophylaxis and treatment of graft-versus-host disease (GVHD).[1]

The heterogeneous nature of SMNs, with differing clinicopathologic characteristics, precludes assessment of risk factors in aggregate. It has become conventional practice to classify SMNs into three distinct groups[12]: (1) myelodysplasia (MDS) and acute myeloid leukemia (AML), (2) lymphoma, including lymphoproliferative disorders, and (3) solid tumors. Although secondary leukemia and lymphoma develop early in the posttransplantation period, secondary solid tumors have a longer latency. In this chapter, the three broad categories of SMNs seen among patients undergoing HCT are discussed, with emphasis on clinical presentation, magnitude of risk and associated risk factors, current insights into pathogenesis, and treatment options and outcome of patients with these malignancies. We will conclude the chapter with a brief summary regarding strategies for early detection of SMNs.

MYELODYSPLASIA AND ACUTE MYELOID LEUKEMIA

Therapy-related MDS (t-MDS) and therapy-related AML have emerged as the major cause of nonrelapse mortality in patients undergoing autologous HCT for Hodgkin lymphoma (HL) and non-Hodgkin lymphoma (NHL).[4,13] The risk of t-MDS/AML approaches 9% after autologous HCT for lymphoma with a median latency of 12 to 24 months after HCT (range, 4 months to 6 years).[4]

Clinicopathologic Syndromes

Two types of t-MDS/AML are recognized in the World Health Organization classification, based on the causative therapeutic exposure: alkylating agent/radiation or topoisomerase II inhibitor.[14]

Alkylating Agent/Radiation-Related Therapy-Related Myelodysplasia/Acute Myeloid Leukemia

In patients exposed to alkylating agents, t-MDS/AML usually appears 4 to 7 years after exposure. Approximately two-thirds of patients present with MDS and the remainder with AML with myelodysplastic features. Patients frequently present with cytopenias. There is a high prevalence of abnormalities involving chromosomes 5 (-5/del[5q]) and 7 (-7/del[7q]).

Topoisomerase II Inhibitor–Related Acute Myeloid Leukemia

AML secondary to topoisomerase II inhibitors presents as overt leukemia, without a preceding myelodysplastic phase. The latency is brief (6 months to 5 years) and is associated with balanced translocations involving chromosome bands 11q23 or 21q22. Other translocations include inv(18)(p13q22) or t(17,19)(q22;q12).[15]

Clinical Diagnosis

The common occurrence of cytopenias after autologous HCT and their nonspecific nature necessitated the need for specific criteria for diagnosing t-MDS/AML developing after HCT. These criteria include (1) significant marrow dysplasia in at least two cell lines, (2) peripheral cytopenias without alternative explanations, and (3) blasts in the marrow defined by French-American-British classification.[16] In patients without blasts, presence of a clonal cytogenetic abnormality in addition to morphologic evidence of dysplasia may aid in making this diagnosis.

Risk Factors for Therapy-Related Myelodysplasia/Acute Myeloid Leukemia After Hematopoietic Cell Transplantation

An increased risk of t-MDS/AML is associated with older age at HCT[1]; pretransplantation exposure to alkylating agents, topoisomerase II inhibitors, or radiation[4]; use of peripheral blood stem cells (PBSC; compared to bone marrow); stem cell mobilization with etoposide; conditioning with TBI; low number of CD34+ cells infused; and multiple transplants (see Table 118.1).[1,4,17]

The impact of pre-HCT chemotherapy and radiation on the risk of t-MDS/AML after HCT points toward an origin of events prior to HCT. A role for pretransplantation exposures is further supported by the observation that specific cytogenetic abnormalities observed posttransplantation have also been observed in the pretransplant marrow or peripheral blood graft among patients who develop t-MDS/AML after HCT, supporting a role for injury induced by prior cytotoxic chemotherapy in the etiology of t-MDS/AML.

TBI at 12 Gy does not increase the risk, whereas an increased risk is observed with TBI at 13.2 Gy.[18] An association with TBI indicates that the disease may arise from residual stem cells that persist in the patient despite myeloablative treatment, rather than from re-infused stem cells, although TBI-induced alteration in the hematopoietic microenvironment may contribute to the development of t-MDS/AML.

TABLE 118.1

Magnitude of Risk and Populations at Increased Risk of Subsequent Malignant Neoplasms After Hematopoietic Cell Transplantation

Study	Study Design	Sample Size/ Number of SMNs	Primary Diagnoses; Type of HCT	Magnitude of Risk and Risk Factors
All Second Malignancies				
Bhatia et al.[1]	Retrospectic cohort study	2,150/53 leukemia, lymphoma, solid malignancies	All hematologic malignancies, inborn diseases of immune system Autologous and allogeneic HCT	11.6-fold increased risk compared with general population Cumulative probability: 9.9% at 13 y for all SMNs; 1.6% at 4 y for PTLD; 5.6% at 13 y for solid malignancies. T-cell depletion, use of ATG, unrelated donor HCT, primary immune deficiency associated with increased risk of PTLD
Baker et al.[75]	Retrospective cohort study	3,372/147 leukemia, lymphoma, solid malignancies	All malignancies and metabolic disorders; immune deficiency; aplastic anemia Autologous and allogeneic	8.1-fold increased risk compared with general population Cumulative incidence: 6.9% at 20 y for any malignancy; 1.4% at 10 y for PTLD; 1.4% at 10 y for MDS/AML; 3.8% at 20 y for solid tumors
Therapy-Related MDS/AML				
Krishnan et al.[4]	Retrospective cohort study Nested case-control study	612/22 MDS/AML	Hodgkin lymphoma Non-Hodgkin lymphoma Autologous HCT	Cumulative probability of MDS/AML: 8.6% at 6 y Stem cell priming with etoposide, pre-HCT radiation associated with increased risk of t-MDS/AML
PTLD				
Landgren et al.[52]	Retrospective cohort study	26,901/127 PTLD	Hematologic malignancies and severe aplastic anemia Allogeneic HCT	T-cell depletion, use of ATG, unrelated donor HLA-mismatched grafts. Cumulative risk increased to 8.1% with more than three risk factors
Curtis et al.[53]	Retrospective cohort study	18,014/78 PTLD	Hematologic malignancies Allogeneic HCT	Cumulative incidence 1% at 10 y Unrelated donor HCT, T-cell depletion, use of ATG, use of anti-CD3 monoclonal antibody
Solid Tumors				
Curtis et al.[3]	Retrospective cohort	19,229/80 solid malignancies	Allogeneic HCT	2.7-fold increased risk of solid tumors compared with the general population Cumulative incidence: 6.7% at 15 y; younger age at HCT associated with increased risk of solid malignancies; chronic GVHD and male sex associated with increased risk of squamous cell carcinoma
Bhatia et al.[11]	Retrospective cohort study	2,129/29 solid malignancies	Hematologic malignancies Autologous and allogeneic HCT	Two-fold increased risk compared with general population Cumulative probability: 6.1% at 10 y
Shimada et al.[76]	Retrospective cohort study	809/19 solid malignancies	All malignancies Autologous and allogeneic HCT	2.8-fold increased risk Cumulative incidence: 4.2% at 10 y Extensive chronic GVHD and older age were associated with increased risk
Gallagher et al.[77]	Retrospective cohort study	926/28 solid malignancies	Hematologic malignancies Allogeneic HCT	10-y cumulative incidence: 3.1%; 1.85-fold increased risk compared with general population Older age at HCT, female donor associated with increased risk
Socie et al.[78]	Retrospective cohort	3,182/25 solid tumors; 20 PTLD	Acute leukemia in childhood	Cumulative risk of solid tumors: 11% at 15y Age <5 y at HCT; TBI were associated with increased risk of solid tumors; chronic GVHD associated with decreased risk Chronic GVHD, unrelated donor HCT, T-cell depleted graft, use of ATG associated with increased risk of PTLD

(continued)

PRACTICE OF ONCOLOGY

Magnitude of Risk and Populations at Increased Risk of Subsequent Malignant Neoplasms After Hematopoietic Cell Transplantation (continued)

Study	Study Design	Sample Size/ Number of SMNs	Primary Diagnoses; Type of HCT	Magnitude of Risk and Risk Factors
Solid Tumors				
Majhail et al.[60]	Retrospective cohort	4,318/66 solid cancers	AML; CML; allogeneic HCT	Cumulative incidence: 1.2% at 10 y; 1.4-fold increased risk compared with general population Chronic GVHD associated with increased risk, in particular oral cavity
Rizzo et al.[6]	Retrospective cohort	28,874/189 solid malignancies	All malignancies/ allogeneic HCT	2.1-fold increased risk Age at exposure to TBI <30 y associated with nine-fold increased risk of nonsquamous cell carcinoma Chronic GVHD, male sex associated with risk of squamous cell carcinoma

SMN, subsequent malignant neoplasm; HCT, hematopoietic cell transplantation; PTLD, posttransplantation lymphoproliferative disorder; ATG, antithymocyte globulin; MDS, myelodysplasina; AML, acute myeloid leukemia; t-MDS, therapy-related MDS; HLA, human leukocyte antigen; GVHD, graft-versus-host disease; TBI, total-body irradiation; CML, chronic myelogenous leukemia.

Recipients of CD34-enriched cells isolated from peripheral blood after chemotherapy priming and growth factors are at a higher risk of t-MDS/AML as compared with recipients of CD34+ cells from the bone marrow.[1,4] Potential explanations include harvesting of hematopoietic precursor cells damaged by chemotherapy at a time before they have completed DNA repair or an overrepresentation of damaged cells in the mobilized product. Supporting this hypothesis is the study[4] demonstrating an increased risk of t-AML with 11q23 abnormalities among patients mobilized with high doses of etoposide for collection of stem cells prior to autologous HCT.

Patients receiving a smaller number of re-infused cells have been reported to be at an increased risk of t-MDS.[17] Reconstitution of bone marrow clearly may result in greater proliferative stress in the setting of low stem cell numbers, increasing susceptibility to irreversible DNA damage associated with t-MDS. These observations are supported by in vitro data suggesting an increased proliferative stress placed on committed progenitors at the expense of primitive progenitors.[19]

Pathogenesis of Therapy-Related Myelodysplasia/Acute Myeloid Leukemia

t-MDS/AML is a clonal disorder that results from acquired genetic or epigenetic changes induced by cytotoxic therapy in hematopoietic stem cells. Improved understanding of the molecular pathogenesis of t-MDS/AML is required to allow development of strategies to identify populations at increased risk. Additionally, t-MDS/AML offers a unique perspective on mutagen-induced carcinogenesis. The clinical and epidemiologic data suggest that t-MDS/AML after autologous HCT results from genetic damage to the stem cell from pretransplant cytotoxic treatment, which may be potentiated by the transplant process itself.

Genetic Lesions Associated with Therapy-Related Myelodysplasia/Acute Myeloid Leukemia

Loss of chromosome 5 or del(5q) and loss of chromosome 7 or del(7q) are recurring abnormalities in t-MDS/AML. This has led to a search for candidate tumor suppressor genes in these regions. The majority of patients with 5q deletions exhibit losses at the 5q31 locus, with deletions in 5q33 being seen in some patients.

Systematic evaluation of all 28 chromosome 5q31.2 genes for heterozygous nucleotide mutations or microdeletions using total exonic gene sequencing and array comparative genomic hybridization[20] did not reveal any somatic nucleotide changes or cytogenetically silent 5q31.2 deletions. The mRNA levels of seven genes in the commonly deleted interval were reduced by 50% in CD34+ cells from del (5q) MDS samples, but complete loss of expression was not seen. These findings suggest that deletion leads to haploinsufficiency of multiple genes, but additional deletions or point mutations in 5q31.2 genes are uncommon. The role of specific genes has been evaluated. For example, the APC gene located in the commonly deleted 5q region has been studied. Mice with the Apcmin allele that results in a loss of APC function showed no abnormality in steady-state hematopoiesis but had reduced long-term stem cell function and developed an MDS phenotype over time,[21] supporting a potential role for Apc haploinsufficiency in the MDS phenotype in patients with del (5q).

Chromosomal segment 7q22 is a common site of chromosome 7 deletions. Molecular analysis of a 2.5-Mb commonly deleted segment of chromosome band 7q22 has failed to uncover a candidate tumor suppressor gene. Mice with deletion of the targeted segment showed normal hematologic parameters and did not spontaneously develop myeloid malignancies.[22] The targeted deletion did not cooperate with oncogenic Kras, Nf1 inactivation, or retroviral mutagenesis to accelerate leukemia development. These results fail to support the hypothesis that the 7q22 deletion contains a tumor suppressor gene. Further, 5q and 7q deletions in familial platelet disorder with leukemia are associated with mutations or deletions of a single AML1 allele.[23] Balanced translocations involving the AML1 gene have also been associated with t-MDS/AML in patients exposed to topoisomerase II inhibitors.[23] Transgenic expression of AML1-ETO leads to immortalization of murine myeloid progenitors but not overt leukemia; additional mutations are required for leukemogenesis.[23] Therefore, altered AML1 function may have a major role in dysregulation of hematopoietic growth and genomic instability and predispose to leukemia through a multistep process.

Thus, although several candidate genes have been identified in these regions, including genes that regulate hematopoietic cell growth and differentiation, identification of a commonly deleted tumor suppressor gene has been elusive. It is possible that haploinsufficiency and reduced gene dosage for critical genes involved in hematopoiesis on 5q, including RPS14, EGR1, APC, NPM1, and *CTNNA1*, may sufficiently alter the balance between growth and differentiation to induce dysplastic hematopoiesis.[24] Alternatively, epigenetic inactivation of the remaining allele or alterations in gene expression through loss of miRNA loci could play a role.

MLL rearrangements can be induced when primary human CD34+ cells are exposed to etoposide; stable genome rearrangements originating within the *MLL* translocation breakpoint hotspot were readily detected in etoposide-treated cells.[25] The *MLL* gene located at chromosome band 11q23 has a major role in developmental regulation. Altered *MLL* function, as with *AML1*, may dysregulate hematopoietic growth and genomic instability and predispose to leukemia through a multistep process.

A second class of mutations in genes regulating cytokine signaling pathways has been recognized in AML. The *RAS* signaling pathway is activated downstream of several cytokine receptors. Constitutively activating point mutations of NRAS are detected in 10% to 15% of patients with t-MDS/AML. In contrast, mutations of the *FLT3* gene (point mutations and internal tandem duplications), commonly seen in de novo AML, are not seen in t-MDS/AML.[26]

Genetic Susceptibility

The observed interindividual variability in risk of t-MDS/AML for a given genotoxic exposure is likely related to common polymorphisms in low-penetrance genes that regulate the availability of active drug metabolite, or those responsible for DNA repair. Knight et al.[27] conducted a genome-wide association study in and identified three single nucleotide polymorphisms (rs1394384 [odds ratio (OR) = 0.3; 95% confidence interval (CI) = 0.2 to 0.6], rs1381392 [OR = 2.1; 95% CI = 1.3 to 3.4], and rs1199098 [OR = 0.5; 95% CI = 0.3 to 0.8]) to be associated with t-MDS/AML with chromosome 5/7 abnormalities.[27] rs1394384 is intronic to *ACCN1*, a gene encoding an amiloride-sensitive cation channel that is a member of the degenerin/epithelial sodium channel; rs1199098 is in LD with *IPMK*, which encodes a multikinase that positively regulates the prosurvival AKT kinase and may modulate Wnt/beta-catenin signaling; rs1381392 is not near any known genes or regulatory elements. The investigators confirmed findings in an independent replication cohort.

Mouse strains resistant or susceptible to t-AML induced by the alkylator ethyl-N-nitrosourea were analyzed to identify genes that regulate t-AML susceptibility. Thirteen quantitative trait loci were significantly associated with ethyl-N-nitrosourea–induced leukemogenesis. These quantitative trait loci contained several genes that could contribute to leukemogenesis, including p53, DNA repair, and apoptosis-regulating genes, suggesting that susceptibility to alkylator-induced leukemia may be a complex trait related to multiple genes.[28] The next section summarizes reports of associations between t-MDS/AML and low-penetrance genes that regulate the availability of active drug metabolite, or are responsible for DNA repair.

Drug Metabolism. Allan et al.[29] examined associations between polymorphisms in the glutathione S-transferase genes (*GSTM1*, *GSTT1*, and *GSTP1*) and t-MDS/AML. Individuals with at least one *GSTP1* codon 105 Val allele were significantly overrepresented in t-AML cases compared with de novo AML cases (OR = 1.8; 95% CI = 1.1 to 2.9). Also, relative to de novo AML, the *GSTP1* codon 105 allele occurred more often among patients with t-MDS/AML with prior exposure to chemotherapy (OR = 2.7; 95% CI = 1.4 to 5.1), particularly among those with prior exposure to known GSTP1 substrates (OR = 4.3; 95% CI = 1.4 to 13.2) and not among patients with t-MDS/AML with exposure to radiation alone.

DNA Repair. Individuals with altered DNA repair mechanisms are likely susceptible to the development of genetic instability that drives the process of carcinogenesis as it relates to t-MDS/AML. Ellis et al.[30] examined the association between patients

with t-MDS/AML and two common functional p53-pathway variants: the *MDM2* SNP309 and the TP53 codon 72 polymorphism. Neither polymorphism demonstrated a significant association. However, an interactive effect was detected such that *MDM2* TT TP53 Arg/Arg double homozygotes, and individuals carrying both a *MDM2* G allele and a *TP53* Pro allele were at increased risk of chemotherapy-related t-MDS/AML.

Mismatch Repair. Defects in the mismatch repair pathway result in genetic instability or a mutator phenotype, manifested by an elevated rate of spontaneous mutations characterized as multiple replication errors in simple repetitive DNA sequences (microsatellites)—functionally identified as microsatellite instability (MSI). Approximately 50% of patients with t-MDS/AML have MSI, associated with methylation of the mismatch repair family member *MLH1*.[31,32]

Double-Strand Breaks. Cellular pathways available to repair double-strand breaks include homologous recombination, nonhomologous end-joining, and single-strand annealing. *RAD51* is one of the central proteins in the homologous recombination pathway, functioning to bind to DNA and promote ATP-dependent homologous pairing and strand transfer reactions. *RAD51-G-135C* polymorphism is significantly overrepresented in patients with t-MDS/AML compared with controls (C allele: OR = 2.7).[33] XRCC3 also functions in the homologous recombination double-strand break repair pathway by directly interacting with, and stabilizing RAD51. The variant *XRCC3-241Met* allele has been associated with a higher level of DNA adducts compared with cells with the wild-type allele, implying aberrant repair[34] and has also been associated with increased levels of chromosome deletions in lymphocytes after exposure to radiation.[35] Although *XRCC3-Thr241Met* was not associated with t-MDS/AML (OR = 1.4; 95% CI = 0.7 to 2.9), a synergistic effect resulting in an eight-fold increased risk of t-MDS/AML (OR = 8.1; 95% CI = 2.2 to 29.7) was observed in the presence of *XRCC3-241Met* and *RAD51-135C* allele in patients with t-MDS/AML compared with controls.[33]

Base Excision Repair. The XRCC1 protein plays a central role in the base excision repair pathway and also in the repair of single-strand breaks, by acting as a scaffold and recruiting other DNA repair proteins. The protein also has a BRCA1 C-terminus (BRCT) domain—a characteristic of proteins involved in DNA damage recognition and response. The presence of variant *XRCC1-399Gln* has been shown to be protective for t-MDS/AML.[36]

Nucleotide Excision Repair. Nucleotide excision repair removes structurally unrelated bulky damage induced by radiation and chemotherapy. The nucleotide excision repair pathway is linked to transcription and components of the pathway comprise the basal transcription factor IIH complex, which is required for transcription initiation by RNA polymerase II. One of the genes involved in the nucleotide excision repair pathway (*ERCC2*) is a member of the basal transcription factor IIH complex. The polymorphic Gln variant (*ERCC2 Lys751Gln*) is associated with t-MDS/AML.[37]

Telomeric Shortening

Telomeres are noncoding regions of DNA that provide a cap at the ends of chromosomes and prevent dicentric fusion and other chromosomal aberrations. Each somatic cell division is associated with a loss of telomere length. Cumulative telomere shortening can impose a limit on cell divisions and lead to cell senescence. Telomere shortening is also associated with genetic instability. Following HCT, the increased replicative demand on stem cells associated with hematopoietic regeneration can lead to accelerated telomere shortening. Telomere shortening could be an important issue in autologous HCT, especially when telomere length in the transplanted cells is already short because of prior chemotherapy, older age at HCT, or increased replicative stress on the stem cells because of a small number of cells transplanted. A prospective, longitudinal study revealed accelerated telomere shortening in patients with t-MDS/AML (preceding the onset of t-MDS/AML) when compared with matched controls who did not develop t-MDS/AML. Patients with t-MDS/AML also showed reduced generation of committed progenitors, suggesting that telomere alterations were related to reduced regenerative capacity of hematopoietic stem cells.[38]

Hematopoietic Abnormalities

Autologous HCT for NHL and HL is associated with hematopoietic abnormalities including marked and prolonged reduction in primitive progenitor long-term culture-initiating cells and committed progenitor colony-forming cell numbers, altered progenitor expansion potential, and microenvironmental defects. These abnormalities may be related in part to damage to hematopoietic cells from pretransplant chemotherapy because hematopoietic defects can also be seen in pretransplant samples.[19] Although committed progenitors recover to pretransplant levels, primitive progenitor capacity is further depleted and does not show evidence of recovery for up to 2 years after HCT, consistent with extensive proliferation and differentiation of the committed progenitors and subsequent depletion of primitive progenitors during hematopoietic regeneration post-HCT.[19] HCT may also be associated with defects in the marrow hematopoietic microenvironment, including reduction in stromal precursor growth and reduced capacity to support growth of myeloid progenitors and B progenitors. These microenvironmental defects may contribute to hematopoietic abnormalities posttransplantation. Extensive proliferation of stem cells bearing genotoxic damage posttransplant may have a role in establishment and amplification of an abnormal clone. Alternatively, the numerous replication cycles imposed on hematopoietic stem cells after HCT may result in excessive shortening of telomeres in descendent cells (as previously discussed). Telomeric shortening may be associated with genomic instability and chromosomal abnormalities, and could contribute to the pathogenesis of t-MDS/AML.[39]

CD34+ cells in the graft from patients with NHL also show reduced migration compared with normal CD34+ cells. In vitro migratory capacity of CD34+ cells in the graft correlated with the speed of hematopoietic recovery after transplantation.[40] Therefore, pretransplant chemotherapy may also lead to reduced engraftment potential of primitive progenitor cells. HCT may also be associated with defects in the marrow hematopoietic microenvironment, including reduction in stromal precursor growth and reduced capacity to support growth of myeloid progenitors and B cell progenitors.[41,42]

Microenvironmental defects may contribute to hematopoietic abnormalities after transplantation. There is evidence supporting the importance of the hematopoietic microenvironment in MDS pathogenesis. Repeated sublethal irradiation of mice was shown to result in bone marrow dysfunction with features of MDS including low white blood cell counts, macrocytic anemia, and reduced platelets and megakryocytes. Bone marrow dysfunction was associated with increased bone marrow angiogenesis, vascular endothelial growth factor, and activation of the transcription factor NFkB. Tumor necrosis factor-α deleted mice were protected from irradiation effects,[43] suggesting that radiation-mediated tumor necrosis factor-α induction may contribute to bone marrow dysfunction and t-MDS/AML. Deletion of the microRNA processing factor Dicer1 in mouse osteoblast progenitors resulted in hematopoietic abnormalities leading to development of MDS and AML, associated with reduced expression of the Sbds gene that is mutated in the Schwachman-Bodian-Diamond syndrome, an inherited human marrow failure disorder.[44] Deletion of Sbds in osteoblast progenitors also induced marrow dysfunction and myelodysplasia. These results support a role for perturbation of microenvironmental cells in hematopoietic defects in t-MDS/AML.

Gene Expression Profiling

Gene expression profiling of acute lymphoblastic leukemia cells at diagnosis has been shown to be predictive of subsequent t-MDS/AML.[45] Gene expression profiling of CD34+ hematopoietic progenitor cells from patients with t-MDS/AML has identified different subtypes of t-MDS/AML with characteristic gene expression patterns.[46] Common to each subgroup were gene expression patterns characteristic of arrested differentiation in early progenitor cells. Li et al.[47] performed microarray analyses of gene expression in patients who developed t-MDS/AML after autologous HCT for HL or NHL (cases) and patients who did not develop t-MDS after autologous HCT (controls). To evaluate gene expression changes pre-HCT, PBSC samples obtained from t-MDS/AML cases and controls before HCT were studied. Patients who later developed t-MDS/AML showed significantly altered gene expression when compared with controls, related to mitochondrial function, ribosomes, DNA repair, and hematopoietic stem cell regulation. Additional alterations in cell-cycle regulatory genes were seen on progression to overt t-MDS/AML. PBSC CD34+ cells from cases that developed t-MDS/AML demonstrated altered mitochondrial function, increased reactive oxygen species (ROS), reduced ROS detoxification, and enhanced DNA damage after therapeutic exposure. These results indicate that genetic programs associated with t-MDS/AML are perturbed long before disease onset and are consistent with previous studies indicating a potential role for abnormalities in stem cell growth, DNA repair, and checkpoint response in t-MDS/AML pathogenesis.

Outcomes of Patients with Therapy-Related Myelodysplasia/Acute Myeloid Leukemia After Autologous Hematopoietic Cell Transplantation

The response of t-MDS/AML to chemotherapy is lower than that seen in de novo leukemia, with an average complete remission rate between 35% and 40%, and poor overall long-term survival. As a result, allogeneic transplantation has been evaluated as a therapeutic modality for t-MDS/AML. Armand et al.[48] applied an optimal cytogenetic grouping (developed for de novo MDS/AML) to patients with t-MDS/AML, and showed that the optimized cytogenetic classification (adverse cytogenetics: abnormal 7 or complex; favorable cytogenetics: 5q- or 20q- or Y- or normal; intermediate: all others) outperformed the established grouping schemes for outcome prediction. Using this new scheme, cytogenetics was the strongest prognostic factor for overall survival through its impact on the risk of relapse. After accounting for cytogenetics, patients with t-MDS/AML had an equivalent outcome to those with de novo disease.[48] Yakoub-Agha et al.[49] analyzed the predictors of survival, relapse, and treatment-related mortality among 70 patients with t-MDS/AML undergoing allogeneic HCT. Older age (>37 years), male sex, positive recipient cytomegalovirus serology, absence of complete remission at HCT, and intensive conditioning schedules were independently associated with poor outcome. Litzow et al.[50] analyzed the outcomes in patients with t-MDS/AML treated with allogeneic HCT between 1990 and 2004. The incidence of treatment-related mortality and relapse was 41% and 27%, at 1 year, respectively, and 48% and 31% at 5 years, respectively. In multivariable analysis, four risk factors had adverse impact on disease-free survival and overall survival: (1) age older than 35 years, (2) poor-risk cytogenetics, (3) t-AML not in remission or advanced t-MDS, and (4) donor other than a human leukocyte antigen (HLA)-identical sibling or a partially or well-matched unrelated donor. Five-year survival for subjects with none, one, two, three, or four of these risk factors was 50%, 26%, 21%, 10%, and 4%, respectively.

These data show that HCT provides potentially curative therapy for t-MDS. The major risk factors for inferior outcome appear to be disease stage and cytogenetics, together with patient age and donor HLA match or mismatch. Treatment of t-MDS/AML should include consideration of the likelihood of success of achieving remission with chemotherapy and, depending on the availability of an appropriate donor, the likelihood of a successful outcome with an allogeneic transplant approach. It is important to follow patients at risk for development of t-MDS/AML closely to identify the early development of MDS. Prompt transplantation should be considered after diagnosis of t-MDS/AML. It is clear, however, that innovative transplant strategies are needed to reduce the high risks of relapse and nonrelapse mortality.

Prediction of Risk of Therapy-Related Myelodysplasia/Acute Myeloid Leukemia

Because of the poor prognosis associated with t-MDS/AML, attempts are under way to identify predictors or early biomarkers to decrease the morbidity associated with this disease. Several studies have attempted to correlate identification of genetically abnormal clones with subsequent risk of t-MDS/AML. Assessment of risk of t-MDS/AML after autologous HCT is complicated by the lack of a single underlying genetic abnormality; development of t-MDS/AML requires acquisition of several mutations. Moreover, t-MDS/AML is a heterogeneous disorder with multiple subtypes characterized by different genetic abnormalities. Therefore, identification of a single genetic abnormality may not necessarily have predictive value for development of t-MDS/AML. Identification of early biomarkers would allow the timely use of appropriate measures to treat the disorder, such as reduced intensity conditioning or other novel agents, rather than waiting for the t-MDS/AML to present in the clinically overt form, when the disease burden would require higher-intensity therapy, with a greater risk of resultant morbidity. In fact, identification of patients at high risk for t-MDS/AML prior to transplantation would allow treatment strategies other than autologous transplantation—such as reduced-intensity allogeneic transplantation—to be considered for such patients to avoid the risk of t-MDS/AML.

Standard Cytogenetics and Fluorescent in situ Hybridization

Abnormal clones are frequently detected after autologous HCT for lymphoma. Significant levels of clonally abnormal cells could be detected by fluorescence in situ hybridization prior to high-dose therapy in samples obtained from 20 of 20 patients who developed t-MDS/AML, but only 3 of 24 patients did not.[51] However, this technique is locus-specific and requires prior selection of markers for analysis and has limited sensitivity of detection.

Polymerase Chain Reaction Assays for Point Mutations

Mutations in genes such as *MLL* or *AML1* or gene rearrangements involving the 11q23 gene may be useful markers for risk of subsequent t-MDS/AML. This method is highly sensitive, but is locus specific, and the specificity and predictive value of such assays is unknown at present.[16]

Gene Expression Analysis

Gene expression microarray analysis of PBSC CD34+ cells from patients who developed t-MDS/AML after autologous HCT for HL or NHL and controls that did not develop t-MDS/AML was used to derive a cross-validated t-MDS/AML gene signature.[47] This 38-gene signature when applied to an independent test set of patients who developed t-MDS/AML after autologous HCT for NHL or HL, and matched controls correctly classified 14 of 16 subjects who developed t-MDS/AML, and 19 of 20 subjects who did not. Clonal abnormalities characteristic of t-MDS/AML were

not seen on cytogenetic analysis of bone marrow samples obtained prior to autologous HCT nor were they seen in fluorescence in situ hybridization analysis of PBSC CD34+ cells, indicating that the gene expression profile of cytogenetically normal hematopoietic cells can potentially identify patients at risk for t-MDS/AML post-HCT.

Reducing Risk of Therapy-Related Myelodysplasia/Acute Myeloid Leukemia After Autologous Hematopoietic Cell Transplantation

Our understanding of the etiology and pathogenesis should help develop potential risk-reduction strategies, such as minimization of pretransplant cytotoxic exposure by bringing high-risk patients to HCT earlier in the course of disease. Standardized screening of patients in the immediate pre-HCT period with marrow pathology and cytogenetics could potentially help identify high-risk populations that would then benefit from an allogeneic rather than autologous HCT. Alteration in hematopoietic cell procurement and conditioning regimens could also be considered. If strategies to develop predictors for patients at high risk prior to HCT are realized, alternative treatment approaches such as allogeneic transplantation or nontransplant modalities may be considered for patients identified at increased risk. Finally, strategies for chemoprevention may be worth exploring in this population.

LYMPHOMAS

Posttransplantation Lymphoproliferative Disorders

Posttransplantation lymphoproliferative disorders (PTLD) are the most common SMN in the first year after allogeneic T-cell–depleted HCT and are related to a compromised immune status and EBV infection.[52,53] Subgroups of patients at elevated risk of PTLD have been clearly defined for whom prospective monitoring of EBV activation and early therapeutic intervention may be particularly useful. The vast majority of PTLDs develop within the first year. The risk of PTLD is strongly associated with T-cell depletion of the donor marrow, antithymocyte globulin use, unrelated or HLA-mismatched grafts, presence of acute or chronic GVHD, older age at HCT, and multiple transplants. The cumulative incidence is low (0.2%) among patients with no major risk factors, but is increased to 1.1%, 3.6%, and 8.1% with one, two, and three or more major risk factors, respectively. The large majority of the PTLDs have a B-cell origin.

B-cell PTLD, a clinically and morphologically heterogeneous group of diseases, usually develops within the first 6 months after HCT, with a cumulative incidence of 1% to 2% at 10 years. Risk factors include in vitro T-cell depletion of the donor marrow, unrelated or HLA-mismatched related donor, use of antithymocyte globulin or anti-CD3 monoclonal antibody, TBI, and primary immunodeficiency (see Table 118.1).[1,54] The risk of PTLD also depends on the method of T-cell depletion, being considerably higher when specific monoclonal antibodies are used for T-cell depletion (11% to 25%) rather than in patients in whom techniques removing both T and B lymphocytes, such as soybean agglutinin or Campath-1 (<1%), are used.[53]

Pathogenesis of B-Cell Posttransplantation Lymphoproliferative Disorder

B-cell PTLD is commonly associated with T-cell dysfunction, occurs in the presence of EBV infection, and is thought to develop because of a combination of depressed EBV-specific cellular immunity and the inherent transforming capacities of EBV.

PRACTICE OF ONCOLOGY

EBV is a ubiquitous herpesvirus that infects 95% of individuals by adulthood. The virus persists as a latent infection in B lymphocytes, where reactivation and replication occur intermittently. The latent membrane protein 1 (LMP-1) is one of the EBV-encoded proteins believed to have an important role in B-cell immortalization by inducing the expression of *bcl-2*, which inhibits programmed death of infected cells. LMP-1 is also considered to be an oncogene, and deletions near the 3′ end of the *LMP-1* gene, in a region that affects the half-life of the LMP-1 protein, have been reported in some PTLDs. Infection of B cells by EBV also induces high levels of cytokines such as interleukin (IL)-1, IL-5, IL-6, IL-10, CD23, and tumor necrosis factor. Some of these factors have been shown to act as autocrine growth factors, stimulating the proliferation of EBV-transformed B cells and inhibiting their susceptibility to apoptosis.

Cytotoxic T-lymphocyte precursor frequencies are low at 3 months after allogeneic HCT, but appear to normalize at 9 to 12 months, thus correlating with the period when B-cell PTLD is most frequently observed. Moreover, the EBV-specific cytotoxic T lymphocytes home preferentially and induce selective regression of autologous EBV-induced B-cell lymphoproliferative lesions in xenografted severe combined immunodeficiency syndrome mice. These studies have formed the basis for clinical trials using adoptive transfer of EBV-specific cytotoxic T lymphocytes.[55] The studies demonstrated long-term persistence of gene-marked EBV-specific cytotoxic T lymphocytes in vivo, which not only restore cellular immunity against EBV but also provide a population of cytotoxic T-lymphocyte precursors that respond to in vivo and ex vivo challenges with the virus for as long as 18 months.[56] These studies have demonstrated that a combination of granulocyte–macrophage colony-stimulating factor and low-dose IL-2 therapy can prevent the immunodeficiency that leads to fatal EBV lymphoproliferative disease in xenografted SCID mice depleted of murine natural killer cells, and thus support a critical role for several human cellular subsets in mediating this protective effect.

Treatment of B-Cell Posttransplantation Lymphoproliferative Disorder

Close monitoring of patients at increased risk for PTLD allows for early institution of appropriate therapy prior to development of overt disease. Therapeutic approaches include B cell–specific monoclonal antibodies and cellular therapy. The efficacy of anti-CD20 monoclonal antibody (rituximab) in the treatment of PTLD has been reported. The drug is more efficacious in patients without mass lesions, forming the basis for recommendations to initiate treatment at an early stage, based on increasing EBV load. Because EBV-associated PTLD results from T-cell dysfunction, reconstitution of "at-risk" patients with EBV-specific cytotoxic T-lymphocyte lines reactivated and expanded in vitro has been shown to be efficacious in controlling PTLD, with a decrease in the EBV DNA concentrations and clinical remission.

Thus, over the past few years, the administration of in vitro–generated EBV-specific cytotoxic T cells or anti–B cell monoclonal antibodies has provided an effective option for the prophylaxis or treatment of PTLD. Advances in quantitative polymerase chain reaction–based assays allow both the precise measurement of EBV load in peripheral blood samples and the identification of high-risk patients for early initiation of therapy. Patients should be monitored weekly by quantitative competitive polymerase chain reaction because viral load is a significant predictor of PTLD. Prevention of EBV PTLD by preemptive therapy based on molecular monitoring of EBV load may be used to decrease the occurrence of PTLD. Preemptive therapy with a single dose of rituximab has been reported to lead to the prevention of PTLD and was first demonstrated by Van Esser et al.[57] The cutoff value of >1,000 EBV genome copies in 10^5 peripheral blood mononuclear cells shows a sensitivity and specificity of 100% and a positive and negative predictive value of 1.00.[58]

In summary, chemotherapy seems not to contribute to improved survival of patients with PTLD after HCT, and antiviral agents are not active against PTLD. On the other hand, preemptive use of rituximab and EBV-cytotoxic T lymphocytes significantly reduces the risk of death due to EBV-PTLD in HCT recipients with survival rates of ~90%. The overall success rates for established PTLD is lower than after preemptive therapy, ranging from ~60% (rituximab) to ~80% (cytotoxic T lymphocytes). A reduction of immunosuppression and/or donor lymphocyte infusion might also reduce the risk of death due to EBV PTLD; the responses range from 40% to 50%.[59]

Hodgkin Lymphoma

HL has also been described after HCT.[5] Mixed cellularity is the most commonly reported subtype, and most of the cases contain the EBV genome. These cases differ from the EBV-PTLD by the absence of risk factors commonly associated with EBV-PTLD, by a later onset (>2.5 years), and relatively good prognosis.

SOLID TUMORS

The cumulative incidence of solid tumors after allogeneic HCT ranges from 7% to 11% at 15 years posttransplantation.[1,3,6,9,11,60] The magnitude of risk of solid tumors after HCT exceeds two-fold that of an age- and sex-matched general population.[3,6,11] The risk increases with time from HCT and, for those who survive ≥10 years after HCT, is reported to be eight-fold that of the general population. Types of solid tumors reported in excess among HCT recipients include melanoma, basal cell carcinoma (BCC) and squamous cell carcinoma (SCC) of the skin, and cancers of the oral cavity and salivary glands, brain, liver, uterine cervix, thyroid, breast, bone, and connective tissue.[3] The risk of solid tumors is higher among those exposed to radiation at a younger age and rises with the dose of radiation (see Table 118.1). Majhail et al.[60] evaluated the risk of solid SMNs after HCT using high-dose busulfan-cyclophosphamide conditioning in 4,318 recipients of allogeneic HCT for AML or chronic myelogenous leukemia. The cumulative incidence of solid cancers at 10 years after HCT was 1.2% among AML and 2.4% after chronic myelogenous leukemia. In comparison to general population, HCT survivors were at a 1.4-fold increased risk. Significantly increased risks were observed for tumors of the oral cavity, esophagus, lung, soft tissue, and brain. Chronic GVHD was an independent risk factor for all solid cancers, and especially cancers of the oral cavity. The risk of specific solid SMNs after HCT are summarized in the following sections and detailed in Table 118.2.

Skin Cancer

The 20-year cumulative incidence of BCC and SCC after allogeneic HCT is reported to be 6.5% and 3.4%, respectively.[7] TBI is a risk factor of BCC, particularly among patients younger than 18 years at HCT. Schwartz et al.[8] demonstrated that the risk of BCC associated with radiation is highest for the youngest ages at exposure, with relative risks exceeding 20 for those transplanted at ages <10 years, and decreasing with increasing age at exposure until age 40 years, above which no excess risk was identified. GVHD (acute and chronic for SCC and chronic for BCC) and male sex are associated with an increased risk of skin cancer.[7]

Breast Cancer

The 25-year cumulative incidence of breast cancer is reported to be 11% after allogeneic HCT. Allogeneic HCT survivors are at a 2.2-fold increased risk of developing breast cancer, when compared

TABLE 118.2

Magnitude of Risk and Populations at Increased Risk of Specific Subsequent Malignant Neoplasms After Hematopoietic Cell Transplantation

Study	Study Design	Sample Size/ Number of SMNs	Primary Diagnoses/ Type of HCT	Magnitude of Risk and Risk Factors
Hodgkin Lymphoma				
Rowlings et al.[5]	Retrospective cohort	18,531/8 Hodgkin lymphoma	Hematologic malignancies and severe aplastic anemia Allogeneic HCT	6.2-fold increased risk; Grade 2 to 4 acute GVHD, treatment for chronic GVHD
Skin Cancer				
Leisenring et al.[7]	Retrospective cohort study design	4,180/237 nonmelanoma skin cancer	All malignancies and metabolic disorders Allogeneic HCT	20-y cumulative incidence: BCC: 6.5%; SCC: 3.4% TBI and younger age at irradiation, light skin color, chronic GVHD associated with BCC Acute and chronic GVHD associated with SCC
Curtis et al.[69]	Case-control	58 SCCs and 125 BCCs; 501 matched controls	Hematologic malignancies, severe aplastic anemia, hemoglobinopathies Allogeneic (matched related and unrelated) HCT	Prolonged and severe chronic GVHD and its therapy (azathioprine, corticosteroids, cyclosporine) were associated with SCCs
Schwartz et al.[8]	Retrospective cohort	6,306/282 BCCs	Hematologic malignancies; severe aplastic anemia; Autologous, matched related and unrelated donor HCT	TBI exposure; youngest age at HCT; increasing attained age; whites; more recent birth cohorts
Breast Cancer				
Friedman et al.[9]	Retrospective cohort	3,337 females/52 breast cancers	Hematologic malignancies Allogeneic HCT	Cumulative incidence: 11% at 25 y Longer time since HCT, use of TBI, younger age at HCT
Thyroid Cancer				
Cohen et al.[10]	Retrospective cohort	78,914/32 thyroid cancer	All malignancies and severe aplastic anemia Autologous, allogeneic	3.26-fold increased risk Young age at HCT, irradiation, female sex, chronic GVHD

SMN, subsequent malignant neoplasm; HCT, hematopoietic cell transplantation; GVHD, graft-versus-host disease; BCC, basal cell carcinoma; SCC, squamous cell carcinoma; TBI, total-body irradiation.

with age- and sex-matched general population. The incidence of breast cancer is higher among those exposed to TBI (17%) than among those who did not receive TBI (3%).[9] The median latency from HCT to diagnosis of breast cancer is 12.5 years. The risk is increased among those exposed to TBI at a younger age.

Thyroid Cancer

HCT recipients are at a 3.3-fold increased risk of thyroid cancer, when compared with age- and sex-matched general population.[10] Age younger than 10 years at HCT, neck radiation, female sex, and chronic GVHD are associated with an increased risk. Thyroid cancer develops after a latency of 8.5 years and is associated with an excellent outcome.

Pathogenesis of Solid Tumors After Hematopoietic Cell Transplantation

Radiation is the single most important risk factor for the development of solid tumors. These radiogenic cancers have a long latent period, and the risk is frequently high among patients undergoing irradiation at a young age. Immunologic alterations may predispose

patients to SCC of the buccal cavity, particularly in view of the association with chronic GVHD.[7] In immunosuppressed patients, oncogenic viruses such as human papillomavirus may contribute to SCC of the skin and buccal mucosa after transplantation.

Chronic tissue stress due to interaction of alloreactive donor cells with host epithelium may cause genomic alterations and increase the risk of SMNs. This hypothesis was tested by analyzing buccal cells from allotransplanted patients for MSI.[61] MSI was observed in 52% of the allotransplant recipients, but not among healthy or autotransplanted controls. SMNs were identified in five of the MSI-positive patients (14%) and only one of the MSI-negative patients. In an in vitro model of mutation analysis, significant induction of frameshift mutations and DNA strand breaks in HaCaT keratinocytes cocultured with mixed lymphocyte cultures were observed, but not after exposure to interferon gamma, tumor necrosis factor-alpha, transforming growth factor-beta, or phytohemagglutinin-stimulated peripheral blood mononuclear cells, suggesting an ROS-mediated mechanism. These data indicate that alloreactions may induce genomic alterations in epithelium.

Patients with a family history of early onset cancers have been shown to be at an increased risk for developing a SMN. The tumor types occurring in excess in close relatives were also observed as SMNs in patients (cancers of the breast, bone, joint, or soft tissue), indicating that the risk of SMN is associated with a familial predisposition.[62] Genetic predisposition also has a substantial impact on risk of SMNs (e.g., sarcomas in patients with hereditary retinoblastoma). This risk is further increased by radiation and increases with the total dose of radiation.[63]

In summary, an interaction of cytotoxic therapy (radiation in particular), genetic predisposition, viral infection, and GVHD with the consequent antigenic stimulation and use of immunosuppressive therapy may play a role in the development of new solid tumors, and needs to be explored comprehensively.

Treatment of Patients with Solid Tumors After Hematopoietic Cell Transplantation

Treatment strategies for patients developing solid tumors after HCT are not well defined. Small case series indicate both ends of the spectrum: favorable outcomes and hence a recommendation for an intensive approach and aggressive tumor growth, and early relapse after standard therapy. A comprehensive study of a large number of patients with second solid tumors will help determine the nature of these tumors and their outcomes as compared to de novo tumors. Until then, patients with solid tumors should be treated with the best available therapy for that tumor, unless there is compelling evidence that they will not be able to tolerate that therapy.

Screening for Subsequent Malignant Neoplasms in Hematopoietic Cell Transplantation Survivors

Theoretically, if screening resulted in an earlier diagnosis of SMNs, then treatment would be more successful and survival rates higher. Additionally, less aggressive treatment could be instituted with less toxicity. The issue of who to screen, how to screen, and when to do it are all important but largely unanswered questions. For the pediatric survivor population, the Children's Oncology Group has developed comprehensive long-term follow-up guidelines that provide risk-adapted, yet consensus-based recommendations.[64] For HCT survivors, screening recommendations must incorporate risks associated with pre-HCT therapy, transplant conditioning therapy, and other HCT-associated conditions such as chronic GVHD. Joint recommendations for screening and preventative practices for long-term survivors after HCT from the European Group for Blood and Marrow Transplantation, the Center for International Blood and Marrow Transplant Research, and the American Society of Blood and Marrow Transplant were published in 2006.[65] This reference provides general guidance for SMN screening for HCT survivors, but recommendations are limited to annual risk awareness counseling and clinical assessments. General recommendations for colorectal, breast, and cervical cancer are provided but are for the most part based on guidelines for the general

population. Screening guidelines developed for use in the general population[66,67] may or may not be sufficient or applicable for use in HCT survivors. For some individuals, additional risk factors, either pre-HCT (exposure to chest radiation, cranial radiation, alkylating agents, topoisomerase II inhibitors) or associated with HCT (TBI, chronic GVHD, duration of immunosuppression, T-cell depletion), may lead to elevated risks and must be considered in the screening strategies. Thus, as summarized by Socie and Rizzo,[68] the following recommendations could be made:

1. Reduce ultraviolet skin exposure through use of high–sun protective factor sunscreens or skin coverage
2. Avoid high-risk behaviors such as avoidance or cessation of tobacco use
3. Annual screening among those at highest risk—these are detailed in the Children's Oncology Group Guidelines as well as the joint ASBMT/CIBMTR guidelines

Risk-Reduction Strategies

While strategies aimed at altering therapeutic exposures (chemotherapy and radiation) will most likely result in a reduction in the risk of subsequent malignancies in some patients, it is unlikely that these exposures are the only factors that convey risk. Furthermore, it is often not feasible to alter therapeutic exposures while preserving clinical outcomes. In HCT recipients, the risk of SMNs associated with chronic GVHD[69] could benefit from efforts to prevent GVHD and to improve immune reconstitution after HCT.

There is increasing concern related to the risk of cancer and cancer death associated with obesity and a sedentary lifestyle.[70] Functional and performance limitations and lower levels of physical activity have been reported in HCT survivors, particularly in those who have chronic GVHD.[71,72] Obesity (as determined by body mass index) is uncommon in HCT survivors[73]; however, preliminary studies of body composition reveal that they have a high percentage of fat mass and a reduction in muscle mass. This state of sarcopenic obesity contributes to the development insulin resistance, hyperinsulinemia, and chronic inflammation—factors that have been implicated in the causal pathway of obesity-associated cancer risk.[74] Thus interventions recommended for the general population aimed at improving nutrition and maintaining a physically active lifestyle are likely of even greater significance for HCT survivors as risk-reduction strategies. Finally, as the pathogenesis of SMNs becomes more clearly elucidated, screening for known genetic susceptibility to cancer could possibly be undertaken and alternative therapeutic options presented to the vulnerable subpopulation. These strategies, as well as those encouraged for all, such as avoidance of tobacco and alcohol, use of sunscreen, and HPV vaccination, may help to reduce the risk of SMNs in HCT survivors.

SELECTED REFERENCES

The full reference list can be accessed at lwwhealthlibrary.com/oncology.

1. Bhatia S, Ramsay NK, Steinbuch M, et al. Malignant neoplasms following bone marrow transplantation. *Blood* 1996;87:3633–3639.
2. Witherspoon RP, Fisher LD, Schoch G, et al. Secondary cancers after bone marrow transplantation for leukemia or aplastic anemia. *N Engl J Med* 1989;321:784–789.
3. Curtis RE, Rowlings PA, Deeg HJ, et al. Solid cancers after bone marrow transplantation. *N Engl J Med* 1997;336:897–904.
4. Krishnan A, Bhatia S, Slovak ML, et al. Predictors of therapy-related leukemia and myelodysplasia following autologous transplantation for lymphoma: an assessment of risk factors. *Blood* 2000;95:1588–1593.
5. Rowlings PA, Curtis RE, Passweg JR, et al. Increased incidence of Hodgkin's disease after allogeneic bone marrow transplantation. *J Clin Oncol* 1999;17:3122–3127.

6. Rizzo JD, Curtis RE, Socie G, et al. Solid cancers after allogeneic hematopoietic cell transplantation. *Blood* 2009;113:1175–1183.
7. Leisenring W, Friedman DL, Flowers ME, et al. Nonmelanoma skin and mucosal cancers after hematopoietic cell transplantation. *J Clin Oncol* 2006;24:1119–1126.
9. Friedman DL, Rovo A, Leisenring W, et al. Increased risk of breast cancer among survivors of allogeneic hematopoietic cell transplantation: a report from the FHCRC and the EBMT-Late Effect Working Party. *Blood* 2008;111:939–944.
10. Cohen A, Rovelli A, Merlo DF, et al. Risk for secondary thyroid carcinoma after hematopoietic stem-cell transplantation: an EBMT Late Effects Working Party Study. *J Clin Oncol* 2007;25:2449–2454.
13. Bhatia S, Robison LL, Francisco L, et al. Late mortality in survivors of autologous hematopoietic-cell transplantation: report from the Bone Marrow Transplant Survivor Study. *Blood* 2005;105:4215–4222.

14. Vardiman JW, Harris NL, Brunning RD. The World Health Organization (WHO) classification of the myeloid neoplasms. *Blood* 2002;100:2292–2302.

16. Gilliland DG, Gribben JG. Evaluation of the risk of therapy-related MDS/AML after autologous stem cell transplantation. *Biol Blood Marrow Transplant* 2002;8:9–16.

17. Friedberg JW, Neuberg D, Stone RM, et al. Outcome in patients with myelodysplastic syndrome after autologous bone marrow transplantation for non-Hodgkin's lymphoma. *J Clin Oncol* 1999;17:3128–3135.

19. Bhatia R, Van Heijzen K, Palmer A, et al. Longitudinal assessment of hematopoietic abnormalities after autologous hematopoietic cell transplantation for lymphoma. *J Clin Oncol* 2005;23:6699–6711.

27. Knight JA, Skol AD, Shinde A, et al. Genome-wide association study to identify novel loci associated with therapy-related myeloid leukemia susceptibility. *Blood* 2009;113:5575–5582.

30. Ellis NA, Huo D, Yildiz O, et al. MDM2 SNP309 and TP53 Arg72Pro interact to alter therapy-related acute myeloid leukemia susceptibility. *Blood* 2008;112:741–749.

32. Seedhouse CH, Das-Gupta EP, Russell NH. Methylation of the hMLH1 promoter and its association with microsatellite instability in acute myeloid leukemia. *Leukemia* 2003;17:83–88.

33. Seedhouse C, Faulkner R, Ashraf N, et al. Polymorphisms in genes involved in homologous recombination repair interact to increase the risk of developing acute myeloid leukemia. *Clin Cancer Res* 2004;10:2675–2680.

36. Seedhouse C, Bainton R, Lewis M, et al. The genotype distribution of the XRCC1 gene indicates a role for base excision repair in the development of therapy-related acute myeloblastic leukemia. *Blood* 2002;100:3761–3766.

38. Chakraborty S, Sun CL, Francisco L, et al. Accelerated telomere shortening precedes development of therapy-related myelodysplasia or acute myelogenous leukemia after autologous transplantation for lymphoma. *J Clin Oncol* 2009;27:791–798.

47. Li L, Li M, Sun CL, et al. Altered hematopoietic cell gene expression precedes development of therapy-related myelodysplasia/acute myeloid leukemia and identifies patients at risk. *Cancer Cell* 2011;20:591–605.

48. Armand P, Kim HT, DeAngelo DJ, et al. Impact of cytogenetics on outcome of de novo and therapy-related AML and MDS after allogeneic transplantation. *Biol Blood Marrow Transplant* 2007;13:655–664.

50. Litzow MR, Tarima S, Perez WS, et al. Allogeneic transplantation for therapy-related myelodysplastic syndrome and acute myeloid leukemia. *Blood* 2010;115:1850–1857.

52. Landgren O, Gilbert ES, Rizzo JD, et al. Risk factors for lymphoproliferative disorders after allogeneic hematopoietic cell transplantation. *Blood* 2009;113:4992–5001.

53. Curtis RE, Travis LB, Rowlings PA, et al. Risk of lymphoproliferative disorders after bone marrow transplantation: a multi-institutional study. *Blood* 1999;94:2208–2216.

55. Heslop HE, Ng CY, Li C, et al. Long-term restoration of immunity against Epstein-Barr virus infection by adoptive transfer of gene-modified virus-specific T lymphocytes. *Nat Med* 1996;2:551–555.

56. Rooney CM, Smith CA, Ng CY, et al. Use of gene-modified virus-specific T lymphocytes to control Epstein-Barr-virus-related lymphoproliferation. *Lancet* 1995;345:9–13.

57. van Esser JW, Niesters HG, van der Holt B, et al. Prevention of Epstein-Barr virus-lymphoproliferative disease by molecular monitoring and preemptive rituximab in high-risk patients after allogeneic stem cell transplantation. *Blood* 2002;99:4364–4369.

58. Meerbach A, Wutzler P, Hafer R, et al. Monitoring of Epstein-Barr virus load after hematopoietic stem cell transplantation for early intervention in post-transplant lymphoproliferative disease. *J Med Virol* 2008;80:441–454.

59. Styczynski J, Einsele H, Gil L, et al. Outcome of treatment of Epstein Barr virus-related post-transplant lymphoproliferative disorder in hematopoietic stemcell recipients: a comprehensive review of reported cases. *Transpl Infect Dis* 2009;11:383–392.

60. Majhail NS, Brazauskas R, Rizzo JD, et al. Secondary solid cancers after allogeneic hematopoietic cell transplantation using busulfan-cyclophosphamide conditioning. *Blood* 2011;117:316–322.

64. Landier W, Bhatia S, Eshelman DA, et al. Development of risk-based guidelines for pediatric cancer: The Children's Oncology Group long-term follow-up guidelines from the Children's Oncology Group Late Effects Committee and Nursing Discipline. *J Clin Oncol* 2004;22:4979–4990.

65. Majhail NS, Rizzo JD, Lee SJ, et al. Recommended screening and preventive practices for long-term survivors after hematopoietic cell transplantation. *Bone Marrow Transplant* 2012;47:337–341.

69. Curtis RE, Metayer C, Rizzo JD, et al. Impact of chronic GVHD therapy on the development of squamous-cell cancers after hematopoietic stemcell transplantation: an international case-control study. *Blood* 2005;105:3802–3811.

PRACTICE OF ONCOLOGY

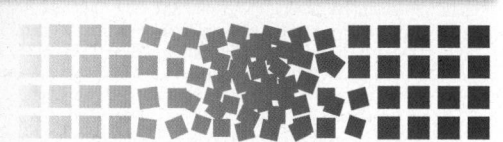

119 Superior Vena Cava Syndrome

Andreas Rimner and Joachim Yahalom

INTRODUCTION

Superior vena cava syndrome (SVCS) is the clinical expression of obstruction of blood flow through the superior vena cava (SVC). Characteristic symptoms and signs may develop quickly or gradually when this thin-walled vessel is compressed, invaded, or thrombosed by processes in the superior mediastinum. Most cases reported in the past were due to syphilitic aneurysms or tuberculosis mediastinitis.[1] Nowadays, malignancy is the most common underlying process in patients with SVCS.[2] With the increased use of intravascular devices such as catheters and pacemakers, thrombosis of the SVC caused by these foreign bodies has been more frequently observed.[3] It is estimated that SVCS develops in 15,000 people in the United States each year.[2]

ANATOMY AND PATHOPHYSIOLOGY

The SVC is the major low-pressure vessel for drainage of venous blood from the head, neck, upper extremities, and upper thorax. It is located in the right mediastinum and is surrounded by the sternum, trachea, right mainstem bronchus, aorta, pulmonary artery, and perihilar and paratracheal lymph nodes. The SVC extends from the junction of the right and left innominate veins to the right atrium, over a distance of 6 to 8 cm. The distal 2 cm of the SVC is within the pericardial sac, with a point of relative fixation of the vena cava at the pericardial reflection. The azygos vein, the main auxiliary vessel, enters the SVC posteriorly, just above the pericardial reflection. The physiologic width of the SVC is 1.5 to 2 cm. The SVC is thin-walled, compliant, easily compressible, and therefore vulnerable to any space-occupying process in its vicinity. The SVC is completely encircled by chains of lymph nodes that drain the right thoracic cavity. Other critical structures in the mediastinum, such as the auxiliary azygos vein, main bronchi, esophagus, and spinal cord, may be involved by the same process that leads to obstruction of the SVC.

When the SVC is fully or partially obstructed, venous collateral circulation may develop if the SVCS gradually develops over time, thus allowing time for collaterals to form. The azygos venous system is the most important alternative pathway. Other collateral systems include the internal mammary veins, lateral thoracic veins, paraspinous veins, and esophageal venous network.[4] Engorgement of collateral subcutaneous veins in the neck and thorax is a typical physical finding in SVCS. Despite these collateral pathways, venous pressure is almost always elevated in the upper compartment if the SVC is obstructed (Fig. 119.1). Venous pressures in the upper extremities have commonly been recorded to be >300 mm saline in severe SVCS.[5]

CLINICAL PRESENTATION AND ETIOLOGY

A subjective sensation of fullness in the head or objective facial swelling and dyspnea are common presenting symptoms

(Table 119.1).[6,7] The characteristic physical findings are venous distention of the neck (66%) and chest wall (54%), facial edema (46%), plethora (19%), and cyanosis (19%). These symptoms and signs may be aggravated by bending forward, stooping, or lying down. SVCS may be the earliest manifestation of invasive involvement of additional critical structures in the thorax such as the bronchi. Pleural effusions are common in SVCS. In one series, effusions were detected in 60% of patients, both in those with malignant etiology and in those with a nonmalignant cause.[8] The majority are exudative and often chylous. Rarely do patients present with life-threatening symptoms like confusion, obtundation, stridor or syncope without precipitating factors, hypotension, or renal insufficiency.

Malignant disease is the most common cause of SVCS. The percentage of patients in different series with a confirmed diagnosis of malignancy varies from 60% to 86% (Table 119.2).[7,9–12] In large series of lung cancer, SVCS was identified in 4% to 8.6% of the patients.[13,14] Small-cell lung cancer (SCLC) and squamous cell carcinoma are the most common histologic subtypes because of their frequent central location.[7,15,16] Lymphoma involving the mediastinum was the cause of SVCS in 2% to 21% (see Table 119.2). In a large series, most patients with lymphoma with SVCS had either diffuse large-cell lymphoma or lymphoblastic lymphoma.[17] The presence of dysphagia, hoarseness, or stridor was a major adverse prognostic factor for patients with lymphoma who presented with SVCS. In a series of patients with primary mediastinal B-cell lymphoma with sclerosis, SVCS was present in 57% of patients.[18] Other primary mediastinal malignancies that may cause SVCS are thymomas and germ cell tumors. SCLC, non-Hodgkin lymphoma (NHL), and germ cell tumors constitute almost half of the malignant causes of SVCS. Hodgkin lymphoma commonly involves the mediastinum, but it rarely causes SVCS. Breast cancer is the most common metastatic disease that causes SVCS in up to 11% of the cases.[9,10] The prognosis of patients with SVCS strongly correlates with the prognosis of the underlying disease.

In recent years, nonmalignant conditions causing SVCS have been more often observed. When the data were collected from general hospitals, as many as 40% of patients had noncancerous causes of SVCS, most commonly due to thrombosis in the presence of central vein catheters or pacemakers.[7,10,12,19] The increasing use of such catheters for the delivery of chemotherapy agents or hyperalimentation in conjunction with a common thromboembolic disposition in many patients with cancer contributes to the development of SVCS.[19]

Obstruction of SVC in the pediatric age group is rare and has a different etiologic spectrum, mainly iatrogenic, secondary to cardiovascular surgery for congenital heart disease, ventriculoatrial shunt for hydrocephalus, SVC catheterization for parenteral nutrition, and mediastinal fibrosis secondary to histoplasmosis.[20,21]

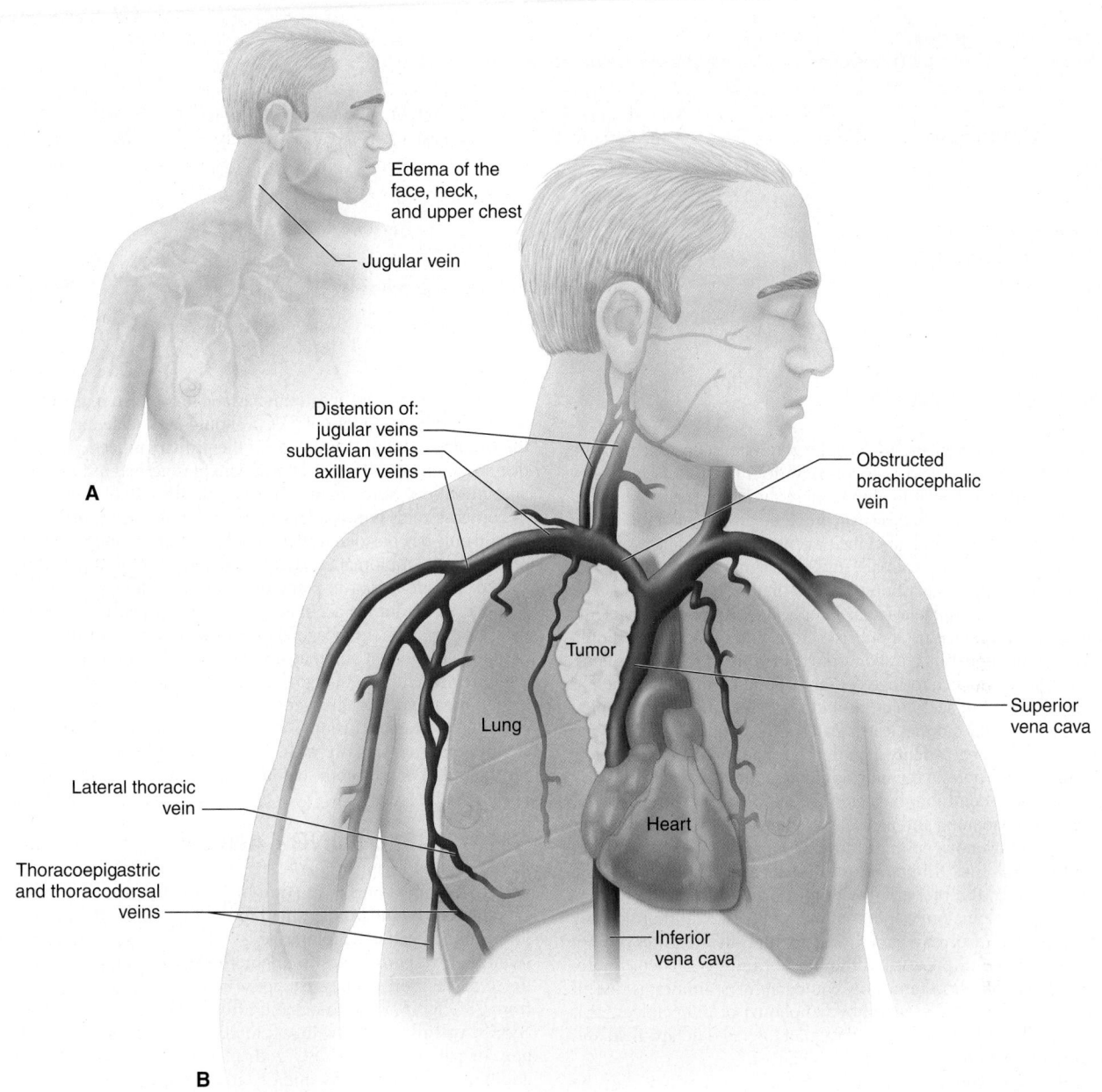

Figure 119.1 Clinical signs of the superior vena cava syndrome. **A** shows facial edema, plethora, jugular venous distention, and prominent superficial vessels in the neck and upper chest. **B** depicts the vascular anatomy and collateral vessel formation in a patient with superior vena cava syndrome. (From Wilson LD, Detterbeck FC, Yahalom J. Superior vena cava syndrome with malignant causes. *N Engl J Med* 2007;356:1862–1869. Copyright © [2007] Massachusetts Medical Society. Reprinted with permission.)

PRACTICE OF ONCOLOGY

TABLE 119.1

Common Symptoms and Physical Findings of Superior Vena Cava Syndrome

Symptoms	Patients Affected[a] (%)	Physical Findings	Patients Affected[a] (%)
Dyspnea	63	Venous distention of neck	66
Facial swelling and head fullness	50	Venous distention of chest wall	54
Cough	24	Facial edema	46
Arm swelling	18	Cyanosis	20
Chest pain	15	Plethora of face	19
Dysphagia	9	Edema of arms	14

[a] Analysis based on data from 370 patients.
Adapted from Schraufnagel DE, Hill R, Leech JA, et al. Superior vena caval obstruction. Is it a medical emergency? *Am J Med* 1981;70:1169–1174. Yellin A, Rosen A, Reichert N, et al. Superior vena cava syndrome. The myth—the facts. *Am Rev Respir Dis* 1990;141:1114–1118; and Rice TW, Rodriguez RM, Light RW. The superior vena cava syndrome: clinical characteristics and evolving etiology. *Medicine (Baltimore)* 2006;85:37–42.

TABLE 119.2

Primary Pathologic Diagnoses for Superior Vena Cava Syndrome

Histologic Diagnosis	Bell et al.[7] 159 Patients (%)	Schraufnagel et al.[10] 107 Patients (%)	Parish et al.[9] 86 Patients (%)	Yellin et al.[11] 63 Patients (%)	Rice et al.[12] 78 Patients (%)
Lung cancer	129 (81)	67 (63)	45 (52)	30 (48)	36 (46)
Lymphoma	3 (2)	10 (9)	8 (9)	13 (21)	6 (8)
Other malignancies (primary or metastatic)	4 (3)	14 (13)	14 (16)	8 (13)	5 (6)
Nonneoplastic	2 (1)	16 (15)	19 (22)	11 (18)	31 (40)
Undiagnosed	21 (13)	—	—	—	—

DIAGNOSTIC WORKUP

The modern treatment of SVCS has become disease-specific from the outset. Therefore, a clear diagnosis prior to initiation of emergency treatment such as mediastinal irradiation should be made. Mediastinal irradiation before a biopsy may preclude proper interpretation of the specimen in almost half of the patients and should be avoided.[22] The safety of modern, minimally invasive diagnostic procedures such as bronchoscopy, mediastinoscopy, computed tomography (CT)-guided biopsy or supraclavicular lymph node biopsy has markedly improved, and concerns about risks from these procedures should not preclude proper diagnostic workup. In contrast to past opinions, there is little evidence to suggest that diagnostic procedures such as venographies, thoracotomies, bronchoscopies, mediastinoscopies, and lymph node biopsies carry an excessive risk in patients with SVCS.[2] Therefore, patients should, if possible, undergo a complete staging workup prior to the initiation of treatment.

The most common radiographic abnormalities are superior mediastinal widening and pleural effusion apparent on chest X-ray. CT with intravenous contrast provides more detailed information about the SVC, its tributaries, and other critical structures, such as the trachea, the bronchi, the esophagus and the spinal cord.[23] The additional anatomic information is necessary to more clearly determine the involvement of these structures that requires prompt action for relief of pressure. Although not fully evaluated, fluorodeoxyglucose-positron emission tomography scanning is useful in patients with SVCS caused by lymphoma or lung cancer, as it may significantly influence the design of the radiotherapy field and treatment intent (definitive versus palliative).[2]

Pathologic confirmation of a thoracic malignancy can be obtained as a cytologic specimen via endobronchial fine needle aspiration, or via CT-guided needle biopsy or mediastinoscopy. Endobronchial fine needle aspirations are as accurate as tissue diagnosis and supply sufficient malignant cells for cytologic evaluation in most cases of lung cancer.[24] Mediastinoscopy has a very high success rate for providing a diagnosis and has a complication rate of approximately 5%.[25] Reports by several authors on using mediastinoscopy for patients with SVCS whose histologic diagnosis could not be established with less invasive techniques confirmed the safety and high diagnostic yield of mediastinoscopy.[25,26] No perioperative mortality was recorded, and the diagnostic yield was excellent. Percutaneous transthoracic CT-guided fine needle biopsy is an effective and safe alternative to an open biopsy or mediastinoscopy.[27] In the presence of a pleural effusion, thoracocentesis can establish the diagnosis of malignancy in 71% of patients with malignancy.[8] A thoracoscopic biopsy or thoracotomy is diagnostic if all other procedures have failed.

DISEASE-SPECIFIC MANAGEMENT AND OUTCOMES

The goal of treatment of SVCS depends on the cause and—in malignancies—the stage of the disease. Malignant tumors are potentially curable if they present at a nonmetastatic stage, even in the presence of SVCS. The treatment of SVCS should be selected according to the histologic disorder and stage of the primary process. During the diagnostic process, the patient can benefit from bed rest and oxygen administration. Some clinicians advocate the use of diuretics and/or corticosteroids if the patient is uncomfortably symptomatic. This should only be considered after pathologic confirmation of the cause of SVCS in symptomatic patients who require urgent palliation, as steroid initiation prior to pathologic confirmation can significantly hamper efforts for an accurate diagnosis, especially with lymphomas. Prophylactic anticoagulation in the absence of thrombosis is of no proven benefit and may interfere with diagnostic procedures.

When the therapeutic goal is only palliation of SVCS, or when urgent treatment of the venous obstruction is required, direct opening of the occlusion should be considered. Endovascular stenting and angioplasty with possible thrombolysis may provide prompt relief of symptoms before more cancer-specific therapy.[3,28]

SMALL-CELL LUNG CANCER

Chemotherapy alone or in combination with thoracic irradiation therapy is the standard treatment for SCLC and is effective in rapidly improving the symptoms of SVCS.[14–16,29] No significant difference in response rates to chemotherapy or radiation has been detected in most studies. Response rates to chemotherapy range from 73% to 93% and to radiation from 43% to 94%.[14,29] Relief of SVCS typically occurs within 7 to 10 days after initiation of therapy. In patients with SCLC with recurrent or persistent SVCS, additional chemotherapy and/or radiotherapy is still likely to relieve symptoms.[29]

NON–SMALL-CELL LUNG CANCER

A review of SVCS in lung cancer indicated that chemotherapy relieved SVCS in 59% of patients with non-SCLS (NSCLC); radiotherapy relieved the obstruction in 63% of patients with NSCLC.[28] Nevertheless, in almost 20% of the patients the obstruction recurred. Response to radiotherapy was higher in patients who had received prior therapy (94% versus 70%).[28]

NON-HODGKIN LYMPHOMA

The primary treatment for NHL is chemotherapy, as it has both local and systemic activity. Local consolidation with radiation therapy is beneficial in patients with early stage diffuse large-cell lymphoma, particularly if the mass is bulky.

In a report of 36 patients with SVCS secondary to NHL, all patients achieved complete relief of SVCS symptoms within 2 weeks of the onset of any type of treatment, whether treated with chemotherapy alone, chemoradiation, or radiotherapy alone.[17]

Eighteen of twenty-two patients (81%) with large-cell lymphoma achieved complete response. However, relapse was common, and the median survival was only 21 months.

NONMALIGNANT CAUSES

Patients with nonmalignant SVCS often have longstanding symptoms before they seek medical advice, and the time to establish the diagnosis and survival are typically markedly longer.[10] The average survival rate has been reported as 9 years for benign causes, compared with 5 months for lung cancer as the cause of SVCS. A total of 12 (75%) of 16 patients with benign SVCS had a mediastinal granuloma that was attributed to histoplasmosis.[30] Ten patients who were available for 1 to 11 years were all doing well at the time of the report. Given the good prognosis of patients with benign SVCS, a need for SVC bypass surgery may not be justified, except for patients in whom SVCS develops, progresses, or persists after 6 to 12 months of observation for possible collateral development.[30] Ketoconazole may prevent recurrent SVCS from active histoplasmosis.

CATHETER-INDUCED OBSTRUCTION

In catheter-induced SVCS, the mechanism of obstruction is usually thrombosis. Streptokinase, urokinase, or recombinant tissue-type plasminogen activator may achieve lysis of the thrombus early in its formation.[31] Heparin and oral anticoagulants may reduce the extent of the thrombus and prevent its progression. Removal of the catheter should be considered, if possible, in combination with anticoagulation to avoid embolization. In patients for whom electrodes of a pacemaker must be changed, the wires should be removed to prevent the risk of developing SVCS.[32] Percutaneous transluminal angioplasty, with or without thrombolytic therapy, and stent insertion have been successfully used to open catheter-induced SVC obstructions.[33]

TREATMENT

Radiation Therapy

Radiotherapy is a treatment option for most patients with malignant SVCS. Radiotherapy does not only provide immediate relief of the obstruction, but will also treat the underlying cause of the obstruction, thus improving symptoms in the long-term and effectively preventing SVCS recurrence. The primary effect of palliative radiotherapy for SVCS is exerted by decreasing the extrinsic pressure on the SVC by the surrounding or invading malignant masses. However, serial venograms and autopsies suggest that the symptomatic improvement may be enhanced by the development of collaterals after the pressure in the mediastinum is eased.

In general, when radiation is given as initial treatment, CT-based simulation and fractions of 1.8 to 2 Gy are recommended for lymphomas. For lung cancers, higher daily fractions of 3 Gy may be considered. However, no data clearly support a particular fractionation scheme. The field and fractionation may be altered after administration of several fractions and achievement of symptomatic relief.[2] In the absence of distant metastatic disease, the radiotherapy course may be extended to a definitive treatment course, in combination with sequential or concurrent chemotherapy when feasible.

A retrospective study evaluated the efficacy of treating patients with SVCS with a regimen of three fractions of 8 Gy once a week to a total dose of 24 Gy compared to two fractions of 8 Gy within 1 week to a total dose of 16 Gy.[34] Transient dysphagia was the main side effect in almost half of the patients in both programs. The 24-Gy regimen resulted in a complete resolution of symptoms in 56% of patients and a partial response in another 40%. The 16-Gy regimen yielded a complete response in only 28% of patients. The mean time for SVCS recurrence and the median overall survival rate were longer in the higher-dose regimen (6 months and 9 months, respectively) compared with the low-dose regimen (3 months and 3 months, respectively). A more recent study reported the experience of using only two fractions of 6 Gy each, delivered 1 week apart, in 23 elderly patients with malignancy-related SVCS.[35] Overall response was 87% with mild toxicity (grade 1-2 dysphagia in six patients, fatigue in four patients, and short-lived systemic side effects consisting of chest pain, rigors, and fever in four patients).

In the definitive treatment setting, the radiation field should encompass all gross disease with appropriate margins for clinical and planning target volumes. In the palliative setting, the radiation field should encompass all gross disease responsible for the SVCS, which may include the hilar, mediastinal, and supraclavicular lymph nodes. Elective nodal irradiation is generally not recommended when treating patients with lymphoma or lung cancer as the cause of malignant SVCS.

Endovascular Stenting and Angioplasty

Percutaneous transluminal angioplasty using the balloon dilatation, insertion of expandable metal stents, or both have been successfully used to open and maintain the patency of SVC obstruction resulting from malignant and benign causes.[3,28,33,36,37] It is an effective initial treatment for obtaining immediate relief of the obstruction if the clinical status of the patient is deteriorating. Median symptom-free survival of 6 months has been reported in a large series of 149 patients with malignant SVCS.[36] However, long-term experience in maintaining patency after stent therapy in patients with SVCS from benign causes who are expected to have long survival is still limited.[33] Complication rates for endovascular therapy range from 0% to 50% and include bleeding, stent migration, stent occlusion, and pulmonary embolus.[3] A recent prospective study examining the outcomes of expanded polytetrafluoroethylene–covered stents found a higher patency and median survival compared to uncovered stents from a historic patient population.[38]

Thrombolysis is often an integral part of the endovascular management of SVCS because thrombosis is frequently a critical component of the obstruction and lysis is necessary to allow the passage of the wire. Most reports have emphasized the use of combination endovascular therapy: thrombolysis, angioplasty, and stent insertion.[3,28] Successful experience with thrombolytic agents was also obtained in the treatment of catheter-induced SVCS.[3,31] The higher yield of thrombolytic therapy in patients with catheters is probably related to the mechanism of obstruction, the ability to deliver the agent directly to the thrombus, and earlier recognition of SVCS in patients with malfunctioning catheters. Early intervention and use of urokinase and recombinant tissue-type plasminogen activator were associated with favorable results.[31]

Surgery

In malignancy-induced SVCS, surgical intervention should be considered only after other therapeutic maneuvers as radiotherapy, chemotherapy, and stenting have been exhausted. Most patients with SVCS of benign origin have long survivals without surgical intervention. However, if the process progresses rapidly or if there is a retrosternal goiter or aortic aneurysm, surgical intervention may be indicated to relieve the obstruction.[39,40]

The experience with successful direct bypass graft for SVC obstruction is limited. It has been recommended that autologous grafts of almost the same size as the SVC should be used.[41] Doty, Flores, and Doty[42] used a composite spiral graft, which was constructed from the patient's saphenous vein. They reported 23 years of experience with this procedure in 16 patients with benign obstruction of SVC; 14 patients maintained patency and 15 were relieved of symptoms of SVCS. Piccione, Faber, and Warren[43] used autologous pericardium to reconstruct the SVC after resection for malignant obstruction. Successful bypasses of obstructed SVCs have used Dacron (DuPont, Wilmington, DE) and polytetrafluoroethylene prostheses.[44-46] The preferred bypass route is between an innominate or jugular vein on the left side and the right atrial appendage, using an end-to-end anastomosis.

The most common surgical approach is via a sternotomy or thoracotomy with extensive resection of the tumor and reconstruction of the SVC. Case series indicate an operative mortality of approximately 5% and patency rates of 80% to 90%.[2]

AREAS OF UNCERTAINTY

Standardized criteria to grade the severity of symptoms in the SVCS are still lacking. More recently, a grading system with an accompanying treatment algorithm has been proposed.[47] It emphasizes that in most patients (>85%) with SVCS, the symptoms are not severe (grades 0, 1, and 2) and cancer-specific treatment could follow appropriate diagnosis and staging. Grade 3 (severe) patients who present with mild or moderate cerebral edema, mild/moderate laryngeal edema, or diminished cardiac reserve may be considered for immediate stent intervention or early radiation therapy, otherwise they should receive disease-specific treatment. Only the rare (<5%) grade 4 (life-threatening) patients, who develop significant cerebral edema or laryngeal edema with stridor or have significant hemodynamic compromise, should undergo stent insertion immediately.

The benefit of either short- or long-term anticoagulation therapy for SVCS is unclear, although thrombolytic agents have been used effectively in patients with vena caval thrombosis.[2] Most experts recommend anticoagulation after thrombolysis (to prevent disease progression and recurrence) and aspirin after stent placement in the absence of thrombosis, but data are limited. The optimal management of recurrent obstruction of the SVC is also controversial. Placement of a stent is often considered because of the limited benefit or the risk of excessive toxic effects from repeat chemotherapy or radiation, but data to guide decision making are limited.

RECOMMENDATIONS

The clinical course of SVCS rarely represents an absolute emergency. In patients without a clear cause of SVCS who do not have life-threatening symptoms, an efficient diagnostic effort should be attempted before any oncologic treatment is given. If all the proposed testing has failed to establish the diagnosis, the location of the suspicious lesion in the chest and the experience of the surgical team should determine whether mediastinoscopy or thoracotomy is performed.

After the cause of SVCS has been established, treatment of the primary process should promptly follow.

Combination chemotherapy with an appropriate regimen is the treatment of choice for SCLC and NHL. Radiation therapy of the lesion and adjacent nodal areas may enhance control after initial response to chemotherapy. NSCLC causing SVCS is best treated with radiation therapy. The incorporation of CT scan and fluorodeoxyglucose-positron emission tomography information into a carefully designed treatment plan may enable the administration of a more definitive total radiation dose of >50 Gy, which may provide long-term local control for some patients when appropriate. Percutaneous endovascular intervention should be considered in severe cases because it relieves symptoms rapidly without masking the diagnosis.

Most patients with nonmalignant causes for SVCS have an indolent course and a good prognosis. Percutaneous transluminal angioplasty or stent insertion should be considered an effective alternative to surgery. However, the long-term maintenance of patency with stent insertion is still unknown. Surgery is indicated only when the process is rapidly progressing or caused by a retrosternal goiter or an aortic aneurysm. If SVCS is induced by a catheter, the catheter should be removed if possible. Heparin should be administered during the removal of the catheter to prevent embolization. In catheter-induced SVCS, urokinase, streptokinase, or recombinant tissue-type plasminogen activator is of value if used early in the thrombotic process.

SELECTED REFERENCES

The full reference list can be accessed at lwwhealthlibrary.com/oncology.

1. Schechter MM. The superior vena cava syndrome. *Am J Med Sci* 1954;227:46–56.
2. Wilson LD, Detterbeck FC, Yahalom J. Clinical practice. Superior vena cava syndrome with malignant causes. *N Engl J Med* 2007;356:1862–1869.
3. Schindler N, Vogelzang RL. Superior vena cava syndrome. Experience with endovascular stents and surgical therapy. *Surg Clin North Am* 1999;79:683–694, xi.
6. Armstrong BA, Perez CA, Simpson JR, et al. Role of irradiation in the management of superior vena cava syndrome. *Int J Radiat Oncol Biol Phys* 1987;13:531–539.
8. Rice TW, Rodriguez RM, Barnette R, et al. Prevalence and characteristics of pleural effusions in superior vena cava syndrome. *Respirology* 2006;11:299–305.
10. Schraufnagel DE, Hill R, Leech JA, et al. Superior vena caval obstruction. Is it a medical emergency? *Am J Med* 1981;70:1169–1174.
11. Yellin A, Rosen A, Reichert N, et al. Superior vena cava syndrome. The myth—the facts. *Am Rev Respir Dis* 1990;141:1114–1118.
12. Rice TW, Rodriguez RM, Light RW. The superior vena cava syndrome: clinical characteristics and evolving etiology. *Medicine (Baltimore)* 2006;85:37–42.
13. Salsali M, Cliffton EE. Superior vena caval obstruction in carcinoma of lung. *N Y State J Med* 1969;69:2875–2880.
14. Sculier JP, Evans WK, Feld R, et al. Superior vena caval obstruction syndrome in small cell lung cancer. *Cancer* 1986;57:847–851.
15. Wurschmidt F, Bunemann H, Heilmann HP. Small cell lung cancer with and without superior vena cava syndrome: a multivariate analysis of prognostic factors in 408 cases. *Int J Radiat Oncol Biol Phys* 1995;33:77–82.
17. Perez-Soler R, McLaughlin P, Velasquez WS, et al. Clinical features and results of management of superior vena cava syndrome secondary to lymphoma. *J Clin Oncol* 1984;2:260–266.
18. Lazzarino M, Orlandi E, Paulli M, et al. Primary mediastinal B-cell lymphoma with sclerosis: an aggressive tumor with distinctive clinical and pathologic features. *J Clin Oncol* 1993;11:2306–2313.
19. Bertrand M, Presant CA, Klein L, et al. Iatrogenic superior vena cava syndrome. A new entity. *Cancer* 1984;54:376–378.
21. Ingram L, Rivera GK, Shapiro DN. Superior vena cava syndrome associated with childhood malignancy: analysis of 24 cases. *Med Pediatr Oncol* 1990;18:476–481.
22. Loeffler JS, Leopold KA, Recht A, et al. Emergency prebiopsy radiation for mediastinal masses: impact on subsequent pathologic diagnosis and outcome. *J Clin Oncol* 1986;4:716–721.
24. Herth FJF, Eberhardt R, Vilmann P, et al. Real-time endobronchial ultrasound guided transbronchial needle aspiration for sampling mediastinal lymph nodes. *Thorax* 2006;61:795–798.
25. Mineo TC, Ambrogi V, Nofroni I, et al. Mediastinoscopy in superior vena cava obstruction: analysis of 80 consecutive patients. *Ann Thorac Surg* 1999;68:223–226.
27. Koegelenberg CF, Bolliger CT, Plekker D, et al. Diagnostic yield and safety of ultrasound-assisted biopsies in superior vena cava syndrome. *Eur Respirat J* 2009;33:1389–1395.
28. Rowell NP, Gleeson FV. Steroids, radiotherapy, chemotherapy and stents for superior vena caval obstruction in carcinoma of the bronchus: a systematic review. *Clin Oncol (R Coll Radiol)* 2002;14:338–351.
29. Chan RH, Dar AR, Yu E, et al. Superior vena cava obstruction in small-cell lung cancer. *Int J Radiat Oncol Biol Phys* 1997;38:513–520.
30. Mahajan V, Strimlan V, Ordstrand HS, et al. Benign superior vena cava syndrome. *Chest* 1975;68:32–35.
31. Gray BH, Olin JW, Graor RA, et al. Safety and efficacy of thrombolytic therapy for superior vena cava syndrome. *Chest* 1991;99:54–59.

33. Kee ST, Kinoshita L, Razavi MK, et al. Superior vena cava syndrome: treatment with catheter-directed thrombolysis and endovascular stent placement. *Radiology* 1998;206:187–193.

34. Rodrigues CI, Njo KH, Karim AB. Hypofractionated radiation therapy in the treatment of superior vena cava syndrome. *Lung Cancer* 1993;10: 221–228.

36. Lanciego C, Pangua C, Chacón JI, et al. Endovascular stenting as the first step in the overall management of malignant superior vena cava syndrome. *Am J Roentgenol* 2009;193:549–558.

37. Fagedet D, Thony F, Timsit JF, et al. Endovascular treatment of malignant superior vena cava syndrome: results and predictive factors of clinical efficacy. *Cardiovasc Intervent Radiol* 2013;36:140–149.

38. Gwon DI, Ko GY, Kim JH, et al. Malignant superior vena cava syndrome: a comparative cohort study of treatment with covered stents versus uncovered stents. *Radiology* 2013;266:979–987.

39. Picquet J, Blin V, Dussaussoy C, et al. Surgical reconstruction of the superior vena cava system: indications and results. *Surgery* 2009;145:93–99.

40. Lanuti M, De Delva PE, Gaissert HA, et al. Review of superior vena cava resection in the management of benign disease and pulmonary or mediastinal malignancies. *Ann Thorac Surg* 2009;88:392–397.

42. Doty JR, Flores JH, Doty DB. Superior vena cava obstruction: bypass using spiral vein graft. *Ann Thorac Surg* 1999;67:1111–1116.

43. Piccione W Jr, Faber LP, Warren WH. Superior vena caval reconstruction using autologous pericardium. *Ann Thorac Surg* 1990;50:417–419.

46. Leo F, Bellini R, Conti B, et al. Superior vena cava resection in thoracic malignancies: does prosthetic replacement pose a higher risk? *Eur J Cardiothorac Surg* 2010;37:764–769.

47. Yu JB, Wilson LD, Detterbeck FC. Superior vena cava syndrome—a proposed classification system and algorithm for management. *J Thorac Oncol* 2008;3:811–814.

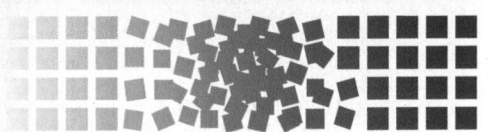

120 Increased Intracranial Pressure

Kevin P. Becker and Joachim M. Baehring

INTRODUCTION

An increase in intracranial pressure (ICP) is a common neurologic complication of patients with cancer involving the nervous system. Various pathomechanisms have to be considered in this patient population. Large cerebral metastases are the most common cause and can give rise to intracranial hemorrhage. Subependymal or leptomeningeal masses located at "bottlenecks" of spinal fluid pathways such as the foramen of Monro or the aqueduct of Sylvius raise pressure by obstructing spinal fluid flow. A cancer-related hypercoagulable state can lead to dural sinus thrombosis or extracranial venous outflow obstruction, and coagulopathies predispose to subdural bleeding. The patient with cancer as an immunocompromised host is at risk for infections of the nervous system such as fungal or bacterial meningitis or a bacterial abscess which can all result in increased ICP. Communicating hydrocephalus reflects decreased reabsorption of spinal fluid, which can be seen in leptomeningeal carcinomatosis or the sequela of prior infection. Dural venous sinus stenosis from dural metastases causes a syndrome resembling idiopathic intracranial hypertension.

This chapter provides an overview of the various mechanisms of increased ICP, the clinical manifestations, diagnosis, and treatment options.

PATHOPHYSIOLOGIC CONSIDERATIONS

Intracranial volume is not expandable in an adult because of its containment by the skull and the dura. The brain itself has an average volume of 1,400 ml, spinal fluid of 52 to 160 ml, and blood 150 ml.[1] An increase in the volume of one compartment occurs at the expense of the other two (Monro-Kellie hypothesis).[2–4] If brain volume increases as a result of a brain tumor, the spinal fluid volume decreases as a compensatory mechanism. Up to an ICP of 200 to 250 mm cerebral spinal fluid (CSF) compartmental volume increase results in only minor increases in ICP as long as CSF flow is not obstructed, the rate between CSF production and reabsorption remains constant, and the dural venous sinuses remain open. However, intracranial compliance decreases with rising ICP (i.e., with rising pressure, increase in volume leads to a disproportionate increase in pressure). This is reflected in the occurrence of plateau waves, which are acute elevations of ICP up to 1,300 mm CSF lasting 5 to 20 minutes. These transient elevations are of pathogenic significance because they further compromise cerebral perfusion in patients with increased ICP.[5] Plateau waves have been suspected to cause intermittent symptoms with orthostasis in patients with brain tumors.[6]

Volume changes within the brain parenchyma that lead to increased ICP in patients with cancer are caused by the direct mass effect of primary or secondary brain tumors, peritumoral edema, or indirect neurologic complications of cancer. Vasogenic edema results from increased leakage of plasma filtrate into brain tissue through leaky capillaries within a brain tumor or surrounding a brain abscess or cerebral hemorrhage. Cytotoxic edema occurs with the breakdown of the adenosine triphosphate–dependent transmembranous ion transport system that leads to the intracellular entrapment of water. This can be seen with ischemic injury, cytotoxic chemotherapy agents, or buildup of toxic metabolites seen in liver failure. Extra-axial mass lesions can arise from neoplastic growth (dural tumors such as metastases, meningioma, or lymphoma), infection (subdural empyema), or hemorrhage (subdural hematoma in the coagulopathic or thrombocytopenic patient).

Increased ICP can also be the consequence of an imbalance between CSF production and reabsorption. Spinal fluid is produced at an average rate of 21 to 22 ml/h or approximately 500 ml/day. CSF represents a plasma filtrate passively diffusing through the choroid plexus of the lateral, third, and fourth ventricles. It is reabsorbed within the arachnoid granulations overlying the cerebral hemispheres. Mass lesions in proximity to bottlenecks of CSF flow (foramen of Monro, cerebral aqueduct, medullary foramina, basilar subarachnoid cisterns) cause obstructive or noncommunicating hydrocephalus. Carcinomatosis or meningitis directly interferes with CSF reabsorption at the arachnoid granulations. Under chronic conditions, the spinal fluid pressure reaches a new equilibrium within the high normal range, and gives rise to a condition called *normal pressure hydrocephalus* (NPH) characterized by ventricular enlargement out of proportion to age-related cortical atrophy. Increased production of CSF is a rare cause of raised ICP. Idiopathic intracranial hypertension (IIH) or pseudotumor cerebri denotes a syndrome characterized by signs of increased ICP in the absence of mass lesions or hydrocephalus. Although poorly defined from a pathophysiologic standpoint, an increasing number of patients with IIH have been found to have partial obstruction of dural venous sinuses. Iatrogenic causes of IIH include all-trans retinoic acid, tetracycline antibiotics, and sulfonamides.

Acute increases in arterial and venous pressure result in an increase in ICP. Cerebral perfusion is kept constant over a wide arterial pressure range (50 to 160 mm Hg). Once this autoregulatory mechanism fails, further increase in arterial blood pressure passively increases ICP. Venous obstruction can be reproduced with the Queckenstedt maneuver (manual compression of both internal jugular veins). Dural venous sinus pressure fluctuates with intrathoracic pressure changes. Thus, coughing, sneezing, and straining (Valsalva maneuver) are accompanied by an increase in ICP. In a patient with increased ICP and decreased intracranial compliance, gagging or coughing can lead to transient decompensation and the acute onset of symptoms (syncope in patients with colloid cyst of the third ventricle, plateau waves).

Depending on the etiology and location of an increase in cerebral parenchymal or extra-axial volume, patients may have relatively few symptoms until herniation ensues. The faster the pathologic process evolves, the more likely is the patient to have symptoms. Cingulate or transfalcian herniation denotes lateral shift of a hemisphere underneath the falx cerebri. Vascular structures (ipsilateral anterior cerebral artery, internal cerebral vein, vein of Galen) can be compromised in this process. In transtentorial herniation, the diencephalon is forced through the tentorial notch as a consequence of a supratentorial mass lesion. Infratentorial masses can result in an upward herniation of posterior fossa structures through the tentorium or downward displacement through the foramen magnum. Uncal herniation, most often encountered in temporal lobe mass lesions, leads to compression of the midbrain at the level of the tentorial notch. When the ICP exceeds 40 to 50 mm Hg, cerebral blood flow is diminished, leading to irreversible brain damage.

EPIDEMIOLOGY AND PATHOGENESIS

Increase in Cerebral Parenchymal Pressure and Cerebral Spinal Fluid Flow Obstruction

Brain metastases are the most common cause of increased ICP in a patient with cancer. In adults, lung cancer and melanoma are particularly prone to seeding to brain.[7] Cerebral metastasis can be further complicated by intratumoral hemorrhage. Although lung cancer is the most common primary tumor leading to hemorrhagic brain seeding, the relative incidence of hemorrhagic transformation of a cerebral metastasis is highest in melanoma, choriocarcinoma, renal cell carcinoma, and papillary thyroid cancer.[8] In children, the brain metastases most commonly associated with intracranial hemorrhage are Ewing sarcoma, rhabdomyosarcoma, and melanoma.[9] Primary brain tumors with a predilection for subependymal or intraventricular locations such as subependymal giant cell astrocytoma, lymphoma, subependymoma, choroid plexus papilloma, ependymoma, meningioma, central neurocytoma, chordoid glioma of the third ventricle, or thalamic tumors can cause spinal fluid obstruction early in their course. Secondary cerebral volume increase in patients with cancer results from hemorrhage, ischemia, infection, or autoimmune inflammatory processes. Cerebral hemorrhage from cancer-related coagulopathies typically occurs in patients with hematologic malignancies such as acute lymphocytic or myelocytic leukemia.[10] Diffuse cerebral edema and increased ICP in patients with leukemia can be the mere result of leukostasis and occurs at blast counts exceeding 4×10^5/mcL. Higher counts are usually required in lymphoblastic leukemia because lymphoid cells are smaller and less adherent than myeloid blasts.[11] An increase in ICP can also be the consequence of diffuse cerebral hemorrhages in disseminated intravascular coagulopathy.

Herpes simplex encephalitis gives rise to extensive vasogenic edema affecting the medial temporal and inferior frontal lobe.

Depending on disease burden, patients with cerebral toxoplasmosis, aspergillosis, or candidiasis can present with signs of increased ICP as well. Brain abscess complicates neurosurgical interventions for resection of metastases, drainage of cerebral hemorrhage, or placement of ventricular catheters. Autoimmune inflammatory encephalomyelitis has been described as a rare entity in patients after stem cell transplantation.

Disorders Affecting Cerebral Spinal Fluid Production or Reabsorption

A syndrome resembling normal pressure hydrocephalus has been observed in long-term survivors of whole-brain or less commonly, partial-brain irradiation. Fibrosis of arachnoid granulations has been suspected to play a role in the pathogenesis of this entity that is also characterized by extensive white matter demyelination and frank necrosis. Selected patients seem to respond favorably to ventriculoperitoneal shunting.[12–14] An acute imbalance between CSF production and reabsorption occurs in neoplastic meningitis and opportunistic meningeal infections in the immunocompromised patient with cancer. *Cryptococcus neoformans* meningitis is almost invariably associated with elevation of ICP. Patients after splenectomy are susceptible to meningitis with encapsulated bacteria. The pathogenesis of communicating hydrocephalus in patients with spinal cord tumors or nonobstructive masses of the cerebellopontine angle is not well understood. Most commonly ependymomas, but also schwannoma, meningioma, neurofibroma, and glioma, might release protein degradation products or cells into CSF that obstruct the arachnoid granulations.[15,16] However, the protein level is rarely elevated in these patients. Others have suspected blockage of the lumbar CSF reservoir,[17–19] arachnoiditis, or increased fibrinogen levels[20] as the cause of this syndrome. All-trans retinoic acid, a differentiating agent used for the treatment of promyelocytic leukemia, has been associated with episodes of communicating hydrocephalus, likely as a consequence of decreased CSF reabsorption.[21,22] Increased ICP is rarely caused by CSF overproduction. Patients with choroid plexus papilloma, especially if they are multifocal, are at risk.[23]

Venous Outflow Obstructions

A hypercoagulable state in patients with cancer can manifest itself as dural venous sinus thrombosis (Fig. 120.1A). The incidence is

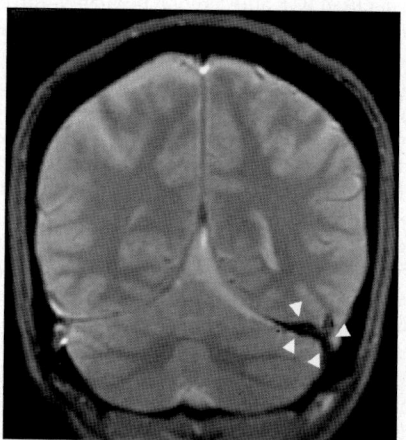 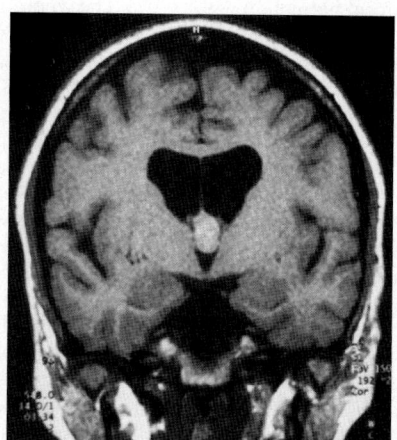 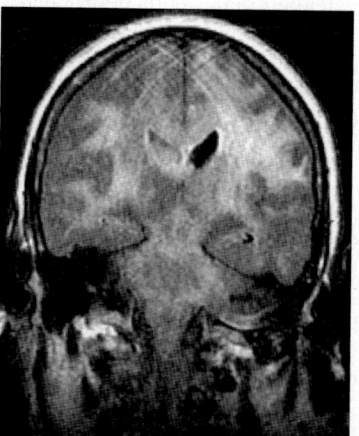

A,B   **C**

Figure 120.1 **(A)** Increased intracranial pressure caused by venous outflow obstruction. A 48-year-old woman with idiopathic myelofibrosis complained of a severe headache. Workup revealed a left transverse sinus thrombosis (gradient echo magnetic resonance imaging, coronal section, intraluminal thrombus outlined by *arrowheads*). **(B)** Intermittent obstructive hydrocephalus caused by the "pressure-valve" effect of a colloid cyst of the foramen of Monro. This 38-year-old patient had experienced several presyncopal episodes and was suffering from positional headaches. The lateral ventricles are dilated (unenhanced T1-weighted magnetic resonance image, coronal section). **(C)** A 78-year-old woman with gliomatosis cerebri. Hyperintense signal on this coronal fluid attenuated inversion recovery magnetic resonance imaging demarcates the extent of cerebral infiltration by neoplastic cells and vasogenic edema. There is extensive effacement of the sulcal pattern and early transtentorial herniation.

increased in patients receiving l-asparaginase therapy. Increased ICP is the only manifestation of cerebral venous thrombosis in more than one-third of patients.[24] Nonthrombotic causes of dural sinus stenosis or occlusion are dural mass lesions such as meningioma or diffuse meningiomatosis of the convexity, metastases from breast or prostate cancer, non-Hodgkin lymphoma, Ewing sarcoma, plasmocytoma, or neuroblastoma that either compress or invade the sinus.[25–27] Venous hypertension can also arise from metastases at the base of the skull, causing obstruction of the internal jugular vein or from compression of the superior vena cava by mediastinal masses. Lesions giving rise to IIH compromise the distal superior sagittal sinus or the torcula Herophili.[28]

CLINICAL PRESENTATION

Headache is the most common complaint of patients with increased ICP. In its classic form, the head pain is severe, resistant to common analgesics, and reaches maximum intensity on awakening in the morning.[29] Decreased venous drainage in the supine position likely accounts for this observation. Patients frequently report immediate relief from their headache by vomiting. However, the majority have nonspecific tension-type or migraine-like headaches. The patient with increased ICP falls easily, particularly backward. With rising pressure, nausea and vomiting ensue. The patient becomes increasingly somnolent and ultimately lapses into a coma.

Funduscopic examination reveals papilledema in about half of patients with increased ICP. Absence of venous pulsations within the center of the optic disc is an early finding, whereas papilledema with blurring of the disc margins or small hemorrhages characterizes later stages. The Foster-Kennedy syndrome—optic nerve atrophy as a result of a sphenoid wing meningioma and contralateral papilledema from increased ICP—is rarely seen in the days of improved neuroimaging methods and earlier diagnosis.

Focal neurologic deficits can help localize the mass accounting for the pressure increase. Cognitive complaints such as slowness to respond and inattentiveness reflect frontal lobe dysfunction. Gaze paresis to the side opposite the lesion indicates involvement of the frontal eye field. Posterior frontal masses cause contralateral hemiparesis. Hemianesthesia or complex neglect syndromes reflect parietal lobe pathology. Temporal and occipital lobe disease causes visual field deficits. An upward gaze paresis occurs in patients with tumors of the tectal region such as pineal neoplasms or metastases. Paresis of extraocular muscles results from stretch injury of the fourth or sixth nerve or uncal herniation with compression of the third nerve. However, the clinician must be aware of "false" localizing signs. Temporal lobe tumors can cause compression of the cerebral peduncle at the tentorial notch on the opposite side, resulting in a hemiparesis on the same side as the mass lesion (Kernohan syndrome).[30]

Symptoms are aggravated by vasogenic edema surrounding intraparenchymal masses and partially or completely resolve with medical management. Hyponatremia as a result of inappropriate secretion of antidiuretic hormone is observed as a metabolic complication of increased ICP. Sphincter incontinence occurs in chronically elevated ICP. Patients with acute meningitis present with classic signs of meningeal irritation, including photophobia, phonophobia, and a Kernig or Brudzinski sign. In meningeal carcinomatosis, these signs are frequently absent.

Elevated ICP in infants results in increased head circumference. Chronic hydrocephalus can be recognized on plain radiographs of the skull as focal thinning of the tabula interna of the skull (Lückenschädel). This is accompanied by personality changes and loss of previously acquired motor skills. Herniation of one cerebellar tonsil causes a head tilt, neck stiffness, and unilateral forced eye closure.[31] Tectal masses result in upgaze inhibition, light-near dissociation of pupillary response, and convergence-retraction nystagmus (Parinaud syndrome). Pressure on the mesencephalic tegmentum leads to pathologic lid retraction and an upward gaze palsy (setting sun sign).

Slowly progressive static ICP changes are accompanied by little or no symptoms. On the other hand, clinical deterioration is profound when dynamic pressure changes such as plateau waves occur or abnormal intracranial compartmentalization or herniation ensues.[32] Signs and symptoms of increased ICP manifest earlier in patients with lesions of the posterior fossa because of the small size of this compartment. A brief bedside assessment including level of consciousness, pupillary size and reflexes, extraocular movements, blood pressure, heart rate, breathing pattern, and motor response to noxious stimuli enables the clinician to determine if herniation is present and which level of the central neuraxis is compromised. The triad of changes in breathing pattern, arterial hypertension, and bradycardia observed with rising ICP is known as the *Kocher-Cushing reflex*.[33] In uncal herniation from temporal lobe masses or herpes encephalitis, ipsilateral compression of the third nerve and associated parasympathetic nerve fibers leads to pupillary dilatation before extraocular dysmotility. With progressive shift of brain substance, complete third nerve palsy ensues and signs of midbrain dysfunction appear. Patients develop contralateral hemiparesis from pressure on the cerebral peduncle and ultimately become stuporous. Increasing pressure from hemispheric or diencephalic mass lesions results in central (transtentorial) herniation. This leads to a progressive syndrome reflecting sequential damage to brainstem structures in a rostrocaudal fashion.[32] At the early diencephalic stage, mild changes in the patient's alertness are accompanied by periodic breathing, yawning, or hiccupping. Pupils are small but remain reactive to light. With further progression of central herniation, the patient becomes obtunded or stuporous. Roving eye movements reflect diffuse cortical dysfunction and preservation of lower brainstem gaze centers. Noxious stimuli elicit flexion of upper extremities and extension of lower extremities (decorticate posturing). Midsize pupils unresponsive to light indicate midbrain dysfunction. Damage to the mesencephalic reticular activating system produces coma. A fast and regular breathing pattern evolves (central neurogenic hyperventilation). Transition to the pontine stage of central herniation is accompanied by extensor posturing of all limbs to noxious stimulation (decerebrate posturing). Absence of the oculocephalic reflex (doll's head maneuver) and horizontal eye movements to caloric stimulation of the vestibular system indicate damage to pontine structures. Breathing becomes apneustic with pontine compression. When the cerebellar tonsils herniate through the foramen magnum, ataxic breathing is observed and the blood pressure drops.[32]

The syndrome of raised ICP and cerebral herniation can evolve slowly over days to weeks or acutely over hours. Rapid progression usually indicates hemorrhage. Subdural hematomas in patients with coagulopathies can evolve so rapidly that signs of cerebral herniation are present before an imaging study can be obtained. Hemorrhage into a metastatic focus is typically characterized by the sudden onset of focal neurologic signs, including seizures. Intraparenchymal hemorrhage as a result of coagulopathy leads to slowly progressive neurologic deterioration.[10]

A peculiar syndrome is associated with tumors or developmental abnormalities causing a pressure valve effect, such as the colloid cyst of the foramen of Monro (Fig. 120.1B). Patients, typically in their late childhood or early adulthood, report sudden onset of severe imbalance, headache, and nausea that is brought on by positional changes (bending down) or Valsalva maneuvers. Sudden deaths have occurred, stressing the need for close observation of these patients until appropriate therapy can be provided.[34,35]

IIH (pseudotumor cerebri) is mostly characterized by nocturnal or hypnopompic headaches aggravated by Valsalva maneuver. Nonspecific visual changes, diplopia due to sixth nerve palsy, or transient visual obscuration are less frequent manifestations. Especially the latter is an ominous sign indicating the need for immediate intervention as the patient's vision is at risk. On physical examination, papilledema is the most striking abnormality.[36] The blind spot is enlarged.

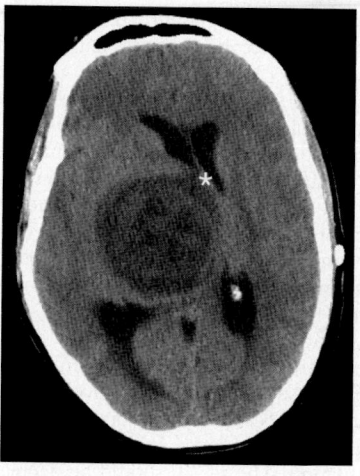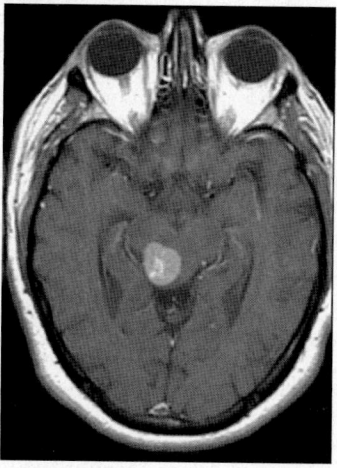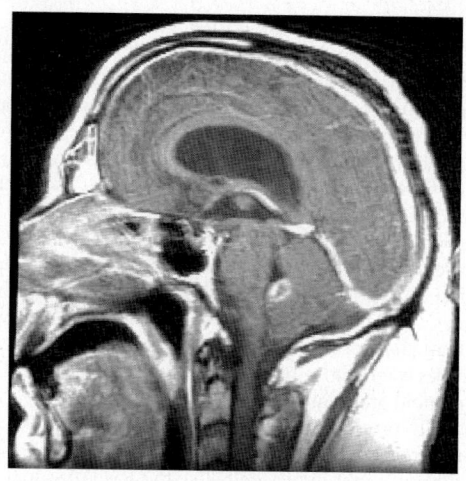

A,B   C

Figure 120.2 (A) A 45-year-old patient with an anaplastic astrocytoma of the right thalamus. Computed tomography revealed obstruction at the level of the foramen of Monro (*asterisk*). **(B)** A 55-year-old patient with a midbrain metastasis from an adenocarcinoma of the lung. There is partial obstruction at the level of the cerebral aqueduct. The temporal horns of the lateral ventricles are dilated (T1-weighted magnetic resonance image with gadolinium). **(C)** A 38-year-old patient with seeding of non–small-cell lung cancer to the floor of the fourth ventricle. He presented with intractable headaches, nausea, vomiting, and severe back pain, indicative of obstructive hydrocephalus and leptomeningeal spread to the spinal canal (T1-weighted magnetic resonance image with gadolinium, sagittal view).

Another characteristic clinical syndrome is recognized in patients with chronic disturbance of spinal fluid reabsorption. These patients, or more likely their family members on their behalf, report a combination of cognitive decline, precipitate micturition, and gait apraxia.[37,38] Dementia is usually of the subcortical type. Precipitate micturition reflects dysfunction of the cortical center for bladder control (paracentral lobule). Minimal bladder filling results in the uncontrollable urge to urinate. The gait disturbance is characterized by difficulty initiating ambulation and postural instability with retropulsion. Strength is preserved.

DIAGNOSIS

The history and clinical examination detect the presence of increased ICP. Imaging studies are helpful in determining its cause and confirming the clinical impression. The most readily available imaging study is unenhanced computed tomography. The study is adequate to determine the presence of intraventricular and subarachnoid CSF flow obstruction (Fig. 120.2), as well as uncal, transfalcian, and transtentorial herniation (Fig. 120.3). The presence of intracranial hemorrhage or a neoplastic or infectious mass lesion can be identified and emergency treatment initiated. Transependymal edema is seen as periventricular hypodensity and indicates CSF flow obstruction.

More detailed neuroanatomic imaging and the distinction between a neoplastic, infectious, inflammatory, or ischemic process requires magnetic resonance imaging. The use of intravenous gadolinium is advised as most conditions associated with increased ICP in patients with cancer cause breakdown of the blood–brain barrier and thus can be better visualized with contrast dye. The use of diffusion-weighted imaging can help identify evolving ischemia or high cellularity suggestive of malignant tumor growth. CSF flow studies (cine magnetic resonance imaging) are helpful to evaluate the functional significance of minute structural lesions within or surrounding the cerebral aqueduct.

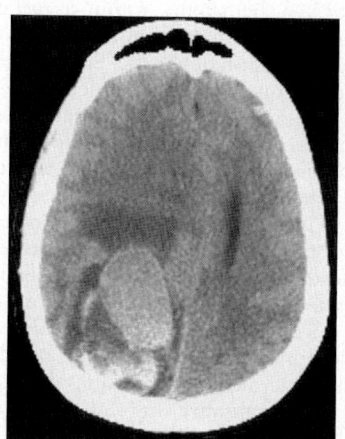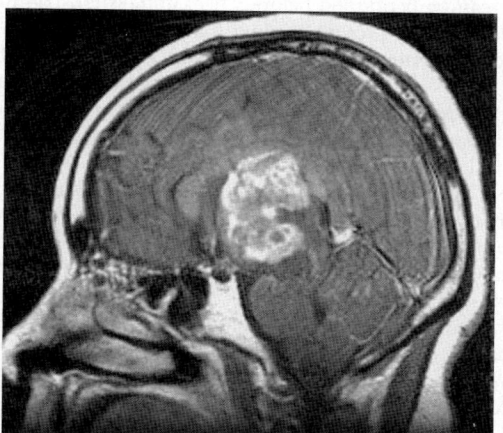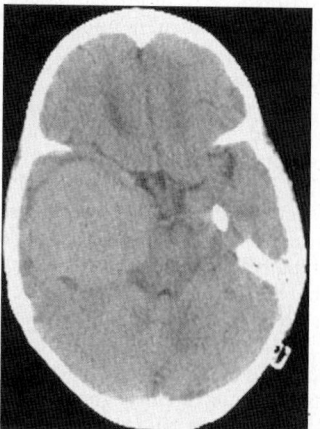

A,B   C

Figure 120.3 (A) This unenhanced computed tomographic scan of the head shows a hemorrhagic brain metastasis in a 42-year-old woman with malignant melanoma. The metastasis exerts mass effect on the right lateral ventricle. There is transfalcian herniation of the right hemisphere. **(B)** A 37-year-old woman with an anaplastic astrocytoma of the diencephalon. There is imminent transtentorial herniation (T1-weighted magnetic resonance image with gadolinium, sagittal view). **(C)** A 25-year-old woman who developed a large right temporal meningioma years after whole-brain radiation therapy for acute lymphoblastic leukemia in early childhood. The tumor compresses the cerebral peduncle and displaces the midbrain (unenhanced computed tomography).

Slit-like ventricles in the correct clinical setting are indicative of IIH. Coronal images through the orbit may reveal dilatation of the optic nerve sheaths in this condition. Ex vacuo ventricular dilatation out of proportion to cortical atrophy is characteristic for NPH. Magnetic resonance imaging of the spine should be considered in patients with unexplained communicating hydrocephalus. Obstruction or infiltration of dural venous sinuses is best visualized with magnetic resonance or computed tomographic venography.[39]

Scintigraphic cisternography can document spinal fluid circulation abnormalities such as NPH. Early ventricular filling with tracer substance after lumbar injection and delayed or absent demarcation of subarachnoid space overlying the cerebral hemispheres is indicative of decreased reabsorption of CSF through the arachnoid granulations.

CSF pressure can be measured directly through a lumbar puncture performed in the lateral decubitus position. Puncture of the subarachnoid space below the level of spinal fluid obstruction bears the risk of initiating or aggravating cerebral herniation. The risk is considerable in mass lesions of the posterior fossa. A computed tomography scan should be obtained prior to lumbar puncture in patients with signs of increased ICP. Compartmentalization (obstructive hydrocephalus at the foramen of Monro or cerebral aqueduct, obliteration of basal cisterns as a result of transtentorial or transforaminal herniation) prohibits puncture of the subarachnoid space below the level of obstruction. When unperturbed communication between the intraventricular and subarachnoid spaces has been determined and the basal cisterns are patent, lumbar puncture should not be delayed if it is deemed necessary for accurate diagnosis.

ICP can be monitored in the intensive care unit with a variety of strain gauge, fiber optic, or pneumatic devices placed into the brain parenchyma, ventricular, subarachnoid, subdural, or epidural space. All these methods require neurosurgical intervention.[40]

Transcranial Doppler sonography is helpful in the intensive care unit for monitoring cerebral perfusion and alteration in cerebrovascular resistance (e.g., in vasospasm or intra-arterial disease) in patients with increased ICP.[41]

TREATMENT

In the majority of cases, the onset of increased ICP in patients with cancer is protracted over days to weeks. After increased ICP is recognized and symptomatic measures have been initiated to lower pressure, a diagnostic procedure can be performed before definitive treatment is provided. Fewer patients present as an emergency but the ones that do require immediate neurosurgical intervention.

The normovolemic patient with increased ICP and suspected decreased intracranial compliance is best positioned with head and upper trunk slightly elevated (~30 degrees). As fever above 100.5°F contributes to elevated ICP, it is common practice to use antipyretics such as acetaminophen above this threshold. Serum osmolality is kept in the high normal range. Isotonic saline solutions are recommended for intravenous hydration, while hypotonic fluids are avoided because free water shifts along an osmolar gradient further exacerbate increased ICP.

Corticosteroids are effective agents for the initial management of increased ICP caused by vasogenic edema. No benefit has been convincingly shown for cytotoxic edema of an acute ischemic stroke, intracranial hemorrhage secondary to remote effects of cancer, or spinal fluid obstruction. Moderate (6 to 10 mg dexamethasone every 6 hours) to high doses (up to 100 mg/d of dexamethasone) are used. A superior therapeutic effect has not been demonstrated for high doses, and the risk of adverse reactions, in particular gastroduodenal ulceration, is considerable. Corticosteroids should be avoided if CNS lymphoma is suspected

before a tissue diagnosis has been established. Dexamethasone and related drugs induce lymphocytic apoptosis and may obscure morphologic diagnosis.

Osmotic diuresis through infusion of hyperosmolar agents such as mannitol or glycerol is an alternative or additional treatment option for the reduction of ICP. Most commonly used are intravenous infusions of 20% to 25% mannitol solutions given at an initial dose of 0.75 to 1 g/kg body weight. Repeat dosing at 0.25 to 0.5 g/kg body weight is possible every 4 to 6 hours but close monitoring of serum osmolality is required. The osmotic effect is transient, and treatment should be stopped if the target serum osmolality is exceeded (~300 to 310 mOsm/L).[42]

Monitoring in the neurologic intensive care unit is required in patients with depressed mental status secondary to ICP elevation. Careful blood pressure adjustment is needed to avoid blood pressure peaks without decreasing cerebral perfusion.

The most rapid method to decrease ICP is intubation with mechanical hyperventilation. The pCO_2 should be decreased to 25 to 30 mm Hg. Lower pCO_2 levels are avoided because cerebral perfusion is reduced. The effect of hyperventilation is transient and thus other measures such as corticosteroid use and osmotic diuresis need to be initiated simultaneously.

Obstructive hydrocephalus constitutes a neurosurgical emergency. Rapid neurologic deterioration with signs of cerebral herniation mandates the immediate placement of an external ventriculostomy. Permanent drainage of CSF through a ventriculoperitoneal shunt or endoscopic placement of a third ventriculostomy may be necessary when the cause of spinal fluid flow obstruction cannot be definitively treated. Although filter systems are available, ventriculoperitoneal shunting is avoided in patients with leptomeningeal tumor in order to prevent peritoneal seeding.

Normal pressure hydrocephalus responds favorably to ventriculoperitoneal shunting. It is the task of the clinician to carefully select patients who may benefit from this procedure. Patients with a short history of the classic clinical triad of gait apraxia, precipitate micturition, and cognitive decline are most likely to respond. Extended lumbar drainage, large-volume spinal fluid releases, or scintigraphic cisternography have been used as objective means to predict outcome of a shunting procedure.[43]

Disease-specific treatment of increased ICP in addition to symptomatic management with corticosteroids or osmotic diuresis is indicated in the majority of cases. Infectious complications are treated with antimicrobial therapy. Patients with a brain abscess undergo surgical drainage and a prolonged course of intravenous antibiotics. A hematoma within a metastatic focus is resected if located in a noneloquent area of the brain and in the absence of widely metastatic disease. Subdural hematoma or empyema requires immediate surgical decompression. Leukostasis in leukemic diseases responds to hydration, leukapheresis, systemic chemotherapy, and low-dose whole-brain irradiation.[44] Systemic intravenous anticoagulation with heparin or fractionated heparinoid is used in dural sinus thrombosis. When l-asparaginase therapy is involved in the pathogenesis of the prothrombotic stage, substitution with fresh-frozen plasma and antithrombin III is often administered prior to anticoagulant use. Petechial hemorrhages due to thrombocytopenia require transfusion of blood platelets. A coagulopathy can be corrected using transfusion of fresh-frozen plasma and substitution of vitamin K. Increased ICP secondary to medication requires dose reduction or discontinuation of the causative drug. All-trans retinoic acid related IIH may be alleviated with acetazolamide.[45] IIH caused by malignant dural sinus compression responds to local surgical treatment or irradiation. Leptomeningeal carcinomatosis is treated with irradiation and intrathecal chemotherapy.[46] CSF flow obstruction prohibits intraventricular injection of cytotoxic agents as it can give rise to a severe, irreversible toxic encephalopathy.

SELECTED REFERENCES

The full reference list can be accessed at lwwhealthlibrary.com/oncology.

1. Fishman RA. *Cerebrospinal fluid in diseases of the nervous system*. Philadelphia: W.B. Saunders Company; 1992.
2. Monro A. *Observations on the structure and function of the nervous system*. Edinburgh: Creech and Johnson; 1783.
4. Mokri B. The Monro-Kellie hypothesis: applications in CSF volume depletion. *Neurology* 2001;56:1746–1748.
5. Lundberg N. Continuous recording and control of ventricular fluid pressure in neurosurgical practice. *Acta Psychiatrica Scand* 1960;36:1–193.
6. Watling CJ, Cairncross JG. Acetazolamide therapy for symptomatic plateau waves in patients with brain tumors. Report of three cases. *J Neurosurg* 2002;97:224–226.
7. Lassman AB, DeAngelis LM. Brain metastases. *Neurol Clin* 2003;21:1–23, vii.
8. Posner JB. *Neurologic complications of cancer*. Philadelphia: FA Davis Company; 1995.
12. DeAngelis LM, Delattre JY, Posner JB. Radiation-induced dementia in patients cured of brain metastases. *Neurology* 1989;39:789–796.
13. Thiessen B, DeAngelis LM. Hydrocephalus in radiation leukoencephalopathy: results of ventriculoperitoneal shunting. *Arch Neurol* 1998;55:705–710.
16. Rifkinson-Mann S, Wisoff JH, Epstein F. The association of hydrocephalus with intramedullary spinal cord tumors: a series of 25 patients. *Neurosurgery* 1990;27:749–754.
21. Colucciello M. Pseudotumor cerebri induced by all-trans retinoic acid treatment of acute promyelocytic leukemia. *Arch Ophthalmol* 2003;121:1064–1065.
22. Kurzrock R, Estey E, Talpaz M. All-trans retinoic acid: tolerance and biologic effects in myelodysplastic syndrome. *J Clin Oncol* 1993;11:1489–1495.
23. Di Rocco C, Iannelli A. Poor outcome of bilateral congenital choroid plexus papillomas with extreme hydrocephalus. *Eur Neurol* 1997;37:33–37.
24. Biousse V, Ameri A, Bousser MG. Isolated intracranial hypertension as the only sign of cerebral venous thrombosis. *Neurology* 1999;53:1537–1542.
25. Gironell A, Marti-Fabregas J, Bello J, et al. Non-Hodgkin's lymphoma as a new cause of non-thrombotic superior sagittal sinus occlusion. *J Neurol Neurosurg Psychiatry* 1997;63:121–122.
26. Kim AW, Trobe JD. Syndrome simulating pseudotumor cerebri caused by partial transverse venous sinus obstruction in metastatic prostate cancer. *Am J Ophthalmol* 2000;129:254–256.
29. Forsyth PA, Posner JB. Headaches in patients with brain tumors: a study of 111 patients. *Neurology* 1993;43:1678–1683.
30. Kernohan JW, Woltman HW. Incisura of the crus due to contralateral brain tumor. *Arch Neur Psych* 1929;21:274–287.
31. Kelly KM, Lange B. Oncologic emergencies. *Pediatr Clin North Am* 1997;44:809–830.
32. Plum F, Posner JB. *The diagnosis of stupor and coma*. Philadelphia: FA Davis; 1980.
33. Cushing HW. Some experimental and clinical observations concerning states of increased intracranial tension. *Am J Med Sci* 1902;124:375–400.
37. Hakim S, Adams RD. The special clinical problem of symptomatic hydrocephalus with normal cerebrospinal fluid pressure. *J Neurol Sci* 1965;2:307–327.
38. Fisher CM. Hydrocephalus as a cause of disturbance of gait in the elderly. *Neurology* 1982;32:1358–1363.
40. Raboel PH, Bartek J Jr, Andresen M, et al. Intracranial pressure monitoring: invasive versus non-invasive methods—a review. *Crit Care Res Pract* 2012;2012:950393.
41. Rasulo FA, De Peri E, Lavinio A. Transcranial Doppler ultrasonography in intensive care. *Eur J Anaesthesiol* 2008;42:167–173.
42. Kaal EC, Vecht CJ. The management of brain edema in brain tumors. *Curr Opin Oncol* 2004;16:593–600.
43. Batra S, Rigamonti D. Idiopathic normal pressure hydrocephalus: the benefits and problems of shunting. *Nat Clin Pract Neurol* 2009;5:80–81.
44. Ferro A, Jabbour SK, Taunk NK, et al. Cranial irradiation in adults diagnosed with acute myelogenous leukemia presenting with hyperleukocytosis and neurologic dysfunction. *Leuk Lymphoma* 2014;55:105–109.
45. Machner B, Neppert B, Paulsen M, et al. Pseudotumor cerebri as a reversible side effect of all-trans retinoic acid treatment in acute promyelocytic leukaemia. *Eur J Neurol* 2008;15:e68–e69.
46. Chamberlain MC. Neoplastic meningitis. *J Clin Oncol* 2005;23:3605–3613.

PRACTICE OF ONCOLOGY

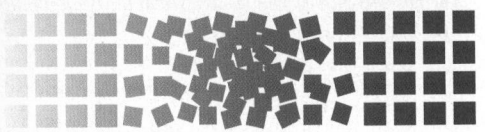

121 Spinal Cord Compression

Kevin P. Becker and Joachim M. Baehring

INTRODUCTION

Compression of the spinal cord is one of the most devastating neurologic complications, affecting 5% to 10% of patients who have cancer.[1–3] The majority of cases result from spine metastases with extension into the epidural space. Pain is the most common initial clinical manifestation of metastases to the axial skeleton. Within weeks, neurologic impairment ensues and is irreversible if treatment is not initiated promptly. Malignant spinal cord compression (MSCC) is a diagnostic challenge, especially in patients without a history of cancer. Back pain is one of the most common ailments in the general population and, in most cases, results from degenerative changes of the spine. Early identification of patients at risk of MSCC is essential as limitation of workup, symptomatic management, and bed rest—common practice in patients with "benign" back pain—almost invariably lead to profound neurologic morbidity.

This chapter describes the clinical syndromes, diagnosis, and treatment of epidural cancer metastases. Metastases below the conus medullaris, corresponding to the level of the first lumbar vertebra in adults and giving rise to isolated radiculopathies or a cauda equina syndrome, are included.

EPIDEMIOLOGY

An estimated 20,000 patients are diagnosed with MSCC per year in the United States.[4,5] The lifetime incidence in cancer patients is 1% to 6%, although autopsy series have revealed higher numbers (5% to 10%).[6–9] The majority of patients with MSCC are older than 50 years of age. However, cumulative incidence decreases with age: 4.4% in 40- to 50-year olds, 3.8% in 50- to 60-year olds, 2.9% in 60- to 70-year olds, 1.7% in 70- to 80-year olds, and 0.54% in patients older than 80 years.[10] The most common types of cancer that account for spinal cord compression are breast, prostate, lung cancer, and lymphoma.[1,6–8,11–14] The cumulative incidence of MSCC is disease specific and is highest in multiple myeloma (8%), prostate cancer (7%), nasopharyngeal cancer (6.5%), and breast cancer (5.5%).[7] The median interval between cancer diagnosis and manifestation of MSCC ranges from 6 to 12.5 months. Late axial bone metastases that cause cord compression are more common in breast cancer (43 months).[6] In only 1 in 500 cancer patients is spinal cord compression part of the presenting oncologic syndrome.[7] However, 20% of MSCC cases lack a history of cancer.[8,15] MSCC as the primary manifestation of a malignancy is more common in non-Hodgkin lymphoma, myeloma, and lung cancer, especially the small-cell variant; it is almost unheard of in breast cancer.[16,17] Two-thirds of MSCC cases affect the thoracic spine and 20% the lumbar spine, whereas cervical and sacral spine are rarely involved (<10% for each site).[1,12,14,18,19] Colon and prostate cancers seem to have a predilection for the lumbosacral spine, whereas lung and breast cancers are more common in the thoracic spine. Multiple epidural metastases are detected on initial presentation in up to one-third of patients in whom the whole axial skeleton is investigated.[20] Local recurrence after irradiation is rare, but 1 in 10 patients develops a second metastatic deposit that causes cord compression at a different spine level within 5 months of the first event.[1,12]

The tumor spectrum that causes cord compression in the pediatric population differs from adults and includes neuroblastoma, Ewing sarcoma, and, less commonly, primary vertebral osteosarcoma, germ cell tumors, and lymphoma. Cord compression as an initial manifestation of the tumor in children occurs more frequently than in the adult population.[21,22]

PATHOPHYSIOLOGY

Bone, particularly the axial skeleton, is one of the most common organ systems involved by metastatic spread. Up to one-third of patients dying of cancer develop metastases to the spine at some point during their illness.[23] Release of bone-derived growth factors and cytokines, capillary structure, and peculiar blood flow phenomena may facilitate deposition and growth of metastases.[24,25] Venous blood from intra-abdominal and intra-thoracic organs is not only drained through the vena cava but also through the vertebral and epidural venous plexus (Batson plexus). This low-pressure circulation without valves and with frequent flow reversal, depending on intrathoracic and intra-abdominal pressure, would appear to be an ideal transportation system for cancer cells.

The most common mechanisms of spinal cord compression are the direct extension of tumor from a hematogenous metastasis to a vertebral body into the epidural space or the pathologic fracture of a vertebral body infiltrated by a metastatic deposit, resulting in cord injury by a bone fragment or spine instability (Fig. 121.1A). Involvement of posterior spine elements with nerve root impingement is less common.[26] Transforaminal progression of paravertebral tumor is encountered in lymphoma and neuroblastoma. Highly aggressive paravertebral tumors such as the Pancoast tumor of the lung apex simply grow through anatomic barriers, including bone, into the epidural space. Primary hematogenous seeding to the epidural space is rare.[11] Spinal cord compression can also result from intradural mass lesions (meningioma, nerve sheath tumors, large leptomeningeal metastases) (Fig. 121.2) or intraneural spread of neurogenic tumors. Nonmetastatic causes are epidural hematoma in patients with coagulopathy or abscess in an immunocompromised host.

The mechanism of cord injury is not entirely understood. The early myelopathy associated with MSCC may be due to impairment of venous drainage, leading to intramedullary vasogenic edema. When the interstitial pressure rises beyond a critical threshold, cord perfusion is compromised, resulting in necrosis. Pathologic fracture of a vertebral body and posterior displacement of bone fragments lead to mechanical cord destruction. On histopathologic examination, demyelination or necrosis of white matter is the predominant finding at the level of cord compression, whereas gray matter is relatively well preserved.[13]

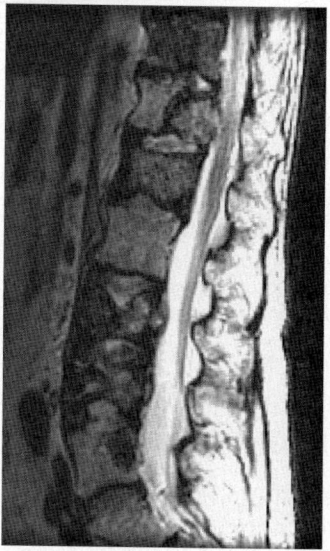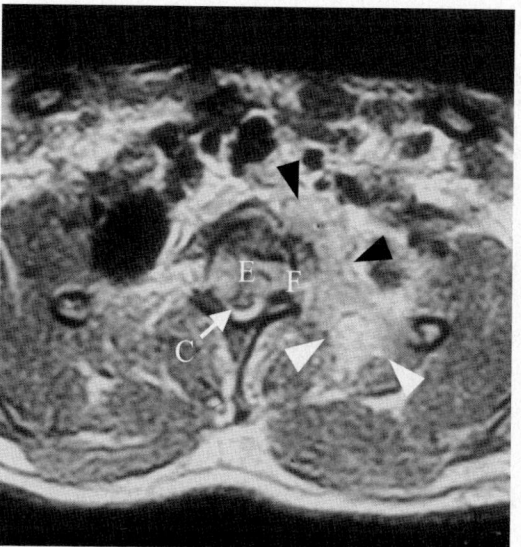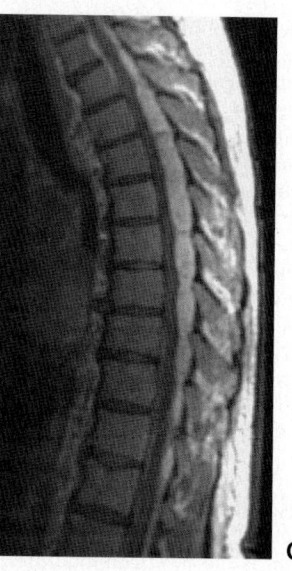

A, B   C

Figure 121.1 (A) A 53-year-old patient with metastatic renal cell cancer. T2-weighted magnetic resonance image (MRI; sagittal view) of the lumbosacral spine shows a pathologic fracture of the T12 vertebral body, posterior dislocation of a bone fragment, and compression of the spinal cord. **(B)** T1-weighted MRI with gadolinium (axial view) of a 19-year-old patient with Ewing sarcoma involving the T2 vertebral body. An enhancing soft tissue lesion is seen in the paravertebral space (*arrowheads*), the intervertebral foramen (*F*) and the epidural space (*E*). The cord (*C, arrow*) is compressed and displaced posteriorly. The patient had noticed that his left pupil had become smaller (Horner syndrome). He then started complaining of intermittent upper back pain aggravated by coughing, difficulty walking up stairs, and initiating urination. **(C)** A 73-year-old man with polycythemia rubra vera complained of progressive leg weakness and back pain. An MRI of the thoracic spine (T1 without contrast dye) revealed a large hyperintense epidural mass lesion compressing the cord posteriorly. A biopsy confirmed the suspected diagnosis of extramedullary hematopoiesis.

The complex syndrome of back pain is composed of local, radicular, and referred components. Pain-sensitive structures of the spine are the vertebral periosteum, the posterior longitudinal ligament, and the synovia of the facet joints innervated by branches of segmental spinal nerves. Pain from metastatic tumor spread to the spine ensues when the cancer infiltrates the periosteum. Radicular pain results from compression or infiltration of a nerve root. Pain

can also be the consequence of irritation of long tracts of the spinal cord (funicular pain) or paravertebral muscle spasm.

Micturition is frequently impaired in patients with MSCC. A brief review of the anatomy of bladder control may help to correctly interpret patients' symptoms. Excitatory input to the detrusor muscle that promotes bladder emptying is parasympathetic and involves sacral spinal cord segments. Relaxation of the

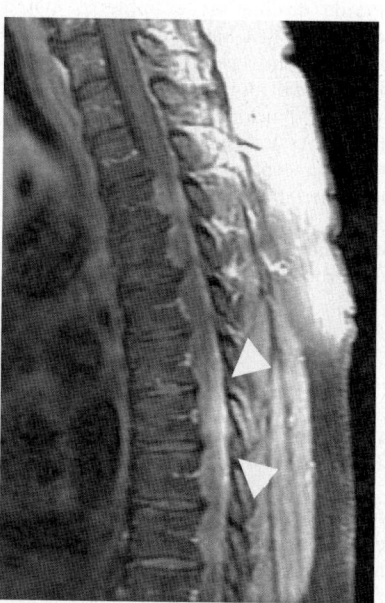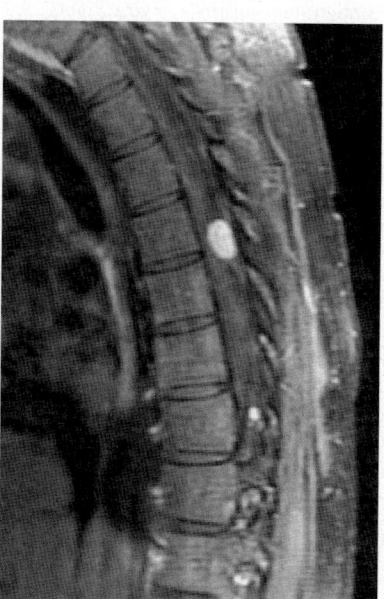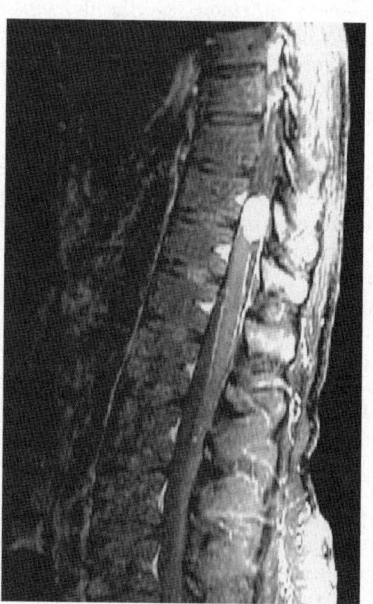

A, B   C

Figure 121.2 Topical differential diagnosis of cord compression. **(A)** Diffuse epidural infiltration by granulocytic sarcoma in a 65-year-old woman, causing cord compression in the lower thoracic spine (*arrowheads*). The tumor originated in the uterus and likely metastasized through the epidural venous plexus (Batson plexus) into the spinal canal (T1-weighted magnetic resonance image [MRI] with gadolinium and fat suppression). **(B)** A 32-year-old woman with neurofibromatosis type 2 and a meningioma of the spinal canal. This T1-weighted MRI with gadolinium and fat suppression (thoracic spine, sagittal view) demonstrates an intradural, extramedullary mass lesion with cord compression. **(C)** Leptomeningeal metastasis with cord infiltration and compression at the level of the T10 vertebral body in a 27-year-old patient with leptomeningeal spread of a diencephalic yolk sac tumor. The tumor infiltrated the thoracic spinal cord, giving rise to a Brown-Sequard syndrome below the level of infiltration (T1-weighted MRI with gadolinium and fat suppression, lower spine, sagittal view).

internal sphincter is transmitted through the sympathetic nervous system. Preganglionic neurons originate from thoracic and upper lumbar cord segments. The external sphincter muscle is innervated by motor neurons located in the anterior horn of the sacral cord (nucleus of Onufrowicz). Voluntary bladder control requires sensory input from stretch receptors within the bladder wall. This is transmitted to the pontine micturition center that also receives descending input from the paracentral lobule of the frontal lobe. The coordinated inhibition of internal and external sphincter muscle is mediated through the pontine micturition center. Spinal cord compression above the conus results in lack of voluntary control of micturition. Reflex emptying is possible but incomplete. When the sacral spinal cord is destroyed, the patient suffers from external sphincter insufficiency, unawareness of bladder fullness, and overflow incontinence. The mechanisms for control of defecation are similar.

CLINICAL PRESENTATION

Pain is the most common presenting symptom in patients with metastases involving the axial skeleton.[6,8,18,19] Any back pain in a patient with cancer known to frequently seed to spine or epidural space should be considered of metastatic origin until proven otherwise. Pain ensues when the richly innervated periosteum is involved. In its early stage, it may be localized to the affected spine segment. The vertebral body is tender to percussion. Pain that results from epidural mass effect is typically exacerbated by sneezing, coughing, or the Valsalva maneuver. Because it is aggravated by the recumbent position, patients experience maximum pain intensity on awakening in the morning; they may even sleep in a sitting position. Compression of a nerve root is associated with lancinating pain in the corresponding radicular distribution provoked by Valsalva maneuver. Radicular pain in the thoracic region is usually bilateral, whereas cervical and lumbar radiculopathies are unilateral.[27] Paravertebral muscle spasm caused by nerve root irritation from a metastasis results in straightening of the physiologic cervical or lumbar lordosis. Straight-leg raising (Lasegue maneuver) or, more specifically, crossed straight-leg raising (passive elevation of the contralateral, pain-free leg), exacerbates a lumbosacral radiculopathy. Referred pain may mimic a radiculopathy. Especially with intraneural tumor spread, neuropathic features (allodynia, hyperpathia, hyperalgesia) may predominate.

Neurologic symptoms typically evolve within weeks to months of the onset of back pain.[15,19] Hyperacute presentation with the evolution of paraplegia within hours to days is not uncommon in bronchogenic carcinoma, while a much slower course is typical for metastases from breast cancer.[13] Motor dysfunction (weakness, spasticity) is the earliest sign and occurs before sensory disturbance. Only one-third of patients report lower extremity weakness as an initial symptom. However, at diagnosis, less than one-third of patients are ambulatory.[6,8,18] Typical early complaints are leg "heaviness" and difficulty climbing stairs or getting up from a chair. As the majority of malignancy-related cord compressions occur at the level of the thoracic spinal cord, most patients present with a paraparesis. The rare patient with a cervical spinal cord metastasis is expected to have quadriparesis of varying degree and, if the high cervical cord is compromised, respiratory insufficiency. Epidural progression of metastases to the upper lumbar spine results in conus medullaris syndrome with distal lower extremity weakness, saddle paresthesia, and overflow leakage from bladder and bowel.

Only few patients report diminished sensation below the level of compression at initial presentation. The level of hypesthesia is usually two to three segments below the metastatic lesion. Discrepancy of up to 10 levels above or below the lesion has been described.[18] Tingling paresthesias radiating down the spine into the extremities on brisk flexion of the neck (Lhermitte sign) indicates an intrinsic or extrinsic spinal cord process. Ataxia in a patient with MSCC reflects compression of spinocerebellar pathways.

Symptoms of neurogenic bladder dysfunction are less common at symptom onset but are frequently overlooked or "rationalized" by the patient. A detailed micturition history is indispensable as patients are unlikely to report their symptoms until their compensatory mechanisms fail. New onset of nocturia or pollakisuria in the correct clinical setting should alarm the physician, and a common explanation by the patient ("I've been drinking a lot") should be disregarded. Alarming symptoms of bladder dysfunction are hesitancy and urinary retention. At diagnosis, almost half of patients with MSCC are incontinent or require catheterization.[8]

Presence of a Horner syndrome (the combination of miosis, ptosis, and enophthalmos) indicates transforaminal progression of tumors located at the level of the cervicothoracic junction and infiltration of the stellate ganglion.

DIFFERENTIAL DIAGNOSIS

Infiltration of the lumbosacral plexus or peripheral nerves originating from it (femoral, sciatic nerve) has to be distinguished from malignant epidural compression of a root or the cauda equina. With unilateral involvement, bladder and bowel symptoms are absent; however, bilateral infiltration of plexus or nerve, giving rise to incontinence, has been seen in neurolymphomatosis and perineural spread from pelvic malignancies. Herpes zoster is encountered at spinal levels previously or concurrently affected by cancer.[13,28]

The cauda equina syndrome is characterized by an asymmetric painful lumbosacral polyradiculopathy, a patchy sensory deficit corresponding to multiple lumbar and sacral nerve roots, and bladder and bowel incontinence. In a patient with cancer, this syndrome raises suspicion for leptomeningeal carcinomatosis. The presence of signs and symptoms referable to intracranial disease (headache, asymmetric cranial neuropathies) facilitates the diagnosis.

Intraparenchymal spinal cord metastases and primary cord tumors are rare but may resemble epidural disease. Metastatic cord tumors predominantly arise from small-cell lung and breast cancers.[29] Infectious (herpes simplex, human T-lymphotropic virus) and autoimmune myelitis are examples of not directly cancer-related myelopathies that have to be distinguished from MSCC. Predominance of transverse myelopathic features in the absence of pain is indicative of an intraparenchymal process.

Spinal cord hemisyndromes indicate intrinsic spinal cord disease. A classic Brown-Sequard syndrome characterized by leg weakness and loss of proprioception on the side of cord infiltration and loss of pain and temperature sensation on the opposite side is rarely seen but incomplete variants exist. Leptomeningeal spread of highly aggressive tumors can lead to spinal cord infiltration, causing an overlap syndrome of extrinsic and intrinsic cord disease (Fig. 121.2C).

DIAGNOSIS

The mere complaint of back pain in a patient with cancer frequently does not lead to an immediate workup for vertebral metastases. Only the occurrence of more severe symptoms such as sphincter dysfunction or paraparesis sets off a comprehensive diagnostic procedure.[6] Despite the availability of sensitive diagnostic tests, the average time between onset of symptoms and definitive diagnosis is still 3 months (range, 37 to 205 days). Two-thirds of this time passes after the patient reports the symptoms to a health professional.[18] An interesting pattern was observed in a Scottish study. The rate of cord compression diagnosis steadily increased throughout the course of the week and reached its peak on Friday.[18]

With the availability of magnetic resonance imaging (MRI), the diagnosis of MSCC has been simplified. The decision to use this tool depends on the clinical evaluation. New onset or change in character of preexisting back pain in a patient with cancer or atypical back pain in the absence of a cancer history warrants measures beyond plain X-ray films and symptomatic therapy. Degenerative spine disease mostly affects the lower cervical and lower lumbar spine, the segments of largest motion. The pain waxes and wanes and responds to bed rest and symptomatic treatment with nonsteroidal anti-inflammatory agents. Pain located in the thoracic spine, progressive pain despite conservative measures, or pain aggravated by supine position should raise the suspicion for MSCC.

MRI of the entire spine is the most sensitive diagnostic test when MSCC is suspected in a patient with cancer. The study can accurately identify the level of the metastatic lesion and guide the radiation oncologist in planning the treatment field. Multiple levels of involvement present in up to one-third of patients with MSCC are recognized.[20,30] Vertebral metastases without protrusion into the epidural space are detected before a potentially irreversible cord syndrome ensues. Metastases can be distinguished from other pathologic processes, involving the axial skeleton, epi- and intradural space, and spinal cord. Bacterial abscesses typically cause end-plate destruction and invasion of the disc space, whereas metastatic deposits leave the latter intact. Leptomeningeal carcinomatosis appears as nodular or linear tumor deposits in the medullary pia and along intradural nerve roots. Intradural extramedullary tumors such as meningioma or nerve sheath tumors can be easily diagnosed by their characteristic appearance and enhancement with contrast dye. Intramedullary metastases or primary tumors cause enlargement of the cord and thus can be distinguished from infectious or inflammatory myelitis that does not expand its transverse diameter.

Plain X-ray films of the spine lack sufficient sensitivity. Series of the pre-MRI era found signs of vertebral metastasis at the level of cord compression on plain X-ray films in only 80% of patients, and multiple levels of involvement were missed.[19] The local extent of metastatic disease is frequently underestimated, and paraspinal tumors with transforaminal extension may be entirely overlooked.

Myelography after intrathecal injection of water-soluble contrast material with or without computed tomography (myelography, computed tomographic myelography) was the diagnostic procedure of choice in the pre-MRI era. Epidural lesions that result in complete block of the subarachnoid space obscure the extent of disease and require a second procedure with cervical or suboccipital injection of dye in order to characterize metastatic deposits rostral to the block. The study remains an option for patients in whom MRI is contraindicated.

Scintigraphic examination of the skeletal system is most useful as a screening procedure for bone metastases. Its resolution, specificity, and sensitivity are inadequate to evaluate a patient with signs or symptoms of epidural metastasis and predict the level of cord compromise.[18] Myeloma may completely evade scintigraphic detection.

Positron emission tomography is likewise most useful as a staging procedure and cannot substitute for more detailed anatomic imaging techniques.

If cancer initially presents with MSCC, a biopsy is mandatory prior to initiation of therapy. This can be done by excisional biopsy of the mass or by computed tomography–guided needle biopsy.

A lumbar puncture is of no diagnostic value in epidural cancer. Complete obliteration of the subarachnoid space by an epidural metastasis results in compartmentation of the spinal canal with the possibility of herniation ("coning") after pressure reduction in the compartment below the level of obstruction by a lumbar puncture. Although cord herniation is a rare event, an MRI scan of the spine is advisable whenever MSCC is suspected before a lumbar puncture is performed.

TREATMENT

Treatment with corticosteroids should be initiated immediately when MSCC is suspected. Corticosteroids not only facilitate pain management but also reduce vasogenic cord edema and may

prevent additional damage to the spinal cord from decreased perfusion. After an initial intravenous bolus, doses of up to 10 mg every 6 hours are most commonly used. Oral bioavailability is excellent and intravenous application is required only in patients who cannot swallow. Protocols using higher doses (initial bolus of 100 mg followed by 96 mg divided into four doses for 3 days and a subsequent rapid taper) may achieve better pain control, but it remains unclear if their use leads to an improvement in neurologic recovery or preservation of motor function and sphincter control.[19,31,32] Complications of steroid use (gastroduodenal ulceration, hallucinations, euphoria, insomnia, generalized burning sensation) are more likely with use of higher doses.[33,34]

At the time of diagnosis, two-thirds of patients are treated with radiotherapy and one in five or six patients with surgical decompression. One-quarter of patients with MSCC are provided comfort care only when there is widespread disease and poor quality of life.[7]

Conventional external beam radiation therapy is the most commonly used treatment modality for patients. Various schedules have been applied with comparable results. Protocols consist of 5 to 10 applications of 3 to 4 Gy (total dose 30 Gy). Others have provided higher daily doses (5 Gy) during a 3-day induction phase followed by daily fractions of 3 Gy over 5 days for consolidation.[19] In the palliative situation, single fractions of 8 Gy may be preferable. Long-course radiotherapy is associated with better local control and similar functional outcome and should be used in patients with a relatively favorable anticipated survival.[35,36] Response to treatment depends on tumor histology. As one would anticipate, patients with relative radiosensitive tumors (breast cancer, lymphoma) have a higher chance of regaining or preserving motor function than patients with less radiosensitive tumors (non-small-cell lung cancer, melanoma, renal cell carcinoma).[19] Dose escalation does not appear to improve outcome.[37] Recently, there has been an increase in the use of stereotactic radiosurgical techniques for spine metastases. A distinct advantage over conventional radiotherapy is the ability to deliver a higher radiation dose without exceeding the tolerance of the spinal cord. Various techniques and dosing schedules are available: linear-accelerator–based stereotactic radiosurgery (SRS), proton beam radiosurgery, or image-guided radiosurgery. SRS is typically administered as an 8 to 24 Gy single fraction. Stereotactic radiation therapy (SRT) is given in three to five fractions of 4 to 9 Gy. To date, radiosurgery has largely been used as salvage therapy for tumor progression in patients who have already been treated with conventional radiotherapy or as an adjuvant therapy following surgery. A role for spinal radiosurgery as a primary modality is seen in patients who are unable to undergo surgery or those with tumors poorly responsive to conventional radiotherapy. Local control rates of 85% to 90% and durable responses even against radioresistant tumors have been reported.[38–40] In 2009, the Spine Oncology Study Group issued a "strong" recommendation to consider radiosurgery over conventional radiotherapy for patients with solid-tumor spinal metastases.[41] In a phase 1/2 trial, SRT as primary or salvage treatment for mechanically stable spinal metastasis led to reductions in patient-reported pain and opioid requirement, satisfactory progression-free survival (72.4% at 2 years), and no late spinal cord toxicities.[42] However, when spinal tumors abut the cord or if there is MSCC, SRS or SRT may not be feasible. Proper prospective evaluation of efficacy, morbidity, and cost-effectiveness as a function of tumor stage is pending and, considering the complexity of the patient population, may only become available for highly selected patient populations.

Strontium-89 is used as palliative treatment for widely metastatic bone metastases from prostate cancer. It provides pain control but cannot reverse the neurologic syndrome from epidural cord compression.

The role of surgical decompression in patients with MSCC remains a controversial subject. For the majority of patients, a benefit from surgical intervention has not been convincingly shown.[43,44] However, in carefully selected patients, tumor resection results in improved functional outcome compared with irradiation. In a prospective randomized trial, the ability to walk was preserved for a longer period of time after surgery compared with radiation therapy (122 days versus 13 days). Patients were eligible only if they did not have certain radiosensitive tumors (lymphomas, leukemia, multiple myeloma, and germ cell tumors) or concomitant neurologic problems not directly related to MSCC (e.g., brain metastases), the duration of paraplegia was <48 hours, MSCC occurred at one level, their general medical status rendered them acceptable surgical candidates, and their life expectancy exceeded 3 months.[45] Other commonly accepted indications for surgery are the lack of a recent history of cancer, involvement of a previously irradiated segment, progressive painful radiculopathy despite irradiation, cord compression resulting from pathologic fracture, and spinal instability.[6,26,30] Younger patients are more likely to undergo surgical debulking.[7] Posterior exposure with laminectomy at the level of cord compression has been a common approach. The metastatic focus, usually located within the vertebral body, cannot be completely visualized and thus at best is only partially removed. Laminectomy may increase the degree of instability in kyphotic deformities resulting from pathologic fracture. Thus, an anterior approach for surgical decompression is favored in selected patients. This procedure, reserved for patients with the possibility of long-term survival, includes resection of the affected vertebral body and implantation of stabilizing instrumentation. Frequently, two surgical sessions are required.[26,46] Surgical morbidity is considerable. A posterolateral transpedicular approach with stabilizing instrumentation is a feasible alternative.[26]

Treatment guidelines are similar in the pediatric population. Surgical intervention is recommended for patients with rapid neurologic deterioration or a severe transverse myelopathy at initial presentation.[21]

Systemic chemotherapy is an appropriate treatment only for patients with MSCC caused by highly chemosensitive tumors such as non-Hodgkin lymphoma or germ cell tumors. Radiation or surgical intervention may not be necessary.[16,47,48]

It is unclear if asymptomatic patients benefit from treatment of incidentally detected epidural metastases. The decision depends on tumor type and the patient's condition. Observation and serial MRI scans may be appropriate until pain ensues.

Bisphosphonates are now widely used, particularly in the treatment of breast cancer and multiple myeloma. Monthly provision of intravenous zoledronic acid or pamidronate in combination with other treatment modalities for the underlying cancer significantly reduces skeletal-related events (SRE; pathologic fracture, MSCC, palliative radiation to bone, or surgery to bone).[24,49–52] The monoclonal antireceptor activator of nuclear factor kappa-B ligand (RANKL) antibody denosumab was found to be noninferior to zoledronic acid in preventing or delaying first on-study SRE in patients with advanced cancer metastatic to bone or myeloma and superior in patients with prostate or breast cancer metastatic to bone.[53–55] The selective androgen biosynthesis inhibitor abiraterone acetate in combination with prednisone prevents SREs in patients with metastatic castration-resistant prostate cancer.[56]

PROGNOSIS

Naturally, the prognosis for the patient with epidural metastasis and cord compression depends on the type and extent of the underlying malignancy. Untreated, patients with MSCC succumb within a month of diagnosis. The median overall survival of patients with MSCC ranges from 3 to 16 months and most patients die of systemic tumor progression.[1,6–8,12,46,57] Patients with therapy-sensitive tumors such as lymphoma or myeloma live longer (lymphoma, 6 to 14 months) than patients with solid tumors.[6,7,12,58] The most important determinant of functional outcome is the severity of neurologic damage at the time treatment is initiated. A total of 80% of patients treated at a time when a significant neurologic deficit is absent, and 50% of those with mild transverse myelopathy, but only 5% of patients who are paraplegic when definitive treatment is initiated remain ambulatory or regain the ability to walk after treatment.[1,8,11,12,14] Late return of function within 6 to 20 months of treatment has been observed in long-term survivors of MSCC in non-Hodgkin lymphoma.[14,16] The faster the neurologic deficit evolves, the lower the chance for recovery of motor function after treatment.[58]

SELECTED REFERENCES

The full reference list can be accessed at lwwhealthlibrary.com/oncology.

1. Helweg-Larsen S, Sorensen PS, Kreiner S. Prognostic factors in metastatic spinal cord compression: a prospective study using multivariate analysis of variables influencing survival and gait function in 153 patients. *Int J Radiat Oncol Biol Phys* 2000;46:1163–1169.
7. Loblaw DA, Laperriere NJ, Mackillop WJ. A population-based study of malignant spinal cord compression in Ontario. *Clin Oncol (R Coll Radiol)* 2003;15:211–217.
9. Loblaw DA, Laperriere NJ. Emergency treatment of malignant extradural spinal cord compression: an evidence-based guideline. *J Clin Oncol* 1998;16:1613–1624.
10. Prasad D, Schiff D. Malignant spinal-cord compression. *Lancet Oncol* 2005;6:15–24.
11. Posner JB. Back pain and epidural spinal cord compression. *Med Clin North Am* 1987;71:185–205.
14. Helweg-Larsen S. Clinical outcome in metastatic spinal cord compression. A prospective study of 153 patients. *Acta Neurol Scand* 1996;94:269–275.
15. Schiff D, O'Neill BP, Suman VJ. Spinal epidural metastasis as the initial manifestation of malignancy. *Neurology* 1997;49:452–456.
19. Greenberg HS, Kim JH, Posner JB. Epidural spinal cord compression from metastatic tumor: results with a new treatment protocol. *Ann Neurol* 1980;8:361–366.
21. Bouffet E, Marec-Berard P, Thiesse P, et al. Spinal cord compression by secondary epi- and intradural metastases in childhood. *Childs Nerv Syst* 1997;13:383–387.
27. Posner JB. Neurological complications of systemic cancer. *Med Clin North Am* 1971;55:625–646.
32. Delattre JY, Arbit E, Rosenblum MK, et al. High dose versus low dose dexamethasone in experimental epidural spinal cord compression. *Neurosurgery* 1988;22:1005–1007.

35. Rades D, Fehlauer F, Schulte R, et al. Prognostic factors for local control and survival after radiotherapy of metastatic spinal cord compression. *J Clin Oncol* 2006;24:3388–3393.
36. Rades D, Lange M, Veninga T, et al. Final results of a prospective study comparing the local control of short-course and long-course radiotherapy for metastatic spinal cord compression. *Int J Radiat Oncol Biol Phys* 2011;79:524–530.
37. Rades D, Freundt K, Meyners T, et al. Dose escalation for metastatic spinal cord compression in patients with relatively radioresistant tumors. *Int J Radiat Oncol Biol Phys* 2011;80:1492–1497.
38. Yamada Y, Lovelock DM, Yenice KM, et al. Multifractionated image-guided and stereotactic intensity-modulated radiotherapy of paraspinal tumors: a preliminary report. *Int J Radiat Oncol Biol Phys* 2005;62:53–61.
39. Gerszten PC, Burton SA, Ozhasoglu C, et al. Radiosurgery for spinal metastases: clinical experience in 500 cases from a single institution. *Spine (Phila Pa 1976)* 2007;32:193–199.
40. Yamada Y, Bilsky MH, Lovelock DM, et al. High-dose, single-fraction image-guided intensity-modulated radiotherapy for metastatic spinal lesions. *Int J Radiat Oncol Biol Phys* 2008;71:484–490.
42. Wang XS, Rhines LD, Shiu AS, et al. Stereotactic body radiation therapy for management of spinal metastases in patients without spinal cord compression: a phase 1-2 trial. *Lancet Oncol* 2012;13:395–402.
44. Rades D, Huttenlocher S, Dunst J, et al. Matched pair analysis comparing surgery followed by radiotherapy and radiotherapy alone for metastatic spinal cord compression. *J Clin Oncol* 2010;28:3597–3604.
45. Patchell RA, Tibbs PA, Regine WF, et al. Direct decompressive surgical resection in the treatment of spinal cord compression caused by metastatic cancer: a randomised trial. *Lancet* 2005;366:643–648.
46. Sundaresan N, Sachdev VP, Holland JF, et al. Surgical treatment of spinal cord compression from epidural metastasis. *J Clin Oncol* 1995;13:2330–2335.

48. Grommes C, Bosl GJ, DeAngelis LM. Treatment of epidural spinal cord involvement from germ cell tumors with chemotherapy. *Cancer* 2011; 117:1911–1916.

49. Terpos E, Morgan G, Dimopoulos MA, et al. International Myeloma Working Group recommendations for the treatment of multiple myeloma-related bone disease. *J Clin Oncol* 2013;31:2347–2357.

50. Morgan GJ, Child JA, Gregory WM, et al. Effects of zoledronic acid versus clodronic acid on skeletal morbidity in patients with newly diagnosed multiple myeloma (MRC Myeloma IX): secondary outcomes from a randomised controlled trial. *Lancet Oncol* 2011;12:743–752.

51. Kohno N, Aogi K, Minami H, et al. Zoledronic acid significantly reduces skeletal complications compared with placebo in Japanese women with bone metastases from breast cancer: a randomized, placebo-controlled trial. *J Clin Oncol* 2005;23:3314–3321.

52. Rosen LS, Gordon D, Tchekmedyian S, et al. Zoledronic acid versus placebo in the treatment of skeletal metastases in patients with lung cancer and other solid tumors: a phase III, double-blind, randomized trial—the Zoledronic

Acid Lung Cancer and Other Solid Tumors Study Group. *J Clin Oncol* 2003;21:3150–3157.

53. Henry DH, Costa L, Goldwasser F, et al. Randomized, double-blind study of denosumab versus zoledronic acid in the treatment of bone metastases in patients with advanced cancer (excluding breast and prostate cancer) or multiple myeloma. *J Clin Oncol* 2011;29:1125–1132.

54. Fizazi K, Carducci M, Smith M, et al. Denosumab versus zoledronic acid for treatment of bone metastases in men with castration-resistant prostate cancer: a randomised, double-blind study. *Lancet* 2011;377:813–822.

55. Stopeck AT, Lipton A, Body JJ, et al. Denosumab compared with zoledronic acid for the treatment of bone metastases in patients with advanced breast cancer: a randomized, double-blind study. *J Clin Oncol* 2010;28:5132–5139.

56. Logothetis CJ, Basch E, Molina A, et al. Effect of abiraterone acetate and prednisone compared with placebo and prednisone on pain control and skeletal-related events in patients with metastatic castration-resistant prostate cancer: exploratory analysis of data from the COU-AA-301 randomised trial. *Lancet Oncol* 2012;13:1210–1217.

PRACTICE OF ONCOLOGY

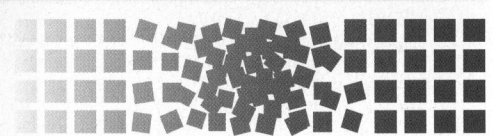

122 Metabolic Emergencies

Antonio Tito Fojo

INTRODUCTION

While increased awareness and improved prophylaxis have helped preempt some metabolic emergencies, their occurrence continues to present challenges to the practicing oncologist. Prompt recognition and the rapid institution of adequate therapy are essential to a successful outcome.

TUMOR LYSIS SYNDROME AND HYPERURICEMIA

General

Tumor cell death with the release of intracellular contents can lead to a constellation of metabolic abnormalities that comprise the tumor lysis syndrome (TLS). While it can occur spontaneously in rapidly proliferating tumors, it occurs most frequently following administration of cytotoxic chemotherapy to patients with hematologic malignancies, with a large percentage of proliferating, drug-sensitive cells (Tables 122.1 and 122.2).[1,2] In these patients, TLS occurs a few hours to a few days after the initiation of therapy. Cell death leads to the release of potassium, phosphate, uric acid, and other purine metabolites overwhelming the kidney's capacity for clearance with resultant hyperkalemia, hyperphosphatemia and secondary hypocalcemia, and hyperuricemia (Table 122.3). Unchecked, TLS can progress to acute renal failure and metabolic acidosis. While established TLS is associated with a high morbidity and mortality, judicious prophylaxis can avoid complications. The higher mortality reported among patients with solid tumors is likely a consequence of less prophylaxis and reduced awareness.

The highest incidence of TLS occurs in patients with rapidly growing, chemosensitive myelo-lymphoproliferative malignancies with high white blood cell counts (acute leukemias) or large bulky adenopathy (high-grade non-Hodgkin lymphomas [NHL], especially Burkitt lymphoma).[3–6] In high-grade NHL, an incidence of TLS as high as 42% has been reported, clinically significant in only 6% of patients.[7] The latter agrees with a Pan-European retrospective chart review that identified TLS in 3.4%, 5.2%, and 6.1%, of patients with acute myeloid leukemia (AML), acute lymphoblastic leukemia (ALL), and NHL, respectively. In an era antedating modern interventions, this review found an overall mortality of 0.9% for all patients and 17.5% for patients who developed TLS.[8] By comparison, TLS occurs infrequently in solid tumors, most likely due to the lower growth fractions, and slower response to treatment—occurring with tumors that are *highly or moderately* sensitive to chemotherapy, or if bulky, metastatic disease is present.[9] TLS has also been reported following ionizing radiation including total-body irradiation in the transplant setting, embolization, radiofrequency ablation, monoclonal antibody therapy, glucocorticoids, interferon, and in the setting of hematopoietic stem cell transplantation. As new therapies emerge, TLS may occur in unanticipated settings, as seen in indolent chronic lymphocytic leukemia treated with flavopiridol.[10] Table 122.2 summarizes the

Cairo and Bishop Classification System for TLS. Table 122.3 summarizes recent guidance from a tumor lysis expert panel.[11]

Hyperuricemia can occur in TLS as noted previously, or more frequently as an isolated finding in patients with cancer. For example, in the Pan-European retrospective chart review previously noted, among 755 patients with ALL, AML, or NHL hyperuricemia without TLS was identified in 13.6% of cases, and with TLS in an additional 5.3%.[8]

Pathogenesis

Cell lysis with the release of contents at a rate exceeding the kidney's clearance capacity is the most important etiologic factor in TLS (see Table 122.3 and Fig. 122.1). Rapidly dividing cells have high nucleic acid turnover, and some cancer cells, particularly lymphoid cells, contain higher levels of phosphate than their normal counterparts.

Hyperkalemia poses the greatest immediate threat. Although release of potassium from dying cells is the principal cause, falling adenosine triphosphate (ATP) levels before cell lysis may lead to potassium leakage, explaining why a rise in serum potassium is often the first sign of TLS.

Hyperphosphatemia, like hyperkalemia, follows cell lysis. The initial adaptation involves increased urinary excretion and decreased tubular reabsorption of phosphate. However, as transport becomes saturated, phosphorus levels rise, the calcium phosphorus multiple exceeds 70, and calcium phosphate precipitates in tissues resulting in hypocalcemia. Hypocalcemia leads to increased levels of parathyroid hormone, with decreased proximal tubule phosphate reabsorption, accentuating hyperphosphaturia and the risk of calcium phosphate crystals in renal tubules (nephrocalcinosis) with tubular obstruction.

While hyperuricemia alone may not be an acute threat, it is the most common finding and contributes to renal failure, a complication that in the setting of tumor lysis is usually multifactorial. Within the cell, there is continuous turnover and salvage of bases (Fig. 122.2). In humans, the end product of purine metabolism is uric acid. Adenine is catabolized to hypoxanthine, and this is converted by xanthine oxidase to xanthine and in turn to uric acid. Guanine forms xanthine that is converted to uric acid by xanthine oxidase. In most mammals, *urate oxidase* catalyzes the oxidation of uric acid to allantoin, a more soluble catabolite. However, a nonsense mutation in the coding region acquired during evolution precludes urate oxidase expression in humans, making uric acid, not allantoin, the final purine metabolite.[12]

Hyperuricemia occurs primarily as a result of accelerated cellular breakdown. Acute uric acid nephropathy occurs when urate and uric acid crystals obstruct renal tubules. Urate is filtered at high concentrations from the plasma and is further concentrated along the course of the tubular system. As the pH becomes more acidic, uric acid can precipitate, obstructing tubules, collecting ducts, and even pelves and ureters. Crystal deposition increases tubular and intrarenal pressure with extrinsic compression of the vasa recta, an increase in renal vascular resistance, and a fall in

TABLE 122.1

Risk Assessment and Initial Management of Tumor Lysis Syndrome

Laboratory TLS[a]	–	–	–	–	–	–	–	–	+	–
Clinical TLS[a]	–	–	–	–	–	–	–	–	–	+
Tumor burden[b]	Small	Medium	Medium	Large	Medium	Large	Medium	Large	–	N/A
Risk of cell lysis[c]	N/A	Low	Mod/Unk	Low	Mod/Unk	Mod/Unk	High	High	–	N/A
Organ function[d]	N/A	N/A	Normal	N/A	Abnormal	N/A	N/A	N/A	N/A	N/A
	↓	↓	↓	↓	↓	↓	↓	↓	↓	↓
Risk of clinical TLS	**Negligible**	**Low**		**Intermediate**				**High**		**Established**

TLS, tumor lysis syndrome; Mod/Unk, moderate/unknown; N/A, not applicable.
[a] At time of diagnosis; see Table 122.2 for definitions.
[b] Bulky disease (hepatosplenomegaly, bulky adenopathy) and/or high leucocyte count, often evidenced by elevated pretreatment lactate dehydrogenase.
[c] Including elevated pretreatment uric acid.
[d] Abnormal = preexisting nephropathy, acidosis, hypotension/volume depletion, or prior/concurrent nephrotoxin exposure.
Adapted from Howard SC, Jones DP, Pui C-H. The tumor lysis syndrome. N Engl J Med 2011;364:1844–1854.

renal blood flow. The elevated tubular pressure and decreased renal blood flow reduce glomerular filtration and can lead to acute renal failure.

Therapy

In the modern era, laboratory abnormalities alert physicians and guide preventive management (see Tables 122.1 and 122.3). In adults, preventive measures include foremost hydration, allopurinol, and oral phosphate binders, beginning preferably 24 hours before chemotherapy administration.

Aggressive hydration, the most important intervention, should begin immediately, administering at least 3,000 mL/m² per day, *when possible delaying tumor therapy so hydration can be administered*. Urine alkalinization remains controversial as it favors precipitation of calcium/phosphate complexes in renal tubules— calcium phosphate, unlike uric acid, becomes less soluble at an alkaline pH. Furthermore, metabolic alkalemia can worsen the neurologic manifestations of hypocalcemia. Administration of 100 mEq sodium bicarbonate will maintain urine pH above 7.5, a pH that is needed not because of uric acid, which has a pKa of 5.4 (so that above a pH of 6.4 >90% is sodium urate), but because of xanthine which as a pKa of about 7.4.

TABLE 122.2

Cairo and Bishop Classification System for Tumor Lysis Syndrome

Laboratory TLS	Clinical TLS
Abnormality in two or more of the following, occurring within 3 d before or 7 d after chemotherapy: ■ Uric acid >8 mg/dL or 25% increase ■ Potassium >6 meq/L or 25% increase ■ Phosphate >4.5 mg/dL or 25% increase ■ Calcium <7 mg/dL or 25% decrease	Laboratory TLS plus one or more of the following: ■ Increased serum creatinine (1.5 × upper limit of normal) ■ Cardiac arrhythmia or sudden death ■ Seizure

TLS, tumor lysis syndrome.
Adapted from Cairo MS, Bishop M. Tumour lysis syndrome: new therapeutic strategies and classification. Br J Haematol 2004;127:3–11.

Hyperkalemia should be treated aggressively. Cation exchange resins should be used, recognizing their value will be delayed. Calcium gluconate antagonizes cardiac effects of hyperkalemia and can be especially helpful if there is concomitant hypocalcemia. Sodium bicarbonate corrects acidemia and shifts potassium back into cells; administering hypertonic dextrose and insulin can augment this. Loop diuretics can eliminate excess potassium in patients without renal failure; hemodialysis is indicated in renal impairment.

Hyperphosphatemia and its resultant hypocalcemia require oral phosphate binders except to manage hyperkalemia avoid calcium administration, because it can promote metastatic calcifications.

Given its central role in acute renal failure, hyperuricemia should be managed aggressively. Allopurinol, an analog of the purine base hypoxanthine, lowers uric acid by inhibiting xanthine oxidase, the enzyme responsible for converting hypoxanthine to xanthine and xanthine to uric acid (see Fig. 122.2). Its active metabolite, oxypurinol, also inhibits xanthine oxidase. Because both allopurinol and oxypurinol inhibit uric acid synthesis, but have no effect on preexisting uric acid, uric acid levels usually do not fall until after 48 to 72 hours of treatment. Furthermore, inhibition of xanthine oxidase leads to an increase in plasma hypoxanthine and xanthine levels, with increased renal excretion of both metabolic products. Like uric acid, xanthine (pKa = 7.4) but not hypoxanthine (pKa = 1.98) may precipitate contributing to acute renal failure. Oral allopurinol has a bioavailability of 50%; alternately, intravenous allopurinol (Aloprim, Bioniche Pharma, Belleville, Ontario, Canada) may be administered. Allopurinol should be discontinued if allergic reactions such as skin rashes and urticaria occur (incidence increased in patients receiving amoxicillin, ampicillin, or thiazides). Finally, the doses of allopurinol should be adjusted for creatinine clearance as follows:

Creatinine clearance	Allopurinol dose
≥20 mL/min	300 mg/d
10–20 mL/min	200 mg/d
3–10 mL/min	100 mg/d
<3 mL/min	100 mg/36–48 h

An alternate approach to the treatment of hyperuricemia involves the use of rasburicase (Fasturtec, Sanofi Synth, Paris, France; Elitek, Sanofi US, Bridgewater, NJ), a recombinant urate oxidase developed to replace uricozyme, a nonrecombinant urate oxidase. Because urate oxidase degrades uric acid rather than prevent its synthesis, as does allopurinol, rapid reduction in uric acid occurs following its administration without the accumulation of

PRACTICE OF ONCOLOGY

TABLE 122.3

Tumor Lysis Syndrome

Complication	Etiology	Manifestations	Management
Hyperkalemia	Intracellular K^+ release rate exceeds renal clearance capacity; K^+ leakage secondary to falling ATP levels	■ Electrocardiographic abnormalities ■ Muscle cramps, weakness, and paresthesias ■ Nausea, vomiting, and diarrhea	■ Aggressive hydration ■ Cation exchange resins ■ Calcium gluconate ■ Sodium bicarbonate ■ Hypertonic dextrose + insulin ■ Loop diuretics
Hyperphosphatemia	Intracellular PO_4 release rate that exceeds renal clearance capacity	■ Acute renal failure ■ Secondary hypocalcemia	■ Aggressive hydration ■ Hypertonic dextrose + insulin ■ Oral phosphate binders
Hypocalcemia	Secondary to hyperphosphatemia and ensuing tissue precipitation of calcium phosphate	■ Muscle twitches, cramps, tetany, carpopedal spasm, or paresthesia ■ Mental status changes, confusion, delirium, hallucinations ■ Rarely seizures ■ Exacerbation of hyperkalemia	■ Manage hyperphosphatemia
Hyperuricemia	Intracellular uric acid release rate exceeds renal clearance capacity	■ Acute renal failure	■ Aggressive hydration ■ Allopurinol ■ Urate oxidase ■ Conventional hemodialysis if acute renal failure develops
Lactic acidosis	Hypovolemia and acute renal failure	■ Acidemia	■ Volume replacement ■ Correct acidosis

ATP, adenosine triphosphate.

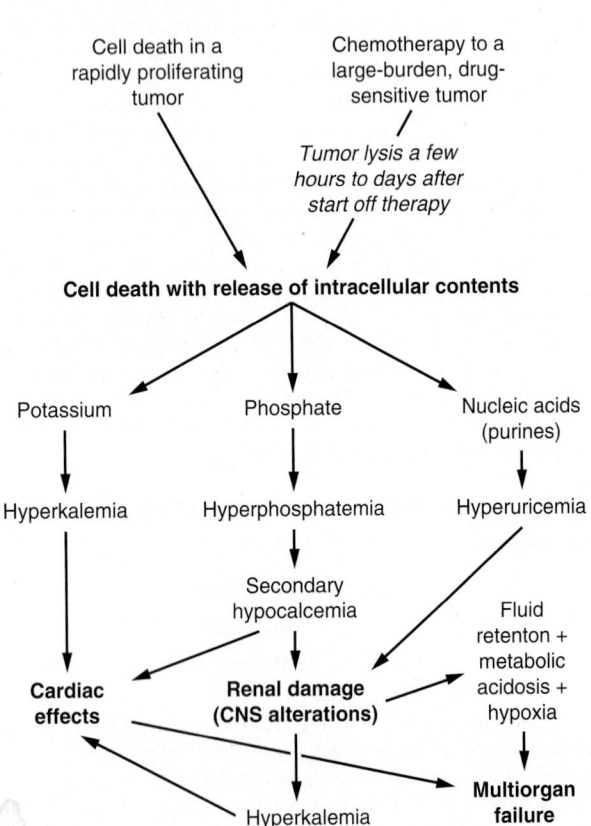

Figure 122.1 Dynamics of tumor lysis syndrome. CNS, central nervous system.

precursors. Studies in adults and children have shown uric acid levels fall to 0.5 to 1 mg/dL within 4 hours of rasburicase injection with low levels maintained throughout treatment. Despite normalization of uric acid levels with rasburicase, a small percentage have required dialysis—a not unexpected observation, given the multifactorial nature of renal failure in TLS and the fact rasburicase affects only one component, albeit an important one.

Table 122.4 contrasts allopurinol and rasburicase, and notes that rasburicase is more expensive.[13] The manufacturer recommends a rasburicase dose of 0.2 mg/kg for up to 5 days (http://products.sanofi.us/elitek/elitek.html). However, except in rare patients with very high serum levels of uric acid, much less is sufficient. A 5-day course of rasburicase is about 15,000 times more expensive than a 5-day course of allopurinol and 15 to 30 times more than intravenous allopurinol, so cost must be factored into decision making. With a 2013 price of ≈$521/mg (Bluebook Average Wholesale Price is $2,345 for three vials containing 1.5 mg each) the 5-day tab for a 70-kg patient receiving the manufacturer's recommended dose of 0.2 mg/kg for 5 days exceeds $36,470. At this price, rasburicase can be justified only if it will prevent acute renal failure, and the existing data is not compelling. While some studies suggest rasburicase can reduce the need for dialysis, no differences or only clinically insignificant differences in serum creatinine have been reported in other studies, and at the present time the data do not definitively proof that less dialysis is required in patients treated with rasburicase.[14–16] It *appears* rasburicase therapy is beneficial in children with hematologic malignancies; however, randomized controlled trials in adults have been less convincing. Nevertheless, rasburicase is approved by the US Food and Drug Administration for use in adults based on a randomized phase 3 trial.[14] Because outcomes other than laboratory parameters were not different, the authors could only conclude "the incidence of laboratory TLS, *which can be regarded as an indicator of the risk of clinical TLS*, was significantly lower with rasburicase than with allopurinol" and "the rapid reduction in uric acid to less than 1.0 mg/dL with rasburicase simplifies uric acid control by reducing the need for

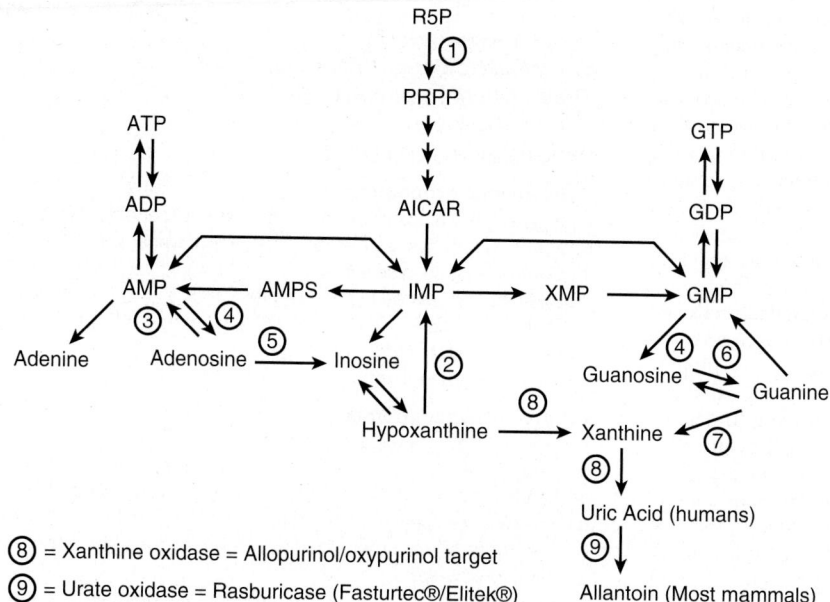

$$R5P$$
$$\downarrow \ \textcircled{1}$$
$$PRPP$$

Figure 122.2 Purine metabolism/catabolism. **(A)** The figure shows the pathways of purine metabolism/catabolism in mammals with an emphasis on pathways involved in purine catabolism and generation of uric acid. The numbers enclosed in circles identify the enzymes involved in catalyzing the reaction. These are (1) PRPP synthetase; (2) hypoxanthine phosphoribosyltransferase; (3) adenosine kinase; (4) 5' nucleotidase; (5) adenosine deaminase; (6) purine nucleoside phosphorylase; (7) guanase; (8) xanthine oxidase, that also catalyzes the conversion of allopurinol to oxypurinol; and (9) urate oxidase or uricase, an enzyme that is present in mammals with the exception of humans and many primates. R5P, ribose 5' phosphate; PRPP, phosphoribosyl pyrophosphate; AICAR, aminoimidazole carboxamide ribonucleotide; IMP, inosine monophosphate; XMP, xanthosine monophosphate; GMP, guanosine monophosphate; GDP, guanosine diphosphate; GTP, guanosine triphosphate; AMPS, adenylosuccinate; AMP, adenosine monophosphate; ADP, adenosine diphosphate; ATP, adenosine triphosphate. **(B)** Structure and dissociation constants of key metabolites in purine metabolic/catabolic pathway.

TABLE 122.4

Allopurinol and Rasburicase: A Comparison

Allopurinol	Rasburicase
Oral, easy to use	Intravenous administration
Slow onset of action: No effect on preexisting uric acid levels	Rapid onset of action: Lowers preexisting uric acid levels without accumulation of precursors; may allow start of chemotherapy without delay
Ineffective in some patients	Lowers uric acid in all patients
1% incidence of allergic reactions[14]	4% to 5% incidence of immunoallergic reactions including anaphylaxis[14]
Can interfere with metabolism of oral but not intravenous 6-mercaptopurine[13]	No effect on drug metabolism
No added risk with G6PD deficiency	**Can lead to hemolysis in patients with G6PD deficiency such as those of African or Mediterranean ancestry**
Comparable efficacy in preventing acute renal failure and need for dialysis[14,16]	Lower incidence of laboratory TLS but not clinical TLS
Inexpensive	Very expensive

TLS, tumor lysis syndrome.

urinary alkalinization in patients who are often critically ill with compromised organ function."[14] An earlier Pan-European multicenter economic evaluation of rasburicase in prevention and treatment of hyperuricemia and TLS in patients with hematologic malignancies concluded rasburicase is economically attractive in the *treatment of hyperuricemia* both in adults and children while in the *prevention of hyperuricemia*, it "has an attractive economic profile in children and is cost-effective in adults with ALL and NHL . . . whereas in adult AML patients, the short average life expectancy and the lower baseline risk of hyperuricemia and TLS limits the cost-effectiveness of rasburicase."[8]

In both children and adults, it appears the manufacturer's recommended dose of 0.2 mg/kg/day for up to 5 days is excessive.[17–20] Evidence indicates a single 3-mg dose is effective in the prophylaxis and treatment of hyperuricemia in adults with uric acid levels up to 12 mg/dL, with uric acid levels continuing to decline beyond 24 hours in most patients without additional treatment.[19] For a 70-kg patient, a 3-mg dose—approximately one-fifth the recommended dose of 0.2 mg/kg—is convenient as vials contain 1.5 mg rasburicase, making it more affordable. Note that as the half-life of rasburicase in serum is approximately 18 to 21 hours, about one-half of the administered dose is still present 24 hours after administration. Given this, a reasonable strategy to consider might be the following: (1) continue to rely on the triad of aggressive hydration, management of electrolyte disturbances, and institution of allopurinol beginning immediately upon presentation; (2) evaluate patients for their TLS risk (see Table 122.1) and *administer a single 3-mg dose of rasburicase at presentation* to patients with "high risk disease"; and (3) follow the levels of uric acid and administer additional rasburicase doses only to patients with uric acid levels above an arbitrary number such as 5 mg/dL 24 hours after a rasburicase dose. Remember a few additional uric acid measurements are far less expensive than a dose of rasburicase. (*Important: Because serum samples contain rasburicase, immediately cool samples obtained for uric acid to 0°C to 4°C, so as to prevent ex vivo enzymatic uric acid degradation that will falsely lower levels. Label test tubes as requiring chilling to avoid removal from ice upon arrival in the laboratory.*)

Finally, if despite aggressive management acute renal failure develops, immediate hemodialysis is recommended. Indeed, in patients presenting with TLS, hemodialysis should be started before cytotoxic therapy is administered. Conventional hemodialysis is more effective in eliminating uric acid and phosphate than peritoneal dialysis.

CANCER AND HYPONATREMIA

General

Water and sodium homeostasis is frequently disordered in patients with cancer. Optimal homeostasis requires a delicate balance between renal free water clearance and renal sodium metabolism. Hyponatremia, commonly defined as serum sodium <130 mEq/L, occurs with a reported incidence of 3.7% in patients with cancer.[21] Clinical manifestations of hyponatremia range from none to impaired consciousness progressing to coma and generalized hypotonia, or seizure activity all secondary to cerebral edema. Less dramatic symptoms, including anorexia, nausea, and asthenia, are often difficult to ascribe to a single cause in patients with cancer.

The differential of hyponatremia is extensive and includes many conditions patients with cancer experience including inappropriate secretion of arginine vasopressin (AVP = antidiuretic hormone = ADH)[22] and sodium depletion secondary to reduced intake and gastrointestinal or renal losses each accounting for about one-third of cases (Table 122.5).[23] Other etiologies more likely to occur in patients with cancer than the general patient population include ectopic atrial natriuretic peptide (ANP) production, hyponatremia associated with third spacing of fluids (ascites),

---

TABLE 122.5

Classification and Differential Diagonsis of Hyponatremia

HYPOTONIC HYPONATREMIA

Hypovolemic hyponatremia

Loss of solutes (sodium or potassium) with secondary water retention. Solute losses may be renal or extrarenal in origin.
1. Gastrointestinal disease
2. Exercise-associated hyponatremia
3. Diuretic therapy
4. Cerebral salt wasting
5. Mineralocorticoid deficiency

Euvolemic hyponatremia

Relative or absolute excess of body water: (a) reduction in electrolyte-free water excretion by kidneys due to AVP effects at the V2R (most common), (b) secondary to overdrinking (rare), (c) non-AVP mechanisms (very rare).
1. Syndrome of inappropriate antidiuretic hormone secretion
2. Primary polydipsia
3. Nephrogenic syndrome of inappropriate antidiuresis
4. Glucocorticoid deficiency
5. Hypothyroidism
6. Exercise-associated hyponatremia
7. Low solute intake

Hypervolemic hyponatremia

Renal sodium/water retention manifest as edema, principally due to AVP effects at the V2R.
1. Heart failure
2. Cirrhosis
3. Acute kidney injury, chronic kidney disease, and nephrotic syndrome

PSEUDOHYPONATREMIA

Artifactual decrease in serum Na$^+$ because excess lipids/proteins occupy a relatively larger proportion of plasma volume. Usually directly measured plasma osmolality will be normal.
1. Elevated lipids
2. Elevated proteins (multiple myeloma and hyperproteinemias)

ISOTONIC OR HYPERTONIC HYPONATREMIA

Hyponatremia with normal or increased osmolality occurring when solutes other than sodium present in the plasma. Initial hyperosmolality causes osmotic shift of water from intracellular to extracellular fluid compartment that, in turn, produces a dilutional decrease in the serum Na$^+$.
1. Hyperglycemia^a is the most common example of this phenomenon. Depending on the severity of hyperglycemia and the duration and magnitude of the accompanying glucose-induced osmotic diuresis, such patients may actually be hypertonic despite hyponatremia.
2. Mannitol.^{b}
3. Radiographic contrast agents.^{b}
4. Glycine from surgical irrigant solutions.^{b}

AVP, arginine vasopressin.
^{a} Assess plasma osmolality directly or correct measured serum Na$^+$ for the glucose elevation.
^{b} Plasma osmolality must be ascertained by direct measurement.
Adapted from Verbalis JG, Goldsmith SR, Greenberg A, et al. Diagnosis, evaluation, and treatment of hyponatremia: expert panel recommendations. *Am J Med* 2013;126:S1–42.

---

and "pseudohyponatremia" as might occur in a patient with multiple myeloma and hyperproteinemia—although one can argue the latter is in fact true hyponatremia with the reduced sodium an adaptation at electrical neutrality imposed by the increase in positively charged myeloma proteins.[24]

Pathogenesis

Only cell membrane impermeable solutes that are "relatively" restricted to either the extracellular or intracellular compartments can effectively function as solutes and create osmotic gradients across cell membranes. Sodium and its accompanying anions are the major cell membrane impermeable plasma solutes, so that hyponatremia is in effect a surrogate for hypoosmolality and these terms are usually synonymous. Under normal circumstances, plasma *osmolality* is closely regulated in the range of 280 to 295 mOsm/kg through (1) thirst perception, (2) control of free water clearance in the kidney by ADH also known as AVP, and (3) renal sodium excretion regulated by ANP and the renin angiotensin system. Understanding this helps one understand the causes of hyponatremia.

In patients with cancer, hyponatremia secondary to inappropriate secretion of AVP (or ADH; syndrome of inappropriate antidiuretic hormone [SIADH] or syndrome of inappropriate antidiuresis) occurs as a paraneoplastic syndrome, or as a complication of therapy.[22] SIADH is defined as a hypo-osmolar or dilutional hyponatremia with excessive natriuresis. Hyponatremia occurs because AVP secretion continues even after plasma osmolality falls below the threshold for AVP release. Key and ancillary features are summarized in Table 122.6.[22,23] The inappropriate secretion of AVP can originate from its normal source, the hypothalamus, as a consequence of dysregulation, or can be ectopic in origin, arising from cancer cells themselves. In cases of ectopic production, AVP is detectable in plasma and correlates with detectable AVP mRNA or immunoreactive peptides in tumor cells. While inappropriate AVP secretion can occur with any cancer, it is most frequently

reported with small-cell lung cancer, head and neck carcinomas, hematologic malignancies, and non–small-cell lung cancer.[25] Drugs reported to cause SIADH include cyclophosphamide and its isomeric analogue, ifosfamide; the vinca alkaloids including vincristine, vinblastine, and vinorelbine; the proteasome inhibitor bortezomib; as well as carboplatin and cisplatin, although the latter more frequently cause renal salt wasting.

Patients with small-cell lung cancer, hyponatremia, and without measurable AVP have also been reported.[25,26] In a fraction of these patients, ectopic production of ANP mRNA and a peptide similar to the bioactive 28-amino acid ANP form present in plasma has been shown in tumors and leads to hyponatremia. Normally, ANP is produced, stored, and released by atrial myocytes and binds to a specific set of receptors increasing renal sodium excretion.

Besides SIADH and syndrome of inappropriate atrial natriuretic peptide (SIANP) production, there is increasing awareness of an alternate mechanism of salt loss referred to as the cerebral salt wasting syndrome (CSWS). Two major criteria must be met for a diagnosis of CSWS: (1) a cerebral lesion and (2) high urinary excretion of Na^+ and Cl^-, in a patient with contraction of the extracellular fluid volume. While the frequency of CSWS is less, it is important to make the correct diagnosis as management is different.

Therapy

The first step is to identify the cause and decide if sodium depletion secondary to either reduced intake, gastrointestinal losses, or renal losses is present. If these are excluded, physicians often proceed with a presumptive diagnosis of SIADH and attempt to restore serum sodium and osmolality to normal. If the hyponatremia is thought to be drug-induced, the offending agent(s) should be discontinued. The rapidity of correction is guided by the severity of the clinical presentation and the pace with which the hyponatremia developed. If the evidence suggests hyponatremia developed slowly, it is likely that some equilibration has occurred and correction *can and should* proceed over several days. Patients in whom hyponatremia develops rapidly are more likely to present with severe clinical symptoms, but can tolerate more rapid correction. Fortunately, most cases present with mild hyponatremia and can be managed with judicious water restriction and intravenous or even oral salt administration. Management options are summarized in Table 122.7. If saline and furosemide prove inadequate so that the hyponatremia fails to improve or worsens after 72 to 96 hours of fluid restriction, plasma levels of AVP and ANP should be measured to discriminate between SIADH [syndrome of inappropriate arginine vasopressin (SIAVP)] and SIANP, especially in patients with SCLC. Unlike patients with SIADH and hyponatremia, patients whose tumors produce ANP experience a persistent decline in serum sodium following fluid restriction, especially if sodium intake is not concomitantly increased. Aquaretic agents, AVP-receptor antagonists, have demonstrated efficacy and safety in clinical trials and represent additional options for managing hyponatremia.[27,28]

LACTIC ACIDOSIS AND CANCER

General

Among patients with cancer, spontaneous lactic acidosis can occur with hematologic and lymphoid malignancies as well as solid tumors having been described in patients with breast, colon, ovarian, and small-cell lung cancer, among others. In some patients with TLS, a metabolic acidosis not accounted by the degree of renal insufficiency can be caused by lactic acidosis. Although most patients with lactic acidosis present or evolve to a more severe acidosis, lactic acidosis is defined as a pH ≤ 7.35, with plasma lactate concentration ≥ 5 meq/L.[29] Not surprisingly, the occurrence of metabolic acidosis in patients with cancer portends a poor prognosis.

TABLE 122.6

Criteria for Diagnosing Syndrome of Inappropriate Antidiuretic Hormone Secretion

Key features:

1. Decreased effective osmolality of the extracellular fluid (<275 mOsm/kg of water)

2. Inappropriate urinary concentration: Urine osmolality >100 mOsm/kg H_2O with normal renal function

3. Clinical *euvolemia* as defined by the absence of signs of hypovolemia (orthostasis, tachycardia, decreased skin turgor, dry mucous membranes) or hypervolemia (subcutaneous edema, ascites)

4. Urine sodium >20–30 mmol/L in the face of normal salt and water intake

5. Normal thyroid and adrenal function

6. Normal renal function and no recent diuretic use

Ancillary features:

1. Plasma uric acid <4 mg/dL

2. Blood urea nitrogen <10 mg/dL (0.357 mmols/L)

3. Fractional sodium excretion >1%

4. Fractional urea excretion >55%

5. Hyponatremia corrected by fluid restriction but not by normal saline

6. Elevated plasma arginine vasopressin levels despite hypotonicity and euvolemia

Adapted from Ellison DH, Berl T. Clinical practice. The syndrome of inappropriate antidiuresis. *N Engl J Med* 2007;356:2064–2072; and Verbalis JG, Goldsmith SR, Greenberg A, et al. Diagnosis, evaluation, and treatment of hyponatremia: expert panel recommendations. *Am J Med* 2013;126:S1–42.

TABLE 122.7

Management of Hyponatremia

High Risk of ODS

- Serum Na$^+$ concentration ≤105 mmol/L
- Alcoholism[a]
- Advanced liver disease[a]
- Hypokalemia[a]
- Malnutrition[a]

Initial Treatment of Hyponatremia

Asymptomatic or serum sodium ≤125 mmol/L and developed over weeks

- Chronic hyponatremia: Neurologic sequelae more likely if correction too rapid
- Increase serum Na$^+$ a maximum of 0.5–2 mmol/L/hr
- High risk of ODS: Correct serum Na$^+$ by 4–6 mmol/L/d not >8 mmol/L/24 h
- Normal risk of ODS: Correct serum Na$^+$ 4–8 mmol/L/d, not >10–12 mmol/L/24 h
- Intravenous normal saline ±20 to 40 mg furosemide when patient is euvolemic

Symptomatic or serum sodium ≤115 mmol/L and developed acutely

- Increase serum sodium 2 mmol/L/hr; 4–6 mmol/L increase in serum Na$^+$ sufficient to reverse most serious manifestations
- Severe symptoms: 100 mL of 3% NaCl over 10 minutes times three as needed
- Mild to moderate symptoms with low risk of herniation: 1 to 2 mL/Kg/hour 3% NaCl then 100 to 250 mL/hour normal saline
- 20 to 40 mg oral or intravenous furosemide when patient is euvolemic

Treatment of Syndrome of Inappropriate Antidiuretic Hormone Secretion

Vaptans[27,28]
Cautions for Using Vaptans to Treat Hyponatremia
- Exclude hypovolemic hyponatremia; approved only for hypervolemic and euvolemic hyponatremia
- Do not use in conjunction with other treatments for hyponatremia or immediately after cessation of other treatments for hyponatremia, particularly 3% NaCl
- Monitor serum Na$^+$ every 6–8 h for the first 24–48 h
- Maintain ad libitum fluid intake during the first 24–48 h of treatment; hyponatremia can correct too quickly with coincidental fluid restriction
- Symptomatic benefit to patients not established
- Do not use a vaptan for severe, symptomatic hyponatremia
- There are insufficient data using vaptans in severe asymptomatic hyponatremia
- Monitor volume status and serum Na$^+$ frequently. Discontinue if hypovolemia, hypotension or rapid rate of rise of serum Na$^+$.

Conivaptan Hydrochloride

- Combined vasopressin V1aR and V2R AVP-receptor.
- Loading dose of 20 mg IV followed by continuous infusion of 20 mg/d over 24 h, for 2–4 d. Following the initial day of treatment, dosage may be increased to 40 mg/d continuous infusion.

Tolvaptan

- Selective vasopressin V2-receptor antagonist.
- Starting dose is 15 mg once daily. Dosage may be increased at intervals ≥24 h to 30 mg once daily, and to a maximum of 60 mg once daily as needed to raise serum Na$^+$. Monitor serum Na$^+$ and volume status.

Demeclocycline

- 300–600 mg twice daily
- Continued several days to achieve maximal diuretic effects; wait 3–4 d before increasing dose
- Monitor renal function carefully

Treatment of Cerebral Salt Wasting Syndrome

1. Aggressive fluid and electrolyte replacement
2. Mineralocorticoid supplementation (fludrocortisone 100–400 mg/d)

ODS, osmotic demyelination syndrome; AVP, arginine vasopressin.
[a]The precise serum K+ concentration nor the degree of alcoholism, malnutrition, or liver disease that renders the brain vulnerable to ODS have not been defined.

Pathogenesis

Lactic acid production normally occurs under conditions of hypoxia in all tissues, and following release into the circulation, 90% of lactic acid is metabolized in the liver, where it is converted to pyruvate, with the remaining 10% metabolized or excreted by the kidney. Unlike normal cells, tumor cells rely on anaerobic glycolysis disproportionately, even in the presence of oxygen, producing large quantities of lactate that can lead to an imbalance between lactate production and its utilization by the liver. The essential role of the liver in lactic acid metabolism explains why patients with compromised liver function are more likely to develop severe lactic acidosis. In patients with cancer, compromise of liver function can occur when extensive hepatic metastases replace a substantial portion of the liver parenchyma. In these patients, once established, lactic acidosis can progress inexorably.

Among patients with leukemias and lymphomas lactic acidosis usually occurs in adults and has an extremely poor prognosis.[29] Liver involvement is frequently present, and in a substantial proportion of patients contributes to hypoglycemia. Indeed, the high frequency of liver involvement in adults with lymphoma and leukemia who develop lactic acidosis supports the possibility reduced hepatic lactate utilization is necessary in the pathogenesis of lactic acidosis. Some have suggested the loss of mitochondrial membrane potential ($\Delta\psi$m) during programmed cell death or apoptosis results in compensatory glycolysis with accumulation of lactic acid and acidosis.[30]

Therapy

Lactic acidosis usually develops in patients with extensive disease and frequently progresses rapidly. Even with maximal supportive therapy, mortality rates of 60% to 90% are common.[31] The developing acidosis can lead to cardiac arrhythmias and hypotension with potential for cardiovascular collapse. Consequently, an aggressive therapeutic approach is indicated including the following: (1) aggressively support blood pressure with fluids and vasopressors to preclude generalized hypoperfusion that will lead to further lactic acid accumulation; (2) use of sodium bicarbonate, though controversial, as no controlled study has shown improvement in outcome but can be supported with acidosis severe enough to impact hemodynamic function and the response to catecholamines; (3) hemodialysis and hemofiltration with a bicarbonate-based replacement fluid; and (4) correction of the underlying causes is essential, but often very difficult if not impossible if the lactic acidosis is a complication of the patient's cancer.

HYPERCALCEMIA AND CANCER

General

Hypercalcemia is the most common paraneoplastic syndrome, occurring in 10% to 30% of patients with advanced cancer.[32] While hypercalcemia has been reported with most tumors, humoral hypercalcemia, discussed subsequently, is most frequently encountered in patients with carcinomas of the breast, lung, kidney, and head and neck, whereas hypercalcemia with skeletal metastases is seen most often in patients with multiple myeloma.

Symptoms of hypercalcemia include nausea, vomiting, constipation, polyuria, and disorientation. Clinical evidence of volume contraction may be apparent. Early and widespread use of bisphosphonates has decreased the frequency and severity of hypercalcemia in patients with cancer.

Pathogenesis

Hypercalcemia can occur as result of focal bone destruction (osteolytic) or more frequently as a humoral paraneoplastic syndrome. Focal bone destruction can be mediated by local (paracrine) fac-

tors secreted by tumor cells infiltrating bone including cytokines and growth factors that stimulate osteoclasts directly or indirectly via osteoblast-mediated upregulation of osteoclast-activating factors. Alternately, hypercalcemia can occur as a paraneoplastic syndrome caused by tumor-produced factors that affect bone resorption and/or tubular calcium reabsorption. The systemic factor most commonly secreted by tumor cells, parathyroid hormone–related protein (PTHrP), mediates a humoral form of malignant hypercalcemia, often referred to as humoral hypercalcemia of malignancy. Circulating PTHrP is found in approximately 80% of hypercalcemic patients with cancer. Although PTHrP shares only limited homology with parathyroid hormone, the common amino terminus binds the same cell surface receptor in bone and kidney and stimulates increases in bone resorption and renal tubular calcium reabsorption leading to hypercalcemia. In addition, PTHrP can synergize local (paracrine) factors including interleukin-1, interleukin-6 and tumor necrosis factor-α further contributing to hypercalcemia.[32,33] Finally, some lymphomas secrete the active form of vitamin D, 1,25 dihydroxyvitamin D–enhancing osteoclastic bone resorption and intestinal calcium absorption.

Hypercalcemia induces an osmotic diuresis, while inhibiting ADH. The resultant polyuria together with nausea and vomiting lead to progressive dehydration, reduced glomerular filtration, and increased calcium resorption further worsening the hypercalcemia.

Therapy

Therapeutic interventions depend on the presentation. Asymptomatic patients with a serum calcium level of ≤3.25 mmol/L can be managed conservatively, whereas symptomatic patients or those with a serum calcium level >3.25 mmol/L require immediate aggressive measures.

Although hydration results at most in only a mild (0.5 mmol/L [~2 mg/dL]) decrease in serum calcium levels, it is a simple, rapid, and effective intervention that can also preclude continued renal calcium reabsorption. *After adequate hydration*, 20 to 40 mg of intravenous furosemide can enhance calcium excretion.

Together with hydration, bisphosphonates are the cornerstone of therapy for malignancy-associated hypercalcemia. Bisphosphonates are based on a phosphorous-carbon-phosphorous backbone, similar to pyrophosphate. The carbon replacing the central oxygen renders the molecules resistant to hydrolysis, but allows the retention of pyrophosphate-like inhibition of bone resorption. Their mechanism of action is complex. Bisphosphonates inhibit both normal and pathologic bone resorption via direct and indirect effects on osteoclasts. The affinity of bisphosphonates for hydroxyapatite leads to their concentration in bone at the interface and they are internalized by osteoclasts at the time of bone resorption. Evidence indicates non–nitrogen-containing bisphosphonates such as clodronate resemble pyrophosphate and are metabolized intracellularly to nonhydrolyzable analogues of ATP that inhibit ATP-dependent intracellular enzymes and are thus cytotoxic. Nitrogen-containing bisphosphonates (aminobisphosphonates), including pamidronate, ibandronate, and zoledronate, impede protein prenylation and bone resorption by osteoclasts by inhibiting the mevalonate pathway (farnesyl diphosphate synthase) disrupting the signaling functions of key regulatory proteins.[34,35] As a group, the biphosphonates are well tolerated with a small incidence of fever, which is the most frequently reported adverse event. Transient hypocalcemia and hypophosphatemia, and a reversible increase in serum creatinine can also occur. Because of poor oral absorption and gastrointestinal discomfort, most are administered intravenously. Several bisphosphonates have been used in the treatment of hypercalcemia of malignancy including the following. (1) Clodronate, a second-generation bisphosphonate of intermediate potency, is usually given orally and achieves normocalcemia in 80% of cases. One-fifth of those treated have an increase in creatinine.[36] In the palliative setting, clodronate can be given subcutaneously with mild local reaction in one-third as the principal side effect.[37] (2) Pamidronate, a nitrogen-containing bisphosphonate, achieves normocalcemia in as many as 90% of patients, for a longer period of time than clodronate.[36,38] (3) Zoledronate, a third-generation bisphosphonate containing a heterocyclic nitrogen, is considered the current best choice, with normalization of serum calcium in 4 to 10 days that lasts 4 to 6 weeks in 90% of patients.[39] A Cochrane Database Review reported no significant adverse effects associated with bisphosphonate administration and found no evidence of superiority of any specific aminobisphosphonate or nonaminobisphosphonate for any outcome, although zoledronate appeared superior to placebo and etidronate in improving overall survival.[39,40]

Bisphosphonates are most effective in the therapy of hypercalcemia associated with multiple myeloma, but are also efficacious in solid tumors with skeletal metastases. They are somewhat less effective in the treatment of patients with humoral-mediated hypercalcemia because they have no effect on tubular calcium reabsorption mediated by humoral factors, including PTHrP.[41] Other agents including gallium nitrate,[42] plicamycin (mithramycin), and calcitonin can be tried in hypercalcemia refractory to bisphosphonates. Plicamycin and calcitonin can effect rapid declines of serum calcium but require frequent administration.

Osteoprotegerin (OPG) is a naturally occurring soluble receptor that inhibits bone resorption by inhibiting osteoclast differentiation. OPG is part of a cytokine system that belongs to the tumor necrosis factor superfamily.[43] The components include the ligand RANKL (receptor activator of nuclear factor-κB ligand), its specific receptor RANK (receptor activator of nuclear factor-κB) and OPG, a soluble "decoy" receptor. By binding to RANK, RANKL enhances bone resorption by (1) increasing osteoclast formation from hematopoietic precursors, (2) increasing osteoclast activity, and (3) inhibiting osteoclast apoptosis. The activity of RANKL, also known as osteoclast differentiation factor (ODF) or OPG ligand, is counterbalanced physiologically by circulating OPG, with the net effect dependent on the local ratio of osteoclast differentiation factor to OPG. By acting as a "decoy," intravenous administration of OPG has potent hypocalcemic effects in murine models of humoral hypercalcemia.

Denosumab, a fully human monoclonal antibody with a high affinity and specificity for RANKL, is approved by the US Food and Drug Administration "for prevention of skeletal-related events in patients with bone metastases from solid tumors . . . but is not indicated for the prevention of skeletal-related events in patients with multiple myeloma." Two phase 3 trials randomized patients with breast cancer or castration-resistant prostate cancer to receive either 120 mg denosumab subcutaneously every 4 weeks or intravenous zometa administered at a dose of 4 mg every 4 weeks.[44,45] Denosumab was superior both in delaying the time to the first on-study "skeletal-related events" (fracture, radiation to bone, surgery to bone, or spinal cord compression) and delaying the time to the first-and-subsequent skeletal-related events. In patients with castration-resistant prostate cancer overall adverse event rates were similar, with hypocalcemia in 13% and 6% of denosumab- and zoledronate-treated patients, respectively, and osteonecrosis of the jaw in 2.3% of patients receiving denosumab and 1.3% of patients treated with zoledronate ($p = 0.09$). While denosumab may garner US Food and Drug Administration approval for hypercalcemia associated with malignancy, it is not currently approved for this indication and data indicate its approval will have at best limited impact. A study of patients with advanced cancer and persistent hypercalcemia after incomplete response or relapse after recent bisphosphonate treatment found that while denosumab effectively lowered serum calcium in 80% of patients, the response was maintained a median of 26 days, compared within a median of 18 days after receiving the last dose of intravenous bisphosphonate.

CANCER-RELATED HEMOLYTIC UREMIC SYNDROME

General

The hemolytic uremic syndrome (HUS) is a microvascular disorder characterized histopathologically by disseminated microthrombi occluding the microvasculature. HUS is often associated with the presence of large von Willebrand factor multimers capable of agglutinating circulating platelets. The hallmark of a Coombs-negative hemolytic anemia with an elevated schistocyte count results from fragmentation of erythrocytes as they pass through clogged arterioles. The disseminated microthrombi lead to ischemic organ damage, most commonly in kidneys and brain, with renal insufficiency, and a range of neurologic symptoms. Although thrombotic thrombocytopenic purpura and HUS represent a spectrum with considerable overlap, renal insufficiency invariably occurs in HUS but is often milder in thrombotic thrombocytopenic purpura, where neurologic symptoms often predominate.

Pathogenesis

In patients with cancer, HUS has been reported: (1) as a manifestation of the cancer itself, (2) as a complication of chemotherapy, (3) in the setting of bone marrow transplantation, and (4) more recently as a problem in patients receiving antibodies and immunotoxins. In untreated patients, HUS has been described primarily with disseminated cancer, although occasionally as a manifestation of occult or early cancers.[47–49] While it has been reported more frequently with adenocarcinomas of the breast, lung, pancreas, prostate, and stomach, it has also been reported in patients with lymphomas as well as other malignancies.[47] In treated patients, a diverse group of chemotherapeutic agents have been implicated in the etiology of HUS. A 1986 review of chemotherapy-related HUS implicated mitomycin-C and 5-fluoruracil as the most frequent culprits.[49] Subsequent reports of gemcitabine-associated HUS reflect the widespread use of this agent.[50] Other agents that have been implicated in the etiology of this syndrome include bleomycin, cisplatin, cytosine arabinoside, daunomycin, deoxycoformycin, estramustine, and methyl-CCNU. The incidence in patients undergoing bone marrow transplant is uncertain, given the difficulty in establishing a diagnosis.[51]

The clinical manifestations of fulminant HUS include the classic pentad of microangiopathic hemolytic anemia, thrombocytopenia, fever, rapidly progressive renal failure, and neurological deficits. Acute respiratory distress syndrome can also develop in some patients. In this setting, a high mortality rate has been reported, because treatment is made even more difficult in a patient with a severe underlying disease. In some patients, a subacute presentation with microangiopathic changes, mild thrombocytopenia, and gradual deterioration of renal function has been described. The main differential is disseminated intravascular coagulopathy. In patients undergoing allogeneic stem cell transplantation, transplant-associated microangiopathy defined as hemolysis and RBC fragmentation, can be found in 25% to 38% of patients. Associated renal dysfunction and neurologic manifestations in patients with more severe forms of this syndrome demonstrate a spectrum of severity that may represent endothelial damage driven by donor-host interactions.[52]

Therapy

A definitive treatment approach for cancer-associated HUS remains to be established.[53–56] When a given therapy is implicated as causative, this should be discontinued. Blood pressure should be controlled. The value of steroids is uncertain precluding their routine use. Hemodialysis is indicated in patients with renal failure. Although the efficacies of therapeutic plasma exchange using fresh frozen plasma as the substitution fluid and of immunoadsorption chromatography are arguable,[56] either or both should be initiated promptly at diagnosis in all patients. These therapies may need to be continued for months. Cryosupernatant plasma has been reported to be at least as effective as fresh frozen plasma. Greater success can be expected in patients with smaller tumor burdens, or those in whom anticancer therapy is effective, and in cases where vigilance has led to an early diagnosis. Some have also suggested that treatment may be more efficacious when HUS occurs as a manifestation of the underlying cancer than as a complication of therapy.

REFERENCES

1. Howard SC, Jones DP, Pui CH. The tumor lysis syndrome. *N Engl J Med* 2011;364:1844–1854.
2. Cairo MS, Bishop M. Tumour lysis syndrome: new therapeutic strategies and classification. *Br J Haematol* 2004;127:3–11.
3. Cohen LF, Balow JE, Magrath IT, et al. Acute tumor lysis syndrome. A review of 37 patients with Burkitt's lymphoma. *Am J Med* 1980;68:486–491.
4. Altman A. Acute tumor lysis syndrome. *Semin Oncol* 2001;28:3–8.
5. Sallan S. Management of acute tumor lysis syndrome. *Semin Oncol* 2001;28:9–12.
6. Fleming DR, Doukas MA. Acute tumor lysis syndrome in hematologic malignancies. *Leuk Lymphoma* 1992;8:315–318.
7. Hande KR, Garrow GC. Acute tumor lysis syndrome in patients with high-grade non-Hodgkin's lymphoma. *Am J Med* 1993;94:133–139.
8. Annemans L, Moeremans K, Lamotte M, et al. Pan-European multicentre economic evaluation of recombinant urate oxidase (rasburicase) in prevention and treatment of hyperuricaemia and tumour lysis syndrome in haematological cancer patients. *Support Care Cancer* 2003;11:249–257.
9. Baeksgaard L, Sorensen JB. Acute tumor lysis syndrome in solid tumors—a case report and review of the literature. *Cancer Chemother Pharmacol* 2003;51:187–192.
10. Byrd JC, Lin TS, Dalton JT, et al. Flavopiridol administered using a pharmacologically derived schedule is associated with marked clinical efficacy in refractory, genetically high-risk chronic lymphocytic leukemia. *Blood* 2007;109:399–404.
11. Cairo MS, Coiffier B, Reiter A, et al. Recommendations for the evaluation of risk and prophylaxis of tumour lysis syndrome (TLS) in adults and children with malignant diseases: an expert TLS panel consensus. *Br J Haematol* 2010;149:578–586.
12. Yeldandi AV, Yeldandi V, Kumar S, et al. Molecular evolution of the urate oxidase-encoding gene in hominoid primates: nonsense mutations. *Gene* 1991;109:281–284.
13. Zimm S, Collins JM, Oneill D, et al. Inhibition of first-pass metabolism in cancer chemotherapy: interaction of 6-mercaptopurine and allopurinol. *Clin Pharmacol Ther* 1983;34:810–817.
14. Cortes J, Moore JO, Maziarz RT, et al. Control of plasma uric acid in adults at risk for tumor Lysis syndrome: efficacy and safety of rasburicase alone and rasburicase followed by allopurinol compared with allopurinol alone—results of a multicenter phase III study. *J Clin Oncol* 2010;28:4207–4213.
15. Navolanic PM, Pui CH, Larson RA, et al. Elitek-rasburicase: an effective means to prevent and treat hyperuricemia associated with tumor lysis syndrome, a Meeting Report, Dallas, Texas, January 2002. *Leukemia* 2003;17:499–514.
16. Goldman SC, Holcenberg JS, Finklestein JZ, et al. A randomized comparison between rasburicase and allopurinol in children with lymphoma or leukemia at high risk for tumor lysis. *Blood* 2001;97:2998–3003.
17. Liu CY, Sims-McCallum RP, Schiffer CA. A single dose of rasburicase is sufficient for the treatment of hyperuricemia in patients receiving chemotherapy. *Leuk Res* 2005;29:463–465.
18. Hutcherson DA, Gammon DC, Bhatt MS, et al. Reduced-dose rasburicase in the treatment of adults with hyperuricemia associated with malignancy. *Pharmacotherapy* 2006;26:242–247.
19. Trifilio S, Gordon L, Singhal S, et al. Reduced-dose rasburicase (recombinant xanthine oxidase) in adult cancer patients with hyperuricemia. *Bone Marrow Transplant* 2006;37:997–1001.
20. Trifilio SM, Pi J, Zook J, et al. Effectiveness of a single 3-mg rasburicase dose for the management of hyperuricemia in patients with hematological malignancies. *Bone Marrow Transplant* 2011;46:800–805.
21. Berghmans T, Paesmans M, Body JJ. A prospective study on hyponatraemia in medical cancer patients: epidemiology, aetiology and differential diagnosis. *Support Care Cancer* 2000;8:192–197.
22. Ellison DH, Berl T. Clinical practice. The syndrome of inappropriate antidiuresis. *N Engl J Med* 2007;356:2064–2072.
23. Verbalis JG, Goldsmith SR, Greenberg A, et al. Diagnosis, evaluation, and treatment of hyponatremia: expert panel recommendations. *Am J Med* 2013;126:S1–S42.
24. Sachs J, Fredman B. The hyponatramia of multiple myeloma is true and not pseudohyponatramia. *Med Hypotheses* 2006;67:839–840.
25. Johnson BE, Chute JP, Rushin J, et al. A prospective study of patients with lung cancer and hyponatremia of malignancy. *Am J Respir Crit Care Med* 1997;156:1669–1678.
26. Chute JP, Taylor E, Williams J, et al. A metabolic study of patients with lung cancer and hyponatremia of malignancy. *Clin Cancer Res* 2006;12:888–896.
27. Peri A. Clinical review: the use of vaptans in clinical endocrinology. *J Clin Endocrinol Metab* 2013;98:1321–1332.
28. Gargani L, Schmidt PH, Gheorghiade M. Tolvaptan for the treatment of hyponatremia secondary to the syndrome of inappropriate antidiuretic hormone secretion. *Expert Rev Cardiovasc Ther* 2011;9:1505–1513.
29. Sillos EM, Shenep JL, Burghen GA, et al. Lactic acidosis: a metabolic complication of hematologic malignancies: case report and review of the literature. *Cancer* 2001;92:2237–2246.
30. Tiefenthaler M, Amberger A, Bacher N, et al. Increased lactate production follows loss of mitochondrial membrane potential during apoptosis of human leukaemia cells. *Br J Haematol* 2001;114:574–580.
31. van der Beek A, de Meijer PH, Meinders AE. Lactic acidosis: pathophysiology, diagnosis and treatment. *Neth J Med* 2001;58:128–136.
32. Esbrit P. Hypercalcemia of malignancy—new insights into an old syndrome. *Clin Lab* 2001;47:67–71.
33. Stewart AF. Clinical practice. Hypercalcemia associated with cancer. *N Engl J Med* 2005;352:373–379.
34. Benford HL, Frith JC, Auriola S, et al. Farnesol and geranylgeraniol prevent activation of caspases by aminobisphosphonates: biochemical evidence for two distinct pharmacological classes of bisphosphonate drugs. *Mol Pharmacol* 1999;56:131–140.
35. Luckman SP, Hughes DE, Coxon FP, et al. Nitrogen-containing bisphosphonates inhibit the mevalonate pathway and prevent post-translational prenylation of GTP-binding proteins, including Ras. *J Bone Miner Res* 1998;13:581–589.
36. Purohit OP, Radstone CR, Anthony C, et al. A randomised double-blind comparison of intravenous pamidronate and clodronate in the hypercalcaemia of malignancy. *Br J Cancer* 1995;72:1289–1293.
37. Walker P, Watanabe S, Lawlor P, et al. Subcutaneous clodronate: a study evaluating efficacy in hypercalcemia of malignancy and local toxicity. *Ann Oncol* 1997;8:915–916.
38. Vinholes J, Guo CY, Purohit OP, et al. Evaluation of new bone resorption markers in a randomized comparison of pamidronate or clodronate for hypercalcemia of malignancy. *J Clin Oncol* 1997;15:131–138.
39. Mhaskar R, Redzepovic J, Wheatley K, et al. Bisphosphonates in multiple myeloma: a network meta-analysis. *Cochrane Database Syst Rev* 2012;5:CD003188.
40. Major P, Lortholary A, Hon J, et al. Zoledronic acid is superior to pamidronate in the treatment of hypercalcemia of malignancy: a pooled analysis of two randomized, controlled clinical trials. *J Clin Oncol* 2001;19:558–567.
41. Walls J, Ratcliffe WA, Howell A, et al. Response to intravenous bisphosphonate therapy in hypercalcaemic patients with and without bone metastases: the role of parathyroid hormone-related protein. *Br J Cancer* 1994;70:169–172.
42. Warrell RP Jr. Gallium nitrate for the treatment of bone metastases. *Cancer* 1997;80:1680–1685.
43. Hofbauer LC, Neubauer A, Heufelder AE. Receptor activator of nuclear factor-kappaB ligand and osteoprotegerin: potential implications for the pathogenesis and treatment of malignant bone diseases. *Cancer* 2001;92:460–470.
44. Cleeland CS, Body JJ, Stopeck A, et al. Pain outcomes in patients with advanced breast cancer and bone metastases: results from a randomized, double-blind study of denosumab and zoledronic acid. *Cancer* 2013;119:832–838.
45. Fizazi K, Carducci MA, Smith MR, et al. Denosumab versus zoledronic acid for treatment of bone metastases in men with castration-resistant prostate cancer: a randomised, double-blind study. *Lancet* 2011;377:813–822.
46. Hu MI, Glezerman I, Leboulleux S, et al. Denosumab for patients with persistent or relapsed hypercalcemia of malignancy despite recent bisphosphonate treatment. *J Natl Cancer Inst* 2013;105:1417–1420.
47. Mungall S, Mathieson P. Hemolytic uremic syndrome in metastatic adenocarcinoma of the prostate. *Am J Kidney Dis* 2002;40:1334–1336.
48. Gordon LI, Kwaan HC. Cancer- and drug-associated thrombotic thrombocytopenic purpura and hemolytic uremic syndrome. *Semin Hematol* 1997;34:140–147.
49. Sheldon R, Slaughter D. A syndrome of microangiopathic hemolytic anemia, renal impairment, and pulmonary edema in chemotherapy-treated patients with adenocarcinoma. *Cancer* 1986;58:1428–1436.
50. Walter RB, Joerger M, Pestalozzi BC. Gemcitabine-associated hemolytic-uremic syndrome. *Am J Kidney Dis* 2002;40:E16.
51. Verburgh CA, Vermeij CG, Zijlmans JM, et al. Haemolytic uraemic syndrome following bone marrow transplantation. Case report and review of the literature. *Nephrol Dial Transplant* 1996;11:1332–1337.
52. Martinez MT, Bucher Ch, Stussi G, et al. Transplant-associated microangiopathy (TAM) in recipients of allogeneic hematopoietic stem cell transplants. *Bone Marrow Transplant* 2005;36:993–1000.
53. Snyder HW Jr, Mittelman A, Oral A, et al. Treatment of cancer chemotherapy-associated thrombotic thrombocytopenic purpura/hemolytic uremic syndrome by protein A immunoadsorption of plasma. *Cancer* 1993;71:1882–1892.
54. von Baeyer H. Plasmapheresis in thrombotic microangiopathy-associated syndromes: review of outcome data derived from clinical trials and open studies. *Ther Apher* 2002;6:320–328.
55. Kaplan AA. Therapeutic apheresis for cancer related hemolytic uremic syndrome. *Ther Apher* 2000;4:201–206.
56. Lechner K, Obermeier HL. Cancer-related microangiopathic hemolytic anemia: clinical and laboratory features in 168 reported cases. *Medicine (Baltimore)* 2012;91:195–205.

PRACTICE OF ONCOLOGY

123 Metastatic Cancer to the Brain

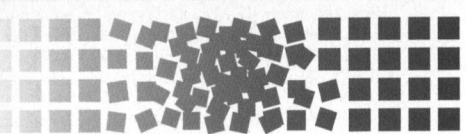

John H. Suh, Samuel T. Chao, David M. Peereboom, and Gene H. Barnett

INTRODUCTION

Brain metastases represent the most common neurologic complication of cancer and affect many patients with cancer. Historically, the outcome for most patients was quite poor. Advances in neuroimaging, neurosurgery, radiation oncology, medical oncology, and supportive care have allowed for earlier detection, better local treatment modalities, and strategies to mitigate potential complications, which have improved survival and quality of life for these patients. As a result, the management of brain metastases has become complex and controversial given the array of treatment options that are currently available.

Epidemiology

The true incidence of brain metastases, which develops in nearly 30% of patients with cancer,[1] is not known although autopsy estimates are as high as 170,000 cases annually in the United States.[2] Brain metastases can be diagnosed at the same time or within 1 month of primary diagnosis, which occurs in about one-third of cases[3] (synchronous) or after the primary tumor has been diagnosed (metachronous). An estimated 30% to 40% of patients present with a solitary lesion, which is defined as a single brain metastasis without any evidence of extracranial disease and controlled primary.[4] Cancers of the lung and breast, which represent 50% and 15-20% of cases, respectively, are the most common primary tumors that spread to the brain.

Clinical Presentation

The clinical presentation can vary widely and may include headache, motor weakness, sensory disturbance, nausea and/or vomiting, cranial nerve abnormalities, change in mental status, seizures, ataxia, speech difficulties, and coordination abnormalities. Historic data from the 1970s to early 1990s showed that 10% of patients diagnosed by computed tomography (CT) or magnetic resonance imaging (MRI) were asymptomatic.[5] Because screening scans are more frequently performed and imaging modalities are more sensitive, most likely an increasing percentage of today's patients present with asymptomatic disease.

Recently, a great deal of attention has been focused on the potential neurocognitive effects of whole-brain radiation therapy (WBRT), which had not historically been examined given the focus on survival rather than quality of life and given the poor outcomes of these patients. The majority of patients have neurocognitive deficits prior to the initiation of WBRT[6–8] with a comprehensive phase 3 trial reporting that >90% of patients have some decline in neurocognitive function (NCF) prior to WBRT.[7] NCF is typically tested with a battery of tests, as listed in Table 123.1. Tumor regression after WBRT appears to correlate with improved NCF.[9]

Imaging and Diagnosis

Imaging is very important in the diagnosis of brain metastases. Although CT scans may be useful in diagnosis, the imaging modality of choice is an MRI as it is more sensitive than CT for determining the number, distribution, and size of lesions.[10] The detection of brain metastases may increase after the use of triple dose contrast.[11] Typically, brain metastases are solid or ring enhancing lesion(s), pseudospherical in shape, multiple in number, occur in the grey-white junction,[12] and occur most frequently in the cerebral hemispheres (80%) followed by the cerebellum (15%) and brain stem (<5%). Hemorrhagic lesions are seen more commonly with germ cell tumors, melanomas, thyroid carcinoma, choriocarcinoma, and renal cell carcinoma. In addition, the leptomeninges can also be involved. The differential diagnosis includes nonmalignant causes such as abscess, infection, demyelination and hemorrhage, and primary brain tumors. If uncertainty exists regarding diagnosis, biopsy or surgery should be performed to confirm diagnosis. For patients with known cancer, restaging scans, which typically include CT scan with and without contrast of the chest, abdomen, and pelvis, should be performed to assess primary and extracranial disease status. The use of fluorodeoxyglucose positron emission tomography alone as the only imaging modality of the brain is not recommended given the high background metabolic use of glucose by the brain.[13] After surgery, postoperative MRIs should be done within 48 hours to differentiate tumor recurrence versus blood. For patients undergoing stereotactic radiosurgery (SRS), the MRI changes can be variable with approximately one-third of lesions experiencing a transient increase in tumor volume.[14] Using diffusion tensor imaging, regional variation in white matter changes can be seen after WBRT, particularly in the inferior cingulum, corpus callosum, and fornix.[15]

Recently, the Response Assessment Working Group, an independent, international, collaborative effort, provided suggestions on the design of trials in patients with brain metastases with emphasis on radiographic response.[16] In addition, the Response Assessment Working Group provided guidelines on neurocognitive, neurologic, and quality-of-life outcomes for patients with brain metastases.[17] The criteria for response rates for patients with brain metastases have been variable between Response Evaluation Criteria in Solid Tumors,[18,19] World Health Organization (WHO),[20] and those used for high-grade gliomas.[21,22]

Prognosis

As the overall survival for patients with brain metastases remains poor, the use of prognostic scales helps to guide therapies. One of the earliest and most useful prognostic scales was based on 1,200 patients from three consecutive Radiation Therapy Oncology Group (RTOG) phase 3 brain metastases trials from 1979 to 1993.[23] Using recursive partitioning analysis (RPA), three well-defined

TABLE 123.1

Neurocognitive Battery of Tests Used in Many Modern Cooperative Group, Consortia, and Industry-Led Trials[a]

Assessment	Domain(s) Tested	
Hopkins verbal learning test-revised	Learning and memory	Test administrator needed. Patient is read a list of words and then asked to verbally repeat the list and identify the words from a word list.
Trail making test, part A and B	Processing speed and executive function	Trained administrator needed. Both parts of the trail making test consist of 25 circles consisting of numbers or letters distributed on a sheet of paper. Patients are asked to draws lines to connect the circles in an ascending pattern.
Multilingual aphasia examination and controlled oral word association	Verbal fluency and executive function	Trained administrator needed. Patients are asked to produce words related to specific letter cues.

[a]Time to complete the entire battery is typically 25 to 30 minutes. Trained administrators (e.g., research coordinator or other study staff) can give the tests. A study neuropsychologist should be involved in the study design and data analysis; however, an onsite neuropsychologist is not needed for test administration. From Lin NU, Wefel JS, Lee EQ, et al. Challenges relating to solid tumour brain metastases in clinical trials, part 2: Neurocognitive, neurological, and quality-of-life outcomes. A report from the RANO group. *Lancet Oncol* 2013;14:407–416, with permission.

prognostic groups (RPA class I, II, and III) were identified based on age (<65 or 65 and older), Karnofsky performance status (KPS) of ≥70 or <70, absence or presence of extracranial metastases, and primary tumor status (Fig. 123.1A).

To develop a less subjective and more quantifiable prognostic system, the graded prognostic assessment (GPA) was developed by analyzing data from five RTOG studies.[24] The GPA, which is stratified into four prognostic groups, is the sum of scores (0, 0.5, or 1.0) based on age, KPS, presence of extracranial metastases, and number of brain metastases (Fig. 123.1B). Given the heterogeneity of outcomes for patients based on tumor type, an updated diagnosis-specific (DS) GPA was developed by combining the databases from 11 institutions, which was the basis for a summary report on 3,940 patients[25] (Fig. 123.1C). Because patients with breast cancer have the best overall survival based on DS-GPA, further stratification incorporates biomarkers such as estrogen receptor (ER), progesterone receptor (PR), and human epidermal growth factor receptor 2 (HER2) status.[26] With advances in the understanding of tumor heterogeneity mediated by biomarkers (e.g., B-raf mutations in melanoma; epidermal growth factor receptor mutations in non–small-cell lung cancer [NSCLC]), molecular features will become more important in assessing the prognosis of patients with brain metastases.

An internally validated prognostic nomogram for survival estimates was developed for 2,367 patients based on seven RTOG randomized trials.[27] The best-fitting model was the Cox proportional hazards survival model, which included primary site and histology, primary disease status, extracranial spread, age, KPS, and number of lesions. The 12-month survival for each RPA class or DS-GPA group varied.

Symptom Management

Corticosteroids

As brain metastases can cause peritumoral edema, corticosteroids are frequently used to help temporarily control brain edema. Dexamethasone, which has low mineralocorticoid effect, is typically used given its long half-life. Based on a prospective randomized trial of patients who were not in danger of cerebral herniation, higher dose (16 mg/day) demonstrated no advantage compared to lower dose (4 mg or 8 mg/day) dexamethasone.[28] Patients receiving higher doses of dexamethasone had more frequent side effects. Common acute side effects may include insomnia, increased appetite, gastritis, fluid retention, mood swings, acne, and elevation of blood sugars. Long-term side effects may include weight gain, facial plethora, pedal edema, immunosuppression, proximal muscle myopathy, cataract formation, aseptic necrosis of the femoral head, and osteoporosis.

Because most brain metastasis trials have not assessed steroid use as endpoints, much controversy exists regarding specific indications and dosing.[29] For patients who are neurologically asymptomatic, routine use of corticosteroids is not necessary.[30,31] For patients with more severe symptoms from increased intracranial pressure, doses of 16 mg/day or higher should be considered.[32] If possible, steroids should be tapered within 1 week of initiation and discontinued within 2 weeks.[31] When tapering dexamethasone, it is important to recognize withdrawal symptoms such as headaches, lethargy, weakness, dizziness, anorexia, diffuse arthralgias, and myalgias. To better understand the therapeutic ratio of corticosteroids, future studies should require better control and record keeping of steroid dose for analysis of response to therapy.[33]

Anticonvulsants

Although seizures are the presenting symptom in 10% of cases and can occur in up to 25% of patients with brain metastases,[34] the role of antiepileptic drugs (AED) in patients with brain metastases has very limited class I evidence.[35] One study of 100 patients with newly diagnosed brain tumors (60 with brain metastases) and no history of prior seizures randomized patients to AEDs versus no AEDs.[36] The primary end point was seizure occurrence at 3 months postrandomization. The trial was terminated early as the seizure rate was only 10%, which was lower than the anticipated rate of 20%.

Given the lack of class I evidence, guidelines on the use of anticonvulsants for patients with metastatic brain tumors have been established.[37,38] For patients without seizures, prophylactic use of AEDs is not recommended. Patients who present with seizures or who develop seizures during therapy should receive AEDs, preferably with agents that do not interact with hepatic cytochrome P450 (e.g., levetiracetam). For patients on dexamethasone, phenytoin levels can be affected by its use. In addition, phenytoin can affect clearance of chemotherapy agents and also can cause Stevens Johnson syndrome, which may be precipitated if radiation is used.[39] The use of anticonvulsants after surgery is controversial given results of a recent study.[40]

Venous Thromboembolism

Because patients with brain tumors and thromboembolism are believed to be at higher risk for intracranial hemorrhage with anticoagulation, guidelines were established by the American Society of Clinical Oncology for prophylaxis and treatment of venous thromboembolism in patients with cancer.[41] Low-molecular-weight heparin is recommended for prophylaxis of hospitalized and higher-risk ambulatory patients given the minimal monitoring of coagulation and rare chance for major bleeding episode.[42]

A

RPA Class	Characteristics	Median Survival (mo)
I	KPS ≥ 70, age < 65, primary controlled, no extracranial metastases	7.1
II	All others	4.2
III	KPS < 70	2.3

B

	0	0.5	1
Age	>60	50–59	<50
KPS	<70	70–80	90–100
# of brain metastases	>3	2–3	1
Extracranial metastases	Present	–	None

Non-small-cell and small-cell lung cancer

GPA Scoring Criteria

Prognostic Factor	0	0.5	1.0	Patient Score
Age, years	> 60	50–60	< 50	_____
KPS	< 70	70–80	90–100	_____
ECM	Present	–	Absent	_____
No. of BM	> 3	2–3	1	_____
Sum total				_____

Median survival (months) by GPA: 0–1.0 = 3.0; 1.5–2.0 = 5.5; 2.5–3.0 = 9.4; 3.5–4.0 = 14.8

Melanoma

GPA Scoring Criteria

Prognostic Factor	0	1.0	2.0	Patient Score
KPS	< 70	70–80	90–100	_____
No. of BM	> 3	2–3	1	_____
Sum total				_____

Median survival (months) by GPA: 0–1.0 = 3.4; 1.5–2.0 = 4.7; 2.5–3.0 = 8.8; 3.5–4.0 = 13.2

Breast cancer

GPA Scoring Criteria

Prognostic Factor	0	0.5	1.0	1.5	2.0	Patient Score
KPS	≤ 50	60	70–80	90–100	n/a	_____
Subtype	Basal	n/a	LumA	HER2	LumB	_____
Age, years	≥ 60	< 60	n/a	n/a	n/a	_____
Sum total						_____

Median survival (months) by GPA: 0–1.0 = 3.4; 1.5–2.0 = 7.7; 2.5–3.0 = 15.1; 3.5–4.0 = 25.3

Renal cell carcinoma

GPA Scoring Criteria

Prognostic Factor	0	1.0	2.0	Patient Score
KPS	< 70	70–80	90–100	_____
No. of BM	> 3	2–3	1	_____
Sum total				_____

Median survival (months) by GPA: 0–1.0 = 3.3; 1.5–2.0 = 7.3; 2.5–3.0 = 11.3; 3.5–4.0 = 14.8

GI cancers

GPA Scoring Criteria

Prognostic Factor	0	1	2	3	4	Patient Score
KPS	< 70	70	80	90	100	_____

C

Median survival (months) by GPA: 0–1.0 = 3.1; 2.0 = 4.4; 3.0 = 6.9; 4.0 = 13.5

Figure 123.1 **(A)** Recursive partitioning analysis class based on analysis of 1,200 patients treated on three consecutive Radiation Therapy Oncology Group trials conducted between 1979 and 1993, testing several different fractionation schemes and radiation sensitizers. Modified from Gaspar L, Scott C, Rotman M, et al. Recursive partitioning analysis (RPA) of prognostic factors in three radiation therapy oncology group (RTOG) brain metastases trials. *Int J Radiat Oncol Biol Phys* 1997;37:745–751, with permission.) **(B)** Graded prognostic assessment (*GPA*) based on analysis of 1,960 patients from five Radiation Therapy Oncology Group studies. (From Sperduto PW, Berkey B, Gaspar LE, et al. A new prognostic index and comparison to three other indices for patients with brain metastases: An analysis of 1,960 patients in the RTOG database. *Int J Radiat Oncol Biol Phys* 2008;70:510–514, with permission.) **(C)** Updated diagnosis-specific graded prognostic assessment based on combining the databases from 11 institutions of 3,940 patients. Karnofsky performance status (KPS), extracranial metastases (ECM), BM (brain metastases). Basal: triple negative; LumA: ER/PR positive, HER2 negative; LumB: triple positive; HER2: ER/PR negative, HER2 positive. ECM, extracranial metastases; ER, estrogen receptor; HER2, human epidermal growth factor receptor 2. (From Sperduto PW, Kased N, Roberge D, et al, Summary report on the graded prognostic assessment (GPA): An accurate and facile diagnosis-specific tool to estimate survival, guide treatment and stratify clinical trials for patients with brain metastases. *J Clin Oncol* 2012;30:419–425.)

Protamine can be used to reverse low-molecular weight heparin in an emergency. For patients with brain tumors and venous thromboembolism, anticoagulation is indicated unless the patient has had an intracerebral bleed or other contraindication for anticoagulation.[41] The insertion of an inferior vena cava filter is an alternative but is associated with a higher risk of thrombosis distal to the filter.[43]

Treatment Options

The optimal management of brain metastases is very controversial given the many factors that influence outcomes, the many modalities available, and the strong opinions that proponents of various treatment modalities have regarding the benefits and risks.[44] Even when "experts" are asked to provide guidance on treatment options, the management recommendations can vary widely.[45,46] The National Comprehensive Cancer Network guidelines for the treatment of brain metastases are not specific as they allow for physician discretion.[47] The guidelines for WBRT, surgery, and radiosurgery for brain metastases by the American Association of Neurological Surgeons and Congress of Neurological Surgeons are more prescriptive, but also allow for flexibility.[48–50]

Whole-Brain Radiation Therapy

WBRT has been the standard treatment for patients with brain metastases since the initial reports from the 1950s.[51] Because WBRT is widely available, is easy to deliver safely and accurately, is effective in providing palliation for the majority of patients, and does not require sophisticated technologies, it has long been considered the gold standard for treatment of brain metastases and represents the most common treatment modality worldwide. Symptomatic improvement has been poorly assessed and is variable. As the response to WBRT is best among patients with small-cell lung cancer, lymphoma, and germ cell tumors, these tumor types are generally excluded from clinical trials due to the relative radiosensitivity of these histologies.

The RTOG has completed numerous phase 3 trials evaluating various fractionation and dose schemes.[52–55] These trials have shown that the majority of patients have partial or complete response of their neurologic symptoms, which range from 40% to 70%, and median survival that averages 3 to 5 months. Extended or hypofractionated WBRT has not shown benefit in terms of survival. As result, the most commonly used fractionation schemes in the United States are 30 Gy in 10 fractions or 37.5 Gy in 15 fractions. For patients with poor prognosis, shortened fractionation schemes of 20 Gy in 5 fractions can be used. Based on an international practice survey of 445 individuals, Tsao et al.[56] reported that 20 Gy in 5 fractions rather than 30 Gy in 10 fractions was preferred fractionation scheme in Canada and Australia/New Zealand. This practice survey also revealed that 88% chose comfort measures for patients previously treated with WBRT and now presented 6 months later with two to four brain metastases all <4 cm in size with poor performance. Seventy-eight percent would use WBRT alone for two to four brain metastases for patients with uncontrolled extracranial disease and KPS of 70. The Medical Research Council has an ongoing trial (QUARTZ) that randomizes patients with inoperable brain metastases from NSCLC to supportive care with dexamethasone versus WBRT and dexamethasone.

The imaging response rates or stabilization of tumors after WBRT are quite variable and can range from 0% to 71%.[57,58] Nieder et al.[59,60] studied the CT responses in 108 patients with 336 measurable lesions following WBRT (30 Gy in 10 fractions) and found the overall response rate at up to 3 months was 59% (lesion complete response rate of 24%, partial response rate of 35%).[59] The complete response rates varied by histology and were 37% for small cell carcinoma, 35% for breast cancer, 25% for squamous cell carcinoma, 14% for nonbreast adenocarcinoma, 0% for renal cell carcinoma, and 0% for melanoma. Smaller tumor volumes and absence of necrosis influenced complete response rates. Higher response rate was obtained with 40 Gy at 2 Gy per fraction with or without a partial boost to 50 or 60 Gy compared with 30 Gy at 3 Gy per fraction.[60]

The most common side effects that occur during or shortly following WBRT include hair loss, mild skin erythema, and fatigue. Other side effects may include headache, nausea, vomiting, loss of appetite, change of taste, serous otitis, and somnolence. Secondary to the effect of opposed tangential radiation beams on skin sparing, hair loss is variable and may be permanent in the top and back of the scalp. Skin reactions typically resolve after several weeks, and fatigue usually improves after 2 to 3 months and may respond to methylphenidate. The long-term and frequency of side effects from WBRT have not been well documented as they were discounted given the short survival of these patients. Long-term side effects may include somnolence, fatigue, hearing loss, memory loss, and, in rare cases, dementia.

Two approaches to minimize the neurocognitive effects of WBRT include innovations in radiation delivery and use of medications. RTOG 0933 was a phase 2 trial evaluating hippocampal avoidance–WBRT (HA-WBRT) for 100 evaluable patients with brain metastases.[61] As the hippocampus dentate gyrus is thought to house neural stem cells responsible for memory, HA-WBRT using intensity-modulated radiation therapy minimizes dose to this stem cell compartment (<10 Gy). Results from this study demonstrated a 7% decline in delayed recall versus 30% from historical study ($p = 0.0003$). RTOG 0614 was a phase 3 trial that randomized 554 patients to WBRT (3,750 cGy in 15 fractions) with or without memantine, an N-methyl-D-aspartate receptor antagonist used for patients with mild to moderate Alzheimer disease.[62] The memantine arm had significantly longer time to cognitive decline ($p = 0.02$), lower median decline on Hopkins Verbal Learning Test-Revised (0 in memantine arm versus -2 in placebo arm at 24 weeks; $p = 0.059$), and fewer patients with decline in Controlled Oral Word Association at 16 weeks ($p = 0.004$) or Trail Making Test Part A at 24 weeks ($p = 0.014$). No difference in overall survival and progression-free survival between the two arms was seen. Based on the results of these trials, a phase 3 study with memantine and HA-WBRT is planned.

Prophylactic Cranial Irradiation

Because patients with small-cell lung cancer (SCLC) have a high propensity to develop brain metastases, prophylactic cranial irradiation (PCI) is commonly used to prevent dissemination to the brain especially for patients who achieve a complete response to induction chemotherapy. The Prophylactic Cranial Irradiation Overview Collaborative Group reported the outcomes in seven previously published PCI trials for patients with complete response to systemic therapy and demonstrated a statistically significant survival advantage favoring the patients treated with PCI and significant reduction in the incidence of new brain metastases from 58.6% to 33.3% at 3 years.[63] Another meta-analysis of PCI efficacy reviewed 12 randomized trials and included 5 studies that evaluated the role of PCI in patients with SCLC who had a complete response after induction chemotherapy.[64] A significant decrease in the incidence of brain metastases was noted when all studies were considered and improvement in survival when PCI was given only to patients who experienced a complete systemic response. A phase 3 international, intergroup study of patients with limited-stage SCLC in complete remission after chemotherapy and thoracic radiotherapy randomized patients to 25 Gy in 10 fractions, 36 Gy in 18 fractions, or 36 Gy in 24 fractions of PCI with the standard dose (25 Gy in 10 fractions) being the recommended fractionation for PCI given the significantly higher risk for mortality seen in the higher dose arms.[65] For extensive-stage patients, 286 patients were randomized to WBRT or observation.[66] The primary end point was development of symptomatic brain metastases, which was decreased with PCI. In addition, PCI increased overall survival at 1 year from 13.3% to 27.1% ($p = 0.003$) and 1-year disease-free survival from 14.6% in the observation group to 40.4% in the treatment group (p <0.001).

The cognitive effects of PCI in patients with SCLC were prospectively studied in 300 patients with SCLC controlled systemically who either received PCI or were observed.[67] Neurocognitive assessment from baseline and 2 years after PCI revealed no significant difference in cognitive status between the observation and PCI-treated cohorts. Another study demonstrated similar results in 136 patients seen at 1 year posttreatment.[68]

RTOG 0214 randomized patients with stage III NSCLC without disease progression after treatment with surgery and/or radiation therapy with or without chemotherapy to PCI (30 Gy in 15 fractions) or observation.[69] The primary end point of the study was overall survival. Unfortunately, the study closed early secondary to slow accrual. The 1-year overall survival and disease-free survival were not significantly different. The 1-year rates of development of brain metastases were significantly less for PCI at 7.7% versus 18.0% for observation ($p = 0.004$). Recently, the impact of PCI on self-reported cognitive functioning and Hopkins Verbal Learning Test were analyzed based on the results of RTOG 0214 and RTOG 0212.[70] At 6 and 12 months, a significant decline in self-reported cognitive functioning and Hopkins Verbal Learning Test was noted after PCI.

Radiation Sensitizers and Modifiers

Given the poor outcomes with WBRT alone, radiation sensitizers have been explored to improve the therapeutic ratio between tumor and normal tissues. Mehta et al.[6] reported on survival and neurologic outcomes in a randomized trial of WBRT (30 Gy in 10 fractions) with or without daily injections of motexafin gadolinium, a redox modulator.[6] Based on the results of subset analysis for NSCLC, a confirmatory trial was performed that showed no significant difference in time to neurologic progression.[71] Suh et al.[72] reported on results of phase 3 randomized trial comparing WBRT (30 Gy in 10 fractions) and supplemental O_2 with WBRT following daily injections of RSR-13 (efaproxiral), an allosteric modifier of hemoglobin.[72] The phase 3 trial showed no significant difference in overall survival between the arms, although the breast subset appeared to do better. Confirmatory phase 3 trial of 360 women with brain metastases from breast cancer showed no survival improvement with RSR-13 and WBRT.[73] A phase 3 trial from the RTOG evaluating thalidomide and WBRT demonstrated no survival benefit over WBRT alone.[74]

Surgery

Surgery plays an important role for some patients with brain metastases as it can provide immediate and effective relief from symptomatic mass effect and can confirm or establish the diagnosis, which is important for those patients who have unknown primary. In addition, patients with larger tumors (diameter >2 cm) may also benefit from surgery more than other treatment modalities. Advances in imaging and image guidance have improved the rates for complete resection.[75] Some of these advances include accurate localization with MRI and CT with stereotaxis, intraoperative imaging with ultrasound, mapping of the important cortices to determine brain function, and fiber tract mapping to avoid damage to important neural pathways to maintain or improve quality of life.

The type of surgical resection also appears to influence the rate of local recurrence. A retrospective review from MD Anderson Cancer Center of 570 patients undergoing surgical resection alone demonstrated that piecemeal resection compared with en bloc resection significantly predicted for higher local recurrence compared to en bloc surgery (hazard ratio = 1.7; $p = 0.03$).[76] Larger tumor volume exceeding 9.71 cm³ compared with smaller tumors also predicted for higher local recurrence (hazard ratio = 1.7; $p = 0.02$). Histologic subtype did not predict for local recurrence. The rate of leptomeningeal dissemination also appears to be higher after

piecemeal rather than en bloc resection of metastases, although larger tumors cannot always be removed without some internal decompression.[77,78] A predisposition for leptomeningeal spread is also seen for surgical resection of metastases of the posterior fossa.[79] For patients with multiple brain metastases, no strong comparative data exists regarding the role of surgery for these patients,[49] but a retrospective report from Bindal et al.[80] showed that survival for patients with multiple metastases where all were surgically removed was equivalent to that of surgery for a single removed lesion and superior to those where some lesions were not removed.

Whole-Brain Radiation Therapy with or without Surgery

The first phase 3 study from the University of Kentucky randomized 48 patients with a single brain metastasis to surgical resection and WBRT versus needle biopsy and WBRT (36 Gy in 12 fractions).[81] The addition of surgery to WBRT significantly improved survival (40 weeks versus 15 weeks, $p < 0.01$), local control (80% versus 48%, $p < 0.02$), and functional independence (38 weeks versus 8 weeks, $p < 0.005$) compared to biopsy and WBRT. Younger age, no extracranial disease, surgical resection, and longer interval from primary diagnosis to diagnosis of brain metastasis were associated with longer survival. The majority of these patients had NSCLC.

The second phase 3 study from Noordijk et al.[82] randomized 63 patients with CT-confirmed brain metastasis to surgical resection and WBRT versus WBRT (40 Gy in 20 fractions). Surgery and WBRT improved median survival (10 months versus 6 months; $p = 0.04$) and functional independence (7.5 months versus 3.5 months; $p = 0.06$) over WBRT alone. Patients with active extracranial disease had no survival benefit with surgery (5 months in each arm). Patients without active extracranial disease had significantly improved median survival in the surgery arm (12 months versus 7 months).

Another phase 3 trial from Mintz et al.[83] showed no benefit for surgical resection and WBRT (30 Gy in 10 fractions) compared to WBRT alone in 84 randomized patients in terms of survival, 30-day mortality, morbidity, or causes of death. The presence of extracranial metastases was an important predictor of mortality (relative risk = 2.3). Unlike the other two randomized trials, a greater percentage of patients had active systemic disease, had lower baseline KPS, and had several gastrointestinal primary tumors in each group.

Surgery with or without Whole-Brain Radiation Therapy

The role of WBRT following surgical resection was addressed in a phase 3 randomized study of 95 patients who had single metastasis to the brain.[84] After gross total resection, patients were randomized to observation versus a protracted course of WBRT (50.4 Gy in 28 fractions). The primary end point was tumor recurrence in the brain with secondary end points of survival, cause of death, and functional independence. The addition of WBRT to surgery decreased the chance for neurologic death (14% versus 44%, $p = 0.003$), decreased local recurrence (10% versus 46%, $p < 0.01$), and decreased tumor recurrence anywhere in the brain (18% versus 70%, $p < 0.001$). The majority of patients (61%) received WBRT at time of recurrence, which resulted in a large crossover of the observation arm to WBRT. Survival was not different, although the study's end point was local control and was not powered to demonstrate a survival advantage.[85]

Kocher et al.[86] reported the results of a phase 3 European Organisation for Research and Treatment of Cancer study of 359 patients comparing SRS (199 patients) or surgery (160 patients) with or without WBRT.[86] The primary end point for this study was time to deterioration of WHO performance status >2. Survival and time to WHO performance status deterioration >2 were not different between the two arms. At 2 years after surgery, WBRT significantly decreased the risk of local and new brain relapse from 59% to 27% ($p < 0.001$) and 42% to 23% ($p < 0.008$), respectively.

Due to the previously discussed concerns of the impact of WBRT on NCF, the use of SRS to the tumor bed has recently gained favor despite lack of class I evidence and is discussed later in this chapter.

Stereotactic Radiosurgery

Unlike WBRT, SRS delivers high dose(s) of ionizing radiation to focal target(s) while minimizing the dose to surrounding brain tissue. Although the concept of SRS dates back to the 1950s, this treatment option did not gain acceptance for many years.[87] Brain metastases have features that make them ideal targets for SRS, which include pseudospherical shape, location in the gray-white junction, and maximum diameter of <4 cm. In addition, the vast majority of brain metastases have distinct pathologic and radiographic margins, which allows for clear delineation of the target.[88] All of these characteristics allow for accurate target delineation, planning, and treatment delivery through the use of multiple intersecting radiation beams, which produce steep dose gradients ("dose falloff"). The linear accelerator, cobalt-60–based units (Gamma Knife; Elekta AB, Stockholm, Sweden), and proton beam unit represent the different types of devices used for SRS. Table 123.2 lists the advantages for SRS and surgery.

Since the 1990s, numerous institutional and multi-institutional studies have been published on the results of SRS as a primary, adjuvant, and salvage treatment for brain metastases. When prescribing doses of 15 to 24 Gy, the local control rates range from 70% to 95%.[89–92] Freedom from local progression depends on dose, volume, histology, and pattern of MRI or CT enhancement at the time of radiosurgery.[93,94] In addition, SRS is effective for all types of primary tumor including radioresistant histologies such as melanoma and renal cell carcinoma.[95,96] The ideal candidate for SRS is subject of debate, but generally consists of patients with controlled or absence of extracranial metastases and excellent KPS. Historically, the number (one to four) of brain metastases was considered a general contraindication, although recent publications refute this.[97–99]

To study the relationship between maximum tolerated radiosurgery dose and maximum diameter of the tumor, RTOG 9005 was a phase 1/2 trial for patients with recurrent primary and metastatic brain tumors.[100] The maximum tolerated doses for >2 cm to 3 cm and >3 cm to 4 cm were 18 Gy and 15 Gy, respectively; maximum tolerated dose was not reached for tumors ≤2 cm given the reluctance to dose escalate beyond 24 Gy. Because the risk of radiation injury increases with increasing tumor volume and diameter,

doses for brain metastases are inversely proportional to the maximum tumor diameter or volume. As a result, the local control rates for smaller targets are generally higher than larger targets, especially when WBRT is not part of the management strategy.[101] As the dose falloff is not as sharp for larger targets, which resulted in higher dose to normal brain tissues, radiosurgery targets are usually limited to maximum diameter of 4 cm. Recently, staged radiosurgery with repeat dose 3–4 weeks after initial treatment has been explored prospectively for larger lesions.[102]

Because the head frame is minimally invasive, there has been growing interest in frameless radiosurgery to allow for fractionation (two to five fractions). This may be helpful for larger tumors and those close to critical structures such as the optic apparatus. The results with frameless radiosurgery appear equivalent to frame-based radiosurgery, although the total number of treated patients is still limited.[103–107] For radioresistant tumors, fractionated SRS may be less effective than single-fraction SRS.[108]

Unlike WBRT, SRS increases the risk for radiation necrosis, which can lead to significant side effects such as steroid dependency. As radiation necrosis can closely mimic tumor recurrence, the diagnosis and treatment of radiation necrosis can be very difficult.[109] A recent questionnaire regarding practice patterns for diagnosis and treatment of intracranial radiation necrosis after SRS revealed variation in the management of steroid refractory radiation necrosis.[110] Figure 123.2 shows a sequence of images from diagnosis, after SRS, images confirming radiation necrosis, and resolution of radiation necrosis after treatment. Figure 123.3 shows an algorithm that we use to diagnose and treat radiation necrosis. In terms of imaging, cerebral blood volume can have high sensitivity and specificity.[111] Based on a double-blind, placebo-controlled phase 3 trial, the use of bevacizumab is the therapy with the best supported evidence for patients who are refractory to steroids.[112] One novel approach for treatment of steroid refractory radiation necrosis that is being explored is focused laser interstitial thermal therapy.[113]

Stereotactic Radiosurgery Versus Surgery

Several attempts at phase 3 trials comparing surgery to SRS have been done with little success. In the 1990s, the Joint Center for Radiation Therapy in Boston attempted to enroll patients onto a phase 3 trial comparing surgery to SRS and enrolled only six patients after 3 years due to patient or physician preference.[114] A prospective randomized trial from Germany compared SRS alone versus surgery and WBRT for patients with a single metastasis.[115] Unfortunately, this study closed early due to poor accrual with 33 patients in the surgery and WBRT arm, and 31 patients in the SRS alone arm. Overall survival, neurologic death, and local recurrence were equivalent. Shorter hospitalizations, less steroid treatment, and lower central nervous system (CNS) grade 1 and 2 toxicities were noted in the patients treated with SRS. Patients treated with SRS alone developed more distant recurrences ($p = 0.04$); however, this difference was lost after adjusting for salvage SRS. Another prospective randomized trial of surgery versus radiosurgery for patients with a single brain metastasis who were considered eligible for either treatment was performed at MD Anderson Cancer Center.[116] A total of 59 patients were entered into the randomized arm (30 underwent surgery and 29 SRS), and 155 patients were entered into the nonrandomized arm (89 chose surgery and 66 chose SRS). Although the results demonstrated higher local recurrence with SRS alone, the statistical analyses used in this study are controversial. However, as radiosurgery was usually effective, SRS remains their primary management approach with surgery as salvage.[117]

Whole-Brain Radiotherapy with or without Stereotactic Radiosurgery

The first randomized trial of WBRT (30 Gy in 12 fractions) with or without SRS boost (16 Gy) enrolled functionally independent patients with two to four brain metastases measuring ≤2.5 cm in

---

TABLE 123.2

Comparison of the Advantages for Surgery and Stereotactic Radiosurgery

Surgery	Stereotactic Radiosurgery
Treatment of larger lesion(s) (>4 cm diameter)	Treatment of small deep lesion(s) or eloquent areas
Immediate removal of mass effect and edema	Minimally invasive
Histologic confirmation	No general anesthesia use
Rapid taper of steroids for symptomatic lesions	Outpatient procedure
Removal of cancer	Treatment of multiple lesions at same session
Minimal risk for radiation necrosis	Short recovery time (<1 wk)
Less intensive follow-up	Potentially avoid whole-brain radiation therapy
Less long-term dependency on steroids	Rapid initiation of systemic therapies
	Fewer immediate complications

From Suh JH. Stereotactic radiosurgery for the management of brain metastases. *N Engl J Med* 2010;362:1119–1127, with permission.

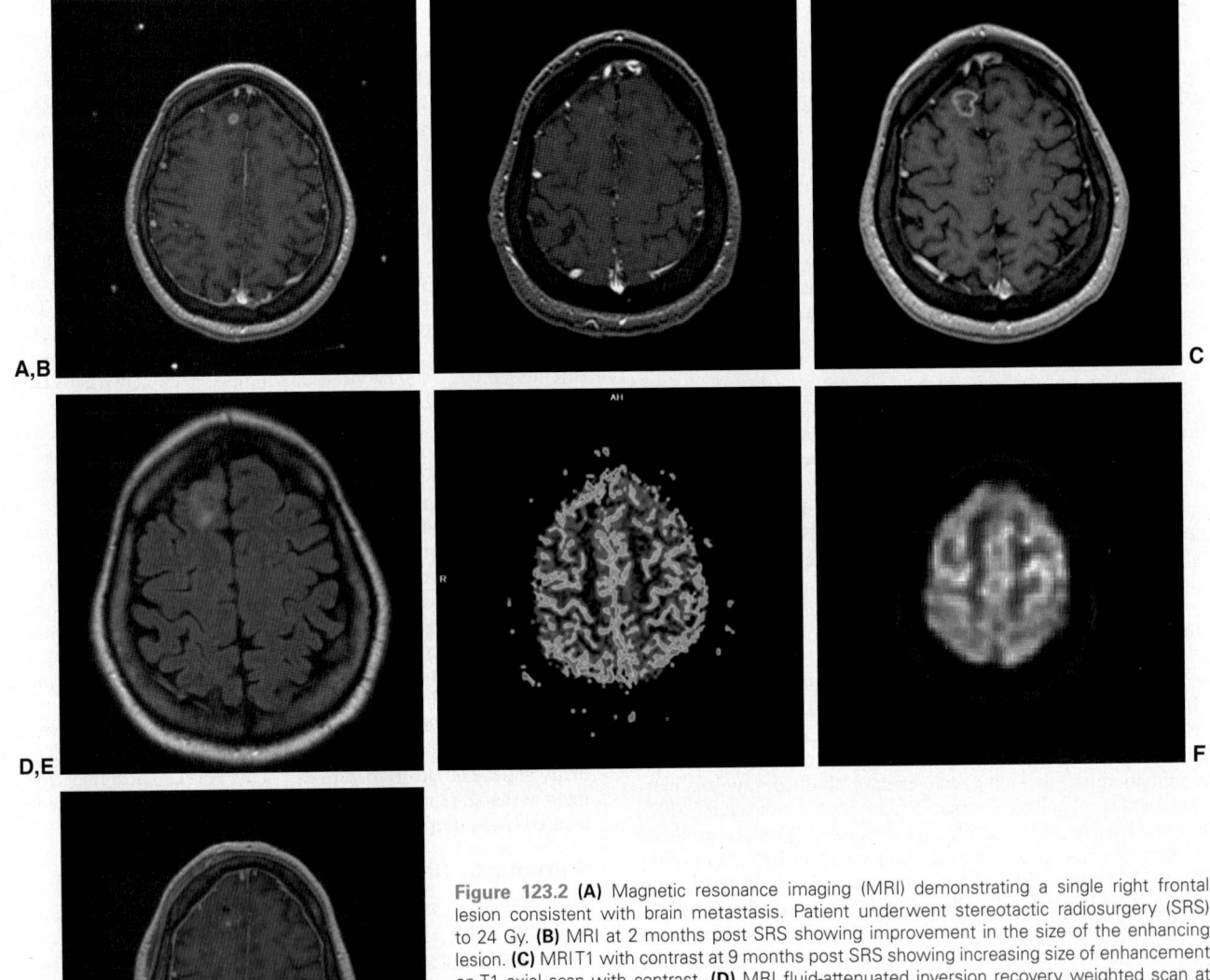

Figure 123.2 (A) Magnetic resonance imaging (MRI) demonstrating a single right frontal lesion consistent with brain metastasis. Patient underwent stereotactic radiosurgery (SRS) to 24 Gy. **(B)** MRI at 2 months post SRS showing improvement in the size of the enhancing lesion. **(C)** MRI T1 with contrast at 9 months post SRS showing increasing size of enhancement on T1 axial scan with contrast. **(D)** MRI fluid-attenuated inversion recovery weighted scan at 9 months post SRS showing edema surrounding enhancing lesion. **(E)** MRI relative cerebral blood volume sequence at 9 months post SRS. Overall lesion does not show elevated cerebral blood volume. There was some question of neovascularity in the anterior portion of the lesion. **(F)** Fluorodeoxyglucose positron emission tomography demonstrating no uptake within the lesion consistent with radiation necrosis. **(G)** Patient underwent NeuroBlate (Monteris Medical, Plymouth, MN) on the Laser Ablation After Stereotactic Radiosurgery (LAASR) protocol since the radiation necrosis progressed and was refractory to steroids. Biopsy was consistent with radiation necrosis. Postoperative MRI is shown.

diameter and >5 mm from the optic chiasm.[57] This trial enrolled only 27 patients secondary to early stopping rules. The two arms were well balanced with respect to known prognostic factors such as age, KPS, and extracranial disease status. The local control was 92% in the WBRT+SRS arm versus 0% in the WBRT arm ($p = 0.002$). Median survival was not significantly different in the two arms (7.5 months for WBRT versus 11 months for WBRT plus radiosurgery; $p = 0.22$).

The next trial, RTOG 9508, was a phase 3 trial of 333 patients with one to three newly diagnosed brain metastases who were randomized to WBRT (37.5 Gy in 15 fractions) with or without SRS boost using maximum doses from the RTOG 9005 trial.[58] Patients with brainstem or metastases located within 1 cm of the optic apparatus, RPA class III patients, and patients who had received systemic treatment within 1 month of enrollment were excluded. Median survival was significantly improved for patients with a single brain metastasis undergoing WBRT + SRS (6.5 months versus 4.9 months; $p = 0.039$) but not for patients with two or three lesions (5.8 months versus 6.7 months; $p = 0.98$). Patients in the SRS arm were more

likely to have stable or improved KPS through 6 months (43% versus 27%; $p = 0.03$) and better local control (82% versus 71%; $p = 0.01$). Neurologic death rate was similar in the two arms (approximately 34%). No survival advantage was noted based on type of radiosurgery unit used (linear accelerator versus Gamma Knife).

Since subset analysis from RTOG 9508 demonstrated benefit for patients with NSCLC, RTOG 0320 was a phase 3 trial of WBRT + SRS, WBRT + SRS + erlotinib, and WBRT + SRS + temozolomide.[118] Primary end point was overall survival. Given poor accrual (126 of 381 patients), this study closed early and showed no significant survival advantage with the addition of erlotinib or temozolomide. The results suggested the best outcomes were achieved in the WBRT and SRS arm.

Stereotactic Radiosurgery with or without Whole-Brain Radiation Therapy

Arguably the greatest area of debate in the management of brain metastases is the routine use of WBRT.[44,119] Sneed et al.[120] found

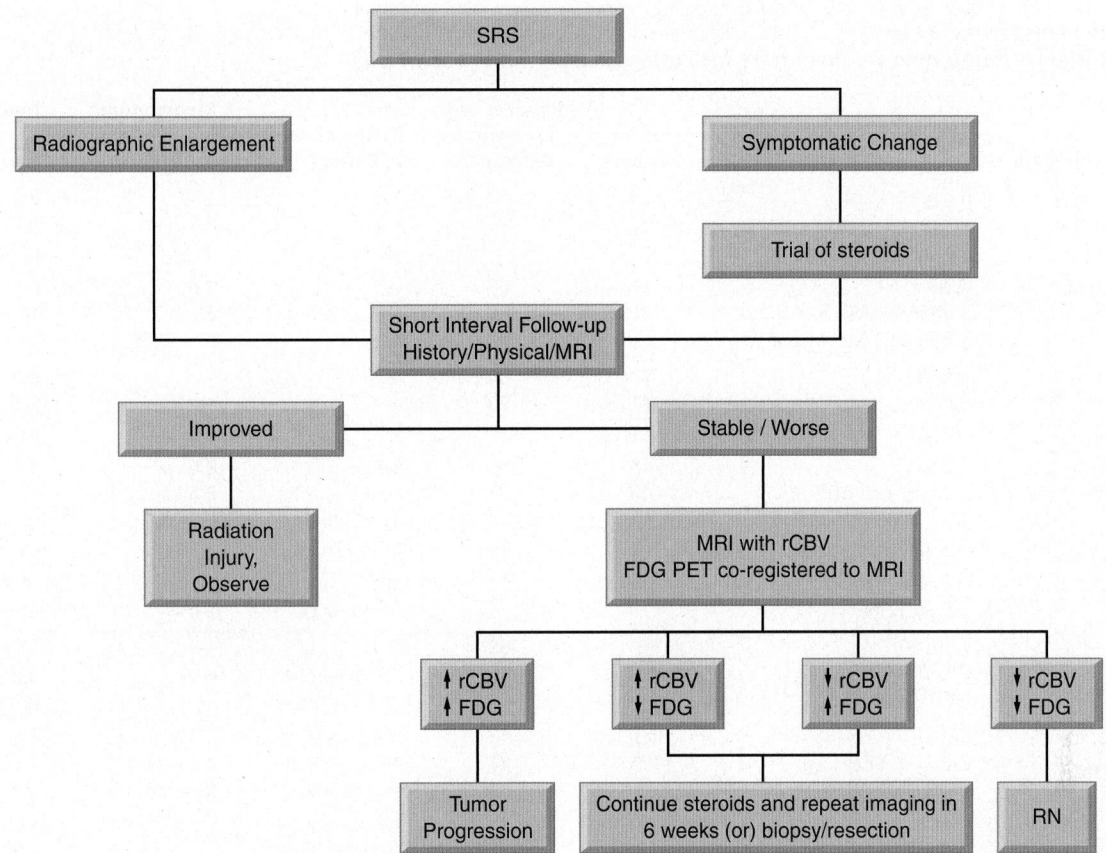

Figure 123.3 Algorithm for diagnosing and managing radiation necrosis at the Cleveland Clinic. SRS, stereotactic radiosurgery; MRI, magnetic resonance imaging; rCBV, regional cerebral blood volume; FDG, fluorodeoxyglucose; PET, positron emission tomography; RN, radiation necrosis. (From Chao ST, Ahluwalia MS, Barnett GH, et al. Challenges with the diagnosis and treatment of cerebral radiation necrosis. *Int J Radiat Oncol Biol Phys* 2013;87:449–457, with permission.)

that omission of WBRT in patients who received initial radiosurgery for up to four brain metastases did not compromise intracranial control, provided salvage therapy information was included in the actuarial outcome analysis, an analysis that is not usually reported. In a multi-institutional analysis, survival is substantially greater in patients who received SRS, with or without WBRT, compared to patients in the RTOG WBRT trials, for each of the three RPA classes.[121]

The Japanese Radiation Oncology Study Group conducted a randomized phase 3 trial of 132 patients with one to four brain metastases, each <3 cm in diameter.[122] Patients were randomized to WBRT and SRS or SRS alone. The primary end point was overall survival. The median and 1-year actuarial survival rate were 7.5 months and 38.5% in the WBRT + SRS group and 8 months and 28.4% for SRS alone ($p = 0.42$), respectively. The 12-month brain tumor recurrence rate was significantly lower in the WBRT plus SRS group (46.8%) than the SRS alone group (76.4%) ($p < 0.001$). Salvage brain treatment was also less frequent in the WBRT plus SRS group compared to SRS alone. No significant differences in systemic and neurologic functional preservation, cause of neurologic death, and side effects of radiation between the two arms were demonstrated. When mini-mental state examination was examined in this study, the average duration until deterioration was 16.5 months in the WBRT and SRS group versus 7.6 months in the SRS alone group ($p = 0.05$), suggesting that control of the brain tumor was the most important factor for stabilizing NCF.[123]

Chang et al.[124] published results of a randomized trial from the MD Anderson Cancer Center to examine NCF as the primary endpoint (Hopkins Verbal Learning Test-Revised) in patients who underwent SRS treatment with or without WBRT (30 Gy in

12 fractions). After accrual of 58 patients, the trial was stopped prematurely based on the early stopping rules because analysis determined that patients treated with SRS plus WBRT were at a greater risk of a significant decline in learning and memory function by 4 months, as shown by Hopkins Verbal Learning Test-Revised, compared with the group that received SRS alone. CNS recurrences were, however, significantly higher in the group receiving SRS alone; 73% of patients in the SRS + WBRT group were free from CNS recurrence at 1 year, compared with 27% of patients who received SRS alone ($p = 0.0003$), although the mortality was higher in the arm that received WBRT.

Kocher et al.[86] reported the results of a phase 3 European Organisation for Research and Treatment of Cancer study of 359 patients comparing SRS (199 patients) or surgery (160 patients) with or without WBRT. The primary end point for this study was time to deterioration of WHO performance status >2. Survival and time to WHO performance status deterioration >2 were not different between the two arms. At 2 years after SRS, WBRT significantly decreased the risk of local and new brain relapse from 31% to 19% ($p = 0.04$) and 48% to 33% ($p = 0.008$), respectively. For all patients, the risk of neurologic death was more frequent in the observation versus the WBRT arm (44% versus 28%; $p < 0.002$).

The recently closed phase 3 intergroup trial led by the North Central Cancer Treatment Group (N0574) randomizing patients with one to three brain metastases to SRS alone or SRS and WBRT will provide additional information about the effect of SRS and WBRT on NCF. Table 123.3 summarizes the randomized trials of surgery or radiosurgery for patients with brain metastases.

Lal et al.[125] compared SRS alone versus SRS + WBRT for patients with three or fewer brain metastases, using actual life years saved (LYS), quality-adjusted life years, and incremental

TABLE 123.3

Phase 3 Trials of Surgery or Radiosurgery for Patients with Brain Metastases

Study (Ref.)/Years	Treatment	No. of Patients	Patients with Extracranial Disease (%)	Median Local FFP (mo)	Median funct indep. Survival (mo)	Median Survival (mo)
Patchell et al.[81] 1985–1988	Biopsy + WBRT Surgery + WBRT (36 Gy/12 fx)	23 25	83 76	4.8 >13.6 (p <0.0001)	1.8 8.7 (p <0.005)	3.4 9.2 (p <0.01)
Noordijk et al.[82] 1985–1990	WBRT Surgery + WBRT (40 Gy at 2 Gy twice a day)	31 32	68 69	— — —	3.5 7.5 (P = 0.06)	6 10 (P = 0.04)
Mintz[83] 1989–1993	WBRT Surgery + WBRT (30 Gy/10 fx)	43 41	84 73	— — —	— — (p = NS)	6.3 5.6 (p = 0.24)
Patchell et al.[84] 1989–1997	Surgery Surgery + WBRT (50.4 Gy/28 fx)	46 49	65 63	6.2 >12.0 (p <0.001)	8.0 8.5 (p = 0.61)	9.9 11.0 (p = 0.39)
Kondziolka et al.[57] 1985–1988	WBRT WBRT + SRS (36 Gy/12 fx)	14 13	71 62	6 36 (p = 0.0005)	— —	7.5 11.0 (p = 0.22)
Andrews et al.[58] 1996–2001	WBRT WBRT + SRS (37.5 Gy/15 fx)	167 164	69 68	[71% 1-y LC] [82% 1-y LC] (p = 0.013)	— —	5.7 6.5 (p = 0.136)
Aoyama et al.[122] 1999–2003	SRS WBRT + SRS (30 Gy/10 fx)	67 65	43 37	[73% at 1-yr LC] [89% 1-y LC] (p = 0.002)	[27% at 1 y] [34% at 1 y] (p = 0.53)	8.0 7.5 (p = 0.42)
Chang et al.[124] 2001–2007	SRS SRS + WBRT	30 28	— —	[67% 1-y LC] [100% 1-y LC] (p = 0.012)		15.2 5.7 (p = 0.003)
Kocher et al.[86] 1996–2007	Surgery or SRS Surgery/SRS + WBRT	179 180	46 51	[41% 2-y LC] [73% 2-y LC] (p <0.001)	[22.3% at 2 y] [22.6% at 2 y]	10.9 10.7 (p = 0.89)

FFP, freedom from progression; funct. indep., functionally independent; WBRT, whole-brain radiotherapy; fx, fractions; SRS, stereotactic radiosurgery; NS, not significant; LC, local control.
Adapted from Larson DA, Rubenstein JL, McDermott MW, et al. Metastatic cancer to the brain. In DeVita VT, Lawrence TS, Rosenberg SA, eds. *Cancer: Principles & Practices of Oncology.* 9th ed. Philadelphia, PA: Lippincott Williams & Wilkins; 2011:2160.

cost effectiveness ratio. Compared to SRS with WBRT, SRS alone has a higher average cost ($74,000 versus $119,000, respectively). However, SRS alone has a higher average effectiveness of 1.64 LYS compared with combined SRS and WBRT (0.60 LYS). The authors conclude that SRS alone without WBRT is more cost-effective, even with salvage treatment delivered down the line.

Stereotactic Radiosurgery to Resection Cavity

Because patients undergoing surgical resection alone are at high risk for local recurrence, the use of radiosurgery rather than WBRT has been explored given the potential side effects of WBRT and the convenience of SRS.[126,127] Choi et al.[128] reported that the 12-month cumulative incidence rates of LF with and without a 2-mm margin around the defined tumor bed were 3% and 16%, respectively (p = 0.042). For most patients, the greatest resection cavity volume change occurred immediately after surgery (postoperative days 0 to 3) with no significant volume change occurring up to 33 days after surgery.[129] Although the risk for leptomeningeal spread after SRS is low, patients with breast cancer histology has been found to have a higher rate of leptomeningeal spread.[130] The North Central Cancer Treatment Group, in collaboration with RTOG, has an ongoing phase 3 trial (RTOG 1270/N107C) of postsurgical SRS compared with WBRT for resected brain metastases for patients with four or fewer brain metastases. The resection cavity

must measure <5 cm in maximal extent on the postoperative MRI (or CT) brain scan obtained ≤35 days prior to preregistration. The primary objective is whether there is improved overall survival in patients who receive SRS to the surgical bed compared to patients who receive WBRT. In addition, neurocognitive progression at 6 months postrandomization is being assessed.

Intraoperative Radiation Therapy and Brachytherapy to the Resection Cavity

Intraoperative radiation therapy has been investigated to decrease local recurrence after resection of brain metastases.[131,132] Brachytherapy has also been investigated using high-activity iodine injected into double lumen balloon that is placed in the surgical cavity.[133] As both intraoperative radiation therapy and brachytherapy increases operating room time and may also increase complications such as radiation necrosis, neither technique has been widely adopted.

Salvage Therapy

A number of therapeutic options may be considered for salvage therapy. Given the various options that are available, the relative frequency of various combinations of first and second therapies are unavailable. If WBRT is given upfront and the patient later develops recurrence of brain metastases, the patient can be safely salvaged with SRS. A retrospective study from Chao et al.[134] reviewed 111 patients treated from 1996 to 2004 who received SRS following failure from WBRT. Local control was 73% at a median time of 15.4 months. Median overall survival time was influenced by time from WBRT to recurrence. Repeat WBRT is not usually done as salvage for patients with better prognosis given concerns about the long-term effects of radiation. For patients with limited prognosis, lower doses and smaller fraction sizes, such as 20 to 25 Gy in 10 fractions or 30 Gy in 30 fractions (1 Gy twice a day), may be considered with outcomes are similar to that obtained following initial WBRT for RPA class II or III patients,[135–137] with symptomatic improvement in most patients. Surgery is not often repeated, although reoperation can be considered for selected patients. Bindal et al.[138] reported median survival following reoperation of 11.5 months, no operative mortality or morbidity, and neurologic improvement in most patients (75%).

Chemotherapy

Although historically chemotherapy has not had a prominent role in the management of brain metastases, several advances have been made. One of the major challenges to success of chemotherapy has been that of drug delivery due to the presence of the blood–brain barrier (BBB).[139] This barrier is comprised of the tight junctions between endothelial cells that line cerebral capillaries. In general, two broad classes of drugs have the potential to cross the BBB. Lipid soluble molecules are able to traverse the endothelial cell membranes and cytosol to reach the brain tumor cell by passive diffusion.[140] Examples of such agents include carmustine or lomustine. Small molecules can pass through the tight junctions. In general, these molecules must be less than approximately 500 kDa.[140] Examples of such molecules are temozolomide and many "small molecule" targeted agents such as lapatinib and erlotinib.[141–144] In addition, several drugs, such as bevacizumab, act on the abluminal side of the capillaries, obviating the need to cross the BBB in order to have activity.[145,146]

Several other factors can limit access of drug to the brain tumor. Protein binding of molecules within the vascular space (e.g., imatinib) leaves only a small percentage of a compound as free drug to reach the tumor.[147] The BBB contains several drug efflux pumps, which reverse the movement of molecules across the barrier.[148] The PgP drug transporter is probably the most prevalent of these pumps.[139] Finally, interstitial pressure within the tumor can create a mechanical barrier to convection of molecules toward the tumor.[149]

While all interventions seek to improve survival, delay progression, and preserve or improve a patient's function and quality of life, several goals are unique to the use of chemotherapy for patients with brain metastases. These goals include the enhancement of efficacy of radiation therapy (radiosensitization), the delay for the need of radiation therapy, the simultaneous control of systemic disease, and the ability to address the entire brain parenchyma in patients who may already have received WBRT. One final goal is to treat the leptomeninges in the setting where intrathecal chemotherapy is likely to be ineffective (e.g., bulky leptomeningeal disease given the limited penetration of intrathecal chemotherapy into leptomeningeal deposits) or unsafe due to unpredictable cerebrospinal fluid (CSF) distribution (e.g., impaired CSF flow related to obstructive hydrocephalus). For example, high-dose intravenous methotrexate for the treatment of breast cancer brain and/or leptomeningeal disease can reach the CSF in cytotoxic concentrations.[150]

The selection of patients appropriate to receive chemotherapy for brain metastases includes a number of considerations, especially in this setting where the goal is largely palliative. As with most interventions in oncology, the patient's performance status has a major impact on the likelihood that a patient might benefit from chemotherapy. The status of the patient's systemic disease matters—a patient whose systemic disease is uncontrolled is unlikely to benefit from a chemotherapy regimen intended for the

CNS. As an increasing number of agents becomes available for the treatment of a patient's systemic disease, the patient may have been heavily pretreated by the time CNS metastatic disease occurs. Thus end organ functional reserve, such as that of the bone marrow, must be evaluated carefully to ensure the safe administration of chemotherapy to such patients. The molecular phenotype of the patient's tumor must be considered as it can have a significant impact on prognosis and selection of treatment.[26] Importantly, the phenotype of the metastasis may differ from that of the primary tumor, an example of which is the loss/lack of HER2 receptor in a patient whose original tumor was HER2 positive.[151] In such a patient, the use of lapatinib would be inappropriate. Therefore, in the occasional patient who has undergone a resection or biopsy of a brain metastasis, one should obtain molecular marker tests in the resected lesion if the results would alter the selection of chemotherapeutic agents.

Despite multiple trials that have evaluated the concurrent use of chemotherapy with WBRT, none have documented a meaningful clinical benefit such as a delay in neurologic decline when compared to WBRT alone. Current trials are incorporating such end points. Currently, however, chemotherapy does not have a standard role as a radiosensitizer. Because CNS imaging of asymptomatic patients with cancer has become more prevalent, the paradigm of preirradiation chemotherapy has become a more active area of investigation. The efficacy of chemotherapy against CNS metastases approximates that against systemic cancer when given in the preirradiation setting.[152,153] The potential advantages of preirradiation chemotherapy include the possibility of delaying the need for radiation therapy, the theoretical possibility of improved drug delivery to unirradiated tumor, the delay of neurocognitive toxicity of radiation therapy in the high-risk patient, and the possibility of simultaneous treatment of systemic disease. Several recent trials have documented the efficacy of preirradiation chemotherapy.[151] This paradigm remains a promising area of research. For patients with progressive brain metastases after radiation therapy, chemotherapy can be used based on nonrandomized trials.[154,155] Prevention strategies are beginning to emerge in clinical trials. Primary prevention refers to the use of chemotherapy with the goal of preventing the emergence of brain metastases in patients at high risk for CNS metastases (e.g., triple negative [ER negative/PR negative/HER2 negative] breast cancer). Secondary prevention refers to the use of chemotherapy to delay or prevent the outgrowth of new metastases following the primary treatment of brain metastases with surgical resection or SRS. This paradigm offers an alternative to WBRT for those patients and providers who wish to delay WBRT. A number of clinical trials will explore the utility of prevention strategies. Although chemotherapy does not yet constitute standard treatment for patients with brain metastases, several strategies are under active investigation and should be supported by enrollment of patients onto clinical trials. A particularly promising area of investigation involves the use of novel targeted agents.[156,157] Table 123.4 lists the possible settings for the use of chemotherapy in brain metastases.

TABLE 123.4

Possible Settings for the Use of Chemotherapy in Brain Metastases

Concurrent with whole-brain radiotherapy
Before the use of radiation therapy
Recurrent or progressive disease after radiation therapy
Primary prevention
Secondary prevention

LEPTOMENINGEAL METASTASES

Leptomeningeal metastases (LM) or neoplastic meningitis represents a devastating, serious complication of the CNS in patients with advanced solid or hematologic malignancies. Because LM is often underdiagnosed, early management can be challenging. As a result, treatment is mostly palliative, although early detection and treatment can result in stabilization and prevention of neurologic deterioration, which may improve quality of life. As LM from solid tumors is often associated with an advanced stage of systemic disease, the prognosis is poor with median survival of 2 to 3 months and 1-year survival of 15%.[158] For patients with leukemic and lymphomatous meningitis, the outcomes are better.

Epidemiology

Although the incidence (0.8% to 8 %) of LM varies depending on the type of primary cancer and stage of disease, approximately 5% to 15% of patients with cancer are diagnosed with this complication. For patients with solid tumors, LM is estimated to occur in 5% to 18% of patients.[159] For patients with hematologic cancers such as leukemia and lymphoma, the incidence is 5% to 15% compared to 1% to 2% for patients with primary brain tumors, who appear to have the lowest incidence.[160] In autopsy series, the estimated rate of LM has been reported as high as 19%.[161]

Clinical Presentation

LM can easily be overlooked given the subtle signs and symptoms. As cranial nerves, spine, nerve roots, and brain may be affected, a number of symptoms and signs may occur such as headache, altered mental status, nausea/vomiting, seizures, difficulty swallowing, visual loss, facial numbness, focal weakness, and abnormalities of bowel and bladder function. Greater than 50% of patients have spinal cord dysfunction as the primary presenting symptom followed by cranial neuropathies, hemispheric defects and nonfocal presentations.[162] For patients with hydrocephalus due to obstruction of the cerebral aqueduct or the arachnoid granulations, placement of an external ventricular drain and/or ventriculoperitoneal shunt may be used.[163]

Diagnosis

Because the diagnosis of LM is difficult, a thorough neurologic history and physical examination, contrast-enhanced MRI of the brain, and examination of the CSF are important in establishing the diagnosis of LM.[164] In addition to history and physical examination, a sign and symptom–directed contrast-enhanced MRI of the spine should be completed. Radiographic presentations may include hydrocephalus without an identifiable intracranial lesion, partial or full obstruction of CSF flow, and leptomeningeal enhancement. Approximately 50% of patients with LM and spinal symptoms have abnormal imaging studies using gadolinium-enhanced MRI.[165] In addition, imaging may be the only positive diagnostic modality in 40% of cases.[165]

Examination of the CSF, which is usually performed via high-volume lumbar puncture, represents the sole diagnostic criteria for LM in approximately one-half of cases. The CSF is examined for opening pressure, appearance, glucose, protein, white and red blood cell counts with differential, and the presence of any abnormal cells by cytology or flow cytometry.[166,167] Unfortunately, cytologic evaluation of the CSF is an insensitive test with 40% to 50% of patients having negative CSF cytology.[168] Given the rapid degradation of malignant cells, CSF samples should be processed quickly.[160] In addition, adequate amounts of CSF (at least 10 mL, 1 to 2 mL, and 1 to 3 mL) should be sent for cytologic examination, flow cytometry, and routine studies, respectively.[160] For patients with leukemia or lymphoma, flow cytometry allows the earlier detection of LM before the onset of clinical symptoms and CSF pleocytosis and has superior sensitivity compared to standard cytology.[167,169] If the initial examination of the CSF is negative, up to two repeat CSF examinations should be performed to increase diagnostic sensitivity. Some biochemical markers such as CA 27.29 for breast cancer and CA-125 for ovarian cancer can be useful to help make diagnosis of LMD.

Radiation Therapy

Radiation therapy provides effective palliation in many cases of LM, particularly in areas of bulk disease, obstruction of CSF flow, and symptomatic sites and regions. It is also useful for patients with cranial neuropathies and cauda equina syndrome.[170] Craniospinal irradiation (CSI) is generally not recommended given the potential toxicities of CSI and previous radiation treatment that may have encompassed the brain or spine. In addition, the volume of bone marrow irradiated with CSI may preclude the use of future bone marrow suppressing chemotherapy. As a result, the use of involved field radiation therapy possibly followed by intrathecal chemotherapy is generally recommended given the complementary nature of both treatments.

Intra–Cerebrospinal Fluid Chemotherapy

Given the BBB, the best approach to administer chemotherapy within the leptomeningeal space without bulky disease is through an intraventricular access device such as an implanted subcutaneous reservoir and ventricular catheter (Ommaya reservoir) with intrathecal delivery via lumbar puncture as an alternative. As intra-CSF chemotherapy with agents such as cytarabine and methotrexate has limited systemic toxicity and allows for more uniform distribution and therapeutic levels of drug in the subarachnoid space, it is used for the treatment and prevention of LM from both solid and hematologic tumors.[170] A limitation of this approach is impaired or obstructed CSF flow from bulky meningeal disease. Bulky meningeal disease, which impairs or obstructs CSF flow, may be reversed with local irradiation. Generally, radiation therapy is delivered prior to intra-CSF therapy. Based on limited and older data, radiation therapy and intra-CSF therapies are not delivered concurrently secondary to concerns of increased neurotoxicity.[171]

Commonly used intrathecal chemotherapy agents include methotrexate, cytarabine, liposomal form of cytarabine, and thiotepa. Complications associated with intra-CSF chemotherapy include treatment-related meningitis that most frequently presents as a chemical arachnoiditis. Fewer than 10% of patients experience bacterial meningitis, usually with Gram-positive organisms. Myelosuppression can occur with high-dose methotrexate and thiotepa. Migration or malposition of the catheter and catheter obstruction can also occur including a 1% risk of postoperative hemorrhage. A small percentage of patients may experience chemotherapy-related leukoencephalopathy, which appears to occur most commonly in patients who receive intrathecal methotrexate following cranial irradiation.

Systemic Chemotherapy and Other Agents

Unlike most water-soluble drugs, high-dose systemic administration of methotrexate results in therapeutic drug levels in the CSF. As a result, high-dose methotrexate is active in neoplastic meningitis in lymphoma and in some solid tumors. High-dose intravenous methotrexate administration is active even when there is obstruction of CSF flow, which can sometimes compromise the subarachnoid administration of drugs. High-dose methotrexate administration requires detailed inpatient monitoring of fluid status and renal function, urine alkalinization, and leucovorin rescue, which makes this approach not appropriate or practical for all patients.[172] Other agents that have been investigated include rituximab for lymphomatous meningitis, topotecan for lung cancer, trastuzumab for breast cancer, and etoposide for SCLC in germ cell tumors.[173]

SELECTED REFERENCES

The full reference list can be accessed at lwwhealthlibrary.com/oncology.

1. Scoccianti S, Ricardi U. Treatment of brain metastases: Review of phase III randomized controlled trials. *Radiother Oncol* 2012;102:168–179.
6. Mehta MP, Rodrigus P, Terhaard CHJ, et al. Survival and neurologic outcomes in a randomized trial of motexafin gadolinium and whole-brain radiation therapy in brain metastases. *J Clin Oncol* 2003;21:2529–2536.
7. Meyers CA, Smith JA, Bezjak A, et al. Neurocognitive function and progression in patients with brain metastases treated with whole-brain radiation and motexafin gadolinium: Results of a randomized phase III trial. *J Clin Oncol* 2004;22:157–165.
9. Li J, Bentzen SM, Renschler M, et al. Regression after whole-brain radiation therapy for brain metastases correlates with survival and improved neurocognitive function. *J Clin Oncol* 2007;25:1260–1266.
14. Patel TR, McHugh BJ, Bi WL, et al. A comprehensive review of MR imaging changes following radiosurgery to 500 brain metastases. *AJNR Am J Neuroradiol* 2011;32:1885–1892.
16. Lin NU, Lee EQ, Aoyama H, et al. Challenges relating to solid tumour brain metastases in clinical trials, part 1: Patient population, response, and progression. A report from the RANO group. *Lancet Oncol* 2013;14:e396–e406.
17. Lin NU, Wefel JS, Lee EQ, et al. Challenges relating to solid tumour brain metastases in clinical trials, part 2: Neurocognitive, neurological, and quality-of-life outcomes. A report from the RANO group. *Lancet Oncol* 2013;14:407–416.
23. Gaspar L, Scott C, Rotman M, et al. Recursive partitioning analysis (RPA) of prognostic factors in three radiation therapy oncology group (RTOG) brain metastases trials. *Int J Radiat Oncol Biol Phys* 1997;37:745–751.
24. Sperduto PW, Berkey B, Gaspar LE, et al. A new prognostic index and comparison to three other indices for patients with brain metastases: An analysis of 1,960 patients in the RTOG database. *Int J Radiat Oncol Biol Phys* 2008;70:510–514.
25. Sperduto PW, Kased N, Roberge D, et al. Summary report on the graded prognostic assessment: an accurate and facile diagnosis-specific tool to estimate survival for patients with brain metastases. *J Clin Oncol* 2012; 30: 419–425.
27. Barnholtz-Sloan JS, Yu C, Sloan AE, et al. A nomogram for individualized estimation of survival among patients with brain metastasis. *Neuro Oncol* 2012;14:910–918.
31. Soffietti R, Cornu P, Delattre JY, et al. EFNS guidelines on diagnosis and treatment of brain metastases: Report of an EFNS task force. *Eur J Neurol* 2006;13:674–681.
33. Ryken TC, McDermott M, Robinson PD, et al. The role of steroids in the management of brain metastases: A systematic review and evidence-based clinical practice guideline. *J Neurooncol* 2010;96:103–114.
35. Mikkelsen T, Paleologos NA, Robinson PD, et al. The role of prophylactic anticonvulsants in the management of brain metastases: A systematic review and evidence-based clinical practice guideline. *J Neurooncol* 2010; 96:97–102.
37. Glantz MJ, Cole BF, Forsyth PA, et al. Practice parameter: Anticonvulsant prophylaxis in patients with newly diagnosed brain tumors. Report of the Quality Standards Subcommittee of the American Academy of Neurology. *Neurology* 2000;54:1886–1893.
41. Lyman GH, Khorana AA, Kuderer NM, et al. Venous thromboembolism prophylaxis and treatment in patients with cancer: American Society of Clinical Oncology clinical practice guideline update. *J Clin Oncol* 2013;31: 2189–2204.
44. Suh JH. Stereotactic radiosurgery for the management of brain metastases. *N Engl J Med* 2010;362:1119–1127.
49. Kalkanis SN, Kondziolka D, Gaspar LE, et al. The role of surgical resection in the management of newly diagnosed brain metastases: A systematic review and evidence-based clinical practice guideline. *J Neurooncol* 2010;96:33–43.
50. Linskey ME, Andrews DW, Asher AL, et al. The role of stereotactic radiosurgery in the management of patients with newly diagnosed brain metastases: A systematic review and evidence-based clinical practice guideline. *J Neurooncol* 2010;96:45–68.
56. Tsao MN, Rades D, Wirth A, et al. International practice survey on the management of brain metastases: Third international consensus workshop on palliative radiotherapy and symptom control. *Clin Oncol (R Coll Radiol)* 2012;24:81–92.
57. Kondziolka D, Patel A, Lunsford LD, et al. Stereotactic radiosurgery plus whole brain radiotherapy versus radiotherapy alone for patients with multiple brain metastases. *Int J Radiat Oncol Biol Phys* 1999;45:427–434.
58. Andrews DW, Scott CB, Sperduto PW, et al. Whole brain radiation therapy with or without stereotactic radiosurgery boost for patients with one to three brain metastases: Phase III results of the RTOG 9508 randomised trial. *Lancet* 2004;363:1665–1672.
61. Gondi V, Mehta M, Pugh S. Memory preservation with conformal avoidance of the hippocampus during whole-brain radiotherapy (WBRT) for patients with brain metastases: Primary endpoint results of RTOG 0933. *Plenary Session of ASTRO 2013, Atlanta, Georgia, Late Breaking Abstract* 2013.
62. Brown PD, Pugh S, Laack NN, et al. Memantine for the prevention of cognitive dysfunction in patients receiving whole-brain radiotherapy: A randomized, double-blind, placebo-controlled trial. *Neuro Oncol* 2013;15:1429–1437.
63. Auperin A, Arriagada R, Pignon JP, et al. Prophylactic cranial irradiation for patients with small-cell lung cancer in complete remission. Prophylactic Cranial Irradiation Overview Collaborative Group. *N Engl J Med* 1999;341: 476–484.
65. Le Pechoux C, Dunant A, Senan S, et al. Standard-dose versus higher-dose prophylactic cranial irradiation (PCI) in patients with limited-stage small-cell lung cancer in complete remission after chemotherapy and thoracic radiotherapy (PCI 99-01, EORTC 22003-08004, RTOG 0212, and IFCT 99-01): A randomised clinical trial. *Lancet Oncol* 2009;10:467–474.
66. Slotman B, Faivre-Finn C, Kramer G, et al. Prophylactic cranial irradiation in extensive small-cell lung cancer. *N Engl J Med* 2007;357:664–672.
69. Gore EM, Bae K, Wong SJ, et al. Phase III comparison of prophylactic cranial irradiation versus observation in patients with locally advanced non-small-cell lung cancer: Primary analysis of Radiation Therapy Oncology Group study RTOG 0214. *J Clin Oncol* 2011;29:272–278.
70. Gondi V, Paulus R, Bruner DW, et al. Decline in tested and self-reported cognitive functioning after prophylactic cranial irradiation for lung cancer: Pooled secondary analysis of Radiation Therapy Oncology Group randomized trials 0212 and 0214. *Int J Radiat Oncol Biol Phys* 2013;86:656–664.
71. Mehta MP, Shapiro WR, Phan SC, et al. Motexafin gadolinium combined with prompt whole brain radiotherapy prolongs time to neurologic progression in non-small-cell lung cancer patients with brain metastases: Results of a phase III trial. *Int J Radiat Oncol Biol Phys* 2009;73:1069–1076.
72. Suh JH, Stea B, Nabid A, et al. Phase III study of efaproxiral as an adjunct to whole-brain radiation therapy for brain metastases. *J Clin Oncol* 2006; 24:106–114.
74. Knisely JP, Berkey B, Chakravarti A, et al. A phase III study of conventional radiation therapy plus thalidomide versus conventional radiation therapy for multiple brain metastases (RTOG 0118). *Int J Radiat Oncol Biol Phys* 2008;71:79–86.
76. Patel AJ, Suki D, Hatiboglu MA, et al. Factors influencing the risk of local recurrence after resection of a single brain metastasis. *J Neurosurg* 2010; 113:181–189.
81. Patchell RA, Tibbs PA, Walsh JW, et al. A randomized trial of surgery in the treatment of single metastases to the brain. *N Engl J Med* 1990;322:494–500.
82. Noordijk EM, Vecht CJ, Haaxma-Reiche H, et al. The choice of treatment of single brain metastasis should be based on extracranial tumor activity and age. *Int J Radiat Oncol Biol Phys* 1994;29:711–717.
83. Mintz AH, Kestle J, Rathbone MP, et al. A randomized trial to assess the efficacy of surgery in addition to radiotherapy in patients with a single cerebral metastasis. *Cancer* 1996;78:1470–1476.
84. Patchell RA, Tibbs PA, Regine WF, et al. Postoperative radiotherapy in the treatment of single metastases to the brain: A randomized trial. *JAMA* 1998;280:1485–1489.
86. Kocher M, Soffietti R, Abacioglu U, et al. Adjuvant whole-brain radiotherapy versus observation after radiosurgery or surgical resection of one to three cerebral metastases: Results of the EORTC 22952-26001 study. *J Clin Oncol* 2011;29:134–141.
89. Likhacheva A, Pinnix CC, Parikh NR, et al. Predictors of survival in contemporary practice after initial radiosurgery for brain metastases. *Int J Radiat Oncol Biol Phys* 2013;85:656–661.
91. Serizawa T, Hirai T, Nagano O, et al. Gamma knife surgery for 1-10 brain metastases without prophylactic whole-brain radiation therapy: Analysis of cases meeting the Japanese prospective multi-institute study (JLGK0901) inclusion criteria. *J Neurooncol* 2010;98:163–167.
99. Grandhi R, Kondziolka D, Panczykowski D, et al. Stereotactic radiosurgery using the leksell gamma knife perfexion unit in the management of patients with 10 or more brain metastases. *J Neurosurg* 2012;117:237–245.
100. Shaw E, Scott C, Souhami L, et al. Single dose radiosurgical treatment of recurrent previously irradiated primary brain tumors and brain metastases: Final report of RTOG protocol 90-05. *Int J Radiat Oncol Biol Phys* 2000; 47:291–298.
106. Muacevic A, Kufeld M, Wowra B, et al. Feasibility, safety, and outcome of frameless image-guided robotic radiosurgery for brain metastases. *J Neurooncol* 2010;97:267–274.
109. Chao ST, Ahluwalia MS, Barnett GH, et al. Challenges with the diagnosis and treatment of cerebral radiation necrosis. *Int J Radiat Oncol Biol Phys* 2013;87:449–457.
110. Stockham AL, Ahluwalia M, Reddy CA, et al. Results of a questionnaire regarding practice patterns for the diagnosis and treatment of intracranial radiation necrosis after SRS. *J Neurooncol* 2013;115:469–475.
112. Levin VA, Bidaut L, Hou P, et al. Randomized double-blind placebo-controlled trial of bevacizumab therapy for radiation necrosis of the central nervous system. *Int J Radiat Oncol Biol Phys* 2011;79:1487–1495.
115. Muacevic A, Kreth FW, Horstmann GA, et al. Surgery and radiotherapy compared with gamma knife radiosurgery in the treatment of solitary cerebral metastases of small diameter. *J Neurosurg* 1999;91:35–43.
118. Sperduto PW, Wang M, Robins HI, et al. A phase 3 trial of whole brain radiation therapy and stereotactic radiosurgery alone versus WBRT and SRS with temozolomide or erlotinib for non-small cell lung cancer and 1 to 3 brain metastases: Radiation Therapy Oncology Group 0320. *Int J Radiat Oncol Biol Phys* 2013;85:1312–1318.

PRACTICE OF ONCOLOGY

121. Sneed PK, Suh JH, Goetsch SJ, et al. A multi-institutional review of radiosurgery alone vs. radiosurgery with whole brain radiotherapy as the initial management of brain metastases. *Int J Radiat Oncol Biol Phys* 2002;53:519–526.

122. Aoyama H, Shirato H, Tago M, et al. Stereotactic radiosurgery plus whole-brain radiation therapy vs stereotactic radiosurgery alone for treatment of brain metastases: A randomized controlled trial. *JAMA* 2006;295:2483–2491.

123. Aoyama H, Tago M, Kato N, et al. Neurocognitive function of patients with brain metastasis who received either whole brain radiotherapy plus stereotactic radiosurgery or radiosurgery alone. *Int J Radiat Oncol Biol Phys* 2007;68:1388–1395.

124. Chang EL, Wefel JS, Hess KR, et al. Neurocognition in patients with brain metastases treated with radiosurgery or radiosurgery plus whole-brain irradiation: A randomised controlled trial. *Lancet Oncol* 2009;10:1037–1044.

125. Lal LS, Byfield SD, Chang EL, et al. Cost-effectiveness analysis of a randomized study comparing radiosurgery with radiosurgery and whole brain radiation therapy in patients with 1 to 3 brain metastases. *Am J Clin Oncol* 2012;35:45–50.

127. Gans JH, Raper DM, Shah AH, et al. The role of radiosurgery to the tumor bed after resection of brain metastases. *Neurosurgery* 2013;72:317–325, discussion 325–326.

140. Neuwelt EA. Mechanisms of disease: The blood-brain barrier. *Neurosurgery* 2004;54:131–140, discussion 141–142.

154. Lin NU, Eierman W, Greil R, et al. Randomized phase II study of lapatinib plus capecitabine or lapatinib plus topotecan for patients with HER2-positive breast cancer brain metastases. *J Neurooncol* 2011;105:613–620.

156. Preusser M, Berghoff AS, Schadendorf D, et al. Brain metastasis: Opportunity for drug development?. *Curr Opin Neurol* 2012;25:786–794.

157. Drappatz J, Batchelor TT. Leptomeningeal neoplasms. *Curr Treat Options Neurol* 2007;9:283–293.

161. Van Horn A, Chamberlain MC. Neoplastic meningitis. *J Support Oncol* 2012;10:45–53.

169. Lombardi G, Zustovich F, Farina P, et al. Neoplastic meningitis from solid tumors: New diagnostic and therapeutic approaches. *Oncologist* 2011;16:1175–1188.

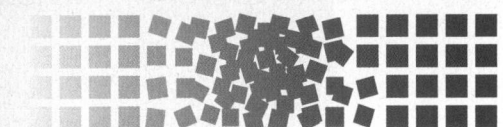

124 Metastatic Cancer to the Lung

Jessica S. Donington and Christopher W. Towe

INTRODUCTION

Ultimately, uncontrolled metastatic disease is the most frequent cause of cancer-related death. Whereas widespread disease is often not amenable to localized therapy, metastatic spread that is limited to the lungs can be successfully treated with localized therapy. Surgical resection of metastatic pulmonary disease gained popularity in the 1960s and 1970s as a result of a series of patients who underwent repeated pulmonary resection for metastatic osteogenic sarcoma and demonstrated a 5-year survival rate >30% relative to 17% in historical controls.[1] Since that time, hundreds of studies have documented improved outcomes among many tumor types. Unfortunately, most studies of pulmonary metastasectomy are small, single-institution retrospective reviews, and large prospective data sets are not available to guide clinical decisions regarding which patients will benefit from resection. Furthermore, the increased efficacy of "targeted" molecular therapies in select histologies requires a continuous evolution of decision making because surgery may no longer be the "only" beneficial treatment option. This chapter discusses the evaluation and management of patients with pulmonary metastases. General issues addressed include the role of diagnostic imaging, surgical approach (video-assisted thoracoscopic surgery [VATS] versus thoracotomy), extent of resection (wedge versus anatomic resection), role of lymph node dissection, and expanding role of image-guided ablative therapies. The chapter will conclude with a review of evidence for metastasectomy by primary tumor type and will include a discussion of tumor-specific multimodality therapy.

PRESENTATION AND DIAGNOSIS OF PULMONARY METASTASES

The majority of pulmonary metastases are asymptomatic and detected radiographically. Approximately 20% of patients with pulmonary metastases are symptomatic, with cough and hemoptysis being the most common. The presence of symptoms usually suggests proximity of tumor to larger airways. True endobronchial metastases are rare, but they can occur in patients with metastases from colorectal, breast, renal, melanoma, and thyroid cancer. Patients may also present with chest pain (a possible sign of chest wall invasion) or constitutional symptoms. Workup should include careful history and physical exam as well as cross-sectional imaging.

Cross-sectional imaging is essential in the evaluation of a patient with pulmonary metastases. The most commonly used method is computed tomography (CT) scanning. Chest CT is accurate, widely available, and is generally associated with a low dose of radiation exposure. CT imaging technology has evolved significantly since its introduction, and modern thin-section low-dose CT is highly effective in imaging pulmonary metastases.[2,3] Fluorodeoxyglucose-positron emission tomography enables identification of extrathoracic tumor sites and simultaneously characterizes pulmonary foci of disease on a metabolic basis. This can be especially important in patients who have a short disease-free

interval and have questionable extrathoracic sites of disease. Magnetic resonance imaging is not good at imaging the lung tissue and is generally not a useful modality for routine imaging pulmonary metastases compared with conventional CT. It is useful for demonstrating tumor invasion of the great vessels, heart, chest wall, or nervous structures including the spine or brachial plexus, and in ruling out synchronous liver metastases.

The classic radiographic appearance of pulmonary metastases is a smooth, well-circumscribed, peripheral nodule, a "gumball" or "cannonball" (Fig. 124.1). Metastases also frequently appear in multiple sites throughout the lungs simultaneously. Despite radiographic appearance, it is important to differentiate suspected metastatic lesions from other pulmonary pathology. Multiple simultaneous lesions may need to be differentiated from infectious processes, while single lesions need to be differentiated from a primary lung cancer. The likelihood of pulmonary metastases relative to new primary malignancy is related to the tissue type of the patient's antecedent cancer, risk factors for lung cancers, as well as the interval between the previous malignancy and presentation. In patients with history of sarcoma or melanoma, a new pulmonary nodule is 10-fold more likely to be a metastases than a new primary lung cancer. If the initial tumor was of genitourinary or colorectal origin, there is equal chance that the tumor is metastasis versus new primary, and if the tumor is of head and neck origin, the newly identified tumor is twice as likely to be a new primary lung cancer.[4] These assumptions reflect relative differences between genetic aberrations and other risk factors (such as tobacco smoking) between lung cancer and the tumors in question. Nowhere is this truer than in patients with history of previous non–small-cell lung cancer (NSCLC). In the first 4 years following curative resection of early stage NSCLC, the risk for recurrence is 6% to 10% per person-year, but recurrence risk then drops to 2% per year, while the risk for a second primary NSCLC ranges from 3% to 6% per person-year and does not diminish over time.[5] In patients with a history of previous lung cancer, new primary lung cancers are more likely after 4 years and usually have a classic radiographic appearance of early tumors, such as a mixed solid and ground-glass nodule. Primary lung cancer risk prediction models, such as the Bach model[6] and model based on the European Prospective Investigation into Cancer and Nutrition data,[7] which takes into account an individual's age, sex, asbestos exposure history, and smoking history (duration, number of cigarettes per day, and time since quitting smoking), can also be used to estimate the probability that a lung nodule is a primary lung cancer as opposed to a metastases.

Ultimately determining whether a new pulmonary nodule in a patient with history of cancer is a metastasis requires histopathologic confirmation. In specific circumstances where surgical removal will not be pursued, nonoperative biopsy is preferable. Techniques such as image-guided percutaneous biopsy, fluoroscopic-guided transbronchial biopsy, endobronchial ultrasound, or navigational bronchoscopy are all reasonable approaches and should be individualized to the location of the nodule, institutional expertise, and patient-specific concerns. Differentiating site of origin can be confounded by the histologic similarity between primary lung

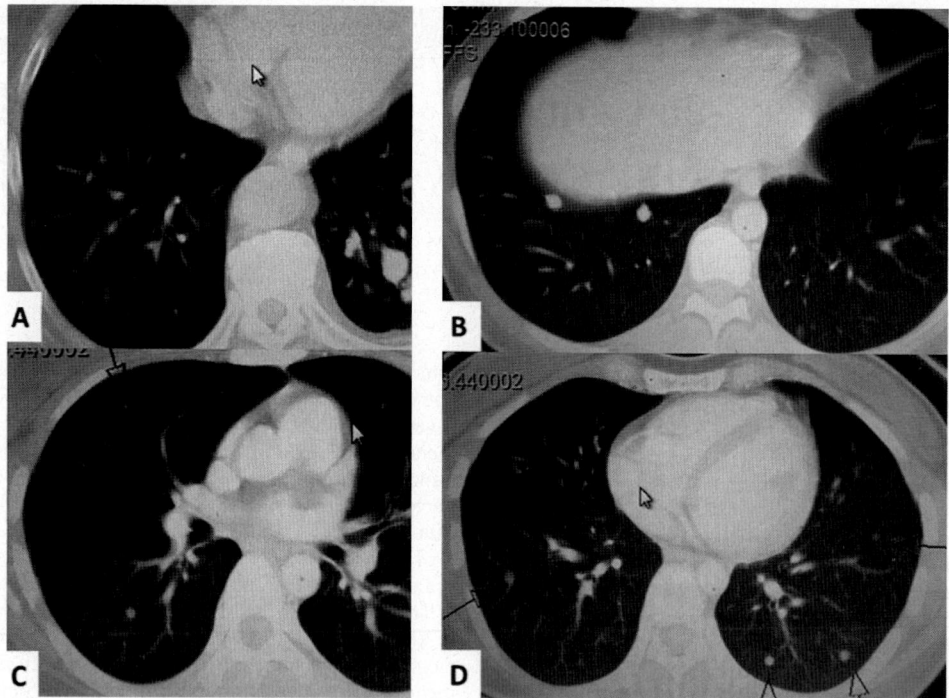

Figure 124.1 **(A–D)** Computed tomography image of pulmonary metastases demonstrates a classic radiographic appearance: circular, well circumscribed, multiple, and peripheral.

cancer and metastatic lesions, most commonly differentiating between primary squamous cell cancers from lung and metastatic head and neck tumors. Molecular analyses may be useful in these circumstances.[8] In patients who cannot be diagnosed by nonoperative means, surgical exploration and biopsy, preferably by VATS or by thoracotomy, is reasonable.

SURGICAL METASTASECTOMY

Criteria for Surgical Resection

Analysis from numerous retrospective studies has led to the following generally accepted criteria for selection of patients for surgical pulmonary metastasectomy: 1) definitive control of the primary tumor has occurred (or is possible), 2) absence of (or ability to control) extrathoracic metastatic disease, 3) the lung metastases are amenable to complete resection, 4) the patient can tolerate the planned procedure, and 5) there is no better treatment alternative.[9] Using these criteria, however, long-term survival after metastasectomy remains uncommon, reflecting the fact that in only a subset of patients does the resected disease represent the entirety of their metastatic burden. Ultimately, the greatest management difficulty is differentiating patients that might benefit from surgical extirpation from those whose disease has already, or will soon, spread beyond the means of surgical control. Studies have used retrospective analyses to help clinicians predict which patients will have good outcome after surgery. By far, the largest such analysis of outcomes after metastasectomy comes from the International Registry of Lung Metastasis (IRLM), which was published in 1997.[10] That project retrospectively analyzed over 5,000 cases of surgical metastasectomy for curative intent for a variety of histologies from 18 institutions around the world. Actuarial overall survival was significantly higher among patients who underwent complete (R0) surgical resection, with 5-, 10-, and 15-year survival of 36%, 26%, and 22%, respectively, compared to 13% at 5 years and 7% at 10 years among patients with incomplete resections. While not as striking as the impact of complete resection, other factors that

had a positive effect on long-term survival in the IRLM analysis were disease-free interval >36 months (5-year survival 45% versus 31% <36 months) and single metastasis (5-year survival 43% versus 34% for two or three and 27% for four or more lesions). Based on their analysis, the outcomes could be differentiated into four groups based on the following risk factors: (1) whether their disease was resectable, (2) single or multiple metastases, and (3) if the disease-free interval was >36 months. Patients with favorable risk in all three criteria could anticipate 50% survival at 5 years compared to <15% for those with unfavorable criteria for each risk factor (Fig. 124.2).

The need to perform a second metastasectomy in the IRLM analysis was associated with remarkably good 5-year survival (44%), which suggested that patients who recur and are still physiologically able should be offered re-resection. Other studies of outcomes after metastasectomy have corroborated the IRLM results and continue to demonstrate the prognostic importance of complete resection, prolonged disease-free interval, and fewer numbers of metastases. Other prognostic factors that have since been proposed include the presence of lymph node metastasis, response to chemotherapy, and size of lesions.

These risk factors alone, however, are not sufficient to solely determine whether a patient should undergo surgery. The decision to operate must be individualized because the risk/benefit relationship is so closely tied to a patient's specific histology, tumor location, and physiologic state. Furthermore, the role of metastasectomy must be tailored to current nonsurgical treatment options, which continue to advance and may offer similar benefit to resection. Breast and renal cell carcinoma exemplify this phenomenon. Several large but older retrospective studies have demonstrated a benefit from pulmonary metastasectomy in these histologies, but patients with pulmonary metastasis from these tumors now have prolonged response to newer systemic therapies and only selected cases are reserved for surgery. As targeted and molecular therapies continue to improve the treatment of solid tumors, the selection criteria for pulmonary metastasectomy will change. The decision to proceed to surgical removal of pulmonary metastases must therefore be part of a multimodality discussion between patients, surgeons, medical oncologists, and radiation oncologists.

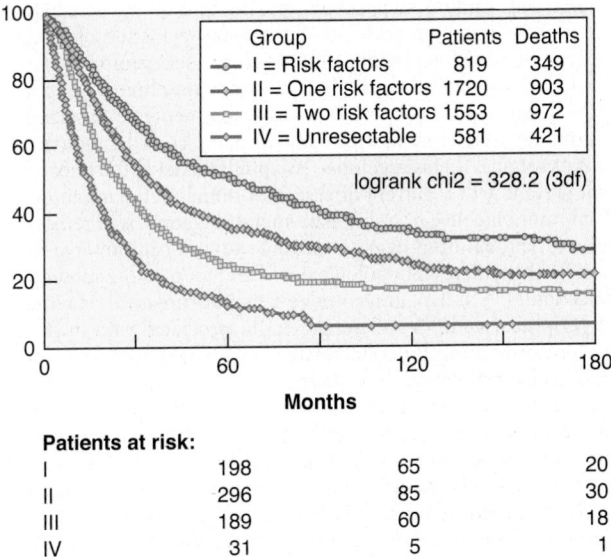

Figure 124.2 Kaplan-Meier survival curves from International Registry of Lung Metastases retrospective review of 5,206 cases of lung metastasectomy. Patient outcomes could be stratified using risk factors of (1) whether their disease was resectable, (2) single or multiple metastases, and (3) if the disease-free interval was >36 months. (Reprinted with permission from Pastorino U, Buyse M, Friedel G, et al. Long-term results of lung metastasectomy: prognostic analyses based on 5206 cases. The International Registry of Lung Metastases. *J Thorac Cardiovasc Surg* 1997;113:37–49.)

Large randomized trials are thought to provide the best evidence to direct efficacious treatment. A large trial of pulmonary metastasectomy for colorectal cancer is under way in Europe and will likely have a significant impact on clinical decision making.[11] Unfortunately, randomized data matures slowly and can be nearly impossible for all clinical scenarios, so the decision to operate often relies upon results of large retrospective series and databases. However, ongoing advances in the treatment of metastatic disease should temper the use of this retrospective data to direct clinical practice.

Open Versus Minimally Invasive Surgery

The surgical approach to metastasectomy is controversial with retrospective studies supporting both open and VATS approaches. The tension between these approaches is based on decreased pain, shorter hospital stay, and increased tolerability in patients with poor pulmonary function associated with VATS[12] relative to improved detection of small metastases afforded by manual palpation of the lung, which is not possible with a minimally invasive approach. As thoracoscopic techniques gain popularity for a wide range of thoracic procedures, surgeons have been keen to apply this technique to metastasectomy. Some historical studies suggested that the lack of manual palpation of the lung leads to small metastatic lesions being missed, and is therefore increasing the risk for incomplete resection. Convincing evidence in favor of an open approach and manual palpation of the lungs came from a series from the Memorial Sloan Kettering Cancer Center in 1996.[13] In this prospective evaluation, 18 patients underwent a VATS resection immediately followed by thoracotomy. Ten patients (56%) had additional malignant lesions found at thoracotomy that were not identified on preoperative imaging or during thoracoscopy. The major findings of the trial were as follows: (1) CT scan of chest underestimated the number of lung metastases (and therefore would be unable to be found thoracoscopically) and (2) thoracotomy after VATS identified nodules missed during VATS. Although this study is criticized for not using "high-definition" imaging and modern thoracoscopic techniques, other studies have subsequently corroborated these

results with a similar percentage of "missed" nodules.[14–16] The rebuttal from VATS supporters is that patients who undergo VATS have similar long-term outcomes relative to thoracotomy.

Modern high-resolution CT scan affords precise diagnostic imaging of patients with pulmonary disease. However, numerous modern series continue to suggest that CT underestimates the number of pulmonary metastases identified during thoracotomy. In a recent study from the John Wayne Cancer Institute in California, additional lesions were identified in 26% of patients undergoing thoracotomy that were not identified by preoperative CT chest scan.[17] In this series, "missed" nodules were more common if multiple nodules were identified preoperatively, and if the preoperative identified nodules were <1.5 cm. Similar results were reported by Cerfolio et al.[16] in a prospective cohort of 152 patients, in which 51 patients (34%) had pulmonary nodules detected at surgery that were not imaged preoperatively and over half were malignant.

An additional concern with minimally invasive approaches is the increased difficulty with intraoperative localization of nodules identified by CT. In a study from Denmark, 37 patients underwent sequential thoracoscopy and thoracotomy for resection of pulmonary metastases. CT scan identified 55 lesions preoperatively, but only 51 were identified using VATS. An additional 29 lesions were found during subsequent thoracotomy, 7 of which (24%) were malignant.[14]

Despite evidence that nodules may be missed by VATS resection, multiple retrospective series have demonstrated that both short-[18,19] and long-term survival are similar between patients undergoing the open and VATS approaches.[20–24] A study that compared VATS to thoracotomy for treatment of sarcoma metastases demonstrated nearly identical 3-year survival without ipsilateral recurrence (44.4% versus 45%).[19] Proponents of the minimally invasive approach argue that ultimately, tumor biology is the factor that most profoundly affects survival after metastasectomy and that patients should be offered the least invasive procedure.

No large or randomized studies exist, or are likely to be performed, to determine which surgical technique is better. Currently, the majority of thoracic surgeons favor the use of thoracotomy for treatment of pulmonary metastases, but minimally invasive techniques are frequently being used with therapeutic intent. This is based on findings from a 2008 survey of the European Society of Thoracic Surgeons (ESTS). A total of 65% of respondents felt that "palpation is considered necessary," relative to 29% who use thoracoscopy with therapeutic intent.[25] There has been a dramatic increase in use of VATS since the 1997 IRLM series, in which only 2% of cases were performed thoracoscopically.[10] An algorithm proposed from Cerfolio et al.[16] to determine which surgical approach to use offers some insight as to the relative strengths and limitations of each technique offer (Table 124.1).

Approach to Open Metastasectomy

The controversy over surgical approach goes beyond the open versus minimally invasive debate. There is also controversy as to which open approach is ideal. In the setting of unilateral nodules, most advocate use of thoracotomy, but the decision is less clear in the setting of bilateral disease. Some advocate a single surgical procedure with a median sternotomy or clamshell for patients with bilateral metastases. Ideologically, it is appealing to limit the patient to one anesthetic and one recovery, but "one-stage" approaches have their drawbacks. Sternotomy affords poor exposure and restricts manual palpation of the posterior aspect of the lower lobes, especially on the left side. The clam shell incision offers improved access to both lung fields, but is associated with increased pain and postoperative recovery. In the 2008 ESTS practitioner survey, only 26.9% of respondents preferred a one-stage sternotomy approach to bilateral disease and only 7.6% preferred the clamshell approach.[25] The most popular approach to bilateral pulmonary metastasectomy is sequential thoracotomy, with contralateral disease being approached by a subsequent thoracotomy after a 3- to 6-week interval.[25,26]

TABLE 124.1

Factors Supporting Use of Minimally Invasive or Open Approach to Pulmonary Metastasectomy

	Favors VATS	Favor Thoracotomy with Manual Palpation
Number of nodules	<3	≥3
Size of largest nodule	<5 cm	>5 cm
Size of smallest nodule	>1.5 cm	<1.5 cm
Location	Peripheral	Central
Histology	Colorectal cancer	Melanoma
Pulmonary function	Marginal	Normal
Previous chest radiation	Never	Yes
Lobar location	Upper or middle	Lower

VATS, video-assisted thoracoscopic surgery.

Role of Lymph Node Dissection

Another controversial aspect of pulmonary metastasectomy involves the decision to perform lymph node dissection or sampling at the time of surgery. The use of systematic lymph node evaluation during metastasectomy varies by institution; no consensus exists. The evidence for lymph node evaluation is supported by a study from Pfannschmidt and colleagues,[27] where 245 patients with metastases from colorectal carcinoma, renal cell carcinoma, and sarcoma underwent routine mediastinal lymphadenectomy. Approximately one-third of patients had lymph node involvement, half were limited to pulmonary and hilar metastases, and the other half had mediastinal nodal disease. Patients with more than one pulmonary metastasis or metachronous disease were more likely to have thoracic lymph node metastases, as were patients with renal cell cancer (42%) and colorectal carcinoma (31%) relative to sarcoma (20.3%). Patients without lymph node involvement demonstrated improved median survival (63.9 months) relative to patients with pulmonary nodal involvement (32.7 months) or mediastinal nodal involvement (20.6 months). Subsequent studies support the premise that intrathoracic nodal disease in conjunction with pulmonary metastasis is a poor prognostic indicator. This message was particularly striking in a Japanese cohort of patients undergoing resection of colorectal metastases; patients without intrathoracic lymph node disease had a 5-year survival of 53.6% compared to 6.2% at 4 years among patients with lymph node involvement (Fig. 124.3).[28]

While the increased prognostic information received from lymphadenectomy appears to support its routine use, many surgeons believe that the primary role for lymphadenectomy is to determine the need for additional oncologic treatment; there are no widely accepted strategies for implementation. The lack of consensus is evident in the ESTS survey, where only 19% of respondents reported routinely performing complete lymphadenectomy, 55% perform lymph node sampling, and 32% do no nodal sampling.[25]

Extent of Resection

In general, the goal of metastasectomy is complete removal of all gross tumor. Oncologic resection is defined further by the "completeness" of resection: An R2 resection involves a partial resection with gross residual disease, an R1 resection is removal of gross

disease but residual microscopic disease, and an R0 resection is a complete resection with no microscopic evidence of disease. In general, an R0 resection is essential for successful metastasectomy, because debulking of disease carries no clinical benefit. A second, but equally important, goal is maintenance of adequate pulmonary function and with that comes the consideration for extent of surgical metastasectomy. As approximately 50% of patients will present with recurrent disease after initial metastasectomy, an important objective of pulmonary metastasectomy is to remove as little functional lung tissue as possible in order to preserve function for the patient's physiologic needs and for possible subsequent resection(s).[10] Nonanatomic wedge resections are ideal for removal of peripheral nodules and are generally associated with improved postoperative lung function relative to a larger anatomic resection (segmentectomy, lobectomy, or pneumonectomy). Lobar and segmental anatomic resections can be safely performed with mortality of <1%, but are usually associated with removal of more functional lung parenchyma than a wedge resection. Although lobectomy has been associated with lower rates of local recurrence in the treatment of primary NSCLC,[29] no such data exists for patients receiving resections for metastatic disease. On the contrary, because patients with pulmonary metastases frequently undergo multiple procedures (and additional other therapies), lung conservation is particularly essential.

Studies of lung function after surgical metastasectomy suggest that these resections are associated with a 10% to 15% decrease in pulmonary function on average. Pulmonary function was significantly reduced among patients receiving bilateral operations and postoperative chemotherapy.[30] For the purposes of metastasectomy, multiple wedge resections are frequently performed and patients can experience a cumulative decrease in lung function that is similar to a lobectomy.[31] The use of VATS/thoracoscopy has been associated with less significant decrease in pulmonary function and fewer complications in patients with marginal lung function.[32,33]

In patients with multiple lesions in a single lobe, central lesions, or involvement of airway or vascular structures, lobectomy may be the only therapeutic option, and therefore appropriate in patients with acceptable physiologic reserve. Pneumonectomy is rarely indicated for the treatment of metastatic disease, and many believe that the morbidity of a pneumonectomy is a relative contraindication to metastasectomy.[25] There are, however, select reports of long-term survival and acceptable morbidity in small case series.[34] Pneumonectomy should therefore be reserved for patients with ideal circumstances: long disease-free interval, single central lesion, and excellent performance status.

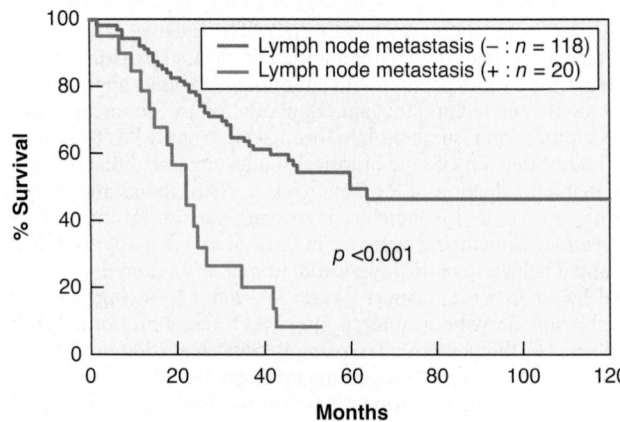

Figure 124.3 Kaplan-Meier survival curves of patients with and without lymph node involvement after pulmonary metastasectomy. (Reprinted with permission from Saito Y, Omiya H, Kohno K, et al. Pulmonary metastasectomy for 165 patients with colorectal carcinoma: A prognostic assessment. *J Thorac Cardiovasc Surg* 2002;124:1007–1013.)

ABLATIVE THERAPIES

Image-guided ablative therapies are being used with great frequency in the lungs and are a popular alternative to surgical metastasectomy. Stereotactic body radiotherapy (SBRT) or stereotactic ablative body radiotherapy is highly precise and dose-intensive form of external beam radiation therapy that has been used to treat metastases in the thorax. Percutaneous technologies include radiofrequency ablation (RFA), microwave ablation, or cryoablation, which uses heat or cold to create cellular destruction with necrosis. Patterns of the use of ablative therapies vary significantly according to practitioner and institutional expertise, but have been applied most consistently in patients whose performance status prevents thoracic surgery, or in whom complete surgical resection is not possible. Studies in those populations have been promising, and accordingly the use of ablative techniques to treat metastatic pulmonary lesions has increased. While, the "gold standard" treatment of pulmonary metastases remains surgical, the growing success of ablative techniques has led to more widespread use of these techniques. Rather than compare the techniques to determine which is superior for all cases, prudent complementary use of all available technologies is appropriate. For example, a patient who has undergone multiple previous thoracotomies for resection of metastases and has decreased lung function may benefit from an ablative technique to reduce toxicities associated with reoperative surgical resection. The specific strengths and weaknesses of each technique underscore the need for a multidisciplinary approach to patients with pulmonary metastases.

Radiofrequency Ablation

RFA is the most widely used and reported of the percutaneous image-guided technologies. It uses current transmitted through CT-guided, percutaneous probes to heat tissues to temperatures $>60°C$, resulting in coagulative necrosis. The pattern of tissue injury is related to the tissue's specific electrical impedance and is modulated by the cooling effect of adjacent tissues such as airways and large blood vessels. In the lung, air-filled pulmonary parenchyma can act as a thermal insulator that protects nearby tissue. RFA is most efficacious for tumors <3.5 cm in diameter, with larger tumors requiring multiple applications. RFA is also less efficacious in areas adjacent to large blood vessels and is not recommended adjacent to central airways; therefore, application is typically limited to the middle and outer third of the lungs. Pneumothorax is the most frequent complication of percutaneous pulmonary RFA and is reported in up to 30% to 50%, less than a

third of which require a chest tube for management.[35–37] Although radiographic evidence of fibrosis and/or cavitation is common after RFA, serious, symptomatic complications (including bronchopleural fistulae formation, hemoptysis, hemorrhage, infection, and pleurisy) are rare. Cutaneous metastases (tumor seeding) at the electrode insertion site have been documented, but are also uncommon.

Percutaneous ablative treatments of pulmonary metastases are gaining in popularity because of evidence of therapeutic similarity to surgical resection. In 2010, a prospective trial of percutaneous RFA of lung metastases demonstrated impressive long-term results among a group of patients with mixed tumor histology.[38] Of 148 patients treated, 26% had complete radiographic response, 20% had partial response, 39% had stable disease, and 16% showed disease progression. The median overall survival was 51 months, and in multivariate analysis, disease-free interval and response to treatment were independent predictors of overall survival. Other small studies have also shown good results of RFA ablation in pulmonary metastases of esophageal, colorectal, breast, and renal cancer[39–41] (Table 124.2).

Stereotactic Body Radiation Therapy

SBRT is another ablative technique being used to treat metastatic lung lesions. Unlike conventional fractionated radiation therapy, SBRT uses highly focused and intensive radiation to deliver ablative doses of radiation to specific areas with less radiation injury to adjacent tissues. The techniques originated for use in the brain. Significant technologic advances were necessary to adaptation to the lung, especially due to the need to compensate for the normal physiologic movement associated with breathing in order to prevent radiation injury to normal tissue without compromising tumor control. Theoretically, the high-dose and tightly focused nature of SBRT provides an ablative response in the target area, which is of particular concern for treatment of pulmonary metastases. In a trial from Kyoto University in Japan, a higher dose of radiation was necessary to treat metastatic pulmonary lesions due to higher rates of local failure (relative to primary NSCLC).[42]

Much of the experience with the use of SBRT for lung tumors was derived from the treatment of medically inoperable NSCLC. Studies in this population have demonstrated successful treatment of early stage NSCLC among patients unfit for surgery with few complications.[43] Although radiation injury to normal tissue can lead to significant toxicities, patients being evaluated for SBRT for lung metastases have few medical contraindications, and even patients with severe emphysema and chronic obstructive pulmonary

PRACTICE OF ONCOLOGY

TABLE 124.2

Outcomes Following Use of Radiofrequency Ablation for Pulmonary Metastasis

Author	No. of Patients	Histology	Overall Survival		
			1 y	3 y	5 y
Ambrogi et al.[83]	24	Mixed ("mostly" CRC)	88%	72%	NR
Simon et al.[37]	18	CRC	87%	78%	57%
Chua et al.[38]	148	Mixed (73% CRC)	NR	60%	45%
Lencioni et al.[84]	53	CRC	89%	66%	NR
	20	Mixed	92%	64%	NR
Petre et al.[85]	45	CRC	95%	50%	0%
Yan et al.[86]	55	CRC	85%	46%	NR

CRC, colorectal cancer; NR, not reported.

disease have tolerated the procedure with few respiratory side effects.[44] In fact, most studies of SBRT have demonstrated no grade 3 or higher toxicities.[45] Treatment of centrally located NSCLC, however, has been associated with increased toxicity[46] and has resulted in the use of altered fractionation schedules for tumors within 2 cm of the central airways.

Based on the success of SBRT in patients with NSCLC, it is now being used to treat foci metastatic disease in the lungs and throughout the body. While not considered the standard of care, it is being used with increased frequency and offers good local control and short-term overall survival. In a recent prospective trial of 32 patients with 47 lung metastases (~30% colorectal cancer), local control rates at 1, 2, and 3 years were 97%, 92%, and 85%, respectively. The median overall survival was 39.6 months. The 1-, 2-, and 3-year overall survival rates were 83%, 76%, and 63%, respectively.[47] Other studies have not documented such favorable results with 3-year survival among mixed group of patients only 16%.[48] Because of its recent introduction, few SBRT studies have mature long-term outcomes for treatment of metastases. A study of SBRT in treatment of various metastases (32% breast) in mixed sites (41% pulmonary) among 121 patients, showed a 6-year overall survival of 20% in the entire study group, and 47% 6-year overall survival among patients with breast cancer[49] (Table 124.3).

TREATMENT CONCERNS AND OUTCOMES FOR INDIVIDUAL HISTOLOGIES

Soft Tissue and Osteogenic Sarcoma

Soft tissue and osteogenic sarcomas are relatively rare malignancies, but they have high rates of pulmonary metastases. Failure to control pulmonary metastatic disease is the most frequent cause of death in these patients. This combined with the young age of patients with sarcoma has resulted in this being the histology in which surgical metastasectomy has been widely studied. Although no formal randomized trials exist, the large numbers of retrospective studies strongly suggest benefit for resection of metastatic disease in these patients. Furthermore, with the lack of efficacious chemotherapeutic options, metastasectomy will likely retain an important role in the treatment of patients with sarcoma for the foreseeable future.

Osteosarcoma is a histologic subtype with high predilection for pulmonary metastases. In 2003, the Cooperative Osteosarcoma Study Group found that, of 202 patients who had metastases at diagnosis, 81% had lung metastases and in 62% the lung was the only site of metastases.[50] Studies have also shown that >50% of cancers recur only in the lung.[51] Patients with osteosarcoma are generally young and healthy and as such are usually excellent candidates for pulmonary resection. Several reports have shown prolonged survival after surgical treatment of pulmonary metastases of osteosarcoma with 5-year overall survivals ranging from 30% to 40%[52] (Table 124.4). While reports have varied, prognostic factors associated with good outcome are prolonged disease-free interval, complete surgical resection, and response to adjuvant therapy.[53,54] Unfortunately, studies of metastasectomy in the pediatric population have documented that new lung metastases frequently recur after resection,[55] and therefore patients should be followed closely postoperatively. Although benign nodules can occur after the initial metastasectomy, recurrent disease ipsilateral to the initial resection is almost always metastatic recurrence, and aggressive surgical management is warranted.[56] Soft tissue sarcomas are a heterogeneous group of tumors with a predilection for metastatic spread to the lungs. Based on multiple retrospective studies, 5-year overall survival of 30% to 40% can be achieved following pulmonary metastasectomy (see Table 124.4). Studies attempting to identify prognostic factors associated with a favorable response to surgery have conflicting results. Generally, solitary pulmonary lesion, prolonged disease-free interval (>2.5 years), low histologic grade, and the ability to perform an R0 resection have been shown to confer a good prognosis.[57] Patients who meet all of these criteria may expect to have ≥70% 5-year survival.

Although adjuvant chemotherapy protocols are not usually associated with significant benefit for treatment of soft tissue sarcoma, some sarcoma subtypes are chemosensitive and emerging therapies should be considered. Despite generally poor responses to chemotherapy, progression after receiving adjuvant chemotherapy is a marker for poor prognosis following metastasectomy. An MD Anderson Cancer Center study from 2011 showed that 5-year overall survival after metastasectomy in patients whose disease progressed after chemotherapy was substantially worse compared with patients without measurable progression (0% versus 32%).[58] The patients with soft tissue sarcoma and reasonable performance status whose disease recurs in the lung should be strongly considered for surgical metastasectomy because of the paucity of effective chemotherapy options.

Melanoma

Disseminated melanoma carries a dismal prognosis, typically with a median survival ≤6 months. While many chemotherapy

---

TABLE 124.3

Outcomes Following Use of Stereotactic Body Radiation Therapy for Pulmonary Metastasis

Author	No. of Patients	No. of Targets	Median Follow-Up (months)	Local Control (%)	Overall Survival (%)
Brown et al.[87]	35	69	18	71 (18 mo)	77 (18 mo)
Stinauer et al.[88]	30	53	28	88 (18 mo)	50 (2 y)
Norihisa et al.[89]	34	43	27	90 (2 y)	84 (2 y)
Rusthoven et al.[90]	38	63	15	96 (2 y)	39 (2 y)
Yoon et al.[91]	53	80	14	81 (2 y)	51 (2 y)
Fritz et al.[92]	25	31	22	80 (3 y)	42 (3 y)
Hof et al.[93]	61	71	14	63 (3 y)	48 (3 y)
Zhang et al.[94]	71	172	25	75 (5 y)	25 (5 y)
Milano et al.[49]	39 (breast)	NA	54	87 (6 y)	47 (6 y)
	82 (other histology)	NA	20	65 (6 y)	9 (6 y)
Dhakal et al.[95]	14 (sarcoma)	74	11	82 (3 y)	50 (2 y)

NA, not available.

TABLE 124.4

Outcomes Following Surgical Metastasectomy for Pulmonary Metastasis by Tumor Histology of Primary Cancer

Histology	Author/Year	No. of Patients	Overall Survival at 5 y (%)	Factors Associated with Improved Prognosis
Osteosarcoma	Pfannschmidt et al., 2006[53]	21	34	CSR
	Diemel, Klippe, and Branseheid, 2009[52]	85	48	CSR
				CSR
	Briccoli et al., 2010[96]	323	37	Unilateral mets
				Fewer than four mets
Soft tissue sarcoma	Billingsley et al., 1999[97]	719	25 (3 y)	CSR
			46 (if CSR)	DFI >12 mo
	Pfannschmidt et al., 2006[98]	50	38	CSR
			53 (if CSR)	
Melanoma	Andrews et al., 2006[99]	86	33	SPM
	Petersen et al., 2007[59]	249	21	CSR
	Schuhan et al., 2011[100]	30	35	Male gender
Renal cell carcinoma	Pfannschmidt et al., 2002[101]	191	37	CSR
			41.5 (if CSR)	pN0
				Fewer than seven mets
				DFI > 23 mo
	Meimarakis et al., 2011[65]	202	39	CSR
			45 (if CSR)	pN0
				Fewer than three mets
				size <3 cm
	Kanzaki et al., 2011[102]	48	47	CSR
			18 (10 y)	DFI >24 mo
Breast cancer	Friedel et al. (IRLM), 2002[71]	467	38	DFI >36 mo
			20 (15 y)	
	Welter et al., 2008[67]	47	36	ER and Her2-neu status
	Chen et al., 2009[69]	41	51	DFI >36 mo
				Fewer than four mets
Germ cell tumors	Pfannschmidt et al., 2006[77]	52	76	CSR
			83 (necrosis/fibrosis or teratoma in resection)	Normal serum tumor markers
	Kesler et al., 2011[75]	154: lung only 133: lung + mediastinum	74 (lung only) 76 (lung and mediastinum)	Younger age Persistent cancer in testes, persistent cancer in mets
Colorectal cancer	Yedibela et al., 2006[103]	153	37	SPM Wedge resection DFI >36 mo Fewer than two units intraoperative blood transfusion
	Welter et al., 2007[104]	169	39 54 (patients undergoing repeated resections)	Shorter DFI Fewer metastases (SPM) Younger age
	Watanabe et al., 2009[105]	113	68	Low prethoracotomy CEA No lymphatic invasion
	Riquet et al., 2010[106]	127	35.1 before 2000 63.5 after 2000–2007	CSR

CSR, complete surgical resection; mets, metastases; DFI, Disease free Interval; IRLM, International Registry of Lung Metastases; ER, estrogen receptor; Her2, human epidermal growth factor receptor 2; SPM, single pulmonary metastasis; pN0, negative nodal status of primary tumor; CEA, carcinoembryonic antigen.

combinations have been attempted, few are successful. Biologic treatments, such as IL-2 and interferon-α, are efficacious but are associated with a survival benefit in only a minority of patients and significant systemic toxicities. Patients with disseminated melanoma often present with disease in multiple sites, and <10% have lung metastases alone.[59] Fluorodeoxyglucose-positron emission tomography is a useful tool for preoperative evaluation of patients and can accurately identify patients with extrathoracic metastasis, thereby avoiding unnecessary thoracic surgery.[60] In patients with isolated pulmonary disease, surgery is a reasonable option.[59] Among appropriately selected patients, resection of pulmonary metastases can result in median survival as high as 20 to 40 months (see Table 124.4). In a large Australian study of 292 patients undergoing pulmonary metastasectomy for melanoma, the progression-free and overall survival were 10 months and 23 months, respectively, with overall 3- and 5- year survival rates of 41% and 34%, respectively.[61] Factors associated with poor overall survival following metastasectomy for melanomas are lesions >2 cm, multiple lesions, disease-free interval <36 months, and involved surgical margins.[59,61] In a review of metastatic melanoma cases from the IRLM, patients with the most favorable prognostic factors had >25% survival at 10 years.[62] Patients frequently recur after pulmonary metastasectomy but can achieve long-term survival despite need for re-resection with 19% surviving 5 years after the second resection in the IRLM database.[62]

Renal Cell Carcinoma

Metastases from renal cell carcinoma are frequently present at the time of diagnosis or can develop after nephrectomy. In autopsy series, metastases to the lung occur in approximately 75% of patients, and the lung is the most common metastatic site.[63] Historically, few chemotherapy options were available, but in the modern era, the majority of patients with systemic disease are treated with targeted therapy.[64] Prior to these targeted therapies, surgical metastasectomy had been used with impressive results for patients with isolated pulmonary disease and may still have a role in selected patients after demonstrating a response to systemic therapy. Most studies of metastasectomy were performed prior to the introduction of targeted therapies and therefore offer limited insight in the modern management of these patients. Those "pretargeted therapy" studies demonstrated several factors that were associated with favorable prognosis: R0 resection, size of metastasis <3 cm, lack of pleural infiltration, fewer than three lesions, and negative mediastinal lymph nodes[65] (see Table 124.4). One study examined metastasectomy after targeted therapy in patients with advanced renal cell carcinoma. It showed that metastasectomy was feasible, safe, and could be associated with long-term survival, but was unfortunately in a small and heterogeneous patient cohort.[66] Current recommendations, therefore, are based on little evidence, but speak to prevailing theories: metastasectomy should be considered in patients with a small number of easily accessible pulmonary metastases who have demonstrated a long disease-free interval after nephrectomy or a partial response in metastases after systemic immunotherapy or targeted chemotherapy.[64]

Breast Cancer

Although metastases from breast cancer frequently occur in the lungs, patients rarely present with isolated pulmonary disease. In a Mayo Clinic series of 13,502 patients with breast cancer, <1% developed isolated pulmonary metastases.[67] Despite the relative infrequency, metastasectomy for isolated pulmonary metastases has been described. Modern studies of metastasectomy demonstrate 5-year survival rates between 30% and 50%, with 5-year survival in excess of 80% in highly selected patients.[68,69] Factors associated with prolonged survival include long disease-free interval (>36 months), R0 resection, hormone receptor positivity, and

fewer than four metastases[67–71] (see Table 124.4). The importance of hormone receptor status on survival after metastasectomy reiterates the need for individualized therapy in breast cancer therapy, and to that end, pulmonary metastasectomy is often used to obtain tissue to further guide treatment due to changes in molecular profile, which has been shown to occur in approximately a quarter of cases.[67] Thoracic surgery intervention can also be indicated for patients with breast cancer who develop extensive chest wall involvement, which can also present with direct pulmonary invasion. In these patients, chest wall resection and reconstruction can be considered and has been associated with improved quality of life and, in rare circumstances, prolonged survival.[72,73]

Germ Cell Tumors (Testicular Cancer)

Survival following pulmonary metastasectomy is highest for germ cell tumors compared to other histologies. This is due the primarily to the efficacy of chemotherapy and the important role surgery plays in the multimodality approach to these tumors. Testicular nonseminomatous germ cell tumors are the most common neoplasm in males younger than 40 years, and many present with supradiaphragmatic metastases. Disease can spread both hematogenously to the lungs (the most common site) and by lymphatic spread to mediastinal lymph nodes. Metastasis to these sites equates to stage III disease and is typically treated with cisplatin-based chemotherapy and surgical resection with excellent results.[74] Complete resection of residual postchemotherapy disease plays a critical part in achieving long-term cure and is another example of the role that surgery can take in a multimodal approach to pulmonary metastases (see Table 124.4). A large review of results in the cisplatin era documented overall median survival after thoracic metastasectomy of 23.4 years, 79% survival at 5 years, and 73% survival at 10 years.[75] The pathology from resection is important to determine the response to therapy and need for subsequent treatment in these patients. The majority will have complete necrosis or only residual teratoma in the resected specimen, each of which portends improved survival compared to those with persistent malignant disease.[75–77] The presence of persistent malignant disease is an indication for additional chemotherapy. Other predictors of poor survival after surgery include older age at diagnosis, elevated preoperative serum tumor markers, and incomplete resections.[75,76,78]

Colorectal Cancer

Lung metastases develop in 5% to 15% of patients with colorectal cancer, and pulmonary metastasectomy has become an integral part in the multimodality treatment of these patients. Colorectal cancer treatment is a rapidly evolving field, and the benefit of metastasectomy in the era of targeted therapy is accepted yet somewhat unproven. To address this question, a randomized trial of metastasectomy for colorectal carcinoma is currently under way in Europe. This trial compares "active monitoring" to "active monitoring plus pulmonary metastasectomy" and evaluates overall survival, relapse-free survival, lung function, and patient-reported quality of life.[11] Until these data are available, there is a considerable volume retrospective data that supports a role for metastasectomy in selected patients. In a recent meta-analysis of lung metastasectomy for colorectal carcinoma, four parameters were associated with poor survival after metastasectomy: short disease-free interval, multiple metastases, positive hilar and/or mediastinal lymph nodes, and elevated prethoracotomy carcinoembryonic antigen level[79] (see Table 124.4). In this analysis, the presence of liver metastases was not associated with poor prognosis. In fact, combined resection of colorectal hepatic and pulmonary metastases has been shown to offer improved outcomes relative to chemotherapy alone, with overall survival in metastasectomy patients more than double that of chemotherapy patients in matched-pair analysis (65 months versus 30 months).[80] After initial resection, some patients will develop recurrent pulmonary metastases. Predictors of lung recurrence include more than three metastases at the first metastasectomy, and interval between primary surgery and first metastasectomy.[81] Second surgery can be beneficial in patients who "re-recur" in the lung, as suggested by a trial that showed improved overall survival among patients receiving a second resection relative to patients who refused surgery and were treated with chemotherapy alone (58 months versus 24 months).[82]

CONCLUSION

The management of patients with pulmonary metastases remains in a state of evolution. Since the initial revelation that long-term survival after metastasectomy was possible, clinicians now have a variety of treatment modalities to offer patients with metastatic solid tumors to the lungs. While the criteria for patient selection to undergo surgical metastasectomy have been stable for several decades, the landscape in which patients are being treated has evolved. As targeted chemotherapies emerge, procuring tissue for genetic and chemosensitivity analyses will likely be an evolving aspect of surgical metastasectomy. After one decides that resection is indicated, it is necessary to consider which approach is appropriate, balancing the risk for missing unrecognized metastases with VATS versus the increased operative complications and recovery associated with thoracotomy. Even as randomized trials slowly define the role of surgical metastasectomy, clinicians should be mindful that the benefit of surgery should always be weighed against less invasive methods of controlling metastases with the goal of offering high-quality long-term survival. Although surgery remains the "gold standard" approach because it is associated with well-documented long-term results, ablative therapies offer impressive results (especially among patients not amenable to surgical resection). More frequently today, a multimodality approach to pulmonary metastases is being used and includes consideration for the patient's specific physiologic status, tumor burden, and histology.

SELECTED REFERENCES

The full reference list can be accessed at lwwhealthlibrary.com/oncology.

1. Martini N, Huvos AG, Mike V, et al. Multiple pulmonary resections in the treatment of osteogenic sarcoma. *Ann Thorac Surg* 1971;12:271–280.
4. Rusch VW. Pulmonary metastasectomy. Current indications. *Chest* 1995;107:322S–331S.
6. Bach PB, Kattan MW, Thornquist MD, et al. Variations in lung cancer risk among smokers. *J Natl Cancer Inst* 2003;95:470–478.
7. Hoggart C, Brennan P, Tjonneland A, et al. A risk model for lung cancer incidence. *Cancer Prev Res (Phila)* 2012;5:834–846.
9. Rusch VW. Pulmonary metastasectomy: a moving target. *J Thorac Oncol* 2010;5:S130–S131.
10. Pastorino U, Buyse M, Friedel G, et al. Long-term results of lung metastasectomy: prognostic analyses based on 5206 cases. The International Registry of Lung Metastases. *J Thorac Cardiovasc Surg* 1997;113:37–49.
11. Treasure T, Fallowfield L, Lees B, et al. Pulmonary metastasectomy in colorectal cancer: the PulMiCC trial. *Thorax* 2012;67:185–187.
13. McCormack PM, Bains MS, Begg CB, et al. Role of video-assisted thoracic surgery in the treatment of pulmonary metastases: results of a prospective trial. *Ann Thorac Surg* 1996;62:213–216, discussion 216–217.
14. Eckardt J, Licht PB. Thoracoscopic versus open pulmonary metastasectomy: a prospective, sequentially controlled study. *Chest* 2012;142:1598–1602.
15. Mutsaerts EL, Zoetmulder FA, Meijer S, et al. Outcome of thoracoscopic pulmonary metastasectomy evaluated by confirmatory thoracotomy. *Ann Thorac Surg* 2001;72:230–233.
16. Cerfolio RJ, McCarty T, Bryant AS. Non-imaged pulmonary nodules discovered during thoracotomy for metastasectomy by lung palpation. *Eur J Cardiothorac Surg* 2009;35:786–791, discussion 791.
17. Kidner TB, Yoon J, Faries MB, et al. Preoperative imaging of pulmonary metastasis in patients with melanoma: implications for minimally invasive techniques. *Arch Surg* 2012;147:871–874.
19. Gossot D, Radu C, Girard P, et al. Resection of pulmonary metastases from sarcoma: can some patients benefit from a less invasive approach? *Ann Thorac Surg* 2009;87:238–243.
20. von Meyenfeldt EM, Wouters MW, Fat NL, et al. Local treatment of pulmonary metastases: from open resection to minimally invasive approach? Less morbidity, comparable local control. *Surg Endosc* 2012;26:2312–2321.
24. Landreneau RJ, De Giacomo T, Mack MJ, et al. Therapeutic video-assisted thoracoscopic surgical resection of colorectal pulmonary metastases. *Eur J Cardiothorac Surg* 2000;18:671–676, discussion 676–677.
25. Internullo E, Cassivi SD, Van Raemdonck D, et al. Pulmonary metastasectomy: a survey of current practice amongst members of the European Society of Thoracic Surgeons. *J Thorac Oncol* 2008;3:1257–1266.
27. Pfannschmidt J, Klode J, Muley T, et al. Nodal involvement at the time of pulmonary metastasectomy: experiences in 245 patients. *Ann Thorac Surg* 2006;81:448–454.
28. Saito Y, Omiya H, Kohno K, et al. Pulmonary metastasectomy for 165 patients with colorectal carcinoma: A prognostic assessment. *J Thorac Cardiovasc Surg* 2002;124:1007–1013.
30. Welter S, Cheufou D, Ketscher C, et al. Risk factors for impaired lung function after pulmonary metastasectomy: a prospective observational study of 117 cases. *Eur J Cardiothorac Surg* 2012;42:e22–e27.
34. Koong HN, Pastorino U, Ginsberg RJ. Is there a role for pneumonectomy in pulmonary metastases? International Registry of Lung Metastases. *Ann Thorac Surg* 1999;68:2039–2043.
37. Simon CJ, Dupuy DE, DiPetrillo TA, et al. Pulmonary radiofrequency ablation: long-term safety and efficacy in 153 patients. *Radiology* 2007;243:268–275.
38. Chua TC, Sarkar A, Saxena A, et al. Long-term outcome of image-guided percutaneous radiofrequency ablation of lung metastases: an open-labeled prospective trial of 148 patients. *Ann Oncol* 2010;21:2017–2022.
42. Nagata Y, Negoro Y, Aoki T, et al. Clinical outcomes of 3D conformal hypofractionated single high-dose radiotherapy for one or two lung tumors using a stereotactic body frame. *Int J Radiat Oncol Biol Phys* 2002;52:1041–1046.
44. Timmerman R, Papiez L, McGarry R, et al. Extracranial stereotactic radioablation: results of a phase I study in medically inoperable stage I non-small cell lung cancer. *Chest* 2003;124:1946–1955.
47. Baschnagel AM, Mangona VS, Robertson JM, et al. Lung metastases treated with image-guided stereotactic body radiation therapy. *Clin Oncol (R Coll Radiol)* 2013;25:236–241.
48. Guckenberger M, Wulf J, Mueller G, et al. Dose-response relationship for image-guided stereotactic body radiotherapy of pulmonary tumors: relevance of 4D dose calculation. *Int J Radiat Oncol Biol Phys* 2009;74:47–54.
49. Milano MT, Katz AW, Zhang H, et al. Oligometastases treated with stereotactic body radiotherapy: long-term follow-up of prospective study. *Int J Radiat Oncol Biol Phys* 2012;83:878–886.
50. Kager L, Zoubek A, Potschger U, et al. Primary metastatic osteosarcoma: presentation and outcome of patients treated on neoadjuvant Cooperative Osteosarcoma Study Group protocols. *J Clin Oncol* 2003;21:2011–2018.
53. Pfannschmidt J, Klode J, Muley T, et al. Pulmonary resection for metastatic osteosarcomas: a retrospective analysis of 21 patients. *Thorac Cardiovasc Surg* 2006;54:120–123.
54. Harting MT, Blakely ML, Jaffe N, et al. Long-term survival after aggressive resection of pulmonary metastases among children and adolescents with osteosarcoma. *J Pediatr Surg* 2006;41:194–199.
57. Kim S, Ott HC, Wright CD, et al. Pulmonary resection of metastatic sarcoma: prognostic factors associated with improved outcomes. *Ann Thorac Surg* 2011;92:1780–1786, discussion 1786–1787.
58. Stephens EH, Blackmon SH, Correa AM, et al. Progression after chemotherapy is a novel predictor of poor outcomes after pulmonary metastasectomy in sarcoma patients. *J Am Coll Surg* 2011;212:821–826.
61. Chua TC, Scolyer RA, Kennedy CW, et al. Surgical management of melanoma lung metastasis: an analysis of survival outcomes in 292 consecutive patients. *Ann Surg Oncol* 2012;19:1774–1781.
62. Leo F, Cagini L, Rocmans P, et al. Lung metastases from melanoma: when is surgical treatment warranted? *Br J Cancer* 2000;83:569–572.
65. Meimarakis G, Angele M, Staehler M, et al. Evaluation of a new prognostic score (Munich score) to predict long-term survival after resection of pulmonary renal cell carcinoma metastases. *Am J Surg* 2011;202:158–167.
66. Karam JA, Rini BI, Varella L, et al. Metastasectomy after targeted therapy in patients with advanced renal cell carcinoma. *J Urol* 2011;185:439–444.
67. Welter S, Jacobs J, Krbek T, et al. Pulmonary metastases of breast cancer. When is resection indicated? *Eur J Cardiothorac Surg* 2008;34:1228–1234.
68. Yhim HY, Han SW, Oh DY, et al. Prognostic factors for recurrent breast cancer patients with an isolated, limited number of lung metastases and implications for pulmonary metastasectomy. *Cancer* 2010;116:2890–2901.
69. Chen F, Fujinaga T, Sato K, et al. Clinical features of surgical resection for pulmonary metastasis from breast cancer. *Eur J Surg Oncol* 2009;35:393–397.
75. Kesler KA, Kruter LE, Perkins SM, et al. Survival after resection for metastatic testicular nonseminomatous germ cell cancer to the lung or mediastinum. *Ann Thorac Surg* 2011;91:1085–1093, discussion 1093.

76. Schirren J, Trainer S, Eberlein M, et al. The role of residual tumor resection in the management of nonseminomatous germ cell cancer of testicular origin. *Thorac Cardiovasc Surg* 2012;60:405–412.
77. Pfannschmidt J, Zabeck H, Muley T, et al. Pulmonary metastasectomy following chemotherapy in patients with testicular tumors: experience in 52 patients. *Thorac Cardiovasc Surg* 2006;54:484–488.
79. Gonzalez M, Poncet A, Combescure C, et al. Risk factors for survival after lung metastasectomy in colorectal cancer patients: a systematic review and meta-analysis. *Ann Surg Oncol* 2013;20:572–579. .
81. Blackmon SH, Stephens EH, Correa AM, et al. Predictors of recurrent pulmonary metastases and survival after pulmonary metastasectomy for colorectal cancer. *Ann Thorac Surg* 2012;94:1802–1809.
82. Brandi G, Corbelli J, de Rosa F, et al. Second surgery or chemotherapy for relapse after radical resection of colorectal cancer metastases. *Langenbecks Arch Surg* 2012;397:1069–1077.
83. Ambrogi MC, Lucchi M, Dini P, et al. Percutaneous radiofrequency ablation of lung tumours: results in the mid-term. *Eur J Cardiothorac Surg* 2006;30:177–183.
84. Lencioni R, Crocetti L, Cioni R, et al. Response to radiofrequency ablation of pulmonary tumours: a prospective, intention-to-treat, multicentre clinical trial (the RAPTURE study). *Lancet Oncol* 2008;9:621–628.
85. Petre EN, Jia X, Thornton RH, et al. Treatment of pulmonary colorectal metastases by radiofrequency ablation. *Clin Colorectal Cancer* 2013;12:37–44.
86. Yan TD, King J, Sjarif A, et al. Treatment failure after percutaneous radiofrequency ablation for nonsurgical candidates with pulmonary metastases from colorectal carcinoma. *Ann Surg Oncol* 2007;14:1718–1726.
87. Brown WT, Wu X, Fowler JF, et al. Lung metastases treated by CyberKnife image-guided robotic stereotactic radiosurgery at 41 months. *South Med J* 2008;101:376–382.
88. Stinauer MA, Kavanagh BD, Schefter TE, et al. Stereotactic body radiation therapy for melanoma and renal cell carcinoma: impact of single fraction equivalent dose on local control. *Radiat Oncol* 2011;6:34.
89. Norihisa Y, Nagata Y, Takayama K, et al. Stereotactic body radiotherapy for oligometastatic lung tumors. *Int J Radiat Oncol Biol Phys* 2008;72:398–403.
90. Rusthoven KE, Kavanagh BD, Burri SH, et al. Multi-institutional phase I/II trial of stereotactic body radiation therapy for lung metastases. *J Clin Oncol* 2009;27:1579–1584.
91. Yoon SM, Choi EK, Lee SW, et al. Clinical results of stereotactic body frame based fractionated radiation therapy for primary or metastatic thoracic tumors. *Acta Oncol* 2006;45:1108–1114.
92. Fritz P, Kraus HJ, Muhlnickel W, et al. Stereotactic, single-dose irradiation of stage I non-small cell lung cancer and lung metastases. *Radiat Oncol* 2006;1:30.
93. Hof H, Hoess A, Oetzel D, et al. Stereotactic single-dose radiotherapy of lung metastases. *Strahlenther Onkol* 2007;183:673–678.
94. Zhang Y, Xiao JP, Zhang HZ, et al. Stereotactic body radiation therapy favors long-term overall survival in patients with lung metastases: five-year experience of a single-institution. *Chin Med J (Engl)* 2011;124:4132–4137.
95. Dhakal S, Corbin KS, Milano MT, et al. Stereotactic body radiotherapy for pulmonary metastases from soft-tissue sarcomas: excellent local lesion control and improved patient survival. *Int J Radiat Oncol Biol Phys* 2012;82:940–945.
96. Briccoli A, Rocca M, Salone M, et al. High grade osteosarcoma of the extremities metastatic to the lung: long-term results in 323 patients treated combining surgery and chemotherapy, 1985-2005. *Surg Oncol* 2010;19:193–199.
97. Billingsley KG, Burt ME, Jara E, et al. Pulmonary metastases from soft tissue sarcoma: analysis of patterns of diseases and postmetastasis survival. *Ann Surg* 1999;229:602–610, discussion 610–612.
98. Pfannschmidt J, Klode J, Muley T, et al. Pulmonary metastasectomy in patients with soft tissue sarcomas: experiences in 50 patients. *Thorac Cardiovasc Surg* 2006;54:489–492.
99. Andrews S, Robinson L, Cantor A, et al. Survival after surgical resection of isolated pulmonary metastases from malignant melanoma. *Cancer Control* 2006;13:218–223.
100. Schuhan C, Muley T, Dienemann H, et al. Survival after pulmonary metastasectomy in patients with malignant melanoma. *Thorac Cardiovasc Surg* 2011;59:158–162.
101. Pfannschmidt J, Hoffmann H, Muley T, et al. Prognostic factors for survival after pulmonary resection of metastatic renal cell carcinoma. *Ann Thorac Surg* 2002;74:1653–1657.
102. Kanzaki R, Higashiyama M, Fujiwara A, et al. Long-term results of surgical resection for pulmonary metastasis from renal cell carcinoma: a 25-year single-institution experience. *Eur J Cardiothorac Surg* 2011;39:167–172.
103. Yedibela S, Klein P, Feuchter K, et al. Surgical management of pulmonary metastases from colorectal cancer in 153 patients. *Ann Surg Oncol* 2006;13:1538–1544.
104. Welter S, Jacobs J, Krbek T, et al. Long-term survival after repeated resection of pulmonary metastases from colorectal cancer. *Ann Thorac Surg* 2007;84:203–210.
105. Watanabe K, Nagai K, Kobayashi A, et al. Factors influencing survival after complete resection of pulmonary metastases from colorectal cancer. *Br J Surg* 2009;96:1058–1065.
106. Riquet M, Foucault C, Cazes A, et al. Pulmonary resection for metastases of colorectal adenocarcinoma. *Ann Thorac Surg* 2010;89:375–380.

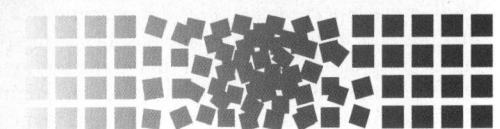

125 Metastatic Cancer to the Liver

Clifford S. Cho, Samuel J. Lubner, and Brian D. Kavanagh

INTRODUCTION

Hepatic metastasis is a unique oncologic event for three reasons. First, the nature of portal venous drainage makes the liver a common hematogenous destination of alimentary tract malignancies. Indeed, the most common metastatic tumors in the liver are derived from primary cancers of the alimentary tract and pancreas. Second, unlike other anatomic locations susceptible to hematogenous seeding (e.g., brain, lungs, bone), the liver is often the sole site of metastatic disease. Third, several aspects of hepatic anatomy and physiology make it particularly accessible to oncologic therapy. As a consequence, the phenomenon of hepatic metastasis deserves special focused attention. In this chapter, we will discuss disease biology and treatment options as they relate to the two types of hepatic metastasis (colorectal adenocarcinoma and neuroendocrine carcinoma) that are most commonly treated with liver-directed therapy, and will briefly discuss a few less-commonly treated forms of hepatic metastasis.

Relevant Hepatic Physiology

The venous drainage of the alimentary tract, pancreas, and spleen comprise the portal venous circulation. Blood flow returning from these sites converges into the portal vein. At the microscopic level, portal venous blood enters into the hepatic sinusoids, where it interfaces with hepatocytes. Once the contents from the portal venous circulation are metabolized and filtered, blood is directed into the hepatic venous system, which then re-enters the nonportal systemic venous circulation at the level of the inferior vena cava. A unique anatomic property of the liver is its dual blood supply. Hepatocytes derive the majority of their blood supply from the portal venous circulation; in contrast, the cholangiocytes that comprise the biliary ductal system derive most of their blood supply from the hepatic arterial circulation. Importantly, it is believed that primary and metastatic tumors within the liver generally derive the large majority of their blood supply from the hepatic arterial circulation. This important physiologic contrast in circulatory perfusion between normal hepatocytes and abnormal cancer cells provides an opportunity for therapeutic intervention; as will be discussed in the following, many liver-directed therapies rely on the delivery of embolic particles, chemotherapy, or radiation into the hepatic arterial circulation, where they will target mostly neoplastic cells while largely sparing normal hepatocytes. The highly metabolic properties of hepatocytes also facilitate liver-directed therapy. Chemotherapeutic agents that undergo first-pass hepatic metabolism can be delivered at unusually high concentrations into the hepatic arterial circulation, with the expectation that hepatocellular metabolism will result in negligible levels of systemic exposure and toxicity.

A unique physiologic characteristic of the liver is its ability to hypertrophy in response to various insults. Indeed, resection of up to 80% of the liver can be safely tolerated in patients with normal hepatic function. As long as the vascular perfusion and biliary and venous drainage of the remnant liver are preserved, it will be capable of rapid hypertrophy that will restore full hepatic functional capacity within weeks. In a similar way, hepatocellular ischemia resulting from deprivation of portal venous inflow to one portion of the liver (e.g., due to venous thrombosis or tumoral invasion) induces a compensatory hypertrophic response in other portions of the liver; as a result, the ischemic atrophy of the affected liver is functionally offset by reactive hypertrophy of the non-ischemic liver. Liver-directed therapies take advantage of both of these physiologic phenomena. The ability of the liver to hypertrophy in response to resection allows surgeons to use aggressive operative procedures to resect even large and multifocal hepatic metastases, as long as a well-functioning liver remnant is preserved. Moreover, in some patients who are not candidates for aggressive surgical resection due to an excessively small future liver remnant (FLR), intentional portal vein embolization of the portions of the liver affected by tumor is commonly employed as a means of inducing sufficient hypertrophy of the anticipated FLR to permit safe surgical resection.

Hepatic Anatomic Nomenclature

A comprehensive understanding of the treatment modalities available in hepatic oncology requires some familiarity with hepatic anatomic nomenclature.[1] The liver is composed of eight segments, four sections, and two hemilivers. The right and left hemilivers are divided by the principal scissura, or Cantlie line, which runs between the inferior vena cava and the gallbladder fossa. The liver is also bisected by the middle hepatic vein, which runs through the principal scissura. The left hemiliver is divided into two sections separated by the umbilical fissure, a natural cleft that houses the left portal vein and remnant of the umbilical vein. The left lateral section, comprised of segments II and III, is situated to the left of the umbilical fissure, and the left medical section, comprised of segment IV, is situated between the umbilical fissure and the principal scissura. The venous drainage of the left hemiliver is via the left hepatic vein, which courses between segments II and III, and the middle hepatic vein. The right hemiliver is separated into a right anterior section and a right posterior section; the anatomic plane between the right anterior and posterior sections is defined by the course of the right hepatic vein. The right anterior section is comprised of segments V and VIII, and the right posterior section is comprised of segments VI and VII. Segment I, or the caudate lobe, is a centrally located structure that lies between the portal vein and inferior vena cava. Operative procedures are named according to the anatomic structures that are being removed. For example, resection of the left hemiliver (i.e., removal of segments II to IV) is referred to as a left hemihepatectomy; a right hemihepatectomy refers to removal of segments V to VIII. Resection of segments II and III is referred to as a left lateral sectionectomy; resection of segments VI and VII is referred to as a right posterior sectionectomy. Resection of segments IV to VIII is a right trisectionectomy. Resection of the caudate lobe is referred to as a segmentectomy I.

Hepatic Imaging

Nearly every aspect of the clinical management of hepatic metastases is dependent on and made possible by high-quality radiographic imaging. At a minimum, the evaluation of patients with hepatic metastases requires high-resolution contrast-enhanced computed tomography (CT) or magnetic resonance imaging (MRI). Ultrasonography and positron emission tomography (PET) are used more selectively, and somatostatin receptor scintigraphy is occasionally employed during the evaluation of neuroendocrine carcinoma.

CT imaging should include so-called triple-phase imaging (consisting of a noncontrast phase, an arterial phase, and a venous phase) to provide maximal characterization of tumors based on their uptake and excretion of intravenous contrast. For example, neuroendocrine carcinoma metastases often appear very intense on arterial-phase imaging, whereas colorectal adenocarcinoma metastases typically have lower attenuation characteristics that are best appreciated on delayed venous phases, when the rest of the hepatic parenchyma has taken up contrast. Current multidetector helical CT scanners provide thin-slice (1 to 2 mm) images that can be reconstructed in coronal and sagittal projections to facilitate accurate tumor localization.

Because of the availability of numerous imaging sequences including T1- versus T2-weighted imaging and diffusion-weighted imaging, and the availability of numerous contrast agents, MRI is particularly useful for characterization of lesions that elude precise characterization by CT. Newer hepatocyte-specific contrast agents like gadoxetate disodium (Eovist, Bayer HealthCare Pharmaceuticals Inc., Whippany, NJ) and gadobenate dimeglumine (Multihance, Bracco Diagnostics, Inc., Munroe Township, NJ), which are taken up by hepatocytes and partially excreted through the biliary system, appear to enhance the sensitivity of MRI in the detection of metastatic lesions.[2,3]

Because of its comparatively weaker sensitivity and specificity, the utility of ultrasonography is largely confined to intraprocedural guidance during tumor ablation, or during intraoperative examination of the liver. Although not yet universally available in the United States, contrast agents for use in ultrasonography may strengthen the sensitivity and specificity of this modality in the detection and characterization of liver metastases.

When used after administration of radiolabeled ^{18}F-fluorodeoxyglucose, PET may be a means of identifying hypermetabolism within liver lesions. Because of its poor anatomic resolution, PET is typically used in conjunction with CT imaging. Several analyses have found that routine use of PET can provide additional information that alters treatment planning in up to a third of patients with hepatic colorectal adenocarcinoma metastases, particularly by detecting extrahepatic disease.[4,5] Two important caveats are that PET is insensitive for the detection of tumor foci that are <1 cm in diameter, and its sensitivity in the detection of colorectal adenocarcinoma is blunted when patients are receiving chemotherapy. Somatostatin receptor scintigraphy can be useful in identifying foci of neuroendocrine carcinoma; however, it does not appear to enhance the level of diagnostic information that can be rendered with CT and MRI alone.[6]

Hepatic Resection

The determination of resectability of hepatic metastases centers around the concept of the FLR, which is defined as the portion of the liver that will remain following hepatic resection. As stated previously, the FLR is generally capable of rapid postoperative hypertrophy; however, the FLR must be capable of a minimum level of function in order to avoid fatal postoperative hepatic failure. In order for hepatic resection to be performed safely, four criteria regarding the FLR must be met: (1) the FLR must be well-vascularized (i.e., the portal venous and hepatic arterial inflow into the FLR must be retained), (2) the FLR must have adequate biliary drainage (i.e., the hepatic duct[s] emanating from the FLR must not be damaged), (3) the FLR must have adequate venous drainage (i.e., the hepatic vein[s] decompressing the FLR must remain intact), and (4) the FLR must be of an adequate size. Using cross-sectional CT or MRI, the volume of the FLR and the volume of the entire liver can be calculated. In this way, the ratio of the FLR volume to the total estimated liver volume (or, alternatively, to the total ideal liver volume based on patient size) can be calculated.[7] The minimal FLR to total liver volume ratio necessary to sustain sufficient postresection liver function and hypertrophy depends on the condition of the underlying liver. In patients with normal liver function, the ratio can be as small as 20%. In patients with severe underlying liver dysfunction (e.g., resulting from cirrhosis), the minimal ratio may be 40% to 50%. As will be outlined subsequently, iatrogenic impairment of hepatic function resulting from prolonged chemotherapy may require a minimal FLR of 30% to 40%. In cases of advanced disease with large or multifocal tumors, adjustments to operative planning may become necessary in order to preserve a sufficient FLR. These so-called parenchymal-sparing approaches to hepatic metastasectomy may invoke the use of adjuncts like thermal ablation or portal vein embolization, as will be discussed in the following.

Although the safety of hepatic surgery has greatly improved in recent decades (with operative mortality risk following major hepatic resections approximating 1% to 3% in large volume centers), it remains a considerable undertaking. The major perioperative risks for hepatic resection are hemorrhage, bile leak, and postoperative hepatic failure. The predominant source of intraoperative hemorrhage results from venous "backbleeding" from the inferior vena cava and hepatic veins; consequently, great effort is expended to minimize central venous pressure to as low as 0 to 3 mm Hg during hepatic parenchymal transection. Patients with underlying comorbidities that render them unable to tolerate the hemodynamics of low central venous pressure are clearly at higher risk of operative blood loss. Hemorrhage during hepatic parenchymal transection can also result from injury to portal venous and hepatic arterial inflow vessels; this risk can be mitigated by transient occlusion of the hepatic inflow at the porta hepatis (the so-called Pringle maneuver). In the absence of significant underlying hepatic functional derangement, the liver can tolerate relatively prolonged periods of hepatic inflow occlusion during hepatic transection, particularly when it is performed during intermittent periods (10 to 20 minutes) interrupted by brief pauses (5 minutes) to restore hepatic perfusion. A number of methods for parenchymal transection have been developed and compared, including direct manual ligation of biliary and vascular structures, thermal energy devices, and cutting staplers, but no single approach has been consistently proven to decrease hemorrhage. In experienced hands, the majority of major hepatic resections can be performed without the need for intraoperative or postoperative blood transfusion. Bile leakage from the cut surface of the liver occurs in <5% to 10% of cases, and, when necessary, can typically be managed with percutaneous drainage. Interestingly, there is evidence that the increasing complexity of hepatic resections that has evolved over time may be associated with an increasing prevalence of bile leakage.[8] The most devastating complication that can occur after hepatic surgery is postoperative hepatic failure. If the remnant liver is incapable of sustaining hepatic function, postoperative demise from hepatic insufficiency typically cannot be averted. For this reason, great attention is devoted to the FLR preoperatively, intraoperatively, and postoperatively. Meticulous care is taken to avoid unnecessary intraoperative dissection of and injury to the vascular and biliary inflow and outflow of the FLR. Minimally invasive approaches to hepatic resection are being adopted with gradually increasing frequency, although to a lesser extent compared with other arenas of surgery. In well-selected cases and in experienced centers, minimally invasive hepatic surgery is a safe alternative to traditional open methods.

Thermal Ablation

An important adjunct or alternative to operative resection is thermal tumor ablation using radiofrequency ablation (RFA) or microwave ablation (MWA). RFA and MWA have largely replaced the older modality of cryoablation and can be applied percutaneously or directly into the liver. Thermal ablation is often used in conjunction with or instead of operative resection. RFA and MWA involve the direct insertion of ablation probes into the region of a tumor, followed by the application of several cycles of hyperthermic energy to induce a zone of cell death that fully encompasses the tumor. For deep-seated tumors that would require resection of a large volume of liver (e.g., deep, centrally located tumors that would require a formal hemihepatectomy), ablation can be useful as a parenchymal-sparing approach to hepatic metastasectomy. As such, the combined use of ablation with surgical resection enables some patients with traditionally unresectable disease to undergo complete tumor eradication. The conduct of thermal ablation requires radiographic guidance, usually with the use of real-time ultrasonography, in order to direct accurate placement of probes into and around the tumor. Ablation can be administered at the time of open or laparoscopic operation, or in a percutaneous fashion.

Stereotactic Body Radiation Therapy

Stereotactic body radiation therapy (SBRT) is a noninvasive technique of providing local therapy for liver malignancies with ablative intent. The historical development of SBRT has been well chronicled.[9,10] In essence, SBRT is an extracranial application of methodologies developed for intracranial stereotactic radiosurgery of benign and malignant brain lesions. As it is defined by the American Society for Radiation Oncology, here the adjective *stereotactic* implies that the target lesion is localized relative to a fixed three-dimensional spatial coordinate system.[11] Multiple non-opposed radiation beams or arcs converge upon the tumor target, thus avoiding a high dose to normal tissues in the entrance and exit paths of the beams while depositing an ablative dose within the target volume. The entire course of therapy is abbreviated into five or fewer treatments, or fractions.

The ideal SBRT treatment delivery plan achieves a high level of dose conformality, implying that the volume receiving the prescription dose closely approximates the intended target volume, thus minimizing the volume of normal tissue exposed to a high dose. Unlike the case in some applications of conventionally fractionated radiation therapy, wherein dose homogeneity within the target volume is clinically valuable for cosmetic or other end points,[12] for SBRT it is usually advantageous to allow for a dose hotspot to be present within the target volume, both for the purpose of increasing the intensity of therapeutic effect and also steepening the gradient of dose falloff into surrounding normal tissues. This latter goal is often best achieved by closely conforming the beam's eye view of the tumor closely to the cross-sectional projection of the tumor, sometimes with even a "negative margin" where the beam is slightly smaller than the tumor projection, thus exploiting the fact that the steepest gradient of dose falloff outside the beam is generally at the midpoint of the lateral penumbra.[13]

SBRT has a range indication as either primary treatment of an early stage cancer or radical therapy of oligometastic disease. Liver SBRT in particular was initially studied in prospective dose escalation studies utilizing a so-called critical volume method that is conceptually similar to the FLR notion mentioned previously with respect to hepatectomy. Initially applied when considering radiation effects on the spinal cord,[14] in principle the critical volume method works backward from the premise that for any given organ, a certain amount of functional tissue must remain after a course of radiation therapy to avoid severe late sequelae. In the case of liver SBRT, the proposed initial good faith estimate was that at least 700 ml of normal liver must receive a dose <15 Gy in

a three-treatment regimen, a threshold below which organ functionality was expected to be preserved. With this type of constraint in place, it was possible to escalate the prescription dose to individual lesions to 60 Gy in three fractions in the initial University of Colorado study[15] and in five fractions in the University of Texas-Southwestern study,[16] thus achieving actuarial rates of local control of 93% to 100% at 18 to 24 months.

A structured review of normal liver tolerance after SBRT or conventionally fractionated radiotherapy is available in the QUAntitative Normal Tissue Effects in the Clinic project report.[17] It should be appreciated, though, that the rate of radiation-induced liver disease after SBRT is extremely low in the absence of preexisting liver disease, primarily because the mean normal liver dose is kept low. In clinical practice, the more concerning dose-limiting structure for liver SBRT is typically the gastrointestinal tract in cases where the treated lesion approaches within <1 cm or so of the medial surface. To minimize the risk of severe mucosal injury, conservative constraints that have been recommended by a leading expert include a maximum point dose to the upper intestine in the range of 24 to 30 Gy in three fractions and slightly higher for a five-fraction regimen.[18] The Mayo Clinic group has reported outcomes from a series of patients treated with SBRT to the liver and other abdominal targets that suggests a higher risk of bowel toxicity in patients receiving abdominal SBRT and a vascular endothelial growth factor inhibitor,[19] though this finding has not yet been observed by other groups.

Portal Vein Embolization

Some patients with multifocal metastases are not candidates for complete tumor eradication if the size of their anticipated FLR is insufficient to sustain hepatic function. For these patients, consideration can be given to preoperative chemotherapy or to operative adjuncts to maximize the size of the FLR. Downsizing of tumors through the use of preoperative systemic chemotherapy may enable a parenchymal-sparing approach to resection and/or ablation that permits a FLR of sufficient volume. Alternatively, portal vein embolization (PVE) can be used as a means of inducing FLR hypertrophy.[20,21] In this approach, embolization of portal venous inflow to the portion of the liver to be resected is performed prior to operative intervention to induce rapid and significant hypertrophy of the nonembolized hepatic segments. For example, some patients may have multifocal or large tumors that can only be completely removed with a right trisectionectomy. If the FLR (segments I to III) is too small to permit safe resection, PVE of segments IV to VIII is undertaken. If hepatic function is normal, this will usually result in a rapid hypertrophy of segments I to III that peaks in 4 weeks. Thus, if repeat imaging and volumetric analysis performed 1 month following PVE identifies sufficient post-PVE hypertrophy, operative therapy can be undertaken immediately thereafter. In circumstances of impaired liver function (e.g., patients with significant chemotherapy-associated hepatotoxicity), the hypertrophic response to PVE can be attenuated. Indeed, absence of post-PVE hypertrophy (<5% increase in FLR volume) is strongly predictive of postresection liver failure. As such, PVE can occasionally be employed as a "stress test" to predict the likelihood that partial hepatectomy could be safely tolerated. Although it had previously been thought that systemic chemotherapy would significantly impair the hepatic hypertrophic response to PVE, recent analyses suggest that chemotherapy may be safely used in patients with aggressive disease during the period between PVE and resection.[22]

Two-Stage Hepatectomy

A common treatment algorithm employed for patients with advanced, multifocal disease is the two-stage hepatectomy.[23] In this approach, two separate operative procedures are used to effect complete clearance of hepatic tumors. In the first stage, operative resection and/or ablation is used to clear the anticipated FLR (most commonly the left hemiliver or left lateral section). This is often undertaken in a minimally invasive manner so as to facilitate recovery and progression to subsequent therapy. Very shortly after this procedure, contralateral PVE is performed to induce hypertrophy of the newly cleared portion of the liver. If post-PVE imaging verifies satisfactory hypertrophy of the FLR, completion hepatectomy is then performed to clear all remaining sites of disease.

Transarterial Therapy

Transarterial therapies take advantage of the aforementioned unique physiologic characteristic of hepatic metastases. Unlike normal hepatocytes, which derive approximately 75% of their blood supply from the portal venous circulation, hepatic metastases derive 80% to 90% of their blood supply from the hepatic arterial circulation. As a result, a number of therapeutic interventions targeting hepatic metastases have been designed to be delivered intra-arterially (via the hepatic arterial system). Hepatic arterial infusion (HAI) chemotherapy involves the delivery of chemotherapeutic agents directly into the hepatic arterial system. HAI typically employs chemotherapeutic agents that undergo high first-pass hepatic metabolism. Once metabolized by hepatocytes, negligible quantities of chemotherapy are then exposed to the rest of the body; in this way, HAI enables the administration of vastly higher concentrations of chemotherapy to hepatic metastases than can be delivered systemically. Transarterial embolization (TAE) involves the selective administration of polyvinyl alcohol or microspheres into the small arterial vessels that perfuse hepatic tumors. Once delivered, these agents induce thrombosis in small-diameter arteries that results in selective ischemia of tumors but not of the surrounding hepatic parenchyma. Transarterial chemoembolization (TACE) is a combination of these two approaches, in which high doses of chemotherapy are selectively delivered into the arteries that perfuse tumor, after which the arteries are embolized.

Selective Internal Radiation Therapy

Selective internal radiation therapy (SIRT) is a targeted approach that delivers glass or resin microspheres labeled with ^{90}Yttrium, primarily a beta particle emitter, into the arteries that perfuse metastatic or primary liver tumors. The rationale for the potential selectivity of the technique is that postinfusion histologic analysis demonstrates that the spheres are preferentially distributed into vessels around the periphery of the tumor, with relative sparing of the normal liver.[24] It is difficult to compare SBRT and SIRT directly; in general, SBRT can likely provide a more intense dose of radiation to individual discrete lesions, whereas SIRT can be used for somewhat larger and more diffuse hepatic involvement. The initial assessment of the appropriateness of SIRT for a given patient involves a consideration of not only performance status and goals of treatment but also an evaluation of the expected distribution of particles within the patient's liver and identification of any potential concerns regarding a pulmonary shunt or anatomic variant that would cause an excess amount of particles to be distributed into nontarget regions.[25]

The pre-SIRT evaluation may be achieved using planar or single photon emission CT scintigraphy of technetium-99m macroaggregated albumin. The scans will provide information useful for determining the appropriate amount of radioactivity to be infused based on the expected ratio of tumor to normal liver distribution as well as the dose-limiting constraint of pulmonary radiation dose in cases with a demonstrable pulmonary shunt. The incidence of radiation-induced liver toxicity after SIRT is typically low,[26] but gastrointestinal toxicities can also occur from exposure to adjacent tissue or nontargeted sphere deposition.[27] The rate of individual tumor control is not commonly reported after SIRT, but intrahepatic control is lower than after SBRT, possibly because the disease burden

treated with SIRT is typically higher. For example, in one series the median liver tumor volume treated was over 300 ml; the progression-free survival was 3.2 months, and half the patients experienced a component of intrahepatic failure.[28] 6 month intrahepatic control rate was. The therapy is often used as sole treatment for liver lesions but can also be positioned as a bridge to transplantation or downstaging method prior to other interventions.[29]

Palliative Whole Liver Radiation Therapy

Less biologically potent than SIRT is the use of palliative whole liver external beam radiation therapy. This form of treatment becomes more appropriate as the goals of treatment move farther away from radical, potentially curative ablation of oligometastatic disease toward symptom relief in patients with limited life expectancy. A high burden of liver disease can sometimes cause nausea, anorexia, and pain presumed to result from stretching of the liver capsule, among other symptoms. A number of prospective studies have addressed this condition, and an American Society for Radiation Oncology–commissioned review of the topic has been published.[30] The major prospective clinical studies of note are the Radiation Therapy Oncology Group studies performed in the late 1970s and early 1980s. The initial Radiation Therapy Oncology Group pilot study enrolled over 100 patients and involved whole liver external beam radiation therapy regimens in the range of 21 to 30 Gy in 7 to 19 fractions.[31] Patient-reported symptom reduction was observed in most patients: 55% had at least partial relief of abdominal pain, 49% experienced reduced nausea and vomiting, and 28% had less anorexia. There was no clear advantage to a dose above 21 Gy in seven fractions. In a subsequent Radiation Therapy Oncology Group study, this regimen was used again (21 Gy in seven fractions) and was confirmed to achieve pain relief in approximately 80% of patients within 2 to 6 weeks following treatment.[32] The pain relief was complete in 54% of patients; toxicity was limited to mild transient nausea in 22% of patients, and 28% of patients enjoyed improved performance status. More recently, the Princess Margaret Hospital group has reported encouraging similar overall results for palliative liver radiotherapy using an even simpler and shorter schedule involving a single fraction of 8 Gy to the whole liver.[33]

HEPATIC COLORECTAL ADENOCARCINOMA METASTASES

Introduction

Like other adenocarcinomas of the alimentary tract (e.g., gastric adenocarcinoma, pancreatic adenocarcinoma), colorectal adenocarcinoma has a proclivity for hepatic metastasis. However, very much unlike other alimentary tract adenocarcinomas, the liver is often the *only* site of metastatic spread for colorectal adenocarcinoma. This nuance of cancer biology makes liver-directed therapy an attractive approach in the management of metastatic colorectal adenocarcinoma. Another impetus for aggressive liver-directed therapy is the broad availability of effective systemic chemotherapy. Indeed, over the past several decades, continual advances in chemotherapy have incrementally but substantively raised the median overall survival for patients with metastatic colorectal adenocarcinoma from 6 months in the era of 5-fluorouracil (5-FU) monotherapy to over 2 years in the contemporary era of combinatorial FOLFOX or FOLFIRI chemotherapy administered in conjunction with so-called targeted biologic agents.

Hepatic Resection

The goal of hepatic metastasectomy for colorectal adenocarcinoma is complete tumoral extirpation with negative resection

TABLE 125.1

Selected Published Series of Outcomes After Hepatic Resection of Colorectal Adenocarcinoma Metastases

Author	Era	N	Operative Mortality	Median FU	Five-y OS	Ten-y OS	Median OS	Five-y DFS	Ten-y DFS	Median DFS
Andreou et al.[35]	1997–2010	378	3%	32 mo	53%	26%	62 mo	NS	NS	NS
House et al.[36]	1999–2004	563	1%	34 mo	51%[a]	37%[a,b]	64 mo	33%	31%[b]	
Wei et al.[37]	1992–2002	423	2%		47%	28%		27%	22%	
Choti et al.[38]	1993–1999	133	<1%	22 mo	58%	NS	NS	28%	NS	19 mo
House et al.[36]	1985–1998	1,037	3%	38 mo	37%[a]	26%[a,b]	43 mo	27%	23%[b]	
Choti et al.[38]	1984–1992	93	<1%	122 mo	31%	NS	36 mo	14%		12 mo
Scheele et al.[39]	1960–1992	1,718	4%		39%	24%		34%		

FU, follow-up; OS, overall survival; DFS, disease-free survival; NS, not stated.
[a] Disease-specific survival.
[b] Eight-year disease-specific survival.

margins. It is evident that a subset of patients who undergo resection of their hepatic colorectal metastases will be cured. Longitudinal analyses indicate that the cure rate is approximately 20% of all patients; these studies also demonstrate that recurrences can occur late, such that the declaration of cure cannot be made until 10 years after surgical resection.[34] Despite decades of accumulating experience with surgical therapy, there are no prospective randomized data to verify that hepatic metastasectomy improves survival for patients with hepatic colorectal adenocarcinoma metastases beyond that which could be expected with systemic chemotherapy alone. However, as shown in Table 125.1, single-institution series have demonstrated steady improvements in actuarial survival estimates that now approximate 5-year overall survival rates of 50% after hepatic metastasectomy.[35–39] As systemic chemotherapy has become more effective, surgical therapy has been implemented more aggressively, being offered to patients who previously might have been deemed poor candidates for operative intervention. Indeed, tumor characteristics that were once considered contraindications to surgical intervention (e.g., bilobar tumor involvement, more than four tumors) are now commonplace among patients undergoing hepatic metastasectomy. As the indications for operative therapy broaden, and as surgical resection is offered to more and more patients with highly aggressive manifestations of metastatic disease, it is unlikely that the chance of actual cure will rise. However, in light of the ever-improving capacity of systemic chemotherapy to prolong survival for patients with advanced disease, it is also likely that aggressive hepatic metastasectomy, when used rationally and in the context of multimodality, multidisciplinary care, may prolong survival.

Extrahepatic Disease

One special circumstance of liberalizing indications for hepatic metastasectomy that deserves mention is that of extrahepatic metastases. The presence of additional foci of metastatic disease outside of the liver (e.g., pulmonary, peritoneal, retroperitoneal) was once universally considered to be an absolute contraindication to hepatic resection. However, there is now accumulating experience with combined hepatic and extrahepatic metastasectomy. Although this experience is derived from highly unique and selected cases, in the context of this careful patient selection, it is apparent that patients undergoing resection of hepatic and pulmonary metastases can experience a median overall survival of 3 to 4 years (recurrence-free survival of approximately 2 years), and patients undergoing resection of hepatic and peritoneal metastases can experience a median overall survival of 2 to 3 years

(recurrence-free survival of approximately 2 years). Interestingly, comparatively worse survival outcomes have been described for patients presenting with hepatic pedicle or retroperitoneal lymph node metastases.[40,41]

Thermal Ablation

Thermal ablation using MWA or RFA has the advantage of allowing greater parenchymal sparing than hepatic resection, particularly for deep-seated, centrally located tumors. As such, ablation is often used instead of or in conjunction with resection. Ablation can be performed intraoperatively during open or laparoscopic procedures, or percutaneously in a nonoperative setting. The less invasive nature of ablation can be attractive for patients who are suboptimal candidates for major operative intervention. Ablation is particularly appealing for cases of colorectal adenocarcinoma metastases that have recurred following previous resection, as it avoids the heightened risks of repeat hepatic resection. A review of single and multi-institutional experiences with thermal ablation for hepatic colorectal adenocarcinoma metastases indicates a risk of local recurrence (i.e., incomplete ablation; Table 125.2).[42–47] In experienced hands, the risk of local recurrence can be <10%. The biggest risk factor for local recurrence is tumor size; for small tumors (<1 to 2 cm), the likelihood of incomplete ablation with modern MWA and RFA is quite small. The overall survival estimates observed in these series is significantly lower than those associated with hepatic resection; however, this is likely reflective of the significant selection bias that is inherent in any decision to undertake ablation over operative resection.

Adjuvant and Perioperative Chemotherapy

Adjuvant chemotherapy has been shown to decrease the risk of recurrence and improve survival for patients with stage III colorectal adenocarcinoma; moreover, systemic chemotherapy clearly prolongs survival for patients with unresectable metastatic colorectal adenocarcinoma. For these reasons, operative resection and systemic chemotherapy are typically used in close conjunction with one another, even for patients with readily resectable hepatic metastases. A fair amount of effort has been expended in an effort to measure the benefit of this multimodal approach to patients with resectable hepatic colorectal adenocarcinoma metastases. The largest multicenter prospective randomized trials evaluating the influence of adjuvant systemic chemotherapy are summarized in Table 125.3.[48–52] Two prospective randomized clinical trials

TABLE 125.2

Selected Published Series of Outcomes After Thermal Ablation of Colorectal Adenocarcinoma Metastases

Author	Era	N (Tumors)	Ablation Type	Median Tumor Size	Median FU	Local Recurrence	Five-y OS	Ten-y OS	Median OS	Five-y RFS	Ten-y RFS	Median RFS
Groeschl et al.[42]	2003–2011	403	MWA	2 cm	19 mo	5%	17%	NS	32 mo	9%	NS	25 mo
Kingham et al.[43]	1996–2011	315	RFA, cryoablation, MWA			11%						
Martin et al.[44]	2004–2009	135	MWA	3 cm			47%	28%		27%	22%	
Siperstein et al.[45]	1997–2006	292	RFA	3.9 cm	24 mo	NS	18%	NS	24 mo	34%		
Abdalla et al.[46]	1992–2002	57	RFA	2.5 cm	21 mo	9%	22%[a]	NS	~25 mo	~5%[b]	NS	~10 mo
Park et al.[47]	1995–2005	30	RFA	3.1 cm		23%			36 mo			

FU, follow-up; OS, overall survival; RFS, relapse-free survival; MWA, microwave ablation; NS, not stated; RFA, radiofrequency ablation.
[a] Four-year OS.
[b] Three-year RFS.
[c] Four-year progression-free survival.

comparing surgical resection alone to surgical resection followed by postoperative 5-FU and leucovorin identified a suggestion of improvement in progression-free survival among patients randomized to receive chemotherapy, but no improvement was seen in overall survival.[48,49] Although some have argued that the combination of 5-FU and leucovorin is largely of historical interest because of the advent of more effective regimens of chemotherapy, a randomized trial comparing adjuvant 5-FU/leucovorin to FOLFIRI showed no differences in survival.[50] Indeed, the more recent European Organisation for Research and Treatment of Cancer 40983 randomized trial comparing patients treated with surgical resection alone versus surgical resection with perioperative FOLFOX4 chemotherapy also only suggested an improvement in progression-free survival on subset analysis.[51,52] It is worth recognizing that patients

TABLE 125.3

Selected Published Multicenter Prospective Randomized Controlled Trials Evaluating the Benefit of Postoperative or Perioperative Chemotherapy in Patients Undergoing Resection of Hepatic Colorectal Adenocarcinoma Metastases

Author	Era	Arm	Median FU	N	Five-y OS	Median OS	P (OS)	Five-y DFS	Median DFS	P (DFS)
Portier et al.[48]	1991–2001	Resection alone	91 mo	100	42%	46 mo		27%	18 mo	
		Resection → 5-FU/leucovorin	85 mo	100	51%	62 mo	0.13	34%	24 mo	0.028
Mitry et al.[49]	1991–2001	Resection alone	NS	135	40%	47 mo		28%	19 mo	
		Resection → 5-FU/leucovorin	NS	292	53%	62 mo	0.095	37%	28 mo	0.058
Ychou et al.[50]	2001–2006	Resection → 5-FU/leucovorin	42 mo	153	72%[a]	NR		46%[b]	22 mo	
		Resection → FOLFIRI	42 mo	153	73%[a]	NR	0.69	51%[b]	25 mo	0.44
Nordlinger et al.[51]	2000–2004	Resection alone	102 mo	182	NS	54 mo		30%[c]	13 mo	
		FOLFOX4 → resection → FOLFOX4	102 mo	182	NS	61 mo	0.3	38%[c]	20 mo	0.068

FU, follow-up; OS, overall survival; DFS, disease-free survival; 5-FU, 5-fluorouracil; NS, not stated; NR, not reached.
[a] Three-year OS.
[b] Two-year DFS.
[c] Three-year progression-free survival.

who eventually develop recurrent metastatic disease after resection are likely to receive systemic chemotherapy, regardless of the nature of perioperative or postoperative treatment. Thus, it is quite possible that the reason these trials did not show differences in overall survival was because systemic chemotherapy was able to "salvage" patients who developed disease recurrence.

Neoadjuvant Chemotherapy

Regardless of these uncertainties, most patients with hepatic colorectal adenocarcinoma metastases are treated in a multimodal manner. Indeed, for patients with radiographic evidence of resectable disease (and whose underlying medical condition permits operative therapy), the decision is generally not whether to give chemotherapy, but when. It is likely that optimal therapy of hepatic colorectal adenocarcinoma metastases involves the multimodal use of systemic chemotherapy and operative tumor resection (or ablation). However, controversy persists regarding the ideal sequencing of treatment for patients with resectable tumors. The routine use of neoadjuvant chemotherapy (administered prior to operative therapy) offers several theoretical advantages: (1) it allows one to measure the chemosensitivity of tumors by observing radiographic evidence of tumoral regression; (2) in circumstances of rapid disease progression, as is the case with synchronous metastases, it allows for a period of safe observation in which other occult foci of metastases may become evident; and (3) it helps to ensure that patients will receive a vital component of multimodality therapy (chemotherapy), even if they develop major postoperative complications that prevent them from completing additional therapy. As the response rate of hepatic colorectal metastases to contemporary chemotherapy has improved to well over 50%, the rationale for using neoadjuvant therapy for drug selection or as a means of monitoring for prognostically adverse disease progression has diminished.[53-55]

Conversion to Resectability

A major advancement in the treatment of metastatic colorectal adenocarcinoma has been in the array of technologies that can occasionally enable patients with initially unresectable disease to eventually undergo complete tumor extirpation. In circumstances where the FLR is insufficient in size, PVE and two-stage hepatectomy are commonly employed. A typical case example is illustrated in Figure 125.1.

On occasion, the extent of tumor burden is so great that PVE and two-stage approaches are not enough to achieve resectability. Fortunately, the steady improvements in response rates to chemotherapy have led to the use of systemic chemotherapy as a means of converting some patients with unresectable disease to resectability.[56] In one illustrative experience of 1,104 patients with unresectable hepatic colorectal adenocarcinoma metastases treated over an 11-year period at the Hôpital Paul Brousse, 138 patients (12.5%) demonstrated sufficient disease regression after an average of 10 cycles of chemotherapy to permit an attempt at resection; potentially curative hepatic metastasectomy was possible in 93% of the 138 patients, resulting in actuarial 5-year survival estimates of 33%.[57] It is important to recognize that this aggressive utilization of surgical resection for patients with advanced disease is unlikely to be curative; over the course of follow-up in this series, 80% of patients eventually developed disease recurrence, and overall survival in this select cohort of patients was significantly poorer than in patients who initially presented with resectable disease. However, it is likely that the outcomes observed following such aggressive surgical interventions might not have occurred following chemotherapy alone. A recent analysis from the MD Anderson Cancer Center compared patients with extensive tumor burden who exhibited a radiographic response to systemic chemotherapy. After controlling for a number of relevant patient and tumor characteristics, they

observed a striking difference in survival between patients who underwent hepatic metastasectomy at some point in their treatment versus patients who did not.[58] Although this study cannot account for all of the selection biases inherent in a retrospective comparison of surgical and nonsurgical patients, the magnitude of difference suggests that operative metastasectomy may likely impart an independent influence on survival duration.

Biological Agents

The armamentarium of systemic treatment options has been greatly expanded by the introduction of so-called biologic agents, which are targeted inhibitors or antibodies that interfere with the function of specific proteins and receptors involved in carcinogenic signaling pathways. Biologic agents such as bevacizumab, which targets the angiogenic vascular endothelial growth factor,[59-61] and cetuximab, which targets the mitogenic epithelial growth factor,[62,63] have been shown to improve response rates and progression-free survival when used in conjunction with traditional chemotherapy. One concern related to the use of bevacizumab is its potential negative influence on wound healing and bleeding. Although the extent to which preoperative administration of bevacizumab affects perioperative complication rates remains uncertain, a preferred approach has been to delay operative intervention until 4 to 8 weeks after the last administration of bevacizumab; when used in this manner, no significant changes in wound-related complications have been observed.[64,65] An important variable to consider when using cetuximab is the tumoral mutational status of the KRAS oncogene; retrospective and prospective analyses have verified that the benefit associated with the use of cetuximab is confined to the KRAS wild-type population.[66,67]

Chemotherapy-Associated Hepatotoxicity

An important argument against neoadjuvant chemotherapy is the risk of chemotherapy-associated hepatotoxicity. As the efficacy of chemotherapeutic agents against colorectal adenocarcinoma has increased, so too has their side effect profile of hepatotoxicity.[68-70] Agents like 5-FU and irinotecan have been associated with a risk of hepatic steatosis, which can evolve into steatohepatitis. Livers afflicted by steatosis appear rounded and pink, and those with steatohepatitis demonstrate fibrotic changes that, over time, can progress to frank cirrhosis; both are associated with higher risks of intraoperative hemorrhage and impaired hepatic regeneration. Oxaliplatin is primarily toxic to endothelial or vascular tissues in the liver, and has been associated with sinusoidal vasodilation and obstruction that appears as a patchy bluish discoloration of the liver; heavy oxaliplatin use has been associated with higher risks of intraoperative hemorrhage. Several retrospective studies have reported higher rates of perioperative morbidity and prolonged hospitalizations in patients undergoing hepatic metastasectomy after prolonged courses of chemotherapy,[71,72] and the aforementioned European Organisation for Research and Treatment of Cancer 40983 prospective trial identified a significantly higher rate of postoperative complications in the perioperative chemotherapy arm versus the operation alone arm (25% versus 16%, $p = 0.04$).[51] As outlined previously, the ability of neoadjuvant or adjuvant chemotherapy to improve overall survival for patients undergoing hepatic metastasectomy remains unclear; whether and how the timing of chemotherapy vis-à-vis resection affects survival is unknown. Because prolonged administration of chemotherapy can induce enough liver damage to challenge the safety of surgical intervention, some clinicians have argued against the routine administration of neoadjuvant chemotherapy for patients with resectable hepatic metastases. At the very least, care should be taken to limit the duration of preoperative chemotherapy so as to minimize the risk of chemotherapy-associated hepatotoxicity; based on retrospective analyses, it appears that the risk of perioperative complications

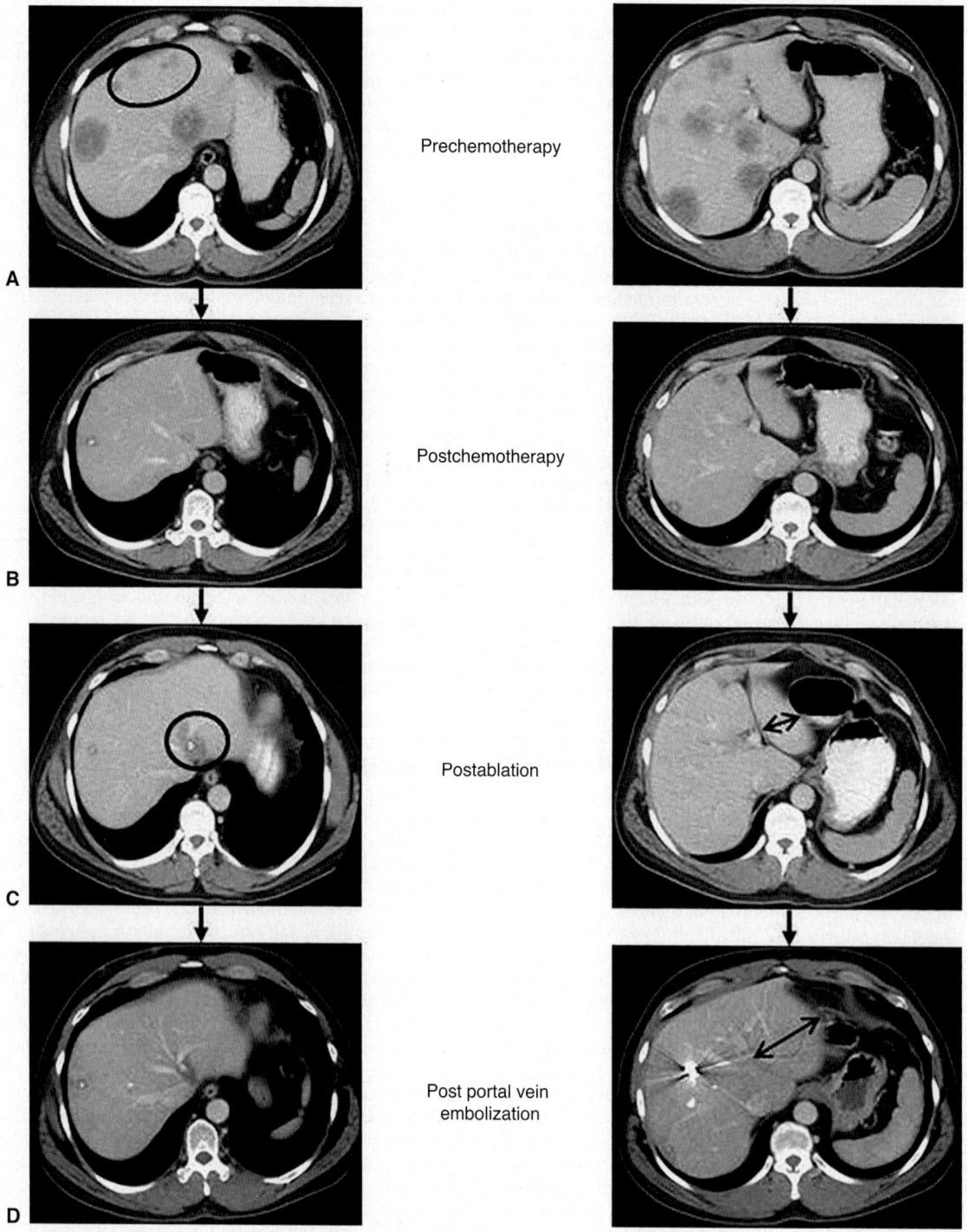

Prechemotherapy

Postchemotherapy

Postablation

Post portal vein embolization

Figure 125.1 Two-stage hepatectomy. A man in his 50s presented with colon adenocacinoma and radiographic evidence of synchronous, multifocal, bilateral hepatic metastases **(A)**. Repeat imaging obtained after six cycles of systemic FOLFOX chemotherapy demonstrated marked regression of his metastases **(B)**. Some of the lesions seen on initial imaging (*circled* in **A**) were no longer evident following chemotherapy. He underwent colectomy and microwave ablation of his solitary segment II metastasis, after which repeat imaging **(C)** and hepatic volumetrics (not shown) verified the presence of a small future liver remnant (segments II/III shown between *arrows* in **C**). Right portal vein embolization was performed, after which postembolization imaging suggested hypertrophy of the future liver remnant (segments II/III shown between *arrows* in **D**). Following verification of satisfactory hypertrophy by postembolization volumetrics (not shown), the patient underwent an extended right hemihepatectomy but subsequently developed intrahepatic and extrahepatic metastases after an interval of 18 months.

increases after six or more cycles of preoperative chemotherapy. Identification of chemotherapy-associated hepatotoxicity can be challenging, as routine laboratory assessment of hepatic function is typically not sensitive enough to identify these changes. Thrombocytopenia can be suggestive of hypersplenism resulting from hepatic fibrosis–induced portal hypertension. Radiographic evidence

of steatosis (as estimated by a decrease in hepatic parenchymal attenuation on CT imaging or signal dropout on in- and out-of-phase MRI sequences) or fibrosis (as indicated by alterations in hepatic segmental atrophy or hypertrophy or irregularities in parencymal contour) can also be suggestive of hepatotoxicity.[73] Because of the inconsistency with which these preoperative diagnostics identify significant hepatotoxicity, some have argued for the routine use of percutaneous liver biopsy (to evaluate for steatosis, fibrosis, or sinusoidal obstruction) in patients who have received intensive systemic chemotherapy.[74]

Hepatic Artery Infusional Chemotherapy

As stated previously, hepatic metastases preferentially derive their perfusion from the hepatic arterial circulation. Floxuridine (FUDR) is a derivative of 5-FU that is rapidly metabolized by the liver. HAI of FUDR has therefore been developed as a means of delivering extremely high doses of chemotherapy to hepatic tumors with negligible systemic exposure. Clinical trials have demonstrated impressive benefits with the use of adjuvant and neoadjuvant HAI chemotherapy.[75–77] However, many of these trials were undertaken prior to the availability of more modern chemotherapeutic agents; as a result, the contemporary role and benefit of HAI chemotherapy is not clear. Use of HAI FUDR has been associated with favorable response rates when used in patients who have been refractory to contemporary chemotherapy, suggesting that there is likely to be a role for this modality of treatment.[77,78] However, its use requires familiarity with proper techniques for infusion pump placement and care. In addition, patients receiving HAI chemotherapy must be closely monitored for signs of biliary sclerosis. Like metastases, cholangiocytes of the biliary tree also derive their blood supply from the hepatic arterial system; as a result, prolonged arterial infusion of chemotherapy can result in biliary strictures. Administration of dexamethasone in conjunction with FUDR has been found to mitigate this risk.

The "Disappearing Metastasis"

Because of the risk of chemotherapy-associated hepatotoxicity, patients with advanced disease undergoing preoperative systemic chemotherapy must undergo serial imaging surveillance so that operative intervention can be undertaken before the onset of liver damage. On occasion, follow-up imaging will identify a complete radiographic disappearance of tumor(s). Appropriate management of the "disappearing metastasis" remains controversial. It is evident that a majority of these tumors have simply become radiographically occult, but will eventually reappear and progress after discontinuation of chemotherapy.[79] Interestingly, longitudinal analyses suggest that a subset of as many as one-fifth of highly selected patients may have durable remission of "disappeared metastases."[80,81] However, it is also noteworthy that most of these patients will eventually shows signs of disease progression elsewhere, attesting to the significant risk of eventual relapse among patients with aggressively advanced hepatic colorectal metastases.

Prognostic Factors

A number of investigations have sought to identify the patient and disease variables that influence outcomes after hepatic metastasectomy. A prognostication system that has been shown to be of some utility is the Memorial Sloan Kettering Cancer Center Clinical Risk Score, which is a simple 0 to 5 scoring system incorporating the presence (or absence) of five prognostic variables related to both the primary and metastatic disease ([1] node-positive primary cancer, [2] disease-free interval [between the time of primary and metastatic cancer diagnosis] <12 months, [3] carcinoembryonic antigen >200 ng/mL, [4] maximal hepatic tumor size >5 cm, and [5] multifocal [>1] hepatic tumors). Developed prior to the introduction of contemporary chemotherapeutic regimens, the Clinical Risk Score has been shown to be useful for stratifying patients in terms of their risk of developing recurrent disease.[82] However, recent analyses have suggested that, in the modern era of highly effective systemic therapy, the dominant variables influencing

outcomes after hepatic metastasectomy may be tumor responsiveness to chemotherapy and technical resectability.[83] This suggests that modern chemotherapy has largely overcome the impact of such traditional prognostic factors as nodal positivity and disease-free interval, largely reducing the decision of whether to undertake surgical intervention to a technical determination of resectability.

The goal of operative therapy is a margin-negative resection. However, the optimal distance of margin clearance remains unclear. As hepatic resections become more aggressive in their efforts to clear multifocal tumors while preserving a maximal amount of hepatic parenchyma, the ability to consistently obtain widely negative resection margins has become more difficult. Interestingly, recent analyses suggest that the critical goal is simply the presence of a microscopically negative margin, with relatively little prognostic impact being associated with the actual distance of margin clearance.[84–86]

Stereotactic Body Radiation Therapy

It is difficult to compare SBRT clinical outcomes with those observed after resection primarily because the SBRT series generally include patients who have been heavily pretreated with systemic therapy for metastatic disease and are, therefore, further along in the disease history. In most of the early liver SBRT pilot trials, an assortment of primary histologic types of cancers were included, though the most common is generally colorectal cancer by virtue of its frequency among cancer types. In 2006, Hoyer and colleagues[87] reported a phase 2 study of SBRT for patients with limited metastatic colorectal cancer. While the trial included patients with metastatic disease in a variety of sites, the majority (44/64 patients) had liver metastases, alone or in combination with other sites.[87] The 45-Gy dose was prescribed to the isocenter and not to the periphery of the tumor, and thus the actual dose received by the periphery of the tumor was likely close to 30 Gy in three fractions. The treatment was administered without the use of daily CT-based image guidance. Over half the patients had received prior chemotherapy, and roughly one-third had had prior surgery or RFA. The 2-year actuarial lesion local control rate was 86%, and the 1-year survival was 67%. One patient died due to hepatic failure possibly related to treatment, and another had surgery for colonic perforation. The toxicity observed was otherwise generally mild.

In 2011, Chang and colleagues[88] reported a pooled experience of liver SBRT restricted to colorectal cancer metastases from three major institutions collected prospectively on prospective clinical trials at each institution. Sixty-five patients with 102 lesions treated from August 2003 to May 2009 were analyzed. The patients were heavily pretreated: 47 (72%) patients had had one chemotherapy regimen prior to SBRT and 27 (42%) patients had had two or more regimens. Daily image guidance was used in all cases; only two patients experienced any late grade 3 toxicity, and none had any grade 4 or 5 toxicity. Local control of individual lesions was correlated with total dose and either of two composite equivalent dose indices taking into consideration the number of fractions and fraction size. When the data were fit to a logistic tumor control probability curve, the dose required to expect ≥90% local control was on the order of 48 Gy or higher in three fractions. On multivariate analysis, active extrahepatic disease was associated with worse overall survival, and the attainment of durable local control was also closely correlated with longer survival. The results support the contention that even for heavily pretreated patients, clearing or cytoreducing the burden of tumor in the liver is associated with longer survival.

Evaluating local control after SBRT requires an understanding that there will be changes on CT scans whereby transiently for a few months after treatment, a hypodense region will be seen that correlates to the volume of liver that received a dose above the threshold to cause local veno-occlusive change, and this region is typically larger than the treated tumor.[89] PET scanning likely

PRACTICE OF ONCOLOGY

offers a more reliable means of evaluating whether active tumor remains after treatment. Transient moderate increases in individual lesion maximum standardized uptake value (SUV_{max}) may be observed after SBRT, but generally the SUV_{max} declines steadily in a manner that can be modeled as exponential decay with a half-life of approximately 2 months, eventually reaching the typical normal liver tissue SUV_{max} of approximately 3.[90] It has been proposed that an SUV_{max} of 6 could serve as a cutoff to score post-SBRT local recurrence after SBRT.

HEPATIC NEUROENDOCRINE CARCINOMA METASTASES

Introduction

Like colorectal adenocarcinoma, neuroendocrine carcinoma arising from the gastrointestinal tract and pancreas commonly metastasizes to the liver via the portal venous circulation. As a result, therapies to target hepatic metastases have been developed and pursued aggressively. Unlike colorectal adenocarcinoma, comparatively little progress has been made in the development of systemic chemotherapy for neuroendocrine carcinoma. The motivation and rationale for aggressive liver-directed therapy for patients with hepatic neuroendocrine carcinoma center on the generally indolent and often highly symptomatic nature of its disease course. Well-differentiated forms of neuroendocrine carcinoma often grow and progress slowly, with median survival of patients with even widely metastatic disease being measured in years. In addition, the hormones that are often elaborated by neuroendocrine neoplasms escape hepatic metabolism when they arise from tumors located in the liver; as a result, patients with hepatic metastases can suffer from occasionally bizarre syndromes of hormonal overproduction that can quickly become refractory to pharmacologic suppression. The effort to prolong survival and/or improve quality of life has led to a variety of treatment options for patients with hepatic neuroendocrine carcinoma metastases.

An important difference between hepatic metastases from colorectal adenocarcinoma and neuroendocrine carcinoma is that neuroendocrine metastases tend to be more diffuse and multifocal in their dissemination. Indeed, it is not uncommon to find innumerable, miliary liver lesions in patients with metastatic neuroendocrine carcinoma. Not surprisingly, the likelihood of performing a complete resection, and the durability of hepatic recurrence-free survival, are much lower for hepatic neuroendocrine metastases. This important difference informs decision making when considering the various treatment options available for this disease.

Hepatic Resection

Hepatic neuroendocrine carcinoma metastasectomy follows the same principles of anatomy, physiology, and surgery that influence hepatic metastasectomy for colorectal adenocarcinoma. As such, assessment of FLR and the use of adjuncts like ablation and PVE are very relevant to the care of hepatic neuroendocrine metastases. Because of the paucity of systemic chemotherapy options for patients with metastatic neuroendocrine carcinoma, neoadjuvant and adjuvant chemotherapy and chemotherapy-associated hepatotoxicity are not particularly relevant.

Analyses of outcomes after hepatic metastasectomy are limited to retrospective series of carefully selected patients.[91–94] An overview of such analyses (Table 125.4) suggests that most patients can expect to survive for years following surgical therapy. However, it is also evident that the likelihood of cure is vanishingly small; in most series with reasonable durations of follow-up, the vast majority of patients experience disease recurrence, most often in the liver remnant.

One very important difference in the approach to hepatic resection for neuroendocrine carcinoma is the concept of operative cytoreduction. Whereas the goal of surgical treatment for hepatic colorectal metastases is invariably a complete resection, subtotal resection (also referred to as "debulking") is occasionally advocated in the management of hepatic neuroendocrine metastases. The circumstance in which this is most appropriately pursued is in the palliation of patients with refractory symptoms of hormonal overproduction. Operative cytoreduction of a majority of hepatic disease burden has been associated with a magnitude and duration of symptomatic improvement that compares very favorably with nonoperative modalities of treatment. When cytoreduction is undertaken for this reason, therapy is typically directed at eliminating the largest tumors and resecting the maximal amount of total disease burden possible. There are no clear data to support the specific manner (e.g., the target tumor size or percentage of tumor bulk elimination) in which cytoreduction should be best performed. Some centers have argued that operative cytoreduction also prolongs survival for patients with metastatic neuroendocrine carcinoma.[93] However, it is important to recognize that patients with even significant hepatic tumor burden often survive for years without any form of tumor-directed therapy. Therefore, in the absence of randomized controlled data, the extent to which operative cytoreduction (resulting in gross residual disease) prolongs survival remains unclear. On the other hand, in light of the often diffuse manner in which neuroendocrine carcinoma metastasizes to the liver, and the near inevitability of hepatic recurrence following surgical resection, one can make the argument that all hepatic resections for metastatic neuroendocrine carcinoma are inherently cytoreductive.

TABLE 125.4

Selected Published Series of Outcomes After Hepatic Resection of Neuroendocrine Carcinoma Metastases

Author	Era	N	Median FU	Operative Mortality	Five-y OS	Ten-y OS	Median OS	Five-y RFS	10-y RFS	Median RFS	Symptom Control	Five-y SFS	Median SFS
Mayo et al.[91]	1984–2009	339			74%	51%	125 mo	6%					
Cho et al.[92]	1990–2006	63	51 mo	4%	65%	26%	108 mo	~8%[a]	NS	19 mo	100%	~15%	39 mo
Sarmiento et al.[93]	1977–1998	170	NS	1%	61%	35%	81 mo	16%	10%	21 mo	96%	41%	46 mo
Chen et al.[94]	1984–1995	15	27 mo	0%	73%	NS	NS	NS	NS	21 mo	NS	NS	NS

FU, follow-up; OS, overall survival; RFS, relapse-free survival; SFS, symptom-free survival; NS, not stated.
[a] Five-year progression-free survival.

Systemic Chemotherapy

Until recently, systemic therapy for patients with metastatic neuroendocrine carcinoma was restricted to somatostatin analogs and cytotoxic chemotherapy.[95] Treatment with somatostatin analogs like octreotide has been shown to delay disease progression when compared with placebo controls. Somatostatin analog therapy can also ameliorate hormonal symptoms in 60% to 90% of patients; however, this effect is typically short-lived, as symptoms typically recur in a refractory fashion about 1 year after initiation of therapy. Combinatorial approaches to cytotoxic chemotherapy using 5-FU, streptozocin, and doxorubicin or cisplatin and etoposide have been associated with response rates of approximately 40% for patients with poorly differentiated carcinoma. Unfortunately, these regimens are also associated with significant treatment-related toxicity.

Targeted therapies with biologic agents that have been used against other malignancies have recently shown promising efficacy and tolerability when used to treat pancreatic neuroendocrine carcinoma. Treatment with sunitinib, a tyrosine kinase inhibitor that targets vascular endothelial growth factor receptors and platelet-derived growth factor receptors, has been shown to prolong median progression-free survival (11.4 months versus 5.5 months) with a significantly higher objective response rate (9% versus 0%) when compared with placebo in the treatment of well-differentiated pancreatic neuroendocrine carcinoma.[96] Treatment with everolimus, an inhibitor of the protein mammalian target of rapamycin, resulted in a similar prolongation of progression-free survival (11 months versus 5.4 months) and improvement in objective response rates (5% versus 2%) compared with placebo in patients with well-differentiated pancreatic neuroendocrine carcinoma.[97] Further investigations will determine the efficacy of these novel agents in the treatment of hepatic neuroendocrine metastases.

Transarterial Therapy

Neuroendocrine carcinoma tumors are highly vascular, and the avidity with which hepatic metastases derive their blood supply from the hepatic arterial circulation has led to a great deal of interest in transarterial therapies. TAE and TACE have both been used to treat advanced cases of hepatic neuroendocrine carcinoma metastases. Despite the theoretical advantage of TACE, comparative studies have not identified a clear advantage of TACE over TAE, with both modalities of therapy improving hormonally referable symptoms in one-third to three-quarters of patients and inducing radiographically objective tumor regression in the majority of patients.[98] Accumulating experience suggests that [90]Yttrium-based SIRT compares favorably with TAE and TACE.[99] Of note, hormonal symptoms can occasionally be paradoxically exacerbating immediately following transarterial therapy; periprocedural administration of octreotide and histamine blockers may alleviate this transient effect.

Prognostic Factors

It is evident that the most informative prognostic variable for neuroendocrine carcinoma is the degree of histologic differentiation. Neuroendocrine carcinoma is characterized into three levels of histologic differentiation based on mitotic activity as assessed by mitotic figures or by Ki-67 immunohistochemical proliferative index. Classification of well-differentiated, moderately differentiated, and poorly differentiated disease permits stratification of oncologic outcomes. The prognosis of poorly differentiated neuroendocrine carcinoma is extremely poor, such that patients whose neuroendocrine metastases are preoperatively determined to be poorly differentiated are typically not subjected to aggressive surgical therapies.[92]

Selective Internal Radiation Therapy

In the consensus report of the 2011 National Cancer Institute Neuroendocrine Tumor clinical trials planning meeting, the limitations on data concerning liver-directed therapy were acknowledged.[100] Specifically, it was noted that patients who undergo either hepatic resection or orthotopic liver transplantation are typically well selected; at the same time, it was acknowledged that randomized controlled trials studying patient outcomes with these treatment modalities would likely be difficult to execute.

A pooled multi-institutional retrospective review of patients who received SIRT for neuroendocrine tumor liver metastases was reported in 2008.[101] A total of 148 patients who underwent 185 separate procedures were analyzed. The median age was 58 years (range, 26 to 95), and the median activity delivered was 1.14 GBq (0.33 to 3.30 GBq). The risk of Common Toxicity Criteria for Adverse Events grade 3 or higher fatigue or nausea was 6.5% and 3.2%, respectively. The 3-month imaging-based response was stable in complete in 3%, partial in 60%, stable in 23%, progressive disease in 5%, and unavailable in the others. No radiation-related liver failure occurred, and the median survival was 70 months.

In a 42-patient prospective study, King and colleagues[102] treated patients with neuroendocrine tumor liver metastases who had failed standard-of-care therapies, defined as progression on octreotide and after resection, ablation, or embolotherapy. SIRT was performed with either [90]Yttrium resin or glass microspheres. Prior treatments included medication (60%), surgery or ablation (55%), and bland or chemoembolization (14%). The overall response rate was approximately 50% for either type of microsphere (resin or glass). Median survival was roughly 2 years for the entire group.

NONCOLORECTAL NONNEUROENDOCRINE HEPATIC METASTASES

Introduction

As stated, liver-directed therapy is often undertaken for colorectal adenocarcinoma and neuroendocrine carcinoma because of nuances related to disease biology and available chemotherapy. The tendency of metastatic colorectal adenocarcinoma and neuroendocrine carcinoma to be confined to the liver, the availability of effective systemic chemotherapy (for colorectal adenocarcinoma), and the relative indolence of disease progression (for neuroendocrine carcinoma) all enable the aggressive implementation of surgical and nonsurgical liver-directed treatments. For noncolorectal and nonneuroendocrine malignancies that do not share these biologic and therapeutic characteristics, the decision to utilize liver-directed therapy is made on a more individualized, case-by-case basis. As a result, it is difficult to provide generalized treatment recommendations for these types of metastatic disease. However, there has been enough experience with some malignancies such as ocular melanoma, breast carcinoma, and sarcoma to share a few observations.

Ocular (Uveal) Melanoma

Like colorectal adenocarcinoma and neuroendocrine carcinoma, ocular melanoma has a biologic tendency to metastasize to the liver. Because of its tendency to metastasize in a miliary, diffuse manner, meaningful surgical intervention is rarely an option. However, because the liver is the predominant site of metastatic disease in 70% to 90% of cases, transarterial therapy like TACE, SIRT, and HAI chemotherapy have been used in carefully selected patients, with over half of patients exhibiting tumoral regression or transient disease stabilization.[103]

Breast Carcinoma

Liver-directed therapy is occasionally contemplated for unusual cases of oligometastatic breast carcinoma in which the metastases are confined to the liver. The preferred therapy for metastatic breast carcinoma is systemic chemotherapy and hormonal therapy. However, in carefully selected patients, hepatic metastasectomy has been associated with median overall survival estimates of 3 to 4 years, with median disease-free survival estimates of nearly 2 years.[104] In the absence of randomized controlled trials, the extent to which these outcomes represent actual improvements beyond those that might have be expected with systemic chemotherapy alone remains uncertain.

Sarcoma

Intraabdominal and retroperitoneal sarcomas occasionally metastasize to the liver. There are relatively few effective systemic chemotherapy options for patients with metastatic sarcoma, and liver-directed therapy is generally undertaken in highly selected cases that exhibit relatively favorable disease biology. One important exception to this is gastrointestinal stromal tumors, which are likely to respond to systemic administration of the tyrosine kinase inhibitors imatinib and sunitinib. Not surprisingly, hepatic metastasectomy can be undertaken more aggressively in patients with metastatic gastrointestinal stromal tumors when used in conjunction with tyrokine kinase inhibition. When used in this manner, hepatic metastasectomy has been associated with median overall survival estimates exceeding 5 years.[104,105]

SELECTED REFERENCES

The full reference list can be accessed at lwwhealthlibrary.com/oncology.

3. Koh DM, Collins DJ, Wallace T, et al. Combining diffusion-weighted MRI and Gd-EOB-DTPA-enhanced MRI improves the detection of colorectal liver metastases. *Br J Radiol* 2012;85:980–989.

7. Vauthey JN, Chanoui A, Do KA, et al. Standardized measurement of the future liver remnant prior to extended liver resection: methodology and clinical associations. *Surgery* 2000;127:512–519.

15. Rusthoven K, Kavanagh BD, Cardenes H, et al. Multi-institutional phase I/II trial of stereotactic body radiation therapy for liver metastasis. *J Clin Oncol* 2009;27:1572–1578.

16. Rule W, Timmerman R, Tong L, et al. Phase I dose-escalation study of stereotactic body radiotherapy in patients with hepatic metastases. *Ann Surg Oncol* 2011;18:1081–1087.

17. Pan CC, Kavanagh BD, Dawson LA, et al. Radiation-associated liver injury. *Int J Radiat Oncol Biol Phys* 2010;76:S94–S100.

20. Abdalla EK, Barnett C, Doherty D, et al. Extended hepatectomy in patients with hepatobiliary malignancies with and without preoperative portal vein embolization. *Arch Surg* 2002;137:675–680.

23. Jaeck D, Bachellier P, Nakano H, et al. One or two-stage hepatectomy combined with portal vein embolization for initally nonresectable colorectal liver metastases. *Am J Surg* 2003;185:221–229.

25. Lau WY, Kennedy AS, Kim YH, et al. Patient selection and activity planning guide for selective internal radiotherapy with yttrium-90 resin microspheres. *Intl J Radiat Oncol Biol Phys* 2012;82:401–407.

34. Tomlinson JS, Jarnagin WR, DeMatteo RP, et al. Actual 10-year survival after resection of colorectal liver metastases defines cure. *J Clin Oncol* 2007;25:4575–4580.

35. Andreou A, Aloia TA, Brouquet A, et al. Margin status remains an important determinant of survival after surgical resection of colorectal liver metastases in the era of modern chemotherapy. *Ann Surg* 2013;257:1079–1088.

36. House MG, Ito H, Gonen M, et al. Survival after hepatic resection for metastatic colorectal cancer: trends in outcomes for 1,600 patients during two decades at a single institution. *J Am Coll Surg* 2010;210:744–752.

37. Wei AC, Greig PD, Grant D, et al. Survival after hepatic resection for colorectal metastases: a 10-year experience. *Ann Surg Oncol* 2006;13:668–676.

38. Choti MA, Sitzmann JV, Tiburi MF, et al. Trends in long-term survival following liver resection for hepatic colorectal metastases. *Ann Surg* 2002;235:759–766.

39. Scheele J, Stang R, Altendorf-Hofmann A, et al. Resection of colorectal liver metastases. *World J Surg* 1995;19:59–71.

42. Groeschl RT, Pilgrim CH, Hanna EM, et al. Microwave ablation for hepatic malignancies: A multiinstitutional analysis. *Ann Surg* 2014;259:1195–1200.

43. Kingham TP, Tanoue M, Eaton A, et al. Patterns of recurrence after ablation of colorectal cancer liver metastases. *Ann Surg Oncol* 2012;19:834–841.

48. Portier G, Elias D, Bouche O, et al. Multicenter randomized trial of adjuvant fluorouracil and folinic acid compared with surgery alone after resection of colorectal liver metastases: FFCD ACHBTH AURC 9002 trial. *J Clin Oncol* 2006;24:4976–4982.

49. Mitry E, Fields AL, Bleiberg H, et al. Adjuvant chemotherapy after potentially curative resection of metastases from colorectal cancer: a pooled analysis of two randomized trials. *J Clin Oncol* 2008;26:4906–4911.

51. Nordlinger B, Sorbye H, Glimelius B, et al. Perioperative chemotherapy with FOLFOX and surgery versus surgery alone for resectable liver metastases from colorectal cancer (EORTC Intergroup trial 40983): a randomised controlled trial. *Lancet* 2008;371:1007–1016.

52. Nordlinger B, Sorbye H, Glimelius B, et al. Perioperative FOLFOX chemotherapy and surgery versus surgery alone for resectable liver metastases from colorectal cancer (EORTC 40983): long-term results of a randomised, controlled, phase 3 trial. *Lancet Oncol* 2013;14:1208–1215.

57. Adam R, Delvart V, Pascal G, et al. Rescue surgery for unresectable colorectal liver metastases downstaged by chemotherapy: a model to predict long-term survival. *Ann Surg* 2004;240:644–657.

58. Broquet A, Abdalla EK, Kopetz S, et al. High survival rate after two-stage resection of advanced colorectal liver metastases: response-based selection and complete resection define outcome. *J Clin Oncol* 2011;29:1083–1090.

61. Saltz LB, Clarke S, Diaz-Rubio E, et al. Bevacizumab in combination with oxaliplatin based chemotherapy as first-line therapy in metastatic colorectal cancer: a randomized phase III study. *J Clin Oncol* 2008;26:2013–2019.

66. Folprecht G, Gruenberger T, Bechstein WO, et al. Tumour response and secondary resectability of colorectal liver metastases following neoadjuvant chemotherapy with cetuximab: The CELIM randomised phase 2 trial. *Lancet Oncol* 2010;11:38–47.

67. Ye LC, Liu TS, Ren L, et al. Randomized controlled trial of cetuximab plus chemotherapy for patients with KRAS wild-type unresectable colorectal liver-limited metastases. *J Clin Oncol* 2013;31:1931–1938.

71. Karoui M, Penna C, Amin-Hashem M, et al. Influence of preoperative chemotherapy on the risk of major hepatectomy for colorectal liver metastases. *Ann Surg* 2006;243:1–7.

72. Vigano L, Capussotti L, De Rosa G, et al. Liver resection for colorectal metastases after chemotherapy: impact of chemotherapy-related liver injuries, pathological tumor response, and micrometastases on long-term survival. *Ann Surg* 2013;258:731–740.

81. Goere D, Gaujoux S, Deschamp F, et al. Patients operated on for initially unresectable colorectal liver metastases with missing metastases experience a favorable long-term outcome. *Ann Surg* 2011;254:114–118.

83. Blazer DG 3rd, Kishi Y, Maru DM, et al. Pathologic response to preoperative chemotherapy: a new outcome end point after resection of hepatic colorectal metastases. *J Clin Oncol* 2008;26:5344–5351.

88. Chang DT, Swaminath A, Kozak M, et al. Stereotactic body radiotherapy for colorectal liver metastases. *Cancer* 2011;117:4060–4069.

91. Mayo SC, de Jong MC, Pulitano C, et al. Surgical management of hepatic neuroendocrine tumor metastasis: results from an international multi-institutional analysis. *Ann Surg Oncol* 2010;17:3129–3136.

92. Cho CS, Labow DM, Tang L, et al. Histologic grade is correlated with outcome after resection of hepatic neuroendocrine neoplasms. *Cancer* 2008;113:126–134.

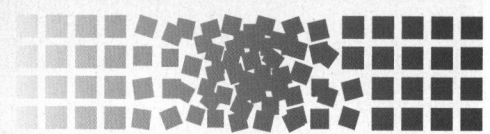

126 Metastatic Cancer to the Bone

Edward Chow, Joel A. Finkelstein, Arjun Sahgal, and Robert E. Coleman

INTRODUCTION

Bone metastases are most frequent in breast and prostate carcinomas, and affect two-thirds to three-quarters of patients with advanced disease from these tumors. In addition, lung, thyroid, and renal carcinoma metastasize to bone in approximately 30% to 40% of cases.[1] Mean survival ranges from a low of 6 months for those with lung carcinoma, to several years for those with bone metastases from prostate, thyroid, or breast carcinoma.[1] If patients have skeletal metastases only, their average survival is even longer.

PRESENTATION

The morbidity associated with metastatic bone disease, often referred to as skeletal-related events (SRE), includes pain that may require opiates, the need for radiotherapy and/or surgery, hypercalcemia, pathologic fractures, and spinal cord compression. The most common symptom is pain. Pain initially may be either a well-localized focus of pain or a diffuse ache, typically worse at night and often not relieved by lying flat. Pain from extremity lesions tends to be well defined, in contrast to spine and pelvic sites, which produce vague, diffuse symptoms. Eventually the pain worsens with weight-bearing activity. Initially, pain results from the physical presence of tumor in the bone; with the release of inflammatory mediators, neuropeptides, and cytokines; as well as elevation of the intraosseous pressure from tumor mass effect, causing irritation of intraosseous and periosteal nerve endings.[2] Functional pain is caused by the mechanical weakness of the bone, which can no longer support the normal stresses of daily activities. Mechanical pain is more typically associated with the focal bone loss within lytic lesions; however, radiographically blastic lesions may also weaken the bone through associated areas of osteolysis that are sufficient to compromise structural integrity. The development of functional pain may be a marker for bone at risk for fracture. Pathologic fractures may be the first sign of metastatic bone disease. In breast carcinoma, as many as 35% of patients with bone disease experience a fracture.[3] Breast, lung, renal, and thyroid cancers have been the most common cancers with pathologic fracture, but even in endocrine-resistant prostate cancer where osteoblastic metastases are typical, annual fracture rates in excess of 20% may be seen.[1]

PATHOPHYSIOLOGY

Historically, Batson[1] described the high-flow, low-pressure, valveless plexus of veins that connects the visceral organs to the spine and pelvis. Recent research has focused on the multistep cellular process of metastases. First, the cancer cell must disengage from its primary site. The loss of expression of E-cadherin, a cell-surface adhesion molecule, has been demonstrated in breast, prostate, colorectal, and pancreatic carcinoma as an early step in cellular disengagement. After invasion of the vascular or lymphatic system, the cancer cell must survive the immune system and then arrest at its final destination. At the distant site, the malignant cell must adhere to the basement membrane, invade the surrounding tissue, induce angiogenesis, and develop into a secondary mass.

However, in addition to these generic steps involved in metastases, tumor cells in the bone marrow require interaction with normal bone cells to establish a metastatic lesion in bone. The growth factor and cytokine expression of the tumor cells leads to an interaction with osteoclasts and osteoblasts, the balance of which determines the nature of the lesion and its corresponding radiographic appearance. Osteoclastic activity has been shown to be increased by tumor expression of interleukins 6 and 11, and parathyroid hormone–related protein.[4] Bone resorption leads to the release of bone-derived growth factors, notably transforming growth factor–beta, that in turn may react with receptors on the tumor cells. This sets up the so-called vicious cycle whereby the stimulation of bone cell activity produces a favorable microenvironment for the neighboring tumor cells and facilitates the metastatic process. The new bone formation associated with osteoblastic lesions has been associated with endothelin-1 and insulin-like growth factor stimulation of osteoblasts, but typically even in osteoblastic lesions there is also an associated increase in osteoclastic bone resorption.[5]

DIAGNOSTIC EVALUATION

Radiographs and bone scans are the first lines of imaging to document the presence or absence of an osseous lesion, and to identify whether these are solitary or multiple lesions. In the spine, plain films classically show absence of a pedicle with the "winking owl sign" (Fig. 126.1).

A computed tomography (CT) scan is the best to define the size of an osseous lesion and to evaluate the extent of cortical involvement. In the spine, CT scan is most useful to evaluate aspects of bony stability as measured by pedicle and/or posterior body wall integrity. These factors are important in establishing risk of burst fracture and for planning and assessing the safety of vertebroplasty as a treatment alternative.[6] CT-guided biopsy can be used for obtaining tissue samples. Magnetic resonance imaging is valuable for evaluating marrow disease and is most sensitive in identifying metastatic deposits in the spine and pelvis. In patients with neurologic compromise, magnetic resonance imaging is best for assessing epidural disease and extent of vertebral involvement (solitary versus multifocal).

THERAPEUTIC MODALITIES

Optimal management requires a multidisciplinary team. Medical treatment, radiation therapy, surgery, and bone-targeted treatment with the bisphosphonates and denosumab are combined depending on the biology of the disease, extent of the skeletal involvement, and the life expectancy of the patient.

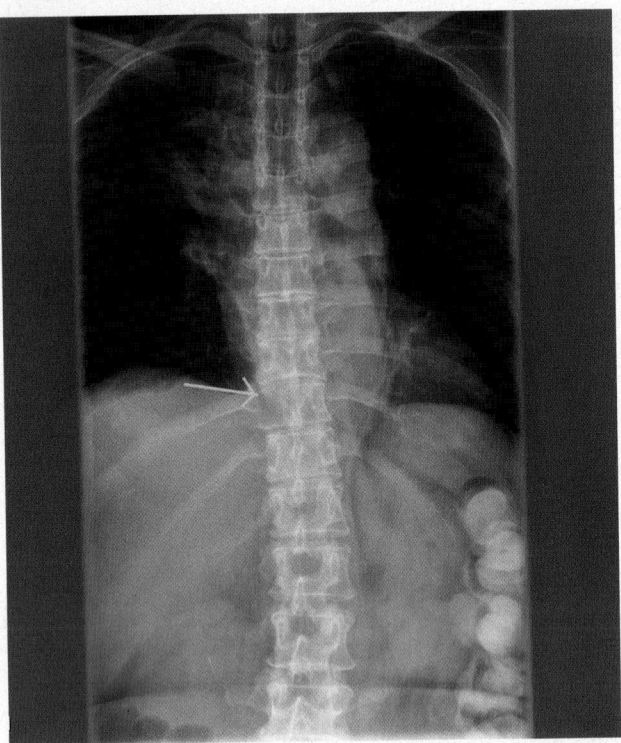

Figure 126.1 Anteroposterior radiograph of thoracolumbar spine. Right-sided T10 pedicle is absent, giving appearance of a winking owl (see *arrow*).

Systemic Therapy

Systemic therapy for bone metastases can be targeted against the tumor cell itself to reduce tumor burden or, alternatively, directed toward blocking the effect of tumor-derived growth factors and cytokines on host cells. Chemotherapy, biologically targeted agents, and endocrine treatments have direct antitumor effects, whereas agents such as the bisphosphonates and denosumab are effective by preventing host cells (primarily osteoclasts) from reacting to tumor products. Systemic therapy, therefore, has either direct or indirect actions. In general, the choice of systemic treatment for metastatic bone disease is based on the same criteria as those used for other metastatic manifestations of the malignancy.[7]

For breast cancer, endocrine therapy is the treatment of choice for the initial treatment of metastatic disease unless the disease is known to be estrogen receptor–negative or there is extensive and/or aggressive visceral disease. Objectively responding patients usually gain relief of symptoms (including bone pain) and might become able to resume their previous activities. Although in general the median duration of response to endocrine therapy is around 15 months, prolonged responses to first-line hormone treatments lasting several years are not uncommon in patients with bone metastases.

There have been many recent developments in cytotoxic and biologic treatments of relevance to the patient with metastatic bone disease from breast cancer. Response in bone to chemotherapy is nearly always only partial, with a median duration of response of 9 to 12 months. Chemotherapy can be more hazardous for patients with extensive bone disease, because of both poor bone marrow tolerance after replacement of functioning marrow by tumor and the effects of previous irradiation. Primary prophylaxis with hematopoietic growth factors may be required to enable chemotherapy to be administered safely.

In prostate cancer, at least 80% of prostate tumors exhibit some degree of hormone responsiveness with a median duration of response of around 2 years. Until recently, treatment to extend survival for castration-resistant prostate cancer (CRPC) was limited to docetaxel. Patients with CRPC tend to be elderly and often of too poor a performance status to receive aggressive systemic therapy. However, the recent introduction of the endocrine agents, such as abiraterone and enzalutamide, and the bone-seeking, alpha particle–emitting radioisotope alpharadin into clinical practice provides well-tolerated additional therapeutic options.

Skeletal morbidity is a major problem in multiple myeloma despite a high rate of response to chemotherapy. Despite the subjective improvement that is seen, bone healing is rare, with lytic lesions persisting despite control of the disease for months or years. Newer agents provide many more options and have transformed the clinical course of multiple myeloma in recent years into that of a chronic disease. Bone involvement in germ cell tumors and lymphoma conveys a worse prognosis, but despite this, cure with chemotherapy is frequent. For relatively chemotherapy-resistant solid tumors such as non–small-cell lung cancer or melanoma, the benefits of current chemotherapy regimens are limited and many patients with skeletal metastases from these tumors derive most benefit from local radiotherapy and bone-targeted agents. However, more effective treatments are emerging, notably the angiogenesis inhibitors in renal cell cancer, and the emergence of a range of targeted treatments for patients with specific mutations (e.g., b-raf in melanoma, epidermal growth factor receptor and alk in lung cancer) that are providing exciting new options for subsets of patients with solid tumors that also involve the skeleton.

Bisphosphonates for Metastatic Bone Disease

Over the past 15 years, bisphosphonates have become established as a valuable additional approach to the range of current treatments. Bisphosphonates are analogues of pyrophosphate, characterized by a phosphorus-carbon-phosphorus–containing central structure that binds to bone and a variable side chain that determines the relative potency, side effects, and the precise mechanism of action.[8] Bisphosphonates bind avidly to exposed bone mineral, and during bone resorption, bisphosphonates are internalized by the osteoclast and subsequently cause apoptotic cell death.

After intravenous administration of a bisphosphonate, the kidney excretes approximately 25% to 40% of the injected dose, and the remainder is taken up by bone where it is retained for months or even years. All bisphosphonates suffer from poor bioavailability when given by mouth and must be taken on an empty stomach, as they bind to calcium in the diet. It is generally accepted that osteoclast activation is the key step in the establishment and growth of bone metastases. Biochemical data indicate that bone resorption is of importance not only in classic "lytic" diseases such as myeloma and breast cancer, but also in prostate cancer.[5] As a result, the osteoclast is a key therapeutic target for skeletal metastases irrespective of the tissue of origin.[9] Although radiotherapy is the treatment of choice for localized bone pain, the bisphosphonates provide an additional treatment approach for the relief of bone pain across a range of tumor types.[9]

Oral Bisphosphonates

The absorption of bisphosphonates from the gut is poor, variable, and dramatically inhibited by food intake. Nevertheless, oral clodronate and ibandronate have been shown in randomized trials to have useful efficacy in breast cancer.[9,10]

Intravenous Bisphosphonates

There is extensive experience with intravenous bisphosphonates in breast cancer, with zoledronic acid, pamidronate, and ibandronate all showing useful clinical activity.[9,10] Comparative data are few but, in a double-blind randomized trial of 1,130 patients with advanced breast cancer, an additional 20% reduction in the risk of SREs was seen with zoledronic acid compared with pamidronate ($p = 0.025$).[11] Ibandronate is licensed in Europe for the treatment of metastatic bone following a placebo-controlled trial of monthly infusions that showed a significant reduction in skeletal-related morbidity.[12]

Intravenous bisphosphonates have become routine clinical management for most patients with multiple myeloma, with zoledronic acid and pamidronate the agents of choice.[11,13] Improved survival with the inclusion of zoledronic acid in first-line myeloma treatment, as well as fewer SREs, has been shown in a large randomized comparison of zoledronic acid to oral clodronate.[14] In advanced CRPC, zoledronic acid was shown to reduce the overall risk of skeletal complications by 36%.[15] Additionally, zoledronic acid significantly reduced the risk for SRE(s) by about 30% ($p = 0.003$) in the management of bone metastases from solid tumors other than breast or prostate cancer.[16]

DENOSUMAB

Denosumab is a fully human monoclonal antibody that binds and neutralizes RANKL with high affinity and specificity to inhibit osteoclast function and bone resorption. Following a single subcutaneous dose, denosumab caused rapid and sustained suppression of bone turnover in patients with multiple myeloma and patients with breast cancer.[17] A subsequent dose-finding phase 2 study defined a subcutaneous 120 mg dose every 4 weeks for phase 3 development.[18] A broad development program in >5,700 patients with metastatic disease has shown superiority of denosumab over zoledronic acid in the time to first SRE in trials encompassing a broad range of solid tumors.[19–21] The hazard rates for first SRE were 0.82 (95% confidence interval [CI] = 0.71 to 0.95),[19] 0.82 (95% CI = 0.71 to 0.95),[20] and 0.84 (95% CI = 0.71 to 0.98),[21] in the trials performed in breast cancer, CRPC, and other solid tumors and myeloma groups, respectively. However, no differences in overall survival or investigator-reported disease progression were found between the two treatment groups in any of the studies.

The safety profiles of denosumab and zoledronic acid are different. Denosumab does not adversely affect renal function, eliminating the need for routine monitoring of renal function. Acute-phase reactions are also less common with denosumab, but hypocalcemia is more frequent.[19–21] As a result, vitamin D deficiency should be corrected and all patients should be encouraged to take calcium and vitamin D supplements throughout the course of their treatment. As with intravenous bisphosphonates, the most important adverse event associated with denosumab in the oncology setting is osteonecrosis of the jaw. This occurs with similar frequency in patients treated with denosumab or zoledronic acid, affecting 0.5% to 1% of patients per year on treatment.[22]

Optimum Use of Bone Targeted Agents in Metastatic Bone Disease

Despite the obvious clinical benefits of bisphosphonates and denosumab, it is clear that only a proportion of events are prevented, while some patients do not experience a skeletal event despite the presence of metastatic bone disease. It is currently impossible to predict whether an individual patient needs or will benefit from a bisphosphonate. Because of the logistics and cost of delivering monthly treatments to all patients with metastatic bone disease, certain empiric recommendations on who should receive treatment are needed. These should take into account the underlying disease type and extent, the life expectancy of the patient, the probability of the patient experiencing an SRE, and the ease with which the patient can attend for treatment (or be

treated by a domiciliary service).[23] The development of an SRE is not a sign of treatment failure or a signal to stop treatment; evidence is now available to confirm that bone-targeted treatments delay second and subsequent complications, not just the first event.

The recent guidelines on the management of metastatic bone disease in breast cancer from the American Society of Clinical Oncology did not recommend one bone-modifying agent (zoledronic acid, pamidronate, denosumab) over another.[24] Although denosumab has some efficacy and convenience advantages, it is much more expensive than zoledronic acid and pamidronate, which are now available as generic formulations. Denosumab or zoledronic acid is appropriate for patients with endocrine-resistant metastatic bone disease from prostate cancer,[25] whereas zoledronic acid or pamidronate are recommended for multiple myeloma.[26] Patients with other tumors and symptomatic metastasis to bone should certainly be considered for treatment with denosumab or zoledronic acid if bone is the dominant site of metastasis, and also if bone is one of multiple involved sites when the prognosis is reasonable (life expectancy >6 months).[9] Bone resorption markers such as N-telopeptide of type 1 collagen may be useful to identify patients at high risk of skeletal complications.[5] Additionally, normalization of bone resorption is associated with improved clinical outcomes including fewer SREs and prolonged survival.[27]

NEW TARGETED THERAPIES IN THE TREATMENT OF METASTATIC BONE DISEASE

A number of targeted agents have entered clinical development. These include radium-223, inhibitors of cathepsin K, an osteoclast-derived enzyme that is essential for the resorption of bone, and Src kinase, a key molecule in osteoclastogenesis. Of all these, radium-223 shows the most promise. Radium-223 is a calcium mimetic that preferentially targets bone metastases and emits high-energy alpha particles resulting in highly localized cytotoxic effects with minimal myelosuppression. In a recent phase 3 study of radium-223 in 921 patients with CRPC and symptomatic bone metastases, radium-223 improved median overall survival by 3.6 months (hazard ratio = 0.70; 95% CI = 0.58 to 0.83; $p < 0.001$) and significantly delayed the time to first symptomatic skeletal event (hazard ratio = 0.66; 95% CI = 0.52 to 0.83; $p < 0.001$).[28]

EXTERNAL BEAM RADIATION THERAPY

Radiotherapy is effective in relieving bone pain, preventing impending fractures, and promoting healing in pathologic fractures. Hematologic or gastrointestinal side effects are usually mild and transient. Numerous randomized trials have been conducted on dose-fractionation schedules of palliative radiotherapy. Despite that, there is still no uniform consensus on the optimal dose fractionation scheme. One of the first randomized studies on bone metastases was conducted by Radiation Therapy Oncology Group (74-02).[29] A total of 90% of patients experienced some relief of pain, and 54% achieved eventual complete pain relief. The trial concluded that the low-dose, short-course schedules were as effective as the high-dose protracted programs. However, this study was criticized for using physician-based pain assessment. A reanalysis of the same set of data, grouping solitary and multiple bone metastases, using the end point of pain relief and taking into account of analgesic intake and retreatment, concluded that the number of radiation fractions was statistically significant related to complete combined relief (absence of pain and use of narcotics). The conclusion was that protracted dose-fractionation schedules were more effective than short-course schedules.[30] This reanalysis was contrary to the initial report, highlighting that the choice of end points are very important in defining the outcomes of clinical trials.[31]

Several large-scale prospective randomized trials were subsequently performed. The United Kingdom Bone Pain Trial Working Party randomized 765 patients with bone metastases to either an 8-Gy single fraction or a multifraction regimen (20 Gy in 5 fractions or 30 Gy in 10 fractions).[32] There were no differences in the time to first improvement in pain, time to complete pain relief, or time to first increase in pain at any time up to 12 months from randomization. Retreatment was twice as common after 8 Gy than after multifraction radiotherapy. There were no significant differences in the incidence of nausea, vomiting, spinal cord compression, or pathologic fracture between the two groups. The study concluded that a single 8 Gy is as safe and effective as a multifraction regimen for the palliation of metastatic bone pain for at least 12 months. The Dutch Bone Metastases Study included 1,171 patients and found no difference in pain relief or the quality of life following a single 8-Gy or 24-Gy dose in six daily radiation treatments.[33] However, the retreatment rates were 25% in the single 8-Gy arm and 7% in the multiple-treatment arm, respectively. In the cost-utility analysis of this randomized trial, there was no difference in life expectancy or quality-adjusted life expectancy. The estimated cost of radiotherapy, including retreatments and nonmedical costs, was statistically significantly lower for the single-fraction schedule than for the multiple-fraction schedule.[34]

One critical review included a systematic search for randomized trials of localized radiotherapy of bone metastases employing different dose fractionations.[35] The authors suggested that protracted fractionated radiotherapy, given over 2 to 4 weeks, results in more complete and durable pain relief. However, two earlier meta-analyses showed no significant difference in complete and overall pain relief between single-fraction and multifraction palliative radiotherapy for bone metastases.[36,37] The meta-analysis reported that the complete response rates (absence of pain) were 33.4% and 32.3% after single-fraction and multifraction radiation treatments, respectively, while the overall response rates were 62.1% and 58.7%, respectively. Most patients will experience pain relief in the first 2 to 4 weeks after radiotherapy, be it single or multiple fractionations.[36] However, the retreatment and pathologic fracture rates were higher in single-fraction treatments.[37]

Since the publication of the two meta-analyses, more randomized trials on bone metastases have been reported. The Radiation Therapy Oncology Group repeated the randomized study in patients with breast or prostate cancer who had one to three sites of painful bone metastases and moderate to severe pain with patient self-assessment.[38] There were 455 patients in the single 8-Gy arm and 443 in the 30-Gy in 10 fractions arm. Grade 2 to 4 acute toxicity was more frequent in the multiple arms (17%) than in the single arm (10%) ($p = 0.002$). Late toxicity was rare (4%) in both arms. The overall response rate was 66%. Complete and partial response rates were 15% and 50%, respectively, in the single-fraction arm compared with 18% and 48%, respectively, in the multiple-fractions arm ($p = 0.6$). Both regimens were equivalent in terms of pain and narcotic relief at 3 months. The single-fraction arm had a higher rate of retreatment (18% versus 9%; $p < 0.001$). Four Norwegian and six Swedish hospitals planned to recruit 1,000 patients with painful bone metastases. Patients were randomized to single 8 Gy or 30 Gy in 10 fractions.[39] The interim analysis indicated that, as in other recently published trials, the treatment groups had similar outcomes. Similar pain relief within the first 4 months was experienced in both groups and this was maintained throughout the 28-week follow-up. No differences were found for fatigue, global quality of life, and survival in both groups.

An updated meta-analysis reporting 25 randomized trials totaling 2,818 and 2,799 randomizations in single-fraction and multiple-fraction arms revealed the overall and complete response rates were 60% and 23%, respectively, in single-fraction

arm versus 61% and 24%, respectively, in multiple-fraction arms, again demonstrating equal efficacy.[40] However, there is some evidence that certain groups of patients would benefit from a protracted schedule. Roos et al.[41] compared a single 8 Gy versus 20 Gy in five fractions for 272 patients with bone metastases causing pain with a neuropathic component. They concluded that a single dose was not as effective as multiple fractions for the treatment of neuropathic pain; however, it was also not significantly worse. They recommended that 20 Gy in five fractions be used as standard radiotherapy for patients with neuropathic pain. However, in patients with short survival, poor performance status, where the cost/inconvenience of multiple treatments was a factor, and in treatment centers with lengthy wait times, single fractions could be used instead.[41]

How, then, are radiation oncologists to prescribe treatment? The answer most likely resides within the clinical circumstances and individual wishes of each patient. There is no doubt that in patients with short life expectancy, protracted schedules are a burden. However, in patients with a longer expected survival, such as patients with breast cancer and patients with prostate cancer with bone metastases only, other parameters need to be taken into account. Because retreatment rates are known to be higher following a single versus multiple fractions, about 25% versus 10%, respectively, patients with good performance status may wish to share in the decision-making process.

What should be an optimal dose for single fraction treatment? A prospective randomized trial on 270 patients with painful bone metastases compared efficacy of 4-Gy or 8-Gy single doses.[42] At 4 weeks, the actual response rates were 69% for 8 Gy and 44% for 4 Gy ($p < 0.001$), but there was no difference in complete response rates at 4 weeks or duration of response between the two arms. It is concluded that 8 Gy gives a higher probability of pain relief than 4 Gy, but that 4 Gy can be an effective alternative in situations of reduced tolerance. Another randomized trial of three single-dose radiation therapy regimens in the treatment of metastatic bone pain consisted of single 4 Gy, 6 Gy, or 8 Gy.[43] The authors confirmed that 8 Gy could be considered as probably "lowest" optimal single-fraction radiation treatment for painful bone metastases, although single 4 Gy should not be easily discarded because of its applicability in specific cases.

Wide-Field or Half-Body External Beam Radiation

Wide-field or half-body irradiation (HBI) differs from localized external beam radiation mainly in the volume of tissues and bone metastases covered as a single treatment field. It is more useful for patients with multiple painful bone metastases. HBI is usually delivered either to the upper half or to the lower half of the body. Single-fraction HBI has been shown in retrospective and prospective phase 1 and 2 studies to provide pain relief in 70% to 80% of patients.[44,45] Pain relief is apparent within 24 to 48 hours, suggesting that cells of the inflammatory response pathway may be the initial target tissue, as tumor cell activities are unlikely to be halted so quickly. Toxicities include minor bone marrow suppression and gastrointestinal side effects such as nausea and vomiting in upper abdominal radiation and may be controlled with ondansetron or dexamethasone.

Pulmonary toxicity is minimal provided the lung dose is limited to 6 Gy.[46] Fractionated HBI was investigated in a randomized phase 2 study involving 29 patients, comparing a single fraction with fractionated HBI (25 to 30 Gy in multiple fractions). Pain relief was achieved in over 94% of patients. At 1 year, 70% in the fractionated and 15% in the single-fraction group had pain control, and repeat radiation was required in 71% and 13% for the single and fractionated group, respectively.[47] Poulter et al.[48] reported results of a randomized trial of 499 patients comparing local radiation alone versus local radiation plus a single fraction of HBI.

The study documented a lower incidence of new bone metastases (50% versus 68%) and fewer patients requiring further local radiotherapy at 1 year after HBI (60% versus 76%). The choice of dose-fractionation schedule for HBI was explored by Salazar et al.[49] among 156 randomized patients. Among the three trial arms of 15 Gy in five fractions over 5 days, 8 Gy in two fractions over one day, and 12 Gy in four fractions over 2 days, the 15-Gy regimen not only provided pain relief as much as the other regimens, but also a longer survival duration in prostate cancer patients.

Reirradiation

As effective systemic treatment and better supportive care result in improved survival, certain subsets of patients have longer life expectancies than before and outlive the duration of the benefits of initial palliative radiotherapy, requiring reirradiation of the previously treated sites.

Among the radiation trials comparing single- versus multiple-fraction schemes, reirradiation rates varied from 11% to 42% following single-fraction and 0% to 24% following multiple-fraction schedules. There are at least three scenarios of "failure" where reirradiation may be considered. Response to reirradiation may be different for each of these scenarios: (1) No pain relief or pain progression after initial radiotherapy, (2) partial response with initial radiotherapy and the hope to achieve further pain reduction with more radiotherapy, and (3) partial or complete response with initial radiotherapy but subsequent recurrence of pain.

Mithal et al.[50] reported a retrospective analysis of 105 patients treated with palliative radiotherapy for painful bone metastases. A total of 280 individual treatment sites were identified, of which 57 were retreated once and 8 were retreated twice. The overall response rate to initial treatment was 84% for pain relief, and at first retreatment this was 87%. Seven of the eight (88%) patients retreated a second time also achieved pain relief. A total of 17 of 23 (74%) patients responded to second radiation that used a number of single-fraction regimens, which was not significantly inferior to 31 of 34 (91%) obtained with more protracted regimens. Jeremic et al.[51] investigated the effectiveness of a single 4 Gy given for retreatment of bone metastasis after previous single-fraction radiotherapy. Of 135 patients retreated, 109 patients were retreated because of pain relapsing, whereas 26 patients were reirradiated after initial nonresponse. Of the 109 patients who were reirradiated for pain relapse, 80 (74%) patients responded (complete response = 31%; partial response = 42%). Among the 26 patients who did not respond initially, there were 12 (46%) responses. The authors concluded that the lack of response to initial single-fraction radiotherapy should not deter repeat irradiation. Toxicity in their series was low and gastrointestinal only. No acute toxicity grade 3 or higher was reported. Pathologic fractures were reported in 3 of 135 (2%) patients and spinal cord compression in 3 of 135 (2%) patients in their series. The same group reported the efficacy of the second single 4 Gy reirradiation for painful bone metastases following the previous two single fractions. The overall response rate of the 25 patients (19 responders and 6 nonresponders to the two prior single fractions) was 80%, with both complete response and partial response being 40%. No acute or late high-grade toxicity (≥3) was observed in their study. No pathologic fractures or spinal cord compression were seen in any of these patients during the follow-up.[52]

The Dutch Bone Metastases Study Group presented the efficacy of reirradiation of painful bone metastases.[53] For patients not responding to the initial radiation who were reirradiated, 66% of patients who initially received a single 8-Gy fraction responded to the retreatment versus 33% of patients who received the initial multifraction regimens. Retreatment for patients with progression was successful in 70% single-fraction patients versus 57% multifraction patients. In general, retreatment was effective in 63% of all retreated patients. A recent intergroup randomized trial on dose fractionations in repeat radiation for painful bone metastases in 850 patients concluded a single 8 Gy appears to be noninferior and less toxic than 20 Gy in multiple fractions with 2-month response rates in evaluable patients of 45% versus 51%, respectively ($p = 0.17$).[54]

SYSTEMIC RADIONUCLIDES

Patients with bone metastases often have diffuse bony disease. Administration of a systemic radionuclide has the advantage of targeting all bony lesions simultaneously, and can be given as a single administration on an outpatient basis. Osteoblastic bone metastases can be detected by a technetium-99 methylenediphosphonate bone scan. Radionuclides react with bone mineral (hydroxyapatite), and the pattern of uptake mirrors that seen on the bone scan. Strontium-89 and samarium-153 are the agents most commonly used in clinical practice; phosphorus-32, rhenium-186, and tin-117 have also been used. These radionuclides emit beta particles with a mean range between 0.2 to 3 mm, thereby minimizing toxicity to surrounding tissue. Retention in the areas of bone metastases is greater than in the normal bone marrow, with a tumor-to-marrow ratio of 10:1. The average time to clinical response is 7 to 14 days, with a median duration of action of 18 weeks. Retreatment is possible, with an interval of 10 to 12 weeks for strontium-89 and 6 to 10 weeks for samarium-153, although a nonresponder is unlikely to respond to subsequent administration. The mechanism of pain reduction is unclear but may include radiation-induced apoptosis of lymphocyte-secreting cytokines and direct cell kill and reduction of mass effect.

Treatment-related toxicity consists mainly of reversible myelosuppression, especially thrombocytopenia. The nadir is 4 to 6 weeks after injection; recovery is completed by 6 to 10 weeks, with severity related to disease burden. Bone marrow toxicity is therefore of concern with the use of systemic chemotherapy. A small percentage of patients (10% to 20%) may experience a pain flare shortly after administration. Contraindications to the use of radionuclides include poor performance status, <2 months' projected survival, extensive soft tissue metastases, platelet count $<60 \times 10^9$/L, recent rapid fall in platelet count even if $>60 \times 10^9$/L, white count $<2.5 \times 10^9$/L, and disseminated intravascular coagulation within 1 month of myelosuppressive chemotherapy and within 2 months of hemibody radiotherapy. Impending or actual pathologic fracture and cord compression are also contraindications for use.

The evidence for use of radionuclides has been reported in several phase 2 and 3 trials. Overall pain reduction rates for the various radionuclides are comparable and similar to localized and hemibody external beam radiotherapy, with an overall response rate of 80% and complete response rate of 20%. The "Trans Canada" study reported on 126 patients with metastatic prostate cancer randomized to strontium-89 or placebo in addition to external beam radiotherapy.[55] Patients receiving strontium showed a significant improvement at 3 months in analgesic use and an improved quality of life. Reduced lifetime requirements for radiotherapy and reduction in development of new painful bone metastases were seen. Hematologic toxicity was acceptable. A lifetime management cost savings of $5,800 in the group receiving strontium-89 was found.[56] A second multicenter trial in patients with prostate cancer compared strontium-89 with either local-field or wide-field radiotherapy and found no significant difference in analgesic efficacy, with a significant increase in time for further radiotherapy and development of new pain sites.[57] Samarium-153 is also licensed for use in the United States and has shown similar efficacy to strontium. Patients with a variety of primary malignancies had an 85% pain response rate, with patients with breast cancer achieving the best palliation. The recent introduction of radium-223 for advanced prostate cancer was discussed earlier.[28]

Controlling Side Effects of Treatment

Radiation treatment planning is the most critical aspect of reducing radiation side effects. Management of the acute effects of radiotherapy requires attentive medical management that prevents expected side effects. Radiation side effects are specific to the area treated. Careful radiation treatment planning that avoids critical structures like mucosal surfaces can prevent most side effects. Patients should be reassured that the unavoidable side effects that they experience will resolve following the completion of radiotherapy. Skin reactions are usually minimal during radiotherapy for bone metastases and are limited only to the radiation portal. Nausea and vomiting, resulting from a radiation portal that includes the abdomen, will usually respond to antiemetic therapy, but ondansetron or dexamethasone also is commonly used, especially if patients have recently received emetogenic chemotherapy. Diarrhea, resulting from abdominopelvic radiation, will respond to antidiarrhea medications such as loperamide. Local irritation from mucositis of the oropharyngeal region may be relieved by soluble aspirin, analgesics, or benzydamine mouthwashes. Secondary infections, like *Candida*, should be treated.

The side effects of electron beam radiation are more limited because they only treat superficial structures like the ribs, skin lesions, and superficial lymph nodes. Underlying structures are spared with the selection of the proper electron beam energy. The most prominent side effect of electron beam radiation is an erythematous skin reaction. Other side effects listed here do not occur with electron beam radiation because the radiation beam does not penetrate to these structures. No side effects, other than a possible flare of pain in the first 2 weeks after administration, are observed with systemic radioisotope therapy because all the radiation is localized to the bone. This is an important consideration for patients who have significant symptoms of the disease or other treatments. Side effects from external beam radiation also are more severe when the radiation fields are large because more normal tissues are treated. Pain flare is common after palliative radiotherapy for osseous metastases.[58] Systemic radioisotopes can have significant advantage over large external beam radiation fields by reducing risk for side effects like nausea and diarrhea.

RADIOTHERAPY FOR COMPLICATIONS OF BONE METASTASES: LOCALIZED EXTERNAL BEAM RADIOTHERAPY FOR PATHOLOGIC FRACTURES

Pathologic and Impending Fractures

Pathologic fractures are handled with orthopedic stabilization whenever possible. Surgery rapidly controls pain and returns the patient to mobility. Elective orthopedic stabilization has reportedly resulted in good pain relief and sustained mobility in up to 90% of patients. Early identification of patients with a high risk of fracture is especially important. A fracture of the weight-bearing long bones can be a devastating event even in a healthy person. Prophylactic orthopedic fixation is often advised to avoid the trauma of a pathologic fracture. The operative procedure has fewer complications and less impact on functional outcome.

In the randomized Dutch Bone Metastasis Study, 14 fractures occurred in 102 patients with femoral metastases. The authors analyzed the pretreatment radiographs of femoral metastases and concluded that fracturing of the femur mostly depended on the amount of axial cortical involvement of the metastases. They recommend treating femoral metastases with an axial cortical involvement of ≤30 mm with a single 8-Gy dose for relief of pain.

If the axial cortical involvement is >30 mm, prophylactic surgery should be considered to minimize the risk of pathologic fracturing or, if the patient's condition is limited, irradiation to a higher total dose.[59]

Although radiotherapy provides pain relief and tumor control, it does not restore bone stability. Postoperative radiotherapy is usually recommended after surgical stabilization of a pathologic fracture. Townsend et al.[60] reported normal use of extremity (with or without pain) in 53% for postoperative radiotherapy versus 11.5% for surgery alone. Second orthopedic procedures to the same site were more frequent in the group that received surgery alone.

Patients who are without visceral metastases and who have a relatively long survival (e.g., >3 months) are more likely to benefit from postoperative radiotherapy. Because the entire bone is at risk for microscopic involvement and the procedure involved in rod placement may seed the bone at other sites, the length of the entire rod used for bone stabilization should be included in the radiation field. When the radiation fields are more limited, instability of the rod, resulting in pain and need for reoperation, can result from recurrent osteolytic metastases outside the radiation portal. When a pathologic fracture has occurred, the primary goal is to provide pain relief. Secondary intentions are to achieve stability and restore function. Unless there are medical contraindications or extremely short life expectancy, surgery is usually recommended. Otherwise, radiotherapy alone may be considered.

Stereotactic Body Radiotherapy of Spinal Metastases

Technological advances in radiation oncology have resulted in the ability to apply stereotactic body radiotherapy (SBRT) to the spine, and the predominant indication has been spine metastases. The Canadian Association of Radiation Oncology defined SBRT as "the precise delivery of highly conformal and image-guided hypo-fractionated external beam radiotherapy, delivered in a single or few fraction(s), to an extra-cranial body target with doses at least biologically equivalent to a radical course when given over a conventionally fractionated (1.8-3.0 Gy/fraction) schedule."[61] For spine metastases, this application represents a major shift in the therapeutic intent as doses such as 16 to 24 Gy in a single fraction, 24 Gy in two to three fractions, and 30 to 35 Gy in five fractions represent two to six times the biologically equivalent dose as those investigated in the conventional radiotherapy literature.[62] With respect to the ideal candidate for spine SBRT, a detailed summary of inclusion and exclusion criteria have been summarized in the American Society for Radiation Oncology International Bone Metastases Guideline.[63]

Although the spine SBRT evidence suggests high rates of local tumor control at >80%[2] and pain control with complete pain relief at ~50%,[64] the data are uncontrolled and a randomized controlled trial (Radiation Therapy Oncology Group O631) is accruing patients with the two arms being 8 Gy in one fraction delivered conventionally and 16 to 18 Gy in one fraction delivered with SBRT.

Beyond the high-dose aspect of SBRT, the aim is to target the gross tumor volume with or without an anatomic clinical target volume while sparing the spinal cord and surrounding normal tissues from the high tumor dose. This is achieved using sophisticated radiotherapy treatment planning and delivery units that allow for intensity-modulated radiotherapy, image guidance, and multiple beams of radiation centered on the target. This is a stark contrast to traditional practice where at least one or two healthy vertebrae beyond the disease is included in a simple one- or two-field treatment, which has the benefit of ensuring the entire target receives the prescribed dose. This fundamental contrast is illustrated in Figures 126.2 and 126.3. There has been progress as to optimal target volume to treat, as described by Cox et al.,[65] that essentially

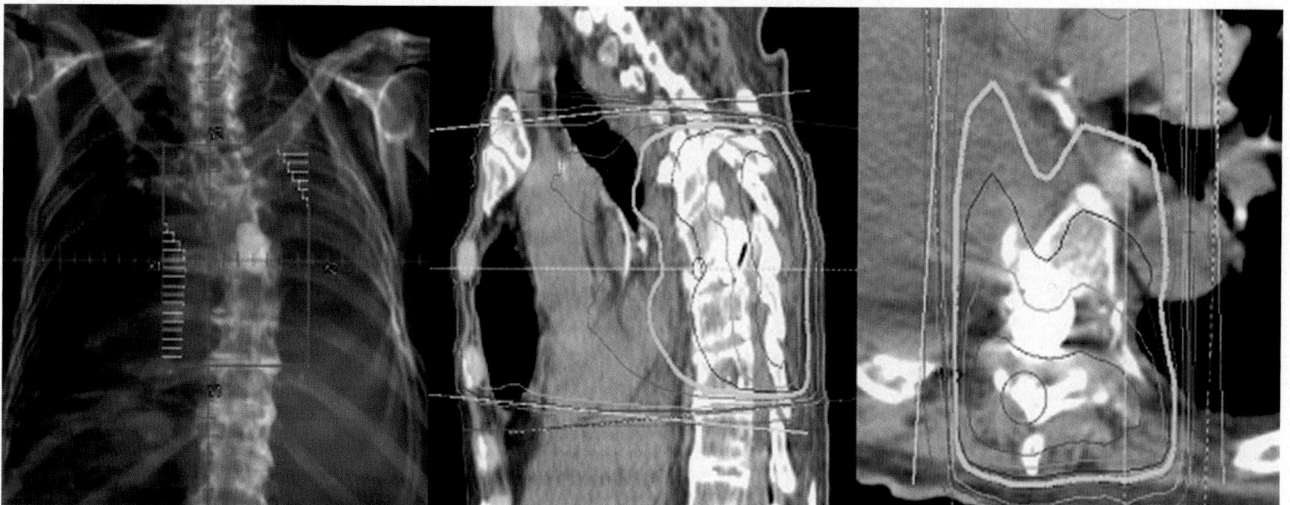

Figure 126.2 A typical radiation field for a seventh thoracic vertebrae metastases where two vertebral bodies above and below the target are included in the radiotherapy field. This patient was treated with 8 Gy in a single fraction, and one can appreciate the entire vertebral column within the field being encompassed by the 8-Gy isodose line in *yellow*.

confirms the practice of taking at-risk spinal anatomy into the target volume. This is critical as it has been shown that the risk of local failure increases if we treat only what we see as gross tumor on imaging.[66]

The treatment of spinal metastases with SBRT is not without risk given the high doses delivered within the bone, millimeters away from tissues such as the spinal cord, esophagus, and kidneys. With respect to acute toxicity, the risk of pain flare has been well documented following conventional radiation,[58] and only recently following spine SBRT. Chiang et al.[67] reported that the majority of patients experienced a pain flare at 68%, and that rescue dexamethasone was effective in reducing the pain response. More importantly, the risk of clinically significant late toxicities with conventional palliative radiotherapy regimens is negligible; however, spine SBRT has resulted in serious adverse events. The most devastating is radiation myelopathy, which can leave the palliative patient paralyzed and is unacceptable considering the goals of treatment for this population. Much progress has

been made, and there are now guidelines for the maximum spinal cord doses that are safe for both the unirradiated and reirradiated patient based on dose-volume histogram analysis of cases and controls.[68,69] What has become more alarming is the risk of SBRT-induced vertebral compression fracture (VCF). A pooled analysis of 410 spinal segments treated with SBRT was recently reported, and the 1-year cumulative incidence of fracture (new or progression of an existing VCF) was 12.4%.[70] From this analysis, we learned that SBRT dose is an independent risk factor, and with ultra-high single fraction doses such as 24 Gy in one dose, the risk of VCF was prohibitive at 39%. When the dose per fraction was kept below 19 Gy, the risk was more reasonable at 10%. The investigators also applied the spine instability neoplastic score criteria to each treated segment and determined that misalignment (kyphotic deformity), preexisting VCF, and lytic tumor were significant risk factors on multivariate analysis. With respect to pathomechanism, it is postulated that radionecrosis is causal as explained by Al-Omair et al.,[71] and a comprehensive

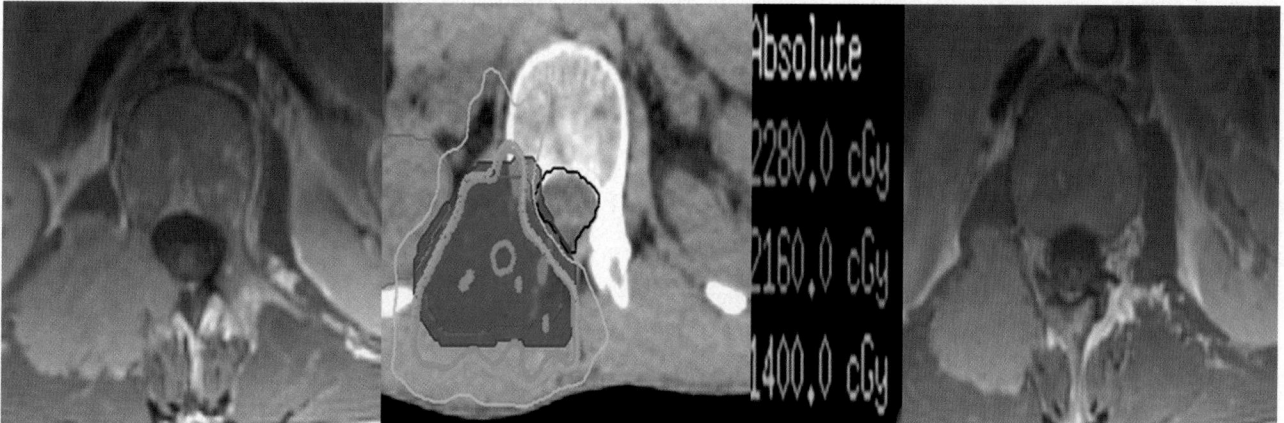

Figure 126.3 A spine stereotactic body radiotherapy treatment plan for a patient with a first lumbar vertebrae hepatocellular paraspinal metastasis that involves the ipsilateral pedicle and lamina. The location of this target is complicated as it is situated between the kidneys. Together with thecal sac sparing, the treatment planning is even more complex. This patient was treated with 24 Gy in three fractions and the high-dose isodose lines in *green* and *orange* conform tightly around the target while the thecal sac and kidneys are spared from the high dose. The lower 14-Gy isodose line skims the left kidney while sparing the spinal cord, hence, reflecting the highly shaped nature of the dose distribution at both the high and lower dose levels. Despite a radioresistant hepatocellular histology, the patient had an excellent response 4 months following therapy with significant regression of the disease, as shown on the right-hand posttreatment axial image.

TABLE 126.1

Summary of Key Issues Comparing and Contrasting Conventional External Beam Radiotherapy with Spine Stereotactic Body Radiotherapy in the Treatment of Spinal Metastases

Conventional External Beam Radiotherapy	Stereotactic Body Radiotherapy
Low BED delivered to the tumor	Two to six times the BED delivered to the tumor
Technique requires at least one or two healthy vertebral bodies to be treated	Targeted treatment to only those areas of disease
Low risk of acute and long-term side effects due to low BED exposure to healthy tissues	Pain flare a high-risk acute event and devastating late toxicities have been reported
Risk of vertebral compression fracture ~5%	Prohibitive risk of vertebral compression fracture with ultra-high single fraction doses (24 Gy in one fraction)
Protracted regimes can include 5 to 20 fractions	Fewer treatments whereby definition SBRT involves one to five fractions
May be less efficacious in radioresistant histologies like sarcoma and renal cell carcinoma	Greater dose may lead to better outcomes for radioresistant tumors
Greater volume of normal tissue exposed to the prescribed tumor dose and potential for greater acute toxicities	Dose to the normal surrounding nontumor tissue much lower than that prescribed to the tumor, which may limit acute toxicities
Short treatment times of 5 to 10 min, which are ideal for the patient in pain	Prolonged treatment times where each treatment takes 45–60 min and requires strict immobilization
If local failure occurs then likely dose- or biology-related as opposed to geographic miss	Potential for geographic miss and if within the epidural space then tumor regrowth can lead to cord compression
Limited doses apply in the retreatment patient, which may preclude efficacy	High doses still possible in the retreatment patient and data suggest efficacy
Standard of care for patients with malignant epidural cord compression with level 1 evidence for efficacy	Contraindicated in the patient with symptomatic malignant epidural spinal cord compression
Indicated for the patient with multiple-level spinal metastatic disease	No more than three consecutive metastases recommended to be treated at once
Deliverable in any radiotherapy department and low cost	Requires sophisticated radiation equipment and quality assurance
Level 1 evidence and well-defined outcomes supporting common palliative treatment regimens	No level 1 evidence to indicate superiority over conventional radiotherapy

BED, biologically effective dose; SBRT, stereotactic body radiotherapy.

review is recommended for the interested reader that also discusses the surgical management of VCF.[72] This toxicity is serious as approximately 50% of patients are then treated with some form of surgical salvage, although the predominant treatment has been a percutaneous cement augmentation procedure.[70,73] It has also been shown that this complication occurs relatively soon after SBRT with a median time to fracture of 2.5 months,[70] which implies that patients should be followed relatively frequently within the first 6 months.

Spine SBRT is still considered an emerging therapeutic option for patients with spinal metastases. It is technically demanding, requires considerable skill, requires close and ongoing follow-up, and there is potential for serious late toxicities that are not otherwise a concern with conventional radiotherapy. Although there is a significant potential to improve long-term pain relief and local control as compared to conventional palliative radiotherapy (Table 126.1), the true value will only become apparent by randomized controlled trials.

Surgical Management of Bone Metastases

Prophylactic stabilization of the appendicular skeleton or decompression of the spine is preferable to a catastrophic unexpected event. Prophylactic or preventative surgery is optimal as it gives clinicians time to optimize patients for surgery from a medical standpoint. The goal of surgery is to allow immediate weight bearing and return to function immediately.[74]

MECHANICAL STABILITY AND FRACTURE RISK

Stability is an important concept to understand. In the spine, this is the ability of the supporting structures of the spine to allow for physiologic loading in order to prevent pain and deformity. Spinal instability may not necessarily result in a catastrophic collapse and paralysis; however with a pathologic burst fracture this can occur. More commonly, the affected spinal segment will develop a gradual loss of architecture resulting in activity related pain. In the appendicular skeleton, instability results in mechanical pain from cortical loss, creating symptoms with use of the extremity or with weight bearing. A pathologic fracture can result when loads applied are greater than the support provided by the normal boney trabeculae. An impending fracture is a bone at risk of fracture if not treated.

The biomechanical effects of osteolytic metastases are of two categories: stress risers and open-section defects.[75] Stress

TABLE 126.2

Mirels System

Variable/score	1	2	3
Site	Upper limb	Lower limb	Peritrochanteric
Pain	Mild	Moderate	Functional
Radiographic appearance	Blastic	Mixed	Lytic
Size	Less than one-third of the cortex	One-third to two-thirds of the cortex	Greater than two-thirds of the cortex

risers are perforations that are smaller than the cross-sectional diameter of the bone that decrease torsional rigidity by 60%. Open-section defects decrease bone strength by almost 90%. Accurate prediction of which metastases are most likely to fracture is essential. Severity of pain and site and size of the metastatic lesion affect risk of fracture. The Mirels system has been used to help predict the risk of pathologic fractures in weight-bearing bones within 6 months (Table 126.2).[76] Risk of fracture increases above a score of 7. Lesions with scores <6 can be treated with radiation; scores >8 should be treated with prophylactic internal fixation.

Lower Extremity

Pathologic fractures of the femur have profound morbidity for the patient as well as considerable issues related to stabilization that would be preventable if treated prior to fracture. A femur at high risk of fracture included cortical bone destruction >50%, lesions >2.5 cm, pathologic avulsion fracture of the lesser trochanter, and persisting pain after radiation. In the absence of these signs, femoral metastases can be treated nonoperatively.[77–79]

The subtrochanteric segment of the femur extends from the lesser trochanter to the junction of the proximal and middle thirds of the diaphysis. This segment of the femur is subjected to very high axial loads of weight bearing and tremendous bending forces because of the eccentric load application to the femoral head. The medial cortex is loaded in compression and the lateral cortex in tension. Ward et al.[80] compared the results of 97 impending fractures of the femur with 85 complete fractures. In the impending group, there was less blood loss (438 ml versus 636 ml), shorter hospital stays (7 days versus 11 days), greater likelihood of discharge home as opposed to an extended-care facility (79% versus 56%), and a greater likelihood of resuming support-free ambulation (35% versus 12%).

For diaphyseal lesions of the femur, the loads are less and the threshold for surgical stabilization is higher. Each case needs to be individualized, taking into consideration the degree of functional impairment, pain, and radiosensitivity of the tumor. The same size lesion in the diaphysis is less of a risk for fracture than in the subtrochanteric region. Recent work at our center on remineralization of bone following radiation may allow us to avoid surgical intervention in the appropriate candidate.[81]

Operative Techniques

Proximal Femur. Impending or pathologic fractures of the femoral neck or head or intertrochanteric region are usually managed with hemiarthroplasty. If there is involvement of the acetabulum, total hip arthroplasty is indicated. Lesions in the intertrochanteric region can also be stabilized with a hip screw and side plate device with consideration for augmentation using polymethylmethacrylate (PMMA) cement. It is imperative to plan preoperatively with a full-length femur radiograph to ensure the plate is able to span the length of disease involvement. With associated diaphyseal or distal femur involvement, an intramedullary device is indicated in order to span the entire length of the femur. Second- and third-generation nails are most commonly used in order to allow fixation into the femoral head (Fig. 126.4).[82]

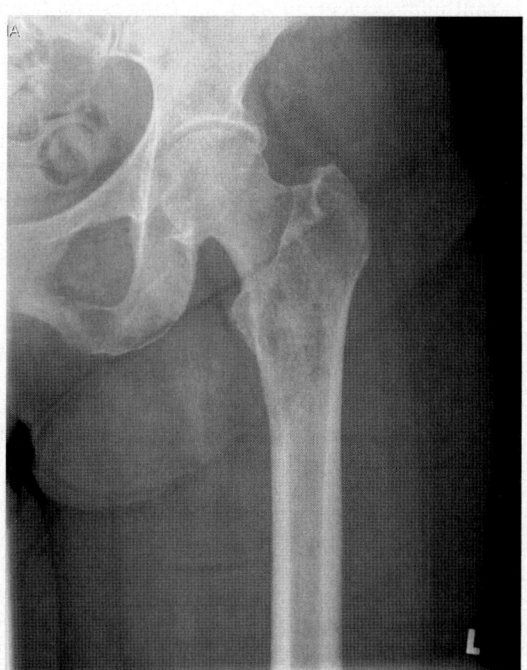
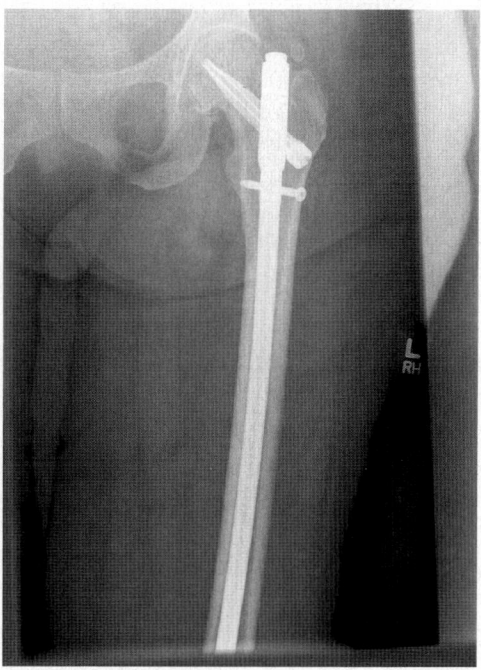

Figure 126.4 (A) Plain anteroposterior radiograph of a lytic metastatic lesion with impending fracture of the peritrochanteric region of the femur. **(B)** Plain anteroposterior radiograph after treatment with reconstruction intramedullary nail providing fixation into the femoral head.

Femoral Diaphysis. Similar to proximal femoral lesions, intramedullary devices are used for fixation. In the case of an impending fracture, a distal vent should be used to allow efflux of marrow contents in order to reduce the risk of fat emboli.[83,84]

Pelvis and Acetabulum. Reconstruction of the proximal part of the femur and the acetabulum is often technically demanding, and hardware failure is not uncommon. The implant is at risk of failure because the forces about the hip are extremely high for most normal activities. Forces on the proximal femur can be 3.5 times body weight during the midstance phase of gait and can increase to 7.7 times body weight during stair climbing.[85,86] Acetabular insufficiency secondary to bone metastases is classified according to location and extent of bone loss. Where the acetabulum is structurally intact, a conventional total hip arthroplasty can be performed. PMMA is often used to provide added support in cases of perforations of the medial wall. When the medial wall has an unconstrained defect, techniques are required that transfer the stress of weight bearing away from the deficiency and onto the intact acetabular rim with use of a protrusion ring. With more extensive bone involvement including both the medial and lateral walls, reconstruction of the acetabular columns requires the use of implants such as Steinmann pins and PMMA to fix the protrusion ring into place.

Preoperative Embolization of Bone Metastases

Metastases from renal cell carcinoma are hypervascular as a result of neovascularization. Other primaries can also be associated with hypervascularity.[87] Historically, stabilization of spinal or appendicular lesions from renal cell carcinoma was associated with excessive bleeding requiring transfusion. Uncontrollable hemorrhage may even result in death. There is growing experience and evidence that preoperative embolization is a safe and reliable method of reducing intraoperative blood loss at the time of stabilization of bone metastases. The methods of embolization include the use of polyvinyl alcohol, coils, and gel foam. The procedure is performed in the angiography suite, and surgery should be performed within 48 to 96 hours of embolization or revascularization will occur.

Roscoe et al.[88] reported on the use of embolization for renal cell carcinoma metastases to the spine before stabilization. Comparing 8 patients who underwent perioperative embolization with 20 patients who did not, the blood loss during stabilization for former group averaged 940 ml compared with 1,975 ml in the nonembolized group. Similar results have been reported by other authors on the safe and effective role of perioperative embolization prior to spinal decompression and stabilization[89,90] (Fig. 126.5).

Upper Extremity

In the upper extremity, the difference in management and patient outcome is less profound between an impending and pathologic fracture. Fractures of the humerus can be managed with plate fixation or with intramedullary devices. Atesok et al.[91] have shown that an unreamed humeral nail provides immediate stability and pain relief with minimum morbidity and early return of function to the arm. Similar conclusions were made by Dijkstra et al.[92] when comparing intramedullary nail with compression plating for humeral pathologic fractures.

Spine

The spine is the most common site of metastatic bone disease. Spinal complications are due to loss of mechanical stability creating pain and spinal cord compression causing paralysis. Neurologic compression occurs due to direct tumor load in the epidural space or from a pathologic fracture causing boney compression or vertebral instability. The goals of spinal surgery in metastatic disease are to preserve or restore spinal stability for pain and to restore or protect neurologic function.

Because of immunosuppression, poor nutritional status, and medical comorbidities, surgery to the spine may be associated with significant complications. Considerations in decision making are life span of the patient, general medical condition, number of spinal levels involved, age, cancer type, and radiation status.[93] The significance of the primary cancer type on survival is well established. After detection by bone scan of spine involvement, Tatsui et al.[94] reported a 1-year survival of 0% and 22% for gastric and pulmonary cancers, respectively, and 78% and 83% for breast and prostate primaries, respectively. In a population-based study, Finkelstein et al.[95] used Cox multivariate regression to model survival as a function of potential predictor variables in a cohort of 987 patients. This study also quantified postoperative complication rates and identified significant risk factors that were associated with poor survival and outcome. There was an overall 1- and 3-month mortality rate of 9% and 29%, respectively. Increasing age and primary lung cancer were significant risk factors for death within 30 days of surgery. For overall survival, each year of advancing age had a 1% increased risk of dying. Lung primary had a 2.65 relative risk of mortality within 30 days.

The effect of a preoperative neurologic deficit on survivorship has been evaluated by a number of authors. In a multicenter study by Argenson et al.,[96] patients with a preoperative deficit had significantly lower mean survival at 1 and 3 years after surgery. We have shown that patients with preoperative neurologic deficits were 71% more likely to get a postoperative infection, likely from the administration of preoperative radiation. Other authors have likewise found increased infection rates and poorer outcomes following surgery in the presence of preoperative radiation.[95,97–99] In 2003, Wai et al.[93] prospectively evaluated the efficacy of surgery in patients with metastatic spinal disease with respect to quality of life using a validated outcome measure specific for palliative patients. This study demonstrated the largest improvement to be in pain following surgery. There were significant improvements in six other domains and trends toward improvement in another one. There was no significant deterioration in any domain. The major benefit of surgery occurs within the first month and remained stable until death or at least 6 months (length of follow-up).

Principles of open surgical techniques and considerations are beyond the scope of this chapter. In general, tumor location within the vertebrae, spinal level, radiation status, neurologic deficit, and number of levels involved affect decision making. Surgery can be from an anterior or posterior approach. Rarely is decompression alone suitable for management of metastatic spinal cord compression. Laminectomy and radiation has been shown to be no better than radiation alone. Unless there is solely posterior epidural disease, posterolateral decompression is required with pedicle screw stabilization.

A more recent approach to management of metastatic spinal disease is percutaneous vertebroplasty (PV) and kyphoplasty. These are minimally invasive approaches and an alternative to open surgery for restoring stability to the spine.[100,101] PV may be applied to a greater number of candidates with pain due to instability. These same patients may not be suitable for invasive spinal surgery because of medical comorbidities, multilevel disease, or having a profound neurologic deficit. PV is performed under intravenous sedation in the radiology suite or in the operating room. Real-time fluoroscopy is used to introduce bone cement (PMMA) into the vertebral body via a parapedicular or transpedicular approach. Commercially available PV kits contain bone cement, mixers, trocars, cannulas, and syringes. PMMA is injected in a

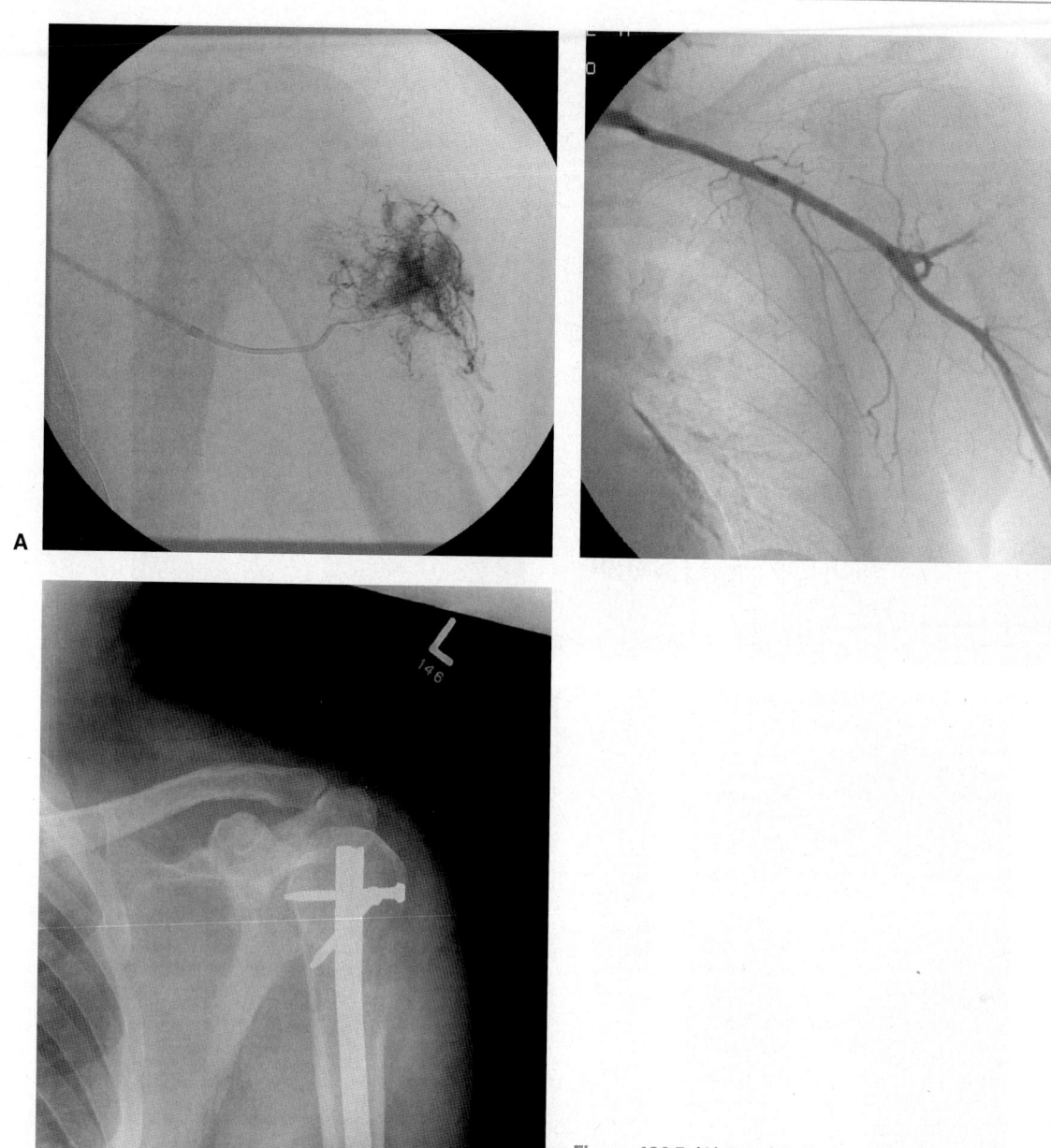

Figure 126.5 (A) Pre-embolization angiogram demonstrating hypervascular renal cell tumor in the proximal humerus. Lytic metastases and impending fracture is present. **(B)** Postembolization angiogram demonstrates significantly reduced neovascularization. **(C)** Postoperative plain radiograph with fracture treated with an unreamed locked intramedullary nail.

semiliquid state such that extravasation and intravertebral pressure is minimized.

Complication rates of PV have been reported to be around 10% in metastatic disease.[102] These complications include cement entering the nerve root foramen or spinal canal, resulting in radiculopathy or spinal cord compression. Systemic complications include embolic events due to marrow fat, tumor fragments, or cement entering the circulation. The use of biplanar fluoroscopy and "live" imaging during injection, the addition of increased concentration of barium to facilitate visualization, intraosseous venogram, limiting the volume of fill, gentle and slow injection, and the use of viscous cement are technical details that have been described to minimize the complications of this procedure.[103] Despite these precautions, extrusion of cement has been commonly reported. The vast majority of

extrusions, however, are minor and do not result in neurologic sequelae.[104]

Vertebroplasty and kyphoplasty more recently have been combined with decompression in an open technique (Fig. 126.6). PMMA is used to provide anterior column support following decompression and in some cases is able to replace the need for posterior instrumentation. In some candidates with or without previous radiation or in the high-risk/poor surgical candidate with multiple-level disease, unifocal decompression can be performed and stabilized in this technique. The concerns for hardware failure as previously noted are eliminated. This minimalistic approach is providing improved outcomes, allowing for greater numbers of patients to be operated on when previously the risks associated with multilevel fixations had unacceptable complication rates.

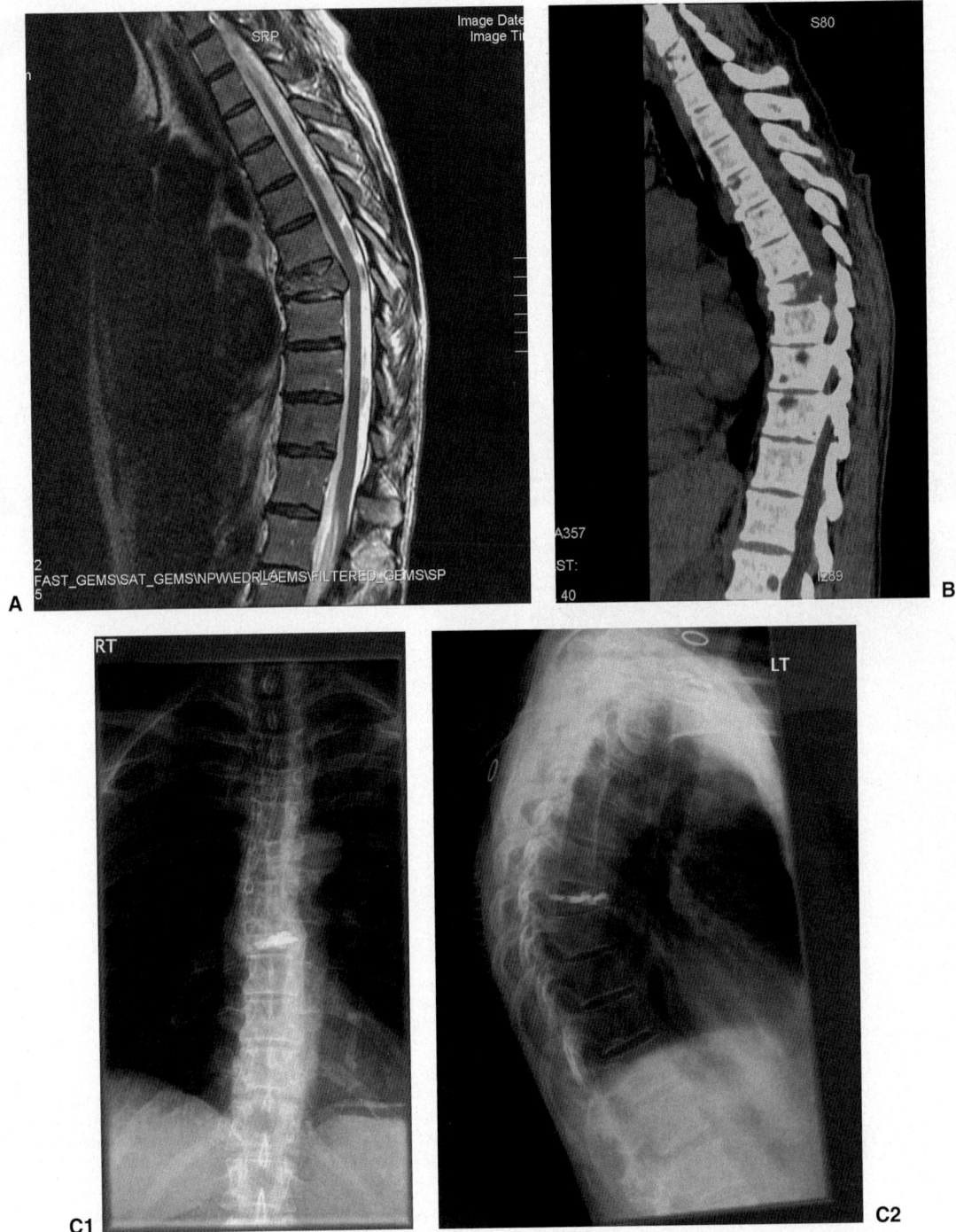

Figure 126.6 (A) Magnetic resonance image of thoracic spine with T8 spinal cord compression. **(B)** Computed tomographic sagittal reformat showing bony destruction of T8 and multiple level metastases. Postoperative anteroposterior **(C1)** and lateral **(C2)** radiographs following open posterolateral decompression and vertebroplasty of T8 vertebra.

SELECTED REFERENCES

The full reference list can be accessed at lwwhealthlibrary.com/oncology.

1. Coleman RE. Clinical features of metastatic bone disease and risk of skeletal morbidity. *Clin Cancer Res* 2006;12:6243s–6249s.
3. Plunkett T, Smith P, Rubens R. Risk of complications from bone metastases in breast cancer: implications for management. *Eur J Cancer* 2000;36: 476–482.
6. Tschirhart CE, Roth SE, Whyne CM. Biomechanical assessment of stability in the metastatic spine following percutaneous vertebroplasty: effects of cement distribution patterns and volume. *J Biomech* 2005;38:1582–1590.

7. Green MC, Hortobagyi GN. Systemic treatments: chemotherapy. In Jasmin C, Coleman RE, Coia LR, et al., eds. *Textbook of bone metastases.* Chichester, England: Wiley; 2005:261.
9. Coleman RE, McCloskey EV. Bisphosphonates in oncology. *Bone* 2011;49:71–76.
14. Morgan GJ, Davies FE, Gregory WM, et al. First-line treatment with zoledronic acid as compared with clodronic acid in multiple myeloma (MRC Myeloma IX): A randomized controlled trial. *Lancet* 2010;376:1989–1999.
16. Rosen LS, Gordon D, Tchekmedyian S, et al. Long-term efficacy and safety of zoledronic acid in the treatment of skeletal metastases in patients with non

small cell lung carcinoma and other solid tumors: a randomized, phase III, double-blind, placebo-controlled trial. *Cancer* 2004;100:2613–2621.

17. Body JJ, Facon T, Coleman RE, et al. A study of the biological receptor activator of nuclear factor-kappa B ligand inhibitor, Denosumab, in patients with multiple myeloma or bone metastases from breast cancer. *Clin Cancer Res* 2006;12:1221–1228.

18. Lipton A, Steger GG, Figueroa J, et al. Extended efficacy and safety of denosumab in breast cancer patients with bone metastases not receiving prior bisphosphonate therapy. *Clin Cancer Res* 2008;14:6690–6696.

19. Stopeck AT, Lipton A, Body JJ, et al. Denosumab compared with zoledronic Acid for the treatment of bone metastases in patients with advanced breast cancer: a randomized, double-blind study. *J Clin Oncol* 2010;28:5132–5139.

20. Fizazi K, Carducci M, Smith M, et al. Denosumab versus zoledronic acid for treatment of bone metastases in men with castration-resistant prostate cancer: a randomised, double-blind study. *Lancet* 2011;377:813–822.

21. Henry DH, Costa L, Goldwasser F, et al. Randomized, double-blind study of denosumab versus zoledronic acid in the treatment of bone metastases in patients with advanced cancer (excluding breast and prostate cancer) or multiple myeloma. *J Clin Oncol* 2011;29:1125–1132.

22. Saad F, Brown JE, Van Poznak C, et al. Incidence, risk factors, and outcomes of osteonecrosis of the jaw: integrated analysis from three blinded active-controlled phase III trials in cancer patients with bone metastases. *Ann Oncol* 2012;23:1341–1347.

23. Aapro M, Abrahamsson PA, Body JJ, et al. Guidance on the use of bisphosphonates in solid tumours: recommendations of an international expert panel. *Ann Oncol* 2008;19:420–432.

24. Van Poznak CH, Temin S, Yee GC, et al. American Society of Clinical Oncology clinical practice guideline update on the role of bone-modifying agents in metastatic breast cancer. *J Clin Oncol* 2011;29:1221–1227.

25. Mottet N, Bellmunt J, Bolla M, et al. EAU guidelines on prostate cancer. Part II: treatment of advanced, relapsing, and castration-resistant prostate cancer. *Eur Urol* 2011;59:572–583.

26. Terpos E, Morgan G, Dimopoulos MA, et al. International myeloma working group recommendations for the treatment of multiple myeloma-related bone disease. *J Clin Oncol* 2013;31:2347–2357.

27. Coleman R, Costa L, Saad F, et al. Consensus on the utility of bone markers in the malignant bone disease setting. *Crit Rev Oncol Hematol* 2011;80:411–432.

28. Parker C, Nilsson S, Heinrich D, et al. Alpha emitter radium-223 and survival in metastatic prostate cancer. *N Engl J Med* 2013;369:213–223.

29. Tong D, Gillick L, Hendrickson F. The palliation of symptomatic osseous metastases: final results of the study by the Radiation Therapy Oncology Group. *Cancer* 1982;50:893–899.

30. Blitzer P. Reanalysis of the RTOG study of the palliation of symptomatic osseous metastases. *Cancer* 1985;55:1468–1472.

31. Chow E, Hoskin P, Mitera G, et al. Update of the international consensus on palliative radiotherapy endpoints for future clinical trials in bone metastases. *Int J Radiat Oncol Biol Phys* 2012;82:1730–1737.

32. Bone Pain Trial Working Party. 8 Gy single fraction radiotherapy for the treatment of metastatic skeletal pain: randomized comparison with multi-fraction schedule over 12 months of patient follow-up. *Radiother Oncol* 1999;52:111–121.

33. Steenland E, Leer J, van Houwelingen H, et al. The effect of a single fraction compared to multiple fractions on painful bone metastases: a global analysis of the Dutch Bone Metastasis Study. *Radiother Oncol* 1999;52:101–109.

34. Van den Hout WB, van der Linden YM, Steenland, et al. Single- versus multiple-fraction radiotherapy in patients with painful bone metastases: cost-utility analysis based on a randomized trial. *J Natl Cancer Inst* 2003;95:222–229.

38. Hartsell WF, Scott CB, Bruner DW, et al. Randomized trial of short- versus long-course radiotherapy for palliation of painful bone metastases. *J Natl Cancer Inst* 2005;97:798–804.

40. Chow E, Zeng L, Salvo N, et al. Update on the systematic review on palliative radiotherapy trials for bone metastases. *Clin Oncol* 2012;24:112–124.

41. Roos DE, Turner SL, O'Brien PC, et al. Randomized trial of 8 Gy in 1 versus 20 Gy in 5 fractions of radiotherapy for neuropathic pain due to bone metastases (Trans-Tasman Radiation Oncology Group, TROG 96.05). *Radiother Oncol* 2005;75:54–63.

42. Hoskin PJ, Price P, Easton D, et al. A prospective randomized trial of 4 Gy or 8 Gy single doses in the treatment of metastatic bone pain. *Radiother Oncol* 1992;23:74–78.

45. Hoskin PJ, Ford HT, Harmer CL. Hemibody irradiation (HBI) for metastatic bone pain in two histologically distinct groups of patients. *Clin Oncol (R Coll Radiol)* 1989;1:67–69.

48. Poulter CA, Cosmatos D, Rubin P, et al. A report of RTOG 8206: a phase III study of whether the addition of single dose hemibody irradiation to standard fractionated local field irradiation is more effective than local field irradiation alone in the treatment of symptomatic osseous metastases. *Int J Radiat Oncol Biol Phys* 1992;23:207–214.

49. Salazar OM, Sandhu T, da Motta NW, et al. Fractionated half-body irradiation (HBI) for the rapid palliation of widespread, symptomatic, metastatic bone disease: a randomized Phase III trial of the International Atomic Energy Agency (IAEA). *Int J Radiat Oncol Biol Phys* 2001;50:765–775.

50. Mithal NP, Needham PR, Hoskin PJ. Retreatment with radiotherapy for painful bone metastases. *Int J Radiat Oncol Biol Phys* 1994;29:1011–1014.

53. van der Linden YM, Lok JJ, Steenland E, et al. Single fraction radiotherapy is efficacious: a further analysis of the Dutch Bone Metastasis Study controlling

for the influence of retreatment. Dutch Bone Metastases Study Group. *Int J Radiat Oncol Biol Phys* 2004;59:528–537.

54. Chow E, van der Linden Y, Roos D, et al. A randomized trial of single versus multiple fractions for re-irradiation of painful bone metastases: NCIC CTG SC.20. *J Clin Oncol* 2013;31:Abstr 9502.

55. Porter AT, McEwan AJ, Powe JE, et al. Results of a randomized phase-III trial to evaluate the efficacy of strontium-89 adjuvant to local field external beam irradiation in the management of endocrine resistant metastatic prostate cancer. *Int J Radiat Oncol Biol Phys* 1993;25:805–813.

58. Hird A, Chow E, Zhang L, et al. Determining the incidence of pain flare following palliative radiotherapy for symptomatic bone metastases: results from three Canadian cancer centers. *Int J Radiat Oncol Biol Phys* 2009;75:193–197.

59. Van der Linden Y, Kroon H, Dijkstra S, et al. Simple radiographic parameter predicts fracturing in metastatic femoral bone lesions: results from a randomized trial. *Radiother Oncol* 2003;69:21–31.

60. Townsend PW, Smalley SR, Cozad SC, et al. Role of postoperative radiation therapy after stabilization of fractures caused by metastatic disease. *Int J Radiat Oncol Biol Phys* 1995;31:43–49.

61. Sahgal A, Roberge D, Schellenberg D, et al. The Canadian Association of Radiation Oncology scope of practice guidelines for lung, liver and spine stereotactic body radiotherapy. *Clin Oncol (R Coll Radiol)* 2012;24:629–639.

62. Sahgal A, Bilsky M, Chang EL, et al. Stereotactic body radiotherapy for spinal metastases: current status, with a focus on its application in the postoperative patient. *J Neurosurg Spine* 2011;14:151–166.

63. Lutz S, Berk L, Chang E, et al. Palliative radiotherapy for bone metastases: an ASTRO evidence-based guideline. *Int J Radiat Oncol Biol Phys* 2011;79:965–976.

65. Cox BW, Spratt DE, Lovelock M, et al. International Spine Radiosurgery Consortium Consensus Guidelines for target volume definition in spinal stereotactic radiosurgery. *Int J Radiat Oncol Biol Phys* 2012;83:e597–e605.

66. Patel VB, Wegner RE, Heron DE, et al. Comparison of whole versus partial vertebral body stereotactic body radiation therapy for spinal metastases. *Technol Cancer Res Treat* 2012;11:105–115.

67. Chiang A, Zeng L, Zhang L, et al. Pain flare is a common adverse event in steroid-naive patients after spine stereotactic body radiation therapy: a prospective clinical trial. *Int J Radiat Oncol Biol Phys* 2013;86:638–642.

68. Sahgal A, Ma L, Weinberg V, et al. Re-irradiation human spinal cord tolerance for stereotactic body radiotherapy. *Int J Radiat Oncol Biol Phys* 2012;82:107–116.

69. Sahgal A, Weinberg V, Ma L, et al. Probabilities of radiation myelopathy specific to stereotactic body radiation therapy to guide safe practice. *Int J Radiat Oncol Biol Phys* 2013;85:341–347.

70. Sahgal A, Atenafu EG, Chao S, et al. Vertebral compression fracture after spine stereotactic body radiotherapy: a multi-institutional analysis with a focus on radiation dose and the spinal instability neoplastic score. *J Clin Oncol* 2013;31:3426–3431.

71. Al-Omair A, Smith R, Kiehl TR, et al. Radiation-induced vertebral compression fracture following spine stereotactic radiosurgery: clinicopathological correlation. *J Neurosurg Spine* 2013;18:430–435.

72. Sahgal A, Whyne CM, Ma L, et al. Vertebral compression fracture after stereotactic body radiotherapy for spinal metastases. *Lancet Oncol* 2013;14:e310–e320.

76. Mirel H. Metastatic disease in long bones: a proposed scoring system for diagnosing impending pathologic fractures. *Clin Orthop Relat Res* 1989;249:256–264.

77. Beals RK, Lawton GD, Snell WH. Prophylactic internal fixation of the femur with metastatic breast cancer. *Cancer* 1971;28:1350–1354.

81. Chow E, Holden L, Rubenstein J, et al. Computed tomography (CT) evaluation of breast cancer patients with osteolytic bone metastases undergoing palliative radiotherapy: a feasibility study. *Radiother Oncol* 2004;70:291–294.

88. Roscoe MW, McBroom FJ, St Louis E, et al. Preoperative embolization in the treatment of osseous metastases from renal cell carcinoma. *Clin Orthop* 1989;238:302–307.

89. Breslau J, Eskridge JM. Preoperative embolization of spinal tumors. *J Vasc Interv Radiol* 1995;6:871–875.

90. Manke C, Bretschneider T, Lenhart M, et al. Spinal metastases from renal cell carcinoma: effect of preoperative particle embolization on intraoperative blood loss. *Am J Neuroradiol* 2001;22:997–1003.

92. Dijkstra S, Stapert J, Boxma H, et al. Treatment of pathological fractures of the humeral shaft due to bone metastases: a comparison of intramedullary locking nail and plate osteosynthesis with adjunctive bone cement. *Eur J Surg Oncol* 1996;22:621–626.

93. Wai EK, Finkelstein JA, Tangente RP, et al. Quality of life in surgical treatment of metastatic spine disease. *Spine* 2003;28:508–512.

95. Finkelstein JA, Zaveri G, Wai E, et al. A population based study of surgery for spinal metastases. Survival rates and complications. *J Bone Joint Surg* 2003;85:1045–1050.

97. Wise JJ, Fischgrund JS, Herkowitz HN, et al. Complications, survival rates, and risk factors of surgery for metastatic disease of the spine. *Spine* 1999;24:1943–1951.

101. Alvarez L, Perez-Higueras A, Quinones D, et al. Vertebroplasty in the treatment of vertebral tumors: post procedural outcome and quality of life. *Eur Spine J* 2003;12:356–360.

102. Chiras J, Depriester C, Weill A, et al. Percutaneous vertebral surgery: techniques and indications. *J Neuroradiol* 1997;24:45–59.

103. Jang JS, Lee SH, Jung SK. Pulmonary embolism of polymethylmethacrylate after percutaneous vertebroplasty: a report of three cases. *Spine* 2002;27:E416–E418.

104. Mousavi P, Roth S, Finkelstein J, et al. Volumetric quantification of cement leakage following percutaneous vertebroplasty in metastatic and osteoporotic vertebrae. *J Neurosurg* 2003;99:56–59.

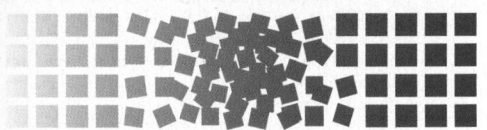

Dao M. Nguyen and Eddie W. Manning, III

MALIGNANT PLEURAL EFFUSION

Malignancy is the second most common cause of exudative pleural effusions and the term malignant pleural effusion (MPE) signifies the identification of cancers cells in the pleural fluid or the pleura of the affected hemithorax.[1] In the absence of positive cytologic or histologic confirmation of malignancy, pleural effusion in association with cancers is termed paramalignant pleural effusion. Over 150,000 cases of MPE are diagnosed annually in the United States.[1] Exudative pleural effusion occurs in 90% of patients with malignant pleural mesothelioma (primary cancer of the pleura with an annual incidence of 3,000 new cases a year in the United States). The vast majority of MPE, however, is caused by metastasis to the pleura with lung and breast cancers accounting for about 50% of cases and lymphoma, gynecologic, and gastrointestinal malignancies responsible for most of the remaining cases while 10% of MPEs have no known primary.[2] MPE is the first presenting sign and symptom in about 10% of patients eventually proven to have metastatic cancers.[2]

The parietal pleura plays a more crucial role than does its visceral counterpart in the homeostasis of pleural fluid in which an equilibrium exists between the rate of fluid production and fluid absorption keeping the intrapleural fluid volume constant. Pleural effusion occurs when there is a disruption of pleural fluid homeostasis with either too much production or too little absorption or more frequently a combination of both. Metastasis of cancer cells to the visceral/parietal pleurae elicits local inflammation/fibrosis, increased permeability of capillaries in pleural surfaces, and physical obstruction of lymphatics that lead to both increased fluid exudation and impaired fluid absorption and the net effect of pleural effusion. Cancer cells may shed into the pleural fluid and be detectable by cytologic examination of the fluid. In many instances, in the absence of positive cytology for malignancy, MPEs are only diagnosed by pleural biopsy at the time of thoracoscopy.

Unilateral pleural effusions in patients with a history of malignancy raise the possibility of MPE. Its presence frequently indicates advanced disease, and the overall prognosis of patients with MPE depends largely on the underlying type of malignancy and the extent of primary disease. Effective chemotherapy exists for lymphoma, breast cancer, or colon cancer affording longer survival for patients with MPE secondary to these cancers than those with MPE from lung cancer. As life expectancy of patients with MPE is often markedly reduced (averaging about 6 to 9 months),[3] the primary goal of its management should be palliation, with an emphasis on employing therapies to prevent reaccumulation of pleural fluid and dyspnea, and those that may be administered with minimal morbidity/mortality and the shortest hospitalization possible.

Clinical Presentation

Moderate to large MPEs are often symptomatic, with dyspnea being the predominant symptom. Chest discomfort can range from dull ache (characterized as heaviness or pressure) to sharp pleuritic pain. Physical examination usually reveals decreased breath sounds with dullness to percussion and diminished tactile fremitus. Tracheal deviation and low cardiac output related to mediastinal compression occasionally may be seen with massive MPEs.

Diagnosis and Evaluation

Radiographic Examinations

As little as 200 ml of pleural fluid, resulting in blunting of the costophrenic angle, can be detected by standard chest radiographs. Upright and lateral decubitus chest radiographs are often performed initially and can demonstrate "free-flowing" pleural effusions. However, MPEs are best assessed radiographically with a computed tomography (CT) scan of the chest performed with administration of an intravenous contrast agent. Particularly in the setting of a newly diagnosed effusion, CT can define fluid loculations, mediastinal and/or hilar lymphadenopathy, pleural-based masses, and any associated parenchymal disease. Complete opacification of the hemithorax occurs in about 15% of MPEs. An opacified hemithorax with mediastinal shift toward the contralateral side indicates massive effusion and raises concern for a tension hydrothorax, which requires urgent percutaneous drainage of the effusion to relieve the intrathoracic pressure. Opacification of the hemithorax from a massive effusion without mediastinal shift is also possible, the etiology of which is the combination effects of pleural fluid accumulation and lung collapse secondary to proximal airway obstruction, or mediastinal fixation by malignant lymphadenopathy, or a diffuse malignant process involving the parietal pleura thus restricting mediastinal movement.

Invasive Diagnostic Maneuvers

After appropriate radiographic assessment of a newly presenting effusion, thoracentesis should be performed to obtain fluid for biochemical and cytologic analyses, to relieve symptoms, and to determine the extent of lung re-expansion following pleural fluid drainage. When a free-flowing effusion is found, thoracentesis can be safely performed at the level of the sixth or seventh intercostal space posteriorly. In the presence of a large pleural effusion occupying >50% of the pleural cavity, gradual drainage of the fluid, vis-à-vis smaller volumes incrementally over time, has traditionally been advocated to avoid re-expansion pulmonary edema (RPE) and subsequent respiratory insufficiency.[4] However, the overall incidence of clinically significant RPE is low and thoracic surgeons routinely remove >1.5 L of pleural effusion without serious sequelae during thoracoscopic procedures to treat various conditions. The widespread availability of small-bore catheters (8-Fr to 14-Fr "pigtail" catheters, which are named for the formation a curve tip after removal of the inner metal stylet once inserted to prevent dislodgement) and their ease of insertion under local anesthetic at the bedside have replaced the use of needle thoracentesis as the initial diagnostic/therapeutic maneuver in the management of pleural effusion including MPE. Slow fluid drainage and gradual expansion of the lung following placement of a small-bore pigtail catheter over minutes are safe and not associated with RPE in our experience. If the pleural fluid collection is loculated, however, ultrasound or CT guidance may be necessary to direct drainage of accessible portions of the effusion. Intrapleural fibrinolytic therapy using recombinant tissue plasminogen activator may be required to facilitate drainage (chemical decortication) and expansion of the lung.

If the diagnosis of MPE has not been previously confirmed, pleural fluid should routinely undergo biochemical analysis, cell counts, cultures, and cytopathologic examination. Frequently, pleural fluid from an MPE is blood-tinged or grossly hemorrhagic because of disruption of capillaries or venules by direct tumor invasion or cytokine-mediated increased vascular permeability resulting in erythrocyte diapedesis. MPEs are typically hypercellular, populated with leukocytes (predominantly lymphocytes and monocytes), reactive mesothelial cells, and exfoliated tumor cells. Identification of malignant cells within the cellular component of the effusion fluid (either via cell smears or cytospin cell blocks) or from a pleural biopsy specimen is diagnostic of the malignant nature of the pleural effusion.

Initial cytology from the pleural fluid is positive in approximately 66% of patients with MPE. If initial cytology has negative results, repeat thoracentesis can be performed (no longer a common practice) or the patient may proceed directly to thoracoscopy if clinical conditions permitted for both diagnostic and therapeutic intents (a favored approach). Repeat thoracentesis can improve the yield of confirming the diagnosis of MPE in an additional 20% of cases.[5] Thoracoscopy performed via direct pleuroscopy under local anesthesia with intravenous sedation or with video assistance under general anesthesia has a diagnostic yield of nearly 100% for malignant disease involving the pleura.[6] Thoracoscopy has obviated the need for "blind" pleural biopsy as a diagnostic procedure for MPE.

Management and Treatment

Because advanced disease states often lead to the development of MPE, the over arching treatment goal should be palliation via selecting therapeutic options associated with the least morbidity and greatest preservation of quality of life for the patient. The initial steps in the management of malignant effusions should be focused on confirming a diagnosis of MPE, within reasonable measures, and relieving to the extent possible the degree of symptoms associated with the newly identified pleural effusion. If the patient is asymptomatic from a respiratory standpoint and the corresponding effusion is small in size in a patient eligible to continue further effective anticancer treatment, then it may be prudent to closely observe the patient for the onset of pulmonary symptoms, deferring drainage of the effusion to a later time point, and thus avoiding delay to further anticancer therapy. In patients with symptomatic or recurrent malignant effusion despite prior drainage procedures, therapeutic intervention is warranted and the optimal choice of palliative treatment is primarily dependent on the performance status of the patients as measured by Eastern Cooperative Oncology Group or Kanofsky scores, the life expectancy, patient's preference, and most importantly whether full lung re-expansion can occur after evacuation of the effusion to restore normal apposition of the visceral and parietal pleurae. The goal of therapy for MPE is complete evacuation of the pleural effusion and prevention of recurrence by means of inducing symphysis of the parietal and visceral pleurae (pleurodesis) using sterile talc. Therapeutic interventions for MPE include thoracentesis, tube thoracoscotomy (large-bore [28-Fr to 32-Fr] or small-bore [8-Fr to 14-Fr] pleural tubes) with or without transcatheter pleurodesis, indwelling tunneled pleural catheter (TPC), thoracoscopy and talc pleurodesis (lung expansion to fill >90% of pleural cavity), or placement

of tunneled catheter (trapped lung with residual pleural space) and rarely pleural decortication (mainly for malignant pleural mesothelioma).

Thoracentesis

Thoracentesis, in addition to being the initial diagnostic procedure for patients with pleural effusion including MPE, is an appropriate treatment for patients with very limited life expectancy or who cannot tolerate more invasive procedures. However, recurrent effusions occur in virtually every cases of MPE following thoracentesis alone and hence this is not a definitive therapeutic option. In general, instillation of chemical pleurodesis agents into the chest without the placement of a pleural drainage catheter is ineffective because residual or reaccumulating pleural fluid will dilute the concentration of the sclerosing agent, thus diminishing its irritant effects on the pleura. Loculated effusions may also form after such treatment, making subsequent definitive therapy of the pleural effusion more complicated. In select patients, particularly those with chemotherapy-responsive malignancies such as breast cancer, presenting with MPE as the initial manifestation, thoracentesis alone followed by immediate systemic chemotherapy may successfully treat the pleural space as well, obviating the need for more invasive procedures. However, the majority MPEs require additional intervention to prevent recurrence.

Complex multiloculated MPEs can pose a therapeutic challenge as they are frequently refractory to complete drainage by thoracentesis or chest tube drainage and thus unsuitable for percutaneous chemical pleurodesis. Some have reported that intrapleural instillation of fibrinolytics such as streptokinase, urokinase, or recombinant tissue plasminogen activator for loculated MPE can be effective in promoting lysis of fibrinous septations and facilitating complete pleural drainage and ultimately successful pleurodesis.[7] This noninvasive approach should be reserved for those patients with poor performance status or who may not tolerate surgical procedures to take down pleural loculations.

Tube Thoracostomy Pleurodesis

Following thoracentesis and confirmation of lung re-expansion, the pleural space should be completely evacuated with a large-bore chest tube (28-Fr or 32-Fr) or pleural catheter (preferably 14-Fr pigtail catheter) to allow for full apposition of the visceral and parietal pleurae. Recurrent effusions occur in 60% to 100% of patients following chest tube drainage alone.[8] Chemical pleurodesis is a preferred treatment for patients with MPE, and its efficacy is dependent on (1) complete drainage of the pleural space and full re-expansion of the lung to allow for apposition of the pleural surfaces, and (2) instillation of an effective sclerosing agent into the pleural space and retention of this agent in the chest for several hours to induce an intense intrapleural inflammatory response and symphysis of pleural surfaces and practically obliterate the pleural space. Once complete drainage is achieved (as confirmed by chest radiograph), the sclerosing agent (suspended or dissolved in 50 ml of normal saline) is instilled into the pleural space via the pleural catheter. The tube is then clamped for up to 4 hours to allow for retention of the sclerosant within the pleural space. Although many practitioners rotate the patient's positioning in bed (lateral decubitus, supine, and prone) to enhance distribution of the sclerosant inside the pleural cavity, there is a paucity of objective data to indicate such maneuvers are necessary for successful pleurodesis.[9] Concurrent intrapleural administration of lidocaine 3 mg/kg (up to 250 mg total) and the sclerosant of choice is recommended, as significant pleuritic chest pain occurs in 7% to 40% of patients having chemical pleurodesis as shown with talc or doxycycline, respectively.[10] Pain, discomfort, and anxiety associated with pleurodesis performed at bedside may also be alleviated with judicious use of intravenous sedatives and narcotics in a monitored setting. Subsequently, the tube is unclamped and the chest drain is connected to suction until the daily drainage is <150 ml, at which point the chest tube can be removed from the patient. This method of treatment requires hospitalization. With regards to whether the size of chest tube used for pleurodesis effect outcome, recent studies involving small numbers of patients have indicated that pigtail catheter drainage and chemical pleurodesis may be as successful as the more traditional chest tube–pleurodesis approach and associated with less discomfort and acceptable results.[11]

Video-Assisted Thoracoscopic Surgery

Thoracoscopic surgery for MPE is performed under either general anesthesia or intravenous sedation/local anesthetics without the need for single lung ventilation. The advantages of thoracoscopy include rapid and complete drainage of pleural fluid, breakdown of fibrinous septations, evaluation for lung entrapment, biopsy of abnormal parietal pleura, and enhanced distribution of chemical pleurodesis via talc insufflation. Video-assisted thoracoscopic surgery (VATS) can simply be performed using a single 1-cm thoracic port site with intermittent apneas for lung deflation using an operating thoracoscope, whereas both pleural biopsy and talc insufflation can be accomplished through the inline working channel of the thoracoscope. If trapped lung is detected, an indwelling tunneled catheter can be placed when the catheter enters the pleural cavity through the camera port. While VATS can be performed rapidly and safely with minimal morbidity for many patients with MPE and with acceptable performance status (Eastern Cooperative Oncology Group 0 to 2), its use is contraindicated in more debilitated patients as other less invasive options are available.

Pleurodesis Agents

Many chemicals have been used to induce pleural symphysis to treat exudative pleural effusions including MPE. Only a few sclerosants (i.e., doxyclycline, beleomycin, and talc) have been extensively evaluated in both randomized and nonrandomized clinical studies for their efficacy as pleurodesis agents; these are further discussed in detail in the following text for academic interests. All sclerosants share a common mechanism of inducing pleurodesis by causing intense pleural inflammation and subsequent adhesive fibrosis of the parietal and visceral pleurae. Among these, only bleomycin is known to possess antitumor activity. Overall, talc is the most frequently used drug to date because it is a safe, effective, and least expensive sclerosing agent. Recent survey of >800 physicians who collectively performed >8,000 pleurodeses annually indicated that the majority preferred talc as the sclerosing agent of choice.[12]

Tetracycline and Doxycycline. Tetracycline has been extensively used as a sclerosant to treat pleural effusions of benign and malignant etiologies because of its efficacy, low cost, and safety. However, tetracycline is no longer commercially available for pleurodesis. The semisynthetic antibiotics, doxycycline and minocycline, are currently used in place of tetracycline in the United States. Response rates range from 67% to 88% following doxycycline pleurodesis.[13] Side effects are similar to those observed with tetracycline, but most patients require repeated doxycycline instillations for successful pleurodesis. Only 15% of patients responded to a single treatment, and 9% required more than four instillations. Doxycycline is administered intrapleural as 500 mg in 100 ml of normal saline; also, doxycycline is light sensitive and care must be taken to avoid exposure of the drug to ambient light.

Bleomycin. Intrapleural administration of bleomycin (60 to 120 U) achieves pleurodesis in about 65% of patients with MPE (range, 62% to 81%).[8,14] Intrapleural bleomycin is well tolerated and associated with few side effects. In one multicenter randomized trial, bleomycin was found superior to tetracycline for pleurodesis; 70% of patients treated with bleomycin had successful control of

their MPE compared with only 47% of patients treated with tetracycline.[11] Unfortunately, bleomycin can be considerably more expensive than its alternatives. Bleomycin has been compared with the less expensive talc in one prospective randomized study of 29 women with MPE secondary to breast cancer—all 10 patients (100%) treated with talc had complete control of their MPE compared with 10 of 15 patients (67%) receiving bleomycin.[14]

Talc. Asbestos-free, gas-sterilized, or heat-sterilized talc may be administered via chest tube as slurry (4 to 5 g in 50 or 100 ml of normal saline), or insufflated as aerosolized powder (4 to 6 g) during thoracoscopy or thoracotomy.[15] Talc pleurodesis is highly effective with overall response rates ranging from 80% to 100%.[16–18] Viallat and colleagues[18] reported on thoracoscopic talc poudrage (dusting of powder) pleurodesis for MPE in 360 cases (88 patients with mesothelioma and 272 individuals with other malignancies). Approximately 3 to 4.5 g of heat-sterilized asbestos-free talc was insufflated via atomizer during thoracoscopy. Pleurodesis was successful in 90% of 327 evaluable patients at 1 month, and 82% of individuals had lifelong pleurodesis. Talc has been consistently shown to be superior to other commonly used sclerosing agents (tetracycline, doxycycline, or bleomycin).[16–18] Many single-institution studies have similarly demonstrated the effectiveness of talc pleurodesis either by thoracoscopic insufflation of dry talc to the pleural cavity or by intrapleural instillation of talc slurry (TS) via chest tubes, but controversies still exist with respect to the cost-effectiveness and the clinical efficacy of each method. A random-assignment phase 3 intergroup clinical trial led by the Cancer and Leukemia Group B (9334) was initiated in 1993 to address this question.[19] The primary end point was 30-day freedom from radiographic MPE recurrence in surviving patients whose lungs initially re-expanded >90%. A total of 501 patients were accrued to this study that compared the efficacy, cost-effectiveness, and quality of life of talc pleurodesis for MPE using either TS via chest tube or thoracoscopic talc insufflation (TTI). There was no difference between study arms in the percentage of patients with successful 30-day outcome (TS 71% versus TTI 78%; $p = 0.169$). However, a subgroup of patients with primary lung or breast cancer had higher success with TTI than with TS (82% versus 67%; $p = 0.022$). The 30-day survival rates were similar in both groups and respiratory complications were greater in the TTI group (13.5%) compared with TS group (5.6%; $p = 0.007$). Quality-of-life measurements demonstrated less fatigue with TTI than TS. Patient ratings for comfort and safety were also higher for TTI, but there were no differences on perceived value or convenience of the procedure. A prospective comparative analysis involving 109 patients with MPEs (77 secondary to breast or lung cancer) of talc poudrage by thoracoscopy (72 patients, 66%) versus TS pleurodesis via 20-Fr chest tube performed at the bedside (37 patients, 33%) demonstrated that 82% of patients having thoracoscopic talc poudrage had lifelong pleurodesis compared to 62% of patients having TS ($p = 0.023$). There was no procedure-related mortality, and both techniques had similar incidences of morbidities, mainly pleuritic pain and fever.[20] The authors concluded that thoracoscopic talc pleurodesis was significantly more effective than chest tube TS. Collective review by Tan and colleagues[21] summarized the current practice of pleurodesis for MPE: talc is associated with less recurrence compared to other sclerosing agents; there is no difference in the effectiveness of tube pleurodesis via small- or large-bore pleural catheters; and TTI is associated with less recurrence than bedside TS pleurodesis via chest tube.[21] The most commonly reported adverse effects of talc pleurodesis are fever (16%) and pain (7%), and less common complications include empyema (thus the common clinical practice of administering empiric broad-spectrum antibiotic prior to talc pleurodesis), pneumonitis (similar to acute respiratory distress syndrome), and respiratory failure.[22] The deleterious pulmonary effects of talc appear related to the use of small rather than large particle–sized talc. Small particle-sized talc (<15 micron) is associated with increased pulmonary inflammation, damage, and impaired gas exchange while large particle–sized talc (>15 micron) is not.[22] Thus, modern formulations of medicinal grade sterile size-calibrated talc should be considered safe in the treatment of MPE.

Indwelling Tunneled Pleural Catheter

Another treatment option for MPE independent from chemical pleurodesis is the use of indwelling TPC. Two types of TPC are approved for clinical application, yet the one manufactured by Denver Biomedicals Inc., Golden, CO (PleurX), is the current industry standard for TPC. The other type of TPC is the Aspira pleural drainage system (Bard Access System, Salt Lake City, UT). Both catheters can be inserted percutaneously and tunneled subcutaneously under local anesthesia and mild intravenous sedation, which can be performed on an inpatient or outpatient basis. The external end of the PleurX catheter has a unidirectional valve to allow for egress of pleural fluid when desired but prevents the inflow of air into the pleural space. Vacuum bottles are connected to the catheter for intermittent drainage of the pleural effusion. The Aspira catheter is connected to a collection bag with a pump in-line. The patient squeezes the pump to initiate pleural fluid drainage to the bag, the flow of which is aided by gravity. The TPC is particularly indicated when the lung cannot re-expand fully to achieve pleural surface apposition despite complete drainage of an effusion, and in such cases pleurodesis is unlikely to be successful irrespective of the chosen sclerosant or approach to pleurodesis. The use of TPC to treat MPE has increased steadily in the last 15 years. Multiple large case series[23–25] and a collective review[26] demonstrated 90% of patients experienced symptomatic relief and required no further intervention. Spontaneous durable pleurodesis occurs in about 45% (28% to 58%) of MPE treated with TPC regardless of the status of lung expansion, and the catheter can be removed without risk of recurrence (median 45 days after insertion).[23–26] The authors have observed pleurodesis in patients with MPE with trapped lung and small residual pleural space (<30% of pleural space volume) who were selectively treated with TPC and eventually had the catheter removed. Complications of TPC include empyema (3.8%), catheter-related complications (3.7%), symptomatic loculations (8%), and cellulitis (3.4%). The successful use of TPC requires a committed third-party payer, patient cooperation, the existence of infrastructure support systems in the community to manage frequent fluid drainage as well as the availability of supplies and health-care providers. Our personal experience is that the majority of patients rely on visiting nurses to perform drainage and catheter maintenance at home, and the initial acceptance of this device decreases significantly over time.

The first prospective multi-institutional random-assignment clinical trial comparing the efficacy of the PleurX pleural catheter versus chest tube doxycycline pleurodesis (not the more superior sclerosing agent talc) for recurrent symptomatic MPE in 144 patients was conducted by Putnam and colleagues (randomization ratio of 2:1, 99 patients with indwelling catheter, 45 patients with doxycycline pleurodesis).[27] The two groups in the study were equivalent with respect to performance status or initial dyspnea scores. After treatment, both groups showed similar improvements of respiratory symptoms and had similar morbidity. Because the study treatments differed markedly between the two arms, the most meaningful measure of success is the long-term absence of recurrent pleural effusion. In this study, there was no difference in the numbers of late failure as defined by recurrence of MPE between treatment groups (13% for pleural catheter group and 21% for doxycycline group, $x^2 = 0.23$; $p = 0.631$). This study is the first to demonstrate that TPC is as safe and effective as chest tube doxycycline pleurodesis but requires less hospitalization (median 1 day versus 6.5 days for tube pleurodesis). A small phase 3 random-assignment clinical trial comparing TPC versus bedside talc pleurodesis (Cancer and Leukemia Group B 30102) for MPE ($n = 57$) demonstrated that TPC achieved superior palliation of unilateral MPE than tube talc pleurodesis, especially in patients

with trapped lung.[28] A patient-centered approach was taken whereby patients with MPE requiring intervention together with their physicians selected TPC versus talc pleurodesis (chest tube or thoracoscopy).[29] While safety profiles and symptom control were similar in both groups, TPC was associated with shorter hospital stay and less re-intervention.[29] Such observation was substantiated by the randomized controlled Therapeutic Intervention in Malignant Pleural Effusion Trial comparing TPC and chest tube talc pleurodesis.[30] Freeman and colleagues[31] performed propensity-matched comparison of thoracoscopic talc pleurodesis or thoracoscopic placement of TPC for MPE. They noted equal efficacy of symptom control by both techniques, yet TPC afforded shorter hospitalization and faster initiation of systemic therapy. A single-institution retrospective analysis of the treatment outcomes of TPC versus thoracoscopic talc pleurodesis ($n = 109$, 59 had TPC and 50 had VATS talc pleurodesis) demonstrated that TPC was associated with shorter postprocedure hospital stay and lower rates of re-intervention for pleural effusion.[32] Long-term TPC is therefore an effective and economical palliative measure for recurrent MPE refractory to pleurodesis or those associated with incomplete lung re-expansion and can decrease the overall in-hospital time for many patients with cancer. Puri and colleagues[33] provided a cost-effectiveness analysis of the treatment modalities of MPE (repeated thoracentesis, bedside tube talc pleurodesis, TPC, and VATS talc pleurodesis) using sophisticated modeling methodology. They demonstrated that TPC is the preferred treatment for patients with MPE with limited survival (<3 months), whereas bedside talc pleurodesis is the most cost-effective treatment for patients with MPE with more prolonged (12 months) survival. All these studies confirm the initial report by Putnam and colleagues[27] that TPC is a useful treatment modality for MPE. None of these studies, however, address the direct cost and quality-of-life assessment associated with postdischarge care of the indwelling catheter. Talc pleurodesis, while associated with longer hospital stay and slightly higher treatment-related morbidities, has a higher rate of durable pleurodesis (>80% for thoracoscopic talc pleurodesis versus about 50% for TPC) and requires no prolonged outpatient care.

Practical Treatment Algorithm for the Management of Malignant Pleural Effusion

Following the diagnosis of MPE, the clinician needs to determine the best treatment option of the patient. There is no "one-size-fits-all" therapy in the management of MPE. Each patient's presentation and underlying malignancy is unique and requires a personalized approach. This starts with assessment of the patient's performance status, estimated survival, expectations, availability of family and community support, as well as insurance status. Patients with marginal performance status should have pigtail catheter and bedside talc pleurodesis or PleurX catheter if there is failed initial talc pleurodesis or the presence of trapped lung. Patients with acceptable performance status, especially in the absence of cytologic diagnosis of MPE, should be offered VATS for pleural biopsy and confirmation of pleural metastasis and talc pleurodesis if lung expands or PleurX if lung is trapped. Patients without access to outpatient care should not have PleurX catheter placement unless such a device is absolutely indicated (recurrence MPE after talc pleurodesis/trapped lung) and should have talc pleurodesis preferably by thoracoscopic technique (Fig. 127.1).

MALIGNANT PERICARDIAL EFFUSION

Malignancy is one of the most common causes of pericardial effusion in the Western world.[34] Pericardial effusion in patients with current or past history of malignancy can be directly caused by the malignancy itself (contiguous extension or metastasis to the pericardium evidenced by identification of cancer cells in the pericardial fluid and/or in the pericardium) or due to inflammatory process such as benign idiopathic pericarditis or radiation-induced

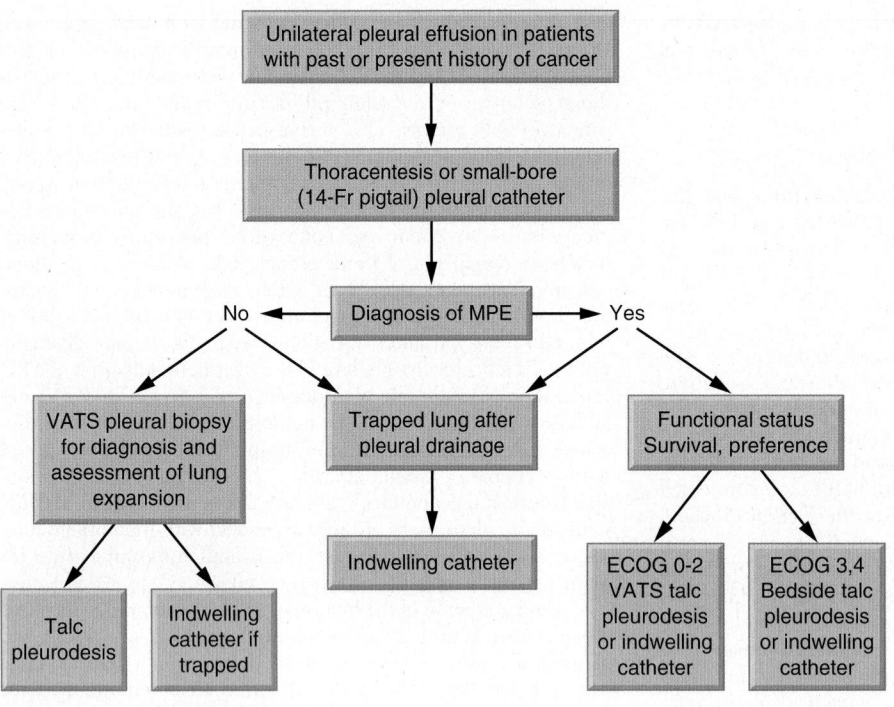

Figure 127.1 Treatment algorithm for malignant pleural effusion. MPE, malignant pleural effusion; VATS, video-assisted thoracoscopic surgery; ECOG, Eastern Cooperative Oncology Group.

pericarditis.[34] Primary cancers of the pericardium, such as mesothelioma, fibrosarcoma, and lymphangioma, are exceedingly rare. Patients with malignant pericardial disease may be asymptomatic or present with a number of manifestations, with pericardial effusion being the most common. Cardiac tamponade due to malignant pericardial effusion (MPCE) accounts for at least 50% of all reported cases of pericardial fluid that require intervention. Only 15% to 25% of patients with documented metastasis to the pericardium have pericardial effusion and only a small percentage of those patients will develop pericardial tamponade.[34] Similar to MPEs, MPCEs are frequently indicative of advanced incurable malignancy, and the overall median survival of patients with MPCE is often <6 months.

Clinical Presentation

In most cases, MPCE is observed in patients with an established diagnosis of cancer, typically at late stages of their disease. MPCE is rarely seen as the initial manifestation of extracardiac malignancy. Nonspecific symptoms are frequent with MPCE; as such, pericardial effusion may remain unsuspected in patients for whom nonspecific symptoms are otherwise attributed to overall disease progression. Whether cardiac tamponade presents as the initial manifestation of MPCE is highly variable and depends on the rate of fluid accumulation, volume of pericardial fluid, and the patient's underlying cardiac function. Classic signs and symptoms of cardiac tamponade include dyspnea, orthopnea, low cardiac output (peripheral vasoconstriction, cold clammy extremities, poor capillary refill, and diaphoresis), jugular venous distention, distant heart sounds, pulsus paradoxus, and narrowed pulse pressure. An electrocardiogram may show low-voltage complexes across all monitoring leads and electrical alternans.

Diagnostic Modalities

Radiographic and Echocardiographic Studies

Pericardial effusion should be suspected in the asymptomatic patient with cancer when an enlarged globular water-bottle pericardial silhouette is found on plain posteroanterior and lateral chest

radiographs or more commonly detected by thoracic CT scans. Once a pericardial effusion is suspected, echocardiography should be performed to confirm its presence, to assess the hemodynamic significance of pericardial effusion, and to determine the presence of pericardial or intracardiac masses. Right atrial and ventricular collapse are the classic echocardiographic signs of cardiac tamponade, with sensitivity ranging from 38% to 60% and specificity ranging from 50% to 100%.[35] Echocardiography-guided pericardiocentesis is a preferred initial approach to alleviate pericardial tamponade.

Cytopathology and Histopathology

The cytology of a pericardial effusion determines definitively its benign or malignant nature. Malignant cells are identified in pericardial fluid from 66% to 79% of MPCE, with the cytology correlating with histologic diagnosis of the underlying malignancy in 100% of these individuals.[36] In contrast, parietal pericardial biopsy is frequently nondiagnostic because the distribution of malignant involvement is not uniform.

Treatment

General goals of treatment for MPCE include relief of immediate symptoms, confirmation of the malignant nature of the fluid, and prevention of recurrence. Therapy for MPCE should be tailored to the performance status and prognosis of each patient. Although simple pericardiocentesis can be life-saving in cases of cardiac tamponade, more definitive treatment options for clinically significant MPCE are indicated to minimize the risk of recurrence. These include surgical procedures such as subxiphoid pericardiostomy (pericardial window), transthoracic pericardial window or pericardiectomy (either by VATS or thoracotomy), and medical interventions such as percutaneous tube pericardiostomy with or without intrapericardial instillation of sclerosing agents.

Pericardiocentesis

Pericardiocentesis is the intervention of choice for patients with hemodynamic instability due to pericardial effusion as removal of as little as 50 ml of pericardial fluid can significantly improve signs and symptoms of acute cardiac tamponade. In patients with cancer with symptomatic pericardial effusion, pericardiocentesis may be performed to stabilize the patient prior to additional drainage procedures, such as percutaneous tube pericardiostomy or subxiphoid pericardial window. Echocardiography-guided percardiocentesis is the preferred technique as it minimizes complications and improves the success of the pericardiocentesis by delineating the size and location of the effusion relative to cardiac structures. Overall rates of complication and success are approximately 2.4% and 100%, respectively, for echocardiography-guided pericardial drainage as compared with 4.8% and 90%, respectively, for unassisted pericardiocentesis.[37]

Percutaneous Tube Pericardiostomy and Pericardial Sclerotherapy

Following pericardiocentesis, the rate of fluid reaccumulation has been reported to range from 44% to 70%.[38] To improve these results, a 9-Fr pigtail draining catheter is now routinely placed into the pericardial space using Seldinger technique, following successful needle pericardiocentesis, to enable more complete evacuation of the effusion and provide access for sclerotherapy. Tetracycline and doxycycline have been most extensively evaluated as pericardial sclerosing agents. Maher and colleagues[38] reported 93 patients with MPCE treated by percutaneous pericardial drainage followed by tetracycline or doxycycline sclerosis. Successful placement of the pericardiostomy tube was achieved in 85 patients (92%). Pericardial effusion was controlled in 75 patients (88%); 10 patients (12%) did not respond to sclerosis, 8 of whom subsequently underwent surgical pericardiostomy. Successful sclerotherapy often requires multiple instillations of tetracycline or doxycycline (range, 1 to 8; median, 3); 50 patients required three or more instillations to control their effusions. Treatment-related complications (in decreasing order of frequency) included pain, catheter occlusion, fever, and atrial arrhythmias. The favorable results of this minimally invasive treatment strategy are offset by the need for repeated instillations of the sclerosing agent in order to achieve pericardial symphysis. Liu and associates[39] conducted a prospective study to evaluate the efficacy and toxicity of bleomycin versus doxycycline as sclerosing agents in MPCE. Bleomycin was found to be as effective as doxycycline in achieving satisfactory control of MPCE but with much less retrosternal pain. As a result, these authors recommend that bleomycin be considered the first-line chemical sclerosing agent for MPCE. Phase 2 random-assignment clinical trial evaluating intrapericardial bleomycin sclerotherapy following pericardial drainage (tube periocardiostomy or subxiphoid periocardiostomy) in 79 patients with lung cancer with MPCE only demonstrated a very modest additional clinical benefit of reducing recurrence of pericardial effusion.[40] Pericardial sclerotherapy, while being reported in these small series, is not a commonly performed procedure.

Percutaneous Balloon-Tube Pericardiostomy

Percutaneous balloon-tube pericardiostomy is an extension of the more commonly performed percutaneous tube pericardiostomy. In balloon-tube pericardiostomy, pericardiocentesis is performed as previously described but 150 to 200 ml of fluid is intentionally left in the pericardial space. Subsequently, dilatation of the needle tract is performed under fluoroscopy using a balloon catheter creating a larger pericardial opening to the subcutaneous space and mimicking surgical pericardiostomy to reduce recurrence. Ziskind and colleagues[41] reported that this technique was effective in relieving pericardial effusions in 46 of 50 patients (92%). Procedure-related complications included fever (six patients), pleural effusion requiring chest tube placement or thoracentesis (eight patients), small pneumothorax (two patients), and right ventricular injury requiring surgery (one patient) for an overall clinically significant complication rate of 18%. This is an effective minimally invasive

technique of pericardial drainage in experienced hands but it is not widely used.

Subxiphoid Pericardiostomy (Subxiphoid Pericardial Window)

Subxiphoid pericardiostomy is the most commonly performed surgical procedure for benign as well as MPCEs. This procedure can be performed under local anesthesia with intravenous sedation or general anesthesia. It can be performed as the initial procedure for MPCE in medically stable patients or following needle pericardiocentesis in unstable patients with signs and symptoms of significant cardiac tamponade. A comprehensive review of >800 patients with effusions of different etiologies who underwent subxiphoid pericardiostomy indicated an overall mortality rate of 0.62% (range, 0% to 2%), an overall morbidity rate of 1.87% (range, 0% to 7%), and a recurrence rate of 3.6% (range, 0% to 9.1%).[42] These results compare favorably with percutaneous pericardiocentesis/pericardiostomy with or without sclerosis (1.03% mortality, 9.48% morbidity, and 13.8% recurrence [cumulative results from nine reported series including 427 patients]).[42]

Partial Pericardiectomy or Pericardial Window via Thoracotomy

Pericardial window or pericardiectomy via thoracotomy is performed uncommonly today. Piehler et al.[43] reviewed surgical management of pericardial effusions in 145 patients and concluded that the extent of pericardial resection influenced incidence of recurrent effusions. However, comparative analysis indicated no difference in recurrence rates of patients treated by subxiphoid pericardiostomy compared with those undergoing transthoracic drainage.[44] The postoperative complications (pneumonia, pleural effusion, respiratory failure, cardiac arrhythmia, deep vein thrombosis, and pulmonary embolism) are much less frequent following subxiphoid pericardial drainage compared with transthoracic pericardial resection (10% versus 50%, respectively). Thus, transthoracic pericardial resection is rarely the initial recommended procedure for drainage of MPCE.

If a transthoracic approach is chosen, VATS should be used if transthoracic pericardial resection is needed for the treatment of recurrent MPCE following subxiphoid pericardiostomy, or for diagnosis and treatment of simultaneous pleural/parenchymal pathology. Compared with thoracotomy, VATS approaches, when feasible, are more suitable interventions in the debilitated patient with cancer. A potential limitation of VATS pericardiectomy for patients is the need for general anesthesia and single-lung ventilation.

Local or Systemic Therapies for Malignant Pericardial Effusion

Radiotherapy is generally reserved for MPCE associated with lymphoma or breast carcinoma. Vaitkus et al.[45] reported 54 patients treated with radiotherapy as the primary mode of therapy for MPCE. Of these patients, 39 (72%) underwent initial pericardiocentesis. The majority received neither systemic nor other direct pericardial intervention. Radiation therapy was successful in controlling MPCE in 36 patients (66.7%). The highest success rates were noted in patients with leukemia/lymphoma and patients with breast cancer (93% and 71%, respectively). Forty-five percent of patients with other solid tumors had adequate control of their effusions as well. Although noninvasive radiotherapy requires repeated visits or even prolonged hospitalization and may theoretically cause acute pericarditis or myocarditis, these potential complications may not be as pertinent in many patients with MPCE because of their limited survival. Patients with MPCE secondary to lymphoma or breast carcinoma may have effusions that respond to systemic chemotherapy. These authors also reported another

PRACTICE OF ONCOLOGY

46 patients with breast (38 patients), lymphoma (2 patients), or other solid tumors (6 patients) treated with systemic chemotherapy. Of this group, 36 patients (78%) underwent initial therapeutic pericardiocentesis. Systemic chemotherapy prevented recurrence of effusion in 31 patients (67%); successful control of effusion was achieved in over two-thirds of these select individuals irrespective of whether pericardiocentesis preceded systemic therapy. Intrapericardial instillation of chemotherapeutic agents (teniposide, 5-fluorouracil, carboplatin, cisplatin) to achieve high local drug concentrations has been reported for MPCE[46] but is considered still too experimental to be discussed here.

Summary

MPCE is frequently an indication of advanced, incurable malignancy. Hence, the goals of intervention include relief of symptoms and prevention of recurrence if possible. The treatment of MPCE should proceed in a stepwise fashion. Surgical (subxiphoid pericardiostomy) or medical (ultrasound-guided percutaneous tube pericardiostomy and sclerotherapy) interventions have acceptable risks and provide excellent results. The choice of treatment for any particular patient should consider the individual's specific medical issues and overall life expectancy.

REFERENCES

1. American Thoracic Society. Management of malignant pleural effusions. *Am J Respir Crit Care Med* 2000;162:1987–2001.
2. Antunes G, Neville E. Management of malignant pleural effusions. *Thorax* 2000;55:981–983.
3. Roberts ME, Neville E, Berrisford RG, et al. Management of a malignant pleural effusion: British Thoracic Society Pleural Disease Guideline 2010. *Thorax* 2010;65:ii32–ii40.
4. Feller-Kopman D, Berkowitz D, Boiselle P, et al. Large-volume thoracentesis and the risk of reexpansion pulmonary edema. *Ann Thorac Surg* 2007;84:1656–1661.
5. Sahn SA. Pleural effusion in lung cancer. *Clin Chest Med* 1993;14:189–200.
6. DeCamp MM Jr, Jaklitsch MT, Mentzer SJ, et al. The safety and versatility of video-thoracoscopy: a prospective analysis of 895 consecutive cases. *J Am Coll Surg* 1995;181:113–120.
7. Davies CW, Traill ZC, Gleeson FV, et al. Intrapleural streptokinase in the management of malignant multiloculated pleural effusions. *Chest* 1999;115:729–733.
8. Kessinger A, Wigton RS. Intracavitary bleomycin and tetracycline in the management of malignant pleural effusions: a randomized study. *J Surg Oncol* 1987;36:81–83.
9. Mager HJ, Maesen B, Verzijlbergen F, et al. Distribution of talc suspension during treatment of malignant pleural effusion with talc pleurodesis. *Lung Cancer* 2002;36:77–81.
10. Robinson LA, Fleming WH, Galbraith TA. Intrapleural doxycycline control of malignant pleural effusions. *Ann Thorac Surg* 1993;55:1115–1121.
11. Patz EF Jr, McAdams HP, Erasmus JJ, et al. Sclerotherapy for malignant pleural effusions: a prospective randomized trial of bleomycin vs doxycycline with small-bore catheter drainage. *Chest* 1998;113:1305–1311.
12. Lee YC, Baumann MH, Maskell NA, et al. Pleurodesis practice for malignant pleural effusions in five English-speaking countries: survey of pulmonologists. *Chest* 2003;124:2229–2238.
13. Heffner JE, Standerfer RJ, Torstveit J, et al. Clinical efficacy of doxycycline for pleurodesis. *Chest* 1994;105:1743–1747.
14. Hamed H, Fentiman IS, Chaudary MA, et al. Comparison of intracavitary bleomycin and talc for control of pleural effusions secondary to carcinoma of the breast. *Br J Surg* 1989;76:1266–1267.
15. Colt HG, Russack V, Chiu Y, et al. A comparison of thoracoscopic talc insufflation, slurry, and mechanical abrasion pleurodesis. *Chest* 1997;111:442–448.
16. Fentiman IS, Rubens RD, Hayward JL. A comparison of intracavitary talc and tetracycline for the control of pleural effusions secondary to breast cancer. *Eur J Cancer Clin Oncol* 1986;22:1079–1081.
17. Hartman DL, Gaither JM, Kesler KA, et al. Comparison of insufflated talc under thoracoscopic guidance with standard tetracycline and bleomycin pleurodesis for control of malignant pleural effusions. *J Thorac Cardiovasc Surg* 1993;105:743–747.
18. Viallat JR, Rey F, Astoul P, et al. Thoracoscopic talc poudrage pleurodesis for malignant effusions: a review of 360 cases. *Chest* 1996;110:1387–1393.
19. Dresler CM, Olak J, Herndon JE, et al. Phase III intergroup study of talc poudrage vs talc slurry sclerosis for malignant pleural effusion. *Chest* 2005;127:909–915.
20. Stefani A, Natali P, Casali C, et al. Talc poudrage versus talc slurry in the treatment of malignant pleural effusion. A prospective comparative study. *Eur J Cardiothorac Surg* 2006;30:827–832.
21. Tan C, Sedrakyan A, Browne J, et al. The evidence on the effectiveness of management for malignant pleural effusion: a systematic review. *Eur J Cardiothorac Surg* 2006;29:829–838.
22. Janssen JP, Collier G, Astoul P, et al. Safety of pleurodesis with talc poudrage in malignant pleural effusion: a prospective cohort study. *Lancet* 2007;369:1535–1539.
23. Suzuki K, Servais EL, Rizk NP, et al. Palliation and pleurodesis in malignant pleural effusion: the role for tunneled pleural catheters. *J Thorac Oncol* 2011;6:762–767.
24. Tremblay A, Michaud G. Single-center experience with 250 tunnelled pleural catheter insertions for malignant pleural effusion. *Chest* 2006;129:362–368.
25. Warren WH, Kalimi R, Khodadadian LM, et al. Management of malignant pleural effusions using the Pleur(x) catheter. *Ann Thorac Surg* 2008;85:1049–1055.
26. Van Meter ME, McKee KY, Kohlwes RJ. Efficacy and safety of tunneled pleural catheters in adults with malignant pleural effusions: a systematic review. *J Gen Intern Med* 2011;26:70–76.
27. Putnam JB Jr, Light RW, Rodriguez RM, et al. A randomized comparison of indwelling pleural catheter and doxycycline pleurodesis in the management of malignant pleural effusions. *Cancer* 1999;86:1992–1999.
28. Demmy TL, Gu L, Burkhalter JE, et al. Optimal management of malignant pleural effusions (results of CALGB 30102). *J Natl Compr Canc Netw* 2012;10:975–982.
29. Fysh ET, Waterer GW, Kendall PA, et al. Indwelling pleural catheters reduce inpatient days over pleurodesis for malignant pleural effusion. *Chest* 2012;142:394–400.
30. Davies HE, Mishra EK, Kahan BC, et al. Effect of an indwelling pleural catheter vs chest tube and talc pleurodesis for relieving dyspnea in patients with malignant pleural effusion: the TIME2 randomized controlled trial. *JAMA* 2012;307:2383–2389.
31. Freeman RK, Ascioti AJ, Mahidhara RS. A propensity-matched comparison of pleurodesis or tunneled pleural catheter in patients undergoing diagnostic thoracoscopy for malignancy. *Ann Thorac Surg* 2013;96:259–263.
32. Hunt BM, Farivar AS, Vallières E, et al. Thoracoscopic talc versus tunneled pleural catheters for palliation of malignant pleural effusions. *Ann Thorac Surg* 2012;94:1053–1057.
33. Puri V, Pyrdeck TL, Crabtree TD, et al. Treatment of malignant pleural effusion: a cost-effectiveness analysis. *Ann Thorac Surg* 2012;94:374–379.
34. Refaat MM, Katz WE. Neoplastic pericardial effusion. *Clin Cardiol* 2011;34:593–598.
35. Chong HH, Plotnick GD. Pericardial effusion and tamponade: evaluation, imaging modalities, and management. *Compr Ther* 1995;21:378–385.
36. Wiener HG, Kristensen IB, Haubek A, et al. The diagnostic value of pericardial cytology: an analysis of 95 cases. *Acta Cytol* 1991;35:149–153.
37. Clarke DP, Cosgrove DO. Real-time ultrasound scanning in the planning and guidance of pericardiocentesis. *Clin Radiol* 1987;38:119–122.
38. Maher EA, Shepherd FA, Todd TJ. Pericardial sclerosis as the primary management of malignant pericardial effusion and cardiac tamponade. *J Thorac Cardiovasc Surg* 1996;112:637–643.
39. Liu G, Crump M, Goss PE, et al. Prospective comparison of the sclerosing agents doxycycline and bleomycin for the primary management of malignant pericardial effusion and cardiac tamponade. *J Clin Oncol* 1996;14:3141–3147.
40. Kunitoh H, Tamura T, Shibata T, et al. A randomised trial of intrapericardial bleomycin for malignant pericardial effusion with lung cancer (JCOG9811). *Br J Cancer* 2009;100:464–469.
41. Ziskind AA, Pearce AC, Lemmon CC, et al. Percutaneous balloon pericardiotomy for the treatment of cardiac tamponade and large pericardial effusions: description of technique and report of the first 50 cases. *J Am Coll Cardiol* 1993;21:1–5.
42. Allen KB, Faber LP, Warren WH, et al. Pericardial effusion: subxiphoid pericardiostomy versus percutaneous catheter drainage. *Ann Thorac Surg* 1999;67:437–440.
43. Piehler JM, Pluth JR, Schaff HV, et al. Surgical management of effusive pericardial disease: influence of extent of pericardial resection on clinical course. *J Thorac Cardiovasc Surg* 1985;90:506–516.
44. Naunheim KS, Kesler KA, Fiore AC, et al. Pericardial drainage: subxiphoid vs. transthoracic approach. *Eur J Cardiothorac Surg* 1991;5:99–103, discussion 104.
45. Vaitkus PT, Herrmann HC, LeWinter MM. Treatment of malignant pericardial effusion. *JAMA* 1994;272:59–64.
46. Lestuzzi C. Neoplastic pericardial disease: Old and current strategies for diagnosis and management. *World J Cardiol* 2010;2(9):270–279.

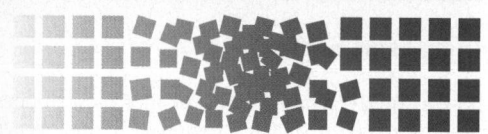

128 Malignant Ascites

Ajay V. Maker

INCIDENCE AND ETIOLOGY

Ascites is the accumulation of serous fluid in the abdominal cavity. Malignant ascites (MA) is a pathologic condition secondary to either primary peritoneal neoplasms or advanced-stage cancers resulting in either increased abdominal fluid production, inhibited reabsorption, or both, accounting for 10% of ascites cases.[1] Abdominal malignancies commonly associated with MA include ovarian, endometrial, appendiceal, colorectal, gastric, primary peritoneal, and pancreatic tumors, whereas breast, lung, and hematologic malignancies are the main nonabdominal tumors responsible. Ascites may be found in 52% of patients at the time of cancer diagnosis,[2] with up to one-third of these patients having nonmalignant etiologies for their accumulation of free peritoneal fluid (e.g., malnutrition, portal hypertension, cirrhosis, congestive heart failure, nephrosis, pancreatitis, infectious processes, or benign gynecologic conditions); however, the majority of patients with newly diagnosed ascites and cancer will be found to have MA.[3] Approximately 15% of all patients with gastrointestinal cancers will develop ascites during the disease process, whereas up to 20% of all MA cases are from an unknown primary.[4,5]

ANATOMY AND PATHOLOGY

Ascitic Fluid Homeostasis

Lining the abdominal cavity is the parietal peritoneum, a thin layer of mesothelium that contains multiple foramina. The amount of fluid and solutes that are secreted through this layer are tightly controlled, first by the capillary endothelium, then the capillary basement membrane, followed by the interstitial stroma between the capillaries and the peritoneum, and then the mesothelial basement membrane.[6,7] The capillary endothelium contains anionic charges within an extracellular glycocalix that discourages anionic proteins and albumin from extravasating. This maintains plasma oncotic pressure. The capillary basement membrane is also lined with negatively charged proteoglycans, acting as a selective barrier against transit of anionic proteins. The interstitial space is a negatively charged filter of connective tissue, fibroblasts, and hyaluronic acid that is lined by the mesothelial cell basement membrane, also coated with anionic glycosaminoglycans. The peritoneal mesothelial cells also maintain a glycocalix of anionic charges, thereby forming a multilayered matrix that functions to inhibit transgression of intravascular proteins into the abdominal cavity.

The total peritoneal surface area is approximately 2 m^2, and fluid is continually secreted into the abdomen. At least two-thirds of peritoneal fluid reabsorbs into the open lymphatic channels of the diaphragm, leaving approximately 100 ml of fluid to lubricate and bathe the serosal surfaces.[8] The free fluid enters through open ends of lymphatic channels, stomata, which connect the abdominal cavity with the submesothelial diaphragmatic lymphatics.[6,7,9] Scintigraphic studies have traced the fluid from this point through mediastinal lymph channels into the right thoracic duct and ultimately the right subclavian vein.[10]

Pathophysiology of Malignant Ascites

MA results from an imbalance in fluid production and absorption by the peritoneal lining, with a net positive balance. The relationship is defined by Starling's law where the amount of fluid leaving the capillary is determined by the hydraulic pressure minus the plasma oncotic pressure multiplied by the product of the porosity of endothelium and its surface area.[11,12] In equation form:

$$\begin{aligned} Net\ filtration &= Capillary\ Porosity \times Surface\ area \times \\ &\quad (\Delta Hydraulic\ pressure - \Delta Oncotic\ pressure) \\ &= Capillary\ Porosity \times Surface\ area\ [(Capillary \\ &\quad hydraulic\ pressure - Interstitial\ hydraulic \\ &\quad pressure) - S(Capillary\ oncotic\ pressure - \\ &\quad Interstitial\ oncotic\ pressure)] \end{aligned}$$

where S is a permeability coefficient.

Therefore, increased net filtration can result from any of the following or a combination of (1) increased capillary permeability, (2) increased surface area, (3) increased hydraulic pressure differences, and (4) decreased oncotic pressure differences.

Increased Capillary Permeability

Murine models of carcinomatosis have revealed increased permeability of proteins compared to control animals, with peritoneal capillary permeability reaching three times normal within a week of intraperitoneal tumor instillation.[13] This permeability is thought to be driven, in part, by tumor angiogenesis, as in the process of neovascularization the basement membrane and stroma are remodeled and there is a period of hyperpermeability during the migration and proliferation of new endothelial cells.[14] Multiple growth factors are critical to the process of angiogenesis, including fibroblast and vascular endothelial growth factor (VEGF), and early murine models of MA found increased VEGF (termed vascular permeability factor at the time) in the ascitic fluid proportional to the amount of neovascularization.[15] The MA could be inhibited by treating mice with anti-VEGF antibodies, which reaccumulated upon withdrawing the antibodies.[16] These findings have been reflected in patients with MA where marked neovascularization of the parietal peritoneum was observed,[17] and ascitic fluids were found to contain high levels of VEGF, especially in patients with gastric, colorectal, and ovarian cancers compared to ascites from patients with nonmalignant ascites due to cirrhosis.[18–20] The effect of VEGF on vascular permeability is estimated to be 50,000 times more potent than histamine.[20]

Another factor that may increase vascular permeability in these patients is the increased production and secretion of matrix metalloproteinases (MMP) by tumor cells. These enzymes, namely gelatinase and stromelysin-3, function to digest extracellular tissue scaffolds to allow tumor in-growth.[21–23] Inhibition of these enzymes can reduce MA formation, and in a murine model of colon and ovarian MA, not only was ascites formation inhibited, but survival was increased.[24,25] Therefore, carcinomatosis appears to increase capillary permeability through a process of growth factor–driven angiogenesis and MMP production, and this may play a role in increasing intraperitoneal fluid and macromolecules.

Increased Surface Area

As the surface area of capillaries increases, so does the potential amount of cell permeate. Secondary to angiogenesis and growth factor–stimulated neovascularization, the size and amount of mesothelial blood vessels is increased in a murine model of MA.[26] Furthermore, in patients with carcinomatosis, studies measuring the sources of ascitic effluent by using plastic rings and absorptive paper on both tumor surfaces and tumor-free surfaces, found an abundance of effluent from nontumor-bearing omentum and small bowel, thus identifying additional surfaces not traditionally considered responsible for ascites formation.[27,28]

Increased Hydraulic Pressure Differences

Increased portal pressures can increase the hydraulic pressure in the mesothelial capillaries. Though this does not seem to play a large role in the formation of MA, increases in portal venous pressure have been seen in patients with ovarian cancer with MA.[28] Furthermore, malignancies that cause liver dysfunction due to excessive hepatic tumor load or form on a background of cirrhosis (e.g., hepatocellular carcinoma) can tip the balance of hydrostatic pressures in the mesothelial capillaries to levels above the interstitium.

Decreased Oncotic Pressure Differences

Chronic or advanced malignancy can result in chronic protein malnutrition. This results in a catabolic state with reduced intravascular protein, thereby creating an oncotic pressure gradient that favors fluid extravasation from the vessels into the peritoneal cavity and lack of fluid reabsorption.[29] In addition, due to the increased capillary permeability in patients with carcinomatosis, proteins and other macromolecules enter the ascitic fluid and accumulate in the intraperitoneal cavity.[20,30] A combination of these forces increases the extravascular oncotic pressure, driving fluid into the interstitium.

Increased Ascitic Fluid Production

Increased fluid production appears to contribute to the formation of MA secondary to increased microvascular permeability, increased surface area, increased hydraulic pressure, and decreased colloid oncotic pressure. Capillary permeability is increased due to cytokine release. Molecules such as VEGF, vascular permeability factor, interleukin-6, and tumor necrosis factor (TNF) are intimately involved.[4] Enhanced vascular permeability leads to secretion of osmotic particles and fluid into the peritoneum, further increasing the intra-abdominal fluid volume. Endocrine homeostasis may also contribute. Intravascular volume is decreased with increasing ascites, which results in pressure-volume feedback loops that stimulate renin and aldosterone secretion. These hormones reduce urinary output and incidentally increase accumulation of ascites.[4,31] Furthermore, due to decreased removal of fluid as a consequence of malignant obstruction of lymphatics, the circulating blood volume is further reduced and this similarly activates the renin–angiotensin–aldosterone system.

Reduction in Fluid Reabsorption

Venous and lymphatic obstruction by visible solid tumors or by microscopic tumor cells is one mechanism that results in impaired drainage of peritoneal fluid content.[32] Fluid kinetic studies performed on patients undergoing peritoneal dialysis identified that the normal rate of lymphatic uptake remains constant at 40 ml/h.[33] This rate would be necessary in the absence of increased production to maintain homeostasis. Murine models of carcinomatosis by intraperitoneal tumor cell injection resulted in diaphragmatic and retrosternal lymph occlusion by 5 days with ascites forming soon thereafter. Lymphoscintigraphy in human patients with MA also documented no radioactive sulfur colloid above the diaphragm in 85% of patients treated with tagged intraperitoneal colloid, implying that diaphragmatic lymphatics were obstructed by malignant invasion.[15,34–36] Additionally, due to increased capillary permeability, proteins and other macromolecules enter the ascitic fluid and these can mechanically obstruct lymphatic drainage channels.[20] Therefore, the rate of lymphatic uptake may be decreased or inhibited in malignancy, contributing to increased intra-abdominal fluid.

DIAGNOSIS

Comprehensive history taking combined with physical exam will diagnose ascites in most patients. In patients with known malignancy, increasing abdominal girth, bloating, abdominal discomfort, or weight gain are concerning for carcinomatosis and MA. Imaging, usually computed tomography (CT) scan or ultrasound,[37] can confirm the presence of ascites (Fig. 128.1). The CT finding of peritoneal nodules, thickening, omental caking, solid organ metastases, or intraperitoneal nodules raise the suspicion that ascites is malignant as opposed to secondary to benign etiologies. In over 100 patients studied with MA or cirrhotic ascites, CT signs significantly associated with a malignant etiology were fluid in the omental bursa, higher ascitic density (11.5 HU versus 6.7 HU), thickening of the parietal peritoneum, and, in patients with at least a moderate amount of ascites, a tethered-bowel sign.[38] As most patients with abdominal pain or malignancy are undergoing cross-sectional imaging as part of the workup or for surveillance, attention to these radiographic signs are important as they can help direct treatment and streamline further workup.

The gold standard to diagnose MA is positive peritoneal cytology, which is present nearly 100% of the time in patients with carcinomatosis.[39] This can be obtained percutaneously and safely under image guidance. For advanced gastrointestinal and hepatopancreaticobiliary malignancies without metastases on cross-sectional imaging, diagnostic laparoscopy is often utilized for evaluation of occult carcinomatosis (see Fig. 128.1). If incidental low-volume ascites is found in these patients, then ascites can be aspirated and set for cytology, as can peritoneal washings. This is now a standard approach for advanced gastric cancer in some centers, including our own, as positive peritoneal cytology carries a prognosis similar to stage IV disease.

For those without carcinomatosis but still with MA, cytology is diagnostic in only 50% to 60% of patients.[40] For these patients, perhaps the most useful single test is the serum to ascites albumin gradient. Calculated as the difference between serum and ascites albumin concentrations, values <1.1 g/dl are suspicious for carcinomatosis as opposed to portal hypertension or other cardiopulmonary causes.[41] The use of ascitic fluid protein and other chemistries to discriminate between malignant and nonmalignant causes is variable and not reliable. If negative for malignancy, cell counts with >250 neutrophils per mm^3 are suggestive of infection and Gram stain should be performed. High levels of ascitic amylase may reflect pancreatic ascites or small bowel perforation.[42] Ascitic fluid fibronectin levels have been reported to be 100% sensitive and specific for malignancy, but this is not a standard test currently, nor is sialic acid, telomerase, or human gonadotropin-beta, all of which have shown discriminatory promise.[43–46]

In the absence of a known primary tumor or imaging revealing evidence of malignancy, serum tumor markers can be helpful. Elevated carcinoembryonic antigen values are traditionally associated with colorectal cancer, but can also be elevated in breast,

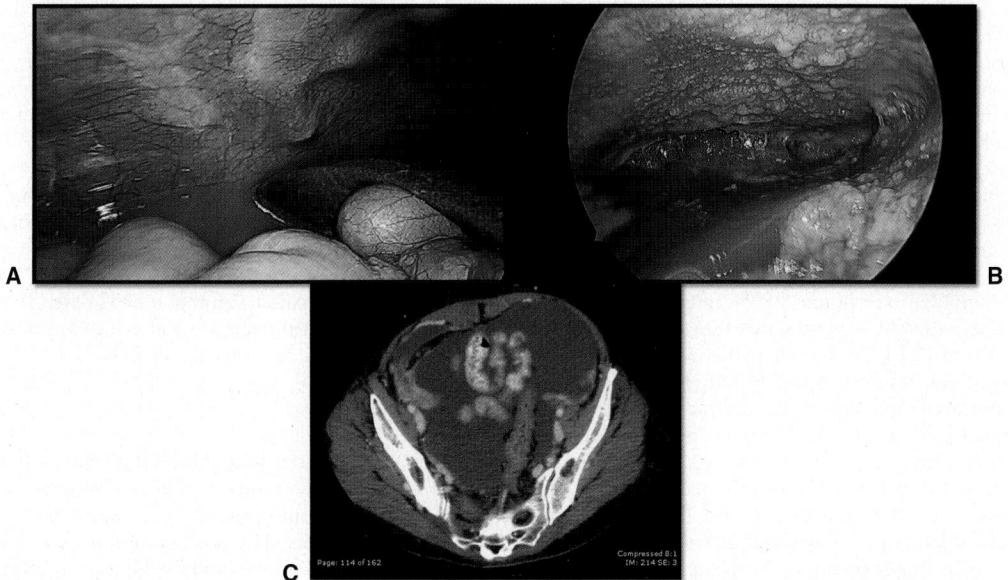

Figure 128.1 (A) Exploratory laparoscopy in a patient with known poorly differentiated gastric cancer but no evidence of metastases on cross-sectional imaging revealed malignant ascites with positive peritoneal cytology. Resection was not performed and the patient was treated with palliative systemic chemotherapy. **(B)** A patient with progressive abdominal pain and an omental nodule on cross-sectional imaging underwent a diagnostic laparoscopy revealing extensive primary peritoneal mesothelioma and cytology positive malignant ascites. The patient was treated with cytoreduction and hyperthermic chemotherapy. **(C)** A patient with node-positive pancreatic adenocarcinoma underwent a successful R0 resection followed by adjuvant chemotherapy; however, the patient presented over a year later with increasing abdominal girth and anorexia. Cross-sectional imaging confirmed recurrence and malignant ascites.

lung, pancreas, gastric, or breast cancers. Hepatopancreaticobiliary tumors can often reveal elevated Ca19-9 levels. Increased Ca125 levels are most suspicious for ovarian carcinoma, though they can be elevated in pancreas, lung, and breast cancers. Alphafetoprotein is another helpful serum marker, which when elevated can be indicative of hepatocellular carcinoma.

MANAGEMENT

The management of MA has evolved from the contributions of many specialties, including surgical oncology, medical oncology, hepatology, palliative care, and interventional radiology. The goals of treatment are to provide symptomatic relief and to either maintain or improve the quality of life. Randomized controlled trials are lacking, and studies evaluating the efficacy of various treatments are difficult to extrapolate to the individual patient. Common end points have included comparisons in time between paracenteses. Therefore, there is no standard approach to these patients and multiple medical and surgical options exist. The mainstays of treatment have been based on non-malignant acsites and include diuretics and paracentesis.[4] A survey of randomly sampled Canadian medical oncologists, gastroenterologists, palliative care physicians, and gynecologic oncologists revealed that 98% employed paracentesis with 89% efficacy, followed by diuretic use 61% of the time and rarely peritoneal shunting—both with unclear advantages.[47] Certainly, systemic antineoplastic therapy should be utilized whenever possible in a malignancy-specific fashion. In the last few years, new systemic agents as well as regional chemotherapy combined with surgical cytoreduction have offered alternative options for palliation. The various options for treatment are reviewed herein.

Removal of Fluid

Perhaps the most utilized treatment strategy in managing MA is by removal of fluid, either by diuresis, paracentesis, or shunting.

Diuretics

The use of diuretics in the management of MA is largely extrapolated from the treatment of cardiogenic or cirrhotic ascites, though it has been advocated as first-line treatment of MA.[48] Its role appears to be most useful when the etiology of ascites involves stimulation of the renin-aldosterone axis.[8,49] As a result, diuretic use is most successful in selected patients with liver dysfunction or portal hypertension secondary to metastatic liver disease or extensive intrahepatic primary tumor burden, as opposed to patients with peritoneal disease or superficial disease of Glisson capsule.[40,49] For this reason, patients with a serum to ascites albumin gradient <1.1 (see the section titled "Diagnosis") have been found to be less responsive to diuretic use, as was identified in a prospective study of patients with MA of various primary tumor etiologies.[49] A review of five studies with >100 patients with MA from a variety of primary tumors found the use of diuretics to be successful in managing symptoms in up to 43% of patients.[50] The agent most commonly utilized is spironolactone with doses ranging from 150 to 450 mg/day.[51] Loop diuretics (e.g., furosemide) can be added to spironolactone.[4] Maximal expected ascitic reabsorption can reach 800 ml with optimized medication doses in selected patients, though it was noted by Pockros et al.[49] that no change in ascitic volume was achieved in patients with MA secondary to peritoneal carcinomatosis or chylous malignant ascites. Complications of diuretic use include dehydration, renal toxicity, and electrolyte imbalances that can result in cardiac arrhythmias. There is no level 1 data evaluating diuretic efficacy in MA and, as a result, its use is controversial and without clear guidelines.[47]

Paracentesis

Paracentesis is the most commonly used treatment for patients with MA with up to 98% of physicians utilizing it for their patients.[47] Improvement in symptoms, although temporary, can be achieved in ~90% of these patients,[24] and its use in palliation is supported by the available literature.[52] There are no randomized trials comparing paracentesis with the use of diuretics in the management of MA.

The volume of drainage per session is limited by the potential complications of hypovolemia and resulting hypotension or renal dysfunction, though hypovolemia and hypotension may be averted with concomitant 5% dextrose infusions or intravenous albumin.[53–57] Randomized studies have demonstrated no difference in survival between patients treated with albumin compared to other plasma expanders, and for patients with MA no definitive trials on this subject have been performed.[58] Reports of 5 L per 1 to 2 hours were demonstrated to be safe without hypovolemia or renal dysfunction,[50] and volumes up to 20 L per session have been reported, though there is no consensus on the rate of withdrawal, ranging from 30 minutes to 24 hours.[54,56,59–61] Forty-eight paracenteses in 44 patients with MA suggested that removal of a mean of 5.8 L (range, 0.8 L to 15 L) can provide palliation of symptoms.[55] Serial paracentesis can result in hypoalbuminemia, a complication possibly minimized with high-protein diets and small volume taps.[62,63] Additional procedural risks of paracentesis include solid and hollow viscous organ injury or perforation, bleeding, fistula, peritonitis, and sepsis. In patients with carcinomatosis and/or prior surgery, there may be extensive scarring and fluid loculations, making ultrasound-guided paracentesis attractive with potentially less complications in this population. As the procedure is often required on multiple occasions,[47] efficacy decreases and complication risks compound. In a study of 67 patients with ovarian, breast, and colorectal cancer, 392 paracentesis, or approximately six aspirations per patient, were required for palliation with other studies reporting mean procedure-free intervals to be 10 to 11 days.[50,64]

To overcome the risks, potential complications, and patient discomfort of serial paracentesis, indwelling peritoneal drainage catheters may be advocated. Furthermore, these catheters offer the option of self-drainage. The utility of catheter placement should be weighed against the patient's condition as survival from catheter placement ranges from 15 days to 18 months.[65] Typically, patients with a life expectancy of >2 to 3 months and requiring serial taps are considered for this procedure.[66] The most frequently used options include tunneled Tenckhoff catheters (Covidien, Mansfield, MA), untunneled or tunneled PleurX

catheters (Denver Biomedicals Inc., Golden, CO), cope-type loop catheters, and tunneled peritoneal Port-a-Caths (Smiths Medical, St. Paul, MN).[65] The greatest risk with indwelling catheters is peritonitis, which occurred in 4.4% of patients with tunneled Tenckhoffs[67] and 2.5% of tunneled PleurX catheters compared to reports of 21% to 34% for untunneled catheters.[68]

Additional complications can occur in ~25% of patients with untunneled catheters including leakage from the insertion site, cellulitis, infections, occlusion, and fatal hypotension.[4,47,64,65,67,69] Tunneled catheters appear to have a superior efficacy and patency rate of >95%.[69] Control of ascites ranges from 83% to 100% of cases with a mean patency duration of 52 days.[4] It should be noted that though these catheters are widely used to treat MA with successful outcomes, it remains off-label use.

Shunting

Shunting involves removal of fluid from the peritoneal cavity and returning it to the venous circulation (superior vena cava) with the goal of maintaining electrolytes and proteins, as compared to drainage procedures. The most commonly employed options include the LeVeen catheter and the Denver shunt (Denver Biomaterials Inc., Denver, CO)[70] (Fig. 128.2). Peritoneovesicular shunts were attempted; however, peritonitis and occlusion limited their utility.[71] There is no level 1 evidence comparing shunt efficacy in MA.[50] Contraindications to shunt placement include hemorrhagic ascites, loculations, heart disease, renal failure, jaundice, portal hypertension, pleural effusion, and clotting disorders.[4,66] Theoretically, there is a risk of systemic seeding from positive peritoneal cytology, but this has not been found to be clinically significant.[66,72] Though shunt placement would be advised only in select patients with prolonged life expectancy, survival has been found to be ~30 days in one study and ranged from 52 to 266 days in a comprehensive review, with perioperative mortality as high as 20%.[66,72] A review of 27 studies evaluating LeVeen and Denver shunts found 78% control of ascites with 70% subclinical and ~3% clinical disseminated intravascular coagulation, a mean patency of

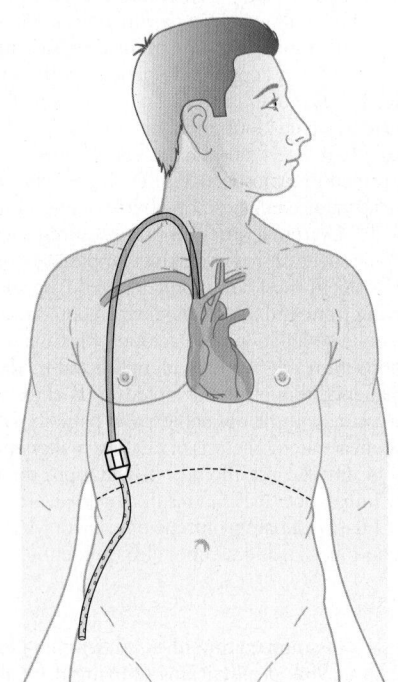

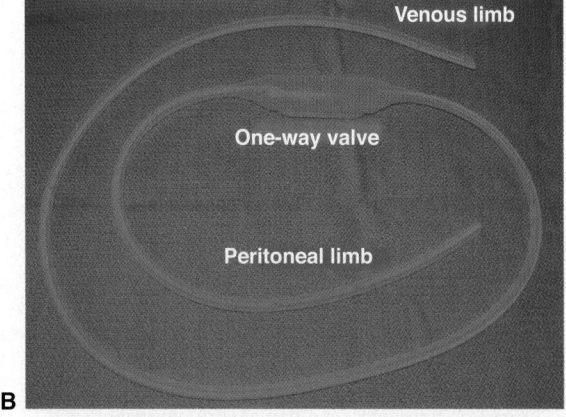

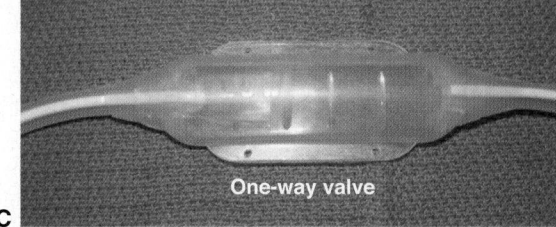

Figure 128.2 (A) Peritoneovenous shunt placement. **(B, C)** Denver shunt showing the compressible chamber and one-way valve. **(A** modified from Millard FC, Powis SJ. Management of intractable malignant ascites using the Denver peritoneovenous shunt. *J R Coll Surg Edinb* 1988;33:138, with permission.)

10 weeks, and lowest response rates in patients with gastrointestinal cancers (10% to 15%).[50] Therefore, their use in gastrointestinal malignancies is relatively contraindicated.[24,66] Complication rates of 25% to 40% are reported with kinking or occlusion occurring in almost one-third of patients.[24,73–75] In summary, in highly selected patients with prolonged life expectancy, surgical shunting may provide palliation with known procedure related morbidity and mortality.

Regional Treatments

Intracavitary Chemotherapy, Cytoreduction, and Hyperthermic Chemotherapy

The goal of intracavitary chemotherapy is to expose tumor cells to higher concentrations of toxic chemotherapy than would otherwise be possible via systemic administration. The theoretical mode of action involves direct cytostatic effects plus ensuing fibrosis and scar formation, inhibiting peritoneal secretion and limiting the free volume of the peritoneal cavity.[8,66] Response rates in controlling MA have varied from 33% to 85% in different histologies and historically using different agents, including mechlorethiamine, thiotepa, bleomycin, mitoxantrone, 5-fluorouracil, cisplatin, and mitomycin C.[60,76–81] Ovarian cancer seems to be the most sensitive to local peritoneal chemotherapy, and success appears improved when limited to microscopic disease.[4]

Penetration of the selected chemotherapeutic agent into the tumor is critical, and optimal tumor bulk <1 mm is recommended[82,83]; therefore, cytoreduction is often required prior to treatment to improve outcomes. This can be an extensive and morbid surgical procedure involving removal of all involved visceral and parietal peritoneal surfaces, and organ resection when stripping is not possible.[84,85] This, combined with heating the chemotherapy, has led to studies evaluating the efficacy of intraperitoneal hyperthermic chemotherapy (HIPEC). Hyperthermia of selected chemotherapeutic agents can enhance cytotoxicity through improved tissue penetration and reduced drug resistance.[86] Agents studied in HIPEC include cisplatin, etoposide, mitomycin C, paclitaxel, taxol, gemcitabine, and 5-fluorouracil. In many tumor histologies studied, improved local control and overall survival can be achieved with this approach. Regarding MA specifically, in one study of 32 patients with gastrointestinal and ovarian cancers, MA was successfully treated in 11/12 patients, and in another report of 39/84 patients with ascites from gastrointestinal-only cancers, 79% of patients achieved control of their ascites.[87,88] Rates of control of MA with HIPEC range from 75% to 100%.[88–91] Studies in patients with ovarian malignancy, primary peritoneal mesothelioma, and pseudomyxoma peritonei in particular have demonstrated promising results, and continued study of additional tumor histologies is warranted.[92,93]

Combining minimally invasive surgery with HIPEC may offer a less invasive approach to achieve similar goals, and in a study of five patients with MA from stage IV gastric cancer, HIPEC with mitomycin C and cisplatin achieved complete response of MA in all patients without morbidity or mortality.[94] In 52 patients with MA secondary to gastric cancer, colorectal cancer, ovarian cancer, breast cancer, peritoneal mesothelioma, and melanoma, laparoscopic HIPEC with cisplatin and doxorubicin or mitomycin C resulted in resolution of ascites in 49/52 patients.[95] In a review of eight studies with 183 patients, the procedure effectively controlled MA in 95% of cases.[96]

This approach often foregoes the extensive cytoreduction of open procedures, and the optimal approach of HIPEC in these patients remains to be determined. Clearly, in highly selected patients with optimal tumor biology, with specific histopathologies, and using select cytotoxic agents, intracavitary chemotherapy plays a significant role in controlling MA, and future treatments will likely involve study of cytoreduction, HIPEC, and minimally invasive surgical techniques.

Immunotherapy: Cytokines, Infectious Agents, and Monoclonal Antibodies

The goal of immunotherapy in MA is to incite an antitumor response within the peritoneal cavity that will reduce tumor burden and decrease ascites formation. Various immunostimulatory agents, both specific and nonspecific, have been administered systemically and locally with varying responses. Cytokines studied have included TNF and interferon (IFN). TNF-α use was promising in preclinical models, but has not been well established in humans. One study demonstrated no objective response in controlling MA in 39 patients with ovarian cancer, while another demonstrated a 76% objective response rate in a phase 1 trial of 29 patients with MA of various histopathologies.[97,98] IFN may increase natural killer cell activity in the peritoneal cavity, and both IFN-α2b and IFN-β reduced MA in some patients when administered intraperitoneally.[99–102]

Infectious agents have also shown an immunologic response resulting in improvement in MA. OK-432 is a penicillin-heat–treated powder of Su-strain *Streptococcus pyogenes* A3 that indirectly enhances cytotoxic T-cell activity.[103] Intraperitoneal OK-432 alone or when combined with other immunostimulatory cytokines has been shown to palliate MA, and in 400 patients with MA of various tumor histologies reduced effusions in 60% of cases.[103–105] *Corynebacterium parvum* has also been administered in a small series of patients resulting in decreased malignant effusion formation.[106]

Monoclonal antibodies, including the antimucin antibody 2G3, have been used in the past to increase the time needed between paracenteses.[107] By specifically targeting VEGF, a growth factor thought to promote ascites formation (see section titled "Incidence and Etiology"), anti-VEGF antibodies have been theorized to improve outcomes in patients with MA. PTK-787, an inhibitor of the VEGF receptor, significantly inhibited MA and the growth of intraperitoneal ovarian cancer cells in a murine model, and also enhanced control of MA in patients with ovarian cancer.[99,108] Further research evaluating the utility of anti-VEGF therapy, such as with SU5416, an anti-VEGF receptor 2 small molecule inhibitor, is undergoing.[109] Bevacizumab, a humanized monoclonal antibody against VEGF-A that has been used systemically in various cancers, has been administered intraperitoneally in a small pilot study of nine patients. Presentation in abstract form revealed resolution of MA in all patients treated.[110]

Recently, a trifunctional monoclonal antibody, catumaxomab, has been engineered with two different antigen-binding sites and a functional Fc domain.[111] One binding site engages EpCAM, an epithelial cell adhesion molecule expressed in 70% to 100% of epithelial tumor cells found in MA from breast, ovarian, gastric, and colon cancers, and the other engages CD3.[112–114] The Fc domain activates phagocytosis and cytotoxicity in various immune effector cells. The use of this antibody in various tumor histologies including ovarian and gastric cancers was found to be safe and resulted in control of MA.[115–118] A recent phase 2/3 clinical trial randomized 258 patients with MA consisting of 129 ovarian and 129 nonovarian primaries into treatment with paracentesis alone or in combination with catumaxomab.[119] Puncture-free survival was improved as was the time to next paracentesis, both by over 1 month. Importantly, signs and symptoms of ascites were improved. Clearly, immunotherapy may have a role in the future management of malignant ascites.

Steroids, Radioisotopes, and Octreotide

Intraperitoneal triamcinolone was used in a phase 2 study of 15 patients with MA of various histologies and improved symptoms and decreased the time between paracentesis by approximately 1 week.[120]

Radioisotopes have been employed in patients with MA to administer local particulate radiation for decades with good effect. In 566 patients treated with intraperitoneal Au-198, ascites was reduced in 47% of patients.[121] Chromic phosphate colloid (32P), which penetrated tissues up to 8 mm compared to 3.8 mm for Au-198,[122] also resulted in clinically significant response rates up to 80%.[66,123,124] Dose escalation in both cases improved control but increased toxicity, including intestinal necrosis. Au-198 is now considered hazardous; however, 32P may still have a role in patients with no adhesions and minimal tumor bulk with only positive cytology.

Though small series of patients treated with octreotide appeared promising, in a pilot study of 33 patients with MA, octreotide did not prolong the time to next paracentesis.[125]

Metalloproteinase Inhibitors

MMPs function to digest extracellular tissue scaffolds to allow tumor in-growth, thus inhibitors of these enzymes may play a role in tumor cell cytostasis and palliation of MA (see section titled "Incidence and Etiology"). Intraperitoneal administration of the MMP inhibitor batimastat after paracentesis in 23 patients with MA of various histologies resulted in no reaccumulation of ascites in 12 patients in a phase 1 study.[21] However, preclinical models have shown variable improvement in MA with this agent, and further studies investigating marimastat and other subsequent-generation MMPs in MA may warranted before MMPs are clinically applicable.

SELECTED REFERENCES

The full reference list can be accessed at lwwhealthlibrary.com/oncology.

1. Runyon BA. Current concepts: Care of patients with ascites. *N Engl J Med* 1994;330:337–342.
4. Smith EM, Jayson GC. The current and future management of malignant ascites. *Clin Oncol* 2003;15:59–72.
8. Cavazzoni E, Bugiantella W, Graziosi L, et al. Malignant ascites: pathophysiology and treatment. *Int J Clin Oncol* 2013;18:1–9.
14. Hanahan D, Folkman J. Patterns and emerging mechanisms of the angiogenic switch during tumorigenesis. *Cell* 1996;86:353–364.
20. Zebrowski BK, Liu W, Ramirez K, et al. Markedly elevated levels of vascular endothelial growth factor in malignant ascites. *Ann Surg Oncol* 1999;6:373–378.
21. Beattie GJ, Smyth JF. Phase I study of intraperitoneal metalloproteinase inhibitor BB94 in patients with malignant ascites. *Clin Cancer Res* 1998;4:1899–1902.
28. Tamsma J. The pathogenesis of malignant ascites. *Cancer Treat Res* 2007;134:109–118.
30. Runyon BA, Hoefs JC, Morgan TR. Ascitic fluid analysis in malignancy-related ascites. *Hepatology* 1988;8:1104–1109.
31. Chung M, Kozuch P. Treatment of malignant ascites. *Curr Treat Options Oncol* 2008;9:215–233.
35. Coates G, Bush RS, Aspin N. A study of ascites using lymphoscintigraphy with 99m Tc-sulfur colloid. *Radiology* 1973;107:577–583.
38. Risson JR, Macovei I, Loock M, et al. Cirrhotic and malignant ascites: differential CT diagnosis. *Diagn Interv Imaging* 2012;93:365–370.
39. Ayantunde AA, Parsons SL. Pattern and prognostic factors in patients with malignant ascites: a retrospective study. *Ann Oncol* 2007;18:945–949.
40. Parsons SL, Lang MW, Steele RJ. Malignant ascites: A 2-year review from a teaching hospital. *Eur J Surg Oncol* 1996;22:237–239.
41. Runyon BA, Montano AA, Akriviadis EA, et al. The serum-ascites albumin gradient is superior to the exudate-transudate concept in the differential diagnosis of ascites. *Ann Intern Med* 1992;117:215–220.
47. Lee CW, Bociek G, Faught W. A survey of practice in management of malignant ascites. *J Pain Symptom Manage* 1998;16:96–101.
49. Pockros PJ, Esrason KT, Nguyen C, et al. Mobilization of malignant ascites with diuretics is dependent on ascitic fluid characteristics. *Gastroenterology* 1992;103:1302–1306.
50. Becker G, Galandi D, Blum HE. Malignant ascites: systematic review and guideline for treatment. *Eur J Cancer* 2006;42:589–597.
52. Keen A, Fitzgerald D, Bryant A, et al. Management of drainage for malignant ascites in gynaecological cancer. *Cochrane Database Syst Rev* 2010;1:CD007794.
55. McNamara P. Paracentesis - an effective method of symptom control in the palliative care setting? *Palliat Med* 2000;14:62–64.
64. Rosenberg S, Courtney A, Nemcek AA Jr, et al. Comparison of percutaneous management techniques for recurrent malignant ascites. *J Vasc Interv Radiol* 2004;15:1129–1131.
66. Adam RA, Adam YG. Malignant ascites: past, present, and future. *J Am Coll Surg* 2004;198:999–1011.
84. Sugarbaker PH. Peritonectomy procedures. In Sugarbaker PH, ed. *Peritoneal Carcinomatosis: Principles of Management.* New York: Springer; 1996:235–253.
88. Loggie BW, Fleming RA, McQuellon RP, et al. Cytoreductive surgery with intraperitoneal hyperthermic chemotherapy for disseminated peritoneal cancer of gastrointestinal origin. *Am Surg* 2000;66:561–568.
92. Elias D, Gilly F, Quenet F, et al. Pseudomyxoma peritonei: a French multicentric study of 301 patients treated with cytoreductive surgery and intraperitoneal chemotherapy. *Eur J Surg Oncol* 2010;36:456–462.
95. Valle M, Van Der Speeten K, Garofalo A. Laparoscopic hyperthermic intraperitoneal peroperative chemotherapy (HIPEC) in the management of refractory malignant ascites: A multi-institutional retrospective analysis in 52 patients. *J Surg Oncol* 2009;100:331–334.
96. Facchiano E, Risio D, Kianmanesh R, et al. Laparoscopic hyperthermic intraperitoneal chemotherapy: indications, aims, and results: a systematic review of the literature. *Ann Surg Oncol* 2012;19:2946–2950.
103. Katano M, Morisaki T. The past, the present and future of the OK-432 therapy for patients with malignant effusions. *Anticancer Res* 1998;18:3917–3925.
119. Heiss MM, Murawa P, Koralewski P, et al. The trifunctional antibody catumaxomab for the treatment of malignant ascites due to epithelial cancer: Results of a prospective randomized phase II/III trial. *Int J Cancer* 2010;127:2209–2221.

129 Paraneoplastic Syndromes

Ramaswamy Govindan, Thomas E. Stinchcombe, and Daniel Morgensztern

INTRODUCTION

Paraneoplastic syndromes are disorders caused by systemic effects occurring remotely from the cancer primary site or metastasis. They are estimated to affect up to 8% of patients with cancer.[1] The most commonly involved systems in paraneoplastic syndromes are the neurologic, endocrine, hematologic, dermatologic, and rheumatologic. Small-cell lung cancer (SCLC) is the most commonly associated malignancy, with lymphoproliferative disorders, thymoma, and gynecologic and breast cancers accounting for the majority of the other causes. The two main mechanisms for paraneoplastic syndromes are ectopic production of humoral factors such as hormones, peptides, or cytokines, and immune cross-response between malignant and normal tissues.

Paraneoplastic syndromes may be the first manifestation of a malignancy, and their timely detection may allow the diagnosis of tumors at an early stage. Therefore, these malignancies that would likely be otherwise clinically occult may be detected at an earlier stage with increased probability of cure. The successful treatment of the underlying malignancy usually results in resolution of the paraneoplastic syndromes caused by ectopic hormone production. However, the tumor-directed treatment is less effective in the immune-mediated syndromes.

PARANEOPLASTIC NEUROLOGIC SYNDROMES

Paraneoplastic neurologic syndromes (PNS) are a rare complication of malignancies, and it is estimated that only 0.01% of all patients with cancer will develop PNS.[1,2] Malignancies that produce neuroendocrine proteins such as SCLC, immunoglobulin (lymphoma or multiple myeloma), or involve immune organs such as thymoma are the most commonly associated with the development of PNS. It is estimated that approximately 5% of patients with SCLC and approximately 10% of patients with lymphoma or multiple myeloma will develop and PNS.[3] In the majority of cases, the neurologic symptoms are detected prior to the diagnosis of the malignancy. This clinical situation creates a diagnostic dilemma as the symptoms of the PNS, including cognitive changes, ataxia, weakness, or numbness, are often nonspecific and may be associated with other nonmalignant syndromes or etiologies.

The presenting symptoms provide insight into the area of the nervous system affected, the type of PNS, and the potential underlying malignancy. PNSs that affect the central nervous system include limbic encephalitis (LE) and paraneoplastic cerebellar degeneration, whereas those affecting the neuromuscular junction include myasthenia gravis (MG) and Lambert-Eaton myasthenia syndrome (LEMS). Involvement of the peripheral nervous system can cause autonomic neuropathy and subacute sensory neuropathy. Approximately 70% of cases with limbic encephalitis and subacute sensory neuropathy are associated with a malignancy. However, only 40% to 50% of cases subacute cerebellar ataxia, LEMS, and MG are associated with a malignancy.[3]

PNSs occur when the immune system cross-reacts with antigens on the tumor cells and proteins expressed in the neurologic system.[4] The two categories of antigens are intracellular antigens and extracellular antigens, with the pathophysiology differing according to the antigen.[5] For syndromes where the antigen is an intracellular, the antibody stimulates antigen-specific T-cell lymphocytes, leading the immune system to attack the neurologic system.[6] In syndromes where the antigen is extracellular, including myelin proteins, gangliosides, ion channels, or cell membrane proteins, the antibodies bind with the target and change the protein expression of the cell or damage the cell membrane by complement activation. The syndromes related to monoclonal antibodies against extracellular antigens respond better to therapy than syndromes associated with cell-mediated mechanisms.[7] Because the tumor cells are not the source of antibody production, successful treatment of the malignancy may not reduce the symptoms associated the PNS and the neurologic damage sustained prior to diagnosis may be permanent. Another mechanism of action for the monoclonal antibodies is a direct interference with the extracellular protein or receptor. An example of this mechanism is LEMS in which the monoclonal antibody interferes acetylcholine binding and postsynaptic signal transduction at the neuromuscular junction, leading the symptoms of muscle weakness. The role of the monoclonal antibody and the pathophysiology in PNSs is unknown in many syndromes.

Diagnosis

The initial diagnostic workup depends on whether the patients have a known malignancy or not. For patients with a known malignancy the workup includes radiologic imaging to evaluate for brain metastases, leptomeningeal disease or spinal cord compression, and a review of previous radiation therapy or chemotherapy treatments that are associated with neurologic toxicity. Once other causes of the neurologic symptoms have been excluded, a workup for PNS is initiated, including additional imaging, cerebrospinal fluid (CSF) analysis, nerve conduction studies, and electroencephalography, or electromyography depending on the symptoms. Lumbar puncture can be performed to evaluate for leptomenigeal disease and inflammatory or infectious etiologies of the symptoms. In PNS, the CSF often reveals pleocytosis and elevated protein consistent with inflammation, elevated immunoglobins (Ig) G and oligoclonal bands.[8] Oligoclonal bands may be the only CSF abnormality in 10% of the cases.[8]

The constellation of symptoms define a syndrome, and the syndromes are often defined as "classical," which are the syndromes commonly associated with an underlying malignancy. An international panel of neurologists established criteria for "definite" and "possible" PNS (Table 129.1).[9] Examples of classical syndromes include encephalomyelitis, LE, subacute cerebellar degeneration, opsoclonus-myclonus syndrome (OMS), subacute sensory neuropathy chronic gastrointestinal (GI) pseudo-obstruction, LEMS, and dermatomyositis (DM).[9] Some syndromes are associated with specific malignancies (Table 129.2).

TABLE 129.1

Diagnostic Criteria for Neurologic Paraneoplastic Syndromes

Definite	Possible
1. A classical syndrome and cancer that develops within 5 years of the diagnosis of the neurologic disorder	1. A classical syndrome, no onconeural antibodies, no evidence of cancer but a high risk of having an underlying cancer
2. A nonclassical syndrome that resolves or significantly improves after cancer treatment without concomitant immunotherapy (provided the syndrome is not susceptible to spontaneous remission)	2. A neurologic syndrome (classical or not) with partially characterized onconeural antibodies and no cancer
3. A nonclassical syndrome with onconeural antibodies (well characterized or not) and cancer that develops with 5 years of the diagnosis of the neurologic disorder	3. A nonclassical syndrome, no onconeural antibodies, and cancer present within 2 years of diagnosis
4. A neurologic syndrome (classical or not) with characterized onconeural antibodies (anti-HU, Yo, CV2, Ri, Ma2, or amphipysin) and no cancer	

TABLE 129.2

Overview of Common Paraneoplastic Neurologic Syndromes

Syndrome Name	Common Clinical Symptoms	Associated Malignancies	Onconeural Antibodies	Potential Diagnostic Studies
Limbic encephalitis	Mood changes, hallucinations, memory loss, seizures, hypothalamic syndromes	1. SCLC (most common) 2. Testicular germ cell 3. Breast 4. Thymoma 5. Teratoma 6. Hodgkin lymphoma	1. Anti-Hu 2. Anti-Ma2 3. Anti-CRMP5 4. Anti-amphiphysin	1. EEG 2. MRI of the brain for hyperintensity in the temporal lobe 3. CSF analysis
Subacute cerebellar degeneration	Ataxia, diplopia, dysphagia, dysarthria, dizziness, nausea/vomiting	1. SCLC 2. Gynecologic 3. Hodgkin lymphoma 4. Breast	1. Anti-Yo 2. Anti-Hu 3. Anti-CRMP5 4. Anti-Ma 5. Anti-Tr 6. Anti-Ri 7. Anti-VGCC 8. Anti-MGluR1	1. MRI of brain for cerebellar atrophy
Lambert-Eaton myasthenia syndrome	Lower extremity proximal muscle weakness, fatigue, diaphragmatic weakness, bulbar symptoms, autonomic symptoms	1. SCLC 2. Prostate 3. Cervical 4. Lymphoma	Anti-VGC	EMG: low muscle action amplitude, decreased response with low-rate stimulation and increased response with high rate stimulation
Myasthenia gravis	Fatigable weakness of voluntary muscles (ocular-bulbar and limbs), diaphragmatic weakness	Thymoma	Anti-AchR	EMG: decreased response to repetitive nerve stimulation
Autonomic neuropathy	Panautonomic neuropathy involving sympathetic, parasympathetic, and enteric systems (symptoms include orthostatic hypotension, GI, or bladder dysfunction, dysphagia, altered pupillary light reflexes, arrhythmias)	1. SCLC 2. Thymoma	1. Anti-Hu 2. Anti-nAchR 3. Anti-CRMP5 4. Anti-amphiphysin	Symptom dependent
Subacute peripheral neuropathy	Paresthesias, pain, ataxia, decreased deep tendon reflexes	1. SCLC 2. Breast 3. Ovarian 4. Sarcoma 5. Hodgkin lymphoma	1. Anti-hu 2. Anti-CRMP5 3. Anti-amphiphysin	1. Nerve conduction studies 2. CSF analysis

SCLC, small-cell lung cancer; EEG, electroencephalogram; MRI, magnetic resonance imaging; CSF, cerebrospinal fluid; EMG, electromyelogram; GI, gastrointestinal.

Frequently, a panel of serum antibodies against neural proteins, referred to as onconeural antibodies, are checked as part of the initial workup, as a single syndrome may be associated with multiple antibodies.[10] These antibodies are useful but have some well-recognized flaws. The association between onconeural antibodies and PNS is variable (Table 129.3).[9] Onconeural antibodies found in both PNS and nonmalignant syndromes include antiacetylcholine receptor, antinicotinic, antivoltage-gated calcium channel (VGCC), and voltage-gated potassium channels (VGKC).[1,4] Among the known VGCC subtypes including L, R, T, N, and P/Q,[11,12] the latter two are expressed in SCLC and are common targets for antibodies in these patients.[13] All these antibodies target extracellular antigens. Importantly, <50% of patients with a clinical syndrome of PNS will have the antibodies detected, and these antibodies can be detected in patients without PNS.[1,10] Therefore, the absence of onconeural antibodies should not exclude the diagnosis of PNS, and the presence of onconeural antibodies alone should not be considered diagnostic. Of note, anti-Tr antibodies associated with cerebellar degeneration can be detected in the CSF but not in the serum.[14] Another clinical dilemma is that onco-neural antibody tests take time and symptomatic patients may require treatment before the results are available.

Patients may present with symptoms consistent with PNS without a known diagnosis of cancer, and a workup for an underlying malignancy is initiated. This should include a history to assess for symptoms and risk factors for an underlying malignancy, a physical exam, and a workup for occult malignancy. Frequently, the initial test is computed tomography scan of the chest, abdomen, and pelvis. Fluorodeoxyglucose positron emission tomography (FDG-PET) is increasingly popular. A small study compared computed tomography and FDG-PET, and the sensitivity for detection of tumor or tumor recurrence in patients with PNS was 30% and 90%, respectively (*p* <0.01).[15]

Specific Syndromes

Numerous neurologic syndromes have reported to be associated with malignancy in case reports. However, several specific syndromes with a common constellation of symptoms have been reported consistently in the literature. This section will focus on the more common PNSs. PNSs that affect the central nervous system include LE, subacute cerebellar degeneration, and OMS. Symptoms associated with LE include short-term memory loss, confusion, psychiatric symptoms such as hallucinations and mood changes, and seizures. The symptoms will present over a period of several days to several months. Magnetic resonance imaging (MRI) reveals hyperintensity of the medial temporal lobe(s), and CSF analysis will reveal pleocytosis, elevated protein, elevated IgG, and oligoclonal bands.[1] LE is associated with onconeural antibodies against the VGKC.[9] Subacute cerebellar degeneration typically presents with symptoms of ataxia, diplopia, dysphagia, and dysarthria. Typically, the first symptoms are isolated gait ataxia and subsequent development of truncal and hemispheric cerebellar dysfunction.[9] The onset of symptoms is generally <12 weeks, and MRI of the brain does not reveal any significant cerebellar atrophy. The P/Q type anti-VGCC antibodies and other antibodies have been reported with this PNS.[1,16] Concurrent cerebellar degeneration and LEMS has been reported as well in patients with SCLC.[17] OMS is characterized subacute onset of opsoclonus, a disorder or saccadic eye movements, chaotic saccades in all directions, and arrhythmic-action myoclonus that predominately involves the trunk, limbs, and head.[18] The pathophysiologic mechanism for this disorder is unclear but may be mediated by disruption of the Nova-1/Nova-2 proteins of the glycine receptor.[19] This disorder has been associated with SCLC in adults and neuroblastoma in children.[19]

Subacute sensory neuropathy and GI dysmotility are two PNSs that affect the peripheral nervous system. The common symptoms

PRACTICE OF ONCOLOGY

TABLE 129.3

Onconeural Antibodies and Associated Syndromes and Malignancies

Onconeural Antibody	Paraneoplastic Syndrome	Malignancy	Antigen Location
Strong Association			
Anti-Hu (ANNA-1)	▪ Limbic encephalitis ▪ Paraneoplastic cerebellar degeneration ▪ Subacute sensory neuropathy ▪ Chronic gastrointestinal pseudo-obstruction ▪ Autonomic neuropathy	SCLC, neuroblastoma, prostate cancer	Nucleus
Anti-Yo (PCA1)	Paraneoplastic cerebellar degeneration	Ovary, breast	Cytoplasmic
Anti-CV2 (CRMP5)	▪ Subacute sensory neuropathy ▪ Chronic gastrointestinal pseudo-obstruction ▪ Paraneoplastic cerebellar degeneration ▪ Limbic encephalitis ▪ Autonomic neuropathy ▪ Chorea	SCLC, thymoma	Cytoplasmic
Anti-Ri (ANNA2)	▪ Brainstem encephalitis ▪ Opsoclonus myoclonus	Breast, SCLC	Nucleus
Anti-Ma2 (Ta)	▪ Limbic encephalitis ▪ Paraneoplastic cerebellar degeneration	Testicular, lung cancer	Nucleus
Anti-amphiphysin	▪ Stiff person syndrome ▪ Sensory neuropathy	Breast, SCLC	Cytoplasmic
Moderate Association			
Anti-Tr(PCA-tr)	Paraneoplastic cerebellar degeneration	Hodgkin disease	Cytoplasmic
Anti-zic4	Paraneoplastic cerebellar degeneration	SCLC	Nucleus
Anti-mGluR1	Paraneoplastic cerebellar degeneration	Hodgkin disease	Cytoplasmic

SCLC, small-cell lung cancer.

of subacute sensory neuropathy are numbness and pain of the extremities, marked asymmetry of symptoms at onset, and loss of proprioception; the onset symptoms is often <12 weeks.[1,9] In the later stages, patients can develop ataxia and multifocal involvement. On physical exam, there is loss of the deep tendon reflexes, and electrophysiologic studies reveal involvement of sensory fibers and absence of sensory nerve action potentials.

Patients with cancer often report GI symptoms, including anorexia, early satiety, nausea, emesis, abdominal pain, diarrhea, or constipation. Among the multiple causes for GI complaints in patients with cancer is a paraneoplastic dysmotility, which may affect either the entire GI tract or isolated segments, where they produce specific syndromes such as achalasia, gastroparesis, and intestinal dysmotility with constipation.[20] Paraneoplastic dysmotility should be suspected in patients with rapid symptom onset, significant weight loss, presence of concurrent autonomic or sensory neuropathy, and risk factors for malignancy such as smoking and strong family history. The onset of GI dysmotility usually precedes the diagnosis of cancer, and the most common associated malignancy is SCLC. The presumed pathophysiology is the presence of tumor antigens that elicit an immune response which cross-reacts with the enteric nervous system. The most common antibody associated with GI dysmotility is the antineuronal nuclear antibody-1, also known as anti-Hu, and approximately 30% of patient with this antibody have symptoms of GI dysmotility.[20,21] Other antibodies associated with GI dysmotility include antineuronal nuclear antibody-2 (anti-Ri), VGCC types N and P/Q, VGKC, and Purkinje cell cytoplasmic (anti-Yo). In a retrospective evaluation of 12 patients diagnosed with malignant tumors and GI motor dysfunction, SCLC was the most common primary malignancy, accounting for 9 cases.[22] The three other patients had lung adenocarcinoma, follicular lymphoma, and ovarian papillary serous adenocarcinoma. The most common presenting symptoms were weight loss, nausea, emesis, and early satiety, which were acute in onset and rapidly progressive in all patients. Although the symptoms preceded the diagnosis of SCLC by a mean interval of approximately 9 months, they developed after the diagnosis in patients with other tumors. Among the 11 patients with serum available, 10 had one or more markers of paraneoplastic immunity including antineuronal nuclear antibody-1, which was detected in all 8 patients with SCLC tested.

MG and LEMS are two PNSs that impact the function of the neuromuscular junction. MG is characterized by muscle weakness of the voluntary muscles that is worsened by exertion. Common symptoms are diplopia and ptosis related to eye muscle weakness. Other symptoms include dysarthria, problems with chewing and swallowing caused by oropharyngeal weakness, and limb girdle weakness, which is generally more pronounced in the proximal than distal muscle groups. Approximately 85% of patients have an onconeural antibody against the muscle acetylcholine receptor (antiacetylcholine receptor), and about 6% of patients will have an onconeural antibody against the muscle specific kinase known as "striational antibodies."[23] MG is associated with thymoma. MG occurs in 30% to 50% of patients with thymoma but only 15% of patients with MG will have thymoma. The presence of antistriational antibodies in a patient younger than 60 years is suspicious for a thymoma.[23] Patients with MG and thymoma may have a better prognosis due to early detection and/or more indolent disease.[24] Importantly, thymectomy will result in an improvement of the symptoms of in the MG, and all thymic tissue should be removed to reduce the rate of recurrence.[25]

Approximately 50% to 60% of patients with LEMS have an underlying tumor, the most commonly SCLC.[26] Clinical symptoms include proximal muscle weakness, autonomic features such as dry mouth, constipation, erectile dysfunction, and less commonly orthostatic hypotension and micturition difficulties, and reduced tendon reflexes. Proximal muscle weakness is frequently the first symptom.[26] Distinguishing MG from LEMS on clinical symptoms can be difficult. In MG, the initial weakness frequently affects the extraocular or bulbar muscles, whereas in LEMS the proximal muscle weakness is frequently the presenting symptom.[27] Patients with LEMS frequently present with leg weakness, whereas limb weakness restricted to the arms is more common in patients with MG. Onconeural antibodies against the P/Q-type VGCC on the presynaptic nerve terminal are characteristic of LEMS and the cause of the muscle weakness. Electromyography studies reveal a low amplitude compound muscle action potential, which becomes lower at low-stimulating frequencies.[26] In order to distinguish LEMS from MG, high-frequency or postexercise stimulation are the diagnostic tests. An increased compound muscle action potential of 60% is considered abnormal and is very sensitive and specific for LEMS.[28] Postexercise stimulation and high-frequency stimulation have a similar sensitivity, but high-frequency stimulation is painful and should be avoided if possible.[26]

Treatment

Given the rarity of PNS, there are no "evidence-based" studies for optimal care. In general, care follows the principles of treating the underlying malignancy, immunosuppression, and symptom-directed supportive care. Many times, the care of a patient with a PNS requires the coordination of care with oncologists, neurologists, and specialists in palliative care. The appropriate care for the type and stage of underlying malignancy should be initiated. Immunosuppression used in the treatment of PNS including corticosteroids, alkylating agents such as cyclophosphamide, intravenous Ig (IVIG), rituximab, and plasmaphaeresis. The prednisone dose frequently employed is 1 mg/kg daily or high-dose intravenous methylprednisolone (1 gm/day for 5 days, followed by weekly therapy of the same dose for 6 to 12 weeks).[10] The dose of oral cyclophosphamide frequently used is 2 mg/kg daily, and azathioprine dose frequently used is up to 2.5 mg/kg daily with adjustments related to toxicity such as myelosuppression.

IVIG is believed to modulate the immune system by interacting with the Fc receptor on immune cells, neutralizing the autoimmune antibody and/or increasing the clearance of the autoimmune antibody, and increasing the regulatory T-cells.[29] PNSs that frequently respond to IVIG include LEMS, MG, Guillain-Barre syndrome, stiff person syndrome, and anti-VGKC limbic encephalitis.[29] IVIG is frequently given 400 to 1,000 mg/day for a total of 2 to 3 g, and the most serious toxicity is nephrotoxicity.[29] Plasmapheresis removes the onconeural antibodies from circulation, and an improvement in symptoms can be observed within days. The effect generally only lasts several weeks, and the concurrent administration of immunosuppressive drugs is required.[1] Rituximab, an anti–B-cell monoclonal antibody, has been used as immunosuppression and case reports of efficacy exist in the treatment of OMS, stiff-person syndrome, paraneoplastic cerebellar degeneration, and LE.[30,31] Rituximab has been mainly studied in patients with PNS who demonstrate the presence of an established onconeural antibody, and the rituximab did not result in consistent effect of serum or CSF antibody titers.[31] The standard dose of rituximab of 375 mg/m² weekly for 4 weeks has been used.

Some PNS benefit from therapies focused on reducing symptoms. The best examples of this are LEMS and MG in which treatment was with the cholinesterase inhibitor pyridostigmine, which inhibitors the degradation of acetylcholine at the neuromuscular juncture and may improve muscle strength.[32] For patients with LEMS, guanidine inhibits the VGKC and enhances the release of acetylcholine. However, the toxicities of myelosuppression and renal insufficiency make the use of this agent problematic, especially if the patient requires cytotoxic chemotherapy.[33] Aminopyridines prolong nerve terminal depolarization, which increases calcium and consequently the release of acetylcholine. Whereas dalfampridine, the first available aminopyridine, is not routinely used due to toxicity concerns, 3,4-diaminopyridine is better tolerated and has been shown to improve motor and autonomic symptoms.[34,35] The common adverse effects include lightheadness, fatigue, epigastric distress, and difficulty sleeping. For patients with autonomic neuropathy and symptomatic hypotension, treatment options include increased water intake, fludrocortisone, midodrine, and caffeine.[36,37] For patients with pseudo-obstruction, neostigmine has been investigated.[38]

Prognosis

Given the rarity of and the multiple different malignancies associated with this PNS, it has been difficult to determine the impact of this PNS of prognosis. In the case of MG associated with thymoma, there is some evidence that patients may have a better prognosis due to more indolent disease and/or earlier detection, and for patients with SCLC with anti-Hu antibody–associated PNS, there is some evidence that they are more responsive to therapy.[24,39] Conversely, patients with a PNS often have poor performance as a consequence of well-advanced malignancy, and many times there are justifiable concerns about the patient's ability to tolerate cytotoxic chemotherapy. If the poor performance status is related to the underlying PNS, cancer-specific therapy is often initiated in an attempt to improve the symptoms. Although the exact impact of a concurrent PNS on prognosis is difficult to assess, survival consistent with the prognosis of the underlying malignancy has been reported with treatment.

PARANEOPLASTIC ENDOCRINOLOGY SYNDROMES

Inappropriate Antidiuretic Hormone Secretion

The syndrome of inappropriate antidiuretic hormone secretion (SIADH) is a disorder of sodium and water balance characterized by a hypotonic euvolemia hyponatremia. The nonapeptide antidiuretic hormone (ADH) or arginine-vasopressin is synthetized in the hypothalamic magnocellullar neurons of the supraoptic and paraventricular nuclei and stored in the posterior lobe of the pituitary gland. There are three known receptors for ADH at the cell membrane: V1a, V1b, and V2.[40,41] V1a receptors are found in the vascular smooth muscle, uterus, platelets, and hepatocytes, where the main functions include vasoconstriction, uterine contraction, platelet aggregation, and glycogenolysis, respectively. V1b receptors are located in the corticotroph cells of the anterior pituitary gland where they are involved in the release of adrenocorticotrophin hormone (ACTH) and beta-endorphin. V2 receptors are located in the basolateral membrane of the renal-collecting duct principal cells, vascular smooth muscle, and vascular endothelium, where they are involved in the synthesis and insertion of aquaporin 2 (AQP-2) channels into the apical membrane, vasodilation, and release of von Willebrand and factor VIII. Binding of ADH to the V2 receptor in the basolateral membrane of the collecting duct cells leads to activation of adenylate cyclase, with increased production of cyclic adenosine monophosphate, which in turn leads to activation of protein kinase A. Protein kinase A phosphorylates vesicles containing preformed AQP-2 vesicles, which leads to their movement to the apical membrane, where AQP-2 is inserted and works as selective water-conducting channel according to the gradient from the tubular lumen to the medullary interstitium. V2 receptor activation also leads to the increased synthesis of AQP-2. The water enters the cells through AQP-2 channels in the apical membrane and exits through the constitutively active AQP-3 and AQP-4 in the basolateral membrane. The two main stimuli for the ADH secretion are the increased plasma osmolality and decreased intravascular volume, which are regulated by the hypothalamic central sensing system and baroreceptors, respectively. Both ADH and thirst maintain the serum osmolality within a narrow range

averaging approximately 285 mOsm/kg, with an increased osmolality above the threshold being the most important stimulus for the ADH secretion. A second stimulus is a decrease in the effective arterial volume caused by extracellular volume depletion or hypotension, which is detected by the volume-sensitive receptors on the left atrium and leads to a restoration of the effective blood volume through V2 receptors and the blood pressure through V1A receptors in the vascular smooth muscle.[42] Stimulation of V1a receptors occur at higher plasma concentrations of ADH compared those needed for V2-dependent antidiuretic effects.

The main etiologies for SIADH can be broadly categorized into malignancies or drug-induced and pulmonary or central nervous system disorders. Both intrathoracic and extrathoracic malignancies have been associated with SIADH, with SCLC usually identified as the most common cause. List and colleagues[43] reported the presence of SIADH in 40 (11%) out of 350 patients with SCLC, without correlation to stage or site of metastases, and no influence, as an independent variable, on response to chemotherapy or survival. SIADH has been described in approximately 3% of patients with head and neck cancer,[44] most commonly in tumors of the oral cavity.[45] Other malignancies that have been rarely associated with SIADH include thymomas,[46,47] lymphoma,[48–50] pancreatic carcinomas,[51] and prostate cancer.[52–54]

Clinical Manifestations

The symptoms from SIADH depend on the degree and rapidity of the change in the serum sodium levels, with the rate of sodium fall considered to be a stronger predictor for morbidity and mortality compared its magnitude.[55,56] Severe hyponatremia is arbitrarily defined as serum sodium concentration <115 mmol/L.[57] Due to hypoosmolality, there is an entry of free water into the cells, with the brain being particularly affected as it has limited space for expansion inside the skull. Therefore, the most common symptoms from hyponatremia are neurologic and result from cerebral edema. The presence of brain edema triggers an adaptive response to restore the brain volume and limit the neurologic complications, with an initial decrease in brain electrolyte content followed by loss of organic solutes such as creatine and amino acids.[58] During acute hyponatremia, defined as the rapid decline of serum sodium over a period of <48 hours, the adaptive brain response is overwhelmed, with the development of severe brain edema and neurologic symptoms including nausea and vomiting and headaches, which may progress to seizures, respiratory arrest, and death. Patients with chronic hyponatremia are usually either asymptomatic or have milder symptoms compared to acute hyponatremia, including fatigue, confusion, falls, and attention deficit.[59]

Diagnosis

The diagnostic criteria for SIADH may be subdivided into essential and supplementary features (Table 129.4).[60–62] The diagnosis of SIADH is usually made after exclusion of other etiologies for hyponatremia through the use of the essential diagnostic criteria. The first step is to measure the plasma osmolality, with values <275 mOsm/kg of water ruling out the causes of hyponatremia with normal or increased plasma osmolality such as translocation by hyperglycemia or pseudohyponatremia caused by hyperlipidemia or hyperproteinemia. The next step is to evaluate the urinary osmolality, which should be >100 mOsm/kg of water during hypotonicity, to define the presence of inappropriate renal dilution and help to exclude the few causes of hyponatremia with decreased urinary osmolality such as beer potomania and polydipsia. Clinical euvolemia is defined as the absence of signs of volume depletion (dry mucous membranes, tachycardia, and orthostasis) caused by renal or extrarenal sodium loss or volume overload (edema and ascites) caused by renal failure, nephrotic syndrome, cirrhosis, and heart failure. The next step is to rule out hypothyroidism and glucocorticoid deficiency, the other two common etiologies that fall into the hypotonic euvolemic hyponatremia.

Diagnostic Criteria for Inappropriate Antidiuretic Hormone Secretion

Essential features	1. Effective osmolality <275 mOsm/kg of water 2. Urine osmolality >100 mg/kg of water during hypotonicity 3. Clinical euvolemia 4. Urine sodium >40 mmol/L with normal dietary salt intake 5. Normal thyroid and adrenal function 6. No recent use of diuretics
Supplemental features	1. Serum uric acid <4 mg/dl 2. BUN <10 mg/dl 3. Fractional sodium excretion >1% 4. Fractional excretion of urea >55% 5. Failure to correct the hyponatremia after infusion of 2 L of 0.9% saline 6. Correction of hyponatremia with fluid restriction 7. Abnormal result on the water test load 8. Elevated plasma ADH levels despite hypotonicity and clinical euvolemia

BUN, blood urea nitrogen; ADH, antidiuretic hormone.

The supplementary features include reduced uric acid and blood urea nitrogen, increased fractional excretion of sodium and urea, correction of hyponatremia with fluid restriction but not after a 2 liter infusion of 0.9% saline, elevated plasma ADH levels despite hypotonicity and clinical euvolemia and abnormal result on the test of water load, which is defined as inability to excrete at least 90% of a 20 mg/Kg water load in 4 hours or failure to achieve an urine osmolality <100 mOsmol per Kg of water. Decreased blood urea nitrogen and uric acid are both indicative of euvolemia although not specific for SIADH, whereas increased values are suggestive of hypovolemia. Because some patients with nonparaneoplastic SIADH may have low or undetectable levels of ADH, the term syndrome of inappropriate diuresis has been proposed as a more accurate description of this condition.[63]

Treatment

The treatment of paraneoplastic SIADH may be broadly subdivided into indirect and direct modalities. In addition to cancer-specific therapy that, if effective, may eventually improve the hyponatremia by reducing the production of ADH by the malignant cells, the initial treatment for nonsevere cases of hyponatremia caused by SIADH is fluid restriction to approximately 800 ml daily in an attempt to induce a negative balance as the urinary excretion plus insensible losses usually exceed 1 L per day.[55] This treatment modality, however, is associated with a slow improvement, has a very low compliance rate, particularly in outpatients, and is often insufficient to improve the hyponatremic symptoms. Therefore, pharmacologic interventions are usually indicated. Oral administration of urea at 30 g daily has been associated with improvement in hyponatremia associated with SIADH by causing osmotic diuresis and increased water excretion.[64–66] The main drawback from urea is the poor palatability, with most patients unable to tolerate it despite being dissolved in strong flavored liquids. Loop diuretics such as furosemide and triamterene have been shown to be effective in patients with SIADH by causing increased excretion of free water.[67] Both demeclocycline and lithium decrease the responsiveness to ADH in the collecting tube, causing nephrogenic diabetes insipidus, with decreased urine concentration despite elevated ADH.[68–71] Demeclocycline is a tetracycline derivative

with unpredictable onset of action and may cause significant side effects including GI intolerance, photosensitivity, and azotemia. The typical doses are from 300 to 600 mg twice daily. Lithium improves hyponatremia through dysregulation of AQP-2[72] but has been abandoned as a treatment for SIADH due to the association with interstitial nephritis and end-stage renal failure as well as decreased efficacy compared to demeclocycline.[69]

Patients with symptomatic acute hyponatremia should be treated with continuous infusion of hypertonic saline (3% NaCl), as the euvolemic hyponatremia is unlikely to respond to normal saline, with a maximal correction rate of 8 to 12 mmol/L during the first 24 hours.[62] The initial infusion rate can be estimated by multiplying the patient's body weight in kilograms by the desired rate of increase of serum sodium in mmol/L per hour.[73] As an example, for a 70-kg patient, an infusion of 3% saline at 70 ml and 35 ml/hour will increase the serum sodium by approximately 1 mmol/L and 0.5 mmol/L per hour, respectively. Patients with known cardiovascular disease should receive 20 to 40 mg of intravenous furosemide to avoid volume overload. The main goal of therapy is to achieve a safe serum levels with symptomatic relief, rather than completely normal levels. Therefore, acute treatment can be discontinued once the symptoms are resolved, a safe serum sodium usually defined as ≥120 mmol/L, or the total magnitude of correction reached 18 mmol/L.

Vasopressine Receptor Antagonists

Vasopressine receptor antagonists (vaptans) are nonpeptide ADH (arginine-vasopressin) antagonists that penetrate deeper into the transmembrane region of V2 receptors compared to ADH, and competitively block the activation of the receptor by endogenous ADH.[74] With the inactivation of the receptor, the synthesis and transport of AQP-2 into the apical membrane of the collecting duct cells is inhibited, resulting in a decrease in the free water reabsorption and increased urine volume.[75] Although the increased diuresis produced by V2 receptor antagonists is quantitatively similar to loop diuretics, the latter produces essentially an aquaresis, which unlike the diuretics, is characterized by decreased urinary osmolality. Vaptans are indicated for patients with either euvolemic or hypervolemic hyponatremia, and should not be used in hypovolemic hyponatremia. During treatment with vaptans, it is very important to monitor the sodium levels to exclude rapid correction rates; there is no need for fluid restriction. Among the four vaptans with reported data from randomized clinical trials, only conivaptan and tolvaptan are currently approved by the US Food and Drug Administration and are available for clinical use (Table 129.5). Conivaptan is the only drug that inhibits both V2 and V1a receptors, while the other vaptans are V2 receptor–specific.[76–78] Another difference between conivaptan and the other vaptans is that although the former was originally developed

Vaptans Tested in Clinical Trials

Name	Receptor Specificity	Administration Route	Dose
Tolvaptan	V2	Oral	15–60 mg once daily
Lixivaptan	V2	Oral	50–100 mg twice daily
Satavaptan	V2	Oral	5–50 mg once daily
Conivaptan	V1a/V2	Intravenous	20–40 mg once daily

as an oral preparation,[79,80] it was subsequently approved by the US Food and Drug Administration and marketed as an intravenous drug.[81] The recommended treatment includes a loading dose of 20 mg over 30 minutes followed by a maintenance dose of 20 to 40 mg daily through continuous infusion for up to 4 days. Due to infusion site complications, including erythema, phlebitis, and swelling, the infusion should be through a large vein with the site changed every 24 hours. There are several medications with potential for significant drug interactions including statins, calcium channel blockers, benzodiazepines, azole antifungals, and chemotherapy agents including vinca alkaloids, doxorubicin, and etoposide, with the latter particularly important given the frequency of SCLC as the SIADH etiology, for which etoposide is commonly the chemotherapy of choice in the first-line setting. Tolvaptan is an oral drug that is 29 times more selective for V2 receptors than V1a and does not have intrinsic agonist effects.[82,83] Schrier and colleagues[84] reported the combined results of two multicenter randomized clinical trials, the Study of Ascending Levels of Tolvaptan in Hyponatremia (SALT) 1 and 2, where 448 patients were randomized to oral tovaptan 15 mg daily or oral placebo. During the first 4 days of therapy, the dose of the study drug could be escalated to up to 60 mg daily according to the serum sodium concentrations. Eligible patients had hyponatremia due to cirrhosis, congestive heart failure, or SIADH. Tolvaptan was associated with a significant increase in the serum levels of sodium during the first 4 days (p <0.001) and after 30 days of therapy (p <0.001). The treatment was well tolerated with increased thirst, dry mouth, and urination as the main side effects. In a subset analysis of 110 patients with SIADH from the SALT trials, the results were similar to the overall population, with a significant improvement in the serum sodium concentration both in the first 4 days and on day 30.[85] The long-term administration of tolvaptan was evaluated by the open-label SALTWATER study, which was an extension of the SALT studies where 111 patients previously assigned to both placebo and tolvaptan arm received tovalptan for an extended period of time.[86] Prolonged treatment was associated with maintenance of normal serum sodium levels and tolerable profile where the most common toxicities were similar to SALT studies, including dry mouth, thirst, polydipsia, and polyuria. The most likely role for vaptans in SIADH is in the treatment of mild to moderate hyponatremia and severe asymptomatic hyponatremia.[87] There is not enough data to support the use of vaptans in patients with symptomatic hyponatremia, who should be treated with hypertonic saline.

One of the main concerns during the treatment of chronic hyponatremia is the overzealous treatment, which may lead to osmotic demyelination.[88–90] This complication, also known as osmotic demyelination syndrome (ODS), occurs when the hyponatremia is corrected too rapidly, outpacing the recapture of lost organic molecules by the brain. During the rapid increase in the serum osmolality, the brain cells try to reverse the loss of solutes by increasing the production of organic osmolytes and inorganic ions.[91] This process, however, causes a significant metabolic strain on glial cells leading to adenosine triphosphate depletion. The shifting of water to outside the cells during the correction of hyponatremia results in shrinkage of the glial cells, cellular damage, and disruption of the blood–brain barrier, with the latter allowing inflammatory mediators to enter the central nervous system where they may cause damage to the oligodendrocytes and demyelination. Some central nervous system areas such as the pons appear to be more vulnerable than others. The main risk factors for the development of ODS are serum sodium ≤105 mmol/L, hypokalemia, alcoholism, malnutrition, and advanced liver disease. ODS usually follows a biphasic course with an initial symptomatic improvement with the correction of the hyponatremia, which is followed by new and progressive neurologic symptoms developing a few days later. The presentation symptoms range from confusion to progressive quadriplegia associated with dysphagia and dysarthria. ODS is best evaluated by MRI where hypodense nonenhancing lesions can be seen on T1-weighted images and hyperdense lesions on T2-weighted images.[92,93]

Ectopic Cushing Syndrome

Cushing syndrome is a constellation of symptoms caused by a sustained exposure to excessive concentrations of circulating glucocorticoids. The most common cause of Cushing syndrome is iatrogenic, due to exogenous administration of glucocorticoids. Endogenous Cushing syndrome may be subdivided into ACTH (or corticotropin) dependent and independent.[94] ACTH-dependent Cushing syndrome is far more common, accounting for approximately 80% to 85% of the cases and subdivided into Cushing disease, which is caused by pituitary adenomas and accounts for 80% of the ACTH-dependent endocrine causes, ectopic secretion of ACTH by nonpituitary tumors in approximately 20% of cases, and the rare ectopic secretion of corticotropin-releasing hormone (CRH). ACTH-independent Cushing syndrome is almost always caused by adrenal adenomas or carcinomas, with <1% of cases caused by macronodular adrenal hyperplasia, primary pigmented nodular adrenal disease, and McCune-Albright syndrome.

The most common tumors associated with ectopic ACTH production are the SCLC and bronchial carcinoids, with each accounting for approximately 22% of cases in the largest series.[95–99] Other reported tumors include GI neuroendocrine tumors, thymic carcinoids, medullary thyroid carcinoma, and pheochromocytoma. Occult tumors have been reported in approximately 13% of cases, ranging from 6.7% to 18.9%. In a retrospective review of 545 patients with SCLC seen at the Toronto General Hospital between 1980 and 1990, there were 23 patients (4.5%) with Cushing syndrome caused by ectopic ACTH production. These patients had low response to chemotherapy, high rate of complications from the chemotherapy, and shorter survival.

The clinical features of Cushing syndrome are variable, with decreased libido, obesity or weight gain, facial plethora or rounding, menstrual changes, hypertension, and hirsutism as the most common manifestations.[100] The characteristic features of increased supraclavicular fat, proximal muscle weakness, and purple striae occur in a minority of patients. When compared to neuroendocrine tumors, SCLC has been shown to be associated with higher frequency of hyperpigmentation and ankle edema, but lower frequency of psychiatric findings.[98] Due to the high percentage of SCLC and other advanced malignancies, which are usually associated with weight loss, weight gain is less common in paraneoplastic than nonmalignant Cushing syndrome.

Diagnosis

Patient with characteristics of glucocorticoid excess should have a biochemical confirmed diagnosis of hypercortisolemic state prior to proceeding to the differential diagnosis of Cushing syndrome.

The initial screening tests for Cushing syndrome are the 24-hour urinary free cortisol, low-dose dexamethasone suppression, and the late-night salivary cortisol tests.[101–103] The measurement of urinary cortisol allows a direct assessment of the circulating free cortisol. In contrast, plasma cortisol levels measure the total cortisol levels, including both free and bound to cortisol-binding globulin or other serum proteins. When the excess of cortisol saturates the serum-binding proteins, it is excreted in the urine in a free or unbound form. Therefore, unlike serum cortisol, urinary levels measure only the biologically active form and are not affected by conditions and drugs that alter cortisol-binding globulin. Urinary free cortisol values higher than four-fold greater than the upper normal limit are rare in disorders other than Cushing syndrome. However, up to three 24 hour collections may be required to exclude intermittent hypercortisolism, and the test is not reliable in patients with creatinine clearance <30 ml/min.

There are two low-dose dexamethasone suppression tests commonly used, based on the fact that in normal subjects, the administration of supraphysiologic doses of glucocorticoids suppresses ACTH and cortisol secretion.[104] In patients with endogenous Cushing syndrome, however, the administration of low-dose dexamethasone does not suppress ACTH. The overnight test involves the administration of 1 mg of dexamethasone between 11 p.m. and 12 a.m. with measurement of fasting serum cortisol between 8 and 9 a.m. of the following day. In the 48-hour test, patients receive 0.5 mg of dexamethasone every 6 hours for eight doses, starting at 9 am on day 1, with serum cortisol measured at the start of the test and 6 hours after the last dose. Serum cortisol levels <1.8 mcg/dl have a sensitivity and specificity rates of >95% and 80%, respectively, in excluding Cushing disease. The late-night salivary cortisol test is based on the high correlation between free serum and salivary cortisol levels, independently of salivary flow rates.[105] Furthermore, unlike the serum counterpart, salivary cortisol is not significantly affected by changes in the serum binding proteins. Due to its easy collection and prolonged stability at room temperature, the late-night salivary cortisol test appears particularly suitable for outpatient screening of Cushing disease. The saliva samples are collected during expected plasma cortisol nadir, between 11 p.m. and 12 a.m., via a cotton swab or by spitting into a tube, which can be sealed and transported at room temperature. Normal reference levels are dependent on the assays used, with cutoff values used in trials ranging from 3.6 to 15.2 mmol/L. Therefore, the values should be validated for each laboratory. The presence of normal salivary cortisol levels from samples obtained in two separate days makes Cushing syndrome very unlikely. The diagnosis of Cushing syndrome is confirmed when two tests are unequivocally abnormal, with additional evaluation required in case of slightly abnormal or discordant test results.

Once the diagnosis of Cushing disease is confirmed, the next step is to establish the cause among the three broad subgroups including the ACTH-independent adrenal etiologies, ACTH-dependent pituitary, and ectopic causes. The workup starts with the measurement of plasma ACTH, with levels <5 pg/mL and >20 pg/mL indicating ACTH independent and dependent, respectively.[106–108] In cases with intermediate values, the CRH stimulation test may help to clarify the ACTH dependency.[109] In this test, 100 mcg of CRH is administered intravenously with measurements of ACTH before and after the infusion. Increase in ACTH suggests ACTH-dependent causes. ACTH responses, however, are more common in Cushing disease than ectopic ACTH secretion. As both pituitary and ectopic causes belong to the ACTH-dependent category, the next task is to rule out Cushing disease, usually by a brain MRI but occasionally with bilateral inferior petrosal sinus sampling, which is considered the gold standard for the differential diagnosis of ACTH-dependent Cushing syndrome.[110–113] In this test, ACTH is collected simultaneously from both inferior petrosal sinuses, which drain directly from the pituitary circulation and blood. CRH stimulation is occasionally used to increase the test sensitivity. Petrosal sinus to serum ACTH ratios >2 in basal condition or 3 after CRH stimulation are consistent with Cushing disease. Despite the very high sensitivity and specificity for this test, its use is limited by the cost and expertise necessary to perform the inferior petrosal sinus collection. Patients with ACTH-dependent Cushing syndrome without evidence of a pituitary cause are likely to have ectopic ACTH production from neuroendocrine malignancies. Therefore, in patients without the established cancer diagnosis, the next step would be to search for the occult malignancy with computed tomography scans of the chest and abdomen. The use of further imaging tests will be guided by the findings from the initial workup.

Treatment

Complete remission of Cushing syndrome may be achieved in the majority of patients where the ectopic source of ACTH is identified and the tumor is treated with curative intent. Nevertheless, curative resection is often not possible and patients require therapies aimed at decreasing the cortisol secretion by the adrenal glands. Although systemic therapy may improve the hypercortisolism, particularly in cases of SCLC, most patients require inhibitors of cortisol secretion. The most commonly used drugs are ketoconazole metyrapone and mitotane.[114] Ketoconazole inhibits several steps in adrenal steroidogenesis, has a rapid onset of action, and is effective in approximately 50% of patients with ectopic ACTH secretion.[115,116] The typical dose ranges from 400 to 1200 mg daily. Metyrapone inhibits 11-beta hydroxylase in the adrenal cortex, blocking the conversion of 11-deoxycortisol to cortisol. Mitotane is adrenolytic and inhibits several steroidogenic steps in the adrenal cortex. An alternative to medical therapy is bilateral adrenalectomy, which induces a rapid resolution of the Cushing symptoms and may be performed through laparoscopic surgery.[117]

Hypoglycemia

Hypoglycemia is most commonly caused by drugs, usually as a complication from treatment with insulin or oral hypoglycemic agents in patients with diabetes mellitus. Hypoglycemia in patients without diabetes mellitus undergoing treatment is rare and may be caused mainly by drugs, ethanol, liver disease, renal disease, congestive heart failure, endocrinopathies, malnutrition, sepsis, and malignancies.[118] Hypoglycemia in patients with cancer may occur due to increased production of insulin by pancreatic insulinomas or ectopic insulin-producing tumors, destruction of the liver and adrenal glands by large metastases, or production of substances interfering with the glucose metabolism such as secretion of insulin-like growth factor (IGF)-I and partially processed precursors of IGF-II, which are collectively known as nonislet cell tumor–induced hypoglycemia (NICTH).[119] Although virtually any type of cancer may cause NICTH, the most common etiologies are sarcomas, hepatocellular carcinoma, and GI carcinomas. The proposed mechanism for the development of NICTH is the increased production of pro-IGF-II that cannot be processed by the tumors, leading to release of the stable and metabolic active intermediate pro-IGF-IIE (68–88) ("big IGF-II") into the circulation. The released big-IGF-II competes with the mature IGF-I and IGF-II for the IGF-binding proteins. Unlike mature IGF-II, big-IGF-II does not allow the formation of a ternary complex with acid-labile subunit, forming mostly a binary complex with IGF-binding protein. There also an increase in free IGF-I and IGF-II due to decreased binding to IGF-binding proteins. Due to the large size, the ternary complexes cannot pass the capillary membrane. However, both the binary complexes and free IGFs cross the capillary membranes, resulting in increased tissue levels of IGF-II and big-IGF-II, which causes hypoglycemia through binding to the insulin receptor B.

Diagnosis

Clinical hypoglycemia is defined as a plasma glucose concentration that is low enough to cause symptoms.[120] As it is unable to either store or generate glucose, the brain relies on a continuous external supply of glucose to meet its energy requirements. The physiologic adaptation to hypoglycemia includes a decrease in insulin secretion and an increase in glucagon and epinephrine secretion. In prolonged cases, there is also an increase in cortisol and growth hormone secretion. The symptoms from hypoglycemia may result from the insufficient supply of glucose to the brain (neuroglycopenia) or the action of the autonomic system.[121] Neuroglycopenic symptoms include cognitive impairment, behavior changes, seizure, and coma, whereas autonomic symptoms include palpitations, tremors, sweating, and hunger. Patients may also have pallor and diaphoresis as the result of adrenergic vasoconstriction and cholinergic activation of the sweat glands, respectively. As the clinical manifestations are nonspecific, the diagnosis may be confirmed by documenting the Whipple triad, which consists of symptoms and signs of hypoglycemia, low plasma glucose

TABLE 129.6

Differential Diagnosis of Hypoglycemia

Diagnosis	Insulin	C Peptide	Circulating Hypoglycemic Agent
Insulinoma	≥3 μU/mL	≥0.2 mmol/L	Absent
NICTH	<3 μU/mL	<0.2 mmol/L	Absent
Oral hypoglycemic	≥3 μU/mL	≥0.2 mmol/L	Present
Exogenous insulin	≥3 μU/mL	<0.2 mmol/L	Absent

NICTH, nonislet cell tumor–induced hypoglycemia.

concentration, and resolution of the symptoms with the increased glucose concentration.

Once the diagnosis of hypoglycemia is established, the next step is to identify the etiology (Table 129.6). In patients with insulinoma or using oral hypoglycemic agents, both insulin levels and C-peptide are elevated. The detection of oral circulating hypoglycemic agents such as sulfonylureas allows the differentiation from insulinoma. In contrast, exogenous administration of insulin and NICTH are associated with low C-peptide levels. Insulin levels, however, are elevated with exogenous insulin and decreased in NICTH.[120]

Treatment

The treatment of hypoglycemic disorders is subdivided into symptomatic relief and correction of the underlying cause. The acute treatment of hypoglycemia is with fast-acting carbohydrate replacement including oral ingestion of glucose tablets, candy, or fruit juice. Patients with severe hypoglycemia should be treated with intravenous dextrose 50% or 1 mg of glucagon by subcutaneous or intramuscular route.[122] After the correction of the glucose levels and symptomatic improvement, further workup with imaging studies should be pursued depending on the initial serologic tests. Surgical resection of the primary malignancy, when feasible, usually provides a resolution of the fasting hypoglycemia. Chemotherapy combinations and radiation therapy may be effective in a variety of unresectable solid tumors associated with NICTH and insulinoma. The combination of diazoxide and a thiazide diuretic may improve the hypoglycemia caused by both NICTH and insulinomas.

Tumor-Induced Osteomalacia

Tumor-induced osteomalacia (TIO), also known as oncogenic osteomalacia, is a rare paraneoplastic syndrome characterized by hypophosphatemia, increased urinary phosphate excretion, reduced 1,25 dihydroxy vitamin D, and osteomalacia.[123] The decrease of both hyphophosphatemia and 1,25 dihydroxy vitamin D appears to be related to fibroblast growth factor 23 (FGF23), which has been identified as the phosphatonin that regulates the phosphate homeostasis.[124,125] When FGF23 binds its FGF receptor, it leads to a reduction of the sodium-dependent phosphate co-transporter 2a in the basal surface of the proximal renal tubule, which ultimately causes an increased urinary excretion of phosphorus and hypophosphatemia.[126] FGF23 also causes downregulation of 1α-hydroxylase and upregulation of 24-hydoxylase, leading to a decrease in 1,25 dihydroxy vitamin D.[127] TIO is caused by mesenchymal tumors that are characteristically slow-growing and polymorphous, and have been subdivided into four groups based on the histology features: phosphaturic mesenchymal tumor mixed connective tissue type (PMTMCT), osteoblastoma-like tumors, ossifying fibrous-like tumors, and nonossifying fibrous-like tumors.[128] PMTMCT is the most common subtype, accounting for approximately 75% of the mesenchymal tumors associated with TIO. Although usually benign, there have been reports of malignant and metastatic PMTMCT.[129,130]

Patient usually present with bone pain, muscle weakness, and fractures for several years prior to the diagnosis.[126] Although hypophosphatemia is the hallmark of TIO, it is often not identified as serum phosphorus measurements are not included in the standard comprehensive metabolic panel.[131] In patients with consistent symptoms and hypophosphatemia, the next step is to confirm the presence of renal phosphate wasting, which can be accomplished by measurements of the percent tubular reabsorption of phosphate or the maximum tubular reabsorption of phosphorus corrected for the glomerular filtration rate.[126] Patients with hypophosphatemia due to increased urinary excretion of phosphorus should undergo additional tests to establish the diagnosis of TIO. Calcium and PTH are usually normal, and 1,25 dihydroxy vitamin D may be low or inappropriately normal. Elevated plasma levels of FGF23 help to confirm the diagnosis.

The treatment of choice for TIO is resection of the tumor with a wide margin, which is curative in the majority of patients. However, as the tumors are often very small and may be located anywhere in the bones of soft tissue, their location may be challenging. Both FDG-PET and [111]Indium octreotide scintigraphy combined with single photon emission computed tomography scan have been recommended as functional imaging studies for the location of the tumors.[132] For patients whose tumors cannot be localized or treated surgically, the mainstay of therapy is phosphorus supplementation, which should be administered in multiple doses per day due to its rapid absorption and clearance.

PARANEOPLASTIC HEMATOLOGIC SYNDROMES

Anemia

Anemia, defined as hemoglobin (Hgb) <12 g/dL and 14 g/dL in women and men, respectively, is a common finding in patients with cancer, with a wide range of prevalence depending on the cancer type, geographic area, and definition of anemia, which has been arbitrarily subdivided in epidemiologic studies according to the Hgb and hematocrit cutoffs into liberal (Hgb >11 g/dl or hematocrit <33%), moderate (Hgb between 9 g/dL and 11 g/dl or HCG between 27% and 33%), and stringent (Hgb <9 g/dl or hematocrit <27%).[133] The etiology of anemia in patients with cancer is usually multifactorial, including a combination of blood loss, hemolysis, and decreased red cell production. Usual factors leading to anemia in patients with cancer include bleeding; treatment-related myelosupression; hemolysis; impaired renal function; deficiency of iron, folate, or vitamin B_{12}; and the anemia of chronic disease (ACD), also known as anemia of inflammation.[134] The main etiologies for ACD include infections, autoimmune disorders, chronic kidney disease, and malignancies.[135] ACD is caused by an increased uptake and retention of iron within the reticuloendothelial cells, with a diversion of iron from the circulation to the storage sites, leading to a state of functional iron deficiency. The production of cytokines such as interleukin (IL) 6, IL-1, tumor necrosis factor-alpha, and interferon-gamma, among others, causes an increase in the production of hepcidin by the liver, in an effect mediated by JAK and STAT3, which decreases the duodenal absorption of iron and binds to ferroportin causing its degradation.[136] Ferroportin is an important transmembrane exporter of iron and its degradation decreases the release of iron into the plasma, resulting in entrapment of iron inside the macrophages and hepatocytes. ACD is usually normochromic and normocytic, with decreased serum iron and transferrin saturation. Ferritin, a marker of iron storage, is usually normal or increased in ACD, in contrast to low values in iron-deficiency anemia. When caused by a malignancy, ACD fits the criteria for paraneoplastic syndrome. Although the treatment of choice for paraneoplastic ACD is directed at the underlying malignancy, this approach is not always possible or successful.[137] Therefore, management of the anemia becomes important in a large fraction of patients. Red blood cell transfusion is indicated in patients with Hgb <8 g/dL, particularly in the presence of coronary artery disease. Use of erythropoiesis-stimulating agents (ESA), including erythropoietin and darbepoetin, are associated with decreased in the transfusion rates and increase in Hgb levels during or shortly after myelotoxic chemotherapy.[138,139] However, there are no other established benefits from this class of drugs, and their indications have become more restricted after reports of increased risk of venous thromboembolism, stroke, tumor progression, and mortality. In a large meta-analysis including 13,933 patients from 53 randomized clinical trials, ESAs were associated with increased mortality by 17% during the treatment period and decrease overall survival.[140] Similar findings were observed in a more recent meta-analysis including 91 trials with 20,102 participants, where ESAs decreased the risk of blood transfusions but caused increased mortality during the study period, hypertension, thromboembolic complications, and thrombocytopenia with hemorrhage.[141] ESAs are recommended only for the treatment of patients undergoing palliative chemotherapy, whereas they are currently not indicated in patients that are either not receiving chemotherapy or treated with curative intent. New therapies under development for ACD include hepcidin antagonists,[142,143] monoclonal antibodies agains IL-6 receptor,[144] and STAT-3 inhibitors.[145]

Pure red cell aplasia (PRCA) is a syndrome characterized by severe normocytic anemia, reticulopenia, and absence of erythroblasts in an otherwise normal bone marrow.[146] PRCA may occur as a congenital or acquired syndrome, with the latter presenting as either an acute self-limited disease occurring mainly in children or as a chronic form most commony seen in adults. There are several causes for PRCA including parvovirus B19 infection, collagen vascular diseases, drugs including erythropoietin, hematologic malignancies, and solid tumors. The diagnosis is made in cases with isolated anemia, characterized by normal white cell and platelet counts as well as normal marrow myeloid cells and megakaryocytes, with an almost complete absence of erythroblasts. Patients with thymoma-associated PRCA may benefit from tumor resection. Several immossupressive drugs have been succesfully used, including corticosteroids, cyclophosphamide, and cyclosporin A. Other options are splenectomy and plamapheresis. For patients with resistant disease, both rituximab and alemtuzumab have been shown to be effective.[147–149]

Polycythemia

Polycythemia is defined by hematocrit >48% and >52% in women and men, respectively. It may be classified as relative, when caused by decreased plasma volume, and absolute, with the latter subdivided into primary and secondary. Primary polycythemias are caused by mutations within the erythroid precursors, with the most common etiology being the polycythemia vera, which is characterized by *JAK2V617F* mutations in 96% of the cases and *JAK2* exon 12 mutations in approximately 3% of the remaining cases.[150] Secondary polycythemias are usually caused by increases in circulating erythropoietin. There are several causes of secondary polycythemias, including hypoxia, endocrine disorders, renal cysts, use of androgens or erythropoietin, and tumors. The most common tumors associated with paraneoplastic erythrocytosis are hepatocellular carcinoma, renal cell carcinoma, cerebellar hemangioblastoma, pheochromocytomas, and uterine leiomyomas.[151,152] Paraneoplastic erythrocytosis is present in approximately 2% to 10% of patients with hepatocellular carcinoma and 1% to

5% with renal cell carcinoma. The treatment for paraneoplastic erythrocytosis is surgical removal of the tumor. There is usually no need for specific therapy of the erythrocytosis, with phlebotomy indicated only in symptomatic cases.

Leukocytosis

Paraneoplastic leukocytosis is frequently observed in patients with cancer, has been reported in a variety of malignancies, is most likely caused by tumor production of granulocyte colony-stimulation factor,[153–155] and is associated with worse prognosis compared to patients without leukocytosis, particularly in gynecologic and lung cancers.[156–158] In a review of 252 patients with nonhematologic malignancies who underwent a complete workup to exclude other possible causes, 77 (30%) had leukocytosis at the time of diagnosis.[159] Absolute monocytosis and eosinophilia were observed in 25% and 4.8% of the patients, respectively. Among patients with non-SCLC, paraneoplastic leukocytosis has been more commonly associated with large cell histology.[155,160] Both tumor-associated tissue eosinophilia and tumor-associated blood eosinophilia have been reported in a variety of cancers including lung, cervical, breast, colon, liver, and pancreatic sarcomas, and hematologic tumors.[161,162] The development of eosinophils is regulated by three cytokines encoded by closely linked genes on chromosome 5q31: IL-3, IL-5, and granulocyte macrophage colony-stimulating factor. IL-5, also known as eosinophil-differentiating factor, is the most specific cytokine for eosinophil lineage and responsible for both selective differentiation of eosinophils and their release from the bone marrow.[162] Several studies have reported the association between intratumoral production of IL-5 and tumor-associated blood eosinophilia.[163–165]

Thrombocytosis is defined as platelet count >450/µL and is usually subdivided into familial, primary, and reactive.[166] In a review of 732 patients with platelet counts ≥500/µL, 643 (87.7%) had secondary thrombocytosis, with 85 (11.6%) of those caused by malignancies, including lymphoma, sarcomas, and GI, lung, breast, and ovarian cancers.[167] Paraneoplastic thrombocytosis is usually associated with poor prognosis.[168] The decreased survival in patients with paraneoplastic thrombocytosis may be related to the tumor-induced platelet aggregation, which correlates with the metastatic potential of cancer cells.[169] Platelet coating protects tumor cells from the physical stressors within the blood vessels and allows evasion from the immune system. Platelets are also a major source of proangiogenic factors such as vascular endothelial growth factor and lymphangiogenesis through vascular endothelial growth factor-C present in the α-granules.

PARANEOPLASTIC DERMATOLOGIC MANIFESTATIONS

The dermatologic manifestations of malignancy are extensive and include cutaneous metastases and changes in the skin due to anatomic obstruction, particularly due to superior vena cava syndrome and rheumatologic changes related to a paraneoplastic endocrine disorder. However, occasionally patients will present with a dermatologic symptom or physical finding that is related to a previously undetected malignancy or during the course of their malignancy. Historically, the criteria for the for paraneoplastic dermatologic syndrome (PDS) are (1) concurrent onset and parallel course of dermatologic condition and malignancy, (2) characteristic type of associated malignancy, (3) statistical association of the dermatosis and the malignancy, and (4) a genetic link between the dermatosis and malignancy.[170] These criteria serve as a "gold standard," but the term PDS is often applied to conditions with a strong association with a specific malignancy. Importantly, the syndrome and cutaneous cells are not malignant, and the pathogenesis of the dermatologic condition is the result of imbalance in cytokines, growth factors, or an aberrant immune response to the underlying malignancy.[171] PDSs are the initial presentation in approximately 1% of internal malignancies and may be initially detected by a dermatologist.[171] This section will focus on the classical PDSs rather than PDSs that have been reported in case reports or where there is a doubt about association between the dermatologic disorder and the malignancy. For simplicity, the disorders are organized by the predominant skin manifestation, although some disorders may have multiple skin manifestations. Many of cutaneous lesions are associated with malignant and nonmalignant conditions. Consultation with a dermatologist is frequently required to assist in the diagnosis and management of PDS. Appropriate treatment of the underlying malignancy is the primary therapy for most PDS, as is supportive care to alleviate the symptoms.

Hyperpigmentation

Polyneuropathy, organomegaly, endocrinopathy, and monoclonal gammopathy and skin changes (POEMS syndrome) is associated with diffuse and homogenous hyperpigmentation. Hyperpigmentation is usually diffuse and homogenous, and generally limited to the extremities or trunk or acral areas. Other cutaneous manifestations of POEMS syndrome include hypertrichosis, digital clubbing, skin thickening or scleroderma-like skin changes, and white spots or streaking of the fingernails (leukonychia).[171]

The initial presentation of malignant acanthosis nigricans is hyperpigmentation of the skinfolds and the posterior neck. The cutaneous lesions are symmetric, hyperpigmented plaques with variable amounts of epidermal hypertrophy that creates a velvety texture.[171,172] As the malignancy progresses, the lesions may involve the oral mucosa and areola, and palmoplantar hyperkeratosis and cutaneous papillomatosis have been observed.[172,173] Generalized pruritus has also been described.[174] The most common malignancy associated with this disorder is gastric adenocarcinoma, accounting for approximately 70% of the cases, with the majority of the remaining cases associated with other GI adenocarcinomas.[172] Malignant acanthosis nigricans may precede the diagnosis of gastric cancer by several years and is believed to be due to the secretion of growth factors by the tumor.[175] Tripe refers to the edible lining of the bovine foregut, and "Tripe palms" describes a condition characterized by rough, velvety appearance of the palms with exaggerated dermatoglyphics (the lines forming the skin pattern of the palms of the hands or the soles of the feet).[171,172] This condition is considered a variant of malignant acanthosis nigricans rather than a separate entity and is most frequently associated with gastric and lung carcinoma.[172]

Leser-Trelat is the sudden increase in the size and number of seborrheic keratosis that is associated with an underlying malignancy. However, there is debate about the validity of this disorder and the association of the disorder with underlying malignancy due to its rarity, the prevalence of seborrheic keratosis and malignancy in the elderly patient population and the inexact definition of "sudden."[172]

Annular Lesions

Erythema gyratum repens is the most common type of erythematous lesion associated with cancer and is characterized by erythematous, scaly, concentric rings that progress at a rate of 1 cm a day and that occur on the trunk or proximal aspect of the extremities.[171] The lesions are pruritic and are frequently described as having a "wood grain" appearance.[176] The face, hands, and feet are generally spared. An underlying malignancy is present in approximately 80% of cases. The most common malignancies are lung cancer, esophagus, and breast.[171,177] The hypothesis is that this condition is caused by deposition of IgG and complement in the skin.[178,179] This disorder may precede the diagnosis, occur at the same time of the diagnosis, or after the diagnosis of malignancy.

The manifestations usually improve or resolve with a successful treatment of the malignancy.[176]

Migratory necrolytic erythema is associated with glucagon-secreting alpha-islet cell tumors and glucagonoma syndrome, which includes diabetes mellitus or glucose intolerance, weight loss, diarrhea, anemia, venous thromboembolism, and neuropsychiatric disorders.[177] Migratory necrolytic erythema is characterized by erythematous annular or arciform lesions that will coalesce into plaques. The edges of the lesions are characterized by blisters, erosions, and crusts. Other mucocutaneous symptoms include cheilosis, atrophic glossitis, oral mucosal inflammation, and alopecia.[176] The lesions are most common in the groin, perineum, buttocks, intertriginous areas, and perioral area.[171,177] The histopathologic features are nonspecific and include epidermal necrosis, subcorneal pustules, confluent parakeratosis, epidermal hyperplasia, and marked papillary dermal hyperplasia in a psoriasiform pattern.[176]

Erythematosquamous and Hyperkeratotic Lesions

Bazex syndrome, also known as acrokeratosis paraneoplastica of Bazex, is a psoriasiform condition that presents with symmetric erythematous and scaling lesions on the hands, feet, elbows, and knees. This condition is considered pathognomonic of an internal malignancy.[180] Patients develop palmoplanter keratoderma with a violaceous color and nail dystrophy, and subsequently develop psoriasiform lesions on the ears, nose, scalp, and trunk.[181] The syndrome may precede the diagnosis of a malignancy by a year and is most closely associated with squamous cell carcinoma of aerodigestive track including larynx, oropharynx, esophagus, and lung.[182] The pathogenesis of this disorder remains unclear with proposed mechanisms including immunologic factors, exogenous production of growth factors for keratinocytes, and vitamin A deficiency. It is important to note there is the unrelated Bazex-Dupre-Christol syndrome, which consists of hypotrichosis, follicular, atrophoderma, and basal cell carcinomas arising at an early age, that is not a paraneoplastic syndrome.[177,183]

Paraneoplastic Pemphigus

The association between pemphigus and malignancy has been controversial and debated, leading to the establishment of diagnostic criteria for paraneoplastic pemphigus (Table 129.7).[184] In order to be considered paraneoplastic pemphigus, all three of the major or two of the major and two of the minor criteria need to be present. The antibodies in a paraneoplastic pemphigus are directed against desmoglein 1 and 3, and against plakin proteins that form

TABLE 129.7

Diagnostic Criteria for Paraneoplastic Pemphigus

Major	Minor
1. Polymorphous mucocutaneous eruption	1. Positive cytoplasmic staining of rat bladder epithelium by indirect immunofluorescence
2. Concurrent internal neoplasia	2. Intercellular and basement membrane zone immunoreactants on direct immunofluorescence or perilesional tissue
3. Characteristic serum immunoprecipitation findings	3. Acantholysis in biopsy specimen from at least one anatomic site of involvement

the intracellular plaques of desmosome and hemidesmosomes, mediating the attachment of cytoskeletal intermediate filaments to transmembrane adhesion molecules.[185,186] These proteins are found in numerous tissues including the epithelium of the respiratory, intestinal, and urinary organs. Histologic evaluation of the skin biopsy reveals interface dermatitis, vacuolization of the basement membrane, necrotic keratinocytes, suprabasal clefting, and acantholysis.[187] Direct immunofluorescence testing reveals IgG and complement 3 deposits in the intercellular epidermal spaces and at the dermal-epidermal junction; however, paraneoplastic pemphigus without evidence Ig deposits is observed.[188]

Paraneoplastic pemphigus is characterized by polymorphous skin lesions that progress to blistering eruptions on the trunk and extremities.[176] Clinically, painful stomatitis is the most characteristic finding, and frequently involves the entire mouth and lips.[177] The stomatitis is often intractable and may involve the esophagus and/or anogenital region. Some patients will have pulmonary involvement and can develop bronchiolitis obliterans–organizing pneumonia; pulmonary involvement portends a poor prognosis.[185] In the majority of the cases, the underlying malignancy is diagnosed before the onset of pemphigus, and the most commonly associated malignancies are non-Hodgkin lymphoma, chronic lymphoid leukemia, Castleman disease, and thymoma.[176,187]

Hypertrichosis Lanuginosa

This disorder is characterized by the development of long, fine nonpigmented hairs ("lanugo hairs") initially on the face and then on the trunk, axillae, and the extremities.[177,187] The palms of the hands, the soles of the feet, and the genital area are characteristically spared. If the tongue is involved, patients develop painful glossitis, hypertrophy of the papillae of the tongue, and disturbance in taste and/or smell.[177] Among men, the most commonly associated malignancies are lung cancer and then colorectal cancer, whereas colorectal cancer, lung cancer, and breast cancer predominate in women.[187] Trichomegaly of the eyebrows and eyelashes and severe hypertrichosis of the face have been reported with agents that target the epidermal growth factor receptor pathway.[189,190]

Ichthyosis Acquisita

Ichthyosis is characterized by the development of dead skin cells that accumulate and present as dry scales on the skins surface. The scales may be delicate and localized to the trunk and legs or diffuse and thickened, and there is generally sparing of the flexures, palms, and soles.[172] The scales are often described as "rhomboid" or "fish-like." Histologically, the defining features are hyperkeratosis and occasional parakaratosis, and decreased granular layer.[172] This condition can be observed in patients with nonmalignant condition such as hypothyroidism and sarcoidosis, and drugs such as butyrophenones used to treat schizophrenia. Nevertheless, it may also be associated with underlying malignancies, particularly Hodgkin lymphoma, which is the most common cause accounting for approximately 70% of the patients with paraneoplastic-acquired ichthyosis.[176] Other associated malignancies include T-cell lymphomas, multiple myeloma, and lung, breast, and cervical cancer. Unlike other PDSs, ichthyotic changes often occur several weeks or months after the detection of the tumor, and the cutaneous symptoms rarely are the presenting sign of an underlying malignancy.[172] Supportive care with moisturizers and keratolytics, and infection prophylaxis in selected cases are valuable.

Sweet Syndrome

Sweet syndrome, also referred to as acute febrile neutrophilic dermatosis, is characterized by the sudden onset of erythematous papules and nodules that coalesce to form irregular, sharply plaques,

and associated elevated neutrophil count and fever. These lesions are painful and are predominantly observed in the face, neck, and trunk. The vesiculated appearance is sometimes seen and related to edema. The histologic appearance is of neutrophilic inflammatory infiltrate that is distributed throughout the upper dermis.[172] Sweet syndrome may be associated with nonmalignant and malignant conditions, with the latter accounting for approximately 20% of the cases.[191] In >60% of the cases of malignancy-associated Sweet syndrome, the diagnosis of Sweet syndrome is either preceded or is made at the time of the diagnosis of malignancy.[191] Among patients with Sweet syndrome, 85% will have an underlying hematologic malignancy, with acute myelogenous leukemia being the most common followed by lymphomas, myelodysplastic syndrome, and chronic myelogenous leukemia. Solid tumors including breast cancer, genitourinary tumors, and GI tumors have also been reported in association with Sweet syndrome.[176,191] Corticosteroid therapy alleviates the symptoms of Sweet syndrome regardless of the response of the underlying malignancy to therapy.[191]

PARANEOPLASTIC RHEUMATOLOGIC MANIFESTATIONS

Hypertrophic Osteoarthropathy

Hypertrophic osteoarthropathy (HOA) is a syndrome characterized by abnormal proliferation of the skin and osseous tissues at the distal extremities. Patients usually have digital clubbing, periostosis of the tubular bones, and synovial effusions.[192] HOA is divided into primary and secondary forms, with the latter most commonly associated with intrathoracic malignancies. Patients may be asymptomatic or complain of bone pain, occasionally deep and excruciating, more prominent in the lower extremities. Periostosis is the radiographic hallmark of HOA and may be detected by radiograph or bone scan. Successful treatment of the underlying malignancy has been associated with significant improvement of HOA.[193] Patients with refractory tumors may benefit from bisphosphonates[194,195] or radiotherapy.[196]

Vasculitis

Cancers may be found in approximately 2% to 5% of patients with vasculitis.[197] The most common types of paraneoplastic vasculitis are the leukocytoclastic vasculitis and Henoch-Schonlein purpura. Leukocytoclastic vasculitis, the most common paraneoplastic vasculitis accounting for 50% to 60% of cases, is associated most commonly with hematologic malignancies. Henoch-Schonlein purpura accounts for 15% of paraneoplastic vasculitis and occurs more commonly in carcinomas of the lung, urogenital, and GI tracts.

Idiopathic Inflammatory Myopathies

Idiopathic inflammatory myopathies are a group of acquired connective tissue diseases that affect mainly the skeletal muscle and may be subdivided according to the characteristic features into DM, polymyositis (PM), and inclusion-body myositis.[198] Cancers may be discovered before, at the same time, or after the diagnosis of the inflammatory myopathy, with the highest risk within the first year of diagnosis and extending up to 5 years in DM.[199] The interval between the appearance of PM and the diagnosis of cancer may be shorter. In a review of case series of inflammatory myopathies, there were 2,439 patients with DM and 947 patients with PM, of which 574 (24%) and 97 (10.2%) had associated malignancy, respectively.[200] The most common malignancies associated with DM were carcinomas of the nasopharynx (21%), breast (15%), lung (15%), ovary (9%), and colon (5%), with no predominant tumor among patients with PM. In a combined analysis of six population-based cohorts, the frequency of malignancies in DM and PM ranged from 9% to 42% and 5% to 18%, respectively. The type of malignancy associated with the inflammatory myopathies depends on the geographic area. In a Scandinavian study, ovarian, lung, and GI cancers were the most commonly associated with DM, while non-Hodgkin lymphoma and bladder cancer were the most common cancers associated with PM.[201] Overall, 70% of associated malignancies for DM and PM combined were adenocarcinomas. In contrast, a study performed in Taiwan showed nasopharyngeal carcinoma as the most common malignancy associated with DM, followed by lung cancer and breast cancer,

whereas there were no dominant tumors in PM.[202] The muscle weakness in patients with cancer-associated myopathy is usually rapidly progressive and severe, leading to a higher frequency of immobility compared to nonparaneoplastic myopathies.[199] The risk for underlying malignancy is increased in older patients, males, and those with more severe disease including more severe or distal muscle weakness, dysphagia, respiratory muscle involvement, and disease refractory to treatment. Screening for malignancies in patients with inflammatory myopathies should be based according to the age, gender, and geographic area, although patients with higher risk may require a more comprehensive screening including tumor markers and imaging studies.

SELECTED REFERENCES

The full reference list can be accessed at lwwhealthlibrary.com/oncology.

1. Pelosof LC, Gerber DE. Paraneoplastic syndromes: an approach to diagnosis and treatment. *Mayo Clin Proc* 2010;85:838–854.
2. Darnell RB, Posner JB. Paraneoplastic syndromes involving the nervous system. *N Engl J Med* 2003;349:1543–1554.
4. de Beukelaar JW, Sillevis Smitt PA. Managing paraneoplastic neurological disorders. *Oncologist* 2006;11:292–305.
5. Lancaster E, Martinez-Hernandez E, Dalmau J. Encephalitis and antibodies to synaptic and neuronal cell surface proteins. *Neurology* 2011;77:179–189.
7. Antoine JC, Camdessanche JP. Treatment options in paraneoplastic disorders of the peripheral nervous system. *Curr Treat Options Neurol* 2013;15:210–223.
9. Graus F, Delattre JY, Antoine JC, et al. Recommended diagnostic criteria for paraneoplastic neurological syndromes. *J Neurol Neurosurg Psychiatry* 2004;75:1135–1140.
13. Lennon VA, Kryzer TJ, Griesmann GE, et al. Calcium-channel antibodies in the Lambert-Eaton syndrome and other paraneoplastic syndromes. *N Engl J Med* 1995;332:1467–1474.
15. Linke R, Schroeder M, Helmberger T, et al. Antibody-positive paraneoplastic neurologic syndromes: value of CT and PET for tumor diagnosis. *Neurology* 2004;63:282–286.
17. Mason WP, Graus F, Lang B, et al. Small-cell lung cancer, paraneoplastic cerebellar degeneration and the Lambert-Eaton myasthenic syndrome. *Brain* 1997;120:1279–1300.
20. DiBaise JK. Paraneoplastic gastrointestinal dysmotility: when to consider and how to diagnose. *Gastroenterol Clin North Am* 2011;40:777–786.
22. Lee HR, Lennon VA, Camilleri M, et al. Paraneoplastic gastrointestinal motor dysfunction: clinical and laboratory characteristics. *Am J Gastroenterol* 2001;96:373–379.
23. Zisimopoulou P, Brenner T, Trakas N, et al. Serological diagnostics in myasthenia gravis based on novel assays and recently identified antigens. *Autoimmun Rev* 2013;12:924–930.
24. Evoli A, Minisci C, Di Schino C, et al. Thymoma in patients with MG: characteristics and long-term outcome. *Neurology* 2002;59:1844–1850.
27. Wirtz PW, Sotodeh M, Nijnuis M, et al. Difference in distribution of muscle weakness between myasthenia gravis and the Lambert-Eaton myasthenic syndrome. *J Neurol Neurosurg Psychiatry* 2002;73:766–768.
35. McEvoy KM, Windebank AJ, Daube JR, et al. 3,4-Diaminopyridine in the treatment of Lambert-Eaton myasthenic syndrome. *N Engl J Med* 1989;321: 1567–1571.
37. Gupta V, Lipsitz LA. Orthostatic hypotension in the elderly: diagnosis and treatment. *Am J Med* 2007;120:841–847.
41. Lehrich RW, Ortiz-Melo DI, Patel MB, et al. Role of vaptans in the management of hyponatremia. *Am J Kidney Dis* 2013;62:364–376.
42. Raftopoulos H. Diagnosis and management of hyponatremia in cancer patients. *Support Care Cancer* 2007;15:1341–1347.
55. Adrogue HJ, Madias NE. Hyponatremia. *N Engl J Med* 2000;342:1581–1589.
57. Gross P, Reimann D, Neidel J, et al. The treatment of severe hyponatremia. *Kidney Int Suppl* 1998;64:S6–S11.
58. Gullans SR, Verbalis JG. Control of brain volume during hyperosmolar and hypoosmolar conditions. *Ann Rev Med* 1993;44:289–301.
60. Schwartz WB, Bennett W, Curelop S, et al. A syndrome of renal sodium loss and hyponatremia probably resulting from inappropriate secretion of antidiuretic hormone. *Am J Med* 1957;23:529–542.
61. Bartter FC, Schwartz WB. The syndrome of inappropriate secretion of antidiuretic hormone. *Am J Med* 1967;42:790–806.
62. Ellison DH, Berl T. Clinical practice. The syndrome of inappropriate antidiuresis. *N Engl J Med* 2007;356:2064–2072.
69. Forrest JN Jr, Cox M, Hong C, et al. Superiority of demeclocycline over lithium in the treatment of chronic syndrome of inappropriate secretion of antidiuretic hormone. *N Engl J Med* 1978;298:173–177.

72. Grunfeld JP, Rossier BC. Lithium nephrotoxicity revisited. *Nat Rev Nephrol* 2009;5:270–276.
73. Verbalis JG, Goldsmith SR, Greenberg A, et al. Hyponatremia treatment guidelines 2007: expert panel recommendations. *Am J Med* 2007;120:S1–S21.
75. Peri A. Clinical review: the use of vaptans in clinical endocrinology. *J Clin Endocrinol Metab* 2013;98:1321–1332.
84. Schrier RW, Gross P, Gheorghiade M, et al. Tolvaptan, a selective oral vasopressin V2-receptor antagonist, for hyponatremia. *N Engl J Med* 2006;355: 2099–2112.
85. Verbalis JG, Adler S, Schrier RW, et al. Efficacy and safety of oral tolvaptan therapy in patients with the syndrome of inappropriate antidiuretic hormone secretion. *Eur J Endocrinol* 2011;164:725–732.
86. Berl T, Quittnat-Pelletier F, Verbalis JG, et al. Oral tolvaptan is safe and effective in chronic hyponatremia. *J Am Soc Nephrol* 2010;21:705–712.
87. Verbalis JG, Goldsmith SR, Greenberg A, et al. Diagnosis, evaluation, and treatment of hyponatremia: expert panel recommendations. *Am J Med* 2013;126:S1–S42.
88. Kleinschmidt-DeMasters BK, Norenberg MD. Rapid correction of hyponatremia causes demyelination: relation to central pontine myelinolysis. *Science* 1981;211:1068–1070.
89. Sterns RH, Riggs JE, Schochet SS Jr. Osmotic demyelination syndrome following correction of hyponatremia. *N Engl J Med* 1986;314:1535–1542.
94. Newell-Price J, Bertagna X, Grossman AB, et al. Cushing's syndrome. *Lancet* 2006;367:1605–1617.
100. Nieman LK. Diagnostic tests for Cushing's syndrome. *Ann N Y Acad Sci* 2002;970:112–118.
104. Nieman LK, Biller BM, Findling JW, et al. The diagnosis of Cushing's syndrome: an Endocrine Society Clinical Practice Guideline. *J Clin Endocrinol Metab* 2008;93:1526–1540.
105. Carroll T, Raff H, Findling JW. Late-night salivary cortisol measurement in the diagnosis of Cushing's syndrome. *Nat Clin Pract Endocrinol Metab* 2008;4:344–350.
106. Newell-Price J, Trainer P, Besser M, et al. The diagnosis and differential diagnosis of Cushing's syndrome and pseudo-Cushing's states. *Endocr Rev* 1998;19:647–672.
108. Arnaldi G, Angeli A, Atkinson AB, et al. Diagnosis and complications of Cushing's syndrome: a consensus statement. *J Clin Endocrinol Metab* 2003;88: 5593–5602.
110. Oldfield EH, Doppman JL, Nieman LK, et al. Petrosal sinus sampling with and without corticotropin-releasing hormone for the differential diagnosis of Cushing's syndrome. *N Engl J Med* 1991;325:897–905.
115. Engelhardt D. Steroid biosynthesis inhibitors in Cushing's syndrome. *Clin Invest* 1994;72:481–488.
118. Guettier JM, Gorden P. Hypoglycemia. *Endocrinol Metab Clin North Am* 2006;35:753–766, viii–ix.
119. de Groot JW, Rikhof B, van Doorn J, et al. Non-islet cell tumour-induced hypoglycaemia: a review of the literature including two new cases. *Endocr Relat Cancer* 2007;14:979–993.
120. Cryer PE, Axelrod L, Grossman AB, et al. Evaluation and management of adult hypoglycemic disorders: an Endocrine Society Clinical Practice Guideline. *J Clin Endocrinol Metab* 2009;94:709–728.
121. Service FJ. Hypoglycemic disorders. *N Engl J Med* 1995;332:1144–1152.
124. Shimada T, Mizutani S, Muto T, et al. Cloning and characterization of FGF23 as a causative factor of tumor-induced osteomalacia. *Proc Natl Acad Sci U S A* 2001;98:6500–6505.
125. Jonsson KB, Zahradnik R, Larsson T, et al. Fibroblast growth factor 23 in oncogenic osteomalacia and X-linked hypophosphatemia. *N Engl J Med* 2003;348:1656–1663.
128. Jan de Beur SM. Tumor-induced osteomalacia. *JAMA* 2005;294:1260–1267.
133. Knight K, Wade S, Balducci L. Prevalence and outcomes of anemia in cancer: a systematic review of the literature. *Am J Med* 2004;116:11S–26S.

135. Weiss G, Goodnough LT. Anemia of chronic disease. *N Engl J Med* 2005;352:1011–1023.

137. Spivak JL. The anaemia of cancer: death by a thousand cuts. *Nat Rev Cancer* 2005;5:543–555.

138. Rizzo JD, Brouwers M, Hurley P, et al. American Society of Clinical Oncology/American Society of Hematology clinical practice guideline update on the use of epoetin and darbepoetin in adult patients with cancer. *J Clin Oncol* 2010;28:4996–5010.

139. Rizzo JD, Brouwers M, Hurley P, et al. American Society of Hematology/American Society of Clinical Oncology clinical practice guideline update on the use of epoetin and darbepoetin in adult patients with cancer. *Blood* 2010;116:4045–4059.

140. Bohlius J, Schmidlin K, Brillant C, et al. Recombinant human erythropoiesis-stimulating agents and mortality in patients with cancer: a meta-analysis of randomised trials. *Lancet* 2009;373:1532–1542.

141. Tonia T, Mettler A, Robert N, et al. Erythropoietin or darbepoetin for patients with cancer. *Cochrane Database Syst Rev* 2012;12:CD003407.

143. Cooke KS, Hinkle B, Salimi-Moosavi H, et al. A fully human anti-hepcidin antibody modulates iron metabolism in both mice and nonhuman primates. *Blood* 2013;122:3054–3061.

146. Sawada K, Fujishima N, Hirokawa M. Acquired pure red cell aplasia: updated review of treatment. *Br J Haematol* 2008;142:505–514.

151. McMullin MF. The classification and diagnosis of erythrocytosis. *Int J Lab Hematol* 2008;30:447–459.

152. Kremyanskaya M, Mascarenhas J, Hoffman R. Why does my patient have erythrocytosis? *Hematol Oncol Clin North Am* 2012;26:267–283, vii–viii.

158. Mandrekar SJ, Northfelt DW, Schild SE, et al. Impact of pretreatment factors on adverse events: a pooled analysis of North Central Cancer Treatment Group advanced stage non-small cell lung cancer trials. *J Thorac Oncol* 2006;1:556–563.

161. Lowe D, Jorizzo J, Hutt MS. Tumour-associated eosinophilia: a review. *J Clin Pathol* 1981;34:1343–1348.

162. Rothenberg ME. Eosinophilia. *N Engl J Med* 1998;338:1592–1600.

167. Griesshammer M, Bangerter M, Sauer T, et al. Aetiology and clinical significance of thrombocytosis: analysis of 732 patients with an elevated platelet count. *J Intern Med* 1999;245:295–300.

169. Bambace NM, Holmes CE. The platelet contribution to cancer progression. *J Thromb Haemost* 2011;9:237–249.

172. Moore RL, Devere TS. Epidermal manifestations of internal malignancy. *Dermatol Clin* 2008;26:17–29, vii.

173. Schwartz RA, Burgess GH. Florid cutaneous papillomatosis. *Arch Dermatol* 1978;114:1803–1806.

174. Brown J, Winkelmann RK. Acanthosis nigricans: a study of 90 cases. *Medicine* 1968;47:33–51.

175. Talsania N, Harwood CA, Piras D, et al. Paraneoplastic acanthosis nigricans: The importance of exhaustive and repeated malignancy screening. *Dermatol Online J* 2010;16:8.

176. Abreu Velez AM, Howard MS. Diagnosis and treatment of cutaneous paraneoplastic disorders. *Dermatol Ther* 2010;23:662–675.

177. Stone SP, Buescher LS. Life-threatening paraneoplastic cutaneous syndromes. *Clin Dermatol* 2005;23:301–306.

179. Eubanks LE, McBurney E, Reed R. Erythema gyratum repens. *Am J Med Sci* 2001;321:302–305.

182. Ellis DL, Kafka SP, Chow JC, et al. Melanoma, growth factors, acanthosis nigricans, the sign of Leser-Trelat, and multiple acrochordons. A possible role for alpha-transforming growth factor in cutaneous paraneoplastic syndromes. *N Engl J Med* 1987;317:1582–1587.

184. Camisa C, Helm TN. Paraneoplastic pemphigus is a distinct neoplasia-induced autoimmune disease. *Arch Dermatol* 1993;129:883–886.

192. Pineda C, Martinez-Lavin M. Hypertrophic osteoarthropathy: what a rheumatologist should know about this uncommon condition. *Rheum Dis Clin North Am* 2013;39:383–400.

195. Jayakar BA, Abelson AG, Yao Q. Treatment of hypertrophic osteoarthropathy with zoledronic acid: case report and review of the literature. *Semin Arthritis Rheum* 2011;41:291–296.

197. Park HJ, Ranganathan P. Neoplastic and paraneoplastic vasculitis, vasculopathy, and hypercoagulability. *Rheum Dis Clin North Am* 2011;37:593–606.

198. Dalakas MC, Hohlfeld R. Polymyositis and dermatomyositis. *Lancet* 2003;362:971–982.

199. Aggarwal R, Oddis CV. Paraneoplastic myalgias and myositis. *Rheum Dis Clin North Am* 2011;37:607–621.

201. Hill CL, Zhang Y, Sigurgeirsson B, et al. Frequency of specific cancer types in dermatomyositis and polymyositis: a population-based study. *Lancet* 2001;357:96–100.

202. Huang YL, Chen YJ, Lin MW, et al. Malignancies associated with dermatomyositis and polymyositis in Taiwan: a nationwide population-based study. *Br J Dermatol* 2009;161:854–860.

130 Autologous Stem Cell Transplantation

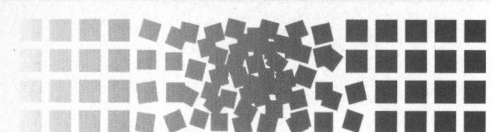

Hillard M. Lazarus, Mehdi Hamadani, and Parameswaran N. Hari

INTRODUCTION

Many decades ago, researchers determined that bone marrow cells transplanted from one animal to another could restore blood production.[1] As these preclinical investigations were taken into the clinical arena, hematopoietic cell transplantation (HCT) evolved as a potentially curative modality for selected malignant and certain nonmalignant diseases. Many malignancies show a steep dose-response to cytotoxic therapy (i.e., small increments in dose of drug or radiation markedly increase the number of cancer cells killed). Cure or effective disease control depends on delivering intensive doses of chemotherapy and/or radiation therapy. This intensity often exceeds the tolerance of bone marrow, necessitating restoration of hematopoietic marrow function in such patients to prevent irreversible and fatal marrow aplasia. This is accomplished by restoring blood production using either autologous ("self") cells (i.e., autologous HCT) or cells collected from another individual (i.e., allogeneic) donor cells (i.e., allogeneic HCT). Autologous HCTs depend entirely upon high-dose therapy to eradicate malignancy, in contrast to allogeneic HCT in which the immunocompetent infused cells exert an "allogeneic effect" against the tumor (i.e., graft-versus-tumor effect).

The phases of autologous HCT include collection of autologous hematopoietic progenitor cells (HPC) and their cryopreservation; administration of high-dose therapy (also called conditioning or preparative regimen); thawing and intravenous administration of the autologous cells; and then vigorous supportive care including antibiotics, blood transfusions, and other measures such as electrolyte replacement while awaiting recovery of hematopoiesis.

Careful patient selection is crucial to successful outcomes after autologous HCT. Patients with poor performance status (Karnofsky performance score ≤60) or significant comorbidities (e.g., poor cardiac reserve [left ventricular ejection fraction <40%], compromised pulmonary function [FEV1 and/or adjusted diffusion capacity <40% of predicted normal], advanced renal insufficiency) are not suitable candidates for high-dose therapies. Similarly heavily pretreated and chemotherapy-refractory patients are unlikely to benefit from this procedure, underscoring the need for timely transplant evaluation for suitable patients.

AUTOLOGOUS HEMATOPOIETIC PROGENITOR CELL COLLECTION

Autologous HPCs can be collected from the patient's bone marrow or blood. The collected bone marrow or blood HPCs are suspended in a balanced salt solution containing a cryoprotectant (often dimethyl sulfoxide [DMSO]) and are cryopreserved in liquid nitrogen. Bone marrow collection involves aspiration of approximately 1,000 ml of marrow (10 to 15 ml/kg patient weight) from the posterior superior iliac crests with the patient in the prone position under spinal or general anesthesia. However, in the last decade, nearly all autografts utilize HPCs collected from blood. HPCs are normally found in low levels in the blood but they can be released or "mobilized" from marrow in large numbers and collected via apheresis instruments. This procedure usually takes 2 to 3 hours and processes three to four blood volumes. The minimum HPC dose to successfully perform an autologous HCT is generally considered to be 2 million CD34+ cells/kg recipient body weight. A dose of ≥4 to 6 million CD34+ cells/kg is considered optimal. This target is based on data showing slower hematopoietic recovery with doses <2 million CD34+ cells/kg and faster platelet recovery with doses ≥5 million CD34+ cells/kg.[2]

HPCs are generally mobilized by serial administration of hematopoietic growth factors such as granulocyte colony-stimulating factor (G-CSF) either alone ("cytokine only" strategy) or in combination with chemotherapy agents such as cyclophosphamide ("chemomobilization" strategy). Another agent, plerixafor, works by disrupting the chemokine receptor type 4 and stromal-derived factor tether between the HPCs and the marrow stromal cells.[3,4] Most patients have an adequate HPCs collected after one or two apheresis procedures. Prior chemotherapy or radiation therapy can impair mobilization, which may affect mobilization or collection strategy.

AUTOLOGOUS HEMATOPOIETIC CELL TRANSPLANTATION TOXICITIES AND SUPPORTIVE CARE

Specific regimens used for high-dose therapy vary depending on the indication for HCT and are discussed in coming sections in detail. HPCs infused after high-dose therapy require time to regenerate hematopoiesis; during this time, the patient requires intensive supportive care to prevent complications arising from prolonged cytopenias and organ damage induced by conditioning regimen. Breakdown of the normal mucosal barriers in the gastrointestinal tract leading to oral mucositis, pain, diarrhea, and increased susceptibility to infectious complications is common. Hematopoietic recovery takes approximately 2 to 3 weeks, and recombinant hematopoietic growth factor support early after HPC infusion can reduce the duration of severe neutropenia by 2 to 4 days. Red blood cell and platelet transfusions are essential to prevent or treat complications and symptoms of profound cytopenias. All blood products must be irradiated to prevent inadvertent engraftment of "contaminating" allogeneic lymphocytes from the transfused unit that may cause lethal transfusion-associated graft-versus-host disease. Major infections encountered in autologous HCT are with gram-negative and gram-positive bacteria; *Clostridia difficile* toxin–associated diarrhea, herpes simplex, and fungi, particularly

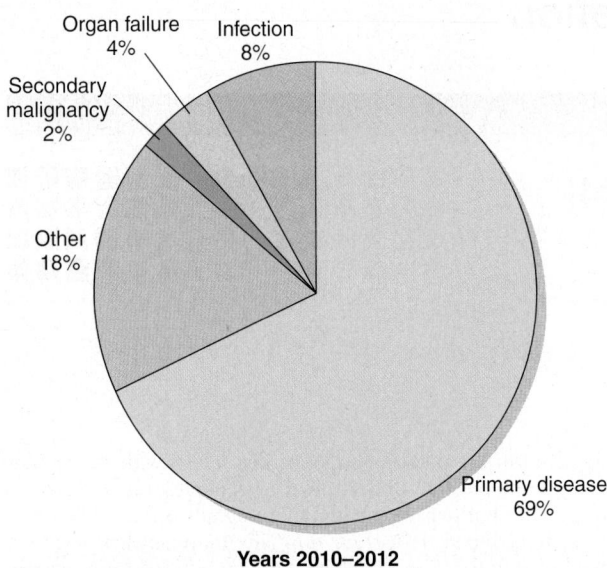

Years 2010–2012

Figure 130.1 Causes of death after autologous hematopoietic cell transplantation (US data).

Candida spp. and *Aspergillus spp.* The use of prophylactic antibacterial, antiviral, and antifungal agents, recombinant hematopoietic growth factors, and blood HPCs have decreased the incidence of severe infections.[5,6] Other common and reversible toxicities include nausea, vomiting, alopecia, poor appetite, rash, edema, and flushing. In patients with myeloma, dose-limiting gastrointestinal toxicities of melphalan (MEL) and a higher risk of posttransplant engraftment syndrome, especially in those receiving novel agent induction, is described.[7,8]

Visceral organs may also be damaged by high-dose therapy. Rare but serious problems include hepatic veno-occlusive disease, also known as sinusoidal obstruction syndrome, idiopathic pneumonia syndrome, and diffuse alveolar hemorrhage.[9,10] Hepatic veno-occlusive disease usually presents within the first 2 to 3 weeks of the HCT and manifests as tender hepatomegaly, jaundice, and fluid retention. Lung injury can present early or later after HCT and may take months to resolve. Compared to allogeneic HCT, treatment-related mortality is low, typically <3% during the first 100 days after transplant; relapse remains the most common cause of death (Fig. 130.1).

INDICATIONS FOR AUTOLOGOUS HEMATOPOIETIC CELL TRANSPLANTATION

The predominant indication for autologous HCT is the treatment of cancer, although it is sometimes performed for nonmalignant diseases (Fig. 130.2). This chapter focuses on the oncologic indications of autologous HCT.

AUTOLOGOUS HEMATOPOIETIC CELL TRANSPLANTATION FOR PLASMA CELL MYELOMA

In the United States, myeloma and other plasma cell disorders are the most common indication for autologous HCT (Figs. 130.3 and 130.4). Two large randomized trials[11,12] and several nonrandomized comparisons[13–15] have demonstrated the efficacy of autologous HCT in prolonging event-free survival (EFS) and overall survival (OS) (in some studies) compared with nontransplant therapies. The majority of autologous HCTs for myeloma are performed as "early or upfront autologous HCT" in newly diagnosed patients after induction therapy. As myeloma is incurable, even those that do not receive an upfront autograft may undergo transplant at relapse ("delayed autologous HCT"). Similarly, those who have benefited from an upfront autograft may receive a second autologous HCT after a subsequent relapse.

Early Experience with Autologous Hematopoietic Cell Transplantation for Myeloma

Randomized trials have compared autologous HCT to conventional chemotherapy in newly diagnosed patients with myeloma. The Intergroupe Francophone Myeloma (IFM)[11] and Medical Research Council[12] led clinical trials that demonstrated that patients randomized to receive autologous HCT had significantly higher complete remission (CR), EFS, and OS rates. Other randomized studies (Table 130.1), however, have not uniformly demonstrated a survival benefit,[16–20] although most show an improvement in EFS with the notable exceptions of Blade et al.[16] and the US Intergroup study.[19] Blade et al.[16] randomized patients responding to induction chemotherapy to autologous HCT versus further chemotherapy. The inability to prove an

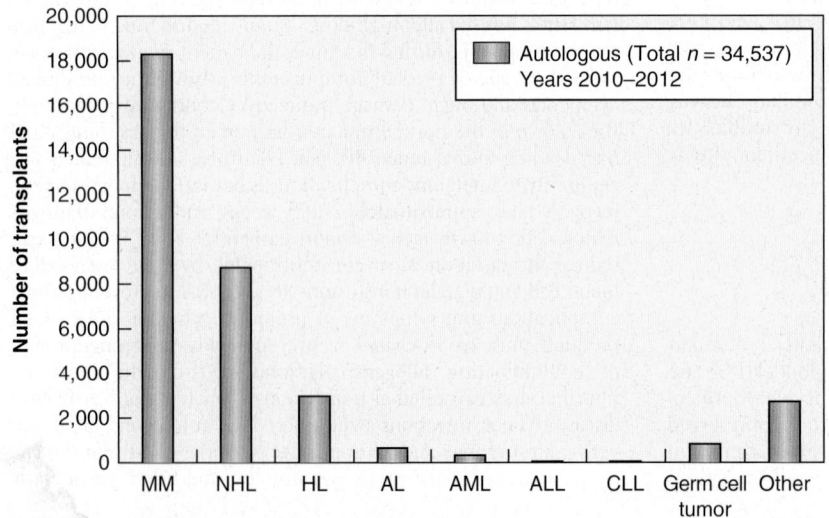

Figure 130.2 Indications for autologous transplantation in the United States. MM, multiple myeloma; NHL, non-Hodgkin lymphoma; HL, Hodgkin lymphoma; AL, amyloidosis; AML, acute myeloid leukemia; ALL, acute lymphoblastic leukemia; CLL, chronic lymphocytic leukemia.

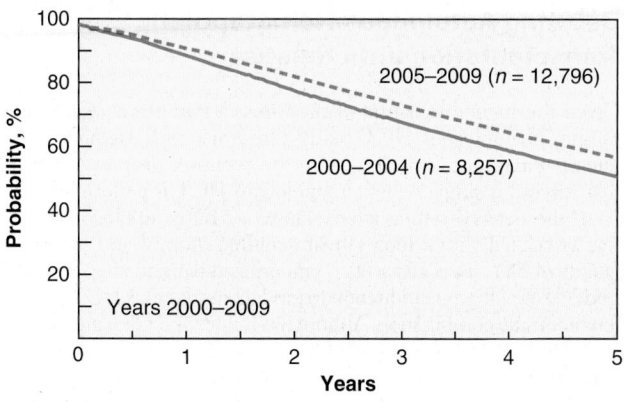

Figure 130.3 Survival after autologous hematopoietic cell transplantation: Myeloma.

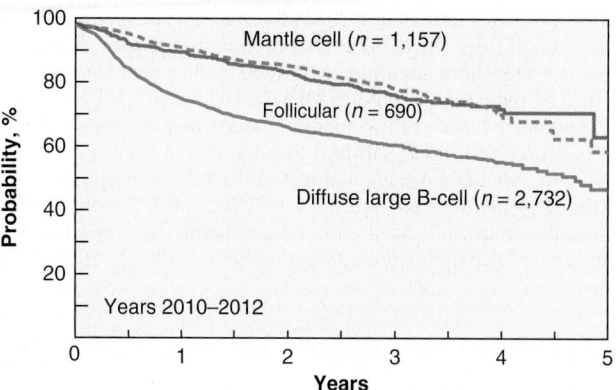

Figure 130.4 Survival after autologous hematopoietic cell transplantation: Common B cell non-Hodgkin lymphoma subtypes.

EFS benefit for autologous HCT in this setting may reflect the relatively lower incremental benefit of high-dose therapy in good responders to induction therapy. In the US Intergroup study, 52% of subjects in the chemotherapy arm received a delayed autologous HCT at the time of relapse, which may have masked differences between the two arms.[19] A prior randomized French study Myeloma Auto Greffe (MAG 95) reported comparable OS between early versus delayed autologous HCT.[17] In general, these studies indicate that autologous HCT improves CR rates and EFS in comparison to conventional chemotherapy. Survival benefit was not seen in studies that permitted or planned for delayed autologous HCT, as well as in studies conducted in later time periods when novel antimyeloma agents were available as an option after relapse.

Conditioning Regimens for Autologous Hematopoietic Cell Transplantation in Myeloma

Several cytotoxic agent combinations and total-body irradiation (TBI) have been evaluated as conditioning regimens for autologous HCT in myeloma. The only randomized phase 3 trial compared intravenous MEL 200 mg/m² (MEL200) to a combination of MEL 140 mg/m² (MEL140) and 8 Gy TBI.[21] The MEL140-TBI regimen caused significantly more mucositis, delayed hematologic recovery, higher transfusion requirements, and longer hospitalization. OS and progression-free survival (PFS) were similar. Current Center for International Blood and Mar-

TABLE 130.1

Selected Randomized Trials of Conventional Chemotherapy Compared to Single Autologous Hematopoietic Cell Transplantation as Upfront Therapy in Multiple Myeloma

Study (Year)	Transplant Arm[a]	No. and Age (y)	CR % Chemotherapy versus Auto-HCT	Comments
Attal et al.[11] (1996)	MEL 140 + TBI 8 Gy	200 ≤65	5 vs. 22[b]	OS and EFS superior for HCT.
Child et al.[12] (2003)	MEL 200	401 ≤64	8 vs. 44[b]	OS and EFS superior for HCT.
Blade et al.[16] PETHEMA (2005)	MEL 200 or MEL 140 + 12 Gy TBI	164 ≤65	11 vs. 30[b]	Only responders randomized. No OS and EFS benefit of HCT.
Palumbo et al.[14] (2005)	MEL 100 × 2 auto-HCT	194 50–70	6 vs. 25[b]	EFS and OS superior for autologous HCT.
Barlogie et al.[19] (2006)	MEL 140 + TBI 12 Gy	899 <70	15 vs. 17	No OS and EFS benefit for HCT vs. conventional chemotherapy; 55% of patients relapsed after conventional chemotherapy received delayed HCT.
Fermand et al.[17] (1998)	CCNU + etoposide + cyclophosphamide + MEL + TBI	185 <56	20 vs. 57	EFS superior for autologous HCT. No OS difference as patients in conventional chemotherapy randomized to HCT at relapse. QOL superior for HCT.
Fermand et al.[18] (2005)	MEL 200 or MEL 140 + busulfan	55–65	20 vs. 36	EFS and OS similar to conventional chemotherapy. QOL superior for early autologous HCT.

CR, complete response; HCT, hematopoietic cell transplantation; MEL, melphalan; TBI, total-body irradiation; OS, overall survival; EFS, event-free survival; CCNU, lomustine; QOL, quality of life.
[a] Chemotherapy doses in mg/m². Definitions of response were based on nonuniform criteria.
[b] Statistically significant difference (p <0.05).

row Transplant Research (CIBMTR) data indicate that most centers (>80%) use MEL200 as conditioning therapy for myeloma. Some groups have attempted to reduce the toxicity of autologous HCT by reducing the dose of MEL to 100 mg/m^2 (MEL100). In a randomized study of two planned, sequential autologous HCT procedures performed within 3 to 6 months of each other (e.g., tandem MEL200 versus tandem MEL100[22]), hospitalization rates, transplant-related mortality (TRM), and OS were similar in both groups, but MEL200 had a superior EFS. MEL200 is considered the standard conditioning before autologous HCT in myeloma.

Older Patients and Those with Comorbidities

The presence of comorbidities and advanced age should be considered when planning autologous HCT for myeloma. While most randomized studies were limited to patients ≤65 years, a survival benefit was shown for MEL100 followed by autologous HCT compared to nontransplant therapy in the 50- to 70-year age group.[23] The IFM 99-06 trial arrived at the opposite conclusion in patients aged 65 to 75 years, showing no superiority for MEL100 over MEL-prednisone (MP); in fact, both approaches were inferior when compared with the combination of MP and thalidomide.[24] For vulnerable elderly patients or those with organ dysfunction, reduced intensity MEL increases treatment tolerability and optimizes efficacy. MEL140 is the preferred conditioning regimen dose in the elderly population in the United States.

Advanced renal impairment is frequent (20% to 30%) in patients with myeloma, with up to 8% requiring long-term renal replacement therapy.[25,26] Autologous HCT is feasible, even in those with advanced renal impairment (defined as a creatinine >3 mg/dl or receiving hemodialysis). MEL200 is associated with severe toxicity, and a dose of 140 mg/m^2 is preferred.[27,28] Residual DMSO in the thawed infusion can cause toxicity including histamine release, abdominal pain, hypotension, and worsening of renal function. Washing the HPC product to remove DMSO prior to infusion is especially important in the context of renal failure.[29]

Tandem Autologous Hematopoietic Cell Transplantation

Barlogie and coworkers pioneered the tandem autologous transplant approach in their Total Therapy program.[15,30] The IFM94 was the first randomized trial[31] comparing single to tandem autologous HCT in patients with previously untreated myeloma. The projected 7-year EFS and OS benefits were significantly better for the tandem autologous HCT arm (10% versus 20% for EFS, and 21% versus 42% for OS, single versus double, respectively). In an unplanned subgroup analysis, there was no benefit for the second autologous HCT for patients who were in a very good partial remission (VGPR) status or better after the first autograft. Another randomized study (Bologna 96) confirmed the observation that the second HCT does not benefit patients in VGPR after the first transplant.[32] More importantly, this study did not show an OS benefit for the tandem HCT. Most recently, in a combined Dutch-Belgian Hemato-Oncology Cooperative Group (HOVON) and the German Multicenter Myeloma Group (GMMG) study (HOVON65/GMMG-HD4), patients receiving tandem autologous HCT in the German (GMMG) component of the study were shown to have superior OS (70% versus 55% at 5 years) over otherwise similarly treated patients receiving a single autologous HCT.[33] Randomized studies show tandem autologous HCT produce superior CR rates and EFS overall but not OS (with the exception of IFM94) compared to single autologous HCT. Moreover, benefits of the second autograft appear to apply to patients who are not in a VGPR after the first autologous HCT.

Delaying Autologous Hematopoietic Cell Transplantation until Relapse

Given the incurable nature of myeloma despite novel agents, the timing of autologous HCT (early versus delayed) warrants reappraisal. Randomized studies (from the prenovel drug era) suggest that survival is similar whether autologous HCT is performed early or in the delayed setting after relapse.[17,19] Early autologous HCT was associated with a longer treatment-free interval and improved quality of life.[17] Boccadoro et al. randomized patients after lenalidomide/dexamethasone induction to tandem autologous HCT or MP/lenalidomide combination. Although CR rates and OS were similar, early HCT provided superior PFS (41 months versus 18 months).[34] Data from this trial caution against abandoning the upfront autologous HCT for myeloma. The depth of response and its duration are increasingly recognized as key prognostic factors in myeloma and the achievement of a minimal residual disease (MRD)–negative CR predicts longer PFS and OS.[35] Currently, the highest rates of MRD negativity are seen in early autologous HCT recipients.[36,37] Moreover, the feasibility of autologous HCT at relapse could be negatively impacted by a decline in patient performance status or the development of comorbid illnesses. The results of ongoing studies of early versus delayed transplantation (e.g., NCT01208662 and NCT01208766) will eventually assist decision making in this setting.

Role of Autologous Transplantation in High-Risk Disease

Myeloma is a biologically diverse disease with clonal heterogeneity and genomic instability.[38,39] The presence of t(4;14), del(17p), or high serum β$_2$-microglobulin concentration predict inferior OS.[40] Autologous HCT has provided suboptimal results in high-risk myeloma,[41] questioning its benefit for these patients. Addition of bortezomib in induction, consolidation, and maintenance phases of therapy programs incorporating tandem HCT support the role of autologous HCT in high-risk myeloma.[33,42,43]

Unique Considerations for Hematopoietic Progenitor Cell Collection in Myeloma

In patients with myeloma who are autologous HCT candidates, it is important to avoid factors that impair HPC mobilization (e.g., MEL-based regimens, prolonged use of lenalidomide, and radiation therapy, to significant volume of bone marrow).[44,45] While plerixafor has improved mobilization yields in difficult to mobilize patients with myeloma,[46] intermediate-dose cyclophosphamide-based mobilization may be an equally effective and less expensive alternative.[47] Given the increasing use of autologous HCT in the salvage setting after relapse from a prior autograft, it is prudent to collect ≥6 to 10 million CD34+ cells/kg at initial mobilization attempt.

Maintenance Therapy for Myeloma after Hematopoietic Cell Transplantation

Various consolidation and maintenance strategies have been evaluated to delay the inevitable post-HCT progression/relapse in myeloma. In general, novel agents have shown superior results as maintenance therapy. Thalidomide maintenance after tandem autologous HCT has been studied in several randomized studies.[48–51] Lenalidomide maintenance was studied in the Cancer and Leukemia Group B 100104 and IFM 05-02 trials.[52,53] Both studies demonstrated a superior PFS and EFS with lenalidomide maintenance, while Cancer and Leukemia Group B 100104 also demonstrated an OS benefit. A two- to three-fold increase in second primary malignancies was seen in both studies associated with the lenalidomide maintenance. Pretransplant bortezomib induction coupled with post-HCT bortezomib maintenance in the HOVON-65/GMMG-HD4 trial was shown to have superior PFS and OS.[33] Based on these data, the risks/benefits and health-care costs of novel agent maintenance should be discussed with autologous HCT recipients.

Salvage Second or Third Transplants at Relapse

Salvage second autologous HCT is an option at relapse following a prior transplant. This is especially true for patients with available cryopreserved HPCs stored from their initial collection. A CIBMTR analysis showed that second salvage autologous HCT, while feasible, mostly benefits individuals relapsing ≥36 months from first autologous HCT.[54] Following an initial tandem autograft, a (third) salvage autologous HCT at relapse while providing acceptable CR rates (29%) resulted in a disappointing 19% OS at 2 years.[55]

Future Directions in Autologous Hematopoietic Cell Transplantation for Myeloma

Recent advances in supportive care have made autologous HCT relatively safe and cost-effective. Current (2009–2011) CIBMTR data suggest a day 100 mortality of 1% in upfront autologous HCT for myeloma. Median 100-day cost for autologous HCT in the United States is approximately $100,000 US dollars, and largely represents the cost of hospitalization.[56] Many institutions routinely perform autologous HCT entirely in the outpatient setting with excellent results.[57,58] Robust quality systems, electronic chemotherapy ordering, and a support team of physicians, nurses, and pharmacists, etc., are essential to setting up an outpatient program.

Current directions being explored in HCT for myeloma include newer conditioning regimens and novel maintenance or consolidation strategies that aim to induce deeper responses. Based on the dose-response relationship of MEL in myeloma, escalated doses have been attempted with a maximum tolerated dose of 280 mg/m^2 (limited by cardiac and gastrointestinal toxicity).[59] Other approaches such as the combinations of busulfan and MEL[60,61]; busulfan and cyclophosphamide[62]; idarubicin and MEL[63–65]; thiotepa, busulfan, and cyclophosphamide[64]; bendamustine and MEL[66]; as well as bortezomib and MEL[67] are without mature results.[68] Approaches at delivering higher doses of radiation therapy to the marrow prior to autologous HCT without increasing overall toxicity are also being explored with helical tomotherapy or bone-seeking radioisotopes.[69,70] Incorporation of modern imaging (positron emission tomography [PET] scans) and MRD detection in response assessment may enhance our ability to predict post-HCT outcomes and prognosis.[71]

AUTOLOGOUS HEMATOPOIETIC CELL TRANSPLANTATION FOR LYMPHOID MALIGNANCIES

Autologous HCT is standard for relapsed, aggressive non-Hodgkin lymphoma (NHL) and classical Hodgkin lymphoma (HL), and is curative in ~40% to 45% of patients.[72–75] The role of HCT in indolent NHL and T-cell NHL is more controversial. The role of autologous HCT in lymphoma has recently been reappraised as conventional therapies have dramatically improved with the advent of monoclonal antibodies[76,77] and radioimmunotherapy (RIT).[78]

Conventional and Novel Conditioning Regimens

Commonly used conditioning regimens for lymphomas include cyclophosphamide, etoposide, and carmustine; carmustine, etoposide, cytarabine, and melphalan (BEAM); carmustine, etoposide,

cytarabine, and cyclophosphamide; and TBI-containing regimens.[79] Limited retrospective data suggest lower TRM and superior outcomes following TBI-free conditioning.[80] Several uncontrolled studies have reported efficacy and feasibility of combining rituximab with high-dose therapy,[81,82] but convincing randomized evidence for this approach is lacking.

RIT with monoclonal antibody-radionuclide conjugates is effective in B-cell NHL. Incorporation of RIT into preautologous HCT conditioning has been studied, either alone or in combination with high-dose therapy.[83–86] Two randomized trials have examined the latter approach. In the Blood and Marrow Transplant Clinical Trials Network (BMT CTN) 0401 trial, iodine-131 tositumomab was prospectively compared against rituximab, both in combination with BEAM conditioning for relapsed diffuse large B-cell lymphoma (DLBCL).[87] Another study compared BEAM plus yttrium-90 ibritumomab tiuxetan to BEAM alone in aggressive NHL.[88] Neither study favored a RIT-based conditioning regimen.

Disease-Specific Indications for Hematopoietic Cell Transplantation in Lymphoid Malignancies

The indications of autologous HCT in lymphoid neoplasia are dependent on patient age, comorbidities, chemosensitivity, histologic subtype, and remission status at the time of HCT.

Hematopoietic Cell Transplantation for Follicular Lymphoma

Hematopoietic Cell Transplantation for Follicular Lymphoma: First Remission. The role of autologous HCT as *consolidation* for advanced-stage follicular lymphoma (FL) in first remission was examined in four randomized trials, including three trials conducted in the prerituximab era[89–91] and one in rituximab era[92] (Table 130.2). Autologous HCT provided a PFS benefit in three out of these four trials. OS, however, was not improved as this therapy was associated with a higher risk of second malignancies,[91] including myelodysplastic syndrome/acute myeloid leukemia (AML).[89,92] With the advent of RIT consolidation[78] and rituximab maintenance[93] or retreatment,[94] the routine use of upfront HCT consolidation in FL is not recommended.

Hematopoietic Cell Transplantation for Follicular Lymphoma: Relapsed Disease. The role of autologous HCT in relapsed FL is controversial. In the prerituximab era, the CUP study compared salvage chemotherapy alone versus chemotherapy followed by either *un*purged or *p*urged HCT for relapsed FL; overall, the investigators reported a PFS and OS benefit with autologous HCT (see Table 130.2).[95] More than a decade later, the superiority of autologous HCT over modern salvage chemoimmunotherapies is debated.[96] Registry data from the European Blood and Marrow Transplant Group (EBMT)[97] and CIBMTR show no plateau in relapse rates post-HCT in FL[98] and a 5% to 15% risk of second malignancies[97,99] (see Table 130.2). Autologous HCT for relapsed FL should be considered in the context of alternative treatment choices, patient age, remission status, comorbidities, and a small but definite risk of secondary cancers. Autologous HCT is best reserved for chemotherapy-sensitive, relapsed FL in those subjects who are not candidates for curative intent allogeneic transplantation.

Hematopoietic Cell Transplantation for Transformed Follicular Lymphoma. An EBMT report of 50 patients receiving autologous HCT for chemotherapy-sensitive transformed FL described 5-year PFS and OS of 30% and 51%, respectively.[100] A prospective Norwegian study also reported 5-year PFS and OS of 32% and 47%, respectively.[101] In the rituximab era, a Canadian cohort analysis suggested an OS benefit for patients undergoing HCT compared with those receiving chemoimmunotherapy alone.[102,103]

TABLE 130.2

Select Studies Addressing the Role of Autologous Hematopoietic Cell Transplantation in Lymphoid Malignancies

Study (Year)	No.	Study Design	TRM	EFS/PFS (y)	OS (y)	Comments
Follicular Lymphoma in First Remission						
GLSG (2004)[89]	307	Phase 3 Auto vs. chemo	<2.5% in both arms	Auto = 64%[a] Chemo = 33% (5)	Not reported	Higher sMDS/AML with autologous HCT (3.5%[a] vs. 0%; p = 0.02)
GELA (2006)[90]	402	Phase 3 Auto vs. chemo	Not reported	Auto = 38% Chemo = 28% (7)	Auto = 76% Chemo = 71% (7)	Second malignancies similar in both groups
GOELAMS (2009)[91]	166	Phase 3 Auto vs. chemo	Not reported	Auto = 64%[a] Chemo = 39% (9)	Auto = 76% Chemo = 80% (9)	Autologous HCT associated with significantly more second malignancies
GITMO (2008)[92]	136	Phase 3 Auto vs. chemo	Auto = 3 Chemo = 2 at day 100	61%[a] vs. 28% (4)	81% vs. 80% (4)	At 4 y sMDS/AML higher with autologous HCT (6.6% vs. 1.7%)
Relapsed Follicular Lymphoma						
CUP (2003)[95]	89	Phase 3 Chemo vs. purged auto vs. unpurged auto	Not reported	Chemo = 26% Unpurged = 58%[a] Purged = 55%[a] (2)	Chemo = 46% Unpurged = 71%[a] Purged = 77%[a] (4)	No benefit of purging; trial in prerituximab era
CIBMTR (2004)[98]	728	Retrospective	Purged = 14% Unpurged = 8% (5)	Purged = 39% Unpurged = 31% (5)	Purged = 62%[a] Unpurged = 55% (5)	OS favored purged autologous HCT
EBMT (2007)[97]	693	Retrospective	9% (5)	31% (10)	52% (10)	9% of patients had second cancers
Mantle Cell Lymphoma in First Remission						
Dreyling et al.[104] (2005)	122	Phase 3 Auto vs. chemo	Not reported	Auto = 54%[a] Chemo = 25% (3)	Auto = 83% Chemo = 77% (3)	Performed in prerituximab era; no survival benefit
Geisler et al.[107,198] (2008)	160	Phase 2	5%	66% (6)	70% (6)	Late relapses seen
Damon et al.[105] (2009)	78	Phase 2	0%	56% (5)	64% (5)	In vivo rituximab purging
Hermine et al.[109] (2012)	455	R-CHOP vs. R-CHOP/R-DHAP induction	4% vs. 4%	49 mo vs. 84 mo[a] (median)	82 mo vs. not reached[a] (median)	Addition cytarabine in induction improved OS
Relapsed Diffuse Large B-Cell Lymphoma						
Philip et al.[72] (1995)	215	Phase 3 Auto vs. chemo	Not reported	Auto = 46%[a] Chemo = 12% (5)	Auto = 53%[a] Chemo = 32% (5)	Performed in prerituximab era
CIBMTR (2009)[143]	994	Retrospective	11% (3)	50% (3)	57% (3)	Pre-HCT rituximab exposure improved survival outcomes
CORAL (2010)[74]	206	Prospective RICE vs. R-DHAP salvage	Not reported	53% (3)	Not reported	Established continued feasibility of autologous HCT for relapsed DLBCL
Relapsed Hodgkin Lymphoma						
CIBMTR (2001)[199]	414	Retrospective	7% at day 100	46%–64% (3)	58%–75% (3)	Patients in second CR had better outcomes
CIBMTR (1999)[150]	122	Retrospective	12% at day 100	38% (3)	50% (3)	Established primary refractory patients can be salvaged by autologous HCT

(continued)

TABLE 130.2

Select Studies Addressing the Role of Autologous Hematopoietic Cell Transplantation in Lymphoid Malignancies *(continued)*

Study (Year)	No.	Study Design	TRM	EFS/PFS (y)	OS (y)	Comments
T-Cell Non-Hodgkin Lymphoma in First Remission						
Corradini et al.[154] (2006)	62	Phase 2	4.8%	30% (12)	34% (12)	ALK-positive anaplastic T-cell patients and ones in CR had favorable outcomes
Reimer et al.[157] (2009)	83	Phase 2	3.6%	36% (3)	48% (3)	66% enrolled patients received autologous HCT
NLG-T-01 (2012)[158]	166	Phase 2	4%	44% (5)	51% (5)	ALK-negative anaplastic T-cell had best outcomes

TRM, Treatment-related mortality; EFS, event-free survival; PFS, progression-free survival; OS, overall survival; GLSG, German Low Grade Lymphoma Study Group; sMDS, secondary myelodysplastic syndrome; AML, acute myeloid leukemia; HCT, hematopoietic cell transplantation; GELA, Groupe d'Etude des Lymphomes de l'Adulte; GOELAMS, Groupe Ouest-Est Leucémies et Maladies du Sang; GITMO, Gruppo Italiano Trapianto di Midollo Osseo; CUP, *chemotherapy alone versus chemotherapy followed by either unpurged or purged HCT for relapsed FL*; CIBMTR, Center for International Blood and Marrow Transplant Research; EBMT, European Blood and Marrow Transplant Group; R-CHOP, rituximab, cyclophosphamide, doxorubicin [hydroxydaunomycin], vincristine [Oncovin] and prednisone; CORAL, Collaborative Trial in Relapsed Aggressive Lymphoma; RICE, rituximab, ifosfamide, carboplatin, etoposide; DLBCL, diffuse large B-cell lymphoma; CR, complete response; ALK, anaplastic lymphoma kinase; NLG, Nordic Lymphoma Group; T-01 refers to their study, number T-01
[a] Statistically significant value.

Autologous HCT is appropriate for transformed FL patients with nonbulky (nodal areas ≤3 cm), chemotherapy-sensitive disease.

Hematopoietic Cell Transplantation for Mantle Cell Lymphoma

The European MCL Network trial randomized patients with mantle cell lymphoma (MCL) after first-line chemotherapy to either upfront autologous HCT consolidation or interferon maintenance (see Table 130.2)[104] and demonstrated a superior PFS but no OS benefit for HCT. Similar randomized trials in the rituximab-era after first-line chemoimmunotherapy are not available. Rituximab-era nonrandomized trials examining upfront HCT in patients with MCL have reported encouraging 5-year PFS and OS of ~60% and 70%, respectively[105–110] (see Table 130.2). Despite the lack of randomized data, autologous HCT for MCL in first remission can be considered *standard* practice as retrospective data suggest that HCT after relapse may not be as effective.[111,112] A CIBMTR analysis reported a 5-year OS of 61% for upfront HCT versus 44% for HCT performed in chemosensitive relapse.[113] In patients with chemotherapy-sensitive, relapsed MCL, who are not candidates for allogeneic transplant, autologous HCT is reasonable; however, it is not recommended for therapy-refractory MCL.

Hematopoietic Cell Transplantation for Waldenström Macroglobulinemia

Prospective data are not available to recommend the use of autologous HCT for Waldenström macroglobulinemia (WM) in first remission. On the other hand, retrospective studies and expert opinion[114] support the role of HCT in patients with relapsed/refractory WM.[115–118] In an EBMT study of 158 patients with mostly chemotherapy-sensitive WM,[119] 5-year PFS and OS were 40% and 68%, respectively. Autologous HCT should be considered in patients with relapsed, chemotherapy-sensitive WM who already have received two or three different therapies.

Hematopoietic Cell Transplantation for Marginal Zone and Small Lymphocytic Lymphoma

Limited retrospective studies for HCT in marginal zone lymphoma[120,121] indicate PFS rates similar to FL and frequent relapses after transplant. In patients with relapsed but chemotherapy-sensitive marginal zone lymphoma, autologous HCT could be considered. Data for autologous HCT for small lymphocytic lymphoma are scant. Extrapolating the data showing lack of a survival benefit for autologous HCT[122–124] in chronic lymphocytic leukemia, HCT is not recommended in patients with small lymphocytic lymphoma.

Hematopoietic Cell Transplantation for Diffuse Large B-Cell Lymphoma

Hematopoietic Cell Transplantation for Diffuse Large B-Cell Lymphoma: In First Remission for High-Risk Disease? Studies using autologous HCT as consolidation after first-line therapies in aggressive (mostly DLBCL) NHL in the prerituximab era have reported contradictory findings. While the majority reported no benefit[125–131] or (in one case) inferior outcomes,[132] a handful of trials reported PFS and/or OS benefit with HCT either in general[133–135] or in patients with high or intermediate-high International Prognostic Index (IPI).[133] Studies from the rituximab-era restricted to higher-risk patients have also reported contradictory outcomes: two reports showed no benefit,[136,137] whereas one intergroup US study suggested improved PFS and OS with autologous HCT consolidation high-risk IPI DLBC.[138] Considering these discordant data and the high cure rates of DLBCL,[139] use of upfront autologous HCT for this histology is not generally recommended.

Hematopoietic Cell Transplantation for Diffuse Large B-Cell Lymphoma: In Relapsed Disease. The role of autologous HCT in relapsed DLBCL is well-defined. The PARMA trial (see Table 130.2)[72] established that salvage chemotherapy plus HCT consolidation provided an OS benefit in subjects with relapsed, chemotherapy-sensitive disease. Several registry[140–143] and prospective studies in the rituximab era[74] (see Table 130.2) have reproduced these results. Autologous HCT is thus the *standard-of-care* for relapsed/chemotherapy sensitive DLBCL.

Hematopoietic Cell Transplantation for Burkitt Lymphoma

Historically, brief induction therapies followed by upfront autologous HCT provided durable disease control in Burkitt lymphoma (5-year OS and PFS of 81% and 73%, respectively).[144] However, the contemporary intense chemoimmunotherapy regimens are curative for majority of patients,[145,146] and autologous HCT in first CR is not necessary. Fortunately, the grim prognosis for the patient with relapsed/refractory Burkitt lymphoma is uncommon. Retrospective studies[147,148] describe 3- to 5-year OS and PFS rates of ~30% and 25%, respectively, after autologous HCT in chemotherapy-sensitive relapses.

Hematopoietic Cell Transplantation for Hodgkin Lymphoma

Hematopoietic Cell Transplantation for Relapsed Hodgkin Lymphoma. Autologous HCT is potentially curative for relapsed HL. The British National Lymphoma Investigation study compared autologous HCT against salvage chemotherapy alone in relapsed HL[149] and reported a PFS benefit in the high-dose therapy arm (53% versus 10%; $p = 0.02$). In another randomized trial, two cycles of chemotherapy were followed by two additional chemotherapy cycles versus autologous HCT.[75] In chemotherapy-sensitive patients, freedom from treatment failure was significantly better with high-dose therapy. An OS benefit was not shown in either of these studies, most likely because those subjects assigned to the chemotherapy arm could still be salvaged by later HCT. Autologous HCT is the *standard-of-care* in chemotherapy-sensitive first relapse of HL.

Hematopoietic Cell Transplantation for Primary Refractory Hodgkin Lymphoma. Primary refractory (<CR after first-line therapy) HL has a poor prognosis. Lazarus and coworkers[150] showed that autologous HCT can cure about a third of patients with primary refractory HL (see Table 130.2). Chemotherapy-refractory disease at autologous HCT is a poor prognostic factor (5-year PFS of <20%).[151] While HCT is curative for HL, the 10-year late relapse rate (after the first 2 years) was 17% accounting for 25% of late mortality in a registry analysis.[152] Autologous HCT is *standard-of-care* for relapsed HL, including those with primary refractory disease.

T-Cell Lymphomas

Relapsed T-cell NHLs have poor prognosis with chemotherapy alone,[153] and autologous HCT has been explored as initial therapy or at the time of tumor progression. Phase 2 studies (with heterogeneous subtypes) examining upfront HCT in T-cell NHL (see Table 130.2)[154–158] suggest a 3- to 4-year PFS of ~30% to 50%. Although randomized data are not available, considering the poor outcomes with conventional therapies, it is appropriate to consider upfront autologous HCT consolidation in T-cell NHL. Because of its excellent prognosis with standard chemotherapies, autologous HCT in first CR is not recommended for anaplastic lymphoma kinase–positive anaplastic large cell lymphoma.[159] Relatively encouraging outcomes for a highly select group of patients with relapsed T-cell NHL with sensitive disease also have been shown with 3- to 5-year PFS and OS rates of approximately 15% to 30% and 30% to 45%, respectively.[160–162] Autologous HCT is also reasonable in those patients with relapsed/chemotherapy-sensitive T-cell NHL not deemed candidates for allogeneic HCT.

Unique Considerations for Hematopoietic Cell Transplantation Mobilization in Lymphomas

While many patients with lymphoma can successfully mobilize HPCs with "cytokine only" strategies, mobilization failure remains a concern in patients with prior radiotherapy, heavily pretreated disease; exposure to hyper-CVAD (fractionated cyclophosphamide, vincristine, doxorubicin, and dexamethasone), fludarabine-containing regimens, or RIT; advanced age; and bone marrow involvement.[174,163–166] In such cases, consideration should be given to chemotherapy- or plerixafor-based mobilization strategies.[167]

Tumor Cell Contamination in Autograft

Relapse after autologous HCT derives usually from proliferation of a chemotherapy-resistant clone of lymphoma cells surviving the high-dose therapy, or rarely from re-infusion of an autograft contaminated by tumor cells. Studies of syngeneic HCT suggest that a "tumor-free" graft may prevent/delay relapse.[168] Ex vivo purging (by monoclonal antibodies, CD34+ cell selection, etc.)[169,170] or in vivo purging (e.g., rituximab therapy during mobilization)[171,172] of autografts appear to reduce or eliminate the risk of tumor-cell re-infusion at HCT. Reduction of tumor cell re-infusion, however, may not lead to improved outcomes. The CUP trial in relapsed FL[95] reported no significant difference in the outcomes of immune-magnetically purged versus unpurged autografts. Similarly, pretransplant in vivo rituximab purging has not been shown to improve HCT outcomes.[173] The lack of clear benefit in randomized data and a possible increase in infectious complications with ex vivo purging[174,175] preclude routine use of this approach.

Posttransplant Maintenance Therapies for Lymphoid Malignancies

Disease relapse following HCT in lymphoid malignancies remains a challenge. Rituximab maintenance, effective in B-cell NHL,[93] has been studied in the post-HCT setting.[174,176] In a randomized EBMT study, rituximab maintenance postautologous HCT in relapsed FL[173] was well tolerated and provided a superior 10-year PFS (54% versus 37%; $p = 0.01$) but no OS benefit. In the Collaborative Trial in Relapsed Aggressive Lymphoma (CORAL) study, post-HCT rituximab maintenance for DLBCL provided no PFS or OS benefit, but was associated with increased risk of adverse events.[177] Routine use of rituximab maintenance after HCT in B-cell NHL is not recommended.

Functional Imaging and Autologous Hematopoietic Cell Transplantation Outcomes

PET scanning is a powerful tool to predict autologous HCT outcomes in lymphoid malignancies. A PET-negative state before HCT either alone[178] or in combination age-adjusted IPI[179] predicts improved PFS and OS. Similarly, conversion from a PET-positive to a PET-negative state, either following pre-HCT salvage therapies[180] or after high-dose therapy,[181] is predictive of improved HCT outcomes.

AUTOLOGOUS HEMATOPOIETIC CELL TRANSPLANTATION FOR RARER PLASMA CELL DYSCRASIAS

Light chain amyloidosis (AL), light chain deposition disease, and POEMS syndrome are rare clonal plasma cell disorders. High-dose therapy with MEL has proven effective in many of these disorders, although randomized trials are lacking.[182,183] Special challenges for HCT in these disorders include higher rates of TRM, engraftment syndrome, and severe fluid retention.[184,185] In AL, cardiac involvement, pleural effusions, and significant fluid retention during G-CSF–based mobilization have emerged as predictors of higher TRM.[184] Careful patient selection, dose-adapted MEL use, and center experience are critical. A randomized multicenter trial failed to show benefit for HCT over conventional chemotherapy in AL,[184,186] whereas experience from specialized centers seems to show a significant benefit, by inducing CRs after HCT that lead to organ function recovery from AL over time.[183]

AUTOLOGOUS HEMATOPOIETIC CELL TRANSPLANTATION FOR ACUTE MYELOID LEUKEMIA AND ACUTE LYMPHOBLASTIC LEUKEMIA

While the majority of younger patients with AML attain CR after induction therapy, postremission treatment is necessary to prevent relapse. The preferred postremission strategy in first CR is largely dependent on patients' cytogenetic risk category. Allogeneic HCT does not add benefit for patients with AML with favorable-risk cytogenetics.[187] This group of patients, as well as those patients with AML in remission who have intermediate-risk characteristics, may benefit from autologous HCT if a suitable donor is not available. On the other hand, patients with unfavorable-risk AML should be discouraged from this approach. There is no evidence that an autologous HCT can replace consolidation or maintenance therapy or allogeneic HCT in any risk group of patients with acute lymphoblastic leukemia.[188] Limited data suggest that tyrosine kinase inhibitors plus sequential chemotherapy can lead to significant cytoreduction in Philadelphia chromosome–positive patients with acute lymphoblastic leukemia, allowing collection of HPCs not contaminated by residual lymphoblasts and thus reducing the likelihood of relapse after autologous HCT for patients without available donors.[189]

AUTOLOGOUS HEMATOPOIETIC CELL TRANSPLANTATION FOR GERM CELL TUMORS

Autologous HCT is potentially curative for relapsed germ cell tumors (GCT).[190] In the first-line setting for high-risk GCT, phase 3 studies have not demonstrated superiority of HCT over conventional chemotherapy.[191,192] For GCTs refractory to initial therapy, however, HCT may be superior as salvage treatment.[193] Several prognostic models have been developed for post-HCT outcomes, and these generally incorporate adverse risk factors such as platinum refractoriness, poor-risk score GCT, and third-line or later use of HCT.[190] Thus, for higher-risk GCT relapsing after or not responding to initial chemotherapy, HCT referral should be considered early.

LATE COMPLICATIONS AFTER AUTOLOGOUS HEMATOPOIETIC CELL TRANSPLANTATION

Autologous recipients of HCT have a reduced life expectancy compared to the general population and are at increased risk for late complications such as opportunistic infections, iron overload, endocrine abnormalities, osteoporosis, and second malignancies.[10,194–197] Recipients should be monitored for these potential maladies at least yearly, including administering all age-appropriate cancer screening and anti-infective vaccinations. Other recommended screenings in long-term survivors include yearly eye examinations for cataracts (especially after TBI), yearly assessment of cardiovascular risk factors, education/counseling on a "heart"-healthy lifestyle, blood pressure monitoring and aggressive management of hypertension to prevent chronic kidney disease, screening for osteopenia/osteoporosis, thyroid function evaluation, sexual/gonadal function and fertility assessment (when appropriate), and periodic psychological evaluations.[197]

SELECTED REFERENCES

The full reference list can be accessed at lwwhealthlibrary.com/oncology.

11. Attal M, Harousseau JL, Stoppa AM, et al. A prospective, randomized trial of autologous bone marrow transplantation and chemotherapy in multiple myeloma. Intergroupe Francais du Myelome. N Engl J Med 1996;335:91–97.

12. Child JA, Morgan GJ, Davies FE, et al. High-dose chemotherapy with hematopoietic stem-cell rescue for multiple myeloma. N Engl J Med 2003;348:1875–1883.

14. Palumbo A, Triolo S, Argentino C, et al. Dose-intensive melphalan with stem cell support (MEL100) is superior to standard treatment in elderly myeloma patients. Blood 1999;94:1248–1253.

17. Fermand JP, Ravaud P, Chevret S, et al. High-dose therapy and autologous peripheral blood stem cell transplantation in multiple myeloma: up-front or rescue treatment? Results of a multicenter sequential randomized clinical trial. Blood 1998;92:3131–3136.

22. Palumbo A, Bringhen S, Bruno B, et al. Melphalan 200 mg/m(2) versus melphalan 100 mg/m(2) in newly diagnosed myeloma patients: a prospective, multicenter phase 3 study. Blood 2010;115:1873–1879.

24. Facon T, Mary JY, Hulin C, et al. Melphalan and prednisone plus thalidomide versus melphalan and prednisone alone or reduced-intensity autologous stem cell transplantation in elderly patients with multiple myeloma (IFM 99-06): a randomised trial. Lancet 2007;370:1209–1218.

31. Attal M, Harousseau JL, Facon T, et al. Single versus double autologous stem-cell transplantation for multiple myeloma. N Engl J Med 2003;349:2495–2502.

33. Sonneveld P, Schmidt-Wolf IG, van der Holt B, et al. Bortezomib induction and maintenance treatment in patients with newly diagnosed multiple myeloma: results of the randomized phase III HOVON-65/ GMMG-HD4 trial. J Clin Oncol 2012;30:2946–2955.

36. Paiva B, Vidriales MB, Cervero J, et al. Multiparameter flow cytometric remission is the most relevant prognostic factor for multiple myeloma patients who undergo autologous stem cell transplantation. Blood 2008;112:4017–4023.

40. Avet-Loiseau H, Attal M, Moreau P, et al. Genetic abnormalities and survival in multiple myeloma: the experience of the Intergroupe Francophone du Myelome. Blood 2007;109:3489–3495.

46. DiPersio JF, Micallef IN, Stiff PJ, et al. Phase III prospective randomized double-blind placebo-controlled trial of plerixafor plus granulocyte colony-stimulating factor compared with placebo plus granulocyte colony-stimulating factor for autologous stem-cell mobilization and transplantation for patients with non-Hodgkin's lymphoma. J Clin Oncol 2009;27:4767–4773.

52. Attal M, Lauwers-Cances V, Marit G, et al. Lenalidomide maintenance after stem-cell transplantation for multiple myeloma. N Engl J Med 2012;366:1782–1791.

53. McCarthy PL, Owzar K, Hofmeister CC, et al. Lenalidomide after stem-cell transplantation for multiple myeloma. N Engl J Med 2012;366:1770–1781.

72. Philip T, Guglielmi C, Hagenbeek A, et al. Autologous bone marrow transplantation as compared with salvage chemotherapy in relapses of chemotherapy-sensitive non-Hodgkin's lymphoma. N Engl J Med 1995;333:1540–1545.

73. Philip T, Armitage JO, Spitzer G, et al. High-dose therapy and autologous bone marrow transplantation after failure of conventional chemotherapy in adults with intermediate-grade or high-grade non-Hodgkin's lymphoma. N Engl J Med 1987;316:1493–1498.

75. Schmitz N, Pfistner B, Sextro M, et al. Aggressive conventional chemotherapy compared with high-dose chemotherapy with autologous haemopoietic stem-cell transplantation for relapsed chemosensitive Hodgkin's disease: a randomised trial. Lancet 2002;359:2065–2071.

79. Kharfan-Dabaja MA, Nishihori T, Otrock ZK, et al. Monoclonal antibodies in conditioning regimens for hematopoietic cell transplantation. Biol Blood Marrow Transplant 2013;19:1288–1300.

87. Vose JM, Carter S, Burns LJ, et al. Phase III randomized study of rituximab/carmustine, etoposide, cytarabine, and melphalan (BEAM) compared with iodine-131 tositumomab/BEAM with autologous hematopoietic cell transplantation for relapsed diffuse large B-cell lymphoma: results from the BMT CTN 0401 trial. J Clin Oncol 2013;31:1662–1668.

97. Montoto S, Canals C, Rohatiner AZ, et al. Long-term follow-up of high-dose treatment with autologous haematopoietic progenitor cell support in 693 patients with follicular lymphoma: an EBMT registry study. Leukemia 2007;21:2324–2331.

99. Rohatiner AZ, Nadler L, Davies AJ, et al. Myeloablative therapy with autologous bone marrow transplantation for follicular lymphoma at the time of second or subsequent remission: long-term follow-up. J Clin Oncol 2007;25:2554–2559.

103. Villa D, Crump M, Panzarella T, et al. Autologous and allogeneic stem-cell transplantation for transformed follicular lymphoma: a report of the Canadian blood and marrow transplant group. J Clin Oncol 2013;31:1164–1171.

104. Dreyling M, Lenz G, Hoster E, et al. Early consolidation by myeloablative radiochemotherapy followed by autologous stem cell transplantation in first remission significantly prolongs progression-free survival in mantle-cell lymphoma: results of a prospective randomized trial of the European MCL Network. Blood 2005;105:2677–2684.

134. Haioun C, Lepage E, Gisselbrecht C, et al. Survival benefit of high-dose therapy in poor-risk aggressive non-Hodgkin's lymphoma: final analysis of the prospective LNH87-2 protocol—a groupe d'Etude des lymphomes de l'Adulte study. J Clin Oncol 2000;18:3025–3030.

136. Schmitz N, Nickelsen M, Ziepert M, et al. Conventional chemotherapy (CHOEP-14) with rituximab or high-dose chemotherapy (MegaCHOEP) with rituximab for young, high-risk patients with aggressive B-cell lymphoma: an open-label, randomised, phase 3 trial (DSHNHL 2002-1). Lancet Oncol 2012;13:1250–1259.

138. Stiff PJ, Unger JM, Cook JR, et al. Autologous transplantation as consolidation for aggressive non-Hodgkin's lymphoma. *N Engl J Med* 2013;369:1681–1690.

142. Lazarus HM, Zhang MJ, Carreras J, et al. A comparison of HLA-identical sibling allogeneic versus autologous transplantation for diffuse large B cell lymphoma: a report from the CIBMTR. *Biol Blood Marrow Transplant* 2010;16:35–45.

150. Lazarus HM, Rowlings PA, Zhang MJ, et al. Autotransplants for Hodgkin's disease in patients never achieving remission: a report from the Autologous Blood and Marrow Transplant Registry. *J Clin Oncol* 1999;17:534–545.

173. Pettengell R, Schmitz N, Gisselbrecht C, et al. Rituximab purging and/or maintenance in patients undergoing autologous transplantation for relapsed follicular lymphoma: a prospective randomized trial from the lymphoma working party of the European group for blood and marrow transplantation. *J Clin Oncol* 2013;31:1624–1630.

190. Einhorn LH, Williams SD, Chamness A, et al. High-dose chemotherapy and stem-cell rescue for metastatic germ-cell tumors. *N Engl J Med* 2007; 357:340–348.

197. Majhail NS, Rizzo JD, Lee SJ, et al. Recommended screening and preventive practices for long-term survivors after hematopoietic cell transplantation. *Biol Blood Marrow Transplant* 2012;18:348–371.

199. Lazarus HM, Loberiza FR Jr, Zhang MJ, et al. Autotransplants for Hodgkin's disease in first relapse or second remission: a report from the autologous blood and marrow transplant registry (ABMTR). *Bone Marrow Transplant* 2001;27:387–396.

131 Allogeneic Stem Cell Transplantation

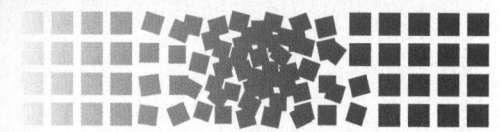

Stanley R. Riddell and Edus H. Warren

PRACTICE OF ONCOLOGY

INTRODUCTION

Allogeneic hematopoietic cell transplantation (HCT) is successful in curing many patients with advanced hematologic malignancies. The premise underlying allogeneic HCT was the observation that the antitumor effects of irradiation and chemotherapy were limited by dose-related hematopoietic toxicity that led to prolonged or permanent pancytopenia and predisposed the patient to fatal infection. Studies in mice demonstrated that the transfer of splenocytes or bone marrow (BM) could rescue animals from the lethal effects of irradiation, which provided the impetus to develop HCT as a means of dose-escalating irradiation and chemotherapy to treat cancer.[1,2] The initial efforts at applying allogeneic HCT to patients with leukemia began in the late 1950s, but were impeded by an incomplete understanding of histocompatibility antigens that imposed an immunologic barrier to durable engraftment of allogeneic donor stem cells or resulted in life-threatening graft-versus-host disease (GVHD), and by the challenges of supporting critically ill immunocompromised patients until donor hematopoietic cell engraftment ensued.[3,4] These barriers were systematically overcome in the 1970s, notably through the work of E. Donnall Thomas, who was awarded the Nobel Prize in 1990 for his contributions to HCT.[5] Advances in supportive care, conditioning regimens, and alternative donor sources have continued to improve outcome and expand the utility of allogeneic HCT. Currently, >8,000 procedures are performed in the United States each year.

CONDITIONING REGIMENS

Conditioning regimens for allogeneic HCT are designed to serve two purposes: to suppress the patient's immune system sufficiently to prevent rejection of donor hematopoietic stem cells and to eradicate malignant cells. The initial approach to allogeneic HCT for hematologic malignancies administered myeloablative doses of systemic chemotherapy alone or combined with total-body irradiation (TBI), and resulted in considerable toxicity to nonhematopoietic organs, which limited its use to younger patients without serious comorbidities. Even with intensive myeloablative conditioning (MAC) regimens, it soon became apparent that the elimination of leukemic cells after allogeneic HCT was partly dependent on a graft-versus-leukemia (GVL) effect mediated by donor immune cells.[6,7] This understanding fostered the development of reduced intensity conditioning (RIC) regimens that provide sufficient immunosuppression to achieve donor cell engraftment and rely to a greater extent on GVL effects for tumor eradication. The use of RIC has made this procedure feasible in older patients and patients with comorbidities that tolerate MAC poorly. RIC is typically most effective in patients with malignancies that are highly responsive to the GVL effect and/or are in remission at the time of HCT.

Myeloablative Conditioning

The most extensively used MAC regimens were developed in parallel in the 1980s, and include cyclophosphamide (Cy) administered intravenously in a dose of 60 mg/kg on two consecutive days combined with TBI typically in a fractionated schedule to a total dose of 12 Gy (2 Gy × 6), which is superior to a single dose of 10 Gy;[8–10] or the combination of oral busulfan (Bu) in a dose of 16 mg/kg over 4 days and Cy in a dose of 120 mg/kg (Bu/Cy).[11,12] A higher dose of fractionated TBI (15.75 Gy) reduced relapse in patients with myeloid leukemia, but was associated with higher nonrelapse mortality and did not provide a survival benefit.[13]

The major acute toxicity of MAC is irreversible damage to recipient hematopoiesis; however, these regimens often cause nausea, vomiting, fever, mild skin erythema, and oral mucositis that typically develop 5 to 7 days after transplant and require narcotic analgesia. Patient-controlled analgesia provides superior patient satisfaction for mucositis pain and results in lower cumulative doses of narcotics. TBI is associated with transient parotiditis during conditioning and a high risk of cataracts later in life. Regimens that include high-dose Cy can result in acute hemorrhagic cystitis, which can usually be prevented by the sulfhydryl compound mercaptoethanesulfonate (mesna). Rarely, Cy causes an acute hemorrhagic cardiomyopathy. As discussed later in this chapter, MAC can result in serious organ toxicity including diffuse alveolar hemorrhage, idiopathic interstitial pneumonia, and hepatic sinusoidal obstruction syndrome.

The choice of MAC regimen is in part based on the patient's underlying malignancy and stage of disease. The Bu/Cy regimen was associated with a high incidence of sinusoidal obstruction syndrome in early studies; however, this complication has been reduced by the use of ursodiol prophylaxis.[14,15] A recent retrospective analysis of data from the Center for International Blood and Marrow Transplantation Research for patients with acute myeloid leukemia (AML) in first complete response (CR) that received HCT from human leukocyte antigen (HLA)-matched related or unrelated donors after conditioning with Cy/TBI, or with oral or intravenous Bu combined with Cy, demonstrate superior outcome with the Bu/Cy regimens.[16] A prospective nonrandomized cohort study in patients with AML, chronic myelogenous leukemia (CML), and myelodysplastic syndrome (MDS) similarly concluded that intravenous Bu/Cy was superior to Cy/TBI.[17] Based on data from older studies, Cy/TBI has been the generally preferred regimen for acute lymphoblastic leukemia (ALL).[18,19] Other myeloablative regimens such as fludarabine/Bu have been developed and gained popularity at some centers, although a survival benefit has not been established.[20,21]

Reduced Intensity Conditioning

The recognition of the immune-mediated GVL effect, both from retrospective analysis of rates of relapse in recipients of allogeneic versus syngeneic HCT and from studies in which donor

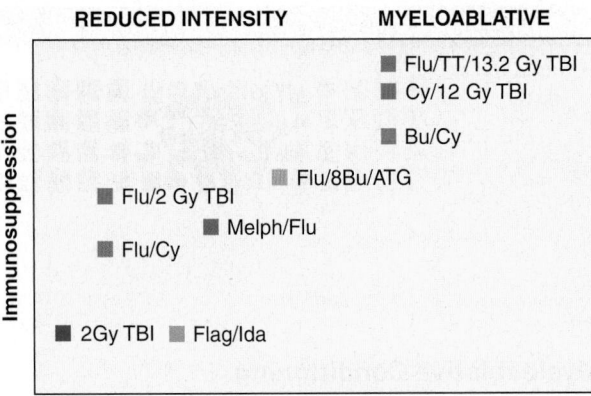

Figure 131.1 Relative intensity of conditioning regimens used for allogeneic hematopoietic cell transplantation. Flu, fludarabine; TT, thiotepa; TBI, total body irradiation; Cy, cyclophosphamide; Bu, busulfan; ATG, antithymocyte globulin; Melph, melphalan; Flag, fludarabine, cytosine arabinoside, granulocyte colony stimulating factor; Ida, idarubicin.

leukocytes were infused to treat relapse after HCT,[6,7,22,23] suggested that RIC might be successfully employed in patients who were less able to tolerate MAC. The objective of RIC is to provide sufficient immunosuppression of the host to achieve engraftment of donor hematopoietic cells and avoid both the severe pancytopenia and nonhematopoietic toxicity of MAC regimens. Many RIC regimens have been developed that provide for donor engraftment but vary in hematopoietic and nonhematopoietic toxicity, and the choice of regimen is in part based on balancing the risks of transplant-related mortality and relapse (Fig. 131.1). A recent large retrospective analysis of >1,000 patients with hematologic malignancies that received a nonmyeloablative RIC regimen consisting of 2 Gy TBI ± fludarabine demonstrated 5-year overall survival rates from 25% to 60% depending on disease risk, comorbidities, and GVHD.[24] At 5 years, the nonrelapse mortality rate was 24% and the relapse mortality rate was 34.5%. Analysis of registry data shows that RIC regimens of higher dose intensity provide for similar overall and disease-free survival as MAC regimens in patients with AML and MDS, whereas the lowest intensity regimens were inferior, due to higher relapse rates.[25] A phase 3 randomized trial conducted by the Blood and Marrow Transplant Clinical Trials Network is in progress to compare outcomes of MAC and RIC in patients 18 to 65 years of age. The benefit of RIC is the ability to offer potentially curative allogeneic HCT to older patients. However, novel approaches to reducing relapse and preventing or diminishing the morbidity and mortality of GVHD in these patients are needed to improve outcome.

Radiolabeled Monoclonal Antibodies

Targeting radiation to leukemic cells with radiolabeled monoclonal antibodies that bind to cell surface molecules could increase the radiation dose at sites of tumor and spare normal organs such as the liver and lung. An iodine-131–labeled anti-CD45 antibody has been used for this purpose in conjunction with conventional MAC in younger patients, or with RIC in patients over the age of 55. These studies have demonstrated that it is feasible to deliver >25 Gy to the BM while limiting liver and lung exposure, and achieve long-term survival in patients with high-risk AML.[26,27] A similar approach using an yttrium-90–labeled anti-CD20 monoclonal antibody combined with RIC for patients with refractory CD20+ B-cell malignancies has shown promise in early phase studies.[28,29] The use of pretargeting and new radioisotopes with more favorable tissue penetration might improve therapeutic efficacy and reduce toxicity.[30]

STEM CELL SOURCES

Donor/recipient genetic nonidentity at loci within the major histocompatibility complex (MHC) on chromosome 6p that encode specific HLA molecules is the most important risk factor for severe GVHD.[4] Thus, hematopoietic cell grafts from donors who are identical with the recipient at the critical HLA loci are the preferred source of hematopoietic stem cells for allogeneic HCT. Although BM continues to be the most common graft source obtained from donors <20 years old in the United States, hematopoietic cells collected from the peripheral blood (PB) by apheresis after stimulation with filgrastim (granulocyte colony-stimulating factor) to mobilize CD34+ stem cells account for a majority of grafts harvested from donors >20 years of age (Fig. 131.2). For the large number of patients for whom a suitably HLA-matched donor cannot be identified, grafts derived from umbilical cord blood (UCB) or harvested from BM or PB of HLA-mismatched or HLA-haploidentical donors can provide a source of hematopoietic stem cells for allogeneic HCT.

Human Leukocyte Antigen–Matched Donors

The preferred donor for any patient who requires allogeneic HCT continues to be a full sibling who is genetically identical with the recipient for specific exons within the *HLA-A*, *-B*, *-C*, and *-DRB1* genes. BM or PB grafts from HLA-identical siblings have been associated with the lowest risks for severe acute and chronic GHVD, and with superior posttransplant hematologic and immunologic reconstitution. Filgrastim-stimulated PB grafts in general contain a several-fold higher number of CD34+ hematopoietic progenitor cells than BM, but also contain a ≥10-fold higher number of T-lymphocytes, which are the central mediators of GVHD. Several large, randomized trials of transplantation with BM or PB grafts from HLA-identical sibling donors have shown that PB provides superior hematopoietic engraftment, but at the cost of a higher risk for both acute and chronic GVHD.[31–35] Some of these studies have shown a decreased rate of relapse and superior survival in recipients of PB as compared with BM grafts, primarily in the subset of patients with high-risk malignancies.[31,34] Donors of BM and PB generally report similar levels of discomfort associated with the stem cell donation, but PB donors report faster resolution of symptoms.[36] Limited data also suggest that the economic cost of BM donation exceeds that of PB donation.[37] Despite the higher risk of GVHD associated with PB grafts, the superior engraftment and lower relapse risk and the strong preference of donors

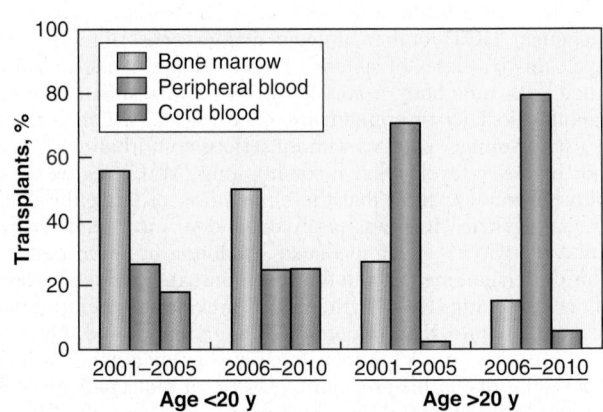

Figure 131.2 Allogeneic stem cell source by recipient age (2001 to 2010). Redrawn with permission from Pasquini MC, Zang Z. Current use and outcome of hemaotpoietic stem cell transplantation: Center for International Blood and Marrow Transplant Research Summary Slides, 2012.

for PB as opposed to BM donation have made PB grafts the preferred and, in fact, the default source of stem cells for patients with HLA-identical sibling donors. BM remains the preferred stem cell source for patients with nonmalignant disorders such as aplastic anemia, in whom there is no need for a GVL effect.

Unrelated Donors

Most patients who are candidates for allogeneic HCT do not have an HLA-identical sibling donor available; for many such patients, suitably HLA-matched volunteer unrelated donors can be identified in worldwide registries that now include more than 22 million individuals (www.bmdw.org; accessed January 5, 2014). The annual number of transplants performed in the United States with grafts from volunteer unrelated donors has exceeded the number performed with grafts from HLA-identical sibling donors since 2005 (Fig. 131.3). Improved understanding of the role of the MHC in allogeneic HCT has driven steady evolution of the laboratory procedures used to establish that patients and prospective donors are suitably "matched." The National Marrow Donor Program currently recommends matching recipients and prospective donors at the DNA sequence level in exons 2 and 3 of the *HLA-A*, *-B*, and *-C* genes, and exon 2 of the *HLA-DRB1* gene.[38] In practice, recipients and prospective donors are also "typed" and matched for exon 2 of the *HLA-DQB1* gene, primarily to ensure optimal donor/recipient matching at *HLA-DRB1*. Retrospective analysis of 3,857 unrelated donor transplants between 1998 and 2003 revealed that donor/recipient matching at *HLA-A*, *-B*, *-C*, and *-DRB1* (termed 8/8 matches) was associated with superior survival, and that a single mismatch at any one of these loci (7/8 matches) was associated with higher mortality.[39] Accumulating evidence suggests that donor/recipient matching at an additional HLA locus, *HLA-DPB1*, also influences the outcome of unrelated donor HCT.[40] Although donor/recipient matching at *HLA-DQB1* is typically achieved with current selection algorithms for unrelated donors, no data demonstrate that *HLA-DQB1* matching is associated with a survival benefit.

The strong preference for utilization of PB grafts in transplants between HLA-identical sibling pairs has profoundly influenced clinical practice in the unrelated donor setting, and PB grafts are currently used in over three-fourths of unrelated donor transplants. Unrelated PB grafts, like PB grafts from sibling donors, are associated with superior hematopoietic engraftment, and unrelated donors who donate PB grafts experience faster resolution of donation-related discomfort than do BM donors.[36] A recent multicenter international randomized trial demonstrated no significant difference in 2-year survival between the recipients of unrelated BM and PB grafts; however, trends toward more graft failure in the BM recipients and more chronic GVHD in the PB recipients were observed.[41]

Although the outcome of allogeneic HCT from unrelated donors was for many years inferior to that of transplants between HLA-identical siblings, advances in donor selection and in transplant practice—particularly conditioning regimens and supportive care—are steadily eliminating this critical differential. Retrospective analyses of HCT between HLA-matched related and 8/8 locus-matched unrelated donor/recipient pairs have shown comparable overall survival between the two groups, albeit with significantly more acute and chronic GVHD after unrelated donor transplant.[42,43] The equivalent outcome of transplantation from HLA-matched related versus unrelated donors is all the more impressive given that patients who are referred for unrelated donor HCT have, on average, more advanced and higher risk disease.

Umbilical Cord Blood

The development and applications of UCB transplantation have been recently reviewed,[44] and this stem cell source provides an increasingly used alternative for patients that do not have a readily available, suitably HLA-matched family or unrelated donor. There are now >131 voluntary banks in 35 countries that house >500,000 UCB units available for searches to identify a suitable UCB unit for patients who need an allogeneic HCT.[45] The advantages of UCB include rapid availability, little or no risk to the

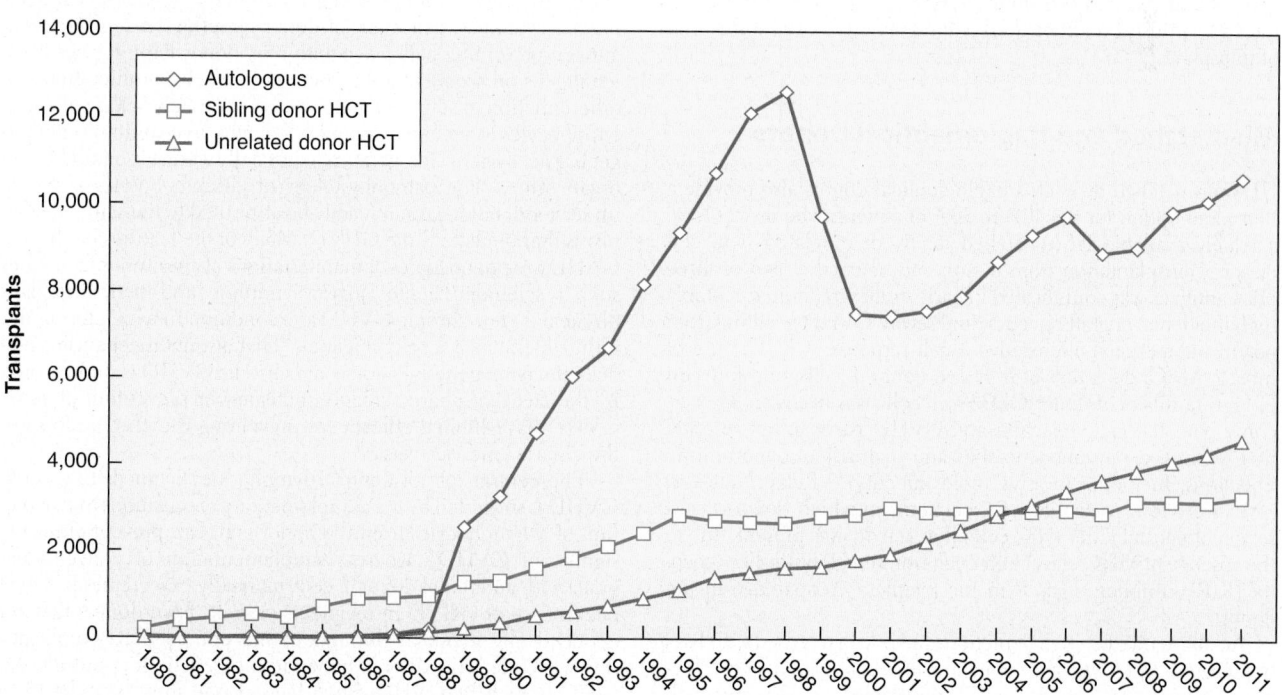

Figure 131.3 Transplant activity in the United States based on source of stem cells (1980 to 2011). (Reprinted with permission from Pasquini MC, Zang Z. Current use and outcome of hemaotpoietic stem cell transplantation: Center for International Blood and Marrow Transplant Research Summary Slides, 2012.)

PRACTICE OF ONCOLOGY

mother or newborn infant, and a low risk of transmitting viruses. There is also a decreased requirement for stringent HLA matching, and UCB transplants that match at only four of six HLA class I and II molecules lead to acceptable rates of GVHD. The disadvantages of UCB include delayed engraftment, especially in patients that receive a nucleated cell dose of $<2.5 \times 10^7$/kg or a CD34+ cell dose of $<1.2 \times 10^5$/kg, and delayed immune reconstitution, which contributes to higher transplant-related mortality.[46] The initial applications of UCB transplant focused on pediatric patients, who because of their size could receive a higher dose of CD34+ cells/kg of body weight. Data from registry studies demonstrate that the overall survival of patients receiving single UCB transplant compares favorably to HLA-matched unrelated donor BM or PB transplants.[47,48]

To overcome the low CD34+ cell dose in a single UCB unit, two UCB units that were matched for at least four of six HLA alleles with the recipient have been administered. Such double UCB transplant improved the time to engraftment in adult recipients,[49,50] even though chimerism analysis revealed that one UCB unit often rapidly dominated engraftment.[51] A comparison of outcomes of double UCB transplant to those using HLA-matched related or unrelated donors has suggested a lower risk of relapse but higher transplant-related mortality with UCB grafts, and a similar overall survival.[50] UCB transplant has also been successfully employed with RIC, providing an option for older patients that could not tolerate MAC and do not have a suitably matched related or unrelated donor.[52,53]

Innovations that may improve the outcome of UCB transplant are the subject of intense research. A promising approach to shorten the duration of neutropenia is to infuse an uncultured UCB unit along with in vitro expanded progenitor cells derived either by culturing UCB CD34+ cells with the Notch ligand delta 1, or with mesenchymal progenitor cells.[54,55] These approaches currently require specialized cell culture facilities, but in the future cryopreserved banks of third-party "off-the-shelf" progenitors could be derived and used for this purpose. Strategies to improving homing of the infused stem cells to hematopoietic niches are also being explored to improve engraftment.[56] Immune reconstitution might be improved by the transfer of virus-specific cells or lymphoid progenitors derived de novo from UCB T cells,[57,58] and GVHD reduced by infusing additional CD4+ regulatory T cells at the time of transplant.[59,60]

Mismatched and Haploidentical Donors

HLA-mismatched or related haploidentical donors also provide a transplant option for the 40% to 50% of patients who do not have a readily available HLA-matched family or unrelated stem cell donor. Transplantation from donors mismatched at two or three HLA antigens was complicated in early studies by an unacceptably high incidence of graft rejection and severe GVHD resulting from potent bidirectional alloreactive T-cell responses.[61–63] The use of intense MAC, depletion of host and donor T cells, and infusion of high numbers of donor CD34+ T cells was necessary to overcome both the graft rejection and GVHD barriers, but resulted in a prolonged immunodeficiency and high risk of opportunistic infections, including invasive mold infection.[64] Relapse rates in AML were low, particularly in recipients in which donor-versus-recipient natural killer (NK) cell alloreactivity was present, due to the absence of MHC class I killer cell immunoglobulin-like receptor (KIR) inhibitory ligands in the recipient compared with the donor.[65]

An alternative to T-cell depletion, and one that is used with RIC to prevent GVHD and graft rejection after haploidentical HCT, is the administration of high-dose Cy posttransplant. This approach has the advantage of selectively eliminating alloreactive T cells that become activated in the recipient, resulting in preservation of immune reconstitution to pathogens, thus avoiding the severe

opportunistic infections that are observed after T-cell–depleted haploidentical HCT.[66–68] A recent Blood and Marrow Transplant Clinical Trials Network study of two parallel phase 2 trials of RIC and haploidentical donor BM transplant with high-dose Cy posttransplant or double UCB transplant demonstrated similar overall and progression-free survival at 1 year (62% and 48% haploidentical HCT; 54% and 46% double UCB transplant), and similar incidence of grade II to IV acute GVHD (32% haploidentical HCT; 40% double UCB transplant).[69] The 1-year cumulative incidences of nonrelapse mortality and relapse, respectively, were 7% and 45% after haploidentical HCT, and 24% and 31% after double UCB transplant. These results illustrate the vast improvements in outcomes after haploidentical HCT and suggest that randomized comparisons of UCB, matched unrelated donor, and haploidentical related donor HCT will be needed to determine if any of these procedures is superior.

IMMUNOBIOLOGY OF ALLOGENEIC HEMATOPOIETIC CELL TRANSPLANTATION

The outcome of allogeneic HCT is in large part determined by recognition of alloantigens expressed on recipient cells by donor lymphocytes. Genetic disparity between donor and recipient is a key to the therapeutic efficacy of allogeneic HCT, but also the root cause of GVHD, which is its primary limitation. GVL and GVHD are mediated primarily by lymphocytes contained in or derived from the donor hematopoietic cell graft. GVL activity is closely linked to the development of GVHD, but clinically significant GVHD is not required for GVL, implying that important mechanistic distinctions exist between the two phenomena.

Graft-versus-Host Disease

GVHD comprises two distinct but variably overlapping clinical syndromes—acute and chronic GVHD—that differ in their time course, clinical manifestations, and response to therapy. The pathophysiology of acute GVHD is complex and involves tissue injury caused by cytotoxic conditioning and subsequent release of inflammatory cytokines, activation of donor lymphocytes and recipient antigen-presenting cells, recognition by donor lymphocytes of alloantigens on recipient antigen-presenting cells, proliferation and differentiation of activated donor lymphocytes, trafficking of donor lymphocytes to secondary lymphoid organs, and infiltration of target organs by activated donor effector cells with subsequent target organ injury. The pathophysiology of chronic GVHD is poorly understood, but it cannot readily be attributed to the same mechanisms that mediate acute GHVD. Many of the features of chronic GVHD are phenocopies of manifestations of autoimmune diseases such as scleroderma and Sjögren syndrome, and many transplant physicians view chronic GVHD as a condition in which loss of immune tolerance is a central feature. That distinct mechanisms mediate the pathogenesis of acute and chronic GVHD is underscored by the fact that pharmacologic strategies for prevention of acute GVHD have limited efficacy for preventing the chronic form of the disease (and vice versa).

The central role of donor T-lymphocytes in mediating acute GVHD is suggested by the complementary observations that depletion of T-lymphocytes from the donor graft can prevent clinically significant GVHD,[7] whereas supplementation of conventional grafts with additional donor T cells markedly exacerbates it.[70] The occurrence of GHVD in recipients of grafts from donors that are genotypically identical throughout the entire MHC implicates donor/recipient disparity at polymorphic genetic loci outside the MHC in causing GVHD. Such loci encode short peptides (8 to 12 residues in length) termed "minor histocompatibility antigens" that are presented on the cell surface by HLA molecules encoded in the MHC. Minor histocompatibility (H) antigens are created by the extensive sequence and structural variation present in the human genome, and all donor/recipient transplant pairs, despite selection for identity at the MHC, will be mismatched for many minor H antigens.[71]

The etiology of chronic GVHD is distinguished from acute GVHD by a significant role for B-lymphocytes and dysregulated B-cell homeostasis. Abnormal levels of naïve B cells are observed in chronic GVHD[72] and are associated with elevated levels of B-cell activating factor,[73] which can promote the survival and activation of autoreactive B cells.[74] Autoantibodies specific for nuclear, mitochondrial, parietal cell, smooth muscle, and parotid gland antigens have been detected in patients with severe symptoms of chronic GVHD.[75,76] Autoantibodies against platelet-derived growth factor have been detected in patients with chronic GVHD with prominent sclerosis and fasciitis.[77]

Graft versus Leukemia

The elimination of malignant cells in recipients of allogeneic HCT is intimately associated with GVHD, but GVL activity is observed in the absence of GVHD, suggesting important distinctions between the two. It is clear that the GVL effect is not a single homogeneous phenomenon, and that the mechanisms that mediate GVL are determined by the genetic disparity between the donor and recipient, the source, composition, and processing of the hematopoietic cell graft from the donor and the recipient tumor type. Donor T-lymphocytes and NK cells are the primary GVL effector cells. Donor T cells specific for minor H antigens expressed on recipient malignant cells are particularly important in patients who receive T-replete grafts from HLA-identical donors. Minor H antigen-specific T cells exhibit potent antileukemic activity both in vitro[78] and in vivo,[79,80] and specifically eliminate the leukemic stem cells that establish human leukemia in immune-deficient mice.[79,80] Minor antigen-specific T cells with reactivity against recipient leukemic cells have frequently been detected in the blood of HCT recipients demonstrating regression of leukemia following donor lymphocyte infusion.[81] It is thought that donor T cells recognizing minor H antigens that are selectively or exclusively expressed on recipient hematopoietic cells—including leukemic cells—may mediate GVL activity without contributing to GVHD.

Donor T cells recognizing nonpolymorphic antigens encoded by genes that are over- or aberrantly expressed in myeloid and lymphoid leukemic cells can contribute to GVL activity. CD8+ T cells recognizing peptides encoded by genes overexpressed in myeloid leukemic cells such as myeloblastin and neutrophil elastase,[82] by the *WT1* oncogene that is expressed in a wide range of leukemic cells,[83] or from the cancer-testis gene *NY-ESO-1* that is often expressed in AML and multiple myeloma[84] have been detected in the blood of HCT recipients. Donor T-cell responses against tumor-specific antigens can also develop in allogeneic HCT recipients and contribute to GVL activity.[85] It is likely that donor T-cell responses against this class of recipient antigens are enabled and facilitated by the immunogenic milieu created by responses against recipient minor H antigens, as they have not in general been detected in recipients of syngeneic transplants.

Alloreactive donor NK cells can be major mediators of GVL in recipients of grafts from multiple HLA-mismatched and haploidentical donors, in whom extensive in vitro or in vivo T-cell depletion of the graft is required to prevent lethal GVHD.[65] The recognition of recipient target cells by cytotoxic donor NK cells in allogeneic HCT is in large part determined by donor and recipient genotypes at the KIR locus on chromosome 19q, as well as at the *HLA-A*, *-B*, and *-C* loci on chromosome 6p. KIR genes encode transmembrane receptors that are expressed selectively or exclusively in NK cells and subsets of $\alpha\beta$ or $\gamma\delta$ T cells; bind to specific subsets of HLA-A, -B, and -C alleles in a manner that is influenced by HLA-bound peptide; and participate in specific recognition of target cells by NK and T cells. In the HLA-haploidentical or multiple

HLA-mismatched setting, cytotoxic donor NK cells can eliminate recipient leukemic cells that express molecules for which they are specific. The interaction of donor NK and recipient leukemic cells is in part determined by the gene content and haplotype of the donor at the KIR locus, but the nature of the interactions have yet to be completely defined. Several models of NK alloreactivity have been proposed, but it is not yet clear which of these models has the greatest accuracy.

Accumulating evidence, much of it indirect, also suggests that donor NK cells may make a significant contribution to the elimination of myeloid leukemias after allogeneic HCT between fully HLA-matched donor/recipient pairs (reviewed in Warren and Deeg[86]). The most compelling data have been provided by several large retrospective studies of MHC and KIR genotype and posttransplant relapse, and have shown significant associations between the presence in the donor of a specific type of haplotype at the KIR locus, or one or more components thereof, and decreased rate of relapse in recipients undergoing unrelated HCT for AML and other myeloid neoplasms.[87,88]

COMPLICATIONS OF ALLOGENEIC HEMATOPOIETIC CELL TRANSPLANTATION AND THEIR MANAGEMENT

Acute and Chronic Graft-versus-Host Disease

The syndrome of acute GVHD is characterized by fever, skin rash, gastrointestinal symptoms referable to involvement of the upper or lower tract, and cholestatic liver dysfunction, often accompanied by elevations in hepatic transaminases. It typically occurs within the first 60 days after HCT, but can occur later, particularly in recipients of RIC. The most important risk factors for the development of acute GVHD are donor/recipient HLA mismatch, donor and recipient age, a filgrastim-stimulated PB graft rather than a BM graft, myeloablative conditioning with a TBI-containing regimen, and donor/recipient cytomegalovirus (CMV) seropositivity. The skin rash of GVHD is most commonly an erythematous, variably pruritic, macular or maculopapular eruption that can involve any part of the body surface. Blistering and desquamation is seen in severe cases (Fig. 131.4A,B). The symptoms of gut GVHD range widely in severity and can include anorexia, nausea, vomiting, abdominal cramping, and diarrhea, the latter of which can be voluminous (measurable in liters per day) and bloody. Endoscopic evaluation of gut GVHD reveals mucosal edema and erythema in mild cases, frankly hemorrhagic epithelium in more severe cases, and pseudomembranes and extensive denudation in life-threatening disease. The pathologic hallmarks of mild to moderate skin and gut GVHD are apoptotic epithelial cells and an infiltrate of inflammatory cells, composed chiefly of lymphocytes and neutrophils, the latter primarily in the gut. Hepatic GVHD is most specifically characterized by damage to bile ducts with bile stasis, often accompanied by inflammatory cell infiltration. Recent studies have identified plasma biomarkers for skin[89] and lower gastrointestinal and liver[90] GVHD, and a plasma biomarker associated with therapy-resistant, life-threatening GVHD.[91]

Chronic GHVD has protean manifestations that can appear in a broader range of target organs than acute GHVD, including the eyes, mouth, skin and nails, gut, liver, lungs, joints, subcutaneous tissue, and genital tract, particularly in women. Symptoms and signs of chronic GVHD include skin tightness and thickening, hypo- or hyperpigmentation (Fig. 131.4C,D), skin erosion or ulcers, pruritus, brittle and/or ridged nails, dry eyes and dry mouth, hair thinning or loss, edema, fatigue, weight loss, anorexia, dysphagia or odynophagia, joint stiffness or contractures, chronic cough, dyspnea, vaginal dryness, and dyspareunia, among others. Laboratory signs include eosinophilia, thrombocytopenia, and hypo- or, less commonly, hypergammaglobulinemia. Biopsy of involved

PRACTICE OF ONCOLOGY

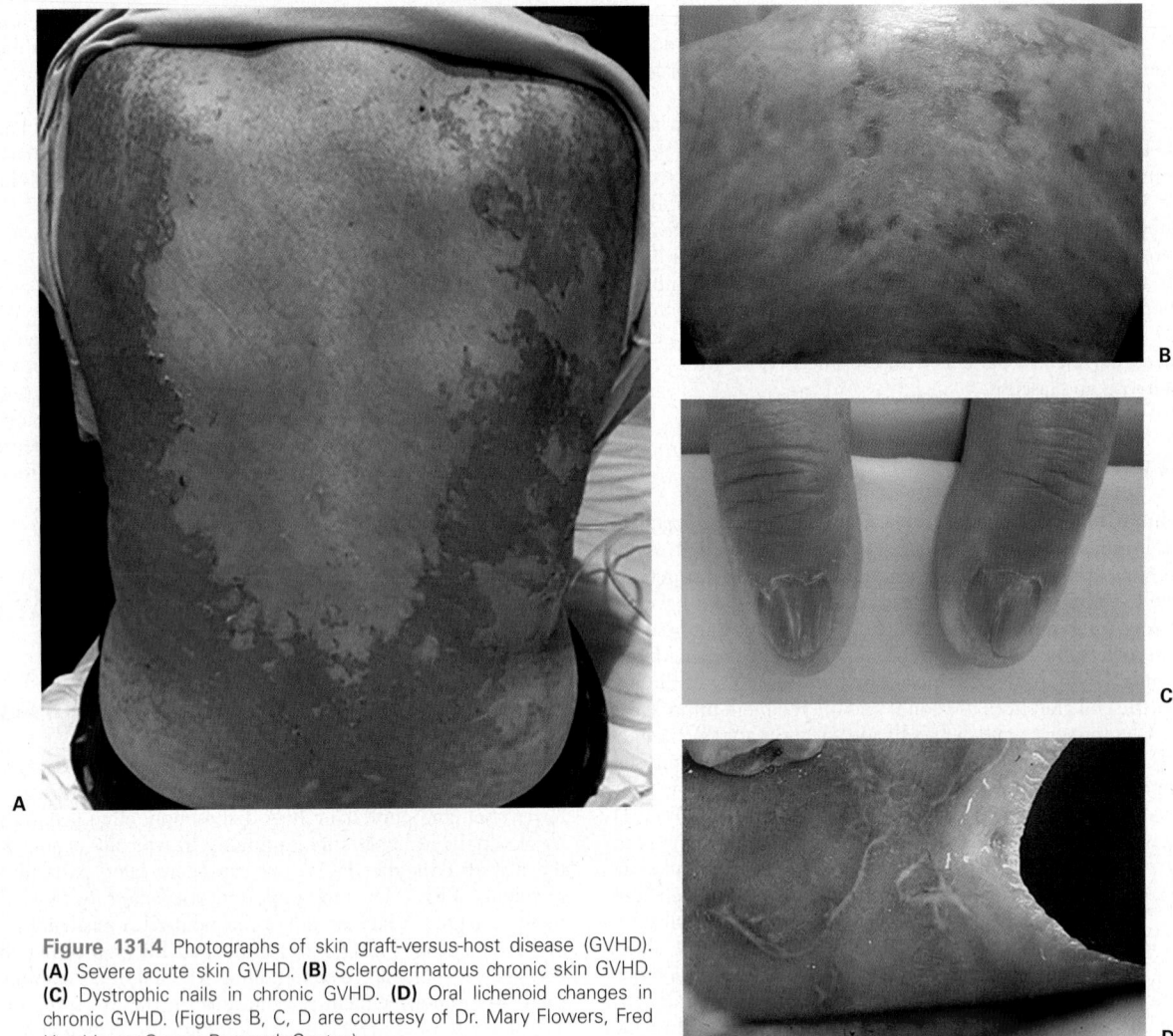

Figure 131.4 Photographs of skin graft-versus-host disease (GVHD). **(A)** Severe acute skin GVHD. **(B)** Sclerodermatous chronic skin GVHD. **(C)** Dystrophic nails in chronic GVHD. **(D)** Oral lichenoid changes in chronic GVHD. (Figures B, C, D are courtesy of Dr. Mary Flowers, Fred Hutchinson Cancer Research Center.)

sites reveals a spectrum of characteristic changes; fibrosis is a common feature. Evaluation of advanced lung involvement often reveals bronchiolitis obliterans. Immune deficiency is a prominent feature of chronic GVHD, and manifests as increased susceptibility to bacterial, fungal, and viral pathogens.

Pharmacologic Prophylaxis/Therapy

The incidence and severity of acute GVHD can be reduced with pharmacologic prophylaxis. Calcineurin inhibitors such as cyclosporine and tacrolimus combined with methotrexate have been the mainstay of prophylaxis in MAC transplants for several decades. Salts of mycophenolic acid have successfully replaced methotrexate in prophylaxis regimens in some RIC regimens. Two- and three-drug regimens combining tacrolimus, or tacrolimus and mycophenolic acid, with sirolimus have been extensively evaluated in clinical trials in both the MAC and RIC settings, with promising results.[92] Novel approaches to preventing GVHD based on donor and/or recipient statin treatment[93] or blockade of lymphocyte chemotaxis[94] also appear to have significant potential. None of the pharmacologic strategies for preventing acute GVHD have yet been shown to be effective at preventing chronic GVHD.

Synthetic corticosteroids such at prednisone or methylprednisolone at 0.5 to 2 mg/kg per day are the cornerstone of therapy for acute and chronic GVHD that requires systemic therapy. Topical tacrolimus or halogenated steroids, and the combination of an oral photosensitizing psoralen with ultraviolet A irradiation can provide useful, steroid-sparing adjuvant therapy for skin GVHD. Similarly, orally administered, poorly absorbed synthetic steroids such as beclomethasone[95] and budesonide are effective agents for mild to moderate gut GVHD, and facilitate a reduction in the intensity of systemic therapy. The treatment of moderate to severe (grade 3 to 4) acute GVHD that is refractory to treatment with 2 mg/kg per day prednisone equivalent continues to be an enormous clinical challenge. Anti–T-cell antibody preparations such as antithymocyte globulin of equine or lapine origin, and monoclonal anti–T-cell antibodies such as daclizumab are commonly used in this setting, but there is no agent that has been shown to be effective in a randomized, double-blind, placebo-controlled fashion.[96]

Alternative Approaches to Prevention of Graft-versus-Host Disease

Several approaches to GVHD prevention have been investigated as adjuncts or alternatives to the traditional combination of a calcineurin inhibitor and methotrexate. Depletion of donor T cells in vitro, using one of several different methodologies, or in vivo, typically using polyclonal or monoclonal anti–T-cell antibodies, is effective prophylaxis for both acute and chronic GVHD, but at the cost of more frequent graft failure, slower immune reconstitution, increased opportunistic infections, and higher rates of relapse in some but not all malignancies.

T-cell depletion has been examined in randomized studies of allogeneic HCT between 8/8 or 7/8 HLA locus-matched donor/

recipient pairs. A multicenter trial in which 405 patients with hematologic malignancies were randomized to receive in vitro T-depleted BM grafts from unrelated donors and posttransplant cyclosporine A, or T-replete marrow grafts with cyclosporine A and standard-dose methotrexate demonstrated a lower rate of grade 3 to 4 acute GVHD in the T-cell depletion arm (18% versus 37%) but no significant difference in 3-year disease-free survival.[97] A subsequent randomized, multicenter trial of standard cyclosporine and methotrexate GVHD prophylaxis with or without in vivo antithymocyte globulin treatment in 202 patients receiving unrelated donor HCT similarly showed a lower cumulative incidence of grade 3 to 4 acute GVHD (11.7% versus 24.5%) and of clinical extensive chronic GVHD (12.2% versus 42.6%) in the antithymocyte globulin group, but no significant difference in overall survival between the two groups.[98]

A novel approach to the prevention of acute and chronic GVHD based on administration of high-dose intravenous Cy within 3 to 4 days of infusion of the hematopoietic cell graft (high-dose Cy posttransplant) has shown promise in the prevention of both acute and chronic GHVD. Long studied in preclinical models of solid organ and hematopoietic cell transplantation,[68] this approach was first tested in the clinic for GVHD prophylaxis in haploidentical HCT.[66] These studies demonstrated that high-dose Cy posttransplant, combined with a calcineurin inhibitor, was comparable if not superior to T-cell depletion for haploidentical transplantation. High-dose Cy posttransplant alone, without additional prophylactic immunosuppression, has subsequently been studied in the setting of HLA-matched HCT from related and unrelated donors, and in both single-center[99] and multicenter studies, and has proved to be strikingly effective in the prevention of chronic GVHD, without compromising GVL activity.

Infectious Complications

Infections, both early after allogeneic HCT during the period of severe pancytopenia and later as a result of persistent immunodeficiency and/or immunosuppressive drug therapy, remain a significant cause of morbidity and mortality. Several strategies for reducing infectious complications are routinely employed, including handwashing policies for patients, families, and healthcare workers; prophylactic antibiotics; screening for respiratory viruses; monitoring and preemptive therapy for CMV infection; and prompt empiric therapy for infections in at-risk patients. The types of pathogens to which the patient is most susceptible varies over time after HCT: The risk of bacterial infections is highest during the early neutropenic phase after HCT, and again later in patients with chronic GVHD. Viral infections occur most often in the first 3 months after HCT when cellular and humoral immunity are impaired by immunosuppressive drug therapy.

Bacterial Infections

Factors that predispose allogeneic HCT recipients to bacterial infections are disruption of oral and gastrointestinal mucosal barriers, neutropenia (absolute neutrophil count <500 cells/μL), indwelling central catheters, glucocorticoid therapy, and alterations in the microbiota from prior antibiotic therapy.[100,101] The degree of mucosal damage and the duration of neutropenia vary depending on the intensity of the conditioning regimen, and RIC is associated with fewer early infections.

Up to 60% of HCT recipients develop a bloodstream infection with a gram-positive or gram-negative bacteria, and bacterial infections are the most common cause of infection-related mortality after allogeneic HCT.[102–104] Antibiotic prophylaxis and prompt evaluation and empiric therapy of patients with neutropenic fever are critical to reduce the risk of life-threatening infections. Prophylaxis with a broad-spectrum antibiotic such as levofloxacin or ceftazidime is typically initiated at the onset

of neutropenia and continued until neutrophil recovery.[105,106] Levofloxacin has broad activity against gram-positive and gram-negative pathogens, an excellent safety profile, and can be administered orally in once daily dosing. Patients that develop a fever should be evaluated by physical exam for potential portals of entry, blood and urine cultures, and a chest X-ray or other imaging studies informed by the clinical presentation. Empiric antibiotic therapy should be initiated promptly and modified depending on the results of cultures. The choice of antibiotics for empiric therapy of febrile neutropenia depends on clinical presentation, results of prior surveillance cultures, local susceptibility patterns, toxicity of individual agents, and allergic history. Typically, a third- or fourth-generation cephalosporin, carbapenem alone or in combination with an aminoglycoside, to provide coverage for pseudomonas and other gram-negative pathogens, are considered in seriously ill patients with neutropenic fever, with adjustment of the antibiotic regimen as culture data becomes available. *Nocardia*, *Legionella*, and *Mycobacterium* infections are uncommon but should be considered in patients with pulmonary infiltrates. The potential for antibiotic-resistant bacteria, such as methicillin-resistant *Staphylococcus* and vancomycin-resistant *Enterococcus*, to cause serious infections in HCT recipients who have often been heavily exposed previously to antibiotics should be carefully evaluated.

Late bacterial infections can occur after recovery from neutropenia, particularly in patients with chronic GVHD who have low serum immunoglobulin levels. Such patients are at risk from serious sinopulmonary infections and systemic infections with encapsulated organisms, and should be treated with daily prophylaxis with penicillin, trimethoprim-sulfamethoxazole, or a suitable alternative.[107]

Clostridium difficile

There is a high incidence of *Clostridium difficile* infection in allogeneic HCT recipients because of frequent hospitalization, use of broad-spectrum antibiotics, and disruption of gastrointestinal mucosal barriers.[108] The incidence of *C. difficile* in allogeneic HCT recipients in one major US transplant center was 12.5%, and infection occurred at a median of 33 days after transplant.[109] This study also identified an association between *C. difficile* infection and acute GVHD, suggesting the possibility that alterations in the microbiome may contribute broadly to transplant outcomes. *C. difficile* infection after allogeneic HCT responds to standard treatment with oral metronidazole.[109] Recurrent *C. difficile* infections in nontransplant patients that do not respond to antibiotic therapy have been treated successfully with fecal microbiota transfer,[110] and this approach has been reported to be effective in an allogeneic HCT recipient with fulminant antibiotic refractory *C. difficile* colitis.[111]

Fungal and *Pneumocystis jiroveci* Infection

Allogeneic HCT recipients, particularly those that require intensive immunosuppression to treat GVHD or that receive a T cell–depleted HCT, are at risk for serious fungal infections. *Candida* and *Aspergillus* are the most common fungal pathogens; however, other organisms may be observed.[112] The incidence of invasive and superficial *Candida* infections is markedly reduced by administration of prophylactic fluconazole,[113–115] and this is now the standard of care in transplant centers. Fluconazole has limited activity against *Candida krusei*, *Aspergillus* spp., and *Torulopsis glabrata*, and patients receiving fluconazole prophylaxis remain at risk for infections with these pathogens. Azole agents such as voriconazole and itraconazole that are active against *Aspergillus* are more effective than fluconazole in preventing *Aspergillus* infection in HCT recipients, but have a higher incidence of side effects.[116–118] Patients that require glucocorticoid therapy for acute GVHD are at high risk for invasive *Aspergillus* and *Zygomycetes* infection, and posaconazole has been shown to be more effective than fluconazole in this subset of patients.[119]

Pneuomcystis jiroveci can cause pneumonia late after allogeneic HCT, and patients should receive prophylaxis with trimethoprim/sulfamethoxazole, or, if not tolerated, an acceptable alternative such as dapsone, atovoquone, or aerosolized pentamidine, until they are off of all immunosuppressive drug therapy.[120]

Herpesvirus Infections

Reactivation of latent viruses of the herpes family occurs frequently in seropositive patients after allogeneic HCT, and in the absence of therapy can cause life-threatening disease. Historically, herpes simplex virus type 1 or 2 infection occurred in approximately 80% of seropositive patients, but is now nearly universally prevented by the administration of acyclovir beginning with conditioning. Varicella zoster virus can present late after HCT, most frequently in patients with GVHD, either as reactivation in dermatomal sites or less commonly as a disseminated infection with hepatitis, pneumonitis, and/or meningoenephalitis. Prolonged administration of prophylactic acyclovir for 1 year after HCT is effective in decreasing varicella zoster virus reactivation.[121]

Latent CMV infection is common in the general population and can reactivate and cause serious life-threatening invasive disease both early and late after allogeneic HCT. Prevention of CMV disease is the most effective management strategy. For patients who are CMV seronegative, it is standard practice to reduce the risk of the patient acquiring the virus by administering "CMV-safe" blood products as transfusion support, either obtained from CMV-seronegative donors or leukocyte reduced by filtration.[122] CMV-seropositive recipients have frequent monitoring of blood for CMV reactivation using polymerase chain reaction to detect CMV DNA, and preemptive antiviral drug therapy to prevent disease is instituted in patients with reactivation to prevent progression of infection.[123,124] Ganciclovir is most commonly used for preemptive therapy; however, foscarnet is a useful agent in patients with neutropenia.[122] UCB transplant recipients are at particularly high risk for serious CMV infection due to the lack of transferred memory T-cell responses to CMV in the graft, the low total T-cell dose, and the delay in immune reconstitution.[125] Moreover, the delayed recovery of neutrophil counts in these patients complicates preemptive therapy with ganciclovir. Thus, some centers have implemented an intensive strategy to prevent CMV disease using ganciclovir during conditioning for UCB transplant, high-dose acyclovir prophylaxis after transplant, and preemptive ganciclovir for any positive CMV DNA polymerase chain reaction.[126] Ganciclovir and foscarnet cause myelosuppression and nephrotoxicity, respectively, and there is need for a safer drug for prophylaxis of CMV. CMX001 is an orally bioavailable acyclic nucleoside phosphonate that is converted intracellularly to cidofovir, and has potent antiviral activity against both herpesviruses and adenoviruses. A multicenter randomized study demonstrated that oral administration of CMX001 was effective as prophylaxis for CMV infection in CMV-seropositive allogeneic HCT recipients without myelosuppression or nephrotoxicity,[126] suggesting that less toxic approaches to controlling CMV infection after allogeneic HCT may be forthcoming.

CMV surveillance and preemptive antiviral drug therapy has reduced the incidence of CMV disease in the first 3 months after allogeneic HCT. However, late CMV disease still occurs in up to 15% of CMV-seropositive recipients, most commonly in the first year after transplant, and has a poor outcome.[127] Patients at high risk include recipients of T cell–depleted or UCB grafts, and those with low CD4+ T cells, absent reconstitution of CMV-specific T-cell immunity and GVHD. Extended monitoring for CMV reactivation and preemptive antiviral therapy is recommended in such patients to reduce late CMV disease.[124]

Epstein-Barr virus (EBV) reactivation in donor B cells and progression to an aggressive lymphoproliferative disorder (LPD) may occur in recipients of T cell–depleted allogeneic HCT or in patients that receive T cell–depleting antibodies to treat GVHD. Strategies for T-cell depletion that also remove donor B cells from the graft reduce the incidence of EBV-LPD.[128] The pathogenesis of LPD is a deficiency of EBV-specific T cells that are necessary to control latent EBV infection. Thus, EBV-LPD can be treated effectively or prevented by infusing donor lymphocytes that contain EBV-specific T cells or are enriched for EBV-specific T cells by in vitro culture prior to infusion.[129–132] An effective alternative to adoptive T-cell therapy for patients at risk for EBV-LPD is to monitor EBV-DNA in blood and preemptively administer rituximab, an anti-CD20 monoclonal antibody that depletes B cells in vivo.[133,134]

Other Viral Infections

Allogeneic HCT recipients have an increased susceptibility to developing lower respiratory tract disease from seasonal respiratory viruses, and mortality from influenza, respiratory syncytial virus, parainfluenza, and human metapneumovirus infections can be significant.[135,136] Systemic or high-dose oral ribavirin therapy may be beneficial in patients with serious respiratory syncytial virus or parainfluenza virus infections, although controlled efficacy trials have not been performed.[137,138] Active surveillance during seasonal outbreaks can identify patients with asymptomatic or symptomatic shedding, and isolation of such patients may reduce spread to health-care workers and other patients.

Adenovirus can cause disseminated infection in allogeneic HCT recipients who received T cell–depleted grafts or develop severe GVHD requiring prolonged immunosuppression. There are no antiviral drugs with proven efficacy for adenovirus; however, this infection may be susceptible to adoptive T-cell therapy with donor-derived adenovirus-specific T cells.[139,140] BK virus is a prevalent latent polyomavirus that is increasingly recognized as a cause of urinary tract infection and hemorrhagic cystitis in allogeneic HCT recipients, particularly those with GVHD.[141,142] The pathogenesis of symptomatic hemorrhagic cystitis associated with BK virus infection remains to be fully elucidated, and therapy is largely symptomatic.

Organ Complications

Organ complications are associated with an adverse outcome after allogeneic HCT; however, mortality has declined in recent years due to prevention strategies, improved supportive care, and the use of RIC.[143]

Early and Late Pulmonary Complications

Pulmonary complications occur in up to one-third of allogeneic HCT recipients and can be divided into infectious and noninfectious etiologies.[144] Pretransplant pulmonary function testing is predictive of early respiratory failure and mortality, and may influence the choice of conditioning regimen in individual patients.[145,146] The incidence of pulmonary infections has been declining due to effective preventive measures. Bacterial pneumonia in the neutropenic phase can be reduced by the use of prophylactic antibiotics. Similarly, the occurrence of CMV pneumonia has been reduced by preemptive antiviral drug therapy. Invasive pulmonary *Aspergillus* and *Zygomycetes* infections remain serious complications, particularly in patients with prolonged neutropenia and/or those who require intensive immunosuppression to treat GVHD, and prophylaxis with newer azoles is indicated in such patients.[146]

Noninfectious pulmonary complications that occur in the first 100 days after allogeneic HCT include periengraftment respiratory distress syndrome, diffuse alveolar hemorrhage (DAH), and idiopathic pneumonia syndrome. Periengraftment respiratory distress syndrome typically develops approximately 1 to 3 weeks after HCT coincident with neutrophil recovery and is characterized by fever, hypoxemia, noncardiogenic pulmonary edema, and erythroderma. This syndrome is thought to result from release of proinflammatory cytokines and influx of neutrophils into the lung, and responds to high-dose corticosteroids.[147] DAH is characterized by damage to pulmonary vasculature and bleeding into the alveolar space. Diagnosis requires bronchoalveolar lavage to exclude coexisting infection. Patients that develop DAH within the first 30 days after HCT and do not require mechanical ventilation have a favorable prognosis.[148] Early diagnosis and treatment with high-dose steroids appear to improve survival in DAH, although prospective trials have not been performed.[149,150] Idiopathic pneumonia syndrome occurs in 1% to 10% of HCT recipients and is defined as evidence of widespread alveolar injury and the absence of an infection, cardiac dysfunction, acute renal failure, or iatrogenic fluid overload.[151,152] The pathogenesis is poorly understood, there are no proven treatments, and the collective mortality in large series of patients is 74%.[153]

Late pulmonary complications occurring >100 days after HCT occur most commonly in patients with chronic GVHD, and include bronchiolitis obliterans (BO) and cryptogenic-organizing pneumonia (COP). BO often presents with cough and dyspnea in the absence of infection on bronchoscopy, and evidence of a mosaic pattern on high-resolution computed tomography scan. In addition to GVHD, risk factors include older age, unrelated donor, TBI dose of >12 Gy, and PB as a graft source.[154] Pulmonary function tests show airflow obstruction, and patients exhibit a variable clinical course typified by slowly progressive airway obstruction with episodes of exacerbation. The management of BO includes high-dose or inhaled corticosteroids, and optimization of the immunosuppressive drugs for chronic GVHD.[155] The clinical course is typically progressive, and overall mortality for patients diagnosed with BO is ~12% at 5 years with a worse prognosis in older patients and those with progressive GVHD.[156]

COP is an idiopathic pneumonia with characteristic histopathology showing proliferation of granulation tissue in small airways and alveolar ducts and chronic inflammation in surrounding alveoli. COP occurs earlier than BO and has a restrictive pattern with low diffusion capacity and minimal airflow obstruction. The diagnosis is established by tissue biopsy and histopathology.[157] Patients with COP have a good response to systemic corticosteroids and the disease stabilizes or resolves in the majority of patients.[144]

Hepatic Complications

Liver complications after allogeneic HCT have become less frequent with improved strategies for preexisting hepatic infections and for preventing sinusoidal obstruction syndrome (SOS) and cholestasis after HCT.[15,158,159] Preexisting fungal liver infections should be diagnosed and treated with antifungal therapy prior to transplant. Patients with chronic liver disease due to cirrhosis or active hepatitis C virus or hepatitis B virus (HBV) infection are at increased risk for transplant-related mortality.[160] Patients infected with HBV should receive antiviral drug therapy.[161] HBV and hepatitis C virus infection of the donor poses a risk of transmission to an uninfected HCT recipient, and pretreatment of HBV-positive donors to reduce viral load and prophylaxis of the recipient post HCT are indicated.

SOS, which was previously often referred to as veno-occlusive disease, is characterized by hepatomegaly, fluid retention, and elevated bilirubin resulting from damage to hepatic sinusoids by high-dose cytotoxic therapy.[162] Cy is the most common offending chemotherapy agent because its metabolism is highly variable, and patients who generate a greater amount of toxic Cy metabolites have a higher risk of fatal SOS.[163] The incidence of SOS is higher with conditioning regimens that include >12 Gy TBI with Cy, and in patients with underlying liver disease. Patients with underlying liver disease should be considered for a RIC regimen that does not contain high-dose Cy. The onset of SOS is typically 1 to 3 weeks after conditioning, and the diagnosis is established by clinical criteria of hyperbilirubinemia, weight gain, and hepatomegaly. Imaging studies of the liver are useful to demonstrate hepatomegaly, ascites, and attenuated hepatic venous flow, and exclude other causes.[164] Transvenous measurement of hepatic venous pressure and biopsy can be useful in difficult cases.

The majority (>70%) of patients with SOS will recover spontaneously, and therapy should be supportive and directed at management of fluid retention, preservation of renal blood flow, and paracentesis to remove ascitic fluid if associated with compromised pulmonary function. Patients with severe SOS who have a rapidly progressive course and develop pulmonary and renal dysfunction may benefit from intravenous defibrotide.[165]

Cholestasis or hyperbilirubinemiaa after allogeneic HCT may be caused by systemic or local infection, medications such as calcineurin inhibitors, antibiotics and antifungal drugs, gallbladder and biliary disease, and acute GVHD. The etiology of cholestasis may be evident after clinical evaluation and imaging studies, and therapy should be directed at the causative factors. The frequency of cholestasis has been reduced by the use of prophylactic ursodeoxycholic acid, which has reduced nonrelapse mortality.[159]

Renal Complications

The etiology of renal dysfunction after allogeneic HCT is often multifactorial and contributing factors include hemodynamic alterations in sepsis and hepatic SOS, nephrotoxic antibiotics, and thrombotic microangiopathies associated with calcineurin inhibitors or GVHD.[166] Early recognition of patients at risk for renal dysfunction, adjusting drug doses based on serum creatinine or drug levels, and the use of less nephrotoxic antibiotics when appropriate are important to mitigate the development of renal insufficiency.

GRAFT FAILURE

In some instances, the allogeneic stem cell graft functions briefly and then after a period of days or weeks, marrow function is lost and myeloid elements are absent on evaluation of a BM biopsy. Failure of the graft usually is the result of the persistence of host immune cells that reject the donor marrow, a phenomenon that is termed graft rejection.[167] Following HCT with HLA-identical donor stem cells, graft rejection occurs most commonly when the patient has received multiple transfusions prior to transplantation, little prior chemotherapy, and/or when the preparative regimen is less immunosuppressive. HLA disparity between donor and recipient and T-cell depletion of the donor graft prior to transplant increase the risk of graft rejection. A limited array of options is available to treat graft rejection. Retransplantation from another donor or the same donor with more immunosuppressive conditioning is sometimes successful for patients with primary graft failure or acute graft rejection.[167]

Some patients may retain donor stem cells and have poor graft function in the absence of immune rejection. In this situation, a search for infectious causes of pancytopenia, or drugs that suppress graft function should be undertaken. These patients sometimes respond to treatment with a hematopoietic growth factor with an increase in the granulocyte count that may be sustained even after discontinuation of the growth factor.

OUTCOME OF ALLOGENEIC HEMATOPOIETIC CELL TRANSPLANTATION FOR HEMATOLOGIC MALIGNANCIES AND SOLID TUMORS

The most common indication for allogeneic HCT in the United States in 2012 was for the treatment of AML (Fig. 131.5). Allogeneic HCT is also commonly used for the treatment of MDS and ALL, and less commonly to treat non-Hodgkin lymphoma and Hodgkin disease, CML in advanced stage, multiple myeloma, chronic lymphocytic leukemia (CLL), and some solid tumors. Allogeneic HCT is potentially curative for aplastic anemia and several other nonmalignant disorders.

Acute Myeloid Leukemia

Allogeneic HCT has been an important component of standard care for AML for over two decades. It is the only therapy with curative potential for patients with primary refractory or relapsed disease, and is increasingly utilized as consolidation therapy for patients in first remission whose disease characteristics are associated with significant risk for relapse. Interpretation of HCT outcome for AML is complicated by significant evolution over the past two decades of the criteria used to define disease risk, from classification based on proportion of marrow blasts to more sophisticated nosologies incorporating cytogenetic, flow cytometrics, and molecular characteristics of the leukemic cells. The use of multicolor flow cytometry to evaluate patients with AML has enabled detection of very low levels of leukemic cells. Consequently, patients who would have been classified a decade ago as being in remission on the basis of <5% marrow blasts could potentially be considered to have persistent or recurrent disease today if the marrow contained ≥0.01% cells with an abnormal surface phenotype identical or similar to the leukemic cells at diagnosis. One consequence of this evolution in diagnostic criteria is the likely inclusion in older transplant studies of patients erroneously classified as being in remission due to the use of the <5% marrow blast criterion.

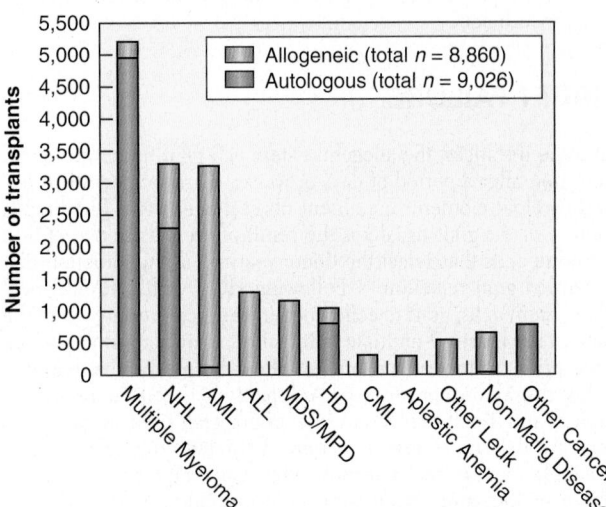

Figure 131.5 Disease indications for hematopoietic stem cell transplants in the United States, 2010. Reprinted with permission from Pasquini MC, Zang Z. Current use and outcome of hematopoietic stem cell transplantation: Center for International Blood and Marrow Transplant Research Summary Slides, 2012. NHL, non-Hodgkin lymphoma; AML, acute myeloid leukemia; ALL, acute lymphoblastic leukemia; MDS, myelodysplastic syndrome; MPD, myeloproliferative disease; HD, Hodgkin disease; CML, chronic myelogenous leukemia; Leuk, leukemia; Non-Malig, nonmalignant.

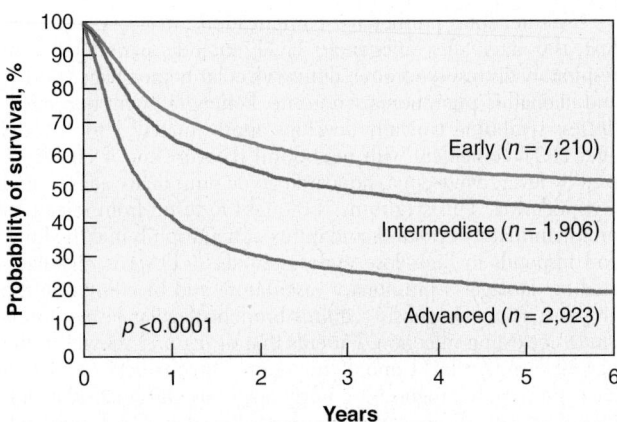

Figure 131.6 Probability of survival after human leukocyte antigen–identical sibling donor transplants for AML, 2000 to 2010 by disease status. (Reprinted with permission from Pasquini MC, Zang Z. Current use and outcome of hematopoietic stem cell transplantation: Center for International Blood and Marrow Transplant Research Summary Slides, 2012.)

This should be kept in mind when comparing AML HCT studies from different decades.

Disease stage and marrow cytogenetics are important variables that influence outcome of HCT for AML. Registry data on transplants performed from 2000 to 2010 demonstrate that overall survival of patients with AML in CR1 undergoing HCT from HLA-identical sibling donors exceeds 50% at 6-years posttransplant, whereas the corresponding survival of patients receiving grafts from unrelated donors is ~40%. Overall survival of patients with advanced disease—those beyond CR2 or not in remission at the time of HCT—is <20% (Fig. 131.6), and there is little effect of donor/recipient relation. Analysis of 560 unrelated donor transplants for patients in CR1 or CR2 suggests that cytogenetics has little influence on the outcome of unrelated HCT in CR1, but a modest influence on the outcome of HCT in CR2.[168] Specific chromosomal abnormalities have been identified that are associated with a poor prognosis. Retrospective analysis of 432 transplants for AML at the Fred Hutchinson Cancer Research Center revealed that a monosomal karyotype—defined as ≥2 autosomal monosomies or a single monosomy in the presence of other structural abnormalities—was associated with markedly inferior 4-year survival: 25% for monosomal karyotype–positive AML and 56% for monosomal karyotype–negative AML.[169]

Patient age has historically been one of the strongest prognostic variables in AML, and this also holds true for patients with AML who undergo allogeneic HCT. The effect of age is not independent of cytogenetics, however, as the proportion of patients with AML with unfavorable cytogenetics increases steadily with age, ranging from 35% of patients <56 years to 51% of patients >75 years.[170] Analysis of registry data for the period 1998 to 2005 demonstrated that the adjusted 5-year overall survival of children (<15 years), adolescents and young adults (15 to 40 years), and older adults (>40 years) transplanted for AML from HLA-matched related donors was 53%, 42%, and 34%, respectively, while the overall survival of those transplanted from unrelated donors was 37%, 28%, and 23%, respectively.[171] The development of RIC regimens has allowed a steadily increasing number of older patients who are not eligible for MAC to undergo HCT, and similar to other hematologic malignancies, the proportion of patients with AML undergoing transplants with such regimens has increased from <5% in 1998 to >30% in 2010 (Fig. 131.7). A retrospective multicenter study of RIC HCT in 274 patients with AML with a median age of 60 reported a 5-year overall survival of 33%, with 37% and 34% survival observed in patients in CR1 or CR2, respectively, and 18% in patients with advanced disease.[172] Limited data indicate

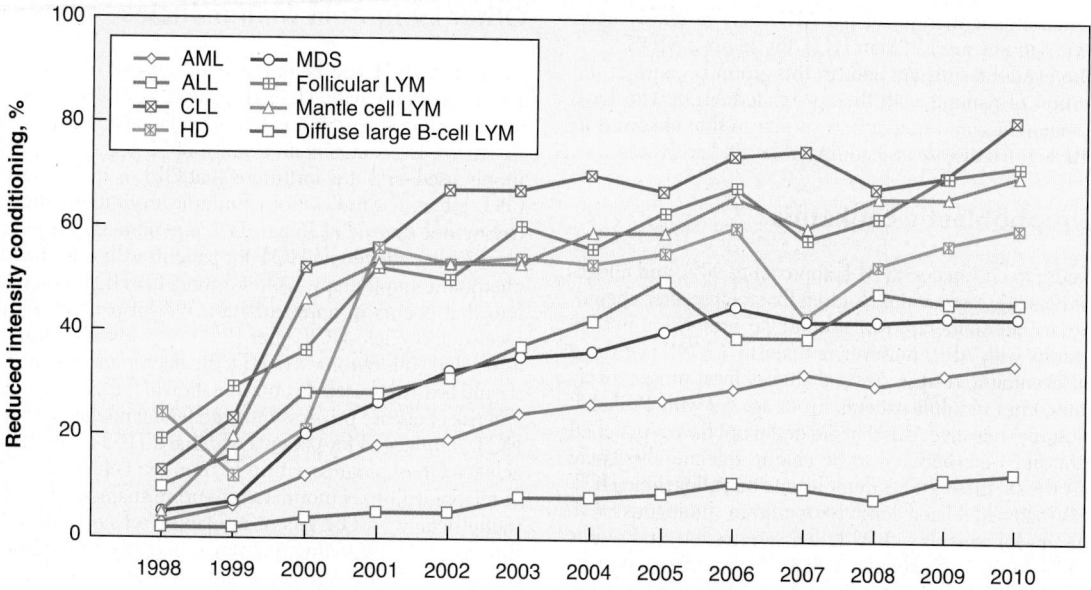

Figure 131.7 Increase in the use of reduced intensity conditioning for allogeneic hematopoietic cell transplantation for acute myeloid leukemia and other hematopoieitc malignancies, 1998 to 2010. Data is shown for year of transplant and disease type. AML, acute myeloid leukemia; ALL, acute lymphoblastic leukemia; CLL, chronic lymphocytic leukemia; HD, Hodgkin disease; MDS, myelodysplastic syndrome; LYM, lymphoma. (Reprinted with permission from Pasquini MC, Zang Z. Current use and outcome of hematopoietic stem cell transplantation: Center for International Blood and Marrow Transplant Research Summary Slides, 2012.)

that carefully selected patients with AML age 70 or older can safely undergo RIC HCT, but relapse in this age group remains a significant challenge.[173]

Myelodysplastic Syndrome

The median age of US patients with MDS at the time of diagnosis is 70 to 75 years[174]; therefore, most MDS patients are not suitable for MAC. Steady refinement of RIC regimens has made an increasing fraction of patients with MDS eligible for allogeneic HCT. A seminal retrospective study of registry data on patient outcomes showed that patients with MDS with int-2 and high-risk International Prognostic Scoring System (IPSS) benefit most from immediate transplantation, whereas those with low and int-1 scores optimize outcomes by delaying HCT until their disease progresses.[175] The central concept of this transplant strategy—immediate transplantation for advanced disease and delayed transplantation for early stage/low-grade disease—has subsequently been espoused by the National Comprehensive Cancer Network and the American Society for Blood and Marrow Transplantation. A recent analysis suggests that this strategy also optimizes outcome in older patients with MDS who undergo HCT following RIC.[176] These events have influenced the utilization of allogeneic HCT for MDS, which has been steadily increasing over the past decade.

The outcome of transplantation for MDS is associated with patient age, IPSS score, cytogenetic risk classification, donor type, conditioning regimen, and etiology of MDS. Retrospective data on 1,007 patients transplanted over two decades at the Fred Hutchinson Cancer Research Center demonstrate ~40% 10-year survival in a subset of generally younger patients with MDS who received myeloablative Bu/Cy conditioning.[177] A major challenge in patients with MDS is posttransplant relapse, even in young patients that receive myeloablative Bu/Cy conditioning, and is particularly challenging in the subset of patients with poor cytogenetic risk.[178] In large part due to a high incidence of relapse, the long-term outcome after HCT using RIC in older patients with MDS and those with significant comorbidities remains inferior to that observed in younger patients, with 5-year survival in remission in the range

of 20%. The poorest survival is observed in patients with int-2 or high IPSS score.[179] Maturing data suggest that combination of fludarabine, treosulfan, and low-dose (2 Gy) TBI may be an effective RIC regimen for MDS, with a low incidence of relapse even in patients with high-risk cytogenetics.[180] HCT for MDS from unrelated, as compared to HLA-matched related, donors has been reported to have inferior survival in numerous trials, particularly among patients with advanced disease (Fig. 131.8). However, more recent studies show progressive improvement of outcome following unrelated donor HCT, which in single-institution studies is approaching the results achieved with related donors. Registry data show a 2-year survival probability increasing from 39% for transplants performed in the period 1999 to 2003 to 47% for patients transplanted in 2008 to 2010.

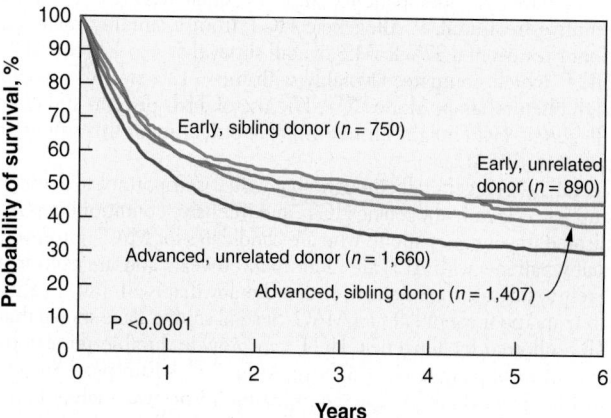

Figure 131.8 Probability of survival after allogeneic hematopoietic cell transplantation for myelodysplastic syndrome (2000 to 2010) by disease status and donor type. (Reprinted with permission from Pasquini MC, Zang Z. Current use and outcome of hematopoietic stem cell transplantation: Center for International Blood and Marrow Transplant Research Summary Slides, 2012.)

Transplantation for therapy-related MDS has generally been associated with poorer survival than HCT for de novo MDS.[181,182] However, the overall results are poor in this group because of the large proportion of patients with therapy-related MDS who have high-risk cytogenetics, and outcome is similar to that observed in patients with de novo disease and comparable risk karyotypes.

Acute Lymphoblastic Leukemia

The rate of cure in children with ALL approaches 90%, and allogeneic HCT is typically reserved for children that relapse after chemotherapy. Primary chemotherapy can also induce a remission in 65% to 85% of adults with ALL; however, a majority (~70%) of these patients will eventually relapse. Several studies have prospectively examined outcomes of adult patients up to age 59 with Philadelphia chromosome–negative ALL that did or did not have a matched related donor and were believed to be able to tolerate allogeneic HCT.[183–185] Overall, these studies demonstrate that allogeneic HCT from an HLA-matched related donor is superior to autologous HCT or chemotherapy for patients with ALL in first remission, and results in cure in 40% to 60% of patients. A retrospective study comparing related and unrelated donors as a graft source showed that the overall survival data for patients that receive a matched unrelated donor is similar to that for related donors,[186] and registry data from the Center for International Blood and Marrow Transplantation Research demonstrates that UCB grafts provide comparable results to 8/8 and 7/8 HLA allele–matched unrelated donor grafts.[48] These results suggest that for Philadelphia chromosome–negative ALL in adults, allogeneic HCT should be considered for eligible patients aged younger than 55 in CR1, particularly if there are adverse prognostic features at presentation such as a high leukocyte count; chromosomal translocations involving (t4:11), t(1:19), or t(8:14); or evidence of minimal residual leukemia at 12 weeks by molecular or flow cytometry monitoring. Advances in the intensity of conventional chemotherapy in adult ALL may improve the outcome for patients with standard risk disease and it is conceivable that in the future, allogeneic HCT may be reserved for the subset of patients that relapse after CR1. Novel approaches such as blinatumomab and adoptive therapy with autologous T cells modified to express a CD19 chimeric antigen receptor[187,188] have shown remarkable efficacy in patients with advanced chemotherapy refractory B-cell malignancies including ALL, and these strategies might also be incorporated earlier in treatment schedules and reduce the need for allogeneic HCT, or after HCT to reduce relapse.

The prognosis for Philadelphia chromosome–positive ALL with chemotherapy and tyrosine kinase inhibitors (TKI) is poor, particularly in older patients, and allogeneic HCT is the only curative treatment.[189] Allogeneic HCT from a suitably matched donor results in a 37% to 54% overall survival at 3 to 10 years after HCT, which compares favorably with the ~12% overall survival with chemotherapy alone.[190,191] The use of TKIs prior to and after allogeneic HCT might further improve outcome for this subset of patients with ALL.[192,193]

It has been generally thought that MAC is important to achieve cure of ALL with allogeneic HCT, and intensive conditioning is indicated in younger patients who are candidates for MAC. However, many patients with ALL are older than 60 years and are both less likely to tolerate the intensive chemotherapy that is curative in children and poor candidates for MAC. Several studies have shown that RIC followed by allogeneic HCT can provide durable remissions in a subset of patients with high-risk ALL.[194,195] A European Society for Blood and Bone Marrow Transplant retrospective analysis compared RIC with conventional MAC and reported a higher relapse rate with RIC ($p = 0.03$; hazard ratio = 0.59), but a correspondingly decreased non-relapse mortality (NRM) ($p = 0.0001$; hazard ratio = 1.98).[196] These studies demonstrate that RIC and the GVL effect can be sufficient to affect cure in a subset of patients with ALL that are in CR at the time of transplant, and that RIC provides a reasonable choice for patients with advanced age or comorbidities.

Other Lymphoid Malignancies

Allogeneic HCT can be curative for a subset of patients with CLL and for patients with Hodgkin disease, non-Hodgkin lymphoma, and mantle cell lymphoma that have failed autologous HCT.[197–203] Because CLL occurs at an average of 72 years of age, RIC is commonly used. and it is fortuitous that CLL is highly sensitive to the GVL effect.[204] Studies from multiple institutions show long-term disease-free survival of 36% to 43%, and nonrelapse mortality of 16% to 23% after allogeneic HCT for patients with CLL that have failed chemoimmunotherapy.[197–200] Chronic GVHD is a significant problem that occurs in approximately 50% of patients with CLL that receive allogeneic HCT after RIC.[197–200] Because of the morbidity associated with chronic GVHD, the decision to proceed with HCT should be made based on consideration of the patient's overall health and risk of disease progression. A general guideline is that allogeneic HCT is indicated for patients who have *TP53* abnormalities, fail to achieve CR or progress within 12 months of chemoimmunotherapy, or relapse within 24 months after purine analogue–based chemoimmunotherapy.[205] The recent availability of novel drugs that target B cell–receptor signaling pathways, adoptive immunotherapy with autologous T cells engineered with CD19-specific chimeric antigen receptors, and novel monoclonal antibodies provide alternatives to allogeneic HCT in individual patients.

Allogeneic HCT for patients with Hodgkin disease, non-Hodgkin lymphoma, and mantle cell lymphoma is usually reserved for those that have failed chemotherapy and a prior autologous HCT, but can be curative even in advanced cases.[201–203,206] Multiple myeloma is susceptible to the GVL effect; however, transplant-related mortality is high in these patients with MAC, and the role of RIC and allogeneic HCT continues to be defined.[207]

Chronic Myelogenous Leukemia

Utilization of allogeneic HCT for the treatment of CML declined precipitously after the advent of TKI therapy in 2000 to 2001. Nonetheless, transplant continues to have therapeutic utility, with 1,197 transplants performed in the United States from 2008 to 2012. TKI failure or intolerance, and disease progression beyond first chronic phase are currently the most common indications for HCT in CML. Survival after HCT for patients with these indications is comparable to that observed before the TKI era. Treatment with TKIs before HCT does not compromise the outcome of transplant,[208] and HCT can effectively salvage many patients who develop TKI resistance due to *bcr-abl* mutations.[209] In a multicenter study of transplants performed in the TKI era, the German CML Study Group observed a 91% 3-year survival in 56 patients who underwent HCT in first chronic phase, and 59% 3-year survival in 28 patients transplanted for advanced disease; 88% of the 84 patients who received a transplant achieved a molecular remission.[210] Collectively, these studies have confirmed that HCT is a highly effective option for second- or subsequent-line therapy of CML in both early and advanced phase.[211] TKIs are widely used for adjuvant therapy following HCT for advanced-phase CML, but there are few randomized data to support this practice.

Solid Tumors

Durable regression of several metastatic solid tumor types has been observed after allogeneic HCT. Most studies of HCT for solid tumors have used RIC regimens with little, if any, tumoricidal activity, and the posttransplant tumor regression observed has thus been attributed to the activity of immune cells contained in or derived from the donor graft. Regression of renal, breast, colorectal, ovarian, and pancreatic cancer has been observed after allogeneic HCT, with the most impressive responses observed in patients with metastatic renal cell carcinoma.[212] Responses are associated with the development of acute and chronic GVHD, or both, and laboratory studies have suggested that donor T cells specific for tumor antigens and/or minor histocompatibility antigens may mediate tumor regression.[85,213] An unacceptably high rate of treatment-related morbidity and mortality, much of it attributable to acute or chronic GVHD, has been observed with allogeneic HCT for metastatic solid tumors, which has dampened enthusiasm for the procedure. Future utilization of allogeneic HCT for solid tumors will require the development of strategies for selectively enhancing graft-versus-tumor activity and limiting GVHD.

MANAGEMENT OF POSTTRANSPLANT RELAPSE

Despite the many advances in allogeneic HCT, later relapse of the underlying malignancy remains a leading cause of death.[214] Relapse occurs because some of the tumor cells are resistant to the cytotoxic effects of the conditioning regimen, and because the immune mechanisms of the GVL effect are insufficient to eradicate all remaining malignant cells, either due to intrinsic resistance or inhibition of donor immune cell function by the immunosuppressive drugs given to prevent or treat GVHD.[215] The prognosis for patients who relapse is poor if relapse occurs in the first 3 months after allogeneic HCT, but many patients who relapse later can be salvaged with donor lymphocyte infusions (DLI) alone or following reinduction chemotherapy.[216,217] The infusion of donor T cells selected for specificity with recipient minor H antigens,

for leukemia-associated antigens such as WT1, or engineered with chimeric antigen receptors has been evaluated in phase 1 trials, and might provide greater selectivity and potency than DLI.[218–220] A variety of preemptive and maintenance strategies to prevent relapse after HCT are also being examined including the use of hypomethylating agents to enhance the GVL effect and combining targeted agents with DLI.[221–223]

FUTURE DIRECTIONS

Allogeneic HCT has provided curative therapy for thousands of patients with hematologic malignancies and has served as a paradigm for translational research efforts that have provided crucial scientific insights in immunobiology, histocompatibility, antitumor immunity, and stem cell biology. Advances including large volunteer unrelated donor registries, UCB banks, improvements in supportive care and management of infections, and the development of RIC regimens have combined to make allogeneic HCT a therapeutic option for increasing numbers of patients with life-threatening malignancies. GVHD and relapse remain the two major causes of failure, and ongoing research in the pathogenesis of GVHD in animal models is identifying novel approaches for preventing this serious complication that can be translated to humans. Moreover, the rapid advances in cancer immunotherapy are providing an increasing number of targeted therapies that are likely to be evaluated for reducing relapse after allogeneic HCT.

SELECTED REFERENCES

The full reference list can be accessed at lwwhealthlibrary.com/oncology.

3. Thomas ED, Storb R, Clift RA, et al. Bone-marrow transplantation (second of two parts). *N Engl J Med* 1975;292:895–902.
4. Thomas E, Storb R, Clift RA, et al. Bone-marrow transplantation (first of two parts). *N Engl J Med* 1975;292:832–943.
7. Horowitz MM, Gale RP, Sondel PM, et al. Graft-versus-leukemia reactions after bone marrow transplantation. *Blood* 1990;75:555–562.
8. Thomas ED, Buckner CD, Clift RA, et al. Marrow transplantation for acute nonlymphoblastic leukemia in first remission. *N Engl J Med* 1979;301: 597–599.
11. Santos GW, Tutschka PJ, Brookmeyer R, et al. Marrow transplantation for acute nonlymphocytic leukemia after treatment with busulfan and cyclophosphamide. *N Engl J Med* 1983;309:1347–1353.
14. Ruutu T, Eriksson B, Remes K, et al. Ursodeoxycholic acid for the prevention of hepatic complications in allogeneic stem cell transplantation. *Blood* 2002;100:1977–1983.
16. Copelan EA, Hamilton BK, Avalos B, et al. Better leukemia-free and overall survival in AML in first remission following cyclophosphamide in combination with busulfan compared with TBI. *Blood* 2013;122:3863–3870.
17. Bredeson C, Lerademacher J, Kato K, et al. Prospective cohort study comparing intravenous busulfan to total body irradiation in hematopoietic cell transplantation. *Blood* 2013;122:3871–3878.
18. Davies SM, Ramsay NK, Klein JP, et al. Comparison of preparative regimens in transplants for children with acute lymphoblastic leukemia. *J Clin Oncol* 2000;18:340–347.
24. Storb R, Gyurkocza B, Storer BE, et al. Graft-versus-host disease and graft-versus-tumor effects after allogeneic hematopoietic cell transplantation. *J Clin Oncol* 2013;31:1530–1538.
27. Pagel JM, Gooley TA, Rajendran J, et al. Allogeneic hematopoietic cell transplantation after conditioning with 131I-anti-CD45 antibody plus fludarabine and low-dose total body irradiation for elderly patients with advanced acute myeloid leukemia or high-risk myelodysplastic syndrome. *Blood* 2009;114: 5444–5453.
31. Bensinger WI, Martin PJ, Storer B, et al. Transplantation of bone marrow as compared with peripheral-blood cells from HLA-identical relatives in patients with hematologic cancers. *N Engl J Med* 2001;344:175–181.
33. Couban S, Simpson DR, Barnett MJ, et al. A randomized multicenter comparison of bone marrow and peripheral blood in recipients of matched sibling allogeneic transplants for myeloid malignancies. *Blood* 2002;100:1525–1531.
39. Lee SJ, Klein J, Haagenson M, et al. High-resolution donor-recipient HLA matching contributes to the success of unrelated donor marrow transplantation. *Blood* 2007;110:4576–4583.
41. Anasetti C, Logan BR, Lee SJ, et al. Peripheral-blood stem cells versus bone marrow from unrelated donors. *N Engl J Med* 2012;367:1487–1496.

42. Robin M, Porcher R, Ades L, et al. Matched unrelated or matched sibling donors result in comparable outcomes after non-myeloablative HSCT in patients with AML or MDS. *Bone Marrow Transplant* 2013;48:1296–1301.
44. Ballen KK, Gluckman E, Broxmeyer HE. Umbilical cord blood transplantation: the first 25 years and beyond. *Blood* 2013;122:491–498.
46. Wagner JE, Barker JN, DeFor TE, et al. Transplantation of unrelated donor umbilical cord blood in 102 patients with malignant and nonmalignant diseases: influence of CD34 cell dose and HLA disparity on treatment-related mortality and survival. *Blood* 2002;100:1611–1618.
48. Eapen M, Rocha V, Sanz G, et al. Effect of graft source on unrelated donor haemopoietic stem-cell transplantation in adults with acute leukaemia: a retrospective analysis. *Lancet Oncol* 2010;11:653–660.
50. Brunstein CG, Gutman JA, Weisdorf DJ, et al. Allogeneic hematopoietic cell transplantation for hematologic malignancy: relative risks and benefits of double umbilical cord blood. *Blood* 2010;116:4693–4699.
52. Peffault de Latour R, Brunstein CG, Porcher R, et al. Similar overall survival using sibling, unrelated donor, and cord blood grafts after reduced-intensity conditioning for older patients with acute myelogenous leukemia. *Biol Blood Marrow Transplant* 2013;19:1355–1360.
54. Delaney C, Heimfeld S, Brashem-Stein C, et al. Notch-mediated expansion of human cord blood progenitor cells capable of rapid myeloid reconstitution. *Nat Med* 2010;16:232–236.
55. de Lima M, McNiece I, Robinson SN, et al. Cord-blood engraftment with ex vivo mesenchymal-cell coculture. *N Engl J Med* 2012;367:2305–2315.
58. Awong G, Singh J, Mohtashami M, et al. Human proT-cells generated in vitro facilitate hematopoietic stem cell-derived T-lymphopoiesis in vivo and restore thymic architecture. *Blood* 2013;122:4210–4219.
59. Brunstein CG, Miller JS, Cao Q, et al. Infusion of ex vivo expanded T regulatory cells in adults transplanted with umbilical cord blood: safety profile and detection kinetics. *Blood* 2011;117:1061–1070.
65. Ruggeri L, Capanni M, Urbani E, et al. Effectiveness of donor natural killer cell alloreactivity in mismatched hematopoietic transplants. *Science* 2002; 295:2097–2100.
66. Brodsky RA, Luznik L, Bolanos-Meade J, et al. Reduced intensity HLA-haploidentical BMT with post transplantation cyclophosphamide in nonmalignant hematologic diseases. *Bone Marrow Transplant* 2008;42:523–527.
69. Brunstein CG, Fuchs EJ, Carter SL, et al. Alternative donor transplantation after reduced intensity conditioning: results of parallel phase 2 trials using partially HLA-mismatched related bone marrow or unrelated double umbilical cord blood grafts. *Blood* 2011;118:282–288.
71. Warren EH, Zhang XC, Li S, et al. Effect of MHC and non-MHC donor/recipient genetic disparity on the outcome of allogeneic HCT. *Blood* 2012;120:2796–2806.
74. Allen JL, Fore MS, Wooten J, et al. B cells from patients with chronic GVHD are activated and primed for survival via BAFF-mediated pathways. *Blood* 2012;120:2529–2536.

79. Bonnet D, Warren EH, Greenberg PD, et al. CD8(+) minor histocompatibility antigen-specific cytotoxic T lymphocyte clones eliminate human acute myeloid leukemia stem cells. *Proc Natl Acad Sci U S A* 1999;96:8639–8644.

81. Marijt WA, Heemskerk MH, Kloosterboer FM, et al. Hematopoiesis-restricted minor histocompatibility antigens HA-1- or HA-2-specific T cells can induce complete remissions of relapsed leukemia. *Proc Natl Acad Sci U S A* 2003;100:2742–2747.

82. Molldrem JJ, Lee PP, Wang C, et al. Evidence that specific T lymphocytes may participate in the elimination of chronic myelogenous leukemia. *Nat Med* 2000;6:1018–1023.

85. Takahashi Y, Harashima N, Kajigaya S, et al. Regression of human kidney cancer following allogeneic stem cell transplantation is associated with recognition of an HERV-E antigen by T cells. *J Clin Invest* 2008;118:1099–1109.

88. Venstrom JM, Pittari G, Gooley TA, et al. HLA-C-dependent prevention of leukemia relapse by donor activating KIR2DS1. *N Engl J Med* 2012;367:805–816.

89. Paczesny S, Braun TM, Levine JE, et al. Elafin is a biomarker of graft-versus-host disease of the skin. *Sci Transl Med* 2010;2:13ra2.

90. Ferrara JL, Harris AC, Greenson JK, et al. Regenerating islet-derived 3-alpha is a biomarker of gastrointestinal graft-versus-host disease. *Blood* 2011;118:6702–6708.

91. Vander Lugt MT, Braun TM, Hanash S, et al. ST2 as a marker for risk of therapy-resistant graft-versus-host disease and death. *N Engl J Med* 2013;369:529–539.

94. Reshef R, Luger SM, Hexner EO, et al. Blockade of lymphocyte chemotaxis in visceral graft-versus-host disease. *N Engl J Med* 2012;367:135–145.

95. Hockenbery DM, Cruickshank S, Rodell TC, et al. A randomized, placebo-controlled trial of oral beclomethasone dipropionate as a prednisone-sparing therapy for gastrointestinal graft-versus-host disease. *Blood* 2007;109:4557–4563.

99. Luznik L, Bolanos-Meade J, Zahurak M, et al. High-dose cyclophosphamide as single-agent, short-course prophylaxis of graft-versus-host disease. *Blood* 2010;115:3224–3230.

101. Taur Y, Xavier JB, Lipuma L, et al. Intestinal domination and the risk of bacteremia in patients undergoing allogeneic hematopoietic stem cell transplantation. *Clin Infect Dis* 2012;55:905–914.

105. Bucaneve G, Micozzi A, Menichetti F, et al. Levofloxacin to prevent bacterial infection in patients with cancer and neutropenia. *N Engl J Med* 2005;353:977–987.

119. Ullmann AJ, Lipton JH, Vesole DH, et al. Posaconazole or fluconazole for prophylaxis in severe graft-versus-host disease. *N Engl J Med* 2007;356:335–347.

122. Pollack M, Heugel J, Xie H, et al. An international comparison of current strategies to prevent herpesvirus and fungal infections in hematopoietic cell transplant recipients. *Biol Blood Marrow Transplant* 2011;17:664–673.

126. Milano F, Pergam SA, Xie H, et al. Intensive strategy to prevent CMV disease in seropositive umbilical cord blood transplant recipients. *Blood* 2011;118:584–592.

127. Boeckh M, Leisenring W, Riddell SR, et al. Late cytomegalovirus disease and mortality in recipients of allogeneic hematopoietic stem cell transplants: importance of viral load and T-cell immunity. *Blood* 2003;101:407–414.

131. Bollard CM, Rooney CM, Heslop HE. T-cell therapy in the treatment of post-transplant lymphoproliferative disease. *Nat Rev Clin Oncol* 2012;9:510–519.

132. Heslop HE, Slobod KS, Pule MA, et al. Long-term outcome of EBV-specific T-cell infusions to prevent or treat EBV-related lymphoproliferative disease in transplant recipients. *Blood* 2010;115:925–935.

134. Blaes AH, Cao Q, Wagner JE, et al. Monitoring and preemptive rituximab therapy for Epstein-Barr virus reactivation after antithymocyte globulin containing nonmyeloablative conditioning for umbilical cord blood transplantation. *Biol Blood Marrow Transplant* 2010;16:287–291.

143. Gooley TA, Chien JW, Pergam SA, et al. Reduced mortality after allogeneic hematopoietic-cell transplantation. *N Engl J Med* 2010;363:2091–2101.

144. Chi AK, Soubani AO, White AC, et al. An update on pulmonary complications of hematopoietic stem cell transplantation. *Chest* 2013;144:1913–1922.

159. Ruutu T, Juvonen E, Remberger M, et al. Improved survival with ursodeoxycholic acid prophylaxis in allogeneic stem cell transplantation: long-term follow-up of a randomized study. *Biol Blood Marrow Transplant* 2014;20:135–138.

163. McDonald GB, Slattery JT, Bouvier ME, et al. Cyclophosphamide metabolism, liver toxicity, and mortality following hematopoietic stem cell transplantation. *Blood* 2003;101:2043–2048.

168. Tallman MS, Dewald GW, Gandham S, et al. Impact of cytogenetics on outcome of matched unrelated donor hematopoietic stem cell transplantation for acute myeloid leukemia in first or second complete remission. *Blood* 2007;110:409–417.

169. Fang M, Storer B, Estey E, et al. Outcome of patients with acute myeloid leukemia with monosomal karyotype who undergo hematopoietic cell transplantation. *Blood* 2011;118:1490–1494.

171. Majhail NS, Brazauskas R, Hassebroek A, et al. Outcomes of allogeneic hematopoietic cell transplantation for adolescent and young adults compared with children and older adults with acute myeloid leukemia. *Biol Blood Marrow Transplant* 2012;18:861–873.

172. Gyurkocza B, Storb R, Storer BE, et al. Nonmyeloablative allogeneic hematopoietic cell transplantation in patients with acute myeloid leukemia. *J Clin Oncol* 2010;28:2859–2867.

173. Brunner AM, Kim HT, Coughlin E, et al. Outcomes in patients age 70 or older undergoing allogeneic hematopoietic stem cell transplantation for hematologic malignancies. *Biol Blood Marrow Transplant* 2013;19:1374–1380.

175. Cutler CS, Lee SJ, Greenberg P, et al. A decision analysis of allogeneic bone marrow transplantation for the myelodysplastic syndromes: delayed transplantation for low-risk myelodysplasia is associated with improved outcome. *Blood* 2004;104:579–585.

176. Koreth J, Pidala J, Perez WS, et al. Role of reduced-intensity conditioning allogeneic hematopoietic stem-cell transplantation in older patients with de novo myelodysplastic syndromes: an international collaborative decision analysis. *J Clin Oncol* 2013;31:2662–2670.

178. Schanz J, Tuchler H, Sole F, et al. New comprehensive cytogenetic scoring system for primary myelodysplastic syndromes (MDS) and oligoblastic acute myeloid leukemia after MDS derived from an international database merge. *J Clin Oncol* 2012;30:820–829.

180. Gyurkocza B, Gutman J, Nemecek ER, et al. Treosulfan, fludarabine and 2 Gy total body irradiation followed by allogeneic hematopoietic cell transplantation in patients with MDS and AML. *Biol Blood Marrow Transplant* 2014; 20;549–555.

182. Litzow MR, Tarima S, Perez WS, et al. Allogeneic transplantation for therapy-related myelodysplastic syndrome and acute myeloid leukemia. *Blood* 2010;115:1850–1857.

183. Goldstone AH, Richards SM, Lazarus HM, et al. In adults with standard-risk acute lymphoblastic leukemia, the greatest benefit is achieved from a matched sibling allogeneic transplantation in first complete remission, and an autologous transplantation is less effective than conventional consolidation/maintenance chemotherapy in all patients: final results of the International ALL Trial (MRC UKALL XII/ECOG E2993). *Blood* 2008;111:1827–1833.

185. Kako S, Morita S, Sakamaki H, et al. A decision analysis of allogeneic hematopoietic stem cell transplantation in adult patients with Philadelphia chromosome-negative acute lymphoblastic leukemia in first remission who have an HLA-matched sibling donor. *Leukemia* 2011;25:259–265.

187. Brentjens RJ, Davila ML, Riviere I, et al. CD19-targeted T cells rapidly induce molecular remissions in adults with chemotherapy-refractory acute lymphoblastic leukemia. *Sci Transl Med* 2013;5:177ra38.

188. Grupp SA, Kalos M, Barrett D, et al. Chimeric antigen receptor-modified T cells for acute lymphoid leukemia. *N Engl J Med* 2013;368:1509–1518.

189. Fielding AK, Rowe JM, Richards SM, et al. Prospective outcome data on 267 unselected adult patients with Philadelphia chromosome-positive acute lymphoblastic leukemia confirms superiority of allogeneic transplantation over chemotherapy in the pre-imatinib era: results from the International ALL Trial MRC UKALLXII/ECOG2993. *Blood* 2009;113:4489–4496.

192. Kebriaei P, Saliba R, Rondon G, et al. Long-term follow-up of allogeneic hematopoietic stem cell transplantation for patients with Philadelphia chromosome-positive acute lymphoblastic leukemia: impact of tyrosine kinase inhibitors on treatment outcomes. *Biol Blood Marrow Transplant* 2012;18:584–592.

196. Mohty M, Labopin M, Volin L, et al. Reduced-intensity versus conventional myeloablative conditioning allogeneic stem cell transplantation for patients with acute lymphoblastic leukemia: a retrospective study from the European Group for Blood and Marrow Transplantation. *Blood* 2010;116:4439–4443.

197. Brown JR, Kim HT, Armand P, et al. Long-term follow-up of reduced-intensity allogeneic stem cell transplantation for chronic lymphocytic leukemia: prognostic model to predict outcome. *Leukemia* 2013;27:362–369.

200. Sorror ML, Storer BE, Sandmaier BM, et al. Five-year follow-up of patients with advanced chronic lymphocytic leukemia treated with allogeneic hematopoietic cell transplantation after nonmyeloablative conditioning. *J Clin Oncol* 2008;26:4912–4920.

205. Dreger P, Corradini P, Kimby E, et al. Indications for allogeneic stem cell transplantation in chronic lymphocytic leukemia: the EBMT transplant consensus. *Leukemia* 2007;21:12–17.

206. Fenske TS, Zhang MJ, Carreras J, et al. Autologous or reduced-intensity conditioning allogeneic hematopoietic cell transplantation for chemotherapy-sensitive mantle-cell lymphoma: analysis of transplantation timing and modality. *J Clin Oncol* 2014;32:273–281.

210. Saussele S, Lauseker M, Gratwohl A, et al. Allogeneic hematopoietic stem cell transplantation (allo SCT) for chronic myeloid leukemia in the imatinib era: evaluation of its impact within a subgroup of the randomized German CML Study IV. *Blood* 2010;115:1880–1885.

212. Demirer T, Barkholt L, Blaise D, et al. Transplantation of allogeneic hematopoietic stem cells: an emerging treatment modality for solid tumors. *Nat Clin Pract Oncol* 2008;5:256–267.

216. Mielcarek M, Storer BE, Flowers ME, et al. Outcomes among patients with recurrent high-risk hematologic malignancies after allogeneic hematopoietic cell transplantation. *Biol Blood Marrow Transplant* 2007;13:1160–1168.

217. Thanarajasingam G, Kim HT, Cutler C, et al. Outcome and prognostic factors for patients who relapse after allogeneic hematopoietic stem cell transplantation. *Biol Blood Marrow Transplant* 2013;19:1713–1718.

218. Warren EH, Fujii N, Akatsuka Y, et al. Therapy of relapsed leukemia after allogeneic hematopoietic cell transplantation with T cells specific for minor histocompatibility antigens. *Blood* 2010;115:3869–3878.

219. Chapuis AG, Ragnarsson GB, Nguyen HN, et al. Transferred WT1-reactive CD8+ T cells can mediate antileukemic activity and persist in post-transplant patients. *Sci Translat Med* 2013;5:174ra27.

132 Infections in the Cancer Patient

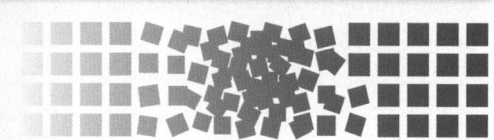

Tara N. Palmore, Mark Parta*, Jennifer Cuellar-Rodriguez,
and Juan C. Gea-Banacloche

RISK FACTORS FOR INFECTIONS IN PATIENTS WITH CANCER AND ANTIMICROBIAL PROPHYLAXIS

RISK FACTORS FOR INFECTION

Cancer patients are at increased risk for infection because of their disease and its treatment. Awareness of the risk factors present in the patient is important for diagnosis and empirical management. Selected host defense defects are presented in Table 132.1.

Intrinsic Host Factors

Hematologic Malignancies

Some hematologic malignancies are associated with increased frequency of infections even in the absence of treatment. For instance, the rate of mycobacterial disease seems to be increased in hairy cell leukemia and Hodgkin lymphoma. Multiple myeloma and chronic lymphocytic leukemia are associated with a high risk of encapsulated bacterial infections due to impaired B-cell immunity. Mutations in GATA2 are associated with myelodysplastic syndrome, acute leukemia, and Epstein-Barr virus (EBV)-associated malignancies, and they result in a particular immunodeficiency syndrome (MonoMac) characterized by viral, mycobacterial, and fungal infections in the setting of monocytopenia, B, natural killer, and CD4 lymphocytopenia.[1]

Solid Tumors

Tumor-related erosion of normal anatomic barriers or obstruction of the respiratory, biliary, and genitourinary tracts contributes to an increased risk of infection. The relief of obstruction remains the primary therapeutic maneuver, with ancillary antimicrobial therapy directed by a knowledge of the normal flora and its alterations in the presence of obstruction. The specific association of colon cancer with bacteremia and/or endocarditis caused by

Streptococcus gallolyticus (formerly *Streptococcus bovis*) should still be noted. Breast tumors increase the risk of mastitis and abscess formation, usually by *Staphylococcus aureus*. Adrenal corticosteroid-producing tumors and ectopic adrenal corticotrophin hormone–secreting tumors are associated with an increased risk of bacterial and opportunistic infections.

Asplenia

Functional or surgical asplenia is a risk for overwhelming sepsis by encapsulated bacteria. Functional asplenia is present after splenectomy, splenic irradiation, and with chronic graft-versus-host disease (GVHD).[2] The most common pathogen is *Streptococcus pneumoniae*, but other pathogens include *Hemophilus influenzae* and *Neisseria meningitidis*. Patients without a functional spleen who present with fever should be started promptly on antibiotics active against *S. pneumoniae*. The drug susceptibility of *S. pneumoniae* now is unpredictable, and local patterns should be taken into consideration. Pathogens associated with animals (*Capnocytophaga canimorsus*) and geographic risks (*Babesia*, *Plasmodium*) should be considered. The US Centers for Disease Control and Prevention (CDC) recommends that asplenic persons be immunized with the pneumococcal polysaccharide and meningococcal vaccines.[3] The conjugated meningococcal vaccine is preferred in adults 55 years of age or younger because it confers longer lasting immunity than the polysaccharide vaccine. Immunization of adults with the *H. influenzae* type B vaccine is also recommended. Immunization is ideally performed at least 2 weeks in advance of splenectomy. If this is not feasible, immunization is still advisable after the procedure. Penicillin prophylaxis is advised in asplenic patients to prevent pneumococcal disease.

Treatment-Related Factors

Mucositis

Chemotherapy and radiation therapy impair mucosal immunity at several different levels. Chronic GVHD may further compromise mucosal immunity, including defective salivary immunoglobulin (Ig) secretion. Compromise of the epithelial lining may result in invasion by local flora, and bacteremia and candidemia may result. Severe mucositis is a known risk factor for viridans-group streptococcal infections,[4] but many pathogens, including oral anaerobes, may cause invasive disease in this setting.

Chemotherapy-Induced Neutropenia

Neutropenia is a major risk factor for infections in cancer patients. Lack of granulocytes facilitates bacterial and fungal infections, and blunts the inflammatory response, allowing infections to progress much faster. The source of bacterial infections is most commonly

*Disclosure Summary:

This project has been funded in whole or in part with federal funds from the National Cancer Institute, National Institutes of Health, under Contract No. HHSN261200800001E. The content of this publication does not necessarily reflect the views or policies of the Department of Health and Human Services, nor does mention of trade names, commercial products, or organizations imply endorsement by the U.S. Government.

This research was supported [in part] by the National Institute of Allergy and Infectious Diseases.

TABLE 132.1

Risk Factors and Infectious Disease Associations in Cancer Patients

Risk Factors	Infection	Comment
MALIGNANCY-RELATED FACTORS		
Hematologic Malignancies		
Myelodysplastic syndrome and acute leukemia	Bacteria, viruses, and fungi	Infectious risk related to prolonged neutropenia
Acute lymphoblastic leukemia	*Pneumocystis jirovecii* pneumonia	Corticosteroid treatment possible confounding factor
Chronic lymphocytic leukemia	Encapsulated bacteria	Infectious risk linked to hypogammaglobulinemia
Multiple myeloma	Encapsulated bacteria	Impaired B-cell immunity, hypogammaglobulinemia
Hairy cell leukemia	Mycobacteria, herpes viruses	Defective T-cell immunity
Hodgkin lymphoma	Mycobacteria, herpes viruses	Defective T-cell immunity
Adult T-cell lymphoma/leukemia	*P. jirovecii, Cryptococcus neoformans*, CMV, *Strongyloides stercoralis*	Defective T-cell immunity
Solid Tumors		
Endobronchial tumors	Postobstructive pneumonia	Mechanical obstruction
Colon carcinoma	*Streptococcal bacteremia*	
	Clostridium bacteremia	
Hepatobiliary tumors	Bacterial infection with enteric organisms	Mechanical obstruction plus abnormal liver function if underlying cirrhosis
Head and neck cancer	Infections with oral flora and anaerobes	Mechanical disruption
Genitourinary tumors	Gram-negative bacilli, *Enterococcus* spp.	Related to obstruction
Asplenia	*Streptococcus pneumoniae, Haemophilus influenzae,* and *Neisseria meningitidis* (encapsulated bacteria), *Salmonella, Capnocytophaga canimorsus, Babesia microti*, malaria	
TREATMENT-RELATED FACTORS		
Neutropenia	Bacterial and fungal infections	
Mucositis	Bacterial infections caused by oral and enteric flora, candidiasis	
Corticosteroids	Bacteria, *P. jirovecii, C. neoformans*, molds, herpes viruses	Decrease signs and symptoms of inflammation
Nucleoside analogues (e.g., fludarabine, 2-chlorodeoxyadenosine, and 2-deoxycoformycin)	Bacteria, *P. jirovecii, C. neoformans*, herpes viruses	Defective T-cell immunity by T-cell depletion
Alemtuzumab	Opportunistic and nonopportunistic infections, including bacteria, viruses (e.g., CMV, VZV), *P. jirovecii*, and fungi	Broad defect in host defense involving depletion of T, B, NK cells, and monocytes Occasional neutropenia
Rituximab	Bacterial infections, VZV, *P. jirovecii*	Impaired B-cell immunity
Daclizumab	Bacterial sepsis	Infections in the setting of steroid-refractory GVHD
Antibodies inhibiting cytokine signaling (e.g., infliximab)	Bacterial infections, tuberculosis, and other mycobacterial infections, mold infections in GVHD, other fungal infections (e.g., histoplasmosis)	Suppression of inflammation may allow infections to progress undetected
Calcineurin inhibitors	*P. jirovecii*, VZV	Defective T-cell immunity
Radiation therapy	Local and systemic bacterial infections, mucosal candidiasis and HSV infection	Damages mucosal surfaces, marrow suppression

CMV, cytomegalovirus; VZV, varicella-zoster virus; NK, natural killer; GVHD, graft-versus-host disease; HSV, herpes simplex virus.

the commensal flora of the gastrointestinal tract. Fungal infections may be related to prior colonization in the case of *Candida* (skin or gastrointestinal flora) or inhalation in the case of molds. Risk of fungal diseases increases with the duration of neutropenia. Aspergillosis is uncommon during neutropenic periods of <10 days, but its incidence increases in direct proportion to the length of neutropenia after 14 days.[5]

Hematopoietic Stem Cell Transplantation

Autologous and allogeneic hematopoietic stem cell transplantation (HSCT) present different infectious disease problems. Autologous transplant may be considered a form of intensive chemotherapy. As such, it is typically associated with a few days or weeks of neutropenia and mucositis, followed by a few weeks or months of defective T-cell–mediated immunity. The duration of the defect in T-cell immunity varies depending on the type of cancer (longer in hematologic malignancies), the manipulation of the stem cells preinfusion (longer with T-cell depletion), and the age of the recipients (shorter immunodeficiency in children). Autologous transplants have fewer infections than allogeneic transplants, but T-cell depletion results in risk for cytomegalovirus (CMV) and other opportunistic infections similar to allogeneic HSCT recipients.[6]

Allogeneic transplant is a more complex procedure. The character and duration of increased risk for infection varies with conditioning, human leukocyte antigen (HLA) matching, source and dose of transplanted cells, and GVHD prophylaxis. Infections after HSCT tend to follow a timeline associated with different predominant immune defects: neutropenia early on, then GVHD disease and its treatment. Active GVHD requires treatment with corticosteroids and other immunosuppressive agents and is associated with increased risk of infection.[7] The specific role of CMV reactivation (which often accompanies GVHD) is also important, not only as a potential disease process, but as a predisposition to bacterial and fungal infections.[8] Defects in cell-mediated immunity persist for several months even in uncomplicated allogeneic HSCT recipients, predisposing to opportunistic infections. Allografts from alternative donors (e.g., HLA-matched unrelated donors, haploidentical family donors, umbilical cord blood) may result in higher risk of infection due to higher risk of GVHD, decreased T-cell function, and delayed immune reconstitution.[9] Recommendations for monitoring and prophylaxis are outlined in Table 132.2.

Immunomodulatory Agents and Infectious Risk

Corticosteroids

High-dose corticosteroids have profound effects on the distribution and function of neutrophils, monocytes, and lymphocytes. Corticosteroids blunt fever and local signs of infection. Patients treated with corticosteroids have impaired phagocytic function (increasing risk of bacterial and fungal infections) and cell-mediated immunity (increasing risk of infections like herpes zoster and *Pneumocystis jirovecii*). The incidence of infectious complications increases when the adult equivalent of prednisone 20 mg per day is administered for longer than 4 to 6 weeks.[10]

Fludarabine

Fludarabine is a lymphotoxic analogue of adenine, primarily affecting CD4+ lymphocytes. The combination of fludarabine and corticosteroids results in a uniform depression of CD4+ cells that may persist for several months after completion of therapy, resulting in opportunistic infections like *P. jirovecii* pneumonia (PCP) or listeriosis, sometimes more than a year after treatment. Mycobacterial and herpes virus infections have also been described.

Interleukin-2

Patients receiving high dose interleukin (IL)-2 for malignancy have an increased risk of bacterial infections, mainly *S. aureus* and coagulase-negative staphylococci, possibly related to indwelling catheters. High-dose, continuous infusion IL-2 causes a profound but reversible defect in neutrophil chemotaxis that may account for the increased frequency of infections. Prophylactic oxacillin led to a reduction in central venous catheter–associated staphylococcal bacteremia in IL-2 recipients in one randomized trial.[11]

Monoclonal Antibodies

Monoclonal antibodies (mAb) that target specific cellular steps or factors have made it possible to manipulate disease pathways in such a way that it has been possible to use "targeted" cancer therapies with astonishing clinical responses.[12] However, many of these agents interfere with natural immunity and have therefore increased rates of both common and uncommon infections.[13] As with many other immunosuppressive drugs, establishing causality is a challenge; only those associated with a probable increase in the risk of infection are described in the following (see Table 132.1).

Rituximab and Ofatumumab. There are now multiple anti-CD20 mAbs available for clinical use. Those approved in oncology are rituximab, a chimeric murine-human mAb that targets CD20 on mature B-lymphocytes, and ofatumumab, an entirely human mAb that targets different CD20 epitopes. Most evidence regarding infectious complications refer to rituximab, but it is likely that similar risks will apply to the newer anti-CD20 mAbs. These agents are used against a variety of B-cell malignancies, as preemptive treatment of EBV-associated lymphoproliferative disorder and also as immunomodulating drugs in the treatment of GVHD.

Rituximab results in rapid and profound depletion of B cells that can last up to several months. In most patients, serum Ig levels remain largely stable, as plasma cells do not express CD20. Some patients, however, develop persistent hypogammaglobulinemia, although its contribution to infection risk is unclear.[14] Initial trials suggested that rituximab had minimal effect on the occurrence of infections; however, more recent meta-analyses have reported a higher relative risk of infections. The increase in the risk infection seems to be more prominent in the setting of repeated administration and in patients with underlying immune defects or concomitant significant immunosuppression.[15] Hepatitis B virus (HBV) reactivation has been consistently associated with rituximab treatment, including reports of fulminant hepatitis and death in patients who experience hepatitis B flare, particularly when used in combination therapy (e.g., rituximab plus cyclophosphamide, doxorubicin, vincristine and prednisone [R-CHOP]). Also a reverse seroconversion phenomenon has been described, with loss of protective HBV surface antibodies and reactivation.[16] Most reactivation occurs within 6 months of therapy, but there are cases up to a year after treatment. The US Food and Drug Administration (FDA) has issued a black-box warning regarding hepatitis B reactivation and rituximab and ofatumumab (http://www.fda.gov/Drugs/DrugSafety/ucm366406.htm). It is recommended to assess the HBV status in *all* patients before rituximab or ofatumumab by hepatitis B surface antigen and hepatitis B core antibody and consider pharmacologic suppression of HBV with lamivudine or lamivudine and tenofovir, and follow all patients for signs of hepatitis B while they are receiving either drug and for several months thereafter, as reactivation has been described well after completion of therapy. Periodic determination of hepatitis B DNA while on treatment should be considered.

Another opportunistic infection reported with both rituximab and ofatumumab is progressive multifocal leukoencephalopathy (PML), also called JC encephalopathy. This is a demyelinating disease caused by JC virus, a ubiquitous virus that is acquired during infancy by most people. Since the initial approval of rituximab, there have been close to 100 cases of PML associated with its use.[17]

PRACTICE OF ONCOLOGY

TABLE 132.2

Prophylaxis of Infections in Cancer Patients

Intervention	Indication	Agent	Comments
PROPHYLAXIS FOR BACTERIAL INFECTIONS			
Prophylaxis for neutropenia	Patients who are expected to be neutropenic for >7 d	Levofloxacin 500 mg orally daily	Start the first day of ANC <1,000 and continue until resolution of neutropenia.
		TMP/SMX may be used	Other agents have been used, but there is less experience.
Prophylaxis for *Streptococcus pneumoniae*	Patients splenectomized	Penicillin V-K, 500 mg orally bid	Patient education related to early recognition of signs and symptoms of infection is imperative; consider having the patient keep systemic antibiotics (e.g., levofloxacin) at home for an emergency.
	Splenic irradiation		
	Chronic GVHD	In penicillin-allergic: TMP/SMX 1 DS tablet daily or azithromycin 250 mg/d	
PROPHYLAXIS FOR FUNGAL INFECTIONS			
Antifungal prophylaxis	Induction therapy for AML and MDS	Posaconazole 200 mg orally tid is drug of choice. In patients unable to take oral medications or who are intolerant to posaconazole, alternatives include itraconazole, voriconazole, lipid formulation of amphotericin B, or an echinocandin.	Posaconazole was superior to fluconazole/itraconazole in a randomized controlled trial, but the risk of aspergillosis in this setting is variable and some institutions may choose to use fluconazole prophylaxis if their incidence of aspergillosis is low. If fluconazole prophylaxis is used, serial monitoring with serum galactomannan and/or β-D-glucan should be considered. Begin with initiation of chemotherapy and continue until resolution of neutropenia.
	Acute lymphoblastic leukemia receiving vinca alkaloid–containing regimen	Fluconazole[a] or an echinocandin	Mold-active azoles are potent inhibitors of cytochrome P-450 isoenzymes, and are expected to interfere with metabolism of vinca alkaloids. Continue prophylaxis for duration of neutropenia.
	Autologous HSCT recipient during neutropenia	Fluconazole[a] or echinocandin	Continue prophylaxis for duration of neutropenia. Consider no antifungal prophylaxis if regimen does not have significant mucosal toxicity.
	Allogeneic HSCT recipient during neutropenia	Fluconazole, a1 itraconazole, voriconazole, and micafungin have each been evaluated in this setting and are acceptable options. Posaconazole has not been evaluated in this setting, but is reasonable.	Continue prophylaxis for duration of neutropenia.
	Allogeneic HSCT with significant GVHD receiving intensive immunosuppressive therapy[b]	Posaconazole 200 mg orally tid is drug of choice. Alternatives include voriconazole, itraconazole, lipid formulation of amphotericin B, or an echinocandin.	Continue prophylaxis for 16 wk and for at least the duration of intensive immunosuppressive therapy,[b] whichever occurs later.
Prophylaxis against *Pneumocystis jirovecii*	Allogeneic HSCT recipients Alemtuzumab recipients Fludarabine recipients	TMP/SMX 1 DS (TMP 160 mg + SMX 800 mg) orally daily or 3 d/wk OR dapsone 100 mg orally daily OR inhaled pentamidine 300 mg every 4 wk OR atovaquone 1,500 mg/d.	TMP/SMX seems effective as long as three or four DS tablets are given every week; daily administration may be more effective.
	Patients with gliomas receiving temozolomide and radiation or corticosteroids (≥20 mg of prednisone equivalent) for ≥1 mo in the presence of other immunosuppression or myelotoxic chemotherapy		In allo-HSCT, continue prophylaxis for 2 mo after stopping immunosuppression. In patients treated with alemtuzumab, continue prophylaxis for 2 mo after the last dose or until the CD4 count is >200, whichever occurs later.

(continued)

TABLE 132.2

Prophylaxis of Infections in Cancer Patients *(continued)*

Intervention	Indication	Agent	Comments
PROPHYLAXIS FOR VIRAL INFECTIONS			
Prophylaxis for HSV	HSCT recipients (HSV-seropositive recipients) Induction chemotherapy for acute leukemia (HSV-seropositive)	Acyclovir 400 mg orally bid or tid OR 800 mg orally bid OR 250 mg/m^2/12 h or valacyclovir 500 mg orally once or twice (higher doses have been used up to 1,000 mg tid) or famciclovir 250 mg orally tid.	In patients with acute leukemia and HSCT recipients, continue prophylaxis for HSV until resolution of neutropenia and mucositis.
	Consider in patients with recurrent HSV reactivation following chemotherapy, or patients receiving fludarabine and corticosteroids		In patients treated with alemtuzumab, continue prophylaxis for 2 mo after the last dose or until the CD4 count is >200, whichever occurs later.
	Patients treated with alemtuzumab		
Prophylaxis for VZV	Allogeneic HSCT recipients with a history of chicken pox or shingles	Acyclovir 800 mg orally bid OR valacyclovir 500 mg orally daily	
Prophylaxis for CMV (preemptive therapy)	Patients requiring CMV surveillance (1) Allogeneic HSCT recipients who are CMV+ or whose donor is CMV+ (standard of care) (2) Autologous SCT recipients receiving a CD34-enriched autograft (should be considered) (3) Patients treated with alemtuzumab (should be considered)	Induction for 1 wk followed by maintenance for 1 wk as follows: Ganciclovir 5 mg/kg IV q 12 h for 7 d (induction), followed by ganciclovir 5 mg/kg IV daily 5 times a wk (maintenance) OR foscarnet^a 60 mg/kg IV q 12 h times 7 d (induction) followed by foscarnet^c 60 mg/kg IV daily (maintenance) Oral valganciclovir (900 mg bid) is an acceptable alternative to IV formulations in patients who do not have severe gut GVHD (see text).	Time for CMV surveillance: (1) Allogeneic HSCT recipients: from day 30 to at least 6 mo after allogeneic HSCT, during periods of GVHD, and until the CD4+ count is >100 mcL. (2) Recipients of CD34-enriched autologous grafts: from day 30 to day 100 and until the CD4+ count is >100 mcL. (3) Alemtuzumab recipients: from the time of initiation until at least 2 mo after completion of therapy and until the CD4 count is >100 mcL, whichever occurs later.
			The level of CMV reactivation that triggers preemptive therapy varies with the method. The CDC recommends any positive CMV antigenemia (pp65) or two consecutive qualitative PCR results within the first 100 d, and five cells per slide after the first 100 d. Some institutions initiate preemptive CMV therapy with any positive antigenemia result as late CMV disease is well established (see text).
			Institutions with quantitative PCR systems must establish their own standards, as the results are quite variable depending on the methodology.
Prophylaxis against CMV		Ganciclovir or foscarnet at the same dose as in preemptive regimen.	Treatment is given for the first 100 d, then weekly or biweekly monitoring and preemptive management is initiated.
			Prophylaxis with ganciclovir is seldom used. The authors recommend preemptive therapy as described.
Prophylaxis against hepatitis B flare	Patients who are HBsAg+ or have detectable HBV DNA in the blood at high risk who are about to receive chemotherapy and are at high risk for hepatitis B reactivation	Lamivudine 100 mg/d	Start 7 d before chemotherapy and continue for 8 wk after completing chemotherapy.

(continued)

PRACTICE OF ONCOLOGY

TABLE 132.2			
Prophylaxis of Infections in Cancer Patients *(continued)*			
Intervention	**Indication**	**Agent**	**Comments**
			Not all cancer treatments are associated with the same risk; lymphoma therapy seems to be the highest risk.
	Patients who are HBsAg+ or have detectable HBV DNA in the blood who are about to receive hematopoietic stem cell transplant	Lamivudine 100 mg/d starting 2–3 wks pretransplant and restart 2 wks posttransplant.	If the transplant may be delayed, start lamivudine and vaccinate the donor so anti-HBV immunity will be transplanted. It is not known how long to continue lamivudine.

ANC, absolute neutrophil count; TMP/SMX, trimethoprim/sulfamethoxazole; bid, twice daily; GVHD, graft-versus-host disease; DS, double strength; AML, acute myelogenous leukemia; MDS, myelodysplastic syndrome; tid, three times a day; HSCT, hematopoietic stem cell transplant; HSV, herpes simplex virus; VZV, varicella-zoster virus; SCT, stem cell transplant; CMV, cytomegalovirus; IV, intravenous; CDC, Centers for Disease Control and Prevention; PCR, polymerase chain reaction; HBsAg, hepatitis B surface antigen; HBV, hepatitis B virus.
[a] Fluconazole is effective as prophylaxis against candidal, but not mold, infections. If prophylactic fluconazole is used in patients with prolonged neutropenia, the authors suggest a strategy of empirical modification to a mold-active drug in patients with persistent neutropenic fever (see text). The benefit versus risk of surveillance laboratory markers for invasive fungal infection (e.g., serum galactomannan or β-glucan) coupled with preemptive antifungal therapy remains to be established (see text).
[b] In the pivotal randomized prophylactic trial by Ullmann et al.,[53] eligibility criteria required either acute grade II to IV GVHD, or chronic extensive GVHD, or treatment with intensive immunosuppressive therapy consisting of either high-dose corticosteroids (1 mg/kg of body weight per day for patients with acute GVHD or 0.8 mg/kg every other day for patients with chronic GVHD), antithymocyte globulin, or a combination of two or more immunosuppressive agents or types of treatment.
[c] Doses apply to adults with normal renal function.

Most cases have been reported in patients with hematologic malignancies; the role of rituximab in the development of PML is not well understood. A few reports of PCP following the administration of rituximab are far from conclusive, given that most patients had received other immunosuppresive therapies. It is unclear whether PCP prophylaxis should be recommended.[18] Other rare infections that have been described in the setting of rituximab use are enteroviral meningoencephalitis, CMV disease, disseminated varicella zoster virus (VZV), refractory babesiosis, parvovirus B19, and nocardiosis.

Alemtuzumab. Alemtuzumab (Campath-1H) is a humanized mAb that targets and lyses cells expressing CD52, a glycoprotein abundantly expressed on most B- and T-lymphocytes, macrophages, and natural killer cells. This results in profound and sustained deficits in cellular and humoral immunity. CD4 and CD8 cell count nadir within weeks and may remain at <25% of baseline for approximately 9 months. Alemtuzumab is increasingly used for a variety of hematologic malignancies. Infections associated with its use include reactivation of latent viruses (herpesvirus like CMV, EBV, VZV, and human herpesvirus [HHV]-6, as well as adenovirus and JC virus), fungal infections (PCP, cryptococcosis, disseminated histoplasmosis, aspergillosis, mucormycosis), and mycobacterial infections (both tuberculosis [TB] and nontuberculous mycobacteria).[19] The incidence of these opportunistic infections varies with the dose and combination with other immunosuppressants. All patients receiving alentuzumab should receive PCP and herpesvirus prophylaxis for a minimum of 2 months after therapy or until CD4 counts are ≥200 cells/μl (Campath package insert). Given the high incidence of CMV reactivation and disease, prophylaxis or preemptive therapy is warranted.

Daclizumab and Basiliximab. Daclizumab and basiliximab are humanized and chimeric mAbs, respectively, that target CD25, the α chain of the IL-2 receptor complex expressed on activated T-lymphocytes. They competitively inhibit IL-2 binding and prevent IL-2–mediated activation of lymphocytes and cytokine release. In hematology/oncology, they are used for steroid-refractory GVHD after allo-HSCT.[20] Infections described in this setting are common bacterial infections, viral reactivations (CMV, BK virus, adenovirus, HSV, RSV, influenza), EBV-associated posttransplant lymphoproliferative disease (PTLD), invasive fungal infections, as well as legionella, nocardia, nontuberculous mycobacteria, TB, and toxoplasmosis.[21] The specific contribution of daclizumab to the infectious risk is impossible to quantify.

Tumor Necrosis Factor-α Inhibitors: Adalimumab, Infliximab, Etanercept, Certolizumab Pegol, and Golimumab

Infliximab, adalimumab, and golimumab are mAbs directed against interferon-α; certolizumab pegol is a pegylated Fab fragment of a humanized anti–tumor necrosis factor (TNF)-α mAb; and etanercept is a soluble receptor for TNF-α.[13] These agents are potent immunosuppressants, but their use in oncology is very limited, mainly GVHD. TNF-α is a cytokine that plays a central role in macrophage and phagosome activation and granuloma formation and maintenance. TNF-α blockade results in increased risk of infection, particularly granulomatous infections such as TB and histoplasmosis, but also multiple others.[22,23] The risk of serious infections appears to be lower with etanercept, than with the other TNF-α blockers. Several cases of severe HBV reactivation in patients with positive surface antigen at the start of treatment have been reported. Patients receiving anti-TNF-α therapy should be screened for TB (latent or active), HBV, and hepatitis C virus before starting treatment.[24]

Cetuximab. Cetuximab is chimeric human-murine IgG1 that targets epidermal growth factor receptor. It is used in the treatment of epidermal growth factor receptor–expressing metastatic colorectal cancer and in advanced or metastatic squamous cell carcinoma of the head and neck. Its use has been associated with slight increase in the risk of serious bacterial infections, mainly pneumonia.[25] There is one case report of a disseminated *Mycobacterium chelonae* infection.[26]

Brentuximab Vedotin. Brentuximab vedotin is an antibody-drug conjugate consisting of a chimeric IgG1 antibody that targets CD30 and the microtubule-disrupting agent monomethyl auristatin E. Brentuximab vedotin results in death of CD30+ cells. It is approved for use in relapsed Hodgkin lymphoma and relapsed systemic anaplastic large cell lymphoma.[27] Its use has been associated with a high frequency of upper respiratory tract infections. More relevant has been the reports of some cases of PML.[28,29]

Bevacizumab. Bevacizumab, an inhibitor of vascular endothelial growth factor, widely used for the treatment of metastatic colon cancer, non–small-cell lung cancer, and other tumors, has been associated with increased risk of gastrointestinal perforation.[30] Anecdotal reports of localized aspergillosis and fusariosis could be related to the potential for reduced angiogenesis to contribute to the pathogenesis of invasive mold infections.[31,32]

PREVENTION OF INFECTIONS

Infections may be prevented by avoidance of exposure, immunization, and chemoprophylaxis. A comprehensive guideline cosponsored by the Center for International Blood and Marrow Research, the National Marrow Donor program, the European Blood and Marrow Transplant Group, the American Society for Blood and Marrow Transplantation, the Canadian Blood and Marrow Transplant Group, the Infectious Diseases Society of America (IDSA), the Society for Healthcare Epidemiology of America, the Association of Medical Microbiology and Infectious Disease Canada, and the CDC makes evidence-based recommendations for HSCT that may be applicable to other cancer patients.[33] The National Comprehensive Cancer Network publishes and continuously updates broad guidelines for prophylaxis.[34,35] A summary is provided in Table 132.2.

In general, antimicrobial prophylaxis reduces the number of episodes of the targeted infection. The question frequently is whether this reduction translates into a survival benefit or a clinically meaningful outcome (e.g., sepsis, hospital admission, shortened hospitalization) that outweighs the toxicities or secondary effects (e.g., generation and spreading of resistant organisms). The number of subjects that need to be treated to prevent one episode of infection and the severity of the infection should be considered.

Prevention of Bacterial Infections

Antibacterial Prophylaxis in Afebrile Neutropenic Patients

Several meta-analyses support a beneficial effect in fever, documented infections, and overall mortality by administering fluoroquinolone prophylaxis to patients who are neutropenic for ≥7 days.[36–39] In high-risk neutropenic patients, prophylactic levofloxacin led to a reduction in infections.[40] In lower-risk neutropenic patients (e.g., those with solid tumors and short-duration neutropenia), prophylaxis showed a modest but significant reduction in febrile episodes.[41] The potential risks of quinolone prophylaxis regarding selection for resistant organisms and *Clostridium difficile* colitis are important questions that have made some experts stay away from recommending levofloxacin prophylaxis except in special circumstances,[42] but the most recent American Society of Clinical Oncology guidelines still endorse their use when neutropenia is expected to last 7 days or more.[43]

Prophylaxis against Pneumococcal Infection

Pneumococcal prophylaxis should be considered in asplenic patients and in allogeneic HSCT recipients with chronic GVHD. The Working Party of the British Committee for Standards in Haematology recommend lifelong prophylactic antibiotics in patients who have had a splenectomy, and particularly in the first 2 years, in children up to age 16, and in patients with other immune impairment.[44] Among allogeneic HSCT recipients, pneumococcal disease typically occurs in the later transplant period, from 3 months to years after transplant. Chronic GVHD is the major risk factor. Vaccination is recommended as in asplenic patients. Penicillin prophylaxis is also recommended.[33] Some experts recommend starting penicillin prophylaxis in all HSCT recipients 3 months after transplant, whereas others reserve it for patients with active

chronic GVHD. Alternative agents may be considered based on local susceptibility patterns, although the risk/benefit ratio is not well defined.

Prevention of Fungal Infections

Candida spp. and molds are the major fungal pathogens in patients with cancer. Systemic antifungal prophylaxis may be mold-active (voriconazole, posaconazole, echinocandins, amphotericin B) or not (fluconazole). *Candida* spp. are part of our endogenous flora; the major risk factors for candidemia in patients with cancer are chemotherapy-related mucositis and central venous catheters. Patients who have undergone gastrointestinal surgeries complicated by anastomotic leaks, total parenteral nutrition, and prolonged admission in the intensive care unit are also risk factors for invasive candidiasis. In contrast, the risk of invasive mold infections is principally related to the duration of neutropenia and, in allogeneic HSCT recipients, amount and duration of corticosteroids used to treat GVHD. The most common mold infections are aspergillosis and mucormycosis, but multiple opportunistic molds can infect neutropenic cancer patients (*Fusarium*, *Paecylomyces*, dematiaceous molds)

Antifungal prophylaxis should be risk-based: different patient groups are at risk for different pathogens, and these should be targeted accordingly.[45] Most cancer patients do not require antifungal prophylaxis. Prolonged neutropenia increases the risk of candidiasis, and this is prevented by the use of fluconazole 400 mg/day[46,47] (which may result in colonization by azole-resistant *Candida* strains).[48] Itraconazole has similar efficacy and may reduce the risk of aspergillosis, but is poorly tolerated and has higher toxicity and worse drug interactions.[49,50] Micafungin, an echinocandin with activity against *Candida* and *Aspergillus*, was as effective as fluconazole in preventing candidiasis and showed a favorable trend to prevent aspergillosis in a randomized, double-blinded study in HSCT recipients.[51] Prevention of aspergillosis has been shown most convincingly with posaconazole, with a survival benefit demonstrated in neutropenic patients[52] and decreased incidence of aspergillosis in transplant patients with GVHD.[53] A randomized trial comparing voriconazole and fluconazole prophylaxis in allogeneic HSCT recipients showed a trend toward reduction of aspergillosis cases in voriconazole recipients, but no difference in overall or fungal infection–free survival.[54] A systematic review and meta-analysis suggests that, overall, mold-active prophylaxis significantly reduces invasive aspergillosis (IA) and invasive fungal infection (IFI)-related mortality, but does not affect overall mortality and has more adverse effects than fluconazole.[55]

In summary, fluconazole is a safe and well-studied agent to prevent invasive candidiasis, but it has no activity against molds. When the risk of aspergillosis is significant, a mold-active drug should be considered, but different institutions may choose different agents.[56] The mold-active azoles (i.e., itraconazole, voriconazole, posaconazole) are potent inhibitors of certain cytochrome P-450 isoenzymes to a greater degree than fluconazole. This may lead to reduced clearance of other drugs, such as calcineurin inhibitors, cyclophosphamide metabolites,[57] and vinca alkaloids with potentially serious adverse effects.[58] Careful monitoring of drug-drug interactions and appropriate dose modifications are required.

Prevention of *Pneumocystis jirovecii* Pneumonia

Defective T-cell immunity is the principal risk factor for PCP. Recommendations for prophylaxis in the non-AIDS setting are based on the expected level of risk of PCP and consensus criteria rather than on randomized clinical trials. The traditional groups of cancer patients at risk have been acute lymphocytic leukemia and allogeneic HSCT. After allo-HSCT, prophylaxis is recommended

PRACTICE OF ONCOLOGY

until at least day 180 after transplant, and longer if immunosuppressive agents are continued.[59] PCP prophylaxis should be considered in patients with cancer who receive prolonged high-dose steroids (i.e., equivalent of prednisone 20 mg daily for ≥1 month). Other candidates for prophylaxis include alemtuzumab recipients (package insert recommends prophylaxis until at least 2 months after completion of alemtuzumab and CD4 count ≥200/mcL, whichever occurs later), patients with chronic lymphocytic leukemia receiving fludarabine, and patients with gliomas receiving temozolomide and radiation or corticosteroids.

The most effective agent is trimethoprim/sulfamethoxazole (TMP/SMX). A variety of dosages seem to be effective (from one double-strength tablet daily, to one double-strength tablet twice daily 2 days per week). When TMP/SMX cannot be administered because of marrow intolerance or hypersensitivity reaction, second-line agents include dapsone (50 mg twice daily or 100 mg orally daily), inhaled pentamidine (300 mg every 4 weeks), and atovaquone (1,500 mg daily) (see Table 132.2). All second-line agents are less effective than TMP/SMX, with the difference increasing with the degree of immune compromise.

Prophylaxis of Viral Infections

Prevention of Herpes Simplex Virus and Varicella Zoster Virus

Among seropositive patients, the incidence of herpes simplex virus (HSV) reactivation following induction chemotherapy for leukemia or conditioning for HSCT is 70% to 80%. HSV and VZV infections are common after alemtuzumab, bortezomib,[60] and lenolidomide.[61] Antiviral prophylaxis (acyclovir, valacyclovir, or famciclovir) against HSV is advised in patients receiving chemotherapy for acute leukemia, in all HSV-seropositive allogeneic HSCT recipients, and in some autologous HSCT recipients at high risk for mucositis during the neutropenic period. Prophylaxis is recommended until mucositis resolves and engraftment takes place.[34] It is also advised in myeloma patients treated with bortezomib or lemolidomide.[60,61] For alemtuzumab recipients, the package insert recommends at least 2 months after completion of therapy and CD4 count ≥200/mcL, whichever occurs later.

Nosocomial transmission of VZV is well documented. Patients with chickenpox, disseminated zoster, and immunocompromised patients with dermatomal zoster should be placed under contact and respiratory isolation. In the absence of varicella zoster immune globulin, oral acyclovir for 2 weeks after exposure has been used successfully for postexposure prophylaxis. The two available live attenuated varicella vaccines are Varivax (used to induce immunity in persons who have not been exposed to varicella; Merck, Inc., Whitehouse Station, NJ) and Zostavax (for older immunocompetent persons with prior exposure to varicella to augment immunity to prevent shingles; Merck, Inc.). Neither vaccine should be used in highly immunosuppressed persons because of the risk of viral disease. Household contacts of immunocompromised patients and health-care workers with no history of varicella and seronegative for VZV should receive the Varivax vaccine to prevent infection by wild-type varicella.[33] If a rash occurs following vaccination, direct contact with immunocompromised persons should be avoided.

Prevention of Cytomegalovirus Disease

CMV is a very important pathogen after allo-HSCT, but CMV disease is uncommon in other cancer patients. It has been reported mainly in patients receiving alemtuzumab (although asymptomatic reactivation without disease seems to be much more frequent) and occasionally in patients receiving therapy for acute leukemia. CMV infection happens early in life and results in viral latency. Most adults (60% to 80%) are infected, as proven by the detection of CMV-specific IgG in their serum. A transplant recipient is at risk for reactivation (if he or she is CMV seropositive) or for primary infection (from the allograft if the donor is CMV seropositive) or from blood products.[62]

Prevention of Cytomegalovirus Disease After Allogeneic Hematopoietic Stem Cell Transplantation

Prevention of Primary Cytomegalovirus Infection. To prevent CMV primary infection, CMV-seronegative HSCT recipients receiving allografts from CMV-seronegative donors should receive transfusion products from only CMV-negative donors or, if this is not feasible, leukocyte-depleted blood products.[63]

Prevention of Cytomegalovirus Disease Following Reactivation. In case of preexisting CMV infection, CMV disease may be prevented by one of two approaches: prophylaxis or preemptive management. In prophylaxis, antiviral agents are administered for a variable period to all allogeneic HSCT recipients in which either the donor or recipient is CMV seropositive. In preemptive management, active surveillance of the patients at risk is followed by initiation of antiviral agents following detection of CMV reactivation.

Prophylaxis for Cytomegalovirus. Ganciclovir prophylaxis for CMV-seropositive allogeneic transplant recipients was highly effective at suppressing CMV during the early transplant period, but was associated with higher rates of neutropenia, bacterial and opportunistic infections, and late CMV disease, without improvement in overall survival.[64,65]

Preemptive Therapy for Cytomegalovirus. CMV infection may be diagnosed early by detection of the CMV pp65 antigen in peripheral blood leukocytes or by measuring CMV DNA by polymerase chain reaction (PCR). A single positive CMV antigenemia or two consecutive positive PCR results are triggers for preemptive antiviral therapy. When compared in a randomized controlled trial, preemptive therapy and prophylaxis resulted in equivalent overall survival, but with different complications: universal prophylaxis had less early CMV disease but more invasive fungal infections, more ganciclovir use, and more late CMV disease. Preemptive therapy (using pp65 antigenemia) resulted in more CMV disease by day 100.[66] The preemptive approach is more commonly used. Foscarnet can also be used preemptively, with similar results but different toxicities (renal toxicity with foscarnet, myelosuppression with ganciclovir). Valganciclovir an orally administered prodrug of ganciclovir is another alternative, although it may result in increased exposure to ganciclovir and potentially more toxicity.[67] Similar CMV recommendations have been made for patients treated with alemtuzumab.[34]

Prevention of Viral Hepatitis

Three etiologic agents of viral hepatitis are a matter of significant concern in cancer patients. Hepatitis B and C have special importance because of their etiologic role in hepatobiliary cancer and the enormous populations affected by with these viruses.

Hepatitis B

Carriers of HBV, even if they are asymptomatic or have undetectable HBV DNA levels, are at risk for hepatitis B flare after immunosuppressive therapy or cytotoxic chemotherapy, particularly with rituximab and high-dose corticosteroids. All patients should be screened for hepatitis B status before receiving cytotoxic chemotherapy by determining hepatitis B surface antigen (HBsAg) and anti–hepatitis B core antibody. Seronegative patients should be vaccinated if possible. HBsAg-positive patients, regardless of their HBV DNA level, should treated with lamivudine or some other of the nucleoside/nucleotide analogues currently available during the duration of chemotherapy and for up to 12 months thereafter.[68] It is unclear what the duration and best method of monitoring are. Treatment of active hepatitis B during cytotoxic chemotherapy is daunting and should be attempted in consultation with an expert in the use or combinations of these newer agents.

Hepatitis C

Chronic hepatitis C infection has a broad worldwide distribution and thus would be expected to occur at baseline in a substantial portion of the cancer patient population. There is little evidence to support concerns for recrudescence of latent disease in patients who are screened and not viremic at baseline, whether by natural evolution or as the result of therapy. The inflammatory disease associated with chronic hepatitis C is variable and has been associated with clinically relevant worsening, predominantly in patients with therapy for hematologic malignancy, but occasionally in solid tumor patients.[69,70] As with hepatitis B, interferon-based therapy has prohibitive toxicities in this context, but the evolution of true antiviral agents may make consultation with an expert in the use of these drugs an important consideration.

Hepatitis E

Hepatitis E, a predominantly water-borne virus, has caused chronic infection in both solid and hematologic transplant patients. No specific antiviral therapies are available, but acquisition and recrudescence should be considered in patients receiving chemotherapy who develop new or worsening hepatic inflammation.[71–73]

DIAGNOSIS AND MANAGEMENT OF INFECTIOUS DISEASES SYNDROMES

FEVER AND NEUTROPENIA

Fever is single oral T $\geq 38.3°C$ or sustained T $\geq 38°C$ for 1 hour.[74] Slightly different definitions may have been used in different trials over the years. Neutropenia is defined as an absolute neutrophil count (ANC) of <500 cells/mm^3 or an ANC that is expected to decrease to <500 cells/mm^3 during the next 48 hours.[74] In neutropenic patients, fever should be considered evidence of infection and treated accordingly.

Bacterial infections may progress quickly in the absence of granulocytes and appropriate antibiotics must be started immediately. Empirical administration of broad-spectrum antibiotics to neutropenic febrile patients showed early on to result in improved outcomes[75] and remains the standard of care. Numerous professional organiztions have issued guidelines for the management of fever during neutropenia in adults and children, inpatient and outpatient.[34,43,74,76,77] The initial evaluation consists of a complete history and physical examination. Important elements of the history include prior infections or known colonization with resistant pathogens, as well as timing of the fever in relation to manipulation of the central venous catheter if one is present. Special attention should be given to the mouth, skin, catheter exit site, and perianal region during the physical exam.

Initial laboratory studies should include complete blood count and differential, serum chemistry including liver function tests, and at least two sets of blood cultures. Other cultures (urine, sputum, stool if diarrhea) should not delay the administration of antibiotics. An initial chest radiograph in the absence of symptoms or signs of pulmonary infection is of low yield in ambulatory adult patients with fever and neutropenia.

Risk Stratification

One of the key current concepts in the management of neutropenic fever involves risk stratification: not all patients who develop fever during chemotherapy-induced neutropenia have the same risk of a poor outcome, and this has practical implications for management

(choice of antibiotics, inpatient versus outpatient setting). Most adult guidelines endorse the use of the Multinational Association for Supportive Care in Cancer (MASCC) index.[78] The pediatric guidelines support the concept of risk stratification, but emphasize the importance of using strategies that have been validated locally.[77] The MASCC index was designed as a tool to identify adult patients at low risk of complications.[78] To obtain a MASCC score, points are allocated and added up. Points are given for burden of illness (no or mild symptoms 5, severe symptoms 3), absence of hypotension (5), absence of chronic obstructive pulmonary disease (4), solid tumor OR no previous fungal infection (4), absence of dehydration (3), outpatient status (3) and age <60 years (2). The points are added up, and patients with a score of ≥ 21 points (of 26 possible) are "low risk" and can be considered for oral therapy. The index has been validated in multiple settings and performs well, although it may do so better in solid tumors than in hematologic malignancies.[79] The IDSA guidelines include "expert" clinical criteria derived from clinical trials: patients with neutropenia expected to last ≥ 7 days, clinically unstable or with significant comorbidities, or high intensity chemotherapy are all "high risk" and should be hospitalized for intravenous antibiotics.[74] Similarly, the American Society of Clinical Oncology guidelines present a list of conditions that makes the outpatients high-risk independently of their MASCC score.[43]

For "low-risk" patients, it is still important to make sure they can tolerate oral agents and have adequate access to medical care before deciding to treat them as outpatients with oral antibiotics. The antibiotics used for adults have been ciprofloxacin + amoxicillin/clavulanic acid[80] and moxifloxacin monotherapy.[81] Quinolones should not be used for treatment if patients were receiving them for prophylaxis. In penicillin-allergic patients, the combination of ciprofloxacin + clindamycin is recommended.[43]

Neutropenic Fever Syndromes

The practical management of fever during neutropenia is easier if every episode is categorized as one of the following: first fever, persistent fever, recrudescent fever, and fever at the time of myeloid recovery.[82,83] Although overlap may exist, these four syndromes represent useful clinical categories that should be managed differently.

First Episode of Fever

Most episodes of fever during neutropenia are supposed to be infectious in origin. Infection, however, is not always documented. The percentages are roughly as follows: fever of unknown origin, 50% to 60%; microbiologically documented infection (frequently bacteremia), 10% to 20%; and clinically documented infection (e.g., typhlitis or cellulitis without any pathogen being isolated), 20% to 30%.[74] The majority of documented infections during neutropenia are caused by the patient's own endogenous bacterial flora. In the absence of localizing symptoms, physical examination findings, or positive cultures, several antibiotic regimens may be used. For high-risk patients, most of the guidelines recommend to start monotherapy with a beta-lactam with activity against *Pseudomonas aeruginosa* (piperacillin-tazobactam, imipenem, meropenem, cefepime, ceftazidime),[34,74,77] with the important caveat that some form of combination therapy should be chosen in patients who are clinically unstable and/or if there is suspicion (or high risk) of infection caused by resistant gram-negative (second gram-negative agent should be added) or gram-positive bacteria (vancomycin or linezolid should be added). The antipseudomonal beta-lactam of choice depends on local resistance patterns; meta-analyses suggest that, unless there is high prevalence of resistant bacteria that make its use unadvisable, piperacillin-tazobactam may offer the best combination of high efficacy and low toxicity.[84] The routine use of combination therapy (typically beta-lactam + aminoglycoside) was shown to be associated with higher toxicity and not superior outcome.[85,86]

The so-called de-escalation approach suggests starting with broader coverage (based on local susceptibility patterns this may consist, for instance, of carbapenem + colistin ± another agent) then de-escalate appropriately.[76] All the guidelines recommend not including vancomycin routinely in the initial regimen and not adding it empirically for persistent fever. The details regarding when to actually use vancomycin are more variable. The IDSA strongly recommends adding vancomycin in cases of hemodynamic instability, pneumonia, clinically evident catheter–related infection, severe mucositis, and known colonization with methicillin-resistant S. aureus (MRSA), although the quality of the evidence is low.[74] Our own approach is presented in Figure 132.1 and Table 132.3. Regarding the use of alternative agents for gram-positive bacteria, linezolid and vancomycin had similar efficacy in a randomized trial where there were no cases of vancomycin-resistant enterococci (VRE), but linezolid resulted in delayed neutrophil and platelet recovery.[87] Regardless of the initial regimen actually chosen, modifications may be required between 30% and 50% of the time, depending on clinical evolution and/or microbiologic results (see Table 132.3). If fever resolves following initiation of empirical therapy, the assumption is that an infection is responding to antibiotics. The standard recommendation is to continue antibiotics until resolution of neutropenia. If the neutropenia persists, older studies showed that 2 weeks may be adequate duration of treatment.[88] More recent data, mainly in children, suggest shorter duration of antibiotic treatment may be associated with similar outcomes as long as the antibiotics are restarted promptly if fever recurs, but it is important to pay attention to the patient population included in these trials.[76]

Persistent Fever

The average time to defervescence in neutropenic fever is 4 days. Modifications of the antimicrobial regimen are not recommended during this period in the absence of new clinical or microbiologic findings. However, the persistence of fever beyond 4 days (96 hours) on broad-spectrum antibiotics identifies a population of patients with higher likelihood of IFI. The majority of persistently febrile neutropenic patients do not harbor an identifiable fungal infection, but several autopsy series in the 1970s documented occult fungal infection as a common cause of death in persistently febrile neutropenic patients.[89] Delay in initiating antifungal therapy was associated with treatment failure and death,[90] and empirical use of amphotericin B seemed to help.[91] Two randomized trials established the benefit of adding amphotericin B (one after 7, the other after 4 days of persistent fever) compared with continuing the antibacterial regimen in terms of preventing fungal infection, although they were not powered to demonstrate a survival advantage.[92,93] Of note, these studies were performed before there was systemic antifungal prophylaxis and identified Candida spp. as the principal fungal pathogen in this situation. Initiation of amphotericin B after 4 to 7 days of fever became standard of care, and most randomized controlled trials have focused on the choice of antifungal agent (liposomal amphotericin B,[94] voriconazole,[95] caspofungin[96,97]). To reduce the perceived unnecessary use of empirical antifungal therapy with its attendant toxicity and cost, an alternative approach to empirical antifungal therapy has been proposed and called "preemptive antifungal therapy."[45] The goal is to use the currently available diagnostic modalities (computed tomography [CT], serum galactomannan, and/or β-D-glucan) to postpone starting antifungal therapy until IFI is more likely. By design, this approach means that patients receiving "preemptive" antifungals are more likely to actually have an IFI than patients receiving "empirical" therapy by the time the antifungal agent is started.[98] The results of this approach are encouraging,[99–101] and it has been endorsed by the IDSA.[74] The details vary according to risk category of the patient, specific antifungal prophylaxis given, and diagnostic modalities available. The basic concept is that a persistently febrile neutropenic patient with no clinical findings, normal CT scans of chest and sinuses (where most mold infections

would start), and repeatedly negative fungal serologic markers (β-D-glucan and galactomannan) is unlikely to have an IFI, and antifungal coverage may be safely delayed. When these diagnostic options are not available, we support the addition of empirical antifungal therapy, typically caspofungin or liposomal amphotericin B, after 5 days of fever.[95]

Recrudescent Fever

Recurrent fever refers to a new episode of fever that takes place after the initial episode has resolved with antimicrobial therapy when the patient remains neutropenic.[82] This is a common occurrence in clinical practice in cases of prolonged neutropenia, and it has not been adequately studied. The one systematic investigation of this syndrome analyzed data on 836 neutropenic patients who had had a first fever that responded to antimicrobials and then had remained afebrile for 4 days.[102] The important result of this analysis is that fungal infections were just as common as breakthrough bacterial infections, suggesting the appropriate management of this situation is to modify both the antibacterial and the antifungal part of the regimen, as well as perform a thorough diagnostic workup. Unfortunately, this scenario is not addressed separately from persistent fever in the guidelines.

Fever After Resolution of Neutropenia

In most cases, an undiagnosed fever that has persisted during neutropenia will resolve around the time of myeloid recovery. In a minority of patients, fever appears or worsens at this time. The three likely causes of this situation are superinfection, immune reconstitution syndrome,[103] and engraftment syndrome.[104] Other noninfectious causes should also be considered (e.g., drug fever, transfusion reactions, and deep venous thrombosis). A systematic, thorough diagnostic workup is more appropriate than empirical therapeutic modifications. Blood and urine cultures, complete blood cell count, serum chemistry, and liver enzyme levels should be obtained. An elevated alkaline phosphatase should prompt consideration of hepatosplenic candidiasis (which is uncommon in patients receiving yeast-active antifungal prophylaxis). A chest X-ray should be obtained. Pulmonary infiltrates identified after neutrophil recovery have a favorable prognosis and may be managed conservatively.[105] In contrast to the neutropenic period, empirical antibiotics can be discontinued after resolution of neutropenia in patients who are stable with fever without apparent source.

Fungal Infections in Patients with Cancer

Pathogenic fungi include yeasts and molds. Candida spp. are yeasts that form part of the normal flora; they gain access to the bloodstream through disruption of anatomic barriers (mucositis or indwelling catheters). Molds are ubiquitous soil inhabitants whose conidia or spores are inhaled on a regular basis. Aspergillosis is the most common mold infection in cancer patients, but other pathogenic fungi (Mucor, Rhizopus, Fusarium, and Scedosporium spp.) have become more common over the past 20 years. In-depth practice guidelines for the management of the different fungal diseases have been issued by the IDSA.[106,107]

Candidiasis

Oropharyngeal and Esophageal Candidiasis. Cytotoxic chemotherapy, corticosteroids, and antibiotics predispose to oral candidiasis. The most common presentation is white adherent plaques on the palate, buccal mucosa, tongue, or gingiva. A wet mount or Gram stain showing pseudohyphae establishes the diagnosis. Therapy includes local treatments such as clotrimazole troches or oral fluconazole. Esophageal candidiasis causes odynophagia. The differential diagnosis includes HSV, CMV (principally in HSCT recipients), and bacteria. Initial therapy should

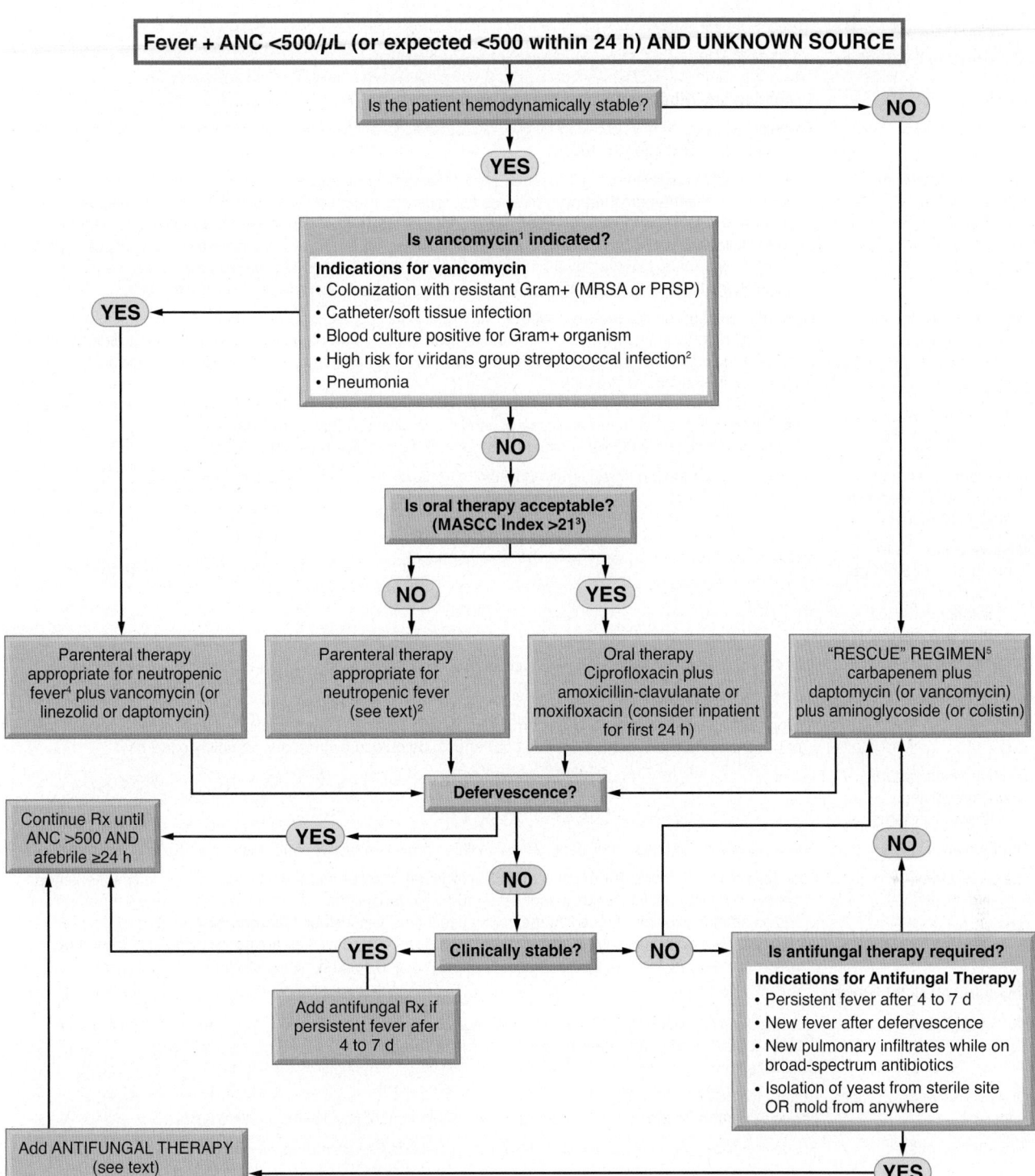

PRACTICE OF ONCOLOGY

Figure 132.1 A general approach to patients with fever and neutropenia without a clinically or microbiologically documented infection. See text for more detailed descriptions. *(1)* Linezolid was comparable to vancomycin in this setting in a single randomized controlled trial. It may be considered instead of vancomycin for patients who are known carriers of vancomycin-resistant enterococcus, but experience is limited, and there are concerns about linezolid use (see text). *(2)* Some experts add vancomycin in patients with neutropenic fever at high risk for viridans streptococci (e.g., prior quinolone prophylaxis, severe mucositis associated with cytarabine-containing regimens); this must be weighed against the significant downside of selection for vancomycin-resistant pathogens. *(3)* Multinational Association for Supportive Care in Cancer (MASCC) index: burden of illness: no or mild symptoms, +5; moderate symptoms, +3; no hypotension, +5; no chronic obstructive pulmonary disease, +4; solid tumor or no previous fungal infection, +4; no dehydration, +3; outpatient status, +3; age <60 years, +2. A MASCC index of ≥21 has been associated with a relatively low frequency of severe complications. *(4)* See text for a detailed discussion. In a stable patient with undifferentiated neutropenic fever who does not require vancomycin, appropriate parenteral monotherapy consists of ceftazidime, cefepime, imipenem, meropenem, or piperacillin/tazobactam. For specific information on each of these agents, see text. *(5)* This "rescue" antibacterial regimen will vary between institutions depending on the local patterns of antibiotic resistance. Carbapenem (imipenem or meropenem) plus vancomycin plus an aminoglycoside is a reasonable initial regimen that should be tailored once culture results are known. A fluoroquinolone may be used instead of an aminoglycoside in patients with significant renal impairment in institutions where fluoroquinolones retain significant activity against the local gram-negative pathogens. In settings in which carbapenem-resistant *Acinetobacter* or carbapenemase-producing *Klebsiella* are prevalent, colistin or polymyxin B should be considered. ANC, absolute neutrophil count; MRSA, methicillin-resistant *Staphylococcus aureus*; PRSP, penicillin-resistant *Streptococcus pneumoniae*.

Diagnostic Evaluation and Modifications of Therapy During Neutropenia

Findings	Evaluation and Modifications
Initial neutropenic fever	Take history, perform physical examination, and order appropriate cultures; initiate empirical antibiotic therapy promptly (see text and Fig. 132.1).
Persistent neutropenic fever (4–7 d)	Look for invasive fungal infection (chest CT recommended, serologic tests depending on the clinical setting). Add empirical antifungal therapy in patients not receiving mold-active prophylaxis. Options include amphotericin B deoxycholate (0.7 mg/kg/d), LAMB (3 mg/kg/d); voriconazole (IV 6 mg/kg q 12 h for two doses, followed by 3 mg/kg q 12 h; switch to oral 200 mg q 12 h may be considered); and caspofungin 70 mg × one dose, followed by 50 mg daily. Caspofungin is in general preferred over amphotericin B formulations based on similar efficacy and reduced toxicity compared with LAMB (see text).
Recurrent neutropenic fever without a source after initial response to empirical antibiotics	Signs of breakthrough sepsis (e.g., hypotension, rigors, tachypnea, decline in urine output) should prompt empirical modification of antibacterial regimen (see text), repeat blood cultures, and a chest radiograph. Consider modification of the antimicrobial regimen to include breakthrough bacterial and fungal infections while awaiting diagnostic results. Consider chest CT scan to evaluate for signs of mold infection. If a nodule or infiltrate is present, consider bronchoscopy or percutaneous biopsy depending on location. Galactomannan and β-d-glucan antigenemia assays should be considered in patients at high risk for invasive mold infections.
Persistent or recurrent fever without a source after ANC recovery	Infections are diagnosed infrequently. Consider chronic disseminated candidiasis (see text).
Positive culture from blood obtained before starting empirical antibiotics for neutropenic fever	
Gram-positive	Add vancomycin (or linezolid or daptomycin if VRE is prevalent or the patient is known to be colonized).
Gram-negative	If patient is stable, continue initial regimen.
	If patient is unstable, switch to imipenem, meropenem, or piperacillin-tazobactam and add an aminoglycoside or ciprofloxacin. The selection of antibiotics should be guided by local susceptibility patterns.
Positive blood culture while receiving antibacterial therapy	
Gram-positive	Add vancomycin (or linezolid or daptomycin if VRE is prevalent or the patient is known to be colonized).
Gram-negative	Suspect a pathogen resistant to initial empirical regimen. If ceftazidime was used initially, suspect extended-spectrum β-lactamase or cephalosporinase-producing organisms; switch to imipenem or meropenem and add an aminoglycoside. If a carbapenem was used initially, consider *Stenotrophomonas maltophilia* or resistant *Pseudomonas* spp.; switch to piperacillin-tazobactam plus an aminoglycoside plus trimethoprim-sulfamethoxazole. Modify regimen once identification and sensitivity are known.
Head and Neck Infection	
Necrotizing gingivitis	If ceftazidime or cefepime was used in initial regimen, change to imipenem, meropenem, or piperacillin-tazobactam, or add metronidazole for anaerobic coverage. Culture for HSV.
Oral ulcerative or vesicular lesions	Culture for HSV. For documented or suspected mucocutaneous HSV infection, acyclovir 5 mg/kg q 8 h.
Sinus tenderness	Suspect aerobic gram-negative rod (Enterobacteriaceae or *Pseudomonas aeruginosa*). Examine palate and nasal mucosa for signs of invasive infection. Perform sinus CT scan to evaluate extent of disease and to guide diagnostic and therapeutic drainage. With prolonged neutropenia or concomitant high-dose corticosteroids, invasive mold infections become more likely and initiation of empirical lipid formulation of amphotericin B (5 mg/kg/d) may be considered to cover both aspergillosis and zygomycosis.
Respiratory Tract	
Upper respiratory tract symptoms	Send nasopharyngeal washing for community respiratory viruses.
New infiltrate after resolution of neutropenia	May be inflammatory response to old infection. Conservative management results in good outcome: If the patient is asymptomatic, observe; if symptomatic and not responding to antibacterial agents, consider BAL.[a]

(continued)

TABLE 132.3

Diagnostic Evaluation and Modifications of Therapy During Neutropenia *(continued)*

Findings	Evaluation and Modifications
Respiratory Tract	
New infiltrate while neutropenic	Suspect resistant bacteria or mold infection.
	Perform chest CT scan to evaluate extent of disease and to detect other lesions. Perform sputum cultures and GM and BG antigenemia assay; if GM and BG assays are unavailable or nondiagnostic, bronchoscopy with BAL or percutaneous biopsy is warranted based on location of lesion.
	If pneumonia developed in hospital, broaden antibiotic regimen to cover nosocomial pathogens. Consider MRSA, resistant gram-negative pathogens, and nosocomial legionellosis. Consider empirical addition of voriconazole (IV 6 mg/kg q 12 h for two doses followed by 4 mg/kg q 12 h).
	Diffuse infiltrates raise concern for community respiratory viruses (particularly during winter), *Pneumocystis jirovecii* (in setting of concomitant corticosteroid therapy), bacterial pneumonia, CMV (in acute leukemia, may infrequently be associated with neutropenia), and noninfectious causes (e.g., hemorrhage, aspiration, drug toxicity, respiratory distress syndrome, congestive heart failure). BAL recommended.
Gastrointestinal Tract	
Retrosternal burning, odynophagia	Consider esophagitis. Suspect *Candida* or HSV esophagitis. Bacterial esophagitis and CMV (primarily in allogeneic HSCT recipients) also possible. Add fluconazole (400 mg oral or IV) and acyclovir (5 mg/kg q 8 h IV) empirically. If no response in 3 d, consider endoscopy.
Acute abdominal pain	Differential diagnosis includes same causes as in nonneutropenic patient (e.g., cholecystitis, appendicitis) plus typhlitis (neutropenic colitis).
	Ensure that antibiotic regimen has adequate anaerobic activity (e.g., imipenem, meropenem, or piperacillin-tazobactam). Provide bowel rest.
	Abdominal and pelvic CT scan. Monitor for need for surgical intervention (see text).
Perianal cellulitis	Consider pelvic CT scan to evaluate extent of disease. Monitor need for surgical drainage. Broaden antibiotic regimen to include anaerobic activity. Provide local care.
Central Venous Catheter (Surgically Implanted)	
Exit-site cellulitis	Add vancomycin.
Tunnel infection	Add vancomycin; remove catheter.
Collection around catheter	Incise and drain; if infected, add appropriate antibiotics and remove catheter.
Infection by molds and mycobacteria	May require excision of tunnel tract.
Catheter-associated bacteremia	Add appropriate antibiotics.
	Remove catheter for infection by *Staphylococcus aureus*, *Candida* spp., and mycobacteria (see text) and for antibiotic-resistant pathogens.

CT, computed tomography; LAMB, liposomal amphotericin B; IV, intravenous; ANC, absolute neutrophil count; VRE, vancomycin-resistant enterococcus; HSV, herpes simplex virus; BAL, bronchoalveolar lavage; GM, serum galactomannan; BG, β-glucan; MRSA, methicillin-resistant *Staphylococcus aureus*; CMV, cytomegalovirus; HSCT, hematopoietic stem cell transplant.

[a] The differential diagnosis of pneumonia in immunocompromised patients is broad, and the authors advise early BAL or percutaneous biopsy (depending on location of the lesion). Studies must be tailored to the individual patient. In highly immunocompromised patients, perform Gram staining; culture for bacteria, mycobacteria, fungi, *Nocardia* spp., *Legionella* spp., herpes viruses, CMV, and community respiratory viruses (particularly during winter); and cytologic analysis for *P. jirovecii*.

be with fluconazole. Options for fluconazole-resistant mucosal candidiasis include an echinocandin, voriconazole, posaconazole, or amphotericin B formulation.

Candidemia. Candida species are the fourth most common cause of nosocomial bloodstream infections in the United States. Clinical findings vary from asymptomatic to full-blown septic shock. The species should be identified. *Candida albicans* is the most common, and it is usually susceptible to fluconazole, but the proportion of nonalbicans *Candida* has been increasing. *Candida tropicalis* is highly virulent in neutropenic hosts but is susceptible to most agents. *Candida krusei* is always resistant to fluconazole, and *Candida glabrata* has variable susceptibility. *Candida parapsilosis* is mostly associated with vascular catheters and is usually susceptible to fluconazole but relatively resistant to echinocandins. A minority of *Candida lusitaniae* and *Candida guilliermondii* isolates are resistant to amphotericin B.

It is recommended to remove all intravascular catheters in patients with candidemia.[106] In neutropenic patients, candidemia

may arise from defects in the gut mucosa rather than the catheter, so the need for catheter removal has been questioned.[108] In general, we remove the catheter where feasible, but sometimes attempt to conserve it when vascular access is limited and thrombocytopenia is present. We immediately remove all intravenous catheters in the setting of clinical instability, lack of resolution of fever within 2 to 3 days, or persistent candidemia after 2 days of appropriate antifungal therapy.

Chronic Disseminated Candidiasis. Chronic disseminated candidiasis (also called hepatosplenic candidiasis) is a complication of intensive chemotherapy regimens, such as those used as induction therapy for acute leukemia. The typical picture is persistent fever after neutrophil recovery with elevation of liver enzymes (particularly alkaline phosphatase). Numerous target lesions in the liver and spleen become apparent by CT scan, ultrasonography, or magnetic resonance imaging (MRI). A liver biopsy is required for a definitive diagnosis. Blood and biopsy cultures are almost always negative, but the pathology is diagnostic. We recommend surgical liver biopsy when the diagnosis is in question. Chronic disseminated candidiasis that is controlled with antifungal therapy is not a contraindication to subsequent chemotherapy or HSCT.[109]

Therapy for Invasive Candidiasis. An echinocandin (caspofungin, micafungin, or anidulafungin) or a lipid formulation of amphotericin B is recommended for candidemia in neutropenic patients.[106,109] In patients receiving an azole who develop breakthrough candidemia, an echinocandin is advised. Azoles (generally, fluconazole) can be used as step-down oral agents or as initial therapy in certain patients at lower risk for mortality and serious complications. Voriconazole does not have a demonstrated advantage over fluconazole, but can be considered for treatment of *C. krusei* (which is intrinsically fluconazole-resistant) and when a mold-active agent is otherwise warranted (e.g., as prophylaxis in a high-risk patient). We reserve amphotericin B products for unusual complicated cases, such as meningitis and endocarditis, in which data to support optimal therapy are lacking. Some authorities still prefer a lipid formulation of amphotericin B in neutropenic patients, particularly in the presence of hemodynamic instability.

Invasive Aspergillosis

Risk Factors and Clinical Manifestations. Prolonged and persistent neutropenia is a critical risk factor for IA.[5] Most cases, however, take place during episodes of active GVHD treated with high doses of corticosteroids. Other risk factors for aspergillosis after allogeneic HSCT include T-cell–depleted transplant, lymphopenia, CMV disease, and respiratory virus infections.[110,111] Aspergillosis can involve virtually any organ in the immunocompromised host, but sinopulmonary disease is the most common. Angioinvasion of hyphae leading to vascular thrombosis and tissue infarction and coagulative necrosis is characteristic. Clinical manifestations are quite variable. During neutropenia, persistent fever, chest pain, and a pleural rub are common, although nonspecific, signs. When steroids are the only risk factor, the manifestations may be subtle, and sometimes a pulmonary infiltrate is found in the absence of symptoms.

Diagnosis of Invasive Aspergillosis. The most common finding on chest CT in early invasive pulmonary aspergillosis in patients with neutropenia and HSCT recipients is the presence of one or more well-circumscribed nodules. These may be inapparent on chest radiographs (Fig. 132.2). Other characteristic findings include the "halo sign," a haziness surrounding a nodule or infiltrate representing alveolar hemorrhage, and the "crescent sign" (cavitation that usually coincides with neutrophil recovery). These signs reflect different stages of hemorrhagic infarction secondary to angioinvasive organisms. Sequential CT scans of neutropenic patients with IA demonstrated that halo signs were common at diagnosis but decreased during the first week of infection as the frequency of the "air crescent sign" increased. The median volume of lesions increased during the first week of therapy and remained stable during the second week.[112] Bronchoalveolar lavage (BAL) cultures have approximately 50% sensitivity in focal pulmonary lesions, and definitive diagnosis often requires an invasive procedure and is usually made only when the disease is advanced. The use of galactomannan antigen seems to be much more sensitive.[113,114] Isolation of an *Aspergillus* sp. from sputum or BAL should be presumed to represent invasive disease in neutropenic patients.

Both the serum *Aspergillus* galactomannan[115] and β-D-glucan[116] assays, immunoassays that detect fungal antigens in peripheral blood, have been accepted as diagnostic adjuncts of invasive fungal infections in the revised European Organisation for Research and Treatment of Cancer/Mycosis Study Group consensus criteria.[117] PCR-based detection is considered investigational.[118] These immunoassays have three potential uses: (1) as a diagnostic adjunct, (2) as a surveillance tool in high-risk patients (e.g., allogeneic HSCT recipients) to detect early aspergillosis prior to clinically overt disease, and

(3) in monitoring response to antifungal therapy.[119] The sensitivity of the galactomannan assay is significantly reduced by concomitant mold-active antifungal agents, and false-positive results may be more common in allogeneic HSCT recipients or with concomitant piperacillin/tazobactam and other antibiotics.[120] Meta-analysis suggest that the galactomannan assay has a sensitivity of 60% to 80% and specificity of 80% to 90% for proven IA, but emphasize the results are fairly heterogeneous.[115,119] A rising serum galactomannan correlates with failure of antifungal therapy, and decreasing galactomannan correlates with a positive outcome in patients with IA.[121]

The serum β-D-glucan assay has recently received FDA approval as a diagnostic adjunct. In patients with acute myeloid leukemia and myelodysplastic syndrome, the assay was highly sensitive and specific in detecting early invasive fungal infections, including candidiasis, fusariosis, trichosporonosis, and aspergillosis.[116] It does not detect mucormycosis.

Therapy for Invasive Aspergillosis. Voriconazole is currently the treatment of choice of IA,[107] because in a randomized controlled trials it was more effective than amphotericin B (successful outcomes: 53% versus 32%) and was associated with significantly improved survival (71% versus 58%).[122] Voriconazole appears to have comparable safety and efficacy in children with invasive mold infections compared to adults, although the doses in children must be higher.[123] Three different lipid formulations of amphotericin B are available: amphotericin B colloidal dispersion, amphotericin B lipid complex, and liposomal amphotericin B. The lipid formulations have less nephrotoxicity than conventional amphotericin B deoxycholate, and are therefore more suitable for long-term administration. A randomized controlled trial has shown that liposomal amphotericin B at a dose of 3 mg/kg per day is at least as effective, and less toxic, than 10 mg/kg per day for IA.[124]

Posaconazole is a broad-spectrum azole, so far only available in oral form, which has been used successfully as salvage therapy for a variety of IFIs refractory to standard therapy. Of note, 5 to 7 days are required before therapeutic serum levels are reached.[125] The overall success rate of posaconazole in patients with IA refractory or intolerant of standard therapy was 42%.[126] Monitoring levels of both posaconazole and voriconazole may be reasonable, particularly when there are questions about absorption or when the response to treatment is inadequate.[127] Echinocandins have not been evaluated as initial monotherapy for IA in controlled trials. Caspofungin as salvage therapy in patients with IA led to a favorable response in 37 of 83 patients (45%).[128]

There has been significant interest in combination antifungal therapy pairing an echinocandin with either an amphotericin B preparation or a mold-active azole. The rationale is that echinocandins target a site (the β-glucan constituent of the fungal cell wall) distinct from the polyenes and azoles that target the fungal cell membrane. In vitro and animal models data have been encouraging, and uncontrolled clinical studies suggest minimal toxicity and potentially improved outcome of aspergillosis. The question of combination is far from settled, but many experts recommend its use, at least early in the course of treatment.[109]

Patients who recover from an episode of IA are at risk for relapse of infection during subsequent immunosuppression. Secondary prophylaxis with a mold-active agent is advised for the entire period of immunosuppression.

Mucormycosis (Formerly Zygomycosis)

Risk factors for mucormycosis include diabetic ketoacidosis, proteincalorie malnutrition, iron overload, desferrioxamine (but not other iron chelators), corticosteroid therapy, and prolonged neutropenia.[129] Mucormycosis typically manifests as rhinocerebral or pulmonary disease following inhalation of spores. In rhinocerebral disease, fever, facial pain, and headache are common. Contiguous extension may lead to orbital involvement with proptosis and extraocular muscle paresis, involvement of hard palate, and spread to the brain. The use

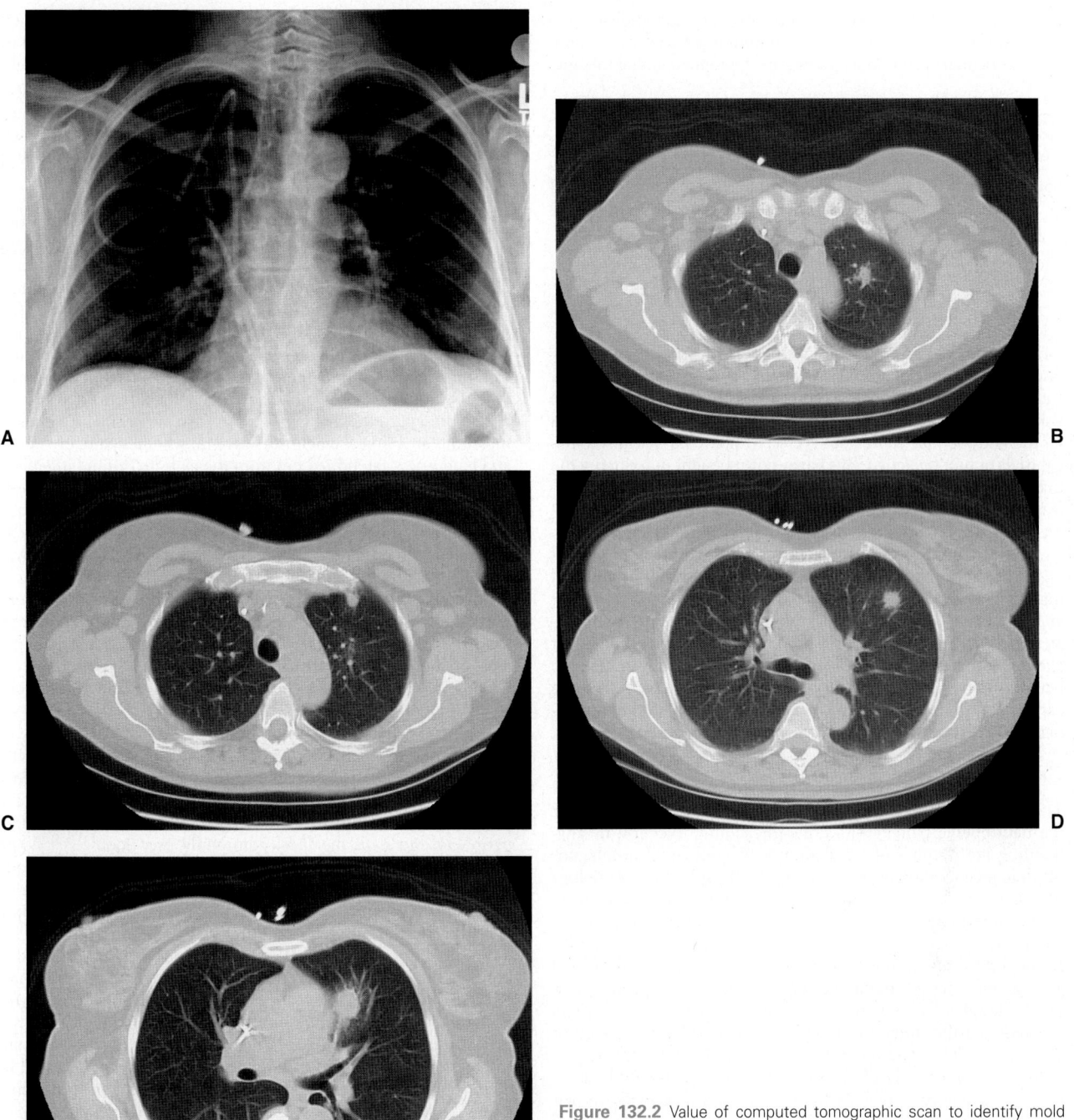

Figure 132.2 Value of computed tomographic scan to identify mold infections during neutropenia. A patient with chronic lymphocytic leukemia who had been neutropenic for 35 days developed a new fever while receiving prophylaxis with fluconazole and ceftazidime for neutropenic fever. The chest radiograph did not show the four nodules evident by computed tomography. Notice the "halo sign" in the largest nodule.

of voriconazole prophylaxis may contribute to increased incidence of mucormycosis.[130] Therapy for zygomycosis involves amphotericin B lipid formulation (5 mg/kg per day) plus early and aggressive surgical debridement in cases of localized cutaneous or sinus disease. Voriconazole and echinocandins are not active against zygomycetes. Posaconazole has shown promising results as salvage therapy.[131]

Less Common Molds

Fusarium, Paecilomyces, Scedosporium, and several dematiaceous molds are increasingly important causes of mortality in leukemia

and in allogeneic HSCT recipients.[132] It is recommended to obtain infectious diseases expertise for the management of these infections. The likelihood of infection by a *Fusarium* spp. is increased by the presence of disseminated cutaneous lesions and isolation of a mold from blood culture. Different species of *Fusarium* have different susceptibilities, and it has been proposed to start empirical voriconazole and amphotericin B until the results of testing are available.[109] *Scedosporium apiospermum* and *Scedosporium* are usually treated with voriconazole. Dematiaceous (dark-walled) molds like *Alternaria, Curvularia,* and *Phaeoacremonium* can cause subcutaneous infection in immunocompetent persons following traumatic inoculation;

pneumonia, central nervous system (CNS) disease, and dissemination can occur in severely immunocompromised persons. Itraconazole, voriconazole, or posaconazole are appropriate initial therapy.

Immune Augmentation

The optimal treatment of fungal infections requires attempting to optimize the host's ability to fight infection. Corticosteroids should be tapered or discontinued if possible, therapeutic levels of the antifungal agents achieved anatomic obstacles, if present, removed. The use of colony-stimulating factors (CSF) and granulacyte transfusions is frequently a consideration.

Colony-Stimulating Factors

Granulocyte-colony stimulating factor (G-CSF) has shown to reduce the incidence of febrile neutropenia and is recommended by European[133] and American[134] professional organizations when the risk of neutropenic fever is ≥20% or if the patient has experienced febrile neutropenia in previous cycles. Multiple randomized clinical trials of prophylactic CSFs have shown benefit in reducing the time to neutrophil recovery and duration of fever and hospitalization. Meta-analyses confirm its efficacy in HSCT[135] and breast cancer,[136] although reductions in mortality has not been shown.

The use of CSFs as treatment of established infection continues to be experimental. The rationale to use CSFs for established infections (as opposed to prophylaxis) stems from the quantitative and qualitative effects of these agents on phagocytic cells. Randomized trials have not shown a benefit of CSFs as adjunct therapy for patients with newly diagnosed fever and neutropenia. Although the benefit of any CSF for established infections is unproven, some experts may consider them in selected cases of profound neutropenia (ANC <100/mcL) and/or with serious documented infections.

Granulocyte Transfusions

The rationale for granulocyte transfusions is to provide support for the neutropenic patient with a life-threatening infection by augmenting the number of circulating neutrophils until autologous myeloid regeneration occurs.[137] In the 1970s, apheresis technology for harvesting large numbers of donor granulocytes became available. Controlled trials of granulocyte transfusions as adjuvant therapy in neutropenic patients at the time produced mixed results. In the 1980s, the enthusiasm for granulocyte transfusions waned as more effective antibiotics became available, survival from serious bacterial infections improved, and recombinant growth factors reduced the duration of neutropenia. In addition, concerns about the toxicity of granulocyte transfusions, including acute pulmonary reactions,[138] HLA alloimmunization (which could render patients refractory to platelet transfusions and potentially impair myeloid engraftment following HSCT), and transfusion-associated infections (particularly CMV), outweighed the perceived benefits.

Today, the impetus to reexamine the role of granulocyte transfusions stems largely from improvements in donor mobilization methods (G-CSF). Currently, the mean absolute neutrophil yield per collection is in the range of 8×10^{10} cells, resulting in higher posttransfusion neutrophil counts that are sustained for 24 to 30 hours following transfusion. The qualitative functions of G-CSF– and steroid-mobilized neutrophils are intact based on in vitro testing. Published single-center experience suggests this procedure may have tolerable safety and can sometimes be helpful,[139,140] but whether it provides overall benefit remains controversial.[141]

Catheter-Related Infections and Bacteremia

Bacteremia is a common complication of antineoplastic cytotoxic chemotherapy. Common sources are the intravenous catheter and the digestive tract. To maximize the detection of bacteremia, it is important to obtain adequate volume of blood.[142] The recommendation of the American Society of Microbiology is between 10 ml and 30 ml of blood per culture.[143] When possible, we recommend sampling all the lumens of multilumen catheters.[144] The importance of peripheral blood cultures obtained by venipuncture (as opposed to blood drawn from preexisting central lines) is related to the ability to determine the source of bacteremia by using a quantitative or semiquantitative method, rather than to sensitivity.[145]

Guidelines from professional societies provide extensive reviews of the available evidence for the prevention and management of intravascular catheter-related infection.[146–148] Organized systems (bundles) that place and manage vascular access should be a part of all cancer center programs.[149] Programs have demonstrated benefit in ambulatory populations, and we believe that this justifies the extension to the inpatient setting.[150]

Several types of catheter-related infections have been defined: exit site infection, tunnel infection (or pocket infection in the case of ports), and catheter-related bacteremia. Bacteremia may or may not be present in the first two types.[151] Exit and tunnel (or pocket) infections are clinical diagnoses based on whether pain, erythema, and tenderness extend >2 cm from the exit site (tunnel infection) or not (exit site infection). Infected short-term catheters should be removed. Tunneled and implanted devices require more thorough investigation. Although some times exit site infections can be treated with systemic antibiotics and local care, signs and symptoms of infection that may reflect associated vascular thrombosis or involvement of a tunneled catheter track >2 cm central to the exit site suggest the need for immediate removal.[152] Purulence from the exit site may be present, although in neutropenic patients, local erythema and tenderness may be the only signs of infection, making it difficult to distinguish from sterile inflammation associated with mild trauma.

Catheter-related bacteremia or fungemia may occur with or without signs of localized infection. Determining whether an episode of bacteremia is associated to the catheter may be difficult, and it has important implications for management. Differential time to positivity (catheter culture positive at 2 hours earlier than peripheral blood) is the most commonly used tool.[153–156] When used as a gold standard, it provides further justification for a modification of existing diagnostic standards for central line–associated blood stream infection.[157] Frequently, however, there is no peripheral blood culture to determine differential time to positivity. In these situations, "host criteria" and "organism criteria" are used to estimate the likely source of bacteremia. Some gram-positive bacteria, such as coagulase-negative *Staphylococcus* spp. and *Corynebacterium* spp. are common blood culture contaminants, but they may also represent true bacteremia in the presence of intravenous catheters. The likelihood of true bloodstream infection caused by these organisms is increased when they are isolated from more than one blood culture. On the other hand, isolation of *S. aureus* from a single blood culture should be considered evidence of true bacteremia and treated accordingly.

Neutropenia, gastrointestinal GVHD, and severe mucositis with diarrhea secondary to the treatment of solid tumors[158] are "host criteria" that affect the assessment of infection source. These factors are associated with different microbiology than that of bacteremias that originate in intravascular catheters.[159,160]

Mucosal-barrier injury–associated bacteremias are the proposed events that are related to specific populations and "organism criteria." Organisms include *Candida* spp., *Enterococcus* spp., Enterobacteracieae, viridans streptococci, and certain anaerobes (*Bacteroides* spp., *Clostridium*, *Fusobacterium*, *Prevotella*, *Peptostreptococcus*, *Veillonella*). This concept applies to patients with grade 3-4 gut GVHD, severe diarrhea, or neutropenia. Although these diagnostic criteria have been developed primarily as reporting tools for attribution of hospital-related events to preventable causes,[161,162] they support the need for a conceptual change.[157,163]

The standard approach for central line–associated blood stream infection is removal of the catheter and treatment of the patient with systemic antibiotics.[151] For permanent catheters in hemodynamically stable patients, catheter salvage may be considered.[164] Microbiologic factors are important in deciding whether a catheter can be saved. Coagulase-negative staphylococci are successfully treated in >93% of cases, although recurrence of infection is markedly increased with catheter retention.[165] Attempts to salvage catheters infected with *S. aureus* usually fail and frequently result in complications.[166] Similarly, catheters infected with *Candida* or mycobacteria should be removed.[151,166] Antibiotic lock techniques are sometimes effective, almost always with concomitant systemic therapy, but failure may occur because the catheter to be salvaged needs to be used, thus limiting the dwell time of antibiotic lock solutions.[167–169] The catheter should be removed if the blood cultures remain positive 3 days after starting appropriate therapy or in case of recurrent bacteremia.

Skin Lesions and Soft Tissue Infections

Consider infectious and noninfectious causes for these lesions. Some noninfectious causes include drug reactions (including chemotherapy-induced hand-foot syndrome), Sweet syndrome, erythema multiforme, vasculitis, leukemia cutis, and (in the case of allogeneic transplant) GVHD.[170] Early biopsy of skin lesions for histology and culture is recommended.[171]

Infections of the skin can either be localized or manifestations of systemic infection. Ecthyma gangrenosum is the most characteristic skin lesion associated with systemic *P. aeruginosa* infection, but can also be caused by *S. aureus*, enteric gram-negative bacilli infection, and molds including *Aspergillus*, zygomycetes, and *Fusarium*. Ecthyma gangrenosum begins as a raised erythematous papule or nodule that progresses to a bluish-black necrotic lesion within 12 to 24 hours. A central area of necrosis surrounded by erythema is typical. Pathologically, ecthyma gangrenosum is a necrotizing process in which masses of bacteria are often observed within the vessel wall and infiltrating white cells are absent.

A needle aspirate of the lesion showing gram-negative bacilli establishes the diagnosis of invasive infection, but a negative aspirate does not rule it out. Parenteral antibiotics with activity against *P. aeruginosa*, MRSA, and anaerobes (e.g., carbapenem + vancomycin ± a second agent against gram-negative bacteria) should be instituted emergently, pending culture results. The presence of a necrotizing process indicates surgical debridement is required.[172] Sometimes surgical exploration is necessary to determine the extent of the infection.

Gram-positive bacteria that cause skin and soft tissue infections include *Streptococcus* (group A and B) and *S. aureus*. Besides *P. aeruginosa*, other gram-negative bacilli with propensity to cause dermatologic infections include *Stenotrophomonas maltophilia* (mucocutaneous ulcerations, primary cellulitis, metastatic nodular cellulitis, and ecthyma gangrenosum), *Aeromonas hydrophila*, and *Vibrio vulnificus* (septicemia with secondary cellulitis with hemorrhagic bullae after ingestion of contaminated seafood, most common in patients with underlying liver disease, or primary cellulitis with bacteremia when an open wound is exposed to seawater). *Clostridium* spp. are gram-positive anaerobes that may cause deep soft tissue infection involving the fascia and muscle. In neutropenic patients, the typical presentation is disseminated soft tissue infection with *Clostridium septicum* bacteremia. Typically, a small dusky or purplish lesion on the leg or abdominal wall rapidly expands, and as infection progresses, the lesions may become necrotic, bullous, and hemorrhagic. Systemic toxicity including fever, malaise, and mental status changes occur early. Because the infection occurs in the deep soft tissue, tenderness and evidence of vascular compromise typically precede the development of cellulitis. A rapidly progressive deep soft tissue infection with gas formation suggests clostridial myonecrosis or polymicrobial necrotizing fasciitis. Needle aspiration characteristically shows the organism in the setting of a mild or absent inflammatory response. Extensive surgical debridement

may be life-saving if initiated early, but the mortality rate is high.[173] Metronidazole plus an antipseudomonal cephalosporin (such as ceftazidime or cefepime) or single-agent therapy with imipenem, meropenem, or piperacillin/tazobactam are reasonable regimens.

The characteristic skin lesions of disseminated candidiasis are raised erythematous discrete papules, measuring about 0.5 to 1 cm in diameter. In their earliest form, the lesions resemble those of heat rash. They are usually not tender. Concurrent myalgias raise the possibility of *Candida* myositis. The yeast is cultured from skin lesions in only about half the cases. Blood cultures are typically positive. Similar lesions may appear with disseminated trichosporonosis.[174]

Cutaneous infection by molds may be primary or result from systemic infection. The hematogenous lesions of *Aspergillus* and *Fusarium* usually begin as discrete subcutaneous nodules that may be tender, whereas traumatic inoculation appears as ulcerations. If a primary cutaneous lesion is isolated and surgically resectable, it has an excellent prognosis. In the neutropenic patient, the likelihood of systemic infection is high, and therefore systemic antifungal therapy is warranted. Clinically, these lesions resemble ecthyma gangrenosum. Histologically, hyphae are present with angioinvasion and infarction. Primary cutaneous fusariosis has a varied appearance, including cellulitis, paronychia, onychomycosis resembling dermatophyte infection, as well as papular and nodular lesions.[175]

HSV and VZV can involve the skin. Oral or genital ulcers should be sampled to rule our HSV by immunofluorescence or PCR. Multiple well-circumscribed disseminated cutaneous ulcers can be manifecstations of disseminated HSV. Disseminated HSV disease should be treated with intravenous acyclovir (10 mg/kg every 8 hours). Acyclovir-resistant HSV is occasionally observed in HSCT recipients. When acyclovir resistance is suspected, the decision to switch therapy (generally to foscarnet) should be made on clinical grounds as antiviral susceptibility testing of the isolate at a reference laboratory takes weeks. VZV presents with maculopapular or vesicular lesions, often but not always in a dermatomal distribution. Secondary bacterial infections, usually due to streptococci or *S. aureus*, may occur. Visceral involvement of VZV can manifest as hemorrhagic pneumonia, encephalitis, retinal necrosis, hepatitis, and small bowel disease. Both viruses can be detected in the blood by PCR in case of disseminated infection; this may be particularly helpful if VZV presents with pain only, with no apparent rash. Intravenous acyclovir is the established treatment for primary varicella or disseminated zoster in immunocompromised patients.

Respiratory Tract Infections

Community-Acquired Respiratory Viruses

Community respiratory viruses include influenza, parainfluenza, respiratory syncytial virus, human metapneumovirus, adenoviruses, rhinoviruses, and coronaviruses. Most respiratory viruses typically cause self-limited infection in healthy persons, but are important causes of morbidity and mortality in immunocompromised patients with hematologic malignancies and in HSCT recipients.[176] Immunocompromised persons with symptoms of respiratory infection should be evaluated for respiratory viruses, among other etiologies, and contact and respiratory precautions should be established. There are no significant differences in clinical presentation that allow predicting the causative virus in any individual case. Rapid immunodiagnostic tests (i.e., enzyme-linked immunosorbent assay) are insensitive: they are useful only to "rule in" these infections but a negative result cannot be used to rule out the disease. PCR is the most sensitive test.

Influenza. Influenza A and B can be treated with neuraminidase inhibitors (zanamivir and oseltamivir); influenza A can also be treated with amantadine and rimantadine. The circulating strain may be susceptible or resistant to these agents; it is important to consult the CDC to find out what is the recommended treatment during each influenza season. The CDC advises annual administration of the inactivated influenza vaccine to immunocompromised persons and their close contacts (e.g., health-care workers and household members). Immunization should be provided ideally 2 weeks before chemotherapy, or if given during chemotherapy, immunization is preferably administered between cycles. The recently approved inhaled live attenuated influenza vaccine, FluMist (MedImmune, LLC, Gaithersburg, MD), should not be used in the severely immunocompromised patient. Use of the injected inactivated vaccine is preferred among close contacts of the immunocompromised persons, including health-care workers.

Respiratory Syncytial Virus. Respiratory syncytial virus infection is most virulent in patients with leukemia and in HSCT recipients. Upper respiratory symptoms (sinusitis, coryza, rhinorrhea) usually precede lower respiratory tract involvement (dyspnea, wheezing) and pneumonia but may be absent. Accumulating evidence suggests that severely immunocompromised HSCT recipients may benefit from treatment with ribavirin.[177,178]

Parainfluenza. Parainfluenza viruses are important community respiratory viruses in leukemia and HSCT patients.[179,180] Given there is no effective antiviral treatment available, emphasis should be placed on infection control measures and diagnosis and treatment of copathogens.[181]

Human Metapneumovirus. Human metapneumovirus is a recently described paramyxovirus that causes upper and lower respiratory tract infection. It occurs mostly during the winter and spring. More severe disease is reported in young children, the elderly, and immunocompromised hosts.[182,183] The treatment is supportive.

Adenovirus

The spectrum of adenovirus in immunocompromised patients extends from asymptomatic shedding to fatal multisystem disease with pneumonia and hepatitis, and includes upper respiratory tract infection, renal parenchymal disease, hemorrhagic cystitis, hepatitis, small and large bowel disease, and encephalitis.[184] Viral shedding from throat secretions, urine, and stool is common, occurring in ~5% to 20% of HSCT recipients, and should not be equated with disease. Gastroenteritis and hemorrhagic cystitis are usually self-limited, whereas pneumonia and disseminated disease are associated with a high mortality rate. Adenovirus is more common in T-cell–depleted transplants and in younger patients and recipients of stem cells from unrelated donors. Cidofovir is the antiviral of choice.

Sinusitis

Congestion, sinus tenderness, and fever are common signs of sinusitis, but are nonspecific. In immunocompetent patients, respiratory bacterial pathogens, including *S. pneumoniae*, *H. influenzae*, and *Moraxella catarrhalis* predominate, and a standard antibiotic regimen, such as amoxicillin-clavulanic acid, or a respirtory fluoroquinolone is appropriate if the diagnosis is properly established. Of note, macrolides, TMP/SMX and second-generation cephalosporins are no longer recommended.[185] In patients with neutropenia or who are otherwise highly immunocompromised, infections by *P. aeruginosa*, *S. aureus*, Enterobacteriaceae, and molds must be considered. We initiate standard agents for fever and neutropenia, and promptly obtain a CT scan of the sinuses and otolaryngologist consultation to obtain samples for culture and, if there are lesions suspicious for invasive mold (e.g., ischemia, necrotic eschar), biopsy. The CT may be suggestive of fungal disease if a heterogeneous mass or bony erosions are seen. *Aspergillus* and agents of mucormycosis (e.g., mucor, rhizopus) are the most common isolates, but less common molds such as *Fusarium* spp., and dematiaceous molds are being recognized more frequently. Pending

microbiologic identification, empirical therapy should include a lipid formulation of amphotericin B (5 mg/kg per day), to ensure coverage of mucormycosis. If the diagnosis of invasive fungal sinusitis is confirmed, surgical resection should be performed because medical therapy alone is unlikely to contain infection in the setting of neutropenia or severe immunosuppression. Antifungal therapy should be continued for weeks or months even if all of the visualized necrotic tissue is fully resected. An etiologic diagnosis will allow choosing the appropriate antifungal (e.g., voriconazole for aspergillosis, amphotericin for mucormycosis). For some causes of mucormycosis, posaconazole may be a useful alternative to amphotericin B for long-term therapy.[186,187]

Pulmonary Infiltrates

There are multiple infectious and noninfectious causes of pulmonary infiltrates in cancer patients. Some noninfectious processes that should be considered include the malignancy, complications of its treatment (drug toxicity, radiation pneumonitis), congestive heart failure, pulmonary hemorrhage, pulmonary embolism with infarction, cryptogenic organizing pneumonia, and acute respiratory distress syndrome. Atypical radiographic appearances and several coexisting pulmonary processes are common in this patient population. We recommend early use of CT scans and diagnostic procedures, including bronchoalveolar lavage, fine needle aspiration, or lung biopsy if required.

Community-Acquired Pneumonia

Sputum and blood cultures should be collected prior to starting therapy if feasible. In patients with malignancies who do not require hospital admission based on a validated pneumonia severity index,[188] either a respiratory fluoroquinolone alone (levofloxacin, moxifloxacin) or a β-lactam plus a macrolide (e.g., high-dose amoxicillin or amoxicillin-clavulanate and azithromycin) is advised. In patients requiring hospital admission, we use monotherapy with a respiratory fluoroquinolone or combine a macrolide with either ceftriaxone, cefotaxime, or, in selected cases, ertapenem. For cancer patients with severe community-acquired pneumonia (e.g., requiring admission to an intensive care unit), we usually institute broad-spectrum coverage with an antipseudomonal β-lactam plus a respiratory fluoroquinolone. In patients with prior MRSA infection or known colonization with MRSA, we add vancomycin or linezolid. A parapneumonic effusion should be sampled for microbiologic studies and cytologic examination.

Legionella Species. *Legionella* infections are associated with compromised cellular immunity. In the cancer population, patients at highest risk include those receiving high-dose corticosteroids, T-cell–depleting agents, and allogeneic HSCT. There are no clinical or radiologic criteria that reliably distinguish legionellosis from pneumococcal pneumonia, although diarrhea, rhabdomyolysis, and lack of response to β-lactam antibiotics have been proposed as suggestive of the diagnosis. A combination of culture (special culture medium required) and urinary antigen test is the optimal diagnostic combination in most situations.[189] The urine legionella antigen assay is sensitive and specific for *Legionella pneumophila* serogroup 1, the isolate responsible for up to 80% of clinical disease; however, it does not detect other serogroups or *Legionella* spp. PCR on respiratory secretions is both sensitive and specific for *Legionella* detection, but standardized assays are not commercially available. Azithromycin or fluoroquinolones (e.g., levofloxacin, moxifloxacin) are standard therapy for legionellosis. Nosocomial legionellosis has been linked to contamination of hospital water.

Hospital-Acquired Pneumonia

Hospital-acquired pneumonia (HAP) is considered "early" when it happens within 4 days of admission or "late" when it occurs 5 days or more after admission. Late HAP is more likely to be caused by multidrug-resistant pathogens. Initial therapy for early onset HAP is similar to that of community-acquired pneumonia, except when there are risk factors for colonization with multidrug-resistant pathogens (e.g., prior antibiotics within the past 90 days, recent hospitalization, nursing home, dialysis center) in which case they should be treated similar to patients with late-onset HAP. In late-onset HAP, the goal is to broadly cover nosocomial pathogens and then to deescalate the antibiotic regimen once culture results and susceptibility are known. A typical initial regimen for late-onset HAP includes an antipseudomonal β-lactam (e.g., ceftazidime, cefepime, imipenem, meropenem, or piperacillin/tazobactam) plus an antipseudomonal fluoroquinolone (e.g., ciprofloxacin or levofloxacin), plus either linezolid or vancomycin (aim for trough vancomycin level of 15 to 20 mcg/ml).[190]

Pulmonary Infiltrates in Neutropenic Patients

In patients with <1 week of neutropenia, pulmonary infections are likely to be caused by Enterobacteriaceae, P. aeruginosa, and S. aureus. Community respiratory viruses should also be considered. Because of neutropenia, physical findings of consolidation and sputum production may be absent. We recommend the early use of CT. A CT scan of the chest may disclose lesions missed by the chest radiograph as well as findings characteristic of invasive fungal disease: well-circumscribed, dense infiltrates, the "halo sign" (see Fig. 132.2), and/or cavitation. Cavitation usually coincides with neutrophil recovery and does not indicate treatment failure. Besides molds, other angioinvasive infections including P. aeruginosa may cavitate. A new or progressive infiltrate developing while on broad-spectrum antibacterial agents in patients with prolonged neutropenia raises the concern about invasive mold infection, and makes the need for definitive diagnosis more pressing. Because radiographic findings are often nonspecific, we recommend early BAL. In patients at risk for invasive mold diseases, a serum galactomannan and β-D-glucan may be considered, although the interpretation of a single value of these tests (as opposed to trends) may be difficult.

In highly immunocompromised patients (e.g., chemotherapy for acute leukemia, HSCT receiving active treatment for GVHD), we suggest the following studies on BAL and lung biopsies: culture and stains for bacteria, including Legionella, mycobacteria, and Nocardia species as well as fungi; special stains or PCR for P. jirovecii; and rapid culture (shell vial) or PCR for virus (HSV, CMV, VZV, community respiratory viruses). Cytologic examination of the BAL may also be diagnostic of pneumocystis, nocardia, fungi, mycobacteria, CMV, and adenovirus, and can suggest diffuse alveolar hemorrhage. BAL galactomannan is more sensitive than serum galactomannan, particularly in neutropenic patients, and should be considered in patients at risk for IA.[125]

The yield of induced sputum for the diagnosis of PCP in non-HIV-infected patients may be only 60%,[191] and early consideration should be given to BAL. The yield of BAL is high for P. jirovecii, Mycobacterium tuberculosis, and respiratory viruses. For focal lesions such as nodules, the diagnostic yield is much lower (15% to 50%), and a percutaneous biopsy may be a better diagnostic choice.[192] Transbronchial biopsy may be helpful in diffuse processes. Video-assisted thoracic surgery has been used successfully in cases with diffuse involvement and with peripheral lesions. Open lung biopsy is the definitive diagnostic method, and it also allows for easier visualization and control of bleeding.

Treatment

Besides the standard antimicrobials used for fever and neutropenia, we include a macrolide or fluoroquinolone to treat Legionella and agents of atypical pneumonia. Vancomycin or linezolid should be added for pneumonia in patients colonized with MRSA and for nosocomial pneumonia. Depending on the clinical scenario and preexistent antifungal prophylaxis, we may add voriconazole or a

lipid formulation of amphotericin B. There is disagreement between experts on which is the best antifungal strategy. Aspergillus spp. are by far the most common mold infections, but mucormycosis may be the cause in any individual case. Voriconazole is the drug of choice for IA,[107] but is inactive in mucormycosis. Amphotericin B is active in both aspergillosis and mucormycosis, but it may be significantly inferior to voriconazole in aspergillosis. Some experts might add both agents and aggressively pursue a diagnosis that will allow de-escalation.

Pulmonary Infiltrates in Patients with Defects in Cellular Immunity

Patients with impaired cellular immunity and those taking corticosteroids are at increased risk for opportunistic infections, including fungi (Cryptococcus neoformans, dimorphic fungi, other molds), Legionella spp., P. jirovecii (Fig. 132.3), M. tuberculosis, nontuberculous mycobacteria, Nocardia spp., and viral pathogens. CMV pneumonia principally occurs in allogeneic HSCT recipients, but can uncommonly occur in other severely immunocompromised patients. Diffuse necrotizing pneumonia by varicella and HSV are also encountered in transplant recipients.

The diagnostic evaluation in patients with impaired cellular immunity and pulmonary infiltrates is similar to neutropenic patients. Typically, broad-spectrum antibiotics for community-acquired pneumonia requiring hospitalization (see previous discussion) will be started, ideally after obtaining respiratory samples for diagnosis. The empirical addition of TMP/SMX for PCP should be considered.

Nocardia **Species.** Patients with hematologic malignancy, allogeneic HSCT recipients, lymphopenia, and receiving corticosteroids are at highest risk.[193] Bronchopneumonia, lobar pneumonia, nodules, or necrotizing abscesses with cavitation are observed. Empyema and extension to the chest wall may occur. Dissemination may include brain abscess, meningitis, osteomyelitis, soft tissue mass, cutaneous abscess, and liver abscess. It is important to alert the microbiology laboratory when nocardiosis is suspected so that a modified acid stain is performed and that appropriate culture conditions are used and culture plates are held for weeks instead of days. Treatment of nocardial infections is based on case series. Most experience is with TMP/SMX, but other agents that have been used include carbapenems, minocycline, ceftriaxone, and linezolid. Identification is important to predict susceptibility.[194] Surgical drainage or resection should be considered in cases refractory to medical therapy. Therapy should be continued for several months to a year.

Pneumocystis jirovecii. P. jirovecii (formerly P. carinii) is more appropriately classified as a fungus than a protozoan based on gene sequence data and cell wall constituents. Defective T-cell immunity is the principal risk factor for PCP, with the risk in people infected with HIV increasing significantly after the CD4 count declines below 200. In patients without AIDS, corticosteroid use is the main risk factor.[195] Fever, cough, and shortness of breath are the most common clinical features.[196] Patients treated with corticosteroids may develop initial clinical manifestations of PCP only during steroid taper. The most common radiographic findings are bilateral interstitial infiltrates, although unilateral or patchy infiltrates are also observed.[197] Nodules, cavitary lesions, and pleural effusions are less common. In a minority of patients, the chest radiograph is normal. Diagnosis of PCP relies on visualization of the organism microscopically or use of melucular methods, as it does not grow in culture. BAL is the standard diagnostic modality for PCP, but induced sputum has acceptable yield in some institutions. Immunofluorescent staining using mAbs is more sensitive than silver staining or Wright-Giemsa staining. Patients with cancer have reduced organism burden compared with people infected with HIV, which decreases the sensitivity of every diagnostic

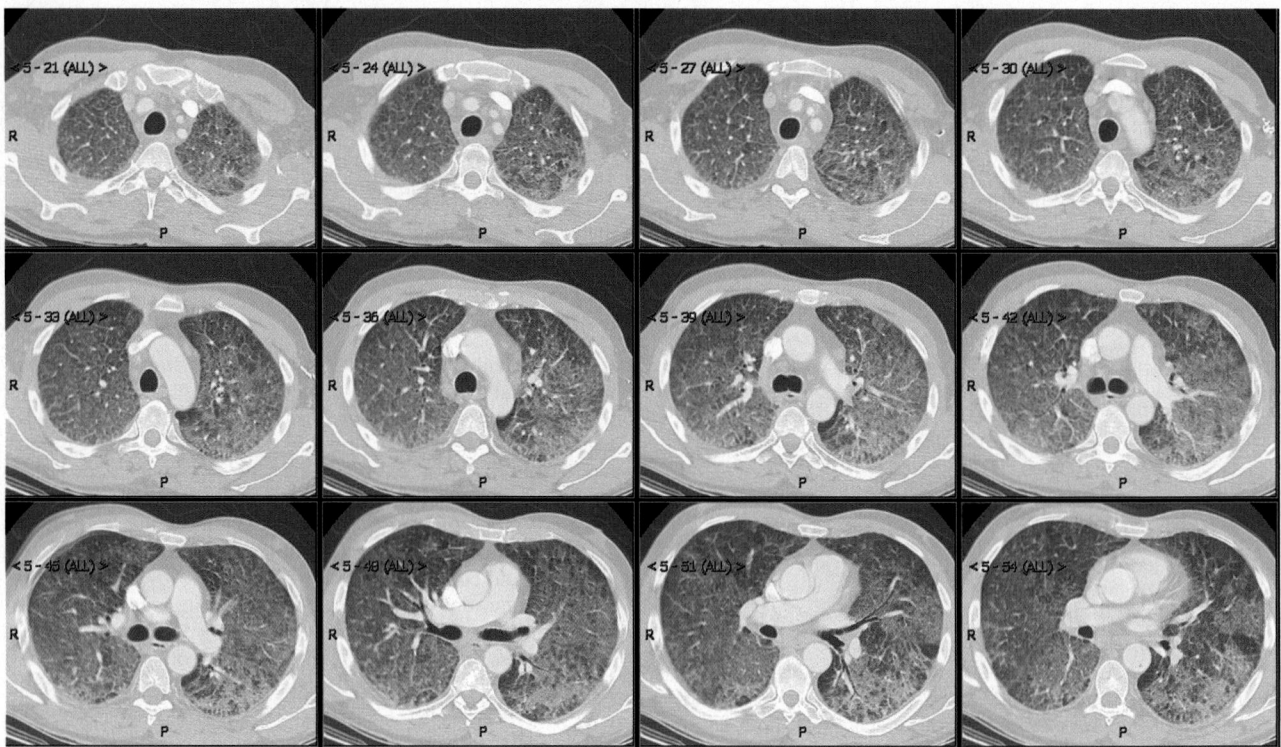

Figure 132.3 *Pneumocystis jirovecii* pneumonia. A patient with chronic lymphocytic leukemia developed fever, hypoxemia, and shortness of breath soon after tapering a prednisone course for hemolytic anemia. He had received multiple courses of fludarabine, rituximab, and corticosteroids. He was receiving inhaled pentamidine as *Pneumocystis jirovecii* pneumonia prophylaxis. His last treatment had taken place 3 weeks prior to this illness.

modality. Quantitative PCR of respiratory samples may be the most sensitive test in this setting.[198,199] The serum β-D-glucan test seems to have very good sensitivity and specificity.[200]

Treatment. TMP/SMX is the treatment of choice for *P. jirovecii*. If TMP/SMX is not feasible because of significant allergy or toxicity, intravenous pentamidine or pyrimethamine plus clindamycin can be used. In cases of mild or moderate PCP (which has been defined as room air Pao_2 >70 torr) in patients intolerant of TMP/SMX, dapsone-trimethoprim, clindamycin-primaquine, and atovaquone are acceptable options, but the efficacy of all these is less than that of TMP/SMX. In patients with moderate or severe PCP (Pao_2 ≤70 torr), corticosteroids should be added based on studies of patients with AIDS-associated PCP. In patients who are not responding to therapy, repeat bronchoscopy should be considered to exclude additional pathogens.

Cytomegalovirus Pneumonitis. Pulmonary disease typically manifests as bilateral infiltrates resembling PCP with hypoxia and progression to respiratory failure. In transplant patients, the diagnosis is established by a compatible clinical syndrome with detection of CMV in BAL (by culture or cytopathology showing characteristic intracytoplasmic and intranuclear inclusions) or tissue (by culture or histologic diagnosis).[201] In nontransplant patients, CMV pneumonia is rare, and the culture alone is not considered sufficient to make the diagnosis as CMV can be shed from pulmonary secretions without causing invasive disease. Demonstration of intracellular CMV inclusions on BAL is diagnostic of disease, but is uncommon. In many cases, other pathogens are found, including *P. aeruginosa, Legionella, Aspergillus* spp., *Mycobacteria* spp., *Nocardia* spp., toxoplasmosis, or respiratory viruses.

We treat CMV pneumonia with ganciclovir or foscarnet plus Ig (either regular intravenous Ig or CMV-specific). The benefit of Ig is based on historical controls and has been questioned.[62] Cidofovir may be considered in cases of CMV disease after failure or intolerance to ganciclovir or foscarnet.

Postobstructive Pneumonia and Pleural Effusion

There are no professional guidelines or professional society guidance statements on the indication for airway stenting to relieve malignant obstruction. There are no outcomes reported in sufficiently large series to answer the question as to whether the risk and consequence of infection outweigh the benefit of the relief of obstruction. Retrospective series suggest that stenting is followed by infection with moderate frequency and (predominantly *P. aeruginsoa*) has increased mortality.

A similar lack of controlled data is present in the evaluation of intrapleural catheters placed for the relief of malignant pleural effusion, although infection as a complication seems to be infrequent.[202]

Epstein-Barr Virus–Induced Posttransplant Lymphoproliferative Disease

Most adults have been infected by EBV. Latent infection persists in B cells and produces no disease in the vast majority of people. EBV-specific cytotoxic T-lymphocytes are the main controllers of the replication of EBV-infected B cells. EBV lymphoproliferative diseases are encountered in patients with severely impaired T-cell immunity, such as AIDS or intensive and prolonged immunosuppressive therapy. EBV-induced PTLD is defined as an abnormal proliferation of EBV-infected B cells in a transplant recipient. The lesions may be composed of polyclonal or monoclonal populations of transformed B cells. PTLD is most common between 1 and 6 months after allogeneic HSCT. Typically, the proliferating B cells are of donor origin. Immunosuppressive therapy for GVHD and T-cell–depleted allografts increases the risk of PTLD. Uncontrolled EBV infection may also cause a hemophagocytic syndrome that is characterized clinically by fever, pancytopenia, and hepatosplenomegaly.[203]

Clinical manifestations of PTLD are varied. Patients may have a mononucleosis-like syndrome with fever and localized adenopathy. Disseminated disease may manifest with generalized adenopathy and extranodal organ involvement, including the bowel, liver, bone marrow, and CNS. A CT/positron emission tomography scan is useful in a high-risk patient with unexplained fever. Diagnosis of PTLD requires a biopsy showing the characteristic histology and evidence of EBV infection by immunohistochemistry or EBV DNA detection.

Whereas PTLD in organ transplant recipients typically responds to a reduction in the intensity of immunosuppression, PTLD in HSCT recipients may not respond to such conservative measures. Antiviral agents may attenuate the lytic cycle of EBV and reduce the frequency of new B-cell clones, but they will not affect the replication of EBV-transformed PTLD B cells, and are not useful. Other strategies include rituximab,[204] low-dose chemotherapy, anti–IL-6, donor lymphocyte infusions, and adoptive immunotherapy using donor-derived EBV-specific cytotoxic T-lymphocyte clones. However, using alloreactive T cells in such unfractionated preparations may induce GVHD. A potentially safer approach involves transfer of EBV-specific donor cytotoxic T-lymphocyte clones. Adoptive transfer of EBV-specific cytotoxic T-lymphocytes has been generally safe and effective in controlling PTLD and in preventing EBV lymphoproliferative disorders when used prophylactically.

Gastrointestinal Tract and Abdominal Infections

Oropharyngeal Infections

Oropharyngeal infections in patients with cancer usually result from the combination of neutropenia and mucositis. The distinction of chemotherapy-induced mucosal erosions and superimposed infection is difficult. HSV may produce mucosal ulcerations resembling chemotherapy-induced mucositis and necrotizing gingivitis, and it should be ruled out by culture or PCR. Oral mucosal candidiasis may present with typical thrush, but also with erosions and erythema; diagnosis is made by a wet mount or Gram stain preparation showing pseudohyphal forms (the culture is not of diagnostic value because *Candida* spp. are part of the normal oral flora). Molds (e.g., *Aspergillus* spp. and zygomycetes) can cause invasive disease of the hard palate and other oral cavity structures, principally in patients with prolonged neutropenia and allogeneic HSCT recipients with GVHD. Severe local bacterial infection may occur with spread to adjacent tissue structures and bacteremia. The antibacterial regimen should cover both common oral flora (gram-positive bacteria and anaerobes) and hospital-acquired gram-negative bacilli.

Esophagitis

Gradual onset of retrosternal chest pain or burning and odynophagia are the most common symptoms of esophagitis. The infectious differential diagnosis includes candidiasis, HSV, CMV (principally in HSCT recipients), bacterial infections, and aspergillosis. *Candida* esophagitis is probably most common, but more than one infection may be present. Radiation therapy to the chest and chemotherapy-induced mucositis may produce an erosive esophagitis that is clinically indistinguishable from infection. The definitive diagnosis requires endoscopy with brushing or biopsy. The endoscopic appearance is often misleading. In neutropenic patients, we recommend empirical therapy with fluconazole, with or without high-dose acyclovir (10 mg/kg every 8 hours) for *Candida* and HSV, respectively, followed by endoscopy if there is no improvement. In the setting of concurrent neutropenic fever, appropriate broad-spectrum antibacterial agents should of course be added. Esophagitis may be complicated by bacteremia by predominantly gram-positive pathogens (viridans group streptococci, *S. aureus, Bacillus* spp.).

Neutropenic Enterocolitis (Typhlitis)

Typhlitis ("inflammation of the cecum") results from a combination of neutropenia and defects in the bowel mucosa related to

cytotoxic chemotherapy. Patients receiving chemotherapy for acute leukemia are at highest risk, but it is also observed in patients with solid tumors receiving taxanes.[129,130] Pathologically, typhlitis is characterized by ulceration and necrosis of the bowel wall, hemorrhage, and masses of organisms. Suggestive signs include fever, abdominal pain and tenderness, and radiologic evidence of right colonic inflammation. Nausea, vomiting, and diarrhea (sometimes bloody) are the most common associated symptoms. Bacteremia with bowel flora, *P. aeruginosa*, and polymicrobial sepsis may occur. Clostridial species are the most common anaerobic pathogens.

A CT scan should be performed in neutropenic patients with suspected typhlitis or undiagnosed abdominal pain. Positive CT scan findings are present in about 80% of cases of typhlitis,[205] and include a right lower quadrant inflammatory mass, pericecal fluid, soft tissue inflammatory changes, localized bowel wall thickening and mucosal edema, and a paralytic ileus (Fig. 132.4). Disease may be limited to the cecum, but more extensive involvement of the large bowel and terminal ileum may occur (*neutropenic enterocolitis*). The differential diagnosis includes *C. difficile* colitis, GVHD of the bowel, CMV colitis, and bowel ischemia.[206]

Treatment of typhlitis requires broad-spectrum antibiotics with activity against aerobic gram-negative bacilli and anaerobes (e.g., ceftazidime plus metronidazole, imipenem, meropenem, or piperacillin/tazobactam) and supportive care, including intravenous fluids and bowel rest. Nasogastric decompression may be indicated. The indications for surgery must be individualized, but include (1) persistent gastrointestinal bleeding after resolution of neutropenia, thrombocytopenia, and clotting abnormalities; (2) perforation; (3) uncontrolled sepsis despite fluid and vasopressor support; and (4) an intra-abdominal process (such as appendicitis) that would require surgery in the absence of neutropenia.[133]

Anorectal Infections

Anorectal infections may be life-threatening in patients who are receiving repeated courses of cytotoxic chemotherapy. Infection may follow the development of an anal fissure. Once anorectal infection is established, fascial extension to the external genitalia, pelvic floor, retroperitoneum, and peritoneal cavity may occur. Anorectal infections, with or without extensive regional spread, may lead to bacteremia. The most common pathogens in neutropenic patients are Enterobacteriaceae, anaerobes, enterococci, and *P. aeruginosa*. In most cases, the infection is polymicrobial.[207]

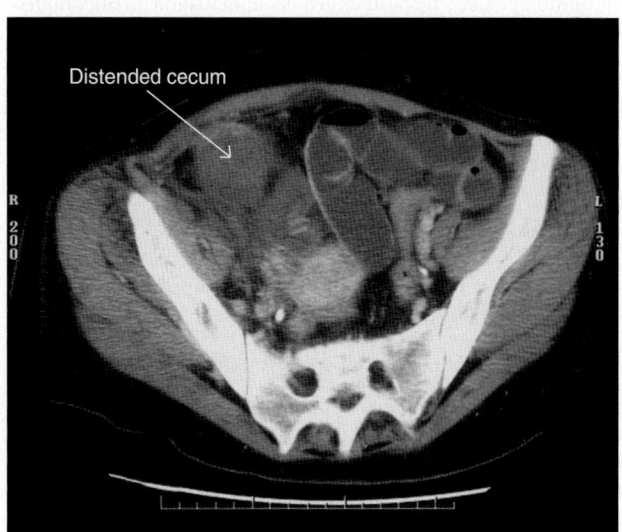

Figure 132.4 Typhlitis (neutropenic enterocolitis). The computed tomographic scan shows edema of the cecal wall and "stranding" of pericolic fat in a neutropenic patient with fever and abdominal pain.

Fever often precedes symptoms and signs suggestive of anorectal infection, and perirectal pain, often exacerbated by defecation, may initially occur in the absence of findings in the physical examination. Therefore, serial examinations of the perianal region are necessary, looking for point tenderness and poorly demarcated induration.[208] Perianal and perirectal infections are distinguished anatomically, clinically, and therapeutically. Among neutropenic patients, perianal infections are common and are usually managed medically, whereas perirectal infections are uncommon and often warrant surgical intervention. Visual inspection should assess for the presence of perianal fissures, fistulas, cellulitis, and induration. Digital rectal examination should be avoided during neutropenia. A CT scan should be obtained to show the extent of perirectal involvement and drainable collections. Stool softeners and analgesics should be provided. Most cases of anorectal infections can be managed with appropriate broad-spectrum antibiotics and supportive measures without surgical intervention.[207] Indications for surgery include progression of disease locally or continued sepsis despite adequate antibiotics.[208]

Surgical Intra-Abdominal Infections

Esophageal Obstruction

The available literature on stents for the relief of malignant esophageal disease and gastroduodenal or colonic obstruction does not suggest an increased risk of infectious complications. Professional guidance does exist for esophageal and upper gastrointestinal malignant obstruction.[209]

Biliary Obstruction

Both gastroenterology and radiology professional guidelines exist related to the placement of devices for the relief of malignant biliary tract obstruction.[210,211] The best current evidence does not support the need for decompression in order to allow for better surgical outcomes.[212]

Infection (cholangitis, cholecystitis, and liver abscess) is a common adverse outcome of device placement. Prior manipulation (endoscopic retrograde cholangiopancreatogram) and incomplete drainage are the most consistently identified risk factors.[213] Infection rates of 22% (percutaneous transhepatic drainage) and 29.5% (endoscopic placement) with self-expanding metallic stents have been reported in unresectable hilar cholangiocarcinoma without a statistically significant difference by procedure.[214] Prophylactic antibiotics are recommended in anticipation of incomplete endoscopic drainage, which occurs most frequently in proximal obstruction.[213,214] There is evidence that neither ursodeoxycholic acid nor antibiotics improve stent patency.[215] Antibiotic choices should be made in consultation with an expert in local susceptibility patterns. No clear evidence relates the type of device used to the risk of infection.

Central Nervous System Infections

CNS infections in patients with cancer can be divided into surgical and nonsurgical.

Infections Related to Neurosurgical Procedures

Devices are placed in the CNS/cranioskeletal system to relieve intracranial hypertension, replace structural defects, and deliver chemotherapy. As such, the dominant infectious events, which have been reported in >10% of cases, are related to contamination at placement or access.[216] Skin flora predominate, with staphylococci (both aureus and coagulase-negative) and other commensals (*Propionibacterium*). CSF indices are helpful but not adequately sensitive and cultures should always be obtained in evaluating signs or symptoms that might represent infection.[217,218] A reasonable

assessment of treatment strategies is difficult as the vast majority of circumstances are treated with removal of the device. Intrathecal administration of antibiotics has some chance of success but should be used with caution when the infecting organism is virulent (*S. aureus*, *P. aeruginosa*).[219] Titanium devices for the correction of cranial defects are associated with infectious complications in 18.5% of cases despite their reported resistance to infection.[220]

Meningitis/Meningoencephalitis

Meningitis and encephalitis in cancer patients are part of a clinical spectrum of CNS disorders causing fever and meningismus. Encephalitis may manifest with signs and symptoms of meningeal inflammation, but is distinguished by the predominance of alterations of consciousness and neurologic deficits. The IDSA has published guidelines on the management of bacterial meningitis[221] and encephalitis.[222]

Initial evaluation generally involves an MRI and lumbar puncture. CSF studies should include cell count with differential; cytology and flow cytometry if appropriate; glucose, protein, and bacterial culture; and Gram stain evaluation. In neutropenic patients, we add fungal culture, β-D-glucan, and galactomannan antigen. In patients with impaired cellular immunity, CSF cryptococcal antigen should be ordered. Noninfectious causes of meningitis include carcinomatous meningitis, nonsteroidal antiinflammatory medications, TMP/SMX, and serum sickness (e.g., associated with antilymphocyte gammaglobulin or intravenous Ig).

A reasonable empirical regimen for suspected bacterial meningitis in patients with cancer is ceftriaxone plus ampicillin plus vancomycin. This regimen will cover common causes of bacterial meningitis, including penicillin-resistant pneumococci and listeriosis. In the penicillin-allergic patient, the combination of vancomycin and TMP/SMX may be used. In patients at risk for *P. aeruginosa* meningitis (e.g., neutropenia, neurosurgery within the past 2 months, allogeneic HSCT, prior history of *P. aeruginosa* infection), cefepime or meropenem should be used instead of ceftriaxone.

In patients with suspected encephalitis (fever, mental status changes, CSF pleocytosis), viral etiologies should be considered and frequently treated empirically until they are ruled out. Intravenous acyclovir should be considered for HSV; it will also treat VZV. After allogeneic HSCT (particularly cord or T-cell–depleted transplants), HHV-6 is a common cause of viral encephalitis, and empirical treatment with ganciclovir or foscarnet may be considered pending PCR results.[223] In patients at risk for TB, nucleic acid amplification methods for the diagnosis of TB should be obtained and adenosine deaminase considered. Mycobacterial culture has low yield and take many days or weeks, but should be obtained. After allo-HSCT and in other settings of impaired T-cell immunity, toxoplasmosis and CMV are possibilities; both may be diagnosed by PCR. Different virus may be considered depending on the region and time of the year; the diagnosis may be made by PCR or, in the case of West Nile virus, by determination of IgM against the virus.

Herpes Viruses. HSV meningoencephalitis has been associated with older age, steroid therapy, and brain irradiation. Typically, there is enhancement of the temporal lobe on MRI. After allo-HSCT, HHV-6 has been associated with a characteristic "limbic encephalitis" consisting of confusion, lethargy, memory loss, seizures, and (late) hippocampal enhancement on MRI fluid-attenuated inversion recovery images.[224–226] The diagnosis is made by detection of HHV-6 DNA in the CSF by PCR.[223] Ganciclovir, foscarnet, and the combination of both may be used, but there are no clinical data to choose one over the other. Detection of high levels of EBV DNA should raise suspicion of EBV-related lymphoproliferative disorder,[227] but encephalitis and myelitis have been described. Adenovirus encephalitis also occurs in HSCT patients and is usually part of disseminated adenoviral infection; treatment with cidofovir may be attempted.

Cryptococcus Neoformans. Host defense against cryptococcal infection is principally dependent on cellular immunity. Among patients with cancer, those with hematologic malignancies, receiving high-dose corticosteroids, and allogeneic HSCT recipients are at highest risk for cryptococcosis. Meningoencephalitis is the most common presentation of cryptococcal infection, but other manifestations include primary pneumonia, pulmonary nodules, fungemia, and cutaneous and visceral dissemination. Diagnosis in disseminated disease may be obtained by determining cryptococcal antigen in the CSF and peripheral blood; in cases of localized disease, tissue must be obtained. In immunocompromised patients, the preferred regimen is amphotericin B (plus 5-flucytosine for the first 2 weeks), followed by maintenance fluconazole therapy. In neutropenic patients, reduction of the dosage of 5-flucytosine may be considered to avoid delay in myeloid recovery. Because fluconazole is well tolerated, continuing therapy with this agent for several months (or longer if intensive immunosuppressive therapy is continued) is reasonable.

Brain Abscess

Brain abscesses usually manifest with headache, focal neurologic findings, or seizures. MRI typically shows single or multiple lesions with edema and ring enhancement. Bacterial abscesses in nonimmunocompromised patients are typically caused by dental flora. In cancer patients, brain abscesses unrelated to surgery occur primarily in patients with prolonged neutropenia or profoundly depressed cell-mediated immunity, and are frequently fungal (92% of 58 cases of brain abscesses following HSCT[152]). Almost all cases of CNS aspergillosis are associated with a pulmonary focus. Most cases of *Candida* brain abscess are associated with candidemia or neutropenia.

Manifestations of CNS aspergillosis include focal seizures, hemiparesis, cranial nerve palsies, and hemorrhagic infarcts due to vascular invasion.[228] Serum and CSF galactomannan and β-glucan testing are also useful to make the diagnosis. Aspergillus brain abscesses are typically multiple, hypodense, and nonenhancing with little mass effect. CT scans with contrast enhancement

initially may reveal no focal lesions, but usually evolve to focal ring-enhancing or hemorrhagic lesions. MRI may show varying patterns depending on the stage of the lesion. In patients with impaired cellular immunity, other etiologies include toxoplasmosis, nocardiosis, cryptococcosis, and mycobacterial infections. Noninfectious etiologies include CNS malignancies, including secondary lymphomas and EBV-associated PTLD in patients with impaired cellular immunity. Given the broad differential diagnosis of new focal CNS lesions in immunocompromised patients, a brain biopsy is recommended if feasible. Cultures and stains should include bacteria, fungi, mycobacteria, and *Nocardia*.

In nonimmunocompromised patients with a bacterial brain abscess, initial therapy with ceftriaxone plus metronidazole is advised. In patients with prolonged neutropenia without corticosteroids or lymphocyte-depleting agents, voriconazole should be added. Voriconazole has important drug–drug interactions with certain antiseizure agents (e.g., phenytoin). In allogeneic HSCT recipients and other patients with severe T-cell impairment or high-dose corticosteroids, addition of high-dose TMP/SMX should be considered to cover toxoplasmosis and nocardiosis, pending a definitive diagnosis. In an analysis of 86 patients with CNS aspergillosis treated with voriconazole either as primary or salvage therapy, 34% had a complete or partial response.[154]

Toxoplasmosis. Reactivation of *Toxoplasma gondii* may cause life-threatening disease in patients with profound deficits in T-cell immunity. Risk factors include therapy with corticosteroids, alemtuzumab, cytotoxic agents and/or radiation therapy, and poorly controlled malignancy. Toxoplasmosis is an uncommon complication of HSCT, occurring in <1% of patients, nearly all seropositive prior to transplantation. It tends to occur in the presence of moderate to severe GVHD (median day of onset of disease was 64 days after HSCT).[229,230]

CNS disease with altered mental status, coma, seizures, cranial nerve abnormalities, and motor weakness are the most common findings.[231] MRI typically shows two or more lesions that may be ring-enhancing (Fig. 132.5). The differential diagnosis

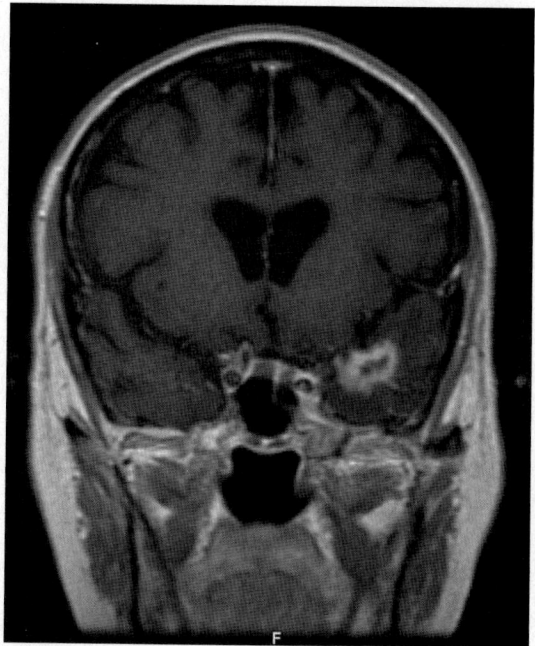
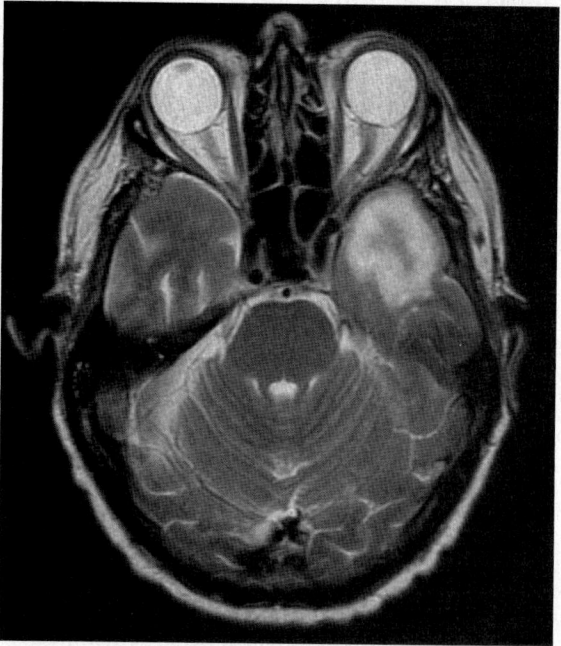

Figure 132.5 Toxoplasmosis. A 58-year-old man developed seizures and aphasia 8 months after allogeneic stem cell transplant for chronic Epstein-Barr virus lymphoproliferative disorder. Brain biopsy showed toxoplasmosis. **(A)** Coronal T1-weighted image shows a necrotic lesion in the left anterior temporal lobe. **(B)** Axial T2-weighted image shows significant edema. The magnetic resonance imaging differential diagnosis included infection, lymphoma, and glioma.

includes bacterial infection, IA, nocardiosis, and malignancy. Differentiating toxoplasmosis from lymphoma is particularly difficult; 18-fluorodeoxyglucose positron emission tomography typically shows increased metabolism in lymphoma.[232] CSF in toxoplasmosis is usually normal; however, a mononuclear pleocytosis and elevated protein may be seen. Besides the CNS, other organs may also be involved (myocarditis, interstitial pneumonitis, culture-negative sepsis, and hemophagocytic syndrome have been described). Although definitive diagnosis of toxoplasmosis relies on demonstration of tachyzoites and cysts in histopathologic sections, PCR applied to serum and CSF has become widely used and may facilitate earlier diagnosis.[229,233] The initial treatment of choice for toxoplasmosis is TMP/SMX or the combination of sulfadiazine and pyrimethamine. Folinic acid (10 to 20 mg daily) should be administered to reduce myeloid toxicity. In patients intolerant of sulfonamides, clindamycin and primaquine may be used instead after verifying normal glucose-6-phosphate dehydrogenase activity. Atovaquone has also been used after exhausting other options.

JC Virus Encephalopathy.

PML is a demyelinating disease associated with lytic infection of oligodendrocytes by the human polyomavirus JC virus. Patients may develop rapidly progressive dementia as well as focal motor or cerebellar findings. PML is occasionally seen in immunocompromised persons with hematologic malignancies and in HSCT recipients. Several cases associated with the use of rituximab[29] have prompted an advisory by the FDA regarding a possible association. There may also be an association with mycophenolate mofetil, an agent used sometimes for GVHD. MRI typically shows multiple white matter lesions without mass effect or enhancement. Diagnosis is generally established by detection of the JC virus in spinal fluid by PCR (90% sensitivity); if the PCR is negative, brain biopsy should be obtained. There is no established therapy for PML. In patients with AIDS, highly active antiretroviral therapy is the best option. By extrapolation, it is logical to try to reduce immunosuppressive therapy in persons with cancer and PML as a means of augmenting cell-mediated immunity. There are reports of improvement following the use of the antidepressant mirtazapine, which may interfere with virus entry.[234]

Genitourinary Infections

Neutropenic patients with a urinary tract infection are less likely to show pyuria and are far more likely to become bacteremic compared with nonneutropenic patients. We usually treat asymptomatic bacteriuria during neutropenia, although evidence is lacking. Asymptomatic candiduria is common in patients with bladder catheters. Removal of indwelling bladder catheters and cessation of antibacterial agents frequently leads to clearing of candiduria. Therefore, routine treatment of asymptomatic candiduria is not warranted. However, because of the risk of candidemia following genitourinary tract manipulations, candiduria should be treated before such procedures are performed. Candiduria should be treated in neutropenic patients with fever because of the possibility of occult invasive candidiasis.

Genitourinary Infections Related to Instrumentation or Devices

The American College of Radiology provides guidance to determine the appropriateness of interventions.[210] Relief of malignant obstruction of the urinary tract is best described in the context of gynecologic malignancy.[235] Acute fever (10.3% to 15%) and pyelonephritis (5.9% to 3.8%) are common, respectively, for internal ureteral stent and percutaneous nephrostomy (no significant difference by procedure). Sepsis and bacteremia are common events in the placement of stents or percutaneous nephrostomy tubes when the urinary tract is infected, with septic shock in 7% to 9% of cases of pyonephrosis.[236] No clear evidence favors any type of device, and

although prophylactic antibiotics are recommended, evidence for efficacy in preventing infection-related complications is lacking.[237]

Cystitis.

Hemorrhagic cystitis is a common consequence of some cytotoxic regimens, particularly cyclophosphamide. A viral etiology should be considered in HSCT recipients and other immunocompromised patients with unexplained hematuria. The polyomavirus BK, adenovirus, and, rarely, CMV have been associated with hemorrhagic cystitis. Adenovirus hemorrhagic cystitis is usually self-limited, and the value of antiviral therapy is unclear. It is recommended to consider the possibility of adenovirus-related obstructive uropathy, hemorrhagic nephritis, and disseminated adenovirus disease.[238] Low-dose cidofovir is sometimes used with the aim of preventing disseminated adenovirus disease.[239] BK virus commonly reactivates after allogeneic HSCT, but only a minority of patients develop hemorrhagic cystitis; high plasma viral load correlates with risk of both BK virus–associated hemorrhagic cystitis and the less commonly seen BK nephropathy.[240,241] A retrospective study suggested that low-dose cidofovir may be effective therapy for BK virus–associated hemorrhagic cystitis,[242] but the disease tends to be self-limited, so the study is inconclusive.

MULTIDRUG RESISTANT ORGANISMS OF INTEREST IN ONCOLOGY

Patients being treated for malignancy or undergoing HSCT are particularly vulnerable to health-care–associated infections. Gram-negative bacterial resistance in particular is a rising challenge that threatens to undermine outcomes of cancer therapy.[243] Twenty percent of nosocomial infections in the United States are caused by multidrug-resistant bacteria.[244] The proportions are even higher in some European and Asian countries.[245] In fact, receipt of health care outside the United States is associated with carriage of highly antibiotic-resistant gram-negative organisms.

Multidrug resistant organisms (MDRO) not only cause serious infections, but leave patients colonized, often for months.[246–248] Colonization refers to asymptomatic carriage on or in the body, without bacterial invasion. MRSA tends to colonize the nares and skin, while VRE and gram-negative bacteria colonize the intestinal tract. Colonization with multidrug-resistant bacteria can hasten death in patients who are already seriously ill with malignancy or HSCT. Under conditions that impair gut mucosal integrity (such as chemotherapy, GVHD, and other causes of colitis), the organisms colonizing the intestinal tract can invade and cause bloodstream or device-associated infections.[249,250] Patients with cancer who develop infections with MDROs have a substantially higher mortality rate than those who have infections with susceptible strains of the same bacteria, due in part to misdirected empiric therapy.[251–253]

Multidrug-resistant bacteria are shed by colonized patients and spread via the health-care environment, hands of health-care personnel, and contaminated equipment. Patients with hematologic malignancies and HSCT are particularly vulnerable to acquisition of certain MDROs because immune suppression, receipt of broad-spectrum antibiotics, and prolonged hospitalization. In addition, patients undergoing HSCT have significant derangement of their intestinal microbiota that diminish colonization resistance and allow long-term establishment of MDROs in the abnormal intestinal flora.[254]

Multidrug-Resistant Gram-Positive Bacteria

Methicillin-Resistant *Staphylococcus Aureus*

MRSA is commonly acquired in the community as well as in health-care facilities, and causes primarily skin and soft tissue infections, central line–associated bloodstream infections, and pneumonia. MRSA has declined in frequency as a cause of invasive infections in hospitalized adults,[255–257] due in part to widespread MRSA surveillance and infection control efforts, as well as improvements in central line care.[256] Nonetheless, MRSA bloodstream infections carry a high mortality rate in patients with cancer.[258] The IDSA has published guidelines for the treatment of MRSA.[259] Though resistant to penicillins and cephalosporins, MRSA is typically susceptible to several oral and intravenous antibiotics. However, recommended empirical therapy for fever and neutropenia does not cover MRSA unless the patient is known to be colonized or presents with sepsis or pneumonia.[74] The value of screening patients before administering cytotoxic chemotherapy has not been addressed recently. Preoperative screening for MRSA and treatment with nasal mupirocin and chlorhexidine gluconate baths prior to oncologic surgery may reduce the risk of postoperative MRSA infection, though this measure has not been studied in a multicenter clinical trial.[260,261] Besides the ongoing relevance of health-care–associated MRSA, there has been a dramatic increase in the incidence of community-acquired MRSA.[262] Community-acquired MRSA strains are generally susceptible to clindamycin, doxycycline, and TMP/SMX. The standard treatment for severe MRSA infections is vancomycin. Vancomycin-intermediate and vancomycin-resistant MRSA is rare.[263] However, vancomycin failure in MRSA bacteremia has been associated with increasing vancomycin minimum inhibitory concentrations well within what is currently considered the susceptible range.[264] Based on these observations, new guidelines on vancomycin dosing and therapeutic monitoring have been published.[265] Minimum serum vancomycin trough concentrations should always be maintained above 10 mg/L to avoid development of resistance.

Linezolid seems at least as effective as vancomycin against MRSA in most published studies,[266,267] and American Thoracic Society guidelines consider both linezolid and high-dose vancomycin (trough level of vancomycin of 15 to 20 mcg/ml) to be acceptable options for suspected or proven MRSA pneumonia. The major concern of linezolid in patients with cancer relates to duration-dependent marrow suppression. Short courses of linezolid appear to delay myeloid recovery only modestly in neutropenic patients with cancer[87]; however, experience with long durations of therapy (e.g., >14 days) is limited. Peripheral and optic neuropathies have also been described with prolonged linezolid administration. Daptomycinis an acceptable option for *S. aureus* bacteremia and MRSA, based on the results of randomized controlled trials.[268,269] Daptomycin is inactivated by lung surfactant and therefore should not be used to treat pneumonia.

Vancomycin-Resistant Enterococcus

VRE is a ubiquitous pathogen in hematology-oncology units. Once colonized, patients can carry VRE for many months, and, as with other colonizing multidrug-resistant pathogens, can cause bloodstream and device-related infections.[270] Patients acquire VRE in health-care facilities, where 30% of nosocomial enterococcal infections are attributable to VRE. The bacteria are hardy and tenacious in the environment, and easily establish colonization in HSCT patients who have had major shifts in intestinal flora due to antibiotics and other aspects of their therapy.[271] Although VRE are less virulent than MRSA and many other MDROs, they can still cause lethal bloodstream infections in immunocompromised patients.[272] Screening for VRE in this high-prevalence population allows for implementation of isolation precautions to limit further spread as well as more effective empiric therapy for fever and neutropenia or sepsis.[272] VREs are resistant to vancomycin and usually ampicillin, but are typically susceptible to at least two other intravenous or oral antibiotics, linezolid, and daptomycin; resistance to those has been reported and may be increasing, making prevention even more crucial.[273] Tigecycline often shows activity in vitro, but there are no good data on efficacy in clinical practice. Quinupristin/dalfopristin is a 30:70 mixture of these two semisynthetic streptogramin antibiotics. It has been shown to be safe and effective in serious

vancomycin-resistant *Enterococcus faecium* infections, but is not active against *E. faecalis*. One randomized controlled trial comparing treatments for VRE bacteremia showed that both quinupristin/ dalfopristin and linezolid have similar (moderate) efficacy.[274] The reported results with daptomycin seem to be similar.[275]

Clostridium difficile

Epidemiology. The incidence of *C. difficile* infection (CDI) has risen steadily since the early 2000s, when a new, hypervirulent strain emerged and became widespread and predominant in many North America hospitals.[276] Since the emergence of the B1/NAP1 strain, the incidence of *C. difficile* has more than quadrupled, resulting in >300,000 infections and 10,000 deaths per year. Hospitalized patients with cancer develop CDI at twice the rate of other inpatients.[270] The reported incidence is highest in allo-HSCT, followed by auto-HSCT and hematologic malignancies, and lower in solid tumors.[270,277–281] Patients with malignancy develop *C. difficile* due to their exposure to the chief risk factors: antibiotics, chemotherapy, neutropenia, advanced age, and hospitalization. Proton pump inhibitors have been implicated as a risk factor, but the evidence is weak.[282]

Diagnosis. *C. difficile* produces exotoxins that cause colitis with a wide spectrum of severity. Mild disease is characterized by diarrhea and abdominal pain; patients with severe infection can become systemically ill, requiring intensive care and, occasionally, emergency colectomy. The disease may occur in outpatients, and patients may develop infection weeks after hospital discharge,[283] or in the absence of hospitalization. Diagnosis is made via detection of bacterial toxin in diarrhea stool by enzyme immunoassay, PCR, or cytotoxin assay.[284,285] Multistep testing using a less specific screening test followed by PCR testing of positive samples is used in some centers for cost savings. Among these methods, PCR is by far the most sensitive and specific, and its use is expanding.[286] *C. difficile* assays should only be applied to diarrheal stools or, in patients presenting with ileus, a swab, in order to avoid detecting asymptomatic carriage.[284,285] Repeat testing by PCR is not necessary, but repeat enzyme immunoassay tests may identify additional cases following a single negative assay in a high-risk patient.[176]

Treatment. Because *C. difficile* is an antibiotic-associated infection, discontinuation of antibiotics, if possible, may improve the chance of cure and reduce risk of recurrence. The American guidelines from the Society for Healthcare Epidemiology of America and the IDSA suggest an expert-opinion clinical classification of the severity of CDI as mild/moderate, severe, and severe/complicated based on leucocytosis, renal dysfunction, and the presence of hypotension, shock, or toxic megacolon.[285] How applicable these criteria would be to cancer patients is unknown. The initial therapy is targeted to the severity: oral vancomycin is recommended for severe *C. difficile*, and metronidazole (oral or intravenous) for initial episodes of mild to moderate infection.[285] A 10- to 14-day course of metronidazole is recommended for mild to moderate infection because of its lower cost and efficacy equivalent to vancomycin for nonsevere disease.[287] There is no need to send additional toxin assays as tests of cure during or following treatment unless there is renewed diarrhea that raises concern for relapse. Severe infection is treated with a 10- to 14-day course of oral vancomycin due to possible higher efficacy in severe cases.[287] Complicated infection leading to critical illness or toxic megacolon is treated with vancomycin administered both orally and per rectum, as well as intravenous metronidazole[285]; patients with fulminant infection may require emergency colectomy. A first recurrence, or second episode, of CDI is typically treated with the same therapy as the first episode, depending on the disease severity. Further recurrences are often treated with progressively long courses and tapers of oral vancomycin, although there are no randomized trials to support the practice.[285] Fidaxomicin, a newer antibiotic, is equivalent to vancomycin in improving symptoms of infection, and may achieve a more enduring cure than vancomycin.[288–291] Patients who have recurrent or refractory infection are treated with fecal microbiota (stool) transplantation, which has a cure rate of at least 80% to 90%.[292,293] This approach has not been routinely attempted in patients with hematologic malignancies.

Probiotics are popular, due in part to the perception that they are harmless and may help prevent initial or recurrent CDI. Although *Lactobacillus* spp. and *Saccharomyces* spp. at varying doses are marketed for these purposes, benefits seen in clinical trials have been inconsistent.[294,295] Furthermore, probiotics must be used with caution in hospitalizedd patients, as both *Lactobacillus* and *Saccharomyces* can translocate from the intestinal tract and cause bloodstream infections in immunocompromised or critically ill patients.[296–298]

Outcome. The majority of patients experience mild to moderate infection, of whom >90% recover when treated with a standard regimen[287]; a significant minority, in particular those who are infected with the B1/NAP1 strain, develop severe disease, often requiring intensive care or emergency colectomy. About 20% to 30% of patients experience relapse,[289] usually within 2 weeks and at approximately equivalent rates among those treated with metronidazole or vancomycin.[299] Relepse rate may be lower in patents treated with fidaxomicin.[289] About 40% of relapsed patients experience additional relapses of infection. A smaller proportion develop refractory disease. Advanced age and continued antibiotic therapy are risk factors for severe, recurrent, and refractory infection.

Patients with cancer have a lower rate of cure and double the time to resolution of symptoms than other patients, but do not have a higher mortality rate from CDI.[278,289,300] HSCT recipients do not experience more severe disease than control patients, and do not have higher mortality than other HSCT patients. Among allo-HSCT recipients, there may be a self-reinforcing cycle between CDI and intestinal GVHD. Gut GVHD is a risk factor for CDI,[278,279] and CDI is strongly associated with subsequent development of gastrointestinal GVHD.[279,301] Allogeneic HSCT patients may also be more vulnerable to bloodstream infections following CDI, possibly due to further impairment of intestinal mucosal integrity.[301]

Prevention. Implementation of facility-wide antimicrobial stewardship programs has been shown to reduce rates of CDI in healthcare facilities and can reduce rates among cancer patients.[302] Several risk factors for CDI (e.g., broad-spectrum antibiotics) may not be modifiable in patients with malignancy and HSCT recipients. However, evidence suggests that much of the CDI that occurs in hospitals is transmitted from other patients via health-care personnel or from the hospital environment. *C. difficile* spores are extremely hardy and remain viable in the health-care environment for weeks to months. Hospitalized patients who experience recurrences of CDI are often reinfected with different strains, possibly from contamination in the health-care environment.[303] Infection control precautions can contribute significantly to prevention and control of *C. difficile* spread within a health-care facility.[304] Empirical isolation of patients while tests for diarrheal pathogens are pending is essential to prevent spread of *C. difficile* and other pathogens from patient to patient, as is effective disinfection of hospital rooms when patients are discharged or have recovered from infection.[285,305] Strict adherence to isolation precautions (glove, gown, and hand hygiene) is crucial.[33] Hand hygiene with soap and water in lieu of alcohol-based hand gel will achieve superior removal of *C. difficile* spores.[306]

Multidrug-Resistant Gram-Negative Bacteria

Extended-Spectrum Beta Lactamase–Producing and Carbapenem-Resistant Enteric Bacteria

Multidrug-resistant gram-negative enteric pathogens, such as *Klebsiella*, *E. coli*, and *Enterobacter*, are of great concern due to both increasing prevalence and increasing risk of treatment failure among oncology and HSCT patients.[243] Enteric bacteria are common causes of bloodstream infections, device-related infections, and deep surgical site infections. Many gram-negative bacteria are resistant to fluoroquinolones, particularly in patients who have received fluoroquinolone prophylaxis.[38,307,308] Extended-spectrum beta lactamase–producing gram-negative enteric bacteria are generally resistant to all cephalosporins and most or all penicillins. For extended-spectrum beta lactamase–producing enteric bacteria, carbapenems are the treatment of choice, but a post hoc study suggests that piperacillin-tazobactam may be used successfully.[309] Unfortunately, resistance to carbapenems is becoming more prevalent. A rapidly expanding subset of carbapenem-resistant bacteria carry a plasmid-mediated carbapenemase enzyme that hydrolyzes the antibiotic.[310] Gram-negative enteric bacteria that have carbapenem resistance may require treatment with nephrotoxic and neurotoxic drug combinations including aminoglycosides and colistin. The dearth of additional effective antibiotics leads to frequent treatment failure even when patients are treated with antibiotic combinations. These pathogens are readily transmitted in hospital wards, and bloodstream infections carry a mortality rate of >50% in hematology-oncology patient populations.[311–313] There are no prospective comparative data to support any particular antibiotic regimen. Frequently, a carbapenem like doripenem is administered together with colistin and tigecycline. Prolonged infusion of meropenem may result in systemic levels above the minimum inhibitory concentration of some bacteria[314,315]; alternatively, it is possible the presence of carbapenem results in synergy.[316]

Pseudomonas Aeruginosa

P. aeruginosa continues to be frequently documented during neutropenic fever.[317] Many cases of *P. aeruginosa* bacteremia now occur in outpatients.[318,319] *Pseudomonas* also causes device-related infections and surgical site infections in patients with solid tumor malignancies. No single antimicrobial is effective against 100% of *Pseudomonas* isolates, which is the reason most authorities recommend combining an antipseudomonal β-lactam antibiotic and an aminoglycoside until results of susceptibility testing become available.[320] Isolates of *P. aeruginosa* in colonized patients who receive antibiotics frequently develop progressive resistance to those antibiotics,[321] resulting in limited treatment options. Approximately 13% of nosocomial *P. aeruginosa* infections are multidrug resistant. Colistin administered parenterally[322] or aerosolized (in infections limited to the lung)[323–325] may be considered as salvage therapy. The continuous infusion of ceftazidime or other β-lactam antibiotics has also been used in attempts to prevent or overcome the emergence of resistance during therapy.[326–328]

Other multidrug-resistant pathogens that are occasional causes of nosocomial infection or even hospital outbreaks include waterborne organisms such as *Acinetobacter baumannii* and *S. maltophilia*. These bacteria can cause bloodstream infections and device-related infections, and can colonize the gastrointestinal tract, skin, and respiratory tract of immunocompromised or critically ill patients. *Acinetobacter* is a pathogen that has become endemic in many health-care facilities.[329] Susceptible strains of *Acinetobacter* are found in water and soil, but health-care–associated isolates are frequently resistant to many classes of antibiotics, often including carbapenems.[330] Although *Acinetobacter* causes 2% to 7% of health-care–associated infections, 63% of *Acinetobacter* isolates are multidrug resistant. *Stenotrophomonas* isolates are intrinsically resistant to carbapenems and cephalosporins, and may be selected out by prior use of broad-spectrum antibiotics, particularly carbapenems.[331] The majority of strains are susceptible to TMP/SMX, which is the preferred initial antibiotic. If TMP/SMX cannot be used, there have been reports of success with ticarcillin-clavulanic acid and fluoroquinolones (particularly moxifloxacin). Tigecycline and colistin are often active in vitro.

The grave danger posed by some highly antibiotic-resistant bacteria to immunocompromised patients warrants heightened infection control efforts to prevent nosocomial acquisition of the pathogens. Surveillance efforts should be targeted identifying patient colonization with the most highly prevalent (e.g., VRE) or most clinically significant pathogens (e.g., carbapenemase-producing enteric bacteria). Rapid molecular assays that detect MRSA, VRE, and some carbapenem-resistant enteric bacteria have lowered the barrier to identification of colonized patients. Once identified, colonized patients are isolated in order to prevent transmission. Meticulous adherence to isolation precautions, rigorous hand hygiene, and effective environmental disinfection are essential to prevent transmission from colonized patients who are isolated and those whose colonization has not yet been discovered. In addition to the infection control rationale, knowledge of MDRO colonization status offers clinicians a chance to tailor empiric antimicrobial therapy to cover the most likely potential pathogens. Important drawbacks of surveillance and isolation are the adverse social and patient safety consequences of isolation.[332]

Several other measures aid in the effort to prevent nosocomial spread of multidrug-resistant pathogens. Improved antimicrobial stewardship both in health-care facilities and the community have been shown to reduce rates of colonization with resistant bacteria. Chlorhexidine gluconate 2% daily baths have been demonstrated repeatedly to reduce the risk of acquisition of multidrug-resistant bacteria, in addition to reducing rates of central line–associated bloodstream infections.[333] This intervention carries an extremely small risk of severe skin reaction and a potential risk of selecting out chlorhexidine-resistant skin flora.[333] Finally, minimizing the duration of use of invasive devices such as central venous lines and urinary catheters reduces the opportunities for introduction of multidrug-resistant bacteria, and therefore the risk of serious infection.

A number of multidrug-resistant bacteria threaten oncology and HSCT patients, who are vulnerable because of impaired immunity, antibiotic use, and frequent contact with the health-care system. Measures to prevent acquisition of these bacteria are essential given the increasing complexity and declining success of managing infections with the most highly resistant pathogens.

SELECTED REFERENCES

The full reference list can be accessed at lwwhealthlibrary.com/oncology.

1. Spinner MA, Sanchez LA, Hsu AP, et al. GATA2 deficiency: a protean disorder of hematopoiesis, lymphatics and immunity. *Blood* 2014;123:809–821.
2. Kalhs P, Panzer S, Kletter K, et al. Functional asplenia after bone marrow transplantation. A late complication related to extensive chronic graft-versus-host disease. *Ann Intern Med* 1988;109:461–464.
3. National Center for Immunization and Respiratory Diseases. General recommendations on immunization — recommendations of the Advisory Committee on Immunization Practices (ACIP). *MMWR Recomm Rep* 2011;60:1–64.
7. Fukuda T, Boeckh M, Carter RA, et al. Risks and outcomes of invasive fungal infections in recipients of allogeneic hematopoietic stem cell transplants after nonmyeloablative conditioning. *Blood* 2003;102:827–833.
13. Salvana EM, Salata RA. Infectious complications associated with monoclonal antibodies and related small molecules. *Clin Microbiol Rev* 2009;22:274–290, Table of Contents.
15. Gea-Banacloche JC. Rituximab-associated infections. *Semin Hematol* 2010; 47:187–198.
19. Martin SI, Marty FM, Fiumara K, et al. Infectious complications associated with alemtuzumab use for lymphoproliferative disorders. *Clin Infect Dis* 2006;43:16–24.
24. Koo S, Marty FM, Baden LR. Infectious complications associated with immunomodulating biologic agents. *Hematol Oncol Clin North Am* 2011;25:117–138.
28. Jalan P, Mahajan A, Pandav V, et al. Brentuximab associated progressive multifocal leukoencephalopathy. *Clin Neurol Neurosurg* 2012;114:1335–1337.
30. Hapani S, Chu D, Wu S. Risk of gastrointestinal perforation in patients with cancer treated with bevacizumab: a meta-analysis. *Lancet Oncol* 2009;10:559–568.
33. Tomblyn M, Chiller T, Einsele H, et al. Guidelines for preventing infectious complications among hematopoietic cell transplantation recipients: a global perspective. *Biol Blood Marrow Transplant* 2009;15:1143–1238.
35. National Comprehensive Cancer Network. Prevention and Treatment of Cancer-Related Infections V 1.2013. http://www.nccn.org/professionals/physician_gls/f_guidelines.asp. Accessed May 18, 2014.
37. Gafter-Gvili A, Fraser A, Paul M, et al. Meta-analysis: antibiotic prophylaxis reduces mortality in neutropenic patients. *Ann Intern Med* 2005;142:979–995.
40. Bucaneve G, Micozzi A, Menichetti F, et al. Levofloxacin to prevent bacterial infection in patients with cancer and neutropenia. *N Engl J Med* 2005;353:977–987.
42. Slavin MA, Lingaratnam S, Mileshkin L, et al. Use of antibacterial prophylaxis for patients with neutropenia. Australian Consensus Guidelines 2011 Steering Committee. *Intern Med J* 2011;41:102–109.
43. Flowers CR, Seidenfeld J, Bow EJ, et al. Antimicrobial prophylaxis and outpatient management of fever and neutropenia in adults treated for malignancy: American Society of Clinical Oncology Clinical Practice Guideline. *J Clin Oncol* 2013;31:794–810.
46. Goodman JL, Winston DJ, Greenfield RA, et al. A controlled trial of fluconazole to prevent fungal infections in patients undergoing bone marrow transplantation. *N Engl J Med* 1992;326:845–851.
51. van Burik JA, Ratanatharathorn V, Stepan DE, et al. Micafungin versus fluconazole for prophylaxis against invasive fungal infections during neutropenia in patients undergoing hematopoietic stem cell transplantation. *Clin Infect Dis* 2004;39:1407–1416.
52. Cornely OA, Maertens J, Winston DJ, et al. Posaconazole vs. fluconazole or itraconazole prophylaxis in patients with neutropenia. *N Engl J Med* 2007;356:348–359.
54. Wingard JR, Carter SL, Walsh TJ, et al. Randomized, double-blind trial of fluconazole versus voriconazole for prevention of invasive fungal infection after allogeneic hematopoietic cell transplantation. *Blood* 2010;116:5111–5118.
55. Ethier MC, Science M, Beyene J, et al. Mould-active compared with fluconazole prophylaxis to prevent invasive fungal diseases in cancer patients receiving chemotherapy or haematopoietic stem-cell transplantation: a systematic review and meta-analysis of randomised controlled trials. *Br J Cancer* 2012;106:1626–1637.
59. Gea-Banacloche J, Masur H, Arns da Cunha C, et al. Regionally limited or rare infections: prevention after hematopoietic cell transplantation. *Bone Marrow Transplant* 2009;44:489–494.
62. Boeckh M, Ljungman P. How we treat cytomegalovirus in hematopoietic cell transplant recipients. *Blood* 2009;113:5711–5719.
66. Boeckh M, Gooley TA, Myerson D, et al. Cytomegalovirus pp65 antigenemia-guided early treatment with ganciclovir versus ganciclovir at engraftment after allogeneic marrow transplantation: a randomized double-blind study. *Blood* 1996;88:4063–4071.
68. European Association for the Study of the Liver. EASL clinical practice guidelines: Management of chronic hepatitis B virus infection. *J Hepatol* 2012;57:167–185.
70. Mahale P, Kontoyiannis DP, Chemaly RF, et al. Acute exacerbation and reactivation of chronic hepatitis C virus infection in cancer patients. *J Hepatol* 2012;57:1177–1185.
73. Versluis J, Pas SD, Agteresch HJ, et al. Hepatitis E virus: an underestimated opportunistic pathogen in recipients of allogeneic hematopoietic stem cell transplantation. *Blood* 2013;122:1079–1086.
74. Freifeld AG, Bow EJ, Sepkowitz KA, et al. Clinical practice guideline for the use of antimicrobial agents in neutropenic patients with cancer: 2010 update by the infectious diseases society of america. *Clin Infect Dis* 2011;52:e56–e93.
76. Averbuch D, Orasch C, Cordonnier C, et al. European guidelines for empirical antibacterial therapy for febrile neutropenic patients in the era of growing resistance: summary of the 2011 4th European Conference on Infections in Leukemia. *Haematologica* 2013;98:1826–1835.
77. Lehrnbecher T, Phillips R, Alexander S, et al. Guideline for the management of fever and neutropenia in children with cancer and/or undergoing hematopoietic stem-cell transplantation. *J Clin Oncol* 2012;30:4427–4438.
79. Klastersky J, Paesmans M. The Multinational Association for Supportive Care in Cancer (MASCC) risk index score: 10 years of use for identifying low-risk febrile neutropenic cancer patients. *Support Care Cancer* 2013;21:1487–1495.
81. Kern WV, Marchetti O, Drgona L, et al. Oral antibiotics for fever in low-risk neutropenic patients with cancer: a double-blind, randomized, multicenter trial comparing single daily moxifloxacin with twice daily ciprofloxacin plus amoxicillin/clavulanic acid combination therapy—EORTC infectious diseases group trial XV. *J Clin Oncol* 2013;31:1149–1156.
82. Bow EJ. Neutropenic fever syndromes in patients undergoing cytotoxic therapy for acute leukemia and myelodysplastic syndromes. *Semin Hematol* 2009;46:259–268.
92. Pizzo PA, Robichaud KJ, Gill FA, et al. Empiric antibiotic and antifungal therapy for cancer patients with prolonged fever and granulocytopenia. *Am J Med* 1982;72:101–111.

93. Empiric antifungal therapy in febrile granulocytopenic patients. EORTC International Antimicrobial Therapy Cooperative Group. *Am J Med* 1989; 86:668–672.

95. Walsh TJ, Teppler H, Donowitz GR, et al. Caspofungin versus liposomal amphotericin B for empirical antifungal therapy in patients with persistent fever and neutropenia. *N Engl J Med* 2004;351:1391–1402.

98. Cordonnier C, Pautas C, Maury S, et al. Empirical versus preemptive antifungal therapy for high-risk, febrile, neutropenic patients: a randomized, controlled trial. *Clin Infect Dis* 2009;48:1042–1051.

100. Maschmeyer G, Heinz WJ, Hertenstein B, et al. Immediate versus deferred empirical antifungal (IDEA) therapy in high-risk patients with febrile neutropenia: a randomized, double-blind, placebo-controlled, multicenter study. *Eur J Clin Microbiol Infect Dis* 2013;32:679–689.

103. Miceli MH, Maertens J, Buvé K, et al. Immune reconstitution inflammatory syndrome in cancer patients with pulmonary aspergillosis recovering from neutropenia: Proof of principle, description, and clinical and research implications. *Cancer* 2007;110:112–120.

104. Spitzer TR. Engraftment syndrome following hematopoietic stem cell transplantation. *Bone Marrow Transplant* 2001;27:893–898.

106. Pappas PG, Kauffman CA, Andes D, et al. Clinical practice guidelines for the management of candidiasis: 2009 update by the Infectious Diseases Society of America. *Clin Infect Dis* 2009;48:503–535.

107. Walsh TJ, Anaissie EJ, Denning DW, et al. Treatment of aspergillosis: Clinical practice guidelines of the Infectious Diseases Society of America. *Clin Infect Dis* 2008;46:327–360.

113. Maertens J, Maertens V, Theunissen K, et al. Bronchoalveolar lavage fluid galactomannan for the diagnosis of invasive pulmonary aspergillosis in patients with hematologic diseases. *Clin Infect Dis* 2009;49:1688–1693.

116. Lamoth F, Cruciani M, Mengoli C, et al. β-Glucan antigenemia assay for the diagnosis of invasive fungal infections in patients with hematological malignancies: a systematic review and meta-analysis of cohort studies from the Third European Conference on Infections in Leukemia (ECIL-3). *Clin Infect Dis* 2012;54:633–643.

122. Herbrecht R, Denning DW, Patterson TF, et al. Voriconazole versus amphotericin B for primary therapy of invasive aspergillosis. *N Engl J Med* 2002;347:408–415.

124. Cornely OA, Maertens J, Bresnik M, et al. Liposomal amphotericin B as initial therapy for invasive mold infection: a randomized trial comparing a high-loading dose regimen with standard dosing (AmBiLoad trial). *Clin Infect Dis* 2007; 44:1289–1297.

127. Hope WW, Billaud EM, Lestner J, et al. Therapeutic drug monitoring for triazoles. *Curr Opin Infect Dis* 2008;21:580–586.

129. Roden MM, Zaoutis TE, Buchanan WL, et al. Epidemiology and outcome of zygomycosis: a review of 929 reported cases. *Clin Infect Dis* 2005;41: 634–653.

132. Walsh TJ, Groll A, Hiemenz J, et al. Infections due to emerging and uncommon medically important fungal pathogens. *Clin Microbiol Infect* 2004;10:48–66.

133. Aapro MS, Bohlius J, Cameron DA, et al. 2010 update of EORTC guidelines for the use of granulocyte-colony stimulating factor to reduce the incidence of chemotherapy-induced febrile neutropenia in adult patients with lymphoproliferative disorders and solid tumours. *Eur J Cancer* 2011;47:8–32.

134. Smith TJ, Khatcheressian J, Lyman GH, et al. 2006 update of recommendations for the use of white blood cell growth factors: an evidence-based clinical practice guideline. *J Clin Oncol* 2006;24:3187–3205.

137. Gea-Banacloche J. Granulocyte transfusions: where is the controversy? *Cytotherapy* 2011;13:389–390.

139. Quillen K, Wong E, Scheinberg P, et al. Granulocyte transfusions in severe aplastic anemia: an eleven-year experience. *Haematologica* 2009;94: 1661–1668.

145. DesJardin JA, Falagas ME, Ruthazer R, et al. Clinical utility of blood cultures drawn from indwelling central venous catheters in hospitalized patients with cancer. *Ann Intern Med* 1999;131:641–647.

146. Mermel LA, Allon M, Bouza E, et al. Clinical practice guidelines for the diagnosis and management of intravascular catheter-related infection: 2009 Update by the Infectious Diseases Society of America. *Clin Infect Dis* 2009;49:1–45.

148. Schiffer CA, Mangu PB, Wade JC, et al. Central venous catheter care for the patient with cancer: American Society of Clinical Oncology clinical practice guideline. *J Clin Oncol* 2013;31:1357–1370.

154. Blot F, Nitenberg G, Chachaty E, et al. Diagnosis of catheter-related bacteraemia: a prospective comparison of the time to positivity of hub-blood versus peripheral-blood cultures. *Lancet* 1999;354:1071–1077.

156. Raad I, Hanna HA, Alakech B, et al. Differential time to positivity: a useful method for diagnosing catheter-related bloodstream infections. *Ann Intern Med* 2004;140:18–25.

157. Freeman JT, Elinder-Camburn A, McClymont C, et al. Central line-associated bloodstream infections in adult hematology patients with febrile neutropenia: an evaluation of surveillance definitions using differential time to blood culture positivity. *Infect Control Hosp Epidemiol* 2013;34: 89–92.

158. Peterson DE, Bensadoun RJ, Roila F, et al. Management of oral and gastrointestinal mucositis: ESMO Clinical Practice Guidelines. *Ann Oncol* 2011;22:vi78–vi84.

162. See I, Iwamoto M, Allen-Bridson K, et al. Mucosal barrier injury laboratory-confirmed bloodstream infection: results from a field test of a new National Healthcare Safety Network definition. *Infect Control Hosp Epidemiol* 2013;34:769–776.

167. Schoot RA, van Dalen EC, van Ommen CH, et al. Antibiotic and other lock treatments for tunnelled central venous catheter-related infections in children with cancer. *Cochrane Database Syst Rev* 2013;6:CD008975.

169. Castagnola E, Ginocchio F. Rescue therapy of difficult-to-treat indwelling central venous catheter-related bacteremias in cancer patients: a review for practical purposes. *Expert Rev Anti Infect Ther* 2013;11:179–186.

170. Falagas ME, Vergidis PI. Narrative review: diseases that masquerade as infectious cellulitis. *Ann Intern Med* 2005;142:47–55.

171. Farmakiotis D, Ciurea AM, Cahuayme-Zuniga L, et al. The diagnostic yield of skin biopsy in patients with leukemia and suspected infection. *J Infect* 2013;67:265–272.

177. Seo S, Campbell AP, Xie H, et al. Outcome of respiratory syncytial virus lower respiratory tract disease in hematopoietic cell transplant recipients receiving aerosolized ribavirin: significance of stem cell source and oxygen requirement. *Biol Blood Marrow Transplant* 2013;19:589–596.

180. Srinivasan A, Wang C, Yang J, et al. Parainfluenza virus infections in children with hematologic malignancies. *Pediatr Infect Dis J* 2011;30: 855–859.

182. Renaud C, Xie H, Seo S, et al. Mortality rates of human metapneumovirus and respiratory syncytial virus lower respiratory tract infections in hematopoietic cell transplantation recipients. *Biol Blood Marrow Transplant* 2013;19:1220–1226.

183. Schlapbach LJ, Agyeman P, Hutter D, et al. Human metapneumovirus infection as an emerging pathogen causing acute respiratory distress syndrome. *J Infect Dis* 2011;203:294–295.

186. Spreghini E, Orlando F, Giannini D, Barchiesi F. In vitro and in vivo activities of posaconazole against zygomycetes with various degrees of susceptibility. *J Antimicrob Chemother* 2010;65:2158–2163.

194. Brown-Elliott BA, Brown JM, Conville PS, et al. Clinical and laboratory features of the Nocardia spp. based on current molecular taxonomy. *Clin Microbiol Rev* 2006;19:259–282.

199. Azoulay E, Bergeron A, Chevret S, et al. Polymerase chain reaction for diagnosing pneumocystis pneumonia in non-HIV immunocompromised patients with pulmonary infiltrates. *Chest* 2009;135:655–661.

200. Karageorgopoulos DE, Qu JM, Korbila IP, et al. Accuracy of β-D-glucan for the diagnosis of Pneumocystis jirovecii pneumonia: a meta-analysis. *Clin Microbiol Infect* 2013;19:39–49.

204. Milpied N, Vasseur B, Parquet N, et al. Humanized anti-CD20 monoclonal antibody (Rituximab) in post transplant B-lymphoproliferative disorder: a retrospective analysis on 32 patients. *Ann Oncol* 2000;11:113–116.

206. Kirkpatrick ID, Greenberg HM. Gastrointestinal complications in the neutropenic patient: characterization and differentiation with abdominal CT. *Radiology* 2003;226:668–674.

207. Lehrnbecher T, Marshall D, Gao C, et al. A second look at anorectal infections in cancer patients in a large cancer institute: the success of early intervention with antibiotics and surgery. *Infection* 2002;30:272–276.

209. Sharma P, Kozarek R, Practice Parameters Committee of American College of Gastroenterology. Role of esophageal stents in benign and malignant diseases. *Am J Gastroenterol* 2010;105:258–273, quiz 274.

210. Ray CEJ, Lorenz JM, Burke CT, et al. ACR Appropriateness Criteria radiologic management of benign and malignant biliary obstruction. *J Am Coll Radiol* 2013;10:567–574.

212. van der Gaag NA, Rauws EA, van Eijck CH, et al. Preoperative biliary drainage for cancer of the head of the pancreas. *N Engl J Med* 2010;362:129–137.

214. Paik WH, Park YS, Hwang JH, et al. Palliative treatment with self-expandable metallic stents in patients with advanced type III or IV hilar cholangiocarcinoma: a percutaneous versus endoscopic approach. *Gastrointest Endosc* 2009;69:55–62.

218. Conen A, Walti LN, Merlo A, et al. Characteristics and treatment outcome of cerebrospinal fluid shunt-associated infections in adults: a retrospective analysis over an 11-year period. *Clin Infect Dis* 2008;47:73–82.

220. Hill CS, Luoma AM, Wilson SR, et al. Titanium cranioplasty and the prediction of complications. *Br J Neurosurg* 2012;26:832–837.

221. Tunkel AR, Hartman BJ, Kaplan SL, et al. Practice guidelines for the management of bacterial meningitis. *Clin Infect Dis* 2004;39:1267–1284.

222. Tunkel AR, Glaser CA, Bloch KC, et al. The management of encephalitis: clinical practice guidelines by the Infectious Diseases Society of America. *Clin Infect Dis* 2008;47:303–327.

223. Ljungman P, de la Camara R, Cordonnier C, et al. Management of CMV, HHV-6, HHV-7 and Kaposi-sarcoma herpesvirus (HHV-8) infections in patients with hematological malignancies and after SCT. *Bone Marrow Transplant* 2008;42:227–240.

229. Martino R, Bretagne S, Einsele H, et al. Early detection of Toxoplasma infection by molecular monitoring of Toxoplasma gondii in peripheral blood samples after allogeneic stem cell transplantation. *Clin Infect Dis* 2005; 40:67–78.

234. Yoshida H, Ohshima K, Toda J, et al. Significant improvement following combination treatment with mefloquine and mirtazapine in a patient with progressive multifocal leukoencephalopathy after allogeneic peripheral blood stem cell transplantation. *Int J Hematol* 2014;99:95–99.

235. Izumi K, Mizokami A, Maeda Y, et al. Current outcome of patients with ureteral stents for the management of malignant ureteral obstruction. *J Urol* 2011;185:556–561.

237. Moon E, Tam MD, Kikano RN, et al. Prophylactic antibiotic guidelines in modern interventional radiology practice. *Semin Intervent Radiol* 2010;27:327–337.

238. Mori K, Yoshihara T, Nishimura Y, et al. Acute renal failure due to adenovirus-associated obstructive uropathy and necrotizing tubulointerstitial nephritis in a bone marrow transplant recipient. *Bone Marrow Transplant* 2003;31:1173–1176.

240. Haines HL, Laskin BL, Goebel J, et al. Blood, and not urine, BK viral load predicts renal outcome in children with hemorrhagic cystitis following hematopoietic stem cell transplantation. *Biol Blood Marrow Transplant* 2011;17:1512–1519.

243. Bow EJ. There should be no ESKAPE for febrile neutropenic cancer patients: the dearth of effective antibacterial drugs threatens anticancer efficacy. *J Antimicrob Chemother* 2013;68:492–495.

244. Sievert DMP, Ricks PP, Edwards JRMS, et al. Antimicrobial-resistant pathogens associated with healthcare-associated infections: summary of data reported to the National Healthcare Safety Network at the Centers for Disease Control and Prevention, 2009–2010. *Infect Control Hosp Epidemiol* 2013;34:1–14.

248. O'Fallon E, Gautam S, D'Agata EMC. Colonization with multidrug-resistant gram-negative bacteria: prolonged duration and frequent cocolonization. *Clin Infect Dis* 2009;48:1375–1381.

252. Kang C-I, Chung DR, Ko KS, et al. Risk factors for infection and treatment outcome of extended-spectrum β-lactamase-producing Escherichia coli and Klebsiella pneumoniae bacteremia in patients with hematologic malignancy. *Ann Hematol* 2012;91:115–121.

253. Huh K, Kang C-I, Kim J, et al. Risk factors and treatment outcomes of bloodstream infection caused by extended-spectrum cephalosporin-resistant Enterobacter species in adults with cancer. *Diagn Microbiol Infect Dis* 2014;78:172–177.

256. Kallen AJ, Mu Y, Bulens S, et al. Health care–associated invasive MRSA infections, 2005-2008. *JAMA* 2010;304:641–647.

257. Iwamoto M, Mu Y, Lynfield R, et al. Trends in invasive methicillin-resistant Staphylococcus aureus infections. *Pediatrics* 2013;132:e817–e824.

259. Liu C, Bayer A, Cosgrove SE, et al. Clinical practice guidelines by the infectious diseases society of america for the treatment of methicillin-resistant Staphylococcus aureus infections in adults and children. *Clin Infect Dis* 2011;52:e18–e55.

261. Schweizer ML, Herwaldt LA. Surgical site infections and their prevention. *Curr Opin Infect Dis* 2012;25:378–384.

265. Rybak M, Lomaestro B, Rotschafer JC, et al. Therapeutic monitoring of vancomycin in adult patients: a consensus review of the American Society of Health-System Pharmacists, the Infectious Diseases Society of America, and the Society of Infectious Diseases Pharmacists. *Am J Health Syst Pharm* 2009;66:82–98.

267. Wunderink RG, Niederman MS, Kollef MH, et al. Linezolid in methicillin-resistant Staphylococcus aureus nosocomial pneumonia: a randomized, controlled study. *Clin Infect Dis* 2012;54:621–629.

268. Rehm SJ, Boucher H, Levine D, et al. Daptomycin versus vancomycin plus gentamicin for treatment of bacteraemia and endocarditis due to Staphylococcus aureus: subset analysis of patients infected with methicillin-resistant isolates. *J Antimicrob Chemother* 2008;62:1413–1421.

269. Fowler VG, Boucher HW, Corey GR, et al. Daptomycin versus standard therapy for bacteremia and endocarditis caused by Staphylococcus aureus. *N Engl J Med* 2006;355:653–665.

270. Kamboj M, Chung D, Seo SK, et al. The changing epidemiology of vancomycin-resistant Enterococcus (VRE) bacteremia in allogeneic hematopoietic stem cell transplant (HSCT) recipients. *Biol Blood Marrow Transplant* 2010;16:1576–1581.

273. Casapao AM, Kullar R, Davis SL, et al. Multicenter study of high-dose daptomycin for treatment of enterococcal infections. *Antimicrob Agents Chemother* 2013;57:4190–4196.

276. Lessa FC, Gould CV, McDonald LC. Current status of Clostridium difficile infection epidemiology. *Clin Infect Dis* 2012;55:S65–S70.

279. Alonso CD, Treadway SB, Hanna DB, et al. Epidemiology and outcomes of Clostridium difficile infections in hematopoietic stem cell transplant recipients. *Clin Infect Dis* 2012;54:1053–1063.

283. Palmore TN, Sohn S, Malak SF, et al. Risk factors for acquisition of Clostridium difficile-associated diarrhea among outpatients at a cancer hospital. *Infect Control Hosp Epidemiol* 2005;26:680–684.

284. Debast SB, Bauer MP, Kuijper EJ, et al. European Society of Clinical Microbiology and Infectious Diseases (ESCMID): update of the treatment guidance document for Clostridium difficile infection (CDI). *Clin Microbiol Infect* 2014;20:1–26.

285. Cohen SH, Gerding DN, Johnson S, et al. Clinical practice guidelines for Clostridium difficile infection in adults: 2010 update by the society for healthcare epidemiology of America (SHEA) and the infectious diseases society of America (IDSA). *Infect Control Hosp Epidemiol* 2010;31:431–455.

287. Zar FA, Bakkanagari SR, Moorthi KM, et al. A comparison of vancomycin and metronidazole for the treatment of Clostridium difficile-associated diarrhea, stratified by disease severity. *Clin Infect Dis* 2007;45:302–307.

288. Cornely OA, Crook DW, Esposito R, et al. Fidaxomicin versus vancomycin for infection with Clostridium difficile in Europe, Canada, and the USA: a double-blind, non-inferiority, randomised controlled trial. *Lancet Infect Dis* 2012;12:281–289.

291. Louie TJ, Miller MA, Mullane KM, et al. Fidaxomicin versus vancomycin for Clostridium difficile infection. *N Engl J Med* 2011;364:422–431.

292. van Nood E, Vrieze A, Nieuwdorp M, et al. Duodenal infusion of donor feces for recurrent Clostridium difficile. *N Engl J Med* 2013;368:407–415.

293. Kassam Z, Lee CH, Yuan Y, et al. Fecal microbiota transplantation for Clostridium difficile infection: systematic review and meta-analysis. *Am J Gastroenterol* 2013;108:500–508.

295. Pozzoni P, Riva A, Bellatorre AG, et al. Saccharomyces boulardii for the prevention of antibiotic-associated diarrhea in adult hospitalized patients: a single-center, randomized, double-blind, placebo-controlled trial. *Am J Gastroenterol* 2012;107:922–931.

305. Siegel JD, Rhinehart E, Jackson M, et al. 2007 Guideline for Isolation Precautions: Preventing Transmission of Infectious Agents in Health Care Settings. *Am J Infect Control* 2007;35:S65–S164.

306. Jabbar U, Leischner J, Kasper D, et al. Effectiveness of alcohol-based hand rubs for removal of Clostridium difficile spores from hands. *Infect Control Hosp Epidemiol* 2010;31:565–570.

310. Gupta N, Limbago BM, Patel JB, et al. Carbapenem-resistant enterobacteriaceae: epidemiology and prevention. *Clin Infect Dis* 2011;53:60–67.

312. Snitkin ES, Zelazny AM, Thomas PJ, et al. Tracking a hospital outbreak of carbapenem-resistant Klebsiella pneumoniae with whole-genome sequencing. *Sci Transl Med* 2012;4:148ra116.

315. Pea F, Viale P, Cojutti P, et al. Dosing nomograms for attaining optimum concentrations of meropenem by continuous infusion in critically ill patients with severe gram-negative infections: a pharmacokinetics/pharmacodynamics-based approach. *Antimicrob Agents Chemother* 2012;56:6343–6348.

316. Jernigan MG, Press EG, Nguyen MH, et al. The combination of doripenem and colistin is bactericidal and synergistic against colistin-resistant, carbapenemase-producing Klebsiella pneumoniae. *Antimicrob Agents Chemother* 2012;56:3395–3398.

324. Kofteridis DP, Alexopoulou C, Valachis A, et al. Aerosolized plus intravenous colistin versus intravenous colistin alone for the treatment of ventilator-associated pneumonia: a matched case-control study. *Clin Infect Dis* 2010;51:1238–1244.

326. Felton TW, Goodwin J, O'Connor L, et al. Impact of Bolus dosing versus continuous infusion of Piperacillin and Tazobactam on the development of antimicrobial resistance in Pseudomonas aeruginosa. *Antimicrob Agents Chemother* 2013;57:5811–5819.

327. Delvallée M, Mazingue F, Abouchahla W, et al. Optimization of continuous infusion of piperacillin-tazobactam in children with fever and neutropenia. *Pediatr Infect Dis J* 2013;32:962–964.

328. Moriyama B, Henning SA, Childs R, et al. High-dose continuous infusion beta-lactam antibiotics for the treatment of resistant Pseudomonas aeruginosa infections in immunocompromised patients. *Ann Pharmacother* 2010;44:929–935.

330. Pogue JM, Mann T, Barber KE, et al. Carbapenem-resistant Acinetobacter baumannii: epidemiology, surveillance and management. *Expert Rev Anti Infect Ther* 2013;11:383–393.

333. Climo MW, Yokoe DS, Warren DK, et al. Effect of daily chlorhexidine bathing on hospital-acquired infection. *N Engl J Med* 2013;368:533–542.

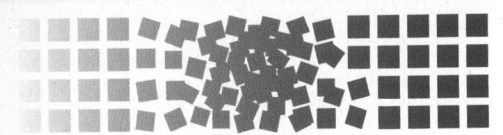

133 Neutropenia and Thrombocytopenia

Lodovico Balducci, Bijal Shah, and Kenneth Zuckerman

INTRODUCTION

Neutropenia and thrombocytopenia are the most frequent manifestations of cytotoxic chemotherapy-induced myelosuppression.[1] During the treatment of acute leukemia, this complication may last several weeks during which the risk of mortality from infection and bleeding is increased.[2] In all circumstances, myelosuppression may impact the antineoplastic treatment in several negative ways that include increased mortality[3,4] from infection or bleeding, more frequent hospitalizations,[5] increased treatment cost,[3,5,6] reduction in dose intensity of chemotherapy,[7–10] and treatment discontinuation.[7,8]

This chapter explores the management of neutropenia and thrombocytopenia in the course of cytotoxic chemotherapy, after a brief review of hematopoiesis.

Hematopoiesis

Hematopoiesis is a hierarchical and compartmentalized process involving early multipotent progenitors, late committed progenitors, and differentiated precursors of the mature blood elements[11] (Fig. 133.1). The early multipotent progenitors include the totipotent hematopoietic stem cells, capable of generating both the lymphoid and the myeloid series, and the myeloid and lymphoid stem cells. The totipotent stem cells include different populations of cells: the most primigenius ones with long-term repopulation capacity and the more mature ones with short-term repopulation capacity. The myeloid stem cell undergoes commitment into the myeloid, erythroid, and megakaryocytic progenitors, from which the differentiated marrow precursors of the circulating blood elements are derived. Both stem cells and early progenitors are indistinguishable from lymphocytes in microscopic preparation of the bone marrow and of the peripheral blood. Their existence was established from the ability to generate hematopoietic colonies containing multiple (multipotent progenitors) or single (committed progenitors) cell lines. Currently, a number of surface markers identify these elements with specific phenotypes (see Fig. 133.1).

The stem cell and to some extent the committed progenitors have high self-renewal potential and low proliferative rate, while the differentiated marrow precursors have a low self-replicative capacity and high proliferation. Low proliferation protects the stem cells and the committed progenitors from cytotoxic chemotherapy that is cycle active and damages preferentially proliferating cells. In addition, the earliest progenitors express the MDR-1 gene that encodes the P-glycoprotein, a calcium channel pump extruding natural genotoxic products from the cell.[12] These include both tumor antibiotics and plant derivatives. Thanks to the preservation of the hematopoietic reserve, the myelodepression of chemotherapy is generally fully reversible. There are exceptions, however. Some alkylating agents including busulfan, melphalan, nitrogen mustards, and the nitrosureas, and the antibiotic mitomycin C are able to overcome the protective mechanisms and to destroy the hematopoietic progenitors.[13,14]

Hematopoiesis requires an intact hematopoietic stroma capable to home the early progenitors, and a network of growth factors that stimulate proliferation, commitment, and differentiation[11,15–18] (Table 133.1). The homing occurs in the so-called hematopoietic niches that bind the hematopoietic progenitors through specific receptors to endothelial cells and osteoblasts. Except for erythropoietin that is produced in the kidney, and thrombopoietin that is produced both in the liver and in the kidneys, the other hematopoietic growth factors are produced by monocytes and by stromal cells of the bone marrow.

Hematopoiesis may be altered due to a reduction in the number of progenitors, the development of abnormal progenitors that have lost their ability to self-replicate or commit, abnormal production of hematopoietic growth factors, and abnormalities in the hematopoietic microenvironment. Some of these changes do occur with aging and include loss of homing, increased concentration of stem cells with reduced self-renewing capacity, and preferential differentiation of the totipotent stem cell toward the myeloid rather than the lymphoid series.[19,20]

Neutropenia and Its Management

Definition of Neutropenia and Its Consequences

According to the Common Terminology Criteria for Adverse Event version 4.0, neutropenia is defined by a granulocyte count that is $\leq 1,500/\mu l$,[21] and neutropenic infection is assumed for any fever episodes occurring when the neutrophil count is $<1,000/\mu l$. When the neutrophil count is $<500/\mu l$, the risk and severity of infection is inversely related to the neutrophil count.[22] The duration of neutropenia also determines the type of infections.[2] Bacterial infections from gram-negative pathogens and *Staphylococcus aureus* are more common during the first week of neutropenia.[23] A number of fungal infections including *Candida*, *Aspergillus*, *Mucor*, and others may develop in patients with more prolonged neutropenia including those receiving treatment for acute leukemia.[24] In addition to the severity, the duration of neutropenia determines the risk of infection. Infections are rare during the first 3 days of neutropenia as the neutrophils may still be present in the tissues.

For management purposes, it is useful to identify two different conditions: the neutropenia that follows marrow ablation for the treatment of some forms of acute leukemia, and the neutropenia that develops during the treatment of solid tumors or lymphomas with cyclic cytotoxic chemotherapy. Following marrow ablation, the neutropenia may last several weeks and the risk of infections is $>90\%$.[22] The main concern in this situation is support of the patient until marrow regeneration.

The neutropenia following noncytotoxic chemotherapy of solid tumors and lymphomas causes two concerns: infectious complication and maintenance of treatment dose intensity. This may be compromised due to treatment delay or dose reductions in order to prevent neutropenia. The relative dose intensity (RDI) is the percentage of the planned treatment dose

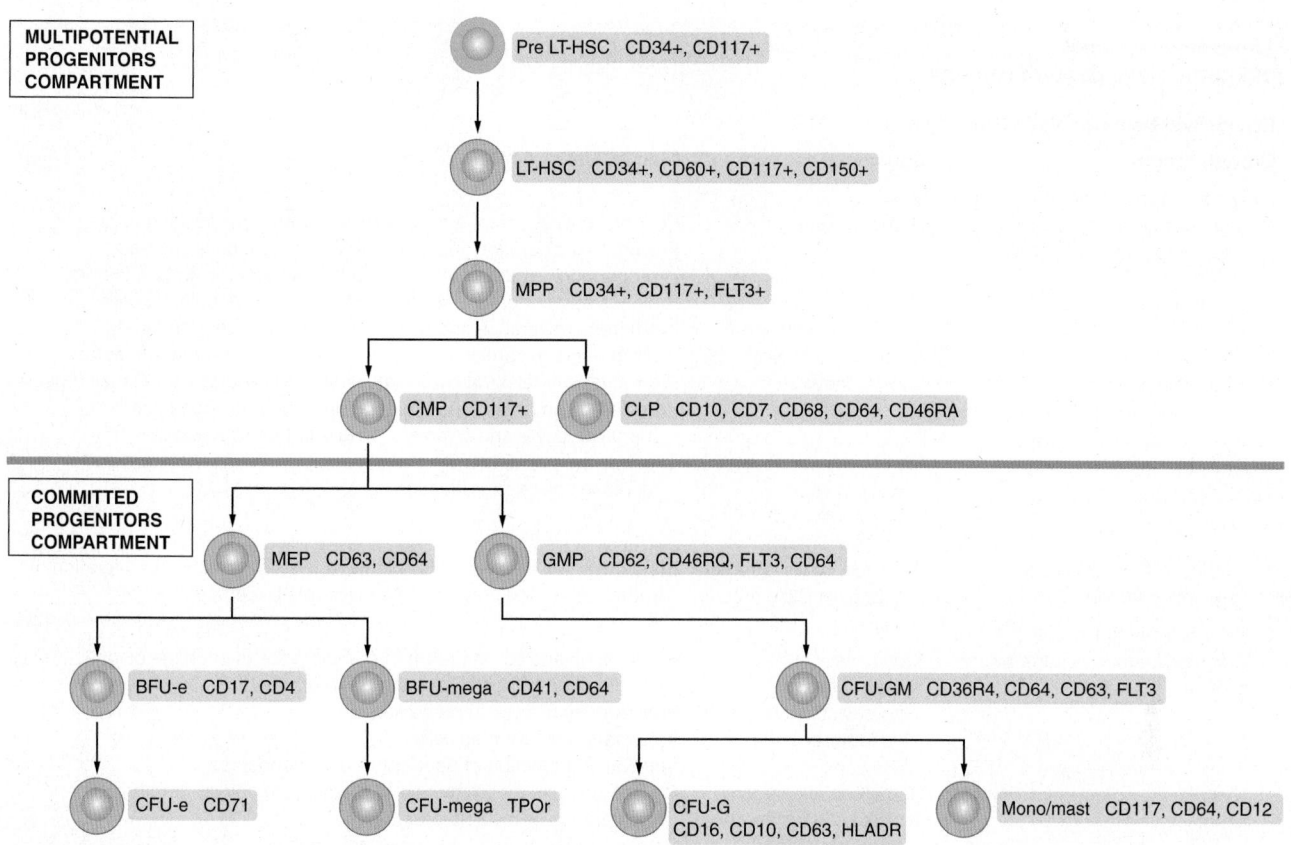

Figure 133.1 Hematopoiesis as a hierarchical compartmentalized process. Lymphopoiesis is not shown beyond CLP as it is not relevant to this chapter. LT-HSC, long-term hematopoietic stem cell repopulation capacity; MPP, multipotent progenitor; CMP, common myeloid progenitor; CLP, common lymphoid progenitor; MEP, megakaryocyte-erythroid progenitor; GMP, granulocyte monocyte progenitor; BFU, burst-forming unit; BFU-mega, burst-forming unit megakaryocyte; CFU-GM, colony-forming unit granulocyte-monocyte; CFU-e, Colony Forming Unit erythroid; CFU-megaTPOr, colony-forming unit megakaryocyte; CFU-G, colony-forming unit granulocyte.

administered during a course of treatment per unit of time and is calculated[25] as:

$$\frac{\text{D/T administered} \times 100}{\text{D/T planned}}$$

where D is the dose and T the time unit.

The effectiveness of chemotherapy may be determined by the RDI, whose preservation is essential in curable diseases. When the dose intensity of adjuvant cyclophosphamide, methotrexate, and fluorouracil was <85%, the treatment was not effective in women with early breast cancer.[25] Likewise, a reduction of the dose density of doxorubicin <85% was associated with reduced response rate and survival in patients with B-cell large-cell lymphoma treated with cyclophosphamide, hydroxydaunorubicin, oncovin, and prednisone (CHOP).[25] Neutropenia has been responsible for at least 50% of the cases in which the chemotherapy dose intensity has been reduced below 85%.[25]

The neutrophil kinetics determines the course of chemotherapy-induced neutropenia.[26] The median survival of mature neutrophils is approximately 12 hours in the circulation and 3 days in the tissues. The bone marrow contains a reserve of mature granulocytes to last approximately 7 days. The development of mature granulocytes from committed myeloid progenitors takes approximately 10 to 14 days. Consequently, the nadir neutrophil count following chemotherapy every 3 or 4 weeks is expected around the 10th treatment day, with recovery beginning around the 14th and completed by the 21st day. The time-honored way to prevent neutropenia and neutropenic infections prior to the introduction

of myelopoietic growth factors included reduction of the doses of myelotoxic agents for a neutrophil count <500/μl at nadir or <1,500/μl at the beginning of the new treatment cycle, whose initiation was delayed until the neutrophil count was completely recovered.

The neutrophil kinetics may be altered by a number of factors. Drugs that affect the pluripotent progenitors, such as mitomycin C and nitrosureas,[27] may cause later, more prolonged and cumulative neutropenia. In the presence of infection, the neutrophil reserve of the bone marrow may be exhausted at an earlier time and neutropenia may be more prolonged due to increased utilization of mature neutrophils. Also, hematopoiesis may be compromised by a number of factors that include age, previous chemotherapy administration, and myelophthisis.

Risk Factors for Chemotherapy-Induced Neutropenia

Clearly, the risk of neutropenia varies from patient to patient and includes both treatment- and patient-related factors. The determination of the individual risk of neutropenia and neutropenic infections is helpful to plan the most effective management of neutropenia. A number of risk factors for febrile neutropenia were identified in several studies[28–30] (Table 133.2).

The risk of neutropenic infections from different treatment regimens is obtained from the original trials of those regimens. It should be underlined that the incidence of neutropenic infections may be higher in patients treated in the community than in those included in clinical trials.[28–30]

TABLE 133.1

Hematopoietic Growth Factors

Recognized Hematopoietic Growth Factors

Growth Factor	Source	Mechanism of Action
Early acting growth factors[15]		
■ Stem cell factor (c-kit ligand, steel factor, mast cell growth factor)	Hematopoietic stroma	Prolongs survival of long-term and short-term repopulating cells Promotes proliferation and self-renewal of stem cells and early progenitors in combination with other hepatocyte growth factors
■ Flt3 ligand	Hematopoietic stroma; hematopoietic stem cell?	Prolongs survival of long-term and short-term repopulating cells Promotes proliferation and self-renewal of stem cells and early progenitors in combination with other hepatocyte growth factors
■ Thrombopoietin	Liver, kidney	Promotes survival of hematopoietic stem cells and promotes their division Promote commitment and proliferation of burst-forming unit megakaryocyte and colony-forming unit megakaryocyte
■ Leukemia inhibitory factor	Fibroblasts, monocyte/macrophages, endothelium, activated T cells	Expands the population of several hematopoietic progenitors and increases platelet production
■ Interleukin-3 (multicolony-stimulating factor)	Activated T cells, stromal cells of multiple organs	Stimulates self-renewal of hematopoietic stem cells and proliferation of most committed progenitors; in vivo role uncertain
Colony stimulating factors[16,67]		
■ Granulocyte-macrophage colony-stimulating factor	Monocyte, macrophages, fibroblasts, and endothelial cells	Proliferation and commitment of granulocyte-macrophage colony-forming unit and granulocyte colony-forming unit Proliferation of myeloid precursors Proliferation of dendritic cells Survival and function of neutrophils and monocytes
■ Granulocyte colony-stimulating factor	Hematopoietic stromal cells and stromal cells from other organs	Proliferation and differentiation of granulocyte colony-forming unit, proliferation of myeloid precursors Release, survival, and function of neutrophils
Erythropoiesis-stimulating agent[17]		
■ Erythropoietin	Kidney	Stimulates proliferation, differentiation and maturation of burst-forming unit, colony-forming unit granulocyte, and erythroid precursors
Thrombopoietic factors[18]		
■ Thrombopoietin	Liver, kidney	Promotes survival of hematopoietic stem cells and promotes their division Promotes commitment and proliferation of burst-forming unit megakaryocyte and colony-forming unit megakaryocyte

Hematopoietic Growth Factors in Clinical Practice

Growth Factor	Preparation	Use
Early hepatocyte growth factors ■ Stem cell factor*	Ancestim	Mobilization of hematopoietic stem cells for transplantation
Colony-stimulating factor ■ Granulocyte macrophage–colony-stimulating factor	Sargramostin Molgramostin[a] Regramostin[a]	■ Prevention of neutropenia and neutropenic infections ■ Stem cell mobilization ■ Dendritic cell proliferation as adjuvant in immunotherapy
■ Granulocyte–colony-stimulating factor Short-acting	Filgrastim Lenograstim[a] Tbo-filgrastim	Prevention of chemotherapy-induced neutropenia and neutropenic infections
Long-acting	Peg-filgrastim Lipegfilgrastim[a]	
Erythropoiesis-stimulating agents ■ Erytrthopoetin	Epoetin α Epoetin β Darbepoetin	Anemia in patients with chronic kidney disease Myelodysplasia Chemotherapy-induced anemia
Thrombopoietic agents ■ Interleukin 11 ■ Thrombopoietin mimetics	Oprelvekin Romiplostin Eltrombopag	Chemotherapy-induced thrombocytopenia Idiopathic thrombocytopenic purpura

[a] Not available in the United States.

TABLE 133.2

Assessment of the Risk of Neutropenic Infections in Individual Patients

Risk Factors for Development of Neutropenic Fever

Type of chemotherapy

Age >60–65 y

Advanced disease

Poor performance status

Previous chemotherapy

Previous episodes of neutropenic infections

Myelophthisis

Number of comorbid condition

Abnormal liver enzymes

Abnormal creatinine clearance

Low neutrophil count at the beginning of the treatment

Lymphopenia

Hemoglobin

Presence of an ongoing infection

Multinational Association for Supportive Cancer Care Risk Index (DeSouza et al.[47] and Innes et al.[48])

Patient Characteristics	Score
Burden of illness	
No or mild symptoms	5
Moderate symptoms	3
No hypotension	5
No chronic obstructive pulmonary disease	4
Solid tumor or lymphoma and no previous fungal infection	4
No dehydration	3
Outpatient status	3
Age <60 y	2

Low-risk score ≥21. High-risk score <21.

Age is probably the best identified patient-related risk factor. It is clear that the risk of neutropenic infections increases with age. A review of 500 patients with large-cell B-cell lymphoma treated in the community with CHOP or cyclophosphamide, novantrone, oncovin, and prednisone showed that the risk of neutropenic infections was 28% for the total population, 18% in the younger individuals and 40% for those 65 and older.[5] Hospitalization for neutropenic infections was 25% longer for older individuals. This finding is important as both treatment cost and risk of deconditioning increase with hospitalization.

In most studies the age threshold was 65, and in some it was 60. The risk of breakthrough infection despite growth factor support[30] and of infectious mortality also increases with age.[3,4]

In the Surveillance, Epidemiology and End Result database, the risk of febrile neutropenia in Medicare recipients increased with the number of comorbid conditions.[31] In other studies, chronic liver and kidney dysfunctions, chronic obstructive lung disease, diabetes, congestive heart failure, osteoarthritis, and thyroid diseases were associated with increased risk of febrile neutropenia.[10,32]

In several studies, anemia was an independent risk factor for the development of chemotherapy-induced neutropenia and neutropenic fever.[33–38] Anemia may represent a sign of chronic diseases, of bone marrow insufficiency, and of malnutrition.[39] Another explanation is suggested by pharmacokinetic considerations.[34] As the majority of cytotoxic agents are bound to the red blood cells, a reduction of hemoglobin may be associated with increased concentration of free drug in the circulation and consequently with increased risk of toxicity.

Protein calorie malnutrition also appears as a risk factor for chemotherapy-induced myelotoxicity.[40–43]

Myelophthisis may occur with most tumors and is particularly common in patients with lymphoma, breast, and prostate cancer.

The relationship between lymphopenia and risk of neutropenic infections is well established albeit poorly explained.[44–46] A drop in lymphocyte count during the first week after chemotherapy seems predictive of febrile neutropenia. A possible explanation is that lymphopenia represents poor nutrition.

A number of models to predict the risk of neutropenia or neutropenic fever in solid tumors and lymphomas were developed. The five models that have been prospectively validated are described here. The Multinational Association for Supportive Cancer Care risk index illustrated in Table 133.2 divides the patients in high and low risk according to a score obtained from the presence of different risk factors.[47] The main advantages include simplicity and reproducibility.[48] Of concern is the fact that the index has been validated prospectively in a small number of patients and only to predict the benefits of prophylactic antibiotics. Another simple index[49] divides patients in four groups according to the original neutrophil (<3,100/μl) and lymphocyte (<1,500/μl) count. When both counts are lowest, the risk of neutropenic fever is the highest. This model was validated in patients receiving adjuvant chemotherapy of breast cancer with docetaxel, doxorubicin, and cyclophosphamide.

Among 266 patients with non-specified hematologic malignancies, Moreau et al.[36] found that aggressive chemotherapy, baseline hemoglobin level, type and stage of disease, body surface area, involvement of the bone marrow, and monocyte count <150/μl were independent risk factors for neutropenic fever during the first course of chemotherapy. Among 240 patients with non-Hodgkin lymphoma, Pettengell et al.[50] found that a model including age, weight, previous chemotherapy, chemotherapy dose, albumin levels, and use of granulocyte–colony-stimulating factor (G-CSF) predicted individual risk of neutropenic fever with 80% accuracy. While of interest, these models have limited use due to the fact that they involve only a small number of patients with specific malignancies.

In a prospective study of 3,760 patients treated for solid tumors and lymphomas in 115 practices in the United States, Lyman et al.[30] were able to derive an individual risk of neutropenia, severe neutropenia, and neutropenic infection based on prior chemotherapy, low neutrophil count, abnormal hepatic and renal function, type of chemotherapy, and planned delivery of ≥85% of the dose intensity. The index has a predictive value positive and negative of 34% and 96%, respectively. Surprisingly, age was not an independent risk factor even though one-third of the patients were 65 and older. This model is interesting for several reasons. First, it was derived and validated from the cohort study of a large number of patients. Second, it included severe neutropenia in addition to neutropenic infections among the outcomes. Severe neutropenia should be avoided, at least in curable diseases, because it may purport a reduction of RDI of chemotherapy.[51–54] Third, it provides a determination of individual risk of neutropenic infections. Fourth, it was derived from a number of community practices and as such it reflects the situation of the majority of patients undergoing cancer chemotherapy. Fifth, it encompasses a wide array of diseases and of chemotherapy regimens. The limits of this model include the need for a calculator and the fact that the age range of the patients was not specified. While we know that one-third of the patients were 65 and older, we don't know how many of them were older than 75 or 80. In the time of electronic health records, the calculation of the index may not represent a problem anymore.

Due to the lack of prospective comparisons, it is premature to recommend a specific model for the prediction of neutropenic infections in individual cases. In a community-based oncology practice,[55] the adoption of an instrument to assess the risk of neutropenic infections prior to the initiation of cytotoxic chemotherapy has led to a marked reduction in the incidence of neutropenic infections and of hospitalization for neutropenic infections. Also, more patients than before received chemotherapy with a RDI ≥85%.

Management of Neutropenia

Prevention of Neutropenic Infections in Patients Receiving Chemotherapy for Solid Tumors and Lymphomas

In the treatment of solid tumors and lymphomas, the management of neutropenia has two goals: reduction in the incidence and severity of infectious complications, and maintenance of the RDI of chemotherapy at ≥85%.

Prior to the introduction of the myelopoietic growth factors, it was recommended that the dose of chemotherapy be reduced in patients experiencing severe neutropenia at nadir or neutropenic infections and that the treatment be delayed for neutrophil counts ≤1,500/μl.[2,22] Prophylactic administration of antibiotics has been a complementary strategy toward the reduction of neutropenic infections. The fluoroquinolones and the combination of sulfamethoxazole/thrimethrophrim reduce the risk of gram-negative infections from enteric pathogens in patients with prolonged neutropenia.[56-59] By causing an anaerobe overgrowth in the colon, these compounds suppress the growth of gram-negative pathogens that are the most common cause of bacterial infections during neutropenia. Most of the studies were performed in patients with acute leukemia and in those undergoing bone marrow transplant, however, so that the information is limited in patients with solid tumors and lymphoma. In two large randomized controlled studies, prophylactic levofloxacin was associated with a reduction of episodes of neutropenic fever of approximately 30% without a reduction of documented infections or of infectious deaths.[56,58] In one of these studies, stool cultures showed emergence of gram-negative organisms resistant to levofloxacin and rose the concern that this practice may lead to antibiotic-resistant hospital infections.[56] According to a meta-analysis of randomized controlled trials, the prophylactic use of fluoroquinolones was associated with a significant reduction in the incidence of neutropenic fever in patients with solid tumors and lymphomas and a nonsignificant reduction in mortality.[59] A Dutch study compared the combination of growth factors and antibiotics versus antibiotics alone in patients receiving treatment for small-cell lung cancer.[60] The combination of colony-stimulating factors and antibiotics was more effective than antibiotic alone in preventing neutropenic fever. According to this study, the role of prophylactic antibiotics is questionable in the case of solid tumors.

Based on these data, no consensus exists on the use of prophylactic antibiotics in patients treated for solid tumors and lymphomas.[61-63] This practice may be justified when the duration of neutropenia is expected to be longer than 7 days.

Myelopoietic Growth Factors

The introduction of recombinant hematopoietic growth factors (see Table 133.1) has provided a new weapon to prevent both neutropenia and neutropenic infections. Both recombinant G-CSF and granulocyte macrophage–colony-stimulating factor (GM-CSF) are available for clinical use.[64-66] Recombinant forms of G-CSF include both short-acting (filgrastim, lenograstim, and tbo-filgrastim) and long-acting (pegfilgrastim and lipegfilgrastim) preparations. Unlike the short-acting preparations, pegfilgrastim and lipegfilgrastin cannot be eliminated from the kidneys. They are metabolized by the neutrophils at the time of recovery from neutropenia. As such, they linger in the circulation until recovery has occurred.

Three different recombinant human GM-CSFs are available and include sargramostim, molgramostim, and regramostim. Of these, sargramostim is the only one approved for use in the United States. Sargramostim is derived from yeast (*Saccharomyces cerevisiae*) and is O-glycosylated; molgramostim is not glycosylated recombinant human GM-CSF and is derived from *Escherichia coli*. Regramostim is fully glycosylated and is derived from Chinese hamster ovary cells. The different formulations appear to have similar pharmacologic activity.

Despite that they have been available now for more than 20 years, a number of controversies linger concerning hematopoietic growth factors. The controversies hinge on three questions: which growth factor should be used, when and how it should be used, and what are short- and long-term complications for their use.

Which Growth Factor Should be Used? In solid tumors and lymphomas, G-CSFs have reduced the incidence of neutropenia and neutropenic infections, as well as the hospitalization for neutropenic infections according to a number of randomized controlled studies examined in six meta-analyses[8,67-71] and a review of its use in clinical practice in patients with lymphoma.[5] In two of these meta-analysis,[8,68] the use of these agents was also associated with reduced mortality from neutropenic infections. In addition, the most recent meta-analysis suggested that the all causes of mortality might have been reduced[8] and that the dose intensity of chemotherapy was better preserved with these agents.[9] At least one meta-analysis of 148 clinical trials failed to see any benefits for the use of myelopoietic growth factors.[72] However, this study included different growth factors and different ways of administration such as delayed administration that was proven ineffective previously. According to a number of meta-analysis and systematic reviews, filgrastim and lenograstim have comparable activities.[8,67,68,73] In a review of the drug approval process in Europe,[74] the activity of the biosimilar Tevagrastim (Teva Pharmaceuticals, North Wales, PA) also appears comparable with that of filgrastim.

A number of randomized controlled studies found that safety and effectiveness of filgrastim and pegfilgrastim were comparable in patients with lymphoma and solid tumors.[75-78] According to a meta-analysis of these trials, pegfilgrastim was superior to filgrastim in reducing the risk of neutropenic infections.[70] Similar conclusions were reached by an analysis of a US claim database involving more than 18,000 patients[79] and by a review of the use of filgrastim and pegfilgrastim in Spain.[80] These results may be explained, at least in part by improved patient compliance with a single injection per cycle. In a randomized controlled trial, pegfilgrastim and lipegfilgrastim, the new long-acting form of filgrastim undergoing clinical trials, had comparable activities and safety.[81]

A number of studies demonstrated that GM-CSF decreases the duration of neutropenia and the risk of neutropenic infections in patients with lymphoma and solid tumors and is a reasonable choice for this purpose.[61,82,83]

At present, the studies comparing filgrastim and sargramostim provided inconclusive and somehow conflicting evidence of the superiority of one drug over the other. In a small randomized controlled study including 181 patients,[84] filgrastim was associated with a shorter duration of neutropenia (1 day), but sargramostim was associated with decreased risk of hospitalization and shorter hospitalization for neutropenic fever. Both agents were equally well tolerated. A retrospective matched control study of national insurance claims indicated that the prophylactic use of sargramostim was associated with decreased risk of neutropenic infections and rehospitalization.[85] In another study of similar design, pegfilgrastim proved superior to both filgrastim and sargramostim in preventing neutropenic infections and hospitalizations.[86,87] According to another report,[88] the substitution on the formulary of filgrastim with sargramostim in a single institution was associated with an increased incidence of infections and hospitalization rates as well as of treatment side effects (pain and fever). A review of 10 US outpatient practices revealed that sargramostim was associated with increased risk of complications including unexplained fever, fatigue, and skin eruptions.[89] In a randomized comparison of filgrastim and sargramostim in patients with febrile neutropenia, sargramostim was also associated with increased risk of side effects.[90] One may conclude that the efficacy of myeloid growth factors in use in the United States is comparable, sargramostim may have increased risk of side effects, and pegfilgrastim at present is the most practical and convenient of the growth factors.

Timing of Use. The questions related to the timing include primary versus secondary prophylaxis, treatment duration with filgrastim and sargramostim, the administration of pegfilgrastim on the same day of chemotherapy, and the effectiveness of growth factors in course of neutropenic infections.

Primary prophylaxis means treatment of patients at high risk of neutropenia or neutropenic infections beginning with the first cycle of chemotherapy treatment; in secondary prophylaxis, growth factors are reserved for those patients who had already experienced an episode of neutropenic fever.

A number of randomized controlled[91–93] and retrospective[94–96] studies demonstrated that primary prophylaxis decreased risk of neutropenic infections throughout treatment, not only during the first course of treatment, and therefore it should be preferred[61,65] in patients at high risk.

Filgrastim and sargramostim are administered daily for a minimum of 7 to 10 days. It is common practice to discontinue filgrastim when the neutrophil count is $\geq 3,000/\mu l$ (though the drug insert recommends $10,000/\mu l$). Several strategies have been employed for reducing the duration of growth factor treatment with inconclusive results. In a randomized controlled study, treatment of patients who had developed afebrile neutropenia did not reduce the risk of neutropenic infections.[97] Another approach included the reduction of the administration of G-CSF to 5 days[98]; though it may be more effective than placebo, this approach may not be optimal. A review of several US practices revealed that administration of G-CSF for a duration shorter than 7 days was associated with increased risk of febrile infections and hospitalizations.[99] As the risk of neutropenic infections is highest during the first two courses of chemotherapy, a study addressed the question of whether the use of filgrastim could be avoided after the first two chemotherapy cycles in patients receiving adjuvant treatment for early breast cancer.[100] The risk of neutropenic infections was >20% during the successive chemotherapy cycles, and the authors concluded that filgrastim prophylaxis should be continued throughout all treatment cycles.

According to the current recommendations pegfilgrastim is administered once per treatment cycles between 24 and 72 hours from chemotherapy. These recommendations are based on the review of four randomized phase 2 studies including patients with breast cancer, lymphoma, nonsmall-cell cancer, and ovarian cancer.[101] In the lymphoma and breast cancer studies, the duration of neutropenia was more prolonged and the neutropenia more severe in patients receiving same-day pegfilgrastim. Up to now, no new evidence has emerged supporting the use of pegfilgrastim on the same day as chemotherapy.

A meta-analysis of 13 randomized controlled studies of growth factors showed that myelopoietic growth factors do reduce the duration of hospitalization and the duration of neutropenia in patients with neutropenic infections.[90] However, they do not affect the overall mortality, though they may have a marginal influence on infectious mortality. The same conclusions were reached by a more recent review of the literature.[102] This use is not recommended in the current guidelines.[61,65]

Complications. The acute complications of growth factors include fever and skin reactions that appear more common with GM-CSF.[90] Bone pain is particularly common with pegfilgrastim, generally occurs during the first 5 days of treatment, and may lead to discontinuation of the treatment.[103] In a randomized controlled study involving 510 patients with different malignancies, naproxen

administered at 500 mg twice daily for 5 days initiated on the day of pegfilgrastim administration significantly reduced the incidence and severity of pain without appreciable side effects.[103] Of interest, the pain was more severe in African American patients who benefited most of the intervention.

The most worrisome long-term side effects of colony-stimulating factors is acute myelogenous leukemia.[104] In a meta-analysis of 25 prospective randomized clinical trials involving >6,000 patients, the risk of acute myelogenous leukemia had doubled with the use of filgrastim. In the same study, however, the overall mortality was reduced by the use of filgrastim, especially in patients treated with dose-intense chemotherapy. The authors concluded that the tradeoff of adverse outcomes was in favor of filgrastim. The risk of acute leukemia appeared mostly elevated in patients 65 and older receiving breast cancer adjuvant chemotherapy with anthracyclines[105,106] and particularly with mitoxantrone.[107] There is no clear evidence that sargramostim or other forms of GM-CSF may induce acute myelogenous leukemia.

Cost should also be considered a complication of myelopoietic growth factors, as their use adds a substantial cost to treatment. It is debated whether and in which circumstances the use of these compounds is cost-effective. The controversy reflects, at least in part, the difficulty to assess cost and cost-effectiveness and the fact that in the cost estimate may be different perspectives (that of the patient, of the third-party payers, and of the healthcare provider). This confusion is well illustrated in a recent review of the pharmacoeconomics of the myeloid growth factors[25] that found that pegfilgrastim is more cost-effective than filgrastim, and primary prophylaxis more cost-effective than secondary prophylaxis in the United States. In Europe, where medical care is less costly, the cost-effectiveness of growth factors is substantially reduced. A number of independent factors may also affect the cost-effectiveness of these agents. For example, neutropenic infections, when treated in the outpatient setting, are less costly than in the hospital setting, which may diminish the cost-effectiveness of growth factors. A recent analysis indicates that primary prophylaxis with growth factors is cost-effective when the risk of neutropenic infections is $\geq 20\%$.[108] In accordance with this finding, current guidelines recommend that myeloid growth factors be used prophylactically when the risk of neutropenic infections is $\geq 20\%$ and not be used when the risk is $\leq 10\%$.[61,65] The use for cases at intermediate risk is trusted to the practitioner's judgment.

Another area of controversy is whether these compounds should be used when the goal of the treatment is palliation instead of cure, and whether it would be wiser in these circumstances to institute a reduction of chemotherapy dose in lieu of growth factors.

As general principles one may state that:

- The cost of healthcare is an increasingly pressing social problem, and it is an ethic duty to use limited resources sparingly.[109]
- The use of growth factors increases the cost of cancer care.
- The cost-effectiveness of these compounds increases when the risk of neutropenic infections is the highest. Practitioners should try to estimate this risk in individual situations based on chemotherapy regimen and patient's characteristics
- Cost-effectiveness considerations are secondary when an intervention may be life-saving as the use of myeloid growth factors may be in the treatment of older individuals.
- Patients receiving palliative chemotherapy should not be automatically excluded from treatment with growth factors. For example, patients with stage III ovarian cancer may enjoy several years free of disease thanks to platinum-based chemotherapy. Likewise, maintenance of adequate chemotherapy dose intensity may be life-saving in face of life-threatening metastases, such as lymphangitic lung metastases.

Conclusions Related to Myeloid Growth Factors Use. From this review, one may conclude that myeloid growth factors reduce the risk of neutropenic infections and hospitalizations in patients receiving chemotherapy, allow the administration of more effective dose intensities of chemotherapy, and may reduce the infectious mortality. In the meantime, there is no evidence that growth factors improve the cancer-related survival. The use of growth factors appear cost-effective in patients in whom the risk of neutropenic infections is ≥20%. Pegfilgrastim may be more effective and certainly appears more cost-effective than the short-acting preparations.

Prevention of Neutropenic Infections in Patients with Acute Leukemia

In the management of acute leukemia, neutropenia may last several weeks, and virtually all patients are susceptible to neutropenic infections. The use of a protected environment including reverse isolation[110] and neutropenic diet[111] are still of common use, though the evidence supporting them is controversial. Three interventions have been studied in randomized controlled studies: antibiotic prophylaxis, myelopoietic growth factors, and granulocyte transfusions.

Antibiotic Prophylaxis. A meta-analysis of 109 trials including 13,579 patients, the majority of whom had acute leukemia or had undergone bone marrow transplant,[57] demonstrated that prophylactic treatment with fluoroquinolones or trimethoprim-sulfamethoxazole was associated with a reduction in infectious mortality, overall mortality, and neutropenic fever without documented infection. This practice is recommended in patients in whom the neutropenia is expected to last 7 days or longer. Though the difference between the two types of antimicrobials was not significant, there was a trend favoring the fluoroquinolones.

Myelopoietic Growth Factors. The use of these agents is controversial. A meta-analysis of 18 randomized controlled trials involving 5,256 patients[112] failed to demonstrate any benefits for the use of growth factors in acute myelogenous leukemia after induction therapy. The same investigators in a previous meta-analysis established that growth factors were safe in acute leukemics.[113] This should dispel concern about growth factor–induced stimulation of the neoplastic growth.

A systematic review of 14 studies established that the use of growth factors led to a decreased duration of neutropenia and early hospital discharge without effect on overall mortality.[114] An early meta-analysis[113] yielded similar results.

Some considerations are necessary prior to being convinced of the conclusion that myeloid growth factors have at best a marginal role in the management of acute myeloid leukemia. These studies were conducted in the 1990s,[115–122] when many prognostic factors of acute leukemia were poorly defined, so they might have compared different patient populations. Some studies utilized GM-CSFs[115,118–122] and other G-CSFs,[116,117] and the source of these compounds was sometimes different. For example, the Eastern Cooperative Oncology Group[115] utilized GM-CSF from *Candida* and the Cancer Acute Leukemia Group B the one from *E. coli*.[119] One of the studies found increased response rates and increased survival with GM-CSF, while the other study found the growth factor ineffective. Also, the treatment with growth factors was started at different times in different studies and induction regimens were different.

In all studies, the growth factors reduced the duration of neutropenia and of antibiotic use in elderly patients (55 and older). In four studies,[115,116,121,122] the use of growth factors after induction chemotherapy was associated with increased remission rate, and in one study with increased survival and reduction of treatment-related death.[115] One can conclude that growth factors at the very least reduce the duration of neutropenia, of neutropenic infections, and of hospitalization in patients aged 55 and over, who are also the patients more vulnerable to the treatment complications.

More recently, other randomized controlled studies have explored the use of growth factors in remission induction of acute leukemia with inconclusive results.[123,124] In one study, the use of G-CSF was associated with shorter disease-free survival in individuals younger than 40,[124] but other factors might have contributed to the poorer outcome.

In a randomized controlled study, G-CSF reduced the duration of neutropenia and the duration of antibiotic treatment, and hospitalization for neutropenic infections in patients receiving consolidation therapy with high-dose cytarabine, but it did not change the overall survival or the infectious death rate.[125] A retrospective analysis of adult acute leukemias treated at a single institution with G-CSF during consolidation therapy reached similar conclusions.[126]

In conclusion, in the management of acute myelogenous leukemia, myeloid growth factors decrease the duration of neutropenia and neutropenic infections after induction chemotherapy in individuals 55 and older, they decrease the duration of neutropenia and hospitalization after consolidation treatment with high-dose cytarabine, and they do not promote the growth of the neoplastic cells. In one study,[115] the use of GM-CSF was associated with improved response rate and survival and decreased mortality, but these results were not confirmed in any of the other studies.

A number of randomized controlled trials demonstrated that both G-CSF and GM-CSF after induction treatment for acute lymphoblastic leukemia reduced the duration of neutropenia and of neutropenic infections, and that they can be safely used in these patients.[127–129] At present, there is no evidence that they affect response rate or survival.

Granulocyte Transfusions. A meta-analysis of 10 studies performed decades ago did not show any reduction in infections related mortality from granulocyte transfusions.[130] However, these studies were conducted at a time when antibiotic treatment was more limited and antifungal treatment almost nonexistent. It would be reasonable to explore the value of granulocyte transfusions in conjunction with modern supportive care.

Thrombocytopenia

Definition, Epidemiology, and Causes. According to the Common Terminology Criteria for Adverse Event, thrombocytopenia is defined as a platelet count $<100^3/\mu l$.[21] The main risk of thrombocytopenia is hemorrhage, which is increased for platelet counts $\leq 50^3/\mu l$. The risk of spontaneous bleeding including intracranial hemorrhage is increased when the platelet count drops to $<10^3/\mu l$.[131–133]

In patients with malignant diseases, there are many causes of thrombocytopenia. The most common is cytotoxic chemotherapy. With most agents, the nadir platelet count is observed 10 to 14 days from the beginning of the treatment cycle and the recovery is completed by 3 weeks. If the platelet count is $<100^3/\mu l$ at the beginning of a new cycle, the chemotherapy is delayed and the successive dose of treatment is decreased.[134]

Thrombocytopenia from drugs that affect the early hematopoietic progenitors, such as the nitrosureas, mitomycin C, busulfan, and melphalan, may be delayed and cumulative. In addition to cytotoxic chemotherapy, some of the new biologic agents may also cause thrombocytopenia. This complication is particularly common with lenalidomide.[135]

Thrombocytopenia is a well-recognized complication of cytotoxic chemotherapy,[136] but its impact on morbidity, mortality, and decrease in chemotherapy RDI is not well established in patients with lymphomas and solid tumors. Among Medicare recipients with breast cancer treated with chemotherapy, thrombocytopenia accounted for only 0.6% of the hospital admission, whereas neutropenia and neutropenic infections accounted for 24%.[137]

Myelosuppression is the most common, albeit not the only mechanism of chemotherapy-induced thrombocytopenia. Some chemotherapy agents, in particular mitomycin C, dacarbazine, and cysplatin, may induce thrombocytopenia as part of a hemolytic uremic syndrome.[138]

The other major cause of thrombocytopenia is myelophthisis. In patients with acute leukemia, thrombocytopenia is almost universal at presentations and hemorrhages represent a common cause of death in these patients.[139]

Other causes of thrombocytopenia may include hypersplenism, idiopathic thrombocytopenic purpura, disseminated intravascular coagulation,[140] and heparin-induced thrombocytopenia,[141] as the use of heparin is becoming common in patients with cancer to maintain vascular access devices and to manage cancer-related thrombosis.

Management. Platelet transfusions remain the mainstay of the management of thrombocytopenia. One may distinguish prophylactic and therapeutic transfusions.[131] Currently, prophylactic transfusions are recommended in patients with decreased platelet productions in two circumstances. In all individuals with a count $\leq 10^{\#}/\mu l$ to prevent spontaneous intracranial bleeding and individuals with a count $<50^{3}/\mu l$ for whom a surgical procedure is planned.[131] Therapeutic transfusions are those administered to actively bleeding patients and are indicated for platelet count $<50^{3}/\mu l$. It should be underlined that the threshold for both prophylactic and therapeutic transfusions are controversial. Two current studies are being conducted in Germany and in the United Kingdom to establish whether the threshold for prophylactic transfusions may be lowered, to prevent the risk associated with the transfusions and especially platelet refractoriness.[142,143]

A recombinant preparation of interleukin-11 has been approved for use in patients with solid tumors or lymphoma.[136] This compound is associated with substantial toxicity including fever, malaise, and fluid retention, which limit its use. It may be indicated in the rare cases when thrombocytopenia is the main factor preventing the administration of adequate RDI of chemotherapy.

None of the currently available thrombopoietin mimetics has been approved as of yet for the management of chemotherapy-induced thrombocytopenia. These include romiplostin, which is a peptide, and eltrombopag, a nonpeptide mimetic that is administered orally.[144,145] Four phase 1 and 2 trials of romiplostin were performed in patients with solid tumor and lymphoma, but the results have not been published. A phase 1/2 study of eltrombopag has been concluded in patients with osteosarcoma and soft tissue sarcoma, but the results are not available at the time of this writing.

In conclusion, thrombocytopenia is associated with risk of severe bleeding and death in patients with acute leukemia. In patients with lymphoma and solid tumors, chemotherapy-induced thrombocytopenia is rarely life-threatening. The current indications for platelet transfusions include a count $<10^{3}/\mu l$ for prophylactic transfusions and $<50^{3}/\mu l$ for therapeutic transfusions for patients undergoing invasive procedure. These thresholds are based on soft data. Ongoing clinical trials explore whether these thresholds could be safely lowered.

Oprevelkin is indicated for the prevention of chemotherapy-induced thrombocytopenia in patients with lymphomas and solid tumors. This compound has a number of adverse effects that limit its usefulness.

SELECTED REFERENCES

The full reference list can be accessed at lwwhealthlibrary.com/oncology.

2. Bodey GP. Infections in cancer patients. *Cancer Treat Rev* 1975;2:89–128.
4. Lyman GH, Michel SL, Reynolds MW, et al. Risk of mortality in patients who experience febrile neutropenia. *Cancer* 2010;116:5555–5563.
6. Lathia N, Mittmann N, DeAngelis C, et al. Evaluation of direct medical cost for hospitalization in febrile neutropenia. *Cancer* 2010;116:742–748.
7. Michele SL, Barron RL, Reynolds MW, et al. Cost associated with febrile neutropenia in the US. *Pharmacoeconomics* 2012;30:809–823.
8. Lyman GH, Dale DC, Culakova E, et al. The impact of the granulocyte colony-stimulating factor on chemotherapy dose intensity and cancer survival: a systematic review and meta-analysis of randomized controlled trials. *Ann Oncol* 2013;24:2475–2484.
11. Shah B, Zuckerman K. Normal and malignant hematopoiesis. In Mufti GJ, Saba HI, eds. *Advances in malignant hematology*. Hoboken, NJ: Wiley-Blackwell; 2011:3–30.
15. Szilvassy SJ. Early acting hematopoietic growth factors: biology and clinical experience. *Cancer Treat Res* 2011;157:11–32.
16. Molineux G. Granulocyte colony stimulating factors. *Cancer Treat Res* 2011;157:33–54.
18. Wei P. Thrombopoietin factors. *Cancer Treat Res* 2011;157:75–94.
19. Pang WW, Price EA, Sahoo D, et al. Human hematopoietic stem cells are increased in frequency and myeloid biased with age. *Proc Natl Acad Sci U S A* 2011;108:20012–20017.
20. Kuranda K, Vargaftig J, de la Rochere P, et al. Age-related changes in human hematopoietic stem/progenitor cells. *Aging Cells* 2011;10:542–546.
22. Bodey GP, Rodriguez V, McKredie K, et al. Neutropenia and infections following cancer chemotherapy. *Int J Radiol Oncol Biol Phys* 1976;1:301–314.
25. Hirsch BR, Lyman GH. Pharmacoeconomics of myeloid growth factors. A critical and systematic review. *Pharmacoeconomics* 2012;30:497–511.
30. Lyman GH, Kuderer N, Crawford J, et al. Predicting individual risk of neutropenic complications in patients receiving cancer chemotherapy. *Cancer* 2011;117:1917–1927.
32. Chia VM, Page GH, Rodriguez R, et al. Chronic comorbid conditions associated with risk of febrile neutropenia in breast cancer patients treated with chemotherapy. *Cancer* 2013;138:621–632.
33. Schrijvers D, Highley M, DeBruyn E, et al. Role of red blood cell in pharmacokinetics of chemotherapeutic agents. *Anticancer Drugs* 1999;10:147–153.
35. Extermann M, Boler I, Reich R, et al. Predicting the risk of chemotherapy toxicity in older patients. The Chemotherapy Risk Assessment Scale for High Age Patient (CRASH). *Cancer* 2012;118:3377–3386.
40. Aaldriks AA, Van Der Geest LG, Giltay EJ, et al. Frailty and malnutrition predictive of mortality risk in older patients with advanced colorectal cancer receiving chemotherapy. *J Geriatr Oncol* 2013;4:218–226.

43. Soubeyran P, Fonck M, Blanc-Bisson C, et al. Predictors of early death risk in older patients treated with first line chemotherapy for cancer. *J Clin Oncol* 2012;20:1829–1834.
47. de Souza Viana L, Serufo JC, Da Costa Rocha MO, et al. Performance of a modified MASCC index score for identifying low risk febrile neutropenic cancer patients. *Support Care Cancer* 2008;16:841–846.
54. Lyman GH. Impact of chemotherapy dose intensity on cancer patient outcomes. *J Natl Compr Canc Netw* 2009;7:99–108.
55. Donohue R. Development and implementation of a risk-assessment tool for chemotherapy induced neutropenia. *Oncol Nurse Forum* 2006;33:347–352.
57. Gafter-Gvili A, Fraser A, Paul M, et al. Antibiotic prophylaxis for bacterial infections in afebrile neutropenic patients following chemotherapy. *Cochrane Database Syst Rev* 2012;1:CD004386.
59. Imran H, Tleyjeh IM, Arndt CA, et al. Fluoroquinolone prophylaxis in patients with neutropenia. A meta-analysis of randomized placebo-controlled studies. *Eur J Clin Miocrobiol Infect Dis* 2008;27:53–63.
61. Aapro MS, Bohlius J, Cameron DA, et al. 2010 update of EORTC guidelines for the use of granulocyte-colony stimulating factor to reduce the incidence of chemotherapy-induced febrile neutropenia in adult patients with lymphoproliferative disorders and solid tumors. *Eur J Cancer* 2011;47:8–32.
65. Crawford J, Armitage J, Balducci L, et al. Myeloid growth factors. *J Natl Compr Cancer Netw* 2013;11:1266–1290.
68. Kuderer NM, Dale DC, Crawford J, et al. Impact of primary prophylaxis with granulocyte colony-stimulating factor on febrile neutropenia and mortality in adult cancer patients receiving chemotherapy: a systematic review. *J Clin Oncol* 2007;25:3158–3167.
69. Bohlius J, Herbst C, Reiser M, et al. Granulopoiesis-stimulating factors to prevent adverse effects in the treatment of malignant lymphoma. *Cochrane Database Syst Rev* 2008;4:CD003189.
70. Cooper KL, Madan J, Whytre S, et al. Granulocyte colony-stimulating factors for febrile neutropenia prophylaxis following chemotherapy: systematic review and meta-analysis. *BMC Cancer* 2011;11:404.
71. Renner P, Milazzo S, Liu SP, et al. Primary prophylactic colony-stimulating factors for the prevention of chemotherapy-induced febrile neutropenia in breast cancer patients. *Cochrane Database Syst Rev* 2012;10:CD007913.
79. Henck HJ, Becker L, Tan H, et al. Comparative effectiveness of pegfilgrastim, filgrastim, and sargramostim prophylaxis for neutropenia-related hospitalization: two US retrospective claims analyses. *J Med Econ* 2013;16:160–168.
80. Almenar D, Mayans D, Juan O, et al. Pegfilgrastim and daily granulocyte colony-stimulating factor: patterns of use and neutropenia-related outcomes in cancer patients in Spain—results of the LEARN Study. *Eur J Cancer Care* 2013;18:280–286.

85. Heaney ML, Toy EL, Vekeman F, et al. Comparison of hospitalization risk and associated costs among patients receiving sargramostim, filgrastim, and pegfilgrastim for chemotherapy-induced neutropenia. *Cancer* 2009; 115:4839–4448.

90. Clark OA, Lyman GA, Castro AA, et al. Colony stimulating factors for chemotherapy-induced febrile neutropenia: a meta-analysis of randomized controlled trials. *J Clin Oncol* 2005;23:4198–4214.

100. Aarts MJ, Peters MP, Mandigers CM, et al. Primary granulocyte colony-stimulating factor prophylaxis during the first two cycles only or throughout all chemotherapy cycles in patients with breast cancer at risk for febrile neutropenia. *J Clin Oncol* 2013;31:4290–4296.

103. Kirshner JJ, Heckler CE, Janelsins MC, et al. Prevention of pegfilgrastim-induced bone pain: a phase III double-blind placebo-controlled randomized clinical trial of the University of Rochester cancer center clinical community oncology program research base. *J Clin Oncol* 2012;30:1974–1979.

104. Lyman GH, Dale DC, Wolff DA, et al. Acute myeloid leukemia or myelodysplastic syndrome in randomized controlled clinical trials of cancer chemotherapy with granulocyte colony-stimulating factor: a systematic review. *J Clin Oncol* 2010;28:2914–2924.

108. Potovsky AL, Malin JL, Kim B, et al. Use of colony-stimulating factors with chemotherapy: opportunities for cost savings and improved outcome. *J Natl Cancer Inst* 2011;103:979–982.

109. Lyman GH. Counting the cost of cancer care. *Lancet Oncol* 2013;14: 1142–1143.

112. Gurion R, Belnik-Plitman Y, Gafter-Gvili A, et al. Colony-stimulating factors for prevention and treatment of infectious complications in patients with acute myelogenous leukemia. *Cochrane Database Syst Rev* 2012;6:CD008238.

113. Gurion R, Belnik-Plitman Y, Gafter-Gvili A, et al. Colony-stimulating factors for prevention and treatment of infectious complications in patients with acute myelogenous leukemia. *Cochrane Database Syst Rev* 2011;9:CD008238.

114. Hauser M, Zapf A, Morgan M, et al. Myeloid growth factors in acute myeloid leukemia: systematic review of randomized controlled trials. *Ann Hematol* 2011;90:273–281.

115. Rowe JM, Andersen JW, Mazza JJ, et al. A randomized placebo controlled phase III trial of granulocyte–macrophage colony stimulating factor in adult patients (>55-70 years of age) with acute myelogenous leukemia. An Eastern Cooperative Oncology Group Study. *Blood* 1995;86:457–462.

123. Wheatley K, Goldstone AH, Littlewood T, et al. Randomized placebo-controlled trial of granulocyte colony stimulating factor (G-CSF) as supportive care after induction chemotherapy in adult patients with acute myeloid leukaemia: a study of the United Kingdom Medical Research Council Adult Leukaemia Working Party. *Br J Haematol* 2009;146:54–63.

124. Löfgren C, Paul C, Aström M, et al. Granulocyte-macrophage colony-stimulating factor to increase efficacy of mitoxantrone, etoposide and cytarabine in previously untreated elderly patients with acute myeloid leukaemia: a Swedish multicentre randomized trial. *Br J Haematol* 2004;124:474–480.

125. Harousseau JL, Witz B, Lioure B, et al. Granulocyte colony-stimulating factor after intensive consolidation chemotherapy in acute myeloid leukemia: results of a randomized trial of the Groupe Ouest-Est Leucémies Aigues Myeloblastiques. *J Clin Oncol* 2000;18:780–787.

130. Massey E, Paulus U, Doree C, et al. Granulocyte transfusions for preventing infections in patients with neutropenia or neutrophil dysfunction. *Cochrane Database Syst Rev* 2009;1:CD005341.

131. Valent J, Schiffer CA. Thrombocytopenia and platelet transfusions in patients with cancer. *Cancer Treat Res* 2011;157:251–265.

134 Cancer Associated Thrombosis

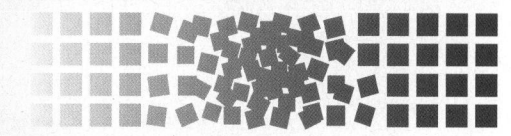

Agnes Y. Y. Lee and Alok A. Khorana

INTRODUCTION

Cancer is a prothrombotic state. Cancer and anticancer therapies are frequently complicated by the development of vascular events, often with devastating clinical consequences. The most frequent vascular events include deep venous thrombosis (DVT) and pulmonary embolism (PE), together described as venous thromboembolism (VTE). Arterial events including stroke and myocardial infarction can also occur, particularly with regimens containing antiangiogenic agents. Subclinical abnormalities in the hemostatic system can be observed in up to 90% of patients with cancer. Recent preclinical and translational data suggest that this prothrombotic state is driven by oncogenic events and the close linkage between regulation of angiogenesis and coagulation, and is integral to cancer growth and metastasis.

The association of cancer with thrombotic events is commonly linked to Armand Trousseau, who was one of the first to comprehensively describe the eponymous syndrome. In one of medical history's great ironies, Professor Trousseau himself developed thrombophlebitis prior to succumbing to gastric cancer. The past decade has seen a renewal of awareness, owing to a rising incidence of cancer-associated thrombosis, particularly in the setting of chemotherapy and antiangiogenic therapy.[1,2]

The occurrence of vascular events has significant clinical consequences: VTE recurs at an annual risk of 21%, requires long-term anticoagulation with a 12% annual risk of major bleeding complications, impacts negatively on patients' quality of life, and consumes health-care resources.[3] Most importantly, thrombosis is the second-leading cause of death in patients with cancer, accounting for 9% of deaths in one study of cancer outpatients receiving chemotherapy.[4] Cancer patients with VTE have a twofold or greater increase in mortality compared with cancer patients without VTE, even after adjusting for stage.[5,6] This impact on prognosis likely reflects the close association between activation of coagulation and an unfavorable tumor biology. In this chapter, we will review the mechanisms underlying the prothrombotic state in cancer and the incidence, risk factors, prevention, and treatment of cancer-associated thrombosis.

MECHANISMS OF CANCER-ASSOCIATED THROMBOSIS

The pathogenesis of the prothrombotic state in cancer is complex, principally involving procoagulant molecules produced by tumor cells, suppression of fibrinolytic activity, and platelet activation (Fig. 134.1). The genetic mechanisms responsible for malignant transformation such as oncogene activation (*RAS* or *MET*) or tumor suppressor gene inactivation (*P53* or *PTEN*) also directly induce the expression of genes regulating hemostasis.[7–9] Extrinsic factors such as antineoplastic therapy, surgery, and vascular access devices further exacerbate this prothrombotic state.

The most important procoagulant expressed by tumor cells is tissue factor (TF), a transmembrane glycoprotein and the physiologic initiator of coagulation. TF is present on neoplastic cells as well as tumor-associated endothelial cells in a variety of cancers. TF expression occurs early in neoplastic transformation, driven by oncogenic mutations in *KRAS* and *TP53* genes.[9] TF may contribute to tumor growth, metastasis, and angiogenesis through a variety of mechanisms including the formation of the TF/VIIa complex and activation of protease-activated receptor 2.[10] TF expression is associated with increased angiogenesis, tumor invasiveness, and worsened prognosis in various malignancies.[11] Secretion of TF-containing microvesicles into the circulation may also account for the systemic coagulopathy of cancer. Emerging reports suggest that the degree of TF expression by tumor cells or elevated levels of circulating systemic TF may be predictive of VTE and mortality in some cancers, particularly pancreatic.[12–14]

Tumor cells also express plasminogen activator inhibitor-1, a potent inhibitor of the fibrinolytic system that has prothrombotic properties and also promotes tumor growth and angiogenesis. Proinflammatory cytokines such as tumor necrosis factor, interleukins-1 and -6, and interferons are elevated in malignancy. Their enhanced expression results from activation of monocytes or direct release from tumor cells, and can in turn activate coagulation. Finally, interactions mediated by platelet P-selectin between circulating carcinoma mucins and platelets lead to platelet aggregation and platelet-rich thrombus formation without accompanying thrombin generation, and this may also contribute to the prothrombotic state in cancer.[15]

Antineoplastic therapy further exacerbates the prothrombotic state in cancer. Several studies have documented changes in the markers of thrombin generation within hours of chemotherapy administration.[16] Chemotherapy can induce endothelial cell activation leading to increased TF expression, elevated levels of plasma von Willebrand factor and factor VIII coagulant protein, and decreased levels of natural anticoagulants antithrombin and proteins C and S.[17] Chemotherapy can induce release of cell-free DNA, with neutrophils as a predominant source and this in turn acts as a trigger for the intrinsic pathway.[18] DNA and RNA from platelets and neutrophils generate neutrophil extracellular traps (NET). These form a specialized extracellular matrix that can activate coagulation. In animal models, cancers can induce an increase in peripheral blood neutrophils that are sensitized toward NET formation and spontaneous thrombosis is associated with NET generation in vivo.[19] Thus, extracellular chromatin released through NET formation is a potential novel cause for cancer-associated thrombosis.

Most recently, scientists are exploring the complex crosstalk between the coagulation cascade, complement pathway, and the immune system in their synergistic roles in tumor growth.[20–22] It is possible that cooperation among these pathways also contributes to the hypercoagulability in malignancy and may explain the high frequency of anticoagulant failure in patients with cancer-associated thrombosis.

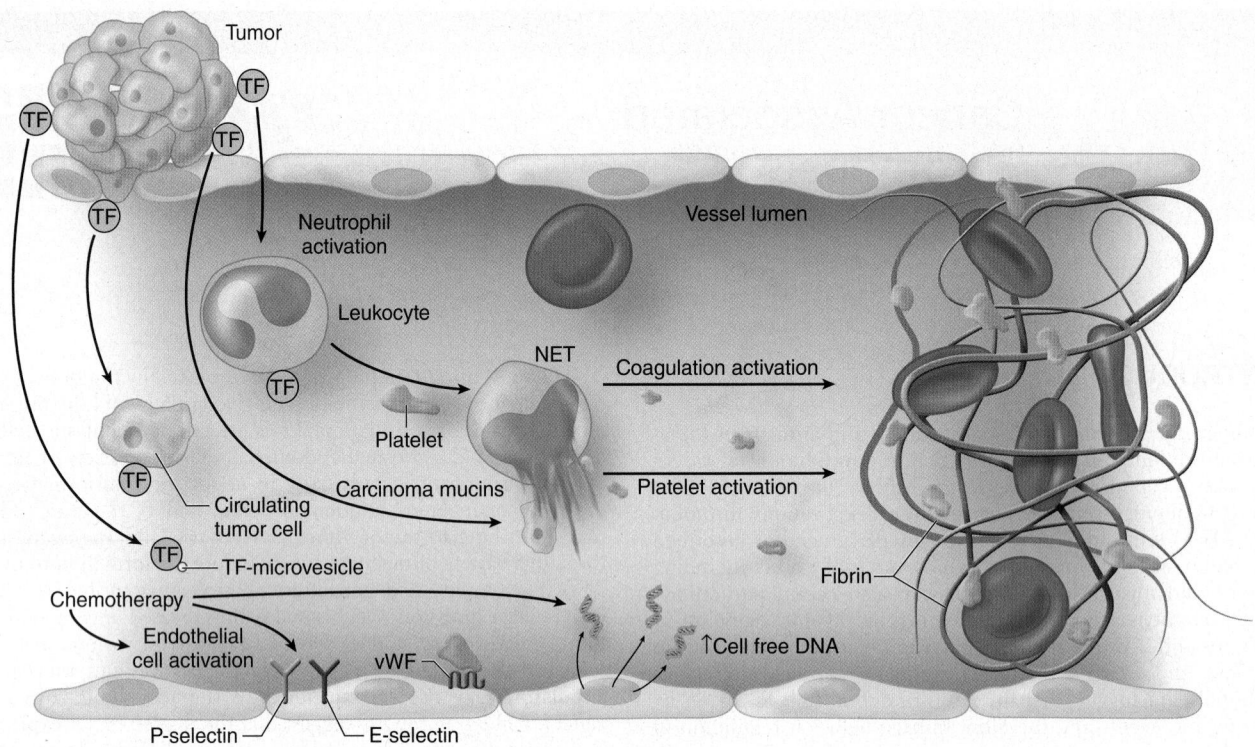

Figure 134.1 Proposed mechanisms for cancer-associated thrombosis. Multiple mechanisms have been postulated including tissue factor upregulation on tumor cell surface as well as release associated with microvesicles into the systemic circulation, platelet activation by carcinoma mucins and other factors, endothelial cell activation by chemotherapy, release of cell-free DNA by chemotherapy, and formation of neutrophil extracellular traps.

EPIDEMIOLOGY OF CANCER-ASSOCIATED THROMBOSIS

Incidence and Prevalence

The incidence of VTE is increased several-fold in patients with cancer when compared with patients without cancer.[1,23–25] In general, the risk among patients with cancer is estimated to be 13 per 1,000 person-years (95% confidence interval [CI] = 7 to 23) in a recent systematic review.[26] However, rates vary significantly depending on specific cancer subgroups, settings, and over time, with more contemporary studies demonstrating higher incidence. Among ambulatory patients, the reported incidence of VTE varies from 7.8% during 26 months (0.3% per month) to 1.93% during a median follow-up of 2.4 months (0.8% per month) to 12% during 8 months (1.5% per month).[27,28] The cause of this increase in the rate of VTE is likely related to improved diagnostic technologies as well as a true increased incidence related to newer antineoplastic drugs and regimens. The advent of highly sensitive multidetector-row computed tomography scans for routine staging has also led to an increased diagnosis of "incidental" PE.[29] The term incidental does not, however, indicate a more benign natural history. Retrospective studies show that the consequences of incidentally discovered PE are no different than those following symptomatic VTE including risk of recurrent VTE and mortality.[30,31]

Rates of arterial thromboembolism (ATE) are less well studied. The use of bevacizumab-containing regimens is clearly associated with a high risk of arterial events.[32] In a pooled analysis of five randomized studies, 4.4% of patients receiving bevacizumab and chemotherapy developed arterial events, compared with 1.9% of patients receiving chemotherapy alone. Rates were particularly high in older patients. In a large meta-analysis of clinical trials with sunitinib and sorafenib, both oral vascular endothelial

growth factor receptor inhibitors, the incidence of ATE was 1.4% (95% CI = 1.2% to 1.6%).[33]

Risk Factors

Patients with cancer comprise a heterogeneous group and include patients undergoing surgery, hospitalization, receiving antineoplastic therapy, or end-of-life care. The risk of VTE differs across these various cancer subpopulations as well as over the natural history of the disease. A recent update by the American Society of Clinical Oncology VTE Guidelines Panel recommends that patients with cancer be assessed for VTE risk at the time of chemotherapy initiation and periodically thereafter (recommendation 6.1).[34] Table 134.1 provides a comprehensive list of cancer-related, treatment-related, and patient-related risk factors and biomarkers for cancer-associated VTE.

Cancer-related risk factors include the primary site, stage, and time after initial diagnosis. The primary site of cancer is historically the best-known and commonly used risk factor. Cancers of the pancreas, stomach, brain, ovary, kidney, and lung have long been associated with VTE; hematologic malignancies, particularly lymphomas, are also strongly associated with VTE.[23,27,28,35] Patients with metastatic disease have a 2- to 20-fold increased risk of VTE.[5,23] VTE is more likely to occur in the initial period after diagnosis. In a population-based study, the adjusted odds ratio for developing VTE in the first 3 months was 53.5 (95% CI = 8.6 to 334.3), declining to 14.3 (95% CI = 5.8 to 35.2) and 3.6 (95% CI = 2.0 to 6.5) in the 3-month to 1-year and 1- to 3-year intervals, respectively.[23]

Treatment-related risk factors include surgical interventions, central venous access devices, hospitalization, and systemic therapy. Patients with cancer undergoing surgery have a two-fold increased risk of postoperative DVT and a three-fold increased risk of fatal PE compared with patients without cancer. The risk

TABLE 134.1

Risk Factors for Cancer-Associated Thrombosis

Cancer-related

Primary site of cancer (gastrointestinal, brain, lung, gynecologic, renal, bladder, lymphoma, myeloma)

Initial period after diagnosis (highest in first 3 to 6 mo)

Histology (higher for adenocarcinoma and high-grade tumors)

Stage (higher with regional and metastatic disease)

Treatment-related

Major surgery

Hospitalization

Chemotherapy

Antiangiogenic therapy (bevacizumab, sunitinib, sorafenib for arterial events)

Immunomodulatory agents (thalidomide- or lenalidomide-based combination regimens)

Certain hormonal therapy agents (e.g., tamoxifen)

Erythropoiesis-stimulating agents

Central venous access devices

Transfusions

Patient-related

Age (higher in older patients)

Race (higher in African Americans, lower in Asian-Pacific Islanders)

Patient comorbidities

Obesity, infection, renal disease, pulmonary disease, arterial thromboembolism

Prior history of thrombosis

Inherited prothrombotic mutations (e.g., factor V Leiden, prothrombin gene mutation)

Performance status

Varicose veins

Biomarkers

Prechemotherapy leukocyte count >11,000/mm^3

Prechemotherapy platelet count ≥350,000/mm^3

Hemoglobin <10 g/dL

Tissue factor (antigen expression, circulating microparticles, antigen, or activity)

D-dimer

C-reactive protein

Soluble P-selectin

Peak thrombin generation

Factor VIII

Biomarkers range from tests as simple as the complete blood count to novel assays that may be predictive of VTE in cancer.[43] Prechemotherapy platelet counts of ≥350,000/mm^3 (odds ratio = 1.8; 95% CI = 1.1 to 3.2) and leukocyte counts >11,000/mm^3 (odds ratio = 2.2; 95% CI = 1.2 to 4.0) have been independently associated with VTE.[44] Other candidate biomarkers predictive of VTE include D-dimer, tissue factor, thrombin generation assays, soluble P-selectin, factor VIII, and C-reactive protein.[43] These are not recommended for clinical use until validation studies have been completed.

Risk factors for arterial events are less well investigated. In hospitalized patients receiving chemotherapy, variables associated with ATE included age 65 years or older; male gender; African American ethnicity; sites of cancer including leukemia, colon, prostate, and lung; and presence of comorbid illnesses.[35] For patients receiving bevacizumab-containing regimens, age over 65 years and prior history of ATE were significant risk factors in a pooled analysis of clinical trials.[40] The relative risk of arterial events associated with sorafenib and sunitinib is 3.03 (95% CI = 1.25 to 7.37; $p = 0.015$) compared with control patients.[33]

Risk Assessment Score

Multiple randomized studies have attempted to evaluate the benefit of thromboprophylaxis in patients with cancer, utilizing one or two risk factors to select a high-risk group.[45,46] Low event rates in the control arms of these studies indicate that a high-risk population was not selected. Hence the updated American Society of Clinical Oncology VTE Guidelines Panel recommends against the use of single risk factors or biomarkers to identify high-risk patients.[34] Instead, the panel recommends the use of a validated risk score that incorporates five variables to identify high-risk patients (Table 134.2). This risk score was originally developed and validated in a US national cohort study.[34,44] Observed rates of VTE over median follow-up of 2.5 months in the development and validation cohorts were 0.8% and 0.3% for low-risk, 1.8% and 2% for intermediate-risk, and 7.1% and 6.7% for high-risk patients, respectively. This model was subsequently externally validated in a prospective European cohort study, with rates of 17.7% in the high-risk cohort as compared to 1.5% in low-risk patients, over a 6-month follow-up period.[47] Multiple other cohort studies have further validated this score, although absolute rates vary between studies based on heterogeneous populations and follow-up periods.[48]

of VTE increases significantly when patients with cancer are hospitalized. Patients with cancer on active therapy are at greater risk for VTE. Specific chemotherapeutic agents are associated with higher rates of VTE. In a prospective study, platinum-based regimens were significantly associated with VTE.[36] Even within this class of agents, rates were higher in patients receiving cisplatin as compared with oxaliplatin.[37] Studies of newer cancer regimens that include drugs such as thalidomide, lenalidomide, and bevacizumab have reported very high rates of VTE and ATE events. For thalidomide-containing regimens, rates of VTE up to 34% in patients with myeloma have been reported.[38,39] Bevacizumab, an antivascular endothelial growth factor antibody, has been clearly associated with an increased risk of ATE; data on its association with VTE are conflicting.[1,32,40,41] Even supportive therapy drugs have been associated with increased VTE. In a large meta-analysis, erythropoiesis-stimulating agents were associated with a 1.6-fold increased risk of thromboembolism.[42]

Finally, *patient-related* risk factors further add to risk. In particular, comorbid conditions including infection, ATE, renal disease, pulmonary disease, and anemia can strongly affect risk.

TABLE 134.2

Predictive Risk Score for Cancer-Associated Venous Thromboembolism[44]

Patient Characteristics	Risk Score
Site of cancer	
Very-high-risk (stomach, pancreas)	2
High-risk (lung, lymphoma, gynecologic, bladder, testicular)	1
Prechemotherapy platelet count ≥350,000/mm^3	1
Hemoglobin level <10 g/dl or use of red cell growth factors	1
Prechemotherapy leukocyte count >11,000/mm^3	1
Body mass index ≥35 kg/m^2	1

High-risk ≥ 3
Intermediate risk = 1–2
Low-risk = 0

PREVENTION OF CANCER-ASSOCIATED THROMBOSIS

Prophylaxis in Major Surgery

Few clinical trials have been conducted to study the efficacy and safety of thromboprophylaxis specifically in patients with cancer having major surgery. Randomized controlled trials of in-hospital prophylaxis in patients having major abdominal surgery for cancer have shown no difference in the incidence of DVT or major bleeding between unfractionated heparin (UFH) administered three times daily and a low-molecular-weight heparin (LMWH) enoxaparin given once daily.[49,50] Overall, up to 15% of patients with cancer will develop DVT following surgery, despite standard prophylaxis with UFH or LMWH. In addition to LMWH and UFH, fondaparinux is approved for prophylaxis following major abdominal surgery. This selective inhibitor of activated factor X is given once daily subcutaneously and is associated with a lower risk of heparin-induced thrombocytopenia compared with UFH and LMWH. In a phase 3 randomized trial, fondaparinux was found to be comparable to LMWH dalteparin in patients undergoing high-risk abdominal surgery.[51] A post hoc analysis of patients with cancer suggested that fondaparinux was associated with a statistically significant reduction in VTE (4.7% versus 7.7%; $p = 0.02$).

Mechanical methods of prophylaxis, such as graduated compression stockings or intermittent pneumatic calf compression devices, can lower the risk of VTE but are less effective than anticoagulants.[52] Their use should be limited to patients in whom anticoagulation is contraindicated. There is weak evidence that combined mechanical and pharmacologic prophylaxis may further reduce VTE, especially in the patients who are at highest risk.

Extending prophylaxis beyond hospitalization can further reduce the risk of VTE in patients with cancer. In a multicenter, placebo-controlled trial, patients undergoing elective, curative abdominal surgery for cancer received LMWH enoxaparin for the first 6 to 10 days after surgery and then were randomized to continue enoxaparin or placebo injections for 4 weeks.[53] Extended prophylaxis with enoxaparin significantly reduced the rate of VTE by 60% (12.0% versus 4.8%; $p = 0.02$) at 1 month, and this benefit was maintained at 3 months. The absolute risk reduction of 7% means that 14 patients must be treated to avoid one case of DVT. Overall, there

was no difference in bleeding during the treatment period and no difference in mortality up to 1 year of follow-up. Similar results were also reported in a subgroup analysis of an open-label randomized trial in which patients having abdominal surgery were randomized to receive LMWH dalteparin once daily and compression stockings, or to stockings alone for 21 days after hospital discharge.[54] Dalteparin significantly reduced the incidence of DVT from 19.6% to 8.8% ($p = 0.03$) as well as that of proximal DVT from 10.4% to 2.2% ($p = 0.02$). Accordingly, 9 patients must be treated to avoid one episode of DVT while 12 must be treated to avoid one episode of proximal DVT.

The increased risk of postdischarge symptomatic VTE has been shown to peak at 3 weeks after cancer surgery in two large prospective studies.[55,56] One study found that 46% of the deaths occurring within the first month after cancer surgery were due to fatal PE, and the other study reported that 1 in 85 women will develop VTE within the first 12 weeks after cancer surgery.[55] The American Society of Clinical Oncology and the American College of Chest Physicians (ACCP) recommend that extended prophylaxis in patients undergoing cancer surgery should be considered, especially in patients with high-risk features.[34,57] These include previous history of VTE, anesthesia lasting ≥2 hours, bed rest for ≥4 days, advanced malignancy, and older age.[55]

Prophylaxis for Central Venous Catheters

Contemporary trials have provided evidence that neither warfarin (dose fixed at 1 mg daily or adjusted to an international normalized ratio [INR] between 1.5 and 1.9) nor prophylactic doses of LMWH is effective in reducing symptomatic catheter-related thrombosis.[58–60] With or without prophylaxis, symptomatic catheter-related thrombosis rates of approximately 4% were reported in these studies, and bleeding may be increased in those who received an anticoagulant. Based on these data, the ACCP guidelines have recommended against routine prophylaxis using LMWH and fixed-dose warfarin.[52] Although high-risk patients may still benefit from prophylaxis, the selection criteria of such patients and the optimal anticoagulant regimen are not defined.

Prophylaxis in Medical Patients

Randomized trials have studied the efficacy and safety of anticoagulant prophylaxis in outpatients receiving chemotherapy (Table 134.3).

TABLE 134.3

Randomized Controlled Trials of Primary Prophylaxis in Patients with Solid Tumors

Study Population (Ref.)	No. of Patients	Anticoagulant Prophylaxis	VTE in Anticoagulant Group (%)	VTE in Control Group (%)	P Value
Stage IV breast cancer[60]		Warfarin 1 mg/d × 6 wk then INR 1.3–1.9	0.7	4.4	0.03
Advanced breast cancer[62]	351	Certoparin 3,000 units once daily	4.0	3.9	NS
Advanced NSCLC[62]	532	Certoparin 3,000 units once daily	4.5	8.3	0.07
Grade III/IV malignant glioma[63]	186	Dalteparin 5,000 units once daily	11.0	17.0	0.3
Advanced cancer of breast, lung, GI, pancreas, ovary, head and neck[44]	1,150	Nadroparin 3,800 units once daily	2.0	3.9	0.02
Advanced cancer of lung, pancreas, stomach, colon or rectum, bladder, or ovary[45]	3,212	Semuloparin 20 mg once daily	1.2	3.4	<0.001
Advanced pancreatic cancer[66]	312	Enoxaparin 1 mg/kg once daily × 12 wk then 40 mg once daily	14.5	5.0	<0.01
Advanced pancreatic cancer[64]	123	Dalteparin 200 U/kg once daily × 4 wk then 150 U/kg × 8 wk	31.0	12.0	0.02

VTE, venous thromboembolism; INR, international normalized ratio; NS, nonsignificant; NSCLC, nonsmall-cell lung cancer; GI, gastrointestinal.

One small randomized trial found that very-low-dose warfarin was effective in reducing symptomatic DVT in women with stage IV breast cancer receiving multiagent chemotherapy,[61] while small, placebo-controlled trials in patients with a number of different solid tumors provided inconsistent evidence for prophylactic doses of LMWH.[62,63] But two large placebo-controlled clinical trials have demonstrated LMWH or an ultra-LMWH are effective in reducing symptomatic thrombosis. The PROTECHT study reported a relative risk reduction of 49% associated with nadroparin prophylaxis and the SAVE-ONCO trial found a relative reduction of 64% associated with semuloparin in patients with locally advanced or metastatic solid tumors. There were no differences in bleeding or overall survival.[45,46]

Two open-label studies in patients with advanced pancreatic cancer reported significant and dramatic reductions in clinically relevant VTE when therapeutic or half-therapeutic doses of LMWH were given in conjunction with standard chemotherapy. In one study, enoxaparin at 1 mg/kg daily for 3 months reduced the incidence of symptomatic VTE by 66% (from 14.5% to 5.0%; $p < 0.01$), whereas dalteparin at therapeutic dosing reduced the incidence from 31% to 12% (relative risk = 0.38; $p = 0.02$).[64–66] In the latter study, the risk of fatal PE was also significantly lowered (relative risk = 0.08; $p = 0.03$). Bleeding was not increased in the LMWH groups in these studies. Overall, the findings suggest that patients with specific tumor types or who have a high risk of thrombosis do benefit from anticoagulant prophylaxis and that doses that are higher than what is used for standard primary prophylaxis are very effective and well tolerated. Identifying high-risk patients using a risk-assessment model will also improve the benefit-risk ratio of anticoagulant prophylaxis.

Another population in whom primary prophylaxis may be beneficial is patients with multiple myeloma who are receiving thalidomide or lenalidomide in combination with chemotherapy or high-dose steroids. Incidences of symptomatic VTE of 20% to 30% have been reported, but the pathophysiologic mechanisms remain elusive.[39] This high risk has prompted the use of aspirin, warfarin, and LMWH in uncontrolled settings and guidelines to recommend anticoagulation prophylaxis in patients receiving thalidomide- or lenalidomide-based regimens.[34,52] Randomized trials are urgently needed to identify a safe and effective prophylaxis regimen, given the potential for serious bleeding in this patient group.

Randomized trials in a cancer-specific population have not been done in acutely ill medical patients admitted to hospital. Recommendations regarding the efficacy and safety of thromboprophylaxis in these patients are based on three large randomized studies that included only a minority (5% to 15%) of patients with cancer. However, post hoc and meta-analysis of these studies do not show a significant reduction with standard LMWH prophylaxis in medically ill cancer patients.[67] Nonetheless, given the known high risk of VTE during hospitalization for patients with cancer and its attendant consequences, all of the guidelines recommend thromboprophylaxis in the absence of contraindications.[34,52] There continue to be ongoing concerns regarding the risk of bleeding in these patients, for which few cancer-specific data are available.

TREATMENT OF CANCER-ASSOCIATED THROMBOSIS

Anticoagulants are the cornerstone agents for the treatment of acute VTE. Although these agents are highly efficacious and have an acceptable safety profile in most patients, patients with cancer have a three-fold higher risk of recurrent VTE and two-fold higher risk of anticoagulant-related bleeding compared with patients without cancer.[68,69] These complications reflect the prothrombotic state associated with malignant diseases and the multiple comorbidities in patients with cancer that may alter their response to anticoagulant therapy and their risk of bleeding. LMWH is the preferred treatment for initial and long-term treatment because of its favorable efficacy, safety, and convenience profile compared with UFH and vitamin K antagonists (VKA).[34,70–72]

Initial Therapy

Formal comparisons of LMWH, UFH, and fondaparinux for initial treatment of VTE in patients with cancer have not been conducted. Based on results extracted from randomized trials that evaluated these agents, LMWH and UFH appear equally effective in reducing recurrent thrombosis in patients with cancer, but LMWH is associated with a 3-month survival benefit over UFH.[73] Furthermore, LMWH can be given safely as once-daily subcutaneous injections in an outpatient setting without the need for laboratory monitoring and have a lower risk of heparin-induced thrombocytopenia. Fondaparinux given once daily is also comparable to heparins for the initial treatment of VTE and may eliminate the risk of heparin-induced thrombocytopenia. However, a post hoc analysis of a randomized trial suggests that it is less effective than enoxaparin for outpatient treatment of DVT in patients with cancer.[74] New oral anticoagulants that inhibit activated factor X (e.g., rivaroxaban, apixaban, edoxaban) or thrombin (e.g., dabigatran) are comparable to traditional therapy with a LMWH followed by a VKA for treatment of acute VTE. In some of these trials, monotherapy with the new oral anticoagulant was compared with LMWH followed by warfarin; however, efficacy and safety data for the initial treatment period have not been published. Because these trials included only a small number of highly selected patients with cancer, further investigation is essential to show efficacy and safety in the general cancer population.[75] The major concerns about these new anticoagulants in patients with cancer include potential interaction with chemotherapeutic agents, altered metabolism in patients with renal dysfunction or hepatic metastases, lack of antidote when patients are actively bleeding, and whether treatment doses in patients without cancer are as effective in these hypercoagulable patients.

Long-Term Therapy

Despite their pharmacologic and practical limitations, VKAs were the mainstay of long-term anticoagulant treatment for VTE in patients with cancer for many years. Although VKAs are highly effectively in reducing recurrent thrombosis in the general population, treatment failures, serious bleeding, and difficulties with maintaining the INR within the therapeutic range are common problems in patients with cancer. A prospective cohort study reported that the 12-month cumulative incidence of recurrent VTE in patients with cancer was 20.7%, versus 6.8% in patients without cancer, and the corresponding estimate for major bleeding was 12.4% versus 4.9%, respectively.[69] Patients with cancer also experience recurrent VTE despite having therapeutic INR levels and suffer serious bleeding complications even without receiving excessive anticoagulation.[68]

Clinical trials have now established LMWH as the preferred long-term treatment for VTE. The CLOT trial randomized 676 patients with cancer with symptomatic proximal DVT, PE, or both, to receive usual treatment with dalteparin initially followed by 6 months of therapy with either VKA or dalteparin alone.[76] In the dalteparin group, patients self-injected therapeutic doses at 200 U/kg once daily for the first month followed by 75% to 80% of the full dose for the next 5 months. The VKA group was treated to maintain a therapeutic INR between 2 and 3. The cumulative risk of recurrent VTE at 6 months was reduced from 17% in the VKA group to 9% in the dalteparin group, resulting in a statistically significant risk reduction of 52% ($p = 0.002$; Fig. 134.2). Accordingly, one episode of recurrent VTE is prevented for every 13 patients treated with dalteparin. Overall, there were no differences in major or any bleeding between the groups. By 6 months, 39% of the patients had died in each group, with 90% of the deaths being from progressive cancer. A post hoc subgroup analysis showed that, among patients who had no known metastatic disease at randomization, those who were randomized to dalteparin had better survival compared with those who had received a VKA.[77]

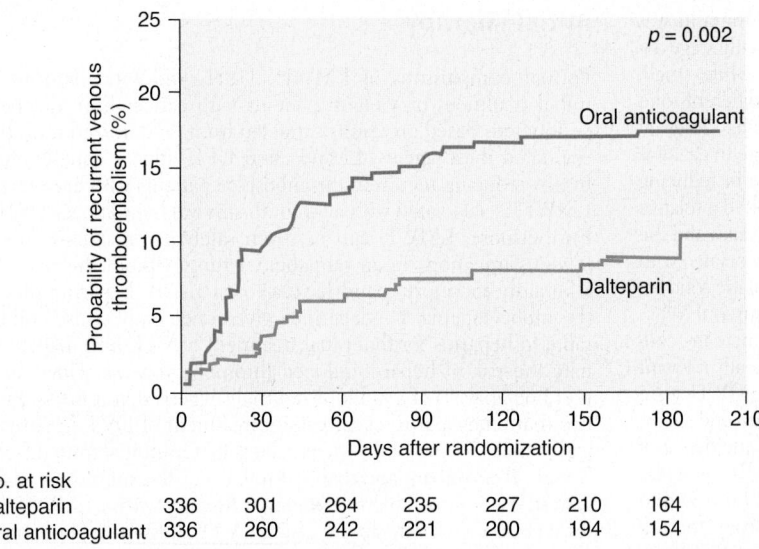

No. at risk

Dalteparin	336	301	264	235	227	210	164
Oral anticoagulant	336	260	242	221	200	194	154

Figure 134.2 The cumulative risks of recurrent venous thromboembolism comparing 6 months of treatment with low-molecular-weight heparin dalteparin versus a vitamin K antagonist (hazard ratio = 0.48; 95% confidence interval = 0.30 to 0.77; p = 0.002). (From Lee AY, Levine MN, Baker RI, et al. Low-molecular-weight heparin versus a coumarin for the prevention of recurrent venous thromboembolism in patients with cancer. *N Engl J Med* 2003;349:146–153, with permission.)

Whether this was the result of an anticoagulant or an anticancer effect remains uncertain. The observation that the separation of the survival curves occurred only after the discontinuation of dalteparin suggests that the survival benefit is not the result of a reduction in fatal PE. Ongoing research is being done to determine if LMWH offers antineoplastic effects in specific cancers and to explore the potential biologic mechanisms. In contrast to the CLOT study, three randomized trials reported nonsignificant reductions in symptomatic VTE with LMWH compared with VKA therapy.[55–57,78–80] It is likely that these other trials were underpowered (two were terminated prematurely prior to achieving target sample size) or that the dosing of other LMWHs were inadequate. Nonetheless, the finding of LMWH superiority over warfarin was consistent in all the trials. This led to major consensus guidelines to recommend LMWH over warfarin therapy.[34,71,72] Fondaparinux has not been evaluated against LMWH for long-term treatment in patients with cancer, but a small study suggests it is effective and well tolerated.[81] Ongoing randomized controlled trials are being conducted to examine the role of novel oral anticoagulants for long-term treatment of cancer-associated thrombosis. As discussed previously, robust data are not yet available to demonstrate that they are comparable to warfarin or LMWH in the oncology setting. Issues unique to patients with cancer such as unpredictable gastrointestinal absorption, drug interaction with chemotherapy, and renal or liver dysfunction may render these novel agents inferior to LMWH.

There is no evidence to guide the choice of anticoagulant after the first 6 months of treatment. For patients who have tolerated LMWH or VKA for the first 6 months, continuing with the same anticoagulant is a sensible option if ongoing anticoagulation is needed. It is recommended that the risks and benefits of LMWH versus VKA therapy are discussed with the patient in order to individualize treatment. Besides the risk of bleeding, there does not appear to be any significant side effects associated with long-term use of LMWH or VKA. Although animal studies suggest that LMWH exposure may reduce bone density, this has not been shown to be a concern in patient populations (e.g., pregnant women with VTE) that also need extended treatment with LMWH.

Based on the evidence to date, long-term treatment with a LMWH for patients with cancer with DVT or PE is recommended by the ACCP Consensus Guidelines, the National Comprehensive Cancer Network Clinical Practice Guidelines in Oncology, and the American Society of Clinical Oncology.[34,71,72]

Therapy for Recurrent Venous Thromboembolism

Although recurrent VTE is frequent in patients with cancer, optimal treatment has not been investigated in clinical trials.[70,82] Insertion of an inferior vena cava filter is commonly used in patients with recurrent thrombosis despite anticoagulation, but evidence supporting this practice is lacking. In fact, studies have shown that patients with filters have a higher risk of recurrent DVT than those without the device, and fatal PE has been reported in patients with cancer following filter insertion. It is recommended that the use of filters be limited to situations in which anticoagulant therapy cannot be used because of serious, active bleeding. Success has been reported with using LMWH in patients who break through VKA therapy and with using higher doses of LMWH in those who break through usual LMWH treatment doses.[70] In a small series of patients with cancer with recurrent thrombosis, 9% of patients treated with dose escalation of LMWH had a second thrombotic event and 1% had a major bleed over a 3-month follow-up period.[83] Mortality in patients who developed recurrent thrombosis was high, with a median time between recurrence and death at 11 months. This observation reinforces the concept that activation of coagulation is associated with unfavorable tumor biology.

Duration of Therapy

Although clinical trial evidence is lacking, it is generally recommended that patients with metastases should continue with "indefinite" anticoagulant therapy after a single thrombotic event because metastatic malignancy is a risk factor for recurrent thrombosis. In patients without metastases, anticoagulant treatment is recommended for as long as the cancer is "active" and while the patient is receiving antitumor therapy. Although this period is sometimes difficult to define, patients who have not experienced any complications often prefer to continue anticoagulant therapy to avoid recurrent thrombosis. Given the complex and changing clinical courses of most patients with cancer, periodic evaluation of the risk-benefit ratio of continuing anticoagulant therapy in individual patients is absolutely essential. The decision should take into consideration the patient's preference, the anticancer treatments, the comorbid conditions, and most importantly, the patient's quality of life and life expectancy.

SELECTED REFERENCES

The full reference list can be accessed at lwwhealthlibrary.com/oncology.

1. Khorana AA, Dalal M, Lin J, et al. Incidence and predictors of venous thromboembolism (VTE) among ambulatory high-risk cancer patients undergoing chemotherapy in the United States. *Cancer* 2013;119:648–655.

4. Khorana AA, Francis CW, Culakova E, et al. Thromboembolism is a leading cause of death in cancer patients receiving outpatient chemotherapy. *J Thromb Haemost* 2007;5:632–634.

6. Sorensen HT, Mellemkjaer L, Olsen JH, et al. Prognosis of cancers associated with venous thromboembolism. *N Engl J Med* 2000;343:1846–1850.

7. Boccaccio C, Sabatino G, Medico E, et al. The MET oncogene drives a genetic programme linking cancer to haemostasis. *Nature* 2005;434:396–400.

9. Yu JL, May L, Lhotak V, et al. Oncogenic events regulate tissue factor expression in colorectal cancer cells: implications for tumor progression and angiogenesis. *Blood* 2005;105:1734–1741.

10. Kasthuri RS, Taubman MB, Mackman N. Role of tissue factor in cancer. *J Clin Oncol* 2009;27:4834–4838.

17. Lee AY, Levine MN. The thrombophilic state induced by therapeutic agents in the cancer patient. *Semin Thromb Hemost* 1999;25:137–145.

19. Demers M, Krause DS, Schatzberg D, et al. Cancers predispose neutrophils to release extracellular DNA traps that contribute to cancer-associated thrombosis. *Proc Natl Acad Sci U S A* 2012;109:13076–13081.

23. Blom JW, Doggen CJ, Osanto S, et al. Malignancies, prothrombotic mutations, and the risk of venous thrombosis. *JAMA* 2005;293:715–722.

26. Horsted F, West J, Grainge MJ. Risk of venous thromboembolism in patients with cancer: a systematic review and meta-analysis. *PLoS Med* 2012;9:e1001275.

27. Khorana AA, Francis CW, Culakova E, et al. Risk factors for chemotherapy-associated venous thromboembolism in a prospective observational study. *Cancer* 2005;104:2822–2829.

29. Khorana AA, O'Connell C, Agnelli G, et al. Incidental venous thromboembolism in oncology patients. *J Thromb Haemost* 2012;10:2602–2604.

31. O'Connell CL, Boswell WD, Duddalwar V, et al. Unsuspected pulmonary emboli in cancer patients: clinical correlates and relevance. *J Clin Oncol* 2006;24:4928–4932.

34. Lyman GH, Khorana AA, Kuderer NM, et al. Venous thromboembolism prophylaxis and treatment in patients with cancer: American Society of Clinical Oncology clinical practice guideline update. *J Clin Oncol* 2013;31:2189–2204.

35. Khorana AA, Francis CW, Culakova E, et al. Thromboembolism in hospitalized neutropenic cancer patients. *J Clin Oncol* 2006;24:484–490.

43. Pabinger I, Thaler J, Ay C. Biomarkers for prediction of venous thromboembolism in cancer. *Blood* 2013;122:2011–2018.

44. Khorana AA, Kuderer NM, Culakova E, et al. Development and validation of a predictive model for chemotherapy-associated thrombosis. *Blood* 2008;111:4902–4907.

45. Agnelli G, Gussoni G, Bianchini C, et al. Nadroparin for the prevention of thromboembolic events in ambulatory patients with metastatic or locally advanced solid cancer receiving chemotherapy: a randomised, placebo-controlled, double-blind study. *Lancet Oncol* 2009;10:943–949.

47. Ay C, Dunkler D, Marosi C, et al. Prediction of venous thromboembolism in cancer patients. *Blood* 2010;116:5377–5382.

49. Efficacy and safety of enoxaparin versus unfractionated heparin for prevention of deep vein thrombosis in elective cancer surgery: a double-blind randomized multicentre trial with venographic assessment. ENOXACAN Study Group. *Br J Surg* 1997;84:1099–1103.

52. Kahn SR, Lim W, Dunn AS, et al. Prevention of VTE in nonsurgical patients: Antithrombotic Therapy and Prevention of Thrombosis, 9th ed: American College of Chest Physicians Evidence-Based Clinical Practice Guidelines. *Chest* 2012;141:e195S–e226S.

53. Bergqvist D, Agnelli G, Cohen AT, et al. Duration of prophylaxis against venous thromboembolism with enoxaparin after surgery for cancer. *N Engl J Med* 2002;346:975–980.

55. Agnelli G, Bolis G, Capussotti L, et al. A clinical outcome-based prospective study on venous thromboembolism after cancer surgery: the @RISTOS project. *Ann Surg* 2006;243:89–95.

56. Sweetland S, Green J, Liu B, et al. Duration and magnitude of the postoperative risk of venous thromboembolism in middle aged women: prospective cohort study. *BMJ* 2009;339:b4583.

57. Gould MK, Garcia DA, Wren SM, et al. Prevention of VTE in nonorthopedic surgical patients: Antithrombotic Therapy and Prevention of Thrombosis, 9th ed: American College of Chest Physicians Evidence-Based Clinical Practice Guidelines. *Chest* 2012;141:e227S–e277S.

60. Young AM, Billingham LJ, Begum G, et al. Warfarin thromboprophylaxis in cancer patients with central venous catheters (WARP): an open-label randomised trial. *Lancet* 2009;373:567–574.

66. Maraveyas A, Waters J, Roy R, et al. Gemcitabine versus gemcitabine plus dalteparin thromboprophylaxis in pancreatic cancer. *Eur J Cancer* 2012;48:1283–1292.

69. Prandoni P, Lensing AW, Piccioli A, et al. Recurrent venous thromboembolism and bleeding complications during anticoagulant treatment in patients with cancer and venous thrombosis. *Blood* 2002;100:3484–3488.

70. Lee AY, Peterson EA. Treatment of cancer-associated thrombosis. *Blood* 2013;122:2310–2317.

71. Kearon C, Kahn SR, Agnelli G, et al. Antithrombotic therapy for venous thromboembolic disease: American College of Chest Physicians Evidence-Based Clinical Practice Guidelines (8th Edition). *Chest* 2008;133:454S–545S.

72. National Comprehensive Cancer Network. *Clinical Practice Guidelines in Oncology Venous Thromboembolic Disease* Version 2.2011. Accessed November 26, 2013. http://www.nccn.org/professionals/physician_gls/f_guidelines.asp#supportive.

73. Akl EA, Rohilla S, Barba M, et al. Anticoagulation for the initial treatment of venous thromboembolism in patients with cancer: a systematic review. *Cancer* 2008;113:1685–1694.

77. Lee AY, Rickles FR, Julian JA, et al. Randomized comparison of low molecular weight heparin and coumarin derivatives on the survival of patients with cancer and venous thromboembolism. *J Clin Oncol* 2005;23:2123–2129.

82. Carrier M, Khorana AA, Zwicker J, et al. Management of challenging cases of patients with cancerassociated thrombosis including recurrent thrombosis and bleeding: guidance from the SSC of the ISTH. *J Thromb Haemost* 2013;11:1760–1765.

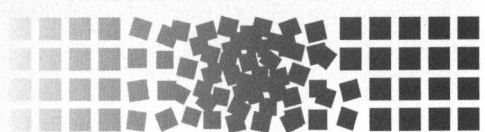
Elizabeth M. Blanchard and Paul J. Hesketh

INTRODUCTION

Nausea and vomiting associated with cancer treatment have historically been among the most difficult side effects that patients face while being treated for cancer. Chemotherapy-induced nausea and vomiting (CINV) in particular remains one of the most dreaded side effects from a patient perspective. Patient surveys have consistently listed CINV as one of the most severe and troublesome adverse events related to treatment.[1] Although intuitive, nausea and vomiting related to chemotherapy have also been shown to negatively impact a patient's functional status as tested by objective measures.[2] In fact, CINV has been shown to negatively impact all aspects of quality of life for patients including emotional, social, and physical functioning as well as global quality of life.[3] The last 20 years have seen tremendous progress in this area, which has significant implications for patients in improving their quality of life as well as compliance with cancer treatment.

In the era before the use of newer antiemetics, nearly 80% of patients would experience an episode of nausea or vomiting during the 5 days following chemotherapy of moderate to high emetogenic potential.[4] The prevalence of CINV has been dramatically decreased with the introduction of the 5-hydroxytryptamine-3 (5-HT$_3$) receptor antagonists in the early 1990s and with the subsequent introduction of a new class of antiemetic, the neurokinin (NK)-1 (NK$_1$) receptor antagonists. Despite the progress, CINV remains suboptimally controlled for a significant minority of patients. An important remaining challenge is the recognition and management of the symptom of nausea following chemotherapy treatment.

Optimizing the control of treatment-induced nausea and vomiting should be a high priority for all health-care providers involved in the care of patients with cancer. Knowledge of the extent of the problem, understanding the basic pathophysiologic principles, recognition of patients at risk, and applying available pharmacologic treatments in an evidence-based manner are all key elements in attaining this goal.

NAUSEA AND VOMITING SYNDROMES

CINV does not describe a single clinical entity but rather three relatively distinct clinical syndromes including acute, delayed, and anticipatory nausea and vomiting. Although these distinctions have limitations and are somewhat arbitrary, they are nevertheless useful in terms of characterizing the problem and optimizing treatment. Acute CINV is defined as nausea and vomiting that develop within the first 24 hours after chemotherapy administration. With most emetogenic chemotherapy agents, in the absence of effective prophylactic therapy, nausea and vomiting will develop within a few hours of chemotherapy administration. Delayed CINV is defined as nausea and vomiting occurring >24 hours after chemotherapy administration. It is generally not as well understood as acute emesis and has been described in association with a number of chemotherapy agents such as cisplatin, carboplatin, cyclophosphamide, and the anthracyclines. It appears to be less severe than acute emesis but can last for a longer period of time.[5,6] Delayed CINV has been best characterized in relation to cisplatin.[7] In the absence

of antiemetic treatment, it will develop in ≥90% of patients receiving this agent. It peaks between 24 and 72 hours after cisplatin and gradually dissipates during the next several days. Anticipatory nausea and vomiting occur as the result of a conditioned response to prior episodes of CINV. Symptoms occur after exposure to a variety of stimuli that remind the patient of their prior emetic experiences such as returning to clinic, seeing health-care personnel, or the apparatus involved with chemotherapy administration.[8]

Unlike CINV, radiation-induced nausea and vomiting (RINV) has not been broken down into distinct clinical syndromes. Risk of nausea and vomiting is generally related to the body area exposed to treatment with fields encompassing small bowel and stomach associated with the greatest risk. This issue is further addressed in the section on defining the risk of nausea and vomiting.

PATHOPHYSIOLOGY OF TREATMENT-INDUCED NAUSEA AND VOMITING

The mechanisms underlying the control of nausea and vomiting are extraordinarily complex and still incompletely understood at the present time. The central nervous system (CNS) is thought to play a critical role in the physiology of nausea and vomiting, serving as the primary site where a variety of emetic stimuli are received and processed. The CNS is also believed to have the primary role in generating the efferent signals to a number of structures in the body that eventually result in the development of nausea and vomiting.

The mechanisms by which chemotherapy causes nausea and vomiting are only partially delineated. Our current understanding of the pathophysiology of this process is based on the pioneering studies of Borison and Wang[9] conducted more than 60 years ago and more recent insights provided during the development process of the newer antiemetic agents.[10] Borison and Wang[9] proposed that two sites within the brainstem were critical in the control of emesis. The first of these sites is the area postrema, which is a circumventricular structure located at the caudal end of the fourth ventricle. It is positioned outside the blood–brain barrier and therefore is accessible to emetic substances borne in either blood or cerebral spinal fluid. Given its central role in processing a variety of emetogens, it has often been termed the *chemoreceptor trigger zone*. The area postrema cannot independently initiate the emetic process but does so indirectly through neural projections to a second site proposed by Borison and Wang: the vomiting center. According to their theory, a vomiting center located in the lateral reticular formation of the medulla is the final common pathway through which efferent signals are generated to initiate the emetic process. It is now appreciated that an anatomically distinct vomiting center does not exist and that the motor outputs are coordinated by a variety of brainstem nuclei such as the parvicellular reticular formation, the Botzinger complex, and the nucleus tractus solitarius.[11,12] These nuclei have been collectively referred to as the *vomiting center*.[10]

In addition to the area postrema, three other sources of afferent input to the vomiting center appear to have importance in the generation of the emetic response.[9,13] Of greatest importance with respect to CINV is the stomach and proximal small bowel.

Chemotherapy agents can either directly or indirectly access the gut mucosa causing release of local mediators from the enterochromaffin cells, stimulating vagal and splanchnic afferent fibers within the bowel wall. These vagal afferents can then transmit afferent signals to the brainstem either directly to nuclei within the vomiting center such as the nucleus tractus solitarius or indirectly via the area postrema initiating the emetic reflex. Direct stimuli arising within the limbic system in the CNS can also apparently trigger emesis by poorly defined mechanisms. This process may be operative in patients experiencing anticipatory emesis. Finally, input from the vestibular system may also induce emesis. This appears to be a predominant mechanism associated with motion sickness but is likely to have a modest role in CINV.

It is now appreciated that a number of neurotransmitters appear to have important roles in the emetic process. More than 30 neurotransmitters have been identified within the area postrema and nuclei of the vomiting center.[14] Some neurotransmitters such as histamine and acetylcholine, which have established roles in certain types of emesis such as motion sickness, appear to have minimal involvement in CINV. The most clinically relevant neurotransmitters involved in CINV include dopamine, serotonin (5-HT), Substance P, and the cannabinoids.[10,15] Much of our current understanding of the neurotransmitters relevant to CINV has come from preclinical studies that preceded the introduction of a number of our current antiemetics. The role of dopamine receptors in CINV forms the basis of some of the earliest interventions in the prevention of emesis related to chemotherapy. Dopamine D2 receptors are found in the area postrema. Stimulation of these receptors has been shown to induce emesis in animal models.[11] Phenothiazines, which are dopamine antagonists, represented the first class of agents with antiemetic efficacy when introduced into clinical practice nearly 50 years ago.

Over the past 25 years, the role of 5-HT has been gradually elucidated and ultimately surpassed dopamine as the most relevant neurotransmitter in the treatment of CINV. Of the more than a dozen known subtypes of 5-HT receptors, the type 3 (5-HT$_3$) receptor has been found to play the most important role in emesis, and antagonism of these receptors has had a significant impact on prevention of acute CINV.[10] 5-HT$_3$ receptors are found on vagal afferent fibers, within the area postrema, and the nucleus tractus solitarius.[16–18] The precise mechanisms of 5-HT involvement in treatment-related emesis are incompletely understood. It appears that the most clinically relevant site of action of 5-HT occurs at the peripheral level by increasing afferent stimuli from the gut to the vomiting center and area postrema. Whether 5-HT has meaningful central activity is unclear.

Another neurotransmitter, Substance P, has emerged during the past decade as playing a major role in the development of acute and delayed emesis. It is part of a class of regulatory peptides belonging to the tachykinins, which bind to NK receptors[19] and was first noted to cause emesis in animal models. Three tachykinin receptors have been identified, of which the NK$_1$ receptor is preferentially bound by Substance P.[19] The NK$_1$ receptors are found in the gastrointestinal tract, the area postrema, and the nucleus tractus solitarius.[20] NK$_1$ receptor antagonists demonstrated wide-ranging antiemetic effects in ferrets, which prompted their development for clinical use.[21,22] Animal models have demonstrated that the site of action of Substance P appears to be mainly central, as experimental NK$_1$ antagonists that do not cross the blood–brain barrier are ineffective in preventing cisplatin-induced emesis.[23]

Unlike dopamine, 5-HT, and Substance P, which all appear to have a "proemetic" role, other neurotransmitters such as the endogenous cannabinoids, enkephalins, and γ-amino butyric acid appear to exert an agonist antiemetic effect. This area of antiemetic research has received much less attention than efforts devoted to the development of neurotransmitter antagonist antiemetics. Of the endogenous neurotransmitters, only the cannabinoids have relevance in the treatment of CINV at present.[24]

There appear to be differences in the relative importance of the various neurotransmitters in the different emetic syndromes. Acute CINV as well as RINV are thought to be primarily due to 5-HT–mediated pathways. The effectiveness of the 5-HT$_3$ receptor antagonists in both of these settings is thought to be primarily secondary to the ability of these agents to antagonize the binding of 5-HT to the 5-HT$_3$ receptors on the afferent fibers of the vagus and splanchnic nerves, stimulating afferent nerves in the upper small intestine. Dopamine also appears to be most relevant to acute CINV and to a lesser extent in RINV given the utility of dopamine D2 antagonists in these settings.

Dopamine and 5-HT appear to be less important in delayed CINV, given the limited clinical utility of the 5-HT$_3$ receptor antagonists and dopamine D2 antagonists in this setting. The mechanisms underlying delayed CINV are very poorly defined. Changes in the gastrointestinal tract as a result of chemotherapy such as altered gastrointestinal secretions and motility may play a role. In addition, chemotherapy-induced enhanced cell breakdown and turnover with the resulting release of cytokines and inflammation may be important contributors to delayed CINV.[25] The clinical utility of the corticosteroids in delayed CINV may be partly due to their anti-inflammatory effect. Of the known clinically relevant neurotransmitters, Substance P may have the most important role in the pathophysiology of delayed emesis. This is strongly supported by the unique preclinical and clinical efficacy of the NK$_1$ antagonists in the delayed emesis setting. In addition, an analysis of the time course of cisplatin-induced emesis demonstrated that 5-HT mechanisms appeared to predominate in the first 8 to 12 hours after cisplatin administration, but thereafter NK$_1$-dependent mechanisms appeared to be more important.[26]

The pathophysiology of RINV likely involves several mechanisms. If the gastrointestinal tract is included in the field of radiation, direct effects are likely with stimulation of afferent pathways in the upper gastrointestinal tract.[25,27] In addition, it is theorized that the chemoreceptor trigger zone in the area postrema may also be involved, possibly from radiation-induced tissue breakdown products.

DEFINING THE RISK OF NAUSEA AND VOMITING

There are a number of factors that can influence the development of CINV, including those related to the patient receiving therapy as well as the chemotherapy treatment itself. The most important patient-related factors include gender, age, history of ethanol consumption, and history of nausea or vomiting with prior chemotherapy treatment.[28–33] Gender is a strong and uniform predictor of difficulty with CINV, with women consistently experiencing poorer control of CINV than men.[28–32] Age is also an important risk factor, with younger patients having more difficulty than older patients.[28,32] A history of chronic alcohol consumption seems to decrease the risk of emesis.[28,30,31] Patients who have experienced CINV with prior chemotherapy treatment are also at greater risk of developing CINV with subsequent treatments.[33] A history of nausea and vomiting associated with pregnancy and a history of motion sickness have been suggested to predict for poor control of CINV, but definitive data are lacking. There is some genetic variation in the metabolism of 5-HT$_3$ receptor antagonists, and patients who are rapid metabolizers are at risk for more significant CINV.[34] In addition, genetic variations in the 5-HT$_3$ receptor may also predispose to a decreased response to this class of medication and more difficulty with CINV.[35]

Treatment-related factors include the actual chemotherapy agent, its dose, rate, and route of administration. Of all the known predictive factors for CINV, clearly the most important is the intrinsic emetogenicity of the chemotherapeutic agent employed. The emetogenicity schema that is most widely used is modified from the Hesketh classification, which was first described in 1997.[36] This system, based on an extensive literature review, classifies chemotherapeutic agents according to their intrinsic emetogenicity and establishes a framework for the development of antiemetic treatment guidelines. What was originally described as five levels of emetogenicity has been subsequently modified to a four-level schema (Table 135.1) classifying agents as having a high, moderate, low, or minimal risk of inducing emesis.[37,38] Oral agents are considered separately and have been classified by emetic risk into four categories.[38,39]

Risk of RINV is defined primarily by the anatomic area receiving treatment as well as the type of treatment.[38] The most commonly employed category includes four levels of risk: high, moderate, low, and minimal.[37,38] High-risk therapy consists of total-body irradiation. Moderate risk includes the upper abdomen, which carries a 60% to 90% risk of emesis without prophylaxis. Low risk includes the lower thoracic region and pelvis as well as the cranium (with radiosurgery) and craniospinal therapy. Minimal risk includes cranium, head and neck, extremities, and breast.

ANTIEMETIC AGENTS

Highest Therapeutic Index

There are several classes of drugs that are effective in the prevention of CINV (Table 135.2). Those of highest therapeutic index include the 5-HT$_3$ receptor antagonists, the NK$_1$ receptor antagonists, and corticosteroids. The most widely available first generation 5-HT$_3$ receptor antagonists include dolasetron, granisetron, ondansetron, and tropisetron. They have been shown to be superior to high-dose metoclopramide[40] and have replaced it as first-line therapy in prevention of acute emesis. They have proven to be most effective in the prevention of acute CINV in the settings of highly and moderately emetogenic chemotherapy. All first-generation 5-HT$_3$ receptor antagonists are considered therapeutically equivalent and are used interchangeably.[37,38,41] Oral formulations of the first-generation 5-HT$_3$ receptor antagonists have similar efficacy to intravenous formulations.[42]

Palonosetron is a second-generation 5-HT$_3$ antagonist that differs from other agents in this class by virtue of a longer half-life of 40 hours and a higher binding affinity to the 5-HT$_3$ receptor. It has been compared with first-generation 5-HT$_3$ antagonists in two randomized phase 3 trials in patients receiving moderately emetogenic chemotherapy.[43,44] Both trials were designed as noninferiority trials and met their primary end point. Post hoc analyses indicated superiority for palonosetron in a number of parameters to the comparator agents. In one trial, palonosetron 0.25 mg was superior to dolasetron 100 mg in complete response (no emesis or use of rescue medications) during the delayed (24 to 120 hours) and overall study periods.[43] In the other trial, palonosetron 0.25 mg was superior to ondansetron 32 mg in complete response during the first 24 hours, delayed period, and overall 5-day study period.[44] A third phase 3 trial in patients receiving highly emetogenic chemotherapy also reached its end point of noninferiority in comparing palonosetron with ondansetron 32 mg.[45] Unlike the moderately emetogenic trials, there was no significant difference between palonosetron and ondansetron in the control of acute or delayed emesis. Approximately two-thirds of patients also received corticosteroids at the discretion of the investigator in the highly emetogenic trial. A post hoc secondary subgroup analysis of the patients receiving dexamethasone demonstrated superior control of acute and delayed emesis in the group receiving palonosetron. In another phase 3 trial,[46] patients receiving either cisplatin or the combination of doxorubicin or epirubicin and cyclophosphamide were randomized in a double blind fashion to either a single dose of palonosetron at a dose of 0.75 mg or a single dose of granisetron (40 µg/kg) on day 1 of chemotherapy. In this trial, steroids for acute and delayed emesis were mandated. Palonosetron was more efficacious than granisetron, with 56.8% of patients in the palonosetron group experiencing an overall complete response (no vomiting or use of rescue medications) compared with 44.5% in the granisetron group ($p < 0.0001$). This was also true for delayed emesis (56.8% versus 44.5%, $p < 0.0001$). Palonosetron was found to be comparable to granisetron in the acute phase, with 75.3% complete response in the palonosetron group versus 73.3% in the granisetron group (difference of 2.29, 95% confidence interval = 2.70 to 7.27; p not done). The results of the phase 3 trials with palonosetron suggest that this agent is superior in efficacy to the first-generation 5-HT$_3$ antagonists when used as a single agent or with dexamethasone. The relative efficacy of palonosetron compared with first-generation 5-HT$_3$ receptor antagonists when used with NK$_1$ antagonists remains unknown given the lack of randomized data. Most of the studies done with palonosetron have used the 0.25 mg dose given intravenously. Boccia et al.[47] compared

TABLE 135.1

Classification of Emetic Risk of Intravenous Antineoplastic Agents

Emetic Risk (Estimated Incidence without Prophylaxis)	Antineoplastic Agent
High (>90%)	Cisplatin
	Mechlorethamine
	Streptozotocin
	Cyclophosphamide ($\geq$1,500 mg/m^2)
	Carmustine
	Dacarbazine
Moderate (30%–90%)	Oxaliplatin
	Cytarabine (>1 g/m^2)
	Carboplatin
	Ifosfamide
	Cyclophosphamide (<1,500 mg/m^2)
	Doxorubicin
	Daunorubicin
	Epirubicin
	Idarubicin
	Irinotecan
	Azacitadine
	Bendamustine
	Clofarabine
	Alemtuzumab
Low (10%–30%)	Paclitaxel
	Docetaxel
	Mitoxantrone
	Doxorubicin HCl liposome injection
	Ixabepilone
	Topotecan
	Etoposide
	Pemetrexed
	Methotrexate
	Mitomycin
	Gemcitabine
	Cytarabine ($\leq$100 mg/m^2)
	5-Fluorouracil
	Bortezomib
	Cetuximab
	Trastuzumab
	Panitumumab
	Catumaxumab
Minimal (<10%)	Bleomycin
	Busulfan
	2-Chlorodeoxydenosine
	Fludarabine
	Vinblastine
	Vincristine
	Vinorelbine
	Bevacizumab
	Rituximab

Modified from Basch E, Prestrud AA, Hesketh PJ, et al. Antiemetics: American Society of Clinical Oncology clinical practice guideline update. *J Clin Oncol* 2011;29:4189.

TABLE 135.2

Doses of Commonly Used Antiemetic Agents

Drug	Prechemotherapy Dose (Day 1)	Postchemotherapy Dose
Highest Therapeutic Index		
Aprepitant	125 mg orally	80 mg orally days 2 and 3
Fosaprepitant	150 mg IV	

Dexamethasone
  With aprepitant or fosaprepitant
  Without aprepitant
	12 mg orally or IV
	20 mg orally or IV[a]
	8 mg orally or IV[b]
		8 mg days 2–4[a]
		8 mg bid days 2–4[a]
		8 mg days 2 and 3[c]

Ondansetron	24 mg orally[a]; 8 mg orally bid[b] 8 mg or 0.15 mg/kg IV	8 mg bid days 2 and 3
Granisetron	2 mg orally 1 mg or 0.01 mg/kg IV	—
Tropisetron	5 mg orally or IV	—
Dolasetron	100 mg orally	—
Palonosetron	0.25 mg IV 0.5 mg orally	—
Lower Therapeutic Index		
Prochlorperazine	10 mg orally or IV	—
Dronabinol	5 mg/m² orally	5 mg/m² orally q2–4 hr p.r.n.
Nabilone	1–2 mg orally	1–2 mg bid or tid p.r.n.
Olanzapine	5 mg orally daily for 2 d preceding chemotherapy; 10 mg on day 1	10 mg days 2–4

IV, intravenously; bid, twice daily; tid, three times a day; p.r.n., pro re nata.
[a] When used with highly emetic chemotherapy, day 4 is optional.
[b] With moderately emetic chemotherapy.
[c] When used with moderately emetic chemotherapy with potential for delayed emesis.

three oral doses of palonosetron to the standard 0.25 mg intravenous dose in 651 patients receiving moderately emetogenic chemotherapy. Patients were also randomized to dexamethasone or placebo. The oral dose of 0.5 mg was found to be noninferior to the intravenous 0.25 mg dose in the acute and overall phase. However, none of the oral doses attained noninferiority to the intravenous dosing in the delayed emesis phase.

Corticosteroids are a mainstay in the prevention of both acute and delayed CINV. In a large meta-analysis that included data from >5,000 patients, dexamethasone, the most commonly employed corticosteroid, was found to significantly improve the prevention of CINV compared with placebo or other antiemetics.[48] Most of the studies involved the use of highly emetogenic chemotherapy. In the acute phase, it was estimated to increase the chance of complete prevention of vomiting by 25% to 30% versus placebo. Similar results were seen with delayed emesis. With moderate to highly emetogenic chemotherapy regimens, corticosteroids are typically not used alone but in combination with other antiemetics. Single-agent use is appropriate with mildly emetogenic regimens. The appropriate doses of dexamethasone for use with highly and moderately emetogenic therapy (in the absence of a NK$_1$ antagonist) are 20 mg and 8 mg, respectively, based on the results of two large phase 3 trials.[49,50]

The most recent advance in CINV prevention has been the introduction of selective antagonists of Substance P's binding to the NK$_1$ receptor. Aprepitant is the first approved agent in this new class of antiemetics. In a phase 3 randomized study that included >500 patients, aprepitant significantly increased the overall 5-day complete response (no emesis or use of rescue) rate (72.7% versus 52.3%) when added to the standard therapy of ondansetron and dexamethasone in patients receiving high-dose cisplatin chemotherapy.[51] Superiority for the aprepitant arm was demonstrated

in both the control of acute and delayed emesis. Similar results were found in an identically designed phase 3 trial enrolling patients from Latin America.[52] The addition of aprepitant may also improve the durability of antiemetic control over multiple cycles of cisplatin-based chemotherapy.[53] Benefit for the addition of aprepitant has also been demonstrated in patients receiving a combination of an anthracycline and cyclophosphamide, a combination now recognized to be highly emetogenic. In a phase 3 trial in patients with breast cancer receiving an anthracycline plus cyclophosphamide, patients were randomized to an aprepitant-containing regimen, which included dexamethasone and ondansetron, or a standard regimen that consisted of dexamethasone and ondansetron.[54] Aprepitant alone was used as delayed emesis prevention in the aprepitant arm, while ondansetron alone was used for delayed emesis protection in the comparison arm. A superior rate of complete response (50.8% versus 42.5%) during the 5-day study period was noted in the aprepitant arm.

A possible benefit for aprepitant in the prevention of CINV associated with moderately emetogenic chemotherapy has been demonstrated. Rapoport et al.[55] reported the results of a phase 3 trial evaluating aprepitant with a variety of moderately emetogenic chemotherapy regimens as well as doxorubicin and cyclophosphamide. Patients were treated with aprepitant or placebo plus ondansetron and dexamethasone on day 1 and either aprepitant (experimental arm) or ondansetron (control arm) for delayed emesis. Overall, patients randomized to the aprepitant containing arm had significantly higher proportions of patients with complete response, including overall (62.8% versus 47.1%, p <0.01), in the acute setting (84.3% versus 72.5%, p <0.01), and in the delayed setting (64.8% versus 52.9%, p <0.01). Retrospective analysis was done comparing patients receiving doxorubicin/cyclophosphamide with those receiving moderately emetogenic combinations, which confirmed the superiority of aprepitant in those patients treated with doxorubicin/cyclophosphamide. For the non–doxorubicin/cyclophosphamide arm, while the addition of aprepitant statistically improved the proportion of patients who did not experience vomiting, the overall complete response rate did not differ between the aprepitant-containing group and the non–aprepitant-containing group. An additional trial prospectively evaluating aprepitant in moderately emetogenic chemotherapy did not demonstrate value for the addition of the NK$_1$ antagonist. Hesketh et al.[56] investigated the use of a single dose of casopitant, an NK$_1$ receptor antagonist, in oxaliplatin-based chemotherapy. All patients were treated with ondansetron starting prior to oxaliplatin administration and continuing until day 3, dexamethasone day 1, and randomized to receive casopitant or placebo day 1. The primary end point was complete response (no vomiting and no use of rescue medications), and a total of 710 patients were included in the intention to treat analysis. Casopitant did not improve outcome compared to the dexamethasone and ondansetron regimen with similar rates of complete response overall (85 % in the placebo arm versus 86% in the casopitant arm; odds ratio = 1.1054; 95% confidence interval = 0.73 to 1.68; $p = 0.6373$), in the acute phase (96% in the placebo arm versus 97% in the casopitant arm), and in the delayed phase (85% in the placebo arm versus 86% in the casopitant arm). Given the limited and somewhat conflicting data on the value of aprepitant in the moderately emetogenic setting, the most recent European Society of Clinical Oncology-Multinational Association of Supportive Care in Cancer[38] and American Society of Clinical Oncology (ASCO) antiemetic guidelines[37] do not recommend the use of aprepitant with moderately emetogenic chemotherapy.

In 2008, an intravenous formulation of aprepitant (fosaprepitant) received regulatory approval for use with moderately and highly emetogenic chemotherapy. A single intravenous dose of fosaprepitant 150 mg was compared with 3-day oral dosing of aprepitant in a randomized double blind active-control designed trial and was found to be equivalent in efficacy in patients treated with cisplatin at doses of at least 70 mg/m^2.[57] This held true for both the delayed emesis period and the overall study period.

Of note, aprepitant is an inhibitor of the cytochrome P450 enzyme CYP3A4, which is involved in the metabolism of many drugs, including dexamethasone and certain chemotherapeutic agents. A pharmacokinetic study demonstrated that the plasma concentration of dexamethasone as measured as the area under the curve was more than two-fold higher with aprepitant compared with the same dose of dexamethasone without concomitant aprepitant.[58] A dose reduction of dexamethasone from 20 to 12 mg (day 1) and 8 to 4 mg (days 2 and 3) yielded similar plasma dexamethasone levels to those in patients not taking aprepitant. The slowed metabolism of dexamethasone in the presence of aprepitant accounts for the recommendation to reduce dexamethasone doses by approximately 50% when administered with aprepitant.[37] However, if the corticosteroids are given as part of the chemotherapeutic regimen rather than for antiemetic prophylaxis, the corticosteroid dose should not be adjusted.[37] There is also a theoretical concern that chemotherapeutic agents that are metabolized by CYP3A4 may have a slowed clearance, leading to higher drug exposure, and increased toxicity. However, analysis of the completed phase 3 trials with aprepitant has not demonstrated a significant increase in adverse events in patients receiving aprepitant.

Recently, data on a new selective NK$_1$ receptor antagonist netupitant has been presented. In a phase 2 study,[59] 694 patients receiving cisplatin-based chemotherapy were randomized to four study arms comparing three oral doses of netupitant (100 mg, 200 mg, 300 mg), all combined with oral palonosetron 0.50 mg, all given on day 1. All patients received oral dexamethasone on days 1 to 4. An exploratory aprepitant + ondansetron/dexamethasone arm was included. The study arm, combining 300 mg of netupitant with palonosetron, was superior to the palonosetron and dexamethasone arm in control of acute and delayed nausea and emesis as

well as complete protection ($p \leq 0.05$). A subsequent phase 3 study including 1,455 patients receiving cyclophosphamide combined with doxorubicin or epirubicin evaluated a fixed-dose tablet containing netupitant 300 mg combined with palonosetron 0.5 mg termed NEPA. Patients were randomized to receive NEPA or oral palonosetron 0.5 mg on day 1 prior to chemotherapy. All patients also received dexamethasone (12 mg NEPA arm; 20 mg palonosetron arm) on day 1. NEPA plus dexamethasone was found to be superior to palonosetron plus dexamethasone in rates of complete response during acute ($p = 0.001$), delayed ($p = 0.047$), and overall ($p = 0.001$) phases as well as in rates of no significant nausea.[60]

Lower Therapeutic Index

Drugs of lower therapeutic index include metoclopramide, butyrophenones, phenothiazines, cannabinoids, and olanzapine (see Table 135.2). These drugs in general are all associated with less efficacy than the high therapeutic index agents and can have troublesome adverse effects. These drugs are most commonly used in patients who are unable to tolerate or who do not respond to 5-HT$_3$ receptor antagonists, aprepitant, or dexamethasone. Of the lower therapeutic index agents, the phenothiazines are probably used most often either as monotherapy with patients receiving mildly emetogenic chemotherapy or as an as-needed agent in patients failing frontline antiemetics. Another class of agents that may have value in selected situations is the benzodiazepines. Although limited in their antiemetic efficacy, the antianxiety properties of these agents can be useful. The most commonly employed agent in the class is lorazepam, which has demonstrated value with anticipatory emesis and can be useful as an adjunct to other antiemetics in patients failing to completely respond to their frontline regimens. Olanzapine, which is an antagonist of multiple neurotransmitter receptors including those of dopamine and serotonin, may be effective in preventing both acute and delayed CINV. Olanzapine has been investigated in place of aprepitant in a phase 3 trial[61] of patients receiving highly emetogenic chemotherapy including both cisplatin (at ≥ 70 mg/m^2) and the combination of doxorubicin and cyclophosphamide. In this trial, 247 patients were randomized to either (1) olanzapine, palonosetron, and dexamethasone given on day 1 with olanzapine 10 mg daily given on days 2 to 4 or (2) aprepitant, palonosetron, and dexamethasone with dexamethasone given on days 2 to 4. Both groups had similar rates of complete response to emesis. In the olanzapine arm, there was a complete response of 97% in the acute phase, 77% in the delayed phase, and 77% overall compared, with the aprepitant arm, which had complete response rates of 87% in the acute phase and 73% in the delayed phase and overall ($p > 0.05$). A majority (87%) of patients in both groups experienced no nausea; however, olanzapine was more effective at controlling nausea in the delayed setting with 69% of patients in the olanzapine arm reporting no nausea compared with 38% in the aprepitant arm ($p \leq 0.01$).

ANTIEMETIC TREATMENT BY CLINICAL SETTING

In planning antiemetic therapy in patients with cancer receiving chemotherapy, it is important to consider a few basic principles: (1) the primary goal should be complete prevention; (2) to minimize the risk of anticipatory emesis, antiemetic therapy should be appropriately maximized from the initial cycle of chemotherapy; (3) antiemetic therapies should be chosen to match the intrinsic emetogenicity of the chemotherapy; and (4) consider prescribing antiemetics for use in the event breakthrough emesis develops. If emesis does develop in the patient receiving chemotherapy, an assessment should be made to exclude nonchemotherapy causes of the patient's nausea and vomiting. These include bowel obstruction or dysmotility; concomitant medications, particularly opioids;

TABLE 135.3

Recommended Antiemetic Therapy for Single-Day Intravenous Chemotherapy

Emetic Risk Category	Prevention of Acute Emesis (Day 1 Prechemotherapy)	Prevention of Delayed Emesis
High[a]	5-HT$_3$ receptor antagonist *plus* dexamethasone *plus* aprepitant or fosaprepitant	Dexamethasone days 2–4[b]
Moderate	Palonosetron *plus* dexamethasone	Dexamethasone days 2 and 3
Low	Dexamethasone *or* prochlorperazine	No preventive measures
Minimal	As needed	No preventive measures

5-HT$_3$, 5-hydroxytryptamine-3.
[a] The combination of doxorubicin and cyclophosphamide is considered highly emetogenic.
[b] Day 4 is optional.

metabolic disturbances such as hyponatremia and hypercalcemia; and occult CNS metastasis.

ASCO guidelines[37] have moved the combination of doxorubicin and cyclophosphamide from the moderate to the highly emetogenic risk category, reflecting a myriad of data on the high intrinsic emetogenicity of this regimen. For patients receiving single-day intravenously administered highly emetogenic chemotherapy such as cisplatin and now including the combination of doxorubicin and cyclophosphamide, recommended prophylaxis involves the use of a 5-HT$_3$ receptor antagonist on day 1, dexamethasone on days 1 to 4, and fosaprepitant day 1 only or aprepitant on days 1 to 3 (Table 135.3). For moderately emetogenic chemotherapy given intravenously, prophylaxis using palonosetron is recommended on day 1, along with dexamethasone on day 1. Patients should also receive either a 5-HT$_3$ antagonist (if palonosetron is not used) or dexamethasone on days 2 to 3 after chemotherapy. For intravenously administered chemotherapy of low emetic potential, single-agent dexamethasone or prochlorperazine is recommended on day 1 with no routine prophylaxis for delayed emesis. For minimal-risk chemotherapy agents, no routine antiemetic prophylaxis is indicated.

SPECIAL CHEMOTHERAPY-INDUCED NAUSEA AND VOMITING PROBLEMS

There are a number of situations in addition to single-day intravenously administered chemotherapy that pose emetic challenges. Regimens containing highly emetogenic chemotherapy, such as cisplatin given on multiple days, require special attention, though there is limited data for this setting. ASCO guidelines[37] suggest antiemetic prophylaxis corresponding to the level of emetogenicity for the duration of the chemotherapy administration plus 2 days after, when applicable, and the use of aprepitant, dexamethasone, and a 5-HT$_3$ antagonist for 5-day cisplatin regimens. In 2008, the U.S. Food and Drug Administration approved the use of a transdermal granisetron patch for use in patients receiving multiple-day regimens of chemotherapy based on a phase 3 multinational, double blind, double dummy, noninferiority study.[62] In this trial, 641 patients receiving chemotherapy regimens of 3- to 5-day duration were randomized to the granisetron patch applied on the day prior to chemotherapy and kept on for 7 days or oral granisetron 2 mg daily prior to chemotherapy. The primary end point of this study was complete control: no vomiting, use of rescue medication, or more than mild nausea. The study met its primary end point of noninferiority with complete control in 60% of patients using the patch and 65% of patients taking single daily oral granisetron (difference of 5%, 95% confidence interval = −13% to 3%). A related problem is noted in patients receiving high-dose chemotherapy in the setting of hematopoietic stem cell transplantation. Chemotherapy regimens are often administered during several days in sequence, and there are data supporting the value of daily 5-HT$_3$ receptor antagonist and dexamethasone in this setting as well.[63] A randomized trial in patients receiving preparative regimens for hematopoietic stem cell transplantation noted improved outcome with the addition of aprepitant to ondansetron

and dexamethasone.[64] No emesis rates of 73.3% and 22.5% were noted for the entire study period in the aprepitant and control arms, respectively ($p = 0.001$). In addition, complete response (no emesis and no mild nausea) was seen in 48.9% versus 14.6% in the aprepitant and control arms, respectively ($p < 0.001$).

Anticipatory nausea and vomiting pose additional special CINV challenges. These symptoms are often poorly responsive to common antiemetics. Fortunately, given the recent improvements noted in the control of CINV in general, anticipatory nausea and vomiting are much less commonly seen. Therapies that have been studied with some success include systemic desensitization and hypnosis. One series showed benefit for alprazolam when combined with a psychological support program.[65]

Oral chemotherapeutic agents are increasingly used in clinical oncology practices and also have a propensity to cause varying degrees of CINV. There is a scarcity of data on the emetogenicity of oral drugs; therefore, the risk of CINV has not been as well defined. The lack of clinical trials addressing the issue of oral agent–induced CINV precludes definitive treatment recommendations.

Finally, if patients receive appropriate evidence-based prophylaxis for CINV and still develop so-called breakthrough emesis, this can also be a troublesome problem. As with oral chemotherapy, there is little prospective data evaluating treatment approaches for this problem. If other causes of nausea and vomiting are excluded, adjunctive medications such as benzodiazepines or dopaminergic antagonists can be added. One double-blind trial in patients who failed initial prophylaxis found that switching from one 5-HT$_3$ receptor antagonist to another afforded significantly higher rates of complete protection compared with those patients remaining on the original 5-HT$_3$ receptor antagonist.[66] Olanzapine has also been studied for breakthrough nausea and vomiting. In a randomized double-blind phase 3 trial,[67] olanzapine was compared with metoclopramide for breakthrough nausea and vomiting after guideline-specific prevention for highly emetic chemotherapy, which included both high-dose cisplatin and the combination of doxorubicin and cyclophosphamide. Breakthrough medications were started at the onset of vomiting or moderate to severe nausea on a visual and numeric scale. Approximately 40% of patients in each arm developed breakthrough vomiting or moderate to severe nausea. In the 72-hour period after breakthrough medications were initiated, 70% of patients using olanzapine for breakthrough had no emesis compared with 31% of patients taking metoclopramide ($p < 0.01$). Nausea after breakthrough antiemetics were given was measured on the MD Anderson Cancer Center Symptom Inventory scale, with 68% of patients reporting no nausea compared with 23% of patients taking metoclopramide ($p < 0.01$).

RADIOTHERAPY-INDUCED NAUSEA AND VOMITING

Radiotherapy can also clearly cause nausea and vomiting in a number of settings and warrants appropriate prophylactic therapy (Table 135.4). Updated guideline recommendations[37,38] have

TABLE 135.4

Recommended Antiemetic Therapy for Radiotherapy-Induced Emesis

Risk Level	Irradiated Area	Antiemetic Guidelines
High (>90%)	Total-body irradiation, total nodal irradiation	Prophylaxis with 5-HT$_3$ antagonists + DEX
Moderate (60%–90%)	Upper abdomen, HBI, UBI	Prophylaxis with 5-HT$_3$ antagonists + optional DEX
Low (30%–60%)	Cranium, craniospinal, H&N, lower thorax region, pelvis	Prophylaxis or rescue with 5-HT$_3$ antagonists
Minimal (<30%)	Extremities, breast	Rescue with dopamine receptor antagonists or 5-HT$_3$ antagonists

5-HT$_3$, 5-hydroxytryptamine-3; DEX, dexamethasone; HBI, half-body irradiation; UBI, upper-body irradiation; H&N, head and neck.
Note: In concomitant radiochemotherapy, the antiemetic prophylaxis is according to the chemotherapy-related antiemetic guidelines of the corresponding risk category, unless the risk of emesis is higher with radiotherapy than chemotherapy.
Adapted with permission from Roila F, Herrstedt J, Aapro M, et al. Guideline update for MASCC and ESMO in the prevention of chemotherapy- and radiotherapy-induced nausea and vomiting: results of the Perugia consensus conference. *Ann Oncol* 2010;21:v232–243.

been provided. Optimal prophylaxis for total-body or total-nodal radiation is the use of a 5-HT$_3$ receptor antagonist plus dexamethasone. Reasonable prophylaxis for radiation of moderate emetic risk would be 5-HT$_3$ receptor antagonist before each fraction with the optional use of dexamethasone for fractions one to five. Prophylaxis or rescue with 5-HT$_3$ antagonists is appropriate for low-risk radiation. Minimal-risk radiation is treated with 5-HT$_3$ receptor antagonists or dopamine antagonists as needed.

SELECTED REFERENCES

The full reference list can be accessed at lwwhealthlibrary.com/oncology.

1. Griffin AM, Butow PN, Coates AS, et al. On the receiving end. V: Patient perceptions of the side effects of cancer chemotherapy in 1993. *Ann Oncol* 1996;7:189–195.
2. O'Brien BJ, Rusthoven J, Rocchi A, et al. Impact of chemotherapy-associated nausea and vomiting on patients' functional status and on costs: survey of five Canadian centers. *CMAJ* 1993;149:296–302.
7. Kris MG, Gralla RJ, Clark RA, et al. Incidence, course, and severity of delayed nausea and vomiting following the administration of high-dose cisplatin. *J Clin Oncol* 1985;3:1379–1384.
9. Borison HL, Wang SC. Physiology and pharmacology of vomiting. *Pharmacol Rev* 1953;5:193–230.
10. Sanger GJ, Andrews PLR. Treatment of nausea and vomiting: gaps in our knowledge. *Auton Neurosci* 2006;129:3–16.
15. Hesketh PJ. Understanding the pathobiology of chemotherapy-induced nausea and vomiting. *Oncology (Williston Park)* 2004;18:9–14.
19. Andrews PLR, Judd JA. The role of tachykinins and the tachykinin NK$_1$ receptor in nausea and emesis. In: Holzer P, ed. *Handbook of Experimental Pharmacology*. New York, Berlin: Springer; 2004:359.
20. Quartara L, Maggi CA. The tachykinin NK$_1$ receptor. Part II: distribution and pathophysiological roles. *Neuropeptides* 1998;32:1–49.
24. Tramer MR, Carroll D, Campbell FA. Cannabinoids for control of chemotherapy induced nausea and vomiting: quantitative systematic review. *BMJ* 2001;7:16–21.
26. Hesketh PJ, Van Bells S, Aapro M, et al. Differential involvement of neurotransmitters through the time course of cisplatin-induced emesis as revealed by therapy with specific receptor antagonists. *Eur J Cancer* 2003;39:1074–1080.
27. Endo T, Minami M, Hirafuji M, et al. Neurochemistry and neuropharmacology of emesis-the role of serotonin. *Toxicology* 2000;16:189–201.
28. Hesketh PJ, Plagge P, Bryson JC. Single-dose ondansetron for prevention of acute cisplatin-induced emesis: analysis of efficacy and prognostic factors. In: Bianchi AL, Grelot L, Miller AD, et al. eds. *Mechanisms and Control of Emesis*. London: John Libbey; 1992:25.
29. du Bois A, Meerpohl HG, Vach W, et al. Course, patterns, and risk-factors for chemotherapy-induced emesis in cisplatin-pretreated patients: a study with ondansetron. *Eur J Cancer* 1992;28:450–457.
30. Osoba D, Zee B, Pater J, et al. Determinants of postchemotherapy nausea and vomiting in patients with cancer. *J Clin Oncol* 1997;15:116–123.
31. Hesketh P, Navari R, Grote T, et al. Double-blind, randomized comparison of the antiemetic efficacy of intravenous dolasetron mesylate and intravenous ondansetron in the prevention of acute cisplatin-induced emesis in patients with cancer. *J Clin Oncol* 1996;14:2242–2249.
32. Pollera CF, Giannarelli D. Prognostic factors influencing cisplatin-induced emesis. *Cancer* 1989;64:1117–1122.
33. de Witt R, Herrstedt J, Rapoport B, et al. Addition of the oral NK$_1$ antagonist aprepitant to standard antiemetics provides protection against nausea and vomiting during multiple cycles of cisplatin-based chemotherapy. *J Clin Oncol* 2003;21:4105–4111.
34. Kaiser R, Sezer O, Papies A, et al. Patient-tailored antiemetic treatment with 5-hydroxytryptamine type 3 receptor antagonists according to cytochrome P-450 2D6 genotypes. *J Clin Oncol* 2002;20:2805–2811.
35. Tremblay P, Kaiser R, Sezer O, et al. Variations in the 5-hydroxytryptamine type 3B receptor gene as predictors of the efficacy of antiemetic treatment in cancer patients. *J Clin Oncol* 2003;21:2147–2155.
36. Hesketh PJ, Kris MG, Grunberg SM, et al. Proposal for classifying the acute emetogenicity of cancer chemotherapy. *J Clin Oncol* 1997;15:103–109.
37. Basch E, Prestrud AA, Hesketh PJ, et al. Antiemetics: American Society of Clinical Oncology clinical practice guideline update. *J Clin Oncol* 2011;29:4189–1498.
38. Roila F, Herrstedt J, Aapro M, et al. Guideline update for MASCC and ESMO in the prevention of chemotherapy- and radiotherapy-induced nausea and vomiting: results of the Perugia consensus conference. *Ann Oncol* 2010;21:v232–243.
39. Grunberg SM, Osoba D, Hesketh PJ, et al. Evaluation of new antiemetic agents and definition of antineoplastic agent emetogenicity—an update. *Support Care Cancer* 2005;13;80–84.
40. Bonneterre J, Chevallier B, Metz R, et al. A randomized double-blind comparison of ondansetron and metoclopramide in the prophylaxis of emesis induced by cyclophosphamide, fluorouracil, and doxorubicin or epirubicin chemotherapy. *J Clin Oncol* 1990;8:1063–1069.
41. del Giglio A, Soares HP, Caparroz C, et al. Granisetron is equivalent to ondansetron for prophylaxis of chemotherapy-induced nausea and vomiting. *Cancer* 2000;89:2301–2308.
42. Perez EA, Hesketh P, Sandbach J, et al. Comparison of single-dose oral granisetron versus intravenous ondansetron in the prevention of nausea and vomiting induced by moderately emetogenic chemotherapy: a multicenter, double-blind, randomized parallel study. *J Clin Oncol* 1998;16:754–760.
43. Eisenberg P, Figueroa-Vadillo J, Zamora R, et al. Improved prevention of moderately emetogenic chemotherapy-induced nausea and vomiting with palonosetron, a pharmacologically novel 5-HT3 receptor antagonist: results of a phase III, single-dose trial versus dolasetron. *Cancer* 2003;98:2473–2482.
44. Gralla R, Lichinitser M, Van Der Vegt S, et al. Palonosetron improves prevention of chemotherapy-induced nausea and vomiting following moderately emetogenic chemotherapy: results of a double-blind randomized phase III trial comparing single doses of palonosetron with ondansetron. *Ann Oncol* 2003;14:1570–1577.
45. Aapro MS, Grunberg SM, Manikhas GM, et al. A phase III double-blind, randomized trial of palonosetron compared with ondansetron in preventing chemotherapy-induced nausea and vomiting following highly emetogenic chemotherapy. *Ann Oncol* 2006;17:1441–1449.
46. Saito M, Aogi K, Sekine I, et al. Palonosetron plus dexamethasone versus granisetron plus dexamethasone for prevention of nausea and vomiting during chemotherapy: a double-blind, double dummy, randomized, comparative phase III trial. *Lancet Oncol* 2009;10:115–124.
48. Ioannidis JPA, Hesketh PJ, Lau J. Contribution of dexamethasone to control of chemotherapy-induced nausea and vomiting: a meta-analysis of randomized evidence. *J Clin Oncol* 2000;18:3409–3422.
49. Italian Group for Antiemetic Research. Double-blind, dose-finding study of four intravenous doses of dexamethasone in the prevention of cisplatin-induced acute emesis. *J Clin Oncol* 1998;16:2937–2942.
50. Italian Group for Antiemetic Research. Randomized, double-blind, dose-finding study of dexamethasone in preventing acute emesis induced by anthracyclines, carboplatin, or cyclophosphamide. *J Clin Oncol* 2004;22:725–729.

51. Hesketh PJ, Grunberg SM, Gralla RJ, et al. The oral neurokinin-1 antagonists aprepitant for the prevention of chemotherapy-induced nausea and vomiting: a multinational, randomized, double-blind, placebo-controlled trial in patients receiving high-dose cisplatin—the Aprepitant Protocol 052 Study Group. *J Clin Oncol* 2003;21:4112–4119.
52. Poli-Bigelli S, Rodrigues-Pereira J, Carides AD, et al. Addition of the neurokinin 1 receptor antagonist aprepitant to standard antiemetic therapy improves control of chemotherapy induced nausea and vomiting. *Cancer* 2003;97:3090–3098.
53. de Wit R, Herrstedt J, Rapoport B, et al. Addition of the oral NK₁ antagonist aprepitant to standard antiemetics provides protection against nausea and vomiting during multiple cycles of cisplatin-based chemotherapy. *J Clin Oncol* 2003;21:4105–4111.
55. Rapoport BL, Jordan K, Boice JA, et al. Aprepitant for the prevention of chemotherapy-induced nausea and vomiting associated with a broad range of moderately emetogenic chemotherapy and tumor types: a randomized, double blind study. *Support Care Cancer* 2010;18:423–431.

57. Grunberg S, Chua D, Maru A, et al. Single dose fosaprepitant for the prevention of chemotherapy-induced nausea and vomiting associated with cisplatin therapy: randomized, double-blind study protocol—EASE. *J Clin Oncol* 2011;29:1495–1501.
63. Einhorn LH, Rapoport B, Koeller J, et al. Antiemetic therapy for multiple-day chemotherapy and high-dose chemotherapy with stem cell transplant: review and consensus statement. *Support Care Cancer* 2005;13:112–116.
64. Stiff PJ, Fox-Geiman MP, Kiley K, et al. Prevention of nausea and vomiting associated with stem cell transplant: results of a prospective, randomized trial of aprepitant used with highly emetogenic preparative regimens. *Biol Blood Marrow Transplant* 2013;19:49–55.e1.
66. de Wit R, de Boer AC, vd Linden GHM, et al. Effective cross-over to granisetron after failure to ondansetron, a randomized double blind study in patients failing ondansetron plus dexamethasone during the first 24 hours following highly emetogenic chemotherapy. *Br J Cancer* 2001;85:1099–1101.

PRACTICE OF ONCOLOGY

Nathan I. Cherny and Batsheva Werman

INTRODUCTION

Constipation and diarrhea are both common problems in patients with advanced cancer. They are a source of major morbidity and distress. Treatment-induced diarrhea can be severe and be associated with life-threatening dehydration and electrolyte abnormalities. Treatment-induced constipation is, as a result of very widespread use of opioid analgesics for cancer pain, more common than diarrhea. Oncologists must be familiar with the common causes of constipation and diarrhea among patients with cancer and the strategies to evaluate and manage these common and distressing symptoms.

DIARRHEA

Diarrhea is defined as the frequent passage of loose stools with urgency. Objectively defined, it is the passage of more than three unformed stools in 24 hours. As with constipation, the patient's definition of diarrhea varies and needs to be clarified by medical staff.

Diarrhea is a common and significant problem among patients with advanced cancer. Increasingly, it is seen as a major treatment complication, particularly among patients receiving fluoropyrimidines and irinotecan.[1] The causes of diarrhea among patients with advanced cancer are diverse and some require specific therapies. Thus, careful evaluation of the underlying cause is necessary.

Severe diarrhea can be debilitating and at times, even life-threatening.[1] It contributes to dehydration, electrolyte imbalance, malnutrition, declining immune function, and pressure ulcer formation.

Chemotherapy-Induced Diarrhea

The chemotherapy agents commonly causing diarrhea include 5-fluorouracil (5-FU), capecitabine, and irinotecan.[1] This is usually a dose-related adverse effect and may be associated with other features of toxicity. Chemotherapy-induced diarrhea appears to be a multifactorial process whereby acute damage to the intestinal mucosa (including loss of intestinal epithelium, superficial necrosis, and inflammation of the bowel wall) causes an imbalance between absorption and secretion in the small bowel.

5-Fluorouracil

Mechanism. 5-FU causes mitotic arrest of intestinal epithelial crypt cells resulting in an increase in the ratio of immature secretory crypt cells to mature villous enterocytes. This results in abnormal absorption and secretion of fluids and electrolytes. Opportunistic infections, causing local inflammation and factors released by necrosis secondary to chemotherapy, directly stimulate intestinal secretion of fluids and electrolytes. The diarrhea associated with 5-FU therapy may be watery or bloody. Disruption of the integrity of the gut lining may permit access of enteric organisms into the bloodstream, with the potential for overwhelming sepsis, particularly if the granulocyte nadir coincides with diarrhea. Severity is variable but it may be severe and at times life-threatening. Pathologic changes range in severity from a mild colitis to severe necrotizing enterocolitis with pneumacystic colitis.

Risk Factors. Diarrhea is most commonly observed when 5-FU is coadministered with leucovorin (LV). It is slightly more common with bolus rather than infusional administration of 5-FU/LV, in particular with high-dose LV (500 mg/m^2),[2,3] but it occurs with all administration schedules.[4] In the initial reports of weekly 5-FU/LV, diarrhea was seen in up to 50% of patients, with one-half of these requiring hospitalization for intravenous fluids[2,3] and, in one study, a 5% mortality rate.[3] Other risk factors have been identified including unresected primary tumor, previous episodes of chemotherapy-induced diarrhea, and female gender.

Dihydropyrimidine Dehydrogenase Deficiency. 5-FU is normally metabolized to inactive dihydro-5-FU after an intravenous dose; 80% of the drug is metabolized to the inactive dihydro-5-FU by dihydropyrimidine dehydrogenase (DPD) in the liver. Administration of 5-FU to patients with DPD deficiency can lead to life-threatening complications, including severe diarrhea, mucositis, and pancytopenia.[5] DPD deficiency is relatively common among Caucasians (3% to 5%).[5] Although the diagnosis can be made by radioimmunometric assay for the DPD enzyme, this test is not readily available. More recently, a simple breath test has been developed, and this may provide an effective screening tool.[5]

Irinotecan

Irinotecan can cause acute diarrhea (immediately after drug administration) or a delayed diarrhea. Immediate-onset diarrhea is caused by acute cholinergic properties, and it is often accompanied by other symptoms of cholinergic excess, including abdominal cramping, rhinitis, lacrimation, and salivation. The mean duration of symptoms is 30 minutes, and it usually responds rapidly to atropine.[6]

Delayed-onset diarrhea usually occurs at least 24 hours after drug administration and can be potentially life-threatening, especially in combination chemotherapy regimens with bolus intravenous fluorouracil and leucovorin.[6] The late diarrhea associated with irinotecan is unpredictable, noncumulative, and occurs at all dose levels. It is more common with 3-weekly dose schedules than with lower weekly dosing.[6] The median time to onset is 6 to 14 days. The mechanism of irinotecan-induced delayed diarrhea is not known, but it is believed to result from the deconjugation of irinotecan's metabolite, 7-ethyl-10-hydroxycamptothecin (SN38) glucuronide, by intestinal bacteria, thus enabling direct effect of the active agent on colonic epithelium. It is suggested that the active agent binds to topoisomerase I and induces apoptosis of intestinal epithelia, leading to the disturbance in the absorptive and secretory functions of mucosa. Additionally, both irinotecan and SN-38 may also stimulate the production of proinflammatory cytokines and prostaglandins, thus contributing to an inflammatory/secretory diarrhea.[7]

Genetic factors may influence the glucuronidation of SN-38, the active metabolite of irinotecan, and thus increase this risk of diarrhea. Polymorphisms that alter UDP-glucuronosyltransferase activities have been identified; the homozygous presence of the UGT1A1*28 polymorphism, leading to less efficient glucuronidation of SN-38, has been identified as a potential risk factor for the occurrence of delayed-type diarrhea and grade 3 to 4 neutropenia.[8] In one study, heterozygote had a two-fold elevation of risk of severe diarrhea.[9]

Capecitabine

Capecitabine, a precursor of 5-FU, is an oral fluoropyrimidine cytotoxic agent developed with the aim of providing a more effective, less toxic alternative to 5-FU, with the added advantage of oral administration. Administered at usual doses (2,000 mg/m² per day for 14 of every 21 days), the prevalence of diarrheas is 30% to 40%; in 10% to 20%, it is severe.[10]

Other Cytotoxics

The taxane docetaxel commonly causes a relatively mild diarrhea. Data from phase 2 and 3 studies indicated a prevalence of approximately 30%.[11] In most cases, the diarrhea is mild; however, cases of severe enteritis and colitis have been reported (see the following).[12,13]

Similarly, the antifolate pemetrexed can also cause mild diarrhea. In phase 2 and 3 trials, mild diarrhea has been reported in about 10% to 15% of patients.[14]

Neutropenic Colitis

Neutropenic enterocolitis (also called necrotizing enterocolitis or typhlitis) is an acute life-threatening complication of chemotherapy that is most commonly observed with high-dose treatments in the setting of myeloablative therapies.[15,16] It is, however, also observed with nonmyeloablative therapies,[17,18] particularly with taxanes.[16,19,20]

Clinical Presentation

Neutropenic enterocolitis usually occurs when the absolute neutrophil count falls to <500/μL. Patients present with fever, abdominal pain, nausea, vomiting, diarrhea, and not uncommonly, sepsis. Abdominal pain may be diffuse or localized to the right lower quadrant. Sometimes pain is absent, particularly if the patient has received steroid therapy.

Pathogenesis

The pathogenesis of neutropenic enterocolitis is multifactorial: mucosal injury by cytotoxic drugs or other means, profound neutropenia, and impaired host defense to invasion by microorganisms.[16,21,22] The microbial infection leads to necrosis of various layers of the bowel wall. Anatomically, the cecum is almost always affected, and the process often extends into the ascending colon and terminal ileum. The predilection for the cecum is possibly related to its dispensability and its relatively diminished vascularization. Various bacterial and/or fungal organisms, including gram-negative rods, gram-positive cocci, anaerobes (e.g., *Clostridium septicum*), and *Candida* spp., are often seen infiltrating the bowel wall. Polymicrobial infection is frequent. Bacteremia or fungemia is also common, usually with enteric organisms such as *Pseudomonas* or yeasts such as *Candida*.

Diagnostic Investigations

The diagnosis is based upon signs and symptoms in the appropriate clinical setting as well as imaging studies. Plain abdominal radiographs may demonstrate dilated loops of bowel, thickening of the bowel wall, "thumbprinting" resulting from bowel wall edema,

or indications of a right lower quadrant mass or phlegmon. Free intraperitoneal air indicates perforation of the bowel wall. Pneumatosis intestinalis is often seen.

Computed tomography scanning is the preferred imaging modality. Computed tomography scanning techniques can evaluate the entire abdomen for pathology, especially in patients with distended loops of bowel and ileus for whom ultrasound would not be possible. Scans commonly demonstrate concentric thickening of the bowel wall, a fluid-filled cecum, pericolic fluid collections or abscesses, pneumatosis intestinalis, and free air if an underlying perforation exists. Bowel wall thickening of >3 mm to 5 mm is considered abnormal and is consistent with, but not diagnostic of, necrotizing enterocolitis.[23] Indeed, *Clostridium difficile*–related colitis in patients with neutropenia may be associated with substantial or even greater wall thickening.[24] *Pneumatosis intestinalis* along with cecal and colonic wall thickening is very suggestive.[24]

Abdominal ultrasonography can identify thickening of the bowel wall that produces a target or halo sign. Indeed, a bowel wall thickening of >5 mm was associated with a higher mortality (29% versus 0%). If one takes a cutoff of >10 mm, the mortality was 60% versus 4.2%.[25] Ultrasound is useful as a follow-up tool to assess the gradual decrease in bowel wall thickening. Additionally, signs of pericolic fluid and intramural or abdominal free air often indicate perforation.

Diagnostic Criteria

Established standardized diagnostic criteria include the presence of neutropenia (absolute neutrophil count <500 × 106 cells/L), bowel wall thickening of >4 mm on radiographic imaging, and the exclusion of other diagnoses such as *C. difficile*–associated colitis, graft-versus-host disease, or other abdominal syndromes.[20,26]

Targeted Therapy–Associated Diarrhea

Almost all of the recently developed small molecule targeted therapies cause diarrhea as a side effect. Diarrhea, which can be severe, has been reported in 30% to 50% of patients receiving bortezomib,[27] erlotinib,[28] gefitinib,[29] sorafanib,[30] sunitinib,[31] and imatininib,[32] and the mammalian target of rapamycin inhibitors temsirolimus[33] and everolimus.[34]

The monoclonal therapies targeting the epidermal growth factor receptors cetuximab[35] and panitumumab[36,37] both cause diarrhea in 10% to 20% of patients, which may be severe in a small subset of patients.

Radiotherapy-Induced Diarrhea

Radiation injury to the lower intestine is usually encountered following treatment of cancers of the anus, rectum, cervix, uterus, prostate, urinary bladder, and testes, and as part of total-body irradiation. Radiotherapy of the abdomen or pelvis damages intestinal mucosa, causing prostaglandin release and bile salt malabsorption. These two factors increase intestinal peristalsis, causing diarrhea.

Acute radiation enteritis/proctitis occurs within 6 weeks of therapy. Symptoms include diarrhea, cramping, rectal urgency or tenesmus, and, uncommonly, bleeding. These symptoms usually resolve without specific therapy within 2 to 6 months.[38,39]

Late radiation enteritis/proctitis generally occurs 8 to 12 months after therapy and in some cases it may be delayed by years.[40] It may manifest as malabsorption and/or diarrhea, with more rapid transit times occurring in the affected bowel. Bacterial overgrowth causes malabsorption and contributes to the nausea, abdominal pain, and diarrhea, and it should be suspected in patients with intestinal strictures or enterocolic fistulae.[40] Although the large intestine is less radiosensitive, some patients can develop a pancolitis that resembles inflammatory bowel disease.[41,42]

Other Causes of Treatment-Related Diarrhea

Clostridium Difficile Diarrhea

C. difficile diarrhea occurs when the normal intestinal flora is altered, allowing *C. difficile* to flourish in the intestinal tract and produce a toxin that causes a watery diarrhea.[43] It can be triggered by repeated enemas, prolonged nasogastric tube insertion, gastrointestinal tract surgery, and the use of antibiotics, especially penicillin (ampicillin), clindamycin, and cephalosporins. Occasionally, however, it is reported after chemotherapy in the absence of antibiotic therapy.[44–46] The most common confirmatory study is an enzyme immunoassay for *C. difficile* toxins A and B, which yields results in 2 to 4 hours. Specificity of the assay is high (93% to 100 %), but sensitivity ranges from 63% to 99%, and this limited sensitivity may require two to three repeat stool samples to document disease.[43] Recently, a Polymerase chain reaction test Xpert C. difficile test (Cepheid, Sunnyvale, CA) has been approved by the US Food and Drug Administration. Limited data indicates that this may have greater sensitivity.[47]

Enteral Feeding

Tube feedings, either by nasogastric tube, gastrostomy, or jejunostomy, may be associated with the development of diarrhea.[48,49] This is a common problem occurring in 10% to 60% of patients.[48,49] Many potential factors may contribute to the problem and indeed it is often multifactorial.[49] Both formula osmolality and rate of delivery may be associated with diarrhea.[49]

Partially hydrolyzed guar gum is a soluble fiber added to enteral formulas and has the largest body of evidence supporting its use in diarrhea prevention when compared against fiber-free formulas.[49] There is some data indicating that partially hydrolyzed guar gum may be preferable to insoluble fiber in this setting. There is conflicting evidence of efficacy of probiotics in preventing diarrhea in patients receiving enteral nutrition, and there is no consensus regarding the use of this approach prophylactically.[49]

Contamination of the enteral formula may be a contributing or causative factor. Recommendations to reduce the risk of contamination include hand washing before handling the feeding system, use of clean equipment to prepare and mix feedings, bag and tubing change at least once a day, limitation of "hanging time" of individual bags to under 6 hours, and refrigerated storage of prepared bags until use.[50]

Celiac Plexus Block

Celiac plexus block is commonly associated with a self-limiting acute diarrhea. Occasionally, diarrhea may be persistent.[51] This diarrhea may be amenable to treatment with atropine.[52]

Assessment

The National Cancer Institute grading for the severity of diarrhea is presented in Table 136.1. For chemotherapy indiced diarrhea, the severity of the diarrhea, as reflected in its grading, is an important consideration in treatment selection (see the following).

Assessment includes a detailed medical history, dietary history, medication review, description of stools, and a physical examination focused on the identification of dehydration abdominal and rectal areas. When appropriate, abdominal radiographs can be ordered to evaluate for abdominal obstruction or fecal impaction. Biochemical parameters should be checked for evidence of dehydration, hypokalemia, or renal impairment. If enteric infections are suspected, stool samples should be sent for fecal leukocytes, *C. difficile* toxins A and B, and culture for organisms including *C. difficile*, *Salmonella*, *Escherichia coli*, *Campylobacter*, and infectious colitis.

As described previously, when neutropenic enterocolitis is suspected, computed tomography or ultrasound imaging of the abdomen should be undertaken and additional prognostic information may be obtained by ultrasound evaluation of bowel wall thickness.

General Principles in the Management of Diarrhea

Patients must be rehydrated either orally or when appropriate by parenteral infusion. In cases of large-volume diarrhea, there is the potential for very rapid dehydration with risk of prerenal impairment or even, in extreme cases, shock. Patients may suffer electrolyte imbalance particularly from hypokalemia. In general, milk products should be avoided if an infectious cause is suspected because a transient lactase deficiency sometimes may occur. Special attention should be given to patients who are incontinent of stool due to the risk of pressure ulcer formation. Skin barriers should be used to prevent skin irritation caused by fecal material.

Antidiarrhea Medications

Opioids

Loperamide is generally the opioid of choice because it has local activity in the gut and is absorbed only minimally (this accounts for the lack of systemic effects). It reduces stool weight, frequency of bowel movements, urgency, and fecal incontinence in acute and chronic diarrhea. Loperamide can be started at an initial dose of 4 mg followed by 2 mg every 2 to 4 hours or after every unformed

---

TABLE 136.1

National Cancer Institute Common Toxicity Criteria for Grading of Diarrhea

Toxicity	0	1	2	3	4
Patients without a colostomy	None	Increase of <4 stools/d over pretreatment	Increase of 4–6 stools/d or nocturnal stools	Increase of ≥7 stools/d	>10 stools/d
	None	None	Moderate cramping, not interfering with normal activity	Severe cramping and incontinence, interfering with daily activities	Grossly bloody diarrhea and need for parenteral support
Patients with a colostomy	None	Mild increase in loose, watery colostomy output compared with pretreatment	Moderate increase in loose, watery colostomy output compared with pretreatment, but not interfering with normal activity	Severe increase in loose, watery colostomy output compared with pretreatment, interfering with normal activity	Physiologic consequences requiring intensive care; hemodynamic

Adapted from National Cancer Institute. Cancer Therapy Evaluation Program Common Toxicity Criteria, Version 2.0. 1999:11.

stool.[53,54] Other opioids, such as tincture of opium, morphine, or codeine, can be used.

Tincture of opium is a widely used antidiarrheal agent. It is often recommended as an alternative to loperamide. Deodorized tincture of opium contains the equivalent of 10 mg/ml morphine, and the recommended dose is 10 to 15 drops in water every 3 to 4 hours. It is important not to confuse this with paregoric, which is a camphorated (alcohol-based) tincture. The latter is a less-concentrated preparation that contains the equivalent of 0.4 mg/ml morphine. The recommended dose is 1 teaspoon (5 ml) in water every 3 to 4 hours.

Somatostatin Analogues

In cases of severe or persistent diarrhea, the somatostatin analogue octreotide should be considered. Octreotide has multiple antidiarrheal actions including suppression of release of insulin, glucagon, vasoactive intestinal peptide, and gastric acid secretion; reduction in motility and pancreatic exocrine function; and increased absorption of water, electrolytes, and nutrients from the gastrointestinal tract. The usual starting dose for octreotide is 100 to 150 μg subcutaneously/intravenously three times a day.[55] As there is a dose response relationship for its antidiarrheal effect, the dose can be titrated up to 500 μg subcutaneously/intravenously three times a day or by continual intravenous infusion 25 to 50 μg/hour.[56] A microencapsulated, long-acting formulation of octreotide has been developed for once-monthly intramuscular dosing. This formulation has demonstrated efficacy in resolving severe diarrhea[57,58] and preventing further episodes of diarrhea in patients receiving ongoing therapy.[57,58]

Other Agents

Budesonide is an orally administered, topically active steroid with high activity in inflammatory bowel disease, a 90% first-pass effect in the liver, and therefore low systemic availability. It is commonly used in the management of diarrhea in patients with low- to medium-grade inflammatory bowel disease. A small study demonstrated efficacy of oral budesonide in the management of chemotherapy-induced diarrhea that was refractory to loperamide[59]; however, studies did not show benefit in prophylactic use to prevent diarrhea induced by irinotecan[60] or ipilimumab.[61]

Specific Management Guidelines

Chemotherapy-Induced Diarrhea

Chemotherapy-induced diarrhea is a major problem in the management of patients with gastrointestinal cancer in which the drugs irinotecan and fluorouracil are commonly used. Diarrhea can be severe and in some cases life-threatening. The most recent American Society for Clinical Oncology guidelines for management of treatment-induced diarrhea were published in 2004.[56] Patients are classified as uncomplicated or complicated on the basis of clinical features, and this classification guides treatment approach.

Prevention. Although a randomized trial did not show any advantage of neomycin in the primary prevention of late irinotecan diarrhea,[9] there is limited evidence supporting its use as secondary prevention in selected patients.[62]

"Uncomplicated" Diarrhea. *Step 1:* Patients with grade 1 or 2 diarrhea with no other complicating signs or symptoms may be classified as "uncomplicated" and managed conservatively with oral hydration and loperamide. Initial management of mild to moderate diarrhea should include dietary modifications (e.g., eliminating all lactose-containing products and high-osmolar dietary supplements), and the patient should be instructed to record the number of stools and report symptoms of life-threatening sequelae (e.g., fever or dizziness on standing). Loperamide should be started at an initial dose of 4 mg followed by 2 mg every 4 hours or after every unformed stool (not to exceed 16 mg/day).

If diarrhea resolves with loperamide, patients should be instructed to continue dietary modifications and to gradually add solid foods to their diet. In the case of chemotherapy-induced diarrhea, patients may discontinue loperamide when they have been diarrhea-free for at least 12 hours.

Step 2: If mild to moderate diarrhea persists for more than 24 hours, the dose of loperamide should be increased to 2 mg every 2 hours, and oral antibiotics may be started as prophylaxis for infection.

Step 3: If mild to moderate chemotherapy-induced diarrhea has not resolved after 24 hours on high-dose loperamide (48 hours total treatment with loperamide), the patient should be seen in the physician's office or outpatient center for further evaluation, including complete stool and blood workup. Stool workup should include evaluation for pathogens. Fluids and electrolytes should be replaced as needed. Loperamide should be discontinued, and the patient should be started on a second-line antidiarrheal agent such as SC octreotide (100- to 150-μg starting dose, with dose escalation as needed) or other second-line agents (e.g., oral budesonide or tincture of opium).

"Complicated" Chemotherapy-Induced Diarrhea. Patients with mild to moderate diarrhea complicated by moderate to severe cramping, nausea and vomiting, diminished performance status, fever, sepsis, neutropenia, bleeding, or dehydration, and patients with severe diarrhea are classified as "complicated" and should be evaluated further and monitored closely and treated aggressively.

Aggressive management of complicated cases usually necessitates admission and involves intravenous fluids; octreotide at a starting dose of 100 to 150 μg subcutaneously three times a day or intravenously (25 to 50 μg/hour) if the patient is severely dehydrated, with dose escalation up to 500 μg subcutaneously three times a day until diarrhea is controlled, and administration of antibiotics (e.g., fluoroquinolone). These patients should be evaluated with complete blood count, electrolyte profile, and a stool workup evaluating for blood, fecal leukocytes, *C. difficile*, *Salmonella*, *E. coli*, *Campylobacter*, and infectious colitis.

Radiation Therapy–Induced Diarrhea

The most recent American Society for Clinical Oncology guidelines for management of treatment-induced diarrhea were published in 2004.[56] The initial management of uncomplicated radiation-induced diarrhea is the same as for chemotherapy-induced diarrhea: starting with low-dose loperamide and then progressing to high-dose loperamide if diarrhea persists beyond 24 hours.

If diarrhea has not resolved after a further 24 hours on high-dose loperamide, continue loperamide (2 mg every 2 hours). In such cases, the patient should be evaluated; in severe cases, octreotide therapy may be indicated.

Patients with mild to moderate diarrhea complicated by moderate to severe cramping, nausea and vomiting, diminished performance status, fever, sepsis, neutropenia, bleeding, or dehydration, and patients with severe diarrhea are classified as "complicated." Complicated radiotherapy-induced diarrhea needs intensive monitoring and aggressive management either in hospital or an intensive home care nursing program or an outpatient facility able to provide a high level of care. Patients with severe symptoms or features suggestive of sepsis should undergo complete stool and blood workup and should be treated with octreotide and intravenous antibiotics.

Management of Neutropenic Enterocolitis

Management of neutropenic enterocolitis is challenging and the risk of mortality is high. There are roles for both medical and surgical interventions.

The initial treatment for neutropenic enterocolitis is medical, with the administration of broad-spectrum antibiotics, granulocyte colony-stimulating factors, nasogastric decompression, intravenous fluids, bowel rest, and serial abdominal examinations.[16,20,22] In most patients, these measures are sufficient, and symptoms resolve after correction of the neutropenia. The administered antibiotics should have a broad spectrum of activity to cover enteric gram-negative organisms, gram-positive organisms, and anaerobes. Causative microorganisms include *Pseudomonas*, *Staphylococcus aureus*, *E. coli*, and group A *Streptococcus*.[20] Reasonable initial choices include monotherapy with piperacillin-tazobactam or imipenem-cilastatin or duotherapy with cefepime or ceftazidime along with metronidazole.[15] In cases that do not respond to antibacterial agents, amphotericin should be considered, because fungemia is common.[20] Blood transfusions may be necessary because the diarrhea is often bloody. Anticholinergic, antidiarrheal, and opioid agents should be avoided as they may aggravate ileus.

The indications for and timing of surgical intervention are controversial. The mortality of patients who fail to respond to medical interventions is high, and many patients may not be salvageable. Nonetheless, in selected patients, surgery may be helpful to avoid progressive bowel necrosis, perforation, and to help control sepsis. Commonly cited indications for surgery include (1) persistent gastrointestinal bleeding after correction of thrombocytopenia and coagulopathy, (2) evidence of free intraperitoneal perforation, (3) evidence of abscess formation, (4) clinical deterioration despite aggressive supportive measures, and (5) to rule out other intra-abdominal processes such as bowel obstruction or acute appendicitis examinations.[16,20,22,63,64]

If exploratory surgery is performed, resection of grossly involved bowel is necessary. All necrotic material must be resected, usually by a right hemicolectomy, ileostomy, and mucous fistula. Failure to remove the necrotic focus in these severely immunocompromised patients is often fatal.[64] Primary anastomosis is not generally recommended in such severely immunocompromised patients because of the increased incidence of anastomotic leak.[64]

Diarrhea Prophylaxis

Prevention of Radiation Diarrhea

Multiple clinical trials have focused on prevention of diarrhea in patients receiving pelvic radiotherapy.[65] There is limited data to support the use of probiotic treatment containing *Lactobacillus*[65–67] and/or prophylactic 500 mg sulphasalzaine administered orally twice a day for prevention of radiotherapy-induced diarrhea.[65,68,69]

Prevention of Chemotherapy Diarrhea

Other than the use of atropine to prevent acute irinotecan diarrhea,[70] prophylactic antidiarrheal treatment is not a standard approach for any chemotherapy regimen. Small studies in the prevention of irinotecan-induced diarrhea have suggested the potential utility of oral alkalinization of the intestinal lumen,[71] activated charcoal,[72] and oral administration of probiotics microorganisms such as *Lactobacillus rhamnosus*.[73]

Negative studies have been reported with prophylactic octreotide,[74] long-acting octreotide,[75] oral racecadotril,[76] and oral neomycin.[9]

CONSTIPATION

Definition

Constipation is the slow movement of feces through the large intestine resulting in infrequent bowel movements and the passage of dry, hard stools. Constipation is a symptom, not a disease. It is usually a temporary condition and is not considered serious.

According to the "Rome 2 Criteria" proposed by a working group of gastroenterologists,[77] the clinical definition of chronic constipation is the presence of any two of the following symptoms for at least 12 weeks (not necessarily consecutive) in the previous 12 months:

- Straining during bowel movements
- Lumpy or hard stool
- Sensation of incomplete evacuation
- Sensation of anorectal blockage or obstruction
- Manual maneuvers to remove stool
- Fewer than three bowel movements per week

Prevalence

The prevalence of constipation in patients who have advanced cancer is approximately 40% to 60%[78]; the greatest prevalence occurs in the opioid-treated population.[79–81] Constipation is a major cause of patient distress and is often underappreciated and undertreated.[82]

Treatment-Related Causes

Medications, in particular opioids, serotonin antagonist antiemetics, and vinca alkaloid chemotherapy agents, are the most common causes of constipation among patients with cancer.

Opioid Analgesics

All opioids cause constipation, and tolerance to this effect is not observed over time. Importantly, the dose response relationship to this effect is very flat and the severity does not appear to be strongly dose-related. There is some data to indicate that the severity is less severe with fentanyl and, possibly, methadone,[83,84] and with oxycodone/naloxone combined formulation tablets.[85,86] Other medications that are commonly implicated are listed in Table 136.2.

Serotonin 5-Hydroxytryptamine-3 Receptor Antagonists

The 5-hydroxytryptamine-3 receptor antagonist antiemetics slow colonic transit, increase fluid absorption, and increase left colon compliance.[87] Overall, these agents are very well tolerated but 2% to 5% of patients report constipation,[88] and laxative therapy is often indicated.

Vinca Alkaloids

All the vinca alkaloids have pronounced neuropathic effects and reduce gastrointestinal transit time. Severity appears to be most pronounced with vincristine and vindesine, less so with vinblastine, and least with vinorelbine. Among patients receiving vincristine,

TABLE 136.2

Drugs Commonly Causing Constipation in Patients with Cancer

Opioids
Serotonin antagonists
Antidepressants
Aluminum- or calcium-containing antacids
Iron supplements
Diuretics
Antihypertensive medications
Anticonvulsants

SELECTED REFERENCES

The full reference list can be accessed at lwwhealthlibrary.com/oncology.

1. Arnold RJ, Gabrail N, Raut M, et al. Clinical implications of chemotherapy-induced diarrhea in patients with cancer. *J Support Oncol* 2005;3:227–232.
4. Meta-Analysis Group In Cancer. Toxicity of fluorouracil in patients with advanced colorectal cancer: effect of administration schedule and prognostic factors. Meta-Analysis Group In Cancer. *J Clin Oncol* 1998;16:3537–3541.
20. Nesher L, Rolston KV. Neutropenic enterocolitis, a growing concern in the era of widespread use of aggressive chemotherapy. *Clin Infect Dis* 2013;56:711–717.
21. Ullery BW, Pieracci FM, Rodney JR, et al. Neutropenic enterocolitis. *Surg Infect (Larchmt)* 2009;10:307–314.
23. Blijlevens NM. Neutropenic enterocolitis: challenges in diagnosis and treatment. *Clin Adv Hematol Oncol* 2009;7:528–530.
26. Gorschluter M, Mey U, Strehl J, et al. Neutropenic enterocolitis in adults: systematic analysis of evidence quality. *Eur J Haematol* 2005;75:1–13.
40. Theis VS, Sripadam R, Ramani V, et al. Chronic radiation enteritis. *Clin Oncol (R Coll Radiol)* 2010;22:70–83.
41. Kountouras J, Zavos C. Recent advances in the management of radiation colitis. *World J Gastroenterol* 2008;14:7289–7301.
43. McFee RB, Abdelsayed GG. Clostridium difficile. *Dis Mon* 2009;55:439–470.
49. Whelan K, Schneider SM. Mechanisms, prevention, and management of diarrhea in enteral nutrition. *Curr Opin Gastroenterol* 2011;27:152–159.
54. Hanauer SB. The role of loperamide in gastrointestinal disorders. *Rev Gastroenterol Disord* 2008;8:15–20.
56. Benson AB 3rd, Ajani JA, Catalano RB, et al. Recommended guidelines for the treatment of cancer treatment-induced diarrhea. *J Clin Oncol* 2004;22:2918–2926.
57. Rosenoff S. Resolution of refractory chemotherapy-induced diarrhea (CID) with octreotide long-acting formulation in cancer patients: 11 case studies. *Support Care Cancer* 2004;12:561–570.
65. Gibson RJ, Keefe DM, Lalla RV, et al. Systematic review of agents for the management of gastrointestinal mucositis in cancer patients. *Support Care Cancer* 2013;21:313–326.
66. Delia P, Sansotta G, Donato V, et al. Prevention of radiation-induced diarrhea with the use of VSL#3, a new high-potency probiotic preparation. *Am J Gastroenterol* 2002;97:2150–2152.
67. Giralt J, Regadera JP, Verges R, et al. Effects of probiotic Lactobacillus casei DN-114 001 in prevention of radiation-induced diarrhea: results from multicenter, randomized, placebo-controlled nutritional trial. *Int J Radiat Oncol Biol Phys* 2008;71:1213–1219.
68. Kilic D, Egehan I, Ozenirler S, et al. Double-blinded, randomized, placebo-controlled study to evaluate the effectiveness of sulphasalazine in preventing acute gastrointestinal complications due to radiotherapy. *Radiother Oncol* 2000;57:125–129.
69. Kilic D, Ozenirler S, Egehan I, et al. Sulfasalazine decreases acute gastrointestinal complications due to pelvic radiotherapy. *Ann Pharmacother* 2001;35:806–810.
70. Yumuk PF, Aydin SZ, Dane F, et al. The absence of early diarrhea with atropine premedication during irinotecan therapy in metastatic colorectal patients. *Int J Colorectal Dis* 2004;19:609–610.
73. Osterlund P, Ruotsalainen T, Korpela R, et al. Lactobacillus supplementation for diarrhoea related to chemotherapy of colorectal cancer: a randomised study. *Br J Cancer* 2007;97:1028–1034.
76. Ychou M, Douillard JY, Rougier P, et al. Randomized comparison of prophylactic antidiarrheal treatment versus no prophylactic antidiarrheal treatment in patients receiving CPT-11 (irinotecan) for advanced 5-FU-resistant colorectal cancer: an open-label multicenter phase II study. *Am J Clin Oncol* 2000;23:143–148.
77. Shih DQ, Kwan LY. All roads lead to Rome: update on Rome III criteria and new treatment options. *Gastroenterol Rep* 2007;1:56–65.
82. Laugsand EA, Jakobsen G, Kaasa S, et al. Inadequate symptom control in advanced cancer patients across Europe. *Support Care Cancer* 2011;19:2005–2014.
83. Staats PS, Markowitz J, Schein J. Incidence of constipation associated with long-acting opioid therapy: a comparative study. *South Med J* 2004;97:129–134.
86. Meissner W, Leyendecker P, Mueller-Lissner S, et al. A randomised controlled trial with prolonged-release oral oxycodone and naloxone to prevent and reverse opioid-induced constipation. *Eur J Pain* 2009;13:56–64.
99. Gray JR. What is chronic constipation? Definition and diagnosis. *Can J Gastroenterol* 2011;25:7B–10B.
100. Nagaviroj K, Yong WC, Fassbender K, et al. Comparison of the Constipation Assessment Scale and plain abdominal radiography in the assessment of constipation in advanced cancer patients. *J Pain Symptom Manage* 2011;42:222–228.
103. Klaschik E, Nauck F, Ostgathe C. Constipation—modern laxative therapy. *Support Care Cancer* 2003;11:679–685.
104. Brandt LJ, Prather CM, Quigley EM, et al. Systematic review on the management of chronic constipation in North America. *Am J Gastroenterol* 2005;100:S5–S21.
108. Twycross R, Sykes N, Mihalyo M, et al. Stimulant laxatives and opioid-induced constipation. *J Pain Symptom Manage* 2012;43:306–313.
117. Thomas J, Karver S, Cooney GA, et al. Methylnaltrexone for opioid-induced constipation in advanced illness. *N Engl J Med* 2008;358:2332–2343.
119. Wald A. Management and prevention of fecal impaction. *Curr Gastroenterol Rep* 2008;10:499–501.

PRACTICE OF ONCOLOGY

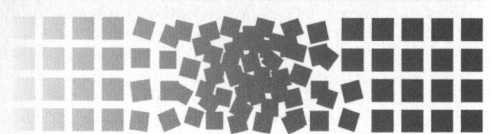

Eliezer Soto, Jane M. Fall-Dickson, and Ann M. Berger

INTRODUCTION

The effectiveness of cancer therapies to improve cure rates and to extend survival time, including chemotherapy (CT), radiation therapy (RT), and conditioning regimens used for hematopoietic stem cell transplantation (HSCT), is tempered by intolerable and quality-of-life (QOL)-impairing side effects. Oral complications are one such side effect, including CT- and RT-related oral mucositis and oral chronic graft-versus-host disease (cGVHD) and associated oropharyngeal pain, xerostomia, and oral infection. Pathogenesis of and management strategies for these oral complications, and future clinical research directions, are presented in this chapter.

ORAL MUCOSITIS

Oral mucositis is an inflammation of the mucous membranes of the oral cavity and oropharynx characterized by tissue erythema, edema, and atrophy, often progressing to ulceration.[1] The clinical significance of CT- and RT-related oral mucositis as a dose- and treatment-limiting side effect is related to pain and impairment in patient's QOL and functional status.[2-4]

The frequency and severity of oral mucositis are influenced by patient- and treatment-related risk factors (Table 137.1).[5,6] Risk factors for CT-related oral mucositis are complex. Although women have reported more frequent severe oral mucositis than men, and children are three times more likely than adults to develop mucositis, Driezen[7] reported no age or gender risk for this oral condition. In a study of 332 ambulatory patients undergoing CT, no increased risk for oral mucositis was seen for outpatients with dental appliances, previous oral lesions, a history of smoking, or diverse oral care practices, than patients who did not.[6] Conflicting study results may derive from lack of defined risk factors for entry into clinical trials.[5] Risk factors include continuous CT infusion therapy for breast and colon cancer (5-fluorouracil [5-FU] and leucovorin); selected anthracyclines, alkylating agents, taxanes, vinca alkaloids, antimetabolites, and antitumor antibiotics; myeloablative conditioning regimens for HSCT (e.g., high-dose melphalan or carmustine, cytarabine, melphalan [BEAM])[8-10]; and RT to the head and neck. Individual drug metabolism affects oral mucositis incidence and severity.

CHEMOTHERAPY-INDUCED MUCOSITIS

Approximately 40% of patients undergoing CT develop oral mucositis,[11] and approximately half of these patients develop painful lesions requiring parenteral analgesia or total parenteral nutrition (TPN) and treatment modification.[12] Incidence rates of 60% are seen in the HSCT setting and 78% for ulcerative oral mucositis.[13] Oral mucositis is a risk factor for life-threatening infections for patients with neutropenia. Oral infections, such as herpes simplex virus (HSV) may increase oral mucositis severity. There is a four times greater relative risk of septicemia in patients with oral mucositis and oral infections due to mucosal barrier injury.

The relationship between severe oral mucositis and clinical outcomes in patients who receive conditioning chemotherapy has been reported.[14,15] McCann et al.[14] conducted an observational study in 197 patients with multiple myeloma (MM) or non-Hodgkin's lymphoma treated with either high-dose melphalan or BEAM chemotherapy, respectively. Severe oral mucositis (World Health Organization grades 3 and 4) increased TPN duration by 2.7 days, opiates by 4.6 days, and antibiotics by 2.4 days. Oral mucositis presents with asymptomatic erythema and progresses from solitary, white, elevated desquamative patches that are slightly painful to large, contiguous, pseudomembranous, painful lesions. Typical oral sequelae of CT agents include epithelial hyperplasia, collagen and glandular degeneration, epithelial dysplasia, atrophy, and localized or diffuse mucosal ulceration. Nonkeratinized mucosa areas are most affected. The loss of basement membrane epithelial cells exposes underlying connective, innervated tissue stroma, which contributes to more severe oropharyngeal pain.

RADIATION-INDUCED MUCOSITIS

Oral mucositis is virtually universal when RT targets the oropharyngeal area, with severity dependent on type of ionizing radiation, volume of irradiated tissue, daily and cumulative dose, and duration. Oral mucositis is a dose- and rate-limiting toxicity of RT for head and neck cancer and of hyperfractionated RT and CT. Atrophic changes in the oral epithelium usually occur at total doses of 1,600 to 2,000 cGy, administered at a rate of 200 cGy/day.[16] Doses >6,000 cGy or concomitant CT are risk factors for permanent salivary gland changes.[16,17] The addition of total-body irradiation to HSCT increases oral mucositis severity through both direct mucosal damage and xerostomia. CT-induced dental effects are related to the treatment field including salivary glands. Teeth in the irradiated field may be desensitized, leading to asymptomatic early caries. Therefore, daily fluoride application is necessary.

Significant health-care costs and resource use are associated with oral mucositis in head and neck cancer.[18,19] In a prospective, longitudinal study of 75 patients with head and neck cancer receiving RT with or without CT,[19] 76% had severe oral pain requiring an increased number of health-care visits, 51% had a feeding tube, and 37% were hospitalized for an average of 4.9 days.

RADIATION THERAPY–RELATED COMPLICATIONS

Long-term effects of head and neck RT include soft tissue fibrosis, trismus, nonhealing or slow-healing mucosal ulcerations, and slow healing dental extraction sites. RT-induced fibrotic changes may occur in the masticatory muscles or the temporal mandibular joint up to 1 year posttherapy. Early phases of fibrogenesis following RT are seen as wound healing characterized by upregulation of tumor necrosis factor (TNF)-α and other proinflammatory cytokines.[20] As radiation fibrogenesis continues, it functions as a nonhealing wound.[20]

TABLE 137.1

Patient- and Treatment-Related Risk Factors for Stomatitis

Patient-Related

Age older than 65 or younger than 20
Gender
Inadequate oral health and hygiene practices
Periodontal diseases
Microbial flora
Chronic low-grade mouth infections
Salivary gland secretory dysfunction
Herpes simplex virus infection
Inborn inability to metabolize chemotherapeutic agents effectively
Inadequate nutritional status
Exposure to oral stressors including alcohol and smoking
Ill-fitting dental prostheses

Treatment-Related

Radiation therapy: dose, schedule
Chemotherapy: agent; dose, schedule
Myelosuppression
Neutropenia
Immunosuppression
Reduced secretory immunoglobulin A
Inadequate oral care during treatment
Infections of bacterial, viral, or fungal origin
Use of antidepressants, opiates, antihypertensives, antihistamines, diuretics, and sedatives
Impairment of renal or hepatic function
Protein or calorie malnutrition, and dehydration
Xerostomia

Adapted from Barasch A, Peterson DE. Risk factors for ulcerative mucositis in cancer patients: unanswered questions. *Oral Oncol* 2003;39:91–100; and Dodd MJ, Miaskowski C, Shiba GH, et al. Risk factors for CT-induced oral mucositis: dental appliances, oral hygiene, previous oral lesion, and a history of smoking. *Cancer Invest* 1999;17:278–284, with permission.

Osteoradionecrosis is a relatively uncommon condition related to hypocellularity, hypovascularity, and tissue ischemia. Higher incidences are reported with total doses to the bone exceeding 65 Gy.[21] Osteoradionecrosis is usually related to trauma and is reported following tooth extractions not timed to allow extraction site healing for 10 to 14 days before the start of RT. Osteonecrosis of the jaw bone is strongly associated with bisphosphonate use.[22,23]

PATHOGENESIS OF CHEMOTHERAPY- AND RADIATION-INDUCED ORAL MUCOSITIS

Current knowledge of oral mucositis pathogenesis is informed by translational research that applies advances in molecular-genetic technique and cell biology to this clinical condition.[24] Cancer therapy affects rapidly dividing cells including oral basal epithelium with a 7- to 14-day cell turnover rate, thus placing them at risk for CT targeting. Sonis et al.[25] reported a "burst" of cyclooxygenase (COX)-2 expression relative to RT-related oral mucositis progression, suggesting that COX-2 plays an amplifying role. In a small pilot study exploring the role of the COX pathway in three patients undergoing autologous HSCT, pain scores significantly correlated with COX-1, microsomal prostaglandin-E synthase, and salivary prostaglandin, suggesting a role for the COX pathway in oral mucositis, possibly via upregulation of proinflammatory prostaglandins.[26]

Sonis[24] has described a five-phase oral mucositis pathogenesis model including initiation, message generation, signaling and amplification, ulceration, and healing. Initiation occurs after administration of CT as a result of DNA damage and generation of reactive oxygen species. The relatively acute inflammatory or vascular phase occurs shortly after CT or RT administration.[12] Message generation involves upregulation of transcription factors, including nuclear factor kB and activation of cytokines and stress response genes. Signaling and amplification involves the production of proinflammatory cytokines from epithelial tissue, including TNF-α, which is related to tissue damage, and interleukin (IL)-1, which incites the inflammatory response and increases subepithelial vascularity that may lead to increased local CT levels. Logan et al.[27] reported preliminary results in 20 patients undergoing CT demonstrating elevated nuclear factor kB and COX-2 after CT, even though histologically the tissue was similar pre- and post-CT. The epithelial phase shows reduced epithelial renewal and atrophy, and typically begins 4 to 5 days after CT administration. The cell cycle S-phase–specific agents, including methotrexate, 5-FU, and cytarabine, are most efficient for this phase. The ulcerative or bacterial phase begins approximately 1 week post-CT in parallel with maximum neutropenia[12]; is the most complex, symptomatic phase; and is probably not CT agent class–specific. Patients often experience acute oropharyngeal pain, leading to dysphagia, decreased oral intake, and difficulty speaking. Bacterial colonization of mucosal ulceration occurs, and gram-negative organisms release endotoxins that induce the release of IL-1 and TNF and production of nitric oxide that may increase local mucosal injury. RT and CT are likely to amplify and prolong this proinflammatory cytokine release, leading to exacerbated tissue response. Genetic expression of cytokines and enzymes critical in tissue damage may be modified by transcription factors.[12] Fall-Dickson et al.[28] described oropharyngeal pain related to oral mucositis in patients undergoing HSCT with CT and measured TNF-α concentration in blood, saliva, and oral buccal brush biopsy samples. Oral mucositis severity was significantly associated with overall intensity of oral pain. TNF-α RNA content in oral buccal brush biopsy samples correlated with worst intensity of oral pain with swallowing. Healing of oral lesions in nonmyelosuppressed patients occurs 2 to 3 weeks after cancer treatment, with decrease in oropharyngeal pain seen in parallel with mucosal healing.

Avivi et al.[29] evaluated salivary antioxidant and immunologic capacities in 25 patients with MM treated with conditioning melphalan for HSCT who developed oral mucositis. Oral mucositis was associated with a reduction in secretory immunoglobulin A and antioxidant activity. The increase in salivary Alb and carbonyl indicated mucosal and oxidative damage, respectively.

CHRONIC GRAFT-VERSUS-HOST DISEASE ORAL MANIFESTATIONS

Patients who have undergone allogeneic HSCT (alloHSCT) frequently develop GVHD, an alloimmune condition derived from an immune attack mediated by donor T cells recognizing antigens expressed on normal tissues. GVHD occurs following alloHSCT due to disparities in minor histocompatibility antigens between donor and recipient, inherited independently of HLA genes.[30] cGVHD was historically defined as occurring at or beyond 100 days post HSCT,[31] and is now classified based on the characteristic clinical presentation.

cGVHD is reported to occur in 30% to 60% of patients more than 100 days post alloHSCT.[32] Approximately 80% of patients with extensive cGVHD have some type of oral involvement[33] that is a major contributing factor to the morbidity seen with alloHSCT. Although oral lesions are most common with extensive cGVHD, patients may also present with disease involving only the oral cavity, thus making comprehensive oral assessment important. Oral cGVHD presents with tissue atrophy and erythema, lichenoid changes, and pseudomembranous ulcerations, occurring typically on buccal and labial mucosa and the lateral tongue, angular stomatitis, and xerostomia.[33] Treister et al.[34] correlated the distribution, type, and extent of oral cGVHD lesions with oral pain and discomfort. The buccal and labial mucosa and tongue were the sites of 93% of ulcerations, 72% of erythematous lesions, and 76%

of reticular lesions. Ulcerations in the soft palate, although uncommon, were associated with increased pain. Functional impact was significant as seen by restriction of oral intake due to discomfort. Decreased oral intake leads to weight loss and malnutrition, which remain serious problems. Despite the importance of oral cGVHD as a major long-term complication of alloHSCT, little is known about its pathogenesis. Imanguli et al.[35] proposed a model of cGVHD pathogenesis in which the production of type 1 interferon by plasmacytoid dendritic cells plays a central role in initiation and continuation of cGVHD. Fall-Dickson et al.[36] analyzed associations among clinical characteristics of oral cGVHD and related oral pain and dryness, salivary proinflammatory cytokine IL-6 and IL-1α concentrations, and health-related QOL. Salivary IL-6 correlated with oral cGVHD severity, oral ulceration, and erythema, suggesting its potential utility as a biomarker for active oral cGVHD.

The importance of oral cGVHD was recognized by the National Institutes of Health (NIH) Consensus Development Project on Criteria for Clinical Trials in cGVHD[37] and the outcomes of a 2009 conference sponsored by the German-Austrian-Swiss working party for bone marrow and blood stem cell transplantation held in Regensburg, Germany.[38] Outcomes of the international conference included a summary of evidence for diagnosis, first- and second-line therapies, topical treatments, and practical treatment guidelines. The authors concurred that a comprehensive, interdisciplinary treatment approach for oral cGVHD must include assessment of mucosa, salivary glands, musculoskeletal tissues, teeth, periodontium, and combined oral function.[38] The Schubert Oral Mucositis Rating Scale was validated under the auspices of this NIH Consensus Development Project.[37] Treister et al.[39] analyzed inter- and intraobserver variability in the component and composite scores using the NIH oral cGVHD Activity Assessment Instrument. Twenty-four clinicians from six major HSCT centers scored high-quality intraoral photographs of 12 patients with a second evaluation 1 week later. Although mean interrater reliability was poor to moderate and unacceptable for the clinical trial setting, greater concordance among the oral medicine experts, high intrarater reliability, and participant feedback suggest formal training may decrease variability. Bassim et al.[40] examined the construct validity and internal consistency of the NIH Oral Mucosal Score (OMS) and its individual components (erythema, lichenoid, ulcers, mucoceles), as well as measures of oral pain, function, and related QOL, nutrition, and laboratory parameters in 198 patients diagnosed with cGVHD. The NIH OMS is based only on clinicians' assessment of oral mucosa in the patient who has undergone peripheral blood stem cell transplantation/bone marrow transplant (BMT). Results supported the construct validity of the discrete components of the NIH OMS as seen through strong associations between erythema and lichenoid and poor oral QOL, function, and nutrition, and lower serum albumin levels. Oral cGVHD ulceration was correlated primarily with oral pain. Validated assessment measures for oral cGVHD are needed to test agents in the clinical trial setting to advance the science of oral cGVHD, and to increase the treatment options.

SEQUELAE OF ORAL COMPLICATIONS

Oropharyngeal Pain

Oral mucositis is the principal etiology of most pain experienced during the 3-week post-BMT time period. This oral pain is often described as the most unforgettable ordeal of BMT. McGuire et al.[41] reported in a sample of patients undergoing autologous and allogeneic BMT that pain was reported before observed mucositis, that pain intensity did not correlate directly with extent of mucosal injury, and that some patients reported limited or no pain after BMT. A descriptive, cross-sectional study of women with breast cancer undergoing autologous HSCT conducted by Fall-Dickson et al.[42] showed a significant positive correlation between oral pain and oral mucositis severity.

The sensory dimension of oral mucositis–related pain reported with general mucosal inflammation and breakdown ranges from mild discomfort to severe and debilitating pain requiring opioids.[43] Oral pain is associated strongly with cGVHD and has been described as severe, burning, and irritating with dryness and loss of taste. Mucositis-related oral pain reported with CT is usually of <3 months' duration, contrasting with the usually chronic oral pain accompanying oral cGVHD.

Gender differences have been reported for pain. Women reported higher pain levels in a study to test capsaicin efficacy for oral mucositis–related pain. Pain management is critical to avoid suffering and psychological distress.[44] Adequate assessment of oral pain requires a comprehensive pain assessment tool such as the Pain-O-Meter (Dola Health Systems, Baltimore, MD),[45] which assesses overall intensity, sensory, and affective dimensions of pain.

Xerostomia

Xerostomia experienced by patients who receive head and neck RT is a major sequela, with severity dependent on RT dosage and location and volume of exposed salivary glands. Patients may also develop xerostomia as a late oral complication of HSCT. Brand et al.[46] reported in a cross-sectional study of patients with history of autologous or alloHSCT significantly higher levels of xerostomia compared to the comparison group. Xerostomia severity was not significantly associated with RT given before HSCT or the type of HSCT. Xerostomia can affect taste, oral comfort, prosthetic fit, speech, swallowing, and promote caries-producing organisms.

A recent cross-sectional study by Imanguli et al.[47] evaluated sicca signs and symptoms in 101 patients with cGVHD using assessment tools used in Sjögren syndrome. Of the 77% of patients reporting xerostomia, those with salivary dysfunction showed histopathologic changes consisting of mononuclear infiltration and fibrosis or atrophy, suggesting that salivary gland involvement is common in cGVHD. A valid, reliable assessment tool is needed to evaluate salivary function in clinical trials. Salivary antioxidant capacity and function were assessed in 30 patients after HSCT by Nagler et al.[48] Salivary gland function was assessed measuring total protein, secretory immunoglobulin A, the antioxidant peroxidase, uric acid, and total antioxidant status in a saliva sample. In patients who developed GVHD, there was a significant decrease in salivary flow rate pre- and post-HSCT with no recovery and a reduction in salivary protein content and salivary antioxidant capacity. In patients without GVHD after HSCT, salivary flow rates returned to normal in 3 to 5 months. Decreased salivary flow rate with related decrease in its protective functions for oral mucosa contribute to oral cGVHD severity. Bassim et al.[49] tested the feasibility of using liquid chromatography tandem mass spectrometry to identify and elucidate protein biomarkers related to oral cGVHD. Pooled saliva from five patients with moderate or severe oral cGVHD was compared to saliva from a gender- and age-matched pool of five patients with GVHD without oral mucosal findings. Reported reduction in salivary lactoperoxidase, lactotransferrin, and several cysteine proteinase inhibitor family proteins suggests impaired oral antimicrobial host immunity in oral cGVHD.[49]

STRATEGIES FOR PREVENTION AND TREATMENT OF ORAL COMPLICATIONS

Pretherapy Dental Evaluation and Intervention

Oral or dental stabilization prior to CT and RT is critically important to avoid serious sequela and requires an experienced dental team and informed patients working together for adequate cleaning, elimination oral infection and trauma, and appropriate oral hygiene.[50]

conflicting results. An extensive literature review performed by Savarese et al.[74] reported that glutamine supplementation may have an impact on incidence and severity of anthracycline-associated oral mucositis. A randomized, double-blind, placebo-controlled trial on glutamine supplementation in patients who underwent autologous HSCT reported increase in severe oral mucositis and opiate, and prolonged hospital stay.[75] Another randomized controlled study comparing oral glutamine supplementation (30 g/day) versus placebo in 58 patients undergoing HSCT reported no difference in length of hospitalization, nutrition, oral mucositis and diarrhea severity, engraftment time, survival, and relapse between both groups.[76]

Other clinical trials have reported more promising data on the use of glutamine.[77,78] A retrospective cohort study including 117 patients treated with RT for cancer of the head and neck or chest tested if oral glutamine prevents oral mucositis or acute radiation-induced esophagitis and favors nutritional status.[79] Overall, glutamine was associated with significant reduction of mucositis, weight loss, and enteral nutrition. The risk difference for developing oral mucositis in patients receiving glutamine when compared with controls was -9.0% (95% confidence interval $= -18.0\%$ to -1.0%). The majority of patients not receiving glutamine developed severe malnutrition. No differences were seen in interruption of RT, hospitalization, opioid use, or death during RT.

In a double-blind, randomized, placebo-controlled trial of oral glutamine in the prevention of oral mucositis in children undergoing HSCT, 120 patients were randomized to receive glutamine or glycine twice a day until 28 days post-HSCT. The glutamine group showed a significant reduction in days of intravenous opiates use and TPN, but no difference in toxicity was observed between the two groups.[80]

A phase 3 study of topical AES-14, which is a novel drug system designed to concentrate delivery of l-glutamine to oral mucosa for ulceration treatment, was conducted with 121 patients at risk for oral mucositis.[81] Patients were randomized to either AES-14 or placebo and received protocol treatment from day 1 of CT until 2 weeks following the last CT dose or oral mucositis resolution. Results showed a potential 20% reduction of moderate-to-severe oral mucositis in the AES-14 group and a 10% increase in grade 0 oral mucositis.

Anti-Inflammatory Agents

Prostaglandins are a family of naturally occurring eicosanoids, some of which have shown cytoprotective activity. Misoprostol, a synthetic analog of prostaglandin E1, has been studied as prevention and treatment option for oral mucositis due to its anti-inflammatory and mucosa-protecting properties. A randomized, double-blind, placebo-controlled, parallel-group study conducted by Lalla et al.[82] evaluated the efficacy of misoprostol oral rinse in reducing the severity of oral mucosal injury caused by high-dose CT. Forty-eight patients receiving myeloablative high-dose CT were randomized to misoprostol ($n = 22$) or placebo rinse ($n = 26$). Results showed no significant effect of misoprostol rinse in mucositis.

Topical dinoprostone was administered four times daily in a nonblinded study to 10 patients with oral carcinomas who were receiving 5-FU and mitomycin with concomitant RT.[83] The control group comprised 14 patients who were receiving identical treatment. Eight of the ten subjects who received dinoprostone were evaluable; no patient developed severe oral mucositis as compared with six episodes in the control arm. A second pilot study was conducted with 15 patients who received RT to the head and neck, showing that an inflammatory reaction was detected in 5 patients in the vicinity of their tumor when treated with topically applied PGE[2], and that no patients developed any bullous or desquamating inflammatory lesions.[84] A double-blind, placebo-controlled study of PGE[2] in 60 patients undergoing BMT showed no significant

differences in incidence, severity, or duration of oral mucositis. Incidence of HSV was higher in the PGE[2] arm. Increase in oral mucositis severity was seen in in patients who developed HSV.[85]

Benzydamine is a nonsteroidal anti-inflammatory drug with reported analgesic, anesthetic, and antimicrobial properties without activity on arachidonic acid metabolism. It has been shown to reduce the severity of oral mucositis and associated pain in patients who undergo RT. Epstein and Stevenson-Moore[86] reported in a double-blind, placebo-controlled trial that benzydamine produced statistically significant relief of pain from RT-induced oral mucositis and a reduction in both the total area and the size of ulceration. Positive responses to benzydamine have been reported in three other studies.[87–89] In a small prospective, double-blind, randomized study comparing the efficacy of chlorhexidine gluconate and benzydamine hydrochloride oral rinse in patients with head and neck cancer to prevent and treat RT-induced oropharyngeal mucositis, a trend showed decrease in mucositis, oropharyngeal pain, and dysphagia in those receiving benzydamine.[90] Given the proposed importance of the prostaglandin pathway in the pathogenesis of oral mucositis, additional studies are warranted.

Current evidence does not support the use of systemic steroids to reduce the frequency or severity of oral mucositis.[91]

BIOLOGIC RESPONSE MODIFIERS

Epidermal Growth Factors

Studies on epidermal growth factor (EGF) as a treatment option for CT- and RT-induced oral mucositis have reported conflicting data. EGF may function as a marker of mucosal damage and could facilitate the healing process.[92] In a phase 1 trial conducted by Girdler et al.,[93] EGF mouthwash used by patients treated with CT showed onset delay and severity reduction of recurrent ulcerations. No statistical difference was seen in resolution of established ulcers. A double-blind, placebo-controlled, prospective phase 2 study reported potential benefit from EGF oral spray for oral mucositis in patients undergoing RT for head and neck cancer. One hundred and thirteen patients were randomized into one of four arms: EGF-treatment groups (10, 50, and 100 mcg/ml doses twice daily) and placebo. The 50 mcg/ml dose showed the best efficacy.[94]

Kim et al.[95] evaluated efficacy and safety of recombinant human EGF (rhEGF) oral spray for CT-induced oral mucositis with HSCT. Fifty-eight patients were randomly assigned to either the rhEGF group or placebo group. The incidence of National Cancer Institutes grade ≥ 2 oral mucositis was higher in rhEGF than placebo group (78.6% versus 50%; $p = 0.0496$), respectively. Duration of mucositis with National Cancer Institutes grade ≥ 2 was shorter in the rhEGF group (8.5 days versus 14.5 days). rhEGF significantly reduced limitations in swallowing and drinking, and reduced hospitalization duration, administration of TPN, and opioid usage, in patients with grade ≥ 3. Results were better for patients with advanced oral mucositis in the rhEGF group for several secondary end points.

Hematopoietic Growth Factors

Hematologic growth factors are standard treatment for patients who are treated with high-dose CT because of well-established efficacy to decrease the duration of CT-induced neutropenia. In vitro studies have demonstrated that EGF is present in saliva with ability to affect growth, cell and migration, and repair mechanisms.[96] The development of increased oral toxicity or mucosal repair may be dependent on timing of EGF administration in relation to CT treatment.[97] Gabrilove et al.[98] reported from a sample of 27 patients with bladder cancer who received escalating doses of granulocyte–colony-stimulating factor (G-CSF) during treatment with methotrexate, vinblastine, doxorubicin, and cisplatin. The patients received the G-CSF during the first of two cycles of CT. Although significantly less oral mucositis was seen during cycle one of G-CSF, positive results may be biased related to possible cumulative CT toxicity with resultant increase in oral mucositis severity. Conversely, Bronchud et al.[99] reported from a study of 17 patients with breast or ovarian carcinoma treated with escalating doses of doxorubicin with G-CSF that G-CSF did not prevent severe oral mucositis. A third study compared clinical outcomes in 55 adult patients who received CT for non-Hodgkin's lymphoma and G-CSF with clinical outcomes in 39 patients who received CT alone. Patients who did not receive G-CSF had neutropenia as the primary cause of treatment delay compared with those patients who did receive G-CSF and experienced oral mucositis as the main cause of treatment delay.[100] Granulocyte macrophage–colony-stimulating factor (GM-CSF) has demonstrated conflicting results in patients who received diverse cancer treatments.[101–104] An open, randomized controlled phase 3 trial conducted by Masucci et al.[102] analyzed the efficacy of GM-CSF in patients with head and neck cancer with RT-induced oral mucositis. A significant reduction in oral mucositis severity was observed in the GM-CSF treatment group. Conversely, results from a Radiation Therapy Oncology Group sponsored a double-blind, placebo-controlled, randomized study ($n = 121$) to analyze efficacy and safety of GM-CSF in reducing severity and duration of oral mucositis and related pain in patients with head and neck cancer receiving RT.[104] GM-CSF had no significant effect on severity or duration of oral mucositis.

Keratinocyte Growth Factors

Palifermin, a recombinant human keratinocyte growth factor and member of fibroblast growth factor family, has shown efficacy in reducing oral mucosal injury related to cytotoxic therapy.[105] Spielberger et al.[105] reported from a double-blind study comparing the effect of palifermin with a placebo for development of oral mucositis in 212 patients with hematologic cancers. Palifermin or placebo was administered intravenously for 3 consecutive days immediately before initiating conditioning therapy with fractionated total-body radiation plus high-dose CT. The palifermin group had significant reductions in grade 4 oral mucositis, soreness of the mouth and throat, opioid use, and incidence of TPN use. Luthi et al.[106] reported lower grade 3 or 4 oral mucositis in 34 patients who received melphalan or BEAM with HSCT and were treated with palifermin (0.06 mg/kg) injections 3 days before conditioning CT and 3 days after HSCT compared with controls. Nasilowska-Adamska et al.[107] reported palifermin 60 mcg/kg per day for 3 consecutive days before and after conditioning therapy for HSCT significantly reduced incidence, severity, and duration of oral mucositis in 106 patients. In a subsequent study,[108] 53 patients with hematologic diseases used the same regimen, also showing a significant reduction in incidence and median duration of oral mucositis, decreased incidence of opioid and TPN use, and less prevalence of acute GVHD.

A randomized, placebo-controlled, double-blind study conducted by Le et al.[109] evaluated efficacy and safety of palifermin to reduce CT-induced oral mucositis in patients with locally advanced head and neck cancer. A total of 188 patients received palifermin (180 mcg/kg) or placebo before chemoradiotherapy and then weekly for 7 weeks. The group receiving palifermin showed a lower incidence of severe oral mucositis when compared with the placebo group (54% and 69%, $p = 0.041$). However, opioid analgesic use, average mouth and throat soreness, and chemoradiotherapy compliance were not significantly different between treatment arms. After median follow-up of 26 months, overall survival and progression-free survival and other secondary outcomes such as opioid use were similar between treatment arms.

A multicenter, double-blind, randomized study investigated the effectiveness of palifermin in reducing severe oral mucositis in patients with postoperative chemoradiotherapy for head and neck cancer.[110] A total of 186 patients with carcinoma of the oral cavity, oropharynx, hypopharynx, or larynx (stages II to IVB) were randomly assigned to receive weekly palifermin (120 mcg/kg) or placebo from 3 days before and throughout radiochemotherapy. A total of 47 of 92 patients (51%) in the palifermin group developed severe oral mucositis versus 63 (67%) of 94 administered placebo ($p = 0.027$). In addition, palifermin decreased the duration and prolonged the time to develop severe mucositis. Although palifermin reduced the occurrence of severe oral mucositis, its role in the management patients with head and neck cancer undergoing postoperative chemoradiotherapy remains to be elucidated.

Palifermin has also been studied in patients with solid tumors. In a randomized controlled trial conducted by Rosen et al.,[111] 64 patients with metastatic colorectal cancer who received 5-FU and leucovorin were randomized to receive palifermin (40 mcg/kg) for 3 consecutive days before each of two cycles of CT. The incidence of oral mucositis World Health Organization grade 2 or higher was significantly lower, and patients reported less severe symptoms in the treatment arm. Brizel et al.[112] compared palifermin (60 mcg/kg) versus placebo in patients with locally advanced head and neck cancer treated with chemoradiation. Patients received two types of RT—standard (total dose of 70 Gy delivered in 2 Gy–daily fractions) and hyperfractionated (total dose 72 Gy delivered in 1.25-Gy fractions twice a day for 7 weeks)—and CT including cisplatin (20 mg/m^2 for 4 days) and continuous infusion of 5-FU (1,000 mg/m^2 per day for 4 days in weeks 1 and 5 of RT). Palifermin was well tolerated and decreased incidence of oral mucositis, dysphagia, and xerostomia in patients treated with hyperfractionated RT but not standard RT. However, palifermin did not reduce the morbidity of concurrent chemoradiotherapy.

A randomized, double-blind, placebo-controlled trial conducted by Vadhan-Raj et al.[113] evaluated efficacy of palifermin as a single dose before each cycle in patients receiving multicycle chemotherapy. Forty-four patients with sarcoma were randomized in a 2:1 ratio to receive palifermin (180 mcg/kg), single dose 3 days before each chemotherapy cycle (maximum of six cycles), or placebo. Palifermin decreased incidence of moderate to severe mucositis (44% versus 88%, $p < 0.001$) and severe mucositis (13% versus 51%, $p = 0.002$). Reported adverse effects include thickening of oral mucosa and altered taste. Eighty-eight percent (seven of eight) patients with severe mucositis in the placebo group received palifermin in an open-label fashion. Palifermin as a single-dose before each chemotherapy cycle reduced incidence and severity of oral mucositis in patients with sarcoma.

Antimicrobials

Antimicrobial approaches have included systemic types such as antibiotics, antivirals (acyclovir, valacyclovir, ganciclovir), antifungal (fluconazole), as well as topical therapy. Donnelly et al.[114] evaluated the evidence regarding the role of infection in the pathophysiology of oral mucositis via a comprehensive review of 31 prospective randomized trials. No clear pattern of patient type, cancer treatment, or type of antimicrobial agent used was seen, and there was a lack of consistent oral mucositis assessment.

Oral candidiasis is a common acute and chronic oral sequela of head and neck RT, with lesions presenting as removable (whitish) chronic or hyperplastic (nonremovable) and chronic erythematous (diffused as patchy erythema), which frequently appear as angular cheilitis (first signs or symptoms). Treatment approaches for oral candidiasis include Mycostatin (troche; Bristol-Myers Squibb Company, New York. NY), nystatin (liquid or ointment), or clotrimazole. Pseudomembranous candidiasis is successfully treated topically. Chronic candidiasis usually requires much longer treatment, and it may be necessary to use oral ketoconazole, fluconazole, or intravenous amphotericin B.

Acyclovir prophylaxis is currently accepted treatment for HSV and patients with are cytomegalovirus seropositive and undergoing HSCT. A randomized controlled clinical trial in patients undergoing HSCT compared fluconazole with placebo showing that that fluconazole prevented systemic fungal infections (7% fluconazole versus 18% placebo) and significantly reduced the incidence of mucosal infection and oropharyngeal colonization by *Candida albicans*.[115]

Conflicting reports have been published regarding chlorhexidine mouthwash for alleviating oral mucositis and reducing oral colonization by gram-positive, gram-negative, and *Candida* species in patients receiving CT, RT, or HSCT. The majority of studies have not demonstrated efficacy of chlorhexidine mouthwash for oral mucositis reduction in patients receiving intensive CT.[116] Dodd et al.[117] tested the efficacy of the PRO-SELF Mouth Aware (PSMA) program combined with randomization to one of two mouthwashes (0.12% chlorhexidine or sterile water) for prevention of CT-related oral mucositis in 222 patients. Although chlorhexidine was no more effective than water regarding oral mucositis incidence, days to onset, and severity, the PSMA program appeared to reduce oral mucositis incidence. A double-blind, placebo-controlled, randomized study of chlorhexidine prophylaxis for 5-FU–based CT-induced oral mucositis in patients with gastrointestinal malignancies conducted by Sorensen et al.[118] suggested a role for chlorhexidine in prevention of oral mucositis. A total of 225 patients were randomized to chlorhexidine mouth rinse three times a day for 3 weeks versus placebo or cryotherapy with ice 45 minutes during CT. The frequency and duration of oral mucositis were significantly improved in the chlorhexidine and cryotherapy arms.

Sutherland and Browman[119] reviewed 59 studies assessing prophylaxis of RT-induced oral mucositis in patients with head and neck cancer. Interventions chosen based on the biologic etiology of oral mucositis were effective. Spijkervet et al.[120] evaluated efficacy of lozenges containing polymyxin E_2 2 mg, tobramycin 1.8 mg, and amphotericin B 10 mg taken four times daily for oropharyngeal flora related to oral mucositis. These researchers compared 15 patients receiving RT using polymyxin E_2 2 mg, tobramycin 1.8 mg, and amphotericin B 10 mg, and two other groups of 15 patients each, one using 0.1% chlorhexidine and the other using placebo. The selectively decontaminated group had significantly reduced severity and oral mucositis extent when compared with the chlorhexidine and placebo groups.

A randomized, double-blind study conducted by Sharma et al.[121] evaluated the effects of administering *Lactobacillus brevis* CD2 lozenges on incidence and severity of oral mucositis and tolerance to chemoradiotherapy in patients with head and neck squamous cell carcinoma. Two hundred patients received daily treatment with lozenge containing either *L. brevis* CD2 or placebo during and for 1 week after completion of chemoradiation therapy. Severe oral mucositis (grades 3 and 4) developed in 52% and 77% of patients in the treatment and placebo arms, respectively ($p < 0.001$). There was a significant difference in anticancer treatment completion rates among groups ($p = 0.001$). *L. brevis* CD2 lozenges were associated with a lower incidence of CT-/RT-induced severe oral mucositis and a higher rate of treatment completion.

Triclosan, an antibacterial agent used commonly in periodontal therapy has also been evaluated in the management of RT-induced oral mucositis. Satheeshkumar et al.[122] conducted a randomized study to determine the effectiveness of this therapy in the management of RT-induced oral mucositis. Twenty-four patients with oral cancer with grade 1 RT-induced oral mucositis were randomized to receive either triclosan mouthwash (0.03%) or sodium bicarbonate (2 mg) mouthwash. The use of triclosan reduced the progression to grade 4 oral mucositis in most patients. Changes were also noticed in food intake and weight loss. Triclosan mouthwash was effective in reducing the severity of RT-induced oral mucositis; however, the small sample size was a major study limitation. Further studies are needed to confirm this observation.[123]

Cryotherapy

Cryotherapy, which is administered as ice chips and flavored ice products, has been used to prevent oral mucositis and to improve patient's overall QOL by decreasing its severity and improving nutritional status. Efficacy of cryotherapy for the reduction of 5-FU–induced oral mucositis severity was seen through a North Central Cancer Treatment Group and Mayo Clinic–sponsored controlled randomized trial.[124] A subsequent study with a sample of 178 patients randomized to 30 minutes versus 60 minutes of oral cryotherapy reported similar severity of oral mucositis in both groups.[125] The study recommended use of 30 minutes of oral cryotherapy prior to bolus administration of 5-FU–based CT. Additional studies have confirmed these results.[126–128] Cryotherapy used to induce vasoconstriction should be considered for patients receiving 5-FU or melphalan[129] administered for short infusion times.

The effectiveness of aggressive oral care in combination with cryotherapy has also been evaluated in the literature. In a pilot randomized controlled study, 46 patients admitted for autologous HSCT were randomly assigned to the experimental arm ($n = 23$) or usual care ($n = 23$).[130] The patients in the experimental arm received an hour regimen of oral cryotherapy. The overall mean of oral mucositis severity for the treatment arm was significantly lower than for the control group: 0.43 versus 1.14, on a 0 to 4 scale ($p < 0.001$). In terms of overall mean pain score, for the treatment arm's mean pain score was significantly lower: 0.30 versus 1.64 ($p < 0.001$). Oral cryotherapy added to aggressive oral care protocols appears to reduce mucositis and related pain severity compared with oral care alone.

Use of intravenous opioids has become a common practice for patients with CT- and RT-induced oral mucositis. Cryotherapy is an important adjuvant technique to opiate analgesia. A randomized controlled trial conducted by Svanberg et al.[131] showed that this technique may alleviate development of oral mucositis and oral pain, resulting in decreased days and total dose of intravenous opiates in patients treated with autologous BMT.

Laser

Several studies have confirmed the effectiveness of low-energy laser for prevention and treatment of CT- or RT-induced oral mucositis.[132–137] A phase 3 double-blind, placebo-controlled randomized study compared two different low level GaA1As diode lasers (650 nm and 780 nm) to prevent oral mucositis in patients undergoing HSCT treated with either CT or chemoradiotherapy.[135] Seventy patients were randomized into treatment with 650 nm or 780 nm laser or placebo. Low-level laser therapy was safe and more effective for decreasing oral mucositis and related oral pain. The efficacy of low-energy He/Ne laser was studied in a sample of 30 and 24 patients in two randomized controlled clinical trials.[133,138] Low-energy He/Ne laser demonstrated a reduction in the severity and duration of oral mucositis.

In a triple-blinded randomized controlled trial conducted by Gautam et al.,[139] prophylactic low-level laser therapy was tested to prevent CT-induced oral mucositis. A total of 221 patients with head and neck cancer scheduled to undergo chemoradiation were randomized into laser ($n = 111$) and placebo ($n = 110$) groups. The laser group received (HeNe) $\lambda = 632.8$ nm, power-density = 24 mW, dosage = 3.0 J/point, total dosage/session = 36 to 40 J, spot-size = 1 cm^2, five sessions/week; and the placebo group received sham treatment daily prior to radiation. In the laser group, there was significant reduction in incidence of severe oral mucositis ($p < 0.0001$), associated pain ($p < 0.0001$), dysphagia ($p < 0.0001$), and opioid use ($p < 0.0001$) when compared to the placebo group. The same researchers demonstrated efficacy of low-level laser therapy in improving patients' subjective experience of oral mucositis and QOL in patients with head and neck cancer.[140]

Miscellaneous Agents

Mangoni et al.[141] analyzed the protective efficacy of a heparan mimetic biopolymer, RGTA-OTR4131, alone or with amifostine, in the management of oral mucositis and evaluated its effects on tumor growth in vitro and in vivo. A single dose of 16.5 Gy was delivered to the snout of mice and the effects of OTR4131 were analyzed by macroscopic scoring and histology. OTR4131 was well tolerated and effective in reducing RT-induced oral mucositis without affecting tumor sensitivity to RT. These results need to be confirmed in clinical trials.

A prospective, randomized, multicenter study conducted by Wu et al.[142] investigated the role of Actovegin (Nycomed Austria GmbH, Linz, Austria), a deproteinized extract of calf blood, in the prevention and treatment of CT-induced oral mucositis in patients with nasopharyngeal carcinoma. A total of 156 patients were randomized to receive Actovegin for prevention ($n = 53$) or treatment ($n = 51$) or to a control group ($n = 52$). Actovegin 30 ml/daily (5 days/week) was given for the duration of the radiotherapy for Group 1 and from the onset of grade 2 mucositis for Group 2. The incidence of grade 3 mucositis was lower in Group 1 versus Group 3 ($p = 0.002$), and Group 2 had a lower progression rate of mucositis (grade 2 to 3) when compared to the placebo group ($p = 0.035$). Thus, Actovegin showed efficacy in the prevention and treatment of CT-/RT-induced oral mucositis.

Rhodiola algida, a traditional Chinese medicine widely used to stimulate the immune system, also has been tested as a treatment option for patients with cancer with oral ulcers. Loo et al.[143] investigated the effect of *R. algida* on healthy lymphocytes in vitro, the homeostasis of patients with cancer, and the healing time of oral ulcers. A total of 462 subjects were treated with 100 ug/ml *R. algida* for 48 hours. Lymphocytes were isolated, and the level of several cytokines and mRNA content were determined. A total of 138 patients with breast cancer were randomized to receive *Rhodiola* (for 14 days after each cycle) and placebo after modified total mastectomy with adjuvant chemotherapy. *R. algida* favored the proliferation of lymphocytes, as well as an increase of IL-2, IL-4, GM-CSF, and the mRNA content of these cytokines. The white blood cell count increased faster in the treatment group. The patients also presented with smaller and fewer oral ulcers. This study suggests that *R. algida* increases immunity of patients receiving adjuvant chemotherapy and decreases the quantity of oral ulcers.

Other therapies such as phenylbutyrate mouthwash and visible-light therapy have also shown to mitigate oral mucositis during CT/RT in patients with head-and-neck cancer or in patients undergoing HSCT, respectively.[144,145] Larger randomized trials are needed to confirm these results.

TREATMENT FOR ORAL CHRONIC GRAFT-VERSUS-HOST DISEASE

Almost all patients with extensive cGVHD require systemic immunosuppressive therapy. Thus, there is a critical need for adjuvant therapies that are both efficacious and avoid the long-term consequences of these corticosteroid therapies. In general, advances in the treatment of cGVHD have been modest, and no standard therapy exists for cGVHD that fails to respond to initial therapy or recurs. Granitto et al.,[32] Imanguli et al.,[146] and Mays et al.[147] have presented comprehensive reviews of available therapies for oral cGVHD. Most commonly recommended therapy for management of mucosal involvement of oral cGVHD is topical high and ultrahigh potency corticosteroids, calcineurin inhibitors, and analgesics.[147] The most common systemic therapy is corticosteroids with or without cyclosporine. Other agents such as tacrolimus, sirolimus, pentostatin, mycophenolate mofetil, and hydroxychloroquine have been used as salvage treatment.[146] Emerging systemic therapies include monoclonal antibodies such as

infliximab, etanercept, daclizumab, and rituximab.[146,148] Extracorporeal photophoresis, a process that separates a patient's mononuclear cells through apheresis and exposes them to ultravioletlight A, has shown promise.

Patients with symptomatic disease limited to the oral cavity have been found to benefit from topical steroids such as dexamethasone elixir (0.5 mg/ml) as a mouth rinse (10 ml) for 2 to 3 minutes at least four times daily.[44,149] Clobetasol 0.05%, which is a topical high-potency steroid, has been administered four times daily for 2 to 3 weeks depending on the severity of the ulcerative oral cGVHD to decrease inflammation and oral pain. If local steroids alone are not adequate to control oral disease, then topical cyclosporine[150] or topical tacrolimus may be tried.[44,151,152] Intraoral psoralen plus ultraviolet A irradiation may be appropriate based on the patient's condition.[44,146] Although topical and local therapy for oral cGVHD offers several advantages to systemic therapy, including fewer side effects, there currently exists no evidence that one topical therapy is superior to another. Most trials have been open label with very small numbers of subjects. Oral topical treatments need further evaluation in multicenter randomized clinical trials such as conducted by Elad et al.,[153] who reported that a new mouthwash formulation using effervescent tablets of budesonide (3 mg/10 ml) improved oral cGVHD and reduced pain in all four treatment arms ($n = 18$).

St. John et al.[154] examined the efficacy of topical thalidomide gel 20 mg in patients with oral ulcerative cGVHD through a phase 2, randomized, placebo-controlled, double-blind clinical trial. Results suggested that topical thalidomide gel 20 mg has single-agent activity for oral ulcerative cGVHD. This therapy also decreased cGVHD-related oropharyngeal pain and decreased TNF-α and IL-6 expression levels in oral saliva and oral ulcer exudate. There is an ongoing randomized, double-blind, placebo-controlled pilot study examining the safety and efficacy of a clobetasol oral rinse in 34 subjects with oral cGVHD who are being randomized to clobetasol 0.05% rinse or placebo at the NIH Clinical Center in Bethesda, Maryland.[155]

SYMPTOM MANAGEMENT

Oropharyngeal Pain

Oral mucositis is the principal etiology of most pain experienced during the 3-week post-HSCT time period. This pain is often described as the most unforgettable ordeal of HSCT. Oral mucositis–related oropharyngeal pain is multidimensional. The sensory dimension of this oral pain has been described with general mucosal inflammation and breakdown as ranging from mild discomfort to severe and debilitating pain, requiring opioids for pain management.[55] Immunocompromised patients with cancer who are also HIV-positive develop larger, more painful lesions than those experienced by patients without cancer. Oral pain associated with cGVHD has been described as severe, with symptoms of burning, irritation, dryness, and loss of taste being reported. In contrast to the often long-lasting oral pain with oral cGVHD, oral mucositis–related oral pain with CT is usually of <3 months' duration.

Sucralfate

Sucralfate is an aluminum salt of a sulfated disaccharide that has shown efficacy in the treatment of gastrointestinal ulcerations and has been tested as a mouthwash for the prevention and treatment of oral mucositis. Sucralfate creates a protective barrier at the ulcer site via the formation of an ionic bond to proteins. Study results with sucralfate are conflicting. A phase 3 study conducted by the North Central Cancer Treatment Group compared sucralfate suspension versus placebo for 5-FU–related oral mucositis. Results demonstrated that in the 50 patients who experienced oral mucositis, the sucralfate suspension provided no beneficial reduction in 5-FU–induced oral mucositis severity or duration, and also had considerable additional gastrointestinal toxicity.[156] Additionally, no efficacy was demonstrated for a sucralfate mouthwash for prevention and treatment of 5-FU–induced oral mucositis in a randomized controlled clinical trial with 81 patients with colorectal cancer who received either sucralfate suspension or placebo four times daily during their first cycle of 5-FU and leucovorin.[157]

A prospective, double-blind study compared the effectiveness of sucralfate suspension to a formulation of diphenhydramine hydrochloride syrup plus kaolin-pectin for RT-induced oral mucositis in patients with head and neck cancer. Results showed no statistically significant differences between the two groups. In a study comparing outcomes between 21 patients who received standard oral care and 24 patients who received sucralfate suspension four times daily, the sucralfate group had a significant difference in mucosal edema, oral pain, dysphagia, and weight loss.[158] Conversely, a double-blind, placebo-controlled study with sucralfate in 33 patients who received RT to the head and neck showed no statistically significant differences in oral mucositis.[159] However, the sucralfate group did experience less oral pain and required a later start of topical and systemic analgesics throughout RT.[159] Dodd et al.[160] used a pilot randomized controlled clinical trial to evaluate the efficacy of a micronized sucralfate mouthwash compared with a salt and soda mouthwash in 30 patients who received RT. All patients also used PSMA, which is a systematic oral hygiene program. Results demonstrated no significant difference in efficacy between the two groups.

Gelclair

Gelclair (Sinclair Pharmaceuticals, Surrey, England) is a concentrated, bioadherent gel that has received US Food and Drug Administration approval as a 510(k) medical device indicated for the management of oral mucositis–related pain. Gelclair adheres to the oral surface, creating a protective barrier for irritated tissue and sensitized nociceptors. The safety and efficacy have been evaluated in small clinical trials with mixed results. Innocenti et al.[161] reported a 92% decrease in oral pain from baseline 5 to 7 hours after Gelclair administration in patients with oral mucositis, severe diffuse oral aphthous lesions, and postoral surgery pain. More than half of these patients reported that the maximum effect of Gelclair lasted longer than 3 hours, and 87% of patients reported overall improvements from baseline for pain with swallowing food, liquids, and saliva following 1 week of treatment. DeCordi et al.[96] reported from a clinical study in which Gelclair was administered to patients with oral mucositis three times daily before meals as a 2- to 3-minute swish and spit for 3 to 10 days. Significant improvements were reported for pain, oral mucositis severity, and function. No adverse effects were reported during either trial. Patients reported that the taste, smell, texture, and use of Gelclair were acceptable. Barber et al.[162] conducted a prospective, randomized controlled trial comparing Gelclair versus standard therapy with sucralfate and oxethazaine (Mucaine, Wyeth, Dallas, TX) in patients with RT-induced oral mucositis. This study showed no significant difference between both therapies in terms of general pain. Gelclair can be an important adjuvant to opiate therapy in the management of oral mucositis–related oral pain, with the caveat that more research in the clinical setting is needed.

Anesthetic Cocktails

Anesthetic cocktails, composed of agents such as viscous lidocaine or dyclonine hydrochloride, have been used with some success for oral mucositis–related oral pain for temporary pain relief. These agents may alter taste perception, which may decrease oral intake. Other analgesics and mucosal-coating agents used for pain control include kaolin-pectin, diphenhydramine, Orabase (Colgate-Palmolive Company, New York, NY), and Oratect Gel (MGI Pharma, Woodcliffe Lake, NJ). Hospital-based pharmacies commonly formulate and dispense topical mixtures containing an analgesic, an anti-inflammatory agent, and a coating agent for use as an oral comfort measure for patients during cancer treatment. One large clinical research center uses a topical formulation containing viscous lidocaine 2% (40 ml), diphenhydramine 12.5 mg/5 ml (40 ml), and Maalox (Norvartis, Basel, Switzerland) 10 mg (40 ml) and prescribes its use every 3 to 4 hours as needed.

Doxepin

Doxepin is a tricyclic antidepressant used for many years in the management of patients with chronic benign or malignant pain. Its topical application is prescribed for pruritus and neuropathic pain. Pilot studies on topical doxepin rinse in patients with oral mucositis pain have shown adequate analgesia for up to 4 hours after application.[163,164] Epstein et al.[165] assessed the effectiveness of oral doxepin rinse for oral mucositis–related pain in patients with head and neck cancer in the RT or HSCT setting. Nine patients rinsed with doxepin (5 ml) three to six times per day during a week and returned for a follow-up visit. Oral mucositis was scored using the OMAS and oral pain was assessed using a visual analog scale. There was a statistically significant reduction in visual analog scale scores for 2 hours following doxepin rinse at the initial visit and also over a 1-week period, showing that repeated dosing continues to bring significant pain relief. Further randomized controlled trials are needed to confirm these results.

Opioids

Severe oral mucositis–related oropharyngeal pain may interfere with hydration and nutritional intake and affect QOL. Management of this pain may require use of opioids, often administered at high doses by patient-controlled analgesia pumps. Other routes of administration are oral, transmucosal, transdermal, and parenteral. The efficacy of oral transmucosal fentanyl citrate was compared with morphine sulfate immediate release in a randomized, controlled clinical trial for the treatment of breakthrough cancer pain in 134 adult ambulatory patients with cancer.[166] Study results showed that oral transmucosal fentanyl was more effective than morphine sulfate immediate release in treating breakthrough pain. Darwish et al.[167] conducted a phase 1 open-label study to investigate the absorption profile of fentanyl buccal tablets in patients with or without oral mucositis. Sixteen patients (50% with oral mucositis), received a single 200 mcg dose of fentanyl buccal tablet, which was well tolerated and showed a similar absorption profile within both groups. Transdermal fentanyl has also shown to be an effective, convenient, and well-tolerated treatment in patients with oral mucositis pain in the RT and in the HSCT setting.[168,169]

Topical morphine for mucositis-related pain was evaluated in 26 patients following chemoradiation for head and neck cancer.[169] Patients were randomized to morphine mouthwash (1 ml 2% morphine solution) or magic mouthwash (equal parts of lidocaine, diphenhydramine, and magnesium aluminum hydroxide). Patients in the morphine group demonstrated both significantly shorter duration and lower intensity of oral pain than the magic mouthwash group. Swisher et al.[170] described an oral mucositis pain management algorithm to promote symptom management for patients undergoing HSCT who are transitioning from inpatient to ambulatory care. A key component of this successful program was use of a multidisciplinary team who could respond to the report of oral pain. No standard treatment has been defined for the prevention or treatment of oral mucositis–related pain; thus, it is essential to continue clinical trials testing promising agents such as sublingual methadone, transdermal buprenorphine, and ketamine mouthwash.[171–173]

Xerostomia

Xerostomia is a major negative sequela for patients who receive RT to the head and neck. Xerostomia severity depends on radiation dosage, location, and volume of exposed salivary glands. Significant xerostomia has not been shown with CT alone. The severity of xerostomia can affect oral comfort, fit of prostheses, speech, and swallowing. Many of the enzymes (mucin) found in patients with xerostomia contribute to the growth of caries-producing organisms. Oral hygiene regimens that include the use of water/saline and daily fluoride application with brushing teeth at least three times daily may reduce colonization of oral pathogens.

Treatment guidelines for the management of xerostomia are designed to increase patient comfort.[174] Sialagogues have been investigated as stimulants for the residual salivary parenchyma (pilocarpine, 5- and 10-mg doses), with reported subjective improvement in some patients.[175] Extreme caution with the use of pilocarpine is warranted because of reported side effects of glaucoma and cardiac problems. A randomized, controlled trial tested the efficacy of amifostine in a sample of 315 patients with head and neck cancer.[176] The patients received standard fractionated radiation with or without amifostine, administered at 200 mg/m^2 as a 3-minute intravenous infusion 15 to 30 minutes before each treatment fraction. Patient eligibility criteria required that the radiation field encompassed at least 75% of both parotid glands. The Radiation Therapy Oncology Group Acute and Late Morbidity Score and Criteria was used to rate the severity of xerostomia. The incidence of grade ≥ 2 acute xerostomia (90 days from start of radiotherapy) and late xerostomia (9 to 12 months after radiotherapy) was significantly reduced in patients receiving amifostine. Whole saliva collection 1 year following RT showed in the amifostine group that more patients produced 0.1 g of saliva (72% versus 49%) and that median saliva production was greater (0.26 g versus 0.1 g). Stimulated saliva collections showed no difference between the treatment arms. Supporting these improvements in saliva production were subjects' reports of oral dryness. Artificial saliva has not demonstrated increased oral cavity comfort. Patients have reported subjective improvement in comfort levels through the frequent use of sugarless gum, mints, or candies.

SELECTED REFERENCES

The full reference list can be accessed at lwwhealthlibrary.com/oncology.

1. Raber-Durlacher JE, Elad S, Barasch A. Oral mucositis. *Oral Oncol* 2010; 46:452–456.
3. Cheng KK, Leung SF, Liang RH, et al. Severe oral mucositis associated with cancer therapy: impact on oral functional status and quality of life. *Support Care Cancer* 2009;18:1477–1485.
4. Elting LS, Keefe DM, Sonis ST, et al. Patient-reported measurements of oral mucositis in head and neck cancer patients treated with radiotherapy with or without chemotherapy: demonstration of increased frequency, severity, resistance to palliation, and impact on quality of life. *Cancer* 2008;113: 2704–2713.
5. Barasch A, Peterson DE. Risk factors for ulcerative mucositis in cancer patients: unanswered questions. *Oral Oncol* 2003;39:91–100.
8. Grazziutti ML, Dong L, Miceli MH, et al. Oral mucositis in myeloma patients undergoing melphalan-based autologous stem cell transplantation: incidence, risk factors and a severity predictive model. *Bone Marrow Transplant* 2006;38:501–506.
14. McCann S, Schwenkglenks M, Bacon P, et al. The prospective oral mucositis audit: relationship of severe oral mucositis with clinical and medical resource use outcomes in patients receiving high-dose melphalan or BEAM-conditioning chemotherapy and autologous SCT. *Bone Marrow Transplant* 2009;43:141–147.
16. Shih A, Miaskowski C, Dodd MJ, et al. Mechanisms for radiation-induced oral mucositis and the consequences. *Cancer Nurs* 2003;26:222–229.
18. Elting LS, Cooksley CD, Chambers MS, et al. Risk outcomes, and costs of radiation-induced oral mucositis among patients with head-and-neck malignancies. *Int J Radiat Oncology Biol Phys* 2007;68:1110–1120.
23. Ruggiero SL, Mehrotra B, Rosenberg TJ, et al. Osteonecrosis of the jaws associated with the use of biphosphonates: a review of 63 cases. *J Oral Maxillofac Surg* 2004;62:527–534.
24. Sonis ST. The pathobiology of mucositis. *Nat Rev Cancer* 2004;4:277–284.
27. Logan RM, Gibson RJ, Sonis ST, et al. Nuclear factor-kB (NF-kB) and cyclooxygenase-2 (COX-2) expression in the oral mucosa following cancer CT. *Oral Oncol* 2007;43:395–401.
28. Fall-Dickson JM, Ramsay ES, Castro K, et al. Oral mucositis–related oropharyngeal pain and correlative tumor necrosis factor-a expression in adult oncology patients undergoing hematopoietic stem cell transplantation. *Clin Ther* 2007;29:2547–2561.
29. Avivi I, Avraham S, Koren-Michowitz M, et al. Oral integrity and salivary profile in myeloma patients undergoing high-dose therapy followed by autologous SCT. *Bone Marrow Transplant* 2009;43:801–806.
31. Mays JW, Sarmadi M, Moutsopoulos NM. Oral manifestations of systemic autoimmune and inflammatory diseases: Diagnosis and clinical management. *J Evid Base Dent Pract* 2012;12:265–282.
32. Granitto MH, Fall-Dickson JM, Norton CK, et al. Review of therapies for the treatment of oral chronic graft-versus-host disease. *Clin J Oncol Nurs* 2013;18:76–81.
35. Imanguli MM, Swaim WD, League SC, et al. Increased T-bet+ cytotoxic effectors and type 1 interferon-mediated processes in chronic graft-versus-host disease of the oral mucosa. *Blood* 2009;113:3620–3630.
36. Fall-Dickson JM, Mitchell SA, Marden S, et al. Oral symptom intensity, health-related quality of life, and correlative salivary cytokines in adult survivors of hematopoietic stem cell transplantation with oral chronic graft-versus-host disease. *Biol Blood Marrow Transplant* 2010;16:948–956.
37. Pavletic SZ, Martin P, Lee SJ, et al. Measuring therapeutic response in chronic graft-versus-host-disease: National Institutes of Health Consensus Development Project on Criteria for Clinical Trials in Chronic Graft-versus-Host Disease: IV. Response criteria working group report. *Biol Blood Marrow Transplant* 2006;12:252–266.
38. Meier JK, Wolff D, Pavletic S, et al. Oral chronic graft-versus-host disease: report from the International Consensus Conference on clinical practice in cGVHD. *Clin Oral Investig* 2011;15:127–139.
39. Treister NS, Stevenson K, Kim H, et al. Oral chronic graft-versus-host disease scoring using the NIH Consensus Criteria. *Biol Blood Marrow Transplant* 2010;16:108–114.
40. Bassim CW, Fassil ZH, Mays JW, et al. Validation of the National Institutes of Health chronic GVHD oral mucosal score using component-specific measures. *Bone Marrow Transplant* 2014;49:116–121.
43. Schubert MM, Williams BE, Lloid ME, et al. Clinical assessment scale for the rating of oral mucosal changes associated with bone marrow transplantation. Development of an oral mucositis index. *Cancer* 1992;69:2469–2477.
47. Imanguli MM, Atkinson JC, Mitchell SA, et al. Salivary gland involvement by chronic graft-versus-host disease: prevalence, clinical significance and recommendations for evaluation. *Biol Blood Marrow Transplant* 2010;16:1362–1369.
49. Bassim CW, Ambatipudi KS, Mays JW, et al. Quantitative salivary proteomic differences in oral chronic graft-versus-host disease. *J Clin Immunol* 2012;32:1390–1399.
50. Berger AM, Kilroy, TJ. Oral complications. In: DeVita VT, Hellman S, Rosenberg SA, eds. *Cancer: Principles and Practice of Oncology.* 6th ed. Philadelphia: JB Lippincott; 1997: 2714.
51. Beumer J, Curtis, T, Morris LR. Radiation complications in edentulous patients. *J Prosthet Dent* 1976;36:193–203.
59. Sonis ST, Oster G, Fuchs H, et al. Oral mucositis and the clinical and economic outcomes of hematopoietic stem-cell transplantation. *J Clin Oncol* 2001;19:2201–2205.
62. Zlotolow IM, Berger AM. Oral manifestations of cancer therapy. In: Berger AM, Portnoy RK, Weissman DE, eds. *Principles and Practice of Palliative Care and Supportive Oncology.* Philadelphia: Lippincott Williams & Wilkins; 2002: 282.
66. Wadleigh RG, Redman RS, Graham MI, et al. Vitamin E in the treatment of chemotherapy-induced mucositis. *Am J Med* 1992;92:481–484.
69. Sangthawan D, Phungrassami T, Sinkitjarurnchai W. A randomized double-blind, placebo-controlled trial of zinc sulfate supplementation for alleviation of radiation-induced oral mucositis and pharyngitis in head and neck cancer patients. *J Med Assoc Thai* 2013;96:69–76.
72. Sasse AD, Clark LG, Sasse EC, et al. Amifostine reduces side effects and improves complete response rate during radiotherapy: results of a meta-analysis. *Int J Radiat Oncol Biol Phys* 2006;64:784–791.
74. Savarese DM, Savy G, Vahdat L, et al. Prevention of chemotherapy and radiation toxicity with glutamine. *Cancer Treat Rev* 2003;29:501–513.
78. Peterson DE, Jones JB, Pettit RG. Randomized, placebo-controlled trial of safaris for prevention and treatment of oral mucositis in breast cancer patients receiving anthracycline-based chemotherapy. *Cancer* 2007;109:322–331.
82. Lalla RV, Gordon GB, Schubert M, et al. A randomized, double-blind, placebo-controlled trial of misoprostol for oral mucositis secondary to high-dose chemotherapy. *Support Care Cancer* 2012;20:1797–1804.
89. Epstein JB, Silverman S, Paggiarino DA, et al. Benzydamine HCl for prophylaxis of radiation-induced oral mucositis: results from a multicenter, randomized, double-blind, placebo-controlled clinical trial. *Cancer* 2001;92:875–885.

92. Hong JP, Lee SW, Song SY, et al. Recombinant human epidermal growth factor treatment of radiation-induced severe oral mucositis in patients with head and neck malignancies. *Eur J Cancer Care* 2009;18:636–641.

96. DeCordi SD, Giorgutti E, Martina S, et al. Gelclair: potentially an efficacious treatment for CT-induced mucositis. *Proceedings from the Italian Antitumor League III Congress of Professional Oncology Nurses.* October 10–12, 2001, Congliano, Italy, (abst).

102. Masucci B, Broman P, Kelly C, et al. Therapeutic efficacy by recombinant human granulocyte/monocyte-colony stimulating factor on mucositis occurring in patients with oral and oropharynx tumors treated with curative radiotherapy: a multicenter open randomized phase III study. *Med Oncol* 2005;22:247–256.

105. Spielberger R, Stiff P, Bensinger W, et al. Palifermin for oral mucositis after intensive therapy for hematologic cancers. *N Engl J Med* 2004;351:2590–2598.

110. Henke M, Alfonsi M, Foa P, et al. Palifermin decreases severe oral mucositis of patients undergoing postoperative radiochemotherapy for head and neck cancer: a randomized, placebo-controlled trial. *J Clin Oncol* 2011;29:2815–2820.

118. Sorensen JB, Skovsgaard T, Bork E, et al. Double-blind, placebo-controlled, randomized study of chlorhexidine prophylaxis for 5-fluorouracil-based chemotherapy-induced oral mucositis with nonblinded randomized comparison to oral cooling (cryotherapy) in gastrointestinal malignancies. *Cancer* 2008;112:1600–1606.

121. Sharma A, Rath GK, Chaudhary SP, et al. Lactobacillus brevis CD2 lozenges reduce radiation- and chemotherapy-induced mucositis in patients with head and neck cancer: a randomized double-blind placebo-controlled study. *Eur J Cancer* 2012;48:875–881.

123. Svanberg A, Ohrn K, Birgegård G. Oral cryotherapy reduces mucositis and improves nutrition—a randomized controlled trial. *J Clin Nurs* 2010;19:2146–2151.

124. Mahoud DJ, Dose AM, Loprinzi CL, et al. Inhibition of fluorouracil-induced stomatitis by oral cryotherapy. *J Clin Oncol* 1991;9:449–452.

132. Bensadoun RJ, Ciais G. Radiation- and chemotherapy-induced mucositis in oncology: results of multicenter phase III studies. *J Oral Laser Appl* 2002;2:115–120.

143. Loo WT, Jin LJ, Chow LW, et al. Rhodiola algida improves chemotherapy-induced oral mucositis in breast cancer patients. *Expert Opin Investig Drugs* 2010;19:S91–S100.

144. Elad S, Luboshitz-Shon N, Cohen T, et al. A randomized controlled trial of visible-light therapy for the prevention of oral mucositis. *Oral Oncol* 2011;47:125–130.

147. Mays JW, Fassil H, Edwards DA, et al. Oral chronic graft-versus-host disease: current pathogenesis, therapy, and research. *Oral Diseases* 2013;9:327–346.

153. Elad S, Zeevi I, Finke ZJ, et al. Improvement in oral chronic graft-versus-host disease with the administration of effervescent tablets of topical budesonide – an open, randomized, multicenter study. *Biol Blood Marrow Transplant* 2012;18:134–140.

154. St. John L, Gordon SM, Childs R, et al. Topical thalidomide gel in oral chronic GVHD, and role of *in situ* cytokine expression in monitoring biological activity. *Bone Marrow Transplantation* 2013;48:610–611.

160. Dodd MJ, Miaskowski C, Greenspan D. Radiation-induced mucositis: a randomized clinical trial of micronized sucralfate versus salt and soda mouthwashes. *Cancer Invest* 2003;21:21–33.

161. Innocenti M, Moscatelli G, Lopez S. Efficacy of Gelclair in reducing pain in palliative care patients with oral lesions. Preliminary findings from an open pilot study. *J Pain Symptom Manage* 2001;24:456–457.

167. Darwish M, Kirby M, Robertson P, et al. Absorption of fentanyl from fentanyl buccal tablet in cancer patients with or without oral mucositis. *Clin Drug Invest* 2007;27:605–611.

170. Swisher ME, Scheidler VR, Kennedy MJ. A mucositis pain management algorithm: a creative strategy to enhance the transition to ambulatory care. *Oncol Nurs Forum* 1998.

176. Brizel DM, Wasserman TH, Strnad V, et al. Final report of a phase III randomized trial of amifostine as a radioprotectant in head and neck cancer. Proceedings of the American Society for Therapeutic Radiology and Oncology 41st Annual Meeting. *Int J Red One Biol Phys* 1999, San Antonio, Texas, Oct. 31–Nov. 4, Texas. (abst).

PRACTICE OF ONCOLOGY

138 Pulmonary Toxicity

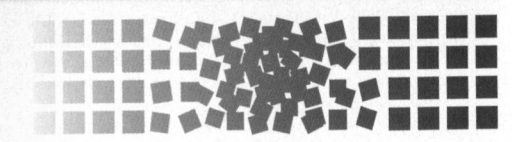

Diane E. Stover, Caroline M. Gulati, Alexander I. Geyer, and Robert J. Kaner

INTRODUCTION

Pulmonary disease can be caused by a wide spectrum of pathogenic mechanisms in patients with cancer. These include a variety of infectious agents and neoplastic disorders as well as pulmonary thromboembolic disease, pulmonary hemorrhage, pulmonary edema (cardiogenic and noncardiogenic), and leukocyte agglutinin reactions. Pulmonary toxicity caused by antineoplastic agents is being recognized more frequently, and the number of drugs known or suspected to cause lung disease is steadily increasing. Because continuing the offending agent may cause death and because withholding the agent may result in resolution of the pulmonary toxicity, it is important to recognize radiation- and drug-induced pulmonary disease. In this chapter, parenchymal lung disease caused by irradiation and chemotherapy is discussed. Mechanisms of lung injury, histopathologic findings, clinical and laboratory features, diagnosis, and treatment of the abnormalities produced by these agents are reviewed.

RADIATION-INDUCED PULMONARY TOXICITY

Mechanisms of Lung Injury and Histology

Radiation can affect dividing and nondividing cells and can cause genetic and nongenetic damage. The first phase of radiation-induced lung injury (RILI) is the production of reactive oxygen species (ROS) and reactive nitrogen species. These species cause oxidative damage to cellular proteins, lipids, and DNA.[1]

Nonlethal ionizing radiation also activates a stress response in cells, which leads to upregulation of specific nuclear transcription factors such as nuclear factor κB and transcription of specific early response genes such as *c-abl, c-jun, egr-1*, and *c-fos*. This leads to sloughing and denudation of type I pneumocytes, which make up 90% of alveolar epithelium, while type II pneumocytes proliferate in an effort to replace dying type I cells. In addition to pneumocyte injury, capillary endothelial cells are also injured, leading to the loss of barrier function. This microvessel damage leads to ongoing tissue hypoxia as well as chronic inflammation.[2]

The second phase of RILI includes inflammation in response to injury. Abnormalities in the intermediate stage (2 to 9 months after radiation) are characterized by obstruction of pulmonary capillaries by platelets, fibrin, and collagen. Alveolar-lining cells (primarily type II pneumocytes) become hyperplastic and the alveolar walls become infiltrated with fibroblasts and mast cells. Inflammatory cells are recruited to the site of radiation injury and perpetuate the inflammatory response. Cellular activation initiates a repair process that involves cytokines and growth factors, such as basic fibroblast growth factor, vascular endothelial growth factor (VEGF), and platelet-derived growth factor, as well as tumor necrosis factor-α, interleukin (IL)-1, IL-6, and transforming growth factor (TGF)-β. Prostaglandin synthesis is also upregulated. This second burst of cytokine release leads to more ROS/reactive nitrogen species damage, tissue hypoxia, and TGF-β1 expression.[2,3]

Impairment of the regulation of the inflammatory response is thought to contribute to late RILI.[1] Although bronchiolitis obliterans with organizing pneumonia (BOOP) is an unusual histopathologic pattern for cancer therapy–related lung injury, radiation damage resulting in BOOP has been reported.[4]

The last stage of RILI is characterized by a process of repair. These cellular changes include capillary regeneration and alveolar epithelium repopulation by type II cells as well as fibrosis, a process that is dominated by TGF-β release. Several cytokines mediate chemoattraction of fibroblasts and recruitment of myofibroblast precursors from the circulation followed by differentiation into myofibroblasts as well as direct epithelial to mesenchymal transition. If the initial injury is severe, damage to extracellular matrix components of the lung, such as basement membrane glycoproteins and proteoglycans, takes place. Due to previous damage from the first phase of RILI, endothelial cells are unable to respond fully to VEGF and continue to die. Hypoxia is thought to be an important component of chronic injury.[5]

If the radiation injury is mild, these changes may subside entirely; however, when the injury is severe, a chronic phase ($\geq$9 months after radiation) ensues that may persist or progress for months or years. The histopathologic appearance is then dominated by dense fibrosis, thickening of the alveolar walls, vascular subintimal fibrosis, and luminal narrowing. In some instances, the lung may shrink to less than half its original size, with a thickened adherent pleura and scarred hilar structures.

Patient Considerations

Certain factors are known to promote the development of classic radiation pneumonitis. These include female sex, lower lobe site of primary lung cancer, concurrent chemotherapy, previous irradiation, and withdrawal of steroids.[6-10] Current tobacco use has been associated with a decreased incidence of injury and relative protection from inflammatory damage.[11] Most of the cases of radiation-related BOOP, however, have occurred in patients receiving radiation treatment to the breast.

Damage to the lung increases as the volume of lung tissue irradiated increases. A threshold effect also appears to occur, such that irradiation of at least 10% of the lung is required to produce significant pulmonary toxicity. This threshold may be reached in the treatment of some patients with breast cancer, depending on the specifics of their individualized treatment program. The toxic effects of radiation as measured by symptoms and signs, radiographic changes, and physiologic tests are proportionate to the total amount delivered to the lung. Radiation pneumonitis seldom occurs with fractionated total doses of <20 Gy but is more likely when doses exceed 60 Gy.

Besides the volume of lung irradiated and the total radiation dose, the number of fractions into which it is divided and, to a lesser extent, the time span over which it is delivered are important factors. The greater the number of fractions in which the radiation is given, the lower is the damaging effect. However, the incidence of radiation pneumonitis exhibits a threshold effect and a steep sigmoidal dose-response curve. Fractionation is different from dose rate, which refers to output of the machine during radiation therapy. Dose rate has an effect on lung tolerance: radiation delivered as 0.05 Gy/min is less damaging than radiation delivered at 0.30 Gy/min. In sum, the incidence and severity of radiation damage to the lungs are related to the volume of lung tissue irradiated, the total dose, the fractions into which the total dose is divided, and the quality of the radiation.

Combined positron emission tomography/computed tomography (CT) imaging offers some advantages in designing the radiation port and in detecting metastases not evident on CT, thus changing the intent of the radiotherapy from curative to palliative.[12,13] Other newer technologies have allowed for refined and localized radiation therapy for the curative treatment of early stage medically inoperable lung cancer and palliation of small pulmonary metastases including minimally invasive image-guided delivery of thermal energies, specifically radiofrequency ablation, microwave ablation, cryoablation, and more conformal stereotactic body radiation therapy (SBRT). These techniques are performed percutaneously under CT guidance and can be done under conscious sedation with a short hospital stay (in the case of radiofrequency ablation) or as an awake outpatient procedure (as in SBRT). Radiofrequency ablation involves the emission of high-frequency alternating currents that cause ion agitation in the surrounding tissue and induce heat production. This heat then causes intracellular protein denaturation, melting of lipid bilayers, and necrosis of nearby tumor cells.[14,15] Some studies have suggested that local control with this modality is comparable to surgery with minimal morbidity; however, pneumothorax has been described.[16,17]

Clinical Features

Signs and Symptoms

The clinical syndrome of radiation pneumonitis develops in 5% to 15% of patients receiving high-dose external beam radiation for treatment of lung cancer. No significant difference is seen in the incidence of radiation pneumonitis between the young and elderly, but the pneumonitis is inclined to be more severe in the latter. Underlying chronic obstructive pulmonary disease does not appear to potentiate radiation damage.

Symptoms of acute radiation pneumonitis usually become evident 2 to 3 months after the completion of therapy; rarely, they occur within the first month and occasionally as late as 6 months after irradiation.[18] Early onset of symptoms often implies a more serious and more protracted clinical course. The cardinal symptom of radiation pneumonitis is dyspnea. It may be self-limited or may progress to severe respiratory distress. Patients may also have a nonproductive cough or a cough productive of small amounts of pinkish sputum. Frank hemoptysis early in the clinical course is distinctly uncommon; massive hemoptysis has been reported as a late complication of pulmonary irradiation. Fever is unusual but can be high and spiking; in severe cases, other constitutional symptoms may occur. Chest pain, which is rarely a prominent feature, may be due to fractured ribs, pleural changes, or coughing. Symptoms of airway obstruction can occur in the first few days of radiation therapy and are usually associated with swelling of a central bronchogenic carcinoma. Severe respiratory distress can result and may be prevented by the administration of steroids the day before and several days after the initiation of radiation therapy. Hemoptysis and other manifestations of radiation pneumonitis may also occur in patients given palliative endobronchial brachytherapy or after surgical implantation of radioactive seeds. Whereas dyspnea is the hallmark of radiation-induced pneumonitis, fever and cough are the predominant features of radiation-related BOOP.

On physical examination, signs of pulmonary involvement are minimal. Occasionally, rales, a pleural friction rub, or evidence of

pleural fluid may be heard over the area of irradiation. In severe cases, tachypnea and cyanosis may be present, and occasionally evidence of acute cor pulmonale appears, usually predicting a fatal outcome. Finger clubbing due to radiation is distinctly unusual and is most likely caused by the underlying malignancy. Skin changes corresponding to the ports of irradiation are often present but provide no clue as to the presence or severity of the pulmonary reaction beneath.

Although patients with acute pneumonitis may show complete resolution of signs and symptoms, most develop gradual progressive fibrosis. In some cases, patients present with radiation fibrosis without a previous history of acute pneumonitis. The permanent changes of fibrosis take 6 to 24 months to evolve but usually remain stable after 2 years. Patients with fibrosis can be asymptomatic or can have varying degrees of dyspnea. The major complications of radiation pneumonitis occur late in the disease and are secondary to persistent fibrosis of a large volume of lung. These include cor pulmonale and respiratory failure.

Diagnostic Imaging

Although radiographic abnormalities are found at the time clinical radiation pneumonitis is present, these changes may be seen in asymptomatic patients as well. Early radiographic changes include a ground glass opacification (GGO), diffuse haziness, or indistinctness of the normal pulmonary markings over the irradiated area. Later, the chest radiograph may show alveolar infiltrates or dense consolidation with or without air bronchograms. As the pneumonitis progresses to fibrosis, the radiographic appearance changes to that of linear streaks radiating from the area of pneumonitis and of contraction toward the hilar, the perimediastinal, or the apical areas. Pleural effusions, if present, are usually small and always coincident with the pneumonitis. They can persist for long periods but often disappear spontaneously and never increase during a period of stability unless secondary complications occur such as radiation-induced pericarditis. Mediastinal or hilar adenopathy and cavitation are almost always due to causes other than radiation pneumonitis. Pneumothorax is occasionally associated with radiation fibrosis but not with acute pneumonitis.

One of the most characteristic features of radiation pneumonitis and fibrosis is that the radiologic changes are confined to the outlines of the field of radiation. In a few cases, extensive changes outside the field, even in the contralateral lung, have been observed. This syndrome, which occurs in a minority of patients, is characterized by a bilateral lymphocytic alveolitis of activated CD4+ T-lymphocytes 4 to 6 weeks after strictly unilateral lung irradiation. Other explanations for this phenomenon include obstruction of lymphatic flow from radiation-induced mediastinal fibrosis and absorption of X-rays by regions outside the irradiated ports. BOOP, which is most commonly seen in patients with breast cancer after radiation to the chest wall, can begin in areas of the lung contiguous with the irradiated soft tissues but progresses outside the portal in approximately 40% of cases and may include the lung contralateral to the irradiated breast.

SBRT changes can differ from those of standard radiation therapy; however, lung toxicity is rare due to the small fields. Several different patterns of early (acute pneumonitis) and late changes (fibrosis) have been described including GGOs, consolidations, and patchy or diffuse patterns, as well as late bronchiectasis and scar formation.[19] Due to the hypofractionated dose of radiation used in stereotactic radiotherapy and the delivery of radiation in a spherical volume with a gradient between the high dose and the low dose within normal adjacent tissue, the shape of the SBRT-induced injury mimics the tumor and does not have a linear pattern that may be seen with conventional radiation therapy. Similar to conventional therapy, late fibrosis may develop after 6 to 9 months without a preceding acute pneumonitis.

PRACTICE OF ONCOLOGY

Pulmonary Function Tests

Prediction of changes in pulmonary function after high-dose irradiation to the lung has proven to be problematic.[20,21] No gross physiologic changes occur in the lung until 4 to 8 weeks after completion of irradiation, usually coincident with the period of clinical pneumonitis. Then, there is a decrease in lung volumes, which can progress. These changes persist indefinitely, with little evidence of recovery. Small changes in spirometric values and gas exchange abnormalities, which include a decrease in diffusing capacity and arterial hypoxemia, especially with exercise, occur at approximately the same time but show some tendency toward recovery after 6 to 12 months.[22] A fall in compliance coincident with the clinical pneumonitis is seen in most subjects. Accordingly, the elastic work of breathing is increased, and dyspnea, resulting from the increased workload, ensues. Air-flow parameters remain close to normal in most studies.[23]

Diagnosis

The diagnosis of radiation pneumonitis can sometimes be made clinically based on the timing of irradiation in relation to symptoms and the typical chest radiographic appearance (i.e., infiltrates corresponding to the margins of the irradiated portal).[20] Differentiation from recurrent malignancy or infection often poses a problem, in which case lung biopsy is necessary. Although histopathologic changes are nonspecific for radiation pneumonitis, when elements of the acute stages (fibrin exudate in the alveoli) are seen adjacent to the more chronic stages (alveolar fibrosis and subintimal sclerosis), this entity can be diagnosed with reasonable certainty.

Several biomarkers have been investigated in order to predict those who may go on to develop RILI. TGF-β has shown mixed results as a potential marker but may predict those at low risk.[24–26] IL-1, -6, -8, and -10 have been evaluated to predict progression of RILI as has surfactant A and D, cytokeratin 19, and thrombomodulin. KL-6, a glycoprotein that is expressed on type II pneumocytes and bronchiolar epithelial cells, was evaluated in 16 patients whom underwent radiation therapy with or without concurrent chemotherapy. Higher levels of KL-6 were associated with more severe RILI that was unresponsive to steroid treatment and lower levels corresponded to RILI in the radiation field alone.[27–29] CD-36, a protein required for TGF-β activation, has been examined and shown to increase with onset of radiation-induced pneumonitis.[30] Other proteins such as TGF-β1 have also been evaluated for their potential role in identifying those who might be susceptible to radiation pneumonitis but have failed to show strong enough predictive values.[27] Currently, research is focusing on patient genotypes that may hold promise in identifying patients in whom radiation pneumonitis is most likely. In particular, single nucleotide polymorphisms for genes encoding DNA repair and response genes have been evaluated and suggest certain single nucleotide polymorphisms are associated with increased risk of severe RILI.[31,32] The TGF-β Leu10Pro and 509CT polymorphisms have also been associated with late RILI in breast cancer.[33]

Treatment

Corticosteroid administration during irradiation in mice markedly improves the physiologic abnormalities and decreases mortality without an effect on late pulmonary fibrosis. No controlled clinical trials in humans are available on the efficacy of steroid therapy in radiation pneumonitis.[34] Nonetheless, clinicians often begin prednisone 1 mg/kg as soon as the diagnosis is reasonably certain. The initial dose is maintained for several weeks and then reduced cautiously and slowly. If steroids are tapered too rapidly, symptoms can be exacerbated, necessitating higher doses for longer periods. Similarly, if corticosteroids are part of a recent chemotherapeutic regimen, stopping them abruptly can precipitate clinically evident radiation pneumonitis. What parameters, if any, to follow during the tapering schedule are not known, and no studies are available. Generally, physicians follow symptoms. Most clinicians agree that corticosteroids have no place in the treatment of radiation fibrosis.

Free radical scavenging agents have also been investigated. Amifostine, a thiophosphate, and captopril, which has a thiol group as well, have been investigated but failed to come to fruition.[35,36] Inhibition of endothelial cell apoptosis by therapeutic administration of basic fibroblast growth factor or VEGF has been beneficial in some animal models, but no human trials have been attempted. Many experimental therapies are being investigated in mouse models including the use of nitric oxide, superoxide dismutase, statins, matrix metalloproteinase inhibitors, growth factors, and other antioxidants.[37] None have as yet been demonstrated to have efficacy in humans.

CHEMOTHERAPY-INDUCED PULMONARY TOXICITY

The list of chemotherapeutic agents reported to cause cytotoxic drug-induced lung disease continues to grow. The true incidence of toxicity is unknown, but the reported frequency of pulmonary toxicity ranges from 10% to 30%. True toxicity must be distinguished from other factors that affect the lung in patients with cancer including cardiac-induced pulmonary edema, infection, lymphangitic carcinomatosis, and diffuse alveolar hemorrhage. With the development of targeted monoclonal antibodies used in cancer treatment, new toxicities are continuously being reported. Classes of drugs added to the list include tyrosine kinase inhibitors, anti-VEGF agents (such as bevacizumab), rituximab, granulocyte–colony-stimulating factor (G-CSF), and the mammalian target of rapamycin inhibitors (Table 138.1).[38–98] There are also reports of lung injury with trastuzumab, ifosfamide, irinotecan/topotecan, oxaliplatin, and temozolomide.[34,99–104] A summary of the mechanisms of lung damage; the pathologic findings; common clinical, radiographic, and physiologic features; and the diagnosis and treatment of the more common chemotherapeutic drugs that cause pulmonary toxicity are discussed in this section (see Table 138.1).

Mechanisms of Pulmonary Injury and Histology

Except for a few chemotherapeutic agents (e.g., bleomycin), the details of the pathophysiology of lung injury are unknown. Various mechanisms of pulmonary toxicity have been proposed based on the mechanisms of action of different classes of therapeutic agents. These include a direct toxic effect on alveolar epithelial cells, the induction of an inflammatory immunologic response and endothelial cell injury, or activation causing capillary leak syndrome. These events can result in a variety of clinical presentations including nonspecific interstitial pneumonitis, hypersensitivity reaction syndrome, noncardiogenic pulmonary edema, infusion reaction, capillary leak syndrome, eosinophilic pneumonia, bronchospasm, acute lung injury, diffuse alveolar damage, or fibrosis.

The histopathologic changes of drug-induced pulmonary toxicity show common features. Similar to radiation-induced damage, abnormalities are seen in endothelial and epithelial cells. The vascular damage is characterized by endothelial swelling with exudation of fluid into the interstitium and the intra-alveolar spaces. Destruction and desquamation of type I pneumocytes occurs with delamellation and proliferation of type II pneumocytes. Mononuclear cell infiltration and fibroblast proliferation with fibrosis are common findings; the character of the inflammatory cellular infiltrate may be a feature that distinguishes the toxicity of one drug from another.

TABLE 138.1

Characteristics of Pulmonary Toxicity Caused by Commonly Used Chemotherapeutic Agents

Drug (Reference)	Mechanism of Injury and Histopathology	Clinical Presentation	Imaging and Diagnosis	Treatment and Prognosis
Alkylating Agents				
Busulfan[38,39]	Direct alveolar epithelial toxicity. Pneumocyte hyperplasia, mononuclear cells, fibrosis.	4% incidence; rare <500 mg dose; XRT enhance toxicity. Onset 8 mo to 10 y. SOB, cough, weight loss, weakness, fever.	Most common bibasilar reticular pattern. Rarely pleural effusion, pulmonary ossification. Definitive dx by SLB.	Withdrawal of drug. Anecdotal reports of response to high-dose steroids. Mean survival 5 mo after dx.
Cyclophosphamide[38,40]	Reactive oxygen species. Endothelial swelling, pneumocyte dysplasia, mononuclear cells, fibrosis.	<1% incidence; no dose dependence. Synergy with O2 and other agents. Acute sx early; subacute up to 8 y.	Commonly bibasilar reticular pattern. Rarely pulmonary edema. Diagnosis of exclusion. May require surgical bx.	Withdrawal of drug. Steroids may hasten improvement. Recovery approximately 65%.
Chlorambucil[41–43]	Unknown mechanism. Histology similar to busulfan. Interstitial pneumonitis, fibrosis.	Rare reports; subacute onset (5 mo to 10 y). Cough, dyspnea, anorexia, bibasilar rales.	Bibasilar reticular pattern. Rarely normal radiograph. Alveolar infiltrates not reported.	Half of reported patients died despite stopping drug and using steroids.
Melphalan[41,44]	Unknown mechanism. Histology similar to busulfan. Pneumocyte dysplasia > fibrosis.	Rare; onset 1 to 48 mo after therapy. Progressive dyspnea.	Reticular and alveolar infiltrates. May require TBBX/SLB.	Despite cessation of drug, three-fifths of reported patients died. Most were already on steroid for tumor Rx.
Antibiotics				
Bleomycin[41,45–60]	Direct endo-/epithelial toxicity via O2 free radicals. TNF-α, inflammation. TGF-β, fibrosis. Endothelial blebbing, interstitial edema, type I cell necrosis, metaplastic type II cell, neutrophilic infiltration; fibroblast proliferation and fibrosis; rare eosinophilic infiltration; rare BOOP.	Incidence up to 10%. Risk factors: older age, higher dose, renal dysfunction, O2 therapy, thoracic irradiation. Occurs during and up to 6 mo after stopping therapy. Cough dyspnea, fever, tachycardia, crepitant rales. Hypersensitivity pneumonitis variant may occur.	Bibasilar reticular pattern; multiple nodules similar to metastases; acinar pattern, especially with hypersensitivity. Rarely localized infiltrates and cavitary nodules. BALF with neutrophilic alveolitis. TBBX or open lung biopsy may be required to rule out other cause.	Drug withdrawal. Excellent response to steroids in hypersensitivity, but less clear efficacy otherwise. Reported mortality between 3% and 50%.
Mitomycin[41,61,62]	Endothelial injury; alveolar macrophage activation, cytokine release. Several patterns: capillary leak and DAD especially with vinca alkaloids; thrombotic microangiopathy; fibrosis.	3%–14% incidence; usually not dose-related. Possible synergy with O2, XRT and other agents, especially vinca. Dry cough, dyspnea. Fever not seen. Bibasilar rales.	Diffuse interstitial and/or alveolar infiltrates. May have normal CXR. Clinical picture is suggestive; lung biopsy may be required to rule out other causes.	Drug withdrawal. Steroids. Mortality 14%–50%.
Nitrosoureas (e.g., carmustine)[41]	Direct injury through oxidative stress; possible involvement of depletion of the antioxidant glutathione. Histology similar to bleomycin. Fibrosis predominates.	20%–30% incidence; dose-related. Increased risk with preexisting lung disease, tobacco use; synergism with other agents. Reported up to 17 y after drug.	Bibasilar reticular pattern. Lung biopsy may be needed. No BALF studies reported.	Recognition and drug withdrawal. Questionably benefit of steroids. Reported mortality 24%–90%. Worst prognosis in patient <5 y of age.
Antimetabolites				
Methotrexate[41,63,64]	Hypersensitivity suggested by T-lymphocytes and eosinophils in BALF. Interstitial and alveolar infiltration with lymphocytes, eosinophils, plasma cells. Occasionally poorly formed granuloma.	2%–8% incidence. Days to weeks after start therapy. Acute: Fever, cough, malaise, headache. Subacute: Dyspnea, cough. Rales on exam. Skin rash in 17%. Blood eosinophilia in 40%. Progression to fibrosis in 10%.	Early: Interstitial infiltrates. Later: Alveolar infiltrates. Hilar and mediastinal adenopathy. Pleural effusions. CXR can be normal. BALF suggestive if T-cell predominance, but biopsy may be required.	Drug withdrawal. Reports of reinstitution without recurrence of abnormalities. Dramatic response to steroids reported. Mortality 1%. Favorable outlook.

(continued)

PRACTICE OF ONCOLOGY

TABLE 138.1

Characteristics of Pulmonary Toxicity Caused by Commonly Used Chemotherapeutic Agents *(continued)*

Drug (Reference)	Mechanism of Injury and Histopathology	Clinical Presentation	Imaging and Diagnosis	Treatment and Prognosis
Cytokine arabinoside[65]	Pulmonary edema; proteinaceous exudate, extravasation of RBCs; no inflammatory cells.	Abrupt onset of dyspnea; coexistent gastrointestinal toxicity.	Diffuse interstitial and alveolar infiltrates. Clinical picture suggests diagnosis.	Supportive therapy. No studies.
Gemcitabine[66–68]	Reports of DAD.	Dyspnea may be severe and progress to respiratory failure and ARDS. Low-grade fever.	Reticular nodular infiltrates or ground glass opacities. Exclude other causes.	Drug withdrawal. Usually, brisk response to steroids, but fatalities have been reported.
Fludarabine[69]	Unknown mechanism. Rare reports of granulomatous or diffuse nonspecific inflammation.	Hypoxemia, fever, CD4 lymphopenia.	Interstitial or nodular infiltrates. Associated with pneumocystis, so must rule out infection.	Drug withdrawal. Probably response to steroids.
Taxanes				
Paclitaxel/ docetaxel[70–73]	(1) AR: Mast cell activation, histamine release. Caused by suspension in Cremophor (BASF Inc., Florham Park, NJ). (2) HP: BALF with lymphocytes, biopsy with mononuclear cells and septal thickening. May also present with DAD or fibrotic NSIP.	AR: up to 5% incidence. Erythematous rash, urticaria, hypotension, bronchospasm during or soon after the infusion. HP: dyspnea and/or cough several days to weeks after treatment. Fever may occur. Crepitant rales or normal chest exam.	AR: normal CXR; highly suggestive clinical picture HP: patchy reticular, nodular, or diffuse alveolar infiltrates. Rule out infection or progression of disease. Bronchoscopy and biopsy may be necessary.	AR: slow infusion; pretreatment with steroids, H1/2 blockers reduces incidence to <2%. HP: Can resolve on its own; If severe, steroids. May not recur with rechallenge.
Tyrosine Kinase Inhibitors				
EGFR inhibitors: Gefitinib, erlotinib[42,74–79]	Augmentation of inflammation, alteration of repair capability, potentiation of damage by other chemo agents. DAD, NSIP, BOOP, DAH, fibrosis.	<1% incidence in Caucasians; 2%–6% in Asians. Usually in first month of Rx. Pulmonary fibrosis is a risk factor. Dyspnea with/without cough and fever.	GGO with/without airspace consolidation. Diagnosis of exclusion. Rule out progression of disease or infection.	Discontinue the drug; steroids; small series report high mortality rates.
Kit/BCR-ABL inhibitors: Imatinib/dasatinib[80–83]	Hypersensitivity suggested by lymphocytic exudate with high CD4/CD8 in plural fluid. Eosinophilic infiltration; interstitial inflammation/fibrosis.	Low-grade fever; dry cough; dyspnea with/without hypoxemia	Pleural effusions; GGO; nodular opacities, consolidation. Clinical picture suggestive, especially if with exudative lymphocytic pleural effusion.	Discontinuation of the drug; may need repeated steroids; may need repeated thoracentesis.
Myeloma Therapies				
Bortezomib[84]	BOOP, DAD, and DAH have been reported.	Rare. ARDS reported only in Asians and African Americans. Rapid onset of dyspnea, hypoxemia, respiratory failure.	Bilateral infiltrates, GGOs, effusions.	May occur even with pretreatment with steroids. Variable response to treatment with high-dose steroids. High mortality.
Thalidomide, lenalidomide, pomalidomide[85]	Antiangiogenic properties may predispose to PE. BOOP, cellular NSIP, HP, and eosinophilic pneumonia have rarely been reported.	8%–12% incidence of PE. ILD very rare; presentation acute or subacute. Increased risk of opportunistic infections especially with dexamethasone.	Pulmonary embolism on CTA. Diffuse bilateral air space and interstitial infiltrates; must rule out infection, especially PJP, if on concurrent steroids.	DVT prophylaxis recommended with thalidomide (black box warning).

Mammalian Target of Rapamycin Inhibitors

Sirolimus, temsirolimus, everolimus[86–91]	May possibly bind to plasma proteins and evoke TH1 response. BOOP.	0.5%–5% incidence. Dyspnea, fatigue, fever. Risk factors include late switch to the drug.	Focal consolidation, GGO. May be waxing and waning.	Stop drug if symptomatic. No data on effectiveness of steroids, but recommended with severe or progressive disease.

Monoclonal Antibodies

VEGF inhibitors: Bevacizumab[92–94]	Effects on vascular integrity and regeneration; procoagulant effects. Pulmonary hemorrhage and venous thromboembolism.	Risk of hemoptysis highest in patients with lung cancer, especially squamous cell carcinoma.	GGO and air space opacification, tumor cavitation, pulmonary embolism.	Withdrawal of the drug. Anticoagulation for PE. Role for steroids, aminocaproic acid, factor VIIa in pulmonary hemorrhage is unknown.
EGFR inhibitors: Trastuzumab[95]	Neutrophilic alveolitis, eosinophilic pneumonia, and organizing pneumonia have been described.	Sx range from exertional dyspnea to rapidly progressive respiratory failure.	Interstitial and alveolar opacities or consolidations can be seen. Diagnosis of exclusion.	Resolution with discontinuation of the drug described. Steroids may speed improvement.

Immunotherapeutic Agents

Ipilimumab[96,97]	Presumably through activation of cytotoxic T cells via inhibition of CTLA4. Sarcoid-like granulomata. BOOP.	May be asymptomatic or present with cough, dyspnea.	Micronodular pattern on CT, hilar and mediastinal LAD; peripheral air space consolidations. Biopsy to rule out POD or infection.	Withdrawal of the drug. Steroids are usually not needed, but highly effective in symptomatic disease.
Nivolumab[98]	Mechanism unknown, but presumably through activation of T-lymphocytes. BOOP.	Reports of pneumonitis. Dyspnea, cough, hypoxemia.	Migratory infiltrates: GGO and consolidations; interstitial opacities. Biopsy to rule out malignancy or infection.	Stop drug and start steroids. Additional infliximab, cyclophosphamide have been used.

XRT, radiation therapy; SOB, shortness of breath; dx, diagnosis; SLB, surgical lung biopsy; O2, oxygen; sx, symptom; bx, biopsy; TBBX, transbronchial biopsy; Rx, treatment; TNF, tumor necrosis factor; TGF, transforming growth factor; BOOP, bronchiolitis obliterans with organizing pneumonia; BALF, bronchoalveolar lavage fluid; DAD, diffuse alveolar damage; XRT, radiation therapy; CXR, chest X-ray; RBC, red blood cell; ARDS, acute respiratory distress syndrome; AR, anaphylactoid reaction; HP, hypersensitivity pneumonitis; NSIP, nonspecific interstitial pneumonitis; EGFR, epidermal growth factor receptor; DAH, diffuse alveolar hemorrhage; GGO, ground glass opacity; PE, pulmonary embolism; ILD, interstitial lung disease; CTA, computed tomography angiography; PJP, *Pneumocystis jirovecci* pneumonia; DVT, deep vein thrombosis; VEGF, vascular endothelial growth factor; CTLA4, cytotoxic T-lymphocyte antigen 4; CT, computed tomography; LAD, lymphadenopathy; POD, progression of disease.

PRACTICE OF ONCOLOGY

Pathways involved in chemotherapy-induced lung disease include apoptosis, impaired repair response, and angiogenesis. Apoptosis pathways include the death receptor pathway and the Fas ligand as well as the mitochondrial pathway and Bcl-2 protein. Both of these lead to activation of caspases, which activate degradative enzymes within the cell. Cells affected can be immune cells, endothelial cells, or epithelial and other parenchymal cells. Impaired pathways involving epidermal growth factor and TGF may contribute to alterations in repair mechanisms; both factors are expressed in type II pneumocytes and epithelial cells.

The older chemotherapy agents are the best described in their mechanism of lung injury. It is thought that a major contributor to the toxicity from these agents results from ROS including superoxide anions, hydrogen peroxide, and hydroxyl radicals, primarily from activated neutrophils.[105] Bleomycin induces reactive oxygen radicals by forming a complex with Fe^{3+}. Consistent with a direct pathologic role for this mechanism, iron chelators ameliorate the pulmonary toxicity of bleomycin in animal models.[45] ROS formed after bleomycin therapy can produce direct toxicity through participation in oxidation-reduction reactions and subsequent fatty acid oxidation, which leads to membrane instability.[46] Oxidants also cause other inflammatory reactions within the lung. For example, the oxidation of arachidonic acid is an initial step in the metabolic cascade that produces active mediators, including prostaglandins and leukotrienes.[47] Because ROS are so highly tied to bleomycin toxicity, high-dose oxygen can exacerbate its effects, and toxicity can be seen years after its administration.[48,49] In addition to ROS direct toxicity, cytokines such as IL-1, macrophage inflammatory protein-1, monocyte chemoattractant protein-1, and TGF-β are released from alveolar macrophages in animal models of bleomycin toxicity resulting in fibrosis.[50,51,105] Through modulation of fibroblast proliferation, bleomycin can cause excessive interstitial and intra-alveolar collagen deposition leading to pulmonary fibrosis.[51] Bleomycin directly upregulates collagen synthesis in fibroblasts by stimulating transcription. There is some evidence to support a role for a mast cell/fibroblast interaction in the generation of this fibrosis as well.[53]

One of the potential determinants of bleomycin toxicity is the bleomycin hydrolase, which is the major enzyme responsible for metabolizing bleomycin to a nontoxic molecule.[54] Interestingly, the two organs that are the most common targets for bleomycin toxicity (lung and skin) have the lowest levels of the enzyme. Studies are needed to determine if genetic variability of this enzyme accounts for individual susceptibility or immunity to bleomycin pulmonary toxicity in humans, as it does in animals.[55–57] Likewise, with linkage and association studies, genetic susceptibility to bleomycin-induced pulmonary fibrosis has been investigated in mice. Polymorphisms in *Cep55*, a gene encoding proteins involved in autophagy, and *Masp2*, a gene encoding complement pathway proteins, as well as several others, have been identified as potentially increasing toxicity susceptibility.[58,59] However, these associations have not been replicated in other studies and are currently not being used clinically.[60]

Because the lung is exposed to many substances that can activate its immune system, there appears to be a pulmonary immune tolerance state to avoid overreactions. This tolerance state in part may be a result of an effector and suppressor cell balance. Cytotoxic drugs can alter the normal balance, which may cause tissue damage.[41] For example, lymphocytic alveolitis is a consistent finding in methotrexate pneumonitis, with an imbalance of the CD4-to-CD8 ratio.[106] Bronchoalveolar lavage studies in patients with methotrexate pulmonary toxicity have shown the presence of a T-lymphocytic alveolitis, whereas studies on some patients with bleomycin toxicity have revealed a polymorphonuclear alveolitis.[106–107] G-CSF is also implicated in pulmonary toxicity through its effects on neutrophil activation. G-CSF toxicity is thought to be secondary to activation of inflammatory pathways and ROS within the neutrophils, causing pulmonary edema and acute respiratory distress syndrome.[108]

IL-2, used to treat metastatic melanoma and renal cell cancer, stimulates the immune system by stimulating CD4+ T cells and increasing natural killer cell activity. These effects likely contribute to a generalized inflammatory state, contributing to the capillary leak syndrome and noncardiogenic pulmonary edema associated with this drug. IL-2 has been shown to directly increase endothelial permeability and indirectly increases vascular leak by increasing cytokine levels, particularly tumor necrosis factor (TNF)-α, leukocyte adhesion, and inflammation, and altering the extracellular matrix.[109]

Tyrosine kinase inhibitors, although generally well tolerated, can show serious pulmonary toxicity. Epidermal growth factor receptor (EGFR) is a target of these newer molecular-targeted chemotherapies including gefitinib and erlotinib. Inhibition of the EGFR pathway can exacerbate damage from other chemotherapy agents or sepsis by altering the repair capability of cells. It has been shown that inhibition of the EGFR pathway can upregulate genes that promote prolonged inflammation.[110] Angiogenesis, which involves VEGF, TNF-α, TGF-β, and platelet-derived growth factor, also are targets of tyrosine kinase inhibitors, and impaired function of these factors likely also contribute to pulmonary toxicity. Inhibition of the platelet-derived growth factor pathway, seen with dasatanib, is thought to contribute to the pathogenesis of pleural effusions, which is seen in up to 54% of patients treated with this agent. Interestingly, pulmonary hypertension can also be seen with this agent, although the mechanism is unclear. Other Abelson gene inhibitors do not show this effect.[111] Dasatinib, axitinib, crizotinib, pazopanib, and sunitinib have been reported to cause pulmonary embolism.[112]

Mammalian target of rapamycin inhibitors, such as everolimus and sirolimus, which inhibit cell proliferation, growth, and angiogenesis by inhibiting phosphatidylinositol kinases, specifically mTORC1, also are thought to cause a pneumonitis by a T-cell–mediated delayed-type hypersensitivity.[87] In bronchoalveolar lavage (BAL) fluid of patients with pneumonitis from sirolimus, a CD4+ T-cell lymphocytosis is found. Re-exposure to sirolimus may result in antigen presentation and the activation of Th1-cells and recruitment of macrophages and production of proinflammatory cytokines.[87,113]

Bortezomib, thalodimide, and lenolinomide are all used to treat multiple myeloma. Bortezomib, a proteosome inhibitor, has been associated with parenchymal changes, organizing pneumonia, and pleural effusions; thalodimide, which downregulates TNF-α and has antiangiogenic properties, is associated with pulmonary embolism, organizing pneumonia, and pneumonitis.[114,115] The mechanism of pulmonary toxicity associated with bortezomib and thalidomide is unclear.

Bevacizumab and other anti-VEGF therapies can cause epistaxis. Pulmonary hemorrhage and pulmonary embolism have been reported. The mechanism of hemorrhage and thrombosis likely reflects the multiple actions of VEGF on vasculature and on the coagulation system. Inhibition of VEGF reduces regeneration of endothelial cells and can cause defects that expose procoagulant phospholipids on the luminal plasma membrane or underlying matrix, leading to thrombosis or hemorrhage.[116] VEGF also increases production of nitric oxide and prostacyclin (prostaglandin I_2); suppresses pathways involved in endothelial cell activation, apoptosis, and procoagulant changes; and inhibits proliferation of vascular smooth muscle cells.[117] Reduction in nitric oxide and prostaglandin I_2 by anti-VEGF agents may predispose to thromboembolic events. A few cases of pulmonary arterial hypertension have been reported with bevacizumab.[85]

Clinical Features

Combination chemotherapy, concurrent radiation treatments, oxygen therapy, renal dysfunction, preexisting pulmonary disease such as idiopathic pulmonary fibrosis, chronic obstructive

TABLE 138.2	
Factors Associated with Increased Risk of Drug-Induced Pulmonary Toxicity	
Risk Factors	**Drugs**
Total dose	Bleomycin Carmustine
Advanced age	Bleomycin Carmustine Methotrexate
Oxygen therapy	Bleomycin Cyclophosphamide Mitomycin
Simultaneous or prior radiation therapy to lungs	Bleomycin Busulfan Mitomycin Gemcitabine
Increased toxicity when given with other drugs	Carmustine Mitomycin Cyclophosphamide Bleomycin Methotrexate Etoposide Gemcitabine Docetaxal
Preexisting pulmonary disease	Carmustine
Renal dysfunction	Bleomycin

pulmonary disease, radiation pneumonitis, extensive pulmonary metastases, and poor functional status and advanced age have been associated with increased pulmonary toxicity. Table 138.2 lists some of the drugs that have been associated with these predisposing factors.[41] Because bleomycin toxicity is relatively common, it deserves special mention. Although toxicity drastically increases with doses in excess of 450 to 500 mg, it can occur with much lower doses, especially when other risk factors are present. Renal damage after cisplatin administration, with subsequent accumulation of bleomycin, was a likely cause of pulmonary toxicity and 67% mortality reported early in its use. If possible, bleomycin should precede cisplatin infusion to minimize the risk. Although supplemental oxygen has been a classic cofactor in bleomycin pulmonary toxicity, there are no large controlled studies.[41] An increased risk of pulmonary toxicity (4 of 12 patients, fatal in 3 of 4) was described in a small uncontrolled study of patients receiving G-CSF in combination with bleomycin-containing chemotherapy for non-Hodgkin's lymphoma.[118]

Long intervals between drug administration and onset of clinical toxicity have been described. Late-onset pulmonary fibrosis has been reported many years after cyclophosphamide and carmustine are discontinued.[41]

Signs and Symptoms

The cardinal symptom of drug-induced pulmonary toxicity is dyspnea; however, symptoms can range from nonproductive cough with low-grade fevers to overt respiratory failure. If bronchospasm occurs, shortness of breath is accompanied by wheeze. Fibrosis typically causes basilar crackles, although clubbing is not found. Increased fremitus and decreased breath sounds are signs of pleural effusion. Other characteristics of chemotherapy-induced pulmonary disease are outlined in Table 138.1. These findings can occur immediately following administration of the drug or over a treatment cycle. Fibrosis may take years to develop. Chest pain has been reported during infusion of bleomycin or immediately after therapy with methotrexate; however, it is an unusual manifestation

of toxicity.[41,55] A syndrome of acute dyspnea, probably resulting from direct toxicity to the pulmonary vasculature, can occur during or shortly after vinca alkaloid infusion when given in combination with mitomycin for treatment of nonsmall-cell lung cancer.[61] Because hemoptysis is an uncommon feature of drug-induced pulmonary toxicity unless treated with an anti-VEGF therapy, when it is present, other diagnoses should be considered.

Capillary leak syndrome can lead to a variety of symptoms. These include pulmonary edema that will manifest as tachypnea, low pulse oximetry readings, or in severe cases which lead to mechanical ventilation, cardiovascular symptoms that include tachycardia and hypotension or shock as well as renal insufficiency and hepatic insufficiency. For IL-2 therapy specifically, weight gain from loss of albumin can be seen after 3 to 4 days of administration of the drug and typically resolve after 2 weeks. However, manifestations can appear later and take longer to resolve as well.

All-trans-retinoic acid treatment of leukemias can induce the retinoic acid syndrome, which consists of fever, dyspnea, weight gain, pulmonary infiltrates, pleural or pericardial effusions, hypotension, renal dysfunction, and leukocytosis.[119] The pulmonary disorder is thought to be mediated by newly differentiated leukemia cells marginating into the pulmonary circulation, increasing capillary permeability and releasing cytokines that induce neutrophil migration into the interstitium. High doses of corticosteroids are the most effective treatment, and steroid prophylaxis has been reported to be useful.

Diagnostic Imaging

The most common radiographic abnormality associated with drug-induced pulmonary toxicity is a reticulonodular or interstitial pattern with thickened septal lines or both, which may be basilar or diffuse. These changes can be seen with many different chemotherapies including antimetabolites, taxanes, and molecular-targeted therapies. Pleural effusions can be seen alone, as with tyrosine kinase inhibitors or thalidomide, or in the setting of heart failure or capillary leak syndrome, which is described with IL-2 therapy, G-CSF, and gemcitabine. Distinguishing capillary leak from heart failure is important as it will affect ongoing therapy and response to steroids. Effusions are also found with treatment from mitomycin, busulfan, methotrexate, and procarbazine toxicity.

EGFR inhibitors are associated with GGOs, which should be distinguished from tumor progression. They can cause dense consolidation with associated GGOs within 1 week to 1 month after initiation of therapy. Other CT patterns include patchy GGOs with interlobular septal thickening, or extensive bilateral GGOs with consolidation and traction bronchiectasis. The latter pattern carries the highest mortality rate.

Bleomycin pulmonary toxicity can have several patterns on chest CT, notably interstitial pneumonitis, cryptogenic organizing pneumonia, or fibrosis. Cavitating and noncavitating nodules, simulating metastatic disease, have been seen with bleomycin toxicity as well.[41]

Methotrexate toxicity often presents with bilateral interstitial and alveolar infiltrates along with pleural effusions. Hilar adenopathy is distinctly unusual in chemotherapy toxicity but has been reported with methotrexate toxicity.[41] These changes can be seen with fever and eosinophilia and will usually not progress to fibrosis if the medication is stopped. These findings typically occur within the first year of therapy.

In some instances, the chest radiograph is normal, even in the presence of histologically proven pulmonary infiltration and fibrosis.[41] Most commonly, methotrexate and carmustine toxicity have been reported, with normal chest radiographic findings. Finally, rituximab can cause interstitial infiltrates with cryptogenic organizing pneumonia in the setting of rapid onset of fever, dyspnea, and cough; however, this is a rare finding. Other CT findings of toxicity are GGO associated with vasculature that proves to be pulmonary hemorrhage. This is most often seen with bevacizumab.

PRACTICE OF ONCOLOGY

Pulmonary Function Tests

The most common abnormalities associated with chemotherapy-induced pulmonary toxicity are a reduced diffusing capacity for carbon monoxide and a restrictive ventilatory defect.[41] Isolated gas transport abnormalities manifested by a decrease in the diffusing capacity and/or arterial hypoxemia, especially with exercise, have been seen. Screening pulmonary function tests to predict which patients receiving chemotherapy are likely to develop toxicity would be helpful but have not been established. In bleomycin toxicity, changes in the diffusing capacity may be transient, whereas decreases in total lung capacity seem to correlate better with radiographic abnormalities.[120,121]

Diagnosis

Lung biopsy is usually necessary for a definitive diagnosis and to rule out other causes of lung injury including infection, tumor progression, or diffuse alveolar hemorrhage. Acute respiratory distress syndrome is suggested by radiographic and physical examination, and lymphangitic spread is suggested by malignant cells within BAL fluid. Cardiogenic pulmonary edema is suggested by echocardiography as well as brain natriuretic peptide values and resolution with diuresis. Through the use of BAL, several studies reported the presence of a characteristic or predominant cell associated with particular drugs.[56,63,106] Although these data might be of value in understanding the pathogenesis of drug-induced lung disorders, their usefulness in diagnosing drug toxicity is limited.

To date, biomarkers for chemotherapy-induced lung injury are research tools more than clinically applicable tests. No serum marker for drug-induced pulmonary toxicity currently exists. KL-6 may be helpful in diagnosis as it is elevated in 53% of patients with drug-induced pneumonitis.[122] It will not be elevated in patients with bacterial pneumonia, pulmonary aspergillosis, asthma, bronchiectasis, emphysema, eosinophilic pneumonia, or organizing pneumonia.[123] It lacks specificity, however, as it can also be elevated in patients with radiation pneumonitis, viral pneumonia, and *Pneumocystis* pneumonia in this patient population. Though elevated levels of TGF-β in plasma after high-dose chemotherapy for breast cancer predicted an increased risk of pulmonary toxicity after autologous bone marrow transplantation, its clinical applicability has been limited.[124]

Treatment

The most effective way to manage pulmonary toxicity associated with chemotherapeutic agents is to prevent it. Animal studies of bleomycin toxicity showed a beneficial preventive effect of dietary supplementation with taurine and niacin; no comparable human studies have been reported.[125] G-CSF should be discontinued as soon as leukocytes reach over 1,000 cell/μL. Hypersensitivity reactions can be mitigated with the administration of steroids and H2 blockers prior to dosing.

If toxicity occurs, withdrawal of the offending agent is the cornerstone of therapy. Although no controlled studies in humans have systematically examined the efficacy of corticosteroids, a trial of these agents is probably warranted in most cases. The optimal dose and duration of therapy are not known; however, 1 mg/kg per day is usually initiated with a slow and careful tapering schedule because clinical deterioration after tapering has been reported. The use of lung transplant in the treatment of advanced drug-induced pulmonary fibrosis should be considered in appropriate patients. One report described the case of a 23-year-old male patient who underwent a single lung transplant because of presumed drug-induced pulmonary fibrosis 12 years after undergoing chemotherapy for acute lymphocytic leukemia.[126]

SELECTED REFERENCES

The full reference list can be accessed at lwwhealthlibrary.com/oncology.

1. Zhao W, Robbins ME. Inflammation and chronic oxidative stress in radiation-induced late normal tissue injury: therapeutic implications. *Curr Med Chem* 2009;16:130–143.
2. Fleckenstein K, Zgonjanin L, Chen L, et al. Temporal onset of hypoxia and oxidative stress after pulmonary irradiation. *Int J Radiat Oncol Biol Phys* 2007;68:196–204.
5. Vujaskovic Z, Anscher MS, Feng QF, et al. Radiation-induced hypoxia may perpetuate late normal tissue injury. *Int J Radiat Oncol Biol Phys* 2001;50:851–855.
7. Robnett TJ, Machtay M, Vines EF, et al. Factors predicting severe radiation pneumonitis in patients receiving definitive chemoradiation for lung cancer. *Int J Radiat Oncol Biol Phys* 2000;48:89–94.
10. Catane R, Schwade JG, Turrisi AT 3rd, et al. Pulmonary toxicity after radiation and bleomycin: a review. *Int J Radiat Oncol Biol Phys* 1979;5:1513–1518.
11. Dehing-Oberije C, De Ruysscher D, van Baardwijk A, et al. The importance of patient characteristics for the prediction of radiation-induced lung toxicity. *Radiother Oncol* 2009;91:421–426.
16. Timmerman R, Paulus R, Galvin J, et al. Stereotactic body radiation therapy for inoperable early stage lung cancer. *JAMA* 2010;303:1070–1076.
18. McDonald S, Rubin P, Phillips TL, et al. Injury to the lung from cancer therapy: clinical syndromes, measurable endpoints, and potential scoring systems. *Int J Radiat Oncol Biol Phys* 1995;31:1187–1203.
20. Poust JC, Woolery JE, Green MR. Management of toxicities associated with high-dose interleukin-2 and biochemotherapy. *Anticancer Drugs* 2013;24:1–13.
27. Madani I, De Ruyck K, Goeminne H, et al. Predicting risk of radiation-induced lung injury. *J Thorac Oncol* 2007;2:864–874.
29. Goto K, Kodama T, Sekine I, et al. Serum levels of KL-6 are useful biomarkers for severe radiation pneumonitis. *Lung Cancer* 2001;34:141–148.
32. Andreassen CN, Alsner K, Overgaard M, et al. Prediction of normal tissue radiosensitivity from polymorphisms in candidate genes. *Radiother Oncol* 2003;69:127–135.
37. Graves PR, Siddiqui F, Anscher MS, et al. Radiation pulmonary toxicity: from mechanisms to management. *Semin Radiat Oncol* 2010;20:201–207.
40. Malik SE, Myers JL, DeRemee RA, et al. Lung toxicity associated with cyclophosphamide. Two distinct patterns. *Am J Respir Crit Care Med* 1996;154:1851–1856.
41. Cooper JA Jr, White DA, Matthay RA. Drug-induced pulmonary disease. Part 1: Cytotoxic drugs. *Am Rev Respir Dis* 1986;133:321–340.
46. Freeman BA, Crapo JD. Biology of disease: free radicals and tissue injury. *Lab Invest* 1982;47:412–426.
48. Waid-Jones MI, Coursin DB. Perioperative considerations for patients treated with bleomycin. *Chest* 1991;99:993–999.
51. Chandler DB. Possible mechanisms of bleomycin-induced fibrosis. *Clin Chest Med* 1990;11:21–30.
53. Veerappan A, O'Connor NJ, Brazin J, et al. Mast cells: a pivotal role in pulmonary fibrosis. *DNA Cell Biol* 2013;32:206–218.
54. Jules-Elysee K, White DA. Bleomycin-induced pulmonary toxicity. *Clin Chest Med* 1990;11:1–20.
56. Nuver J, Lutke Holzik MF, van Zweeden M, et al. Genetic variation in the bleomycin hydrolase gene and bleomycin-induced pulmonary toxicity in germ cell cancer patients. *Pharmacogenet Genomics* 2005;15:399–405.
58. Paun A, Lemay AM, Tomko TG, et al. Association analysis reveals genetic variation altering bleomycin-induced pulmonary fibrosis in mice. *Am J Respir Cell Mol Biol* 2013;48:330–336.
64. Imokawa S, Colby TV, Leslie KO, et al. Methotrexate pneumonitis: review of the literature and histopathological findings in nine patients. *Eur Respir J* 2000;15:373–381.
68. Kouroussis C, Mavroudis D, Kakolyris S, et al. High incidence of pulmonary toxicity of weekly docetaxel and gemcitabine in patients with non-small cell lung cancer: results of a dose-finding study. *Lung Cancer* 2004;44:363–368.
72. Ostoros G, Pretz A, Fillinger J, et al. Fatal pulmonary fibrosis induced by paclitaxel: a case report and review of the literature. *Int J Gynecol Cancer* 2006;16:391–393.
73. Shepherd GM. Hypersensitivity reactions to chemotherapeutic drugs. *Clin Rev Allergy Immunol* 2003;24:253–262.
77. Takano T, Ohe Y, Kusumoto M, et al. Risk factors for interstitial lung disease and predictive factors for tumor response in patients with advanced non-small cell lung cancer treated with gefitinib. *Lung Cancer* 2004;45:93–104.
82. Bergeron A, Rea D, Levy V, et al. Lung abnormalities after dasatinib treatment for chronic myeloid leukemia: a case series. *Am J Respir Crit Care Med* 2007;176:814–818.

84. Miyakoshi S, Kami M, Yuji K, et al. Severe pulmonary complications in Japanese patients after bortezomib treatment for refractory multiple myeloma. *Blood* 2006;107:3492–3494.

87. Pham PT, Pham PC, Danovitch GM, et al. Sirolimus-associated pulmonary toxicity. *Transplantation* 2004;77:1215–1220.

89. Duran I, Siu LL, Oza AM, et al. Characterisation of the lung toxicity of the cell cycle inhibitor temsirolimus. *Eur J Cancer* 2006;42:1875–1880.

91. White DA, Camus P, Endo M, et al. Noninfectious pneumonitis after everolimus therapy for advanced renal cell carcinoma. *Am J Respir Crit Care Med* 2010;182:396–403.

92. Amit L, Beh-Ahatron I, Vidal L, et al. The impact of Bevacizumab (Avastin) on survival in metastatic solid tumors—a meta-analysis and systematic review. *PLoS One* 2013;8:e51780.

94. Liotta M, Rose PG, Escobar PF. Pulmonary hypertension in 2 patients treated with bevacizumab for recurrent ovarian cancer. *Gynecol Oncol* 2009;115:308–309.

95. Charpidou AG, Gkiozos I, Tsimpoukis S, et al. Therapy-induced toxicity of the lungs: an overview. *Anticancer Res* 2009;29:631–639.

107. White DA, Kris MG, Stover DE. Bronchoalveolar lavage cell populations in bleomycin lung toxicity. *Thorax* 1987;42:551–552.

110. Harada C, Kawaguchi T, Ogata-Suetsugu S, et al. EGFR tyrosine kinase inhibition worsens acute lung injury in mice with repairing airway epithelium. *Am J Respir Crit Care Med* 2011;183:743–751.

118. Lei KI, Leung WT, Johnson PJ. Serious pulmonary complications in patients receiving recombinant granulocyte colony-stimulating factor during BACOP chemotherapy for aggressive non-Hodgkin's lymphoma. *Br J Cancer* 1994;70:1009–1013.

120. Rossi SE, Erasmus JJ, McAdams HP, et al. Pulmonary drug toxicity: radiologic and pathologic manifestations. *Radiographics* 2000;20:1245–1259.

122. Ohnishi H, Yokoyama A, Yasuhara Y, et al. Circulating KL-6 levels in patients with drug induced pneumonitis. *Thorax* 2003;58:872–875.

Joachim Yahalom and Matthew A. Lunning

INTRODUCTION

Chemotherapy, immunotherapy, and radiotherapy (RT) may have deleterious effects on the cardiovascular system.[1,2] Within these categories exist agents that have well-described cardiotoxicity: chemotherapeutics (anthracyclines, alkylators, taxanes, fluropyrimidines) and monoclonal antibodies. Each will be discussed in detail. A more comprehensive list is shown in Table 139.1. The effects of RT on the cardiovascular system are detailed in the latter section.

CHEMOTHERAPEUTICS

Anthracyclines

Reversible acute cardiotoxicity and delayed irreversible dilated cardiomyopathy (CM) are uncommonly seen with the use of anthracyclines. The reversible acute toxicity presents as a myocarditis and occasionally with evidence of pericarditis, and may lead to nonischemic CM (NICM) with or without concomitant arrhythmias. This acute toxicity is rarely a fatal complication of anthracycline therapy.

The delayed CM presents as fatigue, dyspnea on exertion, orthopnea with sinus tachycardia, S3 gallop, pedal edema, pleural effusions, and elevated jugular venous distention. Nevertheless, these classic clinical features of NICM are often late manifestations. In order to reduce the incidence and/or severity of delayed CM, keen clinical recognition of factors that may lead toward a NICM include monitoring cumulative dose (CD) of agent used, early detection strategies, limiting total cumulative dose, and the timely use of adjunctive cardioprotective agents or modified infusional or pegylated regimens/drugs are important.

The risk of anthracycline CM depends on CD received. Historically, a 5% risk is seen at 400 to 450 mg/m^2 for doxorubicin, 900 mg/m^2 for daunorubicin, 800 to 935 mg/m^2 for epirubicin, and 223 mg/m^2 for idarubicin.[3] Cofactors for cardiotoxic risk include mediastinal irradiation, which includes the heart, older (particularly >70 years) or younger (<15 years) age, known coronary artery disease, antecedent valvular disease, and hypertension. Concurrent monoclonal antibodies (i.e., HER2 antibodies) appear to potentiate anthracycline-induced CM, whereas other chemotherapeutic agents may have independent or synergistic cardiac effects when used in combination.

The diagnosis of an NICM in the setting of a history of anthracycline exposure is generally made by comparing serial left ventricular function studies. Several modalities can be employed including multigated radionuclide imaging, two-dimensional transthoracic echocardiography, and cardiac magnetic resonance imaging (cMRI).[4-6] Nevertheless, it is imperative that an ischemic CM be excluded. Regardless of the modality employed, a left ventricular ejection fraction (LVEF) of ≥50% is considered within normal range. A threshold CD has not been identified below which left ventricular dysfunction is not seen.[7,8] A low LVEF regardless of symptom burden remains a contraindication for anthracycline use.

Echocardiograms and cMRI can also evaluate other structural changes of the myocardium in the setting of CM. Typical progression on serial imaging includes left ventricular diastolic dysfunction and, later, left ventricular systolic dysfunction, particularly affecting septal wall motion. Initially, the left ventricle is not enlarged or only moderately enlarged; with complete development of CM, there is multisegment hypokinesis and evidence of muscle wall thinning. The electrocardiogram (ECG) findings associated with anthracycline-induced CM include sinus tachycardia, low voltage, poor R-wave progression, and nonspecific T-wave changes. Even sinus tachycardia alone is a relatively late finding, such that serial ECGs are of little value in early detection.

Early detection of anthracycline-induced CM may be important in preventing overt CM. As described above measurement of LVEF by multigated radionuclide imaging, transthoracic echocardiogram, cMRI can be utilized. In two small prospective studies of transthoracic echocardiogram and cMRI, both modalities reported that it was possible to distinguish patients who had developed CM from others by LVEF measures at baseline and at 200 to 300 mg/m^2 of doxorubicin.[9,10] A fall of ≥10% at 200 mg/m^2 had 72% specificity and 90% sensitivity in detecting later CD. At a dose of 300 mg/m^2, 50% had developed a change in LVEF >10% with 25% of patients with evidence of myocardial structure changes. Long-term follow-up data is lacking in the later publication. Others have examined the strategy of serial LVEF retrospectively and demonstrated that the overall costs of early detection were less than the medical costs of overt CM management.[11] Therefore, it is generally accepted that all patients prior to undergoing anthracycline-based regimens should have a baseline measure of LVEF; the modality employed is often left to the physician. Subsequent follow-up evaluation of the myocardium is often driven by symptoms as no large prospective studies have demonstrated an overall survival advantage to surveillance and are unlikely to given the low incidence of CM and high number needed to screen.

Additional serologic methods of CM detection include measurement of levels of brain natriuretic peptide, a peptide synthesized by the myocardium that reflects the degree of heart failure, and cardiac troponin T levels, a measure of active myocardial damage.[12] Brain natriuretic peptide and to a lesser extent troponin T levels are encouraging serologic markers and may correlate with subclinical left ventricular diastolic dysfunction; however, prospective sequential serologic and radiographic studies are lacking. Percutaneous endomyocardial biopsy of the right ventricle, the historic gold standard for anthracycline-induced CM, may demonstrate characteristic histologic features that include loss of myofibrils, distention of the sarcoplasmic reticulum, and vacuolization of the cytoplasm; however, with more conventional technologies, this modality is rarely used.

Aside from early detection, other strategies to reduce the incidence of CM are the use of low-dose or infusional drug schedules in an attempt to reduce peak drug dose delivery, and the use of liposomal formulations.[13,14] Liposomal formulations have been shown to permit higher CD and lower CM at the same dose. Data remains limited, however, regarding tumor response and survival.

TABLE 139.1

Other Less Common Drugs Associated with Cardiovascular Toxicities

Drug	Incidence	Cardiovascular Effects	Onset
Arsenic trioxide	3%–24%	QT, VR	Acute
Busulfan	2%	CHF	Late
Carmustine	Rare	H, AR, CP	Acute
Cisplatin	Rare	H, AR, VR, CP	Acute
Cytarabine	Rare	AR, VR, CP, P, CHF	Acute, subacute
Etoposide	1%–2%	H	Acute
Gemcitabine	Rare	AR, CHF	Acute
Interferon	Rare	H, AR, CP, MI, CHF	Acute, subacute
Interleukin-2	Dose-dependent	H, AR, CP, MI	Acute, subacute
Mitomycin[a]	10%	CHF	—
Pentostatin	3%–10%	AR, VR, CP, MI, CHF	Subacute
Sunitinib	15%–28%; rare	HBP, CHF, MI	Acute, subacute
Sorafenib	20%; rare	HBP, CHF, MI	Acute, subacute
Teniposide	2%	H	Acute
Tretinoin[a]	14%–23%	H, AR	Acute, subacute
Vinca alkaloids	10%;	H	Acute, subacute

QT, prolonged QT; VR, ventricular arrhythmia; CHF, congestive heart failure; H, hypotension; AR, atrial arrhythmia; CP, chest pain; P, pericarditis; HBP, hypertension; MI, myocardial infarction.
[a] Retinoic acid syndrome.

The iron-chelating cardioprotectant dexrazoxane decreases the risk of clinical CM in patients who have received doxorubicin doses of $\geq$300 mg/m^2.[15] The American Society of Clinical Oncology recommends the use of dexrazoxane in this setting.[16] However, American Society of Clinical Oncology guidelines do not advocate dexrazoxane in the several important situations including adjuvant regimens, CD <300 mg/m^2, pediatric patients, or in high-risk disease patients. Clinical data are also insufficient to recommend dexrazoxane with other anthracyclines, except epirubicin in metastatic breast cancer. A pivotal study in pediatric acute lymphoblastic leukemia may serve to change these recommendations. With a median follow-up of 5.7 years, this prospective trial revealed no significant impact on 5-year event-free survival, whereas dexrazoxane reduced serial troponins during therapy.[17]

The management of anthracycline-induced CM is similar to other causes of NICM.[1] Angiotensin-converting enzyme inhibitors, β-blockers, and diuretics are commonly used. As pointed out in long-term pediatric studies, these agents do not cure or permanently control the CM. Rather, the CM may become progressive despite these agents after more than 5 years. The only curative therapy remains cardiac transplantation.

The mechanism of anthracycline CD is not fully elucidated, but there is emerging evidence that cardiomyocyte apoptosis may play a major role.[18] The production of free radicals generated during cardiomyocyte metabolism of the anthracycline results in membrane lipid peroxidation, with the consequent activation of the extrinsic and intrinsic apoptotic pathways. It is thought that free radicals are generated by enzymatic reduction of the anthracycline quinone ring and by formation of iron-anthracycline complexes. The intrinsic antioxidant defense of the cardiomyocyte is more limited than other organs, leading to its apparent selective toxicity profile. In a knockout mouse model suggesting that a deficiency of the *HFE* gene (associated with hereditary hemochromatosis) confers increased susceptibility to doxorubicin CD.[19] They studied wild-type, HFE (+/−), and HFE (−/−) mice that were chronically treated with doxorubicin. Survival was significantly decreased in the HFE-negative mice, and cardiac iron concentration was significantly elevated. Moreover, cardiac ultrastructure changes demonstrated iron-associated mitochondrial damage. Interestingly, in rats the site of cardiac oxidative toxicity was also the mitochondria of the cardiac cell by gene expression profiling, and using cMRI in an anthracycline-exposed mouse model, these lesions demonstrate gadolinium enhancement.[20,21]

Cyclophosphamide

The classic cardiac toxicity of cyclophosphamide (CTX) is an acute myopericarditis associated with high-dose therapy. In the era of stem cell transplantation and vigorous hydration, irreversible hemorrhagic myonecrosis is rare. More commonly, patients develop an acute or subacute congestive heart failure that is generally reversible with medical management.

Prospective monitoring of 16 patients during CTX high-dose administration (7 g/m^2) and serial enzymes (CPK, CPK-MB, and troponin I) did not become elevated using a fractionated drug administration schedule during 13 hours.[22] The only positive findings were four cases of transient, mild diastolic, and systolic left ventricular dysfunction. Moreover, others have reported on early and late cardiac toxicity in a combination regimen using a CTX used in doxorubicin-naïve patients.[23] A total of 6 of 100 patients developed transient NICM. There were no acute cardiotoxic fatalities; late cardiotoxicity was not seen except in those patients requiring anthracycline salvage. Thus, with current administration guidelines used with high-dose therapy, CTX cardiotoxicity is uncommon (<10% of patients treated), generally transient, and reversible.[24]

Ifosfamide

Ifosfamide is an alkylating agent with similar properties to CTX. As a result of possible chemical cystitis, it is always administered with mesna. However, there is no evidence that mesna has any cardioprotective effect for CTX or ifosfamide. Similar to CTX, ifosfamide may cause a dose-related NICM, which is generally transient and reversible. In a small report, no episodes of NICM were seen at 10 g/m^2 (0 of 6 patients), but at $\geq$16 g/m^2, a NICM was more seen in 40% (6 of 15 patients).[25] Clinical symptoms were delayed and presented subacutely (mean, 12 days; range, 6 to 23 days). They often resolved with medical management. These doses are rarely encountered in current clinical practice. A larger study prospectively studied high-dose CTX or ifosfamide-based regimens in 211 patients with metastatic breast cancer.[26] The cardiac effects were similar with the two agents: troponin I became positive in 70 patients (33%) and remained negative in 141. LVEF fell significantly and continuously after the first month among the troponin I–positive patients, and the degree of dysfunction correlated with the troponin I level. Those who developed NICM had prior or concurrent exposure to anthracycline.

Taxanes (Paclitaxel and Docetaxel)

The taxanes (paclitaxel and docetaxel) are important antimicrotubule agents derived from the yew tree (paclitaxel, *Taxus brevifolia*; docetaxel, *Taxus baccata*). The yew tree is known to be poisonous, and the taxine alkaloid byproduct can affect cardiac conduction and automaticity. Although not fully proven, the mechanism of paclitaxel cardiotoxicity appears to be related to its taxane ring structural similarities to yew taxine.

The cardiovascular effects of paclitaxel are multiple: asymptomatic bradycardia may be documented in almost one-third of patients, hypersensitivity reactions associated with the Cremophor EL diluent (which can be ameliorated with corticosteroids, histamine H$_1$, and H$_2$ receptor antagonists), and most importantly, life-threatening atrial and/or ventricular rhythm disturbances and/or conduction abnormalities in approximately 0.5% of patients. Rare ischemic events have also been reported.

Life-threatening arrhythmias may occur acutely during infusion, or delayed up to 14 days after treatment. These tend to occur after two or more treatment exposures, rather than with initial therapy. There does not appear to be a cumulative dosing threshold or limit, unlike that with anthracyclines. The grade 4 and 5 adverse cardiac events, atrial arrhythmias (tachycardia, flutter, and/or fibrillation) occurred in 0.24%, ventricular arrhythmias (tachycardia/fibrillation) in 0.26%, heart block in 0.11%, and ischemia in 0.29%.[27] Paclitaxel does not appear to cause an NICM.

In metastatic breast cancer, the incidence of NICM in patients treated with a taxane and anthracycline in combination has been studied. Eighty-two doxorubicin/taxane-naïve patients received doxorubicin 60 mg/m^2 followed by a 1- or 3-hour paclitaxel 200 mg/m^2 infusion (AT) administered every 21 days for six to seven cycles.[28] The change in LVEF was a median of 10% (to 52.5%) at a CD of doxorubicin 310 to 360 mg/m^2. A later phase 3 trial compared AT, doxorubicin (60 mg/m^2) followed by paclitaxel (175 mg/m^2 in 3-hour infusion) versus doxorubicin/CTX (60/600 mg/m^2; AC) in 375 patients.[29] Similarly, treatment was repeated every 3 weeks for six cycles (maximum doxorubicin, 360 mg/m^2). Overt NICM was not statistically different in the two study arms (3% versus 1%; p = 0.62). However, a fall in LVEF ($\geq$10% fall from baseline or $\geq$5% drop below the normal range) was significantly more frequent for AT (27%) versus AC (14%). Moreover, the risk of LVEF decrease was significantly greater for AT than AC at every cumulative doxorubicin dose level >180 mg/m^2. Importantly, paclitaxel was administered within 30 minutes of preceding doxorubicin. It is now apparent that the enhanced cardiac toxicity of the doxorubicin-paclitaxel combinations is related to prolonged doxorubicin elimination, resulting in a plasma level of up to 30% greater when paclitaxel immediately precedes doxorubicin or follows it by <1 hour. This risk has been shown to be mitigated when the interval between doxorubicin and taxanes was 4 to 24 hours or longer and has remained minimal at 7-years of follow-up.[30–32]

It is known that paclitaxel appears to facilitate the metabolic conversion of doxorubicin to the toxic metabolite doxorubicinol in

a human heart in vitro model.[33] The taxane docetaxel has a similar effect on doxorubicinol generation and both are attributed to allosteric interactions with cytoplasmic aldehyde reductases.

Docetaxel has not been generally associated with clinical cardiac toxicity, NICM, or enhancement of doxorubicin cardiac dysfunction. However, data suggests this is due to a lower cumulative anthracycline level rather than a different mechanism of drug interaction than paclitaxel. Both docetaxel and paclitaxel increase toxic cardiomyocyte doxorubicinol production in vitro. Therefore, the lack of docetaxel effect on doxorubicin clearance and the relatively lower doses of the drug used when combined with doxorubicin are now thought to be the explanation for the prior differences.

Fluoropyrimidines

5-Fluorouracil (5-FU) is a synthetic pyrimidine antimetabolite and an important backbone agent in many common solid tumors regimens. Its cardiac toxicity is manifested as angina, atrial/ventricular arrhythmias, myocardial infarction (MI), and cardiogenic shock. A prior history of coronary artery disease significantly increases the risk of complication (15.1% versus 1.5%, with no coronary artery disease history). Other predisposing factors include prior mediastinal irradiation and prior/concurrent exposure to other cardiac toxic medications. The reported incidence of cardiac toxicity was low at 1.6% among 1,083 patients.[34] Using a continuous infusion of 5-FU noted a higher incidence of cardiac toxicity (6%) as compared with other daily schedules of administration.[35] The addition of leucovorin to the continuous infusion regimen appeared to further increase the cardiotoxicity risk, but this has not been conclusively reproduced.[36]

The oral fluoropyrimidine capecitabine also appears to have similar frequency of cardiotoxicity. In a large retrospective study of the cardiac toxicities (grade 3 to 4) reported in four large metastatic cancer trials, it was demonstrated that in 593 patients who received bolus 5-FU-leucovorin (Mayo Clinic regimen) or capecitabine (596 patients), the incidence of cardiotoxic events was 3% and 1%, respectively.[37]

The mechanism of fluoropyrimidine cardiotoxicity is not well understood. It is possibly related to vascular spasm in reaction to the parent drug and its catabolites (fluoro-beta-alanine and fluoroacetate). In an in vitro model, 5-FU causes vasoconstriction in smooth muscle rings, which is reversible with nitrates.[38,39] On electron microscopy, the changes appear to be in the small arterial endothelium.[39] Although coronary angiography following the 5-FU–induced angina did not reveal ongoing cardiac spasm, and in fact on autopsy evaluation, patients were found to have myocarditis.[40] Brachial artery ultrasound was performed prospectively in 60 patients receiving regimens containing 5-FU (n = 30) versus regimens not containing 5-FU (n = 30).[41] Fifty percent of the patients showed artery contraction with 5-FU and none with other therapy. Interestingly, arterial tone recovered within 30 minutes, but reoccurred with retreatment in a high proportion. Pretreatment with glyceroltrinitrate, a vasodilator, abrogated the contractions in five patients.

Nevertheless, there is no known prophylactic regimen that can be provided to prevent the cardiotoxicity, and despite evidence to the contrary vasodilators do not necessarily relieve the symptoms once apparent. As a result, the optimal treatment is discontinuation of the fluoropyrimidine infusion and supportive measures with keen attention toward likely myocardial damage, with available cardiac support.[42]

Monoclonal Antibodies

Trastuzumab and Lapatinib

Trastuzumab and lapatinib are humanized monoclonal antibodies that target p185^{HER2} (ErbB2 or HER2 receptor), a transmembrane receptor tyrosine kinase of the epidermal growth factor family. This receptor protein is overexpressed or amplified in 20% to 30% of breast cancer and is associated with a poor clinical outcome. These antibodies are important agents in the management of primary and metastatic breast cancer.[43]

Cardiac HER-2 is essential for normal embryonic and adult cardiac development and function, respectively. Using cardiac HER2–deficient mutant mice, a dilated CM begins in the second postnatal month and extends into adulthood of affected mice.[44,45] Moreover, HER2-deficient cardiomyocytes were more susceptible to anthracycline toxicity. However, it was subsequently discovered that no cardiac toxicity was seen when trastuzumab preceded anthracycline-based adjuvant therapy in a prospective study.[46]

Currently, trastuzumab is generally given after an anthracycline-based regimen. Evidence that supported that conclusion came from an independent Cardiac Review and Evaluation Committee that retrospectively evaluated data from seven phase 2/3 clinical trials.[47] They identified 112 patients with a CM (as defined by the Cardiac Review and Evaluation Committee) among 1,219 treated patients. Three studies used trastuzumab alone: 383 patients, of whom 17 (4%) had a CM. Among 114 patients who received single-agent trastuzumab as first-line therapy for metastatic disease, 3% developed a CM. In contrast, concurrent trastuzumab with anthracycline-based regimens or paclitaxel had an increased incidence of CM (27% versus 13%, respectively) as compared to chemotherapy alone (11% versus 1%, respectively) or antibody alone (3%).

The degree of cardiac impairment (New York Heart Association class III or IV) among those with CM was greatest for patients receiving trastuzumab plus concurrent anthracycline (64%) as compared with 20% receiving trastuzumab plus paclitaxel. Moreover, all trastuzumab plus paclitaxel patients had functional cardiac recovery with treatment as compared with only half the trastuzumab plus concurrent anthracycline patients. Risk factors for CM included older age and cumulative doxorubicin 300 mg/m^2 or more. Concurrent anthracycline (doxorubicin or epirubicin) appeared to be more hazardous than temporally separated trastuzumab therapy.

The diagnosis of trastuzumab-induced CM is often made by the detection of an asymptomatic decrease in LVEF and now considered to be an "on-target" adverse event. Similarly to anthracycline-induced CM, tachycardia may be an early clinical indicator, and the late constellation of a dilated and hypokinetic myocardium is a late manifestation. Dissimilar to anthracyclines, trastuzumab-induced CM does not depend on the CD of the antibody and is often self-limited with supportive measure. For example, with echocardiography follow-up, the use of adjuvant trastuzumab had no additive adverse effect when used after anthracycline therapy.[48] To date, there remain no definitive predictive tests other than documenting a low LVEF prior to therapy and no preventive measures to ameliorate the development of trastuzumab-induced CM. Lastly, concurrent trastuzumab-anthracycline exposure is contraindicated. Guidelines have restricted eligibility to those with LVEF of ≥55% and delay of initiation to 1 to 2 months if following anthracyclines.[48] In such criteria, trastuzumab was discontinued in only 4.3% of such patients for CM. In practice, active monitoring of LVEF is recommended every 4 months during therapy and every 6 months thereafter for up to 2 years.

Because of the previously described cardiac toxicity associated with trastuzumab, T-DM1, a recently approved antibody drug conjugate against HER-2 and used in HER-2–positive breast cancer while in development, was carefully assessed for CM by surveillance imaging. In 882 patients treated with T-DM1, defined cardiac-specific events were seen in only 1.5% (13 patients) with nearly all of the events being low grade.[49] Further clinical testing in combination strategies are ongoing, but lessons learned from the trastuzumab era will hopefully reduce the incidence of CM as the drug moves forward into the up-front setting.

Rituximab

Rituximab is a CD20 monoclonal antibody widely used in the management of non-Hodgkin's lymphoma (HL). In early development of the antibody, an initial concern for CM was seen that was felt to be related to the rate of infusion; however, those findings went unfounded when used in combination regimens.[50] There have been no long-term effects from rituximab; however, arrhythmias with cardiac death have been reported related to infusion reaction most commonly seen with the initial infusion but at a rate of <0.07%.[51,52]

Bevacizumab

Bevacizumab is a humanized monoclonal antibody that inhibits the vascular endothelial growth factor. Currently, bevacizumab is approved for use in combination with 5-FU–based chemotherapy in metastatic colon cancer. A recent US Food and Drug Administration black box warning was placed on bevacizumab after an increase in risk of MI, angina, and heart disease. The risk was greatest in those who are older than 65 with prior arterial events. The risk of grade 2 to 4 CM was 1.2% when used as a single agent, but increased to 3.8% in those with prior anthracycline exposure.

RADIOTHERAPY-ASSOCIATED CARDIAC SEQUELAE

In the past, cardiac complications resulting from mediastinal irradiation were considered rare and insignificant.[53] Since the mid-1960s, when follow-up information on a large number of patients who had been cured of HL with higher doses of radiation became available, the heart has no longer been considered radioresistant.[54] Radiation-associated heart disease has now been clinically described and the pathologic features of the damage have been described with regard to the coronary arteries and all three layers of the heart.

Pericarditis and pericardial effusion have been regarded as the most common side effects of cardiac irradiation.[55] However, modern techniques of irradiation, dose decrease, and reduction of the heart volume irradiated in most malignancies have substantially reduced the frequency of this complication. At the same time, evidence has accumulated to suggest that ischemic heart disease resulting from radiation-induced coronary heart disease (CHD) is the most concerning long-term risk of cardiac irradiation, particularly in patients at high-risk for ischemic disease.[56–60]

The clinical spectrum of radiation-induced heart disease involves most structures of the heart and is summarized as follows:

Pericardial disease
Acute pericarditis during irradiation
Delayed acute pericarditis
Pericardial effusion
Constrictive pericarditis
Myocardial dysfunction
Valvular heart disease
Electrical conduction abnormalities
CHD

Although the pathologic and clinical manifestations of radiation-induced heart disease may overlap in many patients, they are discussed separately in the following paragraphs.

Pericardial Disease

Incidence

The risk of radiation-induced pericardial disease depends on the dose given and on the volume of the heart irradiated.[61,62] Even

PRACTICE OF ONCOLOGY

when a large volume of the heart (≥60%) is irradiated ≤40 Gy, the risk for mild pericarditis is <5%, and severe pericarditis is rare.[63] Smaller heart volumes (20% to 30%) may tolerate up to 60 Gy, with an expected 2% risk of mild pericarditis. In the past, when the whole pericardium was irradiated, the pericarditis incidence was 20%, but when most of the left ventricle was excluded, it was reduced to 7%.[64] An updated analysis of these patients showed a sharp decrease in the risk of death from cardiac complications other than acute MI for patients who received mediastinal irradiation after 1972, reflecting the change in cardiac shielding.[59] Indeed, all series that showed a high risk of pericarditis are of patients treated with a radiation technique, energy, and total dose and fractionation that are no longer considered to be an acceptable standard of care in most centers.[58] With current RT techniques for HL and breast cancer, pericarditis is an infrequent event.

Acute Pericarditis During Radiation

Acute pericarditis during the course of RT is rare. It is almost always associated with massive mediastinal tumors adjacent to the heart. The signs and symptoms are of acute nonspecific pericarditis with chest pain, fever, and often ECG abnormalities. It does not lead to a significant risk of late pericardial damage and is not an indication for interrupting the radiation course.[53,56]

Delayed Pericarditis

Radiation-induced pericarditis typically occurs within the first year after mediastinal irradiation. The common range is from 4 months to several years after treatment.[53,65] Pericardial disease presents either as an acute pericarditis, as a pericardial effusion that may be asymptomatic, or as a combination of both. The symptoms of delayed acute pericarditis are indistinguishable from those of other types of pericarditis and usually consist of fever, pleuritic chest pain, pericardial friction rub, ST-T segment changes, and a decrease of the QRS voltage in the ECG. Pericardial effusion may be large and manifest as an enlarged cardiac silhouette.[66] Most cases of radiation-induced pericarditis and pericardial effusion resolve spontaneously, usually within 16 months. Approximately 20% of patients with delayed pericarditis progress within 5 to 10 years to develop symptomatic constriction requiring pericardiectomy. This is very rare in current practice. Radiation-induced hypothyroidism should also be considered in the etiology of pericardial effusion after mediastinal irradiation.[67]

Treatment

Careful cardiac evaluation and monitoring with echocardiography and radionuclide ventriculography should be performed whenever radiation-induced heart disease is suspected.[66–68] Patients with mild symptoms and no hemodynamic compromise can be followed without treatment or can receive symptomatic therapy with salicylates or other nonsteroidal anti-inflammatory agents. Symptomatic pericardial effusion or clinical evidence for hemodynamic compromise warrants a drainage procedure. Pericardiocentesis with or without percutaneous placement of an indwelling catheter is successful in the majority of patients. Failure to relieve tamponade with pericardiocentesis, recurrence of effusion, or the presence of symptomatic constrictive pericarditis requires pericardiectomy. This is rarely required with current RT practice.

Myocardial Dysfunction

When myocardial dysfunction is detected after standard-dose mediastinal irradiation, it is typically mild or subclinical.[52,58,69] In patients who were studied 15 days after mediastinal irradiation, a transient decrease in LVEF was observed. Complete recovery of ejection fraction 2 months after irradiation and no additional change in patients who were also receiving doxorubicin were documented.[70] Noninvasive studies using echocardiographic and radionuclide angiography detected subtle left ventricular dysfunction in patients with HL evaluated a few years after mediastinal irradiation.[70] A study of asymptomatic patients who were treated with mediastinal irradiation for HL at a young age showed reduced average left ventricular dimension and mass suggestive of restricted CM in 42% of patients.[71] The majority of patients with abnormal ventricular function findings, however, do not have clinical heart failure.[71] The magnitude of the potential contribution of cardiac irradiation to the risk of doxorubicin-induced CM is not well established. Some data suggest potentiation of anthracycline-induced cardiotoxicity when combined with RT. Yet the histopathologies of radiation heart disease and anthracycline heart disease are different, and the combined effects are probably additive rather than synergistic.[72] It was reported that doxorubicin-induced decrease in LVEF was aggravated with concurrent mediastinal irradiation.[73,74] In programs of combined modality therapy for HL that included relatively low doses of doxorubicin (up to 300 mg/m²) and mediastinal irradiation of 20 to 40 Gy, no significant clinical myocardial dysfunction was detected.[75]

Symptomatic myocardial dysfunction after a radiation dose that does not exceed 60 Gy is rare. The few cases described with intractable heart failure had myocardial fibrosis as part of pancarditis, a generalized process with damage to all three layers of the heart. The hemodynamic pattern is usually of restrictive CM and is difficult to distinguish from constrictive pericarditis.

Valvular Disease

Clinically significant valvular heart disease resulting from mediastinal irradiation is relatively uncommon.[73] Analysis of 635 patients treated for HL before the age of 21 years revealed 29 patients in whom new murmurs of indeterminate significance developed. Of those, 14 received mediastinal doses of 44 Gy or more, and 2 patients who received high-dose irradiation died of valvular heart disease.[53,54] When echocardiographic studies were performed in asymptomatic patients with HL >7 years after mediastinal irradiation, valvular abnormalities were detected in 25% to 33% of the patients, although there was rarely any clinical significance. An echocardiographic study of 294 asymptomatic patients who received mediastinal irradiation disclosed moderate or severe regurgitation of the aortic valve in 5.0% of patients, of the mitral valve in 3.4%, and of the tricuspid valve in 1.4%. Four percent of the patients had aortic stenosis.[76] Valvular disease, particularly involving the aortic valve, increased with time after irradiation. Of 73 asymptomatic patients evaluated >20 years after mediastinal irradiation, 60% had mild or more aortic regurgitation and 16% had aortic stenosis. It is important to note that radiation dose, volumes, and technique of radiation delivery have markedly changed during the last three decades, and the lower prevalence of valvular disease in patients treated at <20 years may reflect those changes.[77] In a retrospective study of 415 patients that were irradiated from 1962 to 1998, 6.2% of patients developed clinically significant valvular dysfunction at a median of 22 years.[74] Of interest is a report from Norway that showed a significantly higher risk of cardiopulmonary complications for female subjects after radiation for HL.[78,79] The mean interval from irradiation to detection of valvular disease in asymptomatic and symptomatic patients was 11.5 and 16.5 years, respectively.[80] Patients that received mediastinal RT and an anthracycline-containing chemotherapy had significantly more valvular disorders than patients receiving RT with no anthracyclines.[59]

Electrical Abnormalities

Many ECG abnormalities were recorded years after mediastinal irradiation, the most common clinically significant abnormality being complete atrioventricular block.[68,81] Slama et al.[82] reported that radiation-related atrioventricular block was typically infranodal and occurred at long intervals (mean of 12 years), after radiation doses above 40 Gy, most frequently in patients with abnormal conduction on ECG before the advent of complete block, and in those who had other radiation-related cardiac abnormalities.

Another aspect of RT and heart disease relates to the management of patients with implanted cardiac pacemakers.[83–86] Although transient interference from electromagnetic noise (with the exception of betatrons) is not a problem in properly functioning RT equipment, pacemaker-dependent patients should be closely observed during the first treatment with a linear accelerator.[87–90] Placing the pacemaker in an unshielded RT field may cause cumulative damage to the pacemaker components. The absorbed dose to the pacemaker should be estimated before treatment. If the total dose to the pacemaker might exceed 2 Gy, the pacemaker function should be checked weekly to detect any indicator of damage that may require replacement of the device.[87]

Coronary Heart Disease

Experiments in laboratory animals,[91,92] analysis of pathologic specimens,[93] clinical observations,[93–95] and since the 1990s, long-term risk analysis in large series of patients treated for HL[57–59] all indicate that mediastinal irradiation may facilitate the development of CHD.[53]

Stenosis at the origin of the coronary arteries appears to be a common finding for radiation-associated CHD.[57,90–93] After mediastinal irradiation, there is a greater likelihood for right coronary or left main or left anterior descending coronary artery lesions as opposed to circumflex lesions, which might be due to the fact that the former vessels, particularly at their origin, receive more radiation.[95,96] Coronary spasm after RT has also been documented in patients in whom acute MI developed with patent coronary arteries.[94]

Although only approximately 1% to 2% of patients with HL in series that analyzed death from MI after RT for HL actually died of MI, the observed risk in all series was higher than expected (Table 139.2).

Current involved field RT techniques, better fractionation schemes, and modern equipment deliver smaller doses of radiation to the coronary arteries and may have a lower risk of promoting CHD.[79] In a study by Boivin et al.,[97] the relative risk of acute MI was reduced from 6.33 for patients treated during the years 1940 to 1966 to 1.97 (with no significant difference from unity) for patients irradiated from 1967 to 1985.

Hancock et al.[58,59] analyzed the risk of cardiac disease in patients with HL who were treated at Stanford University Medical Center from 1961 to 1991. In patients that were irradiated prior to age 21 years, the relative risk for death from acute MI was 41.5 and that the actuarial risk of fatal or nonfatal MI at 22 years was 8.1%.[58]

Of note, all deaths in this study occurred in patients who received relatively high doses of radiation (42 to 45 Gy) to the mediastinum. When the Stanford analysis was extended to include 2,232 patients with HL (of all age groups), the relative risk for death from acute MI was 3.2.[53] This study showed that patients younger than 20 years who received high-dose irradiation had the highest relative risk, that the risk decreases with increasing age, and that patients older than 50 years had no increased risk. However, these results contrast with data published by other investigators,[93] suggesting an increased risk of acute MI for the older age groups. The small number of patients in the Stanford study who received radiation doses of <30 Gy did not allow an adequate analysis of the dose effect. The average interval between HL treatment and death from acute MI was 10.3 years, but risk was already significant during the first 5 years after treatment and remained elevated throughout the follow-up period (>20 years).[53]

Two European studies analyzed the ischemic heart disease in patients with HL who received standard fractions and dose (30 to 42 Gy) of mediastinal irradiation.[60,61] Both studies demonstrated an increase of ischemic heart disease after mediastinal irradiation. Of importance, a multivariate analysis of risk factors in the Rotterdam study showed that increasing age, gender (male), and a pretreatment cardiac medical history were significant for developing ischemic heart disease. Treatment-related parameters did not affect the risk.[60] In a study from Zurich, a detailed analysis of the effect of other CHD risk factors on the radiation-induced risk was performed. The study showed that, although the risk of CHD after irradiation increased by 4.2 for all patients, in irradiated female patients and in all irradiated patients without other cardiovascular risk factors (smoking, hypertension, obesity, hypercholesterolemia, diabetes), the risk remained as expected in the normal population.[60] In a recent study of 1,474 survivors of HL treated mostly with RT with or without chemotherapy, hypercholesterolemia was the most significant independent risk factor for developing CHD.[57] These data suggest that aggressive modification of CHD risk factors is warranted in patients who received mediastinal RT and/or anthracycline-containing chemotherapy.

Anthracycline-containing regimens like doxorubicin, bleomycin, vinblastine, and dacarbazine (ABVD), and rituximab, CTX, doxorubicin, vincristine, and prednisone, with or without RT, are the mainstay of current treatment of HL and non-HL, respectively. Yet, only recently, serious concerns regarding anthracycline-related risks (with or without RT) to the coronary arteries have been documented.[98] Aviles et al.[98] studied 476 patients with HL with anthracycline-containing chemotherapy and no RT. At a median follow-up of 11.5 years, 9% of patients who received ABVD had a clinical cardiac event and 7% had a cardiac-related death. The standard mortality ratio for cardiac death for patients who received

TABLE 139.2

Relative Risk of Mortality from Myocardial Infarction After Mediastinal Irradiation for Hodgkin's Lymphoma

Study (Ref.)	Center	No. of Patients	Lethal Myocardial Infarctions	Relative Risk	95% Confidence Interval
Boivin et al.[97]	Multiple	4,665	68	2.6	1.1–5.9
Hancock et al.[59]	Stanford (California)	2,232	55	3.2	1.5–5.8
Henry-Amar et al.[121]	European Organisation for Treatment and Research on Cancer	1,449	17	8.8	5.1–14.1
Mauch et al.[57]	Joint Center for Radiation Therapy (Boston)	636	15[a]	2.2[a]	1.2–3.6
Glanzmann et al.[60]	Zurich	352	8	4.2	1.8–8.3
Reinders et al.[100]	Rotterdam	258	12[b]	5.3	2.7–9.3
Swerdlow et al.[64]	Britain	7,033	168	2.5	2.1–2.9

[a] Includes one patient who died of cardiomyopathy.
[b] Myocardial infarction or sudden death.

doxorubicin was 46.4 (95% confidence interval = 28.9 to 70.1), and the absolute excess risk was 39.[98]

Reduction of the radiation volume from even involved-field to the new concept of involved-site RT may have a significant impact on the risk as well the reduction in the recommended dose in HL.[99]

The largest and most recent analysis of MI mortality risk after treatment for HL is a collaborative British cohort study of 7,033 patients.[64] This study included 3,590 patients who received RT without anthracyclines, 3,052 patients who received chemotherapy with supradiaphragmatic RT, and 1,744 patients received anthracycline regimens and no RT. For the whole group of survivors of HL, the death from MI was statistically significantly more than expected: standardized mortality ratio (SMR) of 2.5 with an absolute excess risk of 125.8. The risk was higher for male patients. The relative risk of death from MI decreased sharply with older age at first treatment, but as expected, the absolute excess risk increased with age. The 20-year cumulative risk of MI mortality for patients treated at age younger than 35 was 1.8%. The risk of death during the first year after treatment was four-fold compared with the general population, and it was higher for patients treated before 1980.[100]

Of particular concern are the new data regarding chemotherapy alone.[64,95] In the British study,[64] the risk of death from MI was statistically significantly increased for patients who had received anthracyclines (SMR of 2.9) and especially those treated with ABVD (SMR of 9.5). These data remained significantly elevated for patients who received those chemotherapy regimens and no RT (ABVD, no RT; SMR of 7.8). The authors suggest that the risk was particularly high for ABVD (compared with other doxorubicin-containing regimens) because ABVD alone was virtually always given for a full six cycles. The increased risk for patients treated with anthracyclines was primarily during the first year after treatment and the highest risk was in young patients (≤35 years). MI mortality risk was also significantly increased for treatment with vincristine with or without radiation.

Long-term mortality data from three trials, which randomized patients with breast cancer to receive postmastectomy RT as opposed to no additional treatment, demonstrated a higher incidence of cardiac death in the irradiated group.[101–103] The excess in mortality did not appear until after 10 years posttreatment.[104,105] In one study, the increase in mortality risk was significant only in women who were irradiated for tumors in the left breast.[104] It was also increased in patients treated with orthovoltage irradiation, as opposed to those treated with more modern supervoltage equipment.[70]

A recent study from The Netherlands of 4,414 10-year survivors of breast cancer who were treated from 1970 through 1986 recorded both cardiovascular morbidity and mortality events.[106] It showed that radiation to the breast alone is not associated with increased risk of cardiovascular disease. Similar to other studies,[107,108] it also documented that the increased risk of MI that was noted in patients treated prior to 1980 has disappeared with more recent RT techniques.

Prophylactic irradiation of the internal mammary nodes using a single anterior photon beam (hockey stick technique) or large tangents, which may deliver a high dosage to the heart,[109] is not indicated in most patients irradiated for breast conservation or postmastectomy.[101] Techniques that reduce the risk of irradiating the coronary arteries have been developed; they include the prone breast technique[110] and use of three-dimensional computed tomography planning and intensity-modulated RT.[111] Patients with breast cancer irradiated with modern techniques are unlikely to receive a significant dose of radiation to the coronary arteries.[109–115] Proton therapy may also reduce the exposure of the heart in selected patients with breast cancer.[116]

In patients with breast cancer, conventional-dose doxorubicin-containing chemotherapy used as an adjuvant in combination with local-regional irradiation was not associated with a significant increase in the risk of cardiac events. However, higher doses of adjuvant doxorubicin were associated with a three- to four-fold increased risk of cardiac events. This appears to be especially true in patients treated with higher dose volumes of cardiac irradiation.[117] Interestingly, in one recent large-scale study, patients with breast cancer who were treated with CTX, methotrexate, and 5-FU and RT had a significantly higher risk of congestive heart failure compared with patients treated with RT alone.

The radiation threshold for an increased risk of CHD has not been determined. Lederman et al.[118] reported that patients with seminoma who received a relatively low dose of mediastinal irradiation (median, 24 Gy) had more ischemic heart disease than a similar group of patients whose mediastinums were not irradiated. It should be noted, however, that the observed cardiac risk in the irradiated group did not differ significantly from the expected risk of a comparable normal population.

Monitoring and reduction of other contributing CHD risk factors in patients who received mediastinal irradiation should be part of the follow-up of patients who underwent mediastinal irradiation[119,120] However, the value of routine noninvasive or invasive cardiac studies in asymptomatic patients has not been fully determined. In a recent screening study of 294 patients that received mediastinal radiation (median dose, 44 Gy) from 1960 to 1995, 21% of screened patients had abnormal ventricular images at rest.[59] During stress testing that included ECG and radionuclide perfusion, 14% showed abnormalities in one or both tests. Based on these tests, 40 patients underwent coronary angiography and 55% of them (7% of the screened population) had ≥50% stenosis. The risk of a cardiac event in those patients was significantly related to abnormal stress testing, older age, RT given in early period, and higher RT dose given to the mediastinum.

Early detection of coronary artery disease should be encouraged, particularly in patients irradiated with high RT dose (practiced mostly in the past) and/or those with other CHD risk factors[56,121–123] because angioplastic or surgical intervention may be indicated in special anatomic or clinical situations. Successful treatment of radiation-induced coronary disease with bypass surgery and with stenting or angioplasty has been reported.[120] In some cases, surgery may be technically difficult because of mediastinal and pericardial fibrosis.[89]

CONCLUSION

It is hoped that increased awareness and knowledge about potential cardiotoxicity from chemotherapy and RT will enable physicians to adequately monitor patients and modify therapy so as to minimize serious acute and chronic cardiac sequelae. The growing information about late cardiac effects should facilitate early diagnosis and therapeutic intervention for the benefit of previously treated patients.

SELECTED REFERENCES

The full reference list can be accessed at lwwhealthlibrary.com/oncology.

1. Jones RL, Swanton C, Ewer MS. Anthracycline cardiotoxicity. *Expert Opin Drug Saf* 2006;5:791–809.
2. Jones RL, Ewer MS. Cardiac and cardiovascular toxicity of nonanthracycline anticancer drugs. *Expert Rev Anticancer Ther* 2006;6:1249–1269.
10. Lunning MA, Kutty S, Rome ET, et al. Cardiac magnetic resonance imaging for the assessment of the myocardium after doxorubicin-based chemotherapy. *Am J Clin Oncol* 2013 [Epub ahead of print].

12. Suter TM, Meier B. Detection of anthracycline-induced cardiotoxicity: is there light at the end of the tunnel? *Ann Oncol* 2002;13:647–649.
13. van Dalen EC, Michiels EM, Caron HN, et al. Different anthracycline derivates for reducing cardiotoxicity in cancer patients. *Cochrane Database Syst Rev* 2010;5:CD005006.
16. Hensley ML, Hagerty KL, Kewalramani T, et al. American Society of Clinical Oncology 2008 clinical practice guideline update: use of chemotherapy and radiation therapy protectants. *J Clin Oncol* 2009;27:127–145.

24. Morandi P, Ruffini PA, Benvenuto GM, et al. Cardiac toxicity of high-dose chemotherapy. *Bone Marrow Transplant* 2005;35:323–334.

32. Romond EH, Jeong JH, Rastogi P, et al. Seven-year follow-up assessment of cardiac function in NSABP B-31, a randomized trial comparing doxorubicin and cyclophosphamide followed by paclitaxel (ACP) with ACP plus trastuzumab as adjuvant therapy for patients with node-positive, human epidermal growth factor receptor 2-positive breast cancer. *J Clin Oncol* 2012;30:3792–3799.

34. Labianca R, Beretta G, Clerici M, et al. Cardiac toxicity of 5-fluorouracil: a study on 1083 patients. *Tumori* 1982;68:505–510.

38. Mosseri M, Fingert HJ, Varticovski L, et al. In vitro evidence that myocardial ischemia resulting from 5-fluorouracil chemotherapy is due to protein kinase C-mediated vasoconstriction of vascular smooth muscle. *Cancer Res* 1993; 53:3028–3033.

44. Crone SA, Zhao YY, Fan L, et al. ErbB2 is essential in the prevention of dilated cardiomyopathy. *Nat Med* 2002;8:459–465.

48. Ewer MS, Vooletich MT, Durand JB, et al. Reversibility of trastuzumab-related cardiotoxicity: new insights based on clinical course and response to medical treatment. *J Clin Oncol* 2005;23:7820–7826.

51. Garypidou V, Perifanis V, Tziomalos K, et al. Cardiac toxicity during rituximab administration. *Leuk Lymphoma* 2004;45:203–204.

55. Arsenian MA. Cardiovascular sequelae of therapeutic thoracic radiation. *Prog Cardiovasc Dis* 1991;33:299–311.

56. Adams MJ, Lipshutz SE, Schwartz C, et al. Radiation-associated cardiovascular disease: manifestations and management. *Semin Radiat Oncol* 2003;13:346–356.

58. Hancock SL, Tucker MA, Hoppe RT. Factors affecting late mortality from heart disease after treatment of Hodgkin's disease. *JAMA* 1993;270:1949–1955.

60. Glanzmann C, Kaufmann P, Jenni R, et al. Cardiac risk after mediastinal irradiation for Hodgkin's disease. *Radiother Oncol* 1998;46:51–62.

61. Aleman BM, van del Belt-Dusebout AW, De Bruin M, et al. Late cardiotoxicity after treatment for Hodgkin lymphoma. *Blood* 2007;109:1878–1886.

62. Hull MC, Morris CG, Pepine CJ, et al. Valvular dysfunction and carotid, subclavian, and coronary artery disease in survivors of Hodgkin lymphoma treated with radiation therapy. *JAMA* 2003;290:2831–2837.

63. Heidenreich PA, Schnittger I, Strauss HW, et al. Screening for coronary artery disease after mediastinal irradiation for Hodgkin's disease. *J Clin Oncol* 2007;25:43–49.

64. Swerdlow AJ, Higgins CD, Smith P, et al. Myocardial infarction mortality risk after treatment for Hodgkin disease: a collaborative British cohort study. *J Natl Cancer Inst* 2007;99:206–214.

69. Loyer EM, Delpassand ES. Radiation-induced heart disease: imaging features. *Semin Roentgenol* 1993;28:321–332.

71. Blayney DW, Longo D. Radiation-induced pericarditis. *N Engl J Med* 1982; 306:550.

77. Adams MJ, Lipsitz SR, Colan SD, et al. Cardiovascular status in long-term survivors of Hodgkin's disease treated with chest radiotherapy. *J Clin Oncol* 2004;22:3139–3148.

78. Hequet O, Le QH, Moullet I, et al. Subclinical late cardiomyopathy after doxorubicin therapy for lymphoma in adults. *J Clin Oncol* 2004;22: 1864–1871.

79. Glanzmann C, Huguenin P, Lutolf UM, et al. Cardiac lesions after mediastinal irradiation for Hodgkin's disease. *Radiother Oncol* 1994;30:43–54.

80. Huge TJ, Ballonoff A, Rusthoven KE, et al. Cardiac mortality in patients with stage i and ii diffuse large b-cell lymphoma treated with and without radiation: a Surveillance, Epidemiology, and End-Results analysis. *Int J Radiation Oncol Biol Phys* 2010;76:845–849.

82. Slama M-S, LeGuludec D, Sebag C, et al. Complete atrioventricular block following mediastinal irradiation: a report of six cases. *Pacing Clin Electrophysiol* 1991;14:1112–1118.

86. Lund MB, Kongerud J, Boe J, et al. Cardiopulmonary sequelae after treatment for Hodgkin's disease: increased risk in females? *Ann Oncol* 1996;7: 257–264.

89. Last A. Radiotherapy in patients with cardiac pacemakers. *Br J Radiol* 1998; 71:4–10.

95. Handler CE, Livesey S, Lawton PA. Coronary ostial stenosis after radiotherapy: angioplasty or coronary artery surgery? *Br Heart J* 1989;61:208–211.

98. Aviles A, Neri N, Nambo MJ, et al. Late cardiac toxicity secondary to treatment in Hodgkin's disease. A study comparing doxorubicin, epirubicin and mitoxantrone in combined therapy. *Leuk Lymphoma* 2005;46:1023–1028.

99. Campbell BA, Hornby C, Cunninghame J, et al. Minimising critical organ irradiation in limited stage Hodgkin lymphoma: a dosimetric study of the benefit of involved node radiotherapy. *Ann Oncol* 2012;23:1259–1266.

103. Haybittle JL, Brinkley D, Houghton J, et al. Postoperative radiotherapy and late mortality: evidence from the Cancer Research Campaign trial for early breast cancer. *BMJ* 1989;298:1611–1614.

110. Stegman LD, Beal KP, Hunt MA, et al. Long-term clinical outcomes of whole-breast irradiation delivered in the prone position. *Int J Radiat Oncol Biol Phys* 2007;68:73–81.

111. Landau D, Adams EJ, Webb S, et al. Cardiac avoidance in breast radiotherapy: a comparison of simple shielding techniques with intensity-modulated radiotherapy. *Radiother Oncol* 2001;60:247–255.

113. Borst GR, Sonke JJ, den Hollander S, et al. Clinical results of image-guided deep inspiration breath hold breast irradiation. *Int J Radiat Oncol Biol Phys* 2010;78:1345–1351.

114. Kirova YM. Recent advances in breast cancer radiotherapy: Evolution or revolution, or how to decrease cardiac toxicity? *World J Radiol* 2010;2:103–108.

117. Shapiro CL, Hardenbergh PH, Gelman R, et al. Cardiac effects of adjuvant doxorubicin and radiation therapy in breast cancer patients. *J Clin Oncol* 1998;16:3493–3501.

122. Ng AK. Review of the cardiac long-term effects of therapy for Hodgkin lymphoma. *Br J Haematol* 2011;154:23–31.

123. Carver JR, Szalda D, Ky B. Asymptomatic cardiac toxicity in long-term cancer survivors: defining the population and recommendations for surveillance. *Semin Oncol* 2013;40:229–238.

PRACTICE OF ONCOLOGY

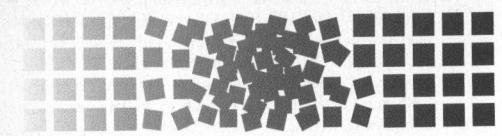

140 Hair Loss

Joyson J. Karakunnel, Ibrahim M. Qazi, and Ann M. Berger

INTRODUCTION

Hair is an important aspect of a person's self-image. During many cancer treatments, hair is adversely affected and this can have a profound negative impact on patients. "The loss of hair is an extremely traumatic experience precisely because it is the symbolic precursor to the loss of self. This raises the psychological terror and consequent fear that the known self will no longer exist."[1] The incidence of alopecia is exceptionally high and is currently ranked third among the most common side effects of chemotherapy, directly behind nausea and vomiting.[2] In addition, cancer-related alopecia is not only due to chemotherapy but also to metastatic disease and the presentation of different malignancies. Also, with the introduction of biologic agents, chemotherapy-induced alopecia is no longer limited to cytotoxics, as anecdotal reports of biologic agents inducing alopecia are increasingly reported.[3]

Hair loss can be an immense burden both psychologically and physically. Currently, there are modalities to help alleviate the physical and emotional issues that are involved with alopecia. In addition, several experimental treatments are being explored. This chapter will focus on chemotherapy-induced alopecia.

ANATOMY AND PHYSIOLOGY

Normal hair is divided into three parts: the infundibulum, the isthmus, and the inferior segment (deepest area). Other structures attached to the hair follicle include the sebaceous gland and arrector pili muscle. The hair follicle consists of the outer and inner sheath, cuticle, hair shaft, hair matrix, dermal papilla, and follicular sheath.

Hair growth is cyclical in nature. The three phases during the hair life cycle are anagen, telogen, and catagen. The majority of the time, most hair is in the anagen phase. During this phase, hair undergoes mitotic changes and rapid cell growth. During telogen, hair is dormant and mitotic activity is arrested. This phase lasts from 3 to 6 months. During the catagen phase, the hair root is separated from the hair bulb, pigment storage is terminated, and the club-shaped root end is pushed out from the bulb. Less than 1% of hair is in this phase at any time.[4] Chemotherapy-induced alopecia frequently occurs during anagen. Hair exposed to chemotherapy during this phase is much thinner and more brittle due to the suppression of cell proliferation.

Several types of alopecia are associated with problems in the transition from anagen to telogen. Hair lost during this period is called *telogen effluvium* or *hair breakage*. The five functional mechanisms of telogen effluvium are immediate anagen release, delayed anagen release, short anagen syndrome, immediate telogen release, and delayed telogen release.[5] Immediate anagen release is the most important mechanism with respect to chemotherapy. Normally, hair bulbs are released 4 to 6 weeks after the onset of anagen. The mechanism consists of hair being prematurely forced into telogen, leading to a greater amount of shedding. This mechanism is seen during drug-induced alopecia and severe illness.

CLASSIFICATION

Classification for hair loss has been divided into several different categories. Telogen effluvium can be subdivided into three categories depending on the amount of time during which hair shedding occurs. These subcategories are acute telogen effluvium, chronic diffuse telogen effluvium, and chronic telogen effluvium. During acute telogen effluvium, hair loss begins to occur approximately 2 to 3 months after the insult. Some of the causes include fever, surgery, or hemorrhage. Hair growth resumes approximately 3 to 6 months after the insult has subsided. Chronic diffuse telogen effluvium is defined by shedding that is present for >6 months. Some of the causes are thyroid disease, acrodermatitis enteropathica, malnutrition, iron-deficiency anemia, pancreatic disease, zinc deficiency, and drug-induced alopecia. Hair loss associated with thyroid disease, zinc deficiency, and iron-deficiency anemia begins to resolve once therapy is initiated. Finally, chronic telogen effluvium is a diagnosis of exclusion once the possibilities for chronic diffuse telogen effluvium have been considered. When evaluating a patient with a possible chronic telogen effluvium, androgenetic alopecia should be excluded.

Chemically induced alopecia is due to immediate anagen release and destruction, known as *hair follicle dystrophy*. Intravenously administered chemotherapy usually leads to greater hair loss compared to orally administered chemotherapy. Hair loss generally begins approximately 2 to 4 weeks after treatment and hair usually begins to return 3 to 6 months later.[2] There are several causes for alopecia, some of which are listed in Table 140.1. In addition, multiple other animal models are being developed to characterize alopecia that is associated with different chemotherapeutic agents.[6] Specifically, doxorubicin has been shown to inhibit angiogenesis in a mouse model, which may play a role in alopecia.

Some malignancies have been directly linked to alopecia. Mixed reports have appeared, indicating an association of prostate cancer with male pattern baldness. Some studies have shown that the risk of prostate cancer is as high as 50% in men who have male pattern baldness.[7] Conversely, other studies have found no association between male pattern baldness and prostate cancer. In addition, follicular mycosis fungoides, a rare disease associated with a poor prognosis, should be differentiated from alopecia mucinosa when considered in the setting of alopecia. These illnesses should be carefully considered when a patient presents with hair loss.

DIAGNOSIS

The diagnosis of alopecia should begin with a thorough history and physical examination. Patients should be asked about the onset of alopecia. Drug-induced alopecia can be differentiated by considering the time elapsed since medication was initiated and alopecia started. In addition, the pattern of the hair loss should be considered as a physical finding that can help in etiology of the hair loss. Clinical examination revealing bitemporal recessions can help to narrow the diagnosis between telogen effluvium and androgenetic alopecia.

TABLE 140.1

Etiologic Classification of Alopecia

Telogen effluvium
Anagen effluvium
Follicular mucinosis (anecdotal reports)
Acute myeloid leukemia
Squamous cell cancer of tongue
T-cell lymphoma
Lung cancer
Alopecia neoplastica (anecdotal reports)
Breast cancer
Gastric cancer
Trophoblastic tumor
Androgenetic alopecia

Several tests can be conducted if a diagnosis of telogen effluvium is being considered. A blood workup should include, but not be limited to, blood count, thyroid function studies, rapid plasma reagin, Venereal Disease Research Laboratory, antinuclear antibody, and zinc or other nutritional deficiencies. In addition, clinical tests can determine whether the patient exhibits telogen effluvium such as hair-pull test and phototrichogram.

The most important test that helps to differentiate chronic telogen effluvium and androgenetic alopecia is the 4-mm punch biopsy. Biopsy is used to obtain a ratio of the amount of hair that is in anagen and telogen. This test has a diagnostic accuracy of 98%.[5] In addition, a biopsy helps to differentiate between a follicular mycosis fungoides and metastatic tumor.

TREATMENT

Several treatments in varying stages of research and with varying efficacies can be used in the treatment of chemotherapy-induced alopecia (Table 140.2). They include scalp cooling, minoxidil, immunomodulator ammonium trichloro-9-dioxoethlyene-O,O′-tellurate (AS101), scalp tourniquet, α-tocopherol, pulsed electrostatic fields (ETG), and various immunomodulating compounds. The therapies fall into three general modes: decreasing blood flow to the scalp, pharmacologically protecting the hair bulb, and inactivating the chemotherapeutic agent locally.

The amount of chemotherapy that reaches the scalp can be reduced in two ways: a scalp tourniquet or scalp hypothermia.

TABLE 140.2

Therapeutic Interventions in Alopecia

Decrease local delivery
  Scalp tourniquet
  Scalp hypothermia

Protection of the hair bulb
  Topical minoxidil
  AS101
  α-Tocopherol

Inhibitors of cyclin-dependent kinase
  Thiol solution

Inactivate chemotherapy locally
  ImuVert
  Epidermal growth factor and fibroblast growth factor
  Topical cyclosporine
  Interleukin-1
  Topical calcitriol
  Liposome-entrapped monoclonal antibody
  Pulsed electrostatic field

Both methods induce vasoconstriction of superficial scalp vessels. For these methods to be effective, the chemotherapeutic agents must have short half-lives and rapid clearance of the drug and its metabolites.

Scalp tourniquets were first used in 1966. They are pneumatic devices placed around the hairline and inflated to a pressure greater than the systolic blood pressure while the patient is receiving the chemotherapy infusion. Several studies have been reported using scalp tourniquets that revealed their effectiveness in preventing hair loss; however, the studies are difficult to interpret due to inadequate sample size, inconsistent criteria of assessing alopecia, and differences in chemotherapy regimens. Side effects of the scalp tourniquet include nerve compression and headaches.[4]

Scalp hypothermia (i.e., scalp cooling), first used in 1978, decreases blood flow to the scalp and may slow uptake of the chemotherapeutic agent by the hair follicles. Several devices, such as bags of ice, molded gel packs, and thermocirculator devices, can be used to achieve scalp hypothermia; however, it is believed that the scalp temperature must be decreased to at least 24°C to effectively prevent alopecia. A common side effect is patient discomfort from heavy caps. Several concerns have been raised about the use of scalp hypothermia in those with liver dysfunction or in hematologic malignancies including leukemia and lymphoma, as well as a concern about the possibility of developing scalp metastases. More recent studies have found that hypothermia was effective, and several studies found no increased incidence of scalp metastases.[8,9] A trial with 238 patients taking docetaxel found that scalp cooling reduced the risk of alopecia by 78%. The most common adverse event was sensation of cold.[10] A study of 1,411 patients found that 50% of patients had good hair preservation. The study also showed positive benefits for almost all patients, except those using the taxotere, adriamycin, and cyclophosphamide regimen.[11]

There are currently no approved or effective pharmacologic treatments for chemotherapy-induced alopecia. Several different medications may reduce or prevent alopecia by pharmacologically protecting the hair bulb from the damaging effects of chemotherapy. These medications include AS101, topical minoxidil, α-tocopherol, thiol, and inhibitors of cyclin-dependent kinase (CDK).

AS101 is a synthetic compound that is structurally similar to cisplatin. Studies initially done with mice revealed that AS101 works as an immunomodulator by stimulating production of interleukin (IL)-1, IL-2, IL-6, colony-stimulating factor, and tumor necrosis factor, thereby potentially being used to minimize cytotoxicity. The mechanism of AS101 may be due to IL-1 because there is an inverse correlation between IL-1 and alopecia.[12] An open-label prospective randomized trial with 44 patients who had unresectable or metastatic nonsmall-cell lung cancer and were receiving carboplatin and etoposide revealed a significant reduction in neutropenia and thrombocytopenia as well as chemotherapy-induced alopecia.[13]

Topical minoxidil has been used for the treatment of androgenetic alopecia and alopecia areata. Two randomized trials have been performed in patients with cancer. The first was in 48 patients with many different solid tumors who were receiving doxorubicin-containing regimens. Minoxidil 2% twice a day did not prevent alopecia as compared with placebo.[14] A second randomized trial with 22 women being treated for breast cancer also found that topical minoxidil did not prevent alopecia; however, there was a statistically significant difference (favoring minoxidil) in the interval from maximal hair loss to first regrowth. Thus, the period of baldness was shortened in the minoxidil group.[15]

Oral α-tocopherol showed some degree of protection from doxorubicin-induced alopecia. α-Tocopherol was tested prospectively in two trials of patients with cancer who were receiving doxorubicin. In both trials, oral α-tocopherol did not prevent alopecia.[16,17]

Several different immunomodulators have been studied for the treatment of alopecia by inactivating the chemotherapy locally.

PRACTICE OF ONCOLOGY

These include ImuVert, epidermal growth factor (EGF) and fibroblast growth factor (FGF), IL-1, topical calcitriol, topical cyclosporine, and liposome-entrapped monoclonal antibodies. All of these agents have been studied only in vitro and in animal models, with no translation into clinical practice.

ImuVert is a biologic response modifier that was initially developed to perform immunomodulating or immunorestorative properties for malignancies and other diseases in which immune system dysfunction is implicated. It is produced by the bacterium *Serratia marcescens*. The mechanism of action is unclear; however, it induces many cytokines, including IL-1, tumor necrosis factor, interferon-α, IL-6, granulocyte macrophage–colony-stimulating factor, and platelet-derived growth factor. In rat studies, ImuVert showed almost complete protection against cytosine arabinoside and doxorubicin-induced alopecia, but offered no protection against cyclophosphamide-induced alopecia. Dose-limiting side-effects were hypotension and flu-like symptoms. No human studies have been reported to date.[18]

Several studies in rat models have been done with other biologic response modifiers, including FGF, EGF, and IL-1. FGF given systemically provided relief only from cytarabine at the site of injection. Topical EGF provided protection in the treated area. EGF given systemically provided relief from cytarabine- but not cyclophosphamide-induced alopecia.[4] Animal studies with IL-1 revealed that it is a potent inhibitor of cytarabine-induced alopecia, in a mechanism similar to that of ImuVert. There was no protective effect with IL-1 on cyclophosphamide-induced alopecia.[18] These results led to the hypothesis that there may be different mechanisms for inducing alopecia, depending on whether the chemotherapeutic agent is cell-cycle specific or cell-cycle nonspecific.

Epidermal growth factor receptor inhibitors may also play a role in reducing the incidence of alopecia. A secondary analysis of nine clinical trials showed that patients taking gefitinib or erlotinib had a lower incidence of alopecia. However, this effect is only noted in small molecule inhibitors as epidermal growth factor receptor–neutralizing antibodies (cetuximab and panitumumab) did not show a similar effect.[19]

Cyclosporine A administered topically protected newborn rats from alopecia induced by cytarabine, etoposide, and a cyclophosphamide plus doxorubicin combination at the site of application. Cyclosporine is a potent inhibitor of P-glycoprotein, as well as a hypertrichotic agent. The mechanism of action is unknown; however, it is thought that it may protect the hair follicle keratinocytes from chemotherapy by the expression of P-glycoprotein.[20]

A study done with a topical liposome-entrapped monoclonal antibody (MAD11) against doxorubicin-induced alopecia revealed that in 31 of 45 rats, alopecia was completely prevented.[21] No human studies have been done with this agent. In addition, this agent would have very little benefit in chemotherapy-induced alopecia from other agents.

Another area of interest that is being investigated is cell-cycle arrest by inhibition of CDK2. Several preclinical models have explored the role of topical small-molecule inhibitors of CDK2. In the neonatal rat chemotherapy-induced alopecia model, the application of the topical CDK2 inhibitor led to areas of less hair loss in 33% to 50% of the animals.[22]

Topical calcitriol (1,25-dihydroxyvitamin D$_3$) has been evaluated in rat models and found to prevent alopecia from a cyclophosphamide-doxorubicin regimen or cyclophosphamide-etoposide regimen. At a dose of 0.2 mcg topical calcitriol, the protection was noted over the entire animal and not just at the site of topical application.[23] However, a phase 1 trial of topical calcitriol in 14 patients with breast cancer showed no efficacy in preventing alopecia.[24]

A pilot project using ETGs was undertaken, with 13 women receiving chemotherapy with cyclophosphamide, methotrexate, and 5-fluorouracil for breast carcinoma. All patients were treated for 12 minutes twice weekly with an ETG. Twelve of the thirteen women had good hair retention throughout the chemotherapy period and afterward. No side effects were reported. The mechanism of ETG is unknown. Randomized, double-blind control studies should be developed using ETG for chemotherapy-induced alopecia.[25]

Inhibition of apoptosis by p53 and caspase is another area of interest that is being explored. Unfortunately, there are drawbacks to each of these experimental theories. Inhibition of caspase has been tested only in etoposide animal models and p53 inhibition would not affect alopecia that is independent of p53. Further studies in this area may yield drugs that have a wider profile, which in the topical setting may be of greater benefit.[2]

Radiation-induced alopecia can be just as concerning for patients as chemotherapy-induced alopecia. One agent that is currently being explored for radiation-induced alopecia is tempol gel. This is a topical agent that has shown efficacy in animal models. Specifically, this agent is a nitroxide that has protective properties in vitro against free radical compounds. In addition, there was no decrease in tumor control in mice. The agent, applied prior to radiation treatments, has been shown to be well tolerated in a phase 1 trial in patients who were found to have metastatic lesions to the brain. Some of the patients in this study were found to have protection against radiation.[26] These results are being further evaluated by ongoing phase 2 trials.

REFERENCES

1. Dorr VJ. A practitioner's guide to cancer-related alopecia. *Semin Oncol* 1998;25:562–570.
2. Wang J, Lu Z, Au JL. Protection against chemotherapy-induced alopecia. *Pharm Res* 2006;23:2505–2514.
3. Tosti A, Pazzaglia M, Starace M, et al. Alopecia areata during treatment with biologic agents. *Arch Dermatol* 2006;142:1653–1654.
4. Hussein AM. Chemotherapy-induced alopecia: new developments. *South Med J* 1993;86:489–496.
5. Harrison S, Sinclair R. Telogen effluvium. *Clin Exp Dermatol* 2002;27:389–395.
6. Amoh Y, Li L, Katsuoka K, et al. Chemotherapy targets the hair-follicle vascular network but not the stem cells. *J Invest Dermatol* 2007;127:11–15.
7. Hawk E, Breslow RA, Graubard BI. Male pattern baldness and clinical prostate cancer in epidemiological follow-up of the first National Health and Nutrition Examination Survey. *Cancer Epidemiol Biomarkers Prev* 2000;9:523–527.
8. Protiere C, Katrin E, Camerlo J, et al. Efficacy and tolerance of a scalp-cooling system for prevention of hair loss and the experience of breast cancer patients treated by adjuvant chemotherapy. *Support Care Cancer* 2002;10:529–537.
9. Ridderheim M, Bjurberg M, Gustavsson A. Scalp hypothermia to prevent chemotherapy-induced alopecia is effective and safe: a pilot study of a new digitized scalp-cooling system used in 74 patients. *Support Care Cancer* 2003;11:371–377.
10. Betticher DC, Delmore G, Breitenstein U, et al. Efficacy and tolerability of two scalp cooling systems for the prevention of alopecia associated with docetaxel treatment. *Support Care Cancer* 2013;21:2565–2573.
11. van den Hurk CJ, Peerbooms M, van de Poll-Franse LV, et al. Scalp cooling for hair preservation and associated characteristics in 1441 chemotherapy patients – results of the Dutch Scalp Cooling Registry. *Acta Oncol* 2012;51:497–504.
12. Sredni B, Xu RH, Albeck M, et al. The protective role of the immunomodulator AS101 against chemotherapy-induced alopecia studies on human and animal models. *Int J Cancer* 1996;65:97–103.
13. Sredni B, Albeck M, Tichler T, et al. Bone marrow-sparing and prevention of alopecia by AS101 in non–small-cell lung cancer patients treated with carboplatin and etoposide. *J Clin Oncol* 1995;13:2342–2353.
14. Rodriguez R, Machiavelli M, Leone B, et al. Minoxidil (Mx) as a prophylaxis of doxorubicin-induced alopecia. *Ann Oncol* 1994;5:769–770.
15. Duvic M, Lemak NA, Valero V, et al. A randomized trial of minoxidil in chemotherapy-induced alopecia. *J Am Acad Dermatol* 1996;35:74–78.
16. Martin-Jiminez M, Diaz-Rubio E, Gonzalez L, et al. Failure of high-dose tocopherol to prevent alopecia induced by doxorubicin. *N Engl J Med* 1986;315:894–895.

17. Perez JE, Macchiavelli M, Leone BA, et al. High-dose alpha-tocopherol as a preventative of doxorubicin-induced alopecia. *Cancer Treat Rep* 1986; 70:1213–1214.

18. Hussein AM. Interleukin 1 protects against 1-beta-D-arabinofuranosylcytosine-induced alopecia in the newborn rat model. *Cancer Res* 1991;51:3329–3330.

19. Bichsel KJ, Gogia N, Malouff T, et al. Role for the epidermal growth factor receptor in chemotherapy-induced alopecia. *PLoS One* 2013;8: e69368.

20. Hussein AM, Stuart A, Peters WP. Protection against chemotherapy induced alopecia by cyclosporine A in the newborn rat model. *Dermatology* 1995; 190:192–196.

21. Balsari AL, Morelli D, Menard S, et al. Protections against doxorubicin induced alopecia in rats by liposome-entrapped monoclonal antibodies. *FASEB J* 1994;8:226–230.

22. Davis ST, Benson BG, Bramson HN, et al. Prevention of chemotherapy-induced alopecia in rats by CDK inhibitors. *Science* 2001;291: 134–137.

23. Jimenenz JJ, Yunis AA. Protection from chemotherapy-induced alopecia by 1,25-dihydroxyvitamin D3. *Cancer Res* 1992;52:5123–5125.

24. Hidalgo M, Rinaldi D, Medina G, et al. A phase I trial of topical topitriol (calcitriol, 1,25-dihydroxyvitamin D3) to prevent chemotherapy-induced alopecia. *Anticancer Drugs* 1999;10:393–395.

25. Benjamin B, Ziginskas D, Harman J, et al. Pulsed electrostatic field (ETG) to reduce hair loss in women undergoing chemotherapy for breast carcinoma: a pilot study. *Psychooncology* 2002;11:244–248.

26. Metz JM, Smith D, Mick R, et al. A phase I study of topical Tempol for the prevention of alopecia induced by whole brain radiotherapy. *Clin Cancer Res* 2004;10:6411–6417.

PRACTICE OF ONCOLOGY

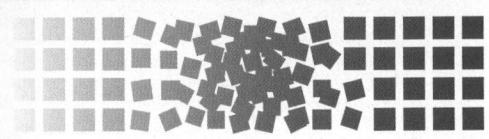

141 Gonadal Dysfunction

George Patounakis, Alan H. DeCherney, and Alicia Y. Armstrong

INTRODUCTION

The increased survival associated with oncologic treatment has made the late-term effects, such as gonadal failure, increasingly important. When the cancer is controlled, quality of life, which often includes the ability to have a normal child, then becomes a major issue.[1,2] Currently, the 5-year survival rate of childhood cancer is over 80%, and more than about 75% will have a 10-year survival.[3] Furthermore, the number of women less than 45 years old, and thus likely premenopausal, who are estimated to be diagnosed with breast cancer in 2013 is 24,430.[4] These statistics signify that gonadal dysfunction from the effects of treatment is becoming even more important.

Both neoplastic disease and its treatment can interfere with normal sexual and reproductive function (Table 141.1). Testicular and ovarian cancers directly involve the gonad and prostate, endometrial, and cervical cancers directly involve the reproductive tract. Surgical treatment for any of these diseases results in damage or loss of these important reproductive organs. Retroperitoneal lymph node dissection (RPLND) for testicular and colon cancer, prostatectomy, and surgery involving the bladder neck may result in loss of the ability to ejaculate. Primary and metastatic tumors in the hypothalamus and pituitary can directly affect gonadotropin secretion, resulting in secondary hypogonadism. Both chemotherapy and radiation cause toxic effects on the male and female gonads. Cytotoxic therapies delivered to women during pregnancy can have teratogenic effects on the fetus. If fertility is maintained or recovers, there remains the concern about the heritability of cancer and at least a theoretical risk of mutagenic alterations to germ cells caused by cytotoxic therapies. The literature on the safety of male reproduction just after and during treatment is still unclear largely because of methodologic differences and different end points assessed by studies.[5] More well-controlled studies are needed in this area to address these concerns. A recent large study of 3,915 cancer survivors looked at adverse birth outcomes of congenital anomalies, preterm birth, perinatal death, and low birth weight.[6] For the offspring of male cancer survivors, they did not find any differences versus controls. For female survivors, there was an increased risk of the preterm birth and low birth weight. They did not find a difference in major congenital abnormalities for either male or female survivors. Another recent retrospective study drawing data from the Childhood Cancer Survivor Study of 4,699 children of male and female cancer survivors showed a prevalence of 2.7% of congenital anomalies, which is similar to the 3% prevalence of congenital anomalies in the United States.[7] Based on these two recent studies, patients receiving cancer treatments can be counseled that it will not affect their offspring in terms of congenital abnormalities.

The reproductive consequences of cancer potentially affect a large number of patients in the United States. Between the years 2006 and 2010, there were 175,214 people between the ages of birth and 45 years old that were diagnosed with cancer in the United States.[8] Of these, 20,506 were diagnosed between the ages of birth and 19 years old. Both males and females share the burden of cancer development from birth to 39 years of age, with males having a risk of cancer in that age group of 1 in 69, whereas females have a risk of 1 in 46.[9] In women, the risk of developing breast cancer specifically within this age range is 1 in 202. The creation of patient advocacy groups such as RESOLVE and LIVESTRONG both underscore the importance of these issues. Furthermore, quality of life committees in professional oncology groups also support the importance of issues such as these to cancer patients.

This chapter will first review the effects of cytotoxic agents in men, women, and children. Next, the effects of cranial irradiation with respect to gonadal dysfunction will be addressed. Subsequently, the preservation of fertility in males and females will be reviewed in the context of both standard of clinical care and experimental technologies. Finally, the genetic and pregnancy outcome concerns after treatment will be addressed.

EFFECTS OF CYTOTOXIC AGENTS ON ADULT MEN

Biologic Considerations

The testis consists of the seminiferous (or germinal) epithelium arranged in tubules and endocrine components (testosterone-producing Leydig cells) in the interstitial region between the tubules. The seminiferous tubules contain the germ cells, which consist of stem and differentiating spermatogonia, spermatocytes, spermatids, sperm, and the Sertoli cells, which support and regulate germ cell differentiation. The testicular vasculature is permeable, and drugs can freely reach the Leydig and Sertoli cells and the spermatogonia, which are at the outer rim of the tubules. Many chemotherapeutic drugs may penetrate the Sertoli cell barrier, albeit at a lower intensity, and damage late-stage germ cells.[10]

Among the germ cells, the differentiating spermatogonia proliferate most actively and are extremely susceptible to cytotoxic agents. In contrast, the Leydig and Sertoli cells, which do not proliferate in adults, survive most cytotoxic therapies. These cells, however, may suffer functional damage. Frequently, after cytotoxic therapies, germ cells appear to be absent and the tubules contain only Sertoli cells, a state described as *germinal aplasia*. This could be a result of killing of the spermatogenic stem cells, the loss of the ability of the somatic cells to support the differentiation of a few surviving stem cells, or a combination of the two.

After cytotoxic treatment, sperm count diminishes with a time course that depends on the sensitivities of the different spermatogenic cells and their kinetics of maturation to sperm.[11] Because the later-stage germ cells (spermatocytes onward) are relatively insensitive to killing and progress through spermatogenesis, sperm count is not immediately affected. However, these later-stage cells are susceptible to the induction of mutagenic damage, and studies in rodents have shown they can transmit mutations induced in their DNA to the next generation.[12] The eventual recovery of

TABLE 141.1

Impact of Cancer and Cancer Therapy on the Reproductive System

Tumor	Direct gonadal involvement Reproductive tract involvement Hypothalamic and pituitary involvement Concern about heritability of cancer susceptibility
Surgery	Removal of gonad Genital mutilation Failure of emission and retrograde ejaculation Impotence and loss of orgasm
Radiotherapy or chemotherapy	Germ cell depletion Loss of gonadal hormones Mutagenic changes in germ cells Teratogenic effects on fetus
Chemotherapy	Seminal transmission of drug
Radiotherapy (cranial)	Loss of gonadotropic hormones

sperm production depends on the survival of the spermatogonial stem cells and their ability to differentiate. Surviving stem cells can remain in the testis but fail to differentiate to sperm for several years after cytotoxic insult.[13] It is important to note that human studies have not necessarily shown an increased rate of congenital anomalies.[6,7]

The loss of germ cells has secondary effects on the hypothalamic–pituitary–gonadal axis. Inhibin secretion by the Sertoli cells declines, and because inhibin limits follicle-stimulating hormone (FSH) secretion by the pituitary, serum FSH rises. Germinal aplasia reduces testis size, and testicular blood flow is consequently reduced, which results in the distribution of less testosterone into the circulation (Table 141.2).[14] Because testosterone is a negative regulator of luteinizing hormone (LH) secretion by the pituitary, and LH is the primary stimulator of testosterone synthesis by the Leydig cells, LH increases to maintain constant serum testosterone levels.

Characteristics of Gonadal Toxicity

Although subnormal semen profiles, ejaculatory dysfunction, and low libido can often be results of cancer treatment, a thorough examination should be done to determine whether symptoms of these problems might have been present before treatment. A sexual and reproductive history should be taken, including information on developmental factors such as ages at testicular descent and puberty; surgery or injury to the genitals; diseases that might affect reproduction; drug, chemical, or heat exposure; and pretreatment fertility and libido status. A physical examination should consist of an examination of the testicles and secondary sexual

characteristics such as beard and hair distribution pattern. If there are indications, a semen analysis and a hormone profile should be done and results should be compared with normal values (see Table 141.2).

Cytotoxic therapies in the form of chemotherapy or radiation can have varying effects on the sperm quantity and quality. A recent study of testicular germ cell cancer patients looked at patients treated with less than or equal to two cycles of chemotherapy, more than two cycles of chemotherapy, and irradiation.[15] For all three groups, the sperm count nadir was at 3 months posttreatment. This is expected because it is the time required for differentiating spermatogonia to become sperm. In the group of patients treated with two or less of bleomycin, etoposide, and cisplatin (BEP), the sperm counts returned to pretreatment levels by 12 months, whereas in the other two groups, it took 24 months to return to pretreatment levels. Another recent study shows similar results with the beginning of normalization of seminal parameters by approximately 18 months posttreatment.[16]

The induced azoospermia can be either temporary or prolonged, depending on the survival of stem spermatogonia and their ability to proliferate, differentiate, and produce spermatozoa, which in turn depends on the nature of the cytotoxic agent and dose (Table 141.3).[17–20] If treatment is limited to the cytotoxic agents that do not kill stem spermatogonia or block their differentiation, normospermia is usually restored within 3 months after the cytotoxic therapy. However, if agents that kill stem spermatogonia or affect differentiation are used, longer periods of azoospermia ensue.[13,21]

To evaluate the effects of cytotoxic therapy, one must consider the initial gonadal status. Men with testicular germ cell tumors have impaired semen quality even before cytotoxic therapy is instituted. Approximately 65% are oligospermic (counts <20 million/mL) and approximately 20% are azoospermic,[22] whereas the values are 9% and 1%, respectively, in control populations. In half of the patients with reduced semen quality, this impaired testicular function is a result of abnormalities in the remaining gonad, such as carcinoma in situ or a history of cryptorchidism. In the other half, it may be a result of reversible factors such as chorionic gonadotropin production by the tumor with resulting increases in estradiol levels or the trauma of the recent orchiectomy.[23] In addition, emission and ejaculation may have been compromised by earlier RPLND so that the sperm density may not accurately reflect gonadal function.[24] In contrast to the severe dysfunction seen in cases of testicular cancer, in Hodgkin's lymphoma, between 16% and 50% of patients are oligospermic, only 2% to 8% are azoospermic, and the distribution of counts in the remainder is not significantly different from normal.[25,26] Poor semen quality was more prevalent in patients with advanced than with early-stage Hodgkin's lymphoma, but specific risk factors have not been identified. In patients with other lymphomas and sarcomas, pretreatment sperm counts tend to be normal except for similar modest increases in the incidence of oligospermia.[13,21]

The age at treatment is not a major factor in recovery from gonadal damage in men. Most studies have failed to show any age effect,[13,21] but a few have indicated increased testicular damage after cytotoxic therapy in older men.[27]

TABLE 141.2

Typical Clinical and Laboratory Features for Diagnosis of Male Reproductive Dysfunction

	Testis Size		Serum Hormone Levels			
	Length × Width (cm)	Volume (mL)	Sperm Count (Millions/mL)	Follicle-Stimulating Hormone (mIU/mL)	Hormone (mIU/mL)	Testosterone (ng/dL)
Normal men	5.0 × 3.0	15–25	20 to >100	1–12	2–12	300–1,200
Germinal aplasia	3.7 × 2.3	8–15	0	>20	>12	200–700

PRACTICE OF ONCOLOGY

TABLE 141.3

Effects of Different Antitumor Agents on Sperm Production in Men

Agents (Cumulative Dose for Effect)	Effect
Radiation (2.5 Gy to testis)	Prolonged azoospermia
Chlorambucil (1.4 g/m^2)	
Cyclophosphamide (19 g/m^2)	
Procarbazine (4 g/m^2)	
Melphalan (140 mg/m^2)	
Cisplatin (500 mg/m^2)	
BCNU (1 g/m^2)	Azoospermia in adulthood after treatment before puberty
CCNU (500 mg/m^2)	
Busulfan (600 mg/kg)	Azoospermia likely, but always given with other highly sterilizing agents
Ifosfamide (42 g/m^2)	
BCNU (300 mg/m^2)	
Nitrogen mustard	
Actinomycin D	
Carboplatin (2 g/m^2)	Prolonged azoospermia not often observed at indicated dose
Doxorubicin (Adriamycin) (770 mg/m^2)	Can be additive with previous agents in causing prolonged azoospermia, but cause only temporary reductions in sperm count when not combined with previous agents
ThioTEPA (400 mg/m^2)	
Cytosine arabinoside (1 g/m^2)	
Vinblastine (50 g/m^2)	
Vincristine (8 g/m^2)	
Amsacrine, bleomycin, dacarbazine, daunorubicin, epirubicin, etoposide, fludarabine, 5-fluorouracil, 6-mercaptopurine, methotrexate, mitoxantrone, thioguanine	Only temporary reductions in sperm count at doses used in conventional regimens, but additive effects are possible
Prednisone	Unlikely to affect sperm production
Interferon-α	No effects on sperm production

BCNU, carmustine; CCNU, lomustine.

Individual Drugs

The most sterilizing drugs are the alkylating agents (with the exception of dacarbazine) and cisplatin. The cumulative dose appears to be more important than the dose rate in determining whether sperm production will recover (see Tables 141.3 and 141.4). Chlorambucil[28] and cyclophosphamide[29] induce prolonged azoospermia when given alone. The gonadal toxicities of other agents have generally been deduced from the effects of combination regimens; the doses given might be underestimates because there may be additive contributions from other drugs in the regimen. Procarbazine[30] and cisplatin in high doses[31] are also highly sterilizing. Busulfan has an additive effect on the sterility resulting from cyclophosphamide treatment.[32] The addition of high doses of ifosfamide (46 g/m^2) to cisplatin-containing chemotherapy regimens significantly reduced the recovery of spermatogenic function.[33] Carboplatin, an analog of cisplatin, appeared in the same combination regimens to produce less sterility than cisplatin.[22] The treatment of boys with carmustine (BCNU) and lomustine (CCNU) produced prolonged azoospermia,[34] and it is likely, but not proven, that the same would occur in adults. The agents that have only temporary effects were also identified from single-agent and combination chemotherapy regimens.

Radiation Therapy

The effects of radiation on the testes depend on the fractionation regimen. Whereas in all other organ systems, fractionation of radiation reduces the damage, radiation doses to the germinal epithelium of the testis given in 3- to 7-week fractionated courses cause more gonadal damage than single doses.[35] In the usual fractionated regimens, doses to the testes above 0.15 Gy are required to produce any reduction in sperm count. Doses between 0.15 and 0.5 Gy cause oligospermia.[36] Above 0.6 Gy, azoospermia occurs. The duration of azoospermia is dose dependent, and recovery can begin within 1 year after doses of less than 1 Gy, but not until more than 2 years after delivery of 2 Gy. Cumulative doses of fractionated radiotherapy of more than 2.5 Gy generally result in prolonged and likely permanent azoospermia. However, after a single dose of 8 Gy or fractionated doses of 10 to 13 Gy, given as total body irradiation in preparation for bone marrow transplantation, sometimes also with cyclophosphamide (4.5 g/m^2), spermatogenesis eventually recovers in 15% of the patients.[20]

Testicular androgen production is relatively resistant to irradiation: doses of over 18 Gy are required before an effect is evident,

TABLE 141.4

Probability of Germinal Aplasia in Men Treated with Different Combination Chemotherapy Regimens

Regimen	Disease	Courses or Dose	Patients with Prolonged Azoospermia (%)
High-Dose or Moderately High-Dose Alkylating Agents			
MOPPd or MVPPd	Hodgkin's lymphoma	≥6 courses	85
CyOPPd	Hodgkin's lymphoma	4–9 courses	100
I, Pl, A, Mx	Osteosarcoma	I = 46 g/m^2 Pl = 560 mg/m^2	75
BuCy + HSCT	Leukemia, lymphoma	Cy = 4.4 g/m^2	50
BuTT + HSCT		Bu = 600 mg/m^2 or TT = 400 mg/m^2	
BcECaMl + HSCT	Lymphoma	Bc = 300 mg/m^2 Ml = 140 mg/m^2 + prior treatment	100
MOPPd/ABVD	Hodgkin's lymphoma	6–9 courses	50
CyOPPd/ABVD, X	Hodgkin's lymphoma	6–9 courses	85
ChlVPPd/EVA	Hodgkin's lymphoma	6–8 courses	95
CyHOPd-Bleo	Lymphoma	Cy < 9.5 g/m^2 Cy > 9.5 g/m^2	17 50
E, Ep, B, Cy, Pd (VEBEP)	Hodgkin's lymphoma	Cy = 8 g/m^2	40
CyVAD or CyAD	Sarcoma	Cy < 7.5 g/m^2 Cy >7.5 g/m^2	30 90
Nonalkylating or Low-Dose Alkylating Agent			
Cy, A, Mx	Sarcoma	Cy = 5.6 g/m^2	20
MOPPd	Hodgkin's lymphoma	2 courses	0
ABVD, X	Hodgkin's lymphoma	6 courses	0
NOVPd, X	Hodgkin's lymphoma	3 courses	0
Bc, Cy, Ca, L, Mp, TG	Leukemia	Cy = 5.1 g/m^2	0
Platinum			
PlVB	Testicular cancer	Pl ≤ 400 mg/m^2 400 mg/m^2	10 50
PlVB-I	Testicular cancer	Pl ≤ 400 mg/m^2 I = 30 g/m^2	55
PlEB	Testicular cancer	Pl ≤ 300 mg/m^2 Pl = 400 mg/m^2	0 25
CbEB	Testicular cancer	Cb = 1.6 g/m^2	20
Pl, A, D	Osteosarcoma	Pl < 600 mg/m^2 Pl ≥ 600 mg/m^2	5 55

M, mechlorethamine (nitrogen mustard); O, vincristine (Oncovin); P, procarbazine; Pd, prednisone; V, vinblastine; I, ifosfamide; Pl, cisplatin; A, doxorubicin (Adriamycin); Mx, methotrexate; B, bleomycin; Cy, cyclophosphamide; Bu, busulfan; HSCT, hematopoietic stem cell transplantation; TT, thioTEPA; E, etoposide; Ca, cytosine arabinoside; Ml, melphalan; Bc, BCNU (carmustine); X, radiotherapy; Bleo, bleomycin; Cb, carboplatin; Chl, chlorambucil; D, dacarbazine; Ep, epirubicin; H, doxorubicin; L,l-asparaginase; Mp, 6-mercaptopurine; N, mitoxantrone (Novantrone); TG, thioguanine.

and major damage does not occur until the dose exceeds 30 Gy.[37] The radiation-associated impotence after such treatments is likely a result of vascular damage.

Combination Regimens

The sterilizing potential of each combination chemotherapy or chemotherapy plus radiotherapy regimen is the additive effects of the doses of the individual agents given (see Table 141.3); there is no evidence for synergistic interactions between the agents. Although it is impossible to predict whether sperm production

in any given man will recover, the probability of prolonged azoospermia has been determined for many combinations (see Table 141.4). The sterilizing potential of new regimens can be predicted from the information in Table 141.3 and the results found with similar combinations. The additive effects of agents can be seen in the case of cyclophosphamide: When cyclophosphamide is given alone, 19 g/m^2 is required to produce prolonged sterility in half the men, but only 15 g/m^2 is required when cyclophosphamide is given with a median doxorubicin dose of 450 mg/m^2 in the cyclophosphamide, doxorubicin, vincristine, and prednisone (CHOP) regimen, and only 11 mg/m^2 is required when it is given with a median doxorubicin dose of 880 mg/m^2 in the cyclophosphamide, vincristine, doxorubicin, and dacarbazine (CY[V]ADIC) regimen.[13,21]

EFFECTS OF CYTOTOXIC AGENTS ON ADULT WOMEN

Biologic Considerations

Gonadal cell kinetics in women are opposite to those in men: the germ cells are nonproliferative, whereas the somatic cells proliferate. Female germ cells only proliferate prenatally, and by birth, are arrested at the oocyte stage. At birth, there are 1 million oocytes, which are reduced to 300,000 at puberty and to fewer than 1,000 oocytes when menopause occurs at approximately age 50 years.[38]

Before recruitment to the process leading to ovulation, oocytes are found in primordial follicles with few pregranulosa cells, surrounded by theca cells of the ovarian stroma. The stimulus for the initiation of follicular maturation depends on local growth factors, not the gonadotropic hormones. Once a follicle is recruited into growth, it develops until it either degenerates or ovulates. Follicular maturation is characterized by proliferation of granulosa cells and the development of steroidogenic potential of both the theca and granulosa cells. Estrogen production involves the stimulation of both these cell types by LH and FSH and causes the LH surge that triggers ovulation. The cyclic variations in FSH, LH, and estradiol are essential for menstrual cycles and reproduction.

Because the destruction of oocytes results in loss of follicles, germ cell loss leads directly to estrogen insufficiency. Radiation and chemotherapy appear to cause this germ cell loss by direct apoptotic action on the oocytes in mouse models.[39] Although the direct action on oocytes may be the dominant mechanism in the most gonadotoxic agents, other mechanisms such as effects on granulosa cells, surrounding stroma, and blood vessels may indirectly affect the oocyte.[40] When maturing follicles are destroyed by cytotoxic therapy, the result is oligomenorrhea or temporary amenorrhea. If the number of primordial follicles is reduced below the minimum necessary for menstrual cyclicity, irreversible *ovarian failure* and menopause (>12 months without a menstrual period) occur.

Characteristics of Gonadal Toxicity

Because the size of the germ cell population in women cannot be determined, menstrual and reproductive histories are important in assessing the effects of cytotoxic therapy on ovarian function. Information on the patient's sexual function and menstrual histories during and after therapy is particularly useful (Table 141.5).[41] Because the mechanisms of temporary and irreversible treatment-related amenorrhea are different, a posttreatment follow-up must be given to evaluate the significance of the outcome. To determine if effects are related to cytotoxic therapy, pretherapy ovarian function should be evaluated from the history of menarche, menses, pregnancies, and oral contraceptive use. The symptoms of recent primary ovarian failure, including hot flashes, night sweats, insomnia, mood swings, irritability, vaginal dryness, dyspareunia, decreased libido, and bladder infection, should be recorded. Laboratory measurements of hormone levels are most definitive in the diagnosis of primary ovarian failure. FSH level is the most sensitive, but LH and estradiol levels are also useful (Table 141.5). Antimüllerian hormone (AMH), a hormone produced by growing follicles from the primary to antral stage, is another hormone that can be used to determine ovarian reserve by inferring the number of primordial follicles present. AMH has been shown to be a useful marker of ovarian reserve in both prepubertal and postpubertal girls after gonadotoxic treatments.[42] The physical symptoms and the changes in hormone levels associated with ovarian failure may be masked by oral contraceptive use or hormone replacement therapy.

Cytotoxic therapy often induces temporary amenorrhea, which may occasionally last several years.[43] Some patients with treatment-induced temporary amenorrhea do display menopausal symptoms. The permanent amenorrhea may begin during chemotherapy or, subsequently, after several years of oligomenorrhea.[44] Factors resulting in temporary amenorrhea during treatment appear to be age independent.[45] In contrast, the incidence of permanent treatment-induced amenorrhea (ovarian failure) dramatically and continuously increases with age at treatment (Tables 141.6 and 141.7), as expected from the decreasing number of follicles with increasing age.

TABLE 141.5

Periodic Evaluation: Children's Oncology Group

	Male	Female
History	Pubertal (onset, tempo) Sexual function (erections, nocturnal emissions, libido) Medication use impacting sexual function *Frequency:* Yearly	Pubertal (onset, tempo) Sexual function (vaginal dryness, libido) Medication use impacting sexual function Menstrual/pregnancy history *Frequency:* Yearly
Physical	Tanner staging Testicular volume by Prader orchidometry *Frequency:* Yearly until sexually mature	Tanner staging *Frequency:* Yearly until sexually mature
Screening	FSH LH Testosterone *Frequency:* Baseline at age 14 *and* as clinically indicated in patients with delayed puberty and/or clinical signs and symptoms of testosterone deficiency Semen analysis *Frequency:* As requested by patient and for evaluation of infertility; periodic evaluation over time recommended as resumption of spermatogenesis can occur up to 10 years after therapy	FSH LH Estradiol *Frequency:* Baseline at age 13 *and* as clinically indicated in patients with delayed puberty, irregular menses, primary or secondary amenorrhea, and/or clinical signs and symptoms of estrogen deficiency

TABLE 141.6

Effects of Different Cytotoxic Agents on Ovarian Function

Agent	Prepuberty	Age 20 Y	Age 35 Y	Age 45 Y
Cumulative Doses to Cause Permanent Ovarian Failure				
Cyclophosphamide	>48 g	20–50 g	6–10 g	5 g
Melphalan	—	>240 mg/m^2	>510 mg/m^2	340 mg/m^2
Busulfan	600 mg/m^2	<600 mg/m^2	<600 mg/m^2	—
Chlorambucil	>3 g	>1.5 g	>1 g	1 g
Mitomycin C	—	—	≥30 g	≥30 g
Radiation	12 Gy	7 Gy	3 Gy	<2 Gy
Incidence of Permanent Ovarian Failure (%)				
Cyclophosphamide (7.4 g/m^2)	0	0	60	—
Radiation (pelvic) (4–5 Gy)	<10	40	90	95
Radiation (total body irradiation) (10 Gy)	40	75	100	100

Childhood cancer survivors who retain ovarian function after treatment have an increased relative risk of 13 for developing premature menopause.[46] When women aged 13 to 19 years are treated with alkylating agent chemotherapy and radiotherapy below the diaphragm, their median age at menopause is 32 years, compared with 44 years for women treated with either radiotherapy or chemotherapy alone and 49 years for controls.[47]

Cytotoxic therapy–induced ovarian failure accelerates bone density loss. However, when only chemotherapy is used, some residual ovarian function may be present despite the menopausal state, and the rate of bone density loss is less than when pelvic radiotherapy is used.[48]

Individual Drugs

In women, as in men, alkylating agents appear to be the most likely to produce permanent gonadal failure (see Table 141.6).

TABLE 141.7

Probability of Ovarian Failure in Postmenarchal Women Treated with Combination Chemotherapy Regimens Containing Alkylating Agents

Regimen	Disease	Courses or Doses	Permanent Age (Y)	Incidence of Ovarian Failure (%)
MOPPd or MVPPd	Hodgkin's lymphoma	Approximately 6 courses P = approximately 6 g/m^2	25 35	15 85
MOPPd/ABVD	Hodgkin's lymphoma	6 courses P = 4.2 g/m^2	25	0
CyOPPd	Hodgkin's lymphoma	Cy = 8 g/m^2 P = 8 g/m^2	<24 >24	28 86
ChlVPPd/EVA	Hodgkin's lymphoma	6–8 courses P = 4 g/m^2 Chl = 300 mg/m^2	25 36	0 100
Cy (alone) + HSCT	Aplastic anemia	Cy = 7.4 g/m^2	13–58	50
BuCy + HSCT	Leukemia	Bu = 600 mg/m^2 Cy = 7.4 g/m^2	14–57	99
BuMl + HSCT	Various	Bu = 600 mg/m^2 Ml = 140 mg/m^2	9–17	100
FACy	Breast cancer	Cy = 13 g/m^2	<34 >39	0 100
CyMxF	Breast cancer	Cy = 34 g/m^2	<30 >35	0 100
CyAMx	Sarcoma	Cy = 5.3 g/m^2	<35 >40	0 100

M, mechlorethamine (nitrogen mustard); O, vincristine (Oncovin); P, procarbazine; Pd, prednisone; V, vinblastine; A, doxorubicin (Adriamycin); B, bleomycin; D, dacarbazine; Cy, cyclophosphamide; Chl, chlorambucil; E, etoposide; HSCT, hematopoietic stem cell transplantation; Bu, busulfan; F, 5-fluorouracil; Ml, melphalan; Mx, methotrexate.

The cumulative dose appears to be more important than the dose rate, as evidenced by similar incidences of ovarian failure in women who received similar total doses of cyclophosphamide, given either daily over several months[49] or within 4 days.[50] High doses of cisplatin ($\geq$600 mg/m^2) also produce permanent ovarian failure.[51] Procarbazine is likely to be highly sterilizing inasmuch as permanent ovarian failure is observed after treatment with several different procarbazine-containing combinations (see Table 141.7).

Nonalkylating agents are thought to be far less likely to induce permanent ovarian failure. No ovarian failure was observed with 5-fluorouracil (30 g),[49] methotrexate (200 g) plus vincristine (40 g),[52] etoposide (5 g),[53] or cisplatin (<450 mg/m^2) plus doxorubicin (<400 mg/m^2)[51] in women aged 15 to 35 years. Doxorubicin (300 mg/m^2), bleomycin, vincristine, and dacarbazine (ABVD) do not appear to induce ovarian failure because none was observed after this treatment of women up to age 41 years.[54]

Radiation Therapy

Radiation therapy induces permanent ovarian failure with marked age dependence in sensitivity (see Table 141.6). Irradiation of the para-aortic nodes for Hodgkin's lymphoma results in cumulative ovarian doses of only 1.5 Gy and does not appear to interfere with menstruation in most patients.[55] Total nodal irradiation for Hodgkin's lymphoma or pelvic radiation for cervical cancer results in an ovarian dose of 4 to 5 Gy when proper transposition (oophoropexy) and shielding of the ovaries are performed, which preserves fertility in some younger women.[56] Total body irradiation in preparation for bone marrow transplantation delivers 8 to 12 Gy to the gonads, which destroys ovarian function in nearly all adult women.[50,57] Ovarian damage from radiation appears to be independent of whether it is given in one or six fractions.[32]

Combination Regimens

All combinations that include procarbazine and other alkylating agents (mechlorethamin, vincristine, procarbazine, prednisone [MOPP]; CHOP; mechlorethamine, vinblastine, procarbazine, and prednisone [MVPP]; and chlorambucil, vinblastine, procarbazine, and prednisone [ChlVPP]) induce ovarian failure in almost all older women and even in some younger ones (see Table 141.7). Ovarian function is maintained better by reducing the doses of these drugs through use of the MOPP/ABVD regimen.[58] Radiation and MOPP chemotherapy have additive, but not synergistic, effects, and the combination results in a higher incidence of ovarian failure than either modality alone.[59]

Similarly, regimens containing cyclophosphamide also produce ovarian failure; however, the age dependence obscures any possible dose dependence. The treatments used for leukemia, which involve lower doses of cyclophosphamide and other agents that do not destroy primordial follicles, allow for the recovery of menses in women under the age of 35 years.[60] Combination chemotherapy regimens without alkylating agents do not produce ovarian failure.

EFFECTS OF CYTOTOXIC AGENTS ON CHILDREN

Extent of Gonadal Toxicity in Boys

The germinal epithelium in the prepubertal testis is not any more resistant to cytotoxic therapy than that in adults. When chemotherapy doses to boys are expressed appropriately on a per-meter-squared basis and radiation doses are calculated, the sterilizing effects of a variety of chemotherapy[61] and radiotherapy[62] regimens can be predicted on the basis of their effects on adult testes (see Tables 141.3 and 141.4).

As in adults, radiation; alkylating agents such as procarbazine, cyclophosphamide, chlorambucil, BCNU, and CCNU; and cisplatin are the most sterilizing and produce prolonged and sometimes permanent azoospermia.[34,51] In addition, high doses of doxorubicin and cytosine arabinoside are additive with the aforementioned agents in producing gonadal damage.[63] Regimens lacking alkylating agents, such as some used for acute lymphocytic leukemia, can even allow pubertal progression of spermatogenesis during treatment.[64]

Most chemotherapy regimens do not affect Leydig cell function, and hence, the timing of pubertal development and postpubertal testosterone levels are generally normal.[65] However, busulfan plus cyclophosphamide, used in preparation for hematopoietic stem cell transplantation, appears to delay puberty in approximately 30% of boys.[43]

Extent of Gonadal Toxicity in Girls

Prepubertal girls appear to be less susceptible than young postpubertal women to cytotoxic therapy–induced ovarian failure (see Table 141.6). Furthermore, girls treated with radiation and alkylating agents after puberty have about a 10 times greater relative risk of developing early menopause versus those treated before puberty.[66] Exposure of the ovaries to high-dose radiation, alkylating agents, and procarbazine are significant risk factors for acute ovarian failure in childhood cancer survivors.[67] Radiation is the most damaging agent to the prepubertal ovary: 20 to 30 Gy induces permanent ovarian failure in nearly all girls.[68] Doses of 8 to 15 Gy, usually with cyclophosphamide or melphalan in preparation for bone marrow transplantation, cause failure of ovarian function and pubertal development in 50% of girls,[69] with younger girls being less sensitive than older ones.[43] Radiation doses of up to 7 Gy do not cause ovarian failure or inhibit puberty[62] but can have additive effects if chemotherapy is also given.

Most chemotherapy regimens do not cause loss of primordial follicles or failure of pubertal development and menarche. This includes high doses of cyclophosphamide of up to 48 g,[70] various combination chemotherapy regimens used to treat leukemia, and the ABVD regimen for Hodgkin's lymphoma.[71] Even MOPP or nitrosourea chemotherapy does not affect pubertal and menstrual function development in 90% of girls.[62,72] However, ChlVPP produces ovarian failure in 25% of girls[73] and busulfan plus cyclophosphamide inhibits puberty in 50% of girls.[43]

Besides causing ovarian damage, irradiation for solid tumors in the abdomen (20 Gy or more for Wilms' tumor) or in preparation for hematopoietic stem cell transplantation produces irreversible damage to uterine growth and blood flow in girls.[74] This damage affects achievement and outcome of pregnancy later in life.[75] If radiation doses are not too high (approximately 10 Gy, as in total body irradiation for transplantation), sex steroid replacement can improve uterine function.

GONADAL DYSFUNCTION AFTER CRANIAL IRRADIATION

Whereas gonadal irradiation causes primary hypogonadism, cranial irradiation is associated with secondary hypogonadism because of damage to the hypothalamus or the gonadotrophs in the pituitary, or both. In patients with pituitary or suprasellar lesions, gonadotropin deficiency is often present before antineoplastic therapy; however, patients with nasopharyngeal cancer or brain tumors have normal hypothalamic–pituitary–gonadal axes until they receive therapeutic irradiation with fields encompassing the hypothalamic–pituitary areas. In contrast, none of the cancer chemotherapeutic drugs directly impairs hypothalamic or anterior pituitary function.

TABLE 141.8		
Reproductive Effects of Cranial Irradiation		
Radiation Dose to Pituitary/ Hypothalamus (Gy)	**Disease**	**Reproductive Effects**
Childhood Cancers		
18–24	Leukemia	Slightly early puberty (girls) Subtle ovulatory disorder (after puberty)
25–49	Retinoblastoma, brain tumors, face and neck cancers	Some with precocious puberty (both genders) Higher doses: delay of puberty, gonadotropin deficiency at later times, failure of puberty
>50	Brain tumors, optic glioma	Some show gonadotropin deficiency (failure to undergo puberty)
Cancers In Adults		
10–13	Leukemia	No deficiencies at <5 y
20	Pituitary tumors	LH/FSH deficiency: 30% at 5 y; 40% at 10 y
35–40	Pituitary tumors	LH/FSH deficiency: 65% at 5 y, 90% at 10 y
40–70	Brain tumors	LH/FSH deficiency: 60% at 7 y
40–70	Nasopharyngeal, paranasal sinus tumors	LH/FSH deficiency: 15%–30% at 5 y, 45% at >10 y

In children, prophylactic cranial irradiation with 24 Gy for leukemia does not affect LH or FSH pulsatile secretion in the first 6 years,[76] but it does produce subtle effects that appear after puberty (Table 141.8).[77] However, in the shorter term, they may indirectly increase LH and FSH levels and cause precocious puberty in both boys and girls.[78] Because irradiation also produces growth hormone deficiency, precocious puberty further exacerbates the risk of decreased adult stature. Treatment with a gonadotropin-releasing hormone (GnRH) analog to delay closure of the epiphyseal growth plates and, with growth hormone, can be given to avoid growth stunting.

In adults, LH and FSH secretion decreases after cranial irradiation, and the decline becomes more severe with increasing treatment dose and time since treatment. This results in oligomenorrhea in women and low testosterone levels in men. Hyperprolactinemia might mediate the observed gonadal dysfunction in some cases.[79]

PRESERVATION OF FERTILITY, HORMONE LEVELS, AND SEXUAL FUNCTION

Choice of Regimens

It is sometimes possible to choose, among nearly equally curative regimens, one that minimizes the doses of the agents that are most sterilizing (see Tables 141.3 and 141.6). The use of ABVD instead of MOPP to treat Hodgkin's lymphoma has dramatically reduced gonadal toxicity in a large group of patients.[80] In the treatment of non-Hodgkin's lymphoma, regimens that minimize the dose of cyclophosphamide, such as doxorubicin, cyclophosphamide, etoposide, vincristine, bleomycin, prednisone (VAPEC-B), produce gonadal failure less often in men than does CHOP with bleomycin.[81]

Gonadal Shielding and Oophoropexy

Except when the gonads must be irradiated because of actual or potential neoplastic involvement, they must be outside the field or shielded from the direct radiation beam. Nevertheless, an appreciable radiation dose from the accelerator head, collimator scatter, or internal lateral scatter may reach the gonads. Although moderately low radiation doses may be achieved, further reductions are desirable because of the possibilities of additive effects from chemotherapy and genetic damage to the sperm.

Gonadal dose depends on the distance from the field edge, field size, and photon energy. Pelvic radiation fields result in significant doses to the testis. Clamshell or other shields and beam blocking can reduce testicular doses two- to fivefold to 2 to 3 Gy for the inverted Y field used for Hodgkin's lymphoma and to 0.2 to 0.8 Gy for the hemipelvic field used for seminoma.[82]

To reduce ovarian dose, an oophoropexy, in which the ovaries are surgically translocated away from the direct beam, can be performed. That region is further shielded using lead blocks. Some investigators report reductions in cumulative ovarian doses to 4 to 5 Gy during total nodal irradiation,[62] which preserves fertility in younger women (see Table 141.6).[56] There is convincing evidence that moving the ovaries outside of the radiation field is beneficial in preserving ovarian function and future fertility in an adult population.[83,84] There is also evidence that this technique can preserve fertility in girls treated with radiation for Hodgkin's lymphoma who were ultimately able to become pregnant.[85] With advancement in the field of endoscopic surgery, these procedures can now be performed laparoscopically[86,87] or robotically,[88] allowing for a shortened hospital stay, earlier mobilization, and earlier return to normal activity.

Sperm Cryopreservation

Semen cryopreservation is an important procedure for preserving the fertility potential of men after cytotoxic treatment for cancer.[89] The significance of notifying the patient of the potential risk of iatrogenic sterility as early as possible cannot be overemphasized.[90] Physicians often are aware early during the diagnostic process that the patient will most likely need to receive potentially sterilizing cytotoxic therapy, although the exact diagnosis, stage, and treatment regimen may not have yet been decided. This time should be used to initiate and complete the cryopreservation procedure.

The number of samples to be banked may depend on how much time is available before starting therapy, sperm quality, and the cost of storing samples. A collection of three or four samples with approximately 48-hour periods of abstinence between sampling (a total of more than 5 days) is ideal. With current assisted reproductive technologies, however, success can be achieved with fewer samples, even with poor-quality semen. It is strongly advisable to complete sperm banking before starting therapy to avoid increased genetic damage in sperm collected after the start of therapy.[12] It is even possible to obtain semen with normal characteristics from 14- to 17-year-old boys by masturbation,[91] penile vibratory stimulation, or electroejaculation.[92] In addition, testicular sperm extraction is successful in 43% of pretreatment cancer patients who are azoospermic,[93] and the sperm obtained in this way can be cryopreserved and used in intracytoplasmic sperm injection (ICSI) procedures.[94] Testicular samples for sperm extraction can be obtained from orchiectomy or biopsy specimens that are routinely taken from testicular cancer patients if the surgeon is aware of the need and the processing procedures required for harvesting the sperm. Although a controversial topic, cryopreservation of immature testicular tissue in prepubertal boys with cancer may prove to be another suitable alternative, but the fear of reintroducing malignant cells through a graft is real, especially given the limitations of current technology.[95]

The success of in vitro fertilization (IVF) and ICSI makes cryopreservation of all samples containing any live sperm worthwhile. Even though 100% of oncologists in a study by Zapzalka et al.[96] reported discussing fertility issues with their patients, Schover et al.[89] found that only 60% of 900 male cancer patients surveyed who replied stated that they were informed about fertility issues and that only 51% stated they had been notified about sperm banking. According to Kohler et al.,[97] only 36% of surveyed pediatric oncologists believe sperm banking is affordable, and the most likely reason to not offer it is poor survival prognosis.[97] The cost of sperm banking three samples, including analysis and storage for 5 years, is between $1,200 (at a university medical school clinic) and $2,500 (at some private sperm banks). Intrauterine insemination is the least expensive assisted reproductive technology method (cost per cycle: $200 to $500, plus $1,200 for superovulation of the female partner, if necessary), but the sperm count and quality after thawing must be high, and conception rates are lower than with IVF. If sperm count or motility is impaired or sample amounts are limited, IVF is necessary. The average cost of IVF, including the medications used, is $15,000 per cycle.

Optimization of Fertility after Treatment

If sperm count recovers after cancer therapy, it usually reaches normospermic levels. However, some men remain oligospermic for many years. Although controlled studies have not been done, men who have recovered sperm production appear to have normal fertility, and their incidence of infertility does not appear to be any higher than the 15% rate among couples in the general population. Furthermore, cancer patients with recovered sperm counts ranging from just below 1 million/mL to 10 million/mL are able to successfully father children.[19] Infertile patients with oligospermia should be managed in the same way as are those in the general population with male factor infertility, including the use of IVF with or without ICSI.[98]

Assisted Reproductive Technologies

Currently, the choices for preserving fertility in chemotherapy patients are limited (Table 141.9). Some are investigational, and all have demonstrated variable success. Fertility preservation can be attempted either with assisted reproductive technologies, gamete cryopreservation, or medical treatment. Assisted reproductive technology refers to in vitro handling of human oocytes and sperm or

TABLE 141.9
Options for Fertility Preservation

Males	Females
Sperm banking prior to chemotherapy Sperm collection via masturbation or surgical retrieval	**Medical treatment** GnRH analogs (agonists, antagonists)
Testicular cryopreservation and future transplantation	**Ovarian cryopreservation and future transplantation** Cortical strip Whole ovary
	Assisted reproductive technology Embryo banking (partner sperm or donor sperm) Oocyte banking (cryopreservation or vitrification)

embryos for the purpose of establishing a pregnancy. Techniques for gamete preservation include sperm cryopreservation, oocyte cryopreservation, ovarian cortical cryopreservation, or whole ovary cryopreservation. Medical therapy includes treatment with hormonal agents such as oral contraceptive pills, progesterone, and GnRH analogs.[99–112]

Assisted reproductive technology is still undergoing rapid advances and provides new options for cancer survivors with gonadal damage to achieve fertility. Previously, intrauterine insemination following cryopreserved sperm had been the only fertility preservation method available, and only 30% of men who had stored high-quality semen samples were able to achieve pregnancy.[113]

Currently, IVF with ICSI is the most successful method for achieving pregnancy from banked sperm. ICSI makes it possible to use a single spermatozoa to achieve oocyte fertilization through IVF. This technology has revolutionized the treatment of male infertility.[114] ICSI is also often used with frozen banked sperm. IVF can be performed to create embryos that can be frozen and stored for later use. Pregnancy outcomes vary by IVF center but are excellent overall with frozen embryo transfers. The downside of IVF is that a single cycle can take 2 to 3 weeks to complete and necessitates a delay in cancer treatment.

Women with estrogen-responsive tumors can undergo ovulation induction with an aromatase inhibitor either as a solo agent or as an adjunct to standard stimulation protocols.[115,116] To avoid the potential risks of rising estradiol levels during ovarian stimulation (sometimes 10 to 20 times levels seen in natural cycles), an increasing number of fertility specialists are using aromatase inhibitors (letrozole or tamoxifen) for ovarian stimulation.[117] To date, the recurrence and survival rates of breast cancer patients undergoing such protocols were comparable with those of unstimulated control breast cancer patients.[118]

Clinical pregnancy rates of 30% to 50% per cycle and live birth rates of 25% to 50% can be expected at most fertility clinics. Cumulative live birth rates after four cycles have been reported between 60% to 80% in patients with male factor infertility, ovulatory dysfunction, endometriosis, and unexplained infertility.[119] Although fresh sperm is preferred to frozen sperm in intrauterine insemination and IVF cycles, studies have shown excellent outcomes using sperm that was frozen and banked prior to cancer treatment.[120] Although insemination with testicular sperm is an acceptable procedure, the use of nuclei from earlier stages (round spermatid nuclear injection) is not currently advisable.[121] Overall, embryo banking is the most successful form of fertility preservation and should be offered to all women who are either in a serious relationship, married, or who are open to the idea of using donor sperm.

Oocyte banking either via cryopreservation (slow freezing) or vitrification (rapid freezing) is an option for single women who are not interested in using donor sperm. Similar to IVF, this entails ovarian hyperstimulation followed by surgical oocyte retrieval and, similar to IVF, also necessitates a delay in treatment ranging from 2 to 6 weeks.[122] Mature oocyte cryopreservation and vitrification were recently changed from experimental treatments to options that can be offered in routine clinical care.[123] There is no statistically significant difference in outcomes for fresh oocytes versus vitrified oocytes in oocyte donation programs.[124] Although oocyte vitrification appears to be a good option for the female cancer patient without a partner, the technology to achieve comparable pregnancy rates is not available at all IVF centers and, thus, may not be available to all patients. Furthermore, when embryo cryopreservation is a viable option, it should be used instead of oocyte preservation because of the greater experience with that method.

A recent meta-analysis[125] showed a 32% increase over baseline risk of birth defects in children born as a result of IVF/ICSI treatment, whereas another study[126] found no significant difference after controlling for confounders in its IVF population but still found an increased risk in its ICSI population. These results should be interpreted with caution in terms of counseling patients for fertility preservation. First, assuming the baseline risk of birth defects is approximately 5%, even a 30% increase risk results in an absolute risk of only 6.5%. Second, subfertile couples, who are the majority undergoing IVF/ICSI, already carry an increased risk of birth defects, which would not apply to the fertility preservation patient.[126] The increased risk of birth defects in ICSI treatment also has to be interpreted with caution in the setting of counseling the fertility preservation patient. There is an increased risk of approximately 3% for chromosomal abnormalities, mostly in the numbers of sex chromosomes, in offspring of ICSI procedures.[127] Most of the chromosome abnormalities were not caused by ICSI, but were already present in the sperm of the infertile male parent. These abnormalities, which are common in cases of primary male infertility, should not be present in cryopreserved sperm from cancer patients.

Female Germ Cell Cryopreservation and Development

In addition to cryopreservation of oocytes, cryopreservation of ovarian tissue can also be undertaken (see Table 141.9). One method entails the surgical removal of ovarian tissue containing numerous primordial follicles, cryopreservation of tissue slices, and subsequent grafting back to the site of the ovary. This was initially successful in restoring ovarian endocrine function and fertility in sheep.[128] There has been some reported success with ovarian tissue transplantation that has resulted in at least 12 patients with 28 subsequent live births in humans.[129,130] These reports have included both fresh transplants from identical twins with discordant ovarian function and frozen transplants because of cancer. Some of the ovarian tissue grafts in these series have been functioning for over 7 years. A potential drawback of ovarian tissue cryopreservation and transplantation is the concern for reintroduction of malignant cells back into the host, particularly for patients treated for leukemia.[131] Overall, this method of surgical conservation of ovarian tissue may prove to be more useful in the future as this concern for occult malignancy gets resolved.

Ovarian tissue cryopreservation is also an attractive alternative for fertility preservation and for restoring ovarian function in the pediatric population because ovarian stimulation is not required. Furthermore, patients do not need to have a partner at the time of treatment, there is no delay in treatment, and the tissue can remain frozen until the patient is ready for conception. Because of the large numbers of immature oocytes in the ovarian cortex, this is an excellent emerging method suitable for premenarchal girls.[132–134]

Does It Work?

Results in various animal models have been encouraging in demonstrating the efficacy of ovarian cryopreservation and reimplantation.[135–138] Silber and Gosden[139] published a case series describing seven pairs of monozygotic twins discordant for ovarian function who underwent ovarian transplantation. Four of seven conceived and one patient conceived twice. On average, the restoration of ovarian function ensued after 2 to 4 months after transplantation. Several other live births have been reported from ovarian cortical transplantation.[140–142]

The first case of heterotopic grafting of cryopreserved ovarian tissue following bilateral oophorectomy for a granulosa cell tumor resulting in an ongoing pregnancy at 26 weeks gestation has also recently been reported.[143] There are some advantages of heterotopic grafting of ovarian tissue to sites such as the abdominal wall, forearm, or breast. These advantages include potentially less invasive procedures for implantation, easy access to the graft, and avoidance of severe pelvic adhesions in the case of prior pelvic irradiation. A disadvantage is that the environment may not be optimal for follicle development in terms of temperature and other paracrine factors.

These cases are undoubtedly the first of many more to come. Ovarian cortical cryopreservation with subsequent reimplantation at this time is considered experimental and should only be performed in centers under institutional review board–approved protocols and necessary expertise. It can be anticipated that many more live births will occur as a result of this novel technique.

An alternate approach to ovarian preservation involves transplantation of the whole ovary as opposed to just cortical strips. The main obstacle facing ovarian cortical strip cryopreservation is the threat of ischemic damage prior to graft reimplantation.[136,144] To combat this threat, maintenance of blood supply via whole-ovary cryopreservation with preservation of vascular pedicles might offer a potential advantage in reducing the large follicular loss. With the use of dimethyl sulfoxide as a cryoprotectant, improved follicular preservation has been noted compared with glycerol, which had been used in the past. Furthermore, recent microsurgical advances to enhance intact ovarian freezing and transplantation have been successful in rodents. Nine of 10 transplanted ovaries had successful restoration of ovarian function and 6 of 10 transplanted rats became pregnant.[145] In sheep, whose ovarian structure is more comparable to that of humans, intact ovaries with vascular pedicles were cryopreserved and later autotransplanted with microvascular anastomosis of the ovarian artery and vein to the branches of deep inferior epigastric vessels.[146] A recent study in sheep demonstrated ovarian function 6 years after transplantation of whole ovaries with the use of unidirectional solidification freezing technology.[147] The sheep underwent superovulation and the ovaries were found to have evidence of follicular growth and development.[147] More experience is needed with whole ovary transplantation for this to be a viable option for fertility preservation.

Another approach to oocyte preservation involves cryopreservation of immature oocytes in the germinal vesicle stage, followed by in vitro maturation (IVM) to meiotic metaphase II. These oocytes can then be fertilized in vitro. The first live birth from IVM was reported in 1991.[148] The application of IVM is becoming more widespread, ranging from the retrieval of immature oocytes in unstimulated or minimally stimulated cycles to reduce the cost of IVF to the retrieval of immature oocytes for fertility preservation.[149–151]

It is possible that in the future stem cells may be used to repopulate the ovary. The derivation of oocytes from mouse embryonic stem cells in culture suggests the eventual power of stem cell technology and nuclear transplantation for the production of oocytes, perhaps even from somatic cell nuclei.[152] Early animal

PRACTICE OF ONCOLOGY

experiments involving human ovarian stem cells obtained from purified ovarian cortical tissue have been xenotransplanted into immunodeficient mice to yield what resemble oocytes.[153] This suggests that human ovarian stem cells may potentially be used for fertility preservation in the future. If this method proves to be successful, it would avoid the risks of reintroduction of malignant cells back into the patient. However, applications of such techniques to human fertility preservation are currently still under early investigation using animal models and should not be discussed with patients as options.

Most women who continue to have menstrual function after cytotoxic therapy for cancer but are infertile should be treated in the same way as similar women in the general population. One important exception is women who have uterine damage from receiving more than 10 Gy of abdominal radiation in childhood. These patients have increased rates of adverse pregnancy outcomes, including fetal or neonatal death, premature delivery, and low–birth-weight babies, and hence, their pregnancies must be closely monitored.[75]

Immature Male Germ Cell Cryopreservation and Development

For the restoration of spermatogenesis, the harvest and cryopreservation of spermatogonial stem cells, which are capable of proliferation, self-renewal, and repopulation of the seminiferous tubules, are under investigation. Transplantation of cryopreserved testicular germ cells from a donor mouse into the seminiferous tubules of a recipient mouse, in which endogenous stem spermatogonia were killed with busulfan, restored spermatogenesis and fertility.[154] There are preliminary indications that this technique might restore spermatogenesis in irradiated macaques.[155] Testicular cells have been harvested from men before sterilizing cytotoxic therapy and later injected back into the testicular tubules after the completion of radiotherapy or chemotherapy. This technique would be most valuable for prepubertal boys, who are too young to produce sperm but have testes enriched in spermatogonia. Similar to female cancer patients, there exists concern that cancer cells may be reintroduced into the recipients. This possibility is a contraindication in cases of leukemia or testicular cancer, but the risks with other cancers may not be high.[156] To date, there has not yet been a report of successful transplantation of testicular tissue in a male patient, but this therapy is likely to first be applied to patients with nonmalignant disease then to those with cancer.[95]

One way to circumvent the problem of the presence of tumor cells is to first transplant the tissue into a xenogeneic host. Human spermatogonial stem cells have been shown to survive and proliferate in seminiferous tubules of mice.[157] Also, subcutaneous transplantation of cryopreserved testicular tissue from immature pigs and goats into nude mice results in the production of functional sperm.[158] However, the risks of transfer of animal DNA or viruses (especially retroviruses) from the host to the human spermatogonial cells must be evaluated before such techniques could be applied.

New experimental approaches to germ cell development could potentially be applied to fertility preservation in men. The in vitro development of human round spermatids into elongated spermatids, which were used to produce normal embryos by ICSI, has been reported.[159] Development of an in vitro cell line derived from genetically modified mouse spermatogonia, which proliferates to produce more spermatogonia and can be stimulated to form haploid cells,[160] holds promise as a very useful resource for optimizing proliferation of spermatogonia and production of spermatids. Furthermore, the development of sperm from mouse embryonic stem cells by a combination of induction of differentiation in vitro and transplantation into host testes[161] might eventually lead to methods for the development of sperm from other stem cell types obtained from a cancer patient.

PHARMACOLOGIC ATTEMPTS AT PRESERVING FERTILITY IN MEN

Hormone treatments have been investigated for their ability to enhance the survival of germ cells and promote recovery after cytotoxic treatments. Treatment of male rats with hormones that suppress testosterone levels or action (gonadal steroids, GnRH analogs, antiandrogens) before and during cytotoxic therapy with radiation or procarbazine enhances the subsequent recovery of spermatogenesis and fertility.[162] The original proposal that these treatments would protect the spermatogonia from killing by suppressing their proliferation is incorrect; rather, the suppression of testosterone levels protects the subsequent ability of the somatic cells of the testis to support the recovery of spermatogenesis from surviving stem spermatogonia.[163] The hormonal treatment can even be given several months after exposure to radiation or procarbazine and still restore spermatogenesis and fertility.[162]

Because stem spermatogonia are indeed present in regions of the testes of some cancer patients during prolonged periods of iatrogenic azoospermia, their recovery could possibly be stimulated. However, only one[164] of eight clinical trials has been able to demonstrate protection of spermatogenesis in humans by hormone treatment before and during cytotoxic therapy.[165] One attempt to restore spermatogenesis by steroid hormone treatment after cytotoxic therapy was unsuccessful[166]; however, the doses of cytotoxic therapy were very high, and the hormonal suppression was given many years after the anticancer treatment. More discouraging was the failure of GnRH antagonist treatment to enhance spermatogenic recovery in a controlled primate study,[167] which suggests that there are important differences in this process in rats and in primates. Hence, pharmacologic preservation of male fertility is currently not effective.

PHARMACOLOGIC ATTEMPTS AT PRESERVING FERTILITY IN WOMEN

Although studies have been performed to assess the efficacy of oral contraceptive pills and GnRH analogs in girls, adolescents, and women, no comparative studies have been done using progestins in these age groups. Most studies do not support the use of hormonal therapy for the prevention of premature ovarian failure in girls and premenarchal adolescents receiving chemotherapy, because prior to the onset of menarche, the ovaries are thought to be quiescent and less likely to be subject to damage by cytotoxic agents. Therefore, there would be no additional benefit to giving hormonal therapy to an already suppressed hypothalamic–pituitary–ovarian axis. Furthermore, the use of estrogen may be associated with an increased risk of venous thrombosis. There is also concern regarding the side effect profile of hormonal therapy in premenarchal girls.

Longhi et al.[99] performed a small, observational study that examined the effects of oral contraceptive pills on ovarian function in premenarchal girls and postmenarchal women undergoing neoadjuvant chemotherapy treatment for osteosarcoma. They concluded that age and alkylant dose were the most predictive factors for early menopause, and that oral contraceptives during high-dose alkylant-based chemotherapy did not prevent chemotherapy-induced premature ovarian failure. The follow-up time of this study was too short to rule out any positive long-term effects on the preservation of ovarian function. In addition, this study did show greater risk than benefit because two patients in the group receiving chemotherapy plus oral contraceptive pills developed thrombophlebitis. Similar findings have been observed in other studies.[100] The majority of the evidence suggests that children and premenarchal adolescents do not benefit from hormonal suppression to preserve their ovarian function while undergoing chemotherapy.

The use of GnRH analogs to preserve fertility, although once thought to have promise, has failed to demonstrate consistent results in human studies. Preservation of ovarian function with the use of GnRH analogs, specifically agonists, prior to cancer treatment, in some studies has been shown to be beneficial.[101,102] It has been proposed that GnRH agonist use prior to chemotherapy has a protective effect via two mechanisms. First, by downregulating the hypothalamic–pituitary–ovarian axis, it might reduce the number of primordial follicles destroyed by toxic agents. Second, it may reduce the blood flow to the ovary and decrease the delivery of toxic chemotherapeutic agents.[103,104] This second theory may also explain the lack of a protective effect with GnRH analogs on ovarian function observed with increasing chemotherapeutic dosages and provide an explanation why this treatment has no effect with radiation therapy.[103,105]

Animal studies have provided very convincing evidence regarding the efficacy of GnRH analogs. Ataya et al.[101] conducted a prospective study looking at the effects of leuprolide on ovarian function in primates exposed to cyclophosphamide. Six adult female rhesus monkeys underwent unilateral oophorectomy and were divided into two groups. One group received cyclophosphamide and monthly injections of leuprolide, and the other received cyclophosphamide and placebo. At the end of treatment, the remaining ovary was removed and compared to the pre-treated ovary. Ovarian follicle number and size were compared. As expected, there was a decline in follicle number with chemotherapy. Cyclophosphamide resulted in a significant reduction of nonprimordial follicles and primordial follicles compared to the leuprolide and cyclophosphamide group. The authors concluded that in rhesus monkeys, leuprolide protected the ovary against cyclophosphamide-induced damage.

Human studies have provided conflicting evidence for the efficacy of GnRH analogs. Two recent randomized studies from patients with breast cancer demonstrated some evidence of a protective effect of GnRH agonist treatment on the preservation of ovarian function.[168,169] However, these studies have been questioned[170–172] and will require larger study populations to definitively conclude the chemoprotective effects of GnRH analog therapy. A meta-analysis of this treatment showed an overall benefit of GnRH analog therapy.[173] This meta-analysis included the widely questioned study[168] and did not include the 24-month follow-up of the ZORO study[174]; therefore, when reanalyzed, there is no difference in premature ovarian failure.[175]

Although there is less evidence in the literature for the use of GnRH antagonists, the experience with ovulation induction and assisted reproductive technologies suggests it may have similar efficacy to GnRH agonists. On administration of GnRH agonists, there is an initial stimulatory *flare* effect prior to pituitary desensitization that ensues after 7 to 14 days. GnRH antagonists work via rapid inhibition of gonadotropin and sex steroids secretion and have an almost immediate downregulation of the pituitary gland. Because desensitization is so rapid, they have the advantage of not causing an initial flare effect. Gonadotropin deprivation halts follicular recruitment and decreases the size of the chemotherapy-sensitive pool.[103]

GnRH antagonists are beginning to be studied further in both animals and humans. Using a mouse model, Meirow et al.[103] administered a GnRH antagonist, cetrorelix, prior to exposure to increasing doses of cyclophosphamide. The aim of the study was to assess the number of surviving primordial follicles in the ovaries of young mice. In each treatment group, half of the females were injected daily with cetrorelix starting 9 days before and 7 days posttreatment with cyclophosphamide. After treatment, ovarian sections were taken and the total number of primordial follicles in both ovaries was counted. A dose-response relationship was observed. Ovaries exposed to cyclophosphamide at dosages of 50 and 75 mg per kilogram had significantly fewer primordial follicles than those in the control group. In each of the cyclophosphamide groups that were pretreated with cetrorelix, there were higher numbers of primordial follicles compared to controls. The administration of the GnRH antagonist cetrorelix to mice significantly decreased the extent of ovarian damage induced by the chemotherapeutic agent. A recent randomized trial in humans comparing a combination of GnRH agonist combined with antagonist to avoid the flare response in patients requiring early cyclophosphamide chemotherapy for hormone insensitive breast cancer (within 1 week of enrollment) versus GnRH agonist treatment for those with delayed chemotherapy (at least 10 days after enrollment) found no protective or harmful effects of the intervention.[176]

Although some of the data seem promising with regard to GnRH analogs, the studies are plagued by low numbers and short follow-up periods. Thus, there is insufficient evidence to definitively recommend this therapy, and further study is needed. At this point, ovarian suppression should be considered and offered to all postmenarchal and reproductive-age women prior to initiating therapy if other, more well-proven options for female fertility preservation are not available or not feasible. Despite these conflicting results about the efficacy in terms of protecting ovarian function, both GnRH agonists and antagonists have the added advantage of menstrual suppression and, therefore, can be used to avoid heavy uterine bleeding often seen with hematologic malignancies.

FERTILITY PRESERVATION IN WOMEN WITH CERVICAL CANCER

Women with early-stage cervical cancer are most often treated with radical hysterectomy or radiotherapy to the pelvis. As women delay their childbearing and as screening programs have become more effective, an increasing number of patients with early-stage cervical cancer seek to preserve their future fertility.[177] Conservative surgery in the form of radical vaginal excision of the cervix (radical trachelectomy) to preserve the uterus in cases of cervical carcinoma has been reported with relatively good outcomes in terms of disease recurrence and pregnancy.[177–180]

EVALUATION OF FERTILITY AFTER TREATMENT

Male and female cancer survivors should undergo timely evaluation when they are attempting conception. For males, it would be reasonable to obtain a semen analysis either before attempting conception or when conception fails to occur after 6 months of unprotected intercourse. Premature ovarian failure can be suspected based on a careful menstrual history. Shortening of the intermenstrual interval is an ominous sign that ovarian reserve is diminished. An evaluation of ovarian reserve with a gynecologist or reproductive endocrinologist is warranted for women who report amenorrhea, shortened menstrual cycles, irregular cycles, or for cancer survivors who have failed to conceive after 6 months of unprotected intercourse. There is no single best test available to measure ovarian reserve, but surrogate markers such as early follicular phase (cycle day 2 through 4) measures of antral follicles, ovarian volumes, FSH, estradiol, and antimüllerian hormone levels can be used. These tests, however, must be interpreted with caution, because the true utility is in predicting ovarian responsiveness and not reserve.

HORMONE REPLACEMENT THERAPY

Information that estrogen with or without progesterone given to postmenopausal women (aged 50 to 79 years) increases the cardiovascular risks[181] has led to the view that the risks of hormone replacement therapy for normal postmenopausal women (cardiovascular disease and breast cancer) outweigh the benefits (increased bone mineral density and reduced incidence of fracture). A further analysis of the Women's Health Initiative (WHI) and long-term follow-up essentially concluded that oral hormone replacement therapy, as given in the WHI, should not be used for the prevention of chronic disease, but this conclusion may be questioned in younger postmenopausal women and with other forms of hormone replacement.[182] However, the physiologic replacement of ovarian hormones still remains appropriate for young, otherwise premenopausal girls who have developed premature ovarian failure as a result of their malignancy or cancer treatment. This is particularly true for adolescent girls and young women in whom bone mineral density is normally increasing.[183] In these cases, it is important to test for ovarian failure shortly after treatment and, if appropriate, to start hormone replacement therapy in a timely manner. If a woman has an intact uterus, estrogen should be combined with progesterone to prevent endometrial hyperplasia and cancer.[183] The use of hormone replacement therapy in survivors of breast cancer to alleviate debilitating postmenopausal symptoms that do not respond to nonhormonal treatments is controversial because of its unclear effects on breast cancer recurrence.[184]

In males, germinal aplasia is often associated with testosterone levels in the low to normal range, and such individuals may experience reduced bone mineral density and a slight reduction in sexual function.[185] However, a controlled trial failed to show any benefit of testosterone treatment on bone mineral density or sexual function, which indicates that this mild hypogonadism is not of clinical importance in most men.[185] Testosterone replacement is, nevertheless, very important in cases of overt Leydig cell failure in prepubertal boys to promote secondary sexual characteristics, growth, and bone density.

PREVENTION AND MANAGEMENT OF ERECTILE AND EJACULATORY DYSFUNCTION

Ejaculation of semen first requires emission (the deposition of semen in the posterior urethra by contractions of the vas deferens, seminal vesicles, and prostate) and then antegrade ejaculation, which involves coordinated tightening of the bladder neck, relaxation of the external sphincter, and expulsion of semen. Most of these processes are controlled by trunks of nerve fibers forming the hypogastric plexus overlying the aorta and sacrum below the origin of the inferior mesenteric artery.[186] Surgery for testicular, prostate, and bladder cancers can produce neurologic dysfunction, resulting in failure of emission, retrograde ejaculation, impotence, and loss of orgasm. However, improvements in surgical techniques have reduced these adverse outcomes without diminishing the efficacy of treating the cancer.[187] Newer RPLND techniques used for nonseminomatous testicular germ cell tumors in addition to bilateral nerve-sparing modification for patients undergoing radical prostatectomies preserves ejaculatory function compared with controls.[24,188] In cases in which the cavernous nerves cannot be spared, the technique of interposition sural nerve grafting has been shown to help preserve postoperative potency.[189]

For men experiencing erectile dysfunction, phosphodiesterase type 5 inhibitors, such as sildenafil, vardenafil, and tadalafil, are clinically effective and safe treatments.[190] For patients who are not responsive to oral administration of these drugs, other treatment options for improving erectile function include intracorporeal injection therapy with a prostaglandin or a mixture of a prostaglandin, an alkaloid, and an α-adrenergic blocker, or penile prosthetic surgery. A penile prosthesis is usually not offered to patients until 2 years after a radical prostatectomy to allow for tissue healing and adequate monitoring of cancer control.

In patients who experience ejaculatory dysfunction after RPLND, the postmasturbation urine should be investigated for the presence of sperm cells.[191] Use of sympathomimetic agents may enhance seminal emission and partially or completely convert the

patient to antegrade ejaculation.[192] Although multiple therapies for retrograde ejaculation exist, a comparison of the therapies is difficult and must be tailored to the individual.[193] Natural pregnancies have been reported, but use of assisted reproductive technologies is often needed. Even when retrograde ejaculation is present, sperm may be recovered from the bladder by direct voiding into a buffering medium or by catheterization and irrigation with a somewhat alkaline solution.[194] When no ejaculation is present, electroejaculation, using a rectal probe under general anesthesia, has been successful in most patients.[195] Although patients will have some antegrade ejaculate, catheterization should always be done to collect the retrograde semen. Sperm obtained by these methods can be used with IVF/ICSI procedures to achieve 15% pregnancy rates per cycle.

GENETIC CONCERNS

Biologic Considerations

Many anticancer agents damage DNA and interfere with its replication and repair and with chromosome segregation in both animal and human cells. These agents induce both single-gene and chromosomal mutations in germ cells of animals,[196] both of which cause genetic disease in the offspring. Mutations induced in stem spermatogonia cause the continued production of mutation-carrying sperm for the lifetime of the male, whereas those induced in later stages of spermatogenesis result in the production of mutation-carrying sperm for only a few months. Radiation and several alkylating agents produce single-gene mutations in murine spermatogonia, whereas other tested chemotherapeutic drugs do not.[196] Radiation is the only agent that effectively induces stable reciprocal chromosomal translocations in stem spermatogonia that can be transmitted to offspring.[197]

In male rodents, meiotic and postmeiotic germ cells are more sensitive to induction and transmission of mutations than are stem spermatogonia.[12] Therefore, mutational risks are highest when a pregnancy occurs within one spermatogenic cycle (time required for stem cells to become sperm) after the male is exposed to the damaging agent. Clinical reports of outcomes of pregnancies in which conception occurred while the man was undergoing cytotoxic therapy are too limited to evaluate the risks, but animal experiments and gamete genetic analyses show a higher risk.[12] In men, this higher risk period extends from the start of cytotoxic therapy until 3 months after the last course. Damage to sperm DNA for up to 2 years after the completion of therapy has been reported in a patient undergoing radiation therapy and chemotherapy for testicular cancer and systemic therapy for Hodgkin's lymphoma.[198,199]

Fewer studies of the mutagenicity of cytotoxic agents have been done in female mice, but the limited results indicate induced mutation frequencies similar to those in male mice. Radiation induces single-gene and chromosomal mutations in developing oocytes.[200] Most alkylating agents and a variety of other chemotherapeutic drugs induce chromosome aberrations or other mutations in developing oocytes that result in embryonic death.[196] There are insufficient data to determine whether primordial or growing oocytes are more sensitive to the induction of mutations.

Pregnancy Outcome

In humans, nearly all of the case reports, small series, and a few large retrospective case studies of the outcomes of pregnancies in, or produced by, survivors of cancer indicated no significant increase in birth defects or genetic disease in offspring conceived after cytotoxic treatment above the background level in the general population of approximately 4% to 5%.[7,200,201] No increase in genetic disease was observed in 630 offspring of patients who were children or adolescents at the time of treatment and received alkylating agents or radiation proximal to the gonads.[202] A study of 368 conceptions in adult women treated previously with methotrexate alone showed no significant adverse effects, as expected.[203] In males, 70 offspring of testicular cancer patients treated with radiotherapy or chemotherapy (most received cisplatin), or both, revealed no apparent increase in congenital malformations.[204] In a case-control study involving 45,000 children with congenital abnormalities, there was no higher incidence of parental exposure to alkylating agents or radiation proximal to the gonads in the parents of children with congenital abnormalities than in the parents of the control group of children.[205] The results from the atomic bomb studies in Japan also show no significant increase in genetic damage in the offspring born to radiation-exposed parents.[206]

These observations should reassure those who wish to have children after treatment for cancer. However, the power of these studies can only rule out twofold or higher increases in abnormalities; the possibility remains of a small genetic risk that would increase genetic abnormalities less than twofold over background levels. Also, these long-term studies do not include as many patients receiving the newer chemotherapeutic agents.

There are significant teratogenic risks from cytotoxic therapy given to a woman during pregnancy. Radiation is highly damaging; doses as low as 0.1 to 0.2 Gy in the first trimester and doses higher than 0.7 Gy in the second trimester cause microcephaly.[207] Almost all cytotoxic chemotherapeutic agents are considered teratogenic; however, some may be safely given in the second and third trimesters of pregnancy.[208] Treatment with fluorouracil, doxorubicin, and cyclophosphamide during this period did not result in any adverse effects. Methotrexate, which is a documented teratogen in the first trimester, was excluded from the combination.

Gamete Genomic Analysis

Because epidemiologic studies of genetic damage in humans require large numbers of offspring, direct analyses of the genetic material of gametes have huge potential advantages for identifying heritable mutations in humans. Such analyses are used only in the male because harvesting female gametes is impractical. These analyses can be used to detect both single-gene and chromosomal mutations.

Chromosomal abnormalities are measured by sperm karyotyping after fusion with hamster eggs or by fluorescence in situ hybridization. Structural chromosomal aberrations were present in sperm more than 5 years after the end of MOPP or radiation therapy, or both, which indicates that they are induced in stem cells.[209] Numerical aberrations (aneuploidy) can show up to a fivefold increase during and shortly after chemotherapy with mitoxantrone, vincristine, vinblastine, prednisone (NOVP) or BEP and then return to baseline within 4 months or 2 years, depending on the study.[210,211] These results demonstrate that there can be significant genetic risks if conception or storage of sperm occurs during cytotoxic therapy, but that this risk declines after the end of such therapy.

Cancer patients should be informed by their physicians about the possibilities of sterility and genetic risk from their disease and its treatment. The probability that sterility will result from the planned cytotoxic therapy should be calculated from the cumulative doses of agents and combinations that cause prolonged azoospermia, ovarian failure, or pituitary damage (see Tables 141.3, 141.4, 141.6, 141.7, and 141.8). They should also be told about psychological and physical effects on sexual desire, erectile function, and the ability to achieve orgasm. Now that a large percentage of reproductive-aged patients are surviving cancer, different methods of fertility preservation (see Table 141.9) should be discussed with both male and female patients, and they should be given information about different education resources. Pretreatment gonadal function testing and referral to a reproductive endocrinologist should be considered.

ACKNOWLEDGMENTS

We acknowledge the contributions of John M. Norian and Eve C. Feinberg for their assistance with the writing of the prior revision of this chapter.

SELECTED REFERENCES

The full reference list can be accessed at lwwhealthlibrary.com/oncology.

1. Loren AW, Mangu PB, Beck LN, et al. Fertility preservation for patients with cancer: American Society of Clinical Oncology clinical practice guideline update. *J Clin Oncol* 2013;31:2500–2510.
6. Stensheim H, Klungsøyr K, Skjaerven R, et al. Birth outcomes among offspring of adult cancer survivors: a population-based study. *Int J Cancer* 2013;133:2696–2705.
10. Bart J, Groen HJ, van der Graaf WT, et al. An oncological view on the blood-testis barrier. *Lancet Oncol* 2002;3:357–363.
12. Meistrich ML. Potential genetic risks of using semen collected during chemotherapy. *Hum Reprod* 1993;8:8–10.
13. Meistrich ML, Wilson G, Brown BW, et al. Impact of cyclophosphamide on long-term reduction in sperm count in men treated with combination chemotherapy for Ewing and soft tissue sarcomas. *Cancer* 1992;70:2703–2712.
16. Di Bisceglie C, Bertagna A, Composto ER, et al. Effects of oncological treatments on semen quality in patients with testicular neoplasia or lymphoproliferative disorders. *Asian J Androl* 2013;15:425–429.
19. Marmor D, Duyck F. Male reproductive potential after MOPP therapy for Hodgkin's disease: a long-term survey. *Andrologia* 1995;27:99–106.
20. Anserini P, Chiodi S, Spinelli S, et al. Semen analysis following allogeneic bone marrow transplantation. Additional data for evidence-based counseling. *Bone Marrow Transplant* 2002;30:447–451.
21. Pryzant RM, Meistrich ML, Wilson G, et al. Long-term reduction in sperm count after chemotherapy with and without radiation therapy for non-Hodgkin's lymphomas. *J Clin Oncol* 1993;11:239–247.
26. Howell SJ, Shalet SM. Effect of cancer therapy on pituitary-testicular axis. *Int J Androl* 2002;25:269–276.
27. Hansen PV, Trykker H, Svennekjaer IL, et al. Long-term recovery of spermatogenesis after radiotherapy in patients with testicular cancer. *Radiother Oncol* 1990;18:117–125.
29. Buchanan JD, Fairley KF, Barrie JU. Return of spermatogenesis after stopping cyclophosphamide therapy. *Lancet* 1975;2:156–157.
31. Hansen PV, Trykker H, Helkjoer PE, et al. Testicular function in patients with testicular cancer treated with orchiectomy alone or orchiectomy plus cisplatin-based chemotherapy. *J Natl Cancer Inst* 1989;81:1246–1250.
32. Sanders JE, Hawley J, Levy W, et al. Pregnancies following high-dose cyclophosphamide with or without high-dose busulfan or total-body irradiation and bone marrow transplantation. *Blood* 1996;87:3045–3052.
35. Meistrich ML, van Beek MEAB. Radiation sensitivity of the human testis. *Adv Radiat Biol* 1990;14:227–268.
39. Tilly JL, Kolesnick RN. Sphingolipids, apoptosis, cancer treatments and the ovary: investigating a crime against female fertility. *Biochim Biophys Acta* 2002;1585:135–138.
40. Morgan S, Anderson RA, Gourley C, et al. How do chemotherapeutic agents damage the ovary? *Hum Reprod Update* 2012;18:525–535.
41. Children's Oncology Group. *Long-Term Follow-Up Guidelines for Survivors of Childhood, Adolescent, and Young Adult Cancers.* Version 3.0. www.survivorshipguidelines.org/pdf/LTFUGuidelines.pdf.
42. Brougham MF, Crofton PM, Johnson EJ, et al. Anti-Müllerian hormone is a marker of gonadotoxicity in pre- and postpubertal girls treated for cancer: a prospective study. *J Clin Endocrinol Metab* 2012;97:2059–2067.
43. Sanders JE. Growth and development after hematopoietic cell transplantation. In: Thomas ED, Blume KG, Forman SJ, eds. *Hematopoietic Cell Transplantation.* Malden, MA: Blackwell Science; 1999.
46. Sklar CA, Mertens AC, Mitby P, et al. Premature menopause in survivors of childhood cancer: a report from the childhood cancer survivor study. *J Natl Cancer Inst* 2006;98:890–896.
47. Byrne J, Fears TR, Gail MH, et al. Early menopause in long-term survivors of cancer during adolescence. *Am J Obstet Gynecol* 1992;166:788–793.
49. Koyama H, Wada T, Nishizawa Y, et al. Cyclophosphamide-induced ovarian failure and its therapeutic significance in patients with breast cancer. *Cancer* 1977;39:1403–1409.
54. Bonadonna G, Santoro A, Viviani S, et al. Gonadal damage in Hodgkin's disease from cancer chemotherapeutic regimens. *Arch Toxicol Suppl* 1984;7:140–145.

56. Morice P, Juncker L, Rey A, et al. Ovarian transposition for patients with cervical carcinoma treated by radiosurgical combination. *Fertil Steril* 2000; 74:743–748.

57. Spinelli S, Chiodi S, Bacigalupo A, et al. Ovarian recovery after total body irradiation and allogeneic bone marrow transplantation: long-term follow up of 79 females. *Bone Marrow Transplant* 1994;14:373–380.

59. Horning SJ, Hoppe RT, Kaplan HS, et al. Female reproductive potential after treatment for Hodgkin's disease. *N Engl J Med* 1981;304:1377–1382.

60. Kreuser ED, Xiros N, Hetzel WD, et al. Reproductive and endocrine gonadal capacity in patients treated with COPP chemotherapy for Hodgkin's disease. *J Cancer Res Clin Oncol* 1987;113:260–266.

62. Ortin TT, Shostak CA, Donaldson SS. Gonadal status and reproductive function following treatment for Hodgkin's disease in childhood: the Stanford experience. *Int J Radiat Oncol Biol Phys* 1990;19:873–880.

63. Siimes MA, Dunkel L, Rautonen J. Risk factors for endocrine testicular dysfunction in adolescent and adult males who have survived malignancies in childhood. *Cancer J* 1992;5:28–31.

66. Thomas-Teinturier C, El Fayech C, Oberlin O, et al. Age at menopause and its influencing factors in a cohort of survivors of childhood cancer: earlier but rarely premature. *Hum Reprod* 2013;28:488–495.

67. Green DM, Sklar CA, Boice JD Jr, et al. Ovarian failure and reproductive outcomes after childhood cancer treatment: results from the Childhood Cancer Survivor Study. *J Clin Oncol* 2009;27:2374–2381.

74. Urbano MT, Tait DM. Can the irradiated uterus sustain a pregnancy? A literature review. *Clin Oncol (R Coll Radiol)* 2004;16:24–28.

75. Critchley HO. Factors of importance for implantation and problems after treatment for childhood cancer. *Med Pediatr Oncol* 1999;33:9–14.

76. Mauras N, Sabio H, Rogol AD. Neuroendocrine function in survivors of childhood acute lymphocytic leukemia and non-Hodgkins lymphoma: a study of pulsatile growth hormone and gonadotropin secretions. *Am J Pediatr Hematol Oncol* 1988;10:9–17.

79. Constine LS, Woolf PD, Cann D, et al. Hypothalamic-pituitary dysfunction after radiation for brain tumors. *N Engl J Med* 1993;328:87–94.

81. Radford JA, Clark S, Crowther D, et al. Male fertility after VAPEC-B chemotherapy for Hodgkin's disease and non-Hodgkin's lymphoma. *Br J Cancer* 1994;69:379–381.

83. Bisharah M, Tulandi T. Laparoscopic preservation of ovarian function: an underused procedure. *Am J Obstet Gynecol* 2003;188:367–370.

90. Schover LR, Brey K, Lichtin A, et al. Oncologists' attitudes and practices regarding banking sperm before cancer treatment. *J Clin Oncol* 2002;20: 1890–1897.

95. Goossens E, Van Saen D, Tournaye H. Spermatogonial stem cell preservation and transplantation: from research to clinic. *Hum Reprod* 2013;28:897–907.

100. Whitehead E, Shalet SM, Blackledge G, et al. The effect of combination chemotherapy on ovarian function in women treated for Hodgkin's disease. *Cancer* 1983;52:988–993.

108. Blumenfeld Z, Dann E, Avivi I, et al. Fertility after treatment for Hodgkin's disease. *Ann Oncol* 2002;13:138–147.

118. Azim AA, Costantini-Ferrando M, Oktay K. Safety of fertility preservation by ovarian stimulation with letrozole and gonadotropins in patients with breast cancer: a prospective controlled study. *J Clin Oncol* 2008;26: 2630–2635.

120. Meseguer M, Molina N, Garcia-Velasco JA, et al. Sperm cryopreservation in oncological patients: a 14-year follow-up study. *Fertil Steril* 2006;85: 640–645.

122. Lobo RA. Potential options for preservation of fertility in women. *N Engl J Med* 2005;353:64–73.

123. Practice Committees of American Society for Reproductive Medicine, Society for Assisted Reproductive Technology. Mature oocyte cryopreservation: a guideline. *Fertil Steril* 2013;99:37–43.

125. Hansen M, Kurinczuk JJ, Milne E, et al. Assisted reproductive technology and birth defects: a systematic review and meta-analysis. *Hum Reprod Update* 2013;19:330–353.

126. Davies MJ, Moore VM, Willson KJ, et al. Reproductive technologies and the risk of birth defects. *N Engl J Med* 2012;366:1803–1813.

129. Donnez J, Silber S, Andersen CY, et al. Children born after autotransplantation of cryopreserved ovarian tissue. A review of 13 live births. *Ann Med* 2011;43:437–450.

131. Bastings L, Beerendonk CC, Westphal JR, et al. Autotransplantation of cryopreserved ovarian tissue in cancer survivors and the risk of reintroducing malignancy: a systematic review. *Hum Reprod Update* 2013;19:483–506.

135. Gosden RG, Baird DT, Wade JC, et al. Restoration of fertility to oophorectomized sheep by ovarian autografts stored at -196 degrees C. *Hum Reprod* 1994;9:597–603.

140. Demeestere I, Simon P, Emiliani S, et al. Orthotopic and heterotopic ovarian tissue transplantation. *Hum Reprod Update* 2009;15:649–665.

143. Stern CJ, Gook D, Hale LG, et al. First reported clinical pregnancy following heterotopic grafting of cryopreserved ovarian tissue in a woman after a bilateral oophorectomy. *Hum Reprod* 2013;28:2996–2999.

153. White YA, Woods DC, Takai Y, et al. Oocyte formation by mitotically active germ cells purified from ovaries of reproductive-age women. *Nat Med* 2012; 18:413–421.

158. Honaramooz A, Snedaker A, Boiani M, et al. Sperm from neonatal mammalian testes grafted in mice. *Nature* 2002;418:778–781.

160. Feng LX, Chen Y, Dettin L, et al. Generation and in vitro differentiation of a spermatogonial cell line. *Science* 2002;297:392–395.

165. Howell SJ, Shalet SM. Fertility preservation and management of gonadal failure associated with lymphoma therapy. *Curr Oncol Rep* 2002;4:443–452.

173. Bedaiwy MA, Abou-Setta AM, Desai N, et al. Gonadotropin-releasing hormone analog cotreatment for preservation of ovarian function during gonadotoxic chemotherapy: a systematic review and meta-analysis. *Fertil Steril* 2011;95:906–914.e1–e4.

176. Elgindy EA, El-Haieg DO, Khorshid OM, et al. Gonadatrophin suppression to prevent chemotherapy-induced ovarian damage: a randomized controlled trial. *Obstet Gynecol* 2013;121:78–86.

178. Gien LT, Covens A. Fertility-sparing options for early stage cervical cancer. *Gynecol Oncol* 2010;117:350–357.

183. Mulder JE. Benefits and risks of hormone replacement therapy in young adult cancer survivors with gonadal failure. *Med Pediatr Oncol* 1999;33:46–52.

186. Lange PH, Narayan P, Fraley EE. Fertility issues following therapy for testicular cancer. *Semin Urol* 1984;2:264–274.

187. Mirone V, Imbimbo C, Palmieri A, et al. Erectile dysfunction after surgical treatment. *Int J Androl* 2003;26:137–140.

191. Magelssen H, Brydoy M, Fossa SD. The effects of cancer and cancer treatments on male reproductive function. *Nat Clin Pract Urol* 2006;3:312–322.

198. Tempest HG, Ko E, Chan P, et al. Sperm aneuploidy frequencies analysed before and after chemotherapy in testicular cancer and Hodgkin's lymphoma patients. *Hum Reprod* 2008;23:251–258.

200. Blatt J. Pregnancy outcome in long-term survivors of childhood cancer. *Med Pediatr Oncol* 1999;33:29–33.

202. Meistrich ML, Byrne J. Genetic disease in offspring of long-term survivors of childhood and adolescent cancer treated with potentially mutagenic therapies. *Am J Hum Genet* 2002;70:1069–1071.

210. Frias S, Van Hummelen P, Meistrich ML, et al. NOVP chemotherapy for Hodgkin's disease transiently induces sperm aneuploidies associated with the major clinical aneuploidy syndromes involving chromosomes X, Y, 18, and 21. *Cancer Res* 2003;63:44–51.

211. Robbins WA, Meistrich ML, Moore D, et al. Chemotherapy induces transient sex chromosomal and autosomal aneuploidy in human sperm. *Nat Genet* 1997;16:74–78.

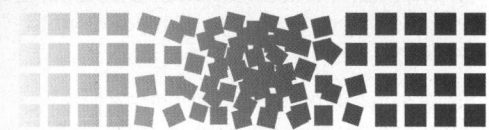

142 Fatigue

Sandra A. Mitchell and Ann M. Berger

INTRODUCTION

Fatigue is recognized as one of the most common symptoms in patients receiving treatment for cancer, often persisting beyond the conclusion of active treatment and at the end of life.[1,2] Longitudinal and comparative studies indicate that fatigue may also be a significant problem for cancer survivors, with many survivors reporting fatigue scores higher than that of an age-matched general population.[3–5] Prevalence estimates of fatigue vary from 25% to 99%, depending on how fatigue is defined and measured.[6–10] Fatigue is often found to occur as a component of a cluster of symptoms such as depression, pain, sleep disturbance, and menopausal symptoms.[11–14]

Cancer-related fatigue (CRF) is a multifaceted condition characterized by diminished energy and an increased need to rest, disproportionate to any recent change in activity level, and accompanied by a range of other characteristics, including generalized weakness, diminished mental concentration, insomnia or hypersomnia, and emotional reactivity.[15–17] Consequences of CRF include decrements in physical, social, cognitive, and vocational functioning[18–20]; mood[21–23] and sleep disturbances[24–26]; as well as emotional and spiritual distress for both the patient and the family members.[27–29]

This chapter reviews the state of the science concerning CRF, and offers guidance for practice and continued research. Major content areas relative to CRF are addressed and include: (1) definition and etiology, (2) explanatory models, (3) screening and evaluation of the patient with CRF, and (4) evidence-based pharmacologic and nonpharmacologic interventions to prevent and manage fatigue during and following cancer and its treatment.

DEFINITION AND ETIOLOGY OF CANCER-RELATED FATIGUE

The etiology and clinical expression of CRF is multidimensional. An inherently subjective condition, fatigue may be experienced and reported differently by each individual. Qualitative studies of fatigue underscore the fact that the cancer fatigue experience is unlike any other fatigue patients have previously experienced,[30] and patients emphasize that its unpredictability and refractoriness to self-management strategies that were previously effective make fatigue a particularly distressing symptom.[31] Personality and coping style may also influence the experience of CRF.[32–34] Some patients complain of a loss of efficiency, mental fogginess, inertia, and that sleep is not restorative; others describe an excessive need to rest, the inability to recover promptly from exertion, or muscle heaviness and weakness.[31,35] Whether these are features of CRF, the cause, or sequelae of fatigue, remains a focus of continued study.[17,36–38] Efforts continue to be directed toward clarifying what are the defining features of fatigue,[39] and determining how CRF may be distinguished from syndromes such as depression, cognitive dysfunction, or asthenia that have overlapping symptoms[20,40–44] or may share neurophysiologic mechanisms.[45,46]

Despite its complex etiology and varied features at presentation, fatigue may be defined quite simply as a distressing, persistent, subjective sense of physical, emotional, and/or cognitive tiredness or exhaustion related to cancer or cancer treatment that is not proportional to recent activity and that interferes with usual functioning.[47] The criteria for a diagnosis of CRF syndrome[15] are provided in Table 142.1.

The relative contributions to CRF of treatment with radiation, chemotherapy, hematopoietic stem cell transplantation, and hormonal, biologic, and molecularly targeted agents have been explored.[6,8,10,39,48–52] Fatigue symptoms are known to fluctuate across the cancer treatment course,[53] although few relationships between treatment-related variables such as dose-intensity, schedule, and time since treatment completion have been observed.[2] Comparatively less is known about the association between surgical treatments and CRF.[54] During a course of fractionated radiation therapy, fatigue is often cumulative and peak severity may occur after radiation is concluded.[55]

Although the precise pathophysiology is poorly understood, studies suggest that fatigue may be related to anemia; mood disorder; concurrent symptoms such as pain, sleep disturbances, electrolyte disturbances, cardiopulmonary, hepatic or renal dysfunction, hypothyroidism, hypogonadism, adrenal insufficiency, infection, dehydration, protein-calorie malnutrition, cachexia, asthenia, and deconditioning; and the side effects of drugs such as opioid analgesics or anticonvulsants that act on a central nervous system.[43,50,52,56–65] Altered energy metabolism within skeletal muscle has been postulated to cause CRF. Both the tumor itself and treatment with radiation or chemotherapy can produce anemia or cachexia, and both of these may contribute to altered skeletal muscle energy metabolism, disrupted mitochondrial synthesis of ATP, or diminished oxygen delivery to muscle cells.[66] Treatment with radiation or chemotherapy can produce anemia or cachexia, and both of these may contribute directly or indirectly to altered skeletal muscle energy. Accumulating evidence also suggests that gene polymorphisms, disruptions in the hypothalamic-pituitary-adrenal (HPA) axis, altered circadian rhythmicity, immune dysregulation, altered proteomic pathways, and proinflammatory cytokine activity may directly or indirectly contribute to CRF.[46,67–73] Associations between the occurrence and severity of CRF and demographic variables such as gender, age, marital status, and employment status have not been consistently identified.[2] In any one individual, the etiology of CRF is likely to be multifactorial, and contributors across the disease trajectory may fluctuate.

CURRENT THEORIES OF CANCER-RELATED FATIGUE

Several different explanatory models of CRF have been proposed. Many of these models use similar constructs. Conceptual models can be organized into four thematic groups: (1) energy balance/energy analysis models, (2) fatigue as a stress response models, (3) neuroendocrine-based regulatory fatigue models, and (4) hybrid models.

TABLE 142.1

International Classification of Diseases, 10th Revision, Criteria for Cancer-Related Fatigue

Six (or more) of the following symptoms have been present every day or nearly every day during the same 2-week period in the past month, and at least one of the symptoms is (A1) significant fatigue.

A1. Significant fatigue, diminished energy, or increased need to rest, disproportionate to any recent change in activity level
A2. Complaints of generalized weakness or limb heaviness
A3. Diminished concentration or attention
A4. Decreased motivation or interest to engage in usual activities
A5. Insomnia or hypersomnia
A6. Experience of sleep as unrefreshing or nonrestorative
A7. Perceived need to struggle to overcome inactivity
A8. Marked emotional reactivity (e.g., sadness, frustration, irritability) to feeling fatigued
A9. Difficulty completing daily tasks attributed to feeling fatigued
A10. Perceived problems with short-term memory
A11. Postexertional malaise lasting several hours
B. The symptoms cause clinically significant distress or impairment in social, occupational, or other important areas of functioning.
C. There is evidence from the history, physical examination, or laboratory findings that the symptoms are a consequence of cancer or cancer therapy.
D. The symptoms are not primarily a consequence of comorbid psychiatric disorders such as major depression, somatization disorder, somatoform disorder, or delirium.

Data derived Cella D, Peterman A, Passik S, et al. Progress toward guidelines for the management of fatigue. *Oncology (Williston Park, N.Y.)* 1998;12:369–377, with permission.

Energy balance/energy analysis models depict energy as the major variable in fatigue and alterations in the balance among intake, metabolism, and expenditure of energy as factors in producing fatigue. Examples of this thematic group of models include the integrated fatigue model of Piper et al.,[74] the energy analysis model of Irvine et al.,[75] and the psychobiologic-entropy model of Winningham.[76] *Fatigue as a stress response* models posit that tiredness, fatigue, and exhaustion form an adaptational continuum of response to stress. Each state along this continuum from tiredness to exhaustion may be distinguished by different behavioral and symptom patterns. Examples of models included in this thematic class include fatigue models proposed by Aistars,[77] Rhoten,[78] Glaus,[79] and Olson.[80] *Neuroendocrine-based regulatory fatigue* models hypothesize that the multiple dimensions of fatigue are explained by dysregulation in the function of neuroendocrine-based regulatory systems including the hypothalamic–pituitary axis, circadian rhythms, and neuroimmune system transmitter secretion and function.[81] Examples of models based on neuroendocrine dysregulation include those that have been proposed by Lee et al.,[82] Payne,[83] and Schubert et al.[71] Models that represent *hybrid* conceptual approaches have also been proposed. Olson et al.[84] have recently proposed a model of CRF suggesting that stressors associated with cancer and its treatment trigger declines in four systems—cognitive function, sleep quality, nutrition, and muscle endurance—and that these declines reduce one's ability to adapt. Al Majid and Gray[85] have also proposed a hybrid model that incorporates biologic, psychobehavioral, and functional variables implicated in the induction of fatigue, and have illustrated the application of this model to define the mechanisms by which exercise may ameliorate CRF.

Models in all four thematic classes may be helpful in generating testable hypotheses for continued research into the problem of

CRF and in guiding the development and evaluation of interventions to limit and manage fatigue, and to reduce its deleterious impact on health-related quality of life.

EVALUATION OF THE PATIENT WITH CANCER-RELATED FATIGUE

Studies suggest that CRF is underdiagnosed, that the assessment of fatigue in patients with cancer is suboptimal, and that health-care professionals may not fully appreciate the degree of distress and functional loss that fatigue produces.[86–90] Identified barriers to communication between patients and their clinicians about fatigue include a tendency to view fatigue as an inevitable consequence of illness, clinicians' failure to offer interventions, patients' lack of awareness of effective treatments for fatigue, a desire on the patient's part to treat fatigue without medications, and a tendency to be stoic about fatigue to avoid being labeled as a *complainer* and to avoid prompting a change in therapy toward less active/aggressive treatments.[86,91–93] Instruments to evaluate patient-derived barriers to fatigue management,[94,95] self-efficacy for fatigue management,[96] and the contributing factors to fatigue[58] have been proposed.

Identifying patients with CRF is the first key step in improving fatigue evaluation and management. Although there is currently no consensus concerning the optimal method or frequency to screen for CRF in the clinical or research setting,[97–99] evidence of the widespread occurrence of CRF suggests that routine screening for CRF at regular intervals throughout treatment, follow-up, and long-term follow-up is warranted. Technologies that use electronic or Web-based assessment routines, including computer-adapted testing (CAT), can streamline screening procedures and integrate fatigue screening into workflow.[100,101]

There is accumulating evidence that single-item measures to screen for fatigue are rapid and sensitive, and can be applied efficiently in the clinic to identify patients who would benefit from more systematic evaluation.[102] Based on National Comprehensive Cancer Network (NCCN) guidelines,[103] fatigue should be assessed quantitatively on a 0 to 10 scale (0 = no fatigue and 10 = worst fatigue imaginable); those patients with a severity of more than 4 should be further evaluated by history and physical examination.

Although a single-item measure may provide for a rapid assessment of general fatigue or serve as a screening tool, evidence suggests that single-item measures do not fully capture all the dimensions of fatigue.[104,105] There is good consensus in the literature that fatigue generally consists of a sensory dimension (fatigue severity, persistence), a physiologic dimension (e.g., leg weakness, diminished mental concentration), and a performance dimension (reduction in performance of needed or valued activities). More than 20 self-report measures (including single-item measures, multi-item unidimensional scales, and multidimensional inventories) have been developed to measure fatigue in patients with cancer.[106–110] Consideration of the measurement properties and strengths and limitations of these instruments, including reliability, validity, specificity, sensitivity to change, recall period, respondent burden, translation in multiple languages, and the availability of normed values to aid interpretation, should be used to guide decisions about the utility of a measure for specific clinical or research purposes.[97,111–113] Ecologic momentary assessment (a technique that offers real-time measurement of a phenomenon as it occurs in a naturalistic setting) may overcome some of the methodologic limitations of fatigue assessment, including recall bias and the influence of current context on the self-report of fatigue.[114]

A detailed history in patients with moderate or severe CRF includes the presence, intensity, and pervasiveness of fatigue, its course over time, the factors that exacerbate or relieve fatigue, and the impact of fatigue on functioning and level of distress. Clinicians can obtain valuable information about the consequences of CRF by exploring the effects of CRF on self-esteem, mood, and the ability to perform activities of daily living; fulfill important roles as parent, spouse, and worker; and relate to family and

TABLE 142.2

Dimensions to Include in an Assessment of Fatigue

Fatigue is a common problem for patients with cancer. It is a feeling of weariness, tiredness, or exhaustion that can include a loss of physical and/or emotional energy. Many factors can contribute to the fatigue that a person with cancer experiences.

- On a scale of 0 to 10, where zero is no fatigue and 10 is the worst fatigue imaginable, how severe has your fatigue been in the past 7 days:
- Would you say that your fatigue is mild, moderate, or severe?
- When did the fatigue start?_____
- Duration of fatigue: _____ Days per week or hours per day: _____
- To what extent have you, because of fatigue, had to limit social activity, had difficulty getting things done, or thought that fatigue was making it difficult to maintain a positive outlook?
- To what extent does fatigue interfere with relationships or fulfilling responsibilities at work or in the home?
- What makes your fatigue better?
- What makes your fatigue worse?
- What do you do to help with fatigue or manage fatigue?
- Does rest relieve your fatigue?
- Do you have any trouble sleeping?
- Do you have other symptoms such as pain, difficulty breathing, nausea, and vomiting?
- Do you experience anxiety? If yes, how often?
- Do you feel discouraged, blue, or sad? If yes, how often?
- Have you discussed your fatigue with anyone on your health-care team?
- Have you ever been given any recommendations for managing your fatigue?

friends. Also important to the evaluation is an assessment of what interventions the patient is using to manage fatigue and the effectiveness of them. The dimensions of the fatigue experience that should be explored when evaluating a patient with CRF are listed in Table 142.2.

In evaluating the patient with CRF, it is important to screen for treatable etiologic or potentiating factors including hypothyroidism, hypogonadism, adrenal insufficiency, cardiomyopathy, pulmonary dysfunction, anemia, sleep disturbance, fluid and electrolyte imbalances, emotional distress, physical inactivity, deconditioning, and uncontrolled concurrent symptoms.[10,57,115–118] The medication profile should also be reviewed to identify specific classes of medications such as opiates, antidepressants, anticonvulsants, antiemetics, antihistamines, and beta blockers, and drug–drug interactions that can also intensify fatigue.[19,103,119,120]

INTERVENTIONS FOR FATIGUE

Because fatigue typically has several different causes in any one patient, the treatment plan needs to be individualized. It is helpful to work with the patient and family caregivers to improve the assessment of fatigue and identify management strategies. Open communication between the patient, family, and caregiving team will facilitate discussion about the experience of fatigue and its effects on daily life. General supportive care recommendations for patients with fatigue include encouraging a balanced diet with adequate intake of fluid, calories, protein, carbohydrates, fat, vitamins, ABD minerals and balancing rest with physical activity and attention-restoring activities such as exposure to natural environments and pleasant distractions such as music.[103]

There have been more than 210 empiric studies of pharmacologic and nonpharmacologic interventions to reduce or manage CRF and a number of meta-analyses or systematic reviews.[121–134] These are summarized in Table 142.3, and selected findings are

TABLE 142.3

Evidence-Based Interventions for Fatigue During and Following Cancer and Its Treatment

Interventions for Fatigue with Strong Evidence Supporting Effectiveness
- Exercise
- Education/information provision and supportive counseling
- Measures to optimize sleep quality
- Energy conservation and activity management
- Structured rehabilitation
- Yoga
- Management of concurrent symptoms

Interventions for Fatigue with Some Evidence Supporting Effectiveness
- Acupuncture
- Massage
- Levocarnitine supplementation
- Corticosteroids
- Ginseng
- Bright light therapy
- Mindfulness-based stress reduction
- Healing touch, hypnosis, relaxation

Interventions for Fatigue for which Effectiveness Has Not Been Established
- Paroxetine, methylphenidate, donepezil, bupropion sustained release, modafinil, etanercept, infliximab, amisulpride, sertraline, venlafaxine
- Correction of anemia less than 10 g/dL with erythropoiesis-stimulating agents
- Essiac, Chinese medicinal herbs, ginseng, mistletoe extract
- High-dose vitamin C, multiple vitamin, omega-3 fatty acid supplementation
- Adenosine 5'-triphosphate infusion
- Beta-hydroxyl beta-methyl butyrate, glutamine, and arginine mixture
- Individual and group psychotherapy
- Animal-assisted therapy, art therapy, expressive writing
- Reiki, aromatherapy, qigong, distraction/virtual reality immersion
- Combination therapy: aromatherapy, foot soak, and reflexology
- Combination therapy: medroxyprogesterone, celecoxib, and enteral food supplementation
- Combination therapy: soy protein supplementation and nutrition counseling following discharge from hospital

Interventions for Fatigue Supported by Expert Opinion
- Work with patient and family to improve assessment of fatigue and identify management strategies
- Promote open communication between patient, family, and caregiving team to facilitate discussions about the experience of fatigue and its effects on daily life
- Consider attention restoring activities such as exposure to natural environments and pleasant distractions such as music
- Encourage a balanced diet with adequate intake of fluid, calories, protein, carbohydrates, fat, vitamins, and minerals

Data derived from Mitchell SA. Cancer-related fatigue: State of the science. *PMR* 2010;2:364–383; Mitchell SA, Beck SL, Eaton LH. ONS Putting Evidence Into Practice (PEP): Fatigue. In: Eaton LH, Tipton JM, eds. *Putting Evidence into Practice.* Pittsburgh: Oncology Nursing Society; 2009; and Mitchell S, Beck S, Hood L, et al. Putting evidence into practice (PEP): evidence-based interventions for fatigue during and following cancer and its treatment. *Clinical J Oncol Nurs* 2007;11:99.

discussed here. Guidelines for the management of cancer-related fatigue have been disseminated by NCCN[103] and the Oncology Nursing Society.[135]

PHARMACOLOGIC MEASURES

Several pharmacologic agents (including paroxetine, venlafaxine, methylphenidate, donepezil, bupropion, and modafinil) have been evaluated for their effectiveness at reducing fatigue during and following cancer treatment.[122,126,136] Four trials have examined the effectiveness of paroxetine in treating fatigue during and following cancer treatment with mixed results. In three multicenter, randomized, double-blind, placebo-controlled trials, paroxetine 20 mg by mouth daily did not demonstrate a beneficial effect on fatigue outcomes, although improvements in depression and overall mood were noted in the paroxetine treatment group.[137–139] However, two small trials show a trend toward a possible benefit for either paroxetine[140] or venlafaxine[141] in treating fatigue in women experiencing hot flashes.

Two recent meta-analyses and a systematic review concluded that there is preliminary evidence supporting the use of methylphenidate to treat CRF, although more study of efficacy and tolerability was warranted.[127,142,143] Recent evidence from a meta-analysis across trials suggests that the D-isomer form of methylphenidate may be more effective than other forms, and that patients with more severe and those demonstrating an improvement in fatigue within the first few days of methylphenidate treatment are the most likely to derive benefit.[144]

Two small trials also suggest that donepezil 5 to 10 mg per day[145,146] or bupropion sustained release at a dose of 100 to 150 mg per day[147,148] may be effective at limiting fatigue. However, in a controlled trial of donepezil, improvements in fatigue outcomes were not observed.[149] Several trials also suggest that modafinil at a dose of 100 mg twice a day may be effective at treating fatigue and improving daytime wakefulness and cognitive function in patients during and following cancer treatment.[150–153] Additional rigorously designed trials of donepezil, bupropion, and modafinil for fatigue appear warranted.

Several nutritional supplements including coenzyme Q10, levocarnitine, lectin standardized mistletoe, omega-3 fatty acid supplements, ginseng, guarana, and valerian have been explored, either as single agents or as part of a combination therapy.[130,154–156] Several trials suggest that levocarnitine supplementation is effective in patients who have low serum carnitine levels.[157–161] However a large double-blind, placebo-controlled trial failed to demonstrate an improvement in fatigue outcomes in patients with malignancy and good performance status, even in those study participants who were levocarnitine deficient.[162] Guarana 50 mg twice daily has been shown to be safe and effective at treating CRF in women with breast cancer in a randomized placebo-controlled cross-over study (n = 75)[163]; however, guarana 75 mg once daily was not effective at treating fatigue in women with breast cancer who were undergoing radiation therapy.[164] The primary active ingredient in guarana is caffeine. A week course of Wisconsin ginseng dosed at 2,000 mg daily was effective at improving fatigue outcomes in cancer survivors and was well-tolerated in a large (n = 364) double-blind, placebo-controlled trial.[165]

Low-dose dexamethasone at a dose of 4 mg twice daily for 2 weeks improved fatigue outcomes in a randomized placebo-controlled trial in 84 patients with advanced cancers.[166] Although adverse events were comparable in the dexamethasone and placebo groups, systemic corticosteroids could be associated with a prominent adverse effects profile in particular subpopulations such as those at the end of life.[167] A pilot, randomized placebo-controlled cross-over study has also shown evidence for the effectiveness and tolerability of thyrotropin-releasing hormone in improving fatigue outcomes in a small sample of cancer patients with significant fatigue.[168] Although male hypogonadism

is hypothesized to adversely affect mood and well-being,[169] a recent blinded, placebo-controlled trial of testosterone replacement therapy in a small sample of men with advanced cancer did not demonstrate positive effectiveness on fatigue end points.[170]

TREATMENT OF ANEMIA WITH ERYTHROPOIESIS-STIMULATING AGENTS

Although data from seven systematic reviews suggest that patients receiving erythropoiesis-stimulating agents (ESA) to correct severe anemia (hemoglobin less than 10 g/dL) may experience diminished fatigue and increased vigor,[171] there is only limited evidence that ESAs improve fatigue when anemia is less severe.[172–176] In addition, a recent systematic review concluded that in many of the trials, the improvement in fatigue outcomes did not exceed the minimally important clinical difference.[177] Importantly, the use of ESAs for fatigue must be considered in light of safety issues, including an increased risk of thrombotic events, hypertension, and pure red cell aplasia, and concerns that ESAs may decrease local–regional disease control and survival outcomes in particular tumor types.[173,175,178]

National clinical practice guidelines[179–181] and product labeling from the U.S. Food and Drug Administration[182] should direct individualized management of patients with cancer- or treatment-associated anemia, including an analysis of the risks and benefits of ESAs versus packed red blood cell transfusions based on cancer treatment goals, and decisions about patient monitoring, treatment thresholds, dose reductions, treatment discontinuation, and the use of supplemental iron in patients receiving ESAs. Particular caution is needed when using ESAs in patients who are not receiving chemotherapy because recent trials report increased thromboembolic risks and decreased survival in this subpopulation.[176,183–185]

EXERCISE

Meta-analyses of randomized trials support the benefits of exercise in the management of fatigue during and following cancer treatment in patients with breast cancer or solid tumors, or who are undergoing hematopoietic stem cell transplantation, although effect sizes are generally small, and positive results for the outcome of fatigue have not been observed consistently across studies.[132,186–189] The exercise modalities that have been applied differ in content (walking, cycling, swimming, resistive exercise, or combined exercise), frequency (ranging from two times per week to two times daily), intensity (with most programs at 50% to 90% of the estimated VO₂ maximum heart rate), degree of supervision (fully supervised group versus self-directed exercise), and duration (from 2 weeks up to 1 year). Knowledge about the type, intensity, and duration of physical exercise that is most beneficial for reducing fatigue at different stages of disease and treatment is not known,[190] and more research is needed to systematically assess the safety of exercise (both aerobic exercise and strength training) in cancer subpopulations.[191]

MANAGEMENT OF CONCURRENT SYMPTOMS

A recent large randomized trial demonstrated that effective management of concurrent symptoms including pain, shortness of breath, insomnia, and depression also produces improvements in CRF outcomes.[38,118] Four other RCTs (n = 200 cancer patients with major depressive disorder[192]; n = 83 cancer survivors with fatigue[193]; n = 45 women with metastatic breast cancer who were depressed[194]; n = 78 advanced cancer patients with fatigue[118] and a small case series (n = 6 women with metastatic breast cancer)[195] as well as a systematic review,[128] confirm that cognitive-behavioral therapy (CBT) interventions for symptoms may also alleviate CRF, including fatigue that occurs as a component of a symptom cluster along with pain and insomnia.

PSYCHOEDUCATIONAL INTERVENTIONS

Several adequately powered randomized controlled trials suggest that educational interventions; cognitive-behavioral treatment for fatigue, depression, and other symptoms; and psychological support have a role in supporting positive coping in patients with fatigue.[121,124,196,197] Psychoeducational interventions that have been shown to be effective include anticipatory guidance about patterns of fatigue and recommendations for self-management, counseling, and supportive psychotherapy, and coordination of care. Energy conservation and activity management is a self-management intervention that teaches patients to apply the principles of energy conservation and activity management and provides coaching to integrate these activities into their daily lifestyle.

INTERVENTIONS TO IMPROVE SLEEP QUALITY

Studies indicate that cognitive-behavioral interventions designed to improve sleep quality also have a beneficial effect on fatigue.[198–201] In contrast, the efficacy of pharmacologic therapies in treating fatigue by reducing insomnia has had very little systematic study.[202] Cognitive-behavioral interventions to improve sleep quality can be delivered individually or in a group setting, and include relaxation training along with sleep-consolidation strategies (e.g., avoiding long or late afternoon naps, limiting time in bed to actual sleep time), stimulus control therapy (e.g., go to bed only when sleepy, use bed/bedroom for sleep and sexual activities only, set a consistent time to lie down and get up, avoid caffeine and stimulating activity in the evening), and strategies to reduce cognitive-emotional arousal (e.g., keep at least an hour to relax before going to bed, establish a presleep routine to be used every night). Morning exposure to bright light has been shown in two small randomized trials to prevent deterioration in CRF during chemotherapy for breast cancer,[203,204] potentially by protecting recipients from circadian rhythm desynchronization during cancer treatment.[205]

STRUCTURED REHABILITATION

Several trials[206–211] and two systematic reviews[212–214] support a conclusion that structured rehabilitation programs delivered formally by a multidisciplinary group result in statistically significant and sustained improvements in fatigue, particularly in patients who have completed treatment and are in the survivorship phase. However, because at least one study[215] suggests that programs that are too intensive may actually worsen fatigue, tailoring based on the patient's current level of energy and stage along the treatment trajectory is important.

INTEGRATIVE THERAPIES

There is preliminary evidence to support the efficacy of integrative approaches to the treatment of fatigue, including yoga, relaxation, mindfulness-based stress reduction, acupuncture, medical qigong, massage, healing touch, and Reiki, and combined-modality interventions that include aromatherapy, lavender foot soaks, and reflexology.[125,128] The design of these studies tend to be open label and/or uncontrolled, with no random assignment, and with sample sizes that were extremely small, making it difficult to draw firm conclusions about efficacy. Despite these limitations, and with acknowledgment that the inclusion of controls such as double-blinding presents methodologic challenges,[216] results suggest that these complementary therapies have potential in the treatment of fatigue in patients with cancer.

Yoga practices have shown particular effectiveness at improving fatigue outcomes in two rigorously conducted RCTs in breast cancer survivors.[217,218] Yoga may also have beneficial effects in reducing fatigue in other populations.[219–224] However, four systematic reviews[223–226] have concluded that the effectiveness of yoga on fatigue outcomes has not been consistently established across a wide range of patient populations and at all points in the cancer trajectory. In addition, the high risk of bias across studies with respect to sample selection and blinding of participants and outcome assessors was also noted.

SUMMARY

A wide range of pharmacologic and nonpharmacologic interventions have been studied, although many have been tested only in uncontrolled or pilot studies. Interventions for fatigue that are supported by one or more well-designed randomized trials include exercise, psychoeducational interventions, measures to optimize sleep quality, as well as integrative and behavioral approaches such as relaxation, mindfulness-based stress reduction, massage, and healing touch. There is preliminary evidence or inconclusive evidence to suggest that pharmacologic agents, including paroxetine, methylphenidate, donepezil, bupropion sustained release, modafinil, and levocarnitine, have a role in the management of fatigue, although systematic drug development studies are needed to define the optimal dosing, gauge the toxicity profile, and determine the effectiveness of these agents in specific populations. Interventions for which there is preliminary evidence of effectiveness include individual and group psychotherapy and complementary therapies such as yoga and acupuncture. Rigorously designed and adequately powered randomized controlled trials of therapies for fatigue that have shown initial promise are urgently needed.

SELECTED REFERENCES

The full reference list can be accessed at lwwhealthlibrary.com/oncology.

4. Goedendorp MM, Gielissen MF, Verhagen CA, et al. Development of fatigue in cancer survivors: a prospective follow-up study from diagnosis into the year after treatment. *J Pain Symptom Manage* 2013;45:213–222.
6. Campos MP, Hassan BJ, Riechelmann R, et al. Cancer-related fatigue: a practical review. *Ann Oncol* 2011;22:1273–1279.
10. Weis J. Cancer-related fatigue: prevalence, assessment and treatment strategies. *Expert Rev Pharmacoecon Outcomes Res* 2011;11:441–446.
16. Barsevick AM, Irwin MR, Hinds P, et al. Recommendations for high-priority research on cancer-related fatigue in children and adults. *J Natl Cancer Inst* 2013;105:1432–1440.
17. Piper BF, Cella D. Cancer-related fatigue: definitions and clinical subtypes. *J Natl Compr Canc Netw* 2010;8:958–966.
31. Scott JA, Lasch KE, Barsevick AM, et al. Patients' experiences with cancer-related fatigue: a review and synthesis of qualitative research. *Oncol Nurs Forum* 2011;38:E191–E203.
32. Lukkahatai N, Saligan LN. Association of catastrophizing and fatigue: a systematic review. *J Psychosom Res* 2013;74:100–109.
35. Hauser K, Rybicki L, Walsh D. What's in a Name? Word descriptors of cancer-related fatigue. *Palliat Med* 2010;24:724–730.
38. de Raaf PJ, de Klerk C, Timman R, et al. Systematic monitoring and treatment of physical symptoms to alleviate fatigue in patients with advanced cancer: a randomized controlled trial. *J Clin Oncol* 2013;31:716–723.

39. Donovan KA, McGinty HL, Jacobsen PB. A systematic review of research using the diagnostic criteria for cancer-related fatigue. *Psychooncology* 2013;22:737–744.

41. Traeger L, Braun IM, Greer JA, et al. Parsing depression from fatigue in patients with cancer using the fatigue symptom inventory. *J Pain Symptom Manage* 2011;42:52–59.

42. Scialla SJ, Cole RP, Bednarz L. Redefining cancer-related asthenia-fatigue syndrome. *J Palliat Med* 2006;9:866–872.

46. Bower JE, Lamkin DM. Inflammation and cancer-related fatigue: mechanisms, contributing factors, and treatment implications. *Brain Behav Immun* 2013;30:S48–S57.

47. Berger AM, Abernethy AP, Atkinson A, et al. Cancer-related fatigue. *J Natl Compr Cancer Netw* 2010;8:904–931.

52. Giacalone A, Quitadamo D, Zanet E, et al. Cancer-related fatigue in the elderly. *Support Care Cancer* 2013;21:2899–2911.

60. Oh HS, Seo WS. Systematic review and meta-analysis of the correlates of cancer-related fatigue. *Worldviews Evid Based Nurs* 2011;8:191–201.

68. Saligan LN, Kim HS. A systematic review of the association between immunogenomic markers and cancer-related fatigue. *Brain Behav Immun* 2012;26:830–848.

81. Miller AH, Ancoli-Israel S, Bower JE, et al. Neuroendocrine-immune mechanisms of behavioral comorbidities in patients with cancer. *J Clin Oncol* 2008;26:971–982.

92. Pertl MM, Quigley J, Hevey D. 'I'm not complaining because I'm alive': barriers to the emergence of a discourse of cancer-related fatigue. *Psychol Health* 2014;29:141–161.

93. Borneman T, Koczywas M, Sun V, et al. Effectiveness of a clinical intervention to eliminate barriers to pain and fatigue management in oncology. *J Palliat Med* 2011;14:197–205.

101. Lai JS, Cella D, Choi S, et al. How item banks and their application can influence measurement practice in rehabilitation medicine: a PROMIS fatigue item bank example. *Arch Phys Med Rehabil* 2011;92:S20–S27.

109. Minton O, Stone P. A systematic review of the scales used for the measurement of cancer-related fatigue (CRF). *Ann Oncol* 2009;20:17–25.

110. Seyidova-Khoshknabi D, Davis MP, Walsh D. Review article: a systematic review of cancer-related fatigue measurement questionnaires. *Am J Hosp Palliat Care* 2011;28:119–129.

113. Barsevick AM, Cleeland CS, Manning DC, et al. ASCPRO recommendations for the assessment of fatigue as an outcome in clinical trials. *J Pain Symptom Manage* 2010;39:1086–1099.

120. Dy SM, Lorenz KA, Naeim A, et al. Evidence-based recommendations for cancer fatigue, anorexia, depression, and dyspnea. *J Clin Oncol* 2008;26:3886–3895.

126. Minton O, Richardson A, Sharpe M, et al. Drug therapy for the management of cancer related fatigue. *Cochrane Database Syst Rev* 2010:CD006704.

127. Minton O, Richardson A, Sharpe M, et al. Psychostimulants for the management of cancer-related fatigue: a systematic review and meta-analysis. *J Pain Symptom Manage* 2011;41:761–767.

130. Finnegan-John J, Molassiotis A, Richardson A, Ream E. A systematic review of complementary and alternative medicine interventions for the management of cancer-related fatigue. *Integr Cancer Ther* 2013;12:276–290.

133. Puetz TW, Herring MP. Differential effects of exercise on cancer-related fatigue during and following treatment: a meta-analysis. *Am J Prev Med* 2012;43:e1–e24.

171. Eton DT, Cella D. Do erythropoietic-stimulating agents relieve fatigue? A review of reviews. *Cancer Treat Res* 2011;157:181–194.

173. Bohlius J, Tonia T, Schwarzer G. Twist and shout: one decade of meta-analyses of erythropoiesis-stimulating agents in cancer patients. *Acta Haematologica* 2011;125:55–67.

187. Mustian KM, Sprod LK, Janelsins M, et al. Exercise recommendations for cancer-related fatigue, cognitive impairment, sleep problems, depression, pain, anxiety, and physical dysfunction: a review. *Oncol Hematol Rev* 2012;8:81–88.

196. Jacobsen PB, Donovan KA, Vadaparampil ST, et al. "Systematic review and meta-analysis of psychological and activity-based interventions for cancer-related fatigue": Correction. *Health Psychol* 2008;27:42.

197. Wanchai A, Armer JM, Stewart BR. Nonpharmacologic supportive strategies to promote quality of life in patients experiencing cancer-related fatigue: a systematic review. *Clin J Oncol Nurs* 2011;15:203–214.

226. Sadja J, Mills PJ. Effects of yoga interventions on fatigue in cancer patients and survivors: a systematic review of randomized controlled trials. *Explore (NY)* 2013;9:232–243.

143 Second Cancers

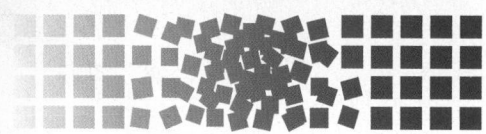

Lois B. Travis, Smita Bhatia, James M. Allan, Kevin C. Oeffinger, and Andrea Ng

INTRODUCTION

The occurrence of second primary cancers (SPC) in cancer survivors is one of the most serious and lethal complications of cancer and its therapy. Subsequent malignancies comprise about 18% of all incident cancers in the United States,[1] superseding first cancers of the breast, lung, and prostate. As such, second-order and higher order cancers are now the most common incident cancer and have been identified as one of the National Cancer Institute's (NCI's) Provocative Questions.[2] Increases in the prevalence of subsequent malignancies mirror advances in cancer survival, and thus reflect improvements in early detection, supportive care, and treatment. For all cancers combined, the 5-year relative survival rate has advanced steadily over the past few decades and is now approximately 66.1% for patients diagnosed between 1999 and 2006.[1] There are presently over 13.7 million cancer survivors in the United States, representing approximately 4% of the population,[3] and this number continues to grow at a rate of about 2% per year.[4] By 2022, it is anticipated that this population will expand to 18 million. Commensurately, it is expected that the number of patients with subsequent and higher order malignancies will increase.

In view of these rising numbers, it is important to recognize that SPC may not necessarily be due to the late sequelae of cytotoxic treatment, but rather reflect shared etiologic influences (including tobacco and excessive alcohol intake), environmental determinants, host factors, genetic predisposition, and combinations of influences including gene–environment interactions.[5,6] Even though treatment can, in part, enable patients to live long enough to develop SPC, therapy in and of itself might not be solely responsible for their occurrence. A population-based survey of the U.S. Surveillance, Epidemiology and End Results (SEER) registries concluded that cancer treatment may cause only a minor proportion of all SPCs after all adult-onset cancers considered together, although it has a considerably larger role in survivors of childhood cancer.[7] Nonetheless, among long-term survivors of selected adult-onset cancers such as Hodgkin lymphoma (HL), SPCs are one of the most common causes of death.[8] Although the carcinogenicity of radiotherapy has long been recognized,[9,10] an increasing body of research points to the importance of the role of chemotherapeutic agents, not only in the development of treatment-related leukemias, but also now in selected solid tumors including cancers of the lungs, sarcoma, thyroid, stomach, bladder, and kidney.[9,10] Although in many patients, the development of SPC can be lethal, outcomes in patients after a SPC are being increasingly studied.[10–16] Moreover, a number of patients may develop third and higher order cancers.[17] The important role of genetic susceptibility in the development of SPC was reviewed in 2006 by Travis et al.,[6] but major advances in genomics now underscore the importance of these factors. Shared genetic pathways for a number of different tumor types were recently highlighted by Sakoda et al.[18] (Fig. 143.1). The focus of this chapter will be treatment-associated malignancies, taking into account new data on radiotherapy and chemotherapy carcinogenicity, genetic underpinnings, and outcomes.

CARCINOGENICITY OF INDIVIDUAL TREATMENT MODALITIES

Radiation Therapy

The leukemogenic and carcinogenic effects of ionizing radiation have long been recognized in atomic bomb survivors[19–25] and individuals exposed to low doses of radiation for diagnostic purposes or therapeutic radiation for benign conditions.[26–30] The relation between radiation dose and cancer risk is well described in these low-dose ranges, with an approximately linear increase in risk with increasing radiation dose up to about 5 Gy for solid tumors,[22,31,32] and up to 1.5 to 2 Gy for leukemia.[10,23,33,34] The traditional view has been that increased cell killing occurs in the higher dose region and, therefore, results in a lowered cancer risk, whereas tissues exposed to intermediate doses are at highest risk for cancer development. A classic radiation dose-response curve plotting the incidence of cancer against the dose of radiation absorbed has a characteristic shape, with the incidence of malignancy increasing with a dose up to a maximum of about 3 to 10 Gy, followed by a decrease in cancer risk with a further increase in dose.[34,35]

Much of the data on the leukemogenic and carcinogenic effects of radiation in the higher dose range were derived from cancer survivors who have received therapeutic radiation.[9,10] In assessing radiation-related SPCs in these patients, it is important to take into consideration other potential contributing factors. These include exposure to cytotoxic drugs (see Chemotherapy section), genetic predisposition,[36–40] immunosuppression,[41,42] infections,[42–44] environmental exposures,[45] and heightened surveillance in cancer survivors.[46] Additional factors can modify the effect of radiotherapy on SPC risk. Patients with certain cancer prone syndromes, including hereditary retinoblastoma (RB), nevoid basal cell carcinoma syndrome, and neurofibromatosis-1 are more susceptible to radiation-induced cancer.[36,47–49] More recently, genome-wide association studies (GWAS) have identified single nucleotide polymorphisms (SNP) associated with sensitivity to radiation-related cancers.[50–52] Tobacco history increases the risk of treatment-related lung cancer in a multiplicative manner as demonstrated in a case-control study of HL survivors.[53] Younger age at irradiation is associated with a significantly increased risk of breast cancer[54–59] and thyroid cancer,[54,60] as shown in survivors of HL, breast cancer, and childhood cancer. On the other hand, early menopause has a protective effect on breast cancer after radiotherapy in HL survivors,[61,62] suggesting that ovarian hormones play an important role in promoting tumorigenesis once an initiating event has been induced by radiation.

More recent studies have addressed the effect of radiation dose in the therapeutic range on SPC risk by estimation of radiation dose at the site of SPC development. The risk of radiation-related cancer has been shown to increase with increasing dose for cancers of the breast,[59,61–63] esophagus,[64] lungs,[53,65] stomach,[66] meningioma,[67] and sarcoma,[68–70] with no evidence of a downturn in risk at high doses within the therapeutic range. Preliminary data also

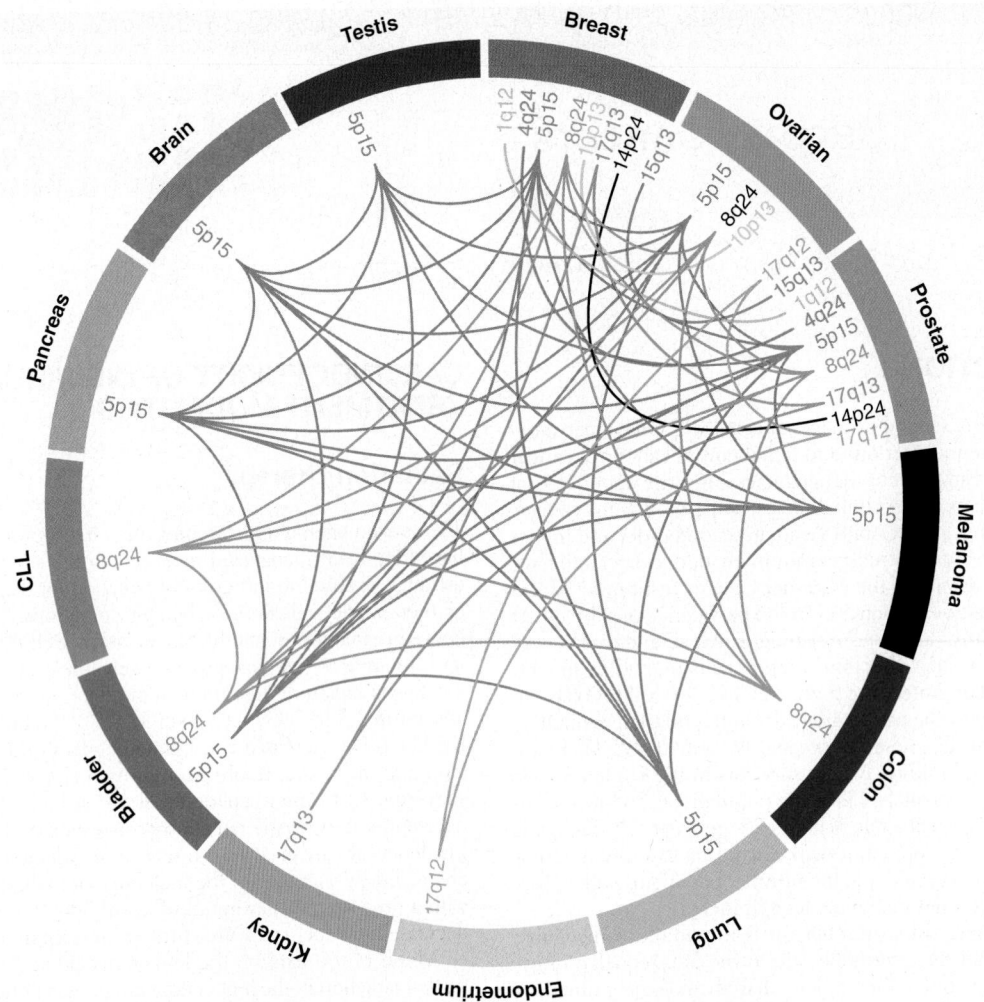

Figure 143.1 Pleiotropy among different cancers detected by the Collaborative Oncological Gene-environment Study (COGS) and previous association studies. Risk-associated loci for each cancer are indicated by chromosomal location, and sharing is indicated by colored lines connecting different cancers. For example, the loci at 8q24 are associated with breast, ovarian, prostate, colon, and bladder cancers and with chronic lymphocytic leukemia (CLL) *(light blue lines)*. (Reprinted with permission from Sakoda LC, Jorgenson E, Witte JS. Turning of COGS moves forward findings for hormonally mediated cancers. *Nat Genet* 2013;45:345–348.)

show an increasing risk of secondary pancreas cancers with increasing radiation dose received during treatment for either HL or testis cancer (LB Travis, personal communication). An exception to these trends is thyroid cancer risk, which has been shown to decrease after doses above 20 to 30 Gy in childhood cancer survivors.[71,72] The radiation dose-response relation in SPC development, therefore, appears to be tissue specific. A recent systemic review on data on the radiation dose–response relationship for 11 second solid cancers found that for most SPCs (except for thyroid cancer), the dose-response curve was linear, even at doses of 60 Gy or higher.[73]

In addition to radiation dose, radiotherapy fields, which directly reflect the volume of normal exposed tissue, can affect SPC risk. The association between more extensive treatment fields and higher SPC risk has been shown in survivors of HL,[74,75] breast cancer,[76,77] and prostate cancer.[78]

Radiotherapy techniques and delivery systems have undergone major transformations over the past few decades.[9] In recent years, highly conformal radiation techniques, including intensity-modulated radiation therapy (IMRT), have been adopted.[79] IMRT uses sophisticated computer technology and dose optimization algorithms to produce precisely shaped dose distributions via multileaf

collimator systems resulting in improved dose conformality in the high-dose region. However, with the use of multiple modulated beams, a larger volume of normal tissue is exposed to low doses of radiation. In addition, more radiation output, or monitor units (MU), are needed to deliver a specified dose to the target than for conventional treatments.[80] Figure 143.2 illustrates the differences in dose distribution using conventional three-dimensional (3D) radiation therapy with anterior–posterior beam versus IMRT approach in a patient with mediastinal disease. The IMRT technique allows improved conformality at high doses, but at the expense of a larger volume of normal tissue exposed to low doses.

There is also increasing momentum for the use of proton therapy, given the physical characteristics of the depth dose curve,[81,82] which peaks at the end of the particle range (Bragg peak). The beam has sharp edges with little side scatter, and the dose drops to zero after the Bragg peak. In addition, the integral dose, or the mean absorbed dose multiplied by the mass of irradiated tissue, is significantly lower with proton than photon beam. However, there have been concerns with regard to the SPC risk associated with ancillary neutron production, especially with the passive scattering technique, which results in dose exposure to the whole body.[83,84] The newer beam scanning technique holds

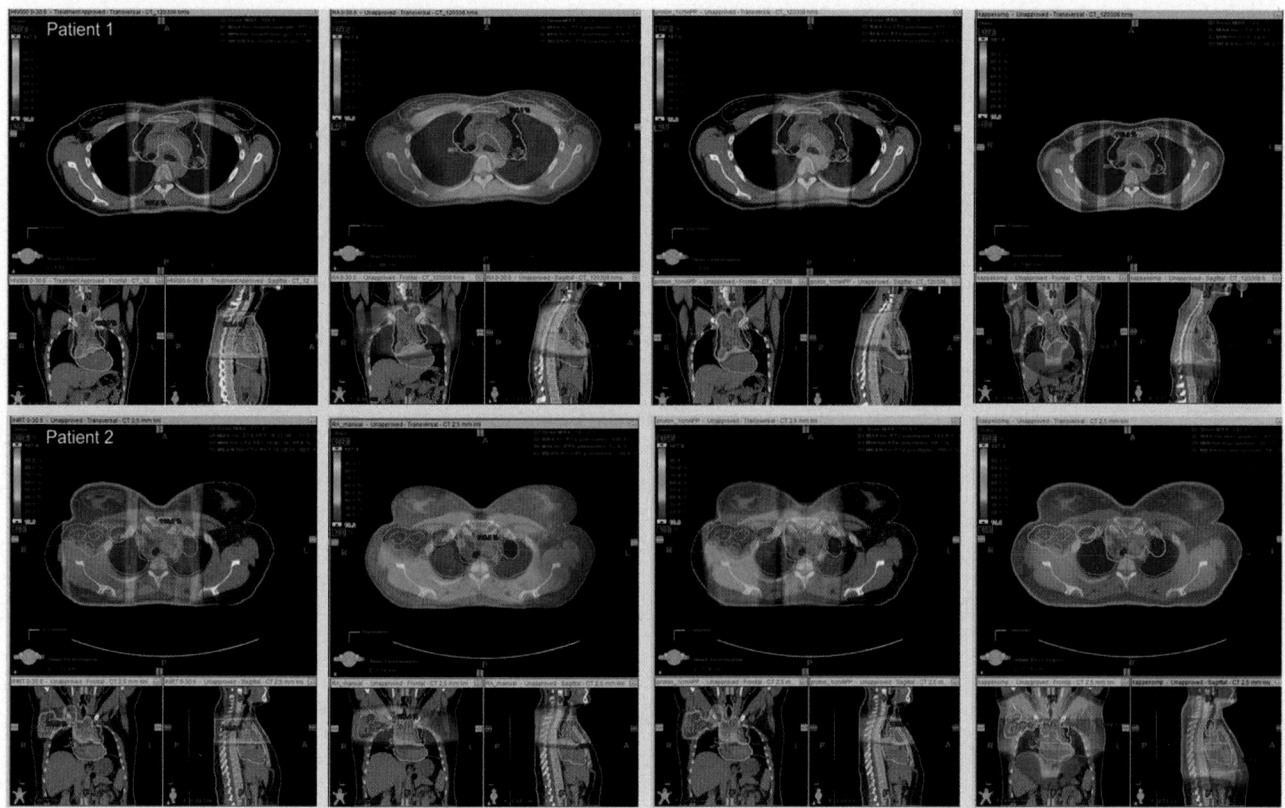

Figure 143.2 Treatment plans with three-dimensional (3D-CRT) *(left)*, VMAT *(middle, left)*, proton therapy (PT) *(middle, right)*, and MF *(right)* treatment for two different patients with mediastinal HL are shown in dose color wash. The *top panels* show the treatment plans for patient 1; the *lower panels* are for patient 2. (With permission from Maraldo MV, Brodin NP, Aznar MC, et al. Estimated risk of cardiovascular disease and secondary cancers with modern highly conformal radiotherapy for early-stage mediastinal Hodgkin lymphoma. *Ann Oncol* 2013;24:2113–2118.)

promise for reducing SPC risk as a result of low neutron contamination.[83,85] This technique utilizes magnetically scanned pencil beams over the target volume, does not require scattering devices, collimation, or compensation, and therefore, is associated with reduced secondary neutron production from the treatment head.

There has been a growing literature on the estimation of SPC risks using radiobiologic modeling of SPC risk with these new radiotherapy techniques and delivery systems,[80,86] some of which focused on specific disease sites, including prostate cancer,[87–90] HL,[91,92] gynecologic malignancies,[93] lung cancer, and childhood malignancies.[90,94] The estimated risks vary considerably depending on the model assumptions.[88,89,92] Several studies estimated the lowest SPC risk with the scanning proton beam technique.[91,94,95] Epidemiologic data for SPC risks in patients treated with modern techniques are currently lacking. Preliminary epidemiologic data on SPC risks following proton beam therapy for 503 patients treated at the Harvard Cyclotron with proton radiotherapy with passive scattering were reported.[96] Compared to a matched cohort of 1,591 photon-treated patients identified in the SEER database,[96] treatment with photon therapy was associated with a significantly increased risk of SPC (hazard ratio, 2.73; *p* <0.0001) after adjusting for age and gender. The median duration of follow-up was 6.1 and 7.7 years, respectively, in the photon and proton cohorts. Additional observation time may be needed to fully assess the long-term SPC risks following proton therapy. In a recent report issued by the National Council on Radiation Protection and Measurements (NCRP),[9] recommendations with regard to future research on treatment-associated SPCs were outlined and are summarized in Table 143.1.

Chemotherapy

The association between alkylating agents and acute myeloid leukemia (AML) has long been recognized. Alkylating agents with known or suspected leukemogenic effects include mechlorethamine, chlorambucil, cyclophosphamide, melphalan, semustine, lomustine, carmustine, procarbazine, prednimustine, busulfan, dihydroxybusulfan, and the platinating agents.[97–100] Of these, the platinating agents are the most commonly used group of cytotoxic drugs worldwide, and the most recently identified class of drugs for which highly significant dose-response relationships with therapy-associated leukemia have been observed.[101,102] Chemotherapeutic topoisomerase II poisons, such as the epipodophyllotoxins (e.g., etoposide), the anthracyclines (e.g., epirubicin), and the anthracenediones (e.g., mitoxantrone), are associated with a clinically and cytogenetically distinct type of AML, which show a relatively short induction period (median 2 to 3 years) and typically present without preceding myelodysplastic syndrome (MDS).[103–105]

Although the risk of treatment-related leukemias following chemotherapy has long been established, the induction of solid tumors is less well understood. Elevated risks of cancers of the bladder,[106] bone,[107] the lungs,[53] gastrointestinal sites,[66,108] and the thyroid[109] following chemotherapy have been reported. There are also suggestions of associations between anthracyclines and excess sarcomas and thyroid cancers.[108,109] Wilson et al.[110] reported a 3.5-fold increased risk of renal cell carcinoma, albeit based on four cases, after cisplatin exposure in childhood cancer survivors. More recently, Fung et al.[111] found a significant threefold (standardized incidence ratio [SIR] 3.37; 95% confidence interval [CI], 1.798 to 5.77; n = 13 cases) risk of renal cell carcinoma

TABLE 143.1

Summary of Conclusions and Research Recommendations of the NCRP 1-17 Report on Second Malignant Neoplasms after Radiotherapy

Conclusions

- Second malignant neoplasm (SMN) after radiotherapy (RT) are experienced by an ever growing number of cancer survivors.
- Quantitative estimates of RT-induced SMN are: (1) derived from studies incorporating comprehensive dose reconstructions, (2) although based on past regimens, are applicable to risk assessment following current RT in terms of organ-specific doses and dose-response relationship.
- Newer RT modalities and treated techniques, which include intensity-modulated radiation therapy (IMRT) and protons, result in different organ dose distributions.
- Computational models are useful for SMN risk assessment and comparisons with other RT modalities.
- Few reports describe survival after SMN.
- For individual and epidemiologic risk assessment, the effective dose (a construct for radiation protection purposes) should not be used. Instead, the organ-specific absorbed dose coupled with the appropriate relative biologic effectiveness for end point of interest and radiation type (e.g. electrons, protons, neutrons) should be used for the risk assessment.

Research Recommendations

- Overarching recommendations:
  a) Long-term large-scale follow-up of extant cancer survivors to characterize the risks of SMNs and to evaluate role of comorbidities and effect modifiers
  b) Follow-up of prospective cohorts of cancer patients to evaluate the life-long risks of SMNs, including:
     - Populations treated with newer RT modalities (including IMRT, tomoTherapy, stereotactic RT, CyberKnife, gamma knife, and protons)
     - Cancer sites for which a reduction in field size and radiation dose have been implemented (e.g., HL, testis cancer), and cancer populations not treated with radiation (e.g., testes cancer patients treated with surgery) to define natural history and baseline risks
     - Collect biologic specimen for an evaluation of genetic factors in survival and development of SMNs
- Specific recommendations:
  a) Given the differing dose-response relationships for various SMNs, analytic studies should continue to address the relationship between dose and risk.
  b) Compare the risks of SMN after different RT modalities.
  c) Address interactions between RT and other risk factors for SMNs.
  d) Particular attention should be given to adolescents and young adult cancer survivors, given the scarcity of data.
  e) Molecular and genetics underpinnings:
     - Investigate genetic contributions of RT associated SMNs.
     - Intensively study patients who develop two or more primary cancers likely associated with RT.
  f) Risk prediction models:
     - Develop comprehensive risk prediction models for SMNs to stratify patients into risk groups to customize follow-up strategies and develop evidence-based interventions.

NCRP, National Council on Radiation Protection and Measurements.
Adapted from: Travis LB, Ng AK, Allan JM, et al. Second malignant neoplasms and cardiovascular disease following radiotherapy. *J Natl Cancer Inst* 2012;104: page 8, Box 1.

in a population-based study of 6,013 testicular cancer survivors treated in the modern cisplatin-based era (also see Testicular Cancer section). Just as the study of chemotherapy-induced leukemia has yielded considerable insight into the molecular mechanisms underlying SPC etiology, it will also be important to determine whether these or other mechanisms might be operant in second solid tumors.

Other agents used in cancer therapy may also have leukemogenic and carcinogenic effects. Immunosuppressants, including azathioprine, a thiopurine pro-drug related to 6-mercaptopurine and 6-thioguanine, is associated with significant excesses of AML,[112] where risk is modified by host genetics (discussed in the Genetics section). In addition, azathioprine is also linked to the development of non-Hodgkin lymphoma (NHL),[113] skin cancer,[114] and brain tumors.[115] There is evidence that granulocyte colony–stimulating factors, which are used in the treatment of lymphoblastic leukemia, breast, and other conditions, may also be associated with an increased risk of therapy-related AML.[116–119] Similarly, the tyrosine-kinase inhibitors, such as imatinib, which is used to treat Philadelphia chromosome–positive cancers, including leukemia and gastrointestinal stromal tumors, might also be leukemogenic.[120–123]

Cancer after Bone Marrow Transplantation

Cancer after bone marrow transplantation is reviewed in Chapter 101. In brief, in survivors of high-dose therapy with bone marrow or stem cell transplantation, the estimated 10-year incidence of MDS/AML is 5% to 20%.[124–126] Risk factors include the use of total body irradiation (TBI) in the conditioning regimen, prior radiotherapy, extent and type of prior chemotherapy, peripheral stem cell source, and low stem cell dose. Increased solid tumor risks are also evident after bone marrow or stem cell transplantation.[127–129] Friedman et al.[130] reported a 25-year cumulative incidence of breast cancer of 11% among 3,337 female 5-year survivors of allogeneic hematopoietic stem cell transplantation. In a multivariable analysis, risk factors included time since transplantation, use of TBI, and age <18 years at transplant. Rizzo et al.[131] found a 3.3% 20-year cumulative risk of solid tumors in 28,874 recipients of allogeneic stem cell transplantation. The use of TBI as conditioning was significantly associated with solid tumor risk, but was restricted to patients age <30 years at transplant. The risk of invasive solid cancers among 4,318 allogeneic hematopoietic cell transplant (HCT) recipients given high-dose busulfan–cyclophosphamide without total body irradiation was 1.4-fold (95% CI,

1.08 to 1.79).[132] Chronic graft-versus-host disease was an independent risk factor for all solid cancers, especially those of oral cavity.

GENETIC SUSCEPTIBILITY TO SECOND PRIMARY CANCERS

The role of chemotherapy and radiation in the development of SPC is well-established,[9,10] although the existence of considerable interindividual variability suggests a role for genetic variation. Proposed mechanisms for susceptibility to the development of SPC after exposure to genotoxic therapy are summarized in Figure 143.3. SPC risk could potentially be modified by mutations in high-penetrance genes that lead to serious genetic diseases such as Li-Fraumeni syndrome,[133] Fanconi anemia,[134–137] and RB (see Pediatric Malignancy section). In fact, clues to the identification of loci important in affecting the risk of SPCs were initially suggested from studies of constitutional human cancer susceptibility syndromes (e.g., neurofibromatosis [NF]), many of which confer acute sensitivity to the mutagenic and cytotoxic effects of chemotherapy and radiotherapy, and where elevated risks of SPC are known or suspected.[47,138] Consistent with this hypothesis, whole-genome sequencing of a patient with therapy-related AML identified a novel constitutional heterozygous deletion of TP53, affecting exons 7 through 9 encoding the DNA-binding domain of the protein. This likely represents a founder mutation in this patient with first primary breast and ovarian cancers and is consistent with a Li-Fraumeni syndrome–like phenotype.[139] However, because of their low frequency, these alleles appear to contribute to only a small fraction of SPC risk at the population level. Nevertheless, this case highlights the possibility that TP53 and other established *cancer susceptibility genes* might harbor other novel low-frequency alleles conferring susceptibility to therapy-induced SPC, either with or without associated familial susceptibility to disease.

Evidence suggests that outside the context of familial cancer susceptibility syndromes, the genetic contribution to chemotherapy and radiotherapy-related cancer risk is multigenic, and likely related to the coinheritance of common low-penetrance polymorphisms in genes that regulate the availability of active drug metabolites, or those responsible for DNA damage signaling and repair. In the multigenic model, penetrance for SPC is predicted to be modulated by gene exposure and gene–gene interactions. For example, Ellis et al.[140] utilized a case-control study design (171 cases) to examine the association of t-MDS/AML with two common functional p53-pathway variants—the mouse double minute 2 homolog (MDM2) SNP309 and the TP53 codon 72 polymorphism.[140] Although neither polymorphism demonstrated a significant association, an interaction was detected such that patients with both *MDM2* G and *TP53* pro alleles were at increased risk of chemotherapy-related t-MDS/AML (interaction term $p = 0.009$). MDM2 is an E3 ubiquitin-protein ligase that recognizes the N-terminal transactivation domain of TP53 and negatively regulates its transcriptional activity in response to DNA damage. As such, interaction at the genetic level to modify SPC risk is plausible.

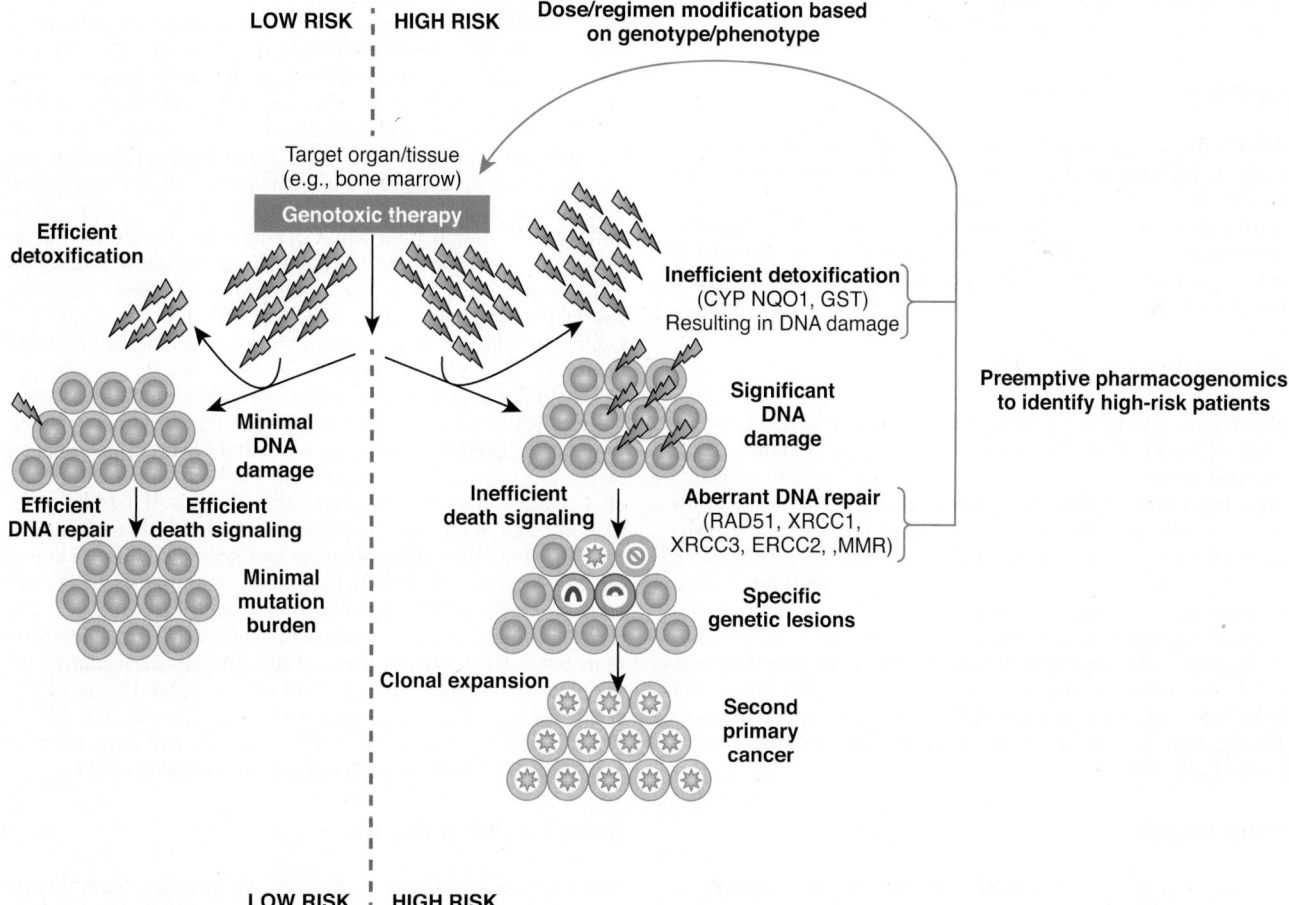

Figure 143.3 Proposed mechanisms of susceptibility to single nucleotide polymorphism (SPC) development after exposure to genotoxic chemotherapy and translational potential for patient care (preemptive pharmacogenomics). Similar principles could be applied for preemptive radiogenomics (refer to text). (Figure adapted and modified from Seedhouse C, Russell N. Advances in the understanding of susceptibility to treatment-related acute myeloid leukemia. *Br J Haematol* 2007;137:513.)

Strengths of this study included the utilization of discovery (n = 80) and replication (n = 91) case sets. However, the investigators utilized healthy controls as a comparison group, thus precluding the ability to assess whether case-control differences reflected differences in susceptibility to primary disease or t-MDS/AML.

Genetic variation contributes 20% to 95% of the variability in cytotoxic drug disposition.[141] Polymorphisms in genes involved in drug metabolism and transport are relevant in determining both disease-free survival and drug toxicity.[142] Variation in DNA damage signaling and repair also plays a role in susceptibility to de novo cancer,[143–145] and likely modifies SPC risk after exposure to DNA-damaging agents. Just as the pharmacology of cancer chemotherapy is impacted by underlying principles of pharmacokinetics, pharmacodynamics, and pharmacogenomics, these influences likely also contribute to SPC risk. Many loci that affect SPC risk encode proteins that metabolize and detoxify human carcinogens in an exposure-specific manner.[146–149]

Drug-Metabolizing Enzymes—Activation/Detoxification Pathways

The metabolism of genotoxic agents occurs in two phases. Phase I involves activation of substrates into highly reactive electrophilic intermediates that can damage DNA, a reaction principally performed by the cytochrome P-450 family of enzymes. Phase II enzymes (conjugation) function to inactivate genotoxic substrates, and include glutathione S-transferase (GST), NAD(P)H:quinone oxidoreductase-1, and others. The high activity of a phase I enzyme and the low activity of a phase II enzyme can result in DNA damage from excess harmful products (see Fig. 143.3).

Cytochrome P-450 Enzymes

The chemotherapeutic substrates of cytochrome P-450 proteins include cyclophosphamide, ifosfamide, thioTEPA, doxorubicin, and dacarbazine.[150] The expression of these enzymes is highly variable among individuals because of several functionally relevant genetic polymorphisms, some of which are suspected to impact on SPC risk in patients treated with DNA damaging chemotherapy for a first primary cancer.[146,147]

Glutathione S-Transferases

Polymorphisms exist in cytosolic subfamilies such as μ [M], π [P], and θ [T]. GSTs detoxify doxorubicin, lomustine, busulfan, chlorambucil, cisplatin, cyclophosphamide, melphalan, and others.[151] A common functional polymorphism in GSTP1 is associated with a significantly increased risk of developing therapy-related AML after exposure to chemotherapy that includes a leukemogenic GSTP1 substrate (chlorambucil, cyclophosphamide, melphalan, or doxorubicin) (odds ratio [OR], 4.34; 95% CI, 1.43 to 13.20), but does not influence the risk of radiogenic leukemia.[152] Fabiani and colleagues[153] also report an association with therapy-related myeloid neoplasia (n = 94 case) in carriers of the GSTP1 codon 105 risk allele (OR, 1.60; 95% CI, 0.95 to 2.69; p = 0.08), although findings were not stratified by treatment modality or exposure to a GSTP1 substrate.

DNA Repair

Variants in pathways that mediate cellular response to genotoxic damage are also likely to influence the risk of chemotherapy and radiotherapy-induced cancer, such as cell death signaling, cell proliferation, and DNA repair (MLH1,[154] MSH2,[155] XPD,[156] XRCC1,[157] XRCC3,[158] NBN,[158] RAD51,[159–161] and P73[162]). DNA repair mechanisms protect cells from mutations in tumor suppressor genes and oncogenes that can lead to cancer initiation and progression, with an individual's DNA repair capacity largely genetically determined.[163] A number of DNA repair genes contain polymorphic variants, resulting in large interindividual variation in repair capacity, which could affect SPC risk.[163] In support of this, a study of HL survivors suggested that those who developed a SPC had higher baseline levels of DNA damage than those who remained cancer free.[164]

Mismatch Repair

Mismatch repair (MMR) functions to correct mismatched DNA base pairs that arise as a result of misincorporation errors that avoided polymerase proofreading during DNA replication.[165] Defects in this pathway result in genetic instability or a mutator phenotype, manifested by an elevated rate of microsatellite instability. Up to 90% of therapy-related AML patients have microsatellite instability, associated with methylation of the MMR family member MLH1,[166,167] low expression of MSH2,[168] or polymorphisms in MSH2.[155,169]

Double-Strand Break Repair

High levels of double-strand breaks follow ionizing radiation and chemotherapy exposures. Cellular pathways available to repair double-strand breaks include homologous recombination, nonhomologous end joining, and single-strand annealing.[170] RAD51 is one of the central proteins in the homologous recombination pathway,[171] and a common variant in the RAD51 gene (G-135C) is significantly overrepresented in patients with therapy-related AML compared with controls (C allele: OR, 2.7; 95% CI, 1.17 to 6.02).[159] XRCC3 also functions in the homologous recombination double-strand break repair pathway by directly interacting with and stabilizing RAD51,[172] and functions to maintain genetic stability.[173,174] A polymorphism at codon 241 in the XRCC3 gene results in a Thr→Met amino acid substitution.[175] The variant Met-encoding allele has been associated with a higher level of DNA damage, and has also been associated with increased levels of chromosome deletions in lymphocytes after radiation exposure,[176] implying aberrant repair.[177] Although the XRCC3 Thr241Met variant was not an independent risk factor for t-MDS/AML, a synergistic interaction with the RAD51-135C variant resulted in an eightfold increased risk of therapy-related AML (OR, 8.1; 95% CI, 2.2 to 29.7).[159] Genes encoding proteins responsible for signaling DNA strand breaks are also predicted to carry risk alleles for therapy-induced SPCs. Prime candidates include those encoding components of the MRE11/RAD50/NBS1 (MRN) heterotrimeric complex responsible for recognition of DNA double-strand breaks in mammalian cells. Consistent with this hypothesis, the Women's Environmental, Cancer, and Radiation Epidemiology (WECARE) study (a population-based, multicenter, case-control study of 708 women with asynchronous bilateral breast cancer and 1,395 women with unilateral breast cancer) identified a haplotype encompassing the RAD50 gene associated with the risk of contralateral breast cancer.[178] The report identified an interaction with radiation dose (interaction term p = 0.006), where carriers of the RAD50 risk haplotype exposed to ≥1 Gy had an increased risk of contralateral breast cancer compared to unexposed carriers (rate ratio 4.31; 95% CI, 1.93 to 9.62). Taken together, these studies highlight the importance of gene–gene and gene exposure interactions in studies of SPC.

Base Excision Repair

Base excision repair corrects individually damaged bases that result from ionizing radiation and exogenous xenobiotic exposure. A common variant at codon 399 of the XRCC1 protein, which is central to the base excision repair pathway and functions as a scaffold for other repair components,[179,180] was associated with an increased risk of developing t-AML,[157] and has also been implicated as a risk factor in numerous other cancers.

Nucleotide Excision Repair

Nucleotide excision repair removes structurally unrelated *bulky* DNA lesions induced by radiation and chemotherapy. The nucleotide excision repair pathway is linked to transcription, and components of the pathway comprise the basal transcription factor IIH complex, which is required for transcription initiation by RNA polymerase II. Polymorphic variation in ERCC2, a component of the transcription factor IIH complex, has been associated with an increased risk of therapy-related AML.[156]

Hypothesis-Generating Genome-wide Association Studies

The associations reported previously were identified based on known gene-exposure interactions and analysis of loci in relevant pathways. Unfortunately, stratification by exposure is not always possible, particularly when a biological role has not been defined or when gene-exposure interactions are speculative. In this case, the application of high-density single nucleotide polymorphism arrays or next-generation sequencing can prove useful in identifying genetic variants and cellular pathways potentially important in causing chemotherapy- and radiotherapy-related cancer,[139,140,181,182] as have genome-wide and whole transcriptome-based studies in laboratory animals.[183,184]

Knight et al.[181] utilized a case-control study design to conduct a GWAS in patients who developed therapy-related leukemia (cases) and healthy controls. The discovery set included 80 cases and 150 controls. The relevant findings were replicated in an independent set of 70 cases and 95 controls. The investigators identified three SNPs (rs1394384 [OR, 0.29; 95% CI, 0.15 to 0.56], rs1381392 [OR, 2.08; 95% CI, 1.29 to 3.35], and rs1199098 [OR, 0.46; 95% CI, 0.27 to 0.79]) to be associated with t-MDS/AML with chromosome 5/7 abnormalities. The SNP rs1394384 is intronic to ACCN1, a gene encoding an amiloride-sensitive cation channel that is a member of the degenerin/epithelial sodium channel; rs1199098 is in linkage disequilibrium with IPMK, which encodes a multikinase that positively regulates the prosurvival protein kinase B (AKT) kinase and may modulate WNT/beta-catenin signaling; rs1381392 is not located near any annotated genes, miRNAs, or regulatory elements, although it lies in a region recurrently deleted in lung cancer. Although the investigators were able to confirm findings in an independent replication cohort, the utilization of a noncancer healthy control group raises concerns about any case-control differences being generated by the genetics of the primary cancer, rather than t-MDS/AML. Nevertheless, this study highlights the potential of GWAS to reveal novel risk alleles for SPC. Moreover, the identification of risk alleles unique to t-MDS/t-AML with somatic chromosome 5/7 abnormalities suggests that some risk alleles for SPCs may be subtype specific. Indeed, subtype-specific risk alleles have been identified for some first primary cancers. For example, Papaemmanuil and colleagues[185] identified a risk allele at the ARID5B gene for pediatric B-cell precursor acute lymphoblastic leukemia that appears to be selective for disease with somatic hyperdiploidy. Likewise, there is compelling evidence that estrogen receptor-positive and estrogen receptor-negative breast cancers have different genetic components to their etiology.[186,187] These data highlight the importance of appropriate stratification to identify the context (e.g., gender, exposure, disease subtype) in which risk alleles for SPCs are operating and where penetrance for SPC is highest, an approach that will facilitate translation into the clinic for patient benefit.

Considering this model, Best et al.[52] performed a GWAS to identify genetic variants associated with radiation-associated solid malignancies in HL survivors. They identified two variants at chromosome 6q21 associated with SPC, but which only modified risk in patients who were exposed to radiation in childhood and had no penetrance for SPC when exposure occurred in adulthood. The variants comprise a risk locus associated with decreased basal expression of PRDM1 and impaired protein induction after radiation exposure. These data suggest a novel gene-exposure interaction implicating PRDM1 in the etiology of radiation therapy-induced SPC, with evidence that age at radiation therapy exposure modifies the association between variants in this gene and SPC risk. Hosking and colleagues[51] also conducted a GWAS for inherited susceptibility to radiation-associated malignancy—specifically, meningioma in patients previously treated for tinea capitis. Although the average radiation dose to the brain was relatively low ($\sim$1.5 Gy), there was a significant increase in the risk of meningioma in exposed individuals (excess relative risk [ERR]/Gy 4.63; 95% CI, 2.4 to 9.1).[188] The high level of natural linkage disequilibrium in the exposed population allowed the authors to identify putative risk haplotypes associated with radiation-induced meningioma at 18q21.1 ($p = 7.5 \times 10^{-5}$), 18q21.32 ($p = 2.8 \times 10^{-5}$), and 10q21.3 ($p = 1.6 \times 10^{-4}$), although none reached GWAS significance and they require validation in independent cohorts with the inclusion of appropriate control groups to exclude an association with meningioma without a radiation etiology. To the extent that carcinogenic pathways operant at very low doses of radiotherapy may also be functional at the high doses given in cancer treatment, these genomic regions may also harbor risk alleles predisposing to meningioma in cancer survivors who were administered cranial radiotherapy.

Although most candidate gene association studies for SPC have focused on pathways involved in regulating cell death or maintaining genetic stability in response to genotoxic therapies, genome-wide approaches also have the potential to uncover risk alleles in novel pathways influencing the risk of therapy-induced malignancy. By conducting a genome-wide linkage study using inbred mice, Boulton et al.[189] identified genomic regions harboring putative risk loci for radiogenic AML. One such locus on chromosome 1 encompassed Scfr1, a gene encoding a key regulator of stem cell frequency, suggesting that the size of the stem cell pool at risk of transformation is genetically defined and a determinant of radiation-induced AML. If validated in human disease, these data would add another dimension to risk models of therapy-induced SPC.

Preemptive Pharmacogenomics and Preemptive Radiogenomics

Regardless of whether identified via candidate gene, genome-wide, or systems biology approaches, accurate estimates of the contribution of single gene variants will require large studies with sufficient power such that specific gene–gene or gene exposure can be identified. Indeed, the identification of the context in which penetrance for a genetic variant for SPC is greatest will facilitate the identification of patients at largest risk. Moreover, precise estimates of the magnitude of the effect(s) are required in order to develop personalized risk-adapted clinical strategies, including dose modification, alternative treatments, and posttherapy surveillance. Risk management could prove particularly important in children or young adults with primary cancers in whom cure rates are high and the risk of a subsequent cancer is associated with substantial morbidity or premature mortality.

In several instances, such as the relation between constitutional thiopurine methyltransferase (TPMT) activity and SPC risk, the goal of clinical translation has already been achieved. For example, children with acute lymphoblastic leukemia (ALL) who received combined-modality therapy that included 6-mercaptopurine at a dose of 75 mg/m^2 and who had high TPMT activity (conferred by constitutional polymorphism in the TMPT gene) had an 8.3% cumulative risk of subsequently developing a brain tumor, whereas children with low TPMT activity had a 42% risk of a posttherapy brain tumor ($p = 0.0077$).[115] It was hypothesized that the deficient TPMT activity resulted in higher exposures to thioguanine nucleotide metabolites of 6-mercaptopurine during the period of radiation. Likewise, patients with lower TPMT activity also had an increased risk of developing AML and other SPC after high-dose thioguanine chemotherapy.[190–192] However, a reduction in 6-mercaptopurine dose (50 mg/m^2), along with other changes adopted as part of the Berlin-Frankfurt-Munster protocol for the treatment of childhood ALL, appeared to attenuate the effect of *TPMT* status on risk of AML after thioguanine-containing chemotherapy.[193]

The gene-exposure interaction between TPMT and chemotherapeutic thioguanine nucleotides is well-established and strongly associated with several life-threatening toxicities (bone marrow, hepatotoxicity) in cancer patients inadvertently *overtreated* with these agents as a consequence of genotype. Indeed, convincing evidence of acute toxicity in TPMT-compromised patients prompted the U.S. Food and Drug Administration (FDA) to add a warning to the drug along with information on genotype frequencies and a recommendation for *TPMT* genetic testing following the administration of 6-mercaptopurine for patients with clinical or laboratory evidence of severe bone marrow toxicity, particularly myelosuppression.[194] Evidence of elevated SPC risk in carriers of *TPMT* null alleles[115,190–192] also underscores the importance of preemptive genotyping within this context, rather than posttherapy response-mode genotyping, particularly because there is now convincing evidence that toxicity and SPC risk can both be ameliorated with appropriate dose modification.[193] Preemptive testing for *TPMT* genotype and/or phenotype status is recommended by the Clinical Pharmacogenetics Implementation Consortium and others prior to initiating therapy that includes thioguanine nucleotides, including 6-mercaptopurine.[192,195–201]

Although it remains to be determined whether the TPMT model can be extended to other gene exposure interactions involving therapeutic agents, dose, and/or regimen modification has the potential to reduce the risk of SPCs in genetically susceptible individuals. Indeed, this principle has also been applied to other populations at risk of therapy-induced SPC, such as patients with NF1. Neurofibromatosis (NF) (caused by mutations in the *NF1* gene) is an autosomal dominantly inherited disorder characterized by a predisposition to benign tumors of the nerve sheath. There is evidence from studies of both laboratory animals[202] and humans[203] that constitutional heterozygosity for *NF1* pathogenic mutations confers susceptibility to radiogenic cancer, such that many investigators now recommend avoidance of radiotherapy whenever possible to treat tumors in NF patients.[204,205]

Preemptive testing of either genotype or phenotype status, such that appropriate dose modification or alternative treatment approaches can be implemented at first treatment, is critical to reducing therapy-induced SPC risk in patients with a strong genetic predisposition. Although not routinely yet considered in the context of SPC risk, preemptive testing based on gene-exposure interactions could potentially be applied in other clinical settings, and the value of this approach as a mechanism to reduce acute adverse drug events is already evident.[206,207] *TPMT* and *NF1* represent two examples where dose/regimen modification can ameliorate the risk of therapy-induced SPC in affected individuals, providing proof of principle of the potential value of preemptive genomics to reduce the risk of therapy-induced malignancy in selected cancer survivors (see Fig. 143.3). Moreover, as additional data are accrued with regard to molecular mechanisms that underlie radiotherapy-associated carcinogenesis,[9,10,52,208] the principles previously outlined can also be expanded to introduce a new field of preemptive radiogenomics.

RISK OF SECOND MALIGNANCY IN PATIENTS WITH SELECTED PRIMARY CANCERS

Lymphoma

The use of combined-modality therapy in patients with both HL and NHL has resulted in significant improvements in survival, but with the attendant risk of SPCs, including leukemia and a number of solid tumors.[209]

Hodgkin Lymphoma

Reports from large, well-characterized cohorts of HL survivors show that the risk of SPC is 2 to 18 times higher than in the general population.[55,56,210–218] Dores et al.[216] reported an analysis of 32,591 HL survivors (1935 to 1994) in 16 population-based registries. A total of 2,153 SPCs (relative risk [RR] = 2.3) was observed, including 1,726 solid tumors (RR = 2.0). The 25-year cumulative incidence of a solid tumor was 21.9%. Temporal trends for cancers of the female breast, thyroid, esophagus, stomach, rectum, bladder, and bone/connective tissue were suggestive of a radiogenic effect.

Hodgson et al.[54] reported on 18,862 5-year survivors of HL in 13 population-based registries from North America and Europe, treated between 1970 and 2001, and identified 1,490 cases of solid tumors (RR = 2.38). Cancers of the lung, breast, and gastrointestinal sites comprised the three most common diagnoses accounting for 21%, 19%, and 17% of the cases, respectively. The RRs of lung and breast cancers were 6.7 and 6.1, respectively, and the RR of gastrointestinal cancers ranged from 1.8 for anorectal cancer to 9.5 for stomach cancer. Other solid tumors with significantly increased risks included cancers of the head and neck, kidney, thyroid, gynecologic organs, soft tissue, bone, and brain.

It is important to recognize that radiation therapy for HL has undergone substantial changes in 4 decades with fields decreasing from total nodal irradiation to involved-field radiation therapy and, most recently, to involved site therapy. Prescribed dose has also decreased from 40 to 44 Gy to as low as 20 Gy in selected early-stage patients as part of combined modality therapy. Modeling studies show significant reduction in SPC with lower dose and smaller fields and with modern radiation therapy techniques. Many currently available epidemiologic studies of SPC after HL were based on patients treated in the earlier era, and long-term follow-up of patients treated with modern techniques will be needed to accurately assess SPC risk.

Non-Hodgkin Lymphoma

Several population-based studies have provided estimates of the risk of SPCs following NHL.[91–95,219–223] In a study by Dores et al.,[223] 5,490 subsequent cancers were observed among 73,958 2-month survivors of NHL, reflecting an overall elevated risk of 14% compared with the general population (observed-to-expected ratio [O/E] = 1.14; 95% CI, 1.11 to 1.7; excess absolute risk [EAR] = 19). The cumulative risk of SPC reached 12.3% within 25 years. Lung cancer accounted for the largest excess of SPCs after NHL. Results from the SEER program[223] corroborated findings in previous surveys of NHL, which reported significant excesses of cutaneous melanoma, Kaposi's sarcoma, HL, AML, and cancers of the buccal cavity, lip, lungs, urinary bladder, and kidneys.[219–221,224]

Radiotherapy for NHL appeared related to the increased risks for bladder cancer, bone sarcoma, and mesothelioma.[223] Chemotherapy for NHL has been associated with an increased risk for leukemia[225] as well as several solid tumors, including bladder cancer[106] with dose-dependent relationships. The immunosuppressive state associated with NHL[226] may contribute to excesses reported for cutaneous melanoma, HL, and lip cancer.[223,224,227,228] Most recently, analyses of the SEER program data reported SPC risk by major histologic groups of NHL,[229] akin to studies of SPC after ovarian cancer.[230] Among patients without known HIV/AIDS, the SIR of SPC after chronic lymphocytic leukemia/small lymphocytic lymphoma (CLL/SLL), diffuse large B-cell lymphoma (DLBCL) and follicular lymphoma (FL) were 1.19 (95% CI, 1.13 to 1.25), 1.11 (95% CI, 1.04 to 1.19), and 1.03 (95% CI, 0.96 to 1.11), respectively. Risks of lung cancer and melanoma were significantly increased in survivors of CLL/SLL and FL, but not DLBCL. Moreover, an elevated risk was observed regardless of whether radiation therapy was given as part of the initial treatment. An increased risk of acute nonlymphocytic leukemia was seen after FL and DLBCL, with a SIR of 4.96 (95% CI, 3.87 to 6.87) and 5.96 (95% CI, 4.15 to 8.29), respectively, but not after CLL/SLL. The increased leukemia risk was restricted to survivors who received chemotherapy initially.

In summary, NHL survivors are at increased risk for a number of SPCs, although to a considerably lesser degree than HL patients. The persistent increase in the risk of all SPCs for more than 20 years after NHL treatment alerts clinicians to the importance of long-term surveillance.

Selected Second Primary Cancers Following Hodgkin Lymphoma or Non-Hodgkin Lymphoma

Breast Cancer

Breast cancer is one of the most common solid tumors after HL. Studies have consistently shown that young age at radiotherapy is associated with a significantly higher risk of breast cancer.[54–57,231] In a population-based cohort study,[54] the absolute risks of breast cancer in women diagnosed with HL at ages 15 through 25 years were higher than the absolute risks of women in the general population between 50 and 54 years, a standard age when mammography screening is recommended. Travis et al.[232] developed estimates of the cumulative absolute risk of breast cancer, taking into account age and calendar year of HL diagnosis, current age, radiation dose, and competing causes of mortality. Thus, for a HL survivor who received a chest radiation dose of ≥40 Gy at age 25 years, the cumulative absolute risks of breast cancer at 10, 20, and 30 years were estimated to be 1.4%, 11% and 29%, respectively. A report from the Childhood Cancer Survivor Study (CCSS) estimated the risk of breast cancer in a cohort of 1,268 female 5-year childhood cancer survivors given chest radiation therapy. The overall cumulative incidence of breast cancer by age 50 years among HL survivors was 30% (95% CI, 25% to 35%).

There is a clear radiation dose-response relation for breast cancer risk after HL. In an international case-control study of breast cancer after HL that included 105 cases of breast cancer and 266 matched controls,[61] radiation dose to the area of the breast where the tumor developed in the case (and a comparable area in controls) was estimated. Breast cancer risk increased significantly with increasing radiation dose to reach eightfold for the highest category (median dose 42 Gy) compared to the lowest dose group (<4 Gy) (p-trend for dose <0.001) (Table 143.2).

A significant radiation dose-response relation was similarly demonstrated in a Dutch study that was included in the previous international investigation.[62] The CCSS also published a case-control study of 120 cases of breast cancer (65% in survivors of HL) matched to 464 controls.[63] Again, a significant linear radiation dose-response was observed (p-trend <0.0001), with an estimated relative risk of breast cancer of 6.4 at 20 Gy and 11.8 at 40 Gy (see Table 143.2). Radiation field size for HL also affects breast cancer risk. A cohort study of 1,122 5-year female HL survivors showed that mantle field irradiation (inclusion of mediastinum, bilateral axillae and neck) was associated with a 2.7-fold increased risk (95% CI:, 1.1 to 6.9) of breast cancer compared with mediastinal irradiation alone.[74] A meta-analysis of SPC after HL found that extended-field radiotherapy was associated with a significantly higher breast cancer risk than involved-field radiotherapy (OR = 3.25; p = 0.04).[75] A study from Yale University evaluated solid tumor risks in 404 HL survivors and observed 10 cases of breast cancer in women who received radiation treatments that included the axillae, but no cases when the axillae were omitted from the field.

Early menopause has been shown to be protective against breast cancer in HL survivors treated with radiotherapy. In particular, the Dutch study clearly documented that breast cancer risk reduction associated with chemotherapy was due to premature menopause.[62] In a more recent HL cohort study from the same group,[74] among women age <41 years at treatment, those women with >20 years of ovarian function post-treatment had a significantly higher risk

of breast cancer compared to patients with 10 to 20 years of intact ovarian function after therapy (hazard ratio = 5.3; 95% CI, 2.9 to 9.9).

Several studies have shown a reduced risk of breast cancer among NHL survivors compared to the general population, likely due to chemotherapy-related early menopause.[233,234] Although breast cancer risk after mediastinal irradiation for NHL has not been specifically assessed, indirect data suggested an increased risk with younger age at irradiation. In a SEER-based study of 77,876 NHL patients,[222] the relative risk of breast cancer was significantly increased among women irradiated at age <25 years (RR = 5.05; p <0.05), whereas breast cancer excesses were not observed in the entire irradiated cohort. Similarly, in a Swedish Cancer Registry–based study of 29,134 patients with NHL,[235] the relative risk of breast cancer was significantly increased only among women diagnosed between age 20 to 39 years (RR = 3.29; 95% CI, 1.91 to 5.67) and not in older patients. The increased breast cancer risk in these young women may have been due to chest radiotherapy, although this cannot be confirmed because the sites of irradiation were not described.

Lung Cancer

Significantly elevated three- to sevenfold relative risks of lung cancer have been reported after HL,[53–56,65,216,217,236] with a dose-dependent relationship documented for antecedent alkylating agent chemotherapy[53,236] and for radiation dose to the area of the lungs in which the cancer developed.[53] The modifying effect of smoking history on treatment-related lung cancer in HL survivors was investigated in a case-control study by Travis et al.[53] Using patients who had minimal radiation or alkylating chemotherapy exposure and who were nonsmokers as the reference group, exposure to >5 Gy of radiotherapy and/or alkylating agent chemotherapy was associated with a 4.3- to 7.2-fold increased risk of lung cancer. The relative risk increased to 16.8 and 20.2, respectively, in patients who had either one of the treatment exposures and who used tobacco. Moreover, the relative risk was 49.1 in patients who had >5 Gy of radiotherapy, received alkylating chemotherapy, and who used tobacco, consistent with a multiplicative effect of tobacco use on the risk of treatment-related lung cancer.

The risk of lung cancer is modestly increased after NHL, with most studies reporting a risk of less than twofold compared to the general population.[219,220,222,233–235,237,238] The increased risk appears to be associated with both chemotherapy and radiotherapy, with significantly increasing risk following higher cumulative doses of chemotherapy.[237] Increased risks for malignant mesothelioma have been reported in survivors of both HL and NHL, although the excesses appear limited to irradiated patients.[236,239,240]

Gastrointestinal Malignancies

Population-based and multi-institutional cohort studies have consistently reported an increased risk, compared to the general population, for cancers of the esophagus, the stomach, the colon, and the rectum among HL survivors.[55,56,215,216,241,242] Van den Belt-Dusebout et al.[66] conducted a nested case-control study of 5,142 Dutch testicular cancer and HL survivors to examine the role of radiation dose and chemotherapy in the etiology of gastric cancer. Because age characteristics of the testicular cancer and HL patients were generally similar, these populations were pooled, although it should be kept in mind that the underlying cancers are distinctly different and that only males were represented in the former group. A 3.4-fold increased risk of gastric cancer was observed compared with the general population. Risk increased with increasing mean radiation dose to the stomach, with an ERR of 0.84 per Gy. Adjusted for radiation, higher doses of procarbazine (≥13,000 mg versus <10,000 mg) were associated with a 5.4-fold increased risk. Smoking more than 10 cigarettes per day was associated with a 1.6-fold increased risk compared with survivors who did not smoke.

PRACTICE OF ONCOLOGY

TABLE 143.2

Relative Risk of Breast Cancer after Chest Radiotherapy According to Radiation Dose to Affected Site in Breast and Alkylating Chemotherapy Exposure

National Cancer Institute-International Study[a]				Childhood Cancer Survivor Study[b]			
Radiation Exposure							
Radiation Dose to Affected Site in Breast (Gy)	Cases/ Controls	Relative Risk	95% Confidence Interval	Radiation Dose to Affected Site in Breast (Gy)	Cases/ Controls	Relative Risk	95% Confidence Interval
0–3.9	15/76	1.0	(Referent)	0	13/127	1.0	(referent)
4.0–6.9	13/30	1.8	0.7–4.5	>0–0.13	6/49	1.4	0.5–4.4
7.0–23.1	16/30	4.1	1.4–12.3	0.14–1.29	7/48	1.9	0.7–5.4
23.2–27.9	9/30	2.0	0.7–5.9	1.30–11.39	11/55	1.9	0.7–5.0
28.0–37.1	20/31	6.8	2.3–22.3	11.40–29.99	34/56	7.1	2.9–17
37.2–40.4	12/31	4.0	1.3–13.4	30.00–60.00	36/54	10.8	3.8–31
40.5–61.3	17/29	8.0	2.6–26.4	—	—	—	—
Alkylating Chemotherapy Exposure							
Number of Cycles of Alkylating Chemotherapy	Cases/ Controls	Relative Risk	95% Confidence Interval	Alkylating Agent Score[c]	Cases/ Controls	Relative Risk	95% Confidence Interval
0	68/132	1.0	(referent)	0	53/163	1.0	(Referent)
1–4	10/20	0.7	0.3–1.7	1	12/63	0.67	0.3–1.5
5–8	17/55	0.6	0.3–1.1	2	12/36	1.40	0.6–3.4
≥9	4/29	0.2	0.1–0.7	3	17/37	1.15	0.6–2.4
Ovarian Radiation Exposure							
Radiation Dose to Ovaries (Gy)	Cases/ Controls	Relative Risk	95% Confidence Interval	Radiation Dose to Ovaries (Gy)	Cases/ Controls	Excess Odds Ratio per Gy of Radiation Dose to Site of Breast Tumor	95% Confidence Interval
<3.0	94/214	1.0		<5	99/342	0.36	0.14–0.93
3.0–4.0	4/13	1.2	(0.3–3.9)	≥5	8/47	0.06	−0.06–0.27

[a] Population included women who were diagnosed with HL at age 30 years or younger and who survived 1 or more years. (Adapted from Travis LB, Hill DA, Dores GM, et al. Breast cancer following radiotherapy and chemotherapy among young women with Hodgkin disease. *JAMA* 2003;290:465–475.)
[b] Population included patients diagnosed with the following primary cancers at age younger than 21 years and who survived 5 or more years: HL (65%), soft tissue sarcoma (7.5%), leukemia (5.8%), non-Hodgkin lymphoma (3.3%), central nervous system tumors (2.5%), kidney tumors (2.5%), and neuroblastoma (0.8%). (Adapted from Inskip PD, Robison LL, Stovall M, et al. Radiation dose and breast cancer risk in the Childhood Cancer Survivor Study. *J Clin Oncol* 2009;27:3901–3907.)
[c] Dose scores were assigned to individual alkylating agents on the basis of the distribution of dose (mg/m^2) of each agent, with scores then summed across agents.

In a nested case-control study of stomach cancer risk in 19,882 HL survivors,[243] 89 cases and 190 matched controls were included, with 19 of the cases and 69 controls previously reported.[66] Risk was significantly associated with radiation dose to the stomach (excess OR, 0.09/Gy; p-trend <0.001) and number of cycles of alkylating chemotherapy (p-trend = 0.02) Patients who received gastric radiation doses of 25 Gy or more to the stomach and cumulative doses of procarbazine of 5,600 mg/m^2 or higher had an OR of 77.5 (95% CI, 14.7 to 1,452). Exposure to dacarbazine was also associated with an increased stomach cancer risk (OR, 8.8; 95% CI, 2.1 to 46.6), after adjustment for radiation and procarbazine dose.

Breast Cancer

Women with breast cancer are at significantly elevated risk for developing SPCs. The largest amount of data have accrued on the risk of contralateral breast cancer (CBC), which is estimated to be increased two- to fivefold. Factors that may modify the increased risk include preexisting breast cancer risk factors such as genetic predisposition, reproductive factors and health habits, as well as treatment exposures.[244–247]

Conflicting data exist on the contribution of radiotherapy to excess risks of CBC.[248–251] In a case-control study by Boice et al.,[250] the overall relative risk of CBC was not significantly increased after radiotherapy (RR, 1.19; 95% CI, 0.94 to 1.15). Among women age <45 years at the time of irradiation, however, the relative risk was significantly elevated at 1.59 (95% CI, 1.07 to 2.36). Hooning et al.[58] assessed the long-term risk of CBC in 7,221 breast cancer survivors, and found a 2.91-fold (95% CI, 2.66 to 3.18) increased risk compared with the general female population (absolute excess risk [AER] = 46.1 out of 10,000 person-years). The risk of radiotherapy-related CBC also increased significantly with decreasing age at treatment; among women who received radiotherapy at age <35 years, the hazard ratio for CBC was 1.78 (95% CI, 0.85 to 3.72), whereas for women irradiated at age ≥45 years, risk decreased to 1.09 (95% CI, 0.82 to 1.45). The Early Breast Cancer Trialists' Collaborative Group reported a significantly increased risk of CBC with radiotherapy, mainly during the period 5 to 14 years after randomization (RR, 1.43; $p = 0.00001$), and the increased risk was significant even among women aged ≥50 years when randomized (RR, 1.25; $p = 0.002$).[252] In a report from the WECARE group,[59] where absorbed doses to quadrants of the contralateral breast were estimated, women <40 years of age who received >1.0 Gy of absorbed dose to the specific quadrant of the contralateral breast had a significantly increased 2.5-fold greater risk for CBC than unexposed women. No excess risk was observed in women >40 years of age. In contrast, in an earlier case-control study from Denmark, a significant difference in CBC risk was not observed in women who did and did not receive radiotherapy, regardless of age at treatment.[253] A study from the Institut Curie, which included 13,472 women also similarly showed no increased risk of CBC when comparing women who did or did not receive radiotherapy (RR, 1.1; 95% CI, 0.96 to 1.27). Currently available data, therefore, support a modest risk of CBC after radiotherapy, mostly limited to younger women at the time of treatment.

Several other solid tumors have been linked to radiotherapy for breast cancer, including lung cancer, sarcoma, and esophageal cancers. Compared to women who did not receive radiotherapy, women given radiotherapy have a 1.5- to 3-fold increased risk of developing lung cancer.[248,254,255] In a case control study by Kaufman et al.,[256] 113 breast cancer patients who developed lung cancer were matched to 364 controls without lung cancer; excess risks of lung cancer following postmastectomy radiotherapy were limited to ever-smokers. Compared with nonsmoking women who did not receive postmastectomy radiotherapy, the adjusted OR for lung cancer among nonirradiated ever-smokers was 5.9 (95% CI, 27 to 12.8) and the adjusted odds ratio among ever-smokers who also received postmastectomy radiotherapy was 18.9 (95% CI, 7.9 to 45.4). Others have shown that the increased risks of lung cancer appeared more related to postmastectomy radiotherapy, in which the radiation target volume often also includes the supraclavicular, axillary, and/or internal mammary nodal regions, thus exposing a larger volume of lung tissue, whereas the risk after postlumpectomy radiotherapy is less clear.[76,77] Similarly, in a population-based study by Zablotska et al.[77] of squamous cell esophageal cancer after adjuvant radiotherapy for breast cancer, the relative risk was significantly increased only among women who received postmastectomy radiotherapy, but not among those who received postlumpectomy radiotherapy. In a recent international population-based nested case-control study of esophageal cancer in breast cancer survivors that included 252 cases and 488 controls, the esophageal cancer risk was 8.3-fold (95% CI, 2.7 to 28) higher in women who received doses of 35 Gy or higher, compared with women who received no radiation dose to the site of esophageal tumor.[64]

Although the occurrence of sarcoma after breast cancer is a rare event, with a 15-year incidence rate of <0.5%, the relative risk has been estimated to be as high as sevenfold, given the low background incidence in the general population.[248,257,258] In a study by Rubino et al.,[70] all sarcomas occurred among women initially given radiotherapy, and in all cases, the sarcomas were located in the irradiated fields or in the upper extremity of the arm ipsilateral to the treated breast. Further, a significant dose-response relationship was demonstrated. In a SEER-based study of 563,155 breast cancer patients, women who received radiotherapy had a 1.5-fold risk (95% CI, 1.3 to 1.8) of all types of sarcomas, and a 7.6-fold risk (95% CI, 4.9 to 11.9) of angiosarcoma, compared to women who did not receive radiotherapy.[259] In addition to radiotherapy, partial mastectomies and lymph node dissections were also independent risk factors for the development of angiosarcoma. Unlike other radiation-related soft tissue sarcomas, angiosarcoma has a short latency and can occur in the first 5 years after therapy.

Endometrial cancer after breast cancer can be linked with both shared etiologic factors and antecedent therapy—in particular, tamoxifen therapy. Several large studies have demonstrated a two- to fourfold increased risk of endometrial cancer after tamoxifen therapy.[30] Earlier studies indicated that endometrial cancer after tamoxifen use may have a more favorable prognosis, although recent data have raised the concern that tamoxifen-related endometrial cancers may have a more aggressive behavior.[260–262] In a study that included 732 women with endometrial carcinoma, 59 patients (8%) had a previous diagnosis of breast cancer, of whom 29 (49%) had used tamoxifen.[263] A longer duration of tamoxifen use (60 versus 46 months; $p = 0.034$) was significantly associated with high-risk histologic type. A Dutch study, which examined endometrial cancer after tamoxifen treatment for breast cancer, found that long-term tamoxifen use was associated with a higher proportion of nonendometrioid tumors than nonusers (32.7% versus 17.4%; $p = 0.004$), especially serous adenocarcinomas and carcinosarcomas; a higher proportion of International Federation of Gynecology and Obstetrics (FIGO) stage III and IV tumors was also observed (20.0% versus 11.3%; $p = 0.049$).[261] The differences in histologic and stage distributions translated to a significantly lower 3-year endometrial cancer-specific survival among long-term tamoxifen users (82% versus 93%; $p = 0.001$).

Testicular Cancer

Significant excesses of solid tumors, leukemia, and contralateral testicular cancer (CTC) have been documented in testicular cancer survivors (TCS).[102,264–275] In an international population-based survey of 40,576 TCS,[264] significantly elevated 1.5- to 4-fold relative risks were noted for malignant melanoma and cancers of the lungs, thyroid, esophagus, pleura, stomach, pancreas, colon, rectum, kidneys, bladder, and connective tissue among 10-year survivors (Table 143.3). By age 75 years, men who were diagnosed with seminomas or nonseminomatous tumors at age 35 years experienced cumulative risks of solid cancer of 36% and 31%, respectively. Among TCS treated with radiotherapy alone, relative risks of SPC at sites included in typical infradiaphragmatic radiotherapy fields were significantly larger than risks at nonexposed sites (RR, 2.7 versus RR, 1.6; $p <0.05$) and remained elevated for ≥35 years. No decrease in the risk of postradiotherapy in-site SPC was observed for seminoma patients diagnosed between 1975 and 2001, although a lowered risk was noted among nonseminoma patients. In a case-control investigation of 23 stomach cancers among TCS,[66] a significant relation with increasing radiation dose was observed. In the international series,[264] the relative risk (RR = 1.8) of solid tumors was significantly elevated after chemotherapy alone, although information on specific cytotoxic drugs was not available. A subsequent investigation[265] showed that cisplatin-based chemotherapy was associated with a significantly elevated twofold risk of solid tumors, confirming other reports.[275]

In a study exploring cause-specific mortality in patients with stage I seminoma using data from the SEER program, with 121,037 person-years of follow-up, the standardized mortality ratio (SMR) of SPC was 1.81 (95% CI, 1.61 to 2.03).[276] The risk was higher among irradiated patients, with an estimated 15-year cumulative risk of 2.64%.

Cytotoxic drugs used to treat testicular cancer (TC) that have been related with excess secondary leukemias include etoposide and cisplatin.[102,271,273,274] Kollmannsberger et al.[274] estimated that the cumulative risk of leukemia for TCS given etoposide at total doses of <2,000 mg/m^2 and >2,000 mg/m^2 was 0.5% and 2%, respectively. A strong dose-response relation ($p <0.001$) between cumulative dose of cisplatin and subsequent leukemia risk was reported by Travis et al.,[102] who also noted a nonsignificant threefold risk following involved-field radiotherapy. Fung et al.[111] recently examined solid tumor risk after surgery and chemotherapy in 12,691 testicular nonseminoma survivors in the SEER program (1980 to 2008). A significantly increased RR of solid tumor of 1.43 (95% CI,

TABLE 143.3

Estimated Relative Risk of Second Cancers According to Time Since Testicular Cancer Diagnosis for Patients Diagnosed with Testicular Cancer at Age 35 Years[a]

| | All ≥10 Y Intervals | | Time Since Testicular Cancer Diagnosis | | | | | | Excess Number (%)[b] |
| | | | 10–19 Y | | 20–29 Y | | ≥30 Y | | |
	Obs.	RR (95% CI)	Obs.	RR (95% CI)	Obs.	RR (95% CI)	Obs.	RR (95% CI)	
Cancer Site									
All solid tumors	1,694	1.9 (1.8–2.1)	802	2.1 (1.9–2.3)	563	2.0 (1.8–2.2)	329	1.7 (1.6–1.9)[c]	698 (100)[d]
Esophagus	26	1.7 (1.0–2.6)	13	2.0 (<1.0–3.8)	7	0.9 (<1.0–2.3)	6	2.1 (<1.0–4.0)	9 (1.3)
Stomach	129	4.0 (3.2–4.8)	64	4.9 (3.7–6.4)	49	4.5 (3.3–5.9)	16	1.9 (1.0–3.2)[e]	88 (12.6)
Colon	153	2.0 (1.7–2.5)	62	1.8 (1.3–2.6)	52	2.1 (1.5–2.8)	39	2.2 (1.6–3.0)	66 (9.5)
Rectum/anus	101	1.8 (1.4–2.3)	60	2.7 (1.9–3.8)	22	1.3 (<1.0–1.9)	19	1.7 (1.1–2.6)	39 (5.5)
Pancreas	95	3.6 (2.8–4.6)	44	4.1 (2.8–5.9)	38	4.3 (3.0–6.0)	13	2.3 (1.3–3.7)	63 (9.0)
Lung	256	1.5 (1.2–1.7)	148	2.2 (1.7–2.7)	73	1.4 (1.1–1.8)	35	1.0 (<1.0–1.4)[e]	65 (9.3)
Pleura	12	3.4 (1.7–5.9)	7	6.0 (2.3–12)	3	2.6 (0.5–6.6)	2	1.9 (0.4–6.1)	8 (1.1)
Prostate	249	1.4 (1.2–1.6)	88	1.1 (<1.0–1.6)	91	1.4 (1.1–1.8)	70	1.5 (1.2–1.8)	52 (7.4)
Kidney	80	2.4 (1.8–3.0)	29	1.7 (1.0–2.6)	30	2.5 (1.7–3.6)	21	3.0 (1.9–4.4)[f]	43 (6.2)
Bladder	211	2.7 (2.2–3.1)	75	2.0 (1.4–2.7)	85	3.2 (2.5–4.0)	51	2.6 (2.0–3.5)	115 (16.4)
Malignant melanoma	70	1.8 (1.3–2.3)	43	1.9 (1.3–2.6)	23	2.1 (1.4–3.1)	4	0.8 (0.3–1.7)	30 (4.2)
Thyroid	16	2.3 (1.0–4.4)	15	4.2 (1.8–8.2)	1	1.0 (<1.0–3.4)	0	—	9 (1.2)
Connective tissue	19	4.0 (2.3–6.3)	9	3.7 (1.7–7.0)	9	6.1 (2.8–11.0)	1	1.6 (<1.0–5.8)	14 (2.0)
Other solid tumors[g]	277	1.6 (1.4–1.9)	145	1.5 (1.2–1.9)	80	1.6 (1.3–2.0)	52	1.9 (1.4–2.4)	98 (14.1)
Radiotherapy Only									
All solid tumors	892	2.0 (1.9–2.2)	399	2.2 (1.9–2.5)	300	2.0 (1.8–2.3)	193	1.8 (1.6–2.1)[h]	387 (100)[d]
Sites in-field[i]	445	2.7 (2.4–3.0)	174	2.6 (2.1–3.2)	165	2.9 (2.4–3.4)	106	2.5 (2.0–3.0)	246 (63.7)
Other sites	447	1.6 (1.4–1.8)	225	1.9 (1.6–2.3)	135	1.5 (1.3–1.8)	87	1.4 (1.1–1.7)[j]	141 (36.3)

Obs., observed number of cases; RR, relative risk; CI, confidence interval.

[a] The table is restricted to those sites for which significantly increased RR were observed in 10-year survivors of testicular cancer. The RR is a decreasing function of age at testicular cancer diagnosis; results are presented for age 35 years, which is the mean age of the cohort.

[b] Percentage contribution to the total excess is shown within the parentheses; percentages may not sum to 100 due to rounding.

[c] P trend (negative) = .007

[d] Obtained as sum of site-specific excesses.

[e] P trend (negative) <0.001

[f] P trend (positive) = 0.02

[g] Includes 172 tumors for which site was specified and 105 tumors of unknown or ill-defined primary site.

[h] P trend (negative) = 0.013

[i] Restricted to those sites that are included in typical infradiaphragmatic radiotherapy fields for testicular cancer: stomach, small intestine, colon, rectum, liver, gallbladder and ducts, pancreas, kidneys, and bladder.

[j] P trend (negative) = 0.005.

Modified from Travis LB, Fossa SD, Schonfeld SJ, et al. Second cancers among 40,576 testicular cancer patients: focus on long-term survivors. *J Natl Cancer Inst* 2005;97:1354–1365.

1.18 to 1.73) was found (median latency period: 12.5 years), with significantly increased site-specific risks for cancers of the kidney (SIR, 3.37; 95% CI, 1.79 to 5.77), thyroid (SIR, 4.40; 95% CI, 2.19 to 7.88), and soft tissue (SIR, 7.49; 95% CI, 3.59 to 13.78).

In a population-based study of 29,515 TCS, the 15-year cumulative risk of CTC was 1.9%, representing a 12.4-fold higher risk than expected in the general population.[272] Chemotherapy may reduce the risk of CTC,[277,278] although the delaying effect and duration of cisplatin-based chemotherapy on CTC incidence should be examined further.

In the future, it will be important to determine whether the decrease in radiation dose and field size in the 1990s,[279,280] along with the use of carboplatin as adjuvant therapy in seminoma patients,[281] will be associated with a reduction in excess SPCs. The long-term influence of cisplatin-based chemotherapy on the site-specific risk of solid tumors, temporal patterns, and the effect of age at exposure and attained age should also be addressed in analytic investigations that control for lifestyle factors, shared etiologic influences, and host determinants.[5,6] Screening strategies for selected SPCs should be considered.[282] The risk of SPCs in TCS initially treated with radiotherapy or chemotherapy should be compared to the risk in patients managed with surgery alone, because the development of cancer at a young age may itself indicate an underlying susceptibility for subsequent malignancy. Similarly, the incidence of SPC among TCS managed with surgery only should be contrasted with cancer incidence in the general male population in order to understand the evolution of cured TC, given its origin from a pluripotent stem cell and the presence of non–germ-cell elements in nonseminomatous TC and its metastases.[283,284] Future research strategies for testicular cancer survivors, including detailed recommendations for the study of SPC, were recently published.[285] These included an evaluation of the role of genetic variants in the development of SPC after testicular cancer and the development of site-specific risk prediction models.

Prevention and Risk Reduction for Second Primary Cancers

Given the increased SPC risk in survivors of adult-onset cancer, screening and early detection strategies have been suggested for this population.[282] In general, survivors should follow applicable national guidelines for cancer screening. Further, earlier or additional screening may be indicated in survivors deemed at high risk due to genetic predisposition, previous treatment history, and/or health habits. Site-specific recommendations regarding screening and prevention are summarized in Table 143.4.

In survivors with a family history suggestive of hereditary nonpolyposis colon cancer (HNPCC), colonoscopy screening starting at age 20 to 30 years, and endometrial sampling in women annually starting at age 35 years, should be considered.[286] For survivors with a strong family history and/or personal or family history of BRCA1 and BRCA2, screening breast magnetic resonance imaging (MRI) as an adjunct to mammograms starting at age 25 years, and serum cancer antigen 125 (CA-125) and transvaginal ultrasound every 6 to 12 months are recommended in women, and serum prostate specific antigen (PSA) with or without digital rectal examination every 1 to 2 years, starting at age 45 years, are recommended in men.[287] Screening breast MRI scans in addition to mammograms are also recommended in female survivors with a history of chest irradiation at a young age, 8 to 10 years after treatment (further discussed in the following paragraphs), and colonoscopy screening is recommended in survivors with a history of pelvic irradiation, starting 10 years after treatment.[288] In survivors with a history of chest irradiation and/or tobacco history, annual low-dose chest computed tomography should be considered.[289,290] Finally, survivors with a family history of early melanoma may benefit from annual skin examination and monthly skin self-examinations.[291]

Data on chemoprevention strategies specifically for SPCs are limited. At this time, there are data to support the use of tamoxifen in pre- and postmenopausal women, and raloxifene in postmenopausal women, as primary breast cancer prevention in high-risk women.[292,293] The role of low-dose tamoxifen as breast cancer chemoprevention in HL survivors is currently being addressed in an ongoing clinical trial.[294] Observational studies have demonstrated a reduction in colon cancer risk with aspirin, which might be considered for high-risk cancer survivors.[295,296] Although preclinical and early clinical studies have shown that retinoids have chemopreventive effects against lung cancer and squamous cell cancer of the head and neck,[297] currently, insufficient data exist to support their use as chemoprevention in high-risk cancer survivors.[298–300]

PEDIATRIC MALIGNANCIES

Survival rates for children with cancer have increased substantially over the past 3 decades, with this rapidly growing population at lifelong risk for the late effects of cancer treatment. In a British population–based study of 17,981 5-year survivors of childhood cancer diagnosed prior to age 15 years and followed for a median of 24.3 years, 1,354 SPCs were ascertained, yielding an overall fourfold risk (SIR, 3.9; 95% CI, 3.6 to 4.2). The cumulative percentage of survivors developing an SPC by age 60 years was 13.8% (95% CI, 12.3% to 15.5%). The AER for attained ages older than 40 years was highest for digestive and genitourinary SPCs; 36% of the total AER was attributable to these two SPCs.[301] In a recent update of 14,359 5-year survivors (diagnosed prior to age 21 years) in the CCSS,[302] the 30-year cumulative incidence was 7.9% for invasive SPC, 9.1% for nonmelanoma skin cancers (NMSC), and 3.1% for meningiomas, with an overall 30-year incidence for all SPCs of 20% (Fig. 143.4). Childhood cancer survivors have a three- to sixfold increased risk of developing an SPC compared with the general population, translating into an EAR ranging from 1 (in early life) to 6 per 1,000 patient-years of observation.[302–304] Furthermore, survivors of childhood cancer have a persistent excess risk of an SPC throughout life, accompanied by continuous changes in the risk of cancers at specific sites.[302–304] The incidence and type of SPC differs with the primary diagnosis, type of therapy received, and presence of genetic conditions.

Influence of Primary Cancer

Among 5-year survivors in the CCSS, the 30-year cumulative incidence of SPC by primary cancer diagnosis was as follows: HL, 18.4%; Ewing sarcoma, 10.1%; soft tissue sarcoma, 8.8%; osteosarcoma, 6.0%; neuroblastoma, 5.9%; NHL, 5.8%; leukemia, 5.6%; central nervous system (CNS) tumor, 5.5%; and kidney tumor, 4.0%. In multiple studies, it is evident that hereditary RB, HL, and soft tissue sarcomas are overrepresented among patients who develop an SPC relative to their incidence in the general population.[48,210,302,305,306] The 40- to 50-year cumulative incidence of a SPC following RB ranged from 28% to 36%,[48,306] reflecting an interaction between genetic predisposition in patients with hereditary RB and radiotherapy,[47,305,307] as observed in familial soft tissue sarcoma. In individuals with other primary malignancies such as HL, the extent to which the primary cancer type may serve as an independent risk factor for SPC in addition to the well-established role of treatment requires further study.

Host-Related Risk Factors

Younger age at diagnosis of a primary cancer is associated with a higher risk of radiation-associated solid tumors.[210,211,308] Conversely for t-MDS/AML, which is strongly linked with specific chemotherapeutic agents, risk appears to increase with age at treatment of primary cancer.[125,309] Female sex is associated with a higher risk

TABLE 143.4

Second Malignant Neoplasm (SMN) Screening and Prevention Recommendations in Cancer Survivors at Moderate to High Risk

SMN Site	Risk Level	Screening Recommendation	Chemoprevention Agents
Breast	Moderate risk: Family history of breast cancer High risk: Personal or family history of *BRCA1*, *BRCA2*, *TP53*, or *PTEN* mutation History of radiation to chest between age 10 and 30 years	Mammogram starting 5 to 10 years before earliest case of cancer in the family; CBE twice yearly; BSE monthly Screening breast MRI, starting at age 25 years (or for women with a history of chest radiation, 5 to 10 years after radiation); annual mammogram; CBE twice yearly, BSE monthly	■ Tamoxifen, raloxifene: Recommended for those at increased risk of first primary breast cancer; recommendations for second tumors are not established ■ Other SERMs (e.g., lasofoxafine): No recommendation ■ Aromatase inhibitors: No recommendation for SMN
Colon	Moderate risk: FDR with colon cancer younger than age 60 years or two SDRs with colon cancer at any age Radiation in which colon/rectum were included in treatment fields High risk: Family history suggestive of HNPCC	Colonoscopy at age 40 years or 10 years before the earliest case of cancer in the family Colonoscopy at age 35 years or 10 years after radiation Colonoscopy every 1 to 2 years, starting at age 20 to 30 years (depending on syndrome)	■ NSAIDs, COX-2 inhibitors, curcumin, difluoromethylornithine, aspirin, isothiocyanates (including sulforaphane), or resveratrol: Not recommended for secondary or tertiary prevention
Ovary	High risk: Family history of ovarian cancer; personal history or family member with mutation in *BRCA1* or *BRCA2* or mismatch repair gene (*MLH1*, *MSH2*, *MSH6*, *PMS2*)	Serum CA-125 and TVUS every 6 to 12 months starting at age 35 years	—
Endometrium	High risk: Family history suggestive of HNPCC	Endometrial sampling annually starting at age 35 years	—
Skin	High risk: Family history of early melanoma	Annual skin examination and monthly skin self-examination	—
Lung	Increased risk: Prior radiation to chest with or without chemotherapy High risk: Current smokers (>30 pack years); former smokers (>30 pack years and quit <15 years ago)	Smoking cessation Annual low-dose spiral CT	■ Isotretinoin, etretinate, vitamin E, retinoids, N-acetylcysteine, or aspirin: Not recommended ■ Budesonide, COX-2 inhibitors, 5-LOX inhibitors, and prostacyclin analogs: Not recommended for individuals who have a history of lung cancer
Prostate	High risk: Family history of early prostate cancer (onset younger than age 65 years); personal or family member with mutation in *BRCA1* or *BRCA2*	Serum PSA with or without DRE every 1 to 2 years, starting at age 45 years	—
Head and neck (upper aerodigestive tract)			■ Isotretinoin, β-carotene: Not recommended

CBE, clinical breast examination; BSE, breast self-examination; MRI, magnetic resonance imaging; SERM, selective estrogen receptor modulator; FDR, first-degree relative; SDR, second-degree relative; HNPCC, hereditary nonpolyposis colon cancer; NSAID, nonsteroidal anti-inflammatory drug; CT, computed tomography; COX-2, cyclooxygenase-2; TVUS, transvaginal ultrasound; 5-LOX, 5-lipoxygenase; PSA, prostate-specific antigen; DRE, digital rectal examination.
Adapted from Wood ME, Vogel V, Ng A, et al. Second malignant neoplasms: assessment and strategies for risk reduction. *J Clin Oncol* 2012;30:3741–3742, Tables 5 and 6

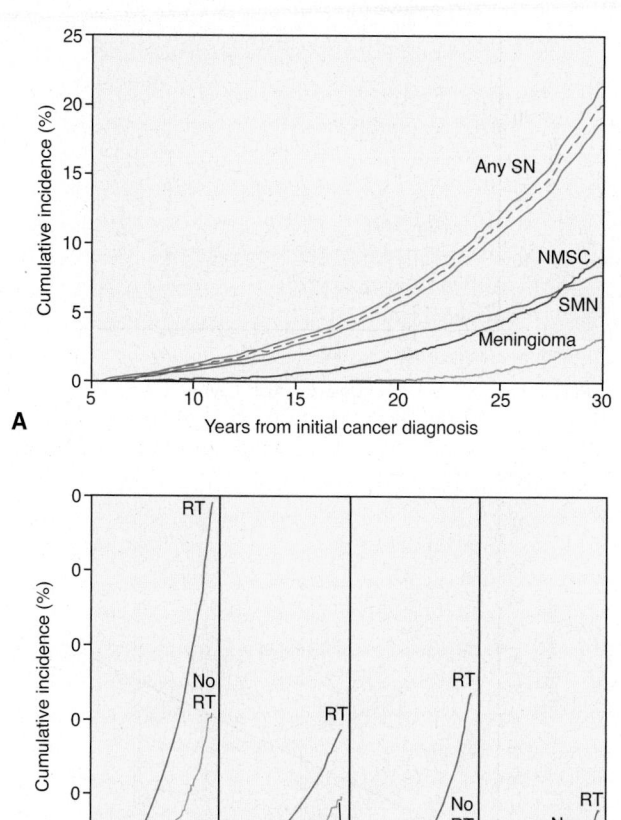

A

B

Figure 143.4 Cumulative incidence at 30 years for second neoplasms. **A:** All second malignant neoplasms. **B:** All second neoplasms by radiotherapy exposure. (With permission from Friedman DL, Whitton J, Leisenring W, et al. Subsequent neoplasms in 5-year survivors of childhood cancer: the Childhood Cancer Survivor Study. *J Natl Cancer Inst* 2010;102:1083–1095.)

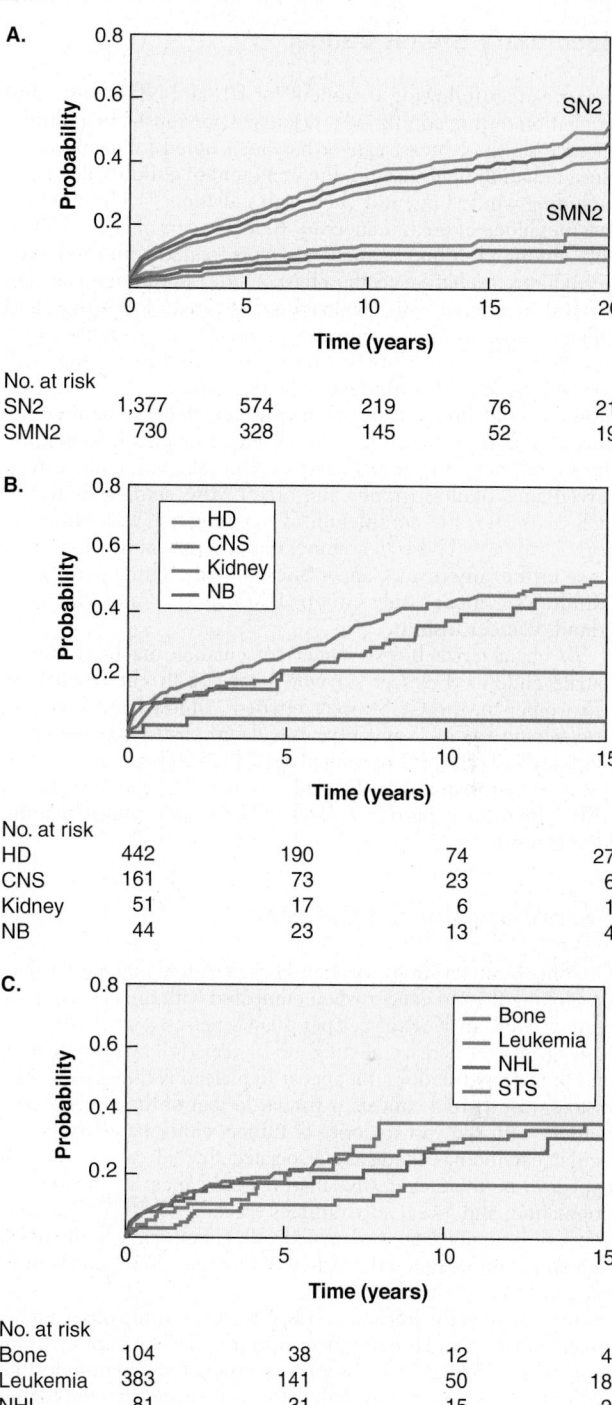

Figure 143.5 A: Cumulative incidence of second subsequent neoplasm (SN2) after the occurrence of first SN *(top line)* with 95% CI and of second subsequent malignant neoplasm (SMN2; *bottom line*) after occurrence of first SMN (SMN1) with 95% CI. **B, C:** Cumulative incidence of SN2 after SN1 by primary pediatric cancer diagnosis. NB, neuroblastoma; STS, soft tissue sarcoma. (With permission from Armstrong GT, Liu W, Leisenring W, et al. Occurrence of multiple subsequent neoplasms in long-term survivors of childhood cancer: a report from the Childhood Cancer Survivor Study. *J Clin Oncol* 2011;29:3056–3064.)

of SPC, primarily contributed to the excess occurrence of secondary breast cancers among female cancer survivors. Moreover, some studies indicate a greater susceptibility of women to known carcinogens such as cigarette smoke, which has been postulated to account for differences in the risk of first primary lung cancers.[310] Possible mechanisms that underlie this greater susceptibility include greater activity of cytochrome P-450 enzymes, enhanced formation of DNA adducts, and the effects of hormones such as estrogen on tumor promotion.[310]

Radiation

Radiation is associated with the majority of excess SPC following therapy for childhood cancer, with a two- to threefold increased risk among irradiated patients compared with those treated with chemotherapy alone.[302,311–313] In order of decreasing incidence, radiation-associated SPCs include NMSC, breast cancer, CNS tumors, thyroid cancer, bone and soft tissue sarcomas, and other carcinomas.[302,312]

Multiple Subsequent Cancers in Long-term Childhood Cancer Survivors

Long-term childhood cancer survivors are at increased risk for multiple SPCs. The cumulative incidence of a third neoplasm was 38.8% at 15 years after a diagnosis of an SPC in the CCSS study and varied by type of first primary cancer (Fig. 143.5). Among

survivors given radiotherapy for a first primary cancer, the cumulative incidence of a third neoplasm was 41.3% at 15 years compared with 25.7% for those not treated with radiation. As noted by Armstrong et al.,[17] limited data with regard to the treatment of SPCs restricted risk factor analyses to primary therapy only.

Secondary Breast Cancer

Breast cancer following treatment for HL and NHL with chest irradiation during adulthood is discussed previously. In addition, an excess risk of breast cancer has been noted following other chest radiation fields used in the treatment of childhood cancer, including whole lung and chest wall radiation.[314] The cumulative incidence of breast cancer by 40 to 45 years of age is 13% to 20% among childhood cancer survivors treated with moderate-to high-dose radiation to the chest.[74,241,315,316] Although overall survival in women with localized breast cancer following chest radiation for childhood cancer may not be as favorable as for women with de novo breast cancer, an early cancer stage still appears associated with favorable outcomes.[15,317,318] Furthermore, second breast cancers can be detected by mammography, although sensitivity is limited. Based on this information, the Children's Oncology Group (COG) recommends annual surveillance mammography and breast MRI, starting at age 25 or 8 years after the completion of radiotherapy, whichever occurs last.[288,314] These recommendations are consistent with those of the American Cancer Society,[319] the United Kingdom Children's Cancer Study Group (UKCCSG),[320] and the Netherlands Cancer Institute.[321]

To characterize breast cancer surveillance practices among female childhood cancer survivors treated with chest radiation, 675 women in the CCSS were queried. Almost half of women between the ages of 25 and 39 years had never had any breast imaging study and only 53% of women aged 40 to 50 years were undergoing regular mammography, and less than 3% reported a breast MRI. The primary barrier was lack of physician recommendation for screening.[322]

Secondary Thyroid Cancer

Childhood cancer survivors are at 11.3- to 18-fold increased risk of developing thyroid cancer when compared with the general population, with an EAR of 1.4 per 10,000 person-years.[211,312,323,324] Risk begins to increase about 8 to 10 years following radiation, and the excess risk does not appear to plateau with age.[71,324] The histology of thyroid cancers is similar to that of the general population, with the vast majority of tumors either papillary or follicular carcinomas. Radiation-associated thyroid cancers do not appear to be more aggressive than thyroid cancer in the general population, and 5-year survival rates exceed 95%.[325,326] The most common primary diagnoses treated with radiotherapy to the neck/thyroid region include HL, ALL, CNS tumors, NHL, and soft tissue sarcoma.[71,323,324]

In contrast to the linear dose-response relationship observed between radiation and breast cancer risks (Fig. 143.6A)[63] or CNS tumors (Fig. 143.6B),[67] there is a linear exponential relation for the risk of thyroid cancer consistent with a cell-killing effect at higher doses (Fig. 143.6C).[71] As illustrated in a nested case-control study (n = 69 cases) conducted in the CCSS, Sigurdson et al.[71] reported a peak risk of thyroid cancer between 10 and 29 Gy with a decrease in the dose-response relation at doses greater than 30 Gy. An update of the CCSS study with 119 pathologically confirmed second thyroid cancers among 12,547 5-year survivors of childhood cancer demonstrated a linear increase in risk with radiation dose up to ~20 Gy, where the relative risk peaked at 14.6-fold (95% CI, 6.8 to 31.5). At thyroid radiation doses >20 Gy, a downturn in the dose-response relationship was observed. Female sex, younger age at exposure, and time since exposure were significant modifiers of radiation-related risk.[72] A pooled analysis of 16,757 childhood cancer survivors with 187 second thyroid cancers also demonstrated a dose-related linear increase in risk for exposures <10 Gy and a leveling off of the risk from 10 to 30 Gy, followed by a decline thereafter. However, the risk remained elevated for doses >50 Gy.[327] Risk was modified by age at first cancer diagnosis, with those

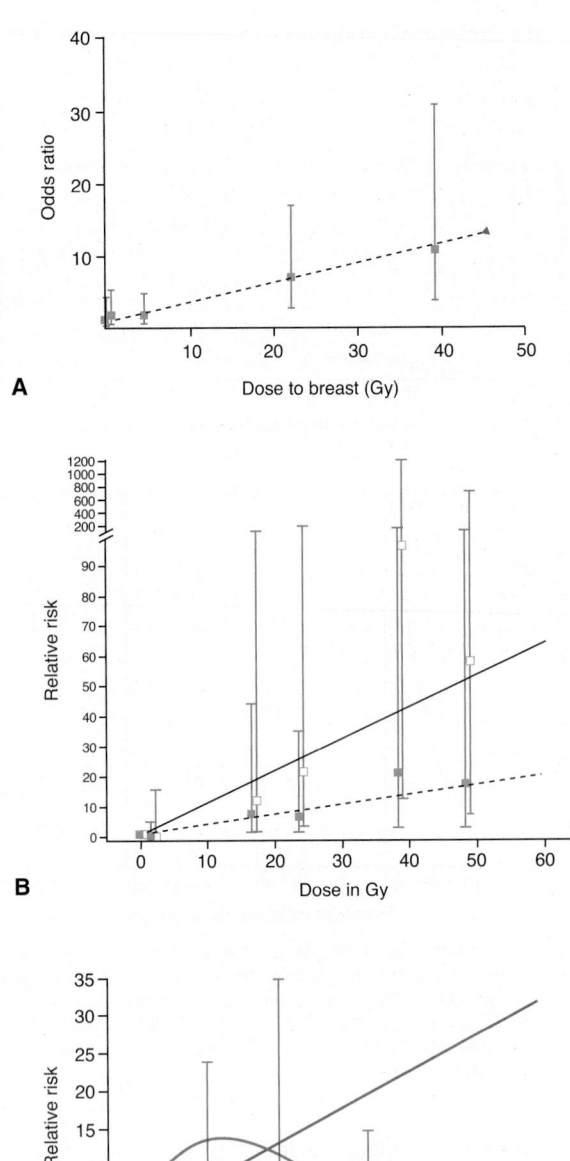

Figure 143.6 **A:** Breast cancer risk by radiation dose to the breast. (From Inskip PD, Robison LL, Stovall M, et al. Radiation dose and breast cancer risk in the Childhood Cancer Survivor Study. *J Clin Oncol* 2009;27: 3901–3907 with permission.) **B:** The relative risk of subsequent glioma and meningioma within the Childhood Cancer Survivor Study cohort by radiation dose (*open boxes*, mean observed relative risk for meningioma; *closed boxes*, mean observed relative risk for glioma; *solid line*, fitted line for meningioma risk; *hatched line*, fitted line for glioma risk). *p* <0.001 (likelihood ratio test, two sided). (From Neglia JP, Robison LL, Stovall M, et al. New primary neoplasms of the central nervous system in survivors of childhood cancer: a report from the Childhood Cancer Survivor Study. *J Natl Cancer Inst* 2006;98:1528–1537 with permission.) **C:** Thyroid cancer risk by radiation dose in cases and controls after adjustment for first cancer. (From Sigurdson AJ, Ronckers CM, Mertens AC, et al. Primary thyroid cancer after a first tumour in childhood [the Childhood Cancer Survivor Study]: a nested case-control study. *Lancet* 2005;365: 2014–2023 with permission.)

treated before age 10 years at highest risk.[71,324] Although some studies report no relationship with chemotherapy,[71,324] others reported an association with anthracyclines (RR = 4.5; 95% CI, 1.4 to 17.8).[327] Although the majority of thyroid cancers occur in females, this reflects the same sex distribution of first thyroid cancers in the general population. Taylor et al.[324] reported a higher SIR for males (26.2) than females (15.1; p = 0.05); however, the AER was higher for females (1.9 per 10,000 person-years) than in males (1.0 per 10,000 person-years). In an effort to reduce the incidence of serious late effects, including breast cancer and coronary artery disease, the dose of radiation has been lowered or omitted in contemporary risk-adapted therapy.[257,328] Although this may achieve these primary goals, the use of reduced radiation doses may in fact lead to an increased incidence of thyroid cancer among certain groups. Based on a small cohort of survivors of childhood HL who were treated with low-dose involved field radiation (15 to 25.5 Gy), O'Brien et al.[329] reported an SIR of 53.2 and an AER of 22.9 thyroid cancers per 10,000 person-years.

Given the indolent nature and excellent long-term survival rates associated with a radiation-related thyroid cancer, the high incidence of thyroid nodules following radiation, and the high rate of false-positive findings with ultrasonography, neither the COG[288] nor the UKCCSG[320] recommend a screening thyroid ultrasound in the follow-up of asymptomatic survivors of pediatric or young adult cancer. Instead, both groups recommend a yearly neck examination. If a thyroid nodule is palpated, it should be further evaluated with an ultrasound and fine-needle aspiration.

Secondary Osteosarcoma and Soft Tissue Sarcoma

In a French–British cohort of 4,400 3-year survivors of a childhood solid tumor (including RB), the 20-year cumulative incidence of a secondary osteosarcoma and soft tissue sarcoma was 1% and 0.6%, respectively.[69,330] In an analysis of 5-year survivors in the CCSS (excluding RB), Henderson et al.[331] reported a 30-year cumulative incidence of 1.1% for secondary sarcoma among those treated with radiation (any location) and 0.5% among those who did not receive radiation. An overall ninefold increased risk existed compared with the general population, with an EAR of 3.3 cases per 10,000 person-years. Risk among survivors who received radiation therapy (SIR = 11.4) was higher than among survivors who did not receive radiotherapy (SIR = 2.7). In general, increased risks for secondary osteosarcoma and soft tissue sarcoma emerge 5 to 8 years after radiotherapy and appear to remain consistently elevated thereafter.[68,69,107,330,331]

Although increased risks of both secondary osteosarcoma and soft tissue sarcoma are associated with radiation, patterns of risk appear somewhat different according to radiation dose. In a nested case-control study set within the French–British cohort (32 cases and 160 controls), the excess risk of secondary osteosarcoma was 1.8 per Gy, with increased risks beginning at low doses (1 to 10 Gy).[330] In two other case-control studies, with 59 and 64 cases (both including RB), no increased risk was associated with lower radiation doses (<10 Gy),[68,107] but an increased risk was observed at higher doses and reached 40-fold after doses to the bone of more than 60 Gy.[68] In another case-control study in the French–British cohort, the excess risk of a soft tissue sarcoma was very low until 10 Gy, with most sarcomas developing after exposure to very high doses of radiation; a quadratic model of the dose-response relationship provided the best fit to the data.[69] In multiple studies, alkylating agent exposure has been independently associated with excess secondary sarcomas in a dose-response fashion[68,69,107,330,331] However, there do not appear to be interactions between radiation and alkylating agent chemotherapy in terms of risk. Gender, race/ethnicity, and age at primary cancer diagnosis did not modify risk in any of the previous studies.[68,69,107,330,331]

There are few data on the long-term prognosis of childhood cancer survivors with secondary sarcoma; however, 5-year survival rates have been less than 50% among other populations with radiation-associated sarcomas.[332] Routine screening with MRI or computed tomography scans of the irradiated field is not recommended.[288,320]

Secondary Central Nervous System Tumors

Secondary gliomas and meningiomas are well-recognized late effects after cranial radiation. In a recent review, childhood cancer survivors were found to be at an 8.1- to 52.3-fold increased risk of secondary CNS tumors. Nearly all cancer survivors who develop CNS neoplasms have been exposed to cranial radiation. Gliomas have a shorter latency than meningiomas. Further, the dose-response relationship between radiation and risk of CNS tumors is steeper for meningiomas.[333] Secondary gliomas occur relatively soon after completion of treatment for the first cancer. Neglia et al.[67] reported that over 50% of secondary gliomas in the CCSS occurred between 5 and 9 years after the first cancer and over 90% occurred before 15 years. The ERR dropped to nearly zero among persons followed past 25 years. There was a linear relationship between radiation dose and glioma risk. Although there was not a difference in risk between males and females, those who were diagnosed at a younger age (<5 years) had a higher risk than those treated in later childhood. Subsequent survival following a secondary glioma is poor: the British CCSS reported 19.5% 5-year survival, with 4.9% for high-grade gliomas and 38.9% for low-grade gliomas.[334]

Secondary meningiomas tend to appear later after radiotherapy and are associated with generally good outcomes. Taylor et al.[334] reported an 83% 5-year survival rate for patients in the British CCSS with a secondary meningioma. Most secondary meningiomas are benign,[302] but may be large or cause significant morbidity depending on location (e.g., seizures, hearing loss). Neglia et al.[67] reported that over 70% of the meningiomas occurring among CCSS survivors were diagnosed 15 years or more after the primary cancer. As with secondary gliomas, there was a strong radiation dose-response relationship for meningioma risk with an excess relative risk per Gy of 1.06, translating to substantial excesses for the majority of CNS tumor survivors treated with 30 Gy or more to the whole brain. The British CCSS also demonstrated a strong linear and independent relationship with radiation dose and intrathecal methotrexate. Those whose meningeal tissue received 0.01 to 9.99 Gy, 10.00 to 19.99 Gy, 20.00 to 29.99 Gy, 30.00 to 39.99 Gy, and ≥40 Gy had risks that were 2-fold, 8-fold, 52-fold, 568-fold, and 479-fold, respectively, compared to those whose meningeal tissue was unexposed.[335] Gender did not modify risk. In contrast to the risk for secondary gliomas, children irradiated after the age of 5 years had a higher risk than those irradiated before 5 years. Genetic susceptibility may also increase the risk of radiation-induced meningiomas.[336]

Five-year survival ranged from zero to 19.5% for subsequent high-grade gliomas and 57.3% to 100% for meningiomas; these rates are similar to those observed in patients with primary gliomas or meningiomas. Despite the poor outcomes associated with secondary gliomas and high frequency of secondary meningiomas following cranial irradiation, there is no evidence that surveillance improves outcomes. Consequently, neither the COG[288] nor the UKCCSG[320] recommend screening brain MRI for asymptomatic patients. However, clinicians should have a heightened index of suspicion for childhood cancer survivors treated with cranial irradiation and who experience new neurologic signs or symptoms.

Secondary Melanoma and Nonmelanoma Skin Cancer

Among the CCSS cohort, the risk of melanoma was 3.3-fold higher than the general population, with a median interval from primary cancer to melanoma of 18.9 years.[302] Similarly, in a Nordic population-based study, the risk of melanoma was 2.6-fold higher than the general population. A systematic review included 151,575 childhood cancer survivors, of whom 212 developed melanoma.[337] Melanomas were most frequently observed after HL, hereditary RB, soft tissue sarcoma, and gonadal tumors. This review identified exposure to radiation as well as the combination of alkylating agents and antimitotic drugs to be associated with an increased risk of melanoma. Although many of these cases of melanoma occurred among patients who received irradiation, to date and to our knowledge, there has not been a study assessing the radiation dose-relation or potentially modifying factors. Moreover, for patients such as those with HL, underlying immunosuppression may also be a factor in excess risks of malignant melanoma.

NMSC is common among childhood cancer survivors following irradiation, exceeding the incidence of all other SPCs combined.[302,304] Indeed, in the recent CCSS update, among 14,359 survivors, there were 1,574 cases of NMSC and 802 cases of invasive or in situ cancer.[302] The 30-year cumulative incidence of NMSC was 9.1%.[302] The vast majority of NMSC was basal cell carcinoma (97%), with a median age of 31 years at occurrence.[338] Radiotherapy was associated with a sixfold increase in risk, and 90% of the tumors occurred within the radiation field. Gender did not appear to modify risk.[302,338] However, older age at radiation exposure (10 to 20 years of age) appeared to be associated with increased risk.[302] Among childhood cancer survivors who received hematopoietic cell transplantation, Leisenring et al.[339] reported that patients given either total-body irradiation or who were light skinned had an increased risk of basal cell carcinoma. Acute graft-versus-host disease was associated with an increased risk of squamous cell carcinoma; chronic graft-versus-host disease was associated with an increased risk of both basal and squamous cell carcinoma. The COG[288] and the UKCCSG[320] recommend annual examination of the skin in irradiated fields.

Other Secondary Carcinomas

The risk of other carcinomas (besides breast, thyroid, and skin) appears to increase with age among childhood cancer survivors. Using CCSS data, Bassal et al.[340] reported that radiation was associated with a significantly increased risk for carcinomas of the head and neck, the colorectum, other gastrointestinal sites, the kidneys, the bladder, and the lungs. The risk for an SPC (excluding breast, thyroid, and skin) was fivefold higher for survivors treated with radiation compared with the general population. In the CCSS update,[302] the number of these other carcinomas increased by 28% in just 4 years. As survivors in the CCSS and similar cohorts (e.g., British CCSS, Dutch LATER[341]) enter mid adulthood, this is an area that warrants further study to better understand modifying risk factors, to quantify radiation dose-response relations, and to identify surveillance approaches. In the following paragraphs, we describe some of the more recent reports of carcinomas among the aging childhood cancer survivor population.

Secondary Tumors of the Digestive Tract

Excess cancers of digestive tract sites have been reported among childhood cancer survivors. A French and British cohort found a 9.7-fold increased risk of SPCs of digestive tract sites compared with the general population.[342] These included esophageal cancer, gastric carcinoma, pancreatic cancer, hepatocellular carcinoma, and colorectal cancer. A strong dose-response relation was identified; compared with those who had not received radiation, survivors with a history of exposure to radiation between 10 and 29 Gy were at 5.2-fold increased risk, and those exposed to doses ≥30 Gy were at 9.6-fold increased risk. The CCSS reported a 4.6-fold increased risk of gastrointestinal cancers among childhood cancer survivors when compared with the US population.[108] The highest

risk was associated with abdominal radiation. In addition, exposure to procarbazine (RR = 3.2) and platinum (RR = 7.6) were identified to be associated with increased risks.

Colorectal cancer has been described as an SPC after successful treatment of childhood cancer. A single institution study found the 40-year cumulative incidence of secondary colorectal cancer to be 1.4%.[343] The cohort was at 10.9-fold increased risk when compared with the general US population. Colorectal carcinomas were more likely to develop in an irradiated colon; the risk increased by 70% with each 10-Gy increase in radiation dose. Increasing radiation volume also increased colorectal cancer risk. Finally, alkylating agent exposure was associated with an 8.8-fold increased risk of secondary colorectal cancer. The population-based British CCSS found the cumulative incidence of colorectal cancer for survivors treated with direct abdominopelvic irradiation to be 1.4% (95% CI, 0.7% to 2.6%) by age 50 years, comparable with the 1.2% risk in individuals with at least two first-degree relatives affected by colorectal cancer.[301] Similarly, the CCSS reported a cumulative incidence of colorectal cancer following abdominal radiation to be 1.2% by 30 years following radiotherapy.[108]

The COG recommends a screening colonoscopy every 5 years in childhood, adolescent, and young adult cancer survivors treated with more than 30 Gy of radiation to the abdomen or pelvis, starting at age 35 years or 10 years after radiation, whichever occurs last.[344] Nathan et al.[345] reported that only 17% of long-term childhood cancer survivors at risk for colorectal cancer reported ever having a colonoscopy.

Renal Cell Carcinoma

An eightfold increased risk of renal cell carcinoma compared with the general population was reported in the CCSS cohort.[110] The highest risk was observed among neuroblastoma survivors. Exposure of the renal bed to radiation as well as exposure to platinum chemotherapy increased the risk.

Salivary Gland Cancer

The incidence of salivary gland cancer among childhood cancer survivors has been reported to be 39-fold that of the general population.[346] Of the 23 salivary gland tumors, 14 were mucoepidermoid carcinomas, 3 were adenocarcinomas, 3 were acinar cell carcinomas, and 3 were miscellaneous other types. The risk increased linearly with radiation dose and remained elevated for 20 years. Exposure to chemotherapeutic agents, tobacco, or alcohol did not appear to increase the risk.

Genetic Conditions

RB is the prototype malignancy in which genetic factors are responsible for a substantial proportion of SPC. Familial RB is caused by inherited mutations of the *RB1* tumor suppressor gene, which has been localized to the long arm of chromosome 13q14.[347] Approximately 90% of hereditary RB patients have bilateral disease. In a large cohort of 1,601 RB survivors in Boston and New York, the risk of SPC was increased 19-fold in hereditary RB survivors; risk was not elevated in nonhereditary patients.[48] The 50-year cumulative incidence of an SPC was 36% and 5.7% for hereditary and nonhereditary patients, respectively. Among the hereditary patients, radiotherapy increased the 50-year cumulative incidence of an SPC to 38.2%, whereas the cumulative incidence was 21.0% for nonirradiated patients. Similar risks among hereditary RB survivors have been reported in the Dutch[306] and British[348] nationwide cohorts. The 50-year cumulative mortality from any SPC for hereditary RB survivors ranged from 17.3 to 25.5%.[349,350]

The majority of SPCs are bone and soft tissue sarcomas occurring in the most heavily irradiated areas (head and neck region). A radiation dose-response relationship exists for sarcomas, with an almost 11-fold risk increase at doses of 60 Gy or greater.[305] Osteosarcomas and soft tissue sarcomas that develop after hereditary RB harbor similar *RB1* mutations as found in RB. Radiation is thus likely to cause the somatic mutations needed to result in sarcomas in carriers of germ-line *RB1* mutations.

Importantly, hereditary RB survivors also have an increased risk in comparison with the general population of second (and third and fourth) cancers in sites distal to the radiation field, suggesting a genetic predisposition independent of radiation exposure.[48,305,306,323,351] Sites for distal cancers include the breast, lung, colon, bladder, uterus, and long bones. In particular, there are excess risks of distal soft tissue sarcomas (leiomyosarcoma, fibrosarcoma, and rhabdomyosarcoma) and osteosarcomas (especially in the lower extremities), suggesting that *RB1* mutation carriers may be inherently predisposed to soft tissue sarcomas and osteosarcomas.[306,351,352] Moreover, the Boston–New York cohort recently reported an increased risk of secondary uterine leiomyosarcomas in hereditary RB survivors.[353] Risk increased from 20 to 27 per 10,000 females for those age 30 to 39 years and 40 or more years, respectively; risk was unrelated to radiation dose for primary RB treatment (ocular radiotherapy). With contemporary therapy largely excluding external beam radiotherapy, it is anticipated that hereditary RB survivors may now live longer without radiation-associated SPC, but with treatment-associated tumors possibly supplanted by increasing uterine leiomyosarcomas in older women.

Childhood sarcoma survivors also have an excess risk of non-radiation-related SPCs, such as breast cancer.[302,315,354] Although many of these patients likely have a *p53* germ-line mutation and are thus classified with Li-Fraumeni syndrome,[355] there may be other genetic factors affecting risk. These issues are discussed in detail elsewhere in the chapter.

Outcomes after Second Primary Cancers

Outcomes among patients who survive SPCs are being increasingly studied.[10–16,356] A comprehensive systematic investigation of factors that affect survival after an SPC diagnosis were recommended as a research priority in the recent NCRP report.[9,10] One large population-based analysis[16] compared mortality after 621 SPCs in testicular cancer survivors with mortality after 12,420 matched first cancers, and found no overall difference between the two groups. Rate ratios for cancer-specific and all-cause mortality were 1.05 (95% CI, 0.90 to 1.23) and 1.09 (95% CI, 0.96 to 1.23), respectively. The exception was among those TC patients treated from 1973 to 1979, during an era when chest irradiation was routinely given and before reductions in infradiaphragmatic radiation fields and doses were implemented; for these patients, all-cause mortality after either a second primary lung cancer or a cancer below the diaphragm (likely to be included in irradiated fields) was significantly higher than in patients with matched first cancers.

Other large population-based studies have systematically evaluated survival after second primary cancers of the breast,[15] the lung,[13] or gastrointestinal sites[14] after HL. In each survey, survival after a second cancer at one of these sites among HL survivors was significantly reduced compared with first primary cancers at the same site. Each of these SPCs has, in part, been linked to antecedent HL treatment. Solomon et al.[11] evaluated overall and cancer-specific survival after second cancers of the breast, colorectum, lungs, and prostate in patients with and without CLL. Although, to date, these cancers have not been associated with CLL treatment, Solomon and colleagues[11] hypothesized that CLL patients who develop these cancers could experience less favorable cancer-specific outcomes, due either to more aggressive biologic characteristics of the second cancers or to less effective immune surveillance and control. Overall, among CLL patients, 892 developed colorectal cancer, almost 1,300 were diagnosed with lung cancer, 608 with female breast cancer, and over 1,200 men later developed prostate cancer. After taking into account age,

gender, and disease stage, the overall age-specific survival for CLL patients was significantly inferior to patients who developed a first primary cancer at one of these sites. Cancer-specific survival was significantly inferior for CLL patients who developed cancers of the breast (HR, 1.41), lung (HR, 1.3), and colorectal sites (HR 1.64), but not prostate (HR, 1.40). These findings have important implications for CLL patients, because cancers of the breast, lung, and colorectal sites represent the three most common cancers in US women and two of the three most common cancers in US men.[12] These data suggest that CLL patients who develop these common cancers experience a more aggressive clinical course and are more likely to die from these cancers, even after adjusting for age, race, and disease stage. Limitations of the SEER data set (a lack of detailed data with regard to initial therapy, other patient-specific factors that may affect prognosis, and a lack of information on subsequent therapy) precluded Solomon et al.[11] from an in-depth probe of various hypotheses. Nonetheless, this study heightens awareness of the importance of the further investigation of outcomes after a SPC diagnosis.[15,16,356] Even if risks, per se, for some of the more common cancers (e.g., cancers of the breast, colorectum, prostate, lungs) are not elevated after a selected first primary cancer, nonetheless these cancers remain common.

At a minimum, all cancer survivors should be encouraged to follow guidelines for cancer screening recommended for the general population, as recently reviewed.[282] The identification of individuals at increased risk for additional primaries due to genetic predisposition, treatment, and other factors can also pinpoint patients who should have earlier and more frequent screening and/or who might be candidates for prevention strategies.[282] Furthermore, it will also now be important to determine optimal *management* strategies for second cancers. Many times, cancer survivors are limited with regard to treatment options, because they have already received large amounts of cytotoxic therapies.[15,16] Further research is needed to understand how to optimize the treatment of not only those SPCs that indeed may reflect the carcinogenic effects of prior therapy, but also those SPCs that represent the operation of other factors.

COMMENTS

Future SPC research areas of importance to cancer survivors include those of etiopathogenesis, optimal management, and subsequent outcomes.[6,9,10,12,282,356,357] Overarching research recommendations in the 2012 NCRP report (see Table 143.1)[9,10] included the long-term, large-scale follow-up of extant cancer survivors and the construction of prospective cohorts of patients given new treatment modalities. One identified need involved the long-term follow-up of survivors successfully treated for tumors at sites for which reductions in field size and radiotherapy dose have been implemented, and the follow-up of populations successfully managed without any type of cytotoxic treatment to define baseline risks. For carcinogenic drugs, pharmacogenomic and pharmacoepidemiologic studies should be carefully considered.[6,356,358,359] It will also be important to follow survivors of adolescent and young adult cancer,[360] given the sparseness of information for this population.

Groups of cancer survivors for whom detailed treatment data information are collected will also be important in providing new insights into a wide range of outcomes,[6,356] including other possible late sequelae, such as cardiovascular disease, neuropathies, and endocrine dysfunction.[9,10,285,356] Furthermore, an enhancement of the understanding of genetic and other influences that contribute to one late effect of cancer and its treatment might inform our understanding not only of other untoward sequelae, but also factors that impact survival. Thus, future investments in research infrastructure should also include the collection of biologic samples to better evaluate the role of genetic factors in not only SPC development,[6,52] but also the occurrence of other outcomes.[356] In addition, future investment should be directed to the application of animal models in unraveling the genetic underpinnings of SPC risk.[356,361] The elucidation of functional genetic variants will also enhance risk assessment[282] and the development of risk-stratification in terms of a cost-effective framework for patient follow-up. Comprehensive SPC risk prediction models could also stratify patients into risk groups to personalize follow-up strategies and develop evidence-based interventions.[6,362]

The database to support various lifestyle recommendations in reducing SPC occurrence is grounded in only a few observational studies and randomized clinical trials conducted in cancer survivors,[363,364] and rests largely on inference from studies conducted in other diseases, such as cardiovascular disease. Therefore, additional research is needed among cancer survivors to understand the relative contribution and interaction of lifestyle factors with the patient's genetic profile and exposure to treatment and environmental factors. Furthermore, additional efforts should be directed to determinate the efficacy of different SPC screening approaches in survivors of adult-onset cancer. Many of the strategies applied to childhood cancer survivors serve as a potential paradigm for future work.[344,365]

As additional information is generated with regard to SPCs,[17,357] it should be recognized that the time of cancer diagnosis and the period that follows are opportune times for healthcare providers to counsel patients about health promotion to not only reduce the risk of cancer recurrence, but also to minimize comorbidities. Health-care providers can play an important role in this process by recommending genetic counseling for selected patients (and family members), and by referring patients to nutrition counselors, exercise trainers, and clinical psychologists to assist with lifestyle change interventions. In particular, the importance of smoking cessation, weight control, physical activity, and other factors consistent with a healthy lifestyle should be consistently conveyed to patients. Given the current investment in cancer survivorship research, further study of the late effects of cancer and its treatment is critical.[356] It will be important to continue to add to our understanding of genetic variants and etiologic influences that increase not only SPC risk, but also factors that influence subsequent management and survival.[6,9,10,12,15,282,356,357]

SELECTED REFERENCES

The full reference list can be accessed at lwwhealthlibrary.com/oncology.

3. Siegel R, DeSantis C, Virgo K, et al. Cancer treatment and survivorship statistics, 2012. *CA Cancer J Clin* 2012;62:220–241.
6. Travis LB, Rabkin CS, Brown LM, et al. Cancer survivorship—genetic susceptibility and second primary cancers: research strategies and recommendations. *J Natl Cancer Inst* 2006;98:15–25.
9. Travis LB, Boice JD Jr, Allan JM, et al. *Report No. 170—Second Primary Cancers and Cardiovascular Disease after Radiation Therapy.* National Council on Radiation Protection & Measurements Web site. http://www.ncrppublications.org/Reports/170.
10. Travis LB, Ng AK, Allan JM, et al. Second malignant neoplasms and cardiovascular disease following radiotherapy. *J Natl Cancer Inst* 2012;104:357–370.
11. Solomon BM, Rabe KG, Slager SL, et al. Overall and cancer-specific survival of patients with breast, colon, kidney, and lung cancers with and without chronic lymphocytic leukemia: a SEER population-based study. *J Clin Oncol* 2013;31:930–937.
15. Milano MT, Li H, Gail MH, et al. Long-term survival among patients with Hodgkin's lymphoma who developed breast cancer: a population-based study. *J Clin Oncol* 2010;28:5088–5096.
16. Schairer C, Hisada M, Chen BE, et al. Comparative mortality for 621 second cancers in 29356 testicular cancer survivors and 12420 matched first cancers. *J Natl Cancer Inst* 2007;99:1248–1256.
17. Armstrong GT, Liu W, Leisenring W, et al. Occurrence of multiple subsequent neoplasms in long-term survivors of childhood cancer: a report from the Childhood Cancer Survivor Study. *J Clin Oncol* 2011;29:3056–3064.
18. Sakoda LC, Jorgenson E, Witte JS. Turning of COGS moves forward findings for hormonally mediated cancers. *Nat Genet* 2013;45:345–348.
30. Adams MJ, Dozier A, Shore RE, et al. Breast cancer risk 55+ years after irradiation for an enlarged thymus and its implications for early childhood medical irradiation today. *Cancer Epidemiol Biomarkers Prev* 2010;19:48–58.
52. Best T, Li D, Skol AD, et al. Variants at 6q21 implicate PRDM1 in the etiology of therapy-induced second malignancies after Hodgkin's lymphoma. *Nat Med* 2011;17:941–943.
53. Travis LB, Gospodarowicz M, Curtis RE, et al. Lung cancer following chemotherapy and radiotherapy for Hodgkin's disease. *J Natl Cancer Inst* 2002;94:182–192.
54. Hodgson DC, Gilbert ES, Dores GM, et al. Long-term solid cancer risk among 5-year survivors of Hodgkin's lymphoma. *J Clin Oncol* 2007;25:1489–1497.
61. Travis LB, Hill DA, Dores GM, et al. Breast cancer following radiotherapy and chemotherapy among young women with Hodgkin disease. *JAMA* 2003;290:465–475.
63. Inskip PD, Robison LL, Stovall M, et al. Radiation dose and breast cancer risk in the Childhood Cancer Survivor Study. *J Clin Oncol* 2009;27:3901–3907.
64. Morton LM, Gilbert ES, Hall P, et al. Risk of treatment-related esophageal cancer among breast cancer survivors. *Ann Oncol* 2012;23:3081–3091.
71. Sigurdson AJ, Ronckers CM, Mertens AC, et al. Primary thyroid cancer after a first tumour in childhood (the Childhood Cancer Survivor Study): a nested case-control study. *Lancet* 2005;365:2014–2023.
74. De Bruin ML, Sparidans J, van't Veer MB, et al. Breast cancer risk in female survivors of Hodgkin's lymphoma: lower risk after smaller radiation volumes. *J Clin Oncol* 2009;27:4239–4246.
91. Maraldo MV, Brodin NP, Aznar MC, et al. Estimated risk of cardiovascular disease and secondary cancers with modern highly conformal radiotherapy for early-stage mediastinal Hodgkin lymphoma. *Ann Oncol* 2013;24:2113–2118.
92. Weber DC, Johanson S, Peguret N, et al. Predicted risk of radiation-induced cancers after involved field and involved node radiotherapy with or without intensity modulation for early-stage hodgkin lymphoma in female patients. *Int J Radiat Oncol Biol Phys* 2011;81:490–497.
96. Chung CS, Keating N, Yock T, et al. Comparative analysis of second malignancy risk in patients treated with proton therapy versus conventional photon therapy. *Int J Radiat Oncol Biol Phys* 2008;72:s8.
101. Travis LB, Holowaty EJ, Bergfeldt K, et al. Risk of leukemia after platinum-based chemotherapy for ovarian cancer. *N Engl J Med* 1999;340:351–357.
108. Henderson TO, Oeffinger KC, Whitton J, et al. Secondary gastrointestinal cancer in childhood cancer survivors: a cohort study. *Ann Intern Med* 2012;156:757–766.
109. Veiga LH, Bhatti P, Ronckers CM, et al. Chemotherapy and thyroid cancer risk: a report from the Childhood Cancer Survivor Study. *Cancer Epidemiol Biomarkers Prev* 2012;21:92–101.
111. Fung C, Fossa SD, Milano MT, et al. Solid tumors after chemotherapy or surgery for testicular nonseminoma: a population-based study. *J Clin Oncol* 2013;31:3807–3814.
115. Relling MV, Rubnitz JE, Rivera GK, et al. High incidence of secondary brain tumours after radiotherapy and antimetabolites. *Lancet* 1999;354:34–39.
131. Rizzo JD, Curtis RE, Socie G, et al. Solid cancers after allogeneic hematopoietic cell transplantation. *Blood* 2009;113:1175–1183.
140. Ellis NA, Huo D, Yildiz O, et al. MDM2 SNP309 and TP53 Arg72Pro interact to alter therapy-related acute myeloid leukemia susceptibility. *Blood* 2008;112:741–749.
145. Han FF, Guo CL, Liu LH. The effect of CHEK2 variant I157T on cancer susceptibility: evidence from a meta-analysis. *DNA Cell biol* 2013;32:329–335.
152. Allan JM, Wild CP, Rollinson S, et al. Polymorphism in glutathione S-transferase P1 is associated with susceptibility to chemotherapy-induced leukemia. *Proc Natl Acad Sci U S A* 2001;98:11592–11597.
164. Lorenzo Y, Provencio M, Lombardia L, et al. Differential genetic and functional markers of second neoplasias in Hodgkin's disease patients. *Clin Cancer Res* 2009;15:4823–4828.
178. Brooks JD, Teraoka SN, Reiner AS, et al. Variants in activators and downstream targets of ATM, radiation exposure, and contralateral breast cancer risk in the WECARE study. *Hum Mutat* 2012;33:158–164.
181. Knight JA, Skol AD, Shinde A, et al. Genome-wide association study to identify novel loci associated with therapy-related myeloid leukemia susceptibility. *Blood* 2009;113:5575–5582.
183. Funk RK, Maxwell TJ, Izumi M, et al. Quantitative trait loci associated with susceptibility to therapy-related acute murine promyelocytic leukemia in hCG-PML/RARA transgenic mice. *Blood* 2012;112:1434–1442.
193. Stanulla M, Schaeffeler E, Moricke A, et al. Thiopurine methyltransferase genetics is not a major risk factor for secondary malignant neoplasms after treatment of childhood acute lymphoblastic leukemia on Berlin-Frankfurt-Munster protocols. *Blood* 2009;114:1314–1318.
202. Chao RC, Pyzel U, Fridlyand J, et al. Therapy-induced malignant neoplasms in Nf1 mutant mice. *Cancer Cell* 2005;8:337–348.
203. Sharif S, Ferner R, Birch JM, et al. Second primary tumors in neurofibromatosis 1 patients treated for optic glioma: substantial risks after radiotherapy. *J Clin Oncol* 2006;24:2570–2575.
207. Dolgin E. Preemptive genotyping trialed to prevent adverse drug reactions. *Nat Med* 2011;17:1323.
208. West C, Rosenstein BS. Establishment of a radiogenomics consortium. *Radiother Oncol* 2010;94:117–118.

215. Constine LS, Tarbell N, Hudson MM, et al. Subsequent malignancies in children treated for Hodgkin's disease: associations with gender and radiation dose. *Int J Radiat Oncol Biol Phys* 2008;72:24–33.

232. Travis LB, Hill D, Dores GM, et al. Cumulative absolute breast cancer risk for young women treated for Hodgkin lymphoma. *J Natl Cancer Inst* 2005;97:1428–1437.

247. Li CI, Daling JR, Porter PL, et al. Relationship between potentially modifiable lifestyle factors and risk of second primary contralateral breast cancer among women diagnosed with estrogen receptor-positive invasive breast cancer. *J Clin Oncol* 2009;27:5312–5318.

264. Travis LB, Fossa SD, Schonfeld SJ, et al. Second cancers among 40,576 testicular cancer patients: focus on long-term survivors. *J Natl Cancer Inst* 2005;97:1354–1365.

265. van den Belt-Dusebout AW, de Wit R, Gietema JA, et al. Treatment-specific risks of second malignancies and cardiovascular disease in 5-year survivors of testicular cancer. *J Clin Oncol* 2007;25:4370–4378.

276. Beard CJ, Travis LB, Chen MH, et al. Outcomes in stage I testicular seminoma: a population-based study of 9193 patients. *Cancer* 2013;119:2771–2777.

280. Jones WG, Fossa SD, Mead GM, et al. Randomized trial of 30 versus 20 Gy in the adjuvant treatment of stage I testicular seminoma: a report on Medical Research Council Trial TE18, European Organisation for the Research and Treatment of Cancer Trial 30942 (ISRCTN18525328). *J Clin Oncol* 2005;23:1200–1208.

282. Wood ME, Vogel V, Ng A, et al. Second malignant neoplasms: assessment and strategies for risk reduction. *J Clin Oncol* 2012;30:3734–3745.

285. Travis LB, Beard C, Allan JM, et al. Testicular cancer survivorship: research strategies and recommendations. *J Natl Cancer Inst* 2010;102:1114–1130.

301. Reulen RC, Frobisher C, Winter DL, et al. Long-term risks of subsequent primary neoplasms among survivors of childhood cancer. *JAMA* 2011;305:2311–2319.

314. Henderson TO, Amsterdam A, Bhatia S, et al. Systematic review: surveillance for breast cancer in women treated with chest radiation for childhood, adolescent, or young adult cancer. *Ann Intern Med* 2010;152:444–455.

318. Elkin EB, Klem ML, Gonzales AM, et al. Characteristics and outcomes of breast cancer in women with and without a history of radiation for Hodgkin's lymphoma: a multi-institutional, matched cohort study. *J Clin Oncol* 2011;29:2466–2473.

322. Oeffinger KC, Ford JS, Moskowitz CS, et al. Breast cancer surveillance practices among women previously treated with chest radiation for a childhood cancer. *JAMA* 2009;301:404–414.

324. Taylor AJ, Croft AP, Palace AM, et al. Risk of thyroid cancer in survivors of childhood cancer: results from the British Childhood Cancer Survivor Study. *Int J Cancer* 2009;125:2400–2405.

327. Veiga LH, Lubin JH, Anderson H, et al. A pooled analysis of thyroid cancer incidence following radiotherapy for childhood cancer. *Radiat Res* 2012;178:365–376.

329. O'Brien MM, Donaldson SS, Balise RR, et al. Second malignant neoplasms in survivors of pediatric Hodgkin's lymphoma treated with low-dose radiation and chemotherapy. *J Clin Oncol* 2010;28:1232–1239.

333. Bowers DC, Nathan PC, Constine L, et al. Subsequent neoplasms of the CNS among survivors of childhood cancer: a systematic review. *Lancet Oncol* 2013;14:e321–e328.

337. Braam KI, Overbeek A, Kaspers GJ, et al. Malignant melanoma as second malignant neoplasm in long-term childhood cancer survivors: a systematic review. *Pediatr Blood Cancer* 2012;58:665–674.

343. Nottage K, McFarlane J, Krasin MJ, et al. Secondary colorectal carcinoma after childhood cancer. *J Clin Oncol* 2012;30:2552–2558.

345. Nathan PC, Ness KK, Mahoney MC, et al. Screening and surveillance for second malignant neoplasms in adult survivors of childhood cancer: a report from the Childhood Cancer Survivor Study. *Ann Intern Med* 2010;153:442–451.

348. Maccarthy A, Bayne AM, Brownbill PA, et al. Second and subsequent tumours among 1927 retinoblastoma patients diagnosed in Britain 1951–2004. *Br J Cancer* 2013;108:2455–2463.

356. Elena JW, Travis LB, Simonds NI, et al. Leveraging epidemiology and clinical studies of cancer outcomes: recommendations and opportunities for translational research. *J Natl Cancer Inst* 2013;105:85–94.

358. Wheeler HE, Maitland ML, Dolan ME, et al. Cancer pharmacogenomics: strategies and challenges. *Nat Rev Genet* 2013;14:23–24.

359. Freedman AN, Sansbury LB, Figg WD, et al. Cancer pharmacogenomics and pharmacoepidemiology: setting a research agenda to accelerate translation. *J Natl Cancer Inst* 2010;102:1698–1705.

363. Rock CL, Doyle C, Demark-Wahnefried W, et al. Nutrition and physical activity guidelines for cancer survivors. *CA Cancer J Clin* 2012;62:243–274.

PRACTICE OF ONCOLOGY

144 Neurocognitive Effects

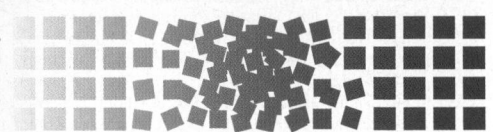

Paul D. Brown, Sanne B. Schagen, and Jeffrey S. Wefel

INTRODUCTION

Patients with central nervous system (CNS) tumors frequently suffer from a number of adverse symptoms, including cognitive impairment. Cognitive dysfunction occurs in most patients with brain tumors, often at presentation, and is frequently progressive even after aggressive treatment. In addition, recent advances in multimodality therapy have led to improvement in survival, raising concerns regarding the long-term effects of these interventions on cognitive function. Treatment options for cognitive deficits remain quite limited; therefore, a thorough understanding of the impacts of brain tumor interventions and an awareness of the cognitive function of patients with adult brain tumors at presentation and over time is necessary to help guide treatment decisions. Finally, in non-CNS cancers, there is a growing understanding of the cognitive impact of the cancer process itself and non-CNS–directed therapies.

ASSESSMENT OF COGNITIVE FUNCTION

Cognitive impairment in patients with primary brain tumors is extremely common at presentation before any interventions have been performed. Several studies report cognitive dysfunction in over 90% of patients with primary brain tumors prior to surgical intervention.[1,2] Memory and executive function are most commonly impaired, which is consistent with the tendency for primary brain tumors to arise in the frontal or temporal regions. Studies of patients suffering from stroke or epilepsy have demonstrated that the nature of the cognitive impairments often relates to the location of a lesion. Although tumor patients have shown typical lateralizing patterns of cognitive impairment (e.g., left hemisphere lesions frequently cause difficulties with verbal learning and memory and language functions),[3] these impairments are often more subtle and diffuse in patients with tumors than are those observed in sudden-onset neurologic conditions such as a stroke.[4] Differences in the pathophysiology of these lesions are believed to underlie these observations; whereas a cerebrovascular accident may rapidly result in tissue destruction, tumors diffusely and often more slowly infiltrate the brain, thereby disrupting normal brain function in networks that are proximal to the visible tumor as well as more distant from the site through mechanisms such as diaschisis. Using magnetoencephalography and functional magnetic resonance imaging (MRI), the abnormal organization of widespread brain networks has been demonstrated in cognitively impaired brain tumor patients.[5,6] Prior to surgery, differences in tumor histology are associated with differences in network organization, which may reflect the adverse effects of seizure and anticonvulsant use on brain organization or the effects of neuroplasticity.[7]

Cognitive impairment is associated with difficulty in daily life more often than physical impairments, and caregivers cite cognitive problems as the most difficult problems to manage.[3] These cognitive deficits cause significant difficulties, such as decreased independence, interference in academic or vocational pursuits, and increased caregiver distress and burden. Even subtle cognitive deficits can significantly limit a patient's ability to perform usual activities, but may not be evident on casual observation or detectable via routine medical examinations. If unrecognized, these cognitive deficits can lead to inaccurate judgment on the part of the medical team regarding the patient's ability for self-care and in the believed safety of the treatments themselves.

A neuropsychological assessment provides quantitative, objective measurement of potentially subtle, yet clinically significant, changes in a patient's cognitive function. Cognitive testing involves the administration of standardized psychometric instruments (i.e., tests) that evaluate various aspects of brain function such as attention, learning and memory, information processing speed, expressive and receptive language function, executive function (e.g., abstract reasoning, planning, decision making), visual perception and construction, and mood and personality. Test results are integrated with the patient's clinical history, observations of the patient's behavior, patient report, and reports of family members and/or caregivers. Interpreting these psychometric instruments and assessments requires a trained neuropsychologist. A brief evaluation with screening instruments such as the Mini-Mental Status Examination are not recommended because these were not developed to assess cognition in brain tumor patients and they provide limited information about domains of cognitive function frequently affected by brain tumors and their treatment (e.g., learning and memory, executive function, processing speed, fine motor control).[8] Similarly, a patient self-report does not routinely correlate with objectively measured cognitive function[9] or functional outcomes.[10]

The neuropsychological assessment may be used to identify and guide interventions for impaired patients, including compensatory strategy training (cognitive rehabilitation), pharmacotherapy, or psychotherapy. This information is critical in designing realistic goals and future plans for patients with cognitive deficits. In addition, repeated assessments can track the patient's response to primary therapy, allowing for careful evaluation of the costs and benefits of a given treatment regimen or supportive therapy (e.g., deterioration of cognitive function predicts tumor progression) and to targeted interventions for cognitive dysfunction.[11]

IMPACT OF TUMOR

Whether the *predominant* cause of cognitive decline in patients with brain tumors is the treatment or the tumor itself is an important question and has a significant impact on treatment recommendations. Older studies have emphasized the late neurotoxicity of treatment, especially radiotherapy.[12] However, these studies have suffered from deficiencies, but most importantly, have lacked baseline cognitive testing because the brain tumor itself is often the primary cause of cognitive difficulties. The importance of baseline testing cannot be overemphasized because, for example, large prospective studies with baseline evaluations have found more than 90% of patients with brain metastases have significant cognitive impairment in one or more cognitive domains at the time of diagnosis (i.e., before whole-brain radiotherapy [WBRT]).[13]

2068

More recent studies that have included prospective baseline and serial cognitive testing have found the tumor to be the dominant cause of cognitive decline in brain metastases,[13,14] patients with low-grade gliomas,[15] and patients with high-grade gliomas.[16] For example, Li et al.[14] divided 135 patients with brain metastases into poor responders and good responders based on the response of their brain metastases on MRI 2 months after WBRT. For all tests, the median time to cognitive deterioration was longer in good than in poor responders and was statistically significant in a number of domains. In long-term survivors, tumor shrinkage was significantly correlated with the preservation of executive function and fine motor coordination.

There is also mounting evidence that cognitive decline in brain tumor patients after therapy may frequently reflect subclinical tumor progression rather than neurotoxicity resulting from treatment. In a North Central Cancer Treatment Group study of 1,244 patients with high-grade gliomas prospectively treated with radiation and nitrosourea-based chemotherapy, cognitive deterioration was noted at evaluations prior to radiographic failure; in contrast, patients without tumor progression had stable cognitive function.[16] In an M.D. Anderson Cancer Center study of 56 patients with recurrent high-grade gliomas treated on phase 1 and phase 2 trials, cognitive deterioration occurred 6 weeks prior to radiographic failure, highlighting the sensitivity and predictive value of cognitive assessments.[17] Similarly, a large randomized phase 3 glioblastoma (GBM) trial studying the effects of standard- versus a dose-dense regimen of temozolomide found cognitive dysfunction at baseline and cognitive decline after concurrent chemoradiation (in progression-free patients) was prognostic for progression-free and overall survival time.[18]

IMPACT OF TREATMENT

Surgery

Nonbrain surgery is known to cause postoperative cognitive impairments, especially in the elderly. The deficits, particularly for memory, may be present for weeks or months.[19] Risk factors besides age includes duration of anesthesia and postoperative complications. In contrast to nonbrain surgery, surgery for brain tumors may lead to focal cognitive deficits.[3] However, relief of mass effect and increased intracranial pressure frequently results in improvement in cognitive function. Variability in frequency of cognitive improvement or decline have been reported, with 24% to 84% demonstrating cognitive improvement and 36% to 38% demonstrating cognitive decline.[1,20,21] There is some preliminary evidence that better preoperative cognitive function (i.e., memory, language) is associated with increased risk for postoperative cognitive dysfunction in patients with high-grade gliomas.[20,21] Potential adverse effects of surgery can be seen in patients with benign tumors, such as pituitary adenomas. Neuropsychological tests performed on a cohort of 69 pituitary tumor patients treated found that a transfrontal approach was associated with greater frequency and severity of cognitive impairment (44% impaired) when compared to the transsphenoidal approach (30% impaired) and even more so when compared to a nonsurgical control group with pituitary tumors.[22]

The balance between attaining a maximal resection and, at the same time, preserving function has been difficult, especially because gliomas are infiltrative and invasive. However, that goal has been advanced by comprehensive evaluations, including neuropsychological assessments and technologic advances such as intraoperative MRI, functional neuroimaging techniques, white matter pathway mapping, and intraoperative stimulation.[23] Recent studies indicate that as many as 80% of patients with low-grade gliomas will experience postoperative cognitive deficits even when using intraoperative-guided imaging and functional mapping in patients

with tumors in eloquent brain locations. However, most of these deficits resolve within a few months. In a report by Duffau,[23] 94% of patients returned to their preoperative functioning by 3 months, presumably owing to the plasticity of the normal brain and recovery from the acute effects of surgery.[24]

Radiotherapy

Radiation therapy plays an important role in the treatment of primary and metastatic tumors located in the CNS. As more effective treatments for intracranial lesions have become available and long-term survival has increased, more attention has been placed on identifying and quantifying the adverse effects of radiation on cognitive function in adult patients. The mechanisms for these adverse effects are not fully understood but include neuroinflammation, alterations in neurogenesis, and direct vascular injury.[25,26]

Because of their relatively long progression-free and overall survival, patients with low-grade brain tumors are an ideal population to study when analyzing the potential cognitive deficits of radiotherapy because cognitive deficits can take years to develop. In addition, patients with low-grade brain tumors are often young and do not have underlying medical comorbidities that may confound the cognitive analysis. A number of retrospective studies have found increased cognitive difficulties after cranial radiotherapy for low-grade brain neoplasms. However, these studies have suffered from many deficiencies such as an absence of baseline cognitive testing because the brain tumor itself is often the primary cause of cognitive difficulties.[12] A retrospective study of patients with low-grade gliomas followed longitudinally highlights some of these shortcomings.[27] With a median follow-up of 12 years, there were declines in attentional functioning in the patients who received radiotherapy, whereas the patients who were observed retained stable cognitive functioning. Although these data are valuable in that they provide long-term follow-up on patients with low-grade gliomas, the study has been criticized for a lack of baseline testing, the inherent selection bias of patients who received radiotherapy having a more aggressive disease, and outdated techniques such as WBRT.[28]

In sharp contrast, a number of studies have prospectively performed extensive neuropsychological testing on adult patients with low-grade neoplasms before (baseline) and after radiotherapy (up to 6 years after radiotherapy) (Table 144.1) and have not found significant cognitive deterioration when compared to either baseline[29–33] or to a cohort of patients with low-grade brain neoplasms not treated with radiotherapy.[15,34] For example, a subset of 20 of the 203 patients with adult low-grade gliomas enrolled on an Intergroup prospective phase 3 trial that randomized patients to 50.4 or 64.8 Gy underwent cognitive testing before and up to 5 years after localized radiation therapy.[32] No significant losses in general intellectual function, new learning function, or memory function were seen. The groups' mean test scores were higher at follow-up evaluations than their initial performances on all psychometric measures, although the improvement was not statistically significant. However, four patients, all in the 64.8-Gy arm, had a mild decline in one or more of the domains assessed. The results of this study are consistent with the weight of evidence that indicates a low incidence of cognitive difficulties after *focal*, conventionally fractionated (i.e., 1.8 to 2 Gy) radiotherapy using modern techniques to deliver moderate doses (i.e., 45 to 54 Gy) in adults.[12,35]

An extreme form of *focal* radiotherapy used to treat many benign and neoplastic cranial conditions is stereotactic radiosurgery (SRS). SRS uses multiple radiation beams and is able to encompass treatment volumes in the high-dose region with small margins because of the stereotactic imaging and immobilization. This results in rapid dose falloff, allowing greater sparing of normal brain tissues, and therefore minimizes risk to the surrounding structures. The cognitive impact of SRS was evaluated in a prospective trial assessing 95 patients with cerebral arteriovenous malformations

TABLE 144.1

Prospective Trials for Low-Grade Neoplasms with Baseline and Serial Neurocognitive Testing

Study (Reference)	Number of Patients	Radiation Total Dose/ Fraction Size (Gy)	Mean Follow-up (Years)	Extensive Neurocognitive Assessment	Neurotoxicity After RT
Glosser[30]	17	Proton RT median 68.4 CGE/1.8	4	Yes	No; mild decline in psychomotor speed with high doses
Vigliani[34]	17	Focal RT 54/1.8	4	Yes	No; transient decline in reaction time
Armstrong[29]	26	Focal RT mean 54.6/1.8–2.0	3	Yes	No; mild decline in visual memory after 5 years
Brown[88]	203	Focal RT 50.4/1.8 or 64.8/1.8	7.4 (median)	No (MMSE and NFS)	5.3% with MMSE decline at 5 years
Torres[15]	15	Focal RT mean 54/1.8	2	Yes	No; decline in memory and attention only if tumor progression
Laack[32]	20	Focal RT 50.4/1.8 or 64.8/1.8	3	Yes	No
Steinvorth[33]	40	SRT median 57.6/1.8	1	Yes	No
Jalali[31]	22	SRT median 54/1.8	2	Yes	No

RT, radiotherapy; CGE, centigray equivalent; MMSE, Folstein Mini-Mental State Examination; NFS, neurologic function scores; SRT, stereotactic radiotherapy.

with extensive neuropsychometric testing before and after SRS (median dose: 20 Gy in one fraction) and found all measures of cognitive function were stable or improved 3 years after SRS.[36]

The impact of WBRT on cognitive function is best addressed by prophylactic cranial irradiation (PCI) trials because, by definition, these patients should not have brain metastases (and, therefore, tumor progression is less of a confounding variable). PCI has been shown to decrease the development of brain metastases and improve cure rates and survival for small-cell lung cancer patients because of the propensity of these patients to develop brain metastases. Similar to low-grade brain tumors, a number of retrospective studies have raised concerns of neurotoxicity after PCI, but these studies have been compromised by the use of large, unconventional fraction sizes, comorbid conditions (known brain metastasis), high total doses (up to 50 Gy), concomitant use of chemotherapy, and, most importantly, lack of baseline neuropsychological testing (prospective cognitive studies have shown up to 97% of limited stage small-cell lung cancer patients have evidence of cognitive dysfunction *prior* to PCI).[37,38] Two of the largest randomized trials of PCI did incorporate prospective neuropsychometric testing and both found a significant proportion of patients had cognitive dysfunction at baseline, but found no differences in cognitive performance between the randomization arms of PCI or no PCI.[39,40] However, higher doses of PCI are associated with worse cognitive outcomes; a randomized trial of different radiation schedules found greater rates of cognitive decline in patients treated with 36 Gy compared to patients treated with 25 Gy.[41] Finally, in patient populations with a low incidence of brain metastases, the risk–benefit ratio of PCI shifts and is less favorable. A phase 3 trial of PCI for patients with non–small-cell lung cancer found worse function on some measures of cognitive function in those patients treated with PCI compared to the observation arm. However, the 1-year rate of brain metastases was only 18% in the observation arm—much lower than would be expected with small-cell lung cancer, where 50 to 60% of patients develop brain metastases if they do not receive PCI.[42,43] Therefore, it should be recognized that PCI does have a risk, but in high-risk populations such as those with small-cell lung cancer, the risk of brain metastases and associated decline has historically intracranial lesions outweighs the cognitive risk of PCI.

More recently, there have also been prospective trials with extensive cognitive testing for patients with brain metastases treated with WBRT. One of these studies, an international phase 3 trial, prospectively evaluated cognitive function in 135 patients with brain metastases before and after WBRT and found tumor progression was the predominant cause of cognitive decline, with stable or improving cognitive function in long-term (i.e., 15-month) survivors.[14] A smaller German trial assessed 15 patients with brain metastases with a 90-minute battery of cognitive tests before and after WBRT (40 Gy in 2-Gy daily fractions) and found stable cognitive function in long-term survivors.[44] On the other hand, in a recent study comparing SRS alone to SRS and WBRT for 58 patients with up to three brain metastasis, 49% of patients in the WBRT group experienced declines in learning and memory at 4 months compared to only 23% in the SRS group.[45] Critics note the small size of the single-institutional study and a substantial difference in survival in the two groups, suggesting that the patients may not have been well-matched for prognostic factors.[46] Additionally, at 4 months, cognitive function after radiotherapy is at a nadir due to subacute or early-delayed effects of radiotherapy that gradually resolve over time.[47] Recognizing the limitations of this trial, it does suggest that for patients undergoing radiosurgery for a relatively small burden of intracranial disease followed closely with MRI, delay or avoidance of WBRT may be reasonable and may result in better cognitive function over time.

Radiotherapy techniques may impact the cognitive risk of WBRT. For example, large fraction sizes, as delivered in many historical studies, have been associated with dementia and cognitive decline in long-term survivors after WBRT; therefore, dose-fractionation schedules should be determined by the patient's estimated prognosis, with more protracted schedules used for patients with the possibility of long-term survival.[38] Another approach is to modify the WBRT to avoid sensitive regions of the brain. It has been suggested that hippocampal neural stem cell injury from WBRT may play a role in memory decline.[48] Intensity-modulated radiotherapy can be used to conformally avoid the hippocampal neural stem cell compartment during WBRT (HA-WBRT). The Radiation Therapy Oncology Group (RTOG) conducted a single-arm phase 2 study of HA-WBRT for 113 patients with brain metastases.[49] Only 4.5% of patients experienced progression within the hippocampal avoidance region consistent with prior retrospective studies.[50] The mean relative decline in verbal memory at 4 months was 7%, which was significantly lower in comparison to the historical control of 30% at 4 months (p = 0.0003).

In summary, although WBRT and PCI prospective trials suggest that, on the whole, any detrimental effects on cognitive function from radiotherapy seem to be balanced by the beneficial cognitive effects of improved tumor control in the brain, this must be balanced with selecting the proper patient population and weighing out the risk–benefit ratio. Modification of WBRT techniques such as hippocampal avoidance presents an intriguing treatment approach, although further study is needed.

Chemotherapy

The last decade has seen a surge in research on cognitive functioning following diagnosis and treatment of non-CNS cancer. An emerging body of data show that a subgroup of cancer patients is vulnerable to posttreatment (mostly but not exclusively chemotherapy related) cognitive decline, which has a significant impact on quality of life and daily function.[51–55] Chemotherapy is widely used in patients with non-CNS cancer and is known to be harmful to multiple organ systems. Traditionally, the CNS has been considered to be less vulnerable to the toxic effects of chemotherapy; however, acute and delayed neurologic complications are being identified with increasing frequency. Human and preclinical studies into the occurrence and determinants of cognitive decline in non-CNS cancer patients have led to a growing consensus that many chemotherapeutic agents for non-CNS cancer can interfere with various neurobiologic processes and can induce cognitive impairment.[56,57]

Incidence and Pattern of Cognitive Decline

Cognitive dysfunction has been particularly well studied in breast cancer patients undergoing adjuvant systemic therapy. The majority of the prospective studies in this patient population have indicated that 20% to 60% of patients have cognitive decline after chemotherapy compared to pretreatment cognitive performance.[54,55] In addition, several neuropsychological studies have demonstrated that cognitive impairment may already be present in cancer patients before the start of treatment.[58–61] Psychological distress, fatigue, or surgical factors (in case the assessment took place postsurgery) do not completely explain the possible link between cancer and cognitive dysfunction. Proposed causes for pretreatment cognitive dysfunction include not only the biology of cancer (inflammatory responses triggering neurotoxic cytokines) and common risk factors for the development of cancer and cognitive decline (e.g., poor DNA repair mechanisms linked to cancer and neurodegenerative disorders), but also methodologic considerations (patients participating in cognitive studies may not represent a random sample of individuals confronted with cancer).[62,63]

Patients show changes from pre- to posttreatment on a wide range of standardized neuropsychological tests. On the basis of studies with comprehensive neuropsychological examinations, a pattern of cognitive impairment can be described. Patients frequently demonstrate learning and memory deficits possibly secondary to impairment of encoding or initial processing of information and the retrieval of stored information, and diminished speed of information processing and reduced executive functioning. These changes in cognitive function have been associated with adverse impacts in cancer survivors' daily life (e.g., work-related disabilities).[64]

Trajectory of Cognitive Decline

The majority of prospective studies have demonstrated cognitive dysfunction up to 1 to 2 years postchemotherapy.[65] Cross-sectional studies with long-term cancer survivors show the presence of cognitive differences between chemotherapy-treated patients and noncancer controls up to 20 years posttherapy, suggesting the persistence of cognitive impairment over the years.[66,67] But, mature follow-up data from prospective studies are lacking to ascertain these changes from the baseline state and to determine the slope of cognitive changes over the course of years. This is relevant, because current insights into the mechanisms of chemotherapy-induced neurologic complications raise the possibility of chemotherapy-associated premature and accelerated cognitive aging.[68] Whether

patients treated with chemotherapy are at risk for developing new late-onset cognitive dysfunction or dementia is not known. Several retrospective studies have been published examining the risk of dementia in breast cancer survivors who completed cytotoxic treatment up to 15 years previously using data from the linked Surveillance, Epidemiology and End Results (SEER)–Medicare database. None of these studies showed clear evidence for the existence of such a relationship, but several important methodologic issues limit the validity and interpretation of the studies.[66]

Risk Factors

The finding that subgroups of patients experience posttreatment cognitive decline has led to the examination of patient- and disease/treatment-related risk factors for cognitive change.[69] There are some indications for a dose-response relationship based on a study that observed more patients with cognitive decline following high-dose chemotherapy compared to conventional dose chemotherapy and on a study showing a linear decline in cognitive performance after each cycle of chemotherapy.[70,71] Also, several studies have pointed to a higher frequency of cognitive dysfunction in breast cancer patients receiving both chemotherapy and endocrine therapy compared to breast cancer patients treated solely with chemotherapy or endocrine treatment.[55] Plausible patient-related risk factors such as age, intelligence quotient (IQ), baseline cognitive function, presence of comorbid conditions, and a host of other factors such as depression, anxiety, stress, fatigue, and treatment-induced menopause have not been identified as strong contributors to the impact of chemotherapy on cognitive function. A limited number of studies also looked at genetic factors (e.g., vulnerable alleles of genes such as APOE and COMT allele) as an explanation for why only a subgroup of patients seem to be more vulnerable for treatment-associated cognitive decline. In a study among lymphoma and breast cancer survivors, it was shown that survivors with at least one E4 allele scored lower on several cognitive tasks as compared to survivors who did not carry an E4 allele.[72] Another study found that breast cancer patients who had the COMT-Val allele and were treated with chemotherapy performed more poorly on several neuropsychological tests as compared to those with the COMT-Met allele.[73]

Based on experimental animal studies, other blood-based biomarkers that may mediate chemotherapy-associated cognitive decline are circulating proinflammatory cytokines. Up to now, studies in cancer patients show only weak correlations between interleukin 1B (IL-1B), IL-6, and tumor necrosis factor alpha (TNF-α) levels and cognitive impairment and suggests that the role of cytokines in postchemotherapy cognitive decline is not well understood and requires further evaluation.[63]

Neural Substrate

Structural, functional, and molecular imaging studies in non-CNS cancer patients are helping to clarify the neural basis and have started to shed light on the brain alterations that may be part of the mechanisms underlying the observed cognitive dysfunction.[74–77] White matter pathology has been observed within months and after 10 years posttreatment, both following high-dose and standard-dose regimens. Studies using voxel-based morphometry have reported volume reductions of white and grey matter 1 year and also at 20 years after the completion of chemotherapy.[78,79] A prospective study observed a decrease in focal gray matter volume 1 month after cessation of chemotherapy, which recovered in some but not in all regions at 1 year posttreatment.[80] The cerebral white matter seems particularly vulnerable to the effects of chemotherapy. Prospective studies investigating cerebral white matter integrity using diffusion tensor imaging reported lower fractional anisotropy (FA) in the genu of the corpus callosum, lower FA in the frontal and temporal white matter, and higher mean diffusivity in the frontal white matter of breast cancer patients who received standard-dose anthracycline-based regimens compared to breast cancer controls and healthy controls.[81] In cross-sectional studies conducted, on average, 10 and 20 years after the completion of chemotherapy, comparable indications for affected white matter tracts in breast cancer patients who received chemotherapy compared to subjects without a history of cancer or breast cancer patients who never received chemotherapy were observed.[78,79] Importantly, several studies have demonstrated a link between the abnormal microstructural properties in white matter regions and the cognitive impairments seen in breast cancer patients treated with chemotherapeutic agents.[81] The observed changes in diffusion tensor imaging (DTI) parameters may be related to demyelination of white matter axons or axonal injury after chemotherapy. Functional MRI (fMRI) studies have demonstrated postchemotherapy changes in brain activation and in resting brain connectivity pattern. The prospective fMRI studies show a complex picture with both hyper- and hypoactivation patterns and inconsistent findings with regard to accompanying changes in fMRI task performance.[76]

Underlying Mechanisms

A large number of studies in rodent models have extended our understanding of the cell biology and molecular basis underlying chemotherapy-associated CNS toxicity. Moreover, patterns of behavioral performance in animals seem to correspond to a significant extent with cognitive patterns in patients, supporting the important role for preclinical research in understanding the cognitive effects of cancer treatments in humans. Using detailed cell lineage–based approaches, it has been shown that neural progenitor cells, which are the direct ancestors of all differentiated cell types in the CNS, and mature postmitotic oligodendrocytes are the most vulnerable cell populations to the effects of multiple chemotherapeutic agents.[48,56,57,82,83] It has been hypothesized that long-term cognitive decline in cancer survivors is the result of a combination of decreased proliferation of neural progenitor cells, impaired hippocampal neurogenesis, and damage to oligodendroglial cells and white matter tracts.

As many different chemotherapeutic agents seems to have similar effects on the CNS, studies are also exploring common indirect mechanisms as etiologic factors of chemotherapy-associated neurotoxicity, such as pro-oxidative effects, toxic neurotranmitters/monoamine release, disruption of blood vessel density and supply, and inflammation.[57] Unraveling the precise mechanisms underlying chemotherapy-related cognitive side effects is necessary to enable the identification of novel treatment strategies. Several animal studies have shown promising interventions such as the prevention of oxidative stress associated with chemotherapy using as N-acetyl cysteine or melatonin, strategies that stimulate neurogenesis using insulin-like growth factor 1 or fluoxetine, and treatments with glutamate receptor antagonists such as dextromethorphan, which ameliorate negative chemotherapy-induced cognitive outcomes.[84–87]

TREATMENT OF COGNITIVE DYSFUNCTION

If cognitive impairment is identified in a patient, it is essential to evaluate for reversible causes such as depression, medications (e.g., changing or, if possible, discontinuing antiepileptics), or endocrine disturbances (i.e., hypothyroidism). For patients with a brain tumor, the most common reversible cause of cognitive dysfunction is tumor progression because a number of studies have shown effective treatment of the tumor can result in improvement in cognitive function.[88]

There are few proven therapies for cognitive dysfunction in patients with a brain tumor, although there are a number of small trials with interesting findings.[89] Methylphenidate is a psychostimulant that has generated clinical and research interest for some time, and several small studies have suggested a benefit for patients with psychomotor slowing, a decline in executive functioning, or

general apathy.[90] Unfortunately, a phase 3, placebo-controlled trial did not confirm a benefit in cognitive function or quality of life in patients receiving radiotherapy for brain tumors.[91,92] Similarly a phase 3 trial of donepezil, an acetyl cholinesterase inhibitor used in the treatment of symptoms of Alzheimer's disease, was no better than placebo at improving overall cognitive function in brain tumor survivors.[93] However, on a subgroup analysis, among patients with more cognitive problems at baseline, there was a significant benefit in verbal memory for patients on donepezil.

Patients with a brain tumor actually represent an ideal population for research in neuroprotection because, unlike stroke patients, patients with a brain tumor typically have *planned* injurious events (i.e., surgery, chemotherapy, radiotherapy) to their brain, providing a golden opportunity for prophylactic treatment. A phase 3 trial of 554 adult patients with brain metastases evaluated the potential neuroprotective properties of memantine, an N-methyl-D-aspartate (NMDA) receptor antagonist that has been shown to be effective and well tolerated in vascular dementia patients.[94] All patients received WBRT and were randomized to either placebo or memantine at the start of radiotherapy and were treated for a total of 24 weeks. Memantine was well tolerated and had a toxicity profile very similar to placebo. Although there was less decline in the primary endpoint of delayed recall at 24 weeks, this lacked statistical significance (p = 0.059), possibly due to significant patient loss over time due to disease progression and death. The memantine arm had significantly longer time to cognitive decline (p = 0.01), and the probability of cognitive function failure at 24 weeks was 53.8% in the memantine arm and 64.9% in the placebo arm. Superior results were also seen in the memantine arm for specific tests of executive function, processing speed, and memory.

Another treatment option is brain injury rehabilitation, using methods developed for traumatic brain injury survivors. Gehring et al.[95] conducted a phase 3 trial of 140 patients with adult brain tumors. Patients were randomly assigned to an intervention group or to a waiting list control group.[95] The intervention involved six weekly 2-hour sessions, self-study for reinforcement, and at 3 months, a telephone-based booster session. The sessions incorporated both computer-based attention retraining and compensatory skills training of attention, memory, and executive functioning. At the 6-month follow-up, the intervention group performed significantly better with attention and verbal memory than the control group and reported less mental fatigue.

Pharmacologic interventions to prevent or intervene against cognitive symptoms in non-CNS cancer patients are still in an early stage of development. Some agents are promising, but rigorous testing with appropriate study designs and sufficient sample sizes necessary to translate and implement these agents in daily practice are either absent or have generated disappointing results. For example, several studies found positive effects of erythropoietin (EPO) on cognitive functioning during or shortly after chemotherapy, but randomized controlled studies at longer follow-ups failed to show positive effects of EPO on cognition. Psychostimulants like methylphenidate and modafinil have been tested in several studies, but the effectiveness of methylphenidate to treat cancer therapy–associated cognitive dysfunction is, at present, not established. Initial small studies with modafinil are slightly more hopeful, but larger studies with longer follow-ups are needed before conclusions about effectiveness can be drawn. Another example of an agent that received attention following initial interesting preclinical findings but for which convincing data from phase 3 studies on the efficacy are lacking is donepezil.[89,96]

Nonpharmacologic interventions like mindfulness-based stress reduction and exercise interventions are gaining increasing attention as potential effective interventions for cancer- and cancer-treatment related cognitive effects, and several large trials are underway that should clarify the value of these behavioral interventions. Multiple behavioral-based studies have proven successful in improving daily life functioning using intact cognitive abilities and strategies together with psychoeducation.[97–101] Finally, interventions focusing on mental stimulation, collectively known as brain training, are frequently accessed by cancer survivors, but limited evidence supports their efficacy,[102] and recent reviews of the current brain training literature indicate that most programs still fail to display fundamental transfer (i.e., generalization of trained skills).[103]

CONCLUSION

Just as recent technologic advances in neurosurgery and radiotherapy have enabled physicians to perform surgery and administer radiation more safely than in prior eras, it is expected that future technologic advances will further improve the therapeutic ratio. Current radiation and chemotherapy doses and regimens are based on populations of patients and not the individual sensitivity of the patient or the tumor. As more research is conducted in this arena, it is likely that, in the future, treatments will be individualized for each unique patient and tumor.

Recent cellular, molecular, and biochemical work has also been instrumental in elucidating the mechanism of the CNS response to injury, and this should lead to the rational development of selective neuroprotective and therapeutic agents. In the meantime, larger prospective, longitudinal studies with well-validated quality of life instruments and neuropsychological batteries are needed to determine the impact of (especially novel) treatment regimens on cognitive function. And, finally, because lack of tumor control remains the predominant cause of cognitive dysfunction and deterioration in brain tumors, it is imperative that the neuro-oncology community continues to focus their scientific endeavors on the ultimate goal of durable tumor control.

SELECTED REFERENCES

The full reference list can be accessed at lwwhealthlibrary.com/oncology.

13. Meyers CA, Smith JA, Bezjak A, et al. Neurocognitive function and progression in patients with brain metastases treated with whole-brain radiation and motexafin gadolinium: results of a randomized phase III trial. *J Clin Oncol.* 2004;22:157–165.

14. Li J, Bentzen SM, Renschler M, et al. Regression after whole-brain radiation therapy for brain metastases correlates with survival and improved neurocognitive function. *J Clin Oncol* 2007;25:1260–1266.

15. Torres IJ, Mundt AJ, Sweeney PJ, et al. A longitudinal neuropsychological study of partial brain radiation in adults with brain tumors. *Neurology* 2003;60:1113–1118.

16. Brown PD, Jensen AW, Felten SJ, et al. Detrimental effects of tumor progression on cognitive function of patients with high-grade glioma. *J Clin Oncol* 2006;24:5427–5433.

17. Meyers CA, Hess KR, Yung WK, et al. Cognitive function as a predictor of survival in patients with recurrent malignant glioma. *J Clin Oncol* 2000;18:646–650.

18. Armstrong TS, Wefel JS, Wang M, et al. Net clinical benefit analysis of radiation therapy oncology group 0525: a phase III trial comparing conventional adjuvant temozolomide with dose-intensive temozolomide in patients with newly diagnosed glioblastoma. *J Clin Oncol* 2013;31:4076–4084.

25. Dietrich J, Monje M, Wefel J, et al. Clinical patterns and biological correlates of cognitive dysfunction associated with cancer therapy. *Oncologist* 2008;13:1285–1295.

32. Laack NN, Brown PD, Ivnik RJ, et al. Cognitive function after radiotherapy for supratentorial low-grade glioma: a North Central Cancer Treatment Group prospective study. *Int J Radiat Oncol Biol Phys* 2005;63:1175–1183.

33. Steinvorth S, Welzel G, Fuss M, et al. Neuropsychological outcome after fractionated stereotactic radiotherapy (FSRT) for base of skull meningiomas: a prospective 1-year follow-up. *Radiother Oncol* 2003;69:177–182.

34. Vigliani MC, Sichez N, Poisson M, et al. A prospective study of cognitive functions following conventional radiotherapy for supratentorial gliomas in young adults: 4-year results. *Int J Radiat Oncol Biol Phys* 1996;35:527–533.

35. Brown PD, Buckner JC, Uhm JH, et al. The neurocognitive effects of radiation in adult low-grade glioma patients. *Neurooncology* 2003;5:161–167.

36. Steinvorth S, Wenz F, Wildermuth S, et al. Cognitive function in patients with cerebral arteriovenous malformations after radiosurgery: prospective long-term follow-up. *Int J Radiat Oncol Biol Phys* 2002;54:1430–1437.

37. Komaki R, Meyers CA, Shin DM, et al. Evaluation of cognitive function in patients with limited small cell lung cancer prior to and shortly following prophylactic cranial irradiation. *Int J Radiat Oncol Biol Phys* 1995;33:179–182.

38. Laack NN, Brown PD. Cognitive sequelae of brain radiation in adults. *Semin Oncol* 2004;31:702–713.

39. Arriagada R, Le Chevalier T, Borie F, et al. Prophylactic cranial irradiation for patients with small-cell lung cancer in complete remission. *J Natl Cancer Inst* 1995;87:183–190.

40. Gregor A, Cull A, Stephens RJ, et al. Prophylactic cranial irradiation is indicated following complete response to induction therapy in small cell lung cancer: results of a multicentre randomised trial. United Kingdom Coordinating Committee for Cancer Research (UKCCCR) and the European Organization for Research and Treatment of Cancer (EORTC). *Eur J Cancer* 1997;33:1752–1758.

41. Wolfson AH, Bae K, Komaki R, et al. Primary analysis of a phase II randomized trial Radiation Therapy Oncology Group (RTOG) 0212: impact of different total doses and schedules of prophylactic cranial irradiation on chronic neurotoxicity and quality of life for patients with limited-disease small-cell lung cancer. *Int J Radiat Oncol Biol Phys* 2011;81:77–84.

42. Gore EM, Bae K, Wong SJ, et al. Phase III comparison of prophylactic cranial irradiation versus observation in patients with locally advanced non-small-cell lung cancer: primary analysis of radiation therapy oncology group study RTOG 0214. *J Clin Oncol* 2011;29:272–278.

43. Sun A, Bae K, Gore EM, et al. Phase III trial of prophylactic cranial irradiation compared with observation in patients with locally advanced non-small-cell lung cancer: neurocognitive and quality-of-life analysis. *J Clin Oncol* 2011;29:279–286.

45. Chang EL, Wefel JS, Hess KR, et al. Neurocognition in patients with brain metastases treated with radiosurgery or radiosurgery plus whole-brain irradiation: a randomised controlled trial. *Lancet Oncol* 2009;10:1037–1044.

49. Gondi V, Mehta MP, Pugh S, et al. Memory preservation with conformal avoidance of the hippocampus during whole-brain radiotherapy for patients with brain metastases: Primary endpoint results of RTOG 0933. *Int J Radiat Oncol Biol Phys* 2013;87:1186.

52. Jansen CE, Miaskowski C, Dodd M, et al. A metaanalysis of studies of the effects of cancer chemotherapy on various domains of cognitive function. *Cancer* 2005;104:2222–2233.

54. Ahles TA, Root JC, Ryan EL. Cancer- and cancer treatment-associated cognitive change: an update on the state of the science. *J Clin Oncol* 2012;30:3675–3686.

55. Wefel JS, Schagen SB. Chemotherapy-related cognitive dysfunction. *Curr Neurol Neurosci Rep* 2012;12:267–275.

57. Seigers R, Schagen SB, Van Tellingen O, et al. Chemotherapy-related cognitive dysfunction: current animal studies and future directions. *Brain Imaging Behav* 2013;7:453–459.

59. Wefel JS, Lenzi R, Theriault RL, et al. The cognitive sequelae of standard-dose adjuvant chemotherapy in women with breast carcinoma: results of a prospective, randomized, longitudinal trial. *Cancer* 2004;100:2292–2299.

66. Koppelmans V, Breteler MM, Boogerd W, et al. Late effects of adjuvant chemotherapy for adult onset non-CNS cancer; cognitive impairment, brain structure and risk of dementia. *Crit Rev Oncol Hematol* 2013;88:87–101.

67. Koppelmans V, Breteler MM, Boogerd W, et al. Neuropsychological performance in survivors of breast cancer more than 20 years after adjuvant chemotherapy. *J Clin Oncol* 2012;30:1080–1086.

70. van Dam FS, Schagen SB, Muller MJ, et al. Impairment of cognitive function in women receiving adjuvant treatment for high-risk breast cancer: high-dose versus standard-dose chemotherapy. *J Natl Cancer Inst.* 1998;90:210–218.

81. Deprez S, Amant F, Smeets A, et al. Longitudinal assessment of chemotherapy-induced structural changes in cerebral white matter and its correlation with impaired cognitive functioning. *J Clin Oncol* 2012;30:274–281.

88. Brown PD, Buckner JC, O'Fallon JR, et al. Effects of radiotherapy on cognitive function in patients with low-grade glioma measured by the Folstein mini-mental state examination. *J Clin Oncol* 2003;21:2519–2524.

90. Khuntia D, Brown P, Li J, et al. Whole-brain radiotherapy in the management of brain metastasis. *J Clin Oncol* 2006;24:1295–1304.

94. Brown PD, Pugh S, Laack NN, et al. Memantine for the prevention of cognitive dysfunction in patients receiving whole-brain radiotherapy: a randomized, double-blind, placebo-controlled trial. *Neuro Oncol* 2013;15:1429–1437.

95. Gehring K, Sitskoorn MM, Gundy CM, et al. Cognitive rehabilitation in patients with gliomas: a randomized, controlled trial. *J Clin Oncol* 2009;27:3712–3722.

98. Ferguson RJ, McDonald BC, Rocque MA, et al. Development of CBT for chemotherapy-related cognitive change: results of a waitlist control trial. *Psychooncology* 2012;21:176–186.

PRACTICE OF ONCOLOGY

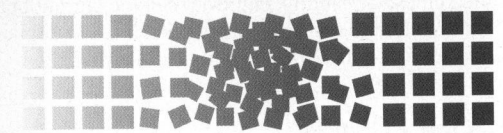

145 Cancer Survivorship

Wendy Landier, Craig C. Earle, Smita Bhatia, Melissa M. Hudson,
Kevin C. Oeffinger, Patricia A. Ganz, and Louis S. Constine

INTRODUCTION

Living beyond cancer into long-term survivorship is now a reality for most children and many adults who are diagnosed with cancer today. However, as the numbers of long-term cancer survivors continue to increase, oncologists and other clinicians must understand and address the complex interplay of their biologic, psychological, and socioeconomic needs. Biologic sequelae disrupt organ function and cause tissue-specific and systemic comorbidities, which can compromise quality of life (e.g., fatigue, infertility) or cause death (e.g., cardiovascular disease, second malignancies). Psychological sequelae, including depression and distress from fear of cancer recurrence, and failure to work effectively and to socially engage with others, are clear detriments to life satisfaction. Socioeconomic consequences such as insufficient income and high costs of medical care and medical bankruptcies may exacerbate the difficulties associated with daily living.

The multifaceted needs of survivors demand a spectrum of actions from clinicians in order to provide them with quality survival. It is necessary that clinicians diagnose and treat the chronic physical effects of cancer and its therapy, promote adaptive and rehabilitative lifestyle changes, and campaign for fair socioeconomic treatment by society. The process begins with communication between the clinician and patient regarding details of the treatment, potential sequelae in all the various domains, and guidance for ongoing care. Table 145.1 outlines the essential components of survivorship care as discerned by the Committee on Cancer Survivorship from the Institute of Medicine (IOM), and Table 145.2 states their 10 recommendations.[1] In this seminal report, specific goals were defined to ensure optimal outcomes for cancer survivors as follows:

- Raise awareness of the medical and psychosocial problems faced by cancer survivors and establish cancer survivorship as a distinct phase of the cancer trajectory during which specific clinical interventions are needed.
- Define quality health care for cancer survivors and identify strategies to achieve it.
- Improve quality of life through policies to ensure cancer survivors' access to psychosocial services, fair employment practices, and health insurance.

There are many unanswered questions about surveillance strategies, models of health-care delivery, research strategies, and education of both patients and health-care providers. This chapter is designed to serve as an introduction to understanding the scope of the survivorship problem.

DEFINITION OF SURVIVORSHIP AND SCOPE OF THE PROBLEM

Cancer survivorship is an evolving concept with multiple definitions. Prior to the recent evolution of curative cancer therapy, *cancer survivors* were defined as family members left behind after a loved one had succumbed to the disease.[2] In the latter half of the 20th century, as survival rates increased, the dramatic impact of life-saving but potentially toxic therapies began to emerge. Izsak and Medalie[3] are credited with first describing the "costs" of cancer survivorship: "Survival rates . . . do not relate to how the patient survives, at what cost to his physical functioning, how he adapted to his condition from a psychological point of view, and how he is fulfilling his roles in his family, at work, among friends, and in the wider society." Three decades ago, Fitzhugh Mullan,[4] a young physician and cancer survivor, challenged the binary concept of illness versus cure and suggested that survivorship was a process with predictable stages, ranging from the acute diagnosis and treatment phase, through the post-therapy phase of watchful waiting, and finally to the phase of permanent survival, when the focus shifts from concerns about risk of recurrence to those impacting long-term quality of survival. Soon after, the National Coalition for Cancer Survivorship (NCCS) was founded, raising awareness of the importance of the survivorship experience and setting the stage for recognition of survivorship as a distinct phase along the cancer control continuum.[5] In the mid 1990s, the National Cancer Institute established the Office of Cancer Survivorship, which was charged with directing and supporting research, training, and education regarding issues relating to cancer survivorship. Over the past decade, many influential groups, including the IOM,[1] the President's Cancer Panel,[6] and the American Society of Clinical Oncology (ASCO),[7] have released reports highlighting issues relating to cancer survivorship. For the purposes of this chapter, the IOM's definition of cancer survivorship will be used, which focuses on the phases of cancer care following the completion of primary treatment and lasting until cancer recurrence or the end of life.[1]

The number of cancer survivors has increased more than threefold since 1975 as a result of improvements in early detection and therapeutic successes (Fig. 145.1).[8] There are currently nearly 14 million cancer survivors in the United States[8] and more than 25 million worldwide.[9] The 5-year relative survival rate has also continued to increase steadily, and has now reached 68% for adults and 83% for children.[10] The number of cancer survivors is expected to increase in the United States by 31% to almost 18 million over the next decade,[8] because of the general population growth and the increasing proportion of older adults in the population for whom cancer prevalence rates are the highest. More than 8 million cancer survivors in the United States are age 65 or older, representing 59% of all cancer survivors.[11] Among survivors, the most common diagnoses are breast cancer (22%) and prostate cancer (20%); survivors of colorectal cancer, hematologic malignancies, gynecologic, urinary, melanoma, lung, and other cancers each represent less than 10% of the population of cancer survivors (Fig. 145.2).[11] Dramatic improvements in childhood cancer survival has resulted in a growing population that now exceeds 379,000 in the United States alone,[12] and multiple studies regarding the impact of cancer therapy on health-related outcomes in this population have been published.[13] In a retrospective cohort of 10,397 childhood cancer survivors diagnosed between 1970 and 1986 (the Childhood Cancer Survivor Study), Oeffinger et al.[14] reported that 62.3% experienced

TABLE 145.1

Essential Components of Survivorship Care

1. **Education** of the cancer survivor, family, health-care providers
   - A plan for care based on the treatment administered and future health risks
   - Promotion of healthy lifestyles
   - Information to assist health-care providers in understanding future risks and to foster an effective interaction with the oncology team
2. **Surveillance** for cancer spread, recurrence, or second cancers and for long-term adverse physical, psychosocial, socioeconomic effects
3. **Intervention** to prevent or treat consequences of cancer or its therapy
4. **Communication** between specialists and primary care providers to ensure that the survivor's health needs are met and detailed records are kept about treatment history
5. **Research** focused on understanding, preventing, and treating adverse consequences of cancer or its therapy
6. **Patient advocacy** to address problems related to employment, insurance, and disability

Modified from Hewitt M, Greenfield S, Stovall E. *From Cancer Patient to Cancer Survivor: Lost in Transition.* Washington, D.C.: National Academies Press; 2006.

at least one treatment-related late effect, 37.6% developed multiple late effects, and 27.5% developed a late effect that was severe or life-threatening. The impact of cancer therapy on health-related outcomes in the rapidly growing population of adult cancer survivors is largely unknown, but the need for ongoing follow-up care and late effects surveillance for all cancer survivors is clear.[1]

GOALS OF SURVIVORSHIP HEALTH CARE

Identifying Late Effects of Cancer Therapy

The modern era of cancer therapy is predicated on the safe intensification of radiation, chemotherapy, and biologic therapies. Malignancies resistant to therapy have demanded an aggressive treatment approach that often resides on the edge of normal tissue tolerance, or even exceeds tolerance to some "acceptable" degree. The potential to ameliorate or prevent such normal tissue damage, or to manage and rehabilitate affected patients, requires an understanding of these persistent long-term or late-onset chronic effects. Because late effects can manifest months or years after the cessation of treatment, therapeutic decisions intended to obviate such effects can be based only on the probability, not the certainty, that such effects will develop.

Determining the frequency and pathogenesis of late effects is difficult for several reasons: (1) Patients must survive long enough for tissue injury to develop, (2) the number of patients both affected and unaffected by therapy must be known, and (3) the latent period to the manifestation of damage compromises discernment of the responsible component of multimodality therapy. Further complicating our understanding of organ tolerance to therapy is that cancer and host factors interact with therapy in the causation of late effects. Cancer factors include direct tissue effects (e.g., from organ invasion such as the lung), systemic effects of cancer-induced organ damage or loss (e.g., hepatic dysfunction or loss of a kidney), and indirect mechanical effects (e.g., renal or airway obstruction). Host factors include genetic (e.g., ataxia-telangiectasia) and comorbid (e.g., vascular disease, diabetes) conditions, the developmental age at treatment, and underlying structural abnormalities (e.g., cardiac). The previously mentioned report by Oeffinger et al.[14] documents the high frequency of chronic health conditions in adult survivors of childhood cancer, many of which

TABLE 145.2

Ten Recommendations for Cancer Survivorship Care

1. Health-care providers, patient advocates, and other stakeholders should work to raise awareness of the needs of cancer survivors, establish cancer survivorship as a distinct phase of cancer care, and act to ensure the delivery of appropriate survivorship care.
2. Patients completing primary treatment should be provided with a comprehensive care summary and a follow-up plan that is clearly and effectively explained. This Survivorship Care Plan should be written by the principal provider(s) who coordinated the oncology treatment. This service should be reimbursed by third-party payors of health care.
3. Health-care providers should use systematically developed evidence-based clinical practice guidelines, assessment tools, and screening instruments to help identify and manage the late effects of cancer and its treatment. Existing guidelines should be refined, and new evidence-based guidelines should be developed through public and private sector efforts.
4. Quality of survivorship care measures should be developed through public/private partnerships and quality assurance programs implemented by health systems to monitor and improve the care that all survivors receive.
5. The Centers for Medicare and Medicaid Services (CMS), the National Cancer Institute (NCI), the Agency for Healthcare Research and Quality (AHRQ), the Department of Veterans Affairs (VA), and other qualified organizations should support demonstration programs to test models of coordinated, interdisciplinary survivorship care in diverse communities and across systems of care.
6. Congress should support the Centers for Disease Control and Prevention (CDC), other collaborating institutions, and states in developing comprehensive cancer control plans that include the consideration of survivorship care and promoting the implementation, evaluation, and refinement of existing state cancer control plans.
7. The NCI, professional associations, and voluntary organizations should expand and coordinate their efforts to provide educational opportunities to health-care providers to equip them to address the health care and quality of life issues facing cancer survivors.
8. Employers, legal advocates, health-care providers, sponsors of support services, and government agencies should act to eliminate discrimination and minimize adverse effects of cancer on employment while supporting cancer survivors with short-term and long-term limitations in their ability to work.
9. Federal and state policy makers should act to ensure that all cancer survivors have access to adequate and affordable health insurance. Insurers and payors of health care should recognize survivorship care as an essential part of cancer care and should design benefits, payment policies, and reimbursement mechanisms to facilitate coverage for evidence-based aspects of care.
10. The NCI, CDC, AHRQ, CMS, VA, private voluntary organizations such as the American Cancer Society (ACS), and private health insurers and plans should increase their support of survivorship research and expand mechanisms for its conduct. New research initiatives focused on cancer patient follow-up are urgently needed to guide effective survivorship care.

Modified from Hewitt M, Greenfield S, Stovall E. *From Cancer Patient to Cancer Survivor: Lost in Transition.* Washington, D.C.: National Academies Press; 2006.

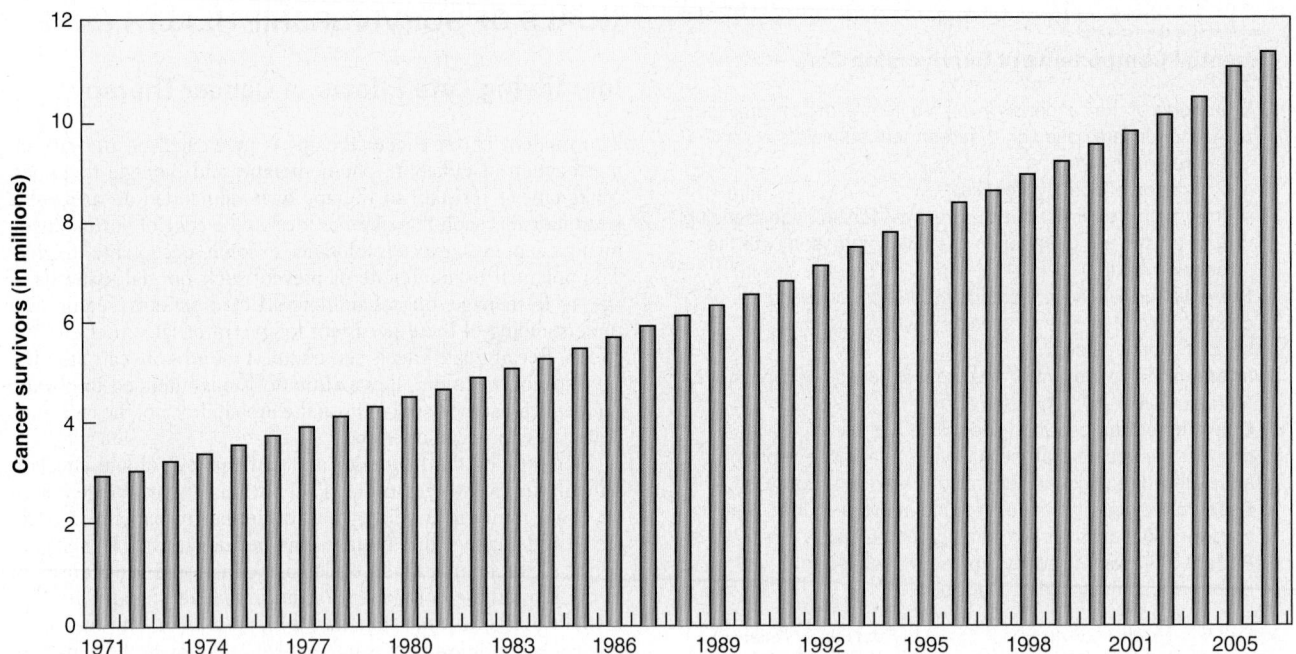

Figure 145.1 Estimated number of cancer survivors in the United States over time as of January 1, 2012. (Data from http://cancercontrol.cancer.gov/ocs/prevalence/prevalence.html#survivor, based on modeling provided by Angela Mariotto, PhD as described in Mariotto AB, Yabroff KR, Shao Y, et al. Projections of the cost of cancer care in the United States: 2010-2020. *J Natl Cancer Inst* 2011;103:117–128. Accessed November 5, 2013.)

are severe or life-threatening. At 30 years, almost three-fourths of survivors had a chronic health condition, more than 40% had a serious health problem, and one-third had multiple conditions. Additionally, Yeh et al.[15] have recently developed a model based on Childhood Cancer Survivor Study data to estimate cumulative excess mortality in a simulated cohort of 5-year survivors of childhood cancer. These investigators predict a substantial decrement in life expectancy of 10.4 years (range: 4 to 17.8 years) for the childhood cancer survivors, compared with the general population.[15,16] Moreover, the model estimates that the reduction in life expectancy is up to 28%, and that approximately one in four survivors will die of either a late recurrence or late effects related to secondary cancer and cardiopulmonary conditions. These data underscore the importance of understanding the toxic effects of our therapy. Several chapters in this text provide detailed information on the long-term physical effects of cancer therapy for each organ system.

Surveillance/Guidelines for Late Effects

Treatment-related sequelae can manifest at any time during or after therapy, and may be clinically silent at times when a diagnosis might lead to effective interventions. Some chronic or late effects can evolve during normal development or aging. Healthcare providers need to anticipate these effects as well as evaluate those that are overt in order to optimize measures that can enhance quality of life. The need for standardized guidelines to direct follow-up care after cancer treatment and surveillance for late effects of therapy has been recognized as an important component of cancer care for over a decade.[1,5,17,18] However, the development of evidence-based long-term follow-up guidelines has proven to be a challenging endeavor. The Children's Oncology Group (COG) developed the *Children's Oncology Group Long-term Follow-up Guidelines for Survivors of Childhood, Adolescent, and Young Adult Cancers*, a set of risk-based, exposure-related screening recommendations to guide the long-term follow-up care of pediatric cancer survivors with the goals of improving quality of life and decreasing complication-related health-care costs.[19]

The COG guidelines (available at www.survivorshipguidelines.org)[20] exemplify a hybrid of evidence-based and consensus-driven approaches to guideline development. The strength of the evidence linking specific therapeutic exposures with adverse outcomes is considered for the inclusion of a therapeutic agent or modality. Screening recommendations in these guidelines were initially determined by consensus from a panel of experts in the late effects of pediatric cancer treatment; evidence is now emerging

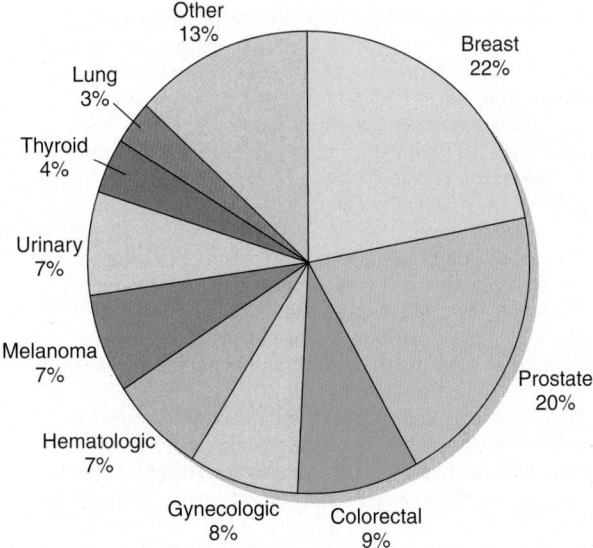

Figure 145.2 Estimated proportion of cancer survivors in the United States by site as of January 1, 2012. (Data from http://cancercontrol.cancer.gov/ocs/prevalence/prevalence.html#survivor, based on modeling provided by Angela Mariotto, PhD as described in Mariotto AB, Yabroff KR, Shao Y, et al. Projections of the cost of cancer care in the United States: 2010-2020. *J Natl Cancer Inst* 2011;103:117–128. Accessed November 5, 2013.)

regarding the yield and utility of these recommendations, and further guideline refinement is in process.[21,22] The screening recommendations outlined in the COG guidelines are organized by therapeutic exposure and are appropriate for asymptomatic survivors presenting for routine exposure-based medical follow-up 2 or more years following the completion of therapy for a pediatric malignancy, and can be customized for individual patients based on age, gender, and treatment history. Multidisciplinary task forces continue to monitor the literature to ensure that guideline recommendations reflect emerging knowledge about late effects; version 1.0 of the COG guidelines was published in 2003, and version 4.0 was released in 2014.

Guidelines for follow-up of pediatric cancer survivors have also been developed by the Scottish Intercollegiate Guidelines Network (SIGN),[23] the United Kingdom Children's Cancer and Leukemia Group (CCLG),[24] and the Dutch Childhood Oncology Group (DCOG).[25] An international effort is currently underway to harmonize these guidelines.[26] Joint European–American guidelines for follow-up after hematopoietic cell transplantation were released in 2006[27,28] and updated in 2012.[29–31]

The lack of standardized guidelines to direct the care of adult cancer survivors with regard to health promotion and the early detection of treatment-related complications is an ongoing focus of concern, particularly given the IOM's recommendation for the development of such guidelines in their 2006 report.[1] In 2011, ASCO formed a Cancer Survivorship Committee, which has recently partnered with ASCO's Clinical Practice Guidelines Committee to develop consensus-based guidance documents, informed by evidence, to address long-term effects in cancer survivors.[7] Two ASCO guidance documents have now been released.[32,33]

Intervention to Prevent Potential Late Effects

In the past decade, a growing number of studies have been designed and conducted with the intent of treating health conditions that are identified during or after the completion of therapy as well as preventing later occurring conditions. Randomized clinical trials have tested the effectiveness of a wide range of interventions, including ones aimed at increasing levels of physical activity, promoting healthy diets and smoking cessation, and reducing adverse psychosocial outcomes.

To illustrate the evolution of survivor-focused intervention studies, one can look at studies of breast cancer survivors. In the general population, it has been well documented that physical inactivity and obesity are associated with an increased risk of all-cause mortality, several cancers, cardiovascular disease, insulin resistance, hypertension, osteoporosis, and diminished quality of life. Women with pre- or postmenopausal breast cancer who are obese and physically inactive usually experience lower 5-year survival rates, increased rates of recurrence, and increased all-cause and cancer-related mortalities. Several randomized clinical trials conducted in breast cancer survivors have demonstrated that increasing levels of physical activity are associated with improved cardiorespiratory fitness, weight management, decreased fatigue, and quality of life.[34] A prospective trial now in progress is designed to assess the feasibility of a cognitive–behavioral intervention on achieving sustained weight loss in overweight/obese women with early stage breast cancer and to examine the impact of weight loss on comorbidities and quality of life.[35] Similar interventions designed to promote physical activity and weight management are also being tested in other populations of cancer survivors.[36,37]

Although many interventions have been found to be effective at reducing psychosocial morbidities such as depression and anxiety in patients undergoing therapy for cancer, Stanton[38] notes that relatively few studies have focused on long-term survivors. Kazak et al.,[39] Pai and Kazak,[40] and Alderfer et al.[41] have published an elegant series of studies describing post-traumatic stress symptoms

experienced by childhood and adolescent cancer survivors and testing interventions to reduce these symptoms.

With this experience in survivor intervention studies, a growing survivor-based data set and increased sophistication in study design, it is becoming more feasible to compare outcomes across trials. Important challenges remain, including the ability to test specific interventions in survivor populations that are relatively small in number, and to recruit and retain long-term survivors in these studies.[42] Several potentially helpful interventions have yet to be studied, such as the use of statins to reduce the progression of radiation-associated atherosclerosis or chemoprevention to reduce the incidence of breast cancer in women who were treated with chest radiation.

Promotion of Adjustment and Healthy Lifestyles

The importance of providing appropriate support to facilitate positive psychosocial adjustment following treatment for cancer has been a central facet of the survivorship movement since its inception.[18] The rates of depression and other types of psychosocial distress in cancer survivors (such as anxiety, anger, and feelings of isolation) have been found to exceed those in the general population, and unmet psychosocial needs often persist following the completion of cancer treatment.[38] The oncology health-care provider should play a key role in screening for psychosocial distress in cancer survivors, and appropriate referrals to psychosocial professionals or other resources should be provided. Numerous print and online materials are available to address patient concerns, including: *Facing Forward: Life after Cancer Treatment*, from the National Cancer Institute (www.cancer.gov/cancertopics/life-after-treatment.pdf); the Cancer Survivor Toolbox, from the NCCS (www.canceradvocacy .org/resources/cancer-survival-toolbox/); and online resources from the Office of Cancer Survivorship (http://cancercontrol.cancer.gov/ ocs/) and the American Cancer Society's (ACS) Cancer Survivors Network (http://csn.cancer.org/).

The potential for positive modification of lifestyle behaviors following a cancer diagnosis and treatment in adulthood has been recognized as a window of opportunity during which cancer survivors may be open to making significant changes in their health habits oriented toward decreasing the likelihood of cancer recurrence and enhancing their overall health status.[43] In a study of more than 1.2 million records from the Surveillance, Epidemiology, and End Results Program, cancer-specific death rates were found to underestimate the mortality associated with a cancer diagnosis; death rates from non–cancer-related causes were noted to be higher among persons with a history of cancer than among the general population.[44] Taking advantage of the *teachable moment*, which occurs when patients transit from active cancer therapy to follow-up care, is an important role for oncology health-care professionals who are poised to serve as powerful catalysts in promoting behavioral change and modifying adverse health risks.[45] Although a substantial proportion of cancer survivors may be willing to initiate positive lifestyle changes at this juncture, there are known groups of survivors who are less likely to adopt healthy lifestyle changes, including males, those with lower educational levels, and those who live in urban areas.[46] Additional support and intervention may be required in order to achieve positive lifestyle modification in these subgroups.

Survivors of childhood cancer often lack a distinct teachable moment for lifestyle modification such as that experienced by survivors of adult-onset cancers, given the wide range of ages and developmental stages of patients treated for pediatric malignancies. They are known to be at increased risk for multiple chronic health conditions such as obesity and cardiovascular disease.[14] Several suboptimal health behaviors, including smoking and unhealthful dietary and exercise habits, have been observed in subsets of these survivors.[46] The importance of health promotion in this population should be emphasized, and attention should be given to providing targeted health counseling appropriate to each patient's cancer history, therapeutic exposures, age, gender, and developmental stage.

CARE PLANS

Providing high-quality care for cancer survivors presents several challenges. Cancer care is often fragmented among many different specialists, and traditionally, there has been inadequate communication between physicians about the diagnosis and treatments a patient received. Primary care providers (PCP) often have limited contact with patients undergoing active cancer treatment and lack details regarding their experience at its completion. Furthermore, there is limited information about the types and severity of potential long-term and late effects from cancer treatments, and a paucity of guidelines for surveillance for both recurrence and late effects. Most nononcology physicians will only have a handful of cancer survivors in their practice, and each survivor will likely have had a different disease and exposures. Consequently, it is not reasonable to expect PCPs to have knowledge of all of the potential survivorship scenarios these patients could face in the future.

The IOM[1] recommended that "upon discharge from cancer treatment . . . every patient should be given a record of all care received and important disease characteristics" and went on to assert that every patient should receive "a follow-up plan that is clearly and effectively explained." (See Table 145.3 for details regarding the IOM recommendations for survivorship treatment summary and care plan content.) These documents are intended to communicate the survivor's treatment history, to delineate a plan to ensure that the survivor receives appropriate follow-up care, and to specify which caregivers will provide which services.[1,7] To date,

only two randomized controlled trials have evaluated outcomes related to use of survivorship care plans in clinical practice. One trial reported no effect,[47] and the other reported a decrease in self-reported health worry in the group receiving care plans.[48] This has sparked lively dialogue, particularly with regard to the patient-reported outcome variables measured,[49] as well as the appropriateness of focusing on the care plan document, rather than on the process of care planning.[50]

Several organizations have developed standardized treatment summaries and survivorship care plans to guide post-therapy follow-up care. Important components include surveillance for the recurrence of the primary cancer, the identification of potential long-term complications resulting from specific therapies employed during treatment of the primary cancer, and a plan for psychosocial support and coordination of cancer survivorship care.[1] Downloadable survivorship care plan templates are available from ASCO (www.asco.org/treatmentsummary), COG (www.survivorshipguidelines.org), Journey Forward (www.journeyforward.org), and the LIVESTRONG Survivorship Network (www.livestrongcareplan.org).

Creating a survivorship care plan as outlined here requires time and energy.[51] Despite the barriers this presents, leading groups such as the IOM, LIVESTRONG, COG, and ASCO are promoting the idea that treatment summaries and survivorship care plans should be the standard of care in oncology. This is now a specific quality metric in the ASCO quality of care certification program (Quality Oncology Practice Initiative),[52,53] and was also recently adopted as an American College of Surgeons Commission on Cancer Program Standard, with required implementation by 2015.[54] The information contained within well-developed care plans is intended to facilitate necessary communication between the patient and their oncology, primary care, and specialty providers, thereby maximizing the likelihood that high-quality survivor care can occur.

TABLE 145.3

The Institute of Medicine Survivorship Care Plan

On discharge from cancer treatment, every patient should be given a record including:
1. Contact information for each treating institution and key individual providers
2. Dates of treatment initiation and completion
3. Diagnostic tests and results
4. Tumor characteristics
5. Surgery or other therapies provided, including specific agents, regimens, dosage, number and title of clinical trials (if any), treatment response, and toxicities experienced
6. Psychosocial and nutritional services provided
7. Identification of a coordinator of continuing care

On discharge from cancer treatment, every patient and his or her primary health-care provider should receive a written follow-up care plan including:
1. The likely course of recovery from treatment
2. Recommended periodic testing and examinations by whom and on what schedule
3. Possible late and long-term effects of treatment and symptoms
4. Possible signs of recurrence and second tumors
5. Possible effects of cancer on daily life (personal relationships, work, mental health) and available resources for support
6. Potential insurance, employment, and financial consequences of cancer and referrals to counseling, legal aid, and financial assistance if needed
7. Recommendations for healthy behaviors that should also be shared with first-degree relatives to minimize their potential risk of cancer
8. As appropriate, information on genetic counseling and testing to identify high-risk individuals who could benefit from more comprehensive cancer surveillance
9. As appropriate, information on known effective chemoprevention strategies for secondary prevention (e.g., tamoxifen for breast cancer, aspirin for colorectal cancer)
10. Referrals to specific follow-up care providers
11. A listing of cancer-related print or online information resources and support organizations

Modified from Hewitt M, Greenfield S, Stovall E. *From Cancer Patient to Cancer Survivor: Lost in Transition.* Washington, D.C.: National Academies Press; 2006.

DELIVERY OF FOLLOW-UP CARE AND BEST PRACTICE MODELS

There is no consensus on the best strategy for providing follow-up care to the growing number of cancer survivors. Most children with cancer are treated at pediatric oncology referral centers where, on termination of cancer therapy, they are seen in a follow-up clinic or program.[55] Because of the diverse ages at diagnosis (infancy to adolescence), childhood cancer survivors may be under the care of pediatric oncologists for a decade or more. However, once they become young adults and leave home for college or work, they may need to transition to care outside of the pediatric referral center.[56] This poses a substantial challenge, because few PCPs will be knowledgeable about the exposures and risks from prior cancer therapy.[57,58] Thus, arming the young adult survivor with a treatment summary and care plan with specific surveillance recommendations can facilitate subsequent care with generalist physicians.[55]

Delivery of high-quality care to survivors is not without challenges.[59] Although PCPs given explicit instructions about the necessary components of surveillance and follow-up have been shown to produce the same outcomes as specialist follow-ups,[60] they have also expressed concerns about the lack of adequate training to provide survivorship care and report being more likely than oncologists to order tests/treatments as malpractice protection.[61] Although oncologists are able to provide primary noncancer care to patients,[43] many report uncertainty regarding responsibility for general preventive care,[61] and only a minority appear to want to regularly assume this role.[62] Most survivors experience some form of shared care, in which PCPs collaborate with cancer specialists. The role of oncologists in a shared care model is to provide or guide periodic surveillance and to be available to evaluate patients when potential cancer-related concerns arise, and the PCP continues to carry out routine prevention and health maintenance interventions and manage comorbid conditions.[62–65]

Based on the IOM report, better coordination is needed and direct communication among providers is critical to ensure that that appropriate follow-up care is provided. Current adult survivorship care models include tertiary care centers with consultative services, free-standing cancer centers that integrate survivorship care within their disease-oriented teams using advanced practice nurses and/or PCPs, hybrid models, and community-based models.[65,66] A recent systematic review of models of care for post-treatment follow-up for adult cancer survivors identified a global consensus among cancer-focused organizations that the oncologist/cancer center-based follow-up model is not sustainable and that, given the burgeoning survivor population, a reconfiguration of care models is needed.[67]

EDUCATIONAL CONSIDERATIONS

Educating the cancer survivor, health-care provider, and family is critical to promoting cancer survivorship. Studies evaluating health knowledge among childhood cancer survivors have revealed significant knowledge deficits and misconceptions regarding diagnosis, treatment, and therapy-related health risks.[68] Studies of survivors of adult cancers report similar knowledge deficits regarding risks of and surveillance for disease recurrence or therapy-related late effects, such as risks for infertility or second malignancies.[1,69] Many health-care professionals are also ill-equipped to provide cancer survivorship care, primarily because of the lack of experience in caring for cancer survivors and a deficit of relevant information in professional and/or continuing education curricula.[1,7]

COG has developed a set of health education materials specifically targeted to childhood cancer survivors.[70] These materials, known as Health Links, address 43 key topics within the COG *Long-term Follow-up Guidelines* and are designed to enhance health knowledge and improve compliance with guideline-specific recommendations. Each Health Link provides an overview of the

potential therapy-related complication, a review of relevant risk factors, recommendations for screening, and an explanation of applicable health-protective behaviors. They are designed to be used in conjunction with the COG *Long-term Follow-up Guidelines* and are available to download from www.survivorshipguidelines.org.

COG, working collaboratively with Baylor College of Medicine, developed an Internet-based decision support system for COG institutions that provides up-to-date screening and health information from the COG guidelines that can be individually tailored to each patient's specific treatment exposures.[71] This technology-driven system, known as Passport for Care, will also empower survivors to assume greater control of their own health care via a planned survivor portal that will allow direct access to information that will assist in making decisions regarding individual lifestyle behaviors and follow-up care. When comprehensive guidelines for follow-up care are available for adult cancer survivors, similar Internet-based systems may prove valuable in disseminating this information to survivors and their health-care providers. In addition to providing education to cancer survivors, the incorporation of cancer survivorship care into the objectives for medical school core curricula, along with development and dissemination of continuing education programs for practicing health-care professionals, are imperative in order to optimize care for survivors.[1,7]

ENHANCING RESEARCH

The growing and rather heterogeneous population of cancer survivors provides novel opportunities for research in many domains, including the etiopathogenesis, screening, and early detection of adverse outcomes and their impact on quality of life. This population lends itself to research regarding these issues because of the ability to assess therapeutic exposures accurately, both in terms of the type of exposure and its timing, and to examine the role of host characteristics.

Reports demonstrating the risks of adverse outcomes in childhood cancer survivors were published beginning more than 4 decades ago and have subsequently proliferated.[72–84] Outcomes include premature death, second neoplasms, organ dysfunction, impaired growth and development, decreased fertility, impaired intellectual function, and overall reduced quality of life. Extended follow-ups of large cohorts of survivors has demonstrated the emergence of adverse outcomes at a younger age than would be expected in the general population. There remains a critical need for systematic follow-ups of large cohorts of adult cancer survivors to identify the role of host and clinical characteristics along with comorbidities in the health and well-being of this rapidly growing population.

The focus of investigation thus far has been on the magnitude of risk and the identification of demographic and treatment-related risk factors. Attention needs to be devoted to understanding the underlying etiopathogenesis, such as the role of genetic susceptibility, or the mechanism of action of specific therapeutic exposures associated with the development of the adverse event. In addition, specific research initiatives focusing on the utility of surveillance and interventional strategies need to be mounted. These include the efficacy of agents designed to protect normal tissues from the toxic effects of specific therapeutic agents (e.g., dexrazoxane and anthracycline-induced cardiomyopathy), the use of chemopreventive agents for the prevention of second malignancies, the use of afterload-reducing agents for the prevention of further progression of myocardial dysfunction, lifestyle and behavior modifications, and education to increase awareness of the need for screening. Follow-ups for extended periods of time are required to assess the efficacy of these strategies. The efficiency and cost-effectiveness of competing models of survivorship care and community-based services also require study.

Several challenges persist in the conduct of survivorship research. The multiple etiologies that can influence long-term sequelae often demand large sample sizes in order to address the research questions effectively. Incompleteness of follow-up of cancer survivors results in surveillance bias, which can significantly compromise the quality of research; this may be particularly problematic in younger survivors due to the mobility of this population. Resources are therefore needed to establish the necessary infrastructure to conduct cancer survivorship research effectively.

SURVIVORSHIP ADVOCACY

Employment

Cancer survivors face challenges that go beyond medical issues. Work and ongoing access to health care are primary areas of difficulty, and not just in the United States. A study based on the 2000 National Health Interview Survey found that 18% of cancer survivors were unable to work because of residual health problems, compared with only 10% of matched controls.[85] A further 27% were limited in the amount or kind of work they could do. Such employment problems can impact many other people if the survivor was the main breadwinner. A recent prospective cohort study similarly showed that long-term labor force departures attributable to cancer occurred in 17% of lung and colorectal cancer survivors who were employed at diagnosis.[86] Even among those who are able to return to work, there may be discrimination that is either overt or an unstated undercurrent based on a perception by others that the cancer survivor is not well enough to perform his or her job at the highest level or would be unable to tolerate the added responsibilities entailed by a promotion. The situation has definitely improved over the years because of federal laws like the Americans with Disabilities Act (1990) and the Family and Medical Leave Act (1993) and several state regulations that have done much to protect the rights of workers such as those with a history of cancer.

Insurance

To be effective, health insurance options must be available, affordable, and adequate in coverage.[1] Historically, health insurance options for cancer survivors in the United States have often been deficient on one or more of these criteria. The implementation of the Patient Protection and Affordable Care Act (ACA) in the United States promises to remove restrictions, such as lifetime limits and denial of coverage for preexisting conditions, for those with a history of cancer.[87] Additionally, this new health-care law provides coverage for preventive care and certain services of particular relevance to survivors, such treatment of infertility, that have not been consistently covered previously. Cancer survivors over the age of 65 years have almost all been covered by Medicare and this will not change, but provisions in the ACA will now address gaps in outpatient medication coverage for Medicare recipients. Despite the increased access to coverage that will occur with full

implementation of the ACA, there are nevertheless unanswered questions of potential concern for cancer survivors, such as the scope of coverage for screenings beyond those typically offered for the general population, and coverage for other specialized post-treatment needs. An analysis by the American Cancer Society has identified 160 provisions within the ACA that have significant implications for those affected by cancer.[88] Life insurance applications by people with a personal history of cancer are often rejected or the plans come with very high premiums unless it is part of an employer-based group insurance.

Advocacy

Several nonprofit organizations have formed to provide advocacy for the issues that affect cancer survivors. Some, like the ACS and CancerCare, are not exclusively for survivors of cancer but have survivorship as one of their main areas of interest, whereas the NCCS and LIVESTRONG clearly make survivorship their focus. In addition to advocating for more research funds and resources for survivor care, several of these organizations provide education, counseling, links to legal contacts, and other types of assistance to help survivors with employment, insurance, or economic issues. They also provide assistance in navigating the Social Security Disability system. The ACS reports that about 13% of the calls to an information line it operates are about employment concerns.[1]

There are a few programs of limited financial assistance run through government and charitable organizations that assist with expenses incurred during cancer treatment or transportation to medical appointments. Programs are also offered by several pharmaceutical companies to help provide expensive long-term outpatient medications to cancer patients and survivors. Providing information about resources available to cancer survivors to help them deal with these nonmedical issues is a recommended component of the survivorship care plans discussed earlier in this chapter.

CONCLUSION

The English word "cure" derives from the Latin *cura*, which means "care." Survivorship care is a young science, although substantial progress has been made over the past decade in our understanding of the multifaceted needs of our ever growing and vulnerable population of cancer survivors. The sobering physical, psychosocial, and socioeconomic correlates of successful therapy are their long-term consequences that can compromise quality and quantity of life for our patients and their families, friends, and society. It is the obligation of health-care providers to critically assess and study these adverse effects, intervening when possible. We must also advocate for societal adjustment to our patients' needs in order to provide care in the broadest sense. Celebrating cancer survival is no longer sufficient, and we are fortunate to embrace the associated challenges with our patients.

SELECTED REFERENCES

The full reference list can be accessed at lwwhealthlibrary.com/oncology.

1. Hewitt M, Greenfield S, Stovall E. *From Cancer Patient to Cancer Survivor: Lost in Transition.* Washington, D.C.: National Academies Press; 2006.
2. Leigh S. Cancer survivorship: a consumer movement. *Semin Oncol* 1994;21: 783–786.
4. Mullan F. Seasons of survival: reflections of a physician with cancer. *N Engl J Med* 1985;313:270–273.
5. Rowland JH, Hewitt M, Ganz PA. Cancer survivorship: a new challenge in delivering quality cancer care. *J Clin Oncol* 2006;24:5101–5104.
7. McCabe MS, Bhatia S, Oeffinger KC, et al. American Society of Clinical Oncology statement: achieving high-quality cancer survivorship care. *J Clin Oncol* 2013;31:631–640.

8. de Moor JS, Mariotto AB, Parry C, et al. Cancer survivors in the United States: prevalence across the survivorship trajectory and implications for care. *Cancer Epidemiol Biomarkers Prev* 2013;22:561–570.
12. Smith MA, Seibel NL, Altekruse SF, et al. Outcomes for children and adolescents with cancer: challenges for the twenty-first century. *J Clin Oncol* 2010;28:2625–2634.
13. Hewitt M, Weiner SL, Simone JV. *Childhood Cancer Survivorship: Improving Care and Quality of Life.* Washington, D.C.: The National Academies Press; 2003.
14. Oeffinger KC, Mertens AC, Sklar CA, et al. Chronic health conditions in adult survivors of childhood cancer. *N Engl J Med* 2006;355:1572–1582.
19. Landier W, Bhatia S, Eshelman DA, et al. Development of risk-based guidelines for pediatric cancer survivors: the Children's Oncology Group

Long-Term Follow-Up Guidelines from the Children's Oncology Group Late Effects Committee and Nursing Discipline. *J Clin Oncol* 2004;22:4979–4990.

26. Kremer LC, Mulder RL, Oeffinger KC, et al. A worldwide collaboration to harmonize guidelines for the long-term follow-up of childhood and young adult cancer survivors: a report from the International Late Effects of Childhood Cancer Guideline Harmonization Group. *Pediatr Blood Cancer* 2013;60:543–549.

29. Majhail NS, Rizzo JD, Lee SJ, et al. Recommended screening and preventive practices for long-term survivors after hematopoietic cell transplantation. *Bone Marrow Transplant* 2012;47:337–341.

32. Meyerhardt JA, Mangu PB, Flynn PJ, et al. Follow-up care, surveillance protocol, and secondary prevention measures for survivors of colorectal cancer: American Society of Clinical Oncology clinical practice guideline endorsement. *J Clin Oncol* 2013;31:4465–4470.

33. Khatcheressian JL, Hurley P, Bantug E, et al. Breast cancer follow-up and management after primary treatment: American Society of Clinical Oncology clinical practice guideline update. *J Clin Oncol* 2013;31:961–965.

36. Schmitz KH, Holtzman J, Courneya KS, et al. Controlled physical activity trials in cancer survivors: a systematic review and meta-analysis. *Cancer Epidemiol Biomarkers Prev* 2005;14:1588–1595.

38. Stanton AL. Psychosocial concerns and interventions for cancer survivors. *J Clin Oncol* 2006;24:5132–5137.

39. Kazak AE, Alderfer MA, Streisand R, et al. Treatment of posttraumatic stress symptoms in adolescent survivors of childhood cancer and their families: a randomized clinical trial. *J Fam Psychol* 2004;18:493–504.

43. Ganz PA. A teachable moment for oncologists: cancer survivors, 10 million strong and growing! *J Clin Oncol* 2005;23:5458–5460.

47. Grunfeld E, Julian JA, Pond G, et al. Evaluating survivorship care plans: results of a randomized, clinical trial of patients with breast cancer. *J Clin Oncol* 2011;29:4755–4762.

48. Hershman DL, Greenlee H, Awad D, et al. Randomized controlled trial of a clinic-based survivorship intervention following adjuvant therapy in breast cancer survivors. *Breast Cancer Res Treat* 2013;138:795–806.

59. Forsythe LP, Parry C, Alfano CM, et al. Use of survivorship care plans in the United States: associations with survivorship care. *J Natl Cancer Inst* 2013;105:1579–1587.

61. Virgo KS, Lerro CC, Klabunde CN, et al. Barriers to breast and colorectal cancer survivorship care: perceptions of primary care physicians and medical oncologists in the United States. *J Clin Oncol* 2013;31:2322–2336.

67. Howell D, Hack TF, Oliver TK, et al. Models of care for post-treatment follow-up of adult cancer survivors: a systematic review and quality appraisal of the evidence. *J Cancer Surviv* 2012;6:359–371.

69. Kent EE, Arora NK, Rowland JH, et al. Health information needs and health-related quality of life in a diverse population of long-term cancer survivors. *Patient Educ Couns* 2012;89:345–352.

73. Bhatia S, Yasui Y, Robison LL, et al. High risk of subsequent neoplasms continues with extended follow-up of childhood Hodgkin's disease: report from the Late Effects Study Group. *J Clin Oncol* 2003;21:4386–4394.

78. Haupt R, Fears TR, Robison LL, et al. Educational attainment in long-term survivors of childhood acute lymphoblastic leukemia. *JAMA* 1994; 272:1427–1432.

80. Kremer LC, van der Pal HJ, Offringa M, et al. Frequency and risk factors of subclinical cardiotoxicity after anthracycline therapy in children: a systematic review. *Ann Oncol* 2002;13:819–829.

85. Yabroff KR, Lawrence WF, Clauser S, et al. Burden of illness in cancer survivors: findings from a population-based national sample. *J Natl Cancer Inst* 2004;96:1322–1330.

86. Earle CC, Chretien Y, Morris C, et al. Employment among survivors of lung cancer and colorectal cancer. *J Clin Oncol* 2010;28:1700–1705.

87. Patient Protection and Affordable Care Act. 124 USC § 119–1024 (2010).

PRACTICE OF ONCOLOGY

PART VI

Palliative and Alternative Care

146 Management of Cancer Pain

Thomas W. LeBlanc and Amy P. Abernethy

INTRODUCTION

Advances in the diagnosis and treatment of cancer, coupled with advances in understanding the anatomy, physiology, pharmacology, and psychology of pain perception, have led to improved care of the patient with pain of malignant origin. Specialized methods of cancer diagnosis and treatment provide the most direct approach to treating cancer pain by facilitating the treatment of its underlying cause. However, prior to the initiation of antitumor therapy, when primary cancer treatment has failed, or when injury to bone, soft tissue, or nerve has occurred as a result of therapy, appropriate pain management remains essential. Patients with cancer are managed most effectively through a multidisciplinary approach that draws on the expertise of a wide range of health-care professionals.[1–3] The goal of pain therapy for patients receiving active treatment is to provide them with sufficient relief to tolerate the diagnostic and therapeutic approaches required to treat their cancer and to improve or maintain quality of life. For patients with advanced disease, pain control should be sufficient to allow them to function at an achievable level of their choosing and to die in relative comfort.

Effective pain management is only one component of a broad palliative care approach for cancer patients.[4–8] The American Society of Clinical Oncology now recommends palliative care as an essential component of comprehensive cancer care for all patients with advanced solid tumors.[9] Early palliative care, along with high-quality comprehensive cancer care, may even prolong patients' survival, while improving quality of life.[10] Control of other symptoms, treatment of psychological distress, and attention to the religious, spiritual, and existential dimensions of the patient's illness experience should be concurrently addressed to maintain the patient's quality of life throughout the cancer illness course from diagnosis to death. Palliative care interdisciplinary teams specialize in providing this type of care. The World Health Organization (WHO) has published international guidelines for cancer pain relief and palliative care.[6–8] In the United States, the National Comprehensive Cancer Network has published specific guidelines that provide a best practice approach for both the provision of pain treatment and palliative care; the American Pain Society, the British Pain Society, and the European Society of Medical Oncology (ESMO) have also published specific pain guidelines.[11–16]

EPIDEMIOLOGY

Numerous national and international surveys, supplemented by WHO estimates, suggest that moderate to severe pain is experienced by one-third of cancer patients who receive active therapy, and by 60% to 90% of patients with advanced disease.[17] There are over 19 million new cases of cancer diagnosed worldwide each year and more than 7 million cancer deaths, many of whom suffer from cancer pain.[18] Pain related to direct tumor involvement is the most common cause, occurring in as many as 85% of patients according to one pain service study, or in 65% of cases, as demonstrated through an outpatient cancer center pain clinic survey.[19–21] Bone pain is the most common type, with tumor infiltration of nerve and hollow viscera as the second and third most common pain sources. Cancer therapy causes pain in 15% to 25% of patients receiving chemotherapy, surgery, or radiation therapy. Up to 10% of patients with cancer have pain caused by non–cancer-related problems, with pain syndromes reflecting the common causes of pain in the general population. Chronic pain is also prevalent in cancer survivors, with prevalence rates ranging from 5% to 40% of patients, varying by tumor and treatment type.[22,23]

Patients with cancer often have multiple causes of pain, involving multiple sites.[24–31] Based on a variety of survey data, up to one-third of patients have more than one type of pain, and 81% of patients report two or more distinct pain complaints; 34% report three types of pain.

Studies to date have explored not only the prevalence of pain, but also its intensity, the degree of pain relief, and its effect on quality of life in patients with various malignancies, including the lungs, colon, and ovarian cancers.[25,26,28–30] These studies highlight that pain is prevalent in both ambulatory patients and those who are hospitalized, and that it compromises function in approximately one-half of those who experience it.

A series of studies have focused on the seriously ill and nursing home cancer population and have identified a high prevalence of pain in these groups as well. The Study to Understand Prognoses and Preferences for Outcomes and Risks of Treatments (SUPPORT) showed that 50% of adults who die in the hospital experience moderate to severe pain in their last 3 days of life.[31] A study of 4,000 elderly nursing home residents with cancer revealed that 24%, 29%, and 38% of those over age 85 years, 75 to 84 years, and 65 to 74 years, respectively, reported daily pain.[24] Twenty-six percent of these elderly in daily pain did not receive any medication. Those older than 85 years who reported pain were most likely to receive no analgesic. Similar studies of children report that 54% to 85% of pediatric inpatients and 26% to 35% of pediatric outpatients experience pain. Up to 62% to 90% of children experience pain at the end of life.[27]

Such studies have led to an assessment of the factors that influence the prevalence of cancer pain. Primary tumor type is one factor. Tumors that commonly metastasize to bone such as breast or prostate tumors are associated with a higher incidence of pain (60% to 80%) than lymphoma and leukemia.[19] Stage of disease is a contributing factor, with pain prevalence increasing as disease progresses. For example, fewer than 15% of patients with nonmetastatic disease report pain, whereas pain is the most common symptom in patients in the last months of life.[32,33] Tumors that occur in close proximity to neural structures also produce a higher incidence of pain. Patient variables such as anxiety, depression, and history of previous substance abuse also influence the patient's report and experience of pain.[34,35]

DEFINITION OF PAIN

The definition of pain, as proposed by the International Association for the Study of Pain, is as follows: "an unpleasant sensory and emotional experience associated with actual or potential tissue damage or described in terms of such damage."[36] Because pain is a subjective experience, there is no definitive way to distinguish pain that occurs in the absence of tissue damage from pain that results from such damage. Pain as a somatic delusion or masked depression is rare in cancer patients; the presence of pain usually implies a pathologic process.

Types of Pain

Three major categories of pain have been described based on the neuroanatomy and neurophysiology of pain pathways: (1) somatic, (2) visceral, and (3) neuropathic. Each type results from the activation and sensitization of nociceptors and mechanoreceptors in the periphery by either mechanical stimuli (e.g., tumor compression, infiltration) or chemical stimuli (e.g., epinephrine, serotonin, bradykinin, prostaglandin, histamine).

Somatic Pain

When nociceptors are activated in cutaneous or deep tissues, somatic pain results, typically characterized by a dull or aching but well-localized pain. Metastatic bone pain, postsurgical incisional pain, and myofascial and musculoskeletal pain are common examples of somatic pain.

Visceral Pain

Visceral pain results from the activation of nociceptors due to infiltration, compression, extension, or stretching of the thoracic, abdominal, or pelvic viscera. This typically occurs in patients with intraperitoneal metastases and is common with pancreatic cancer. This type of pain is poorly localized; is often described as deep, squeezing, and pressure like; and, when acute, it is often associated with significant autonomic dysfunction, including nausea, vomiting, and diaphoresis. Visceral pain is often referred to cutaneous sites that may be remote from the location of the lesion itself (e.g., shoulder pain with diaphragmatic irritation). It may also be associated with tenderness in the referred cutaneous site. Recent data demonstrate the role of kappa-opioid receptors in modulating visceral pain.[37]

Neuropathic Pain

Neuropathic pain results from injury to the peripheral or central nervous system as a consequence of tumor compression or infiltration of peripheral nerves or the spinal cord, or from chemical injury to the peripheral nerve or spinal cord caused by surgery, radiation therapy, or chemotherapy. Examples of neuropathic pain include both metastatic and radiation-induced brachial and lumbosacral plexopathies, chemotherapy-induced peripheral neuropathies, paraneoplastic peripheral neuropathies, and postmastectomy, postthoracotomy, and phantom limb pain.[38] Pain from nerve injury is often severe and is described as burning or dysesthetic, with a viselike quality. The pain is typically most common in the site of sensory loss and may be associated with hypersensitivity to nonnoxious (*allodynia*) and noxious stimuli. Intermittently, patients complain of paroxysms of burning or electric shock–like sensations. The latter symptoms result from the phenomenon of central sensitization.

These three types of pain may occur alone or together in the same patient. Experimental models of bone and nerve pain provide great insight into the mechanisms underlying these clinical pain states. Clohisy and Mantyh,[39] Lindsay et al.,[40] and Peters et al.[41] have developed both a bone tumor model and a chemotherapy-induced peripheral neuropathy model in animals that have helped to elucidate the mechanisms of pain and their biologic correlates. These correlative studies with animal models provide the opportunity to test both bone and nerve pain model responses to clinical treatments. For example, opioids, gabapentin, and nonsteroidal anti-inflammatory agents produce analgesic efficacy in the bone tumor model.[39]

Temporal Aspects of Pain

Acute Pain

Acute pain is characterized by a well-defined temporal pattern of pain onset, generally associated with subjective and objective physical signs and with hyperactivity of the autonomic nervous system. These signs provide the physician with objective evidence that substantiates the patient's complaint of pain. Acute pain is usually self-limited and responds to treatment with analgesic drug therapy and to treatment of its precipitating cause. This type of pain can be further subdivided into subacute and episodic categories. Subacute pain arises over several days, often with increasing intensity, and represents a pattern of progressive symptomatology. Episodic or intermittent pain occurs during confined periods of time on a regular or irregular basis. Subacute pain is also generally accompanied by autonomic hyperactivity.

Chronic Pain

Chronic pain is pain that persists for more than 3 months, with a less well-defined temporal onset. The autonomic nervous system adapts, and chronic pain patients lack the objective signs common to those with acute pain. Chronic pain often leads to significant changes in personality, lifestyle, and functional ability. Treatment of chronic pain in the cancer patient is especially challenging because it requires a careful assessment of not only the intensity of the pain, but also its broad multidimensional aspects. Evidence suggests that the persistence of pain has a major negative effect on patients' quality of life.

Investigators have developed a nomenclature to describe a series of specific pains in cancer patients with both acute and chronic pain states. *Baseline pain* is the average pain intensity experienced for 12 or more hours during a 24-hour period. *Breakthrough pain* is a transient increase in pain to greater than moderate intensity that occurs on a baseline pain of moderate intensity or less. Various epidemiologic studies provide a range of prevalence of breakthrough pain from 23% to as high as 90% of cancer patients.[42–45] Breakthrough pain has a diversity of characteristics. In this and other series, the transitory increase in pain marks the onset or worsening of pain at the end of the dosing interval or the regularly scheduled analgesic. In other patients, it is caused by an action of the patient, referred to as *incident pain*. Sometimes the incident pain has a nonvolitional precipitant, such as flatulence. Clinical trials have focused attention on the clinical management of breakthrough pain and dosing guidelines.[42]

Intensity of Pain

Pain may also be defined on the basis of intensity, but there are limitations to a concept of pain based solely on intensity. Specific categorical scales of pain intensity have been used in which patients are asked to describe their pain as mild, moderate, severe, or excruciating. Visual analog scales (VAS) have also been used. These are presented on a 10-cm line anchored at either end by two points, signifying *no pain* and *worst possible pain*. The patient is asked to mark the intensity of the pain on the line. Numeric scales are also commonly used, and patients are asked to rate their pain between 1 (no pain) and 10 (worst possible pain). These scales have their limitations, but they are part of a series of validated instruments that include a measure of pain intensity as one of the components of the pain experience to be defined.

Measurement of Pain

The multidimensional pain assessment is the recommended approach to the study of pain prevalence and pain intervention. Several validated instruments for pain measurement attempt to look at it in a multidimensional way. The use of such methods can provide a rapid evaluation in clinical settings of the major aspects of the pain experienced by cancer patients. The Joint Commission for the Accreditation of Healthcare Organizations require the use of pain scales in routine care.[46]

Brief Pain Inventory

The Wisconsin Brief Pain Inventory (BPI) is a self-administered, easily understood, brief method to assess pain.[47] It addresses the relevant aspects of pain (history, intensity, location, and quality) and the ability of the pain to interfere with the patient's activities, and helps to provide an understanding of its cause. The history of pain and its relation to the patient's disease are assessed initially. If the patient admits to pain in the past month, he or she answers questions about current manifestations of pain. If the patient has no pain, he or she skips to the end of the questionnaire to complete the demographic information. For patients with pain, a human figure drawing is provided on which the patients shade the area corresponding to the pain. Patients are asked to rate their pain at its worst, their usual pain, and their pain at the time they are completing the questionnaire. The pain scales consist of numbers from 0 to 10; 0 is labeled *no pain* and 10 is labeled *pain as bad as you can imagine*. Patients are asked to report the medications or treatments they receive for pain, the percentage relief that these medications or treatment provide, and their belief about the cause of their pain. Finally, they are asked to rate how much the pain interferes with their mood, relations with other people, and functional ability (walking, sleeping, working, enjoying life). All patients, including those without pain, are asked for basic demographic information about marital status, education, occupation, spouse's occupation, and months since diagnosis. This inventory has been translated into numerous languages and has been used to assess pain in cancer patients in various settings.

McGill Pain Questionnaire

The McGill Pain Questionnaire (MPQ) is an extensively used pain assessment instrument that produces scores on four empirically derived dimensions, as well as several summary scores.[48] The instrument consists of 78 adjectives that cluster in 20 categories. Within each category, the adjectives are arranged in order of intensity from low to high. The categories are divided into four dimensions: sensory, affective, evaluative, and miscellaneous. The patient is asked to choose one adjective from each applicable category that describes an aspect of his or her current pain, and the score for each dimension is obtained by adding the rank values of the selected adjectives. Adding the scores across the four dimensions derives a total summary score, and a total word count is also obtained. Finally, a rating of present pain intensity is made on a five-point scale. Studies with this instrument have demonstrated that the factors derived reflect specific sensory qualities and combined emotional and sensory dimensions. This tool has also been used to assess distinct score profiles according to the nature of pain. For instance, patients with acute pain tend to use more sensory words, but patients with chronic pain tend to use more affective and reaction word subgroups. The MPQ offers a methodologic approach to assessing the sensory, affective, and evaluative

components of pain, but it may be more difficult and cumbersome for patients to understand and complete than some other pain assessment tools and may also be limited by its language constraints.

Patient-Reported Outcome Measures

Assessing symptoms by direct patient self-report is an increasingly common and desirable method for collecting data on important patient-centered outcomes like pain.[49] These so-called *patient-reported outcome* (PRO) measures avoid clinicians' bias in their assessments and allow for reproducible collecting and trending of self-reported items over time. A growing body of literature demonstrates that electronic methods for data collection are quite robust and at least equivalent if not superior to paper options. PROs are increasingly included as outcome measures in oncology clinical trials, and several instruments have been directly developed as PROs, including the M. D. Anderson Symptom Inventory (MDASI) and the Patient Care Monitor (PCM).[50,51] Others include the following.

Memorial Symptom Assessment Scale

The Memorial Symptom Assessment Scale (MSAS) is a validated, patient-rated measure that provides multidimensional information about a diverse group of common symptoms. Thirty-two physical and psychological symptoms are characterized in terms of intensity, frequency, and distress. The MSAS provides a Global Distress Index (MSAS-GDI), a 10-item subscale that reflects global symptom distress and separate subscales that measure physical (MSAS-Phys) and psychological (MSAS-Psych) symptom distress. Ongoing studies have confirmed its value in patients with various types of cancer, and studies of its reliability and validity with repeated administration are currently under way. The use of the MSAS allows the concurrent measurement of pain and various other symptoms, psychological distress, and psychological factors; overall, it represents a useful, patient-accepted method to measure the multidimensional issues facing cancer patients with pain.[52] Newer studies have identified the usefulness of a short form for a rapid assessment.[53]

Functional Assessment of Cancer Therapy – General

The Functional Assessment of Cancer Therapy – General (FACT-G) is a 27-item PRO that assesses cancer-related symptoms across four major domains: physical, social, emotional, and functional. Patients are asked to rate each item as it applies to the past 7 days. Each question is anchored to a five-point scale from zero to four (*not at all, a little bit, somewhat, quite a bit, very much*). It includes a specific question on pain, and also explores the impact of pain and other symptoms on the patient's overall well-being.

European Organization for Research and Treatment of Cancer Quality of Life Questionnaire-C30

The European Organization for Research and Treatment of Cancer has included specific pain questions in its Quality of Life Questionnaire-C30 (QLQ-C30) scale. The pain scale measures pain intensity and interference with function. The pain scale has a four-level verbal rating scale (*not at all, a little, quite a bit, very much*), measuring the presence of pain and pain interference with daily activities. The responses are summed to a composite score and transformed to a 0 to 100 pain scale of severity. The pain severity composite score better represents the cancer pain experience than the intensity score alone. In published studies, it has been shown to reliably predict functional status, toxicity, and chemotherapy response. Because of their multiple scales, the QLQ-C30 and the FACT-G require more time, attention, and cooperation on the part of patients, which makes them less useful as routine measurement tools, and more useful in the context of research.[54]

TABLE 146.1

Tumor-Related Chronic Pain Syndromes

Bone Pain
Multifocal or generalized bone pain
Multiple bony metastases
Marrow expansion
Vertebral syndromes
Atlantoaxial destruction and odontoid fractures
C7 to T1 syndrome
T12 to L1 syndrome
Sacral syndrome
Back pain and epidural compression
Pain syndromes of the bony pelvis and hip
Hip joint syndrome
Acrometastases
Arthrides
Hypertrophic pulmonary osteoarthropathy
Other polyarthritides
Muscle pain
Muscle cramps
Skeletal muscle tumors

Headache and Facial Pain
Intracerebral tumor
Leptomeningeal metastases
Base of skull metastases
  Orbital syndrome
  Parasellar syndrome
  Middle cranial fossa syndrome
  Jugular foramen syndrome
  Clivus syndrome
  Sphenoid sinus syndrome
Painful cranial neuralgias
  Glossopharyngeal neuralgia
  Trigeminal neuralgia
Eye and Ear syndromes
  Otalgia
  Eye pain

Tumor Involvement of the Peripheral Nervous System
Tumor-related radiculopathy
Post therapeutic neuralgia
Cervical plexopathy
Brachial plexopathy
Malignant brachial plexopathy
Idiopathic brachial plexopathy associated with Hodgkin's lymphoma
Malignant lumbosacral plexopathy
Tumor-related mononeuropathy
Paraneoplastic painful peripheral neuropathy
Subacute sensory neuropathy
Sensorimotor peripheral neuropathy

Pain Syndromes of the Viscera and Miscellaneous Tumor-Related Syndromes
Hepatic distention syndrome
Midline retroperitoneal syndrome
Chronic intestinal obstruction
Peritoneal carcinomatosis
Malignant perineal pain
Malignant pelvic floor myalgia
Adrenal Pain Syndrome
Ureteric obstruction
Ovarian cancer pain
Lung cancer pain

Paraneoplastic Nociceptive Pain Syndromes
Tumor-related gynecomastia

From Cherny NI, Portenoy RK. Cancer pain: principles of assessment and syndromes. In: Wall PK, Melzack R, eds. *Textbook of Pain*. London: Churchill Livingstone; 1994:787, with permission.

Edmonton Symptom Assessment Scale

The Edmonton Symptom Assessment Scale (ESAS) is a nine-item patient-reported symptom visual analog scale developed to assess symptoms in patients who receive palliative care. The scale has been validated in cancer patients and correlated closely with the MSAS and BPI measurement tools.[55]

COMMON PAIN SYNDROMES

Pain in the cancer patient results from direct tumor infiltration and from the various cancer treatments and can occur unrelated to the cancer and cancer therapy. Tables 146.1 and 146.2 list the common wide range of both acute and chronic pain syndromes in patients with cancer. These lists are a compendium of various sources and serve to summarize the broad and now well-recognized pain syndromes that occur often uniquely in this population of patients.[1,5,19–21,25]

Clinical Assessment of Pain

Certain general principles should be followed in evaluating cancer patients with pain.[56] Lack of attention to these general principles is the major cause for misdiagnosis of a specific pain syndrome. Adequate assessment is a critical component for defining the appropriate therapeutic strategy for each patient. The general principles are the following:

- Believe the patient's complaint of pain.
- Take a careful history of the patient's pain complaint.
- Evaluate the patient's psychological state.
- Perform careful medical and neurologic examinations.
- Order the appropriate diagnostic studies and personally review the results.

TABLE 146.2

Treatment-Related Chronic Pain Syndromes

Postchemotherapy Pain Syndromes
Chronic painful peripheral neuropathy
Avascular necrosis of femoral or humeral head
Plexopathy associated with intra-arterial infusion
Raynaud's Phenomenon

Chronic Pain Associated with Hormonal Therapy
Gynecomastia with hormonal therapy for prostate cancer

Chronic Postsurgical Pain Syndromes
Postmastectomy pain syndrome
Postradical neck dissection pain
Postthoracotomy pain
Postoperative frozen shoulder
Phantom pain syndromes
  Phantom limb pain
  Phantom breast pain
Phantom anus pain
  Phantom bladder pain
  Stump pain
Postsurgical pelvic floor myalgia

Chronic Post Radiation Pain Syndromes
Plexopathies
Radiation-induced brachial and lumbosacral plexopathies
Radiation-induced peripheral nerve tumors
Chronic radiation myelopathy
Chronic radiation enteritis and proctitis
Burning perineum syndrome
Osteoradionecrosis

Adapted from Cherny NI, Portenoy RK. Cancer pain: principles of assessment and syndromes. In: Wall PK, Melzack R, eds. *Textbook of Pain*. London: Churchill Livingstone; 1994:787.

■ Treat the pain to facilitate the appropriate workup.
■ Reassess the patient's response to therapy.
■ Individualize the diagnostic and therapeutic approaches.
■ Discuss advance directives with the patient and family.

Critical to the management of the patient with cancer pain is the establishment of a trusting relationship with the physician. The complaint of pain is a symptom, not a diagnosis. Pain perception is not simply a function of the amount of physical injury sustained by the patient but is a complex state determined by multiple factors. The diagnosis of a specific pain syndrome and a complete understanding of the patient's psychological state are not always accomplished during the initial evaluation. In fact, it may take several weeks to define its nature because of the lack of radiologic or pathologic verification. It may take a similar period to fully comprehend each patient's psychological makeup.

Take a Careful History of the Patient's Pain Complaint

A careful history of the patient's pain complaint should include the patient's description of site of pain, quality of pain, exacerbating and relieving factors, temporal pattern, exact onset, associated symptoms and signs, interference with activities of daily living, effect on the patient's psychological state, and response to previous and current analgesic therapies.[56] Patients should be asked to describe the intensity, frequency, and severity of their baseline pain and episodes of breakthrough pain. Routine pain assessment tools should be provided to patients and families to record the patient's pain experience and provide easy recording of analgesic drug use and the use of rescue medications. Multiple pain complaints are common in patients with advanced disease and must be ranked, classified, and recorded.

Evaluate the Patient's Psychological State

The patient's current level of anxiety and depression must be clarified and his or her past history of such symptoms must be defined. Knowledge of the patient's previous psychiatric history and need for past hospitalization for psychiatric care helps to clarify the patient's potential psychological risk. Information on how the patient has handled previous painful events may provide insight into whether the patient has demonstrated chronic illness behavior or has a past history of a chronic pain syndrome. It is important to know about a personal or family history of alcohol or drug dependence to understand why the patient may be fearful of taking or refuses to take opioid drugs.

Because each patient has his or her own understanding of the meaning of pain, it is useful to have the patient elaborate this meaning.[57-60] Does he or she think it represents a recurrent tumor, or is he or she convinced it is simply arthritis? Evidence suggests that when patients have a clear understanding of the meaning of their pain as representing a recurrent tumor, they have increased psychological distress.

The importance of defining the psychological makeup of the patient with pain is supported by a variety of studies that have focused on the effect of suffering in patients with pain.[57-62] Psychological factors play a significant role in accounting for the differences in pain experiences in cancer patients. A series of psychiatric syndromes have been described for cancer patients, with depression occurring in as many as 25% of patients.[57,62] The depression presents either as an acute stress response or as a major depression. Awareness of the common psychiatric syndromes when evaluating the pain complaint expands the physician's understanding of such a complaint.

Although it is critical to know as much as possible about each patient with pain, some information may not be readily available in the first interview; in some instances, it may never be available because of some patients' inabilities to clearly define the various components of their pain. It is often necessary to verify the history by consulting a family member who may provide additional information. The family may be more objective in assessing a disability of a patient who underreports symptoms. Similarly, in a patient who is a poor historian, family may be able to provide essential information that may alter the diagnostic approach. All attempts should be made to compile a careful history and define the medical, neurologic, and psychological profile of the pain complaint. In geriatric patients with compromised cognitive function, geriatric pain and symptom scales should be used.[24]

It is critical to define the goals of any pain treatment. Some patients harbor unreasonable expectations, whereas others fail to critically consider the various options available to them. Complete relief is typically impossible, and the degree of relief must be balanced with any treatment's adverse effects. Before starting any intervention, review carefully with patients the risks and benefits to provide them with a reasonable expectation of the potential outcome of this approach. As patients become more active in defining advance directives and as they focus on the quality of life, it is critical to ask them to define what they would do if the pain were intractable or intolerable.[62] Did the patient have a family member who died a painful death? In the authors' experience, patients who have had such an experience are particularly fearful of their own deaths. Does the patient have suicidal thoughts or a pact with a family member? Does the patient have a family history of suicide? Does the patient have drugs in reserve or a gun in the house that he or she might use in desperation? In a study by Chochinov et al.,[62] pain alone did not correlate with patients' suicidal ideation. Significant depression appeared to be the major correlating factor, although pain clearly played a role in the development of depression in some patients. This series of questions allows patients to discuss openly their fears of death and their intention to take matters into their own hands rather than trust the health-care professional. Such open discussions can allow the physician to better define for the patient the options for care and to reassure the patient of the physician's commitment to care. Because patients rarely offer this information unless requested, it is critical to develop specific questions that can be readily integrated into the initial history taking by the physician. Discussing with the patient how he or she would die and engaging the patient in a discussion of his or her concerns and desires can address the commonly heard comment of patients, "I have never died before, how do I do it?"

Perform Careful Medical and Neurologic Examinations

Medical and neurologic examinations help provide the necessary data to substantiate the history. They also provide a direct assessment of the cognitive status of the patient. Knowledge of the referral patterns of pain and the common cancer pain syndromes can direct the examinations. For example, the commonly described pain syndromes associated with postmastectomy states can readily be defined as separate from tumor infiltration of the brachial plexus.[63]

The physical and neurologic examinations allow a physician to visually inspect and palpate the site of pain and to look for the associated physical and neurologic signs that might help to better define the nature of the pain symptom. Defining the degree of motor or sensory changes can help identify the specific site in the nervous system that may be involved. Similarly, in patients with sensory loss, the presence of allodynia and hyperesthesia can further identify the nature of the sensory problem and define a neuropathic pain syndrome. Moreover, the degree of muscle spasm, gait instability, and impaired coordination can only be fully assessed by such an evaluation. In patients with neuropathic pain, the use of quantitative sensory testing can help define the underlying mechanism and determine selection of drug therapy.

Order the Appropriate Diagnostic Studies and Personally Review the Results

Diagnostic studies confirm the diagnosis and define the site and extent of tumor infiltration, when applicable. Computed tomography (CT) and magnetic resonance imaging (MRI) are the most useful diagnostic procedures for evaluating cancer patients with pain. Positron-emission tomography (PET) helps to further define the tumor and differentiate the tumor from radiation injury and postsurgical injury. The bone scan is a useful screening device and is more sensitive for demonstrating abnormalities in the bone before changes appear on a plain radiograph. However, a negative finding on bone scan does not rule out bony metastatic disease, nor does a positive finding on bone scan confirm the diagnosis of metastatic tumor. In patients with collapsed vertebral bodies, an MRI can distinguish osteoporotic from tumor-induced bony changes. The physician should review the results personally with the radiologist to correlate any pathologic change with the site of pain. Also, the measurement of tumor markers such as carcinoembryonic antigen (CEA), cancer antigen 125 (CA-125), and prostate-specific antigen, among others, can be useful in a patient in whom a recurrent tumor is suspected. In certain pain syndromes, the presence of recurrent disease is closely associated with the onset of pain (e.g., the appearance of late postthoracotomy pain syndrome in a patient after initial resolution of the postoperative pain).[19]

Treat the Pain to Facilitate the Appropriate Workup

Inadequate evaluations sometimes occur in the setting of severe pain. Early aggressive pain management while the source is investigated markedly improves the patient's ability to participate in any necessary diagnostic procedures. During the initial evaluation, early consideration of the use of alternative methods of pain control, including anesthetic and neurosurgical approaches, should be considered (e.g., the temporary use of a local anesthetic via an epidural catheter to manage sacral pain).

Reassess the Patient's Response to Therapy

A continual reassessment of the patient's response to the prescribed therapy provides the best method to validate the initial diagnosis as correct. If relief is less than predicted or if the pain worsens, a reassessment of the treatment approach or a search for a new cause of the pain should be considered. Ideally, use the same assessment instrument at each time point; for example, if you are monitoring pain using a 0 to 10 numerical rating scale, continue to use that for each follow-up visit.

Individualize the Diagnostic and Therapeutic Approaches

An evaluation of the patient must be closely linked to the patient's level of function, ability to participate in the diagnostic workup, willingness to undergo the necessary diagnostic approaches, objective evidence that treatment approaches may be beneficial, and life expectancy. Careful judgment is required to select diagnostic approaches that will have a direct effect on the choice of the therapeutic strategy or will answer a specific question. The random use of diagnostic procedures in these patients, particularly those with advanced cancer and significant pain, is inappropriate and costly. Open discussion with the patient about the need for assessment as well as the therapeutic options is critical to allow the patient to be part of the decision-making process. For some patients, diagnostic procedures such as an MRI are inappropriate because they simply confirm the existence of a disease for which no treatment is available, or for which the treatment would be a major surgical procedure (e.g., vertebral body resection) that would be inappropriate for a dying patient. Patient refusal of an evaluation or treatment must be respected when the physician has fully explained the options and is convinced that the patient has an accurate understanding of the implications of undertaking no further workup or treatment.

Discuss Advance Directives with the Patient and Family

When treatment approaches are being developed, there must be an open discussion about advance directives so that the physician has a clear understanding of the patient's goal for therapy. The physician must have unconditional positive regard for the patient, placing the control of symptoms of pain and treatment of psychological distress in the highest regard. Knowledge of the patient's decisions about resuscitation, living wills, and symptom management should he or she become incapacitated improves the physician's ability to appropriately and humanely care for the dying patient with advanced disease.[59]

MANAGEMENT OF CANCER PAIN

Evidence-based cancer pain management follows a systematic strategy of applying demonstrated interventions in the context of individual needs, circumstances, and preferences. The basic approach employs three categories of agents: opioid analgesics, non-opioid analgesics, and adjuvant therapies. The foundation of this approach is an individualized combination of opioid and nonopioid drugs; to this foundation is added tailored care that selects from a broad array of adjuvant interventions to achieve maximum comfort for the individual patient. Guidelines are available to assist the clinician in determining a foundation treatment plan (the reader is referred to the National Comprehensive Cancer Network, the American Pain Society guidelines, ESMO guidelines, and the British Pain Society as excellent sources of cancer pain management guidelines).[8,11-16] To enhance the effectiveness of this foundation, many pharmacologic and nonpharmacologic options exist for tailoring adjuvant care to individual exigencies.

The sections that follow will emphasize the principles of pharmacologic, nonpharmacologic, procedural, and manual management of cancer pain and briefly describe anesthesia and neurosurgical approaches to pain management to which the oncologist might refer a patient for specialized procedures.

Pharmacologic Management of Cancer Pain

Analgesic Drug Therapy: The Mainstay of Cancer Pain Management

Cancer pain management combines treatment of the primary disease with (1) analgesic drug therapy and (2) specific approaches that may include anesthetic, neurosurgical, rehabilitative, psychological (cognitive–behavioral), psychiatric, or complementary and alternative methods. The clinician begins with determining a patient-specific appropriate analgesic drug plan. Titration to effective pain relief and individualization of treatment represent hallmarks at this stage in the therapeutic approach. In recent years, standard analgesic drug therapy has become more effective due to increased sophistication in the use of analgesic drugs, coupled with research to understand the underlying mechanisms of pain. These new and more effective analgesic practices include the use of novel means of drug administration, particularly transdermal and transmucosal delivery; novel methods, such as the use of bisphosphonates and calcitonin for bone pain, radiopharmaceuticals, and novel approaches to neuropathic pain, such as antidepressants and anticonvulsants; and anesthetic, neurosurgical, psychological, and psychiatric approaches concurrently applied in the overall continuum of care.

As noted previously, numerous guidelines for the management of cancer pain have been issued by various organizations and researchers.[8,11-16] These guidelines have each defined analgesic drug therapy as the mainstay of treatment and have articulated the aims of drug therapy as the achievement of adequate pain relief safely within an acceptable time frame, minimization of side effects of treatment, and ongoing analgesia by the most convenient and least noxious means available. Yet, despite available guidelines and an agreed upon approach to cancer pain management, determination of the best treatment path for the individual patient remains a complex, individualized process.

The World Health Organization Cancer Pain Guidelines

Although frequently debated, the WHO guidelines on cancer pain continue to provide a framework approach for pharmacologic management of cancer pain management. Field testing of these guidelines, as well as clinical experience, has shown that 70% to 90% of cancer patients' pain can be controlled using a simple and inexpensive method described as the *three-step analgesic ladder*.[64,65]

The ladder describes a process for combining nonopioid, opioid, and adjuvant drugs, titrated to meet the individual needs of the patient according to the severity of pain and its pathophysiology. A randomized controlled trial of an algorithm based on the WHO ladder demonstrated that a standardized approach to cancer pain management using the algorithm provided more effective analgesia than routine oncology care.[66] These new studies suggest that a two-step ladder is equally effective for cancer pain management, and the WHO is beginning a process of guideline revision and updates.[67]

Step 1 of the WHO ladder focuses on analgesic drug therapy for patients with mild-to-moderate cancer pain. Such patients should be treated with a nonopioid analgesic that may or may not be combined with an adjuvant drug, depending on the specific pain pathophysiology. For example, in a patient with mild pain from a peripheral neuropathy, the combination of a nonopioid with a tricyclic antidepressant or an anticonvulsant drug would be appropriate.

Step 2 of the WHO ladder focuses on patients with moderate pain who do not experience adequate pain relief from a nonopioid analgesic. These patients are candidates for a combination of a nonopioid, such as aspirin, acetaminophen, cyclooxygenase 2 (COX-2) inhibitors, or other nonsteroidal anti-inflammatory drug (NSAID), and low doses of opioid analgesics, such as codeine, oxycodone, or morphine, usually dosed at less than 60 mg oral morphine equivalents (OME) daily. These patients often require adjuvant drugs, depending on the pain pathophysiology.

Step 3 pertains to patients who report either severe pain (often gauged as greater than 7 on a 0 to 10 scale) or moderate pain that is inadequately managed after appropriate administration of drugs at the second step of the WHO ladder. For these patients, nonopioids are often used in combination with more potent doses of opioids to mitigate the opioid effect, and adjuvants are administered depending on the pain pathophysiology or need to control other concurrent symptoms in the individual patient. Opioid doses on step 3 are commonly greater than 60 mg OME daily.

In short, the analgesic drug ladder of the WHO defines a method for using drug combinations in three categories: nonopioids, opioids, and adjuvants; it is based on previously well-tested pharmacologic principles. However, controversy in the application of the WHO ladder continues to surround the choice of analgesic drug for the individual patient.[63–66] For example, one meta-analysis of the role of NSAIDs in bone pain found them to be no more or less effective than opioids, although they are commonly used.[68]

Cancer Pain Management Using the World Health Organization Three-Step Analgesic Ladder

Nonopioid Analgesics for Cancer Pain Management. The nonopioid analgesics include acetaminophen and the NSAIDs, of which aspirin is the prototypic agent. These compounds are most commonly administered orally. Their analgesia is limited by a ceiling effect, such that increasing the dose beyond a certain level (900 to 1,300 mg per dose of aspirin) produces no increase in peak effect. Tolerance and physical dependence do not occur with repeated administration. Aspirin and the other NSAIDs have analgesic, antipyretic, anti-inflammatory, and antiplatelet actions. Some NSAIDs, such as choline magnesium trisalicylate, lack the antiplatelet effects of aspirin and may have less collateral toxicity in cancer patients already at risk of bleeding. Others (e.g., ibuprofen) appear to produce fewer gastrointestinal side effects than aspirin. The COX-2 inhibitors potentially offer less gastrointestinal (GI) toxicity and without affecting platelet function. However, the drug currently marketed as a COX-2 inhibitor—celecoxib—has not been systematically studied in cancer patients to define its particular role in pain management; concerns regarding cardiovascular side effects have limited use of this class of agents.[69] More recently, cardiovascular effects have been recognized across even nonselective COX inhibitors, including ibuprofen; naproxen

may pose a slightly lower risk.[70] Acetaminophen, an analgesic and antipyretic agent equipotent to aspirin, is much less effective as an anti-inflammatory agent but does not interfere with platelet function or pose cardiovascular risk.

The nonopioid analgesics are generally thought to produce analgesia by inhibiting activation of peripheral nociceptors through their prevention of the formation of prostaglandin E$_2$, a known sensitizer of peripheral receptors to nociceptive stimulation from tissue injury. The NSAIDs differ from one another both in duration of their analgesic action and in their pharmacokinetic profile. Ibuprofen and fenoprofen have short half-lives and the same duration of action as aspirin, whereas diflunisal and naproxen have longer half-lives and are longer acting. Because clinical experience has found that some patients respond better to one NSAID than to another, each patient should be given an adequate trial of one drug on a regular basis before switching to another. Survey data from the WHO demonstration projects suggest that 20% to 40% of patients obtain pain relief with the use of nonopioid analgesics alone.[71]

These drugs are thought to play a special role in the management of bone pain because numerous studies have shown that aspirin inhibits tumor growth in an animal model of metastatic bone tumor. A meta-analysis of studies using NSAIDs to treat bone pain did not demonstrate them to be more effective than weak opioids such as codeine, oxycodone, and propoxyphene.[68] Recent data that detail cancer-related bone pain as a neuropathic pain model have challenged the dogma of NSAIDs for bone pain.[39]

Numerous studies have elucidated the major risk factors for GI toxicity, particularly ulcerative complications, associated with NSAIDs. These risk factors include advanced age, higher doses, concomitant administration of corticosteroids, and history of either ulcer disease or previous GI complications from NSAIDs. Various prophylactic therapies are administered to prevent GI complications. Misoprostol is the only U.S. Food and Drug Administration (FDA)–approved medication for this indication; a Cochrane systematic review supports its use for the prevention of NSAID-induced GI complications.[72] More commonly, proton-pump inhibitors are prescribed, which have been associated with significantly decreased frequency of NSAID-related dyspepsia and fewer ulcers diagnosed by endoscopy.[73] Whether this leads to fewer GI bleeds and reduced health-care utilization is still being debated. An empiric approach at this time is to administer misoprostol or a proton-pump inhibitor to all patients who are receiving NSAIDs with significant risk factors for GI complications.[74]

Nonopioid drugs represent the front-line approach for cancer pain management, but the choice and use of nonopioids must be individualized. Although several NSAIDs are FDA approved for use as analgesics for mild to moderate pain (Table 146.3), guidelines for the use of NSAIDs in patients with cancer are largely empirical. According to a 2004 Cochrane systematic review of 42 trials involving cancer pain patients, the evidence demonstrated at best a nonstatistically significant trend toward improvements when NSAIDs and opioids were combined; conclusions were limited by the short duration of the studies.[75] The clinician must select an agent based on evidence, individual patient history, and patient-specific considerations, and then must give the patient an adequate trial of that nonopioid analgesic before switching to an alternative one. Such a trial should include the administration of the drug to maximum levels at regular intervals. Because there is a great variability among patient responses to different drugs, patients may require trials with several NSAIDs before finding an effective drug and dose regimen. If pain relief is not obtained, adding an opioid to a nonopioid provides additive analgesia.

Combinations containing codeine, oxycodone, and propoxyphene are available, but these combinations often contain less than the full dose of 650 mg of aspirin or acetaminophen. Prescribing each drug separately provides a better method for individualizing pain control; this is particularly important when the patient requires escalation of the combination to provide analgesia,

TABLE 146.3

Nonopioid Analgesics for Mild to Moderate Pain

Class	Generic Name	Half-Life (h)	Dosing Schedule	Recommended Starting Dose (mg)	Maximum Starting Dose (mg)
Salicylates	Aspirin	3–12	q4–6h	2,600	6,000
	Choline magnesium trisalicylate	9–17	q12h	200	600
	Diflunisal	8–12	q12h	1,500 × 1, then 1,000 q12h	4,000
p-Aminophenol derivative	Acetaminophen (paracetamol)	2–4	q4–6h	2,600	4,000
Propionic acids	Ibuprofen	1.8–2	q4–8h	1,200	3,200
	Fenoprofen	2–3	q4–6h	800	3,200
	Ketoprofen	2–3	q6–8h	150	300
	Naproxen	13	q12h	550	1,100
	Naproxen sodium	13	q12h	550	1,100
Acetic acids	Etodolac	7	q6–8h	600	1,200
	Ketorolac	4–7	q6h	15–30 q6h IV, IM	120 IV, IM
				10 q6h PO	40 PO
Fenamates	Meclofenamic acid	1.3	q6–8h	150	400
	Mefenamic acid	2	q6h	500 × 1, then 250 q6h	1,000
COX-2 inhibitor	Celecoxib	11	qd–q12	100	200

IV, intravenous; IM, intramuscular; PO, by mouth.

in which case the additional amount of the NSAID or acetaminophen may become excessive.

Opioid Drugs for Cancer Pain Management. The opioid analgesics, of which morphine is the prototype, vary in potency, efficacy, and adverse effects. These drugs produce their analgesic effects by binding to discrete opiate receptors in the peripheral and central nervous systems. In contrast to the nonopioid analgesics, opioid analgesics, at least the opioid pure agonists, do not appear to have a ceiling effect (i.e., as the dose is escalated on a log scale, the increment in analgesia is linear to the point of loss of consciousness). There are also series of drugs that are pure antagonists (i.e., they block the effect of morphine at the receptor). The antagonist drug most commonly used in clinical practice is naloxone, which is administered to reverse respiratory depression and other complications associated with opioid overdose.

Effective use of opioids requires the balancing of the most desirable effects of pain relief with the undesirable effects of nausea, vomiting, mental clouding, sedation, constipation, tolerance, and physical dependence. These undesirable effects impose a practical limit on the dose useful for a particular patient and have led to the concept of opioid responsiveness.

The use of opioids in the management of cancer pain remains controversial.[5,76–90] Some of the controversies include their role in the management of neuropathic pain, which has been suggested to be *opioid resistant*, the specific choice of opioid drug, the use of sequential trials of opioids, routes of administration, the development of tolerance, risk of addiction, economic factors influencing these controversies, and the concern that opioids are agents of physician-assisted suicide and euthanasia. The following principles take into account these controversies while laying out a basic approach to the use of opioids in cancer pain management (Table 146.4).

1. Start with a specific drug for a specific type of pain. As defined by the WHO three-step analgesic ladder, the specific drug chosen depends in part on the degree of pain intensity and the type of pain. Cancer patients commonly have multiple sites and types of pain. A continuum of opioid responsiveness, rather than an all-or-none phenomenon, has been clearly observed. *Opioid responsiveness* is defined as the degree of analgesia achieved during dose escalation to either intolerable side effects or adequate analgesia. Patient characteristics and pain-related factors, as well as drug-selective effects, influence this variable response.[89]

It has been suggested that neuropathic pain, which accounts for 15% to 20% of pain problems that are difficult to manage, is opioid resistant and that opioid drugs should not be used in this patient population.[82] In fact, studies that explored reasons for inadequate pain treatment have identified that up to two-thirds of cancer pain patients have some contribution of neuropathic pain to their global pain syndrome[66]; when the concept of bone pain as a neuropathic pain syndrome is included, this number increases.[39] Studies of cancer patients with both nociceptive and neuropathic pain, as well as controlled studies of nonmalignant neuropathic pain, demonstrate the variable responsiveness of neuropathic pain to opioid analgesics. Hence, the contribution of neuropathic pain must be considered when assessing opioid responsiveness.

A wide range of adjuvant analgesics has been suggested to provide analgesia alone or in combination with opioid drug therapy, and there are specific adjuvants for bone pain and neuropathic pain. The choice of a specific drug is dictated not only by pain intensity and type of pain, but also by the patient's prior opioid exposure and history of allergy or side effects.

The WHO's Cancer Pain Relief Program has developed cancer pain guidelines that designate morphine as the drug of choice based on practical, not scientific, considerations. The introduction of the WHO program rapidly demonstrated the limited availability of morphine worldwide for the oral treatment of chronic cancer pain.[6,17] Morphine consumption worldwide is now used as an indicator of the success of the WHO Cancer Pain Relief Program.[18] Controlled-release oral morphine is currently available in a wide range of doses from 15 to 200 mg; differing products provide options for every 8-, 12-, and 24-hour administration. These preparations

TABLE 146.4

Guidelines for the Rational Use of Analgesics in the Management of Cancer Pain

Start with a Specific Drug for a Specific Type of Pain
Know the pharmacology of the drug prescribed.
Know the relative potency of the drug.
Know the duration of the analgesic effect.
Know the pharmacokinetics of the drug.
Know the equianalgesic doses for the drug and its route of administration.

Administer Analgesic on a Regular Basis
Gear the route of administration to the patient's needs
Oral
Buccal
Rectal
Subcutaneous
Intrathecal
Sublingual
Transmucosal
Transdermal
Intravenous
Intraventricular

Use a Combination of Drugs to Provide Additive Analgesia
Narcotic plus nonnarcotic (aspirin, acetaminophen, nonsteroidal anti-inflammatory drugs)
Narcotic plus adjuvants

Anticipate and Treat Side Effects
Sedation
Respiratory depression
Nausea and vomiting
Constipation
Multifocal myoclonus and seizures

Management of the Tolerant Patient
Use combinations of nonopioid and opioid drugs.
Use combinations of drug therapy, anesthetic, and neurosurgical procedures.
Switch to an alternative opioid analgesic, starting with one-half the equianalgesic dose.
Use epidural local anesthetics.
Reassess the nature of the pain.

Prevent and Treat Acute Withdrawal
Taper drugs slowly.

Anticipate Complications
Overdose
Psychological dependence

provide analgesia comparable to that of immediate-release forms and offer increased convenience, improved compliance, and a reduction in the duration of pain. Historically, the dogma was to titrate patients to adequate pain relief using 4-hourly doses and then combine into sustained-release doses that provide an equal amount of opioid in 24 hours. In a recent randomized clinical trial, it was demonstrated that for cancer pain patients receiving greater than 60 mg OMEs daily, titration with a sustained release product was equally efficacious and yielded fewer side effects.[91]

The clinician's armamentarium for managing cancer pain now encompasses a series of opioid alternatives to morphine, including congeners of morphine—hydromorphone, oxycodone, and oxymorphone—as well as methadone, levorphanol, fentanyl, and buprenorphine. The choice of agent depends on the clinician's knowledge about how to use the drug, patient factors such as age and renal function, route of delivery, opioid availability, and cost (Tables 146.5 and 146.6). Recently, new formulations of these drugs have been marketed with various combinations to deter tampering and to reduce their diversion.[92]

Hydromorphone has poor oral availability and a short half-life. Its high solubility and availability in high-potency parenteral form (10 mg per milliliter) make it a useful choice for chronic subcutaneous administration. Because of its short half-life, it is commonly used in the elderly patient. Myoclonus has been reported after high doses, possibly due to an accumulation of its metabolites (3-0 methyl-glucuronide and hydromorphone-6-glucuronide).[93] When compared in a double-blind trial of patient-controlled analgesia, no differences in analgesia or side effects were noted between morphine and hydromorphone; these findings have been confirmed in several settings.[94,95] Although cognitive performance was poor in the hydromorphone group, patients reported better mood than those who received morphine. A slow-release 24-hour formulation was recently released, but clinical experience thus far remains limited, and its cost is high.

Oxycodone, which is commonly administered in a 5-mg dose at the second step of the WHO analgesic ladder, can also be used in the third step at higher doses. It is available in a slow-release preparation.[96] Its half-life is 3 to 4 hours. Oxymorphone is its active metabolite. Oxymorphone is currently available in oral sustained

release, intravenous, and rectal preparations and serves as an alternative to morphine and its other congeners. Oxymorphone has a reduced histamine effect and may be of use in patients who complain of headache or itch after the administration of other opioids.

Levorphanol has high bioavailability but a long plasma half-life (12 to 16 hours). It should be used cautiously because, with repeated administration, accumulation may occur.

The role of methadone in managing cancer pain also remains controversial.[5,76,87,88,90] Methadone represents a second-line drug for cancer pain patients who have had prior exposure to opioids. It is a relatively inexpensive oral analgesic, but its name has negative connotations for cancer patients, who view methadone as a

TABLE 146.5

Relative Single-Dose Potencies of Commonly Used Opioid Drugs for Pain and Their Oral–Intravenous Ratios

Drug	Equianalgesic Intravenous or Intramuscular Dose (mg)	Oral–Intravenous Ratios
Morphine	10	3
Oxycodone	Not available	Not available
Oxymorphone	1	10–15
Hydromorphone	1.5	5
Methadone[a]	10	1–2
Levorphanol	2	2
Fentanyl	100 µg	1 (transdermal intravenous)

This table should be used as a guide only. Individual dosing and drug selection depend on each patient's particular situation and comprehensive assessment.
[a] Refer to Table 146.6 for rotation to methadone for long-term administration.

TABLE 146.6

Variability in Dose Ratios When Switching Oral Morphine, Oral Hydromorphone, and Transdermal Fentanyl to Methadone

Dose	Morphine–Methadone Ratio
Morphine (mg/24 h)	
30–90	4:1
91–300	9:1
≥300	12:1
Hydromorphone (mg/24 h)	Hydromorphone–methadone ratio
<330	0.95:1
≥330	1.6:1
Fentanyl	Fentanyl–methadone ratio
50–2,500 [mu] g/h	250 [mu] g/h:1 mg/h

Based on direct morphine to methadone, hydromorphone to methadone, and fentanyl to methadone conversion studies, when the clinician needs to rotate to methadone convert all opioids first to intravenous (IV) morphine (see Table 146.5 for equianalgesic dose ratios) and then convert the IV morphine dose to an IV methadone dose using a 10:1 ratio. The resulting methadone dose may be higher in less opioid-tolerant patients and lower in highly opioid-tolerant patients (see Moryl et al.[5]).

drug used to treat addicts. The bioavailability of methadone is higher than that of morphine (85% versus 35%, respectively). Its analgesic potency also differs, with a parenteral to oral ratio of 1:2 in contrast to 1:6 for morphine. Moreover, the plasma half-life of methadone is 17 to 24 hours, with reports of up to 50 hours in some cancer patients, but with an analgesic duration of only 4 to 8 hours. Significant adverse effects have been reported in cancer patients receiving methadone by various routes. Most notably, reports of drug-induced long QT syndrome have increased concern, especially in cancer patients who may be on multiple agents that can prolong the QT interval.[97–99] The discrepancy between the analgesic duration and plasma half-life of methadone has made it a difficult drug to use in the naïve patient because of the need for careful titration. In a randomized trial, the initial treatment of cancer pain with morphine versus methadone provided equal analgesic efficacy.[100]

A number of case reports have highlighted the possibly greater analgesic potency of methadone than the often quoted 1:1 equivalency with morphine.[76,87,88,90] Studies of interindividual differences in response to opioid analgesics have demonstrated that dramatically reduced dosages of methadone are required to produce analgesia in patients chronically taking morphine or hydromorphone. Several authors have shown marked reductions in the equianalgesic dose of methadone when patients with either uncontrolled pain or extreme side effects were switched to methadone.[5,90] These clinical survey studies suggested up to a 75% reduction in the methadone equianalgesic dose when switching from hydromorphone to methadone (see Table 146.6).

In a prospective study, Ripamonti et al.[90] developed a specific dose ratio based on the patients' morphine doses. For patients taking 30 to 90 mg of morphine, the dose ratio is 4:1; for those taking 90 to 300 mg daily, the dose ratio is 6:1; and for those taking 300 mg or more, the dose ratio is 8:1. Bruera et al.[76] developed a similar ratio for hydromorphone based on survey data. In patients who received more than 330 mg of hydromorphone, the dose ratio is 1.6:1.0; and in those who received less than 300 mg, the dose ratio is 0.95:1.0.

Studies of the use of methadone by experienced clinicians in caring for advanced cancer patients at home report fewer dose escalations and good pain control, which supports the use of methadone in home settings.[87] Methadone can be administered

by a variety of routes, but the subcutaneous route is associated with adverse effects, including cutaneous hypersensitivity.[101] Due to its long half-life, some offer the suggestion that methadone be administered every 8 to 12 hours, whereas others have demonstrated analgesic efficacy and safety in acute 3- to 4-hour dosing intervals.[102] Ongoing studies are attempting to better elucidate the clinical pharmacology of methadone to facilitate its broader use.

Meperidine is a drug that should not be used chronically in the management of patients with cancer pain. Meperidine has a poor parenteral to oral ratio (1:4). It is available in oral and intramuscular preparations, but repetitive intramuscular administration is associated with local tissue fibrosis and sterile abscess. Repetitive dosing of meperidine (more than 250 mg per day) can lead to the accumulation of normeperidine, an active metabolite that can produce central nervous system hyperexcitability.[103] This hyperirritability is characterized by subtle mood effects followed by tremors, multifocal myoclonus, and occasional seizures. It occurs most commonly in patients with renal disease but can also occur after the repeated administration in patients with normal renal function. Naloxone does not reverse meperidine-induced seizures, and its use in meperidine toxicity is controversial. There have been some case reports that the use of naloxone has precipitated generalized seizures in individual patients. In rare instances, central nervous system toxicity characterized by hyperpyrexia, muscle rigidity, and seizure has been reported after the administration of a single dose of meperidine to patients receiving treatment with monoamine oxidase inhibitors. Recent reports of potentially fatal serotonin syndromes due to concurrent use of meperidine with selective serotonin reuptake inhibitors (SSRI) or with the antimicrobial linezolid raise further concern about the safety profile of this medication.[104–106]

The availability of transdermal patches and various transmucosal preparations facilitates the use of fentanyl for the management of both acute and chronic pain.[107] The half-life of fentanyl is 1 to 2 hours. Published guidelines for fentanyl use summarize available data.[85] In chronic cancer pain management, relative potency comparisons have not been fully established, but the common dosing guideline is that 10 mg of intravenous morphine is equivalent to 100 μg of intravenous fentanyl (see http://www.aahpm.org/pdf/equianalgesictable.pdf). The uniqueness of the available fentanyl preparations facilitates the management of patients who are unable to take drugs by mouth by providing them with continuous opioid analgesia. Patches are currently available in 12.5 to 100 μg per hour doses and are changed every 72 hours. When a patient is started on the fentanyl patch, there is up to a 12- to 15-hour delay in the onset of analgesia, and a 24- to 72-hour equilibration period; alternate approaches must be used to maintain pain control during this early period. Patients should be cautioned about factors that can impact the absorption rate of the drug from the patch, such as heating pads, sweating, or fever; deaths likely relating to these issues led to an FDA advisory. Proper disposal is also paramount, given the risk posed by unintentional exposure to caregivers or children. Of note, reliable drug absorption requires adequate subcutaneous fat to be present; topical fentanyl may not be appropriate in the setting of cachexia. Specific guidelines for switching to the fentanyl patch after an intravenous infusion of fentanyl have been developed and are based on use of a 1:1 conversion ratio.[85] Fentanyl can also be used as an anesthetic premedication, as well as intravenously for pain control. Oral transmucosal and sublingual formulations have demonstrated effectiveness in treating breakthrough pain in cancer patients.[85,108,109]

Buprenorphine, a mixed agonist/antagonist opioid drug, is used to treat chronic noncancer pain and drug addiction and is also available in a transdermal preparation for cancer pain management. It is reported to be a useful agent in patients with moderate to severe pain, and it does not accumulate in patients with renal dysfunction. Its place in the management of cancer pain among the other opioids is not yet fully clarified.[110]

PALLIATIVE AND ALTERNATIVE CARE

2. Know the equianalgesic dose of the drug and its route of administration. Knowing the equianalgesic dose (i.e., the dose of one analgesic drug that is equivalent in the pain-relieving potential of another analgesic drug) can ensure more appropriate drug use. The equianalgesic dose guides the recommended starting dose, with the optimal dose for each patient determined by dose adjustment. *Relative potency* is the ratio of the doses of two analgesics required to produce the same effect. Estimates of relative potency allow for a calculation of the equianalgesic dose, which provides the basis for selecting the appropriate dose when switching drugs or changing the route of administration of the same drug. The values in Table 146.5 are based on studies using 10 mg of morphine as the standard dose.[111] There is now evidence to suggest that relative potency may differ in single-dose and repeated-dose studies. For example, for morphine, a 1:6 relative analgesic potency ratio should be used for patients with acute pain, whereas a 1:2 or 1:3 ratio is more appropriate in patients treated with repeated doses on a chronic basis. Lack of attention to differences in drug dose is the most common cause of undermedication of pain.

3. Administer analgesics regularly after initial titration. Medication should be given regularly to maintain the plasma level of the drug above the minimum effective concentration for pain relief. In the initial titration, patients should be advised to take their medication as needed to determine their total 24-hour requirements. During this time, the patient should reach the steady-state level of drug, which depends on the drug's half-life. For morphine, a steady state can be reached in 24 hours; with methadone, it may take up to 5 to 7 days to reach a steady state. In patients on a fixed schedule, rescue medications equivalent to one-half of the standing dose should be available for breakthrough pain.

Continuous intravenous and subcutaneous opioid infusions to manage both acute and chronic cancer pain are commonly administered using a patient-controlled analgesic pump programmed to the patient's need with a set *lock-out time* to prevent overdosing. This method of drug administration is especially useful in managing patients with breakthrough pain. It is a significant advance in facilitating adequate titration of analgesics in chronic cancer patients, allowing discharge to home and hospice settings.

4. Gear the route of administration to the patient's needs. Various methods of opioid drug delivery have been developed in order to maximize pharmacologic effects and minimize side effects. Most patients require at least two routes of drug administration, and 20% need up to four approaches during the course of their cancer pain treatment.

The oral route is preferable and easy. Orally administered drugs have a slower onset of action, delayed peak time, and longer duration of effect. Drugs given parenterally have a rapid onset of action but a shorter duration of effect. Slow-release preparations of morphine, hydromorphone, and oxycodone allow more convenient dosing every 8 to 12 hours, or every 24 hours.

For cancer pain management by the sublingual route, well-absorbed drugs include fentanyl and methadone.[112] Oral transmucosal fentanyl citrate preparations and intranasal sprays have been widely studied for the management of breakthrough pain and are increasingly available.

For the rectal route, oxymorphone, hydromorphone, and morphine are available in suppository form. Oxymorphone suppositories produce analgesia equivalent to 10 mg of parenteral morphine. Slow-release oxycodone and morphine preparations have also been demonstrated to be effective rectally, and ongoing studies with rectal methadone suggest that this drug is well absorbed by the rectal route.

The transdermal route is a convenient way to deliver a potent short-acting opioid on a continuous basis. Drug is released through the skin patch at a nearly constant amount per unit time with a concentration gradient from patch to skin. Serum fentanyl concentrations increase and steady-state levels are approached at 12 to 24 hours.[109] After patch removal, the drug persists in the skin, with falling blood levels over 24 hours. Innovative transdermal delivery systems are in phase 3 testing, which include systems for immediate-dose delivery using iontophoresis and drug reservoirs. Iontophoresis is the transfer of ionic solutes through biologic membranes under the influence of an electric field. It offers an alternative system for parenteral administration and has been shown to allow for comparatively rapid achievement of fentanyl dose levels using a transdermal system.

Various parenteral routes include intermittent and continuous subcutaneous, intravenous, epidural, intraventricular, and intrathecal infusions. The use of intermittent and continuous subcutaneous infusions is most appropriate for patients who cannot tolerate oral analgesics because of GI obstruction or intractable nausea and vomiting, and for those who do not have intravenous access. The utility of this technique has been demonstrated using morphine, heroin, hydromorphone, levorphanol, and fentanyl. The administration of methadone by this route is associated with the development of a cutaneous hypersensitivity syndrome.[101]

Patient-controlled analgesic pumps designed to infuse continuously but with options for bolus administration are connected to a 27-gauge butterfly needle that the patient can insert into a new subcutaneous site every 3rd to 6th day. Limited pharmacokinetic studies have demonstrated that, for example, systemic absorption of the drug at a steady state reaches 87% bioavailability from subcutaneous infusion of hydromorphone.[95] Intermittent and continuous intravenous infusions are used if intravenous access is available and more commonly in patients who are hospitalized. Specific guidelines for the use of continuous infusions have been developed.[5,113]

The use of intermittent and continuous epidural and intrathecal opioid infusions is based on the demonstration of opioid receptors in the dorsal horn of the spinal cord and the availability of opioid drugs to suppress noxious stimuli at the spinal cord level. Localized selective analgesia is produced without motor or sensory blockade. An analysis of the pharmacokinetics of epidural opioid administration demonstrates that there is significant systemic uptake after epidural injection, comparable with that after an intramuscular injection of the same drug and dose. However, distribution of the drug directly into the cerebrospinal fluid is 10 to 100 times greater. Existing studies demonstrate that this approach is used with approximately 10% of cancer patients to maximize analgesia and minimize side effects. This technique is commonly used in patients who have mixed nociceptive neuropathic pain syndromes and in whom combinations of local anesthetics and opioids are administered epidurally. A 3-year retrospective outcome study of the use of epidural catheters in the management of chronic cancer pain identified the occurrence of technical problems and infection, including epidural abscesses, in a significant number of patients. The study suggests that epidural catheters be used in patients with limited life expectancy.[114]

Smith et al.[115] completed a randomized clinical trial in which an implantable drug delivery system was compared to comprehensive medical management of refractory cancer pain. The patients using the implantable system reported better pain relief with fewer drug side effects and improved survival. Cost-effectiveness studies have not been done, but there is clearly the added cost of the pump, and the costs of the system need to be compared to the costs of nonpump medicines, with the potential savings from prevention of hospitalizations for pain management analyzed. Rarely, intraventricular opioid infusion has been used to manage patients with pain in the cervical and craniofacial region from tumor infiltration.[116] Doses between 1.0 and 7.5 mg per 24 hours have been used, and excellent results have been reported in 70% of patients. At present, there is not a clear indication that this intraventricular route offers special advantages over systemic approaches.

5. Use a combination of drugs. By using a combination of drugs, the physician can increase analgesic effects without escalating the opioid dose. Combinations that produce additive analgesic effects include an opioid plus a nonopioid, an opioid plus an antihistamine (100 mg of intramuscular hydroxyzine), and an opioid plus an amphetamine (10 mg of intramuscular dextroamphetamine).[117-119]

6. *Anticipate and treat side effects.* The side effects of the opioid analgesics often limit their effective use. The most common side effects are sedation, respiratory depression, nausea, vomiting, constipation, and multifocal myoclonus and seizures.

Sedation and drowsiness vary with the drug and dose and may occur after both single and repeated administration. They are mediated through activation of opiate receptors in the reticular formation and diffusely throughout the cortex. Management of these effects includes reducing the individual drug dose while giving the drug more frequently, or switching to an analgesic with a shorter plasma half-life. In controlled trials, amphetamine, methylphenidate, and caffeine have been demonstrated to counteract opioid-induced sedative effects. It is important to discontinue all other drugs that might exacerbate the sedative effects of opioid analgesics, including a wide variety of medications such as cimetidine, barbiturates, and other anxiolytics.

Respiratory depression is the most serious adverse effect of the opioid drugs. It occurs most commonly after short-term administration of an opioid and is usually associated with other signs of central nervous system depression, including sedation and drowsiness. The opioid agonist drugs act on brain stem respiratory centers to produce, as a function of dose, increasing respiratory depression to the point of apnea. Tolerance to this effect develops rapidly with repeated drug administration, which allows for prolonged use without significant risk of respiratory depression. Respiratory depression can be reversed by giving the short-acting opioid antagonist naloxone (suggested dose: 0.4 mg per milliliter). Repeated administration, including an intravenous drip, may be necessary to prevent respiratory arrest in such patients. In patients receiving opioids for prolonged periods who develop respiratory depression, diluted doses of naloxone (0.4 mg in 10 mL of saline) should be titrated carefully to prevent the precipitation of severe withdrawal symptoms while reversing the respiratory depression. A useful dosing nomogram for continuous intravenous infusion of naloxone has been developed in which two-thirds of the initial bolus is started on an hourly basis and titrated against the patient's symptoms.[120]

In some patients, the use of naloxone to reverse drug-induced respiratory depression can be dangerous. An endotracheal tube should be placed in the comatose patient before giving naloxone to prevent aspiration from excessive salivation and bronchial spasm induced by naloxone administration. In patients receiving meperidine over a longer period, naloxone may precipitate seizures by lowering the seizure threshold and by allowing the convulsant activity of the active metabolite, normeperidine, to become evident. In this instance, special attention must be given to the potential seizure effect of naloxone. If naloxone is used, diluted doses, slow titration, and appropriate seizure precautions are advised. There is insufficient clinical evidence to make more specific recommendations. If respiratory support can be affected by other means (i.e., continuous stimulation to maintain the patient's wakefulness), such an approach may place the patient at less risk and clearly in less discomfort.

The opioid analgesics produce nausea and vomiting by an action limited to the medullary chemoreceptor trigger zone. The incidence of nausea and vomiting is markedly increased in ambulatory patients. Tolerance develops to these side effects with repeated administration. The occurrence of nausea with one drug does not mean that all drugs will produce it. Switching to alternative opioid analgesics and using an antiemetic together with the opioid analgesic are ways to obviate this effect. Lack of controlled trials to identify a specific first-line agent has supported the practice of using sequential trials of agents, beginning with prochlorperazine concurrently with the opioid, to clarify a useful regimen. Droperidol has also been noted to be effective against opioid-induced nausea and vomiting.[121] Low doses of haloperidol may also be effective.

Constipation results from the action of these drugs at multiple sites in the GI tract and in the spinal cord to produce a decrease in the intestinal secretions and peristalsis, which leads to dry stools and constipation. When opioid analgesics are started, a regular bowel regimen, including use of cathartics and stool softeners, should also be instituted. Laxative bowel regimens have been suggested because of their specific ability to counteract the effects of the opioid drugs, but none has been studied in a controlled way. Anecdotal surveys suggest that doses far above those used for routine bowel management are needed, that senna derivatives are effective, and that careful attention to dietary factors along with the use of a bowel regimen can reduce patient complaints dramatically. Tolerance to this effect develops over time, but relatively slowly. Oral naloxone has been shown to be effective in treating constipation, but its use is variable depending on the degree of opioid exposure of the patient; oral naloxone may reverse the analgesic effect of the opioid.[122] Clinical trials of two peripherally acting opioid antagonists, methylnaltrexone and alvimopan, have proved the concept that these drugs prevent opioid-induced constipation by targeting mu opioid receptors in the gut without interfering with analgesia and are available for clinical use in selected patients; only methylnaltrexone is FDA-approved for the indication of opioid-induced constipation.[122,123]

Multifocal myoclonus may occur with high doses of all of the opioid drugs. Multifocal myoclonus and seizures have been reported in patients receiving multiple doses of meperidine (250 mg or more per day), although signs and symptoms of central nervous system hyperirritability may occur with toxic doses of all the opioid analgesics. In a series of cancer patients receiving meperidine, accumulation of the active metabolite normeperidine was associated with these neurologic signs and symptoms. However, in a similar group of cancer patients with pain, subtle mood effects were noted after meperidine administration, which suggests a spectrum of central nervous system effects. Management of this hyperirritability includes discontinuing the meperidine, using intravenous diazepam if seizures occur, and substituting morphine to control the persistent pain. Because the half-life of normeperidine is 16 hours, it may take 2 or 3 days for the signs of central nervous system hyperirritability to clear completely. As previously, meperidine may also result in a fatal serotonin syndrome when used in conjunction with monoamine oxidase inhibitor (MAOI) drugs or possible even SSRIs. Its use is contraindicated in patients with chronic renal disease, but these complications as noted in cancer pain treatment occurred in patients with normal renal function.[103] Morphine and hydromorphone at high doses produce myoclonus, which has not been directly associated with their known active metabolite such as M6G and hydromorphone-6-glucuronide. In dying patients with myoclonus, the use of benzodiazepines or barbiturates has been reported anecdotally to suppress this sign, improving the patient's comfort.

Opioid hyperexcitability has been reported with the use of increasing opioid doses by the parenteral and epidural routes. They have most often been observed in patients on high doses of morphine and hydromorphone and are characterized by uncontrolled pain, hypervigilance, total body hyperalgesia, and allodynia. They are best managed by rapid dose reduction and substitution with an alternative opioid such as methadone. The mechanism of action is unclear.

7. *Manage tolerance.* The earliest sign of developing tolerance is the patient's complaint that the duration of effective analgesia has decreased. For reasons not yet understood, cancer patients develop tolerance at vastly different rates. Some demonstrate tolerance within days of initiating opioid therapy; others experience pain control for many months on the same dosage. Studies in an outpatient clinic population, a hospitalized population, and a home care population revealed three patterns of drug use: a rapid increase in opioid requirements, stabilization at one dose for several weeks or months, and a decrease or elimination of opioids.[124] Increased opioid requirements are most commonly associated with

disease progression rather than with tolerance alone. With the development of tolerance, increases in the frequency of the dose of the opioid are required to provide continued pain relief. Because the analgesic effect is a logarithmic function of the dose of opioid, a doubling of the dose may be needed to restore full analgesia. There appears to be no limit to the development of tolerance, and with appropriate dose adjustments patients can continue to obtain pain relief. Tolerance to the respiratory effects of opioid doses occurs. This degree of tolerance makes it safe for patients to increase their opioid doses for analgesia.

Tolerance to one opioid does not lead to complete tolerance to another opioid. This phenomenon of so-called *incomplete cross-tolerance* is best exemplified in the dramatic reduction in dosages needed to provide analgesia when patients are switched from, for example, morphine or hydromorphone to methadone, as previously discussed.[76,87,88,90] Further data elucidating the mechanism of opioid tolerance demonstrate that the N-methyl-D-aspartate (NMDA) receptor plays a critical role in opioid tolerance and analgesia.[125] These findings have focused new attention on methadone's opioid and nonopioid mechanisms of action and its potential role in the management of neuropathic pain. The use of analgesic combinations can reduce the amount of opioid required. Similarly, the use of bolus or continuous epidural local anesthetics in patients with perineal pain can dramatically reduce the need for systemic opioids and reverse tolerance.

8. *Taper drugs slowly.* The long-term administration of opioid analgesics is associated with the development of physical dependence; thereafter, the sudden cessation of the opioid analgesic produces signs and symptoms of withdrawal: agitation, tremors, insomnia, fear, marked autonomic nervous system hyperexcitability, and exacerbation of pain. Slowly tapering the dose of the opioid analgesic prevents such symptoms. The appearance of abstinence symptoms from the time of drug withdrawal is related to the elimination half-life for the particular drug. For example, with morphine, withdrawal symptoms occur within 6 to 12 hours after drug cessation. Reinstituting the drug in doses of approximately 25% of the previous daily dose suppresses these symptoms.

9. *Anticipate complications.* An overdose with opioid analgesics occurs either intentionally, when a patient takes an excessive amount of drug in a suicide attempt, or unintentionally, when the recommended dose accidentally produces excessive sedation and respiratory depression. In both instances, the complication can be treated effectively with naloxone. Intentional overdose in cancer patients occurs rarely, and concern for this is overemphasized. An overdose in patients previously stabilized on an opioid regimen for cancer pain rarely is caused by drug intake alone. More commonly, the cause is the medical deterioration of the patient with a superimposed metabolic encephalopathy. Reducing the opioid drug dosage and carefully assessing the patient's metabolic status usually provide the differential diagnosis.

Psychological dependence or addiction is characterized by a concomitant behavioral pattern of drug abuse evidenced by craving a drug for other than pain relief and overwhelming involvement in the use and procurement of the drug. This is a state distinct from tolerance and physical dependence, which are responses to the pharmacologic effects of long-term opioid administration. The profound fear of causing psychological dependence plays a major role in a physician's reluctance to prescribe opioid analgesics, particularly in cancer patients in the early phase of their disease. Patients may share this fear, consistently taking less analgesic drug than is effective to control their pain. Increasing evidence suggests that cancer patients with pain can take opioid analgesics for prolonged periods but can discontinue such drugs when adequate pain relief is achieved using other approaches. In almost all instances, a dramatic escalation of drug intake is associated with the progression of disease and subsequent death. Few patients with cancer and pain become psychologically dependent on the drugs and participate in drug seeking and illicit drug use. A careful evaluation of patients who might be at risk for

this complication is necessary, but such concern should not be punitive to the patient with severe cancer pain.

Out-of-control, aberrant drug taking among oncology patients with or without a prior history of substance abuse represents a serious and complex clinical occurrence. Passik and Portenoy[35] have developed guidelines for the management of such patients. The most difficult situations present themselves in the patient who is actively abusing illicit or prescription drugs or alcohol while concurrently receiving medical therapies. Such patients need a multidisciplinary approach usually focused on a harm-reduction concept that attempts to enhance social support for the patient to maximize treatment compliance. Passik and Portenoy have outlined a series of approaches to maximize the effectiveness of strategies for promoting compliance, including the consideration of a written contract between the team and patient, the inclusion of spot urine toxicology screens to assess compliance, set expectations regarding attendance at the clinic, and the patient's management of medication supplies. It is often most useful to see the patient on a regular basis, often every several days, and to limit prescribing opioids on that basis until the patient has demonstrated his or her willingness to be compliant and to follow an appropriate drug regimen. In an inpatient setting when patients demonstrate manipulative behaviors in the inappropriate use of medication, directing discussion with the patient about the drug use in an open manner is a first step. Providing the patient with a private room near the nurses' station to monitor the patient, discouraging attempts to leave the hospital for the purchase of illicit drugs, and requiring visitors to check in with the nursing staff before visitation are additional steps. Underlying all of this is the attempt to provide the patient with a supportive environment that respects the patient's pain symptomatology and serious medical illness and attempts to limit harm to the patient or others by the aberrant drug use and behaviors.

Adjuvant Drugs

Adjuvant drugs are used to enhance opioid analgesia, provide analgesia for certain types of pain (e.g., neuropathic pain, bone pain, visceral pain), and treat opioid side effects or other symptoms associated with pain.[126] They are an integral part of the WHO three-step analgesic ladder. Because of the lack of well-defined guidelines for their use, sequential drug trials are necessary to identify the most useful drug and dose titration to find a safe and effective dose.

Adjuvants to Enhance Analgesia

Adjuvants to enhance analgesia have been previously discussed in this chapter. Acetaminophen, NSAIDs, hydroxyzine, and dextroamphetamine have been demonstrated to provide additive analgesia to patients chronically receiving opioids.

Adjuvant Analgesics for Neuropathic Pain

The common neuropathic pain syndromes in patients with cancer include injury to the peripheral nerves and the plexus by tumor invasion, chemotherapy, surgery, or viral agents. Cancer-related bone pain may be a neuropathic pain syndrome as well.[39] Depending on the intensity of pain, nonopioid and opioid analgesics are the first-line agents. However, neuropathic pain has a variable responsiveness to opioid drug regimens and may be less responsive than other types of pain.[89] Some of the commonly used adjuvant drugs for managing this population of patients are described in the following sections.

Antidepressants

The tricyclic antidepressants (TCA) have historically been one of the most useful classes of psychotropic drugs applied in pain management.[127,128] Their analgesic effects are mediated by the enhancement of serotonin activity. Data from controlled trials indicate that both the tertiary amine TCAs (amitriptyline, doxepin, imipramine, and clomipramine) and the secondary amine compounds (desipramine and nortriptyline) have analgesic effects. Another major class of antidepressants, the SSRIs, is increasingly used as adjunctive therapies, given their preferable side effect profile compared to TCAs. Paroxetine, for example, has been shown to have analgesic properties in patients with neuropathic pain.[128] Similarly, duloxetine, a balanced and potent dual reuptake inhibitor of serotonin and norepinephrine, has recently been demonstrated to be an active analgesic for the management of diabetic peripheral neuropathic pain.[129] It was also shown to be superior to placebo in treating painful chemotherapy-induced peripheral neuropathy, yielding improvements in pain, function, and quality of life at a dose of 60 mg daily.[130]

These drugs have been reported to be effective in treating continuous dysesthesias as well as intermittent lancinating dysesthetic pain. The doses used for analgesia are far below those needed to produce an antidepressant effect, and the analgesic properties appear to be independent of the mood-altering effects. Patients should be started on low doses—for example, amitriptyline at 25 mg nightly—and the dose titrated up to achieve adequate analgesia in a 2- to 4-week trial. Blood levels should be measured to determine both patient compliance and drug absorption because of wide individual variation. Patients who are unable to tolerate amitriptyline or who are predisposed to experiencing its sedative, anticholinergic, or hypotensive effects should be considered for a trial with a secondary amine tricyclic antidepressant, an SSRI such as paroxetine, or duloxetine. In the management of cancer patients with pain, antidepressant drugs are the first-line therapeutic approach for neuropathic pain, and every attempt should be made to provide the patient with a several-week trial before discontinuing these drugs.

Anticonvulsants

The role of anticonvulsants in the management of patients with neuropathic pain is based, in part, on the fact that the mode of action is to stabilize membranes and alter sodium and calcium influx.[131] Many patients with neuropathic pain complain of paroxysmal, brief, and lancinating pains. To date, clinical experience with the anticonvulsants has been positive. The drugs most commonly used include gabapentin, carbamazepine, and phenytoin and pregabalin. Survey studies have suggested the usefulness of valproic acid, clonazepam, lamotrigine, topiramate, and oxcarbazepine.[132] A systematic review confirms these findings.[133,134] Gabapentin is considered the first-line anticonvulsant to manage neuropathic pain, although some meta-analyses suggest that it is equivocal with the other anticonvulsants.[133] Controlled trials in patients with diabetic neuropathy, postherpetic neuralgia, and AIDS neuropathy demonstrate the effectiveness of this agent in reducing pain. Dosages range from 900 to 1,800 mg per day.[134] The major drug side effect is sedation. Patients should be started at 300 mg per day and rapidly titrated to 900 mg per day; some patients may need to start at even lower doses, such as 100 mg per day, to avoid sedation. Pain relief in up to 30% to 50% of patients has been suggested.

Clinical studies with carbamazepine demonstrate efficacy, but the usefulness of this drug in the cancer population is limited by its potential to produce bone marrow suppression, particularly leukopenia. The dosing guidelines used for the treatment of seizures are suggested in managing neuropathic pain. Each of the drugs should be initiated at low doses and gradually titrated upward. There is anecdotal experience to suggest that administering intravenous loading doses of phenytoin to patients in an acute crisis with severe lancinating pain may be of clinical value. Both valproate and clonazepam have been reported anecdotally to be useful

in managing neuropathic pain, but these are considered third-line agents in this patient population.[132] Currently, there are no high-quality data relating the plasma level and pain relief for any of these drugs. In patients with persistent neuropathic cancer-related pain, pregabalin is another option; in a randomized controlled trial of patients with noncancer neuropathic pain, over half of the patients treated with pregabalin experienced a decrease in their mean pain intensity over 50%.[135] However, a recent systematic review highlights the absence of conclusive, high-quality data on the efficacy of pregabalin in treating neuropathic cancer pain.[136] Sequential trials of different agents are necessary to identify the most useful treatment for each patient.[127]

Local Anesthetics

The use of both brief intravenous local anesthetic infusions (lidocaine) and maintenance oral anesthetic drugs has demonstrated some efficacy in the management of chronic neuropathic pain, particularly in those patients with both lancinating and continuous dysesthesias. Mexiletine is the oral local anesthetic for which there are pilot data to support analgesic efficacy.[137] The initial dosage of mexiletine is low, at 150 mg per day, with gradual upward dose titration. Electrocardiograms should be monitored at higher doses, and measurement of blood levels of mexiletine may be useful to prevent toxicity. Currently, there are no good data available to predict which patients might respond to the use of oral local or intravenous anesthetics. A recent Cochrane review suggests that lidocaine and oral analogs are safe and superior to placebo; these agents should be tested further in the population of patients with neuropathic cancer pain.[138]

Epidural local anesthetics (bupivacaine, lidocaine) have been most widely used to manage neuropathic pain, either alone or in combination with an opioid. Alternatively, the use of brief intravenous infusions of lidocaine may be helpful in patients who have an opioid-refractory continuous dysesthesia that has not responded to an antidepressant or anticonvulsant.[139] These drugs clearly serve as a second-line approach, with individualized therapy the rule. An anesthesia pain specialist or palliative medicine specialist should be called to assist with these complex and potentially dangerous medications.

Cutaneous Local Anesthetics

The use of cutaneous anesthesia has been suggested to be most helpful in patients who have significant allodynia and marked hyperesthesia. The topical application of a local anesthetic, such as an eutectic mixture of local anesthetics, has been demonstrated to be efficacious in patients who undergo painful procedures, especially children.[140] The cream should be applied under an occlusive dressing to increase skin penetration and augment analgesic efficacy. The use of high-concentration lidocaine (5% and 10%) has also been reported to be effective in patients with significant allodynia associated with postherpetic neuralgia.[141] Current indications for its use include peripheral nerve injury, peripheral neuropathy, ischemic pain, peripheral vascular disease, and unstable angina. Few cancer patients have been treated using this approach and, therefore, it is not possible to fully assess its role in cancer pain management.

Corticosteroids

A series of controlled and uncontrolled surveys have demonstrated that the use of chronic corticosteroid therapy to reduce pain in patients with breast and prostate cancer improves quality of life.[142,143] In a controlled study of corticosteroid use in patients with far-advanced disease, transient improvement in appetite, analgesia, and mood were noted, but they were not sustained after the initial effect. The major pain-related indications for corticosteroid use include refractory neuropathic pain, bone pain, pain associated with capsular expansion or duct obstruction, and headache due to increased intracranial pressure. In certain cancer pain syndromes, such as epidural cord compression, 85% of patients who received 96 mg of dexamethasone as part of their radiation therapy protocol reported significant pain relief associated with a marked reduction in analgesic requirements.[144] Similarly, in patients with tumor infiltration of the brachial and lumbosacral plexus, corticosteroids provided additive analgesic effects. The risk of adverse effects associated with corticosteroid therapy varies with the duration. Long-term use may be associated with GI toxicity and acute psychosis. A wide range of dosages has been suggested, including a dose of 30 mg per day in patients with prostate cancer, which was effective at providing improved quality of life and reduced pain. With epidural cord compression, initial doses of 96 mg of dexamethasone with maintenance doses of 96 mg, with subsequent tapering in 10 days, have been associated with effective analgesia.[144] However, more recent data suggest that lower doses are similarly efficacious, with reduced toxicity. Giving between 6 and 10 mg of dexamethasone intravenously or orally every 6 hours is reasonable and appears to be just as effective, with a lower rate of anxiety, restlessness, insomnia, hyperglycemia, and delirium.[145]

Other Adjuvant Drugs

A wide variety of other drugs have been used to manage neuropathic pain, including benzodiazepines, neuroleptics, α_2-adrenergic agonist drugs, NMDA antagonists, and peptides. Of the benzodiazepines, clonazepam is commonly used in patients with lancinating or paroxysmal pain. The use of these drugs must be balanced with their potential to cause somnolence and cognitive impairment. They serve as second- to third-line therapy in patients who have not responded to antidepressant or anticonvulsant drug therapy. Of the neuroleptics, pimozide has been reported to be analgesic in patients with trigeminal neuralgia.[146] Methotrimeprazine has been demonstrated to have analgesic properties comparable to those of morphine.[147] This drug has sedative, anxiolytic, and antiemetic properties and is commonly used in patients who have excessive opioid side effects. It provides analgesia by a nonopioid mechanism.

The coadministration of these drugs with opioids can often be effective in patients with neuropathic pain. Of the α_2-adrenergic agonist drugs, clonidine has been demonstrated to be analgesic in controlled trials.[148] It can be administered by either the oral or transdermal route and has been reported to be specifically effective in patients with dysesthetic pain, who demonstrate sympathetic hyperactivity. After intrathecal administration, clonidine was reported to improve pain in patients with intolerable neuropathic pain. Dextromethorphan and ketamine are two commercially available NMDA antagonists. The mechanism of action relates to the fact that the NMDA receptor reduces the development of the wind-up phenomenon, which occurs as a result of changes in the response of central dorsal horn neurons with neuropathic pain. Ketamine has demonstrated analgesic effects in observational studies, but an adequately powered randomized trial failed to show that ketamine infusion led to improved analgesia beyond that offered by opioids plus nonopioid coanalgesics.[149–153] Calcitonin has been reported to provide analgesia in patients with sympathetically maintained pain and in patients with acute phantom pain.[154] The mechanism underlying these analgesic effects is unknown, but it has suggested the empiric use of calcitonin in patients with refractory neuropathic pain.

Adjuvant Drugs for Bone Pain

Metastatic disease to bone is the most common cause of pain in patients with cancer. Analgesic drug therapy is commonly used to manage pain during the initial treatment with either chemotherapy or radiation therapy. Numerous investigators have identified a management approach for bone pain, which includes the use of specific surgical palliative approaches, radiotherapeutic approaches, hormonal therapies, and bone resorption inhibitors. Patients with multifocal metastatic bone disease that is refractory to routine treatments may benefit from the use of a series of agents, including the bisphosphonate compounds, gallium nitrate, calcitonin, and radiopharmaceuticals. The newer models of metastatic bone pain as neuropathic pain imply that more traditional neuropathic pain drugs may have an important role in managing bone pain.[39] For example, in a murine bone pain model, opioids and tricyclic antidepressants demonstrated analgesic efficacy.[155] The selection of any one of these treatments to manage metastatic bone pain needs to be individualized.

Bisphosphonate drugs such as pamidronate, zoledronate, clodronate, and etidronate bind to bone hydroxyapatite, inhibiting osteoclast activity, and are highly effective in the management of bony metastatic disease and in multiple myeloma.[156–160] The major indication for these drugs is to prevent skeletal morbidity, with data in breast cancer patients and patients with multiple myeloma showing efficacy in reducing fractures and bone pain. Pamidronate is usually administered as a brief infusion in a starting dose of 60 to 120 mg. Analgesia, if it occurs, usually appears within days but may accrue for many weeks with repeated infusions. In two studies, pamidronate at dosages of 30 to 60 mg every 2 weeks produced relief of pain in 30% to 60% of patients.[157,160] The analgesic effect of bisphosphonates appears to be dose dependent. Current recommendations include a regimen of intravenous pamidronate, 60 mg every 2 weeks for at least two or three treatments. If no response is obtained, therapy can be discontinued. If the drug is effective, a biweekly regimen can be continued. Zoledronate is administered at 4 mg intravenously over 15 minutes every 3 to 4 weeks. A systematic review suggests that it may be the most effective bisphosphonate in prostate cancer.[156] Clodronate may be administered orally (1,600 mg per day) and has been demonstrated to be efficacious in patients with breast cancer and multiple myeloma.

Calcitonin has also been reported anecdotally to be useful in patients with malignant bone pain, but the appropriate dose and dosing frequency have not been well defined.[161] Gallium nitrate has also been used with some efficacy in patients with metastatic bone pain, but due to limited experience, appropriate dosing guidelines have not been well defined, and nephrotoxicity has been reported.[162]

A new class of bone-modifying agents targets the so-called RANK ligand, or receptor activator of nuclear factor kappa B. High-quality clinical trials data suggest that denosumab, a monoclonal antibody against this new target, provides further reductions in skeletal-related events in patients with metastatic breast and prostate cancers beyond that provided by zoledronic acid.[163,164] Although there appeared to be less bone pain in breast cancer patients who received denosumab, research has focused on fracture rates; further research is needed to explore the impact of denosumab on pain itself, especially in light of its modest impact beyond traditional bisphosphonates and its significant cost.

Strontium-89 and samarium-153 are bone-seeking radiopharmaceuticals that have been recognized as useful in the treatment of bone pain secondary to metastatic disease.[165–167] Their use is indicated in patients with refractory multifocal pain due to osteoblastic lesions who have a life expectancy of longer than 3 months, who have sufficient bone marrow reserve (i.e., a platelet count above 60,000 and a white blood cell count above 2,400), and for whom there is no further planned myelosuppressive chemotherapy. The onset of effect is slow and may require several weeks, with peak effects at 2 to 3 months. Bone marrow suppression is the major adverse effect, with irreversible thrombocytopenia. Both radiopharmaceuticals have similar analgesic efficacy and side effects. More recently, radium-223, a novel alpha-particle–emitting compound, was shown to have significant efficacy in metastatic castrate-resistant prostate cancer.[168] It improved survival by 3.6 months and did so without significant myelosuppression or other adverse events. Early studies with this agent suggest a significant palliative effect on bone pain.[169] Patients with advanced prostate cancer and bone pain should be considered for treatment with this agent.

Adjuvants to Treat Side Effects

Nausea and vomiting, confusion, sedation, and constipation are common opioid-induced side effects. Side effects should be managed expectantly, rather than waiting until patients are experiencing negative consequences of analgesic therapy that aggravate the pain and suffering of cancer. The use of drugs to manage these effects has been discussed previously. The uses of caffeine, methylphenidate, and dextroamphetamine to reduce opioid-induced sedation have all been demonstrated in clinical trials. Haloperidol is the treatment of choice to manage hallucinations and agitated delirium in patients receiving opioid analgesics. The use of bowel regimens to manage depressed GI motility is critical. Because nearly all patients have some constipation when receiving opioids, a bowel regimen should be prescribed along with all opioid therapies, unless there is a serious contraindication.

PSYCHOLOGICAL APPROACHES

Psychological approaches should be an integral part of the care of the cancer patient with pain.[170] Studies strongly support an association between cancer pain and psychological distress, predominantly manifested as mood disturbance, anxiety, and depression.[171] Pain catastrophizing (i.e., the tendency to ruminate about pain and negatively evaluate one's ability to deal with pain) leads to increased pain intensity, pain interference, and anxiety. Similarly, patients who lack confidence in their ability to control pain experience lower quality of life and higher psychological distress. Worse pain leads to decreased social interactions, reduced social functioning, and poor social networks. At the other end of the spectrum, increased self-efficacy and active coping manifested by the sense of ability to control or decrease pain is associated with improved pain control. Given these psychological factors, it follows that psychological approaches would be effective adjuvant interventions for cancer pain.

Established behavioral therapies for cancer pain fall into three categories: (1) comprehensive cognitive behavioral therapy (CBT); (2) hypnosis and imagery-based CBT; and (3) psychoeducational interventions.[172] Comprehensive CBT comprises varied packages of adaptive strategies taught to a patient to maximize coping. There are several basic components, namely: (1) providing patients with a rationale that emphasizes pain as a complex experience influenced by thoughts, feelings, and behavior; (2) providing systematic training in one or more cognitive or behavioral strategies for controlling pain (e.g., progressive relaxation, imagery, goal setting, activity pacing) typically carried out over a series of sessions; and (3) emphasizing that the skills can only be mastered through home practice. In hypnosis-based CBT, a trained therapist helps the patient achieve a relaxed state and then actively provides specific hypnotic suggestions designed to enhance pain control and relaxation. In imagery-based CBT, also called *guided imagery*, the patient is taught how to intentionally focus his or her attention on specific mental images so as to divert attention from pain. Psychoeducational interventions combine patient education with behavioral techniques such a skills training, personal interaction with the learner, and repeat visits to reinforce key messages and skills. Biofeedback and caregiver-assisted approaches have been advocated and studied as well, but to date, most evaluations of these methods have been uncontrolled or preliminary.[170]

Behavioral therapies have a defined role in the management of nonmalignant pain,[173] but their role in cancer pain is less clear. A systematic review of behavioral interventions for cancer pain that compared their relative efficacy was conducted in 2005.[170] Cognitive behavioral interventions were effective in the management

of cancer-related pain. Imagery and hypnosis-based interventions were most effective. Education-focused interventions with brief CBT were intermediate, with 56% of the studies positive. Comprehensive CBT interventions were least effective, with less than half of studies positive and no obvious relationships between components of the comprehensive CBT package, intensity of the intervention, and outcome. It appears that psychological approaches that incorporate therapeutic hypnosis and guided imagery have a role in the management of cancer-related pain, especially pain associated with acute situations such as a lumbar puncture or oral mucositis in the setting of bone marrow transplant. Psychoeducational interventions may have a role, especially nursing-based education programs with skills training for the patient and caregivers. Clearly, more studies are needed to better define when these approaches are indicated.

ANESTHETIC AND NEUROSURGICAL APPROACHES

Anesthetic and neurosurgical approaches are most effective at treating patients with well-defined localized pain. Tables 146.7 and 146.8 outline the indications for their use. Of cancer pain patients, 10% to 20% require these approaches, together with pharmacologic approaches, to obtain adequate analgesia.

Several factors are important in selecting the appropriate procedure for each patient. Diffuse pain problems are more common in cancer patients, whereas most neurosurgical and anesthetic procedures are useful for the management of well-defined and localized pain, thus the role of these approaches is limited at best. Further complicating their use is the small number of professionals who have expertise in these procedures. As patients become more cognizant of their disease and treatment options, they are often hesitant to undergo neurodestructive procedures. Patients may consider their pain to be an important marker for their disease and are frightened of the potential, although unlikely, complications of these procedures. As a result, these procedures are often performed late in the illness, and a full evaluation of their effectiveness and duration of action is limited by patients' overriding medical problems.

Local Anesthetics

Anecdotal reports and several controlled studies support the use of cutaneous, subcutaneous, intravenous, intrapleural, and epidural local anesthetics in the management of patients with somatic, visceral, and neuropathic pain.

Intravenous lidocaine can be considered as both a diagnostic and therapeutic approach in patients with neuropathic pain.[174] If such patients obtain an analgesic response, a trial of oral mexiletine or the use of continuous subcutaneous lidocaine should be considered to determine whether prolonged relief may be possible, as previously discussed. Case reports suggest that continuous subcutaneous infusions of lidocaine may have a role in improving neuropathic cancer pain, but a small, randomized study did not support these findings.[175]

Intrapleural local anesthetics have been used for acute pain in the chest wall and have been adapted for the management of chronic cancer pain.[176] Anesthetic delivered via a subcutaneously tunneled intrapleural catheter offered long-term relief of right upper quadrant pain from hepatic metastases in a patient with significant pain from tumor infiltration of the liver. This novel method offers an alternative approach for patients with local or regional pain in the pleural and abdominal regions.

Epidural local anesthetics are used to manage localized pain syndromes, usually below the waist. Intermittent and continuous epidural infusions of local anesthetics have been used to manage the difficult chronic pain associated with metastatic disease below the waist, often involving the sacrum and lumbosacral plexus.[177]

TABLE 146.7

Types of Anesthetic Procedures Commonly Used in Cancer Pain

Type of Procedure	Most Common Indications
Inhalation therapy with nitrous oxide	Breakthrough pain, incidental pain in patients with diffuse poorly controlled pain
Intravenous barbiturates (sodium pentobarbital)	Diffuse body pain and suffering inadequately controlled by systemic opioids
Local anesthetic by intravenous, subcutaneous, or transdermal application	Neuropathic pain in any site with local application to the area of hyperesthesia or allodynia
Trigger point injections	Focal muscle pain
Nerve Block	
Peripheral	Pain in discrete dermatomes in chest and abdomen or in distal extremities
Epidural	Unilateral lumbar or sacral pain; midline perineal pain; bilateral lumbosacral pain
Intrathecal	Midline perineal pain; bilateral lumbosacral pain
Autonomic	
Stellate ganglion	Reflex sympathetic dystrophy
Lumbar sympathetic vascular insufficiency of the lower extremity	Reflex sympathetic dystrophy of the lower extremities; lumbosacral plexopathy
Celiac plexus	Mid-abdominal pain from tumor infiltration
Intermittent or continuous epidural infusion with local anesthetics	Unilateral and bilateral lumbosacral pain; midline perineal pain; neuropathic pain from the mid-thoracic region down
Intermittent or continuous epidural or intrathecal with local opioid analgesics	Unilateral and bilateral pain below the mid-thoracic region; often combined with local anesthetics
Intermittent or continuous intraventricular infusions with opioid analgesics	Head and neck pain and upper chest pain
Chemical hypophysectomy	Diffuse bone pain

This method consists of infusing a local anesthetic via a subcutaneous infusion pump or reservoir to a catheter temporarily or permanently placed in the epidural space. If the amount and concentration of the anesthetic are varied, effective pain relief can be achieved without interrupting significant motor or autonomic function. The risk of infection is minimized because local anesthetics have antimicrobial effects. The use of continuous low-dose infusions of local anesthetics is associated with minimal systemic side effects. Further studies on the use of this technique in comparison with standard therapies are needed to define its place in the management of the cancer patient. Its major advantages are that the resultant analgesia is not cross-tolerant with the analgesia produced by the opioid analgesics, and that temporary use of this technique allows for reducing the amount of systemic opiate drugs and, therefore, partially reversing tolerance. This has been a useful preliminary approach in patients for whom the use of spinal opiate analgesia is considered but who have developed tolerance from large doses of systemic opiates. This approach is also most useful

TABLE 146.8

Neuroablative and Neurostimulatory Procedures for Relief of Pain from Cancer

Site	Procedure	Indications
Neuroablative Procedures		
Nerve root	Rhizotomy	Useful in somatic and neuropathic pain from tumor infiltration of the cranial and, rarely, intercostal nerves
Spinal cord	Dorsal root entry zone lesion	Useful in unilateral neuropathic pain from brachial, intercostal, and lumbosacral plexopathy and postherpetic neuralgia
	Cordotomy	Useful in unilateral pain below the waist; often combined with local neurolytic blocks in perineal and bilateral lumbosacral plexopathy; may be performed bilaterally
	Myelotomy	Useful in midline pain below the waist but rarely used because it involves extensive surgery
Brain stem	Mesencephalic tractomy	Useful in pain in the nasopharynx and trigeminal region
Thalamus	Thalamotomy	Useful in unilateral neuropathic pain in the chest and lower extremity
Cortex	Cingulotomy	Useful through a stereotactic approach for diffuse pain
Pituitary	Transsphenoidal hypophysectomy	Useful in pain control of bone metastases in endocrine-dependent tumors, breast, and prostate
Neurostimulatory Procedures		
Peripheral nerve	Transcutaneous and percutaneous electrical nerve stimulation	Useful in reducing painful dysesthesias from tumor infiltration of nerve or trauma (e.g., neuroma)
Spinal cord	Dorsal column stimulation	Of limited use in neuropathic pain in the chest, midline, and lower extremities
Thalamus	Thalamic stimulation	Of rare use in neuropathic pain in the chest, midline, or lower extremity

in patients who experience an acute pain crisis, such as the patient with a pathologic hip fracture who is not a surgical candidate; this approach would allow the patient to move about in bed.

Peripheral Nerve Block

Peripheral nerve blocks are used both diagnostically to localize the nerve distribution and therapeutically to interrupt pain transmission within a determined nerve distribution. This technique is limited to areas of the body in which the interruption of both motor and sensory function will not interfere with the patient's functional status. It is most commonly used in patients who have pain in the head, chest, or abdomen.[178] This technique is also limited by the fact that each peripheral nerve subserves sensory function over many levels, and usually several nerves must be blocked to provide adequate analgesia. These techniques are most useful in patients with somatic pain; neuropathic pain is rarely controlled by peripheral nerve blocks alone. Examples of successful blocks include gasserian ganglion blocks for craniofacial pain, intercostal blocks for chest wall infiltration from a tumor, and paravertebral blocks for radicular pain. In patients with somatic pain who respond to a local anesthetic block, neurolytic blockade with either alcohol or phenol may provide more prolonged relief. A block produced by phenol tends to be less profound and of shorter duration than that produced by alcohol. Phenol has local anesthetic as well as neurolytic effects.

The most common peripheral neurolytic block is a paravertebral block for localized intercostal pain. Fluoroscopic, ultrasonic, or computed tomographic localization assists in more accurately interrupting the individual intercostal nerve.

Epidural and intrathecal neurolytic blocks have been used primarily to manage patients with far-advanced disease whose pain is either unilateral in the chest or abdomen or midline in the perineum. These approaches are less useful in managing upper and lower limb pain associated with brachial and lumbosacral plexopathy because of the high risk of motor weakness associated with effective neurolytic blockade by this route. Epidural phenol blocks are useful in the management of chest wall pain over several dermatomes. Such an approach obviates the need for multiple paravertebral injections. Phenol is injected in small increments (1 to 2 mL per segment) over 2 or 3 days by an epidural catheter, and preliminary data demonstrate 80% pain relief in patients with documented somatic pain. Epidural and intrathecal phenol blocks have been used to manage perineal pain, but no studies have delineated the superiority of one approach over the other. Case series reviews suggest that an average of 60% of patients experience good relief, 21% achieve fair relief, and 18% obtain poor relief.[177] The duration of pain relief is poorly documented; the overall estimate for relief of pain with both subarachnoid alcohol and phenol blocks suggests a mean duration of pain relief of between 2 weeks and 3 months.

The selection of patients for management with epidural or intrathecal neurolytic agents is based on the following criteria: exhaustion of appropriate antitumor approaches; clear clinical and radiologic definition of the pain; poor candidacy for percutaneous cordotomy; failure of nonopioid, opioid, and adjuvant analgesics to produce adequate analgesia without significant side effects; a favorable response to diagnostic or epidural or intrathecal blocks producing at least 75% pain relief; and an MRI of the spine or myelography done before the procedure that rules out tumor infiltration of the subarachnoid space. Complications are of two kinds. With an intrathecal injection, a self-limiting spinal headache may occur. Complications that result from the action of neurolytic substances on nerve fibers include motor paresis, loss of sphincter function, impairment of touch and proprioception, and troublesome dysesthesias. Injection in the thoracic region has a lower complication rate. If a patient already has both motor and autonomic dysfunction before the use of neurolytic blockade, these often remain the same or may worsen. Patients should be informed of the risk of these procedures, with particular attention

given to the fact that they may develop motor paresis and bladder dysfunction—specifically, incontinence—after the blockade.

Celiac Plexus Block

A sympathetic block is effective in conditions with vasomotor or visceromotor hyperactivity. This hyperactivity accompanies many of the cancer-related pain syndromes such as visceral pain or plexopathies. The most commonly used sympathetic block is that of the celiac ganglion for pain due to abdominal malignancy, including cancer of the pancreas, stomach, duodenum, liver, gallbladder, adrenal gland, and colon. Nociceptive fibers of the splanchnic, sympathetic, vagal, phrenic, and somatic nerves converge on the celiac ganglion, which is amenable to a regional block; this block successfully treats 70% to 85% of patients.[179]

Standardized approaches for the use of this technique have been described using computed tomographic monitoring or fluoroscopic control. After placement of the needle, 25 mg of absolute alcohol mixed with local anesthetic and contrast is injected. The major side effect of the procedure is transient hypotension; patients must be well hydrated and monitored carefully during the procedure and for 4 to 6 hours afterward. Significant neurologic complications occur in less than 1% of patients if proper technique is used. Complications include paraparesis, postural hypotension, and urinary difficulties.

Although there has been debate about the usefulness of this procedure in patients with pancreatic cancer, it should be considered as one option, together with pharmacologic approaches, in managing these patients. A recent systematic review of five randomized trials of celiac plexus block for advanced pancreatic cancer demonstrated that overall the procedure led to less pain, opioid use, and constipation, albeit with small effect size of questionable clinical significance.[180] The use of a thoracic endoscopy to perform sympathetic blockade in patients with cancer may replace the standard celiac plexus approach.

Lumbar Sympathetic Block

A lumbar sympathetic block may provide significant relief of intractable urogenital pain or pain due to carcinomatous invasion of local nerves and the plexus in the perineum and lower extremity.[181] This ganglion conveys visceral nociceptive afferents from the pelvic viscera. Pain caused by cancer of the sigmoid colon or rectum may be relieved by a bilateral lumbar sympathetic block if the disease is confined to those viscera. Similarly, pain caused by cancer of the seminal vesicles or prostate, and pain caused by uterine cancer confined to the body of the uterus, may be relieved by this block. In many instances, however, the block must be extended to the T12 ganglion. A lumbar sympathetic block alone is usually not useful in patients with lumbosacral plexopathy; therefore, the role of this procedure is limited to the management of pain at specific anatomic sites.

Stellate Ganglion Block

A stellate ganglion block may sometimes be useful for pain in the face, upper neck, ear, and hemicranium. However, the potential complications of the stellate ganglion block limit the use of neurolytic solution with this technique, because there is a high risk of spillage of the neurolytic material into the brachial plexus, with secondary nerve injury and focal pain.

NEUROPHARMACOLOGIC APPROACHES

Epidural and Interspinal Approach

Epidural and intraspinal analgesia, using opioids alone or in combination with (1) local anesthetics, (2) clonidine, (3) both local anesthetics and clonidine, or (4) experimental agents, is used to manage chronic cancer pain in patients with a reasonable (1-year) expected survival.[182] In all instances, patients should have a trial of an epidural or intraspinal drug combination before permanent implementation is considered. It is advised that patients have a continuous intrathecal trial lasting as long as possible before permanent implementation. A wide array of external and implantable catheters and pumps is available with specific indications and uses. Both computer-controlled battery-operated pumps and continuous fixed-infusion pumps are used. The cost of the pump, the patient's psychosocial status and social support systems, and the patient's ability to care for the pump and port are important considerations in the decision to use such devices. As discussed previously, a randomized clinical trial of intrathecal opioids compared to comprehensive medical management reported improved pain relief, less drug toxicity, and improved survival.[115]

NEUROABLATIVE AND NEUROSTIMULATORY PROCEDURES FOR THE RELIEF OF PAIN

Table 146.8 summarizes the commonly used neurosurgical approaches to cancer pain. A detailed review of these procedures is beyond the scope of this chapter. A review of the current literature suggests the limited use of most of these ablative and stimulatory procedures. The integration of these procedures is often dependent on the specific training of the consultant neurosurgeon, and medical oncologists need to work effectively in a team to decide the optimal use of these approaches.[183,184]

TRIGGER POINT INJECTION AND ACUPUNCTURE

Patients with significant musculoskeletal pain often identify specific tender trigger point areas, and injection of these trigger points with either saline or local anesthetic is associated with significant pain relief. Effective relief of pain from trigger point injections is not by itself diagnostic of musculoskeletal pain, however, and an evaluation of the cause of the pain is still necessary to rule out other specific sources.

Acupuncture has been used to treat both acute and chronic pain. The selected acupuncture points are manually or electrically stimulated with a needle until the patient feels the sensation. A wide variety of acupuncture techniques are available, ranging from a traditional Chinese approach to a Western adaptation. Laser acupuncture with external laser probes has also been used. Randomized and systematic data are emerging in support of acupuncture to manage pain; however, a lack of detailed pain assessments with specific acupuncture techniques and lack of a critical review of the patient population make it difficult to interpret these observations.[185,186] Based on its current empiric use, this approach is relatively safe, but its benefit in cancer patients with pain remains undefined.

PHYSIATRIC APPROACHES

Rehabilitation medicine plays an important role in the multidisciplinary approach to the patient with cancer pain.[187] Physiatrists are concerned with a patient's physical functioning and provide expertise in assessing how impairment in a patient's physical capacity affects his or her ability to function. A wide variety of interventions are available, including transcutaneous electrical nerve stimulation (TENS), diathermy (heating pads, ultrasound treatments, and hydrotherapy), and cryotherapy (ice and vapocoolants). Assistive devices and braces, as well as therapeutic exercise and massage, are important. Trigger point injections and acupuncture have also been used. These interventions are commonly used

in combination with other pain therapy approaches, particularly behavioral and pharmacologic approaches. Rehabilitation approaches are discussed throughout the text specific to the cancer patients' needs. A large body of data supports the use of rehabilitative interventions in acute and chronic nonmalignant pain, but similar studies have not addressed the rehabilitation needs of the cancer pain patient. Neurologic dysfunction is one of the common components in patients with cancer pain, and aggressive neurorehabilitation is necessary to promote ambulation in these patients and provide them with functional independence.

ALGORITHM FOR CANCER PAIN MANAGEMENT

An algorithm has been developed that integrates all of these management approaches for cancer pain. It attempts to integrate assessment techniques, drug therapy, behavioral approaches, and anesthetic and neurosurgical approaches and stresses continuity of care. Treatment begins with a diagnostic evaluation that addresses the medical, psychological, and social components of pain. A plan is developed to treat the cancer and pain. If the anticancer treatment is effective, pain relief usually occurs and the drugs used for analgesia can be discontinued without difficulty. Pain treatment begins with the use of analgesic drugs, starting with nonopioid drugs alone or in combination. If these drugs are successful, no further therapy is necessary. If severe, persistent pain does not respond to analgesic drugs, or if the side effects of the drugs are not tolerated, the physician should consider switching analgesics (e.g., from oral morphine to methadone), changing the route of administration (e.g., from oral to subcutaneous), or performing a cordotomy for localized pain. A trial of an adjuvant drug together with the opioid and nonopioid drug would also be appropriate. In patients with excessive sedation or confusion, the use of a neurostimulant or haloperidol provides adequate treatment of the side effects of the opioid drugs and maintains the patient's analgesia while markedly reducing concurrent side effects. Alternatively, epidural or intrathecal opioids may be considered if systemic analgesics produce excessive side effects such as confusion or sedation. If the pain is localized (e.g., intercostal pain from tumor infiltration of the chest wall), neurolytic blocks are indicated. If the pain is unilateral and below the waist, a cordotomy should be considered. For diffuse pain, nitrous oxide inhalation may be tried. Behavioral approaches, including guided imagery, should be integrated from the onset of treatment and used along with the medical and surgical approaches.

FUTURE DIRECTIONS

The study of pain in cancer patients offers a unique opportunity to use clinical observations to advance biologic knowledge. There is a critical need to expand both the research and educational efforts in cancer pain to improve the control of pain in these patients. Information on the basic mechanisms of pain modulation can be culled only from a careful study of these clinical pain problems. These studies can teach us the physiologic and psychological differences between acute and chronic pain problems, the importance of the evolution of psychological factors, the difference between pain and suffering, the clinical pharmacology of analgesic drugs, and the behavioral mechanisms humans use to suppress pain. The use of innovative approaches based on sound scientific principles and advances in research technology offers the opportunity to understand the complex phenomenon of pain. The development of animal models to test new therapies, the new insights learned from the molecular genetics of opioid receptors, and the increasing knowledge base of the molecular mechanisms of neuropathic pain, bone pain, and visceral pain offer the promise for translating these discoveries into the improved care of the patient with pain.

SELECTED REFERENCES

The full reference list can be accessed at lwwhealthlibrary.com/oncology.

1. Foley K, Gelband H, eds. *Institute of Medicine. National Cancer Policy Board. Improving Palliative Care for Cancer.* Washington, DC: National Academies Press; 2001.
3. National Institute of Health. Improving end-of-life care. *NIH Consens State Sci Statements* 2004;21:23.
5. Moryl N, Coyle N, Foley KM. Managing an acute pain crisis in a patient with advanced cancer: "this is as much of a crisis as a code". *JAMA* 2008;299:1457–1467.
6. Stjernsward J, Foley KM, Ferris FD. The public health strategy for palliative care. *J Pain Symptom Manage* 2007;33:486–493.
7. World Health Organization. *Cancer Pain Relief and Palliative Care: Report of a WHO Expert Committee.* Geneva: World Health Organization; 1990.
8. World Health Organization. *Cancer Pain Relief.* 2nd ed. Geneva: WHO; 1996.
9. Smith TJ, Temin S, Alesi ER, et al. American Society of Clinical Oncology Provisional Clinical Opinion: The Integration of Palliative Care into Standard Oncology Care. *J Clin Oncol* 2012;30:880–887.
10. Temel JS, Greer JA, Muzikansky A, et al. Early palliative care for patients with metastatic non-small-cell lung cancer. *New Engl J Med* 2010;363:733–742.
11. Gordon DB, Dahl JL, Miaskowski C, et al. American Pain Society recommendations for improving the quality of acute and cancer pain management: American Pain Society Quality of Care Task Force. *Arch Intern Med* 2005;165:1574–1580.
12. Jost L, Roila F. Management of cancer pain: ESMO Clinical Practice Guidelines. *Ann Oncol* 2010;21:v257–v260.
13. Raphael J, Ahmedzai S, Hester J, et al. Cancer pain: part 1: Pathophysiology; oncological, pharmacological, and psychological treatments: a perspective from the British Pain Society endorsed by the UK Association of Palliative Medicine and the Royal College of General Practitioners. *Pain Med* 2010;11:742–764.
14. Sanft TB, Von Roenn JH. Palliative care across the continuum of cancer care. *J Natl Compr Canc Netw* 2009;7:481–487.
15. Swarm RA, Abernethy AP, Anghelescu DL, et al. Adult cancer pain. *J Natl Compr Canc Netw* 2013;11:992–1022.
16. Ripamonti CI, Santini D, Maranzano E, et al. Management of cancer pain: ESMO Clinical Practice Guidelines. *Ann Oncol* 2012;23:vii139–vii154.
18. Foley KM. How well is cancer pain treated? *Palliat Med* 2011;25:398–401.
19. Foley KM. Acute and chronic cancer pain syndromes. In: Doyle D, Hanks G, Cherny N, Calman K, eds. *Oxford Textbook of Palliative Medicine.* 3rd ed. New York: Oxford Unversithy Press; 2004: 298.
20. Gonzales GR, Elliott KJ, Portenoy RK, et al. The impact of a comprehensive evaluation in the management of cancer pain. *Pain* 1991;47: 141–144.
25. Cherny NI, Portenoy RK. Cancer pain: principles of assessment and syndromes. In: Wall PK, Melzack R, eds. *Textbook of Pain.* London: Churchill Livingstone; 1994: 787.
26. Cleeland CS, Gonin R, Hatfield AK, et al. Pain and its treatment in outpatients with metastatic cancer. *N Engl J Med* 1994;330:592–596.
29. Portenoy RK, Miransky J, Thaler HT, et al. Pain in ambulatory patients with lung or colon cancer. Prevalence, characteristics, and effect. *Cancer* 1992;70:1616–1624.
30. Schuit KW, Sleijfer DT, Meijler WJ, et al. Symptoms and functional status of patients with disseminated cancer visiting outpatient departments. *J Pain Symptom Manage* 1998;16:290–297.
31. The SUPPORT Principal Investigators. A controlled trial to improve care for seriously ill hospitalized patients. The study to understand prognoses and preferences for outcomes and risks of treatments (SUPPORT). *JAMA* 1995;274:1591–1598.
33. Coyle N, Adelhardt J, Foley KM, et al. Character of terminal illness in the advanced cancer patient: pain and other symptoms during the last four weeks of life. *J Pain Symptom Manage* 1990;5:83–93.
34. Chochinov H, Breitbart W, eds. *Handbook of Psychiatry in Palliative Medicine.* New York: Oxford University Press; 2009.
35. Passik S, Portenoy R. Substance abuse issues in palliative care. In: Berger A, et al, eds. *Principles and Practices of Supportive Oncology.* Philadelphia: Lippincott–Raven Publishers; 1998.
36. Pain terms: a list with definitions and notes on usage. Recommended by the IASP Subcommittee on Taxonomy. *Pain* 1979;6:249.
38. Elliott K, Foley KM. Neurologic pain syndromes in patients with cancer. *Crit Care Clin* 1990;6:393–420.
39. Clohisy DR, Mantyh PW. Bone cancer pain. *Cancer* 2003;97:866–873.
42. Hagen NA, Fisher K, Victorino C, Farrar JT. A titration strategy is needed to manage breakthrough cancer pain effectively: observations from data pooled from three clinical trials. *J Palliat Med* 2007;10:47–55.
43. Petzke F, Radbruch L, Zech D, et al. Temporal presentation of chronic cancer pain: transitory pains on admission to a multidisciplinary pain clinic. *J Pain Symptom Manage* 1999;17:391–401.
44. Portenoy RK, Hagen NA. Breakthrough pain: definition, prevalence and characteristics. *Pain* 1990;41:273–281.
48. Graham C, Bond SS, Gerkovich MM, et al. Use of the McGill pain questionnaire in the assessment of cancer pain: replicability and consistency. *Pain* 1980;8:377–387.

49. Basch E, Abernethy AP, Mullins CD, et al. Recommendations for incorporating patient-reported outcomes into clinical comparative effectiveness research in adult oncology. *J Clin Oncol* 2012;30:4249–4255.
51. Miriovsky BJ, Abernethy AP. Measurement of quality of life outcomes. In: Berger AM, Shuster JL, Von Roenn JH, eds. *Principles and Practice of Palliative Oncology and Supportive Oncology.* Philadelphia: Wolters Kluwer/Lippincott Williams & Wilkins; 2013.
56. Foley KM. The treatment of cancer pain. *N Engl J Med* 1985;313:84–95.
57. Block SD. Perspectives on care at the close of life. Psychological considerations, growth, and transcendence at the end of life: the art of the possible. *JAMA* 2001;285:2898–2905.
58. Cherny NI, Coyle N, Foley KM. Suffering in the advanced cancer patient: a definition and taxonomy. *J Palliat Care* 1994;10:57–70.
59. Cherny NI, Coyle N, Foley KM. Guidelines in the care of the dying cancer patient. *Hematol Oncol Clin North Am* 1996;10:261–286.
60. Foley KM. The relationship of pain and symptom management to patient requests for physician-assisted suicide. *J Pain Symptom Manage* 1991;6: 289–297.
61. Cassel EJ. The nature of suffering and the goals of medicine. *N Engl J Med* 1982;306:639–645.
62. Chochinov HM, Wilson KG, Enns M, et al. Desire for death in the terminally ill. *Am J Psychiatry* 1995;152:1185–1191.
64. Ventafridda V, Caraceni A, Gamba A. Field-testing of the WHO Guidelines for Cancer Pain Relief: summary report of demonstration projects. In: Foley K, Bonica J, Ventafridda V, Callaway M, eds. *Second International Congress on Cancer Pain. Advances in Pain Research and Therapy.* Vol 16. New York: Raven Press; 1990: 451.
65. Zech DF, Grond S, Lynch J, et al. Validation of World Health Organization Guidelines for cancer pain relief: a 10-year prospective study. *Pain* 1995;63:65–76.
66. Du Pen SL, Du Pen AR, Polissar N, et al. Implementing guidelines for cancer pain management: results of a randomized controlled clinical trial. *J Clin Oncol* 1999;17:361–370.
67. Fallon M, Hanks G, Cherny N. Principles of control of cancer pain. *BMJ* 2006;332:1022–1024.
68. Eisenberg E, Berkey CS, Carr DB, et al. Efficacy and safety of nonsteroidal antiinflammatory drugs for cancer pain: a meta-analysis. *J Clin Oncol* 1994;12:2756–2765.
71. Ventafridda V, De Conno F, Panerai AE, et al. Non-steroidal anti-inflammatory drugs as the first step in cancer pain therapy: double-blind, within-patient study comparing nine drugs. *J Int Med Res* 1990;18:21–29.
76. Bruera E, Pereira J, Watanabe S, et al. Opioid rotation in patients with cancer pain. A retrospective comparison of dose ratios between methadone, hydromorphone, and morphine. *Cancer* 1996;78:852–857.
77. Cherny N, Chang V, Frager G, et al. Opioid pharmacotherapy in the management of cancer pain: a survey of strategies used by pain physicians for the selection of analgesic drugs and routes of administration. *Cancer* 1995;76:1283–1293.
79. Foley KM. Changing concepts of tolerance to opioids. What the cancer patient has taught us. In: Chapman C, Foley K, eds. *Current and Emerging Issues in Cancer Pain: Research and Practice.* New York: Raven Press; 1993: 331.
81. Foley KM. Competent care for the dying instead of physician-assisted suicide. [see comment]. *N Engl J Med* 1997;336:54–58.
82. Foley KM. Opioids and chronic neuropathic pain. [see comment][comment]. *N Engl J Med* 2003;348:1279–1281.
83. Jadad AR, Browman GP. The WHO analgesic ladder for cancer pain management. Stepping up the quality of its evaluation. *JAMA* 1995;274: 1870–1873.
86. McQuay H. Opioids in pain management. *Lancet* 1999;353:2229–2232.
91. Klepstad P, Kaasa S, Jystad A, et al. Immediate- or sustained-release morphine for dose finding during start of morphine to cancer patients: a randomized, double-blind trial. *Pain* 2003;101:193–198.
92. von Gunten CF, Bruera E, Pirrello RD, et al. New opioids: expensive distractions or important additions to practice? *J Palliat Med* 2010;13: 505–511.
94. Moulin DE, Johnson NG, Murray-Parsons N, et al. Subcutaneous narcotic infusions for cancer pain: treatment outcome and guidelines for use. *Can Med Assoc J* 1992;146:891–897.
98. Fredheim OM, Borchgrevink PC, Hegrenaes L, et al. Opioid switching from morphine to methadone causes a minor but not clinically significant increase in QTc time: A prospective 9-month follow-up study. *J Pain Symptom Manage* 2006;32:180–185.
99. Krantz MJ, Mehler PS. QTc prolongation: methadone's efficacy-safety paradox. *Lancet* 2006;368:556–557.
100. Bruera E, Palmer JL, Bosnjak S, et al. Methadone versus morphine as a first-line strong opioid for cancer pain: a randomized, double-blind study. *J Clin Oncol* 2004;22:185–192.
102. Morley J, Makin M. The use of methadone in cancer pain poorly responsive to other opiates. *Pain Rev* 1998;5:51–58.
108. Coluzzi PH, Schwartzberg L, Conroy JD, et al. Breakthrough cancer pain: a randomized trial comparing oral transmucosal fentanyl citrate (OTFC) and morphine sulfate immediate release (MSIR). *Pain* 2001;91:123–130.

PALLIATIVE AND ALTERNATIVE CARE

113. Portenoy RK, Moulin DE, Rogers A, et al. I.V. infusion of opioids for cancer pain: clinical review and guidelines for use. *Cancer Treat Rep* 1986;70: 575–581.

114. Devulder J, Ghys L, Dhondt W, et al. Spinal analgesia in terminal care: risk versus benefit. *J Pain Symptom Manage* 1994;9:75–81.

115. Smith TJ, Staats PS, Deer T, et al. Randomized clinical trial of an implantable drug delivery system compared with comprehensive medical management for refractory cancer pain: impact on pain, drug-related toxicity, and survival. *J Clin Oncol* 2002;20:4040–4049.

119. Bruera E, Fainsinger R, MacEachern T, Hanson J. The use of methylphenidate in patients with incident cancer pain receiving regular opiates. A preliminary report. *Pain* 1992;50:75–77.

120. Goldfrank L, Weisman RS, Errick JK, Lo MW. A dosing nomogram for continuous infusion intravenous naloxone. *Ann Emerg Med* 1986;15:566–570.

121. Apfel CC, Cakmakkaya OS, Frings G, et al. Droperidol has comparable clinical efficacy against both nausea and vomiting. *Br J Anaesth* 2009;103:359–363.

122. Thomas J, Karver S, Cooney GA, et al. Methylnaltrexone for opioid-induced constipation in advanced illness. *N Engl J Med* 2008;358:2332–2343.

123. Holzer P. Opioid antagonists for prevention and treatment of opioid-induced gastrointestinal effects. *Curr Opin Anaesthesiol* 2010;23:616–622.

124. Kanner RM, Foley KM. Patterns of narcotic drug use in a cancer pain clinic. *Ann N Y Acad Sci* 1981;362:161–172.

126. McQuay HJ, Tramer M, Nye BA, et al. A systematic review of antidepressants in neuropathic pain. [see comment]. *Pain* 1996;68:217–227.

127. Finnerup NB, Otto M, McQuay HJ, et al. Algorithm for neuropathic pain treatment: an evidence based proposal. *Pain* 2005;118:289–305.

128. Sindrup SH, Gram LF, Brosen K, et al. The selective serotonin reuptake inhibitor paroxetine is effective in the treatment of diabetic neuropathy symptoms. *Pain* 1990;42:135–144.

130. Smith EM, Pang H, Cirrincione C, et al. Effect of duloxetine on pain, function, and quality of life among patients with chemotherapy-induced painful peripheral neuropathy: a randomized clinical trial. *JAMA* 2013;309:1359–1367.

131. Backonja M, Beydoun A, Edwards KR, et al. Gabapentin for the symptomatic treatment of painful neuropathy in patients with diabetes mellitus: a randomized controlled trial. [see comment]. *JAMA* 1998;280:1831–1836.

132. Stute P, Soukup J, Menzel M, et al. Analysis and treatment of different types of neuropathic cancer pain. *J Pain Symptom Manage* 2003;26:1123–1131.

133. Wiffen P, Collins S, McQuay H, et al. Anticonvulsant drugs for acute and chronic pain. [update of Cochrane Database Syst Rev 2000;(3):CD001133; PMID: 10908487]. *Cochrane Database Syst Rev* 2005:CD001133.

134. Wiffen PJ, McQuay HJ, Edwards JE, et al. Gabapentin for acute and chronic pain. *Cochrane Database Syst Rev* 2005:CD005452.

135. Freynhagen R, Strojek K, Griesing T, et al. Efficacy of pregabalin in neuropathic pain evaluated in a 12-week, randomised, double-blind, multicentre, placebo-controlled trial of flexible- and fixed-dose regimens. *Pain* 2005;115:254–263.

136. Bennett MI, Laird B, van Litsenburg C, et al. Pregabalin for the management of neuropathic pain in adults with cancer: a systematic review of the literature. *Pain Med* 2013;14:1681–1688.

138. Challapalli V, Tremont-Lukats IW, McNicol ED, et al. Systemic administration of local anesthetic agents to relieve neuropathic pain. *Cochrane Database Syst Rev* 2005:CD003345.

141. Galer BS, Rowbotham MC, Perander J, et al. Topical lidocaine patch relieves postherpetic neuralgia more effectively than a vehicle topical patch: results of an enriched enrollment study. *Pain* 1999;80:533–538.

144. Sorensen S, Helweg-Larsen S, Mouridsen H, et al. Effect of high-dose dexamethasone in carcinomatous metastatic spinal cord compression treated with radiotherapy: a randomised trial. *Eur J Cancer* 1994;30A:22–27.

145. Abrahm JL, Banffy MB, Harris MB. Spinal cord compression in patients with advanced metastatic cancer: "all I care about is walking and living my life". *JAMA* 2008;299:937–946.

149. Bell RF, Eccleston C, Kalso E. Ketamine as adjuvant to opioids for cancer pain. A qualitative systematic review. [see comment]. *J Pain Symptom Manage* 2003;26:867–875.

151. Hardy J, Quinn S, Fazekas B, et al. Randomized, double-blind, placebo-controlled study to assess the efficacy and toxicity of subcutaneous ketamine in the management of cancer pain. *J Clin Oncol* 2012;30:3611–3617.

156. Berry S, Waldron T, Winquist E, et al. The use of bisphosphonates in men with hormone-refractory prostate cancer: a systematic review of randomized trials. *Can J Urol* 2006;13:3180–3188.

158. Ernst DS, Brasher P, Hagen N, et al. A randomized, controlled trial of intravenous clodronate in patients with metastatic bone disease and pain. *J Pain Symptom Manage* 1997;13:319–326.

159. Pavlakis N, Stockler M. Bisphosphonates for breast cancer. [update in Cochrane Database Syst Rev. 2005;(3):CD003474; PMID: 16034900]. *Cochrane Database Syst Rev* 2002:CD003474.

160. Gralow J, Tripathy D. Managing metastatic bone pain: the role of bisphosphonates. *J Pain Symptom Manage* 2007;33:462–472.

163. Fizazi K, Carducci M, Smith M, et al. Denosumab versus zoledronic acid for treatment of bone metastases in men with castration-resistant prostate cancer: a randomised, double-blind study. *Lancet* 2011;377:813–822.

164. Stopeck AT, Lipton A, Body JJ, et al. Denosumab compared with zoledronic acid for the treatment of bone metastases in patients with advanced breast cancer: a randomized, double-blind study. *J Clin Oncol* 2010;28:5132–5139.

166. Bauman G, Charette M, Reid R, Sathya J. Radiopharmaceuticals for the palliation of painful bone metastasis-a systemic review. *Radiother Oncol* 2005;75:258–270.

167. Finlay IG, Mason MD, Shelley M. Radioisotopes for the palliation of metastatic bone cancer: a systematic review. [see comment]. *Lancet Oncol* 2005;6:392–400.

168. Parker C, Nilsson S, Heinrich D, et al. Alpha emitter radium-223 and survival in metastatic prostate cancer. *N Engl J Med* 2013;369:213–223.

169. Nilsson S, Strang P, Aksnes AK, et al. A randomized, dose-response, multicenter phase II study of radium-223 chloride for the palliation of painful bone metastases in patients with castration-resistant prostate cancer. *Eur J Cancer* 2012;48:678–686.

170. Keefe FJ, Abernethy AP, Campbell LC. Psychological approaches to understanding and treating disease-related pain. *Annu Rev Psychol* 2005;56:601–630.

171. Zaza C, Baine N. Cancer pain and psychosocial factors: a critical review of the literature. *J Pain Symptom Manage* 2002;24:526–542.

172. Devine EC. Meta-analysis of the effect of psychoeducational interventions on pain in adults with cancer. *Oncol Nurs Forum* 2003;30:75–89.

175. Bruera E, Ripamonti C, Brenneis C, et al. A randomized double-blind crossover trial of intravenous lidocaine in the treatment of neuropathic cancer pain. *J Pain Symptom Manage* 1992;7:138–140.

177. Cherny NI, Arbit E, Jain S. Invasive techniques in the management of cancer pain. *Hematol Oncol Clin North Am* 1996;10:121–137.

178. Kim PS. Interventional cancer pain therapies. *Semin Oncol* 2005;32: 194–199.

179. Patt R. Peripheral neurolysis and the management of cancer pain. In: Patt R, ed. *Cancer Pain*. Philadelphia: Lippincott; 1993: 359.

182. Staats PS. Neuraxial infusion for pain control: when, why, and what to do after the implant. *Oncology* 1999;13:58–62.

183. Benedetti C, Ibinson J, Adolph M. Cancer pain: anesthetic and neurosurgical approaches. In: Walsh D, Caraceni AT, Fainsinger R, et al., eds. *Palliative Medicine*. Philadelphia: Saunders Elsevier; 2009 : 1394.

184. Raslan AM, Burchiel KJ. Neurosurgical advances in cancer pain management. *Curr Pain Headache Rep* 2010;14:477–482.

185. Alimi D, Rubino C, Pichard-Leandri E, et al. Analgesic effect of auricular acupuncture for cancer pain: a randomized, blinded, controlled trial. *J Clin Oncol* 2003;21:4120–4126.

186. Bardia A, Barton DL, Prokop LJ, et al. Efficacy of complementary and alternative medicine therapies in relieving cancer pain: a systematic review. *J Clin Oncol* 2006;24:5457–5464.

187. Sliwa JA, Marciniak C. Physical rehabilitation of the cancer patient. In: von Gunten CF, ed. *Palliative Care and Rehabilitation of Cancer Patients*. Boston: Kluwer Academic; 1998:76.

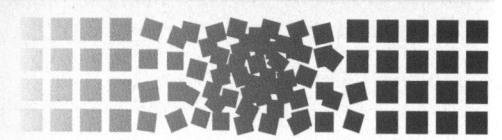

Laleh G. Melstrom, Vadim P. Koshenkov, and David A. August

BACKGROUND

Nutrition and diet play a major role in cancer. Dietary factors are a significant component of the identifiable attributable risks of cancer.[1-3] Cancer-related malnutrition and cancer cachexia are prominent elements that cause signs and symptoms of cancer and are major contributors to patient distress. Comparable historically to tuberculosis (*consumption*) or even AIDS, cancer is often thought of as a *wasting disease*. Furthermore, malnutrition and weight loss often contribute to the death of cancer patients.[4,5] More recently, the role of overnutrition in cancer pathogenesis and prognosis has been identified.

Undernutrition is a hallmark of cancer. Approximately 40% of cancer patients present with weight loss, and cancer cachexia syndrome (CCS), with its profound implications for quality of life and survival, may develop in as many as 80% of patients with advanced malignancies.[6,7] A loss of more than 10% of usual body weight at the time of diagnosis is prognostic for survival; a rate of weight loss of greater than 2.75% per month also confers a poor prognosis.[7,8] Weight loss in cancer patients is associated with symptom distress (including fatigue, depression, and social withdrawal), poor quality of life, and increased surgical morbidity.[9-16] In fact, many cancer patients may not be candidates for potentially curative life-prolonging treatment because of the risk of life-threatening complications that their malnutrition confers.

Overnutrition (body mass index greater than 30 kg/m^2) is becoming a more frequently recognized problem in cancer patients, in part because of the obesity epidemic in the United States. Obesity is an attributable cause in more than 15% of cancer deaths in the United States, including cancers usually associated with wasting (such as liver cancer, pancreas cancer, gastric cancer, and esophageal cancer) and in *female cancers* such as uterine cancer, cervix cancer, and breast cancer.[17] Hypothesized links between the pathophysiology of cancer mortality and obesity include: delayed detection on physical exam and screening studies; the difficulty of administering precise surgery, radiation therapy, and chemotherapy in obese patients resulting in decreased efficacy and increased side effects; the role of lipocytes in steroid and sex-hormone metabolism; the altered cytokine milieu in obese patient; and the proinflammatory/pro-oxidant effects of obesity.[18]

Despite our current understanding of the role of malnutrition in cancer pathogenesis, pathophysiology, and patient outcomes, the ability to avoid the consequences of under- and overnutrition in cancer patients remains a work in progress. The nutrition care of cancer patients should focus on the goals of recognizing the presence and/or risk of malnutrition; assessing nutritional needs and requirements; defining and implementing appropriate nutrition interventions while avoiding ineffective and potentially harmful therapies; maintaining function and quality of life; and improving the ability to administer effective anticancer treatments.

CAUSES OF MALNUTRITION IN CANCER PATIENTS

Metabolic, cytokine, and clinical factors contribute to the development of malnutrition in cancer patients (Table 147.1). The role of each of these factors varies from patient to patient. Anorexia is a prominent contributor to weight loss in many cancer patients. Although multiple factors contribute to cancer-associated anorexia, it primarily results from cytokine and metabolic derangements.[19,20] Although many factors may diminish nutrient intake, the underlying problem is a metabolic milieu that prevents the effective utilization of nutrients. Supporting this contention are a number of observations: parenteral nutrition support may be used to overcome diminished nutrient intake or gut failure, but this only rarely reverses the weight loss and clinical stigmata of CCS; the clinical and metabolic features of simple starvation in humans differ markedly from those seen in cancer patients, suggesting decreased intake is not the underlying cause of cancer-associated weight loss; cancer weight loss may precede changes in appetite; and in some situations, the perceived anorexia is actually an adaptive decrease of food intake in response to weight loss.[21-23] Therefore, even with an effective treatment of other causes of weight loss in cancer patients, the metabolic and clinical consequences of cancer cachexia may not resolve.

Other factors that contribute to weight loss in cancer patients include symptom distress and psychosocial factors, alterations in taste (dysgeusia), gastrointestinal dysfunction, and side effects of cancer therapy. The symptom-related and psychological factors associated with cancer that may alter food intake include pain, nausea, vomiting, anxiety, depression, and social isolation. Dysgeusia may be a direct side effect of chemotherapy, radiation therapy, and surgery, but it may also be psychological in origin (including food aversions and anticipatory nausea and vomiting).[24,25] Gastrointestinal dysfunction is common in cancer patients; it may relate to direct effects of tumor (i.e., obstruction, compression of hollow viscuses), or to side effects or complications of therapy. Cancer surgery is invariably accompanied by a temporary catabolic state and decreased nutrient intake, and this may be prolonged by the development of complications such as obstruction, infection, and fistula formation. These may cause symptom distress, including alterations in taste, early satiety, pain, cramps, vomiting, diarrhea, and constipation. Chemotherapy often induces transient nausea and vomiting or injury to gastrointestinal mucosa with resultant stomatitis, mucositis, diarrhea, and/or typhlitis, all of which may be exacerbated by neutropenia. Radiation therapy can cause acute gastrointestinal injury accompanied by many of the previously mentioned symptoms and also chronic radiation enteritis with malabsorption and stricture formation.

CANCER CACHEXIA SYNDROME

The word "cachexia" comes from the Greek words *kakos* (bad) and *hexis* (condition). It is not surprising that the development of CCS confers a worse prognosis. The clinical features of CCS include

TABLE 147.1

Causes of Weight Loss and Malnutrition in Cancer Patients

A. Metabolic Factors
    a. Cytokine-, peptide-, and hormone-induced metabolic changes
    b. Cytokine-mediated anorexia
B. Symptom Distress
    a. Depression and other psychosocial factors
    b. Pain, nausea, diarrhea, constipation, fatigue, and other symptoms
C. Alterations in taste (dysgeusia), conditioned food aversion
D. Gastrointestinal dysfunction
    a. Obstruction, dysmotility, fistula, and malabsorption
E. Side Effects of Cancer Therapies
    a. Nausea, vomiting, diarrhea, fatigue, mucositis, enteritis, infection, etc.

weight loss, anorexia, fatigue, anemia, and hypoalbuminemia. Cancer cachexia can be present at any stage of disease, although it is more common with advanced malignancy. Weight loss is a central component of the undernutrition that occurs in cachectic patients. It varies between tumor types, and is most profound for tumors of the pancreas and the upper gastrointestinal tract.[7]

The etiology of CCS is multifactorial. Anorexia of malignancy is defined as a spontaneous decrease in food intake,[26] and is most often mediated by cytokines.[24] An abnormal metabolic rate; altered cellular metabolism of lipids, proteins, and carbohydrates; and a deranged cytokine milieu (Table 147.2) are the other causes of cancer cachexia. The interplay of these factors varies from patient to patient.

Energetics

Early studies that evaluated resting energy expenditure (REE) in cancer patients concluded that it is increased.[27,28] However, these investigations did not account for fat-free mass (FFM) when calculating the REE. Weight-losing patients initially lose fat mass, and body composition should be accounted for when estimating REE.[29,30] Even with these adjustments, inaccuracies still exist in the estimation of REE in cancer patients.[31–33]

The type of malignancy and the host response have been hypothesized to result in the variability of the metabolic rate that has been observed in cancer patients.[31,32,34–39] For example, although patients with hepatobiliary neoplasms are mostly hypometabolic, gastric and lung cancer patients are frequently hypermetabolic.[40–42] Factors

TABLE 147.2

Cytokine Milieu and Effects in Cancer Cachexia

Cytokine	Effects
TNF-α	Lipolysis, muscle degradation, increased glucose turnover
Interferon-γ	Potentiates lipolysis, decreases protein synthesis
Interleukin-1 (IL-1)	Induces anorexia, early satiety, peripheral proteolysis, potentiates release of IL-6
IL-6	Severe wasting
Proteolysis-inducing factor	Skeletal muscle degradation
Lipid mobilizing factor	Lipolysis

such as increased acute phase reactants, prolonged duration of illness, and advanced cancer have been associated with an elevated REE, whereas the stage of the tumor has not.[32,35–38] Additionally, because of anorexia and other factors, cancer patients may not adjust their food intake to compensate for the altered REE.[26] The hallmark of REE in cancer patients is its variability and unpredictability.

Intermediary Metabolism

Increased turnover (cycling) of proteins and lipids is a feature of CCS, leading to decreased skeletal muscle mass and depleted fat stores. Augmented proteolysis and attenuated peripheral protein synthesis cause severe muscle loss in weight-losing patients with advanced cancer, which can result in respiratory complications and death.[43,44] Proteolysis-inducing factor (PIF) is a major mediator of protein catabolism in cancer patients; it activates nuclear factor kappa B (NF-κB), which then turns on the ubiquitin-proteasome proteolytic pathway.[20] By mass, most of the weight loss in cancer cachexia occurs from the depletion of fat stores. The primary mechanism behind this is elevated fat cell lipolysis. Similar to PIF, lipid-mobilizing factor (LMF) is central to the process of adipocytic lipolysis via regulation of hormone-sensitive lipase (HSL).[43] Interestingly, both proteolysis and lipolysis are not suppressed with the administration of exogenous nitrogen[45] and glucose.[46] With respect to the metabolism of carbohydrates, multiple aberrations stem from the Warburg effect, an early 20th century observation that glycolysis is the main process for energy generation in cancer cells.[47] This energy-inefficient process leads to an increase in hepatic gluconeogenesis and can cause the normal tissues to be energy starved.

Cytokines and Hormones

In CCS, many of the processes that have just been described are driven by an altered cytokine milieu (see Table 147.2). Both tumor cell production and host responses contribute to the deranged cytokine milieu.[48]

Although integral to local host defenses in the face of inflammation or infection, tumor necrosis factor-α (TNF-α) can have harmful systemic effects.[49] These include muscle breakdown mediated by the ubiquitin-proteasome pathway and nitric oxide synthase expression, fat depletion that occurs because of increased lipolysis through the activation of HSL and decreased lipogenesis, and anorexia that is induced when TNF is produced or administered in the brain.[50] Evidence for the role of TNF in cachexia comes from multiple animal models.[51,52] Similar to TNF, interferon-γ (IFN-γ) is an important contributor to muscle wasting and fat burning through the activation of these same processes.[53] Antibodies to these two key cytokines have been developed with some success in suppressing the metabolic changes of CCS, but no single agent has been able to prevent most of its features.[49,53]

Interleukin-1 (IL-1) and interleukin-6 (IL-6) are two proinflammatory cytokines that further contribute to CCS. IL-1 induces anorexia, increases peripheral breakdown of muscle, and promotes the release of IL-6.[53,54] In turn, IL-6 has been demonstrated to elevate the rate of hepatic gluconeogenesis and peripheral proteolysis, and can result in more profound wasting than TNF.[53,55] Despite the almost indistinguishable effects of TNF and IL-6, the latter (unlike TNF) is easily found in the serum of cancer patients with cachexia, and likely works through different mechanisms.[53]

Besides cytokines, several hormones and tumor-derived proteins have been implicated in CCS. These include leptin, serotonin, PIF, and LMF. Proteolysis-inducing factor and LMF are predominantly produced by tumor cells, whereas leptin and serotonin are generated by host tissues. PIF contributes to peripheral muscle wasting and to decreased protein synthesis, whereas LMF is central to lipolysis. Interestingly, LMF is detectable in weight-losing cancer patients, but not weight-stable cancer patients.[50]

The key function of leptin, an adipocyte-derived hormone, is to regulate body fat mass by reducing appetite and increasing REE.[56] It does so via hypothalamic neuropeptides.[48] When there is an increase in food intake, leptin levels are elevated. This leads to the suppression of appetite stimulants ghrelin and neuropeptide Y (NPY) and the stimulation of appetite suppressors corticotropin-releasing factor (CRF) and melanocortin. Persistently decreased levels of leptin have been identified in cachectic patients, indicating that tumors are capable of mimicking leptin and causing sustained anorexia and weight loss.[48,55] Another hormone that has been found to contribute to the anorexia of cancer cachexia is serotonin.[48] Several mechanisms have been proposed for this, including the depression of appetite and the inhibition of ghrelin secretion.[57,58]

The multiplicity of factors, both clinical and metabolic, that underlie CCS have, to date, frustrated most attempts to reverse its devastating clinical sequelae.

NUTRITION SCREENING AND ASSESSMENT

Nutrition screening to identify cancer patients at risk for malnutrition and a nutrition assessment to elucidate their nutrient requirements are the first step in the nutrition care of cancer patients.[18] Objective parameters such as albumin, transferrin, and body weight changes are used in various formulae to predict preoperative risk in malnourished cancer patients (Table 147.3). The Prognostic Nutritional Index (PNI) has been validated prospectively and calculates the percentage risk of an operative complication in an individual. It can differentiate patients at low risk for nutrition-related complications (<10%) from those that are at high risk (>50%).[59] The Nutrition Risk Index (NRI) was utilized to stratify nutrition risk in the Veterans Affairs Total Parenteral Nutrition Cooperative Study Group trial of perioperative parenteral nutrition and classifies individuals as either well nourished or malnourished.[60] The Hospital Prognostic Index (HPI) identifies high-risk patients and evaluates the efficacy of hospital therapy.[61]

As effective, and more generalizable and practical, are various questionnaire-based tools; they can effectively and reproducibly categorize nutrition risk in cancer patients. The most frequently utilized and validated tool is the Patient Generated Subjective Global Assessment (PG-SGA). Prognostic factors such as weight loss, performance status, and nutrition-related symptoms are assessed in the PG-SGA. The clinician combines physical examination findings (especially loss of subcutaneous fat and the presence of muscle wasting, ankle and sacral edema, and ascites) with historical factors such as weight change, change in dietary intake, presence of gastrointestinal symptoms, functional capacity (performance status), and primary diagnosis to establish a global assessment of nutrition status (A: well nourished, B: moderately malnourished, C: severely malnourished). A numerical score can be added to the global rating creating the *scored PG-SGA*, which is the standard tool utilized by Oncology Dietetics Practice Group of the American Dietetics Association. The PG-SGA is practical, cost-effective, validated, and considered by some to be a *gold standard*.[62]

PHARMACOTHERAPY OF CANCER-ASSOCIATED WEIGHT LOSS AND MALNUTRITION

Cancer cachexia and the associated weight loss cause symptom distress and impair quality of life in cancer patients. They are associated with fatigue, anorexia, early satiety, and social isolation, as well as other symptoms.[63,64] Furthermore, cancer treatments are often accompanied by gastrointestinal symptom distress relating either to the underlying cancer or, more generically, to the hormonal and cytokine milieu that accompanies the CCS. Qualitative research suggests an important role for psychosocial interventions directed at both the patient and family members to address these symptoms.[65] Much of the focus, to date, however, has been on pharmacologic interventions.

Progestational agents have been the mainstay of the pharmacotherapy of cancer-associated anorexia and weight loss. Megestrol acetate and medroxyprogesterone acetate have been shown to improve appetite and to ameliorate weight loss in studies of patients with cancer and cachexia.[66,67] Improved quality of life has been demonstrated in prospective studies in patients with cancer cachexia treated with megestrol acetate, with minimal side effects.[68,69] Doses studied ranged from 160 to 1,280 mg per day, and maximal weight gain was generally seen within 8 weeks. The mechanism of action may, in part, be mediated via alterations in IL-6 levels.[70] One study suggests that combining megestrol acetate with a cocktail of anti-inflammatory and antioxidant nutrients may have an additional benefit.[71] Dronabinol, a marijuana derivative, has been shown to improve appetite and cause weight gain in small studies. Combined therapy with megestrol acetate dronabinol is not superior to megesterol acetate as a single agent.[72]

Anabolic steroids have no proven efficacy. In human trials, corticosteroids produce transient improvement in nutritional parameters and appetite, but continued use is associated with a negative nitrogen balance, net calcium loss, glucose intolerance, and immunosuppression.[73] Agents such as growth hormone, insulin-like growth factor I, insulin, ghrelin, and melatonin, although promising in rodent models, have not been shown to be helpful in humans in improving nutrition status or quality of life.[73–80] Cyproheptadine, an antihistamine and serotonin antagonist, can reduce diarrhea and reverse weight loss in patients with carcinoid syndrome.

Cytokine-directed therapies offer the promise of potentially reversing the cascade of metabolic and hormonal events that result in cancer cachexia. Animal studies are promising. However, although some agents have demonstrated effects in humans, none have been demonstrated to be clinically effective.[18] Thalidomide and pentoxifylline have been shown to inhibit TNF-α, but have not demonstrated clear efficacy in clinical trials.[81,82]

Eicosapentanoic acid (EPA) and docosahexaenoic acid (DHA) are α-3 omega fatty acids found in high concentrations in fish oils that have anti-inflammatory properties.[83,84] Unfortunately, they have not been shown to be effective in clinical trials in patients with cancer cachexia.[84,85]

Medications to relieve cancer- or treatment-related symptoms that impair oral intake can be important adjuvants to reduce or even eliminate the need for nutrition support in many cancer

TABLE 147.3

Nutrition Screening Tools

A. Prognostic Nutritional Index: % risk of perioperative complication = 158 − 16.6 (albumin; grams per deciliter [g/dL]) − 0.78 (triceps skin fold thickness; mm) − 0.2 (serum transferrin; g/dL) − 5.8 (delayed type hypersensitivity reaction; mm)

B. Nutritional Risk Index: 1.519 × the serum albumin (grams per liter) + 0.417 × (current weight/usual weight) × 100
  a. Patients are characterized as malnourished if they had a score of 100 or less on the Nutritional Risk Index

C. Patient Generated Subjective Global Assessment (PG-SGA)
  a. Patient History: weight change, change in dietary intake, gastrointestinal symptoms, change in functional capacity, diagnosis
  b. Physical Exam: loss of subcutaneous fat, muscle wasting, ankle edema, sacral edema, ascites
  c. The previous are combined to create a numerical score to categorize patients as mildly, moderately, or severely malnourished.

patients.[86] Nausea, vomiting, diarrhea, and constipation are common. They can lead to an aversion to eating, with resultant weight loss. When these symptoms are present, a formal evaluation to look for an underlying cause and intervention by a registered dietitian has been shown to be helpful.[87] General approaches include the use of antiemetics, promotility agents, antidiarrheals, fiber, laxatives, and (when pancreatic insufficiency is suspected) pancreatic enzyme replacement.[88,89] Depression occurs in 25% to 45% of patients with cancer and can lead to a loss of appetite and weight loss.[90,91] Antidepressant medications can help.[90–93]

NUTRITION SUPPORT OF CANCER PATIENTS

Because malnutrition is associated with a poor prognosis in cancer patients, it seems intuitive that nutrition support should improve cancer outcomes. Unfortunately, this notion is an oversimplification. The mere provision of nutrition support does not guarantee that the cancer patient will optimally utilize the nutrients to improve clinical outcomes. However, evidence does suggest that some form of nutrition support can be effective and can improve clinical outcomes in cancer patients who are currently undergoing anticancer treatment (surgery, chemotherapy, and/or radiation) AND who are moderately or severely malnourished OR who are anticipated to be unable to meet their nutrition needs orally for a period greater than 7 to 14 days in perioperative patients and greater than 14 days in nonsurgical patients.[94] Guidelines that specify the cancer patients who are likely to benefit from nutrition support (i.e., the provision of nutrients other than orally) have been published by major nutrition organizations.[94,95] Evidence-based guidelines published by the American Society for Parenteral and Enteral Nutrition for nutrition support during anticancer treatment and in hematopoietic cell transplantation are summarized in Table 147.4.

The *routine* use of nutrition support in cancer patients is not indicated. More than 35 clinical trials, some of them prospective and randomized, including more than 5,500 patients, have been summarized.[96] In adequately nourished patients, nutrition support by the enteral or parenteral route does not improve outcomes in patients receiving chemotherapy or radiation therapy or who are undergoing cancer surgery, and in fact, nutrition support may actually harm these patients.[96] Nutrition support should be reserved for those patients who are actively receiving anticancer treatment and who are malnourished or who are at high risk of becoming acutely malnourished because of an anticipated inability to take in adequate oral nutrition for 7 to 14 days or longer.

Optimal Route of Administration of Nutrition Support

On the initial presentation, dietary counseling and oral supplementation is often the best approach to support the nutrition needs of cancer patients.[97–100] However, this may not be feasible secondary to side effects of cancer therapy, generalized cancer cachexia, abnormal physiology secondary to the malignancy, or anatomic factors that preclude oral intake. When oral supplementation is not an option, enteral nutrition (EN) is preferred. The enteral route is more physiologic, has fewer associated complications (especially infection), has a decreased incidence of associated hyperglycemia, and is more cost effective than parenteral nutrition (PN).[101–103] EN can improve nitrogen balance and stimulate weight gain in cancer patients.[104] EN is generally contraindicated in patients with bowel obstruction, abdominal distention, ileus, severe diarrhea, gastrointestinal bleeding, and high output external fistulas.

If use of the gastrointestinal tract is not feasible, then PN should be used. PN can facilitate weight gain; however, this is primarily in the form of fat.[105] Historically, it was thought that the use of PN may mitigate morbidity and decrease mortality in the periop-

---

TABLE 147.4

Nutrition Support Guideline Recommendations During Adult Anticancer Treatment (A.S.P.E.N. Clinical Guidelines)[94]

1. **Nutrition Support Therapy During Anticancer Treatment**
   a. Patients with cancer are nutritionally at risk and should undergo nutrition screening to identify those who require a formal nutrition assessment with development of a nutrition care plan.
   b. Nutrition support therapy should not be used routinely in patients undergoing major cancer operations.
   c. Perioperative nutrition support therapy may be beneficial in moderately or severely malnourished patients if administered for 7–14 days preoperatively, but the potential benefits of nutrition support must be weighed against the potential risks of the nutrition support therapy itself and of delaying the operation.
   d. Nutrition support therapy should not be used routinely as an adjunct to chemotherapy.
   e. Nutrition support therapy should not be used routinely in patients undergoing head and neck, abdominal, or pelvic irradiation.
   f. Nutrition support therapy is appropriate in patients receiving active anticancer treatment who are malnourished and who are anticipated to be unable to ingest and/or absorb adequate nutrients for a prolonged period of time (7–14 days).
   g. The palliative use of nutrition support therapy in terminally ill cancer patients is rarely indicated.
   h. Omega-3 fatty acid supplementation may help stabilize weight in cancer patients on oral diets experiencing progressive, unintentional weight loss.
   i. Patients should not use therapeutic diets to treat cancer.
   j. Immune-enhancing enteral formulas containing mixtures of arginine, nucleic acids, and essential fatty acids may be beneficial in malnourished patients undergoing major cancer operations.

2. **Nutrition Support Therapy in Hematopoietic Cell Transplantation**
   a. All patients undergoing hematopoietic cell transplantation with myeloablative conditioning regimens are at nutrition risk and should undergo nutrition screening to identify those who require formal nutrition assessment with development of a nutrition care plan.
   b. Nutrition support therapy is appropriate in patients undergoing hematopoietic cell transplantation who are malnourished and who are anticipated to be unable to ingest and/or absorb adequate nutrition.
   c. Enteral nutrition should be used in patients with a functioning gastrointestinal tract in whom oral intake is inadequate to meet nutrition requirements.
   d. Pharmacologic doses of parenteral glutamine may benefit patients undergoing hematopoietic cell transplantation.
   e. Patients should receive dietary counseling regarding foods that may pose infectious risks and that require safe food handling during the period of neutropenia.
   f. Nutrition support therapy is appropriate for patients undergoing hematopoietic cell transplantation who develop moderate to severe graft versus host disease accompanied by poor oral intake and/or significant malabsorption.

---

erative setting in gastrointestinal malignancy patients. However, many studies suggest that in adequately nourished patients, the perioperative use of PN in patients with gastrointestinal malignancies actually increases the incidence of infections and does not improve survival.[94] However, severely malnourished patients can benefit because the use of PN in the perioperative setting in these patients can reduce the incidence of surgical complications and can improve survival in comparison to standard isotonic fluids.[106]

Optimal Timing for Initiation of Nutrition Support

Once the ideal route of nutrition is established, the timing of initiation of nutrition support must be considered. Historically, enteral feeding was discouraged following abdominal surgical procedures; *bowel rest* was thought to promote anastomotic healing and prevent nausea and vomiting. More recently, it has been recognized that early oral and enteral feeding can promote healing and reduce length of stay.[107] Failure to consider nutrition and diet issues perioperatively can result in lost opportunities to maintain nutrition status and to avoid nutrition-related complications. In contrast, a delay in the initiation of PN may be appropriate, even in those patients in whom oral or enteral feeding is not possible. In a prospective, randomized trial, critically ill patients, including cancer patients, patients in whom EN was attempted early but in whom the initiation of PN was delayed for 7 days had a shorter length of intensive care unit (ICU) stay and also had reductions in the incidence of infectious complications, organ dysfunction, and hospital length of stay compared to patients in whom PN was initiated on day two.[108]

Perioperative PN appears to beneficial in moderately or severely malnourished patients if administered for 7 to 14 days prior to an operation.[106] In mildly or borderline malnourished patients, there is no demonstrable benefit to preoperative PN.

Prescribing Nutritional Support

Energy requirements are determined by a patient's age, gender, body composition, and energy expenditure. Multiple formulas have been suggested to determine caloric requirement, but none has been demonstrated to be more reliable.[18] Typically, non-physiologically stressed patients require approximately 1.0 g per kilogram of body weight per day of protein and 25 kcal per kilogram of body weight per day of nonprotein calories. Essential fatty acids (linoleic and linolenic acids are generally used in the United States) are provided, approximately 1 to 2.0 g per kilogram per day, to supplement calories and to prevent essential fatty acid deficiency. There are additional fluid, electrolyte, vitamin, and trace mineral requirements (Table 147.5). Enteral formulas come premixed and contain all of the required nutrients. PN is generally individually prescribed, and vitamins and trace elements must be added.

Enteral Nutrition

The selection of a formula for EN is based on an assessment of both nutrient and fluid requirements. The calorie concentration in balanced formulae can range from 1.0 to 2.0 kcal per milliliter. The nonprotein component is derived from carbohydrates and lipids. Those diets with more carbohydrates have a higher osmolarity than isocaloric diets containing lipids.

Access for EN can be via percutaneous gastrostomy, operative gastrostomy, feeding jejunostomy (placed endoscopically or operatively), or via a nasojejunal tube.[109] Feeding rates should start at 30 mL per hour and increase at set intervals (12 to 24 hours) to achieve an assessed caloric goal.

Hyperosmolar formulas are generally not administered to the jejunum directly. If patients develop symptoms of diarrhea (most frequent) or constipation, changes should be made to either the rate or formulation of the tube feedings; antimotility agents and/or fiber can often be added to feedings to treat these symptoms. Additionally, with diarrhea, it is reasonable to check a *Clostridium difficile* toxin prior to making other changes.

TABLE 147.5

Vitamin and Mineral Requirements[139]

Vitamin and Mineral	Units	Recommended Dietary Allowance (RDA) for Daily Oral Intake	Daily Amount Provided (Recommended) by Standard Intravenous Preparations
Vitamin A (retinol)	IU	1,760 (females); 3,300 (males)	3,300
Vitamin D (ergocalciferol)	IU	200	200
Vitamin E (tocopherol)	mg TE	8–10	10
Vitamin K (phylloquinone)	μg	20–40	0
Vitamin C (ascorbic acid)	mg	60	100
Thiamine (vitamin B_1)	mg	1.0–1.5	3.0
Riboflavin (vitamin B_2)	mg	1.2–1.7	3.6
Niacin	mg	13–19	40
Pyridoxine (vitamin B_6)	mg	2.0–2.2	4.0
Pantothenic acid	mg	4–7 (adults)	15
Folic acid	mg	0.4	0.4
Vitamin B_{12}	mg	3.0	5
Biotin	μg	100–200	60
Zinc	mg	15	5
Copper	mg	2–3	1
Manganese	mg	2.5–5	0.5
Chromium	mg	0.05–0.2	0.1
Iron	mg	10 (males); 18 (females)	3

Regardless of the route of EN, all tubes need to be flushed at least daily with 20 to 25 mL of saline or water to ascertain tube patency. Tubes can also be dislodged, and patients should present urgently back to the clinician to reinsert a tube into an established track prior to scarring and closure.

Parenteral Nutrition

Central venous access is necessary to administer PN because of its hyperosmolarity. Commonly, PN is comprised of hypertonic glucose (25%), amino acids (4.25%), lipids, electrolytes, and essential vitamins, minerals, and trace elements. The caloric density of these formulae is usually 1 kcal per milliliter and, therefore, 2 to 2.5 L of volume a day provides 2,000 to 2,500 kcal and all essential nutrients. To prevent essential fatty acid deficiency, patients should receive at least 500 mL of a 20% fat emulsion containing both linoleic and linolenic fatty acids weekly.

Specialty Nutrition Formulas: Immune Enhancing and Formulas for Organ Failure

In order to address special needs based on physiologic deficiencies, there are multiple specialty nutrition formulas. There have been numerous studies evaluating the potential benefits of immune-enhancing formulas. These are enteral formulas that have been tested both in the perioperative and ICU setting and contain various combinations of arginine, glutamine, RNA, and/or omega-3 fatty acids. Although findings are variable, in general, these formulas result in fewer infectious complications and perhaps shorter lengths of stay in the postoperative setting.[110–116]

EFFECT OF NUTRITION SUPPORT ON TUMOR GROWTH

Historically, concern has been voiced concerning the potential for nutrition support to stimulate tumor growth and metastasis.[117] In murine models, PN provided in excess of energy requirements can more than double tumor growth rate.[118–120] In humans, the provision of nutrition support may stimulate tumor cell proliferation and protein synthesis, but this finding is not consistent.[121–124] There are no clinical outcomes data that suggest a deleterious effect of nutrition support when used in malnourished patients on tumor growth and spread. These data emphasize the sensibility of using nutrition support in cancer patients when malnutrition or the risk of malnutrition is clearly demonstrated.[96,117]

GLYCEMIC CONTROL IN PATIENTS WITH CANCER

Hyperglycemia is frequently observed in stressed, critically ill patients and in patients receiving nutrition support. Multiple factors (many of which are present in cancer patients) contribute to this, including elevated levels of stress hormones, systemic activation by inflammatory cytokines that promote insulin resistance, and the administration of carbohydrate-rich nutrition support.[125] In seriously ill patients, including cancer patients, the occurrence of hyperglycemia is associated with increased morbidity and mortality.[126] Five major trials have investigated the role of tight glycemic control in critically ill patients receiving nutrition support.[126–131] They have been nicely summarized.[131,132] Many of the patients in these trials were cancer patients. In these trials, intravenous insulin was used in the experimental groups to maintain blood sugars below approximately 100 mg per deciliter, and in the conventional treatment groups, the blood sugar target was higher (140 to 200 mg per deciliter). In general, mortality was increased in the tight glucose control groups. All of these trials observed a higher incidence of hypoglycemia in the stringent control groups than in the conventional therapy groups. It seems prudent in critically ill cancer patients receiving nutrition support to target a blood sugar in the 140 to 180 mg per deciliter range to attain at least some of the benefits of more stringent glucose control but without risking the possible increase in mortality that may result from overly tight control.[133,134]

PALLIATIVE NUTRITION SUPPORT IN PATIENTS NOT RECEIVING ANTICANCER TREATMENT

The use of PN support in patients with advanced cancer and not actively receiving anticancer treatment remains controversial.[94] This is despite evidence that PN support in this setting is often futile and may be harmful. In a palliative setting, a patient's quality of life should be the primary factor addressed when considering the use of home PN.[135,136]

In determining the utility of palliative home PN, important considerations include the patient's estimated survival, potential risks and benefits, and the patient's and family's wishes. The goals of nutrition support in this particular setting are to prolong life and to ameliorate nutrition-related symptoms that cause undue suffering.[137] A review of home PN in cancer patients who are terminally ill noted that the most frequent indications were obstruction, malabsorption, fistula, and radiation enteritis.[138] Overall, there is some suggestion of a survival benefit. The patients that are potential beneficiaries of home PN are those with a good performance status (Karnofsky score >50); those with inoperable bowel obstruction; those with minimal symptoms from a disease involving major organs such as brain, liver, and lungs; and those with indolent disease progression. Guidelines suggest PN support should only be offered if a patient is a candidate for active anticancer therapy and/or the patient is expected to have a survival greater than 40 to 60 days.[110] Additionally, in the context of home PN, patients must have caretaker support nearly 24 hours per day. There are few patients that meet the previous criteria for home PN. Honest and compassionate discussions are necessary with these patients, their families, and their referring physicians in order to optimize decision making and the delivery of palliative care in this end-of-life setting.

SELECTED REFERENCES

The full reference list can be accessed at lwwhealthlibrary.com/oncology.

3. Polednak AP. Estimating the number of U.S. incident cancers attributable to obesity and the impact on temporal trends in incidence rates for obesity-related cancers. *Cancer Detect Prev* 2008;32:190–199.

7. Dewys WD, Begg C, Lavin PT, et al. Prognostic effect of weight loss prior to chemotherapy in cancer patients. Eastern Cooperative Oncology Group. *Am J Med* 1980;69:491–497.

12. Ravasco P, Monteiro-Grillo I, Vidal PM, et al. Cancer: disease and nutrition are key determinants of patients' quality of life. *Support Care Cancer* 2004;12:246–252.

14. August D, Huhmann M. Nutritional care of cancer patients. In: Norton JA, Barie P, Bollinger RR, et al., eds. *Surgery: Basic Science and Clinical Evidence.* 2nd ed. New York: Springer Publishing; 2008: 2123–2149.

17. Calle EE, Rodriguez C, Walker-Thurmond K, et al. Overweight, obesity, and mortality from cancer in a prospectively studied cohort of U.S. adults. *N Engl J Med* 2003;348:1625–1638.

18. August DA, Huhmann MB. Nutritional support of the cancer patient. In: Ross CA, Caballero B, Cousins RJ, et al., eds. *Modern Nutrition in Health and Disease.* Philadelphia, PA: Lippincott, Williams and Wilkins; 2013: 1194–1213.

24. Laviano A, Meguid MM, Rossi-Fanelli F. Cancer anorexia: clinical implications, pathogenesis, and therapeutic strategies. *Lancet Oncol* 2003;4:686–694.

27. Hyltander A, Drott C, Korner U, et al. Elevated energy expenditure in cancer patients with solid tumours. *Eur J Cancer* 1991;27:9–15.

32. Johnson G, Salle A, Lorimier G, et al. Cancer cachexia: measured and predicted resting energy expenditures for nutritional needs evaluation. *Nutrition* 2008;24:443–450.

34. Falconer JS, Fearon KC, Plester CE, et al. Cytokines, the acute-phase response, and resting energy expenditure in cachectic patients with pancreatic cancer. *Ann Surg* 1994;219:325–331.

45. Jeevanandam M, Legaspi A, Lowry SF, et al. Effect of total parenteral nutrition on whole body protein kinetics in cachectic patients with benign or malignant disease. *JPEN J Parenter Enteral Nutr* 1988;12:229–236.

48. Suzuki H, Asakawa A, Amitani H, et al. Cancer cachexia—pathophysiology and management. *J Gastroenterol* 2013;48:574–594.

62. Bauer J, Capra S, Ferguson M. Use of the scored Patient-Generated Subjective Global Assessment (PG-SGA) as a nutrition assessment tool in patients with cancer. *Eur J Clin Nutr* 2002;56:779–785.

63. Andrew IM, Waterfield K, Hildreth AJ, et al. Quantifying the impact of standardized assessment and symptom management tools on symptoms associated with cancer-induced anorexia cachexia syndrome. *Palliat Med* 2009;23:680–688.

70. Yeh S, Wu SY, Levine DM, et al. Quality of life and stimulation of weight gain after treatment with megestrol acetate: correlation between cytokine levels and nutritional status, appetite in geriatric patients with wasting syndrome. *J Nutr Health Aging* 2000;4:246–251.

71. Mantovani G, Maccio A, Madeddu C, et al. Randomized phase III clinical trial of five different arms of treatment for patients with cancer cachexia: interim results. *Nutrition* 2008;24:305–313.

73. Ottery FD, Walsh D, Strawford A. Pharmacologic management of anorexia/cachexia. *Semin Oncol* 1998;25:35–44.

83. Tisdale MJ. Cachexia in cancer patients. *Nat Rev Cancer* 2002;2:862–871.

84. Fearon KC, Barber MD, Moses AG, et al. Double-blind, placebo-controlled, randomized study of eicosapentaenoic acid diester in patients with cancer cachexia. *J Clin Oncol* 2006;24:3401–3407.

86. Licitra L, Spinazze S, Roila F. Antiemetic therapy. *Crit Rev Oncol Hematol* 2002;43:93–101.

90. Fisch M. Treatment of depression in cancer. *J Natl Cancer Inst Monogr* 2004:105–111.

91. Valente SM, Saunders JM, Cohen MZ. Evaluating depression among patients with cancer. *Cancer Pract* 1994;2:65–71.

94. August DA, Huhmann MB, American Society for Parenteral and Enteral Nutrition (A.S.P.E.N.) Board of Directors. A.S.P.E.N. clinical guidelines: nutrition support therapy during adult anticancer treatment and in hematopoietic cell transplantation. *JPEN J Parenter Enteral Nutr* 2009;33:472–500.

95. Bozzetti F, Arends J, Lundholm K, et al. ESPEN Guidelines on Parenteral Nutrition: non-surgical oncology. *Clin Nutr* 2009;28:445–454.

96. Huhmann MB, August DA. Review of American Society for Parenteral and Enteral Nutrition (ASPEN) Clinical Guidelines for Nutrition Support in Cancer Patients: nutrition screening and assessment. *Nutr Clin Pract* 2008;23:182–188.

104. Bozzetti F. Rationale and indications for preoperative feeding of malnourished surgical cancer patients. *Nutrition* 2002;18:953–959.

105. Shike M, Russel DM, Detsky AS, et al. Changes in body composition in patients with small-cell lung cancer. The effect of total parenteral nutrition as an adjunct to chemotherapy. *Ann Intern Med* 1984;101:303–309.

106. Perioperative total parenteral nutrition in surgical patients. The Veterans Affairs Total Parenteral Nutrition Cooperative Study Group. *N Engl J Med* 1991;325:525–532.

108. Casaer MP, Mesotten D, Hermans G, et al. Early versus late parenteral nutrition in critically ill adults. *N Engl J Med* 2011;365:506–517.

109. Itkin M, DeLegge MH, Fang JC, et al. Multidisciplinary practical guidelines for gastrointestinal access for enteral nutrition and decompression from the Society of Interventional Radiology and American Gastroenterological Association (AGA) Institute, with endorsement by Canadian Interventional Radiological Association (CIRA) and Cardiovascular and Interventional Radiological Society of Europe (CIRSE). *Gastroenterology* 2011;141:742–765.

112. Marik PE, Zaloga GP. Immunonutrition in high-risk surgical patients: a systematic review and analysis of the literature. *JPEN J Parenter Enteral Nutr* 2010;34:378–386.

114. Beale RJ, Bryg DJ, Bihari DJ. Immunonutrition in the critically ill: a systematic review of clinical outcome. *Crit Care Med* 1999;27:2799–2805.

115. Heyland DK, Novak F, Drover JW, et al. Should immunonutrition become routine in critically ill patients? A systematic review of the evidence. *JAMA* 2001;286:944–953.

125. Kavanagh BP, McCowen KC. Clinical practice. Glycemic control in the ICU. *N Engl J Med* 2010;363:2540–2546.

126. NICE-SUGAR Study Investigators, Finfer S, Chittock DR, et al. Intensive versus conventional glucose control in critically ill patients. *N Engl J Med* 2009;360:1283–1297.

127. van den Berghe G, Wouters P, Weekers F, et al. Intensive insulin therapy in critically ill patients. *N Engl J Med* 2001;345:1359–1367.

128. Van den Berghe G, Wilmer A, Hermans G, et al. Intensive insulin therapy in the medical ICU. *N Engl J Med* 2006;354:449–461.

132. Huhmann MB, August DA. Perioperative nutrition support in cancer patients. *Nutr Clin Pract* 2012;27:586–592.

138. Mackenzie ML, Gramlich L. Home parenteral nutrition in advanced cancer: where are we? *Appl Physiol Nutr Metab* 2008;33:1–11.

139. Rolandelli RH, Gupta D, Wilmore D. Nutritional support. In: Souba WW, Fink MP, Jurkovich GJ, et al., eds. *ACS Surgery Principles and Practice*. New York: WebMD Professional Publishing; 2007: 1789–1809.

PALLIATIVE AND ALTERNATIVE CARE

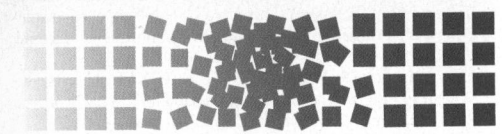

Veronica Sanchez Varela, Eric S. Zhou, and Sharon L. Bober

INTRODUCTION

Rapid and recent advances in cancer care now mean that the majority of newly diagnosed cancer patients will "live beyond cancer." This shift has resulted in a consistently increasing focus on maintaining and/or restoring quality of life for cancer survivors. Despite widespread acknowledgment that sexual function is often profoundly disrupted by cancer treatment, there is still a deafening silence when it comes to addressing this quality of life issue for a majority of cancer patients and survivors. Often, oncologists do not feel comfortable addressing sexual problems and instead focus on treatment outcomes related to survivorship rather than quality of life.[1] However, several studies have shown that patients, both male and female across diseases, are often disappointed by the lack of information, support, and practical strategies provided by their clinicians to help manage the sexual changes secondary to cancer and cancer treatments.[2-4]

Although there are real barriers to bringing frank conversation about sexuality into the routine clinical oncology encounter, we would like to begin this chapter by clarifying why it is important for clinicians to address this topic with patients and survivors. Sexuality and intimacy have been shown to help lessen emotional distress and improve psychosocial adjustment in the face of cancer.[5] Acknowledging the importance of sexuality to patients' quality of life, the World Health Organization has recently declared that maintaining sexual health indeed falls under the purview of physicians. For patients who endure so many losses as a result of cancer, including social, financial, physical, and emotional disruptions, the loss of sexual function adds a burden that is only magnified by the shame and embarrassment that this aspect of life is not only changed, but also feels unspeakable. Moreover, patients worry that their experience of "damage" cannot be undone and often wrongly assume that sexual dysfunction cannot be adequately addressed. Many of these assumptions are unwittingly reinforced by clinicians who, by not addressing the topic, mistakenly give patients the message that "nothing can be done"—an unfortunate occurrence because the majority of typical sexual problems facing cancer patients and cancer survivors can indeed be effectively treated.

Several studies have examined medical professionals' barriers to communication about sexual health needs with their patients. It has recently been suggested that these barriers appear to fall into three categories: issues related to patient characteristics, provider characteristics, and systems issues.[6] Patient characteristics refer to a range of assumptions about a patients' sexuality based on age, gender, partner status, sexual orientation, prognosis, economic and social class, as well as religious, cultural, and ethnic backgrounds that may deter clinicians from asking about sexual health. For example, doctors may assume that an older person who is widowed or divorced is no longer sexually active or that if a patient is from another culture it would be inappropriate to ask about sexual concerns. Provider characteristics refer to the training, experience, knowledge, and attitudes of the provider that may either deter or facilitate conversations about sexuality after cancer.

Lack of experience and lack of knowledge have repeatedly been shown to explain why sexuality is not addressed[7,8] with cancer patients and survivors. Finally, systems issues are often reported as major barriers to this topic. Oncologists will aver that there is no time to address sexuality when there is barely enough time to manage more pressing concerns.[7] Oncologists are also concerned about the lack of available resources for patients if a patient were to endorse a problem.[1]

The aim of this chapter is threefold: (1) to familiarize clinicians with the most common sexual problems for men and women that are related to specific cancers and their particular treatments; (2) to review intervention options for sexual problems including acknowledgment of current resources that are readily available to both clinicians and patients, and (3) to provide clear and straightforward language that clinicians can use to initiate a brief discussion about sexuality with their patients as well as to overview some brief and previously validated measures of sexual dysfunction that can be incorporated into standard practice in order to assess sexual dysfunction more systematically.

CANCER IN MEN

Prostate

The relative 5-year survival rate for those diagnosed with localized stage disease approaches 100%.[9] The combination of the increase in diagnosed cases, increasing survival rates, and the decreasing age at diagnosis has made sexual dysfunction following prostate cancer treatments a progressively more pressing issue.[10,11]

Surgery

One of the primary treatment options for men diagnosed with early stage disease is a prostatectomy, which can have a major impact on the sexual functioning of the patient.[10,12] During surgery, the seminal vesicles are removed and the vas deferens is cut, which causes dry orgasms and urinary incontinence during orgasm. This is associated with poor satisfaction with orgasms, and the avoidance of sexual activities.[13-17] In addition, the cavernous nerves may be affected during surgery, which can cause erectile dysfunction in up to 90% of men.[18-20] Therefore, nerve-sparing surgical approaches are preferred because they are proven to be effective in helping patients sustain erectile function postsurgery, especially if bilateral nerve-sparing surgery is feasible.[19,21-25] Age, ethnicity, preoperative sexual and overall physical function, extent of neurovascular bundle preservation, and the surgeon's level of experience are factors related to postsurgical sexual function.[23,26-33] The recovery period for the nerves related to erectile function is approximately 18 to 24 months.[27] Additionally, the denervation caused by surgery may result in smooth muscle atrophy, erectile tissue apoptosis, and/or hypoxia-induced tissue damage, all of which can contribute to reduction in penile length and circumference.[34-37]

There are currently a variety of treatments for erectile dysfunction. With the advent of sildenafil, the first-line treatments for erectile dysfunction are oral medications because they are effective and noninvasive.[38] However, they may be ineffective in men who are older, and men who had low erectile functioning prior to surgery, as well as for men who have neurovascular bundle damage as a result of surgery.[39–41] Oral agents also may result in physical side effects (e.g., headache, muscle pain) and psychological side effects (e.g., concern about medication use).[42,43] Because oral medications may not be effective for 18 to 24 months postsurgery, alternative treatment options can be considered and include intracavernous injection therapy, transurethral alprostadil, and vacuum erection devices. Intracavernous injection therapy is effective in the majority of patients,[44–46] although its use can be anxiety provoking. Up to half of patients who are offered injection therapy either refuse or stop treatment within first 6 months.[47,48] Transurethral alprostadil is also effective.[49] The use of vacuum erection devices can be beneficial for men who experience penile shortening,[50–52] although approximately 1 in 5 men discontinue use due to discomfort, difficulty with operating the device, penile bruising, and social inconvenience.[52] Finally, the use of a penile prosthesis can be a helpful treatment for erectile dysfunction,[53–56] although it is typically reserved for patients who fail other treatments given its invasive and irreversible nature.[57] Combination treatments (e.g., both phosphodiesterase type 5 inhibitor [PDE-5] and vacuum erection devices) may provide the most hope for the recovery of erectile function.[58,59]

From a rehabilitation, rather than a treatment, perspective, oxygenation preserving strategies including the use of vacuum erection devices,[50,51] daily low-dose PDE-5 inhibitor use,[60] intracavernous injection of vasoactive agents,[61] and hyperbaric oxygen therapy[62] can help to reduce tissue fibrosis.[63] This penile rehabilitation therapy can be helpful with the preservation of erectile tissue and is associated with improved erectile function.[64,65] There is some debate regarding the efficacy of penile rehabilitation therapy,[66–69] including questions regarding the use of on-demand, rather than daily, dosing of PDE-5 inhibitors,[70] dosing, and timing of rehabilitation therapy.[71,72] Recent evidence suggests that there may be subsets of patients who would benefit from penile rehabilitation.[73,74]

Radiation

External beam radiation and brachytherapy are also treatment options for men with early stage prostate cancer. Patients may believe that radiation therapy will have less of a negative impact on sexual function, and often times may choose radiation therapy over surgery as a way to preserve sexual health. However, radiation therapy, in all forms, is associated with sexual dysfunction, although radiation therapy patients experience different functional trajectories compared to prostatectomy patients.[23,75] Radiation patients report their highest sexual functioning immediately posttreatment, and then proceed to decline subsequently, which is in direct contrast to surgery patients, where their sexual function tends to improve over time.[76–80] Although there are better outcomes for younger men (≤60 years),[81] up to a third of radiation therapy patients become impotent 3 years posttreatment.[82] This progressive decline in sexual function is caused by fibrosis that continues to develop after radiation treatment is completed.[76] Although brachytherapy tends to be associated with a less severe side effect profile compared to external beam radiation, sexual function is still likely to be compromised as a result of treatment. Brachytherapy patients report changes to their overall sexual function,[83] reduced ejaculate volume, premature or diminished orgasms,[84] and declines in erectile function.[85] Risk factors for erectile dysfunction after brachytherapy include greater age, poorer pretreatment functioning, and prostate volume.[86]

Treatment for erectile dysfunction in radiation therapy patients is similar to surgery patients, with first-line therapy being oral treatment.[87] However, the scar tissue that builds up over time on the nerves may limit the effectiveness of oral medication, and patients who achieve potency after radiation therapy may experience a slow decline in function.[88,89]

Hormone Therapy

In men diagnosed with late stage disease as well as high-risk disease, androgen deprivation therapy is the most common course of treatment. It is also associated with a range of side effects, including marked sexual dysfunction, such as decreased libido, elevated erectile dysfunction, and lower levels of sexual activity.[90–94] Additionally, treatment-related side effects such as body feminization, hot flashes, fatigue, and decreased mood and self-esteem also greatly impact sexual health among men who choose hormone therapy.[95] Treatment for erectile dysfunction associated with hormone therapy is consistent with options used after surgery and radiation. However, the more difficult sexual dysfunction to treat is the low libido. Medical options, such as increasing testosterone levels, are counter to androgen-deprivation therapy. There has been recent research evaluating the role of estrogen in restoring libido among men undergoing hormone therapy.[96] Use of targeted cognitive-behavioral interventions designed to improve communication, reduce relationship distress, and improve coping skills and self-esteem have shown promise in terms of improving adjustment and reducing distress for men on androgen deprivation therapy.[97–101]

Quality of Life Implications of Sexual Dysfunction

All active treatment options for prostate cancer are associated with compromised sexual functioning,[102] which has been identified as the most common cause of disease-specific distress among survivors.[11,102–105] Even if sexual function returns to baseline levels, prostate cancer survivors often continue to report sexual bother.[106] Men who struggle with sexual dysfunction are at risk for mood-related disturbances, which impacts their posttreatment adjustment and quality of life.[107,108] Sexual dysfunction presents a multidimensional challenge that requires multidisciplinary support from physicians, nurses, physical therapists, and psychologists who work together in treating both the physical and psychological impact of treatment.[109–111] In any intervention work, it is important to consider the relational context,[112–114] although this is often overlooked.[115,116]

Testicular

Testicular cancer is the most common cancer among men between the ages of 20 and 34 years.[117] These statistics signal to the fact that these men are in their sexual prime and at a likely age to start a family, making the sexual and fertility aspects of testicular cancer treatment an important topic.[118] Most commonly, these men report that treatment for their cancer impacts their orgasm intensity and frequency (20% to 38%), causes problems with ejaculation (6% to 51%), lowers libido (20% to 35%), and causes erectile dysfunction (17% to 40%).[119–122] As a result, up to 43% of testicular cancer patients report decreased sexual activity, and approximately 1 in 5 are dissatisfied with their sexual experience following treatment.[123,124] For these patients, their sexual function appears to reach a low point about 3 months posttreatment, and tends to recover over the course of 1 year,[125–127] although there are survivors for whom treatment-related sexual side effects can last for up to 5 years.[128]

The primary concern for many men with testicular cancer is fertility. Although there are variations, abnormal sperm concentrations can be seen in up to half of testicular cancer survivors.[120,129] Testicular cancer survivors have various fertility options, including sperm cryopreservation and intracytoplasmatic sperm injection.[130,131] Patients benefit greatly from receiving information about reproductive options[120] as well as a discussion about broader sexual health issues (Table 148.1).[132]

PALLIATIVE AND ALTERNATIVE CARE

TABLE 148.1

Medications for Sexual Problems (Men)

Medication	Purpose	Notes	References
Oral PDE-5 inhibitor	Erectile dysfunction	First-line treatment. Ineffective in some men (older, lower function previously, treatment-related nerve damage), and immediately posttreatment. Both physical (e.g., headache, dizziness) and psychological (dependence) side effects can occur. Daily low-dose use may help repair damaged blood vessel endothelium and improve erectile function.	38, 40, 42, 43, 60
Intracavernosal injection therapy	Erectile dysfunction	Effective treatment. Patient adherence is a significant challenge. Patients benefit from effective training, and psychoeducation about proper use.	44, 47, 48
Estrogen therapy	Libido	Consideration of parenteral estrogen add back. Preliminary research. May be helpful in improving libido in androgen-deprived men.	96
Testosterone replacement therapy	Erectile dysfunction, libido, vitality	Effective in treating symptoms of hypogonadism. Lack of controlled studies to document its safety in prostate cancer survivors.	285–289

CANCERS THAT AFFECT MEN AND WOMEN

Bladder

The most common presentation of bladder cancer is in the form of transitional cell carcinoma, and although most cases tend to be superficial when first diagnosed, repeated treatments may be required to treat recurrences. Treatments for bladder cancer mainly include surgery, radiation therapy, immunotherapy, and chemotherapy, with surgery used in most of the cases. From a sexual health perspective, treatment of bladder cancer by radical cystectomy is the procedure that has received the most attention given its likely negative implications on sexual functioning.[133] The efficacy of laparoscopic surgery in terms of oncologic control has been recently studied,[134–136] but it is not clear if it differentially impacts sexual functioning.[137]

Male Sexual Function

A standard radical cystectomy for treating bladder cancer in men involves the removal of the bladder as well as the prostate, seminal vesicles, vasa deferentia, and the removal or damage of the neurovascular bundles, leaving the patient with the likely consequent loss of sexual function.[138] Alternatively, a nerve-sparing cystectomy is associated with a temporary decrease in function after surgery, commonly followed by a return to function.[139–143] Unfortunately, oncologic failure rates for nerve-sparing cystectomies are higher.[144–146] This has resulted in a debate regarding the minimization of cancer risk, while maximizing sexual function preservation.[142,147–150] In addition, men report body image issues as a result of their need for urinary diversion following surgery,[133,151] which is associated with sexual dissatisfaction.[152]

For men who are treated with radical or nerve-sparing cystectomy, erectile dysfunction prevails at similar rates to those seen after prostatectomy or nerve-sparing prostatectomy, respectively, and its treatment follows the standard of care for erectile dysfunction in men treated with a prostatectomy. Early PDE-5 inhibitor intervention is associated with improved sexual function and satisfaction.[153] However, almost half of male bladder cancer patients do not seek treatment for their sexual dysfunction postsurgery.[138,154]

Female Sexual Function

The standard radical cystectomy for bladder cancer in women involves the removal of the bladder, urethra, anterior vaginal wall, uterus, and ovaries and it is likely to result in sexual dysfunction,[155–157] including weakened libido, dyspareunia, decreased lubrication, and diminished ability or inability to achieve orgasm.[158,159] Consequently,

many women who undergo non–nerve-sparing cystectomies report discontinuing sexual intercourse following surgery.[157] The use of nerve-sparing surgical procedures has recently been evaluated in an attempt to reduce the impact of treatment on the significant sexual dysfunction caused by a radical cystectomy.[157] Women who undergo nerve-sparing surgery retain sexual function comparable to presurgical levels,[141,157,160] as well as increased potential of fertility preservation.[161] However, there has been limited exploration of the oncologic impact of nerve-sparing surgeries for these women.

Treatment for sexual dysfunction amongst female bladder cancer survivors is similar to recommendations for female survivors of breast, gynecologic, and colorectal cancers. For women who experience physical and/or psychological difficulties resulting from the extent of their cystectomy, vaginal reconstruction surgery may be a viable option.[162]

Head and Neck

Head and neck cancers are considered to be among the most impactful with regard to the patient's posttreatment quality of life. Treatment for head and neck cancer can include surgery, radiation therapy, targeted therapy, and/or chemotherapy. Even when function-sparing approaches are utilized, treatment can still result in facial alterations, as well as changes to saliva quality and/or quantity, breathing, and speech,[163] which cannot be completely corrected with follow-up treatments.[164,165] Head and neck cancer survivors report lowered self-esteem and body image as a result of these treatment-related side effects, which negatively impact their intimate relationships.[166–168] These survivors report feeling less attractive, a reduced libido, and decreased overall satisfaction with their sexual relationships.[169–173] In particular, females, and those who were diagnosed with more advanced stage disease, who underwent surgery, or whose treatment caused more extensive disfigurement are at elevated risk for sexual dysfunction.[169,174,175]

The majority of these patients do not discuss implications of their disease and treatment on body image and sexual health with their medical providers.[172] Sexual health rehabilitation is not well understood in this population.[176,177] Open communication about possible sexual side effects of treatment between providers and patients is associated with improved psychosocial adjustment.[175,178]

Blood, Bone Marrow, and Lymphatic System

Treatment of systemic disease often involves intense interventions with chemotherapy, whole-body irradiation, and/or bone marrow transplant and may cause side effects, including sexual dysfunction. In particular, preparative regimes of high-dose chemotherapy and total body irradiation may result in ovarian failure and low-estrogen levels for women, and gonadal and cavernosal arterial insufficiency in men.[179] Sexual problems in bone-marrow transplant patients may still be present several years after the procedure and include difficulty obtaining an erection, ejaculation, and orgasm for men and concerns about body appearance, vaginal dryness, and painful intercourse and orgasm for women.[180] Moreover, a longitudinal study of sexual function in long-term survivors of hematopoietic cell transplantation documented that at 5 years after treatment, sexual dysfunction is a major problem for this population, with male survivors continuing to have lower sexual function and female survivors having lower scores for sexual activity and function compared to controls.[181] Another important issue that often develops for females after transplant is genital graft-versus-host disease (GVHD). Female genital GVHD after transplant is a complication that tends to receive little attention despite the significant impact it has on the survivor's quality of life. Female tract GVHD may manifest in several forms, from irritation of the vagina or the vulva to ulceration and vaginal stenosis, and it has been found to be present in at least 25% of the transplant survivor population.[182,183] Research studies suggest that an early detection of genital GVHD is highly treatable with steroids and vaginal dilators, and therefore, education on active self-surveillance should be given to patients in addition to a plan for regular gynecologic follow-up posttransplant.[183,184]

Studies that investigate the effectiveness of interventions for sexual dysfunction in women after bone-marrow transplantation are scarce, but therapies including vaginal lubricants, dilators, and vibrators can be recommended to improve some of the sexual side effects of treatment. In men, there is evidence to support that a number of patients recover sexual function over time,[181] and that testosterone cypionate and sildenafil have shown to improve erectile dysfunction in this population.[179] More importantly, many survivors and their partners may feel hesitant or even fearful to resume sexual activity after bone marrow transplantation given concerns about immunosuppression, such as coming in contact with germs. These concerns may prevail even after survivors have been cleared by their medical team to resume sexual activity. It is important, therefore, to anticipate and openly discuss these concerns with survivors and their partners while offering gentle guidance and reassurance about their eligibility to resume sexual activity.

Colorectal

Treatments for colorectal cancer mainly include surgery, radiation therapy, and chemotherapy, with surgery used in most of the cases.[9] Colorectal cancer surgery often causes damage to the sympathetic and parasympathetic nerves and results in erectile and ejaculatory disorders in men and dyspareunia, decreased libido, and changes in the orgasm experience in women.[185] And although the impact of radiotherapy in colorectal cancer survivors has rarely been addressed, the available research suggests that radiation is associated with sexual dysfunction in both men and women.[186]

Because most colorectal cancer patients are over 50 years of age and may presumably have a higher incidence of non–cancer-related sexual dysfunction, studies that use a longitudinal design to assess the prevalence of sexual dysfunction in these survivors are of particular interest. In a longitudinal study by Jayne et al.,[187] the authors compared treatment outcomes in patients who underwent a laparoscopic-assisted surgery versus open surgery for colorectal cancer, including quality of life and sexual functioning. The authors assessed functioning preoperatively and at 2 weeks and 3, 6, 18, and 36 months after surgery and found that although there was no change from baseline in sexual functioning or enjoyment for men and women in both arms, men tended to report more sexual problems from 3 months onward in the laparoscopic arm and from 6 months onward in the open surgery arm. The authors also found

that body image was worse than at baseline from 2 weeks onward for all patients. Therapies recommended for prostate cancer survivors, such as the use of sildenafil,[188] appear to be adequate for a number of male colorectal cancer survivors who suffer from erectile dysfunction following treatment. Likewise, therapies recommended for breast and gynecologic cancer survivors, such as the use of water-based lubricants, vaginal moisturizers, and vaginal dilators, can also be recommended for female colorectal cancer survivors who suffer from vaginal dryness and/or stenosis after radiation.[186] More specific to colorectal cancer survivors are the negative emotional reactions to the colostomy, such as poor body image and reduced self-esteem, which are commonly present and may negatively impact intimacy. But patients and their partners can and do learn how to manage the impact of an ostomy on sexuality, and there are resources available for this purpose. Patients with ostomies should receive information on deodorants to minimize odor, as well as on foods that are likely to cause stronger odors, gas, or diarrhea. Patients should also receive information on pouch covers, and suggestions such as changing positions to avoid pain during intercourse and emptying the stoma before sexual activity.[189] Additional information for patients and their partners can also be found through the United Ostomy Associations of America, Inc.

CANCER IN WOMEN

Breast

Difficulty with sexual function, loss of desire, changes in body image, and disruption of emotional relationships are primary sexual complications of breast cancer from diagnosis through all stages of treatment and into survivorship. Chemotherapy, radiation, surgery, and adjunctive hormonal therapy, whether delivered alone or in combination with each other, all have the potential to negatively impact sexual function. The survival rates of breast cancer for localized disease continue to improve and are now 95% or better.[9] Not only will the majority of breast cancer survivors go on to become long-term cancer survivors, but studies have also shown that the majority of partnered women will remain sexually active either after diagnosis or at the end of treatment.[190,191]

A number of factors have been identified regarding who is at risk for developing sexual problems after breast cancer. Women who have premorbid sexual dysfunction,[192] negative self-concept,[193] depression, and relationship discord[194] are all more likely to struggle with sexual problems. In one recent prospective study assessing the impact of breast cancer on women's sexuality, a younger age was found to be the most salient predictor of lower sexual function in addition to a lack of partner status.[195] Unfortunately, there is a wide range of sexual problems that are related to breast cancer, and reports of sexual problems range from 30% to 100%.[196] More specifically, 23% to 64% of women report problems with desire, 20% to 48% report arousal or lubrication problems, 16% to 36% report problems with orgasm, and 35% to 38% report problems with pain or dyspareunia.[197–199] Problems with body image are also quite common both during and after treatment, although there is some evidence that certain areas of distress such as feeling feminine or perceived attractiveness tend to improve over time.[190,200,201]

Surgery

Conceptually, losing one or both breasts would seem to be one of most dramatic ways to damage a woman's core sense of femininity, body integrity, and attractiveness. Concern about body image in the face of breast surgery and potential breast changes and breast loss is prevalent with approximately 30% to 67% of women reporting concern with body image.[194,202] Breast-conserving surgical procedures and reconstructive surgery have become a standard part of breast cancer care, and it is generally assumed that breast-conserving surgery (lumpectomy versus mastectomy) as well as breast reconstruction is essential in helping women maintain a positive body image.[203] Several studies have shown that women who undergo modified radical mastectomies have poorer body image than those who have had breast-conserving procedures. In Moyer's meta-analysis[204] of 40 studies comparing quality of life differences between breast-conserving surgery and mastectomy between 1980 and 1995, it was shown that patients undergoing breast conservation had a better body image compared to mastectomy patients.

However, aside from body image and maintaining body integrity, breast surgery can still have a significantly negative impact on sexuality. In particular, women who undergo breast reconstruction are typically left with a complete lack of sensation, including nipple sensation. The nipple has been shown to be the most sensitive area of the breast and loss of nipple sensation is akin to losing a key erogenous zone for many women.[205] Although their breast shape may be restored, the loss of feeling is not. In addition to the use of saline-filled or silicone gel–filled implants, women may also have tissue flap procedures where tissue from a woman's body may be harvested from her abdomen, back, thighs, or buttocks in order to reconstruct a breast. These surgeries, although more intensive than implant surgery, offer the advantage of reconstruction that often feels and looks more natural without the concern about implant rupture or the need to replace implants over time. However, flap procedures necessitate a second surgical site and additional scars. There is growing attention now being paid to the use of nipple-sparing mastectomy; however, although the nipple and areola may be left in place and breast tissue is removed, sensation is no longer intact.[206]

Chemotherapy

Disruption of sexual function after breast cancer seems to be significantly related to whether a woman undergoes chemotherapy as part of her treatment.[190,194,196,197,200,207] Ganz[191] looked at the impact of breast cancer treatment on sexual function and found that women who had either a lumpectomy or mastectomy followed by chemotherapy were more likely to report negative sexual outcomes than patients who had surgery alone. Schover[207] has noted that younger women who undergo abrupt chemotherapy-related menopause are at the highest risk for sexual problems, and that the rates of sexual dysfunction in these women are clearly higher than would be expected in a healthy, community-based sample. In particular, the intensive estrogen deficiency that comes with chemotherapy-induced menopause often leads to severe vaginal dryness and vaginal atrophy, which makes penetration painful. Painful intercourse due to vaginal dryness is one of the most common sexual problems after breast cancer, and it is one of the primary factors also implicated in women's experience of decreased desire, another common and often vexing problem for breast cancer survivors.[207,208] Testosterone deficiency related to premature ovarian failure has also been discussed as a factor related to a loss of desire after breast cancer, but research has not uniformly supported this hypothesis.[209,210] Rather, a loss of desire appears to be multidimensional, with causes that span a bio–psycho–social continuum.

Hormonal Therapy

Endocrine therapy including selective estrogen receptor modifiers (SERM) and aromatase inhibitors (AI) now play an important role in breast cancer treatment for both premenopausal as well as postmenopausal women. Tamoxifen has been used as systemic adjuvant treatment for over 20 years and primary side effects are hot flashes, fatigue, and nausea. Regarding sexual function, tamoxifen use has been associated with vaginal dryness and low desire,[211] although in the large-scale Breast Cancer Prevention Trial, there were no differences found in the frequency of sexual activity between those using tamoxifen versus placebo.[212] Raloxifene, another SERM, does not appear to confer a significant difference from tamoxifen in patient-reported outcomes on physical health

and depression, but sexual function has been reported as being slightly better than in women taking tamoxifen.[213] More recently, sexual side effects of raloxifene treatment have been examined and no deleterious effects were found.[214] The third-generation AIs (anastrozole, letrozole, and exemestane) have become an integral component in the care of postmenopausal women with estrogen-receptor–positive breast cancer and are currently being evaluated for use in chemoprevention.[215] A significant and distressing exacerbation of postmenopausal gynecologic symptoms such as extreme vaginal dryness and dyspareunia has been reported in several studies investigating the quality of life of women taking AIs, including in the first and largest Arimidex and Tamoxifen Alone or in Combination (ATAC) trial with over 9,000 participants.[216] It has been noted that as use of AIs has become the gold standard of care for postmenopausal breast cancer survivors, it is imperative to explore comprehensive management of these gynecologic symptoms that impair sexual function.[217]

Radiotherapy

Radiation therapy for breast cancer is generally localized to the breast. Radiation can result in skin fibrosis, additional loss of sensitivity in the skin, and fatigue, all which can contribute to low desire. However, there has hardly been any research conducted that specifically examines the effects of breast cancer–related radiotherapy on sexuality.

Intervention

Several approaches for addressing sexual problems after breast cancer have been identified. Most approaches focus on individually based information and education about the management of sexual side effects, such as vaginal dryness. The minority of interventions have been developed aimed at working with couples to establish new norms for intimacy after cancer. Ganz and colleagues[218] demonstrated that nurse-delivered individually based counseling was more successful in managing menopausal and sexual side effects from treatment over a 4-month period than usual care. Alternatively, it has been suggested that interventions need to actively involve women's partners in order to produce lasting benefits on sexual functioning.[219] It is our perspective that optimal intervention is essentially based on "two tracks" and addresses sexuality in both an individual and relational context.

Track 1: Focus on the Individual. It is imperative that women receive information and education about how to maintain and restore good sexual health in the context of maintaining good vaginal health as well as overall well-being after breast cancer. In anticipation of the common side effects of both chemotherapy-induced menopause as well as adjuvant hormonal therapies, we believe that all women should receive information as part of their overall treatment planning about (1) nonhormonal vaginal moisturizers, (2) water-based vaginal lubricants, (3) pelvic floor strengthening (Kegel) exercises, and (4) the value of maintaining blood flow to vaginal tissue to prevent vaginal atrophy. This kind of information is readily available to patients through a number of resources, including a free, recently updated booklet by the American Cancer Society called "Sexuality and Cancer: For the Woman Who Has Cancer and Her Partner." This booklet is free to patients and can be obtained in hard copy or online. In addition, the National Cancer Institute as well as the Lance Armstrong Foundation have information about sexuality on their Web sites.

Track 2: Focus on the Relational Context. For the majority of breast cancer patients who are in a partnered relationship, it may also be important to acknowledge that sexuality is experienced in a context. Often, patients do not realize that partners may benefit from looking at some of the same educational resources, and many popular books and Web sites about sexuality after breast cancer actually have sections that are specifically written for partners.

It can be a great relief to patients to get the message that not only are sexual problems common after breast cancer, but also that although the majority of partners want to be helpful when it comes to reconnecting sexually, they too may be unsure of how to proceed and may need guidance. For patients that are not currently in a relationship, sexuality is, in part, still a relational experience whether based on past relationships or in the context of hopes for future relationships. Patients who are not partnered are frequently unsure of how to proceed in terms of dating and lack of confidence in initiating new sexual relationships after their treatment. Often, these patients gain enormous benefit from being able to talk about these challenges and strategize about communication with a new potential partner.

Gynecologic Cancers

Treatments for gynecologic cancer often result in sexual dysfunction that may affect a substantial number of patients and can persist for many years after diagnosis. The effect of surgeries on the genitals can impact a patient's self-esteem and body image and can create significant physical barriers, such as pain, to satisfactory sexual experiences. In addition, women who receive radiation therapy are at risk for developing vaginal fibrosis and stenosis, and hormonal interventions are likely to result in an abrupt development of menopausal symptoms, all of which can considerably disrupt sexual functioning.[220] For instance, Carmack et al.[221] found that sexual problems were quite prevalent in ovarian cancer patients, with 80% reporting problems with vaginal dryness, 75% reporting problems reaching orgasm, and 62% reporting pain or discomfort during penetration. Moreover, research has found that ovarian cancer survivors report significantly less sexual pleasure than disease-free controls.[222]

In a cross-sectional study of women diagnosed with early-stage cervical carcinoma, Bergmark et al.[223] noted that long-term survivors reported sexual function changes that appear to persist over time, including decreased lubrication and genital swelling during arousal, reduced perceived elasticity during intercourse, and distress over these changes. Moreover, the authors[223] found that the changes in sexual function reported by the survivors were associated with the effects of surgery, whether or not the treatment included radiotherapy. Later results obtained by Jensen et al.,[224] who studied early-stage cervical cancer survivors longitudinally, suggest that although low sexual interest and vaginal dryness seem to persist for years after a radical hysterectomy, other changes such as distress by a reduced vaginal size and problems completing sexual intercourse after surgery are likely to resolve over time. In contrast, research also suggests that women treated with radiation for advanced, recurrent, or persistent cervical cancer report sexual problems including low sexual interest, lack of lubrication, dyspareunia, and inability to complete sexual intercourse throughout the first 2 years after treatment and with little improvement over time.[225]

Even though most women who are diagnosed with cervical cancer are younger, Bergmark et al.[223] found that women of all ages included in their study are likely to consider sexuality an important aspect of their lives, and therefore, providers should feel particularly encouraged to discuss with their patients possible disease- and treatment-related sexual changes that may occur.

There is limited information of the sexual outcomes associated with vulvar cancer treatment. However, the available research suggests that vulvar cancer survivors experience significant sexual dysfunction.[226,227]

Intervention

Research studies on interventions that may be used for women treated for gynecologic cancers and who experience subsequent sexual dysfunction are limited, and mostly focus on information giving and suggestions to manage specific symptoms.[228] For instance, for women who experience vaginal dryness, silicone-based or water-based lubricants may be recommended. The use of vaginal dilators a few times per week, and even in combination with Kegel exercises, help stretch the vaginal tissue after radiation. As a general recommendation, vaginal dilation should start as soon as the woman is comfortable, but usually within 4 weeks after completion of radiotherapy.[228] Of note, research has suggested that psychoeducational interventions that combine information with motivational and behavioral skills are more effective than information alone in improving adherence to the use of vaginal dilators in younger women treated for gynecologic cancer.[229] Moreover, psychoeducation may be particularly useful at decreasing some of the distress associated with sexual changes following gynecologic cancer treatment.[230] For women who experience vaginismus after radiation therapy, a combined approach of pharmacotherapy and sex therapy should be recommended.[228] In addition, information should be given to patients on techniques to restore the blood flow to the clitoris and the vagina.[231] It is important to also consider that sexuality is more than the ability to complete sexual intercourse. For survivors who feel unable to have intercourse, either due to physical or psychological factors, counseling may facilitate the exploration and broadening of sexual and intimate interactions that feel comfortable to the survivors and their partners.

BRCA Mutation Carriers

Related to the sexual problems that both breast and gynecologic cancer patients face, women with a *BRCA1* or *BRCA2* mutation represent a vulnerable population that has received very little attention regarding sexual dysfunction. The hereditary cancer genes, *BRCA1* and *BRCA2*, confer a remarkably high lifetime risk of both breast (55% to 85%) and/or ovarian cancer (15% to 44%).[232] A prophylactic bilateral mastectomy (PBM) has been shown to reduce the risk of breast cancer in mutation carriers by over 90%,[233] and a prophylactic bilateral salpingo-oophorectomy (BSO) significantly reduces both ovarian cancer risk over 80% and the risk of breast cancer by at least 50%.[234] Although BSO and PBM are the most effective options to reduce cancer risk in BRCA carriers, their impact on sexual functioning should not be underestimated. It is recommended that female *BRCA1* carriers have their ovaries and fallopian tubes removed prophylactically by age 35 to 40 years, whereas *BRCA2* carriers may be able to defer this surgery until their mid 40s because the average time for developing ovarian cancer in *BRCA2* carriers is somewhat later. However, for both groups, recommendations for BSO is long before the average age of natural menopause, meaning that these women will face an abrupt, surgically induced onset of menopause with all of the related sexual side effects such as vaginal dryness and irritation, pain with penetration, decreased arousal, and loss of desire. Like breast cancer patients who undergo breast surgery, mutation carriers who opt for PBM will face similar issues regarding surgical scars, loss of sensation, and changes in perceived self-image secondary to potentially significant body changes. However, unlike other cancer patients, often, BRCA carriers identify their genetic mutation in a context in which they themselves do not have cancer, and may have to wrestle with the decisions about surveillance versus risk-reducing surgery with moderate to little support and a paucity of adequate counseling and guidance, including regarding management of sexual side effects of surgery.[235]

Regarding intervention, BRCA carriers should receive the same information and education regarding the management of premature menopause as is given to other cancer patients, including recommendations for managing vaginal dryness using vaginal moisturizers and water-based lubricants. In contrast to women who have already had breast cancer, it has been shown that short-term hormone replacement therapy does not appear to negate the risk-reduction benefit gained by prophylactic surgery,[236] thus making systemic hormone replacement as well as localized vaginal estrogen both reasonable options to be explored (Table 148.2).

TABLE 148.2

Medications For Sexual Problems (Women)

Medication	Purpose	Notes	References
Nonestrogenic vaginal moisturizer	Vaginal atrophy	Can decrease symptoms of vaginal dryness and dyspareunia. For some women, vaginal moisturizer use alone is insufficient because its impact on vaginal tissue health is limited.	228, 290, 291
Local estrogen replacement (intravaginal)	Vaginal atrophy/ urogenital atrophy	Estrogen replacement is contraindicated for some female cancer survivors. Use of local estrogen replacement therapy may be contraindicated for patients receiving aromatase inhibitors because of increased systemic estradiol levels. Various systems of delivery; use of creams can be messy.	292–294
Intravaginal DHEA	Vaginal atrophy, arousal, orgasm	DHEA is an androgen, but the specific mechanism of action on its role in sexual function has not been clarified. Only intravaginal, and not oral, DHEA has been shown to improve sexual function.	196, 295–297
Ospemifene (Selective estrogen receptor modulator)	Vaginal atrophy/ dyspareunia	FDA approved. Acts as an estrogen agonist in the endometrium. Preliminary research findings. No safety data for cancer patients.	298–300
Testosterone replacement therapy	Libido	Can be effective in improving libido, although many other bio–psycho–social factors contribute to libido that are not addressed by this therapy (e.g., relationship function, physical health comorbidities).	210, 301

DHEA, dehydroepiandrosterone; FDA, U.S. Food and Drug Administration.

CANCER IN CHILDREN AND YOUNG ADULTS

Cancer during childhood and adolescence can have a tremendous impact on the patient's psychosexual development.[237] Treatment puts these young patients at risk for significant sexual dysfunction and infertility,[238–242] as well as impairing their normal social development, which can result in increased isolation, more limited sexual behavior (e.g., less frequent masturbation, communication with friends about sex), longer delays before dating, and decreased interest in and satisfaction with sex.[243–246] In light of these potential challenges in their psychosexual maturation, about one-third of survivors report at least one distressing long-term sexual problem, with females more likely to report sexual dysfunction.[247] Problems with sexual function are associated with poorer psychological and quality of life.[247,248]

Adolescent and young adult cancer survivors do not receive adequate age-appropriate information and counseling regarding issues related to their sexual development.[246,249–251] Limited intervention research has demonstrated that a psychosocial intervention can help to improve sexual knowledge and body image and can decrease anxiety related to sexual issues.[252] Furthermore, survivors report limited (and, often, inaccurate) knowledge about fertility issues following treatment,[253,254] which is concerning because the majority of patients who are childless at diagnosis report a desire for future offspring.[255] For both genders, there are medical options for fertility preservation that should be discussed with the patient as soon as is feasible.[256]

RELEVANT SOCIOCULTURAL CONSIDERATIONS

It is now well documented that specific racial and ethnic groups in the United States have a higher risk for developing certain cancer diagnoses that directly affect sexual organs. For instance, African American men have a higher risk of developing prostate cancer compared to Caucasians,[257] and Latinas have twice the risk

of developing cervical cancer compared to non-Hispanic Caucasians.[258] But beyond gaining knowledge on the cancer facts and figures for different racial and ethnic groups, becoming aware of the impact that culture has on the development of sexual beliefs, attitudes, and practices may be one of the best tools for providers when understanding and helping cancer patients of diverse backgrounds who are coping with sexual dysfunction.

Guidelines for what constitute normative sexual behaviors and gender-specific role prescriptions are greatly influenced by consensus within particular communities,[259] and it has been found that certain prescribed gender roles can intensify sexual problems.[260] The following are some of the differences that have been observed in sexual attitudes and quality of life in cancer patients and survivors of diverse ethnicities and their implications for medical practice.

Special Considerations for Male Patients

Recent findings on issues related to sexual functioning for African American prostate cancer patients report results that are worth noting. Although having erectile dysfunction is likely to lead to psychological consequences for men across races and cultures, it has been found that African American men are significantly more likely than Caucasian men to consider sexual side effects when choosing treatment for prostate cancer.[261] In the same study by Jenkins et al.,[261] African American men were more likely than their Caucasian counterparts to indicate that an erection is an essential element to sex and to seek help for sexual problems. According to Johnson et al.,[262] African American men, in spite of showing better recovery of sexual function at 12 and 60 months after diagnosis and treatment with prostatectomy, were more likely than non-Hispanic Caucasians to report that sexual function continued to be a moderate to big problem. Knowledge of these reported differences, and specific factors such as the fact that African American prostate cancer patients seem likely to have positive attitudes about seeking treatment for an erectile problem, may assist providers in framing a culturally sensitive discussion with prostate cancer patients of African American origin with regard to their options for treatment and management of sexual side effects.

Special Considerations for Female Patients

A few studies document special considerations for minority, female cancer patients, and survivors with regard to their sexual functioning. For African American breast cancer survivors, particular concerns about body image are reported, such as keloid formation and total body hair loss,[263] and body image concerns in general appear to be greater for African American than for Caucasian women.[264] Although findings suggest that African American breast cancer survivors view their sex lives as less disrupted by cancer compared to their Caucasian counterparts,[265] feeling sexually attractive has been found to be predictive of subsequent psychological well-being for this population.[266] Similar to breast cancer survivors of other ethnicities, African American breast cancer survivors report a need to receive more information from their health-care providers regarding sexual dysfunction as a possible side effect of treatment.[263] However, research suggests that African American women may prefer to address their sexual health concerns in a one-to-one context rather than in group settings.[263,266] Moreover, a randomized trial of peer counseling in African American breast cancer survivors documented that brief psychoeducational interventions can be effective at addressing informational needs on sexual health for this population.[267]

For Latino, Asian, and Native American women, the literature on sexual outcomes in cancer treatment and appropriate interventions for treatment-related sexual dysfunction continues to be limited. However, Asian and Latina cervical cancer survivors have reported great concern with the effects of treatment on their appearance, with Latinas expressing more negative feelings about the impact of treatment on their bodies and their relationships compared to Asian, African American, and Caucasian survivors.[268] Moreover, cultural factors such as the language barrier for Latinas,[268] and the perception of sex as taboo for women from many Asian societies[269] ought to be considered as prevalent impediments in accessing services and to address treatment-related sexual dysfunction. In spite of these challenges, however, the available research findings suggest that psychoeducational interventions may be appropriate for Latinas,[270] and factual information on sexuality after cancer, preferably delivered by nurses or doctors, is often sufficient and acceptable to Asian and African American women cancer survivors as a way to address their concerns.[263,271]

DISRUPTION OF INTIMACY AND RELATIONAL CONSIDERATIONS

In addition to the myriad of physiologic changes that can disrupt sexual function after cancer diagnosis, it is important to acknowledge the significant interpersonal shifts that may take place and subsequently affect sexuality. For instance, women's perceptions of their partner's reactions to their appearance after cancer consistently predict their own acceptance of their self-image and of their sense of femininity.[272] Moreover, women often do not feel comfortable voicing this aspect of their cancer experience with their partners out of a fear of rejection, and partners are afraid to broach the subject out of fear of causing distress.[273] Similarly, male patients tend to avoid conversations with their wives about their sexual challenges that result from cancer treatment[274] and speculate how their wives feel about their sexual functioning.[275]

This interpersonal silence can quickly become the *elephant in the room* and, over time, disruptions in intimate functioning can become more difficult to address, with either one or both partners misperceiving each other's feelings and intentions. Consistent with this understanding, levels of relationship distress and emotional well-being have been found to be more related to variables such as arousal, orgasm, and sexual satisfaction than hormonal levels in women.[276] From a provider perspective, what seems most relevant is that providers are particularly well-positioned to assist couples in communicating more openly about their fears and to answer questions regarding sexual dysfunction, by providing them with available resources on social support and information on cancer treatments that affect sexuality.[277] Research shows that psychoeducational group interventions targeting communication training and sex therapy show promise in improving women breast cancer survivors' relationships and sexual functioning even without including a partner in the intervention.[278] Moreover, Manne and Badr[279] have proposed an integrative theoretical framework for understanding and addressing the challenges that couples face during and after cancer. By focusing on relationship processes that contribute to intimacy, this framework can help providers facilitate a discussion of the illness as something that happens to the relationship, rather than to individual partners.

Communication about Sexual Problems

Although the optimal time to initiate discussion about sexual concerns may vary, it is essential that clinicians prepare patients for potential changes that may be encountered and to let them know that they welcome discussions about sexual health concerns. This allows patients to prepare for managing side effects and potentially may help patients make better informed decisions about treatment options. It is our belief that clinicians should learn to address this topic as though they would any other topic. Along with setting expectations, practical information should be provided, and this information can be offered at multiple time points across the continuum of cancer care.

Asking about Sexual Problems

One straightforward model that has been proposed is the BETTER Model,[280] which stands for: (1) **B**ring up the topic; (2) **E**xplain that you are concerned with quality of life, including sexual health; (3) **T**ell patients that you will help find appropriate resources as needed; (4) **T**iming needs to be taken into consideration, including letting patients know that they can ask for information at any time point; (5) **E**ducate patients about expected sexual side effects; and (6) **R**ecord your assessment in the patient's medical record. Specific language that clinicians can use to "bring up the topic" includes phrases such as: "How has your treatment affected your sexual health?" or "Tell me how your sexual function has been since you started treatment." Although clinicians often worry that patients will be offended or embarrassed if asked about sexual health, multiple studies clearly indicate that patients want to talk about this topic with their doctors and that they desire more information about possible sexual side effects of treatment. Furthermore, patients will rarely initiate conversation on this topic for fear of embarrassing their doctor and also out of concern that their symptoms are not treatable. For a majority of patients, it is invaluable to receive a brief, yet clear message that serves to normalize their symptoms and reassure them that they are not alone and that resources are available.

Use of Validated Assessment Tools

The overwhelming majority of cancer patients do not receive any kind of standardized screening for sexual dysfunction. One method of gaining information and assessing how patients are doing relative to others is to use a brief screening inventory in one's oncology practice. Recently, Jeffery and colleagues[281] published a large-scale review article of sexual function measures to be used with cancer patients. The large majority of published articles relevant to measurements were focused on prostate cancer (76%), followed by breast (9%) and then gynecologic cancer (7%). Upon review, the authors identified three measures that, after undergoing extensive psychometric testing including trial administration in a clinical oncology setting, were deemed psychometrically valid for broad use. These measures are the University of California, Los Angeles Prostate Cancer Index/Expanded

Prostate Cancer Index Composite (UCLA PCI/EPIC),[282] the International Index of Erectile Function (IIEF),[283] and the Female Sexual Function Index (FSFI).[284] The 20-item UCLA PCI is a measure of quality of life after prostate cancer and the IIEF is a measure specifically of sexual function after prostate cancer. Both are available at no cost, and the IIEF is self-administered in 5 to 10 minutes and may be easiest to use in a clinic setting. The 19-item FSFI is a general measure of sexual functioning for women, and it was the only measure for women that met the authors' criteria for being a "standard-setting" instrument. The FSFI is also readily available free of charge and takes less than 15 minutes to complete. This measure has been used with a broad range of female cancer patients, including breast, gynecologic, urologic, and rectal cancers.

Intervention

For the majority of cancer patients, a moderate amount of information and education, such as getting information about personal lubricants and vaginal moisturizers, is often adequate to address their needs. For others, more intensive consultation and/or referral may be necessary. For example, oncology practices often have educational *tip sheets* about managing fatigue, diet, and emotional changes that offer some basic information and usually give additional resource information; it is reasonable to add sexual health to such a roster.

For some patients, it may be valuable and/or necessary to make a referral for more intensive therapy. Additional intervention may include counseling with a licensed therapist who specializes in sex therapy and/or couples counseling. Other relevant referrals may be for urology, gynecology, endocrinology, psychiatry, and physical therapy, including pelvic physical therapy in particular. Collaborative relationships should be developed across disciplines and within the community so that when a problem is identified, established resources are available. Often, it can be useful within an oncology practice to identify one clinician—either a physician, nurse, social worker or psychologist—who can serve as the primary resource person for sexual health issues and who can be responsible for updating available resources and maintaining relevant contacts with community referral sources. It is important to note that several professional organizations, such as the American Psychosocial Oncology Society (APOS, www.apos-society. org), the Society for Sex Therapy and Research (SSTAR, www. sstarnet.org), and the American Association of Sexual Educators, Counselors and Therapists (AASECT, www.aasect.org), all have directories and resources for locating professionals who specialize in working with sexual dysfunction.

SELECTED REFERENCES

The full reference list can be accessed at lwwhealthlibrary.com/oncology.

1. Mercadante S, Vitrano V, Catania V. Sexual issues in early and late stage cancer: a review. *Support Care Cancer* 2010;18:659–665.

2. Hordern A, Street A. Issues of intimacy and sexuality in the face of cancer: the patient perspective. *Cancer Nurs* 2007;30:E11–E18.

6. Park ER, Norris RL, Bober SL. Sexual health communication during cancer care: barriers and recommendations. *Cancer J* 2009;15:74–77.

12. Litwin MS, Flanders SC, Pasta DJ, et al. Sexual function and bother after radical prostatectomy or radiation for prostate cancer: multivariate quality-of-life analysis from CaPSURE. Cancer of the Prostate Strategic Urologic Research Endeavor. *Urology* 1999;54:503–508.

19. Dubbelman YD, Dohle GR, Schroder FH. Sexual function before and after radical retropubic prostatectomy: a systematic review of prognostic indicators for a successful outcome. *Eur Urol* 2006;50:711–718.

23. Sanda MG, Dunn RL, Michalski J, et al. Quality of life and satisfaction with outcome among prostate-cancer survivors. *N Engl J Med* 2008;358:1250–1261.

29. Penson DF, Mclerran D, Feng Z, et al. 5-year urinary and sexual outcomes after radical prostatectomy: results from the Prostate Cancer Outcomes Study. *J Urol* 2008;179:S40–S44.

38. Yuan J, Zhang R, Yang Z, et al. Comparative effectiveness and safety of oral phosphodiesterase type 5 inhibitors for erectile dysfunction: a systematic review and network meta-analysis. *Eur Urol* 2013;63:902–912.

53. Stephenson RA, Mori M, Hsieh YC, et al. Treatment of erectile dysfunction following therapy for clinically localized prostate cancer: patient reported use and outcomes from the Surveillance, Epidemiology, and End Results Prostate Cancer Outcomes Study. *J Urol* 2005;174:646–650.

65. Mulhall J, Land S, Parker M, et al. The use of an erectogenic pharmacotherapy regimen following radical prostatectomy improves recovery of spontaneous erectile function. *J Sex Med* 2005;2:532–540.

72. Mulhall JP, Parker M, Waters BW, et al. The timing of penile rehabilitation after bilateral nerve-sparing radical prostatectomy affects the recovery of erectile function. *BJU Int* 2010;105:37–41.

95. Elliott S, Latini DM, Walker LM, et al. Androgen deprivation therapy for prostate cancer: recommendations to improve patient and partner quality of life. *J Sex Med* 2010;7:2996–3010.

101. Chisholm KE, Mccabe MP, Wootten AC, et al. Review: psychosocial interventions addressing sexual or relationship functioning in men with prostate cancer. *J Sex Med* 2012;9:1246–1260.

110. Wittmann D, Foley S, Balon R. A biopsychosocial approach to sexual recovery after prostate cancer surgery: the role of grief and mourning. *J Sex Marital Ther* 2011;37:130–144.

118. Carpentier MY, Fortenberry JD. Romantic and sexual relationships, body image, and fertility in adolescent and young adult testicular cancer survivors: a review of the literature. *J Adolesc Health* 2010;47:115–125.

120. Kuczyk M, Machtens S, Bokemeyer C, et al. Sexual function and fertility after treatment of testicular cancer. *Curr Opin Urol* 2000;10:473–477.

122. Jonker-Pool G, Van De Wiel HB, Hoekstra HJ, et al. Sexual functioning after treatment for testicular cancer—review and meta-analysis of 36 empirical studies between 1975-2000. *Arch Sex Behav* 2001;30:55–74.

125. Tuinman MA, Hoekstra HJ, Vidrine DJ, et al. Sexual function, depressive symptoms and marital status in nonseminoma testicular cancer patients: a longitudinal study. *Psychooncology* 2010;19:238–247.

138. Zippe CD, Raina R, Massanyi EZ, et al. Sexual function after male radical cystectomy in a sexually active population. *Urology* 2004;64:682–685.

141. Horenblas S, Meinhardt W, Ijzerman W, et al. Sexuality preserving cystectomy and neobladder: initial results. *J Urol* 2001;166:837–840.

143. Hekal IA, El-Bahnasawy MS, Mosbah A, et al. Recoverability of erectile function in post-radical cystectomy patients: subjective and objective evaluations. *Eur Urol* 2009;55:275–283.

148. Richards KA, Parks GE, Badlani GH, et al. Developing selection criteria for prostate-sparing cystectomy: a review of cystoprostatectomy specimens. *Urology* 2010;75:1116–1120.

157. Bhatt A, Nandipati K, Dhar N, et al. Neurovascular preservation in orthotopic cystectomy: impact on female sexual function. *Urology* 2006;67:742–745.

163. Bjordal K, De Graeff A, Fayers PM, et al. A 12 country field study of the EORTC QLQ-C30 (version 3.0) and the head and neck cancer specific module (EORTC QLQ-H&N35) in head and neck patients. EORTC Quality of Life Group. *Eur J Cancer* 2000;36:1796–1807.

165. El-Deiry M, Funk GF, Nalwa S, et al. Long-term quality of life for surgical and nonsurgical treatment of head and neck cancer. *Arch Otolaryngol Head Neck Surg* 2005;131:879–885.

168. Low C, Fullarton M, Parkinson E, et al. Issues of intimacy and sexual dysfunction following major head and neck cancer treatment. *Oral Oncol* 2009;45:898–903.

181. Syrjala KL, Kurland BF, Abrams JR, et al. Sexual function changes during the 5 years after high-dose treatment and hematopoietic cell transplantation for malignancy, with case-matched controls at 5 years. *Blood* 2008;111:989–996.

184. Hirsch P, Leclerc M, Rybojad M, et al. Female genital chronic graft-versus-host disease: importance of early diagnosis to avoid severe complications. *Transplantation* 2012;93:1265–1269.

185. Havenga K, Maas CP, Deruiter MC, et al. Avoiding long-term disturbance to bladder and sexual function in pelvic surgery, particularly with rectal cancer. *Semin Surg Oncol* 2000;18:235–243.

186. Donovan KA, Thompson LM, Hoffe SE. Sexual function in colorectal cancer survivors. *Cancer Control* 2010;17:44–51.

189. Sprunk E, Alteneder RR. The impact of an ostomy on sexuality. *Clin J Oncol Nurs* 2000;4:85–88.

191. Ganz PA, Kwan L, Stanton AL, et al. Quality of life at the end of primary treatment of breast cancer: first results from the moving beyond cancer randomized trial. *J Natl Cancer Inst* 2004;96:376–387.

199. Burwell SR, Case LD, Kaelin C, et al. Sexual problems in younger women after breast cancer surgery. *J Clin Oncol* 2006;24:2815–2821.

204. Moyer A. Psychosocial outcomes of breast-conserving surgery versus mastectomy: a meta-analytic review. *Health Psychol* 1997;16:284–298.

207. Schover LR. Premature ovarian failure and its consequences: vasomotor symptoms, sexuality, and fertility. *J Clin Oncol* 2008;26:753–758.

210. Barton DL, Wender DB, Sloan JA, et al. Randomized controlled trial to evaluate transdermal testosterone in female cancer survivors with decreased libido; North Central Cancer Treatment Group protocol N02C3. *J Natl Cancer Inst* 2007;99:672–679.

216. Cella D, Fallowfield L, Barker P, et al. Quality of life of postmenopausal women in the ATAC ("Arimidex", tamoxifen, alone or in combination) trial after completion of 5 years' adjuvant treatment for early breast cancer. *Breast Cancer Res Treat* 2006;100:273–284.

221. Carmack Taylor CL, Basen-Engquist K, Shinn EH, et al. Predictors of sexual functioning in ovarian cancer patients. *J Clin Oncol* 2004;22:881–889.

223. Bergmark K, Avall-Lundqvist E, Dickman PW, et al. Vaginal changes and sexuality in women with a history of cervical cancer. *N Engl J Med* 1999;340:1383–1389.

227. Likes WM, Stegbauer C, Tillmanns T, et al. Correlates of sexual function following vulvar excision. *Gynecol Oncol* 2007;105:600–603.

228. Katz A. Interventions for sexuality after pelvic radiation therapy and gynecological cancer. *Cancer J* 2009;15:45–47.

235. Matloff ET, Barnett RE, Bober SL. Unraveling the next chapter: sexual development, body image, and sexual functioning in female BRCA carriers. *Cancer J* 2009;15:15–18.

244. Van Dijk EM, Van Dulmen-Den Broeder E, Kaspers GJ, et al. Psychosexual functioning of childhood cancer survivors. *Psychooncology* 2008;17:506–511.

245. Sundberg KK, Lampic C, Arvidson J, et al. Sexual function and experience among long-term survivors of childhood cancer. *Eur J Cancer* 2011;47:397–403.

247. Bober SL, Zhou ES, Chen B, et al. Sexual function in childhood cancer survivors: a report from Project REACH. *J Sex Med* 2013;10:2084–2093.

252. Canada AL, Schover LR, Li Y. A pilot intervention to enhance psychosexual development in adolescents and young adults with cancer. *Pediatr Blood Cancer* 2007;49:824–828.

261. Jenkins R, Schover LR, Fouladi RT, et al. Sexuality and health-related quality of life after prostate cancer in African-American and white men treated for localized disease. *J Sex Marital Ther* 2004;30:79–93.

263. Wilmoth MC, Sanders LD. Accept me for myself: African American women's issues after breast cancer. *Oncol Nurs Forum* 2001;28:875–879.

268. Ashing-Giwa KT, Kagawa-Singer M, Padilla GV, et al. The impact of cervical cancer and dysplasia: a qualitative, multiethnic study. *Psychooncology* 2004;13:709–728.

273. Wimberly SR, Carver CS, Laurenceau JP, et al. Perceived partner reactions to diagnosis and treatment of breast cancer: impact on psychosocial and psychosexual adjustment. *J Consult Clin Psychol* 2005;73:300–311.

274. Boehmer U, Clark JA. Communication about prostate cancer between men and their wives. *J Fam Pract* 2001;50:226–234.

279. Manne S, Badr H. Intimacy and relationship processes in couples' psychosocial adaptation to cancer. *Cancer* 2008;112:2541–2555.

280. Mick J, Hughes M, Cohen MZ. Using the BETTER Model to assess sexuality. *Clin J Oncol Nurs* 2004;8:84–86.

281. Jeffery DD, Tzeng JP, Keefe FJ, et al. Initial report of the cancer Patient-Reported Outcomes Measurement Information System (PROMIS) sexual function committee: review of sexual function measures and domains used in oncology. *Cancer* 2009;115:1142–1153.

PALLIATIVE AND ALTERNATIVE CARE

David Spiegel and Michelle B. Riba

INTRODUCTION

Coping, distress, and support are crucial psychological issues that every cancer patient faces with his or her health-care team. The diagnosis of cancer is a life-altering experience for anyone. The nature of the patient's response to it will affect mood, adherence to treatment, and the quality of his or her social support. Effective coping with the disease involves dealing with its direct and indirect effects, ranging from managing the details of medical appointments to handling existential dread. Facing the illness and its consequences requires acknowledging and managing strong but inevitable emotions that can interfere with medical care,[1] family and vocational engagement, sleep, diet, and exercise.[2]

A wide range and prevalence of psychiatric and psychological problems affect patients and families before, during, and after cancer care and treatment. Recent studies in adults treated in outpatient cancer clinics demonstrate a 40% to 50% clinically relevant level of distress.[3,4] Some have even called for screening for distress to be the *sixth vital sign*, especially in certain patient groups, such as those with head and neck and neurologic cancers.[5]

In addition, there are also physical symptoms of the cancer and its treatments that overlap with the somatic symptoms that are included in many psychiatric conditions. For example, it is often very difficult for even skilled clinicians to determine the extent to which fatigue, decreased appetite, or sleep problems are related to depression or anxiety versus certain types of cancer and targeted therapies and their side effects. It is thus easy to misattribute the symptoms of a mood disorder to the cancer itself and fail to notice important opportunities for treatment. Despite the complexity involved in coping with serious medical and psychiatric problems, there are some guiding principles for understanding patient dynamics and potential psychological issues.

COMMON PSYCHIATRIC CONDITIONS

Although there are many psychiatric conditions that occur in patients with cancer, the more commonly diagnosed are depression, anxiety (panic, post-traumatic stress disorder [PTSD], phobias), adjustment disorders, and delirium.

Although many would like to maintain a positive view of the diagnosis and treatment for cancer, it still is for many a trauma analogous to experiencing an assault, accident, or natural disaster. Patients can often remember the date and time they received their cancer diagnosis. They can remember exactly where it was discussed, who said it, the specific words that were used, and how they felt. These are life-altering, life-changing moments that are, psychologically, often transformative. In the initial stages of diagnosis and early treatment, the use of the term *acute stress disorder* (ASD) or *post-traumatic stress disorder* (PTSD) may best encapsulate the psychological problems that occur. In one study of breast cancer patients after treatment, 5% to 10% met diagnostic criteria for PTSD,[6] and there was little change in their status over the ensuing year.[7] Often, patients experience disbelief, inability to sleep, fears, and intrusive thinking. Lives and schedules change from the mundane routine of going to work or school, to being in a whirlwind of doctors' appointments, receiving news and data in technical language, making appointments for surgery, blood draws, chemotherapy, and radiotherapy.

As patients move through the various stages of cancer care, so too does the trauma response—from acute stress to a more chronic PTSD.[8–10] The adjustment to the trauma can also become chronic. Even the cessation of acute treatment can be fraught with anxiety about recurrence. At the same time, many patients and their families also experience what has been called post-traumatic growth, an altered perspective on what matters in life that comes from facing and dealing with major life stressors.[11] This ability to come to terms with trauma and enhancing domains that include relating to others, appreciation of life, and spiritual change occurs in a substantial proportion of cancer patients[12,13] and, in some cases, predicts better long-term adjustment.[14]

Often, patients have mixed states or combinations of symptoms, such as depression and anxiety. Furthermore, there are symptoms that often are not diagnosed but are quite difficult for patients to manage, such as difficulties with falling asleep and staying asleep and problems adhering to complex and lengthy medication regimens. This is especially difficult when patients have cognitive changes related to the underlying cancer (as in brain tumors) or to the chemotherapeutic agents (cisplatin, steroids). Some of these regimens alter the efficiency with which the brain processes information storage and retrieval.[15]

SCREENING FOR PSYCHOLOGICAL PROBLEMS

As part of good, routine clinical care, it is important to obtain a working diagnosis and treatment plan for each patient regarding psychiatric problems. There are numerous screening tools that are available for clinical as well as research purposes.[16–18] A regular, ongoing evaluation of emotional distress affects management and treatment of psychiatric issues and contributes to better patient outcome, satisfaction, doctor–patient communication, and improved overall oncologic care.[19] Approximately one-third of patients in outpatient oncology clinics experience significant levels of distress, with greater degrees of distress in patients who have tumors with poorer prognosis and outcomes.[20] This means that any screening tool must include a routine, systematized method for busy clinicians to review the measures and provide clinical assessment, treatment, and referral as appropriate. The patient data should be included in the medical record and should provide sufficient diagnostic information to guide mental health care. The diagnostic criteria in the American Psychiatric Association's *Diagnostic and Statistical Manual* (DSM-5) provide the essential definitions of specific mental disorders utilized in practice.[21]

In 1997, the National Comprehensive Cancer Network published the Distress Management Guidelines as a tool for oncology clinicians to develop a differential diagnosis of distress, including common psychiatric disorders and psychosocial and spiritual problems. The panel addressed the issue of the difficulty of psychiatric symptoms that overlap with underlying oncologic disease and treatments and noted that using the term *distress* was a good starting point for clinicians, patients, and families to talk about problems. Using an algorithmic approach, clinicians are guided by the presenting symptoms, possible interventions, evaluation, and treatment options. As a self-report method of measuring and screening for distress, patients are asked to mark their level of distress on a visual analog tool, called the distress thermometer. Along with the distress thermometer is a problem list the patient uses to indicate possible causes of distress such as practical, emotional, family, spiritual, or physical. Using a cutoff of 4 or 5 out of a possible score of 10 provides an indication of distress and has been validated against other screening tools for psychological distress.[4] Psychosocial screening provides an opportunity to determine baseline distress and then prospectively evaluate response to psychosocial treatments.[22]

COPING

Cancer patients and their families are confronted with new situations arising from the illness itself or from the demands of the treatment (Table 149.1). Moos and Schaeffer[23] summarize these challenges as the need to preserve a reasonable emotional balance, maintain a sense of competence and mastery, sustain relationships with family and friends, and prepare for an uncertain future. Cancer patients benefit from help in improving their coping skills or in learning new and more adaptive ones. Previous coping strategies may no longer be appropriate to the new situation. Social support directed at the expression of emotion helps cancer patients to maintain realistic optimism and mitigate distress.[24–28] The adaptive tasks that are necessary in order to adjust to the illness involve several different kinds of coping skills: the evaluation of novel information, decision making, learning to express emotions, mobilizing social support, and increasing role flexibility. Adaptive coping has been divided into three types: information focused, emotion focused, and problem focused.[29,30] Problem-focused coping skills are important to help the cancer patient live with the illness and manage its treatment. However, emotional adjustment to the illness is also essential. Some studies have shown that avoidant strategies may be less adaptive in the long run than task-oriented and approach strategies,[31] although in the context of medical illness, coping is situation specific.[30,32,33] A broad coping-skills repertoire, consisting of both problem- and emotion-focused strategies, increases the probability of matching the response to the particular demands of a given stressful medical situation (Table 149.2).

TREATMENT INTERVENTIONS

Psychosocial

The appropriate treatment for psychological symptoms associated with cancer can be determined by clarifying the nature of emotional distress (anxiety, depression, psychosis), the use of pharmacotherapy to relieve acute and chronic symptoms, and the selection of appropriate psychosocial interventions for treating problems related to anxiety, depression, existential concerns, somatic symptoms, and social or communication problems.[32–34]

TABLE 149.1

Principles of Adaptive Coping with Cancer

Stressors are best handled by:
Facing rather than fleeing
Altering perception
Coping actively
Expressing emotion
Social support

TABLE 149.2

Stage-Specific Coping Challenges and Medical Responses

Stage of Cancer	Coping Challenge	Physician Response
Initial diagnosis	Existential anxiety	Rapid and clear evaluation
Acute treatment	Helplessness	Invite participation in treatment decisions
	Fatigue/disruption of social roles	Invite involvement of family/friends
End of acute treatment	Increased sense of vulnerability/anxiety about relapse and long-term treatment effects	Treatment summary and long-term follow-up plan Survivorship program
	Medical isolation	
Relapse	Anxiety about disease progression/ treatment effects	Clear communication Compassion
	Truncated future	Commitment to providing care
	Loss of social contacts	Reordering priorities Group and other support

The efficacy of psychosocial treatments for depression and anxiety in medically ill patients, particularly brief psychodynamic, educational, supportive, and interpersonal therapies, hypnosis, and behavioral and cognitive-behavioral methods, has been supported by numerous outcome studies.[35–39]

Psychoeducational Interventions

Principles of Psychoeducational Intervention

Medical knowledge enhances the sense of control and mastery a person has over his or her disease, and educational interventions generally yield positive outcomes. Interventions for medical patients are usually more effective when they provide patients with cues for using the knowledge related to their disease and daily management[29] or with some emotion-focused components, which helps them to adjust and live through the different phases of the illness. Anticipatory guidance is an important component of these interventions, helping patients to prepare to respond to future as well as current disease-related problems. The evaluation of outcomes of psychoeducational interventions indicates consistent if modest improvement.[38,40–46]

Coping Skills Training

Education-based group interventions that provide informational support can facilitate the initial adjustment of early stage breast cancer patients by improving self-esteem, body image, and perceived control and by reducing uncertainty about the illness.[47,48] Women who lack personal resources and support benefit the most. Many of these approaches have demonstrated benefit in controlled trials. One cognitive-behavioral stress management group program proposed a multimodal type of intervention combining 20 therapy hours of relaxation training, coping skills training, cognitive restructuring, assertiveness and anger management training, and social support for women with breast cancer. Patients improved in self-reports of benefits from cancer, but no improvement on the distress measures was found.[49] In this study, the greatest changes in positive benefits were reported by women who were low in optimism. An eight-session educational intervention, providing training in stress management, problem solving, goal setting, and assertiveness, produced improvements in general quality of life, as well as specific competence in managing emotional, financial, and legal problems.[50] A five-session family intervention for women with recurrent breast cancer, designed to improve communication, enhance information seeking, improve coping, and manage symptoms, did not affect overall quality of life but did reduce negative appraisal of the cancer and reduced hopelessness.[51] A multidimensional cancer rehabilitation program produced improvements in physical functioning and reductions in distress.[52] A more existentially oriented approach emphasized finding ways to develop a sense of meaning and has been shown to enhance self-efficacy, optimism, and self-esteem among breast and colorectal cancer patients.[53] It is quite clear that facing the existential threat posed by cancer in a supportive way improves coping and reduces distress rather than demoralizing cancer patients.[34,54–56]

Mindfulness Training

Mindfulness-based stress reduction is an adaptation of Zen Buddhist meditation techniques taught in weekly courses. The focus is on enhancing the ability to live in the moment and to tolerate stresses as real but transient phenomena, while more comfortably relating to one's body, and often employing gentle yoga exercises as well.[57] Such techniques have been used to good effect with cancer patients. A meta-analysis of 10 studies documented a significant (moderate effect size; $d = 0.48$) overall improvement in quality of life and possible benefit for various aspects of physical health.[58] A 7-week group training for patients with a variety of cancers resulted in significantly reduced distress.[59] Other studies have shown that a combination of such techniques with more traditional group therapy produced reductions in intrusive thinking and other post-traumatic stress symptoms[60] as well as reduced depression and fear of recurrence and produced higher energy levels[61] among women with breast cancer. A recent study of mindfulness for primary breast cancer patients demonstrated greater reductions in stress symptoms than in an intervention involving emotional expression or a control group, and that both treatment conditions resulted in normalization of diurnal cortisol levels.[62] Similar mindfulness interventions have also been shown to result in lower mean cortisol, reduced Th1 (proinflammatory) cytokines, and lower systolic blood pressure,[62] as well as improved natural killer cell cytotoxicity.[63]

Electronic Technology-Based Interventions

Technology-assisted interventions have proven highly effective. A peer-modeling videotape shown to patients shortly after diagnosis produced increases in vitality and post-traumatic growth and decreases in depression and intrusive thoughts.[64] A combined home visiting and telephone intervention resulted in reduced pain.[65] Computer-based patient support tools provided information, decision support, and interaction with other patients and produced not only increments in knowledge, but also better patient–doctor interactions and enhanced social support.[66] Support groups have been adapted to the Internet with remarkably good effect. Online-mediated social support for cancer-related fatigue have proven very beneficial as well.[67] Real-time leader-conducted groups for breast cancer patients have produced significant reductions in depression and pain.[68]

Excellent Internet resources for information about various types of cancer and their treatments, as well as supportive services, are now available. These include the National Cancer Institute's Web site, its database of cancer treatments, and its associated phone information line. Web sites with authoritative information about supportive care services include those sponsored by the American Cancer Society. The Wellness Community Web site is maintained by the Cancer Support Community, a collaboration of the Wellness Community and Gilda's Clubs, which maintain a network of facilities that provide free community supportive services, including classes and support groups. Another excellent example is the Breast Cancer Connections Web site.

Cognitive-Behavioral Therapy

The cognitive-behavioral approach[69] is built on the assumption that previous social learning, developmental history, and significant experiences lead people to form a unique set of meanings and assumptions, or cognitive schemas, about themselves, the world, and their future. These schemas are then used to organize perception and to govern and evaluate behavior.[70] When specific schemas are activated, they directly influence the content of a person's perceptions, interpretations, associations, and memories from a given time. Cognitive-behavioral therapy (CBT) was developed as a short-term (12 to 20 sessions) intervention for depression, targeting patients' thoughts and their relation to behavior and their affect. CBT for cancer patients generally features a multicomponent intervention integrating coping skills training, stress management, and an intervention designed to enhance cognitive and behavioral processes that will be useful in adjusting to illness.[36] The CBT therapist seeks to identify maladaptive cognitions, turn them into testable hypotheses, and submit them to empirical investigation, so the patient can then reject, modify, or retain these thoughts based on the evidence. Alternatively, more adaptive cognitions and behaviors are similarly examined and tested. In the early sessions, the goal of CBT is to establish a therapeutic relationship, identify primary problems, produce symptom relief, and educate the patient about the process of psychotherapy, CBT, and the role of thoughts, images, and beliefs on emotions and behavior. Together, the therapist and patient decide on the treatment goal, a plan for subsequent therapy sessions, and homework assignments intended to augment the therapy and direct structured practice. The initial homework might require the patient to identify and record maladaptive cognitions (e.g., automatic thoughts). As therapy progresses, verbal techniques are employed to trigger automatic thoughts and associated assumptions and reveal core beliefs or schemas. In an environment of collaborative empiricism, the patient learns to identify, logically and empirically evaluate, and justify the usefulness of systematic biases, cognitive distortions and dysfunctional assumptions, and thoughts, images, and beliefs that underlie emotional distress. The therapist helps the patient challenge cognitive distortions such as overgeneralization, catastrophizing, "should" statements, magnification, minimization, dichotomous thinking, and the fallacies of control, worry, fairness, and attachment. Cognitive restructuring techniques and guided discovery help the patient choose more adaptive cognitions and behaviors. Cognitive techniques used in CBT include thought stopping, self-instruction, distraction, direct disputation, labeling distortions, and development of replacement imagery. Behavioral techniques such as activity scheduling, relaxation training, social skills training, mastery and pleasure ratings, assertiveness training, bibliotherapy, homework, behavioral rehearsal, and in vivo exposure are also employed.

The efficacy of CBT as a treatment for depression is well established.[71] A review of empirically supported treatments for psychosomatic disorders determined that CBT is efficacious for chronic pain management and some cancers.[36]

Group Psychotherapy

Group intervention in a variety of forms has become an increasingly popular, effective, and efficient means of providing psychosocial support for cancer patients.[72,73] Groups of different types may encompass theoretical approaches that include the psychodynamic, existential, educational, and cognitive-behavioral, among others.[72] Although some cancer patients are disinclined to join a support group, most are initially reluctant to undertake other aspects of cancer treatment as well. Factors associated with reluctance include less favorable views of such groups, feeling less control over their cancer, using less active coping styles, and having less distress.[74,75] Although men may initially be more reluctant than women to openly discuss emotional problems relating to cancer, cognitive aspects of coping can be a good starting point, and men with prostate cancer report information sharing with other patients as a helpful aspect of group experience. Although reactions to catastrophic illness may differ for individuals with preexisting psychopathology, most cancer patients share with their emotionally healthy counterparts the need for support in dealing with diagnosis and treatment, changes wrought by disease, social isolation, and existential issues.

Common elements of group psychotherapeutic intervention include the following:[73]

1. *Social support.* Psychotherapy, especially in groups, can provide a new social network with the common bond of facing similar problems. At a time when the illness makes a person feel removed from the flow of life and when many others withdraw out of awkwardness or fear, group psychotherapeutic support provides a new and important social connection. Indeed, the very thing that damages other social relationships is the ticket of admission to such groups, providing a surprising intensity of caring among members from the very beginning. Furthermore, members find that the process of giving help to others enhances their own sense of mastery of the role of *patient* and increases their self-esteem, imbuing the experience of illness with a new meaning.

2. *Emotional expression.* The expression of emotion is important in reducing social isolation and improving coping. Yet patients often believe that they are controlling the psychological and even physical impact of the disease by suppressing their emotional reaction to it. This attitude is often reinforced by friends and family who are made anxious by a display of appropriate fear or sadness in the patient, and by medical professionals as well, who perceive a patient's sadness as an indication of nihilism about treatment or loss of hope. Persistent negative affect, as is seen in depression, often elicits anger in those involved with the patient, because the patient seems unwilling rather than unable to modulate his or her feelings. However, normal anxiety and sadness related to having cancer is phasic and is better managed through expression and discussion. Indeed, there is evidence that emotional expression actually facilitates the resolution of long-term negative emotion.[25,54] Encouragement of emotional expression can enhance intimacy in families, providing opportunities for direct expression of affection and concern. The use of the psychotherapeutic setting to deal with painful affect also provides an organizing context for handling its intrusion. When unbidden thoughts involving fears of dying and death intrude, they can be better managed by patients who know that there is a time and a place during which such feelings will be expressed, acknowledged, and dealt with. Furthermore, disease-related dysphoria is more intense when amplified by isolation, leaving the patient to feel that he or she is deservedly alone with the sense of anxiety, loss, and fear that he or she experiences. Being in a group where many others express similar distress normalizes their reactions, making them feel less alien and overwhelming.

3. *Detoxifying dying.* Processing existential concerns by facing rather than avoiding issues such as dying and death, which could be considered likely to exacerbate depression, actually helps to reduce it. This approach encourages patients to face what they most fear and find some aspect of it they can do something about (e.g., control the process of dying when death is unavoidable). This helps patients to feel more active and less helpless, even in the face of dying. Others have combined principles of cognitive therapy with a focus on existential concerns,[73] finding it an effective approach to reduce symptoms of distress. Death anxiety, in particular, is intensified by isolation, in part because patients often conceptualize death in terms of separation from loved ones. This can be powerfully addressed by psychotherapeutic techniques that directly confront such concerns in a supportive social setting. Yalom[76] has described the ultimate existential concerns as death, freedom, isolation, and meaninglessness. Rather than avoiding painful or anxiety-provoking topics in attempts to "stay positive," this form of group therapy addresses these concerns head-on with the intent of helping group members make better use of the time they have left. The goal is to help those facing the threat of death to see it from a new point of view. Facing even life-threatening issues can directly help patients shift from emotion-focused to problem-focused coping.[29,30,77]

The process of dying is often more threatening than death itself. Direct discussion of death anxiety can help to divide the fear of death into a series of problems: loss of control over treatment decisions, fear of separation from loved ones, anxiety about pain, and control of the manner of one's own dying. Discussion of these concerns can lead to means of addressing, if not completely resolving, each of these issues. Even the process of grieving can be reassuring at the same time that it is threatening. The experience of grieving for others who have died of the same condition constitutes a deeply personal experience of the depth of loss that will be experienced by others after one's own death.

4. *Reorganizing life priorities and living in the present.* The acceptance of the possibility of illness shortening life carries with it an opportunity for reevaluating life's priorities. Facing the threat of death in a way that facilitates a sense of active coping can aid in making the most of what remains in life.[78] This can help patients take control of those aspects of their lives they can influence, while grieving and relinquishing those they cannot. Progress in life goal reappraisal, reorganization of priorities, and perception of benefits may also mediate improvement in symptoms and enhance quality of life.[79]

5. *Enhancing family support.* Psychotherapeutic interventions can also be quite helpful in improving communication, identifying needs, increasing role flexibility, and adjusting to new medical social, vocational, and financial realities.[80] The group format is especially helpful for such a task, in that problems expressing needs and wishes can be examined among group members as a model for clarifying communication in the family.

6. *Improving communication with physicians.* Support groups can be quite useful in facilitating better communication with physicians and other health-care professionals.[81,82] Groups provide mutual encouragement to get questions answered, to participate actively in treatment decisions, and to consider alternatives carefully.

7. *Symptom control.* Many group and individual psychotherapy programs teach specific coping skills designed to help patients reduce cancer-related symptoms such as anxiety, anticipatory nausea and vomiting, and pain. Techniques used include specific self-regulation skills such as self-hypnosis, meditation, biofeedback, and progressive muscle relaxation. Hypnosis is widely used for pain and anxiety control in cancer to attenuate the experience of pain and suffering and to allow painful emotional material to be examined.[83] Group sessions that involve instruction in self-hypnosis provide an effective means of reducing pain and anxiety and consolidate the major themes of discussion in the group.[84,85] Hypnosis is an altered state of consciousness, composed of heightened absorption in focal attention, dissociation of peripheral awareness, and enhanced responsiveness to social cues.[81] It has a long tradition of effectiveness in controlling somatic symptoms such as pain and anxiety. Patients with the requisite hypnotic capacity can be taught to utilize self-hypnosis to reduce or eliminate pain and the tension that accompanies it. Hypnotic techniques have been shown to effectively reduce cancer pain[81,84,85] and to facilitate medical procedures.[86] Hypnotic intervention actually alters perceptual processing in the brain, with reduced response to painful stimuli as measured by event-related potentials[87] and positron-emission tomography.[88]

OUTCOME

Clinical trials have demonstrated the benefit of group therapy for breast cancer patients,[76,89–91] with notable reductions in pain[84,85] and emotional distress.[54,92] A systematic review of the literature that included two meta-analyses and nine well-designed randomized controlled trials indicated that psychoeducational interventions not only enhance patient knowledge about their cancer and its treatments, but also reduce depression, anxiety, nausea, and pain.[38] A Cochrane database review concluded that group psychotherapy for cancer patients significantly reduces depression, even in the setting of advanced disease.[93]

PALLIATIVE AND ALTERNATIVE CARE

IMPLICATIONS FOR CANCER PROGRESSION AND MORTALITY

There are literature that raises the possibility that psychotherapeutic intervention may affect survival time as well as quality of life.[94–98] Eight of 15 published randomized trials demonstrate such an effect.[99] Spiegel et al.[94] initially reported that a year (minimum) of supportive-expressive group psychotherapy resulted in a significant 18-month increase in survival time in metastatic breast cancer patients. A 6-week cognitive behavioral group intervention composed of education, stress management, coping skills training, and psychological support for malignant melanoma patients found significantly lower death rates at 10-year follow-ups in the treatment group.[100] A study of individual psychotherapeutic support offered at the bedside early in the course of disease to a group of gastrointestinal cancer inpatients also had favorable results on survival,[97] which has been confirmed at 10-year follow-ups.[97] A randomized replication trial of supportive-expressive group psychotherapy among 125 women with metastatic breast cancer found positive effects on mood,[54] but no overall survival advantage,[101] although there was a significant interaction with tumor type, such that women with estrogen receptor–negative tumors who had been randomized to the group condition lived significantly longer than estrogen receptor–negative controls. An educational group intervention among 227 women with primary breast cancer demonstrated that those who were randomized to receive group support had significantly lower rates of relapse and mortality at 11-year follow-ups.[102] A randomized trial of a palliative care intervention involving an average of four visits that focused on choices about resuscitation preference, pain control, and quality of life among 151 patients with non–small-cell lung cancer demonstrated a significant reduction of depression and pain, and also a significant 2.7-month improvement in survival time (median survival, 11.85 versus 8.9 months; $p = 0.02$).[103]

However, seven other trials found no effect of psychosocial intervention on survival time.[55,90,104–108] One large multicenter trial that utilized supportive-expressive group psychotherapy with metastatic breast cancer patients showed reduced distress and pain but no survival advantage.[104] However, the treatment arm in this study was more depressed than the controls at the beginning of the study, which indicated a risk for shorter survival prior to intervention.[109] In another three of these trials, psychotherapy produced no psychological benefit[90,106,107]; therefore, a survival improvement would be unlikely. Taken together, these studies suggest that psychosocial effects on survival time are most pronounced when medical treatments have become less effective.[91] No study has found that psychotherapy, even involving direct confrontation with dying and death, shortens survival. The potential benefit of psychotherapeutic support on cancer progression remains an open research question, but receives further support from evidence that being married is associated with a 12% to 33% improvement in overall survival.[110] This study involved analysis of Surveillance, Epidemiology, and End Results (SEER) data in the United States from 2004 to 2008 involving 734,889 cancer patients with lung, colorectal, breast, pancreatic, prostate, liver/intrahepatic bile duct, non-Hodgkin lymphoma, head/neck, ovarian, or esophageal cancer. Being married was associated with better outcome with each of these cancer types, independent of demographics, stage, and treatment. Thus, social support would seem to have a tangible effect on disease progression and survival time.

PSYCHOTROPIC MEDICATION

Antidepressants

It is becoming increasingly clear that, as is the case with major depression in general, depression that arises in the context of cancer is responsive to antidepressant treatment.[111] Using various measures of depression and outcome, studies indicate that paroxetine,[111] mianserin,[112] fluoxetine,[113] amitriptyline,[111] and desipramine[114] are useful in treating depression in patients with cancer (Table 149.3). Antidepressants decrease depressive symptoms, improve functional capacity, reduce cachexia, ameliorate some menopausal symptoms, and reduce pain.[115]

Fisch et al.[116] found that treatment with fluoxetine significantly improved depressive symptoms and some measures of quality of life when compared to placebo in cancer patients with a variety of tumors with an expected survival of 3 to 24 months. Importantly, these patients were recruited based on reporting that they were bothered by a depressed mood at a severity of "somewhat" or greater and not by meeting criteria for full major depression. Another large trial compared paroxetine to placebo in cancer patients with fatigue and found that the antidepressant significantly lowered depressive (but not fatigue) symptom scores.[117]

In double-blind trials, fluoxetine, paroxetine, and venlafaxine have been shown to reduce hot flashes,[118] and mirtazapine and the anticonvulsant gabapentin have been reported to decrease pruritus in cancer patients.[119] Venlafaxine, bupropion, and the tricyclic antidepressants have been shown to relieve neuropathic pain, which frequently accompanies cancer and its treatment.[120] Trazodone, a tetracyclic antidepressant, which in low doses (50 to 150 mg) is often used as a sedative hypnotic that does not produce dependency, has also been used to treat a variety of adjustment disorders among breast cancer patients.[121]

Cancer patients treated with cytokines such as interferon-α often become significantly depressed, with a substantial increase in suicidal ideation and acts.[122] Pretreatment of such patients with selective serotonin reuptake inhibitors (SSRI) actually reduces the risk of developing depression.[123] There are increasing data that suggest that depression-specific symptoms may disproportionately contribute to the relationship between depression and morbidity or mortality in the context of medical illness.[109,124,125]

These findings may also provide an explanation for the oft-repeated observation that agents with catecholaminergic activity are generally more effective than SSRIs in the treatment of neurovegetative and somatic symptoms, such as pain and fatigue, even when these symptoms occur outside the context of a diagnosable mood disorder.[117] Combination treatment may also be especially helpful in more severe depressions.[126] Evidence that proinflammatory cytokines contribute to the development of depression, even in medically healthy individuals,[99] may explain the utility of combined serotonin–norepinephrine or dopamine treatment, such as adding desipramine or bupropion with an SSRI or using a serotonin–norepinephrine reuptake inhibitor, such as venlafaxine or duloxetine. These approaches may be more effective than selective serotonergic agents alone in the treatment of major depression, especially when comorbid pain is present. Stimulants such as amphetamine, methylphenidate, and modafinil can also be used effectively either alone or in combination with antidepressants, especially to provide more rapid onset. They rarely trigger anorexia in this population,[127] and they are also agents of choice for cancer patients with short expected survival periods.

Tamoxifen and Selective Serotonin Reuptake Inhibitors

Tamoxifen continues to be used as an important selective estrogen receptor modulator (SERM) to reduce the risk of recurrence in estrogen receptor–positive postmenopausal breast cancer patients. In order to be clinically active, tamoxifen is converted to 4-hydroxy-tamoxifen (endoxifen) and other active metabolites by cytochrome P450 (CYP) enzymes. Over 80 different major alleles of CYP2D6 genes have been identified, many of which confer decreased or absent CYP2D6 activity, and patients can be divided into poor, intermediate, extensive, and ultrarapid metabolizers based on their genotype.[128]

TABLE 149.3

Antidepressants: Selective Serotonin Reuptake Inhibitors and Newer Antidepressants

Generic	Brand Names	Starting Dose	Maximal Suggested Dose (24 h)	Sedating	Forms Available	Comments
Bupropion	Wellbutrin, Zyban	75 mg	300 mg	✓	SR (twice per day); XL	Use <150 mg per dose except XL; fewer sexual side effects; risk of seizures; also for smoking cessation
Citalopram	Celexa	10 mg	40 mg	SolTabs		
Duloxetine	Cymbalta	20 mg	60 mg	✓		Also for neuropathic pain; taper slowly
Escitalopram	Lexapro	5 mg	20 mg			Isomer of citalopram
Fluoxetine	Prozac, Sarafem	5 mg	60 mg			Moderate benefit for hot flashes, premenstrual syndrome
Mirtazapine	Remeron	15 mg	45 mg	✓✓	SolTabs	Very sedating; stimulates appetite
Paroxetine	Paxil	5 mg	40 mg	✓		Also for hot flashes; slow taper
Sertraline	Zoloft	25 mg	200 mg			
Trazodone	Desyrel	50 mg	300 mg	✓		Primarily for insomnia
Venlafaxine	Effexor	25–37.5 mg	375 mg		XR	Also for hot flashes and neuropathic pain; slow taper

SR, sustained release; XL, extended release; XR, sustained release.
Adapted from Holland JC, Greenberg DB, Hughes MK, et al., eds. *Quick Reference for Oncology Clinicians: The Psychiatric and Psychological Dimensions of Cancer Symptom Management.* Charlottesville, VA, US; International Psycho-Oncology Society (IPOS) Press; 2006, with permission.

Breast cancer patients treated with tamoxifen who were homozygous for a poor metabolizer genotype had significantly lower serum concentrations of endoxifen than those with an active genotype.[129] In a review of retrospective studies evaluating the effect of *CYP2D6* genotype on breast cancer outcomes, Goetz et al.[130] found that patients with estrogen receptor–positive breast cancer, homozygous for the poor metabolizer genotype and treated with tamoxifen monotherapy, were more likely to experience a recurrence of breast cancer than those patients who carried an allele coding for active enzyme. Stearns et al.,[131] in a prospective clinical trial, evaluated the effects of the coadministration of tamoxifen and paroxetine, a selective serotonin reuptake inhibitor, at the time, commonly used to treat depression and hot flashes. The authors found that the use of paroxetine, which inhibits *CYP2D6*, decreased the plasma concentration of endoxifen, suggesting that the *CYP2D6* genotype and drug interactions should be considered in patients treated with tamoxifen.

More recently, Kelly et al.,[132] in a population-based cohort study, studied postmenopausal women aged 66 years or older living in Ontario who had been treated between 1993 and 2005 with tamoxifen for breast cancer and overlapping treatment with a single SSRI, finding that, after adjustment for age, duration of tamoxifen treatment, and other potential confounders, absolute increases of 25%, 50%, and 75% in the proportion of time on tamoxifen with overlapping use of paroxetine were significantly associated with 24%, 54%, and 91% increases in the risk of death from breast cancer, respectively. The authors concluded that paroxetine use during tamoxifen treatment is associated with an increased risk of death from breast cancer, supporting the hypothesis that "paroxetine can reduce or abolish the benefit of tamoxifen in women with breast cancer."

In addition to paroxetine, sertraline and venlafaxine have also been noted to reduce the metabolism of tamoxifen.[129] Lash et al.[133] found no reduction of tamoxifen effectiveness among patients using citalopram. With the accumulation of studies, Desmarais et al.,[134] in an important review, provide recommendations that clinicians who are treating patients with breast cancer should carefully evaluate the best and safest options for treatment of depression, reviewing pharmacologic profiles, while being very mindful of the risks of untreated depression. In an interesting study regarding the prevention of depression in patients receiving treatment for head and neck cancer, Lydiatt et al.[135] studied the prophylactic use of escitalopram oxalate to determine if the incidence of depression could be reduced in patients receiving primary therapy for head and neck cancer. Results in the nondepressed group showed that prophylactic escitalopram reduced the risk of developing depression by more than 50%. Quality of life was also improved for 3 consecutive months in the nondepressed group after the cessation of escitalopram.

Antianxiety Agents

It is becoming increasingly clear that the antidepressants, as discussed previously, have antianxiety properties as well and can be utilized effectively for the frequent problem of mixed anxiety and depression. Benzodiazepines can provide immediate short-term relief of anxiety symptoms, but generally are not a good strategy for long-term treatment, in part because of the problem of habituation and a tendency to produce dependence. Withdrawal from high doses can be a serious medical problem. Although many of the newer benzodiazepines such as lorazepam are relatively short acting, the problem of symptom recurrence may be addressed in the future with longer acting formulations.[136] In addition, many of the antianxiety agents are used for insomnia with good effect and, after, are used in the short term for symptom management (Tables 149.4 and 149.5).

Antipsychotics

Neuroleptics are rarely used among cancer patients, but they can be highly effective at managing symptoms of delirium, which can occur during worsening of medical status, with metabolic disequilibrium associated with cachexia, mood disorders, and psychosis associated with steroid treatment and as a preterminal event (Table 149.6). Disorientation to time, place, and person coupled with agitation can be misunderstood as a sign of poor pain management, but increases in opiates and other analgesics, which can be very useful when pain is the problem, may contribute to further delirium. Initially small but increasing doses of antipsychotics such as haloperidol either orally or intravenously can be very helpful in controlling delirium and agitation.[137]

TABLE 149.4

Antidepressants: Tricyclics

Generic	Brand Name	Starting Dose	Maximal Suggested Dose (24 h)	Comments
Amitriptyline	Elavil	10 mg	300 mg	25–50 mg for pain
Desipramine	Norpramin	10 mg	300 mg	
Doxepin	Sinequan	10 mg	150 mg	Very antihistaminic; sedating; also for itching
Imipramine	Tofranil	10 mg	300 mg	
Nortriptyline	Pamelor	10 mg	150 mg	25 mg for pain

Adapted from Holland JC, Greenberg DB, Hughes MK, et al., eds. *Quick Reference for Oncology Clinicians: The Psychiatric and Psychological Dimensions of Cancer Symptom Management*. Charlottesville, VA, US; International Psycho-Oncology Society(IPOS) Press; 2006, with permission.

TABLE 149.5

Hypnotics

Generic	Brand Name	Starting Dose	Maximal Suggested Dose (24 h)	Half-Life Short/Med	Comments
Eszopiclone	Lunesta	1 mg	3 mg	Half-life short	For sleep
Oxazapam	Serax	10 mg	30 mg	Half-life short	For sleep, also for alcohol withdrawal
Temazepam	Restoril	7.5 mg	30 mg	Med	For insomnia
Triazolam	Halcion	0.125 mg	0.5 mg	Half-life short	For insomnia
Zaleplon	Sonata	5 mg	20 mg	Half-life short	For sleep
Zolpidem	Ambien	2.5 mg	10 mg	Half-life short	For sleep, technically nonbenzodiazepine but shares properties (dependence, withdrawal)

Adapted from Holland JC, Greenberg DB, Hughes MK, et al., eds. *Quick Reference for Oncology Clinicians: The Psychiatric and Psychological Dimensions of Cancer Symptom Management*. Charlottesville, VA, US; International Psycho-Oncology Society(IPOS) Press; 2006, with permission.

TABLE 149.6

Antipsychotic Medications: Major Tranquilizers

Generic	Brand Name	Starting Dose	Maximal Dose	Forms Available	Administration Routes	Comments
Chlorpromazine	Thorazine	10 mg	200 mg			Parenteral; postural hypotension; sedation; hiccups
Haloperidol	Haldol	0.25 mg	30 mg	IV, PO	IV, PO	Antiemetic; risk of extrapyramidal side effects; parenteral
Olanzapine	Zyprexa (Zydis)	2.5 mg	20 mg	Wafer, PO		Wafer form (Zydis); weight gain; antiemetic sedation; long-term risk of diabetes; can cause restlessness
Perphenazine	Trilafon	2 mg	32 mg			
Quetiapine	Seroquel	25 mg	500 mg		PO	Antihistamine associated somnolence; 5-hour half-life
Risperidone	Risperdal	0.25 mg	8 mg			Postural hypotension; smaller risk of Parkinson's than typical agents

IV, intravenous; PO, by mouth.
Adapted from Holland JC, Greenberg DB, Hughes MK, et al., eds. *Quick Reference for Oncology Clinicians: The Psychiatric and Psychological Dimensions of Cancer Symptom Management*. Charlottesville, VA, US; International Psycho-Oncology Society(IPOS) Press; 2006, with permission.

SELECTED REFERENCES

The full reference list can be accessed at lwwhealthlibrary.com/oncology.

1. Grube M. Compliance and coping potential of cancer patients treated in liaison-consultation psychiatry. *Int J Psychiatry Med* 2006;36:211–229.
2. Spiegel D. A 43-year-old woman coping with cancer [comments]. *JAMA* 1999;282:371–378.
4. Jacobsen PB, Donovan KA, Trask PC, et al. Screening for psychologic distress in ambulatory cancer patients. *Cancer* 2005;103:1494–1502.
5. Bultz BD, Groff SL, Fitch M, et al. Implementing screening for distress, the 6th vital sign: a Canadian strategy for changing practice. *Psychooncology* 2011;20:463–469.
6. Jacobsen PB, Widows MR, Hann DM, et al. Posttraumatic stress disorder symptoms following bone marrow transplantation for breast cancer. *Psychosom Med* 1998;60: 366–371.
7. Andrykowski MA, Cordova MJ, McGrath PC, et al. Stability and change in posttraumatic stress disorder symptoms following breast cancer treatment: a 1-year follow-up. *Psychooncology* 2000;9:69–78.
8. Green BL, Rowland JH, Krupnick JL, et al. Prevalence of posttraumatic stress disorder (PTSD) in women with breast cancer. *Psychometrics* 1998;32: 102–111.
10. Cordova MJ, Andrykowski MA, Kenady DE, et al. Frequency and correlates of posttraumatic stress disorder-like systems following treatment for cancer. *J Consult Clin Psychol* 1995;63:981–986.
12. Cordova MJ, Cunningham LL, Carlson CR, et al. Social constraints, cognitive processing, and adjustment to breast cancer. *J Consult Clin Psychol* 2001;69: 706–711.
13. Cordova MJ, Cunningham LL, Carlson CR, et al. Posttraumatic growth following breast cancer: a controlled comparison study. *Health Psychol* 2001;20: 176–185.
14. Carver CS, Antoni MH. Finding benefit in breast cancer during the year after diagnosis predicts better adjustment 5 to 8 years after diagnosis. *Health Psychol* 2004;23:595–598.
15. Kesler SR, Bennett FC, Mahaffey ML, et al. Regional brain activation during verbal declarative memory in metastatic breast cancer. *Clin Cancer Res* 2009;15:6665–6673.
19. Holland JC, Andersen B, Breitbart WS, et al. Distress management. *J Natl Compr Cancer Netw* 2010;8:448–485.
25. Giese-Davis J, Koopman C, Butler L, et al. Change in emotion-regulation strategy for women with metastatic breast cancer following supportive expressive group therapy. *J Consult Clin Psychol* 2002;70:916–925.
32. Rosenbaum E, Gautier H, Fobair P, et al. Cancer supportive care, improving the quality of life for cancer patients. A program evaluation report. *Support Care Cancer* 2004;12:293–301.
34. Spiegel D. A 43-year-old woman coping with cancer [clinical conference] [see comments]. *JAMA* 1999;282:371–378.
39. Grunfeld E. Looking beyond survival: how are we looking at survivorship? *J Clin Oncol* 2006;24:5166–5169.
49. Antoni MH, Lehman JM, Kilbourn KM, et al. Cognitive-behavioral stress management intervention decreases the prevalence of depression and enhances benefit finding among women under treatment for early-stage breast cancer. *Health Psychol* 2001;20:20–32.
50. Rummans TA, Clark MM, Sloan JA, et al. Impacting quality of life for patients with advanced cancer with a structured multidisciplinary intervention: a randomized controlled trial. *J Clin Oncol* 2006;24:635–642.
51. Northouse L, Kershaw T, Mood D, et al. Effects of a family intervention on the quality of life of women with recurrent breast cancer and their family caregivers. *Psychooncology* 2005;14:478–491.
58. Ledesma D, Kumano H. Mindfulness-based stress reduction and cancer: a meta-analysis. *Psychooncology* 2009;18:571–579.

61. Lengacher CA, Johnson-Mallard V, Post-White J, et al. Randomized controlled trial of mindfulness-based stress reduction (mbsr) for survivors of breast cancer. *Psychooncology* 2009;18:1261–1272.
62. Carlson LE, Speca M, Faris P, et al. One year pre-post intervention follow-up of psychological, immune, endocrine and blood pressure outcomes of mindfulness-based stress reduction (MBSR) in breast and prostate cancer outpatients. *Brain Behav Immun* 2007;21:1038–1049.
63. Witek-Janusek L, Albuquerque K, Chroniak KR, et al. Effect of mindfulness based stress reduction on immune function, quality of life and coping in women newly diagnosed with early stage breast cancer. *Brain Behav Immun* 2008;22:969–981.
67. Wagner-Johnston N. Computer/online-mediated social support for cancer-related fatigue. *J Natl Compreh Cancer Netw* 2013;11:1211–1217.
68. Lieberman MA, Golant M, Giese-Davis J, et al. Electronic support groups for breast carcinoma: a clinical trial of effectiveness. *Cancer* 2003;97:920–925.
73. Spiegel D, Classen C. *Group Therapy For Cancer Patients: A Research-Based Handbook Of Psychosocial Care.* New York: Basic Books; 2000.
82. Fallowfield LJ, Jenkins VA, Beveridge HA. Truth may hurt but deceit hurts more: communication in palliative care. *Palliat Med* 2002;16:297–303.
85. Butler LD, Koopman C, Neri E, et al. Effects of supportive-expressive group therapy on pain in women with metastatic breast cancer. *Health Psychol* 2009;28:579–587.
86. Lang EV, Benotsch EG, Fick LJ, et al. Adjunctive non-pharmacological analgesia for invasive medical procedures: a randomised trial. *Lancet* 2000;355: 1486–1490.
89. Carlson LE, Doll R, Stephen J, et al. Randomized controlled trial of mindfulness-based cancer recovery versus supportive expressive group therapy for distressed survivors of breast cancer (mindset). *J Clin Oncol* 2013;31: 3119–3126.
91. Spiegel D. Mind matters in cancer survival. *JAMA* 2011;305:502–503.
93. Akechi T, Okuyama T, Onishi J, et al. Psychotherapy for depression among incurable cancer patients. *Cochrane Database Syst Rev* 2008:Cd005537.
94. Spiegel D, Bloom JR, Kraemer HC, et al. Effect of psychosocial treatment on survival of patients with metastatic breast cancer. *Lancet* 1989;2:888–891.
101. Spiegel D, Butler LD, Giese-Davis J, et al. Effects of supportive-expressive group therapy on survival of patients with metastatic breast cancer: a randomized prospective trial. *Cancer* 2007;110:1130.
102. Andersen BL, Yang HC, Farrar WB, et al. Psychologic intervention improves survival for breast cancer patients: a randomized clinical trial. *Cancer* 2008;113:3450–3458.
103. Temel JS, Greer JA, Muzikansky A, et al. Early palliative care for patients with metastatic non-small-cell lung cancer. *N Engl J Med* 2010;363: 733–742.
109. Giese-Davis J, Collie K, Rancourt KM, et al. Decrease in depression symptoms is associated with longer survival in patients with metastatic breast cancer: a secondary analysis. *J Clin Oncol* 2011;29:413–420.
110. Aizer AA, Chen MH, McCarthy EP, et al. Marital status and survival in patients with cancer. *J Clin Oncol* 2013;31:3869–3876.
132. Kelly CM, Juurlink DN, Gomes T, et al. Selective serotonin reuptake inhibitors and breast cancer mortality in women receiving tamoxifen: a population based cohort study. *BMJ* 2010;340:C693.
134. Desmarais JE, Looper KJ. Interactions between tamoxifen and antidepressants via cytochrome P450 2d6. *J Clin Psychiatry* 2009;70:1688–1697.
135. Lydiatt WM, Bessette D, Schmid KK, et al. Prevention of depression with escitalopram in patients undergoing treatment for head and neck cancer: randomized, double-blind, placebo-controlled clinical trial. *JAMA Otolaryngol Head Neck Surg* 2013;139:678–686.

PALLIATIVE AND ALTERNATIVE CARE

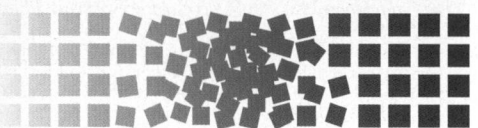

150 Communicating News to the Cancer Patient

Eric J. Cassell

INTRODUCTION

Helene Fink was a 56-year-old woman with stage IV breast cancer. Toward the end of the course of the disease, her bone marrow was filled with tumor cells, with all the usual hematologic sequelae. Her pain was well-controlled and she continued an active life in seeming disregard of her disease. Her oncologist was concerned that Mrs. Fink did not appreciate the gravity of her situation, so she explained to the patient in detail what was happening and how serious it was. The patient stopped her activities and became bedridden. The oncologist explained to me at length that she believed in telling patients the truth and that truth-telling was essential for the patient's well-being, especially in the contemporary scene. She also called the patient's husband to explain the importance of telling the truth. It took considerable effort to get the patient back to her previous level of activity, which continued until shortly before her death 3 months later.

This scenario is quite common. Apparently, the physician's goal in such settings is to make sure the patient knows the truth. The emphasis is on telling the truth. All clinical actions, all actions meant to have an impact on the patient—in oncology, as elsewhere—should have a goal. For example, diagnostic actions have a goal-specific therapy; chemotherapy, radiation, or other modalities have a goal, usually curative, palliative, or local control of disease. The goal of cancer treatment, in general, has long been to improve survival. Recently, this has been modified by the addition of the goal to treat without decreasing quality of life. A general statement of these goals is that they are meant to help the patient.

Patient communication—talking with patients—is a clinical action. Therefore, talking with patients should also have a goal: As with the other clinical acts, it should help the patient be better. In the case of Helene Fink, the communication of her oncologist had a negative impact. Truth-telling is not a primary goal; telling the truth is a moral imperative. With rare exceptions, it is obvious that you should tell the truth. Put another way, your communication with the patient should be truthful, but that should be only one of several functions that that communication serves.

PREVENTING ILLNESS

The goal of increasing length of survival in the treatment of cancer has achieved considerable prominence over the past several decades. Although this is understandable, people do not get up in the morning just to survive; when they do—like soldiers in battle—survival is in the service of living a life. People get up in the morning to live their lives, to work, to play, to take care of their families, to become famous, or to achieve their goals in life, just like you and your family. Perhaps you believe your patients cannot do that because they are too sick. It is true that many patients with advanced disease are sick. By *sick*, the author means requiring care in bed, or, if out of bed, requiring regular skilled care. Most people (including doctors) think patients are sick because of the symptoms or because of their advanced disease. Symptoms are often very unpleasant, but the medical community has become

very good at symptom relief; still, the patients are sick. Ask them, and they will tell you (whatever their other symptoms may be) that they are "weak," that they have "no energy," or that they have "run out of gas." They have all the characteristics of the sick: They are disconnected from their world, they have the feeling that they have no control over their lives, they have lost the normal feeling of indestructibility, their cognitive function is not what it was, they are filled with uncertainties, and they do not really understand (as hard as they try) what is happening to them. These features and others characterize the phenomenon called *the state of illness*.

The state of illness is usually brought on by the symptoms and presence of serious disease, but the state of illness is an independent phenomenon. It is not a necessary accompaniment of serious disease. Many clinicians have known patients with serious disease who are not as sick as described here. This was true of Mrs. Fink before the conversation about her bone marrow. They have also known others who were similarly sick, but in whom the disease and symptoms were not serious. The state of illness is an independent phenomenon. It is a state of being. The *Oxford English Dictionary* definition of a *state* is, "A combination of circumstances or attributes belonging for the time being to a person . . . a particular manner of existing as defined by the presence of certain circumstances or attributes; a condition." (For example, the state of love, the state of grief, or a state of helplessness.) States of being are not psychological or physical alone. States of being are physical, psychological, social, and personal. States of being are pervasive, with effects ranging from the molecular to the social. The state of illness can be worsened independently of the disease, and it can be improved independently of the disease. A state of illness is aggravated by pain and other symptoms, but particularly by inadequately controlled pain. The state is also activated or worsened by uncertainty and fear (the two are often related), and it is made worse by actions that remove independence or increase dependence on the staff. (Like the ubiquitous intravenous bag and pole.) Patients can leave the state of illness even though the disease is not better. An important therapeutic goal is ending a state of illness. The primary modalities for the relief of the state of illness are symptom relief and talking with the patient—communication.

COMMUNICATION

The spoken language is the most important tool in medicine; almost nothing happens in its absence. Physicians commonly train themselves to meet very high standards of expertise, but this everyday tool gets about as much respect and training in its use as paperwork.[1,2] Yet the most common complaint that patients have now and have had for decades past is that doctors do not talk to them. It has been repeatedly shown that patients who understand what is happening to them and why, are more cooperative and compliant with physician's suggested regimens. The implication is that what you say to patients really matters. Every word matters. Sometimes physicians say, "I can't watch every word," but that would be like a surgeon saying, "I can't watch my scalpel every moment." Physicians are all so accustomed to talking and using words in their everyday life that they forget the impact of words on the listener. And they forget that doctor–patient communication is not ordinary conversation. The spoken language acts on the person, and what acts on the person acts on every part of the person. In talking with patients, physicians themselves are the primary therapeutic agent. The vehicle through which virtually everything that physicians do to and with patients is the relationship between the patient and the physician. That relationship is best that is built on trust, and trust is best engendered by the truth. That is not the end of the story; it is the beginning.

Talking to patients necessarily transmits information, and in communication, it is the information that counts; therefore, physicians should be aware that they are involved in information control. There are specific tasks that should be accomplished by information flowing to patients. First, it should reduce uncertainty. Second, it should improve the patient's ability to act. Finally, it should improve the relationship between the physician and patient. It follows that information that you provide to patients should meet certain tests. Does it reduce the patient's uncertainty now or in the future? Does it improve the patient's ability to act? Does it improve your relationship with the patient (now or in the future)? If information wisely used can do those things, then information poorly used can create uncertainty, paralyze action, and destroy the relationship. Going back to the example of the patient Helene Fink, explaining to her the entire nature of her disease had all those negative effects, *even though it was true.*

Here follows a small tangent about death and the issue of denial. Most patients receiving treatment for cancer are aware of the possibility of dying. It has been on their minds since their diagnosis, but not always within awareness. They are often afraid of the subject, or of talking about it; like many people (maybe even you), patients are afraid of dying. It is usually not dying (ceasing to be) that they are afraid of; instead, the author believes it is separation from others. One way in which worries about death are handled is denial. Is denial in and of itself a bad thing? This author personally does not believe that it is, especially as the opposite face of denial may be panic. The important question is whether the denial is getting in the way of anything else important; for example, treatment or family relationships. Further, the author thinks you should be very cautious if you decide to break through denial. For this reason, the author usually does not tell people things, but rather answers their questions. When they do not ask the questions, the author can usually stimulate the question wanting to be answered. Telling Helene Fink the truth scared her and got her angry at her physician.

In giving information to a patient, a statement is only complete when it includes (1) what it is (the facts), (2) what it means, and (3) what is to be done about it. Here is an example:

What it is: "Your platelet count is lower today, which is why you are not getting your chemotherapy."

This is what it means: "The platelet count drops because of the action of the chemotherapy on your body. Today's platelet count is the expected reaction to the drugs and will cause you no harm. There is nothing unusual about it. It will not reduce the effect of your treatment if you do not get chemotherapy today."

This is what we are going to do about it: "There is no need to do anything about your platelet count. Because the platelet count is one way we decide how much medicine you should get, we will be testing it regularly. It usually comes back to a point where you can get your chemotherapy in about a week."

Patients frequently ask questions about what something is—for example, a pain, a new symptom, something on their skin, or a swelling somewhere. Physicians commonly give an "it is a this or that" answer. For example, "Oh that is a bruise," or "The swelling is some edema in your foot." The same rule applies as previously, the answer should not be it is a this or a that, but this is what it is,

this is what it means, and this is what is going to be done about it. "The black and blue mark is just a bruise. Because your platelet count is low from the chemotherapy you are going to bruise more easily than you used to. When your platelet count is normal again after the chemotherapy, that will stop happening. We don't have to do anything because it doesn't require any treatment."

EXPLANATIONS

Explanations should be brief, clear, unambiguous, and jargon free. The test of the adequacy is not what you say, but what the patient understands. The best way to find that out is to ask the patient to repeat what you just said. Remember, the explanation is focused on the patient's need for information. And the enemy of clarity is ambiguity.

Here is an example from an actual interaction (with a physician who prided himself on his communication skills). "It looks as though we'll probably get out of the woods. Most of the bad stuff seems pretty well gone and I doubt if we'll have trouble again if things hold the way they are."

Think what these phrases really mean:

- ". . . probably get out of the woods." Will we or won't we?
- ". . . most of the bad stuff . . ." Is it gone or is it not? And what about the rest?
- ". . . I doubt if we'll . . ." Do you believe it or not?

This is the way physicians commonly talk to patients. This is supposedly done this way because physicians do not want to commit themselves. If challenged, physicians may say, "I'm not God. I don't know what is going to happen." Or, "I don't have a crystal ball." Patients know both statements are true. But such statements are beside the point. The physician may not have a crystal ball, but he or she knows better than the patient what can happen and what will probably happen. It has been shown repeatedly that people do not understand clearly what percentages mean such as, "You have a 30% chance of recurrence." Cognitive psychologists have demonstrated that people understand information better if it has been translated into natural frequencies. (You have a 3 in 10 chance of recurrence, or there is a 7 in 10 chance that you will not have a recurrence.) It is not necessary to pretend or lie. Here is a possible way to say the same thing that does not suggest omniscience, but that, at the same time, is reassuring. "These tests show regression of your cancer. You are getting a very good response to treatment and I believe you're going to do well." You can stop there; there is no reason to express doubt. If you believe you are not being truthful because you have not shared the whole truth, ask whether the patient has any questions. If there are questions, answer them honestly but briefly and wait for more questions. Do not answer a question that has not been asked. If the patient wonders whether things could turn bad again, here is a possible response. "You and I both know that I can't promise that this good response will keep up, but I expect it to. And even though that may leave you with some doubt or maybe you find it worrisome, don't make bad news out of good news. This is good news. We're doing well. Let's keep it up."

UNCOMFORTABLE QUESTIONS

If the patient asks a question that you do not want to answer, you can buy some time to find out what the patient is really asking by, "What do you mean by that?" Or, "I'm not sure I understand what you're asking me, say it again in a different way." If it is a direct difficult question that does not mince words, then answer it in the same manner in clear, unambiguous, spare, jargon-free, truthful language. Say no more than you must say to answer the question, and then wait for the next question. The same rules apply here as outlined previously: Say what it is, say what it means, and say what you are going to do about it. Do not leave the patient hanging in the air with statements like, "Let's wait a month and see how things stand." Be more specific. "In a month, we will repeat your CT scan. I expect that it will still show a good response. If you've had some growth of your tumor, we will decide what that means and then, if necessary, modify your treatment." You will notice that the author has repeatedly used the words "we," "we'll," "we're," and "let's" (as in, "let us"). In each instance, you are telling the patient that you and the patient are a team, that the patient is not alone, and that you are right there with him or her.

Earlier, the author said that he did not believe that fear of death is a fear of ceasing to exist, but a fear of separation from others. He does not know if that is a correct interpretation, but he does know that patients greatly fear being abandoned by or distanced from their doctors. It does not take many words to express your continued connection to the patient, no matter what happens.

INFORMATION

Information can be conveyed in different quantities ranging from terse to fulsome. It has degrees of detail, complexity, or sophistication and should be tailored to the patient's ability to understand. It has timing. There is a big difference between conveying information to a patient in a recovery room or to someone who has come to the office specifically to discuss a diagnosis or treatment. It has timing. Choose your place and choose your time. If the patient wants information before you are ready, tell him or her that you are going to discuss this in detail at such and such a time and ask if that will be all right. If the patient insists on talking at that moment, then be brief and again refer to future discussion. Information has relevance; stay on the subject. And, finally, information has truth content.

Information is flowing all the time from multiple sources. Information comes to the patient from the environment. For example, a patient in a radiation suite in most hospitals is getting a lot more information than you may wish from simply looking around the waiting area. He or she gets information from knowledge stored in memory. Needs, wishes, desires, fears, or fantasies are another source of information. Other people may also provide information, such as family, friends, nurses, attendants, technicians, and other doctors. Everybody! And everybody is talking all the time. Patients get information from their bodies as they interpret the feelings they have as well as what they see. Remember, you are only one source of information among many. Information is flowing all the time. Even no information is information.

The Internet represents a special problem. It seems that everyone goes to the Internet to find out about their disease, treatment, doctors, and the institutions in which they get care. Whatever the question, the Internet overflows with information. As of the time of this writing, if you enter "ingrown toenail" into Google, more than 440,000 sites become accessible. If you search Google about cancer of the breast, more than 59 million sites become accessible. Diverse sources of information inevitably bring conflict, and disagreement between sources of information produces uncertainty. The more pressing the need to act, the less tolerable is uncertainty.

Increased uncertainty often makes patients more fearful. Their fear increases the difficulty they experience when decisions have to be made, which also increases fearfulness. Uncertainty and fear reinforce the state of illness. One solution to the problem of uncertainty is increased trust in doctors. That is one of the reasons why patients put so much faith in their doctors' words and actions. This may make it uncomfortable for physicians who know that they are far from invulnerable, but it is much easier for patients. Also, it is one of the reasons that it is so important to maintain strong doctor–patient relationships. Too many times, doctors react to the amount

of trust that patients lay on them by insisting that the patient make his or her own decision (see later discussion). This makes it more difficult for the patients in situations wherein they need support and in whom they should invest their trust. "Thank you—together we'll do the best we can," is much better than, "You know that I'm not infallible and that I can't make your decisions for you."

MEANING

The topic of meaning, in general, is complicated, but some things about it are straightforward. Physicians do not act directly because of events, objects, or relations; they act because of the meaning of these things. Information does its work because it acts on meaning. Meaning has two characteristics that are important to this discussion. The first is significance. For example, "Dark clouds signify rain" or "Postmenopausal bleeding means I have cancer." Meaning also conveys importance. For example, "Rain will ruin the picnic" or "I could die from that kind of cancer." Importance is another way of saying value. And values, although they may be shared, are always personal; importance is always importance to someone. These two characteristics of meaning are present whenever you are talking and whenever the patient is listening. That is why it is so important to find out what significance the patient is giving to your explanation and what its importance is to the patient.

Another characteristic of meaning is that it can be changed. Sometimes, when you can do nothing else for a patient, you can change the meaning that the patient has assigned to objects, relations, events, or the words that you have used. For example, when someone presented in 1950 with what we now identify as stage I Hodgkin's lymphoma, after the diagnosis he or she was met with lies and pessimism. Now, the same patient is met with smiles and optimism. But for the individual patient, on first being diagnosed, death is still possible because you do not know for sure what the outcome will be. Why the smiles? For this patient, on first diagnosis, only the meaning of the disease has changed, but that is enough to change the physician's attitude and hearten both patient and family. To change the significance of the events, you must change the patient's meaning—the patient's objective knowledge of the world. To change the importance of events, you must address their impact on the patient—how they will affect the patient in the present and in the future.

Meaning is also used here in the sense of purpose. This was popularized by Viktor Frankl[3] in his book, *Man's Search for Meaning*. Here, patients may search for the meaning of the fact of their cancer, or use the disease as a spur to find a new meaning in their life. This not the sense in which the author has been using the word. Meaning is important to physicians because words do not simply have a denotation, a dictionary meaning, or a personal or connotative meaning, but because every meaning has cognitive, emotional, physical, and spiritual dimensions. Words act on the body to the molecular level. As a simple example, if somebody tells you something with a meaning that induces fear in you, the fear may be felt like a gripping in the chest and may be accompanied by all the physiologic manifestations of fear.[4] The words do not cause the fear; rather, the fear is part of the meaning of the words. In the same way, the physiologic events are not caused by fear; they are a part of fear itself.

CAFETERIA EXPLANATIONS

It cannot be said too strongly: Give up, get past, eschew, and forget about cafeteria information and decision making. Simply laying out the information and asking the patient to make the decisions is not fair to the patient and it takes away from you one of your important therapeutic options: control of the information. Cafeteria decisions abandon the patient when he or she needs you most. You can honor the patient's autonomy and honor the realistic need for clinicians to maintain the control of the case by helping patients make decisions that you believe are in their best interests because they know those interests. Ask yourself how well you would be able to make a decision if you were frightened, uncertain, and fundamentally ignorant about the issues involved in the decision. If just knowing the medical facts was enough to make decisions, doctors, when they are patients, would be the best decision makers of all. Doctors know that that is not true. Sick people need help expressing their best interests.

Communication, as with all other therapeutic agents, should be goal directed. The goal is to help the patient be better, whatever the outcome. The spoken language is a powerful tool toward that end and worth learning how to use effectively.

REFERENCES

1. Cassell EJ. *Talking with Patients. Vol. 1. The Theory of Doctor-Patient Interaction.* Cambridge, MA: MIT Press; 1985.
2. Cassell EJ. *Talking with Patients. Vol. 2. Clinical Technique.* Cambridge, MA: MIT Press; 1985.
3. Frankl V. *Man's Search for Meaning.* New York: Pocket Book; 1959.
4. Cassell EJ. *Mind and Body: The Nature of Suffering and the Goals of Medicine.* 2nd ed. New York: Oxford University Press; 2004:221.

PALLIATIVE AND ALTERNATIVE CARE

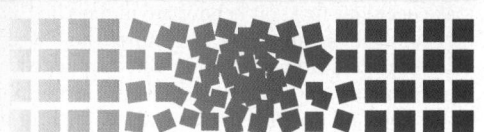

151 Specialized Care of the Terminally Ill

Robert S. Krouse and F. Amos Bailey

INTRODUCTION

The evolution of cancer care has led to survival advantages for many cancer patients. Some cancers, such as breast and colorectal, may be considered a chronic disease in many settings. Nonetheless, clinicians must be prepared for the specialized care for cancer survivors and those living with progressive cancer whose suffering is unique, complex, and multifaceted as described by Eric Cassel in his essay "The Nature of Suffering".[1] Now, recognition of the needs of patients has propelled the development of programs to provide concomitant palliative and supportive care with cancer treatment to help address the myriad concerns for both patients and their family and caregivers.

INTERDISCIPLINARY CARE FOR PATIENTS WITH ADVANCED CANCER

Specialized care for terminally ill cancer patients requires appropriate interdisciplinary care. Members of the interdisciplinary team (IDT) will include physician providers representing medical, surgical, and radiation oncology. Importantly, palliative medicine specialists, who work in tandem with nursing, social work, pastoral care, and other providers, can develop and lead integrated holistic care plans that reflect the goals of care and the values of patients.

Palliation is increasingly becoming recognized as an important component of care of the cancer patient for specialties treating cancer patients with advanced disease. In the terminally ill patient, chemotherapy, surgery, and radiation therapy may have the potential to provide palliation of symptoms and improve health-related quality of life (HRQOL) and extend survival. Decisions related to disease-modifying treatments must take into account the patient's functional status, often as expressed by performance status, and the goals of care. The intent of treatments must be clear, because patients and families will often have unrealistic goals based on the potential outcomes for treatments offered.[2,3]

Clearly, all providers caring for patients with advanced cancer should work closely together to ensure that the patient and family are able to maximally benefit from our interventions while minimizing iatrogenic harm. Importantly, as death becomes more imminent, patients and families often benefit from the IDT support during this stressful time.

EARLY PALLIATIVE CARE

Recent studies of concomitant palliative care with standard oncologic care have demonstrated that patients with concomitant treatment had improved HRQOL, a reduction in symptom burden, and the potential to reduce use of aggressive treatment at end of life,[4] while having an improvement in survival.[5] Therefore, ideally, patients who present with advanced stage cancers and those experiencing progressive disease despite treatment will have access to concomitant palliative care early in their treatment course. This can allow for better support as described previously, but can make the transition from a focus on disease-modifying treatment to more symptom-focused care less jarring. This also recognizes that the complex issues of suffering with its physical as well as psychosocial and spiritual dimensions are most often present from the time of diagnosis and may vary in intensity and distress throughout the course of disease. Certainly, patients, families, as well as providers experience increased intensity of suffering near the end of life and practical expertise in the care of the dying is recognized as one of several important themes of care in order to achieve a "Good Death".[6] To do this, the team must engage in new types of conversations with patients and their families and among themselves and broaden their assessments to be able to ensure physical comfort, address psychological needs, and identify goals of care and social and spiritual sources of distress.

COMMUNICATION

Communication skills are key for all providers to have successful interactions with patients and families. Communication skills can be learned and honed. Patient and family perceptions of quality and satisfaction with medical care are closely linked to the ability to effectively communicate the clinical situations, treatment options, and empathic support for all involved. There are a number of communication skill training programs, and all providers should work to continuously improve communication skills and consider specific training. When providers can communicate their clinical situation effectively with patients and families, they are better equipped to make decisions that focus on achievable goals of care in the terminally ill cancer patient.

SPECIFIC PROBLEMS IN THE SETTING OF ADVANCED CANCER

There are many specific issues that require attention in the terminally ill beyond pain and psychological distress. When patients present with these issues, the evaluation of the extent of disease, overall performance status, and treatment options may take some time to ascertain.

Aggressive palliative treatment of symptoms should be undertaken. At this point, discussions with the patient, their family or caregivers, and the medical team should then review the patient's goals of care and align them with available treatment options. Some patients may opt for a more palliative focused approach, whereas others may choose, if potentially feasible, operative or interventional approaches. Patients must be supported in that interventions are not always successful to relieve symptoms, and the problem may recur. It may be difficult to weigh the risk and benefits of interventions. Involvement of the IDT is important because the patient will need support in the provision of complex medical information in such a way as to be able to make an informed decision.

Regardless of the outcome of any intervention, the patient is likely to have a limited survival such that ongoing palliative/hospice support in the hospital or after discharge is needed.

DYSPNEA

Dyspnea, the uncomfortable sensation or awareness of breathing or needing to breathe (i.e., shortness of breath), is a commonly encountered symptom in cancer patients, which results from multiple disease processes and can lead to limited function and poor HRQOL. The prevalence of dyspnea among cancer patients has been reported to be between 21% to 90%, depending on the type and stage of cancer.[7]

The pathophysiology of dyspnea is multifactorial and incompletely understood.[8] Researchers believe the cerebral cortex integrates this sensory input with other cognitive and emotional factors as well as motor information from the respiratory center.[9]

The *gold standard* for the diagnosis of dyspnea is the self-report of the patient. There are no other reliable, objective measures of dyspnea. Respiratory rate, oxygen saturation, and arterial blood gas determinations do not necessarily correlate with, or measure dyspnea. Hypoxemic patients may not be dyspneic, and those with dyspnea are often not hypoxic or remain dyspneic when hypoxemia is resolved. The severity scales developed for pain (numerical, visual analog scale) have been reliably used to assess dyspnea.[10]

The goal of the symptomatic management of dyspnea is to relieve the patient's sense of breathlessness. Specific therapy to manage underlying causes (e.g., bronchodilators, stent placement to relieve focal obstruction), is appropriate in selected patients. To manage the experience of shortness of breath, both pharmacologic and nonpharmacologic interventions have been shown to be effective.

Oxygen supplementation has a perceived benefit by patients who are dyspneic that far exceeds the number who have hypoxemia.[11] There is likely a placebo effect of oxygen, partially based on the medical symbolism inherent in its administration. It is recommended to use the least confining oxygen supplement possible for the comfort of the patient and the ability to communicate with the family. In the imminently dying, if the patient is comfortable with nasal prong oxygen, fans, and opioids, it is not necessary to monitor the oxygen saturation or escalate oxygen therapy for relatively asymptomatic hypoxia. It has also been observed that similar relief is experienced from cool air blowing on the face, such as from a breeze or a fan.

Opioids are the most effective medication for the symptomatic control of dyspnea.[12,13] In opioid-naïve individuals, small amounts of morphine can relieve dyspnea.[14] For those on baseline opioids, start by increasing the opioid dose by 25%.[13] Patients frequently report anxiety concurrent with dyspnea, and these symptoms can reinforce each other. Dyspnea frequently leads to anxiety, and anxiety can also exacerbate dyspnea. Opioids alone may break the cycle by relieving dyspnea, but they do not have a direct anxiolytic effect. Anxiolytics (e.g., benzodiazepines) are frequently prescribed for anxiety related to dyspnea. However, when tested, the evidence for their effectiveness is not persuasive.[15] Therefore, benzodiazepines should not be used alone as first-line therapy for dyspnea.

MALIGNANT BOWEL OBSTRUCTION

Malignant bowel obstruction (MBO) is defined as: (1) clinical evidence of a bowel obstruction via history, physical exam, or radiographic examination, (2) bowel obstruction beyond the ligament of Treitz, (3) intra-abdominal primary cancer with incurable disease, or (4) non–intra-abdominal primary cancer with clear intraperitoneal disease.[16] It occurs most frequently with ovarian and colorectal cancers, but occurs with other abdominal and, occasionally, with nonabdominal malignancies. MBO may be related to tumor, its treatment (e.g., radiation enteritis), or benign etiologies

(e.g., adhesions, internal hernia). The goals of treatment include relieving nausea and vomiting, allowing oral intake, alleviating pain, and permitting the patient to return to their chosen care setting.

When patients are admitted to the hospital, conservative measures (e.g., nasogastric tube, decompression, intravenous hydration, nothing by mouth [NPO]) is typically initiated. Palliative pharmacologic therapies have the goals of reducing intestinal inflammation and edema and/or controlling pain, nausea, vomiting, and dehydration. Pharmacologic options include: (1) antisecretory agents (e.g., somatostatin analog, steroids, scopolamine); (2) pain medications (e.g., morphine, fentanyl, hydromorphone, methadone); and (3) antiemetic therapy (e.g., haloperidol, prochlorperazine). Opioids act both directly to relieve pain related to intestinal obstruction, as well as to reduce painful bowel contractions against the obstruction. Antiemetics can be given through a variety of nonoral routes to control vomiting,[17] although complete relief of emesis is achieved in a minority of patients through antiemetics alone. Hormonal manipulation of gut activity has substantially added to the armamentarium of MBO management. Octreotide, a synthetic analog of the gut hormone somatostatin, dramatically decreases gastrointestinal (GI) secretions and reduces bowel motility, often markedly reducing or resolving MBO symptoms.[18] Duration of treatment may be short lived (median: 9.4 to 17.5 days),[18] although symptoms are frequently relieved for the life of the patients. Anticholinergic medications, such as scopolamine, can decrease peristalsis and secretions and can lead to improved control of vomiting and intestinal colic for malignant GI obstruction. Although direct comparisons of these agents have not yielded clear recommendations,[19,20] a combination of these medications may offer synergistic benefits. Finally, corticosteroids are commonly used as adjunctive agents or alone in MBO management, with the goals of decreasing tumor-associated bowel edema and of providing antiemetic benefits. Although a meta-analysis has suggested no statistical benefit of corticosteroid use, a subset of patients may benefit from them, and medication-related morbidity is low,[21] particularly in patients in the terminal stages of their disease. If surgery is being considered, it has been shown that somatostatin or its analogs are likely not a risk to an operation. Steroids may carry operative risks and should be initiated with caution.

Persistent obstructions in the face of palliative treatments or evidence of complete obstructions are indications that a surgical procedure should be considered unless actively dying. Many patients are deemed inoperable (6.2% to 50%).[22] This may be due to poor operative risk or contraindications to surgery. Poor operative risk must be assessed based on comorbidities (e.g., cardiac and pulmonary function), the amount and location of metastatic disease (e.g., overwhelming metastasis to the liver causing malfunction), and current functional status (e.g., Karnofsky score: <50%). Potential contraindications for surgery in patients with incurable cancer and MBO include ascites (greater than 3 L) and, in particular, ascites that rapidly recur after drainage, carcinomatosis, multiple obstructions, or a palpable intra-abdominal mass.[17,23]

The optimal procedure is that which is the quickest, safest, and most efficacious in alleviating the obstruction. Although bowel resection may lead to the best outcome,[24,25] a bypass may be a safer option, and the placement of a gastrostomy tube for intermittent venting might be optimal in some settings. In addition, an intestinal stoma may be necessary after resection or to adequately bypass the blockage. Cytoreductive procedures (e.g., resection of an intraperitoneal tumor) frequently carry a high morbidity and usually are only considered with very low-grade tumors, such as pseudomyxoma peritonei.

Although it is recognized that improvement in HRQOL after surgery is variable (42% to 85%),[22,26] there is no consistent parameter used to determine this clinical outcome; operations *may* offer an advantage of an increased survival. Surgical risks must be carefully considered prior to an operation, because morbidity (42%)[27] and mortality (5% to 32%)[22,25,27] are common, and the reobstruction rate is high (10% to 50%).[22]

Endoscopic procedures are suitable for patients who are poor operative candidates or who decline an open operative intervention. The major approaches include stenting and percutaneous endoscopic gastrostomy (PEG) tube placement. Stenting may include procedures to initially canalize the lumen (e.g., laser or balloon dilatation). PEG tubes are generally well-tolerated *venting* procedures that can alleviate symptoms of intractable vomiting and nausea for upper GI obstructions.[28] A study from M.D. Anderson Cancer Center found that percutaneous gastrostomy tubes were utilized for palliation in 23% of small bowel obstructions in patients with advanced malignancy.[29] Complications related to PEGs are rare, even when puncturing other organs.[28] The presence of significant ascites is a relative contraindication. In combination with other medical techniques, both open and percutaneous gastrostomy offers the possibility of intermittent oral intake. Endoluminal wall stents have a high success rate for relief of symptoms (64% to 100%) in complete and incomplete colorectal obstructions,[30] and in over 70% of upper intestinal malignant obstructions including gastric outlet, duodenal, and jejunal obstructions.[31] Although risks include perforation (0% to 15%), stent migration (0% to 40%), or reocclusion (0% to 33%), stents can frequently lead to adequate palliation for long periods of time.[30] Stent occlusion by tumor in-growth is usually amenable to another endoscopic intervention.

MALIGNANT BILIARY OBSTRUCTION

Malignant biliary obstruction is an obstruction of the biliary tract due to cancer. Malignancies associated with MBO are pancreatic cancer, cholangiocarcinoma (most commonly ampullary cancer, followed more uncommonly by lymphoma, duodenal cancer, and metastatic disease). Hyperbilirubinemia may become symptomatic, leading to pruritus, bleeding diathesis, and liver failure. Patients need prompt relief of the biliary obstruction before embarking on any other palliative treatments. Two major treatment approaches are currently available: (1) surgical bypass and (2) stent management (via gastroenterology or interventional radiology).

There are multiple studies comparing methods, especially stenting versus surgery.[32] Endoscopic stenting has been shown to have similar success rates as surgery. Although most patients receive stents, recurrence rates are higher and subsequent hospitalizations may be lower for patients who have surgical bypass.[32] Metal stents have improved patency compared to plastic stents with lower recurrent obstruction rates, although this may require a second procedure if not placed initially. One approach is to perform endoscopic stent placement in patients considered to have short life spans with a limited potential for recurrent obstruction and to perform surgical bypass for patients with less aggressive tumors, longer expected life expectancy, or limited access to endoscopic expertise for treatment of recurrent obstruction.

If the bile duct is entered via an endoscopic retrograde cholangiopancreatography (ERCP) but a stent could not be placed, it may necessitate a relatively urgent surgical procedure due to the potential cholangitis risk. If urgent surgery is not realistic due to patient comorbidities, overall status, or operating room availability, a transhepatic drain placed by an interventional radiologist is indicated. If a laparoscopic exploration is first undertaken for a potentially resectable mass and metastatic disease is noted, it is reasonable to abort the procedure with the hope that a less morbid endoscopic stenting can be accomplished. Also, if endoscopic stenting fails or is unavailable, an open or laparoscopic bypass is warranted. If, at open exploration, the patient is found to be unresectable, it is reasonable to proceed with a surgical bypass.

There are multiple options to surgically bypass the biliary system (e.g., cholecystojejunostomy, choledochojejunostomy, choledochoduodenostomy). The overall morbidity of surgical bypass is almost 20%, and the recurrence rate is 0% to 15%.[32] It has been shown that choledochoduodenostomy has the fewest complications at only 3%.[33] Of course, the ability to mobilize the duodenum may not be possible in all patients. A laparoscopic biliary bypass might be performed in expert hands.[34]

GASTRIC OUTLET OBSTRUCTION

Gastric outlet obstructions typically occur in the setting of gastric, peri-pancreatic, and duodenal tumors. Procedures are considered in the setting of persistent nausea, vomiting, eructation, and early satiety. They also may be considered when there is evidence of duodenal compression on radiographic or endoscopic evaluations.

Although few centers have the technical expertise, endoscopic stents for gastric outlet obstruction may be quite successful (approximately 90%) with rare complications.[35,36] In addition, if the stent fails due to tumor in-growth or migration (around 10%), another stent can often be placed.[35,36]

Another endoscopic option is percutaneous gastrostomy, with some centers reporting use in almost a quarter of their patients with gastric outlet obstruction and advanced malignancy.[26] Unfortunately, this will not allow the patient to eat, and should only be considered in patients for whom a stent fails or is unavailable and who would not tolerate a surgical procedure.

If endoscopic stenting fails for the gastric outlet blockage or is unavailable, an open or laparoscopic bypass is warranted. There are several technical variations of a surgical bypass procedure (gastrojejunostomy), but the results are similar. This can be achieved safely via open or laparoscopic techniques. For an unresectable gastric cancer, the laparoscopic technique has been shown to have less suppression of immune function, less pain, shorter hospital stays, lower postoperative morbidity, and earlier recovery of bowel movements than an open procedure.[37] Additionally, there might be slightly better emptying if this is done to the posterior wall of the stomach. A distal gastric tumor may also be resected with a palliative intent.

It has been shown that symptomatic patients (e.g., vomiting prior to operation) typically have a poor outcome (approximately 90% did not have relief of symptoms) to gastric bypass. In comparison, if patients were not symptomatic but had evidence of impending obstruction, only about 40% had a poor outcome.[33] One consideration as to the reason for this is that symptomatic patients are potentially sicker with a greater tumor burden.

Antrectomy along with gastrojejunostomy in the setting of unresectable pancreatic cancer has been shown to have excellent results until death in one small series.[38] There is limited evidence in the literature to support this procedure in the setting of gastric outlet obstruction, and a simpler bypass may be more reasonable.

Finally, in the setting where a surgical biliary bypass is planned, there is some controversy as to whether a preemptive gastric bypass (gastrojejunostomy) in the asymptomatic patient is warranted. Because a late gastric obstruction occurs from 9% to 23%,[39–41] a duodenal bypass should be considered at the time of biliary bypass, especially if the patient is of good performance status with limited disease (no or minimal metastasis).

MALIGNANT ASCITES

Ascites in the terminally ill cancer patient may be due to overwhelming liver metastasis, cirrhotic liver disease, or carcinomatosis. It can be a difficult problem to manage, and treatment may be determined by the extent of the ascites, the condition of patient, or etiology. If ascites are minimal, no therapy is indicated. Larger volumes of ascites can lead to discomfort, fullness, or respiratory problems. Diuretics along with paracentesis is typically the primary treatment option. Typically, spironolactone is used in combination with furosemide. Alternative options should be considered if diuretics no longer are of benefit or if percutaneous aspirations become painful and frequent. Chemotherapy has been shown to be efficacious in certain settings.[42,43] Intraperitoneal verapamil may enhance chemotherapy response.[44] Intercavitary chemotherapy may also have efficacy, especially in the setting of ovarian cancers. Multiple agents have been used, and ascites can be controlled in 33% to 85% of patients.[45] Targeted agents, such as catumaxomab[46] and aflibercept[47,48] may also play a role in treating malignant ascites.

There are multiple more invasive treatments for malignant ascites. If the patient has very advanced disease, simpler approaches should be initiated. If the patient has a longer life span, more invasive techniques may be considered. Probably the simplest intervention is the insertion of permanent intraperitoneal drainage catheters. This will allow for the serial drainage of fluid by the patient or their caretaker. Catheters can be placed surgically or by the interventional radiology team via computed tomography[49] or ultrasound guidance.[50] Multiple types of catheters have been used, including a pigtail catheter, peritoneal dialysis catheters (e.g., a Tenckoff catheter), pleural cavity catheters (e.g., a PleurX catheter), fenestrated port-a-catheters, and even a Foley catheter.[51-55] The patient and/or caregiver can be trained to drain excess peritoneal fluid when the patient is symptomatic. The success rates for permanent intraperitoneal catheters functioning until death is quite high (90%).[50,51] There is low procedural morbidity. The major complications are obstruction and infection and are around 17%,[50,51] although catheter sepsis has been reported to be 35%.[56] To avoid infection, there must be meticulous insertion technique, close patient follow-up, and liberal use of antibiotics. In fact, many catheter-related infections can be treated with antibiotics.[50,57] Sometimes the catheters may need to be removed due to infection, occlusion, or leakage around the catheter. Leakage has been reported to be alleviated by continuous drainage[51] or a suture around the drain.[56]

Another option for malignant ascites is a peritoneovenous shunt. The two most common are the LeVeen and the Denver shunt. Ascitic fluid travels from the peritoneal cavity into the venous circulation due to higher peritoneal pressures. Complications include sepsis, disseminated intravascular coagulation (DIC), heart failure, and pulmonary embolism leading to a rapid death. Although the incidence of major complications may be less common than previously reported for peritoneovenous shunts, the overall complication rate can be quite high (14% to 51%).[58-61] DIC is the major complication that most frequently will lead to a patient's death. It has been reported to occur from 5% to 10% in these procedures. Congestive heart failure is another major complication. The more common complication is shunt occlusion. The advantage of the Denver shunt over the LeVeen shunt is that the Denver shunt has a pump to help the shunt remain patent (26% Denver versus 50% LeVeen shunt occlusion rates).[60] Denver shunts have been shown to have a quite high function rate until death (96%).[59] The risk of infection is variable (0% to 18%),[59] and this may lead to shunt removal if not relieved with antibiotics. Importantly, relief of symptoms can be as high as 87.5%.[59] Therefore, a peritoneovenous shunt may be an excellent option in properly selected patients.

Hyperthermic intraperitoneal chemotherapy (HIPEC), without cytoreduction, is an accepted approach for the palliation of malignant ascites with good early data. In addition, this procedure can be performed laparoscopically in an attempt to minimize complications.[62] A much more invasive surgical technique includes a major debulking of carcinomatosis followed by intraperitoneal hyperthermic chemotherapy. This procedure is only available at specialized institutions, but will likely be infrequently performed for palliation in the future based on the results emerging from HIPEC without cytoreduction and laparoscopic HIPEC.[63] In the carcinomatosis patient, cytoreduction and intraperitoneal chemotherapy can have dramatic effects on ascites. In one report, 79% of patients did not have recurrence for the remainder of their life (median survival: 7.6 months).[64] Surprisingly, their group has also shown that this procedure can lead to an acceptable HRQOL and return-of-function status for many patients.[65] Palliative treatment of malignant ascites with cytoreduction and HIPEC may be of historical interest only because the contribution from cytoreduction

may be minimal based on reports of laparoscopic HIPEC. Laparoscopic HIPEC without cytoreduction is a less technically demanding procedure with a shorter length of stay and a decreased risk of surgical complications. A recent systematic review of 76 patients undergoing palliative laparoscopic HIPEC reported that the procedure was considered successful in 72 patients (95%), defined as a complete regression of ascites with no deaths and a morbidity rate of 12%.[60] Laparoscopic HIPEC appears to be safe and highly effective for the treatment of malignant ascites. The morbidity, although low, suggests that this procedure is best utilized in settings of ascites refractory to less aggressive treatments.[45,66] The improvement in ascites and the lack of a need for catheters or follow-up procedures is encouraging, but it should be noted that none of the studies of palliative laparoscopic HIPEC have included symptom assessment or HRQOL outcomes measures. HIPEC has also been shown to be accomplished via ultrasound guidance, further making this technique possible for patients with advanced disease.[67]

WOUNDS

There are multiple different kinds of wounds related to advanced cancer. These are often directly related to tumors, but may be due to treatments such as surgical procedures (e.g., lymph node dissections, tumor resections) or radiation therapy (e.g., nonhealing ulcers). Primary cancers that frequently lead to wound problems include breast cancer, skin cancers, soft tissue sarcomas, or soft tissue manifestations of other cancers (e.g., lung cancer). Special consideration must be taken related to the primary tumor type, and interdisciplinary decision making is imperative. Finally, due to debilitation, patients may have pressure sores, which complicate their overall course and lead to suffering. In the debilitated patient, pressure sores are more likely to occur. The prevention of pressure sores, as well as other wounds, is of primary importance.

Many wounds, especially related to radiation injury or in the severely malnourished, may not heal. Therefore, this should not be a goal of treatment, but focus should be on control of pain, odor, and mess. Wound care is of primary importance. This may include local debridement as indicated to keep the wound as clean as possible. Although surgical options for wounds are limited, operative intervention has been reported in 38% and primarily involves incision and drainage or debridement.[68] Only a minority of patients are able to undergo wide excision and closure of tumors causing wound problems.

One example of a chronic wound problem is chest wall complications of breast tumors. IDT care is imperative to recommend optimal therapy. Even in the terminally ill, chemotherapy, especially if the patient is chemo naïve, may have a role. Radiation therapy is unlikely to have a great effect with a very large tumor. Surgical resection, or *toilet* mastectomy, may be utilized in the setting of a fungating incurable breast cancer to remove the tumor with the intent of wound control. It is always important to know the previous treatments to better understand possible success. This will also help to identify the optimal reconstruction alternatives as well as the extent of resection that is possible. The surgical literature is not very helpful in directing the extent of resection, and this must be based on surgeon judgment. Reconstruction options include primary closure, skin grafts, and an omental flap with skin graft, musculocutaneous flaps, or free flaps. The major surgical complications that must be considered include infection, open wounds, and flap loss. The extent of procedure must be considered along with the patient's overall medical status and likely survival. The recurrence rates in this setting may be high. In one small series, it was noted to be 73%,[69] and 20% to 52% in some of the larger series.[70-73] The majority of these recurrences were quite small, however, and could be locally excised or observed in patients who already had other major metastatic disease. Local wound morbidity is variable, and most are quite minor, such as local skin necrosis in a skin graft, which will not have great impact on the patient's life. Importantly, if there is major local wound morbidity, this could have a profound effect on the patient for the remainder of his or her life.

Related to amputation, there are multiple small reports that do indicate good to excellent palliation.[74] Complications may be over 50%, including flap necrosis, infection, and death. Complication rates will depend on the extent of amputation. In addition to amputation, limb perfusion most commonly utilizing melphalan with or without tumor necrosis factor alpha (TNF-α) has been advocated in some centers for melanoma or sarcoma recurrences. Complete response rates are 45% to 72%, usually greater if TNF-α was used.[75] Importantly, it has been shown that HRQOL can be excellent, with reasonable long-term function.[75]

Additional morbid options are possible based on the site of the tumor and medical status of the patient. These may include amputations, limb perfusions, and major head and neck resections. Although these options may seem quite radical in the setting of palliation, they may be reasonable solutions based on symptoms and if the patient can withstand a large procedure. There have been many reports concerning local wound care for tumor-related wounds.

Finally, local wound care for tumor-related wounds is extremely important, and has been shown to have great impact on HRQOL. For example, controlling odor and seepage has been shown to lead to less isolation, greater comfort, and increased psychosocial well-being.[76] This straightforward approach to some wounds will lead to the best outcomes for many patients facing the end of life.

BLEEDING

Tumor-related bleeding is a difficult problem for terminally ill cancer patients. Bleeding may be related to superficial tumors such as recurrent breast, head and neck, or sarcomas. Symptoms related to deeper tumors include hemoptysis (e.g., primary or metastatic lung tumors), hematemesis (e.g., gastric cancer), melena or hematochezia (e.g., colorectal tumors), vaginal bleeding (e.g., cervical or endometrial carcinomas) or hematuria (e.g., renal or bladder tumors). In addition, patients may have a coagulopathy related to illness or treatments. Surgical intervention for GI bleeding is infrequently required. If surgery is indicated, the optimal surgical option will depend mainly on the location and reason for bleeding, along with the least morbid and most efficacious procedure possible. Nonsurgical options include radiation therapy, arterial embolization, and endoscopic procedures. For bronchial bleeding, bronchoscopic techniques may be warranted.

The IDT should be involved if possible to discuss the best therapeutic algorithm. Surgical options may be quite simple (e.g., local excision) or quite complex (e.g., gastrectomy).

One example where the IDT involvement may be helpful is with rectal tumor bleeding. Surgical options are typically complex with high morbidity. In addition, intestinal stomas would likely be needed. Local excision may be considered, although this procedure may be technically difficult or not possible in this setting. Therefore, patients would likely be better served with nonsurgical attempts to stop bleeding, which can be highly efficacious (e.g., radiation therapy, interventional radiology embolization). Again, the success of alternative approaches will be based on the availability and expertise at each institution.

Finally, it is a well-known strategy in hospice care for a patient with a known massive bleeding risk but no optimal or indicated intervention for the patient and family to be prepared for this outcome with dark sheets and sedation. Dark sheets are recommended so that blood will be less visible and disturbing for the patient and family. Medication for sedation should be immediately available and provided in adequate doses if exsanguination is a potential complication of the cancer to mitigate distress for the patient at that time. If sedation should be required for longer period (i.e., hours to short days), palliative sedation is often appropriate and emergent consultation with palliative medicine would be appropriate.

IMPENDING DEATH

Patients in the last days or hours of life often have unrelieved physical suffering, as well as significant emotional, spiritual, and social distress. Recognizing that a person is entering the imminently dying or terminal phase of their illness is critical to appropriate care planning, with a shift to comfort care. Defining when this phase begins is not always straightforward. Patients at the end of life are frequently not recognized as dying. As a result, suffering may not be properly appreciated or managed, and the patient's overall condition may even be exacerbated by the continuation of standard medical treatments. Palliative medicine providers in the hospital are an important resource to provide for care of the imminently dying by employing the best practices of end-of-life care from the home hospice setting, which are not routinely available in in-patient settings. The involvement of a palliative IDT will benefit not only patients and their family, but also their oncology team, because providing care to actively dying patients presents unique challenges that often require special expertise. Patients in their final days require careful symptom management, and families need support and coaching as death approaches.

Preparing the Family for the Dying Process

Patients and families are usually unaware of the changes that typically occur during the last hours of life and the actual moment of death. Health-care professionals should explain the expected changes in cognition and physical function before they occur in order to alleviate distress and to prevent panic. This is particularly useful for families planning a home death, or for those closely involved in institutional care. Frequent points for education to families/friends that are sitting in vigil with a patient may include:

- The interpretation of purposeless bodily movements or grimaces as expressions of physical discomfort or emotional distress.
- The *death rattle*—a loud wet rattling respiration due to small amounts of secretions in the back of the throat—may be interpreted as dyspnea or choking by family members.
- Encouragement of those present to speak to, touch, and comfort their loved one. Although it is not possible to know the patient's experience, it is often observed that a familiar voice, touch, and music may have a calming presence for some patients.

Among the issues that are important to resolve, if not previously discussed, are preferences for location of care and for limits on invasive or aggressive resuscitative therapies that often are ineffective in a patient with end-stage disease. Communication between caregivers and patients/families is particularly important for seriously ill hospitalized patients in whom there is a considerable mismatch between what patients prefer and what treatments they actually receive.[77,78] Finally, clinicians should review and discontinue orders that may no longer be necessary, including nonessential medications, scheduled laboratory tests, radiographic studies, and telemetry or other monitoring.

Nonessential drugs (i.e., those that are no longer consistent with the overall care plan) should be discontinued if possible.[79–81] These may include antihypertensives, lipid-lowering medications, calcium and iron supplements, vitamins, diabetic medications, and prophylaxis for thrombus with injections of heparin compounds. The continuation of medications for angina or heart failure should be guided by a clinical assessment of need; poor control of these conditions may adversely impact HRQOL during the final weeks, although this is unlikely in the final days.

The management of patients with diabetes at the end of life must be tailored to the individual patient's needs and the severity of the illness. In general, the risks and consequences of hypoglycemia are greater than those of hyperglycemia in patients at the end of life; looser control of blood sugars is appropriate. If at all possible, sliding scale insulin, which requires painful finger sticks to assess blood sugars, should be avoided.

Anticonvulsants are generally maintained; however, the need for the initial prescription should be scrutinized; ongoing treatment may not be needed if the anticonvulsant was started for neuropathic pain or seizure prophylaxis. If the patient has a documented seizure disorder, it is imperative that an alternative route of administering such as intravenously (IV) or subcutaneously (SQ) for lorazepam and levetiracetam or diazepam per rectum be instituted if and when the oral route is lost to prevent the recurrence of seizures.

Most medications can be stopped abruptly; however, certain medications should be gradually stopped (tapered) to prevent complications. As a general rule, this includes cardiovascular medications and those affecting the central nervous system (e.g., beta-blockers, clonidine, antidepressants, benzodiazepines).

It is recommended that a comfort care order set or guide be used to formulate care plans to ensure that there are environmental orders for the comfort and support of both the patient and the family; nonpharmacological interventions such as fans; eye, mouth, and skin care; as well as orders for comfort medications such as an opioid, antipsychotic, anxiolytic in usually lower but frequent doses. The care order should also take into account that the oral and intravenous routes may not be practical during the dying process. In almost all cases, symptoms can be managed with sublingual, subcutaneous, or per rectal routes. As *required* drugs for common symptoms (including pain, dyspnea, nausea, delirium, anxiety, and noisy respiratory secretions) should be prescribed according to an agreed upon protocol. This ensures that needed medications are available for comfort care at any time, without the delay in obtaining an order.

Providing care to actively dying patients presents unique challenges for the clinician. Patients in their final days require careful symptom management, and families need support and coaching as death approaches.

SELECTED REFERENCES

The full reference list can be accessed at lwwhealthlibrary.com/oncology.

1. Cassel EJ. The nature of suffering and the goals of medicine. *N Engl J Med* 1982;306:639–645.
4. Bakitas M, Lyons KD, Hegel MT, et al. Effects of a palliative care intervention on clinical outcomes in patients with advanced cancer: the Project ENABLE II randomized controlled trial. *JAMA* 2009;302:741–749.
5. Temel JS, Greer JA, Muzikansky A, et al. Early palliative care for patients with metastatic non-small-cell lung cancer. *N Engl J Med* 2010; 363:733–742.
6. Steinhauser K, Clipp EC, McNeilly M, et al. In search of a good death: observations of patients, families, and providers. *Ann Intern Med* 2000; 132:825–832.
7. Muers MF, Round CE. Palliation of symptoms in non-small-cell lung cancer: a study by the Yorkshire Regional Cancer Organisation Thoracic Group. *Thorax* 1993;48:339–343.
9. Peiffer C, Poline J, Thivard L, et al. Neural substrates for the perception of acutely induced dyspnea. *Am J Respir Crit Care Med* 2001;163: 951–957.
12. Light RW, Muro JR, Sato RI, et al. Effects of oral morphine on breathlessness and exercise tolerance in patients with chronic obstructive pulmonary disease. *Am Rev Respir Dis* 1989;139:126–133.
14. Mazzocato C, Buclin T, Rapin CH. The effects of morphine on dyspnea and ventilator function in elderly patients with advanced cancer: a randomized double-blind controlled trial. *Ann Oncol* 1999;10:1511–1514.
15. Mitchell-Heggs P, Murphy K, Minty K, et al. Diazepam in the treatment of dyspnea in the 'pink puffer' syndrome. *QJ Med* 1980;49:9–20.
16. Anthony T, Baron T, Mercadante S, et al. Report of the clinical protocol committee: development of randomized trials for malignant bowel obstruction. *J Pain Symptom Manage* 2007;34:S49–S59.
18. Mercadante S, Caraceni A, Simonetti MJ. Octreotide in relieving gastrointestinal symptoms due to bowel obstruction. *Palliative Medicine* 1993; 7:295–299.
20. Mercadante S, Ripamonti C, Casuccio A, et al. Comparison of octreotide and hyoscine butylbromide in controlling gastrointestinal symptoms due to malignant inoperable bowel obstruction. *Support Care Cancer* 2000; 8:188–191.
21. Feuer DJ, Broadley KE. Systematic review and meta-analysis of corticosteroids for the resolution of malignant bowel obstruction in advanced gynecological and gastrointestinal cancer. *Ann Oncol* 1999;10:1035–1041.
22. Feuer DJ, Broadley KE, Shepherd JH, et al. Systematic review of surgery in malignant bowel obstruction in advanced gynecological and gastrointestinal cancer. *Gynecol Oncol* 1999;75:313–322.
23. Ripamonti C, Twycross R, Baines M, et al. Clinical-practice recommendations for the management of bowel obstruction in patients with end-stage cancer. *Support Care Cancer* 2001;9:223–233.
26. Miner TJ, Jaques DP, Shriver CD. A prospective evaluation of patients undergoing surgery for the palliation of an advanced malignancy. *Ann Surg Oncol* 2002;9:696–703.
27. Makela J, Kiviniemi H, Laitinen S, et al. Surgical management of intestinal obstruction after treatment for cancer. *Eur J Surg* 1991;157:73–77.
28. Campagnutta E, Cannizzaro R. Percutaneous endoscopic gastrostomy (PEG) in palliative treatment of non-operable intestinal obstruction due to gynecologic cancer: a review. *Eur J Gynaecol Oncol* 2000;21:397–402.
29. Badgwell BD, Contreras C, Askew R, et al. Radiographic and clinical factors associated with improved outcomes in advanced cancer patients with bowel obstruction. *J Palliat Med* 2011;14:990–996.

30. Harris GJ, Senagore AJ, Lavery IC, et al. The management of neoplastic colorectal obstruction with colonic endoluminal stenting devices. *Am J Surg* 2001;181:499–506.
31. Soetikno RM, Carr-Locke DL. Expandable metal stents for gastric outlet, duodenal, and small intestinal obstruction. *Gastrointest Endosc Clin N Am* 1999;9:447–458.
32. Glazer ES, Hornbrook MC, Krouse RS. A meta-analysis of randomized trials: immediate stent placement vs. surgical bypass in the palliative management of malignant biliary obstruction. *J Pain Symptom Manag* 2014;47: 307–314
33. Potts JR III, Broughan TA, Hermann RE. Palliative operations for pancreatic carcinoma. *Am J Surg* 1990;159:72–78.
35. Kaw M, Singh S, Gagneja H, et al. Role of self-expandable metal stents in the palliation of malignant duodenal obstruction. *Surg Endosc* 2003; 17:646–650.
37. Choi YB. Laparoscopic gastrojejunostomy for palliation of gastric outlet obstruction in unresectable gastric cancer. *Surg Endosc* 2002;16:1620–1626.
38. Lucas CE, Ledgerwood AM, Bender JS. Antrectomy with gastrojejunostomy for unresectable pancreatic cancer-causing duodenal obstruction. *Surg* 1991;110:583–590.
39. Coene PPLO, Huibregtse K, van Gulk TM, et al. Duodenal obstruction requiring surgery following endoscopic palliation in patients with pancreatic local tumors. *Neth J Med* 1994;45:A28.
40. Holbrook AG, Chester JF, Britton DC. Surgical palliation for pancreatic cancer: will biliary bypass alone suffice? *J R Soc Med* 1990;83:12–14.
41. Huguier M, Baumel H, Manderscheid JC, et al. Surgical palliation for unresected cancer of the exocrine pancreas. *Eur J Surg Oncol* 1993;19:342–347.
44. Jia W, Zhu Z, Zhang T, et al. Treatment of malignant ascites with a combination of chemotherapy drugs and intraperitoneal perfusion of verapamil. *Cancer Chemother Pharmacol* 2013;71:1585–1590.
45. Cavazzoni E, Bugiantella W, Graziosi L, et al. Malignant ascites: pathophysiology and treatment. *Int J Clin Oncol* 2013;18:1–9.
50. O'Neill MJ, Weissleder R, Gervais DA, et al. Tunneled peritoneal catheter placement under sonographic and fluoroscopic guidance in the palliative treatment of malignant ascites. *Am J Roentgenol* 2001;177:615–618.
56. Lee A, Lau TN, Yeong KY. Indwelling catheters for the management of malignant ascites. *Support Care Cancer* 2000;8:493–439.
58. Smith DA, Weaver DW, Bouwman DL. Peritoneovenous shunt (PVS) for malignant ascites. *Am Surg* 1989;55:445–449.
59. Zanon C, Grosso M, Apra F, et al. Palliative treatment of malignant refractory ascites by positioning of Denver peritoneovenous shunt. *Tumori* 2002;88:123–127.
60. Bieligk SC, Calvo BF, Coit DG. Peritoneovenous shunting for nongynecologic malignant ascites. *Cancer* 2001;91:1247–1255.
61. Sugawara S, Sone M, Arai Y, et al. Radiological insertion of Denver peritoneovenous shunts for malignant refractory ascites: a retrospective multicenter study (JIVROSG-0809). *Cardiovasc Intervent Radiol* 2011;34:980–988.
62. Valle M, van der Speeten K, Garofalo A. Laparoscopic hyperthermic intraperitoneal preoperative chemotherapy (HIPEC) in the management of refractory malignant ascites: A multi-institutional retrospective analysis in 52 patients. *J Surg Oncol* 2009;100:331–334.
64. Loggie BW, Fleming RA, McQuellon RP, et al. Cytoreductive surgery with intraperitoneal hyperthermic chemotherapy for disseminated peritoneal cancer of gastrointestinal origin. *Am Surg* 2000;66:561–568.
65. McQuellon RP, Danhauer SC, Russell GB, et al. Monitoring health outcomes following cytoreductive surgery plus intraperitoneal hyperthermic chemotherapy for peritoneal carcinomatosis. *Ann Surg Oncol* 2007;14:1105–1113.

PALLIATIVE AND ALTERNATIVE CARE

67. Cui S, Ba M, Tang Y, et al. B ultrasound-guided hyperthermic intraperitoneal perfusion chemotherapy for the treatment of malignant ascites. *Oncol Rep* 2012;28:1325–1331.

68. Badgwell BD, Smith K, Liu P, et al. Indicators of surgery and survival in oncology inpatients requiring surgical evaluation for palliation. *Support Care Cancer* 2009;17:727–734.

69. Cheung KL, Willsher PC, Robertson JF, et al. Omental transposition flap for gross locally recurrent breast cancer. *Aust N Z J Surg* 1997;67:185–186.

70. Flook D, Webster DJ, Hughes LE, et al. Salvage surgery for advanced local recurrence of breast cancer. *Br J Surg* 1989;76:512–514.

71. Sweetland HM, Karatsis P, Rogers K. Radical surgery for advanced and recurrent breast cancer. *J R Coll Surg Edinb* 1995;40:88–92.

72. Downey RJ, Rusch V, Hsu FI, et al. Chest wall resection for locally recurrent breast cancer: is it worthwhile? *J Thorac Cardiovasc Surg* 2000;119:420–428.

73. Henderson MA, Burt JD, Jenner D, et al. Radical surgery with omental flap for uncontrolled locally recurrent breast cancer. *Aust N Z J Surg* 2001;71:675–679.

74. Paz IB. Major palliative amputations. *Surg Oncol Clin N Am* 2004;13:543–547.

78. Hardin SB, Yusufaly YA. Difficult end-of-life treatment decisions: do other factors trump advance directives? *Arch Intern Med* 2004;164:1531–1533.

81. Plonk WM Jr, Arnold RM. Terminal care: the last weeks of life. *J Palliat Med* 2005;8:1042–1054.

152 Rehabilitation of the Cancer Patient

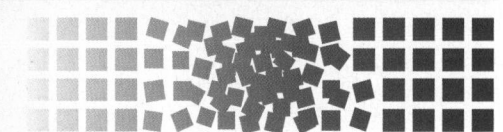

Michael D. Stubblefield

INTRODUCTION

Physical medicine and rehabilitation, also known as rehabilitation medicine or physiatry, is the medical specialty concerned with restoring and/or maintaining the highest possible level of function, independence, and quality of life. This relatively new specialty has evolved into a number of subspecialties to meet the needs of patients from all age groups whose primary medical issues may be cardiac, pulmonary, amputation, spinal cord injury, traumatic brain injury, sports injury, or pain to name a few. Cancer rehabilitation is a rapidly emerging subspecialty of rehabilitation medicine whose primary focus is the evaluation and management of neuromuscular, musculoskeletal, pain, and functional disorders that result from cancer and/or its treatments, including surgery, chemotherapy, and radiation. This chapter will discuss the principles of a safe and effective evaluation and rehabilitation of many of the common disorders encountered by cancer patients throughout the cancer continuum. The full scope of a cancer survivor's rehabilitation needs is vast and cannot be adequately addressed in one chapter due to space limitations. A comprehensive reference on the topic of cancer rehabilitation is available.[1]

The American Cancer Society estimates that in 2013 there were 13.7 million cancer survivors, 1.7 million new cancer patients, and 580,000 cancer deaths in the United States (Fig. 152.1).[2] The number of cancer survivors is expected to grow to 18.1 million by the year 2020.[3] The rapidly growing number of cancer survivors is more than 50 times the relatively stable estimate of 273,000 US spinal cord injury survivors in 2013.[4] Despite this marked disparity in numbers, there are more than 20 fellowship programs to train spinal cord injury physicians but only 2 to train cancer rehabilitation physicians.[5] This translates into scores of well-trained spinal cord injury physicians but only a handful of cancer rehabilitation physicians to take care of the millions of patients who need their services. More should be done to increase the ranks of well-trained cancer rehabilitation physicians.

COMPLICATIONS OF CANCER AND ITS TREATMENT

The complications of cancer and its treatment represent a broad and diverse group of disorders that are covered in detail throughout this textbook. In the context of cancer rehabilitation, several specific disorders are of interest because they can heavily impact the safety and effectiveness of rehabilitative efforts. It is imperative for the clinician to fully understand that there are no absolutes in oncology and that every decision made with or on behalf of a patient has an implicit cost-benefit analysis underlying it. This is as true for the physical or occupational therapist deciding if it is safe to ambulate a patient as it is for the neurosurgeon deciding whether to attempt resection of metastatic disease compressing the spinal cord. Poor outcomes are common in cancer and can happen at any time, often unexpectedly and occasionally dramatically. The challenge for the rehabilitation specialist is to maximize

function and quality of life while minimizing, to the best of their ability and knowledge, any potential adverse outcomes.

Direct Effects of Cancer

The direct effects of cancer are often obvious, with the clinical impact on function being dependent largely on the location and extent of disease. Examples are a large lung mass compromising pulmonary function and, subsequently, endurance and stamina, or an epidural metastasis to the spine compressing the spinal cord causing weakness and pain. A working understanding of several of the direct complications of cancer including its effects on the central and peripheral nervous system and on bony integrity, are of great importance in cancer rehabilitation and will be discussed in detail in subsequent sections.

Paraneoplastic Effects

Paraneoplastic syndromes (PNS) are rare disorders (<1% of cancer patients) that cause tissue or organ damage via remote effects of a primary or metastatic cancer.[6] Most PNS occur because the tumor secretes a substance that mimics normal hormones or that interferes with circulating proteins. Systemic paraneoplastic disorders include cancer cachexia, hypercalcemia, Cushing syndrome, and Trousseaus syndrome.[7–10] A number of PNS affect the central nervous system (CNS) (limbic encephalitis, encephalomyelitis, cerebellar degeneration, opsoclonus-myoclonus, optic neuropathy/retinopathy, brain stem encephalitis, stiff person syndrome, motor neuron disease, necrotizing myopathy) and peripheral nervous system (sensory neuronopathy, acute sensorimotor neuropathy, chronic sensorimotor neuropathy, neuromyotonia, chronic gastrointestinal pseudo-obstruction/autonomic neuropathy, Lambert-Eaton myasthenic syndrome, myasthenia gravis, inflammatory myopathy) with potentially devastating impacts on function and quality of life.[11] These disorders, although relatively rare, represent a significant therapeutic challenge to the rehabilitation specialist.

Chemotherapy

Chemotherapy is a cornerstone of cancer treatment for many malignancies and may be given either with intent to cure or to prolong life. The myriad complications of the ever growing number of agents are discussed at length in other chapters. The impact of these complications on function and quality of life depends on the specific derangement or complications induced by the agent. Anemia, neutropenia, thrombocytopenia, myopathy, cardiomyopathy, neuropathy, contracture, fatigue, thromboembolism, nausea, and edema are just a few of the common disorders resulting from chemotherapy that can have a major impact on rehabilitation efforts. Several of these complications and their specific implications for rehabilitation will be discussed in subsequent sections.

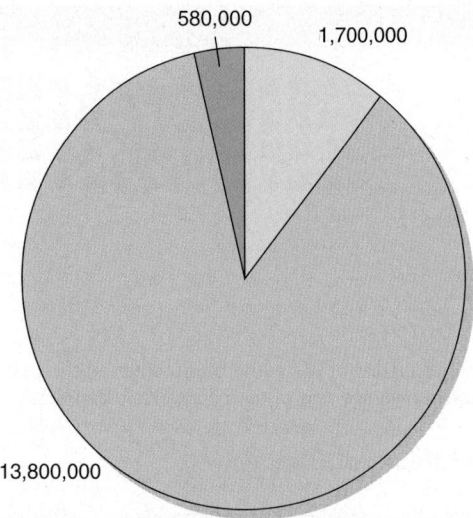

580,000

1,700,000

13,800,000

Figure 152.1 Pie chart illustrating the number of cancer survivors (13,800,000), new cancer cases (1,700,000), and cancer deaths (580,000) in 2013. (From Cancer Facts & Figures 2013. American Cancer Society Web site. http://www.cancer.org/research/cancerfactsfigures/cancerfactsfigures/cancer-facts-figures-2013.)

Radiotherapy

Approximately 50% of cancer patients will be treated with radiation therapy at some point during the course of their disease, and radiation may play a critical role in as many as 25% of cancer cures.[12] Despite the important beneficial effects of radiation in cancer care, its adverse effects on normal tissue are a major source of disability for both patients with active cancer and cancer survivors.[13] Evaluations and treatment of the long-term complications of radiation are extremely important components of the clinical activities of the cancer rehabilitation specialist and will be discussed in detail in the following paragraphs.

Surgery

Postsurgical impairments depend not only on the anatomic site and extent of the procedure, but also on any medical comorbidity the patient has. Surgical complications are common in the cancer setting and impact heavily on overall outcome as well as rehabilitation needs. Rehabilitation is often instrumental in returning function and quality of life to patients following surgery. Efforts may be directed at the restoration of functional disorders ranging from diminished stamina following prolonged bed rest to restoration of a limb following hemipelvectomy. The postsurgical rehabilitation needs of any given patient are unique.

Thromboembolism

There is considerable and high quality data available on the prevention and treatment of thromboembolism, including comprehensive guidelines specific to the cancer and rehabilitation settings.[14,15] There is comparatively little data concerning the safe and effective rehabilitation of patients with thromboembolism. The dogma from the not too distant past was to immobilize patients with deep vein thrombosis (DVT) and range of motion (ROM) exercises for anywhere from 2 to 10 days presumably to allow the clot to mature by the formation of fibrin cross-links and to thereby decrease the risk of dislodging the clot to form a pulmonary embolism (PE).[16] This commonly followed, long-held, and nonevidence-based recommendation was ultimately supported by a limited study suggesting that immobilization of the affected limb

for at least 48 to 72 hours while the patient is anticoagulated was justified and prudent to prevent PE.[17] Partsch[16] describes a survey of 31 international experts who gave the recommendation to immobilize patients for 4 to 5 days prior to intensifying physical activity. The development of low–molecular-weight heparin (LMWH) prompted a reevaluation of the bed rest recommendation as patients with acute DVT treated with LMWH injections at home did at least as well in terms of recurrent thromboembolism and bleeding as did patients treated in the hospital with unfractionated heparin delivered intravenously.[18,19] Although not directly applicable to patients in either the inpatient or outpatient rehabilitation setting, the realization that no increase in morbidity or mortality was seen in patients with acute DVT treated with LMWH injections served as justification for liberalization of the bed rest recommendation that had inhibited rehabilitation efforts, particularly on inpatient rehabilitation units.

Although the question of when a patient with lower extremity DVT can begin to ambulate has not been answered with the same evidence-based rigor as other questions concerning thromboembolism, there is a growing body of clinical trials on the topic that support the safety and potential benefits of early mobilization.[16,20–25] Several reviews and one meta-analysis are also available and support the safety and benefits of early mobilization following both DVT and PE while dispelling the recommendation for bed rest as part of the early management of thromboembolism.[16,26–31]

Upper extremity DVT (UEDVT) represents about 10% of DVTs and can be idiopathic but is more often associated with central venous catheter use, pacemakers, or cancer.[32] The relative incidence of UEDVT may be rising due to increased use of central venous catheters and is associated with PE in up to one-third of patients. Other conditions associated with UEDVT include postthrombotic syndrome, superior vena cava syndrome, septic thrombophlebitis, thoracic duct obstruction, and brachial plexopathy.[33] Despite the high incidence of conversion of UEDVT to PE, no studies are available to address the multitude of questions concerning the rehabilitation of patients with UEDVT. This lack of data concerns such basic issues as the safe timing and type of exercise that can be safely done following the diagnosis of UEDVT as well as if and when decongestive therapy (massage, wrapping, pumps) for upper extremity swelling disorders such as lymphedema can be performed. Lack of even basic data on these matters represents a major shortcoming in our overall knowledge on the topic of cancer rehabilitation and challenges our ability to guide risk–benefit analyses for patients with UEDVT who will likely benefit from physical therapy (PT), occupational therapy (OT), or decongestive therapy.

Although not strictly evidence based due to major shortcomings in the literature concerning the rehabilitation of patients with thromboembolism, the guidance developed by the author and used at the Memorial Sloan-Kettering Cancer Center (MSKCC) is presented in Table 152.1. It is critical to remember that each patient and situation is unique and that these recommendations are only starting points that should not supersede clinical judgment and assessment of the risks and benefits to the patient of engaging in a given activity.

Other Medical Disorders

The evidence base for the safe and effective rehabilitation of patients with a variety of general medical disorders is also limited. Despite this limitation, guidance with widespread clinical use has evolved on such issues as thrombocytopenia, anemia, neutropenia, cardiac dysfunction, pulmonary dysfunction, and electrolyte abnormalities. In general, these recommendations applied to rehabilitation are based on indirect evidence from the medical literature. Exercise precautions for cancer patients with a variety of disorders are presented in Table 152.2. Again, the potential risks and benefits of pursuing any course of therapy must be carefully weighed.

TABLE 152.1

Guidelines for Physical, Occupational, and Lymphedema Therapy in Patients with Venous Thromboembolism

■ Lower Extremities

1. For patients with acute lower extremity deep vein thrombosis (DVT), with or without pulmonary embolism (PE), and no inferior vena cava (IVC) filter, therapy (including physical, occupational, and lymphedema with bandaging and manual lymphatic drainage [MLD]) can be initiated once they are <u>therapeutic</u> on an anticoagulant. Resistive exercises should generally be deferred for 48–72 hours. Definition of therapeutic anticoagulation by modality:

   ■ Low–molecular-weight heparin (LMWH) preparations are preferred because they are therapeutic immediately following the first injection. Monitoring is not required. Common preparations include: enoxaparin (Lovenox), dalteparin (Fragmin), and tinzaparin (Innohep).

   ■ Unfractionated heparin may take 1–2 days to become therapeutic but patients on heparin are more prone to bleeding complications than with LMWH. The adjusted partial thromboplastin time (APTT) should be monitored and therapy can begin when it is between 50 and 70.

   ■ Warfarin (Coumadin) may take several days to become therapeutic. The International Normalized Ratio (INR) should be monitored and therapy can begin when it is between 2 and 3.

2. For patients with acute lower extremity DVT (with or without PE) and an IVC filter, therapy can be initiated <u>immediately</u> regardless of their anticoagulation status.

3. For patients with acute lower extremity DVT who cannot be anticoagulated and an IVC filter cannot be placed, therapy can be started immediately but should be <u>functional</u> in nature (ambulation, balance, ADL training) and avoid resistive and repetitive exercises. Such patients are at very high risk for PE and death. Therapists are advised to discuss therapy interventions with the patient's primary or rehabilitation medicine physician so that the relative risks and benefits of therapy can be better delineated.

■ Upper Extremities

1. Upper extremity DVT carries the same risk for PE and death as lower extremity DVT. IVC filters are not protective. For patients with acute upper extremity DVT with or without PE, therapy (including physical, occupational, and lymphedema with bandaging and MLD) can be initiated once they are <u>therapeutic</u> on an anticoagulant. Resistive exercises should generally be deferred for 48–72 hours. (See anticoagulation guidelines previously.)

2. For patients with acute upper extremity DVT who cannot be anticoagulated therapy should be <u>functional</u> in nature (ambulation, balance, ADL training) and should avoid resistive and repetitive exercises. Such patients are at very high risk for PE and death. Therapists are advised to discuss therapy interventions with the patient's primary or rehabilitation medicine physician so that the relative risks and benefits of therapy can be better delineated.

TABLE 152.2

Exercise Precautions for Cancer Patients

Medical Problem	Laboratory Values	Recommendations
Thrombocytopenia Normal values: platelets 150,000–450,000/m³	30,000–50,000/m³	ROM, aerobic activity, light weights (1–2 lb; no heavy resistance or isokinetic exercise); ambulation
	20,000–30,000/m³	Self-care, gentle passive/active ROM, aerobic activity, ambulation
	<20,000/m³	Ambulation and self-care with assistance as needed for safety; minimal/cautious activity; essential ADLs only
Anemia Normal values: hematocrit 37%–47%; hemoglobin 12–16 g/dL	Hematocrit <25%, hemoglobin <8 g/dL	ROM exercise, isometrics; avoid aerobic or progressive programs
	Hematocrit 25%–35%; hemoglobin 8–10 g/dL	Light aerobics, light weights (1–2 lb)
	Hematocrit >35%; hemoglobin >10 g/dL	Activity as tolerated
Neutropenia Normal values: ANC >1.500/mm³	ANC 500–1,000/mm³	Infection risk moderate; consider increased hygiene procedures and limited contact with other patients, particularly if further nadir anticipated
	ANC <500/mm³	Infection risk high; strict hygiene and limit contact with other persons
Pulmonary Dysfunction Pulmonary function tests, chest radiograph	Maintain pulse oximetry >90% 50%–75% of predicted FEV₁ or diffusion capacity	Titrate O₂ supplementation Light aerobic exercise
	75%+ of predicted FEV₁ or diffusion capacity	Most programs fine
	Large plural effusions or pericardial effusions or multiple metastases to lungs	ROM; few submaximal isometrics; consult cardiologist and oncologist
Cardiac Dysfunction Ejection fraction, electrocardiogram	Recent PVCs; fast atrial arrhythmia; ventricular arrhythmia; ischemic pattern	No aerobics; consult cardiologist
Electrolyte Abnormalities Na K⁺	Below 130 Below 3.0 or above 6.0 requires treatment	No exercise No exercise

ADLs, activities of daily living; ANC, absolute neutrophil count; FEV$_1$, forced expiratory volume in 1 second; PVCs, premature ventricular contractions.

NEUROMUSCULAR COMPLICATIONS OF CANCER AND CANCER TREATMENT

The treatment of neuromuscular complications of cancer is a major component of the services offered by both the rehabilitation medicine physician and the physical and occupational therapists. Such disorders include those of the brain, spinal cord, nerve roots, plexus, peripheral nerve, and muscle.[34]

Brain Dysfunction

The brain, along with the myriad cognitive and physical functions that it serves, is often compromised in the cancer setting. Such dysfunction can result from direct effects of the tumor, radiation, radiation necrosis, paraneoplastic effects, or other medical disorders.

Brain tumors vary widely in aggressiveness and prognosis. Even a benign or relatively low-grade lesion may have severe functional consequences depending on its location. It is unclear to what extent tumor type or location impacts rehabilitation prognosis; however, some studies suggest a tendency for better gains in meningioma patients and in those with left hemispheric lesions.[35,36]

The most common neurologic deficits in brain tumor patients undergoing acute rehabilitation include impaired cognition (80%), weakness (78%), and visual–perceptual impairment (53%) with most patients having multiple impairments.[37] Although overall prognosis may be a factor, most rehabilitation disposition decisions are guided by the patient's neurologic status, clinical course, and activity tolerance. A patient whose neurologic status is actively worsening will likely not benefit from intensive rehabilitation.

Specific rehabilitation interventions depend on the combination of deficits and are generally similar to measures used for patients with other etiologies of brain disorders, such as traumatic brain injury or stroke. Rehabilitation efforts are directed toward such goals as the improvement of bed mobility, transfers, self-care, ambulation, and if necessary, wheelchair training. Strategies are employed to promote functional cognition, clear communication, bowel and bladder continence, safe swallowing, adequate nutritional intake, optimal sensory input (including vision and hearing), and restorative sleep. Attention must be paid to the prevention of complications of impaired mobility such as skin breakdown or DVT. Similarly, complications related to the primary tumor and other comorbidities such as pain, neurologic decline, seizure, and depression should be evaluated and treated. The hemiplegic patient will generally benefit from gait training with an assistive device and a brace such as an ankle–foot orthosis (AFO) when appropriate. Proper arm positioning, with support of the shoulder to prevent pain in a flaccid or spastic limb, should be used. A variety of adaptive equipment are available for individuals who must perform tasks one handed, such as reachers, sock donners, and elastic shoelaces.

Cognitive strategies often rely on compensations such as keeping a regular routine and maintaining a journal or *memory notebook*. The patient's insight into cognitive deficits may be impaired, and education regarding these deficits can allow the patient to more effectively compensate and allow family, friends, and caregivers to have appropriate expectations. In some cases, especially those in which cognitive status is anticipated to remain fairly stable, in which functional expectations are high, or where conflict or confusion exists about the patient's abilities, neuropsychological testing helps to more fully define the extent of cognitive deficits and also to elucidate cognitive strengths. For example, determining whether an individual learns best with auditory, written, or nonverbal presentations can facilitate the most efficient compensation for cognitive deficits. Pharmacologic and nonpharmacologic therapies to address pain, spasticity, mood, bowel/bladder, and sleep/wake issues are often indicated.

Functional recovery is similar in patients with brain tumors as compared with acute stroke.[38] Better functional improvement is a significant predictor of longer survival in patients with brain metastases and glioblastoma multiforme (GBM). The literature suggests that the length of stay for inpatient rehabilitation for brain tumor patients is generally shorter than patients with other brain disorders such as traumatic brain injury and stroke.[35,36] This may relate to better initial functional status; other possible contributing factors include fewer behavioral sequelae, better social supports, and expedited discharge planning due to prognostic factors.[39] In one study, although functional status improved during rehabilitation, quality-of-life scores did not improve until the discharge home. The functional independence measure (FIM) and the disability rating scale are more sensitive than the Karnofsky performance status scale in detecting changes in functional status.[40]

Spinal Cord Dysfunction

Symptomatic spinal cord injury (SCI) due to spinal metastasis occurs in up to 5% of all cancer patients.[41] Patients with cancer can develop SCI as a direct result of their cancer, its treatment (e.g., radiation), and other preexisting or acquired conditions. SCI in the cancer setting can present a significant decision-making and management challenge.[42] This challenge is compounded as cancer-related SCI most often occurs as a late complication when poor overall prognosis and declining medical status can significantly and adversely impact rehabilitation interventions and functional prognosis.

Life expectancy following spinal surgery varies with cancer type. One study demonstrated a median survival of 7.7 months for all cancer types combined, with colon cancer patients surviving only 3.3 months and lung cancer patients only 3.6 months. Sarcoma, prostate, renal cell, and breast carcinoma did better, with median survival ranging from 7.8 to 15.4 months.[43] A retrospective evaluation of patients with neoplastic SCI admitted for inpatient rehabilitation demonstrated a combined median overall survival time of only 4.1 months from the date of rehabilitation admission to death. Patients with gastrointestinal cancer had an even poorer prognosis with a median survival of only 0.6 months.[44] The phase of cancer treatment can have a profound impact on survival and prognosis for functional recovery. A patient with metastatic prostate or breast cancer, for instance, whose initial presentation is with SCI and has not received systemic therapy, can be expected to have a much better prognosis for survival and functional restoration than a patient who has undergone and failed multiple treatment options.

SCI in the cancer setting can result directly from the cancer (epidural, leptomeningeal, or intramedullary tumor; Fig. 152.2), indirectly from the cancer (paraneoplastic phenomenon), or from treatment of the cancer (radiation, chemotherapy, surgery). Other causes of SCI in the cancer setting may include infection (meningitis, epidural abscess, discitis/osteomyelitis), vascular disorders (hemorrhage, infarct), degenerative disorders (cervical spinal stenosis), and even metabolic disorders (osteoporotic compression fractures).

The vertebral body is the most common site of metastasis within the spine, largely reflecting its volume relative to other spinal structures. Metastatic tumors of the spine are more common than primary spine tumors. Cancers that commonly metastasize to the spine are those of the breast, lungs, prostate, and kidneys.[45] Epidural tumors are the most common cause of SCI in cancer and can arise from the vertebra, enter the spinal canal through the neural foramen or be deposited hematogenously in the epidural space. Leptomeningeal metastases occur in 3% to 8% of all cancer patients and can be associated with significant neurologic dysfunction. The most common tumors that metastasize to the leptomeninges include leukemia, lymphoma, melanoma, and breast and lung cancers.[46] Intramedullary tumors are the rarest of the tumors that affect the CNS but can produce profound neurologic deficits that vary depending on the location and pathology of the tumor.

SCI from epidural-based tumors generally affects all spinal tracts either completely or to varying degrees. Asymmetric compression does occur and can have unpredictable patterns in early

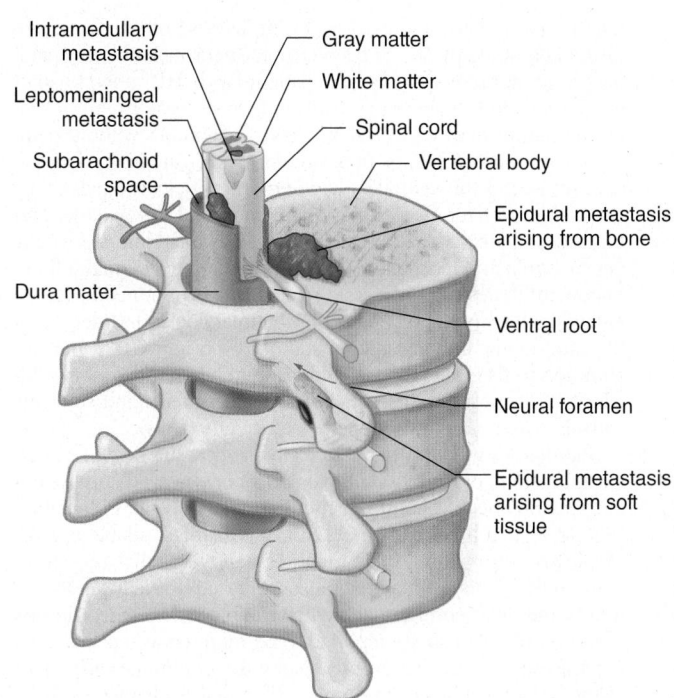

Figure 152.2 The spinal cord and nerve roots can be affected by metastatic or primary tumors arising from epidural, intramedullary, or leptomeningeal spaces.

compression but generally progresses to affect all components of the spinal cord. Clinically, such patients present with weakness, bowel and bladder dysfunction, and multimodal sensory loss including light touch, pain, vibration, and proprioception. Pain, if present, is usually local.

The level of injury significantly affects the potential for functional recovery. It should be noted that the degree of functional recovery anticipated in a patient with a nonmalignant cause of SCI (such as trauma from a motor vehicle accident) is generally greater than that anticipated in malignant SCI. This is because patients with cancer tend to develop SCI later in their disease and usually progress in their cancer and other medical comorbidities.

The care of patients with acute SCI includes the maintenance of ventilation in those with high levels of injury. It also includes the treatment of pain, autonomic dysregulation, and bowel and bladder dysfunction. Patients are at risk of developing DVT, PE, pulmonary and urinary tract infections, fecal impaction, decubiti, immobilization hypocalcemia, spasticity, contractures, and osteoporosis. A comprehensive treatment plan includes DVT and PE prophylaxis, spirometry, and chest physiotherapy; the initiation of intermittent urinary catheterization every 4 to 6 hours when urine volumes are less than 2,000 mL per day; the initiation of a bowel program; turning every 2 hours; and use of high-airflow mattresses, use of heel protectors, and daily PT and ROM.[15,47]

The use of LMWH is currently recommended for DVT and PE prophylaxis during the acute management phase of SCI.[15] The independent use of low-dose unfractionated heparin, elastic compression stockings, and intermittent pneumatic compression devices is not recommended. When used alone, they appear to be relatively ineffective. It is recommended that LMWH be continued or converted to full-dose oral anticoagulation for a minimum of 3 months or at least until completion of the rehabilitation phase.[48]

Patients with injuries above the T6 level are at risk of developing autonomic dysreflexia, which is defined as an increase in blood pressure of greater than 20 mm Hg above baseline. It results from stimulation of the splanchnic division of the sympathetic nervous system by a noxious stimulus below the level of the lesion and causes the sympathetic responses of vasoconstriction and hypertension. Autonomic dysreflexia constitutes a medical emergency and must be evaluated and treated immediately.

The patient's ability to participate in rehabilitation therapies while undergoing further treatments must be considered when an acute or subacute inpatient rehabilitation program is sought. Rehabilitation programs for those with SCI due to spinal tumors have been shown to improve mobility and self-care.[49] Research indicates that clinical and functional status is a valuable prognostic factor for survival of those with SCI due to metastatic tumor disease.[50] The rehabilitation program should be started as early as possible and should be of short duration.[44] Thus, the selection of patients who have the potential to improve function may improve survivability as well as quality of life and ability to perform activities of daily living (ADL) and mobility.

Peripheral Nervous System Dysfunction

Radiculopathy can result from a variety of disorders that affect one or more nerve roots and is a very common cause of pain and disability in the cancer setting. Radiculopathy can occur from compressive or less common noncompressive etiologies. Although the incidence of radiculopathy in cancer patients and survivors is unknown, it is likely that most nerve root pathology results from the same degenerative disorders, largely spondyloarthropathies, that affect the general population with a prevalence of 3% to 5%.[51] One large study on the epidemiology of cervical radiculopathy in a population of patients in Rochester, Minnesota placed the average annual age-adjusted incidence at 83.2 per 100,000.[52] Degenerative causes of radiculopathy can be discogenic (e.g., herniated nucleus pulposus), from hypertrophy of ligaments and other soft tissues (e.g., ligamentum flavum), or from excess bone formation (e.g., osteoarthritis). The narrowing of the spinal canal or neural foramen with subsequent compression of neural and vascular structures resulting from one or more degenerative processes is called spinal stenosis. Lumbar spinal stenosis is estimated to affect 1 in 1,000 persons older than 65 years of age.[53]

Compressive radiculopathy resulting directly from cancer most commonly results from an epidural tumor that can arise from the vertebral body, paravertebral structures, or the epidural space itself.[54] Intramedullary tumors, including leptomeningeal and intramedullary disease, can also cause compressive radiculopathy. Of these, compression by leptomeningeal disease is far more common affecting 5% to 8% of patients with cancer.[54]

Noncompressive causes of radiculopathy include radiation, chemotherapy, and paraneoplastic syndromes as well as disorders such as acute idiopathic demyelinating polyradiculoneuropathy (AIDP), a subtype of Guillain-Barré syndrome (GBS), chronic idiopathic demyelinating polyradiculoneuropathy (CIDP), amyloidosis, sarcoidosis, diabetes mellitus, and rheumatologic disorders (Fig. 152.3).[1] *Herpes zoster* is also a common cause of radiculopathy in the cancer setting causing a dermatomal vesicular rash known as shingles.[55] *Herpes zoster* causing dermatomal pain without a rash is termed zoster sine herpete.[56] An eruption of *Herpes zoster* is related to immunosuppression from cancer, steroids, and chemotherapy with 1% to 2% of cancer patients having at least one infection during the course of their disease.[57] Polyradiculopathy from radiation may mimic a leptomeningeal tumor because the cauda equina may demonstrate enhancement on magnetic resonance imaging (MRI; see Fig. 152.3).[58] Although relatively uncommon, radiculopathy from radiation has been reported as sequelae of testicular cancer, vertebral metastases, and lymphoma.[59–64] In the author's clinical experience, radiation-induced radiculopathy is most commonly seen in Hodgkin lymphoma (HL) survivors who have received mantle field (MF) or periaortic radiation and head and neck cancer patients often in conjunction with plexopathy. Additionally, in rare instances, radiculoplexopathy can result from single fraction (2,400 cGy) radiation. Neurotoxic chemotherapy can also adversely affect the nerve root as part of a more generalized neuropathy. Patients with preexisting radiculopathy from a degenerative or other cause

may be particularly predisposed to the adverse effects of neurotoxic chemotherapy.[65,66] Subacute motor neuronopathy is a paraneoplastic disorder described in patients with HL, non-Hodgkin lymphoma, and thymoma as a subacute lower motor neuron syndrome that primarily involves the lower extremities without pain, significant sensory loss, or upper motor neuron findings. Secondary thinning of the ventral nerve roots and widespread patch segmental demyelination of spinal nerve roots and the brachial and lumbosacral plexus can be seen histologically in addition to patchy degeneration and loss of anterior horn cells and occasional inflammatory infiltrates.[67] Non–cancer-related causes of noncompressive radiculopathy including diabetes, rheumatologic disorders, and idiopathic radiculoneuropathies such as GBS and CIDP not uncommon in the general population should be included in the differential diagnosis when evaluating cancer patients and survivors with signs and symptoms suggestive of radiculopathy.

Plexopathy affects as many as 1% of cancer patients.[68] The cervical, brachial, or lumbosacral plexus can be involved and the etiology can be neoplastic or radiation induced as well as idiopathic (idiopathic brachial neuritis, CIDP, GBS), diabetic (diabetic radiculoplexus neuropathy), or traumatic (surgery). Malignancy most commonly affects the brachial plexus followed by the lumbosacral plexus and, least commonly, the cervical plexus.[69] Benign tumors of the plexus are usually reported to be more common than malignant ones.[70–72] Radiation plexopathy is a common component of the radiation fibrosis syndrome (RFS) that is characterized by

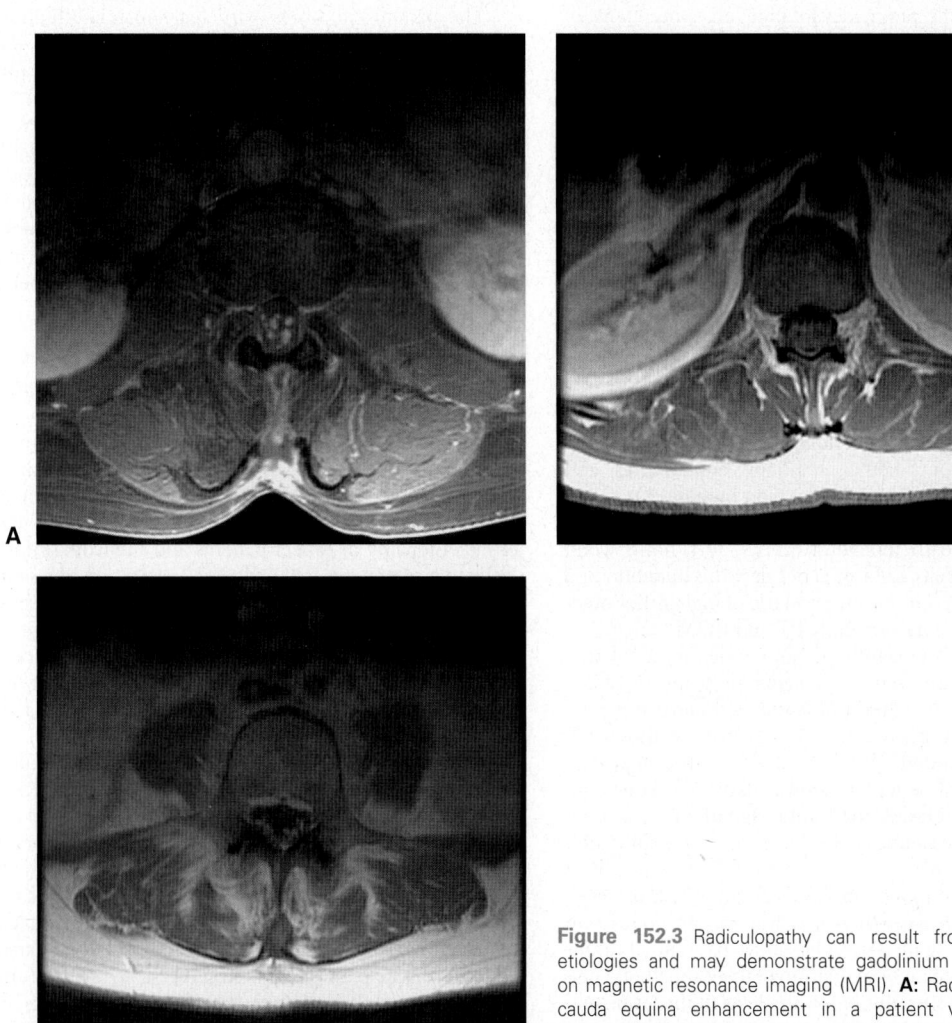

Figure 152.3 Radiculopathy can result from variety of etiologies and may demonstrate gadolinium enhancement on magnetic resonance imaging (MRI). **A:** Radiation-induced cauda equina enhancement in a patient with testicular cancer. **B:** Cauda equina enhancement from Waldenstrom macroglobulinemia. **C:** Cauda equina enhancement from leptomeningeal metastases in a patient with breast cancer.

insidious fibrosis with axonal demyelination and, ultimately, axonal loss. Radiation plexopathy is commonly seen with radiculopathy. Radiation to the plexus can rarely cause a mild reversible syndrome but is more commonly a delayed and progressive one.[73] The risk of brachial plexopathy in the adjuvant breast cancer setting is <1% when the dose per fraction is 2 Gy and the total dose is 50 Gy or the dose per fraction is 2.2 Gy to 2.5 Gy and the total dose is 34 Gy to 40 Gy. However, if the dose per fraction is 2.2 Gy to 4.58 Gy and the total dose is 43.5 Gy to 60 Gy, the brachial plexopathy risk increases to 1.7% to 73%.[74] Delayed radiation-induced brachial plexopathy usually occurs after a latent interval that can vary from a few months to several years with a peak onset of neurologic symptoms occurring between 2 and 4 years after radiation.[75] The upper plexus is commonly affected preferentially in HL survivors treated with MF radiation and head and neck cancer patients possibly due to the longer course of the upper trunk and lateral cord of the brachial plexus through the neck as well as the pyramidal shape of the thorax providing less protective tissue. Additionally, the upper plexus may represent the most caudal extent of radiation delivered for some head and neck cancer patients.

Differentiating radiation induced from malignant plexopathy is a diagnostic challenge and both etiologies may be present together. Imaging with gadolinium-enhanced MRI is the diagnostic test of choice when excluding a tumor of the brachial plexus.[76] Positron-emission tomography/computed tomography (PET-CT) has a role to play in selected cases. Malignant etiologies of plexopathy are generally more painful than radiation-induced plexopathy, although either can manifest severe pain.[77] Myokymia on needle electromyography is suggestive of a radiation-induced etiology but does not exclude a malignant component.[78]

Idiopathic brachial neuritis (IBN), also known as neuralgic amyotrophy, Parsonage-Turner syndrome, and other synonyms, have an incidence of approximately 2 to 3 per 100,000 person-years.[79] The disorder can be idiopathic or hereditary. The idiopathic form is often precipitated by antecedent events such as infection, immunization, strenuous exercise, surgery, and a variety of other causes.[79] Clinically, IBN is classically characterized by severe and acute burning pain in the shoulder and arm that may last for several days or weeks and is followed by muscle weakness, atrophy, and sensory loss. IBN may go unrecognized in cancer patients if only the obvious cancer and treatment-related causes of brachial plexopathy are considered. Similarly, diabetic radiculoplexus neuropathies can affect the cervical, thoracic, and lumbosacral nerve roots as well as the brachial and lumbosacral plexus. Perhaps the best known of these disorders is diabetic lumbosacral radiculoplexus neuropathy (DLRPN), also known as diabetic amyotrophy among other synonyms. DLRPN usually presents clinically with unilateral acute to subacute and severe lower extremity pain in the thigh or leg that may spread to the entire extremity.[80] Like IBN, DLRPN may go unrecognized in the cancer setting if only neoplastic or treatment-related etiologies are considered and can occur even with relatively low blood glucose levels as might be seen with steroid-induced hyperglycemia.

Neuropathy is any condition arising from the damage and dysfunction of the peripheral nerves including the motor, sensory, and autonomic nerves that connect the CNS (brain and spinal cord) to the rest of the body.[81] The peripheral nerve includes the nerve root and plexus as well as the peripheral nerve proper. Peripheral neuropathy is common in the cancer setting as a result of neurotoxic chemotherapy or radiation as well as from direct and paraneoplastic effects of cancer. Neuropathy is also very common in the general population with diverse etiologies that can affect cancer patients even if unrelated to malignancy or its treatment. Such etiologies include toxic or metabolic derangements (diabetes mellitus, vitamin B-12 deficiency, alcoholism), inherited disorders (Charcot-Marie-Tooth), paraprotein disorders (monoclonal gammopathy of unknown significance [MGUS]), critical illness neuropathy, and idiopathic disorders such as CIDP or GBS just to name a few.[82] The clinical manifestations of neuropathy may

include any combination of weakness, sensory deficits, pain, and autonomic dysfunction with resultant gait and other functional deficits. Often, multiple peripheral nervous system disorders such as radiculopathy and neuropathy coexist, compounding the clinical features of each disorder. It is important to remember that, as described previously, any preexisting pathology at any part of the neuron (nerve root, plexus, or peripheral nerve), even if asymptomatic, may predispose the patient to the development of weakness, paresthesias, pain, and other signs and symptoms commonly described as *neuropathy* when challenged with a neurotoxic chemotherapy or another insult to the peripheral nervous system. This phenomenon is termed *neuronal predisposition*.[65,66]

Peripheral neuropathy is one of the most common chronic complications of cancer and its treatment. It may be caused by a variety of chemotherapeutic agents including the taxanes (paclitaxel, docetaxel), the vinca alkaloids (vincristine, vinorelbine, vinblastine), the platinum analogs (cisplatin, carboplatin, oxaliplatin), bortezomib, thalidomide, and others.[65,83–85] The clinical, pathophysiologic, and electrodiagnostic features of the various neurotoxic chemotherapeutics vary significantly. The taxanes and vinca alkaloids are tubulin inhibitors and cause a predominately length-dependent motor and sensory axonal polyneuropathy in a distal symmetric distribution.[83] Clinically, this causes paresthesias, pain, sensory ataxia, and potentially, weakness during and immediately following treatment that usually improves when the treatment is stopped. The platinum analogs, however, damage the cell body of the sensory nerves in the dorsal root ganglion, and at higher doses can damage the anterior horn cell within the spinal cord. It is the accumulation of the platinum analogs within the neuron cell body with subsequent DNA damage and altered cellular activities that underlie the toxicity.[86] The clinical manifestations include severe sensory deficits including sensory ataxia and pain usually without significant weakness. Because the platinum analogs accumulate in the cell body, the deficits can progress for months following treatment, a phenomenon known as *coasting*. Electrophysiologically, neuropathy due to platinum analogs, may demonstrate a widespread decrease in sensory nerve action potential (SNAP) amplitudes *without* a proximal to distal gradient. In such cases of non–length-dependent neuropathy, it is possible to see an electrophysiologic pattern wherein the SNAP amplitudes in the upper extremities (shorter nerves) are lower than those in the lower extremity nerves (longer nerves).[87] This pattern is useful not only in differentiating non–length-dependent from length-dependent neuropathies associated with tubulin inhibitors, but also from other causes of peripheral nervous system dysfunction likely to be encountered in the oncology setting including radiculopathy, chronic idiopathic demyelinating polyradiculopathy, and diabetic neuropathy.

The need for an evaluation of neuropathy is largely dependent on the context in which a patient develops neuropathic signs and symptoms. If a patient develops the expected signs and symptoms from chemotherapy or other treatment that is expected to produce those symptoms, then no further investigation is generally indicated. It is when a patient develops signs and/or symptoms that exceed what is generally anticipated, or at a time when they would not have been expected to have complications of treatment that a work-up is indicated. For instance, a patient with metastatic prostate cancer who develops lower extremity pain and weakness on hormonal therapy needs an evaluation as opposed to one who develops the same symptoms on paclitaxel. In the former case, it is prudent to consider a very broad differential diagnosis and eliminate possibilities systematically and logically because many of the causes of such symptoms are curable or highly treatable. Oncologic causes such as epidural spinal cord compression, leptomeningeal metastases, intramedullary metastases, and paraneoplastic disorders should be considered along with degenerative causes of lower extremity pain and weakness such as spinal stenosis, disk herniation, facet arthropathy, and compression fracture. Similarly, idiopathic and acquired causes of neuropathy should be considered including disorders such as diabetic amyotrophy, vitamin B-12 deficiency, Lyme disease, alcoholism, paraprotein neuropathies (MGUS), and CIDP. As with the nerve root and plexus, radiation can cause damage to any peripheral nerve in the radiation field. Such damage is usually obvious when it affects one or more named nerves in an extremity but may be less obvious when it affects nerves on the trunk such as the dorsal scapular nerve to the rhomboid muscles or the supraspinatus nerve to the supra and infraspinatus muscles. These nerves are commonly affected by MF radiation and radiation for head and neck cancer. Radiculopathy mimicking peripheral neuropathy is an extremely common cause of lower extremity symptoms in cancer patients due to their often advanced age and predisposition to spinal degenerative disease. Acquired neuropathy, including MGUS and CIDP, are also relatively common and should be considered in the evaluation of patients with idiopathic neuropathies.[82,88]

A prospective neuropathy assessment algorithm intended to be used before and during the administration of neurotoxic chemotherapy in breast cancer patients is presented in Figure 152.4.[66] Although intended for breast cancer patients, this algorithm, including the evaluation and assessment outlined, is widely applicable.

Myopathy

Myopathy in the cancer setting can occur as a result of a variety of processes including direct invasion by a primary or metastatic tumor, paraneoplastic disorders, inflammatory disorders (polymyositis, dermatomyositis, inclusion body myositis), infiltrative disorders (amyloid), toxins, or more commonly as a result of corticosteroid use or critical illness. Radiation can cause a focal nemaline rod myopathy.[89] Skeletal muscle metastases are relatively rare but can occur from a variety of tumor types including lung, breast, melanoma, thyroid, and liver.[90] Paraneoplastic necrotizing myopathy characterized by rapidly progressive proximal muscle weakness that occurs over months can be seen in association with breast, small cell lung, gastrointestinal, genitourinary, bladder, ovarian, and prostate carcinomas as well as melanoma, multiple myeloma, and head and neck cancer.[91] Each of the inflammatory myopathies has a distinct clinical phenotype and unique myopathologic features.[92] Amyloid myopathy is rare but can be seen as a complication of multiple myeloma or primary amyloidosis.[93,94] Vincristine, alcohol, and a variety of other agents can cause a toxic myopathy.[95]

By far, the most common therapy-induced myopathy is steroid myopathy from glucocorticoid use. Steroid-induced myopathy is

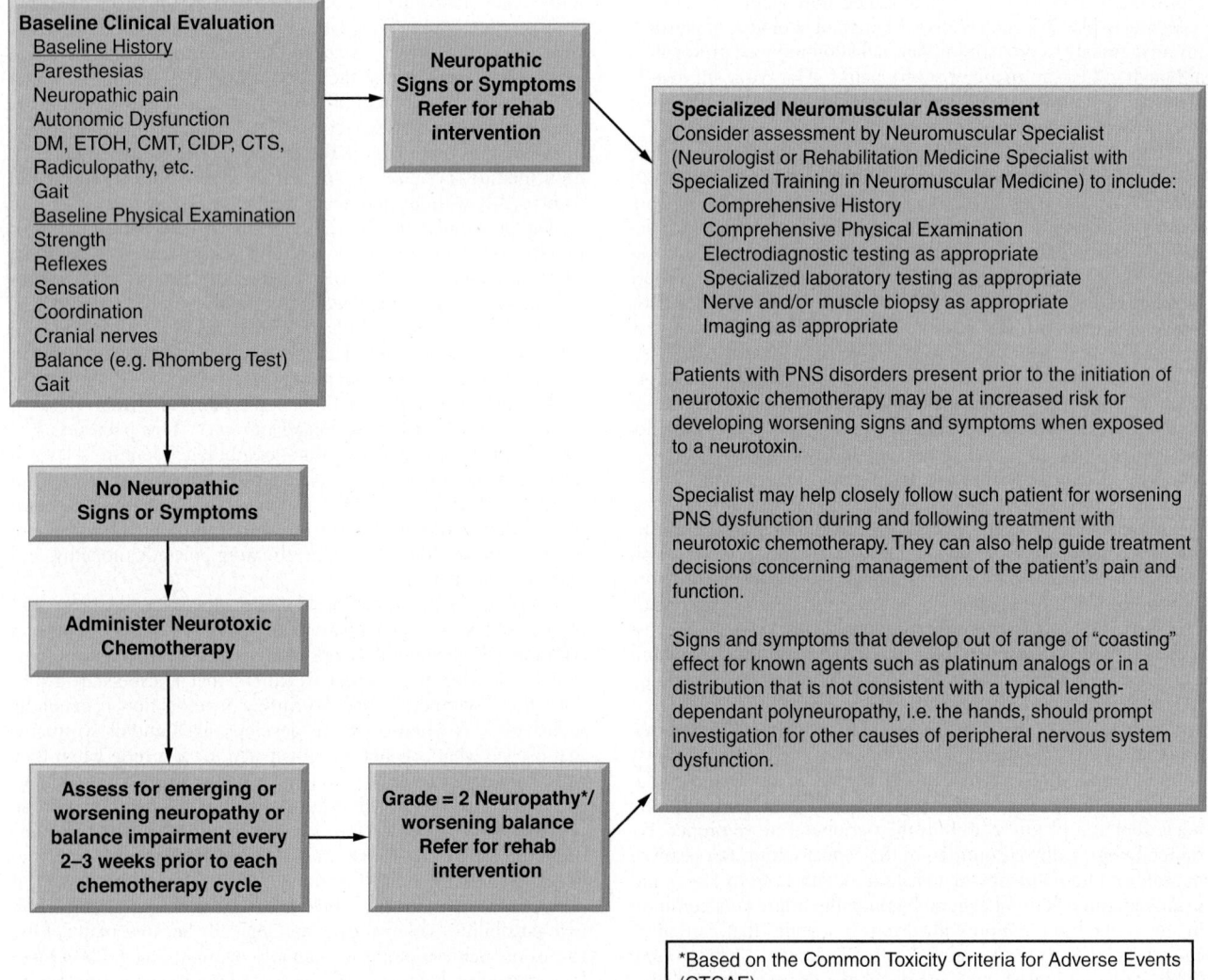

Figure 152.4 A neuropathy assessment algorithm intended to be used before and during the administration of neurotoxic chemotherapy in patients with breast cancer. This algorithm is likely useful for other cancer types as well. DM, diabetes mellitus; ETOH, alcohol abuse; CMT, Charcot-Marie-Tooth disease; CTS, carpal tunnel syndrome. (Adapted Stubblefield MD, McNeely ML, Alfano CM, Mayer DK. A prospective surveillance model for physical rehabilitation of women with breast cancer: chemotherapy-induced peripheral neuropathy. *Cancer* 2012;118:2250–2260.

characterized by fast-twitch or type II muscle fiber atrophy with decreased fiber cross-sectional areas and reduced myofibrillar protein content.[96] Steroid use is associated with a variety of adverse side effects that are related to the total and daily dose, duration of therapy, and poorly understood patient susceptibility factors.[97] In one small prospective study, glucocorticoid use was found to contribute to proximal muscle weakness in 9 out of 15 (60%) patients and was severe enough to interfere with ADLs in 6 out of 15 (40%) treated patients.[98] The development of steroid myopathy was rapid, occurring within 15 days in 8 out of 9 patients who developed weakness. Of 16 patients, 10 (63%) also demonstrated a significant decline in respiratory function. Steroid myopathy is painless and usually demonstrates proximal weakness most evident on physical examination to affect the shoulder and hip girdle muscles with relative preservation of distal muscle strength. This pattern of weakness helps differentiate steroid myopathy from most types of neuropathy, which cause distal relative to proximal weakness. In addition, sensation and reflexes should be preserved in steroid myopathy but which is abnormal in neuropathy. Although most cases of steroid myopathy are mild to moderate, at its extreme measure, it can cause complete tetraplegia and respirator dependence. Most patients with steroid myopathy recover, some completely; however, the course of resolution can be on the order of months to years.

Critical illness myopathy is not unique to the cancer setting, but due to the nature of cancer, is commonly seen. Critical illness myopathy is often associated with critical illness polyneuropathy. Often, the first sign of these disorders is difficulty in weaning a patient from a ventilator that is not explained by pulmonary, cardiovascular, or another disorder.[99] The clinical features and time course for resolution of critical illness myopathy are similar to those of steroid myopathy.

Evaluation of Neuromuscular Disorders

The key components of neuromuscular evaluation are history and physical examination. The etiology of most disorders can be elucidated with accuracy and specificity by a skilled clinician in the majority of instances, even in the cancer setting. Additional evaluations with imaging and electrodiagnostic and laboratory testing is indicated when competing diagnoses are being considered and require exclusion. Imaging is extremely useful to exclude a tumor as a source of nerve compression, particularly of the spinal cord and nerve root. Although a variety of tests have utility in select situations, magnetic resonance imaging (MRI) is usually the modality of choice for imaging the central and peripheral nervous systems.[100,101] Intravenous gadolinium is useful in the identification of peripheral nerve and plexus tumors, leptomeningeal disease, and intramedullary spinal cord tumors as well as to differentiate scar from tumor, exclude infection, and identify radiation changes.[46,102] Nerve roots may enhance with gadolinium in AIDP and CIDP as well as radiation-induced radiculopathy (see Fig. 152.3).[59–64,82] Electrodiagnostic testing is often extremely useful in clarifying the etiology of symptoms (radiculopathy versus plexopathy versus neuropathy versus myopathy), clarifying the type of neuropathy (i.e., axonal versus. demyelinating, polyneuropathy versus mononeuropathy multiplex versus mononeuropathy), localizing a lesion (i.e. femoral mononeuropathy at the inguinal ligament versus intrapelvic). Electrodiagnostic testing can also assist in chemotherapeutic or radiotherapeutic decision making, predict neurologic prognosis, and exclude disorders in the differential diagnosis. Specialized expertise is useful in the electrophysiologic assessment of cancer patients.[81] Laboratory testing is often indicated in the evaluation of peripheral nervous system dysfunction, particularly neuropathy. Such tests may include complete blood count, erythrocyte sedimentation rate or C-reactive protein, vitamin B-12, folate (methylmalonic acid with or without homocysteine for low

normal vitamin B-12 levels), a comprehensive metabolic panel (fasting blood glucose, renal and liver function), thyroid function tests, serum protein immunofixation electrophoresis, glucose tolerance test if indicated to evaluate for impaired glucose tolerance, and urine protein electrophoresis with immunofixation.[103] Specialized laboratory investigations may also be indicated depending on other clinical features exhibited or expressed by the patient. Evaluations may include but are not limited to those for connective tissue diseases with vasculitis (antinuclear antigen profile, rheumatoid factor, anti-Ro/SSA, anti-La/SSB, antineutrophil cytoplasmic antigen antibody, cryoglobulins), infections (hepatitis B and C, HIV, cytomegalovirus), sarcoidosis (serum angiotensin converting enzyme), dysimmune disorders (antiganglioside antibody profile [GM1, GDla, GDlb, GD3, GQ1b GT1b, antimyelin-associated glycoprotein]), and a paraneoplastic panel (anti-Hu, anti-CV2).[103]

Treatment of Neuromuscular Disorders

The treatment of peripheral nervous system disorders can be highly specific (e.g., injection of a median mononeuropathy at the wrist) or extremely general (e.g., prescription of opioids for pain). The most common impairments experienced by patients with peripheral nervous system dysfunction include pain and weakness with subsequent disorders of mobility and ADLs. Skin breakdown, secondary musculoskeletal derangements (i.e., Charcot joint, rotator cuff tendonitis/adhesive capsulitis), contracture, osteoporosis, and other conditions can also result. Dysfunction of the peripheral components of the autonomic nervous system can cause orthostatic hypotension, gastroparesis, constipation, urinary retention, erectile difficulties, and a variety of other autonomic derangements.

Specific treatments depend largely on accuracy of diagnosis of the underlying disorder. For instance, severe and disabling hand pain may be from a CNS cause (thalamic or funicular pain), radiculopathy, plexopathy, a polyneuropathy, or a mononeuropathy such as the median mononeuropathy responsible for carpel tunnel syndrome. In addition to neuromuscular causes of pain, a variety of musculoskeletal disorders such as osteoarthritis and tenosynovitis, as well as infections and neoplasms, should be considered in the differential diagnosis because they can coexist with or mimic neuromuscular dysfunction.

A primary responsibility of the cancer rehabilitation physician is to be a diagnostician. An accurate diagnosis of pain and functional disorders is often instrumental in guiding oncologic colleagues on such matters as whether to continue neurotoxic chemotherapy or if a lesion requires chemotherapy. For instance, the treatment of hand pain that is due to carpel tunnel syndrome is very different from the treatment offered for a metastasis to the brachial plexus. A guide to the expected physical examination findings (pain/sensory abnormalities, weakness pattern, reflex abnormalities) anticipated from the various common central and peripheral nervous system abnormalities are listed in Table 152.3. A full accounting of the specific treatments for each of these disorders is beyond the scope of this chapter due to space limitations.

A comprehensive discussion on the management of neuropathic pain is discussed elsewhere in this textbook. Again, the first step in the effective treatment of neuropathic pain is its identification. Treatments may include behavior modification, PT and/or OT, modalities such as transcutaneous electric nerve stimulation (TENS) or ultrasound, splints and braces, injections, and other procedures and medications. Weakness and difficulties with ADLs can often be improved with PT and/or OT. Bracing may be required to compensate for weakness such as foot dorsiflexors where an AFO is often indicated. Discussions on nonpharmacologic pain management and orthotic use are presented in the following section.

PALLIATIVE AND ALTERNATIVE CARE

TABLE 152.3

Physical Examination Findings in Painful Neurologic Disorders

Location	Pain/Sensory Abnormalities	Weakness Distribution	Reflex Abnormality
Brain			
Thalamus	Contralateral to lesion, varies from discrete (i.e., arm only) to entire side of body	None (unless other structures involved)	None (unless other structures involved)
Spinal Cord			
Ascending spinothalamic tracts	Contralateral if small lesion or bilateral if larger lesion, varies from discrete (i.e., arm only) to entire side of body	None (unless other structures involved)	None (unless other structures involved)
Root			
C-5	Posterior–lateral shoulder, lateral arm, lateral forearm	Rotator cuff, shoulder abduction > elbow flexion	Biceps tendon > brachioradialis tendon
C-6	Posterior–lateral shoulder, lateral arm, lateral forearm, thumb, index finger	Rotator cuff, shoulder abduction < elbow flexion, forearm pronation, wrist extension	Biceps tendon < brachioradialis tendon, pronator teres tendon
C-7	Posterior arm, posterior forearm, index/middle fingers	Elbow extension, wrist extension, finger extension	Triceps tendon
C-8	Posterior–medial arm, posterior–medial forearm, little/ring fingers	Long finger extensors, long finger flexors > hand intrinsics	Finger flexors
T-1	Anterior–medial arm, anterior–medial forearm (little/ring fingers generally spared)	Long finger extensors, long finger flexors < hand intrinsics	Finger flexors
T-2 to T-12	Corresponding thoracic dermatome (i.e., T4 nipples, T10 navel)	Corresponding thoracic myotome (rarely clinically evident)	None
L-1	Upper low back, lateral hip, groin	None	None
L-2	Upper/middle low back, lateral hip, groin, high anterior and medial thigh	Hip flexion > knee extension	Patellar tendon
L-3	Middle low back, lateral hip, middle anterior and medial thigh	Hip flexion < knee extension, hip adduction	Patellar tendon
L-4	Middle/low back, lateral hip, lateral thigh, knee, medial leg	Knee extension > ankle dorsiflexion	Patellar tendon
L-5	Low back, buttock, lateral hip, posterior/lateral thigh, lateral leg, dorsal foot, big toe	Hip abduction, knee flexion, ankle and toe dorsiflexion, foot inversion and eversion	Medial hamstring tendon
S-1	Low back, buttock, lateral hip, posterior thigh, posterior leg, lateral and plantar foot	Hip extension, knee flexion, plantar flexion, toe flexion	Achilles tendon, lateral hamstring tendon
S-2 to S-5	Posterior leg (S2), saddle anesthesia	None	None
Cauda equina syndrome	Varies, all lumbar roots possible, saddle anesthesia common	Varies, all lumbar roots possible	Varies, all lumbar roots possible
Conus medullaris	Varies, all lumbar roots possible, loss of bladder function common	Varies, all lumbar roots possible	Varies, all lumbar roots possible
Plexus			
Cervical	Anterior neck, ear lateral occiput, upper chest, and upper back	None	None
Upper trunk brachial	Shoulder, lateral arm, lateral forearm, lateral hand	Rotator cuff, shoulder abduction, elbow flexion, radial wrist extension (rhomboid and serratus anterior spared)	Biceps tendon, brachioradialis tendon
Middle trunk brachial	Posterior arm and hand	Elbow extension (partial), wrist extension, finger extension (brachioradialis spared)	Triceps tendon

(continued)

TABLE 152.3

Physical Examination Findings in Painful Neurologic Disorders *(continued)*

Location	Pain/Sensory Abnormalities	Weakness Distribution	Reflex Abnormality
Posterior cord brachial	Posterior arm and hand	Shoulder abduction (past first 30 degrees), elbow extension, wrist extension, finger extension	Triceps tendon
Lower trunk brachial	Medial arm, medial forearm, little/ring fingers	Long finger extensors, long finger flexors, hand intrinsics	Finger flexors
Lumbar	Anterior thigh	Hip flexors, knee extensors, leg adductors	Patellar tendon
Lumbosacral trunk	Buttock, lateral leg, dorsum of foot	Hip extensors (variable), knee flexors (variable), dorsiflexion, ankle inversion, ankle inversion, toe flexion	Medial hamstring tendon
Sacral	Buttock, lateral hip, posterior thigh, posterior leg, lateral and plantar foot	Anal sphincter (variable), hip extensors, knee flexors, plantar flexors	Achilles tendon
Nerve			
Occipital	Posterior head	None	None
Trigeminal	Face	Masticatory muscles (rarely clinically evident)	None
Intercostobrachial	Axilla, medial arm	None	None
Axillary	Lateral arm	Shoulder abduction, external rotation	None
Musculocutaneous	Lateral forearm	Elbow flexion, supination	Biceps tendon
Radial	Distal posterior arm, posterior forearm, posterior–lateral hand	Elbow extension (spared if lesion below spiral groove), wrist extension, finger extension, supination	Triceps tendon (if above spiral groove), none (if below spiral groove)
Ulnar	Anterior–medial hand, posterior–medial hand	Finger flexion (4th–5th digits), finger abduction (spares thumb abduction)	Finger flexors
Median	Anterior–lateral hand	Forearm pronation, wrist flexion, finger flexion (2nd–3rd digits), thumb abduction (spares finger abduction)	None
Lateral femoral cutaneous	Anterior–lateral thigh (spares medial thigh)	None	None
Femoral	Anterior–medial thigh (spares lateral thigh), medial leg, medial foot	Hip flexion (if intrapelvic lesion, spared if at inguinal ligament), knee extension	Patellar tendon
Sciatic	Posterior buttock, posterior thigh, posterior–lateral leg, plantar foot	Hip extension < knee flexion, dorsiflexion, plantar flexion, foot eversion and inversion, toe flexion	Achilles tendon, hamstring tendons
Peroneal	Anterior–lateral leg, dorsum of foot	Dorsiflexion, foot eversion	None
Tibial	Plantar foot	Plantar flexion, foot inversion	None
Polyneuropathy	Generally distal symmetric in a "stocking and glove" distribution	Generally in distal muscle groups	Varies, generally distal tendon reflexes
Mononeuropathy multiplex	Varies by nerves affected	Varies by nerves affected	Varies by nerves affected
Small fiber neuropathy	Generally distal symmetric in a "stocking and glove" distribution (affects pain/pinprick and temperature sensation but spares light touch, vibration and proprioception)	None	None

PALLIATIVE AND ALTERNATIVE CARE

MUSCULOSKELETAL COMPLICATIONS OF CANCER AND CANCER TREATMENT

Musculoskeletal disorders represent a diverse group that includes derangement of muscle, ligament, tendon, joint, cartilage, bone, and associated tissues. Included are arthritis, tendonitis, tenosynovitis, bursitis, myofascial pain, and countless other disorders. The pain associated with musculoskeletal disorders is somatic from activation of nociceptors in affected structures as opposed to neuropathic. There may be considerable overlap as when neuromuscular disorders (e.g., C-5 radiculopathy) play a causal role in the development of musculoskeletal disorders (e.g., rotator cuff tendonitis).[104] As with neuromuscular disorders, musculoskeletal disorders are extremely common in the general population as well as in the cancer setting. The accurate assessment of musculoskeletal disorders, including the differentiation of benign from malignant etiologies of pain, is an important component of the cancer rehabilitation physician's duties. It is often the case that benign musculoskeletal disorders cause as much morbidity as malignant ones. The successful identification and treatment of these disorders can help improve the function and quality of life of cancer patients and survivors. A full accounting of the assessment and treatment of the countless musculoskeletal disorders is not possible due to space limitations.

Bony Metastases

Bone metastases are a common complication of cancer, occurring in 69% of patients with advanced breast cancer.[105] The primary risk of bony metastases is fracture with subsequent pain and disability. A long-bone fracture poses perhaps the greatest risk to the patient because it may prevent their ability to ambulate and perform ADLs. Preventing fractures before they occur is instrumental to maintaining function and quality of life in cancer patients. Improvements in oncologic treatments, such as hormonal and biologic therapies, have changed the time course to fix many bony metastases because patients with certain malignancies may go for months or even years with widely metastatic disease and no bony pain. When they do ultimately progress, the treatment of symptomatic bony metastases is radiation and/or surgery depending on where the lesion is located.

The concept of prophylactically fixing impending fractures was first presented by Griessman in 1947.[106] Although unproven, the potential benefits include a technically easier operation, decreased operating time and blood loss, fewer complications, reduced pain, and convenience. Several strategies have been developed to predict the risk of sustaining a pathologic fracture. These predictive models are only useful in the long bones.[107] Mirels proposed a scoring system to quantify the risk of sustaining a pathologic fracture through a metastatic lesion in a long bone based on the site (upper limb, lower limb, peritrochanter), pain (mild, moderate, functional), lesion type (blastic, mixed, lytic), and size relative to the diameter of affected bone (<1/3, 1/3 to 2/3, >2/3).[108] Each of these four variables was given a score of 1, 2, or 3 according to the degree of risk. It was determined that lesions with a cumulative score of 7 or lower could be safely irradiated without risk of fracture, but lesions with a score of 8 or higher required prophylactic internal fixation prior to irradiation. A more recent study comparing various methods found only axial cortical involvement of more than 30 mm and circumferential cortical involvement as predictive of fracture; the former measure has the advantage of being accessible via plain x-ray.[109] In practice, the actual lesion size may be difficult to delineate because of an infiltrative, permeating pattern and surrounding osteopenia. Factors such as histology (with highly vascular or lytic lesions perhaps at highest risk) and location (importance to weight bearing) are also considerations.[110] Perhaps the best practical determinant of fracture risk is the degree of pain experienced by the patient both spontaneously and with evocative

maneuvers such as the FABER (Flexion Abduction External Rotation) test for intrinsic pathology of the hip joint. Patients with symptomatic lesions without systemic or radiotherapeutic treatment options are likely to progress and should generally have long-bone lesions corrected surgically.

Spine stability in the oncology setting is handled very differently from the traumatic setting. The Spine Oncology Study Group (SOSG) defines spinal instability as the "loss of spinal integrity as a result of a neoplastic process that is associated with movement related pain, symptomatic or progressive deformity, and/or neural compromise under physiologic loads."[111] The assessment of spinal instability is determined based on clinical and radiographic criteria. SOGS has developed an 18-point Spinal Instability Neoplastic Score (SINS) to aid clinicians in the diagnosis of neoplastic spinal instability. This grading scheme includes elements from six parameters: location, pain, alignment, osteolysis, vertebral body collapse, and posterior element involvement. Lesions with a low SINS (0 to 6) are considered stable and do not require surgery. Lesions with a high SINS (13 to 18) are considered unstable and likely need surgery. Lesions with an intermediate SINS require a further assessment. In an analysis, the SINS demonstrated excellent inter-and intraobserver reliability for detecting clinically relevant spinal stability.[112]

Bilsky has developed a conceptual framework to guide therapeutic decision making with respect to surgical, radiotherapeutic, and chemotherapeutic options for spine tumors.[113,114] This tool for an individual patient assessment is known as the NOMS criteria and is based on an evaluation of the neurologic (N), oncologic (O), mechanical instability (M), and systemic disease (S) status of the patient. In this model, mechanical instability is defined simply as movement-related pain referable to a focus of the tumor. Instability pain is distinguished from biologic or tumor-related pain in that it does not respond to steroids. A tumor involving the atlantoaxial complex (C1–2) usually presents with rotational pain. Such patients are considered unstable if they have a fracture subluxation greater than 5 mm or angulation greater than 11 degrees with a greater than 3.5-mm subluxation. Patients meeting these radiographic criteria are generally offered surgery at presentation, whereas those with less than a 5-mm subluxation can be irradiated in a hard collar (usually a Miami J design because it comes in a variety of sizes, is more adjustable, and is more comfortable than other designs) and weaned 6 weeks following the completion of radiation. Bracing is rarely used to treat instability of the subaxial cervical, thoracic, and lumbar spine for instability because surgery is the treatment of choice in those instances. In cases where surgery is indicated but is unable to be performed because of other clinical contraindications or patient refusal, a thoracolumbar corset can provide limited support and pain relief. Used in combination with gait aids, such as a walker, the thoracolumbar corset minimizes torque across the spine. Bed rest should be avoided because additional functional loss will occur, and thromboembolic disease may complicate the course.

RADIATION FIBROSIS SYNDROME

Radiation therapy uses high-energy radiation to kill rapidly proliferating tumor cells. The less mitotically active normal body cells are relatively spared. The acute effect of radiation on tissues is mediated through the induction of apoptosis or mitotic cell death from free radical–induced DNA damage. Radiation fibrosis (RF) is the insidious pathologic tissue sclerosis that occurs in response to radiation treatment.[13] The mechanism underlying RF is complex and involves interactions between multiple cell types that is dependent on the organ system involved.[115] RF is associated with increased collagen synthesis, altered remodeling, and sequential activation of key fibrinogenic growth factors and cytokines such as transforming growth factor beta 1 (TGFβ1) and connective tissue growth factor (CTGF).[115] Important to the process of RF is the activation of fibroblasts by fibrogenic cytokines. Once activated, myofibroblasts may not require continued paracrine stimulation by fibrogenic cytokines. Autocrine stimulation may perpetuate fibrogenesis without continued inflammation or other external stimuli.[115] This may explain the immortalization of the process of RF in cancer survivors wherein the progressive decline of organ function due to RF can continue, albeit at differing rates, indefinitely.

RF can damage any tissue type including skin, muscle, ligament, tendon, nerve, viscera, and even bone.[116] The effects of radiation can be acutely experienced during or immediately following treatment. Radiation effects can also be early delayed (up to 3 months) or late delayed (more than 3 months) following the completion of treatment.[117] Fatigue is generally an acute or early-delayed complication of radiation therapy. RF is generally a late complication, and may manifest years after treatment, progress rapidly or insidiously, and is not generally reversible.[118]

The term *radiation fibrosis syndrome* (RFS) describes the clinical manifestations that result from the progressive fibrotic sclerosis that follows radiation treatment.[13] RFS occurs locally at the treated site, but may also cause distant effects when a neural, vascular, lymphatic, or other structure passing through a radiation field is damaged.[119] The radiation field can be sharply localized or extensive.[120] The mantle radiation field used to treat supradiaphragmatic HL, for instance, involves all lymph nodes in the neck, chest, and axilla. The inverted-Y radiation field involves the periaortic and ilioinguinal lymph nodes. The combination of mantle and inverted-Y radiation is known as total nodal irradiation (Fig. 152.5). Such broad radiation fields can result in widespread neuromuscular sequelae including myelopathy, radiculopathy, plexopathy, neuropathy, and myopathy, either individually or in combination. This syndrome is termed *myelo-radiculo-plexo-neuro-myopathy*.[13] Other well-known late effects of radiation for HL include secondary malignancies, cardiovascular disease, pulmonary disease, thyroid dysfunction, infertility, fatigue, and psychosocial issues.[121]

Radiation damage to the CNS is also classified temporally as acute, early delayed, and late delayed. Acute encephalopathy occurs days to weeks after the initiation of treatment, and early-delayed encephalopathy at 1 to 6 months likely represents transient demyelination. Clinical manifestations include irritability, loss of appetite, exacerbation of tumor-like symptoms, Lhermitte's sign, and in children, somnolence syndrome.[117,118] Late-delayed encephalopathy, caused by irreversible white matter necrosis, may rarely occur. Early-delayed encephalopathy usually responds well to corticosteroids, but late-delayed encephalopathies respond less consistently. Memory loss or cognitive dysfunction may result from brain atrophy after whole-brain irradiation. Other side effects of cranial irradiation include fatigue, loss of taste, decreased salivation, impaired gag reflex, and decreased hearing.[122]

Radiation-induced myelopathy can manifest as a transient syndrome that usually occurs within 4 to 6 months of treatment. Delayed radiation myelopathy usually occurs 1 to 2 years after radiation, but may occur as soon as 3 months or more than 10 years later. It usually presents with lower extremity sensory symptoms (numbness, paresthesias, or dysesthesias), followed by weakness and loss of bowel and bladder dysfunction. It may progress over weeks to months in a stepwise fashion leading to paraplegia or quadriplegia in at least 50% of patients. Patients may rarely show spontaneous recovery but most continue to progress. Pain is not generally a prominent feature of radiation myelopathy.[73]

RF can damage any peripheral nervous system structure.[123] Such injury can cause focal paraspinal muscle spasms, distant muscle spasms, referred pain, local pain, and weakness.[104] The upper brachial plexus may be more prone to damage than other plexus structures, arguably because of its superior location within the pyramid shaped chest where it is less protected by overlying tissue.[68] Muscle cramps commonly occur as a result of radiation damage and are thought to arise from spontaneous discharges at any level of the motor nerve with resultant volleys of neural activity being sent to and across the neuromuscular junction thereby involuntarily activating the muscle.[124] Myokymic discharges are common (but not pathognomonic) in radiation damage to the peripheral nervous system and are responsible for some of the

PALLIATIVE AND ALTERNATIVE CARE

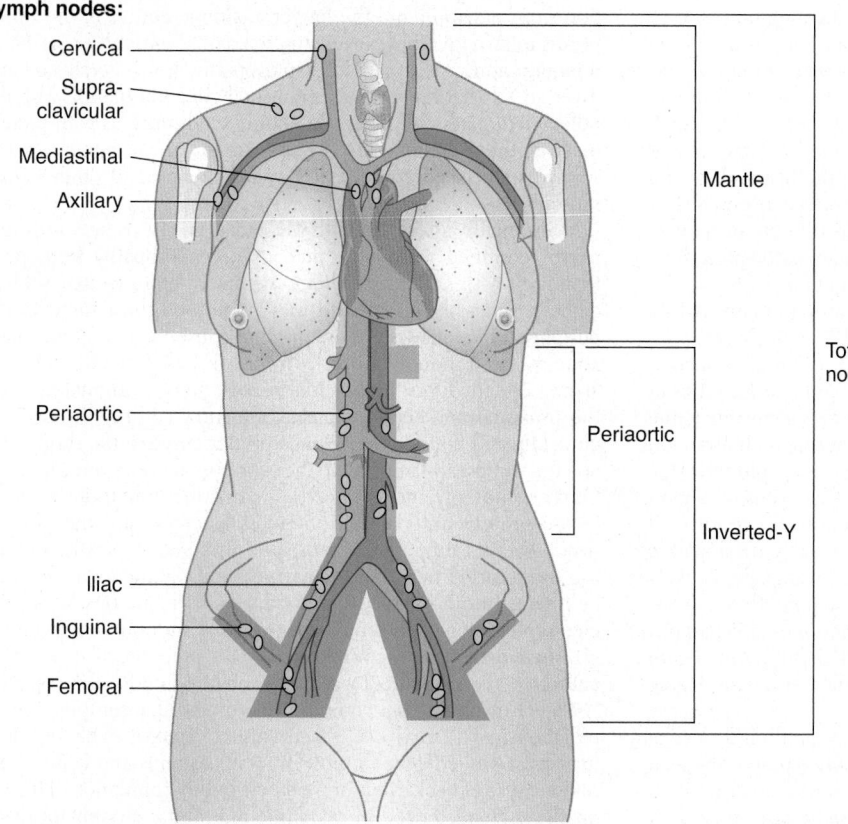

Lymph nodes:
- Cervical
- Supra-clavicular
- Mediastinal
- Axillary
- Periaortic
- Iliac
- Inguinal
- Femoral

Mantle

Total nodal

Periaortic

Inverted-Y

Figure 152.5 Radiation fields historically used in the treatment of Hodgkin lymphoma include the mantle, periaortic, and inverted-Y among others. When all nodes are radiated, this is known as total nodal irradiation. The late-term morbidity experienced by Hodgkin lymphoma survivors often depends on the extent of their radiation treatment. Contemporary treatment of Hodgkin lymphoma primarily involves chemotherapy and, when necessary, more targeted involved site radiation therapy, which generally uses smaller doses and affects less normal tissue.

muscle spasms seen in the RFS. Myokymia is seen clinically as vermiculations (wormlike movements under the skin) and have a characteristic sound and appearance on needle electromyography. Myokymia is thought to result from ephaptic cross-talk between motor nerves that have been focally demyelinated.[125] Progressive fibrosis in muscle fibers within the radiation field can cause a focal myopathy that is associated with nemaline rods.[89] Myopathic muscles are weak relative to normal muscle and prone to spasm and pain.

Although RFS can potentially result from treatment with radiation for any cancer type, it is commonly encountered in head and neck cancer and HL patients and survivors.

Radiation Fibrosis Syndrome in Hodgkin Lymphoma

No group of cancer survivors better typifies the potential for long-term radiation complications than those treated for HL.[13,126] The high doses of radiation historically used in this group of patients are responsible for a variety of complications that can affect any organ system. The complications likely to be encountered in these patients depends largely on the radiation port used (MF, inverted-Y, total nodal), and thus the structures involved by radiation (see Fig. 152.5). Contemporary treatment regimens for HL have evolved considerably in recent years and now utilize chemotherapy as the primary modality and involved site radiation therapy (ISRT) if needed. Late radiation sequelae are less likely with ISRT because the amount of tissue treated and total doses used are generally smaller.

Although the majority of neuromusculoskeletal complications result from late effects of radiation, other morbidities such as cardiotoxicity may result from anthracycline exposure or a combination of radiation and anthracycline exposure.[126] The list of morbid non-neuromusculoskeletal conditions ascribed to HL is long and includes, but is not limited to, arterial disease (coronary artery disease, myocardial infarction, valvular heart disease, congestive heart failure, pericardial disease, electrical conduction abnormalities, carotid artery disease, peripheral arterial disease), lung disease (pulmonary fibrosis, pulmonary hypertension, chest wall restriction), autonomic dysfunction (carotid barrow receptor failure, orthostasis, gastric dysmotility, impotence), endocrine dysfunction (hypothyroidism, infertility), as well as a variety of gastrointestinal, genitourinary, and sexual disorders.[121,126] Second primary malignancy followed by cardiovascular disease are the first and second leading causes of mortality for HL survivors, respectively.[126] The clinician who evaluates and treats HL survivors should be acutely aware of the vast potential for individual variation in the presenting symptoms and disorders in this complex group of patients.

Subacute myelopathy is estimated to occur in as many as 15% of patients treated with MF irradiation for HL[122]; plegia rarely results. Brisk reflexes may be seen in the lower extremities accompanied by depressed or absent reflexes in the upper extremities in patients treated with MF radiation. This pattern is likely due to the combination of central and peripheral nervous system dysfunction in HL survivors treated with MF radiation. Detrusor-sphincter dyssynergia, bowel dysfunction, spasticity, weakness, sensory abnormalities, ataxia, movement disorders, and abnormal gait have all been seen in the author's clinical practice as likely myelopathic manifestations of distant radiation. Subacute myelopathy is likely a contributing factor to the fatigue seen in many HL survivors. Myelopathy in HL rarely occurs in isolation and is usually part of a myelo-radiculo-plexo-neuro-myopathy. An MRI of the spinal cord rarely demonstrates parenchymal abnormalities, although degenerative changes are often seen in the elderly.

Radiculopathy in HL survivors is often part of a myelo-radiculo-plexo-neuro-myopathy but it is more commonly seen without clinically overt myelopathy. Neuronal predisposition from preexisting or emergent degenerative spine disease is likely

an extremely important etiologic factor in the development of radiculopathy. Radiculopathy can be seen in isolation, particularly when degenerative spinal disease at the affected level is present, but is more commonly part of a radiculo-plexopathy or a radiculo-plexo-neuro-myopathy. Patients treated with MF irradiation generally develop radiculopathy in the upper (C5, C6) roots but may have more widespread or patchy involvement. Patients treated with periaortic or inverted-Y radiation may develop radiculopathy at any lumbosacral root, but the L5 or S1 levels are most frequently involved, likely due to their coexistence with degenerative changes such as disk herniations and central or neuroforaminal spinal stenosis. A diffuse polyradiculopathy is commonly seen. Radiation-induced cauda equina syndrome should be suspected when no degenerative or other compressive etiologies are present on MRI to explain the nerve root dysfunction documented clinically and/or on electrophysiologic testing.

The electrophysiologic pattern of radiculopathy resulting from radiation is similar if not identical to radiculopathy seen from other causes. If the entire cauda equina is involved, the findings are more widespread and involve the distribution of multiple nerve roots. Myokymia may or may not be present and its absence does not exclude radiation as an etiologic contributor.[125] An electrophysiologic assessment of radiculopathy in HL survivors treated with radiation may be complicated due to the coexistence of plexopathy, neuropathy, and/or myopathy.

Plexopathy can affect both the brachial and lumbosacral plexus in HL survivors depending on the extent of radiation they received (e.g., MF, inverted-Y, total nodal). Brachial plexopathy is rarely seen without a component of radiculopathy, neuropathy of the nerves within the radiation field, and localized myopathy. Plexopathy, however, can be a prominent feature of radiation in HL survivors. Plexopathy seems less common in the author's clinical experience than radiculopathy. One possible reason for this observation is that the plexus is not directly affected by degenerative changes. Plexopathy from MF irradiation generally affects the upper brachial plexus (upper trunk and/or lateral cord) more severely than the rest of the plexus, but a pan-plexopathy can be seen. The pyramidal shape of the thorax provides less protection from radiation and the longer anatomic course of the upper plexus relative to other plexus structures may arguably explain this phenomenon.[127] Lumbosacral plexopathy from periaortic and inverted-Y radiation may be seen, usually in combination with the polyradiculopathy of the cauda equina syndrome. As with radiculopathy, the electrophysiologic assessment of plexopathy in HL survivors is usually complicated by the presence of other neuromuscular disorders.

Neuropathy associated with MF radiation affects only proximal nerves confined within the field. A polyneuropathy from prior treatment with neurotoxic chemotherapy or other causes, such as diabetes, may be present and may predispose the patient to the peripheral nervous system dysfunction caused by radiation. Radiation-induced mononeuropathy from MF radiation affects nerves arising directly form the brachial plexus. Nerves originating from the proximal and superior plexus are most commonly involved clinically and include the dorsal scapular nerve to the rhomboids and the suprascapular nerve to the supraspinatus and infraspinatus. Other commonly affected nerves include the long thoracic nerve to the serratus anterior, the intercostal nerves, and the phrenic nerve. Nerves originating from the lumbosacral plexus, including the femoral nerve and lateral femoral cutaneous nerve, can be affected from inverted-Y and total nodal radiation. Again, the electrophysiologic assessment of proximal mononeuropathies in HL survivors is usually complicated by the presence of a coexistent pathology such as radiculopathy, plexopathy, and focal myopathy.

Focal myopathy is a common neuromuscular complication of radiation in HL survivors. Given enough time, it likely develops to at least some degree in most if not all patients and is likely the major cause of neck extensor weakness in this population. The myopathy is characterized by nemaline rods and is sharply localized

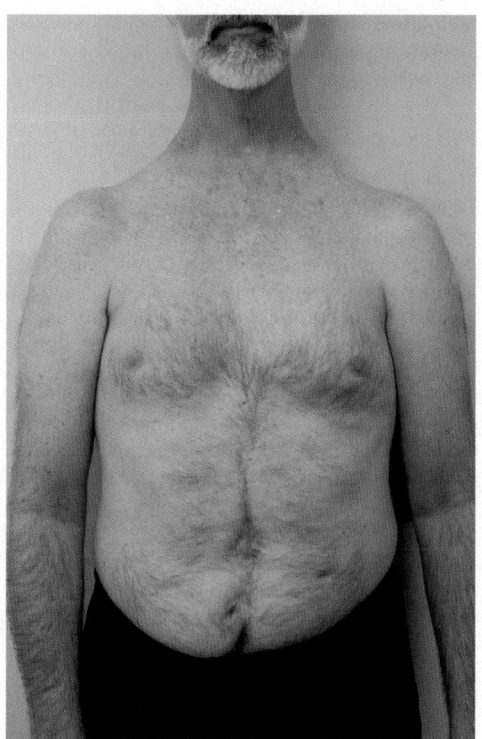
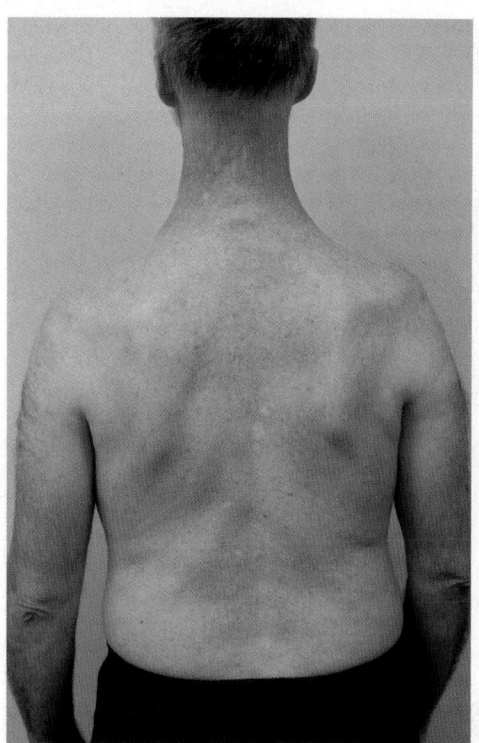

Figure 152.6 A 50-year-old Hodgkin lymphoma survivor treated in 1982 with staging laparotomy, splenectomy, and radiation including Mantle (4,020 cGy), Waldeyer's ring (3,990 cGy), para-aortic/splenic pedicle (3,570 cGy), and right preauricular (800 cGy) as well as nitrogen mustard, vincristine, procarbazine, and prednisone. Although he is without evident disease, he suffers from a host of late effects of treatment including myelo-radiculo-plexo-neuro-myopathy with subsequent severe upper and lower extremity weakness and gait disturbance requiring ankle–foot orthoses and a gait aid for ambulation. He has neck extension weakness. Note the marked atrophy of the cervicothoracic musculature including the cervical and thoracic paraspinal muscles, the rhomboids, and supraspinatus, and infraspinatus. The scapulae are protracted. His pectoral muscles are relatively spared due to shielding designed to protect the lungs.

to muscle fibers within the radiation field such as the cervical and thoracic paraspinal, rhomboid, supraspinatus, and infraspinatus muscles.[89]

One of the most clinically obvious, ubiquitous, and disabling disorders afflicting HL survivors is cervicothoracic atrophy and neck extensor weakness (Fig. 152.6). At its worst, this usually painful condition can result in an inability to maintain the head in a normal upright posture long enough to participate meaningfully in ADLs or even complete neck drop. Atrophy of the cervicothoracic musculature is essentially universal in HL survivors treated with MF radiation. The underlying pathophysiology is likely various components of the myelo-radiculo-plexo-neuro-myopathy (described previously) with myopathy being the major contributor. Needle electromyography (EMG) of the cervical paraspinal muscles in HL survivors treated with MF radiation generally shows mixed neuropathic and myopathic motor units.

Although there is no way to reverse the fibrosis and resultant cervical and thoracic atrophy that results from MF radiation, the function and quality of life of these patients can be meaningfully improved with PT to improve core as well as neck strength, posture, body mechanics, and endurance. Myofascial techniques are employed to release the anterior pectoral girdle. Proprioception of the neck and shoulders are often severely impaired. Lymphedema is almost universally present in the neck, thorax, and extremities and should be treated to improve proprioception and facilitate myofascial release. Emphasis on a lifelong home exercise program is of paramount importance if a durable benefit is to be achieved. In cases where neck weakness and pain impair ADLs despite adequate PT, the use of a cervical collar to assist elevation of the chin is recommended. The Headmaster Cervical Collar, manufactured by Symmetric Designs in Salt Spring Island, British Columbia, is smaller, lighter, and more comfortable than other collars

(Fig. 152.7). Some patients (i.e., those with anterior chest wall abnormalities) may prefer other designs, such as a soft cervical collar, and their preferences should be accommodated whenever possible. The cervical collar is not intended to be used at all times but as an energy conservation device. Patients who experience pain due to cervicothoracic muscle overload and/or fatigue as the day progresses are encouraged to use a collar whenever possible. Such activities include housework, meals, time spent in front of the computer, watching television, or reading. Use of the collar during such activities may rest the neck muscles so the patient can tolerate and enjoy activities that occur later in the day without wearing the collar. For instance, using the collar during work might make it possible to comfortably attend and enjoy dinner with family or friends after work without the aid of the collar.

Shoulder pain and dysfunction in HL survivors is usually causally related to their radiation treatment. Although the shoulder joint is largely outside of the direct effects of the radiation field, the nerves and muscles that actuate the shoulder are not. Directly radiated structures include the cervical nerve roots, brachial plexus, rotator cuff muscles, and nerves such as the suprascapular nerve that innervate the rotator cuff. Any damage to the C5 or C6 cervical nerve roots or upper brachial plexus can denervate and weaken the rotator cuff muscles and refer neuropathic pain to the lateral shoulder and arm. If rotator cuff weakness results in anterior translation of the humerus within the glenohumeral joint, then impingement of the rotator cuff tendons may develop and cause a secondary rotator cuff tendonitis and, potentially, a tertiary adhesive capsulitis due to the local inflammation within the shoulder capsule.[104,128]

Imaging of the rotator cuff is only necessary if the clinical assessment, including physical examination, is not consistent with what is expected. For instance, an MRI is indicated if a palpable

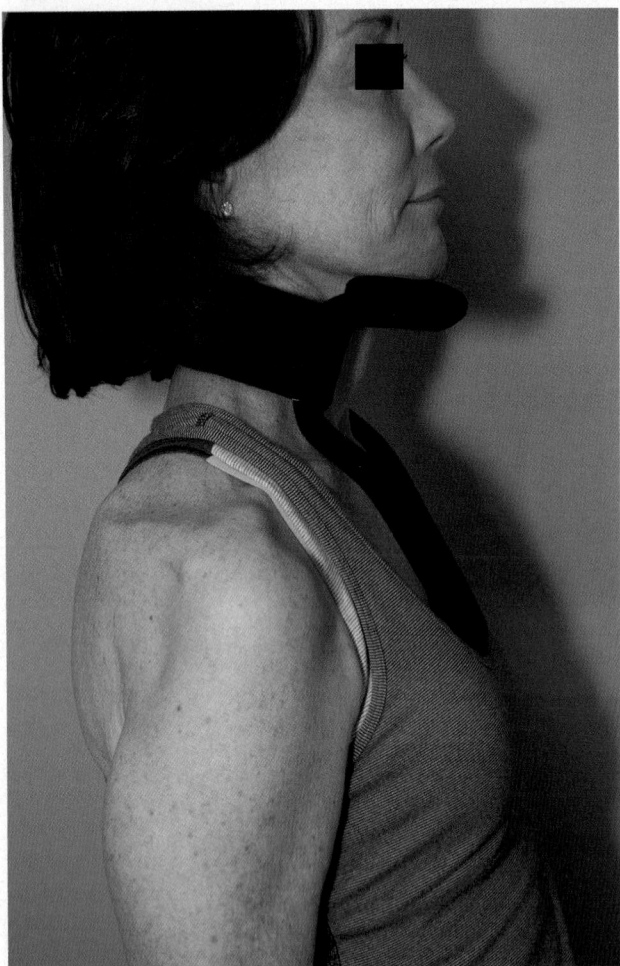

Figure 152.7 The Headmaster Cervical Collar (Symmetric Designs Ltd., Salt Spring Island, British Columbia, Canada) is a simple and comfortable way to support the head in patients with weakened cervical paraspinal muscles from radiation and other cancer-associated causes. It is being modeled by a Hodgkin lymphoma survivor with severe cervicothoracic atrophy and neck extensor weakness.

mass is present or if the pain elicited is atypical (e.g., sharply localized to the spine of the scapula suggesting malignancy or fracture). Imaging is also useful if a patient has not responded to initial treatment measures and surgical intervention is contemplated. As a general rule, shoulder surgery should be avoided in RFS patients because it is unlikely to impact the progressive neuromuscular disorders that precipitated the shoulder dysfunction and will continue to drive the shoulder pathology. Conservative measures are the mainstay of treatment for shoulder pathology in HL survivors. PT is the primary modality and is the only treatment to confer a durable benefit. Therapy should address, among other disorders, rotator cuff weakness and tightness of the pectoral girdle with the goal of restoring the normal anatomic alignment of the shoulder at the glenohumeral joint and, thus, the rotator cuff tendons within the coracoacromial arch. Anti-inflammatory medications and/or nerve stabilizing agents are often indicated. Subacromial injection, although not curative, may facilitate PT efforts and comfort.

HEAD AND NECK CANCER

Treatment and disease-related neuromuscular and musculoskeletal complications are common in head and neck cancer survivors. Common complications requiring rehabilitation include shoulder dysfunction, trismus, radiation-induced cervical dystonia, lymphedema, a variety of nerve injuries, and speech and swallowing dysfunction.

Shoulder pain is one of the most common sequelae of head and neck cancer treatments, being present in as many as 70% of patients following nonselective neck lymph node dissection.[129] Radical neck dissection (RND) involves the removal of all the ipsilateral cervical lymph node groups (from levels I to V) as well as the spinal accessory nerve (SAN), the internal jugular vein, and the sternocleidomastoid muscle (SCM).[130] Modified radical neck dissection (MRND) involves the excision of all lymph nodes routinely removed by RND but with preservation of one or more of the nonlymphatic structures (e.g., the SAN, internal jugular vein, or the SCM).[130] In selective lymph node dissection (SND), nonlymphatic structures are spared, whereas the excision of lymph node groups is based on the pattern of metastases.[130] In addition to pain, neck dissection can cause reduced ROM in the neck and shoulder, loss of sensation, and loss of neck and shoulder function.[131]

The role of exercise for the treatment of shoulder dysfunction in patients treated for head and neck cancer has been subject to investigation with several randomized prospective trials.[132–134] A Cochrane review of these trials concluded that progressive resistance training is more effective than standard PT treatment for shoulder dysfunction in patients treated for head and neck cancer in terms of improving pain, disability, and shoulder joint ROM.[135] Quality of life, however, was not improved. Although statistically significant, the relative benefits were small compared to traditional PT.

In addition to PT, medications including nonsteroidal anti-inflammatory drugs (NSAIDS), nerve stabilizers, and in some cases, opioids have a role in the treatment of chronic shoulder pain associated with neck dissection in head and neck cancer survivors. Subacromial corticosteroid injections can be useful for severe exacerbations of pain or to facilitate therapy but only offer temporary relief.

The prevalence of trismus in treated head and neck cancer patients ranges from 5% to 38%.[136] Impairment in mouth opening may have an adverse effect on quality of life by compromising functions such as chewing, swallowing, respiratory function, oral hygiene and health, the ability to survey for recurrence, and intimacy. Normal mouth opening for an adult ranges from 23 to 71 mm as measured between the incisors.[137] The wide variation in reported incidence reflects the lack of uniform criteria for the definition of trismus.[138] Trismus in the head and neck cancer setting can result from tumor invasion into critical structures of mastication including the masseter and pterygoid muscles and/or their neural innervation, the temporal mandibular joint (TMJ), and/or other supportive tissues.[139] Surgery and radiation therapy are well-known causes of trismus. Radiation can result in trismus in up to 45% of patients who received curative doses.[140] Trismus evolves most rapidly 1 to 9 months after the completion of radiation therapy.[141] The mandibular opening worsens as the dose of radiation delivered to the pterygoid muscles increases, and the probability of developing trismus is reported to increase 24% for every 10 Gy of additional radiation delivered.[142,143] Noncancer- and cancer treatment–related causes of trismus are also common in the cancer setting and include infection, trauma, and osteoradionecrosis of the jaw.[144]

Multiple modalities have been used in the treatment of trismus. PT is the mainstay of trismus treatment and is often used alone or in combination with other modalities. Despite widespread and accepted use, the use of PT to treat trismus in the head and neck cancer population has not demonstrated the ability to improve trismus.[145–147] A more recent prospective randomized trial, however, did demonstrate the benefit of exercise in slowing the progression of trismus and improving swallowing function in nasopharyngeal carcinoma patients treated with radiation.[148] Hyperbaric oxygen and pentoxifylline have shown modest efficacy.[149,150] Forced mouth opening under general anesthesia can improve trismus, but the effect is often short lived and potentially complicated by alveolus fracture and rupture of adjacent soft tissues. Surgical coronoidectomy has demonstrated significant efficacy in a noncontrolled study of head and neck cancer patients who had failed PT but is not in widespread clinical use.[151] Botulinum toxin injection has been reported to have potential benefit in treating selected complications of the RFS including trismus.[152] A study of the efficacy of botulin toxin injection into the masseters of head and neck cancer patients with radiation-induced pain and trismus did not demonstrate significant improvement of trismus, but did demonstrate significantly reduced local pain.[153]

A variety of jaw opening devices are available to treat trismus (Fig. 152.8).[154] Devices commonly used in clinical practice include stacked tongue depressors, corkscrew devices, the Thera-Bite (TB) Jaw Motion Rehabilitation System, and the Dynasplint Trismus System (DTS). The TB demonstrated efficacy in a small trial (seven patients) when used within 6 weeks of surgery for oropharyngeal carcinoma.[155] A larger trial demonstrated that TB increased mouth opening an average of 5.4 mm, but the odds of increasing mouth opening 5 mm or more was reduced as the time from oncologic treatment to the start of exercise lengthened.[156] TB combined with unassisted exercise also demonstrated efficacy in patients who had undergone radiation therapy within the preceding 5 years (most within the preceding year) when compared with unassisted exercise and mechanically assisted mandibular mobilization using stacked tongue depressors combined with unassisted exercise.[147]

The fabrication and/or use of dynamic jaw opening devices to treat both benign and oncologic causes of trismus have been detailed in reports as early as 1968.[157–162] The DTS is a commercially available dynamic jaw opening device that operates on the principle of low-torque, prolonged duration stretches. It has demonstrated efficacy in achieving improved jaw opening in a retrospective evaluation of 48 patients with trismus from four cohort groups including radiation therapy for head and neck cancer, dental treatment, oral surgery, and stroke.[163] Although the 20 patients in the head and neck cancer cohort improved their maximal interincisal distance by a mean of 13.6 mm, little demographic and oncologic information was given save that they all received radiation therapy. A retrospective cohort study demonstrated the efficacy of the DTS as part of a multimodal treatment strategy with improvement in the maximal interincisal distance from 16 mm to 27 mm ($p < 0.001$).[164]

In clinical practice, the devices of choice are the TB and DTS. Stacked tongue depressors and corkscrew devices are relatively ineffective. The TB may be effective early in the course of trismus development, is inexpensive, is easy and intuitive to use, and is readily available. The device is inserted in the mouth and activated to near tolerance by squeezing leveraged handles for seven repetitions of 7 seconds. This is usually repeated seven times per day. Though often effective at improving mouth opening, this regimen may cause rebound spasm of the masseter and pterygoid muscles. If the patient has had trismus for more than 3 months, the DTS may be a better option because it works on the principle of low-torque, prolonged stretches, which have been demonstrated to be more effective at improving ROM in an experimental model involving contracted rat knees than high-torque, short duration stretching.[165] A custom bite plate is fabricated for the device and its use is progressed until the patient is able to tolerate the device for 30 minutes three times per day. PT is usually used in collaboration with a jaw stretching device to ensure its proper use, to provide and teach muscle massage techniques, and to address other neuromuscular

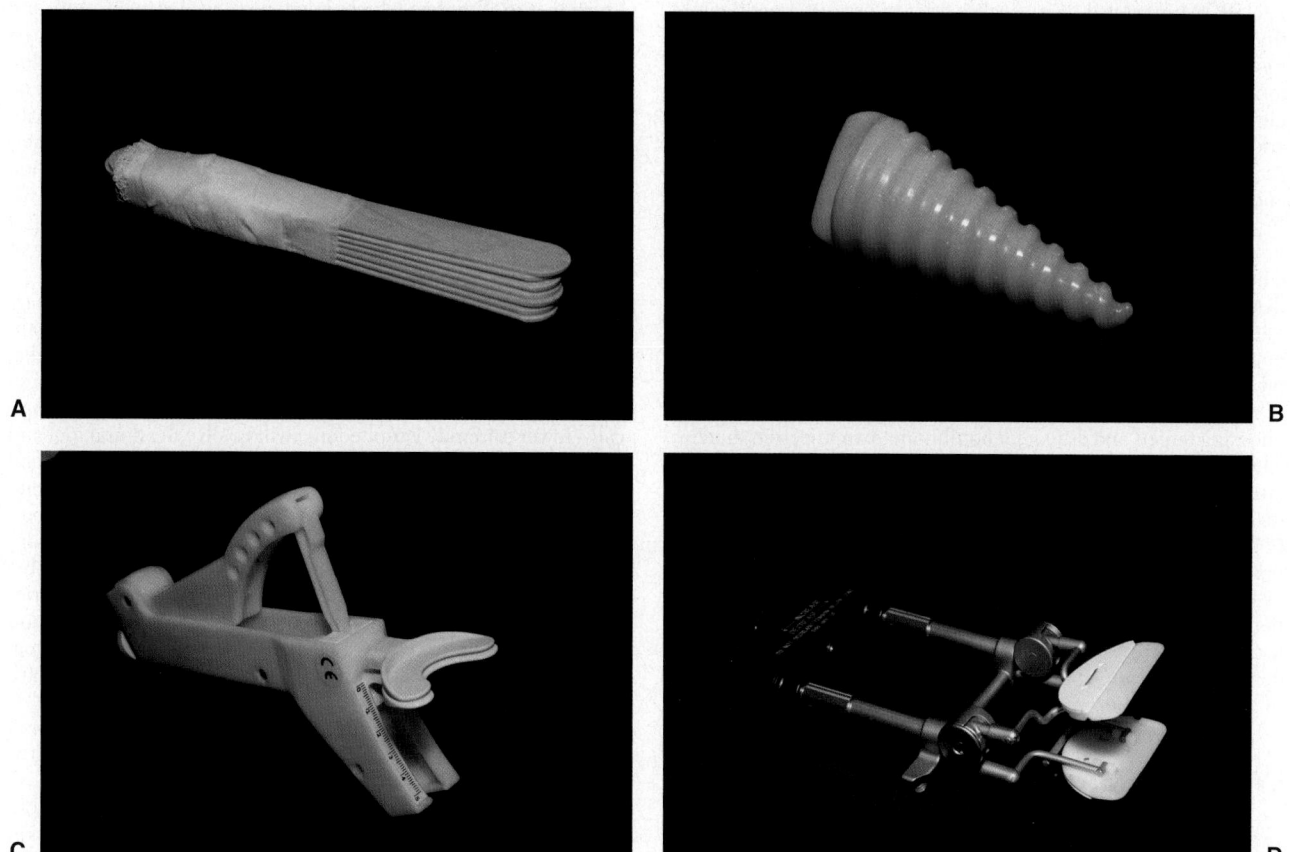

A   B

C   D

Figure 152.8 Jaw stretching devices use to treat trismus include **(A)** stacked tongue depressors, **(B)** corkscrew devices, **(C)** the TheraBite Jaw Motion Rehabilitation System (TB), and **(D)** the Dynasplint Trismus System (DTS). (From Stubblefield MD, O'Dell MW. *Cancer Rehabilitation Principles and Practice.* New York: Demos Medical Publishers; 2009, with permission.)

and musculoskeletal issues such as neck pain, stiffness, or weakness that often accompany trismus. Pain medications may be necessary to diminish the pain and spasm of mastication muscles. Generally, nerve stabilizing agents such as pregabalin, gabapentin, or duloxetine are used initially. Botulinum toxin injections will not improve oral opening in isolation, but may decrease the dynamic muscle spasm that contributes to trismus and makes other therapeutic interventions, including PT and jaw opening devices, more effective.

Radiation-induced cervical dystonia can result not only from the treatment of head and neck cancers, but from the treatment of any tumor treated with radiation that involves the occiput, cervical spine, or upper thoracic spine including metastatic disease from any cancer type, sarcomas, lymphomas such as HL, or thyroid cancer.[166] Idiopathic cervical dystonia is broadly defined as a movement disorder characterized by involuntary contractions of the head and shoulders that may be twisted into abnormal positions including torticollis, laterocollis, retrocollis, and anterocollis.[167] In radiation-induced cervical dystonia, RF likely contributes to ectopic activity in the distribution of the cervical plexus, the spinal accessory nerve, and the cervical nerve roots. This ectopic activity may be asymmetric or contribute to pain, soreness, tightness, or aberrant positioning of the head and neck characteristic of cervical dystonia. More often, symptoms are at least partially bilateral. As RF progresses, posturing of the head and neck becomes less pronounced and fixed contractures can develop. Most patients complain of neck tightness, which progresses slowly and insidiously and is almost always accompanied by varying degrees of pain. Inability to position the head due to progressive fibrosis can affect swallowing, phonation, and ADLs such as driving and work-related tasks important to one's quality of life.

The natural history of radiation-induced cervical dystonia is usually one of progression. Aggressive PT with an emphasis on a lifelong home exercise program designed to maintain head and neck ROM is critical. It is usually easier to prevent a contracture than to treat one. Medications may be useful in treating the symptoms of radiation-induced cervical dystonia but are not a substitute for ROM exercises. Medications of potential benefit include muscle relaxants such as baclofen, nerve stabilizers such as pregabalin, and analgesics.

Botulinum toxin injections can be effective at treating the pain and spasms associated with radiation-induced cervical dystonia. Botulinum toxin injections will not directly treat fixed contracture, but may facilitate the progression of ROM through PT and a home exercise program. Techniques used in the treatment of radiation-induced cervical dystonia are very similar to those used for idiopathic cervical dystonia. A clinical evaluation with particular emphasis on the patient's anatomy, which may have been compromised by neck dissection, and the patient's historical account of symptoms, as well as physical examination are instrumental in choosing targets and dosing for botulinum toxin injection therapy. The dosages and technique are often modified on subsequent visits to maximize efficacy. Potential complications of botulinum toxin injection include bleeding and infection, especially if injections are near recent or active injection sites, spinal stabilization hardware, or tumor. Neck drop can occur when injecting weak or liminal cervical paraspinal muscles or the trapezius. Precipitation or worsening of dysphagia is particularly problematic because patients with RFS that involves the neck often have preexisting deficits. Overtreatment with botulinum toxin can potentially result in aspiration or the need for a feeding tube.

LYMPHEDEMA

Lymphedema is the abnormal accumulation of protein-rich lymphatic fluid in an extremity, face, neck, trunk, or genitalia. Primary lymphedema is due to aplastic or hypoplastic development of the lymphatics, whereas secondary lymphedema is usually the result of infection, tumor, or lymphatic injury. Risk factors for

lymphedema include the extent of surgery (e.g., axillary lymph node dissection, the number of lymph nodes dissected, mastectomy) and being overweight or obese.[168] Radiation therapy involving the lymph nodes is also a well-known factor in the development of lymphedema.[169] In addition to breast cancer, lymphedema can result from any type of cancer in which the lymph nodes are involved directly or by treatments such as radiation or surgery. Pelvic, colorectal, and head and neck cancers are commonly associated with lymphedema. If untreated, the accumulation of protein-rich lymphatic fluid can result in fibrotic deposition with progressive sclerosis further worsening the lymphedema and ultimately resulting in elephantiasis.[170] Lymphedema is not usually a painful condition but can cause the sensation of extremity heaviness or constriction. Increased weight, traction, and altered biomechanics can contribute to secondary neuromuscular and musculoskeletal pain disorders in patients with lymphedema.[104]

The reported incidence of lymphedema in breast cancer varies depending on the diagnostic criteria used and the means of assessment. For instance, a recent systematic review and meta-analysis of unilateral arm lymphedema in breast cancer survivors measured an incidence of 16.6% for all of the 72 studies that met their inclusion criteria, 21.4% for the 30 included prospective cohort studies, and 28.2% for the 9 studies that used more than one diagnostic method to measure lymphedema.[168] The authors also found that lymphedema was approximately four times higher (19.9%) in women who had axillary lymph node dissection than those who underwent sentinel node biopsy (5.6%).

Swelling can occur immediately following surgery and resolve spontaneously without necessarily heralding the onset of lymphedema. Axillary web syndrome is characterized by palpable cords in the breast, underarm, medial arm, antecubital fossa, forearm, and/or abdomen that develop following axillary lymph node dissection (38% to 72%) or sentinel lymph node biopsy (20%). Fortunately, the disorder, which is often associated with pain and shoulder ROM limitations, is usually self-limited. New onset lymphedema that develops after the acute treatment phase of the primary disease should prompt an evaluation for recurrence. Imaging is the modality of choice to exclude a recurrence. An MRI with gadolinium is usually sufficient, but a PET-CT scan may be necessary in borderline cases. A duplex Doppler ultrasound is often indicated to exclude deep venous thrombosis.[170] CT scans of the chest, abdomen, and pelvis commonly used by the primary oncologist as screening for visceral recurrences will likely miss an axillary or brachial plexus recurrence.

Peripheral edema from fluid overload, heart failure, pulmonary hypertension, hypoalbuminemia, and other causes are common in the cancer setting and require differentiation from lymphedema. This differentiation is made on clinical grounds by a history, physical examination, and laboratory evaluation when necessary. Typically, lower extremity lymphedema will involve the dorsal foot and spare the metatarsal–phalangeal joints and will not have peripheral vascular disease stigmata, vascular distention, or ulceration. Studies such as lymphoscintigraphy, which evaluates lymphatic transport and abnormalities, can clarify the etiology of venous edema from mixed or lymphatic edema. Lymphoscintigraphy is rarely done because it is very dependent on the skill of the examiner and carries considerable morbidity without providing significant information over a comprehensive clinical evaluation. Impedance plethysmography is a noninvasive technique that uses small changes in electrical resistance to evaluate and follow lymphedema.[171]

Improved cancer treatment approaches diminish but do not prevent the development of lymphedema.[172,173] Lymphedema is not curable and must be managed as a chronic condition. At-risk patients should be educated about lymphedema and its complications, especially cellulitis. Risk-reduction strategies include skin care and protection and avoiding venipuncture, blood pressure measurements, or constricting clothing to the affected region. The current research regarding airline travel in at-risk individuals is limited and controversial. One study concluded that domestic air travel (less than 4.5 hours) is low risk and that compression devices may actually contribute to increased swelling.[174]

A variety of therapies have been trialed for the management of lymphedema including complex physical therapy (CPT), low-level laser therapy (LLLT), pharmacotherapy, and surgery.[175] CPT (also known as complex decongestive therapy, complex decongestive therapy, or comprehensive decongestive therapy) is by far the most commonly used modality and consists of manual lymphatic drainage (MLD), exercise, nonelastic wrapping, application of compression garments, and skin care. The application of low stretch bandaging followed by compression stockings was found to be superior to compression stockings alone in a randomized, controlled, parallel-group trial for patients with both upper and lower limb lymphedema.[176] LLLT was found to reduce the volume of the affected arm, extracellular fluid, and tissue hardness in approximately 33% of postmastectomy patients in one study and to reduce limb volume and increase shoulder mobility and hand grip strength in approximately 93% of postmastectomy lymphedema patients in a more recent study.[177,178] Diuretics may have a role in treating lymphedema of mixed origin (e.g., cardiogenic plus lymphedema) but are not recommended for long-term use because, although they may reduce the intravascular fluid volume, they cannot effectively remove the elevated interstitial protein that characterizes lymphedema resulting in an osmotic gradient that facilitates rapid fluid reaccumulation. The benzopyrones (e.g., Coumarin (5,6-benzo-[a]-pyrone, or 1,2-benzopyrone) have had controversial findings and are not currently approved by the U.S. Food and Drug Administration.[179] Flavonoids have been reported to reduce stage 2 and 3 lymphedema; however, trials have been limited and they are not widely used in clinical practice.[180] Antibiotics, including second-generation cephalosporins and penicillins, are commonly used to treat cellulitis associated with lymphedema. Patients who have had multiple cellulitic infections may need to receive prophylactic antibiotics. A variety of surgical options exist for the management of lymphedema. These techniques can be categorized as physiologic (flap interposition, lymph node transplantation, lymphatic bypass, lymphaticovenous bypass) or reductive (direct excision, liposuction).[181] In general, the data supporting these various options are limited and suffer from short follow-up intervals.[175] External pneumatic compression pumping alone or in combination with CPT is controversial.[172]

The question of whether patients with lymphedema could exercise or lift weights was controversial until recently. Considerable high-quality data are now available to affirm that resistance exercise including weight lifting does not increase the risk of or exacerbate symptoms of lymphedema.[182–184] In contradiction to the long-held dogma that weight lifting is not safe for patients with lymphedema, those in the weight lifting group of the Schmitz study demonstrated a decreased incidence of exacerbations of lymphedema as well as reduced symptoms and increased strength.[184] A later randomized prospective trial by Schmitz et al. demonstrated not only that women at risk for breast cancer–related lymphedema who lifted weights did not see an increased incidence of lymphedema, but also that the women in the highest risk group actually saw a decreased risk of lymphedema compared with the control group.[185] Comprehensive treatment of lymphedema should address weight control because of the association between increased body mass and lymphedema.[172,182,183] Although the women in the majority of the trials evaluating the effects of resistive exercises wore compression garments, it is not clear that they are necessary for safe exercise.[186]

REHABILITATION INTERVENTIONS

Therapeutic Exercise

The benefits of exercise in cancer patients during and after treatment, as well as for cancer survivors, are perhaps the best studied topic in cancer rehabilitation. Several systematic reviews and meta-analyses have exhaustively evaluated the available evidence concerning the role of exercise in cancer.[187–191] Physical activity has been shown to have positive effects on physiology, body composition, physical functions, psychological outcomes, and quality of life after treatment for breast cancer.[190] When other cancer types are included, physical activity is also associated with reduced body mass index and body weight, increased peak oxygen consumption, peak power output, as well as improved quality of life.[190] Exercise also has a modest positive effect on depressive symptoms in cancer survivors.[189] The American College of Sports Medicine has issued guidelines on the safety and efficacy of exercise during and after cancer treatments and concluded that exercise results in improvements in physical functioning, quality of life, and cancer-related fatigue for several cancer groups.[192]

Among the multiple rationales of exercise in the cancer setting are avoiding effects of deconditioning, which include muscle weakness and atrophy, loss of cardiopulmonary fitness, and improving efficiency of energy metabolism at a cellular level. Improved immune effects have also been reported with exercise in cancer survivors, including increases in natural killer cell cytolytic activity, monocyte function, proportion of circulating granulocytes, and decreases in the duration of neutropenia.[193] Appropriate precautions should be incorporated into the exercise program (see Tables 152.1 and 152.2). A physician recommendation to exercise improves compliance.[194] The program should incorporate interventions for strength, endurance, and flexibility, and should be individualized. When possible, the form of exercise should be one that is enjoyable and sustainable.

Another strong justification for exercise in cancer patients is weight reduction. Body mass index is directly proportional to tumor recurrence rates and all-cause mortality.[195] Obesity is also a risk factor for lymphedema.[196] Weight control and weight reduction require a limitation of caloric intake, but patients in the active treatment phase may have side effects that interfere with adequate nutrition, and in this setting, promoting increased caloric intake may be an integral part of management. The use of anabolic steroids has been described to augment weight gain and the building of muscle mass but is rarely used in clinical practice.[7] Hydration must be adequate to prevent orthostatic hypotension.

An appropriate exercise program should be discussed with all cancer patients, with the exception of those with cachexia. Cachexia is defined as more than a 25% loss of lean bone mass or a body mass index 10% or less below normal range. Most cachectic patients are not consuming adequate amounts of protein or calories to meet basal needs and rehabilitation efforts should focus on maintaining basic functional skills and quality-of-life priorities. Any activity program that is attempted should be individualized, taking into account the patient's comfort and the incorporation of rest periods.

It is estimated that 50% to 90% of patients experience fatigue at some point during the continuum of the cancer experience.[197] Although much of the initial fatigue and the extremely pervasive nature of this disorder is likely due to primary treatment with chemotherapy and radiation, the disorder can persist for months or even years after treatment. The pathogenesis of cancer-related fatigue (CRF) is not well understood. A variety of pathogenic mechanisms are likely to contribute including tumor-related effects, effects of cancer treatment on the central or peripheral nervous system, muscle energy metabolism, comorbid medical conditions (anemia), hypothyroidism, cytokines, sleep disturbances (circadian rhythms), mediators of inflammation and stress, immune activation, hormonal changes related to effects on the hypothalamic pituitary axis, premature menopause in women, androgen deprivation in men, psychological factors (anxiety, depression), or other unknown factors.[197,198] A Cochrane review concluded that aerobic exercise is beneficial for individuals with CRF during and after cancer therapy, specifically for those with breast and prostate cancer, but not for those with hematologic malignancies.[198] Another Cochrane review noted preliminary evidence for the use of psychostimulants to treat CRF but acknowledged that the number of trials was small

PALLIATIVE AND ALTERNATIVE CARE

(5) and more data are needed before definitive recommendations concerning their usage and safety could be made.[199]

Therapeutic Modalities

Physical modalities are nonpharmacologic agents used to produce a therapeutic effect in tissues.[200] They include heat, cold, and electrotherapy. They are frequently used to reduce pain, facilitate stretch, aid in wound care, and introduce medications such as corticosteroids.

Heat includes superficial and deep-heating modalities. Superficial heat is applied to the surface of the skin to achieve the maximum tissue temperatures in skin and subcutaneous fat. Heat should not be applied to an area of acute trauma and inflammation and in patients with bleeding diatheses, edema, peripheral vascular disease, large scars, impaired sensation, or cognitive or communication deficits that impair their ability to report pain. Superficial heat is applied using heating pads, moist compresses, hydrocollator packs, paraffin baths, and whirlpool baths. Deep heat is directed to heat muscle, tendons, ligaments, or bone. It is most commonly applied using ultrasound waves. Deep heat modalities are generally avoided to an area where active regional malignancy exists for fear of causing tumor growth.[201–203] This recommendation, however, is based on in vitro studies of tumor growth in mice subjected to ultrasound at intensities 10 times higher than are possible by standard machines.[204] There is contradictory evidence that ultrasound at various intensities can actually have an antitumor effect.[202] It is unclear if this phenomenon represents a real clinical concern and if it can be extrapolated to other heating modalities such as laser or moist heat. Because of the reported risk of increasing tumor growth with such modalities, they are generally avoided, particularly in primary tumors subject to potentially curative treatment, unless the potential benefit is substantial and outweighs the unknown risks. In patients with metastatic disease, and in areas well away from a primary tumor, the risks of contributing significantly to tumor growth or spread, if any, are likely minimal.

Medication such as 1% lidocaine or corticosteroids can be applied using ultrasound. This technique is known as *phonophoresis*, which is often used to treat tendonitis, bursitis, scar tissue, neuromas, and adhesions that may be complications associated with cancer or its treatment.[205]

Cold modalities, also known as *cryotherapy*, are often used to treat acute pain and inflammation associated with musculoskeletal disorders, as well as myofascial pain, spasticity, and emergent care of minor burns. Cryotherapy is the treatment of choice for acute trauma and inflammation. It can also be used in patients with bleeding diathesis and large scars. Cryotherapy should not be used in cold-intolerant patients or those with cryoglobulins, cold hypersensitivity, and Raynaud's disease.

TENS is the most common form of electroanalgesia and enjoys widespread use, although its effectiveness in both acute and chronic pain conditions remains controversial in both benign and malignant conditions.[206–208] It has been used to help reduce neuropathic and nociceptive pain conditions, depending on the type of TENS unit and parameters chosen. It is applied by placing one to four electrode pads surrounding the area of pain. A small stimulating unit is connected and specific frequency, pulse width, and amplitude settings are selected based on the type of pain and the patient's response. The analgesic effect of TENS may be the result of a combination of mechanisms, including acting as a counterirritant in the CNS to inhibit activity of dorsal horn nociceptive neurons, activating the production of endogenous opioids, and possibly activating other neurotransmitter systems, including the serotonergic and substance P systems. As with deep heating modalities such as ultrasound, it is recommended that TENS should not be delivered over or near a malignancy unless it is being used in patients with terminal cancer. As with ultrasound, however, there is little evidence to support this recommendation.

Orthotics and Prosthetics

Patients with weakness or impaired balance often need equipment such as assistive devices for ambulation, bath equipment such as a tub bench and raised toilet seat, and other equipment for self-care such as reachers. A wheeled walker usually suffices for individuals with balance impairment or with mild weakness and allows for a quicker cadence than a standard walker, which must be manually lifted between steps. However, a standard walker is needed when more severe weakness is present or when protected weight bearing is needed.

Foot drop (weakness of dorsiflexion) is often seen in the cancer setting as a result of a brain, spinal cord, cauda equina, L-5 root, lumbosacral trunk, sciatic nerve, or most commonly, peroneal nerve injury. Patients with foot drop will often benefit from an AFO, which helps to restore a more normal gait pattern by allowing the foot to clear the ground without hiking the hip. A number of AFO designs exist. If the patient has some residual dorsiflexor strength, a relatively normal-shaped limb, and normal skin integrity, a prefabricated posterior leaf-spring orthosis may be adequate. For most patients, a custom-molded AFO or posterior leaf-spring orthosis is the brace of choice because of its better fit and more durable design. For patients with weakness of plantar flexion as well as dorsiflexion, a higher medial–lateral trim line will increase medial–lateral stability and help prevent ankle sprain. This modified AFO design may compromise the optimal gait, however, because it is generally too stiff to allow for passive dorsiflexion in the terminal stance phase of the gait cycle. This can be overcome by using a hinged AFO design with free dorsiflexion or a dorsiflexion stop at 15 degrees and a plantar flexion stop at neutral. This will provide excellent medial–lateral stability without significantly affecting terminal stance. For patients with severe spasticity or pain on ankle motion, a solid AFO is indicated. For most patients, a plastic orthotic is preferred because it is relatively aesthetic, lightweight, and can be used with different pairs of shoes. In instances in which lower extremity pain, fluctuating edema, skin fragility, deformity, or other circumstances prohibit the use of a plastic molded AFO, a double-metal upright AFO may be an option. There are a variety of other orthotics available to optimize deficits arising from other peripheral nervous system dysfunction. Knee-immobilizers, for instance, are often useful to control knee flexion in patients with femoral neuropathy or lumbar plexopathy.[63]

NONPHARMACOLOGIC PAIN MANAGEMENT

Rehabilitation medicine typically emphasizes nonpharmacologic interventions in addition to medications to address pain associated with musculoskeletal and neuromuscular syndromes. The primary goal of this approach is to limit the impact of pain on function and to minimize disability. The emphasis of nonpharmacologic pain management may be of particular benefit in elderly patients who may not tolerate medications well. Historically, direct tumor spread is thought to account for most cancer pain.[209] As treatments for cancer have improved and an emphasis has been placed on cancer survivorship, more pain disorders encountered in the cancer setting are related to causes other than the direct effects of a tumor. These disorders include treatment effects and degenerative diseases of various types.

The appropriate treatment depends on the nature and type of pain. The identification and treatment of depression, anxiety, fatigue, quality of sleep, and mood can have a marked impact on pain and should be considered as part of multimodal treatment where appropriate in all patients.[210,211] Psychological strategies such as guided imagery, hypnotherapy, biofeedback, and deep breathing can be effective.[212] Pain may respond to PT to improve muscle strength and condition as well as to improve joint ROM. Physical modalities including heat, cold, and electrotherapy may be of benefit where appropriate.[200] Aerobic exercise has been shown to improve mental outlook and may result in an improved ability to cope with pain in a variety of clinical settings including cancer.[213] Pain of muscle or bone etiology is usually worse on weight bearing or other mechanical stress and improves with rest. Splinting or assistive devices may help achieve protected weight bearing. Neuropathic pain may benefit from desensitization measures such as vibration or tapping. Topical agents such as anesthetic (lidocaine) patches or chili pepper extract–based ointments (capsaicin) can be tried (the latter should not be applied to the face). A local injection of anesthetic into trigger or tender points can be effective at relieving pain in select patients, although there is no clear evidence to support either the benefit or ineffectiveness of such procedures.[214] Similarly, the injection of corticosteroids or viscosupplements into arthritic or inflamed joints may help decrease pain and improve function.[215] Complimentary therapies such as acupuncture, mind–body techniques, and massage therapy may help with a variety of cancer- and cancer treatment–related symptoms including pain.[216,217] In severe cases, neurosurgical procedures, such as intrathecal pumps, dorsal column stimulation, and neuroablative procedures (neurectomy, rhizotomy, cordotomy) can be considered.

SELECTED REFERENCES

The full reference list can be accessed at lwwhealthlibrary.com/oncology.

1. Stubblefield MD, O'Dell MW. *Cancer Rehabilitation Principles and Practice.* New York: Demos Medical Publishers; 2009.
2. Cancer Facts & Figures 2013. American Cancer Society Web site. http://www.cancer.org/research/cancerfactsfigures/cancerfactsfigures/cancer-facts-figures-2013.
3. Mariotto AB, Yabroff KR, Shao Y, et al. Projections of the cost of cancer care in the United States: 2010-2020. *J Natl Cancer Inst* 2011;103:117–128.
11. Toothaker TB, Rubin M. Paraneoplastic neurologic syndromes: a review. *Neurologist* 2009;15:21–33.
12. Hauer-Jensen M, Fink LM, Wang J. Radiation injury and the protein C pathway. *Crit Care Med* 2004;32:S325–S330.
13. Stubblefield MD. Radiation fibrosis syndrome: neuromuscular and musculoskeletal complications in cancer survivors. *PM R* 2011;3:1041–1054.
14. Clinical Practice Guidelines in Oncology. Venous thromboembolic disease V.1.2010. National Comprehensive Cancer Network Web site. http://www.nccn.org.
15. Kelly BM, Yoder BM, Tang CT, et al. Venous thromboembolic events in the rehabilitation setting. *PM R* 2010;2:647–663.
16. Partsch H. Bed rest versus ambulation in the initial treatment of patients with proximal deep vein thrombosis. *Curr Opin Pulmonary Med* 2002;8:389–393.
17. Kiser TS, Stefans VA. Pulmonary embolism in rehabilitation patients: relation to time before return to physical therapy after diagnosis of deep vein thrombosis. *Arch Phys Med Rehabil* 1997;78:942–945.
20. Partsch H, Kechavarz B, Kohn H, et al. The effect of mobilisation of patients during treatment of thromboembolic disorders with low-molecular-weight heparin. *Int Angiol* 1997;16:189–192.
21. Schellong SM, Schwarz T, Kropp J, et al. Bed rest in deep vein thrombosis and the incidence of scintigraphic pulmonary embolism. *Thromb Haemost* 1999;82:127–129.
22. Partsch H, Blattler W. Compression and walking versus bed rest in the treatment of proximal deep venous thrombosis with low molecular weight heparin. *J Vasc Surg* 2000;32:861–869.
23. Aschwanden M, Labs KH, Engel H, et al. Acute deep vein thrombosis: early mobilization does not increase the frequency of pulmonary embolism. *Thromb Haemost* 2001;85:42–46.
24. Partsch H. Therapy of deep vein thrombosis with low molecular weight heparin, leg compression and immediate ambulation. *Vasa* 2001;30:195–204.
25. Junger M, Diehm C, Storiko H, et al. Mobilization versus immobilization in the treatment of acute proximal deep venous thrombosis: a prospective, randomized, open, multicentre trial. *Curr Med Res Opin* 2006;22:593–602.
28. Partsch H. Ambulation and compression after deep vein thrombosis: dispelling myths. *Semin Vasc Surg* 2005;18:148–152.
29. Kahn SR, Shrier I, Kearon C. Physical activity in patients with deep venous thrombosis: a systematic review. *Thromb Res* 2008;122:763–773.
30. Gay V, Hamilton R, Heiskell S, et al. Influence of bedrest or ambulation in the clinical treatment of acute deep vein thrombosis on patient outcomes: a review and synthesis of the literature. *Medsurg Nurs* 2009;18:293–299.
31. Aissaoui N, Martins E, Mouly S, et al. A meta-analysis of bed rest versus early ambulation in the management of pulmonary embolism, deep vein thrombosis, or both. *Int J Cardiol* 2009;137:37–41.
34. Custodio CM. Neuromuscular complications of cancer and cancer treatments. *Phys Med Rehabil Clin N Am* 2008;19:27–45.
36. O'Dell MW, Barr K, Spanier D, et al. Functional outcome of inpatient rehabilitation in persons with brain tumors. *Arch Phys Med Rehab* 1998;79:1530–1534.
38. Geler-Kulcu D, Gulsen G, Buyukbaba E, et al. Functional recovery of patients with brain tumor or acute stroke after rehabilitation: A comparative study. *J Clin Neurosci* 2009;16:74–78.
40. Kirshblum S, O'Dell MW, Ho C, et al. Rehabilitation of persons with central nervous system tumors. *Cancer* 2001;92:1029–1038.
41. Parsch D, Mikut R, Abel R. Postacute management of patients with spinal cord injury due to metastatic tumour disease: survival and efficacy of rehabilitation. *Spinal Cord* 2003;41:205–210.
42. Stubblefield MD, Bilsky MH. Barriers to rehabilitation of the neurosurgical spine cancer patient. *J Surg Oncol* 2007;95:419–426.

43. Wang JC, Boland P, Mitra N, et al. Single-stage posterolateral transpedicular approach for resection of epidural metastatic spine tumors involving the vertebral body with circumferential reconstruction: results in 140 patients. Invited submission from the Joint Section Meeting on Disorders of the Spine and Peripheral Nerves, March 2004. *J Neurosurg Spine* 2004;1:287–298.
44. Guo Y, Young B, Palmer JL, et al. Prognostic factors for survival in metastatic spinal cord compression: a retrospective study in a rehabilitation setting. *Am J Phys Med Rehabil* 2003;82:665–668.
49. McKinley WO, Conti-Wyneken AR, Vokac CW, et al. Rehabilitative functional outcome of patients with neoplastic spinal cord compressions. *Arch Phys Med Rehabil* 1996;77:892–895.
54. Posner JB. *Neurologic Complications of Cancer.* Philadelphia: F.A. Davis Company; 1995.
55. Chamberlain MC. Neurotoxicity of cancer treatment. *Curr Oncol Rep* 2010;12:60–67.
58. Hsia AW, Katz JS, Hancock SL, et al. Post-irradiation polyradiculopathy mimics leptomeningeal tumor on MRI. *Neurology* 2003;60:1694–1696.
61. Kristensen O, Melgard B, Schiodt AV. Radiation myelopathy of the lumbosacral spinal cord. *Acta Neurol Scand* 1977;56:217–222.
63. Lamy C, Mas JL, Varet B, et al. Postradiation lower motor neuron syndrome presenting as monomelic amyotrophy. *J Neurol Neurosurg Psychiatry* 1991;54:648–649.
64. Bowen J, Gregory R, Squier M, et al. The post-irradiation lower motor neuron syndrome neuronopathy or radiculopathy? *Brain* 1996;119:1429–1439.
65. Stubblefield MD, Slovin S, MacGregor-Cortelli B, et al. An electrodiagnostic evaluation of the effect of pre-existing peripheral nervous system disorders in patients treated with the novel proteasome inhibitor bortezomib. *Clin Oncol (R Coll Radiol)* 2006;18:410–418.
66. Stubblefield MD, McNeely ML, Alfano CM, et al. A prospective surveillance model for physical rehabilitation of women with breast cancer: chemotherapy-induced peripheral neuropathy. *Cancer* 2012;118:2250–2260.
67. Dropcho EJ. Remote neurologic manifestations of cancer. *Neurol Clin* 2002;20:85–122.
68. Jaeckle KA. Neurological manifestations of neoplastic and radiation-induced plexopathies. *Semin Neurol* 2004;24:385–393.
73. Dropcho EJ. Neurotoxicity of radiation therapy. *Neurol Clin* 2010;28:217–234.
74. Galecki J, Hicer-Grzenkowicz J, Grudzien-Kowalska M, et al. Radiation-induced brachial plexopathy and hypofractionated regimens in adjuvant irradiation of patients with breast cancer—a review. *Acta Oncol* 2006;45:280–284.
75. Kori SH, Foley KM, Posner JB. Brachial plexus lesions in patients with cancer: 100 cases. *Neurology* 1981;31:45–50.
77. Thomas JE, Colby MY Jr. Radiation-induced or metastatic brachial plexopathy? A diagnostic dilemma. *JAMA* 1972;222:1392–1395.
78. Ferrante MA. Brachial plexopathies: classification, causes, and consequences. *Muscle Nerve* 2004;30:547–568.
81. Stubblefield MD, Burstein HJ, Burton AW, et al. NCCN task force report: management of neuropathy in cancer. *J Natl Compr Canc Netw* 2009;7:S1–S26.
83. Lee JJ, Swain SM. Peripheral neuropathy induced by microtubule-stabilizing agents. *J Clin Oncol* 2006;24:1633–1642.
84. Umapathi T, Chaudhry V. Toxic neuropathy. *Curr Opin Neurol* 2005;18:574–580.
85. Kocer B, Sucak G, Kuruoglu R, et al. Clinical and electrophysiological evaluation of patients with thalidomide-induced neuropathy. *Acta Neurol Belg* 2009;109:120–126.
86. Quasthoff S, Hartung HP. Chemotherapy-induced peripheral neuropathy. *J Neurol* 2002;249:9–17.
87. Lauria G, Pareyson D, Sghirlanzoni A. Neurophysiological diagnosis of acquired sensory ganglionopathies. *Eur Neurol* 2003;50:146–152.
88. Ramchandren S, Lewis RA. Monoclonal gammopathy and neuropathy. *Curr Opin Neurol* 2009;22:480–485.
89. Portlock CS, Boland P, Hays AP, et al. Nemaline myopathy: a possible late complication of Hodgkin's disease therapy. *Hum Pathol* 2003;34:816–818.
97. Owczarek J, Jasinska M, Orszulak-Michalak D. Drug-induced myopathies. An overview of the possible mechanisms. *Pharmacol Rep* 2005;57:23–34.

98. Batchelor TT, Taylor LP, Thaler HT, et al. Steroid myopathy in cancer patients. *Neurology* 1997;48:1234–1238.

100. Stoll G, Bendszus M, Perez J, et al. Magnetic resonance imaging of the peripheral nervous system. *J Neurol* 2009;256:1043–1051.

101. van Es HW, Bollen TL, van Heesewijk HP. MRI of the brachial plexus: A pictorial review. *Eur J Radiol* 2010;74:391–402.

102. Huang JH, Johnson VE, Zager EL. Tumors of the peripheral nerves and plexuses. *Curr Treat Options Neurol* 2006;8:299–308.

103. England JD, Gronseth GS, Franklin G, et al. Evaluation of distal symmetric polyneuropathy: the role of laboratory and genetic testing (an evidence-based review). *Muscle Nerve* 2009;39:116–125.

104. Stubblefield MD, Custodio CM. Upper-extremity pain disorders in breast cancer. *Arch Phys Med Rehabil* 2006;87:S96–99.

105. Coleman RE, Rubens RD. The clinical course of bone metastases from breast cancer. *Br J Cancer* 1987;55:61–66.

107. Bunting RW, Shea B. Bone metastasis and rehabilitation. *Cancer* 2001;92:1020–1028.

108. Mirels H. Metastatic disease in long bones. A proposed scoring system for diagnosing impending pathologic fractures. *Clin Orthop Relat Res* 1989:256–264.

109. Van der Linden YM, Dijkstra PD, Kroon HM, et al. Comparative analysis of risk factors for pathological fracture with femoral metastases. *J Bone Joint Surg Br* 2004;86:566–573.

111. Fisher CG, DiPaola CP, Ryken TC, et al. A novel classification system for spinal instability in neoplastic disease: an evidence-based approach and expert consensus from the Spine Oncology Study Group. *Spine (Phila Pa 1976)* 2010;35:E1221–1229.

112. Fourney DR, Frangou EM, Ryken TC, et al. Spinal instability neoplastic score: an analysis of reliability and validity from the spine oncology study group. *J Clin Oncol* 2011;29:3072–3077.

113. Bilsky MH. New therapeutics in spine metastases. *Expert Rev Neurother* 2005;5:831–840.

114. Laufer I, Rubin DG, Lis E, et al. The NOMS framework: approach to the treatment of spinal metastatic tumors. *Oncologist* 2013;18:744–751.

115. Yarnold J, Brotons MC. Pathogenetic mechanisms in radiation fibrosis. *Radiother Oncol* 2010;97:149–161.

117. New P. Radiation injury to the nervous system. *Curr Opin Neurol* 2001;14:725–734.

121. Thompson CA, Mauck K, Havyer R, et al. Care of the adult Hodgkin lymphoma survivor. *Am J Med* 2011;124:1106–1112.

122. Cross NE, Glantz MJ. Neurologic complications of radiation therapy. *Neurol Clin* 2003;21:249–277.

123. Pradat PF, Delanian S. Late radiation injury to peripheral nerves. *Handb Clin Neurol* 2013;115:743–758.

126. Baxi SS, Matasar MJ. State-of-the-art issues in Hodgkin's lymphoma survivorship. *Curr Oncol Rep* 2010;12:366–373.

127. Jaeckle KA. Neurologic manifestations of neoplastic and radiation-induced plexopathies. *Semin Neurol* 2010;30:254–262.

128. Herrera JE, Stubblefield MD. Rotator cuff tendonitis in lymphedema: a retrospective case series. *Arch Phys Med Rehabil* 2004;85:1939–1942.

129. Dijkstra PU, van Wilgen PC, Buijs RP, et al. Incidence of shoulder pain after neck dissection: a clinical explorative study for risk factors. *Head Neck* 2001;23:947–953.

131. Speksnijder CM, van der Bilt A, Slappendel M, et al. Neck and shoulder function in patients treated for oral malignancies: a 1-year prospective cohort study. *Head Neck* 2013;35:1303–1313.

132. McNeely ML, Parliament M, Courneya KS, et al. A pilot study of a randomized controlled trial to evaluate the effects of progressive resistance exercise training on shoulder dysfunction caused by spinal accessory neurapraxia/neurectomy in head and neck cancer survivors. *Head Neck* 2004;26:518–530.

133. McNeely ML, Parliament MB, Seikaly H, et al. Effect of exercise on upper extremity pain and dysfunction in head and neck cancer survivors: a randomized controlled trial. *Cancer* 2008;113:214–222.

134. Lauchlan DT, McCaul JA, McCarron T, et al. An exploratory trial of preventative rehabilitation on shoulder disability and quality of life in patients following neck dissection surgery. *Eur J Cancer Care (Engl)* 2011;20:113–122.

135. Carvalho AP, Vital FM, Soares BG. Exercise interventions for shoulder dysfunction in patients treated for head and neck cancer. *Cochrane Database Syst Rev* 2012;4:CD008693.

136. Dijkstra PU, Kalk WW, Roodenburg JL. Trismus in head and neck oncology: a systematic review. *Oral Oncol* 2004;40:879–889.

141. Wang CJ, Huang EY, Hsu HC, et al. The degree and time-course assessment of radiation-induced trismus occurring after radiotherapy for nasopharyngeal cancer. *Laryngoscope* 2005;115:1458–1460.

148. Tang Y, Shen Q, Wang Y, et al. A randomized prospective study of rehabilitation therapy in the treatment of radiation-induced dysphagia and trismus. *Strahlenther Onkol* 2011;187:39–44.

152. Stubblefield MD, Levine A, Custodio CM, et al. The role of botulinum toxin type A in the radiation fibrosis syndrome: a preliminary report. *Arch Phys Med Rehabil* 2008;89:417–421.

153. Hartl DM, Cohen M, Julieron M, et al. Botulinum toxin for radiation-induced facial pain and trismus. *Otolaryngol Head Neck Surg* 2008;138:459–463.

155. Cohen EG, Deschler DG, Walsh K, et al. Early use of a mechanical stretching device to improve mandibular mobility after composite resection: a pilot study. *Arch Phys Med Rehabil* 2005;86:1416–1419.

156. Kamstra JI, Roodenburg JL, Beurskens CH, et al. TheraBite exercises to treat trismus secondary to head and neck cancer. *Support Care Cancer* 2013;21:951–957.

163. Shulman DH, Shipman B, Willis FB. Treating trismus with dynamic splinting: a cohort, case series. *Adv Ther* 2008;25:9–16.

164. Stubblefield MD, Manfield L, Riedel ER. A preliminary report on the efficacy of a dynamic jaw opening device (dynasplint trismus system) as part of the multimodal treatment of trismus in patients with head and neck cancer. *Arch Phys Med Rehabil* 2010;91:1278–1282.

167. Costa J, Espirito-Santo C, Borges A, et al. Botulinum toxin type A therapy for cervical dystonia. *Cochrane Database Syst Rev* 2005:CD003633.

168. DiSipio T, Rye S, Newman B, et al. Incidence of unilateral arm lymphoedema after breast cancer: a systematic review and meta-analysis. *Lancet Oncol* 2013;14:500–515.

172. Cheville AL, McGarvey CL, Petrek JA, et al. Lymphedema management. *Semin Radiat Oncol* 2003;13:290–301.

175. Paskett ED, Dean JA, Oliveri JM, et al. Cancer-related lymphedema risk factors, diagnosis, treatment, and impact: a review. *J Clin Oncol* 2012;30:3726–3733.

177. Carati CJ, Anderson SN, Gannon BJ, et al. Treatment of postmastectomy lymphedema with low-level laser therapy: a double blind, placebo-controlled trial. *Cancer* 2003;98:1114–1122.

178. Ahmed Omar MT, Abd-El-Gayed Ebid A, El Morsy AM. Treatment of post-mastectomy lymphedema with laser therapy: double blind placebo control randomized study. *J Surg Res* 2011;165:82–90.

181. Mehrara BJ, Zampell JC, Suami H, et al. Surgical management of lymphedema: past, present, and future. *Lymphatic Res Biol* 2011;9:159–167.

182. Ahmed RL, Thomas W, Yee D, et al. Randomized controlled trial of weight training and lymphedema in breast cancer survivors. *J Clin Oncol* 2006;24:2765–2772.

183. Sagen A, Karesen R, Risberg MA. Physical activity for the affected limb and arm lymphedema after breast cancer surgery. A prospective, randomized controlled trial with two years follow-up. *Acta Oncol* 2009;48:1102–1110.

184. Schmitz KH, Ahmed RL, Troxel A, et al. Weight lifting in women with breast-cancer-related lymphedema. *N Engl J Med* 2009;361:664–673.

185. Schmitz KH, Ahmed RL, Troxel AB, et al. Weight lifting for women at risk for breast cancer-related lymphedema: a randomized trial. *JAMA* 2010;304:2699–2705.

186. Kwan ML, Cohn JC, Armer JM, et al. Exercise in patients with lymphedema: a systematic review of the contemporary literature. *J Cancer Surviv* 2011;5:320–336.

188. McNeely ML, Campbell KL, Rowe BH, et al. Effects of exercise on breast cancer patients and survivors: a systematic review and meta-analysis. *CMAJ* 2006;175:34–41.

190. Fong DY, Ho JW, Hui BP, et al. Physical activity for cancer survivors: meta-analysis of randomised controlled trials. *BMJ* 2012;344:e70.

191. Jones LW, Alfano CM. Exercise-oncology research: past, present, and future. *Acta Oncol* 2013;52:195–215.

192. Schmitz KH, Courneya KS, Matthews C, et al. American College of Sports Medicine roundtable on exercise guidelines for cancer survivors. *Med Sci Sports Exerc* 2010;42:1409–1426.

197. Campos MP, Hassan BJ, Riechelmann R, et al. Cancer-related fatigue: a practical review. *Ann Oncol* 2011;22:1273–1279.

201. Sicard-Rosenbaum L, Danoff J. Cancer and ultrasound: a warning. *Phys Ther* 1993;73:404–406.

202. Sicard-Rosenbaum L, Lord D, Danoff JV, et al. Effects of continuous therapeutic ultrasound on growth and metastasis of subcutaneous murine tumors. *Phys Ther* 1995;75:3–11.

203. Sicard-Rosenbaum L, Danoff JV, Guthrie JA, et al. Effects of energy-matched pulsed and continuous ultrasound on tumor growth in mice. *Phys Ther* 1998;78:271–277.

204. Robertson VJ, Ward AR. Dangers in extrapolating in vitro uses of therapeutic ultrasound. *Phys Ther* 1996;76:78–79.

153 Complementary, Alternative, and Integrative Therapies in Cancer Care

Catherine E. Ulbricht

BACKGROUND

Definitions

In the United States, complementary and alternative medicine (CAM) is defined by the National Center for Complementary and Alternative Medicine (NCCAM) as a group of diverse medical and health-care systems, practices, and products that are not normally considered to be conventional medicine.[1] Other terms used to refer to CAM include folkloric, holistic, irregular, nonconventional, non-Western, traditional, unconventional, unorthodox, and unproven medicines. NCCAM classifies CAM therapies into five categories or domains: alternative medical systems, mind–body interventions, biologically based therapies, manipulative and body-based methods, and energy therapies (Table 153.1).[1–3]

Recently, the term *integrative medicine* has come into common use. The Consortium of Academic Health Centers for Integrative Medicine has defined this term as the practice of medicine that reaffirms the importance of the relationship between practitioner and patient, that focuses on the whole person, is informed by evidence, and makes use of all appropriate therapeutic approaches, providers, and disciplines to achieve optimal health and healing.

Prevalence

In the United States, an estimated 44% of the population used at least one CAM therapy in 1997.[2,4–6] According to the 2007 National Health Interview Survey (NHIS), the prevalence of CAM use in the United States was approximately 38% for adults and 12% for children.[7]

Surveys published since 1999 suggest that between 25% and 83% of US adult cancer patients have used CAM therapies at some point after diagnosis, with variations in utilization rates depending on geographic area and type of cancer.[8–25] Earlier studies generally report lower overall prevalence of CAM use (9% to 54%), possibly due to increasing rates of use or broadening of the definition of CAM.[26,27] Initial studies of CAM prevalence during the 1970s and 1980s focused on the toxicity of the anticancer therapy laetrile. The reported prevalence of CAM was 9% to 16%,[27] but surveys within the past decade estimated the prevalence of use in pediatric oncology to be 31% to 87%; moreover, in many cases, the treating physician was unaware that their patients were using CAM.[28–31] Use of CAM is also prevalent among cancer patients outside the United States in all regions of the world, with significantly varying use among different regions.[26,32,33]

In the West, CAM use appears to be more common among those with higher education levels and higher incomes. CAM use is also higher among young females who have had surgery, used chemotherapy, or had a history of CAM use before diagnosis.[19,32,34,35]

ESTABLISHING AN INTEGRATIVE ONCOLOGY APPROACH WITH PATIENTS

Integrative Oncology Model

An integrative approach to cancer should be comprehensive, personalized, evidence-based, and safe. The conventional model of cancer treatment involves three different disciplines (surgery, radiation, chemotherapy), and integrative oncology aims to expand the interdisciplinary approach to include therapies such as acupuncture, yoga, meditation, diet, exercise, and other modalities. This is in response to the concept of treating the whole patient in all domains. Engel's biopsychosocial model of health care, first published in *Science* more than 30 years ago, describes one conceptual model of these domains of patient care and its importance in the treatment of all patients.[36] The Integrative Medicine Program at M. D. Anderson Cancer Center provides one example of how this framework may assist in creating comprehensive integrative care plans (Fig. 153.1). Without a comprehensive assessment and appropriate attention given to their needs, patients may perceive gaps in their care. Although symptoms such as severe pain or nausea are typically thought of as purely physical symptoms, if symptoms remain severe and chronic, they will often impact the psychosocial dimensions of health as patients may become more irritable, socially inactive, and fatigued due to insomnia. With comprehensive care plans, patients will have cancer treatments that address all of their needs in a more seamless manner. These plans will also have the greatest potential for improving the overall health and well-being of cancer patients. These basic comprehensive evaluations are aggregates of many different components; by addressing issues of nutrition, physical activity, symptom control, and other factors, these plans will help improve the performance of cancer patients throughout the continuum of care.

Physical Well-Being

Growing evidence supports the important role of physical activity and nutrition in the health of cancer patients, and these factors

TABLE 153.1	
National Institutes of Health: National Center for Complementary and Alternative Medicine Categories	
Whole medical systems	Traditional Chinese medicine, Ayurvedic medicine
Biologically based therapies	Herbs, supplements, special diets
Mind–body therapies	Meditation, prayer, yoga
Body manipulation	Chiropractic, massage
Energy therapies	Qi gong, Reiki, magnetic

have been correlated with improved clinical outcomes. Moreover, several phytochemicals demonstrate pharmacologic effects on molecular targets in known cancer signaling pathways.[37] The Women's Intervention Study reported that a 24% reduction in fat intake resulted in lower cancer recurrence rates.[38] Participants were randomized to increase fruit and vegetable intake and reduce dietary fat, but a significant reduction in breast cancer events was not found; however, when secondary analyses were performed, including physical activity, an increased survival of approximately 50% was found among women who were physically active and maintained a diet high in fruits and vegetables.[39,40] Similar associations are beginning to be reported in colon cancer patients.[39–42] The American Institute for Cancer Research (AICR) and the World Cancer Research Fund (WCRF) have created a combined report for guidelines regarding nutrition and physical activity to prevent cancer; the American Cancer Society (ACS) has also published guidelines for those with cancer.[43–48] Additionally, a recent study examining obesity during neoadjuvant chemotherapy for breast cancer patients found obesity was correlated with decreased survival,[49] and a different study found that obesity predicts a second primary tumor on the contralateral breast.[50] Patients need to be encouraged to follow the ACS guidelines and the AICS/WCRF guidelines for cancer prevention and encouraged to adopt healthful behaviors in regard to physical activity and diet.

Psychosocial Well-Being: The Mind–Body Connection

The mind–body connection is an important aspect of integrative oncology, as emphasized in the recent Institute of Medicine (IOM) report "Cancer Care for the Whole Patient."[51] This comprehensive report states that "cancer care today often provides state-of-the-science biomedical treatment, but fails to address the psychological and social (psychosocial) problems associated with the illness. These problems—including . . . anxiety, depression or other emotional problems . . .—cause additional suffering, weaken adherence to prescribed treatments, and threaten patients' return to health." Extensive research has documented that mind–body interventions appear to address many of the issues mentioned in the IOM report.

The belief that what we think and feel can influence our health and healing dates back thousands of years.[52] The importance of the role of the mind, emotions, and behaviors in health and well-being has been a part of medical traditions of the world, such as Chinese, Tibetan, and Ayurvedic medicine. Many patients with cancer turn to CAM therapies as a way to reduce stress; substantial evidence now shows the negative health consequences of sustained stress on health and well-being. The profound psychological and behavioral effects of stress may include post-traumatic stress disorder, increased health-impairing behaviors (e.g., poor diet, lack of exercise, substance abuse), poor sleep, and decreased quality of life.[53–57] Research has shown that stress can also decrease compliance with regular health screening.[58,59]

Many stress-induced physiologic changes can have direct effects on health, including persistent increases in sympathetic nervous system activity and the hypothalamic–pituitary axis that can cause increased blood pressure, heart rate, catecholamine secretion, and platelet aggregation.[60–65] Furthermore, research has associated stress with increased latent viral reactivation, upper respiratory tract infections, and wound-healing time.[66–70] Stress also deregulates a variety of immune indices, as shown in both healthy subjects and cancer patients.[71] Such stress-induced physiologic changes can affect cancer progression, treatment, recovery, recurrence, and survival.[72,73] Spiegel et al.[76] first published on the possible impact of a psychosocial intervention on breast cancer survival,

Integrative Oncology Clinical Model

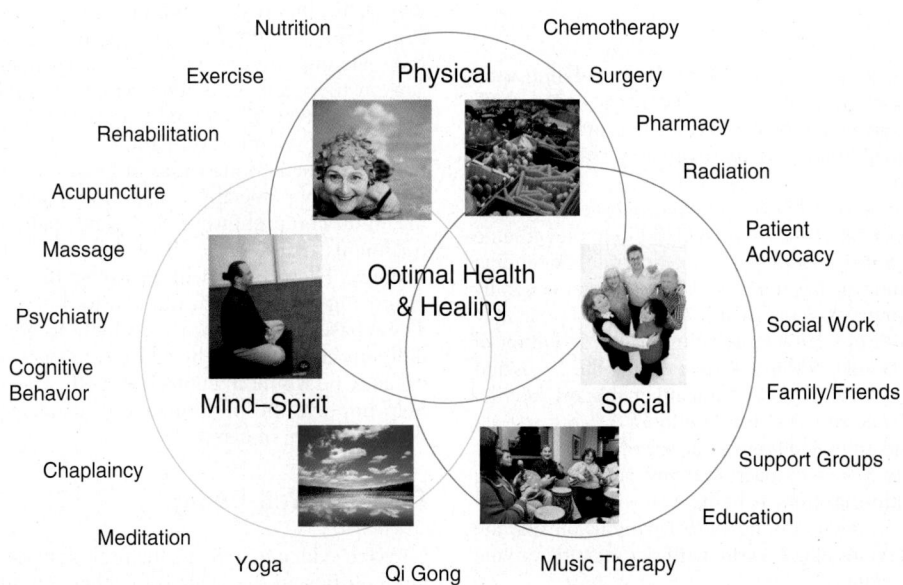

Figure 153.1 Guiding model for integrative medicine at M. D. Anderson Cancer Center.

but subsequent studies have not consistently reproduced these results.[74,75,77] However, recent research has demonstrated a survival advantage among breast cancer patients who received psychological intervention with more than 10 years of follow-up[78] as well as improved mood and quality of life during and after radiotherapy.[79] These studies underscore the importance of psychosocial intervention in cancer treatment.

Patient–Clinician Communication Regarding Complementary and Alternative Medicine

Research indicates that neither adult nor pediatric patients receive sufficient information or discuss CAM therapies with physicians, pharmacists, nurses, or CAM practitioners.[21,28] Most patients do not bring up the topic of CAM because no one asks; thus, patients may believe it is unimportant to disclose. It is estimated that 38% to 60% of patients with cancer are taking complementary medicines without informing their health-care team.[8,80] This lack of discussion is of grave concern because biologically based therapies (such as herbs) may interact with cancer treatments. Patients are commonly unaware of the differences between U.S. Food and Drug Administration (FDA)–approved medications (which require evidence of efficacy, safety, and quality control in manufacturing) and supplements, which are governed not by the FDA but by the Dietary Supplement Health and Education Act (DSHEA) of 1994. Supplements under this legislation are exempt from the same scrutiny the FDA imposes on medications; furthermore, these supplements are not intended to treat, prevent, or cure diseases. The common belief by patients that *natural* means safe needs to be addressed with education as some herbs and supplements have been associated with multiple drug interactions[81] as well as increased cancer risk and organ toxicity. These specific concerns are addressed later in this chapter.

Existing research suggests that the majority of cancer patients desire communication with their doctors about CAM,[82] and there is general agreement within the oncology community that in order to provide optimal patient care, oncologists must not only be aware of CAM use, but also be willing and able to discuss all therapeutic approaches with their patients.[83,84] It is the health-care professional's responsibility to ask patients about their use of complementary medicines,[85] and the discussion should ideally take place before the patient starts using a complementary treatment—whether it is a nutritional supplement, mind–body therapy, or other CAM approach.

A number of strategies can be used to increase the chance of a worthwhile dialogue.[86] One approach is to include the topic of CAM as part of a new patient assessment. For example, when asking about medications, physicians should inquire about everything the patient ingests—including over-the-counter products, vitamins, minerals, herbs, and even the patient's diet. Physicians may consider having the patient bring in the actual bottles of herbs and supplements for evaluation. When asking about a patient's past medical history, physicians may ask other health-care professionals to determine if the patient has visited with naturopathic or chiropractic practitioners. If the issue of CAM arises, clinicians need to develop an empathic communication strategy that addresses the patient's needs while maintaining an understanding of the current state of the science. In other words, this strategy needs to be balanced between clinical objectivity and bonding with the patient so that it can benefit both the patient and the health-care provider. These patients need reliable information on CAM from evidence-based resources such as Natural Standard Research Collaboration (www.naturalstandard.com), as well as adequate time to discuss this information with their oncologists.

Safety Concerns

Many CAM therapies can potentially cause adverse outcomes, and are thus a major concern among health-care professionals.[87–90] Nonbiologically based CAM therapies, such as massage or acupuncture, often have minimal risks when performed by trained health professionals. In contrast, herbs and supplements should be considered more similar to prescription medications in that they have the potential to have powerful effects on the natural biologic processes of the body. This is especially true when natural plants are processed into concentrated formulations. The pathways by which CAM therapies may lead to negative clinical outcomes include metabolic interactions, treatment interactions, direct organ toxicity, direct biologic effects on the cancer, and unregulated low quality manufacturing of biologically based CAM. Some of these topics are briefly reviewed here.

Metabolic Interactions

Many botanical agents are pharmacologically active, raising concerns about pharmacodynamic effects that can lead to changes with conventional therapy, such as cytotoxic agents.[87] Published data are available regarding potential interactions between specific herbs or vitamins and prescription drugs.[87,88,91–97] Overall, there is substantial clinical evidence of herb–drug interactions in general.[81] Therefore, negative interactions should be considered prior to integrating herbs, vitamins, or nutritional supplements during chemotherapy.

Common chemotherapy agents metabolized through the cytochrome P-450 system and the specific isoenzymes responsible for their metabolism are a starting point to consider possible interactions. St. John's wort (*Hypericum perforatum*) is of particular concern, with multiple well-documented drug interactions. This herb appears to inhibit the hepatic enzyme cytochrome P-450 3A4 acutely, then induce it with repeated administration. A study of individuals given irinotecan (CPT11) reports a greater than 50% reduction in serum levels of the active metabolite SN38 after concomitant administration of St. John's wort.[98] Imatinib levels appear to be altered by similar mechanisms.[99] St. John's wort and similar herb–chemotherapy combinations should be used with extreme caution because of the potential for alterations in drug metabolism.

The common practice by patients of combining compounds, in which there is a lack of data regarding the pharmacodynamics and pharmacokinetics, creates a dangerous situation that may lead to inadvertent detrimental impact on clinical outcomes. This possible negative impact must be evaluated and discussed with patients whenever considering the use of untested natural products with other therapies.

Treatment Interactions

Antioxidant Interference with Chemotherapy or Radiation. Because oxidative damage to cells may increase the risk of cancer, the use of antioxidant herbs and vitamins has been proposed for cancer treatment or prevention. Examples include vitamins A, C, and E, as well as lycopene, green tea, soy, grape seed extract, melatonin, and selenium. Concern has been raised that antioxidants may interfere with radiation therapy or some chemotherapy agents (e.g., alkylating agents, anthracyclines, or platinums), which themselves can depend on oxidative damage to tumor cells for their cytotoxic effects. Studies of the effects of antioxidants on cancer therapies have yielded mixed results, with some reporting antagonistic effects, others noting synergism (i.e., benefits), and most suggesting no significant interaction.[89,90,100,101] A large randomized trial of head and neck cancer patients evaluated the use of beta-carotene and vitamin E for the reduction of radiation side effects.[102] Results found a reduction in side effects, but also found decreased survival among patients taking beta-carotene and vitamin E. Additionally, the use of these antioxidants seemed to correlate to an increase in second primary cancer.[103] Whether antioxidants are beneficial or harmful is a critical question without a clear scientific answer at this time; rather, it remains an area of continuing study and controversy.[104,105]

Direct Organ Toxicity

Hepatotoxicity and Nephrotoxicity. The long-term use of concentrated natural products is an increasing concern. A recent report evaluating the risk for end-stage renal disease in Taiwan found that chronic use of traditional Chinese medicine herbs carried an increased risk of kidney failure.[106] Multiple herbs and supplements may cause hepatotoxicity or transaminitis based on human research or known hepatotoxic constituents and should be used cautiously in combination with other hepatotoxic agents (Table 153.2).

Hematologic Toxicity

Many herbs and supplements carry an increased risk of bleeding. Multiple case studies have reported clinically significant bleeding with the use of *Ginkgo biloba* (either alone or with aspirin or warfarin), and isolated case reports of bleeding with the use of saw palmetto (*Serenoa repens*), fish oil, and garlic (*Allium sativum*).[81] The suspected mechanism for increased bleeding is interference with platelet function. Because herbal supplementation is common among cancer patients, surgical staff should screen patients presurgically for use of herbal and other dietary supplements. These agents should be discontinued before surgical procedures, and should be used cautiously with other agents that increase the risk of bleeding. Clinicians should also be cautious about taking natural products concurrently with warfarin, which is known to be sensitive to vitamin K intake and possible drug interactions. Numerous other herbs and vitamins may increase bleeding risk based on known constituents, preclinical data, or traditional use (Table 153.3).

Direct Biologic Effects on Cancer

A common concern is the potential for herbs and supplements to have procancerous effects. One clear example comes from Sidney Farber from Harvard University and the discovery of antifolate agents such as methotrexate, which came from the observation that folic acid supplementation actually promoted disease progression.[107] Until appropriate clinical trials have been completed on herbs and supplements for individual types of cancer, the resulting impact—whether beneficial, harmful, or neither—will remain unknown, and thus, caution will always be considered a prudent approach.

Phytoestrogens. Phytoestrogens are plant-based compounds structurally similar to estradiol and capable of binding to estrogen receptors as agonists or antagonists. Multiple popular herbs contain phytoestrogens, such as black cohosh (*Cimicifuga racemosa*), red clover (*Trifolium pratense*), and soy (*Glycine max*) (Table 153.4).

Although some epidemiologic evidence has found reduced breast cancer risk associated with *the* consumption of phytoestrogens,[108,109] effects of these agents in hormone-sensitive cancers remain unclear, and use in patients with estrogen receptor–positive breast cancer is controversial (see *the* Soy *section, which follows*, for further discussion).

STANDARDIZATION AND QUALITY

The preparation of herbs and supplements can vary from manufacturer to manufacturer and from batch to batch within one manufacturer. Because the active components of a product are often not clear, standardization may not be possible, and the clinical effects of different brands may not be comparable. There may also be harmful contaminants in products not manufactured under good manufacturing practice (GMP). One example includes PC-SPES, an herbal formula for the treatment of prostate cancer. This product was taken off the market in 2002 by the FDA because different lots were found to contain warfarin, indomethacin, and estrogen diethylstilbestrol.[110]

SPECIFIC COMPLEMENTARY AND ALTERNATIVE MEDICINE THERAPIES

Many cancer therapies used are the same as those used in the general population for common noncancer indications such as St. John's wort (*Hypericum perforatum*) for depression, kava (*Piper methysticum*) for anxiety, *Echinacea purpurea* for common cold symptoms, or yoga, massage, and tai chi for overall well-being. This chapter lists some of the more common therapies about which oncologists might be questioned by their patients; this only represents a small sample of therapies. Several resources are available that can provide a summary of the available evidence regarding CAM therapies.

Biologically Based Therapies Used for Cancer Treatment and Secondary Prevention

Beta-Carotene

Two large randomized trials have been completed for the prevention of lung cancer: the Alpha-Tocopherol and Beta-Carotene Cancer Prevention Trial (ATBC) and the Beta-Carotene and Retinol Efficacy Trial (CARET).[111] Neither trial showed any efficacy of beta-carotene to prevent lung cancer among patients at elevated

TABLE 153.3

Herbs and Supplements that May Increase the Risk of Bleeding or Clotting

Agents Reported to Cause Clinically Significant Bleeding in Case Report(s)
Garlic (*Allium sativum*), *Ginkgo biloba*, saw palmetto (*Serenoa repens*).

Agents that May Increase the Risk of Bleeding Based on Mechanism of Action, Preclinical Data, or Traditional Use
Acacia (*Acacia* spp.), acerola (*Malpighia emarginata*), aconite (*Aconitum* spp.), agrimony (*Agrimonia* spp.), alfalfa (*Medicago sativa*),[a] aloe (*Aloe vera*), alpha-linolenic acid, alpinia (*Alpinia* spp.), American ginseng (*Panax quinquefolius*), andrographis (*Andrographis paniculata*), angelica (*Angelica archangelica*),[a] angel's trumpet (*Brugmansia* and *Datura* spp.), anise (*Pimpinella anisum*),[a] annatto (*Bixa orellana*), aortic acid, arabinogalactan, arginine (L-arginine), aristolochia (*Aristolochia* spp.), arnica (*Arnica montana*), asafoetida (*Ferula foetida*),[a] ashwagandha (*Withania somnifera*), aspen (*Populus* spp.),[b] astragalus (*Astragalus membranaceus*), avocado (*Persea americana*), babassu (*Attalea speciosa*), banaba (*Lagerstroemia speciosa*), barley (*Hordeum vulgare*), bear's garlic (*Allium ursinum*), beta-sitosterol, bilberry (*Vaccinium myrtillus*), birch (*Betula barosma*),[b] black cohosh (*Cimicifuga racemosa*),[b] black currant (*Ribes nigrum*), bladderwrack (*Fucus vesiculosus*), blessed thistle (*Cnicus benedictus*), bogbean (*Menyanthes trifoliata*), boldo (*Peumus boldus*), borage seed oil (*Borago officinalis*), bromelain (*Ananas comosus*), bupleurum (*Bupleurum*), burdock (*Arctium lappa*), calamus (*Acorus calamus*), calendula (*Calendula* spp.), capsicum (*Capsicum* spp.), cat's claw (*Uncaria tomentosa*), celery (*Apium graveolens*),[a] chamomile (*Matricaria recutita*),[a] chaparral (*Larrea tridentata*), chia (*Salvia hispanica*), chlorella (*Chlorella* spp.), chondroitin sulfate, cinnamon (*Cinnamomum* spp.),[a] clove (*Eugenia aromaticum*), codonopsis (*Codonopsis* spp.), coenzyme Q10, coleus (*Coleus forskohlii*), coltsfoot (*Tussilago farfara*), cordyceps (*Cordyceps sinensis*), cowhage (*Mucuna pruriens*), cranberry (*Vaccinium* spp.), daisy (*Bellis perennis*), dandelion (*Taraxacum officinale*),[a] danshen (*Salvia miltiorrhiza*), datura (*Datura* spp.), dehydroepiandrosterone (DHEA), desert parsley (*Lomatium dissectum*), devil's claw (*Harpagophytum procumbens*), diallyl trisulfide, dong quai (*Angelica sinensis*), echistatin, eicosapentaenoic acid (EPA), elder (*Sambucus* spp.), evening primrose oil (*Oenothera biennis*),[c] fennel (*Foeniculum vulgare*), fenugreek (*Trigonella foenum-graecum*),[a] feverfew (*Tanacetum parthenium*),[c] fig (*Ficus carica*), fisetin, fish oil, flavonoids, flaxseed (*Linum usitatissimum*), gamma-linolenic acid, gamma-oryzanol, garlic (*Allium sativum*),[c] genistein, ginger (*Zingiber officinalis*),[c] ginkgo (*Ginkgo biloba*),[c] ginseng (*Panax* spp.),[c] globe artichoke (*Cynara scolymus*), goldenseal (*Hydrastis canadensis*), grape seed (*Vitis vinifera*), grapefruit (*Citrus* x *paradisi*), ground ivy (*Glechoma hederacea*), guarana (*Paullinia cupana*), guggul (*Commiphora mukul*), gymnema (*Gymnema sylvestre*), hawthorn (*Crataegus* spp.), heartsease (*Viola tricolor*),[b] hirudin, holy basil (*Ocimum tenuiflorum*), horny goat weed (*Epimedium* spp.), horse chestnut (*Aesculus hippocastanum*),[a] horseradish (*Radicula armoracia*), jackfruit (*Artocarpus heterophyllus*), jequirity (*Abrus precatorius*), jiaogulan (*Gynostemma pentaphyllum*), juniper (*Juniperus* spp.), kava (*Piper methysticum*), kelp (Laminariales), kinetin, kiwi (*Actinidia deliciosa*), kudzu (*Pueraria lobata*), lady's mantle (*Alchemilla* spp.), lavender (*Lavandula* spp.), lemongrass (*Cymbopogon* spp.), licorice (liquorice) (*Glycyrrhiza glabra*),[c] lotus (*Nelumbo* spp.), lovage (*Levisticum officinale*), male fern (*Dryopteris filix-mas*), marjoram (*Origanum majorana*), meadowsweet (*Spirea/Filipendula ulmaria*),[b] melatonin (N-acetyl-5-methoxytryptamine), methylsulfonylmethane (MSM), mistletoe (*Viscum album*), modified citrus pectin, mugwort (*Artemisia vulgaris*), mullein (*Verbascum* spp.), nettle (*Urtica dioica*), niacin (vitamin B3), nopal (*Opuntia* spp.), nordihydroguaiaretic acid (NDGA), octacosanol, omega-3 fatty acids, onion (*Allium cepa*), oregano (*Origanum vulgare*), pagoda tree (*Styphnolobium* spp.), pantethine, papain, papaya (*Carica papaya*), parsley (*Petroselinum crispum*), passion flower (*Passiflora incarnata*), pawpaw (*Asimina* spp.), PC-SPES, peony (*Paeonia* spp.), policosanol, polypodium (*Polypodium* spp.), poplar (*Populus* spp.),[b] prickly ash (*Zanthoxylum* spp.),[a] propolis, polysaccharide K (PSK) (*Trametes versicolor*, formerly *Coriolus versicolor*), Pycnogenol (*Pinus pinaster* subsp. *atlantica*), quassia (*Picrasma excelsa*),[a] quercetin, quinine, red clover (*Trifolium pratense*),[a] red yeast rice (*Monascus purpureus*), rehmannia (*Rehmannia* spp.), reishi (*Ganoderma* s spp.), resveratrol, rhubarb (*Rheum rhabarbarum*), Roman chamomile (*Anthemis nobilis*), rose hip (*Rosa* spp.), rosemary (*Rosmarinus officinalis*), rue (*Ruta* spp.), rutin, safflower (*Carthamus tinctorius*), sage (*Salvia officinalis*), sarsaparilla (*Smilax regelii*),[b] sassafras (*Sassafras* spp.), savory (*Satureja* spp.), saw palmetto (*Serenoa repens*), schisandra (*Schisandra* spp.), scotch broom (*Cytisus scoparius*, syn. *Sarothamnus scoparius*), sea buckthorn (*Hippophae* spp.), seaweed, selenium, shea (*Vitellaria paradoxa*, syn. *Butyrospermum parkii*, *B. paradoxa*), shiitake mushroom (*Lentinula edodes*), Siberian ginseng (*Eleutherococcus senticosus*), skullcap (*Scutellaria* spp.), sorrel (*Rumex acetosa*), soy (*Glycine max*),[c] Spanish bayonet (*Yucca* spp.), spirulina (*Arthrospira* spp.) St. John's wort (*Hypericum perforatum*), star anise (*Illicium verum*), stinging nettle (*Urtica dioica*), strawberry (*Fragaria* x *ananassa*), sweet birch (*Betula lenta*),[b] sweet clover (*Melilotus* spp.),[a] sweet pea (*Lathyrus* spp.), sweet woodruff (*Galium odoratum*), tamanu (*Calophyllum inophyllum*), tamarind (*Tamarindus indica*), tarragon (*Artemisia dracunculus*), taurine, tea (*Camellia sinensis*), thyme (*Thymus vulgaris*), tonka bean (*Dipteryx odorata*), turmeric (*Curcuma longa*), usnea (*Usnea* spp.), vanilla (*Vanilla* spp.), verbena (*Verbena* spp.), vitamin A, vitamin C,[c] vitamin E,[c] wasabi (*Wasabia japonica*), watercress (*Nasturtium officinale*), wheatgrass (*Triticum aestivum*), wild carrot (*Daucus carota*), wild lettuce (*Lactuca virosa*), willow (*Salix* spp.),[b] wintergreen (*Gaultheria* spp.),[b] yarrow (*Achillea millefolium*), yew (*Taxus* spp.), yohimbe (*Pausinystalia yohimbe*, formerly *Corynanthe yohimbe*).

Possible Procoagulant Agents
Abuta (*Abuta* spp.), acerola (*Malpighia emarginata*), aconite (*Aconitum* spp.), African wild potato (*Hypoxis hemerocallidea*), agrimony (*Agrimonia* spp.), alfalfa (*Medicago sativa*), annatto (*Bixa orellana*), apricot (*Prunus armeniaca*), arnica (*Arnica montana*), astragalus (*Astragalus membranaceus*), bael (*Aegle marmelos*), bilberry (*Vaccinium myrtillus*), black haw (*Viburnum prunifolium*), blessed thistle (*Cnicus benedictus*), cat's claw (*Uncaria tomentosa*), chlorella (*Chlorella* spp.), coenzyme Q10, *cordyceps* (*Cordyceps sinensis*), DHEA (dehydroepiandrosterone), dong quai (*Angelica sinensis*), ginseng (*Panax* spp.), goldenrod (*Solidago* spp.), goldenseal (*Hydrastis canadensis*), guggul (*Commiphora mukul*), horsetail (*Equisetum* spp.), jequirity (*Abrus precatorius*), jiaogulan (*Gynostemma pentaphyllum*), lime (*Citrus aurantifolia*), melatonin, milk thistle (*Silybum marianum*), mistletoe (*Viscum album*), myrcia (*Myrcia* spp.), nopal (*Opuntia* spp.), ginseng (*Panax ginseng*), psyllium (*Plantago* spp.), raspberry (*Rubus* spp.), rhubarb (*Rheum rhabarbarum*), sage (*Salvia officinalis*), Scotch broom (*Cytisus scoparius*, syn. *Sarothamnus scoparius*), shepherd's purse (*Capsella bursa-pastoris*), skunk cabbage (*Symplocarpus foetidus*), stinging nettle (*Urtica dioica*), tamanu (*Calophyllum inophyllum*), tea (*Camellia sinensis*), white oak (*Quercus alba*), white water lily (*Nymphaea alba*), yarrow (*Achillea millefolium*).

Note: This is not an all-inclusive list. Because passionflower, hydroalcoholic extracts, juniper, spinach, plants in the cabbage family (Brassicaceae, such as kale and broccoli), and verbena supply variable quantities of vitamin K, they may lessen the effect of oral anticoagulant therapy.
[a] Agents with coumarin constituents.
[b] Agents with salicylate constituents.
[c] Agents that inhibit platelets.

TABLE 153.4

Herbs and Supplements Containing Potential Phytoestrogens or Phytoprogestins

Herbs Containing Potential Phytoestrogens (constituents reported to act as estrogen receptor agonists and/or to exhibit estrogenic properties in basic science studies, animal research, or human trials)

Aconite (*Aconitum* spp.), agrimony (*Agrimonia* spp.), alfalfa (*Medicago sativa*), alizarin (1,2-dihydroxyanthraquinone), allspice (*Pimenta dioica*), alpha-linolenic acid, amaranth (*Amaranth* spp.), anise (*Pimpinella anisum*), apple cider vinegar, arabinogalactan, arginine (L-arginine), arnica (*Arnica* spp.), ashwagandha (*Withania somnifera*), astragalus (*Astragalus* spp.), avocado (*Persea americana*), bay leaf (*Laurus nobilis*), bee pollen, belladonna (*Atropa belladonna*), beta-sitosterol, betel nut (*Areca catechu*), betony (*Stachys* spp.), bilberry (*Vaccinium* spp.), black cohosh (*Cimicifuga racemosa*),[c] black currant (*Ribes nigrum*), black haw (*Viburnum prunifolium*), black hellebore (*Veratrum nigrum*), black horehound (*Ballota nigra*), black seed (*Nigella sativa*), bladderwrack (*Fucus vesiculosus*), blessed thistle (*Cnicus benedictus*), bloodroot (*Sanguinaria canadensis*), blue cohosh (*Caulophyllum thalictroides*), blue flag (*Iris versicolor*), boldo (*Peumus boldus*), boneset (*Eupatorium* spp.), borage (*Borago officinalis*), boron, boswellia (*Boswellia* spp.), bromelain, bugleweed (*Lycopus* spp.), bupleurum (*Bupleurum* spp.), burdock (*Arctium lappa*), butterbur (*Petasites* spp.), calabar bean (*Physostigma venenosum*), calendula (*Calendula* spp.), camphor, Canada balsam (*Abies balsamea*), cannabis (*Cannabis indica*), carrot (*Daucus carota*), cat's claw (*Uncaria tomentosa*), chamomile (*Matricaria recutita*), chasteberry (*Vitex agnus-castus*), cherry (*Prunus* spp.), chia (*Salvia hispanica*), chicory (*Cichorium intybus*), cinnamon (*Cinnamomum* spp.), cleavers (*Galium aparine*), comfrey (*Symphytum* spp.), cordyceps (*Cordyceps* spp.), cornflower (*Centaurea cyanus*), daisy (*Bellis perennis*), damiana (*Turnera diffusa*), dandelion (*Taraxacum officinale*), danshen (*Salvia miltiorrhiza*), deer velvet, devil's claw (*Harpagophytum procumbens*), dill (*Anethum graveolens*), dogwood (*Cornus* spp.), dong quai (*Angelica sinensis*), echinacea (*Echinacea* spp.), Essiac, eucalyptus (*Eucalyptus* spp.), evening primrose oil (*Oenothera biennis*), false pennyroyal (*Hedeoma* spp.), fennel (*Foeniculum vulgare*), fenugreek (*Trigonella foenum-graecum*), feverfew (*Tanacetum parthenium*), flax (*Linum usitatissimum*), fo-ti (*Polygonum multiflorum*), gamma-linolenic acid, gamma-oryzanol, garcinia (*Garcinia* spp.), garlic (*Allium sativum*), ginger (*Zingiber officinale*), ginkgo (*Ginkgo biloba*), ginseng (*Panax* spp.), goji (*Lycium barbarum*), goldenseal (*Hydrastis canadensis*), gotu kola (*Centella asiatica*), ground ivy (*Glechoma hederacea*), guggul (*Commiphora wightii*), hawthorn (*Crataegus* spp.), hop (*Humulus lupulus*),[a] horny goat weed (*Epimedium* spp.), horse chestnut (*Aesculus hippocastanum*), horsetail (Equisetum spp.), hyssop (*Hyssopus* spp.), ignatia (*Strychnos ignatia*), jointed flatsedge (*Cyperus articulatus*), kava (*Piper methysticum*), kelp (Laminariales), kudzu (*Pueraria lobata*),[b] lady's mantle (*Alchemilla* spp.), lady's slipper (*Cypripedium* spp.), lavender (*Lavandula spica*), lemongrass (*Cymbopogon* spp.), licorice (liquorice) (*Glycyrrhiza glabra*),[a] lotus (*Nelumbo nucifera*), lovage (*Levisticum officinale*), maca (*Lepidium meyenii*), meadowsweet (*Spirea/Filipendula ulmaria*), melatonin (*N*-acetyl-5-methoxytryptamine), milk thistle (*Silybum marianum*), mistletoe (*Viscum album*), mugwort (*Artemisia vulgaris*), muira puama (*Ptychopetalum olacoides*), mullein (*Verbascum thapsus*), neem (*Azadirachta indica*), niacin, noni (*Morinda citrifolia*), nux vomica (*Strychnos nux-vomica*), oleander (*Nerium oleander, Thevetia peruviana*), oregano (*Origanum vulgare*), ovaraden, passion flower (*Passiflora incarnata*), peony (*Paeonia* spp.), peppermint (*Mentha* x *piperita*), pleurisy (*Asclepias tuberosa*), pokeweed (*Phytolacca americana*), pomegranate (*Punica granatum*),[a] Pycnogenol, pygeum (*Pygeum spp.*), quassia (*Quassia* spp.), quercetin, raspberry (*Rubus idaeus*), red clover (*Trifolium pratense*),[b] rehmannia (*Rehmannia* spp.), resveratrol, rhodiola (*Rhodiola* spp.), rhubarb (*Rheum officinale*), rose hip (*Rosa* spp.), rosemary (*Rosmarinus officinalis*), safflower (*Carthamus tinctorius*), sage (*Salvia officinalis*), sarsaparilla (*Smilax regelii*), saw palmetto (*Serenoa repens*), schisandra (*Schisandra chinensis*), Scotch broom (*Cytisus scoparius*, syn. *Sarothamnus scoparius*), sea buckthorn (*Hippophae* spp.), seaweed, shepherd's purse (*Capsella bursa-pastoris*), Siberian ginseng (*Eleutherococcus senticosus*, formerly *Acanthopanax senticosus*), sitosterol, skullcap (*Scutellaria* spp.), slippery elm (*Ulmus rubra*), soy (*Glycine max*),[b] St. John's wort (*Hypericum perforatum*), star anise (*Illicium verum*), stinging nettle (*Urtica dioica*), sweet almond (*Prunus amygdalus dulcis*), sweet marjoram (*Origanum majorana*), sweet woodruff (*Galium odoratum*), tansy (*Tanacetum vulgare*), tea (*Camellia sinensis*), thyme (*Thymus vulgaris*), tribulus (*Tribulus* spp.), turmeric (*Curcuma longa*), verbena (*Verbena* spp.), white horehound (*Marrubium vulgare*), wild ginger (*Asarum* spp.), yucca (*Yucca* spp.).

Herbs and Supplements Containing Potential Phytoprogestins (constituents reported to exhibit progestin-like activity in basic science and/or animal studies).

Bloodroot (*Sanguinaria canadensis*), chasteberry (*Vitex agnus-castus*), damiana (*Turnera diffusa*), ephedra/ma huang (*Ephedra sinica*), oregano (*Origanum vulgare*), PC-SPES, saw palmetto (*Serenoa repens*), wild yam (*Dioscorea villosa*), yohimbe (*Pausinystalia yohimbe*, formerly *Corynanthe yohimbe*), yucca (*Yucca* spp.).

[a] Estriol, estrone, estradiol, or estrogen constituents.
[b] Isoflavone constituents.
[c] Estrogen and isoflavone constituents.

risk, primarily smokers or those with secondhand smoke exposure. Additionally, the ATBC study showed a trend toward increased risk for lung cancer. Both trials found a higher mortality rate among those randomized to beta-carotene supplementation. A meta-analysis of nine randomized clinical trials of beta-carotene supplement also indicated an increase in stomach cancer with daily supplementation of 20 mg or higher.[112] Supplementation with beta-carotene is generally discouraged as a result of these studies.

Coenzyme Q10 (Ubiquinol/Ubiquinone)

Clinical Studies. Coenzyme Q10 (CoQ10) has been studied for the prevention of anthracycline cardiotoxicity based on purported antioxidant effects, but without conclusive results. Cortes et al.[113]

observed 10 patients who received adriamycin and received CoQ10 at a dose of 50 mg per day. A decreased incidence of cardiac dysfunction was reported. In another study, 20 children with acute lymphoblastic leukemia (ALL) or non-Hodgkin's lymphoma (NHL) who were treated with anthracyclines were randomized to CoQ10 therapy.[114] There was decreased fractional shortening in both the CoQ10 treated and untreated groups, but no comparison was made between these two groups. The small sample size and poor study design limit the ability to draw firm conclusions.

Safety. High doses (greater than 300 mg per day) for long periods may elevate liver enzymes (aspartate aminotransferase and lactate dehydrogenase).[115] Concern also exists when CoQ10 is used with antihyperglycemic,[116,117] psychiatric and cardiovascular agents, and warfarin or anticoagulants,[118,119] based on conflicting evidence and secondary sources.[120-122]

Polysaccharide K

Clinical Studies. An uncontrolled trial of polysaccharide K (PSK; *Trametes versicolor*, formerly *Coriolus versicolor*) reported improved survival in cancer patients compared with historical controls.[123] PSK has been reported to improve survival in colorectal,[124] gastric,[125,126] breast,[127-130] esophageal,[131-133] lung,[134-136] hepatocellular,[137] nasopharyngeal carcinoma,[123,138] and in acute leukemia.[139,140] However, other studies have reported no survival benefit with PSK as an adjuvant therapy.[123,130,139,140] Preoperative carcinoembryonic antigen (CEA), Purified Protein Derivative (skin test agent; tuberculosis) (PPD), human leukocyte antigen A2 (HLA-A2), and human leukocyte antigen B40 (HLA-B40) have been reported to be associated with response to PSK therapy.[127,141-148]

Safety. PSK generally seems to have a low incidence of mild and tolerable side effects.[124,129] Cases of liver impairment and toxicity have been noted with PSK use, and gastrointestinal upset, darkening of the fingernails, leucopenia, thrombocytopenia, and coughing have been reported with extended use of PSK.[138,149-151] Theoretically, concomitant use of PSK with anticoagulants or antiplatelets could increase the risk of bleeding, although clinical evidence of this interaction is lacking.

Essiac Herbal Combination Tea

Clinical Studies. The original proprietary formula of Essiac contained burdock root (*Arctium lappa*), sheep sorrel (*Rumex acetosella*), slippery elm inner bark (*Ulmus fulva*), and Turkish rhubarb (*Rheum palmatum*). There is a lack of reliable research available on Essiac. Mouse studies at Memorial Sloan-Kettering Cancer Center in the 1970s were not formally published, and 86 human case reports collected retrospectively in 1988 by the Canadian Department of National Health and Welfare yielded unclear results.[152]

Safety. Concern has been raised about Essiac herbal tonic's potential to stimulate the growth of human breast cancer cells through estrogen receptor–mediated as well as estrogen receptor–independent mechanisms of action. A 2004 systematic review did not identify any published clinical trials to evaluate this herbal complex in patients with cancer.[152] Despite this lack of evidence, Essiac and Essiac-like products (which may contain additional herbs) remain popular among cancer patients. Rhubarb and sheep sorrel contain oxalic acid, which is known to cause hepatic and renal damage in high doses.

Ginger

Clinical Studies. Although some evidence supports the use of ginger (*Zingiber officinale*) for nausea or emesis during pregnancy,[153-162] ginger's effects on other types of nausea or emesis, such as chemotherapy-induced postoperative nausea or motion sickness, remain undetermined.[163-169] Several randomized trials that utilized different doses of ginger along with standard antiemetics have found mixed results,[166,169,170] although overall, the studies suggest that ginger is more effective than placebo.[171] Thus, more studies are needed to further examine ginger therapy for chemotherapy-induced nausea and vomiting.

Safety. The most frequent side effects associated with ginger use are gastrointestinal upset, heartburn, gas, and bloating. Estrogen receptor–positive patients should be cautious because ginger may also exert high estrogenic potency, based on *in vitro* evidence.[172] Ginger may inhibit platelet aggregation or decrease platelet thromboxane production, thus theoretically increasing bleeding risk. When ginger was used in patients who were taking nifedipine, antiplatelet aggregation was increased, which suggests a synergistic effect on the inhibition of platelet aggregation.[173]

Ginseng

Clinical Studies. Ginseng (*Panax ginseng*, *Panax quinquefolius*) is a common ingredient in traditional Chinese medicine herbal formulas, but few clinical trials have evaluated the use of ginseng alone as an anticancer agent. A clinical trial evaluating American ginseng to treat cancer-related fatigue found nonsignificant trends toward benefit in higher doses compared to placebo.[173,174] Similarly, an improvement in quality of life was found in another smaller randomized clinical trial utilizing sun ginseng.[175] A small study utilizing an American ginseng extract found a decreased length of respiratory symptoms.[176] Further clinical trials are needed to determine if ginseng will be beneficial for cancer patients without interfering with cancer treatments.

Safety. The most frequent side effects associated with ginseng include headache, insomnia, and gastrointestinal toxicities.[177] Concern exists when used in combination with diabetes medications (due to possible hypoglycemic properties), anticoagulants (due to increased risk of bleeding), monoamine oxidase inhibitors, and stimulants. Caution should be used when ginseng is taken with medications that are metabolized by cytochrome P-450 2D6.

Green Tea

Clinical Studies. Several large case-control and cohort studies have mainly focused on the prevention of gastrointestinal and breast cancers with green tea (*Camellia sinensis*). Results are variable, with some suggesting chronic tea consumption may decrease cancer risk and others reporting no benefits.[178-187] Overall, the epidemiologic evidence suggests that green tea consumption may protect against cancer; however, these studies have been mostly observational, and other lifestyle choices of tea drinkers may confound these results. A few studies of green tea have shown some clinical benefits. A decreased occurrence of prostate cancer was reported among healthy men treated with green tea extract (GTE) versus placebo in a recent randomized, placebo-controlled study in 60 volunteers with high-grade prostate intraepithelial neoplasia.[190] The study reported a reduction in tumor development (9 of 30 versus 1 of 30) after 1 year of therapy compared to placebo. GTE has also been evaluated to treat premalignant oral lesions. Patients were randomized to three doses of GTE or placebo for 12 weeks. The two higher dose levels were associated with a higher response rate.[178] In a breast cancer study, green tea ingestion was associated with improved prognosis in stage I and II cancers, but no effect was seen on grade III cancers.[183] Additional human research is needed before a recommendation can be made for or against the use of green tea in cancer prevention or treatment.

Safety. Studies of the specific side effects of green tea are limited. However, green tea, a source of caffeine, is known to act as a central nervous system (CNS) stimulant and diuretic; it may also increase the production of stomach acid, worsen ulcer symptoms, increase heart rate, and raise blood pressure. One cup of green tea contains approximately 30 to 50 mg of caffeine, and excessive tea consumption may lead to adverse effects or toxicity. Green tea supplement capsules usually contain less caffeine (approximately 5 mg of caffeine per 500 mg extract).

Lycopene

Lycopene is a carotenoid present in human serum, the liver, adrenal glands, lungs, prostate, colon, and skin at higher levels than other carotenoids. Most dietary lycopene is derived from tomatoes and tomato-based products. Lycopene is also present in many other fruits and plant products, including apricots, pink grapefruit, guava, rose hip, palm oil, and watermelon. Antioxidant and antiproliferative properties have been reported in preclinical research, and there are more than 75 case-control or cohort studies of the association between increased tomato/tomato-based product intake or serum lycopene levels with cancer risk. Approximately two-thirds of these studies suggest benefits in the range of 40% risk reduction, although fewer than half of the studies are statistically significant, and numerous studies provide negative results.[191] A study that evaluated the association between intake of lycopene and specific tomato products and prostate cancer risk among 29,361 men during an average of 4.2 years of follow-up reported that lycopene intake was associated with a reduction of prostate cancer risk among men with a family history of prostate cancer, but not in the male population overall.[192]

Maitake

Clinical Studies. In a small 2002 case series, therapy with Maitake (*Grifola frondosa*) powder and a proprietary Maitake extract (MD fraction) was associated with tumor regression in greater than 50% of patients with stages II to IV breast, lung, and liver cancer, whereas no improvements were observed in leukemia, gastric cancer, or brain tumors.[193] This series had limited information, particularly regarding patient baseline characteristics. A recent report from Memorial Sloan-Kettering Cancer Center found that Maitake mushrooms had a mixed response on a profile of immune cells; thus, the belief that these mushrooms are purely immunostimulatory is likely incorrect.[194]

Safety. Although Maitake has not been well studied, a long history of dietary use suggests that it is safe in low doses. Possible adverse effects of concentrated extracts, based on animal research, include hypoglycemia and hypotension. It is not clear if this agent interacts with chemotherapy regimens.

Milk Thistle

Clinical Studies. One randomized clinical trial in children with acute lymphoblastic leukemia found a lower incidence of liver toxicity among children randomized to milk thistle (*Silybum marianum*) therapy.[195] Several other trials have evaluated milk thistle, but in combination with several other herbs or supplements; therefore, further study using milk thistle alone is needed before it can be recommended as an anticancer treatment.

Safety. Milk thistle has been investigated for anticancer effects in preclinical and clinical trials; the pharmacokinetics and its mechanisms, effectiveness, and adverse effects reported to date have been reviewed.[196] In clinical trials and traditional use, oral milk thistle has generally been reported as well tolerated in recommended doses for up to 6 years of use. Several studies report mild gastrointestinal symptoms, including nausea, heartburn, diarrhea, epigastric pain, abdominal discomfort, dyspepsia, flatulence, and loss of appetite. Urticaria, eczema, and headache have also been reported. Hypersensitivity and anaphylactic reactions have been associated with milk thistle ingestion in case reports. Because many patients in available clinical trials have liver conditions, it is unclear whether adverse effects are caused by milk thistle or by the underlying liver condition; the rates of adverse effects are often similar to placebo. Data from *in vivo* and *in vitro* studies suggest the inhibition of cytochrome p-450 (CPY450) 3A4 and 2C9 to varying levels.

Mistletoe

Clinical Studies. Multiple case series, retrospective analyses, and prospective trials of mistletoe (*Viscum album*, Iscador) extracts in humans have been published; these studies were largely conducted in Europe and have examined patients with breast, lung, cervical, colorectal, gastric, ovarian, and pancreatic cancers, as well as renal cell carcinoma and glioma. A 1994 systematic review included 11 controlled clinical trials, not all randomized, and

concluded that overall methodologic quality of studies was poor and results were indeterminate.[197] Subsequent publications have not provided definitive evidence of efficacy but have suggested survival advantages in patients with colorectal, gastric, or breast cancers.[198–200] Negative results have been reported in patients with melanoma.[201] According to a 2006 reanalysis of previously published nonrandomized studies on mistletoe therapy, breast cancer patients showed increased survival; however, this required a further evaluation in a well-designed randomized controlled trial.[202] In another randomized trial of mistletoe, researchers evaluated the potential side effects from chemotherapy among breast cancer patients and concluded that patients randomized to mistletoe reported fewer side effects. No long-term evaluation was performed to explore the impact on efficacy of treatment.[203]

Safety. Mistletoe is contraindicated in patients with protein hypersensitivity or chronic progressive infections (e.g., tuberculosis). The most common reactions are erythema and hyperemia.[197] Other possible side effects include anorexia, general malaise, depressive moods, fever, local skin inflammation or pain at injection site, mydriasis and miosis/myalgia, and elevated liver enzymes.

Omega-3 Fatty Acids

Clinical Studies. Several population (epidemiologic) studies report that dietary omega-3 fatty acids (alpha-linolenic acid) or fish oil may reduce the risk of developing breast, colon, or prostate cancer.[204–210] There is evidence from epidemiologic studies and randomized controlled trials that an intake of recommended amounts of docosahexaenoic acid (DHA) and eicosapentaenoic acid (EPA) in the form of dietary fish or fish oil supplements lowers triglycerides and reduces the risk of death from cardiovascular disease. Two randomized controlled trials report no significant benefits of supplementation with omega-3 fatty acids or fish oil in cancer patients with cachexia.[211,212] Questions have been raised, however, about the proportion of DHA to EPA used in these trials. An ongoing National Cancer Institute (NCI)–sponsored clinical trial is examining the effects of fish oil alone or in combination with vitamin D_3 in cancer prevention.

Safety. The FDA classifies intake of up to 3 g per day of omega-3 fatty acids from fish as "generally recognized as safe." Caution may be warranted in diabetic patients (due to potential hyperglycemic effects), patients at risk of bleeding, or those with low blood pressure or high low-density lipoprotein (LDL) cholesterol levels.[213] DHA may have greater effects than EPA.

An increased risk of bleeding is one of the primary concerns with fish oil supplementation.[213] Diets containing salmon oil, mackerel, or cod liver oil have been reported to prolong bleeding times significantly in healthy volunteers. However, in other studies of omega-3 fatty acid supplementation, no adverse effects on bleeding time have been observed. Increased bleeding time is suggested to result from either less thromboxane or higher prostacyclin levels. It is unclear if omega-3 fatty acids affect coagulation. Anecdotal evidence suggests that fish oil may increase the international normalized ratio (INR), a measure of bleeding time. However, clinical evidence suggests that fish oil does not affect coagulation, even when taken with anticoagulant therapy. Nevertheless, caution is warranted when omega-3 fatty acids (from plants or fish) are taken with anticoagulant agents. Some species of fish carry a higher risk of environmental contaminants, such as with methylmercury or other heavy metals.

Reishi

Clinical Studies. Treatment with reishi (*Ganoderma lucidum*) mushroom extract (GanoPoly) for 12 weeks resulted in a significant increase in plasma levels of interleukin 2 (IL-2), interleukin 6 (IL-6), and interferon gamma (IFN-γ), decreased IL-1 and tumor necrosis factor alpha (TNF-α) levels, and increased natural killer (NK) cells in advanced-stage cancer patients.[214,215] Well-designed, long-term studies are needed to confirm these results and to examine potential side effects.

Safety. Caution is recommended when reishi is used in patients with bleeding disorders/coagulopathies or in those taking anticoagulants, as reishi mushroom may alter platelet aggregation and prolong bleeding time.[216] Caution is also advised in patients with low blood pressure, diabetes, or in those taking antidiabetic agents or antihypertensives.

Resveratrol

Clinical Studies. Resveratrol is a naturally occurring hydroxystilbene identified in more than 70 plant species, including nuts, grapes, pine trees, and certain vines, as well as in red wine. Although there are several observational studies that correlate the consumption of wine with a decrease in cancer or cardiovascular disease risk,[217,218] high-quality human trials supporting the efficacy of resveratrol for any indication are currently lacking in the available literature. Ongoing research is examining resveratrol and a possible role in increasing longevity and how it interacts with sirtuins.

Safety. Laboratory study suggests that resveratrol has antiaggregating and antithrombin activity, and may have additive effects when taken with other agents with the same actions[219]; thus, use of resveratrol with antiplatelets could cause increased risk of bleeding, although clinical reports of drug interactions are lacking. Resveratrol apparently has the potential to act as an estrogen agonist or antagonist, depending on such factors as cell type and estrogen receptor isoform (ER-α or ER-β).[220–222] Resveratrol has also been shown to inhibit vitamin D3 receptor expression through estrogenic regulation.[223] Clinical evidence of estrogen interactions is lacking. Some *in vitro* and *in vivo* studies suggest that resveratrol might interfere with paclitaxel.[224] Resveratrol inhibited all of the cytochrome P-450 (CYP) tested (1A1, 1A2, 1B1, 2A6, 2B6, 2E1, 3A4, 4A), except for 2E1.[225]

Selenium

Clinical Studies. Initial evidence has suggested that selenium supplementation reduces the risk of developing prostate cancer in men with normal baseline prostate-specific antigen (PSA) levels and low selenium blood levels. This is the subject of large, well-designed studies, including the Nutritional Prevention of Cancer (NPC) trial and the Selenium and Vitamin E Cancer Prevention Trial (SELECT),[226–240] as well as prior population and case-control studies.[241,242]

The NPC trial with 1,312 Americans reported that 200 mg of daily selenium reduces the overall incidence of prostate cancer, although these protective effects only occurred in men with baseline PSA levels less than or equal to 4 ng per milliliter and those with low baseline blood selenium levels (less than 123.2 ng per milliliter).[229–231,243] The NPC trial was primarily designed to measure the development of nonmelanoma skin cancers and not other types of cancers; therefore, these prostate cancer results cannot be considered definitive.

SELECT was started in 2001 with 32,400 men with serum PSA levels less than or equal to 4 ng per milliliter. The study was ended early due to an interim analysis that determined that the study could not meet its expected end point of a 25% reduction in prostate cancer. Subset analyses indicated selenium supplementation was associated with increased development of diabetes mellitus.

Safety. The level of selenium exposure that will cause chronic toxicity is not clear. Selenium toxicity may cause gastrointestinal symptoms (nausea, vomiting, abdominal pain, diarrhea, garlic-like breath odor, and metallic taste), neuromuscular–psychiatric disturbances (weakness/fatigue, lightheadedness, irritability, hyperreflexia, muscle tenderness, tremor, and peripheral neuropathy), dermatologic changes (skin rash/dermatitis/flushing, fingernail loss/thickening/blotching/streaking/paronychia, and hair changes/loss), liver dysfunction, kidney dysfunction, thrombocytopenia (low blood platelets), immune alterations (NK cell impairment), thyroid dysfunction (decreased T3), reduced sperm motility, or growth retardation.

Soy

Clinical Studies. Preliminary research using soy (*Glycine max*) to control hot flashes in women with breast cancer suggests that it is possibly safe,[244] although the pending results of ongoing research in this area may provide more definitive safety data. Recent studies have indicated that moderate dietary soy intake (observed in most traditional Asian diets—no more than three servings daily) shows no risk and may have possible benefits to breast cancer patients, even among women with estrogen-positive breast cancers.[245,246] However, because higher doses of soy may have estrogenic effects, which clearly increase the risk for progression of estrogen receptor–positive breast cancer, it is prudent for breast cancer survivors to avoid the high doses of soy and soy isoflavones that are provided by more concentrated sources (such as soy powders and isoflavone supplements).[43] Preliminary clinical evidence suggests that the short-term use of soy isoflavones does not elicit endometrial hypertrophy.

Safety. Soy is "generally regarded as safe" according to the FDA, and has long been a staple of Asian diets. Current epidemiologic and laboratory evidence suggests there are unlikely to be harmful effects when soy is provided in the diet consistent with amounts in a typical Asian diet.[245]

Turmeric

Clinical Studies. A phase 1 trial found limited toxicity with doses of turmeric (*Curcuma longa*, curcumin) as high as 8 g daily. A phase 2 clinical trial in pancreatic cancer found a limited response rate with 3 of 25 patients with either stable disease or a reduction in tumor size.[247] Multiple clinical trials are ongoing to evaluate the use of turmeric and associated compounds for the treatment of cancer.

Safety. The most common side effect with turmeric reported in humans is gastrointestinal upset, including epigastric burning, dyspepsia, nausea, and diarrhea.[247,248] High doses of turmeric are thought to be safe based on toxicology studies.[247] The turmeric constituent curcumin has been reported to induce liver function test abnormalities in rats, and may be mildly hepatotoxic in high doses.[248] Caution is warranted when using turmeric with hepatotoxic agents. Increased bleeding risk is a concern with high doses of curcumin.[248] There is evidence that turmeric may interfere with cytochrome P-450 (CYP450) enzymes, which are responsible for breaking down various agents in the liver.[250]

Vitamin A

Vitamin A is comprised of retinol and its carotenoid precursors. All-*trans* retinoic acid, a retinol analog, is well established as a differentiation agent in patients with acute promyelocytic leukemia.[251] However, there is little evidence to support the use of nonprescription vitamin A supplements for cancer treatment or prevention. Trials have yielded variable results, suggesting no reduction in prostate cancer risk and possible increased risk of lung cancer in high-risk patients.[252] Due to the possibility of hypervitaminosis A with supplementation of this fat-soluble vitamin, chronic intake of large doses is discouraged.

Vitamin C

Limited clinical research has been conducted on vitamin C (ascorbic acid) for cancer prevention. In the 1980s, there was initial excitement over epidemiologic evidence correlating high dietary vitamin C intake with reduced rates of cancer, although use of vitamin C in observed populations may have correlated with other healthy lifestyle choices (e.g., diet, exercise) that confounded findings. A subsequent prospective trial found no reduction in rates of breast cancer. Preclinical evidence of reduced platelet aggregation suggests that risks may outweigh potential benefits. Patients may experience scurvy symptoms after abrupt withdrawal of chronic megadoses. Two randomized controlled trials of high-dose intravenous vitamin C in cancer patients found no benefits.[253,254]

Vitamin D

Vitamin D is one of four fat-soluble vitamins and is traditionally linked with calcium metabolism and bone health. Vitamin D_2 (ergocalciferol) and vitamin D_3 (cholecalciferol) are precursors to calcitriol, the active form of vitamin D. Exposing skin to natural sunlight is the most common manner by which the body produces vitamin D. Growing evidence indicates the importance of vitamin D for immune processes. Additionally, studies in cancer populations indicate a possible worse outcome in those with vitamin D deficiency.[255–257] Appropriate supplementation should be considered for those with documented deficiency or those at risk for bone fractures due to poor bone health (i.e., osteoporosis). Prolonged high-dose use of vitamin D may lead to hypercalcemia.

Vitamin E

Vitamin E (α-tocopherol) is a fat-soluble vitamin with antioxidant properties. Epidemiologic studies suggest a possible reduced breast, lung, and prostate cancer risk with intake. However, prevention trials report no reduction in risk of lung, breast, or colon cancers. Several reviews and meta-analyses have also found a higher mortality rate in doses of 400 IU or less daily.[258–261] Additionally, a large randomized trial among head and neck cancer patients investigated vitamin E and beta-carotene and found that these agents were associated with decreased survival among subjects taking both. Some have hypothesized that the agents may have acted as an antioxidant and thus reduced the efficacy of the radiation treatment, leading to increased recurrence rates and, ultimately, decreased survival. Several studies have evaluated the potential to protect against chemotherapy-induced peripheral neuropathy with such agents as platinums and taxanes with positive results.[262–266] However, these studies were not designed to assess for alterations in chemotherapy effectiveness. Preclinical evidence of reduced platelet aggregation has been shown.

Other Therapies

Other herbs and supplements that are used in cancer treatment without reliable evidence include aloe, antineoplastons, barley, bitter melon, bladderwrack, bromelain, calendula, chamomile, clay, danshen, dehydroepiandrosterone (DHEA), echinacea, evening primrose oil, eyebright, flaxseed, Gerson therapy and coffee enemas, ginseng, ginkgo, goldenseal, guggul, gymnema, hops, horsetail, kava, lactobacillus, laetrile, lavender, marshmallow, passion flower, pennyroyal, peppermint, propolis, red clover, sorrel, St. John's wort, sweet almond, white horehound, numerous types of mushroom extracts, and various combinations of Chinese herbal medicine.

Numerous therapies have also been used for cancer prevention, but they have not been well studied. These include aloe, black tea, bromelain, cranberry, eucalyptus oil, ginseng, grape seed extract, lactobacillus (colon cancer risk reduction), oleander, omega-3 fatty acids/fish oil, psyllium (colon cancer risk reduction), red clover, and spirulina.

Nonbiologically Based Therapies

Nonbiologically based therapies generally fall into the categories of mind–body techniques, massage, acupuncture, and energy techniques. These techniques are generally used to support overall well-being or specific treatment-related side effects.[267–276]

Mind–Body Techniques

Background. Mind–body modalities, including meditation, hypnosis, relaxation techniques, cognitive–behavioral therapy, biofeedback, yoga, tai chi, qigong, and guided imagery, have increasingly become part of mainstream care over the years. Mind–body practices are defined as a variety of techniques designed to enhance the mind's capacity to affect bodily function and symptoms.[1]

Clinical Studies. Techniques of stress management that may be helpful include progressive muscle relaxation,[277,278] diaphragmatic breathing,[279,280] guided imagery,[281–283] social support,[284,285] and meditation.[286,287] Participating in stress management programs prior to treatment has enabled patients to tolerate therapy with fewer reported side effects.[288–291] Supportive expressive group therapy has also been found to be useful for patients with cancer.[292–294] Psychosocial interventions have been shown to specifically decrease depression and anxiety and increase self-esteem and active-approach coping strategies.[295–298]

There is some evidence that when incorporated into cancer care, yoga, tai chi, and meditation may help to improve aspects of quality of life, including improved mood, sleep quality, physical functioning, and overall well-being.[296,299–301] Hypnosis, and especially self-hypnosis, has been found to be beneficial for reducing distress and discomfort during difficult medical procedures.[281] A National Institutes of Health (NIH) Technology Assessment Panel found strong evidence for hypnosis in alleviating cancer-related pain.[302] Hypnosis effectively treats anticipatory nausea in pediatric[303] and adult cancer patients,[304] reduces postoperative nausea and vomiting,[305] and improves adjustment to invasive medical procedures.[306–308]

A meta-analysis of 116 studies found that mind–body therapies may reduce anxiety, depression, and mood disturbance in cancer patients and aid their coping skills.[309] Newell et al.[310] reviewed psychological therapies for cancer patients and concluded that interventions involving self-practice and hypnosis for managing nausea and vomiting may be recommended. More recently, Ernst et al.[311] examined the change in the state of the evidence for mind–body therapies for various medical conditions between 2000 and 2005 and found that there is now maximal evidence for the use of relaxation techniques for anxiety, hypertension, insomnia, and nausea due to chemotherapy.

Massage

Clinical Studies. Research to date suggests that massage is helpful for increasing relaxation and relieving pain, anxiety, fatigue, and distress.[269,312–314] The obvious challenge in conducting massage therapy research is the difficulty achieving a placebo control group. It is, therefore, not clear what the exact mechanisms are for the benefits of massage in an oncology setting. Despite some of the imperfections in research design, the current findings are encouraging.

Safety. Massage therapy is generally safe when practiced by credentialed practitioners who have also had some training in cancer patient care. Serious adverse events are rare and tend to be associated with exotic types of massage or untrained or inexperienced practitioners.[315] In general, cancer patients should not receive deep tissue massage, and patients with bleeding tendencies should only receive a light touch. Obviously, areas that have recently had surgery or radiation should be avoided. A therapeutic benefit may also be derived from simply receiving a massage to the feet, hands, and head, because these areas are especially sensitive to tactile stimulation and may result in providing relaxation and an increase in general well-being.[316]

Acupuncture

Background. Acupuncture is a common treatment modality in many cultures. It is a form of traditional Chinese medicine (TCM) and has been practiced in China for thousands of years. Acupuncture is one of the most popular TCM therapies outside of China and is used in at least 78 countries.[317] According to traditional theory, the placement of needles, heat, or pressure at specific places on the body can help to regulate the flow of qi (vital energy). The most common form of acupuncture involves the placement of solid, sterile, stainless steel needles into various points on the body.[318,319] Different techniques can be used to stimulate the needles, including manual manipulation or electrical stimulation.[318-320]

Clinical Studies. There is good scientific evidence that acupuncture is effective for managing both postoperative and chemotherapy-related nausea and vomiting.[44-47] An NIH consensus statement in 1998 supported this use, stating that the level of evidence was sufficient.[321] Further research has substantiated this

claim, and the American Cancer Society now states that clinical studies have found acupuncture may help treat nausea caused by chemotherapy drugs and surgical anesthesia. There is also good evidence that certain types of acupuncture are effective for both postoperative and chronic pain in cancer patients.[321-323]

A growing number of clinical trials, both controlled and uncontrolled, suggest that acupuncture is beneficial for radiation-induced xerostomia, hot flashes, and aromatase-induced arthralgias.[324-327] For the management of other treatment- or cancer-related symptoms, the evidence is not as strong. Nevertheless, there is some preliminary and anecdotal evidence to suggest that acupuncture may be useful in the treatment of anxiety, depression, fatigue, constipation, loss of appetite, peripheral neuropathy, insomnia, dyspnea, and leucopenia.[328,329] However, the overall quality of the evidence for these symptoms remains weak, and further studies are needed.

Safety. When performed correctly, acupuncture has been shown to be a safe, minimally invasive procedure with very few side effects. The most commonly reported complications are fainting, bruising, and mild pain. Infection is also a potential risk, although very uncommon.[330,331] Acupuncture should only be performed by a health-care professional with an appropriate license and preferably one who has had experience in treating patients with malignant diseases.

PALLIATIVE AND ALTERNATIVE CARE

SELECTED REFERENCES

The full reference list can be accessed at lwwhealthlibrary.com/oncology.

8. Richardson MA, Sanders T, Palmer JL, et al. Complementary/alternative medicine use in a comprehensive cancer center and the implications for oncology. *J Clin Oncol* 2000;18:2505–2514.

37. Aggarwal BB, Shishodia S. Molecular targets of dietary agents for prevention and therapy of cancer. *Biochem Pharmacol* 2006;71:1397–1421.

43. Doyle C, Kushi LH, Byers T, et al. Nutrition and physical activity during and after cancer treatment: an American Cancer Society guide for informed choices. *CA Cancer J Clin* 2006;56:323–353.

46. Lee A, Done ML. The use of nonpharmacologic techniques to prevent postoperative nausea and vomiting: a meta-analysis. *Anesth Analg* 1999;88: 1362–1369.

48. Wiseman M. The second World Cancer Research Fund/American Institute for Cancer Research expert report. Food, nutrition, physical activity, and the prevention of cancer: a global perspective. *Proc Nutr Soc* 2008;67:253–256.

73. Lutgendorf SK, Sood AK, Antoni MH. Host factors and cancer progression: biobehavioral signaling pathways and interventions. *J Clin Oncol* 2010;28: 4094–4099.

79. Guo Z, Tang HY, Li H, et al. The benefits of psychosocial interventions for cancer patients undergoing radiotherapy. *Health Qual Life Outcomes* 2013;11:121.

81. Ulbricht C, Chao W, Costa D, et al. Clinical evidence of herb-drug interactions: a systematic review by the natural standard research collaboration. *Curr Drug Metab* 2008;9:1063–1120.

83. Berk LB. Primer on integrative oncology. *Hematol Oncol Clin North Am* 2006;20:213–231.

86. Frenkel M, Ben Arye E, Baldwin CD, et al. Approach to communicating with patients about the use of nutritional supplements in cancer care. *South Med J* 2005;98:289–294.

87. Palmer ME, Haller C, McKinney PE, et al. Adverse events associated with dietary supplements: an observational study. *Lancet* 2003;361:101–106.

90. Weiger WA, Smith M, Boon H, et al. Advising patients who seek complementary and alternative medical therapies for cancer. *Ann Intern Med* 2002;137:889–903.

99. Smith P, Bullock JM, Booker BM, et al. The influence of St. John's wort on the pharmacokinetics and protein binding of imatinib mesylate. *Pharmacotherapy* 2004;24:1508–1514.

103. Bairati I, Meyer F, Jobin E, et al. Antioxidant vitamins supplementation and mortality: a randomized trial in head and neck cancer patients. *Int J Cancer* 2006;119:2221–2224.

105. Lawenda BD, Kelly KM, Ladas EJ, et al. Should supplemental antioxidant administration be avoided during chemotherapy and radiation therapy? *J Natl Cancer Inst* 2008;100:773–783.

106. Lai MN, Lai JN, Chen PC, et al. Risks of kidney failure associated with consumption of herbal products containing Mu Tong or Fangchi: a population-based case-control study. *Am J Kidney Dis* 2010;55:507–518.

107. Frei E 3rd, Jaffe N, Tattersall MH, et al. New approaches to cancer chemotherapy with methotrexate. *N Engl J Med* 1975;292:846–851.

108. Zaineddin AK, Buck K, Vrieling A, et al. The association between dietary lignans, phytoestrogen-rich foods, and fiber intake and postmenopausal breast cancer risk: A German Case-Control Study. *Nutr Cancer* 2012;64: 652–665.

109. Anderson LN, Cotterchio M, Boucher B, et al. Phytoestrogen intake from foods, during adolescence and adulthood, and risk of breast cancer by estrogen and progesterone receptor tumor subgroup among Ontario women. *Int J Cancer* 2013;132:1683–1692.

112. Druesne-Pecollo N, Latino-Martel P, Norat T, et al. Beta-carotene supplementation and cancer risk: a systematic review and meta-analysis of randomized controlled trials. *Int J Cancer* 2010;127:172–184.

119. van Dalen EC, Caron HN, Dickinson HO, et al. Cardioprotective interventions for cancer patients receiving anthracyclines. *Cochrane Database Syst Rev* 2008;(2):CD003917.

120. Landbo C, Almdal TP. [Interaction between warfarin and coenzyme Q10]. *Ugeskr Laeger* 1998;160:3226–3227.

123. Go P, Chung CH. Adjuvant PSK immunotherapy in patients with carcinoma of the nasopharynx. *J Int Med Res* 1989;17:141–149.

124. Sakamoto J, Morita S, Oba K, et al. Efficacy of adjuvant immunochemotherapy with polysaccharide K for patients with curatively resected colorectal cancer: a meta-analysis of centrally randomized controlled clinical trials. *Cancer Immunol Immunother* 2006;55:404–411.

125. Oba K, Teramukai S, Kobayashi M, et al. Efficacy of adjuvant immunochemotherapy with polysaccharide K for patients with curative resections of gastric cancer. *Cancer Immunol Immunother* 2007;56:905–911.

127. Yokoe T, Iino Y, Takei H, et al. HLA antigen as predictive index for the outcome of breast cancer patients with adjuvant immunochemotherapy with PSK. *Anticancer Res* 1997;17:2815–2818.

132. Ogoshi K, Satou H, Isono K, et al. Possible predictive markers of immunotherapy in esophageal cancer: retrospective analysis of a randomized study. The Cooperative Study Group for Esophageal Cancer in Japan. *Cancer Invest* 1995;13:363–369.

134. Hayakawa K, Mitsuhashi N, Saito Y, et al. Effect of Krestin as adjuvant treatment following radical radiotherapy in non-small cell lung cancer patients. *Cancer Detect Prev* 1997;21:71–77.

137. Suto T, Fukuda S, Moriya N, et al. Clinical study of biological response modifiers as maintenance therapy for hepatocellular carcinoma. *Cancer Chemother Pharmacol* 1994;33:S145–S148.

138. Chung CH, Go P, Chang KH. PSK immunotherapy in cancer patients— a preliminary report. *Zhonghua Min Guo Wei Sheng Wu Ji Mian Yi Xue Za Zhi* 1987;20:210–216.

139. Ohno R, Yamada K, Masaoka T, et al. A randomized trial of chemoimmunotherapy of acute nonlymphocytic leukemia in adults using a protein-bound polysaccharide preparation. *Cancer Immunol Immunother* 1984;18: 149–154.

146. Ito K, Nakazato H, Koike A, et al. Long-term effect of 5-fluorouracil enhanced by intermittent administration of polysaccharide K after curative resection of colon cancer. A randomized controlled trial for 7-year follow-up. *Int J Colorectal Dis* 2004;19:157–164.

152. Kaegi E. Unconventional therapies for cancer: 1. Essiac. The Task Force on Alternative Therapies of the Canadian Breast Cancer Research Initiative. *CMAJ* 1998;158:897–902.

165. Mahesh R, Perumal RV, Pandi PV. Cancer chemotherapy-induced nausea and vomiting: role of mediators, development of drugs and treatment methods. *Pharmazie* 2005;60:83–96.

169. Pillai AK, Sharma KK, Gupta YK, et al. Anti-emetic effect of ginger powder versus placebo as an add-on therapy in children and young adults receiving high emetogenic chemotherapy. *Pediatr Blood Cancer* 2011;56:234–238.

170. Zick SM, Ruffin MT, Lee J, et al. Phase II trial of encapsulated ginger as a treatment for chemotherapy-induced nausea and vomiting. *Support Care Cancer* 2009;17:563–572.

171. Ernst E, Pittler MH. Efficacy of ginger for nausea and vomiting: a systematic review of randomized clinical trials. *Br J Anaesth* 2000;84:367–371.

172. Kang SC, Lee CM, Choi H, et al. Evaluation of oriental medicinal herbs for estrogenic and antiproliferative activities. *Phytother Res* 2006;20:1017–1019.

173. Young HY, Liao JC, Chang YS, et al. Synergistic effect of ginger and nifedipine on human platelet aggregation: a study in hypertensive patients and normal volunteers. *Am J Chin Med* 2006;34:545–551.

174. Barton DL, Soori GS, Bauer BA, et al. Pilot study of *Panax quinquefolius* (American ginseng) to improve cancer-related fatigue: a randomized, double-blind, dose-finding evaluation: NCCTG trial N03CA. *Support Care Cancer* 2010;18:179–187.

175. Kim JH, Park CY, Lee SJ. Effects of sun ginseng on subjective quality of life in cancer patients: a double-blind, placebo-controlled pilot trial. *J Clin Pharm Ther* 2006;31:331–334.

179. Sun CL, Yuan JM, Koh WP, Yu MC. Green tea, black tea and colorectal cancer risk: a meta-analysis of epidemiologic studies. *Carcinogenesis* 2006;27:1301–1309.

184. Imai K, Suga K, Nakachi K. Cancer-preventive effects of drinking green tea among a Japanese population. *Prev Med* 1997;26:769–775.

190. McLarty J, Bigelow RL, Smith M, et al. Tea polyphenols decrease serum levels of prostate-specific antigen, hepatocyte growth factor, and vascular endothelial growth factor in prostate cancer patients and inhibit production of hepatocyte growth factor and vascular endothelial growth factor *in vitro*. *Cancer Prev Res (Phila Pa)* 2009;2:673–682.

191. Giovannucci E. Tomatoes, tomato-based products, lycopene, and cancer: review of the epidemiologic literature. *J Natl Cancer Inst* 1999;91:317–331.

192. Kirsh VA, Mayne ST, Peters U, et al. A prospective study of lycopene and tomato product intake and risk of prostate cancer. *Cancer Epidemiol Biomarkers Prev* 2006;15:92–98.

193. Kodama N, Komuta K, Nanba H. Can Maitake MD-fraction aid cancer patients? *Altern Med Rev* 2002;7:236–239.

194. Deng G, Lin H, Seidman A, et al. A phase I/II trial of a polysaccharide extract from Grifola frondosa (Maitake mushroom) in breast cancer patients: immunological effects. *J Cancer Res Clin Oncol* 2009;135:1215–1221.

195. Styczynski J, Wysocki M. Alternative medicine remedies might stimulate viability of leukemic cells. *Pediatr Blood Cancer* 2006;46:94–98.

196. Cheung CW, Gibbons N, Johnson DW, et al. Silibinin—a promising new treatment for cancer. *Anticancer Agents Med Chem* 2010;10:186–195.

197. Kleijnen J, Knipschild P. Mistletoe treatment for cancer: review of controlled trials in humans. *Phytomedicine* 1994;1:255–260.

202. Grossarth-Maticek R, Ziegler R. Randomised and non-randomised prospective controlled cohort studies in matched-pair design for the long-term therapy of breast cancer patients with a mistletoe preparation (iscador): a re-analysis. *Eur J Med Res* 2006;11:485–495.

203. Semiglasov VF, Stepula VV, Dudov A, et al. The standardised mistletoe extract PS76A2 improves QoL in patients with breast cancer receiving adjuvant CMF chemotherapy: a randomised, placebo-controlled, double-blind, multicentre clinical trial. *Anticancer Res* 2004;24:1293–1302.

205. Rose DP, Connolly JM. Omega-3 fatty acids as cancer chemopreventive agents. *Pharmacol Ther* 1999;83:217–244.

213. Bays HE. Safety considerations with omega-3 fatty acid therapy. *Am J Cardiol* 2007;99:35C–43C.

214. Gao Y, Zhou S, Jiang W, et al. Effects of ganopoly (a Ganoderma lucidum polysaccharide extract) on the immune functions in advanced-stage cancer patients. *Immunol Invest* 2003;32:201–215.

215. Gao Y, Tang W, Dai X, et al. Effects of water-soluble Ganoderma lucidum polysaccharides on the immune functions of patients with advanced lung cancer. *J Med Food* 2005;8:159–168.

219. Guerrero RF, Garcia-Parrilla MC, Puertas B, Cantos-Villar E. Wine, resveratrol and health: a review. *Nat Prod Commun* 2009;4:635–658.

224. Fukui M, Yamabe N, Zhu BT. Resveratrol attenuates the anticancer efficacy of paclitaxel in human breast cancer cells *in vitro* and *in vivo*. *Eur J Cancer* 2010;46:1882–1891.

230. Duffield-Lillico AJ, Dalkin BL, Reid ME, et al. Selenium supplementation, baseline plasma selenium status and incidence of prostate cancer: an analysis of the complete treatment period of the Nutritional Prevention of Cancer Trial. *BJU Int* 2003;91:608–612.

234. Klein EA, Thompson IM, Lippman SM, et al. SELECT: the selenium and vitamin E cancer prevention trial. *World J Urol* 2003;21:21–27.

244. Quella SK, Loprinzi CL, Barton DL, et al. Evaluation of soy phytoestrogens for the treatment of hot flashes in breast cancer survivors: a North Central Cancer Treatment Group Trial. *J Clin Oncol* 2000;18:1068–1074.

245. Shu XO, Zheng Y, Cai H, et al. Soy food intake and breast cancer survival. *JAMA* 2009;302:2437–2443.

247. Dhillon N, Aggarwal BB, Newman RA, et al. Phase II trial of curcumin in patients with advanced pancreatic cancer. *Clin Cancer Res* 2008;14:4491–4499.

251. Ravandi F, Estey E, Jones D, et al. Effective treatment of acute promyelocytic leukemia with all-trans-retinoic acid, arsenic trioxide, and gemtuzumab ozogamicin. *J Clin Oncol* 2009;27:504–510.

252. The Alpha-Tocopherol and Beta Carotene Cancer Prevention Study Group. The effect of vitamin E and beta carotene on the incidence of lung cancer and other cancers in male smokers. *N Engl J Med* 1994;330:1029–1035.

255. Goodwin PJ, Ennis M, Pritchard KI, et al. Prognostic effects of 25-hydroxyvitamin D levels in early breast cancer. *J Clin Oncol* 2009;27:3757–3763.

256. Mezawa H, Sugiura T, Watanabe M, et al. Serum vitamin D levels and survival of patients with colorectal cancer: post-hoc analysis of a prospective cohort study. *BMC Cancer* 2010;10:347.

260. Bjelakovic G, Nikolova D, Gluud LL, et al. Antioxidant supplements for prevention of mortality in healthy participants and patients with various diseases. *Cochrane Database Syst Rev* 2008;(2):CD007176.

266. Pace A, Giannarelli D, Galie E, et al. Vitamin E neuroprotection for cisplatin neuropathy: a randomized, placebo-controlled trial. *Neurology* 2010;74:762–766.

310. Newell SA, Sanson-Fisher RW, Savolainen NJ. Systematic review of psychological therapies for cancer patients: overview and recommendations for future research. *J Natl Cancer Inst* 2002;94:558–584.

311. Ernst E, Pittler MH, Wider B, Boddy K. Mind-body therapies: are the trial data getting stronger? *Altern Ther Health Med* 2007;13:62–64.

316. Myers CD, Walton T, Small BJ. The value of massage therapy in cancer care. *Hematol Oncol Clin North Am* 2008;22:649–660.

323. Park J, Linde K, Manheimer E, et al. The status and future of acupuncture clinical research. *J Altern Complement Med* 2008;14:871–881.

329. Lewith G, Berman B, Cummings M, et al. Systematic review of systematic reviews of acupuncture published 1996–2005. *Clin Med* 2006;6:623–625.

Note: Page locators followed by *f* and *t* indicate figure and table, respectively.